Appendix D and the Glossary are located on the Student Resources site at nursing.pearsonhighered.com.

MEDICAL-SURGICAL NURSING

Preparation for Practice

SECOND EDITION

Kathleen S. Osborn, RN, MS, EdD
Professor Emeritus, California State University, Sacramento, California
University of California, Davis Medical Center, Coordinator, Nurse Residency Program
Educator, ReSurge International

Cheryl E. Wraa, RN, MSN
Trauma Care After Resuscitation (TCAR), Programs Director
Educator, ReSurge International

Annita B. Watson, RN, MS, PhD
Professor Emeritus, California State University, Sacramento, California

Renée Holleran, APRN, FNP-BC, PhD, CEN, CCRN, CFRN, CTRN, FAEN
Nurse Practitioner, Palliative Care
Staff Nurse, Emergency Department, Intermountain Medical Center
Salt Lake City, Utah

PEARSON

Boston Columbus Indianapolis New York San Francisco Upper Saddle River
Amsterdam Cape Town Dubai London Madrid Milan Munich Paris Montreal Toronto
Delhi Mexico City São Paulo Sydney Hong Kong Seoul Singapore Taipei Tokyo

Publisher: Julie Levin Alexander
Publisher's Assistant: Regina Bruno
Executive Acquisitions Editor: Pamela Fuller
Development Editor: Laura Horowitz, Hearthside Publishing Services
Editorial Assistant: Cynthia Gates
Managing Production Editor: Patrick Walsh
Production Liaison: Cathy O'Connell
Production Editor: Emily Bush, S4Carlisle Publishing Services
Manufacturing Manager: Lisa McDowell
Art Director/Cover and Interior Design: Mary Siener
Director of Marketing: David Gesell
Senior Marketing Manager: Phoenix Harvey
Marketing Manager: Deborah Doyle
Marketing Specialist: Michael Sirinides
Marketing Assistant: Crystal Gonzalez
Assistant Editor for Media: Sarah Wrocklage
Media Project Managers: Rachel Collett and Michael Dobson
Composition: S4Carlisle Publishing Services
Printer/Binder: Courier/Kendallville
Cover Printer: LeHigh Phoenix Color/Hagerstown
Cover Image: @ Ingram Publishing/Alamy

Credits and acknowledgments for content borrowed from other sources and reproduced, with permission, in this textbook appear on appropriate page within text.

A Note about Nursing Diagnoses: Nursing Diagnoses in this text are taken from *Nursing Diagnoses—Definitions and Classification 2012–2014*. Copyright © 2012, 1994–2012 by NANDA International. Used by arrangement with John Wiley & Sons Limited. In order to make safe and effective judgments using NANDA-I nursing diagnoses it is essential that nurses refer to the definitions and defining characteristics of the diagnoses listed in this work.

Notice: Care has been taken to confirm the accuracy of information presented in this book. The authors, editors, and the publisher, however, cannot accept any responsibility for errors or omissions or for consequences from application of the information in this book and make no warranty, express or implied, with respect to its contents.

The authors and publisher have exerted every effort to ensure that drug selections and dosages set forth in this text are in accord with current recommendations and practice at time of publication. However, in view of ongoing research, changes in government regulations, and the constant flow of information relating to drug therapy and drug reactions, the reader is urged to check the package inserts of all drugs for any change in indications of dosage and for added warnings and precautions. This is particularly important when the recommended agent is a new and/or infrequently employed drug.

Library of Congress Cataloging-in-Publication Data
Medical-surgical nursing: preparation for practice/Kathleen S. Osborn . . . [et al.]. — 2nd ed.
p. ; cm.
Rev. ed. of: Medical-surgical nursing/Kathleen S. Osborn, Cheryl E. Wraa, Annita B. Watson. c2010.
Includes bibliographical references and index.
ISBN-13: 978-0-13-270669-8
ISBN-10: 0-13-270669-5
I. Osborn, Kathleen S. II. Osborn, Kathleen S. Medical-surgical nursing.
[DNLM: 1. Perioperative Nursing—methods. 2. Nurse's Role.
3. Nursing Care—methods. WY 161]
610.73—dc23

2012024533

10 9 8 7 6 5 4 3 2 1

PEARSON

ISBN-10: 0-13-270669-5
ISBN-13: 978-0-13-270669-8

ABOUT THE AUTHORS

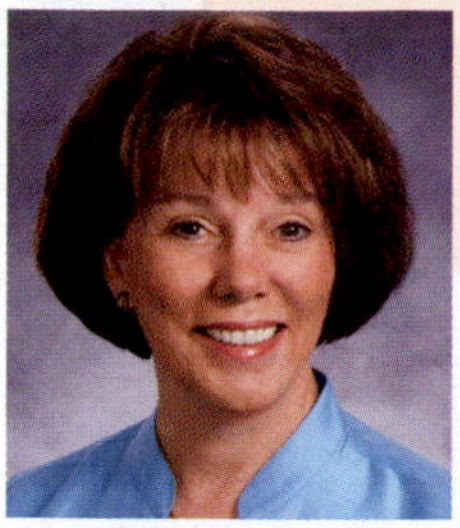

KATHLEEN S. OSBORN

Dr. Kathleen Osborn was first introduced to the profession of nursing at St. Francis School of Nursing in San Francisco, where she received her diploma. She went on to obtain a bachelor's degree in nursing from Sacramento State University; a Master of Science degree from the University of California, San Francisco; and a doctorate in educational leadership from the University of Southern California. Her clinical practice is in critical care, including cardiac, burn, neurological, and respiratory specialties. She has more than 31 years of experience teaching bachelor and master's degree students, as well as teaching nurses in hospital in-service and continuing education programs. Dr. Osborn's expertise includes program and course development, didactic lecturing, and clinical supervision of undergraduate and graduate students. Her areas of practice include medical–surgical nursing, and critical care, including medical, cardiac, surgical, and burns. She also has been actively involved in nursing research and publication throughout her clinical and teaching career. Dr. Osborn is currently the coordinator of the New Graduate Nurse Residency program at the University of California, Davis Medical Center.

Since 1999, Dr. Osborn has volunteered her services with ReSurge International and has participated on surgical/educator humanitarian missions to Laos, Mali, Ghana, Vietnam, Honduras, Bangladesh, Ecuador, and Nepal. She received the "Heroes in Healthcare" Community Service Award for her humanitarian work from the Coalition for Excellence in Healthcare, a division of the Health Communication Research Institute of Northern California. She also received the Community Service Award from Sacramento State University for her humanitarian work and her service to student development. In 1995, a perpetual faculty award was begun in her honor by the graduating class: The Guiding Light Award for Outstanding Performance by a Nursing Faculty.

This book is dedicated to the important people in my life. I want to thank my husband John for his devotion, patience, and understanding during this project. I also want to thank our children, Christopher and his wife Toni, Patrick, Staci, and Mike, for their ongoing understanding of my time away from them. Finally, I want to thank all of the nursing students whom I have had the pleasure of teaching and the patients around the world whom I have cared for. You have made my career fulfilling and happy.

—Kathleen Osborn

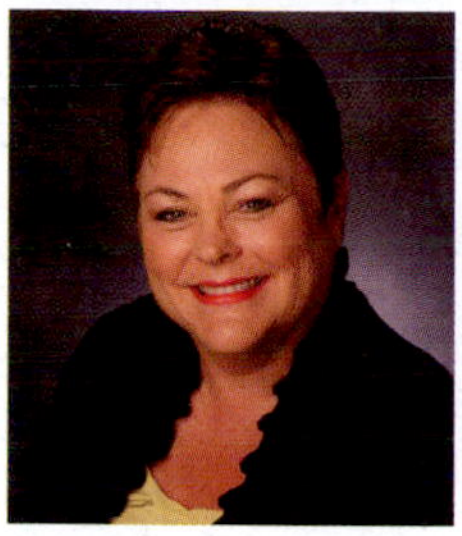

CHERYL E. WRAA

Cheryl Wraa received her nursing diploma from the Kaiser Foundation School of Nursing in Oakland, California. She went on to obtain a bachelor's degree and master of science degree in nursing from California State University, Sacramento. Her clinical career has focused on critical care nursing, leadership, and education. Ms. Wraa's clinical practice includes the medical intensive care unit, emergency department, and flight nursing. She recently retired as the trauma program manager at a level 1 trauma center and clinical faculty for advanced medical–surgical nursing students in a baccalaureate program. She currently is the programs director for the Trauma Care After Resuscitation (TCAR) courses. Ms. Wraa is also an educator for ReSurge International and has participated on surgical/educator missions to Vietnam, Bangladesh, Ghana, and Nepal. She has been active in education and publication throughout her career and is currently a senior clinical editor for the *Journal of Emergency Nursing.* She is past president of the Air and Surface Transport Nurses Association, as well as the Trauma Managers Association of California. Ms. Wraa received the Barbara A. Hess Award for her contributions to education in the air medical and ground transport field.

I dedicate this book to my parents for sharing their incredible faith, zest for life, and unconditional love—I miss you. To my mentors for sharing their wisdom—I would not be where I am without you. To my students for keeping the thirst for knowledge alive and, most importantly, to my family and friends for their unending support and love—I would not have survived this without you.

—Cheryl Wraa

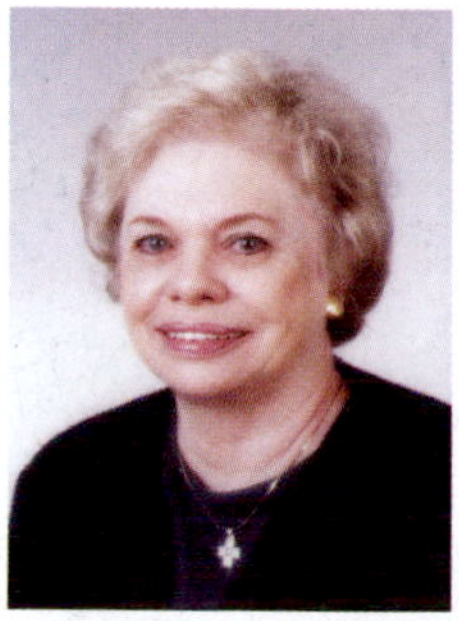

ANNITA B. WATSON

Dr. Annita Watson began her nursing career in Jamestown, New York, at WCA Hospital School of Nursing. She completed her bachelor's degree at Teachers College, Columbia University, and her master's and doctorate in nursing at the University of California, San Francisco. Her graduate focus was medical–surgical nursing and leadership and administration in service and educational settings. Dr. Watson began her teaching career in 1970 at California State University, Sacramento, where she taught at both the undergraduate and graduate levels. Her areas of practice include medical–surgical nursing, intensive care, long-term care, and community health. Throughout her career, she has served as a national consultant to health care agencies and educational programs on topics related to development of management systems, quality improvement of patient care, curriculum development and evaluation, and implementation of accreditation processes. She has published in like areas, and made numerous professional preparations. Her research interests focus on the measurement of patient and student outcomes. Currently Dr. Watson assumes a leadership role on several local and regional community boards, focusing on health services for vulnerable populations, for example, children, the elderly, and people who have been abused. Nationally, she serves as an accreditation site evaluator for the Commission on Collegiate Nursing Education. In 2008, she was awarded the Life Time Achievement Award for community service by California State University, Sacramento, recognizing her contributions to the health of the community and her ability to foster community-based learning experiences for students.

To my family, friends, colleagues, and students who supported me in completing this project. Thank you for always being there and your patience, endurance, and encouragement. I could not have completed this project without you. Your inspiration and guidance remain with me always. Thank you.

—Annita Watson

RENÉE HOLLERAN

Dr. Renée Holleran, inspired by her grandmother's years of service to the nursing profession, studied nursing at her father's alma mater, Kent State University. During her career, she has served in various roles, including critical care, emergency, and transport nurse. Dr. Holleran is past president of the Emergency Nurses Association, former editor of the *Air Medical Journal,* and current editor of the *Journal of Emergency Nursing.* Her hope is that her vast experiences and clinical background will contribute to student nurses' knowledge and inspire them to be "excellent" nurses.

As always, I thank my family—Michael, my husband, and Erin and Sara, my daughters—for putting up with my dedication to nursing. Nursing has provided me with many friends and colleagues. As I have found, "nursing is a way of life."

—Renée Holleran

THANK YOU

We extend a heartfelt thanks to our contributors, who gave their time, effort, and expertise so tirelessly to the development and writing of chapters and resources that helped foster our goal of preparing student nurses for evidence-based practice.

Text Contributors

Sally J. Brush, MSN, FNP
Lead Nurse Practitioner, Heart Failure Prevention and Treatment Program
Utah Cardiac Transplant Program
Intermountain Medical Center
J.L. Sorenson Heart & Lung Center
Salt Lake City, Utah
Chapters 10, 11

Ann Cashion, RN, PhD
Chair and Associate Professor, Acute and Chronic Care Department
Robert Wood Johnson Executive Nurse Fellow
Director, Center for Health Evaluation and Lifestyle Promotion
University of Tennessee Health Science Center
Memphis, Tennessee
Chapter 7

Patricia Caudle, DNSc, CNM, FNP
Faculty
Frontier Nursing University
Heber Springs, Arizona
Chapters 40, 41, 42, 43, 44

Joyce V. Colobong, RN, MS, ACNP-BC, CCRN, CNRN
Nurse Practitioner II, Trauma and Emergency Surgery
University of California, Davis
Chapters 21, 23, 24

Christi DeLemos, CNRN, MSN, ACNP-BC
Associate Clinical Professor UCSF
Nurse Practitioner III, Department of Neurological Surgery
University of California, Davis
Chapters 20, 22, 24

Lucie S. Elfervig, DNS, MSN, BSN, APRN-CS, CRNO, FAAN
Ophthalmic Consultant, Clinician, Researcher, Educator, and Electrophysiologist
Eye Specialty Group
Memphis, Tennessee
Chapter 64

Leslie Flynn, RN, DNP
Clinical Nurse Analyst, Optime and Anesthesia Clinical Information Systems—EMR Team
UC Davis Health System
Sacramento, California
Chapters 17, 18

Kara L. Gasiorowski, RN, MSN, CNOR, ONC
Clinical Manager, Orthopedic Surgery
Perioperative Patient Safety Specialist
New York Presbyterian-Weill Cornell Medical Center
New York, New York
Chapters 48, 49, 50, 51

J. Carolyn Graff, PhD, RN, FAAIDD
Associate Professor, College of Nursing
Chief of Nursing, Boling Center for Developmental Disabilities
University of Tennessee Health Science Center
Memphis, Tennessee
Chapter 7

Rebecca J. Graves, MSN, NP-C
Instructor
Adult Health Nursing
University of South Alabama, College of Nursing
Mobile, Alabama
Chapter 7

Dea Kent, RN, MSN, NP
Manager, Inpatient Wound Program and Outpatient Wound Ostomy Clinic
Riverview Hospital, Indiana
Chapter 58

Jean Klein, PhD, RNCS
Psychiatric/Mental Health Specialist
West Chester, Pennsylvania
Chapter 9

Dawn Lambie, RN, MSN, CHPN
Executive Director, Bristol Hospice, Sacramento LLC
Sacramento, California
Chapter 57

Brenda McCulloch, RN, MSN, CNS
Sutter Heart and Vascular Institute
Sutter Medical Center
Sacramento, California
Chapters 29, 30, 31, 32, 33, 34, 35

John M. Osborn, MD, FACS
Surgeon
Clinical Professor, School of Medicine
University of California, Davis Medical Center
The Plastic Surgery Center
Sacramento, California
Chapters 44, 59

Cynthia Parkman, RN, MS, PhD
University of Nevada, Las Vegas
Professor Emeritus, California State University, Sacramento
Sacramento, California
Chapters 1, 2, 3, 4, 5, 6

Joyce Pittman, PhD, RN, FNP-BC, CWOCN
Nurse Practitioner, Team Lead Wound/Ostomy Team
Indiana University Health—Methodist
Adjunct Assistant Professor
Indiana University School of Nursing
Indianapolis, Indiana
Chapters 59, 60

Laurie Quinn, BSN, MSN, PhD
Clinical Associate Professor, College of Nursing
University of Illinois
Chicago, Illinois
Chapters 45, 46, 47

Carol Rhoades, RN, MSN, CFRN, CTRN
Manager, Adult Services
Intermountain Life Flight
Salt Lake City, Utah
Chapters 25, 26, 27, 28

Len Sterling, MBA, BSN, RN
Nurse Manager, Firefighters Burn Institute Regional Burn Center
University of California, Davis Medical Center
Sacramento, California
Chapter 61

Pamela Stetina, RN, PhD
Professor, Northern Arizona University School of Nursing
Flagstaff, Arizona
Chapters 36, 37, 38, 39

Jacqueline C. Stocking, RN, MSN, MBA
Program Director, Quality and Safety
UC Davis Medical Center, Patient Care Services
Sacramento, California
Nursing Process Care Plan features

Judith Tanner, RN, MSN, Certified School Nurse
School Nurse at Sacramento City College
Part-Time Faculty at Sacramento City College
Sacramento, California
Chapters 62, 63

Gail Thurkauf, RN, MS
Director of the Department of Nursing Quality
Georgetown University Hospital
Washington, DC
Chapters 12, 13, 14, 15, 16
Sheila Tucker, MA, RD
Nutritionist, Dining Services
Part-Time Faculty, School of Nursing and Lynch School of Education
Boston College
Boston, Massachusetts
Chapter 8
Kimberly Yates, RN, BSN
Nurse Manager
Fremont Surgery Center
Fremont, California
Chapter 19
Nancy J. Yilk
Integrative Healthcare Consultant and Author
Optimum Health
Sacramento, California
Complementary & Alternative Therapies features

REVIEWERS. Our heartfelt thanks go out to our colleagues from schools of nursing across the country who have given their time generously to help create this exciting new medical–surgical nursing textbook. These individuals helped us plan and shape our book and resources by reviewing chapters, art, design, and more. *Medical–Surgical Nursing: Preparation for Practice* has reaped the benefit of their collective knowledge and experience as nurses and teachers, and we have improved the materials due to their efforts, suggestions, objections, endorsements, and inspiration. Among those who generously gave their time to help us are the following:

Sheila A. Alexander, PhD, RN
Assistant Professor, University of Pittsburgh
Pittsburgh, Pennsylvania
Deborah Becker, PhD, ACNP, BC, CCNS
Assistant Professor, University of Pennsylvania School of Nursing
Philadelphia, Pennsylvania
Diana Blum, MSN
Full-time Instructor, Metropolitan Community College
Omaha, Nebraska
John Brion, PhD, RN
Professor, Duke University School of Nursing
Durham, North Carolina
Robin Brown, MS, RN
Professor, University of South Dakota
Watertown, South Dakota
Susan E. Caulkins, MSN, APRN, BC
Nursing Instructor, Central Carolina Technical College
Sumter, South Carolina
Sharon Coulter, MSN, RN
Professor, Southern University
Baton Rouge, Louisiana
Stephanie DeBoor, PhD, RN, CCRN
Graduate Coordinator, University of Nevada
Reno, Nevada
Deb Filer, RN, PhD, CNE
Professor, St. Catherine University
St. Paul, Minnesota
Barbara Giguere, EdD, RN
Professor, Worcester State University
Worcester, Massachusetts
Eleanor Green, RN, BSN, MSN
Professor, Bucks County Community College
Bucks County, Pennsylvania
Yolanda Green, RN, MSN
Professor, Chattanaooga State Community College
Chattanooga, Tennessee
Anna Gryczman, DNP, RN, AHN-BC, CNE
Course Coordinator, Century College
White Bear Lake, Minnesota
Misty Hobart, RN, MSN, CNE
Full-Time Instructor, Spokane Community College
Spokane, Washington
Jan Holbrook, MSN, RN, CCRN, FBN/FPN
Professor, Goldfarb School of Nursing at Barnes-Jewish College
St. Louis, Missouri
Karen Hughes, MSN, RN, CNE
Professor, Columbus State Community College
Columbus, Ohio
Heather Jacobs, RN, MSN, FNP-C
Full-Time Instructor, Robeson Community College
Pembroke, North Carolina
Tamela Kisner, RN, MSN
Assistant Professor, University of South Dakota
Rapid City, SD
Wanda K. Lawrence, PhD, RN
Associate Professor, Winston Salem State University
Winston Salem, North Carolina
Katherine Logan, RN, MSN, QMHP
Professor, University of South Dakota
Rapid City, South Dakota
Regan Luken, RN, MSN
Professor, University of South Dakota
Vermillion, South Dakota
Dorothy Mathers, DNP, RN, CNE
Professor, Pennsylvania College of Technology
Williamsport, Pennsylvania
Kimberly McCoy, MSN, RN
Full-Time Instructor, Southern University A & M College
Baton Rouge, Louisiana
Belle M. McGinty, MED, RN
Nursing Instructor, Brunswick Community College
Supply, North Carolina
Cheryl Miller, EdD, MSN, BSN
Professor, Chattanooga State Community College
Chattanooga, Tennessee
Peter Miskin, MSN, RN, PHN
Assistant Professor, Samuel Merritt University
San Mateo, California
Cindy Mulder, RNC, MS, MSN, CNP
Professor, University of South Dakota
Vermillion, South Dakota
Bridget Nichols, RN, MSN, CCRN
Professor, University of South Dakota
Sioux Falls, South Dakota
Joan Niederriter, PhD, MSN, CMSRN, RN-BC
Professor, Cleveland State University
Cleveland, Ohio
Susan Olson, RN, MSN
Professor, McLennan Community College
Waco, Texas
Joan Owens, RN, MSN
Full-Time Instructor, Spokane Community College
Spokane, Washington
Nancy Pares, RN, MSN
Program Coordinator, Metro Community College
Omaha, Nebraska
Jean Phelan, MS, RN
Full-Time Instructor, Metropolitan Community College
Omaha, Nebraska
Erlene Pickett, MN, RN
Program Coordinator, Spokane Community College
Spokane, Washington
Anita K. Reed, MSN, RN
Assistant Professor, St. Elizabeth School of Nursing/Saint Joseph's College
Lafayette, Indiana
Debra Rice, RN, MSN
Full-Time Instructor, Spokane Community College
Spokane, Washington

Pamela Rowsey, PhD, RN
Associate Professor, University of North Carolina
Chapel Hill, North Carolina

Carol R. Sando, RN, PhD, CNE
Assistant Professor, Delaware State University
Dover, Delaware

Deborah Jane Schwytzer, RN, MSN, CEN
Associate Professor, University of Cincinnati
Cincinnati, Ohio

Allison Shields, MS, RN
Professor, Fitchburg State College
Fitchburg, Massachusetts

Jeannie Short, MSN, RN
Assistant Professor, Indiana Wesleyan University
Marion, Indiana

Amy Sneed, MSN, RN, CNE
Course Coordinator, Brunswick Community College
Supply, North Carolina

Linda Steeg, RN, MS, ANP-BC, DNP-c
Assistant Professor, University at Buffalo
Buffalo, New York

Nancy Steffen, RN, MSN
Full-Time Instructor, Century College
White Bear Lake, Minnesota

Sharon Stewart, RN, CPHQ
Pasadena, Maryland

Christine Tesch, MSN, RN
Professor, University of South Dakota
Sioux Falls, South Dakota

Karen Tetreault, RN, MS
Professor, NHTI Concord's Community College
Concord, New Hampshire

Heather Walsh, MSN (Ed), RN
Full-Time Instructor, UCLA
Los Angeles, California

Lisa Williams, DNP, MSN/Ed, MSM, APRN, FNP-BC
Professor, University of South Carolina
Columbia, South Carolina

Aimee Woda, PhD (c), RN, BC
Full-Time Instructor, Marquette University
Milwaukee, Wisconsin

Michael Zychowicz, DNP, ANP-C, ONP-C, FAANP
Professor, Duke University School of Nursing
Durham, North Carolina

PREFACE

As nursing moves forward in the 21st century, greater emphasis is being placed on the nurse's role as a major member of the health care delivery system. The Institute of Medicine report *The Future of Nursing: Leading Change, Advancing Health* emphasizes the importance of nursing as a vital component in the future of health care delivery. The authors used this proclamation as a foundation for restructuring the content of the book and explaining the nurse's role as a member of the interdisciplinary care team. This focus is exemplified in discussions of providing care to patients with multiple disorders and in guiding the learner in providing the preventive aspects of patient care. Safety of patient care, reflective of the Quality and Safety Education for Nurses (QSEN) project (2011), also is incorporated into discussions of treatment and prevention. Nursing core competencies are identified in the nursing process discussions throughout the text.

This journey forward into nursing for the future is an exciting one for those learning to become nurses, as well as those advancing their careers in nursing. This is an era of opportunity for nurses to establish career goals by becoming leaders in health care and exploring multiple opportunities for practice in a variety of settings. Nurses are being prepared to expand their role and to meet current and future challenges in health care. Challenges of the past, such as rapid changes in environmental factors, remain a constant for the future. The multicultural population continues to expand, as do life spans. Some continue to experience poor health conditions and others experience new, rarely treated health conditions. Explosive advances in technology, ever-changing work settings, and a costly and complex health care environment continue to contribute to nursing's evolving environment. The burgeoning level of information affects decision making, and newer, faster modes of communication add to the environment's complexity, as does the rapid growth in scientific advancements in technologies and pharmacy. These advances, coupled with changes in patients' expectations and knowledge, add to the demands of nursing. However, these demands also present opportunities to develop and expand the nursing role of integrator of patients into health care systems, and to advance in nursing practice from novice to expert through experiential learning with a scientific and caring perspective.

With the advent of health care reform, the patterns for health care delivery are uncertain; however, the diversity and adaptability of nursing remains a constant with one certainty: Nurses will continue to be a critical component of health care delivery and the career opportunities are limitless for those who join the ranks of the nursing profession.

With these opportunities and issues, nursing education is challenged to be innovative in preparing nurses for practice now and in the future. The challenge is to prepare nurses who can provide cognitively skilled care, in a caring manner, with a diverse patient population, and in innovative health care settings. The authors' vision for this textbook is to meet that challenge. This textbook prepares the learner to be a knowledgeable, caring health care professional. It is a foundation on which to build the nursing practice of today and tomorrow, incorporating the cognitive, affective, and psychomotor skills necessary to practice. This book is not a destination to be achieved, but the beginning of lifelong learning.

Goals

The goal of this book is to expose the learner to concepts basic to the practice of nursing. To that end, 58 underlying concepts of the book have been identified and defined. Key overriding concepts of professional nursing, including caring, critical thinking, research, nursing process, and health promotion, are threaded throughout the text. Caring is the foundation of nursing practice because of its impact on patients and their families. The authors have adopted Roach's (1984) theory of caring, which includes six components: compassion, competence, confidence, conscience, commitment, and comportment. Within the chapter features the authors have applied these six components when describing the nursing care needed for each of the physical disorders. This helps learners develop their understanding of how to be a caring nurse and makes them aware of these qualities in fellow health care professionals' practice, as well as when advocating for the patient.

The nursing process is used to develop critical thinking and clinical reasoning skills, providing the framework for applying evidence-based practice. Research is discussed throughout the text, providing opportunities for the reader to examine current research topics and their application to nursing practice.

Health promotion, one of the nurse's primary roles, is woven throughout the book, so learners will understand the importance of educating the patient/family about healthy habits and lifestyles that prevent illnesses and injuries.

Readers will become active participants in learning about nursing as they progress through the book's contents. The goal is for the learners to demonstrate an understanding of the concepts of medical–surgical nursing in a variety of settings by collaborating with the authors in defining requisite content for patient care, arriving at patient diagnoses, and developing plans of care.

The concepts of experiential learning shape the book's contents. The intention is that learners will engage in reflective thought and analysis as they apply the principles and concepts incorporated in the book to clinical practice, using the book as a resource for validating perceptions, expanding their knowledge base, and evaluating their approaches to patient care. The book is organized to introduce learners to the basic concepts of health care in general, and to nursing specifically, before moving on to the concepts underlying health promotion and disease management and the common physiological disorders that are encountered in medical–surgical nursing practice.

The units and chapters are grouped to lead the learner from general concepts to the more complex concepts and challenges of disease management. The information is sequenced to enhance critical thinking skills, thereby promoting the development of clinical judgment.

Knowledge acquisition is enhanced by analysis, evaluation, and creation. Thus, this text provides numerous opportunities for learners to participate in activities designed to develop critical thinking and problem-solving skills in collaboration with the nursing experts from a variety of clinical backgrounds who have contributed to the book. These learning activities include preparing clinical preparation guides, establishing priorities for care, developing patient care plans, and evaluating knowledge in the affective, cognitive, and psychomotor domains of practice. As learners complete these experiential and interactive activities, they will achieve a holistic, scientific, and caring approach to professional nursing practice for now and the future.

What's New in this Edition

In concert with the previous goals, the authors have made the following changes in the second edition of this textbook:

- Restructured the book into 15 units and 67 chapters by realigning and combining some chapters and increasing content in specific practice areas.
- Strengthened the conceptual approach to nursing by defining 58 concepts on which the content of the book is developed, and identified relevant concepts per each unit.
- Edited the content to be the most relevant and current, with increased emphasis on prevention, community-based care, and collaboration.
- Updated evidence to 2007–2012.
- Focused the content on the Institute of Medicine findings: *The Future ofNursing: Leading Change, Advancing Health*; the Quality and Safety Education for Nurses (QSEN) project; and Nursing Core Competencies.
- Increased emphasis on collaborative care with nurses as a key member of the health care team.
- Restructured the Nursing Process/Patient Care Plans to align with key concepts in the book and Gordon's Functional Health Patterns.
- Strengthened focus on nursing care as the essential element of learning and applying the underlying concepts of nursing.

Organization

The book consists of 15 units sequenced from simple, basic concepts to complex, medical–surgical disorders. Units 1 and 2 introduce the reader to general concepts related to health care delivery, followed by basic concepts related to nursing practice. The next two units cover physiological concepts and the theoretical basis of skills that are germane to all areas of nursing practice. Units 5 through 15 focus on physiological disorders common to medical–surgical nursing. Each disorder unit opens with an assessment chapter that provides a template to assess the presenting patient within the specific body system.

Text Features

THE TEXT FEATURES were designed to highlight the concepts that form the framework for this textbook and that are basic to professional nursing: **caring, research, critical thinking, the nursing process,** and **health promotion.** The capstone feature in each disorder chapter, **Clinical Preparation,** offers learners the opportunity to bring all of the concepts into one summary exercise and thus prepares learners for safe and knowledgeable clinical practice in their future work as professional nurses.

Competency Tables. Tables are included at the beginning of each unit that guide the reader in finding specific content on the Institute of Medicine competencies, Nursing Core Competencies, Quality and Safety Education for Nurses (QSEN) competencies, and the 58 concepts for concept-based learning that are used in this edition.

Clinical Preparation Assignments. These assignments help the learner develop a problem-solving approach to nursing care. By completing the assignments presented at the end of the chapters, the learner will gain experience in critical thinking skills and develop a systematic method for determining a patient's health problem, devising a plan of care, developing evaluation criteria, and determining expected outcomes. The Clinical Preparation assignments also help the learner articulate the patient's needs and learn how to write effective evaluation statements. This, in turn, significantly improves documentation skills and the ability to communicate with other health care team members to provide the safest, most effective, and holistic care for the patient.

The Clinical Preparation exercise is presented at the end of each disorder chapter to present the learner with a reality-oriented approach to patient assessment and diagnosis. The interactive forms needed to complete this assignment are accessed from the Pearson eText.

CLINICAL PREPARATION READ DOCUMENT APPLY

READ: **History of Present Illnesses** >> Laboratory Study Results >> Critical Thinking Questions

Philip Arnott is a 52-year-old man admitted to your unit with a diagnosis of pneumonia with increasing shortness of breath during the past several days. He is admitted from the emergency department receiving oxygen via nasal cannula at 6 L/min. Three days ago, Mr. Arnott stated that he "didn't feel right" and stayed home from work. He thought he had a cold and was congested and sneezing. He reported not being able to sleep lying flat. Last night he was awakened by an episode of severe shortness of breath. He called 911 and was transported to the hospital. On admission to the emergency department, he was febrile at 39.4°C (102.9°F) with a pulse oximeter of 88% on room air. Oxygen via nasal cannula was instituted, which increased the pulse oximetry reading to 92%. A portable chest x-ray demonstrated consolidation of the right middle and lower lobe. Blood, sputum, and urine cultures were obtained, and antibiotics were initiated. The patient was admitted to the special respiratory unit for further treatment. Continuous pulse oximetry, coughing and deep breathing encouragement, and Tylenol for fever are the nursing priorities for Mr. Arnott on admission. Careful attention to the timing of his antibiotic doses also is a priority.

Medical–Surgical History

Mr. Arnott has never been hospitalized before but has a history of hypertension that is being treated with the angiotensin-converting enzyme inhibitor irbesartan (Avapro), 150 mg, and hydrochlorothiazide, 12.5 mg, each once a day.

Social History

Mr. Arnott is a sedentary business executive who is 6 ft 3 inches (76 inches) tall and weighs 250 pounds. He lives by himself and has no close relatives locally.

Physical Examination

On physical exam, Mr. Arnott is alert and oriented but anxious. His cardiac exam reveals bounding pulses with normal heart sounds and no jugular venous distention. He denies any chest pain or any type of pain except discomfort related to breathing and shortness of breath. His respiratory rate is rapid, but his chest excursion is equal bilaterally. He is using accessory muscles for respiration and is sitting straight up in bed. On auscultation, he has decreased breath sounds on the right side with wet crackles heard posteriorly over the entire right lung field. His cough is productive for sputum that is thick, yellow, and tenacious. His blood pressure is 150/90; heart rate is 100 beats per minute with a respiratory rate of 34 to 36 per minute; and pulse oximetry fluctuating between 90% and 92% on 6 liters nasal cannula. His temperature is running 38° to 40°C (100.4° to 104°F). His abdomen is large but soft and nontender. He denies any problems with urination or defecation. His last bowel movement was yesterday. Skin is warm and dry with no areas of breakdown noted. An intravenous infusion is present in his left forearm with antibiotics infusing.

READ: History of Present Illnesses >> **Physical Exam** >> Admitting Medical Records >> Laboratory Study Results

Admitting Medical Orders

Admit to MIC
Service: MICU
Condition: guarded
Admitting diagnosis: pneumonia
Allergies: no known drug allergies
Vital signs and O_2 sats q1h
Activity: bed rest
Diet: regular
Daily weight
Continuous cardiac monitor
Continuous pulse oximetry
Call house officer: HR < 60 or >120, systolic blood pressure < 90 or >160, RR < 12 or > 30, temperature > 38.5°C, urinary output less than 30 mL/hr × 2, O_2 sat < 92%
IV: D5 1/2 NS @ 50 mL/hr
Strict I/O q1h
Oxygen: via 6 liters nasal cannula; maintain oxygen saturation > 92%
Respiratory care: incentive spirometer q1 hours when awake
Sequential compression stockings to lower extremities while in bed

Scheduled Medications

Irbesartan (Avapro) 150 mg PO once a day
Hydrochlorothiazide 12.5 mg PO once a day
Ceftazidime 2 grams every 8 hours IV

PRN Medications

Tylenol 650 mg po q4h for fever
Morphine 0.3 to 5 mg IV q4h prn pain
Temazepam 15 to 30 mg po at bedtime prn insomnia

Ordered Laboratory Studies

CPK-MB q8h ∞ 3
Chemistry panel, CBC, and magnesium daily
ABGs daily and prn for respiratory distress

Ordered Diagnostic Studies

Chest x-ray q a.m.

Nursing Priorities

Six hours later, the nurse is called to Mr. Arnott's room. His dinner tray is on his bedside stand. He is cyanotic with a pulse oximetry reading in the 70s. He is coughing sporadically with a respiratory rate in the high 40s. Lung sounds are decreased, but bronchial sounds are heard throughout the lung fields except for the right side, which is very decreased. The health care provider is called, and an emergency chest x-ray is ordered. Oxygen is changed to a face mask, 100% nonrebreather. Mr. Arnott's pulse oximetry increases to 85%. ABGs are obtained. (The ABGs are listed in the table with the laboratory results.)

The chest x-ray reveals a new infiltrate in the posterior segment of the left upper lobe and an increasing pattern of consolidation in the right lung. A presumptive diagnosis of worsening pneumonia with possible aspiration pneumonia is considered. On questioning, Mr. Arnott states that he had difficulty swallowing his dinner and remembers that after drinking some of the milk his coughing increased and he vomited. Soon he can barely talk because he is so short of breath and is increasingly anxious with nasal flaring. His respiratory rate has increased to 45 breaths/min, his heart rate has increased to the 120s, and his blood pressure is

COMPLEMENTARY & ALTERNATIVE THERAPIES Cupping

Nancy Yilk

CUPPING REFERS TO AN ANCIENT CHINESE PRACTICE in which cups are applied to the skin to suck out noxious materials. The therapy has been used in China for thousands of years. The technique involves the use of small glass cups, into which a small cloth saturated with alcohol or an herbal mixture is inserted and then ignited. The cup is then pressed against the skin to create a vacuum. The cups are placed on specific acupuncture points and remain for a period of time or are moved across the skin in a dragging motion to follow specific terrains. The cupping often results in a purpling to the skin in round circles mimicking the placement of the cups. There is typically no pain and the purple areas fade in a few days.

Cupping has been used historically for a wide range of health complaints. It was primarily a home remedy that was performed by midwives and family members for respiratory complaints, pain, and fevers. This therapy was used widely in the United States in the 18th and 19th centuries. In fact, as late as 1931 it was indicated in the treatment of bronchopneumonia and acute myelitis. Cupping was included in U.S. medical textbooks prior to 1940 and performed in sanatoriums for tuberculosis. In fact, the therapy is still used today in many cultures.

Cupping fell out of use in the medical field with the onset of newer applications of drugs and surgeries, but remained a mainstay in cultural teachings in Traditional Chinese Medicine (TCM). Currently there is an upsurge in its use within the United States from immigrating families from Pacific Rim countries where family members practice it as a natural medicine.

Between 1959 and 2008, 550 clinical studies were conducted regarding the practice of cupping, including 73 randomized controlled trials (RCTs), 22 clinical controlled trials, 373 case series, and 82 case reports. RCTs on cupping therapy appear to have improved during the past 50 years in China, and the majority of studies show potential benefits for pain conditions, herpes zoster, and other diseases, though increasing an unbiased approach to results will improve the understanding of cupping's benefits and risk (Huijuan et al., 2010).

Researchers explored various distinctions regarding techniques that were employed in cupping patients for the common cold at its early stages and the time duration that the cups were applied. In a randomized trial, 60 patients who were starting to experience colds were assigned to either an observational or control group. The technique of flash cupping, in which the cup is applied to the skin and suctioned in a quick pumping of the cupping tool, was applied to five acupoints historically used for colds. The therapeutic effects were compared after applying the treatments twice to the back. The total effect rate was 93.3% (28/30) in the experimental group, which was superior to the results of 66.7% (20/30) found in the control group ($P < 0.01$) (Ye, Zhang, & Pang, 2011).

The results demonstrated that, in the instances of the common cold, the longer applications were more beneficial. With such a simple treatment, even people who do not know the classic names of the application points can learn the techniques and use them in their families. However, the need still exists to define proper use of cup application and the correct location of cups among both practitioners and participants who want to learn the technique and don't benefit from the oral teachings of an elder in their community.

References

Adapted from Huijuan, C., Mei, H., Xun, L., Shangjuan, D., Yongmei, S., Qian, W., et al. (2010). Clinical research evidence of cupping therapy in China: A systematic literature review. *Complementary and Alternative Medicine, 10,* 70.

Ye, X. F., Zhang, H. F., & Pang, Z. W. (2011). Therapeutic effects of common cold of wind-cold type at early stage treated by different cupping duration. *Zhongguo Zhen Jiu, 31*(4), 357–359.

Complementary & Alternative Therapies. This content introduces the learner to a variety of therapies used by patients that augment mainstream medicine. An understanding of the interactions of these therapies with more traditional therapies is essential for patient safety.

CULTURAL CONSIDERATIONS
Cultural Practices Related to Respiratory Disorders

Cultural Practice	Nursing Considerations
Use of amulets (many cultures)	May interfere with diagnostic testing such as x-rays, MRI, and ultrasound. Suggest alternate placement of amulet for test duration or placement of amulet within eye contact.
Cupping (Southeast Asia, Greece)	May be mistaken for signs of abuse; may delay medical treatment. Burns or skin infections may occur and necessitate medical treatment.
Coining (Southeast Asia, Italy, and Russia)	May be mistaken for signs of abuse; may delay medical treatment. Burns or skin infections may occur and necessitate medical treatment.
Herbal remedies (used in many cultures)	Herbal remedies may be related to allergies because they are derived from plants that are associated with allergens. Herbal remedies may also interfere with the actions of medications and antibiotics or increase bleeding tendencies.

Cultural Considerations. These topics teach the learner to be sensitive to the needs of patients with different ethnic/cultural backgrounds, religious practices, and beliefs about health care and end of life, thereby enabling the learner to develop a multicultural approach to care.

Laboratory and Diagnostic Tests. These tables inform the learner about the relevant diagnostic tests for the disorder under discussion. Normal result ranges are included, as well as expected abnormalities with rationales.

LABORATORY AND DIAGNOSTIC TESTS for ARDS and ALI

Test with Description, Rationale, and Normal Values	Expected Abnormality
Brain Natriuretic Peptide (BNP)	
0–99 pg/mL *BNP is a hormone in the blood that is secreted from the ventricles of the heart in response to increased pressure that occurs with heart failure. The level is higher in women and increases with age. It is used to differentiate cardiac (congestive heart failure) versus pulmonary etiology (ARDS/ALI) of respiratory failure.*	In patients with respiratory failure: BNP < 100 pg/mL = ARDS/ALI etiology BNP > 500 pg/mL = cardiac etiology BNP 100–500 pg/mL = nondefinitive and requires further work-up.
Echocardiology	
Normal heart wall movement, and normal heart chambers and valve function. Ejection fraction 55% to 65%. *An echocardiogram uses sound waves to project images of the heart and determine the size of the heart, pump (ejection) strength, heart muscle motion, and heart valve function. It is used to identify heart function and differentiate cardiac versus pulmonary etiology of respiratory failure when BNP is inconclusive.*	Normal or close to normal in patients with ARDS/ALI. Compromised left ventricular function is suggestive of the cardiac etiology of respiratory failure.
Right Heart Catheterization	
Cardiac index: 2.8–4.2 L/min/body surface area Pulmonary systolic pressure: 17–32 mmHg Pulmonary mean pressure: 9–19 mmHg Pulmonary diastolic pressure: 4–13 mmHg Pulmonary capillary wedge pressure: 4–13 mmHg Right atrial pressure: 0–7 mmHg *A Swan-Ganz catheter is inserted through a vein (usually subclavian or jugular) into the right side of the heart and threaded into the pulmonary artery. The pressures obtained indicate the pressures of the right heart, pulmonary vasculature, and left heart and identify and monitor cardiac function and blood flow, including cardiac output/index. Cardiac output/index is reduced and pulmonary wedge pressure increased in cardiac compromise. ARDS/ALI should demonstrate a normal wedge pressure.*	Pulmonary wedge pressure >18 mmHg is associated with cardiac etiology of respiratory failure. Pulmonary wedge pressure < 18 mmHg is associated with pulmonary etiology of respiratory failure.
Arterial Blood Gases (ABGs)	
pH 7.35–7.45; $PaCO_2$ 35–45; PaO_2 75–100; HCO_3 24–28 *Measures the degree of hypoxemia and hypercarbia* *Identifies acid–base imbalance*	pH < 7.35 = academia PaO_2 < 60 mmHg = hypoxemia $PaCO_2$ > 45 mmHg = respiratory acidosis HCO_3 < 24 = metabolic acidosis A low HCO_3 identifies the metabolic source of respiratory failure, such as sepsis. An elevated $PaCO_2$ identifies a respiratory cause of respiratory failure, such as COPD.
Chest Radiography	
Normal: clear, no trauma, good lung markings *Used to identify possible etiology of ARDS/ALI.*	Abnormalities in CXR can help to identify the source of respiratory failure. These may include pneumonia, pulmonary edema, pneumothorax, abscess, cancer, emphysema, or chest trauma. The progression of ARDS/ALI usually appears on the CXR as diffuse bilateral pulmonary infiltrates.
Sputum and Blood Cultures	
Normal: no growth *Used to identify the possible etiology of ARDS/ALI.*	May identify pathogens such as bacteria, fungus, or mycobacterium as a source of infection leading to respiratory failure.

ETHICAL ISSUES in Nonmalignant Pain Management

Historically, the treatment of chronic nonmalignant pain has been controversial. This controversy is pervasive in those cases where the quality or state of the pain exceeds the expected norm for the diagnosis, as well as in cases where there is medical uncertainty regarding the etiology of the chronic pain (Vallerand & Nowak, 2010). These concerns are, in part, the reason that chronic pain is undertreated. In 2011, the American College of Physicians (ACP) established Clinical Practice Guidelines for the treatment of chronic pain, taking into account recent studies of patients' responses to chronic pain and patient satisfaction with pain assessment and management (Topolovec-Vranic et al., 2010). The Guidelines are directed toward the management of chronic pain precipitated by a variety of causes (e.g., low back pain, fibromylagia, osteoarthritis) and the ethical issues associated with treatment (ACP, 2012; Bolen, 2008). The guidelines can be seen on the following website: www.acponline.org/ckunucak_information/guidelines/guidelines/.

Ethical Issues. This feature highlights the diverse ethical dilemmas that nurses face in clinical practice daily.

EVIDENCE-BASED PRACTICE Noninvasive Positive Pressure Ventilation

Clinical Problem

There are some patient characteristics and some absolutes with regards to patient selection. But how does the health care provider, nurse, or respiratory therapist decide who would be a good candidate for NPPV? It is difficult to predict which patients will tolerate NPPV. For example, some patients who are agitated and anxious when placed on NPPV become calm and relaxed; in these cases, the cause of the agitation is hypoxemia that is resolved by application of the NPPV. If the patient does have any potential contraindications to NPPV, attempting a trial of this therapy is probably the best course for deciding whether the patient will tolerate NPPV. However, there is some research that could assist the team in this regard.

Research Findings

The use of NPPV has long been accepted in patients with obesity hypoventilation syndrome and sleep apnea. In addition, over the past decade its use has become more popular in treating acute respiratory diseases in an attempt to prevent intubation with mechanical ventilation and its sequelae. A meta-analysis report demonstrated a consistent, positive effect on mortality, ICU days, and ventilator-associated pneumonia when using NPPV as a weaning strategy in patients with COPD (Burns, Adhikari, Keenan, & Meade, 2010). A large, multicenter randomized controlled study comparing traditional oxygen therapy against NPPV in patients presenting to the emergency department with acute cardiogenic pulmonary edema showed that NPPV provided earlier improvements in the resolution of breathlessness, reduction of respiratory distress, and reduced hypercarbia and acidosis when compared to the oxygen therapy group (Gray et al., 2009). Because of the complications of intubation in asthmatic patients, interest has been shown in using NPPV in patients with severe acute asthma. Scala (2010) reported on the review of the literature pertaining to NPPV in asthma. The available random controlled trials are few and the study groups small, leaving the application of NPPV in asthmatic patients unclear. This is an area where random controlled trials are clearly needed to identify efficacy in clearly defined patient parameters.

The use of NPPV in hypoxemic respiratory failure remains controversial. The cause of the hypoxemia appears to dictate its success. Agarwal, Aggarwal, and Gupta (2010) reviewed 13 studies (540 patients) on the efficacy of NPPV in patients with ALI/ARDS. They found an almost 50% NPPV failure rate and cautioned against its use in ALI/ARDS. They identified a need for a uniform NPPV protocol for use in patients with ALI/ARDS.

Evidence-Based Practice. This feature presents examples of evidence and how the studies impact nursing interventions, patient teaching, skills, and professional guidelines. Learners have an opportunity to test their understanding by responding to the critical thinking questions provided for each Evidence-Based Practice feature.

Genetic Considerations. In addition to the extensive information presented in the genetics chapter, the Genetic Considerations boxes found throughout the book contribute vital information about risk factors, therapies, research, legal implications, and counseling/screening, as appropriate.

GENETIC CONSIDERATIONS Cystic Fibrosis

Cystic fibrosis is an autosomal recessive genetic disorder that causes the body to produce thick, sticky mucus in the lungs and digestive tract. The mucus builds up in the lungs and pancreas, leading to life-threatening infections and digestive problems. The thickness of the mucus is related to a defect in the cystic fibrosis transmembrane regulator (CFTR). CFTR affects the movement of sodium and water across epithelial tissues, producing thick mucus. Thick mucus is difficult to expectorate from the airways and promotes colonization of bacteria.

Most patients with cystic fibrosis are diagnosed in childhood. Pulmonary complications are the primary cause of death. In the 1980s, children born with cystic fibrosis had a median predicted survival age of 26 years. According to data collected by the Cystic Fibrosis Foundation, however, infants born in 2008 in the United States have a life expectancy of 37.4 years (Cystic Fibrosis Foundation, 2008). Refer to Chapter 27 for more information on cystic fibrosis.

National Guidelines. These guidelines are integrated throughout the chapters where appropriate to provide pertinent, specific objectives to increase the learner's awareness of the need for uniformity of care on national and international levels (i.e., *Healthy People 2010,* the Health Insurance Portability and Accountability Act [HIPAA], and American Heart Association [AHA]).

NATIONAL GUIDELINES for the Prevention of Health Care–Associated Bacterial Pneumonia

Recommendations for Nursing Care

1. Wash hands after contact with mucous membranes, respiratory secretions, or objects contaminated with respiratory secretions. Wash hands before and after patient contact.
2. Educate health care workers about nosocomial bacterial pneumonias and infection control procedures used to prevent these pneumonias. Involve workers in implementing strategies for intervention.
3. Wear gloves when handling respiratory secretions or objects contaminated with respiratory secretions.
4. Provide subglottic suctioning before deflating the cuff of an endotracheal tube or before moving the tube.
5. Elevate the head of the bed to 30° to 45° if not contraindicated.
6. Develop and implement a comprehensive oral hygiene program to provide oropharyngeal cleaning and decontamination with or without an antiseptic agent.
7. Use chlorhexidine gluconate antiseptic rinse during the perioperative period in adult patients who undergo cardiac surgery.

Source: Adapted from Cason, C .L., Tyner, T., Saunders, S., & Broome L. (2007) Nurses' implementation of guidelines for VAP from the CDC. *American Journal of Critical Care, 16,* 2–37.

Nursing Process: Patient Care Plan. The Nursing Process: Patient Care Plan provides the learner with an easy-to-follow, easy-to-apply, succinct way of organizing nursing care, guided by nursing diagnosis, assessment, intervention, and outcome evaluation. It is designed to assist the learner in developing a plan of care specific to the patient with desired patient outcomes and specific nursing interventions for a given diagnosis.

NURSING PROCESS: Patient Care Plan for Patient Receiving Noninvasive Positive Pressure Ventilation

Assessment of Ventilatory Status Using Gordon's Functional Health Patterns:

- Health Perception Health Management Pattern
- Nutrition Metabolic Pattern
- Activity Exercise Pattern
- Cognitive Perceptual Pattern
- Self-Perception Self-Concept Pattern

Subjective Data	Objective Data
Assessment for Selection, Initiation, and Assessment of Patient on NPPV	**Assessment for Selection, Initiation, and Assessment of Patient on NPPV**
Do you think you could attempt a trial of NPPV? Which interface would you prefer? Are you experiencing any episodes of nausea or vomiting? Have you ever had problems with claustrophobia?	Level of consciousness Hemodynamic stability Ventilation Work of breathing Oxygen saturation Abdominal and genitourinary assessment Vital signs ABGs
Assessment for Level of Consciousness, Patient's Ability to Communicate, and Procedural Tolerance	**Assessment for Level of Consciousness, Patient's Ability to Communicate, and Procedural Tolerance**
What is your name, where are you, what is the date, and why are you here?	Glasgow Coma Scale Follow commands
Assessment of Level of Comfort	**Assessment of Level of Comfort**
What is your pain level at, using the 1–10 scale? A 1 is very little pain and a 10 is the worst imaginable pain. What is your experience with pain? Do you routinely take pain medications at home; if so, what for and what kind? Are you allergic to any pain medication? Do you have any cultural or religious beliefs that impact your pain control? Does the pain get worse with deep inspiration? Describe the pain: burning, sharp, aching, or any other term that is descriptive of it.	Grimacing on movement Restlessness and irritability Taut facial expression
Assessment of Hemodynamic Stability	**Assessment of Hemodynamic Stability**
Do you become light-headed or pass out? Do palpitations or light-headedness occur at the same time? Do your feet swell and, if so, under what circumstances?	Vital signs: BP and HR Oxygen saturation Level of consciousness ECG Lab values: electrolytes and measures of acidosis Cardiac output Lung/cardiac Urine output
Assessment of Respiratory Effort	**Assessment of Respiratory Effort**
Do you feel short of breath? Is it becoming worse or better? How long have you been experiencing shortness of breath? Do you have it at rest or just with activities?	Oxygen saturation ABGs Skin color and temperature Respiratory rate Lung sounds

Patient Teaching & Discharge Priorities. These tables help identify priorities for discharge planning while integrating patient teaching with home and community care.

PATIENT TEACHING & DISCHARGE PRIORITIES for a Patient with ARDS

Need	Teaching
Awareness of medications	• Teach the purpose and possible side effects of all medications and which side effects require medical attention. • Have the patient demonstrate proper use of an inhaler. • If home oxygen is ordered, teach proper use of oxygen therapy and safety measures in handling oxygen tanks. Provide information or coordinate through home health care to arrange for oxygen delivery.
Knowledge of continuing home care	• Explain the use of pulse oximetry if prescribed, as well as acceptable values and when to call a health care provider or seek emergency care. • Have the patient demonstrate proper use of an incentive spirometer and identify its frequency of use. • Have the patient demonstrate breathing exercises such as pursed-lip breathing or diaphragmatic breathing. • Provide written instructions of when to notify a health care provider or seek emergency care: fever, bloody sputum, increased shortness of breath, wheezing, or swelling in the legs, feet, or abdomen. • Describe the importance of keeping all follow-up appointments.
Understanding of disease recovery	• Stress that it may take 6 to 12 months or longer to regain normal lung function. • Explain that there may be some memory loss because of poor oxygen supply to the brain. • Anxiety, fear, and depression are normal feelings. Encourage the patient to talk to family, friends, or the health care provider about these feelings. • Inform the family or primary caregivers that they may also experience stress and depression. Encourage them to seek counseling if these feelings become overwhelming. • Encourage the patient to participate in an activity or exercise program under the guidance of the health care provider. • For patients who developed ARDS, provide information of ARDS support groups.
Promote ongoing health and disease prevention	Explain to the patient and family that they can reduce their chance of getting lung infections and other illnesses by doing the following: • Wash hands or use antimicrobial gel frequently. • Do not smoke. • Stay inside when air pollution or pollen count is high. • Stay inside during very cold or hot weather. • Avoid people with flu or cold. • Maintain a healthy diet.

PHARMACOLOGY Summary of Medications Used to Treat Complex Respiratory Disorders

Medication Category and Action	Application/Indication	Nursing Responsibilities
Diuretics Furosemide (Lasix) ***Action:*** Forces increased urine output by the kidney.	Increases water excretion. Used in cardiogenic pulmonary edema and noncardiogenic pulmonary edema to reduce pulmonary congestion, reduce systemic congestion, and decrease the workload to the heart.	Monitor for signs of dehydration: hypotension, dry mucous membranes, decreased urine output, and poor skin turgor. Overdiuresis will depress cardiac output and affect cellular perfusion. Monitor potassium levels. Measure urine output to gauge response to the drug.
Bronchodilators Short-acting beta-2 agonists (albuterol) Anticholinergics (Atrovent) ***Action:*** Relaxes smooth muscle of the bronchi and bronchioles.	Short-acting bronchodilators are fast-acting and used in acute respiratory failure associated with exacerbation of COPD, acute asthma attacks, or other diseases associated with bronchospasm.	Monitor signs and symptoms before and after treatment to identify presence of bronchospasm (wheezes) and response to therapy. Monitor for increased heart rate, palpitations, tremors, headache, nervousness, or dizziness that are associated with sympathomimetic stimulation. Obtain electrocardiogram in patients with chest pain or severe tachycardia. Beta-blockers may be ordered for symptomatic tachycardia or refractory hypotension unresponsive to fluid. Benzodiazepines may be administered for severe agitation or seizures.
Dexamethasone ***Action:*** A synthetic adrenocortical steroid. Has anti-inflammatory effects.	Prophylaxis of high altitude pulmonary edema. Mechanism of action is unknown.	Monitor for signs of infection. Corticosteroids decrease infection resistance and may mask signs of infection. Monitor for hypertension. Anaphylactic reactions have been reported; monitor vital signs after initial dosing.
Nifedipine ***Action:*** A nonspecific calcium-channel blocker that reduces pulmonary vascular resistance and pulmonary pressures; reduces systemic resistance and blood pressure.	Used in high altitude pulmonary edema when oxygen is unavailable and rapid descent is not possible.	Watch for hypotension. Have IV fluid available. Monitor for chest pain, especially in patients with severe obstructive coronary artery disease. May cause dizziness or headache. Patients should be advised to avoid activities that require coordination.
Phosphodiesterase Inhibitors Sildenafil Tadalafil ***Action:*** Inhibits PDE-5 in pulmonary vascular smooth muscle causing vasodilation and reduction in arterial hypertension.	Used in the prophylaxis and treatment of high altitude pulmonary edema (when oxygen and descent to a lower altitude are not options) to reduce hypoxic pulmonary vasoconstriction and pulmonary hypertension.	Assess for epistaxis, headache, dyspnea, flushing, insomnia, and dyspnea. Instruct the patient to report sudden decrease or loss of hearing or vision. Assess for improvement in signs and symptoms of pulmonary hypertension.
Naloxone (Narcan) ***Action:*** An opioid antagonist that competes with the opiate receptor sites in the central nervous system.	Reversal of opiate activity and respiratory depression.	Monitor blood pressure, heart rate, and respiratory rate. Monitor for withdrawal symptoms in patients with known or suspected opioid dependence. They will occur within minutes of naloxone administration and then subside in about 2 hours. Respiratory depression may then recur. Patients should be monitored for at least 2 hours after last dose.
Inotropes Dobutamine Milrinone Dopamine (at lower dosage) ***Action:*** Increase ventricular contractility and decrease ventricular afterload by inducing pulmonary and systemic vasodilation.	Helpful in patients with cardiogenic pulmonary edema associated with heart failure due to severe left ventricular dysfunction and low cardiac output. Unresponsive to diuretics or vasodilator therapy.	These drugs are administered via continuous IV infusion and require monitoring of blood pressure and ECG. Monitor for hypotension and tachydysrhythmias. Blood pressure should be stabilized with a vasopressor, or dopamine used as the initial agent, prior to initiation of these medications, then patient off the vasopressor as blood pressure tolerates.

Pharmacology Summary Tables. These three-column tables offer a comprehensive overview of the pharmacology for the chapter disorders, organized by drug categories, and include medications and actions, applications, and indications, as well as the nursing responsibilities.

RESEARCH OPPORTUNITIES Related to Complex Respiratory Disorders

Research Area	Clinical Impact
Effectiveness of prone ventilation in adults with ARDS	May improve promotion of alveoli and movement of secretions
Ventilator management for the treatment of ARDS: Ventilator settings Mode selection Pressure versus volume High frequency oscillatory ventilation (HFOV)	Improving oxygenation and preventing further lung injury
Liquid ventilation	
Extracorporeal membrane oxygenation (ECMO)	
Appropriate fluid management in ARDS	Effective support of cardiovascular status without increase in alveolar secretions
Ventilated-associated pneumonia (VAP)	Increased prevention of VAP
Role of mouth care in decreasing pathogenic organisms in the oral plaque biofilm	Decrease amount of pathogens from mouth to lungs
Other methods of preventing VAP:	
Patient positioning	Recruitment of alveoli
Use of subglottic endotracheal tube	Decrease amount of pathogens from oral cavity to lungs
Antibiotic-coated endotracheal tube	
Use of NPPV and weaning	Improving weaning
Incorporate this mode of ventilation into weaning strategies	
NPPV and indications for instituting this mode of ventilation in cardiac failure and respiratory failure	Wider use of NPPV for many types of cardiac and respiratory failure
NPPV interfaces (face mask, nasal mask, helmet, etc.)	Improved interfaces that will improve patient comfort and compliance

Research Opportunities. Current research topics and their clinical impact introduce the learner to prospective research needs that are designed to potentially improve patient care. The purpose is to help the learner focus on future research needs and potential projects to improve patient care.

Risk Factors. These boxes highlight particular items in the patient history and interview that should alert the nurse to possible problems.

RISK FACTORS That Cause or Predispose a Patient to ALI/ARDS

Sepsis	Bacteremia
Aspiration	Pneumonia
Severe trauma	Burns
Massive transfusion	Transfusion-related acute lung injury (TRALI)
Near drowning	Lung and hematopoietic stem cell transplantation
Drugs and alcohol	Pancreatitis
Fat embolism	Genetic determinants

Source: Adapted from TenHoor, T., Mannino, D. M., & Moss, M. (2001). Risk factors for ARDS in the United States: Analysis of the 1993 national mortality followback study. *Chest, 119*(4), 1179–1184.

Safety Alert *If an acutely ill patient exhibits any signs or symptoms of inadequate oxygenation or ventilation, the patient history and interview process should be curtailed until the patient's condition is stabilized.*

Safety Alerts. This feature alerts the learner to the immediate need for a nursing intervention that will prevent complications and promote learning. The learner will differentiate the critical nature of various clinical situations and determine the need to prioritize interventions.

Gerontological Considerations. The special needs of the fastest growing population are considered in order to help prevent complications and improve the prognoses for elderly patients.

Health Promotion. Found as appropriate in many chapters, Health Promotion sections call the learner's attention to one of the nurse's primary roles, that of educating the patient and family about healthy habits and lifestyles, thereby preventing or ameliorating unhealthy conditions.

Nursing Management. The Nursing Management sections describe the nurse's responsibilities and in many cases detail the steps of the nursing process that are specific to the disorder. These sections range from a brief paragraph to a full page that covers the nursing process for the disorder.

Collaborative Management. These sections appear in almost every chapter and describe the work of the health care team for patients with particular disorders. For instance, these sections describe working with occupational therapists and physical therapists to recover from trauma, or working with respiratory therapists for a patient with COPD, or working with a team of nurses on a complex case.

ACKNOWLEDGMENTS

In addition to the individuals mentioned in our dedications, we would also like to thank people who were instrumental in the development of the book. The following people assisted us in bringing this project to fruition:

- *Laura Horowitz, the development editor, for being the glue that kept the project moving in a positive direction. We deeply appreciate her patience with our never-ending list of needs. We could not have done it without her.*
- *Charlotte Miller for her precise review of chapters that ensured the accuracy and consistency of content.*
- *Mary Ann Shahdi, Jennifer FitzGerald, Andrea Perry, Sonia Garcia, Kathleen Budesa, and Jolie Tietz, nursing students, who generously shared their thoughts and feelings about caring behavior observed in nurses, presented in Chapter 1.*

CONCEPTS

Fifty-eight concepts, which define the meaning of an idea or theme, are covered in the second edition of *Medical–Surgical Nursing: Preparation for Practice.* The concepts covered in each unit are listed on the unit-opening page. Here we list the concepts with the definitions used in the book:

1. ***Aging.*** The process of becoming older, a process that is genetically determined and environmentally modulated.
2. ***Acid–base balance.*** The maintenance of hydrogen ion concentration in body fluids to maintain a pH range of 7.35–7.45 (North Carolina Concept Based Learning Editorial Board, 2011).
3. ***Addiction behavior.*** The compulsive, problematic patterns of action resulting in psychologic and/or physiologic dependence.
4. ***Body image.*** How a person perceives his physical self, including size, appearance, and functioning of his body parts. Body image includes both affective and cognitive aspects (North Carolina Concept Based Learning Editorial Board, 2011).
5. ***Caring.*** In 1988, Jean Watson identified human care as an inter-subjective human process and a moral ideal for nursing. She stated that the necessary conditions for caring to occur are knowledge and awareness about the need for care, an intention to act, actions based on knowledge, and a positive change that results from caring (Watson, 1988).
6. ***Cell development/abnormalities.*** When there is a change or disturbance of any of the common features of the cell (membrane, cytoplasm, nucleus, nucleolus, ribosomes, endoplasmic reticulum, mitochondria, Golgi apparatus, lysosomes, and DNA), abnormal replication of development can occur (North Carolina Concept Based Learning Editorial Board, 2011).
7. ***Cell division.*** Human cells divide in two ways: mitosis and meiosis. Mitosis is cell division that results in new cells. Meiosis is the reduction division of the cell, and only takes place in the sex cells of the ovaries and testes. Meiosis causes the formation of sperm and oocyte (North Carolina Concept Based Learning Editorial Board, 2011).
8. ***Cell proliferation/regulation.*** Cell reproduction, proliferation, and growth are regulated by the body. Alterations in cell regulation can have devastating effects on the body (North Carolina Concept Based Learning Editorial Board, 2011).
9. ***Clinical judgment.*** The outcomes of critical thinking in nursing practice. Clinical judgments begin with an end in mind. Judgments are about evidence, meaning, and outcomes achieved (Pesut, 2001).
10. ***Cognition.*** A complex process that includes learning, memory, retrieval, and use of information (North Carolina Concept Based Learning Editorial Board, 2011).
11. ***Collaboration/Interprofessional.*** Working across health care professions to cooperate, collaborate, communicate, and integrate care in teams to ensure that care is continuous and reliable. The team consists of the patient, the nurse, and other health care providers as appropriate (Institute of Medicine [IOM], 2003).
12. ***Comfort.*** Much more than just the absence of pain, comfort is the immediate experience of being strengthened by having needs for relief, ease, and transcendence met in four levels: physical, psychospiritual, social, and environmental (Kolcaba, 2003).
13. ***Communication.*** An exchange of information between individuals through a common system of signs, symbols, or behavior (*Merriam-Webster,* 2011).
14. ***Critical thinking.*** All or part of the process of questioning, analysis, synthesis, interpretation, inference, inductive and deductive reasoning, intuition, application, and creativity (American Association of Colleges of Nursing [AACN], 1998). Critical thinking underlies independent and interdependent decision making.
15. ***Culture sensitivity.*** Cultural sensitivity is experienced when neutral language, both verbal and nonverbal, is used in a way that reflects sensitivity and appreciation for the diversity of another. Cultural sensitivity may be conveyed through words, phrases, and categorizations that are intentionally avoided, especially when referring to any individual who may be interpreted as impolite or offensive (American Academy of Nursing Expert Panel on Cultural Competence, 2007).

16. ***Diversity.*** The range of human variation, including age, race, gender, disability, ethnicity, nationality, religious and spiritual beliefs, sexual orientation, political beliefs, economic status, native language, and geographical background (AACN, 2008).
17. ***Ethics.*** Ethics is the science relating to moral actions and individual value systems. It is the systematic study of what a person's conduct and actions ought to be with regard to self, other human beings, and the environment (Izumi, 2010).
18. ***Evidence-Based Practice.*** EBP is "the careful and practical use of current best evidence to guide health care decisions" (Omery & Williams, 1999, p. 51). Care that integrates the best research with clinical expertise and patient values for optimum care (IOM, 2003).
19. ***Elimination.*** The secretion and excretion of body wastes from the kidneys, intestines, and skin.
20. ***Experiential learning.*** Experiential learning is knowledge, skills, and/or abilities attained through observation, simulation, and/or participation. This type of learning engages the mind and/or body through activity, reflection, and application. It provides for affective and behavioral, as well as cognitive learning. Experiential learning is a less abstract learning tool that allows the participant to test theory while demanding that the learner articulate her own questions and seek her own answers.
21. ***Fear.*** A negative emotion that is induced by a real or perceived threat.
22. ***Fluid balance.*** The body's ability to balance fluid. A fluid imbalance in the body is either isotonic, when water and electrolytes are lost or gained in equal proportions and osmolality remains constant, or osmolar, when there is loss or gain of only water and the osmolality of the serum is altered (North Carolina Concept Based Learning Editorial Board, 2011).
23. ***Fluids and electrolyte balance.*** The body's ability to maintain fluid and electrolytes. The kidneys play a major role in maintaining balance, and renal disease causes significant imbalance. Fluid and electrolyte imbalance is a broad term, as fluid or any electrolyte may become deficient or excessive, causing an imbalance (North Carolina Concept Based Learning Editorial Board, 2011).
24. ***Gas exchange.*** The diffusion of oxygen from the alveoli into the pulmonary circulation and the release of carbon dioxide from the circulation into the alveoli.
25. ***Genetics.*** All hereditary material is carried on coiled strands of DNA known as chromosomes. The chromosomes carry the smallest units of inheritance known as genes. The Human Genome Project determined the exact DNA sequence of human genes, allowing the precise genes that are associated with certain abnormalities to be identified (North Carolina Concept Based Learning Editorial Board, 2011).
26. ***Global communication.*** An academic–practitioner partnership reaching across borders and supporting communications scholarship in the service of democratic values (Center for Global Communication Studies, 2012).
27. ***Grief and loss.*** Grief is the human response to loss. Loss is the actual or potential unavailability of something or someone who is valued or loved. This can include loss of family or friends, change in body image, job loss, or destruction of passions.
28. ***Health care systems.*** Health care systems are composed of individuals and organizations that aim to meet the health care needs of target populations.
29. ***Immunity.*** The protective process of response to a foreign substance.
30. ***Infection.*** Infection occurs when a microorganism enters the body and is able to colonize and multiply, leading to an infection and subsequent immune response.
31. ***Inflammation.*** Inflammation is a nonspecific, complex response to anything the body perceives as harmful. It is a protective mechanism that is necessary for normal healing to occur.
32. ***Ingestion.*** The process of taking food and other substances by mouth into the body for digestion or absorption.
33. ***Informatics.*** Informatics is a combination of computer science, information science, and health care science designed to assist in the management and delivery of health care.
34. ***Intracranial regulation.*** The processes that affect intracranial compensation and adaptive neurologic function. The neurologic system regulates and integrates all body functions (North Carolina Concept Based Learning Editorial Board, 2011).

35. ***Metabolism.*** Biochemical reactions occurring in the cells that are necessary to produce energy, repair cells, and maintain life (American Academy of Nursing Expert Panel on Cultural Competence, 2007).
36. ***Mobility.*** The body's function of movement. The musculoskeletal system is composed of the bones that serve as the body's framework and attachment sites of muscles, tendons, and ligaments. Innervated by the nervous system, contraction and relaxation of muscles allow movement at the joints (North Carolina Concept Based Learning Editorial Board, 2011).
37. ***Mood and affect.*** Emotions are feeling responses to stimuli. Mood is a sustained emotional state and how a person subjectively feels. Mood is communicated through affect, the immediate and observable emotional expression communicated verbally and nonverbally (North Carolina Concept Based Learning Editorial Board, 2011).
38. ***Multisystem failure.*** The failure of two or more systems in the body. Multisystem failure is also known as multiple organ failure (MOD).
39. ***Nursing process.*** According to the American Nurses Association (ANA), the nursing process is defined as a variation of scientific reasoning and is used to diagnose and to treat human responses to potential and actual health problems (ANA, 2007).
40. ***Nutritional balance.*** The healthy balance between nutrient intake and nutritional requirements.
41. ***Outcome.*** Broad performance indicator, related to the knowledge, skills, and attitudes needed by a baccalaureate graduate.
42. ***Oxygenation.*** Relates to the body's mechanisms and ability to supply and maintain oxygen to all of its cells.
43. ***Pain.*** An unpleasant and highly subjective sensory experience. There are both emotional and physiological components to pain.
44. ***Patient-centered care.*** Includes actions to identify, respect, and care about patients' differences, values, preferences, and expressed needs; relieve pain and suffering; coordinate continuous care; listen to, clearly inform, communicate with, and educate patients; share decision making and management; and continuously advocate disease prevention, wellness, and promotion of healthy lifestyles, including a focus on population health (IOM, 2003).
45. ***Perception.*** The way a person interprets his environment.
46. ***Reproduction.*** The biologic process by which individual organisms are produced from parents.
47. ***Research.*** A formal, systematic, and organized method used to answer a question or solve a problem. This systematic inquiry provides a forum to facilitate the ongoing process of questioning and evaluating practice, informing practice based on available data, and guiding the development of new practices through experimental learning.
48. ***Safety.*** The methods used to protect patients, families, and staff from self-injury or harm. It is a fundamental concept of nursing and nursing practice.
49. ***Self.*** A person's mental image of herself as a human being. Self includes self-concept, self-awareness, and self-esteem.
50. ***Sensory perception.*** A process that involves the conscious organization and translation of data or stimuli into meaningful information. Four components must be present for this process to occur: a stimulus, a receptor or a nerve cell, impulse conduction, and perception or interpretation of the stimuli.
51. ***Sexuality.*** How one expresses his sexual beliefs. This is influenced by physiological, psychological, and cultural factors.
52. ***Skin integrity.*** The skin, which is a part of the integumentary system, is the largest organ of the body. It assists in maintaining physiologic homeostasis and prevention of infection.
53. ***Stability.*** A state of maintenance of homeostasis, for example, a measurement of a patient's intake and output indicating that the patient is receiving adequate fluid and the kidneys are functioning normally.
54. ***Stress and coping.*** Stress is the body's reaction to a stimulus in the environment that demands change or disrupts homeostasis. The body's response to stress is known as coping.
55. ***Stress and adaptation.*** Stress is a condition in which people respond physiologically, psychologically, and socially to life changes. Stress can be viewed as a sequence of events that begins with a stimulus (stressor), which is recognized by the brain (stress perception), and that results in

the activation of physiological fight/flight/fright systems within the body (stress response). The desired outcome of stress is adaptation. Adaptation refers to the reaction to stress that signifies that the person is able to cope with the stressor or change.

56. ***Thermoregulation.*** Maintenance of a constant internal body temperature independent of the environmental temperature. The body process that balances heat production and heat loss to maintain the body's temperature.
57. ***Tissue perfusion.*** A term that describes the amount of blood that a tissue is receiving from the circulation. Tissue perfusion is measured by the volume of blood that flows through a unit quantity of the tissue, and is often expressed as mL blood/100 g tissue (Biology online, 2008).
58. ***Violence.*** An extreme form of aggression, such as assault, rape, or murder. Violence has many causes, including frustration, exposure to violent media, violence in the home or neighborhood, and a tendency to see other people's actions as hostile even when they are not. Certain situations increase the risk of aggression, such as drinking, insults and other provocations, and environmental factors like heat and overcrowding (adapted from the *Encyclopedia of Psychology*, 2000 [/pubs/books/4600100.aspx]).

References

American Academy of Nursing Expert Panel on Cultural Competence (2007). Retrieved from http://www.aannet.org/ep-cultural-competence

American Nurses Association (ANA). (2007). American Academy of Nursing Standards of Cultural Competence. *Journal of Transcultural Nursing,18*(2), 95–102. *PubMed.* Retrieved from http://www.ncbi.nlm.nih.gov/pubmed/17416710

American Association of Colleges of Nursing (AACN). (2008). *The essentials of baccalaureate education for professional nursing practice.* Washington, DC: Author.

Biology online. (2008). Tissue perfusion. Retrieved from http://www.biology-online.org/dictionary/Tissue_perfusion

Center for Global Communication Studies (2012). Retrieved from http://www.global.asc.upenn.edu/events.html

Encyclopedia of Psychology. (2000). A. E. Kazdin, Ed. Oxford University Press: American Psychological Association.

Institute of Medicine. (2003). *Health professions education: A bridge to quality.* Washington, DC: National Academies Press.

Izumi, S. (2010). Ethical practice in end-of-life care in Japan. *Nursing Ethics, 17*(4), 457–468.

Kolcaba, K. (2003). *Comfort theory and practice. A vision for holistic health care and research.* New York: Springer.

Merriam-Webster Dictionary. (2011). Retrieved from http://www.merriam-webster.com/

North Carolina Concept Based Learning Editorial Board. (2011). *Nursing: A concept-based approach to learning.* Upper Saddle River, NJ: Pearson Education, Inc.

Omery, A., & Williams, R. P. (1999). An appraisal of research utilization across the United States. *Journal of Nursing Administration, 29*(12), 50–56.

Pesut, J. (2001). Clinical judgment: Foreground/background. *Journal of Professional Nursing, 17*(5), 215.

QSEN, Quality and Safety Education for Nurses, 2011. Competency KSAs (Pre-licensure). Retrieved from http://www.qsen.org/ksas_prelicensure.php

Roach, M. (1984). Caring: The human mode of being: Implications for nursing. Toronto, Canada: University of Toronto Press.

Watson, J. (1988). *Nursing: Human science and human care. A theory of nursing.* New York: The National League for Nursing.

CONTENTS

UNIT 7

Nursing Management of Patients with Cardiovascular Disorders 830

UNIT 11

Nursing Management of Patients with Musculoskeletal Disorders 1465

UNIT 12

Nursing Management of Patients with Immunologic, Inflammatory, and Hematologic Disorders 1593

UNIT 13

Nursing Management of Patients with Integumentary Disorders 1829

Appendix D and the Glossary are located in the Student Resources site at nursing.pearsonhighered.com.

Concepts Related to Health Care Delivery and Nursing Practice

UNIT 1

Content in Unit 1 that addresses the **Institute of Medicine (IOM)** competencies, **Nursing Core Competencies (NCC)**, the **Quality and Safety Education for Nurses (QSEN)** competencies, and **Concepts** for concept-based learning is listed below.

Competencies	Feature or Text	Location
IOM, QSEN, NCC Providing patient-centered care	Six Components of Caring Critical Thinking, Decision Making, and Clinical Judgment Care Delivery Models Providing Safe Patient Care Nursing Process Nurse–Patient Relationship Steps of the Nursing Process Assessment of Health	Chapter 1, page 11 Chapter 2, page 52 Chapter 4, page 82 Chapter 4, page 90 Chapter 5, page 95 Chapter 5, page 95 Chapter 5, page 96 Chapter 6, page 115
IOM, QSEN, NCC Working in teams	Looking Toward the Future Nursing Care Delivery Systems: Past to Present Care Delivery Models	Chapter 1, page 16 Chapter 4, page 79 Chapter 4, page 82
IOM, QSEN, NCC Employing evidence-based practice	Health Care Trends Research Opportunities Related to Professional Concepts Research Utilization and Evidence-Based Practice Future Perspectives on Nursing Research	Chapter 2, page 31 Chapter 2, page 53 Chapter 3, page 64 Chapter 3, page 76
IOM, NCC Applying quality and safety improvement	Framework for Nursing Practice Looking Toward the Future Health Care Trends Critical Thinking, Decision Making, and Clinical Judgment Providing Safe Patient Care Critical Thinking and the Nursing Process Critical Thinking	Chapter 1, page 49 Chapter 1, page 16 Chapter 2, page 31 Chapter 2, page 52 Chapter 4, page 90 Chapter 5, page 102 Chapter 6, page 133
IOM, QSEN, NCC Using informatics	Looking Toward the Future Health Care Trends, Information Technology Informatics Nursing Documentation	Chapter 1, page 16 Chapter 2, page 34 Chapter 3, page 71 Chapter 5, page 105
NCC Applying ethical and legal responsibilities	Ethical and Legal Aspects of Nursing Ethics and Nursing Legal Concepts in Nursing Preventing Possible Liability National Guidelines for Interpretation of Ethical and Legal Issues Research and Ethics in Health Care Nursing Documentation	Chapter 2, page 37 Chapter 2, page 38 Chapter 2, page 42 Chapter 2, page 50 Chapter 2, page 52 Chapter 3, page 66 Chapter 5, page 105
NCC Developing professionally	Components of the Nursing Role Dreyfus Model of Skill Acquisition Roles of the Nurse Licensure, Regulation, and Accreditation	Chapter 1, page 3 Chapter 1, page 6 Chapter 1, page 13 Chapter 2, page 36
NCC Education patients	Health and Wellness Promotion National Guidelines: Healthy People 2020	Chapter 1, page 12 Chapter 6, page 114
Concepts covered in Unit 1 include:	Caring Clinical judgment Collaboration/interprofessional Communication Culture sensitivity Diversity Ethics Evidence-based practice Experiential learning Health care systems	Informatics Nursing process Patient-centered care Research

CHAPTER

1 Preparation for Practice

Cynthia Parkman
Patricia Benner
Annita Watson

Outcome-Based Learning Objectives

After studying this chapter, the learner will be able to:

1. Distinguish among the characteristics of nursing as defined in the roles of caregiver, advocate, educator, researcher, and leader.
2. Determine how the six components of caring as defined by Roach can be applied to nursing practice.
3. Critique the roles of the professional nurse within the health care delivery system according to the specified setting.
4. Differentiate the characteristics of the nursing role in the care delivery models for nursing practice.
5. Evaluate the components of cultural competence related to health care professionals, as defined by Campinha-Bacote.
6. Distinguish and analyze how and why the nurse's moral agency might change with experience, according to the Dreyfus model of skill acquisition.
7. Discriminate among the three distinct differences between competent and expert clinical nursing practice as defined by Benner.

KEY TERMS

academic nurse educator p.16
acute care nurse p.13
advanced practice nursing p.15
allopathic medicine p.20
alternative therapy p.20
assisted living p.14
caring p.3
clinical judgment p.10
clinical knowledge p.5
Code of Ethics p.4
community-based nurses p.16
complementary therapy p.20
cultural competence p.18
cultural diversity p.17
culture p.18
Dreyfus model of skill acquisition p.6
ethos p.9
experience p.7
experiential learning p.7
Health System Reform Agenda p.2
moral agency p.6
nursing process p.4
phronesis p.9
practical knowledge p.9
salience p.7
skills of involvement p.6
techne p.7

AS A PROFESSION, nursing is unique in its diversity of practice and opportunities for lifelong learning. The relatively fluid nature of this profession allows nurses to move from one setting to the next, expanding their knowledge, skills, and interest in their profession. The goal of nursing is to mobilize human and environmental resources to support healing, maintain well-being, prevent illness, and promote health. In every setting or specialty, the core of practice is the nursing process: assessment, diagnosis, planning, implementation, rationales, and evaluation (Carpenito-Moyet, 2007). The American Nurses Association (ANA) states that "the essence of nursing is that nurses combine the art of caring with the science of health care. Nursing places its focus not only on a particular health problem, but on the whole patient and his or her response to treatment. Care of the patient and a firm base of scientific knowledge are indispensable elements" (ANA, 2008, p. 1).

Registered nurses represent the largest health care occupation, accounting for nearly 2.6 million jobs in 2008, with hospitals employing 60% of RNs (Bureau of Labor Statistics, U.S. Department of Labor, 2011). In addition to hospitals, nurses deliver care in clinics, nursing care facilities, patients' homes, and other workplaces. Patients within the health care system often turn to nurses for assistance, because nurses are the health care providers that patients are most likely to encounter and the individuals with whom patients spend the greatest amount of time. As America moves forward to improve the health care delivery system, nurses will contribute in many ways. The ANA publication ***Health System Reform Agenda*** (2008a, p. 5) states: "Nursing, as the pivotal health care profession, is well positioned to advocate on behalf of, and in concert with, individuals, families, and communities who are in desperate need of a well-financed, functional, and coordinated health care system that provides safe, high-quality care."

Weblink: Occupational Outlook: Registered Nurses

Medical–Surgical Nursing

The Academy of Medical–Surgical Nurses (AMSN) is a professional organization committed to promoting nursing practice in the areas of health promotion and prevention of illness in adults. Within its position statement, *Identification of the Registered Nurse in the Workplace* (AMSN, 2011), the organization offers a description of medical–surgical nursing:

> Medical–surgical nursing is the foundation of all nursing practice. Once upon a time and not so very long ago, all nurses practiced the art and science of nursing on wards, everyone was a medical or surgical nurse—that is where all nursing started. Today many nurses choose to work in the specialty of medical–surgical nursing. Medical–surgical nursing has evolved from an entry-level position to an adult health specialty. It is no longer viewed as a stepping-stone but is the solid rock and the backbone of every institution. It is the largest group of practicing professionals. Medical–surgical nurses care for adult patients in many settings, such as inpatient care units, clinics, HMOs, ambulatory care units, home health care, long-term care, skilled nursing homes, urgent care centers, surgical centers, and universities, just to name a few.

Nurses play a pivotal role in health care, and in 2010 the Institute of Medicine (IOM) released the report *The Future of Nursing: Leading Change, Advancing Health*. The four key messages of the IOM report (2010) are listed in Chart 1–1. The report emphasized the need for nurses to advance their practice through education, leadership, and partnership with other health care professionals. Advances in health care and technology have allowed more patients to receive care in venues other than the hospital. Regardless of the nurse's practice setting, a renewed emphasis upon nursing practice, quality, and safety has reinforced the focus of this profession. Recently, the Robert Wood Johnson Foundation sponsored the Quality and Safety Education for Nurses (QSEN) (Cronenwett, Sherwood, & Gelmon, 2009) as an initiative to improve the quality and safety in prelicensure nursing programs. This initiative advised that quality and safety education must become core competencies embedded in all programs preparing nurses for basic practice (Cronenwett et al., 2009; QSEN, 2011). The six competencies critical to the nursing role are patient-centered care, teamwork and collaboration, evidence-based practice, quality improvement, safety, and informatics (Anderson, 2010; QSEN, 2011). The overall goal of the QSEN program is to address the challenge of preparing future nurses with the knowledge, skills, and attitudes (KSA) necessary "to continuously improve the quality and safety of the health care systems in which they work" (Anderson, 2010, p. 4).

CHART 1–1 IOM Report Key Messages

- Nurses should practice to the full extent of their education and training.
- Nurses should achieve higher levels of education and training through an improved education system that promotes seamless academic progression.
- Nurses should be full partners, with physicians and other health care professionals, in redesigning health care in the United States.
- Effective workforce planning and policy making require better data collection and information infrastructure.

Source: Adapted from Institute of Medicine (IOM). (2010). *The future of nursing: Leading change, advancing health.* Washington, DC: Author. Retrieved from http://www.iom.edu/Reports/2010/The-Future-of-Nursing-Leading-Change-Advancing-Health.aspx.

By practicing to the full extent of education and training, nurses assure that patients receive quality care. Achieving higher levels of education helps address a commitment to lifelong learning that also promotes a more culturally and ethnically diverse workforce (Hertel, 2011).

Components of the Nursing Role

In the professional nursing role, the nurse develops a partnership with the patient and assists patients in learning how to cope with circumstances in order to develop an environment that promotes health, prevents illness, and facilitates recovery (Figure 1–1 ◆) (Doss, DePascal, & Hadley, 2011). There are specific characteristics or commonalities within every nursing role: caregiver, advocate, educator, researcher, and leader. These characteristic components of the role are discussed next.

Caregiver

The nurse provides care to patients and families based on current research, nursing judgment, and careful analysis of each individual patient's unique situation. The nursing process is the decision-producing model for the selection of nursing interventions (AMSN, 2011). **Caring** is the most central and unifying concept in nursing. In 1988, Jean Watson identified human care as an intersubjective human process and a moral ideal for nursing. She stated that the necessary conditions for caring to occur are knowledge and awareness about the need for care, an intention to act, actions based on knowledge, and a positive change that results from caring (Watson, 1988). Based on Watson's definition, caring can be interpreted to mean feeling and exhibiting concern and empathy for patients by acting to protect, enhance, and preserve their dignity, humanity, wholeness, and inner harmony (Watson, 1988).

Advocate

As patients enter the health care system, they are often overwhelmed and unprepared to make informed decisions regarding their care.

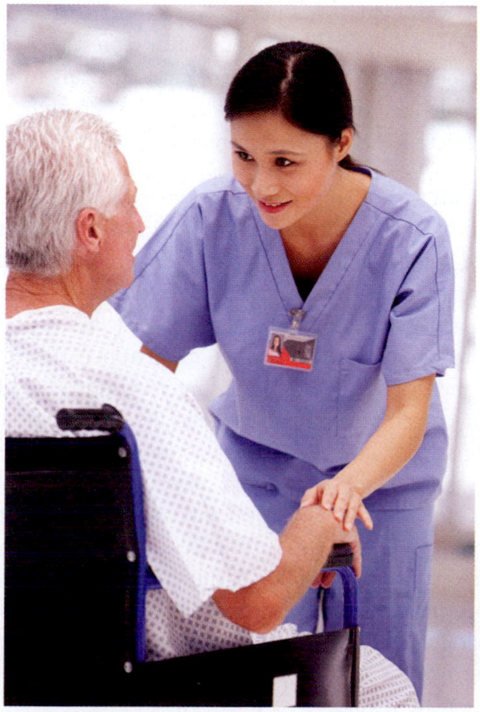

FIGURE 1–1 ◆ The nurse–patient partnership is critical to help the patient cope with illness.

Source: Monkey Business/Fotolia

Weblink: Institute of Medicine Report

Some patients may be so ill that they are unable to communicate their wishes. Part of the nurse–patient relationship is the nurse's assessment of the patient's and family's understanding regarding the diagnosis and plan of care, identification of educational needs, and communication with other members of the health care team as an advocate for the patient's rights to autonomy, free choice, and the ability to make informed decisions.

Nurses play a key role by serving as change agents within the health care system. Advocacy is more than just understanding an issue; it requires involvement and collaboration to provide a strong unified voice for nursing through legislative and regulatory representation. The American Nurses Association has federal and state advocacy web pages that track the status of current issues that are affecting health care. The ANA has also developed the Nurses Strategic Action Team (N-STAT), a grassroots network for nurses that alerts members to the progress of key bills as they move through Congress and whom to contact regarding support or opposition (ANA, 2007a). The nurse as advocate supports excellence of care through patient, family, and community education; communication with other health care team members; and participation in health policy development.

Educator

The nurse not only provides education for patients and families, but also participates in the education of the community. Health education determines how well patients, families, and communities are able to develop behaviors that are beneficial to optimal self-care. The ANA's *Standards of Clinical Nursing Practice* (2010) and all state nurse practice acts include teaching as a function of nursing practice.

The emphasis in nursing education is on health promotion and maintenance. Nurses promote health by teaching, by modeling lifestyles that promote wellness, and by providing information regarding the characteristics and consequences of diseases, including risk factors and ways to decrease health risks. The U.S. Department of Health and Human Services (DHHS) has published national health objectives for the year 2020 (DHHS, 2011). The focus areas represent an opportunity for healthy lifestyle choices and encourage clinicians to incorporate prevention into their practice. A detailed discussion of the focus areas of *Healthy People 2020* occurs in Chapter 6.

Researcher

The American Nurses Association (2010) has adopted a standard wherein the registered nurse integrates research findings into practice. One way of measuring this standard is the active participation of nurses in research activities at various levels appropriate to the nurse's level of education and position. These activities range from participating in data collection and designing the study to interpreting the results. Nurses not only investigate issues of relevance to the practice of nursing, but also participate in interdisciplinary collaborations to research common health care issues. Collaborative and interdisciplinary research fosters communication and mutual respect and enhances collaborative practice. The National Institute of Nursing Research (NINR, 2011) believes that with more interdisciplinary collaborations, nursing can provide a more comprehensive approach to research in health promotion, illness, and disabling conditions. Chapter 3 explores the role of research in nursing practice.

Leader

There are many definitions of the word *leadership*. One definition states that leadership refers to the use of personal traits and personal power to constructively and ethically influence patients, families, and others toward an end point vision or goal (Yoder-Wise, 2011). All nurses are leaders as they model time management, priority setting, patient and family teaching, evaluation of the quality of care, precepting of students, mentoring of colleagues, and development of community outreach programs. A leader has the ability to tie together the support, collaboration, and enthusiasm of people to meet specific goals and objectives, whether it is a patient and his family or an entire organization.

Throughout this book, the learner is presented with a body of knowledge and skills that, with experience, will assist the nurse to create relationships and environments that are healing, humane, and caring. Professional nurses practice with compassion and respect for the inherent dignity, worth, and uniqueness of every individual, despite social or economic status, personal attributes, or the nature of health problems.

Framework for Nursing Practice

The foundational framework for nursing practice is that it is an evidence-based profession which is guided by the ANA **Code of Ethics** for nurses (ANA, 2001). In addition, the concept-oriented approach to nursing includes the QSEN initiatives, the findings from the IOM study, and nursing core competencies as defined in the AACN *Essentials of Baccalaureate Education for Professional Nursing Practice*. Today, nursing practice has expanded to include a focus on leadership and multidisciplinary collaboration. Experiential learning and reflection are key elements of preparing nurses for practice (Benner, Hooper-Kyriakidis, & Stannard, 2011).

The practice of nursing requires knowledge, critical thinking skills, and clinical judgment, and uses the nursing process to apply these concepts to patient care situations. All aspects of nursing practice are shaped and guided by a caring approach to patient care. Additionally, nurses have a responsibility to promote health and wellness for individuals and communities. The nursing profession was among the first groups to understand the need for primary health care and prevention. As gaps in health care have occurred over the years, nurses have been able to fill them and provide high-quality service. This is true in all areas of nursing: acute care, specialty nursing, advanced practice, community nursing, and education. The nursing profession also has actively cared for disadvantaged socioeconomic groups. Because the breadth of nursing practice is so great, the profession is in a good position to impact health care policy and decisions. In this time of tremendous health care transition, nurses must rise to the challenge of providing accessibility to quality patient care. The tenets of the framework for nursing practice are discussed in this chapter.

Nursing Process

The **nursing process** is a thinking and doing approach to patient care that provides the nurse with a systematic means of identifying, preventing, and treating actual and potential health problems in patients (Carpenito-Moyet, 2007). According to the American Nurses Association (2012), the nursing process is defined as a variation of scientific reasoning and is used to diagnose and treat human responses to potential and actual health problems. The nursing process provides an essential patient-centered approach to the patient care plan. This framework provides nurses with a concise method of organizing patient care. The nursing process promotes communication and collaboration with the health care team because it is an established approach that is understood and used by nurses to identify and treat patients' problems. The nursing process includes the following steps: assessment, diagnosis, outcome identification, planning, implementation, and evaluation. These steps are ordered to facilitate the process of identifying patient problems and desired outcomes in an efficient, consistent manner. Chapter 5 contains an in-depth discussion of the nursing process.

Critical Thinking

Nursing is a highly complex and challenging profession that exists within a rapidly changing health care environment. The essence of nursing lies not in the special environments or amid the special equipment, but in the nurse's professional care of the patient, which requires a decision-making process and willingness to act on these decisions. In other words, the nurse must have the ability to think critically, must possess sound clinical judgment, and must be able to apply these concepts effectively in multiple health care arenas and complex patient care situations. Critical thinking is not a separate body of knowledge to be learned; however, like reading and writing, critical thinking is a process that occurs in all areas of life and learning. Critical thinking is typically described as a purposeful, two-dimensional, goal-directed, self-regulatory process that is context bound (Kaddoura, 2010). An international group of nursing experts consisting of 72 participants from nine countries developed a landmark definition of critical thinking as it applies to nursing:

> Critical thinking in nursing is an essential component of professional accountability and quality nursing care. Critical thinkers in nursing exhibit these habits of the mind: confidence, contextual perspective, creativity, flexibility, inquisitiveness, intellectual integrity, intuition, open-mindedness, perseverance, and reflection. Critical thinkers in nursing practice the cognitive skills of analyzing, applying standards, discriminating, information seeking, logical reasoning, predicting and transforming knowledge. (Gendrop & Eisenhauer, 1996)

Two dimensions are necessary for the development of critical thinking: the cognitive, which entails reflective, reasoned thinking, and the affective, which consists of being open-minded to divergent perspectives and having an inquisitive spirit (Kaddoura, 2010). In addition to the cognitive and affective abilities, effective critical thinking skills evolve with time, knowledge, professional practice, and structured feedback (Benner, Tanner, & Chesla, 1996). Critical thinking skills develop in tandem with intellectual and ethical development (L'Eplattenier, 2001). Chart 1–2 identifies key critical thinking skills.

Critical thinking is necessary to begin the problem solving required for complex patient care situations. Critical thinking, however, is not *just* problem solving; it is also an application of logic that evolves from an understanding of the need to question conventions and habits and to base decisions on sound reasoning (D'Amico & Barbarito, 2010; Kaddoura, 2010; Lipe & Beasley, 2006). Critical thinking is cultivated by questioning the norms and avoiding an acceptance of the biases. According to D'Amico and Barbarito (2010), five essential elements are involved in the critical thinking process:

- Collection of information
- Analysis of the situation
- Generation of alternatives
- Selection of alternatives
- Evaluation.

Critical thinking skills are needed in order to observe, gather, organize, and analyze data accurately, because interpretation of a patient's symptoms can be complex and diverse. When applied to patient care situations, critical thinking promotes health and assists the patient to achieve the desired outcomes of care (Kaddoura, 2010). When applying critical thinking to patient care situations, it is important to remember that the patient's sociocultural context (beliefs, values, living and working environments) provide important data that inform the decision-making process.

The process of developing critical thinking skills begins during the nurse's education process. The American Association of Colleges of Nursing (2007) requires that critical thinking be reflected within academic nursing programs as a core competency for program accreditation. However, the evolution and refinement of critical thinking continue as the nurse gains experience through practice (Finn, 2011; Kaddoura, 2010). To think critically, the nurse needs to apply experience and knowledge to patient care situations. Benner (2001) asserts that as nurses gain experience and knowledge in practice, they progress through five distinct stages of skill acquisition, from novice to expert nurse. A complete description of these stages is discussed in the next section.

CHART 1–2 Critical Thinking Skills

- Be inquisitive by asking pertinent questions.
- Assess what information is necessary to determine a solution to the problem.
- Gather the facts and validate the information.
- Consider available options.
- Be flexible and open-minded about all options.
- Draw on past experiences and knowledge.
- Formulate creative decisions and test their effectiveness.
- Be open-minded to dissonance and ambiguity.

Source: Adapted from Finn, P. (2011). Critical thinking: Knowledge and skills for evidence-based practice. *Language, Speech, and Hearing Services in Schools, 42*, 69–72.

Becoming a Nurse

> Nursing like medicine, involves a rich, socially embedded clinical know-how that encompasses perceptual skills, transitional understandings across time, and understanding of the particular in relation to the general. **Clinical knowledge** is a form of engaged reasoning that follows modus operandi thinking, in relation to patients' and clinical populations' particular manifestations of disease, dysfunction, response to treatment and recovery trajectories. Clinical knowledge is necessarily configurational, historical (by historical, I mean the immediate and long-term histories of particular patients and clinical populations), contextual, perceptual, and based upon knowledge gained in transitions. . . . [Through articulation], clinical understanding becomes increasingly articulate and translatable at least by clinical examples, narratives and puzzles encountered in practice. *(Benner, 1994, p. 139)*

Becoming a nurse requires more than mastery of technical and scientific knowledge. It also requires ongoing experiential learning, reflection on practice, and continuous improvement in practice as science, technology, and experiential knowledge change. A metaphor of "mastery" is somewhat misleading in any professional endeavor, because it projects the imagined possibility that the field is stable and can be completely "mastered" or learned at any one point in time. Fields like nursing and medicine, however, are constantly changing and self-correcting, and the study of these fields never completely covers what actually might be encountered in clinical practice. Clinical practice knowledge includes learning directly through experience by engaging in practice situations. Relational knowledge (skills of engaging with patients and patient situations), skilled know-how in actual practice situations, and patient interventions based on patients' responses to their illnesses and therapies are all examples of experiential clinical learning.

To make good clinical judgments, the nurse must be skillful in moral and clinical perception (Benner & Wrubel, 1982; Benner, Hooper-Kyriakidis, & Stannard, 2011; Dunne, 1997; Vetleson, 1994). Although conceptual knowledge is essential, it is not sufficient to ensure that the nurse will form relationships with patients that lead to salient, or noticeable, disclosures. Conceptual knowledge also does not ensure that the nurse will notice and correctly identify an instance of pulmonary edema, despair, or pain when the nurse sees it, even though the nurse may know conceptually what the formal characteristics of these patient conditions are in principle. Perceptual recognition skills, **skills of involvement** (commitment and concern), and **moral agency** (defined as the ability to effect and influence situations) are required for good clinical judgment and acting on behalf of the patient based on that judgment.

In the practice of medicine and nursing, science and technology are used to increase certainty about the measurement of signs and symptoms. The practice of objective measurement of signs and symptoms reduces errors and improves clinical judgment. For example, no one would recommend going back to guessing body temperatures by palpation alone. However, even the most formal measurements cannot replace the clinician's perceptual skill in recognizing when a particular measurement is relevant or its meaning at that point in time. Also, following the course of a patient's development of signs and symptoms (the trajectory or evolution of signs and symptoms) improves the clinician's understanding of the meaning of the signs and symptoms. This may seem patently obvious to any practicing clinician, yet current strategies for applying algorithms or making particular clinical judgments based on aggregate outcomes data alone ignore the clinical know-how, relational skills, and need for clinical judgment as reasoning across time (Halpern, 2001).

Good nursing practice requires ongoing development of clinical knowledge through experiential learning. Experiential learning is not automatic; it requires openness, attentiveness, reflection on practice, and active, engaged learning on the part of the practitioner. Here a distinction is being made between detached, disengaged reflection and engaged thinking-in-action (Guignon, 1983). Standing outside of a situation and reflecting back on it is a powerful critical-thinking strategy for improving practice, especially in situations of breakdown and error (Schon, 1987). However, being emotionally attuned to the patient and family and the demands of the situation in the immediate moment also is required for well-timed expert performance.

The clinician must always intelligently appraise the relevance of the best evidence for a particular patient in addition to critically evaluating the "best evidence" itself. Qualitative distinctions must be made about the patient's concerns, actual responses to therapies, and the disease or injury processes. If a nurse recognizes early signs of deterioration in a patient's clinical condition, she must be able to document and communicate the evidence for the changes. This requires social skills and experiential wisdom in communicating with other clinicians so that the evidence can be verified.

Dreyfus Model of Skill Acquisition

The **Dreyfus model of skill acquisition** is based on determining the level of practice evident in particular situations (Benner, 2001; Dreyfus, 1979; Dreyfus & Dreyfus, with Athanasiou, 1986). It elucidates strengths as well as problems. Situated practice capacities (skills representative of the profession that are learned through experience in a practice setting) are described rather than traits or talents of the practitioners. At each stage of experiential learning (novice, advanced beginner, competent, proficient, expert), clinicians can perform at their best. For example, a clinician can be the best advanced beginner possible, typically during the first year of practice. However, no practitioner can be beyond experience regardless of the level of skill acquisition in most clinical situations, despite the necessary attempts to make practice as clear and explicit as possible. If the nurse has never encountered a particular clinical situation, experiential learning is required. For example, referring to critical pathways is not the same as recognizing when and how these pathways are relevant or must be adapted to particular patients. Experiential learning that leads to individualization and clinical prioritization is required to make the use of critical pathways sensible and safe. Such individualization requires clinical judgment based on personal and direct experience with past actual clinical situations. The ability to make clinical comparisons between the entire clinical scenario without decomposing the whole situation into its analytical components is a hallmark of expert clinical nursing practice (Benner & Wrubel, 1982; Ruddick, 1989).

Experiential learning presents an opportunity to gain new knowledge and new ways of practicing, thus enabling the nurse to consistently develop and change as a practitioner. New skills are constantly being worked out and extended through experiential learning in local and larger practice communities. Practice is a way of knowing, as well as a way of being in the world (Dunne, 1997; Ruddick, 1989; Taylor, 1993, 1994). A self-renewing practice directs the development, implementation, and evaluation of science and technology. Clinical judgment requires moral agency, relationship with the patient, perceptual acuity, skilled know-how, and narrative reasoning across time about particular patient transitions (Benner & Wrubel, 1982; Guignon, 1983). As Joseph Dunne notes:

> A practice is not just a surface on which one can display instant virtuosity. It grounds one in a tradition that has been formed through an elaborate development and that exists at any juncture only in the dispositions (slowly and perhaps painfully acquired) of its recognized practitioners. (Dunne, 1997, p. 378)

Nursing, like other practice disciplines, is not merely an "applied" field in the sense that the practice is complex, varied, and underdetermined. Good practice requires that the nurse develop skillful ethical comportment as a practitioner and that the nurse use good clinical judgment informed by scientific evidence and technological development. The sciences of medicine and nursing are broad and multidisciplinary and require translation into each particular practice situation. Basic sciences such as biochemical, physical, biological, and physiological processes; research and development of specific therapies and technologies; clinical trials; and more make up a broad range of relevant science used in the practice of medicine and nursing.

Monitoring the quality of care and preventing imminent breakdown in practice quality require social communication skills and effective moral agency, both of which are the patient's frontline defense against errors and the hazards of hospitalization. For example, anyone in the operating room (OR) is required to immediately and verbally identify a break in sterile technique, just as it is the nurse's job to provide early warnings of changes in a patient's clinical condition. Moral agency requires more than the intent to do good or to *be* a good practitioner; it requires the experiential skill to recognize when an ethical breach in practice has occurred and the social and communication skills to effectively intervene on behalf of the patient.

Skill Acquisition and Experiential Learning

The clinician's capacity for moral agency literally changes with the growth of clinical judgment, perceptiveness, communication skills, and skillful comportment. The skill of involvement, both with the patient and through engagement with the clinical situation, is learned developmentally over time and changes with the level of skill acquisition. The stages of skill acquisition as uncovered in research on clinical nursing practice are described in this chapter, with a focus on the development of the clinician's relational skills of involvement and moral agency.

Experience, as defined here, is an active process in which a clinician bases current practice on events from a previous situation (Gadamer, 1960/1975). **Experiential learning** requires individuals to turn around their preconceptions, or add nuances to their understanding. Experiential learning also requires learners to remain engaged and be willing to learn, rather than appearing as an expert in **techne,** or technique, who skillfully applies well-established knowledge in prespecified, clear circumstances. To improve practice over time, experiential learning requires openness and responsiveness by the learner. The learner who develops an attuned, response-based practice learns to recognize whole situations in terms of past concrete (actual) experiences as pointed out by the Dreyfus model.

The researchers found that recognizing the situation as an "instance of particular concerns" is central to the logic of excellent practice. For example, consider a situation of heart "pump" failure or fluid depletion (Benner, 2001; Benner, Hooper-Kyriakidis & Stannard, 1999). Deciding which intervention to implement depends on clarifying and confirming the nature of the clinical situation at hand. The skillful practitioner learns to keep background understandings fluid or semipermeable so that he can recognize when these tacit expectations are not met. For example, a nurse with expertise in detecting heart arrhythmias on a unit where all patients' cardiac functioning is monitored will only notice aberrations in sound patterns, rather than attending to the familiar sounds in the foreground of attention. Recognizing the unexpected—that is, recognizing when tacit global expectations of patients' recovery are not met—is a hallmark of expert practice.

Major Shifts in the Style of Practice with the Development of Expertise

As noted earlier, the nurse's capacity for effective moral agency changes as the nurse develops practice skills and insights from experience. In addition, the skills of engaging with both patients and with problems or situations grow more attuned. The development of moral agency and skills of involvement should be considered at each stage of skill acquisition, from novice to expert. The nurse increasingly is able to recognize when she does not have a good grasp of the clinical situation, and this lack of a sense of understanding guides the nurse's questioning and problem solving. Over time, an increased grasp of the nature of particular clinical situations, including opportunities and constraints, guides the nurse's actions and interactions. Consequently, responses to patients become more contextualized and attuned.

Recognition of clinical situations moves from abstract textbook accounts of general features to comparisons with past whole actual cases. These real comparisons can include qualitative distinctions and more subtle variations. Having a grasp of the situation, with all of its various possibilities and constraints, enables the nurse to move from rule-governed thinking to an intuitive grasp of the situation (Dreyfus & Dreyfus with Athanasiou, 1986). This intuitive grasp is based on experience and not based on "extrasensory" powers or wild hunches. It is situated in the clinician's understanding of the situation based on experience with prior similar situations. Improved skills of involvement create disclosive spaces where all patients and families are able to express their concerns, and allow the nurse to notice and respond to the most plausible actions to be discovered and taken in particular situations. Relational skills develop as the nurse learns to be "at home" in a highly differentiated clinical world where some actions are plausible and effective, and others are experienced as "ill timed" or implausible. A sense of **salience** (ability to sense the order or noticeable characteristics of a situation) develops over time so that some things stand out as more plausible and appropriate than others.

The practitioner develops a richer sense of the possibilities of practice based on shared notions of good practice within the profession (Rubin, 1996). Because the Dreyfus model of skill acquisition is a situated and descriptive narrative account of lived experiences that detail skill development over time, it does not consider isolated competencies nor individual enabling traits or talent. Consequently, a practitioner may be at different levels of skill in different areas of practice based on the particular practitioner's background experience and knowledge. For example, a practitioner skilled in caring for adults at an expert level will not be at that level of skill when caring for young children or premature infants. The patient populations that nurses care for determine the nurses' opportunities for experiential learning. The stages of skill acquisition in the Dreyfus model are discussed in the following subsections.

Novice: First Year of Education

The novice stage of skill acquisition occurs in areas where the student has no experiential background on which to base an understanding of clinical situations. For example, the art and skill required for a range of medical and nursing interventions will be new. The educator must offer good descriptions of features and attributes of the situation that the novice can recognize. For example, to determine fluid balance students are given clear parameters and guidelines:

> To determine fluid balance, check the patient's morning weights and daily intake and output for the past three days. Weight gain and an intake that is consistently greater than 500 mls could indicate water retention, in which case fluid restriction should be started until the cause of the imbalance can be found. (Benner, 2001, p. 21)

An experienced clinician can immediately think of the many situations where this evaluation would be inappropriate or too stringent. But the novice is given clear directions about safe ways to proceed until the significance of fluid balance for different clinical conditions can be learned. Levels of practice, as defined by Benner and Chesla, continue to be recognized in current literature as nursing practice is defined (Benner, Hooper-Kyriakidis, & Stannard, 2011; Stokowski, 2011).

Note that the rules and guidelines must not require prior experience for their recognition. They must provide a safe beginning point for specific, situated learning in a clinical situation. Fluid balance is salient, but what must be learned is the particular salience for particular patients. The rule-governed behavior of the novice is extremely limited and inflexible due to lack of direct experience. The student is coached in comparing and matching textbook examples with actual clinical cases. Skills that are performed easily on a mannequin in a skills lab require adaptation, along with communication and reassurance skills, when performed on patients whose attitudes range from calm to highly anxious. Students have a limited ability to forecast immediate futures (e.g., potential responses of the patient) because they have not yet lived through many of them; usually they must rely instead on textbook forecasts.

The best clinical educators give students access to the culture and expectations of the clinical units where they are gaining clinical experience. Clinical educators should offer broad guidelines and timelines to guide their students' understanding of the task world and the expectations of each particular unit (Figure 1–2◆). Good informants are identified as resources for the new students on the unit. In addition, the clinical supervisor is "on call" to deal with questions or emergencies encountered by the student.

Advanced Beginner: New Graduate

The newly graduated nurse usually functions very close to the level of a beginning staff nurse in his final year of nursing education. Typically, newly graduated nurses will not have experienced any administrative or managerial functions, though they will have studied principles and practices related to these roles. The striking change for newly graduated nurses is that they now have full legal and professional responsibility for patients. This new level of responsibility and entitlement brings with it changes in the way nurses experience themselves and their practice environments. They no longer feel that they can always look to other nurses to tell them what to do or to bear their responsibility. This level of individual and team professional responsibility brings new nurses a heightened sense of engagement with patients and their clinical problems. Nurses look to patients and family members to fill in expectations of them in their newly forming role. This heightened and qualitatively different kind of engagement encourages experiential learning and spurs the development of a sense of moral agency in the professional role (Benner et al., 1996, p. 93).

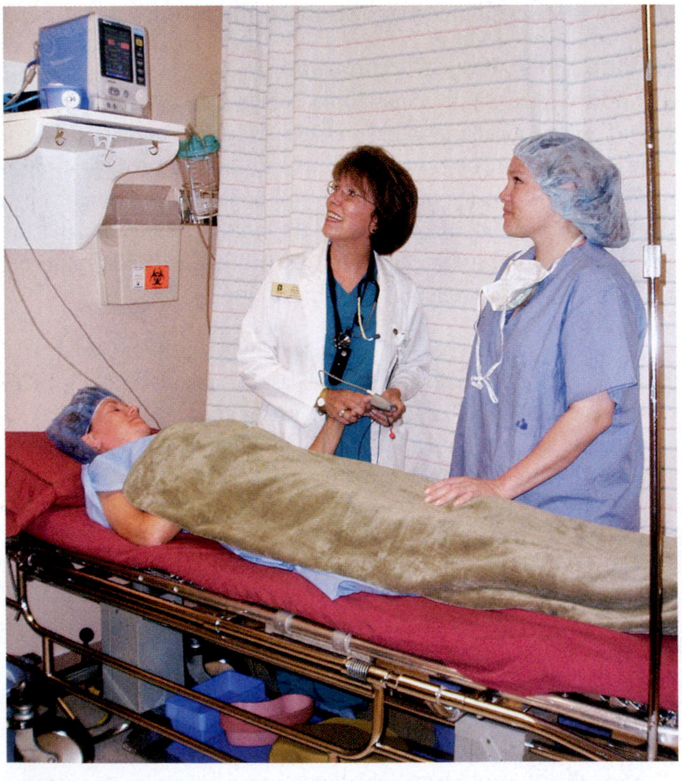

FIGURE 1–2 ◆ A clinical educator presents a broad overview of the experiences students can expect in a particular unit.
Source: John M. Osborn, MD, FACS.

The advanced beginner can experience each situation as a myriad of competing tasks, all of which the new nurse may view as of equal priority. Anxiety and excessive fatigue are frequently experienced by new nurses. Worry and anxiety tend to be more global at this stage, because the advanced beginner does not yet have a sense of salience in a range of situations, and the anxiety of learning to perform new tasks is ever present.

Much of the experiential learning required of an advanced beginner has to do with developing a perspective on particular situations and developing a sense of salience in particular clinical assignments and situations. In coaching an advanced beginner, strategies for keeping anxiety at bay and staying calm enhance performance capacity because the anxiety is so general. The sense of foreboding and anxiousness over particular clinical situations is not yet very attuned to the demands, possibilities, and constraints of the situation simply due to a lack of experience.

Advanced beginners rely on textbook accounts of patient signs and symptoms related to diseases, injuries, and therapies, but they may have difficulty recognizing subtle variations. In addition, they cannot gauge the level of severity based on past experiences simply because they have not had enough experiences. For example, advanced beginners collect their assessment data carefully and then consult about the meanings of the numbers, signs, and symptoms in a particular case. They will need to ask: "Is this the usual amount of bleeding or is this a frank hemorrhage in a postoperative or obstetrical patient?" Drainage from wounds and tubes must be evaluated in relation to the "usual" quantities and qualities. However, the "usual" quantities may vary with specific procedures, patient conditions, and characteristics. The range and variations in clinical signs and symptoms cannot be captured fully in textbooks.

Like the novice, the advanced beginner is dependent on others to provide him with experience-based comparisons, interpretations, and qualitative distinctions. In a later section, this episode is contrasted with the account from the expert's perspective.

Competent Stage: 1 to 2 Years of Practice

Developing skill and clinical judgment in particular cases is dependent on experiential learning. Consequently, how fast someone can gain competence depends on how varied and complex his patient population is. Obviously, nurses working in a high-volume heart surgery center where the patient population is the same will gain more experience sooner about typical patterns in a specific patient population than a nurse working on a general medical–surgical floor. But even in the high-volume center, it usually takes some time before the newer nurse is assigned complete responsibility for complicated postoperative patients.

Competence with particular patient populations will develop unevenly depending on experience with that population and with the quality of clinical teaching available in the institution. The competent stage of skill acquisition is typically a time of heightened planning for what are now more predictable immediate futures. The competent nurse tries to limit the unexpected through planning and analysis and by forecasting the needs and contingencies of the immediate future. Anxiety is no longer just general anxiety; it is now more attuned to the particular situation. The anxiety responses serve as reminders to help the nurse remember or recognize similar past situations.

Nurses at this stage feel exhilarated when they perform well, and remorse when they recognize that their performance could have been more effective or more prescient. These emotional responses are the formative stages of aesthetic appreciation of good practice. Feelings of satisfaction and uneasiness with performance act as a moral compass that guides experiential ethical and clinical learning. There is a built-in tension between the strategies of organizing, planning, and prediction and the development of a more response-based practice as pointed out in our study of critical care nurses:

> Not needing help, ordering the task world, and planning based on goals and predictions structure what the nurse notices, and what are considered issues. It is not accidental that this vision of performance and agency is institutionally rewarded and encouraged as "standard."

Structuring the day by goals and plans, however, interferes with perceiving the demands of the situation and with timing interventions in response to the patient's responses and readiness. The competent nurse seldom sees changing relevance in a clinical situation. The nurse's lack of prior experience with this particular situation calls for new experiential learning in order for her to realize the correct procedure. For example, the nurse may turn a patient so that his good (or less compromised) lung is compressed from lying on his right side, not realizing his left lung (compromised lung), when placed up, is not able to compensate for the loss of aeration from the right lung (Benner et al., 1996). In the future, this common problem with postoperative heart patients will undoubtedly be more recognizable to this nurse.

Experiential learning based on past patient care enables the nurse to develop a greater sense of salience or ability to notice the order of a situation. As illustrated in the preceding nurse's statement, there is an increasing sense of when the nurse has or does not have a good clinical grasp of the situation. Nurses can use their sense of confusion or questioning to propel their understanding of the clinical situation. Because they have now lived through more clinical futures, they can better predict immediate likely events and the resulting patient needs and better plan for them.

Toward the upper limits of competent performance, nurses may begin to apprehend the limits of formal and **practical knowledge** (knowledge learned through actual clinical practice). Nurses can now recognize that not everyone is a proficient or expert clinician, but rather are at the point in which they realize that, in order to perform well in the situation, they must develop a perspective on that situation. Nurses functioning at this level typically buy more comprehensive reference works and medical and nursing textbooks because loss of confidence in the advice of specific others may be overgeneralized; consequently, the nurse may feel hyper-responsible. This inability to trust colleagues can be aggravated if incompetence, accompanied by a lack of social integration and informal coaching, is encountered on a particular clinical unit.

Proficiency: A Transition to Expertise

The proficient nurse perceives the situation as a *whole* and performance is guided by experience and recent events. This nurse possesses an enhanced ability to read a situation. Whereas skill development up until this point has been incremental, now, in order to progress, learners must make a qualitative leap in the way they engage and perform in any given situation. They must literally learn to situate themselves differently in relation to their work. At this stage, recalling experiences in first-person narratives often takes the form of describing changes in their perspectives on a situation. The narrative structure is often something like "I went into the situation thinking that I knew what was going on or that this particular thing was going on," only to have it changed by the patient's responses to their assessment. The nurse is now synthesizing the meaning of the patient's responses through time. She imagines that a computer could capture all of her readings, but she fails to recognize that her understanding of the patient is now situated and based on a practical understanding of the patient's responses and qualitative changes made over time rather than a collection of data points (Benner, 2001).

Though difficult to articulate, this practical grasp is not mystical. It reflects the skill of seeing the practical manifestations of changed physiological states and patient responses and engaging in practical reasoning about these changes. The nurse actively interprets the direction of the change and keeps track of what possibilities can be ruled in or ruled out. Practical grasp of the situation is based on the nurse's perception and the actual patient's response. This requires the nurse to be open to correction and to having his thinking change as the situation unfolds. The clinician (nurse) is always in the situation with some practical understanding, and it is that practical understanding that is revised or confirmed.

In situations where patterns and trends are clear and have definitive interventions associated with the clinical trend, the practitioner can make quick decisive responses. When the practitioner's grasp of the patient's clinical situation is jarred by changes or unexpected patient responses, the practitioner searches for a new grasp; if all goes well, experiential clinical learning occurs. Engaged reasoning through transitions requires being open to correction and disconfirmation. An **ethos** (culture) of openness, rather than one of prediction and control, and fidelity to what one sees and hears, rather than excessive suggestibility and confusion, are embodied and linked to emotional responses to the situation. Thus, the nurse's skilled (developed over time) emotional responses to situations guide her development of perceptual acuity *and* ability to respond to changes in the situation (Benner et al., 1996).

This change is based on procedural knowledge and protocols, but the transition being described is the flexible recognition of patient changes in particular situations. These decisions cannot be based on quantitative physiological measures alone, but must be based on understanding the relationship between the numbers and the way the patient looks and responds. This form of response-based action is crucial for performing well in a rapidly changing emergency (Benner et al., 1996, p. 232).

Expertise: Phronesis

Once a nurse has progressed to proficiency, he becomes a more situated, response-based performer. This self-confidence propels his experiential learning; instead of taking for granted his tacit expectations, he focuses on aspects of the situation that are changing and creates an altered sense of the situation. The expert nurse's actions are response based in using techne (technical) and **phronesis** (wise and skillful decisions that are similar to clinical judgment). The expert now has an intuitive grasp of situations that is based on an enormous background of experience. This is why observation and informal interviewing in actual situations are required to discover and describe all levels of practice, but particularly proficient and expert levels of practice. As noted in our research, ways of seeing the situation increasingly just call for appropriate actions.

Intuitive links develop between seeing and responding to the most relevant issues. This is revealed by observing the nurse in the situation, and is partially captured in the following account of an emergency situation in which a patient who was hemorrhaging stopped breathing. The links between the patient's condition and action are sufficiently strong that the nurse attends primarily to actions rather than assessment of signs and symptoms. This is reasonable since, in extreme circumstances, the possible responses are fewer, but experience is required to make this shift in performance:

> *Nurse:* So we didn't even call the code. We just called the doc[tor] stat [emergency] and got him up there. [They had sufficient people available to resuscitate the patient, so no formal page for additional help was needed.] I looked at his heart rate and I said: "O.K. he is bradying down. Someone want to give me some atropine?" I just started calling out the drugs that I needed to get for this guy, so we started to push these drugs in. In the meantime, I said, "Can we have some more blood?" I was just barking out this stuff [the things that were needed and had to be done]. I can't even tell you the sequence. I was saying, "We need this." I needed to anticipate what was going to happen and I could do this because I had been through this a week before with this guy and knew what we had done [and what had worked]. The anesthesiologist came in and did a good intubation. He asks: "What kind of [IV] lines do we have?" I said, "We have a triple lumen and we have blood. All [IV] ports are taken. We need another kind of line. He's got no veins left." He goes, "O.K., fine, give me a cut-down tray. . . ."

The recognition and assessment language are minimal, in part, because the number of actions per problem are limited, but also because recognition and assessment language become so linked with actions and outcomes that they become self-evident or "obvious" for the expert practitioner. In this situation, the response was fluid and knowing because this nurse had taken care of this patient during a previous successful resuscitation where she had learned, firsthand, what worked and what did not. This is not just a rote repetition of the previous resuscitation; rather, her responses are based on the understanding gained in the previous situation (Benner et al., 1996, pp. 142–143).

Based on enriched experiential learning spawned by an increasing ability to read the current situation in terms of past whole concrete (actual) cases, nurses develop a sense of whether or not they have a good (better or poorer) grasp of the situation. They describe the frustrating situation of "chasing a problem" and never being quite "in synch" with the situation when they do not have a good perceptual grasp of the situation at hand (Benner et al., 1996, pp. 146–147; 1999, pp. 23–87). Skilled "know-how" now allows for more fluid and rapid performance of procedures. Narratives often focus on new clinical learning, troubling moral dilemmas, or conflicts in the situation. Qualitative distinctions associated with nuanced responses allow nurses to know and do more than they can tell or think to describe (Polanyi, 1958/1962).

Attunement, or establishing a harmonious relationship with the patient, strengthens the possibility that patients and family members will disclose or reveal their concerns and fears to the nurse, thereby allowing the nurse to notice changes in the patient/family across time. Establishing a relationship in which the clinician is attentive to the patient creates different disclosive spaces and moods for the patient and family. This, in turn, allows different clinical issues to be noticed. These elements of attunement also facilitate the development of interpersonal core competencies and interdisciplinary collaboration (Essentials of Baccalaureate Education, 2008b; IOM, 2010).

Expert practice, by its very nature, comprises local specific knowledge, know-how, and technical and scientific knowledge, which are transferable to other practice contexts. By sharing this knowledge with beginning practitioners in local settings, clinicians can potentially improve the practice of nursing by articulating the cumulative wisdom they have gained from experiential learning.

Clinical Judgment

The goal of nursing education is to provide the learner with both the necessary critical thinking skills and socialization to the role of nursing. Central to role socialization is the development of **clinical judgment,** which is defined as a complex skill involving several cognitive phases and integrative processes. Critical thinking skills overlap with the conceptual boundaries of clinical judgment (Finn, 2011). Christine Tanner (1983), an identified expert in the study of clinical judgment (Benner et al., 2009), defines clinical judgment skills as follows:

- Making decisions regarding what to observe in the patient situation
- Making inferential decisions by deriving meaning from data observed
- Making decisions regarding actions to be taken that will be of optimal benefit to the patient.

After reviewing more than 200 studies on clinical judgment, Benner et al. (2009) identified five conclusions about a nurse's ability to develop and refine clinical judgment skills:

- Clinical judgment is more influenced by what nurses bring to the situation than the objective data about the situation at hand.
- Sound clinical judgment rests to some degree on knowing the patient's typical pattern of responses, as well as an engagement with the patient and her concerns.
- Clinical judgments are influenced by the context in which the situation occurs and the culture of the nursing care unit.
- Nurses use a variety of reasoning patterns alone or in combination.
- Reflection on practice is often triggered by a breakdown in clinical judgment, and therefore is critical in the development of clinical knowledge and improvement in clinical reasoning skills.

Benner et al. (2009) have stated that nurses' backgrounds, the context of situations, and nurses' relationships with their patients are central to what they notice and how they interpret findings, respond to those findings, and reflect on their responses. Assumptions basic to developing an integrated critical thinking model for clinical judgment are that it is a multidimensional concept and that every act of clinical judgment in nursing has diagnostic, therapeutic, and ethical dimensions. Therefore, sound clinical judgment, which is a requirement for expertise in nursing, is derived from an ability to think critically. It also is critical to expand the nursing role in providing collaborative, interdisciplinary health care (IOM, 2010).

Development of Critical Thinking Skills

As stated earlier, the acquisition of both critical thinking and subsequent clinical judgment skills begins with the education process. During all phases of nursing education, learners are initially taught theory in the classroom followed by psychomotor skill demonstrations, which are practiced in simulated situations. To further refine decision-making and problem-solving skills, the student must then transfer and apply the theoretical knowledge to the clinical setting in a variety of patient care situations (Taylor-Haslip, 2010). Reflective practice is an integral part of the learning process (Ng, 2009). It is imperative for the nurse to reflect on attitudes such as curiosity, fair-mindedness, humility, courage, and perseverance, which facilitate critical thinking in each patient care situation. Additionally, it is beneficial to nurses to reflect on previous patient care situations in which decisions were made and to assess the outcome of those decisions. This reflective thinking process identifies areas of strengths and weaknesses in a given situation, and gives direction to the nurse for future development and refinement of critical thinking and clinical judgment skills. Being open-minded to dissonance and ambiguity is essential if the nurse is going to expand critical thinking skills. If possible, any final decision should be suspended until all sides of an issue have been evaluated; note, however, that emergency situations do not allow for delay. This is why experienced nurses typically function more effectively in emergent situations—they have the thinking and judgment skills to function effectively with minimal delay.

Creating an environment where critical thinking is encouraged and nurtured is the responsibility of the nursing leadership. Differences in opinions and examination of various solutions must be tolerated and encouraged. Independent, individual, and divergent thinking skills are necessary to avoid "group thinking" and the pressure to defer to group decisions. If nurses are aware of their critical thinking skills *while* they are doing the thinking, they can detect errors in judgment. Experiencing both negative and positive outcomes promotes the development of these skills. One example of clinical setting analysis occurs in some trauma centers, where emergency resuscitation situations are videotaped and subsequently analyzed by the staff to determine the effectiveness of the resuscitation efforts. This is an excellent way of reflecting on the thinking and decision making that was done in a high-stress, complex patient care situation. The purpose of this reflective effort is to promote more effective patient care outcomes. But it also presents an opportunity to enhance and refine high-level critical thinking and clinical judgment skills through experience. In addition, it is recognized by the American Organization of Nurse Executives (AONE) as an essential means of preparing the nurse of the future to function as an equal partner, collaborator, and manager in the complex patient care environment of the future (AONE, 2004; Cronenwett, 2010).

Six Components of Caring

When a family member is being treated, families often do not remember the medications and the machines as much as they remember the caring spirit of the nurses. Nursing is a caring discipline with a foundation of nursing science guided by the application of moral and ethical principles of care and responsibility. Caring, which is directly derived from the ethical principle of beneficence, is the core of nursing and constitutes the essence of nursing regardless of the level at which nursing is practiced and conceptualized. Caring represents the unique aspect of nursing and is reflected in conscience, confidence, compassion, commitment, competence, and comportment (Roach, 1984). Without these components, nursing is merely a scientific and technical skill-based body of knowledge. Adding the components of caring to this body of knowledge enables nursing to be identified as a holistic profession. Without caring, the nurse will not see the psychological and spiritual sufferings of the patient (DeWolf-Bosek & Savage, 2007). The definition of each component of caring is outlined here:

- *Conscience* is possessing a moral sense of what is right and wrong. The nurse's conscience guides the nurse's practice and serves as a strong deterrent to providing minimal or inappropriate care. Conscience is not easily displayed, but the nurse's every action is led by her conscience. The conscience helps nurses decide right from wrong and guides the *care* nurses give to patients.
- *Confidence* is defined as having a full belief in the trustworthiness or reliability of a person. Self-confidence is the belief in your own knowledge and skills and the ability to use them when necessary. Confidence in a fellow nurse means that you are totally secure in the accuracy and efficiency of your colleague. Being confident in both yourself and your colleagues minimizes conflict and provides an optimal working environment that ultimately benefits the patient.
- *Compassion* is having a sympathetic feeling for another with an aspiration to help that individual. This is not just a feeling someone possesses; it is accompanied by an action to do good. Effective holistic nursing requires a feeling of compassion for people who are sick and injured.
- *Commitment* means being obligated to see something through to completion. Nurses must value their profession and be committed to delivering the highest level of nursing care. Professional commitment is manifested in different ways. To achieve positive outcomes, nurses must be committed to their patients as well as their institution. The institution also has a duty to be supportive of its nurses, to assist them in increasing their knowledge and skills, and to provide current monitoring equipment that promotes a safe patient care environment.
- *Competence* refers to being capable and qualified to perform a job. Caring as it relates to nursing is not simply a matter of good intentions or warm regard; there also must be a foundation of knowledge. The nurse has a responsibility to the patient to be knowledgeable about the disease process and about the skills necessary to ensure safe patient care.
- *Comportment* means that an individual is aware of his conduct and behavior around others. Professional comportment is an essential aspect of nursing because it is representative of the level of professionalism being exhibited. Additionally, it instills confidence in the patient and provides an atmosphere that alleviates anxiety. Nurses must conduct themselves professionally with their patients as well as their fellow health care workers. Being respectful of each other is germane to creating a positive work environment that promotes team building (Roach, 1984).

The nurse manifests caring as she assists health care consumers in preventing or adapting to actual and potential health problems. Without caring, nursing becomes mechanical and lacking in warmth. The nurse employs much skill and devotion to ensure that every patient is afforded the components just listed, thereby ensuring that patient care is as nurturing and positive as possible. The manner in which nurses choose to implement the six components of caring in clinical practice greatly influences how well the patient is able to adapt to the environment. Caring "sets up the conditions of a trusting relationship that supports the emotional aspects of care" (Papastavrou, Georgios, & Charalambous, 2011, p. 1195).

Development of Caring Skills

During the educational process, it is essential that learners perceive caring as critical to their socialization to the professional nursing role. Therefore, it is incumbent on educators to incorporate the concept of caring with its component parts in all aspects of the curriculum. It is not enough to incorporate the content of caring into didactic materials; the concept also must be communicated as a guide for practice and modeled by the faculty. Caring must become a measurable outcome of learner performance comparable to the measurement of scientific knowledge and psychomotor skills. To illustrate this point, excerpts from learners' clinical assignments in which they were asked to observe an example of nurses demonstrating caring behaviors are listed here:

- ***Conscience***
  An example of staff working by their conscience during my shift was when a young patient came in and we had to treat him. He was brought in after driving drunk, hitting a car, and fleeing the scene. After hitting the first car, he hit a second car and attempted to flee that scene as well and was finally caught. We knew the damage he had done and we knew that when he was released, he was being released to the police and placed under arrest. However, this did not stop us from providing him with the best treatment we could. We did a full assessment, cleaned him up, and controlled his pain just as we did with all of the other patients that we cared for.

Source: Courtesy of Jennifer Fitzgerald, Sacramento, CA

- ***Confidence***
  In the emergency department all of the nurses displayed confidence in their skills and procedures. The nurse established a level of trust right from the beginning. A patient displayed confidence in the nurse when he asked for something and the nurse answered that she could not do that. The patient was not happy with the answer but he had confidence in the nurse to know that she knew what needed to be done for his treatment, and he accepted the answer without question.

Source: Courtesy of Sonia Garcia

- ***Compassion***
  Possibly one of the most important components of caring is compassion. As a medical professional it may become easy to simply detach oneself from the plight of patients in pain or in need; however, remaining compassionate is crucial to good patient care. It is the best way to build trust with your patient and to facilitate a caring environment, which is especially important in the emergency department where patients are often afraid and in severe pain. I saw many people exhibit compassion throughout the shift; for example, when a patient complained of severe leg pain that did not respond to the two doses of morphine his nurse had already given him, the RN went to the physician and requested a stronger pain medicine which finally put the patient at ease.

Source: Courtesy of Maryam Shahdi, Sacramento, CA

- ***Commitment***
  The nurse that I worked with in the Post Anesthesia Care Unit (PACU) had actually been called in that day after another nurse had called in sick. I guess he had been called in because nobody from the night shift wanted to stay and they were anticipating a very busy day in surgery. Since the level of acuity is so high in the PACU, it is necessary to have plenty of nurses on every shift. He told me he did not mind coming in on his day off though, because he really enjoyed his job and liked to come to work. One could say with absolutely no hesitation that this employee was very committed to his job and to his patients.

Source: Courtesy of Jolie Tietz, Sacramento, CA

- ***Competence***
  The nurse I was assigned to in the emergency department had four patients within a half hour that needed IVs placed. In previous experiences, I have seen nurses try three or four times, wiggling the needle around in the poor patient's arm before finding a vein. However, this nurse efficiently and almost painlessly started the IVs one after the other. I know the patients appreciated her accuracy, and she probably did not even think about how simply she had started the things.

Source: Courtesy of Andrea Perry

- ***Comportment***
  The Post Anesthesia Care Unit (PACU) nurse I worked with showed comportment to our patients, especially when they were first waking up. When the patient with a nasopharyngeal tube became more awake, he began to move and flail his arms around. He then began to try to take out the nasopharyngeal tube. The nurse and I carefully took his arms and held them so he would not pull out any lines or hurt himself. My nurse very calmly explained to the patient that the surgery was over, that it went well, and that he was in the PACU. He also explained who we were, what time it was, and why there was a tube in his nose. The nurse's demeanor helped the patient to calm down. The nurse also explained to the patient that the "spacey feeling" he was having was due to the anesthesia because of the fact that our bodies are not used to it. He reassured the patient that the feeling would soon wear off. My nurse handled the situation beautifully, and his caring behavior positively impacted the patient.

Source: Courtesy of Kathleen Budesa, Sacramento, CA

Health and Wellness Promotion

In the last two decades, the concept of health and wellness promotion has come to the forefront of health care issues. The focus has shifted from disease treatment to a holistic approach of disease prevention and promotion of wellness. People are more aware than ever before how the relationship between healthy lifestyles and habits impacts disease prevention. For example, most individuals regularly monitor their cholesterol and triglycerides and understand that lifestyle changes are necessary when the levels become elevated. Regular exercise programs and a well-balanced healthy diet have become a way of life for many individuals.

In 1979, the surgeon general's office published its first health promotion and disease guidelines in *Healthy People.* This first report was followed in 1990 by a second edition, titled *Healthy People 2000,* which emphasized health promotion, health protection, and preventive service strategies (DHHS, 1990). The report was once again updated in the year 2000, and again in 2011 for *Healthy People 2020.* These indicators are discussed in length in Chapter 6.

As discussed in the foundational practice area in this chapter, the IOM Report (2010) outlines the role nurses must take in practicing within a patient-focused system of care that includes health education and promotion, as well as initiatives to promote a more culturally diverse nursing workforce (Hertel, 2011). In addition, the AACN's recommendations on restructured academic curricula will develop renewed high-level competences for the future of nursing practice.

A vital part of the nurse's role today is to promote health and wellness through teaching and modeling of healthy behaviors based on the health indicators. For consistency and comprehensiveness, it is helpful to develop a template for health education. The components of this template include an understandable description of the cause of the disease or disorder, what habits will slow or stop progression, medication actions and side effects, and prognosis. As part of the plan, the nurse should provide written material and other resources, such as websites and support organizations. It is important to provide the patient and family with an opportunity to ask questions and air feelings about the diagnosis. The nurse also needs to tailor the education to be culturally sensitive. This is especially true when it comes to dietary teaching, because food selection is heavily dependent on cultural customs. In summary, teaching as a function of the nursing role is included in the ANA's *Nursing: Scope and Standards of Practice*, 2nd Edition (2010) and in all state nurse practice acts (ANA, 2010). Cultural sensitivity has been identified as a major curricular element in the American Association of Colleges of Nursing's (AACN) *The Essentials of Baccalaureate Education for Professional Nursing Practice* (Sanner, Baldwin, Canella, Charles, & Parker, 2010).

Roles of the Nurse

As stated, the professional nurse embodies many roles. Throughout history, nursing has continuously adapted to the ever-changing needs of patients and the health care delivery system. Some roles interface with patients throughout the entire health care continuum, and these roles continue to grow. The spectrum of nursing roles includes practice in acute and nonacute care, advanced practice, and practice in a number of new and evolving arenas. All nursing practice roles rely on the nursing process as a framework for patient care delivery.

Acute Care Nurses

Acute care nurses practice in the hospital setting. These nurses care for patients with actual and potential health problems related to any body system and any age group. The types of patients an acute care nurse works with will vary depending on the individual hospital's mission, goals, and specialty areas provided.

Staff Nurse

The staff nurse has the primary responsibility to care for a specific patient or group of patients for an assigned period of time. Patient care assignments vary among organizations depending on the nursing care delivery model being used. The nursing care delivery models are discussed in Chapter 4. These models define the workload distribution and job description for each member of the nursing health care team. Organization and coordination are inherent in the role of the nurse regardless of the type of patient care delivery model due to the variety of diagnoses and complexity of patient care. Therefore, the staff nurse uses critical nursing judgments to determine patient interventions according to assigned responsibilities. Regardless of which care delivery model is used, certain components are common to all of them, including nursing management and administration, which are described next.

Nurse Manager

The role of nurse managers is to coordinate and ensure the delivery of quality nursing care in their area of responsibility. Their role encompasses handling personnel management and staff development, as well as ensuring the availability of supplies, other resources, and processes that allow the nurses they manage to provide care. In most settings, a nurse manager has 24-hour accountability for a specific patient care arena.

Nurse Administrator

Nurse administrators have a greater scope of responsibility than nurse managers. The ultimate role of a nurse administrator is to support the achievement of the standards that the organization has set for nursing practice and the guidelines of care that outline how care is to be delivered in a setting.

Nurse Researcher

Research is the never-ending quest for information and validation that lead to evidenced-based nursing practice. Nurse researcher roles are multifaceted and involve many aspects of pharmaceutical, medical, and nursing research. Nurses serve as investigators, monitors, auditors, data managers, clinical coordinators, or research professionals. Research nurses monitor patient responses and other critical parameters.

Factors to consider as a research nurse include regulatory developments and trends, clinical research management, protocol design and implementation, and ethical issues in human research. Educational preparation varies depending on the role and setting in which a nurse practices. Some nurses involved in research may be educationally prepared as ADN, diploma, or BSN nurses. Some nurses accomplish PhD preparation and serve as primary scientific investigators. Chapter 3 provides a complete description of the role of nurses in research.

Nurse Educator

Nurse educators are a critical component to the success of nurses and their patients. The role of educator varies from organization to organization and department to department. Many in-hospital educator roles include responsibilities such as teaching of patients and staff, research, and direct patient care. Core competencies for the role of educator are strong clinical skills and effective teaching skills.

The nurse educator may be responsible for developing educational content for presentation, written delivery, or multimedia applications. Nurse educators also participate in the evaluation of learners (staff or patients) and serve as consultants to staff and patients. The ultimate goal of a nurse educator is to ensure quality patient care by providing education to patients and nurses and assessing the competency of those who practice.

Nonacute Care Nursing

Nonacute nurses practice outside of a hospital setting, and will find their roles continuing to expand with more accountability due to the IOM report and new expectations for nurses related to chronic disorders (2010). For example, nurses perform a variety of roles in the community setting. Each role requires special training and expertise, which can be acquired through formal education and on-the-job training. With the goal of providing nursing care and preventive health care, nurses in these settings have to be flexible and creative when providing their nursing care. Examples of common nonacute nursing roles are discussed in the following subsections.

Community-Based Home Health Nurse

Community-based home health nurses are employed by government agencies, private enterprises, hospitals, and a myriad of other clinics or health care-focused organizations. These nurses provide care to patients in the community by making home visits to patients, operating mobile clinics, and staffing various types of health screening events. Home health nurses concentrate on providing care and educating patients and their significant others regarding health care issues (Figure 1–3 ◆).

These nurses may be specialists who focus on specific populations or generalists who work with families to improve the overall health of communities. Each agency operates with the concepts of disease prevention, nutrition, child care, and the care of older adults as constructs on which to build healthy communities. Home health nurses integrate into the community and work in concert with community

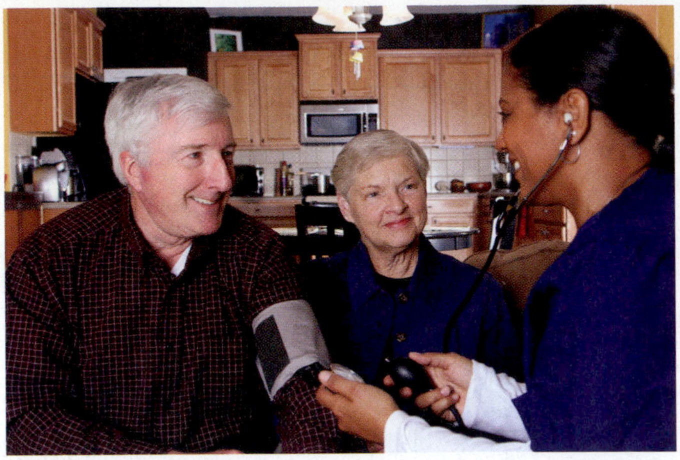

FIGURE 1–3 ◆ Home health nurses visit patients in their homes and concentrate on providing care and education.
Source: Rob/Fotolia

leaders, teachers, and parents, as well as physicians and other health care providers, to promote community health education.

Parish Nurse

Parish nursing is a form of community nursing that concentrates on the population of a church and the members of its congregation. The health care provided by a parish nurse is very similar to that provided by a home health/community health nurse. The parish nurse serves as a consultant and facilitator for the health care needs of the parish's congregation. Many parish nurse programs provide preventive health screening, such as blood pressure and cholesterol clinics.

Long-Term Care Nurse

Long-term care is not a subset of acute care; it is a distinct entity with special needs, functions, and care providers. A variety of medical and social services are provided to help people who have disabilities or chronic care needs. Services may be short or long term and may be provided in a person's home, in the community, or in residential facilities (e.g., nursing homes or assisted living facilities). Care is provided in the form of medical and support services to persons who have lost some or all of the capacity to function due to an illness or disability. Most long-term care clients are older and require care due to diagnoses such as stroke or Alzheimer's disease. However, long-term care is not limited to those who are elderly. Younger patients may require long-term care for a chronic disease, such as multiple sclerosis, or conditions resulting from trauma, such as spinal cord injury or traumatic brain injury. A source for more information on long-term care is the American Society for Long-Term Care Nurses.

Assisted Living Nurse

Assisted living is defined as a setting in which patients are provided long-term assisted care in a residential location. Assisted living settings provide care to patients who have needs that are beyond the scope of home care, but do not require the level of services provided in nursing homes. Assisted living programs take on many forms; however, the most encompassing description is any group residential program not licensed as a nursing home that provides care to residents through trained staff who are available to respond to unscheduled calls for assistance.

Assisted living services support the resident in all activities of daily living (ADLs). Examples of activities where staff assist residents include bathing, grooming, taking medications, transferring assistance, and toileting. The assisted living setting provides a "homey" environment for people requiring or potentially requiring assistance with ADLs, but for which 24-hour nursing care is not a necessity.

Nurses' roles in assisted living facilities are multifaceted. Nurses provide direct care in some situations, oversee medication administration, and participate with the staff in evaluating and planning to meet the needs of residents. Unlike their acute care counterparts, nurses who care for residents in assisted living facilities are often called on to participate in decisions that impact the resident's quality of care and quality of life (Baddeloo, 2010).

Occupational Health and Industrial Nurse

Occupational health and *industrial nursing* are terms that have been used interchangeably. This practice integrates concepts of public health nursing theory, holistic evaluation, primary prevention, surveillance, and compliance. The American Association of Occupational Health Nurses describes occupational nursing as a practice that focuses on promotion and restoration of health, prevention of illness and injury, and protection from work-related and environmental hazards.

The occupational health nurse has two primary objectives: (1) participating in the management of workers' health to mitigate health issues that may adversely affect work productivity and (2) ensuring that the employer's practices are compliant with the requirements of the Occupational Safety and Health Act.

The occupational health nurse practices in many settings, including factories, corporations, and hospitals. This type of nurse may provide direct nursing care to employees, manage workers' compensation records, conduct environmental surveillance for health hazards, and provide health education or counsel employees.

School Nurse

School nursing practice strives to advance the well-being, academic performance, and lifelong achievement of students. School nurses interact with students to foster positive responses to normal growth and development and promote health and safety practices. School nurses get involved with actual and potential health problems. In some situations, a school nurse may be called on to provide case management services. These nurses actively collaborate with the student, administration, teachers, parents, other health care providers, and legal entities to build student and family capacity for adaptation to health care needs and self-management of issues, to promote self-advocacy, and to foster learning of health-related concepts. A source of information regarding school nursing is the National Association of School Nurses.

Clinic Nurse

Clinic nurses provide patient care and support within the setting of an office building, a clinic, or a surgery center. They are routinely responsible for preparing patients for examination, administering injections, and performing clerical duties. Clinic nurses are the physician's most important professional adjunct. In this role, nurses facilitate the delivery of care to patients and manage the daily operation of the office. A source of information regarding clinic nursing is the American Association of Office Nurses.

Hospice Nurse

Hospice nurses provide care for the physical and emotional needs of dying patients and their significant others. Interventions may include pain management, palliative care, symptom management, and emotional support. A source of information regarding hospice nursing is the Hospice and Palliative Nurses Association. Chapter 11 provides a detailed description of the role of hospice nurses.

Gerontological Nurse

Gerontological nurses provide for the physical and psychosocial needs of older adults both in the acute care and community settings. These specialized nurses work with their patient's insurance carrier, such as health maintenance organizations, to maximize functional ability while working with the patient to maintain and restore the patient's physical and mental health. The arena of gerontologic nursing is growing because older adults have begun to represent an increasingly greater component of the population (Karasik, 2009).

Age-related health issues and typically a limited ability to navigate the health care system may result in inadequate health maintenance, especially for the frail elderly. Gerontological nurses are specially trained to deal with the special needs of this population. This training can be either in the form of an advanced degree or on-the-job training. Care specific to the older adult patient is discussed in Chapter 10. One source of information regarding gerontological nursing is the National Gerontological Nurses Association.

Advanced Practice Nursing Roles

Advanced practice nursing roles have grown in response to a societal need to improve the distribution of health care services and to decrease the costs of health care. Such roles will continue to be needed as nursing continues to step up to the IOM expectations of expanded practice (Ruel & Motyka, 2009). The development of advanced practice roles, such as nurse practitioners, clinical nurse specialists, certified nurse midwives, certified registered nurse anesthetists, and academic nurse educators, occurred as a direct response to patient needs, specifically the need for access and cost-effective care (Ruel & Motyka, 2009).

Research has demonstrated that the use of advanced practice nurses has improved patient outcomes and reduced health care costs. Key factors that led to this success were the interpersonal skills of the nurse, knowledge and expertise in the area of practice, and a level of trust when working with physicians, nursing staff, vendors, pharmacists, insurance companies, and other health care providers. Successful enactment of the role required being a facilitator for patients and families with the health care team (Black, 2010).

These nurses provide direct care to patients through independent practice, practice within a health care agency, or practice in collaboration with a health care provider. As in all professions, advancements in technology and the incredible access to information have resulted in the various advanced practice roles becoming more and more specific. The most rapidly growing sectors of advanced practice nursing are the roles of nurse practitioner and clinical nurse specialist.

Nurse Practitioner

Nurse practitioners (NPs) focus on individualized care. They interact with patients of all ages as they examine the impact of illness on the lives of patients and their support networks. NPs practice in both acute and nonacute care settings, are eligible for Medicare reimbursement, and, in some states, have prescriptive authority.

NPs formulate their actions and interventions with a focus on prevention, wellness, and patient education. The impact of these priorities often results in fewer prescriptions and potentially less expensive medical care. NPs collaborate with their patients by fostering the acquisition of knowledge and encouraging participation in decision making related to their health care needs. The role of the NP is not limited to the delivery of health care; many are active participants in research, whereas others are active in patient advocacy work, such as development of support groups for a specific diagnosis.

Nurse practitioner programs classically specialize in an area such as family practice, internal medicine, or women's health. The advanced practice degree can be granted by a number of academic institutions. The variety of educational paths for NPs is a result of the role's development through history. In 1965, the profession of nurse practitioner was introduced with a requirement of a master's degree. After successful completion of the education program, the NP candidates must achieve licensure in the state in which they plan to practice. The state boards of nursing regulate nurse practitioners, and each state has its own licensing and certification criteria. In general, the criteria include completion of an accredited advanced practice program and clinical experience. Depending on the requirements of the various state boards, nurse practitioners may have to fulfill additional requirements such as certification by the American Nurses Credentialing Center (ANCC) or a specialty nursing organization. Terms of licensure also vary from state to state.

Clinical Nurse Specialist

The National Association of Clinical Nurse Specialists (NACNS) defines a clinical nurse specialist (CNS) as a licensed registered nurse who has graduate preparation (master's degree or doctorate) in nursing as a CNS. CNS practice usually takes place in a hospital setting and involves interactions with patients all across the health care continuum. CNSs practice within a prescribed area of care, and define their role as having five components: clinical practice, education, management, consultation, and research. These advanced practice nurses deliver direct patient care, educate staff and patients, consult with other health care professionals, do research, and provide leadership and supervision in the workplace. Depending on the state in which they practice, the institutional policies, and the clinical specialty they choose, clinical nurse specialists may have extended scope of practice authority.

CNSs are expert nurses in a specialized area of clinical practice. According to the NACNS (2011), the specialty may be identified in different ways. The CNS practice may be focused on a specific type of problem (e.g., pain, wounds, and stress), a defined patient population (e.g., pediatrics, geriatrics, women's health), or a setting (e.g., critical care, emergency department). Other practice focuses include medical subspecialty (e.g., diabetes, oncology) and types of care (e.g., psychiatric, rehabilitation). Although most CNSs do practice in the hospital setting, some practice in other health care settings.

In addition to providing direct patient care, the CNS influences care outcomes by providing expert consultation for nursing staff and by implementing improvements in health care delivery systems. The practice of a CNS integrates expert nursing practice, which focuses on assisting patients in the prevention or resolution of illness, with a medical diagnosis and treatment of disease, injury, and disability. It is believed that CNSs improve outcomes such as better pain management, reduced medical complications in hospitalized patients, and reduced frequency of emergency visits.

As advanced practice roles continue to grow, more need for clarification of roles and responsibilities has been required. Many states have amended their nurse practice acts to authorize nurses to perform functions that were previously restricted to the practice of physicians. Examples of these expanded functions include diagnosis, treatment, performance of selected invasive procedures, and prescription of medications and treatments. Each state regulates practices differently. In all states, the board of nursing controls these functions.

The differences in the role of nurse practitioner and clinical nurse specialist are often unclear, especially in hospital settings. This lack of distinction is very confusing to the health care consumer, other health care providers, and nurses. There is a need for clear universal definitions of the roles and responsibilities of advanced practice nurses. Nurses who pursue these roles often discuss the benefits in terms of interdependent function with other health care professionals and the establishment of peer relationships with physicians. As health care systems continue to develop, the roles of these advanced practice nurses will continue to adapt and change.

Nurse-Midwife

A nurse-midwife is defined as a nurse who has special training and certification in child birthing (labor and delivery). Nurse-midwives can perform most of the same tasks as physicians, although they typically have emergency physician backup when they deliver a baby.

Nurse-midwives have been contributing to the birth process of millions of women and families during the past 300 years. The American College of Nurse-Midwives (ACNM) reported in 2010 that there were 11,546 nurse-midwives (CNM/CM) in clinical practice and 39 accredited ACNM nurse-midwifery programs in the United States and Puerto Rico. Of these programs, 4 are postbaccalaureate certificate programs and 39 are graduate degree programs. The advanced practice role of CNM is lawful in all 50 states and in the District of Columbia, whereas the newer CM role is not yet recognized by all state legislatures (2010).

Certified Registered Nurse Anesthetist

The American Association of Nurse Anesthetists (2007) states: "Nurse anesthesia is an advanced clinical nursing specialty. As anesthesia specialists, certified registered nurse anesthetists (CRNA) administer approximately 65% of the 26 million anesthetics given to patients in the United States each year." CRNAs provide care to patients in collaboration with other health care professionals including anesthesiologists, surgeons, and dentists.

The consistent functions of a CRNA include providing care of a patient's anesthesia needs before, during, and after surgery or the delivery of a baby. The CRNA's responsibilities are to assess, participate in operative teaching, prepare the operative area for anesthetic management, administer anesthesia, and maintain anesthesia during the operative procedure.

A CRNA is a registered nurse who is prepared through a formal nurse anesthesia didactic and clinical program. This education process prepares the CRNA candidate to sit for a national certification examination. This exam is administered by the Council on Certification of Nurse Anesthetists (CCNA). The mission of CCNA is to protect the public by ensuring that individuals who are credentialed have met predetermined qualifications or standards for providing nurse anesthesia services. All nurse anesthesia programs are graduate or postgraduate degree programs.

It is clear that initial care, ambulatory health care, and anticipatory guidance are all becoming increasingly important in nursing practice. Advanced practice roles enable nurses to function interdependently with other health care professionals and to establish a more collegial relationship with physicians. As changes in health care delivery continue, the role of advanced practice nurses, especially in primary care settings, is expected to increase in terms of scope, responsibility, and recognition.

Academic Nurse Educator

College and continuing education nursing instruction must be provided by nurses prepared at the master's or doctoral level. All **academic nurse educators** practice as faculty in colleges, universities, hospital-based schools of nursing or technical schools, or as staff development educators in health care facilities. The continuum of students these educators instruct ranges from entry into nursing practice, professional nurses in pursuit of advanced degrees, and practicing nurses interested in expanding their knowledge and skills related to care of individuals, families, and communities (Nurses for a Healthier Tomorrow, 2007).

Community-Based Nurses

While nurses work in multiple areas of acute care, as well as academic roles, they also assume roles in community-based care. Several key issues, such as the necessity for cost containment, role conflicts between health care professions, nursing shortages, and organizational difficulties of health care organizations (Swiadek, 2009), have promoted a shift in focus from acute care hospital-oriented provisions to community-based public health orientations. It is predicted that this evolution will result in improved health outcomes, less need for tertiary treatment, and savings for hospitals and insurance companies (IOM, 2010; Swiadek, 2009). **Community-based nurses** work beyond the confines of the acute care environment and are challenged as patients with complex nursing care needs are discharged from acute care settings early in the recovery process. Such patients include those who are elderly and have multiple-system problems. Medical technologies that were once thought to be useful in the hospital setting only have been adapted to the home and community settings. As a result, the community-based care setting is becoming one of the largest practice areas for nursing. Within these settings, nurses often deliver care without direct supervision or the support of other health care personnel (Stanhope & Lancaster, 2010). Models of community-based nursing care are discussed in Chapter 4.

Looking Toward the Future

Population Demographics

Population changes in general are having a direct impact on health care delivery. The 2010 U.S. Census data determined that the United States population is 308.7 million people. This figure indicates that people are living longer, possibly due to improved health services and improved nutrition. Most sources agree that not only is the population increasing and living longer, but it is also changing in composition. The decline in birth rate and the increase in life span attributed to improved health care have resulted in fewer school-age children and more senior citizens, most of whom are women. People reside in areas dictated by age and ethnicity. Much of the population resides in highly congested urban areas, with a steady migration of minority groups to the inner cities and migration of middle-class people to suburban areas. The culturally diverse population is growing, as is the homeless population (Shelton, Taylor, Bonner, & van den Bree, 2009).

These population shifts, joined by major concerns about emerging infectious diseases, trauma, and bioterrorism, are changing the focus of health care and, therefore, the roles of health care providers. The focus is shifting more to prevention, health promotion, and management of chronic conditions than in the prior century. This shift in focus coincides with a nationwide emphasis on cost control and resource management directed toward providing cost-effective and efficient health services for all (Rakel et al., 2009).

Aging Population

Advances in technology, discoveries of cures for diseases, new treatment modalities, and the push for wellness have all had an impact on life span, significantly increasing the proportion of the population who grow to old age. However, as the population of older adults dramatically increases, a few signs indicate that adequate resources will not be available to meet the challenge of providing health care and good quality of life for these older adults and their families. The older population—persons 65 years or older—numbered 39.6 million in 2009 (the latest year for which data is available). They represented 12.9% of the U.S. population, about one in every eight Americans. By 2030, there will be about 72.1 million older persons, more than twice their number in 2000. People 65+ represented 12.4% of the population in the year 2000 but are expected to grow to be 19% of the population by 2030.

In 2008, the 65–74 age group (20.8 million) was 9.5 times larger than in 1900. In contrast, the 75–84 age group (13.1 million) was 17 times larger and the 85+ group (5.6 million) was 46 times larger (U.S. Census Bureau, 2010).

Also important to note is that many older adults will be from ethnically diverse cultures. Hispanic elders, now 5.7% of the older adult population, will increase to 16.4% of the older adult population in the next 50 years (CDC, 2010). These trends are important to those planning health care services for the future because they suggest an increasing demand on formal services, a pattern already in evidence during the past decade. The health care needs of the aging, the availability of health care resources, and the nurse's role in caring for the aging are discussed in detail in Chapter 10.

Informed Consumers

In addition to age, other demographic factors are developing that will affect health care in the 21st century. The majority of the consumers of health care will be well educated and, hence, better able to obtain and use the information needed for maintaining health (Davies, Hayes, & Quintner, 2011). They will be able to use the Internet to assist them in learning about their illness or health issues, and they will be better able to make informed decisions regarding their health care. Consumers also will be more diverse, requiring a multicultural sensitivity.

The roles of women and the family will change. There will be an increase in single-parent families and an increase in multiple-family combinations. Parents will be older with fewer children. More women will work outside the home and choose to remain in the workplace after having children. Society will place a higher value on children. Such demographic variables have a significant impact on health care, economics, public policy, and quality of life, including the delivery of health care (Tamborini, Iams, & Whitman, 2009).

Cultural Diversity

Diversity is a word that means something different to each and every person. **Cultural diversity** refers to the variations among groups of people with respect to the habits, values, preferences, beliefs, taboos, and rules determined to be appropriate for individuals and social interaction (Huber, 2010). It represents the variety and differences in the customs and practices of defined social groups. The changing demographics and economics of our growing multicultural world and the long-standing disparities in the health status of people from culturally diverse backgrounds have challenged health care providers and organizations to consider cultural diversity as a priority.

As with aging, cultural diversity is increasing at a rapid rate (Figure 1–4◆) (U.S. Census Bureau, 2010). Some projections indicate that by 2030, racial and ethnic minority groups will make up 40% of the U.S. population. With increased immigration, this figure could rise to 50% by the year 2030 (U.S. Census Bureau, 2010). As the cultural composition of the population changes, it becomes increasingly important to address cultural considerations in the delivery of health care. Patients from diverse sociocultural groups bring different health care beliefs, values, and practices to the health care setting, as well as different risk factors for some disease conditions. They also respond to treatment uniquely. These factors significantly affect the way one responds to health care problems or illness, to those who provide the care, and to the care itself. It is understood that an appreciation of the diverse characteristics and needs of individuals from varied ethnic and cultural backgrounds is important in health care and nursing. Unless these factors are understood and respected by health care providers, the care delivered may be ineffective and health care outcomes may be negatively affected.

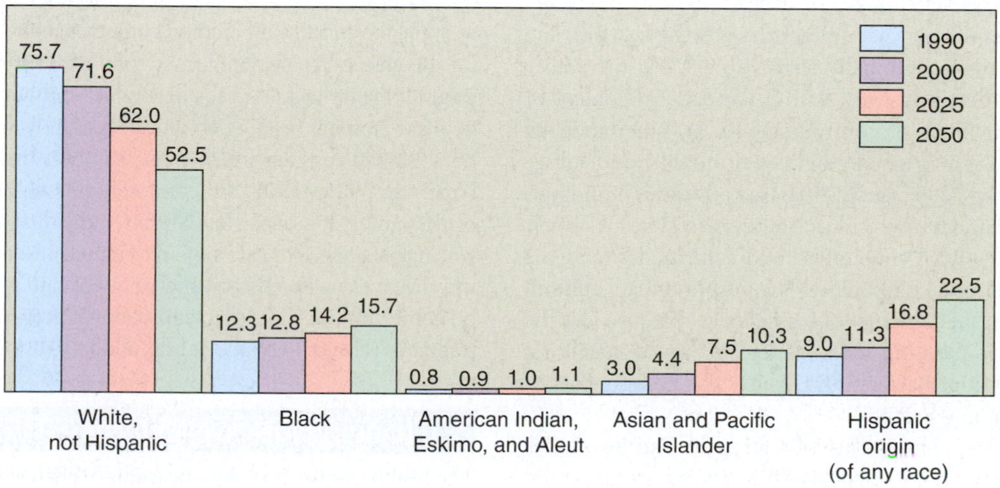

FIGURE 1–4 ◆ Percent of population, by race and Hispanic origin: 1990, 2000, 2025, and 2050.
Source: U.S. Census Bureau.

Video: Cultural Competence

In addressing cultural diversity, health care providers must realize that doing so goes beyond knowing the values, beliefs, customs, and practices of racial groups, such as African Americans, Asians, Hispanics/Latinos, Native Americans, and Pacific Islanders. Religious affiliation, language, physical size, gender, sexual orientation, age, disability, political orientation, socioeconomic status, occupational status, and geographic location also represent a few of the faces of diversity (Wikberg & Eriksson, 2008).

To understand cultural diversity, it is necessary to understand **culture.** Culture refers to a combination of learned patterns of behavior, beliefs, and values that can be attributed to a particular group of people (Wikberg & Eriksson, 2008). These learned behaviors, beliefs, and values guide thinking, decisions, and actions. Included among the many characteristics that distinguish cultural groups are the manner of dress, language spoken, values, rules or norms of behavior, gender-specific practices, economics, politics, laws and social control, artifact, technology, dietary practices, and health beliefs and practices. Health promotion, illness prevention, causes of sickness, treatment, coping, caring, dying, and death are all a part of the health-related component of every culture. Individuals have a unique belief and value system, which has, in part, been shaped by their cultural environment. This value system influences and guides the individual's response to illness and to health care. It is incumbent on the health care delivery system to consider these individual needs by providing practitioners who are culturally competent and providing organizational structures that are sensitive to cultural diversity.

Cultural Competence

Health care service policies, protocols, and regulations call for **cultural competence,** which is the act of providing care effectively to persons from a multiplicity of cultures. Cultural competence is an ongoing evolution of knowing, respecting, and incorporating the values of others. It means being open to the cultural beliefs and behaviors of others, bringing attitudes, knowledge, and skills necessary for providing quality care to diverse populations (American Association of Colleges of Nursing, 2008a). It is a crucial link to practicing empathy, understanding, communicating, valuing, and caring in health care (Health Research and Education Trust, Institute for Diversity in Health Management, 2011).

Campinha-Bacote (2011) has defined the process of cultural competence in the delivery of health care services as "a culturally conscious model of care that defines the process in which the health care professional continually strives to achieve the ability and availability to effectively work within the cultural context of a client (family, individual, or community" (p. 1). This model of cultural competence was originally developed in 1991 and subsequently revised in 1998, 2002, and 2010 based on research findings. Campinha-Bacote's model views cultural awareness, cultural knowledge, cultural skill, cultural encounters, and cultural desire as the five constructs of cultural competence. She purports that: "cultural encounters is the pivotal construct of competence that provides the energy source and foundation for one's journey towards cultural competence" (Campinha-Bacote, 2011, p. 1). The components of the model are shown in Chart 1–3.

Consistent with the components of Campinha-Bacote's model, it is necessary to possess a set of congruent behaviors, attitudes, and policies that come together in a system, agency, or among professionals and that enables the system, agency, or those professionals to work effectively in cross-cultural situations to achieve cultural competence.

Weblink: Cultural Competence

CHART 1–3 Components of Campinha-Bacote Model of Cultural Competence

Cultural Awareness	The process of an individual conducting self-examination of her own biases towards other cultures and an exploration of her cultural and professional background.
Cultural Knowledge	The process in which the health care professional seeks and obtains a sound education base about culturally diverse groups. The health care professional must focus on the integration of health-related beliefs, practices, and cultural values; disease incidence; and prevalence.
Cultural Skill	The ability to conduct a cultural assessment to collect culturally relevant data regarding the client's/patient's presenting problem as well as accurately conducting a culturally based physical exam.
Cultural Encounters	The process which encourages the health care provider to engage in face-to-face cultural interactions and other types of encounters with those from other culturally diverse backgrounds. Done to modify existing beliefs and possible stereotypes.
Cultural Desire	The motivation to want to engage in the process of becoming culturally aware, knowledgeable, and skillful; seeking cultural encounters, not having to.

Source: Campinha-Bacote, J. (2011). The process of cultural competence in the delivery of healthcare services. *Transcultural Care Associates.* Retrieved from http://www.transculturalcare.net/Cultural_Competence-Model.htm.

The word *competence* implies having the capacity to function effectively (Wikberg & Eriksson, 2008). Because cultural differences are learned, cultural sensitivity and competence as a process also can be learned.

It is critically important for the health care delivery system to recognize the increasing diversity of those who seek care and make provisions for those who practice in the system to become culturally competent (Parnell et al., 2011). It is equally important for health care professionals to apply the concepts of cultural competence to the patients they care for. Because every person comes from a unique and different background, the individual needs and values must be taken into account to make hospital stays as comfortable as possible. For example, the nurse should consider which room numbers mean bad luck to Asian Americans, what foods are comfort foods to Hispanics, or how to bring comfort and caring to a Muslim individual. Cultural competence will enable the health care system to reduce health care disparities and improve the quality, efficacy, and equity of care as measured by patient outcomes, and to meet state and national licensure and accreditation standards (Health Research & Educational Trust, 2011).

Changing Disease Patterns

The health problems of Americans have changed significantly during the past 50 years. Many infectious diseases have been controlled or eradicated; others, such as tuberculosis, acquired immunodeficiency syndrome (AIDS), and sexually transmitted infections, are on the rise. An increasing number of infection agents are becoming resistant to antibiotics. Conditions that once were treated easily have become complex and difficult to treat—some have even become life threatening (CDC, 2010).

The increasing life span of the general population is contributing significantly to the increase in chronic disease and disability (CDC, 2010). Also, the successful treatment options for conditions such as cancer and human immunodeficiency virus (HIV) allow people with these conditions to live decades longer than in earlier years. People with chronic illnesses are the largest group of health care consumers in the United States (CDC, 2010). Due to the heavy incidence of chronic conditions, many people are learning how to protect and maximize their health within the constraints of chronic illness and disability. As chronic conditions increase, health care broadens from a focus on cure and eradication of the disease to include the prevention or rapid treatment of exacerbations of chronic conditions. The shifting changes in disease patterns support the need for increased emphasis on community-based care, rather than acute care (IOM, 2010).

In discussing changing disease patterns, it is necessary also to address globalization and health for all. Those entering the United States through travel and immigration are bringing many new diseases with them. Current society exists in a world where global infectious disease cannot be controlled by border patrols. One of the relatively new diseases, West Nile virus, was first detected in the United States in 1999. By 2002, West Nile virus had spread to most of the continental United States. The first human case of this virus was reported in early July 2003, with three deaths due to the virus reported by August. In 2005, there were 3,000 human cases and 119 deaths linked to infection, up from 2,539 cases and 100 deaths in 2004; however, only 1,021 cases were reported in the United States in 2010 (CDC, 2011d).

Severe acute respiratory syndrome (SARS), another example of a new viral disease, was first identified in China, Hong Kong, and Vietnam in 2003. This disease has spread to the United States; at the time of this writing, there were fewer than 200,000 people in the United States with SARS (PubMed Health, 2011). According to the World Health Organization, 8,098 people worldwide became sick with SARS during the 2003 outbreak. Of these, 774 died. In the United States, only 8 people had laboratory evidence of SARS-CoV infection, no deaths were reported, and there have been no reported cases of SARS since 2005 (CDC, 2011c). However, SARS remains a vivid example of how quickly world travel can spread a disease. In the opinion of many, SARS should be recognized as a severe respiratory syndrome that is here to stay (PubMed Health, 2011).

Now, society is faced with the avian flu and methicillin-resistant *Staphylococcus aureus* (MRSA). Avian influenza virus refers to influenza A viruses found chiefly in birds, but infections with these viruses can also occur in humans. Although the risk for human infection is low, confirmed cases of human infection from several subtypes of avian influenza infection have been reported since 1997. Most cases of avian influenza infection in humans have resulted from contact with infected poultry (e.g., domesticated chicken, ducks, and turkeys) or surfaces contaminated with secretions/excretions from infected birds.

Of the few avian influenza viruses that have crossed the species barrier to infect humans, H5N1 has caused the largest number of detected cases of severe disease and death in humans. However, it is possible that those cases in the most severely ill people are more likely to be diagnosed and reported, while milder cases go unreported (CDC, 2011a). Of the human cases associated with the ongoing H5N1 outbreaks in poultry and wild birds in Asia and parts of Europe, the Near East, and Africa, more than half of the people who were reported infected with the virus have died. Most cases have occurred in previously healthy children and young adults and have resulted from direct or close contact with H5N1-infected poultry or H5N1-contaminated surfaces.

Although there has been some human-to-human spread of H5N1, it has been limited, inefficient, and unsustained. Nonetheless, because all influenza viruses have the ability to change, scientists are concerned that one day the H5N1 virus could be able to infect humans and spread easily from one person to another. Because these viruses do not commonly infect humans, there is little or no immune protection against them in the human population. If the H5N1 virus were to gain the capacity to spread easily from person to person, an influenza pandemic (worldwide outbreak of disease) could begin. No one can predict when a pandemic might occur. However, experts from around the world are watching the H5N1 situation in Asia and Europe very closely and are preparing for the possibility that the virus may begin to spread more easily and widely from person to person.

Methicillin-resistant *Staphylococcus aureus* (MRSA) joins avian flu, West Nile virus, SARS, and HIV as a potentially deadly infectious disease that has become prevalent in hospitalized patients and in the community as a whole (Mayo Clinic, 2010). Worldwide, an estimated 2 billion people carry some form of *S. aureus*; of these, up to 53 million (2.7% of carriers) are thought to carry MRSA. In the United States, 95 million carry *S. aureus* in their noses; of these, 2.5 million (2.6% of carriers) carry MRSA (Gorwitz, 2008).

Increasing numbers of outbreaks of community-acquired MRSA colonization and infection through skin contact in locker rooms and gymnasiums, even among healthy populations, have been reported. MRSA causes as many as 20% of *S. aureus* infections in populations that use intravenous drugs. These out-of-hospital strains, or community-acquired (CA)-MRSA, are more easily treated, even though they are more virulent, than hospital-acquired (HA)-MRSA. CA-MRSA apparently did not evolve *de novo* in the community but represents a hybrid between MRSA that spread from the hospital environment and strains that were once easily treatable in the community. Most of the hybrid strains also acquired a factor that increases their virulence, resulting in the development of deep tissue infections from minor scrapes and cuts as well as many cases of fatal pneumonia.

Reducing MRSA in both health care and community settings is a priority for the CDC (2011b). A 2010 CDC study revealed that invasive MRSA infections in health care settings are declining (CDC, 2011b). However, community-acquired MRSA infections increased rapidly during the past decade (CDC, 2011b).

The spread of HIV/AIDS and other catastrophic illnesses threatens both personal and political viability. Lack of access to safe reproductive health puts hundreds of millions of people at risk and also contributes to the burgeoning global population growth and migration. Poor child health and nutrition rob future generations of human potential and years of life. Health for all continues to be a call for equity and social justice, a global issue that must be dealt with at the local level in communities around the world.

Complementary and Alternative Therapy

Health care in the 21st century requires that nurses not only care for the critically ill, elderly, and infirm, but also that they recognize and incorporate new and evolving methods to enhance the health of those who choose alternative or complementary therapies. This evidence-based,

Weblink: MRSA Statistics
Weblink: Severe Acute Respiratory Syndrome (SARS)
Weblink: West Nile Virus Statistics
Weblink: Avian Influenza

integrative style of care originates from holistic nursing, a precursor and philosophical framework for many of the now popular alternative and complementary therapies. Holistic nursing is simply defined as caring for the whole person—body, mind, and spirit—in an ever-changing environment.

Complementary or Alternative: What Is the Difference?

The words *complementary* and *alternative* are sometimes used interchangeably, but they are not the same. **Complementary therapy** refers to a therapy used in addition to a conventional therapy. For example, a nurse might use touch therapies, music, or guided imagery for pain control in addition to the prescribed drug therapy.

Alternative therapy, sometimes called *unconventional therapy*, refers to a therapy used instead of conventional or mainstream therapy. An example is the use of acupuncture instead of analgesics.

Some reputable sources for information on complementary and alternative therapies are:

- The National Center for CAM, www.nccam.nih.gov
- American Holistic Nurses Association, www.ahna.org

Integration of Complementary and Alternative Systems into Traditional American Health Care

Until recently, the primary system of medicine in North America was simply called *medicine*, although some refer to it as **allopathic medicine.** In the past two decades, a number of schools of thought and philosophies have become intertwined with traditional medicine. Some of the most frequently seen new systems include Ayurvedic, Chinese, chiropractic, naturopathic, Native American, and osteopathic medicine. Each of these systems can stand alone, or be used in combination with other systems (Chart 1–4).

Safety and Effectiveness of Alternative Therapies

Safety generally is interpreted to mean "freedom from danger" in which the benefits of alternative therapy outweigh the risks. If the patient is interested in using an alternative or complementary therapy, the nurse should first counsel the person about the benefits and risks and advise her to ask the practitioner of the therapy about the treatment's safety and effectiveness.

Complementary and alternative medicine (CAM) therapies can be dangerous if used improperly. As for any medical endeavor,

CHART 1–4 Systems of Health Care Services

System	Description
Allopathic/Western medicine	The most common name for allopathic medicine is *Western medicine*. Other terms for Western medicine are *conventional medicine* and *mainstream medicine*. Many people have not heard the term *allopathic* because most health care professionals do not use this term to refer to themselves or their practice. Practitioners of other systems of medicine more often use the term when referring to what can be called Western medicine or mainstream medicine. Allopathy is a method of treating disease with remedies that produce effects different from those caused by the disease itself. This system of medicine uses scientific data to determine the validity of a diagnosis and the effectiveness of treatment. It is evidence-based medicine. Practitioners use a variety of therapies, including drugs, surgery, and radiation therapy. Western medicine practitioners have made most of the significant advances and developments in modern medicine.
Ayurvedic medicine	Ayurveda is the ancient Hindu system of medicine from India. Its main goals are to maintain the health of healthy people and cure the illnesses of sick people. Ayurveda maintains that illness is the result of falling out of balance with nature. Diagnosis is based on three metabolic body types call *doshas*. The Ayurvedic doctor identifies the dosha type as vata, pitta, or kapha. Treatment usually involves prescribing a diet, herbal remedies, breathwork, physical exercise, yoga, meditation, massage, and a rejuvenation or detoxification program.
Traditional Chinese medicine	Traditional Chinese medicine is thousands of years old and involves such techniques and practices as acupuncture, acupressure, herbs, massage, and qi gong. The diagnosis and treatment of disturbances of qi (pronounced "chee")—or vital energy—are distinctive characteristics of Chinese medicine. Acupuncturists, one type of traditional Chinese medicine practitioner, access patients' health by checking pulses, looking at the color of the tongue, checking facial color, assessing voice and smell, and asking a variety of questions. To treat patients, acupuncturists insert a needle(s) along the meridians (pathways) where qi flows. Many acupuncturists also prescribe herbs.
Chiropractic	The main treatment modality of chiropractors is manual adjustment and manipulation of the vertebral column and the extremities. They use direct hand contact and mechanical and electrical treatment methods in the course of treatment. Chiropractors primarily treat back pain, neck pain, and headaches. They do not perform surgery, nor do they prescribe drugs.
Homeopathic medicine	Homeopathy is based on the principle that "like cures like," in which tiny doses of a substance that create the symptoms of disease in a healthy person will relieve those symptoms in a sick person.
Naturopathic medicine	Naturopathy primarily uses natural therapies such as nutrition, botanical medicine, hydrotherapy, counseling, physical medicine, and homeopathy to treat disease, promote healing, and prevent illness. Naturopathic physicians have a doctor of naturopathy (ND) degree and must be licensed.
Native American healing	Native American medicine practices vary from tribe to tribe. In general, Native American medicine is a community-based system with rituals and practices: the sweat lodge, use of herbal remedies, the medicine wheel, sacred hoop, the "sing," and shamanistic healing. For example, an ill person may be placed in a small, enclosed sweat lodge. While singing or chanting is done outside the lodge, it is believed that toxic substances will come out in the sweat of the person inside the lodge. After the ceremony, the ill person may be placed on a cot outside and be prayed over.
Osteopathic medicine	This practice of medicine emphasizes the interrelationship of the body's nerves, muscles, bones, and organs. The osteopathic philosophy involves treating the whole person, recognizes the body's ability to heal itself, and stresses the importance of diet, exercise, and fitness with a focus on prevention.

practitioners must be trained and, with some therapies, licensed or certified. The most prevalent deficit of CAM therapies is seen when patients use them instead of conventional therapy and do not also seek traditional diagnosis and treatment. People who choose CAM therapies first and continue to use them for symptom treatment may delay diagnosis of treatable cancers as well as a huge array of curable conditions. Thus, most CAM therapies are best used alongside conventional medicine. The positive effects of these therapies used to augment allopathic medicine are presented in the Complementary & Alternative Therapies feature boxes such as the one found in this chapter and others in many of the forthcoming disorder chapters in this text.

When assessing patients, the nurse should ask if they use any nontraditional therapies and, if so, what their response is to them. The nurse should try to eliminate any preconceived notions she may have about a certain therapy. Patients typically will feel more comfortable discussing nontraditional therapies if they feel the nurse understands the treatment and why they have decided to use it. If patients are unfamiliar with alternative or complementary therapies (Chart 1–4), they may ask the nurse questions about specific treatments or therapies. Following are some sample questions that patients may ask:

- What will this therapy do for me?
- What are the advantages of this therapy?
- What are the disadvantages?
- Are there side effects?
- What risks are associated with this therapy?
- How much will it cost?
- How long will it take? How many treatments will be necessary?
- How will it interact with my other therapies?

The use of alternative and complementary therapies is proliferating. Nurses who have additional training in specific CAM therapies can use many of them to provide better care for patients. When patients use complementary therapies, nurses should consider the usage an attempt to increase potential health benefits and not as signs of distress or dissatisfaction with their current care. Throughout this text in the chapters that cover disorders, Complementary & Alternative Therapies features highlight single or occasionally multiple therapies that will work with one of the conditions referred to in the chapter. These boxed features may be used as an example of how nurses can incorporate CAM into their care.

Advances in Technology and Genetics

Advances in technology and genetics have occurred with greater frequency in the last several decades than ever before. They are causing changes in all health care settings and in the roles and responsibilities of all health care providers.

Technological Changes

Biomedical technology, information technology, telecommunications, and the Internet have changed the delivery of health care into a national and even international system. The previous state of the art technology is being replaced by new high-tech developments at an ever-increasing rate. The advances have enabled practitioners to make faster diagnoses, treat illnesses more quickly, make decisions faster, and communicate more quickly and effectively with all members of the health care team.

Genetics

Within the last decade, the body of knowledge called genetics has exploded, largely due to identifying the human genome through the Human Genome Project (HGP). The HGP was funded by Congress in 1988, and is the result of a collaborative, coordinated research effort in human genetics planned by the Department of Energy and the National Institutes of Health (De Sevo, 2010). The HGP has been instrumental in fostering a multidisciplinary approach to research with an expectation of openness and sharing of discoveries via information technology. The achievement of uncovering the full genome sequence is regarded as a historic scientific event. The HGP has provided knowledge and insights into many diseases and development of improved methods for diagnosis and prevention.

As the pace of genetic knowledge continues to progress at a rapid rate, the private and public sectors have become increasingly interested. The private sector is interested in building markets on the information available from the HGP and offering commercialization of genetic diagnostics and services. Molecular medicine and information-based targeted health care are attracting entrepreneurial companies to consider the role of proactive prediction and prevention of disease risk based on an individuated genetic profile. Optimum goals of the HGP for 2009 and beyond include a catalog of variations in the human DNA sequence, faster/cheaper technology, a focus on gene function, and continued attention to the implications of such knowledge for society.

The new discoveries in genetics are being publicized in all forms of mass media. Health care consumers are becoming more aware of gene-based tests and therapies and the technologies that make them possible. As genetic-based testing becomes more commonplace, individuals and their families will approach health care providers with questions about testing, resources for having testing done, interpretation of results, and requests for specialized services in genetic centers. Because nurses are widely accessible to the public, they are regarded as a group of health care providers who can begin to provide basic information and referrals for appropriate assistance. De Sevo (2010) suggests that nurses must understand genetics and integrate this concept into their current practice. Chapter 7 contains a complete discussion of genetics.

Summary

Nursing is a practice discipline that comprises both practical and theoretical knowledge. Nursing, like medicine, is an underdetermined complex practice that requires clinical judgment and discernment in particular situations. Clinical reasoning calls for reasoning across time about changes in the patient and changes in the clinician's understanding of the situation. Nursing and medicine cannot be reduced to techne (or technique), but must include phronesis, wise and skillful judgment, and practice by excellent practitioners.

Every professional nurse is engaged in ongoing experiential learning, clinical inquiry, and clinical knowledge development. Clinicians need to keep track of their experiential learning over time, reflect on it, and make it public and accessible for examination and further studies.

Even the expert nurse must stay attuned to each situation and remain open to the unexpected. Practitioners must remain open to experiential learning and reading changes in transitions in fast-paced, open-ended environments. In the Dreyfus model, the practitioner is

 Health Locus of Control

COMPLEMENTARY and alternative medicine involves a wide range of therapies including philosophical beliefs about health and illness. These perspectives of health choices are then supported with treatment therapies and practices of lifestyle choices. Over the last decade, a greater acceptance has developed in both the public and health care systems for the use of these therapies as an integrative model. This new acceptance, noted in public dialogue as integrative or functional medicine, is influencing an updated terminology to those who are practitioners and the public seeking its modalities. Research into health locus of control (HLOC) gives insight into which life perspectives may lend a person to seek out the use of integrative health care (IH).

Health locus of control is a psychological concept concerning control beliefs in relationship to an individual's illness, injuries, and health. Developed as a social learning theory in 1954 by Rotter, this concept is based on the general approach of locus of control (LOC). The root word for authority is *author*, as in "who authors one's life," which could be used to shed light on understanding the original terms used in considering a person's access of control in his decision making. *Internal* LOC places authority within the person; he believes his thoughts and actions are the greatest influences in his life; *external* LOC places the authority with other people and their influences, and *chance* LOC gives authority to fate as the determinate of an individual's life blessings or challenges (i.e., their fate).

In an effort to add depth to the use of HLOC in understanding patient decision making, the results of a German study further defined the external expression of HLOC. Previous analysis of HLOC was predominantly done in a health care setting of patients receiving care, while nonclinical studies of general population sampling have been rare in regards to public health care. In sampling 4,075 participants in northern Germany, individuals ages 18 to 64 were randomly selected from registration office files and completed the standardized German questionnaire, which assesses HLOC. This model revealed a breakdown of external LOC into two additional latent variables, formal help and informal help. The following statements provide examples of patient HLOC decision making in seeking both formal and informal assistance (Otto et al., 2011).

HLOC	Statement of Belief/Perspective of One's Decision Making Regarding Health
Internal	"My health is influenced by my actions even when I don't feel well."
	"When I know enough about myself I can help myself when I am sick."
	"It is up to me whether or not I get better when I am sick."
	"It's my responsibility to take the steps to remain healthy."
Formal Help	"When I have a medical concern, I usually go to the doctor."
	"Medical testing will help doctors know how to get me better when I'm sick."
	"Regarding my health, I only do what my doctor tells me to do."
Informal Help	"When I feel physically well, I owe this to all the advice and help of others."
	"When I don't feel well, I seek out the advice of others."
	"I can avoid getting sick when I take the advice of my friends and family."
	"When I don't feel well, others know better than me how I feel."
Chance	"No matter what I do, I'm just going to get sick again."
	"If I didn't have bad luck I wouldn't have any luck at all."
	"Being sick is my cross to bear, there isn't anything I can do, it's God's plan."
	"Being ill is payback for what I do in my life as my destiny."

In a study of 65 healthy graduate students measured by using the Multidimensional Health Locus of Control Scale (MHLC), those with a greater internal HLOC were more likely to believe that their own actions directly related to their health than those attributing their health to external factors (to others or chance). Having greater control over personal health is a commonly reported reason for seeking CAM treatment, with previous studies finding a positive correlation between internal HLOC and CAM use.

Specifically, the study explored whether having a philosophical congruence with CAM, or being dissatisfied with conventional medicine, influences the choice to use CAM treatments. Philosophical congruence with CAM was measured with items such as "Most complementary therapies stimulate the body's natural therapeutic powers," and "I believe complementary medicine enables me to take a more active part in maintaining my health." Dissatisfaction with conventional medicine was measured with items such as "I don't trust medical doctors and hospitals, so I use them as little as possible," and "I have a lot of confidence in the medical doctor I see most often."

Three factors emerged during factor analysis rather than the anticipated two: (1) philosophical congruence with CAM, (2) dissatisfaction with conventional methods, and (3) holistic balance that life is holistic in its nature. The holistic balance factor represents the more holistic views associated with CAM and includes the views that "Physical and mental health are maintained by an underlying energy or vital force," "Health and disease are a reflection of balance between positive life-enhancing forces and negative destructive forces," and "The body is essentially self-healing and the task of a health care provider is to assist in the healing process."

The holistic balance score was significantly correlated with the philosophical orientation congruent with CAM. Dissatisfaction with conventional health care was mostly influenced by the increased belief in holistic balance, which avails greater congruence with CAM (McFadden et al., 2010).

Integral to the use of integrative health is the coaching of patients in adopting lifestyle changes in exercise, diet, and continued healthy behavior. These changes feel more natural to those individuals with internal HLOC who proactively seek out solutions to their health behavior. The success of this group's use of integrative CAM could be explained within the transtheoretical model of change, which organizes change in five stages:

1. *Precontemplation.* Individual has the problem (whether he/she recognizes it or not) and has no intention of changing.
2. *Contemplation.* Individual recognizes the problem and is seriously thinking about changing.
3. *Preparation for action.* Individual recognizes the problem and intends to change the behavior within the next month. Some behavior change efforts may be reported, such as taking supplements when they remember, eating better than they did before, and exercising on weekends. However, the defined behavior change criterion has not been reached (i.e., consistent healthy eating and exercise).
4. *Action.* Individual has enacted consistent behavior change (i.e., consistent healthy eating and active exercise) for less than 6 months.
5. *Maintenance.* Individual maintains new behavior for 6 months or more.

Internal HLOC individuals are more inclined to be in the action phase when they first begin integration of complementary health practices into their daily lives. For external HLOC, the influence of family and friends serves as a factor in the use of integrative health.

Sources: Hirai, K., Komura, K., Tokoro, A., Kuromaru, T., Ohshima, A., Ito, T., Sumiyoshi, Y., & Hyodo, I. (2008). Psychological and behavioral mechanisms influencing the use of complementary and alternative medicine (CAM) in cancer patient. *Annals of Oncology, 19*(1):49–55.

McFadden, K.L., Hernández, T.D., & Ito, T.A. (2010). Attitudes toward complementary and alternative medicine influence its use. *Explore (NY), 6*(6):380–388.

Otto, C., Bischof, G., Rumpf, H.J., Meyer, C., Hapke, U., & John, U. (2011). Multiple dimensions of health locus of control in a representative population sample: ordinal factor analysis and cross-validation of an existing three and a new four factor model. *BMC Medical Research Methodology, 12*(11):114.

Rotter, J.B. (1954). *Social learning theory and clinical psychology.* New York: Prentice Hall.

Rotter, J.B. (1982). *The development and application of social learning theory. Selected papers.* New York: Praeger.

assumed to dwell with increasing skill and finesse in a meaningful, intelligible, but changing world.

Nursing offers a career path in which opportunity abounds for all interested. As the population ages and the need for nurses continues to skyrocket, the practice of nursing will grow and evolve. The work of nurses will continue to change. Many hypothesize that nurses will become much more active in the fields of prevention and health screening as they reach further out into the fabric of the community in which patients live. Others suggest that nursing will continue to grow in the technology of interventional patient care, translating the high-tech information and educating those involved to care for those who have received these interventions in the home environment. The nurse will become a leader in collaborative patient care and provide leadership in policies to reflect the health care needs of our population (IOM, 2011). This is and will be the future of nursing.

This also is a time of incredible tension as the need for change in the U.S. health care delivery system continues to expand. What will nursing be in 10 years? Advancements in the science of clinical practice—including imaging, pharmaceutical agents, and technology—keep adding to the demands of nursing. These advancements also result in changes in patients' expectations and knowledge. Nurses continue to serve the role of integrator of patients into health care systems. Their practice will be based on scientific and caring concepts, and they will develop from novice to expert through experiential learning. In addition, nursing practice will continue to change as the IOM recommendations are integrated into academic and clinical practices.

The future is unclear, but the diversity and adaptability of nursing is a constant. There is one certainty: Nurses will continue to be a critical component of health care delivery and the opportunities are limitless for those who join the ranks of the nursing profession.

NCLEX® PRACTICE

1. One of the characteristics of nursing is defined in the role of nursing education. In providing information regarding the characteristics and consequences of disease, as well as promoting and modeling a healthy lifestyle, the professional nurse is emphasizing which of the following?

1. Health promotion and maintenance
2. Advocacy
3. Complementary therapies
4. Physiological adaptation

2. Roach identified six components of caring: conscience, confidence, compassion, commitment, competence, and comportment. Without caring, the nurse will not see what type of patient needs?

1. Physical and comfort
2. Psychological and spiritual
3. Physiological
4. Ethics and moral

3. A nurse completing the first year of practice has reached a level of competent practice. The level of expert practice has been achieved when the nurse: (select all that apply)

1. experiences daily anxiety over the work situation.
2. recognizes the limitations of formal knowledge.
3. views the work of the nurse as a series of competing tasks.
4. skills are related to the particular patient situation.
5. makes decisions based on the signs and symptoms that the patient displays.

4. The nurse is doing an assessment on a patient and asks about health practices specific to the patient's cultural group. The nurse is demonstrating:

1. a cultural encounter.
2. cultural desire.
3. cultural skill.
4. cultural awareness.

5. After assisting with care for a patient with a sudden gastrointestinal bleed, the student nurse states: "I learned so much from watching all of the other nurses and doctors help this patient." Which of the following levels of experience is this nurse most likely to be?

1. Novice
2. Advanced beginner
3. Competent
4. Proficient

6. The nurse is aware that the types of disease processes that require treatment and nursing care are changing. Which of the following statements about the change in disease is true? (select all that apply)

1. Increases in the life span are resulting in more conditions requiring chronic management.
2. Lack of cure for conditions such as cancer and HIV/AIDS has resulted in reduction in the life span.
3. More people are learning to live healthy lives with chronic health problems.
4. Disease patterns in the United States are influenced by current immigration patterns.
5. Use of antimicrobial drugs has caused infectious disease to be a problem of minimal significance.

Answers to NCLEX Practice Questions can be found in Appendix D in the Osborn Student Resources at nursing.pearsonhighered.com. Practice additional NCLEX questions online at the Student Resources site.

REFERENCES

Academy of Medical–Surgical Nurses. (2011). What is medical-surgical nursing? Retrieved from http://www.amsn.org/cg bin/WebObjects/AMSNMain.woa/1/wa/viewSection?s_id=1073744083&ss_id=536873248&wosid=ARjx6dVQV2ln2hr49DF7bY1UQh7

American Association of Colleges of Nursing. (2007). The essentials of baccalaureate education for professional nursing practice (draft). Retrieved from http://www.aacn.nche.edu/Education/pdf/BEdraft8-1-07.pdf

American Association of Colleges of Nursing. (2008a). *Cultural competency in baccalaureate nursing education.* Washington, DC: American Association of Colleges of Nursing.

American Association of Colleges of Nursing. (2008b). *The essentials of baccalaureate education for professional nursing practice. Washington, DC: American Association of Colleges of Nursing.* Retrieved from http://www.aacn.nche.edu/Education/pdf/BEdraft8-1-07.pdf

American Association of Nurse Anesthetists. (2007). *About AANA.* Retrieved from http://www.aana.com

American College of Nurse-Midwives. (2010). *Essential facts about midwives.* Retrieved from http://www.midwife.org/siteFiles/factsheet/EssentialFactsAboutMidwives_2007.pdf

American Nurses Association. (2001). *Code of ethics for nurses with interpretive statements.* Retrieved from http://www.nursingworld.org/ethics/code/protected_nwcoe303.html

American Nurses Association. (2007). Let's make nurses' voice heard! Sign up for N-STAT today. Retrieved from http://rnaction.org/politicalpower/join.html

American Nurses Association. (2008a). ANA's health system reform agenda. Silver Spring, Maryland: American Nurses Association. Retrieved from http://ana.nursingworld.org/MainMenuCategories/HealthcareandPolicyIssues/HealthSystemReform/Agenda/ANAsHealthSystemReformAgenda.aspx

American Nurses Association. (2008b). What is nursing? Retrieved from http://nursingworld.org/EspeciallyForYou/StudentNurses/WhatisNursing.aspx

American Nurses Association. (2010). *Nursing: Scope and standards of practice* (2nd ed.). Silver Spring, Maryland: American Nurses Association. Retrieved from http://nursesbooks.org/Main-Menu/Standards/H--N/Nursing-Scope-and-Standards-of-Practice.aspx

American Nurses Association. (2012). The nursing process. *Nursing World.* Silver Spring, Maryland: American Nurses Association. Retrieved from http://www.nursingworld.org/EspeciallyForYou/What-is-Nursing/Tools-You-Need/Thenursingprocess.html

American Organization of Nurse Executives. (2004). Position statement on pre-licensure supervised clinical instruction. Retrieved from http://www.aone.org/aone/advocacy/PositionStatementPre-licensureclinicalexperience formatted.pdf

Anderson, C. A. (2010). QSEN: Quality and safety education for nurses. *DEAN's Notes, 31*(5), 4.

Baddeloo, C. (2010). Role of the assisted living nurse and medication management. *Iowa Nurse Reporter, 23*(1), 1, 20.

Benner, P. (1994). The role of articulation in understanding practice and experience as sources of knowledge in clinical nursing. In J. Tully (Ed.), *Philosophy in an age of pluralism: The philosophy of Charles Taylor in question* (pp. 136–155). New York: Cambridge University.

Benner, P. (2001). *From novice to expert: Excellence and power in clinical nursing practice. A commemorative edition.* Upper Saddle River, NJ: Pearson Prentice Hall.

Benner, P., Chesla, C., Dreyfus, H. L., Dreyfus, S. E., & Rubin, J. (1996). *Expertise in nursing practice: Caring, clinical judgment & ethics.* New York: Springer Publishing Company.

Benner, P., Hooper-Kyriakidis, P., & Stannard, D. (1999). *Clinical wisdom and interventions in critical care: A thinking-in-action approach.* Philadelphia: W. B. Saunders.

Benner, P., Hooper-Kyriakides, P., & Stannard, D. (2011). *Clinical wisdom and interventions in critical care: A thinking-in-action approach,* (2nd ed.). Philadelphia: W. B. Saunders.

Benner, P., Tanner, C. A., & Chesla, C. A. (1996). *Expertise in nursing practice: Caring, clinical judgment, and ethics.* New York: Springer.

Benner, P., Tanner, C., & Chesla, C. A. (2009). *Expertise in nursing practice: Caring, clinical judgment, & ethics* (2nd ed.). New York: Springer.

Benner, P., & Wrubel, J. (1982). Clinical knowledge development: The value of perceptual awareness. *Nurse Educator, 7,* 11–17.

Benner, P., & Wrubel, J. (1989). *The primacy of caring: Stress and coping in health and illness.* Menlo Park, CA: Addison-Wesley.

Black, K. (2010). Correlates of case managers' advance care planning practices. *Clinical Gerontologist, 33,* 124–135.

Bureau of Labor Statistics, U.S. Department of Labor. (2011). *Occupational outlook handbook, 2010–11 edition, Registered Nurses.* Retrieved from http://www.bls.gov/oco/ocos083.htm

Campinha-Bacote, J. (2011). The process of cultural competence in the delivery of healthcare services. *Transcultural Care Associates.* Retrieved from http://www.transcultural care.net/Cultural_Competence-Model.htm

Carpenito-Moyet, L. J. (2007). *Nursing diagnosis: Application to clinical practice* (12th ed.). Philadelphia: Lippincott Williams & Wilkins.

Centers for Disease Control and Prevention. (2010). *Health care in America: Trends in utilization* (DHHS Publication No. 2004-1031). Washington, DC: U.S. Government Printing Office.

Centers for Disease Control and Prevention. (2011a). Avian flu statistics. Retrieved from http://www.cdc.gov/flu/avian/outbreaks/current.htm

Centers for Disease Control and Prevention. (2011b). MRSA statistics. Retrieved from http://www.cdc.gov/mrsa/statistics/index.html

Centers for Disease Control and Prevention. (2011c). Severe acute respiratory syndrome (SARS). Retrieved from http://www.cdc.gov/ncidod/sars/situation.htm

Centers for Disease Control and Prevention. (2011d). West Nile virus statistics. Retrieved from http://www.cdc.gov/ncidod/dvbid/westnile/surv&controlCaseCount10_detailed.htm

Cronenwett, L. R. (2010). The future of nursing education. Paper commissioned by the Committee on the RWIF Initiative on the Future of Nursing, at the IOM.

Cronenwett, L. R., Sherwood, G., & Gelmon, S. B. (2009). Improving quality and safety education: the QSEN learning collaborative. *Nursing Outlook, 57,* 304–312.

D'Amico, D., & Barbarito, C. (2010). *Health and physical assessment in nursing* (2nd revised ed.). Upper Saddle River, NJ: Pearson Prentice Hall.

Davies, S. J., Hayes, C., & Quintner, J. L. (2011). System plasticity and integrated care: Informed consumers guide clinical reorientation and system reorganization. *Pain Medicine, 12*(1), 4–8.

De Sevo, M. R. (2010). Genetics and genomics resources for nurses. *Journal of Nursing Education, 49*(8), 470–474.

DeWolf-Bosek, M. S., & Savage, T. A. (2007). *The ethical component of nursing education.* Philadelphia: Lippincott Williams & Wilkins.

Doss, S., DePascal, P., & Hadley, K. (2011). Patient-nurse partnerships. *Nephrology Nursing Journal, 38*(2), 115–125.

Dreyfus, S. E., & Dreyfus, H. L. (1979, February). *The scope, limits, and training implications of three models of aircraft pilot emergency response behavior.* Unpublished report supported by the Air Force Office of Scientific Research, USAF (Grant AFOSR-78-3594), University of California at Berkeley.

Dreyfus, H. L., & Dreyfus, S. E., with Athanasiou, T. (1986). *Mind over machine, the power of human intuition and expertise in the era of the computer.* New York: The Free Press.

Dunne, J. (1997). *Back to the rough ground, practical judgment and the lure of technique.* Notre Dame, IN: University of Notre Dame Press.

Finn, P. (2011). Critical thinking: Knowledge and skills for evidence-based practice. *Language, Speech, and Hearing Services in Schools, 42,* 69–72.

Gendrop, S., & Eisenhauer, L. (1996). A transactional perspective on critical thinking. *Scholarly Inquiry into Nursing Practice: International Journal, 10,* 329–342.

Gadamer, H. (1960/1975). *Truth and method* (G. Barden & J. Cumming, Trans.). New York: Seabury.

Gorwitz, R. J. (2008). Understanding the success of methicillin-resistant Staphylococcus aureus strains causing epidemic disease in the community. *The Journal of Infectious Diseases, 197*(2), 179–182.

Guignon, C. B. (1983). *Heidegger and the problem of knowledge.* Indianapolis, IN: Hackett.

Halpern, J. (2001). *From detached concern to empathy. Humanizing medical care.* Oxford: Oxford University Press.

Health Research & Educational Trust, Institute for Diversity in Health Management. (2011). *Building a culturally competent organization: The quest for equity in health care.* Chicago, IL: Health Research & Educational Trust.

Hertel, R. A. (2011). The IOM report from a legislative standpoint: Addressing the quality of health care. *Med-surg Matters, 3,* 12–13.

Hirai, K., Komura, K., Tokoro, A., Kuromaru, T., Ohshima, A., Ito, T., Sumiyoshi, Y., & Hyodo, I. (2008, Jan.). Psychological and behavioral mechanisms influencing the use of complementary and alternative medicine (CAM) in cancer patients. *Annals of Oncology, 19*(1), 49–55. Epub October 26, 2007.

Huber, D. (2010). *Leadership and nursing care management* (4th ed.). Philadelphia: W. B. Saunders.

Institute of Medicine (IOM). (2010). *The future of nursing: Leading change, advancing health.* Washington, DC: Author. Retrieved from http://www.iom.edu/Reports/2010/The-Future-of-Nursing-Leading-Change-Advancing-Health.aspx

Kaddoura, M. (2010). Effect of the essentials of critical care orientation (ECCO) program on the development of nurses' critical thinking skills. *The Journal of Continuing Education in Nursing, 41*(9), 424–432.

Karasik, R. J. (2009). Maximizing the potential of internships in gerontology and geriatrics. *Gerontology and Geriatrics Education, 30*(4), 281–299.

L'Eplattenier, N. (2001). Tracing the development of critical thinking in baccalaureate nursing students. *Journal of the New York State Nurses Association, 32*(2), 27–32.

Lipe, S., & Beasley, S. (2006) *Critical thinking in nursing: a cognitive skills workbook.* Philadelphia: Lippincott Williams & Wilkins.

Mayo Clinic Staff. (2012). *MRSA infection.* Retrieved from http://www.mayoclinic.com/health/mrsa/ds00735/dsection=symptoms>

McFadden, K. L., Hernández, T. D., & Ito, T. A. (2010, Nov.-Dec.). Attitudes toward complementary and alternative medicine influence its use. *Explore (NY), 6*(6), 380–388.

NACNS. (2011). Clinical nurse specialist core competencies. Retrieved from http://nacns.org/LinkClick.aspx?fileticket=s5bvR1QrNLw%3d&tabid=36

National Institute of Nursing Research. (2011). *Mission statement.* Retrieved from http://www.nimhd.nih.gov/strategicmock/our_programs/strategic/pubs/NINR-Rev.pdf

Ng, S. (2009). *An introduction to reflective practice for audiologists.* Retrieved June 28, 2009, from http://www.audiologyonline.com/articles/pf_article_detail.asp?article_id=2248

Nurses for a healthier tomorrow. (2007). Retrieved from http://www.nursesource.org/nurse-educator.html.

Otto, C., Bischof, G., Rumpf, H. J., Meyer, C., Hapke, U., & John, U. (2011, August). Multiple dimensions of health locus of control in a representative population sample: Ordinal factor analysis and cross-validation of an existing three and a new four factor model. *BMC Medical Research Methodology, 12*(11), 114.

Papastavrou, E., Georgios, E., & Charalambous, A. (2011). Nurses' and patients' perceptions of caring behaviours: Quantitative systematic review of comparative studies. *Journal of Advanced Nursing, 67*(6), 1191–1205. doi: 10.1111/j.1365-2648.2010.05580

Parnell, L., Davidhizar, R. E., Giger, J. N., Strickland, O. L., Fishman, D., & Allison, D. M. (2011). A guide to developing a culturally competent organization. *Journal of Transcultural Nursing, 22*(1), 7–14.

Polanyi, M. (1958/1962). *Personal knowledge: Towards a post-critical philosophy.* Chicago: University of Chicago Press.

PubMed Health. (2011). Severe acute respiratory syndrome (SARS). *A.D.A.M., Inc.* Retrieved from http://www.ncbi.nlm .nih.gov/pubmedhealth/PMH0004460/

QSEN– Quality & Safety Educaton for Nurses. (2011). Competency KSAs (pre-licensure). Retrieved from http:// www.qsen.org/ksas_prelicensure.php

Rakel, D., Bolles, S., Knutson, L., Herman, P. M., Piza, D., & Weeks, J. (2009). Defining cost effective health care teams. *Alternative and Complementary Therapies, 15*(5), 248–250.

Roach, M. (1984). *Caring the human mode of being: Implications for nursing.* Toronto, Canada: University of Toronto Press.

Rotter, J. B. (1954). *Social learning theory and clinical psychology.* New York: Prentice Hall.

Rotter, J. B. (1982). *The development and application of social learning theory. Selected Papers.* New York: Praeger.

Rubin, J. (1996). Impediments to the development of clinical knowledge and ethical judgment in critical care nursing. In P. Benner, C. Tanner, & C. Chesla (Eds.), *Expertise in nursing practice, caring, clinical judgment and ethics* (pp. 170–192). New York: Springer.

Ruddick, S. (1989). *Maternal thinking: Toward a politics of peace.* New York: Ballantine.

Ruel, J., & Motyka, C. (2009). Advanced practice nursing: A principle-based concept analysis. *Journal of the American Academy of Nurse Practitioners, 21*, 384–392.

Sanner, S., Baldwin, D., Canella, K. A., Charles, J., & Parker, L. (2010). The impact of cultural diversity forum on students' openness to diversity. *Journal of Cultural Diversity, 17*(2), 56–61.

Schon, D. (1987). *The reflective practitioner: How professionals think in action.* New York: Basic Books.

Shelton, J. H., Taylor, P. J., Bonner, A., & van den Bree, M. (2009). Risk factors for homelessness: Evidence from a population-based study. *Psychiatric Services, 60*(4), 465–472.

Stokowski, L. A., (2011). Looking out for our new nurse grads. *Medscape Nurses,* http://www.medscape.com/viewarticle/ 744221_print

Stanhope, M., & Lancaster, J. (2010). *Foundations of nursing in the community: Community-oriented practice.* Philadelphia: Mosby/Elsevier.

Swiadek, J. W. (2009). The impact of healthcare issues on the future of the nursing profession: The resulting increased influence of community-based and public health nursing. *Nursing Forum,44*(1), 19–24.

Tamborini, C. R., Iams, H. M., & Whitman, K. 2009. Marital history, race, and Social Security spouse and widow benefit eligibility in the United States. *Research on Aging 31*(5): 577–605.

Tanner, C. (1983). Research on clinical judgment. In W. Holzemer (Ed.), *Review of research in nursing education.* Thorofare, NJ: Charles B. Slack.

Tanner, C. (2006). *Thinking like a nurse: A research-based model of clinical judgment in nursing. Journal of Nursing Education, 45*(6). 2004–2011.

Taylor, C. (1993). Explanation and practical reason. In M. Nussbaum & A. Sen (Eds.), *The quality of life.* Oxford: Clarendon Press.

Taylor, C. (1994). Philosophical reflections on caring practices. In S. S. Phillips & P. Benner (Eds.), *The crisis of care: Affirming and restoring caring practices in the helping professions.* Washington, DC: Georgetown University Press.

Taylor-Haslip, V. (2010). Guided reflective journals depict a correlation to the academic success of nursing students. *Teaching and Learning in Nursing, 2*, 68–72.

U.S. Census Bureau. (2010). *2010 Census data.* Retrieved from http://2010.census.gov/2010census/data/

U.S. Department of Health and Human Services. *Healthy people 2000.* (1990): National Health Promotion and Disease Prevention Objectives. Washington, DC: Government Printing Office.

U.S. Department of Health and Human Services. (2011). *Healthy people 2020.* Retrieved from http://www .healthypeople.gov/2020/

Vetleson, A. J. (1994). *Perception, empathy, and judgment: An inquiry into the preconditions of moral performance.* University Park, PA: Pennsylvania State University Press.

Watson, J. (1988). *Nursing: Human science and human care. A theory of nursing.* New York: National League for Nursing.

Wikberg, A., & Eriksson, K. (2008). Intercultural caring—an abductive model. *Scandinavian Journal of Caring Sciences 22,* 485–496. Retrieved from www.onlinelibrary.wiley.com

Yoder-Wise, P. S. (2011). *Leading and managing in nursing* (5th ed.). St. Louis: Elsevier Mosby.

CHAPTER 2

Regulatory, Ethical, and Legal Aspects of Health Care Delivery

Cynthia Parkman
Annita Watson

Outcome-Based Learning Objectives

After studying this chapter, the learner will be able to:

1. Determine how major trends in health care quality and patient safety are related to nursing practice.
2. Critique the types of managed care plans: health maintenance organizations, preferred provider organizations, Medicare, and Medicaid.
3. Differentiate between the three types of standards used to measure quality in health care settings.
4. Analyze the impact of licensure, regulation, and accreditation on health care delivery systems.
5. Explain how ethical theories and principles influence nursing practice in a clinical setting.
6. Differentiate the types of laws that typically affect nursing practice: common, civil, tort, contract, and criminal, as well as the importance of the doctrine of informed consent as it relates to the use of implied consent in nursing settings.
7. Analyze the types of advance directives for health care and describe the nurse's responsibility in advocating and documenting the patient's wishes related to an advance directive.

KEY TERMS

HEALTH CARE at the federal and state level is highly regulated to ensure that care is delivered safely, access to care is available, and patient rights are secure. Consumers' demands for assurances about the quality of the care they receive and the right to choose their care providers have greatly influenced legislation regarding health care funding and programs. It is important for nurses to understand, from a global perspective, the forces at work in the health care environment that affect nursing practice, patient care, delivery of service, and advancements in science and technology. As will be discussed in Chapter 4, nurses play a vital role in managing these challenges by providing leadership in the management of patient care and design of patient care delivery models.

This chapter provides an overview of ethical, legal, financial, and social forces that influence the way health care is provided in organizations and how it is delivered to patients. The issues discussed directly and indirectly affect the practice of nursing, the way in which nurses contribute to the health of patients, the organizations for which they work, and the communities in which they live.

Hospital Organizations

In 2010 the American Hospital Association (AHA) identified three categories of hospital organizations: community hospitals, systems, and networks. Community hospitals include all nonfederal, short-term general, and other special hospitals (American Hospital Association, 2012). The other *special hospitals* include obstetrics and gynecology; eye, ear, nose, and throat; rehabilitation; orthopedic; and other individually described specialty services such as psychiatry and rehabilitation. *Community hospitals* also include academic medical centers or other teaching hospitals if they are nonfederal short-term hospitals (AHA, 2012). Excluded from this category are hospitals not accessible by the general public, such as prison hospitals or college infirmaries. A *system* refers to a multihospital or a diversified single hospital system (AHA, 2012). This might include two or more hospitals owned, leased, or contract managed by a central organization. Last, *networks* are a group of hospitals, physicians, other providers, insurers, and/or community agencies that work together to coordinate and deliver a broad spectrum of services to their community. Network participation does not preclude system affiliation. Examples of health care networks are Adventist Health System, Ketering Health Network, and Kaiser Health.

Rehabilitative and chronic disease facilities provide care for people who have disabilities caused by long-term problems such as stroke or severe injuries. Their patients receive restorative or adjustive care on either a short-term or long-term basis. Examples of these types of agencies include Alzheimer's and memory loss care centers and skilled nursing or long-term care centers. Finally, *psychiatric care facilities* provide inpatient and outpatient care for psychiatric-related illnesses (American Hospital Association [AHA], 2007). These are freestanding facilities that may or may not be associated with an acute care facility; they may be representative of a community hospital, a health care system, or a health care network.

Health Care Costs

In 2008, national health care spending grew at the slowest pace seen in almost 50 years. The 4.4% increase over prior year spending extended a slowing trend that has been underway since 2003 (California Health Care Foundation, 2010). However, with the nation in the grip of a recession, 2008's modest growth in health spending still outpaced the economy, and health care's share of the gross domestic product (GDP) rose to 16.2%. Total health care spending in 2008 reached $2.3 trillion, or $7,681 per person (California HealthCare Foundation, 2010).

As a result of these increasing health care spending costs, many employers have decreased the amount of coverage provided to employees and/or increased the amount that employees contribute toward their health care costs, thereby increasing the numbers of uninsured and underinsured Americans. On the other hand, even as health care costs have escalated, so have patients' demands for health care services, due largely in part to the growing numbers of elderly and the request for the latest technological and pharmaceutical advances in medical care (U.S. Census Bureau, 2011). Health care organizations are striving to meet patients' expectations in order to survive in a very competitive marketplace.

Historical Development of Health Care Economics

The current economics of health care have developed as a result of the historical impact of social, cultural, political, and economic issues in the United States. Since the 1940s, several major legislative acts have led to an increased role for the federal government. Market forces also have helped to replace fee-for-service plans with prospective contracted insurance plans, referred to as managed care, for most working Americans. Enacted in 1946, following World War II, the Hill-Burton program was established to fund the construction of hospitals. The program required facilities that received federal funds to make their services available to all persons residing in the facility's service area without discrimination. Although the Hill-Burton program meant that health care services would be available to all who lived in that community, it did not dictate how hospitals would charge for their services or how people would pay for them (Medical-Dictionary, 2010).

In the 1960s, Medicare and Medicaid legislation was passed as an amendment to the Social Security Act. The **Medicare** portion of the act provides insurance for people over age 65 and payment for their hospitalization, physicians' fees, and diagnostic tests. Medicare also provides coverage for persons with disabilities and those with permanent kidney failure. As an entitlement for older adults, Medicare essentially provides universal coverage for hospitalization and outpatient care. Together, these services account for more than half of all Medicare expenditures (Centers for Medicare & Medicaid Services [CMS], 2007; Robinson, 2010). The other portion, **Medicaid,** is a state-administered program that provides medical assistance for certain individuals and families (dependents) with low incomes and resources. The federal agency that is responsible for oversight of the programs is the Centers for Medicare and Medicaid Services (CMS). CMS also establishes guidelines for state Medicaid programs; however, program requirements are set by the individual states and administration of the state program may differ by county. These coverage plans may be administered by a managed care contract through a health maintenance organization (HMO) or a preferred provider organization (PPO) to provide care for patients (CMS, 2007).

In the 1980s public attention became focused on the spiraling costs of health care. The philosophy that all citizens had the right to comprehensive quality health care prompted governmental concerns about the spiraling costs and the wide variation in charges among providers. The government was no longer able to pay for care that was delivered without defined limits or costs (Robinson, 2010). In the face of huge budget deficits, the federal government moved to gain control of spiraling Medicare costs by enacting legislation to change Medicare payments from retrospective fee-for-service schedules to prospective fee schedules based on diagnostic categories, termed diagnostic-related groups (DRGs), as a reimbursement method for hospitalized Medicare patients. Through this method, hospitals are paid a certain capped amount per DRG category. A fixed payment has been predetermined for more than 470 possible diagnostic categories, covering the majority of medical diagnoses of all patients admitted to hospitals (CMS, 2007, 2012).

The purpose of the DRG system was, and still is, to ease the burden of Medicare financing and to control delivery of care. The advent of DRGs has served as an incentive for hospitals to place greater emphasis on reduction of costs, utilization of services, and length of patient stay. Under the DRG prospective payment system, hospitals and extended care facilities have had to develop length-of-stay (LOS) estimates for a variety of diagnoses. These estimates help determine, on average, the LOS beyond which the facility will not be reimbursed for the patient's care. A subspecialty of nursing, called *discharge planners,* has evolved to help plan patient discharges in a timely manner. Discharge planning nurses also help provide some assurance that the patient's needs will be met after discharge. At discharge, arrangements are made for family teaching, home care, or extended care. Hospital readmissions became an industry concern due to data showing patients were returning to the ED with problems due to lack of patient-centered discharge planning (Jweinat, 2010).

Managed Care and the Current Status of Reimbursement Practices

Within the complex American health care system, changes in reimbursement practices have led to changes in the way health care is delivered or "managed." *Managed care* is a generic term for a system that attempts to control and influence the way health care is financed and delivered. Managed care has affected the health care industry significantly since the early 1980s by changing the standards, the cost structure of medical care, and many aspects of access to care (Robinson, 2010). The development of managed care has been aimed at balancing the three elements of access, cost, and quality. Under the fee-for-service system, health care costs increased dramatically due to high utilization of services. Other factors that have continued to contribute to high costs include new technology, cost shifting, the aging population, legal pressures, and administrative costs (California HealthCare Foundation, 2010).

Discussions and debate over time have tried to determine the effect of managed care plans on the quality of health care in light of managed care's cost-cutting strategies and tight controls on utilization of services. The National Committee for Quality Assurance (NCQA) reported in 2010 that health plans that spend the most on care do not always deliver the best quality. However, trends indicated that consumers were demanding more choice in the selection of health care providers and seemed to be willing to pay higher premiums for this flexibility.

It is important to understand the basic plan designs that provide coverage for health care within the United States. Plans differ in the aspects of care that are covered and funding for that care. Chart 2–1 defines the types of insurance plans that are common throughout the country.

Forms of Managed Care

A number of abbreviations are used to describe the various forms of managed care: HMO, IPA, PPO, and EPO. An HMO refers to a health maintenance organization, IPA refers to an independent/individual practice association, PPO refers to a preferred provider organization, and EPO refers to an exclusive provider organization. An EPO has a contract with a single entity or group of physicians, unlike a PPO, which uses a network of independent providers (Robinson, 2010).

Health Maintenance Organizations

Health maintenance organizations (HMOs) were the earliest form of managed care, and are now the most common. HMOs deliver comprehensive health services for fixed, prepaid fees or capitation (Bailey, 2008). Comprehensive health care usually includes procedures that focus on preventive care and early detection, such as annual physicals, mammography, proctoscopy, immunizations, and well-baby visits. HMOs manage services and costs through utilization review/management, restriction of access to a specific network of providers, and incentives for physicians.

CHART 2–1 Definitions of Health Insurance Plans

Type of Health Plan	Definition
Traditional insurance	*Indemnity:* The insured individual is indemnified against financial losses for health care costs. The insured is not restricted in terms of which providers they can access and they are reimbursed directly for any costs.
	Service plans: The plan contracts with providers to accept payment based on a fee schedule. The insured may have some restrictions on providers, and the provider is paid directly by the plan.
Government programs	*Medicare:* National health insurance program for individuals age 65 or older, under age 65 with disabilities, and those with end-stage renal disease.
	Medicaid: Medical assistance for individuals and families with low incomes. Each state sets regulations about eligibility and services.
	Military, civil service, federal employees, and veterans programs also fall under this category.
Self-funded plans	Under the Employee Retirement Income Security Act, companies can cover their employees for medical costs instead of providing commercial insurance plans.
Health maintenance organization (HMO)	The organization provides comprehensive health care to individuals who prepay through premiums for the coverage. A primary care physician generally directs care within a network of providers.
Preferred provider organization (PPO)	The organization has a network of providers under contract. The insured can use the network providers or—for a higher deductible—access providers outside the network.

Source: Bailey, E. (2008). There are four main medical plans available for consumers to choose. Retrieved from http://www.suite101.com/content/types-of-health-insurance-a40494#ixzz1Ih1bQ8Ku.

Weblink: Definitions of Health Insurance Plans

Various HMO models and structures are available based on the relationship of the HMO and the providers. A group model is one in which a medical group or organization contracts to provide care exclusively to the HMO's members. In return, the HMO pays the medical group on a capitated basis, which is a set amount per member per month. An example of this model is Kaiser Permanente. In a network model, the HMO has a nonexclusive contract with two or more physician groups and allows the physicians to treat HMO as well as non-HMO patients (Bailey, 2008).

Independent Practice Association

An **independent practice association (IPA)** contracts on the behalf of individual physicians or groups of physicians to provide health care to the members of an HMO. In this model, the physicians remain independent contractors with separate practices. Another model is a staff model in which the HMO employs physicians to provide care to its members (Bailey, 2008).

Preferred Provider Organization

A **preferred provider organization (PPO)** differs from an HMO in several ways (Bailey, 2008). PPOs provide a coordinated care plan that provides medical care by contracting with a network of providers. These providers agree to accept a set reimbursement rate for care covered by the plan. PPOs also provide reimbursement for covered care to out-of-network providers, but the level of reimbursement may differ from their contracted providers, and the member may have to pay a higher deductible.

PPOs also differ from HMOs in that they do not rely on strict utilization management and other controls common with HMOs (Bailey, 2008). Instead, they usually attempt to contain costs by negotiating with individual providers and health care organizations to provide certain kinds of health care at an agreed-upon price. This price is usually lower than the price that a patient would pay for the same medical services outside of the PPO.

Many managed care organizations, regardless of whether the member uses the hospital, physician, or other services, have inducements for maintaining wellness through health screenings and patient education. This emphasis is believed to decrease the number of inpatient hospital days per admission and can have a positive effect on a hospital margin.

Another way in which managed care plans control costs is to require prior approval for many types of care. Referrals by an individual's primary care provider also are often required. Although "true emergencies" are covered, many visits to the emergency department fall into nonemergent categories, in which case coverage for these visits can be denied. The issue of prior approval also can arise before a patient can receive prescription drug benefits for certain drugs. Formularies of lists of drugs that are covered actually help to decrease skyrocketing drug costs by providing therapeutic, cost-effective choices for the practitioner. However, these limits also may delay care as providers or pharmacists attempt to get approval for nonformulary drugs, and patients may be required to pay any costs not covered by the insurance plan (Robinson, 2010). These additional costs are based on the contract prices and selections health care providers have negotiated with the pharmaceutical distributors. Additionally, practitioners in groups often are given financial incentives for keeping their members healthy and out of the hospital.

Managed care today is in the mode of creating a delivery system that manages both costs and care along with methods of documenting cost-effective care. As such, quality improvement activities are now mandated, and health care organizations must meet the standards of the NCQA with the Health Plan Employer Data and Information Set.

Future Economic Projections

Managed care as a model for health care delivery is not going to go away (Marquis & Huston, 2011). It permeates the current health care delivery system and is likely to grow in magnitude in terms of the numbers of subscribers to its plans as well as its impact on the entire health care system. Although managed care continues to dominate markets, it is evolving in ways that have diminished its potential to control costs and promote quality. As health care premiums continue to rise and labor markets slacken, consumers are likely to face a growing financial burden for the cost of care. These developments could have the positive effect of making consumers more cost conscious in their use of health care services. Conversely, they may result in increased disparities in the health system, with further stratification based on the ability to pay and a greater burden on those who have chronic illnesses for the cost of their care (Marquis & Huston, 2011).

It is expected that out-of-pocket costs, or those expenses not covered by health plans, will grow rapidly for consumers. This is primarily due to higher premiums for health plan coverage, which are based on higher medical care costs. These higher premiums have forced employers to share the added burden with their employees. To combat these competing cost structures, which seem to be increasing without end, reform initiatives are being proposed on many fronts. Certainly the government is looking at reducing expenses within the Medicare and Medicaid programs. Additionally, coverage programs are being developed to give consumers more choice about what their health plan will include; however, Medicare beneficiaries are facing increased levels of financial burden due to increasing health care costs (Riley, 2008).

Safety Alert *Patients may express concern about their financial situation and whether or not they have current and adequate health care coverage. This concern can cause significant stress that may affect the patient's ability to rest and recover. Referrals may be made to the hospital's financial department or social services to assist in resolving any payment or coverage issues.*

The cost and financing of health care will continue to drive the development of health care delivery models based on the premise that more should be provided for less. This focus will influence how health care professionals, including nurses, are used in the future. This pressure to determine how, when, where, and by whom health care is delivered will continue until the consumers (individual, employer, and insurance provider) are comfortable that the health care product (service) they are receiving is balanced by its availability and cost. Along with changes in health care finances and managed care, other important trends, such as technological advances, new diseases or recurring old diseases, and new medical specialties, affect the future of health care delivery systems and the financial configuration of health care organizations.

Health Care Reform

In 2011, two major pieces of legislation were signed into law: the Affordable Care Act (P.L. III-148) and the Health Care Education and Reconciliation Act of 2010 (P.LO. III-152) (American Academy of Nursing, 2010). The goals of these health care reform measures are directed toward expanding access to cost-effective, high-quality care, and to encourage a shift in the U.S. health system toward a greater emphasis on primary and preventive care. "The new health reform laws provide a complex series of changes in health care delivery, payment, coverage, and education—some of them immediate and others to be introduced or phased in over five years" (American Academy of Nursing, 2010, p. 1).

The directions taken in the new reform laws are consistent with priorities established by the nursing profession. In 2006, the Academy of Nursing introduced its "Raise the Voice" campaign, which emphasized the roles that nursing can play in transforming health care delivery. The directions set forth in this campaign parallel those established by the Institute of Medicine/Robert Wood Johnson 2010 study on the future of nursing. The Academy's campaign featured innovative, nurse-led models of care that expanded access and extended improved care to communities (American Academy of Nursing, 2010). Participating nurses often encountered barriers such as inadequate payment for advanced practice nursing services, troublesome health plan policies, and government regulations often requiring duplicative oversight by other health professionals (American Academy of Nursing, 2010).

Several provisions in the health care reform legislation broaden the roles of nurses, particularly advanced practice registered nurses (APRN), in expanding access to primary care and other health services. Others provide new funding for nurse-managed health clinics. Several provisions authorize new resources for expanding the health care workforce, particularly APRNs and other registered nurses, to meet growing health care needs (American Academy of Nursing, 2010). "National goals cannot be achieved without maximizing the contributions of nurses" (American Academy of Nursing, 2010, p. 2).

Financial Aspects of Health Care Organizations

Health care organizations, especially hospitals, are structured financially in one of two ways. **For-profit or investor-owned organizations** focus their mission and structure on earning a profit from their operations. The profits are then distributed to the owners of the organization or to investors who have purchased shares of the organization (Health First, 2010). The excess earnings of a **not-for-profit (or nonprofit) organization** must be used for public rather than private gain. The mission of the not-for-profit organization is to earn a profit, but those profits are generally used to improve the physical facility and services offered by the agency (Health First, 2010).

Regardless of whether a hospital uses a for-profit or not-for-profit structure, it cannot turn patients away who require emergency care services and it cannot refuse to care for patients. The **Emergency Medical Treatment and Labor Act (EMTALA)** was enacted in 1986 to ensure public access to emergency services regardless of patients' ability to pay. When patients are not able to pay for care, they fall under the hospital's charity care policy. Charity care is accounted for in annual budgets based on the organization's history and the demographic projections for the population they serve. Charity care is considered a loss from the organization's operations. Programs are available to assist hospitals that are adversely affected by their patient population's inability to pay; however, this assistance does not cover all costs incurred by the organization. Charity care can contribute to higher costs for insured or self-pay patients if the hospital has to structure its financial plan to make up for large losses. Under EMTALA, private hospitals may refuse care if they do not receive federal or state funds. Chapter 66 includes an in-depth discussion on the application of EMTALA laws in the emergency department.

Budgeting Process for Health Care Institutions

Budgets have three main components:

1. Revenue is the money an organization receives or is entitled to receive to cover the costs of providing services or goods.
2. Expenses are costs of operating the organization and include salaries, benefits, supplies, utilities, purchased services, and administrative costs.
3. Capital refers to equipment purchased by the organization or construction projects.

A budget basically is a plan for a future period that is defined in measurable terms and expected outcomes. The process begins with the forecasting of revenue and expense projections for the next budget period. This period, referred to as a fiscal year, is generally a calendar year, but may begin at any time during the year and lasts for 12 consecutive months. For instance, some organizations budget January through December, whereas others may define their fiscal year as July through June.

Forecasting involves a review of the organization's assets, which includes property, equipment, cash on hand, and the amount of money calculated as outstanding from billing. Organizations will next look at the trends in reimbursement for services and population demographics for growth or change. Reimbursement is the payment received for health or medical care from a health plan (insurance) or payer source. The amount of payment is often discounted from the actual charges for the service. Historical data also are reviewed for volume trends and patterns of service that may be seasonal in nature such as higher patient admissions during winter months.

All of this information is calculated to provide a projection for potential revenue, which must be compared to the estimated expenses. The comparison takes into account the bottom line, which is the outcome of revenue subtracted by expense (also referred to as net income). Usually this is a positive outcome, but at times organizations will project a loss or a break-even scenario based on their analysis of all of these factors. The administration and the governing body of the organization generally approve budgets before they are implemented. The budget is monitored continuously throughout the year and appropriate adjustments are made as necessary.

Capital budgets determine the organization's ability to purchase equipment and to upgrade or expand facilities. The capital budget is based on a calculation from the operating budget, or an estimate of what the organization can afford. Projections range from the next fiscal year to multiple years out into the future. Capital equipment needs generally fall into the categories of needing replacement, upgrading of existing equipment or systems, or purchasing of a new business or service opportunity. Facility needs usually are based on the age of the building, technology, and expansion for population growth or new services (Manos, 2010).

Funding for the capital budget comes from the estimated revenue from operations or a percentage of expected income or loans. Some capital equipment can be leased to avoid an outright purchase if purchasing funds are not available. Some leases allow the organization to rent equipment with an option to buy for a discounted price at the end of a set period or to allow payments for large pieces of equipment to be billed over several years.

Nursing professionals play an important part in the budget process through their observations of the environment, equipment, and changing needs of patients. Their input to the management structure provides important information for making decisions about the allocation of resources, the control of expenses, and planning for future growth. It also is important for nurses to take an active role in containing costs through judicious use of supplies, awareness of equipment safety and maintenance, and appropriate adjustments to staffing and workload.

Health Care Trends

Several major trends are affecting and changing health care in the United States:

- Evidence-based practice guidelines and research are creating a shift in approach to care that is clearer and more systematic.
- Quality and patient safety standards, which have been a main focus of consumer watchdog groups and regulatory bodies, are influencing the purchase of health care insurance and the selection of medical care providers.
- Threats of potential major events, such as bioterrorism attacks or widespread epidemics, are requiring health care organizations to set priorities and plan their responses.
- Advancements in technology and science are continuing to enhance medical care.

These and other trends are discussed in the following subsections.

Evidence-Based Practice

Evidence-based practice can be described broadly as an approach that integrates current research evidence with clinical expertise and patients' needs. Evidence-based practice has come about as a response to the demand for grounded clinical decision making that critically examines the benefits and costs of treatments and interventions.

Factors that form a framework for decision making with this approach include understanding patients' needs, concerns, and values; building on the clinical expertise or experience of the professional nurse; and seeking relevant clinical data and best practices (Kotzer & Arellana, 2008). *Best practices* are defined as proven processes that produce consistent, high-quality results. In nursing, there are many sources of knowledge that guide critical thinking about care, including the applicability of nursing interventions and intuition about approaches and interactions with patients. Data and research also are becoming more available through the use of Internet resources in the practice arena. Internet resources provide instant access for caregivers. Information systems used in health care organizations often provide immediate access to concise resources and guidelines for practice. It is important for nurses to keep current with relevant literature in their area of practice and to be competent in accessing available resources. EBP is discussed further in Chapters 3 and 4, and is one of the key concepts on which this text is based.

Hospital Report Cards

Consumer-oriented hospital report cards are available to the public through periodicals and on the Internet. They provide a wealth of information on quality outcome measurements and the experience of organizations in providing care (Chicago Tribune editors, 2009). The development of these tools was intended to help improve the quality of care by providing feedback and benchmarking practice standards. Benchmarking offers qualitative or quantitative measurement of specific data related to reported outcome information. Benchmark information often is displayed as a range and includes the best practice reported by participants. This can be of interest to patients or patient groups with specific health problems or chronic diseases who are making a selection of physicians or health care institutions. Information on hospitals, doctors, and nursing homes regarding ratings and quality of care can be obtained at these websites: www.healthgrades.com/ and www.hospitalcompare/hhs:gov/.

Weblink: Ratings and Quality of Care

Patient Safety Standards

There is heightened awareness in the United States regarding the safety of patients in the health care environment. Major efforts are underway to focus on measuring, reporting, and improving patient safety. Organizations conducting such research include the Institute of Medicine, the Leapfrog Group, and The Joint Commission. Current patient safety goals can be obtained at The Joint Commission and Centers for Disease Control websites: www.spectrumhealth.com/shr_providers/education/SHR_Ed/2012_JointCommissionl.pdf and www.cdc.gov/cliac/pdf/addenda/cliac0904/Addendum_V.pdf.

Weblink: Ratings and Quality of Care

The **Institute of Medicine (IOM)** provides science-based advice on medicine and health in an effort to improve health. It provides unbiased, evidence-based, and authoritative information to policy makers, professionals, and the public at large (IOM, 2010). In 1999, IOM produced the classic study, *To Err Is Human: Building a Safer Health System*, which indicated that preventable errors in hospitals are the eighth leading cause of death in the United States. Following the recommendations of the IOM report, hospitals were required to assess their practices and institute changes to ensure the reduction of preventable errors. Reports from the investigation of medical errors found that errors were not necessarily the result of carelessness, but were instead the result of systems and processes that did not provide the appropriate checks to prevent the errors (Leapfrog Group, 2010).

Weblink: Patient Safety Goals

The **Leapfrog Group** was established by a coalition of public and private organizations that provide health care benefits. The group focuses on collecting data about medical errors and setting standards that will reduce errors. In addition, information is provided to consumers that assists them in making more informed choices about hospitals and health care systems. The Leapfrog Group has developed platforms for improving patient safety including (1) computer physician order entry (CPOE), (2) evidence-based hospital referral, (3) intensive care unit (ICU) physician staffing or the use of intensivists, and (4) National Quality Forum-endorsed safe practices.

Weblink: Patient Safety Goals

CPOE is aimed at eliminating errors from the process of transcribing physician orders that are handwritten or given verbally. CPOE requires that the prescribing physician or allied health care provider personally enter orders into the computer system. It is well known that illegible handwriting has been one of the root causes of medication and therapy error (Institute of Medicine, 2007). According to the Leapfrog Group, if CPOE were implemented in all urban hospitals in the United States, as many as 907,600 serious medication errors could be prevented each year. In addition, CPOE has been shown to reduce patient length of stay and duplicate orders for procedures and tests (Leapfrog Group, 2010). Computer system software programs also are available that help to prevent prescribing errors by providing alerts regarding incompatibilities with medications.

Evidence-based hospital referral is aimed at guiding patients to hospitals and clinical teams that are more likely to produce better outcomes for specific treatments and procedures. Information provided on Leapfrog Group web pages offers data on hospital volume, geographic specifics, risk-adjusted outcomes, and benchmarking among providers. Currently, the Leapfrog Group collects data on eight high-risk conditions or procedures and three maternal high-risk delivery outcomes.

Weblink: Quality and Safety Education in Nursing

The group also advocates for dedicated physician staffing in intensive care units (ICUs). This type of program provides physicians who specialize in critical care and managing complex patients. Studies have shown that when this system is in place, there is a 30% reduction in overall hospital mortality and a 40% reduction in mortality in the intensive care environment (Leapfrog Group, 2010). These intensivist programs in the ICU also can be used to provide remote monitoring of acutely ill patients (Ekeland, Bowes, & Flottorp, 2010). Remote coverage is provided via computer monitoring of clinical data from specific diagnostic equipment and the ongoing review of test results and recorded documentation. Some systems provide video surveillance of the patient from the bedside linked to intensivists at a central location. Benefits of using an intensivist model include reduced mortality rates, reduced inappropriate admissions, shorter ICU stays, faster weaning from mechanical ventilators, early detection of hemodynamic complications, fewer consultations with other specialists, and an overall reduction in hospital/patient care costs (Ekeland et al., 2010).

The National Quality Forum is a public–private partnership created to develop and implement a national strategy for health care quality measurement and reporting. The organization has established an agenda to implement proven patient safety practices (National Quality Forum, 2010). National patient safety goals and practices have been endorsed by other organizations such as The Joint Commission and the Leapfrog Group, who have formed a partnership to collaborate on patient-safety standards. In addition, the CMS has also joined with the Leapfrog Group to provide information for their consumers about the initiatives and hospital-specific ratings that are now available (American Hospital Association, 2011).

The Joint Commission, the accrediting body for hospitals and health care organizations, is an independent, private, not-for-profit organization. The Joint Commission focuses on setting standards for patient care and safety, competency of staff, and responsibilities of the administration and governing board. It evaluates and certifies or accredits health care organizations and programs in the United States. The Joint Commission's patient safety standards took effect in July 2001, and are generally updated or expanded on an annual basis. Hospitals must take all of these standards and initiatives into consideration as they plan quality activities and develop policies and procedures (The Joint Commission, 2012).

In addition to the previously mentioned regulatory agencies that monitor patient safety, the American Association of Colleges of Nursing (AACN) (2009), in conjunction with the Robert Wood Johnson Foundation (RWJF), initiated a project, **Quality and Safety Education in Nursing (QSEN)** in 2009 (Cronenwett, Sherwood, & Gelmon, 2009; QSEN, 2012). This project focuses on improving the safety of nursing care and is designed to enhance the ability of nursing professionals to deliver high quality and safe nursing care. Using the 2003 Institute of Medicine competencies for nursing, QSEN faculty have defined quality and safety standards for nursing. They also have proposed targets for the knowledge, skills, and attitudes to be developed in prelicensure programs. The competencies are:

- Patient-Centered Care
- Teamwork and Collaboration
- Evidence-Based Practice
- Quality Improvement
- Safety
- Informatics.

These competencies are integrated into undergraduate and graduate nursing curricula and are woven throughout this text through incorporation in numerous chapters. The focus consistently is to provide safe patient care and to conform with the standards and goals provided by regulatory agencies. Additional information on QSEN may be obtained from http://www.aacn.nche.eduqsenec/overview.html.

Emergency Preparedness

Hospitals must develop disaster or emergency preparedness plans to ensure that the organization can respond rapidly and function under extreme conditions. These plans are required by licensing and accreditation agencies. Accreditation agencies evaluate and certify organizations on specific standards or regulations. The plans must address fire, utility failures, terrorism, and natural disasters. A committee generally oversees the development and periodic revision of the plan, as well as the conduction of drills to test the training and readiness of the staff to respond (Ablah et al., 2010).

Nurses have a vital role in the response to these emergency situations. Patients in the hospital may need to be evacuated to a safe area or triaged based on their current status. Triage involves skilled evaluation of the patient's condition, stability, and ongoing need for treatment. In a community-wide disaster, beds in the acute care hospital will need to be made available for patients with immediate life-threatening needs. To ensure maximum bed capacity, patients may be discharged to lower levels of care or be sent home to recover. Assessment of the patient's home environment and evaluation of the competency of surrogate caregivers are essential functions of the nurse in these instances. The triage process is discussed in detail in Chapter 66.

With the advent of the September 11, 2001, terrorist attacks in New York City and Washington, D.C., and the events surrounding the mailing of anthrax to citizens, the standards for hospital emergencies have changed dramatically. They now must engage in training and readiness planning for all types of bioterrorism, natural disasters, and mass casualties (Ablah et al., 2010). Disasters and bioterrorism are discussed in detail in Chapter 65.

Scientific and Technological Advancements

Telemedicine refers to systems or programs that use video or computer-based equipment to link providers or to monitor patients electronically. Telemedicine was first given a trial in the 1930s when television technology began. Now it is used throughout the world to provide videoconferencing in a variety of health care settings. This technology is used to improve access to higher levels of care for advice and direction, especially in rural areas, prison health care, psychiatry, and home health.

Telecommunication capabilities for diagnostic imaging examinations, such as digital x-rays and computerized tomography (CAT) scans, are common in institutions. These capabilities are particularly useful for emergency departments, which use them to link physicians remotely to diagnose patient conditions or obtain specialty consultations (Ekeland et al., 2010).

Other applications for telemedicine include its use in accessing consultations in distant clinical settings, which saves the patient time and expense for travel to specialists. Through videoconferencing, physicians and technicians can engage in assessment, view procedures, and review data concurrently while communicating directly with the patient.

Minimally Invasive Surgery

Minimally invasive surgery describes a surgical technique that uses laparoscopic or video equipment to perform procedures without directly opening the body's cavities. Small incisions are made to introduce probes, video devices, and instruments. The technique has been described as telemanipulation, because the surgeon is physically separated from the surgical site and operates equipment using tactile cues and intuitive dexterity (Tchartchian, Dietzel, Bojahr, Hackethal, & De Wilde, 2011). It has been estimated that in the near future 70% of all surgical procedures will involve minimally invasive techniques. Surgeries now being performed in this manner include removal of esophageal tumors, treatment of morbid obesity, excision of malignant liver tumors, removal of gallbladders and colon tumors, and a variety of gynecologic procedures (Tchartchian et al., 2011). Benefits of minimally invasive surgery include reduced pain, quicker return to oral intake, and less scarring. This results in shorter hospitalizations and an increased use of outpatient centers for these procedures (Tchartchian et al., 2011).

Robotics

Robotics as used in surgery is described as computer-controlled manipulators that have artificial sensatory abilities (Figure 2–1◆). These manipulators can be programmed to perform surgical tasks using tools or instruments (Tchartchian et al., 2011). Surgical robots are used passively to consistently hold a position or to actively move instruments in the surgical area. Benefits of using robotics include minimized surgical trauma, improved precision, decreased invasiveness, and fewer complications. It also is estimated that patients recover faster following the use of robotics techniques over other traditional or open procedures. Surgical procedures can be performed long distance, and the same type of robotics has been used to perform nonsurgical procedures in space (Tchartchian et al., 2011).

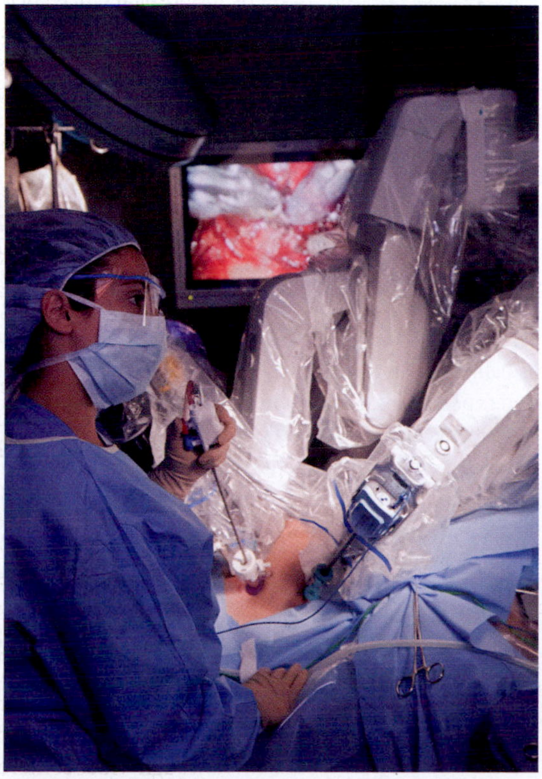

FIGURE 2–1 ◆ Robotic equipment used in surgery.
Source: Jim West/Alamy

Robotics also are being used to perform internal examinations through the use of pills or capsules that contain video cameras and light sources. One such device, a video pill, can perform endoscopic examinations for the small and large bowel (Jayaraman, Davies, & Schlachta, 2009). Robots are being used for multiple types of surgeries internationally, with success reported by studies (Jayaraman et al., 2009).

Gene Therapy

Genes are located in the nuclei of all cells and control hereditary traits and cell functions. Genes are attached end to end in long, double-stranded helical molecules of DNA. The study of genes has been aimed at identifying them individually through their functions, how they work, and what happens when they do not work. Scientists have been able to identify the human genetic code and the sequencing of 100% of the human genome (National Human Genome Research Institute, 2008). This research is helping to determine gene function and even how to stop a gene from functioning if it produces disease or adverse conditions. For example, recent studies have explored cell transplantation and gene therapy for degenerative Parkinson's disease (Wakeman, Dodiya, & Kordower, 2011).

Ethical and legal issues surround the field of gene therapy and the ongoing research in this area. Patients undergoing gene research face social dilemmas, especially if there is the potential to predict a debilitating disease. Personal conflicts may arise when disease is detected, but not yet manifested. Although gene therapy will continue to be a major part of future health research, it is extremely expensive; thus, questions arise about the access to therapy and payment for associated services. See Chapter 7 for a complete discussion on genetics.

Inpatient to Outpatient Shift

As mentioned earlier, one overall trend in health care service is a shift from inpatient care to outpatient care settings for many procedures and treatment modalities. Factors affecting this shift include population growth, aging of the population, new technologies to manage chronic diseases, and less invasive procedures that reduce length of stay. Specialty centers are becoming more prevalent and are offering alternatives to the acute care hospital. This shift also is being endorsed by the 2010 Institute of Medicine/Robert Wood Johnson (IMO/RWJ) study on the Future of Nursing. Outpatient settings have advantages over the hospital in that they provide increased efficiency and reduced costs per procedure. Outpatient specialty centers have been developed for spine surgery, incontinence treatment, diagnostic testing, endoscopic procedures, surgical specialties like orthopedics, and cardiac services (Highbeam Business, 2012).

Health Care Worker Shortages

Shortages of physicians, nurses, and other health care specialists are affecting the delivery of care and services in the United States and elsewhere in the world. In hospitals, shortages of nurses, radiology technicians, pharmacists, medical record personnel, housekeepers, and food service personnel are becoming severe. A report released by the American Hospital Association in 2006 indicated that the many open nursing positions in hospitals in the United States equate to an 8.5% vacancy rate. California hospitals say they may face a shortage of health care workers across specialties in the next five years due to the state's aging workforce (Vesely, 2011).

In 2008, for the first time in the past three decades, the rate of aging of the nursing workforce slowed (HRSA, 2010). In 1988, half of the working population of RNs was less than 38 years of age; by 2008, however, the median age remained steady at 46 years of age. Hospitals are implementing strategies to retain and recruit health care staff; however, the benefits and overall effect of these strategies will not be felt for years. In addition, nursing education programs and health care service organizations are collaborating on new models for boosting the enrollment in and graduation from nursing schools (HRSA, 2010). At this time, many nursing education programs have waiting lists for admission; others use a lottery system to determine admissions, while still others have specific criteria that generate points used to determine admissions. All programs must post their admission criteria for public viewing.

Nurse Residency Programs

There is a growing trend by hospitals across the United States to provide nurse residency programs, which have been shown to reduce turnover rates for new graduate RNs, reduce costs, increase stability in staffing levels, and help first-year nurses develop critical competencies in clinical decision making and autonomy in providing patient care (IOM, 2011). Nurse residency programs provide a series of learning and work experiences that support new graduates as they transition from school into their first professional roles. These programs:

- Emphasize the development of clinical and leadership skills necessary for the advanced beginner nurse to be a successful member of the health care team.
- Promote the development of effective decision-making skills related to clinical judgment and performance.
- Provide clinical nursing leadership at point of care.
- Strengthen beginning nurses' commitment to nursing as a professional career choice and help them develop individual career goals.
- Bring evidence-based practice to the bedside.
- Improve patient safety and quality of care (University Health System Consortium, 2012).

Hospitalist Programs

Inpatient hospital care has become a specialty for physicians, called **hospitalists,** who concentrate their practice in the acute care environment. The use of hospitalists is designed to provide 24-hour coverage for patients. Hospitalists may be contracted to provide care to inpatients by primary care physicians who do not provide inpatient care or by patients who do not have a physician at the time of hospitalization. Internists and family practice physicians are turning the care of their patients who need hospitalization over to these specialists (Buser, 2010).

The benefits of using a hospitalist program include shorter lengths of stay, improved outcomes, and enhanced efficiency (Buser, 2010). Continuity of care is improved, and there is increased development and adherence to critical/clinical pathways and guidelines because the hospitalist is readily available to assess the patient's progress and make adjustments to the medical plan of care. Hospitalists help reduce inpatient costs and provide a higher level of inpatient care. Hospitalists become assimilated as part of the hospital staff, working collaboratively with the nursing staff and other providers to develop relationships and trust (Buser, 2010).

Information Technology

The growth of information management technology in health care has been an ongoing trend. New systems span the continuum of care and provide resources that are immediately available to practitioners and patients. Electronic health records and clinical information systems that integrate departmental functions and facilitate reporting and tracking of data and observations continue to be implemented in a variety of settings. Clinical information systems also link providers to individual patient data and appropriate clinical reference materials (Wells, Whittaker, Dorey, & Bullen, 2010). Some of these systems allow patients to schedule appointments for therapy and follow up, and some systems allow patients to communicate directly with health care professionals regarding their questions or concerns.

Connections through the Internet or a telephone also are used to monitor and interact with patients who have chronic disease disorders/illnesses, such as heart failure and diabetes. Disease management programs are successful in reducing emergency department visits and acute admissions to the hospital. In the future, most data collection and documentation will be electronic and integrated for use in caring for patients. Integrated electronic documentation is expected to improve quality, reduce costs, and enhance work flow. It also creates better clinical collaboration and fosters evidence-based decision making and the use of best practices (Wells et al., 2010). Chapter 5 discusses the use of electronic medical records and documentation in detail.

Demand for Quality Care

Four driving forces underlie health care system policies and decisions: cost, equity, access, and quality. Thus, quality is an important factor in public policy regarding health care delivery. Quality, its definition and interpretation, has become critically important as the general public has become increasingly aware of health care options and as health care moves forward in the 21st century (Marquis & Huston, 2011).

Quality Defined

Quality refers to both the characteristics of, and the pursuit of, excellence. Excellence may be established by determining whether the outcomes compare favorably to the standards that were set. **Quality of care** is the degree to which health services for individuals and populations increase the likelihood of desired health outcomes and are consistent with current professional knowledge. Classic writings by Donabedian (1980) defined health care–related quality as the balance of health benefits and harms to a patient. Quality also may be defined in terms of effectiveness and efficiency, or appropriateness of care, as is the case in a service setting. Quality has been described as consisting of two interdependent parts: quality in fact and quality in perception. **Quality in fact** is defined as an individual conforming to standards and meeting his own expectations. **Quality in perception** is defined as meeting the client's/patient's expectations. Within the framework of continuous quality improvement, quality is defined as meeting or exceeding client/patient requirements. The Joint Commission has identified quality as a factor that increases the probability of desired outcomes being met and reduces the probability of undesired outcomes (Huber, 2010; The Joint Commission, 2007).

Quality processes in which health care delivery systems engage have been categorized as quality assurance programs, quality improvement programs, total quality management, and continuous quality improvement. Each of these terms and its current state of utilization are described next in order to explain the impact of quality demands on health care delivery systems.

- Quality assurance generally refers to an organization's effort or ability to provide services according to accepted professional standards and in a manner acceptable to the patient. Quality assurance activities are intended to guarantee or ensure quality of care (Huber, 2010). Most health care organizations do not use this interpretation of quality anymore because they do not endorse the concept that quality can be assured. The term *quality assurance* generally has been replaced with *quality improvement* or *quality management*.

- Quality improvement programs function as organizational umbrellas that extend into many areas for the purpose of accountability to the consumer and payer. The program is a continuous, ongoing measurement and evaluation process that includes structure, process, and outcomes. The quality improvement process uses preestablished criteria and standards and then follows the evaluation of care with an appropriate change for the purpose of improvement. Thus, quality improvement is a process of attaining a new level of performance that is superior to the previous level (Marquis & Huston, 2011). Many health care organizations have endorsed the concept of quality improvement and have adopted standards of care designed to improve quality of care.
- Total quality management (TQM), sometimes referred to as the total quality process, is a way to ensure client/patient satisfaction by involving all employees in the improvement of the quality of every product or service. Through TQM, all systems and processes are evaluated and improved. The goal of TQM is to reduce the waste and cost of poor quality. TQM has been defined as a structured system for involving an entire organization in a continuous quality improvement process targeted to meet and exceed client/patient expectations (Marquis & Huston, 2011). Many health care systems subscribe to this process of defining and measuring quality.
- Continuous quality improvement (CQI) is a process of continuously improving a system by gathering data on performance and using multidisciplinary teams to analyze the system, collect measurements, and propose changes. The four main principles are (1) a client/patient focus, (2) the identification of key processes to improve quality, (3) the use of quality tools and statistics, and (4) the involvement of all people and departments in problem solving (Huber, 2010). CQI is endorsed by many health care agencies.

With the paradigm shift from quality assurance to quality improvement, there has been a value shift from a focus on the provider's values to a focus on the client's (patient's) values. At the level of the individual nurse and patient, the quality improvement process is an appraisal of how the nurse is performing in taking care of patients. At the unit level, concurrent and retrospective audits (reviewing charts to determine compliance with standards), clinical pathway variances (evaluating patients' progress according to established pathways), and other data analyses (e.g., examining compliance with isolation procedures) may be used to examine the process and outcomes of care (Huber, 2010).

Regulatory Agency Impact

Standard setting occurs outside the professional arena (outside the care setting by external agencies, such as state licensing boards and The Joint Commission) in three areas: (1) federal and state government regulation (via Medicare and Medicaid reimbursement regulations), (2) state licensure, and (3) private accreditation. All are concerned with quality, usually at a minimum level. Federal reimbursement regulations for Medicare, discussed previously, are administered through the Centers for Medicare and Medicaid Services. Individual states promulgate Medicaid rules and regulations. They also regulate segments of the health care system, such as skilled nursing facilities or capital expenditures. Since The Joint Commission's founding in 1951, it has become the principal, but not exclusive, standard setter for health care facilities (The Joint Commission, 2007).

Other major accreditation initiatives are those of the National Committee for Quality Assurance (NCQA). The NCQA, a not-for-profit accrediting body for managed care organizations, has developed a core set of 60 health plan performance measures. These are measures that cover the areas of quality access, patient satisfaction, membership, utilization, and finance, as found in the 1993 version of the Health Plan Employer Data and Information Set (HEDIS). HEDIS represents a major effort to standardize and systematize the quality measurement process, thereby allowing for national comparison of performance and benchmarking. Technical quality of care, access to services, and enrollee satisfaction are measured. HEDIS measures are evaluated every 3 years, and new standards are added as appropriate. NCQA has a national database for comparison and benchmarking, referred to as the Quality Compass (NCQA, 2011).

The CMS has mandated the use of the standardized Outcome and Assessment Information Set (OASIS) for home health care for both Medicare and non-Medicare patients. OASIS is a series of questions for collecting data on the quality of home care. Clinical, financial, and administrative data are included. For all of the accreditation and regulation systems, the goals are to improve the quality of care and collect data for comparisons.

Quality Measurement

The measurement of quality is founded on several principles: (1) Quality can be measured; (2) Quality measures results against a standard or some degree of excellence; and (3) Excellence is determined either by validating standards of care or by measuring professional actions in caring for patients. Standards essentially define quality, against which outcomes and performance are measured. Because standards establish the baseline against which an evaluation is conducted, they need to be reliable and valid. Standards take three different approaches or forms: structure, process, and outcomes (Huber, 2010). Chart 2–2 provides a definition of the three types of standards and examples corresponding to each.

In measuring quality, both structure and process parameters are important, but they are not sufficient in determining whether the care made a difference or whether the patient learned, recovered, or improved his health status. It is important for the care to make a difference and that the care is not above a certain cost. In addition, measuring nursing care outcomes as related to cost would assist in establishing the value of nursing care. It would validate the economic value or worth of nursing care.

Quality Improvement and Research Studies

Research and quality assessment/management both rely on evaluation and are applications of the problem-solving process. However, they are distinct and separate processes. Highly controlled experimental research is on one end of the spectrum, and day-to-day quality assessment evaluation is on the other. Research studies manipulate variables, may introduce new nursing procedures, and may not have an immediate application to practice. In contrast, quality improvement studies do not withhold an intervention to see if it has made a difference. In a quality improvement study, an intervention that is not commonly accepted would not be introduced.

Quality improvement studies are necessary for the institution's patient care management. They are not designed to manipulate variables, withhold interventions, or introduce new techniques. They are designed for measuring existing care-related interventions and activities

CHART 2–2 Quality Standards and Measurement Examples

Type of Standard	Measurement Example
Structure standards focus on the internal characteristics of the organization and its personnel. These standards regulate the environment to ensure quality and answer the question: "Is a structure in place that will allow quality to exist?"	Nursing department provides in-service opportunities for staff development. Agency will staff at least one RN for every six patient visits.
Process standards focus on whether the activities within an organization are being appropriately conducted. These standards target behaviors, activities, interventions, and the sequence of caregiving events.	A nursing assessment will be completed on each patient within 2 hours of admission. Vital signs will be taken every hour.
Outcome standards refer to whether the services provided make any difference. These standards address physical health status, mental health status, social and physical function, health attitudes/knowledge/behavior, utilization of services, and the patient's perception of care.	Ambulates without assistance. Breath sounds are clear, free of rales and rhonchi.

with the idea of determining how they measure against standards, so that patient care can be managed and improved. The purpose of nursing research is generalizable knowledge; the purpose of quality improvement is determining effectiveness, efficiency, and appropriateness of care. Research utilization and other research activities can contribute to quality improvement, whereas the contribution of quality assessment to the research process is through problem identification. A key challenge for the future is to integrate research, clinical practice, and evaluation methods. Chapter 3 includes a complete description of research and quality assessment.

Licensure, Regulation, and Accreditation of Health Care Organizations

Licensure refers to the process for approving a health care organization to provide medical care and services. Licensing is generally accomplished at the state level through a department of health services. The purpose of the licensure process is generally to ensure access to care and monitor the quality of care provided. Regulations on licensure differ from state to state, as does the process for credentialing an organization. Requirements generally cover business practices, building codes, facility maintenance, aspects of safety, evaluation and planning activities, delivery of care, and the credentials and competency of employees. States also determine licensure for professionals and describe the scope of practice for various levels of caregivers.

The state agency responsible for licensing will survey the organization periodically for compliance with regulations. Regulations are rules or laws that govern delivery of care or maintenance of the facility or work environment. A compliance survey focuses on all aspects of the facility's operations in addition to the quality improvement program. State agencies are enforcement bodies that can levy fines and other restrictions on health care organizations that do not meet the intent of the regulations or that show a history of deficiencies or noncompliance with requirements or the organization's own policies.

Federal and state governmental agencies regulate the delivery of health care in specific areas, such as safety, facility structural requirements, and disease prevention and control. These agencies have some jurisdiction over hospitals and other health care delivery organizations to ensure compliance with standards and to assist with problems that may occur in those environments.

Occupational Safety and Health Administration

The **Occupational Safety and Health Administration (OSHA)** is an agency that oversees environmental safety. It was established under the U.S. Department of Labor by the Occupational Safety and Health Act of 1970. This agency works through federal and state partnerships to inspect and enforce safety standards in the workplace. OSHA oversees numerous health and safety requirements within health care facilities. Examples of this oversight include bloodborne pathogen control programs, control of biological hazards, ergonomic health/safety issues, and chemical and radiological safety. OSHA also is concerned with medical equipment, mechanical maintenance, food and laundry services, and housekeeping standards.

OSHA produces guidelines and reports that help hospitals and other care facilities meet state and national regulatory standards. OSHA personnel provide consultation services on health and safety issues, and they survey or inspect facilities if complaints are received regarding regulations under their jurisdiction. If facilities do not meet OSHA regulations, the organization can be fined or have its licensure affected (OSHA, 2011).

Fire and Life Safety Standards

Health care facilities also must meet fire and life safety standards and regulations. Life safety standards refer to a set of fire protection requirements designed to provide a reasonable degree of safety from fire. These standards cover construction, protection, and operational features designed to provide safety from fire, smoke, and panic. These regulations vary by state and community. Inspections are generally made on a routine basis by the fire marshal, or other appropriate officials, to check for building code compliance and the training of staff to respond to emergency situations. Inspections also occur whenever new regulations or standards are enacted, during construction and remodeling, or after any significant structural damage. Facilities must maintain compliance with regulations or be subject to evacuation of employees and patients, as well as the possible closure of affected areas.

Infection and Disease Control

The **Centers for Disease Control and Prevention (CDC),** an agency under the U.S. Department of Health and Human Services, focuses on protecting the health and safety of people within and outside of health care environments. The CDC accomplishes this charge through the development and application of disease prevention and control, promotion of environmental health, and education. The CDC provides guidelines and alerts that are communicated to health care organizations, usually through the infection control department of a health agency. These communications are aimed at assisting organizations with policy development, screening of patients, and reporting requirements if specific diseases are detected. The CDC responds to significant outbreaks and threats to assist health care organizations in taking appropriate actions (CDC, 2010). Chapter 14 provides a full discussion of infection control policies and procedures.

Professional Practice Oversight

Certain agencies oversee the practice of professionally licensed care providers. For example, there are professional licensing boards for physicians, nurses, pharmacists, and radiology and laboratory technicians. These boards set the specific requirements for initial licensure, ongoing or continuing education hours and courses, the scope of practice for the particular discipline, and the disciplinary action processes should a professional act outside of the scope of practice or behavioral requirements.

The requirements may differ from state to state as to the curriculum and number of clinical hours required from educational programs and the acceptable scores for passing licensing examinations. Compliance with licensing standards is reviewed with the professional's periodic recertification or renewal of license and during surveys of the organization by regulatory and accreditation agencies.

Accreditation

Accreditation is the process whereby a professional association or nongovernmental agency grants recognition to a school or health care institution for demonstrated ability to meet predetermined criteria for established standards (Mosby's Medical Dictionary, 2009). The leading accreditation body for health care providers in the United States is The Joint Commission. The Joint Commission accredits about 80% of the nation's health care organizations, which includes hospitals, home health agencies, health care networks, ambulatory care facilities, long-term care facilities, behavioral health agencies, and clinical laboratories (The Joint Commission, 2012).

An approved accrediting body must certify hospitals and other health care organizations that want to participate in the federal Medicare and state Medicaid programs. This requirement from the CMS is termed *conditions of participation.* Through the accreditation process, organizations must develop and maintain a quality assessment and performance improvement program. Organizations also must provide ongoing monitoring of key clinical indicators and be able to demonstrate assessment of the data and appropriate actions taken to improve results (*Federal Register*, 2010).

The Joint Commission generally conducts accreditation surveys every 3 years. Prior to 2004, these surveys were prescheduled and consisted of reviewing written material provided by the health care organization on policies, procedures, and data regarding compliance with standards, in addition to a site inspection of the organization to look at current practice and retrospectively review past practice. Beginning in 2004, a new process was implemented using a "tracer" methodology, which is designed to monitor a specific patient through his or her hospitalization and evaluate policies along with the patient's interactions and experience with all services. In 2005, The Joint Commission initiated unannounced survey visits (The Joint Commission, 2006). Standards for accreditation are organized into functions of the organization, which delineate specific criteria that must be met. Chart 2–3 outlines the functional areas for which The Joint Commission has developed standards.

Hospitals are held to The Joint Commission patient safety standards and national indicators called *core measures.* Hospital-specific data regarding compliance with these criteria are incorporated into the survey process. Hospitals are required to collect data and report performance

CHART 2–3 The Joint Commission's Hospital Standards

Section	Standards
1. Patient-focused functions	• Ethics, rights, and responsibilities • Provision of care, treatment, and services • Medication management • Surveillance, prevention, and control of infection
2. Organization functions	• Improving organization performance • Leadership • Management of the environment of care • Management of human resources • Management of information
3. Structures with functions	• Medical staff • Nursing

Source: © Joint Commission Resources. (2010). *Hospital accreditation standards.* Oakbrook Terrace, IL: Joint Commission on Accreditation of Healthcare Organizations. Retrieved from http://www.jointcommission. Reprinted with permission.

Weblink: Hospital Standards

outcomes from sets of identified core measures. Examples of categories of current core measures set by The Joint Commission include acute myocardial infarction, heart failure, community-acquired pneumonia, prenatal care, venous thromboembolism, and other conditions. These core measures are part of The Joint Commission's initiative focusing on the integration of outcomes and performance measurement into the accreditation process (The Joint Commission, 2012).

The Joint Commission also publishes sentinel event alerts that advise hospitals of process or system failures that have resulted in significant errors. **Sentinel events** are unexpected occurrences that have the potential to cause, or actually result in, death or serious physical or psychological injury. Serious injury specifically includes loss of limb or function. The hospital must review the sentinel event alerts, then address its own policies and procedures to be sure it has measures in place to reduce risk. Examples of recent alerts from The Joint Commission include prevention of fires in surgical areas, misadministration of concentrated potassium chloride, prevention of ventilator-related infections, and prevention of deaths, including inpatient suicide (Tishler & Staats, 2009). The alerts contain a root-cause analysis that defines actual causes of errors or events that threaten patient and staff safety. Risk reduction strategies are provided to assist hospitals with policy and procedure development to prevent error (The Joint Commission, 2012).

Ethical and Legal Aspects of Health Care

In this section, the discussion centers on the continuing influence that ethical and legal concepts have on the professional practice of nursing. Professional accountability and responsibility continue to gather additional prominence, especially as nurses become more autonomous; as practice settings expand from acute care facilities to community, ambulatory, and long-term settings; and as consumers of health care become more knowledgeable about their rights and options for care.

It is not sufficient, though, to know and understand ethical and legal concepts. Nurses must blend these important aspects with competent, skilled nursing diagnoses and interventions (U.S. Legal, 2010). To perform this high-quality nursing care, nurses must also understand the concepts of critical thinking and clinical judgment, for without these latter concepts nurses cannot fully appreciate the application of legal and ethical concepts in professional practice settings. Thus, this chapter first explores ethics and legal concepts and issues that impact professional nursing practice and concludes with a section on critical thinking and clinical judgment. By knowing about and using these concepts and issues, nursing moves from merely a "hands-on" skills performance role to that of a truly professional practice.

Ethics and Nursing

Ethics is the systematic study of what a person's conduct and actions ought to be with regard to self, other human beings, and the environment (Izumi, 2010). From a nursing perspective, a broader conceptual definition of ethics is that ethics is concerned with motives and attitudes and the relationship of these attitudes to the overall care of the individual. It is the justification of what is right or wrong, and the study of what an individual's life and relationships ought to be, not what they are (Marquis & Huston, 2011).

Applied ethics requires application of normative ethical theory to everyday problems. Normative ethical theory for each profession provides the foundation and filter from which ethical decisions are made (Marquis & Huston, 2011).

Morality concerns the social nature of the community, codes of behavior, and community expectations (Stanford Encyclopedia of Philosophy, 2010). Morality provides the means for ascertaining if certain actions are right or wrong and whether the consequences of actions are good or bad. Thus, morals are ways of behaving to accomplish ethical practices. Ethics is the broader, more reflective endeavor and begins when a person goes beyond the acceptance and internalization of traditional rules, or normative behaviors, of the social group. The ultimate goal of ethics is to provide a reasoned and best solution to situations that arise in everyday clinical practice.

As a beginning step in the application of ethics to everyday clinical practice, nurses should first determine the essential or underlying issue. Does the issue concern a situation that the patient or the patient's family views as wrong, such as the discontinuance of nonextraordinary life-support measures? For many, the removal of a feeding tube that is delivering essential fluids and nutritional support to the patient would be considered a violation of a moral duty. Or does the issue involve a treatment or therapy that could or could not be instituted, such as whether to initiate full life-support measures in a geriatric patient who is terminally ill?

The implementation of ethics is internal to an individual's self, looks to the good of an individual rather than society as a whole, and concerns the "why" of an individual's actions. Ethics asks questions about motives and actions: Why did the person act as she did, and what was the final outcome of acting as she did? Was the outcome satisfactory to the individual?

Ethical Theories

Many different ethical theories have evolved to justify existing moral principles. These theories are considered normative because they describe the norms or standards of behavior and value that are ultimately applied to daily life (Responsible Nurse, 2010). Normative ethics concerns human actions and the outcomes of those actions. Most normative approaches to ethics fall under the three broad theoretical categories discussed next (Stanford Encyclopedia of Philosophy, 2010).

Deontological Theories

Deontological (from the Greek *deon*, or "duty") **theories** derive norms and rules from the duties human beings owe to one another by virtue of commitments made and roles assumed. Generally, deontologists hold that a sense of duty consists of rational respect for the fulfilling of one's obligations to other human beings, rather than looking at the rewards of one's actions. The greatest strength of this theory is its emphasis on the dignity of human beings. Deontological theory looks not to the end or consequences of an action, but to the intention of the action. It is one's good intentions—the intentions to do a moral duty—that ultimately determine the praiseworthiness of the action.

Duty-based, rights-based, and intuitionist ethical reasoning derive their framework from deontological theory. Deontological ethics have sometimes been subdivided into situation or "love" ethics, wherein the *decision making* takes into account the unique characteristics of each individual, the caring relationship between the person and the caregiver, and the most humanistic course of action given the circumstances (Park, 2009; Quaghebeur, Casterle, & Gastmans, 2009). Examples of this theory in action in the health care setting abound:

- Decisions about forgoing life-sustaining treatment that may conflict with religious beliefs
- Decisions not to pursue aggressive treatment while waiting to see what outcome God wants or trusting that conservative treatment will work if God so intends
- Decisions to bow to a higher order, given by divine command, such as in the case of Jehovah's Witnesses, who do not ingest blood and, therefore, refuse blood transfusions even if they will lose their lives or the lives of their children (DeWolf-Bosek & Savage, 2007).

Teleological Theories

Teleological (from the Greek *telos*, for "end") **theories** derive norms or rules for conduct from the consequences of actions. Right consists of actions that have good consequences, and wrong consists of actions that have bad consequences. Teleologists disagree, though, about how to determine the goodness or badness of the consequences of actions. Teleological theories support decisions that favor the common good (Izumi, 2010). An alternate way of viewing this theory is that the usefulness of an action is determined by the amount of happiness it brings. An example of a decision using this approach is that of allowing individual family members to make the difficult choices for their loved ones rather than mandating that all patients in persistent vegetative states must be given parenteral nutrition.

This theory frequently is referred to as utilitarianism; what makes an action right or wrong is its utility, and useful actions bring the greatest amount of happiness and satisfaction into existence (Stanford Encyclopedia of Philosophy, 2010). Teleological theories are used to support utilitarianism. Utilitarian ethics can be subdivided into rule and act utilitarianism. Rule utilitarianism seeks the greatest happiness for all; it appeals to public agreement as a basis for objective judgment about the nature of happiness. Act utilitarianism tries to determine in a particular situation which course of action will bring about the greatest happiness, or the least harm and suffering, to a single person. As such, act utilitarianism makes happiness subjective, basing decisions on what is the best for the greatest number of people (Izumi, 2010; Marquis & Huston, 2011).

Principlism

A third ethical theory has slowly been evolving over the past 25 years and, although not yet given the full status of a *theory*, it does assist nurses and health care providers who are struggling with difficult ethical issues. Called **principlism**, this emerging theory incorporates existing ethical principles and attempts to resolve conflicts by applying one or more of those ethical principles (Stanford Encyclopedia of Philosophy, 2010). Ethical principles actually control ethical decision making much more than do ethical theories, since principles encompass the basic premises from which rules are developed. Principles are moral norms that nurses demand and strive to implement daily in clinical settings. In the case of principlism, four principles form the basis for decision making: respect for autonomy, nonmaleficence, beneficence, and justice. Each of the principles can be used individually, although it is much more common to encounter two or more ethical principles used in concert or to see two or more principles coming into conflict in a specific patient situation.

Ethical theories are important because they form the essential base of knowledge from which to proceed (Fowler, 2008). Without ethical theories, decisions revolve around personal emotions. Because most health care providers do not ascribe to either deontology or teleology exclusively, principlism is growing in popularity among health care professionals in today's society.

Ethical Principles

There are eight ethical principles that nurses encounter when making decisions in clinical settings. A description of each principle follows.

Autonomy

The principle of **autonomy** addresses personal freedom and the right of an individual to choose what will happen to herself (Lachman, 2009). The legal doctrine of informed consent is a direct reflection of this principle. Autonomy involves health care providers' respect for patients' rights even if the health care provider does not agree with the decisions made. For example, autonomy issues often arise when an elderly patient insists that she be discharged home after recovering from a fall and fractured hip or ribs. Most health care providers would advocate for the placement of the elderly patient in a protected environment with available help to perform activities of daily living and to prevent complications from occurring that might lead to another hospital admission.

Beneficence

The principle of **beneficence** states that the actions a person takes should promote good. In caring for patients, *good* can be defined in many ways, including allowing a person to die without advanced life support and in the company of loved ones (Lachman, 2009). Good may prompt the nurse to encourage the patient to undergo extensive, painful treatment procedures, especially if these procedures will increase both the quality and quantity of life. Good also may extend to the patient's family by prompting family members to leave a patient's bedside so that both patient and family members can get some needed rest.

Nonmaleficence

The corollary of beneficence, the principle of **nonmaleficence,** states that a person should do no harm (Responsible Nurse, 2010). Many nurses find it difficult to follow this principle when performing treatments and procedures that bring discomfort and pain to patients. Health care providers often use the concept of a detrimental-benefit analysis when the issue of nonmaleficence is raised. Using this analysis, the focus of the projected treatment or procedure is on the consequences of the benefits to the patient and not on the harm that occurs at the time of the intervention. For example, the nurse may use this analysis when medicating a postoperative patient. Even though the injection causes some level of discomfort and suffering, the overall benefit to the client is less postoperative pain. A second example is the need to change and reapply dressings for patients who have sustained severe burns. Though changing dressings is extremely painful to patients, not performing this needed intervention would cause more serious complications. Thus, the principle of nonmaleficence may be chosen at times when pain and suffering can bring about a desirable outcome for the patient.

Veracity

Veracity concerns truth telling and incorporates the concept that individuals should always tell the truth (Lachman, 2009). This principle also compels that the truth be told completely. Nurses and other health care providers exemplify this principle when they give all of the facts of a situation truthfully and then assist patients and their loved ones to make appropriate decisions. For example, patients must be told of all their treatment options in terms that they can understand and then be allowed to make their own decisions.

The principle of veracity compels health care members to fully inform patients about all aspects of care, both the desirable effects as well as any negative effects. Without the entire truth, patients cannot make informed choices. This also is true of nursing management. For instance, a manager who believes deception is morally acceptable if it is done with the objective of beneficence may tell all rejected job applicants that they were highly considered, whether they had been or not. Another management example is that of the nurse manager who, in the event of a low patient census (i.e., a slow period on a unit), relays all of the options to staff and lets them make their own decisions about floating to other units, taking vacation time, or taking a day without pay, contingent on agency policy.

Justice

Justice concerns the ideal that persons should be treated equally and fairly (Responsible Nurse, 2010). This principle usually arises in times of short supplies or when there is competition for resources or benefits. This principle most often is considered when patient census is high and two patients are equally qualified to be cared for in a specific unit, such as an intensive care or cardiac care unit, or when there is an organ available for transplantation and two patients are equally appropriate candidates for the organ transplant.

Justice also demands that the same quality of care be given to all patients, regardless of their ethnicity, socioeconomic status, or lifestyle. Thus, the health care team must be vigilant concerning decisions that are made about why one candidate would be the more appropriate recipient of an available transplant organ and how the care of the second potential recipient will be delivered. Acceptable reasons for selecting one candidate over a second potential recipient could include compliance with recommended therapies and the supportive role of family members.

Paternalism

The principle of **paternalism,** sometimes referred to as parentalism, allows one to make decisions for another; it often has been viewed as a negative or undesirable principle (Milton, 2008). Used appropriately, however, paternalism assists persons to make decisions when they do not have sufficient data or expertise to make a decision. Staff members frequently use some degree of paternalism when they assist patients and their family members to decide if surgical procedures should be undertaken or if medical management is a better option. Paternalism becomes undesirable when the entire decision is taken from the patient or family member.

Fidelity

Fidelity means keeping one's promises or commitments (Responsible Nurse, 2010). Staff members know not to make promises to patients that they may not be able to keep, such as assuring the patient that no code will be performed before consulting with the patient's physician for such an order or that the patient will be able to return home within a specific time frame. Fidelity also prevents health care providers from promising that the patient will be given sufficient pain medication to be totally pain free following a surgical procedure. Rather, nurses reinforce that freedom from pain is a goal that the health care team will work to achieve.

Milton (2008) explored the codes and standards of professional practice and noted that nurses have multiple fidelity duties to the patient, physician organization, profession, and self that at times may conflict with one another. The American Nurses Association (ANA) Code of Ethics (2008) is clear that one duty "dominates" over all others, namely, the nurse's commitment to the patient.

Respect for Others

Many think the principle of **respect for others** is the highest principle and incorporates all other principles (Milton, 2008). Respect for others acknowledges the right of individuals to make decisions and to live by these decisions. Respect for others also transcends cultural differences, gender issues, and racial concerns. Nurses positively reinforce this principle daily when giving competent nursing care to all patients for whom they care. Nurses also reinforce these principles when they incorporate Watson's (Chapter 1) theory of caring into their interactions with patients and peers (Lukose, 2011). For example, caring for a very demanding, verbally abusive patient is difficult, and nurses might elect not to be as attentive to her needs as to those of a patient who is pleasant and cooperative. The principle of respect for others, however, demands that appropriate and competent care be given to both patients; caring is a central theme in Watson's theory (Lukose, 2011).

Ethical Decision Making

In clinical practice, ethical principles may differ among the individuals involved in patient care settings. Just as frequently, the ethical principles and values of family members may differ from patients' values or from health care providers' values. For example, an elderly, but independent patient may value his independence and ability to remain in an independent living situation (autonomy), whereas his family and the staff caring for him may feel that he needs closer supervision and desire that the patient be relocated to an assisted living center (beneficence) (Osborn, Day, Komesaroff, & Mant, 2009). Resolving such issues is the goal of understanding ethical dilemmas and ethical decision making.

Ethical Dilemma

When such disagreements occur, an ethical dilemma emerges. **Ethical dilemmas** by definition involve two or more unfavorable alternatives to a given situation (Von Dras, Flittner, Malcore, & Pouliot, 2009). For example, in the preceding scenario, the elderly gentleman may be at risk for injury when living by himself at home, but his ability to be independent will be hampered by living at an assisted living center. One means of addressing such situations is to use ethical decision-making models. **Ethical decision making** involves asking the following questions (ANA Code of Ethics for Nurses, 2008):

1. Who should make the choices?
2. What are the possible options or courses of action?
3. What are the available and reasonable alternatives?
4. What are the consequences, both positive and negative, of all possible options?
5. Which rules, obligations, and values should direct the choices?
6. What are the desired goals and outcomes in the given situation?

When making decisions, health care providers must use an orderly, systematic, and objective method to find the best solution. Various ethical decision-making models are available to assist with ethical decision making. These models are based on a process of steps and vary from 5 to 20 steps, depending on the specific model. The decision maker moves from step to step in an attempt to decide the best course of action given the specifics of the situation. Perhaps one of the easiest ethical decision-making models to use in clinical settings is the now classic **MORAL model.** The MORAL model was developed by Thiroux (1977) and then subsequently applied to nursing situations. Since that time, the MORAL model was further refined and utilized by Crisham (1990). The MORAL model of decision making is shown in Chart 2–4.

Ethical decision making is always a process, and the steps of the process remain fluid and flexible. As health care providers move through any model's various steps, they may find that they need to return to a previous step and redefine the issue, or they may discover that a major player's values were not taken into consideration when making the final decision. Sufficient time must be allowed for making decisions so that all players in the dilemma reach a conclusion that they can support.

Accountability and responsibility for making ethical decisions varies depending on the dilemma encountered. For the ethical decisions that must be addressed on a daily basis, such as helping family members understand the full extent of their loved one's prognosis or assisting a patient with understanding why a nurse cannot give more pain medication when the patient continues to have pain, the nurses working directly with the patients are generally responsible for these ethical dilemmas (Von Dras et al., 2009). For issues that involve the entire health care team, such as assisting family members to determine

CHART 2–4 MORAL Model of Ethical Decision Making

The letters of the acronym remind users of the steps of the model

Acronym Request	Example
Massage the dilemma.	Issues are identified and defined, taking into consideration the value systems and principles of all major players in the dilemma.
Outline the options.	Options are fully examined, including those that are less realistic.
Resolve the dilemma.	Issues and options are reviewed and basic ethical principles are applied to each of the identified options. A decision is made concerning the plan of action that will be taken.
Act by applying the chosen option.	Requires implementation by all members of the health care team, the patient, and family members.
Look back and evaluate.	Process of reviewing and reexamining whether desired outcomes were attained and whether new options need to be implemented.

if a feeding tube should be placed for nutritional support in an elderly patient who is terminal, the hospital ethics committee may be consulted, particularly if the family members disagree with one another.

Safety Alert *It is not uncommon in the practice of nursing to encounter situations in which a patient and family members must make decisions about lifesaving measures: Should they or should they not be used? It is essential that nurses know what the patient and family wishes are and what resources are available within the agency to help them solve this dilemma and meet the normal standard of care for the given situation.*

Ethics Committees

With the increasing complexity of ethical issues in health care, ethics committees have been created to assist in making ethical decisions in clinical settings (Salas & Cameron, 2010). Ethical committees can:

1. Provide structure and guidelines for potential problems.
2. Serve as an open forum for discussion and debate.
3. Function as a patient advocate by placing the patient at the core of the committee's deliberations.

Committee Structures

Ethics committees generally follow one of three distinct structures, though in some institutions these structures are blended. The autonomy model facilitates decision making for the competent patient. The patient benefit model uses **substituted judgment** (what the person would have done if she were capable of making a decision) and facilitates decision making for the incompetent patient. The social justice model considers broad social issues that may arise within the institution; in this model, many ethics committees hold ethical grand rounds (Salas & Cameron, 2010).

In many agencies, ethical grand rounds are conducted on a monthly basis and allow staff members to begin to be more involved in ethical decision making by presenting cases that involve a variety of ethical issues. The purpose of ethical grand rounds is to assist health care providers with future ethical decision making by making them more knowledgeable about ethical principles and the MORAL model. For example, presenting the case of the elderly gentleman who desires to remain in his own home rather than move to an assisted living center helps nurses to fully examine both sides of the issue. The nurses are then able to more quickly and competently address this same type of issue in the future. Such case presentations also allow nurses to become more fully versed on both sides of controversies and better understand their own ethical values and principles (Salas & Cameron, 2010).

Advance Directives

Advance directives are instructions individuals can give, in advance of a health problem, to guide caregivers in the event the individuals are no longer able to speak for themselves. Advance directives were enhanced with the federal Patient Self-Determination Act of 1989, which was implemented in December 1991. This act requires that individuals under Medicare and Medicaid be provided with information about their rights to determine health care decisions. It was the intention of this legislation to increase the use of advance directives, thus improving appropriateness of care and ensuring the patient's right to make decisions (American Medical Association, 2010; Medline Plus, 2010).

With advancements in medical knowledge and technology, end-of-life decisions have become more and more complex. For patients who are considering making decisions regarding medical care, there are three possible goals: cure, stabilization of functioning, and preparation for a comfortable and dignified death. These goals may change over a person's lifetime, depending on health status and age. Advance directives can be used at any time to establish a plan to meet goals regarding medical care. For example, a young, healthy person may establish an advance directive to guide decisions should she suffer an irreversible condition following a catastrophic event. Another person who has been diagnosed with a potentially terminal disease may document choices about pain management, terminal care, or life-sustaining measures. Advance directives can be changed as the individual's needs and goals change. Chart 2–5 discusses the differences between the various types of advance directives.

CHART 2–5 Types of Health Care Advance Directives

Type of Directive	Key Points
Health care advance directive	Documented instructions about health care to be used if the individual is unable to speak for himself. *Written:* Witnessed document that requires the individual's signature and those of the witnesses. *Oral:* Instructions given to the individual's physician during the course of treatment, illness, or stay in a hospital. This directive is documented in the patient's medical record.
Living will	Formal written documents that communicate the wishes of the individual about life-sustaining medical treatments should she become terminally ill. They are dependent on the caregiver's willingness to follow the wishes stated and they may have no legal effect.
Health care power of attorney, durable health care power of attorney	Legal document that establishes a surrogate decision maker to make medical treatment decisions for the individual should he become incapacitated.
Do-not-resuscitate order	Organizations will usually have policies that describe resuscitation orders and options. These can be implemented by the patient surrogate or family telling the physician, by an advance directive, or by a durable power of attorney for health care.

Sources: Data from Cohen et al. (2010). Exploring attitudes toward advance care directives in two diverse settings. *Journal of Palliative Medicine, 13*(12), 1427–1432. Medline-Plus. (2010). Advance directives. Retrieved from http://www.nlm.nih.gov/medlineplus/advancedirectives.html.

Patient and Caregiver Issues and Concerns

The nurse should be aware of certain issues and concerns for patients establishing advance directives, including the ability of family members and health care providers to carry out the directives (Lachman, 2009). First, not all health care professionals are comfortable or knowledgeable about advance directives. Some providers fail to discuss this aspect of care with the patient. The nurse should query patients regarding any discussions or decisions they may have made. If a patient has not dealt with this issue, it should be brought to the attention of the attending health care professionals. A lack of formal education, barriers to communication, or personal opinions may also interfere with the process. Not all patients wish to be fully informed about their diagnosis or condition. It may be helpful to determine the patient's preferences for receiving information (Lachman, 2009). The patient or family can be given a referral to appropriate resources, such as social services, to aid them in understanding these issues.

Weblink: Health Care Advance Directives

Second, cultural or situational factors may influence an individual's decision about executing an advance directive. This seems to be more prevalent in the younger, healthy population than in the elderly or those dealing with disabilities or chronic illness (Lachman, 2009). Although considerable information has been presented to the public about advance directives, a significant number of individuals have not completed the process. For those dealing with disabilities or chronic illness, knowledge about treatments and alternatives is necessary before they can articulate appropriate choices, including the desire to have an advance directive. For example, an individual may need to choose among palliative care, aggressive chemotherapy, or refusing treatment altogether. In order to make an informed choice, the individual needs complete information about each option and its possible consequences. In the latter case, an advance directive should be executed.

Third, the advance directive may not be present at the time it is needed due to an emergency situation, or the patient may not have given a copy of it to the health care provider. Patients should be encouraged to have documents readily available in their home to guide prehospital caregivers, such as emergency medical technicians (EMTs), should they respond to an emergency situation for the patient. The documentation contained within the patient's medical record and the placement of the advance directive in the record affect the ability of the physician and other caregivers to use the information at critical times (Resnick, Hickman, & Foster, 2012).

In some situations, family members may disagree with the treatment plan and the patient's stated wishes. This can present an ethical dilemma for the nurse in advocating for the patient while simultaneously assisting the family through appropriate decision making. At this point, the nurse should seek consultation with the health care provider and an administrative representative of the organization regarding a plan of action.

If the patient is not able to advocate for himself, the case may need to be referred to social services or the appropriate committee within the organization for discussion and counsel. *Bioethics,* or biomedical ethics, involves obtaining relevant factual information, assessing its reliability, identifying moral problems, and recommending alternative solutions to problems that have been identified. In medicine, this specifically relates to problems identified with making decisions about a patient's care and treatment. The bioethics process in most hospital organizations includes a committee (which could be the ethics committee previously described) or an ad hoc group that can quickly assemble to review a case and provide advice and counsel on a course of action. A case conference with the caregivers, family, and patient, if appropriate, can be called to discuss openly all of the facts. Nurses can be integral to this process because they may have firsthand knowledge of the patient's wishes and can offer information regarding the patient's present condition. Health care providers are obligated to follow an advance directive or the patient's wishes regarding care and treatment. If there is any doubt or conflict, it should be referred to the appropriate authority for resolution (Cohen et al., 2010).

Safety Alert *It is the nurse's responsibility to know the policies and procedures for identifying and referring a bioethical issue. The nurse must notify the health care provider and the organizational leadership when disputes arise and be prepared to participate in conferences to discuss a case and advocate for the patient per her assessment and knowledge of the patient's wishes.*

Documentation and Legal Requirements

Health care directives are legal in all states, but the requirements for their content and authorization may differ. An advance directive has two parts: appointment of an agent or surrogate decision maker and specific instructions about care and treatment preferences. The patient has the option to complete either or both parts. Most states have legal forms and witnessing requirements. An advance directive can be canceled or changed at any time. If an advance directive is changed, all copies of the previous directive should be destroyed and replaced with the new ones to avoid confusion. In the acute care setting, the nurse has a key role in ensuring that documentation is completed regarding the presence of a directive, actions taken if no directive is available, and any ongoing issues regarding the status of the patient's wishes. Chart 2–6 shows the nurses' responsibilities regarding advance directives.

CHART 2–6 Nurses' Responsibilities with Advance Directives

Nursing responsibilities include:

- Query the patient regarding the existence of an advance directive.
- Document the existence in the medical record:
  a. If there is a pre-standing directive from a previous admission, the nurse should query the patient regarding any changes and confirm the date of the directive.
  b. If the patient is submitting the document to a health care provider for the first time, it should be placed in the medical record per policy.
  c. If the patient has a directive, but did not bring it with him, it should be documented as such and efforts should be made to have the document brought in as soon as possible.
- If the patient wishes to make an oral directive, the health care provider should be notified.
- After discussion with the patient, the health care provider must document in the medical record the results of the discussion with the patient.
- If the patient does not have a directive, information should be given to the patient and, if appropriate, a referral made to a resource such as social services. The actions taken should be clearly documented in the medical record.

Legal Concepts in Nursing

Legal concepts are equally as important as ethical concepts in forming a framework for practice in health care settings. A general definition of *law* is that it concerns rules and regulations by which a society is governed (Lewenson & Truglio-Londrigan, 2008). These rules and regulations are made by individuals and are capable of being changed or modified. Legal issues differ from ethical issues in that laws are external to the individual because they entail the rules and regulations of society as a whole, and laws are concerned with one's conduct and actions as opposed to the motives and values of the individual. Law asks the question "What did the person do or fail to do?" rather than "Why did the person act as he did?" Finally, the enforcement of laws is much stronger than the enforcement of ethics; laws are enforced through courts of law, statutes, and state boards of nursing.

Sources of Law

Constitutional law is a system of fundamental laws or principles for the governance of a nation, society, or other aggregates of individuals (US Legal, 2010). *Statutory laws* are those rules and regulations enacted by the legislative branch of the government. The nurse practice act is an example of statutory law. *Administrative laws* are enacted through the decisions and rules of administrative agencies, which are specific governing bodies charged with implementing selected legislation

(US Legal, 2010). When statutory laws are enacted, administrative agencies are given the authority to implement the specific intentions of the statutes, creating rules and regulations that enforce the statutory law. Boards of nursing are examples of administrative law agencies. Finally, *judicial laws* are created by courts of law, interpreting legal issues that are in dispute. For example, a nurse who questions the authority of the state board of nursing may file a court action if the nurse has cause to believe that there has been a legal or procedural error on the part of the board's action against him (Guido, 2010). All laws, regardless of origin, are subject to change. Constitutional laws may be amended; statutory laws may be amended, repealed, or expanded; administrative agencies may be dissolved, expanded, or redefined; and judicial laws may be modified or completely altered by subsequent court decisions (US Legal, 2010).

Nurse Practice Acts

An example of statutory and administrative law is the state **nurse practice act,** which is the single most important piece of legislation for nursing because the practice act affects all aspects of nursing practice (Jarrin, 2010). The act defines nurses' **scope of practice,** those actions and duties that are allowable by a profession, and establishes standards for nurses in a given state or territory (Lewenson & Truglio-Londrigan, 2008). Requirements for licensure and entry into practice, empowerment of a board of nursing to oversee practice, and means for disciplinary action are part of the nurse practice act. The act is the law within the state or territory, and state boards of nursing cannot grant exceptions, waive the act's provisions, or expand practice outside the act's specific provisions.

Nurse practice acts typically define three categories of nurses: licensed practical or vocational nurses (LPN/LVN), licensed registered nurses (RN), and advanced practice nurses (APRN). The nurse practice act, in concert with common law, sets educational and examination requirements, provides for licensing by individuals who have met these requirements, defines the functions of each category of nurse, and may include a section on mandatory continuing education hours for renewal of licenses (Jarrin, 2010). Additionally, nurse practice acts state any exceptions that may occur, such as allowing nursing students to function in clinical settings as an exception to required licensure. The state nurse practice act also may include help for those affected by addiction; for example, diversion programs for registered nurses with drug and alcohol and mental illness problems. Many acts also provide assistance for nurses undergoing rehabilitation for a chemical dependency.

Each state practice act establishes a board of nursing. This board ensures enforcement of the act, regulation of those who come under its provisions, prevention of those not addressed by the act from practicing nursing, and protection of the public. Qualifications for board members, terms of office, and specific duties of board members are defined in the state practice act (Jarrin, 2010).

Although the nurse practice act is a statutory law, judicial law may become involved in its application (Jarrin, 2010). The application of judicial law actually helps define the meaning of the act for practicing nurses. In selected court decisions, the interpretation of the nurse practice act has assisted nurses in understanding the full application of the law. For example, landmark court cases in 1983 upheld the right of nurses to practice as advanced nurse practitioners (*Sermchief v. Gonzales*) and in 1985 allowed a board of nursing to set educational standards for advanced nurse practitioners (*Bellegie v. Board of Nurse Examiners*).

Nurses should be aware that when courts or legislatures expand the nurse's role, the legal accountability of nurses also increases. Thus, nurses have an obligation to continually remain current on issues that affect their practice. Means of remaining current include reading professional nursing journals, accessing the state board of nursing website for changes in the state nurse practice act, and being active in professional nursing organizations. Many states require mandatory continuing education in order to renew the registered nurse license (Jarrin, 2010).

Divisions or Types of Law

There are different types or divisions of law that affect nursing practice. Each type or division of law uses different processes to determine guilt or innocence.

Common and Civil Law

Common law is the system of deciding cases that originated in England and which was later adopted in the United States. Common law is based on precedent (legal principles developed in earlier case law) instead of statutory laws. It is based on justice, reason, and commonsense. Common law represents the traditional law of an area or region created by judges when deciding individual disputes or cases. These case-by-case decisions are used again and again in similar cases, thereby becoming customary or "common" to all people living under the authority of the court of law. Common law in modern America continues to be the product of generations of judicial decisions (US Legal, 2010). Principles that govern the use of human subjects in research and the composition and function of an institutional review board are examples of common law (Stanford Encyclopedia of Philosophy, 2010).

Civil law, or continental law, is the predominant system of law in the world. In contrast to common law, civil law was promulgated after the French Revolution in France and is based on rules and regulations that became normative principles. These normative principles are codified in codes and statutes. In countries with civil law, legislation is seen as the primary source of law. Civil law is enforced by the courts when disputes among parties arise. By default, courts base their judgments on the provision of codes and statutes from which solutions in particular cases are to be derived. The terms *common law* and *civil law* often are used interchangeably to describe law that affects individuals rather than state entities. However, there are differences (Cueto, 2010). Common law develops rules based on the outcomes of specific cases, whereas civil law starts with already developed rules, which are then applied to individual cases (Stanford Encyclopedia of Philosophy, 2010). For example, the features of civil law are compiled and codified into a collection for ready reference, in contrast to common law, which has its rules and regulations administered by judges and vary on a case to case basis. The main difference between common and civil law is that customs dictate common law, whereas civil law is written and has to be abided by the courts. Common and civil law are divided into a variety of legal specializations, including tort law and contract law (Stanford Encyclopedia of Philosophy, 2010).

Tort Law

A tort is a wrongful act committed against another person or the person's property. These wrongful acts result in an injury or harm, thereby constituting the basis for a claim by the injured party. Although some torts are crimes punishable by imprisonment—for example, assault—the primary aim of **tort law** is to provide relief for the damages incurred by the injured party and to deter others from committing the same harms. The injured person may sue for an injunction to prevent the continuation of the tortuous conduct or for monetary damages (Stanford Encyclopedia of Philosophy, 2010). Examples of such tort actions include negligence, malpractice, assault and battery, false imprisonment, defamation, invasion of privacy, and breach of confidentiality. Each of these types of actions is covered in subsequent sections.

Lawsuits involving tort law usually are broken down into intentional, nonintentional, or quasi-intentional wrongs. *Intentional torts* are those that occur when the person acting knew or should have known that a wrong would result from his conduct. A *nonintentional tort* is the result of a person's negligent conduct. A tort becomes *quasi-intentional* when intent is lacking, but there is a volitional or willful action and direct causation (Responsible Nurse, 2010). Examples of quasi-intentional torts are invasion of privacy and defamation. Invasion of privacy might be using patients' pictures without their consent or in a manner not authorized by them. Another example is giving out information about the patient's condition to a person who has not been authorized to receive such information.

Contract Law

Contracts are promises that the law will enforce. Contract law is that which governs the formation of promises or agreements between two or more parties, in relation to a particular subject. Contracts can cover a broad range of matters, including the sale of goods or real property, the terms of employment or of an independent contractor relationship, the settlement of a dispute, and ownership of intellectual property developed as part of a work for hire situation (Stanford Encyclopedia of Philosophy, 2010). The law provides remedies if a promise is breached or recognizes the performance of a promise as a duty. Contracts arise when a duty does or may come into existence because of a promise made by one of the parties. To be legally binding as a contract, a promise must be exchanged for *adequate consideration*. Adequate consideration is a benefit or determinant that a party receives which reasonably and fairly induces him to make the promise (i.e., contract).

Contracts are mainly governed by state statutory and common (judge-made) law and private law. Private law principally includes the terms of the agreement between the parties who are exchanging promises. This private law may override many of the rules otherwise established by state law. Statutory law may require some contracts to be put in writing and executed with particular formality. In certain situations, the parties may enter into a binding agreement without signing a formal written document. Typically, in order to be enforceable, a contract must involve the following elements: mutual consent, offer and acceptance, mutual consideration, performance or delivery, good faith, and no violation of public policy (US Legal, 2010). Given these stipulations, it is important to remember that an agreement, or contract, between parties can be a verbal agreement. This is referred to as an oral contract.

Because contracts are promises that the law will enforce, the law provides remedies if a promise is breached or the court recognizes the performance of a promise as a duty. Though an oral contract is legal, it can be very difficult to prove that an oral contract exists. Absent proof of the terms of the contract, a party may be unable to enforce the contract or may be forced to settle for less than the original bargain. Thus, even when there is no opportunity to draft a formal contract, it is always good practice to put something in writing, signed by both parties, to capture the key terms of an agreement. Nurses, as professionals, are subject to the same penalties for breach of contract as other professionals. These include damage of professional reputation, severance of a professional relationship, incurrence of legal fees, and possible resumption of duties if having been fired and if reinstated by order of the courts. Failure to meet licensure regulation is a breach of contract, as is failure to provide patient care according to agency policy and job description. There are many additional ways in which nurses may breach a contract and be held responsible for same (Responsible Nurse, 2010; US Legal, 2010).

Criminal Law

Criminal law, sometimes called public law, refers to laws that affect the state in its political capacity as well as society as a whole (US Legal, 2010). Criminal law involves prosecution by the government of persons who commit acts classified as crimes. In a criminal case, the state, through a prosecutor, initiates the suit (Kurban, Savas, Cetinkaya, Turan, & Kartal, 2010). A crime is any act or omission to act that violates public law. Most crimes are established by local, state, and federal governments; thus, criminal laws vary from state to state. Criminal law may be divided into misdemeanors, or lesser crimes, and felonies, more serious crimes that involve fines of more than $1,000 and are punishable by prison terms of greater than 1 year or death (Kurban et al., 2010).

Sources of Civil or Criminal Litigation for Nurses

Nurses and other health care professionals may become involved with either the civil or criminal justice systems (Kurban et al., 2010). The most frequent means by which a nurse incurs criminal action is by failing to renew the nursing license in a timely manner. If the nurse continues to practice once a nursing license has expired, the nurse is in direct violation of state nurse practice acts. Actions against nurses that fall under criminal law frequently involve substance abuse, particularly if the nurse is illegally acquiring medications from clinical settings (e.g., when patients' prescribed narcotics are diverted to support a nurse's substance abuse and the patients are given placebos instead) (Responsible Nurse, 2010). Less frequently, nurses have been charged with either intentionally or unintentionally causing the death of a patient.

Negligence and Malpractice

Negligence and malpractice are the common terms for nonintentional torts (US Legal, 2010). **Negligence** is the commission of an act that a reasonable and prudent person would not perform or the failure to do something that a reasonable and prudent person would do in a given situation (Negligence, 2007). In these situations, *reasonableness* is described as acceptable and according to common sense or normal practice. It connotes sensibility and rational thought. Negligence thus denotes conduct that is lacking in care and is usually seen as carelessness on the part of the care provider.

Malpractice, sometimes referred to as professional negligence, evolves from negligence law and the premise that all individuals are responsible for the consequences of their actions or inactions (Negligence, 2007). It refers to any misconduct or lack of skill in carrying out professional responsibilities in a reasonable and prudent manner. Issues of malpractice have become increasingly important to nurses as their authority, accountability, and autonomy have increased (Responsible Nurse, 2010). As roles have expanded, nurses have begun performing duties traditionally reserved for medical practice. As a result of an increased scope of practice, many nurses now carry individual malpractice insurance, which is considered by some to be a double-edged sword. Nurses need malpractice insurance because of their expanded role, but they also incur a greater likelihood of being sued if they have malpractice insurance, because injured parties tend to seek damages from as many individuals with financial resources as possible (Marquis & Huston, 2011).

In all liability suits, there is a *plaintiff* and a *defendant*. In malpractice cases, the plaintiff is the injured party and the defendant is the

CHART 2–7 Elements of Malpractice and Examples of Nursing Actions That May Result in Malpractice

Element	Explanation	Examples of Nursing Actions
Duty owed the person	Care should be given under the circumstances (what the prudent nurse would have done).	Failing to monitor a patient for postoperative bleeding
Breach of duty owed the patient	Not giving the care that should be given under the circumstances.	Failing to observe and report changes in a patient's condition
Foreseeability of harm	The nurse must have reasonable access to information about whether the possibility of harm exists.	Failing to act as a patient advocate; for example, the drug handbook specifies that the wrong route of dosage may cause injury. The nurse fails to act on behalf of the patient to clarify the correct route of administration.
Causation (a direct relationship exists between failure to meet the standard of care and injury and can be proven)	Patient is harmed because proper care is not given.	Failing to question an inappropriate order
Injury	Actual harm results to patient.	Failing to provide patient education and discharge planning
Damages	Based on pain and suffering, expenses, emotional damages, or malicious damages.	Giving the patient incorrect medications

professional who is alleged to have caused the injury. Essentially, six elements must be presented in a successful malpractice suit: duty owed the patient, breach of the duty owed the patient, foreseeability of harm, causation, injury, and damages. All of these factors must be proven before a court will find liability against the nurse and/or institution (US Legal, 2010). Chart 2–7 outlines these elements in greater detail; in addition, each of these elements is further expanded in the subsections that follow.

Elements of Malpractice

To understand how the law applies each element of malpractice to specific court cases, we use the following scenario: A nurse employed by a state medical center has been assigned to care for Mr. Gee, a patient admitted for a right hip replacement. Mr. Gee is 89 years old, weighs 255 pounds, is in relatively good health, and is competent mentally. He is to have surgery tomorrow and requires assistance in ambulating to and from the bathroom. While caring for Mr. Gee, the nurse fails to obtain the assistance of a second person when walking him to the bathroom, and he falls. Mr. Gee sustains a broken left hip and a mild concussion. He will be hospitalized for several additional days because he must now undergo bilateral hip replacement and physical therapy. Additionally, he will spend 2 days in the neurological step-down unit because of the concussion.

Duty Owed the Patient

The first element of malpractice, duty owed the patient, involves both the existence of the duty and the nature of the duty (Responsible Nurse, 2010). The fact that a nurse owes a duty of care to a patient usually is not hard to establish. Often this is established merely by showing the valid employment of the nurse within the institution. The more difficult part is the nature of the duty, which involves standards of care that represent the minimum requirements that define acceptable practice (internal standards). In the preceding scenario, the applicable standard of care is taken from the institution's policy and procedure manual and concerns the standard of care owed the elderly patient regarding safety issues. In this instance, the specific standard of care relates to the need for two attendants to safely assist Mr. Gee to the bathroom. Standards of care are established by reviewing the institution's policy and procedure manual, the individual's job description, and the practitioner's education and skills, as well as the pertinent standards as established by professional organizations, journal articles, standing orders and protocols, and national and community expectations (or standards) for this type of care (Rosen, Porath, Pawlson, Chassin, & Benbassat, 2011).

Several sources can be used to determine the applicable standard of care. The American Nurses Association, as well as a cadre of specialty organizations, publishes standards for nursing practice. The overall framework of these external standards is the nursing process. In 1988, the ANA first published its standards for nurse administrators, a series of nine standards incorporating the responsibilities of nurse administrators across all practice settings. Since that time, additional standards have been published that describe nursing care for a variety of patient populations and in selected nursing settings (ANA, 2008). A list of current ANA nursing practice standards is shown in Chart 2–8. Accreditation standards, especially those published yearly by The Joint Commission (2007), also assist in establishing the acceptable standards of care for health care facilities.

Breach of the Duty Owed the Patient

The second element of malpractice is breach of the duty of care owed the patient, or failure to meet the standard of care (Responsible Nurse, 2010). Once the standard of care has been established, the breach of, or failure to provide, the standard of care is often easy to show. However, establishing the standard of care may be difficult because the various parties to the suit may not be able to agree on the applicable standard of care, depending on whether the injured party or the hospital's attorney is trying to establish the standard of care for the given circumstances. The injured party will attempt to show that the acceptable standard of care is a higher standard of care than that shown by the defendant hospital and staff. Each of these two sides of the dispute help determine the standard of care through the testimony of expert witnesses. These individuals give testimony in court to determine the applicable and acceptable standard of care on a case-by-case basis and to assist the judge and jury in understanding nursing standards of care. In the scenario involving Mr. Gee, the injured party's expert witness would quote the institution's policy manual, and the nurse's expert witness would note any viable exceptions to the stated policy.

An example case that remains the standard for the distinction in standards of care is *Sabol v. Richmond Heights General Hospital* (1996).

CHART 2–8 American Nurses Association Standards of Professional Nursing Practice

ANA Standards of Practice

Standard 1. Assessment The registered nurse collects comprehensive data pertinent to the healthcare consumer's health or the situation.

Standard 2. Diagnosis The registered nurse analyzes the assessment data to determine the diagnoes or issues.

Standard 3. Outcome Identification The registered nurse identifies expected outcomes for a plan individualized to the healthcare consumer or the situation.

Standard 4. Planning The registered nurse develops a plan of care that prescribes strategies and interventions to attain expected outcomes.

Standard 5. Implementation The nurse implements the interventions identified in the plan.

- **Standard 5A.** Coordination of Care
- **Standard 5B.** Health Teaching and Health Promotion
- **Standard 5C.** Consultation (Graduate Prepared Specialty or Advanced Practice Nurse)
- **Standard 5D.** Prescriptive Authority and Treatment (Advanced Practice Nurse)

Standard 6. Evaluation The registered nurse evaluates progress toward attainment of outcomes.

ANA Standards of Professional Performance

Standard 7. Ethics The registered nurse practices ethically.

Standard 8. Education The registered nurse attains knowledge and competence that reflects current nursing practice.

Standard 9. Evidence-Based Practice and Research The registered nurse integrates evidence and research findings into practice.

Standard 10. Quality of Practice The registered nurse contributes to quality nursing practice.

Standard 11. Communication The registered nurse communicates effectively in a variety of formats in all areas of practice.

Standard 12. Leadership The registered nurse demonstrates leadership in the professional practice setting and the profession.

Standard 13. Collaboration The registered nurse collaborates with the healthcare consumer, family and others in the conduct of nursing practice.

Standard 14. Professional Practice Evaluation The registered nurse evaluates her or his own nursing practice in relation to professional practice standards and guidelines, relevant statutes, rules and regulations.

Standard 15. Resource Utilization The registered nurse utilizes appropriate resources to plan and provide nursing services that are safe, effective and financially responsible.

Standard 16. Environmental Health The registered nurse practices in an environmentally safe and healthy manner.

Source: American Nurses Association (ANA). (2010). *Scope and Standards of Nursing Practice.*

In *Sabol*, a patient was admitted to a general acute care hospital for treatment after attempting suicide by drug overdose. While in the acute care facility, the patient became increasingly paranoid and delusional. A nurse sat with the patient and tried to calm him. Restraints were not applied because the staff feared this would compound the situation by raising his level of paranoia and agitation. The patient got out of bed, knocked down the nurse who was in his room, fought his way past two nurses in the hallway, ran off the unit, and jumped from a third-story window, fracturing his arm and sustaining other relatively minor injuries.

Expert witnesses for the patient introduced standards of care pertinent to psychiatric patients, specifically those patients hospitalized in psychiatric facilities or in acute care hospitals with separate psychiatric units. The court ruled that the nurses in this general acute care situation were not negligent in this patient's care. The court stated that the nurses' actions were consistent with basic professional standards of practice for medical–surgical nurses in an acute care hospital. They did not have, nor were they expected to have, specialized psychiatric nursing training and would not be judged as if they did.

Foreseeability of Harm

The third element of malpractice, foreseeability of harm, involves the concept that certain events may reasonably be expected to cause specific results (Responsible Nurse, 2010). The nurse must have prior knowledge or information that failure to meet a standard of care may result in harm. The challenge is to show what was foreseeable given the facts of the case at the time of the occurrence, not when the case finally comes to court. In the scenario involving Mr. Gee, it was foreseeable that the patient could fall and harm himself if fewer than two people attempted to assist him with ambulation.

Causation

The fourth element of malpractice is causation, which means that the nurse's action or lack of action directly caused the patient's harm and not merely that the patient experienced some type of harm. There must be a direct relationship between the failure to meet the standard of care and the patient's injury (Responsible Nurse, 2010). Stated differently, causation means that it is not sufficient that a patient was harmed (Responsible Nurse, 2010; US Legal, 2010)—the patient must be able to show that the nurse's action or lack of action was the direct reason for the injury that resulted.

Injury

The resultant injury, the fifth element of malpractice, must be physical, not merely psychological or transient (Responsible Nurse, 2010). In other words, the patient must incur some physical harm before malpractice will be found against the health care provider. In the scenario about Mr. Gee, the patient was harmed as a direct result of ambulating to the bathroom, and he incurred the physical injuries of both a broken hip and a concussion.

Damages

Finally, the injured party must be able to prove damages, the sixth element of malpractice. The term *damages* refers to financial harm incurred by the injured party (US Legal, 2010). The ability to prove damages is vital in a malpractice suit because malpractice is nonintentional and unintended (US Legal, 2010). Thus, the patient must show financial harm before the courts will allow a finding of liability against the defendant nurse and/or hospital. Mr. Gee would be able to show damages that include additional hospital costs related to the second hip replacement surgery, physical therapy needs, and admission to the step-down unit. In addition, further medical needs may arise based on these injuries, such as a need for long-term physical therapy and temporary admission to a skilled nursing facility.

Liability for Negligence by Students

Nursing students have the ultimate responsibility for their own actions and may be liable for their own negligence. Student liability holds true even if the student is not an adult under state law (Omansky, 2010). The often used adage that a student practices under the instructor's license is not a true or valid statement because only the individual awarded the license practices on the license (Omansky, 2010; Responsible Nurse, 2010). The individual student always retains accountability, and nurse practice acts allow students to perform professional actions without being awarded a license to practice nursing, thus according them the opportunity to learn how to practice nursing.

The standard of care to which the nursing student is held is the same as that for the reasonably prudent practicing professional nurse. As such, the student and the instructor must know hospital policies and procedures and remain current in medical and nursing knowledge. The licensure exception further requires that unprepared nursing students or those who need additional supervision inform the faculty instructor of their special needs or lack of preparedness for clinical practice. Thus, nursing students remain accountable for their knowledge and skills, and faculty or staff may become accountable for individual student incompetence or lack of preparedness (Omansky, 2010: Responsible Nurse, 2010).

Regional and National Norms for Standards of Care

Sometimes the issue of whether standards of care follow a *regional (locality) rule* or national norm becomes an issue in courts of law (US Legal, 2010). **National standards of care** are based on reasonableness and are the average degree of skill, care, and diligence exercised by members of the same profession (Smith, Soriano, & Boal, 2007). Such national standards mean that nurses in all settings, urban and rural, must meet the same standards when caring for patients in clinical settings.

National standards of care have slowly replaced the previously used regional or locality standard of care, which allowed the standard of care to be viewed from the perspective of care within a given geographical area or "similar community" (Guido, 2010). There are two important reasons for national standards of care. With the advent of educational programs and videos; a greater ability to transport individuals to national conferences or to consult in small, more rural areas; and the use of telemedicine and virtual diagnostics, all areas with health care delivery systems have access to the same information and educational opportunities. A second reason is that all patients have the right to quality health care, whether hospitalized in a small community setting or in a major medical center (Guido, 2010).

Intentional Torts

Nurses also may be found liable for intentional torts, which are generally defined as actions that violate another person's rights (Responsible Nurse, 2010). In these cases, the nurse's actions must intend to interfere with the patient or property, the nurse must intend to bring about the consequences of the act, and the act must be a substantial factor in bringing about the consequences or outcomes. Note that, unlike negligence and malpractice, no actual harm is necessary for this tort; it is the violation of another person's rights that creates the cause of action. The more commonly seen intentional torts in health care settings are assault, battery, and false imprisonment (Milton, 2008; Responsible Nurse, 2010), as discussed next.

Assault

Assault causes the patient to feel apprehensive or fearful of being touched in an offensive, insulting, or physically injurious manner, such as when a clinician threatens the patient with an injection or the placement of a nasogastric tube. With assault, no actual touching of the person is required; it is the fear or apprehension of being touched that constitutes the intentional tort—the patient's knowledge of the action is required. Thus, a nurse cannot assault a sleeping or unconscious patient, because no matter how angry or violent the nurse might be or how irrational the nurse's actions might be, the patient has no knowledge of the potential contact and is, therefore, not apprehensive of the potential contact (Responsible Nurse, 2010).

Battery

Battery is the actual contact with another person or the person's property (Responsible Nurse, 2010). Examples of battery include forcing patients to ambulate against their wishes and restraining a patient in order to implement a procedure. With battery, however, a single touch, regardless of how fleeting or faint, is sufficient for a tort to have occurred. The patient does not need to experience any harm, injury, or pain in order for battery to occur. Also, in contrast to assault, the patient need not be aware of the battery for tort to have occurred. Taking the pulse of a sleeping person, for example, could be considered battery. The nurse also may commit battery by the unwarranted touching of the patient's clothes or an article held by the patient, such as a purse or suitcase. For purposes of battery, anything that is connected with the patient's person is viewed as part of the person (Responsible Nurse, 2010). For assault or battery to occur, there must be an absence of legal consent on the part of the patient.

False Imprisonment

False imprisonment is the unjustified detention of a person without the legal right to confine the person, such as when a clinician prevents a patient from leaving against medical advice or when nurses restrain a person in a confined space. Use of medications that alter a patient's ability to leave the health care setting can also create this tort. As with assault and battery, consent is a vital element of this tort; patients who are compromised mentally and restrained to prevent their harm are not falsely imprisoned because consent is implied (US Legal, 2010).

The patient must be aware of the detention or restraint (the act) for a successful false imprisonment lawsuit. False imprisonment also may occur if the act is directed at the patient's family or possessions, such as keys, clothing, or a purse. Sedated patients who are incapable of realizing their confinement do not have a suit for false imprisonment. Likewise, future threats are not enough to sustain the tort of false imprisonment. It is, however, prudent to realize that state law must be followed to the letter when a person's liberty is at stake; if it is not, the person can sue for false imprisonment.

Quasi-Intentional Torts

Tort law also recognizes quasi-intentional torts. The difference between quasi-intentional and intentional torts is that there is no intent to injure or cause distress to another person; there is, however, an intentional (volitional) action that causes injury or distress. Two quasi-intentional torts are recognized in health care settings: defamation of character and invasion of privacy, which includes the subset of breach of confidentiality.

Defamation of Character

Defamation of character, also known as libel and slander, is harming another's reputation by diminishing the esteem, respect, goodwill, or level of confidence that others have for that person. Individuals have the right to their good name (US Legal, 2010). Since defamation often occurs in medical record documentation, nurses are cautioned about what and how to record patient data and descriptions in the medical record. For example, documenting in the health record that a patient is a prostitute or acts "crazy" may raise potential liability issues for the nurse and agency. If there is no reason to include a statement, such as the comment about a person's lifestyle or occupation, then it should not be included in the official record. If, however, a record is needed to validate a patient's mental state or actions, the nurse should document actual patient behaviors or statements rather than making a subjective appraisal of the patient. The nurse should state exactly what the patient said and not the nurse's interpretation of the statement. A rule that assists nurses in this area is to document in the health record as though the patient and her family will be reading the record (Hader & Brown, 2010). Documentation is fully discussed in Chapter 5 (p. 94).

Invasion of Privacy

Invasion of privacy is a violation of a person's right to protection against unreasonable and unwarranted interference with his personal life (Gold, Phillip, McIver, & Komesaroff, 2009; Hader & Brown, 2010). To show that invasion of privacy has occurred, the person must show that the nurse intruded on the patient's privacy, the intrusion would be objectionable to a prudent and reasonable person, the intrusion concerns private or unpublished facts or pictures of a private nature, and that public disclosure of private facts occurred. Examples of invasion of privacy include taking photographs without the patient's permission, disclosing medical facts to persons not entitled to those facts, and publishing information that misrepresents the patient's condition.

Breach of Confidentiality

Breach of confidentiality, a type of invasion of privacy, concerns facts that are presented in the medical record (Hader & Brown, 2010; Kerr, 2009). The majority of the cases concerning breach of confidentiality concern privileged conversations that are included in the patient's medical record and the faxing or electronic conveyance of medical records. Health care professionals are cautioned to put procedures in place that allow for the disclosure of confidential data; the patient's written authorization to reveal selected information prevents a cause of action concerning invasion of privacy and breach of confidentiality.

Health Insurance Portability and Accountability Act (HIPAA)

A newer application of invasion of privacy is the recently enacted **Health Insurance Portability and Accountability Act (HIPAA)** of 1996 (Public Law 104-191), which is further elaborated in Chapter 3, Research Foundations for Nursing Practice (p. 56). The HIPAA regulations greatly expand the patient's right to confidentiality in all health care settings. Prior to the enforcement of this act, federal law did not protect patient confidentiality in the health/medical record, and individual states offered only limited protection of these records.

The HIPAA legislation includes comprehensive standards regarding the transmission of medical data, administrative records, and financial records. Significant fines and penalties are included to enable enforcement of the act against those who violate its provisions, so organizations must take the implementation of and compliance with HIPAA standards seriously (Hader & Brown, 2010; Kerr, 2009). Only "covered entities" come under the HIPAA regulations; covered entities include health care providers, health care cleaning houses, and health care plans that employ greater than 50 participants and who transmit health care information in an electronic format (Code of Federal Regulations, Sections 160.102 and 160.103, 1996).

One of the most important reasons for HIPAA is to ensure that patients retain a right to their medical information. Before HIPAA was enacted, information could be shared with other entities; now, patients have the right to allow or deny the disclosure (Neamatullah et al., 2008). To ensure that medical information is protected, the act defines protected health information (PHI), which recognizes 18 possible identifiers that relate to the past, present, or future physical or mental health of the person. PHI includes the following: names and initials of the individual; addresses, including street, e-mail, and Internet addresses; dates, including birth dates and dates of services received; telephone and fax numbers; Social Security or other personal identification numbers; medical record numbers; health plan identification numbers; license or certificate numbers; medical device identifiers; biometric identifiers such as fingerprints or photographic images; or any other unique identifying characteristic or code (45 Code of Federal Regulations, Section 160.103, 1996).

The HIPAA standards limit how information will be used or shared, mandate safeguards for the protection of health information, and shift control of health information from providers to the patient (Hader & Brown, 2010). Covered health care facilities must provide patients with a document entitled Notice of Privacy Practices, which explains how the PHI will be used or shared with other entities. The document also alerts patients to the process for filing complaints if they determine that their information rights were violated.

It is imperative that health care agencies follow the HIPAA rules that do not allow social media usage for patient information (Hader & Brown, 2010). "In addition to breaches of confidentiality claims, providers who betray patient confidences may also face civil claims for negligent and/or intentional infliction of emotional distress and invasion of privacy" (Hader & Brown, 2010, p. 272).

Consent

Generally, the health care provider's right to treat a patient, barring true emergency conditions or unanticipated occurrences, is based on a contractual relationship that arises through the mutual consent of the parties to the relationship (Paasche-Orlow, Jacob, Hochhauser, & Parker, 2009). This relationship is formed when the health care provider performing the therapy or treatment provides the patient with needed information and the patient voluntarily consents to the therapy or treatment. This fulfills the provisions of contracts: (1) agreements made between two or more persons or entities for the performance of an action; (2) mutual understanding of the terms and meanings of the contract; (3) compensation in the terms of something of value; and (4) fulfillment of a lawful purpose (Paasche-Orlow et al., 2009).

Consent is the voluntary authorization by a patient or the patient's legally recognized representative to do something to the patient. It is based on the mutual consent of all parties involved, and the *key* to true and valid consent is patient comprehension. Consent may be given orally or in writing. Unless state law mandates written consent, the law views oral and written consent as equally valid. As a precaution, health care providers should recognize that oral consent is much more difficult to prove should consent or lack of consent become a legal issue. As a convenience and to prevent such court issues, most health care institutions require written consent, primarily for invasive procedures, surgical interventions, blood product administration, and selected medication regimens.

Consent becomes an important issue from a legal perspective in that the patient may sue for a battery (unconsented touching) if she does not consent to the procedure or treatment and the health care provider goes ahead with the procedure or treatment (Paasche-Orlow et al., 2009). This means that the patient may bring a lawsuit and be awarded damages even if the patient benefitted from the procedure or treatment. The more current trend, though, is to argue consent under a negligence or malpractice cause of action because, in most of these cases, the patient has given consent for the procedure, an adverse outcome has occurred, and the issue of consent is argued secondary to the adverse outcome (harm) that occurred.

The right to consent and the right to refuse consent are based on a long-recognized, common law right of persons to be free from harmful or offensive touching of their bodies. Consent is not contingent on a request for information or clarification by the patient, but must be actively given by the patient. Information necessary to obtain consent is listed in Chart 2–9.

Consent may be obtained in a variety of ways. Perhaps the easiest means of obtaining informed consent is when the consent is *expressed* (Responsible Nurse, 2010). Expressed consent is consent given by direct words, either written or oral. For example, after the nurse informs the patient that she is going to start an intravenous

CHART 2–9 Information Necessary for Informed Consent

1. A brief but complete explanation of the treatment or procedure to be performed.
2. The name and qualifications of the person who will perform the procedure and, if others will assist, the names and qualifications of those assistants.
3. An explanation of any serious harm that may occur during the procedure, including death if that is a realistic outcome. Pain and discomforting side effects that may occur during the procedure and following the procedure also should be discussed.
4. An explanation of alternative therapies to the procedure or treatment, including the risk of doing nothing at all.
5. An explanation that the patient can refuse the therapy or procedure without having alternative care or support discontinued.
6. The fact that the patient can still refuse, even after the procedure or therapy has begun. For example, all of the suggested radiation treatments need not be completed (Paasche-Orlow et al., 2009).

infusion, the patient says, "Okay, but could you put the needle in my left hand, as I am right-handed?" As a rule, expressed consent is the type most often sought and received by health care providers, particularly nurses.

Informed Consent

Consent, technically, is an easy yes or no: "Yes, I will allow the surgery" or "No, I want to try medications first, then maybe I will allow the surgery." The law concerning consent in health care situations is based on informed consent. The doctrine of **informed consent** developed from negligence law as the courts began to realize that although consent may have been given, not enough information was being imparted to form the foundation of an informed decision (Gold et al., 2009). Informed consent mandates to the physician or independent health care provider the separate legal duty to disclose needed material facts in terms that the patient can reasonably understand so that the patient can make an informed choice (Lansimies-Antikainen, Laitinen, Rauramaa, & Pietila, 2009). Patients also should receive a description of the available alternatives to the proposed treatment and the risks and dangers involved in each alternative. Failure to disclose the needed facts in terms the patient can understand does not negate the consent, but it does place potential liability on the practitioner for malpractice. To be informed, the patient must receive, in terms he can understand and comprehend, specific information (American Medical Association, 2007), as shown in Chart 2–9.

Nurses may become involved in the process of obtaining informed consent in one of several ways. When a nurse realizes that consent must be obtained for all procedures and treatments, not just medical procedures, he realizes the vast impact of this doctrine (Gold et al., 2009). This does not mean that nurses have to obtain written consent each time they give an injection or turn a patient. Most nursing interventions rely on oral expressed consent or implied consent that may be readily inferred through the patient's actions.

The doctrine of informed consent means that nurses must continually communicate with patients. It also means that nurses must respect the patient's refusal to allow a certain procedure. If the patient is unable to communicate, permission may be derived from the patient's admission to the hospital or obtained from the patient's legally recognized representative.

A second way to enhance understanding is to allow time between the actual giving of information and when the patient must make a decision. Such time intervals allow patients to consider what has been suggested, to put into words their questions and concerns, and then to make the final decision and sign the informed consent forms, provided the physician has talked with the patient.

Implied Consent

Implied consent is consent that may be inferred by the patient's conduct or that may legally be presumed in emergency situations. For example, many patients hold out their arm and roll up their sleeve when the nurse approaches with a stethoscope and blood pressure cuff. This is an example of implied consent because a reasonable person would infer by the patient's action that she is consenting to the procedure (Lansimies-Antikainen et al., 2009). Another example is the patient extends his left shoulder for an injection after the nurse explains why the medication is being given. Nurses most often obtain implied consent for minor procedures and routine care.

Implied consent may be presumed to exist in true emergency situations; this is known as the **emergency doctrine.** For such consent, the patient must not be able to make his wishes known, and a delay in providing care would result in the loss of life or limb (Lansimies-Antikainen et al., 2009). An important element in allowing emergency consent is that the health care provider must not have any reason to know or believe that consent would *not* be given were the patient able to deny consent. For example, a health care provider cannot wait until a patient loses consciousness to order treatment that the patient had previously refused, such as a blood transfusion for a patient who is known to be a Jehovah's Witness. Implied consent is frequently relied on during surgery or in critical care units when an untoward event occurs and an immediate decision must be made to prevent further injury to the patient. Consent in emergency situations is discussed in Chapter 66.

Revocation of Consent

The nurse also has an important role if the patient subsequently decides to revoke his or her prior consent or if it becomes obvious that the patient's already signed, informed consent form does not meet the institution's standards for informed consent (Milton, 2008). Most nurses have been faced with the problem of what to do when it becomes all too clear that the patient does not understand the procedure to be performed or believes that there are no major risks or adverse consequences inherent to the procedure.

Safety Alert *It is important to remember that the nurse and the hospital may incur liability if there is reason to believe that the standards of informed consent have not been met. In such a case, it is the nurse's responsibility to contact his immediate supervisor and the responsible physician. Both entities need to be informed of the patient's change of mind or lack of comprehension (Lansimies-Antikainen et al., 2009).*

Signing of a Consent Form

Equally as important as the patient being given all material facts necessary for making an informed choice is that the correct person(s) consents to the procedure or therapy (Lansimies-Antikainen et al., 2009). Informed consent becomes a moot point if the wrong signature is obtained. The basic rule is that if the patient is a competent adult according to state law, only that adult can give or refuse consent. Most states recognize 18 as the age at which an individual becomes an adult, although some actions might serve to classify the person as an adult prior to the legal age; for example, marriage or termination of parental rights. The adult giving or refusing consent must be competent to either sign or refuse to sign the necessary consent forms. Competency at law means that (1) the court has not declared the person to be incompetent and (2) the person is generally able to understand the consequences of her actions. There is a strong legal presumption of continuing competency.

Some persons are never adjudicated or judged to be incompetent by a court of law, but they become incompetent to give informed consent based on their current medical condition (Gold et al., 2009). Many states allow the patient's family members to make decisions for the incompetent patient. For example, an automobile accident may render the patient incapable of making decisions and giving consent; in these situations, the physician will frequently ask the family about medical matters for the unconscious patient. The order of selection for most states usually is (1) spouse, (2) adult children or grandchildren, (3) parents, (4) grandparents, (5) adult brothers and sisters, and (6) adult nieces and nephews (Gold et al., 2009).

Most states recognize the child under 18 as a minor. Parental or guardian consent is necessary for medical therapies performed on a minor unless (1) the emergency doctrine applies, (2) the individual is an emancipated (liberated) minor or mature minor, (3) there is a court order to proceed with the therapy, or (4) the law recognizes the minor as having the ability to consent to the therapy (Gold et al., 2009). Some states also follow the *in loco parentis* doctrine, which refers to the ability of a person or the state to stand in the place of the parents. Look to the individual state's statutory laws to see who may consent in the absence of a parent and what constitutes emancipated status, because there is no general consensus on these issues. Such laws can be accessed through the individual state's governmental website. If there is a family consent doctrine, it will generally be a grandparent, adult brother or sister, or adult aunt or uncle.

Emancipated minors are persons under the legal age of an adult who are no longer under their parent's control and regulation and who are managing their own financial affairs (US Legal, 2010). Some states require the parent to completely surrender the right of care and custody of the child to prevent runaways from coming under this classification. Such emancipated minors may validly consent for their own medical therapies. Examples of emancipated minors are married persons, underage parents, or those in the armed service of their country. In some states, pregnant adolescents are considered emancipated for the purposes of giving or refusing medical treatment for themselves and their fetuses. However, after the infant is born, the adolescent mother may only make decisions for the infant or for herself if she is married (Guido, 2010). Some states allow college students living away from their parents to fall in the category of emancipated minor. Individual nurses should consult agency policies and state regulations for information regarding emancipated minors.

Mature minors also may consent to some medical care. The concept of a mature minor, although a relatively new one, is gaining legal recognition (DeWolf-Bosek & Savage, 2007). The mature minor is a minor between the ages of 14 and 17 who is able to understand the nature and consequences of the proposed therapy, is making his own decisions on a daily basis, and is independent. In contrast to the emancipated minor, the mature minor can be determined during an interview by the provider in which the minor answers questions that verify that he has the maturity to provide his/her own consent for treatment. The Mature Minor Rule enables the provider to ask questions of the young person in order to determine whether or not the minor has the maturity to provide his or her own consent for treatment.

In most circumstances, the health care provider is encouraged to seek parental consent along with the consent of the mature minor. Such a practice aids in limiting potential liability and encourages family involvement. It is necessary to consult agency policy for further information regarding this concept and the state statutes that govern the interpretation of mature minors.

The law also recognizes the right of the minor to consent to some selected therapies without informing parents of the treatment (DeWolf-Bosek & Savage, 2007). Selection of chosen therapies is contingent on the situation and state law. The reason for these exceptions is to encourage the minor to seek necessary treatment, especially when informing the parents of the treatment might prevent the minor from receiving the necessary therapy. Instances for which the minor may give valid consent include (1) diagnosis and treatment of infectious, contagious, or communicable diseases; (2) diagnosis and treatment of drug dependency, drug addiction, or any condition directly related to drug usage; (3) obtaining birth control devices; and (4) treatment during a pregnancy as long as the care concerns the pregnancy. There is no foolproof method for determining maturity among minors. It is a subjective and arbitrary process depending to a great degree on the perceptions of the evaluator. Also, state courts are inconsistent in the use of a standard of proof that is required for application of the mature minor.

Preventing Possible Liability

Nurses and other health care providers often ask what they can do to prevent potential lawsuits. Understanding and applying the legal concepts involved are two means of preventing possible liability. For example, ensuring that standards of care are fully implemented each time a nurse administers nursing care will help prevent potential lawsuits. Two other areas where nurses can take action to reduce their potential legal liability involve the nurse–patient relationship and patient rights.

Nurse–Patient Relationship

One of the most fundamental aspects of malpractice law involves relationships. For a duty to be owed the patient, an existing nurse–patient relationship must be established (Lachman, 2009). This may be accomplished by showing that a reliance relationship exists: One person (the patient) is depending on another person (the nurse) for competent, quality nursing care.

The core of any reliance relationship is trust and communication. Establishing rapport with patients, informing patients honestly and openly of all aspects of their care, and allowing patients to make decisions for themselves have always been credited to nurses as one means of preventing potential liability. Nursing is a caring profession; part of caring is maintaining communications and ensuring that trust is established and continues throughout the interactions between the nurse and the patient (Milton, 2008).

Patient Rights

Health care providers are becoming increasingly more aware and respectful of patient rights. In 1959, the National League for Nursing wrote one of the earliest statements regarding patients' rights (National League for Nursing, 1959). In the early 1970s, the American Hospital Association (AHA) published *A Patient's Bill of Rights*, enumerating 12 rights that were to be afforded to all hospitalized patients. These rights primarily concerned the patient's right to considerate and respectful care; informed consent concepts, including making treatment decisions based on informed choice; considerations of privacy; the right to know who will provide care; and the right to information about advance directives. The document was revised in 1992, and more recently in 2008. It is no longer called only a Bill of Rights, but "The Patient Care Partnership" and uses simple language to help consumers to understand their rights (AHA, 2008). The latest document (2008), which is offered in multiple languages, emphasizes a collaborative approach to patient care in which the patients' responsibilities are explicit. In return, patients may expect a certain level of care delivery. This statement is entitled The Patient Care Partnership: Understanding Expectations, Rights, and Responsibilities and may be obtained from the American Hospital Association's *A Patient's Bill of Rights* (AHA, 2008) or at http://www.aha.org/advocacy-issues/communicatingpts/pt-care-partnership.shtml.

Today, nurses are much more cognizant of the rights of patients, including those rights not enumerated on the various published documents (Milton, 2008). For example, the patient has the right to be cared for in a facility that ensures the safety rights of the patients. Observing and enforcing these patient rights prevents possible lawsuits. In this regard, nurses serve as patients' advocates by defending their legal and ethical rights.

Nursing has identified three models of advocacy that are employed in clinical practice settings. In the *rights protection model,* which is perhaps the best known model of advocacy, nurses assist patients in asserting their autonomy rights; for example, a nurse might help an individual patient successfully convince health care providers that he does not desire surgical intervention for coronary artery disease, but will comply with medical management. The third principle in the ANA's Code of Ethics (2008) reinforces this mandate: "The nurse promotes, advocates for, and strives to protect the health, safety, and rights of the patient."

A second approach to advocacy is the *values-based decision* model. Using this approach, the nurse assists the patient by discussing her needs and desires and helps the patient make choices that are most consistent with the patient's values, lifestyle, and desires. This model is predicated on sharing information and assisting the individual to become empowered to speak on her own behalf. Using this approach, the nurse assists the patient to exert her right to autonomy and self-determination.

The third model is the *respect for persons* model, which is sometimes known as the patient-advocate model. This approach centers on the inherent human dignity that is deserving of respect. In this model, the nurse acts to protect the rights, dignity, and choices of the patient. If the patient cannot assist in making decisions about his care and treatments, the nurse advocates for the patient's best interests. The ultimate goal of this model is to promote the autonomy and individual uniqueness of the patient (Milton, 2008).

Defenses Against Torts

In the event that a legal claim or lawsuit is filed, nurses and other health care providers can use certain legal defenses to negate liability. *Defenses* are arguments in support of or arguments used for justification. Defenses may be based on statutory law, common law, or the doctrine of precedent, in which decisions are left to stand based on prior decisions made by a court (Lewenson & Truglio-Londrigan, 2008). Defenses also can be classified by the type of cause of action, or tort, filed against the health care personnel: intentional, quasi-intentional, or nonintentional.

Defenses Against Intentional Torts

Defenses against intentional torts are most commonly consent, self-defense, defense of others, and necessity. Consent, as previously discussed, may be oral, implied by law, or expressed. Self-defense and defense of others may be justifiable to protect oneself and others from harm: for example, in the case of a combative patient. Defense of others can be extended to include the patient as well. The overriding caveat is that a nurse can only use reasonable force—that which is necessary to defend herself or others from injury. Necessity allows the nurse to interfere with the patient's property rights to avoid threatened injury: for example, an attack with a knife. The two overriding caveats in this situation are that a defense of necessity (1) does not allow the nurse the right to search the patient's property and (2) stipulates that the patient's property must be the threatening factor (Lewenson & Truglio-Londrigan, 2008).

Defenses Against Quasi-Intentional Torts

The primary defenses against quasi-intentional torts are consent, truth, privilege, qualified privilege, and disclosure statutes. Consent may be a defense against the quasi-intentional torts of defamation and invasion of privacy, as well as a defense against the intentional torts. Truth is a valid defense against defamatory statements; however, nurses should be aware that in using this defense, the entire statement must be true, not merely parts of the statement (Lansimies-Antikainen et al., 2009).

Privilege is a disclosure that might otherwise be considered defamatory under different circumstances; however, such disclosure may be allowable to protect or further private or public interests recognized by law. An example of such would be the legal mandate to report persons with certain diagnoses or diseases or those suspected of abusing others. Qualified privilege prevails when the person making the allegedly defamatory statements has a legal duty to do so, as in the case of a manager reporting the professional performance of an employee. Qualified privilege legally negates any inference of malice because of the overriding public policy interest (Lansimies-Antikainen et al., 2009). When the quality of medical care is at issue, the reputation rights of health care professionals may concede to the greater social need. Liability will not be imposed, even if the communications are false, as long as there is no malice and the communications are made in good faith to those persons who need to know such facts. Three caveats of qualified privilege need to be observed: First, the communication must be made through appropriate channels to persons needing the information; second, liability may be granted for untruthful communications released with malice: and third, the communications should be worded in objective and observable behavioral terms rather than judgmental descriptions.

Both federal and state laws require the reporting of certain types of health-related information to protect the public at large (Gold et al., 2009). These laws are referred to as disclosure statutes. These statutes require that health care providers submit certain information to the proper agency. The most common example of reporting statutes is vital statistics. All states require births and deaths to be reported, and a majority of states require an accounting of neonatal deaths and abortions. Public health agencies may require a variety of disease states to be reported: for example, communicable and venereal disease must be reported to protect the public. In addition, some states require that patients suffering any type of seizure disorder be reported to the state driver's licensing agency. Also, cancer and other related diseases are to be reported in some states. If providers disclose only the limited information they are required to disclose by law, there is no liability for the disclosure under either a defamation or invasion of privacy lawsuit. Thus, the statutes serve as a defense against both defamation and invasion of privacy (Yakov, Shilo, & Shor, 2010).

Defenses Against Nonintentional Torts

Defenses against nonintentional torts or negligent actions include release, contributory or comparative negligence, assumption of the risk, unavoidable accident, defense of the fact, and immunity statutes. A release may be signed during the process of settling a claim to prevent any and all future claims arising from the same incident. Once signed, the release bars future suits. In medical malpractice claims, a release is frequently a part of the "out-of-court" settlement. Effectively, the plaintiff states that the agreed-upon settlement is the only compensation for the negligent action. Contributory and comparative negligence serve as defenses and, in essence, hold injured parties accountable for their part in the injury. Contributory or comparative negligence may be found if, for example, the patient failed to follow prescribed treatments or if incorrect treatment was given based on the patient providing false information to the physician. Similarly, the assumption of risk defense states that plaintiffs are partially responsible for consequences if they understood the risk involved when they proceeded with the action (Yakov et al., 2010).

The defense of unavoidable accident comes into play when nothing other than an accident could have caused the person's injury. An unavoidable accident is an inevitable occurrence that cannot be foreseen or prevented by vigilance, care, and attention and not occasioned by or contributed to in any manner by an act or omission of the party claiming the accident was unavoidable (Dawson, 2007; Starr, 2010). The defense of the fact is used when there is no indication, direct or otherwise, that the health care provider's actions were the cause of the patient's injury or untoward outcome (e.g., the patient who receives an injection in his right arm and then begins to experience numbness and tingling in his left leg). There is no connection between the two events; thus, the defense is a defense of fact.

Immunity

Some states have enacted immunity statutes that serve to dismiss certain causes of action. A good example of a state immunity statute is the Good Samaritan statute. Good Samaritan laws are enacted to allow health care personnel and citizens who are trained in first aid to deliver needed medical care in an emergency without unnecessary fear of incurring criminal and civil liability (Figure 2–2◆). Because of these laws, negligent actions against health care providers at scenes of accidents are rare (Time, Payne, & Gainey, 2010). Most states require that the care be given in good faith and that it be gratuitous. Guidelines that govern the interpretation of Good Samaritan laws are shown in Chart 2–10.

Critical Thinking, Decision Making, and Clinical Judgment

Nurses in today's professional world must do more than merely understand legal, ethical, and regulatory concepts. Nurses must blend

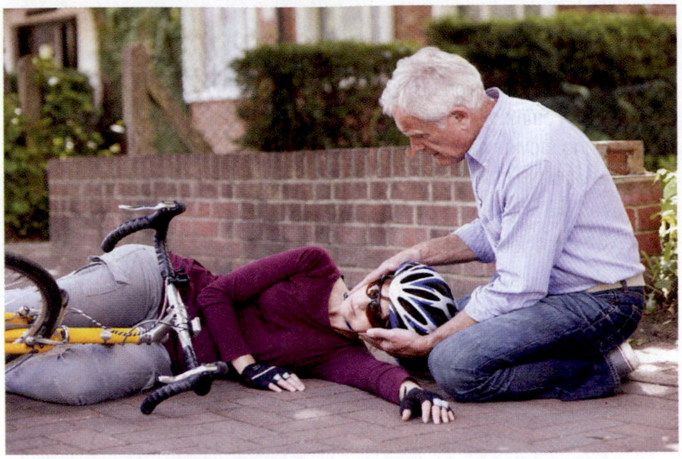

FIGURE 2–2 ◆ Good Samaritan laws allow health care personnel to aid emergency victims without unnecessary fear of liability.
Source: Science Photo Library/SuperStock

these important aspects with competent, skilled nursing diagnoses and interventions. To perform such high-quality nursing care, nurses must understand the concepts of critical thinking and clinical judgment, for without these concepts they are not able to fully appreciate the application of legal, ethical, and regulatory concepts in professional practice settings. For this reason, the concepts of critical thinking, decision making, and clinical judgment are discussed in depth in Chapters 1 and 5. National guidelines that may be used to assist nurses with making legal, ethical, and regulatory decisions are shown in the National Guidelines box. Research possibilities for ethics and legal concepts are suggested in the Research Opportunities and Clinical Impact box.

Summary

It is evident from a historical and current perspective that the types and availability of health care delivery systems are dependent on social and economic factors. Health care delivery systems and health care professionals also are subject to perform according to existing regulatory practices, ethical principles, and legal interpretations. As the health care reform initiative moves forward, consumers/patients, though vulnerable to these influences and practices, are in a position to influence, dictate, and determine how the future of health care should be delivered. The new consumer-driven health care model that is emerging focuses on the quality of services as well as their costs. In developing new models of health care delivery, nurses will play a key role in determining how the future evolution of health care will meet the needs of a changing society.

NATIONAL GUIDELINES for Interpretation of Ethical and Legal Issues

- American Hospital Association *A Patient's Bill of Rights* (1992)
- American Medical Association statement of informed consent (2007)
- American Nurses Association Code of Ethics (2008)
- American Nurses Association Nursing Practice Standards (2010)
- Health Insurance Portability and Accountability Act (HIPAA) (1996)
- Joint Commission *Accreditation Manual for Hospitals* (2012)

CHART 2–10 Good Samaritan Laws

1. Make your decision quickly as to whether you will stay and help. There is no common law duty to stop and render aid; however, once you begin to provide care, you incur the legal duty to maintain a standard of reasonable emergency care.
2. Ask the injured person or family members for permission to help. Do not force your services once refused.
3. Care for the injured party where you can do so safely, in the vehicle or at the exact site where the injured person is found. Only move the injured party if you must do so without causing further harm and as needed to prevent further harm.
4. Apply the rules of first aid. Assess for and prevent major bleeding, assess for the need to initiate cardiopulmonary resuscitation, cover the injured party with a blanket or coat, and so forth.
5. Assess and reassess the person continuously for additional injuries, and communicate findings of your assessment to the injured person and family.
6. Have someone call or go for additional help while you stay with the injured person.
7. Stay with the injured person until equally or more qualified help arrives. Prevent unskilled persons from treating or moving the injured party.
8. Provide the police or emergency medical personnel with as complete a description as possible of the care that you have rendered so that continuity of care exists. Give family members or police any personal items such as dentures, eyeglasses, and the like.
9. Do not accept any compensation of any kind offered by the injured party or family members as this may change your status into a fee-for-service situation and cause you to lose your Good Samaritan protection.
10. Should you choose not to stop and render aid, stop at the nearest phone and report the accident to proper authorities so that the injured party may be aided.

Sources: Guido, G. (2010). *Legal and ethical issues in nursing* (5th ed.). Upper Saddle River, NJ: Prentice Hall. Starr, L. (2009).Attending to those in need: Duty to care or free to go? *Australian Nursing Journal, 17*(6), 32. Time, V., Payne, B. K., & Gainey, R. R. (2010). Don't help the victims of crime if you don't have the time: Assessing support for the Good Samaritan laws. *Journal of Criminal Justice, 38*, 790–795.

RESEARCH OPPORTUNITIES Related to Professional Concepts

Research Opportunity	Clinical Impact
Ethical Concepts	
Means by which nurses make ethical decisions.	Improve the knowledge base of nurses concerning ethical principles so that they can make more effective ethical decisions in clinical practice settings.
Identification of ethical dilemmas by nurses in clinical practice settings.	
Knowledge base of nurses regarding ethical principles.	Explore why nurses are not on ethics committees and the vital need to include nurses in this aspect of patient care.
Involvement of nurses in institutional ethics committees.	
Legal Concepts	
Knowledge base of practicing nurses regarding legal issues.	Understand the extent of lawsuits filed against nurses, the causes of actions in the filed lawsuits, and the legal knowledge of practicing and student nurses to hopefully prevent further lawsuits.
Numbers of malpractice lawsuits in which nurses are named as defendants.	
Numbers of legal courses in schools of nursing.	
Critical Thinking, Decision Making, and Clinical Judgment	
Descriptive and qualitative studies on how nurses make decisions and their critical thinking abilities.	Improve nurses' decision-making and critical thinking skills with the goal of improving patient outcomes.
Use of critical/clinical pathways and clinical judgment in multiple clinical practice settings.	Determine the effectiveness of critical/clinical pathways currently being used and the need for modifications, as applicable.
Patient outcome studies to determine the effectiveness of critical/clinical pathways.	

NCLEX® PRACTICE

1. A nurse is planning the care for a patient using the best practice approach. Which of the following best describes this approach?
   1. It integrates current research evidence with clinical expertise and patient's needs.
   2. It is a proven process that produces consistent high-quality results.
   3. It offers qualitative or quantitative measurement of specific data related to reported outcome information.
   4. It focuses on collecting data about medical errors and setting standards that will reduce errors.
2. When reviewing information about a patient to be admitted the nurse finds little information except that the patient is a Medicare recipient. This information tells the nurse that the patient may be: (select all that apply):
   1. a federal employee
   2. disabled
   3. a veteran
   4. over 65 years old
   5. an end stage renal disease patient

3. Individuals from an accrediting body arrive at a health care organization with the intent of following a patient throughout the hospital admission and evaluate policies and all service encounters. The accrediting body is most likely:
   1. OSHA.
   2. The Joint Commission.
   3. the CDC.
   4. the state board of nursing.
4. A patient tells the nurse that he has a paper that says his wife is supposed to make decisions about his health care if he becomes unable to do so himself. This patient is describing a(n):
   1. living will.
   2. oral advance directive.
   3. health care power of attorney.
   4. written advance directive.
5. During the course of one day, a nurse will support one patient's decision to not receive a particular medication, suggest family members of another patient go home to get rest, promise one patient that the injection will only pinch for a second, and will spend equal amounts of time with each patient on her assignment. Which ethical theory is this nurse demonstrating?
   1. Deontology
   2. Principlism
   3. Rule utilitarianism
   4. Act utilitarianism
6. The hospital ethics committee is currently applying ethical principles to all of the options available to them to address an ethical dilemma. The nurse is aware that the committee is functioning in a stage of the MORAL model. Which stage is the committee in?
   1. Identify issues
   2. Resolve
   3. Options
   4. Evaluate

Answers to NCLEX Practice questions can be found in Appendix D in the Osborn Student Resources at nursing.pearsonhighered.com. Practice additional NCLEX questions online at the Student Resources site.

Pearson Nursing Student Resources Find additional review materials at: **nursing.pearsonhighered.com**

REFERENCES

Ablah, E., Konda, K. S., Konda, K., Melbourne, M., Ingoglia, J. N., & Gebbie, K. M. (2010). Emergency preparedness training and response among community health centers and local health departments: Results from a multi-state survey. *Journal of Community Health, 35*, 285–293.

American Academy of Nursing. (2010). Implementing health care reform: Issues for nursing. Retrieved from http://www.aannet.org/i4a/pages/index.cfm?pageid=4455

American Association of Colleges of Nursing AACN–QSEN Education Committee. (2009). About QSEN education consortium. Retrieved from http://www.aacn.nche.edu/qsenec/overview.html

American Hospital Association. (1992). *A patient's bill of rights.* Chicago, IL: Author.

American Hospital Association. (2006). Healthcare consumer research. Retrieved from http://www.aha.org

American Hospital Association. (2007). *Guide to the health care field—2007 edition* (page A3). Chicago, IL: Author.

American Hospital Association. (2008). The patient care partnership: Understanding expectations, rights, and responsibilities. Retrieved from http://www.aha.org/aha/issues/Communicating-With-Patients/pt-care-partnership.html

American Hospital Association. (2011). Hospital value-based purchasing program: the final rule. Regulatory Advisory. American Hospital Association. Retrieved from http://www.americangovernance.com/americangovernance/webinar/policy/pdf/final_rule_vbp_regulatory_advisory.pdf

American Hospital Association. (2012). Fast facts on US Hospitals. *Health Forum LLC.* Retrieved from http://www.aha.org/reserach/rc/stat-studies/fast-facts.shtml

American Medical Association. (2007). Informed consent. *AMA Legal Issues.* Retrieved from http://www.ama-assn.org/ama/pub/category/print/4608.html

American Medical Association. (2010). Resources/standards, policy statement on provision of life-sustaining medical treatment. Retrieved from http://www.ama-assn.org

American Nurses Association. (2008). *Code of ethics with interpretive statements.* Silver Spring, MD: Author.

American Nurses Association. (2010). *Scope and standards of practice – Nursing* (2nd ed.). Silver Spring, Maryland, American Nurses Association.

Bailey, E. (2008). Types of health insurance. Retrieved from http://eileen-bailey.suite101.com/types-of-health-insurance3-a40494

Buser, M. (2010). Hospitalist programs in the age of healthcare reform. *Journal of Healthcare Management, 55*(6). Retrieved from www.todayshospitalist.com/index.php?b=articles_read&cnt=1233

Caplan, D. (2008). Management accounting: Concepts and techniques. Oregon State University. Retrieved from http://classes.bus.oregonstate.edu/spring07/ba422/Management%20Accounting%20Chapter%205.htm

Centers for Disease Control and Prevention. (2010). Occupational sentinel health events. Retrieved from http://www.cdc.gov/niosh/topics/SHEO/

Centers for Medicare and Medicaid Services. (2007). Brief summaries of Medicare, Medicaid, Title XVIII and Title XIX of the Social Security Act as of November 1, 2007. Retrieved from http://search.cms.hhs.gov/search?q+Ependitures+2002+reference&site=cms_collection&...

Centers for Medicare & Medicaid Services. (2012). Acute care hospital inpatient prospective payment system. Department of Health and Human Services. The Medicare Learning Network. Retrieved from http://www.cms.gov/MLNGeninfo

Chicago Tribune Editors. (2009). How does your hospital check out? Online "report cards" let you compare costs, quality ratings and a whole lot more. *Chicago Tribune.*

Code of Federal Regulations, Sections 160.102 and 160.103. (1996). General administrative requirements. Retrieved from http://www.hhs.gov/OCR/regtext.html

Cohen M. J., McCannon, J.B., Edgman-Levitan, S., & Kormos, W.A. (2010). Exploring attitudes toward advance care directives in two diverse settings. *Journal of Palliative Medicine, 13*(12), 1427–1432.

Crisham, N. (1990). Living wills: Controversy and certainty. *Journal of Professional Nursing, 6*(6), 321.

Crowenwett, L., Sherwood, G., & Gelmon, S. B. (2009). Improving quality and safety education: The QSEN learning collaborative. *Nursing Outlook, 57*(6), 304–312.

Cueto, S. A. (2010). International basics: What's the difference between common law and civil law? *International Business Law Advisor.* Retrieved from http://www.internationalbusinesslawadvisor.com/2010/05/articles/international-litigation/international-basics-whats-the-difference-between-common-law-and-civil-law/

Dawson, J. (2007). Negligence oversimplified. University of Vermont website. Retrieved from http://asci.uvm.edu/equine/law/articles/neg12.htm

DeWolf-Bosek, M. S., & Savage, T. A. (2007). *The ethical component of nursing education.* Philadelphia: Lippincott Williams & Wilkins.

Donabedian, A. (1980). *Explanations in quality assessment and monitoring: The definition of quality and approaches to its assessment* (Vol. 1). Ann Arbor, MI: Health Administration Press.

Ekeland, A. G., Bowes, A., & Flottorp, S. (2010). Effectiveness of telemedicine: A systematic review of reviews. *International Journal of Medical Informatics, 79*, 736–771.

Fowler, M. D. (2008). *Guide to the code of ethics for nurses.* American Nurses Association. Silver Spring, Maryland.

Federal Register. (2010). Medicare and Medicaid programs; hospital conditions of participation: Quality assessment and performance improvement final rule. *Federal Register, 68*(16), 3435–3455.

Gold, M., Phillip, J., McIver, S., & Komesaroff, P. A. (2009). Between a rock and a hard place: Exploring the conflict between respecting the privacy of patients and informing their caregivers. *Internal Medicine Journal, 39*, 582–587.

Guido, G. (2010). *Legal and ethical issues in nursing* (5th ed.). Upper Saddle River, NJ: Prentice Hall.

Hader, A. L., & Brown, E. D. (2010). Patient privacy and social media. *AANA Journal, 78*(4), 270–274.

Health First. (2010). What are not-for-profit/community-minded hospitals? Retrieved from http://www.health-first.org/about_us/not_for_profit.cfm

Health Resources and Services Administration. (2010). What is behind HRSA's projected supply, demand, and shortage of registered nurses? Retrieved from http://hrsa.gov

Highbeam Business. (2012). Specialty outpatient facilities, NEC. The Gale Group, Inc. Retrieved from http://business.highbeam.com/industry-reports/business/specialty-outpatient-facilities-not-elsewhere-classified

Huber, D. (2010). *Leadership and nursing care management* (4th ed.). Philadelphia: W. B. Saunders. Retrieved from http://www.ornl.gov

Institute of Medicine/Robert Wood Johnson Grant. (2010). The future of nursing: Leading change, advancing health consensus report. Retrieved from http://www.iom.edu/Reports/2010/The-Future-of-Nursing-Leading-Change-Advancing-Health.aspx

Institute of Medicine. (2007). *Preventing medication errors.* Washington, DC: National Academy Press.

Institute of Medicine. (2011). The future of nursing: Focus on education. Retrieved from http://iom.edu/Reports/2010/The-Future-of-Nursing-Leading-Change-Advancing-Health/Report-Brief-Education.aspx?page=2

Izumi, S. (2010). Ethical practice in end-of-life care in Japan. *Nursing Ethics, 17*(4), 457–468.

Jarrin, O. F. (2010). Core elements of U.S. nurse practice acts and incorporation of nursing diagnosis language. *International Journal of Nursing Terminologies and Classifications, 21*(4), 166–176.

Jayaraman, S., Davies, W., & Schlachta, C. M. (2009). Getting started with robotics in general surgery with cholecystectomy: The Canadian experience. *Canadian Journal of Surgery, 52*(5), 374–378.

Joint Commission on Accreditation of Healthcare Organizations. (2007). *Setting the standard.* Oakbrook Terrace, IL: Author.

Jweinat, J. J. (2010). Hospital readmissions under the spotlight. *Journal of Healthcare Management, 55*(4), 252–264.

Kerr, P. (2009). Protecting patient information in an electronic age: A sacred trust. *Urologic Nursing, 29*(5), 315–319.

Kotzer, A. M., & Arellana, K. (2008). Defining an evidence-based work environment for nursing. *Journal of Clinical Nursing, 17*(12), 1652–1659.

Kurban, N. K., Savas, H., Cetinkaya, B., Turan, T., & Kartal, A. (2010). Evaluation of nursing students' training in medical law. *Nursing Ethics, 17*(6), 759–768.

Lachman, V. D. (2009). Practical use of the nursing code of ethics: Part II. *MEDSURG Nursing, 18*(3), 191–194.

Lansimies-Antikainen, H., Laitinen, T., Rauramaa, R., & Pietila, A. (2009). Evaluation of informed consent in health research: A questionnaire survey. *Scandinavian Journal of Caring Sciences, 24*, 56–64.

Lewenson, S. B., & Truglio-Londrigan, M. (2008). *Decision-making in nursing.* Massachusetts: Jones and Bartlett.

Lukose, A. (2011). Developing a practice model for Watson's theory of caring. *Nursing Science Quarterly, 240*, 27–30.

Manos, D. (2010). Hospitals look to revive capital expenditures. *Healthcare Finance News.* Retrieved from http://www.healthcarefinancenews.com/news/hospitals-look-revive-capital-expenditures-according-premier

Marquis, B. L., & Huston, C. J. (2011). *Leadership roles and management functions in nursing theory & application* (7th ed.). Philadelphia: Lippincott Williams & Wilkins.

Medical-Dictionary. (2010). Retrieved from http://medical-dictionary.thefreedictionary.com/Hill-Burton+Act"> Hill-Burton Act

Mosby's Medical Dictionary, 8th ed. (2009). Accreditation. *Elsevier.* Retrieved from http://medical-dictionary.thefreedictionary.comaccreditation

Medline Plus. (2010). Advance directives. Retrieved from http://www.nlm.nih.gov/medlineplus/advancedirectives.html

Milton, C. L. (2008). Reflecting on ethical codes and professional standards of nursing practice from a global perspective. *Nursing Science Quarterly, 21*(4), 300–303.

National Committee for Quality Assurance. (2006). Measurement improves healthcare quality for 70 million Americans, but gaps remain. Retrieved from http://ncqa.org

National Human Genome Research Institute. (2008). International consortium announces the 1000 Genomes Project. *National Institutes of Health Services NIH News.* Retrieved from http://www.genome.gov/26524516

National League for Nursing. (1959). *Patients' rights.* New York: Author.

National Quality Forum. (2010). Health care quality measurement and reporting. Retrieved from http://www.qualityforum.org

National Committee for Quality Assurance (NCQA). (2011). HEDIS 2010. Retrieved from http://www.ncqa.org/tabid/1044/Default.aspx

Neamatullah, I., Douglass, M. M., Lehman, L. H., Reisner, A., Villarroel, M., Long, W. J., et al. (2008). Automated de-identification of free-text medical records. *BMC Medical Informatics and Decision Making, 8*(32), 1–17.

NCQA. (October 2010). News release. Retrieved from http://www.ncqa.org/tabid/1259/Default.aspx

Negligence. (2007). *The Columbia electronic encyclopedia* (6th ed.). New York: Columbia University Press.

Omansky, G. L. (2010). Staff nurses' experiences as preceptors and mentors: An integrative review. *Journal of Nursing Management, 18*, 697–703.

Osborn, M., Day, R., Komesaroff, P., & Mant, A. (2009). Do ethical guidelines make a difference to decision-making? *Internal Medicine Journal, 39*, 800–805.

OSHA. (2011). Safety and health regulations and guidelines. Retrieved from http://www.osha.gov/pls/oshaweb/owadisp.show_document?p_table=NEWS_RELEASES&p_id=19533

Paasche-Orlow, M. K., Jacob, D. M., Hochhauser, M., & Parker, R. M. (2009). *Journal of General Internal Medicine, 24*(4), 489–494.

Park, M. (2009). The legal basis of nursing ethics education. *Journal of Nursing Law, 13*(4), 106–111.

QSEN—Quality & Safety Education for Nurses. (2012). Competency KSAs (pre-licensure). Retrieved from http://www.qsen.org/ksas_prelicensure.php

Quaghebeur, T., Casterle, B. D., & Gastmans, C. (2009). Nursing and euthanasia: A review of argument-based ethics literature. *Nursing Ethics, 16*(4), 466–486.

Resnick, H.E., Hickman, S., & Foster, G.L. (2012). Documentation of advance directives among home health and hospice patients: United States, 2007. *American Journal of Hospice Palliative Care, 29*(1), 26–35.

Responsible Nurse. (2010). Retrieved from responsiblenurse@officeliveusers.com

Riley, G. F. (2008). Trends in out-of-pocket healthcare costs among older community-dwelling Medicare beneficiaries. *American Journal of Managed Care, 14*(10), 692–696.

Robinson, J. C. (2010). Applying value-based insurance design to high-cost health services. *Health Affairs, 29*(11), 2009–2016.

Rosen, B., Porath, A., Pawlson, L. G., Chassin, M. R., & Benbassat, J. (2011). Adherence to standards of care by health maintenance organizations in Israel and the USA. *International Journal for Quality in Healthcare, 23*(1), 15–25.

Sabol v. Richmond Heights General Hospital, 676 N.E.2nd 958 (Ohio App. 1996).

Salas, A. S., & Cameron, B. L. (2010). Ethical openings in palliative home care practice. *Nursing Ethics, 17*(5), 655–665.

Smith, K. L., Soriano, T. A., & Boal, J. (2007). Brief communication: National quality of care standards in home-based primary care. *Annals of Internal Medicine, 146*, 188–192.

Stanford Encyclopedia of Philosophy. (2010). Multiple legal references. Retrieved from http://plato.stanford.edu/entries/tort-theories/

Starr, L. (2009). Attending to those in need: Duty to care or free to go? *Australian Nursing Journal, 17*(6), 32.

Tchartchian, G., Dietzel, J., Bojahr, B., Hackethal, A., & De Wilde, R. (2011). Decreasing strain on the surgeon in gynecologic minimally invasive surgery by using semi-active robotics. *International Journal of Gynecology and Obstetrics, 112*, 72–75.

The Joint Commission. (2012). 2012 Joint Commission national patient safety goals. Retrieved from http://www.spectrumhealth.com/shr_providers/education/SHR_Ed/2012_JointCommission.pdf

The Leapfrog Group. (2010). Leapfrog group report on CPOE evaluation tool results June 2008 to January 2010. Retrieved from www.lealpfroggroup.org

Thiroux, J. (1977). *Ethics: Theory and practice.* Philadelphia: Macmillan.

Time, V., Payne, B. K., & Gainey, R. R. (2010). Don't help victims of crime if you don't have the time: Assessing support for the Good Samaritan laws. *Journal of Criminal Justice, 38*, 790–795.

Tishler, C. L., & Staats, N. (2009). Inpatient suicide: Preventing a common sentinel event. *General Hospital Psychiatry, 31*, 103–109.

University Health System Consortium. (2012). UHC/AACN nurse residency program TM. Retrieved from http://www.uhc.edu/16807.htm

U.S. Census Bureau updates. (2011). The 2011 statistical abstract. Retrieved from http://www.census.gov/prod/2011pubs/11statab/pop.pdf

U.S. Department of Health and Human Services. (2006). Medical privacy—National standards to protect the privacy of personal health information. Retrieved from http://www.hhs.gov

US Legal. (2010). Legal terms. Retrieved from http://definitions.uslegal.com/n/nursing

Vesely, R. (2011). California hospitals face worker shortage: Survey. Modern Healthcare.com. Retrieved from http://www.modernhealthcare.com/article/20110209/NEWS/302099962#ixzz1Ihsud5R8

Von Dras, D. D., Flittner, D., Malcore, S. A., & Pouliot, G. (2009). Workplace stress and ethical challenges experienced by nursing staff in a nursing home. *Educational Gerontology, 35*, 321–339.

Wakeman, D. R., Dodiya, H. B., & Kordower, J. H. (2011). Cell transplantation and gene therapy in Parkinson's disease. *Mount Sinai Journal of Medicine, 78*, 126–158. doi: 10.1002/msj.20233

Wells, S., Whittaker, R., Dorey, E., & Bullen, C. (2010). Harnessing health IT for improved cardiovascular risk management. *PLoS Medicine, 7*(8), 1–4.

Yakov, G., Shilo, Y., & Shor, T. (2010). Nurses' perceptions of ethical issues related to patients' rights law. *Nursing Ethics, 17*(4), 501–510.

CHAPTER 3

Research Foundations for Nursing Practice

Cynthia Parkman
Annita Watson

Outcome-Based Learning Objectives

After studying this chapter, the learner will be able to:

1. Differentiate between basic and applied research.
2. Describe the first step of the research process and its relevance to the selection of the research design.
3. Differentiate between research utilization and evidence-based practice.
4. Plan a research study using the three ethical principles that guide nursing practice.
5. Determine the impact of HIPAA on nursing research studies.
6. Distinguish between the stages of completing a quantitative research critique versus a qualitative research critique.

KEY TERMS

analytical preciseness p.72
applied research p.57
auditability p.72
basic research p.57
convenience sampling p.72
correlational research design p.60
data saturation p.63
descriptive research design p.60
descriptive vividness p.62
ethnography p.61
evidence-based practice (EBP) p.64
experimental research design p.60
grounded theory p.61
heuristic relevance p.72
hypothesis p.60
informatics p.71
literature review p.59
methodological congruence p.72
network sampling p.62
nonexperimental research design p.60
nonprobability sampling p.62
phenomenology p.61
pilot study p.62
population p.62
power analysis p.63
probability sampling p.62
purposive sampling p.62
qualitative research p.57
quantitative research p.57
quasi-experimental research design p.60
quota sampling p.62
random assignment p.63
reliability p.75
research p.56
research critique p.71
research design p.60
research problem p.59
research process p.57
research purpose p.59
research question p.59
research utilization (RU) p.64
sample p.62
sampling p.62
selection (sampling) bias p.62
setting p.62
simple random sampling p.62
statistical significance p.63
stratified random sampling p.63
theoretical connectedness p.72
variables p.60
validity p.75

RESEARCH IS a formal, systematic, and organized method used to answer a question or solve a problem. This systematic inquiry provides a forum to facilitate the ongoing process of questioning and evaluating practice, informing practice based on available data, and guiding the development of new practices through experimental learning. **Research** is essential for defining the nursing profession, determining best practices, and advancing the science of nursing practice. The 2010 Institute of Medicine (IOM)/Robert Wood Johnson Foundation (RWJF) Initiative on the Future of Nursing provides impetus for changing health and nursing practice. Nursing research, independently as a profession and collaboratively with others, provides a means by which to improve patient care, nationally and globally (IOM, 2011). This chapter focuses on the process and outcomes of research and the manner in which it is used by nurses to promote clinical practice. Specific examples of research intended to change and improve medical–surgical nursing practice are discussed in the specific disorder chapters within the text.

Nursing Research

Nursing research is similar to research conducted by other professional groups or disciplines in that the same rigorous steps must be followed, and the research design and method of investigation must be appropriate to the problem or question being studied. It is, however, suggested that nursing research is distinguished by the diversity of the human experience (Burns & Grove, 2009; Polit & Beck, 2012). In comparison to other fields, nursing practice requires greater flexibility in defining and interpreting research in order to provide for the variations that occur across professional practice settings. This has become particularly evident as globalization of the world community has highlighted the differences in nursing practice and contexts across countries.

Defining nursing research requires determining how the research will be relevant to nursing. Since Florence Nightingale's era, nurses have expanded their professional practice foundation through research efforts designed to develop and test knowledge. In 1976, the American Nurses Association (ANA) adopted the following definition, which remains broad enough today to encompass globalization of the world community:

> Nursing research is investigation into the area of knowledge in which the physical and behavioral sciences meet and influence one another in an effort to study how health problems relate to human behavior and how behavior relates to health and illness. It addresses the human and behavioral questions that arise in the treatment of disease, in the prevention of illness, and in the promotion and maintenance of health. (ANA, 1976, p. 1)

Nursing research also may be viewed as research into phenomena that are predominantly and appropriately the responsibility of nurses in their professional practice. Nurses are responsible for provision of patient care, administration of nursing and health care services, and education of practitioners. Therefore, research in nursing encompasses systematic inquiry into each of these areas. With this interpretation, nursing research not only adds to the knowledge base of nursing, it also influences changes for patients, their futures, and their environments. Nursing research also impacts the health care delivery system and related costs of health care.

A large portion of nursing knowledge is not generated through research. Nurses typically draw on knowledge from a variety of sources, each offering something unique to holistic nursing practice. These include tradition, authority, trial and error, personal clinical experience, intuition, logical reasoning, medical information, assembled information such as benchmarking, and disciplined research. However, nurses can no longer rely on the assumptions that come only from experience and trial and error. Information that is supported by data is critical to improving the clinical care provided to patients. The difficulty with knowledge that is not supported by a research base is that it has limited scientific predictability and cannot be used to justify nursing actions or provide new scientific information to direct practice.

Evidence from research must be applied to nurses' practices to assure patients that they have the best knowledge available for safe and compassionate care. In addition, research findings must be shared with others in the profession in order to broaden the current knowledge base that is available to all nurses. Increased knowledge provides opportunities to solve problems in different ways, to challenge the status quo of why practice is performed in a certain way, and to understand phenomena that occur in the professional sphere. In this era of rapid change, it is critical for research to be used as a tool to provide caring, compassionate, and scientific care.

Research Approaches

The general purpose of nursing research is to answer questions or solve problems relevant to the nursing profession. In terms of the intent of the research, a distinction is made between basic and applied research. **Basic research** is traditionally undertaken to extend the knowledge base in a discipline or to formulate or refine a theory. **Applied research** focuses on finding solutions to existing problems, such as studying the effectiveness of a nursing intervention to ease pain. Practicing nurses are more likely to be involved in applied research, which is the focus of this chapter.

Research typically takes one of two methological forms: quantitative or qualitative. **Quantitative research** is the investigation of phenomena that lend themselves to precise measurement and quantification (Polit & Beck, 2012). This often involves a rigorous and controlled research design. Control involves imposing conditions on the research situation so that biases are minimized and precision and validity are maximized. Quantitative research collects data by questionnaires, inventories, and measurements. **Qualitative research** is the investigation of phenomena through the collection of narrative materials using a flexible research design (Polit & Beck, 2012). Qualitative research often involves interviews, observations, and notations of behavior.

"The general purpose of nursing research is to answer questions or solve problems of relevance to nursing" (Polit & Beck, 2012, p. 16). The specific purposes of nursing research include identification, description, exploration, explanation, prediction, and control (Polit & Beck, 2012). *Identification* refers to clearly identifying the phenomenon to be studied. In quantitative research, researchers begin with a phenomenon that has been previously studied or defined, sometimes in a qualitative study (Polit & Beck, 2012). In contrast, with qualitatative research the phenomenon has yet to be clearly identified or named, or has been inadequately defined. *Description* identifies or describes the phenomenon being studied. With quantitative research, description focuses on the incidence, size, and measurable attributes of the phenomenon; in qualitative research, however, the investigators describe the dimensions, meanings, and importance of the phenomenon. *Exploration* indicates that the phenomenon is being fully explored, notes how it is being manifested, and identifies other factors to which it is related. *Prediction* refers to the ability to predict the outcomes of the research study, and *control* implies that in some instances the outcomes of the study can be controlled. In many quantitative studies, prediction and control are key objectives. These studies are critical in helping clinicians make decisions.

Although this chapter highlights the current status of research in nursing, particularly in relationship to evidence-based practice, it is necessary for nurses to understand the research process before participating in it. A description of the research process, the conditions under which research is conducted, and the types of research typically used by nurses and other health care professionals provides the foundation for the discussion of research utilization and evidence-based practice.

The Research Process

The **research process** is very similar to the nursing process in that it proceeds through discrete, unconnected, linear steps in order to answer a question. In some studies the steps overlap, and in others certain steps are unnecessary; however, a general flow of activities in a leaner fashion is typical in a quantitative study. Nurses perform similar activities every day when they engage in critical thinking, reflect on their practice, and apply the nursing process. For example, nurses engage in data collection about patients when they read the patient's medical record; receive reports; and engage in dialogue with colleagues, the patient, and the family. Based on this information and observations, the nurse formulates a diagnosis of the patient's health need and identifies objectives for care. This stage is similar to Phase 1 of the research process, identifying researchable phenomenon and generating a purpose for the research study. This phase contains several steps, as do all of the phases of the research process. Next, the nurse develops a plan of care specific to the patient's identified needs; the plan is based on assisting the patient to achieve objectives/desired outcomes with the expectation that specific nursing actions will produce desired patient results. This step is similar to Phase 2 (the Design and Planning Phase) of the research process, which includes the steps of selecting a research design, developing protocols for the intervention, identifying the population to be studied, and developing the sampling process. Phase 2 of the research process also is predicated on the belief that the research design and methodologies selected will produce the expected outcomes of the research study.

Next, the nurse implements the identified nursing interventions that were developed in the planning phase of the nursing process; this is comparable to Phase 3 of the research process, the Empirical Phase, in which data are collected and prepared for analysis. In other words, the sampling plan is actualized. In the next stage of the nursing process, the nurse evaluates the patient's response to the planned interventions to determine if the patient is achieving the desired outcomes of care, and then recommends modifications to the plan as new evidence becomes available. This stage of the nursing process correlates with Phase 4 of the research process, which includes analyzing and interpreting the data. This is similar to interpretation of findings and the recommendation stage of the research process. The last step in the research process is Phase 5, the Dissemination Phase, in which the findings of the study are reported. Ideally, plans are then made to use the research findings as evidence in practice. An analogy can be made to the last stage of the nursing process, in which the patient's status is evaluated and new plans are made for the patient. Beyond that, this phase could represent a sharing of the information as to what worked and what did not work. These data can be summarized and passed on to others in the field as evidence-based practice.

As problem solving is the basis of the nursing process, a relationship also exists between problem solving and research. For some, understanding the research process becomes easier when presented in the context of problem solving and the nursing process. Chart 3–1 shows a comparison of the three processes: nursing process, problem solving, and research. Please note that the research process is presented in steps, as each phase consists of multiple steps.

CHART 3–1 Comparison of the Steps in the Nursing Process, the Problem-Solving Process, and the Stages of Nursing Research

Steps of the Nursing Process	Steps of the Problem-Solving Process	Phases and Steps of Nursing Research
1. Assessment Assess to determine the degree of discrepancy between what is and what should be in relation to the optimum health of an individual patient. This includes data collection, analysis/synthesis of data, and arriving at a preliminary nursing diagnosis. 2. Nursing Diagnosis Validate the nursing diagnosis; make a clinical judgment about the patient's response to actual or potential health conditions or needs. Make goals in collaboration with the patient, and formulate the desired outcomes for problem resolution in the form of behavioral objectives. 3. Outcomes and Planning Based on the assessment and diagnosis, set measurable and achievable short- and long-term goals for the patient (the behavioral objectives). 4. Implementation Implement nursing care with the specific rationale for doing so. 5. Evaluation Evaluate both the patient's status and the effectiveness of the nursing care that was implemented. Revise the plan by redesigning the behavioral objectives that have not been attained; by selecting and implementing other action alternatives; and by collecting and analyzing more data to evolve new nursing diagnoses, new behavioral objectives, and other action alternatives, all in collaboration with the patient.	1. Identify a particular problem or condition of the patient or family or a problem in the setting that requires change. 2. Analyze the various aspects of the problem (e.g., the need for immediate or long-term change), the type of approach that is needed, the need to involve other people in the problem-solving process, and the resources that are available. 3. Collect data about the patient or family, the setting, related facets of the problem, and possible solutions to the problem through the use of observations, interviews, discussion with experts, and a review of the literature. 4. Analyze the information collected using the analysis as a guide for appropriate actions. Establish a plan for change and a means for evaluating the success of the change. 5. Implement the plan of change. 6. Evaluate the effects of the change as determined by the evaluation plan developed. If the actions fail to solve the problem, begin again, looking for alternative solutions to the problem.	Phase 1, Step 1 Identify a research problem and purpose, from clinical observations or from the literature and current theoretical thought, or from a combination of the two. Delineate the problem clearly and delimit the problem to a manageable research question or hypothesis. Phase 1, Steps 2–5 Collect essential facts pertaining to the problem. Review the literature, validate the significance of the problem selected, or develop the theoretical or conceptual framework for the problem to explain it and its possible solution(s). Formulate hypotheses. Phase 2 Steps 6–12 The Design and Planning Phase Develop an appropriate design to answer the question(s) or test the hypotheses, which includes measurement instruments, setting, sample, protocol, methodology, and statistical analysis design and the rationale for each. Phase 3, Steps 13–14 Collect the essential data. Prepare the data for analysis. Phase 4 Analytic Phase Steps 15–16 Analyze the data, interpret the findings, and generalize the results in terms of the framework, the theoretical perspective, and the sampling rationale. Phase 5 Disseminate the research findings.

Sources: Adapted from American Nurses Association. (2012). The nursing process. Retrieved from http://www.nursingworld.org/ExpeciallyForYou/What-is-Nursing/Tools-You-Need/Thenursingprocess.html
Burns, N., & Grove, S. K. (2009). *The practice of nursing research: Appraisal, synthesis, and generation of evidence* (6th ed.). Elsevier.
Polit, D. F., & Beck, C. T. (2012). *Nursing research: Principles and methods* (8th ed.). Philadelphia: Lippincott Williams & Wilkins.
Roy, Sr., C., & Jones, D. A. (2007). *Nursing knowledge development and clinical practice.* New York: Springer.

Conducting Research

Discrete (nonconnected) steps must be taken in order to conduct research. These steps may or may not progress in a linear way depending on whether the researcher is conducting quantitative or qualitative research. With quantitative research, the steps do progress in a linear fashion; they do not necessarily do so in qualitative research. However, some of the basic elements of the process apply to both types of research approaches. These commonalities between the two types of research, such as identifying the problem and purpose, conducting a literature review, collecting and analyzing data, and drawing conclusions, are presented next.

Research Problem and Purpose

Research Problem

The first step in any research process is to identify a researchable problem, defined as a situation in need of a solution, alteration, or improvement. It is an area of concern for a particular population that requires investigation, and it is derived from a topical area. Not all problems are researchable. For instance, problems or questions of a moral or ethical nature are incapable of being researched because there is no right or wrong answer, only points of view that reflect an individual's values. For example, a researcher might question the right of parents to withhold medical treatment for their children. This represents an ethical dilemma; therefore, there is no right or wrong answer.

The topical area of concern, also referred to as the problem concept, typically is very broad and generally contains numerous potential research problems. The actual research problem is a very small piece of the entire topical area. This may be thought of as a very small piece of a large puzzle or a very small slice of a very large pie. For example, pain is a general research topic/concept, and one researchable question (problem) related to pain is "Does fatigue exacerbate pain in cancer patients?" Figure 3–1◆ reflects the minuteness of the research problem in relation to the problem topic. The study or **research problem** is a very specific and precise statement of the phenomenon to be studied. The study problem also may be phrased as a **research question.** Examples of research topics/concepts with related research problems are shown in Chart 3–2.

Research problems may be developed from a variety of sources, such as nursing practice, researcher and peer interactions, literature review, theory, and research priorities identified by funding agencies and

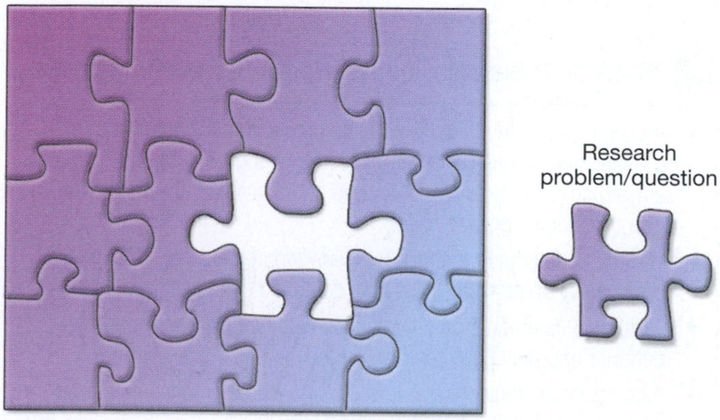

FIGURE 3–1 ◆ The problem concept or topical area of concern typically is very broad, whereas the actual research problem is a very small piece of the entire topical area.

CHART 3–2 Research Topics/Concepts and Related Research Questions

Research Topic/Concept	Research Question
Pregnancy in teenage girls	Does adaptation to pregnancy in teenage girls vary according to ethnic culture?
Discharge planning in acute care settings	What is the role of the staff nurse in discharge planning?
Falls in acute care setting	Do fall prevention programs affect the number of falls in acute care settings?
Evidence-based practice	Is the use of evidence-based practice influenced by the level of education of the registered nurse?
Staffing in acute care settings	Does staffing in acute care settings affect patient outcomes?

specialty groups. The researcher should keep in mind that the problem selected must meet four criteria. Problems must be:

- Significant to nursing (someone must benefit from the evidence that is produced)
- Researchable (amenable to scientific inquiry)
- Feasible to address (time to complete, available study participants, cooperation of others, faculties and equipment, money, experience of the researcher, and ethically sound)
- Of interest to the researcher (genuine interest in and curiosity about the problem).

Research Purpose

The **research purpose,** which researchers generate from the problem, identifies the study's goal or goals and directs its development. In the research process, the purpose usually is stated after the problem has been determined. Since the problem identifies the gap in knowledge in a selected area, it needs to be identified before the purpose, which then clarifies the knowledge a study will generate. One research problem may be the basis for several research purposes. The research purpose usually is a single declarative statement that focuses on the study and clearly identifies what the researcher wants to do. In quantitative research, the problem identifies an area of concern and the purpose reflects the type of study to be conducted: descriptive, correlational, quasi-experimental, or experimental. An example of a quantitative purpose statement is, "This study sought to elicit views of nurses on assignment to monitor the use of evidence-based practice." In qualitative research, the problem identifies an area of concern, and the purpose indicates the focus of the investigation: a subjective concept, an event, a phenomenon, or a fact of a culture or society (Polit & Beck, 2012). An example of a qualitative purpose statement is, "This qualitative study explored the meaning of a supportive environment by patients when receiving a life-threatening medical diagnosis."

Literature Review

After a researcher identifies a researchable problem and states or poses it as a research question, she completes a **literature review.** This critical step can be quite time consuming; however, it is essential and serves several purposes, one of the primary functions being to further clarify the problem identified for study. The review also helps to specify the study problem and set limits for the target population (the entire population in which a researcher is interested and to which she would like to generalize the study results). Another function of the literature review is to verify that this is an important clinical problem that needs to be answered in order to improve patient care. Thus, the literature review should be used to determine (1) if other studies similar to the one to be conducted have been done previously, (2) if prior findings would be helpful in defining the proposed study, and (3) if it would be possible to replicate (copy or redo) a prior study. Other purposes of the literature review include finding gaps in existing knowledge that can help inform the current study design, selecting a research design and identifying instruments to measure the central aspects of the design, and helping the researcher interpret the findings from the study.

Literature searches may be conducted by reviewing references in a library and by conducting computer searches of electronic databases. Computer searches are now the most common way to conduct literature searches, but they can yield vast amounts of data. Therefore, nurses searching electronic databases will find it necessary to limit the search to reasonable time periods and credible websites. Literature searches also may be limited by using only primary resources. Primary resources are those written by investigators who conducted the studies. Secondary sources, such as review articles, are those in which a writer describes or summarizes studies done by others. However, these can be valuable in guiding a researcher to appropriate primary literature. They also may be helpful in reviewing theoretical or conceptual material that assists the researcher in establishing a design and methodology.

Conceptual or Theoretical Framework

A framework is the overall conceptual underpinnings of a study. Although not every study is based on a conceptual or theoretical model, every study has a framework based on conceptual rationale (Polit & Beck, 2012). In a study based on a theory, the framework is identified as a *theoretical framework*. If the framework is based on a conceptual model, it is called a *conceptual framework*. These terms are at times used interchangeably. Most nursing studies do not have an explicit theory or conceptual model; frameworks are built around key constructs at the conceptual level. The concepts are abstractions of observable phenomena that are shaped by both a worldview and a view on nursing. It is important for researchers to make clear the conceptual definition of their key variables, thereby providing information about the study's framework. Researchers may draw on concepts and theories both from within and outside of nursing. Many choose to use sociological concepts and theories to explain the basis of their research. The literature review often is helpful in providing access to concepts and theories that may be useful to the researcher, in addition to helping with their interpretation. Conceptual frameworks may be derived from the literature review.

Examples of conceptual models used in nursing research include socialization, caring (which some consider a theory), therapeutic touch, pain, and health promotion. Models and theories gained from other disciplines, and ones which are used frequently, include self-efficacy (Bandura, 2001) and the health belief model, which has become popular with nurses studying patient compliance and preventative health care practices (Becker, 1978). The researcher should remember that the conceptual or theoretical framework provides an interpretation of behavior, which in turn provides a rationale for your study.

Research Design

The next major step in the research process is selecting the type of research that will answer the question and determine the appropriate **research design.** The design, which is the overall plan or blueprint for the study, should be described in detail and include the methods used for data collection and analysis. A number of research design strategies may be employed to answer the research question, so the researcher should use the strategy that is most likely to achieve accurate information in the results. The design for the study is dictated by the research problem/question, also known as a **hypothesis,** and assumptions of the theoretical framework.

It is helpful to begin the design section by writing an overview in which the theoretical or conceptual framework is stated, if such a framework is used. The overview is an extension of the research problem. It states how and where the study will be conducted, who is going to be studied, and how the study question(s) will be evaluated (measured). Different designs are used for describing phenomena, exploring relationships, or searching for effects of **variables,** attributes that vary and take on different values (e.g., body temperature, heart rate, time to complete a task, and length of time to complete a procedure).

Among the various types of nursing research, the most common types are quantitative and qualitative. The following descriptions provide broad distinctions between these two main types of research.

Quantitative Research

Quantitative research is characterized by the collection of numerical values, under a controlled situation, that yield data that can be generalized. Quantitative designs typically are descriptive, correlational, quasi-experimental, or experimental. **Descriptive research designs** often search for associations among certain variables. Chart 3–3 shows examples of descriptive research. A **correlational research design** is aimed at examining linear relationships between two or more variables. A **quasi-experimental research design** uses an intervention, but one in which it is difficult to manipulate or control the setting, subjects, or variables as needed for a true experimental study. An **experimental research design** is used to determine the effects of an intervention, and it is highly controlled. Experimental research most often occurs in a laboratory setting, and is used to determine the effects of an intervention or the manipulation of an independent variable. In contrast, a **nonexperimental research design,** which is not a specific type of design, consists of studies in which the researcher collects data without introducing an intervention. Quantitative research uses subjects that represent certain groups.

CHART 3–3 Examples of Descriptive Research Problems

- A comparison study to determine the differences in caregiver fatigue between two groups of caregivers, those caring for patients with amyotrophic lateral sclerosis disease and those caring for patients with myasthenia gravis.
- A study to determine the factors elderly women identify as impacting their quality of life when living with comorbid chronic illness.
- A study to determine the effects of diabetes education on self-care behavior and metabolic control.
- A comparison study of care provided by a nurse practitioner versus a medical doctor.
- A study to determine the effects of the quantity and quality of nursing staff on a patient's capabilities for hygiene self-care.

Research is not value free; that is, the background and biases of the researcher have an influence on study outcomes. The term *bias* means to slant away from the true or expected. A biased opinion fails to include both sides of the question. Bias is of great concern in research because anything that deviates or causes a deviation from the true measure in a study leads to distorted findings. In quantitative studies, the researcher strives to control as much bias as possible through design decisions. Understanding what biases can influence certain design decisions can be useful in the data analysis phase of the study.

In a quantitative study, the researcher moves from the beginning point of a study (posing a research question) to the end point (finding an answer). The researcher passes through five phases from the beginning to the end of the study: the conceptual phase, the design and planning phase, the empirical phase, the analytic phase, and the dissemination phase (Polit & Beck, 2012). The conceptual phase consists of thinking about the study and discussing the possibility of the study with colleagues. During this phase, the researcher calls on creativity and deductive reasoning to arrive at a researchable problem. In the second phase, the design and planning phase, the researcher develops methods to be used in conducting the study and to gather data. The third phase, the empirical phase, involves the collection of research data and preparation of those data for analysis. During the fourth phase, the analytic phase, the researcher analyzes and interprets the data to determine the answer to the questions originally posed in the study. The fifth and final stage of the process is the dissemination phase. The researcher disseminates the results of the study and makes recommendations regarding how the results of the study could be incorporated into nursing practice. The sequential steps that occur during each phase of the research process are shown in Chart 3–4.

CHART 3–4 Steps in the Quantitative Research Process

Phase 1: The Conceptual Phase	1. Identify a researchable problem.
	2. Establish a purpose for the study.
	3. Conduct a literature review.
	4. Develop a theoretical/conceptual framework.
	5. Formulate research objectives, questions, and hypotheses.
Phase 2: The Design and Planning Phase	6. Select a research design.
	7. Identify the population to be studied.
	8. Design the sampling plan.
	9. Specify methods to measure the research variables.
	10. Finalize and review the research plan.
	11. Conduct a pilot study (if possible) and make revisions.
Phase 3: The Empirical Phase	12. Collect the data.
	13. Prepare the data for analysis.
Phase 4: The Analytic Phase	14. Analyze the data.
	15. Interpret the results.
Phase 5: The Dissemination Phase	16. Communicate the findings.
	17. Use the findings.

Qualitative Research

Qualitative research describes events as they occur naturally. This process involves the use of a systematic, subjective approach to describe life experiences and give them meaning (Porter, 2007; Speziale & Carpenter, 2010). Compared to quantitative research, qualitative research uses methods that are more subjective, a smaller sample size, and fewer research controls. Qualitative research studies generally use phenomenology, grounded theory, or ethnography to explore personal meaning within a given context.

Phenomenology describes the meaning of a lived experience through the perspective of the participant. **Grounded theory** refers to the idea that the conclusion of a qualitative study should be grounded in the data, that is, based on direct and careful observations of everyday life within the group. **Ethnography** focuses on the culture of a group of people, with an effort to understand the worldview of those under study. Chart 3–5 shows examples of qualitative research questions.

This type of research is important when little is known about a topic because it can identify factors of influence (factors that have the potential to influence data collected and outcomes of the study). Often the discoveries of qualitative research generate hypotheses to be used in quantitative research. For example, the last qualitative research question from Chart 3–5—What type of feelings do women experience when first told that they have breast cancer?—can be used to develop a future hypothesis for quantitative study: If women are told that they have breast cancer in a supportive environment, they will feel less frightened. With the sample hypothesis, the terms *supportive environment* and *frightened* need to be defined, possibly from concepts used in a conceptual framework. Many times a combination of the two methods yields a better understanding of human phenomena as seen every day in nursing. The design of the qualitative study is not specified in advance as it is in quantitative research; instead, the design tends to evolve over time during the study. Decisions about the best ways to gather data, how to schedule and record data, how many subjects will be used in the study, and so on, are all decisions made during the study. This has been called an *emergent design*—a design that becomes clear during the study as the researcher makes decisions about what she has learned (Cooper, Endacott, & Chapman, 2009). Because qualitative studies involve researchers directly, and because the design emerges during the study, the researcher's biases must be carefully examined before the study begins.

Qualitative studies do not follow the same linear progression of quantitative studies. Their process tends to resemble a circle more than a line. The researcher is continually examining and interpreting data and making decisions about how to proceed based on what has already been discovered. There are, however, some major activities in which the researcher engages, and these also occur in phases similar to those described for quantitative research: phase 1, conceptualizing and planning

CHART 3–5 Examples of Qualitative Research Questions

- What is the meaning of serenity for survivors of a life-threatening illness or traumatic event?
- How do patients act or change behaviors when waiting in the emergency department to be seen over a period of 4 hours?
- How is vigilance displayed by families caring for hospitalized patients?
- What are the expectations of nursing students as they prepare to go into the clinical setting and care for patients the first time?
- What type of feelings do women experience when first told that they have breast cancer?

CHART 3–6 Activities Inherent in Qualitative Research

Phase 1: Conceptualizing and Planning the Study

1. Clarify the topic area.
2. Proceed with a broad research question that may be delineated after the study is underway.
3. Conduct a literature review.
4. Identify a study site.

Phase 2: Conducting the Study

5. Develop a sampling plan.[a]
6. Collect data.[a]
7. Analyze and interpret the data.[a]
8. Identify themes and categories.
9. Confirm that findings accurately reflect the feelings and experiences of participants.

Phase 3: Disseminating the Findings

10. Share findings with other nurses and health care specialists.

[a]These activities are cyclical and may be revised as the study progresses. Analysis and interpretation are ongoing and concurrent activities, used to guide the people to the next sample and the questions or observations to make. Sampling also is guided by the data.

the study; phase 2, conducting the study; and phase 3, disseminating the findings. These activities are discussed further in Chart 3–6.

Research Setting

The **setting** in which the study is conducted also will influence the type of research design selected. This is an important consideration when planning a study, because the setting and the dynamics within the setting can greatly influence the outcomes. Settings can be natural or field settings, in which no attempt is made to control elements of the setting; partially controlled, meaning that the setting/environment has been manipulated or modified in some way by the researcher to strengthen the research design; or highly controlled artificial settings, in which case a laboratory setting is usually used, such as with animal research. Many research studies use quasi-natural settings such as hospitals, clinics, or other care facilities where the researcher modifies the environment.

Sample Selection

Studies rarely gather information from an entire population of interest, referred to as a target population. A **population** is the entire aggregation of cases in which a researcher is interested; for example, all registered nurses with a master's degree in nursing who are currently practicing nursing in northern California. Because gathering information from such a large population would be difficult for a variety of reasons, researchers use a process called sampling. **Sampling** is the process of selecting a portion of the population to represent the entire population. A **sample,** then, is a subset of the population.

A major concern when selecting a sample is how representative the sample is of the population; that is, how closely the sample mirrors the characteristics of the entire population of interest. In a representative sample, the key characteristics closely approximate those of the population. Sampling strategies are classified as either probability sampling or nonprobability sampling (Polit & Beck, 2012). **Probability sampling** involves random selection when choosing the elements. **Nonprobability sampling** means that the elements are selected in a nonrandom fashion (not every element of the population has an opportunity to be included in the sample). Common sampling strategies are explained in this chapter.

Convenience Sampling

With **convenience sampling,** the most available persons or units are selected for inclusion in the study. Also referred to as *accidental sampling* (Polit & Beck, 2012), this type of sampling is easy and usually inexpensive. However, it is a weak strategy to use because the researcher has no control over the characteristics of the sample. As a result, the sample may be quite different from the population to which the study results are expected to be relevant. Thus, if this sampling strategy is used, it is wise to build in some limiting characteristics that the sample population must possess. Consider factors that might influence the outcome of the study—for example, socioeconomic status, gender, age, and cultural differences—and decide whether these should be included or excluded. Approaching people in a supermarket to conduct an interview is an example of convenience sampling. This may be a good strategy to use for a **pilot study** (a small preliminary study done prior to conducting a larger study) or when no other alternative is available.

Quota Sampling

Quota sampling involves nonrandom selection of the participants in which the researcher pre-specifies characteristics of the sample to increase its representation. Dividing a convenience sample into two subgroups in order to increase the potential for the sample to be representative of the total population may achieve this. For example, if a researcher were interested in determining how many nurses were willing to work on a unit that cared exclusively for AIDS patients, the total number of participants might be divided between males and females, thus providing quotas (Polit & Beck, 2012).

Purposive Sampling

Purposive sampling implies that certain people or elements are deliberately selected for the study. Subjects, also called participants or informants, are purposively selected for qualitative studies. They are individuals experiencing a common problem or sharing a common circumstance. Usually very few participants are needed since data collection is done through extensive interviews and observations. Purposive sampling may be used when researchers want a sample of experts (Polit & Beck, 2012).

Network Sampling

In **network sampling,** sample participants refer other participants who meet the eligibility criteria to the study. Polit and Beck (2012) also refer to network sampling as *snowball sampling*. This type of sampling works well for hard-to-find participant groups.

Simple Random Sampling

The **simple random sampling** strategy gives each person in a population an equal chance of being selected for the study. For example, if a researcher were going to study a set of characteristics of breast cancer patients seen in a clinic during the past 2 years, the entire population who meet the study criteria would be listed. The researcher would then randomly select a sample from this population.

Random samples may be selected in a number of ways. One way is to put names or patient record numbers in a container and draw the names or numbers randomly. The researcher also may flip a coin. If the toss is heads, the person is selected; if it is tails, the person is not selected. A more sophisticated method is to use a table of random numbers, which may be found in most research books. Random numbers also may be generated through computer programs. Random sampling greatly strengthens the design of the study by reducing potential selection biases. **Selection biases,** sometimes referred to as **sampling biases,** refer to the systematic overrepresentation or underrepresentation of some segment of the population in terms of a characteristic relevant to the research question (Polit & Beck, 2012).

A difference exists between random sample and random assignment that should be noted. As explained, a random sample means that every person within the category has an equal chance of being in the study. A **random assignment,** however, means that subjects are randomly assigned to treatment versus control groups. For example, if the category was "all cancer patients in California," and every patient in California had an equal chance of being in the study, that would constitute random sampling. However, because sampling such a large group would be too costly and time-consuming, a random assignment of subjects would be done. For example, every other woman diagnosed with breast cancer in the clinic could be assigned to the treatment group for an educational intervention and every other woman assigned to the control group. The control group represents subjects in an experiment who do not receive the experimental treatment and whose performance provides a baseline against which the effects of the treatment can be measured (Polit & Beck, 2012). In some cases, random assignment may not be possible (e.g., if the control group is in another location, or if there are ethical issues, such as withholding treatment from the control group may cause undue pain or suffering).

Stratified Random Sampling

Stratified random sampling means that the population is first divided into two or more strata or subpopulations; for example, participants younger than 30 years of age, those between 30 and 45, and those 46 years or older. As with quota sampling, the aim is to enhance representation. Polit and Beck (2012) note that stratified sampling designs subdivide the population into homogeneous subsets from which an appropriate number of elements, such as demographic attributes like age, gender, and income level, are selected at random.

Regardless of the sampling strategy used, it is essential to keep a careful record of the sampling decisions and identify how many people began the study, how many completed it, and why subjects left the study before completing it. This type of record also is very helpful in identifying potential biases in study results and providing a clear narrative of the sampling strategy.

Sample Size

Determining sample size is a major consideration in developing a research study. If subjects are hard to get or expensive to enroll in the study, it is prudent to use as few as possible as long as you maintain the minimum amount needed to still have a credible study. However, too few subjects could result in sampling error. Studies with too few subjects to reliably "determine" an effect have low "power," meaning that tests of **statistical significance** are less likely to indicate significance even if the study has a real effect. This is particularly true if the effect is small relative to the variability of the sample.

There are no simple formulas that can advise how large a sample is needed in a given quantitative study; however, using the largest sample possible is suggested (Polit & Beck, 2012). The larger the sample, the more representative of the population it is likely to be. The process of drawing a sample may vary according to the type of research design employed. However, a general outline of procedures may be employed: (1) identify the population, (2) specify the eligibility criteria, (3) specify the sample plan, and (4) recruit the sample (Polit & Beck, 2012). These steps are shown with limited explanation in Chart 3–7. Because practical constraints such as time, subject availability, and resources often limit sample size, many nursing studies are based on relatively small samples, which can lead to misleading or inconclusive results. For clinical studies that deal with biophysiological processes in which variation is limited, a small sample may adequately represent the population. For most nursing studies, however, it is safer to assume that a fair degree of heterogeneity within the sample will lead to greater representation of the population, unless there is evidence from prior research to the contrary.

Qualitative studies almost always use small, nonrandom samples. Whereas quantitative research is concerned with measuring attributes, the aim of qualitative studies is to discover meaning and to uncover multiple realities. Thus, unlike quantitative studies, in which measurements must accurately reflect and be generalizable to the population, generalizability is not a guideline in qualitative studies. A critical first step in qualitative sampling is selecting settings with high potential for information richness. The qualitative researcher may begin with the following types of sampling questions in mind: Who would be an information-rich data source for my study? Who should I talk to or what should I observe first, so as to maximize my understanding of the phenomenon? There are no criteria or rules for sample size in qualitative research. Sample size is largely a function of the purpose of the inquiry, the quality of the informants, and the type of sampling strategy used. Samples are usually small, probability sampling is almost never used, and final sampling decisions usually take place in the field during data collection (Speziale & Carpenter, 2010). The main consideration for sample size is **data saturation,** which refers to sampling to the point at which no new information is obtained and redundancy is achieved (Polit & Beck, 2012). Saturation depends on a number of factors (e.g., the broader the scope of the research question, the more participants will likely be needed). Data quality also affects sample size. If participants are able to reflect on their experiences and communicate effectively, saturation can be achieved with a relatively small sample. If longitudinal data are collected, fewer participants may be needed, as each provides more information over the length of the study.

In qualitative studies, the sampling plan is evaluated in terms of adequacy and appropriateness. Adequacy refers to the sufficiency and

CHART 3–7 Sampling Steps for Quantitative Studies

Identify the population	Identify an accessible population, and then decide how best to define the target population.
Specify eligibility criteria	The criteria should be as specific as possible with respect to characteristics that might exclude potential subjects (e.g., inability to read Spanish).
Specify sampling plan	Once the accessible population has been identified, decide the method for drawing the sample and how large it will be. If possible, perform a **power analysis** to determine the desired number of subjects. If probability sampling is an option for selecting a sample, it should be exercised.
Recruit the sample	Recruit prospective study participants according to the plan and after needed institutional permissions have been obtained.

Source: Polit, D. G., & Beck, C. T. (2012). *Nursing research: Generating and assessing evidence for nursing practice* (8th ed.). Philadelphia: Wolters Kluwer/Lippincott Williams & Wilkins, pp. 351 and 352, http://lww.com.

quality of data retrieved. In an appropriate sample, the participants can best supply the information according to the study's conceptual requirements. There are similarities and differences among the various qualitative approaches with regard to sampling. The similarities include the following: Sample size is generally small, probability sampling is almost never used, and final sampling decisions usually take place in the field during data collection.

Research Utilization and Evidence-Based Practice

Florence Nightingale may be considered the first nursing researcher, as she wrote down her observations of nursing care during the formative years of the nursing profession. In her writings, she documented her research approach. Nightingale observed what events and occurrences were going on, developed hypotheses, collected and analyzed the data, and then reached conclusions (Burns & Grove, 2009). Essentially, she used the research process to decrease the loss of lives from disease. Based on her skillful analyses of the factors affecting soldier mortality and morbidity during the Crimean War, she was successful in effecting some changes in nursing care and, more generally, public health. Nightingale's landmark publication, *Notes on Nursing* (1859), described her early research interest in environmental factors that promote physical and emotional well-being, an interest of nurses that continues today, nearly 150 years later. For many years after Nightingale's work, there was little reference to research in the nursing literature. It was not until the early 1900s that nursing research began to emerge with a focus primarily on nursing education: characteristics of nurses, the supply and demand of nurses, and the amount of time required in performing certain nursing activities. A shift in focus emerged in the 1950s, accelerating the development of nursing research in the direction of clinical nursing problems. In the 1960s, practice-oriented research emerged in the literature. And now, the emphasis on research has magnified. The Institute of Medicine's (IOM's) study on *The Future of Nursing: Leading Change, Advancing Health* (2010) called for the transformation of the health care system, with nursing playing a fundamental role in this transformation.

The advance of nursing research has continued through the last several decades, highlighted by several publications, including *Advances in Nursing Science, Research in Nursing & Health, Nursing Research,* the *Western Journal of Nursing Research,* and the *Journal of Advanced Nursing.* These journals contribute to the dissemination and use of nursing research and the increased emphasis on improving patient care through research.

Research Utilization

The need for a systematic approach for using research to change practice was recognized in the early 1970s and led to publication of the first model for research utilization by Stetler and Marram (Burns & Grove, 2009; Stetler, 1994). Subsequently, through the next several decades, much of the progress in using research in practice was based on that model and on work completed by the Western Interstate Commission for Higher Education's Regional Program for Nursing Research Development and the Conduct and Utilization of Research in Nursing (CURN) Project (Burns & Grove, 2009). The major emphasis of the CURN project was to increase the use of research results by direct-care nurses through facilitating organizational change. Since that time, there has been a growing emphasis on using research findings to improve nursing practice. This emphasis has grown in importance with the push in the United States to achieve cost-effective, high-quality patient care based on sound scientific evidence coupled with the global emphasis on quality. Though nursing has a long history of using research to make practice decisions, it has not been well used, nor has it been well documented or labeled evidence-based practice.

The formation and adoption of the National Institute of Nursing Research's (NINR's) position in 1993 solidified the recognition of nursing research as a major component of nursing practice and moved nursing into the mainstream research path enjoyed by other health disciplines. At present, **research utilization (RU)** is perceived as the purposeful application of research findings to the clinical setting to improve patient care. RU is important for the bedside nurse whose patients may benefit from implementation of research findings. Nurses in direct patient care are the best resource for determining if a change of practice will be successful on their respective nursing unit and benefit the patients they serve. Because they are the individuals taking care of patients, nurses must use the newest research findings to keep their practice current and to provide the highest standard of care to patients. RU is one method or source for achieving evidence-based practice.

Evidence-Based Practice

In some settings, evidence-based practice and research utilization are used interchangeably; however, there are some distinct differences (Polit & Beck, 2012). In contrast to research utilization, **evidence-based practice (EBP)** is a broader concept and relies on more than research to support and improve practice. It extends beyond research utilization and involves making clinical decisions on the basis of the best possible evidence. Though the best evidence usually comes from rigorous research, EBP also uses other sources of credible information. Some experts have differentiated between RU and EBP by explaining that RU is part of EBP and is a prescribed task of summarizing and using research findings to address a particular practice problem. In contrast, EBP is "the careful and practical use of current best evidence to guide health care decisions" (Omery & Williams, 1999, p. 51). As seen in both examples of differentiation, EBP is broader than RU and is the interpretation generally chosen by agencies adopting EBP as a practice model.

The definition of EBP posed by Omery and Williams (1999) asserts that current best evidence includes clinical practice guidelines usually developed nationally by expert researchers, clinicians, and theorists in their areas of excellence. EBP involves the interpretation and implementation of these clinical guidelines by health care providers based on their clinical expertise, the needs and views of the patient and family, and the resources of the health care system.

Although evidence-based practice has been emphasized in medicine for years, and expert researchers, clinicians, and theorists have developed numerous evidence-based guidelines for the prevention of illness and diagnosis and management of chronic and acute illnesses (Burns & Grove, 2009), EBP is in its initial stages of development in the nursing field. Now that EBP is the recommended standard in health care and nursing, it is important for nurses to understand EBP and how it is used to de-emphasize ritual, isolated clinical experiences, ungrounded opinions, and tradition as a basis for nursing practice. Not only does EBP stress the use of research findings, it also stresses, as appropriate, the use of quality improvement data, other operational and evaluation data, the consensus of recognized experts, and affirmed experience to substantiate practice (Burns & Grove, 2009; Stetler, 1994). EBP calls for nurses to question their practice, to seek reliable evidence to improve and evaluate outcomes, not to do things as they have always been done (Wolf, 2010).

EBP is, in effect, a problem-solving approach to clinical decision making that incorporates a search for the best and latest evidence, clinical expertise and assessment, and a patient's preferences and values within a context of caring, as discussed in Chapter 1. This decision-making approach integrates clinical expertise with the best available evidence from systematic research, in contrast to opinion-based health care decision making that is based primarily on values and resources. Factors that form a framework for decision making with this approach include understanding the patient's needs, concerns, and values; building on the clinical expertise or experience of the professional nurse; and seeking relevant clinical data and best practices (The Joanna Briggs Institute, 2009). Best practices are those proven processes that produce consistent, high-quality results.

Development of Evidence-Based Practice

Five steps are involved in developing evidence-based nursing practice: (1) defining the question, (2) collecting evidence, (3) making a critical appraisal, (4) integrating the evidence and patient factors to make and carry out the decision, and (5) evaluating the whole process (Burns & Grove, 2009). Also, hierarchies or levels of evidence used in practice have been identified (Figure 3–2◆) (Polit & Beck, 2012). The lowest and least powerful evidence is provided by opinions of reviewers that are based on their experience and knowledge and constitute clinical practice guidelines. Somewhat stronger evidence is derived from opinions that come from well-known experts and respected authorities. Even more compelling evidence comes from the results of research studies. Four levels of evidence are derived from research. These are listed in order of increasing strength: non-experimental studies (e.g., correlational, descriptive, and qualitative); quasi-experimental studies such as time series or matched case-control studies; individual experimental studies; and meta-analysis of controlled studies. Large randomized controlled trials and meta-analyses of studies providing evidence in a specific area are considered the "gold standards" as they provide the strongest, most powerful evidence for clinical practice.

Safety Alert *Having defined the question and collected the evidence, it is critical to evaluate the data carefully before adding it into practice in order to prevent patient care errors from occurring.*

As a problem-solving approach to clinical decision making, EBP incorporates a search for the best and latest evidence, clinical expertise and assessment, and patient preferences and values within a context of caring. The search for evidence in an attempt to answer a burning clinical question related to the effectiveness of a clinical intervention or treatment should begin with databases that contain systematic reviews of randomized controlled trials. Critical appraisal of these reviews for validity, strength of the findings, and applicability is a necessary step in evidence-based decision making and quality patient care.

Implementation of Evidence-Based Practice

Government mandates, consumer demands for accountability, professional efforts to improve quality, and organization requirements for fiscally responsible patient care all promote EBP. Alarming reports of medical errors and poor safety practices have and continue to inspire a social and professional mandate to improve care quality. As a result, health care institutions are seeking to implement evidence-based nursing practice, often including it in strategic plans. Many are linking their efforts to the national accrediting body, The Joint Commission. However, two questions remain: Are health care agencies ready to provide the necessary resources to implement a best-practices model, and are nurses ready to meet the challenge?

Barriers to Evidence-Based Practice

Although a laudable and critical goal, EBP within the health care setting is not easily accomplished due to human and organizational barriers. Nurses often act on experiential knowledge, rather than research evidence, in their day-to-day clinical decision making. They tend to rely most frequently on personal experience, information learned about the patient, manuals, information learned in nursing school, fellow nurses, and nonresearch nursing journals and texts. Nurses' reluctance to use research is compounded by lack of time, access, and skills (Drury, 2010; Smith & Donze, 2010). Although most agencies have incorporated computers into the normal work environment, many nurses still have difficulty using computers to conduct literature searches. This often is due to a hectic work environment and lack of time to practice database searching. Nurses' primary responsibility rightfully remains patient care, so taking time away from the bedside to perform literature searches or participate in research projects is not only challenging, but also may be discouraged by peers and managers.

Other types of barriers to implementing EBP are human and institutional barriers. For example, nurses may be attached to historical practice; therefore, they may wake patients during the night to weigh them on standing scales versus using the hospital's newly acquired bed scales because the nurses judge the bed scales to be inaccurate. Absence of support from other clinicians constitutes a barrier, as does lack of manager/director support. Lack of manager support may result in the unit manager going to the hospital education session to foster staff nurses' interest in research and keeping the staff on the unit. Institutional structure and processes (i.e., red tape) also are obstacles. A staff nurse pursuing new, evidence-based protocol at the time of an antibiotic administration must first gain approval from numerous agency committees and

Hierarchy of Research

Least powerful evidence	Somewhat stronger evidence	More compelling evidence comes from research studies				Gold standard
Opinions of reviewers that are based on their experience and knowledge	Opinions that come from well-known experts and respected authorities	Non-experimental studies: correlational, descriptive, qualitative	Quasi-experimental studies: time series, matched case-controls	Individual experimental studies	Meta-analysis of controlled studies	Large randomized controlled studies and meta-analyses of controlled studies

FIGURE 3–2 ◆ Hierarchy of research.

Weblink: Evidence-Based Report Topics and Disease Categories
Weblink: Evidence-Based Nursing and Midwifery
Weblink: AHRQ: Evidence-Based Practice Centers
Weblink: Evidence-Based Staffing and Scheduling

administrative personnel. Lack of funding for research is another barrier, particularly as attempts are made to reduce health care costs.

The role and support of the nurse researcher, if there is one in the agency, also is considered. The nurse researcher position often becomes a position of isolation in which the researcher lacks peer and mentor support. This isolation, when coupled with weak or nonexistent leadership support, prohibits effective use of the nurse researcher and often leads to the nurse researcher leaving the agency, thereby absenting a role model and coordinator for nursing research. Finally, the nurses' skills, or lack thereof, may lead to the collection of unreliable data. For instance, if the unit is participating in a study on skin integrity using the Braden scale, nurses collecting the data must know how to "code" pressure ulcers correctly using the scale, as improper coding will compromise the data.

From the barriers identified, it is obvious that research-based practice initiatives need dedicated expertise, leadership support, and grassroots enthusiasm to thrive. In many situations, this means changing an organization's practice culture.

Strategies to Promote Evidence-Based Practice

Numerous strategies to overcome the barriers of using research and clinical evidence in practice are noted in the literature; some of these are listed in Chart 3–8. The key is to stimulate nurses' interest and enthusiasm so they will want to understand and use research, to captivate their interest and engage them in seeing the excitement of changing practice through research.

EBP is expected to increase as nursing students are taught to use research findings as a basis for interventions and as nurses' perceptions of priority and attitudes about research change. If a nurse does not perceive research findings to be important or relevant to his particular work setting, he will not be as likely to read research or seek out research-related outcomes to improve practice. It is absolutely necessary that nurses know that the nursing administration and the health care organization endorse the concept of EBP. Only then is it probable that the perceptions of priority will change for the nurse. They will be supported by the recommendations of the 2010 Institute of Medicine (IOM) study, *Future of Nursing: Leading Change, Advancing Health*, which strongly endorses EBP in the clinical setting as a necessary change for the future.

Lack of access to information is perhaps the most difficult barrier to overcome. Internet access and current valid literature databases must be available. Personal digital assistants (PDAs, tablets, and smart phones) can provide quick reference, but are not yet practical for most nurses, although they are becoming more useful. An on-site library is helpful, but it is not the entire solution. Information must be available and easy to access at the point of care, and such a resource will only become available when nurses demand it and incorporate it into their practice. Research has shown that using best practices is cost effective and reduces both complications and lengths of stay (Anderson & Kerfoot, 2011; Carlson, 2009; Hasmiller, 2010).

CHART 3–8 Strategies to Promote Evidence-Based Practice

- Establish a research committee.
- Survey nurses to determine their interest in research activities.
- Form a group to look at inconsistencies in practice and varied patient outcomes.
- Increase staff participation in EBP through research clubs.
- Conduct continuing education and in-service programs on EBP.
- Create self-study packets, newsletter, journal club, or other media ideas.
- Provide funding for replacement staff for nurses participating in research.

CHART 3–9 Examples of Ways in Which Research and Clinical Evidence Have Changed Practice

- Use of heat only for acute muscle strain (Flaugher, 2012)
- Managing pain at the end of life: guidelines for palliative care (Ferrell, 2010)
- Chlorhexidene gluconate added to VAP kits (Scannapieco et al., 2009)
- Music as an intervention in hospitals (The Joanna Briggs Institute, 2009)
- Fall risk assessment, prevention, and management (Poe, Cvach, Gartrell, Radzik, & Joy, 2005)
- Assessing and managing pain in older adults (Ardery, Herr, Titler, Sorofman, & Schmidt 2003)
- Development of a heart failure center (Crowther, 2003)
- Use of saline versus heparin to maintain patency of peripheral intravenous access (DeBourgh, 2001)
- Use of Trendelenburg position for hypotension in emergencies (DeBourgh, 2001)
- Use of normal saline when suctioning endotracheal tubes (DeBourgh, 2001)
- Maintaining oral hygiene in older people (The Joanna Briggs Institute, 2001)

Nurses must strive to base their practices on research in order to improve patient outcomes. Nursing manuals, policies, procedures, and protocols should reflect current research-based knowledge. In the future, accrediting agencies will likely require that nursing care interventions be research based. It follows that research utilization should be actively promoted in all health care agencies. Examples of ways in which research and clinical evidence have been used to change practice are shown in Chart 3–9. Additional examples are available on The Joanna Briggs Institute for Evidence-Based Nursing and Midwifery (2012) website at http://www.joannabriggs.edu.au.

As of February 2011, there were 14 evidence-based practice centers (EPCs) across the United States and in Canada funded by the Evidence-Based Practice Program of the Agency for Healthcare Research and Quality (AHRQ) that were continuing 5-year contracts that began in 2007. These agencies are funded to review all relevant scientific literature on clinical, behavioral, organizational, and financing topics to produce evidence reports and technology assessments. The EPCs also conduct research on methodologies to determine the effectiveness of their implementation, to provide technical assistance in translating the reports and assessments into quality improvement tools, and to help inform coverage policies.

Evidence-based report topics and disease category listings may be obtained via the Internet at www.ahrq.gov/clinic/epcindex.htm. More than 100 reports have been released (AHRQ, 2010).

Research and Ethics in Health Care

The practice of ethics guides health care professionals when they are making decisions concerning life and death situations. As discussed in Chapter 2, the term *ethics* is concerned with motives and attitudes and the relationship of these attitudes to the overall care of the individual. It is the justification of what is right or wrong, and the study of what an individual's life and relationships ought to be, not what they are (Marquis & Huston, 2011). The intent of ethics is to develop methods for clarifying confusing questions even if final solutions remain elusive.

At every stage of the research process, there are ethical considerations for nurse researchers to consider. This consideration may start with the selection of a research problem; from an ethical viewpoint, should the problem be studied or not? For example, should subjects with mental impairments who may not be able to give informed and voluntary consent be studied? As more and more nurses participate in research activities, it is imperative for the profession to operate from a sound ethical knowledge base. Because research is central to the evolution of nursing care, avoiding conducting nursing research altogether might be considered unethical. Similarly, the failure to engage in evidence-based practice—in other words, to base practice decisions solely on tradition or intuition rather than on empirical finding—denies patients access to the best available care and, thus, also might be considered unethical.

Nurses are involved in a variety of research efforts, including research specific to nursing, multidisciplinary research, and research of other disciplines on patients receiving nursing care. In all situations, nurses are expected to engage in ethical research behavior. With this expectation a nurse may question how nurse researchers can make ethical decisions: What characterizes ethical research, what are the rights of study participants, and how does the nurse researcher guard those rights? An exploration of ethical decision making addresses these questions (Langone, 2008).

Ethical Frameworks

Western society has proposed two ethical frameworks to assess the ethical acceptability of a research project. These are the utilitarian and the deontological perspectives. Each articulates ethical norms that transcend disciplinary boundaries (Resnik, 2010).

Utilitarian Perspective

The utilitarian perspective suggests that ethical judgments about a research project should be made by evaluating its consequences for the participants, for society, and for the academic discipline. This view entails the belief that the benefit of a research project is defined by the consequences of its results, and that actions should be taken to promote the greatest good for the greatest number of people. In other words, the utilitarian perspective considers that the end justifies the means. From this perspective, a research project is judged ethical if it produces the greatest good for the greatest number. The problem is in determining what is good. Small-scale studies with little ability for generalization of findings to the larger society may be judged to be unethical from a utilitarian perspective. For example, research into liver transplantation that has the potential to influence quality of life for a small number of participants who receive costly medical intervention may not be considered ethical unless it can be shown that the results will benefit a large number of people in the future. Conversely, research into the prevention of liver disease through lifestyle change is justifiable because lifestyle change is more likely to benefit many more people than will costly surgical procedures available to only a few. When discussing the utilitarian perspective, it is necessary to recognize that each researcher may have a different definition of what is good for the majority (Internet Encyclopedia of Philosophy (IEP), 2009).

Deontological Perspective

The deontological approach to research ethics proposes absolute moral imperatives that must never be violated. In taking the deontological view, a researcher might propose absolutes, such as never using deception, never making participants' identity known, and never putting any pressure on respondents to participate in a study. Rather than assessing the consequences of a given research procedure, the deontological approach, in its extreme form, may propose that deception in experiments is never justified, regardless of what the positive contributions to the knowledge base might be. Deontologist Immanuel Kant supported the categorical imperative: Basic laws apply without exception (e.g., telling an untruth is always wrong, regardless of the consequences). If a conflict exists, the patient's welfare must always be placed above the integrity of the research. Some deontologists are more flexible; they accept more than one basic law, consider context and circumstances in determining priority, and argue that types of harm can be distinguished among a participant's interest, wrongdoing, and a moral harm. It is noted that harms can be compensated for, but wrongs cannot be; if doing a wrong is essential to conducting a research project, then the project should be banned (Resnik, 2010).

Codes and Guidelines for Ethical Decision Making

Historically, the field of nursing has been sensitive to the ethical dimension of nursing research. Thus, many professional organizations have developed codes of ethics to guide nurses in their research endeavors. These codes articulate the level of ethical behavior expected of nurse researchers and provide a standard for nurses working through ethical conflicts that may arise in research, practice, education, and administration.

Since the mid-20th century, various codes of ethics have been developed, largely in response to human rights violations. One of the first internationally recognized efforts to establish ethical standards is referred to as the Nuremberg Code, which was developed after the Nazi atrocities of World War II were made public in the Nuremberg trials. Several other international codes of ethics have been developed since then, the most notable being the Declaration of Helsinki, which the World Medical Association adopted in 1964 and most recently revised in 2000.

Nursing is one of many disciplines that has established its own code of ethics. The American Nurses Association's Code of Ethics was adopted in 1985 and is discussed in Chapter 1. In 1995, the ANA put forth a document entitled *Ethical Guidelines in the Conduct, Dissemination, and Implementation of Nursing Research.* This document presents nine ethical principles to guide nursing research. These principles are shown in Chart 3–10.

In 1978, the United States adopted an important code of ethics that was created by the National Commission for the Protection of Human Subjects of Biomedical and Behavioral Research (1978). The commission issued a report that served as the basis for regulations affecting research sponsored by the federal government. This report, referred to as the Belmont Report, also served as a model for many of the guidelines adopted by specific disciplines. The Belmont Report articulated three primary ethical principles on which standards of ethical conduct in research are based: respect for persons, beneficence, and justice. Information about various codes of ethics and ethical requirements for government-sponsored research can be found in the web links for this chapter on Pearson Nursing Student Resources.

Principles of Ethical Research

At times, the ethics of deontology or utilitarianism may not be adequate to guide nurses in ethical decision making. In these situations, ethical principles, rather than theories, may prove more

CHART 3–10 Ethical Principles Used to Guide Nursing Research

The Investigator

1. Respects autonomous research participants' capacity to consent to participate in research and to determine the degree and duration of that participation without negative consequences.
2. Prevents harm, minimizes harm, and/or promotes good to all research participants, including vulnerable groups and others affected by the research.
3. Respects the personhood of research participants, their families, and significant others, valuing their diversity.
4. Ensures that the benefits and burdens of research are equitably distributed in the selection of research participants.
5. Protects the privacy of research participants to the maximum degree possible.
6. Ensures the ethical integrity of the research process by use of appropriate checks and balances throughout the conduct, dissemination, and implementation of the research.
7. Reports suspected, alleged, or known incidents of scientific misconduct in research to appropriate institutional officials for investigation.
8. Maintains competency in the subject matter and methodologies of his or her research, as well as in other professional and societal issues that affect nursing research and the public good.
9. If involved in animal research, maximizes the benefits of the research with the least possible harm or suffering to the animals.

Source: From Silva, M. C. (1995). *Ethical guidelines in the conduct, dissemination, and implementation of nursing research* (pp. v–vi.) Washington, DC: American Nurses' Association. Printed in Polit, D. F., & Beck, C. T. (2012). *Nursing research: Principles and methods* (8th ed.). Philadelphia: Lippincott Williams & Wilkins, http://lww.com.

helpful. The three principles from the Belmont Report are useful for ethical decision making.

Respect for Persons

Inherent in the principle of respect for persons are the concepts of autonomy, dignity, uniqueness, freedom, and choice. This principle forms the foundation of the participants' rights to informed consent, privacy, and confidentiality, and involves respecting people's autonomy or right to choose freely for themselves. Participants have choices based on their own values and beliefs and have the right to be free from undue pressure or coercion by others. Participants must be made aware of risks and benefits of the study, and be guaranteed protection of their anonymity.

Beneficence

Two concepts are inherent in the principle of beneficence: nonmaleficence, or the duty to do no physical or emotional harm, and beneficence, the duty to promote or do good. To apply the concepts of beneficence, researchers must provide a standard of care. Standards of care usually are established by society and by professional role expectations. For example, nurses' duties to act as patient advocates require that nurses intervene if a research intervention produces more harm than benefit to a patient.

It is the researcher's responsibility to minimize risks and maximize benefits to participants; not doing so would violate the ethical principle of beneficence. When a nurse researcher is a care provider, the potential for conflict between the duty to provide care and the duty to advance knowledge may be imminent. Some refer to this as the research imperative, the advancement of knowledge versus the duty to care (Polit & Beck, 2012). Sometimes it is difficult to determine at what point the therapeutic imperative is being compromised by the research imperative. When doubt is evident, the therapeutic imperative must take precedence over the research imperative for the nurse as caregiver: The nurse must always act as the patient's advocate (Keren & Willemsen, 2009).

Justice

The principle of justice requires that people be treated fairly. The protection of participants from incompetence and the right to receive research treatments are expectations of the justice principle. Justice is an important principle to follow in the selection of subjects for research studies. The risks and benefits of a study should be fairly distributed among participants based on the subjects' efforts, needs, and rights. Random selection of participants avoids potential sources of bias and unfairness in sample selection.

Nurses involved in any aspect of the process have a responsibility to see that research complies with the principles of respect for persons, beneficence, and justice. This is true for nurses' own research as well as for research conducted by others that affects their patients.

Methods of Protecting Human Subjects

Two methods of protecting human subjects have been developed during the past three decades: obtaining informed consent and the review of research proposals by an ethics committee or an institutional review board.

Informed Consent

Informed consent is based on the principle of respect for persons. It incorporates the ethical concept of autonomy or the client's right to self-determination. The key elements of informed consent include disclosure of sufficient and appropriate information, understanding of information, and voluntary participation. Comprehension of information is essential to informed consent. The researcher must determine that the participants understand the information provided to them. It is incumbent on the researcher to make sure that the participants understand the risks involved as well as the benefits. They also must be fully informed about the research protocol so that they can make informed choices. Voluntary participation implies that participants agree to be part of a study of their own free will without coercion of any kind.

Safety Alert *In obtaining informed consent, it is imperative that participants have adequate information to make a decision as to whether or not to participate. To avoid coercion, participants must be mentally capable of making a decision independently.*

In qualitative investigations, the idea of process consent is suggested rather than a traditional consent, which is signed at the beginning of a study and not reconsidered. In process consent, the researcher renegotiates the consent with participants as unforeseen circumstances arise, thereby allowing participants to be part of the decision making as the study unfolds.

Institutional Review Boards

Research involving humans is submitted for approval to an ethics committee, commonly referred to as an institutional review board (IRB) or an ethics review committee. The purpose of the review is to ensure that ethical principles are appropriately applied to research involving human subjects. Most institutions, hospitals, governmental agencies, and universities in which research involving human subjects is carried out require specific information to make informed and responsible decisions regarding the ethical acceptability of a proposal. These individual (organizational) mandates are derived from the Code of Federal Regulations, 1991, § 46111, which spells out the main requirements governing IRB decisions. Information typically included in an IRB submission includes: purpose of the study; study design and methodology; potential research participants; a description of the selection process; risks and benefits to the participants; steps to ensure participant choice, confidentiality, and anonymity protection; and areas of potential conflict of interest (Burns & Grove, 2009). Further information on IRBs is included in agency policy and also is found in research texts.

Vulnerable Subjects

When engaging in research, it is necessary to be aware of the populations described as vulnerable subjects. Federal regulations have described possible subjects that require additional consideration of protection as vulnerable subjects. These subjects may be incapable of giving informed consent (e.g., cognitively impaired people), or may be at high risk of unintended side effects because of their circumstances (e.g., pregnant women). These subjects include (Institutional Review Board for Health Sciences Research, 2008):

- ***Pregnant Women, Fetuses, and Neonates:*** The purpose of the research must "meet the needs" of the pregnant woman. There must be minimal risk to the fetus and the pregnant woman.
- ***Prisoners:*** Prisoners are a captured population. They may feel coerced into thinking they have no choice and they may be exposed to abuse.
- ***Children:*** Children are not competent to give informed consent, either legally or ethically. Informed consent must be obtained from the parent or guardian. Assent (agreement) from the child should be obtained, if appropriate. If the child is able to understand, written informed consent should be obtained.
- ***Cognitively Imparied Persons:*** Mentally or emotionally disabled individuals (senility, unconsciousness) cannot legally or ethically provide informed consent. Written consent should be obtained from the legal guardian.
- ***Students and Employees:*** Students and employees may feel coerced or threatened to participate since they have unequal power. They may feel compelled to participate, feeling that failure to participate may affect their grades or performance rewards.
- ***Minorities, Economically and/or Educationally Disadvantaged:*** Minorities may be impoverished and economically dependent. In addition, they may have language barriers that prohibit them from understanding the intent of the research. They may also be decisionally impaired.
- ***AIDS/HIV+ Subjects:*** These individuals are vulnerable due to the nature of their disease and there may be more risks than benefits. They may be subject to needless suffering.
- ***Terminally Ill Subjects.*** The risk/benefit ratio must be considered because there is most likely not a benefit to the individual. The patient's comfort must also be considered. Special procedures must be followed if the patients are mentally or physically incapacitated.

Specific issues that need to be carefully considered with these vulnerable subjects include informed consent, risk/benefit assessment, and research procedures. Research should be conducted only in the following circumstances: The risk is low and benefit is high, or there are no possible alternatives to the study.

Ethical research is guided by the principles of justice, respect for persons, and beneficence. Vulnerable subjects should be included in research, but only if special protections are provided to them. Researchers must take steps to ensure that their rights and welfare are protected. The institutional review board, previously discussed, has the responsibility to review research proposals to ensure that the rights and welfare of vulnerable subjects are protected.

Rules for Conducting Ethical Research

There are ethical rules that serve as guidelines for conducting research. These are organized around two themes: (1) nurse researchers' ethical responsibility to participants and (2) nurse researchers' responsibility to the discipline of nursing and society (Polit & Beck, 2012). These rules are summarized in Chart 3–11 (p. 70).

Rules for Socially Responsible Nursing Research

In addition to having ethical responsibilities to research participants, nurses also have responsibilities to society at large and the nursing discipline in particular. Research-minded practitioners, educators, administrators, nursing students, and other health care professionals expect nurse researchers to do ethical research. The end result of nursing studies is to shape nurses' practice and promote excellence in nursing care. To this end, researchers should conduct unbiased studies and report results in trustworthy manners; the seven rules that guide this process are explained as follows:

1. Researchers should distinguish between science and advocacy.
2. Do not hunt through data looking for pleasing findings.
3. Be aware of potential sources of bias.
4. Represent research literature fairly.
5. Do the best research possible.
6. Acknowledge all sources.
7. Seek advice on ethical issues (Polit & Beck, 2012).

Privacy and the Health Insurance Portability and Accountability Act

One of the rules of conducting ethical research is that of maintaining the privacy and confidentiality of participants. "Privacy is the right an individual has to determine the time, extent, and general circumstances under which personal information will be shared with or withheld from others" (Burns & Grove, 2009, p. 200). Personal information consists of an individual's attitudes, beliefs, behaviors, opinions, and records. The research subject's privacy is protected if the subject is informed and consents to participate in a study and voluntarily shares private information with the researcher. An invasion of privacy occurs when private information is shared without an individual's knowledge or against her will. This most frequently occurs during the data collection phase of the research process (e.g., when invasive or irrelevant questions are asked during an interview, an interview is taped without the subject's consent, or hidden cameras or mirrors are used to observe the subjects).

The Privacy Act of 1974 was enacted to safeguard subjects' privacy rights, and has led to scrutiny of data collection methods by an IRB or committee formed to review all research proposals. Improvements in technology were a precipitating factor for the Privacy Act as it became easier to collect and transmit data without the subject's knowledge or control. With the advent of the Internet and increased access to

Weblink: HIPAA Terms and Explanations

CHART 3–11 Rules for Conducting Ethical Research

Rule	Interpretation
Protect the confidentiality of participants.	Confidentiality is to be treated as a sacred trust, based on the ethical principle of respect for persons. If researchers need to identify individuals' names with particular questionnaires, then number codes, rather than names, should be used. If data are released to other researchers, steps should be taken to mask the individual identities of participants.
Do not put pressure on participants.	Based on the principle of respect for persons, pressure should not be put on participants to cooperate in the study. Respondents must feel free to refuse participation, to withdraw at any time, or to refuse to answer any particular question.
Make the subjects' participation painless and free from discomfort.	Researchers must not expose participants to needlessly long experimental trials or questionnaires or ask questions that pry unnecessarily into personal matters; only relevant information should be collected. Maintaining the comfort, safety, and self-esteem of the participants should be a central concern of researchers. This is based on the principle of beneficence, which requires one to do good and, above all, do no harm.
Identify sponsors.	Participants must be informed about who is doing the study.
Disclose the basis on which participants have been selected.	Participants have the right to know how they were selected for participation in a study. Respondents need to know if the selection was made by means of a probability sampling procedure or if it was based on special characteristics related to the research problem or phenomenon under investigation (e.g., age, health status, medical diagnosis). Selection of participants is based on the ethical principle of justice.
Place no hidden identification codes on questionnaires.	Do not place hidden identification codes on questionnaires to aid in the identification of those who have or have not returned questionnaires. If individuals are to be identified, this information should be placed directly on the questionnaire and discussed in a cover letter. The identification corresponding to participant names should be kept in a secure area to protect the identity of participants. Only the researcher should have access to this information.
Honor promises to provide participants with research reports.	When a promise to provide participants with a copy of the research report is made, this promise should be fulfilled to reinforce the idea of a reciprocal contract.
Informed consent is a key concern.	In dealing with competent adults, participation should be based on informed consent; potential participants must be informed about the nature of the study, what kinds of issues will be explored, how participants were selected, what the risk and benefits to the participants are, and who is sponsoring the research. Prospective participants also should be informed about confidentiality and anonymity; they should feel free to withdraw from the study at any time without prejudice. Any time selective nondisclosure of information or deception is used in a research study, the researcher must question how acceptable it is to do so. With deception, the risks to the participants should be minimal and outweighed by the benefits.
Debrief subjects.	When experiments or field studies involve deception, subjects should have the study explained to them after the session, informing them of what the deception was and why it was necessary.

information on individuals, including health information, the federal government enacted the Health Insurance Portability and Accountability Act (HIPAA) of 1996 (U.S. Department of Health and Human Services, 2011). HIPAA's privacy requirements are intended to guarantee individuals new rights and protections against the misuse or unauthorized disclosure of their health records. Though the law does not specifically target research, it does affect the manner in which research is conducted.

The HIPAA privacy regulations constitute an extensive reform of the way health care information is handled. While HIPAA allows for the disclosure of health information for research, it regulates disclosure beyond the common-rule regulations currently monitored by IRBs, making HIPAA a concern for everyone participating in research activities. There are three points at which the HIPAA privacy regulations impact nursing research: (1) accessing data from a covered entity (e.g., reviewing medical records of subjects), (2) creating data (e.g., an intervention study), and (3) disclosing data (e.g., with a colleague from another institution).

- ***Accessing Data:*** The covered organization has an obligation not to disclose information improperly when a researcher seeks data that includes private health information. A covered organization transmits information in an electronic form and includes health plans, health care clearinghouses, and health care agencies. All covered entities are required to comply with the Privacy Rule (Green, 2008). Researchers are expected to work closely with clinical agencies used as research sites to ensure that both sides meet HIPAA obligations. Individually identifiable health information (IIHI) data may be accessed for research under specific conditions. Pertinent access terms and explanations for IIHI can be found at www.hhs.gov/ocr/hipaa/pivruletxt.txt.
- ***Creating Data:*** Researchers also may be creating IIHI data. If the researcher is part of a covered entity, any protected health information obtained by any means is covered by HIPAA, and the researcher and his or her institution are bound by HIPAA regulations. When obtaining IIHI directly from the subject, the subject must authorize the use of the information. Essential elements of disclosure must be included in the authorization: Who will be receiving the information, what further disclosures the researcher anticipates, and what information will be disclosed to the researcher.
- ***Disclosing Data:*** Nurse researchers must be aware that sharing data with colleagues and students might constitute disclosures of IIHI, according to HIPAA regulations. The researcher is the holder of the IIHI and can disclose it only under appropriate conditions. When the researcher creates and holds IIHI, he must track any further disclosures made through waiver of authorization or in a review preparatory for research for 6 years and be prepared to report these to the former patient (LoBiondo-Wood & Haber, 2010; Wipke-Tevis & Pickett, 2007).

Safety Alert *HIPAA governs privacy in accessing data, creating data, and disclosing data. Violation of HIPAA may cause cessation of ongoing research study.*

A nurse may conclude that privacy of health information is widely accepted as an essential element of the researcher's obligation to respect the autonomy of subjects. To do this effectively, the nurse must understand HIPAA and its privacy provisions. They are of critical importance for current investigations as well as future research endeavors. The primary focus of HIPAA modifications in research protocols is in the area of informed consent. Additional information on HIPAA can be obtained from the HIPAA website. HIPAA also is discussed at length in Chapters 2 and 5.

Informatics

As has been noted, evidence-based practice is characterized by using the best available information when making clinical decisions, in lieu of intuition and unmethodical clinical experience. EBP is the current recommended standard in health care; many agree that it has the potential to improve patient care and outcomes. In order for EBP to be effective, however, information must be available and accessible, and practitioners must be skilled at using resources such as computers. Government mandates, consumer demands for accountability, professional efforts to improve quality, and organizational requirements for fiscally responsible patient care have all helped develop evidence-based practice. However, questions remain: "Are health care facilities ready to provide the resources that will enable nurses to participate in this best-practices model? And are nurses ready to meet the challenge?" Access to and skill in using informatics is essential to participating in evidence-based practice.

Informatics can be interpreted as a combination of computer science, information science, and health care science designed to assist in the management and delivery of health care. It encompasses the knowledge necessary to use the computer and programs effectively to retrieve, input, and use knowledge to assist in decision making. In the case of nursing research, informatics is used to retrieve information to support an identified problem, conduct a literature review, input data for analysis, complete statistical analyses, and share findings with colleagues (Ozbolt, Nahm, Roberts, & Wilson, 2007). A variety of computer programs, including specific research-oriented programs, may be used to analyze both quantitative and qualitative data. Research texts typically identify computer programs that may be used for data analysis (Burns & Grove, 2009). Every nurse is expected to have fundamental information management and computer literacy skills, although it is recognized that the level of skill needed may vary among nurse researchers. Skills may range from those of beginning nurses who have fundamental information management and computer technology skills to experienced nurses with proficiency in their domain of interest and information specialists. Information specialists are generally prepared at the baccalaureate or higher level of education and possess additional knowledge and skills specific to information management and computer technology. They focus on information needs for the practice of nursing, including education, administration, research, and clinical practice, and use critical thinking, data management skills, and computer skills in their practice (American Nurses Association, 2007).

The need for nurses to be skilled in informatics has been recognized in the IOM study on *The Future of Nursing: Leading Change, Advancing Health* (2010) as well as the Quality and Safety Education for Nurses (QSEN) project. QSEN has identified vital knowledge and skills undergraduate nurses are expected to have concerning the use of information and technology to communicate, manage knowledge, mitigate error, and support decision making (QSEN, 2010). Chart 3–12 describes these essential aspects of informatics skills.

CHART 3–12 QSEN Important Knowledge and Skills Concerning Informatics

Knowledge	Skills
Explain why information and technology skills are essential for safe patient care.	Seek education about how information is managed in care settings before providing care. Apply technology and information management tools to support safe processes of care.
Identify essential information that must be available in a common database to support patient care.	Navigate the electronic health record. Document and plan patient care in an electronic health record.
Contrast beliefs and limitations of different communication technologies and their impact on safety and quality.	Employ communication technologies to coordinate care for patients.
Describe examples of how technology and information management are related to the quality and safety of patient care.	Respond appropriately to clinical decision-making supports and alerts. Use information management tools to monitor outcomes of care processes.
Recognize the time, effort, and skill required for computers, databases and other technologies to become reliable and effective tools for patient care.	Use high-quality electronic sources of health care information.

Source: QSEN website. (November 2010). http://www.qsen.org/ksas_prelicensure.php

The Research Critique

Applying research findings to practice is now recognized as essential to developing scientifically based nursing practice. A key step in this process is the ability of nurses to read nursing research studies and determine their usefulness for practice. To determine if the research is useful and applicable, the nurse must evaluate the completed research, identifying areas of adequacy and inadequacy and virtues as well as faults. This **research critique** is an intellectual process of a careful, complete examination of a study to judge its strengths, weaknesses, logical links, meaning, and significance (Coughlan, Cronin, & Ryan, 2007). The critique involves a high level of critical thinking and an analysis of each component of the study. A quality study focuses on a significant problem, demonstrates sound methodology, produces credible findings, and is easily replicated by other researchers. A critique appraisal involves judging whether or not a research study meets these quality standards and if the study is described clearly and comprehensively enough to decide if the findings and implications are logical and believable, generalizable to other populations, and should be seriously considered in practice.

Generally, research is critiqued to broaden understanding, summarize knowledge for use in practice, and provide a base for the conduct of a study (Polit & Beck, 2012). Research critiques are performed by nursing students, nursing instructors, practicing nurses, and nurse researchers. Each may have a different intent and focus; however, they all follow a similar process. For example, in nursing education, a critique often is seen as the first step in learning the research process. Students develop critical thinking skills, strengthen their knowledge base, and increase their use of research findings in practice. Critiques of studies by practicing nurses are essential for the implementation of evidence-based practice. These critiques tend to focus on the scientific merit of the study and on its implications for nursing practice. Educators conduct research critiques to expand their knowledge base and improve the educational process; researchers conduct critiques to plan and implement a study. This section focuses on the general guidelines that can be used by any group to conduct a research critique.

Specific elements must be considered when critiquing a research study. Both quantitative and qualitative studies are used to improve nursing practice. Critiques of both are discussed.

Quantitative Research Critique

The following criteria may be used to evaluate quantitative research studies:

1. A relevant and clearly articulated statement of purpose
2. Consistency between the stated purpose and problem statement or question or hypothesis
3. A comprehensive literature review that identifies gaps in the research area and logically leads to the research questions under study
4. A theoretical or conceptual framework that provides a rationale for the study
5. A congruent match between the purpose, design, and method
6. An appropriate sample and sample selection procedures
7. Statistical procedures appropriate to the type of data collected and research questions posed
8. Adequate reliability and validity to accept findings and generalize to right populations
9. Significance of study for nursing is apparent (LoBiondo-Wood & Haber, 2010).

The actual review of a quantitative study uses the criteria just set forth and divides the critique into four stages of review:

- Stage 1 refers to a review of the purpose, problem statement, and congruency with design and methodology. The reviewer must gain a clear understanding of the meaning of the purpose and problem statement and determine if the research design and methodology are consistent with the study purpose.
- Stage 2 focuses on the conduct of the research. This refers to studying the manner in which the research was conducted and includes determining if the methodology was applied correctly.
- Stage 3 refers to studying the findings of the research and assessing if the outcomes and conclusions are believable and supported by the findings. The focus is on the research outcomes.
- Stage 4 summarizes the overall quality of the study, identifying the strengths and limitations of the study, and evaluating the contributions of the study to nursing. At this point, the reviewer also looks for suggestions for improving the work of the researcher.

Chart 3–13 (p. 73) shows key questions that can be asked by the reviewer when critiquing quantitative designs.

Qualitative Research Critique

Critical evaluation of qualitative studies uses different standards than those of quantitative research due to the nature of the study. Qualitative studies emerge from the naturalistic-inductive paradigm and, as such, are based on a different set of assumptions and a different worldview; they also have a different purpose than quantitative studies. Qualitative research hopes to promote understanding of phenomena. A scholarly critique of qualitative studies includes a balanced evaluation of a study's strengths and weaknesses. Five standards have been proposed to evaluate qualitative studies (Burns & Grove, 2009; Speziale & Carpenter, 2010):

- ***Standard 1: Descriptive Vividness***—With **descriptive vividness,** the site, participants, experience of collecting data, and thinking of the researcher are described so clearly that the reader has the sense of personally experiencing the event.
- ***Standard 2: Methodological Congruence***—**Methodological congruence** has four dimensions: documentation rigor, procedural rigor, ethical rigor, and auditability (Burns & Grove, 2009). All elements of the study must be clearly documented: the study subject, significance, purpose, research questions, assumptions, ethical implications, sampling methods, data gathering and analysis strategies, theoretical development, conclusions, and implications for practice. Documentation regarding these study elements must be clear and complete. Procedural rigor should be evident in that the researcher should clearly state the steps taken to ensure that data were accurately recorded and that the data obtained were representative of the data as a whole. Ethical rigor is reflected in the researcher's discussion of the ethical implications related to the study, informed consent, and protection of participants' rights. **Auditability** refers to a *decision trail.* The research report should be sufficiently detailed to allow a second reader, using the original data and the decision trail, to arrive at conclusions similar to those of the original researcher.
- ***Standard 3: Analytical Preciseness***—**Analytical preciseness** requires the researcher to make the effort needed to identify and record the decision-making processes through which concrete data are transformed into a theory or explanation of the phenomenon being studied.
- ***Standard 4: Theoretical Connectedness***—**Theoretical connectedness** requires that the theoretical schema developed from the study be clearly expressed, logically consistent, reflective of the data, and compatible with the practice of nursing. The reviewer must be able to follow the researcher's logical flow of thought and be able to analyze and evaluate the adequacy of the resulting theoretical schema that emerges from the research, as well as its connection to theory development within the discipline of nursing.
- ***Standard 5: Heuristic Relevance***—The results of the study should have **heuristic relevance** for the reader. "This value is reflected in the reader's ability to recognize the phenomenon described in the study, its theoretical significance, its applicability to nursing practice situations, and its influence on future research activities" (Burns & Grove, 2009, p. 613). Relevance includes intuitive recognition, relationship to existing body of knowledge, and applicability.

Key questions can be used to critique a qualitative research report (Burns & Grove, 2009; Ryan, Coughlan, & Cronin, 2007). They are grouped in four stages consistent with a review of quantitative research and are shown in Chart 3–14.

CHART 3–13 Key Questions Asked When Critiquing Quantitative Designs

STAGE 1 QUESTIONS: CRITICAL APPRAISAL OF PURPOSE, PROBLEM STATEMENT, AND CONGRUENCY WITH DESIGN AND METHODOLOGY

Purpose or Problem Statement

- Are the study problem and purpose statement clearly articulated?
- Are the reasons for conducting the study stated?
- Is the study's potential contribution to nursing knowledge stated?
- Are the research objectives or research questions or hypotheses stated clearly and researchable (answerable through the collection of empirical data)?
- Are terms defined conceptually and operationally?

Literature Review

- Does the literature review or theoretical framework provide evidence that the classic and current literature has been synthesized, and placed the research question in the proper context?
- Does the literature review identify gaps in knowledge, suggest how the current study extends the knowledge base in this area, and point out contradictions in the current knowledge base?
- Does the researcher summarize the literature review, provide a rationale for the current study, and show how this study will extend previous research?

Design

- Is the study design specified, including its advantages and limitations for the research problem?
- Is there evidence a pilot study had been conducted and findings used to enhance the design?
- Is the design (overall plan of research) appropriate to the research purpose and capable of answering the research question?
- How does the design control for extraneous variables?

Sample

- Was probability or nonprobability sampling used and the reason for the choice specified?
- Is the population to whom results will be generalized described?
- Are precautions taken to avoid collecting a biased sample that would limit generalizability of the findings?
- Are the demographic characteristics of the sample described?
- Is the sample representative of the population?
- Are inclusion and exclusion criteria identified?
- Is the sample size appropriate to meet assumptions of statistical tests?

Data Collection

- Are data collection methods appropriate to meet the study purpose and answer the questions or hypotheses?
- What evidence is provided that data collection procedures are valid and reliable?
- Are adaptations to data collection tools described?
- Are data collection instruments described in sufficient detail to enable readers to ascertain the method of scoring and range of values and what a particular score means?

Data Analysis

- Are data analysis procedures described?
- Are the statistical techniques appropriate for the study methodology (i.e., the type of data collected and analysis)?
- Do the statistical tests answer the research questions and specify the level of significance?
- If results are nonsignificant, is a power analysis conducted to explore nonsignificant findings?

STAGE 2 QUESTIONS: CRITICAL APPRAISAL OF THE CONDUCT OF THE RESEARCH

Human Rights

- How are the rights of research participants protected?
- Are ethical issues anticipated and handled appropriately?

Procedures

- Are techniques used to ensure that there is consistency in the data collection process?
- What procedures were used to keep research conditions the same for all participants?
- Are there strategies to limit errors in data collection, recording, and analysis?
- Did any unplanned circumstances influence the results?
- In experimental designs, is there evidence of manipulation of independent variables, randomization in selection of sample and assignment to experimental and control groups, and control of extraneous variables?

STAGE 3 QUESTIONS: CRITICAL APPRAISAL OF RESEARCH OUTCOMES

Findings

- Are the findings presented clearly and correctly, and are they related to the theoretical framework?
- Is there a clear statement of whether or not the data support the hypotheses or answer each research question?
- Are tables and graphs clearly labeled, easy to comprehend, and congruent with results?
- Are findings presented in an unbiased manner?

Discussion

- Are alternative approaches offered for the findings?
- Does the researcher discuss both the clinical and statistical significance of the findings?
- Does the researcher overgeneralize the findings beyond the appropriate population?
- Are limitations of the study such as sample size, inadequate instruments, sources of bias, and so on, identified and their implications discussed?

Implications and Conclusions

- Does the researcher identify important implications of the study for practice, education, or research (if appropriate)?
- How do the findings of the study advance nursing knowledge?
- Do new research questions emerge from the study?

STAGE 4 QUESTIONS: CRITICAL APPRAISAL OF THE OVERALL STUDY

Overall Quality

- What are the major strengths of the study?
- What are the major limitations of the study?
- Was the study described in sufficient detail to facilitate a replication study?
- What are the major contributions of this study to knowledge development in nursing?
- What suggestions might enhance the study and correct the limitations?

Sources: Adapted from Coughlan, M., Cronin, P., & Ryan, F. (2007). Step-by-step guide to critiquing research. Part 1: Quantitative research. *British Journal of Nursing, 16*(11), 658–664. LoBiondo-Wood, G., & Haber, J. (2010). Nursing research: Methods and critical appraisal for evidence-based practice. St. Louis: Mosby. Polit, D. F., & Beck, C. T. (2008). *Nursing research: Principles and methods* (8th ed.). Philadelphia: Lippincott Williams & Wilkins.

CHART 3–14 Key Questions for Critiquing Qualitative Designs

STAGE 1 QUESTIONS: CRITICAL APPRAISAL OF PURPOSE, STATEMENT OF RESEARCH PHENOMENON, AND CONGRUENCE WITH DESIGN AND METHODOLOGY

Purpose or Statement of the Phenomenon of Interest

- Is the research phenomenon of interest clearly stated?
- Is rationale provided for approaching the study in an inductive, qualitative manner?
- Is the philosophy of the research tradition described?
- Is a statement of self-understanding included?
- Is there a single broad research question? Are their subquestions?
- Does the initial question become more focused as data are collected and analyzed?
- Is the study purpose clearly stated (e.g., discovery, description, theory building, and so on)?

Literature Review

- Does the qualitative method used call for a literature review before data collection?
- Does the review indicate that the researcher has expertise in the chosen area, know where gaps exist, and show how this study will eliminate such gaps?
- If a review is appropriate only after data collection, is there evidence that this is done?
- Is a framework appropriate? If so, is it presented clearly?

Design

- Is the design (i.e., overall plan for the research) appropriate to the research purpose?
- Is there congruency between the methodology and the research question?
- Is the context for the study adequately described?
- Is the researcher–participant relationship understood?

Sample

- Is purposive sampling used?
- Are informants capable of informing the study?
- Is the selection of participants appropriate to allow for saturation of data?

Data Collection

- Is data collection congruent with study purpose, research question, and qualitative custom?
- Are prolonged engagement and persistent observation in the field used to build trust with participants and ensure validity of data collection?
- Are data collection strategies and procedures described in sufficient detail?

Data Analysis

- Are data analysis procedures clearly described and appropriate to the research tradition?
- What evidence is provided that data collection and analysis are concurrent and ongoing?
- Is there evidence of decision rules for analyzing data; does the researcher remain true to rules?
- What evidence is there of narrowing the coding as categories are systematically discarded when they are unsupported by the data and the researcher becomes more focused on data collection and analysis?
- Is there evidence of "theoretical saturation?"

STAGE 2 QUESTIONS: CRITICAL APPRAISAL OF THE CONDUCT OF THE RESEARCH

Human Rights

- How are the rights of research participants protected?
- Are ethical issues anticipated and handled appropriately?

Procedures

- What evidence is provided that research meets the criteria of rigor (credibility: findings must be understood and viewed as credible by the informants; trustworthiness: an individual can believe the findings are true; and usefulness: findings shed light on an important phenomenon)?
- Creswell (2007) identifies eight procedures for testing the truth value (appropriate representation of multiple realities) and notes that researchers should use at least two of these in any given study. The critic should ask which of the following the researcher uses:
  1. Prolonged engagement and persistent observation in the field to build trust with participants, learn about culture and context, and correct distortions introduced by researcher's presence.
  2. Triangulation for purpose of corroborating evidence from different sources to shed light on a theme or perspective.
  3. Peer review as an external check of the research process; this person asks hard questions about the method, meanings, and interpretations and keeps the researcher honest.
  4. Negative case analysis, in which the researcher reworks the hypothesis until all cases fit it.
  5. The researcher articulates researcher bias so that the reader knows what prejudices, biases, or past experiences have shaped the researcher's approach to the study.
  6. Member checks to solicit informants' opinions of the accuracy and credibility of the findings and conclusions. Some methods, however, such as hermeneutic analysis, do not always conduct member checks because their emphasis is on the research team's interpretation of the meaning of the participants' experience in the research project.
  7. External audits in which a consultant examines both the process and product of the qualitative study to assess accuracy and determine if the findings, interpretations, and conclusions are supported by the data.
  8. Rich, in-depth descriptions of participants and setting are provided so that the reader can make decisions regarding transferability of findings to other settings.

STAGE 3 QUESTIONS: CRITICAL APPRAISAL OF THE RESEARCH OUTCOMES

Findings

- Are the findings contextualized (i.e., presented within the context of the circumstances that influence their interpretation)?
- Do readers of the report recognize the phenomenon or vicariously experience it?
- Are the findings true to the data?
- Do the themes, categories, or theoretical statements present a comprehensive, plausible, and meaningful picture of the phenomenon?
- If models, diagrams, or figures are used, are they effective?

(continued)

CHART 3–14 Key Questions for Critiquing Qualitative Designs, *continued*

- Are the findings compatible with the field of nursing's knowledge base?
- Are reasons for incompatible findings explored by the researcher?

Discussion, Implications, and Conclusions

- Does the researcher identify implications of the study for nursing (i.e., in practice, theory building, instrument development, education, and research)?
- Is a context provided in which to use the findings?
- Do the implications and conclusions follow logically from the findings?
- Do new research questions emerge from the findings?

STAGE 4 QUESTIONS: CRITICAL APPRAISAL OF THE OVERALL QUALITY OF THE STUDY

- What are the major strengths of the study?
- What are the major limitations of the study?
- What are the major contributions of this study to knowledge development in the field of nursing?
- What suggestions might enhance the study and correct the limitations?

Sources: Adapted from Burns, N., & Grove, S. K. (2009). *The practice of nursing research: Appraisal, synthesis, and generation of evidence* (6th ed.). Elsevier. Ryan, F., Coughlan, M., & Cronin, P. (2007). Step-by-step guide to critiquing research. Part 2: Qualitative research. *British Journal of Nursing, 16*(12), 738–744.

Incorporated in both types of research critique is an assessment of the validity and reliability of the study conducted. **Validity** refers to the extent to which a concept, conclusion, or measurement is well-founded and corresponds accurately to the real world. *Internal validity* refers to the extent to which it is possible to make an inference that the independent variable of the study truly is causing or influencing the dependent variable and that the relationship between the two is not the spurious effect of an extraneous variable. *External validity* refers to the generalizability of the reserach findings to other settings or samples. **Reliability** is the consistency of a set of measurements or of a measuring instrument, often used to describe a test. Reliability is inversely related to random error. Each research study, when critiqued, should be examined for validity and reliability. Chart 3–15 explains types of validity, internal and external, and their effects on the reliaibility of a study.

CHART 3–15 Validity in Research

Type of Validity and Characteristics	Threats to Validity
Internal Validity The extent to which an inference can be made that the independent variable has caused or influenced the dependent variable.	Temporal ambiguity: Ambiguity of whether the independent variable preceded the dependent variable and vice versa. Selection threat: Selection bias in randomness of subjects, or subjects who do not select a treatment in a study. History threat: Events happening concurrently with the independent variable. Mortality: Arises from attrition in groups being compared.
Internal Consistency The extent that an instrument's items measure the same trait. Most widely used by nurse researchers.	Measurement error: Sampling of items that do not focus on the same trait.
Equivalence Concerns the degree to which two or more independent observers or coders agree about the scoring on an instrument. High level of agreement assumes that measurement errors have been minimized.	Poor interrater reliability: *Interrater reliability* is a measure used to examine the agreement between two people (raters/observers) on the assignment of categories of a categorical variable. It is an important measure in determining how well an implementation of some coding or measurement system works. Acceptable levels of interrater reliability fall between 70% and 100%.
External Validity Concerns inferences about the extent to which relationships observed in a study hold true across different situations and contexts. This has become a major concern in EBP. Replication of studies is important to external validity. Multisite studies are powerful with more confidence in generalizability of the results.	The lack of controlled research settings. The ability to generalize findings to the larger population is impacted by sample characteristics.
Construct Validity Exemplars of treatments, outcomes, and settings are stand-ins for general constructs. Inference is made from the particulars of the study to the higher-order construct they are intended to represent.	Construct errors result in the risk that the evidence will be misleading.

Source: Polit, D. F., & Beck, C. T. (2012). *Essentials of nursing research: Appraising evidence for nursing practice* (7th ed.). Philadelphia: Wolters Kluwer/Lippincott Williams & Wilkins, pp. 246–249, 375–376.

Future Perspectives of Nursing Research

Research is critical to acquiring new knowledge and developing the practice of nursing. Knowledge provided through research changes practice, education, and health policy. Applying research findings to practice helps ensure the highest possible quality care is delivered in a cost-effective manner. This is critical to the future of nursing and health care. If nursing is to assume its "rightful" role in transforming the health care system and improving patient care across the continuum from health promotion to disease prevention, to coordination of care, to cure and/or palliative care, research must become an integral role of all nurses (IOM, 2010).

Because knowledge is the foundation for the evolution of nursing practice, all nurses can and must develop and apply research skills in practice. Research begins at the bedside. As a professional nurse, the level of educational preparation will influence the role each nurse plays in research. Though the trend is toward an expanded researcher role with advanced education, nurses at all levels of roles and responsibilities assume a role when it comes to nursing research.

The vision for nursing in the 21st century is to narrow the gap between research and practice by helping nurses base their decisions and practice strategies on the best available evidence, thereby improving nursing care and patient outcomes. As the levels of sophistication and complexity in nursing increase, use of the scientific process to improve patient care and outcomes becomes more crucial, as does educational preparation for engaging in research activities. Thus, research utilization is a critical step in improving nursing care and ultimately patients' outcomes. It is, therefore, incumbent on all nurses to understand and use the research process, and to participate in the critical process of research review and utilization. This chapter has presented the basic guidelines for assisting learners to garner that knowledge, and has provided a background for interpreting research findings and future research goals presented throughout this book.

Future Research Goals

It is apparent that research and evidence-based practice are an integral part of nursing's future. The profession has been challenged to conduct and participate in independent and collaborative research endeavors. Only when nursing steps up to this challenge can the profession improve the health care delivery system and the patients that are cared for. The national research themes for the future endorse the concepts of improving patient care. Additionally, the profession of nursing is looking for individual and collective endorsement of research and evidence-based practice to improve future practice. The National Institute for Nursing Research developed a plan for 2001–2010 research themes; the plan continues on into 2012 and is shown in Chart 3–16.

The Robert Wood Foundation, in concert with the American Association of Colleges of Nursing, also developed a research agenda based on the findings of the Institute of Medicine (IOM) report, *The Future of Nursing: Leading Change, Advancing Health*. Their research questions focused on education, leadership, interprofessional collaboration, and data. A sampling of research questions under each of these broad categories is shown in Chart 3–17.

CHART 3–16 Research Themes for the Future

1. Changing lifestyle behaviors for better health
2. Managing the effects of chronic illness to improve health and quality of life:
   - Health care practice
   - Self-management of chronic illness symptoms and treatment
   - Informal (family) caregiving.
3. Identifying effective strategies to reduce health disparities
4. Harnessing advanced technologies to serve human needs
5. Enhancing the end-of-life experience for patients and their families

Source: National Institute of Nursing Research. (2005–2010). *Research themes for the future.* Bethesda, MD: National Institutes of Health.

CHART 3–17 Sample of Research Questions Derived from the Institute of Medicine (IOM) Report *Future of Nursing: Leading Change, Advancing Health* (2010)

Education
- How effective are various interprofessional education models?
- What is the opportunity cost of adding new different modules to the nursing curriculum?

Leadership
- How can nurses best be prepared and enabled to lead change to advance health?
- What new technologies support nursing decision making and care delivery?

Interprofessional Collaboration
- How do independently practicing APRNs collaborate with primary care or specialist physicians?
- What policies and procedures foster teamwork and professional collaboration?

Data
- What percent of APRNs go into primary care?
- Are there differences in documented care errors, newer events, or malpractice claims between states with independent APRN practice and those with barriers to independent practice?

Full information on all potential research questions can be obtained from the source listed below.

Source: Research Agenda at http:www.thefutureofnursing.org/research.

Summary

This chapter is based on the premise that research is an integral part of nursing practice. Within this context the learner is provided with an explanation of nursing research, the various types of research, and the research process. The steps that are taken to conduct research are explained with the differences between quantitative research and qualitative research exemplified. Major emphasis is placed on research utilization and evidence-based practice within a changing health care environment. Research and ethics in health care are discussed, and the learner is guided through the development of a research critique for use with quantitative and qualitative studies.

NCLEX® PRACTICE

1. The nurse is planning a study using basic research. This nurse is most likely going to be studying:
   1. the effectiveness of a type of wound dressing.
   2. the frequency of side effects from one particular medication.
   3. how Orem's theory can be applied to the nursing process.
   4. the effectiveness of teaching self-insulin administration to a patient diagnosed with diabetes mellitus.
2. The nurse researcher is conducting a quantitative research study. Which of the following will most likely be done during this study?
   1. Change the study design as information is collected.
   2. Approach the process in a circular method rather than a straight line.
   3. Collect numerical values within a controlled situation.
   4. Use a small sample size.
3. The nurse researcher is completing a critique of a quantitative research study. In stage 3 of this critique the nurse will include which of the following questions to guide the critique. (select all that apply)
   1. Does the literature review identify gaps in knowledge, suggest how the current study extends the knowledge base in this area, and point out contradictions in the current knowledge base?
   2. Are the findings presented clearly and correctly, and related to the theoretical framework?
   3. Is there a clear statement of whether or not the data support the hypotheses or answer each research question?
   4. Are tables and graphs clearly labeled, easy to comprehend, and congruent with results?
   5. Do the themes, categories, or theoretical statements present a comprehensive, plausible, and meaningful picture of the phenomenon?
4. The Nursing Quality Improvement Committee is planning to conduct a research study that will involve the collection of patient data. The group plans to share the results with the members of the clinical staff of other community agencies. To ensure compliance with HIPAA regulations the group must ensure what process is followed before sharing data?
   1. Ask the staff members to sign a non-disclosure agreement.
   2. Review with all staff the procedure for gathering data.
   3. Remove all information that may identify a subject from reports and data display.
   4. Include a list of all patients who gave consent to have their information included.
5. A nurse researcher is determining the best design to use for a research project. Which of the following can be used as a guide for this design?
   1. Identify methods used to collect data.
   2. Identify approaches used to analyze the data.
   3. Determine if the study is a quantitative or qualitative research study.
   4. Write out the research problem or question.
6. The nurse is teaching a group of students about the importance of nursing research. In this instruction, the nurse should include which statement(s)? (select all that apply)
   1. Nursing research has influence on how care is delivered.
   2. Cost of care may be the topic of nursing research studies.
   3. Good nursing research must use quantitative methods.
   4. Nursing research develops the foundation of nursing practice.
   5. Compared to other fields, nursing research is relatively inflexible in terms of interpretation.

Answers to NCLEX Practice questions can be found in Appendix D in the Osborn Student Resources at nursing.pearsonhighered.com. Practice additional NCLEX questions online at the Student Resources site.

Pearson Nursing Student Resources Find additional review materials at: **nursing.pearsonhighered.com**

REFERENCES

Agency for Healthcare Research and Quality. (2010). Evidence-based practice centers. Retrieved from http://www.ahrq.gov/clinic/epc

American Nurses Association. (1976). *Preparation for nurses for participation research.* Kansas City, MO: Author.

American Nurses Association. (1994). Education for participation in nursing research. Retrieved from http://www.AmericanNursesAssociation.org

American Nurses Association. (2007). *Scope and standards of nursing informatics practice.* Washington, DC: Author.

American Nurses Association. (2012). The nursing process. Retrieved from http://www.nursingworld.org/EspeciallyForYou/What-is-Nursing/Tools-You-Need/Thenursingprocess.html

Anderson, R., & Kerfoot, K. (2011). The time has come for evidence-based staffing and scheduling. *Nursing Economics.* Press Room. Retrieved from http://www.ncbi.nlm.nih.gov/pubmed/19927442

Ardery, G., Herr, K. A., Titler, M. G., Sorofman, B. A., & Schmitt, M. G. (2003). Assessing and managing acute pain in older adults: A research base to guide practice. *MedSurg Nursing, 12*(il), 7, 13.

Bandura, A. (2001). Self-efficacy and health. In N. J. Smelser & P. B. Baltes (Eds.), *International encyclopedia of the social and behavioral sciences* (Vol. 20, pp. 13815–13820). Oxford: Elsevier Science.

Becker, M. (1978). The Health Belief Model and sick role behavior. *Nursing Digest, 6,* 35–40.

Burns, N., & Grove, S. K. (2009). *The practice of nursing research: Appraisal, synthesis, and generation of evidence* (6th ed.). Philadelphia: Elsevier.

Carlson, C. L. (2009). Use of three evidence-based postoperative pain assessment practices for registered nurses. *Pain Management Nursing, 10*(4), 174–187.

Cooper, S., Endacott, R., & Chapman, Y. (2009). Qualitative research: Specific designs for qualitative research in emergency care? *Emergency Medicine Journal, 25*(10), 773–778.

Coughlan, M., Cronin, P., & Ryan, F. (2007). Step-by-step guide to critiquing research. Part 1: Quantitative research. *British Journal of Nursing, 16*(11), 658–664.

Creswell, J. (2007). *Qualitative inquiry and research design: Choosing among five approaches* (2nd ed.). Thousand Oaks, CA: Sage.

Crowther, M. (2003). Evidence-based development of a hospital based heart failure centre. *Evidence-Based Nursing, 6,* 4–6.

DeBourgh, G. A. (2001). Champions for evidence-based practice: A critical role for advanced practice nurses. *AACN Clinical Issues, 12*(4), 491–508.

Drury, P. (2010). Barriers to evidenced-based nursing care: Listen to the clinicians. Retrieved from http://www.ciap.health.nsw.gov.au/hosppolic/stvincents/stvin98/a9.html

Ferrell, B. R. (2010). Palliative care research: Nursing response to emergent society needs. *Nursing Science Quarterly, 23*(3), 221–225.

Flaugher, M. (2012). Quoted in EBP and nursing research: Avoiding confusion. Adapted from HCPro's Advisor to the ANCC Magnet Recognition Program, February 2010, HCPro, Inc. Retrieved from http://www.strategiesfornursemanager.com/content.cfm?content_id=248282&oc_id=602

Green, S. M. (2008). *Impact of the HIPAA privacy rule in the HMO research network.* Washington, DC: National Academy of Sciences.

Hasmiller, S. (2010). Nursing's role in healthcare reform. *American Nurse Today, 5*(9). Retrieved from http://www.americannursetoday.com/article/aspx?id=7086a&fid=6850

International Review Board for Health Sciences Research. (2008). *Vulnerable subjects. University of Virginia IRB-HSR Research Guidance.* Retrieved from http://www.virginia.edu/vpr/irb/hsr/vulnerable_subjects.html

Institute of Medicine (IOM). (2011). *The future of nursing: Leading change, advancing health.* Washington, DC: The Academic Press.

Internet Encyclopedia of Philosophy (IEP). (2009). Ethics. Retrieved from http://www.iep.utm.edu/ethics/

Keren, G., & Willemsen, M. C. (2009). Decision anomalies, experimenter assumptions, and participants' comprehension: Revaluating the uncertainty effect. *Journal of Behavioral Decision Making, 22*(3), 301–317.

Langone, M. (2008). The use of ethical inquiry as a theoretical basis for qualitative research. Retrieved from http://voices.yahoo.com/the-ethical-inquiry-as-theoretical-basis-1831188.html

Marquis, B. L., & Huston, C. J. (2009). *Leadership roles and managment functions in nursing: theory and application.* (6th ed.). Philadelphia: Wolters Kluwer Health/Lippincott Williams & Wilkins.

LoBiondo-Wood, G., & Haber, J. (2010). *Nursing research: Methods and critical appraisal for evidence-based practice.* St. Louis: Mosby.

National Commission for the Protection of Human Subjects of Biomedical and Behavioral Research. (1978). *Belmont Report: Ethical principles and guidelines for research involving human subjects.* Washington, DC: U.S. Government Printing Office.

National Institute of Nursing Research (NINR). (2001–2010). Focus on NINR and NIH roadmap. Retrieved from http://www.ninr.nih.gov/NR/rdonlyres/2C476ABF-E1F7-4BA3-B6F5-06EDF71225DE/0/RoadmapFocusFINAL113006.pdf

Nightingale, F. (1859). *Notes on nursing: What it is and what it is not.* Philadelphia: J. B. Lippincott.

Omery, A., & Williams, R. P. (1999). An appraisal of research utilization across the United States. *Journal of Nursing Administration, 29,* 50–56.

Osboldt, J., Nahm, E. S., Roberts, D., & Wilson, M. (2007, September). How about a career in nursing informatics? *American Nurse Today, 2*(9). Retrieved from http://www.americannursetoday.com/assets/0/434/436/440/5492/5494/5540/5542/040897ed-4278-4f83-ac66-e015676e38d7.pdf

Poe, S. S., Cvach, M. M., Gartrell, D. G., Radzik, B. R., & Joy, T. L. (2005). An evidence-based approach to fall risk assessment, prevention and management. *Journal of Nursing Care Quality, 20*(2),107–116.

Polit, D. F., & Beck, C. T. (2012). *Nursing research: generating and assessing evidence for nursing practice.* Philadelphia: Wolters Kluwer/Lippincott Williams & Wilkins.

Porter, S. (April 16, 2007). Validity, trustworthiness and rigour: Reasserting realism in qualitative research. *JAN (Journal of Advanced Nursing) Research Methodology,* 79–86.

QSEN. (2010). Knowledge, skills, attitudes concerning informatics. Retrieved from http://www.qsen.org/ksas_prelicensure.php

Resnik, D. G. (2010). What is ethics in research & why is it important? National Institute of Environmental Health Sciences. Retrieved from http://www.niehs.nih.gov/research/resources/bioethics/whatis.cfm

Roy, Sr., C., & Jones, D. A. (2007). *Nursing knowledge development and clinical practice.* New York: Springer.

Ryan, F., Coughlan, M., & Cronin. (2007). Step-by-step guide to critiquing research. Part 2: Qualitative research. *British Journal of Nursing, 16*(12), 738–744.

Scannapieco, F. A., Yu, J., Raghavendran, K., Vacanti, A., Owens, S. I., Wood, K., & Mylotte, J. M. (2009). A randomized trial of chlorhexidine gluconate on oral bacterial pathogens in mechanically ventilated patients. *Critical Care, 13,* R117. doi:10.1186/cc7967

Silva, M. C. (1995). *Ethical guidelines in the conduct, dissemination, and implementation of nursing research.* Washington, DC: American Nurses Publishing of the ANA.

Smith, J. R., & Donze, A. (January–March 2010). Assessing environmental readiness: First steps in developing an evidence-based practice implementation. *Journal of Perinatal and Neonatal Nursing, 24*(1), 61–71.

Speziale, H. J. S., & Carpenter, D. R. (2010). *Qualitative research in nursing: Advancing the humanistic imperative* (5th ed.). Philadelphia: Lippincott Williams & Wilkins.

Stetler, C. B. (1994). Refinement of the Stetler/Maram model for application of research findings into practice. *Nursing Outlook, 42,* 15–35.

The Joanna Briggs Institute (JBI). (2001). Music as intervention in hospitals. *Best Practice: Evidence-Based Information Sheets for Health Professionals, 5*(4), 1–6.

The Joanna Briggs Institute (JBI). (2009). Music as intervention in hospitals. *Best Practice: Evidence Based Information Sheets for Health Professionals, 13*(3), 13–16.

The Joanna Briggs Institute for Evidence Based Nursing and Midwifery. (2012). Retrieved from http://www.joannabriggs.edu.au/

U.S. Department of Health and Human Services, Office for Civil Rights. (2003). Standards for privacy of individually identifiable health information. *Code of Federal Regulations,* Title 45, Parts 160 & 164. Retrieved from http://www.hhs.gov/ocr/hipaa/privruletxt.txt

U.S. Department of Health and Human Services. (2011). Understanding health information privacy. Retrieved from http://www.hhs.gov/ocr/privacy/hipaa/understanding/index.htm

Wipke-Tevis, D. D., & Pickett, M. A. (2007). Impact of HIPAA on subject recruitment and retention. *Western Journal of Nursing Research, 30*(1), 39–53.

Wolf, K. A. (2010). Moving nursing beyond ritualistic practice. Retrieved from http://www.nursetogether.com/tabid/102/itemid/1436/Moving-Nursing-Beyond-Ritualistic-Practice.aspx

Nursing Care Delivery Systems

4 CHAPTER

Cynthia Parkman
Annita Watson

Outcome-Based Learning Objectives

After studying this chapter, the learner will be able to:

1. Distinguish among the four types of nursing care delivery systems most commonly used in health care settings, their effect on nurses, and their impact on quality of care.
2. Determine the differences of the nursing role in the four traditional care delivery models for nursing practice.
3. Outline the delegation and leadership responsibilities of the registered nurse for each of the four traditional nursing care delivery systems.
4. Explain the economic variables influencing the selection of a nursing care delivery system.
5. Differentiate the roles of advanced practice nurses and case managers within the context of the four traditional nursing care delivery systems identified in this chapter.
6. Design modifed approaches to nursing care delivery systems based on the findings of the Institute of Medicine (IOM)/Robert Wood Johnson (RWJ) study on the future of nursing.

KEY TERMS

acuity p.80
advanced practice nurse (APRN) p.81
assignment p.82
associate caregiver p.87
associate nurse p.87
case manager p.81
case method p.84
certified nurse midwife (CNM) p.81
certified registered nurse anesthetist (CRNA) p.81
clinical nurse leader (CNL) p.81
clinical nurse specialist (CNS) p.81
community-based care p.89
community health nursing p.89
delegation p.81
functional nursing p.84
licensed vocational/practical nurse (LVN/LPN) p.84
magnet hospital p.88
medication nurse p.84
modular nursing p.86
nurse practitioner (NP) p.81
nursing care delivery systems p.79
patient-centered care p.89
population-based care p.90
primary nursing p.86
registered nurse (RN) p.81
team nursing p.85
total patient care p.84
unlicensed assistive personnel (UAP) p.80

Nursing Care Delivery Systems: Past to Present

Nursing and health care agency administrators have struggled for more than 100 years with the question of how to deliver appropriate nursing care to patients in an efficient and effective manner. **Nursing care delivery systems** were developed to describe a structure for the organization of nursing work, to identify the types of health care workers providing the nursing care, and to define the boundaries for the delegation of authority.

Registered nurses work in several different settings and have many different job titles, responsibilities, and credentials. (As new roles for nurses develop in the health care setting, many nursing professionals describe these innovations in care modalities as nursing care delivery systems.) This chapter will discuss the innovations and advancements in health care delivery as evolutionary adaptations of the four basic nursing delivery systems using Marie Manthey's (1990) definition of a nursing care delivery system. Manthey describes nursing care delivery systems as ". . . a set of concepts defining four basic organizational elements. The definitions of these elements are based on principles that are in turn based on fundamental values. These fundamental values will ultimately determine the quality of the product. These four fundamental values or elements are clinical decision making, work allocation, communication, and management" (Manthey, 1990, p. 203). Duffield, Roche, Diers, Catling-Paull, and Blay (2010) explored the meaning of a model of care, and found that models of care are not prescriptive, but vary according to nursing unit circumstances and staffing levels based on complex clinical decision-making skills. This finding needs to be considered as delivery systems and models of care are discussed.

Historical Influence

Nursing care delivery systems are complex and subject to the economic, social, political, and technological influences of the time period. World wars, the Industrial Revolution, the Great Depression, and the development of diagnosis-related groups (DRGs) and managed care have sparked changes in health care delivery and challenged the way the profession of nursing is practiced (Marquis & Huston, 2011).

Weblink: Comprehensive Accreditation Manual for Hospitals, The Official Handbook

The pressure to reduce unnecessary costs resulted in the development of several different types of managed care organizations. Managed care is a form of health care delivery that uses financial incentives to direct patients to the most cost-effective and efficient treatment center. Chapter 2 discusses managed care in depth. The financial considerations of health care and the variations in models of nursing care have resulted in increased pressure to prove that the care nurses provide is efficient and an appropriate use of health care funding. However, the "attempts to describe what nursing care involves have not yet resulted in a generally accepted articulation that is fully up to this task" (Adams & Nelson, 2009, p. 3). Chapter 2 discussed health care finance issues.

Current Influence

The nursing shortage has influenced the types of nursing care delivery systems used in many health care settings and continues to drive the search for the ideal nursing care delivery system. It is predicted that there may be a shortage of as many as 800,000 nurses by the year 2020, and an unprecedented shortage of registered nurses by 2030 if dramatic interventions are not taken (Allen, 2008). The decision to implement a particular nursing care delivery system will increasingly depend on the complexity and variability of the health care setting. The availability of the labor pool, the acuity of patients, and the financial health of the institution are important variables to consider when selecting a nursing care delivery system. The term **acuity** refers to the measurement of the patient's severity of illness and the amount of nursing care required by the patient (Hoi, Ismail, Ong, & Kang, 2010). It is an important variable that must be considered when determining the skill level needed to provide appropriate care, and it takes into account patients' needs, the technology required to care for patients, and the amount of interdisciplinary support needed by the nurse (Hoi et al., 2010; Kiekkas et al., 2008).

In response to nursing shortages, institutions tend to implement or modify nursing care delivery systems that use a variety of licensed nurses and **unlicensed assistive personnel (UAP)** (health care workers who are not licensed to perform nursing tasks, but who may be trained and certified) (Meyer, Wang, Li, Thomson, & O'Brien-Pallas, 2009). Because RN salaries have increased due to the decreased supply of nurses and the increased demand for nurses, many health care institutions have changed the skill mix by hiring UAPs in an effort to reduce labor costs. Organized labor unions responded to managements' cost savings efforts by introducing legislation in several states to enact mandatory staffing ratios as a patient safety initiative and to force hospitals to increase the number of licensed nurses. In January 2004, California was the first state to mandate licensed nurse staffing ratios (Aiken et al., 2010). Aiken et al. (2010) explored nurse workloads and patient outcomes across three states (California, Pennsylvania, and New Jersey) and found that the lower ratios in California were associated with significantly lower mortality. In contrast, a literature review covering 10 years (1998–2008) revealed that "while there may be an association between models of nurse staffing and outcomes, there is insufficient evidence to establish a causal relationship between these factors" (Flynn & McKeown, 2009). The legislation by the state of California opened debate and fueled a call for more research to clearly identify the relationship of quality patient outcomes to skill mix. In the meantime, many states continue to introduce legislation in an attempt to attract and retain RNs in the face of increasing acuity and the nursing shortage. Laws and regulations enacted at the state level are not the only standards regarding nurse staffing. The Joint Commission, the national accrediting body for hospitals and health systems, has set standards for nurse staffing and assignment of patient care. Hospitals and health systems must adhere to these guidelines to maintain accreditation and to meet quality of care standards. These guidelines are described in the National Guidelines box.

> **NATIONAL GUIDELINES from The Joint Commission**
>
> The Joint Commission is an accrediting body for hospitals and health systems. Information on staffing requirements can be found in the September 2009 document titled *Comprehensive Accreditation Manual for Hospitals, The Official Handbook,* which can only be accessed through an organization that has purchased the reference. Limited free information can be found on the Joint Commission's official website: http://www.jointcommission.org.

The physical design of patient care areas and the experience and competency of personnel also might influence the choice or modification of a nursing care delivery system (Stichler, 2009). Nursing units designed in circles, squares, or rectangles with central or decentralized medication and supply services may require different configurations of staff to safely provide observation and care. The creation of smaller sections where patient care is delivered may increase the ability of staff to obtain assistance when needed (Stichler, 2009). In 2010, the National Institute of Building Sciences published design standards that emphasize safety for patients and staff. These guidelines recommend a unit layout that promotes patient and staff safety as well as restful recovery for patients (Carr, 2010). Work is currently under way to evaluate the influence of technology upon safe patient care (Institute of Medicine [IOM], 2010).

Evidence-Based Management Practices

Traditional delivery systems form a framework that can be modified to meet the uniqueness of the particular agency setting; however, measuring the effectiveness of such a system is complex and difficult. The efficiency and effectiveness of any system usually are evaluated by measuring four factors: quality of patient care, patient satisfaction, nursing job satisfaction, and cost effectiveness for the health care organization. The Joint Commission has begun focusing on patient safety standards called "National Patient Safety Goals" that list critical areas to assure provision of safe and quality patient care (2010). Improving the accuracy of patient information and improving the safety of using medications are two of these important patient safety standards.

The California Alliance for Nursing Outcomes (CALNOC; formerly known as the California Nursing Outcomes Coalition) is a self-funded organization that was created by the Association of California Nurse Leaders and the American Nurses Association. The organization has been active in collecting a database of patient outcomes and hospital statistics. CALNOC has had more than 30 hospitals volunteer to be study sites to assist in affecting changes in aggregated patient outcomes (Donaldson et al., 2008). A recent study noted that the change in California's nurse staffing ratio did not improve the incidence of falls or prevalence of bed sores (Robertson, 2008). These findings are consistent with another 2008 study conducted by the American Nurses Association/California and the Association of California Nurse Leaders, which was sponsored by CALNOC (William D Ruckelshaus Center, 2009). The outcome variable of patient satisfaction is used to measure the degree of coordination of care, the degree to which emotional and spiritual needs are met, and the degree of safety in the care provided. The outcome variable of nurse job satisfaction measures the degree to which nursing care delivery systems acknowledge, nurture, and protect the practice of the professional nurse. Common indicators of nurse job satisfaction are the degree of job autonomy, the accountability of the professional nurse, and the presence of meaningful work (Hayes et al., 2011). A survey of more than 95,000 nurses found that nurses providing direct patient care and working in hospitals and nursing homes were more likely than other nurses to express job dissatisfaction and burnout, which may lead to patient safety issues, a concern expressed by some of the study participants (Hitt, 2011).

The cost-effective measurement of nursing care delivery systems is difficult to achieve. Identifying the best care for the lowest cost may be deemed a cost-effective choice (Finkler, Kovner, & Jones, 2007). The Quality and Safety Education for Nurses (QSEN, 2012) project funded by the Robert Wood Johnson Foundation has identified safety of patient care as a vital competency for clinical staff and students, thereby influencing the selection of a nursing care delivery system. The selected delivery system determines the type and amount of staffing needed. This, in turn, may influence safety measures in patient care.

Classical work conducted by Houser (2003) tested a model of demands on nursing in an attempt to measure the multivariate nature of the nursing work environment. This research was a first step toward evaluating the complex issues of maintaining a competent, satisfied workforce and providing acceptable patient care at a reasonable cost. Further evidence relating nursing workload to patient outcomes is needed to make the management decisions necessary to achieve the desired results of patient outcomes. While past nursing researchers have contributed to a body of knowledge about the work environment, patient outcomes, and educational preparation, recent studies continue to attempt to identify if these multiple variables can answer some of management's questions about professional practice. Kramer and Schmalenberg (2008) argued that establishing the health of the work environment from the staff nurse perspective is the first step in improving the environment and the quality of care for patients. Recent work has focused on nurse staffing models and the outcomes of patient care. In one study, nurse staffing was associated with an impact on quality of care and job outcomes (satisfaction, autonomy, control) in the context of Korean intensive care units (Cho et al., 2009).

Integration of RN Roles in Care Delivery Systems

There are four well-defined and widely used traditional nursing care delivery systems encountered in acute, outpatient, and long-term health care settings. Each of these systems—the case method, functional nursing, team nursing, and primary nursing—takes advantage of a variety of caregivers with licenses or certifications and different education levels. The 2010 Institute of Medicine (IOM) report on The Future of Nursing: Leading Change, Advancing Health calls for nurses' roles to be expanded significantly over the next 10 years to help meet the increased demand for primary care that is expected as a result of health care reform. Changes include introducing residency training for nurses, increasing the percentage of nurses who attain bachelor's degrees to 80% by 2020, and doubling the number who pursue doctorates. One section also discusses broadening the roles of nurse practitioners. Nurses' roles as primary care providers will expand under the proposed health care reform, especially outside hospital settings, in homes, and through nurse-led health centers. Positive outcomes with the expanded role are anticipated, and heretofore have been documented. A recent study noted that the expanded NP role in elder care provides positive outcomes (Dias, 2008).

Different roles for **registered nurses (RNs)** have been developed over the years to complement and support nurses and physicians delivering care at the bedside. For example, an **advanced practice nurse (APRN),** as previously referenced, is a registered nurse with advanced education, knowledge, and skills. APRNs also may have additional certifications, and their practice may vary depending on the scope of practice defined by the board of registered nursing in the state where they work. APRNs increasingly are being used in the clinical setting and may be used in all nursing care delivery systems without changing the delivery system's basic structure or philosophy. Advanced practice nurses include nurses with the titles **certified registered nurse anesthetist (CRNA), clinical nurse specialist (CNS), certified nurse midwife (CNM),** and **nurse practitioner (NP).**

Weblink: Fact sheet: The Clinical Nurse Leader

A new bedside role for an RN currently is being evaluated. The role of **clinical nurse leader (CNL)** is intended to manage patient services across multidisciplinary boundaries at the bedside and to be a resource to the bedside nurse. The need for clinical nurse leadership to improve the quality of health care systems while controlling costs is recognized in reports internationally. The CNL was developed in response to such reports. The American Association of Colleges of Nursing's (AACN) 2005 position paper envisioned CNLs as nurse leaders responsible for evaluating outcomes and leading change at the point of care (2005). Professional preparation for CNLs is consistent with the curriculum proposed by AACN in 2006. They are master's level nurse graduates (although not necessarily recruited from a nursing background) with the skills and knowledge to create change within complex systems and improve outcomes while they remain direct care providers (Baernholdt & Cottingham, 2011). CNLs are envisioned as coordinators of care and leaders with the authority to function as part of the clinical health care team, thereby serving as catalysts for quality improvement and patient safety (Stanley et al., 2008). Several institutions are piloting this role; however, research is not complete as to its effectiveness (Begun, Hamilton, Tornabeni, & White, 2006). Another, more widely accepted approach to coordinating and managing complex systems has been the delegation of these responsibilities to administrative nurses without direct clinical care duties.

Weblink: Clinical Nurse Leader Competencies

Weblink: Nursing Case Management

The introduction of managed care in the early 1990s resulted in a new position of **case manager** being created within the health care setting. Managed care requires close coordination of care across all health care settings and therefore affects the role of the RN in the delivery of care. Some institutions, however, do not always use RNs (Huber, 2010). The chief function of the case manager is to collaboratively plan, coordinate, and evaluate services in a cost-effective manner. Nurse case managers interact with health care team members to reduce fragmentation and improve outcomes. In many settings, case managers do not provide direct patient care (American Nurses Credentialing Center, 2012). In others, case management is considered to be a care delivery model.

Delegation

Delegation, a process inherent in patient care delivery systems, is defined as being accountable for outcomes of work that is shared with others (Potter, Deshields, & Kuhrik, 2010). Delegation includes important leadership skills such as communication, collaboration with various team members, and conflict negotiation among those to whom the licensed staff member delegates (Potter et al., 2010). This process, though historically driven, currently is being studied as a major component of the future of nursing care under the Institute of Medicine (IOM) (2010).

Video: Delegating Weblink: Delegation Model

In 2010, the American Nurses Association (ANA) affirmed its 2005 statement on the Principles of Delegation. The ANA definition of delegation is consistent with that more recently defined by Potter et al. (2010) and that defined by the National Council of State Boards of Nursing (NCSBN) in 2006 and 2010. Basically, all agree that delegation is "the transfer of responsibility for performance of a task from one individual to another while remaining accountable for the outcome." This represents a transfer of authority for completing selected nursing tasks/activities/functions to a competent individual. Inherent in all definitions is the assumption that delegation is a leadership function of the licensed nurse, in most cases that being the registered nurse (RN).

The RN must consider qualifications, job descriptions, and competency when delegating tasks to various caregivers. Qualifications are generally determined by state licensure or certification, agency policies and procedures, job descriptions, published state practice acts, and unit guidelines on which the RN can rely to determine qualifications and competency (Potter et al., 2010). For instance, an LVN/LPN may be permitted by license to draw blood in some states. In other states, the LVN/LPN must have an additional certification to draw blood. This also is true of agency policy, as some agencies allow LVNs/LPNs to start intravenous solutions, and others do not.

State practice acts address these qualifications in published regulations, and hospital job descriptions delineate the roles and responsibilities of individuals within a specific agency. Many workers may be unlicensed and have only basic training in health care. The nurse needs to be familiar with each job description and confident about the competency of the worker before assigning tasks. The authority and accountability for the outcome of the worker's performance still rests with the RN (Potter et al., 2010). (The functions of state nursing practice acts are discussed in more detail in Chapter 2.)

Competency to perform a task or procedure may be measured by tests, clinical observation, or certification by a training facility. Nursing assistants may be certified by the state or may have a certificate from a training facility. Certifications specifically identify the types of procedures or tasks that the individual has been trained to perform. RNs and LVNs/LPNs also may be certified to perform specific procedures. The RN must be knowledgeable about the competence of the individual before delegating tasks, and the hospital must keep records documenting the competence of the individuals performing those tasks.

Safety Alert *Delegation by an RN requires clinical judgment and knowledge of the applicable state's nurse practice act, which authorizes the scope of responsibility and grants the authority to delegate. All RNs must know how to prioritize patients' needs and assign tasks based on the competency of the personnel, but they also must know how to communicate clearly and to supervise the personnel and intervene when necessary.*

Delegating a task to an individual who is not competent has serious implications for the RN, the RN's license, and the institution should the patient suffer an adverse outcome. The RN should assess the patients' needs and consider situations where the outcome is uncertain or the potential for harm is high. The RN should not delegate tasks under those circumstances. Nursing assessment and judgment may not be delegated. In addition to considering qualifications, job descriptions, competence, and patient needs, the RN must evaluate the effectiveness of the delegation and whether the desired outcome was achieved. The NCSBN and the ANA released a joint position on delegation in 2006, which still holds importance in nursing practice guidelines (NCSBN, 2006). The principles of delegation as outlined by the ANA also continue to be used in establishing nursing practice guidelines. The principles of delegation are shown in Chart 4–1. Additional information on practice strategies for using delegation can be found in the ANA document. The process of delegation is depicted in Figure 4–1◆, Delegation Model.

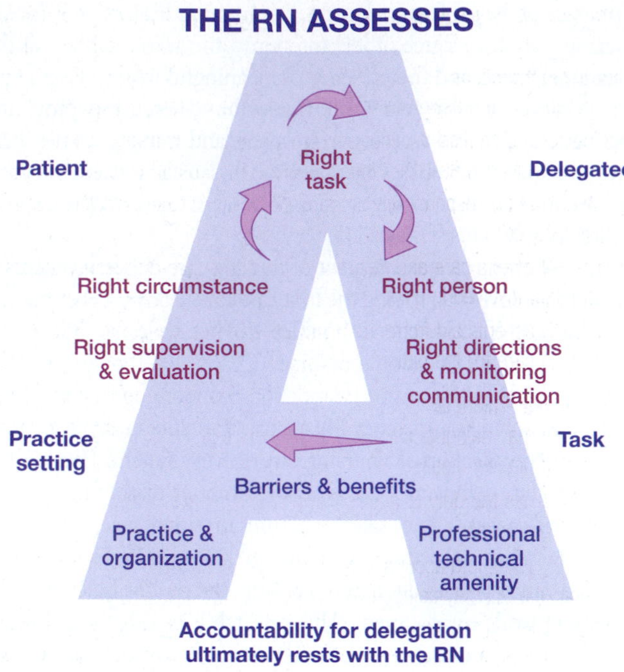

FIGURE 4–1 ◆ Delegation model.

Source: American Nurses Association (ANA). (2005, 2010). ANA principles for delegation, http://www.safestaffingsaveslives.org/WhatisSafeStaffing/SafeStaffingPrinciples/Principle.

Care Delivery Models

The delivery of health care to the patient is a multidisciplinary process that must take into account the availability of resources, the educational preparation of the nurse, the competencies of the staff, the needs of the patient, and the cost implications for the institution or health system (Fernandez, Tran, Johnson, & Jones, 2010). The recent Institute of Medicine (IOM) report must be considered as care delivery models are discussed or changed, and the role of the nurse is defined. Recommendations from the IOM report hold nurses more accountable for assuming a leadership role in developing and evaluating health care delivery systems. This recommendation encompasses the basic activity of assigning nursing care staff to patients. **Assignment** is defined as the transfer of a task and the accountability for the outcome (Huber, 2010). Assignments are the method by which the division of labor is accomplished within the structure of a health care system. *Delegation* is a determination of the parts of an assignment that will be transferred from an RN to an assistant. Organizations use the concept of delegation in nursing when determining the nursing care model, or system of nursing care delivery, that will be established for the work unit. The concept and principles of delegation are discussed further under the functional model of patient care delivery on page 84.

Nurses deliver and coordinate patient care within the framework of the organizational structure and model of the nursing care delivery system. The model of care selected has a direct correlation to the allocation of control over decisions about patient care. This, in turn, has

CHART 4–1 ANA Principles for Delegation

Overarching Principles

- The nursing profession determines the scope of nursing practice.
- The nursing profession defines and supervises the education, training, and utilization for any assistant roles involved in providing direct patient care.
- The RN takes responsibility and accountability for the provision of nursing practice.
- The RN directs care and determines the appropriate utilization of any assistant involved in providing direct patient care.
- The RN accepts aid from nursing assistive personnel in providing nursing care for the patient.

Nurse-Related Principles

- The RN may delegate elements of care but does not delegate the nursing process itself.
- The RN has the duty to answer for personal actions relating to the nursing process.
- The RN takes into account the knowledge and skills of any individual to whom the RN may delegate elements of care.
- The decision of whether or not to delegate or assign is based upon the RN's judgment concerning the condition of the patient, the competence of all members of the nursing team, and the degree of supervision that will be required of the RN if a task is delegated.
- The RN delegates only those tasks for which she or he believes the other health care worker has the knowledge and skill to perform, taking into consideration training, cultural competence, experience, and facility/agency policies and procedures.
- The RN uses critical thinking and professional judgment when following The Five Rights of Delegation:
  1. Right task
  2. Right circumstances
  3. Right person
  4. Right directions and communication
  5. Right supervision and evaluation (NCSBN, 1995).
- The RN acknowledges that there is a relational aspect to delegation and that communication is culturally appropriate and the person receiving the communication is treated respectfully.
- Chief nursing officers are accountable for establishing systems to assess, monitor, verify, and communicate ongoing competence requirements in areas related to delegation, both for RNs and delegates.
- RNs monitor organizational policies, procedures, and position descriptions to ensure there is no violation of the nurse practice act, working with the state board of nursing as necessary.

Organization-Related Principles

- The organization is accountable for delegation through the allocation of resources to ensure sufficient staffing so that the RN can delegate appropriately.
- The organization is accountable for documenting competencies for all staff providing direct patient care and for ensuring that the RN has access to competency information for staff to whom the RN is delegating patient care.
- Organizational policies on delegation are developed with the active participation of all nurses (staff, managers, and administrators).
- The organization ensures that the educational needs of nursing assistive personnel are met through the implementation of a system that allows for nurse input.
- Organizations have policies in place that allow input from nurses indicating that delegation is a professional right and responsibility.

Source: American Nurses Association (ANA, 2005, 2010.). ANA principles for delegation, http://www.safestaffingsaveslives.org/WhatisSafeStaffing/SafeStaffingPrinciples/Principle.

implications for job satisfaction, the character of professional practice, and the amount of authority that is actually transferred to the staff (Huber, 2010).

A nursing care model (sometimes referred to as a practice model) is a method of organizing and delivering nursing care to meet patients' needs. The basic elements of nursing care delivery models are work allocation, clinical decision making, communication, and management. The four traditional models of nursing care delivery systems are: case method, functional nursing, team nursing, and primary nursing. The nursing care practice model also may be thought of as a link between the problems presented by the patient population, the purposes of professional occupations, and the purposes of health care organizations.

For any practice model, there needs to be consistency between the degree of integration of the nursing care given to a patient, the degree of continuity in assignment of care to a patient, and the type of coordination used to plan or organize the patient's care based on general patient characteristics, available nursing resources, and the organizational support available to nursing (Huber, 2010). There is no one correct way of structuring patient care delivery. All models have advantages and disadvantages, and any specific model may be better suited to one set of environmental circumstances than another. It is, therefore, important to have an understanding of the models of patient care delivery. Models of care delivery are continually being modified to adjust for the many variables in the health care setting. The traditional models are presented next to provide a baseline understanding of the structured work of nursing in a health care setting.

Models of Organizing Patient Care

The four traditional means of organizing nursing care for patient care delivery are (1) case method, (2) functional nursing, (3) team and modular nursing, and (4) primary nursing (Duffield et al., 2010). Each of these basic types has undergone many modifications, often resulting in new terminology. For example, *primary nursing* now is frequently referred to as a *professional practice model*, and *team nursing* often is termed *partners in care, patient service partners,* or other similar names.

When closely examined, many of the newer models of patient care delivery systems are recycled, modified, or retitled versions of older models. In fact, it is difficult to find a "pure" delivery model; the models have become blended, with most having parts of others in their design. Choosing the most appropriate organizational model for delivering patient care for any unit or organization depends on the skill and expertise of the staff, the availability of RNs, the economic resources of the organization, the acuity of the patients, and the complexity of the tasks to be completed. These factors may change over time within an organization, contingent on external environmental factors (e.g., the nursing shortage, technological advances, population factors), in which case the nursing care delivery model also may change.

The four primary and historical or traditional means of organizing patient care mentioned previously are discussed in the following subsections. Other recognized methods and new or evolving methods follow.

Case Method

Case method is the oldest model of organizing care. In this method, nurses assume total responsibility for meeting all of the needs of assigned patients during their time on duty. Initially, case method, sometimes referred to as case management, was provided in the patient's home, and the nurse was responsible for cooking, house cleaning, and other activities specific to the patient and family, in addition to traditional nursing care (Huber, 2010). This type of care also historically was called *private duty nursing*. During the Great Depression of the 1930s, as people could no longer afford home care, they began using hospitals for care that had previously been performed by private duty nurses in the home. As hospitals grew during the 1930s and 1940s, case method continued as the primary means of organizing patient care.

The case method of delivering nursing care is simply defined, and sometimes referred to, as **total patient care.** The RN is responsible for the patient and has total care responsibility for the patient during the shift worked.

Work Allocation

All patients have an RN assigned to them, so this type of delivery system requires exclusive use of an all RN staff. There is no assignment requirement that the RN have the same patient day after day, nor is there a consistent coordinator to ensure continuity of care during the course of the patient's hospitalization. The case method is frequently practiced in the intensive care setting or in the home health setting (Huber, 2010). The charge nurse may have a patient load or may assist where needed. The role of the charge nurse is to manage the shift activities, provide consultation to staff, and make patient assignments according to the resources available.

Clinical Decision Making

The RN assumes responsibility for the patient's total care and may have several assigned patients. In addition to being responsible for the nursing process, the RN is responsible for all indirect and direct patient care functions. Care planning and goal setting occur between family, patient, and nurse during the specific shift.

Communication

The RN communicates changes, needs, and requests for assistance to the charge nurse. The RN is generally expected to communicate with physicians and other disciplines regarding patient care needs. Communication and coordination of care between shifts is dependent on the efforts of the individual shift nurse.

Management

Holistic and comprehensive care delivered by a registered nurse is considered the primary advantage of the case method. The cost of RNs, the lack of continuity between shifts, and the dependence on an adequate supply of nurses are considered to be disadvantages of this system (Stanley et al., 2008).

The disadvantages to the case method of nursing care delivery can be mitigated through the use of advanced practice nurses and case managers. Advanced practice nurses typically work side by side in settings where the case method is implemented. The clinical nurse leader serves to coordinate care between the other disciplines in this delivery care system. The use of the CNS or NP in the intensive care unit may provide specialty expertise and education for the nursing staff or extend the physician's capabilities and provide additional consultative support for the bedside nurse (Stanley et al., 2008). The use of advance practice nurses as part of the health care team provides continuity of care and can reduce the length of stay and mortality rate (Stanley et al., 2008). Case managers may place patients with a specific diagnosis on a clinical pathway. In situations where case managers are used, the responsibilities for planning, coordinating, and evaluating care are assumed by the case manager. The bedside nurse then is responsible for the assessment and intervention components of patient care (Huber, 2010). A collaborative effort between the bedside nurse, the case manager, and the physician ensures continuity of care for the patient as the patient progresses to different levels of care. This collaborative partnership is outcome driven and offers the added benefit of providing care to a defined group of patients with limited resources (Huber, 2010). (Case management is discussed in more detail in Chapter 2.)

Functional Nursing

Functional nursing has been defined as work assignment by functions or tasks, such as administering medications, performing dressing changes, giving baths, or taking vital signs. Philosophically, functional nursing is not oriented to individualized and holistic patient care, but is more oriented to task accomplishment, as patterned after the industrial concepts of scientific management. Under functional nursing, the nurse identifies the tasks to be done for a shift. The work is then divided up and assigned to personnel who focus on completing the assigned tasks. Functional nursing has the advantage of being efficient for taking care of the tasks related to handling a large number of patients. It also is considered to be an economical means of providing care with efficiency (Marquis & Huston, 2011).

The functional nursing care delivery system was first developed in response to the increasing demand for hospital nursing in the late 1800s, and it resurfaced due to the sporadic nursing shortages resulting from World War II (Daditch, 2003). A functional nursing care delivery system is defined as a task-oriented system in which individual caregivers are not given patient assignments, but are expected to perform specific assigned tasks within their capability for all patients in a given area. This method of providing care to the patient involves both licensed nursing staff and unlicensed assistive personnel. "Unlicensed assistive personnel (UAP) are health care personnel who are not licensed and may be technicians or certified nurses' aides or nursing assistants" (Daditch, 2003, p. 255). Several variations may be used in health care settings today, but all functional models depend on a hierarchical structure that requires strict definition of roles and responsibilities and control of tasks (Tomey, 2004).

Work Allocation

Figure 4–2◆ shows a standard flowchart for the functional nursing care delivery system. The charge nurse may be responsible for both administrative and clinical functions such as taking orders, contacting physicians for patient needs, assisting personnel with difficult or emergent patient care needs, adjusting staffing schedules, and evaluating or orienting staff. The task of medication administration is usually assigned to an RN in the role of **medication nurse.** The use of a medication nurse is not a common practice in acute care facilities today, but it is a useful function in long-term care facilities. This role may be assigned in acute care settings, however, during disasters or other emergent situations when the patient-to-staff ratio is higher than usual.

In situations where there is a shortage of RNs, a **licensed vocational/practical nurse (LVN/LPN)** may be assigned to administer oral and parenteral medications while the charge RN administers the IV medications (Daditch, 2003). LVNs/LPNs receive 1 to 2 years of practical training to deliver basic nursing care and are licensed according to state practice acts.

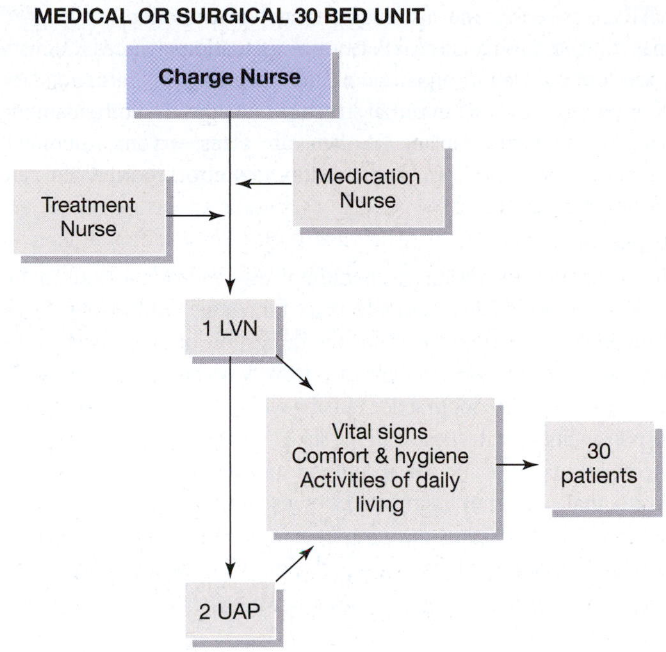

FIGURE 4–2 ◆ Sample staffing assignments for the functional method of nursing care delivery.

In the functional model, a treatment nurse is assigned the responsibility of providing treatments, such as dressing changes, hygiene tasks, administering oral medications, and assessment of vital signs. This nurse is frequently an LVN/LPN and the assignment of tasks is dependent on the scope of practice of the LVN/LPN and the complexity of patients' needs. The scope of practice may change according to state law and regulations. It also is dependent on agency policy, wherein the agency may be more restrictive than the law allows.

UAP are assigned to take vital signs, assist the patients with basic hygiene tasks, and provide comfort measures. This variation in the functional delivery system has been seen as critical in home care and in nursing homes (Siegel, Young, Mitchell, & Shannon, 2008).

Clinical Decision Making

In a typical functional model, an RN is assigned to be in charge and to coordinate the care of all patients. The clinical decision making for all patients rests with the charge nurse because that individual is responsible for collecting all pertinent information about the patients. The RN is responsible for delegating tasks to personnel consistent with the applicable state nurse practice act and agency policies. Delegation, as previously defined, is being held accountable for outcomes of work that is shared with others (Potter et al., 2010). This interpretation of delegation is based on the premise that the RN possesses important leadership skills such as communication, collaboration, and conflict negotiation (Potter et al., 2010).

Communication

The members of the staff are responsible for communicating changes to the charge nurse. It is the charge nurse's ultimate responsibility to communicate patient needs and coordinate patient care with other disciplines. On busy or large patient care units, there is a possibility that patient needs will be overlooked (Huber, 2010). The increased number of personnel performing specific tasks for the individual patient intentionally fragments care. The functional nursing model is an industrial efficiency model that demands a high level of coordination and communication. The overall assessment of the patient from beginning to end may be incomplete and cause critical changes to go unnoticed (Potter et al., 2010).

Management

Functional care delivery systems are implemented by management when efficiency in completing a large number of tasks is the desired outcome. The ability to train unskilled personnel to complete limited specific tasks in order to avoid high labor costs by using lower-paid workers is an incentive for health care facilities interested in the industrial model of efficiency (Huber, 2010). Institutions that embrace the industrial model of efficiency do not tend to modify the nursing care delivery system to provide better coordinated care by using advanced practice nurses or case managers. Nurse practitioners or nurse midwives might be used as physician extenders in these facilities.

The disadvantages of functional nursing are fragmented patient care, low job satisfaction, and low patient satisfaction. Nurses working in the functional model report a lack of satisfaction with their work because tasks are boring or because there is difficulty identifying the effect their work has on their patients. Functional nursing resembles assembly-line tasking, and the fragmentation of tasks results in a perceived lack of accountability and increased frustration (Tomey, 2004). Reduced patient satisfaction is linked to fragmented care and the resulting lack of confidence in the caregivers (Huber, 2010).

Charge nurses working with a functional nursing care delivery system must be knowledgeable about the RN and LVN/LPN practice laws in the state in which they are practicing. The delegation of tasks must be consistent with the state training and licensure or certification regulations. The UAP performing patient care tasks may face misdemeanor charges or penalties for practicing nursing without a license in states where mandatory licensure protects the title of registered nurse and the actions are protected by the state nursing practice act (Potter et al., 2010). The nursing practice act and its functions as related to regulations are discussed at length in Chapter 2.

Team Nursing

Team nursing is a care model that involves a group of people led by a knowledgeable nurse. Team nursing was developed in the early 1950s in response to complaints that functional nursing created a fragmented care delivery system and resulted in nursing and patient dissatisfaction with care (Fairbrother, Jones, & Rivas, 2010; Marquis & Huston, 2011). In team nursing, ancillary personnel collaborate in providing care to a group of patients under the direction of a professional nurse. As the team leader, the nurse is responsible for knowing the conditions and needs of all patients assigned to the team and for planning individual care.

This care delivery model usually is associated with democratic leadership and allows team members to contribute their own special expertise. Group members are given as much autonomy as possible when performing assigned tasks, although the team shares responsibility and accountability collectively. Team leaders use their knowledge about each member's abilities when making patient assignments. Recognizing each member's worth and giving team members autonomy results in high job satisfaction.

In the team nursing care delivery system, patients are assigned to a nursing team, which usually is led by an RN. The team may include RNs, LVN/LPNs, respiratory therapists, dietitians, and UAP (Figure 4–3◆). Small teams may be assigned to care for patients. These teams include an LVN/LPN and UAP. These types of teams may be called care partners, modular teams, patient-focused teams, or any name that incorporates the concept of a work redesign with the skill mix intended to be used.

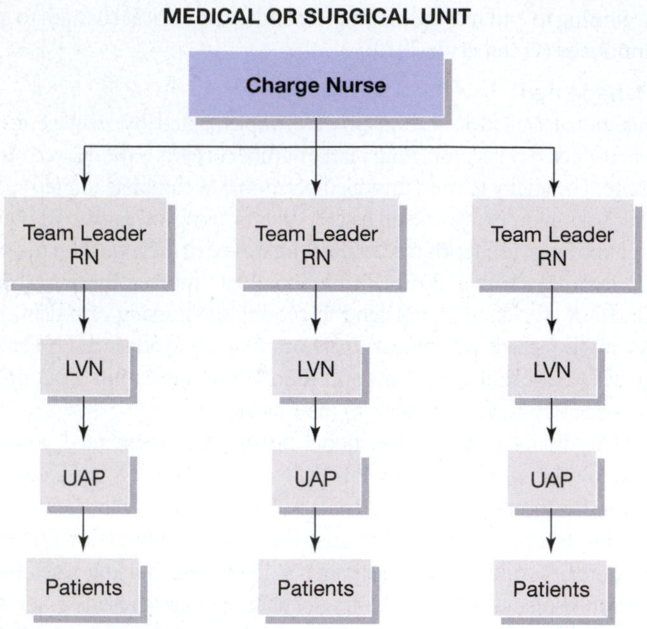

FIGURE 4–3 ◆ Sample staffing assignments for the team method of nursing care delivery.

Work Allocation

A typical unit with 30 patients may have a charge nurse, two team leaders, and usually two to four team members per team (Figure 4–3), but no more than five members per team (Fernandez et al., 2010). Assignments are based on the acuity of the patients and the skill level and experience of the caregivers (Huber, 2010). The team leader assigns all patients to team members and may delegate additional tasks according to the team members' competence (Fairbrother et al., 2010). The team assignments may sometimes mirror a functional approach to care when the team leader is the only RN or licensed person on the team (Fernandez et al., 2010). In that case, the team leader assumes responsibility for administering all medications and IV solutions to patients on the team and delegates the remaining responsibilities to the team members. Effective communication skills and consideration of the skills of each team member have been identified as vital to successful team leadership in acute care areas (Fairbrother et al., 2010).

Clinical Decision Making

The charge nurse is responsible for assigning groups of patients and caregivers to the team leaders and for facilitating communications between multidisciplinary caregivers. Decision making is delegated to several team leaders versus a single charge nurse, and team members work collaboratively toward common goals. Team leaders are responsible for making the individual patient assignments to their team members. Team leaders plan the care, delegate tasks, and monitor the work of the team to ensure quality. As time permits, the team leader may coordinate care conferences for patients with complex health care needs. Daily conferences are the ideal, but frequently time constraints prevent completion of conferences.

Communication

Team nursing is difficult to implement without extensive team communication (Fairbrother et al., 2010). Nursing shortages and high turnover among unlicensed assistive personnel can make communication between ever-changing team members a challenge. Research has documented RN dissatisfaction with communication and teamwork when UAP are used. Research also suggests that how personnel are assigned may mitigate these concerns (Potter et al., 2010). Experienced RNs with good communication, organization, and leadership skills are necessary. Numerous formal and informal structures for communication among team members are available. Written care plans, written assignment responsibilities, and team conferences encourage coordinated care (Yoder-Wise, 2011).

Management

Team nursing has advantages because it uses individual team members' strengths to the greatest advantage for a large number of patients (Huber, 2010). Responsibility for the delegation of tasks remains the same as in the functional nursing care delivery system. Unlicensed assistive personnel may not practice nursing without a license, and nursing responsibilities are delineated in the state nursing practice act. All team members need specific role definition and communication skills to ensure that care is not fragmented, because fragmentation of care may decrease job satisfaction and contribute to decreased quality of care. It also has been reported that high-level teams working toward common goals and focused missions can experience increased job satisfaction (Fairbrother et al., 2010).

Complex, time-intensive training is essential to ensure that team members can function within a team structure and effectively communicate. Clinical nurse specialists and nurse practitioners can provide consultative support in a team nursing care delivery system. The clinical nurse leader (CNL) role could be useful in this type of delivery system, because the CNL can provide coordination within multidisciplinary teams and provide consistent information to the patient as well as the team. The use of APRNs can complement nursing care of patients with complex needs and provide advanced educational support (Baernholdt & Cottingham, 2011).

Recent attempts to refine and improve team nursing have resulted in the concept of "modular" nursing, as discussed next (Marquis & Huston, 2011).

Modular Nursing

Modular nursing is a type of team nursing that involves a small team of two to three persons. It is predicated by a facility's layout and actual structural and spatial changes that enable nurses to stay near the bedside. Nurses are stationed near their patients, and a wider range of responsibility is delegated to them. The open designs and convenient access architectures of modular nursing provide for geographic decentralization of care delivery and enhanced communication (Huber, 2010).

Primary Nursing

Primary nursing was developed as a nursing care delivery system in the late 1960s or early 1970s in response to the unhappiness of professional nurses with the lack of autonomy and the declining quality of patient care (Kjornsberg, Karlsson, Babra, & Wadensten, 2010). **Primary nursing** is defined as a system in which each patient is assigned to a nurse who has 24-hour responsibility for the nursing care delivered to the patient (Kjornsberg et al., 2010). Primary nursing uses some of the concepts of case method to bring the registered nurse back to the bedside to provide clinical care (Marquis & Huston, 2011). This goes along with a societal trend toward accountability and nursing's rising level of professionalism. As originally designed, primary nursing requires a nursing staff comprised totally of RNs. The RN primary nurse assumes 24-hour responsibility for planning the care of one or more patients from admission, or the start of treatment, to discharge, or the treatment's end.

Work Allocation

The primary nurse is responsible for planning the patient's care and delegating the care during the hours that the nurse is not present. The primary nurse also is accountable for the coordination and continuity of care from admission to discharge. The nurse who assists the primary nurse during off-duty hours is called an **associate nurse** or **associate caregiver.** The associate nurse follows the plan of care, communicates pertinent information or changes in the patient status to the primary nurse, and provides direct patient care when the primary nurse is not present. An associate caregiver may be an LVN/LPN or UAP (Fairbrother et al., 2010). A nurse may be a primary nurse for a small caseload of patients and also an associate nurse for other patients.

Clinical Decision Making

The three major responsibilities of the primary nurse can be simplified into (1) clear communication among all care disciplines, (2) development of a plan of care using the nursing process, and (3) discharge planning from the time of admission to discharge (Kjornsberg et al., 2010). The primary nurse is held accountable for collecting and communicating important patient information during the patient's hospitalization. The primary nurse provides direct patient care because this nurse is in the best position to plan the care (Fairbrother et al., 2010). Involving the patient in the collection of information, eliciting patient expectations for the outcomes of care, and encouraging patient participation in the development of goals is a significant part of the process (Fernandez et al., 2010).

The nurse develops the plan of care using whatever documentation method the health care facility has developed to direct all care providers. Instruments such as Kardex care plans, care pathways, care maps, nursing admission forms, guidelines, electronic health records, and multidisciplinary education forms can be used. Planning for the discharge of the patient is facilitated by the process of fulfilling the first two responsibilities: identifying the expected outcomes on admission and keeping the health care team on target with the plan of care (Fairbrother et al., 2010). The primary nurse may use institutional resources, such as discharge planning nurses, case managers, or social services, to assist the patient in discharge from the health care facility.

Communication

Consistent and accurate communication of information between shifts and appropriate delegation of care planning activities between associate nurses and primary nurses eliminate the need for a charge nurse in the communication chain between physician and caregiver (Fernandez et al., 2010). Direct communication improves the rapport and trust between the primary nurse, the patient, and the physician, creating a therapeutic relationship. The charge nurse is then able to support the activities of the unit and provide consultation for the primary nurse.

Management

The use of an associate caregiver is not inconsistent with the intent of the primary nursing care delivery system, which is to provide patient-focused care in an environment where the professional nurse is held accountable for practice. The associate caregiver may be task focused, but the care continues to be coordinated and monitored on a 24-hour basis by the primary nurse.

The advantages of the primary nursing care delivery system are the increased nurse perception of autonomy, the continuity of care provided to the patients, and the increase in focus on the patient. Research also suggests that primary nursing care results in better care outcomes and higher nurse satisfaction (Cho et al., 2009). Although the research does not support a specific patient care delivery model, many studies suggest that richer RN staffing levels result in lower lengths of stay, fewer patient deaths, and lower failure-to-rescue rates (Cho et al., 2009; Furukawa, Raghu, & Shao, 2010; Meyer et al., 2009). Patient satisfaction has been correlated with nurse satisfaction and quality of care in several basic studies (Meyer et al., 2009; Wagner & Bear, 2008). Recent studies suggest a link between nurse burnout and decreased patient satisfaction (Wagner & Bear, 2008). Other research suggests that higher levels of nurse satisfaction, greater continuity of care, positive patient outcomes, and improved nurse retention are associated with the use of primary nursing care delivery systems (Cho et al., 2009; Huber, 2010).

The primary nursing care delivery system uses many hospital resources, but places the control and authorization of such resources in the hands of the primary nurse. The primary nurse is responsible for developing the plan of care and prioritizing the daily activities to achieve the mutually agreed-upon goals in the plan. For instance, because the primary nurse understands the sleeping and eating preferences of a particular patient who has cancer, the nurse can adjust routines and treatments to meet the patient's basic needs. If the patient and family need complex information from the physicians or other members of the health care team about the prognosis and treatment options of chemotherapy and radiation, the primary nurse may coordinate a care conference and identify the desired outcomes to realize a productive meeting. The primary nurse may advocate for scheduling placement of central lines for chemotherapy with patient and family schedules so that chemotherapy treatments may be managed to coincide with family support. All of these activities are the responsibility of the primary nurse providing care at the bedside.

Nurse practitioners can function within this system as physician extenders and consultants to the primary nurse. Clinical nurse specialists are valuable in providing clinical expertise and education to the primary nurse. The use of case managers may be redundant because of the primary nurse's accountability for the entire patient experience. This also may be true of the clinical nurse leader role, depending on the interpretation of primary nursing used, as the primary nurse is responsible for all of the functions that a clinical nurse leader normally would assume in one of the other types of nursing care delivery models. This may not be true in all agencies, depending again on the interpretation and usage of primary nursing.

A primary nursing care delivery system may not be the preferred system during downturns in the economy and cyclical nursing shortages. There is a perception that labor costs are high because primary nursing requires a large number of RNs, although cost studies dispute this perception (Fernandez et al., 2010; Flynn & McKeown, 2009). Additional research is needed to determine whether a primary nursing care delivery system shields an institution from the impact of a nursing shortage by attracting and retaining nurses and improving patient outcomes.

Although designed for use in hospitals, this structure lends itself well to home health nursing, hospice nursing, and other health care delivery systems. An integral responsibility of the primary nurse is to establish clear communication among the patient and family, the physician, associate nurses, and other team members. Although the primary nurse establishes the plan of care, the nurse seeks input from others in coordinating the patient's care. Clear and consistent communication among the group and consistent, direct patient care by relatively few nursing staff allows for holistic, high-quality patient care.

Relationship-Based Care

Primary care is enjoying renewed popularity as a nursing care delivery system because of an evolution described as *relationship-based care.* Relationship-based care incorporates the structure of primary nursing with the principles and values of a professional nursing practice environment. Relationship-based care was designed to establish a therapeutic relationship between nurses, patients, and their families during their episode of care, and to promote the collaborative interdisciplinary practice associated with primary nursing (Schneider & Fake, 2010). The four components of primary care (work allocation, clinical decision making, communication, and management) are consistent with those of relationship-based care.

It is documented that patient outcomes are improved with relationship-based care (Gerri & Nebel, 2010). An orthopedic nursing unit adopted such a model and reported increased ability to provide quality care in a safe and trusting environment (Schneider & Fake, 2010). A magnet-designated hospital integrated primary and relationship-based care and renamed the model "Integrated Primary Nursing" (Jost, Bonnell, Chacko, & Parkinson, 2010).

While the professional nursing practice environment was defined by research conducted in the early 1990s, more recent research has provided findings that are important in any discussion of nursing care models. Flynn, Liang, Dickson, and Aiken (2010) explored the effect of nursing practice models in nursing homes, with findings that a supportive environment was related to fewer pressure ulcers. Friese, Lake, Aiken, Silber, and Sochalski (2008) examined the outcome of a nursing model on cancer patient care and found a poor practice environment was associated with a higher incidence of patient deaths. A professional nursing practice environment facilitates professional autonomy and control over individual practice while encouraging collaborative relationships. It is an environment in which relationship-based care is supported and allowed to thrive, as well as a situation in which nurses feel valued and respected with increased opportunities for independence and collaboration. These researchers and many others identified specific professional nursing practice attributes in hospitals that were successful in retaining and attracting nurses. These hospitals supported a professional nursing practice environment and subsequently were recognized as **magnet hospitals** (Armstrong, Laschinger, & Wong, 2009). Magnet status exemplifies excellence in nursing care delivery services that are provided in a professional practice environment, promote quality, and achieve positive patient outcomes (St. Luke's Hospital, 2011).

Research on magnet hospitals indicates that improved quality of care, improved patient satisfaction, and improved nursing satisfaction exist within hospitals meeting the magnet standards (Armstrong et al., 2009). The magnet designation means that the hospital has created an environment that supports nursing practice and focuses on professional autonomy, decision making at the bedside, nursing involvement in determining the nursing work environment, professional education, career development, and nursing leadership. The standards for magnet hospitals are shown in the National Guidelines box. An updated magnet model released in 2008 provides greater clarity and direction and aligns the 14 forces of magnetism with five overarching model components (Grant, Colello, Riehle, & Dende, 2010). The five new components are shown in Chart 4–2.

The primary nursing care delivery system that has evolved using the principles of relationship-based care reinforces the professional practice environment. This system builds on healing relationships that can be tailored to individual units with varying staffing patterns or standardized health care settings to meet the unique needs of patients and families. This structure may be attractive to health care settings trying to attract and retain nurses while improving the quality of care, improving patient satisfaction, and improving patient safety. There is increasing pressure from third-party payers to reduce medical errors, hospital-acquired infections, patient falls, and pressure ulcers, and the search has begun to discover the links between the environment and the safe delivery of health care (Duffield et al., 2010; Fernandez et al., 2010).

CHART 4–2 The Overarching Model Components

The five components of the new magnet model are:

1. Transformational Leadership
2. Structural Empowerment
3. Exemplary Professional Practice
4. New Knowledge, Innovation, & Improvements
5. Empirical Quality Results

Source: Detailed information on the magnet recognition program can be found at the following website: http://www.nursecredentialing.org/Magnet.aspx.

NATIONAL GUIDELINES for Magnet Hospitals

Hospitals are recognized and formally designated by the American Nurses Credentialing Center as magnet hospitals when they demonstrate, to the satisfaction of specially trained external appraisers, that the 14 forces of magnetism or standards are evident throughout the facility. Designation is valid for 4 years and hospitals must provide annual documentation of continued compliance with the forces.

The 14 forces of magnetism are:

1. Quality of nursing leadership
2. Organizational structure
3. Management style
4. Personnel policies and programs
5. Professional models of care
6. Quality of care
7. Quality improvement
8. Consultation and resources
9. Autonomy
10. Community and the hospital
11. Nurses as teachers
12. Image of nursing
13. Interdisciplinary relationships
14. Professional development

Source: Detailed information on the magnet recognition program can be found at the following website: http://www.nursecredentialing.org/Magnet.aspx.

New Types of Care Delivery Models

Both evolving and new types of nursing care delivery models also can be found in the literature. In general, these are mixed models, revisited primary care, or professional practice models that emphasize outcomes management, collaboration, use of a variety of caregivers with variable competencies and preparation, and integrated practice. The terms *case management* and *managed care* are integrated by major overriding concepts: accountability, cost containment, efficacy, continuum of care, interdisciplinary collaboration, new caregiver roles, changes in skill mix, and new assignment systems (Huber, 2010). All seek to reconfigure nursing's work within resource constraints, care needs, and current ideas about professional nursing practice.

Among the new types of models are partnership models, such as interdisciplinary teams and patient-focused care. These patient-centered models are designed to meet the needs of organizations that are being redesigned to be more cost effective and competitive. Due to the nature of complex knowledge, work models are needed that enhance the professional practice of all disciplines, clarify accountability for outcomes, and focus decision making at the point of service. As organizations integrate, partnership concepts become important as a way to create relationships and horizontal links that will make the system effective. Teams are no longer simply a mechanism for assigning work, nor are they composed of just nursing personnel. Rather, they form the core strategy for managing interdependency to address the complexity of health care service delivery. These newer models of care reflect the future direction of nursing as depicted in the IOM project (2010). Interdependency is, in effect, interdisciplinary and depends on open communication and trust among the interdependent team of professional caregivers. The structure of the team is contingent on the organization and management of individual agencies.

Patient-Centered Care

The **patient-centered care** model, also referred to as *patient-focused care*, is part of a redesign effort to realign the structure and processes involved in delivering care that centers around the patient while improving efficiency and use of resources. This approach adopts the perspective of the person receiving care and strives to establish mutual goals to meet that person's unique needs. The advantage of patient-centered care redesigns is that they center systems and services closer to the patient. This strong customer focus tends to increase patient satisfaction and safety, which can conserve resources (Marquis & Huston, 2011).

Case Management

Case management is the latest work design proposed to meet patient needs. It is a collaborative process that assesses, plans, implements, coordinates, monitors, and evaluates options and services to meet an individual's health needs through communication and available resources to promote quality, cost-effective outcomes (Huber, 2010; McCullough, 2009). The focus in case management is on individual patients, not populations of patients. Case managers handle each case individually, identifying the most cost-effective providers, treatments, and care settings for insured individuals (Ireland et al., 2010; McCullough, 2009).

Some health care organizations use the term *case management* to define a patient-centered model of care. Case management within the hospital setting is seen as a way to incorporate the strengths of earlier care models yet provide a professional practice model. Case management in acute care hospital nursing has been defined as a system of patient care delivery that focuses on the achievement of patient outcomes within effective and appropriate time frames and resources (Marquis & Huston, 2011). In the hospital setting, the case manager role will likely expand under health care reform (Gutbezahl & Mullahy, 2010). Zander (2010) further asserts that case management is vital for smooth and sustained transitioning of patient care. Case management focuses on an entire episode of illness, crossing all sections in which the patient receives care. A case manager directs care; however, the case manager may or may not be a nurse.

Community-Based Care

A community is a "locally-based entity composed of formal organizations reflecting societal institutions, informal groups, and aggregates. These components are interdependent, and function to meet a wide variety of collective needs" (Bull et al., 2010, p. 1013). The community is considered to be the client when the nursing focus is on the collective or common good rather than the health of an individual. Thus, **community-based care,** also called *community-based nursing practice*, is directed toward health changes for the whole community's benefit. The unit of service may be individuals, families, groups, aggregates, institutions, or communities, but the purpose is to affect the entire community. The term *community* denotes a local entity, whereas the term *population* refers to an aggregate with any common characteristic, not necessarily tied to a place (Berman, Snyder, Kozier, & Erb, 2008).

Within this context, community-based nursing describes a setting for practice and a philosophy of care applicable to all nurses in all settings. It reflects how nursing care is provided, is typically not confined to one practice setting, is directed toward individuals and families within any community setting, and is designed to assist patients as they move among health care settings. Community-based nursing occurs in places where people spend their time: in the home, in shelters, in long-term care residences, at work, in senior citizen centers, in ambulatory settings, and in hospitals (Berman et al., 2008; South, Darby, Bagnall, & White, 2010).

Legislative, regulatory, and social changes in the health care system have increased the need to move services out of the hospital and into community-based alternative health care settings. The numbers and kinds of agencies that provide care in the home and community have expanded because of the increasing needs of patients. As more health care delivery shifts into the community, more nurses are working in public health and community-based settings.

Community-based nurses are challenged as patients with complex nursing care needs are discharged from acute care settings early in the recovery process. The aging and those with multiple-system problems must rely independently on technologies for care that once were used only in hospital settings under nursing supervision. Nurses in community settings must be self-directed, flexible, adaptable, and tolerant of various lifestyles and living conditions. A team implementing a community-based self-care initiative found that there needs to be flexibility in response to the needs of participants in different settings (South et al., 2010). Expertise in independent decision making, critical thinking, assessment, health education, and competence in basic nursing care are essential to function effectively in community-based settings. Individuals with chronic care needs also improve with community-based care (Bull et al., 2010). The IOM has placed renewed emphasis upon chronic care, and professionals are stepping up to meet this vital need, particularly for patients in HIV care, palliative care, and others with chronic or terminal illnesses (Bull et al., 2010; Chu, Umanski, Blank, Grossberg, & Selwyn, 2010; South et al., 2010).

Community Health Nursing

The phrase *community-based nursing* often is interchanged with *community health nursing*, but a distinction should be made between them. The phrase **community health nursing** has generally been equated with *public health nursing*, a specialty focused on special populations, although care may be given to individuals. Within this context, the nurse may provide care to an individual with chronic long-term pulmonary obstructive disease or assist in the development of a community-wide program to abate flu development. The term *community health* means meeting the collective needs of a group by identifying problems and managing interactions both within the community and among communities that make up the larger society. An example of community health means working within the community setting to establish health preventive programs such as an immunization program. Community-based nursing is broader and may incorporate community health/public health nursing.

Population-Based Care

Population-based care is focused on aggregates and communities (Truglio-Londrigan & Lewenson, 2010). A population refers to a collection of individuals who have in common one or more personal or environmental characteristics. Also called an aggregate, the members of a community are defined in terms of geography, special interest, disease state, or other common characteristics. The research-related term is target population. In community health, population-focused practice is directed toward care for defined populations or subpopulations. With population-based care, interventions are aimed at disease prevention and health promotion that affect an entire population and extend beyond medical treatment by targeting underlying risk, such as tobacco, drug, and alcohol use; diet and sedentary lifestyles; and environmental factors. Population-based case management is defined as the integration and coordination of health services for a specified population such as those with cerebral palsy or multiple sclerosis, This concept is implemented by providing a continuum of care from many health care organizations, and it is sometimes referred to as disease management.

Disease Management

More typically, the term *disease management* refers to a comprehensive, integrated approach to care and reimbursement based on a disease's natural course. The goal is to address the disease condition with maximum effectiveness and efficiency. Huber (2010) describes this as addressing a high-cost, chronic illness or condition, such as diabetes, with maximum efficiency across treatment settings regardless of typical reimbursement patterns. Thus, a continuum of chronic illness care is established that includes early detection and early intervention. This prevents or reduces exacerbation of the disease, acute episodes, and the use of expensive resources such as hospital inpatient care. Prevention and proactive case management are two major aspects of disease management programs. Additionally, disease management programs include comprehensive tracking of patient outcomes. Thus, the goals for disease management are focused on integrating components and improving long-term outcomes (Marquis & Huston, 2011; McCullough, 2009).

Community-Based Care Versus Acute Care

Although there are notable differences between community-based care and acute care, there also are similarities. Practice in the acute care setting, where the patient is defined by disease or condition, typically takes place in specialized units where family access and patient autonomy are regulated by agency policies. Health is viewed as the opposite of illness, and the focus of care is to eliminate illness. Nursing activities are geared toward short-term interventions. In the community setting, the patient is seen within the context of family and social network, and is treated in his own environment, typically where the patient is more at ease. Illness is seen as a part of life, and the purpose of care is to limit patient disability and to improve functional capacity and quality of life. Nursing practice in the community has greater autonomy with therapeutic interventions, and is usually defined by clinician and patient, both of whom hold the patient's values central to the care performed.

Although traditional values and ways in which we think about each area of practice differ, nursing in the community-based setting does not require widely different skills and knowledge than nursing in the acute care setting. In both settings, nurses apply principles of interpersonal communication and caring skills to the patient, family, and other caregivers. Similarly, in each setting, nurses use leadership skills to plan, organize, coordinate, delegate, and evaluate patient care. In both, nurses provide effective physical care. General principles of community-based care include advocating self-care; focusing on prevention; respecting family, culture, and community; and promoting continuity of care. Within the framework of these principles, when patient self-care, prevention, collaboration, continuity, and care within the context of family, culture, and community are emphasized, the nurse is participating in community-based nursing. Community-based nursing truly becomes a philosophy of care about *how* nurses practice—not *where* they work—and can be incorporated into any type of work setting. Initiatives on the future of nursing from the Institute of Medicine (IOM) 2010 report will provide updated roles to support current and future patient care in hospitals and community-based care.

Providing Safe Patient Care

In 2004 the IOM published a critical consensus report titled *Keeping Patients Safe: Transforming the Work Environment of Nurses.* This report spoke to the importance of providing safe patient care in a complex health system. Six years after the IOM report, in 2010, the National Quality Forum (NQF) published an updated report that adds to the evolution of these practices and acknowledges their ongoing value to the health care community. The 2010 report identified 34 areas of safe practices (evidence-based) for all acute care areas, including prevention of patient falls and prevention of other areas of risk and patient safety.

Four nursing care delivery systems have historically provided a basic structure for organizing and delivering nursing care, but the research appears to support a model that uses a richer mix of RNs. The primary nursing model previously discussed in this chapter uses a richer mix of RNs, and, with its emphasis on relationship-based care, creates new possibilities for collaborative success. Leaders in health care are searching for the components and processes to make patient care safe, and the ability of the RN to coordinate, communicate, and manage the multidisciplinary team of health care workers will be very important.

The Future and Workplace Design

The preceding discussion allows the reader to conclude that there is no one single way to organize patient care delivery systems. The method of workplace design depends on the internal and external environmental factors currently in play. They are not static, but in a constant state of flux.

It is well known that forces and pressures outside of nursing influence nursing care delivery models; however, it is not known which form is the best care model for each setting (Huber, 2010; Marquis & Huston, 2011). Although there is information about the advantages of different model types, there is a lack of research evidence about which setting is most appropriate for which care model, where each is most cost effective, or which one is going to produce a higher quality of care delivery. Restructuring today means looking at new care models as they relate to a cost–quality balance. In the restructuring process, the desired outcomes are that patient care be delivered more safely and efficiently, people be more satisfied, and costs be minimized. What is clear is that with all models, nurses must collaborate with each other and other members of the health care team in order to provide health care to the current and future generations (Lavoie-Tremblay et al., 2010).

A Robert Wood Johnson Foundation–funded research project by Health Workforce Solutions LLC (HWS) identified and profiled new models of care that could be widely replicated throughout the United States (Joynt & Kimball, 2008). A team-oriented primary nursing model was one example that provided a new basis for high-quality nursing care.

Collaborative Care

Collaboration, a key focus of the 2010 IOM report, has become increasingly important among health care professionals as their roles and boundaries change and merge. The manner in which health care professionals work together affects the quality of the patient care that they provide. Problems in communication and interactions with one another may precipitate problems in patient care. "Interprofessional collaboration (IPC) practice-based interventions are strategies put into place in healthcare settings to improve work interactions and processes between two or more types of healthcare practitioners" (Zwarenstein, Goldman, & Reeves, 2009). As the focus on collaboration and IPC practice-based interventions continue to develop and as roles change, it is imperative that practitioners have realistic expectations of each other. Some practitioners have begun to limit their specialized areas of expertise, whereas others are assuming a more generalized approach. Over time, the legal scope of practice of each health care profession, including nursing, may change (Zwarenstein et al., 2009). The 2010 IOM report calls for nurses to become more involved in making health care policy and patient care decisions and to expand their role in a variety of health care settings. As these projections or goals of the report materialize, changes in job descriptions, professional expectations, and licensure requirements for nurses at all levels of practice may result. To deliver optimum comprehensive care to the patient, nurses must work as members of a team, collaborating in a collegial manner with other health care professionals. This specifically requires discussing patients' diagnoses and cooperating in the management and delivery of care (Jost et al., 2010).

Nurses as collaborators in patient care delivery also may be involved in determining and resolving bioethical issues, speaking out on legislation, participating in health-related research, and working with professional organizations. In fulfilling a collaborative role, nurses need to assume accountability and increased authority in practice areas. Key elements necessary for collaboration include effective communication skills, mutual respect and trust, and a decision-making process.

Some institutions use the collaborative practice model. Nurses, physicians, and ancillary health personnel function within a decentralized organizational structure and collaborate with each other and the patient when making clinical decisions. A joint practice committee, with representation from all care providers, may function at the unit level to monitor, support, and foster collaboration (Berman et al., 2008; Marquis & Huston, 2009). The collaborative model of care, or some variation of it, should be a primary goal for nursing. This model promotes shared participation, responsibility, and accountability in a health care environment that is striving to practice patient-centered care and meet the complex health care needs of the public with an increasing array of health care workers.

Influences in Health Care Delivery

In 2008, the Robert Wood Johnson Foundation (RWJF) and the IOM launched an initiative to study the need to assess and transform the nursing profession (IOM, Consensus Report, 2010). This initiative will affect nursing care delivery now and in the future. During the 2-year study, an expert panel reviewed innovative models of nursing care and education and reported the panel's findings in the fall of 2010. Findings of the study have been referenced earlier in the chapter in relationship to delegation, collaboration, increasing focus on chronic illness and community-based care, and interdisciplinary practice. Essentially, the role of the nurse becomes the focus of the key messages of the report. Recommendations include higher levels of nursing education as well as nurses practicing to the full extent of their education and training (IOM, Consensus Report, 2010).

Health care settings that employ more nurses have been shown to have fewer medical errors, lower rates of hospital-acquired infections, shorter hospital stays, and lower patient mortality (Reis, 2009). The Committee of the IOM and RWJF suggested that nurses are uniquely trained to provide case management of patients with chronic diseases, helping them avoid high-cost acute care. In addition, nurse-led efforts in health promotion and screening are at the heart of preventive care and wellness, which can reduce the burden of illness (Reis, 2009). In conjunction with physicians and other health providers, advance practice nurses can provide primary care services to patients.

With the expert findings, it is apparent that the United States has the opportunity to continue to transform the health care system as well as the roles of nurses and care delivery. Improved nursing care delivery models will improve patient care.

Summary

This chapter has covered a wide range of topics, all directed at explaining nursing's role in the health care delivery system. Moving from the historical influence of environmental changes to the current influence of health care reform, nursing's role and functions in acute care delivery models and community based care are explained. Models explained include the case method, functional nursing, team nursing, primary nursing, relationship-based care, patient-centered care, case management and aspects of community based care, such as population-based care and disease management. Providing safe patient care is discussed within the context of future perspectives of work place design and the impetus to engage in collaborative care to best meet future health care needs.

NCLEX® PRACTICE

1. A nurse is responsible for providing total care to a patient during the entire scheduled shift. The nurse is functioning within which of the following care delivery systems?

1. Case method
2. Functional
3. Team
4. Primary

2. Which of the following statements would the nurse use to best describe the quality of care patients receive on a unit that utilizes functional nursing?

1. Holistic and comprehensive
2. Maximum use of individual caregivers' strengths for a large number of patients
3. Better care outcomes and greater nurse satisfaction
4. Intentional fragmentation of care

3. In a functional nursing care delivery system, a registered nurse is in charge and is responsible for delegating activities and tasks to unlicensed assistive personnel. This same approach to delegating tasks to unlicensed assistive personnel is seen in which of the following care delivery systems?

1. Case method
2. Team
3. Primary
4. Primary care

4. An organizational committee is considering changing the current care delivery system to one that is more cost effective. Which of the following characteristics should the nurse consider when asked to provide a statement about selecting a cost-effective method to provide patient care?

1. Highest quality for the lowest cost
2. Amount of job autonomy
3. Nurse accountability
4. Patient acuity

5. Which of the following care areas would be the least likely to utilize advance practice nurses or case managers to assist with patient care needs?

1. Case method
2. Functional
3. Team
4. Primary

6. A health care system is planning to incorporate the recommendations of the IOM report, The *Future of Nursing,* into its plan to redesign the delivery of patient care, particularly to those with chronic conditions. The nurse wishes to advocate for a model that allows the patient maximum participation in setting goals and participating in care. Which new methods of care delivery should the nurse present as models that would meet these requirements? (select all that apply)

1. Team nursing
2. Patient-centered care
3. Disease state management
4. Case management
5. Population-based care

Answers to NCLEX Practice questions can be found in Appendix D in the Osborn Student Resources at nursing.pearsonhighered.com. Practice additional NCLEX questions online at the Student Resources site.

Pearson Nursing Student Resources Find additional review materials at: **nursing.pearsonhighered.com**

REFERENCES

Adams, V., & Nelson, J. A. (2009). The economics of nursing: Articulating care. *Feminist Economics, 15*(4), 3–29.

Aiken, L. H., Sloane, D. M., Cimiotti, J. P., Clarke, S. P., Flynn, L., Seago, J. A., Spetz, J., & Smith, H. L. (2010). Implications of the California nurse staffing mandate for other states. *Health Research and Educational Trust, 45*(4), 904–921.

Allen, L. (2008). The nursing shortage continues as faculty shortage grows. *Nursing Economics, 26*(1), 35–40.

American Association of Colleges of Nursing. (2005). Fact sheet: The clinical nurse leader. Retrieved from http://www.aacn.nche.edu/Media/FactSheets/CNLFactSheet

American Association of Colleges of Nursing. (2006, March). Clinical nurse leader competencies. Retrieved from http://www.aacn.nche.edu/CNL/pdf/TVHCompetencies.pdf

American Nurses Association. (2005). Principles for Delegation. Retrieved from www.nursingworld.org/MainMenuCategories/ThePracticeofProfessionalNursing/workplace/PrinciplesofDelegation.aspx

American Nurses Association. (2010). *Scope and standards of practice: Nursing.* (2nd ed.). Silver Spring, MD: American Nurses Association.

American Nurses Credentialing Center. (2012). *Nursing case management.* Retrieved from http://www.nursecredentialing.org/Certification/NurseSpecialties/CaseManagement.aspx

Armstrong, K., Laschinger, H., & Wong, C. (2009). Workplace empowerment and magnet hospital characteristics as predictors of patient safety climate. *Journal of Nursing Care Quality, 24*(1), 55–62.

Baernholdt, M., & Cottingham, S. (2011). The clinical nurse leader—new nursing role with global implications. *International Nursing Review, 58*(1), 74–78.

Begun, J. W., Tornabeni, J., & White, K. R. (2006). Opportunities for improving patient care through lateral integration: The clinical nurse leader. *Journal of Healthcare Management American College of Healthcare Executives, 51*(1), 19–25. Retrieved from http://www.ncbi.nlm.nih.gov/pubmed/16479747

Berman, A. J., & Snyder, S. (2012). *Kozier & Erb's fundamentals of nursing* (9th ed). Upper Saddle River, NJ: Pearson.

Bull, J., Zafar, Y., Wheeler, J. L., Harker, M., Gblokpor, A., Hanson, L., Hulihan, D., Nugent, R., Morris, J., & Abernethy, A. P. (2010). Establishing a regional, multisite database for quality improvement and service planning in community-based palliative care and hospice. *Journal of Palliative Medicine, 13*(8), 1013–1020.

Carr, R. F. (2010). Health care facilities. National Institute of Building Sciences. Retrieved from www.wbdg.org/design/health_care.php

Cho, S-H., June, K. J., Kim, Y. M., Cho, Y. A., Yoo, C. S., Youn, S-C., & Sung, Y. H. (2009). Nurse staffing, quality of nursing care and nurse job outcomes in intensive care units. *Journal of Clinical Nursing, 18,* 1729–1737.

Chu, C., Umanski, G., Blank, A., Grossberg, R., & Selwyn, P. A. (2010). HIV-infected patients and treatment outcomes: An equivalence study of community-located, primary care-based HIV treatment vs. hospital-based specialty care in the Bronx, New York. *AIDS Care, 22*(12), 1522–1529.

Daditch, K. (2003). Care delivery strategies. In P. S. Yoder-Wise (Ed.), *Leading and managing in nursing* (3rd ed.). St. Louis: Mosby.

Dias, B. (2008). A case for expanded roles for NPs in aged care. *Australian Nursing Journal, 15*(7), 39–42.

Donaldson, N. E., Rutledge, D. N.,& Geiser, K. (2008). The role of the external coach in advancing research translation. In K. Henricksen, J. B. Battles, M. A. Keyes & M. L. Grady (Eds.), *Advances in patient safety: New directions and alternative approaches* (pp. 285–302). Rockville, MD: Agency for Healthcare Research and Quality.

Duffield, C., Roche, M., Diers, D., Catling-Paull, C., & Blay, N. (2010). Staffing, skill mix and the model of care. *Journal of Clinical Nursing, 19,* 2242–2251.

Fairbrother, G., Jones, A., & Rivas, K. (2010). Changing model of nursing care from individual patient allocation to team nursing in the acute inpatient environment. *Contemporary Nurse, 35*(2), 202–220.

Fernandez, R., Tran, D. T., Johnson, M., & Jones, S. (2010). Interdisciplinary communication in general medical and surgical wards using two different models of nursing care delivery. *Journal of Nursing Management, 18,* 265–274.

Finkler, S. A., Kovner, C. T., & Jones, C. (2007). *Financial management for nurse managers and executives* (3rd ed.). Philadelphia: Saunders.

Flynn, L., Liang, Y., Dickson, G. L., & Aiken. L. (2010). Effects of nursing practice environments on quality outcomes in nursing homes. *Journal of the American Geriatrics Society, 58*(12), 2401–2406.

Flynn, M., & McKeown, M. (2009). Nursing staffing levels revisited: A consideration of key issues in nurse staffing levels and skill mix research. *Journal of Nursing Management, 17,* 759–766.

Friese, C. R., Lake, E. T., Aiken, L. H., Silber, J. H., & Sochalski, J. (2008). Nurse staffing and patient outcomes. *Health Services Research, 43*(4), 1145–1163.

Furukawa, M. F., Raghu, T. S., & Shao, B. M. (2010). Electronic medical records, nurse staffing, and nurse-sensitive patient outcomes: Evidence from California hospitals, 1998–2007. *Health Research and Educational Trust, 45*(4), 941–962.

Gerrie, J., & Nebel, A. (2010). Improving patient outcomes with relationship-based care. *Nurse Leader, 8*(6), 51–54.

Grant, B., Colello, S., Riehle, M., & Dende, D. (2010). An evaluation of the nursing practice environment and successful change management using the new generation magnet model. *Journal of Nursing Management, 18*(3), 326–331.

Gutbezahl, C. D., & Mullahy, C. M. (2010). Case management role is likely to expand under health care reform. *Hospital Case Management, 18*(6), 81–96.

Hayes, L.J., et al. (2011). Nurse turnover: a literature review – an update. *International Journal of Nursing Studies.* Retrieved from http://www.sciencedirect.com/science/article/pii/S0020748911003798

Hitt, E. (2011). Nurses involved in patient care report greater job dissatisfaction. *Medscape Medical News.* Retrieved from http://www.medscape.com/viewarticle/737528

Hoi, S. Y., Ismail, N., Ong, L. C., & Kang, J. (2010). Determining nurse staffing needs: The workload intensity measurement system. *Journal of Nursing Management, 18*(1), 44–53.

Houser, J. (2003). A model for evaluating the context of nursing care delivery. *Journal of Nursing Administration, 33*(1), 39–47.

Huber, D. (2010). *Leadership and nursing care management* (3rd ed.). Philadelphia: W. B. Saunders.

Institute of Medicine. (2004). *Keeping patients safe: Transforming the work environment of nurses.* Washington, DC: National Academies Press.

IOM Executive Office. (2010). Consensus report: The future of nursing: Leading change, advancing health. Retrieved from http://www.iom.edu/Reports/2010/The-Future-of-Nursing-Leading-Change-Advancing-Health.aspx

Ireland, S., MacKenzie, G., Gould, L., Dassinger, D., Koper, A., & LeBlanc, K. (2010). Nurse case management to improve risk reduction outcomes in a stroke prevention clinic. *Canadian Journal of Neuroscience Nursing, 32*(4), 7–13.

Joint Commission. (2010). National patient safety goals. Retrieved from www.patientsafety.gov/TIPS/Docs/TIPS_JanFeb10Poster.pdf

Jost, S. G., Bonnell, M., Chacko, S. J., & Parkinson, D. L. (2010). Primary nursing: A care delivery model for the 21st-century knowledge worker. *Nursing Administration Quarterly, 34*(3), 208–216.

Joynt, J., & Kimball, B. (2008). Innovative care delivery models: Identifying new models that effectively leverage nurses. White paper. Retrieved from http://www.healthws.com/pdfs/cdm_whitepaper_012008.pdf

Kiekkas, P., Sakellaropoulos, G. C., Brokalaki, H., Manolis, E., Samios, A., Skartsani, C., & Baltopoulos, G. I. (2008). Association between nursing workload and mortality of intensive care unit patients. *Journal of Nursing Scholarship, 40*(4), 385–390.

Kjornsberg, A., Karlsson, L., Babra, A., & Wadensten, B. (2010). Registered nurses' opinions about patient focused care. *Australian Journal of Advanced Nursing, 28*(1), 35–44.

Kramer, M., & Schmalenberg, C. (2008). Confirmation of a healthy work environment. *Critical Care Nurse, 28*(2), 56–64.

Lavoie-Tremblay, M., Paquet, M., Duchesne, M. A., Santo, A., Gavrancic, A., Courcy, F., & Gagnon, S. (2010). Retaining nurses and other hospital workers: An intergenerational perspective of the work climate. *Journal of Nursing Scholarship, 42*(4), 414–422.

Manthey, M. (1990). Definitions and basic elements of a patient care delivery system with an emphasis on primary nursing. In G. G. Mayer, M. J. Madden, & E. Lawrenz (Eds.), *Patient care delivery models* (pp. 201–211). Rockville, MD: Aspen Publishers.

Marquis, B. L., & Huston, C. J. (2011). *Leadership roles and management functions in nursing* (5th ed.). Philadelphia: Lippincott Williams & Wilkins.

McCullough, L. (2009). The case manager: An essential link in quality care. *Creative Nursing, 15*(8), 124–126.

Meyer, R. M., Wang, S., Li, X., Thomson, D., & O'Brien-Pallas, L. (2009). Evaluation of a patient care delivery model: Patient outcomes in acute cardiac care. *Journal of Nursing Scholarship, 41*(4), 399–410.

National Council of State Boards of Nursing. (1995). *Concepts and decision-making process. National Council Position Paper.* Retrieved from http://www.ncsbn.org/public/resources/ncsbn_Delegation.htm

National Quality Forum (NQF). (2010). *Safe Practices for Better Healthcare–2010 Update: A Consensus Report.* Washington, DC: NQF; 2010.

Potter, P., Deshields, T., & Kuhrik, M. (2010). Delegation practices between registered nurses and nursing assistive personnel. *Journal of Nursing Management, 18*, 157–165.

QSEN—Quality & Safety Education for Nurses. (2012). Competency KSAs (pre-licensure). Retrieved from http://www.qsen.org/ksas_prelicensure.php

Reis, S. (2009). Robert Wood Johnson Foundation, Institute of Medicine launch unprecedented initiative on the future of nursing in America. Retrieved from http://www.thefutureofnursing.org

Robertson, K. (2008). Study: Nurse staffing ratio hasn't improved patient care. *Sacramento Business Journal.* Retrieved February 25, 2011, from http://www.bizjournals.com/sacramento/stories/2008/03/24/story5.html

Schneider, M. A., & Fake, P. (2010). A relationship-based care model on a large orthopaedic/neurosurgical hospital unit. *Orthopaedic Nursing, 29*(6), 374–380.

Siegel, E. O., Young, H. M., Mitchell, P. H., & Shannon, S. E. (2008). Nurse preparation and organizational support for supervision of unlicensed assistive personnel in nursing homes: A qualitative exploration. *Gerontologist, 48*(4), 453–463.

South, J., Darby, F., Bagnall, A., & White, A. (2010). Implementing a community-based self care training initiative: A process evaluation. *Health & Social Care in the Community, 18*(6), 662–670.

Stafford, E. (2008). Study examines impact of managed care on stroke prevention surgery. Retrieved from http://insciences.org/article.php?article_id=1068

Stanley, J. M., Gannon, J., Gabuat, J., Hartranft, S., Adams, N., Mayes, C., Shouse, G. M., Edwards, B. A., & Burch, D. (2008). The clinical nurse leader: A catalyst for improving quality and patient safety. *Journal of Nursing Management, 16*, 614–622.

St. Luke's Hospital, Cedar Rapids, Iowa. (2011). What are characteristics of a magnet hospital. Retrieved from http://www.stlukescr.org/about-us/proud-to-be-a-magnet-hospital/characteristics-of-a-mag

Stichler, J. F. (2009). Wicked problems in designing healthcare facilities. *Journal of Nursing Administration, 39*(10), 405–408.

Tomey, A. M. (2004). *Guide to nursing management and leadership* (6th ed.). St. Louis: Mosby.

Truglio-Londrigan, M., & Lewenson, S. B. (2011). *Public health nursing; Practicing population-based care.* Sudberry, MA: Jones & Bartlett Publishers.

Wagner, D., & Bear, M. (2008). Patient satisfaction with nursing care: A concept analysis within a nursing framework. *Journal of Advanced Nursing, 65*(3), 692–701.

William D. Ruckelshaus Center. (2009). Nurse staffing— a summary of current research, opinion and policy. Retrieved from http://www.ruckelshauscenter.wsu.edu/projects/healthcareproject.html

Yoder-Wise, P. S. (2007). Delegation: An art of professional practice. In P. S. Yoder-Wise (Ed.), *Leading and managing in nursing* (4th ed.). St. Louis: Mosby.

Zander, K. (2010). Case management accountability for safe, smooth, and sustained transitions: A plea for building "wrap-around" case management services now. *Professional Case Management, 15*(4), 188–201.

Zwarenstein, M., Goldman, J., & Reeves, S. (2009). Interprofessional collaboration: Effects of practice-based interventions on professional practice and healthcare outcomes. *Cochrane Database of Systematic Reviews 2009, 3*(CD000072). DOI: 10.1002/14651858.CD000072.pub2.

CHAPTER 5

Nursing Process and Documentation

Cynthia Parkman
Annita Watson

Outcome-Based Learning Objectives

After studying this chapter, the learner will be able to:

1. Distinguish between the roles in nursing as specified by the American Nurses Association.
2. Organize the five steps of the nursing process, their relationship to each other, and the cognitive, affective, and psychomotor skills necessary to implement the process.
3. Distinguish among nursing diagnoses and collaborative problems.
4. Critique the relationship between critical thinking and the nursing process.
5. Interpret regulatory and professional standards for patient care documentation.
6. Summarize general principles that guide documentation.
7. Implement the nursing process within the Preparation for Practice exercises.

KEY TERMS

assessment p.96
collaborative problems p.99
critical pathways p.101
critical thinking p.102
dependent activities p.94
evaluation p.101
goal p.100
health record p.98
implementation p.101
independent activities p.94
interdependent activities p.94
intervention p.100
medication reconciliation p.110
nurse–patient relationship p.94
nurse practice act p.106
nursing diagnosis p.99
nursing process p.94
objective data p.97
outcome p.99
patient care plan p.101
planning p.99
subjective data p.97

Weblink: The Nursing Process

FOR THE PAST 30 YEARS, the American Nurses Association (ANA) has published many standards of nursing practice. These standards and the social policy statement adopted by the ANA (2010c) serve as national guidelines for nursing practice. An overview of both is shown in the National Guidelines box (p. 95).

In nursing practice, nurses' roles are defined as *independent, interdependent,* and *dependent* (ANA, 2007b). **Independent activities** are those that nurses perform, prescribe, and/or delegate based on their education and skills. Examples of independent activities are assessing, analyzing and diagnosing, planning, implementing, and evaluating. **Interdependent activities** are those that overlap with the activities of other health team members, physicians, social workers, pharmacists, nutritionists, and therapists (e.g., physical, speech, occupational) and require coordination and planning with these various health team members. **Dependent activities** are those prescribed by the physician and carried out by the nurse. They include implementing the physicians' orders to administer medications or treatments. The nursing process, a concept coined in 1967 by Yura and Walsh (1988) and subsequently adopted by the ANA (2007b), and updated again in 2007, enhances each of the three roles for the patient's benefit and is the means for nurses to demonstrate accountability and responsibility to patients.

Nursing Process

The **nursing process** is defined as a variation of scientific reasoning and is used to diagnose and to treat human responses to potential and actual health problems (ANA, 2007b). As the operational framework for nursing practice, the nursing process is the vehicle through which the nurse applies knowledge and skills in a systematic, goal-directed fashion to achieve the outcomes desired for the patient (ANA, 2007b). By using the nursing process, the nurse approaches and responds to clinical situations consciously and deliberately. Such an approach avoids nursing care based on imitation ("That's how the others do it"), intuition ("This seems like a good way to do it"), or tradition ("We've always done it that way").

Nurse–Patient Relationship

The **nurse–patient relationship** is the means for applying the nursing process (Figure 5–1◆). This relationship is the mechanism by which the nurse works with the patient (Carpenito-Moyet, 2009).

NATIONAL GUIDELINES for Nursing Practice

Nursing Scope, and Standards of Practice

Scope of Nursing Practice

The scope of practice statement describes the "who," "what," "where," "when," "why," and "how" of nursing practice. The components listed below are described in the Scope of Practice:*

Definition of Nursing	Professional Trends and Issues
Evolution of Nursing Practice	The Professional Registered Nurse
Advanced Practice Registered Nursing	Registered Nurses in Role Specialties
Settings for Nursing Practice	Continued Commitment to the Profession
Integrating the Science and Art of Nursing	

*For full definitions, go to the source publication: American Nurses Association (2010b). *Nursing: Scope and standards of practice* (2nd ed.). Silver Spring, MD: Author.

Standards of Professional Nursing Practice

The standards of professional performance describe a competent level of behavior in the professional role, including activities related to ethics, education, evidence-based practice and research, quality of practice, communicational leadership, collaboration, professional practice evaluation, resource utilization, and environmental health. All registered nurses are expected to engage in professional role activities, including leadership, appropriate to their education and position. Registered nurses are accountable for the professional action to themselves, their healthcare consumers, their peers, and ultimately to society.

Standard 1. Assessment The registered nurse collects comprehensive data pertinent to the healthcare consumer's health and/or the situation.

Standard 2. Diagnosis The registered nurse collects comprehensive data pertinent to the healthcare consumer's health and/or the situation.

Standard 3. Outcomes Identification The registered nurse analyzes the assessment data to determine the diagnoses or the issues.

Standard 4. Planning The registered nurse develops a plan that prescribes strategies and alternatives to attain expected outcomes.

Standard 5. Implementation The registered nurse implements the identified plan.

Standard 5A. Coordination of Care The registered nurse coordinates care delivery.

Standard 5B. Health Teaching and Health Promotion The registered nurse employs strategies to promote health and a safe environment.

Standard 5C. Consultation The graduate level prepared specialty nurse or advanced practice registered nurse provides consultation to influence the identified plan, enhance the abilities of others, and effect change.

Standard 5D. Prescriptive Authority and Treatment The advanced practice registered nurse uses prescriptive authority, procedures referrals, treatments, and therapies in accordance with state and federal laws and regulations.

Standard 6. Evaluation The registered nurse evaluates progress toward attainment of outcomes.

Standard 7. Ethics The registered nurse practices ethically.

Standard 8. Education The registered nurse attains knowledge and competence that reflects current nursing practice.

Standard 9. Evidence-Based Practice and Research The registered nurse attains knowledge and competence that reflects current nursing practice.

Standard 10. Quality of Practice The registered nurse communicates effectively in all areas of practice.

Standard 11. Communication The registered nurse communicates effectively in all areas of practice.

Standard 12. Leadership The registered nurse collaborates with healthcare consumer, family, and others in the conduct of nursing practice.

Standard 13. Collaboration The registered nurse demonstrates leadership in the professional practice setting and the profession.

Standard 14. Professional Practice Evaluation The registered nurse evaluates her or his own nursing practice in relation to professional practice standards and guidelines, relevant statistics, rules, and regulations.

Standard 15. Resource Utilization The registered nurse utilizes appropriate resources to plan and provide nursing services that are safe, effective, and financially responsible.

Standard 16. Environmental Health The registered nurse practices in an environmentally safe and healthy manner.

Nursing's Social Policy Statement

Nursing's Social Policy Statement describes the essence of nursing. The following information is included in the revised statement adopted by the American Nurses Association in 2010.

Content

- Role and characteristics of nursing
  - What nursing is
  - Societal implications
  - Human responses (Phenomena)
  - Theory application (Science)
  - Nursing actions (Evidence-Based Practice)
  - Outcomes
- Nursing and society
  - Social context of nursing
    - Relationship of society to nursing
    - Nursing's social contract
  - Nursing implications
- Standards
  - Definition and purpose of standards
  - Types of standards
    - Standards of practice: assessment, diagnosis, outcomes identification planning, implementation, and evaluation
    - Standards of professional performance: quality of practice, education, professional practice evaluation, collegiality, collaboration, ethics, research, resource utilization leadership
- Model of Professional Nursing Practice (each level is defined and examples are provided)
  - Scope of standards of practice and code of ethics
  - Rules and regulations provided by society
  - Policies and procedures of individual institutions
  - Nurse's self-regulation of duties and responsibilities as he or she provides care
- Competency and autonomy
  - Competency
    - Certification
    - Advanced practice roles
  - Autonomy
    - Relationship to accountability.

Sources: American Nurses Association. (2010c). *Standards of clinical nursing practice.* Washington, DC: Nursebooks.org; American Nurses Association. (2010a). *Nursing's social policy statement* (2nd ed.). Washington, DC: Nursebooks.org.

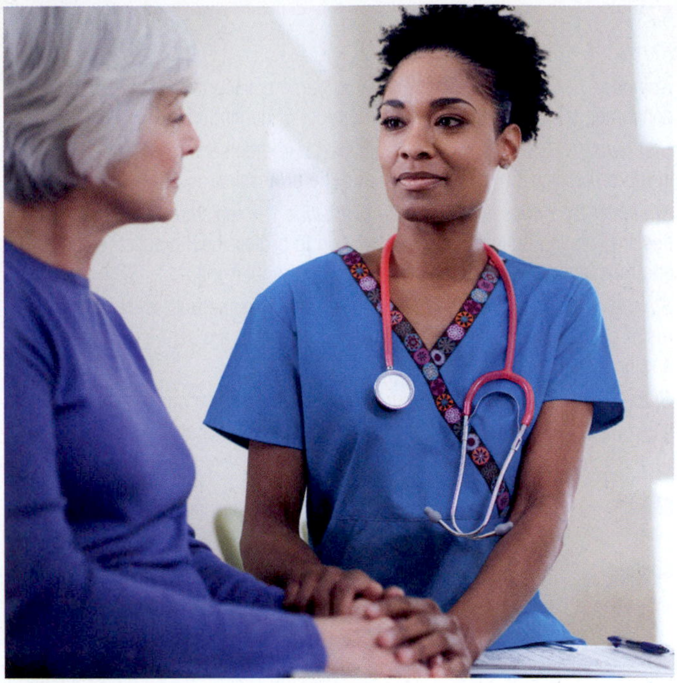

FIGURE 5–1 ◆ Nurse interacting with a patient.
Source: Corbis Super RF/Alamy

Three attributes are necessary to achieve a successful nurse–patient relationship: (1) genuineness, the ability to be aware of his or her own feelings, or being real; (2) unconditional respect for and acceptance of the other; and (3) a continuing desire to understand and empathize with the other. Effective nurse–patient relationships can be obtained when nurses are willing to examine their own values, prejudices, strengths, and limitations. Nurses must be open to the discovery of their own motivations and feelings through experience and relationships with others (Peplau, 1952; Rogers, 1970). Nurses continue to use the work of classic authors such as Peplau and Rogers to help examine their own values and beliefs when entering nurse–patient relationships.

Steps of the Nursing Process

The steps of the nursing process are progressive and successive—each step builds on previous steps and influences subsequent steps. For example, the nurse cannot develop a plan of care and select nursing interventions from that plan until valid nursing diagnoses have been formulated from an adequate database, which includes the patient's perspective and input (Carpenito-Moyet, 2009). The nurse cannot evaluate outcomes of care unless the desired outcomes have been specified as patient goals or objectives in the care plan.

The nursing process generally consists of five successive and interrelated steps: (1) assessment, (2) diagnosis, (3) planning, (4) implementation, and (5) evaluation (Berman & Kozier, 2012). In 1999, however, the ANA added "outcome identification" as a discrete step of the process, although this component is often incorporated into the diagnosis phase and is presented as such in this chapter. The components of the five steps in the nursing process follow:

1. Assessment
   - Data collection
   - Analysis/synthesis of data
   - Nursing diagnosis
2. Nursing diagnosis and outcome identification
3. Planning of goals and objectives
   - Plans
   - Priorities
   - Scientific rationale
4. Implementation
5. Evaluation

These five steps and their components are depicted in more detail in Figure 5–2◆, which illustrates the dynamic, cyclical, interdependent, and often overlapping nature of the steps of the nursing process. For example, while the nurse implements a planned intervention, such as pain relief measures, additional data may be collected that further validate and support the nursing diagnosis of pain, while also leading to the development of additional nursing diagnoses, such as a disturbance in the patient's usual sleeping patterns. Thus, during any nurse–patient interaction, the nurse is continuously collecting data that may be helpful in planning, implementing, evaluating, or revising nursing care.

The nursing process, classically defined, is flexible and is, therefore, capable of being adapted to a variety of situations. It may be used in any type of clinical setting and with patients of varying ages, health status, and cultural backgrounds (Berman & Kozier, 2012; Carpenito-Moyet, 2009). The nursing process also can be used with families and communities as well as with individual patients. Each phase (step) of the nursing process is individually discussed next.

Assessment

In general terms, **assessment** is defined as the act of evaluating or appraising. Yura and Walsh (1988) provide a classic definition that is clear, concise, and useful in assessment as it relates to nursing: "The act of reviewing a situation for the purpose of diagnosing the patient's problems" (p. 110). Assessment actions include "examining the patient and identifying cues, collecting and analyzing the data, and reaching conclusions" (p. 110). These assessment actions remain relevant today in implementing the nursing process (Carpenito-Moyet, 2009).

The nursing assessment begins the moment the nurse establishes initial contact with a patient. The nurse collects data through formal and informal interviews and a variety of other methods including observation, inspection, palpation, percussion, auscultation, and consultation with the patient and other health care providers. Data collection is a foundation of the nursing process; therefore, the nurse must strive for accuracy, completeness, and objectivity. An accurate assessment leads to identification of the patient's health status, concerns, and nursing diagnoses.

The purpose of data collection is to identify and obtain pertinent data about the patient. The classic authors suggest that nurses should consider patients in a multidimensional way; that is, the biophysical, psychological, spiritual, and sociocultural elements of the patient must be considered to ensure a comprehensive and accurate assessment (Henderson, 1966; Johnson, 1980; Watson, 1988, 2003). The work of these theorists continues to guide nurses in assessing and evaluating patients from a multidimensional perspective (Carpenito-Moyet, 2009).

Data Sources

The nurse uses two kinds of data sources: primary and secondary. The primary source of data is the patient. Secondary data sources include family, friends, other health care professionals, the patient's current health care record, and the nurse's own knowledge base. These secondary data sources should be viewed as a supplement to the data supplied

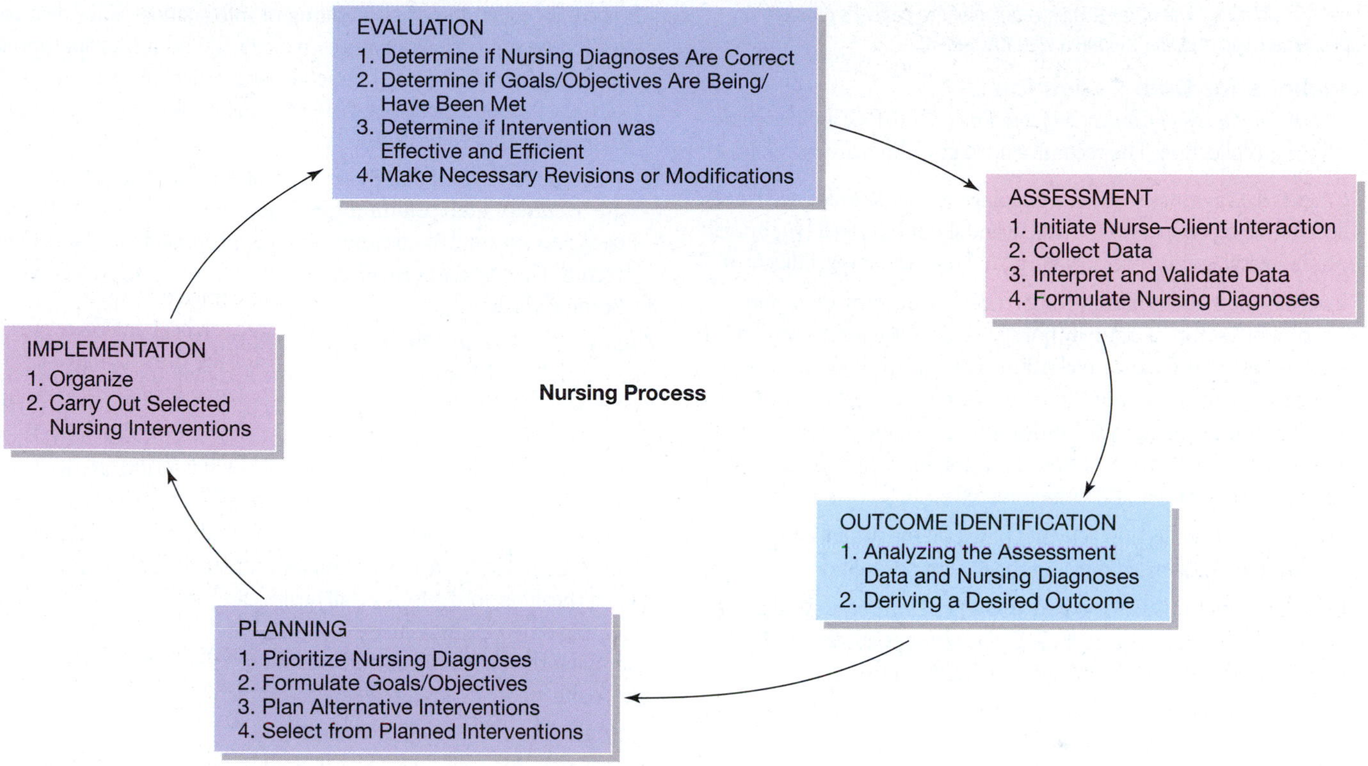

FIGURE 5–2 ◆ The nursing process.

by the primary source (i.e., the patient). The information obtained from secondary sources is useful in clarifying, amplifying, or substantiating the data the nurse obtains from the patient.

Data Types

The nurse gathers two types of data: subjective data and objective data (Berman & Kozier, 2012; Carpenito-Moyet, 2009). **Subjective data** are the information that can be perceived only by the patient and not by the observer. One of the primary sources of subjective data is the nursing or health history. Because the patient is the informant, the information collected while taking a health history is subjective. **Objective data** consist of behaviors, activities, and events that can be observed or measured by another person using the five senses. Objective data are factual; they can be seen, heard, touched, smelled, or tasted. Vital signs, laboratory reports, rashes, and body posture are some examples of objective data.

Objective and subjective data are equally important in a comprehensive nursing assessment. When assessing a patient, the nurse should try to elicit objective data that correspond with the subjective data, and subjective data that correspond with the objective data. By categorizing data as subjective and objective, the nurse is better able to validate data, identify and resolve discrepancies, and accurately report information to assist in communication and establish nursing diagnoses.

Data Collection Process

The process of data collection is influenced by how the data are presented by the patient and how they are perceived by the nurse. The nurse and patient are influenced by their respective:

- Physical, mental, and emotional states and needs
- Cultural, social, and philosophical backgrounds
- Number and functional ability of senses
- Past experiences associated with the present situation
- Meaning of the event
- Interest, preoccupations, preconceptions, and motivational levels
- Knowledge or familiarity with the situation
- Environmental conditions and distractions
- Presence, attitudes, and reactions of others.

The factors in the previous list, such as cultural, social, and philosophical backgrounds, create a situation in which both patient and nurse automatically assign personal meaning or interpretations to situations: "What does cultural background mean to each of them, the patient and the nurse?" Problems arise when the nurse's perception or interpretation is used as fact without validating it with the patient. The nursing diagnosis is the end product of the nursing assessment. The nurse analyzes the data gathered and reaches a conclusion about the patient's health status. A patient may have one or more nursing diagnoses. Once the diagnoses have been formulated, the nurse is ready to develop a plan of care. Therefore, skill is needed in differentiating actual data from personal interpretation. The nurse's interpretation must be validated with the patient in order to determine if the nurse's interpretation is correct, or if it is totally based on her interpretation of cultural background. Chart 5–1 provides examples of objective data versus personal interpretations of them.

CHART 5–1 Objective Data Versus Personal Interpretation

Objective Data	Personal Interpretation
"I'd rather be left alone."	Patient is angry
Shoulder-length dark brown hair	Long, dirty brown hair
Blood pressure: 130/76	Normal blood pressure
Smiles frequently	Appears to be happy

Safety Alert *The nurse's interpretation of the patient's problem (diagnosis) always must be validated with the patient.*

Guidelines for Data Collection

The ANA *Standards of Clinical Nursing Practice* (2010c) are the guidelines for data collection. The recommended guidelines are as follows:

- Collects data in a systematic and ongoing process. The data need to reflect the life experiences of the patient and should consider biophysical, psychological, spiritual, sociocultural, and socioeconomic influences.
- Involves the patient, family, other health care providers, and environment as appropriate, in holistic data collection. A variety of sources are used for data collection. The patient is clearly the primary source for data collection, but because perceptions of events and circumstances can vary, other sources should be used as well. Some general examples of sources are family, significant others, health care personnel, and written records.
- Prioritizes data collection activities based on the patient's immediate condition or anticipated needs of the patient or situation.
- Uses appropriate evidence-based assessment techniques and instruments in collecting pertinent data. The appropriateness of the tool used depends on the patient's age and health status.
- The data collected are objective and nonjudgmental. Data are collected through the use of observation, measurement, and interaction with the patient. Personal interpretations or perceptions of a situation may lead to further data collection, but must never be stated as data themselves.
- A systematic format is used for data collection. Theoretical and conceptual frameworks provide guides for data collection. The nurse begins data collection by assessing the patient's major concern, including multifocal influences on the concern. Then a more general assessment of the patient's health status is included as appropriate.
- The data collected reflect updating of information. Since data collection is continuous in nature, the data should reflect appropriate updating of information obtained from a variety of data sources. As new data are obtained, any changes in the health concerns or status of the patient must be noted.
- Documents relevant data in a retrievable format. The data collected are recorded and communicated appropriately. Data collection is useless unless it is communicated appropriately in the patient's record. Therefore, information must be kept in a retrievable record-keeping system.

Data Collection and the Patient's Health Record

The patient's **health record** is a document containing (1) the patient's medical history; (2) the findings from the physical examination; (3) the reports of laboratory tests; (4) the findings and conclusions from special examinations; (5) the findings and diagnoses of consultants; (6) the diagnoses of the responsible physician; (7) notes on treatment, including medication, surgical operations, radiation, and physical therapy; and (8) progress notes by physicians, nurses, and others. The purpose of the patient's health record is to assist all health care providers (nurses, physicians, and others) with accurate communication and information, thus improving the patient's care and treatment (Yaqub & Barroso, 2010). The health record also is discussed in Chapter 2.

Frameworks for Data Collection

Frameworks for data collection include a health history, a physical format, a functional instrument such as a behavioral assessment, activities of daily living (ADLs), and instrumental ADLs for older adults. Some examples of data collection tools for ADLs are provided in Charts 5–2 and 5–3.

Nursing Diagnosis and Outcome Identification

The assessment process is applicable to all groups of patients: individuals, families, and communities.

CHART 5–2 Activities of Daily living

Toileting

________ Cares for self at toilet completely; no incontinence (lack of bladder/bowel control).
________ Needs to be reminded or needs help in cleaning self, or has rare (weekly at most) accidents.
________ Soiling or wetting while asleep more than once a week.
________ Soiling or wetting while awake more than once a week.
________ No control of bowel or bladder.

Feeding

________ Eats without assistance.
________ Eats with minor assistance at mealtimes and/or with special preparation of food; helps cleaning up after meals.
________ Feeds self with moderate assistance for all meals.
________ Requires extensive assistance for all meals.
________ Does not feed self at all and resists efforts of others to feed him/her.

Dressing

________ Dresses, undresses, and selects clothes from own wardrobe.
________ Dresses and undresses self with minor assistance.
________ Needs moderate assistance in dressing or selection of clothes.
________ Needs major assistance in dressing, but cooperates with efforts of others to help.
________ Needs total grooming care, but can remain well groomed after help from others.

Physical Walking

________ Goes about grounds or city.
________ Walks with assistance of (check one—none may apply):
____ Another person ____ Railing ____ Cane ____ Walker
________ Uses a wheelchair (gets in and out without help).
________ Uses a wheelchair (needs help getting in, out).
________ Sits unsupported in chair or wheelchair, but cannot propel self without help.
________ Bedridden more than half the time.

Bathing

________ Bathes self (tub, shower, sponge bath) without help.
________ Bathes self with help getting in and out of tub.
________ Washes face and hands only, but cannot bathe rest of body.
________ Does not wash self, but is cooperative with those who bathe him/her.
________ Does not try to wash self, and resists efforts to keep himself/herself clean.

CHART 5–3 Instrumental Activities of Daily Living

Ability to Telephone

______ Operates telephone on own initiative (looks up and dials numbers, etc.).
______ Selects a few well-known numbers.
______ Answers telephone, but does not initiate call.
______ Does not use telephone at all.

Shopping

______ Takes care of all shopping needs independently.
______ Shops independently for small purchases.
______ Needs to be accompanied on any shopping trip.
______ Completely unable to shop.

Food Preparation

______ Plans, prepares, and serves adequate meals independently.
______ Prepares adequate meals if supplied with ingredients.
______ Heats and serves prepared meals, or prepares meals but does not maintain adequate diet.
______ Needs to have meals prepared and served.

Housekeeping

______ Maintains house alone or with occasional assistance (i.e., heavy work done by others).
______ Performs light daily tasks such as dish washing and bed making.
______ Performs light daily tasks, but cannot maintain acceptable level of cleanliness.
______ Needs help with all home maintenance tasks.
______ Does not participate in any housekeeping tasks.

Laundry

______ Does personal laundry completely.
______ Launders small items: rinses socks, stockings, etc.
______ All laundry must be done by others.

Mode of Transportation

______ Travels independently on public transportation or drives own car.
______ Arranges own travel via taxi, but does not otherwise use public transportation.
______ Travels on public transportation when assisted or accompanied by another.
______ Travels limited to taxi or automobile, with assistance of another.
______ Does not travel at all.

Responsibility for Own Medication

______ Is responsible for taking medication in correct dosages at correct time.
______ Takes responsibility if medication is prepared in advance in separate dosages.
______ Is not capable of dispensing own medication.

Ability to Handle Finances

______ Manages financial matters independently (budgets, writes checks, pays rent and bills, goes to bank).
______ Manages day-to-day purchases but needs help with banking, major purchases, etc.
______ Incapable of handling money.

Nursing Diagnoses

After all data have been collected, they are sorted, organized, interpreted, and validated. Conclusions are then drawn about the patient's health status. These conclusions, called **nursing diagnoses,** are clinical judgments about an individual, family, or community response to actual or potential health problems and life processes (North American Nursing Diagnosis Association [NANDA], 2007).

Nursing diagnoses are different from **collaborative problems** such as medical diagnoses (diabetes, hypertension, coronary artery disease) because nurses' accountability differs for nursing diagnoses and collaborative problems. Nurses ultimately are accountable for formulating nursing diagnoses and intervening appropriately. With regard to a collaborative problem, the nurse is accountable for monitoring changes in the problem's status and initiating the appropriate interventions, whether they are nurse prescribed or physician prescribed. Nursing diagnoses and collaborative problems are equally important and are determined by the severity of the patient's illness at a particular point in time (Carpenito-Moyet, 2009). According to Carpenito-Moyet, there are four types of nursing diagnoses: actual, high risk, wellness, and syndrome. Each type has a specific purpose and unique components, as shown in Chart 5–4 (p. 100). The same method for identifying types of nursing diagnoses may be used to formulate population or community health diagnoses. This also is shown in Chart 5–4 (p. 100).

Outcome Identification

Outcome identification is accomplished by analyzing the assessment data and the nursing diagnosis and deriving a desired outcome for a given problem. The **outcome** is a statement of how the patient's status will change once interventions have been successfully instituted. This individual measurable patient objective, or measurable criterion, specifically indicates that the patient care objective has been met.

Planning

Once nursing diagnoses are formulated, the **planning** phase begins. The nurse is seldom able to resolve all of the patient's nursing diagnoses simultaneously; therefore, these diagnoses must be prioritized. Several factors must be considered when establishing the priority of the patient's nursing diagnoses. These include the patient's needs for biological survival and functioning, the urgency of the need, the patient's perceptions and values, and the nature of the nurse–patient relationship (Berman & Kozier, 2012; Carpenito-Moyet, 2009).

Certain basic human needs, such as oxygenation, fluid and electrolyte balance, temperature regulation, pain avoidance, nutrition, elimination, and protection from injury, take precedence over needs such as activity, sexual needs, emotional security, attachment, and self-esteem. A patient's basic survival needs are based on Maslow's hierarchy of needs (Maslow, 1954). For example, a patient with burn injuries has certain needs—a patent airway, prevention of hypovolemic shock, and pain control—that must be attended to immediately. Concerns about the patient's alteration in body image and possible interferences with sexuality and self-esteem are dealt with when the patient's physiological functioning has been stabilized.

The urgency of the nursing diagnosis also must be considered. The potential threat to safety of an orthopedic fall-risk hospitalized patient whose bed is left in a high position, or to an elderly disoriented patient

CHART 5–4 Types of Nursing Diagnoses and Population (Community) Diagnoses

Actual	High Risk	Wellness	Syndrome
Nursing Diagnoses			
A state that has been clinically validated by identifiable major defining characteristics having four components: label, definition, defining characteristics, and related factors.	A clinical judgment that a patient is more vulnerable to develop the problem than are others in the same or similar situation having four components: label, definition, risk factors, and related factors.	A patient's clinically validated desire to move from a specific level of wellness to a higher level of wellness having only one component: the label.	A cluster of actual or high-risk nursing diagnoses that are predicted to be present because of a single event or situation having one component: the label, which contains the etiology or contributing factors to the diagnosis.
Population (Community) Diagnoses			
A state of the community (e.g., economic, social, and/or health) that has been validated by identifiable major characteristics having four components: label, definition, defining characteristics, and related factors.	Identified community problems are prioritized by a team of community representatives. A judgment is made as to which identified problem puts the community at the greatest risk for suffering more serious outcomes, carrying the highest risk of harm to the community. The identified problem should have four components: a label (e.g., Compromised Health Status of Disabled Population), definition, risk factors, and related factors.	The community agrees to move from a specific economic, social, or health level based on the label, definition, and scope of the problem	A cluster of actual or high-risk community diagnoses are predicted to be present because of a single event or situation having one component: the label which contains the etiology or contributing factors to the diagnosis (e.g., Compromised Health Status of Disabled Population related to limited access to health services).

who tries to leave a nursing home unattended, takes precedence (at least temporarily) over the patient's nutritional needs or the elderly patient's nursing diagnosis of pain resulting from arthritis.

The patient's perceptions and values are important determinants in setting priorities for nursing care—when the patient's perceptions of priority are ignored, the desired outcomes of care are not likely to be achieved (Berman & Kozier, 2012). For example, a daughter brings her elderly mother in for a health checkup. The daughter expresses much concern and frustration about her mother's belligerent behavior and "acting out" by eating only candy on a regular basis. The nurse also notes that the mother has lost weight since her last visit and appears undernourished and dehydrated. Although the mother has pressing nutritional needs, the nurse realizes that the daughter is most concerned about her mother's behavior. Unless the nurse focuses first on the daughter's perceived priority need relating to her mother's behavior, his success in changing the mother's nutritional habits will be thwarted.

The nature of the nurse–patient relationship also will determine the order in which the nurse attempts to deal with the patient's diagnoses (Lachman, 2009). For example, suppose the patient's problem is interpersonal or sexual. Effective intervention will depend on a close and trusting relationship between the nurse and the patient. Such relationships take time to develop. Consequently, the nurse may assign these nursing diagnoses a lower priority until mutual rapport, trust, and respect have developed.

After nursing diagnoses have been assigned priorities, patient goals and objectives are established to clearly outline expected outcomes of care. A **goal** is a broad statement of purpose that describes the aim of nursing care—for example, "To alleviate pain and promote comfort" or "To facilitate adequate oxygenation" or "To promote acceptance of altered body image." Objectives for the individual patient should then be formulated for each goal, in terms of changes in patient behaviors that should result from nursing interventions. Objectives must include measurable criteria that provide parameters for determining whether objectives have been achieved. For example, if a hospitalized patient's nursing diagnosis is "Sleep Disturbance related to environmental noise and interruptions for nursing care," the goal may be "To promote adequate rest and sleep." The objective (or outcome), then, may state, "The patient will sleep for at least two uninterrupted periods of 3 hours each during the night." It is important to formulate patient objectives that are both measurable and realistic. An objective that specifies a hospitalized patient will sleep for an 8-hour uninterrupted period is probably quite unrealistic. A realistic objective must take into account the patient's usual pattern and motivation; the health care setting; resources available to the patient and nurse; and the patient's age, cultural background, and health status. Goals and objectives that are inconsistent with the patient's cultural practices, for example, will probably not be achieved (Berman & Kozier, 2012).

Safety Alert *Goals for patient care are based on the nurse's perspective and are differentiated from measurable objectives or outcomes, which are the patient's response to care. To assess the patient's response to care or the outcome, the nurse must identify evaluation parameters that can be observed and measured.*

Objectives may be short term or long term. Short-term objectives can facilitate ongoing evaluation of the patient's progress toward long-term objectives. For example, a long-term objective for an obese woman might be "Patient will lose 50 pounds in 1 year." A short-term statement might be "Patient will lose approximately 1 pound per week."

Objectives are useful and effective when they are:

- Mutually acceptable to nurse, patient, and family
- Appropriate in terms of nursing and medical diagnoses and therapy
- Realistic in terms of patient's capabilities, time, energy, and resources
- Specific enough to be understood clearly by the patient and other nurses
- Measurable enough to facilitate evaluation.

Once goals and objectives have been identified, the next step is to formulate interventions for achieving the stated goals and objectives. **Interventions** are planned nursing actions that are likely to facilitate desired outcomes. For example, alternatives for a postoperative patient experiencing pain may include distraction and relaxation techniques, positioning for comfort, or administration of a prescribed analgesic.

After identifying nursing actions (interventions), the nurse then selects from the alternatives. In a sense, selection of nursing actions parallels the process of prioritizing the nursing diagnoses. The actions the nurse selects, and the order in which they are implemented, depend on the following factors:

- Patient preferences
- Known effectiveness of the action (based on prior knowledge, experience, and evidence)
- Time and resources available
- Possible side effects of treatments or medications.

In the case of pain relief, for example, the nurse might decide to help the patient learn conscious relaxation techniques. This action requires time, however, and if the patient is having acute, intense pain and is requesting "a pain medication," the nurse probably will choose to administer the prescribed analgesic first and then teach the patient relaxation techniques once pain relief has been achieved. This will help the patient cope with recurrence of the pain; for instance, if the pain recurs, the nurse may select distraction as the first alternative nursing action.

Implementation

Implementation is the "doing" or intervening phase of the nursing process. It involves organization and actual delivery of nursing care, which leads to achievement of stated goals and objectives. Nursing interventions are actions designed to facilitate the achievement of positive patient outcomes. They must be purposeful and must be supported by a rationale. A sound rationale is derived from the nurse's knowledge base, prior experience, and the individualized assessment of the patient. Safe and effective nursing interventions are based on an in-depth assessment and individualized care plan (American Nurses Association [ANA], 2007b). NANDA has developed standardized nursing interventions, referred to as the Nursing Intervention Classification (NIC), that correspond with the NANDA nursing diagnoses (Ackley & Ladwig, 2011; NANDA, 2011).

Standards of care are based on research and provide an efficient method for identifying predicted problems that occur in a particular situation. **Critical pathways** are examples of implementation tools that anticipate and describe (in advance) the care of patients within a specified timeline (Carpenito-Moyet, 2009; Kinsman, Rotter, James, Snow, & Willis, 2010). The critical pathway is based on research and consists of evidence-based or benchmark practices. These practices provide rationales for care and serve to assist nurses in providing answers to the patients' questions as to why proposed interventions are the best approach to their health care. Their advantages include improved patient outcomes, streamlined documentation, facilitation of quality assessment, improved patient education, and enhanced communication among health care providers (Kinsman et al., 2010) Critical pathways are discussed in Chapter 6 as guidelines for health assessments.

Evidence-Based Practice

Evidence-based practice (EBP) is the recommended standard in health care used by nurses (Benner, Tanner, & Chesla, 2009; Polit & Beck, 2012). Quality Safety Education for Nurses (QSEN, 2012) was developed by high-level faculty to establish guidelines for nursing students' clinical practice based upon evidence-based practice. QSEN, in their description of pre-licensure competencies, has defined EBP as integrating best current evidence with clinical expertise and patient/family preferences and values for delivery of optimal health care. With this definition "current best evidence" includes clinical practice guidelines developed nationally by expert researchers, clinicians, and theorists in their areas of excellence. EBP involves the interpretation and implementation of these clinical guidelines by health care providers based on their clinical expertise, the needs and values of the patient and family, and the resources of the health care system. Thus, EBP is essential in establishing nursing interventions as part of the nursing process. As a problem-solving approach to clinical decision making, it is inherent in the nursing process and incorporates a search for the best and latest evidence, clinical expertise and assessment, and a patient's preferences and values within a context of caring (Benner et al., 2009). Chapter 3 fully discusses EBP.

Weblink: What is a Clinical Pathway? Weblink: The Nursing Process

Evaluation

Evaluation focuses on a patient's behavioral changes and compares them with the criteria stated in the objectives. It consists of both the patient's status and the effectiveness of the nursing care. Both must be evaluated continuously, with the care plan modified as needed (ANA, 2007b). Thus, evaluation is ongoing through all phases of the nursing process. As the nurse works with a patient, the patient's responses to the nursing interventions are appraised to determine if the desired outcomes (objectives) have been achieved. For example, if the outcome states that the patient "will ambulate with assistance for 15 minutes four times a day," this intervention can easily be evaluated by confirming it with the patient and reviewing the nurses' documentation. However, if the objectives are not achieved, the nurse must determine:

- If the nursing diagnosis was correct
- If the goals and objectives were realistic and reasonable
- If nursing interventions were appropriate
- If any revisions and modifications in the plan are indicated.

It may be that an incorrect nursing diagnosis was made from incomplete or inaccurate data or that the goals and objectives were unacceptable to the patient (unreasonable) or unrealistic in terms of the patient's usual patterns and lifestyles, as well as the available resources (Benner et al., 2009). Nursing interventions must be evaluated in terms of their effectiveness. If the selected intervention did not achieve the intended outcome, another intervention should be attempted.

Patient Care Plan

The **patient care plan** is a documented record of the nursing process. Nursing diagnoses, outcomes with evaluation parameters, and interventions with supporting rationales are recorded on the care plan to communicate with the health care team and to guide patient care. The care plan also needs to be evaluated on the basis of information obtained from the patient evaluation. Evaluation of the patient care plan is necessary to follow a patient's increased or decreased ability to provide self-care, thus allowing for appropriate modifications. The steps of the nursing process are summarized in Chart 5–5. In addition, an example of how the nursing process is used with a patient care plan is shown in the Nursing Process box (p. 103).

CHART 5–5 Nursing Process

- **Assessment** is the collection of both objective and subjective data about the patient. The nurse collects physical evidence; for example, lung sounds, blood pressure, and presence or absence of peripheral pulses. The subjective data are derived from talking with the patient and family about the clinical manifestations that necessitated the need for health care. These data also include the medical history, allergies, and significant previous medical or surgical interventions. Both the subjective and objective data are then organized and documented on the patient's medical record and the patient care plan.
- *Nursing diagnoses* are derived from an analysis of the data collected during the patient's assessment. Diagnoses include both actual and potential health problems (problems that the patient is at risk for developing). For example, a patient may actually have fluid imbalance or the patient may be at risk for fluid imbalance. These diagnoses are then prioritized and categorized into those that can be managed independently by nursing and those that require a collaborative approach to management. Nurses are pivotal in coordinating the other health care professionals who contribute to positive patient outcomes.
- *Outcome identification*, often considered a part of the diagnosis step, consists of analyzing the assessment data and nursing diagnoses and deriving a desired outcome for a given problem. The outcome is a statement of how the patient's status will change once the interventions have been successfully instituted. Seganfredo and Almeida (2011) validated the standardized vocabulary and classifications of nursing outcomes as they relate specifically to nursing interventions—the Nursing Outcomes Classification (NOC).
- *Planning* is the phase of the nursing process in which interventions are planned that will achieve the identified outcomes associated with each nursing diagnosis. The interventions need to be prioritized to ensure patient safety. The planning phase may or may not be documented in the patient record. Often it is a mental process of choosing the appropriate interventions in collaboration with the patient, if possible. The patient may or may not be an active participant in the planning process, dependent on the clinical situation.
- *Implementation* is the carrying out of the plan identified in the previous step of the nursing process. Communication is a critical piece of the implementation process. This phase requires that the nurse identify which interventions can be accomplished independently and which require collaboration with other members of the health care team. The nurse needs to ensure that all members have received clear communication about the patient's needs. There also is a standardized classification of nursing interventions referred to as the Nursing Interventions Classifications (NIC) (Authors, 2010). These standards provide a list of interventions associated with each nursing diagnosis. The final step of the implementation phase is recording the interventions on the patient record.
- *Evaluation* requires that the nurse compare the patient status to the desired outcomes. If an outcome is unmet, the care plan is revised and the process begins again until positive outcomes are achieved, if at all possible.

Critical Thinking and the Nursing Process

Critical thinking and the nursing process are interrelated aspects of judgment and clinical reasoning. These processes influence and empower the nurse to demonstrate accountability to the patient through the independent, interdependent, and dependent roles inherent in nursing practice. Critical thinking has become a popular phrase in nursing circles during the past decade. Essentially, **critical thinking** is a different way of viewing the information that a clinician knows or learns. Critical thinking demands that a clinician examine information in a variety of ways, exploring means of considering what is important and why some information is more important than other aspects of information, and then taking what is most important and using that information to make decisions and solve problems.

Critical thinking is essential to competent, skillful nursing care. When caring for patients, especially in stressful situations, critical thinking enables nurses to recognize important cues, respond quickly, and adapt interventions as needed (Benner et al., 2009). Nurses accomplish critical thinking by: (1) analyzing the situation to discover what issues are involved and what actions are appropriate, (2) applying standards according to established personal and professional rules, (3) discriminating by recognizing the similarities and differences among patients and diagnoses, (4) seeking additional information by searching for knowledge and gathering relevant data about the patient and her condition or diagnosis, (5) drawing conclusions that are supported by the data, (6) creating a plan of action, and (7) transforming knowledge into action. It is essential when analyzing each situation that nurses consider the ethical and legal principles involved. Critical thinking is discussed extensively in Chapter 1.

Decision Making

The application of critical thinking is decision making, or effective clinical judgment (Potter, Deshields, & Kuhrik, 2010). In decision making, a subset of problem solving, the individual selects a course of action from among two or more choices, using a variety of strategies to determine the best course of action. As such, decision making is synonymous with the act of choosing, of converting information into action.

A critical aspect of decision making surrounds the decision to delegate patient care. In the previous nursing care plan, the nurse could delegate interventions that support the patient's need to improve his "activity intolerance." A nursing assistant could walk with the patient and be sure the patient monitors his distance and any symptoms. Likewise, the nursing assistant can remind the patient to use a call bell before getting out of bed, or trying to use the bathroom, for safety at the hospital and at home. These types of care items can be delegated by the nurse to a nursing assistant. In this situation, the nurse has reviewed the principles of delegation and made an informed decision to assign patient care activities to an unlicensed assistive person. This decision is the result of an immediate care problem (Potter et al., 2010).

Elements of making an informed decision include (1) identification of a problem, (2) establishment of criteria to evaluate potential solutions, (3) a search for alternative solutions or actions, (4) evaluation of alternative choices, and (5) selection of a course of action.

The four phases of decision making are deliberation, judgment, choice, and evaluation of the effectiveness of the outcomes. Perhaps the most time-consuming phase is the deliberation phase, in which an individual determines that there is a decision to be made, begins to establish criteria for evaluating the effectiveness of potential solutions, and searches for possible solutions. The judgment phase involves a thorough understanding of the possible choices at hand and evaluation of these choices. Once these two phases have been explored, the third phase involves the selection and implementation of what has been determined to be the best choice of action. Finally, evaluation of the outcomes' effectiveness occurs, which may begin the process anew if desired outcomes are not attained.

NURSING PROCESS: Patient Care Plan for Acute Coronary Syndrome

Assessment of Cardiac Status Using Gordon's Functional Health Patterns:

- Activity Exercise Pattern
- Cognitive Perceptual Pattern
- Nutritional Metabolic Pattern
- Coping-Stress Tolerance Pattern

Subjective Data	Objective Data
Assessment of Cardiac Output	**Assessment of Cardiac Output**
Do you ever feel your heart beat fast, beat irregularly, or skip beats? Do you ever feel light-headed? Do you get short of breath when you walk distances?	Assess heart rate and rhythm for abnormalities. Compare monitor to central and peripheral pulses. Note quality of pulse (weak, bounding) at radial site. Monitor medications given and evaluate the patient's response, especially those given for tachycardia, bradycardia, or any dysrhythmias. Monitor blood pressure. Monitor respirations and SpO_2.
Assessment of Fluid Status	**Assessment of Fluid Status**
Are you short of breath? Do you monitor your weight? Do you eat a lot of salt? Do your feet swell; if so, when and under what circumstances?	Assess lung sounds for rales or crackles. Monitor blood pressure, jugular venous distention (JVD), vital signs, urine output, daily weight, and peripheral edema.
Assessment of Pain	**Assessment of Pain**
Do you have chest pain? Does your jaw hurt or throat hurt? Does it radiate anywhere else on your body? Does it go away with a deep breath? What makes the pain better or worse?	Use pain scale (0–10) to quantify pain level. Assess cultural or religious impact on the patient's response. Assess location, duration, and onset of pain and what provokes and relieves it.
Assessment of Activity Tolerance	**Assessment of Activity Tolerance**
Are you able to complete your activities of daily living without fatigue or chest pain? Are you able to walk up a flight of stairs without getting short of breath or experiencing chest pain? Do you exercise on a regular basis? Are you able to walk in the hall without experiencing fatigue, shortness of breath (SOB), chest pain, or dizziness?	Monitor vital signs (heart rate, blood pressure in both arms, mean arterial pressure, respiratory rate, oxygen saturation) before and after activity. Assess heart sounds. Assess lung sounds.
Assessment of Patient Ability to Cope	**Assessment of Patient Ability to Cope**
How are you feeling about your heart attack? What are your thoughts about your future health?	Evaluate patient response to written and verbal teaching materials about the patient's heart attack. Evaluate patient response to discussion about current and future health concerns. Observe for manifestations of anxiety: restlessness, apprehension, withdrawal.
Assessment of Patient/Family Knowledge of Disease and Treatment	**Assessment of Patient/Family Knowledge of Disease and Treatment**
Tell me what you know about your problems with your heart. Tell me what you are doing about your risk factors. Tell me about your dietary intake and your exercise program. When do you develop chest pain and what makes it go away? What medications are you on, when are you supposed to take them, and what are the side effects you should watch for? When are you supposed to see your doctor? Are you consistently participating in a cardiac rehabilitation program? Has anyone explained your health problems to you? Would you tell me what you know about your disease? How does this disease affect your daily life? Do you feel anxious about your health problems? Do you have family members or close friends who provide emotional support? Do you see your health care provider on a regular basis?	Patient/family may be anxious, confused, and need repeated information. Mistakes being made with treatment plan. Self-care deficit due to clinical manifestations.

(*continued*)

NURSING PROCESS: Patient Care Plan for Acute Coronary Syndrome, *continued*

Outcomes and Evaluation Parameters	Planning and Interventions with *Rationales*
1. NURSING DIAGNOSIS: *Decreased Cardiac Output* related to dysrhythmias secondary to acute myocardial ischemia and infarction (NANDA-I © 2012)	
Outcome: Patient maintains normal and regular heart rate and rhythm. Patient verbalizes less fear and anxiety. ***Evaluation Parameters:*** Vital signs within normal limits. Exercise endurance increases. No anginal-type chest pain. Cardiac output within normal limits. No clinical manifestations of heart failure. Alert and oriented. Lungs clear.	Monitor heart rate and rhythm. Treat symptomatic dysrhythmias as ordered by health care provider. Teach patient about antidysrhythmic medications ordered by health care provider, *to ensure proper dosages, time intervals, and evaluation of side effects.* Provide comfort measures to patient and assurance *to decrease fear and anxiety.*
2. NURSING DIAGNOSIS: *Excess Fluid Volume* related to fluid retention secondary to impaired myocardial contractility (NANDA-I © 2012)	
Outcome: Patient's body weight is within normal range; electrolytes will be maintained in normal range. ***Evaluation Parameters:*** Weight. Electrolyte values daily until stable. Lungs clear. No peripheral edema. Neck vein distention not present. Cardiac index and ejection fraction within normal limits.	Administer diuretics as ordered and teach patient rationale and side effects of medication. Weigh patient daily and stress to patient the importance of daily weights. Instruct patient to notify health care provider with greater than 2–3 pound gain. *This will allow the patient to identify weight gain from fluid.* Fluid restriction and low-sodium diet as ordered in order *to decrease excess fluid accumulation.*
3. NURSING DIAGNOSIS: *Acute Pain* related to cardiac ischemia (NANDA-I © 2012)	
Outcome: Pain free or controlled with medication. ***Evaluation Parameters:*** Patient notifies nurse immediately on experiencing pain. Patient's electrocardiogram (ECG) is normal and pain is relieved with sublingual nitroglycerin (NTG.) Patient is able to verbalize how to take sublingual NTG and its side effects.	Instruct patient to notify nurse immediately of chest pain. Implement health care provider's orders (i.e., ECG, sublingual NTG, morphine, oxygen). Teach patient about how to take sublingual nitroglycerin and its side effects. *This encourages the patient to participate in his own care and teaches one of the most important interventions for patients with coronary artery disease (CAD).*
4. NURSING DIAGNOSIS: *Activity Intolerance* related to insufficient oxygenation secondary to decreased cardiac output (NANDA-I © 2012)	
Outcome: Patient enrolls in cardiac rehabilitation program and attends post-MI lectures. ***Evaluation Parameters:*** Patient regularly uses exercise log to record distances walked and symptoms experienced. Patient is able to monitor vital signs and adjust activity accordingly.	Encourage participation in cardiac rehabilitation program. Teach patient to use exercise log to monitor distances walked and symptoms. Teach patient how to monitor heart rate, blood pressure, and respirations as response to activity. *To increase endurance and strength and prevent weight gain.*
5. NURSING DIAGNOSIS: *Ineffective Coping* secondary to denial related to decreased physical status after MI (NANDA-I © 2012)	
Outcome: Patient verbalizes a decrease in problems and concerns. ***Evaluation Parameters:*** Vital signs within normal limits. Denies apprehension. Able to state an understanding of disease process.	Determine degree of denial; do not directly confront patient's denial; support patient's behavior. Provide active listening *to assure patient you are working with her, not against her.*
6. NURSING DIAGNOSIS: *Deficient Knowledge* related to disease and treatment plan (NANDA-I © 2012)	
Outcome: Patient/family have an understanding of and comply with treatment plan. ***Evaluation Parameters:*** Patient and family understand treatment plan and safely become compliant. Patient and family understand the importance of risk factor control in preventing a progression of the disease. Patient and family participate in a cardiac rehabilitation program.	Describe the required diet, medications, activity, and limitations *to increase knowledge of disease and treatment.* Describe what clinical manifestations need to be reported to the health care provider and when to access the emergency medical system *to ensure immediate care when necessary.* Have patient/family repeat instructions *to assess understanding.* Provide information about the type, setting, cost, and location of a cardiac rehabilitation program, and assist with contacting the program *to decrease anxiety about the process.*

Source: Adapted from Wilkinson, J. M., & Ahearn, N. R. (2009). *Prentice Hall nursing diagnosis handbook* (9th ed.). Upper Saddle River, NJ: Prentice Hall.

A nurse can employ any of several strategies when deciding the best course of action to take. These strategies include trial-and-error methods, pilot projects, brainstorming, group input, cost–benefit analyses, cause and effect, worst-case scenarios, and the more recently endorsed EBP model (see earlier discussion). The appropriateness of different strategies will vary depending on the immediacy of the situation and the potential severity of outcomes.

National Standards and Guidelines

National standards and guidelines also assist with decision making in clinical areas and reducing variance in professional practice patterns. National standards and guidelines have been promulgated by regulatory agencies and professional organizations. The Joint Commission promotes the use of appropriate, measurable clinical indicators in clinical settings. These measures promote quantitative criteria to monitor and evaluate the quality of care. Professional organizations such as the American Association of Critical Care Nurses or the Emergency Nurses Association promote standards of care for patients served in various types of practice settings. Other standards promote care for a specialization, such as the ANA's standards of care for hospice and palliative care nursing or its standards of care for ambulatory nursing care (ANA, 2007a). National standards are discussed in detail in Chapter 2.

Clinical Judgment

Clinical judgment, sometimes referred to as reflective thinking or clinical reasoning, is the process of drawing conclusions based on a comparison of the patient's current data with specific outcome data and giving meaning to data based on that comparison. For example, clinical judgment is involved when a nurse notes that the patient's potassium level is 6.8 compared to a "normal" potassium level of 3.6 to 5.0. Thus, clinical judgment involves comparing the patient's current health status to the expected or desired status and deciding which measures are the most appropriate given that comparison. If the comparison is essentially the same, the nurse can conclude that current interventions are successful. If the comparison varies, the nurse can conclude that further interventions are required. The nurse would then use critical thinking and decision making to determine the next course of action.

Using Critical Thinking with the Nursing Process

The use of critical thinking with the nursing process enhances the validity, reliability, and effectiveness of outcomes for patients. Critical thinking is essential in nursing when the nurse is assessing, diagnosing, implementing, and evaluating the patient and developing the care plan (Benner et al., 2009). Chart 5–6 depicts the relationship between critical thinking and the nursing process.

Nursing Documentation

Nurses collect data from multiple sources; they then analyze and integrate that data to formulate nursing care plans, implement care decisions, evaluate patient response, and communicate the information to other members of the health care team. The most familiar way in which the information is conveyed is through the patient's health record, which is the legal document for all information regarding a patient's hospital course and evidence for the extent of care provided and the outcome of that care. The health record also describes anticipated treatment and educational needs (Bonander & Gates, 2010). The patient's health record is used not only to verify the care given, but to convey the quality of care, ensure continuity of care, assist with reimbursement, demonstrate compliance with regulations and policies, provide evidence in a court of law, and provide data for research and education (Bonander & Gates, 2010).

Documentation Standards

Accrediting organizations, federal and state agencies, and professional organizations and institutions all set standards that guide nursing documentation in the particular places in which nurses practice. These are discussed as follows.

Accreditation Standards

Nursing documentation must comply with the standards established by accrediting and licensing organizations, such as The Joint Commission,

Weblink: ANA's Scope and Standards of Practice

CHART 5–6 Critical Thinking, Nursing Process Actions, and Nursing Process Phases (Steps)

Critical Thinking	Nursing Process Action	Nursing Process Phase
Get a better understanding of something or someone else.	Initiate nurse–patient interaction. Collect data. Interpret and validate data.	Assessment
Identify actual and potential problems.	Formulate nursing diagnosis. Derive a desired outcome.	Nursing diagnosis and outcome identification
Make decisions about an action.	Prioritize nursing diagnosis. Formulate goals/objectives. Select planned interventions.	Planning
Reduce risk of getting undesirable results.	Organize interventions. Carry out selected nursing interventions.	Implementation
Increase likelihood of achieving beneficial results.	Determine if nursing diagnosis is correct. Determine if goal/objectives are/have been met. Make necessary revisions and modifications.	Evaluation
Find ways to improve (even when no problem exists).	Repeat the process to gain optimal independence, sense of well-being, or peaceful death.	Nursing process continues

formerly known as the Joint Commission on Accreditation of Healthcare Organizations or JCAHO. The commission surveys facilities to measure compliance with its standards for safe health care. This accreditation can be jeopardized by inadequate or poor documentation. Loss of accreditation can affect reimbursement eligibility for Medicare, Medicaid, and managed care plans. The Joint Commission's (2001; 2012) standards do not require traditional nursing care plans, but do require documentation of an individualized plan of care for each patient, as well as clear communication to all team members regarding patient care in the 2011 Hospital National Safety Goals. The following list highlights some selected standards that should be reflected within the nursing documentation:

- Staff members integrate the information from various patient assessments to identify and assign priorities to their care needs.
- A registered nurse assesses the patient's need for nursing care in all settings where nursing care is provided.
- The assessment process for an infant, a child, or an adolescent patient is individualized.
- The assessment process addresses the special needs of patients who are receiving treatment for alcoholism or other drug dependencies.
- The assessment process addresses the special needs of patients who are receiving treatment for emotional or behavioral disorders.
- The assessment process addresses the special needs of patients who are possible victims of abuse.
- Each patient is reassessed at points designated by hospital policy.
- Care is planned and provided in an interdisciplinary, collaborative manner by qualified individuals.
- Care, treatment, and rehabilitation are planned to ensure that they are appropriate to the patient's needs and severity of disease, condition, impairment, or disability.
- The patient's progress is periodically evaluated against care goals and the plan of care; when indicated, the plan or goals are revised.
- Continuing care at the time of discharge is based on the patient's assessed needs.
- Functional rehabilitation status is assessed to determine the current level of functioning, self-care, self-responsibility, independence, and quality of life.
- Restraint or seclusion use is limited to situations with adequate, appropriate, clinical justification.
- Patients are educated about pain and pain management.

Accrediting organizations will periodically review medical records to ensure that the standard of care is consistent throughout. The Joint Commission also requires that health care facilities regularly monitor, evaluate, and explore ways to improve the quality of care given to patients.

Each year The Joint Commission publishes current patient safety goals that need to be addressed by health care facilities to improve patient care (The Joint Commission, 2011), which are listed on The Joint Commission website. One example of a patient safety goal is the 2011 goal to "improve the effectiveness of communications among caregivers, to get important test results to the right staff person on time" (NPSG.02.03.01).

State, Federal, and Professional Standards

Documentation must also follow guidelines set by state and federal agencies such as the Health Care Financing Administration (HCFA), insurance companies, professional organizations such as the American Nurses Association, and the policies of the institution where the nurse is employed. In general, these state and federal agencies require documentation to include initial and ongoing assessments, any change in the patient's condition, therapies given and the patient's response, patient teaching, and relevant statements made by the patient (Paans, Sermeus, Nieweg, & van der Schans, 2010).

State boards of nursing control the practice of nursing through developing state **nurse practice acts** that establish guidelines to ensure safe practice. The standards set by the practice acts are based on the nursing process, which is a systematic method of planning and providing care to the patient that requires compliance as evidenced in documentation. State nurse practice acts are revised frequently and, as such, documentation requirements also may change. What the nurse documents in the medical record shows compliance with the standards set by the health care facility, state law, and professional organizations (Paans et al., 2010).

Health Insurance Portability and Accountability Act

The Health Insurance Portability and Accountability Act (HIPAA) of 1996 requires the Department of Health and Human Services (DHHS) to adopt standards for electronic health care transactions. DHHS published a Privacy Rule in December 2000 that became effective on April 14, 2001. This Privacy Rule, which set national standards for the protection of health information, was modified in March 2002 and again in August 2002. Further information is found in Chapters 2 and 3.

The rule affects documentation in that only the patient or those health care team members involved with the patient's care have a legal right to review the health record. Release of patient information without the patient's consent is a violation of the patient's privacy and a violation of HIPAA.

Documentation Principles

To be effective, documentation needs to be systematic, timely, and accurate and give a clear account of the nursing care that was provided. The standards and guidelines for documentation differ among health care facilities and specific patient populations; however, certain fundamental principles guide all forms of documentation:

- Write legibly.
- Date and time each entry.
- Use only approved abbreviations.
- Document in chronological order.
- Document information promptly.
- Document all observations objectively.
- Use institutional policy to correct documentation errors.
- Ensure that documentation is complete, concise, and accurate.
- Sign all documents per your institutional policy and include your professional credentials.

Complete, Concise, and Accurate

It is important to document observations as clearly as possible. The nurse must document only facts—what she sees, hears, and does—and describe precisely what she sees without being vague. For example, "Drainage from the surgical wound soaked three 4×4s in 10 minutes. Surgeon notified" is more accurate than "Drainage from surgical wound increased."

The nurse must document relevant information that relates to the patient's care and the nursing process. The documentation should clearly differentiate the nurse's actions from those of the other health care team members, as well as reflect nursing actions and the patient outcomes indicating the patient's progress. Incomplete documentation negates the purpose of performing documentation. If incomplete, the document cannot stand as sound evidence in a court of law, quality of care cannot be evaluated, continuity of care may be broken, coordination of care may be compromised, and reimbursements may be rejected. Since the patient record is a legal document, the nurse should never:

- Document procedures or medication administration in advance.
- Chart for another person without signing his name.
- Add information at a later date unless the nurse indicates that he did so.
- Add inaccurate information.
- Refer to staff conflicts or staffing problems.
- Document that you filed an "incident report."
- Destroy records.

Objectivity

The nurse must document accurately what happened and state her findings. She should describe the factual occurrences that she can see, hear, smell, or touch. The nurse must be objective and avoid vague, subjective statements. For example, instead of documenting that a patient "appears short of breath" or "breathing appears labored," the nurse should document statements such as these:

- Patient is complaining of shortness of breath.
- Patient is able to speak only in 1- or 2-word sentences.
- Inspiratory and expiratory wheezes heard.

The example "patient appears short of breath" is subjective and could be manipulated later should the nurse's treatment or judgment be challenged. Instead of using the word "appears" as a shortcut, nurses should factually describe what they see that leads them to conclude that the patient "appears" short of breath. For example, "Patient noted to have increased respiratory rate with use of accessory muscles and nasal flaring."

Any information nurses obtain from the patient or family should be documented in that context to preserve their credibility. For example, if the nurse writes "Patient fell from standing position," but did not observe this actually happening, it is not accurate. It should be documented as follows: "Per patient (or witness), patient walking on uneven surface, fell from standing position." Complete, factual, accurate documentation is difficult to misinterpret and gives a clear account of the patient's care.

Timeliness

Documentation should flow so that the person reading it can picture exactly what is occurring (Paans et al., 2010). Timeliness includes the following aspects: (1) Document as soon as possible after an observation is made or care is provided. Documentation that is done concurrently with the care provided is more likely to be accurate and complete (Paans et al., 2010). (2) Document date and time of each entry. Documenting the sequence of events and changes in patient condition is essential. Timed occurrences followed by nursing actions and patient response can help prevent misinterpretation. Failure to act or improper action and/or negative patient outcomes can lead to a malpractice suit. The expectation is that you practice at the same level as any other competent registered nurse in the same situation. Deviation from the standard of care or poor documentation of care can lead to allegations of negligence. Frequent, accurate updates verify the nursing care that was given. If you have forgotten to document something, or need to add important information, add the entry on the first available line and record the current date and time, label it *late entry,* and record the date and time when the entry should have been made.

The 24-hour clock, also referred as military time, is used by many facilities to alleviate confusion over a.m. and p.m. entries. Time is expressed in 24 one-hour-long periods per day, rather than two sets of 12 one-hour periods. For example, 11:00 a.m. is written as 1100, noon is written as 1200, and 1:00 p.m. is written as 1300.

Legibility

One of the main purposes of the patient health record is to communicate with other members of the health care team. Documentation that is sloppy, making it difficult to read and interpret, wastes time and puts the patient in jeopardy because critical information may be missing or misinterpreted. Incorrect grammar and misspelled words can create the same negative impression. Even if excellent care was given to the patient, the attorney or jury in a court of law may interpret it as below the acceptable standard of care if the documentation is sloppy or incomplete (Guido, 2010). The health record is a legal, permanent document.

Abbreviations

Accrediting bodies and state regulation stipulate that health care facilities must develop an approved list of abbreviations to be used for documentation. Use of unapproved abbreviations can lead to serious errors. For instance, what does the abbreviation "BS" mean? Is the nurse documenting information regarding the patient's breath sounds or their bowel sounds? Does "pt" stand for patient, physical therapy, or prothrombin time? In 2001 The Joint Commission issued a "Sentinel Event Alert" regarding the use of abbreviations in accredited agencies. Subsequently, the concern over the use of abbreviations became one of the National Patient Safety Goals of The Joint Commission. They created a "do not use" list of abbreviations and mandated hospitals to comply with this goal through their Information Management standards. For an up-to-date list, go to The Joint Commission website at: http://www.jointcommission.org/facts_about_the_official_/.

Safety Alert *It is imperative that you know and use your institution's approved abbreviations. If you are not sure the abbreviation is correct, spell out the word.*

Corrections

Documentation errors may occur. Therefore, when a nurse makes a documentation error, she needs to correct it. Electronic health record (EHR) systems have specific mechanisms built in to provide a means to correct these errors immediately by drawing a single line through the entry, identifying it as an error, and adding the date, time, and the nurse's signature. In the event that documentation is hand written, the nurse should never try to obliterate the error with ink or correction fluid because this appears as if she is trying to hide something (Guido, 2010). The nurse must follow the protocol developed by the health care facility for correction of entries. As with handwritten entries, once notes are entered into the EHR, they become a part of that permanent record and should not be deleted or changed without explanation, date, time, and signature. If using an electronic health record, the date, time, and signature will be placed automatically.

Safety Alert *Changing a patient care record in any way is illegal and constitutes tampering.*

Effective documentation is clear, concise, objective recording of the care given, including any significant events, presented in a legible, organized manner that is representative of the nursing process.

Documentation in Legal Situations

Certain procedures or legal situations in which the nurse is involved require special documentation. The nurse should be aware of these and know how to document them. A full discussion of legal principles as applied to nursing practice is discussed in Chapter 2.

Consent Forms

Prior to most procedures or treatments, the clinician must explain the procedure to the patient and the patient must agree to have the procedure or treatment. Included in this explanation are the risks and benefits of the procedure, as well as include alternatives to the procedure or treatment or risk of doing nothing at all (Guido, 2010). Most facilities have a standard form that is used to obtain consent. Consent and documentation of consent are addressed in Chapter 2.

Safety Alert *Patients who have received sedation or pain medication should never be allowed to sign a consent for a procedure or surgery. The patient may not be able to understand the risks and benefits associated with the procedure. Any consent made after sedation or pain medication is administered will be invalid and will put the institution and the nurse at legal risk.*

Advance Directives

The Patient Self-Determination Act requires that health care facilities provide information about the patient's right to refuse treatment. It is the nurse's responsibility to document that the patient received the information. The facility also is required to ask if the patient has advance directives, which are legal documents that state the patient's wishes regarding life-sustaining medical care. Documentation surrounding advance directives is addressed in Chapter 2.

Using Restraints

Most facilities have special forms for physical restraint orders. Such orders must contain the date and time of the order, reason for restraint use, duration of restraint use, type of restraint, and the physician's signature (Paans et al., 2010; Voyer, Cole, McCusker, St-Jacques, & Laplante, 2008). The order must be reviewed and renewed every 24 hours. It is the nurse's responsibility to observe the patient frequently for any problems that arise from the restraint, such as skin breakdown or decreased distal circulation. Additionally, the nurse should perform range-of-motion exercises on all extremities, and document his observations and care.

Leaving Against Medical Advice

A patient who is mentally competent has the right to refuse treatment and leave the hospital at any time. If a patient chooses to leave, it should be clearly documented that the patient has been advised that she is leaving against medical advice (AMA), understands the risks of leaving, and understands that she can come back (Voyer et al., 2008).

An AMA form should be signed by the patient and include the following information:

- Names of those notified of the patient's decision
- The risks of leaving as told to the patient
- Name of person accompanying the patient and any discharge instructions given
- The patient's destination, if known.

This protects the facility, physician, and nurse if problems arise after the patient leaves. If the patient refuses to sign or leaves without telling anyone, the clinician should complete an incident report.

Incident Reports

Whenever an adverse event occurs, the clinician should complete an incident report. An incident report is not part of the patient's medical record, but rather a mechanism for informing administration about an incident (Paans et al., 2010). The incident report can alert the administration to a potential claim and, therefore, the need to gather more detail. It also assists the administration in identifying possible areas for performance improvement. Only those who witnessed the incident should complete and sign the form, and each witness should file a separate form. When completing the form, each witness should include, in quotes, any statements made by the patient or family members regarding the incident.

Documentation of the incident in the patient's health record should be factual and include follow-up treatment and the patient's response. Do not document in the patient record that an incident report was completed, because this negates the confidential nature of the report. Most facilities have specific forms for certain legal situations. If the nurse is not familiar with the form, she should ask for assistance in order to protect herself and the facility.

Documentation Systems

Health care facilities select documentation systems to meet the needs of their specific patient care areas and to comply with legal and regulatory requirements. An acute care facility may have multiple systems in different areas of the hospital. Chart 5–7 provides brief comparisons of the different documentation systems.

Narrative System

Narrative documentation is used across many health care settings. It consists of narrative progress notes that describe a chronological account of the patient's status, interventions performed, and the patient's response to interventions. Advantages to narrative documentation are that it is flexible, descriptive, and gives the reader a picture of what has occurred over an extended period of time. Key elements of this system are knowing when to document, what to document, and how to organize the data. A disadvantage to narrative documentation is the tendency to document everything that happens. This can make the documentation long and repetitive.

Flow sheets often are used in conjunction with narrative documentation to document routine observations such as assessments. This allows the reader to observe significant changes or trends. Exercises to practice documentation skills are located online in the Pearson Nursing Student Resources.

Problem-Oriented Medical Record

The problem-oriented medical record (POMR) is most effective in acute and long-term settings (Wraa, 2010). This system consists of five components: a database, problem list, a plan of care for each problem, multidisciplinary progress notes, and a discharge summary. Components of POMR are included in electronic health records, discussed next.

Database

In most cases, nurses complete the database or admission assessment, which is the basis for the patient's plan of care. The database includes the reason for hospitalization, past medical history, allergies, current medications, physical assessment, psychosocial findings, self-care abilities, educational needs, and discharge planning needs. From this information, the nurse forms the problem list.

Problem List

The problem list contains the patient's current medical problems in chronological order of when each was identified, not in order of severity or priority. The list provides the nurse with an overview of the patient's

CHART 5–7 Documentation Systems Comparison

System	Parts of Record	Description	Nurse's Notes Format
Narrative	Nurse's notes Flow sheets to supplement care plan	Each discipline writes narrative progress notes in segregated areas of the medical record.	Narration with time of entry
Problem-oriented medical record (POMR)	Nurse's notes Database Nursing care plan Problem list Discharge summary	Consists of gathering baseline data and creating a problem list and plan of care for each identified problem.	SOAP, SOAPIE, or SOAPIER
Problem, intervention, evaluation (PIE)	Nurse's notes Assessment flow sheets Problem list	Uses a problem, intervention, evaluation format to describe patient problems, intervention, and evaluation of responses to interventions.	Problem Intervention Evaluation
Charting by exception (CBE)	Nurse's notes Flow sheets with patient teaching records and discharge notes Care plan Graphic record	Only requires documentation of abnormal or significant findings and events.	SOAPIE or SOAPIER
Electronic health record (EHR)	Nurse's notes Flow sheets Nursing care plan Database Teaching plan	Uses a database, outcome-based plan of care.	Evaluative statements Expected outcomes Learning outcomes

Source: From Daulong, M. (2010). The spectrum of documentation: A resources guide to better ensure compliance. *PT in Motion,* 51–54.

health status. Each problem is then given a number. Documentation on the initial plan, progress notes, and discharge summary will correspond to these numbers. Even when a problem has been resolved, it remains on the list; however, it is then highlighted to show that it has been resolved.

Initial Plan

From the problem list, an initial plan is developed that includes expected outcomes, plans for further data collection, patient care, and teaching plans. The nurse should include the patient in goal setting as the plan is developed.

Progress Notes

Progress notes are written using the SOAP, SOAPIE, or SOAPIER format. This format documents the following information for each problem:

- ***Subjective Data:*** Information that the patient or significant others tell the nurse. It can be stated as a complaint or, if from someone other than the patient, an impression.
- ***Objective Data:*** Measurable information the nurse gathers during the assessment, such as vital signs, laboratory test results, and signs and symptoms noted.
- ***Assessment Data:*** This is stated as the patient problem or nursing diagnosis that the nurse derived from the gathered subjective and objective data. This is a dynamic process and changes as more information is gathered.
- ***Plan:*** The plan describes the interventions planned to resolve each problem. The plan should include short-term and long-term goals.
- ***Interventions:*** This documents the measures that are taken to achieve an expected outcome. Teaching and documentation of the patient's understanding of the plan is included here.
- ***Evaluation:*** Evaluation of the patient's response to the interventions is noted.
- ***Revision:*** Documentation is recorded of any change of plan for a particular problem.

Discharge Summary

The discharge summary notes whether each problem on the list is resolved. This is the place in the SOAPIE note for the nurse to discuss unresolved problems and document the plan for addressing these problems after discharge. It also is the place to note any communication with an outside facility, agency, or the patient's family.

One disadvantage of the problem-oriented system is that it lists the problems in chronological order, rather than by priority.

Problem, Intervention, Evaluation System

The problem, intervention, evaluation (PIE) system works well in areas where the patient's condition can change rapidly. This system lists the patient's problem first, followed by the interventions taken to alleviate the problem, and, last, the evaluation of the patient's response to the intervention. This system organizes the information according to the patient's problems and integrates the plan of care into the progress notes. A daily assessment flow sheet is used to document routine care and monitoring measures, with detailed information documented in the progress note.

Problem

After performing an initial assessment, nurses identify the nursing diagnoses and form the "problem" piece of the documentation system. Most facilities will develop a list of accepted nursing diagnoses that usually correspond to those approved by the North American Nursing

Diagnosis Association (NANDA). Each problem is then numbered for future reference.

Intervention

Nursing actions that are taken to alleviate a problem are documented for each nursing diagnosis. Each "I" should be labeled with the corresponding problem number.

Evaluation

Following the interventions, the patient's responses should be documented. As with the interventions, the "E" should be labeled with the corresponding problem number.

One disadvantage of the PIE system is that each problem needs to be evaluated once each shift. The PIE system also does not document the planning step in the nursing process, which addresses expected outcomes.

Documenting by Exception System

Documenting by exception (DBE) is used to eliminate lengthy or repetitive documentation. It departs from traditional types of systems by documenting only significant or abnormal findings (Jaffe, 2011). To use the DBE system, the nurse must be using critical pathways or interdisciplinary plans of care that address every possible patient problem. The format contains baseline data and a problem-oriented plan of care. Preprinted guidelines are prepared for each body system and the initial and ongoing assessments are documented only as exceptions to these guidelines. Flow sheets provide a normal assessment to chart against. For each body system, the nurse documents within normal limits or documents what is not normal. The different types of flow sheets needed for the DBE system are:

- Physician's order flow sheet
- Nursing order flow sheet
- Graphic form
- Patient teaching record
- Patient discharge note
- Supplemental nurse's progress notes.

The DBE system saves time and decreases the amount of documentation needed. The flow sheets are nursing focused and improve documentation because the format highlights care interventions and requires a documented evaluation of the patient's response. A disadvantage of the DBE system is the time it takes to develop the guidelines and standards of care. These must be in place and taught to all nursing staff for this system to be effective.

Electronic Health Record

One of the most significant recent changes in documentation has been the introduction of computerized documentation systems. The ability to have universal access to patient records is necessary for the delivery of safe and effective health care (Christensen & Grimsmo, 2008). For example, a patient's medication history is readily accessible throughout the health care system and each change can be updated whether the change is made by telephone or via an office visit. The electronic health record (EHR) (also referred to as the electronic medical record (EMR) in the literature) is legible, decreases recording time and costs, decreases errors, improves communication between health care providers, and provides better access to medical data for patient care, education, performance improvement activities, and research (Christensen & Grimsmo, 2008). Another advantage to the EHR is the use of standard terminology, which promotes better communication among providers.

As stated, the EHR allows a patient's medication history to be accessible throughout the health care system. Complications from drug reactions account for approximately 4.7% of admissions to hospitals in the United States, with the estimated associated costs being $3.8 million per hospital per year (Christensen & Grimsmo, 2008; Varkey et al., 2007). Because of these adverse reactions, the Institute for Healthcare Improvement's 100,000 Lives Campaign and The Joint Commission identified the prevention of adverse drug reactions as a priority for national action and have required institutions to perform **medication reconciliation,** which is the process of identifying an accurate list of all medications the patient is taking and using this list to provide correct medications for the patient anywhere in the health care system. The initial list is developed by either the primary care provider or on admission to the hospital. When a patient is admitted to the hospital, any new medication prescribed is added to her record, and any medication stopped during her hospitalization is marked as deleted. The EHR medication list is then reconciled daily by the health care team. It is of great importance to reconcile the medication list prior to the patient's discharge. The nurse will review the list and be sure that the patient understands all changes.

Depending on the type of computer and software that is used by a facility, patient information may be accessed by voice recognition, keyboard, light pen, touch screen, or mouse. Most facilities place computers or terminals at workstations or patient bedsides to allow quick access to patient information by the health care team.

Privacy rights and confidentiality need to be addressed through institutional policies specific to the EHR. Security can be monitored by assigning electronic log-in names to each user and creating audit trails.

Nursing Care Documentation

Most EHRs (or EMRs: electronic medical records) provide a menu of words and phrases that ensure documentation is provided in a standard format. The nurse can further elaborate on a problem or clarify flow sheet documentation in the comment section of the form.

Clinical nursing information systems (CNIS) software programs have been developed that allow the user to select and record nursing actions in the EHR (Heinzer, 2010). These systems contain most of the components of the nursing process and therefore adhere to The Joint Commission standards for documentation. Most CNIS have features that allow customization of forms to allow for specific institutional requirements. Some newer systems are interactive; as data are entered, they will prompt you with questions and suggestions regarding your data. These systems will also suggest nursing diagnoses for the care plan based on the entered assessment data.

An advantage of an EHR is its ability to retrieve information quickly and easily. The system helps to link different sources of patient information such as clinic notes, laboratory results, consults, and diagnostic results. The EHR uses standard terminology and the documentation is legible, which improves communication among health care providers. However, a number of disadvantages are also present: not all health care providers are comfortable with computer technology, so extensive training may be necessary to fully utilize it; lack of security measures can threaten patient confidentiality; if the system is "down," then information is unavailable unless hard copies are used and readily accessible; and initial implementation of the system is expensive.

Since various EHR programs are available, it provides choices for agencies that are searching for their first EHR program or needing to update their current programs. It is wise to check with other agencies using EHRs to validate a specific system's usefulness and discover any perceived problems with its implementation and use.

Electronic health records have become more common in the past decade in many health care agencies. Information technology has dramatically transformed the delivery of health care, making it safer and more effective and efficient (Thielst, 2007). Such programs not only benefit the care providers, but also patients, who can now manage and share their personal health information and interact with their clinicians more effectively. To become effective, providers have learned that those who must use the technology must be trained to implement all of the potential areas (Ovretveit, Scott, Rundall, Shortell, & Brommels, 2007). In addition, personnel time is often diverted from clinical work during implementation of new programs or updates; this provides time for the staff to learn correct use of the EHR program. Senior management must make implementation of an EHR a priority for their agency, and assure resources are available for integration of the EHR program (Ovretveit et al., 2007).

Regardless of the type of EMR or EHR program an agency plans to implement, it is vital to learn from those who have already completed such work. Sharing organizational climate characteristics and culture (the values, beliefs, and norms of the organization) by defining the type or model of patient care delivery system used, the organizational structure, and how staff relate to one another according to policies and precedents paves the way for organizational comparison. It also is relevant to know what limitations, barriers, and challenges were perceived or experienced by comparable organizations that have integrated EHR. These factors can help an organization prevent errors or unnecessary expenditures of resources due to an agency's own work context. In addition to an individual staff member's change capacity, organizations also have different formal systems for managing organizational changes, such as EHR integration (Ovretveit et al., 2007).

Many countries have established policies for use of EHR, and many hospitals are continuing to select, plan, implement, and update their EHR systems. Findings from studies of those who have integrated EHR show that success depends upon many prior and concurrent organizational factors, as discussed in the preceding paragraph (Ovretveit et al., 2007). Additional practical implementation guidelines are listed in the previously cited reference.

Regardless of the system that is used, knowing the components of that system and understanding the basic principles of documentation are essential. The patient's health record demonstrates that the care given was based on accepted professional and regulatory standards. The nurse needs to evaluate if the following questions were answered upon completion of documentation.

- Is it factual?
- Does it document all the care given?
- If it is read 2 years from now, will it demonstrate that the care given met the standard of care?
- Does it show the sequence of events accurately, including the patient's response to treatment?
- Does it contain subjective statements or personal opinions?
- Does it clearly identify when information was obtained from the patient, family, or others?
- Are errors corrected in the approved manner?

It is important to note that the use of EHRs has received strong emphasis through the American Recovery and Reinvestment Act (ARRA) of 2009 (EHRs). This legislation includes a substantial commitment of federal resources toward improving health care delivery through the use of EHRs (U.S. Department of Health and Human Services, 2010). Specifically, the Health Information Technology for Economic and Clinical Health Act (HITECH) provides for federal incentive payments to doctors and hospitals when they adopt EHRs and demonstrate their use in ways that can improve quality, safety, and effectiveness of care. Eligible professionals can receive incentive payments through Medicare and Medicaid by using EHRs in a "meaningful" way, generally interpreted as securing patient information and reducing health care costs (CMS Centers for Medicare and Medicaid, 2012). If agencies, including physician offices and health care agencies, are not in compliance with these new Medicare and Medicaid rulings, they may be fined. Thus, the potential exists that this legislation will affect the manner in which documentation systems are implemented. It may, in fact, negate many of the documentation systems previously discussed in this chapter. At the time of this writing, it is too soon to determine how this legislation actually will play out in the vast arena of health care settings.

Documentation, no matter the type used, reflects the quality of the care given, the outcome of that care, and collaboration among the members of the health care team. It also describes future interventions and education needed. Documentation that is accurate and complete protects both the patient and the caregiver.

Preparation for Practice

As stated earlier, the development of a nursing plan of care using the nursing process requires critical thinking skills to evaluate findings, identify assumptions, examine alternatives, and understand various points of view. Critical thinking is an integral part of each step of the nursing process. To assist the learner in the development of critical thinking skills, each chapter that covers a disorder has a real-life Clinical Preparation vignette at the end, followed by several questions to stimulate critical thinking. Using the same Clinical Preparation vignette, you will proceed to online Pearson Nursing Student Resources:

1. ***The Patient Care Kardex:*** The Kardex contains information regarding the patient's name, age, religion, medical diagnoses, past medical history, surgeries and major procedures since admission, current medications, treatments, diet, intravenous therapy, diagnostic tests, and procedures. The Kardex also will include the permitted level of activity, functional limitations, and assistance that may be needed.
2. ***Three Days of Laboratory Results:*** This will allow the learner to look for abnormal values and trends. From this information, the learner will be asked to complete several forms that would help prepare for caring for the patient.
   - ***Summary of Hospitalization:*** This includes pertinent information about the patient, such as age, admitting diagnosis, past medical history, surgeries or major procedures since admission, history of current illness or injury, vital signs and physical findings from the previous 24 hours, and the basic nursing care needed for the patient.
   - ***Pathophysiology:*** This includes detailed pathophysiology for the current illness. Included are common signs and symptoms, as well as possible complications. This will help the learner anticipate the patient's needs, possible complications, and knowledge deficits.
   - ***Laboratory Results Explanations:*** All abnormal lab values or significant trends should be listed. Next to the result, the learner will write a brief explanation of what the

cause of the abnormality might be for this patient and the significance of the finding. This will help the learner to become familiar with trends for specific disease processes and hone interpretive skills.

- *Medication Administration Record:* This form includes the usual dose, route, frequency, class, and action of the drug; the rationale for administration; side effects with nursing implications; and assessment data that indicate effectiveness. This will help the learner to become familiar with different classes of drugs, the nursing interventions and assessments necessary for safe administration, and the evaluations necessary to determine effectiveness.
- *Concept Map:* The concept map assists the learner in the development of the nursing plan of care using the nursing process by listing the primary and secondary diagnoses. For the primary diagnosis, list the critical assessments that are a priority for the patient. Follow the primary and secondary nursing diagnoses with high-risk potential problems. For each nursing diagnosis, list all assessment findings that support the diagnosis such as vital signs, laboratory results, and physical assessment findings. Then list medical and nursing interventions aimed at improving the problem. Each concept map contains the nursing diagnosis: knowledge deficit. This is where the learner lists the educational needs for the patient and family. In the last section, describe what the patient must be able to do before discharge or transfer, including appropriate community referrals.

The assignment assists the learner in the development of a problem-solving approach to nursing care. By doing this, the learner will gain experience in critical thinking skills and develop a systematic method for determining a patient's health problem, devising a plan of care, developing evaluation criteria, and knowing expected outcomes. The Preparation for Practice assignments also will help the learner to articulate the patient's needs and learn how to write effective evaluation statements. This, in turn, will significantly improve documentation skills and the ability to communicate with other health care team members to provide the safest most effective and holistic care for the patient.

Summary

The nursing process is a patient-centered method for structuring the delivery of nursing care. As such, it is the common thread that unites different types of nurses who work in varied areas; it serves as the essential core of practice for the registered nurse (ANA, 2007b). The nursing process is the vehicle through which the nurse applies intuitive and scientific knowledge, critical thinking, and nursing skills in a systematic, goal-directed fashion to achieve the outcomes desired for the patient. The nursing process entails gathering and analyzing data in order to identify patient strengths, potential or actual problems, and goals, as well as developing and evaluating a plan of nursing interventions to achieve mutually agreed-upon outcomes. At every stage of the five-step process, the nurse works closely with the patient to individualize care and build a relationship of mutual respect. Implementation of the nursing process requires accurate and complete documentation in the patient's health record. Accurate, concise documentation takes practice. Remember, the patient's medical record is not only used to verify the care given, but to convey the quality of care. The record ensures continuity of care, assists with reimbursement, demonstrates compliance with regulations and policies, provides evidence in a court of law, and provides data for research and education. The patient's health record is a powerful communication tool. Developing the ability to articulate the patient's condition and potential problems assists in creating a collaborative plan of care that promotes achievement of desired patient/family outcomes (Institute of Medicine [IOM], 2010).

NCLEX® PRACTICE

1. The nurse is conducting independent nursing activities with a patient. Which of the following is this nurse doing? (select all that apply)

1. Assessing a wound
2. Documenting intake on a calorie count form
3. Assisting the patient to use a walker
4. Administering medication
5. Listening to breath sounds

2. The nurse is reviewing the results of the patient's health history, physical examination, and recent laboratory studies. This nurse is conducting which phase of the nursing process?

1. Assessment
2. Planning
3. Implementation
4. Evaluation

3. The nurse does a finger stick to check a patient's current blood glucose level before determining the dose of insulin he will receive. Which of the following best describes this according to nursing process?

1. This is an evaluation of the patient before developing a diagnosis.
2. This is implementation of nursing care after setting a goal.
3. This is a patient assessment that will be used to plan care.
4. This is an evaluation of care and future assessments will be based on this.

4. At the completion of a patient's assessment, the nurse creates a clinical judgment about a potential health problem. This clinical judgment is considered:

1. goal setting.
2. planning interventions.
3. determining collaborative problems.
4. determining a nursing diagnosis.

5. The nurse is making a decision about a future action with patient care. This critical thinking activity is equated with which of the following steps of the nursing process?

1. Assessment
2. Planning
3. Implementation
4. Evaluation

6. The nurse is reviewing the latest National Patient Safety Goals. The regulatory body that publishes these goals is:

1. Medicare.
2. Medicaid.
3. The Joint Commission.
4. the State Board of Nursing.

Answers to NCLEX Practice questions can be found in Appendix D in the Osborn Student Resources at nursing.pearsonhighered.com. Practice additional NCLEX questions online at the Student Resources site.

Pearson Nursing Student Resources Find additional review materials at: **nursing.pearsonhighered.com**

REFERENCES

Ackley, B. J., & Ladwig, G. B. (2011). *Nursing diagnosis handbook: An evidence-based guide to planning care* (8th ed.). St. Louis: Mosby.

American Nurses Association. (2007a). *Hospice and palliative nursing: Scope and standards of practice.* Retrieved from http://www.geronurseonline.org/Homepages/HomeLeftMiddle/HospiceandPalliativeNursing.aspx

American Nurses Association. (2007b). *The nursing process: A common thread amongst all nurses.* Retrieved, from http://nursingworld.org/ExpeciallyForYou/StudentNurses/Thenursingprocess.aspx

American Nurses Association. (2008). *Code of ethics with interpretive statements.* Silver Spring, MD: Author.

American Nurses Association. (2010a). *Nursing's social policy statement* (3rd ed.). Washington, DC: Author.

American Nurses Association. (2010b). *Scope and standards of practice, Nursing* (2nd ed.). Silver Spring, MD: Author.

American Nurses Association. (2010c). *Standards of clinical nursing practice.* Silver Spring, MD: Author.

Authors. (2010). Competency profile for registered nurses: NIC in medical-surgical nursing. *Alberta RN, 66*(2), 16–17.

Benner, P., Tanner, C. A., & Chesla, C. A. (2009). *Expertise in nursing practice: Caring, clinical judgment, and ethics* (2nd ed.). New York: Springer.

Berman, A. J., & Snyder, S. (2012). *Kozier & Erb's fundamentals of nursing* (9th ed). Upper Saddle River, NJ: Pearson.

Bonander, J., & Gates, S. (2010). Public health in an era of personal health records: opportunities for innovation and new partnerships. *Journal of Medical Internet Research, 12*(3), e33.

Carpenito-Moyet, L. J. (2009). *Nursing diagnosis: Application to clinical practice* (13th ed.). Philadelphia: Lippincott Williams & Wilkins.

Centers for Medicare & Medicaid Services. (2012). HER incentive programs. CMS.gov. Retrieved from https://www.cms.gov/Regulations-and-Guidance/Legislation/EHRIncentivePrograms/index.html?redirect=/EHRIncentivePrograms/

Christensen, T., & Grimsmo, A. (2008). Expectations for the next generation of electronic patient records in primary care: A triangulated study. *Informatics in Primary Care, 16*(1), 1–28.

Daulong, M. (2010). The spectrum of documentation: A resources guide to better ensure compliance. *PT in Motion,* 51–54.

Guido, G. W. (2010). *Legal and ethical issues in nursing* (5th ed.). Upper Saddle River, NJ: Prentice Hall.

Heinzer, M. M. (2010). Essential elements of nursing notes and the transition to electronic health records. *Journal of Healthcare Information Management (JHIM), 24*(4). Retrieved from http://www.himss.org/content/files/jhim/24-4/13_HEINZER.pdf

Henderson, V. (1966). *The nature of nursing.* New York: Macmillan.

IOM (Institute of Medicine). (2010). *The future of nursing: Leading change, advancing health.* Washington, DC: The Academic Press.

Jaffe, S. E. (2011). Nursing practice & skill: charting by exception. *Clinical Information Systems.* Philadelphia: F.A. Davis Co. Retrieved from atlantis.mendocino.edu/nursing/N%20126/charting%20JAFFE%202011.pdf

Johnson, D. E. (1980). The behavioral system model for nursing. In J. P. Riehl & C. Roy (Eds.), *Conceptual models for nursing practice* (2nd ed.). New York: Appleton-Century-Crofts.

Kinsman, L., Rotter, T., James, E., Snow, P. L., & Willis, J. (2010). BioMed Central Medicine, 8:31. Retrieved from http://www.biomedcentral.com/1741-7015/8/31

Lachman, V. D. (2009). Practical use of the nursing code of ethics: Part II. *MEDSURG Nursing, 18*(3), 191–194.

Maslow, A. H. (1954). *Motivation and personality.* New York: Harper and Row Publishers.

North American Nursing Diagnosis Association. (2007). *Nursing Diagnoses: Definitions and Classification 2012-14,* 9th Edition. (2011). NANDA International ISBN 978-0-470-65482-8 Somerset, NJ: Wiley-Blackwell.

Ovretveit, J., Scott, T., Rundall, T. G., Shortell, S. M., & Brommels, M. (2007). Implementation of electronic medical records in hospitals: Two case studies. *Health Policy, 84,* 181–190.

Paans, W., Sermeus, W., Nieweg, R. M. B., & van der Schans, C. P. (2010). Prevalence of accurate nursing documentation in patient records. *Journal of Advanced Nursing, 66*(11), 2481–2489. doi: 10.1111/j.1365-2648.2010.05433.x

Peplau, H. E. (1952). *Interpersonal relations in nursing.* New York: G. P. Putnam's Sons.

Polit, D. F., & Beck, C. T. (2010). *Essentials of nursing research: Appraising evidence for nursing practice* (7th ed.). Philadelphia: Lippincott Williams & Wilkins.

Potter, P., Deshields, T., & Kuhrik, M. (2010). Delegation practices between registered nurses and nursing assistive personnel. *Journal of Nursing Management, 18,* 157–165.

QSEN. (2010). Knowledge, skills, attitudes concerning evidence-based practice. Retrieved from http://www.qsen.org/ksas_prelicensure.php

Rogers, M. E. (1970). *The theoretical basis of nursing.* Philadelphia: F. A. Davis.

Seganfredo, D. H., & Almeida, M. (2011). Nursing outcomes content validation according to Nursing Outcomes Classification (NOC) for clinical, surgical, and critical patients. *Rev. Latino-Am. Enfermagem, 19*(1), 34–41.

The Joint Commission. (2001). Facts about the official "do not use" list of abbreviations. Retrieved from http://www.jointcommission.org/facts_about_the_official_/

The Joint Commission. (2008). Facts about the 2008 National Patient Safety Goals. Retrieved April 22, 2008, from http://www.jointcommission.org/PatientSafety/NationalPatientSafetyGoals/08_npsg_facts.htm

The Joint Commission. (2011). National patient safety goals. Retrieved from www.jointcommission.org/assets/1/18/2011-2012_npsg_presentation_final_8-4-11.pdf

The Joint Commission. (2012). About our standards. Retrieved from http://www.jointcommission.org/standards_information/standards.aspx

Thielst, C. B. (2007). The new frontier of electronic, personal, and virtual health records. *Journal of Healthcare Management, 52*(2), 75–79.

U.S. Department of Health and Human Services. (2010). Center for Medicare & Medicaid Services; Medicare and Medicaid incentives and administrative funding. Retrieved from http://www.hhs.gov/recovery/reports/plans/pdf20100610/CMS_HIT%20Implementation%20Plan%20508%20compliant.pdf

Varkey, P., Cunningham, J., O'Meara, J., Bonacci, R., Desai, N., & Sheeler, R. (2007). Multidisciplinary approach to inpatient medication reconciliation in an academic setting. *American Journal of Health-System Pharmacists, 64*(8), 850–854.

Voyer, P., Cole, M. G., McCusker, J., St-Jacques, S., & Laplante, J. (2008). Accuracy of nurse documentation of delirium symptoms in medical charts. *International Journal of Nursing Practice, 14,* 165–177.

Watson, J. (1988). New dimensions of human caring theory. *Nursing Science Quarterly, 1*(4), 175–181.

Watson, J. (2003). Jean Watson and the theory of human caring. Retrieved from http://www.uchsc.edu/son/caring/content/sct.asp

Wilkinson, J. M., & Ahearn, N. R. (2009). *Prentice Hall nursing diagnosis handbook* (9th ed.). Upper Saddle River, NJ: Prentice Hall.

Wraa, C. (2010). Chapter 6. In K. Osborn, C. Wraa, & A. Watson, *Medical-surgical nursing: Preparation for practice.* Upper Saddle River, NJ: Pearson Prentice Hall.

Yaqub, E., & Barroso, A. (2010). Distributed guidelines (DiG): a software framework for extending automated health decision support to the general population. *Perspectives in Health Information Management.* Summer 2010, 1–15. Retrieved from http://perspectives.ahima.org/index.php?option=com_content&view=article&id=191:distributed-guidelines-dig-a-software-framework-for-extending-automated-health-decision-support-to-the-general-population2&catid=46:personal-health-records&Itemid=90

Yura, H., & Walsh, M. B. (1988). *The nursing process* (5th ed.). New York: Appleton-Century-Crofts.

CHAPTER 6

Health Assessment

Cynthia Parkman
Annita Watson

Outcome-Based Learning Objectives

After studying this chapter, the learner will be able to:

1. Differentiate among the components of the health assessment as applied to patient assessment.
2. Determine the steps of the patient interview for the health history and analyze its relationship to the nursing process.
3. Compare and contrast verbal and nonverbal responses that enhance the collection of information.
4. Explain how the techniques of inspection, palpation, percussion, and auscultation are used in the physical assessment of the major body systems.
5. Apply the critical thinking process to health assessment.

KEY TERMS

auscultation p.133
blunt percussion p.132
chief complaint p.122
comprehensive exam p.129
direct percussion p.132
direct question p.120
dullness p.133
flatness p.133
focused exam p.129
hyperresonance p.133
indirect percussion p.132
inspection p.130
metabolic equivalent level (MET) p.115
objective data p.114
open-ended questions p.120
palpation p.131
percussion p.132
resonance p.133
sequelae p.123
subjective data p.114
tympany p.133
vital signs p.127

THE FOCUS of health care in the United States is currently evolving beyond treatment of illness and injury to include prevention of illness and promotion of wellness as well. This newer model requires the development of a comprehensive plan of care that will guide the patient and family toward a healthy lifestyle and away from risk factors that can increase illness and injury (Linden, Jackson, Rutledge, & Nath, 2010). The nurse takes an active role in care plan development and execution. The nursing process guides the nurse when gathering and analyzing information. The nursing process is an effective method of problem solving that provides a framework on which to make informed decisions regarding the patient's plan of care.

Assessment, the first step of the nursing process, is when the nurse gathers initial data. The assessment includes data about the physical, emotional, mental, spiritual, and cultural factors that impact a patient's health. It consists of both **objective data** (collected by using the senses: observation, palpation, auscultation, percussion, and smell) and **subjective data** (information the patient or caretaker tells the nurse). Both types of data are used to formulate a nursing diagnosis. The nursing diagnosis, which evolves from the assessment data, describes conditions treated by nurses (North American Nursing Diagnosis Association, 2011). Ultimately, a thorough health assessment allows the nurse to collaborate with the health care team in developing a plan that integrates personal health care with prevention efforts to reach the national goal of increasing the population's quality and years of healthy life.

National Guidelines: *Healthy People 2020*

Each decade, the Department of Health and Human Services (DHHS) issues a national agenda aimed at improving the health of all Americans. The DHHS establishes health benchmarks and monitors how well people are reaching them over time. Additionally, the DHHS has requested that the Institute of Medicine (IOM) review the *Healthy People 2020* objectives and recommend leading health indicators (IOM, 2011). In particular, the DHHS asked the IOM to identify 12 key topics, 24 key objectives, and 24 leading indicators that are critical to the nation's health needs. Of the indicators, 13 new indicators are listed for *Healthy People 2020.* See the National Guideline feature that follows.

The IOM identified a set of basic principles for *Healthy People 2020* and developed a conceptual framework within which the topics, identified indicators, and objectives would be developed (IOM, 2011). The IOM concluded that the indicators for *Healthy People 2020* should prove valuable in eliciting interest and awareness among the general population, and thereby motivate diverse population groups to engage in activities that will exert a positive impact on improving the overall health of the nation.

NATIONAL GUIDELINES ***Healthy People 2020*** **Leading Health Indicators**

These 13 *leading health indicators* reflect the major public health concerns of the 21st century for Americans:

1. Adolescent Health
2. Blood Disorders and Blood Safety
3. Dementias, Including Alzheimer's Disease
4. Early and Middle Childhood
5. Genomics
6. Global Health
7. Healthcare-Associated Infections
8. Health-Related Quality of Life and Well-Being
9. Lesbian, Gay, Bisexual, and Transgender Health
10. Older Adults
11. Preparedness
12. Sleep Health
13. Social Determinants of Health

Assessment of Health

Health assessment is a systematic method of collecting data about a patient for the purpose of determining the patient's current and ongoing health status, predicting risks to health, identifying actual and potential health problems, and identifying areas for health promotion (D'Amico & Barbarito, 2012; Estes, 2010). Health assessment is the first phase of the nursing process, and it provides a framework on which to make informed decisions regarding the patient's health status and plan of care. The collected data includes physical, social, cultural, environmental, and emotional factors that impact the individual's overall well-being. If certain components or characteristics of health (e.g., physical activity, weight) are treated negligently by the individual, they may become risk factors to the health status. Risk factors have the potential of compromising the individual's health status.

These general components are shown as risk factors in the Risk Factors box on this page. Risk factors for specified disorders are discussed in the assessment and disorder chapters throughout the book.

RISK FACTORS **Indicators of Risk Factors Affecting Health**

Decreased or no physical activity
Overweight and obesity
Tobacco use
Substance abuse
Risky unprotected sexual behavior
Mental illness
Injury and violence
Environmental quality
Insufficient recommended immunizations
Lack of access to health care

Decreased or No Physical Activity

Regular physical activity helps maintain physical and psychological well-being. It also plays a significant role in reducing the incidence of many diseases including cardiovascular disease, diabetes mellitus, hypertension, colon cancer, depression, and anxiety. Physical activity is important at all ages to maintain muscle strength and decrease body fat, and it is an important component of weight control.

When assessing a patient's physical activity, it is essential to determine the level, frequency, and type of exercise. A pattern of physical activity is regular activities (running, walking, bicycle riding) that are performed as follows:

- Five or more days of the week of moderate-intensity activities (in bouts of at least 10 minutes for a total of at least 30 minutes per day); or
- Three or more days a week of vigorous-intensity activities (for at least 20 to 60 minutes per session) (Centers for Disease Control and Prevention [CDC], 2008).

One measurement of the level of exercise intensity is the **metabolic equivalent (MET) level.** The MET, which increases as physical activity increases, establishes the amount of oxygen used for physical activity. A second method of determining physical activity intensity is the Borg Rating of Perceived Exertion (RPE) (CDC, 2011b). Perceived exertion is how hard an individual feels like his or her body is working. It is based on the physical sensations a person experiences during physical activity, including increased heart rate, increased respirations, increased sweating, and muscle fatigue. Although this is a subjective measure, a person's exertion rating may provide a fairly good estimate of the actual heart rate during physical activity. The third method for measuring physical activity intensity is by determining the number of calories burned. This is accomplished by counting the intake of calories from food on a daily basis. According to the CDC (2008), adults should strive to meet either moderate-intensity physical activity or vigorous-intensity physical activity. Moderate-intensity physical activity refers to a level of effort in which a person should experience one or more of the following:

- Some increase in breathing or heart rate
- A "perceived exertion" of 11 to 14 on the Borg RPE scale (e.g., the effort a healthy individual might expend while walking briskly, mowing the lawn, dancing, swimming, or bicycling on level terrain)
- Reaching the level of 3 to 6 METs
- Any activity that burns 3.5 to 7 calories per minute (kcal/min). One may measure calories used during various physical activities by using an "Activity" or Calories Burned" calculator. These are available on the Internet and via recommendation of your primary health care provider.

Vigorous-intensity physical activity may be intense enough to represent a substantial challenge to an individual and refers to a level of effort in which a person should experience one or more of the following:

- A large increase in breathing or heart rate (conversation is difficult or "broken")
- A "perceived exertion" of 15 or greater on the Borg RPE scale (e.g., the effort a healthy individual might expend while jogging, participating in high-impact aerobic dancing, swimming continuous laps, bicycling uphill, carrying more than 25 lbs up a flight of stairs, standing or walking with more than 50 lbs)

Weblink: Cigarette Smoking Weblink: Secondhand Smoke

- Greater than 6 METs
- Any activity that burns more than 7 kcal/ min (CDC, 2008).

Overweight and Obesity

Overweight and obesity both describe ranges of weight that are greater than what is generally considered healthy for a given height (CDC, 2010). The terms also identify ranges of weight that have been shown to increase the risk for certain diseases and other health problems, such as diabetes mellitus, stroke, arthritis, and serious sleep disorders. The number of obese persons has risen dramatically since the 1980s and has become a leading health problem in the United States. Obesity is more prevalent among women and proportionately higher in African American and Mexican women (D'Amico & Barbarito, 2012). For adults, overweight and obesity generally are determined by using weight and height to calculate a number referred to as the "body mass index" (BMI). BMI is used because, for most people, it correlates with their amount of body fat. An adult who has a BMI between 25 and 29.9 is considered overweight, whereas an adult who has a BMI of 30 or higher is considered obese (CDC, 2010). Other measures of estimating body fat and body fat distribution include measurements of skinfold thickness and mid-arm or waist circumference. The most common measurement sites for measuring skinfold are the triceps, the subscapular, and the suprailiac skinfolds. The normal measurement of the triceps skinfold should fall between the 5th and 95th percentiles on a standard table of Triceps Skinfold Percentiles (Estes, 2010). Mid-arm measurement provides information on skeletal muscle mass. The National Heart, Lung, and Blood Institute (NHLBI) considers waist circumference greater than 102 cm in males and greater than 88 cm in females indicative of a health risk (D'Amico & Barbarito, 2012). Techniques such as ultrasound, computed tomography, and magnetic resonance imaging (MRE) also may be used to determine the amount of body fat (CDC, 2010).

Nutrition and exercise training are important factors in preventing weight gain and maintaining a healthy weight. Nutrition related to weight maintenance is discussed in detail in Chapter 8.

Tobacco Use

Tobacco use is responsible for nearly one in five deaths in the United States (American Cancer Society, 2011). Because cigarette smoking and tobacco use are acquired behaviors—activities that people choose to do—smoking is the most preventable cause of death in our society. The Centers for Disease Control and Prevention (CDC) reported that more than 46 million U.S. adults were current smokers in 2009 (McClave, Rock, & Thorne, 2010). That is 20.6% of all adults (23.5% of men, 17.9% of women)—about one out of every five people.

In 2009, cigarette smoking prevalence among adults in the United States and territories varied from 6.4% to 25.6%, and smokeless tobacco use ranged from 0.8% to 9.1%. Both cigarette smoking and the use of smokeless tobacco were more frequently reported by men, young adults age 18–24 years, adults with a high school education or less, and adults in states with high smoking prevalence (McClave, Rock, & Thorne, 2010).

The carcinogenic effect of tobacco is demonstrated in several different agents that produce deleterious health conditions. The American Cancer Society has recognized over 19 known chemical carcinogens in cigarette smoke (American Cancer Society, 2011). There appears to be a direct relationship between the numbers of years a person has been smoking, number of cigarettes smoked per day, the age when smoking began, and the development of cancer. Smokers are six times more likely than nonsmokers to develop these cancers. Tobacco smoke from cigarettes, cigars, or pipes can cause cancers anywhere in the oral cavity (oropharynx) and larynx (Figure 6–1◆). Pipe smoking creates a particularly significant risk for cancers in the area of the lips that contact the pipe stem.

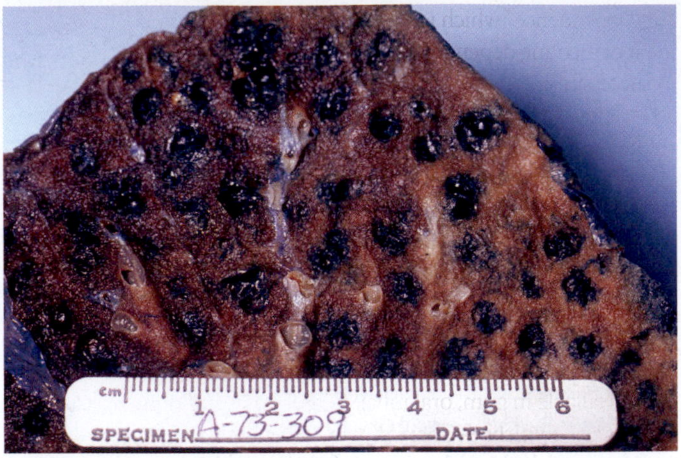

FIGURE 6–1 ◆ Gross pathology of lung showing centrilobular emphysema characteristic of smoking. Cavities lined with deposits of black carbon are easily seen.
Source: CDC/Dr. Edwin P. Ewing, Jr.

Choosing to indulge in smokeless tobacco is not without risk. The use of chewing tobacco places a person at higher risk for developing head and neck cancer. Approximately 90% of people with oral cavity and oropharyngeal cancer use tobacco, and the risk increases with the amount smoked or chewed and duration of the habit. Smokeless tobacco ("snuff" or chewing tobacco) increases the risk of cancer by about 50 times and is associated with cancers of the cheek, gums, and inner surface of the lips.

Exposure to secondhand smoke (called passive or involuntary smoking) also is a risk factor. Some harmful effects of secondhand smoke inhalation include cough, nausea, headache, eye irritation, sore throat, dizziness, and difficulty in breathing in those already suffering from asthma. Long-term involuntary smoking increases the risk of developing smoking-related diseases, such as lung cancer, ischemic heart disease, and other harmful effects on the cardiovascular system, thereby increasing the chances of a heart attack (American Cancer Society, 2011). There is no risk-free level of exposure to secondhand smoke. By eliminating smoking as a lifestyle choice, a person can live longer and reduce the risk of lung cancer by approximately 50% (Rowa-Dewar & Ritchie, 2010).

The past several years have seen a unique twist on the effect of publicity associated with tobacco use, as smoking cessation campaigns across the country have become more prevalent. The American Cancer Society (ACS) has identified school health education as critical to the effort to assist young people in developing and maintaining health practices that reduce cancer risk. Litigation by lung cancer victims or families against tobacco companies also has increased the public's attention to this dangerous and life-threatening behavior.

Smoking cessation decreases the risk of cardiovascular morbidity and mortality to levels that approach those who have never smoked. Abstinence from smoking for as little as 8 weeks causes a gradual normalization of blood and plasma viscosity. The Agency for Healthcare Research and Quality (AHRQ, 2008) published "Treating Tobacco Use and Dependence," which is a set of evidence-based guidelines for treatment of nicotine dependence. The major steps of the AHCR guidelines to successful intervention are termed the "five As": ask, advise, assess, assist, and arrange. Ask your patient if she smokes or is routinely around secondhand smoke. If the patient is not a current smoker, ask about a past history of smoking or tobacco use. If she is currently smoking, advise the patient to quit in a clear, strong, nonjudgmental manner. Assess her willingness to stop. Assist with counseling and pharmacotherapy. Arrange follow up, preferably within the first week of quitting.

Smokers trying to quit should receive pharmacotherapy and counseling. Approved medications for aiding smoking cessation include bupropion (Zyban), a nontricyclic antidepressant; nicotine replacement, available in gum, oral inhaler, nasal spray, and transdermal patch forms; and varenicline (Chantix), a drug that binds to nicotine receptors in the brain, blocking the full reinforcing effects of inhaled nicotine. Additionally, varenicline slows the release of dopamine, which normally provides the feelings of pleasure from smoking. Nicotine replacement therapy is well tolerated and safe. The use of these agents doubles the rate of successful smoking cessation.

The nurse should elicit the number of cigarettes smoked per day and the time in years a patient has smoked (pack-years) from the patient, although patients may be reluctant to accurately describe their smoking history to the nurse. Patients ages 50 or older who have smoked a pack of cigarettes (20) per day are at highest risk of pulmonary complications (Rowa-Dewar & Ritchie, 2010). The disorders associated with smoking, such as chronic obstructive pulmonary disease, are discussed in Chapter 27. It is essential that the nurse refer the patient to a smoking cessation program. The nurse educates the patient regarding the hazards of smoking and provides counseling opportunities as needed.

Substance Abuse

Substance abuse of alcohol and illicit drugs has been linked to many health problems, including injuries from accidents, sexually transmitted infections, cardiac and liver disease, violence, and a disruption of families. The term *substance abuse* also includes abuse of prescription drugs such as pain relievers, sedatives, tranquilizers, and stimulants.

Identification and diagnosis of drug abuse begins with a screening assessment. A questionnaire developed by Ewing (1984) uses the mnemonic CAGE to help professionals remember these four screening questions:

- Have you ever wanted to **C**ut down on alcohol/prescription drug use?
- Have you ever felt **A**nnoyed when remarks are made about alcohol/prescription drug use?
- Have you ever felt **G**uilty about alcohol/prescription drug use?
- Have you ever used alcohol/prescription drugs as a way to change your mood or feeling of **E**nergy?

These questions have assisted professionals with patients in many areas, including free urban clinics (Cadzow & Servoss, 2009). Questions about the amount and type of alcohol/prescription drug used are included in the social history section of a health assessment.

Risky, Unprotected Sexual Behavior

Unprotected sexual activity increases the risk for sexually transmitted infections (STIs) and pregnancy. According to *Healthy People 2020*, individuals must understand how STIs are transmitted in order to help change their risky behaviors. Chapter 43 discusses the transmission of the various STIs.

Health care providers have a pivotal role in assessing behaviors and educating individuals about prevention. It is important to provide privacy when taking a sexual health history (Peate, 2010). Effective questions for a health assessment include the following:

- Are you sexually active?
- When was the last time you had sexual activity (oral, vaginal, anal)?
- When you had sexual activity, was a condom used?
- Do you now have or have you ever had more than one sexual partner?
- Have you ever been treated for STIs?
- Have you ever had sexual activity with a partner who used intravenous drugs?

Mental Illness

Mental illness affects not only individuals, but also families and communities. According to *Healthy People 2020*, approximately 13 million American adults suffer with debilitating mental illness (1 in 17) each year. Mental disorders include depression, schizophrenia, bipolar disorder, obsessive compulsive disorder, and panic disorder. Depression accounts for the majority of these cases and significantly contributes to disability and suicide (National Institute of Mental Health, 2010). Screening for depression may be difficult because the common symptoms of fatigue, sleep disorders, and pain are vague and can be related to many conditions. Screening for depression is accomplished through patient interviews and the use of screening questions such as these:

- Have you felt down, depressed, or hopeless in the last two weeks?
- Have you had little interest or pleasure in doing things?

When a patient answers yes to one or both of these questions, to confirm the diagnosis of depression, the nurse needs to inquire about the presence of the symptoms outlined here:

- Significant weight loss or gain
- Disturbed sleep patterns
- Agitation or slowness
- Fatigue
- Feelings of guilt or worthlessness
- Inability to concentrate or make decisions
- Thoughts of death or suicide.

If the patient answers yes to the presence of four or more of these symptoms, the clinician can confirm a diagnosis of depression. The nurse should then assess for a family history of depression or other mental disorders, two or more chronic illnesses, stress in the home or at work, and loss of interest in sexual activity.

Injury and Violence

Serious injuries occur as a result of motor vehicle and motorcycle crashes, falls, drowning, fires, poison, guns, and knives. Other types of injury include homicides from firearms, domestic violence, intimate partner violence, and elder abuse. The greatest number of injuries occurs from motor vehicle crashes, with the greatest number of deaths from motor vehicle crashes occurring in individuals between 17 and

24 years old (D'Amico & Barbarito, 2012). According to the National Institute on Alcohol, Abuse, and Alcoholism, alcohol has been associated with 40% to 50% of all motor vehicle fatalities (About.com, 2011a). Increased use of safety equipment and decreased driving after alcohol consumption are considered the best ways to decrease fatalities.

When assessing the patient who admits to drinking and then driving, it is important to stress the effects of alcohol on driving. Alcohol is a depressant drug that slows down the activity of the central nervous system. It impairs driving; in fact, the impairment of the most important skills can occur at a very low blood alcohol concentration (BAC). The skills involved in driving a motor vehicle include psychomotor skills, vision, perception, tracking (steering), information processing, and attention. All of these functions are impaired by alcohol, although they differ in the extent of impairment at any given BAC. Alcohol affects driving by causing impaired vision, reduced reaction times, reduced concentration and vigilance, feelings of being more relaxed and drowsy, difficulty in understanding sensory information, difficulty in doing several tasks at once, failure to obey road rules, and overconfidence that may lead to risk taking. The more alcohol a driver consumes, the more impaired that driver becomes. Young people between the ages of 21 and 24, motorcyclists, and drivers with prior driving while impaired (DWI) convictions are at a greater risk of being involved in a motor vehicle accident (Centers for Disease Control and Prevention, 2011a). It is, however, prudent to reinforce the fact that crashes are not limited to drivers with high BACs; rather, there is a significant risk that extends to low and moderate BACs. Drivers need to know that they are impaired and are at increased risk of crash when they have consumed even small amounts of alcohol.

Domestic violence is another type of abuse that involves injuring someone, usually a spouse or partner, although the recipient can also be a parent, child, or other family member (MedlinePlus, 2011). Domestic violence represents a pattern of behavior in any relationship that is used to gain or maintain power and control over a partner or family member (American Psychiatric Association, 2011). Domestic violence is a serious problem and a common cause of injury that can happen to anyone of any race, age, sexual orientation, religion, or gender. It affects people of all socioeconomic backgrounds and education levels. This type of abuse may take the form of physical, sexual, emotional, economic, or psychological actions or threats of actions that influence another person, including any behaviors that frighten, intimidate, terrorize, manipulate, hurt, humiliate, blame, injure, or wound someone. Sexual abuse is discussed in Chapter 41.

Victims of domestic violence may suffer physical injuries such as broken bones and bruises. Their injuries may progress in severity as abuse continues to occur over time (e.g., internal bleeding, or brain injury resulting in disabilities and even death). Victims also may suffer emotionally from depression, anxiety, or social isolation. They may have trauma symptoms, including flashbacks, panic attacks, and trouble sleeping. Victims often have low self-esteem. They may have a hard time trusting others and being in relationships. The anger and stress that victims feel may lead to eating disorders and depression. Some victims even think about or commit suicide. Domestic abuse is linked to harmful health behaviors as well. Victims may try to cope with their trauma in unhealthy ways, such as smoking, drinking, taking drugs, or having risky sex (CDC, 2011d).

It is difficult to determine the exact incidence of domestic violence since in many instances it is not reported; however, the CDC (2011c) indicates that the number of reported incidences is increasing nationally. Each year, women experience about 4.8 million intimate partner-related physical assaults and rapes. In addition, men are the victims of about 2.9 million intimate partner-related physical assaults (CDC, 2011c). In 2007, for example, 2,340 deaths occurred as a result of physical assaults; 70% of these victims were female and 30% were male.

When completing a health assessment, the nurse should determine if the patient is, or has been, subject to domestic violence and/or exposed to risks of abuse. Physical indicators of abuse the nurse may observe when conducing a health examination include bruises and other signs of impact on the skin, such as burns or cuts; broken bones or evidence of old fractures; a black eye; broken or bent eyeglasses; and a battered hand. Emotional effects of abuse should also be noted if apparent: patient expressions of guilt and shame, hopelessness, and low self-esteem. The nurse should also explore the patient's exposure to the following risk factors for perpetration (hurting by a partner). Is, or has, the partner of the patient:

- Been violent or aggressive in the past
- Seen or been a victim of violence as a child
- Used drugs or alcohol, especially drinking heavily
- Been without a job or experiencing other life events that cause stress (CDC, 2011c).

Note: Additional discussion of risk factors can be found at www.cdc.gov/violenceprevention.

Elder abuse, also considered a form of domestic violence, is a growing problem in the country. Elder abuse occurs in a variety of forms: physical, mental, sexual, financial, neglect, and self-neglect. Physical abuse is defined as the use of physical force that may result in bodily injury, physical pain, or impairment. Physical abuse may include but is not limited to such acts of violence as striking (with or without an object), hitting, beating, pushing, shoving, shaking, slapping, kicking, pinching, and burning (National Center on Elder Abuse, 2011). Additionally, inappropriate use of drugs and physical restraints, force-feeding, and physical punishment of any kind are other examples of physical abuse.

Sexual abuse is described as nonconsensual sexual contact of any kind with an older adult, as well as sexual contact with any person incapable of giving consent. It includes unwanted touching and all types of sexual assault or battery, such as rape, sodomy, coerced nudity, and sexually explicit photographing (National Center on Elder Abuse, 2011).

Emotional or psychological abuse assumes the infliction of pain, anguish, or distress through verbal or nonverbal acts. Emotional/psychological abuse includes verbal assaults, insults, threats, intimidation, humiliation, and harassment. Additionally, treating an older adult like an infant; isolating an adult from family, friends, or regular activities; giving her the "silent treatment;" and enforcing social isolation are examples of emotional/psychological abuse (National Center on Elder Abuse, 2011).

Neglect is defined as the refusal or failure to fulfill any part of a person's obligations or duties to an older adult. It typically refers to the refusal or failure to provide a person with life necessities such as food, water, clothing, shelter, personal hygiene, comfort, personal safety, and other essentials when an implied or agreed-upon responsibility exists to an older adult. Neglect also may include failure of a person who has fiduciary responsibilities to provide care for an older adult (e.g., pay for necessary home care services) or the failure on the part of an in-home service provider to provide necessary care (National Center on Elder Abuse, 2011).

Weblink: Domestic Violence **Weblink:** Cost of Violence Against Women **Weblink:** Alcohol and Trauma **Weblink:** Risk Factors for Domestic Violence

Abandonment is classified as the desertion of an older adult by an individual who has assumed responsibility for providing care or who has physical custody of the individual (National Center on Elder Abuse, 2011).

Financial or material exploitation is defined as the illegal or improper use of the funds, property, or assets of an older adult. Examples include "cashing an older adult's checks without authorization or permission; forging an older adult's signature; misusing or stealing an older adult's money or possessions; coercing or deceiving an older adult into signing any document (e.g., contracts or will); and the improper use of conservatorship, guardianship, or power of attorney" (National Center on Elder Abuse, 2011, p. 2).

Self-neglect is characterized as the behavior of an older adult that threatens his own health or safety. Self-neglect generally manifests itself in an older adult as a refusal or failure to provide himself with adequate food, water, clothing, shelter, personal hygiene, medication (when indicated), and safety precautions (National Center on Elder Abuse, 2011).

Signs and symptoms of elder abuse are shown in Chart 6–1.

Conservative estimates of abuse in the United States assume as many as 3.5 million victims annually, with only 15% to 20% of abusive situations reported (National Center on Elder Abuse, 2011). The occurrence of abuse is predicted to grow as several factors come together: aging baby boomers and their insufficient retirement savings, decreased federal funding, and Americans' increasing longevity. The stakes are high: Older adults who experience abuse, neglect, or exploitation are at considerably greater risk for premature death (Deshmukh, 2011). The most common abusers of the elderly are family members, especially spouses and adult children (National Center on Elder Abuse, 2011). The low reporting rate of elder abuse therefore makes unfortunate sense: Victims would often prefer to endure the abuse rather than risk the loss of independence, being removed from their family, or possibly being forced to move into a nursing home.

Risks for elder abuse include behaviors of caregivers and the older adult's condition and history. Significant risk factors for abuse of older adults among caregivers include inability to cope with stress, depression, lack of support from other potential caregivers, caregiver's perception that caring for the older adult is burdensome and without psychosocial reward, and substance abuse. Factors that concern older adults themselves influence whether they are at greater risk for abuse. These include the intensity of illness or dementia, social isolation, the older adult's role as an abusive parent or spouse at an earlier time, a history of domestic violence in the home, and the older adult's own tendency toward verbal or physical abuse (Robinson, de Benedictis, & Segal, 2011).

CHART 6–1 Signs and Symptoms of Elder Abuse, Categorized According to Type of Abuse

Physical Abuse

- Bruises, black eyes, welts, lacerations, and rope marks;
- Bone fractures, broken bones, and skull fractures;
- Open wounds, cuts, punctures, untreated injuries in various stages of healing;
- Sprains, dislocations, and internal injuries/bleeding;
- Broken eyeglasses/frames, physical signs of being subjected to punishment, and signs of being restrained;
- Laboratory findings of medication overdose or underutilization of prescribed drugs;
- An elder's report of being hit, slapped, kicked, or mistreated;
- An elder's sudden change in behavior; and
- The caregiver's refusal to allow visitors to see an elder alone.

Sexual Abuse

- Bruises around the breasts or genital area;
- Unexplained venereal disease or genital infections;
- Unexplained vaginal or anal bleeding;
- Torn, stained, or bloody underclothing; and
- An elder's report of being sexually assaulted or raped.

Emotional Abuse

- Being emotionally upset or agitated;
- Being extremely withdrawn and noncommunicative or nonresponsive;
- Unusual behavior usually attributed to dementia (e.g., sucking, biting, rocking); and
- An elder's report of being verbally or emotionally mistreated.

Neglect

- Dehydration, malnutrition, untreated bed sores, and poor personal hygiene;
- Unattended or untreated health problems;
- Hazardous or unsafe living conditions (e.g., no heat, no running water);
- Unsanitary or unsafe living conditions/arrangements (e.g., dirt, fleas, soiled bedding); and
- An elder's report of being mistreated.

Abandonment

- Desertion of an elder at a hospital, nursing facility, or other similar institution;
- Desertion of an elder at a shopping center or other public location; and
- An elder's self-report of being abandoned.

Financial or Material Misrepresentation

- Sudden changes in bank account or banking practice;
- Inclusion of additional names on an elder's bank signature card;
- Unauthorized withdrawal of elder's funds using an ATM card;
- Unexplained disappearance of funds or valuable possessions (e.g., jewelry);
- Bills unpaid or substandard care being provided;
- Forged elder's signature; and
- Previously uninvolved relatives claiming their rights to elder's affairs.

Self-Neglect

- Dehydration, malnutrition, untreated medical conditions, poor personal hygiene;
- Hazardous or unsafe living conditions (e.g., no indoor plumbing, no heat or running water);
- Unsanitary or unclean living conditions;
- Inappropriate or inadequate clothing; and
- Grossly inadequate housing or homelessness.

Source: National Center on Elder Abuse. (2011). Major types of elder abuse. Retrieved from http://www.ncea.aoa.gov/Main_Site/FAQ/Basics/Types_Of_Abuse.aspx.

Environmental Quality

The environment includes the physical air, water, and soil. The social environment includes housing, transportation, land use, development, and agriculture. Health risks related to the physical environment include exposure to chemical, biological, and physical agents that lead to respiratory and cardiovascular diseases and cancer. Health risks associated with the social environment include those in the physical environment as well as stress, injury, and violence.

Government programs and laws have been enacted that dictate standards for water treatment, food safety, and waste management. Policies vary and are more stringent in some areas, such as urban settings, than others. When assessing patients, it is important to determine risks they may face based on their physical and social environments. *Healthy People 2020* provides information about environmental issues.

Lack of Recommended Immunization

When immunizations are consistently given to a population, they can prevent diseases, disabilities, and the spread of infection. Recommendations for childhood immunizations have been developed; when followed, these will reduce the incidence of many childhood illnesses. Immunizations for diseases such as pneumonia and influenza are considered an effective way to decrease death or complications from infectious diseases in older adults. Chapter 14 includes an in-depth discussion of immunizations. When conducting a health assessment, the health care provider needs to determine what immunizations the patient has had and the approximate date they were given. The health care provider can offer a list of immunizations to the adult patient, which may include influenza; tetanus, diphtheria, pertussis; varicella; measles, mumps, rubella; hepatitis A; hepatitis B; zoster; human papillomavirus; pneumococcal; meningococcal (CDC, 2011d).

Lack of Access to Health Care

Health insurance is the major component of this leading health care indicator. When individuals have health insurance, they tend toward regular and preventive health care practices. Higher education and income also influence health and health promotion. A significant number of individuals in the United States under the age of 65 are without health insurance, and those between 18 and 24 years old are most commonly found to lack ongoing health care (D'Amico & Barbarito, 2012).

The Health History

The health history is a detailed account of the patient's perception of his current and past health, provided in his own words. In the case of a young child or infant, the nurse will have to rely on the subjective perceptions of the patient's adult family member who cares for the child. In the case of an adult who is too ill to give an accurate account of her health history, it is acceptable to rely on the subjective perceptions of a family member or close friend. In some instances, such as a severe car crash, total strangers may be the only source of information for an unconscious patient. To ensure the accuracy of information gathered under these circumstances, the nurse must then use other sources to substantiate the information.

Older adults need carefully obtained health histories (National Institute on Aging, 2011). Therefore, the varied needs of older patients may require different interviewing techniques. The nurse must be flexible in approaching the older patient, and recognize that the deteriorating effects of aging have a wide range. There are 90-year-olds with remarkable cognitive and physical abilities and, conversely, 65-year-old patients with noticeably impaired memory and affected physiological functions. Consequently, the first goal when interviewing an older adult is to make an initial assessment of the person's age-related functions. In particular, the nurse needs to assess the patient's orientation and memory function (John E. Reid & Associates, 2008; Robertson & Hale, 2011). The nurse should not approach the patient with any expectations of physical or mental impairment; however, the nurse should have a heightened awareness of the patient's possible sensory limitations and be prepared to adjust the interviewing techniques accordingly.

The detailed nursing health history differs from the health care provider's medical history in that nurses are focusing on what effect the patient's current health status will have on being able to function independently in providing for activities of daily living (ADLs). For example, if an older adult patient is admitted for a hip fracture, the health care provider is concerned with the surgical intervention needed to repair the fracture. The nurse, however, is focused on what the patient needs to be able to perform his ADLs while in the hospital and once cleared for discharge. The nurse ascertains what the patient's level of functioning was before the event, and applies the new limitations into a plan of care. The nurse needs to assess issues such as whether the patient requires assistive devices and whether the patient has family members or friends who are able to provide assistance once the patient goes home. The nurse also teaches the caretakers all aspects of care and when to seek medical attention.

Conducting the Health Interview

When beginning the interview, nurses should address patients using their surnames and then introduce themselves and their role in the agency. They should state if they are a student. Finally, nurses should tell patients the purpose for the interview.

During the data collection phase of the interview, the nurse uses two types of questions: open ended and direct or closed. **Open-ended questions** ask for narrative information by stating the topic in general terms. This type of question is useful for introducing a subject, such as: "What brought you to the hospital?" A **direct** or *closed* **question** is used to elicit specific information and clarify specific details. For instance, if the patient stated that she is experiencing abdominal pain, a direct question would be: "Is the pain sharp or dull?" If older adults cannot answer open-ended questions well, using several "yes" and "no" questions will provide information about their health concerns (National Institute on Aging, 2011). In addition, it is important not to interrupt an older patient while he is answering the questions.

To encourage free expression, the nurse should listen carefully, not interrupt, and respond in a way that encourages the patient to provide more information. Responses that are helpful include the following:

- ***Silence:*** Quietness allows the patient time to think and allows the nurse to observe for nonverbal cues.
- ***Facilitation:*** Comments such as "Please continue" or nodding the head encourages the patient to tell the nurse more.
- ***Explanation:*** Using factual information to explain an issue helps to clarify it for the patient. For example, telling the patient how a specific procedure is performed may decrease the patient's anxiety regarding the test.

- ***Interpretation:*** Interpretive responses link events or imply cause. "From what you have told me, it appears that whenever you have a meal high in fat you begin to have abdominal pain."
- ***Clarification:*** If patients describe an issue using ambiguous language, the nurse should ask them to clarify, such as: "Please describe for me what 'feeling weird' means."
- ***Empathy:*** Acknowledging patients' feelings with a statement of understanding helps patients to feel more comfortable discussing the issue and to feel more accepted. An example of an empathetic response is: "Not being able to do your normal activities must be frustrating for you."
- ***Summary:*** At the end of the interview, the nurse summarizes his perceptions of the patient's health problem from what he has learned during the interview. This acknowledges agreement between the nurse and the patient regarding the patient's health status.

Nonproductive responses that should be avoided by the nurse include providing false reassurance; using authoritarian language; giving unwanted advice and not allowing the patient to make decisions regarding her own solution; talking too much; using professional jargon that the patient will not understand; and using avoidance language or euphemisms to avoid reality.

An awareness of body language is an important factor during the interview. Positive nonverbal messages enhance the relationship with the patient and show attentiveness and acceptance. Examples of positive nonverbal messages are a professional appearance, a relaxed open posture, appropriate eye contact, equal-status seating, a moderate tone of voice and rate of speech, and appropriate touch. Examples of negative nonverbal messages are a tense posture, critical gestures such as pointing or finger-tapping, yawning, speaking too quickly, avoiding eye contact by focusing on notes, and inappropriate touch. Note that it is important for the nurse to understand the different cultural norms regarding appropriate eye contact and appropriate touch as well as other related issues. Various communication norms for different cultures are discussed in the Cultural Considerations box (Doutrich, Campbell, & Wros, 2010; Estes, 2010).

The components of the health history are consistent from one health care agency to another. The six main components of the health history are (1) biographical data; (2) present health/illness, including health patterns and beliefs; (3) past medical history, including a medication history; (4) family history; (5) psychosocial history; and (6) a review of body systems (i.e., physical assessment). The parts of the health history follow a standardized sequence, differing only in small details from one institution to another. The sequence shown in Chart 6–2 is an example used for adult patients. A different order is usually preferred by pediatricians, who set the birth history and the past history ahead of the present illness.

CULTURAL CONSIDERATIONS for Communication Customs

Native American: Family may request spiritual healers. They may associate a loud voice with aggression. Avoiding eye contact is respectful.

Cambodian: It is inappropriate to touch the head without permission. They consider it impolite to disagree so may say "yes" but not mean it. It is very important to speak softly and be polite.

Chinese: Eye contact with authority figures is avoided as a sign of respect. Chinese language is expressive and loud. Need to assess understanding of conversations because the patient or family may not ask questions as a sign of respect. Privacy is very important.

Gypsies: It is important to establish trust. Very respectful of elder authority; therefore, they will have greater respect for older health care providers and dismiss younger team members. Tone of voice is commonly loud and argumentative. They are very modest; nurses should never ask personal questions in mixed company.

Hmong: Very polite and aware of disrespectful and prejudicial behavior. Prolonged eye contact is considered disrespectful. Communication may be indirect; will not say "no" but may say "I will think about it." Interpreters employed by the hospital are considered to be loyal to the institution and therefore not trusted. The family may request a bilingual family member be present during discussions. Language structure is different; make sure the interpreter understands the intent of the discussion. The Hmong language has almost no medical terms. Have great respect for authority. Elders of the family will meet to make decisions regarding the patient's care. Immediate family members and female relatives may not have exclusive decision-making power.

Japanese: They may not ask questions; defer to health care team to provide care. Illness is not discussed outside of the family. Soft voice is considered polite with direct conflict avoided. Facial expressions are controlled and prolonged direct eye contact is considered disrespectful. Promptness is very important. Cleanliness of the body is important, as is modesty and preservation of dignity.

Mexican: Direct eye contact with authority figures is avoided. Silence may show lack of agreement with the plan of care. Touching by a stranger is considered disrespectful, although therapeutic touch is an integral part of traditional healing.

Russians: Direct eye contact is used. They are respectful of elders. Tone of voice may be loud.

South Asians (India, Pakistan, Bangladesh, Sri Lanka, Nepal, Fiji, East Africa): Touching is not common; caring is expressed through the eyes. Prolonged direct eye contact is considered rude. Modesty, humility, tolerance, and silence are emphasized. Tone of voice should be soft. Loudness is considered disrespectful.

Vietnamese: Head may be considered sacred and feet profane; do not touch the feet and then the head. Avoiding eye contact is a sign of respect. Using both hands when giving a person something shows respect. Tone of voice should be soft. A loud voice or pointing of the finger is a sign of disrespect.

Biographical Data

Biographical data that provides baseline information about the patient contains the following elements:

- ***Name and Address:*** This is usually the first biographical data to be obtained. By having the patient state her name, the nurse is able to hear the patient speak. The patient's response will indicate whether the patient can hear, interpret direction accurately, and respond to the request appropriately. This facilitates assessment of hearing and orientation.
- ***Age and Date of Birth:*** By establishing the patient's chronological age, the nurse is then able to assess certain characteristics that occur over the age continuum. For example, a 20-year-old male will exhibit a developed musculature and his skin will be smooth and without wrinkles, whereas a 70-year-old male will exhibit aging skin with wrinkling and may have muscle wasting secondary to inactivity.

CHART 6–2 Sequence of Taking a Health History

I. Identification and vital statistics
II. Informant, relation to the patient
III. Chief complaints (CC)
IV. Present illness (PI)
V. Medications and allergies
VI. Past history (PH)
  A. General health
  B. Infectious diseases
  C. Operations and injuries
  D. Previous hospitalizations
  E. Review of systems (ROS)
    1. Integument
    2. Lymph nodes
    3. Bones, joints, and muscles
    4. Hematopoietic system
    5. Endocrine system
    6. Allergic and immunologic
    7. Head
    8. Eyes
    9. Ears
    10. Nose
    11. Mouth
    12. Throat
    13. Neck
    14. Breasts
    15. Respiratory system
    16. Cardiovascular system history
    17. Gastrointestinal system
    18. Genitourinary system
    19. Nervous system
    20. Psychiatric history
VII. Social history (SH)
VIII. Family history (FH)
IX. Physical examination
X. Laboratory
XI. Summary

- ***Gender:*** The patient's gender in association with his age gives the nurse clues as to his physical development and the presence of secondary sex characteristics. Adult males will typically have greater muscle mass and possess facial hair, whereas a female of the same age will not have these characteristics.
- ***Birthplace:*** A patient's birthplace can provide the nurse with evidence of environmental or cultural factors that may have contributed to the patient's current state of health. For example, a patient born and raised in the Central Valley of California may have signs and symptoms of reactive airway disease as a result of exposure to pesticides and dust in the region.
- ***Geography:*** Geography refers to the country, region, section, community, or neighborhood in which the patient was born and raised or currently resides. Geography affects family life and general customs practiced by the individual. The availability of community resources, including schools, churches, health care facilities, social systems, transportation, and support services, differs depending on the region. For example, urban areas typically offer more services than rural areas.
- ***Marital Status:*** By determining if the patient is single, married, widowed, divorced, or in a relationship with a significant other, the nurse establishes whether or not there is a significant person involved in this patient's life. It is also important to ask the patient if he or she has ever been in a committed relationship; this question may precipitate the patient's disclosure of a same-gender relationship.
- ***Race:*** By determining the patient's race, the nurse can assess for certain characteristics that are known about certain races. For example, Caucasians have less melanin than Hispanics or African Americans and are, therefore, more prone to skin cancers. There are also certain health-related characteristics associated with race. For example, Mexican Americans have a higher rate of adult-onset diabetes than other races (Kaushik et al., 2007).
- ***Religion:*** Determining the religious affiliation to which the patient ascribes is an important part of an assessment. Belonging to a religious faith can dictate whether a patient will accept the medical/nursing interventions offered. For example, a devout Jehovah's Witness will not permit blood transfusions. Persons belonging to the Jewish or Muslim faiths may not eat pork. Patients who are Roman Catholic may not eat meat on Fridays during the period of Lent.
- ***Occupation:*** By determining the patient's occupation, the nurse can determine if there are health-related conditions inherent in the type of work the patient performs. For example, if a patient works in a factory around loud machines, there may be resultant hearing loss from repeated exposure to noise. Occupation can also be a socioeconomic indicator of the patient. Some jobs for unskilled workers often do not pay enough for the patient to have adequate housing, insurance for health care, and adequate nutrition.
- ***Health Insurance:*** Although information about health insurance is often obtained by the registration staff, it is an important assessment of the nurse. The type of health insurance the patient has is often a predictor of her health-seeking behaviors. For example, some health insurance plans cover the preventive aspect of health and emphasize regular health screenings along the age continuum.
- ***Source of Information:*** As part of the data collection process, the person providing the information must be identified. If the patient is providing the health information, this is considered the primary source. In contrast, a person other than the patient who provides health information about the patient is considered a secondary source. The nurse should note on the questionnaire if an interpreter is used in obtaining the health history. In either case, it is the nurse's responsibility to determine the reliability of the person giving the information.

Present Health/Illness

The history of the present illness includes information about what brought the patient to the health care provider. The reason is usually written verbatim in the health record and is referred to as the **chief complaint.** A leading open-ended question the nurse may ask is: "Why did you come in today?" For example, the patient may say, "I have lost 15 pounds in the last 2 weeks." The nurse can then ask further questions to elicit further subjective data such as: "How has your appetite been?"

Health Patterns

It is important to assess the patient's health patterns because this can be a determinant of his current state of health. For example, sleep is a health pattern, and any sleep disturbances should be evaluated. Open-ended questions can be used to gather this information: "How much sleep do you normally get each night?" "Is your sleep interrupted during the night?" "How many times do you have to get up to go to the bathroom during the night?" The responses that the patient provides will be a good predictor of whether or not he is getting the required 8 to 10 hours of sleep each night. Sleep patterns will usually be addressed in the neurological portion of the body system review.

Other health patterns to assess are the patient's access to preventive health maintenance. Questions such as "When was the last time you had an eye examination?" "How often do you see a dentist?" "When was your last physical exam?" "How often do you exercise?" will assist the nurse in determining the patient's normal routine or preventive measures.

Health Beliefs and Practices

An individual's beliefs about health are based on knowledge, heritage, and experiences. Culture also influences these beliefs. With information so readily available in the mass media and on the Internet, people tend to be more informed about health issues. An increase in information about preventive medicine has made people better informed about lifestyles and habits that promote health.

The following questions and statements will assist the nurse in learning more about the patient's health care beliefs:

- What do you think it means to be healthy?
- Tell me about your own health.
- Do members of your family have the same beliefs about health as you do?
- What do you do to remain healthy?
- Do you have any behaviors that you believe are unhealthy?
- Where do you get your health information?
- Do you have a regular health care provider?
- How often do you have a complete physical examination?
- Do you have any home remedies that you use regularly?

Past Medical History

The past medical history is a timeline of the patient's health that includes childhood illnesses, immunizations, allergies, surgeries, hospitalizations, pregnancies and births, injuries, major illnesses, and any mental, emotional, or psychiatric illnesses. If the patient has a chronic illness, it is important to establish when it first occurred, what has been the progression of the illness to this point, and whether there are any **sequelae** (residual problems as a result of the illness) (National Institute on Aging, 2011). By determining this, the nurse can establish what effect the chronic illness has had on the patient's daily life. Repeated hospitalizations, numerous doctor visits requiring invasive tests, and multiple medications can affect the patient's perception of her quality of life when living with a chronic illness such as diabetes. The past medical history also is the place to discuss whether the patient uses tobacco, alcohol, or drugs. Typical questions include:

- Are you currently under the supervision of a health care provider for a medical condition?
- What diseases have you experienced, beginning with childhood?
- Have you ever been hospitalized? If so, tell me why, when, and for how long?
- Have you been told you have any diseases that are not curable?
- Have you experienced any complications (sequelae) from diseases or injuries?
- Do you have any disabilities or special needs? If so, please describe.
- Have you ever been involved in an accident in which you were injured? If so, please describe.
- Have you ever had a blood transfusion? If so, when and where?
- Has any disease or injury affected your ability to lead a normal life?
- Have you ever suffered from any mental illnesses, such as depression?

Medication History

The nurse must obtain a complete medication history for every patient. The medication history must include both prescription and nonprescription, or over-the-counter (OTC), medications that the patient may be taking. It is important to get the name, dose, and dosage times for each medication and why the patient is taking that particular medication.

While obtaining the medication history, the nurse can determine from the patient's responses how much he knows about the medication regime. The more complete and precise the obtained answers, the greater the indication that the patient has a comprehensive understanding of his medications. It also is important during this time to determine if the patient is taking any home remedies, vitamins, or herbs. Because many medications have the potential for reacting adversely when taken simultaneously, it is important to have a complete and accurate medication history from the patient. General questions about the safe handling of medications also are important to ascertain. Consider these sample questions:

- How long do you save unused drugs and are you aware of discard dates?
- How do you dispose of unused, outdated drugs?
- Where do you keep or store your medications?
- Do you check to see if the medication needs refrigeration?
- Do you take the entire prescription of antibiotics when prescribed?
- Do you share medications or needles with anyone?

Family History

Obtaining a detailed family history from the patient is important because this history serves as a predictor of potential health problems that the patient may encounter later in life. If, for example, the family history reveals that the parents and all of the siblings have diabetes, the nurse could then question the patient about potential signs and symptoms of diabetes, such as weight loss, hunger, and frequent urination.

Because many conditions occur more frequently in specific ethnic backgrounds, the family history must also include information about the patient's ethnic background. Examples include thalassemia in Southeast Asians and Tay-Sachs in Ashkenazi Jewish populations (Gene Clinics, 2008). Some familial illnesses do not occur in every generation; therefore, it is important to ask the patient about relatives in other generations. Typical questions that will illicit the needed information include the following:

- Please tell me about your family members and their health, including your spouse, children, siblings, parents, aunts, uncles, and grandparents.

- Do any of these individuals have medical illnesses or diseases? If so, what are they?
- Have there been any deaths in the immediate family? If so, what was the cause?
- How old were your parents/siblings when they died and what was the cause?

Psychosocial History

Evaluating the patient's behaviors during the health assessment will give the nurse cues to the patient's sense of self-esteem. Assessing the patient's dress, body language, and tone of voice during the interview can aid the nurse in determining the patient's emotional state at that particular time. Note, however, that the nurse must be careful not to formulate a conclusion based solely on one factor such as how the patient dressed for the interview; instead, any conclusions should be based on a variety of factors. The nurse will assess for the presence of eye contact during the interview and posture while seated: Was it relaxed or did the patient appear tense? Did the patient show signs of anxiety about answering the health assessment questions?

The psychosocial history includes information about the patient's occupational history, level of education, financial history, familial roles, relationships and interdependent relationships, cultural identity, and self-concept. The information gathered regarding a patient's occupational history, level of education, and financial history will alert the nurse to possible health risks, both present and future. For example, a patient may work in a job that has actual or potential health hazards associated with it, such as a farmworker who has worked in the fields and has been exposed to prolonged ultraviolet radiation from the sun and pesticides used on the crops.

By obtaining information regarding the patient's level of education, the nurse will gain insight into whether the patient can read and understand prescriptions or instructions given to her by a health care provider. Questions regarding the patient's financial background will give the nurse opportunities to determine the patient's health-seeking behaviors. For example, a patient who is financially secure often will have an established health care provider who is seen on a regular basis versus a patient in a job that does not offer basic health coverage and who only seeks health care when ill.

In determining the patient's perception of role and family identity, the nurse might ask: "Is there someone significant in your life?" This person may be a spouse, significant other, or a trusted friend. Then, the nurse can ask about siblings and other family members that the patient may be close to.

A patient's self-concept can be elicited by such open-ended questions as: "How are you feeling about yourself?" or "Where do you see yourself in the next 5 years?" By gathering subjective and objective data to either support or refute a patient's perception of his self-concept, the nurse can determine if the patient has a good or a distorted view. An example would be a patient who states verbally that he feels good about himself, yet his appearance is unkempt and he does not maintain eye contact with the nurse. All of these observable signs will point toward a person who has a low self-concept. When patients have a positive self-concept, they often will have coping mechanisms in place to deal with stressors in their lives. A leading question the nurse may ask is: "How do you handle stress?"

Sexuality is another component of a person's self-concept. Patients who are in a committed relationship and have a strong self-concept usually will report that their sexuality is complete or strong. The issue of sexuality is a delicate topic that patients may be reluctant to talk about, so it is important to establish a trusting and supportive rapport with the patient before attempting to discuss issues pertaining to sexuality. Once a level of trust and rapport has been established, open-ended questions such as "Are you dating?" or "Are you and your spouse engaging in sexual intimacy on a regular basis?" can be asked.

One final question that the nurse is required to ask of patients is whether or not they have been at risk for abuse. This may be difficult for a patient to answer if a family member or spouse is also in the exam room. Therefore, the nurse may need to ask this question while performing the physical exam or while alone with the patient, so that the patient is able to be more forthright when answering.

Stress and Coping

Stress is a physical or psychological stressor and coping is the individual's physical and emotional response to the stressor (Galbraith & Brown, 2011). Stress is not the event itself, but the individual's interpretation of the event and its meaning. What may be a stressor for one person may not be for another. The immediate physical response to acute stress is the fight-or-flight response, which is due to catecholamine release. This produces a variety of manifestations, such as sweaty palms and a pounding heart. The manifestations of long-term stress are different, and include habitually cold hands and suppressed immune function. Emotional reactions may include difficulty sleeping, inability to concentrate, and anxiety.

The nurse should assess the patient for the physical signs of stress including:

- Increased and pounding heart rate
- Decreased blood clotting time
- Increased rate and depth of respirations
- Dilated pupils
- Elevated glucose levels
- Dilated skeletal blood vessels
- Elevated blood pressure.

Stress in and of itself is not always bad and can, in fact, be a motivator to enhance performance. It is the coping skills or strategies that an individual uses that determine the impact and long-term effect of stress (Galbraith & Brown, 2011). Coping is a learned behavior that develops over a person's lifetime. Chapter 9 provides a complete discussion of stress and adaptation.

Cultural Beliefs and Practices

When inquiring about the patient's cultural identity, the nurse can open with a leading question such as: "What culture do you identify with most?" Cultural identity can determine how patients view themselves and how they seek health services (Garcia, Gilchrist, Vasquez, Leite, & Raymond, 2011). Patients who identify themselves as Hispanic may have a strong sense of family and may be guided by familial desires when making health care decisions. Hispanics also may have a strong sense of spirituality that will lead them to resort to prayer for their concerns. Patients' ethnic identities might also influence their dietary habits. For example, many Asian cultures will have rice as a component with each meal.

Most Americans, when ill, seek out a health care practitioner and then comply with the traditional "Western medicine" approach to treatment. As the influx of emigrants from countries that do not practice

Western medicine increases, it is important for the nurse to assess what health-seeking beliefs and behaviors the patient may favor (Garcia et al., 2011). For example, when a Southeast Asian patient is ill, the family will often perform a "coining" ritual by rubbing a coin forcefully over the person's body in order to rid the person of the spirit causing the ailment. Chinese emigrants may use herbalists to treat many ailments. People from some Hispanic cultures may use a curandera (folk healer) to cast the evil from the body of the ill person.

Some leading questions that the nurse can use to determine if a patient uses alternative forms of medicine to treat illnesses are:

- Do you use any cultural or religious practices to treat illnesses?
- Do you use any home remedies to treat illnesses?
- Do you use any holistic remedies, such as meditation, yoga, or herbs, to treat illnesses?

It is then necessary to document any alternative practices that the patient may use on the health assessment (Garcia et al., 2011).

National standards for culturally and linguistically appropriate services (CLAS) have been issued by the Department of Health and Human Services' (DHHS's) Office of Minority Health (Diamond, Wilson-Stronks, & Jacobs, 2010). These standards are aimed at helping individuals who enter the health care system receive equitable and effective treatment in a culturally and linguistically appropriate manner. The CLAS standards can be found at www.minorityhealth.hhs.gov.

Spiritual Beliefs

As nurses continually strive to assist patients and families with their health needs, they must also attend to their spiritual needs, because a nurse cannot truly assess a patient/family without assessing its spirituality (Borneman, Ferrell, & Pulchalski, 2010). Although there are very few standardized spirituality history tools, a tool called FICA (Faith, Importance and Influence, Community, and Address) was piloted and found to be a feasible tool for clinical assessment of spirituality (Borneman et al., 2010). The purpose of obtaining information about a patient's spiritual beliefs is to better understand the patient and the impact, if any, that these beliefs have on her health. As the interview is being conducted, the nurse should be alert for spiritual clues. For example, if the patient says she is a vegetarian (Hindu) or her hair has never been cut (women: Orthodox Jews), it is appropriate to inquire about the basis for these practices.

While obtaining the spiritual history, the nurse should also inquire about an advance directive (living will or durable medical power of attorney). The patient's answer may involve spiritual beliefs. An example would be a patient who believes that it is up to God to decide when he dies, not anyone else.

Ethical Issues

When conducting the health history, it is important to consider any ethical issues that may arise during the course of the interview. Nurses are guided by ethical principles as expressed in the ANA Code of Nursing Ethics. Examples of these principles are shown in the Ethical Issues box.

Genetic Information

Nurses must also consider the patient's genetic information when completing the health history. According to the Genetic Information Nondiscrimination Act (GINA) of 2009, this information consists of information about an individual's genetic tests; the genetic tests of the individual's family members; the manifestation of a disease or disorder in the individual's family members; any request for, or receipt of, genetic services; or information about participation in clinical research that includes genetic services, by the individual or any family member of the individual (Groom Law Group, 2009). Genetic information does not include any information about the individual's sex or age. Often questions about the family and past family illnesses will lead to discovery of genetic issues. Assessment and disorders chapters in this book identify genetic considerations appropriate to the physiological system being discussed and generally present these as a special feature. For example, a Genetic Considerations feature specific to the chapter on diabetes follows.

ETHICAL ISSUES to Consider When Conducting a Health Assessment

- Is informed consent necessary?
- How is confidentiality maintained?
- Is privacy of the patient protected?
- Are patient rights protected?
- Is the nurse competent to perform the assessment/evaluation?
- Is the assessment performed in a manner compliant with current nursing standards?
- Has the nurse followed an established code of conduct?
- Has the nurse acted in a nondiscriminatory manner?
- Is the nurse's judgment influenced by his own history and current perceptions of self?
- Has the nurse upheld the patient's rights and dignity?

Weblink: Genetics of Diabetes **Weblink:** CLAS Standards

GENETIC CONSIDERATIONS for Diabetes

There is a genetic predisposition for diabetes; a person having a medical history of diabetes, either in first-degree relative (parents or siblings) or second-degree relative (uncle, aunt, cousins), has an increased risk for developing the disease (American Diabetes Association, 2012).

Components of the Physical Assessment

Prior to conducting the physical assessment, the nurse should make sure that the examination area allows for privacy and the physical environment is comfortable and conducive to developing a rapport with the patient. For example, the temperature in the area should be at a comfortable level; lighting should be sufficient to see, but not glaring; distracting objects should be removed; the noise level should not be loud or distracting; and the room should be large enough to allow for 4 or 5 feet of space between the nurse and the patient.

In reviewing the body systems, some nurses use a head-to-toe approach to obtain data about each body system. Usually this is done by asking the patient a series of questions from a preprinted questionnaire regarding each body system. The assessment questionnaire will include a review of biophysical systems such as integument, head and neck, respiratory, cardiovascular, musculoskeletal, neurological, genitourinary (female/male), and reproductive (female/male).

Finally, it is important for the nurse to consider the patient's age when performing a physical assessment. For example, aging patients'

Video: Body Systems—Anatomy and Physiology

body weight will decrease during their 70s and 80s, and the distribution of fat changes with the subcutaneous fat being lost in the face and forearms and additional fat deposited in the abdomen.

Functional Assessment

The functional assessment uses observation to gather data while the patient is performing common or routine activities (D'Amico & Barbarito, 2012). As a part of the general survey, the nurse will observe such things as how patients enter the exam room; their dress, how they seat themselves, and their arm movements when straightening their clothing once seated; their hand gestures while talking; and facial expressions and facial symmetry. The nurse will interpret this information as she begins to formulate assessment data on this patient.

Physical Assessment

In conducting the physical assessment, the nurse starts with a general survey that begins at the time he first encounters the patient and then moves on to a specific examination of the body systems. During the general survey, the nurse observes the patient while performing the interview (described earlier) during the health assessment (Demirustu, Binboga, Oner, & Ozdamar, 2009). As the nurse asks questions, he observes the patient and formulates a mental picture of the patient. The nurse can observe any distinguishing features, such as the presence or absence of facial hair in an adult male (secondary sex characteristics). During this time, the nurse will observe all that can be seen, heard, or smelled while conducting the interview. This will then set the course for the nurse when performing the physical examination. The major components of the survey are physical appearance, nutritional status, mental status, mobility, and behavior of the patient.

Physical Appearance

By observing the patient, the nurse can formulate various impressions related to the patient. If the patient looks older than her stated age, this is an important observation (Demirustu et al., 2009). The patient who appears emaciated may be experiencing intentional or unintentional weight loss, which could be related to an underlying pathology. By looking at the patient, the nurse can observe body symmetry. Is the patient's upper and lower torso the same distance from head to pelvis as pelvis to feet? Does the patient's head appear to be in proportion to the rest of her body? By observing body shape and size, the nurse can determine potential abnormalities or disorders, which the nurse might confirm or disconfirm through a more focused assessment. For example, extreme thinness or obesity may indicate an eating disorder.

Nutritional Assessment

A nutrition assessment, another component of the health assessment, provides insight into the individual's dietary habits and typical food consumption. This leads the examiner into exploring any actual and/or potential problems related to body metabolism and the development and course of chronic diseases, Leading questions such as "How many meals do you normally eat each day?" "What time do you eat your last meal of the day?" and "Do you have any dietary restrictions?" will give the nurse some insight into the patient's dietary habits. A more reliable nutrition assessment is obtained, however, by having the patient fill out a journal of the eating times and amount and type of food eaten for a 3-day period. This requires that the patient be able to write and makes the assumption that he will be honest in keeping and recording the food diary. This technique also requires the patient to make a subsequent visit so the diary can be added to his health assessment. Nutrition is discussed in detail in Chapter 8.

Mental Status

The nurse assesses the patient's mental status to determine the patient's current state of mental and emotional health. If the nurse detects a problem, he must ascertain the patient's behavioral response to the problem. The nurse can assess the patient's mental status while the patient is responding to the various questions during the health history. While asking the health questions, the nurse will note the patient's affect, mood, and demeanor. At this time, the nurse can determine if the patient is oriented to person, place, and time by virtue of how the patient responds to the questions. If the patient appears confused, the nurse can further determine the patient's mental status by asking such questions as "Do you know what day it is today?" or "What time is it?" If the patient has difficulty answering these questions, the nurse will need to conduct a more detailed assessment.

Mobility

The nurse assesses the patient's mobility to determine her functional ability and any deviations that exist from the norm, such as weakness, stiffness, or involuntary motor activities. This assessment provides information about the patient's musculoskeletal system. The nurse can observe how the patient moves when the patient enters the office area or walks to the exam room: Are the patient's movements fluid and purposeful? Is her posture erect and is she moving with a steady stride? The nurse can observe for deviations in movement and assess whether or not the patient has full range of motion in her extremities. An older adult female with advanced osteoporosis may walk with a "stooped over" posture and it may appear that she also is experiencing pain or is laboring to perform movements. Relative to mobility, the nurse also observes whether the patient is using any ambulatory aids such as a walker, cane, wheelchair, leg braces, or special orthotic shoes.

Behavior

The nurse assesses patient behavior to gain a general impression of how the patient is feeling and what, if anything, is bothering the patient physically and psychologically. The nurse can observe the patient's affect and response to questions. Is the patient's response appropriate, or does the patient under- or overreact to the situation? For example, if the patient is telling the nurse about the death of someone close, is there an emotional response? Lack of an appropriate response is referred to as "flat affect" and should be documented in the health record. At the other end of the spectrum, is the patient overreacting or visibly uncomfortable with unemotional queries?

Measuring Height and Weight

The nurse measures the patient's height and weight as a means of obtaining baseline data. In obtaining the patient's actual height and weight, the nurse can account for any differences in what the patient may have subjectively told the nurse during the patient interview.

The most common method of obtaining an adult patient's height and weight is with the platform scale. The nurse measures the patient's weight and then directs the patient to turn his back to the scale. The nurse then slides a height bar up above his head, folds out the right-angled arm, lowers the arm until it barely touches the patient's head, and takes the height measurement.

Many standard height and weight charts for both men and women have been developed by insurance companies and the Department of Health and Human Services (DHHS). The nurse should make sure to use whichever chart is approved by her health system. A common measure of weight to height is the body mass index (BMI). BMI is a person's weight in kilograms divided by the square of his height in meters, giving a measure of kg/m^2. The BMI ranges are as follows:

- Normal range: <18.5– 24.9
- Overweight: 25.0–29.9
- Obese: >30.

Weight, as it is related to cardiac risk factors, is discussed in Chapter 32.

Measuring Vital Signs

Temperature, pulse, respirations, blood pressure, and pain level are the **vital signs** that the nurse will measure during the health assessment. The vital signs are the most immediate indicators that something is wrong, since altered or abnormal vital signs are clues to illness. The patient's temperature is often obtained with an electronic thermometer and recorded in either degrees Fahrenheit or Celsius. The most common route for obtaining a temperature is via the oral cavity. Other routes are rectal, axillary (under the arm), and tympanic (ear).

Obtaining the adult patient's pulse is most commonly done by palpating the radial artery and counting the pulse for 15 seconds, then multiplying by 4 to arrive at a 60-second pulse rate. During the assessment, the nurse evaluates the apical, bilateral radial, and bilateral pedal pulses (Figure 6–2◆). While the nurse is recording the pulse rate, he will simultaneously be assessing the character of the patient's pulses for such descriptors as weak, thready, bounding, regular, or irregular. If there are irregularities in the pulse rate, then the nurse should

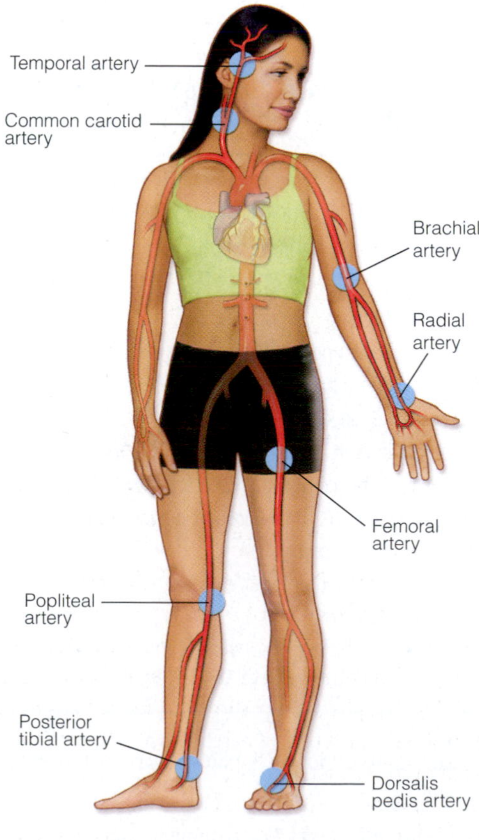

FIGURE 6–2 ◆ Apical, bilateral radial, and bilateral pedal pulse locations.

check the pulse rate for a full 60 seconds to get an accurate pulse rate. Abnormalities related to the pulse are discussed in Chapter 30.

The nurse will usually assess the patient's respiratory rate while obtaining the pulse rate. Once the nurse has obtained the pulse rate, she will observe the patient's chest movement and count the number of times the patient inhales in a 15-second interval, then multiply this amount by 4 to achieve a 1-minute respiratory rate. The nurse should also observe the character and movement of the patient's chest while obtaining the respiratory rate. She will be observing for a rhythmic inhalation and exhalation and for nasal flaring or use of accessory muscles on inhalation. A more detailed examination of the patient's breathing will occur when auscultating the lungs with a stethoscope. The detailed respiratory examination is further explained in Chapter 25.

The nurse obtains the patient's blood pressure by using a cuff, sphygmomanometer, and a stethoscope. It is important for the nurse to select a cuff that is the appropriate size for the patient's upper arm circumference. The width of the cuff should equal 40% of the circumference of the extremity used, and the length of the cuff should equal 80% of the circumference. Using a cuff that is too narrow will give a falsely high blood pressure. The nurse must also palpate the brachial artery (Figure 6–2) and align the arrows of the cuff so that they are over the artery. The assessment will take place while the patient is in a sitting position.

Blood Pressure Measurement

The blood pressure is properly measured using both arms on two or more different occasions, when the patient has been seated for at least 5 minutes prior to measurement (Parker & Glasziou, 2009). Guidelines for consistent, uniform technique for measuring blood pressure are shown in Chart 6–3.

The nurse exerts pressure on the main artery of the patient's arm through the inflated blood pressure cuff. The stethoscope is used to listen for Korotkoff's sounds, which change in tone and volume as the cuff is deflated and blood flow is gradually restarted. The first sound heard is the systolic blood pressure, which represents the highest blood pressure that occurs each time the heart beats. The second recording is the diastolic blood pressure, which represents the lowest blood pressure that occurs when the heart relaxes between beats.

This procedure for blood pressure monitoring describes the manual approach. There is, however, a growing trend to use an electronic blood pressure monitoring system (Haynes, 2011). The stethoscope and gauge are combined in a digital machine. An electronic blood pressure monitor will have an inflatable cuff that is wrapped around a person's upper arm to restrict the flow of blood. This cuff is accompanied by a manometer to determine the blood pressure. The electronic system comes equipped with a built-in stethoscope that listens to the heart as the blood pressure cuff is inflated. When considering an electronic blood pressure monitor, it is imperative to consider the size of the cuff as the tightness of it may give inaccurate readings. This is especially so when using a regular-sized cuff on individuals with larger or smaller than average arms. Electronic blood pressure monitors normally come with a LCD display on a screen of varying sizes.

Most electronic blood pressure monitors can be powered with batteries or an AC adapter. If one needs to use the machine when traveling or moving between locations, a battery powered electronic blood pressure monitor is ideal. Some models also come with a memory function that stores one or many previous readings so that a fluctuation in readings is recorded and can be evaluated. The monitors also may be set to maintain a record for more than one person.

CHART 6–3 Guidelines for Assessing Blood Pressure in Adults

Questions to be Asked Before a Blood Pressure Assessment is Done

- Have you drunk any caffeinated beverages within the last hour?
- Have you eaten any chocolate within the last hour?
- Have you smoked within the last 15 minutes?
- Are you using any nasal decongestants? (If yes, assess whether the decongestant contains phenylephrine.)
- Do you use eyedrops for pupillary dilation?
- Does the environment feel cold to you?
- Have you just eaten a meal?
- Do you need to use the restroom?
- Do you exercise? If so, what do you do, for how long, and how many times per week?

Environment

- A quiet, warm, and comfortable setting.
- Home readings.

Equipment

- *Cuff Size for Adult* The bladder should encircle and cover two-thirds of the length of the arm. If the bladder is too small, a high reading may result.
- *Manometer* Aneroid gauges should be calibrated every 6 months against a mercury manometer.
- *Infants and Children* Use a Doppler method.

Posture

- *Initial Assessment* For patients over age 65 receiving antihypertensive therapy or a diabetic check for postural changes in blood pressure, the first reading is taken after the patient has been supine for 5 minutes, and then both immediately and 2 minutes after the patient stands.
- *Follow-Up* For a follow-up, a sitting pressure is recommended. The patient should be seated quietly for 5 minutes with the back supported. The arm is then supported at the level of the heart.

Technique

- Initially, the blood pressure assessment is taken in both arms. The findings are recorded, identifying the arm and the pressure reading.
- On each occasion, take at least two readings. These should be separated by as much time as practical. When readings vary more than 5 mmHg, take additional readings until two readings are close.
- When making the diagnosis of high blood pressure, obtain three sets of readings at least 1 week apart.
- When the arm pressure is elevated in a patient younger than 30, take the blood pressure in the leg.

Performance

- Find the brachial artery.
- Inflate the bladder quickly to a pressure at least 20 mmHg above the systolic pressure. This can be checked by determining that the radial pulse has disappeared.
- Deflate the bladder at about 3 mmHg every second.
- Record the Korotkoff phase V (disappearance) in adults. In children use phase IV (muffling).
- If the Korotkoff's sounds are weak, have the patient raise the arm, open and close the hand 5 to 10 times, and then inflate the bladder quickly.
- Recording the findings:
  - Note the pressure obtained.
  - Note which arm was used.
  - Note the patient's position.
  - Note the cuff size.

Example: 140/90, seated, right arm, large adult cuff

Source: Andreoli, T. E., Carpenter, C. C. J., Griggs, R. C., & Localzo, J. (2004). *Cecil essentials of medicine* (6th ed.). Philadelphia: Saunders, pp. 38–39.

Many newer blood pressure monitors can be operated single handedly, and come with cuffs that can accommodate nearly any size. When wrapped around the arm, readings are displayed automatically at the touch of a button. Electronic monitors are useful for people who have hearing disabilities and/or impaired vision. They also are advantageous for those who have trouble remembering when to take readings, as many electronic blood pressure monitors have alarms to let one know when to take the blood pressure. Other beneficial features that may be included are capacity to record readings for two individuals and to store them on one unit, extra or adjustable cuffs, and the ability to measure irregular heartbeats (ChristiaNet, 2009).

Accuracy in the measurement of blood pressure is imperative because these data often guide medical and nursing practice. Many therapeutic decisions are made based on BP recordings. Although the skill of measuring blood pressure appears simple, there are many possible causes of errors and inaccuracies (Chart 6–4). Inaccuracies in BP assessment can lead to underestimation or overestimation of blood pressure, causing errors in the diagnosis and treatment of cardiovascular conditions. Chart 6–5 reviews other factors that could affect the blood pressure as well.

CHART 6–4 Inaccuracies in Blood Pressure Measurement

Inaccuracies in blood pressure measurement are common clinical problems and can occur due to human error or device error for numerous reasons:

- Inappropriately sized cuffs (too wide or too narrow)
- Incorrect cuff positioning
- Incorrect cuff wrapping (too loose or uneven)
- Failure to allow a rest period before measurement
- Deflating the cuff too quickly or too slowly
- Inaccurate inflation level
- Not measuring in both arms
- Failure to palpate maximal systolic pressure before auscultation
- Improper position of the arm (above or below heart level)
- Poor observer concentration
- Lack of repeated measurements
- Poorly fitting stethoscope.

Source: Parker, E., & Glasziou, P. (2009). Use of evidence in hypertension guidelines: Should we measure in both arms? *British Journal of General Practice, 59*(560), e87–92.

Pain

The assessment of pain, often referred to as the fifth vital sign, is essential for the nurse to obtain with each assessment of the patient (D'Amico & Barbarito, 2012; Oliver, 2010). The presence of pain—whether acute or chronic, severe or mild—is a subjective experience solely unique to that individual. A pain history includes the following data (Oliver, 2010):

- ***Location:*** The nurse asks the patient to point to the location of the pain source. Often the nurse will ask the patient to use a body

CHART 6–5 Clinical Factors That Affect Blood Pressure

Clinical Awareness and Monitoring

- Anticipate adherence problems for young men.
- Ask about smoking history.
- Ask about use of "Smoke Ender" or a similar program.
- Obtain history of success in quitting smoking.
- Consider nonadherence as a cause of:
  Failure to reach goal blood pressure
  Resistant hypertension
  Sudden loss of control.
- Encourage patients to bring all medications from all health care providers and other sources, whether prescription, complementary, or over the counter, to each visit.
- Ask if the patient is taking anything for pain and, if so, why.
- Recognize depression and other psychiatric illnesses, including panic attacks that may impact blood pressure.
- Be willing to change unsuccessful regimens and search for those more likely to succeed.

Source: Adapted from Berman, A., & Snyder, S. (2010); D'Amico, D., & Barbarito, C. (2012).

diagram to help locate the pain. The nurse then identifies the locus of the pain using the nearest anatomic landmarks (e.g., sharp pain in right patellar region posterior and medial).

- ***Intensity:*** The nurse asks the patient to rate the level of pain that she is experiencing using a pain scale. For most adults, a numerical pain scale of 0 to 10 can be used where 0 is no pain and 10 is the highest level of pain.
- ***Quality:*** Asking the patient to describe the pain as dull, throbbing, sharp, piercing, aching, and so on, gives the nurse a sense of the quality of the pain that the patient is experiencing. When using the patient's exact words to describe the quality of the pain, the nurse puts the patient's words in quotation marks.
- ***Pattern:*** The onset and duration of pain is noted as the pattern. The nurse assesses whether the pain is constant or intermittent. If it is intermittent, the nurse also asks about duration, that is, when the pain subsides and returns. The nurse records the patient's response in the narrative.
- ***Precipitating Factors:*** The nurse attempts to learn from the patient what brings on the pain. A precipitating factor could be, for example, ascending three flights of stairs (after which the patient experiences substernal chest pain).
- ***Relief Methods:*** Along with assessing for the presence of pain, the nurse also asks the patient what she has done to attempt to relieve the pain. Here the nurse lists all prescription treatments and OTC remedies that the patient may have utilized, as well as any alternative health providers such as an herbalist, massage therapist, chiropractor, or acupuncturist. The nurse also notes which of these methods has helped in relieving the pain and for how long.
- ***Impact on ADLs:*** By assessing how the pain is impacting the patient's ability to perform her ADLs, the nurse can obtain a clearer picture of how the pain may be affecting this particular patient's quality of life.
- ***Coping Strategies:*** Coping strategies include yoga, meditation, relaxation exercises, prayer, support groups, or withdrawal. Each of these strategies is unique to the individual patient and will also be a reflection of the patient's age, culture, and belief system.

Refer to Chapter 12 for a thorough discussion of pain.

Documentation of the Health History

In the acute care setting, specific forms or page screens on an electronic health record (EHR) guide the nurse in documentation of the health history. Figure 6–3◆ shows examples of EHR screens for documentation of a health history in the acute care setting. Of note is the importance of documenting *who* is answering the questions. Detailed information on documentation is discussed in Chapter 5.

Physical Examination

There are two types of physical examinations (exam). The **comprehensive exam** (head-to-toe exam) is usually performed on new patients who will be seen on a routine basis by various clinicians. A **focused exam** is performed in emergent or urgent situations and is focused on a specific problem (Demirustu et al., 2009). Regardless of the type of exam to be done, an organized and systematic examination is necessary to obtain pertinent data in the shortest amount of time. An organized approach creates trust and encourages patient cooperation. The information that was gathered during the health history will help to guide aspects of the physical examination. At all times during the exam, nurses show consideration for the patient's physical and psychological comfort. It is important to explain all aspects of the examination to the patient; this will enhance the patient's experience and decrease his anxiety during the examination.

Incorporating the head-to-toe examination into a nurse's routine takes practice and repeated examinations in order for the process to flow in a natural manner that is comfortable for both the nurse and the patient (Demirustu et al., 2009). This routine helps ensure the nurse will not omit any pertinent data during the examination. Expertise comes with practice, and the ability to interpret findings develops with experience. There is no one correct way to perform the head-to-toe examination. The main goal is to have a sequence that flows smoothly and allows for patient comfort and privacy. The examination of specific systems is discussed in detail throughout the book in each unit's assessment chapter.

Preparation for the Physical Examination

The environment where the physical examination takes place must be private, quiet, and at a comfortable temperature. The room needs to have adequate lighting, and the nurse needs to use standard precautions throughout the entire physical examination. The nurse should assemble all the equipment needed for the exam in the room prior to the beginning of the examination. It is helpful to assemble the equipment in order of use. Figure 6–4◆ shows the instruments used for a physical examination.

The patient must be prepared both physically and psychologically for the physical examination. Before beginning, the nurse should ask the patient if she needs to empty her bladder. If a urine specimen is needed, she will instruct the patient on the technique for collection. Then nurse will also provide the patient with a gown and instruct her to remove all necessary clothing, ensuring a drape is available for use during the examination.

During the examination, the patient will have to assume various positions to facilitate the assessment and will need to be draped properly with each position change (Figure 6–5◆). The nurse must be

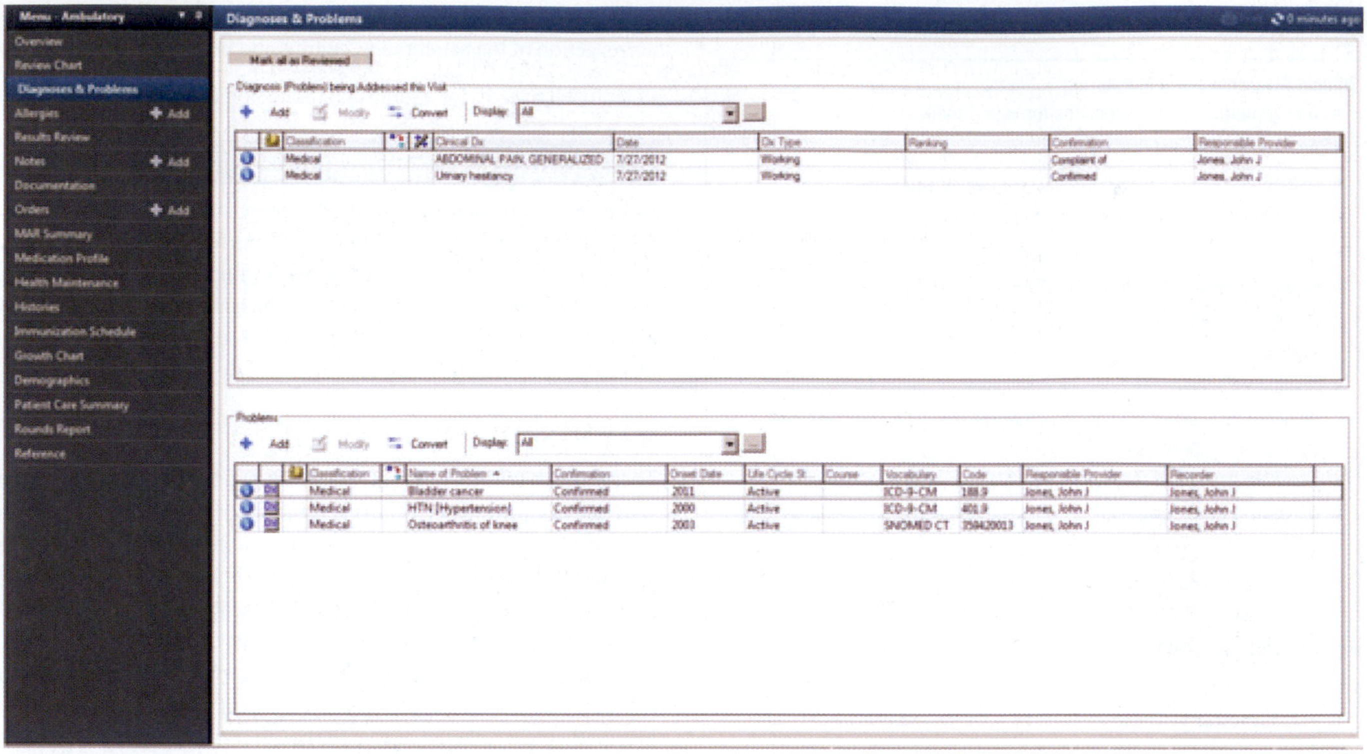

FIGURE 6–3 ◆ Past medical history.

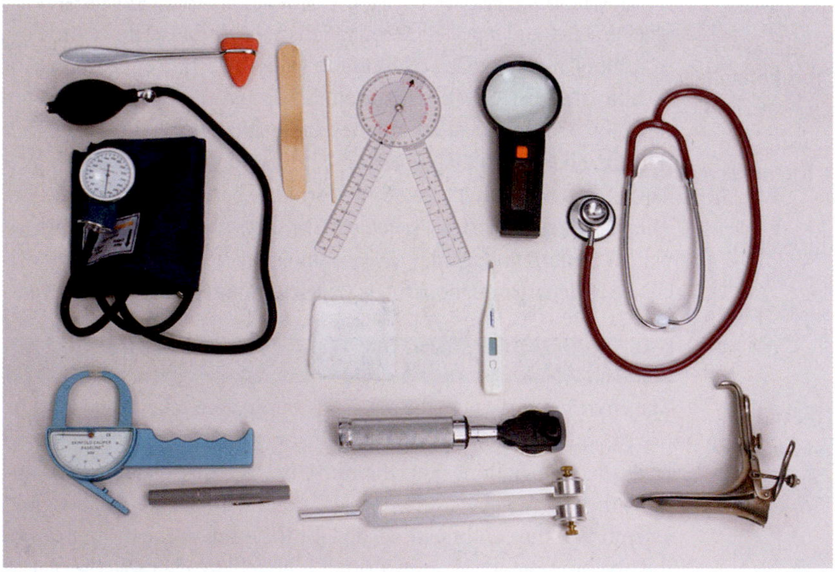

FIGURE 6–4 ◆ Equipment used for physical assessment.

sure to consider any limitations the patient may have that would prevent the usual positioning, including arthritis, weakness, fractures, or joint deformities. This is particularly relevant to the aging patient.

To prepare the patient psychologically for the examination, the nurse should assume a calm, professional demeanor and explain each step of the process in general understandable terms. The nurse must be sensitive to any discomfort created by exposing various parts of the patient's body, and be culturally sensitive when dealing with people from cultures other than her own. In some cultures, women are restricted from revealing their bodies to males other than their husbands. When a person of the same gender is requested for an examination, if at all possible, that request should be honored.

Techniques of Physical Examination

During the physical examination, the nurse will utilize each of his senses while examining the patient. Techniques such as inspection, palpation, percussion, and auscultation are implemented to assess the patient objectively (Demirustu et al., 2009).

Inspection

Inspection is the deliberate, systematic examination of the patient using both sight and smell. It begins with the first encounter and continues the entire time the nurse is with the patient. The nurse observes gait, mannerisms, stature, and other physical attributes. The inspection begins by assessing the patient's appearance and comparing the right and left side of the body for symmetry. Inspection of each region of the body includes observing color, warmth, size, symmetry, contour, movement, or drainage (D'Amico & Barbarito, 2012). For example, the nurse assesses the color of the nail beds and the temperature of the fingers on each side and then compares the right versus left. Under normal conditions, the finger temperature and nail bed color are the same in both hands. A cold dusky blue appearance of only one hand

POSITION	AREAS EXAMINED	RATIONALE	CONTRAINDICATIONS
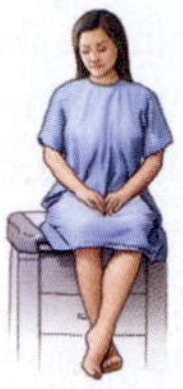 Sitting	Vital signs, head and neck, back, posterior and anterior thorax and lungs, breasts, axillae, heart, upper and lower extremities, reflexes	Sitting upright allows for full lung expansion and better visualization of upper body symmetry.	Older and weak clients may be unable to sit without support. An alternate position is supine with the head of the bed elevated.
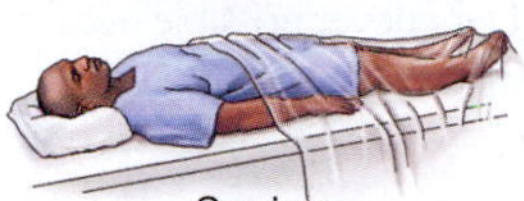 Supine	Vital signs, head and neck, anterior thorax and lungs, breasts, axillae, heart, abdomen, extremities, peripheral pulses	This is a relaxed position for most clients. It provides access to pulse sites and prevents contracture of abdominal muscles, especially if a small pillow is placed under the knees.	Clients with cardiovascular and respiratory problems may be unable to lie flat without becoming short of breath. An alternate position is to raise the head of the bed. Clients with lower back pain may be unable to lie flat without flexing the knees.
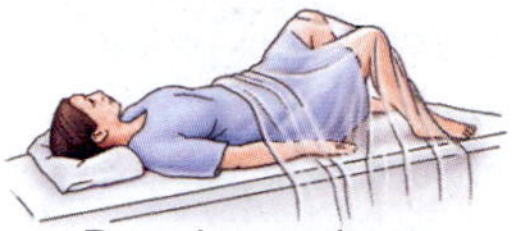 Dorsal recumbent	Abdomen and external genitalia	Flexed knees reduce tension on lower back and abdominal muscles and increase client comfort.	Same as for supine. The client should not raise the arms over the head or clasp the hands behind the head because this increases contraction of the abdominal muscles.
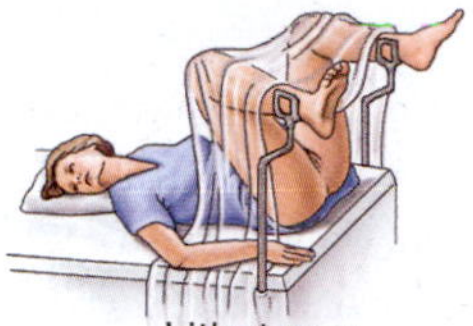 Lithotomy	Female genitalia, reproductive tract, and rectum	This position maximally exposes the genitalia and facilitates the insertion of a vaginal speculum.	This position is assumed immediately before it is needed because it is embarrassing and uncomfortable. The client is kept draped. Clients with arthritis or joint deformity may be unable to assume this position. Alternate positions are dorsal recumbent and Sims'.
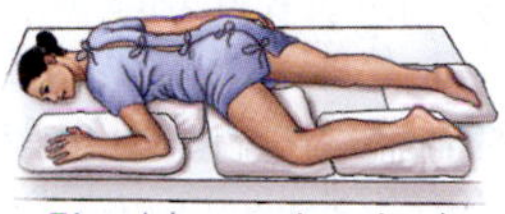 Sims' (posterior view)	Rectum, vagina	Flexion of the upper hip and knee improves exposure of the rectal area.	Clients with deformities of the hip or knee may be unable to assume this position. Older and obese clients may be uncomfortable.
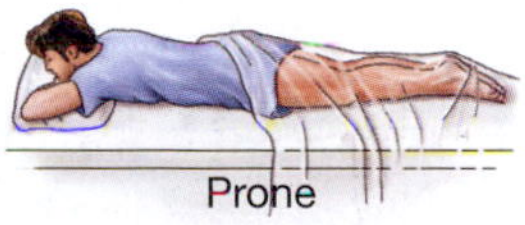 Prone	Posterior thorax, hip movement, popliteal pulses	This position is used to assess hip extension. Sometimes popliteal pulse palpation is facilitated in this position.	This position is not well tolerated by older clients or clients with cardiovascular or respiratory problems.
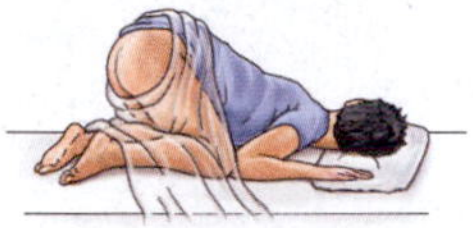 Knee-chest	Rectum, prostate	This position provides maximal exposure of the anal and rectal areas and facilitates insertion of instruments into the rectum.	Poorly tolerated by clients with cardiovascular or respiratory problems. Clients with difficulty flexing hips or knees may be unable to assume this position.
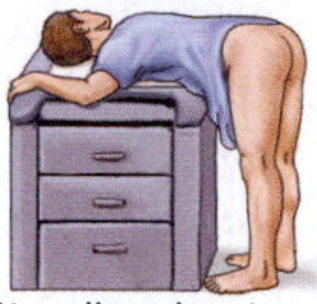 Standing, bent over examining table	Rectum, prostate	This is a more comfortable position than knee-chest and allows for palpation of the prostate gland.	This position is assumed immediately before it is needed because it is embarrassing. Clients with back problems may need assistance.

FIGURE 6–5 ◆ Patient positioning during physical examination.

indicates a problem with the blood supply to that area. The nurse also should note any unusual odor and determine its cause.

During most of the patient inspection, no instruments are needed, but some parts of the assessment require special tools that will assist the nurse. The instruments include the following:

- Ophthalmoscope to inspect the inner aspects of the eye
- Otoscope to inspect inner ear structures
- Tongue blade to inspect the inside of the mouth, tongue, and throat
- Vaginal speculum to dilate the vaginal canal and inspect the cervix
- Vision chart to test near- and farsightedness
- Stethoscope to listen to lungs, bowel sounds, and blood pressure
- Blood pressure cuff
- Penlight to provide direct light source and to test pupillary responses
- Thermometer to check body temperature.

Palpation

Through **palpation,** the nurse uses touch to collect data to determine specific characteristics of the patient's body. This process is described as a vital skill for health care staff (Eberman & Finn, 2010). Characteristics such as temperature, texture, moisture, tenderness, pain, vibrations, and edema are assessed using palpation. Additionally, the size, shape, and mobility of a body part can be palpated. Each specific area of the body is palpated to evaluate underlying structures, pulses, lymph nodes, and specific organs such as the kidney and liver.

In palpating, the nurse will use the fingertips, finger pads, base of the fingers, palmar surface of the fingers, and the dorsal and ulnar surfaces of the hands, using slow, intentional movements (D'Amico & Barbarito, 2012) (Figure 6–6◆). The nurse can minimize discomfort to the patient by warming his hands, having his nails cut short, and not wearing any jewelry. The nurse may wear gloves when the patient's skin has open or exposed areas. When using latex gloves, it is necessary to ask patients if they have any allergies to latex.

Palpation is characterized as being light, moderate, or deep. The nurse always begins with light palpation and culminates with deep palpation to evaluate such organ structures as the kidney and liver (Eberman & Finn, 2010). The use of light palpation first will aid the nurse in assessing the texture, temperature, and any painful or reddened area on the surface of the patient's skin (Figure 6–7◆). Moderate palpation is used to assess major areas of the patient's anatomy, especially the abdominal organs. The nurse uses the palmar aspect of the fingers and gently press down about 1 to 2 centimeters while rotating the fingers in a circular motion (D'Amico & Barbarito, 2012) (Figure 6–8◆). Deep palpation is used to assess an organ that lies deep within the abdominal cavity, such as the liver and/or kidneys (Figure 6–9◆). The level of palpation is usually 2 to 4 cm. The nurse must explain the procedure to the patient, because deep palpation could cause some discomfort if the patient already experienced pain upon light to moderate palpation. It is important for the patient to be relaxed during palpation of the soft tissue areas. It is better to use the dominant hand whenever possible because it is more sensitive than the nondominant one.

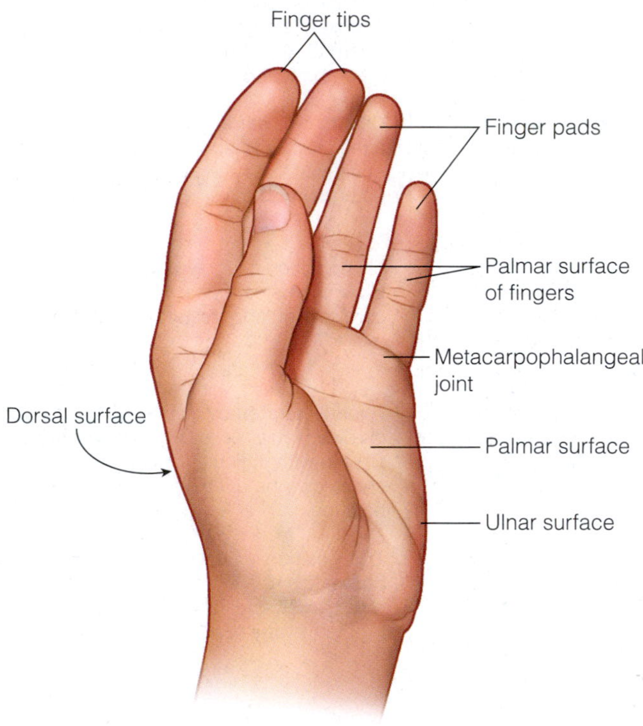

FIGURE 6–6 ◆ Palpation.

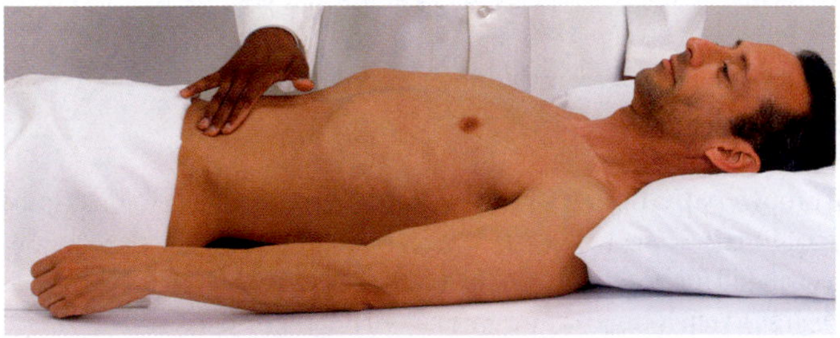

FIGURE 6–7 ◆ Light palpation.

Percussion

Percussion is the creation of sound vibrations by pushing, tapping, or using a device to generate a vibration. The vibrations produced will help the nurse in determining the position of organ structures. The three types of percussion are direct, blunt, and indirect (D'Amico & Barbarito, 2012). **Direct percussion,** used to examine areas such as the sinuses, is gentle tapping to illicit the presence or absence of fluid. Direct percussion results in a dull sound.

Blunt percussion involves placing the palm of the nondominant hand over a body area (such as the kidney) and striking the palm with the closed fist of the dominant hand (Figure 6–10◆). This method is used to assess for pain or tenderness of the liver, gallbladder, or kidneys. The patient is usually sitting upright and the blunt percussion is performed from behind (D'Amico & Barbarito, 2012).

Indirect percussion involves using the hyperextended middle finger of the nondominant hand (pleximeter) and the fingertip of the middle finger of the dominant hand (plexor) to strike the pleximeter

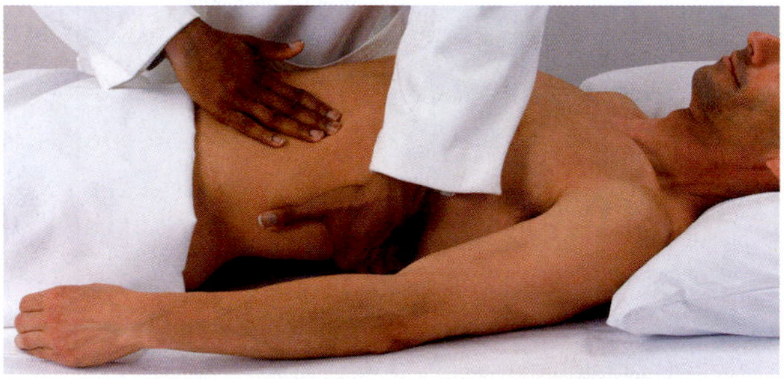

FIGURE 6–8 ◆ Moderate palpation.

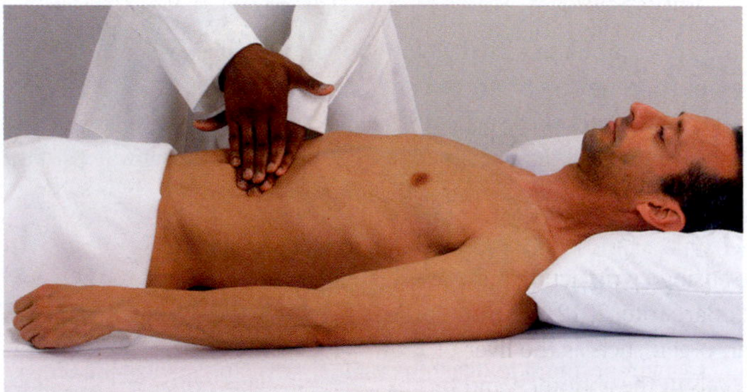

FIGURE 6–9 ◆ Deep palpation.

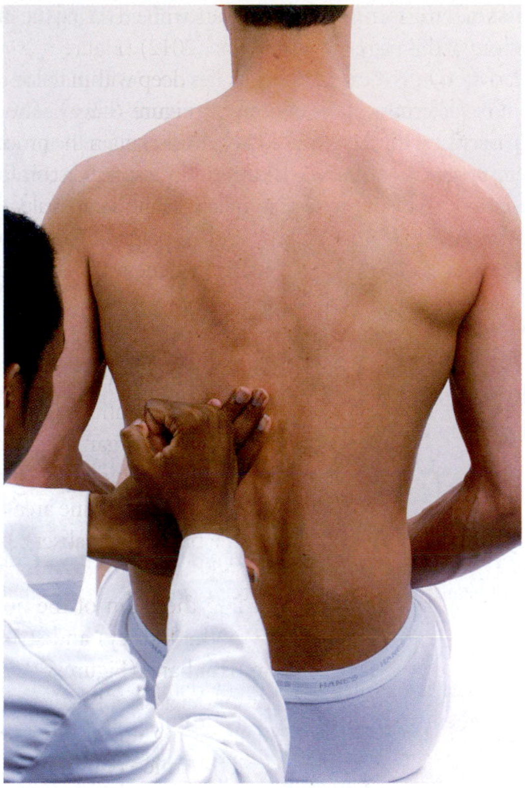

FIGURE 6–10 ◆ Blunt percussion.

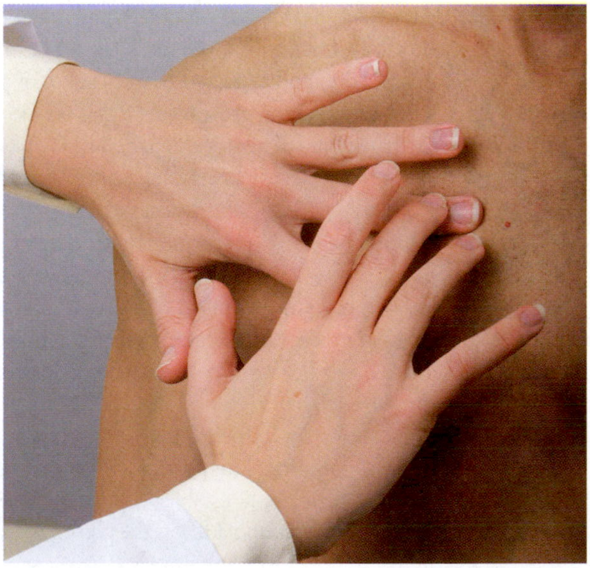

FIGURE 6–11 ◆ Indirect percussion.

by using a wrist action that will elicit a sound (Figure 6–11 ◆) (D'Amico & Barbarito, 2012). This method is used to determine the location of an organ such as the liver or kidney and also to determine fluid air levels in the abdomen and thorax. Organs will produce a dull sound, whereas air and fluid will have a higher, more tympanic sound when percussed. The sounds produced by percussion are as follows:

- **Tympany** is a high-pitched, drumlike tone of medium duration. It is commonly heard over the air-filled intestines.
- **Resonance** is a loud hollow tone of long duration. It is commonly heard over the lungs.
- **Hyperresonance** is a loud low tone with a longer duration than resonance. It is heard when air is trapped in a space such as the lungs.
- **Dullness** is a high-pitched tone of short duration and is soft in quality. It is heard over the large organs such as the liver and kidney.
- **Flatness** is a soft, high-pitched tone with a short duration. It is heard over muscle and bone.

Percussion sounds have characteristic features that the nurse must become familiar with through experience and practice. These features include intensity, pitch, duration, and quality. *Intensity* is the amplitude or the loudness and softness of the sound. The intensity is influenced by the amount of air present and the ability of the structure to vibrate. *Pitch* refers to the frequency of vibrations of sound per second. Slow vibrations produce a low-pitched sound, whereas fast vibrations produce a high-pitched sound. The length of time that the sound can be heard is referred to as *duration*, and it can be very short to very long. *Quality* refers to the type of sound and is described as clear, hollow, muffled, or dull (D'Amico & Barbarito, 2012).

Auscultation

Auscultation is the technique of listening to body sounds (Maude, Lawson, & Foureur, 2010). The nurse must use both the unassisted sense of hearing and, where needed, a stethoscope. Body sounds that can be heard unassisted include speech, coughing, respirations, and the percussion tones just described. The stethoscope (Figure 6–4, p. 130) is used to assess the lungs, heart, and abdomen. The stethoscope has two end pieces, a bell and a diaphragm. The bell has a cuplike shape and is best for hearing low-pitched sounds, such as heart murmurs. In contrast, the diaphragm or flat end piece is best for high-pitched sounds such as bowel, lung, and normal heart sounds. The diaphragm should be held firmly against the patient's skin. When sounds are very soft and difficult to hear with a normal stethoscope, a Doppler ultrasound stethoscope is useful. It uses ultrasound waves to detect sounds such as fetal heart tones and peripheral pulses. Interference with the Doppler can be eliminated by applying gel to the skin.

Safety Alert *Do not press the bell end piece of the stethoscope into the skin. This causes the skin to act as a diaphragm and will reduce audible vibratory sensations.*

When listening with the stethoscope, the environment should be as quiet as possible. Rubbing against the patient's clothing or the bed sheets or touching the stethoscope tubing will produce sounds that will interfere with body sounds. While listening, it is important to focus on only one sound at a time. Closing the eyes often assists the nurse to focus. Sounds are described in the same terms as the percussion sounds described earlier: intensity, pitch, duration, and quality.

Critical Thinking

Critical thinking is a cognitive skill that is needed for every aspect of a health assessment. The nursing process provides an effective framework for applying critical thinking to patient care situations. Critical thinking helps the nurse resolve problems and develop ways to manage situations. Critical thinking requires that the nurse apply logic, question the norm, and problem solve in patient care situations. The nurse must learn to recognize the relative significance of the visual, auditory, or palpable *cues* that occur during the assessment. Cues are bits of information that may hint at the possibility of a health problem (e.g., nasal flaring or inflammation). Taking advantage of the information offered by these cues necessitates the development of critical thinking skills.

The nurse uses critical thinking in the collection of information, analysis of the situation, generation of alternatives, selection of alternatives, and evaluation. *Collection of information* begins with the interview and continues throughout the entire health assessment. If the patient is in acute distress, the nurse's critical thinking skills will assist her in altering the assessment as appropriate to maintain patient safety. For example, if the patient is in respiratory distress, it is imperative to assess airway management and oxygenation first.

As the nurse is collecting data, she must verify the reliability of the information. This is done by determining the patient's ability to be a reliable historian. The nurse should look for inconsistencies and inappropriate information. This is the component where the nurse applies logic and critically assesses information. If the nurse is concerned, it is sometimes helpful to ask the same question twice during the interview, and if possible check with family members for verification (D'Amico & Barbarito, 2012).

The second skill is *analysis of the situation*. During this phase, the nurse must distinguish normal from abnormal. The patient's age, gender, genetic background, and culture affect the analysis. The nurse must utilize laboratory findings, diagnostic tests, charts, and measures related to development and aging. For example, some findings may be normal for an 80-year-old male but not for a 30-year-old female. When using critical thinking skills, the nurse clusters related information to assist in identifying patterns in the information. At this point, the nurse identifies missing information and retrieves it (D'Amico & Barbarito, 2012).

Generation of alternatives includes identifying options and establishing priorities. It begins with identification of options, after which the nurse and patient work together to establish the priorities. The nurse needs to assess the patient's understanding of the situation and provide more information about the advantages and disadvantages of each option so the patient can make an informed decision.

Once informed about options, the next step is the *selection of alternatives*. The critical thinking skill needed for this step is the ability to develop outcomes and plans. The outcome is the final result of what the patient will attain, and the plan is the activities that will lead to that outcome. Some components of the plan are developed in conjunction with the health care team, whereas others are done by the patient independently.

Upon completion of the physical examination and health history assessment, the clinician may order diagnostic tests. In each of the disorder chapters that follow in this book, diagnostic tests related to the disorder are included as a feature of the text. The Diagnostic Tests feature assumes the format shown in the sample Diagnostic Tests box at the bottom of this page.

The last step in critical thinking is *evaluation*. Evaluation requires that the nurse determine if the expected outcomes have been achieved. Each step of critical thinking is used here to determine if any omissions or misinterpretations occurred. It is essential to ensure that decisions were based on all of the facts and that reliable recourses were used (D'Amico & Barbarito, 2012).

Gerontological Considerations

The number of people 65 years of age and older is increasing as a result of the demographic aging of the population, thus increasing the need for skill development in the care of older adults. As of 2009, those over 65 years of age made up 13% of the U.S. population (U.S. Census Bureau, 2011). This segment of the population has a higher percentage of chronic illnesses, such as diabetes or cardiac illnesses, as compared to younger adults (NDIC, 2011). Although the majority of older adults are in good health and report high levels of well-being, the incidence of a variety of illnesses and invalidity increase substantially for adults over 75 years of age (NDIC, 2011).

While collecting health assessment data, a nurse also needs to review the patient's history of acute or chronic illnesses that will influence self-care, as well as the patient's understanding of medications and other care concerns In addition, it is essential to consider older adults' abilities with respect to basic activities of daily living, so that full and individualized care can be provided and the patient's remaining autonomy can be preserved (Deschodt, Dierckx de Casterle, & Milisen, 2010).

Specifically, when completing a health assessment, the older adult patient is measured, weighed, examined, observed, and questioned about physical, functional, and behavioral changes. Chart 6–6 shows specific body areas of inspection and expected characteristics of aging that serve as a guide to the examination process.

In addition to the aging characteristics described in Chart 6–6, the nurse, when completing a health assessment or examination, also should be alert to the possibilities of decreased lung capacity; reduced peripheral perfusion; exertional dyspnea; or deviation of the trachea, especially if scoliosis is present. A decreased resting heart rate and cardiac output, and increased diastolic and systolic blood pressure, also may be evident. The patient's sense of position, smell, touch, and sensitivity to heat and cold may be decreased, as may his deep tendon reflexes (The Free Dictionary, 2011).

When completing an assessment of the elderly person, it is important to make the individual as comfortable as possible. The nurse should face the patient during the examination, establish eye contact, repeat questions if necessary, avoid shouting, and address the person by name.

DIAGNOSTIC TESTS for Hearing and Balance Disorders

Test with Description, Rationale, and Normal Values	Expected Abnormality
Voice and Watch Tick	
Used to test high-frequency hearing loss. The examiner stands 1 to 2 feet behind and to the side of the patient, while the patient occludes each ear sequentially and the examiner whispers four unrelated words near each ear. Normal results are that the patient can hear the words in each ear.	If the patient is unable to hear whispering, there is some degree of hearing loss present. The loss of the ability to hear a watch ticking is considered to be a loss of high-frequency sounds.

CHART 6–6 Physical Assessment of the Elderly with Characteristics of Aging

Skin	Dryness, wrinkles, sagging, thinning over the back of hands, areas of vitiligo, keratoses, warts, changes in appearance of freckles and moles, skin tags.
Nose and Ears	Lack of luster.
Eyes	Possible enlargement relative to face size.
	Dryness, opacity of lens, discoloration of the sclera and iris, an opaque ring near the edge of the cornea, decreased pupil size, and diminished peripheral vision.
Hair	Thinning or loss of hair on scalp and in axillary and pubic areas.
Mouth	Loss of teeth, gum recession, diminished salivation, and diminished taste perception.
Ears	Hearing loss, particularly of high-frequency tones.
Muscles	Decreased muscle mass, osteroarthritic joints, Heberden's or Bourchard's nodes at finger joints, contracture of lateral fingers, osteoporosis, a broad based stance, and slow voluntary movements.

If the patient's visual perception and tactile sense are diminished, the nurse can use color contrasts and items of marked textural differences in the assessment (The Free Dictionary, 2011).

Nursing education programs continue to explore ways to prepare the faculty for teaching gerontology to students, as well as ways to prepare students for the care of older adults (Deschodt et al., 2010). As our society continues to age, attention must be given to gerontology-related competencies for students as well as current nursing staff. Of particular concern are the skills for interviewing elderly adults, for example, as discussed in this chapter. For more information on gerontological considerations, refer to Chapter 10.

Summary

Health assessments allow the nurse to gather information regarding the patient's past and current state of health, along with health promotion behaviors that are being utilized. This information, in conjunction with the physical examination, gives the nurse data to develop a plan of care to assist the patient in reaching optimum health. The development of evidence-based guidelines that assist the nurse in performing appropriate and effective health histories for specific populations is essential.

NCLEX® PRACTICE

1. The nurse is conducting a health assessment with a newly admitted patient. Which of the following should be included in this assessment?

1. Subjective data only
2. Data about the patient's physical, social, cultural, environmental, and emotional statuses
3. Objective data only
4. A list of nursing diagnoses and goals

2. The nurse is preparing to conduct a patient interview. Which of the following should the nurse do first?

1. Introduce him-/herself.
2. Measure the patient's vital signs.
3. Assist the patient into a hospital gown.
4. Address the patient by name, including the patient's surname.

3. During an interview, the patient asks the nurse if she thinks he has cancer. Which of the following should the nurse say in response?

1. "Probably, because your hemoglobin is low and you are exsanguinating from your rectal orifice."
2. "What makes you think that you have cancer?"
3. "I'm not the doctor but I will tell you this, it's a good thing you came into the hospital while you still could because you never know what they are going to find with all of their tests and procedures."
4. "What a silly thing to say! You know, if you believe you have cancer you probably do!"

4. A patient walks with two canes but is stable when ambulating and changing clothes. Which of the following assessment techniques was used to collect this data?

1. Auscultation
2. Palpation
3. Inspection
4. Percussion

5. After completing a health assessment and physical examination with a patient, the nurse begins to review the information and group similar data into clusters. In which step of the critical thinking process is this nurse functioning?

1. Analysis of the situation
2. Generation of alternatives
3. Selection of alternatives
4. Evaluation

6. The patient is a 50-year-old male who has told the nurse that he considers himself physically sedentary. Which of the following can the nurse suggest to assist the patient to comply with guidelines for physical activity? (select all that apply)

1. Walk at a moderate pace 3 times per day for 10 minutes at least 5 days per week.
2. Jog at a moderate pace for 10 minutes 1 or 2 days per week.
3. Play tennis 1 or 2 times per month for 1 hour.
4. Ride a bike at a vigorous pace for 60 minutes 3 days per week.
5. Take a golfing vacation every winter.

Answers to NCLEX Practice questions can be found in Appendix D in the Osborn Student Resources at nursing.pearsonhighered.com. Practice additional NCLEX questions online at the Student Resources site.

REFERENCES

About.com. (2011a). Alcohol and trauma, alcohol alert from NIAAA. Retrieved from http://alchoholism.about.com/cs/alerts/l/blnaa03.htm

About.com. (2011b). CDC reports costs of violence against women. *US Government Info.* Retrieved from http://usgovinfo.about.com/cs/healthmedical/a/violencecosts.htm

About.com. (2011c). Secondhand smoke. Retrieved from http://quitsmoking.about.com/cs/secondhandsmoke/a/secondhandsmoke.htm

Agency for Healthcare Research and Quality, U.S. Department of Health and Human Services. (2008). Treating Tobacco Use and Dependence: 2008 Update. Retrieved from www.ahrq.gov/path/tobacco.htm

American Cancer Society (ACS). (2011). Cigarette smoking. Retrieved from http://www.cancer.org/Cancer/CancerCauses/TobaccoCancer/CigaretteSmoking/cigarette-smoking-who-and-how-affects-health

American Diabetes Association. (2012). Genetics of diabetes. Retrieved from http://www.diabetes.org/diabetes-bsics/genetics-of-diabetes.html

American Psychiatric Association. (2011). Domestic violence. Healthy minds, healthy living. Retrieved from http://healthyminds.org/Main-Topic/Domestic-Violence.aspx

Andreoli, T. E., Carpenter, C. C. J., Griggs, R. C., & Localzo, J. (2004). *Cecil essentials of medicine* (6th ed.). Philadelphia: Saunders, pp. 38–39.

Berman, A. J., & Snyder, S. (2012). *Kozier & Erb's fundamentals of nursing* (9th ed). Upper Saddle River, NJ: Pearson.

Borneman, T., Ferrell, B., & Puchalski, C. M. (2010). Evaluation of the FICA tool for spiritual assessment. *Journal of Pain & Symptom Management, 40*(2), 163–173.

Cadzow, R. B., & Servoss, T. J. (2009). The association between perceived social support and health among patients at a free urban clinic. *Journal of the National Medical Association, 101*(3), 243–250.

Centers for Disease Control and Prevention. (2008). Physical activity for everyone. Retrieved May 6, 2008, from http://www.cdc.gov/nccdphp/dnpa/physical/everyone/recommendations/index.htm

Centers for Disease Control and Prevention. (2010). Defining overweight and obesity. Retrieved from http://www.cdc.gov/obesity/defining.html

Centers for Disease Control and Prevention. (2011a). Impaired driving: Get the facts. Retrieved from http://www.cdc.gov/MotorVehicleSafety/Impaired_Driving/impaired-drv_factsheet.html

Centers for Disease Control and Prevention. (2011b). Perceived exertion (Borg rating of perceived exertion scale). Retrieved from http://www.cdc.gov/physicalactivity/everyone/measuring/exertion.html

Centers for Disease Control and Prevention. (2011c). Understanding intimate partner violence. CDC. Retrieved from http://www.cdc.gov/violenceprevention

Centers for Disease Control and Prevention. (2011d). Recommended adult immunization schedule—United States 2011. *Morbidity and Mortality Weekly Report.* Washington, DC: U.S. Department of Health & Human Services, Centers for Disease Control and Prevention.

ChristiaNet. (2009). Electronic blood pressure monitors. Retrieved from http://www.christianet.com/cholesterol/electronicblood pressuremonitors.htm

D'Amico, D., & Barbarito, C. (2012). *Health and physical assessment in nursing* (2nd ed.). Upper Saddle River, NJ: Pearson Prentice Hall.

Demirustu, C., Binboga, D., Oner, S., & Ozdamar, K. (2009). The relationship between the Ways of Coping with Stress Inventory and the General Health Questionnaire-12 scores among university students. *Turkiye Klinikleri Journal of Medical Sciences, 29*(1), 70–76.

Deschodt, M., Dierckx de Casterle, B., & Milisen, K. (2010). Gerontological care in nursing education programs. *Journal of Advanced Nursing, 66*(1), 139–148. doi: 10.1111/j.1365-2648.2009.05160.x.

Deshmukl h, N. R. (2011). Common signs and symptoms of elder abuse. Buzzle.com. Retrieved from http://www.buzzle.com/articles/common-signs-and-symptoms-of-elder-abuse.html

Diamond, L. C., Wilson-Stronks, A., & Jacobs, E. A. (2010). Do hospitals measure up to the National Culturally and Linguistically Appropriate Services standards? *Medical Care, 48*(12), 1080–1087.

Doutrich, D., Campbell, P. P., & Wros, P. (2010). Nurturing cultural competence in nursing: Collaboration and promising practices. *Communicating Nursing Research, 43*, 463–467.

Eberman, L. E., & Finn, M. E. (2010). Enhancing clinical evaluation skills: Palpation as the principal skill. *Athletic Training Education Journal, 5*(4), 170–175.

Estes, M. E. Z. (2010). *Health assessment and physical examination* (4th ed.). Clifton Park, NY: Delmar Learning.

Ewing, J. A. (1984). Detecting alcoholism: The CAGE questionnaire. *Journal of the American Medical Association, 252*, 1905–1907.

Galbraith, N. D., & Brown, K. E. (2011). Assessing intervention effectiveness for reducing stress in student nurses: Quantitative systematic review. *Journal of Advanced Nursing, 67*(4), 709–721.

Garcia, C., Gilchrist, L., Vasquez, G., Leite, A., & Raymond, N. (2011). *Journal of Immigrant & Minority Health, 13*(3), 500–509.

Gene Clinics. (2008). Gene tests. Retrieved February 3, 2008, from http://www.geneclinics.org

Groom Law Group. (2009). Memorandum to clients: New interim final regulation on Genetic Information Nondiscrimination Act (GINA) (including new restrictions on health risk assessment). Retrieved from http://www.groom.com/resources-89.html

Haynes, D. (2011). Blood pressure machine and blood pressure monitor: What you need to know. Retrieved from http://darrenhaynes.hubpages.com/hub/Blood-Pressure-Machine-Guide

Healthy People 2020. (2011). Mental health and mental disorders. Retrieved July 11, 2011, from http://www.healthypeople.gov/2020/topicsobjectives2020/overview.aspx?topicid=28#one

Institute of Medicine. (2011). Leading health indicators for *Healthy People 2020*—Letter Report. Retrieved June 13, 2011, from http://www.iom.edu/Reports/2011/Leading-Health-Indicators-for-Healthy-People-2020.aspx

John E. Reid & Associates. (2012). Interviewing elderly subjects. Retrieved from http://www.reid.com/educational_info/r_tips.html?serial=10892152163604&print=%5Bprint%5D

Kaushik, V. P., Snih, S. A., Ray, L. A., Raji, M. A., Markides, K. S., & Goodwin, J. S. (2007). Factors associated with seven-year incidence of diabetes complications among older Mexican Americans. *International Journal of Experimental, Clinical, and Behavioral Gerontology, 53*(4).

Linden, T. C., Jackson, C., Rutledge, S., Nath, C., & Lof, L. N. (2010). The Heart of Grinnell: A Community-Wide Rural Health Wellness Initiative: A pilot observational study and a prospective study design. *Alternative Therapies in Health & Medicine, 16*(4), 46–49.

Maude, R., Lawson, J., & Foureur, M. (2010). Auscultation—the action of listening. *New Zealand College of Midwives Journal.* Retrieved from http://findarticles.com/p/articles/mi_6845/is_43_43/ai_n57558650/pg_8

McClave, A., Rock, V., & Thorne, S. (2010). State-specific prevalence of cigarette smoking and smokeless tobacco use among adults—United States, 2009. *MMWR, 59*(43), 1400–1406

MedlinePlus. (2011). Domestic violence. Retrieved from http://www.nlm.nih.gov/medlineplus/domesticviolence.html

National Center on Elder Abuse. (2011). Major types of elder abuse. Retrieved from http://www.ncea.aloa.gov/NCEAroot/Main_Site/FAQ/Basics/Types_Of_Abuse.aspx

National Diabetes Information Clearinghouse (NDIC). (2011). National diabetes statistics, 2011. Retrieved July 11, 2011, from http://www.diabetes.niddk.nih.gov/dm/pubs/statistics/

National Institute of Mental Health (NIMH). (2010). Major depressive disorder among adults. National Institutes of Health, US Department of Health and Human Services. Retrieved from http://www.ninh.nih.gov/statistics/IMDD_ADULT.shtml

National Institute on Aging. (2011). Obtaining the medical history. Retrieved June 13, 2011, from http://www.nia.nih.gov/HealthInformation/Publications/ClinicianHB/03_history.htm

North American Nursing Diagnosis Association. (2007). *Nursing diagnoses: Definitions and classifications 2007–2008.* Philadelphia: Author.

Oliver, D. (2010). The assessment and management of pain in neurological disease. *British Journal of Neuroscience Nursing, 6*(2), 70–72.

Parker, E., & Glasziou, P. (2009). Use of evidence in hypertension guidelines: Should we measure in both arms? *British Journal of General Practice, 59*(560), e87–92.

Peate, I. (2010). Privacy please: Taking a sexual health history. *British Journal of Health Assistants, 4*(2), 71–74.

Robertson, L., & Hale, B. (2011). Interviewing older people: relationships in qualitative research. *The Internet Journal of Allied Health Sciences and Practice, 9*(3), 1–8.

Robinson, L., de Benedictis, T., & Segal, J. (2011). Special issue: Elder abuse. Mayor's Office to Combat Elder Abuse. Retrieved from http://www.nyc.gov/html/ocdy/html/issues/elder.shtml

Rowa-Dewar, N., & Ritchie, D. (2010). Smoking cessation for older people: Neither too little nor too late. *British Journal of Community Nursing, 15*(12), 578–582.

The Free Dictionary. (2011). Assessment of the aging patient. Google. Retrieved from http://medical-dictionary.thefreedictionary.com/assessment+of+ the+aging+patient

U.S. Census Bureau. (2011). State and county QuickFacts. Retrieved from http://quickfacts.census.gov/qfd/states/00000.html

Vance, D. E. (2010). Aging with HIV: Clinical considerations for an emerging population. *American Journal of Nursing, 110*(3), 41–49.

Concepts Essential to Nursing Practice

UNIT 2

Content in Unit 2 that addresses the **Institute of Medicine (IOM)** competencies, **Nursing Core Competencies (NCC)**, the **Quality and Safety Education for Nurses (QSEN)** competencies, and **Concepts** for concept-based learning is listed below.

Competencies	Feature or Text	Location
IOM, QSEN, NCC Providing patient-centered care	Cultural Considerations for Genetics Nutrition Assessment Cultural Considerations in Nutrition Assessment Psychosocial Theories Therapeutic Relationships The Psychodynamics of Illness and Hospitalization Health Assessment of the Aging Patient Ensuring the Patient's Comfort (at end of life)	Chapter 7, page 151 Chapter 8, page 158 Chapter 8, page 161 Chapter 9, page 214 Chapter 9, page 221 Chapter 9, page 230 Chapter 10, page 241 Chapter 11, page 261
IOM, QSEN, NCC Working in teams	Collaborative Management (Stress) Innovations in Caring for the Aging Patient Collaborative Management (End-of-Life Care)	Chapter 9, page 228 Chapter 10, page 255
IOM, QSEN, NCC Employing evidence-based practice	Gene Therapy and Stem Cell Therapy Pharmacogenomics Evidence-Based Practice: Reducing Aspiration Risk During Tube Feeding Administration Oxidative Stress Evidence-Based Practice: Promoting Resilience Through Self-Care Evidence-Based Practice: Management of Bowel Routines Evidence-Based Practice: Mammogram Screenings in Older Adults Evidence-Based Practice: Medication Administration for Aging Patients Evidence-Based Practice for End-of-Life Care	Chapter 7, page 153 Chapter 7, page 153 Chapter 8, page 196 Chapter 9, page 213 Chapter 9, page 220 Chapter 10, page 245 Chapter 10, page 249 Chapter 10, page 252 Chapter 11, page 260
IOM, NCC Applying quality and safety improvement	Stress at the Cellular Level Cardiovascular Assessment (of the aging patient) Influenza Vaccine (for the aging patient)	Chapter 9, page 211 Chapter 10, page 244 Chapter 10, page 248
IOM, QSEN, NCC Using informatics	Pharmacology and the Aging Patient Innovations in Technology for the Aging Patient	Chapter 10, page 250 Chapter 10, page 255
NCC Applying ethical and legal responsibilities	Ethical, Legal, and Social Issues of Genetic Information Legal and Ethical Issues of Aging Ethical Issues at End of Life Ethical Issues for Pain Management at End of Life	Chapter 7, page 150 Chapter 10, page 253 Chapter 11, page 261 Chapter 11, page 262
NCC Developing professionally	Chart 7–2 Essential Nursing Competencies for Genetics and Genomics	Chapter 7, page 148
NCC Educating patients	Genetic Testing The Teaching–Learning Process	Chapter 7, page 147 Chapter 9, page 229
Concepts covered in Unit 2 include:	Genetics Nutritional balance Infection Grief and loss Metabolism Mood and affect	Self Stress and coping Violence

CHAPTER 7

Genetics

Carolyn Graff
Ann Cashion
Rebecca Graves
Cheryl Wraa

Outcome-Based Learning Objectives

After studying this chapter, the learner will be able to:

1. Exemplify the role of genetics in health care and nursing.
2. Summarize the events of cell division that result in chromosomal abnormalities.
3. Explain the organization of the human genome and the DNA sequence.
4. Illustrate the influence of the genome on differences among patients.
5. Explain patterns of inheritance and variables influencing interpretation of inheritance patterns.
6. Summarize the role of nurses in detection, management, and care of patients with genetic disorders.
7. Recall emerging molecular technologies and genetic therapies.

KEY TERMS

allele p.139
aneuploidy p.143
autosomal dominant inheritance p.142
autosomal recessive inheritance p.142
autosome p.139
centromere p.139
chromosome p.139
chromosome disorder p.143
codon p.140
copy number variation (CNV) p.142
cytogenetics p.139
deletions p.144
diploid p.140
epigenetics p.140
exon p.140
expressivity p.147
gamete p.139
gene p.139
gene therapy p.153
genetic variance p.141
genome p.140
genomic imprinting p.143
genomics p.138
genotype p.141
germ line cells p.139
haploid p.140
heterozygous p.139
homozygous p.139
human genome p.138
Human Genome Project (HGP) p.138
inherited cancer syndrome p.145
intron p.140
karyotype p.139
monosomy p.143
mosaicism p.144
mutation p.141
nondisjunction p.144
pedigree p.147
penetrance p.142
pharmacogenetics p.153
pharmacogenomics p.153
phenotype p.141
polymorphism p.141
sex chromosome p.139
single-gene disorder p.142
single nucleotide polymorphism (SNP) p.141
telomere p.139
transcription p.140
translocation p.144
trisomy p.143
X-linked dominant p.143
X-linked recessive p.143
wild type p.140
zygote p.143

GENETICS FOCUSES on variation and heredity in all living beings. A great deal of genetics information derives from the work of many researchers, including Gregor Mendel, who is attributed with discovering the laws of genetics in 1865, and James Watson and Francis Crick, who described the double-helix structure of DNA (Watson & Crick, 1953). Fifty years after the structure of DNA was described, researchers mapped each human gene and completely sequenced the **human genome,** that is, all of the DNA in human cells. This was accomplished through an international research effort known as the **Human Genome Project (HGP).** The HGP has provided information about and insights into many diseases and development of improved methods for diagnosis and prevention.

The completion of the HGP has been described as the beginning of the genomic era (Collins, Green, Guttmacher, & Guyer, 2003). Integrating genomics into health care is critical because the use of genetic information may improve the health of individuals. **Genomics** is the field of genetics that focuses on translating the knowledge of the human genome into health benefits, including the molecular analysis of the human genome in health and illness. In addition to educating nurses and health professionals about genetic and environmental factors affecting health, findings from genetic research can be used by patients and family members to improve their own health and prevent illness. Both nurses and patients must be knowledgeable and informed so they can communicate effectively with each other and engage in discussion about the implications of genomics for health.

Foundations for Genetics

An introduction to genetics requires a foundational understanding of cells, chromosomes, and the human genome. More extensive, in-depth information can be found in genetics textbooks, such as those by Klug, Cummings, Spencer, and Palladino (2009) and Nussbaum, McInnes, and Willard (2007), and appropriate websites.

Cells and Chromosomes

A typical cell has two major parts, the nucleus and the cytoplasm. The nucleus is separated from the cytoplasm by a nuclear membrane and the cytoplasm is separated from the surrounding fluids by a cellular membrane. The nucleus is the cell's primary control center. **Chromosomes,** which house most *deoxyribonucleic acid (DNA)*, are located within the nucleus (Figure 7–1◆). Each species can be characterized by its chromosome number and morphology. For example, humans have 23 pairs of chromosomes, whereas dogs have 39 pairs and tomatoes have only 12 pairs. The number of chromosomes is not associated with intelligence level. The entire chromosome complement within a cell is known as the **karyotype** and is visible microscopically when cells are dividing (Figure 7–2◆). **Cytogenetics** is the study of chromosomes, their structure, and inheritance.

Chromosomes contain genes organized into linear structural units. **Genes** are the fundamental units of heredity that carry traits from one generation to the next. Each gene has a specific location, or locus, on the chromosome (Figure 7–3◆). Each chromosome carries a different subset of genes; however, pairs of chromosomes carry matching genetic information in the same sequence. Because one chromosome of each pair is inherited from each parent, individuals have alternative copies of each gene, called **alleles,** one on each chromosome. For example, if an individual has type AB blood, he has an A allele from one parent and a B allele from the other. Alleles are considered **homozygous** when they are identical (i.e., type AA blood) and **heterozygous** when different (i.e., type AB blood).

Genes are found in the nucleus of almost all human cells, with a notable exception being red blood cells, which have no nucleus. Small subsets of genes are also found in the mitochondria located outside the nucleus in the cytoplasm. Mitochondrial genes exclusively exhibit maternal inheritance, which means an individual can only inherit these genes from his mother.

Chromosomes are divided into two arms by the **centromere,** a constriction in the chromosome (see Figure 7–3). The short or petite arm is designated *p* and the long arm is designated *q*. To identify the locus on a chromosome, both the number of the chromosome and the arm are identified. For example, the gene associated with cystic fibrosis is known as the cystic fibrosis transmembrane conductance regulator (*CFTR*) gene and is located at 7q31.2. This means that the gene is located on the long arm (q) of chromosome 7 at locus 31.2. The end of the chromosome is called the **telomere** and is thought to ensure the integrity of the chromosomes during cell division, in addition to being associated with the aging process.

Of the 23 pairs of human chromosomes, 22 are classified as **autosomes** and are alike in both males and females. Only one pair is designated as the **sex chromosomes** and these differ by gender: Females have two X chromosomes (XX) and males have an X and a Y chromosome (XY).

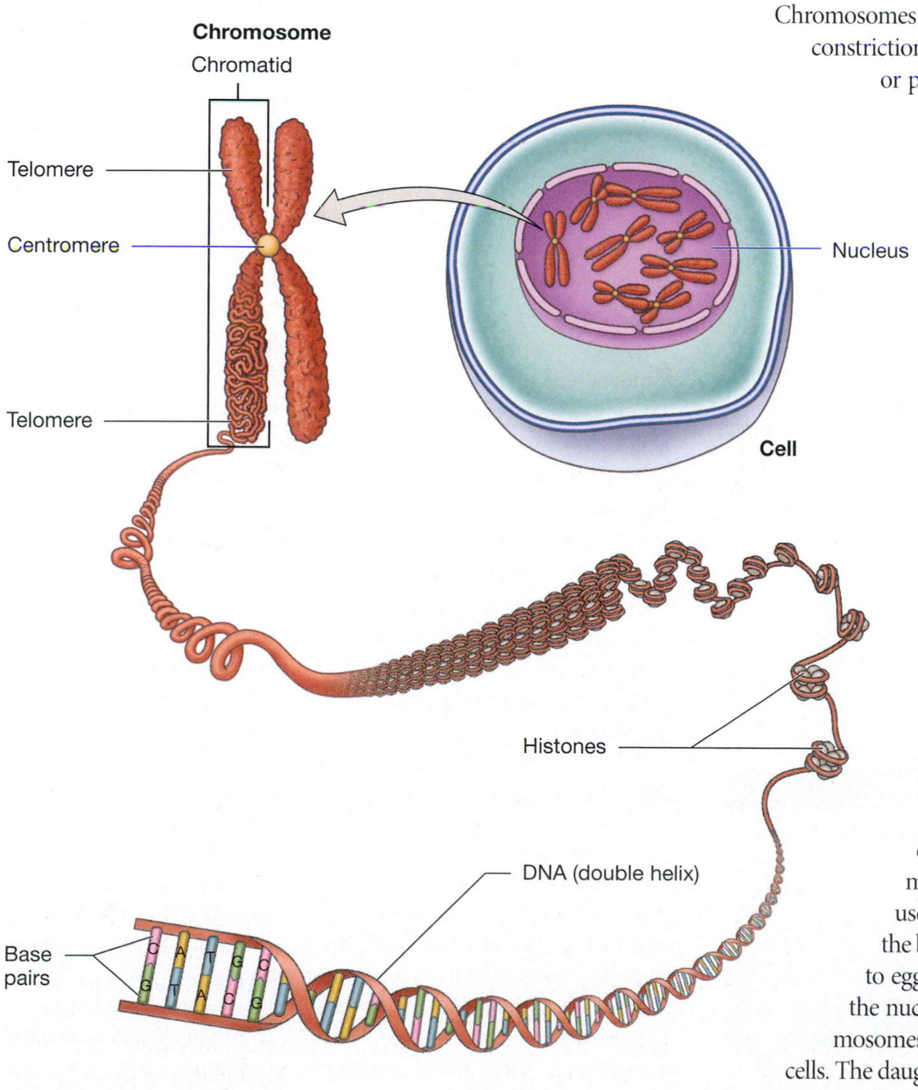

FIGURE 7–1 ◆ The chromosome.

Source: Courtesy of Darryl Leja, National Human Genome Research Institute, National Institutes of Health, Bethesda, MD.

Cell Division

Cell reproduction is controlled by DNA and occurs through one of two processes—mitosis or meiosis. Mitosis is the normal replication process used by somatic cells, which are basically all cells in the body excluding **germ line cells** (cells that give rise to egg and sperm reproductive cells). Mitosis begins in the nucleus with the duplication of all DNA in the chromosomes and ends with the formation of two new daughter cells. The daughter cells are exact copies of the parent cell.

Meiosis is the replication process that occurs in germ line cells. The product of meiosis differs from that of mitosis in that it results in the production of reproductive cells (**gametes**), which have only half

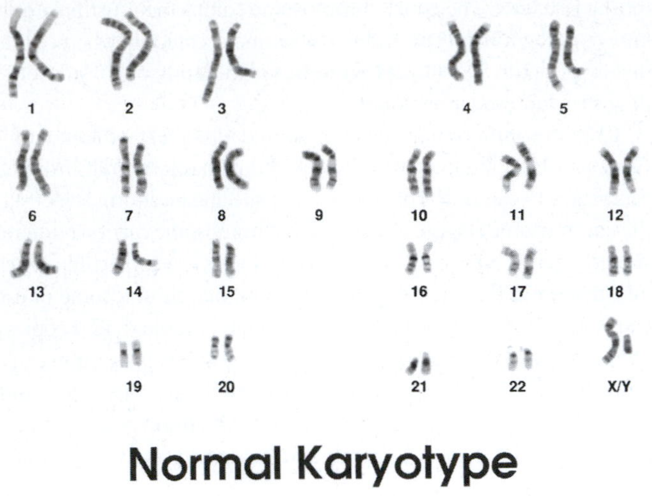

FIGURE 7–2 ◆ Male karyotype, 46xy.
Source: © Mediscan/CORBIS All Rights Reserved.

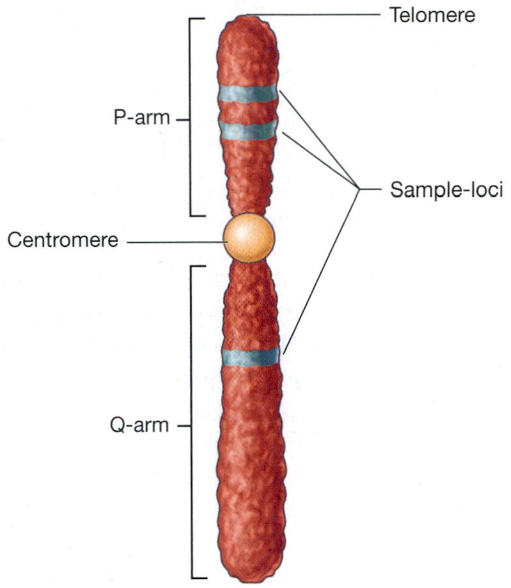

FIGURE 7–3 ◆ Structure of a chromosome.

the chromosomes of a somatic cell. Gametes have only one of each pair of the 23 chromosomes and are **haploid** (single chromosomes), whereas somatic cells have 46 chromosomes and are considered **diploid** (pairs of chromosomes).

The Human Genome

The human **genome** is the total set of genes carried by an individual. Genes are made of DNA.

DNA and RNA Structure

DNA is composed of four nucleotide bases: adenine (A), cytosine (C), guanine (G), and thymine (T), with the addition of sugar (deoxyribose) and phosphate (refer back to Figure 7–1). The four bases, known as the building blocks of DNA, are of two types: purines and pyrimidines. The purine bases are A and G, and the pyrimidine bases are C and T. In DNA, purines and pyrimidines always pair in a complementary nature so that A always binds to T and C always binds to G. The bases align into two polynucleotide chains to create a double-helix form. Because of the complementary nature of DNA's purines and pyrimidines, the base sequence of each single strand can be deduced from that of its partner. The nature of DNA was originally identified by James Watson and Francis Crick in 1953. Together, the DNA macromolecules compose the approximately 20,000 to 25,000 genes in the human genome.

The "central dogma" of molecular biology is contained in the flow of genetic information from DNA to RNA to protein. More specifically, this means that DNA in the nucleus encodes ribonucleic acid (RNA), which then crosses the nuclear membrane into the cytoplasm where it attaches to ribosomes. Once attached to ribosomes, proteins are formed using the pattern originally established by DNA. The chemical structure of RNA is similar to that of DNA, except that each nucleotide in RNA has a ribose sugar component instead of the deoxyribose sugar. In addition, uracil (U) replaces thymine as one of the pyrimidine bases. As new molecular methodologies and tools are developed and we discover more about the flow of genetic information, the "central dogma" is being challenged.

Gene Expression

Each gene has coding regions known as **exons** and noncoding regions known as **introns.** The coding regions make up less than 10% of the human genome. A primary function of exons is to code for about 60,000 to 80,000 proteins. This is accomplished by two processes known as transcription and translation (Figure 7–4◆). **Transcription** occurs when messenger ribonucleic acid (mRNA) is formed using DNA as a template. In DNA, each successive section of three nucleotide base pairs forms a **codon** that codes for a single amino acid. The mRNA uses DNA as a template to transfer the genetic information from the DNA in the nucleus to the protein-forming apparatus in the cytoplasm. Once in the cytoplasm, mRNA is decoded, or translated, to produce the protein that has been designated by the gene. Physiologically, when genes increase transcription of mRNA (sometimes known as up-regulation), their expression or activity increases, resulting in the production of more proteins.

Clinical and research endeavors are targeted toward identifying genetic variations, quantifying gene activity, and ultimately understanding protein formation. Emerging research is focused on the role of **epigenetics** as a regulatory process that controls transcription (formation of mRNA). Epigenetics refers to factors that influence the function of genes but do not change the phenotype. Epigenetic factors, including DNA methylation and histone modifications, vary from tissue to tissue and are altered by aging. It is important to note that they are influenced by environmental factors that are associated with disease risk, such as nutrition, smoking, and alcohol intake. Epigenetic factors can be inherited.

Polymorphisms and Mutations

During the process of conception, individuals obtain one chromosome from each parent, resulting in cells having matched pairs of chromosomes. Although pairs of chromosomes carry corresponding genetic information in similar sequences, the genetic sequence for each pair of genes may not be identical. Alternative copies of each gene are known as alleles. Each individual will have two alleles (one maternal, one paternal), one on each chromosome. The most common version of an allele is considered "normal" and is called the **wild type.** Alleles that differ from the wild type are known as polymorphisms or mutations. Because molecular and genetic technologies are evolving, an increasing number of specific alleles associated with disease are being identified. The

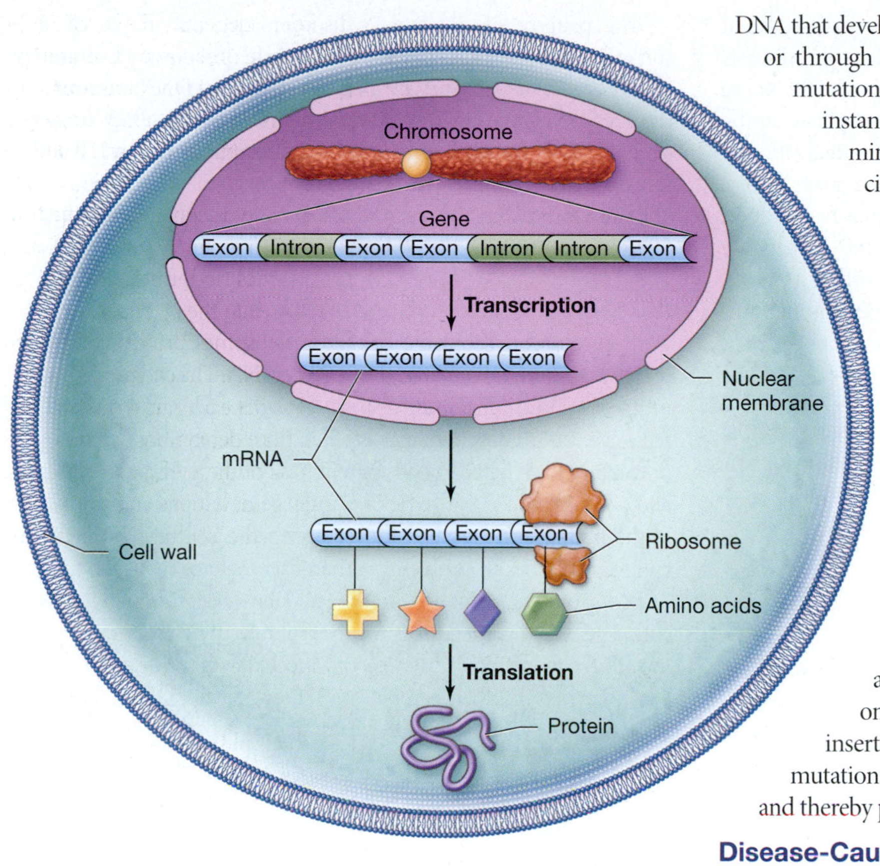

FIGURE 7–4 ◆ Transcription and translation.

genetic makeup of an individual, most specifically the allelic makeup, is that individual's **genotype.**

Polymorphisms

Polymorphisms differ from mutations in that they are observed more frequently in the general population than mutations. Polymorphisms and mutations are key determinants of an individual's observable traits, or **phenotype,** and clinical status. Whether the gene variation is identified as a mutation or polymorphism has more to do with how often the allele is observed than whether the allele is harmful or beneficial. A **mutation** is a change in DNA sequence that has been identified in less than 1% of the population. A **polymorphism** is a change in DNA sequence that has been identified in more than 1% of the population and is, thus, more commonly observed than a mutation. A **single nucleotide polymorphism (SNP)** is present when a single nucleotide (A, T, C, or G) varies between two alleles. For example, one allele may have the DNA sequence of AACTCG while the second allele may have AATTCG. The SNP would be a C to T variation. SNPs occur normally within an individual's DNA. SNPs are useful when exploring genetic variation associated with disease and in understanding the concept of personalized medicine.

Mutations

Mutations can either be inherited or acquired. Inherited mutations are generally germ line mutations that are passed down through families. Examples of diseases caused by hereditary mutations are cystic fibrosis and hemophilia A. Acquired or somatic cell mutations are changes in DNA that develop throughout the life span during normal cell mitosis or through environmental stresses such as radiation. Acquired mutations generally cannot be inherited, for example, in many instances of cancer. Completing a family history to determine genetic patterns of inheritance can assist the clinician in differentiating between inherited and acquired mutations.

Types of Mutations

Mutations can be categorized into several types including *missense, nonsense,* and *frameshift.* A missense mutation, the most common gene mutation, occurs when one DNA nucleotide base is substituted for another. This changes the triplet nucleotide coding section (codon) and results in the production of an alternate amino acid. Nonsense mutations occur when one DNA nucleotide base is inserted for another and protein production is stopped. Both missense and nonsense mutations are also known as *point mutations* or SNPs (Figure 7–5◆). Frameshift mutations are categorized as insertion or deletion mutations. They occur when one or a sequence of nucleotide bases is either deleted or inserted into the gene. As with point mutations, frameshift mutations can alter the nucleotide bases in the coding section and thereby produce a different protein.

Disease-Causing Mutations

In general, disease-causing mutations can be categorized into four groups based on the protein outcome: (1) loss of protein function, (2) gain of protein function, (3) a new protein function, or (4) expression of the protein at the wrong time or place (Nussbaum et al., 2007). The effect of the mutation on an individual depends on what biochemical role the protein performs in the normal biology of the human body. For example, a mutation in the *HBB* gene causes sickle cell anemia, an autosomal recessive inherited blood disorder characterized by chronic anemia and periodic pain. The gene mutation produces an altered protein, resulting in changes in the structure of the hemoglobin molecule. The hemoglobin molecule functions normally except in conditions of low oxygen tension (i.e., stressful situations), at which time the hemoglobin molecule forms a sickle shape, which can produce a medical emergency.

Genetic Variance and Phenotype

The associations between **genetic variance** (variations in genotypes) and phenotype are important. When considering genetic variation and its association with disease, a note of caution is required. It is important to differentiate between a gene and a mutation of a gene.

Individual	DNA sequence	Product
Person 1	GTTACC ↑	Normal protein
Person 2	GTAACC ↑	Low or nonfunctioning protein

FIGURE 7–5 ◆ Point mutations.

It is commonly thought that if a person has the gene associated with a disease, then that individual is predisposed to the disease. This is not the case. All humans have essentially the same 20,000 to 25,000 genes. Therefore, it is the mutation or polymorphism in the gene, not the gene itself, which predisposes some individuals for disease. For example, each individual has a gene named the cystic fibrosis transference regulator (*CTFR*) gene. Only those who have a mutation in that gene will develop cystic fibrosis disease. Some cancers are associated with what is known as **copy number variation (CNV).** When the number of copies of a particular gene varies among individuals, they are said to have a CNV, which can lead to either a gain or loss of genetic material.

Safety Alert *Knowledge of which mutation the patient has (genotype) and how that influences the clinical presentation (phenotype) is essential for effective nursing management of the patient. Knowing the genotype and phenotype allows the nurse to be anticipatory of the progression and treatment of the patient's disease process.*

Types of Genetic Disorders

Just about any illness is the result of some combination of genetic and environmental activity, but the role of genetics varies from small to large. The disorders caused to some extent by genetic factors are placed into three major categories: single-gene, chromosome, and complex or multifactorial disorders.

Single-Gene Inheritance Patterns

Single-gene disorders are caused by a mutation in a single gene that may be on one or both chromosomes of a pair. A mutation is a permanent structural change in DNA. Single-gene disorders occur with a minimum frequency of 3.6 per 1,000 by age 25 years; 16.4 per 1,000 after 25 years of age; and 20 per 1,000 over a person's lifetime (Korf, Rimoin, Connor, & Pyeritz, 2007). Commonly identified examples of single-gene disorders include cystic fibrosis, Huntington disease, and Duchenne muscular dystrophy.

Mendelian Inheritance

Single-gene characteristics are called Mendelian in recognition of Gregor Mendel's work. Mendel, an Austrian monk, is attributed with founding the principles of heredity, or Mendel's laws of inheritance. He studied the traits of garden peas and their offspring and conceived the idea of heredity units or "factors" (later called genes) in which one factor is recessive and the other dominant. He asserted that each individual has two factors for a trait; one factor from each parent. If two factors have identical information, the individual is called homozygous for the trait. If the two factors have different information, the individual is heterozygous.

Mendel believed that a single gene was responsible for one single trait. Today, it is known that individuals inherit genes from their parents and many genes have control over the production of traits. Genes behave as separate units and traits are the product of complex gene–gene and gene–environment interactions.

Online Mendelian Inheritance in Man® (OMIM®) is an online version of Victor McKusick's (1998) listing of single-gene phenotypes. OMIM® is a continuously updated catalog of human genes that includes primarily inherited genetic disorders and is considered the phenotypic companion to the Human Genome Project. It is an excellent resource for clinicians and researchers.

The patterns of single-gene disorders depend on the chromosomal location of the gene and whether the phenotype is dominant or recessive. The gene may be located on an autosome (autosomal) or the X chromosome (X-linked). The patterns of inheritance for single-gene disorders are autosomal recessive, autosomal dominant, X-linked recessive, and X-linked dominant. (Depictions of the patterns of inheritance for single-gene disorders are presented later in this chapter in Figures 7–7 through 7–10, p. 147 and 149.)

Autosomal Recessive Inheritance

With **autosomal recessive inheritance,** the mutant gene is located on an autosome rather than the X chromosome. The most common mechanism for transmitting a single-gene disorder with an autosomal recessive pattern of inheritance is when both parents are heterozygotes or carriers. Each heterozygous parent has one copy of the mutant gene and one copy of the wild-type or normal gene. Parents who are carriers of the mutant gene are usually asymptomatic and have no increased risk for other health problems. When each heterozygous parent gives one copy of the mutant gene to the child, however, the child is affected with a genetic disorder. Risks for the children of heterozygous carriers include the following: (1) they can be affected with the disorder, (2) they can be carriers like their parents, or (3) they may not inherit the mutant gene at all. The risk that a child will be affected with the autosomal recessive disorder is 1 out of 4. However, the risk that phenotypically normal children will be carriers is 2 out of 3. This is true for each pregnancy. Examples of autosomal recessive disorders include cystic fibrosis (CF), phenylketonuria (PKU), and Friedreich ataxia.

Autosomal Dominant Inheritance

With **autosomal dominant inheritance,** the mutant gene is on an autosome and only one copy of the dominant gene is necessary for the effects to be seen. The affected individual is heterozygous and no offspring are carriers. Homozygous individuals, or individuals who have inherited two genes for the disorder, are thought to be so severely affected that they die *in utero* or infancy. The presence of an autosomal dominant disorder in a child may indicate that one parent also has the disorder, although this is not always the case. Exceptions to this may include the following: (1) the gene can be present but nonpenetrant (**Penetrance** is the proportion of individuals with an abnormal genotype who actually manifest the disease or trait), (2) the gene expression (the activity of the gene as measured by the amount of mRNA produced) may be minimal and go undetected due to variable expression, (3) the disorder can be caused by a new mutation, or (4) the child is not the biological offspring of the parents. A gene is nonpenetrant when an individual carries the mutant gene but does not manifest the disorder caused by the gene.

When a child has one typical parent and one parent with the disorder, the risk for the child to inherit the gene is 50%, regardless of the child's gender. The chance of having a typical child without the disorder is also 50%. This is true with each pregnancy produced by these parents. Children who do not inherit the disorder have no greater risk of having an affected child than the general population, unless nonpenetrance has occurred in the child. If two individuals with the same autosomal dominant disorder have children, the risk is 25% for having a child who is an affected homozygote, 50% for having a child who is an affected heterozygote like the parents, and 25% for having a child without the mutant gene. These risks hold true for each pregnancy. The homozygote is usually severely affected and dies *in utero* or infancy. Examples of autosomal dominant disorders are Huntington disease and neurofibromatosis.

X-Linked Inheritance

In X-linked inheritance, the mutant gene is located on the X chromosome. Males have only one X chromosome with no counterpart for its genes. Therefore, the gene is expressed when it is present in males regardless of whether it is recessive or dominant in the individual's mother. A female receives one X chromosome from each parent for a pair of sex chromosomes (XX). A male receives the X chromosome from his mother and the Y chromosome from his father for a pair of sex chromosomes (XY). Males cannot be carriers of an X-linked disorder.

In **X-linked recessive** disorders, the most common pattern of transmission is when the mother is a heterozygous carrier for the mutant gene. If the father is normal, then the parents have a 25% chance, with each pregnancy, for their child to be either (1) a female carrier like the mother, (2) a typical female without the mutant gene, (3) a typical male without the mutant gene, or (4) a male who is affected with the disorder. A mother who is a carrier usually has no obvious clinical manifestations of the mutant gene, unless X inactivation (inactivation of genes on one X chromosome in somatic cells of females early in embryonic life) is skewed. In skewed X inactivation, the mutant allele is located on the active X and the normal allele is located on the inactive X. Variation in expression of X-linked disorders is seen commonly in heterozygotes and can range from no expression to complete expression. X-linked disorders that are manifesting heterozygotes include color blindness, hemophilia A, hemophilia B, and Duchenne muscular dystrophy.

X-linked dominant disorders are seen less frequently than the other patterns of single-gene inheritance. The mutant gene is dominant, so only one is necessary for the phenotype to manifest. Both males and females can be affected and transmit the gene. In X-linked dominant disorders, an affected male usually has an affected mother because males inherit their X chromosome from their mother, and some affected females may be less severely affected than males because of X inactivation. There may be an excess of female offspring in the family because some X-linked dominant genes are lethal in males. Male-to-male transmission is not seen because males transmit their X chromosome only to their daughters, not to their sons.

When a female with an X-linked dominant disorder and an unaffected male have offspring, a 25% chance exists at each pregnancy that they will have an affected female, an affected male, an unaffected female, or an unaffected male, respectively. There is a 50% chance that the offspring of each pregnancy will be affected regardless of the child's sex. When a male with an X-linked dominant disorder and unaffected female have offspring, there is a 50% chance for having an affected female and a 50% chance for having an unaffected male. If both the male and female had an X-linked dominant disorder, there would be a 25% chance for an affected homozygous female (probably resulting in miscarriage), a 25% chance for an affected heterozygous female, a 25% chance for an affected male, and a 25% chance for an unaffected male. Examples of X-linked dominant disorders are hypophosphatemic rickets and vitamin D-resistant rickets.

Atypical Patterns of Inheritance

Most patterns of inheritance follow Mendel's laws of inheritance; however, exceptions do occur. Genomic imprinting and mitochondrial mutation inheritance are examples. Originally the sex of the parent was thought to have little effect on the expression of the genes each parent transmits. For some genetic disorders, the expression of the phenotype depends on whether the mutant allele has been inherited from the father or from the mother. Differences in gene expression between the allele inherited from the mother and the allele inherited from the father result from **genomic imprinting.**

Imprinting is caused by an alteration in chromatin that affects the expression of a gene but not its DNA sequence. Examples of genomic imprinting are Prader-Willi syndrome (PWS) and Angelman syndrome. Approximately 70% of individuals with PWS have a deletion of the proximal long arm of chromosome 15 that is inherited from the individual's father only (Prader-Willi Syndrome Association, 2010). Characteristics of PWS include obesity, excessive and indiscriminant eating, small hands and feet, short stature, hypogonadism, and mental retardation. In Angelman syndrome, there is a deletion of approximately the same region on chromosome 15 inherited from the individual's mother. Angelman syndrome is characterized by unusual facial appearance, short stature, severe mental retardation, spasticity, and seizures.

The mitochondrial chromosome (mtDNA) is located in the mitochondrial organelle, not inside the nucleus. The mother's ovum or egg supplies the **zygote,** or fertilized ovum, with its mitochondria. A mother having a mutation in mtDNA passes the mutation to all of her children, and the father carrying the same mutation passes it on to none of his children. Therefore, defects in mtDNA are inherited maternally. With cell division, mtDNA replicates and sorts randomly among newly synthesized mitochondria, which are distributed randomly between the daughter cells. Each daughter cell receives different proportions of mitochondria that carry normal and mutant mtDNA. Mitochondrial function is essential to nearly all cells. The phenotypic expression of a mutation in mtDNA depends on the proportions of normal and mutant mtDNA in the cells of different tissues. Reduced penetrance, variable expression, and multiple phenotypic effects of a single gene or gene pair are typical in mitochondrial disorders. Examples of genetic disorders caused by mtDNA are Leber's hereditary optic neuropathy, Leigh disease, and progressive sensorineural deafness.

Chromosome Genetic Disorders

Chromosome disorders are caused by an excess or deficiency of genes contained in whole chromosomes or segments of chromosomes. Chromosome disorders make up a major category of genetic disorders, affect about 7 of 1,000 live-born infants, and account for almost half of all spontaneous first-trimester abortions (miscarriages). The frequency of chromosome disorders is 1.8 per 1,000 before age 25 years; 2 per 1,000 after age 25 years; and 3.8 per 1,000 over a lifetime (Korf et al., 2007).

Chromosome abnormalities are related to an abnormal chromosome number or structural rearrangements. They may involve one or more autosomes, sex chromosomes, or both. The most common and clinically significant type is aneuploidy, which occurs in 3% to 4% of all clinically recognized pregnancies. **Aneuploidy** is an abnormal chromosome number due to an extra or missing chromosome. It is usually due to an error during meiosis in which cell division results in a sperm or egg with too many or too few chromosomes.

Most individuals with aneuploidy have trisomy or monosomy, which can be associated with mental or physical developmental problems, or both. **Trisomy** refers to the presence of a third or extra chromosome instead of the normal pair of a particular chromosome. The most common type of trisomy in infants is trisomy 21 or Down syndrome. The chromosome number and structure seen in 95% of individuals with Down syndrome is 47, XX or 47, XY. **Monosomy** refers to the presence of only one chromosome instead of the normal pair of chromosomes. Monosomy for an entire chromosome usually results in death, except in Turner syndrome which is monosomy for the X chromosome (45, X).

Nondisjunction

The failure of a pair of chromosomes to separate properly during meiosis, **nondisjunction,** is the most common chromosomal mechanism leading to aneuploidy. Nondisjunction can also occur in a mitotic division after formation of the zygote. A zygote with an additional chromosome 21 might lose the extra chromosome in a mitotic division, resulting in **mosaicism.** Mosaicism occurs when an individual has at least two cell lines that are different in karyotype or genotype. Mosaicism is difficult to study because an individual's karyotype is rarely done without some clinical indication to do so. Because phenotypic effects of mosaicism may not be present, clinically normal mosaic persons are seldom identified. Individuals who are mosaic for Down syndrome or Turner syndrome are usually thought to be less affected than individuals who are nonmosaic.

Deletions

Structural rearrangements of chromosomes may result from **deletions** or loss of a chromosome segment or piece. The loss of a chromosome tip is the most common deletion in humans. Occurring less commonly are two breaks in one chromosome, with rejoining of the two ends and resulting loss of the piece between the two breaks (National Institutes of Health, 2010). If the deletions occur at both ends of the chromosome, the end pieces are lost and the two broken ends unite, forming a ring chromosome. Most deletions are new, meaning that individuals with normal chromosomes have a child with a deletion. The chance that these parents will have another child who is affected similarly is probably less than 0.5%. Deletions can be large and detectable by cytogenic methods. Smaller deletions, called microdeletions, are detectable by high-resolution banding methods. Very tiny deletions are detectable only by fluorescence *in situ* hybridization (FISH) or other molecular methods, and submicroscopic deletions involving the loss of a single locus are detectable only by molecular methods.

Loss of the short arm of chromosome 5 or 5p– (read "5 p minus") is a cytogenetically visible deletion. It is known as *cri du chat* syndrome or the "cat-cry syndrome" because newborns usually have a high-pitched cry like that of a kitten. Most individuals with 5p– live beyond childhood and have moderate to severe mental retardation. Other syndromes resulting from deletions include Williams syndrome (deletions in 7q) and Prader-Willi syndrome (deletions in 15q).

Translocations

Translocations occur when there are breaks in two or more chromosomes, with reattachments in new combinations. Reciprocal or balanced translocations occur when two chromosomes exchange segments and no chromosomal material is lost. Reciprocal translocations are found in approximately 1 in 600 newborns. They are generally harmless even though these translocations are more common among individuals with intellectual disabilities. Although translocations may not affect an individual's health, carriers of translocations may produce children with an unbalanced amount of chromosome material. These children are at increased risk for mental and physical disabilities, and there is increased risk of spontaneous abortions.

Robertsonian translocations involve the loss of the short arm of chromosomes 13, 14, 15, 21, or 22. Since the short arm (p) is very short on these chromosomes, this loss seems to have little or no effect. Robertsonian translocations are fairly common, occurring in 1 of 900 newborns. Robertsonian translocations between chromosomes 13 and 14 result in trisomy 13 or Patau syndrome, which is characterized by abnormalities of the brain structure and abnormalities in most of the major organ systems. Translocations between chromosome 14 and 21 can result in trisomy 21 or Down syndrome (Ferguson-Smith & Simonic, 2007).

Complex or Multifactorial Disorders

Complex disorders are caused by a combination of small variations in genes that together, with environmental factors, result in or increase susceptibility to a disorder or illness. These illnesses may be caused by single-gene mutations, yet they are not single-gene disorders. They result from complex interactions between predisposing factors to include the genotype at one or more loci and varied environmental exposures that trigger, increase, or worsen a disease process. The pattern of inheritance of the disorder or illness is not Mendelian, but follows a complex or multifactorial pattern (Nussbaum et al., 2007).

Complex disorders are considered to be disorders of adulthood. The frequency of complex disorders by age 25 years is 46.4 per 1,000; after 25 years is 600 per 1,000; and over an individual's lifetime is 646.4 per 1,000 (Korf et al., 2007).

A complex pattern of inheritance is the basis for conditions such as Alzheimer disease, cancer, cardiovascular disease, diabetes, and obesity. Although these conditions often occur in more than one member of a family, they do not follow clear Mendelian patterns of inheritance.

Alzheimer Disease

Alzheimer disease (AD) is a neurodegenerative disease characterized by chronic, progressive loss of memory and other intellectual functions. Other traits of AD include personality changes, death of neurons, development of amyloid neuritic plaques, and formation of neurofibrillary tangles within affected neurons. Alzheimer disease is the most common form of dementia in late life, with about 25% of AD being familial. Less than 2% of these families have early-onset familial AD (EOFAD) in which symptoms occur before age 65. Three genes have been identified as a cause of EOFAD:

1. *PSEN1,* located on chromosome 14 (a precursor for presenilin-1)
2. *AD1,* located on chromosome 21 (a precursor for amyloid beta A4 protein)
3. *AD4,* located on chromosome 1 (a precursor for presenilin-2).

EOFAD appears to follow an autosomal dominant transmission.

The majority of familial AD (FAD) occurs after age 65 or is considered to be late-onset FAD. This complex disorder is thought to involve several susceptibility genes. One of these susceptibility genes is the *APOE e4* gene on chromosome 19. Other genes located on chromosomes 2, 9, 10, 12, and 15 are being investigated for contributing to late-onset FAD. Trisomy 21 or Down syndrome appears to be related to AD because essentially all individuals with trisomy 21 will develop signs of AD after age 40. The reason for this is thought to be accelerated neurofibrillary degeneration due to the lifelong overexpression of the *DYRK1A* gene on chromosome 21 (Weigel et al., 2011).

The majority of AD (approximately 75%) is due to unknown causes. This nonfamilial or sporadic AD is thought to be multifactorial and resulting from the combination of aging, genetic predisposition, and exposure to one or more environmental influences. An association has also been made with ApoE genotype and nonfamilial AD, but the exact nature of this relationship is still under investigation (Kukull & Bowen, 2002). Factors such as head trauma have been investigated for their influence on AD (Magnoni & Brody, 2010).

Cancer

Cancer, a group of diseases that share common characteristics, is a disorder of somatic cells. Specifically, cells experience uncontrolled growth as a result of mutations that affect a limited number of genes. Cancer cells have two characteristics that are not found in normal cells. In normal cells, cell-to-cell contact inhibits further growth and division, a process called contact inhibition. Cancer cells do not have contact inhibition; instead, they continue to grow and divide and may even pile on top of each other. If normal cells are badly damaged or starved for nutrients, they undergo apoptosis, or programmed cell death, and self-destruct. Cancer cells do not undergo apoptosis. Normal cells experience cell senescence or stop dividing in culture after about 50 divisions. Cancer cells in culture divide indefinitely. Additional information about the molecular basis of cancer and conversion of normal somatic cells to cancer cells can be found in Nussbaum et al. (2007) and the National Cancer Institute's website.

About one-third of the 569,490 cancer deaths expected to occur in the United States in 2010 will be related to nutrition, physical inactivity, and obesity or overweight. More than 171,000 cancer deaths are expected to be caused by tobacco use. Although anyone can develop cancer, risks increase as individuals age. About 77% of all cancers are diagnosed in individuals 55 years and older. Cancer researchers refer to the lifetime risk of developing cancer as the probability that an individual will, over the course of his or her lifetime, develop cancer or die from it. Relative risk is a measure of the strength of the relationship between risk factors and a particular cancer. Relative risk compares the risk of developing cancer in individuals with a certain exposure or trait to the risk in persons who do not have this exposure or trait. Male smokers are about 23 times more likely to develop lung cancer than lifelong nonsmokers, so their relative risk is 23. Female smokers are 13 times more likely to develop lung cancer than lifelong nonsmokers, resulting in a relative risk of 13 (American Cancer Society [ACS], 2010).

About 5% of individuals with cancer have familial cancer, cancer in which there is clear evidence that an inherited gene predisposes the individual to very high risk for a particular cancer (ACS, 2010). The remaining 95% are sporadic or cancers that occur as a result of genetic changes in somatic cells. These changes occur over the lifetime and are due to internal factors such as hormones or digestion of nutrients in cells. They may also be caused by external factors, such as tobacco, chemicals, and sunlight. Inheriting a cancer-causing gene usually does not indicate a 100% chance that cancer will develop, but it may indicate a significant risk that an individual will develop cancer at some point over his or her lifetime. Knowing this, a careful surveillance program can be instituted that will identify cancer early and decrease morbidity and mortality.

Nurses should carefully examine the family history and pedigree for clues associated with an **inherited cancer syndrome** or clinical manifestations associated with a mutation that increases cancer susceptibility (Chart 7–1). Cancers with a familial basis often occur at a younger age than sporadic cancers; they are usually bilateral in paired organs (e.g., breasts and kidneys), and multifocal, or occur in multiple sites in a single organ (National Cancer Institute, 2010). Following analysis of the family history and pedigree, nurses should look for the presence of these clues. If an inherited cancer syndrome is suspected and if any of the clues are present, the patient and family should be referred to a nurse, physician, or genetic counselor with advanced professional training in cancer genetics.

CHART 7–1 Clues Suggesting an Inherited Cancer Syndrome

- Multiple cancers in close relatives
- Early age of onset; younger than 40 to 50 years for adult-onset cancers
- Multiple cancers in a single individual
- Bilateral cancer in paired organs (e.g., breast, kidney)
- Recognition of the known association between etiologically related cancers in the family
- Presence of congenital anomalies or precursor lesions that are known to be associated with increased cancer risk (e.g., presence of atypical nevi and risk of malignant melanoma)
- Recognizable Mendelian inheritance pattern

Source: National Cancer Institute. (2010, November 24). Cancer genetics risk assessment and counseling PDQ® health professional version: Components of the risk assessment process. Retrieved from http://www.cancer.gov/cancertopics/pdq/genetics/risk-assessment-and-counseling/HealthProfessional/page3.

Weblink: Clues Suggesting an Inherited Cancer Syndrome

Coronary Artery Disease

Coronary artery disease (CAD) is caused by atherosclerosis or thickening and hardening of the inside walls of arteries. Some hardening of the arteries occurs normally as individuals grow older. In atherosclerosis, plaque deposits build up in the arteries. Plaque is made of fat, cholesterol, calcium, and other substances found in the blood. This buildup of plaque can narrow the arteries, resulting in less blood and oxygen flowing to the heart muscle. This blockage can eventually completely block the arteries and flow of blood. Blood clots may also form and block the arteries. This can lead to angina or a myocardial infarction. Risk factors for CAD include the following: age, family history of early heart disease, high blood cholesterol, high blood pressure, cigarette smoking, diabetes, obesity, and lack of physical activity. All factors except age and family history can be altered by an individual to prevent or delay onset of CAD. Individuals with a family history of early heart disease include those individuals with heart disease diagnosed before age 55 in a father or brother, and before age 65 in a mother or sister. An in-depth review of CAD is provided in Chapter 32.

Several genetic disorders have been associated with premature CAD and myocardial infarctions. A common single-gene disorder is familial hypercholesterolemia which leads to an increase in the low density lipoprotein (LDL) or 'bad' cholesterol beginning at birth. Early detection can lead to treatment, lifestyle changes, and closer surveillance that may decrease the risk of morbidity and mortality. The efficacy of genetic testing to determine those at risk is being pursued. Other genetic disorders leading to CAD include enzyme defects, such as lipoprotein lipase deficiency, and defects in transfer proteins, such as cholesterol ester transfer protein deficiency. Large population-based studies are showing some genes may be associated with multifactorial CAD; however, the impact of each individual gene on an individual person is not fully understood.

Diabetes

The two major types of diabetes are type 1 (insulin-dependent diabetes) and type 2 (non-insulin-dependent diabetes). Of the adults in the

United States who have diabetes, 90% to 95% have type 2 while only 5% to 10% have type 1 (National Institute of Diabetes and Digestive and Kidney Disease [NIDDK], 2008). Both type 1 and type 2 are complex disorders because both genetic and environmental factors are necessary for their expression.

Type 1 diabetes is an autoimmune disorder that is attributed to both an inherited risk and external triggers or factors including viruses, nutrition, and toxins. About 18 regions in the human genome are linked to influencing type 1 diabetes risk. These regions, labeled IDDM1 to IDDM18, each may contain several genes that contribute to this risk. The most studied is IDDM1, which contains human leukocyte antigen (HLA) genes, located on chromosome 6. Inheriting certain alleles of the HLA genes increases the likelihood that immune cells will attack the body's healthy cells. One of the non-HLA genes, *IDDM2,* is the insulin gene, located on chromosome 11. Inheritance of the *IDDM1* HLA genes can account for a greater than 50% genetic risk, and inheritance of the *IDDM2* gene can contribute another 10% genetic risk (Dean & McEntyre, 2004).

Type 2 diabetes has a stronger genetic basis than type 1 and is also affected by environmental factors, such as a diet high in fat and low in fiber and carbohydrates. Risk factors include obesity and a positive family history of diabetes. Although many genes appear to be involved in the occurrence of type 2 diabetes, they have not been well defined. A rare form of diabetes called maturity-onset diabetes of the young (MODY) accounts for 1% to 5% of diabetes in the United States and has a phenotype that is similar to type 1 and type 2 diabetes. MODY is caused by a number of different mutations, many of which are dominant mutations (NIDDK, 2007).

Obesity

It is estimated that 30% or more of U.S. adults are obese (body mass index >30 kg/m^2), which increases their risk for other chronic diseases such as heart disease, diabetes, and cancer. Obesity results from a chronic state of energy imbalance (energy intake exceeds energy expenditure). In a few rare cases, gene mutations have been found to cause morbid obesity regardless of the environment. However, common forms of obesity are due to susceptibility genes acting within a receptive environment to create an obesity phenotype. According to the "thrifty gene" hypothesis, evolution has favored genes that promote weight gain to protect humans against an environment that was unreliable in providing food. Unfortunately, our thrifty genes are maladaptive in today's environment of excess foods and diminished physical activity.

Studies of monozygotic and dizygotic twins have shown that estimated inheritability for obesity is 50% to 90%. For most forms of common obesity, however, individual genes appear to have a small effect. Common variants of genes including melanocortin 4 receptor (MC4R), fat mass and obesity (FTO), and the insulin induced gene2 (INSIG2) are emerging as potential genes of interest in common obesity (Hinney, Vogel, & Hebebrand, 2010).

Clinical studies are exploring the genetic determinants of obesity and identifying critical biologic pathways involved in maintaining energy balance. These studies could point the way toward therapeutic interventions and identify those at risk or responsive to environmental modulations, but they will take time.

Hemoglobinopathies

Two hemoglobinopathies, sickle cell disease and thalassemias, are good examples of disorders of hemoglobin. Both are molecular diseases in which the primary disease-causing event is an inherited or acquired mutation. A genetic disease occurs when there is an alteration in the DNA of an essential gene that changes the amount, function, or both, of the messenger RNA (mRNA) and protein. Single-gene disorders almost always result from mutations that change protein function.

Sickle Cell Disease

Sickle cell disease is an example of a change in the amino acid sequence that causes pathology. This is accomplished by the protein developing a new characteristic, without changing the protein's normal function. Sickle cell disease, originally identified by Linus Pauling, was the first molecular disease to be recognized. The amino acid substitution in sickle cell disease changes the shape of hemoglobin from a round to a distorted sickle shape. The sickled cells' shortened life span (usually a few weeks) results in anemia. Sickle cells become trapped in small blood vessels and cause tissue damage, infections, and periodic episodes of intense pain.

Sickle cell disease is an autosomal recessive disorder occurring most frequently in equatorial Africa, South and Central America, the Caribbean islands, Mediterranean countries, India, and Saudi Arabia, as well as in countries to which people from these regions have migrated. The sickle cell gene has been described as protecting individuals against malaria, which accounts for its high frequency in areas of the world where malaria occurs. About 1 in 500 African Americans are born with sickle cell disease. Although many individuals with this disorder die in early childhood, the life span of individuals with sickle cell disease is increasing with improved treatment and health care (National Heart Lung and Blood Institute, October 2010).

Thalassemias

Mutations also cause loss of protein function, the most common consequence of mutation. Although the mutations are in the same gene as the mutation that causes sickle cell disease, the red blood cells do not sickle in thalassemia. The severity of the thalassemia that results from loss-of-function mutations is generally related to the amount of function lost. When the thalassemias are grouped together, they are the most common single-gene disorder.

Thalassemia was first discovered in persons of Mediterranean origin and offers protection against malaria to individuals who are carriers. Both alpha- and beta-thalassemia have a high frequency in many populations, although alpha-thalassemia is more prevalent among individuals of Southeast Asian, Indian, Chinese, and Filipino ancestry. Beta-thalassemia most often affects individuals of Mediterranean, African, or Asian ancestry (National Heart Lung and Blood Institute, August 2010).

Nursing Role in Detection, Management, and Care of Individuals with Genetic Disorders

The field of genetics influences all aspects of nursing, from the application of genetic principles in patient care to employing cutting-edge molecular and genetic methodologies in research protocols. As may be expected, the specific role played by the nurse depends on several factors, including the patient's needs and the nurse's expertise and knowledge of genetics. A nationwide effort has been under way to increase the genetic content in all health care curricula (e.g., nursing, medicine, and pharmacy). Nurses are on the front line of patient care where the timely integration of genetic knowledge, skills, and attitudes into routine patient care is warranted to provide effective care to individuals and their families. Several organizations, including the International Society of Nurses in Genetics (2007), the National Coalition for Health Professional Education in Genetics (NCHPEG) (2007), and the Consensus Panel on Genetic/Genomic Nursing Competencies (2009), have recommended genetic core competencies and standards for nurses and other health care professionals (Chart 7–2). Principal among these are the abilities to identify who may benefit from genetic services and to make appropriate genetic referrals. As genetic content increases in nursing curricula and as more is learned about genomic determinants of common diseases, nurses will be increasingly involved in the management, interpretation, and decision making related to genetic information and services. In addition, nurses must also consider the ethical, legal, and social issues related to privacy and discrimination of genetic information. These will be discussed in a later section.

Pedigrees

Recognizing patterns of inheritance and clustering of diseases within families is a *key* skill needed to determine genetic risk assessment. These can be determined based on a thorough family history that is organized into a family tree, called a **pedigree.** Pedigrees enable the health care provider to visualize how diseases and characteristics are clustered within a family and through generations.

Three-generation pedigrees are used by geneticists, advanced practice genetic nurses, and genetic counselors, among others, to identify disease risk and to develop a personalized prevention program for chronic conditions as well as single-gene disorders (Consensus Panel on Genetic/Genomic Nursing Competencies, 2009). Once an accurate family history has been established and genetic disorders or health care risks identified, it may be appropriate to refer the patient to a geneticist or genetic counselor for follow up.

Tools have been developed to assist health care providers in conducting a thorough family history and to draw a pedigree (Bennett et al., 1995; Centers for Disease Control and Prevention, 2010). For each family member, the most important information to record is the current age (or age at death), ethnicity, and relevant medical conditions with onset or duration. Commonly used pedigree symbols are listed in Figure 7–6◆ and used in Figures 7–7◆ through 7–10◆ (p. 149) as examples of the types of inheritance patterns for single-gene disorders.

To encourage all Americans to learn more about their family health history, the U.S. Surgeon General, in cooperation with other agencies, has launched a national public health campaign called the U.S. Surgeon General's Family History Initiative, My Family Health Portrait. This is a patient-friendly website designed for the general public to create a personalized family health history report from any computer with an Internet connection and an up-to-date web browser. Using the website software, the patient can create a three-generation pedigree that can be printed and shared with health care professionals (U.S. Department of Health and Human Services, n.d.).

For some disorders, cluster patterns in a pedigree do not appear to follow an autosomal dominant, recessive, or X-linked pattern of inheritance. Occasionally this is due to either reduced penetrance or varied expressivity. These features are most commonly seen in autosomal dominant conditions. Penetrance is the proportion of individuals with an abnormal genotype who actually manifest the disease or trait. It is considered an all-or-none concept. Neurofibromatosis type 1 (NF1), an autosomal dominant disorder that affects the nervous system, eyes, skin, and other parts of the body, can illustrate penetrance. One family member with NF1 is severely affected with multiple neurofibromas while another family member with NF1 has only a few neurofibromas. Adults with NF1 almost always have some signs of this disorder (e.g., café-au-lait spots or neurofibromas). So, penetrance is 100%.

Expressivity is the degree to which an individual with a specific genotype is affected. For example, in two family members with the same genotype, one may have all of the symptoms of the disorder, while the second one has relatively few symptoms. This is known as variable expressivity. Using the previous NF1 example, the degree to which NF1 is expressed in these two family members varies. One is severely affected while the other is mildly affected.

Weblink: Family Health History

Genetic Testing

The explosion in genetic knowledge and molecular technologies has led to a heightened public awareness of the genetic components of disease. Because of public access to cutting-edge research, patients are

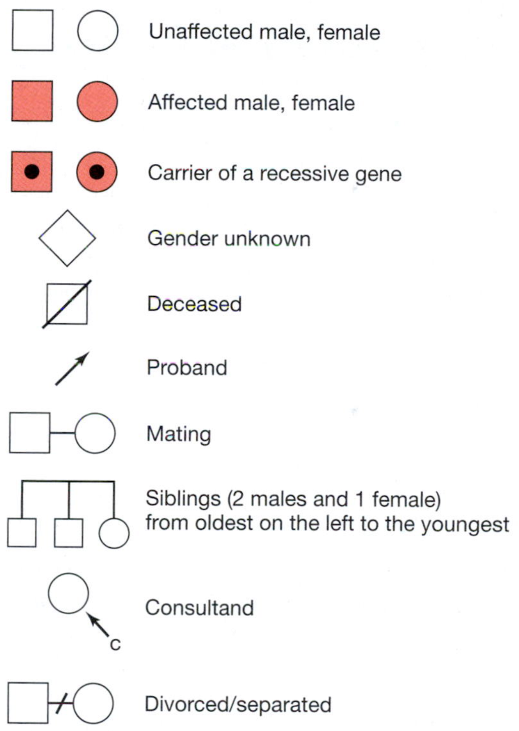

FIGURE 7–6 ◆ Pedigree symbols.

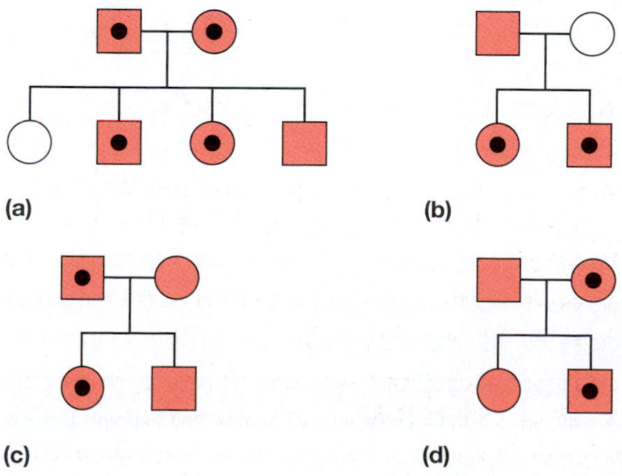

FIGURE 7–7 ◆ Autosomal recessive inheritance pedigree.

CHART 7–2 Essential Nursing Competencies for Genetics and Genomics

PROFESSIONAL RESPONSIBILITIES

All registered nurses are expected to engage in professional role activities that are consistent with *Nursing: Scope and Standards of Practice* (American Nurses Association, 2010). In addition, competent nursing practice now requires the incorporation of genetic and genomic knowledge and skills in order to:

- Recognize when a nurse's own attitudes and values related to genetic and genomic science may affect care provided to patients.
- Advocate for patient's access to desired genetic/genomic services and/or resources including support groups.
- Examine competency of practice on a regular basis, identifying areas of strength, as well as areas in which professional development related to genetics and genomics would be beneficial.
- Incorporate genetic and genomic technologies and information into registered nurse practice.
- Demonstrate in practice the importance of tailoring genetic and genomic information and services to patients based on their culture, religion, knowledge level, literacy, and preferred language.
- Advocate for the rights of all patients for autonomous, informed genetic- and genomic-related decision making and voluntary action.

PROFESSIONAL PRACTICE DOMAIN

Nursing Assessment: Applying/Integrating Genetic and Genomic Knowledge

The registered nurse:

- Demonstrates an understanding of the relationship of genetics and genomics to health, prevention, screening, diagnostics, prognostics, selection of treatment, and monitoring of treatment effectiveness.
- Demonstrates the ability to elicit a minimum of three-generation family health history information.
- Constructs a pedigree from collected family history information using standardized symbols and terminology.
- Collects personal, health, and developmental histories that consider genetic, environmental, and genomic influences and risks.
- Conducts comprehensive health and physical assessments which incorporate knowledge about genetic, environmental, and genomic influences and risk factors.
- Critically analyzes the history and physical assessment findings for genetic, environmental, and genomic influences and risk factors.
- Assesses patients' knowledge, perceptions, and responses to genetic and genomic information.
- Develops a plan of care that incorporates genetic and genomic assessment information.

Information

The registered nurse:

- Identifies patients who may benefit from specific genetic and genomic information and/or services based on assessment data.
- Identifies credible, accurate, appropriate, and current genetic and genomic information, resources, services, and/or technologies specific to given patients.
- Identifies ethical, ethnic/ancestral, cultural, religious, legal, fiscal, and societal issues related to genetic and genomic information and technologies.
- Defines issues that undermine the rights of all patients for autonomous, informed genetic- and genomic-related decision making and voluntary action.

Referral Activities

The registered nurse:

- Facilitates referrals for specialized genetic and genomic services for patients as needed.

Provision of Education, Care, and Support

The registered nurse:

- Provides patients with interpretation of selective genetic and genomic information or services.
- Provides patients with credible, accurate, appropriate, and current genetic and genomic information, resources, services, and/or technologies that facilitate decision making.
- Uses health promotion/disease prevention practices that:
  - Consider genetic and genomic influences on personal and environmental risk factors.
  - Incorporate knowledge of genetic and/or genomic risk factors (e.g., a patient with a genetic predisposition for high cholesterol who can benefit from a change in lifestyle that will decrease the likelihood that the genetic risk will be expressed).
- Uses genetic- and genomic-based interventions and information to improve patient outcomes.
- Collaborates with health care providers in providing genetic and genomic health care.
- Collaborates with insurance providers/payers to facilitate reimbursement for genetic and genomic health care services.
- Performs interventions/treatments appropriate to patients' genetic and genomic health care needs.
- Evaluates the impact and effectiveness of genetic and genomic technology, information, interventions, and treatments on patients' outcome.

Source: Consensus Panel on Genetic/Genomic Nursing Competencies. (2009). *Essentials of genetic and genomic nursing: Competencies, curricula guidelines, and outcome indicators* (2nd ed.). Silver Spring, MD: American Nurses Association.

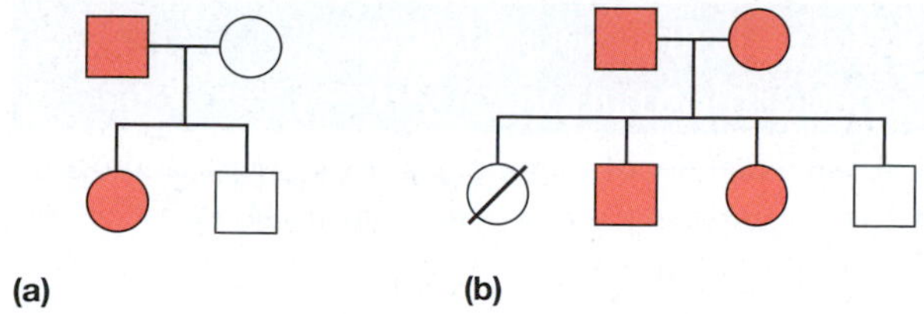

FIGURE 7–8 ◆ Autosomal dominant inheritance pedigree.

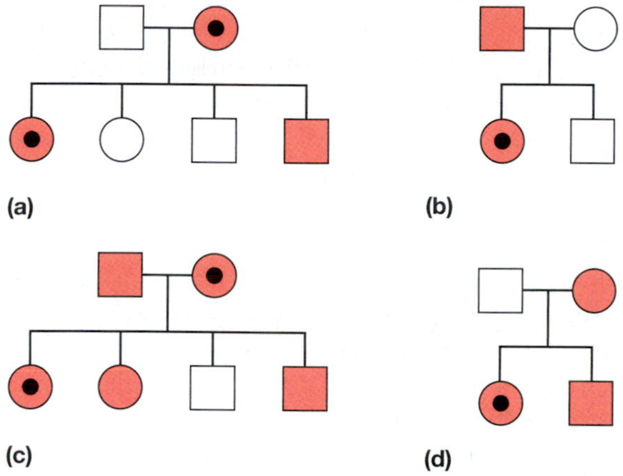

FIGURE 7–9 ◆ X-linked recessive inheritance pedigree.

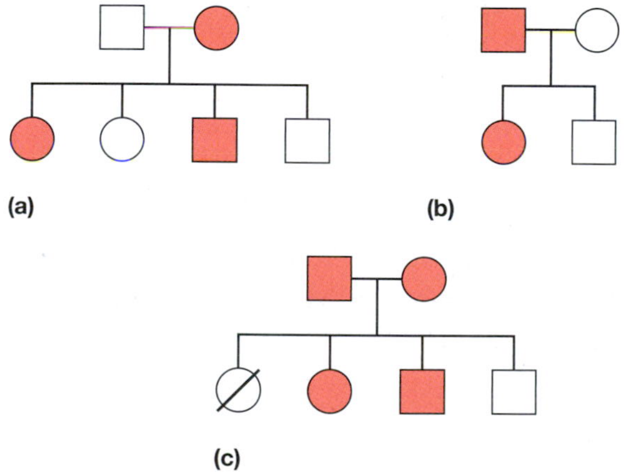

FIGURE 7–10 ◆ X-linked dominant inheritance pedigree.

approaching their primary health care providers with requests for genetic testing for conditions ranging from rare genetic disorders to colon cancer. In the past, genetic counselors have provided guidance and counseling for genetic testing; however, there are not enough genetic counselors to meet the needs of patients referred for genetic testing. Therefore, it has become the nurses' responsibility to become knowledgeable about genetic testing and the ethical, legal, and social issues pertaining to them.

An accurate family history is a powerful initial method for determining genetic risk and can be followed up with appropriate laboratory genetic testing. Currently, clinicians can test for more than 1,900 diseases using genetic tests. Genetic tests include prenatal testing, newborn screening, and carrier, diagnostic, and predictive testing. Specimens for genetic tests include blood, urine, saliva, stool, body tissues, bone, or hair. Genetic tests include molecular analysis of DNA and RNA, linkage analysis, biochemical testing of certain proteins, and cytogenetic testing on chromosomes (GeneTests: Medical Genetics Information Resource, 1993–2011).

Prenatal Testing and Newborn Screening

Prenatal genetic testing is usually offered when there is increased risk of having a child with a genetic condition. This may be due to maternal age, family history, ethnicity, multiple marker screen, or fetal ultrasound. Biochemical, chromosomal, or molecular-based approaches are used to identify individuals with genetic disorders such as Down syndrome. Because of risks to the fetus and the mother, informed consent is required prior to conducting prenatal testing.

Each year, newborns in the United States are screened using heelstick blood spots to detect genetic disorders that can be treated if found early, such as cystic fibrosis and sickle cell anemia. With the increase in new technologies such as tandem mass spectrometry, many states have expanded their newborn screening programs. Up-to-date information on what tests are required in each state can be located at the National Newborn Screening and Genetic Resource Center website (http://genes-r-us.uthscsa.edu/).

Weblink: Newborn Screening

Weblink: Medical Genetics Information Resource

Carrier Genetic Tests

Carrier genetic tests are conducted to determine if an unaffected, relatively healthy individual is carrying a disease-causing gene that could potentially be transmitted to offspring. This can be valuable information in common recessive disorders such as cystic fibrosis and sickle cell disease, or X-linked disorders such as hemophilia A. Knowledge of carrier status in autosomal recessive disorders is important information to use in family planning. If both parents are carriers of a recessive gene, then there is a 25% risk that each child will have the disease and a 50% chance that the child will be a carrier.

Diagnostic Genetic Tests

Diagnostic genetic tests are conducted on symptomatic individuals to identify the genetic disorder and assist with specific treatment and prognosis. For example, if a mother reports to her pediatrician that her 3-year-old son is becoming progressively weak, a DNA test can be conducted to confirm the suspected diagnosis of Duchenne muscular dystrophy. To assist with treatment or prognosis in hereditary cancers, the clinician can test for a mutation in the P53 tumor-suppressor gene. Based on the findings, a decision can be made to treat the cancer more assertively because it is more likely to grow aggressively.

As the clinical validity and utility of genetic testing is demonstrated, increasing numbers of prognostic indicators will be more closely associated with the specific mutation (e.g., BRCA1) instead of the disorder (e.g., breast cancer). Molecular approaches have largely replaced biochemical methodologies for genetic testing. In general, age is not a factor when determining whether or not to conduct a diagnostic genetic test.

Predictive Genetic Tests

Predictive genetic tests are offered to asymptomatic individuals who are at risk for a genetic disorder. The availability of predictive tests is increasing dramatically in association with the explosion in molecular and genetic technologies. Predictive tests are categorized into two groups: presymptomatic and susceptibility.

Susceptibility testing is conducted to identify individuals who are predisposed or at risk for developing the genetic disorder, but it is not certain they will develop the disorder even when the mutation is present. Results can be useful for health care decision making (i.e., potential lifestyle changes or increased surveillance). An example of this is hereditary nonpolyposis colorectal cancer (HNPCC), which has been associated with mutations in five genes responsible for repairing

DNA. Individuals with these mutations have an 80% lifetime risk of developing colorectal cancer. Lifestyle changes and early detection and treatment are associated with better outcomes. Because of the ethical and psychological issues involved with predictive genetic testing, many molecular laboratories require documentation of patient-informed consent and counseling.

An inherited gene mutation will be in the DNA of any cells in the body. Therefore, there are many sources from which to obtain samples appropriate for predictive genetic testing of an inherited disorder. DNA analysis is usually conducted using blood specimens, buccal cells (cheek cells), or skin cells because these specimens are relatively easy to obtain via noninvasive means.

Presymptomatic testing is conducted on individuals who will eventually develop the symptoms when the gene mutation is present. An example of this is an individual who has the mutation for Huntington disease, an autosomal dominant, fatal neurodegenerative genetic disorder resulting from a mutation in the Huntington gene located on the short arm of chromosome 4.

Benefits and Limitations of Genetic Testing

Genetic tests differ from other medical tests because they provide genetic information about the health of individuals *and their families* and also identify asymptomatic individuals who are at risk. Benefits can include medical management that is more appropriate for the particular diagnosis and opportunities for counseling and healthy lifestyle changes. For example, activities to reduce disease risk, increase longevity, and improve quality of life may be prescribed. Genetic testing results can be useful when making future decisions regarding children, financial planning, career choices, and lifestyle. In addition, for some individuals, knowing the test results may decrease stress and anxiety by eliminating uncertainty—even if the test is positive.

Limitations of genetic testing depend on the type of genetic test conducted. For example, a limitation of predictive testing is that it does not provide a diagnosis; instead, it identifies if the patient is "at risk." Just as a positive result does not always mean that the patient will develop a disease, a negative result does not mean the patient will not develop the disease or disorder. Furthermore, diagnostic tests may provide a diagnosis, yet there may or may not be a therapeutic intervention for the genetic disorder.

Another significant limitation is that most molecular tests examine for a mutation at a specific locus (i.e., SNP) and do not identify mutations in other areas of the gene or the genome. For example, cystic fibrosis can be diagnosed by a mutation in the cystic fibrosis gene. However, more than 1,400 different mutations have been identified in that one gene. Over 70% of individuals with cystic fibrosis have the Delta F508 mutation, resulting in most laboratory assay panels testing for only a few of the most frequently identified mutations. Therefore, individuals with one of the other more than 1,300 mutations would not be identified and the disorder would go undiagnosed.

Concerns about the effects of information obtained from genetic testing on the patient and family members and implications for the future should be considered. Although universal guidelines have not been developed for genetic testing, all nurses should handle information obtained from genetic testing carefully. They should honor privacy, informed consent, and confidentiality. Patients have the right to privacy regarding test results to avoid future discrimination or questions about their employability or insurability. Patients and health care providers should have adequate knowledge of the risks, benefits, and alternatives to genetic testing so that they understand the implications.

Ethical, Legal, and Social Issues of Genetic Information

The Ethical, Legal and Social Implications (ELSI) research program began in 1990 as an essential component of the Human Genome Project. The purpose of the program was to address the ethical, legal, and social consequences of the mapping and sequencing of the human genome. The intent was to stimulate discussion on these issues and develop policy options that would ensure that the information gained was used to benefit individuals and society. Funds from the National Human Genome Research Institute (NHGRI) are designated to fund ELSI research (NHGRI, 2010). A particular emphasis is placed on genetic issues related to discrimination, privacy, psychological impact and stigmatization, as well as uncertainties associated with interpretation of predictive genetic tests. In addition, issues surrounding the availability and access to testing and treatment and their cost are being addressed.

Genetic discrimination is the concern that genetic information may be used by employers against employees, or to screen potential employees. Another example involves insurance companies using information to deny or limit insurance. In May of 2008, the Genetic Information Nondiscrimination Act (GINA) was signed into law. The landmark legislation provides protection against discrimination based on an individual's genetic information in health insurance coverage and employment settings and should allow fuller use of genetic testing. In addition, the Health Information Portability and Accountability Act (HIPAA), discussed in Chapter 2, addresses privacy issues by affording genetic information increased confidentiality.

Of primary concern is the psychological impact and emotional response of the individual and family to test results. It is important to recognize that an individual's cultural background influences how she will interpret genetic information, make decisions, and adapt to genetic conditions (McGrath & Edwards, 2009). This cultural and ethical context should be considered when preparing the individual and family to receive genetic results. The Cultural Considerations box provides examples of this.

Careful patient assessment, counseling, and follow up are integral to the nurse's role in the genetic testing process. Genetic information can influence future reproductive decisions and medical treatment. The results may have significant psychological ramifications. For example, it is possible for test results to inadvertently uncover a paternity or adoption issue.

Increasingly, predictive genetic testing for conditions ranging from breast cancer to cardiovascular disease is marketed directly to consumers and is available over the Internet. Because of the complexity of the interpretation of genetic tests, particularly for multifactorial diseases and predictive genetic tests, and the potential lack of counseling and follow up, there are emerging concerns about these marketing techniques.

Emerging Molecular Methodologies and Genetic Therapies

Emerging molecular technological and methodological advances are based on gene expression and the complementary binding nature (A binds to T and C binds to G) of DNA bases. Loescher and Merkle (2005) have described a framework for understanding these technologies. Most genetic variation occurs in only 0.1% of the human genome, and it is there that researchers test for an association

CULTURAL CONSIDERATIONS for Genetics

African American	• Greeting and addressing patients should be formal, without using first names unless requested to do so by the patient or family. • Avoid imitating jargon because this may be viewed as ridicule. • Patient's fear of admitting carrier status with sickle cell disease may be a holdover from negative experiences with mass screening in the 1970s when carriers were denied health and life insurance. • Stressing the positive, such as protection against malaria, is important when providing information about sickle cell trait. • Support systems provided by the family may be more important than support systems outside the family. • During the first counseling session, explain the session, follow up, and give suggestions related to the present. Address the future at a later time (Telfair & Nash, 1996).
Amish	• Introductions of providers should be informal, such as "Dr. Barbara" or "Nurse David." • Decisions are made equally by husband and wife, so provide information directly to both parents. • Because of their religious beliefs, the topics of birth control, DNA storage, abortion, and artificial insemination by a donor are irrelevant. • Carrier screening may be unacceptable. Communities are aware of problems related to consanguinity and may look outside their community for a marriage partner. • Taking photographs of a patient is usually unacceptable, but may be allowed if the patient and family understand its importance in establishing a diagnosis. • Consent for autopsy is usually refused. • A lack of health insurance, which may be common in the community, can result in deciding not to proceed with extensive diagnostic testing. • Written consent may not be well understood because an individual simply giving his word is accepted in the community. • Printed visual aids may be helpful in counseling sessions (Francomano, 1996).
Traditional Asian Indian	• Explain the importance of an in-depth family history. • Explain diagnostic tests thoroughly. Carrier testing can result in discrimination and problems if marriages are arranged. • Because decision making may be done by all family members, schedule two clinic visits so tests can be done at the second visit after family members have made a decision about the suggested tests. • Adoption is well accepted. • Autopsies may be declined by Sikhs and Hindus, whereas Muslims may consent if necessary legally, as with a homicide. • Explain informed consent. • Visual aids may be helpful. • Surgical procedures are not readily accepted so detailed information should be given. • Results of tests that Westerners consider bad news may not be as stressful if fatalism is a strong belief (Patil & Fisher, 1996).
Traditional Chinese	• Family members make decisions in a group and consult other family members, if necessary. The oldest male has the most authority in traditional families. • Adoptions are rare. • Autopsies are viewed as irrelevant and expensive. • Carrier testing and use of other technologies may create the potential for blame, especially toward the mother. Stress the importance of "no fault." • The use of visual aids may be appropriate and helpful. • Family histories may be incomplete and mental illness may not be acknowledged or well recognized (Jung, 1996).
Deaf	• Avoid referring to deafness as a disability because some patients do not consider it to be disabling. When this is the case, giving birth to a child who is deaf will likely not be considered a problem. • Determine how the patient prefers to be referred to (as being deaf, hard of hearing, or hearing impaired) and refer to the patient in that way. • Avoid using terms such as *abnormal* or *affected* when referring to patients who are deaf. Describe genes as altered. • Visual aids can be very helpful. Avoid communicating while the patient is looking at the pictures. • A family history form may need to be sent before clinic visits. The family history may need to be obtained through medical records or hearing family members (Israel, Cunningham, Thumann, & Arnos, 1996).

(*continued*)

CULTURAL CONSIDERATIONS for Genetics, *continued*

Traditional Japanese	• Introductions should include titles when greeting the patient and addressing family members as Mr. or Mrs. • Adoptions, autopsies, and organ transplants are rare. • Assure the family of confidentiality and privacy. • Explain the need for consent forms. • With carrier testing and other testing, explain the importance of "no fault." • The family needs take precedence over the individual's needs. • The family members may make major decisions, so allow time for the family to consult family elders, if necessary. • Photographs may be refused, especially if a child has a visible disability. The disability may be viewed as shameful (Strazar & Fisher, 1996).
North American Jewish	• Use of prenatal diagnosis varies widely, depending on the religious orientation. • In Orthodox families, the male is often the decision maker, but will need to consult with a rabbi. Schedule prenatal testing early enough in the pregnancy to allow for this consultation to occur. • Families may have their own internal support groups, especially if they are practicing Orthodox Jews. Others may use support groups outside their immediate community. • Autopsy is usually discouraged unless it is strongly recommended. Discussion with and advice from a rabbi may be necessary (Greenstein & Bernstein, 1996).
Latino	• The eldest male is greeted first. Shake hands and ask about family to establish rapport. • Prenatal testing should be offered even though many Latinos are Catholic. • Disclosure of carrier status or a child's disability to other family members may be viewed as a loss of dignity. • Couples and patients need time to consult with other family members because family members participate in all decisions. • Loss of pregnancy is viewed as loss of a child. • Folk healers and Western physicians may be used by families and couples, so asking what other treatments are being used is important. • Visual aids may help in explaining genetic concepts. • If the patient needs to see a counselor more than once, schedule the patient with the same counselor (Lopez-Rangel, 1996).
Native Americans of the Southwest	• Amniocentesis may be acceptable but if prenatal care begins later in pregnancy, it is not an option. • Prenatal procedures may be more acceptable if the health provider's hands are blessed by a native healer before the procedure. • Adoption for infertile couples occurs along matrilineal lines; the couple adopts a sister's or cousin's child. • Diagnostic tests such as venipuncture, skin biopsies, and specimen samples usually present no problems. • Family planning is considered an individual's choice and may be used infrequently. • Acceptance of carrier testing is not known. • When greeting the entire family, address the maternal grandmother first. • The amount of eye contact that is comfortable for a patient may vary, so adjust accordingly. • Patients may not answer questions immediately, so allow for silence and do not consider it inattentiveness (Hauck & Knoki-Wilson, 1996).
Countries of Southeast Asia	• If blood tests are done, avoid drawing extra blood. Use microtubes if possible. • Respect the patient's right to refuse procedures by not assuming that refusal indicates a lack of understanding. • Ask the patient or family for permission to use visual aids (Fisher & Lew, 1996).

Source: Fisher, N. L., & Lew, L. (1996). Culture of the countries of Southeast Asia. In N. L. Fisher (Ed.), *Cultural and ethnic diversity: A guide for genetics professionals* (pp. 113–128). Baltimore, MD: The Johns Hopkins University Press.

between genetic variation (gene sequence) and disease susceptibility. These technologies allow professionals to identify disease susceptibility genes and monitor gene activity, thus bringing applied genetics to the clinical practitioner.

Polymerase Chain Reaction, Microarrays, and Sequencing

Although polymerase chain reaction (PCR) has been successfully employed since 1983 to replicate, or amplify, as few as one copy of a gene into billions of copies of that gene, real-time PCR and microarrays are relatively new technologies, and next generation sequencing technologies are rapidly emerging. The many exact copies of a gene made by PCR enable researchers and clinicians to identify and study that gene. Real-time PCR allows for the detection and quantification of a small fragment of replicating DNA or RNA during the amplification process. It is an improvement over PCR because it offers more rapid and sensitive quantification of the gene of interest. Clinically, real-time PCR is used to obtain viral load levels of many different viruses including cytomegalovirus and hepatitis C.

Microarray analysis is primarily used in the research setting although it is transitioning into clinical practice, specifically in the area of cancer prognosis and treatment stratification. When conducting a microarray analysis, specialized equipment that uses sophisticated computer programs simultaneously evaluates up to 33,000 genes that have been placed on a small 2.5-cm (1-in.) solid support (usually glass) chip. An application of this would be to identify a genetic pattern that demonstrates which genes are most active in disease states such as leukemia. In addition, clinicians and researchers may use gene expression patterns that emerge to obtain a more specific diagnosis and to better manage patient care.

The ability to determine the precise order of the nucleotide bases (adenine, guanine, cytosine, and thymine) in a molecule of DNA is known as DNA sequencing. Sequencing of small sections of DNA has been possible since the early 1970s. However, the recent advent of "next generation sequencing" has made whole genome sequencing possible. Ultimately, the goal of this technology is to allow for the interrogation of all possible genetic variations and regulatory processes and associate them with biology and disease in order to develop predictive testing and treatments. These technologies are able to sequence DNA and RNA more quickly (i.e., days instead of weeks or months) and at a fraction of the cost.

Gene Therapy and Stem Cell Therapy

Since the 2001 publication of the sequencing of the human genome (Venter et al., 2001), focus has shifted from sequencing the genome to applying this knowledge to treat diseases. Gene therapy and stem cell therapies are two applications that are currently in clinical development. **Gene therapy** is the correction of a genetic mutation by the introduction of healthy DNA into a cell as a treatment modality to improve the patient's health. Gene therapy has been used in clinical research trials to treat X-linked severe combined immune deficiency, a life-threatening disorder of the immune system. However, complications, such as the short-lived nature of the treatment and significant adverse effects related to a heightened immune response, have arisen in these trials. As a result of the additional research required, no human gene therapy products have been approved for commercial use. Ethical considerations, such as those related to the general availability of gene therapy due to excessive costs, are also issues. For further information on gene therapy, refer to the Human Genome Project Information, Ethical, Legal, and Social Implications website.

In general, stem cells are unspecialized cells that have the potential to divide without limit and to develop into specialized cells. Examples of the specialized cells are neurons, muscle cells, or insulin-producing cells of the pancreas. Research is conducted on embryonic stem cells and adult stem cells. Embryonic stem cells can develop into cell types from anywhere in the body, whereas adult stem cells typically specialize into cell types based on the tissue in which they originated.

Studies using human embryonic stem cells may provide information about complex aspects of human development including birth abnormalities and diseases such as cancer and Parkinson's disease. The focus of stem cell research is learning how undifferentiated cells become differentiated. Learning more about this process can lead to an understanding about how these conditions and diseases occur and strategies for treatment. For additional information, visit the Stem Cell Information website, an official National Institutes of Health (NIH) resource for stem cell research. Although there is hope for the treatment potential of stem cell therapies, ethical and political issues remain to be addressed. The NIH Research Ethics and Stem Cells website provides links and information to explore the issues surrounding the differing views on stem cell research.

As genomic health care expands into the clinical setting, nurses will be required to understand the concepts, principles, and ethical issues underpinning emerging molecular technologies and genetic therapies. Having a basic understanding of these concepts allows the nurse to recognize the benefits, limitations, and applications of each therapy. More importantly, the nurse can translate this knowledge for the patient, thereby improving patient care.

Pharmacogenomics

Pharmacogenomics refers to the application of genomic information and methods to pharmacogenetic problems. **Pharmacogenetics** refers to the area of genetics that focuses on the variability of responses to medications due to genetic variation. These genetic variations can alter the body's ability to absorb, transport, metabolize, or excrete medications or their metabolites. Pharmacogenetics may include any genetically determined variation in response to drugs. As the influence of genetic variation on drug metabolism is determined, a patient profile can be developed to allow health care providers to choose a medication and dosage that are genetically appropriate for the patient.

The HGP has led to the understanding that genomic information can be applied successfully to pharmacogenetic problems. Two facets of pharmacogenomics to consider are (1) the likelihood that the design of new drugs will be influenced by knowledge of all genes, and (2) that a pharmacogenetic profile of each individual who is a candidate to receive a medication can be developed, with two possible benefits. The first benefit is that clinicians should be able to predict those individuals who are likely to have an adverse response to a medication. This may be accomplished even without knowledge of the drug's metabolism or of the specific alleles that modulate responses to it. A second benefit may come from the development of abbreviated pharmacogenetic profiles, so that a clinician may be able to predict the efficacy of the medication in an individual before the drug is administered.

The origin of polymorphisms for drug response and the mechanisms that maintain them are a challenging problem. The response to medications requires specific biochemical reactions, and the enzymes involved may participate in the metabolism of ordinary food substances. The theory that polymorphisms for drug response may have resulted from the different diets in different populations is supported by the geographical distribution of many of these alleles. Recognizing this normal variation in response to drugs, the "potency" of a drug is defined by the dose that produces a given effect in 50% of the population. This variation is thought to be best explained by a combination of genetic and environmental factors or multifactorial inheritance.

Cytochrome P450 (CYP) enzymes are a family of liver enzymes that help break down more than 30 classes of medications. CYP polymorphisms or DNA variations in genes that code for these liver enzymes affect their ability to metabolize certain medications. When CYP enzymes are less active or inactive in terms of breaking down or eliminating medications from the patient's body, overdose can occur (U.S. Department of Energy Genome Programs, 2010). CYP polymorphisms affect patients' responses to medications that are used to treat depression, psychosis, cancer, cardiovascular disorders, ulcers and gastrointestinal disorders, pain, and seizure disorders (Pulczynska et al., 2011). For example, research findings show strong evidence that CYP polymorphisms in genes affect patient responsiveness to Coumadin and clearly improve prediction of therapeutic dosage over clinical predictors (Burmester et al., 2011). Clinical trials are being conducted by researchers who test for variations in CYP genes to determine associations with responsiveness to pharmaceutical therapies. In addition, pharmaceutical companies are screening chemical compounds in medications to determine how well they are broken down by the various CYP enzymes.

Malignant hyperthermia and serum cholinesterase and succinylcholine sensitivity are two genetics-related concerns that can occur during anesthesia. Malignant hyperthermia is an autosomal dominant condition that occurs in 1 out of 12,000 children and 1 out of 100,000 adults. The ratio of malignant hyperthermia in males to females is 2.5 to 1. The condition results in a dramatic adverse response to inhalational anesthetics such as halothane and muscle relaxants such as succinylcholine chloride, which can lead to death. Individuals can experience a very high temperature, sustained muscle contraction, and accompanying increased catabolism. Most cases of malignant hyperthermia are associated with mutations in a gene called *RYR1,* which maps to chromosome 19. Special precautions must be taken when individuals at risk need anesthesia. Dantrolene sodium prevents or reduces the severity of the response if an unsuspected attack occurs and alternative anesthetics can be given to patients at risk.

Overall, the role of drug metabolism in many pathophysiological processes is important. The management of patients with toxic reactions to drugs should include evaluation of the pharmacogenetic status of both the patient and members of the family, and appropriate genetic counseling about potential risks of certain drugs. The application of knowledge from the HGP to pharmacogenetics should usher in an era of "individualized medicine" in which appropriate medications and therapies consider not only the presentation and course of the disease, but also the individual's specific genetic makeup.

Nursing Management

The nursing management tips in this section were derived from the *Genetics/Genomics Nursing: Scope and Standards of Practice* (International Society of Nurses in Genetics, 2007) and the *Essentials of Genetic and Genomic Nursing: Competencies, Curricula Guidelines, and Outcome Indicators* (Consensus Panel on Genetic/Genomic Nursing Competencies, 2009). The nurse assesses the patient at risk for a genetic disorder and uses assessment data to identify diagnoses and expected outcomes. The nurse then develops interventions to achieve expected outcomes, implements interventions, and evaluates the progress made toward those outcomes. Collaboration among the nurse, patient, family, and health care providers is critical during all phases of the nursing process.

Assessment

The nurse assesses the patient and family at risk for or affected by a genetic disorder to identify risk factors and to determine their needs for information, referral, and genetics-related services and interventions. In addition to the routine physical examination and laboratory testing, a physical examination for dysmorphology and genetic testing may be indicated. The expectations of the patient and family must be taken into consideration. These may include their cultural views, values, and beliefs; environmental risk factors; and the patient's health history. The family history is a critical element in the assessment, which can be organized in a pedigree format that includes at least three generations.

Nursing Diagnosis

The nurse analyzes the data collected to identify the nursing diagnoses related to the actual or potential genetic disorder and the patient's and family's responses. Careful attention is given to the patient's knowledge of the risks for and associated with a genetic disorder; the ethical, legal, and social implications of the disorder; and the patient's decisions about managing the genetic disorder. Asking patients to communicate back to the nurse their understanding of a genetic disorder and its implications for the patient and family members can reveal gaps in knowledge, fear of the disorder, and misconceptions about the disorder.

The specific nursing diagnosis for genetic disorders would be related to the clinical manifestations of the genetic disease. For example, with Duchenne muscular dystrophy the typical diagnoses would be:

- *Alteration in mobility*
- *Potential for injury*
- *Grief.*

NANDA-I © 2012

Planning

The nurse and patient work together to develop a plan of care that may include family members, genetic nurses, genetic counselors, geneticists, other specialists, and special laboratories. Clarifying the patient's understanding of the genetic disorder can help ensure that the patient makes decisions with a full understanding of the treatment and related consequences. For example, when genetic testing is pursued, results of the tests can have implications not only for the patient but also for family members.

Interventions and Outcomes

Implementation of interventions may include identifying those persons who have or are at risk for inheriting or transmitting genetic disorders; promoting healthy lifestyles through health teaching; promoting and maintaining the patient's health; and using knowledge of genetic therapeutics to improve the patient's health or prevent health problems and disability. Interventions may also include using counseling interventions to assist patients and their family members in adjusting to and using genetic information; using knowledge of genetic therapeutics to improve the patient's health or prevent health problems and disability; and coordinating services to ensure continuity of health care.

The ability to effectively carry out interventions is directly related to a nurse's genetic and genomic knowledge. Therefore, the nurse must have current and accurate information and knowledge of resources, services, technologies, and therapeutic interventions for broad and specific genetic disorders.

The nurse considers ethical, legal, cultural, religious, and societal issues surrounding genetic and genomic information and technologies and works to define the issues that undermine the rights of each patient to make an informed decision and voluntarily take action based on that decision. The nurse refers patients as needed for routine and specialized services.

Discussion of the pedigree can lead to mutual identification of the patient's educational needs and opportunities for the nurse to share information about factors that place the patient at increased risk for genetic disorders and risk factors that are associated with the genetic disorder. The nurse considers personal and environmental risk factors, interprets information, and identifies services that are available to each patient. Genetic and genomic risk factors are incorporated into the patient's plan of care and interventions are developed with each patient to improve the patient's outcomes. The plan of care may require collaboration with other health care providers and collaboration with insurance providers/payers to facilitate reimbursement for genetic and genomic health care services.

Advanced practice nurses (APNs) use counseling interventions to promote patients' and families' understandings of the genetic disorder and promote their adjustment to the disorder. APNs who provide genetic counseling services discuss the risk for a genetic disorder, results of genetic testing, and options for genetic therapy when this is feasible. The APN may be the case manager for the patient and provide consultations to the patient and family, other nurses, and other health care providers to ensure that proper care is provided to patients and their families.

Evaluation

The nurse carefully evaluates the impact and effectiveness of genetic and genomic technology, information, interventions, and treatments on the patient's outcomes and reassesses and revises the plan of care as changes occur.

The nurse uses current genetic and genomic information to promote the patient's health, educate the patient and family, prevent illness and injury, and promote informed decision making. The patient and family who understand a genetic disorder can make better use of genetic technology and services and more actively participate in maintaining and promoting their own health.

Health Promotion

The *Healthy People 2020* initiative has added objectives that pertain to genomics. This new topic area demonstrates the increase in scientific evidence supporting the health benefits of using genetic testing and family histories to guide clinical and public health interventions. The objectives listed in *Healthy People 2020* for genomics include:

1. Genetic counseling for women with a family history of breast and/or ovarian cancer
2. Genetic testing for persons with colorectal cancer to detect Lynch syndrome (or familial colorectal cancer syndromes).

Research

Determining genetic patterns of inheritance can be a powerful way to establish genetic risk and to initiate health promotion activities that are designed to prevent the onset or lessen the severity of disease. As previously discussed, many diseases of adulthood, such as diabetes and obesity, are a result of gene–gene and gene–environment interactions. Knowing that an individual is susceptible to disease potentially provides a motivation for that individual to make lifestyle changes. In addition, genetic testing provides an opportunity for counseling and health promotion activities that reduce at-risk behaviors. However, for these things to occur, nurses and patients must be knowledgeable and informed so that they communicate effectively with each other and engage in discussion about the identification, monitoring, and treatment of disease using emerging molecular methodologies and genetic therapies. Refer to the Research Opportunities box for research ideas in the area of genetics.

Summary

Nurses should continue to increase their knowledge and integrate research findings into practice to assure the patient and family will benefit from advances in genetics and genomics. The nurse should develop a caring relationship with the patient and family that will take into account ethical, legal, and social issues associated with the genetic disorder (International Society of Nurses in Genetics, 2007).

RESEARCH OPPORTUNITIES Related to Genetics

Physiological Research	Clinical Impact
• Translational research to integrate basic science and clinical research	• Emerging technologies and treatments would be incorporated into clinical care more rapidly.
• Pharmacogenomic research to investigate biologic pathways influencing drug metabolism	• Medications would be individualized based on genotype, and dosage would be calculated based on genotypic response rather than weight and height.
• Quantifying gene activity and subsequent protein formation in genetic disorders	• Innovative assessment and monitoring methods and treatment therapies would emerge.
• Developing animal models to investigate the interaction of genetic and environmental factors on complex disorders	• Hypotheses related to biologic pathways in complex disorders would be tested in the animal models and moved more rapidly into human testing.
Psychosocial, Ethical, and Legal Research	**Clinical Impact**
• Access and barriers to genetic services	• New challenges may be addressing factors such as education, economics, health care resources, values, and beliefs that facilitate or impede access to genetic services.
• The public and policy makers use information about a genetic disorder or predisposition to a genetic disorder	• Ensure policies are developed and followed that protect patients from stigmatization and discrimination.
• Perceptions of genetics, genetic testing, and the use of genomics by individuals and groups from varied cultural and religious backgrounds	• Awareness of the patient perceptions is essential for planning and developing appropriate nursing care with patients and their families.
• Strategies for providing information about the risk for complex disorders	• Patients should be educated about the risk for complex disorders and recommended behavior or lifestyle changes to decrease risk.
• Patient, family, and professional communication about a genetic disorder or predisposition for a genetic disorder	• Patients and their family members should be provided with up-to-date information by appropriately trained professionals to facilitate patient and family communication with themselves and others.

NCLEX® PRACTICE

1. A nurse has made an effort to learn about and include genetics in the care of clients. The nurse's coworker says, "I don't know why you spend so much time on this. How can it help our clients?" Which response is best?

1. "The information gained through genetic testing can often help individuals find health insurance more easily."
2. "I can advise couples whether or not they should have children based upon their genetic testing."
3. "If a client has a genetic disorder, I can tell them exactly what caused it."
4. "Clients who know they are heterozygous for coronary artery disease can initiate medications and lifestyle changes to help lower cholesterol."

2. A client asks how chromosomal abnormalities occur. What is the most appropriate response by the nurse?

1. "With approximately 25,000 genes per chromosome, things statistically go wrong."
2. "There is always either an abundance or deficiency of genes within the chromosome."
3. "The genes of the red blood cells change."
4. "There is a hereditary alteration within an individual gene."

3. Which statement by the student nurse would indicate the need for further instruction regarding the human genome?

1. "The primary function of introns is to code for proteins using transcription and translation."
2. "When genes upregulate the mRNA, their expression also increases and forms more proteins."
3. "A codon specifies for a single amino acid that will eventually aid in production of protein."
4. "The alignment of purines and pyrimidines forms polynucleotide chains that form a double helix."

4. When planning the care of a client, the nurse understands the importance of obtaining the information contained in a pedigree. Which statement best describes the rationale for using this tool during the planning phase?

1. To help determine if unaffected or healthy individuals are carriers of disease-causing genes
2. To locate the genotypic differences among maternal and paternal alleles caused by imprinting
3. To assist in identifying disease risk and developing a customized prevention program for some conditions
4. To recognize core genetic disorders that can be treated if found early in clients with increased risk

5. The medical team suspects that a client has inherited cancer syndrome. Which findings support this suspicion? (select all that apply)

1. Many of the client's close relatives have had multiple cancers.
2. The client developed cancer at age 60.
3. The client has had unrelated cancers of the thyroid, lung, and bowel.
4. The client has cancer in both kidneys.
5. The client has cancer in multiple sites in the bowel.

6. A couple has one child who has cystic fibrosis (CF). The couple asks the nurse what the risk is for their second pregnancy to result in a child with CF. How should the nurse respond?

1. "Your chance for a second child with CF is very small."
2. "Your chance is 1 in 4."
3. "You have a 2 out of 3 chance to have another child with CF."
4. "Your chance is 100%."

Answers to NCLEX Practice questions can be found in Appendix D in the Osborn Student Resources at nursing.pearsonhighered.com. Practice additional NCLEX questions online at the Student Resources site.

Pearson Nursing Student Resources Find additional review materials at: **nursing.pearsonhighered.com**

REFERENCES

American Cancer Society. (2010). *Cancer facts and figures 2010*. Atlanta, GA: Author.

American Nurses Association. (2010). *Nursing: Scope and standards of practice* (2nd ed.). Retrieved from http://nursesbooks.org/Main-Menu/Standards/H-N/Nursing-Scope-and-Standards-of-Practice.aspx

Bennett, R. L., Steinhaus, K. A., Uhrich, S. B., O'Sullivan, C. K., Resta, R. G., Lochner-Doyle, D., et al. (1995). Recommendations for standardized human pedigree nomenclature. Pedigree Standardization Task Force of the National Society of Genetic Counselors. American Journal of Human Genetics, 56(3), 745–752.

Burmester, J. K., Berg, R. L., Yale, S. H., Rottscheit, C. M., Glurich, I. E., Schmelzer, J. R., & Caldwell, M. D. (2011). A randomized controlled trial of genotype-based Coumadin initiation. Genetics in Medicine: Official Journal of the American College of Medical Genetics, 13(6), 509–518.

Centers for Disease Control and Prevention. (2010, November 18). Family health history. Retrieved from http://www.cdc.gov/genomics/famhistory/index.htm

Collins, F. S., Green, E. D., Guttmacher, A. E., & Guyer, M. S. (2003). A vision for the future of genomics research. Nature, 422(6934), 835–847.

Consensus Panel on Genetic/Genomic Nursing Competencies. (2009). Essentials of genetic and genomic nursing: Competencies, curricula guidelines, and outcome indicators (2nd ed.). Silver Spring, MD: American Nurses Association.

Dean, L., & McEntyre, J. (2004). The genetic landscape of diabetes. Retrieved from http://www.ncbi.nlm.nih.gov/books/NBK1667/

Ferguson-Smith, M. A., & Simonic, I. (2007). Cytotic analysis. In D. L. Rimoin, J. M. Connor, R. E. Pyeritz, & B. R. Korf (Eds.), Emery and Rimoin's principles and practice of medical genetics (5th ed., Vol. 1, pp. 567–600). Philadelphia, PA: Churchill Livingstone Elsevier.

Fisher, N. L., & Lew, L. (1996). Culture of the countries of Southeast Asia. In N. L. Fisher (Ed.), *Cultural and ethnic diversity: A guide for genetics professionals* (pp. 113–128). Baltimore, MD: The Johns Hopkins University Press.

Francomano, C. A. (1996). Amish culture. In N. L. Fisher (Ed.), *Cultural and ethnic diversity: A guide for genetics professionals* (pp. 176–197). Baltimore, MD: The Johns Hopkins University Press.

GeneTests: Medical Genetics Information Resource (database online). (1993–2011). Copyright, University of Washington. Retrieved June 2011 from http://www.genetests.org

Greb, A. (1998). Multiculturalism and the practice of genetic counseling. In D. L. Baker, J. L. Schuette, & W. R. Uhlmann (Eds.), A guide to genetic counseling (pp. 171–198). New York: Wiley-Liss.

Greenstein, M. A., & Bernstein, B. A. (1996). Jewish culture in North America. In N. L. Fisher (Ed.), Cultural and ethnic diversity: A guide for genetics professionals (pp. 198–219). Baltimore, MD: The Johns Hopkins University Press.

Hauck, L., & Knoki-Wilson, U. M. (1996). Culture of Native Americans of the Southwest. In N. L. Fisher (Ed.), Cultural and ethnic diversity: A guide for genetics professionals (pp. 60–87). Baltimore, MD: The Johns Hopkins University Press.

Hinney, A., Vogel, C. I., & Hebebrand, J. (2010). From monogenic to polygenic obesity: Recent advances. European Child and Adolescent Psychiatry, 19(3), 297–310.

International Society of Nurses in Genetics. (2007). Genetics/genomics nursing: Scope and standards of practice. Silver Spring, MD: American Nurses Association.

Israel, J., Cunningham, M., Thumann, H., & Arnos, K. S. (1996). Deaf culture. In N. L. Fisher (Ed.), Cultural and ethnic diversity: A guide for genetics professionals (pp. 220–239). Baltimore, MD: The Johns Hopkins University Press.

Jung, J. H. (1996). Traditional Chinese culture. In N. L. Fisher (Ed.), Cultural and ethnic diversity: A guide for genetics professionals (pp. 86–97). Baltimore, MD: The Johns Hopkins University Press.

Klug, W. S., Cummings, M. R., Spencer, C. A., & Palladino, M. A. (2009). Essentials of genetics (7th ed.). San Francisco, CA: Benjamin-Cummings Publishing.

Korf, B. R., Rimoin, D. L., Connor, J. M., & Pyeritz, R. E. (2007). Nature and frequency of genetic disease. In D. L. Rimoin, J. M. Connor, R. E. Pyeritz, & B. R. Korf (Eds.), Emery and Rimoin's principles and practice of medical genetics (5th ed., Vol. 1, pp. 49–52). Philadelphia, PA: Churchill Livingstone Elsevier.

Kukull, W. A., & Bowen, J. D. (2002). Dementia epidemiology. The Medical Clinics of North America, 86, 573–590.

Loescher, L. J., & Merkle, C. J. (2005). The interface of genomic technologies and nursing. Journal of Nursing Scholarship, 37, 111–119.

Lopez-Rangel, E. (1996). Latino culture. In N. L. Fisher (Ed.), Cultural and ethnic diversity: A guide for genetics professionals (pp. 19–35). Baltimore, MD: The Johns Hopkins University Press.

Magnoni, S., & Brody, D. (2010). New perspectives on amyloid-b dynamics after acute brain injury. Archives of Neurology, 67(9), 1068–1073.

McGrath, B. B., & Edwards, K. L. (2009). When family means more (or less) than genetics: The intersection of culture, family, and genomics. Journal of Transcultural Nursing, 20, 270–277.

McKusick, V. A. (1998). Mendelian inheritance in man. Baltimore, MD: The Johns Hopkins University Press.

National Cancer Institute. (2010, November 24). Cancer genetics risk assessment and counseling PDQ® health professional version: Components of the risk assessment process. Retrieved from http://www.cancer.gov/cancertopics/pdq/genetics/risk-assessment-and-counseling/HealthProfessional/page3

National Coalition for Health Professional Education in Genetics. (2007). *Core competencies in genetics essential for all health care professionals.* Retrieved from http://www.nchpeg.org/

National Heart Lung and Blood Institute. (2010, August). Thalassemias. Retrieved from http://www.nhlbi.nih.gov/health/dci/Diseases/Thalassemia/Thalassemia_WhatIs.html

National Heart Lung and Blood Institute. (2010, October). Sickle cell anemia. Retrieved from http://www.nhlbi.nih.gov/health/dci/Diseases/Sca/SCA_WhatIs.html

National Human Genome Research Institute. (2010). ELSI planning and evaluation history. Retrieved from http://www.genome.gov/10001754

National Institute of Diabetes and Digestive and Kidney Disease (NIDDK). (2007). Monogenic forms of diabetes: Neonatal diabetes mellitus and maturity-onset diabetes of the young. Bethesda, MD: U.S. Department of Health and Human Services, National Institutes of Health. Retrieved from http://diabetes.niddk.nih.gov/dm/pubs/mody/

National Institute of Diabetes and Digestive and Kidney Diseases (NIDDK). (2008). National diabetes statistics, 2007 fact sheet. Bethesda, MD: U.S. Department of Health and Human Services, National Institutes of Health. Retrieved from http://diabetes.niddk.nih.gov/dm/pubs/statistics/

National Institutes of Health. (2010). Handbook: Help me understand genetics. Retrieved from http://ghr.nlm.nih.gov/handbook/mutationsanddisorders/structuralchanges

Nussbaum, R. L., McInnes, R. R., & Willard, H. F. (2007). Thompson & Thompson genetics in medicine (7th ed.). Philadelphia, PA: Saunders Elsevier.

Patil, S. R., & Fisher, N. L. (1996). Traditional Asian Indian culture. In N. L. Fisher (Ed.), Cultural and ethnic diversity: A guide for genetics professionals (pp. 142–155). Baltimore, MD: The Johns Hopkins University Press.

Prader-Willi Syndrome Association. (2010). *Research: The symbiotic world of PWSA (USA) research.* Retrieved from http://www.pwsausa.org/research/index.htm

Pulczynska, A., Lukaszkiewicz, J., Wojnar, M., Tomaszewski, P., Kubiak-Tomaszewska, G., & Pachecka, J. (2011). Cytochrome P450 polymorphism-molecular, metabolic, and pharmacogenetic aspects. IV. Application of long polymerase chain reaction for identification of CYP2D6 gene duplication. Acta Poloniae Pharmaceutica, 68, 9–13.

Strazar, M. D., & Fisher, N. L. (1996). Traditional Japanese culture. In N. L. Fisher (Ed.), Cultural and ethnic diversity: A guide for genetics professionals (pp. 98–112). Baltimore, MD: The Johns Hopkins University Press.

Telfair, J., & Nash, K. B. (1996). African American culture. In N. L. Fisher (Ed.), Cultural and ethnic diversity: A guide for genetics professionals (pp. 36–59). Baltimore, MD: The Johns Hopkins University Press.

U.S. Department of Energy Genome Programs. (2010). Human Genome Project information: Pharmacogenomics. Retrieved from http://www.ornl.gov/sci/techresources/Human_Genome/medicine/pharma.shtml

U.S. Department of Health and Human Services. (n.d.). Surgeon General's Family Health History Initiative. Retrieved June 2011 from http://www.hhs.gov/familyhistory/

Venter, J. C., Adams, M. D., Myers, E. W., Li, P. W., Mural, R. J., Sutton, G. G., et al. (2001). The sequence of the human genome. Science, 291(5507), 1304–1351.

Watson, J. D., & Crick, F. H. (1953). Molecular structure of nucleic acids; a structure for deoxyribose nucleic acid. Nature, 171(4356), 737–738.

Weigel, J., Kaczmarski, W., Barua, M., Kuchna, I., Nowicki, K., Wang, K., et al. (2011). Link between DYRK1A overexpression and several-fold enhancement of neurofibrillary deration with 3-repeat tau protein in Down syndrome. *Journal of Neuropathology and Experimental Neurology, 70,* 36–50. doi: 10.1097/NEN.0b013e318202bfa1

CHAPTER 8

Nutrition

Sheila Tucker
Cheryl Wraa

Outcome-Based Learning Objectives

After studying this chapter, the learner will be able to:

1. Distinguish components of a comprehensive nutrition assessment as part of the nursing care process.
2. Examine the nutritional component of national standards for disease prevention and treatment.
3. Analyze the metabolic effects of physiological stress and the potential impact on nutrition status.
4. Critique the nutrition therapy guidelines for patients with physiological stress, such as postoperative wound healing and burn injury.
5. Differentiate among the principles of medical nutrition therapy in treating general medical conditions.
6. Evaluate the indications and nursing interventions associated with enteral and parenteral nutrition support.
7. Distinguish the important role of nursing care in successful medical nutrition therapy.

KEY TERMS

aerophagia p.192
anthropometric measurements p.159
binge-eating disorder (BED) p.172
cachexia p.164
cardiac cachexia p.178
celiac sprue p.183
dysphagia p.180
enteral nutrition p.195
glycemic index p.179
hypercatabolism p.164
hypermetabolism p.164
hypertonic formula p.196
indirect calorimetry p.193
isotonic formula p.196
lanugo p.171
lipodystrophy p.190
malnutrition p.163
overnutrition p.158
parenteral nutrition p.197
peripheral parenteral nutrition (PPN) p.197
physiological stress p.163
pica p.161
protein-calorie malnutrition p.163
pulmonary cachexia p.192
refeeding syndrome p.172
respiratory quotient (RQ) p.192
steatorrhea p.184
therapeutic lifestyle changes (TLC) p.175
total parenteral nutrition (TPN) p.197
undernutrition p.158
xerostomia p.199

NUTRITION PLAYS a crucial role in both the prevention and treatment of disease. Both overnutrition and undernutrition can lead to negative health outcomes. For example, **overnutrition** from excess intake of nutrients can result in weight gain, elevated blood lipids, and risk of hypertension, diabetes, and some cancers. **Undernutrition,** in which dietary intake is less than the body's requirement, can result in impaired wound healing, poor response to medical treatment, and loss of functional capacity.

Medical nutrition therapy is an integral part of the health care process. Proper nutrition, whether accomplished through a therapeutic diet, nutrition support, or general healthy eating, is associated with positive outcomes. The nurse is uniquely positioned to take an active role in the nutrition care process of medical and surgical patients. The nutrition care process involves assessment, evaluation, and setting of patient goals and objectives in a manner that complements the nursing care process. The registered dietitian is the health care professional with the primary responsibility for overseeing medical nutrition therapy in most settings. However, the nurse's active position on the front line of patient care presents an important opportunity for improving nutritional care with efficient screening and assessment of nutrition status, appropriate and timely referrals, reinforcement of patient education, and close monitoring of nutrition intervention.

Nutrition Assessment

The cornerstone of all nutritional care is based on the foundation of an in-depth nutrition assessment. Objective and subjective data gathered as part of the nursing assessment can be evaluated to determine a patient's existing or potential risk for undernutrition or overnutrition. Appropriate nursing diagnoses and interventions can then be developed based on findings from the nutrition assessment.

Nutrition Assessment Parameters

No one parameter or single piece of data should be used in isolation as an indicator of nutrition status. Data gathered during the physical exam and laboratory assays together with subjective data from the focused interview provide a comprehensive set of information on which to base a nutrition assessment. A nutrition assessment based on limited data has limited clinical value because many parameters used in a nutrition assessment can be influenced by a variety of factors. When compiling a nutrition assessment, the nurse should use as many sources of data as are available, along with sound clinical judgment.

Physical Assessment

The physical assessment portion of a nutrition assessment includes the clinical exam along with anthropometric measurements. Pertinent data from the medical history and treatment plan should be considered for any influence they may have on nutrition status because of alterations in physical health. Physical factors that can have negative effects on nutritional status include the presence of pain, gastrointestinal symptoms, medication side effects, and impaired cognition or mobility.

Observations from the clinical examination can be incorporated into the nutrition assessment. Nutritional deficiencies can have few, if any, clinical symptoms until nutrient status is compromised for a length of time. The nurse should not dismiss suspicion of poor nutrition health simply because no physical findings are apparent. Physical changes associated with altered nutrition status also occur for medical or environmental reasons and so deserve further investigation when discovered. Chart 8–1 outlines physical findings that can be indicative of altered nutrition health.

Anthropometric measurements are an important component of the assessment and include any scientific measurement of the body. Examples include height, weight, body mass index, circumference measurements, and body composition. Current weight and height should be measured during an initial assessment. Weight should be obtained at regular intervals thereafter. Self-reported height and weight are not considered accurate and are subject to overreporting and underreporting bias by both adolescents and adults (Urden, 2009). Use of self-reported weight in a patient with undetected weight loss will result in an unaddressed clinical change and subsequent delayed intervention. A patient should be weighed

CHART 8–1 Physical Findings Associated with Altered Nutrition

	Finding	Potential Altered Nutrient
Hair	Dull, sparse, brittle, dyspigmented	Protein, iron, zinc, biotin
Face	Puffy/moon face, temporal wasting	Protein
	Pallor	Iron
Eyes	Sunken	Water
	Dry mucosa, night blindness	Vitamin A
	Pale conjunctiva	Iron
	Fatty deposits around lids	Elevated serum cholesterol
Mouth	Long tongue furrows	Water
	Cracked corners, lips, magenta tongue	Niacin, vitamin B_6, riboflavin
	Atrophic papillae	Iron
	Spongy, bleeding gums	Vitamin C
	Lack of taste (hypogeusia)	Zinc
Glands	Enlarged thyroid (goiter)	Iodine
Skin	Poor wound healing	Protein, zinc, vitamin C
	Dry, scaly	Vitamin A, zinc, fat
	Bruising	Vitamins C and K
	Pinpoint hemorrhages (petechiae)	Vitamin C
	Photosensitive symmetric rash	Niacin
	Tenting, dry mucous membranes or axillae	Water
Skeleton/trunk	Ascites	Protein
	Beading on ribs, bowed legs	Vitamin D
	Loss of fat, muscle wasting	Protein and calories
Limbs	Edema, loss of muscle, fat	Protein and calories
Nails	Spoon shaped, ridges	Iron
Central nervous system	Confusion, headache, lethargy	Water
	Confabulation, hyporeflexia	Thiamine
	Dementia, ataxia, neuropathy	Vitamin B_{12}
Cardiac	Arrhythmias	Magnesium, potassium

Weblink: Body Frame Size Weblink: BMI Table

with a minimal amount of clothing and after voiding. Presence of edema or ascites and any unremoved casts or appliances should be noted. Additionally, adjustments in weight should be made for missing limbs following established guidelines (Urden, 2009).

A weight history should be obtained and confirmed by checking medical records. An unplanned weight loss of >5% in 1 month or >10% in 6 months is clinically significant and warrants attention. Patients who cannot stand to be measured or weighed can be measured using alternative methods. For example, chair and bed scales can be used to obtain current weight while arm span, knee height, or recumbent measures will provide estimates of height.

Body mass index (BMI) is used to calculate an individual's appropriate weight for his height using the formula weight (kg)/height^2 (m). Morbidity and mortality statistics have been employed to determine cutoff points to define overweight, obesity, underweight, and healthy weight. A table from the National Institutes of Health (NIH) that can be used as a tool to determine BMI can be found at http://www.nhlbi.nih.gov/guidelines/obesity/bmi_tbl.htm. Because BMI calculations use simple height and weight measurements, its use does not take into account body composition. Individuals with large bone structure determined by measuring the circumference of the wrist and breadth of the elbow (refer to the tables on www.fitnessandfreebies.com/fitness/bodyframe.html) or those with ample muscle mass, such as body builders, can be categorized erroneously as overweight using this single assessment tool. The nurse should discover this discrepancy when conducting a physical exam.

Waist circumference is used in a nutrition assessment, especially when cardiovascular disease risk is suspected or known. Deposition of excess abdominal fat is considered to be an independent risk factor for heart disease in adults (National Heart, Lung, and Blood Institute [NHLBI], 2007). A waist circumference of >102 cm (40 in.) in men or >88 cm (35 in.) in women is associated with risk. Measurement should be made following proper technique with use of bony landmarks. Waist circumference measurements are not of nutritional value in patients who are pregnant or have ascites or other fat-free mass increases in abdominal girth because of disease.

Body composition—the percentages of fat, bone, and muscle in the body—is tested using a variety of techniques. Examples include skinfold measurements, bioelectrical impedance analysis, near-infrared, and dual x-ray absorptiometry (DEXA). Bone mineral content and fluid composition can be estimated with more sophisticated technology. The nurse must take care to ensure that the most accurate measurements are performed, realizing even then that most methods have a margin of error associated with them.

Reference values for all body composition measurements should be current and age and gender specific. The best use of composition measurements is in the serial monitoring of a patient, with the patient's own baseline measures serving as the initial point of reference.

Laboratory Measurements

Laboratory values can be a useful adjunct to other parameters used in a nutritional assessment. No single laboratory value is uniquely indicative of current nutritional status because confounding variables exist for each. Disease, infection, and the inflammatory process can alter laboratory values. Varying half-lives and the body's pool size of plasma proteins will yield differences in the snapshot of nutrition status reflected by their values. Albumin, with its long half-life, provides an older picture of nutrition status than prealbumin with its shorter half-life. Chart 8–2 outlines laboratory testing used in a nutrition assessment.

Nutrition History

A nutrition history can conveniently be incorporated into the focused interview done during a nursing assessment. The nutrition history may include a 24-hour diet recall and a food frequency questionnaire. A food record or diary can be a useful adjunctive tool to evaluate nutrition intervention for patients who receive ongoing care.

A 24-hour diet recall provides a 1-day snapshot of the patient's intake on which to base an assessment. All meals, snacks, liquids, and nutrition supplements should be recorded with estimates of preparation method and portion size. Because no single day usually illustrates all dietary habits, it is best to ask the patient about other general nutrition habits. For example, the nurse could query the patient about intake on a workday and a non-workday. Chart 8–3 outlines data to be considered when conducting a nutrition history.

A food frequency questionnaire is used to supplement the limited data of a 24-hour recall. The patient provides information on the frequency of consumption of different food groups by filling out a questionnaire or answering questions during the nutrition history. For example, a nurse may find no fruit intake on the limited recall, but a food frequency questionnaire might reveal that the patient eats 10 pieces of fruit a week.

CHART 8–2 Laboratory Tests Used in Nutrition Assessment

Laboratory Test Normal Finding	Expected Abnormality with Mild Malnutrition	Expected Abnormality with Moderate Malnutrition	Expected Abnormality with Severe Malnutrition	Rationale
Albumin 3.5–5 g/L	2.8–3.4 g/L	2.1–2.7 g/L	<2.1 g/L	↓ w/liver disease, inflammation, infection, renal losses
Transferrin >200 mg/L	180–200 mg/L	160–180 mg/L	<160 mg/L	↓ w/renal losses, liver disease; ↑ w/infection, inflammation, iron deficiency
Prealbumin 150–350 mg/L	110–150 mg/L	50–109 mg/L	<50 mg/L	↓ w/liver disease, inflammation, infection, renal losses
Total lymphocytes 2,000–3,500 cells/m^3	1,200–1,500 cells/m^3	800–1,200 cells/m^3	<800 cells/m^3	↓ w/steroid, immunosuppression, cancer treatment

Source: Tucker, S. B., & Dauffenbach, V. (2011). *Nutrition and diet therapy for nurses.* Upper Saddle River, NJ: Pearson.

CHART 8–3 Nutrition History Data

Diet Recall and Food Frequency
- All meals and snacks
- All liquids, including alcohol, water, and caffeinated beverages
- Location of meals (home, school, restaurant, car, work, etc.)
- Preparation methods (convenience food, added fat, salt, etc.)
- Portion size
- Meal patterns: number of meals, missed meals

Supplement and Medication Use
- Vitamin and mineral use; include dose, frequency, and ingredients
- Herbal supplements use; include dose, frequency, ingredients, interactions with medications
- Weight loss and sports supplements; include dose, frequency, ingredients, interactions with medications
- Assess over-the-counter and prescription medications for drug–nutrient interactions

Food Beliefs and Practices
- Use of therapeutic diet for allergy, food intolerance, or medical nutrition therapy
- Lifestyle nutrition choices and food faddism: avoidance of certain foods or food groups, trendy nutrition practices, vegetarianism or vegan diet
- Cultural or religious dietary influences
- **Pica:** consumption of nonfood items or unusual intake of single foods

Other Influences on Nutrition
- Education and literacy as it relates to nutrition knowledge and cooking skills
- Social environment: isolation, food security, access to cooking facilities and refrigeration, presence of substance abuse
- Economics: adequate funds for food
- Functional capacity related to ADLs and I-ADLs: cooking, shopping, self-feeding, meal preparation, general activity level

During the nutrition history, the nurse should ask open-ended questions and make no assumptions about types and patterns of intake. Asking a question such as "What did you have for breakfast?" assumes the patient had breakfast or appears to judge that breakfast consumption is expected. This type of questioning can lead the patient to craft an answer to meet the nurse's perceived expectations rather than answer factually. A better choice to begin the recall would be "What was the first thing you had to drink or eat yesterday? When/what was that?" followed by "When was the next time that you had something?"

Underreporting bias exists in giving a nutrition history. Patients who are seeking the social approval of the interviewer or want to avoid disapproval may under- or overreport their intake of various foods. For example, intake of fruits and vegetables may be overreported because of the perceived social approval of such an answer (Miller, Abdel-Maksoud, Crane, Marcus, & Byers, 2008). Patients who smoke, are obese, or are of lower socioeconomic or educational level underreport intake more than others (Scagluisi et al., 2008). In addition, alcohol intake can be underreported. Cultural influences on the nutrition assessment are outlined in the Cultural Considerations box. See the Gerontological Considerations section at the end of the chapter for information on assessing nutrition in older adults.

CULTURAL CONSIDERATIONS in Nutrition Assessment

- Cultural and religious beliefs and traditions can affect dietary habits and practices in many ways. Preparation methods, food choices, and patterns of intake can be based on beliefs of a group or individual interpretation.
- Explore the influence of cultural interpretations and religious beliefs on individual nutrition habits and beliefs. Diversity exists within groups, and it is best to discuss an individual's personal practices rather than make assumptions based on generalities.
- Ask about religious dietary laws, food preparation methods, food practices for special occasions (including whether fasting is practiced), and beliefs related to food and health. Inquire about medicinal herb use as it varies among cultures and can play an important role.

Nutrition Assessment Tools

Data from a nutrition assessment can be gathered following a protocol, the nursing care process, or by using a validated tool. No one screening or assessment tool is universally accepted as the gold standard for evaluating nutrition status in adults. Thus, many tools exist and will continue to be developed. Examples include the Mini Nutrition Assessment (MNA) and the Malnutrition Universal Screening Tool (MUST). When choosing a tool, it must be validated for use in the intended population. Most assessment tools have cutoff points as part of a scoring system. However, the nurse should be mindful of any change in the patient's nutrition status whether or not it meets established cutoff points. Poor nutrition health occurs along a continuum and sound clinical judgment is needed with any nutrition assessment tool in order to avoid missed opportunities for intervention and improved outcome.

The Mini Nutrition Assessment (MNA), the Subjective Global Assessment (SGA), and the Malnutrition Universal Screening Tool (MUST) have been validated as nutrition assessment tools (Anthony, 2008; Guigoz, 2008; Makhijas & Baker, 2008). All three tools are for use in adults, with the MNA specifically intended for the older adult.

Health Promotion

Health promotion includes nutrition education on both preservation of wellness and disease prevention through diet. The nurse can assist the patient in the development of strategies for lifestyle modifications aimed at improving nutrition health. Several national standards exist with supporting educational tools to guide the nurse in nutrition health promotion.

The *Dietary Guidelines for Americans, 2010 Edition* (U.S. Department of Health and Human Services [DHHS], 2011), are national standards that can be used when advising patients about health maintenance and disease prevention. These science-based general recommendations are targeted to the general population age 2 years and older and serve as the foundation for other federal nutrition guidelines and information, such as the development of the *Healthy People* objectives for the nation (U.S. Department of Health and Human Services, 2011). These guidelines are translated for the public into key messages that provide diet and physical activity guidance. These messages can become a template for general nutrition education as well as more specific advice about disease prevention. The National Guidelines box outlines the major messages of the *Dietary Guidelines for Americans, 2010 Edition*.

Weblink: Dietary Guidelines for Americans

NATIONAL GUIDELINES Dietary Guidelines for Americans, 2010 Edition, Key Recommendations

Balancing Calories to Manage Weight

- Prevent and/or reduce overweight and obesity through improved eating and physical activity behaviors.
- Control total calorie intake to manage body weight. For people who are overweight or obese, this will mean consuming fewer calories from foods and beverages.
- Increase physical activity and reduce time spent in sedentary behaviors.
- Maintain appropriate calorie balance during each stage of life—childhood, adolescence, adulthood, pregnancy and breastfeeding, and older age.

Foods and Food Components to Reduce

- Reduce daily sodium intake to less than 2,300 milligrams (mg) and further reduce intake to 1,500 mg among persons who are 51 and older and those of any age who are African American or have hypertension, diabetes, or chronic kidney disease. The 1,500 mg recommendation applies to about half of the U.S. population, including children, and the majority of adults.
- Consume less than 10% of calories from saturated fatty acids by replacing them with monounsaturated and polyunsaturated fatty acids.
- Consume less than 300 mg per day of dietary cholesterol.
- Keep *trans* fatty acid consumption as low as possible by limiting foods that contain synthetic sources of *trans* fats, such as partially hydrogenated oils, and by limiting other solid fats.
- Reduce the intake of calories from solid fats and added sugars.
- Limit the consumption of foods that contain refined grains, especially refined grain foods that contain solid fats, added sugars, and sodium.
- If alcohol is consumed, it should be consumed in moderation—up to one drink per day for women and two drinks per day for men—and only by adults of legal drinking age.

Foods and Nutrients to Increase

Individuals should meet the following recommendations as part of a healthy eating pattern while staying within their calorie needs.

- Increase vegetable and fruit intake.
- Eat a variety of vegetables, especially dark-green and red and orange vegetables and beans and peas.
- Consume at least half of all grains as whole grains. Increase whole-grain intake by replacing refined grains with whole grains.
- Increase intake of fat-free or low-fat milk and milk products, such as milk, yogurt, cheese, or fortified soy beverages.[a]
- Choose a variety of protein foods, which include seafood, lean meat and poultry, eggs, beans and peas, soy products, and unsalted nuts and seeds.
- Increase the amount and variety of seafood consumed by choosing seafood in place of some meat and poultry.
- Replace protein foods that are higher in solid fats with choices that are lower in solid fats and calories and/or are sources of oils.
- Use oils to replace solid fats where possible.
- Choose foods that provide more potassium, dietary fiber, calcium, and vitamin D, which are nutrients of concern in American diets. These foods include vegetables, fruits, whole grains, and milk and milk products.

Recommendations for Specific Population Groups

Women capable of becoming pregnant:[b]

- Choose foods that supply heme iron, which is more readily absorbed by the body, additional iron sources, and enhancers of iron absorption such as vitamin C-rich foods.
- Consume 400 micrograms (mcg) per day of synthetic folic acid (from fortified foods and/or supplements) in addition to food forms of folate from a varied diet.[c]

Women who are pregnant or breastfeeding:[b]

- Consume 8 to 12 ounces of seafood per week from a variety of seafood types.
- Due to their high methyl mercury content, limit white (albacore) tuna to 6 ounces per week and do not eat the following four types of fish: tilefish, shark, swordfish, and king mackerel.
- If pregnant, take an iron supplement, as recommended by an obstetrician or other health care provider.

Individuals ages 50 years and older:

- Consume foods fortified with vitamin B_{12}, such as fortified cereals, or dietary supplements.

Building Healthy Eating Patterns

- Select an eating pattern that meets nutrient needs over time at an appropriate calorie level.
- Account for all foods and beverages consumed and assess how they fit within a total healthy eating pattern.
- Follow food safety recommendations when preparing and eating foods to reduce the risk of foodborne illnesses.

Source: U.S. Department of Health and Human Services. (2010). *Dietary guidelines for Americans, 2010 edition.* Retrieved February 25, 2011, from http://www.cnpp.usda.gov/dietaryguidelines.

[a] Fortified soy beverages have been marketed as "soymilk," a product name consumers could see in supermarkets and consumer materials. However, FDA's regulations do not contain provisions for the use of the term *soymilk*. Therefore, in this document, the term *fortified soy beverage* includes products that may be marketed as soymilk.

[b] Includes adolescent girls.

[c] "Folic acid" is the synthetic form of the nutrient, whereas "folate" is the form found naturally in foods.

Nutrition health promotion also includes the elimination of health disparities that affect nutrition status. The DHHS, along with the U.S. Department of Agriculture, developed the *Healthy People 2020* document to establish goals and objectives for the nation aimed at improving quality and years of life as well as reducing health disparities (U.S. Department of Health and Human Services, 2011). The *Healthy People 2020* objectives can help the nurse to target appropriate interventions for specific population groups. Another National Guidelines box outlines the objectives from *Healthy People 2020* that relate to nutrition health.

Special Considerations Affecting Nutrition Care

Both malnutrition and physiological stress place additional nutritional requirements on the medical–surgical patient. Existing malnutrition can compromise medical treatment and contribute to adverse medical and surgical outcomes. The presence of physiological stress increases nutritional requirements in the patient who may already be at nutritional risk because of a medical condition or disease.

NATIONAL GUIDELINES ***Healthy People 2020***
Nutrition Objectives

- Increase the number of states with nutrition standards for foods and beverages provided to preschool-aged children in child care.
- Increase the proportion of schools that offer nutritious foods and beverages outside of school meals.
- Increase the number of states that have state-level policies that incentivize food retail outlets to provide foods that are encouraged by the Dietary Guidelines.
- Increase the proportion of primary care physicians who regularly measure the body mass index of their patients.
- Increase the proportion of physician office visits that include counseling or education related to nutrition or weight.
- Increase the proportion of worksites that offer nutrition or weight management classes or counseling.
- Increase the proportion of adults who are at a healthy weight.
- Reduce the proportion of adults who are obese.
- Reduce the proportion of children and adolescents who are considered obese.
- Prevent inappropriate weight gain in youth and adults.
- Eliminate very low food security among children.
- Reduce household food insecurity and, in doing so, reduce hunger.
- Increase the contribution of fruits to the diets of the population age 2 years and older.
- Increase the variety and contribution of vegetables to the diet of the population age 2 years and older.
- Increase the contribution of whole grains to the diets of the population age 2 years and older.
- Reduce consumption of calories from solid fats and added sugars in the population age 2 years and older.
- Reduce consumption of saturated fat in the population age 2 years and older.
- Reduce consumption of sodium in the population age 2 years and older.
- Increase consumption of calcium in the population age 2 years and older.
- Reduce iron deficiency among young children and females of childbearing age.
- Reduce iron deficiency among pregnant females.

Source: U.S. Department of Health and Human Services. (2011). *Healthy People 2020.* http://www.healthypeople.gov

RISK FACTORS for Malnutrition

Decreased Intake
Anorexia
Gastrointestinal symptoms: nausea, vomiting, diarrhea
Medication side effects
Pain
Dysphagia
Poor dental health or chewing difficulties
Sensory changes: loss of vision, taste, neuropathy
Depression, anxiety, cognitive impairment, or other neuropsychological symptoms
Socioeconomic issues: lack of finances, food insecurity, social isolation, bereavement, dependency on others for food or feeding
Alcoholism

Increases Nutrient Losses
Malabsorptive disease
Short bowel syndrome
Alcoholism
Drug–nutrient interactions

Increases Nutrient Requirements
Fever
Infection or sepsis
Wounds
Fracture
Hypermetabolic disease
Increased energy expenditure from increased physical activity

Weblink: Healthy People 2020: Nutrition Objectives

Malnutrition

Malnutrition can be defined as a deficiency of one or more nutrients. The terms *undernutrition* and *malnutrition* are used interchangeably. A deficiency of macronutrients (carbohydrate, protein, and fat) can result in muscle wasting and weight loss from insufficient energy intake. Often the general term *malnutrition* is synonymous with the specific term **protein-calorie malnutrition.** Deficiency of any micronutrient may initially be less physically evident than with macronutrient deficiency because a lack of vitamins and minerals can take many weeks or months to manifest clinical symptoms.

Malnutrition occurs because of decreased intake, increased losses, or unmet increased needs for energy or any nutrient. Decreased intake occurs for a number of medical and psychosocial reasons. Malabsorptive disease and drug interactions, including alcohol, are examples of conditions that cause nutrient loss. Hypermetabolism during physiological stress; increased energy needs because of growth and development; and physical activity all cause increased nutritional needs that must be met or malnutrition will develop. The accompanying Risk Factors box outlines the many contributing risk factors to malnutrition.

Malnutrition has adverse consequences, including poor wound healing, increased risk for infection and disease complications, altered pharmacokinetics, and ultimately increased risk of mortality (Norman, Pichard, Lochs, & Pirlich, 2008). Successful treatment of malnutrition is contingent on discovering the underlying etiology. Provision of adequate nutrition in a well-tolerated form is best based on the recommendations of a registered dietitian who is trained to assess the impact of physiological stress, disease, and alterations in metabolism on baseline nutritional requirements across the life span. Specific nutrition interventions are presented in later discussions in the chapter of medical nutrition therapy.

Physiological Stress

A hypermetabolic response to injury or disease can have significant nutritional ramifications. Major surgery, thermal injury, sepsis, and trauma are examples of **physiological stress.** Unlike periods of inadequate energy intake that result in weight loss and some muscle wasting, a hypermetabolic response because of physiological stress can lead to rapid protein catabolism even when it seems energy and protein intake are sufficient. The body's response to this metabolic stress leads to a cascade that includes release of catecholamines and cortisol, and a systemic inflammatory response (Wanek & Wolf, 2007). The result can be catabolization of skeletal muscle to provide a substrate for gluconeogenesis and a degradation of plasma proteins, such as albumin, that are considered acute-phase reactant proteins. Resting energy needs are elevated, which is referred to as **hypermetabolism.** Thus, physiological stress results in hypermetabolism and hypercatabolism. **Hypercatabolism** occurs when catabolism exceeds normal physiological rates. Each of these represents a nutritional challenge that is compounded when present together. The patient who is already malnourished before surgery, injury, or disease will have less available body stores to draw on during a metabolically challenging circumstance. In severe circumstances, the rate of protein degradation exceeds the body's ability to replenish muscle and plasma stores and, thus, physical and biochemical evidence of malnutrition ensues.

The severe muscle wasting seen with physiological stress is referred to as **cachexia.** The muscle loss found in cachexia is disproportionate to the loss of muscle and fat seen in starvation (Evans et al., 2008). When cachexia becomes evident, nutritional repletion is difficult because of the confounding chronic systemic inflammatory response. High energy and protein intake alone often does not overcome the effects. Considerable research has focused on supplementation with so-called "conditionally essential" amino acids, such as glutamine and arginine. Researchers believe that these nonessential amino acids become essential during extreme metabolic stress, such as with trauma or burns (Graves, Saffle, & Cochran, 2009). More recently, resistance training, pharmacological intervention with anabolic agents, cytokine inhibitors, and other metabolic regulators have all been under investigation for a potential role in cachexia treatment (Dodson et al., 2011). Further discussion of the nutritional effects of physiological stress under specific circumstances is provided later in this chapter. The effects of malnutrition on older adults are presented in the Gerontological Considerations section (p. 199).

Medical Nutrition Therapy

Medical nutrition therapy (MNT) plays a central role in the care of the medical or surgical patient. MNT includes the use of specific nutrition guidelines, nutrients, or therapeutic diets to treat an illness or medical condition. Therapeutic diets are used in the treatment of many diseases and conditions. Descriptions of specific diets are contained within the discussion of each disease state outlined in this chapter. Nutrition support in the form of tube feedings or intravenous nutrition is a type of MNT and is also discussed. Both hospitals and long-term care institutions are required by accrediting agencies to have a diet manual specific to their organization available in each medical unit. Diet manuals describe the specifics of all therapeutic diets and texture-modified diets offered at the institution. The nurse should refer to this manual to become familiar with the modified diets available for patients.

Many patients may not require a therapeutic diet while hospitalized; in this case, a "regular" diet is ordered for them. Some patients have a temporary or permanent need for a texture-modified or liquid diet while hospitalized. Clear liquid diets can be used postoperatively or as part of preparation for some diagnostic testing. A clear liquid diet contains little in the way of adequate nutrition for the patient and should not be used for more than a day or two without considering additional nutrition intervention. Many institutions require daily renewable prescriptions for a clear liquid diet in the hope that it fosters regular reevaluation of the need for the diet. A registered dietitian should be consulted when patients remain on a clear liquid diet as the sole form of nutrition for more than a few days. Difficulties with either chewing or swallowing warrant a nutrition evaluation for the appropriateness of a texture-modified diet. Chart 8–4 outlines various hospital diets prescribed for transitional and texture-modified diets.

Weight Management

The approach to medical nutrition therapy in the area of weight management is constantly evolving and requires maintaining a current knowledge base. Both overweight and underweight states can lead to additional health risks in the medical–surgical patient.

Overweight and Obesity

Overweight and obesity are linked with a multitude of comorbidities, including cardiovascular disease, hypertension, type 2 diabetes,

CHART 8–4 Transitional and Texture-Modified Diets

Diet	Definition	Sample Contents	Indications	Special Concerns
Clear liquids	Liquid at room or body temperature that can be seen through clearly	Clear juices, such as apple and cranberry, Popsicles, gelatin, clear broth, tea	Preparation for diagnostic testing, transition from NPO to reintroduction of oral intake (e.g., after an acute gastrointestinal [GI] event or postoperatively)	Provides hydration and some electrolytes and carbohydrate, but nutritionally inadequate. Limit duration of use.
Full liquids	Pourable consistency at room or body temperature	All liquids, including milk and nutrition supplement drinks, ice cream, cooked cereal	Fractured mandible, difficulty chewing or swallowing other consistencies	Ensure safety of this consistency in patients at risk for aspiration; avoid overmodifying texture unnecessarily. Can be modified to exclude lactose-containing foods.
Mechanical soft	Soft or chopped foods without connective tissue, casings, or tough skins	Full range of soft foods; can be chopped or mashed	Chewing or swallowing difficulties	Vary texture to patient tolerance. Avoid overly chopped or mashed consistency when not necessary.
Puree	Foods mechanically blended to spoon-thick consistency	Mashed potato, pureed hamburger, pureed peas, pudding	Chewing or swallowing difficulties	Avoid more texture modification than is needed. Ensure attractive eating environment to improve visual appeal of diet.
House or regular	All foods	Full choice of available menu items in all food groups	No condition requiring diet modification	Provides complete nutrition. Monitor tolerance and intake.

degenerative joint disease, some pulmonary disease, and cancers (NHLBI, 2007). The prevalence of overweight and obesity is increasing among all population groups in the United States, where 68% of all adults 20 to 74 years of age are considered overweight or obese (Flegal, Carroll, Ogden, & Curtin, 2010).

Many factors are suspected of contributing to the prevalence of overweight and obesity. For example, genetic, metabolic, psychological, and environmental causes have been cited (American Dietetic Association, 2009; NHLBI, 2007). Hormones that affect appetite and satiety, such as leptin and peptide YY, are being investigated for a potential role in the metabolic link to obesity (Kushner, 2007). Certain medications, such as atypical antipsychotics, can foster weight gain (Gentile, 2009). Although genetic and metabolic contributors to obesity are important, most researchers agree that energy imbalance is a more significant contributor (American Dietetic Association, 2009). Increased dietary intake, decreased physical activity, or a combination of both can lead to an imbalance in which energy expenditure is less than energy consumption and weight gain follows.

A nutrition assessment focusing on parameters to measure weight status is an intuitive step before determining treatment interventions for the overweight patient. Overweight is defined as a BMI of 25 to 29.9. Obesity is defined as a BMI greater than 30. Additional stratification exists to denote different classes of obesity. In the past, height–weight tables were used to determine appropriate weight and to diagnose overweight. These tables have been replaced by the BMI table in the clinical setting.

Other considerations to include in the assessment process are the presence of obesity risk factors, weight and dieting history (including failures and successes), and patient readiness to attempt weight loss. The nurse needs to assess the patient's readiness for weight loss based on the Stages of Change model. This model can be used to assess readiness for any behavior change, including weight management, and categorizes individuals according to where they are on a spectrum of thinking or action about new behavior using the terms *precontemplation*, *contemplation*, *action*, and *maintenance* (Cresci & Rotella, 2009). Patients not ready or unwilling to attempt weight loss should be encouraged to prevent further weight gain (NHLBI, 2007). Figure 8–1◆ shows an algorithm developed by the NIH for weight loss treatment. Chart 8–5 outlines important factors to consider when assessing a patient before weight loss intervention.

The nurse can guide the patient in establishing a reasonable weight loss goal. Generally, a goal of 5% to 10% loss of weight is recommended over a 6-month period and is associated with a reduction in health risks associated with obesity (NHLBI, 2007). Many patients wish to attempt a larger weight loss, but this should be discouraged because weight loss maintenance of larger losses can prove frustrating and difficult, and may lead to weight regain (American Dietetic Association, 2009). The nurse should encourage the patient to attempt weight loss by stressing the associated health benefits with even modest loss.

An energy deficit of 500 to 1,000 kilocalories per day can result in weight loss of between 1 to 2 pounds per week. This deficit can be accomplished with a combination of decreased intake and increased energy expenditure (NHLBI, 2007). Individuals who have lost weight and maintained that loss for at least a year cite ongoing attention to diet, engaging in physical activity most days, weight monitoring, and not skipping breakfast as contributors to their success (van Wormer et al., 2009). Any diet with a lower calorie intake than at baseline will produce weight loss. Most current research supports the idea that macronutrient composition (amount of carbohydrate, protein, or fat) does not play a major role, but rather overall calorie deficit does (Kushner, 2007). Fad

CHART 8–5 Assessing the Overweight Client Before Nutrition Intervention

Assessment Component	Parameters
Physical	BMI: measure height and weight
	Waist circumference
	Waist-to-hip ratio
	Body fat percentage
Medical History	Existing comorbidities to overweight
	Medical contributors to weight gain: active mental illness, metabolic disorders, limited mobility
	Medications that contribute to weight gain
	Weight history, pattern of weight gain, contributors/triggers to weight gain or regain after loss, maximum and minimum adult weights, family weight history
	Physical activity level and ability
Nutrition	Nutrition history: diet recall, meal and snack patterns, food preparation methods, skipped meals, meals away from home, time available for meals, dietary supplement use
	Dieting history: methods of weight loss (types of diets, programs, products used), success and failures, length/weight loss is maintained
	Knowledge about nutrition, meal preparation skills, sources of health information
Motivation and Readiness for Change	Personal reasons for weight control
	Personal goals regarding weight and health
	Personal readiness and willingness to manage weight (vs. being told by others)
	Barriers to success: poor social support system, poor finances, food insecurity, substance abuse, eating disorder (binge eating, bulimia), active mental illness, barriers to physical activity

Source: Tucker, S. B., & Dauffenbach, V. (2011). *Nutrition and diet therapy for nurses.* Upper Saddle River, NJ: Pearson.

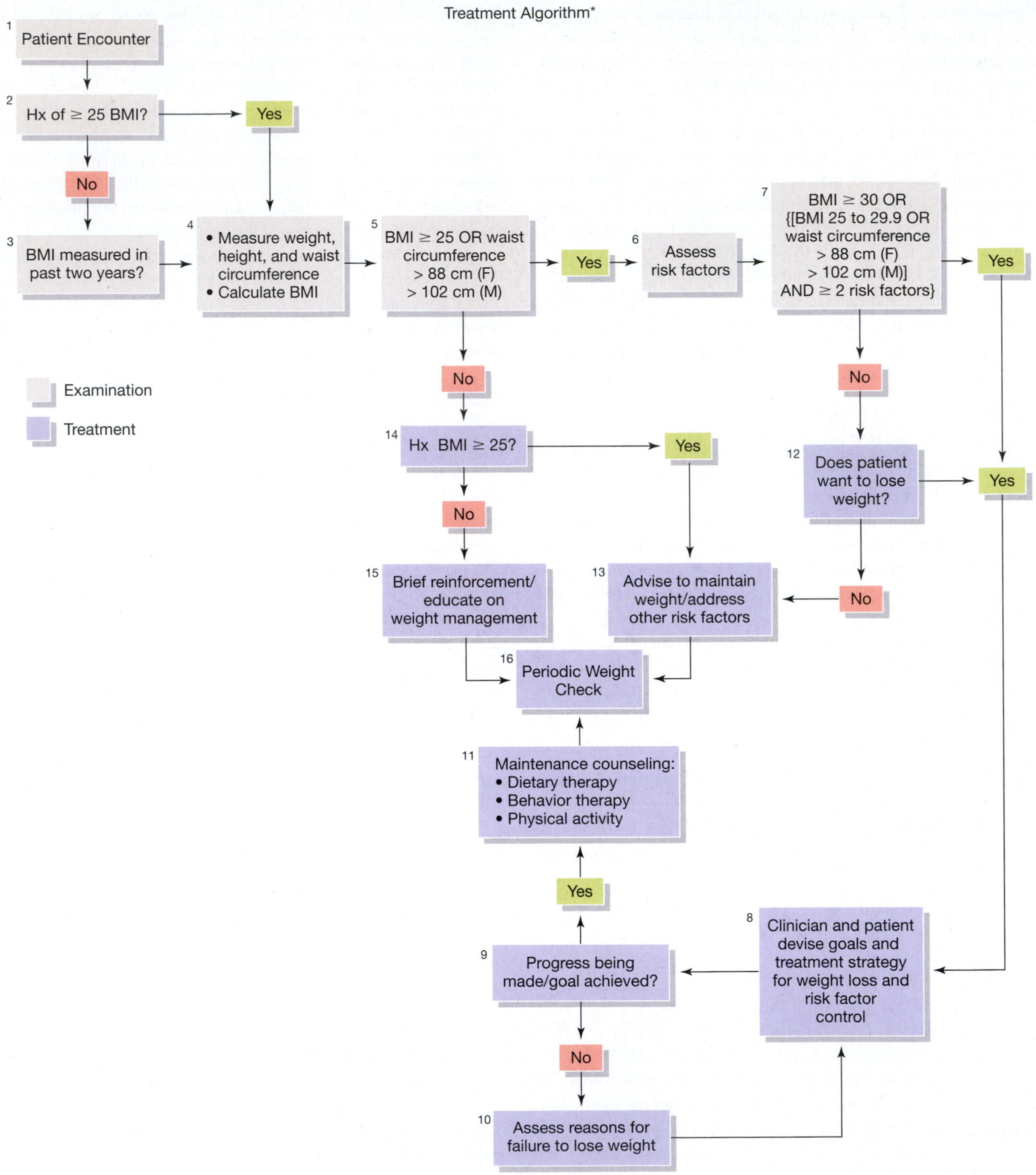

*This algorithm applies only to the assessment for overweight and obesity and subsequent decisions based on that assessment. It does not include any initial overall assessment for cardiovascular risk factors or diseases that are indicated.

FIGURE 8–1 ◆ Obesity treatment algorithm.

Source: From National Institutes of Health website: http://www.nhlbi.nih.gov/guidelines/obesity/ob_gdlns.pdf.

CHART 8–6 Calorie-Saving Examples for Weight Loss Intervention

Original Food	Alternative Food Suggestion	Approximate Calories Saved
1 C whole milk	1 C skim milk	65
1 C premium ice cream, vanilla	1 C low-fat soft-serve frozen yogurt, vanilla	300
2 TBSP cream cheese	2 TBSP fat-free cream cheese	70
2 TBSP half-and-half coffee creamer	2 TBSP fat-free half-and-half creamer	30
3-oz chicken thigh w/skin, roasted	3-oz chicken breast, skinless, roasted	90
4-oz pork sparerib, braised	4-oz pork tenderloin, trimmed, braised	233
Bagel, 4-1/2-in. diameter	2 English muffin halves	100
Yellow cake, no frosting, 1/12 of 8-in. cake	Angelfood cake, no frosting, 1/12 of 10-in. cake	115
Vanilla crème cookie, 1-3/4 in.	Vanilla wafers, 1 medium	30
1 TBSP oil for sautéing	Cooking spray for sautéing	100
2 TBSP mayonnaise	2 TBSP reduced-calorie mayonnaise	100
2 TBSP Ranch salad dressing	2 TBSP fat-free Ranch salad dressing	100

Note: Not all fat-free or reduced fat foods are lower in calories than the original version. The nurse should instruct patients to compare labels.
Source: USDA Nutrient Data Laboratory. (2011). http://www.nal.usda.gov/fnic/foodcomp/search

and fringe diets may target macronutrient composition or the "magical" combining powers of foods. Those that lead to successful weight loss do so because of calorie reduction and the self-limiting nature of their diet restrictions.

Low-calorie diets occur along a continuum from starvation or fasting to the recommended modest calorie reduction of 500 to 1,000 kilocalories per day. Extreme calorie reduction can lead to unhealthy loss of muscle mass, minerals, electrolytes, and water. In select obese patients, extremely low calorie diets (those with <1,000 kilocalories per day) are used, but with close medical supervision to monitor fluid and electrolyte status as well as general health. Such diets are not recommended for long-term success (American Dietetic Association, 2009). Targeting high-fat foods and empty calorie foods with little nutritional content can accomplish a 500- to 1,000-kilocalorie daily reduction in intake. Foods can be replaced with lower calorie foods or omitted. The choices should be realistic and sensible and not contribute to an overall sense of deprivation. Chart 8–6 outlines some examples of lower calorie food swaps.

Some patients want or need the structure of a more formal diet when attempting weight loss. The nurse can educate patients about the components of a healthy diet and guide them in an evaluation of any popular diet they are considering. Chart 8–7 outlines the components of a healthy weight loss diet. Patients who need extensive nutrition guidance and education should be referred to a registered dietitian. Commercial programs are also available for the patient who may benefit from the weekly social support. The nurse can guide the patient to an appropriate individual treatment choice.

Physical activity and a reduction in sedentary activity should be encouraged. Physical activity has a positive effect on energy balance and can improve body composition and cardiovascular fitness. Additionally, regular physical activity assists in the prevention of weight gain (American Dietetic Association, 2009). The nurse should emphasize the importance of physical activity in preventing weight regain. Exercise can be initiated slowly to eventually accumulate at least 30 minutes of moderate intensity exercise on most days (NHLBI, 2007). Even activities such as walking can replace sedentary activities such as riding an elevator or driving. The nurse can explore any barriers to increasing activity with the patient and offer suggestions tailored to the patient.

CHART 8–7 Components of a Healthy Weight Loss Diet

- Contains foods from all the major food groups.
- Diet is practical and realistic; can be adhered to without social interruption.
- Fosters no more than a 2 lb per week weight loss on average; higher losses can yield loss of muscle, fluid, and electrolytes.
- Emphasis on lean sources of protein: skinless poultry, fish, lean meats, legumes, fruits, vegetables, and whole grains.
- Low-fat sources of calcium including nonfat or low-fat milk, yogurt, cheese, or dairy alternatives such as fortified soy milk.
- Limit empty calories from excess sugary or fatty foods and alcohol.
- Minimize intake of saturated and trans fat, total fat, cholesterol, and sodium.
- Place emphasis on portion sizes.
- No skipped meals; avoids becoming overly hungry and overeating as a result.
- Physical activity is encouraged.

Behavior modification is essential for long-term weight loss maintenance and relapse prevention. Weight loss maintenance is a bigger challenge than the initial weight loss for many patients. A lifestyle approach to weight maintenance and healthy social support and coping mechanisms are important. Chart 8–8 outlines behavior modification use in weight loss.

Approved pharmacological treatment for obesity is reserved for patients with a BMI $\geq$ 30 with no obesity comorbidities or a BMI $\geq$ 27 if comorbidities exist. Lifestyle diet and exercise modifications should be attempted for at least 6 months before considering adjunctive medication (NHLBI, 2007). Some individuals choose to take over-the-counter dietary supplements to bolster weight loss. The nurse should assess the patient for use of these supplements during the nursing assessment, since some supplements that are marketed for weight loss, such as bitter orange, can cause dangerous increases in blood pressure and heart rate

CHART 8–8 Behavior Modification in Weight Management

Behavior Component	Behavior Example
Self-monitoring: conducting self-checks and keeping records	Monitoring calorie or fat intake.
	Keeping a food diary.
	Monitoring activity level.
	Logging weight weekly.
	Measuring portion size of snack foods.
Stimulus control: targeting cues to undesired behaviors and controlling them	Planning meals ahead of time to avoid stopping at fast food restaurants when pressed for time.
	Keeping high-calorie foods in the cupboard instead of out in view.
	Placing fruit in a bowl on the table instead of hidden in the refrigerator.
	Carrying alternative snack foods in the car or backpack to avoid the vending machine.
	Eating breakfast to avoid being overly hungry and overeating at lunch.
	Preparing smaller amounts of a recipe to avoid consuming bigger single servings.
	Having portioned desserts or fatty snacks sitting at the dinner table to avoid absent-mindedly munching in front of the television.
	Meeting a friend for a walk rather than at a restaurant.
Cognitive restructuring: reframing thinking about behaviors and enhancement of self-reliant skills	Using self-talk, motivational quotes, books, or other meaningful approaches to reinforce the idea that weight loss requires practicing new behaviors over time.
	Developing problem-solving approaches to slip-ups and barriers instead of abandoning efforts or being self-critical.
	Developing new coping skills to prevent poor diet or lack of exercise resulting from stress, boredom, frustration, or other emotional challenges.
	Developing positive outcomes that are not tied to weight as part of goal setting.
	Brainstorming individual rewards when small and large milestones are reached.

Source: Tucker, S. B., & Dauffenbach, V. (2011). *Nutrition and diet therapy for nurses.* Upper Saddle River, NJ: Pearson.

(NIH, 2010). Caffeine and other stimulants such as yerba mate, kola nut, and guarana may also be present in these products. Additionally, the nurse should be aware of the many alternative approaches to weight loss that a patient may pursue. Nutrition and herbal supplements, fad diets, and various devices are marketed to the patient as alternative and often "no effort" methods to lose weight. Federal regulation of supplements is minimal, because these products are regulated as food and not medicine by the Food and Drug Administration (FDA). The Federal Trade Commission regulates the advertising of such products, however, and can pursue a manufacturer for engaging in flagrantly misleading advertising. Patients need to be educated to view such products with a critical eye. Educational pointers for evaluating alternative products can be found at the website for the Federal Trade Commission, http://www.ftc.gov/bcp/edu/microsites/redflag/.

Bariatric surgery is a treatment option available for select clinically severe obese patients (BMI $\geq$ 40 or $>$35 with comorbidities). Gastric reduction surgeries, including vertical banded gastroplasty, and gastric bypass surgery, such as the Roux-en-Y procedure, are types of bariatric surgery. Weight loss occurs over many months postoperatively. Bypass procedures produce greater weight loss than simpler gastric reduction surgery (American Dietetic Association, 2009). Patients undergoing bariatric surgery require intensive presurgical screening and lifelong medical monitoring because of possible short- and long-term health complications. Nutrition guidelines following bariatric surgery are discussed later in this chapter.

Weight management for older adults is presented in the Gerontological Considerations section at the end of this chapter and a patient care plan for obesity is presented in the Nursing Process feature.

Disordered Eating

Disordered eating consists of behavioral, psychological, and physical symptoms that surround abnormal perceptions regarding food and body weight. Disordered eating patterns occur along a continuum from minor alterations in food-related behaviors to a clinical eating disorder that meets all established diagnostic criteria. Clinical eating disorders include anorexia nervosa, bulimia nervosa, and eating-disorders-not-otherwise-specified (EDNOS), which include binge-eating disorder and disordered eating not meeting the strict criteria for anorexia or bulimia. Criteria for clinical diagnoses are outlined in the *Diagnostic and Statistical Manual of Mental Disorders, Fourth Edition, Text Revision* (DSM-IV) (American Psychiatric Association [APA], 2000a).

Eating disorders affect up to 8 million Americans (American Dietetic Association, 2011). While the disorders occur primarily in females, the prevalence among males and younger children is increasing (Rosen and the Committee on Adolescence, 2010). Much debate surrounds the etiology of these complex disorders. Biology (including genetics), psychology, and sociocultural influences have all received attention as contributors. More than half of the patients with bulimia and almost half of the patients with binge-eating disorder have a substance abuse disorder. Obsessive-compulsive disorder, anxiety, depression, and other mood disorders are prevalent in all forms of eating disorders (APA, 2000b; Setnick, 2011). Chart 8–9 lists population groups thought to be at higher risk for an eating disorder. When conducting a nursing assessment, these groups should be screened for eating disorder signs and symptoms.

NURSING PROCESS: Patient Care Plan for Obesity

Assessment of Nutrition Status Using Gordon's Functional Health Patterns:

- Health Perception Health Management Pattern
- Nutrition Metabolic Pattern
- Activity Exercise Pattern
- Cognitive Perceptual Pattern

Subjective Data

Assessment of Nutritional Status

Have you recently gained or lost weight?

Do you prepare your own meals?

How often do you eat in restaurants?

Do you live/eat alone?

Do you have a regular meal schedule? What is it?

Do you eat during the night?

Assessment of Current Nutritional and Dietary Intake

24-hour and possibly 3-day recall of all meals, snacks, liquids

Location of meals

Method of food preparation

Portion size

Meals missed

Other factors that may influence intake, such as recent acute illness or cultural or religious influences on food intake patterns.

Alcohol intake

Assessment of Disease Risk Factors Influenced by Overweight Status

Do you have diabetes?

Is there a history of diabetes in your family?

When was the last time you had your blood sugar tested and what were the results?

Do you have high blood pressure?

When was the last time you had your blood pressure checked and what was the reading?

Do you have any problems with your heart?

When was your last physical examination?

What medications do you take?

Assessment of Changes That Can Be Made in Food Intake to Lower Caloric Intake, Including Patient Readiness to Change Food Intake

List the foods you typically eat daily.

Is there a particular food that you eat in excess when you are stressed, sick, or disturbed about something?

What activities do you do when you are stressed?

Do you increase your food intake when stressed?

Do you feel a need to change your dietary habits?

Are you motivated to learn new habits and try instituting them?

Do you have an exercise program?

Are you interested in starting an exercise program?

Assessment of Activity Level

Do you exercise; if so, what type?

How many times per week do you exercise?

Do you take your pulse during and after exercise?

Assessment of Knowledge Regarding Surgical Methods of Weight Loss

What are your thoughts on surgical intervention for weight loss?

Do you have questions about the various procedures?

Objective Data

Assessment of Nutritional Status

Current measured weight in pounds/height with minimal clothing and after urination

Serial weights from medical records

Presence of abdominal adiposity

Assessment of Current Nutritional and Dietary Intake

Ask spouse or significant other to validate data if patient agrees.

Assessment of Disease Risk Factors Influenced by Overweight Status

Cholesterol level

Triglyceride level

Blood glucose level

Blood pressure

Medication evaluation

Assessment of Changes That Can Be Made in Food Intake to Lower Caloric Intake, Including Patient Readiness to Change Food Intake

Caloric intake per 24 hours based on above food diary

Cholesterol and fat grams in food

Carbohydrate counting

BMI

Daily, weekly, and/or monthly weigh-ins

Assessment of Activity Level

Pedometer readings

Documented visits to personal health trainer

Assessment of Knowledge Regarding Surgical Methods of Weight Loss

Patient inquires of health provider about suitability of these methods for himself.

Patient attends a surgical information session.

(continued)

NURSING PROCESS: Patient Care Plan for Obesity, *continued*

Outcomes and Evaluation Parameters	Planning and Interventions with *Rationales*
1. NURSING DIAGNOSIS: Imbalanced Nutrition: More Than Body Requirements ***related to imbalance in dietary requirements and energy requirements*** **(NANDA-I © 2012)**	
Outcome: Balanced nutrition. ***Evaluation Parameter:*** Maintaining BMI within normal range.	Perform a complete physical assessment and nutritional history on admission *to assess current nutritional status and to provide a nutritional baseline of data.* Calculate BMI to determine overweight/obesity status. Current weight is compared to BMI charts, height/weight charts, and waist measurement *to determine degree of overweight status, overweight, obese, or morbidly obese.* Measure waist circumference *to determine cardiovascular disease risk.* Differentiate weight gain of obesity from weight gain of edema and other nonadiposity causes *to determine cause of weight gain.*
2. NURSING DIAGNOSIS: Imbalanced Nutrition: More Than Body Requirements ***related to individual factors and patterns in food preparation and eating styles*** **(NANDA-I © 2012)**	
Outcome: Patient lists all foods honestly so that a true intake record is gathered. ***Evaluation Parameters:*** Patient is aware of sources of intake and eating habits. Patient states motivation to change unhealthy habits.	List food intake for the past 24 hours and the past 3 days *to determine patterns, frequency of certain foods, location of meals, and intake patterns that place patient at high risk for increased nutritional intake.* Observe and identify possible patterns of food intake such as nighttime eating, eating while driving, eating while watching television *to determine total calorie intake and patient's awareness, or lack thereof, about the amount of intake.* Keep a food diary of frequency of intake of high-calorie items *to determine calorie intake.*
3. NURSING DIAGNOSIS: Health Maintenance Ineffective Risk ***related to known risk factors for chronic diseases based on overweight status*** **(NANDA-I © 2012)**	
Outcomes: Patient is able to verbalize risk for cardiac disease. Patient establishes a short-term and a long-term weight loss goal that is realistic. ***Evaluation Parameters:*** Verbalization allows the patient to admit that weight is problematic in terms of health status. Verbalizes understanding of impact of excess weight on health status.	Ask patient what disease *risk factors are related to overweight status. This question elicits the patient's understanding of how overweight status may affect health status.* Establish a weight goal that is reasonable and achievable *to reduce disease risks.*
4. NURSING DIAGNOSIS: Impaired Home Maintenance ***related to changes in eating patterns that may affect lifestyle, planning, and financial matters*** **(NANDA-I © 2012)**	
Outcomes: Begins and maintains a change in eating habits. Develops healthy choices to deal with stress. ***Evaluation Parameters:*** Patient can write down changes in food intake that he/she is willing to do in order to lose weight. Keeps weight loss records and measures body circumference area for progress toward goal. Writes daily weight in a weight loss calendar/diary. Loses 1–2 lb(s) of weight per week.	Determine caloric intake for 24-hour period based on patient's size and weight goals. *Weight loss of 7%–10% has been recommended to be a manageable level to achieve and maintain and will also provide a benefit in glucose levels for those who have pre-diabetes or overt diabetes.* Provide some simple ways to lower caloric counts (e.g., removing skin from chicken, avoiding fried foods, avoiding extra fat and caloric intake such as butter and jelly). *Most nutritious foods can be reduced in terms of calories by the method of preparation and the patient will not feel deprived.* Recommend using a support group *to provide emotional support while losing weight.* Teach patient to eat nutritious foods when hungry at regular times. *This strategy will help patient avoid food items with high caloric value and little to no nutritional value (e.g., cake, donuts, chips, etc.).* Teach the patient who wants a structured diet to count calories, carbohydrates, and/or fat grams in food. *Some patients benefit more from a structured weight loss plan, whereas others prefer less structure.* Teach patient recommendations regarding cholesterol and saturated fat intake. Discuss an exercise program and set realistic goals *to increase calorie burning and promote a healthy lifestyle.* Encourage cues to weight loss action, such as keeping a food diary and putting reminders on the refrigerator regarding physical activity. *Cues to action serve as reminders for health promotion behaviors.* Teach patient to avoid triggers to overeating *to prevent weight gain.* Increase activities that are enjoyable other than eating *to minimize food intake.*

(*continued*)

NURSING PROCESS: Patient Care Plan for Obesity, *continued*

Outcomes and Evaluation Parameters	Planning and Interventions with *Rationales*
5. NURSING DIAGNOSIS: Activity Intolerance ***related to lack of motivation and current health status*** **(NANDA-I © 2012)**	
Outcome: Patient walks at least 30 minutes per day at least four times per week. ***Evaluation Parameters:*** Activity log shows daily entries of time engaged in activity. Activity levels show a steady increase in time and distance achieved.	Encourage 30 minutes of physical activity most days of the week, *which will tone the body and assist in weight loss.* If patient has been physically inactive previously, activity levels should gradually increase *to prevent activity intolerance and cardiac stress.*
6. NURSING DIAGNOSIS: Deficient Knowledge ***regarding surgical weight loss methods*** **(NANDA-I © 2012)**	
Outcome: Patient verbalizes knowledge regarding various surgical techniques. ***Evaluation Parameter:*** Patient states he will continue to consider surgical means if weight loss is unsuccessful.	Discuss the surgical means of weight loss, including lap band surgery and intestinal bypass *to help patient understand the new concepts of surgical intervention.* Discuss the pros and cons of weight loss surgery *to assist the patient in being well informed.* Emphasize the importance of using medical means of weight loss until a decision is reached about the appropriateness of surgery for the patient. *The patient needs to understand that surgical interventions take time to consider and that surgery is more successful with fewer complications if about 10% of body weight has been lost prior to surgery by conventional means.*

Source: Adapted from Wilkinson, J. M., & Ahearn, N. R. (2009). *Prentice Hall nursing diagnosis handbook* (9th ed.). Upper Saddle River, NJ: Prentice Hall.

CHART 8–9 Populations at Risk for Eating Disorders

Athletes in sports with

- Subjective scoring (e.g., figure skating, gymnastics)
- Performance thinness philosophy (e.g., dance, distance running)
- Contour-revealing clothing (e.g., cheerleading, swim, dance)
- Emphasis on prepubescent body (e.g., gymnastics, figure skating)
- Weight categories (e.g., rowing, wrestling).

Fashion models

People who are obese

Young people with limited diets because of disease (e.g., diabetes)

Family history of mood, anxiety disorder, substance abuse

Family environment of adverse, critical, controlling, or distance parenting; family dieting; comments on physical appearance

Sources: American Dietetic Association. (2011). Position of the American Dietetic Association: Nutrition intervention in the treatment of eating disorders. *Journal of the American Dietetic Association, 111,* 1236–1241.; Halmi, K. A. (2009). Perplexities and provocations of eating disorders. *The Journal of Child Psychology, 50,* 163–169; Rosen, D. S., and the Committee on Adolescence. (2010). Identification and management of eating disorders in children and adolescents. *Pediatrics, 126,* 1240–1253.

CHART 8–10 Symptoms of Eating Disorders

Disorder	Potential Physical Findings
Anorexia/ Restrictive Eating	Alopecia
	Lanugo (soft, light hair growth on body)
	Dry skin
	Cold intolerance, loss of subcutaneous fat
	Hypotension
	Bradycardia
	Amenorrhea in nonpregnant women
	Muscle mass and strength loss
	Fatigue
	Pedal edema
	GI complaints: bloating, constipation
Bulimia/ Binge–Purge Behavior	Swollen parotid glands
	Dental enamel erosion
	Poor or absent gag reflex
	Bloodshot eyes, broken blood vessels on face
	Hoarse voice
	Scarred knuckle calluses on dorsal surface of hand
	Weight fluctuations
	GI complaints: reflux, bloating, constipation

Although eating disorders are considered a psychiatric diagnosis, medical and nutritional complications often place the patient in the medical care setting. It is important for the nurse to recognize the physical symptoms when assessing patients and to be involved in the medical and nutritional interventions of any treatment.

Anorexia Nervosa

Patients with anorexia nervosa are at 85% or less of expected body weight yet have an intense fear of gaining weight and a disturbed body image. Weight loss can have occurred as a result of restrictive dieting, excessive exercise, or a combination of both. Physical symptoms that may be present on a physical exam are listed in Chart 8–10. During the focused interview, the nurse can use established screening tools to assess for disordered eating or simply rely on informal questions on eating and exercise patterns, dieting behaviors, perception of body weight, and proper nutrition. A vegetarian diet is used by some as a method of masking restrictive eating (Robinson-O'Brien, Perry, Story, & Neumark-Sztainer, 2009). Suspicion of disordered eating accompanied by a new vegetarian lifestyle should be investigated further.

Anorexia nervosa is treated either in the inpatient or outpatient setting depending on the severity of symptoms. Outpatient care is preferred unless the patient is refractory to treatment with a weight of less than 75% expected or has an emergent mental health event or severe cardiovascular risk, such as bradycardia (<40 beats/min), hypotension (<60 systolic) or hypokalemia (<3 mg/dL). Hypothermia (36°C [<97°F]) is also indicative of the need for inpatient treatment (American Dietetic Association, 2011; Williams, Goodie, & Motsinger, 2008). A team approach to treatment is recommended because of the complex medical, psychiatric, and nutritional issues; no one clinician or profession is solely able to provide the scope of care required. Goals for treatment include cessation of weight reduction and weight reduction behaviors, weight restoration, improved behaviors related to food and eating, and improvement of any medical or psychiatric conditions).

Nutrition intervention in anorexia initially focuses on cessation of weight loss and then restoration of body weight. Outpatient weight restoration is recommended at 1 to 2 pounds per week; inpatient restoration of 2 to 3 pounds per week can be safely monitored (American Dietetic Association, 2011). Determination of the appropriate meal plan and its progression is the responsibility of the dietitian (American Dietetic Association, 2011). The nurse plays an important role in educating the patient on the physiological symptoms and consequences of starvation, reinforcing and monitoring the nutrition plan (including assessing for excessive exercise or squirreling away uneaten food in the inpatient setting), monitoring for changes in vital signs and body weight, and assessing for symptoms of refeeding syndrome. **Refeeding syndrome** can occur following starvation and reintroduction of fuel in any medical or surgical situation, including eating disorders. As fuel substrate is reintroduced to the body and metabolism increases, fluid and electrolyte shifts can occur. Serum phosphorous and potassium levels can become dangerously low as new ATP is generated. The Safety Alert outlines essential assessment data when refeeding begins. The Nursing Process Patient Care Plan outlines nursing management of the weight loss patient.

Safety Alert *Patients with refeeding syndrome are at risk for cardiac dysrhythmia and sudden death. The nurse needs to assess the patient for the following symptoms:*

- *Hypophosphatemia*
- *Hypokalemia*
- *Hypomagnesemia*
- *Cardiac dysrhythmia, specifically prolonged QT interval*
- *Edema (can be normal part of refeeding; monitor for presence with other symptoms)*
- *Heart failure.*

Regardless of treatment setting, gradual increase of food intake will help avoid refeeding syndrome and allow the patient to become comfortable physically and emotionally with increased intake. This approach allows for addressing food phobias and assists with eating behavior change. Prescriptive limits or avoidance of exercise is included in the treatment of those patients who exercise excessively. As the patient's condition improves, exercise limitations are lifted slowly.

The treatment team determines which clinician is most appropriate to monitor ongoing weight and whether the patient will learn weight measurements or be "blinded" (weighed while standing backwards on the scale). These determinations are made for each individual patient. When weighing patients, the nurse should ensure that weights are done in a private setting and not in a common area. The patient should wear minimal clothing and void before the weight measure, since some patients will drink excessive amounts of liquids before being weighed. The voided urine can be assessed for specific gravity to determine if this is happening. An assessment should be done for any hidden weights in or under clothing or undergarments.

Bulimia Nervosa

Bulimia nervosa is characterized by chaotic eating patterns such as binge eating and compensatory purging, and is accompanied by a sense of loss of control as a result. Patients with bulimia often have a personal set of "rules" governing "good" and "bad" foods and amounts of food. It is not uncommon for patients with bulimia to be restrictive eaters when not bingeing. Binges can be triggered by a perception of breaking such a "rule," hunger from restrictive eating, perceived fullness, or an emotional cause. Compensatory action can be purging with self-induced vomiting, laxative use, diuretic use, or excessive exercise. At-risk patients should be assessed for use of over-the-counter, prescription, and alternative medicine versions of laxatives and diuretics. Assessment should also include whether syrup of ipecac is used, because it has negative cardiovascular effects such as cardiomyopathy (Rosen and the Committee on Adolescence, 2010). Type, duration, and frequency of exercise should be ascertained as well.

DSM-IV criteria call for binge–purge behavior at least twice a week for 6 months. The nurse may find on assessment that patients engage in this behavior more frequently but not for 6 months. Any binge–purge behavior is deserving of further evaluation. Symptoms of bulimia are subtler than those of anorexia. Patients with bulimia are often of normal weight or slightly overweight, making assessment more difficult. Signs and symptoms of bulimia nervosa are listed in Chart 8–10.

Nutrition intervention for bulimia centers on normalizing eating patterns to interrupt the binge–purge cycle. This includes avoidance of hunger and chaotic eating patterns and slow reintroduction of forbidden foods. Generally, the dietitian prescribes a more structured eating pattern to help the patient meet this goal. Finger foods are avoided because portion control is difficult. When excessive exercise is used as a compensatory purging method, prescriptive limits are generally placed on activity. The nurse can be instrumental in reinforcing the meal pattern to encourage avoidance of long time spans between eating. A food record also can be helpful to assess this.

Corrections of misconceptions about weight and nutrition are also important. The nurse can educate the patient about normal transient symptoms to expect with the normalization of eating patterns. These include water retention (which will worsen if fluid is restricted or diuretics or laxatives abused) and bloating from delayed gastric emptying or from constipation with laxative reliance. Additionally, the nurse can be effective in counseling the patient who abuses laxatives or diuretics as to the ineffectiveness of those treatments in eliminating calories or fat from the body, in addition to their medical dangers. A high-fiber and high-fluid diet should be encouraged for the patient who is weaning from laxative abuse (bulimia.com, 2012).

Binge-Eating Disorder

Binge-eating disorder (BED) is characterized by the same type of binge eating as bulimia nervosa but without the compensatory purging. Binge-eating disorder should not be confused with overeating, especially associated with social activity; it is generally secretive and associated with a negative mood (Sim et al., 2010). Researchers' focus is pointing to increased prevalence in some families of the effects of chronic restrained eating, and depression and other psychiatric diagnoses as contributing to binge eating (Meno, Hannum, Espelage, & Douglas Low, 2008). The nurse should screen obese patients who may be at risk for binge-eating disorder (Sim et al., 2010). Binge eaters often eat 5,000 to 15,000 calories at one sitting, frequently snack between the three meals they eat, and overeat throughout the day between binges (Zieve, 2011).

Treatment of binge-eating disorder involves medical treatment of any complications of obesity, psychological treatment of any underlying

GENETIC CONSIDERATIONS Implications for Weight Management

Speculation about the genetic implications in weight management has existed for some time. The specific roles of genetics as related to risk of obesity and eating disorders are being investigated. Risk factors for the development of eating disorders have been linked to genetic phenotypes for other disorders, such as the traits for obsessive-compulsive disorder and disturbances of dopamine systems.

The role of genetics and the possibility of genetic manipulation have been heavily researched in the hope of identifying obesity risk factors and treatment options. Substances involved in appetite regulation (e.g., neuropeptide Y and ghrelin, proteins involved in thermogenesis, and leptin) and their relation to obesity are among the areas of research. Although the topic of genetic influence on the development of both eating disorders and obesity is intriguing, it is difficult to draw firm conclusions without further research into these areas.

Sources: American Dietetic Association. (2009). Position of the American Dietetic Association: Weight management. *Journal of the American Dietetic Association, 109,* 330–346; Bellar, A., Jarosz, P. A., & Bellar, D. (2008). Implications of the biology of weight regulation and obesity on the treatment of obesity. *Journal of the American Academy of Nurse Practitioners, 20,* 128–135; Kushner, R. F. (2007). Obesity management. *Gastroenterology Clinics of North America, 36,* 191–210.

mental health issues, and nutrition treatment to normalize eating patterns. It is under debate whether any attempt at weight loss should occur during binge-eating treatment or be delayed until the patient's behaviors are stabilized (Sim et al., 2010). The Genetic Considerations box discusses speculation about the roles genetics may play in weight management.

Nutrition and Cardiovascular Disease

Nutrition intervention can play a significant role in reducing the risk of cardiovascular disease. Lifestyle modifications, which include nutrition, can help prevent or manage hypertension and coronary artery disease. Medical nutrition therapy is also indicated in the treatment of heart failure.

Hypertension

Lifestyle modifications, including diet, have been shown to have both clinical and public health significance in reduction of blood pressure in people with hypertension and those with high normal blood pressure, or prehypertension (Maruther, Wang, & Appel, 2009).

Several nutrition-centered modifications and regular physical activity are recommended for the prevention and management of high blood

NURSING PROCESS: Patient Care Plan for Malnutrition (Undernutrition)

Assessment of Cardiac Status Using Gordon's Functional Health Patterns:

- Health Perception Health Management Pattern
- Nutrition Metabolic Pattern

Subjective Data	Objective Data
Assessment of Current Nutritional Status Have you lost weight in the last 3 months? If so, how much? Have you changed your eating habits in the last 3 months? Do you have any discomfort such as pain or bloating after you eat? Does it occur with any particular type of food? Ask patient or family how long nutritional intake has been reduced to help determine severity of malnutrition.	**Assessment of Current Nutritional Status** Patient has experienced an unintentional weight loss of >5% or more in 1 month or >10% in 3 months. Current measured weight and height compared to standardized tables of measurement. BMI < 18.5 kg/m^2. Gastrointestinal symptoms including constipation, diarrhea, pain, or cramping. List of current medications that can cause nutritional side effects (diarrhea, loss of appetite, etc.).
Assessment of Current Nutritional and Dietary Intake What is your normal daily dietary intake? How much alcohol do you drink weekly? What types of food do you use for snacks? How many meals a day do you eat and at what time? Do you use vitamin, herbal, and over-the-counter (OTC) medications? Have you taken any weight loss medications or used laxatives for weight loss? Do you have any difficulty with swallowing or chewing?	**Assessment of Current Nutritional and Dietary Intake** Serial weights from medical records. Assess muscle wasting. Assess for acute and/or chronic disease states (e.g., kidney, liver, diabetes, anorexia, cancer). Test serum albumin level, serum prealbumin level, serum creatinine level, total lymphocyte count, and transferrin level.
Assessment of Disease Risk Factors That Are Influenced by Underweight Status Do you have any acute or chronic diseases? When was the last time you had a complete physical examination?	**Assessment of Disease Risk Factors That Are Influenced by Underweight Status** Assess for cachexia, renal dysfunction, fever, infection, wounds, diabetes mellitus, gastrointestinal pain, and bloating.
Assessment of Changes That Can Be Made in Food Intake to Increase Caloric Intake, Including Readiness to Change Food Intake List the foods you enjoy eating and eat frequently.	**Assessment of Changes That Can Be Made in Food Intake to Increase Caloric Intake, Including Readiness to Change Food Intake** Caloric intake per 24 hr based on above food diary. Write down each food consumed along with portion size for calculation of food intake by dietitian.

(continued)

NURSING PROCESS: Patient Care Plan for Malnutrition (Undernutrition), *continued*

Outcomes and Evaluation Parameters	Planning and Interventions with *Rationales*
1. NURSING DIAGNOSIS: Imbalanced Nutrition: Less Than Body Requirements *related to inability to eat adequate amounts of food to maintain weight* (NANDA-I © 2012)	
Outcome: Normal intake of a balanced diet without side effects. ***Evaluation Parameters:*** Weight is at recommended level for the patient's height and musculature. Treatment of gastrointestinal clinical manifestations is effective.	Perform a complete physical assessment and nutritional history on admission *to assess current nutritional status and to provide a nutritional baseline of data for plan development.* Instruct patient to weigh daily before breakfast, after urination, using the same scale *to monitor weight gain.* Consult registered dietitian *for detailed nutritional analysis and specialized planning.*
2. NURSING DIAGNOSIS: Imbalanced Nutrition: Less Than Body Requirements *related to factors inhibiting successful eating patterns to maintain weight* (NANDA-I © 2012)	
Outcome: Maintain normal nutrition. ***Evaluation Parameters:*** Current weight is compared to BMI charts and height–weight charts to determine level of malnutrition (mild, moderate, or severe). The nurse must use the evaluation parameters that correlate with the etiology of the nutritional deficit. See charts in this chapter for specific deficits in specific disease processes. Food intake is less than energy expenditure.	Ask patient/family to list the foods and portion sizes consumed for the last 24 hours and the past 3 *days to assess adequacy of calorie intake.* Explore nutritional beliefs, cultural and religious attitudes toward food, food taboos, use of alcohol, medication and OTC use, and problems with dentition or self-feeding difficulties *to determine factors that impact food intake.* List the calorie count for each food consumed *to determine adequacy of calorie intake.* Measure triceps skinfold, mid-arm muscle circumference in the younger but not the older patient *to determine baseline for muscle wasting.*
3. NURSING DIAGNOSIS: Ineffective Health Maintenance *related to disease factors that can result in loss of weight* (NANDA-I © 2012)	
Outcome: Identification and management of disease/s that caused weight loss. ***Evaluation Parameters:*** Prealbumin levels within normal limits. BMI within normal limits.	Assess patient for risk factors for malnutrition *to determine problem priority.* Risk factors include acute and chronic illness, depression in the elderly, functional status, polypharmacy, and frailty. Assess patient for signs of impaired wound healing (e.g., pressure ulcers, fistulas), burns, muscle wasting, muscle weakness, loss of calcium, increased risk for falls leading to increased risk for fractures. *These factors indicate patient has high risk for malnutrition.* *In oncology patients, assess for weight loss >5%, which can result in increased mortality, poor response to chemotherapy, and treatment complications.*
4. NURSING DIAGNOSIS: Imbalanced Nutrition: Less Than Body Requirements *related to need to increase caloric intake* (NANDA-I © 2012)	
Outcome: Patient verbalizes changes to increase food intake. ***Evaluation Parameter:*** Weight gain of 1–2 lb per month for 6 months.	Reassess hospitalized patients weekly for nutritional status. Encourage balanced nutrition *to assess progress toward normal BMI.* Measure upper arm and thigh monthly *to assess growth in muscle mass.* Encourage small, frequent meals of foods that patient enjoys. *Potentially increases calorie intake.* For hospitalized patients: Monitor tolerance for prescribed tube feedings, total parenteral nutrition (TPN), and other nutritional support as needed, including electrolytes and vitamins *to prevent malnutrition.* Provide feeding assistance if needed; if assistance is provided, do not hurry the patient and sit down while feeding *so patient doesn't feel rushed to eat.* Place patient in an upright position while eating and for 30 minutes afterward *to prevent regurgitation.* Provide a pleasant environment for mealtime *to encourage the appetite.* Encourage communal environment for mealtime *to encourage social milieu and appetite.* Avoid prolonged NPO status while inpatient *because this contributes to further loss of intake.*

Source: Adapted from Wilkinson, J. M., & Ahearn, N. R. (2009). *Prentice Hall nursing diagnosis handbook* (9th ed.). Upper Saddle River, NJ: Prentice Hall.

Weblink: Lowering Your Cholesterol with TLC

pressure. Decades of research have shown the individual and additive effects on blood pressure reduction that occur due to weight reduction in overweight people, as well as by limiting sodium, alcohol, and total and saturated fat intake while consuming a diet rich in fruits, vegetables, and low-fat dairy products (Parikh, Lipsitz, & Natarajan, 2009). Current national guidelines recommend lifestyle modifications for all people for the primary prevention and management of high blood pressure using the Dietary Approaches for Stopping Hypertension (DASH) diet (USDHHS, 2010). Specific guidelines are outlined in Chart 8–11.

The nurse is uniquely positioned to be instrumental in detecting elevated blood pressure and educating patients on prevention and management of hypertension. In addition to weight management methods discussed in this chapter, the nurse can be involved in patient education and monitoring of other nutrition-related lifestyle modifications.

The primary source of sodium in the American diet is from packaged and processed foods, such as ready-to-eat foods or meals prepared by food manufacturers (American Heart Association, 2010b). The nurse should question the patient about eating patterns and preparation methods during the nutrition portion of a nursing assessment. Specifically asking about frequency of restaurant meals and use of table salt and convenience products is important to estimate sodium intake. Chart 8–12 lists sources of high-sodium foods.

The NIH's Dietary Approaches to Stopping Hypertension (DASH) diet has taken nutrition intervention for high blood pressure beyond the single low-sodium diet approach. The DASH diet emphasizes fruits, vegetables, nuts, and low-fat dairy while also containing reduced fat and saturated fat levels. The specific diet is associated with a reduction in blood pressure and risk of coronary heart disease (Chen, Maruther, & Appel, 2010). The DASH diet recommends the use of foods to attain its goals and remains silent on the use of supplements. Chart 8–13 outlines the DASH diet. The nurse should note that the DASH diet contains various calorie levels that can be used or modified as a weight reduction plan for the overweight patient.

Alcohol intake above one drink a day for women and small men or two drinks a day for men has been shown to have a negative effect on blood pressure (Goldstein et al., 2011). Although some patients tout the reputed cardioprotective effects of alcohol consumption, intake beyond the recommended limit is not conferring additional benefit. Overweight or obese patients trying to lose weight should be made aware of the significant calorie content that alcoholic beverages can contribute to the diet.

Coronary Heart Disease

Aggressive management of serum lipids is recommended as a primary strategy in the prevention and treatment of cardiovascular disease. Management of elevated serum low-density lipoprotein (LDL) cholesterol should receive priority attention because of its established association with increased risk of coronary heart disease (Kuller, 2011). Total cholesterol and high-density lipoprotein (HDL) cholesterol levels are also important predictors of cardiac risk.

The general population as well as those patients with established coronary heart disease can benefit from dietary approaches aimed at reducing serum lipids, controlling blood pressure, and managing body weight in an effort to reduce cardiac risk (Kuller, 2011). Diet modifications, called **therapeutic lifestyle changes (TLC),** are recommended as an initial strategy for treating elevated LDL cholesterol or in conjunction with pharmacologic intervention when indicated. Medical nutrition therapy for hyperlipidemia and coronary heart disease targets reduction of both lipid and nonlipid cardiac risk factors. A fat-controlled diet coupled with weight management and increased physical activity comprises the foundation of the therapeutic lifestyle changes. Therapeutic lifestyle changes are outlined in Chart 8–14.

Saturated Fats and Cholesterol

The NCEP guidelines focus on reducing dietary saturated fat and cholesterol. A dose response exists between saturated fat intake and serum LDL cholesterol (NHLBI, 2007). Saturated fats exist primarily in fats from animal-based foods such as fatty meats or whole-milk dairy products. Tropical fats are also saturated fats and include palm oil, coconut oil, and cocoa butter. Hydrogenated and *trans* fats are included in the recommendation to reduce saturated fat intake. These fats originate as *un*saturated oils, but become saturated during food processing when the manufacturer removes hydrogen molecules to make a fat that is more solid at room temperature. Examples include fats used in shortening, stick margarine, and many baked goods and snacks. High intake of dietary cholesterol is associated with increased LDL cholesterol. Dietary cholesterol is present only in foods of animal

CHART 8–11 Lifestyle Modifications for Hypertension

Lifestyle Component	Recommendation
Weight Management	Practice weight reduction or management of normal weight.
Diet	Eat a diet rich in fruits, vegetables, and low-fat dairy foods that is low in saturated and total fat.
	Reduce sodium intake to not more than 2,400 mg or 6 g NaCl daily.
	Limit alcohol to not more than 2 drinks a day for men and not more than 1 drink a day for women and small men. One drink is 12 oz beer, 5 oz wine, or 1-$^1/_2$ oz 80-proof spirits.
Physical Activity	Engage in physical activity at least 30 minutes most days.

Source: National Heart, Lung, and Blood Institute. (2007). Your guide to lowering your cholesterol with therapeutic lifestyle changes. Retrieved September 15, 2011, from http://www.nhlbi.nih.gov/health/public/heart/chol/chol_tlc.pdf.

CHART 8–12 Dietary Sources of High Sodium

- In general, processed, preserved, and convenience foods are high in sodium. Terms such as *pickled, cured, dehydrated, smoked, seasoned, ready-to-eat,* and *added sauce* hint at a high sodium content.
- Plain forms of most foods have low or moderate sodium content. Fresh fruit, juice, fresh or plain frozen vegetables, plain grains and breads, milk, plain meat, poultry, fish, and dried beans, peas, and lentils are not naturally high in sodium.
- Canned vegetables, frozen vegetables with sauce, canned tomato products, grain mixes, cured or luncheon meats, cheeses, canned meat, fish, beans and poultry, and boxed or frozen meals are higher in sodium than their fresh or plain counterparts.
- Foods labeled "reduced sodium" have 25% less sodium than the original, but may not be low in sodium. Foods labeled "low sodium" have 140 mg sodium or less per serving.

CHART 8–13 DASH Eating Plan: Number of Daily Servings for Other Calorie Levels

Food Groups	Servings/Day		
	1,600 Calories/Day	2,600 Calories/Day	3,100 Calories/Day
Grains*	6	10–11	12–13
Vegetables	3–4	5–6	6
Fruits	4	5–6	6
Fat-free or low-fat milk and milk products	2–3	3	3–4
Lean meats, poultry, and fish	3–6	6	6–9
Nuts, seeds, and legumes	3/week	1	1
Fats and oils	2	3	4
Sweets and added sugars	0	≤2	≤2

*Whole grains are recommended for most grain servings as a good source of fiber and nutrients.

Source: U.S. Department of Health and Human Services. (2010). *Dietary Guidelines for Americans, 2010 edition.* Retrieved February 25, 2011, from http://www.cnpp.usda.gov/dietaryguidelines.

CHART 8–14 Therapeutic Lifestyle Changes for Cardiovascular Disease

Lifestyle Component	Recommendation
Diet	Saturated fat: <7% total daily calorie intake. *Trans* fatty acids should also be limited.
	Monounsaturated fat: up to 20% total daily calorie intake.
	Polyunsaturated fat: up to 10% total daily calorie intake.
	Total fat: 25% to 35% total daily calorie intake.
	Cholesterol: <200 mg/day.
	Fiber: 20–30 g/day with consideration given to include 10–25 g soluble fiber daily.
	Carbohydrate: 50% to 60% of total daily calorie intake.
	Emphasize whole grains, fruits, and vegetable sources.
	Protein: approximately 15% of total daily calorie intake.
	Energy intake to maintain desirable weight and prevent weight gain.
Weight Management	Maintain desirable weight, avoid weight gain, lose weight if indicated.
Physical Activity	Increase physical activity. Energy balance to include at least 200 calories of energy expenditure from moderately intense activity most days.

Source: National Heart, Lung, and Blood Institute. (2007). Your guide to lowering your cholesterol with therapeutic lifestyle changes. Retrieved September 15, 2011, from http://www.nhlbi.nih.gov/health/public/heart/chol/chol_tlc.pdf.

origin. Fatty and organ meats, egg yolks, and shellfish are among the higher sources of dietary cholesterol.

Unsaturated Fats

Unsaturated fats, which are liquid at room temperature, are not associated with elevated LDL cholesterol. The monounsaturated fats present in olive, peanut, and canola oils and most nuts and avocado have been shown to lower LDL cholesterol when substituted for saturated fats in the diet (NHLBI, 2007). Polyunsaturated fats also can foster a decrease in saturated fats when substituted for saturated fats but can adversely contribute to a small decrease in beneficial HDL cholesterol as well (NHLBI, 2007). Sources of polyunsaturated fats include corn, safflower, sunflower, and soybean oils; these, and others, appear in Chart 8–15, which lists practical interventions that can be used to make therapeutic lifestyle changes.

Carbohydrate and Fiber

Carbohydrate can be substituted for saturated fat as a strategy for decreasing LDL cholesterol (NHLBI, 2007). However, high carbohydrate intake exceeding 60% of the diet's energy value has been associated with a decrease in HDL cholesterol and an increase in serum triglycerides, neither of which is beneficial to cardiac risk (NHLBI, 2007). Carbohydrate-containing plant foods that contain fiber, specifically soluble fiber, are recommended for their cholesterol-lowering capabilities (Anderson et al., 2009). Soluble fiber is associated with a 3% to 5% reduction of LDL cholesterol when 5 to 10 grams are consumed daily (NHLBI, 2007). Soluble fiber is present in several plant foods such as oats, oat bran, legumes, and barley. Chart 8–15 lists additional sources of soluble fiber.

Plant Sterol and Stanol Esters

Plant sterol and stanol esters are poorly absorbed derivatives of soybean and wood oils that have been reported to lower total and LDL cholesterol up to 20% with maximum effective intake of 2 g/daily (Cleveland Clinic, 2011). Several brands of margarine and salad dressings exist that have sterol or stanol esters listed as ingredients on the label.

CHART 8–15 Practical Interventions to Achieve Therapeutic Lifestyle Changes (TLC)

Choose	Limit
Monounsaturated and polyunsaturated fats, oils, and margarines to replace saturated fat ingredients: • Olive oil, canola oil, peanut oil = mono • Sunflower, soybean, safflower, corn, sesame = poly Lower fat and saturated fat protein foods: Dried beans, peas, lentils, soy (these also contain soluble fiber) Skinless poultry Fish Lean, trimmed cuts of meat (round/loin) Fat-free and low-fat dairy foods Omega-3 polyunsaturated fat sources: Fish: deep, cold-water fish such as salmon, tuna, bluefish, mackerel Flaxseed Canola oil Nuts Soy Low-fat food preparation methods: Bake, grill, sauté w/ broth or cooking spray Remove fat/skin from meat and poultry before cooking Use low-fat marinades Substitute low-fat ingredients in recipes for high fat version Five or more fruits and vegetables daily. Soluble fiber sources include fruit and vegetables w/edible skins. Whole grains, including soluble fiber sources such as oats, oat bran, barley.	Saturated fat and cholesterol sources Fats that are hard at room temperature tend to be saturated fats: Fatty meats, luncheon meats, organ meats Poultry w/skin Whole-fat dairy products Commercial baked goods made with *trans* and hydrogenated fats or lard Tropical oils found in processed foods: palm oil, cocoa butter, coconut oil Stick margarine, shortening, lard High-fat food preparation methods: Deep-fat or pan frying Adding sauces, gravies, creams, creamy dressings, or mayonnaise to foods Leaving on poultry skin or visible meat fat during cooking Recipes with high oil, butter, margarine, lard, cream, or full-fat cheese content

Source: National Heart, Lung, and Blood Institute. (2007). Your guide to lowering your cholesterol with therapeutic lifestyle changes. Retrieved September 15, 2011, from http://www.nhlbi.nih.gov/health/public/heart/chol/chol_tlc.pdf.

Soy Protein

Soy protein has been investigated for its role in lowering plasma LDL cholesterol, especially when consumed with soluble fibers and used to replace animal proteins. While early research results found an important link between soy intake and cholesterol, more recent research has found that the effect is less significant than originally reported (Taku, Umegaki, Taki, Endoh, & Watanabe, 2007). Soy protein can be found in soybeans, tofu, soy milk, and many soy "meat" alternatives.

Omega-3 Fatty Acids

Omega-3 fats are associated with decreased risk of cardiac events and prevention of coronary heart disease (O'Keefe, Carter, & Lavie, 2009). Reduction of plasma triglycerides, decreased platelet aggregability, reduction in cardiac dysrhythmias, and improvement in endothelial dysfunction all play a role in the mechanism (Riediger, Othman, Suh, & Moghadasian, 2009). The American Heart Association recommends intake of oily fish twice a week for the general adult population and 1 g/day of omega-3 fats from fish or a fish oil supplement in those with existing atherosclerosis (American Heart Association, 2010a). One serving of a fatty fish such as salmon or bluefish has 900 mg of omega-3 fat. Plant sources of omega-3 fats contain smaller amounts of these fats in a serving and include flaxseed and canola oil. The nurse should caution patients who choose to take supplemental forms of omega-3 fats about negative side effects as outlined in the Safety Alert.

Safety Alert *Omega-3 supplements decrease platelet aggregability. Take care to assess patients for any interaction with medications such as Coumadin or aspirin therapy that potentiate this effect. Additionally, assess for other dietary supplements and herbs with antiplatelet action, such as garlic, feverfew, ginkgo biloba, and vitamin E. Make sure the patient respects proper dosage recommendations of any omega-3 fat supplements.*

Alcohol

A moderate intake of alcohol can reduce the risk of coronary heart disease in adults (Goldstein et al., 2011). Moderation is described as no more than one drink per day for a woman and two per day for a man. Wine, specifically red wine, has received great focus when researching the potential cardioprotective effects of alcohol, yet most studies do not support reduced cardiac risk with a specific type of alcohol (Goldstein et al., 2011). Red wine is singled out by some because of its antithrombolytic action and antioxidant content, perhaps contributing additional benefits over other types of alcohol. Higher intake of alcohol does not confer additional cardioprotection, can be the source of excess calorie intake, and can contribute to an elevated triglyceride level in addition to other medical risks (O'Keefe, Carter, & Lavie, 2009). There is little justification to recommend drinking alcohol to patients who do not already do so.

Other Dietary Supplements and Botanicals

Antioxidant vitamins such as vitamins E and C have been investigated for a possible role in reducing coronary heart disease. To date, observations made in epidemiologic studies regarding these antioxidants have not illustrated a reduction in cardiac risk when investigated in controlled clinical trials, and in some cases are associated with increased risk (Sesso et al., 2008).

Many other dietary supplements, including herbs, have received attention for possible roles in the reduction of cholesterol or other cardiac risk factors. Red yeast rice may have modest benefits in those individuals who are intolerant to statin drugs used to treat hypercholesterolemia, but there is marked variability in the content and quality of commercially available products (Becker et al., 2009; Gordon, Cooperman, Obermeyer & Becker, 2010). Supplemental garlic has been investigated for a mild cholesterol-lowering effect compared to placebo in some trials, but not others (Frishman, Beverol, & Carosella, 2009). These examples serve as reminders of the uncertainty of using dietary supplements without clinical evidence of efficacy. Controlled research on supplements is limited, making it difficult to make a good clinical recommendation when queried by patients seeking to avoid or augment the use of pharmacologic therapies. Current lack of research and limited knowledge regarding safety does not support the use of these products in treating coronary heart disease. Additionally, standardization of supplement dosing and ingredients is lacking in the United States, creating uncertainty when choosing underresearched products. Despite the lack of standardization and research, many consumers are willing to try these supplements and may not volunteer this information to their health care providers. The nurse should assess patients for use of supplements and discuss the lack of clinical studies, any safety concerns, and the potential for drug–supplement interactions.

Weight Management

Overweight and obesity are associated with an increased risk of coronary heart disease, among other comorbid conditions (American Heart Association, 2011). Weight management is included in the TLC recommendations for targeting LDL cholesterol reduction. Weight loss of even a few pounds has been reported to reduce LDL cholesterol (NHLBI, 2007). The NCEP and the American Heart Association encourage weight loss through decreased energy intake and increased physical activity. Prevention of weight gain is emphasized (American Heart Association, 2011; NHLBI, 2007). A balanced low-fat diet containing all food groups is stressed for long-term benefit and overall health. A reduction in sedentary time and the addition of moderate physical activity on most days is also encouraged. Weight reduction was discussed earlier in the chapter.

Metabolic Syndrome

Recently a cluster of cardiovascular risk factors, referred to as *metabolic syndrome,* has been defined as having three out of the five following conditions: (1) abdominal obesity, (2) high triglycerides, (3) low HDL-C, (4) high blood pressure, and (5) fasting glucose (≥110 mg/dL). The presence of metabolic syndrome can place the overweight patient at additional cardiac risk. Overweight patients with abdominal obesity (apple shape), elevated triglycerides, low HDL cholesterol levels, high blood pressure, or elevated fasting glucose should be assessed for the metabolic syndrome as discussed in Chapter 32. Treatment recommendations begin with a 3-month trial of standard TLCs emphasizing LDL cholesterol reduction and weight loss. If parameters of metabolic syndrome are still present after 3 months, intensified weight loss efforts are indicated. Elevated triglycerides of ≥500 mg/dL should be attended to urgently because of an associated risk of pancreatitis (NHLBI, 2007). A very-low-fat diet (≤15% of daily calorie needs from fat), weight loss, physical activity, and possible pharmacologic intervention are indicated with this level of hypertriglyceridemia (NHLBI, 2007).

Much attention has been given to the concept of carbohydrate-containing foods and elevated postprandial plasma glucose levels, especially in individuals with insulin resistance at risk for metabolic syndrome. Diets that are high in carbohydrate (>60%) are associated with elevated triglycerides and lowered HDL cholesterol. Individuals with metabolic syndrome or insulin resistance can benefit from replacement of dietary saturated fat with unsaturated fats, specifically monounsaturates, as an alternative to adding carbohydrate food sources to replace needed calories (Finley, Barlow, Halton, & Haskell, 2010).

Additionally, the nurse should encourage high-fiber fruits, vegetables, and whole grains as choices for needed carbohydrate sources, nutrient composition, and to promote satiety. Fiber intake has been shown to have benefit in postprandial glycemic control and improvement of blood lipid levels in diabetic patients (Finley, Barlow, Halton, & Haskell, 2010).

Heart Failure

A low-sodium diet is prescribed as medical nutrition therapy for cardiac failure. Reduction of dietary sodium along with pharmacologic intervention can help reduce extracellular fluid burden and reduce cardiac workload. Commonly, a 2-g sodium restriction is recommended (see Chart 8–12 for a list of high-sodium foods). A 2-g sodium restriction requires the elimination of table salt use and replacement of high-sodium processed foods with unprocessed versions. The use of low-sodium specialty foods is not necessary to comply with the diet unless the patient's situation requires ongoing use of processed foods.

Patients who are on loop diuretics to manage fluid balance should also have thiamin supplementation from a multivitamin. This recommendation is important because loop diuretics cause thiamin loss in the urine and thiamin deficiency symptoms mimic those of heart failure (Wooley, 2008).

Advanced cardiac failure can place increased metabolic needs on the patient when lung function becomes compromised and respiration is altered. Increased respiratory rate and use of auxiliary muscles for labored breathing can increase the body's caloric requirement. Fatigue, early satiety, restrictive diet, and medication side effects can hamper appetite and put the patient at further risk for malnutrition. The term **cardiac cachexia** describes the consequences and physical symptoms seen in advanced cardiac failure when nutritional needs go unmet and muscle and fat wasting ensue.

The nurse should monitor patients for signs of weight loss that can be masked by edema. Temporal wasting, loss of adipose muscle, and lack of strength can be indicative of malnutrition. The patient should be encouraged to consume small, frequent meals to minimize early satiety and difficulty with breathing. Nutrient-dense foods high in protein and calories should be encouraged to maximize intake and "make every bite count." In patients consuming insufficient calories, it is prudent to evaluate their intake of sodium. Sodium intake in these cases may be extremely low because of the lack of general intake. Appropriate consideration can be given to allowing intake of some higher sodium foods to promote intake while remaining within the parameters of an overall sodium-restricted diet. Chart 8–16 lists food suggestions for improving intake in patients at risk for cardiac cachexia.

CHART 8–16 Suggested Nutrition Interventions for Cardiac Cachexia

Add "More Calories per Bite"	Add calorie sources to existing foods: • Butter, gravy,* sauces,* dressings* • Grated cheese* • Powdered milk mixed into regular milk • "Double milk" in baking recipes, desserts, soups,* milkshakes.
Increase Intake of Nutrient-Dense Foods	• Encourage more intake at the start of the day or start of the meal when intake is best • Limit mealtime liquids to avoid fullness • Consume high-protein desserts made w/egg or milk such as pudding, custard, ice cream • Frequent snacks of high energy, protein foods like yogurt, peanut butter on crackers,* cheese* • Cream soup* vs. clear soup, juice vs. water.

Monitor overall sodium intake and urge lower-sodium versions if intake is high.

Diabetes Mellitus

Medical nutrition therapy is an essential lifestyle component in the management of diabetes mellitus. Nutrition choices and habits following recommended guidelines can improve glycemic control and reduce the risk of diabetic complications, such as macrovascular disease, in patients with existing disease (American Diabetes Association, 2008). Additionally, lifestyle modifications, including diet, have a positive effect on disease reduction in those with impaired glucose tolerance and at risk for type 2 diabetes from developing the disease. Goals of medical nutrition therapy for diabetes include maintenance of blood glucose and blood lipids, as well as maintaining blood pressure in the normal range to prevent complications from diabetes while providing adequate nutrition (American Diabetes Association, 2008).

The nutrition recommendations for diabetic patients have evolved beyond the old-school "ADA" diet (named for the American Diabetes Association), in which a specific calorie level was prescribed by the health care provider based on an exchange list of foods according to carbohydrate, protein, and fat content. The ADA (2008) no longer recommends any single type of meal plan for all type 1 or type 2 diabetic individuals and urges that this terminology no longer be used.

Current recommendations call for attention to a healthy diet that is mindful of carbohydrate content, matching food choices and consistency of intake to individual needs. The overall diet also should incorporate TLCs known to reduce risk of coronary heart disease through the prevention of dyslipidemia, overweight, and high blood pressure. Rather than provide a blanket recommendation of a specific diet, the focus is now on individual management decisions. The patient is to be included in decision making along with the treatment team. The ADA (2008) recommends that the registered dietitian be the treatment team member who provides the medical nutrition therapy, but that all team members are knowledgeable about its parameters.

Carbohydrate Recommendations

Carbohydrates are an essential component of a healthy diet. Diabetic patients are urged to include carbohydrates in the form of whole grains, fruits, vegetables, and low-fat milk products. Together with monounsaturated fats, combined intake of carbohydrate and monounsaturated fats should be 60% to 70% of total energy intake (ADA, 2008). The carbohydrate content of the diet and any given meal is determined individually. Some patients with type 1 diabetes adjust premeal insulin based on the meal's carbohydrate content, whereas others who are on a fixed dose of insulin keep a consistent pattern of day-to-day carbohydrate intake (ADA, 2008). Additionally, physical activity can require an adjustment of insulin or carbohydrate intake by some individuals because exercising muscle causes an increased uptake of plasma glucose. The treatment team and patient determine initial parameters for carbohydrate intake based on the registered dietitian's assessment of nutritional needs. Adjustments are made over time to further individualize intake. Patients are educated to read carbohydrate content on food labels and to use a basic system of carbohydrate counting based on a food exchange system. Chart 8–17 provides an example of this system.

It is recommended that patients be educated to recognize their individual glycemic responses to varying foods, levels of activity, and any hypoglycemic agents and to incorporate this into the advice given by the treatment team. The nurse is instrumental in this educational effort.

The ADA (2008) reports that monitoring the glycemic index of foods may offer a modest benefit to glucose control over just monitoring carbohydrate intake. **Glycemic index** is a term that refers to how quickly the food raises blood glucose compared to an equal amount of

CHART 8–17 Sample Carbohydrate Counting for Diabetes Management

Food Group	Serving Size Examples	Grams of Carbohydrate
Starches (grains, breads, cereals, legumes, starchy vegetables)	1/2 cup cooked pasta or rice, 1-oz slice equivalent (bread, rolls, and buns), 3/4 cup cold cereal, 1/4 potato	15
Fruit	1 small piece, 1/2 cup canned or frozen	15
Vegetables	1 cup raw or 1/2 cup cooked greens	5
Dairy	1 cup milk or 2/3 cup plain yogurt	12
Miscellaneous foods w/carbohydrate (snack foods, desserts, etc.)	Read label for portion	15

Note: An RD would help determine an individual carbohydrate recommendation for a patient. Patients monitor grams of carbohydrate in their diet or use a system of "carbohydrate choices." One carbohydrate choice is the serving of a food with ~15 g of carbohydrate. Portions are important to accurately judge intake. Patients learn to manage the diet by reading labels and utilizing the generic exchange system in this chart for carbohydrate-containing foods. Foods not containing carbohydrate (meats, fish, poultry, cheese, fats) must be monitored to avoid cardiovascular risk, but are not part of the carbohydrate-counting system.

Sources: American Diabetes Association & American Dietetic Association. (2010). *Count your carbs: Getting started.* Eat Right: Academy of Nutrition and Dietetics; American Diabetes Association & American Dietetic Association. (2010); American Diabetes Association (2008).

carbohydrate from glucose or white bread. Foods that have a higher glycemic index cause a higher postprandial glucose response compared to those with a lower glycemic index. When asked for glycemic index advice by patients, the nurse can encourage intake of recommended plant sources of carbohydrate such as high-fiber fruits, vegetables, and whole grains. High-fiber carbohydrates, especially soluble fiber sources, have been shown to benefit glycemia, and a high-fiber diet may be a de facto form of a low-glycemic index diet (ADA, 2008).

While glycemic index may be helpful, no type of carbohydrate is prohibited from the diet. Sucrose (table sugar) and other traditionally taboo, empty-calorie "sweets" sources of carbohydrate are allowed, but within the context of an overall healthy diet. The carbohydrate content of these foods should be calculated and considered along with all other carbohydrates in the diet.

Fat Recommendations

Aggressive lipid management and prevention of coronary heart disease are important goals for diabetics (ADA, 2008). Saturated fat and cholesterol intake should be limited to assist the patient with management of LDL cholesterol levels. Guidelines outlined under medical nutrition therapy for coronary heart disease in this chapter should also be followed for the patient with diabetes. Monounsaturated fats or carbohydrates should be encouraged as calorie replacements for displaced saturated fat in patients seeking to maintain energy balance and body weight. Patients attempting weight loss doubly benefit from reduced saturated fat intake by not replacing saturated fat with equivocal calorie sources, therefore fostering a deficit of energy intake. Substitution of monounsaturated fats over carbohydrates is preferred for individuals with elevated triglycerides, elevated postprandial glucose, or low HDL cholesterol. However, this recommendation should be assessed on an individual basis because excess calorie intake from fats and weight gain can ensue if fat is taken *ad libitum* (ADA, 2008). Consumption of fatty fish is encouraged for the cardiovascular disease benefits associated with omega-3 fats as discussed earlier.

Vitamin and Mineral Recommendations

The position of the ADA is that no clear evidence exists to support any different advice on vitamin and mineral intake specific to people with diabetes than already exists for the general population. Research on antioxidants for their potential effects on clinical outcome has yielded no conclusion specific to people with diabetes. Chromium has also been investigated for its role in blood glucose control, but results are limited and seem to apply only to those who have a chromium deficiency, which is uncommon. Thiamine, pyridoxine (B_6), and vitamin B_{12} are used by some to treat diabetic neuropathy, but the efficacy of this is not clear and the ADA does not support this practice (ADA, 2008).

Alcohol Recommendations

Like much of the nutritional advice for people with diabetes, alcohol recommendations coincide closely with those for the general adult population. People with diabetes must be aware of the potential hypoglycemic and hyperglycemic effects of alcohol and consume any intake along with food (ADA, 2008). Moderate intake is stressed in those who do choose to consume alcohol.

Special Considerations

Additional dietary considerations need to be made for the patient with diabetes who is acutely ill, having surgery, or experiencing other specific circumstances. Changes in diet and insulin needs occur under special circumstances.

Overweight and Obesity

Patients with diabetes who are also overweight or obese can benefit from weight management. Weight loss specifically in people with type 2 diabetes can lessen insulin resistance and decrease the risk of coronary heart disease (ADA, 2009). The nurse can encourage and support even small amounts of weight loss in these patients. Lifestyle changes for weight reduction outlined earlier in the chapter coincide with recommendations for the patient with diabetes (ADA, 2008).

Exercise and Type 1 Diabetes

Glucose uptake is increased by exercising muscle. A patient can compensate for this effect by reducing insulin before planned exercise or with consumption of carbohydrate. Patients with diabetes should consult with their treatment team before starting a new or different exercise regimen. A registered dietitian could advise the patient on suitable food or beverage choices to fit the intensity, type, and duration of exercise given these parameters for glucose uptake.

Hypoglycemia

Blood glucose levels of ≤50 mg/dL require immediate treatment, whereas those in the range of 60 to 80 mg/dL can follow a decision-making process determined by the health care team. Glucose is the preferred form of carbohydrate replacement to treat hypoglycemia because of its quick glycemic response compared with other sources, but any carbohydrate source can be used. Guidelines call for an initial 15- to 20-g ingestion of carbohydrate followed by a reevaluation of blood glucose approximately 60 minutes later (ADA, 2009). The nurse can guide the patient in pinpointing potential contributors to low blood sugar and suggest interventions to avoid future episodes.

Special considerations for older adults with diabetes are discussed in the Gerontological Considerations section at the end of the chapter.

Disorders of the Gastrointestinal Tract

Disorders of the gastrointestinal (GI) tract can affect overall health by altering digestion or absorption of food and nutrients. Minor GI complaints are commonplace and may have little impact on nutrition health if short term. Chronic GI conditions or disease can lead to altered intake of food or compromised absorption. Medical nutrition therapy plays a central role in the treatment of most GI diseases.

Swallowing Dysfunction

Dysphagia, or difficulty swallowing, can occur for a number of reasons. Dysphagia is associated with head and neck trauma or disease, neuromuscular disease, stroke, and dementia. Sedation and other medication side effects can impact swallowing directly or indirectly because of diminished saliva production. Difficulty swallowing can lead to an inability to handle oral liquid boluses. Aspiration or loss of fluid volume from drooling or spitting liquids can also lead to dehydration because of diminished intake. Patients can become fearful of drinking liquids and voluntarily self-restrict fluid. Similarly, chewing and swallowing more solid foods can be risky or difficult, so patients may be unable to safely consume adequate nutrition orally. Unmanaged dysphagia can lead to aspiration pneumonia, dehydration, weight loss, and asphyxiation (Bottino-Bravo & Thomson, 2008).

The nurse should conduct a bedside evaluation to screen for dysphagia. The presence or absence of a gag reflex is not considered an accurate assessment tool. Silent aspiration can occur with few overt symptoms and requires a formal assessment to diagnose (Bottino-Bravo & Thomson, 2008). Warning signs of dysphagia during feeding include drooling or food spilling from the mouth; pocketing of food in the cheek or under the tongue or palate; repeated attempts to swallow a single food bolus; complaints of food sticking or heartburn while eating; and frequent throat clearing or coughing while eating.

Patients with symptoms of dysphagia should be referred to the interdisciplinary team for a thorough evaluation. Speech/language pathologists (SLPs) and advanced practice nurses are the experts in management of swallowing problems and typically guide the team in treatment. A dietitian works closely with the team to accommodate appropriate texture modifications to the diet to ensure safe swallowing and provision of adequate fluid and nutrition. The goal of medical nutrition therapy is to reduce choking risk while providing adequate nutrition.

Without attention to preparation, texture modification to the diet can be presented in an unattractive fashion. Pureed or chopped meals can be made more attractive with sauces, gravies, colorful garnishes, and casseroles rather than being served as lumpy mounds with an ice cream scoop. The nurse should help ensure that the patient has meals in as attractive a surrounding as possible to improve the eating environment. To improve nutrition, whenever possible, the patient should not be interrupted during mealtime for tests or procedures.

When patients with dysphagia are evaluated and transition through various diet modifications, the nurse should monitor the patient for tolerance to texture changes. Foods that form a cohesive bolus are most easily handled and are often attempted first; thin liquids are generally most easily aspirated (Garcia, 2010). The nurse should become familiar with hospital protocol for the dysphagia diet, and learn which foods are permitted with each transitional stage. *Pureed, mechanically altered,* or *mechanical soft* are common terms for food consistency. Each patient should have an individualized prescription based on the hospital's dysphagia protocol, since an inadvertent mistake in meal delivery could lead to aspiration. The patient should be watched closely for signs of aspiration, food pocketing, or other dysphagia symptoms. Fluid status should be monitored to ensure adequate intake. Commercial products are available to thicken liquids or foods as appropriate. The nurse can also assist the patient with compensatory swallowing techniques or exercises prescribed by the SLP.

When patients are not able to safely consume adequate food or fluid, enteral nutrition support with a feeding tube is indicated. It is important to note that risk of aspiration still exists, as does the possibility of gastroesophageal reflux. Nursing interventions to minimize aspiration risk are outlined later in this chapter in the discussion on enteral nutrition support.

Gastroesophageal Reflux Disease, Hiatal Hernia, Esophagitis, and Ulcer Disease

Lifestyle modifications, including dietary manipulation, are used as an adjunct to other treatment throughout the course of therapy for disorders of the upper GI tract. Nutrition therapy is targeted to relieve symptoms from gastroesophageal reflux and mucosal irritation by gastric acid. Additionally, certain foods can precipitate reflux from specific effects on reducing lower esophageal sphincter (LES) pressure in some patients. For example, alcohol increases gastric acid production, decreases LES pressure, and delays gastric emptying (Vemulapalli, 2008). The nurse should assess the patient for intake of foods or habits that affect LES pressure or intra-abdominal pressure. Chart 8–18 provides general guidelines for adjunctive dietary treatment for gastroesophageal reflux disease (GERD). Individual patient food intolerances should be added to these guidelines. The nurse should assess the nutritional adequacy of the diet of patients who seem intolerant to many foods or those who have broadly eliminated any major food group, assuming intolerance to all of its constituents. An example of this would be patients who do not consume fruits due to poor tolerance of a citrus juice. Such patients need encouragement to try other foods within the food group to ensure adequate intake.

CHART 8–18 Nutrition Therapy for GERD

Limit foods that predispose to decreased lower esophageal sphincter pressure:	Fat Alcohol Coffee, tea, cola Chocolate Carminatives (mint).
Limit foods that irritate esophagus:	Citrus Tomato Spicy
Limit gastric pressure:	Avoid tight clothing, belts. Avoid large meals and excessive carbonated drinks. Avoid recumbency after meals. Lose weight if indicated.

Sources: American Gastroenterological Association. (2008). American Gastroenterological Association medical position statement on the management of gastroesophageal reflux disease. *Gastroenterology, 135,* 1383–1391; National Institute of Diabetes and Digestive and Kidney Diseases. (2007a). Heartburn, gastroesophageal reflux, and gastroesophageal reflux disease. Retrieved February 18, 2011, from http://digestive.niddk.nih.gov/ddiseases/pubs/gerd/; Vemulapalli, R. (2008). Diet and lifestyle modifications in the management of gastroesophageal reflux disease. *Nutrition in Clinical Practice, 23,* 293–298.

Dumping Syndrome

Dumping syndrome is a condition often resulting from full or partial gastric resection or the removal of the pyloric sphincter. Symptoms include abdominal cramping, diarrhea, sweating, and shakiness following a meal because of rapid emptying of gastric contents into the small intestine. Dumping syndrome can also result following bariatric surgery for morbid obesity. Postoperative nutrition guidelines for bariatric surgical patients are discussed later in this chapter.

The goals of nutrition treatment of dumping syndrome include the prevention of rapid gastric emptying and the reduction of hyperosmolar intestinal contents. Foods high in simple sugars have a concentrated, or hyperosmolar, content that will draw fluid into the gut because of a concentration gradient between plasma and the intestine. This rapid entry of fluid into the gut can contribute to the symptoms of dumping syndrome (NIDDK, 2007c). Large meals, fluids with meals, and extreme food temperatures (very hot or very cold) can promote more rapid gastric emptying than usual. Eating smaller meals, avoiding liquids at mealtime, and lying down following a meal can be helpful. Chart 8–19 outlines the nutrition guidelines for treating dumping syndrome.

Lactose Intolerance

Lactose is the principal disaccharide present in milk products that requires the small intestine enzyme lactase for digestion. Insufficient production of lactase can foster maldigestion of lactose-containing foods with resultant intestinal complaints, including bloating, cramping, and diarrhea. The nurse should help educate the patient that lactose intolerance is not an allergy to milk. Lactose maldigestion or intolerance is a common complaint among people with gastrointestinal symptoms. The prevalence of lactose-intolerance symptoms is high among many

Weblink: Rapid Gastric Emptying Weblink: Lactose Intolerance Weblink: Celiac Disease

CHART 8–19 Nutrition Guidelines for Dumping Syndrome

- Limit consumption of simple sugars and carbonated drinks.
- Avoid extremes of hot or cold foods.
- Eat small meals.
- Save liquid for between meals.
- Lie down if needed after eating.

Source: National Institute of Diabetes and Digestive and Kidney Diseases (NIDDK). (2007c). Rapid gastric emptying. Retrieved February 18, 2011, from http://digestive.niddk.nih.gov/ddiseases/pubs/rapidgastricemptying/index.htm.

ethnic groups with the exception of those of Northern European descent (Eadala, Waud, Matthews, Green, & Campbell, 2009). Insufficient lactase production can occur from birth, which is uncommon, or develop later in life. Secondary lactose intolerance can occur from damage to the small intestine mucosa, such as with infection, small bowel disease, chemotherapy, or intestinal radiation, and may be temporary. Individuals vary in their tolerance to different amounts of lactose, with some tolerating lactose better if it is consumed with foods or in smaller amounts.

A general consensus exists that most people who complain of lactose intolerance are capable of tolerating some lactose in their diets. Additionally, it is believed that tolerance to lactose can be improved with the continual consumption of some lactose-containing foods. Some milk-based foods, such as aged cheeses, naturally contain less lactose than others do. Many yogurts and other fermented dairy products have reduced lactose content and advantageous probiotic bacteria that have a lactase-producing ability that benefits digestion of lactose content (NIDDK, 2007b).

Because each patient with lactose intolerance has a different ability to produce lactose, medical nutrition therapy occurs along a continuum. The nurse should assess the patient for lactose tolerance among different milk-based foods and under different patterns of consumption. Lactose-containing foods tend to be better tolerated with a meal than when consumed alone. The patient's diet should be assessed for adequate calcium and vitamin D sources, especially for those who have broadly eliminated dairy foods from their diets. Chart 8–20 lists suggestions for improving tolerance to lactose and adequate intake of calcium and vitamin D.

CHART 8–20 Nutrition Guidelines for Lactose Intolerance

- Try 1/2 to 1 cup milk with meals.
- Gradually increase milk intake in small increments.
- Try cultured and fermented dairy products: yogurt with active cultures, buttermilk, aged cheese.
- Use digestive aides as needed: oral lactase enzyme products or enzyme-incubated milk.
- Monitor diet for adequate calcium and vitamin D intake.
- Be mindful of hidden lactose in baking mixes, processed foods, instant soups, mashed potato mix, cold cuts, commercial sauces, and medicines.
- Read labels for "nonfat milk solids" or "milk by-products" because lactose may be present.

Source: National Institute of Diabetes and Digestive and Kidney Diseases (NIDDK). (2007b). Lactose intolerance. Retrieved February 18, 2011, from http://digestive.niddk.nih.gov/ddiseases/pubs/lactoseintolerance/.

Inflammatory Bowel Disease

A diagnosis of either Crohn's disease or ulcerative colitis can place a patient at risk for malnutrition. Crohn's disease manifests itself through deeper layers of the intestinal mucosa than ulcerative colitis and thus predisposes the patient to higher risk of malnutrition. Active inflammatory bowel disease can cause diminished nutrient intake, increased gut nutritional losses, and additional metabolic requirements (Aghdassi, Wendland, Stapleton, Raman, & Allard, 2007). Together, or singly, these disease consequences present nutritional challenges to the patient and the clinician. Pain, anorexia, fever, and medication side effects can lead to poor intake in the face of the increased metabolic needs required for tissue healing and to compensate for malabsorptive losses. Patients with inflammatory bowel disease require a comprehensive nutrition assessment on which to base the foundation of nutrition therapy. Chart 8-21 lists common nutrition problems association with Crohn's disease.

Physical symptoms and disease severity will dictate the nutrition care plan. Small bowel disease in Crohn's can lead to malabsorption of multiple nutrients, depending on the specific location of the disease. Calcium, magnesium, iron, and other minerals are generally absorbed in the proximal small intestine, whereas vitamin B_{12}, fat, and fat-soluble vitamin absorption occur in the ileum. Fat malabsorption can lead to

RISK FACTORS for Malnutrition in Inflammatory Bowel Disease

Risk Factor	Etiology of Malnutrition Risk
Decreased Intake	Nausea, vomiting, diarrhea
	Pain or fear of pain
	Discomfort associated w/certain foods
	Anorexia
Increased Nutrient Losses	Malabsorption; depends on disease site
	Drug–nutrient interactions (sulfasalazine and folic acid, steroids and calcium, vitamin D)
	Iron losses w/bleeding
Increased Nutrient Needs	Hypermetabolism from inflammation
	Fistula healing requirements

CHART 8–21 Dietary Sources of Gluten

Label reading is essential. In addition to more obvious sources of barley, rye, and wheat, fillers and additives contain hidden sources of gluten that can be discovered by reading ingredient panels. Dietary sources of gluten include:

- Barley, including beer, malt beverages, and cereal
- Rye
- Wheat, including all wheat flour products (pastas, cereals, baked goods, pizza crust, etc.), wheat or food starch, couscous, durum flour, kamut, spelt, triticale, semolina, and some brands of soy sauce. Wheat or food starch is used in fillers in many products, including instant mixes, sauces, condiments, hot dogs, and sausages.
- Individuals should consult with their health care provider regarding an individual recommendation for the consumption of oats.

Source: National Institute of Diabetes and Digestive and Kidney Diseases (NIDDK). (2008). Celiac disease. Retrieved February 18, 2011, from http://digestive.niddk.nih.gov/ddiseases/pubs/celiac/index.htm.

a cascade of other nutritional problems, such as vitamin A, D, E, and K and calcium malabsorption; increased absorption of oxalates (with subsequent increased risk of oxalate kidney stones); and loss of the valuable energy derived from fat. Losses from diarrhea can compromise fluid and electrolyte status. Inadequate absorption of calcium and vitamin D can lead to bone disease and further complicate the nutritional consequences of the steroid therapy often used in these patients (O'Sullivan, 2009).

Anemia from blood losses and poor iron, folate, and vitamin B_{12} absorption can contribute further to the fatigue experienced from inadequate intake and the disease process. Enteric fistula formation can cause intestinal losses of crucial nutrients, as well as fluid and electrolytes. Surgical resection of diseased intestine can result in the loss of crucial absorptive surface and further place the patient at nutritional risk. Short bowel syndrome can result and is discussed in a later section. Knowledge of the extent and location of disease, along with a complete nutrition history, is essential to identify nutrition risk and goals.

Nutrition treatment of inflammatory bowel disease focuses on correction of malnutrition and provision of adequate nutrients and energy to promote disease remission. Patients with severe fulminant disease can require nutrition support in the form of a low-fat elemental or polymeric enteral nutrition formula, which is discussed later. These formulas can be taken orally or delivered via a feeding tube. Such formulas require minimal digestion for absorption and may be a more easily tolerated mode of providing nutrition than a usual diet, though palatability of some formulas is low. A registered dietitian will determine the appropriate type and amount of enteral nutrition support and make a recommendation for treatment.

The nurse should monitor intake and tolerance as described in the chapter discussion on enteral nutrition. Unless a patient has developed a bowel obstruction, perforation, or severe short bowel syndrome, there is no specific need for parenteral nutrition in disease treatment as compared with enteral support.

A low-fiber diet with adequate energy and protein is indicated as patients recover from a disease flare and transition to their usual diet. Fibrous fruits and vegetables, whole grains, seeds, and nuts are avoided to decrease fecal residue and stool frequency. Lactose-containing foods may need to be limited in patients for whom secondary lactose intolerance has developed. Due to a lack of small bowel involvement, patients with ulcerative colitis are not likely to benefit from altering lactose intake. As the patient improves, the diet can be liberalized as tolerated.

Nutrient supplementation is often indicated for patients unable to tolerate adequate variety in the diet or with active disease. Anemia should be treated with the appropriate dose of iron, folic acid, or vitamin B_{12}, depending on anemia type. Calcium supplementation to meet the federal Recommended Dietary Allowance (RDA) of 1,000 to 1,200 mg is indicated for patients with a limited diet, steroid therapy, or malabsorption. Adequate vitamin D is needed as well. Zinc is lost when there is high-volume intestinal output as with diarrhea or an enteric fistula. Wound healing, including fistula repair, requires zinc. Zinc replacement of 12 to 15 mg/day per liter of stool output or 20 to 40 mg/day zinc gluconate is recommended (Aghdassi et al., 2007). The nurse should routinely assess patients with inflammatory bowel disease for inadequate or overly restrictive intake and refer appropriate patients for nutritional counseling.

Celiac Sprue

Celiac sprue, celiac disease or gluten-sensitive enteropathy, is a lifelong condition affecting the small intestine in which the villi morphology is damaged from the presence of gluten in the diet. Gluten is a protein found in grain products, specifically wheat, rye, and barley. The presence of gluten in the intestine leads to villi atrophy and loss of absorptive surface. Diarrhea with malabsorption of most nutrients can follow with risk of weight loss and malnutrition.

Medical nutrition therapy is essential for the resolution of symptoms and return of normal villi morphology. Gluten-containing foods must be avoided to eliminate disease symptoms (NIDDK, 2008). There is agreement that foods made from wheat, rye, and barley should be eliminated, but considerable debate exists about several other grains. Oats have traditionally been excluded in the diet as well, but more recent evidence exists that oats do not exhibit toxicity and can be well tolerated (NIDDK, 2008). The chance of wheat contamination has led some to recommend avoidance of oats until disease remission and then only consumption of oat products from a trustworthy source (Dickey, 2008). Chart 8–21 outlines common dietary sources of gluten.

The patient with celiac sprue has to be dedicated to label reading and attentive to the diet at all times. Wheat, rye, and barley are present in both obvious and hidden sources in the diet. Some patients with celiac sprue also have secondary lactose intolerance and must adhere to guidelines for that treatment as well. Product reformulation can lead to changes that add or delete ingredients, so continued label reading is essential. The nurse should warn patients to be suspect of labels touting "new and improved" versions because ingredients could be altered. The nurse can be empathetic about the need for restrictions and stress the role of diet in avoiding ill health and correcting existing deficiencies.

Gluten-free versions of grain foods can replace the displaced wheat, rye, and barley products. Corn, potato, rice, and soy flours can be used to make alternative breads, pasta, and baked goods. Gluten-free recipes and products are increasingly available, both through local stores and Internet retailers. A local or online celiac sprue support group and a knowledgeable dietitian can provide patients with lists of available products. It is important to note that wheat flour products are commonly fortified with iron, folic acid, and other B-complex vitamins. Alternative gluten-free products often are not routinely fortified with these nutrients. Therefore, alternative sources of iron and B-complex vitamins should be encouraged. The limited diet warrants a recommendation of a gluten-free multivitamin supplement.

Short Bowel Syndrome

Short bowel syndrome (SBS) describes a set of symptoms that can result from a large surgical resection of any combination of small intestine and colon. Most commonly, the resection is a result of a single or several surgical interventions for inflammatory bowel disease. Bowel infarct, gastric bypass surgery, neoplastic disease treatment, and congenital abnormalities are among other etiologies of SBS. In some forms of gastric bypass surgery for morbid obesity, the loss of small intestine absorptive surface is initiated in a deliberate attempt to have malabsorption contribute to weight loss efforts. Such surgery and its related nutrition interventions are discussed later in the surgical nutrition section of this chapter. Symptoms of SBS can include rapid gut transit time, diarrhea, altered fluid and electrolyte status, malabsorption, and subsequent weight loss and malnutrition. Loss of absorptive surface and the presence of unabsorbed substrate in the colon are responsible for the symptoms.

A patient with <200 cm (6.5 ft) of small intestine is at risk for short bowel syndrome. Patients with <100 cm (3.3 ft) of remaining small intestine most likely will have some symptoms of this syndrome, especially if losses include the terminal ileum or the remaining bowel is diseased (Cagir, 2009). The terminal ileum is the site of reabsorption of bile salts that are responsible for fat and fat-soluble vitamin absorption. Additionally, vitamin B_{12} and some water and electrolyte absorption occur here. When all of these substances remain unabsorbed and pass into the colon, their hyperosmolar content draws fluid from the plasma that leads to diarrhea, malabsorption, and altered hydration. If both ileum and colon have been resected, an end jejunostomy is the result and has compromised absorptive ability (Cagir, 2009). Postsurgical intestinal adaptation can occur over the course of 1 to 2 years and improve absorptive capability. The ileum can adapt to compensate for the absorptive needs previously met by a resected jejunum, but conversely, the jejunum is less able to compensate for a resected ileum (Cagir, 2009).

Medical nutrition therapy for SBS is essential. Patients must receive adequate nutrition to promote wound healing and prevent malnutrition in the postoperative period. Initially, patients will require at least a 7- to 10-day course of parenteral nutrition to meet fluid, electrolyte, and nutritional demands while potential bowel function begins to return (Cagir, 2009). Gradual conversion to enteral nutrition occurs according to patient tolerance. Intestinal absorptive adaptation takes time and requires tolerance to some enteral nutrition in order to occur. When the patient is hemodynamically stable and bowel sounds return, sips of isotonic liquids can be attempted. Isotonic enteral formula and rehydration solutions are recommended (Cagir, 2009). Hypertonic liquids, such as elemental nutrition formula and sugary drinks, or hypotonic liquids (water or overly diluted drinks), are not recommended initially because of potential intestinal fluid and electrolyte shifts compensating for a concentration gradient. Sorbitol should be avoided in sugar-free beverages because of its laxative effect. The nurse should monitor the patient's fluid intake and tolerance with a careful comparison to measured fluid output. Laboratory values, such as sodium and potassium, should also be monitored to assess hydration and electrolyte status. Sodium, potassium, magnesium, and zinc losses can be substantial and may require replacement (Cagir, 2009). Patients will vary in their ability to successfully attempt this stage of diet transition. Some may require months of parenteral support first.

After several months of tolerance to enteral formula, the patient with SBS can begin the challenging process of further intestinal adaptation with a more solid diet. A modified diet is encouraged as tolerated following the parameters outlined in Chart 8–22. The diet may be modified to include less lactose and low oxalate content, but not low fat. Altering fat has little effect on symptoms and deprives the patient of needed calories. A lactose-modified diet is recommended only if lactose maldigestion in known. Patients with SBS and an existing colon are at risk for increased absorption of oxalate (Cagir, 2009). Oxalate, a substance found in foods such as spinach, chocolate, tea, and rhubarb, is normally bound with calcium and poorly absorbed. However, during fat malabsorption, calcium binds with free fats, leaving oxalates unbound and more apt to be absorbed by the intestine. Eventually such elevated oxalate absorption can lead to calcium oxalate kidney stones.

Nutrient supplementation is often necessary if the ileum has been resected. Fat-soluble vitamins A, D, E, and K are needed in a liquid form if **steatorrhea,** or diarrhea from fat malabsorption, is present. Steatorrhea can be confirmed with a laboratory analysis using a Sudan stain of a stool sample. Zinc replacement is also necessary. Calcium supplements are needed if a lactose modification is needed or fat malabsorption is present. Calcium supplements can assist with lessening oxalate absorption. The need for magnesium replacement should also be assessed with blood analysis. Vitamin B_{12} injections are needed in

CHART 8–22 Nutrition Therapy for Short Bowel Syndrome

Early Diet	• Use isotonic feedings to minimize diarrhea. • Replace fluid and electrolyte losses. • Determine nutrients at risk for malabsorption based on resection site.
Adaptation	• Maximize intake of energy (including fat) and protein, adjust to tolerance. • Give frequent meals w/liquids separately. • Dilute sugary drinks.
General Recommendations	• Limit caffeine, oxalates, lactose, sugar alcohols (such as sorbitol, mannitol). • Monitor and replace electrolytes/minerals, including zinc, potassium, and magnesium. • Replace fat-soluble vitamins and B_{12} if ileum resected/fat malabsorbing.

patients without an ileum (Cagir, 2009). Patients who experience SBS require long-term monitoring by an experienced health care team to prevent malnutrition, dehydration, and altered electrolyte status.

Constipation

A high-fiber diet with adequate fluid intake is recommended for the treatment of most types of constipation. A low-fiber diet and sedentary lifestyle contribute to the occurrence of constipation in adults (Blackmer & Farrington, 2010). Fiber is present only in plant foods and can be removed during processing. Adequate fiber intake benefits intestinal motility by contributing to stool bulk and shortening intestinal transit time. The nurse should advise the patient to gradually add fiber to the diet in order to minimize intestinal bloating. Chart 8–23 outlines sources of fiber to recommend.

Diverticular Disease

Patients with uncomplicated diverticulosis should be encouraged to consume adequate fiber to lessen symptoms and potentially avoid diverticulitis. Although there is no evidence that a high-fiber diet will decrease intraluminal pressure and subsequent development of diverticula, the recommendation to consume sufficient fiber is felt to be a reasonable approach to ameliorate symptoms of this condition (NIDDK, 2008). Traditionally, most fiber sources have been recommended with the exception of seeds and nuts, which may foster diverticulitis when trapped in diverticulum. Current research suggests that these substances do not contribute to the risk of diverticular complications (Marcason, 2008).

Nutritional management of an episode of diverticulitis requires a short course of a clear liquid diet while medical treatment is given; symptoms typically abate within a few days. Patients who require surgical intervention, an extended course of no food or fluid intake (nil per os [NPO]), or more prolonged intake of clear liquids need close nutritional assessment and monitoring with appropriate referral to the registered dietitian as needed. Once diverticulitis is resolved and the patient is free of symptoms, the high-fiber diet should be resumed.

Chronic Diarrhea

Chronic diarrhea can occur for many reasons. Appropriate nutrition intervention is determined by the etiology of the diarrhea, if known. Patients in whom pancreatic exocrine function is compromised may require a low-fat diet as outlined in the nutrition treatment of pancreatic

CHART 8–23 Fiber Content of Selected Foods*

≤1 g Fiber	2 g Fiber	3 g Fiber	4 g Fiber	≥5 g Fiber
1-oz white bread	1-oz whole-wheat bread	1 med banana	1 C brown rice	1 C bran flake cereal
1 dinner roll, average	2 C popcorn	1 C corn	1/2 C cooked barley	1/2 C dried fruit
1 boiled potato without skin	1 C couscous	1/2 C winter squash	1 C cooked oatmeal	1/2 C cooked beans, peas, or lentils
1 C iceberg lettuce	1 medium peach	1/4 C soy nuts	1 med apple or pear with skin	1 C cooked collards
1 C mushrooms	1/2 C cooked carrots		1 med baked potato with skin	1 kiwi
			1 C cooked spinach	
			2 TBSP almonds	

*The nurse should advise the patient that fiber content is listed on the "Nutrition Facts" panel of the food label.

Source: USDA Nutrient Data Laboratory. (2011). http://www.nal.usda.gov/fnic/foodcomp/search.

disease. Small bowel disease and lactose intolerance can also result in chronic diarrhea if not adequately treated. (Nutrition therapy for each of these causes was discussed in an earlier section.) The nurse can assess the patient for excessive intake of sugar alcohols, such as sorbitol, which can contribute to diarrhea. The presence of eating disorder symptoms can cause the nurse to suspect laxative abuse, which can lead to chronic diarrhea. Patients with chronic diarrhea should be routinely assessed for fluid, electrolyte, weight loss, and nutrition depletion.

Irritable Bowel Syndrome

Irritable bowel syndrome (IBS) is characterized by abdominal pain, constipation, or diarrhea that has no known coexisting organic cause. Nutrition treatment is largely trial and error according to the individual patient's situation. Often a symptom diary is helpful to guide the patient in finding any lifestyle factors, including offending foods that trigger symptoms. No single food or food group has proven to universally contribute to symptoms, though a significant placebo effect was noticed in many research trials. Caffeine, alcohol, fat, and sorbitol are the most commonly mentioned trigger foods. Sorbitol is a sugar alcohol present in dietetic candies and foods that has a laxative effect.

Many patients with IBS can benefit from a psychosocial assessment and appropriate intervention because coexisting stress, coping difficulties, depression, and anxiety occur in these patients (Clark & DeLegge, 2008). The nurse can guide the patient in recognizing any individual foods that trigger symptoms and suggest experimenting with limiting caffeine, alcohol, sorbitol, and fat in the diet. Lactose intolerance is often a complaint because of similar symptoms, but can be unfounded. Lactose should be managed only in patients known to have lactase deficiency.

Liver Disease

The liver performs various functions related to the storage, metabolism, or excretion of most nutrients. Liver disease impacts nutrition status by decreasing nutrient storage and interfering with efficient metabolism. The body's ability to maintain nutritional health is altered when any aspect of nutrient metabolism is compromised by liver disease.

Fatty Liver

Deposition of fatty deposits in the liver can occur from excessive alcohol intake but can also be associated with etiology unrelated to alcohol. Many cases of fatty liver, or steatosis, are associated with nutritional contributors. Daily intake of more than 20 to 30 g of alcohol, obesity, severe weight loss (as in starvation or following gastric bypass surgery for obesity), total parenteral nutrition, elevated blood triglyceride levels found in type 2 diabetes, and metabolic syndrome are associated with steatosis (Tiniakos, Vos, & Brunt, 2010). Abstinence from alcohol, weight loss if overweight, and control of plasma glucose and lipids are the primary therapies for uncomplicated fatty liver.

Alcohol and Nutrition Status

Both primary and secondary malnutrition can occur from excessive alcohol intake. Poor quality food, infrequent food intake, and anorexia are examples of risk factors for primary malnutrition. Secondary malnutrition can occur because of indirect effects, such as the effects of alcohol on nutrient malabsorption and altered metabolism. Alcohol contains significant calories (7.1 per gram), which can be a concern for the casual drinker trying to maintain or lose weight. However, when intake of alcohol is excessive, weight loss occurs when significant food calories are replaced by alcohol. Chart 8–24 lists the contributing causes of both primary and secondary malnutrition with excessive alcohol intake.

The nurse should perform a careful assessment of the patient's nutritional status when excessive alcohol intake is suspected. Unfortunately, an accurate diet history is difficult to obtain if the patient has suffered periods of altered consciousness. Physical assessment of the patient should focus on skin integrity, presence of muscle or fat wasting, and edema or ascites. Altered fluid status can mask changes in body weight, making weight or BMI unreliable assessment tools for nutrition status. If liver disease is present, plasma protein production can be diminished

CHART 8–24 Effect of Alcohol on Nutrition Status

Primary Malnutrition	Replaces nutrient and food intake with alcohol. Appetite can be suppressed.
Secondary Malnutrition	Decreased nutrient absorption: • Thiamin • Vitamin B_{12} • Folate • Protein. Increased urinary losses of nutrients: • Folate • Zinc • Magnesium • Nitrogen. Decreased nutrient storage: • Folate • Vitamin B_6. • Riboflavin

unrelated to nutrition. Malnutrition can also lower serum albumin, prealbumin, or transferrin levels, but it is impossible to differentiate the major cause with the compounded effects of liver disease and poor nutrition status.

Nutrition supplementation is recommended for several nutrients when excessive alcohol intake is suspected or known and nutrition intake is poor. Special attention should be given to thiamin and folic acid as both nutrients are poorly absorbed in the presence of alcohol. Thiamin supplementation in the alcoholic patient is crucial to avoid development of Wernicke-Korsakoff syndrome (brain damage caused by a lack of vitamin B_1 [thiamine]). Thiamin is routinely administered on admission to patients suspected or known to abuse alcohol. Trace mineral status should be assessed, and deficiencies replaced accordingly. Abstinence from alcohol is the primary goal.

Hepatitis

Anorexia, fatigue, and gastrointestinal complaints are common symptoms with hepatitis that can place a patient at increased risk for malnutrition. Fever and hypermetabolism require closer than usual attention to energy intake and hydration. Nutrition care of a patient with hepatitis should stress the need for calories and protein to enhance hepatocyte regeneration and prevent weight loss. Patients can require an additional 40% more calories than normal (Amini & Runyon, 2010). Lack of appetite and nausea make meal consumption difficult. Small, more frequent, nutrient-dense meals can promote overall increased intake and help with nausea, which is often worsened by an empty stomach. A multivitamin supplement should be considered in patients with poor intake. Importantly, high doses of some vitamins, such as vitamin A, are hepatotoxic and should be avoided.

The nurse should assess the patient for self-prescribed use of supplements and provide education about consuming excesses. Additionally, the patient should be assessed for use of alternative medicine supplements. Many herbal supplements are hepatotoxic. Chaparral, comfrey, and mistletoe are examples of hepatotoxic herbs. Others, like milk thistle, are touted by some for their ability to improve liver function (Seeff et al., 2008). The nurse should consult with a pharmacist knowledgeable about herb safety and review the latest medical research when questions arise. Few recommendations exist on herbal remedies for liver disease, and this should not be misinterpreted to mean untested herbs are efficacious or safe.

Cirrhosis

Malnutrition can be a common complication in patients with cirrhosis. Poor nutrition is more likely to occur in cirrhosis from alcoholic liver disease than nonalcoholic liver disease. Nutrition status is related to the etiology of the liver disease as well as the severity of the disease. An accurate nutrition assessment is often complicated by the presence of edema and ascites, as well as decreased production of plasma proteins—all secondary to liver disease. Digestion, absorption, metabolism, and storage of nutrients are all negatively affected by cirrhosis. Poor glycogen storage with enhanced breakdown of fat and protein occurs and resembles metabolic alterations seen in short-term starvation. Decreased production of bile salts by the liver can cause energy loss from fat because of steatorrhea. Pancreatic exocrine insufficiency is found in alcoholic liver disease and can impact fat absorption. Ascites can cause the sensation of early satiety because of abdominal pressure and lead to diminished intake at meals.

Nutrition therapy in cirrhosis should include adequate protein to foster potential hepatic regeneration (Tsiaousi, Hatzitolios, Trygonis, & Savopoulos, 2008). Frequent meals and snacks should be offered to compensate for hypermetabolism and poor glycogen storage. Hypermetabolism has been reported in some, but not all, patients with cirrhosis. The reason for this increase is not fully understood but can contribute to malnutrition if energy needs go unmet. Adequate intake of calories is essential to spare protein from use as an energy source. Smaller, more frequent meals help if early satiety is an issue. A low-sodium diet (2 g) is indicated in decompensated cirrhosis when ascites or edema is present. The nurse should monitor and encourage intake, stressing the importance of the dietary intake to avoid further nutrition risk and compromised health.

Hepatic Encephalopathy

Many theories exist as to the pathogenesis of hepatic encephalopathy, but it is agreed that unmetabolized ammonia in the intestinal tract is the major precipitating factor. Ammonia is normally metabolized by the liver and skeletal muscle, but this can be compromised with liver damage leading to elevated ammonia levels reaching the brain. Ammonia is produced in response to excessive protein from the diet and from metabolism of protein compounds, including blood, found in the intestine. Intestinal bacteria contribute to this metabolic effect. Traditionally, a chronic low-protein diet has been used to treat hepatic encephalopathy, but this approach is now considered to contribute to encephalopathic symptoms when maintained over time because it leads to ammonia production from the catabolism of skeletal muscle.

Current recommendations for medical nutrition therapy of hepatic encephalopathy do not call for a blanket recommendation for protein, though a short-term protein restriction is still used by many (Schulz, Campos, & Coehlo, 2008). Depending on the patient's level of consciousness, nutrition can be administered as an oral diet or tube feeding. Enteral feeding is contraindicated in patients with active gastrointestinal bleeding. Protein intake should reach up to 1.5 g/kg ideal weight per day. Therefore, a 70-kg (about 150-lb) ideal-weight patient would need up to 105 g of protein. Some patients have improved protein tolerance when a portion of their intake is derived from plant protein sources (Chadalavada, Sappati, Maxwell, & Mullen, 2010). It is believed that the fiber content of these foods quickens gut transit time and alters the intestinal pH environment by providing substrate for beneficial bacteria action.

As a last resort in the patient who seems chronically intolerant of protein, enteral formula with enhanced branch chain amino acid (BCAA) content may be tried. BCAA may be better tolerated than other protein sources in some patients. These formulas are expensive and do not contain complete nutrition, but may be of some benefit in this limited population (Chadalavada et al., 2010). These nutrition-based treatments are used to augment pharmacologic management aimed at lowering ammonia production in the lower GI tract, such as with lactulose or neomycin.

Adequate calorie intake is an essential component of the diet to ensure that energy needs are met. Inadequate energy intake can lead to catabolism of skeletal tissue to provide protein substrate for gluconeogenesis. Altered metabolism of glucose and lipids, or overall hypermetabolism, compounds the difficulty of providing adequate nutrition. Ensuring the delivery of proper nutrition to patients with hepatic encephalopathy can be a challenge for the nurse. Patients have varying levels of somnolence, restlessness, disorientation, agitation, and tremor that can affect their ability to take an oral diet safely. Aggressive or inappropriate behavior in advanced stages of encephalopathy can lead to removal of any feeding tube in place. Family and other visitors who bring gifts of food need to be educated about the incremental protein prescription in order to avoid inadvertent dietary noncompliance that can affect the assessment of protein tolerance. Chapter 38 provides a complete description of hepatic encephalopathy.

Pancreatitis

Most patients who present with acute pancreatitis experience resolution of their symptoms within 5 to 7 days and do not require aggressive nutritional intervention. However, some patients exhibit severe disease and need multidisciplinary intervention, including nutritional support. Symptoms of acute pancreatitis, such as pain, nausea, and vomiting, can preclude oral intake by patients before they seek medical attention. Hypermetabolism and hypercatabolism occur with severe disease because of the body's local and systemic inflammatory responses. The combination of inability to consume adequate oral nutrition in the face of a hypermetabolic and hypercatabolic state places these patients at high risk for malnutrition and related complications. The patient who goes on to develop further infection, sepsis, abscess, or pancreatic fistula—all complications of acute pancreatitis—will be at even greater risk.

Medical nutrition therapy for acute pancreatitis centers on the widely held belief that stimulation of the exocrine pancreas needs to be avoided in order to minimize pain and enzyme secretion. Pancreatic rest through bowel rest and provision of nutrition via the parenteral route were treatments of choice for decades. More recently, debate has arisen about the use of enteral versus parenteral nutrition in achieving pancreatic rest and providing adequate nutrition while minimizing complications. This debate holds only for patients with a functioning gut and not for those in whom an ileus prevents enteral support. It has been demonstrated that use of the enteral feeding route is superior to the parenteral route because of fewer medical complications (Spanier, Bruno, & Mathus-Vliegen, 2011). Elemental or semi-elemental small peptide formulas are used that have negligible fat and free amino acids or di- and tripeptides versus intact whole proteins. Such formulas require no pancreatic enzyme secretion for absorption and do little to stimulate the exocrine pancreas.

A reasonable approach to providing nutrition care to the patient with acute pancreatitis is to begin with a jejunal feeding early in the course of severe disease. Patients with evidence of severe disease are most likely to require nutrition support. A small-bore jejunal tube should be placed distal to the ligament of Trietz. After confirmation of tube placement, an elemental or small peptide enteral formula can begin. A registered dietitian should be consulted to recommend the needed volume of feeding and a protocol for advancing the rate and concentration of the formula. Such formulas are hyperosmolar and should not be started at a full-strength concentration or full volume. The nurse should monitor the patient closely for tolerance to the formula and rate changes. An increase in pain, nausea, vomiting, or diarrhea can indicate intolerance and deserves evaluation. Further elevation of the serum pancreatic enzymes, amylase or lipase, indicates intolerance to enteral nutrition. The patient should also be monitored at the bedside with a stethoscope for signs of tube migration. Movement of the tube into the proximal jejunum or duodenum may precipitate pancreatic stimulation and feeding intolerance. A pharmacist should be consulted relative to the administration of medications via a jejunal tube because the site may bypass the point of absorption of many drugs. Additionally, small-bore tubes are prone to clogging and a precipitate from medications can form. When administering medication, the nurse needs to ensure adequate flushing of the system to maintain patency.

Parenteral nutrition support is indicated when the patient is unable to tolerate enteral support or has an ileus. The nutrition support team will recommend an appropriate parenteral formula to meet the patient's nutritional and fluid and electrolyte needs. The patient should be monitored for hyperglycemia and hypertriglyceridemia because both can occur with pancreatitis and be exacerbated by total parenteral nutrition.

Patients with mild pancreatitis may only require a short period of time NPO and no aggressive nutritional support before resumption of a low-fat oral diet. Fat is minimized to reduce stimulation of the pancreas. Patients transitioning from nutrition support should also receive a low-fat diet.

Chronic pancreatitis can lead to longer term weight loss and malabsorption when the disease affects the majority of the pancreas. Permanent glucose intolerance can also occur. In addition to oral enzyme replacement therapy, many patients will require a modified fat diet. Bone disease and clotting abnormalities have been noted from malabsorption of fat-soluble vitamins D and K, respectively. Vitamin B_{12} may also need to be supplemented if insufficient protease production prohibits the cleaving of vitamin B_{12} from its protein. Medium-chain triglycerides do not require pancreatic lipase for absorption and can be prescribed to provide needed calories for patients who have poor intake. Patients with endocrine pancreas dysfunction will also require modification of the carbohydrate content as outlined in the medical nutrition therapy of diabetes.

Renal Disease

The kidney plays an important role in maintaining homeostasis in the body. Regulating nutrition processes and excreting nutrient by-products of metabolism, such as nitrogen, are among the crucial functions performed by the kidney. Kidneys also regulate fluid and electrolyte balance and are responsible for orchestrating the delicate balance between calcium, phosphorus, and vitamin D in the body. Vitamin D reaches its metabolically active form after being hydroxylated in the kidney.

Nephrotic Syndrome

Damage to the capillary walls of the glomeruli can cause significant losses of protein in the urine. Following significant proteinuria, decreases in plasma albumin can result with subsequent edema formation. Medical nutrition therapy for nephrotic syndrome focuses on replacement of protein losses to prevent malnutrition, slow the disease progression, and minimize edema. Dietary sodium is limited to control edema (Hull & Goldsmith, 2008).

The nurse can educate the patient and reinforce the importance of a low-sodium diet in reducing edema. Adequate, but not high, protein is recommended to provide needed protein without contributing to disease progression. A patient should have a 24-hour urine protein assessment to determine the amount of protein replacement needed in addition to the RDA for protein baseline requirement. A registered dietitian would calculate this recommendation for the patient and outline suitable food choices. Adequate nonprotein sources of calories are needed to provide energy and prevent malnutrition because of catabolism of skeletal muscle for gluconeogenesis. If inadequate energy intake occurs, the protein intake will be sacrificed by the body for use as energy instead of as a substrate for anabolic functions.

Renal Failure

Medical nutrition therapy for both acute and chronic renal failure is determined by whether or not dialysis is part of the patient's treatment

CHART 8–25 Medical Nutrition Therapy for Chronic Renal Disease

	Hemodialysis	Peritoneal Dialysis	No Dialysis	Nephrotic Syndrome
Protein (g/kg dry weight)	1.2 g	1.2–1.3 g	0.6–0.8 g	0.8 g
Sodium (g)	1–3*	2–4*	1–3*	2–3*
Potassium (g)	2–3*	3–4*	2–3*	No restriction
Fluid (mL)	500–1,000 + UOP volume	Assess individually	500–1,000 + UOP volume	No restriction
Calories (kcal/kg)*	30–35	25–30	35–50	35

*Emphasis should be placed on individual diet recommendations based on overall renal function, nutrition status, and general health. All parameters outlined in this chart are general and should be adapted to meet patient requirements.

Source: Adapted from Aase, S. (2010). Kidney friendly: What the National Kidney Disease Education Program Strategic Plan means for dietetic practice. *Journal of the American Dietetic Association, 110*(3), 346–351.

strategy. Additionally, current laboratory values, amount of urine production, and any underlying disease will dictate an individualized diet prescription. Uremia results from the buildup of metabolic by-products in the body that are normally excreted via the kidneys. Uremia can predispose the patient with renal failure to malnutrition. Anorexia, nausea, and altered taste perception can lead to decreased intake. Medication side effects and a restricted diet can further the potential for nutrition risk.

The short-term goals of medical nutrition therapy are to minimize uremia, manage fluid status, and provide adequate nutrition. Long-term nutrition care is focused on prevention of disease progression and malnutrition. Patients who also have comorbid conditions, such as diabetes or hypertension, must also receive appropriate nutrition intervention for those diseases. Overall, the resultant diet prescription can be quite stringent, and patients require close monitoring. Nutrition assessment is essential before an individualized diet prescription can be tailored to fit established guidelines. Parameters normally used to assess nutrition status can require adjustment in this population. A postdialysis edema-free body weight is used in calculating nutritional needs. The dietitian will rely on nursing expertise to make a determination of dry weight based on such factors as blood pressure, heart rate, postdialysis symptoms, and edema. Plasma samples obtained to assess albumin or other proteins should be taken before dialysis to avoid the effect of interdialytic protein losses. Creatinine index and serum creatinine can be employed to assess for loss of muscle mass or poor protein intake.

Dietary protein is responsible for the development of nitrogenous by-products that contribute to uremia. Thus, a controlled protein diet is recommended to control uremia. Because of protein losses during dialysis, patients receiving hemodialysis or peritoneal dialysis as part of treatment can consume more protein than those not dialyzed (Dukkipati & Kopple, 2009). Chart 8–25 outlines recommended protein levels for the treatment of renal failure.

To achieve the most efficient metabolism, the majority of protein consumed should be of high biological value, having all essential amino acids, such as animal proteins (meats, poultry, fish, dairy) and soy. Adequate nonprotein calorie intake is essential to support energy needs and not have protein wasted as an energy source. The dietitian can recommend appropriate individual adjustments to this recommendation for patients who are sedentary, obese, or hypermetabolic. Nutrition management of altered fluid status and plasma electrolyte and mineral abnormalities is recommended with renal failure. General guidelines are presented in Chart 8–26, but it should be understood that each patient should have a customized diet prescription that fits his or her individual needs and laboratory parameters (Aase, 2010). A registered dietitian provides this individualized assessment and diet recommendation. Nonetheless, the nurse can be instrumental in reinforcing the immediate importance of low-potassium food choices in this population. Noncompliance with a potassium restriction can result in quick deleterious consequences with elevated blood potassium, leading to lethal cardiac dysrhythmias and cardiac arrest. Chart 8–27 outlines high-potassium foods. Sodium and fluid restrictions correspond to the amount of urine production and accumulation of fluid between dialysis treatments. Generally, fluid intake is 500 to 1,000 mL plus volume of 24-hour urine output. Patients with acute renal failure who are in the diuretic phase need to have fluid intake reevaluated to match changes in output. For patients receiving dialysis, large interdialytic fluid gains present medical risk and dialysis difficulties and should be avoided. Interdialytic weight gain should be limited to 2–3 kg to reduce the effects of chronic fluid overload on the heart. Compliance with the

CHART 8–26 General Guidelines for Chronic Kidney Disease

1. Medical nutrition therapy by a registered dietitian is recommended
2. Eat the proper amount of calories and protein
3. Carbohydrates—fruits, grains, and vegetables
4. Fats—monounsaturated and polyunsaturated (olive oil, safflower oil, canola oil)
5. Important nutrients
   a. Sodium—decrease intake
   b. Phosphorus—decrease intake
   c. Calcium—add supplement
   d. Vitamin D—add supplement
   e. Potassium—decreased or may need supplement
   f. Fluid—depending on stage of kidney disease may limit intake
   g. Vitamins and minerals—may need supplements
6. Maintain a healthy body weight

Sources: American Dietetic Association. (2010). Chronic kidney disease evidence-based nutrition practice guideline. Retrieved from http://www.guidelines.gov/content.aspx?id=23924; Lin, H.Y. (2011). Diet—chronic kidney disease. Retrieved from: http://www.nlm.nih.gov/medlineplus/ency/article/002442.htm.

CHART 8–27 High Potassium Food Sources

- Banana
- Dried fruit: apricots, raisins, prunes, dates, figs
- Green leafy vegetables: Swiss chard, spinach, mustard greens
- Legumes: dried beans, peas, lentils
- Melon: cantaloupe, honeydew
- Oranges, orange juice
- Potato
- Tomato
- Whole grains, bran.

Note: Check labels on salt substitutes. Many contain potassium.

fluid restriction can be difficult for many patients. The nurse can offer suggestions for helping with thirst, such as mouth care or rinses and sucking on hard candy, and suggest low-potassium fluid choices within restriction parameters.

Chronic renal failure and ongoing dialysis treatment can result in additional nutritional concerns.

Safety Alert *Water-soluble vitamins are lost in the dialysate and require replacement. Dietary restrictions and poor intake also contribute to poor vitamin status. The nurse should educate the patient that formulations are available specifically for renal failure use.*

Kidney endocrine function becomes compromised and final synthesis of active vitamin D is diminished. Calcitriol, an oral supplement of active vitamin D, is given. Without adequate vitamin D, calcium absorption is lowered, predisposing the patient to bone disease. Plasma phosphorous levels are often elevated and complicate the intricate feedback mechanisms among vitamin D, calcium, and parathyroid hormone. Dietary restriction of phosphorus is indicated but only to the level achieved by the simultaneous protein restriction. Phosphorus is found primarily in milk products, nuts, and legumes. Overreliance on dietary restriction of phosphorus could result in insufficient intake of high-quality protein. Further reduction in plasma phosphorus is achieved with binding medications, such as calcium carbonate. These are consumed along with a meal. Erythropoietin (a hormone produced by the kidney that is critical for the formation of red blood cells by the bone marrow) production is diminished with resultant anemia because of lowered red blood cell production by the bone marrow. Patients receive an erythropoiesis-stimulating agent, but additional contributors to anemia should also be investigated. Transferrin saturation and ferritin are assessed to determine appropriate intervention for iron deficiency. Intravenous iron replacement is the preferred route of administration in this anemic population (NKUDIC, 2011).

The patient with end-stage renal disease has unique dietary restrictions that make consumption of adequate nutrition a challenge. Patients on low-protein diets without dialysis treatment are at high risk of malnutrition. Restrictions accompanying comorbid conditions such as diabetes present additional considerations. The nurse can provide much needed reinforcement of the importance of dietary compliance in both short-term well-being and long-term disease management.

Renal Stones

Supersaturation of urine favors nucleation and growth of crystals that can cause nephrolithiasis. Medical nutrition therapy of kidney stones focuses first on adequate fluid intake to promote ample urine volume and flow, which will in turn lessen the risk of a precipitate forming because of a patient's concentrated urine. Consumption of enough fluid to produce between 2 and 3 L of urine daily is recommended. Tailoring intake is required if changes in fluid balance occur, such as when insensible fluid losses increase and urine output is lessened because of increased sweating or fever.

Calcium oxalate stones are the predominant type of kidney stone, comprising up to 70% of all stones (Worcester & Coe, 2008). In the past, a low-calcium diet was recommended in an attempt to decrease hypercalciuria and the likelihood of stone precipitation. However, although this advice resulted in decreased urinary excretion of calcium, it also fostered increased absorption of oxalate from the intestine, increased oxalate in urine, and risk of bone disease with insufficient calcium intake. Current recommendations advise adequate calcium intake and avoidance of excess oxalate intake (spinach, rhubarb, nuts, beets, chocolate, tea, and wheat bran are significant absorbable sources) (Goldfarb, 2009). Additionally, excess intake of nondairy animal proteins and sodium has been shown to contribute to stone formation. Excessive animal protein promotes an acid environment in the body to which the body responds by buffering with calcium released from bone. Sodium excretion is associated with calcium excretion in the urine and thus is a target for control of calciuria. Patients at risk for calcium stones should be educated to avoid high dose vitamin D and C supplements. Vitamin D causes calcium absorption. Vitamin C promotes increased oxalate because it is a precursor to oxalate produced by the body.

Less common uric acid, cystine, and struvite kidney stones require medical management and ample fluid intake to avoid urine supersaturation. Additional dietary manipulations are not common modes of treatment in the prevention of these stones. Purines in meats and organ meats contribute to uric acid formation if consumed in significant quantities on a regular basis. However, management generally involves manipulation of urine pH rather than changes in diet for uric acid nephrolithiasis (Pak, 2008).

Patients at risk for kidney stones should have a nutrition history done to assess for fluid intake and urine output, use of vitamin supplements (vitamins C and D, calcium), and excessive intake of protein and sodium. The nurse should educate the patient to consume adequate fluid to produce between 2 and 3 L of urine daily. Patients who exercise or live in climates where insensible losses are increased should be educated to tailor fluid intake accordingly. Nonnutritional risk factors for kidney stone formation are discussed in Chapter 39.

Acquired Immunodeficiency Syndrome (AIDS)

Nutritional problems, from malnutrition to dyslipidemia, occur in human immunodeficiency virus (HIV) infection. Malnutrition occurs for a variety of reasons, such as opportunistic infection. For example, oral candidiasis can lead to inadequate intake because of pain and dysphagia accompanying inflammation. Other infections can lead to anorexia, fatigue, malabsorption, hypermetabolism from fever and inflammation, nausea and vomiting, or altered cognition and functional status (Colecraft, 2008). AIDS is discussed in detail in Chapter 53.

Pharmacologic treatment of infection can cause gastrointestinal side effects and food and drug interactions. Often, complicated medication schedules and food interactions can make adequate intake a challenge. Chemical dependency and socioeconomic issues present additional challenges to nutrition status. These factors, in combination or alone, can predispose patients with HIV infection to malnutrition.

Development of malnutrition can diminish immunocompetence and leave the patient at further risk of opportunistic infection (American Dietetic Association, 2010b). Thus, a vicious cycle of malnutrition and infection can follow. Weight loss, loss of muscle and adipose tissue, and nutrient deficiencies lead to further negative consequences. Up to 10% of adults with HIV in the United States are malnourished, with a higher prevalence found in the populations of underdeveloped countries (Berger, Fields-Gardner, Wagle, & Hollenbeck, 2008; Siddiqui et al., 2009). Some wasting occurs despite a clear single etiology. In addition to suspected contributors to malnutrition such as inadequate intake and malabsorption, wasting occurs because of changes in metabolism, hypogonadism, and excessive cytokine production associated with HIV (Chang, Sekhar, Patel, & Balasubramanyam, 2007). No matter what the etiology, the health impact resulting from loss of lean muscle and total body weight is significant.

Current medical treatment of patients with HIV infection using highly active antiretroviral treatment (HAART), discussed in Chapter 53, has presented clinicians with additional sequelae of potential nutritional problems. Hyperlipidemia, insulin resistance, and body fat redistribution have been associated with the use of protease inhibitors. Lifestyle modifications, including diet and exercise, do not appear to influence this condition (Cofrancesco, Freedland, & McComsey, 2009). Patients may present with elevated plasma cholesterol, triglyceride, glucose intolerance, and unique lipodystrophy. **Lipodystrophy** is characterized by loss of adipose tissue in the face and extremities and excess fat deposition in the abdomen and over the dorsocervical spine. Such alterations in morphology may lead some patients to alter their diet or medication strategies in an attempt to deal with body image conflicts. This, in turn, may place these patients at risk for poor nutrition or ineffective medication concentration (American Dietetic Association, 2010a). Some patients may experiment with alternative medicine in place of, or in addition to, HAART to counteract the metabolic effects. Not all nutritional and herbal supplements can be safely used by patients with HIV infection and some may compromise effective treatment.

Medical nutrition therapy for HIV infection is based on an up-to-date comprehensive nutrition assessment. Standard nutrition assessment parameters should all be used, but tailored for specificity with this population. Anthropometric measurements are important to obtain at baseline for potential future estimations of any lipodystrophy. Serial weights should be monitored as well as measures of body composition, such as skinfold thickness measurements (American Dietetic Association, 2010a).

Laboratory parameters such as plasma proteins may be reflective of nutrition status or infection-related inflammation and cannot be solely relied on to assess nutrition (American Dietetic Association, 2010a). Vitamin and mineral levels are often diminished in both symptomatic and asymptomatic patients, a finding that is associated with increased risk of disease progression (American Dietetic Association, 2010a).

During the focused interview and the physical examination, the nurse should closely assess the patient for the presence of any factor known to influence nutrition health. Knowledge regarding HIV-related nutrition risk factors is important for nurses because the nurse is often first in line to assess a patient. Existing opportunistic infections, oral and digestive symptoms, medication, use of alternative medicines and supplements, and functional status are among the many parameters that are essential to the assessment. Chart 8–28 outlines essential components of the nutritional assessment of patients with HIV infection.

CHART 8–28 Nutrition Assessment in HIV Infection

The nutrition assessment of the patient with HIV infection should include the standard components of an assessment. Particular attention should be paid to include the following:

Nutrition History

General diet history

Note baseline nutrition knowledge and sources of information

Cultural influences on nutrition and diet

Note any issues of food insecurity

Dietary supplement use, including vitamins, mineral, herbs, and other natural products

Physical Exam

Height and weight

Weight history

Body composition measurements: circumference measurements, waist-to-hip ratio, body fat assessment

Visual assessment for lipodystrophy: note subcutaneous fat pattern, presence of temporal or extremity fat loss, existence of central fat accumulation

Laboratory Values

Plasma proteins

Indices for anemia

Lipid levels

Testosterone, if wasting apparent

Fasting glucose

Bone density, if metabolic bone disease suspected from HAART

Medical History

Presence of opportunistic infections: note symptoms, treatment, and side effects

Presence of comorbid conditions: malignancies, metabolic disease

Presence of anxiety, depression, altered cognition, or other psycho-neurological symptoms

Over-the-counter and prescription drugs: note any food–medication instructions, interactions with food, dietary supplements or nutrients.

Self-prescribed treatment for any medical symptoms

Psychosocial History

Alcohol intake

Use of illicit drugs, substance abuse

Body image

Living arrangements

Ability for self-care

Source: Tucker, S. B., & Dauffenbach, V. (2011). *Nutrition and diet therapy for nurses.* Upper Saddle River, NJ: Pearson.

Patients in whom lipodystrophy is evident may require nutrition intervention for any glucose intolerance or hyperlipidemia. Current recommendations advise the prescription of the same diet treatment as for any patient with hyperlipidemia or hyperglycemia (American Dietetic Association, 2010a). This area requires more research to determine the efficacy of nutrition therapy in treating these metabolic changes when they occur in this population. Nutrition intervention to alter the effects of fat redistribution or to specifically increase muscle mass in wasting has little reported effect.

The findings from the nutritional assessment will determine the extent of needed nutrition intervention. Nutrition care and education are central to management of HIV infection. Asymptomatic patients

CHART 8–29 Guidelines for Safe Food and Water Handling

Prepare foods safely:

- Clean surfaces and utensils.
- Wash hands before preparing food and after handling raw meats, poultry, or fish.
- Wash surfaces and utensils after preparing raw meat, poultry, and fish. Use separate cutting board if possible for raw products.
- Cook foods until done and proper temperature; meats, poultry >165°F internally; fish should be opaque and flaky. Reheat leftovers to 165°F. Bring leftover soup, gravy, or sauce to a boil. Only keep leftovers for 3 to 4 days in refrigerator.

Do not consume raw or undercooked eggs, meat, fish, or poultry:

- Avoid sushi or raw bars, real eggnog, dressings made with raw egg, and runny eggs.
- Do not taste test marinades used for tenderizing proteins.

Consume pasteurized juices, milk, and dairy foods.
Wash and peel fruits and vegetables.
Do not drink water from streams, lakes, springs, or rivers.
Boil tap water if advised by the local health department.
Store foods safely:

- Place raw meat, poultry, and fish in lower shelf of refrigerator to avoid drips onto other food.
- Separate raw products in grocery cart and when bagged in store.
- Keep stored perishable foods out of the 40°–140°F danger zone. Cool hot foods quickly in a shallow dish. Keep foods properly refrigerated or frozen.

Source: U.S. Department of Agriculture. (2011). *Food safety education.* Retrieved from http://www.fsis.usda.gov/Food_Safety_Education/index.asp.

may benefit from general nutrition education about a healthy diet to maintain important muscle mass and body weight. It is important for the nurse to discuss the use of herbal and nutritional supplements that may impact medical management. For example, it has been shown that St. John's wort interacts with protease inhibitors (American Dietetic Association, 2010a). Education about the importance of food and water safety is also important to prevent or decrease the risk of foodborne illness. Improperly handled foods and water from unsafe sources each pose a risk to patients who are immunocompromised. Many pathogens identified in patients with opportunistic infection are recognizable as having potentially originated in a food or water source. Salmonella, listeria, cryptosporidia, and *Vibrio vulnificus* are examples. Chart 8–29 outlines important aspects of food and water sanitation.

Patients with malnutrition or at risk for malnutrition require quick intervention to prevent further deterioration of nutrition health. Underlying factors responsible for malnutrition must be identified and treated or controlled. Nutrition intervention should be tailored to maximize nutrient repletion while minimizing side effects and symptoms. Chart 8–30 outlines common causes of malnutrition in HIV infection and sample nutrition strategies the nurse can suggest.

Cancer

Patients diagnosed with cancer are at risk for poor nutrition status because of the effects of the disease as well as the treatment. Anorexia, nausea, vomiting, changes in taste perception, dysphagia, mucositis,

CHART 8–30 Nutrition Strategies for Common Problems with HIV Infection and Cancer

Problem	Nutrition Intervention
Anorexia	Eat small, frequent meals.
	Choose nutrient-dense foods: peanut butter, cheese, meal replacement or breakfast-type drinks, smoothies.
	See Chart 8–17 on pg. XXX for "more calories per bite" food recommendations.
Nausea and Vomiting	Nibble on dry carbohydrates: toast, crackers, dry cereal.
	Eat small meals to avoid empty stomach or feeling too full.
	Avoid greasy foods and strong odors.
	Sip flat ginger ale, weak ginger, or mint tea.
Diarrhea	Limit fat, caffeine, and fiber.
	Assess for lactose intolerance.
	Replace fluids.
Oral Pain or Dysphagia	Eat smooth, cool foods: pudding, ice cream, cooled soup, liquid supplement drinks.
	Avoid citrus, tomato, and hot foods.
	Use a straw to bypass mouth.
Altered Taste	Eat tart candy, juice, or seasonings.
	Practice good oral care.
	Eat room temperature or cool foods, especially proteins.
Fatigue	Keep ready-to-eat and convenience foods in stock.
	Eat nutrient-dense foods early in the day and meal when energy level is best.

diarrhea, and fatigue can predispose a patient to malnutrition whether the symptoms are caused by tumor effects, radiation, or chemotherapy. Malnutrition that begins from disease alone may be worsened with treatment side effects. A baseline nutrition assessment at diagnosis followed by reassessment periodically through treatment will allow for early intervention when nutrition risk is evident. The nurse who is part of the treatment team during chemotherapy, radiation, or surgery can be instrumental in identifying symptom changes that prevent adequate intake and planning appropriate intervention. Chart 8–30 lists nutrition interventions that the nurse can recommend to patients and caregivers.

The nurse should be knowledgeable regarding current recommendations regarding use of nutritional supplements during active treatment with chemotherapy or radiation. To date, limited research has provided little on which to build the foundation of evidence-based clinical advice. A theoretical concern exists that the use of antioxidants during radiation or with certain types of chemotherapy may interfere with the intended cytotoxic effects of those therapies (Hardy, 2008). Antioxidants have been investigated for their potential in minimizing oxidative damage to cells and therefore preventing or slowing cancer. Examples of antioxidant nutrients include beta-carotene (vitamin A precursor), vitamins C and E, and selenium. Patients may take these supplements, hoping to minimize disease and spare healthy cells the effects of treatment. The controversy arises in that antioxidants may also theoretically spare diseased tissue from the cytotoxic effects of treatment, thereby diminishing treatment efficacy.

Patients may also choose to use herbal remedies, such as ginger for nausea, to lessen the severity of treatment side effects. The nurse should query the patient for use of all supplements and educate the patient about any known interactions with treatment or medications, possible anticoagulant effects, or other contraindications to use. The safety and efficacy of nutrition and herbal supplement use before, during, and after cancer treatment are areas deserving future research.

Chronic Obstructive Pulmonary Disease and Mechanical Ventilation

Chronic obstructive pulmonary disease (COPD) symptoms, such as dyspnea and fatigue, can predispose patients to malnutrition by altering diet consumption. Patients may experience shortness of breath that precludes sufficient intake if chewing and swallowing alter breathing patterns and potentially affect arterial oxygen saturation. Early satiety can occur if gastric filling affects perceived or real breathing capacity. **Aerophagia,** or swallowing of air, may occur while eating and lead to bloating and early satiety as well. Fatigue can impair adequate intake when meal preparation and even simple tasks like cutting meats or opening lids prove too exhausting. Medications such as glucocorticoids may cause appetite stimulation as well as gastrointestinal upset and altered intake.

COPD can lead to an increase in energy expenditure due in part to inefficient respiratory mechanics and the increased work of the respiratory muscles. This effect is noted at rest and increases further during activity or exacerbation of respiratory symptoms (If the increased need for calories goes unmet, weight loss will occur). Weight loss may occur slowly or be exacerbated during acute disease or infection when nutritional needs are further increased.

Patients with elevated resting energy needs have also been reported to have increased protein turnover in the body, resulting in disproportionate loss of muscle mass or "wasting." Loss of muscle does not spare respiratory muscle; diaphragmatic and auxiliary respiratory muscle can be lost. In some patients, this loss of muscle occurs even with maintenance of body weight. The muscle wasting seen in this subpopulation is referred to as **pulmonary cachexia.** Patients with pulmonary cachexia may suffer from loss of respiratory strength and endurance as well as functional capacity. A vicious downward spiral can occur when this in turn leads to further decreased intake and malnutrition. Malnutrition can alter immunocompetence, leaving the patient more susceptible to infection. A reduced BMI in COPD is associated with reduced survival (Celli, 2010).

The goal of medical nutrition therapy for COPD is to prevent malnutrition and weight loss that may occur with advanced disease. In patients who have hypercapnia, nutrition therapy should also focus on minimizing carbon dioxide (CO_2) production from nutrient metabolism. Each macronutrient produces a given amount of CO_2 for each molecule of O_2 consumed. This is called its **respiratory quotient (RQ).** Carbohydrates have a higher RQ than do protein and fat and thus have the potential to produce more CO_2 at a given intake. Overfeeding a patient in total calories or carbohydrate will produce more CO_2 than feeding adequate calories and is therefore not recommended for the patient with hypercapnia (Dickerson, 2011). Nutrition intervention should focus on providing optimal nutrition in a well-tolerated form. For patients with dyspnea, the nurse should encourage consumption of nutrient-dense foods with "more calorie per bite." When fatigue is a problem, the nurse can encourage intake of higher calorie sources first in the meal (and also earlier in the day) to optimize intake before the patient becomes too tired to eat. The patient should be offered assistance with opening cartons or other tasks when in the hospital to conserve energy for eating. Patients experiencing early satiety can be advised to consume many small meals and to minimize filling up on empty-calorie liquids. Supplementation with an oral liquid nutrition supplement can be helpful between meals, but it is important that it not simply become a meal replacement. Chart 8–31 outlines nutrition interventions for the patient with COPD. The patient should be monitored for overall intake and routinely screened for weight loss and muscle wasting.

CHART 8–31 Suggested Nutrition Interventions for COPD

Dyspnea, early satiety, bloating, and fatigue all contribute to poor intake. Suggested interventions include the following:

- Consume higher-calorie, higher-protein foods first.
- Get more "calories per bite," especially by adding fat to foods with butter, margarine, mayonnaise, sauces, cream, dressings, and gravy.
- Consume frequent small meals.
- Save liquids for between meals.
- Limit intake of carbonated beverages.
- Keep convenient and ready-to-eat nutrient-dense foods available.

Nutrition and Wound Healing

The presence of a cutaneous wound places metabolic demands on the body that must be met in order for healing to progress. Each stage of wound healing requires an adequate nutritional substrate and is contingent on the successful outcome of the prior healing phase. As a result, delayed wound healing may occur in patients with malnutrition. Poor baseline nutrition status prior to wound development or subsequent inadequate intake may predispose a patient to weight loss and poor vitamin, mineral, and protein status that can impact healing and increase the risk for infection (Kavalukas & Barbul, 2011). Inadequate fluid intake, if further offset by wound exudative fluid losses, fever, diarrhea, or excessive insensible losses, can lead to dehydration. Decreased blood volume will not only impair needed oxygen delivery to the wound but also slow the arrival of essential nutrients required for tissue repair.

Knowledge of the role nutrition plays in wound healing is beneficial to the nurse when completing an assessment of patients with existing wounds or those at risk of pressure ulcers. The early stages of wound healing require adequate protein stores to provide substrate for the inflammatory process. Diminished plasma protein levels before injury may worsen during this acute reaction. Edema can result with decreased plasma proteins, which can impact healing. Collagen synthesis and tissue repair require adequate protein, vitamins C and A, and zinc, among other nutrients (Kavalukas & Barbul, 2011). Protein is also essential for maintaining immune function and preventing infection. Sufficient calorie intake is needed to prevent the use of crucial protein as energy instead of as a building block for tissue repair. Inadequate calorie intake can delay healing and also lead to skeletal muscle catabolism. The dietitian should be consulted to assess the patient's calorie, protein, and general nutrition needs. The size of the wound, amount of exudate (which can contribute to protein losses), presence of fever, coexisting injuries or disease, and the patient's baseline nutrition status will all affect nutritional recommendations.

The nurse should assess the patient for baseline nutrition status, paying close attention to protein status, physical signs of malnutrition including overall skin integrity, and diet history. The patient should be monitored for adequate intake of calories, protein, and fluid. The routine use of vitamin supplements in wound healing is a common practice, yet benefits of this practice have only been reported for those patients who have existing nutritional deficiencies (Bluestein & Javaheri, 2008). Vitamin C is necessary for collagen formation and is found in many fruits and vegetables, especially citrus or tropical fruit and green leafy vegetables. Zinc supplements are prescribed for the zinc-deficient patient because of the mineral's role in collagen formation. However, there is no benefit to prescribing doses greater than 40 mg zinc/day for this purpose (Posthauer, Dorner, & Collins, 2010). Long-term or excessive use of zinc supplementation can precipitate an imbalance in copper status and gastrointestinal upset. Zinc is found in most foods that contain protein, such as meats, poultry, legumes, and nuts. Fluid status should be monitored to provide at least the recommended 2.7 or 3.7 liters of water daily for women and men, respectively. Adjustments should be made for excessive fluid losses from the gastrointestinal tract, wounds, or other insensible losses.

Pressure Ulcers

Malnutrition is among the many potential risk factors for development of a pressure ulcer (Bluestein & Javaheri, 2008). As with the presence of any wound, adequate nutrition can benefit the healing process by providing necessary nutrients for each phase of tissue repair. Elderly and malnourished patients with a decubitus ulcer require close monitoring to ensure that their nutritional needs are met. Individual consideration should be given to the liberalization of any dietary restrictions in these patients to encourage intake. Supplementation with oral nutrition formula may be beneficial if it does not replace normal intake. Multivitamin use is reasonable with consideration given to extra vitamin C and zinc in those found to be deficient (Posthauer, Dorner, & Collins, 2010).

Burns

Medical nutrition therapy for the patient with a thermal injury focuses on two important management aspects. Both the metabolic response to a burn and the healing process require special attention with aggressive nutrition support. Severe burns cause both a catabolic and hypermetabolic response by the body from hormonal and inflammatory responses to the injury (Jeschke et al., 2008). The nutritional requirements for tissue repair must be met in addition to those that result from catabolism and hypermetabolism. With a severe burn, the result is a daily requirement for high levels of calorie and protein intake.

Early enteral feeding is recommended for the burn patient (Mosier et al., 2011). Oral nutrition, continuous tube feedings, or supplemental nocturnal tube feedings can be utilized to deliver adequate nutrition in the patient who has a functioning gastrointestinal tract. Patients with gastric stasis may tolerate postpyloric enteral feeding in the duodenum or jejunum rather than via a basic nasogastric tube. Parenteral nutrition may be necessary in patients with ileus or intolerance to a sufficient volume of enteral nutrition support. The large dextrose content of parenteral nutrition can supply fodder for bacterial growth; thus, strict aseptic technique is required for the parenteral nutrition intravenous site in order to avoid a disastrous infection.

Nutritional recommendations focus on modulating tissue catabolism and providing sufficient nutrition for tissue repair. Many different equations exist to estimate calorie and protein needs in a burn patient. None is universally accepted due to differences such as the technique for factoring the effects of varying degree and percentage of body surface area burned. Typically 35 to 40 calories/kg per day are required for adults; this can be adjusted if **indirect calorimetry** technology is available to estimate the patient's energy needs based on oxygen consumption and carbon dioxide production. Along with adequate energy intake, protein intake of 1.5 gm/kg of body weight is recommended for tissue repair (Demling, 2009). Adjustments can be made based on wound healing progress. Supplemental amino acids in the form of glutamine and arginine have been investigated for their role in mediating catabolism postburn. The research supports the use of glutamine in burn therapy, but data is lacking to support the use of arginine in this population (Kurmis, Parker, & Greenwood, 2010). Supplemental vitamins and minerals are prescribed to support tissue synthesis and the needs of a hypermetabolic state. Chapter 61 includes a description of the hypermetabolic state.

The nurse should monitor the patient's tolerance to enteral or parenteral nutrition. Close attention should be given to the amount and type of intake and fluid balance. Serial weights should be monitored to assess for weight loss, since loss of >10% body weight will impair healing. Larger losses of lean muscle mass are associated with increased mortality (Demling, 2009). Some patients are able to tolerate adequate oral intake, whereas others require nocturnal supplementation with a tube feeding. The nurse can help optimize intake by facilitating a comfortable eating environment. Dressing and wound care, venipuncture, and any major repositioning are best avoided near mealtime to minimize discomfort. Optimal pain management during meals is also helpful. Depression, pain, and medication side effects, including sedation, can lead to diminished intake. The patient with a thermal injury requires close monitoring and reevaluation of nutrition status throughout the course of injury and recovery.

Nutrition and the Surgical Patient

Malnutrition is associated with poor surgical outcome and increased postoperative mortality (Garth, Newsome, Simmance, & Crowe, 2010). Impaired wound healing, infection, and reduced strength for postoperative rehabilitation can result because of poor baseline nutrition status. Every effort should be made to ensure that a patient is in good nutritional health preoperatively. Lengthy hospitalization with multiple diagnostic tests requiring withholding liquids or clear liquid feeding can contribute to iatrogenic deterioration of the patient's nutrition status. Trauma as a precursor to surgery leads to preoperative metabolic stress with characteristic hypercatabolism and hypermetabolism compromising nutrition status. Chronic disease existing before surgery, such as organ failure requiring transplantation, can place a patient at risk for malnutrition because of medication side effects, the need for a restrictive diet, and depression and anxiety, as well as a host of other medical symptoms. A nutrition assessment should be routinely included in the preoperative work-up of any patient when possible. Patients found to be at risk for poor nutrition status should receive appropriate referral for further evaluation and intervention.

An assessment of preoperative nutrition and medication use is essential. The nurse should inquire about use of nutrition and herbal supplements during the preoperative nutrition assessment. The Safety

Weblink: Gastric Bypass

Alert outlines herbal and nutritional supplements that should be noted during preoperative screening.

Safety Alert *The following are examples of supplements that can alter coagulopathy or sedation:*

Borage	*Bromelain*	*Danshen*
Devil's claw	*Dong quai*	*Evening primrose*
Feverfew	*Fish oil*	*Garlic*
Ginger	*Ginkgo*	*Ginseng*
Kava kava	*Papaya*	*Red clover*
St. John's wort	*Vitamin E*	*Willow bark*
Valerian	*Flaxseed*	

Adequate nutrition in the postoperative period is essential to contend with the increased metabolic demands caused by the physiological stress of the surgery. Additionally, wound healing, preservation of nutritional stores, and immunocompetence require sufficient energy, protein, and micronutrient intake. Patients should be transitioned to diet or enteral feeding as quickly as possible. Parenteral nutrition support may be indicated following some surgeries. Prolonged NPO status, reliance on only peripheral dextrose intravenous fluid, or extended use of a clear liquid diet postoperatively will not provide sufficient energy to meet even baseline needs; nutrition health can become compromised, beginning with weight loss. The nurse should know that 2 L of a 5% dextrose solution provides only 340 calories! Nurses are uniquely positioned to closely monitor patients for lack of intake or poor intake and to ensure communication of prolonged NPO, clear liquid, and other forms of inadequate intake to the health care provider and nutrition staff. It is not uncommon for hospitalized patients to have periods of continuous or significantly cumulative NPO or poor quality intake slip by without intervention when good communication patterns have not taken place.

Some specific surgeries require additional postoperative nutrition intervention. Generally, a registered dietitian with specialized training in the care of these patients is an active member of the treatment care team. It is important for the nurse to understand the nutrition protocol prescribed and participate in the team effort to ensure adequate nutrition contributes to good surgical outcome.

Bariatric Surgery for Morbid Obesity

Gastroplasty or gastric bypass surgery is indicated for weight loss treatment in some patients with morbid obesity. Gastroplasty is called a gastric restrictive procedure because the goal is to simply reduce gastric volume and therefore limit the amount (and energy content) of intake without causing malabsorption. In contrast, gastric bypass surgery involves reduction of the gastric volume but also causes deliberate malabsorption by bypassing the absorptive surface in the small intestine. A Roux-en-Y procedure is the most commonly used bypass configuration; it bypasses the gastric fundus, duodenum, and proximal jejunum (Figure 8–2◆) (Tucker, Szomstein, & Rosenthal, 2007). Postoperative care of patients who have undergone bariatric surgery follows careful steps to reintroduce nutrition to the patient. Patients must learn to accommodate the reduction in gastric volume without precipitating nausea, vomiting, or dumping syndrome. Diets are advanced slowly over weeks and months from just liquids to texture modified foods until tolerance improves.

Patients with malabsorptive procedures or protracted vomiting must be closely monitored for nutrition risk. Commonly, the following supplements are recommended: a chewable multivitamin, multimineral; thiamin in the patient experiencing postoperative vomiting; and vitamin B_{12}, iron, and calcium because of the reduced acid environment required in the stomach for digestion and absorption of these nutrients (Shankar, Boylan, & Sriram, 2010). Chart 8–32 provides a sample diet recommendation and discharge instructions following bariatric surgery.

Transplant Surgery

Patients presenting for organ, intestinal, or bone marrow transplant are often already nutritionally at risk because of preexisting disease. Postoperative recovery requires adequate nutrition for wound healing, repletion of nutrition stores, and support for the hypermetabolic demands of surgery. Patients undergoing renal or hepatic transplantation may have been on a restrictive diet that generally is liberalized following surgery when organ function improves. These recommendations are made on an individualized basis according to metabolic changes following surgery. Therapeutic use of immunosuppressive medications requires careful attention to risk factors for infection, including foodborne illness. The patient and family should be instructed about safe food handling.

Patients undergoing intestinal transplant most commonly have been on some parenteral nutrition support preoperatively because of short bowel syndrome. The postoperative goal is to support the patient with enteral nutrition. Patients are closely monitored for the return of their intestinal motility and function. Enteral nutrition progresses according to patient tolerance and may consist of an oral diet, enteral formula, or a combination of both.

Following allogeneic bone marrow transplant, patients routinely receive parenteral nutrition because of treatment-induced mucositis. The ability to take adequate enteral nutrition may not occur for several weeks and requires close monitoring by the team.

Safety Alert *Educate patients about the deleterious effects of combining some nutritional and herbal supplements with medications. St. John's wort has been reported to decrease crucial plasma levels of cyclosporine therapy, leading to graft rejection (Gardener, Phillips, & Shaughnessy, 2008).*

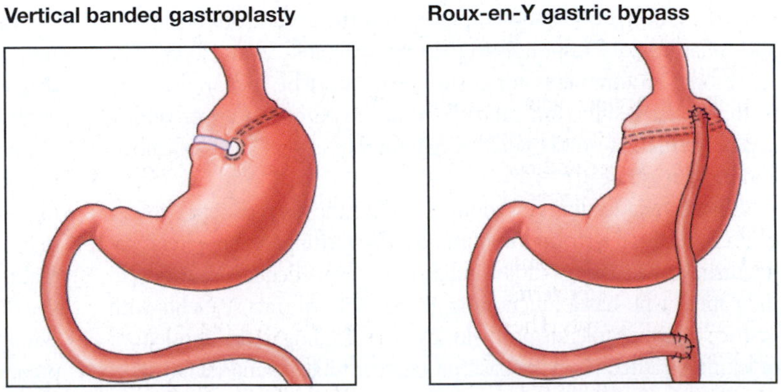

FIGURE 8–2 ◆ Gastric bypass line drawing.

Source: National Institutes of Health. (2000). The practical guide: Identification, evaluation, and treatment of overweight and obesity in adults. Retrieved from http://www.nhlbi.nih.gov/guidelines/obesity/prctgd_c.pdf.

CHART 8–32 Diet Progression and Discharge Planning Following Bariatric Surgery for Weight Loss

DIETARY CHANGES

Liquids for 1–2 weeks postoperatively:

- Begin with clear liquids and add full liquids as tolerated.
- Avoid sugary beverages.
- Avoid carbonation.
- Sip liquids slowly between meals.
- Slowly work toward intake of 64 oz daily.

Progress to pureed and soft foods 1 month postoperatively:

- Start with 2 TBSP and increase as tolerated per meal.
- Consume many small meals.
- Eat slowly. Eating too much or too fast will cause nausea and vomiting.

Follow guidelines for dumping syndrome if present. Dumping syndrome refers to abdominal pain, nausea, and bloating that occur after eating foods high in sugar, such as ice cream and milkshakes, following a bariatric procedure. Diarrhea, sweating, and fainting can also occur. Avoid foods that could cause this.

Eat slowly and chew well.

Save liquids for between meals.

Drink liquids in smaller amounts than prior to surgery. Continue to drink liquids to prevent dehydration. Signs of dehydration include dry mouth and dark urine.

Because of the smaller amounts of food, the types of food selected should be high quality offering high protein, low carbohydrate and low fat.

Use a chewable or liquid multivitamin. Bypass patients require vitamin B_{12}, iron, folic acid, and fluid and electrolyte monitoring.

ACTIVITY

Keep in mind that recovery takes several weeks.

It is normal to feel tired. Rest as needed.

Walk as often as able. Increase activity slowly.

Do not lift anything heavier than 10 pounds.

Avoid strenuous chores, such as vacuuming or lifting full bags of garbage, until the surgeon says it is safe to do so.

Climb stairs slowly and pause after every few steps.

Avoid swimming until incisions have healed completely.

Start an exercise program 1 week after discharge. You can benefit from simple activities such as walking or gardening. Swimming (after incisions have healed) is generally a well-tolerated form of exercise as it is low impact. Ask your surgeon how to get started.

Ask your surgeon when you can expect to return to work.

HOME CARE

Continue the coughing and deep-breathing exercises you learned in the hospital.

Shower as needed. But avoid baths, swimming pools, and hot tubs for 2 weeks after going home. This helps prevent infection of the incision site.

Keep the incision clean and dry. Wash the incision gently with mild soap and warm water. Then gently pat the incision dry with a towel.

Follow your surgeon's instructions about caring for the dressing covering your incisions.

Do not wear tight clothing that rubs against the incision.

Take medications in crushed or liquid form for 3 weeks after surgery and as instructed.

Keep in mind that medications and dosages may need to be adjusted with weight loss.

Do not drive for 2 weeks after surgery.

WHEN TO CALL THE SURGEON

Call the surgeon if the following are present:

- Cloudy or smelly drainage from the incision site
- Fever of 100.4°F or higher, or shaking chills
- Fast pulse
- Night sweats
- Persistent pain, nausea, or vomiting after eating
- Diarrhea beyond the first week after discharge
- Pain in your upper back, chest, or left shoulder
- Persistent hiccups
- Confusion, depression, or unusual fatigue
- Signs of bladder infection (urinating more often than usual; burning, pain, bleeding, or hesitancy when urinating).

Sources: MedlinePlus. (2012). Gastric bypass surgery—discharge. Retrieved from http://www.nlm.nih.gov/medlineplus/ency/patientinstructions/000172.htm; Cloe, A. (2010). Meal plans after bariatric surgery. Retrieved from http://www.livestrong.com/article/325784.

Weblink: Discharge Planning Following Bariatric Surgery for Weight Loss   Weblink: Meal Plans After Bariatric Surgery

Trauma

Patients who sustain major trauma are at nutritional risk because of the hypermetabolic and hypercatabolic metabolic response that follows injury. Blunt or penetrating trauma and head injuries are examples of trauma associated with high nutritional risk. Early and aggressive nutrition support is indicated once the patient is generally hemodynamically stable (Doig, Heighes, Simpson, & Sweetman, 2011). Enteral nutrition support is the preferred route unless bowel obstruction or other contraindication exists. The preservation of gut function and potential reduction of bacterial translocation and septic complications are commonly cited as benefits of enteral over parenteral nutrition support in trauma patients. Longer length feeding tubes, such as those used with a jejunostomy, may be required to deliver nutrition in the distal intestine following abdominal surgery or because of altered gastric emptying associated with physiological stress.

Nutrition Support

Nutrition support with enteral or parenteral feeding is indicated when patients cannot or will not take adequate nutrition to meet their individual needs. Enteral nutrition utilizes the intestinal tract for feeding. In contrast, parenteral nutrition is delivered intravenously and is generally reserved for situations where intestinal function is severely compromised.

Enteral Nutrition

Enteral nutrition is the preferred route of delivery for nutrition support (Kulick & Deen, 2011). Much has been written on the beneficial effects of maintaining gastrointestinal tract (GI [gut]) integrity and function through continued use, even when only small amounts of enteral feeding supplement are tolerated. Increased intestinal permeability and atrophy of intestinal villi occur when the gut is not used. Risk of bacterial translocation and sepsis may be reduced when patients receive enteral nutrition support compared to parenteral support (Kulick & Deen, 2011). Enteral nutrition support is also less costly than parenteral support. Although in the past many clinicians were quick to institute parenteral nutrition for many gastrointestinal or abdominal conditions, it is now realized that enteral nutrition may be tolerated and beneficial to these patients. Acute pancreatitis, postoperative bowel surgery, and active inflammatory bowel disease are examples of situations where enteral nutrition may be used effectively in most patients, replacing the older practice of using parenteral nutrition. Other indications for enteral nutrition include situations where a patient cannot or will not take an adequate oral diet, but has a functioning GI tract. Anorexia, dysphagia, head and neck surgery or tumor, and mechanical ventilation are examples of conditions that may prevent adequate oral intake.

Types of Enteral Formulas

A wide variety of enteral nutrition formulas exist. Most fall into the category of a complete formula (a formula that contains all essential nutrients). Modular feedings are also available that can be used to supplement a complete formula with a single nutrient (for example, fat or protein) or to build a customized formula that comprises all modular components. The latter use is less common.

Complete formulas are further categorized by nutrient composition, density, and form. Some are marketed specifically for a certain disease state, but whether they are superior to generic formulas of similar composition is unknown. Standard complete formulas contain intact nutrients and require full digestive and absorptive ability by the patient. For example, protein is present in its intact form as found in foods, such as soy protein or casein from milk. Some standard formulas contain lactose or added fiber. Fiber in enteral feedings may be beneficial for normal bowel function, especially in patients on long-term feeding. Elemental formulas contain nutrients in a hydrolyzed form such that the patient does not need full digestive or absorptive ability to benefit from the feeding. Instead of whole proteins, an elemental formula may have protein already broken down to amino acids or di- and tripeptides. Generally, these formulas have a minimal fat content as well. An elemental formula may be used with a patient with malabsorptive disease, bowel resection, or impaired pancreatic enzyme function. Both standard and elemental formulas contain between 1 and 2 kilocalories/mL. Many are also available in a high-protein version. Higher and lower calorie and protein contents allow for patients with increased or decreased fluid and/or nutritional needs.

When the composition of a 1 kilocalorie/mL formula is made of intact nutrients, the formula is usually isotonic in concentration. An **isotonic formula** has a concentration similar to that of the plasma and therefore should not contribute to an osmotic draw of fluid into the gut. When fluid is drawn into the gut to dilute a concentrated solution, cramping, bloating, and diarrhea can occur. Other types of formulas can be **hypertonic formulas** because they have a higher concentration of electronically active particles, as in the case of elemental formulas that have many small amino acids instead of large protein molecules. Higher-calorie or higher-protein formulas are also hypertonic because of their increased concentration. Hypertonic formulas may cause an osmotic draw of fluid into the gut in some patients and are often begun at a diluted strength to avoid this consequence initially. The choice of appropriate formula will be driven by whether the patient has full or compromised digestive and absorptive ability and her overall nutrition and fluid requirements.

Routes of Delivery

Enteral nutrition formula may be taken orally or delivered via a small-bore feeding tube of varying lengths. The oral route is used when the patient is able to tolerate liquid intake safely and requires a supplement to the diet, a liquid diet, or an elemental diet. For example, patients with short bowel syndrome may take minimal food and instead consume an elemental formula because of altered absorption. When a tube feeding is indicated, nasogastric, nasoduodenal, or nasojejunal tubes are available. The longer length tubes are used when the upper GI tract is dysfunctional or to reduce risk of aspiration compared with a nasogastric tube. Longer tubes do not remove the risk of aspiration, but they may lessen the risk. The Evidence-Based Practice guidelines discuss the reduction of aspiration risk during tube feeding administration.

Surgical placement of a gastrostomy or jejunostomy feeding tube is used when long-term enteral support is anticipated. Permanent tubes have the advantage of avoiding the irritation and discomfort of a nasal tube. Permanent tubes do not hold open the lower esophageal sphincter

EVIDENCE-BASED PRACTICE Reducing Aspiration Risk During Tube Feeding Administration

Clinical Problem

Tube feedings are often stopped or held in patients at high risk of aspiration if gastric residuals are elevated. As a result, the patient does not receive the goal volume of feeding needed to obtain nutritional requirements.

Research Findings

Tube feedings are stopped or held for gastric residual volumes of 150 mL or more out of fear of aspiration. DeLegge (2011) reports that a cutoff volume for holding feedings can be up to 500 mL without negative effect if there are no other signs of intolerance to the feeding. An evidence-based review of gastric residual volume urges acceptance of an isolated residual of 250 mL followed by clinical evaluation when two or more consecutive volumes exceed 250 mL (Kattlemann et al., 2006). They report that when single residuals of 250 mL are accepted, greater formula delivery results without altered aspiration risk.

Postpyloric placement of the feeding tube tip has been shown to decrease gastric residual volume and gastric reflux of formula, which are both risk factors for aspiration (Kattlemann et al., 2006; Metheny, Davis-Jackson, & Stewart, 2010). In turn, reduction of gastric residuals allows for reduced interruptions to feeding and closer approximation to prescribed feeding volume (Turner, 2010). Aspiration risk is diminished with proper patient positioning. When possible, elevating the head of the bed to a 30- to 45-degree angle during feedings will lessen the risk of reflux of gastric contents (Guenter, 2010). Positioning patients in this fashion is reported to decrease risk of aspiration pneumonia compared with patients in the supine position during feedings (Bankhead et al., 2009).

Implications for Nursing Practice

Critically ill patients are often at high risk of malnutrition. Promoting improved tube feeding tolerance and reduction in risk of aspiration pneumonia through patient positioning and feeding tube placement may offer an additional benefit of increased delivery of crucial nutrition.

Critical Thinking Questions with answers can be found in the Osborn Student Resources at nursing.pearsonhighered.com.

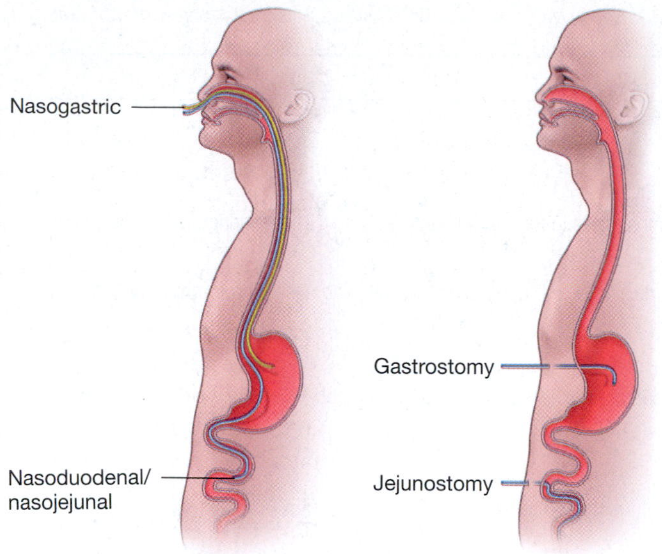

FIGURE 8–3 ◆ Feeding tube placement.

or pylorus, which potentially lessens the risk of aspiration. When a feeding tube is placed in the jejunum, an elemental formula must be used because the site of the tube has bypassed the natural sites for digestion of intact nutrients and enzyme secretion. Figure 8–3◆ demonstrates the various placements and lengths of feeding tubes.

Administration of Feedings

Enteral feedings may be administered in a variety of ways. Bolus feedings can be given several times during the day, mimicking normal food or fluid intake, when the patient is alert and not at risk of aspiration. This would not be unlike a patient consuming an oral diet who consumes a 240-mL cup of a beverage at one sitting. An example of this is a patient with a G-tube secondary to a resected head and neck tumor who is otherwise well and is now receiving long-term enteral feedings.

Patients with longer feeding tubes reaching the small bowel will not tolerate bolus feedings because of the osmotic load of the formula. Intermittent or continuous feedings are more common in the acute care setting. Intermittent feedings are delivered at a set rate for intermittent periods of time (for example, all night), whereas continuous feedings are delivered around the clock. Intermittent feedings may be the sole nutrition provided or they may be used to augment oral intake or parenteral nutrition. For example, a patient recovering from burns or a head injury may take an oral diet during the day with no tube feedings to impede appetite, and then receive intermittent feeding during the night in order to meet her high nutritional needs. Slower delivery of the formula results in avoidance of large gastric or intestinal volumes, minimizing the effect on aspiration risk and intolerance to hypertonic concentration. Feedings may be administered via gravity drip or with a feeding pump. Gravity drip delivery runs the risk of an accidental bolus occurring and should be avoided in patients at risk of aspiration.

The registered dietitian generally will recommend the appropriate formula and volume to meet the patient's needs. Depending on the formula content, the location of the feeding tube, and the patient's medical condition, feedings may be initiated at a diluted concentration or at full strength. Isotonic feedings may be initiated at full-strength concentration in some patients, but hypertonic formulas routinely are initiated at one-quarter to one-half strength. The concentration is gradually increased to full strength over one or more days depending on patient tolerance. The rate of formula delivery begins at about 50 mL/hr and is also increased as tolerated until recommended volume is achieved. Individual rate and concentration recommendations should be made for each patient.

Nutrition support requires close monitoring by the nurse. Tolerance to formula, amount delivered, and the fluid balance are crucial factors in determining the effectiveness of treatment. Starting and stopping feedings for various interventions and repositioning can result in inadequate delivery of feeding and should be monitored for cumulative effect. The nurse must monitor the patient for symptoms such as high gastric residuals of formula, diarrhea, nausea, or vomiting. Severe vomiting or coughing can cause nasal tube displacement and warrants reassessment of placement. Diarrhea is commonly blamed on enteral formula even when other factors contribute more significantly. Medications including antibiotics, infection, or bowel edema from hypoalbuminemia may be to blame and deserve investigation. Loose stools are to be expected with tube feeding and can be erroneously diagnosed as diarrhea. Formulas with added fiber are helpful in normalizing bowel function in appropriate patients. To minimize the risk of aspiration, patients should be fed with the head of the bed up at a 30- to 45-degree angle (Bankhead et al., 2009).

Some medications can be administered through the feeding tube, but not all. Longer tubes may bypass drug absorption sites. Liquid suspension of some medications is not available and crushing medication can alter its action. A pharmacist should be consulted to determine the compatibility of medication with the tube feeding delivery. Tubes should be flushed before, between, and after medication delivery to avoid formation of precipitates that will clog the tube and inconvenience both the nurse and the patient. Taking the time to ensure that medication delivery does not lead to tube obstruction is time well spent. Handling of the equipment and formula requires fastidious sanitation to avoid the risk of feeding contamination. Chart 8–33 outlines nursing interventions for common problems related to tube feedings.

Parenteral Nutrition

Parenteral nutrition support is indicated in the patient who is unable to tolerate adequate enteral nutrition. Bowel obstruction, severe intolerance to enteral feeding (such as can occur with short bowel syndrome), and bone marrow transplant are situations where parenteral nutrition is used. Parenteral formula delivered via a central line is referred to as **total parenteral nutrition (TPN).** This is indicated in patients requiring support for at least 10 days. Formula delivered via a peripheral vein is called **peripheral parenteral nutrition (PPN)** and must be isotonic. PPN is used as a short-term nutrition intervention to offset nutritional requirements until transition to alternative enteral nutrition is initiated. TPN is able to meet most patients' complete nutritional requirements. PPN is limited by the volume of fluid that can be tolerated peripherally and the lower concentration of nutrients that is required to maintain an isotonic concentration. Thus, it may not provide complete nutrition for some patients and is only a short-term solution.

Formula Composition

Parenteral formulas consist of a mix of carbohydrate, protein, fat, micronutrients, and electrolytes in amounts that are individually determined for each patient. Carbohydrate is in the form of dextrose and can be a 5% to 70% solution. Solutions that are more than 10% dextrose are

CHART 8–33 Nursing Interventions in Enteral Nutrition Support

Problem	Intervention
Potential for Foodborne Illness	• Wash hands before handling formula and equipment. • Wipe off top of formula container before opening. • Label, cover, and store open formula in refrigerator for not >24 hours. • Limit "hang time" to 4 hours if water or other additions made to formula. Otherwise, 8- to 12-hour hang time is allowed if canned formula w/no additives is being used.
Aspiration	• Check gastric residuals. Hold feeding for large volume (>150 mL but treat individually and according to physician's order). • Elevate head of bed to at least a 30-degree angle. • Avoid bolus feedings. • Consider smaller bore or longer tube if nasally intubated. Routinely confirm tube placement. • Consider G-tube or J-tube if long-term feeding is required.
Clogged Tube	• Administer feeding with pump vs. gravity drip. • Administer room temperature feeding. High-temperature storage or heating of formula will cause protein content to coagulate. • Follow guidelines for medication administration: 1. Flush tube with 20 to 30 mL water before, between, and after each single medication. 2. Consult pharmacist regarding suitability of crushing medication with a small amount of water and availability of medication elixirs. *Note: If using longer feeding tubes, ensure medication absorption site is not bypassed by tube.*
Diarrhea	• Administer feeding at room temperature. Cold feeding increases gut peristalsis. • Consider lactose-free formula. • Consider formula with fiber. • Consider medications w/cathartic effect: antibiotics, magnesium, potassium, digoxin, theophylline, acetaminophen elixir, and others. • Administer continuous drip vs. bolus. • Consult registered dietitian regarding temporarily altering formula concentration or rate of delivery. • Rule out infection (i.e., *Clostridium difficile*).
Constipation	• Consider formula with added fiber. • Monitor hydration; ensure adequate intake. • Encourage ambulation as indicated. • Assess for contributing medications (e.g., narcotics, some antacids). • Consider obstruction or medical causes.
Dehydration	• Monitor hydration: weight, intake & output, physical signs. • Ensure adequate free water intake. Need 1 mL water per 1 kcal of intake. Most formulas are 50% to 75% free water (formula with >1 kcal/mL or high protein content have less free water).

Source: Winkelman, C., & Best, K. (2009). Formula for success: Deliver enteral nutrition using best practices. *American Nurse Today*, *4*(3), 18–23; Yantis, M. A., & Velander, R. (2011). Untangling enteral nutrition guidelines. *Nursing 2011*, *41*(9), 32–38.

hypertonic and cannot be delivered peripherally. Protein is in the form of amino acids and begins at concentrations of 5%. A 5% amino acid solution, but not greater, can be tolerated peripherally. Fat can be administered centrally or peripherally and is an important calorie-dense component, a useful benefit when fluid volume is an issue. Both 10% and 20% solutions are available. Vitamins, minerals, and electrolytes are also administered with the formula admixture and can be customized to meet patient needs.

The nutrition support team makes recommendations on formula choice after a thorough assessment of the patient's nutritional, metabolic, and medical needs. Parenteral support is initiated at a low rate (about 50 mL/hr) and increased gradually to reach the recommended volume. Maximum rates and volumes for both dextrose and fat administration are individually adjusted to avoid hyperglycemia, poor lipid clearance, and fatty liver. Blood glucose and triglyceride levels are monitored to assess tolerance to formula composition of dextrose and lipid loads, respectively.

The nurse is involved in the close monitoring of parenteral nutrition, whether as a member of the nutrition support team or as a staff nurse. Most hospitals or institutions have clinical pathways or protocols that dictate the frequency and type of nursing interventions in the care of patients on parenteral support. The nurse should become familiar with the specific protocol. Meticulous care of the access site for parenteral nutrition is imperative to avoid local or systemic infection risk because the high dextrose load of the feeding is fuel for bacteria. Accurate fluid balance calculations along with daily weights are essential. A short-term weight gain of >1 kg is more likely associated with fluid gain than accumulation of lean or adipose tissue. Clinical protocols will also outline metabolic monitoring for hyperglycemia and frequency of required laboratory assays. Close attention is paid to overall fluid and electrolyte status, and the nurse can make formula adjustments accordingly.

Patients continuing parenteral nutrition to the home care setting will require regular nursing care and monitoring following modifications of the in-hospital monitoring parameters. Before parenteral nutrition is discontinued, it should be documented consistently that the patient is able to tolerate a diet or enteral formula and consume two-thirds or more of his estimated nutritional needs. Parenteral nutrition may be weaned to allow for appetite stimulation. Institutional policy will also outline nursing guidelines for stopping parenteral support. Some advocate substitution of a peripheral dextrose solution to avoid hypoglycemia once a high-dextrose central solution has been discontinued, whereas others call for a reduced rate of delivery before stopping the solution altogether. The nurse should become knowledgeable about the institutional protocol for discontinuing parenteral nutrition.

Gerontological Considerations

Nutrition Assessment

Nutrition assessment of the older adult should utilize the same parameters outlined for the general population. However, because of the prevalence of malnutrition in older adults, specific attention should be paid to assessment of contributing factors to unintentional weight loss and malnutrition.

Physical Exam and Focused Interview

Assess:

- Signs of malnutrition during clinical exam as outlined in Chart 8–1
- Signs of dysphagia or chewing difficulties; note pocketed food, drooling, mouth sores, dental health, fit of dentures, and **xerostomia** (lack of saliva)
- Cognitive impairment or dependency on others for feeding or meal preparation
- Altered functional status: immobility, loss of strength, fatigue
- Gastrointestinal, appetite, or oral complaints from disease or medication side effects
- Pain
- Psychosocial health: depression, bereavement, isolation, dependency, food security
- Sensory losses and neurological symptoms: vision, hearing, taste, neuropathy, tremors
- Medical conditions or treatment that alters intake, absorption, or nutritional requirements
- Hypermetabolic conditions: fever, infection, sepsis, fracture, wounds, cachexia, burns.

Anthropometric Measurements

Assess:

- Measured height and weight
- Serial weights; check medical record for weight history to confirm
- Body composition measurements must use age and gender-specific references because alterations in skin elasticity, muscle mass, fat distribution, bone density, and water content can change with age.

Nutrition History

Assess:

- Nutrition data as outlined in Chart 8–3
- Whether use of therapeutic diet is appropriate
- Use of alcohol
- Access to personal, cultural, or religious food preferences (especially hospitalized or dependent elderly)
- Iatrogenic malnutrition risk: assess days NPO, on clear liquid, or other insufficient diet; inadequate delivery of supplements or tube feedings; overuse of restricted diet resulting in poor intake

Malnutrition

The prevalence of malnutrition among older adults is disproportionately high compared to younger adults. Almost 60% of hospitalized elderly or those under dependent care are malnourished (Suominen, Sandelin, Soini, & Pitkala, 2009). In adults, malnutrition is associated with an increased mortality rate compared with those who are well-nourished (Lee & Berthelot, 2010).

Alterations in pharmacokinetics from malnutrition are especially pertinent in older adults because of the probability of polypharmacy. Low plasma protein levels affect drug binding for certain classes of medications, leaving an increased circulating free fraction of those drugs. Polypharmacy further complicates this when multiple drugs compete for diminished protein binding sites, increasing the likelihood of an adverse drug reaction. Enzymes required for drug metabolism can be affected by inadequate protein and micronutrient status. Malnutrition can affect pharmacokinetics at both the absorptive and cell level for drug and herb metabolism. Unintentional weight loss and signs of malnutrition among older adults should not be considered a normal part of the aging process and always deserve full consideration and attention to determine the etiology and provide appropriate intervention.

Weight Management

Adults over age 65 years can benefit from weight management with improved day-to-day functioning and reduced cardiovascular risk. Before weight loss is recommended or attempted, however, a thorough nutrition assessment should be considered because of the high prevalence of malnutrition among older adults. Improper dieting attempts could unwittingly contribute to increased risk of malnutrition. Patients should be evaluated for their individual risks and benefits associated with potential weight loss. Specific attention should be given to the preservation of muscle mass with physical activity. Appropriate referrals should be made for monitoring nutrition and exercise in the elderly.

Nutrition for Older Adult Patients with Diabetes

There is no evidence to support the use of any dietary restrictions in older adults with diabetes who reside in long-term care (American Dietetic Association, 2010b). Older adults in long-term care should receive the least restrictive diet possible because the benefits to nutrition status outweigh the risks in this population. In institutionalized older adults, a restricted diet does not provide superior blood glucose control and can lead to diminished intake.

Research

The importance of nutrition as it relates to wellness and diseases has increased. Current topics are presented in the Research Opportunities feature.

RESEARCH OPPORTUNITIES Related to Nutrition

Research Area	Clinical Impact
Nutrigenetics/nutrigenomics: The study of the relationship between gene expression and nutrition. Patients may be genetically predisposed to types of illnesses. Expression of these genes may be influenced a great deal by food.	Knowing which plant-based, nutritionally dense diets positively influence genetic expression could decrease the incidence of certain diseases.
Studying the fact that the way foods are prepared affects the therapeutic benefit.	Plants are the main source of micronutrients. Nutrient content can be altered if cooked or handled improperly. For instance, fruits and vegetables picked before peak ripeness contain fewer phytochemicals. Cooking and processing can further destroy properties of phytochemicals and antioxidants.

CLINICAL PREPARATION READ DOCUMENT APPLY

READ: **History of Present Illness** >> Laboratory Study Results >> Critical Thinking Questions

A 57-year-old unmarried female office worker was admitted to the telemetry unit through the emergency department (ED) after presenting in the early hours of the morning with a complaint of several hours of severe chest pain. On interview, the patient, Ms. Nance, reports that she was experiencing intermittent, nonradiating chest pain during the late evening after returning home from an elaborate dinner party. She relates that she has had this type of pain in the evening multiple times during the last year, and it eventually goes away on its own; for this reason she tolerated this episode of pain for several hours, and it eventually became constant in nature. She then waited several more hours before calling a friend who urged her to seek medical help and drove her to the hospital.

On admission to the ED, she was found to be in sinus tachycardia with no ST segment changes. Initial serial cardiac enzymes were within normal limits (WNL). Nonfasting laboratory values were WNL with the exception of serum cholesterol of 215 mg/dL and blood glucose of 162 mg/dL. Ms. Nance's blood pressure was found to be elevated at 175/110 mmHg and she was begun on antihypertensive medication. The admitting health care provider assessed that her chest pain might be related to gastroesophageal reflux and treated her with a proton pump inhibitor. She was admitted for overnight observation with a diagnosis of acute coronary syndrome due to continued, though milder, chest pain with mid-epigastric tenderness.

Medical–Surgical History

Her medical history is unavailable because Ms. Nance has not had a physical examination or other health care intervention in more than 20 years. Ms. Nance reports no prior physical complaints. She reports NKA, no prescribed or OTC medications, and no surgical history. Both of her parents died in their mid-70s of CAD.

Physical Exam

On physical examination, significant findings include a blood pressure of 170/105 mmHg and a complaint of moderate mid-epigastric tenderness. Ms. Nance is 5'5" in height and weighs 198 pounds. Fasting laboratory values reveal serum cholesterol of 209 mg/dL with LDL cholesterol of 151 mg/dL and HDL cholesterol of 35 mg/dL. Her fasting blood glucose is 130 mg/dL. Cardiac enzymes remain normal. You find the following after eliciting her history:

- Ms. Nance is unable to give a good weight history because she does not own a scale, but you discover that her dress size has climbed by one or two sizes a year for the last 5 years.
- Ms. Nance attempted to lose weight 1 year ago before a nephew's wedding by following a high-protein, very-low-carbohydrate diet. She was able to fit into a dress two sizes smaller after dieting for 6 weeks, but also reported that her chest pain symptoms began while on the diet, leading her to stop adhering to it.
- Her nutrition history reveals that she eats two meals per day, lunch and dinner, plus frequent snacks. She has her first meal at work at noon, but does drink several cups of coffee with cream in the morning. She has four or five cups of coffee a day. She buys her lunch at the office, choosing a meat with gravy or other sauce or a stir-fried dish and a potato or fried rice. She does not eat vegetables because she does not like how they are prepared by the office restaurant. Ms. Nance eats dinner out in a restaurant about four times a week with a preference for steak house establishments. Again, she tends to order red meat or chicken and a potato, plus dessert. When home for dinner, she heats a ready-made meal in her microwave or has instant soup. She always has at least one glass of wine with dinner, two if she is at a restaurant. Her snacks consist of chips or pretzels and crackers and cheese. A food frequency assessment reveals that her only fruit intake is orange juice on occasion when she feels she is getting a cold. Her only dairy intake is cream in her coffee. She takes no dietary supplements of any sort.
- Ms. Nance walks to and from her car in the office parking lot 5 days a week. This is her only exercise and takes approximately 5 minutes each way. On weekends, she remains indoors doing sedentary activities around her apartment and dining out in the evening with friends.

Allergies:	NKA
Medications:	None
Illness:	None reported
Surgeries:	None

Social History

Both parents died in their 70s of CAD. No siblings. Single, never married, lives alone, sedentary office worker. Active social life revolving around dining out with friends.

Physical Exam

Oxygen saturation 94% on RA
BP: 170/105 HR: 90 RR: 20 Temp: 37.1°C (98.9°F)
HEENT: nearsighted, glasses
Skin color: ruddy
Mucous membranes: pink
Sclera: white, no masses
Teeth: partial bridge, no obvious decay
Heart: regular rhythm, with no murmurs/rub, tachycardia
Lungs: clear, reports mild DOE
Abdomen: obese, soft, +BS, mild mid-epigastric tenderness
Pulses: −1 + radial and pedal
Extremities: no edema, warm and dry, no clubbing of fingers
Neuro exam: alert and oriented 4; speech clear and coherent
Skin: good skin turgor, no rashes, no bruising
ECG: NSR, mild tachycardia, no elevated ST segments

Admitting Medical Orders

Admit to cardiology service
Type of floor: telemetry
Condition: good
Admitting diagnosis: acute coronary syndrome, GERD
Final diagnosis: GERD, HTN, obesity, hypercholesterolemia
No known allergies
Vital signs and oxygen saturation q2h
Activity bed rest, with bathroom privileges
Diet: low fat, saturated fat and cholesterol, 2 g sodium, no caffeine; nutrition consult
Call house officer: Pulse 130/minute; BP 160 systolic; temperature >38.5°C (101.3°F); urine output <30 mL/hour; oxygen saturation <92%
IV: saline lock; flush with NS q8h
Strict in/out
Sequential compression devices (SCD) to lower extremities
Oxygen 2 L nasal cannula
ECG continuous monitoring
12-lead ECG daily
Daily weight

Scheduled Medications

Omeprazole 20 mg po daily
Vasotec 10 mg po daily

PRN Medications

Phenergan 25 mg IV q6h prn nausea
Triazolam 0.125–0.25 mg q noc, prn sleep
Ativan 0.5–2 mg IV q6–8h prn anxiety (not to exceed 10 mg/24 hours)
Tylenol 650 mg po/pr q4h for pain

Ordered Laboratory Studies

Troponin I q3h × 3
CPK–MB q8h × 3
Chemistry 20 and PO_4 on admission and chemistry 7 q12h for first 2 days, then daily
CBC q a.m.
$Mg^{2}+$ q a.m.
UA

Ordered Diagnostic Studies

Chest x-ray on admission and with adverse changes in O_2 saturation, increased shortness of breath, and/or increasing rales
GI consult for endoscopy

READ: History of Present Illnesses >> **Laboratory Study Results** >> Critical Thinking Questions

Test	Day 1	Day 2	Day 3
Sodium	142 mEq/L	137 mEq/L	140 mEq/L
Potassium	4.0 mEq/L	3.5 mEq/L	3.4 mEq/L
Chloride	106 mEq/L	100 mEq/L	102 mEq/L
Calcium	9.5 mg/dL		
Venous carbon dioxide	24 mEq/L	29 mEq/L	29 mEq/L
Blood urea nitrogen (BUN)	15 mg/dL	10 mg/dL	12 mg/dL
Creatinine	1.1 mg/dL	0.6 mg/dL	0.8 mg/dL
Blood glucose	162 mg/dL	130 mg/dL	129 mg/dL
Total proteins	5.2 g/dL		
Magnesium	2.1 mEq/L	2.0 mEq/L	2.1 mEq/L
Phosphorus	3.2 mg/dL		
Troponin I	0.26/0.23/ 0.28 ng/mL		
Myoglobin	0.5 μg/L		
Albumin	4.5 g/dL		
GOT	15 units/L	20 units/L	19 units/L

Test	Day 1	Day 2	Day 3
T. bilirubin	0.5 mg/dL		
CPK total	10 units/L	15 units/L	7 units/L
CPK MB	1.8%		
LDH	80 units/L	90 units/L	87 units/L
WBC	6,000/mm^3	5,200/mm^3	5,400/mm^3
Hemoglobin	16 g/dL	12 g/dL	14 g/dL
Hematocrit	45%	38%	40%
RBC	5/mm^3		
Platelets	395/mm^3	325/mm^3	250/mm^3
ABGs			
PO_2	80 mmHg	90 mmHg	91 mmHg
O_2 saturation	94%	97%	97%
pH	7.32	7.40	7.39
PCO_2	35 mmHg	40 mmHg	41 mmHg
HCO_3	22 mEq/L	26 mEq/L	24 mEq/L

Pearson Nursing Student Resources *Log on to* **nursing.pearsonhighered.com** *to download forms*

DOCUMENT:

- >> Summary of Hospitalization
- >> Pathophysiology Form
- >> Laboratory Values
- >> Laboratory Results Explanation

APPLY:

- >> List of Potential Nursing Diagnoses
- >> Concept Map
- >> Critical Thinking Questions and Concept Map

READ: History of Present Illnesses >> Laboratory Study Results >> **Critical Thinking Questions**

1. What are this patient's risk factors for hypertension? Coronary artery disease?
2. What nutrition advice would you give to improve her blood pressure control and decrease her risk of coronary artery disease?
3. What components of the patient's diet may contribute to her symptoms of gastroesophageal reflux?
4. What nutrition advice for cardiac risk reduction should also help with management of reflux symptoms?

Answers to Critical Thinking Questions can be found in Appendix D in the Osborn Student Resources at nursing.pearsonhighered.com.

NCLEX® PRACTICE

1. The nurse should plan to include which anthropometric measurements when assessing a patient's nutritional status?
   1. Body mass index (BMI), weight, and waist circumference
   2. Body mass index (BMI), blood pressure, and pulse
   3. A weight diary and food frequency diary
   4. A 24-hour food recall and blood pressure

2. The nurse should include which nursing intervention when caring for a patient with bulimia?
   1. Offer the patient frequent small servings of finger foods.
   2. Instruct the patient to avoid eating unless hungry.
   3. Encourage frequent periods of vigorous exercise.
   4. Explain the importance of adhering to scheduled mealtimes.

3. A client states, "Now that I am pregnant I want to help my family eat a more balanced diet." Which statements would the nurse evaluate as following the Dietary Guidelines for Americans 2010 recommendations? (select all that apply)
   1. "The adults in our family can have a glass of wine after work and 2 glasses with dinner."
   2. "I should cook with oil rather than using solid shortening."
   3. "We should eat tuna or swordfish 3 to 4 times each week instead of red meat."
   4. "At least half of our grains should be whole grains."
   5. "Our goal should be to take in less than 300 mg of dietary cholesterol daily."

4. The nurse and physician are working together to bring the office practice into line with *Healthy People 2020* nutritional objectives. Which new policy will help meet this objective?
   1. Each client will be weighed at each visit.
   2. Each client will be required to complete a 2-week food diary.
   3. Body mass index measurement will be measured on each office visit.
   4. Weight loss materials will be placed in the office waiting room.

5. Which clients would the nurse assess as being at risk for nutritional imbalances due to physiological stress? (select all that apply)
   1. A client who experienced 20% total body surface burns in an industrial fire
   2. A client who had a laparoscopic cholecystectomy this morning
   3. A client admitted with the diagnosis of urosepsis
   4. A client who sustained multiple fractures in a roll-over motor vehicle accident
   5. A client admitted for labor and delivery of a term infant

6. Refeeding is beginning with a client with a long history of anorexia nervosa. Which nursing interventions are necessary? (select all that apply)
   1. Restrict foods that are high in phosphates.
   2. Monitor for prolonged QT syndrome.
   3. Monitor for shortness of breath.
   4. Notify physician if any edema occurs.
   5. Encourage intake of foods containing potassium.

Answers to NCLEX Practice questions can be found in Appendix D in the Osborn Student Resources at nursing.pearsonhighered.com. Practice additional NCLEX questions online at the Student Resources site.

REFERENCES

Aase, S. (2010). Kidney friendly: What the National Kidney Disease Education Program Strategic Plan means for dietetic practice. *Journal of the American Dietetic Association, 110*(3), 346–351.

Aghdassi, E., Wendland, B. E., Stapleton, M., Raman, M., & Allard, J. P. (2007). Adequacy of nutritional intake in a Canadian population of patients with Crohn's disease. *Journal of the American Dietetic Association, 107*(9), 1575–1580.

American Diabetes Association. (2008). Nutrition recommendations and interventions for diabetes: A position statement of the American Diabetes Association. *Diabetes Care, 31,* S61–S78.

American Diabetes Association. (2009). Standards of medical care in diabetes. *Diabetes Care, 32,* S13–S61.

American Diabetes Association & American Dietetic Association (2010). *Count your carbs: Getting started.* Eat Right: Academy of Nutrition and Dietetics.

American Dietetic Association. (2009). Position of the American Dietetic Association: Weight management. *Journal of the American Dietetic Association, 109,* 330–346.

American Dietetic Association. (2010a). Position of the American Dietetic Association: Nutrition intervention and human immunodeficiency virus. *Journal of the American Dietetic Association, 110,* 1105–1119.

American Dietetic Association. (2010b). Practice paper of the American Dietetic Association: Individualized nutrition approaches for older adults in health care communities. *Journal of the American Dietetic Association, 110,* 1554–1563.

American Dietetic Association. (2011). Position of the American Dietetic Association: Nutrition intervention in the treatment of eating disorders. *Journal of the American Dietetic Association, 111,* 1236–1241.

American Gastroenterological Association. (2008). American Gastroenterological Association medical position statement on the management of gastroesophageal reflux disease. *Gastroenterology, 135,* 1383–1391.

American Heart Association. (2010a). Diet and lifestyle recommendations. Retrieved from http://www.heart.org/HEARTORG/GettingHealthy/Diet-and-Lifestyle-Recommendations_UCM_305855_Article.jsp

American Heart Association. (2010b). Sodium. Retrieved February 9, 2011, from http://www.americanheart.org/presenter.jhtml?identifier=4708

American Heart Association. (2011). Obesity information. Retrieved from http://www.heart.org/HEARTORG/GettingHealthy/WeightManagement/Obesity/Obesity-Information_UCM_307908_Article.jsp

American Psychiatric Association (APA). (2000a). *Diagnostic and statistical manual of mental disorders* (4th ed., text revision). Washington, DC: Author.

American Psychiatric Association (APA). (2000b). Practice guidelines for the treatment of patients with eating disorders. *American Journal of Psychiatry, 157*(s), 1–39.

Amini, M., & Runyon, B. A. (2010). Alcoholic hepatitis 2010: A clinician's guide to diagnosis and therapy. *World Journal of Gastroenterology, 16,* 4905–4912.

Anderson, J. W., Bair, P., Davis, R. H., Ferreri, S., Knudsen, M., Koraym, A., et al. (2009). Health effects of dietary fiber. *Nutrition Reviews, 67,* 188–205.

Anthony. P. S. (2008). Nutrition screening tools for hospitalized patients. *Nutrition in Clinical Practice, 23,* 373–382.

Bankhead, R., Boullata, J., Brantley, S., Corkins, M., Guenter, P., Krenitsky, J., et al. (2009). Enteral nutrition practice recommendations. *Journal of Parenteral and Enteral Nutrition, 33,* 122–167.

Becker, D. J., Gordon, R. Y., Halbert, S. C., French, B., Morris, P. B., & Rader, D. J. (2009). Red yeast rice for dyslipidemia in statin intolerant patients: Randomized trial. *Archives of Internal Medicine, 150,* 830–839.

Bellar, A., Jarosz, P. A., & Bellar, D. (2008). Implications of the biology of weight regulation and obesity on the treatment of obesity. *Journal of the American Academy of Nurse Practitioners, 20,* 128–135.

Berger, M. R., Fields-Gardner, C., Wagle, A., & Hollenbeck, C. B. (2008). Prevalence of malnutrition in human immunodeficiency virus/acquired immunodeficiency syndrome orphans in the Nyanza province of Kenya. *Journal of the American Dietetic Association, 108,* 1014–1017.

Blackmer, A. B., & Farrington, E. A. (2010). Constipation in the pediatric patient: An overview and pharmacologic considerations. *Journal of Pediatric Health Care, 24*(6), 385–399.

Bluestein, D., & Javaheri, A. (2008). Pressure ulcers: Prevention, evaluation, and treatment. *American Family Physician, 78,* 1186–1194.

Bottino-Bravo, P., & Thomson, J. (2008). When it's hard to swallow: Dysphagia in home care. *Home Healthcare Nurse, 26,* 244–250.

Bulimia.com. (2012). Eating disorders recovery—laxative abuse. Retrieved from http://www.bulimia.com/client/client_pages/laxativeabuse.cfm

Cagir, B. (2009). Short-bowel syndrome. *Medscape.* Retrieved from http://emedicine.medscape.com/article/193391-overview#a0104

Celli, B. R. (2010). Predictors of mortality in COPD. *Respiratory Medicine, 104,* 773–779.

Chadalavada, R., Sappati, R. S., Maxwell, J., & Mullen, K. (2010). Nutrition in hepatic encephalopathy. *Nutrition in Clinical Practice, 25,* 257–264.

Chang, E., Sekhar, R., Patel, S., & Balasubramanyam, A. (2007). Dysregulated energy expenditure in HIV-infected patients: A mechanistic review. *Clinical Infectious Diseases, 44,* 1509–1517.

Chen, S. T., Maruther, N. M., & Appel, L. J. (2010). The effect of dietary patterns on estimated coronary heart disease: Results from the Dietary Approaches to Stopping Hypertension (DASH) trial. *Circulation. Cardiovascular Quality & Outcomes, 3,* 484–489.

Clark, C., & DeLegge, M. (2008). Irritable bowel syndrome: A practical approach. *Nutrition in Clinical Practice, 23,* 263–267.

Cleveland Clinic. (2011). Phytosterols: Sterols & stanols. *Women's Cardiovascular Center.* Retrieved from http://my.clevelandclinic.org/heart/women/sterolstanol.aspx

Cloe, A. (2010). Meal plans after bariatric surgery. Retrieved from http://www.livestrong.com/article/325784

Cofrancesco, J., Freedland, E., & McComsey, G. (2009). Treatment options for HIV-associated central fat accumulation. *AIDS Patient Care and Standards, 23,* 5–18.

Colecraft, E. (2008). HIV/AIDS: Nutritional implications and impact on human development. *Proceedings of the Nutrition Society, 67,* 109–113.

Cresci, B., & Rotella, C. M. (2009). Motivational readiness to change in lifestyle modification programs. *Eating and Weight Disorders, 14,* e158–162.

DeLegge, M. H. (2011). Managing gastric residual volumes in the critically ill patient: An update. *Current Opinion in Clinical Nutrition and Metabolic Care, 14,* 193–196.

Demling, R. H. (2009). Nutrition, anabolism, and the wound healing process: An overview. *Eplasty, 9,* e9.

Dickerson, R. N. (2011). Optimal caloric intake for critically ill patients: First, do no harm. *Nutrition in Clinical Practice, 26,* 48–54.

Dickey, W. (2008). Making oats safer for patients with celiac disease. *European Journal of Gastroenterology and Hepatology, 20,* 494–495.

Dodson, S., Baracos, V. E., Jatoi, A., Evans, W. J., Cella, D., Dalton, J. T., et al. (2011). Muscle wasting in cancer cachexia: Clinical implications, diagnosis, and emerging treatment strategies. *Annual Review of Medicine, 62,* 265–279.

Doig, G. S., Heighes, P. T., Simpson, F., & Sweetman, E. A. (2011). Early enteral nutrition reduces mortality in trauma patients requiring intensive care: A meta-analysis of randomized controlled trials. *Injury, 1,* 50–56.

Dukkipati, R., & Kopple, J. D. (2009). Causes and prevention of wasting in chronic kidney failure. *Seminars in Nephrology, 29,* 39–49.

Eadala, P., Waud, J. P., Matthews, S. B., Green, J. T., & Campbell, A. K. (2009). Quantifying the hidden lactose in drugs used for the treatment of gastrointestinal conditions. *Alimentary Pharmacology Therapeutics, 29,* 677–687.

Evans, W. J., Morley, J. E., Argiles, J., Bales, C., Baracos, V., Guttridge, D., et al. (2008). Cachexia: A new definition. *Clinical Nutrition, 27,* 793–799.

Federal Trade Commission. (n.d.). *Red flag bogus weight loss claims.* Retrieved from http://www.ftc.gov/bcp/edu/microsites/redflag/

Flegal, K. M., Carroll, M. D., Ogden, C. L., & Curtin, L. R. (2010). Prevalence and trends in obesity among U.S. adults, 1999–2008. *Journal of the American Medical Association, 303,* 235–241.

Finley, C. E., Barlow, C. E., Halton, T. L., & Haskell, W. L. (2010). Glycemic index, glycemic load, and prevalence of the metabolic syndrome in the Cooper Center Longitudinal study. *Journal of the American Dietetic Association, 110,* 1820–1829.

Frishman, W. H., Beverol, P., & Carosella, C. (2009). Alternative and complementary medicine for preventing and treating cardiovascular disease. *Disease a Month, 55,* 121–192.

Garcia, J. M. (2010). Managing dysphagia through diet modifications. *American Journal of Nursing 110*(11), 26–33.

Gardener, P., Phillips, R., & Shaughnessy, A. F. (2008). Herbal and dietary supplement-drug interactions in patients with chronic conditions. *American Family Physician, 77,* 73–78.

Garth, A. K., Newsome, C. M., Simmance, N., & Crowe, T. C. (2010). Nutrition status, nutrition practices and post-operative complications in patients with gastrointestinal cancer. *Journal of Human Nutrition & Dietetics, 23,* 393–401.

Gentile, S. (2009). Contributing factors to weight gain during long-term treatment with second generation antipsychotics: A systematic appraisal and clinical implications. *Obesity Review, 10,* 527–542.

Goldfarb, D. S. (2009). Prospects for dietary therapy of recurrent nephrolithiasis. *Advances in Chronic Kidney Disease, 16,* 21–29.

Goldstein, L. B., Bushnell, C. D., Adams, R. J., Appel, L. J., Braun, L. T., Chaturvedi, S., et al. (2011). Guidelines for the primary prevention of stroke: A guideline for healthcare professionals from the American Heart Association. *Stroke, 42,* 517–584.

Gordon, R. Y., Cooperman, T., Obermeyer, W., & Becker, D. J. (2010). Marked variability of monacolin levels in commercially available red yeast rice products: Buyer beware. *Archives of Internal Medicine, 170,* 1722–1727.

Graves, C., Saffle, J., & Cochran, A. (2009). Actual burn nutrition care practice: An update. *Journal of Burn Care Research, 30,* 77–82.

Guenter, P. (2010). Safe practices for enteral nutrition in critically ill patients. *Critical Care Nursing of North America, 22,* 197–208.

Guigoz, Y. (2008). The Mini Nutrition Assessment review of the literature—what does it tell us? *Journal of Nutrition, Health, & Aging, 10,* 466–485.

Halmi, K. A. (2009). Perplexities and provocations of eating disorders. *The Journal of Child Psychology, 50,* 163–169.

Hardy, M. L. (2008). Dietary supplement use in cancer care: Help or harm? *Hematology Oncology Clinics of North America, 22,* 581–617.

Hull, R., & Goldsmith, D. (2008). Identifying and managing nephritic syndrome in adults. *The Practitioner, 252,* 32–34.

Jeschke, M. G., Chinkes, D. L., Finnerty, C. C., Kulp, G., Suman, O. E., Norbury, W. B., et al. (2008). Pathophysiologic response to severe burn injury. *Annals of Surgery, 248,* 387–401.

Kattlemann, K. K., Hise, M., Russell, M., Charney, P., Stokes, M., & Compher, C. (2006). Preliminary evidence for a medical nutrition therapy protocol: Enteral feedings for critically ill patients. *Journal of the American Dietetic Association, 106,* 1226–1241.

Kavalukas, S. L., & Barbul, A. (2011). Nutrition and wound healing. *Plastic and Reconstructive Surgery, 127,* 38S–43S.

Kulick, D., & Deen, D. (2011). Specialized nutrition support. *American Family Physician, 83*, 173–183.

Kuller, L. H. (2011). The great fat debate; reducing cholesterol. *Journal of the American Dietetic Association, 111*(5), 663–664.

Kurmis, R., Parker, A., & Greenwood, J. (2010). The use of immunonutrition in burn injury care: Where are we? *Journal of Burn Care & Research, 31*, 677–691.

Kushner, R. F. (2007). Obesity management. *Gastroenterology Clinics of North America, 36*, 191–210.

Lee, M. R., & Berthelot, E. R. (2010). Community covariates of malnutrition based on mortality among older adults. *Annals of Epidemiology, 20*, 371–379.

Makhijas, S., & Baker, J. (2008). The Subjective Global Assessment: A review of its use in clinical practice. *Nutrition in Clinical Practice, 23*, 405–409.

Marcason, W. (2008). What is the latest research regarding the avoidance of nuts, seeds, corn, and popcorn in diverticular disease? *Journal of the American Dietetic Association, 108*, 1956.

Maruther, N. M., Wang, N. Y., & Appel, L. J. (2009). Lifestyle interventions reduce coronary heart disease risk: Results from the PREMIER trial. *Circulation, 119*, 2026–2031.

MedlinePlus. (2012). Gastric bypass surgery—discharge. Retrieved from http://www.nlm.nih.gov/medlineplus/ency/patientinstructions/000172.htm

Meno, C. A., Hannum, J. W., Espelage, D. E., & Douglas Low, K. S. (2008). Familial and individual variables as predictors of dieting concerns and binge eating in college females. *Eating Behaviors, 9*, 91–101.

Metheny, N. A., Davis-Jackson, J., & Stewart, B.J. (2010). Effectiveness of an aspiration risk-reduction protocol. *Nursing Research, 59*, 18–25.

Miller, T. M., Abdel-Maksoud, M. F., Crane, L. A., Marcus, A. C., & Byers, T. E. (2008). Effects of social approval bias on self-reported fruit and vegetable consumption: A randomized controlled study. *Nutrition Journal, 27*, 18.

Mosier, M. J., Pham, T. N., Klein, M. B., Gibran, N. S., Arnoldo, B. D., Gamelli, R. L., et al. (2011). Early enteral nutrition in burns: Compliance with guidelines and associated outcomes in a multicenter study. *Journal of Burn Care and Research, 32*, 104–109.

National Heart, Lung, and Blood Institute. (2007). Your guide to lowering your cholesterol with therapeutic lifestyle changes. Retrieved September 15, 2011, from http://www.nhlbi.nih.gov/health/public/heart/chol/chol_tlc.pdf

National Institute of Diabetes and Digestive and Kidney Diseases. (2007a). Heartburn, gastroesophageal reflux, and gastroesophageal reflux disease. Retrieved February 18, 2011, from http://digestive.niddk.nih.gov/ddiseases/pubs/gerd/

National Institute of Diabetes and Digestive and Kidney Diseases (NIDDK). (2007b). Lactose intolerance. Retrieved February 18, 2011, from http://digestive.niddk.nih.gov/ddiseases/pubs/lactoseintolerance/

National Institute of Diabetes and Digestive and Kidney Diseases (NIDDK). (2007c). Rapid gastric emptying. Retrieved February 18, 2011, from http://digestive.niddk.nih.gov/ddiseases/pubs/rapidgastricemptying/index.htm

National Institute of Diabetes and Digestive and Kidney Diseases (NIDDK). (2008). Celiac disease. Retrieved February 18, 2011, from http://digestive.niddk.nih.gov/ddiseases/pubs/celiac/index.htm

National Institutes of Health (NIH), National Center for Complementary and Alternative Medicine. (2010). Bitter orange. Retrieved February 9, 2011, from http://nccam.nih.gov/health/bitterorange/D390_Herbs.pdf

National Kidney & Urologic Diseases Information Clearinghouse. (2011). Anemia in kidney disease and dialysis. Retrieved from http://kidney.niddk.nih.gov/kudiseases/pubs/anemia/#treatment

Norman, K., Pichard, C., Lochs, H., & Pirlich, M. (2008). Prognostic impact of disease-related malnutrition. *Clinical Nutrition, 27*, 5–15.

O'Keefe, J. H., Carter, M. D., & Lavie, C. J. (2009). Primary and secondary prevention of cardiovascular disease: A practical evidence-based approach. *Mayo Clinic Proceedings, 84*, 741–757.

O'Sullivan, M. (2009). Session 3: Joint Nutrition Society and Irish Nutrition and Dietetic Institute Symposium on Nutrition and Autoimmune Disease: Nutrition in Crohn's disease. *Proceedings of the Nutrition Society, 68*, 127–134.

Pak, C. Y. (2008). Medical stone management: 35 years of advances. *Journal of Urology, 180*, 813–819.

Parikh, A., Lipsitz, S. R., & Natarajan, S. (2009). Association between a DASH-like diet and mortality in adults with hypertension: Findings from a population-based study. *American Journal of Hypertension, 22*, 409–416.

Posthauer, M. E., Dorner, B., & Collins, N. (2010). Nutrition: A critical component of wound healing. *Advances in Skin & Wound Care, 23*, 560–572.

Riediger, N. D., Othman, R., Suh, M., & Moghadasian, M. H. (2009). A systematic review of the roles of n-3 fatty acids in health and disease. *Journal of the American Dietetic Association, 109*, 668–679.

Robinson-O'Brien, R., Perry, C. L., Story, M., & Neumark-Sztainer, D. (2009). Adolescent and young adult vegetarianism: Better dietary intake and weight outcomes but increased risk of disordered eating behaviors. *Journal of the American Dietetic Association, 109*, 648–655.

Rosen, D. S., and the Committee on Adolescence. (2010). Identification and management of eating disorders in children and adolescents. *Pediatrics, 126*, 1240–1253.

Scagluisi, F. B., Ferriolli, E., Pfrimer, K., Laureano, C., Sanita Cunha, C., Gualano, B., et al. (2008). Underreporting of energy intake in Brazilian women varies according to dietary assessment: A cross-sectional study using doubly labeled water. *Journal of the American Dietetic Association, 108*, 2031–2040.

Schulz, G. J., Campos, A. C., & Coehlo, J. C. (2008). The role of nutrition in hepatic encephalopathy. *Current Opinion in Clinical Nutrition and Metabolic Care, 11*, 275–280.

Seeff, L. B., Curto, T. M., Szabo, G., Everson, G. T., Bonkovsky, H. L., Dienstag, J. L., et al. (2008). Herbal products used by persons enrolled in the Hepatitis C Antiviral Long-term Treatment Against Cirrhosis (HALT-C) Trial. *Hepatology, 47*, 605–612.

Sesso, H. D., Buring, J. E., Christen, W. G., Kurth, T., Belanger, C., MacFayden, J., et al. (2008). Vitamins E & C in the prevention of cardiovascular disease in men: The Physicians' Health Study II randomized controlled study. *Journal of the American Medical Association, 300*, 2123–2133.

Setnick, J. (2011). *Eating disorders.* American Dietetic Association.

Shankar, P., Boylan, M., & Sriram, K. (2010). Micronutrient deficiencies after bariatric surgery. *Nutrition, 26*, 1031–1037.

Siddiqui, J., Phillips, A. L., Freedland, E. S., Sklar, A. R., Darkow, T., & Harley C. R. (2009). Prevalence and cost of HIV-associated weight loss in a managed care population. *Current Medical Research and Opinion, 25*, 1307–1317.

Sim, L. A., McAlpine, D. E., Grothe, K. B., Himes, S. M., Cockerill, R. G., & Clark, M. M. (2010). Identification and treatment of eating disorders in the primary care setting. *Mayo Clinic Proceedings, 85*, 746–751.

Spanier, B. W., Bruno, M. J., & Mathus-Vliegen, E. M. (2011). Enteral nutrition and acute pancreatitis: A review. *Gastroenterology Research and Practice.* doi: 10.1155/2011/857949

Suominen, M. H., Sandelin, E., Soini, H., & Pitkala, K. H. (2009). How well do nurses recognize malnutrition in elderly patients? *European Journal of Clinical Nutrition, 63*, 292–296.

Taku, K., Umegaki, K., Taki, Y., Endoh, K., & Watanabe, S. (2007). Soy isoflavones lower serum total and LDL cholesterol in cholesterol: A meta-analysis of 11 randomized controlled trials. *American Journal of Clinical Nutrition, 85*, 1148–1156.

Tiniakos, D. G., Vos, M. B., & Brunt, E. M. (2010). Nonalcoholic fatty liver disease: Pathology and pathogenesis. *Annual Reviews of Pathology, 5*, 145–171.

Tsiaousi, E. T., Hatzitolios, A., Trygonis, S., & Savopoulos, C. (2008). Malnutrition in end stage liver disease: Recommendations and nutrition support. *Journal of Gastroenterology and Hepatology, 23*, 527–533.

Tucker, S. B., & Dauffenbach, V. (2011). *Nutrition and diet therapy for nurses.* Upper Saddle River, NJ: Pearson.

Tucker, O. N., Szomstein, A., & Rosenthal, R. J. (2007). Nutritional consequences of weight loss surgery. *Medical Clinics of North America, 91*, 499–514.

Turner, P. (2010). Providing optimal nutritional support in the intensive care unit: Key challenges and practical solutions. *Proceedings of the Nutrition Society, 69*, 574–581.

Urden, L. D. (2009). *Critical care nursing: Diagnosis and management* (6th ed.). St. Louis: Elsevier.

U.S. Department of Agriculture. Nutrient Data Laboratory. (2011). Retrieved from http://www.nal.usda.gov/fnic/foodcomp/search

U.S. Department of Agriculture. (2011). *Food safety education.* Retrieved from http://www.fsis.usda.gov/Food_Safety_Education/index.asp

U.S. Department of Health and Human Services. (2010). *Dietary guidelines for Americans, 2010 edition.* Retrieved from http://www.cnpp.usda.gov/dietaryguidelines

U.S. Department of Health and Human Services. (2011). *Healthy People 2020.* Retrieved from http://www.healthypeople.gov

Van Wormer, J. J., Martinez, A. M., Martinson, B. C., Crain, A., Benson, G. A., Cosentino, D. L., et al. (2009). Self-weighing promotes weight loss of obese adults. *American Journal of Preventative Medicine, 36*, 70–73.

Vemulapalli, R. (2008). Diet and lifestyle modifications in the management of gastroesophageal reflux disease. *Nutrition in Clinical Practice, 23*, 293–298.

Wanek, S., & Wolf, S. E. (2007). Metabolic response to injury and role of anabolic hormones. *Current Opinion in Clinical Nutrition and Metabolic Care, 10*, 272–277.

Wilkinson, J. M., & Ahearn, N. R. (2009). *Prentice Hall nursing diagnosis handbook* (9th ed.). Upper Saddle River, NJ: Prentice Hall.

Williams, P. M., Goodie, J., & Motsinger, C. D. (2008). Treating eating disorders in primary care. *American Family Physician, 77*, 187–195.

Winkelman, C., & Best, K. (2009). Formula for success: Deliver enteral nutrition using best practices. *American Nurse Today, 4*(3), 18–23.

Wooley, J. A. (2008). Characteristics of thiamin and its relevance to the management of heart failure. *Nutrition in Clinical Practice, 23*, 487–493.

Worcester, E. M., & Coe, F. L. (2008). Nephrolithiasis. *Primary Care: Clinics in Office Practice, 35*, 369–391.

Yantis, M. A., & Velander, R. (2011). Untangling enteral nutrition guidelines. *Nursing 2011, 41*(9), 32–38.

Zieve, D. (2011). Binge eating. Retrieved from http://www.nm.nih.gov/medlineplus/eatingdisorders.html

The Biophysical and Psychosocial Aspects of Nursing

9 CHAPTER

Jean Klein
Cheryl Wraa

Outcome-Based Learning Objectives

After studying this chapter, the learner will be able to:

1. Compare and contrast the physiological components of the general adaptation syndrome (GAS).
2. Explain the relationship of oxidative stress (OS) to the disease process.
3. Generate a nursing management plan for patients with physiological stress.
4. Differentiate the nursing assessment criteria for patients experiencing stress.
5. Utilize the nursing process to assist hospitalized patients and their significant others to deal with stress that is presented in anger, anxiety, depression, frustration, or loss.
6. Apply culturally competent principles of therapeutic communication for the care of patients and significant others.
7. Apply the principles of teaching and learning to the care of patients and significant others.

KEY TERMS

accommodation p.215
acculturative stress p.221
acute stress p.211
acute stressor p.206
adaptation p.206
affective learning p.229
assimilation p.215
chronic stress p.211
cognitive reappraisal p.208
compromised family coping p.225
ego p.215
ego defense mechanisms p.215
eustress p.207
external locus of control p.231
external stressor p.206
general adaptation syndrome (GAS) p.207
holism p.216
hypothalamic–pituitary–adrenal (HPA) axis p.217
id p.215
internal locus of control p.231
internal stressor p.206
local adaptation syndrome (LAS) p.207
locus of control p.231
maladaptive coping mechanisms p.206
mind–body connection p.205
oxidative stress (OS) p.213
psychomotor learning p.229
reactive oxygen species (ROS) p.214
schema p.215
sick role p.231
stress perception p.206
stress response p.206
superego p.215
therapeutic alliance p.221
therapeutic communication p.222

WHEN PATIENTS ARE ILL OR SUFFER AN INJURY, their bodies respond physiologically and emotionally. There is a bidirectional interaction between the body systems and the brain that affects both physical and mental health, known as the **mind–body connection** (Esler et al., 2008; Mahoney, Palyo, Napier, & Giordano, 2009; Koithan, 2009; Taylor, Goehler, Galper, Innes, & Bourguignon, 2010). Messages travel across autonomic and neuroendocrine pathways and connect the central nervous system to the body to elicit affective, hormonal, immune, and autonomic responses. The way patients manage these responses can have a profound impact on their health. It is well accepted that psychological stress and peripheral inflammation are contributors that lead to heart disease and other chronic conditions. One way to mitigate the impact of stress on physical health is to teach patients and ourselves how to control and enhance the mind–body connection. For instance, mind–body therapies such as mental imagery, yoga, Tai Chi, and meditation are effective in reducing insomnia, anxiety, irritable bowel syndrome, depression, and acute and chronic pain. These therapies are thought to promote homeostasis. In this chapter, we will cover five aspects of the mind–body connection and the ways that nurses can intervene to promote health.

STRESS AND ADAPTATION

Stress, a universal phenomenon, is considered to be a condition in which people respond physiologically, psychologically, and socially to life changes. The term *stress* also is used to describe a variety of feelings and reactions that accompany actual and perceived threatening or challenging situations. Stress can be positive or negative.

When an individual experiences an actual or perceived threat or challenge, a physiological stress reaction occurs that helps the individual adapt to the situation's demands. This stress reaction maximizes the expenditure of energy, which helps prepare the body to meet the threatening or challenging situation. The individual mobilizes a great deal of effort in order to deal with the event, thereby engaging both the sympathetic/adrenal and pituitary/adrenal system (Taylor et al., 2010). Within this context, stress is viewed as a subset of the concept of adaptation, or the processes of maintaining psychobiological equilibrium during interaction with the environment.

Although a certain amount of stress is necessary for survival, prolonged stress can affect health adversely. Because stress and adaptation are interactive processes by which people respond to daily stimuli, it is important for nurses to understand the concept of stress, its effects on the total person, how individuals respond to stress, and how nursing can assist patients in coping with stressful situations.

Stress, Adaptation, and Coping

Stress can be viewed as a sequence of events that begins with a stimulus (stressor), which is recognized by the brain (**stress perception**), and that results in the activation of physiological fight/flight/fright systems within the body (**stress response**). This stress response is needed in short-term situations, but if an individual is constantly in a stress response, the negative effect on the body and brain will contribute to dysfunction, including autonomic dysfunction, depression, and cognitive impairment (Taylor et al., 2010).

The desired outcome of stress is adaptation. **Adaptation** is a response to stress that allows the individual to cope with the stressor in a way that promotes return to normal functioning. Coping is a compensatory process with physiological and psychological components that allows the individual to adapt to the stressor. Stressful conditions are factors that disrupt behavioral organization, signal a disruption has occurred, and trigger coping responses to restore balance (Sauls & Warise, 2010). Recognizing that admission to a hospital is a stressful situation for both patients and families, many hospitals provide written instructions on what to expect during the hospitalization regarding when the visiting hours are or how to get in touch with the primary health care practitioners. This written information assists the patients and families in coping with the stress of a hospitalization.

The goals of adaptation are physical health, psychological health, and enhanced social functioning, which includes the ability to work and engage in positive family relationships. Adaptive coping seeks to preserve important relationships during stressful situations and minimize the impact of the stressor, while **maladaptive coping mechanisms** are ineffective responses to stress and may be precursors to disease. These responses generally are chronic, recurrent responses or patterns that do not promote the goals of adaptation or reduce the impact of the stressor. This section explores the concepts of stress, adaptation, and coping as they impact the health and well-being of individuals.

Classifications of Stressors

Stress can be caused by internal or external sources (stressors) and can produce adaptive responses or maladaptive responses. Stress also can be classified as acute or chronic, depending on the length of time that the individual experiences stress or responds to the stressor. Additionally, stress is classified according to the type of human response stimulated by the stressor: physical, physiological, or psychosocial. Stressors can be developmental or situational.

Internal and External Stressors

Internal stressors originate within a person. They include lifestyle choices, such as the use of caffeine; an overloaded schedule; negative self-talk, such as self-criticism; unrealistic expectations, taking things personally, or rigid thinking; and stressful personality traits, such as being a perfectionist or a workaholic. Internal stressors are exaggerated by physiological or psychological stimuli, such as cancer, depression, and anxiety.

External stressors originate outside the body and are precipitated by changes in the external environment. They can be triggered by the actual physical environment, such as noises or bright lights; the social environment, such as rudeness or aggressiveness; the organizational environment, such as rules; major life events, such as the birth of a baby; or trauma, such as experiencing a severe burn, a motor vehicle crash, or a catastrophic event such as a hurricane or flood.

Acute Versus Chronic Stressors

Acute stressors are brief and involve a tangible threat that is readily identified as a stress, such as an initial admission to the hospital or studying for an examination. In contrast, chronic stressors are not readily identified as stressors because the person has been living with the source of the stress for some time and on the surface may "appear" to be adjusting to the source of the stress. Chronic stressors, such as poverty, malnutrition, long-time unemployment, or changes in economic status, have become such a part of modern life that they may be taken for granted and, therefore, may pose a serious health risk if they are not recognized and properly managed.

Human Response Stressors: Developmental and Situational

Sometimes stressors are classified according to the type of human response they generate: physical, physiological, or behavioral. More often they are considered within the domains of developmental and situational stressors.

Developmental stressors predictably occur at various points of development throughout the life span and correspond to Erikson's eight developmental stages, which are discussed later in this chapter. *Situational stressors* are precipitated by various unexpected situations, including a new job, being hospitalized for a myocardial infarction, or the death of a child. Situational stressors are unpredictable, may occur at any time during life, and as such can be more problematic because the person may be the only one experiencing the event at that time.

Contemporary Interpretations of Stress

Current theories typically portray stress as a (1) stimulus, (2) response, and (3) transaction or process. These three views of stress are complementary in nature and provide the framework in which stress is studied, diagnosed, and treated. Nurses use these theories to identify the stressor in a particular situation, to predict the patient's responses, and to assist patients to strengthen health and coping responses and to adjust unhealthy, unproductive responses.

Despite the differentiation made in the types of stress theory, nurses should recognize that stress is ever present, is inevitable, and is a familiar aspect of life. Because stressors originate from different sources, serving as a stimulant in some instances and as a burden in others, it is recognized that the fight-or-flight response, the general adaptation syndrome, and one's mental response to stress are separate mechanisms that fit together in a single integrated stress response.

Stress as a Stimulus

According to the stimulus-based theory of stress, stress is defined as a stimulus, a life event, or a set of circumstances that arouses physiological and/or psychological reactions that result in a response that may increase the individual's vulnerability to illness. Historically, this theory evolved from attempts to develop questionnaires to measure stress in terms of life changes or life events (Holmes & Masuda, 1966; Holmes & Rahe, 1967; Horowitz, Schaefer, Hiroto, Wilner, & Levin, 1977).

Holmes and Rahe (1967) developed *The Social Readjustment Rating Scale* (SRRS) to discover what effects life changes or events had on people. The researchers gave the SRRS to patients who presented in an emergency room and to the people who accompanied them, and then compared their scores. The researchers assigned 43 numerical values to the responses from the participants according to the amount of adjustment required for each event. The highest rated event on the scale was the death of a spouse. Other events included marriage, loss of a job, starting school, and bankruptcy. The results astounded the world of psychology and medicine: sick people had experienced far more of these life events in the year prior to their illness than did the healthy people who brought them to the hospital emergency room. The items included in Holmes and Rahe's SRRS, with the assigned numerical values can be seen at the following website: http://www.mindtools.com/pages/article/newTCS_82.htm.

Research has demonstrated a significant relationship between number and intensity of life events and the resulting probability of physical and emotional illness following the events (Holmes & Masuda, 1966). However, the relationships often are weak, and findings contrary to these studies also have been reported. Therefore, nurses must consider other factors, such as hardiness, when assessing an individual's response to stress.

Research has demonstrated that some individuals who experience high scores in terms of changing life events do not experience illness. A mediating factor in this process, which may act as a predictor of illness, is the condition termed hardiness (Deng, Weber, Sood, & Kemper, 2010). The hardy person has (1) a clear sense of personal values and goals, (2) a strong tendency toward interaction with the environment, (3) a sense of meaningfulness, and (4) control over what she can do. However, the effect hardiness has on an individual continues to be researched.

Stress as a Response: The General Adaptation Syndrome

Selye (1936) introduced stress as a response in the early 1900s. His theory suggests that stressors from different sources produce a similar physical response pattern. He called these physical responses to stress the **general adaptation syndrome (GAS).** Stressors also may result in a local response called the **local adaptation syndrome (LAS),** which proceeds through the same three stages as the GAS. Selye coined the term **eustress** to refer to stress associated with positive events, such as winning a race or a tennis match. The health consequences of eustress were never fully explained.

The GAS is composed of three stages: alarm, resistance, and exhaustion:

- ***Alarm Stage:*** The first stage of the stress response is the alarm reaction of the GAS, in which the individual experiences a physical or mental stressor. During this stage the fight-or-flight response is initiated. When the stressor is of sufficient intensity to threaten the homeostasis of the individual, a reallocation of energy is required so that adaptation can occur. This temporarily decreases an individual's resistance and may even result in disease or death if the stress is prolonged and severe (as in the case of burns or extreme temperature changes).
- ***Resistance Stage:*** The individual quickly moves from the alarm stage to the resistance stage. At this time, adaptation may occur as the body attempts to cope with the stressor by acting to minimize the stressor's impact as much as possible. For example, in the event of an injury, the body's inflammatory processes engage to limit the impact to the injured area. The amount of resistance varies depending on the individual's level of physical functioning, coping abilities, and total number and intensity of stressors experienced.

  There are fewer signs and symptoms at this stage compared to the alarm stage; essentially, the bodily symptoms of the alarm reaction disappear and resistance rises above normal. Throughout the resistance stage, the person is expanding energy in an attempt to adapt in order to return to a normal or near-normal state of functioning. This adaptive response is limited by the individual's resources. When resources are adequate, the individual may successfully recover from a stressor and return to homeostasis. When resources are ineffective, the person may move to the next stage of the GAS, exhaustion.
- ***Exhaustion Stage:*** Exhaustion is the final stage of the GAS. If the adaptation that the body made during the second stage cannot be maintained, the means used to cope with the stressor are depleted. This stage occurs when the stress is overwhelming or not removed, or the person is ineffective in dealing with the stressor.
  - Physical symptoms of the alarm reaction may reappear briefly as the body makes a final attempt to survive. This is exemplified by a terminally ill person whose vital signs become stronger just before death. This stage can be reversed by external sources of adaptive energy such as medication, blood transfusion, and/or intensive psychotherapy. The end of this stage largely depends on the adaptive energy resources of the individual, the severity of the stressor, and the external adaptive resources that are provided. Death may be the ultimate consequence of this phase.

Because stress is a state of the body, it can be observed only by noting the changes it produces in the body. Once the stressor or stimulus is integrated into the central nervous system (CNS), multiple responses occur because of activation of the hypothalamic–pituitary– adrenal axis and the autonomic nervous systems. It is necessary to understand these bodily responses in the individual experiencing stress. With prolonged stress, the adrenal glands enlarge; the lymphatic structures, such as the thymus, spleen, and lymph nodes, atrophy; and deep rugae appear in the lining of the stomach. The body also can react locally. An example of the LAS is inflammation. Figure 9–1◆ depicts these three stages of adaptation to stress.

Weblink: Social Readjustment Rating Scale (SRRS)

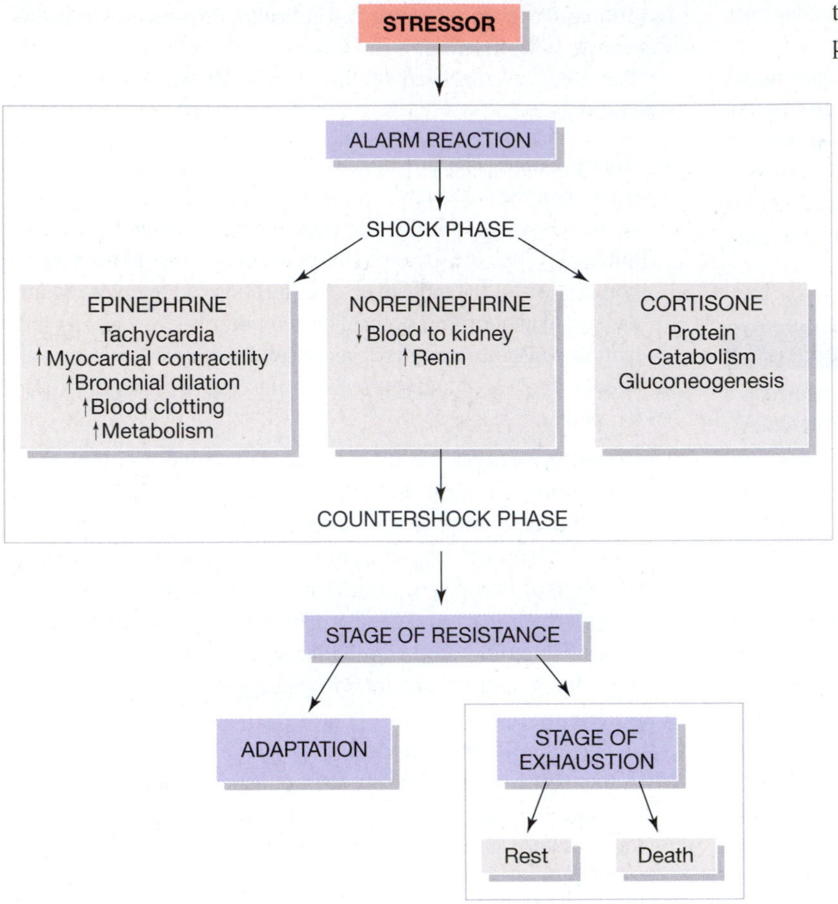

FIGURE 9–1 ◆ The three stages of Selye's adaptation to stress model.

Stress as a Transaction

Transactional theories of stress are based on the work of Lazarus (1966). Lazarus focused on the person–environment transaction and the cognitive appraisals of demands and coping options (Lazarus & Folkman, 1984). The way in which a person appraises or interprets (cognition) his relationship with the environment (objects, persons, and situations in the surroundings) determines whether or not the individual perceives the situation as stressful (Lazarus & Folkman, 1984).

According to Lazarus (1966) psychological stress consists of the demands that tax or exceed available resources (internal and external) as perceived by the individual involved. Stress is generated from the mutual influence that occurs between the person and the environment the person interacts with during the course of an encounter. The emphasis is on the process of what is happening in any given stressful event and how changes are occurring during the event. The transaction is a dynamic one.

Lazarus emphasized that people and groups differ in their sensitivity and vulnerability to certain types of events, as well as in their interpretations and reactions. Lazarus included mental and psychological components or responses as part of the concept of stress. His theory encompasses a set of cognitive, affective, and adaptive responses that arise out of person–environment transactions. Lazarus proposed that multitudes of data are received at the neurocognitive level, and that these are interpreted during the process of cognitive appraisal. Primary and secondary appraisals are the two major forms available to individuals to help them with potential or actual demands.

- *Primary appraisal* is the process of evaluating the significance of the transaction as it relates to a person's well-being. During the primary appraisal, the individual classifies the stressor or transaction as (1) irrelevant; (2) good, or benign-positive; or (3) stressful. If demands are appraised as stressful, they can be classified as representing harm or loss, threat, or challenge. Harm or loss demands involve actual damage, and threat demands involve anticipated harm or loss. Challenges are viewed as a potential for personal growth. Stress results when the demands exceed the individual's adaptive resources.
- *Secondary appraisal* is the process of evaluating the significance of the transaction between the person and the environment as it relates to available coping resources and options. Primary and secondary appraisals often occur simultaneously and interact with each other in determining stress. They are equally important in the person's cognitive assessment of an event. Secondary appraisals include feelings of being able to deal with the problem, such as a diagnosis of cancer by seeking a second opinion, altering lifestyle, or not being able to deal with the problem, such as not going back to the health care practitioner. Figure 9–2 ◆ shows a diagram of stress as a transaction.

- **Cognitive reappraisal** develops from the feedback of changes in the person–environment relationship and from reflection about the coping process. Reappraisal allows for changes in the person's evaluation of the event, or a relabeling of the cognitive appraisal. The event may be reappraised and evaluated as nonstressful due to changes in the relationship between the person and someone

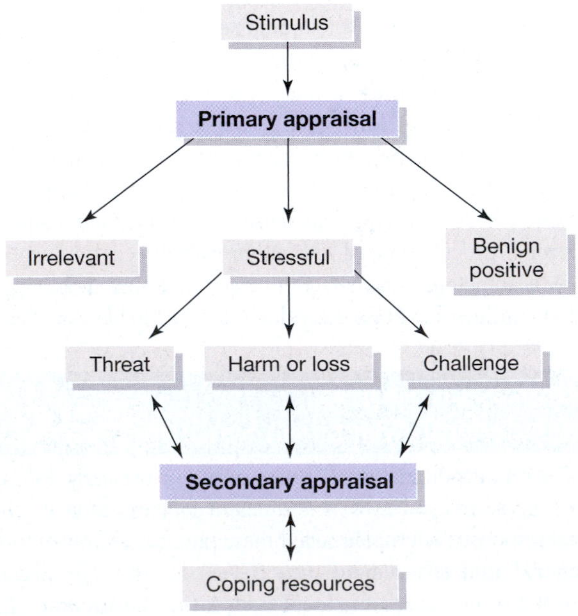

FIGURE 9–2 ◆ Stress as a transaction.

in his environment. For example, a hospitalization initially may be deemed stressful by the individual, based on primary and secondary appraisal. The event may be reappraised and evaluated as nonstressful, because of teaching or explanations the patient received from the primary nurse; these may have caused a change in the relationship between the person and the nurse in the environment, resulting in a positive outcome of improved health from the hospitalization.

Personal factors that lead to stressful appraisals include intellectual, motivational, and personality characteristics. People who have high self-esteem are likely to believe that they have the resources to meet demands and more likely to see stressful events as challenging rather than as threatening (Deng et al., 2010). Events that involve very strong demands and are imminent tend to be seen as stressful. Life transitions—starting school, moving a household, starting or changing a career, becoming a parent, losing a spouse, or retiring—also can be stressful.

Ambiguity, such as role and harm ambiguity, is stressful because people are uncertain about what actions and decisions to make. Role ambiguity can occur in the workplace, for instance, when people are working without clear guidelines, no standards for performance, or no clear consequences. This is stressful because people are uncertain about what actions and decisions to make. Harm ambiguity can occur when people are not sure what to do to avoid harm. A person who is seriously ill and does not have clear information might draw hope from this ambiguity, believing that he will get well, whereas another person in the same situation may believe that people are deliberately giving ambiguous information because the prognosis is poor.

How much control a person has over the situation also is an important factor. Generally, if people have control over an event, or internal locus of control, they may perceive the event as less stressful. People who have limited or no control over an event are more likely to see the event as stressful (Kravits, McAllister-Black, Grant, & Kirk, 2010). There are two types of control a person uses: behavioral and cognitive. Behavioral control means performing some action; for example, taking acetaminophen for a headache to make experiencing a headache less stressful. Cognitive control means using a mental strategy, such as guided deep breathing and positive intention practices.

Anger is another emotional reaction to stress. Anger often results when an individual perceives the situation as harmful or frustrating. When stress is accompanied by anger, negative behaviors tend to increase. An example of this is the patient who yells at the nurse immediately after receiving the negative results from a test or procedure.

Physiological Responses to Stress

Physiological responses to stress should be considered within the context of the body as an open living system with an internal and external environment, with information and matter being exchanged continuously between these two environments. When stress causes a body function to deviate from its stable range, processes are initiated to restore and maintain homeostasis. When these compensatory processes are not adequate, the steady state is threatened, function becomes disordered, and pathophysiological mechanisms occur that can lead to disease. Disease is an abnormal variation in the structure or function of any part of the body that occurs within a living system when the sum of stressors acting on that living system exceeds the system's ability to adapt.

The physiological components involved in the stress response include the central nervous system (CNS), the hypothalamus, the sympathetic nervous system, the anterior and posterior pituitary glands, the adrenal medulla, and the adrenal cortex. The physiological components and their secretions (hormones and catecholamines) are responsible for the neuroendocrine response to stressors (the nervous system, the endocrine system, and the immune system). Because these three systems are interrelated, the ultimate responses of the person to stress reflect the integration of the three systems.

Nervous System

The body responds physiologically to actual and perceived stressors. The hypothalamus participates in both the emotional and physical response to stressors. Other parts of the CNS, including the cerebral cortex, limbic system, and reticular formation, also are involved in the neural control of emotions and the physiological responses to stress. The functions of these structures are interrelated.

- ***Cerebral Cortex:*** The somatic, auditory, and visual associative areas of the cerebral cortex receive input from the peripheral sensory fibers, and then interpret them. The prefrontal area serves to reduce the speed of the associative functions so that the person has time to evaluate the information in light of past experiences and future consequences (primary and secondary appraisal) and to plan a course of action. The temporal lobes of the cerebral cortex contain the auditory association areas, which produce the sensation of fear when stimulated. Stimulation of the temporal lobes can result in sounds that seem louder or softer, visual displays that seem nearer or further, and experiences that seem familiar or strange. These effects modify the perception of stress (Anonymous Harvard Mental Health Letter, 2011).
- ***Limbic System:*** The limbic system is thought to be responsible for emotions and behaviors. When stimulated, behaviors can occur that ensure survival and self-preservation, such as feeding or sexuality. Endorphins are found in structures of the limbic system and are known to reduce the perception of painful stimuli (Levy, 2010).
- ***Reticular Formation:*** The reticular formation is located between the lower end of the brainstem and the thalamus. This structure relays input to and from the thalamus to the cerebral cortex. This network of neurons, which is involved with arousal and consciousness, is called the reticular activating system (RAS). When stimulated by stress, the RAS increases its output of impulses, leading to wakefulness (Fernández-Gil, Palacios-Bote, Leo-Barahona, & Mora-Encinas, 2010).
- ***Hypothalamus:*** The hypothalamus, which lies just above the pituitary gland, integrates autonomic nervous system mechanisms that maintain the chemical constancy of the body's internal environment. Together with the limbic system, it regulates emotions and many visceral behaviors necessary for survival. The hypothalamus receives information regarding traumatic stimuli via the spinothalamic pathway, pressure-sensitive input from the baroreceptors via the brainstem, and emotional stimuli via the limbic system.

  Because the hypothalamus secretes peptide hormones and factors that regulate the release of hormones by the anterior pituitary, it is central to the connection between the nervous and endocrine systems in responding to stress. The hypothalamus regulates the function of both the sympathetic and parasympathetic branches of the autonomic nervous system. When an individual perceives the presence of a stressor, the hypothalamus mediates both the neural and endocrine responses by activating the sympathetic nervous system, and by releasing corticotropin-releasing hormone (CRH), which stimulates the pituitary to release adrenocorticotropic hormone (ACTH). When the parasympathetic nervous system is stimulated, an increased gastrointestinal motility, flushing, or bronchial constriction may occur (Anonymous Harvard Mental Health Letter, 2011).

The sympathetic nervous system response to stress is rapid and short lived. Norepinephrine is released at nerve endings that are in direct contact with the respective end organs to cause an increase in function of the vital organs. Heart rate increases and peripheral vasoconstriction occurs, raising the blood pressure. Blood is shunted away from abdominal organs in order to provide better blood supply to the vital organs, brain, heart, and skeletal muscles. Blood glucose is increased, supplying a more readily available energy. Pupils are dilated, mental activity is increased, and a greater sense of awareness exists (Anonymous Harvard Mental Health Letter, 2011).

Constriction of the blood vessels of the skin limits bleeding in the event of trauma. The person is likely to experience cold feet, clammy skin and hands, chills, palpitations, and a knot in the stomach. Typically, the person appears tense, with the muscles of the neck, upper back, and shoulders tightened, and respirations may be rapid and shallow, with a tense diaphragm. Figure 9–3◆ depicts the increased sympathetic activity present in a stress response.

Endocrine System

Once the hypothalamus is activated in response to stress, the endocrine system becomes involved. The sympathetic nervous system also stimulates the medulla of the adrenal gland to release epinephrine and norepinephrine (catecholamines) into the bloodstream. The effect of catecholamines and the sympathetic nervous system, including the adrenal medulla, is referred to as the sympathoadrenal response. These hormones prepare the body for the fight-or-flight response, which is depicted in Figure 9–3. This response is activated by physical stressors such as hypovolemia and hypoxia or emotional states such as anger, excitement, and fear. Catecholamines can be measured in the blood and urine.

The Hypothalamic–Pituitary–Adrenal Response

As previously stated, ACTH stimulates the adrenal cortex to produce glucocorticoids. Glucocorticoids, particularly cortisol, are essential for the stress response. Cortisol stimulates protein catabolism, releasing amino acids; stimulates liver uptake of amino acids; and inhibits glucose uptake (anti-insulin action) by many body cells, but not those of the brain or heart. Cortisol also potentiates the action of catecholamines on blood vessels and inhibits the inflammatory response. These cortisol-induced metabolic effects provide the body with a ready source of energy during a stressful situation. These effects are important to consider in relation to people experiencing stress; they catabolize body protein and frequently need supplements (Kudielka & Kirschbaum, 2005).

The antidiuretic hormone (ADH) from the posterior pituitary and aldosterone from the adrenal cortex also are released. ADH promotes water reabsorption by the distal and collecting tubules of the kidneys, and aldosterone acts to increase sodium reabsorption in the kidney tubules. ADH and aldosterone increase extracellular fluid (ECF) by promoting water and sodium retention, an adaptive mechanism in the event of hemorrhage or loss of fluids through excessive perspiration.

Stimulation of both the adrenal medulla and cortex results in an increased blood glucose level, which provides the additional fuel for the increased metabolism needed for fight or flight. The increased cardiac output, increased blood glucose levels, and increased metabolic rate make the physical responses possible. The dilation of skeletal muscle blood vessels and resulting increased blood supply to the large muscles and the brain provides for quick movement and increased alertness. The increased blood volume and increased clotting time function to help maintain adequate circulation to vital organs in case of traumatic blood loss. These responses to stress illustrate the complexity and interrelated nature of the processes involved.

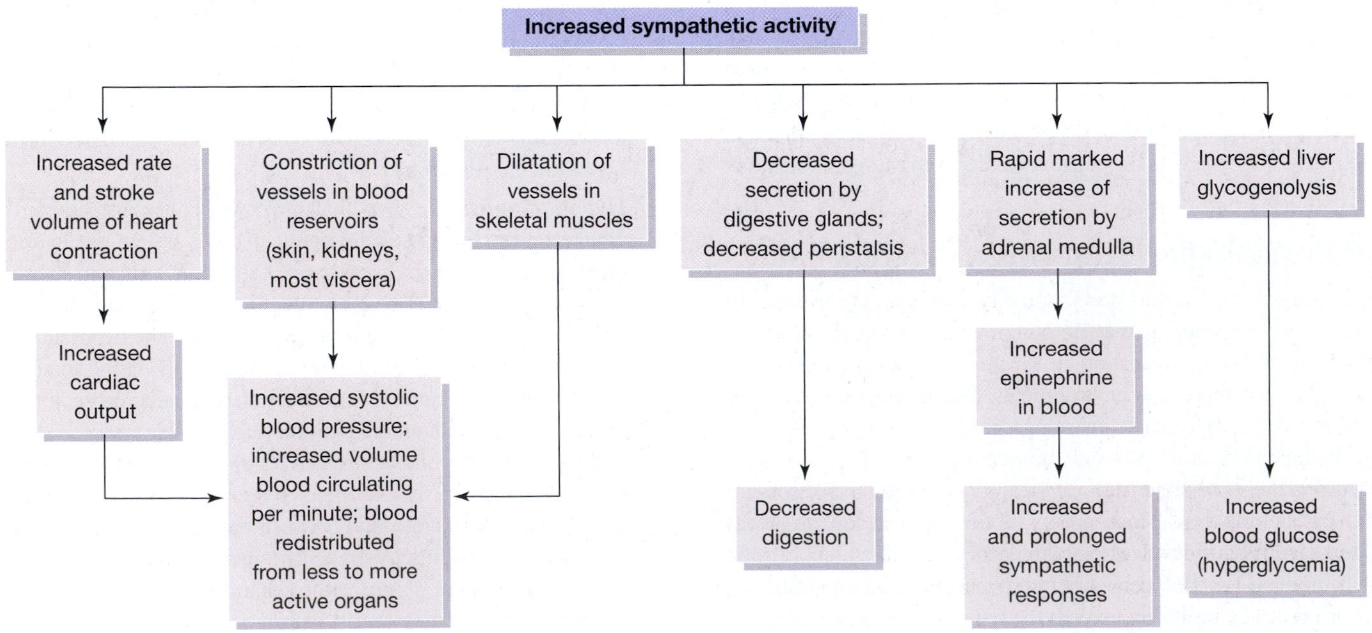

FIGURE 9–3 ◆ Alarm reactions resulting from increased sympathetic activity. These responses commonly are referred to as the "fight-or-flight" reaction.

Immune System

The immune system is the body's surveillance system. It detects and battles foreign invaders, such as bacteria, viruses, and tumor cells. The immune system comprises several organs, including bone marrow, spleen, thymus, and the lymph nodes. The most important elements of the immune system are lymphocytes, which are specialized white blood cells that fight bacteria, viruses, and other foreign invaders. Lymphocytes are originally manufactured in the bone marrow and then migrate to the other immune system organs, where they develop and are stored until needed.

Research has demonstrated the connection of the immune system to the neuroendocrine and autonomic systems and with the development of post-traumatic stress disorder (Gill, Saligan, Woods, & Page, 2009). Negative stressors lead to alterations in immune function in humans through processes involving the hypothalamic–pituitary–adrenal (HPA) axis and the autonomic nervous system that affect immune function (Marshall, 2011). In return, the immune system also affects endocrine and CNS responses. Both corticosteroids and catecholamines are known to suppress immune function.

Physiological Responses of Acute Versus Chronic Stress

With **acute stress,** catecholamines suppress activity in areas at the front of the brain concerned with short-term memory, concentration inhibition, and rational thought. This sequence of mental events allows a person to react quickly to the stressful event, to either fight or flee. It also hinders the person's ability to handle the complex social or intellectual tasks and behaviors associated with the event.

The body actually responds to the stressful event by:

- Breathing more rapidly so that the lungs take in more oxygen, priming the muscles, lungs, and brain for added demands.
- Diminishing parts of the immune system so that infection or other immune molecules can be redistributed. These immune-boosting cells are sent to the injured or infected part of the body.
- Diverting blood flow away from the skin to support the heart and muscle tissues. The physical effect is cool, clammy, sweaty skin.
- Slowing down digestive activity or nonessential body functions during a crisis.

Once the threat has passed, the stress hormones return to normal. This phenomenon is known as the relaxation response.

In contrast, **chronic stress,** which occurs on a daily basis, suppresses the urge to act (fight or flee). Chronic stressors, such as ongoing highly pressured work situations, long-term relationship problems, loneliness, homelessness, or caring for a chronically ill loved one, can contribute to long-term health problems. Additionally, living with a chronic illness such as diabetes, asthma, or coronary artery disease may fatigue the body's response to stress, making individuals more susceptible to the development of other illnesses. The entire concept of the body's physiological response to stress is shown in Figure 9–4◆ (p. 212).

Stress at the Cellular Level

Stress also affects the body at the cellular level, with alterations in cellular structure and function contributing to changes in homeostasis. Thus, the processes of health or adaptation and disease or maladaptation all can occur at the cellular level. Cells are complex units that dynamically respond to the changing demands and stresses of daily life. They exist on a continuum of structure and function. Changes from one state to another can occur rapidly and may not be easily discernible.

Cells possess maintenance and specialized functions (Porth & Matfin, 2009). The maintenance function refers to activities that the cell must perform with respect to itself; specialized functions are those that the cell performs in relation to the tissues and organs of which it is a part. Individual cells may cease to function without negatively affecting the organism; however, if the specialized functions of the tissue are altered, health is threatened.

Cells adapt to environmental stress through structural and functional changes. Some of these adaptations are hypertrophy, atrophy, hyperplasia, dysplasia, and metaplasia:

- *Hypertrophy* and atrophy lead to changes in the size of cells and, therefore, the size of the organs they form. Compensatory hypertrophy occurs in skeletal and cardiac muscles.
- *Atrophy,* a reduction in the size of the cell, can be the consequence of disease or decreased use, decreased blood supply, loss of nerve supply, or inadequate nutrition.
- *Hyperplasia* is an increase in the number of new cells in an organ or tissue. This represents a mitotic response to change that is reversible when the stimulus is withdrawn.
- *Dysplasia* is a change in the appearance of cells after they have been subjected to chronic irritation.
- *Metaplasia* is a cell transformation in which a highly specialized cell changes to a less specialized cell, which is more resistant to the stress that stimulated the change.

These adaptations allow the survival of the organism, and they reflect the changes of the cell in response to stress. If the stress is unremitting, the function of the adapted cell may succumb, and cell injury will occur.

Cellular Injury

Any stressor that alters the cell's ability to maintain optimal balance of its adjustment processes will lead to injury. Structural and functional damage will occur. In some cases, this may be reversible, permitting recovery; in other cases, the damage may be irreversible, leading to disability. With adaptive changes, compensation occurs and a steady state is achieved. With injury, steady-state regulation is lost.

Causes of changes in the system (cell, tissue, organ, body) may arise from either the internal or external environment. The presence of one injury may precipitate another, and a ripple effect may occur. For example, inadequate oxygenation and nutritional deficiencies make the system vulnerable to infection. These agents act at the cellular level by damaging or destroying the integrity of the cell membrane necessary for the cell to synthesize enzymes and necessary proteins to grow and reproduce. Common causes of changes in the system include:

- *Hypoxia,* a lack of oxygen for the cell to use, may be caused by several factors, including decreased hemoglobin which carries oxygen to the cell, a respiratory problem which interferes with delivery of oxygen into the blood, or an acid-base problem which makes the cell unable to use the oxygen delivered to it. Inadequate cellular oxygenation interferes with the cell's ability to transform energy. Ischemia, a decrease in blood supply to the cell, occurs when arterial blood flow is decreased because of atherosclerotic narrowing of blood vessels, as occurs in myocardial cell injury. Ischemia also results from intravascular thrombi or emboli that may form and interfere with

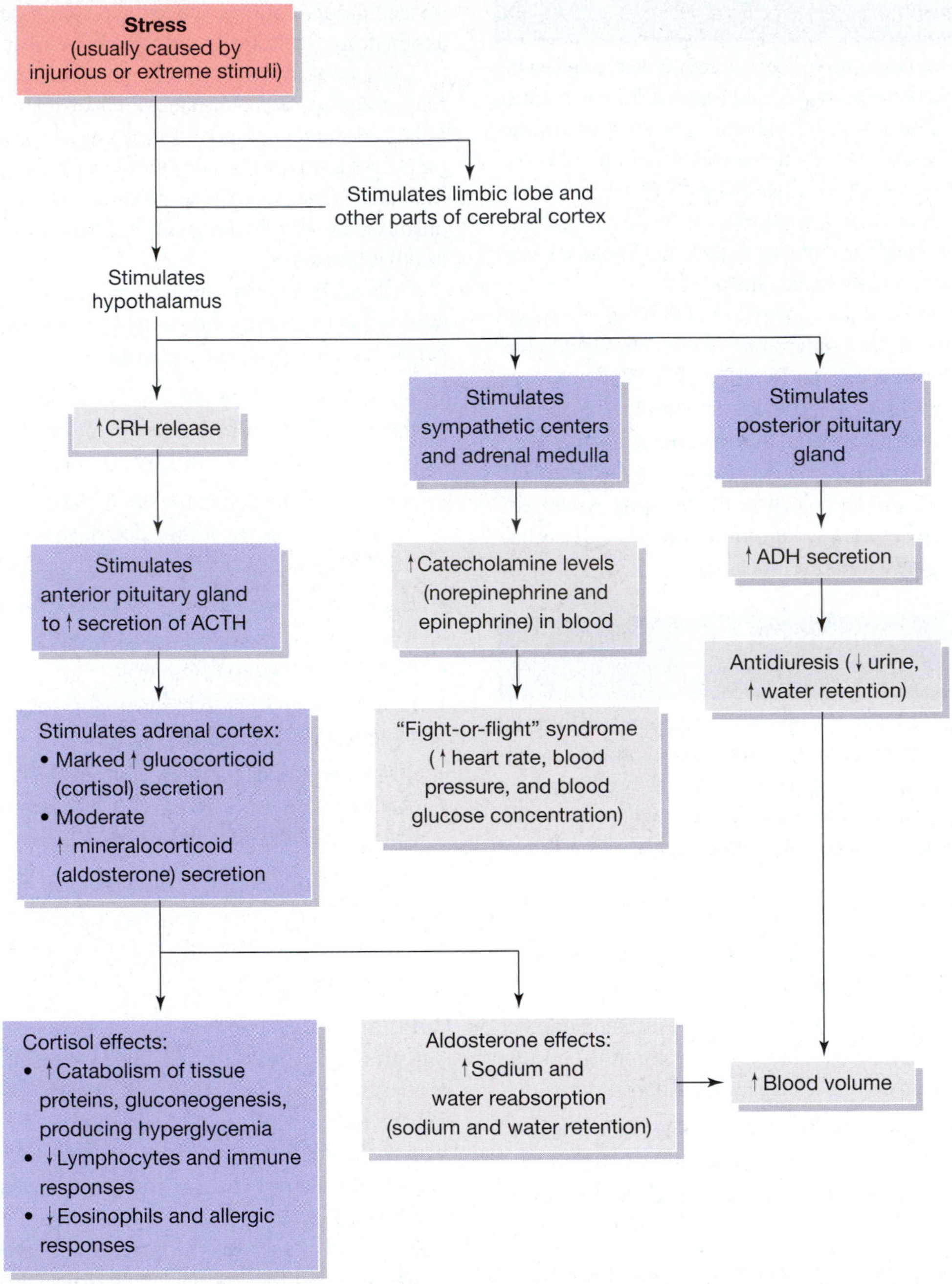

FIGURE 9–4 ◆ Current concepts regarding the body's response to stress syndrome. *ACTH*, Adrenocorticotropic hormone; *ADH*, antidiuretic hormone; *CRH*, corticotrophin-releasing hormone.

the blood supply to the cells, as occurs in cerebral vascular accidents (strokes). The amount of time tissues can survive without oxygen varies; however, if the ischemia is slow and progressive, collateral circulation may develop.

- Nutritional imbalance refers to a deficiency or excess of one or more essential nutrients. This imbalance results from inadequate nutrition (calories) or too much nutrition (calories). Caloric excess leads to obesity and overloads the cells in the body. Obesity places a strain on the body because it requires more energy to maintain the extra tissue and is associated with the development of disease, especially cardiovascular and pulmonary disease.

  Specific diseases can result when an essential nutrient is absent or when there is an imbalance of nutrients. For example, an energy deficit leading to cell injury can occur if there is insufficient glucose or insufficient oxygen to transform the glucose into energy. Conversely, a lack of insulin, or the inability to use insulin, may prevent insulin from entering the cell from the blood. See Chapters 8 and 47, respectively, for more information on nutrition and diabetes.

- Physical agents that can cause stress sufficient to induce injury to the cells include temperature extremes, radiation and electrical shock, and mechanical trauma. Extremely high temperatures precipitate hypermetabolism as manifested by an increase in respiratory rate, heart rate, and basal metabolic rate. With fever induced by infections, the hypothalamic thermostat may be reset. The local response to thermal or burn injury is similar. There is an increase in metabolic activity, heat increases, protein coagulates, enzyme systems are destroyed, and, in the extreme, charring or carbonization occurs. See Chapter 61 for information on burn injuries.

Safety Alert *Extremely high temperatures of 41°C (106°F) cause hyperthermia, which results in cell protein coagulation and cell death. Extremely low temperatures cause vasoconstriction, leading to ischemia in involved tissues.*

- Radiation and electrical shock, though used for diagnosis and disease treatment, also may cause injury. Radiation decreases the cell's protective inflammatory response, creating a favorable environment for opportunistic infections. Electrical shock may produce burns as a result of the heat generated when an electrical current travels through the body.
- Mechanical trauma can result in wounds that disturb the cells and tissues. The outcome of mechanical trauma is dependent on the severity of the wound and the extent of nerve damage.
- Chemical agents, such as lye, or heavy metals, such as mercury or arsenic, cause injuries that have a corrosive action on epithelial tissues. Many other chemicals are toxic in specific amounts and in certain people. Large amounts of glucose can cause osmotic shifts, which affect the fluid and electrolyte balance. In addition, too much insulin can cause subnormal levels of blood glucose and lead to coma.

  Drugs also can cause chemical poisoning. The individual's drug tolerance must be carefully assessed when prescribing medications to prevent toxic reactions to the usual or customary dosages, since aging tends to decrease tolerance to medications. Alcohol, a chemical irritant, breaks down into acetaldehyde in the body. This substance has a direct toxic effect on liver cells that leads to a variety of liver abnormalities, including cirrhosis. Disordered liver cell function leads to complications in other body organs.

Safety Alert *The elderly are susceptible to polypharmacy. Many elderly are on multiple medications that can interact with each other.*

- **Infectious agents** known to cause diseases in humans are viruses, bacteria, rickettsiae, mycoplasmas, fungi, protozoa, and nematodes. The severity of the infectious disease depends on the number of microorganisms entering the body, their virulence, and the host's defenses (e.g., health, age, immune defenses). Typically, an inflammatory response and immune reaction are the body's physiological responses to the presence of infection. These processes are discussed at length in Unit XII.

Cellular Response to Injury

Cells may be injured or killed from the many agents just discussed. When this happens, an inflammatory response occurs in the tissues surrounding the injury. Inflammation is a defensive mechanism, or compensatory response, intended to neutralize, control, or eliminate the offending agent to prepare the site for repair. Thus, the mechanism of inflammation basically is the same regardless of the injuring agent. The intensity of the response depends on the extent and severity of injury and on the reactive capacity of the injured person.

Contrary to a popular misconception, inflammation is not the same as infection. Inflammation always is present with infection, but infection is not always present with inflammation. An infection involves invasion of tissues or cells by microorganisms such as bacteria, fungi, and viruses. In contrast, inflammation can be caused by nonliving agents such as heat, radiation trauma, and allergens. If infection is present, it is from a superimposed invasion of microorganisms. An infectious agent is only one of several agents that may trigger an inflammatory response. An infection exists when the infectious agent is living, growing, and multiplying in the tissues and is able to overcome the body's normal defenses.

The mechanism of inflammation basically is the same regardless of the injuring agent. The intensity of the body's response to the injury, or stressor, depends on the extent and severity of injury and on the injured person's reactive capacity. The inflammatory response involves changes in the microcirculation. The five cardinal signs of inflammation are produced: redness, heat, swelling, pain, and loss of function. Initially, transient vasodilation results in hyperemia, which raises filtration pressure. The pain produced is attributed to the pressure of fluids or swelling on nerve endings and to the irritation of nerve endings by chemical mediators released at the site. Bradykinin is one of the chemical mediators suspected of causing pain. Loss of function is most likely related to the pain and swelling; however, the exact mechanism is not known.

As blood flow increases and fluid leaks into the surrounding tissues, red blood cells, white blood cells, and platelets remain in the blood, causing it to become more viscous. Leukocytes collect in the vessels and migrate to the site of injury to engulf offending organisms and to remove cellular debris (phagocytosis). Fibrinogen in the leaked plasma fluid coagulates, serving to wall off the injured area and prevent the spread of infection.

Injury initiates the inflammatory response, but chemical substances (histamine and kinins) released at the site induce the vascular changes. Histamine is responsible for the early stages of vasodilation and vascular permeability. Kinins increase vasodilation and vascular permeability and attract neutrophils to the area. Prostaglandins also cause increased permeability.

The inflammatory response often is confined to the site, causing only local signs and symptoms. However, systemic responses also can occur. Fever is the most common sign of a systemic response to injury, and it is most likely caused by endogenous pyrogens released from neutrophils and macrophages. The systemic inflammatory response is discussed fully in Chapter 54.

Safety Alert *Fever should not be ignored, because it signifies a systemic response to an infectious agent.*

Cellular Healing

The reparative process of cellular injury, which begins at approximately the same time as the injury itself, is linked with inflammation. Healing progresses after the inflammatory debris has been removed and may occur by regeneration or by replacement. In regeneration, gradual repairs of the defect occur by proliferation of cells of the same type as those destroyed. During replacement, typically connective tissue will fill in the tissue defect, resulting in scar formation.

The condition of the host, the environment, and the nature and severity of the injury affect the processes of inflammation and cell repair. Any of the previously discussed injuries can lead to death of the cell. For information on wound healing, see Chapter 60.

Oxidative Stress

Oxidative stress is rapidly becoming the nutritional and medical buzzword for the 21st century. It is receiving attention as a way of interpreting the body's physiological response to stress, and it is implicated in a growing list of diseases, from cataracts to cancer. Health-conscious people taking heed of the news about oxygen free radicals, are taking steps to prevent themselves from these substances that are sabotaging health.

Oxidative stress (OS) is a physiological response to both internal and external stressors. Although it is not a disease, it can lead to or accelerate disease development. OS occurs when the available supply of the body's antioxidants is insufficient to handle and neutralize free radicals, molecules produced in cells either as a by-product of metabolism or deliberately as in phagocytosis. The molecules are unstable because they have an unpaired electron on the shell of the molecule and bond to other molecules to increase stability. The result of free radicals bonding to other molecules is massive cell damage, which can result in cellular mutations, tissue breakdown, and immune compromise. The increasing focus on OS makes it increasingly important that nurses understand and appreciate the concept of oxidative stress, both from a treatment perspective and a preventive/educational perspective.

Reactive oxygen species (ROS), a major contributing factor in diseases in critically ill patients, is the by-product of mitochondria. It uses oxygen to oxidize other molecules and generates energy in the form of adenosine triphosphate. ROSs are controlled by a defense system that depends on the activity of enzymes and other nonenzyme substances. The imbalance between ROSs and the body's defense system is called oxidative stress.

Formation of ROS

During chemical processes, molecules can be reduced or oxidized. Reduction and oxidation can leave the reduced molecule unstable and free to react with other molecules to cause damage to cell membranes, proteins, and DNA. These reduced substances are called *free radicals* (Urden, Stacy, & Lough, 2009). In homeostasis, the rates of reduction and oxidation are equal. The reduction–oxidation (redox) balance is maintained by physiological defenses, such as specialized enzymes and antioxidants that remove or inactivate the free radicals. The enzymes and antioxidants can become overwhelmed by an increase in reduced molecules or by a decrease in the defense system, thereby allowing the accumulation of free radicals (Urden, Stacy, & Lough, 2009).

Free radicals are involved in many cellular functions and are a normal part of living. White blood cells use free radicals to attach and destroy bacteria, viruses, and virus-infected cells. The detoxifying actions of the liver also require free radicals. Although free radicals have useful functions in the body under controlled conditions, they are extremely unstable molecules that can damage cells if left uncontrolled. Oxygen free radicals are neutralized by antioxidants such as vitamin E or enzymes such as superoxide dismutase. In some patients, oxygen free radicals become a problem when either a decrease in the removal of, or an overproduction of, the radicals occurs. When the body is overwhelmed by increased production of oxidative agents and defense against these agents is decreased, the ensuing damage contributes to cellular derangements, cell injury, and death. The free radicals tend to accelerate aging and contribute to the development of many diseases, such as cancer, and systemic inflammatory response (Urden, Stacy, & Lough, 2009).

Evidence-based research confirms the link between oxidative stress and pathophysiological syndromes and diseases, including cardiogenic shock, sepsis, acute respiratory distress syndrome (ARDS), diaphragm fatigue, burns, septic shock, disseminated intravascular coagulation, multiple organ dysfunction, cardiovascular disease, diabetes mellitus, and trauma, as well as nonhereditary degenerative diseases such as Parkinson's and Alzheimer's (Urden, Stacy, & Lough, 2009).

Psychological or emotional stress can contribute to OS. When the body is under stress, it produces hormones that generate free radicals. Everyone is exposed to free radicals from a variety of sources. Poor nutrition also contributes to OS. When the body is fed poorly, it starves and all of its systems suffer. Weak organ systems are prime targets for free radical attack. Because oxidative stress is associated with a variety of illnesses, the care of patients depends on preventing and controlling production of ROS. Collaborative care, including nutritional counseling, is an essential component of the patient's care and is focused on removing as many stressors as possible.

PSYCHOSOCIAL THEORIES

Many people who seek health care have psychosocial issues in addition to the physiological reason that brought them to the hospital or clinic. Illness and hospitalization are stressful events for patients and their families. As was just discussed, stress in and of itself can affect the homeostasis of the patient. Therefore, it is important for nurses to care for the psychological needs of their patients in addition to their physiological needs.

During a person's life span, experiencing periods of both health and illness is inevitable. These experiences influence how people perceive themselves in relation to their own health belief model as well as the health care delivery system. Nurses play a pivotal role in shaping these experiences, and it is often through their influence that patients are able to give meaning to their experiences. In the process, patients are empowered to assume more autonomy for their health care decisions. To achieve a positive health care outcome, nurses need to monitor and respond to the holistic needs of patients and their families. This means acknowledging patients as biopsychosocial spiritual beings who are more than the sum of their parts. Developing a knowledge base in the principles of psychosocial nursing helps the nurse holistically apply the nursing process to the psychosocial concerns of their patients.

An array of theoretical perspectives informs the practice of psychosocial nursing. Theories provide a scientific basis for practice and further aid the nurse in conceptualizing practice situations. Theories also offer a road map for predicting what may happen in a particular practice situation and often provide guidance about what has been effective in the past. A wide variety of theories are applicable to psychosocial nursing. Some of these theories have been borrowed from other disciplines; others are shared theories and have been modified for nursing practice; and yet others are theories specific to the discipline of nursing. This section introduces the reader to some of the theories that are most relevant to the practice of psychosocial nursing.

Psychoanalytical Perspective

The psychoanalytical perspective is attributed to the work of Sigmund Freud (1935). He was one of the first scientists to suggest a mind–body interaction and to recognize the importance of the unconscious in mental functioning. He divided aspects of the conscious into three categories:

- Conscious, which includes all things a person easily remembers, such as her mother's name, her address, or her favorite food.
- Subconscious, which includes those things that have been forgotten but can easily be brought to consciousness, such as an old address, the feelings a man had on his wedding day, or the feeling of wonder at the birth of a first child.

- Unconscious, which encompasses all of those things that cannot be remembered or brought to conscious thought.

Freud also conceptualized three components of personality. He called these the id, ego, and superego:

- The **id** represents all of a person's biological and psychological drives. Drives are inborn psychological tensions that call for mental action in order to obtain instant gratification of needs. The id is primitive and instinctual and is often associated with sexual and aggressive impulses. The id does not consider reality or morality as it attempts to reduce psychic tension.
- The **ego** mediates the urges of the id with the demands of the superego. It helps individuals to make a connection between the realities of the real world and the demands of the id in a way that promotes well-being and survival. Additionally, the ego protects the mind against conflict-laden impulses coming from the id while obeying a reality principle. The ego does not concern itself with morality or social norms.
- The **superego** is really an extension of the ego and represents individuals' early moral training and ideal values imparted by societal norms. The emphasis of superego functioning is on the ideal. The superego tells a person what is right and what is wrong and acts as a control system to help the ego assist the id in choosing objects of gratification that are not immoral.

The concept of anxiety is a thread that runs through the psychoanalytical perspective. Freud conceptualized anxiety as a feeling of discomfort and tension that alerts the ego to a perceived threat or loss of inner control. Once warned, the ego can then undertake a wide variety of rational defenses to decrease the feelings of discomfort and tension. If, however, the anxiety is overwhelming and the ego is unable to cope, the ego resorts to less rational coping mechanisms. These processes are called the **ego defense mechanism** and are utilized to help alleviate anxiety by denying, distorting, and misinterpreting reality. Although the ego defense mechanisms are helpful for a time, their overuse does not constitute healthy coping. For the most part, the ego defense mechanisms operate at an unconscious level.

Developmental Perspective

Erik Erikson (1963) is best known for his theory on how humans develop across the life span. He embraced some of Freud's conceptualizations and expanded them to include the influence of culture and society on human development. He felt that the determinants of personality development were not just instinctual and biological, as Freud theorized, but social and cultural as well.

Erikson conceptualized eight developmental stages, starting at birth and ending at death. Each of these stages is characterized by a developmental task that must be achieved in order for the person to develop in a healthy manner. Erikson did believe that if a task was not met at an earlier developmental stage, a person could later go backwards and meet the task of that stage successfully. Erikson's developmental stages and tasks and their defining characteristics can be seen on the following website: http://psychology.about.com/od/psychosocialtheories/a/psychosocial.htm.

Humanistic Perspective

The work of Abraham Maslow represents what is known as the "third force" in the field of psychology. He wished to provide an alternative to the somewhat mechanistic view of the psychoanalytical and behaviorist perspectives. The humanistic perspective believes that behavior is shaped by people's own perceptions of themselves, their subjective views of the world, and the need of all human beings to experience growth.

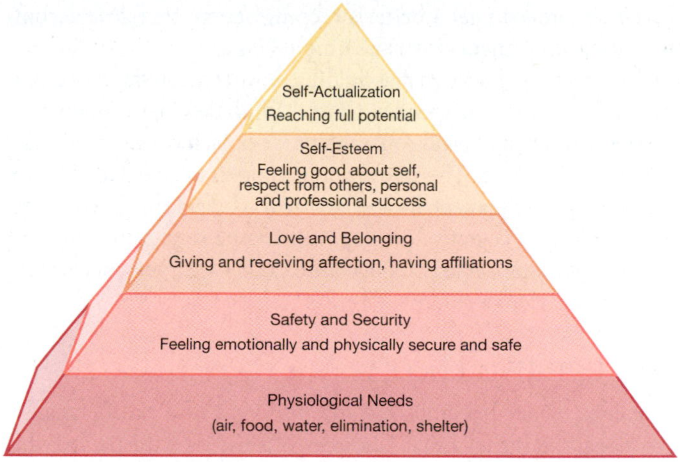

FIGURE 9–5 ◆ Maslow's hierarchy of needs.

Maslow theorized a hierarchy of human needs in which some needs are perceived as more prevailing than other needs. The physiologic needs, such as air, water, and food, are placed on the bottom rung of the hierarchy. The next rung is the need of individuals to feel safe and secure, followed by the need for love and belonging. Further toward the top of the hierarchy is the need for self-esteem. Needs on the first four rungs of the hierarchy are labeled **basic human needs.** Maslow labeled these lower rung needs as *deficit needs*. The next group on the hierarchy is the group of **growth needs.** Maslow identified these as the need to know and understand, aesthetic needs, and self-actualization and transcendence needs. He believed that the higher needs are met only after the lower needs have been satisfied. For example, if a person is without food, it is unlikely that the person will be concerned about her aesthetic needs. Figure 9–5◆ illustrates Maslow's hierarchy of basic human needs.

Cognitive Development

Jean Piaget (1969) was interested in the cognitive development of children. He theorized that children develop cognitively through their exposure to the world around them. The basic mental structure of Piaget's theory is called a **schema.** Schemas are coordinated patterns of recurring action and are created for the purpose of organizing and interpreting information. As such, children's ability to think matures through two processes, assimilation and accommodation. **Assimilation** occurs when a child incorporates new knowledge into an already existing schema. **Accommodation** occurs when a child must modify an existing schema because the incorporation of new knowledge does not fit into his existing schema. For example, a child is given a broom to sweep the floor. He has never really swept a floor before, but has watched his father do it and knows that to sweep he has to move the broom back and forth over the floor. He assimilates his behavior into what schemas he already has. But the broom is too big for him and he is holding it up close to the top, so he adjusts his hands lower on the broom

Weblink: Piaget's Stages of Cognitive Development

handle in order to get a better sweeping action, therefore accommodating adjustments to his existing schema.

Piaget further theorized that children move through stages of cognitive development. The speed at which a child develops cognitively is variable and often depends on a multitude of factors such as genetics and the environment. This information is important to the nurse when considering developmentally appropriate teaching–learning strategies. Piaget's stages of cognitive development can be seen at the following website: http://psychology.about.com/b/2008/04/21/key-concepts-in-cognitive-development.htm.

Cognitive Theory

Cognitive theory has impacted the treatment of a broad range of emotional and mental health disorders. It is based on the premise that mental health symptoms are related to how individuals view themselves and the world around them. Cognitive theory posits that individuals develop a set of core beliefs as a result of interacting with the environment. These beliefs or schemas can be positive or negative. A positive example could be the belief that women are strong and powerful. A negative belief could be the belief that women are weak and helpless. Schemas influence how individuals interpret and evaluate experiences, and behaviors are often the result of these interpretations.

Another construct in cognitive theory is that of the cognitive triad. The cognitive triad is influenced by schemas that influence how people (1) see themselves, (2) interpret an experience, and (3) view the future. These schemas may be viewed positively or negatively. Beck and Freeman (1990) suggest that being stuck in the negative cognitive triad leads to the development of cognitive distortions, which in return may result in the development of mental health symptoms. See Chart 9–1 for examples of cognitive distortions.

Assessing the cognitive distortions of patients and identifying how their cognitive triads influence the ways in which they are evaluating their health care situation can help the nurse design more effective interventions. One way to challenge cognitive distortions is to provide education that assists patients and families in examining all available evidence about a situation so that they are informed about options and alternatives. This helps them develop problem-solving strategies that take the focus away from the most negative extremes of the situation.

CHART 9–1 Cognitive Distortions

Arbitrary inference	Coming to a specific conclusion without having any supporting evidence or in the face of contradictory evidence.
Selective abstraction	Conceptualizing a situation while ignoring contradictory information.
Overgeneralization	Taking specific information and generalizing it broadly to unrelated situations.
Magnification	Seeing something as being far more important than it is.
Minimization	Seeing something as being far less important than it is.
Personalization	Attributing external events to oneself without evidence to support the causal relationship.
Dichotomous thinking	Categorizing experiences with all-or-none reasoning.

Family Systems

In the practice of nursing, it is inevitable that the care of patients will call for the family's inclusion. In today's culture, "family" includes all of those significant others in a person's life such as life partners, friends, or roommates. The family is the mediator between the individual and society. Family assumes the role of helping its members meet their needs, including health care needs. The family often wishes to be involved in all aspects of health care delivery to its individual members. It is important that nurses acknowledge the importance of patients' families in achieving desirable health care outcomes.

Hospital policies often apply traditional definitions of family to include only those individuals who are related by marriage, blood, or adoption. Although this definition applies to many families, it also serves to exclude those families that have chosen variant family forms. Wright and Leahey (2009) define family as "a group of individuals who are bound by strong emotional ties" (p. 50) and encourage nurses to think beyond the traditional definition of family to include all whom the family says is their family.

One theoretical approach that has influenced how to look at families is systems theory. Systems theory examines a unit and describes its relationship to a greater whole. Families are considered to be open social systems because they interact with the environment around them and have discrete boundaries that separate them from the environment. These boundaries allow the family to control how much input the family receives from the environment. Families must continually adapt in order to maintain equilibrium. When families are faced with stress, such as the unexpected hospitalization of a loved one, they must mobilize their adaptive resources in order to maintain a steady state. Stress places more strain on the family unit and creates a situation in which they may need help from outside resources in order to maintain equilibrium. Health care problems are stressful for families; the nurse is in a good position to offer assistance to encourage healthy adaptations. Systems theory helps nurses realize that patients and their families are connected to the outside world and what happens to one member has an effect on the whole.

The Biopsychosocial Model

The biopsychosocial model was formalized by George Engel (1980). Engel believed that mental disorders could not be adequately explained by reducing them to biological causations. The biopsychosocial model offered an alternative to the mechanistic, biomedical model and provided a holistic perspective. The stress diathesis model takes this concept further and postulates that illness is a result of both genetic and biological factors and environmental influences. For example, a person may have a genetic predisposition to develop heart disease, but by embracing a heart-healthy lifestyle may avoid the development of heart problems.

Nursing has embraced the biopsychosocial model and the concept of holism. **Holism** is based on the "interrelationship of body, mind, and spirit in an ever-changing environment" (Burkhardt & Keegan, 2009, p. 125). This means that patients cannot be reduced to a variety of subsystems. When nurses care for people holistically, they consider all aspects of their care. The biopsychosocial model and holism are compatible with systems theory. Individuals as open systems are in constant interaction with their environment; therefore, change in one area of life affects the total system. In providing care, nurses should consider not only the individual, but also family and social support systems.

The theories provide a framework within which psychosocial nursing care can be conceptualized. They provide a rationale for the way to frame nursing problems and apply the nursing process for effective patient-centered care. All nursing care takes place in the context of interpersonal relationships and effective communication. It is through the nurse–patient relationship, therapeutic communication, and patient education that persons are empowered to take an active role in their own health care decisions. The following sections provide an overview of the therapeutic nurse–patient relationship, therapeutic communication, and principles of patient education.

Negative Effects of Stress

In prehistoric times, the physical changes in response to stress were an essential adaptation for meeting natural threats. In current times, the stress response can be an asset for raising levels of performance during critical events such as sports activities, an important meeting, or situations of actual danger or crisis. If stress becomes persistent, all parts of the body's stress apparatus (the brain, heart, lungs, vessels, and muscles) become chronically over- or underactivated. This may produce psychological or physical damage over time.

Acute stress also can be harmful in certain situations. Stress-related conditions that are most likely to produce negative physical effects include:

- An accumulation of persistent stressful situations, particularly those that a person cannot easily control (e.g., high-pressure work plus an unhappy relationship)
- Persistent stress following a severe acute response to a traumatic event, such as an automobile crash
- An inefficient or insufficient relaxation response
- Acute stress in people with serious illness, such as heart disease, COPD, or cancer.

Physiological Effects of Stress

Some evidence suggests that repeated release of stress hormones produces hyperactivity in the HPA axis and disrupts normal levels of serotonin, the nerve chemical that is critical for feelings of well-being. Stress can diminish an individual's quality of life by reducing feelings of pleasure and accomplishment. Stress can also threaten relationships in any area of a person's life.

Stress and Illness

Stress may increase an individual's vulnerability to almost any illness. A threat to his life or safety is considered stressful and triggers a primal physical response by the body. Concentration becomes more focused, reaction time faster, and strength and agility increase. When the stressful situation ends, hormonal signals switch off the stress response and the body returns to normal. But in modern society, fraught with stressful daily events, hassles, and relationships, and also contingent on the individual's hormonal response, stress does not always let up. The stress hormones continue to wash through the system at high levels, never leaving the blood and tissues. Research now shows that long-term activation of the stress system can have a hazardous, even lethal effect on the body, increasing the risk of obesity, heart disease, depression, and a variety of other illnesses.

The stress response results from the complex interplay between the nervous system and stress hormones, or the hormonal systems known as the **hypothalamic–pituitary–adrenal (HPA) axis** (Figure 9–5). As described earlier, the HPA axis is a feedback loop by which the brain triggers the release of hormones needed to respond to stress. Because of its function, the HPA axis also is referred to as the *stress circuit.* The HPA axis affects the autonomic nervous system, regions of the brain, and glandular systems. The short-term response to the stress may be helpful, allowing biochemical resources to be diverted to deal with the threat. However, the long-term response can result in exacerbations of chronic conditions or major disorders.

The HPA axis also can alter its functioning in response to environmental influences. For example, it may be permanently altered in response to extreme stress during the life cycle. If a person experiences major stresses in early childhood, the HPA feedback loop becomes stronger with each new stressful period. This usually results in an adult individual who overreacts hormonally to comparatively minor situations. Certain chronic conditions, such as pain and fatigue, mood and anxiety, or addiction and substance abuse, have a close link to stress. Research also has shown that stress plays an integral part in many disease processes that affect specific organs, body systems, and/or behavioral phenomena (Taylor et al., 2010). Figure 9–6◆ illustrates some disorders that may be caused or aggravated by stress.

- ***Cardiovascular System:*** An impaired ability to adapt to physiological and psychological stress may contribute to the pathogenesis

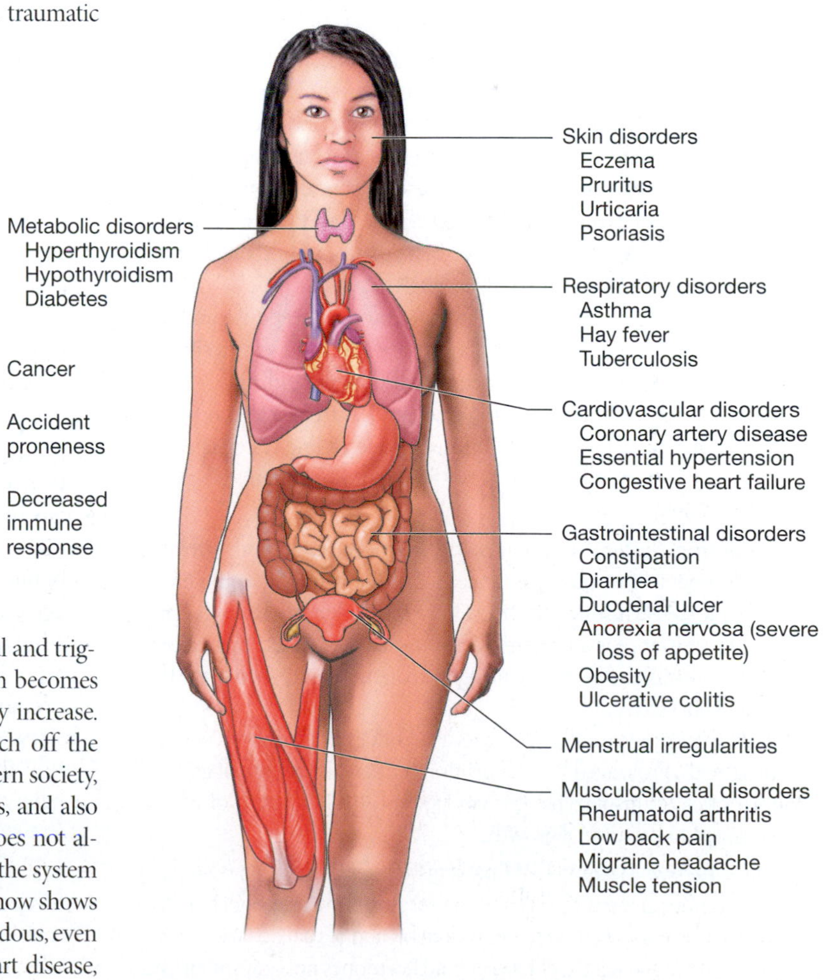

FIGURE 9–6 ◆ Disorders caused or aggravated by stress.

of cardiovascular disease, because the cardiovascular system is particularly vulnerable to stress (Goble & LeGrande, 2008; Lin, Tsai, Linn, & Tsay, 2010; Puustinen, Koponen, Kautianen, Mantyselka, & Vanhala, 2010; Salomon, Clift, Karlsdottir, & Rottenberg, 2009; Shirom, Toker, Berliner, & Shapira, 2008; Whipple et al., 2009). Excessive exposure to uncontrollable stressors and/or the inability to adapt to stress are implicated in the pathogenesis of several different disorders, including hypertension and atherosclerotic vascular disease. Moreover, acute stressors can trigger myocardial infarctions and strokes, and are a major trigger for angina (Bonde et al., 2009; Kibler, Joshi, & Ma, 2009; Koh, 2010).

- ***Cerebrovascular System:*** In some people, prolonged or frequent mental stress causes an exaggerated increase in blood pressure (Kibler et al., 2009; Puustinen et al., 2010).
- ***Gastrointestinal System:*** Many of the same hormones stimulate the brain and the intestine. Although stress does not cause gastrointestinal problems directly, it can be a trigger (Myers & Greenwood-Van Meerveld, 2009; Park, Jarrett, Cain, & Heitkemper, 2008). Prolonged stress can disrupt the digestive system, irritating the large intestine and causing diarrhea, constipation, cramping, and bloating. Excessive production of digestive acids in the stomach may cause a painful burning. Conditions of the digestive system strongly related to stress are irritable bowel syndrome, peptic ulcers, and inflammatory bowel disease. Psychological stress probably functions most often as a cofactor with *H. pylori* by stimulating the production of gastric acid or by promoting behavior that causes a risk to health.
- ***Immune System:*** Physiological responses to stress involve the pituitary–adrenal axis and the autonomic nervous system through the release of corticosteroid hormones and catecholamines. It has been postulated that the relationship between the immune system and the CNS provides confirmation that the autonomic and physiological pathways through which stress passes can modulate an immune response (Kang, Rice, Turner-Henson, & Downs, 2010). Stress can cause wounds to heal more slowly and cause people to become more susceptible to infections, colds, and other illnesses (Solowiej, 2010; Upton & Solowiej, 2010).

  Chronic stress appears to blunt the immune response and increase the risk for infections. It may even impair a person's response to immunizations. Cognitive behavioral therapy and mind–body interventions such as relaxation and guided imagery techniques have been found to influence immune functioning (Crepaz et al., 2008; Lengacher et al., 2008; Scott-Sheldon, Kalichman, Carey, & Fielder, 2008).
- ***Endocrine System:*** Chronic stress has been associated with the development of insulin resistance, a condition in which the body is unable to use insulin effectively to regulate glucose (blood sugar). Insulin resistance is a primary factor in diabetes. Stress can exacerbate existing diabetes by impairing the patient's ability to manage the disease effectively.

  The hormones of the HPA axis also influence hormones needed for growth. Prolonged HPA activation hinders the release of growth hormone and insulin-like growth factor 1, (IGF-1), both of which are essential for normal growth.
- ***Reproductive System:*** CRH prevents the release of gonadotropin-releasing hormone (GnRH), the master hormone that signals a cascade of hormones that direct reproduction and sexual behavior. Similarly, cortisol and related glucocorticoid hormones not only inhibit the release of GnRH, but also inhibit the release of luteinizing hormone, which prompts ovulation and sperm release. Stress can lead to diminished sexual desire and an inability to achieve orgasm in women or can cause temporary impotence or prevent erection in men.
- ***Cancer:*** Based on a review of the literature to date, there is no current evidence to support the idea that stress causes cancer. However, recent studies have indicated that stress may play a role in the outcomes of patients with breast cancer, colorectal cancer, and prostate cancer (Ashing-Giwa & Lim, 2009; Fitzell & Pakenham, 2010; Remmers, Holtgrawe, & Pinkert, 2010; Segrin & Badger, 2010). Research also has focused on ways by which nurses and patients with cancer can have some control over the disease, including the fatigue many cancer patients experience (Faul, Jim, Williams, Loftus, & Jacobsen, 2010; Mok et al., 2010; Swanson & Koch, 2010). Although these studies are promising, more research is warranted. More information on cancer can be found in Chapter 57.
- ***Pain:*** Pain is common in patients who are critically ill. The stress response causes neurohumoral elevations of plasma catecholamine, cortisol, glucose, ADH, and acute-stage protein levels, which may result in tachycardia, hypertension, vasoconstriction, increased oxygen consumption, salt and water retention, and blunting of the immune response. The primary goal of analgesia is to relieve pain to attenuate the stress response. In the acute phase of pain relief, a profound stress response may require higher doses of analgesics. When a plateau is reached, analgesic requirements may decrease. In the recovery phase, analgesics are tapered or discontinued.

  Stress may intensify chronic pain caused by arthritis and other conditions. Tension-type headaches are associated with stress and stressful events. Some research suggests that tension-type headache sufferers may actually have some biological predisposition for translating stress into muscle contraction. Emotional stress is among the range of possible migraine triggers.
- ***Eating Problems:*** Stress can have varying effects on eating problems and weight. When stressed, many people develop cravings for salt, fat, and sugar to counteract tension and, thus, gain weight. Martin-Nemeth et al. (2009) found a relationship between stress and eating behaviors. Eating calorie-rich food seems to calm the nerves, but eating too much can lead to obesity, depression, and more stress.

  Weight gained in the abdominal area is a predictor of diabetes and heart problems. The release of cortisol, a major stress hormone, appears to promote abdominal fat and may be the primary connection between stress and weight gain in people. It has been demonstrated that a hormonal cascade causes hunger (Torres & Nowson, 2007). When a stress response is activated, the brain releases CRH, which suppresses the appetite. The adrenal glands then secrete their powerful fight-or-flight stress hormones, adrenaline, and cortisol, which propel sugar into the bloodstream for a short-term energy rush. After that rush, cortisol sparks ravenous hunger for carbohydrates and fat. If under continuous stress, the result is prolonged, thus elevating cortisol levels that spur the release of insulin, the hormone that directs the body to hang on to the fat it has and store more. If an individual has many stressors, she has many periods of rebound insulin secretion. The cumulative effect is a push toward obesity.
- ***Sleep Disturbances:*** The tensions of unresolved stress frequently cause insomnia, generally keeping the stressed person awake or causing awakening in the middle of the night or early morning. Researchers also have theorized that persistent insomnia may

result from a disorder of the stress system (NIH, 2009). They found that, when compared to a group of people who did not have difficulty falling asleep, the insomniacs had higher ACTH and cortisol levels, both in the evening and in the first half of the night. Their ACTH and cortisol levels indicated that the insomniacs had nervous systems that were on overdrive, alert, and ready to deal with a threat, when they actually should otherwise be quieting down. Therefore, family nurse practitioners may have more success in prescribing antidepressants to help calm an overactive stress system as opposed to prescribing hypnotics to regulate the sleep system. Behavior therapy also can assist with developing good sleep patterns.

- ***Memory, Concentration, and Learning:*** Cognitive changes occur in response to acute, uncontrollable stress. When this happens, an individual can become distracted and disorganized, and the working memory abilities decline.
- ***Other Disorders:*** Other disorders that may be precipitated by stress include allergies, skin disorders, hair loss, periodontal disease, or depression. Stress may be a cause of the so-called "sick-building syndrome," which produces allergy-like symptoms, such as eczema, headaches, asthma, and sinus problems (NIH, 2009). It may play a role in exacerbating some skin conditions including hives, psoriasis, acne, or rosacea. Stress may cause unexplained itching or unexplained hair loss (alopecia areata) that may occur in localized patches. Stress also has been implicated in increasing the risk for periodontal disease.
- ***Depression:*** Melancholic depression has been found to be a major disorder characteristic of an overactive HPA axis. The body turns on the fight-or-flight response, but cannot turn it off again, thereby producing anxiety and overreaction to stimulation. This is followed by the paradoxical response called "learned helplessness." This form of depression manifests itself in anxiety, loss of appetite, loss of sex drive, rapid heartbeat, high blood pressure, and high cholesterol and triglyceride levels. However, rather than producing higher amounts of ACTH in response to CRH, depressed people produce smaller amounts of this substance, presumably because their hippocampi have become less sensitive to the higher amounts of CRH. In an attempt to switch off excess CRH production, people with melancholic depression also produce high levels of cortisol. The by-products of the cortisol serve as sedatives and perhaps contribute to the overall feeling of depression.

  Other conditions, such as anorexia nervosa, malnutrition, obsessive-compulsive disorder, anxiety disorder, alcoholism, alcohol and narcotic withdrawal, and hyperthyroidism (NIH, 2009) are associated with high levels of CRH and cortisol. Most patients with these conditions share psychological symptoms including sleep disturbances, loss of libido, and loss of appetite, as well as physical problems, such as an increased risk for accumulating abdominal fat, hardening of the arteries, and other forms of cardiovascular disease. Many patients are likely to have their life spans shortened by 15 to 20 years if they remain untreated due to their increased risk for other health problems.
- ***Unhealthy Lifestyles:*** People under chronic stress often use unhealthy means to relieve the stress, such as drug or alcohol abuse, tobacco use, abnormal eating patterns, or watching television for more than 5 to 6 hours/day. The damage caused by these self-destructive habits under ordinary circumstances is exacerbated by the physiological effects of stress itself. The cycle becomes self-perpetuating. A sedentary routine, an unhealthy diet, alcohol abuse, and smoking promote heart disease, interfere with sleep patterns, and lead to increased rather than reduced tension levels.

Safety Alert *The nurse should assess for these unhealthy practices and develop education for the patient and family to recognize unhealthy lifestyle practices and develop support systems and healthy practices.*

Although many disorders result from an overactive stress system, some result from an underactive stress system. This occurs in the case of Addison's disease due to the lack of cortisol. Lack of the hormone CRH also results in the feelings of extreme tiredness common to people suffering from chronic fatigue syndrome. In addition, CRH is central to seasonal affective disorder (SAD), the feelings of fatigue and depression that plague some patients during winter months.

Risk Factors for Stress

At some point in everyone's life, stressful events develop that overwhelm their usual coping mechanisms. Job-related stress is particularly likely to become chronic because it is such a large part of daily life. Stress may reduce a worker's effectiveness by impairing concentration, causing sleeplessness, and increasing the risk for illness, back problems, accidents, and lost time. Extreme stress, such as harassment or violence on the job, places a burden on the heart and the cardiovascular system (Franke, Kohut, Russell, Ekkekakis, & Ramsey, 2010; Koh, 2010; Ramey, Downing, & Knobauch, 2008). From a biological perspective, some people exhibit an absent or inadequate relaxation response to stress. In these individuals, stress hormones remain elevated instead of returning to normal levels, possibly leading to illnesses. The types of individuals at higher risk for stress are listed in the Risk Factors box.

RISK FACTORS for Stress

Younger adults	Young adults are relatively stress free (Boardman & Alexander, 2011). Stress may go unnoticed in the very young or very old.
Women in general	Because women may be more emotionally reactive in stressful situations, they may be at higher risk than men for stress-related chest pain, but men's hearts may be more vulnerable to adverse effects from long-term stress.
Working mothers	Working mothers face higher stress levels and possibly adverse health effects, most likely because they bear a greater and more diffuse workload than men or other women.
Divorced or widowed individuals	Unmarried people generally do not live as long as their married contemporaries.
The unemployed	Being unemployed is an environmental stressor that threatens security.
Isolated individuals	Usually lack support systems.
People who are targets of discrimination	Discrimination is an environmental stressor that is beyond individual control.
Those without health insurance	This threat to an individual's health can lead to stress.
People who live in cities	City dwellers may be more stressed as a result of external stressors beyond their control.

Coping

Stress from any source provokes a change in the person's homeostasis or balanced state of being. Adaptive mechanisms promote adjustment to these changes, in the form of coping, to restore the individual to a balanced state so that he has the resources to meet new demands.

Coping is a compensatory process with both physiological and psychological components. Strategies for coping are learned patterns of behavior and are affected by patterns of relationships, situational stressors, and personality traits (Kravits, McAllister-Black, Grant, & Kirk, 2010). Coping is promoted by believing in personal power to control the circumstances of life, setting achievable goals, and creating a positive mood.

Coping Strategies for Stress

It has long been thought that how a person adjusts to life stresses is a major component of his ability to lead a fulfilling life. It was not until the 1980s that coping became a discrete topic of psychological inquiry. Since then, coping has risen to a position of prominence in the modern psychological discourse, especially within the personality, cognitive, and behavioral spheres. The concept of coping has been defined as a compensatory mechanism wherein cognitive and behavioral efforts change constantly to manage specific external or internal demands that are appraised as taxing or exceeding the person's resources (Lazarus & Folkman, 1984).

Coping is influenced by the amount of control the individual is able to exert over the situation. The more control a person has over a situation, the better she copes. Individuals perceive they have greater control when a stress is internal, transient, and specific. Lack of control stems from stressors that are external, or stable.

Cognitive appraisal and coping are affected by internal characteristics such as health, energy, personal belief systems, commitments or life goals, self-esteem, control, mastery, knowledge, problem-solving skills, and social skills. To date, nursing research has focused on health promotion and hardiness. In many circumstances, it has been found to be more feasible to promote a healthy lifestyle than to alter the stressors. The research often is guided by the transactional model of stress and coping as developed by Lazurus and Folkman (1984), which was presented earlier in this chapter. This model provides a framework for evaluating the processes of coping with stressful events. Within this framework, stressful experiences are construed as person-environment transactions; these transactions depend on the impact of the external stressor. The impact is mediated by the person's appraisal or perception of the stressor and the individual's availability of social and cultural resources with which to deal with the stressor.

Coping strategies, also referred to as stress management, refer to the specific efforts, both behavioral and psychological, that people employ to master, tolerate, reduce, or minimize stressful events (Mayo Clinic, 2011). A distinction is often made in the coping literature between active and avoidant coping strategies. *Active* coping strategies are either behavioral or psychological responses designed to change the nature of the stressor itself or how one thinks about it. *Avoidant* coping strategies lead people into activities that are considered unhealthy, such as alcohol or drug abuse, overeating, or smoking. Generally speaking, active coping strategies, whether behavioral or emotional, are thought to be better ways to deal with stressful events. Avoidant coping strategies may become maladaptive ways to deal with stress or stressful events.

Coping resources are defined as characteristics or actions that an individual can draw on to manage stress. For example, as a newly diagnosed diabetic begins to deal with the recent diagnosis, different modes of coping occur that may include the following:

- Information seeking (gathering data about the problem and possible solutions to the problem), searching the Internet.
- Direct actions (performing concrete acts to alter self or environment), beginning an exercise regime.
- Inhibition of action (refraining from an action), not checking BGs as recommended.
- Intrapsychic processes (reappraising the situation; initiating cognitive activity aimed at improving feelings), attending a diabetic support group.
- Obtaining emotional support by turning to others, discussing dietary modifications with loved ones.
- Escaping or avoiding, continuing with previous dietary intake.

The choice of coping strategies depends on various factors, such as degrees of uncertainty, threat, or helplessness, and the presence of conflict (Seaward, 2009). If the degree of threat is severe, additional unhealthy coping modes, such as panic, are more likely to occur. In the presence of conflict, an individual may not be able to take direct actions. Helplessness promotes immobilization. The coping strategy an individual chooses also may be influenced by the outcome of the individual's cognitive appraisal of the stressor as harm or loss, threat, or challenge.

Cultural Background

Culture plays an important role in the choice of a person's coping strategies. Cultures and societies have their own set of rules about what they perceive to be stressful or not. For example, educational systems vary from culture to culture, with some cultures placing greater emphasis on how students do in schools. Access to higher education—and ultimately the better jobs—is determined solely through academic performance, causing high levels of stress.

Stressful life events, as described by Holmes and Rahe (1967), will vary among cultures due to different norms and values. Therefore,

EVIDENCE-BASED PRACTICE Promoting Resilience Through Self-Care

Clinical Problem

As presented earlier in the chapter, hardiness and resilience may be a mediating factor for patients who experience stressful life events but do not become ill. A hardy person has a sense of meaningfulness, personal values, an internal locus of control, and a clear sense of values.

Research

Studies are beginning to show that resilience can be enhanced through mind–body exercises such as visual imagery, meditation, yoga, Tai Chi, Qi gong, group support, and spirituality. Resilience can also be enhanced through spiritual practices such as cultivating gratitude, forgiveness, and compassion (Deng et al., 2010).

Implications for Nursing Practice

It is important for the nurse to evaluate a patient and family's ability to cope. By educating the patient and family to healthy lifestyle changes that include stress reduction activities, the nurse may help to prevent the worsening or development of a chronic condition. Being aware of the types and advantages of mind–body exercises will assist the nurse in guiding the patient and family.

Critical Thinking Questions with answers can be found in the Osborn Student Resources at nursing.pearsonhighered.com.

CULTURAL CONSIDERATIONS
Responses by Individualist and Collectivist Cultures to Stress

Individualist cultures (most Western cultures) tend to emphasize personal autonomy and personal responsibility when dealing with problems. They tend to emphasize the importance and value of exerting control over stressful situations. Therefore, members of this type of culture are less likely to seek social support in stressful situations than are people from collectivist cultures (generally Asian and other Eastern countries). Collectivist cultures tend to be more oriented toward their social group, family, or community and toward seeking help with their problems. However, in collectivist cultures, a greater emphasis is placed on controlling one's personal reactions to a stressful situation rather than trying to control the situation itself. It stands to reason then that the learned component of coping, which is arrived at through experiential and reinforcement situations, may stem from cultural and societal values and beliefs (Finkelstein, 2011).

nurses must consider cultural and societal norms when assisting those from different cultures to identify stressors, stressor resources, and strategies to reduce the stress. The Cultural Considerations box discusses two types of cultures, individualist and collectivist, and how they respond to stress.

Safety Alert *Cultural assessment is instrumental in identifying stressors, stress resources, and coping strategies. Perceptions of stressful life events vary among cultures and are dependent on different norms and values. Nurses must consider cultural norms in order to meet desired outcomes.*

Workplace Culture

Cultural influence also is applicable when discussing work-related stress. Culture has been described as a "defining force" in understanding work habits. Each organization or work setting has its own unique culture. When there is discord in the work setting or when a person's values and beliefs are at odds with the culture of the setting, stress develops. In fact, work stressors can be identified in almost all aspects of a person's job. In most work situations, stress responses cause performance to suffer. As workers become uncomfortably stressed, distractions, difficulties, anxieties, and negative thinking begin to crowd their minds. Concentration suffers and focus narrows as the brain becomes overloaded. The more overloaded the brain becomes, the more performance can suffer. The more performance suffers, the more new distractions, difficulties, anxieties, and negative thoughts develop.

Both decision making and creativity are impaired when people are unable to take account of all of the information available. This inability accounts for the frequent observation that highly stressed people will persist in a course of action even when better alternatives are available. It also explains why anxious people perform best when they are not put under a lot of additional stress, whereas calm people may need additional pressure to produce a good performance. People perform at their best when they are able to concentrate normally and can focus all of their attention on the important task at hand.

Acculturative Stress

In the fast-paced world of today, job-related stress is becoming increasingly recognized as a nontrivial malady that impacts the well-being of both the employees and the organization. Globalization, an irreversible trend of the 21st century, has been widely acknowledged as having a stress-producing impact on the work setting. The increasing permeability of international borders, cross-border transfers of people and technology, and international mergers and partnerships that fuel globalization are influencing the culture of work settings.

When diverse cultures come together for collective effort in an organization, culture shock may be experienced. **Acculturative stress** occurs when individuals try to adapt to a new culture (Berry, 2005).

THERAPEUTIC RELATIONSHIPS

The public has consistently ranked nursing as the most honest and ethical of all the health care professions (Gallup Poll, 2009). For the patient, being able to establish a trusting relationship promotes a healing environment and decreases anxiety, depression, and anger surrounding medical conditions. Developing a therapeutic relationship requires an understanding of the biological, psychological, social, and spiritual factors that affect the patient's health and a belief in her capacity to heal with the goal of integrating the mind, body, spirit, and energy (Mahoney et al., 2009).

Certain actions foster the nurse–patient relationship. Patients need to feel safe, secure, and understood. Nurses accomplish this through the building blocks of the therapeutic nurse–patient relationship: by conveying respect for a person's uniqueness, being nonjudgmental, showing attentiveness, and being empathetic.

The Nurse–Patient Relationship

Hildegard Peplau (1952), a nurse theorist, conceptualized the nurse–patient relationship as moving through three phases: introductory (orientation), working, and termination. During each of the phases, particular goals are achieved and particular events take place. These phases often overlap.

Phases of the Nurse–Patient Relationship

- ***Introductory (Orientation) Phase:*** The introductory phase begins when the therapeutic relationship is initiated. Introductions take place and the patient is given initial information pertinent to her circumstances. During this phase, the nurse and the patient establish an agreement—and in some cases, a contract—about the purposes and direction of the relationship. This agreement or contract is usually verbal in nature; in some settings it will be informal, and in others it will be more formalized.

  An initial assessment takes place in this phase, leading to the identification of nursing diagnoses and mutual goals. The nurse is constantly reassessing the relationship throughout the entire experience. During this phase, mutual goal setting is initiated. It is important that the nurse and the patient mutually agree upon the goals and that they are continually renegotiated.
- ***Working Phase:*** During the second phase, called the working phase, the **therapeutic alliance** is established. A therapeutic alliance is one in which the nurse and the patient consciously work together to reach mutually agreed-upon goals. Application of the nursing process during this stage is continuous; in addition, it is sometimes necessary to seek additional assessment data, realign

goals, try new interventions, and reevaluate outcomes. Because new information and unanticipated events occur, problem solving is also continuous during this phase. Most patient education takes place during the working phase, and trust and rapport continue to grow during this stage as well. Patients begin to reach clarity and learn to explore all of the resources that are available to them.

- ***Termination:*** The third phase of the therapeutic nurse–patient relationship, termination, should begin during the introductory phase and is often discussed during the working phase. Depending on the nature, length, and intensity of the therapeutic relationship, the termination phase can be difficult for patients. During this phase, the nurse and patient review what occurred during the working phase, what goals have been met, and what progress was made. It is important for the nurse to understand that patients often feel a sense of loss and insecurity during this phase. These feelings might cause patients to display hostility or regress backward in their treatment. This is normal, self-protective behavior during this stage and needs to be worked through.

Self-Awareness in the Nurse–Patient Relationship

Hildegard Peplau expressed the importance of each nurse taking on the responsibility of expanding his or her own insight. She believed that the nurse's personality was an important factor in the development of an interpersonal relationship. According to Peplau (1987), the basic task of nursing education should be the development of nurses who want to help patients make positive changes in their lives.

Caring

The nurse–patient relationship also takes place in a context of caring. Watson (2008) feels that caring is one of the most fundamental attributes in nursing. She believes that caring serves to advance health in individuals and families and allows for the development of human potential and health autonomy. She has identified 10 *carative* factors, which are listed in Chart 9–2.

Interpersonal relationships between patients and nurses are strengthened when patients perceive the nurse as interpersonally competent.

CHART 9–2 Watson's Carative Factors

1. Forming a humanistic–altruistic value system
2. Instilling faith and hope
3. Cultivating sensitivity to oneself and to others
4. Developing a helping, trusting relationship
5. Promoting expression of positive and negative feelings
6. Systematically using the scientific problem-solving method for decision making
7. Promoting interpersonal teaching–learning
8. Providing support of a protective or corrective mental, physical, sociocultural, and spiritual environment
9. Assisting with gratification of human needs
10. Allowing for existential phenomenological forces

Source: Watson, J. (2008). *Nursing: The philosophy and science of caring* (Revised ed.). Boulder, CO: The University Press of Colorado.

Bruderle (2002) found that when nursing students begin their education, they are able to describe nurse caring behaviors and that faculty need to build upon their perceptions of nurse caring behaviors during the educational process. More recently, Livsey (2009) found that clinical faculty can influence nursing students' caring.

Nurses enter into therapeutic relationships with persons of diverse beliefs and values; therefore. it is very important to pay attention to cultural influences that may affect the nurse–patient relationship. Providing culturally sensitive care requires a responsible relationship between health care providers and patients, their families, and communities that is based on trust and respect. Camphina-Bacote (2008) charges nurses to become more culturally competent when she ponders if nurses have "ASKED" the right questions. ASKED stands for awareness, skill, knowledge, encounters and desire. By asking the right questions, nurses begin the journey toward cultural competence, the basis for their care.

The Office of Minority Health (2001) has developed the *National Standards on Culturally and Linguistically Appropriate Services in Health Care*. These standards, referred to as the CLAS standards and listed in the National Guidelines box , have been cross-referenced to The Joint Commission standards for accreditation of hospitals.

Therapeutic Communication

Having the ability to communicate skillfully is essential to good nursing care. Communication entails a two-way interaction in which a message is sent by the sender, heard and interpreted by the receiver, and a response is given. Effective communication calls for active listening skills and allows for feedback and clarification.

Communication also involves nonverbal messages. Nonverbal messages can be delivered through voice tone, rate and volume of speech, the use of silence, the use of touch, and body language. For instance, patients may verbally relate that they feel fine, but they may appear to be very sad. If the verbal and nonverbal message are not consistent, then the message is considered a mixed or an incongruent message. Incongruent messages are confusing for the receiver.

Therapeutic communication is purposeful communication that is designed to convey openness and caring. Skillful use of therapeutic communication requires the nurse to have an awareness of the patient's feeling environment. It consists of those words and actions that enhance the nurse–patient relationship and empower patients to make informed choices about their health care. At times, without realizing it, nurses communicate in ways that create barriers to effective communication. Developing an understanding of therapeutic and nontherapeutic communication techniques helps the nurse avoid communication pitfalls. Chart 9–3 (p. 224) provides a summary of therapeutic and nontherapeutic communication techniques. Culture also plays a role in therapeutic communication, as discussed in the Cultural Considerations box.

Nursing Management

Knowledge of stress, adaptation, and coping theories provides a framework for practice that is applicable to every stage of the nursing process. In caring for patients, nurses need to be aware of situations that are likely to be stressful. In addition, they must be able to assess the patient's appraisal of the situation and response to the stressor. Nurses also need to determine the patient's coping resources and strategies, as these impact the patient's physiological and psychosocial response to stressors.

NATIONAL GUIDELINES for the CLAS Standards

Standard 1: Health care organizations should ensure that patients/consumers receive from all staff members effective, understandable, and respectful care that is provided in a manner compatible with their cultural health beliefs and practices and preferred language.

Standard 2: Health care organizations should implement strategies to recruit, retain, and promote at all levels of the organization a diverse staff and leadership that are representative of the demographic characteristics of the service area.

Standard 3: Health care organizations should ensure that staff at all levels and across all disciplines receive ongoing education and training in culturally and linguistically appropriate service delivery.

Standard 4: Health care organizations must offer and provide language assistance services, including bilingual staff and interpreter services, at no cost to each patient/consumer with limited English proficiency at all points of contact, and do so in a timely manner during all hours of operation.

Standard 5: Health care organizations must provide to patients/consumers in their preferred language both verbal offers and written notices informing them of their right to receive language assistance services.

Standard 6: Health care organizations must assure the competence of language assistance provided to limited English proficient patients/consumers by interpreters and bilingual staff. Family and friends should not be used to provide interpretation services (except on request by the patient/consumer).

Standard 7: Health care organizations must make available easily understood patient-related materials and post signage in the languages of the commonly encountered groups represented in the service area.

Standard 8: Health care organizations should develop, implement, and promote a written strategic plan that outlines clear goals, policies, operational plans, and management accountability/oversight mechanisms to provide culturally and linguistically appropriate services.

Standard 9: Health care organizations should conduct initial and ongoing organizational self-assessments of CLAS-related activities and are encouraged to integrate cultural and linguistic competence-related measures into their internal audits, performance improvement programs, patient satisfaction assessments, and outcomes-based evaluations.

Standard 10: Health care organizations should ensure that data on the individual patient's/consumer's race, ethnicity, and spoken and written language are collected in health records, integrated into the organization's management information systems, and periodically updated.

Standard 11: Health care organizations should maintain a current demographic, cultural, and epidemiological profile of the community as well as a needs assessment to accurately plan for and implement services that respond to the cultural and linguistic characteristics of the service area.

Standard 12: Health care organizations should develop participatory, collaborative partnerships with communities and utilize a variety of formal and informal mechanisms to facilitate community and patient/consumer involvement in designing and implementing CLAS-related activities.

Standard 13: Health care organizations should ensure that conflict and grievance resolution processes are culturally and linguistically sensitive and capable of identifying, preventing, and resolving cross-cultural conflicts or complaints by patients/consumers.

Standard 14: Health care organizations are encouraged to regularly make available to the public information about their progress and successful innovations in implementing the CLAS standards and to provide public notice in their communities about the availability of this information.

Source: Office of Minority Health. (2001). *National standards for culturally and linguistically appropriate services in health care. Final report.* Rockville, MD: Author.

Assessment

Three major areas—demands (stressors), the human response to stress, and coping—serve as a useful guide in the assessment process. The manifestations of stress vary among individuals, and the nurse should assess all patients for the signs and symptoms of stress that occur as a result of bodily changes. The patient's age and culture also should be considered.

Stressors on the patient may include major life changes, events, or situations, such as changes in family constellations or daily hassles that the patient is experiencing. These stressors also may be classified as internal or external. Internal demands may include physical demands resulting from disease or injury, whereas external demands may include loss of family or friends, or a change in financial status. The nurse should also assess the number of simultaneous demands, the duration of those demands, and the patient's previous experience with similar demands. It is essential to determine the patient's primary appraisal or perception of the demands to determine if they represent harm or loss, threat, or challenge. Family responses to the patient's demands also should be assessed.

The physiological effects of demands (stressors) that are appraised as stressful are mediated primarily by the sympathetic nervous system and the HPA system. Behavioral responses include observable actions and cognition of the patient. Signs and symptoms of behavioral responses and physiological responses to stress are shown in Chart 9–4.

In assessing the patient, it is critical to remember that objective signs and subjective symptoms are the primary indicators of the physiological processes that are occurring. Further signs of change are indicated in diagnostic studies such as computed tomography (CT) and magnetic resonance imaging (MRI). Objective data also may be obtained from laboratory data (e.g., blood glucose, electrolytes, and urinalysis). In making a diagnosis, the nurse must relate the symptoms or complaints expressed by the patient to the physical and behavioral signs that are present.

Nursing Diagnoses

Many nursing diagnoses are possible for patients suffering from stress. Emotions such as anxiety, frustration, and anger, as well as feelings of inadequacy, helplessness, or powerlessness, often are associated with stress. In the presence of these emotions, the customary activities of daily living may be disrupted. For example, a sleep disturbance may be present, activity and eating patterns may be altered, and family processes and roles may be changed.

According to Carpenito (2009), a coping–stress–tolerance pattern has been identified as 1 of 11 functional health patterns. Assessment of the health pattern elicits a description of the patient's coping–stress–tolerance level, and enables the nurse to identify stressors at the individual or family level. Two overriding diagnoses related to stress have been identified: *Ineffective Coping* and *Compromised, Family Coping*. *Ineffective Coping* is defined as an inability to manage internal or environmental stressors appropriately as a result of inadequate resources (physical, psychological, behavioral, or cognitive). Potential etiologies include disruption of emotional bonds, unsatisfactory

CHART 9–3 Selected Therapeutic and Nontherapeutic Communication Techniques

Techniques	Rationale	Examples
Therapeutic Techniques		
Using silence	Gives the patient the opportunity to collect and organize thoughts, to think through a point, or to consider introducing a topic of greater concern than the one being discussed.	When discussing difficult subjects, such as sexual history or possible abusive situations.
Accepting	Conveys an attitude of reception and regard.	"Yes, I understand what you said." Eye contact, nodding.
Giving recognition	Acknowledging; indicating awareness.	"I see you attended therapy today" or "I see you made your bed."
Offering self	Making himself or herself available, increases the patient's feelings of worth.	"I'll stay with you for awhile," "Let me sit with you awhile," or "I'll be here with you."
Giving a broad opening	Engages the patient in conversation. Emphasizes the importance of her role in the interaction.	"What would you like to talk about today?" or "Tell me what you are thinking."
Offering general leads	Offers the patient encouragement to continue.	"Go on," "Yes, I see," or "And after that?"
Placing the event in time or sequence	Clarifies the relationship of events in time so that the nurse and patient can view them in perspective.	"What seemed to lead up to this," "Was that before or after?" or "When did that happen?"
Making observations	Verbalizing what is observed or perceived. Encourages the patient to recognize specific behaviors and compare perceptions with the nurse.	"You seem tense," "I notice you are pacing a lot," or "You seem uncomfortable."
Encouraging description of perceptions	Asking the patient to verbalize what is being perceived. Often used when a patient is experiencing hallucinations.	"Tell me what is happening now," "Are you hearing the voices now?" or "What do the voices seem to be saying?"
Encouraging comparison	Asking the patient to compare similarities and differences in ideas, or experiences. Helps the patient to recognize life experiences that tend to recur as well as aspects of life that are changeable.	"Was this something like . . . ," "How does this compare to the time when . . . ," or "What was your response the last time this situation occurred?"
Focusing	Taking notice of a single idea or word. Works well with a patient who is moving rapidly from one thought to another. This technique is not therapeutic for someone who is very anxious.	"This point seems worth looking at more closely. Perhaps you and I can discuss it together."
Seeking clarification and validation	Striving to explain that which is vague or incomprehensible and searching for mutual understanding. Clarifying the meaning of what has been said facilitates and increases understanding.	"Tell me if my understanding agrees with yours" or "Do I understand correctly that you said . . . ?"
Presenting reality	When a patient has a misperception of the environment, the nurse defines reality or indicates his or her perception of the situation for the patient.	"I understand that the voices seem real to you, but I do not hear any voices," or "I can only see you and me in the room right now."
Voicing doubt	Expressing uncertainty as to the reality of the patient's perceptions. Often used with patients who are experiencing delusional thinking.	"I find that unusual" or "That seems rather doubtful to me."
Nontherapeutic Techniques		
Giving reassurance	Indicates to the patient that there is no cause for anxiety, thereby devaluing the patient's feelings. May discourage the patient from further expressions of feelings.	"I wouldn't worry about that" or "Everything will be all right." Better to say: "We will work on that together."
Rejecting	Refusing to consider or showing contempt for the patient's ideas or behavior. This may cause the patient to discontinue interaction with the nurse for fear of further rejection.	"Let's not discuss . . ." or "Let's not talk about that now." Better to say: "Let's look at that a little closer."
Giving approval or disapproval	Sanctioning or denouncing the patient's ideas or behavior. Implies that the nurse has the right to pass judgment on whether the ideas or behaviors are good or bad. The nurse's acceptance of the patient is then seen as conditional depending on the patient's behavior.	"That's good, I'm glad that you . . ." or "That's bad. I'd rather you wouldn't." Better to say: "Let's talk about how your behavior at dinner invoked anger in the other patients."
Giving advice	Telling the patient what to do and how to behave implies that the nurse knows what is best and the patient is incapable of self-direction. Nurtures the patient in the dependent role and discourages independent thinking.	"I think you should" or "I wouldn't do it like that." Better to say: "What do you think you should do?"

(continued)

CHART 9–3 Selected Therapeutic and Nontherapeutic Communication Techniques, *continued*

Techniques	Rationale	Examples
Probing	Persistent questioning of the patient. Pushing for answers to issues the patient does not wish to discuss. Causes the patient to feel defensive, used, and valued for only what he or she shares.	"Tell me about your abuse" or "How come you were drinking and driving?"
Defending	Attempting to protect someone from verbal attack. To defend what the patient has criticized is to imply that she or he has no right to express ideas, opinions, or feelings. Defending may cause the patient to think the nurse is taking sides with those being criticized.	"No one here would lie to you" or "You have a very capable doctor, I'm sure he has your best interest at heart." Better to say: "I will try to answer your questions and clarify some issues regarding your treatment."
Requesting an explanation	Asking "why" a patient did something or feels a certain way can be very intimidating and implies that the patient must defend his or her behavior or feelings.	"Why do you think that?" "Why do you feel that way?" or "Why did you do that?" Better to say: "Describe what you were feeling just prior to this occurrence."
Using denial	When the nurse is uncomfortable with a patient's problem, he or she avoids helping the patient identify or explore areas of difficulty.	*Pt:* "I've amounted to nothing in my life." *Nurse:* "Everyone has some accomplishments." Better to say: "Let's talk about how you have come to that conclusion."
Interpreting	The nurse attempts to tell the patient the meaning of her or his experience.	"What you really mean is . . ." or "Unconsciously you feel. . . ." Better to say: "What do think is going on?"

CULTURAL CONSIDERATIONS for Therapeutic Communications

Tamparo and Lindh (2008) state there is a need for multicultural therapeutic communication as approximately one third of the U.S. population is from a culture other than mainstream American. Nurses need to develop the ability to communicate with individuals of other cultures while taking into account their own personal cultural biases and putting them aside. Tamparo and Lindh (2008) list three actions that promote multicultural communication: (1) becoming knowledgeable about the beliefs and values of different cultures, (2) developing techniques that build and foster communication, and (3) recognizing the barriers to multicultural communication (p. 30).

support system, sensory overload, and inadequate psychological and physical resources (Carpenito, 2009). ***Compromised Family Coping*** refers to the usually supportive primary person (family member or friend) providing insufficient, ineffective, or compromised support, comfort, assistance, or encouragement that may be needed by the patient to manage the adaptive strategies related to the health challenge (Carpenito, 2009).

NANDA International (NANDA-I) has identified nursing diagnoses related to stress, adaptation, and coping (NANDA-I, 2009). Some of these appear in alphabetical order in the following list:

- ***Anxiety:*** A vague, uneasy feeling of discomfort or dread, the source of which may not be known. It is an alerting signal that warns of impending danger and enables the individual to take measures to deal with a threat.
- ***Compromised Family Coping:*** Primary supportive person provides insufficient, ineffective, or compromised support, comfort, or assistance that may be needed by the patient to manage adaptive tasks.
- ***Decisional Conflict (Specify):*** Uncertainty about the course of action to take when the choice involves risk, loss, or challenge to personal life values.
- ***Defensive Coping:*** Repeated projection of falsely positive self-evaluation based on a self-protective pattern that defends against underlying perceived threats to positive self-regard.
- ***Disabled Family Coping:*** Behavior of significant person that disables his or her capacities and the patient's capacities to effectively address tasks essential to adaptation of the health challenge.
- ***Fear:*** Response to perceived threat that is consciously recognized as a danger.
- ***Ineffective Coping:*** Inability to form a valid appraisal of the stressors, inadequate choices of practiced responses, and/or inability to use available resources.
- ***Post-Trauma Syndrome:*** Sustained maladaptive responses to a traumatic, overwhelming event.
- ***Relocation Stress Syndrome:*** Physiological and/or psychosocial disturbance following transfer from one environment to another.
- ***Risk Prone Health Behavior:*** Inability to modify lifestyle/behavior in a manner consistent with a change in health behavior.

  NANDA-I © 2012

Other applicable diagnoses dealing with stress include *Caregiver Role Strain, Social Isolation, Risk for Impaired Parenting, Spiritual Distress, Readiness for Enhanced Family Coping, Situational Low Self-Esteem,* and *Powerlessness*. Because human responses to stress are so varied, as are the sources of stress, arriving at an accurate diagnosis allows nursing interventions and goals to be more specific and leads to improved outcomes.

CHART 9–4 Behavioral and Physiological Indicators of Stress

Physiological

- Pupils dilate to increase visual perception when serious threats to the body arise.
- Diaphoresis increases to control elevated body heat due to increased metabolism.
- Heart rate and cardiac output increase to transport nutrients and by-products of metabolism.
- Skin pales due to constriction of peripheral blood vessels, an effect of norepinephrine.
- Sodium and water retention increase due to the release of mineralocorticoids.
- Rate and depth of respirations increase because of dilated bronchioles.
- Urinary output decreases.
- Dryness appears in the throat or mouth.
- Peristalsis of intestines decreases, resulting in possible constipation and flatus.
- Muscle tension increases in preparation for the fight-or-flight response.
- Blood sugar increases due to the release of glucocorticoids and gluconeogenesis.

Behavioral

- Elevated blood pressure
- Tachycardia
- Mobilization of energy stores
- Peripheral vasoconstriction
- Decreased gastric emptying
- Suppressed or stimulated appetite
- Depression
- Anger
- Anxiety
- Apathy
- Alienation
- Increased alcohol consumption
- Increased smoking

Source: From Berman, Audrey J., & Snyder, Shirlee J. (2012). *Kozier & Erb's Fundamentals of Nursing: Concepts, Process, & Practice,* 8th edition, © 2012. Electronically reproduced by permission of Pearson Education, Inc., Upper Saddle River, New Jersey.

Outcomes and Evaluation Parameters

Stress management is directed toward reducing and controlling stress and improving coping. The desired patient outcomes of nursing interventions are illness prevention, improved quality of life as defined by the patient, and fewer maladaptive responses to stress. Specific parameters of success in meeting these goals include identification of stressors, identification of stress resources, and use of adaptive coping strategies. These serve as measurable parameters on which to evaluate the patient's responses to nursing interventions. Examples of how one could respond to stress may be found in Chart 9–5.

Interventions

Interventions are based on the plans developed in collaboration with the patient; significant support people, if possible; and other members of the health care team. They are dependent on the patient's state of health, level of anxiety, support resources, coping mechanisms, and sociocultural and religious affiliation. The nurse and patient need to set goals to change the existing responses to the stressor or stressors.

CHART 9–5 Stress Responses

Healthy Responses = Stress Reduction	Unhealthy Responses = Potential Problems
Sleeping 7 to 8 hours/night	Sleeping less than 6 hours or more than 8 hours
Following a balanced diet	Eating more calories, carbohydrates, or fats than needed
Doing relaxation or visual imagery techniques	Watching 6 or more hours of TV/day
Being happy	Smoking
Increased concentration or staying focused on task	Decreased concentration or staying focused on task
Doing yoga or meditation	Nail biting
Exercising	Physically striking someone
Interacting with a variety of people	Staying by yourself

Although stress occurs daily in one form or another, it also is highly individual. Therefore, it is important to tailor stress reduction approaches to the individual patient. Interventions that seem to be universal in reducing stress include adequate rest and sleep, time management, optimal nutrition, relaxation techniques, and physical exercise. Specific nursing interventions, which already have been discussed, include promoting a healthy lifestyle, providing stress management education, and recommending support and therapy groups to assist in stress reduction.

Regular exercise promotes both physical and emotional health. Physiological benefits include improved muscle tone, improved cardiopulmonary function, and weight control. Psychological benefits include relief of tension, a feeling of well-being, and relaxation. Good nutrition is essential in increasing the body's resistance to stress. Reducing caffeine, salt, sugar, and fat intake and increasing vitamin and mineral intake will minimize the negative effects of stress, irritability, hyperactivity, and anxiety. Rest and sleep restore the body's energy levels and are an essential element of stress management. Effective time management helps patients experience less stress because they feel more in control of their situation. The nurse may need to help patients in both inpatient and outpatient settings to prioritize tasks and to consider whether modifications can be made to decrease role demands. Patients experiencing pain may need additional interventions.

Minimizing anxiety and mediating anger are helpful and appropriate nursing interventions. Nurses carry out measures to reduce patients' anxiety on a daily basis, and these activities should be reinforced. These activities include such measures as explaining procedures before they are performed, administering a massage to help the patient relax, controlling the environment to make it less stressful, providing emotional support to the patient and family, providing an atmosphere of caring and trust, and listening to and validating the patient's perceptions of what is happening and how she is feeling. Anger will be discussed again later in the chapter.

Crisis intervention is a short-term helping process of assisting patients to work through a crisis to its resolution and helping them restore their pre-crisis level of functioning. Those in crisis are experiencing an acute, time-limited state of disequilibrium. Thus, they are incapable of coping with the stressor by using previous methods of problem solving. They generally have a distorted perception of the event, may not have adequate situational support, or are using coping mechanisms inadequately. A crisis is a temporary situation usually requiring intervention from a professional individual, such as the clinical nurse specialist, physician, psychologist, clergy, or social worker.

The traditional steps of the nursing process closely correspond to the steps of crisis intervention. In the assessment phase, the nurse must focus on the person and the problem, collecting data about the patient, his coping style, the precipitating event, the situational supports, the patient's perception of the crisis, and the person's ability to handle the problem. The patient's perception of the event and personal response will determine the nursing diagnoses. Nursing diagnoses such as *Risk for Self-Directed Violence, Risk for Other-Directed Violence, Rape-Trauma Syndrome,* and *Hopelessness* may be appropriate for a patient experiencing a psychological crisis. Nursing diagnoses for patients experiencing a physiological crisis, such as *Altered Health Maintenance, Risk for Infection, Risk for Injury, Noncompliance,* or *Altered Nutrition,* may be appropriate. Effective planning for crisis intervention is based on assessment and active collaboration with the person in crisis and his significant others. Implementation involves crisis counseling and crisis home visits. Crisis counseling focuses on solving immediate problems, because the focus is on a general problem. Incorporating Maslow's hierarchy of needs might be too limiting as the counseling involves individuals, groups, or families. Resolution of the crisis is based upon the utilization of new coping strategies so that the person can return to her pre-crisis level of function or equilibrium.

Education to Promote Coping

The goals of nursing educational interventions are to reduce stress and improve the patient's coping ability. These generally are met by providing procedural information, such as preoperative teaching. Teaching specific content, such as a review of cardiovascular anatomy for the cardiac patient or a description of sensations the patient will experience during cardiac catheterization, is one type of preparatory education. This education may alter the person–environment relationship such that something that might have been viewed as threatening becomes perceived more positively. Providing patients with written information also tends to reduce their emotional response so they can concentrate and problem solve more effectively.

Enhancing Social Support

Social support, which is helpful in mediating life stress, tends to make people feel loved, appreciated, and valued. This can elevate the person's sense of self-worth. The critical qualities within a social network are the exchange of intimate communications and the presence of solidarity and trust. These social support qualities facilitate an individual's coping behaviors and create a sense of sharing the stress burden with the individual. Being involved in a social support system provides people with the ability to talk with someone, express feelings openly, and allow the person to gain control of the situation. Nurses can provide this support; however, it is important to help the person identify social support systems and encourage their use. Persons who are loners, are isolated, or withdraw in times of stress have a high risk of coping failure.

Anxiety also can alter a person's ability to process information. It helps to seek information and advice from others who can assist with analyzing the threat and developing a strategy to manage it. This assists the person in maintaining control and retaining self-esteem. Social networks assist with management of stress by providing the individual with:

- A positive social identity
- Emotional support
- Material aid and tangible services
- Access to information
- Access to new social contacts and new social roles.

Support and Therapy Groups

Support groups are formed for people in similar stressful situations; for example, cancer survivors, people with ostomies, mastectomy patients, parents of autistic children, those with chronic illnesses or disabilities, drug abusers, and alcoholics. By being a member of a group of people who share similar problems or goals, a person is helped to realize that he or she is not the only one experiencing this problem. Although not all individuals benefit from membership in such groups, many do. It is the nurse's responsibility, when assessing an individual's stressors and coping resources and strategies, to determine if such an intervention might be helpful to the individual.

Intervention Summary

A person's psychological and physiological health, internal and external sources of stress management, and relationships with the environment are predictors of health outcomes. These factors are related directly to the individual's health patterns. The nurse plays a significant role in identifying the health patterns of the individual receiving care. If the patient's health patterns are not achieving physiological, psychological, and social balance, the nurse works with the patient to seek ways to promote balance through nursing interventions. Examples of stress reduction techniques are shown in Chart 9–6. Interventions designed to mediate physiological stress and its effect on the body systems are addressed in greater depth in other chapters of this book.

Evaluation

Desired outcomes provide a guide for evaluating the patient's response to nursing interventions. They serve as indicators of accomplishment or lack of accomplishment in helping the patient reduce the stressors or manage the stressful situation. If outcomes are not achieved, the nurse and the patient, in concert with other members of the health care team, need to explore the reasons and revise the interventions as appropriate. Questions such as the following need to be considered:

- How does the patient perceive the problem?
- What underlying problems have not been identified?
- How does the patient perceive the effectiveness of new coping strategies?
- What prevented the patient from implementing new coping strategies?
- Did the patient access and use available resources?
- Have the family and significant others provided effective support?

Additionally, the nurse should assess physiological indicators of stress, including vital signs, heart rate, blood pressure, and

CHART 9–6 Stress Reduction Techniques

Maintain a healthy lifestyle by looking after your body.	Maintain regular exercise and eat a healthy diet rich in a variety of whole grains, vegetables, and fruits, and avoid excessive alcohol, caffeine, and tobacco.
	Exercise helps by creating a distraction from stressful events and releasing nervous energy.
Discover how to relax.	Relaxation is the polar opposite of the stress response. Deep-breathing exercises may help. If persistently unable to relax, try yoga or tai chi. Therapeutic massage also may loosen taut muscles and calm frazzled nerves.
Reduce stress through cognitive–behavioral methods.	Identify sources of stress and question those sources. Whose goals do the stressful activities meet? Can the assumed tasks be reasonably accomplished?
Restructure priorities; add stress-reducing activities.	Shift the balance from stress-producing to stress-reducing activities. Consider as many relief options as possible (e.g., walks, recreation).
Discuss feelings.	Explain your feelings and needs to a trusted individual, in a positive way, or use a journal or letter to express feelings. In return, listen to others.
Keep perspective and look for the positive; shift your outlook.	Focus on positive outcomes; this helps reduce tension and achieve goals. Choose to look at a situation in a more positive way. Step back from the conflict or worry that has put you in knots and ask what part of it is troubling you most. Are you afraid of losing face, or are you so angry that you are in danger of losing self-control. Is your reaction out of proportion? Take a break, talk to someone close, and get a different perspective on your troubles.
Use humor.	Use humor and laughter to release pent-up feelings and keep perspective. Laughter can have physical effects that reduce stress hormone levels.
Get help.	Seek professional help from psychiatric clinical nurse specialists, psychiatric nurse practitioners, psychiatrists, psychologists, or licensed clinical social workers if unable to change your habitual patterns of thought and behavior that trigger your stress response. They are professionals trained to help you break free of these patterns.

respiratory rate measurements; level of pain; sleep and rest patterns; and dietary habits.

Collaborative Management

Humans experience stress as an intrinsic part of life and in conjunction with many standard diagnostic, clinical, and surgical experiences. Intended and unintended stressors may significantly affect the patient's diagnostic and clinical measures and overall health outcomes. Responding to the signs and symptoms of stress and creating a plan of care requires collaboration with all members of the health care team. In order to meet desired patient outcomes, it is essential that this interdisciplinary team communicate openly with one another in developing and evaluating care of the patient and family (Institute of Medicine, 2010).

Acute physiological responses to stress in which the patient is experiencing signs and symptoms of critical illness will require close collaboration with the physician in planning, treating, and monitoring care. Other members of the health care team will play an active part in treating respiratory problems, cardiovascular problems, pain, and nutritional imbalances. If stress manifestations are psychological and/or behavioral, it would be prudent for the nurse to collaborate with the psychiatric clinical nurse specialist. If the patient has a nutritional imbalance or eating habit problems, the nutritionist or dietitian becomes a key player in the patient's care.

In preparing a patient for discharge from an acute care hospital, the nurse would need to coordinate with, and rely on, the expertise of many other members of the health care team in order to provide a comfortable transition from acute care to the home or extended care environment. The most important need is for the nurse to coordinate with the patient and the patient's family or significant others. These people play a key role in providing coping resources and in developing coping strategies. The nurse uses these resources as key elements in implementing the nursing process and developing the plan of care for patients.

Health Promotion

Stress can be a factor in a variety of physical and emotional illnesses. Many stress symptoms are managed with over-the-counter medications; for example, aspirin, acetaminophen, or ibuprofen for tension headache, and antacids and antidiarrhea medications for mild stomach distress. However, a nurse practitioner or physician should be consulted for physical symptoms that are out of the ordinary, particularly those which progress in severity or awaken the patient at night. The psychiatric clinical nurse specialist or practitioner should be consulted for unmanageable acute stress or for severe anxiety or depression.

Health and energy aid individuals with their coping strategies; thus, a health-promoting lifestyle provides resources and helps buffer the impact of stressors. Health risk questionnaires estimate the likelihood that a person with a given set of characteristics will become ill. If provided this information, individuals may alter their activities to improve their health. Reports of health can vary according to socioeconomic class and age (Dowd & Zajacova, 2010; Martin-Nemeth et al., 2009).

In choosing specific strategies for treating stress, the nurse should consider several factors:

- No single method is uniformly successful.
- What works for one person does not necessarily work for someone else.
- Stress can be positive as well as negative. Appropriate and controllable stress can enhance an individual's interest and excitement and motivate the individual to greater achievement. A lack of stress may lead to boredom and depression.
- Stress may play a part in making people vulnerable to illness. Patients should be referred to the appropriate health practitioner when there are indications for accompanying medical or psychological conditions, such as cardiac symptoms, significant pain, anxiety, or depression.

Stress Reduction and Impact on Health

An individual's reaction to a specific stressor is different from anyone else's. Some people are naturally laid-back about almost everything, whereas others react strongly at the slightest hint of stress; most fall somewhere between those extremes. Genetic variations may partly explain the differences. The genes that control the stress response keep most people on a fairly even keel, only occasionally priming the body for fighting or fleeing. Overactive or underactive stress responses may stem from slight differences in these genes. The availability of genetic information and technology enables health care providers to perform screening, testing, and education (Schwartz, 2010) for patients with genetic concerns. Knowledge obtained from the Human Genome Project also has created opportunities for assessing a person's genetic profile and preventing or treating disease.

Life experiences may increase the individual's sensitivity to stress as well. Strong stress reactions sometimes may be traced to early environmental factors. People who were exposed to extreme stress as children tend to be particularly vulnerable to stress as adults.

As explained, stressors develop when the demands of life exceed the individual's ability to cope with them. It follows, then, that stress can be managed by:

- Changing the environment so that the demands are not so high
- Learning how to better cope with the demands in the environment
- Doing both.

It is emphasized that treating stress cannot cure medical problems. Stress management is not a substitute for standard medical treatments, but it can be an important component of a medical regimen. Various stress management techniques such as mindfulness, meditation, massage, relaxation and visual imagery, yoga, and spiritual interventions have been found to assist patients in their recovery from various illnesses (Bauer et al., 2010; Delaney & Barrere, 2008; Fang et al., 2010; Griffiths, Camic, & Hutton, 2009; Klein & Hoffman, 2010; Olivo, Dodson-Lavelle, Wren, Fang, & Oz, 2009; Ulger & Yagli, 2010).

Stress management requires continuous practice as one goes through life and deals with often unexpected change. Even if frustrations are taken in stride, the stress response can surge up when dealing with something big, such as illness, job loss, or bereavement. The body's fight-or-flight reaction has strong biological roots. If stress becomes difficult and is potentially causing long-term effects, it is necessary to take action by learning how to recognize the symptoms and by seeking help to mediate the effects of the stress.

THE TEACHING–LEARNING PROCESS

The teaching–learning process is important to understand because the nurse teaches a variety of learners, such as patients and families, professional colleagues, and the community. Most often, the nurse teaches the patient and family regarding the plan of care, medications, how to perform self-care, and changes in lifestyle behaviors in order to create a healing, healthy environment. In a pilot study, Klein and Hoffman (2010) found that by teaching burn patients relaxation and visual imagery techniques, patients were able to reduce their hypermetabolic status.

Teaching is defined as any deliberate act that involves the planning, implementation, and evaluation of instructional strategies that meet expected learner outcomes. Learning occurs when there is a change in behavior (cognitive, affective, or psychomotor) as a result of being exposed to environmental stimuli. Learning is divided into three domains: cognitive, affective, and psychomotor. Cognitive learning involves the storing and recalling of new knowledge and information in the brain. **Affective learning** involves changes in attitudes, values, and feelings. **Psychomotor learning** involves learning that occurs when a physical skill has been acquired. It is helpful for the nurse to have an understanding of adult learners. Factors that apply to adult learners include the following:

- The adult's previous life experiences can be used as a resource.
- The adult's social role may affect readiness to learn.
- The adult's readiness to learn is increased when the material is useful immediately. (North Carolina Concept-Based Learning Editorial Board, 2011)

The teaching–learning process is facilitated by the existence of a therapeutic nurse–patient relationship. The nurse as teacher needs to be able to communicate effectively with individuals, families, and groups. The teaching–learning process can be conceptualized into four steps: assessment of learning needs, developing a teaching plan, implementation of a teaching plan, and evaluation of the teaching plan.

Assessment of Learning Needs

When nurses assess the learning needs of an individual, group, or family, they should use all appropriate information available to them. Patients and families can provide the most accurate information. Unfortunately, there are times when a patient or family member is not a good historian. In such cases, it is necessary to get information from additional sources, such as old medical records. During the assessment process, the nurse must identify the particular knowledge, skills, and attitudes that are needed by the patient or family. Once this is accomplished, the nurse must assess the emotional and experiential readiness of the patient or family to learn. The following factors should be considered when assessing emotional and experiential readiness to learn:

- The level of emotional health
- Motivation to learn
- Self-concept and body image
- Social and economic stability
- Past experiences with learning
- Attitude toward learning.

Assessing the patient's ability to learn is necessary so an appropriate teaching plan can be designed. The following factors need to be considered:

- Physical condition of the patient and acuity of the illness
- Acuity of the patient's senses
- Level of education
- Literacy
- Communication skills
- Primary language
- Pain level
- Prognosis.

Developing and Implementing a Teaching Plan

The teaching–learning process is more effective when mutual goal setting takes place. Unless the patient values the learning objectives, it is unlikely that much learning will occur. It is also important for all learning goals to be realistic and appropriate for the patient and situation. The following are important steps when designing a teaching plan:

- Identify short- and long-term goals.
- Prioritize the goals.
- Determine who should be included in the teaching.
- Match content with appropriate teaching strategies and learner activities.
- Relate teaching content to the patient's interests, resources, and patterns of everyday living.
- Decide on group versus individual teaching or formal versus informal teaching.
- Design a plan that is realistic for time constraints.

The implementation of the teaching plan should include varied teaching strategies delivered in an organized manner. The strategies should be appropriate for the type of learning that is desired.

Teaching Special Populations

When developing a teaching plan, consideration for special populations is very important. Teaching techniques must fit the patient's abilities to learn. The following populations should be considered:

- ***Older Adults:*** Slow down and give the older adult time to comprehend. When possible, give the older adult written materials to assist those with short-term memory loss. Due to visual changes that occur with aging, use large-print material on no-glare paper. To maximize hearing, face the patient; some older adults use lip reading to enhance understanding.
- ***Visually Impaired:*** Use large-print material without highlighting or visual cues as color discrimination may be impaired. If the patient is blind, convert materials to Braille or auditory formats.
- ***Hearing Impaired:*** Have the patient sit closer to the speaker. Make sure assistive devices are working properly. Use a sign language interpreter, if available. Use written materials and visual aids.
- ***Developmental Disability:*** Teach to the patient's developmental stage rather than to chronological age. Use simple and concrete examples. Demonstrate the material and have the patient do a return demonstration.

Evaluating a Teaching Plan

The mutually agreed-upon learning goals provide the basis for evaluating whether learning has occurred.

If the learning objectives have not been met, the learning content and teaching strategies may need to be reassessed. New goals must be agreed upon, and the teaching repeated or modified.

The Impact of the Internet on Teaching and Learning

Most patients have access to the Internet and use it to obtain information quickly. This has increased most patients' knowledge regarding health care issues and their treatment. It has also allowed nurses to elicit information quickly regarding a patient's diagnosis and treatment. Many health care systems now use the Internet to communicate with their patients and share information with them, including laboratory and radiographic results. Not only can the patient research information regarding specific diseases and treatment, there are many sites where other patients' experiences related to particular health issues are shared. When evaluating patients' knowledge and ability to learn, inquire if they have access to the Internet and can use it to receive and research information. Ask patients who have already researched a subject to share the information with you to check the validity. Give patients a list of credible websites to ensure that they are receiving accurate information and to enhance the teaching you have provided.

THE PSYCHODYNAMICS OF ILLNESS AND HOSPITALIZATION

Many complex factors can influence a patient's perception of a serious illness or hospitalization. Understanding these different factors and providing appropriate nursing care will improve a patient's and family's outlook on health and illness and possibly improve patient outcomes. As stated earlier in the chapter, a perceived stress will have the same physiological response as an actual stressor. By listening carefully to the patient and family, the nurse will be better able to understand their perception of the disease and the plan of care. Teaching the patient and family about the disease process and what to expect from the plan of care helps to create a healing environment.

Crisis

For many people, any illness or hospitalization constitutes a crisis. A crisis can develop when an event or series of events occurs that creates a situation that is perceived as threatening. A *maturational crisis* occurs when the stressors are related to developmental events, such as an adolescent who develops an identity crisis. A *situational crisis* occurs from the stress of an unexpected event, such as the development of an acute illness. An *adventitious crisis* is one that results from unexpected natural disasters such as tornadoes or plane crashes.

A crisis develops in response to a series of events. Both the situation and the individual's perception and response to the event lead to the development of a crisis state. A crisis is self-limiting (Caplan, 1964), usually resolving in 4 to 6 weeks. The development stages of a crisis are as follows:

- The individual or family is in a state of homeostasis or equilibrium.
- A stressful event or events occur.
- The event is perceived as a threat.
- Well-known coping skills are applied but fail to reduce the threat.
- A period of disequilibrium occurs with a decrease in problem-solving ability and an increase in feelings of anxiety and depression.
- The problem is either resolved (return to equilibrium) or personal disintegration occurs (crisis).

Nurses are often in contact with individuals and families when they are in a crisis and therefore become a valuable resource. Early intervention is essential to reduce the effects of the crisis; by providing information and resources, the nurse may prevent a full-blown crisis from occurring. Interventions should meet the level of disorganization that the patient is experiencing and should be done as quickly as possible. Because crisis is about the perception of the problem, it is essential that information be described from the patient's perspective. It is important for the nurse to understand the meaning the event has for the patient. Allowing for free expression of feelings can be cathartic in itself.

Once the problems have been defined, the nurse and the patient develop an initial plan of action. During this time, the nurse can provide the patient with practical, concrete help. The nurse may have to do some things for the patient that under different circumstances the patient would do for himself. It is helpful to have the patient make a list of his needs and concerns from most important to least important. This can help the nurse plan interventions that will decrease the sense of disequilibrium, reduce feelings of anxiety and depression, and mobilize supportive resources. The nurse provides emotional support through this process because the change can be very anxiety producing. If there is a concern about self-harm, the nurse should act to protect the patient and initiate an immediate referral.

Once the crisis has been stabilized, the nurse can help the patient problem solve and explore alternatives. At this point, new coping skills can be taught. Teaching new coping skills empowers patients to better handle future crisis events. For this reason, a crisis is often seen as an opportunity for growth.

Sick Role Behavior

Illness and hospitalization are often perceived as stressful and make patients more vulnerable to experiencing a crisis. When individuals are hospitalized, they are expected to behave in certain ways and assume a sick role. A **sick role** is a set of expectations that people who are ill must meet and which society, including caregivers, expects of them. When a person enters the hospital, that person is immediately oriented to hospital rules, regulations, policies, and procedures. For example, the patient is expected to be cooperative, dependent, and nondemanding. Patients, as well as their families, are expected to adhere to these rules.

Patients often perceive that they are losing control when they are hospitalized. This feeling of losing one's autonomy is more disturbing to some patients than to others. The term **locus of control** refers to the perception people have about how much control they exert over the events that happen in their lives. People with an **internal locus of control** believe that events in their lives are controlled by their own actions and decisions. People with an **external locus of control** believe that events in their lives are controlled more by fate, luck, and external circumstances.

Even though health professionals are strangers, they ask patients to entrust themselves to their care. Because of a strong need to control their own autonomy, patients with an internal locus of control may find this paternalism in health care frustrating. In contrast, patients with an external locus of control may need assistance in being more involved in their own health care decision making. Creating a healing environment includes integration of mind, body, and spirit. It also includes the cultivation of healing relationships that enhance caring, compassion, empathy, and social support. As discussed earlier under Therapeutic Relationships and Therapeutic Communication, the patient, by being able to establish a trusting relationship, promotes a healing environment and decreases anxiety, depression, and anger surrounding medical conditions. The following list features ways in which nurses can demonstrate interpersonal competence and empower patients to be more involved in their health care decisions:

- Answer questions honestly and knowledgeably.
- Do mutual goal setting, and make sure the goal is realistic for the patient to meet.
- Inform patients in advance of procedures.
- Prepare patients for procedures.
- Let patients know what to expect.
- Listen patiently to expressions of concern.
- Do not treat patients as children.

Relationship-based nursing care allows for the collaboration between the patient and the health care team, with the nurse's role to include advocating for the patient. Collaborative medicine promotes healing and self-recovery using both conventional and complementary therapies.

Loss and Grief

When patients and significant others are confronted with a serious illness, they often experience feelings of loss and grief. The amount of loss that is perceived by the patient and significant others is individual and should be assessed. The grieving process can be initiated by any loss. Although impending death represents a major loss, other types of losses can trigger the grieving process as well. Illness can cause the loss of physiological functioning, familiar roles, relationships, financial security, self-esteem, autonomy, and other losses individual to each situation. How each patient and significant other adapts to his losses depends on the individual's perception of the significance of the loss, his coping skills, his support systems, and the significance of the loss. Each will also go through a grief response process. Chart 9–7 presents the stages of grief response as identified by Kübler-Ross and Kessler (2005) and possible responses from Mrs. Mary Jones, a 74-year-old diagnosed with breast cancer. The amount of time a patient spends in each stage will vary from patient to patient.

CHART 9–7 Kübler-Ross's Stages of Grief and Mourning

Denial	Individuals react with a shocked "No, not me, I could not possibly have cancer because I live a healthy lifestyle!" This is healthy and allows individuals and significant others time to gather coping resources.
Anger	Individuals say "Why me?" or "Why us?" or "What did I do wrong?" During this stage, people sometimes blame others, including God.
Bargaining	Individuals say "Yes me, but . . ." or "If you just give me enough time to see my daughter married, I'll be ready."
Depression	Individuals say "Yes me." This acknowledgment of the reality of the situation brings feelings of depression. Mrs. Jones should be assessed for any suicidal feelings and possibly started on antidepressant therapy.
Acceptance	Facing the loss or death peacefully. In the case of death, individuals tend to withdraw into themselves.

Source: Kübler-Ross, E., & Kessler, D. (2005). *On grief and grieving: Finding the meaning of grief through the five stages of loss.* New York: Scribner.

Nursing Management

Nurses are often in the best position to offer support to patients and significant others as they move through the grieving process. It is very important for nurses to provide a safe environment for grieving to be expressed. Nurses need to be sensitive to individual and cultural differences in expressing grief. Some people grieve quietly, some loudly, some verbalize a great deal, some not at all, and some are very stoic. Nurses should provide a quiet acceptance of all grieving practices. Grant and Hanson (2010) found that nurses are uniquely qualified to develop and lead palliative care programs that improve patient care.

Assessment

The nurse should answer the following questions when assessing a patient experiencing grief and loss:

- What is the perceived or observable loss experienced by the individual or significant others?
- How does the individual or significant others explain or describe the loss?
- Is the individual or significant others able to identify their own feelings about the loss?
- Is the individual or significant others in denial about the loss?
- Is the individual or significant others expressing feelings of helplessness or hopelessness?
- Are there observable symptoms of depression?
- In what stage of the grieving process is the individual or significant others?

Nursing Diagnosis

Possible nursing diagnoses for patients experiencing grief and loss include:

- *Grieving*
- *Coping Ineffective*
- *Spiritual Distress*
- *Knowledge Deficit* related to feelings of loss and grief
- *Hopelessness*.

NANDA-I © 2012

Planning

The plan of care should facilitate a healthy grieving process.

Outcomes and Evaluation Parameters

An outcome for the grieving patient is the ability to work through the grieving process. This is evaluated by the patient's ability to:

- Verbalize an awareness of the loss.
- Verbalize the significance of the loss.
- Verbalize an awareness of the grieving process.
- Accept support while moving through the grieving process.
- Move toward acceptance of the loss.

Interventions and Rationales

The following interventions and rationales would be appropriate for the patient experiencing loss and grief:

- Assess the individual's and/or significant others' stage in the grief and loss process. *Identify any issues that may be hindering the grieving process. The patient and family members are frequently at different phases of grieving and should be treated appropriately.*
- Provide nonjudgmental support. *Allowing patients to express feelings openly may allow them to move through the phases of grieving more easily. Nonjudgmental listening allows patients to express their feelings without the fear of rejection.*
- Provide a safe environment in which the individual and/or significant others can express all feelings. *When the nurse spends time with the patient and significant others it may assist with the necessary review and processing of the loss. Being truly present with them can decrease feelings of loneliness and reassure them that caregivers perceive the loss as significant.*
- Educate the individual and/or significant others about the grieving process. *Understanding of the grief process allows the patient and significant others to move through the process more easily.*
- Help individuals and/or significant others to identify and reach out to additional support systems. *Assist the patient to identify resources. Referrals to appropriate support groups will help to meet emotional needs.*
- Help individuals and/or significant others problem solve. *Providing the patient and significant others with accurate information prevents misconceptions and may decrease their fears. Allowing patients to make decisions whenever possible enables them to maintain control.*

Evaluation

The patient will be able to move through the grief process in a healthy manner and exhibit effective coping mechanisms.

Depression

Experiencing feelings of depression is a predictable response to illness and hospitalization and may accompany loss and grief. The DSM-IV-TR (American Psychiatric Association [APA], 2000) provides diagnostic criteria for Major Depressive Disorder, Bipolar Disorder, and Dysthymic Disorder. Specific exploration of these disorders is beyond the scope of this chapter. The focus for this discussion is on depression as a psychological response to the losses associated with illness and hospitalization.

Patients are more vulnerable to developing depressive symptoms when they are experiencing severe, prolonged stress or crisis. The ability to adapt to stressors is dependent on the effectiveness of the individuals' coping mechanisms and the amount of perceived stress. The depression can act as a protective mechanism when people exhaust their coping abilities. Even individuals with excellent coping skills can become overwhelmed when the amount of stressors transcends their ability to cope with them. Depression may occur when patients are diagnosed with cancer (Irving & Lloyd-Williams, 2010), cardiovascular disease (Salomon et al., 2009), diabetes (Anderson, 2010), hepatitis C (Erim et al., 2010), or rheumatoid arthritis (Sinclair & Wallston, 2010). Therefore, it is imperative that nurses be mindful of the psychological responses to an illness that their patients may exhibit.

Nursing Management

Nurses often provide the frontline care for individuals who are experiencing feelings of depression. However, at times nurses might want to avoid depressed patients. After all, intervening with patients who are depressed can sometimes be difficult because dealing with others' pain can be depressing in itself. In addition, the fast pace of the hospital environment is counterproductive to the slower pace of the depressed patient. Sometimes health care providers view depressed individuals as not doing enough to help themselves, thinking that, if these patients would just try harder, they could pull themselves out of their depressed mood. It is important to understand that depression is a clinical diagnosis and needs to be assessed and treated just like any other disease.

Assessment

Depression is an uncomfortable psychological and physical experience of sadness. To a degree ranging from mild to severe, individuals experience behavioral, physical, affective, and cognitive changes as follows:

Behavioral Changes:

- Loss of interest in usually enjoyed activities
- Body posture slumped, dejected looking
- Difficulty making eye contact
- Difficulty carrying out activities of daily living
- Crying.

Physical Changes:

- Weight loss or weight gain
- Appetite changes
- Loss of sexual desire
- Somatic symptoms
- Sleep disturbances
- Fatigue
- Lack of energy
- Change in bowel habits.

Affective Changes:

- Feelings of emotional sadness
- Low self-esteem
- Labile mood
- Feelings of helplessness or hopelessness
- Pessimistic outlook
- Ambivalence.

Cognitive Changes:

- Cognitive distortions
- Slowing of thought processes
- Inability to concentrate
- Indecisiveness
- Loss of memory
- Difficulty problem solving
- Feelings of guilt
- Possible suicidal ideation
- Difficulty looking into the future.

Nursing Diagnoses

Possible nursing diagnoses for a person with depression include:

- *Coping, Ineffective*
- *Impaired Verbal Communication*
- *Social Isolation*
- *Ineffective Health Maintenance*
- *Self-Care Deficits*
- *Sleep Deprivation*
- *Self-Esteem Disturbance*
- *Ineffective Role Performance*
- *Knowledge Deficit*
- *Spiritual Distress*
- *Risk for Self-Directed Violence.*

NANDA-I © 2012

Planning

Nursing priorities for the patient with depression include establishing rapport and trust, identifying threat and coping resources, providing interventions to optimize coping skills, and evaluating the effectiveness of interventions.

Outcomes and Evaluation Parameters

Outcomes for the patient with depression include identification of ineffective coping or the ability to participate in developing a plan of care. This will be exhibited by the patient's ability to:

- Identify significant losses.
- Verbalize the significance of losses.
- Verbalize factors that he or she can control.
- Participate in his or her own health care decision making.
- Exhibit reduced symptoms of depression.
- Remain free from self-harm.

Interventions and Rationales

The following interventions and rationales would be appropriate for the patient experiencing depression:

- Validate the presence of the depression. *Acceptance by the nurse allows the patient to feel positive about the therapeutic relationship. This helps with healing, decreases isolation, and increases coping ability.*
- Provide emotional support through empathetic listening. *Empathetic listening helps to build trust and strengthens the therapeutic relationship.*
- Encourage the expression of feelings both positive and negative. *Patients may not fully understand what is happening to them. If they can express feelings freely, the nurse can plan specific actions to assist the patient to see the situation clearly.*
- Avoid excessive cheerfulness and false reassurance. *This will not help patients to work through their problems.*
- Encourage the patient to be involved in his care. *The ability to control aspects of his life helps to allay feelings of helplessness.*
- Assist the patient in goal setting and problem solving. *Patients may be overwhelmed by their situation. Assisting them to view the problem in its component parts will reduce anxiety and assist with effective coping behaviors.*
- Assess for suicidal ideation and, if present, ensure safety and make a referral. *Involve the health care team if you suspect that the patient is suicidal.*
- If necessary, refer for psychotherapy and pharmacological intervention. *It is important to ensure safety and prevent patients from harming themselves.*

Evaluation

The nurse should frequently reevaluate the patient's coping mechanisms and feelings of wanting to hurt himself or others. The patient should be able to describe his emotional state, participate in developing a plan of care, and use support offered by caregivers.

Anxiety

Anxiety is a universal psychological response. Without anxiety, individuals would not be able to accomplish goals or meet challenges. When faced with illness and possible hospitalization, most people will experience increased feelings of anxiety. They often become worried about their diagnosis, prognosis, and ability to cope with their illness. Anxiety is a primary emotion from which other emotions, such as anger, stem. As with depression, the DSM-IV-TR (APA, 2000) provides diagnostic criteria for an array of anxiety disorders, including Panic Disorder, Generalized Anxiety Disorder, and Post-Traumatic Stress Disorder. An explanation of these specific anxiety disorders is beyond the scope of this chapter. The focus for this discussion is on anxiety as a predictable psychological response to the stress of illness and hospitalization.

Anxiety is an uncomfortable feeling of discomfort, dread, apprehension, and unease, the cause of which can be specific or nonspecific. Oftentimes individuals are unable to identify what is making them feel anxious. The symptoms of anxiety are physiological, psychological, and behavioral. Several factors affect the severity of the anxiety: the strength and intensity of the stressors, the duration of the stressors, the individual's coping abilities, and the individual's perceived sense of helplessness. Variables such as culture, religion, education, and past experiences can also influence how well individuals cope with a particular situation. Many variables affect the development of anxiety, including perceived threats to biological integrity, perceived threats to self-esteem, frustration of needs or motives, the inability to control or influence meaningful events, or mental association with previous anxiety-producing events. Waiting for test results, waiting for a diagnosis, losing time from work, anticipating the outcome of treatment, and experiencing lifestyle changes can all lead to increased anxiety for the hospitalized patient.

Anxiety is both physiological and psychological. This is an important fact because the mind will perceive a stressor as a threat. The physiological response causes the feelings of tension and discomfort. This is because the anxiety response is a sympathetic nervous system response, causing symptoms such as increased heart rate, increased respirations, increased blood pressure, and increased glucose. When this occurs, individuals want relief from the uncomfortable feelings that the anxiety produces, and if they are unable to apply anxiety-reducing interventions that decrease the physiological arousal, their anxiety tends to increase in severity. In the case of chronic anxiety, the increased arousal of the sympathetic nervous system causes dangerous wear and tear on the body. This is why early assessment and intervention to decrease the anxious symptoms is vital.

Anxiety can be conceptualized on a continuum moving from mild to moderate to severe to panic. The higher the level of anxiety, the more uncomfortable the symptoms will feel. Interventions that are designed to decrease the physiologic arousal are of utmost importance. The longer the symptoms go unchecked, the more anxious the person will feel.

Nursing Management

Allred, Byers, and Sole (2010) studied the effects of music and rest on postoperative pain and anxiety experienced by patients undergoing knee arthroplasty. The authors concluded that, since neither intervention provided a risk to the patients, nurses could confidently offer the use of music and rest to help decrease postoperative pain and anxiety. Ylinen, Vehvilainen-Julkunen, and Pietila (2009) found that women were more anxious than men during a colonoscopy. The higher levels of anxiety experienced by the women interfered with their perceptions of the procedure. Seer, Crichton, Tullen, Smith, and Saunders (2008) found that teaching orthopedic patients jaw relaxation provided them with relief from pain. Therefore, nurses are in an optimal environment for teaching patients anxiety reducing techniques.

Assessment

The nurse should assess for the following types of anxiety:

Mild Anxiety:

- Alert, attentive, confident
- Open to new experiences
- Good problem-solving abilities
- Perceptual fields open, can deal with more than one thing at a time
- Can apply coping mechanisms.

Moderate Anxiety:

- Signs and symptoms are beginning to become noticeable
- Ability to pay attention is narrowed
- Perceptual fields begin to narrow
- Verbalization is increasing
- Problem solving is more rigid
- Increased respiratory rate, heart rate, and muscle tension
- Dry mouth, clammy palms, and sometime palpitations
- General feeling of restlessness.

Severe Anxiety:

- Anxiety is obvious
- Cognitive functioning is impaired
- Perceptual fields extremely narrowed
- Can only focus on one detail at a time
- Ability to concentrate decreased significantly
- Learning cannot occur
- Pacing, need for motor activity
- Hyperventilation, tachycardia, sweating
- Tremors, numbness, tingling
- Nausea, headache, dizziness.

Panic:

- Chest pain, breathlessness, tachycardia
- Feelings of impending death
- Extreme discomfort
- Perceptual fields closed
- Unrealistic or distorted perceptions
- Inability to communicate clearly
- Must be resolved quickly.

Nursing Diagnoses

Possible nursing diagnoses for the patient experiencing anxiety include:

- *Anxiety*
- *Coping Ineffective*
- *Social Isolation*
- *Sleep Deprivation*
- *Hopelessness*
- *Powerlessness*
- *Knowledge Deficit.*

NANDA-I © 2012

Planning

Priorities for nursing management for the patient with anxiety should include providing appropriate health information, assisting the patient with applying the information to her current health situation, and promoting identification of methods to cope with anxiety. The plan should also identify ways to minimize or prevent the escalation of the patient's anxiety and promote the patient's overall well-being.

Outcomes and Evaluation Parameters

The patient will be able to recognize the symptoms of anxiety resulting from identified fears by:

- Acknowledging to the nurse the presence of the anxiety.
- Demonstrating the appropriate use of coping mechanisms.

- Demonstrating increased problem solving.
- Verbalizing feeling less anxious.
- Exhibiting a decrease in the symptoms of anxiety.

Interventions and Rationales

The following interventions and rationales would be appropriate for the patient experiencing anxiety:

- Acknowledge the presence of the anxiety. *Recognition of the anxiety helps the patient to feel accepted and strengthens the therapeutic relationship.*
- Ask the patient to perform deep-breathing exercises. *Deep breathing assists the body to relax and the mind to be focused. Learning new techniques allows the patient to participate in promoting personal well-being.*
- Offer music. *Music can distract the patient and help to focus her thoughts.*
- If possible, identify the stimulus for the anxiety. *Identifying the stimulus helps the patient to clarify realistic and unrealistic perceptions and develop appropriate ways of handling the distress.*
- Provide the patient with needed information. *Written materials give the patient information for discussion with the health care team and significant others. The materials can also be used as a reference when questions arise.*
- Remove anxiety-producing environmental stimuli. *When anxious, the patient may have increased sensitivity to environmental stimuli.*
- Stay with the patient and provide support. *Acceptance by the nurse allows the patient to feel positive about the therapeutic relationship. This helps with healing, decreases isolation, and increases coping ability.*
- Encourage the expression of feelings. *Patients may not fully understand what is happening to them. If they can express feelings freely, the nurse can plan specific actions to assist the patient to see the situation clearly.*
- Explore with the patient her usual coping mechanisms. *Understanding the patient's baseline ability allows the nurse to start interventions from the place where the patient is comfortable. It also identifies unhealthy coping skills that need to be changed.*
- Acknowledge to the patient the effective use of coping mechanisms. *Positive reinforcement.*
- Assist the patient in problem solving. *The patient may be overwhelmed by his or her situation. Assisting the patient to view the problem in its component parts will reduce anxiety and assist with effective coping behaviors.*
- Provide opportunities to give the patient more control. *The patient's ability to control aspects of her life helps to allay feelings of helplessness.*
- **In panic levels of anxiety:**
  - Do not leave the patient, do not touch the patient.
  - Do not ask the patient for explanations.
  - Assure the patient you will stay with her.
  - Allow the patient to rest after the panic attack is over.
  - Refer the patient for further evaluation.

Evaluation

It is important for the nurse to assess the effectiveness of the patient's coping strategies. As the patient improves, she will be able to identify effects of increasing anxiety, understand the sources of her anxiety, learn useful coping skills, and differentiate between healthy and unhealthy coping strategies.

Anger

The emotions of anger and anxiety are often related. When individuals feel anxious, they also experience accompanying feelings of frustration or helplessness. These feelings can cause individuals to feel powerless to control their own autonomy. Anger develops as a response to feelings of powerlessness or helplessness. Anger is a powerful feeling that helps individuals feel in control. For some people, the feeling of anxiety is replaced with the more powerful feeling of anger. This is effective as a temporary coping mechanism, but not meant to be the only coping strategy. Long-standing feelings of anger do not promote health. Stephens et al. (2008) found that incorporating anger management assisted some patients with their cardiovascular disease.

It is important to recognize that anger is a natural emotion and can be appropriate for some situations. Nurses often are the recipients of angry feelings, and at times it is difficult for them not to personalize their responses to these expressions of anger. When patients are angry, such as when they have to have a test repeated, nurses may respond to the patients' anger with their own anger. This serves to escalate the angry feelings of both parties. When nurses are able to conceptualize anger as anxiety, nurses feel more in control and are able to intervene professionally and rationally.

Nursing Management

The expression of anger can be blatant, such as when someone yells or throws something, or subtle, such as when someone is a little sarcastic or refuses to speak much. It is important to pick up the early signs of anger because angry feelings tend to increase if the cause for the anger is not dealt with. The earlier the nurse intervenes to reduce the anger and accompanying anxiety, the better the chance for a positive outcome. If a patient's expression of anger is not rational, the nurse will need to set clear limits.

Assessment

Anger can be conceptualized on a continuum ranging from mild, to moderate, to severe, to rage.

Mild Anger:

- Feeling tense
- Feeling irritable
- Argumentative
- Scowling facial expression
- Sarcasm.

Moderate Anger:

- Increasing rumination
- Angry behavior more obvious
- Motor agitation
- Voice pitch increases
- Potential for acting-out behavior.

Severe Anger:

- Signs of acting-out behavior
- Cursing
- Distinct danger of becoming out of control.

Rage Anger:

- Rage is an out-of-control situation and appropriate interventions to protect the safety of the patient and staff must be implemented immediately.

Nursing Diagnoses

Possible nursing diagnoses for an angry person include:

- *Coping Ineffective*
- *Noncompliance with Treatment*
- *Social Isolation*
- *Powerlessness*
- *Risk for Other-Directed Violence.*

NANDA-I © 2012

Weblink: How useful is a Cognitive Interview?

Planning
Nursing planning begins with establishing rapport and trust with the patient. The next steps are to identify the cause of the anger, intervene and identify coping strategies, and evaluate the effectiveness of the interventions.

Outcomes and Evaluation Parameters
The patient will be able to recognize the cause of the anger and use effective coping strategies as evidenced by the ability to:

- Verbalize the presence of anger.
- Demonstrate decreased symptoms of anger.
- Demonstrate decreased symptoms of anxiety.
- Verbalize that he or she feels less angry.

Interventions and Rationales
- Prevention and anger reduction techniques can be useful. *Acceptance by the nurse allows the patient to feel positive about the therapeutic relationship. This helps with healing, decreases isolation, and increases coping ability.*

Prevention:
- Listen when patients talk to you.
- Do not dismiss people's concerns.
- Talk to patients, not at them.
- Respect patients' privacy.
- Do not make rules that treat adults as children.
- Recognize when patients are feeling anxious and intervene to reduce the anxiety.

Anger Reduction:
- Help the patient verbalize angry feelings.
- Avoid defensive responses.
- Use therapeutic communication skills.
- Assist the patient to identify the source of anger.
- Allow the patient an outlet for angry feelings.
- Do mutual problem solving.
- Allow the patient more control over health care decisions.
- Teach the patient techniques such as deep breathing and relaxation.

Evaluation
As the patient develops healthy coping strategies, he should exhibit the ability to describe his emotional state to the nurse, articulate an accurate understanding of the current situation, and accept support offered by caregivers.

Gerontological Considerations
Due to the normal physiologic changes of aging, the older adult may have a more difficult time responding and adapting to stressful situations. Also, older patients are more likely to have comorbidities and be on medications that can alter the response to stress.

Physiological Responses to Stress in Older Adults
The ability to achieve a relaxation response after a stressful event becomes more difficult as people age. Elderly people appear to have an impaired resiliency of the HPA axis response to the acute effects of stress (Hatzinger, Brand, Herzig, & Holsboer-Trachsler, 2011). Aging may simply wear out the systems in the brain that respond to stress, so that they become inefficient.

Chronic stress may accelerate the aging process by causing overactivity of the HPA axis. Other physiological responses vary as one ages, such as a decrease in the thickness of the skin and a decline in height, sense of smell, or visual acuity. It has been demonstrated that the cardiovascular response to stress is increased in the elderly (Robinson, 2009), including such factors as the heart rate, systolic and mean arterial pressure, peripheral resistance and rate pressure product, and lower cardiac output and stroke volume.

Safety Alert *In assessing stress among the elderly, the nurse must consider that the elderly very often are exposed to major stressors such as medical problems, the loss of a spouse and friends, a change in a living situation, and financial worries.*

Physiological changes that appear in the elderly also impact their coping responses to stress. Coping styles vary with age; when people age, they may shift from an active coping style to more passive ones. In addition to the physiological responses to stressors that change, some of the behavioral and cognitive responses change as well. Many elderly have mastered hassles or demands placed upon them by developing the resources necessary to cope with stress. However, many live alone, have a limited social support system in place, and have limited financial resources, all of which can deplete their ability to cope. Cognitive problem-solving skills also may decrease due to ongoing wear and tear on the body, past diseases, or slowing down of responses to a new stimulus.

Communicating with Older Adults
Due to the physiologic changes experienced by older adults, specific techniques can be used to ensure effective communication with this population (Wright & Holliday, 2007).

- Allow time for interaction. Older adults may have difficulty comprehending, and if rushed may feel that they are not important.
- Be aware of the environment. Have conversations in a well-lit room without background noise.
- Before speaking with an older adult, check to see if he has any visual or hearing impairment.
- Be aware of your cultural beliefs and attitudes regarding older adults to avoid personal bias.
- Introduce yourself by name and role and ask patients how they would like to be addressed.
- Avoid the use of slang. Use simple and exact language so you are understood. Do not talk down to patients.
- Ask for feedback from patients to make sure they understood what you have said. Whenever possible, provide information in writing.
- At the end of the conversation, summarize what you have discussed and ask if the patient has any questions.

Research
The biophysical and psychosocial aspects of nursing present many opportunities for research.

Summary
This chapter discussed the biophysical and psychosocial aspects of nursing. They are the concepts that nurses often forget when the pressures exerted by the health care delivery system take precedence. They are also the aspects of nursing care that make nursing a

RESEARCH OPPORTUNITIES Related to the Biophysical and Psychosocial Aspects of Nursing

Research	Clinical Impact
Psychosocial Nursing	
What interventions will help to relieve the "compassion fatigue" described by nurses?	Developing interventions to relieve the discomfort surrounding the care of patients and families will improve the care given to the patients.
What is the best teaching methodology for therapeutic communication?	Best teaching practices would enhance relationship-based care.
What interventions can be done to support culturally appropriate care?	The promotion of cultural customs and rituals surrounding illness can enhance patient care.
Stress	
Determine types of sedation and analgesics that can best alleviate the stress response and attenuate pain and anxiety.	Provide for appropriate use of sedation and analgesic to improve compliance with care.
Identify the effect of repressed stressful emotions on the psychoneuroimmune axis and the predisposition to illnesses.	Develop treatments specific to the stress-related illnesses.
	Educate patients about themselves and the body's response to stress.
Determine the effect of stress on wound healing.	Develop wound-healing protocols that include stress reduction techniques.
Identify the possible potentiation of oxidative stress by nursing care activities.	Develop guidelines for care of patients who are critically ill that minimize oxidative stress.
Determine the effect of integrative patient care models, recognizing that patients and providers use alternative medicine.	Evaluate the role of complementary alternative medicine (CAM) and the potential cost savings with these forms of treatment.
Examine the effect of therapeutic time spent with patients to support lifestyle changes.	Evaluate the effect of therapeutic time and communication with patient acceptance of lifestyle changes to promote their health.
Examine social support and its relationship to personality, health, and adjustment.	Evaluate the role of social support as a coping resource.

patient-centered and holistic profession. Creating an optimal healing environment takes into consideration maintaining the physical environment, developing awareness and intentions, cultivating healing relationships, practicing healthy lifestyles, experiencing personal wholeness, and allowing for collaborative medicine. Stress is universal. It is important that nurses recognize the signs and symptoms of stress, both within patients and within themselves. The nurse must be able to recognize and treat the physical, psychological, and social manifestations of stress to promote positive outcomes. To do so, nurses must become familiar with stress theories; understand the physiological, behavioral, and psychosocial responses to stress; and engage in evidence-based practice. Collaborative health care practices are integral to achieving these outcomes and to applying research findings to practices designed to foster improved patient outcomes. Future research opportunities and their impact on clinical practice are shown in the Research Opportunities box.

NCLEX® PRACTICE

1. During a focused health interview, a patient identifies a number of stressors. Which statement does the nurse identify as reflecting an external source of stress?

1. "I smoke a few cigarettes every day."
2. "My hair is so frizzy and ugly."
3. "My commute to work is an hour each way."
4. "I have to work at least 14 hours every day to do my job correctly."

2. During a routine health assessment, a patient reports a recent job loss and divorce. The patient has no health issues to report or discuss. How does the nurse interpret this patient's ability to handle stress?

1. As disrupted
2. As personal hardiness
3. As having the ability to handle daily hassles
4. As focusing on situational uplifts

3. A patient tells the nurse that she needs to be discharged from the hospital soon because she has a job to go to and a family who needs her. The nurse realizes this patient is at most risk for additional illnesses for which reason?

1. She hasn't fully recovered from her current hospitalization.
2. It is too early for her to return to work.
3. The additional stresses of daily life add more stress hormones to the body, which can lead to disease.
4. She isn't focused on her own health.

4. Which recommendation should the nurse provide to a patient demonstrating signs of oxidative stress?

1. Strive to remove all free radicals from the body.
2. Limit the ingestion of water-based foods.
3. Ingest high doses of vitamin C.
4. Improve nutritional intake including foods containing vitamin E.

5. The patient states, "My stress level is getting way too high." What would the nurse anticipate in this patient's assessment? (select all that apply)

1. Increased heart rate
2. Cool skin
3. Respiration rate of 12 per minute and regular
4. Bowel present, but diminished in one quadrant
5. Increased blood pressure

6. A patient is ambivalent about the types of treatment available for a disease process. Which statements would support a therapeutic nurse–patient relationship? (select all that apply)

1. "You should probably do what your doctors recommend."
2. "I'll let you figure out what you want to do and then let me know your decision."
3. "Do you need more information to help in your decision making?"
4. "You know lots more about your illness than I do."
5. "Let's talk about the treatment options again."

Answers to NCLEX Practice questions can be found in Appendix D in the Osborn Student Resources at nursing.pearsonhighered.com. Practice additional NCLEX questions online at the Student Resources site.

Pearson Nursing Student Resources

Find additional review materials at: **nursing.pearsonhighered.com**

REFERENCES

Allred, K. D., Byers, J. F., & Sole, M. L. (2010). The effect of music on postoperative pain & anxiety. *Pain Management Nursing, 11*, 15–25.

American Psychiatric Association. (2000). *Diagnostic and statistical manual of mental disorders, text revision* (4th ed.). Washington, DC: Author.

Anderson, B. J. (2010). From research to practice/diabetes and depression: Challenges and some opportunities. Living with depression and type 1 or type 2 diabetes in late adolescence and young adulthood: Lessons from research. *Diabetes Spectrum, 23*(1), 32–37.

Anonymous. (2011). Understanding the stress response. *Harvard Mental Health Letter, 27*(9), 4–5.

Ashing-Giwa, K. T., & Lim, J. (2009). Examining the impact of socioeconomic stress on physical and mental quality of life among breast cancer survivors. *Oncology Nursing Forum, 36*, 79–88.

Bauer, B. A., Cutshall, S. M., Wentworth, I. J., Engen, D., Messner, P. K., Wood, C. M., et al. (2010). Effect of massage therapy on pain, anxiety, and tension after cardiac surgery: A randomized study. *Complementary Therapies in Clinical Practice, 16*, 70–75.

Beck, A. T., & Freeman, A. (1990). *Cognitive theory of personality disorders*. New York: Guilford Press.

Berman, A. J., & Snyder, S. (2012). *Kozier & Erb's fundamentals of nursing* (9th ed.). Upper Saddle River, NJ: Pearson.

Berry, J. W. (2005). Acculturation: Living successfully in two cultures. *International Journal of Intercultural Relations, 29*, 697–712.

Boardman, J. D., & Alexander, K. B. (2011). Stress trajectories, health behaviors and the mental health of black and white young adults. *Social Science & Medicine 72*(10), 1659–1666.

Bonde, J. P., Munch-Hansen, T., Agerbo, E., Suadicani, P., Wieclaw, J., & Westergaard-Nielsen, N. (2009). Job strain and ischemic heart disease: A prospective study using a new approach for exposure assessment. *Journal of Occupational & Environmental Health, 51*, 732–738.

Bruderle, E. (2002). *Incoming undergraduate nursing students' perceptions of nurse caring behaviors*. Retrieved from UMI# TX5-761-126.

Burkhardt, M. A., & Keegan, L. (2009). Holistic ethics. In B. M. Dossey & L. Keegan (Eds.), *Holistic nursing: A handbook for practice* (5th ed.). Sudbury, MA: Jones & Bartlett.

Camphina-Bacote, J. (2008). Cultural desire: "caught" or "taught"? *Contemporary Nurse: Advances in Contemporary Transcultural Nursing, 28*, 141–148.

Caplan, G. (Ed.). (1964). *Principles of preventive psychiatry*. New York: Basic Books.

Carpenito, L. J. (2009). *Nursing care plans and documentation: Nursing diagnosis and collaborative problems* (5th ed.). Philadelphia: Wolters Kluwer Health/Lippincott Williams & Wilkins.

Crepaz, N., Passin, W. F., Herbst, J. H., Rama, S. M., Malow, R. M., Purcell, D. W., & Wolitski, R. J. (2008). Meta-analysis of cognitive-behavioral interventions on HIV-positive persons' mental health and immune functioning. *Health Psychology, 27*, 4–14.

De, R., Zemel, A., & Safran, S. A. (2010). Theoretical concepts and models of cellular mechanosensing. *Methods of Cell Biology, 98*, 143–175.

Delaney, C., & Barrere, C. (2008). Blessings: The influence of a spirituality-based intervention on psychosocial outcomes in a cardiac population. *Holistic Nursing Practice, 22*, 210–219.

Deng, G., Weber, W., Sood, A., & Kemper, K. J. (2010). Research on integrative health care: Context and priorities. *The Journal of Science and Healing, 6*(3), 143–158.

Dowd, J. B., & Zajacova, A. (2010). Does self-reported health mean the same across socioeconomic groups? Evidence from biomarker data. *Annals of Epidemiology, 20*, 743–749.

Engel, G. L. (1980). The clinical application of the biopsychosocial model. *American Journal of Psychiatry, 137*, 535–544.

Erikson, E. (1963). *Childhood and society* (2nd ed.). New York: Norton.

Erim, Y., Tagay, S., Beckmann, M., Bein, S., Cicinnati, V., Beckebaum, S., et al. (2010). Depression and protective factors of mental health in people with hepatitis C: A questionnaire survey. *International Journal of Nursing Studies, 47*, 342–349.

Esler, M., Schwarz, R., & Marlies, A. (2008). Mental stress is a cause of cardiovascular diseases: From skepticism to certainty. *Stress & Health 24*(3): 175–180.

Faul, L. A., Jim, H. S., Williams, C., Loftus, L., & Jacobsen, P. B. (2010). Relationship of stress management skill to psychological distress and quality of life in adults with cancer. *Psycho-Oncology, 19*, 102–109.

Fang, C. Y., Reibel, D. K., Longacre, M. L., Rosenzweig, S., Campbell, D. E., & Douglas, S. D. (2010). Enhanced psychosocial well-being following participation in a mindfulness-based stress reduction program is associated with increased natural killer activity. *Journal of Alternative & Complementary Medicine, 16*, 531–538.

Fernández-Gil, M. Á., Palacios-Bote, R., Leo-Barahona, M., & Mora-Encinas, J. P. (2010). Anatomy of the brainstem: A gaze into the stem of life. *Seminars in Ultrasound CT & MRI, 31*(3), 196–219.

Finkelstein, M. (2010). Correlates of individualism and collectivism: Predicting volunteer activity. *Social Behavior & Personality: An International Journal, 39*(5), 597–606.

Fitzell, A., & Pakenham, K. I. (2010). Application of a stress and coping model to positive and negative adjustment outcomes in colorectal cancer caregiving. *Psycho-Oncology, 19*, 1171–1178.

Franke, W. D., Kohut, M. L., Russell, D. W., Ekkekakis, P., & Ramey, S. P. (2010). Is job related stress the link between cardiovascular disease and the law enforcement profession? *Journal of Occupational & Environmental Medicine, 52*, 561–565.

Freud, S. (1935). *A general introduction to psychoanalysis*. New York: Simon and Schuster.

Gallup poll. (2009). Honesty/ethics in professions. Retrieved from: http://www.gallup.com/poll/1654/honesty-ethics-professions.aspx.

Gill, J. M., Saligan, L., Woods, S., & Page, G. (2009). PTSD is associated with an excess of inflammatory immune activities. *Perspectives in Psychiatric Care, 45*, 262–277.

Goble, A., & LeGrande, M. (2008). Do chronic psychological stressors accelerate the progress of cardiovascular disease? *Stress & Health, 24*, 203–223.

Grant, M., & Hanson, J. (2010). Nursing contributions to the development of palliative care programs. *Journal of Hospice & Palliative Nursing, 12*, 319–325.

Griffiths, K., Camic, P. M., & Hutton, J. M. (2009). Participant experiences of a mindfulness-based cognitive therapy group for cardiac rehabilitation. *Journal of Health Psychology, 14*, 675–681.

Hatzinger, M., Brand, S., Herzig, N., & Holsboer-Trachsler, E. (2011). In healthy young and elderly adults, hypothalamic-pituitary-adrenocortical axis reactivity (HPA AR) varies with increasing pharmacological challenge and with age, but not with gender. *Journal of Psychiatric Research, 45*(10), 1373–1380, 8p; DOI: 10.1016/j.jpsychires.2011.05.006

Holmes, D., & Rahe, R. (1967). The social readjustment rating scale. *Journal of Psychosomatic Research, 11*, 213–218.

Holmes, T. A., & Masuda, M. (1966). Magnitude estimations of social readjustments. *Journal of Psychosomatic Research, 11*, 219–225.

Horowitz, M., Schaefer, C., Hiroto, D., Wilner, N., & Levin, B. (1977). Life event questionnaires for measuring presumptive stress. *Psychosomatic Medicine, 39*(6), 413–431.

IOM (Institute of Medicine). (2010). *The future of nursing: Leading change, advancing health*. Washington, DC: The Academic Press.

Irving, G., & Lloyd-Williams, M. (2010). Depression in advanced cancer. *European Journal of Oncology Nursing, 14*(5), 395–399.

Kang, D. H., Rice, M., Park, N. J., Turner-Henson, A., & Downs, C. (2010). Stress and inflammation: A biobehavioral approach for nursing research. *Western Journal of Nursing Research, 32*, 730–760.

Kibler, J. L., Joshi, K., & Ma, M. (2009). Hypertension in relation to posttraumatic stress disorder and depression in the US National Comorbidity Survey. *Behavioral Medicine, 91*, 337–342.

Klein, J. M., & Hoffman, C. A. (2010). Relaxation and visual imagery techniques: Do they work? Can they really help burn patients? *MEDSURG Nursing, 19*, 169–175.

Koh, Z. M. (2010). A literature review: Shift work as a contributor to cardiovascular disease in female nurses who work shifts. *Singapore Nursing Journal, 37*, 23–24, 26–28, 30.

Koithan, M. (2009). Mind-body strategies for health. *Journal for Nurse Practitioners, 5*(5), 374–375.

Kravits, K., McAllister-Black, R., Grant, M., & Kirk, C. (2010). Self-care strategies for nurses: A psycho-educational intervention for stress reduction and the prevention of burnout. *Applied Nursing Research, 23*, 130–138.

Kübler-Ross, E., & Kessler, D. (2005). *On grief and grieving: Finding the meaning of grief through the five stages of loss.* New York: Scribner.

Kudielka, B. M., & Kirschbaum, C. (2005). Sex differences in HPA axis responses to stress: A review. *Biological Psychology, 69*, 113–132.

Lazarus, R. S. (1966). *Psychological stress and the coping process.* New York: McGraw-Hill.

Lazarus, R. S., & Folkman, S. (1984). *Stress, appraisal, and coping.* New York: Springer Publishing.

Lengacher, C. A., Bennett, M. P., Gonzalez, L., Gilvary, D., Cox, C. E., Cantor, A., et al. (2008). Immune responses to guided imagery during breast cancer treatment. *Biological Research for Nursing, 9*, 205–224.

Levy, F. (2010). Internalizing versus externalizing comorbidity: Neural circuit hypothesis. *Australian & New Zealand Journal of Psychiatry, 44*(5), 399–409.

Lin, H., Tsai, Y., Lin, P., & Tsai, P. (2010). Effects of a therapeutic lifestyle-change programme on cardiac risk factors after coronary artery bypass graft. *Journal of Clinical Nursing, 19*, 60–68.

Livsey, K. R. (2009). Clinical faculty influences on student caring self-efficacy. *International Journal of Caring, 13*(2), 52–58.

Mahoney, J. S., Palyo, N., Napier, G., & Giordano, J. (2009). The therapeutic milieu reconceptualized for the 21st century. *Archives of Psychiatric Nursing, 23*(6), 423–429.

Marshall, G. D. (2011). The adverse effects of psychological stress on immunoregulatory balance: Applications to human inflammatory diseases. *Immunology & Allergy Clinics of North America, 31*(1), 133–140.

Martin-Nemeth, P., Peckofer, S., Gulanick, M., Velsor-Friedrich, S., & Bryant, F. (2009). The relationships among self-esteem, stress, coping, eating behaviors and depressive mood and adolescents. *Research in Nursing & Health, 32*, 96–109.

Mayo Clinic. (2011). Stress basics. Retrieved from http://www.mayoclinic.com/health/stress-management/MY00435

Mok, E., Lau, K., Lam, W., Chan, L., Ng, J. S., & Chan, K. (2010). Healthcare professionals' perceptions of existential distress in patients with advanced cancer. *Journal of Advanced Nursing, 66*, 1510–1522.

Myers, B., & Greenwood-Van Meerveld, B. (2009). Role of anxiety in the pathophysiology of irritable bowel syndrome: Importance of the amygdala. *Frontiers in Neuroscience, 3*, 47.

NANDA International. (2009). *NANDA nursing diagnoses: Definitions and classification 2009–2011.* Philadelphia: Author.

National Institutes of Health. (2009). Stress system malfunction could lead to serious, life threatening disease. Retrieved from http://www.nih.gov/news/pr

North Carolina Concept-Based Learning Editorial Board. (2011). *Nursing: A concept-based approach to learning, vol 2.* New Jersey:Prentice Hall.

Office of Minority Health. (2001). *National standards for culturally and linguistically appropriate services in health care. Final report.* Rockville, MD: Author.

Olivo, E. L., Dodson-Lavelle, B., Wren, A., Fang, Y., & Oz, M. C. (2009). Feasibility and effectiveness of a brief meditation-based stress management intervention for patients diagnosed with or at risk for coronary heart disease: A pilot study. *Psychology, Health & Medicine, 14*, 513–523.

Park, H. J., Jarrett, M., Cain, K., & Heitkemper, M. (2008). Psychological distress and GI symptoms are related to severity of bloating in women with irritable bowel syndrome. *Research in Nursing & Health, 32*(2), 98–107.

Peplau, H. E. (1952). *Interpersonal relations in nursing.* New York: Putnam.

Peplau, H. E. (1987). Interpersonal constructs for nursing practice. *Nursing Education Today, 7*, 201–208.

Piaget, J., & Inhelder, B. (1969). *Psychology of the child.* New York: Basic Books.

Piazza, J. R., Almeida, D. M., Dmitrieva, N. O., & Klein, L. C. (2010). Frontiers in the biomarkers of health in research on stress & aging. *Journals of Gerontology Series: Psychological Services & Social Science, 65*(B), 513–525.

Porth, C. M. & Matfin, G. 2009, C. M. (2008). *Essentials of pathophysiology: Concepts of altered health states* (8th ed.). Philadelphia: Lippincott Williams & Wilkins.

Puustinen, P. J., Koponen, H., Kautianen, H., Mantyselka, P., & Vanhala, M. (2010). Gender specific association of psychological distress with cardiovascular risk scores. *Scandinavian Journal of Primary Health Care, 28*, 36–40.

Ramey, S. L., Downing, N. R., & Knobauch, A. (2008). Developing strategic interventions to reduce cardiovascular disease risk among law enforcement officers. *AAOHN, 56*(2), 54–62.

Remmers, H., Holtgrawe, M., & Pinkert, C. (2010). Stress and nursing care needs of women with breast cancer during primary treatment: A qualitative study. *European Journal of Oncology Nursing, 14*(1), 11–16.

Robinson, J. G. (2009). Lipid-lowering therapy for the primary prevention of cardiovascular disease in the elderly: Opportunities and challenges. *Drugs & Aging, 26*(11), 917–931.

Salomon, K., Clift, A., Karlsdottir, M., & Rottenberg, J. (2009). Major depressive disorder is associated with attenuated cardiovascular reactivity and impaired recovery among those free of cardiovascular disease. *Health Psychology, 28*, 157–165.

Sauls, J. L., & Warise, L. F. (2010). Interventions for anxiety in the critically ill: A guide for nurses and families. *Nursing Clinics of North America, 45*, 555–567.

Schwartz, R. R. (2010). Ripples from a stone skipping across the lake: A narrative approach to the meaning of Huntington's Disease. *American Association of Neuroscience Nurses, 42*, 157–168.

Scott-Sheldon, L. A., Kalichman, S. C., Carey, M. P., & Fielder, R. L. (2008). Stress management for HIV+ adults: A meta-analysis of randomized controlled trials, 1989–2006. *Health Psychology, 27*, 129–139.

Seaward, B. L. (2009). *Managing stress: Principles and strategies for health and well-being* (6th ed.). Sudbury, MA: Jones and Bartlett.

Seer, K., Crichton, N., Tutton, L., Smith, L., & Saunders, T. (2008). Effectiveness of relaxation for postoperative pain and anxiety: Randomized controlled trial. *Journal of Advanced Nursing, 62*, 681–688.

Segrin, C., & Badger, T. A. (2010). Psychological distress in different social network members of breast and prostate cancer survivors. *Research in Nursing & Health, 33*, 450–464.

Selye, H. (1984). *The stress of life* (revised). New York: McGraw-Hill.

Selye, H. A. (1936). Syndrome produced by diverse nocuous agents. *Nature, 138*, 32.

Shirom, A., Toker, S., Berliner, S., & Shapira, I. (2008). The job demand-control-support model and stress relate low grade inflammatory responses among healthy employees: A longitudinal study. *Work & Stress, 22*, 138–152.

Sinclair, V. G., & Wallston, K. A. (2010). Psychological vulnerability predicts increases in depressive symptoms in individuals with rheumatoid arthritis. *Nursing Research, 59*(2), 140–146.

Solowiej, K. (2010). Take it easy: How the cycle of stress and pain associated with wound care affects recovery. *Nursing & Residential Care, 12*, 443–444, 446.

Stephens, T., Braithwaite, H., Johnson, L., Harris, C., Katkowsky, S., & Troutman, A. (2008). Cardiovascular risk reduction for African-American men through health empowerment and anger management. *Health Education Journal, 67*(3), 208–218.

Swanson, J., & Koch, L. (2010). The role of oncology nurse navigator in distress management of adult inpatients with cancer: A retrospective study. *Oncology Nursing Forum, 37*, 69–76.

Tamparo, C. D., & Lindh, W. Q. (2008). *Therapeutic communications for health care* (3rd ed.). Clifton Park: Delmar.

Taylor, A. G., Goehler, L. E., Galper, D. I., Innes, K. E., & Bourguignon, C. (2010). Top-down and bottom-up mechanisms in mind-body medicine: Development of an integrative framework for psychophysiological research. *Explore, 6*(1), 29–41.

Torres, S. J., & Nowson, C. A. (2007). Relationship between stress, eating behavior, and obesity. *Nutrition, 23*, 887–894.

Ulger, O., & Yagli, N. V. (2010). Effects of yoga on the quality of life in cancer patients. *Complementary Therapies in Clinical Practice, 16*(2), 60–63.

Upton, D., & Solowiej, K. (2010). Pain and stress as contributors to delayed wound healing. *Wound Practice & Research, 18*(3), 114–122.

Urden, L. D., Stacy, K. M., & Lough, M. E. (2009). *Critical care nursing: Diagnosis and management* (6th ed.). St. Louis Missouri: Mosby.

Watson, J. (2008). Nursing: The philosophy and science of caring (revised ed.). Boulder, Colorado: The University Press of Colorado.

Wright, L. M., & Leahey, M. (2009). *Nurses and families: A guide to family assessment and intervention.* Philadelphia, PA: FA Davis.

Wright, A. M., & Holliday, R. E. (2007). Interviewing cognitively impaired older adults. How useful is a Cognitive Interview? *Memory, 15*(1), 17–33. Retrieved from http://www.tandfonline.com/doi/abs/10.1080/09658210601047351

Whipple, M. O., Lewis, T. T., Sutton-Tyrrell, K., Mathews, K. A., Barinas-Mitchell, E., Powell, L. H., & Everson-Rose, S. A. (2009). Hopelessness, depressive symptoms, and carotid atherosclerosis in women: The Study of Women's Health Across the Nation (SWAN) heart study. *Stroke, 40*, 3166–3172.

Ylinen, E., Vehvilainen-Julkunen, K., & Pietila, A. (2009). Effects of patients' anxiety, previous pain experience and non-drug interventions on the pain experience during colonoscopy. *Journal of Clinical Nursing, 18*, 1937–1944.

CHAPTER 10

The Aging Patient

Sally J. Brush
Cheryl Wraa

Outcome-Based Learning Objectives

After studying this chapter, the learner will be able to:

1. Compare and contrast theories of aging.
2. Identify normal age-related changes of the head, neck, respiratory, cardiovascular, gastrointestinal, genitourinary, musculoskeletal, integumentary, and neurological systems when completing a nursing assessment.
3. Explain the rationale for recommended immunizations and screening exams as proposed by the U.S. Preventive Services Task Force for the patient over 65 years of age.
4. Discuss medications contraindicated in the aging patient as identified by the Beers criteria.
5. Generate a plan when signs and symptoms of elder mistreatment are present to determine appropriate referrals.
6. Differentiate between residential, assisted living, and skilled nursing care in accordance with the type of patient care services provided.
7. Critique the implications of technological advancements in providing care to older adults.

KEY TERMS

activity theory of aging p.241
adverse drug event (ADE) p.250
adverse drug reaction (ADR) p.250
aging p.240
biological aging theory p.240
continuity theory of aging p.241
delirium p.247
dementia p.247
disengagement theory of aging p.241
Folstein Mini-Mental State Exam p.248
gerontological nurse practitioner (GNP) p.254
insomnia p.244
kyphosis p.244
polypharmacy p.251
psychosocial theories of aging p.241
sleep apnea p.244

OLDER ADULTS represent nearly 13% of the U.S. population (AOA, 2009). The rate of growth of the elderly population during this century has exceeded the growth rate of the population as a whole. In 1994, approximately 1 in 8 Americans were elderly, but by 2030, estimates suggest 1 in 5 will be elderly (Hobbs, 2011). As this population grows, it is incumbent on nursing and society as a whole to recognize this group's unique needs and provide special consideration for the care of these individuals. This chapter discusses the physiological and behavioral changes that occur with aging, methods of assessing for these changes, and available health care options, including future innovations in caring for older adults.

Aging is defined as the process of growing old or maturing. An individual is a composite of his chronological, physiological, and functional age. Chronological age is the number of years lived. Physiological age is the determination of age by body function, and functional age is the ability to contribute to society and to benefit self and others. In some cultures, the older adult, or elder, is an individual who has gathered wisdom over a lifetime; this individual is to be respected. The legal definition of an older adult is any individual 65 years of age and older.

Theories of Aging

There are several theories of aging; however, no single theory can answer all of the questions about this process. Two aging theories—biological and psychosocial—attempt to explain the physical and emotional changes that take place as an individual progresses through life.

Biological Aging Theories

Biological aging theories fall into two groups: programmed death theory and error theory, also known as mutation accumulation/modification theory. All of the biological theories of aging can be classified as evolutionary theories. The knowledge base of cellular function and dysfunction with age has grown exponentially over the past 10 years with the mapping of the human genome. In general, the August Weismann theory of programmed death recounts that aging exists to benefit the species and not the individual. On a cellular level, it has been found that each cell has only a preprogrammed number of processes available during its lifetime. Mutation/modification theory points out that environmental conditions can exert selective pressure on genes to alter rates of growth, development, and rejuvenation. This may be seen in the cumulative effects of free radicals on our bodies. Oxygen-derived free radicals are highly reactive and often cause indiscriminate destructions of protein, fat, and DNA molecules (Urden, Stacy, & Lough, 2009). Aging is cumulative, universal, progressive, intrinsic, and detrimental to the human body. The research of the future will focus on methods to change the biologic imperatives of aging (Ljubunic & Reznick, 2009).

Psychosocial Theories of Aging

Psychosocial theories of aging describe the changes that take place emotionally and socially as an individual enters the later years of life. These changes involve roles and social relationships that impact older adults. Three examples of psychosocial theories are activity theory, disengagement theory, and continuity theory. The **activity theory of aging** proposes that the more active older adults are, the greater their satisfaction with life; decreased activity leads to feelings of meaninglessness and dissatisfaction with life. To maintain a positive sense of self, older adults must substitute new roles for those lost in old age; thus, successful aging is achieved by staying active and extending activities enjoyed in middle age. Life care communities and senior retirement communities are designed to promote the activity theory. Such amenities as golf courses, swimming pools, and clubhouses that provide group activities not only help support healthy aging, but also help bring individuals together to develop new relationships and interests.

The **disengagement theory of aging,** introduced in 1961, contradicts the activity theory (Harwood, 2007). It asserts that later in life, age-related changes bring about a mutual and reciprocal withdrawal of the individual and society. Older adults slow down by retiring and not being as socially active as they once were. It is thought that the social withdrawal benefits both individuals and society.

The **continuity theory of aging** proposes that those who successfully age are able to substitute new roles for lost ones. This requires a lifelong ability to engage in the community and to adapt physical changes to the current environment. An elderly individual should maintain the values, habits, and behaviors from his younger adult life. Older age should not be a time for major life changes, but instead a time to maintain the usual activities, but at a slower pace as needed. Some older individuals would never consider a life care community or senior community because of the major changes of such a move. These adults choose to live in their established homes, along with the diversity of a neighborhood that houses both younger and older individuals, rather than living in an "all over age 65" environment (Rantz et al., 2011).

Age stratification theory examines the movement of successive birth cohorts across time, known as *cohort flow.* Each cohort is unique in that it has its own characteristics (e.g., size, gender, and social class distribution). Each cohort experiences particular historical events that affect its members' attitudes and behaviors (Pool, 2007). Modernization theory argues that the role and status of the aged are inversely related to the level of societal industrialization (Harwood, 2007). New technologies and systems lead to a more homogenized society. Modernization theory includes the world of globalization, where culture and ideas are easily spread throughout the world, leading to a more universal culture that becomes the baseline for all cultures.

Lastly, exchange theory indicates that older adults have less power in relation to younger people because they possess fewer resources, and continued interaction with the younger population becomes more costly. Social interaction between the old and the young tends to decrease because older people have fewer resources to bring to the exchange—lower income, poorer health, and less education. Declining resources strain their possibilities for continued interaction with others (Roy & Russell, 2005).

Demographics of the Aging Population

In 2008, 12.8% of adults in the United States were over the age of 65. Older adults were fairly evenly distributed throughout the United States. Alaska has the youngest population of the U.S. states, but the number of adults over age 65 continues to increase. Florida has the largest percentage of residents age 65 and older, with 17.3% of the population falling into this age group. This large percentage is attributed to the many older adults who move there for the sunshine and mild climate. The percentage of adults age 65 and older fell somewhere between these two ranges for all of the other states at 13% in 2010 (U.S. Census Bureau, 2011). Elders 85 years or older are expected to be the fastest growing part of the elderly population during this century (Hobbs, 2011).

Women have always outlived men in the past, and the trend continues among all age groups age 65 and older. At the 2008 U.S. Census, there were 22.4 million women to 16.5 million men over age 65. Older men were much more likely to be married (72%) than older women (42%). These numbers correlate with percentages of women who are widowed. Among women ages 65 to 84, 42% are widowed; 79% of women age 85 and older are widowed. In 2008, 19.8% of the respondents over age 65 claimed minority status (8.3% African American, 6.8% Hispanic origin). Older Americans have attained higher levels of education than the generation before them, and this trend continues. In 1950, 17% of older adults had a high school education; only 3% had at least a bachelor's degree. By 2003, 78% were high school graduates, and at least 20.8% had a bachelor's degree (Administration on Aging [AOA], 2009). In 2008, 6.2 million Americans age 65 and over were in the labor force or actively looking for work. Often, older adults were heads of households containing adult children and grandchildren. This trend has increased over the past 10 years (AOA, 2009).

During the mid-nineties, the racial and ethnic diversity among the elderly population was approximately 29.8 million White; 2.7 million Black; 137,000 American Indian, Eskimo, and Aleut; 615,000 Asian and Pacific Islander; and 1.5 million Hispanic (Hobbs, 2011). It is expected that the elderly population will become more racially and ethnically diverse in the future. By the year 2050, the proportions of elderly are estimated to increase from 13% to 23% for Whites; 8% to 14% for Blacks; 6% to 13% for American Indians, Eskimos, and Aleuts; 6% to 15% for Asians and Pacific Islander; and from 5% to 14% for Hispanics (Hobbs, 2011).

Health Assessment of the Aging Patient

The nurse should view the health assessment of the aging patient as not just an opportunity to gather needed medical information, but as an opportunity to become acquainted with an individual who possesses a lifetime of experience. The health assessment includes both the health history and physical examination.

Interviewing the Older Patient to Obtain a Health History

Interviewing an older patient to collect patient health data is identified by the American Nurses Association (ANA) as a standard for clinical gerontological nursing care. The interview, as part of a comprehensive health assessment, is essential to developing a comprehensive plan of care for the aging adult (ANA, 2010; Congdon et al., 2001).

Weblink: Administration on Aging Profile of Older Americans

Interviewing and obtaining a health history from the aging patient can be both a challenging and rewarding experience. The experience can be challenging for a number of reasons related to the complexity of the health history, as well as the impact of normal changes of aging, such as hearing and visual deficits. Eliciting a health history from an individual with memory deficits presents special challenges. In 2008, 39.1% of noninstitutionalized older adults assessed their own health as excellent or very good. Most older adults will have at least one chronic condition and most will have multiple (AOA, 2009). Obtaining information from this group, who are more likely to be encountered during hospitalization, can be time consuming, yet it is essential to providing quality nursing care (Figure 10–1◆). The American Nurse Association sets the scope and standards of gerontological nursing practice. Refer to Chart 10–1 for further information regarding these standards.

Cultural Considerations

Nurses must also take cultural considerations into account when interviewing and obtaining a health history from the aging patient. Many times the nurse will become involved with patients and families whose cultures are different and whose traditions seem strange and foreign. It is important for the nurse to be sensitive to the needs and customs of patients in any health care setting. Cultural variances that nurses who work with aging patients should be aware of are discussed in the following subsections and the Cultural Considerations feature.

CHART 10–1 Scope and Standards of Gerontological Nursing Practice

One of the responsibilities of the American Nurses Association (ANA) is to define the scope and standards of nursing practice. The *Standards of Clinical Nursing Practice* published in 1998 apply to all professional nurses. The *Scope and Standards of Gerontological Nursing Practice* contain criteria for expectations and competent care associated with the basic and advanced clinical practice of gerontological nursing (American Nurses Association, 2010). This includes nursing care demonstrated through assessment, diagnosis, outcome identification, planning, implementation, and evaluation. These processes form the foundation of clinical decision making that applies to all gerontological nurses. The print version was revised in 2010 and is available through the publishing program of the American Nurses Association, nursesbooks.org. It is also available as a digital download.

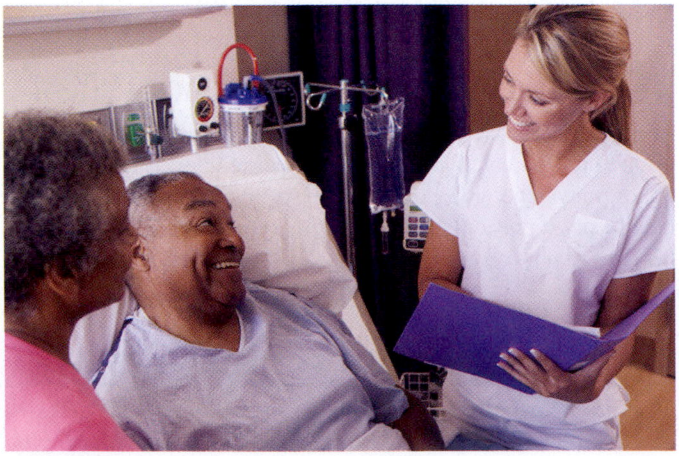

FIGURE 10–1 ◆ Obtaining a thorough health history from an older patient is essential to quality nursing care.

CULTURAL CONSIDERATIONS for the Aging Patient

African American	The family is very important, and values related to the family are rooted in African traditions (Galanti, 2008). The elderly are highly valued in African American families.
Asian	Family authority and structure are defined by family position, which is defined by age and gender. Elders are venerated in Asia, assuming a place of great respect. Males hold higher positions than females. Mutual support, cooperation, and interdependence also characterize the family. Problems generally are solved within the family, and a sense of family honor and pride limits the amount and type of information to be shared with counselors or other professionals. As Asian immigrants grow older in the United States, they are exposed to a health care system that is very different from how they were socialized. Elderly Asians become more culturally and linguistically isolated, particularly as related to health care. Prior health status, such as nutritional imbalance, plays a greater role in healthy aging in the Asian population (Mui & Shibusawa, 2008).
Hispanic/Latino	Family is of paramount value and is influenced by both Catholicism and indigenous values. Family is an extended system that includes blood relations, marriage, and fictive kin adopted through relationships. Mutual help, protection, and caregiving are provided. Elders are not expected to be self-sufficient. Children are obligated to provide care and to respect their elderly parents and grandparents (Falicov, 1998; Lipson & Dibble, 2005).
Native Americans	Native Americans encompass people with many different languages, religions, organizations, and relationships with the U.S. government. Family is regarded as the cornerstone for emotional, social, and economic well-being for individuals (Lipson & Dibble, 2005; Red Horse, 1981). Extended family members assume many different roles. The primary relationship may not be with parents, but with grandparents who assume the caregiver and disciplinarian role. Elder tribal members are highly regarded. The aged are believed to be the repository of wisdom, and their role is to teach traditions, customs, legends, and myths of the tribe. The tribe frequently takes responsibility to care for the elder. Consensus decision making is important and often consumes a great deal of time in an effort to reach harmony within the family/tribe.

One can conclude from the brief discussion of four different cultures in the Cultural Considerations feature, and the role of society in each one of them, that their responses to aging and health care may be quite different. The roles of the family, the environment, and the manner of caring for patients vary. A full discussion of cultural competence and the role of the health care provider is discussed in Chapter 1.

Culturally competent health care systems are those that provide culturally and linguistically appropriate services. An inability to communicate with a patient or insensitivity to cultural differences can result in a compromise in the quality of health care. It is important for the nurse to be cognizant of the cultural values of the patient and family related to aging. It is crucial that, as health care professionals, nurses understand that cultural values often are the driving forces guiding daily behavior. Cultural norms of family life and the role of elderly family members will have an impact on appropriate health care of the older adult. Cultural competence demands that nurses look at patients through both their own eyes and the eyes of patients and family members.

People over the age of 65 in the United States account for more than one-third of all hospital stays. Most nurses will care for an aging patient on a typical medical–surgical nursing unit, necessitating the need for obtaining a health history in the hospital environment. It is useful to inquire initially about the individual's present health problem, which usually is the reason the individual has been hospitalized. It is important to determine the patient's perceptions of his health status and then obtain corroborating information from the medical record. It also is important to find out how the hospitalization and illness have affected the older adult's life, as well as the lives of family members.

Past Medical History

The next step is to interview the individual to obtain the past medical history. Collecting patient health data is essential to developing a comprehensive plan of care as identified by the ANA scope and standards of gerontological nursing care, which were discussed in Chart 10–1. If the patient is unable to give her medical history, the information from the medical record may be referenced and family members may be interviewed to fill in the "information gaps." In addition to recording medical diagnoses, obtaining information as to the length of time an individual has had a medical condition is useful. For example, the nursing management and teaching of a patient who is newly diagnosed with diabetes and has been prescribed oral medications are quite different than the management and teaching of an individual who is hospitalized with diabetic complications and has been on insulin for more than 20 years. Chart 10–2 includes the essential questions to ask when obtaining the past medical history.

Psychosocial History

A psychosocial history is an essential component of the health history. The nurse should keep in mind that education and socioeconomic status may play a role in a patient's vocabulary, self-expression, ability to comprehend, and ability to learn (Fitzsimmons, 2011). Some questions a nurse might ask when obtaining the psychosocial history are outlined in Chart 10–3.

CHART 10–2 Past Medical History Questions

What medical problems do you have?

How long have you had these problems?

What treatment have you sought in the past?

Have you had any past surgeries? If so, when (the date), and were they successful?

What medications are you taking?

Do you have any history of communicable diseases such as tuberculosis (TB), hepatitis, HIV?

CHART 10–3 Psychosocial History Questions

- Where do you live? Do you live alone? Are you married?
- Do you have any history of accidents or falls?
- If you require assistance with your grooming, hygiene, or other activities of daily living (ADLs), who is available to help you?
- If you had an emergency such as falling or feeling ill, who would you contact?
- What did you do for employment when you were younger?
- Do you have children? Where do they live? Are they involved in your life/care?

Health habits must be explored as well. Questions to ask may include the following:

- Do you currently smoke tobacco? How many packs per day for how many years?
- If you have quit smoking, what was the date you quit? Have you ever had any abnormal chest x-rays?
- Do you prepare your own meals? If so, please describe common dishes you prepare.
- If you do not prepare your meals, who does?
- Do you drink alcohol? If so, how much and how often?
- Do you take any over-the-counter medications or herbal preparations?
- Do you exercise? If so, how much and how often?
- Do you have any problems sleeping at night?
- Do you have any problems with your bowels or urinary incontinence?

Physical Assessment of the Older Patient

Nursing assessments in older adults, as with all patients, are best carried out using a systematic approach to the physical examination. This may be done using the head-to-toe approach or by body systems. Whatever approach is chosen, it is best to stay with the same method during every assessment, so that critical elements are not overlooked and in order to identify trends and changes more clearly.

General Impression

When assessing the older adult, it is important to get an overall picture of the individual by looking at his general appearance:

- Is the individual clean; thin or obese?
- Is his behavior and affect appropriate?
- Does the individual seem easily angered, restless, or agitated?
- Do the facial expressions match his speech? Many illnesses affect the speaker's facial expressions, so it is important to identify a correlation, or lack thereof, of expression with speech. For example, people with Parkinson's disease often display a "masked face," which means that their expression looks as if they are wearing a mask. People who have a long history of neuroleptic drug use may exhibit lip smacking, tongue thrusting, and other facial dystonias. These are irreversible side effects attributed to a history of prolonged use of this class of medications. When the medications are discontinued, these movements often remain. Such abnormal facial muscle movements also are seen in individuals with a wide variety of neurological conditions, such as Huntington's disease, Wilson's disease, head injury, and tumors (Tovey, 2007).

Assessment of the Head and Neck

When assessing the head and neck, typical changes may be found with the aging adult. Hair becomes thinner and finer with age, but the size and shape of the skull do not change. The eyes undergo many changes as the body ages. The eyelids relax, often giving the eyes a droopy appearance. Common eyelid problems seen in older adults include ptosis, where the eyelids partially or completely cover the pupil. The lower eyelid can turn inward, called an entropion, or may turn extremely outward, called an ectropion, exposing the tissue of the conjunctiva. Because this pinkish red tissue is normally not visible, when an ectropion develops it is often misinterpreted as an eye infection. If the lower eyelid becomes excessively dry, irritated, or infected, the ectropion can be surgically repaired. Decreased tear production may cause dry eyes, which are easily treated with artificial eyedrops or lubricants. Cataracts also are common and are caused by clouding of the crystalline lens; these can be surgically repaired if they impair vision. Vision problems, even with glasses or contact lenses, affect nearly 20% of the older population (AOA, 2009). See Chapter 64 for more information on disorders of the eye.

When assessing the pupils for light reflex response, one may note a thin, grayish-white ring at the margins of the cornea. This normal finding is called arcus senilis. The lens becomes less transparent and the eyelids may appear dry due to decreased lacrimal duct production. The cornea clouds with aging, and individuals lose peripheral vision. Chapter 64 describes eye disorders in detail.

Changes in the ears are related to normal age-related hearing losses. The auricle of the ear becomes less elastic; the lobes elongate and often develop linear wrinkles. Increased hair growth is seen in the auditory canals of males. The tympanic membrane may appear dull, and atrophy of the membrane itself may make the landmarks appear more prominent. Cerumen may be harder and drier, occluding the auditory canal. Cerumen impaction can become a chronic problem in the aging patient if not addressed on a routine basis. Impacted cerumen can cause hearing loss as well as vertigo. Therefore, removal should be facilitated using a softening agent, such as Debrox or regular mineral oil, and irrigation by medical personnel if wax cannot be removed during showering with warm water. Accurate hearing tests cannot be conducted unless the patient's canals are free of cerumen and the tympanic membrane can be visualized readily using an otoscope. Scarring and chronic perforation of the tympanic membrane resulting from years of occupational exposure to loud sounds and ear infections contribute to hearing loss as well. In 2002, almost one-half of all older men and one-third of older women reported trouble hearing without a hearing aid (AOA, 2009). With the increase in use of personal music players with ear buds that are inserted into ear canals, the need for hearing aids in the next generation is expected to increase.

A decreased sense of smell, along with reduced taste sensation, may be noted with advanced age due to atrophy of papillae on the outer edges of the tongue. Dry oral mucosa along with cheilosis (dry scaling) of the mouth can be indicative of dehydration, vitamin deficiencies, or poorly fitting dentures, or can be the result of medication side effects. Oral assessments should always include removal of dentures, because this is an area where cancerous lesions can appear.

Respiratory Assessment

Structural changes of the thoracic cavity are often seen with aging and can affect respiratory function. **Kyphosis,** which gives the patient a "stooped over" appearance, is caused by osteoporosis and collapse of the patient's vertebrae. The chest wall becomes less compliant, and changes in the breathing pattern are seen. Inspiration tends to be shallower, and expiration requires the use of accessory muscles. As a result, the measured vital capacity is decreased, and increased residual capacity will be seen if pulmonary function tests are conducted. The ciliary function of the lungs is reduced, producing a decreased cough reflex.

Some common disorders of the respiratory system seen in older adults include chronic obstructive pulmonary disease (COPD), pulmonary edema due to congestive heart failure, and pulmonary emboli. Due to physiological changes, the normal PaO_2 should be corrected for age using the formula $109 - 0.43 \times$ patient's age. The PaO_2 and pH may be outside the normal range, but the response to such change is blunted. See Chapter 28 for information on complex respiratory disorders.

An increase in sleep disorders and **sleep apnea** occurs with older adults. This includes both types: (1) obstructive, which is an involuntary pause in breathing, and (2) central, which is caused from a periodic lack of signaling from the brain to make the body breathe. Although older adults need as much sleep as younger people, the sleep they get occurs during the lighter stages of sleep, so is not as restorative as sleep that occurs during the deeper stages of sleep (Fitzsimmons, 2011). The most common sleep disorder in the older adult is **insomnia,** defined as difficulty falling asleep or staying asleep with a negative impact on daytime alertness. Sleep apnea is a sleep disorder with partial or complete obstruction of airflow. The patient must awaken to resume breathing. Diagnosis is usually made after an overnight sleep study. Treatment involves wearing a nasal positive airway pressure mask at night to keep airways open and facilitate unobstructed airflow while sleeping. Sleep apnea is discussed at length in Chapter 26.

Cardiovascular Assessment

The heart of the aging patient undergoes normal, age-related changes. A slower heart rate often is seen due to a decrease in the normal number of pacemaker cells, and may be asymptomatic. The heart valves become thicker and more rigid, and the heart muscle itself experiences decreased elasticity and increased rigidity. The point of maximal impulse (PMI) may be displaced and palpated at the fifth or sixth left intercostal space at the midclavicular line. Murmurs in the older patient do not necessarily produce symptoms and are caused by heart valves that become stiff from fibrosis and calcification. These murmurs are best heard at the base of the heart or the aortic area. The arterial walls are more irregular in size and shape, and they feature an increase in calcium and collagen deposits. The walls themselves are thicker, less distensible, and less pliable.

Cardiovascular disorders are not specific to older adults; however, heart disease is the number one cause of death in older people (Heron & Smith, 2007). Disorders commonly seen may include systolic hypertension, valvular disease (most commonly aortic stenosis), coronary artery disease with acute myocardial infarction (MI), systolic and diastolic heart failure, dysrhythmias, and stroke. These specific disorders are discussed at length in Unit 7 of this text.

Safety Alert *Atrial fibrillation is the most common sustained dysrhythmia seen in the older patient. New-onset atrial fibrillation can be caused by other illnesses such as hyperthyroidism, electrolyte disturbances, or a myocardial infarction. Any patient reporting "palpitations" or "skipped beats" while hospitalized should be reported to the health care provider for further evaluation.*

Gastrointestinal Assessment

Some of the normal age-related changes in the gastrointestinal system contribute to the perception that older adults are fixated on their bowels. For example, the abdominal muscles of the aging patient weaken and peristalsis decreases. The liver itself becomes smaller in size, and its storage capacity is reduced. Alterations in insulin release often are seen as well.

Some of the age-related disorders in digestion are caused by *dysphagia,* difficulty swallowing. Dysphagia may be caused by poorly fitted or absent dentures. Even tooth decay can cause difficulty swallowing, resulting in decreased oral intake, weight loss, and undernutrition. Dyspepsia, gastroesophageal reflux disease (GERD), and upper gastrointestinal malignancies occur more often after age 55, and affect about one in four aging patients (Elsavy & Higgins, 2011). GERD is caused by the backflow of gastric or duodenal contents, or both, into the esophagus and past the lower esophageal sphincter. The reflux causes acute epigastric pain that can radiate to the chest or arm. Pain usually occurs after meals or when the patient lies down—the increased abdominal pressure causes reflux (Elsavy & Higgins, 2011). Upper endoscopy is recommended for aging patients with symptoms that trigger an alarm, new-onset GERD, or long-standing disease. Aging patients are at risk for more severe complications from GERD. Based on safety profiles and success in general, proton pump inhibitors (PPIs) are considered to be the first-line medication treatment for GERD in the elderly (Poh, Navarro-Rodriguez, & Fass, 2010).

Constipation is partially caused by the decreased peristalsis mentioned earlier, but it is also caused by many other contributing factors. A decreased thirst sensation leads to decreased fluid intake, and the use of narcotics for chronic pain management leads to slowed peristalsis, all of which results in constipation. Prolonged constipation can lead to intestinal obstruction, a medical emergency due to the potential for bowel perforation. Constipation also may be caused by a tumor. The incidence of colon cancer affects men and women equally, most commonly between the ages of 60 and 80 years (Tovey, 2007). See the Evidence-Based Practice feature discussion regarding the importance of management of constipation in older adults.

Genitourinary Assessment

As an individual ages, her pubic hair thins and grays, and her bladder capacity decreases. In females, vaginal mucosa atrophies from a decrease in estrogen, which also results in a decrease in size and elasticity of the vagina and a decrease in vaginal secretions. In males, slight testicular atrophy is seen, while the prostate gland enlarges. The scrotal sac elongates as well.

Common disorders of the genitourinary system seen in the aging patient include urinary tract infections (UTIs) and urinary incontinence. More frequent UTIs are thought to be caused by changes in the urinary tract. Urinary incontinence can be caused by stress incontinence, urge incontinence, overflow incontinence, or any combination of the three. Stress incontinence, the result of weakened bladder muscles, is most commonly seen. Urge incontinence, the second most common cause, is the result of bladder spasms, a syndrome often referred to as *overactive bladder,* which can be treated with medication. Overflow incontinence is the result of a bladder that is no longer able to contract efficiently to release urine. Incontinence occurs when urine exceeds the bladder capacity. Atrophic vaginitis, the result of decreased estrogen in the vaginal tissues, can be treated with hormone replacement, although this is controversial. Application of estrogen vaginal cream to the labia also is sometimes helpful.

The prostate enlarges as a normal part of aging due to a decrease of androgen and increase of estrogen, resulting in an imbalance. The increased estrogen receptors trigger the androgen receptors in the prostate gland to increase. An overgrowth of normal cells begins around the urethra and can cause partial bladder neck obstruction (Porth & Matfin, 2009). The result is urinary frequency and retention. Medications in the alpha$_1$ blocker drug class work by relaxing smooth muscle in the bladder neck and prostate. The result is an improvement in urine flow. If the prostate becomes too enlarged, surgical intervention using a transurethral approach may be indicated.

Musculoskeletal Assessment

In the aging patient, the nurse will see normal age-related changes of the musculoskeletal system. A slower reaction time, along with poorer coordination and decreased muscle strength, can all contribute to difficulties with gait. A loss of bone beginning during the fourth decade of life can affect posture and place an individual at risk for developing osteoporosis.

Age-related disorders of the musculoskeletal system include disabilities caused by osteoarthritis, rheumatoid arthritis, gout, osteoporosis, bunions, and hammertoes. Osteoarthritis is the most common type of arthritis, affecting women more than men, with joints of the hand being the most common site affected (Figure 10–2◆). Hip joints and knee joints also can be affected. Rheumatoid arthritis affects women and men over the age of 65 equally, and complications can affect the older person's mobility and ability to carry out ADLs, such as feeding.

Gout is a syndrome caused by deposition of urate crystals in joints and the skin. It causes acute monoarthritis and crystal deposits, called tophi, in the skin. It is more common in older people, specifically men. Other risk factors include non-White ethnicity; obesity; consumption of alcohol, meat, and fish; and use of diuretics. The Mayo Clinic reported that among Black men, the annual incidence of gout was 3.1/1,000 versus 1.8/1,000 in White men (Mayo Clinic, 2007a, 2007b; Tovey, 2007).

EVIDENCE-BASED PRACTICE Management of Bowel Routines

Clinical Problem

Management of bowel routines in the acute care setting often is inadequate. Establishing bowel routines also may be complicated for the patient with dementia. If a patient with dementia is agitated, could the agitation be related to the discomfort associated with constipation?

Research Findings

Constipation and/or difficulty passing stool affects approximately 26% of men and 34% of women over the age of 65. Some elders with chronic constipation believe it diminishes their quality of life. Complications from chronic constipation include fecal impaction, colonic dilatation, incontinence, and, in severe cases, bowel perforation. Patients who have chronic constipation may overuse laxatives, which can become habit forming (Fitzsimmons, 2011).

Implications for Nursing Practice

Constipation is a problem often overlooked in the acute care setting. The nurse can play a role in intervention by advocating for preprinted bowel care orders, as well as thorough documentation and tracking of bowel movements during hospitalization. Such simple interventions may reduce the incidence of physical aggression in elderly patients with dementia.

Critical Thinking Questions with answers can be found in the Osborn Student Resources at nursing.pearsonhighered.com.

Source: Fitzsimmons, S. (2011). Healthy aging. *Western Schools CE Express*, 67–118.

Weblink: Bunions Weblink: AHRQ National Healthcare Quality & Disparities

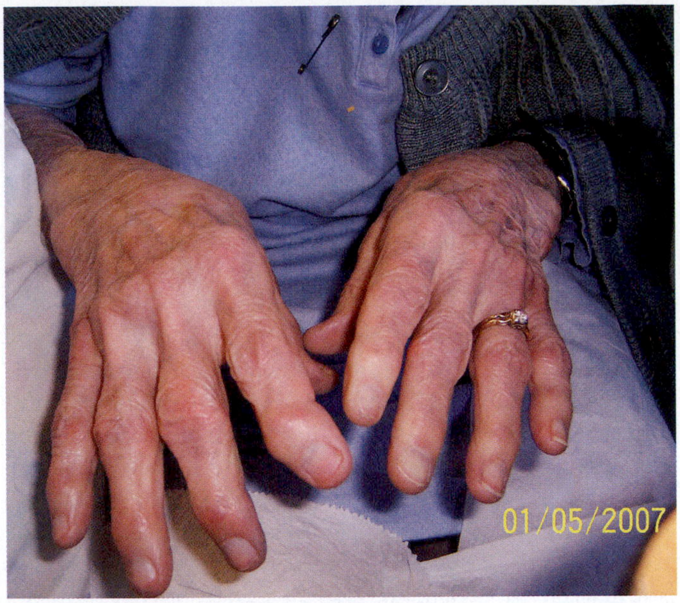

FIGURE 10–2 ◆ Osteoarthritic hands.

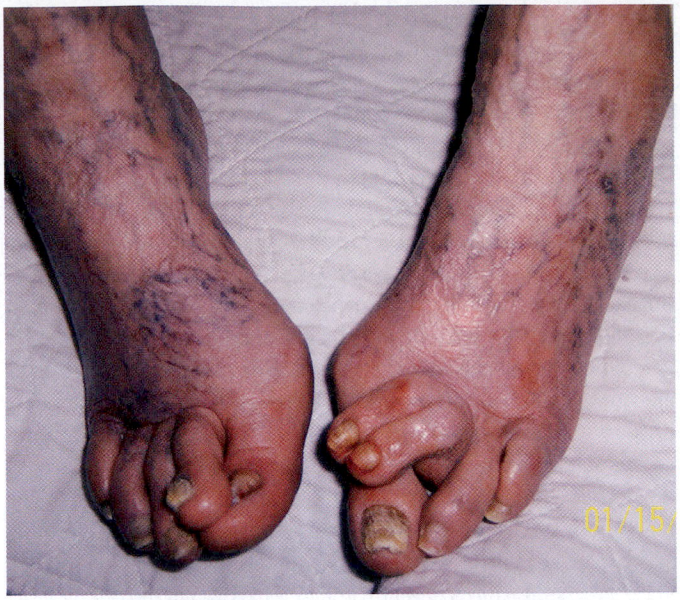

FIGURE 10–3 ◆ Bunion feet.

Osteoporosis is a skeletal disorder characterized by compromised bone strength that places an individual at increased risk for fracture (National Osteoporosis Foundation [NOF], 2007). Fractures due to osteoporosis can permanently affect the older person's function and quality of life. With the advent of bone mineral density (BMD) screening studies, health care providers are able to diagnose osteoporosis before a fracture occurs. The U.S. Preventive Services Task Force (USPSTF), sponsored by the Agency for Healthcare Research and Quality (AHRQ), is an independent panel of private sector experts in prevention and primary care. This panel develops recommendations about which preventive services should be incorporated routinely into primary medical care and for which populations. These are considered to be the "gold standards" for clinical preventive services based on documented evidence regarding effectiveness and outcomes of screening, counseling, and preventive medications. The USPSTF recommends bone mineral density screening at least once at age 65, with no recommendations as to how often the test should be repeated (National Guideline Clearing House, 2007). The universal recommendations for management of osteoporosis include oral calcium 1,200 mg/day, oral vitamin D 800 international units/day, fall prevention, tobacco avoidance, weight-bearing exercise, and no more than moderate alcohol consumption. Pharmacologic management should be considered based on risk factors for osteoporosis and BMD screening results. Bisphosphonates also have been shown to increase bone mineral density in the spine and hip (Reuben et al., 2007).

Bony deformities of the feet often are seen as a result of years of poorly fitting footwear, especially for women who regularly wear tight-fitting, high-heeled shoes (Figure 10–3◆). The bones of the toes take on an angled appearance and, in severe cases, the first toe of the foot will be permanently pushed over the second and third toe. These deformities can only be corrected surgically, where the bones of the feet are essentially "broken" and recast and reset into their proper alignment (American Academy Orthopedic Surgery, 2012).

Falls Assessment

It is important to determine whether older patients are at risk of falling by asking and observing whether they have fallen recently or if they have unsteady walking. A positive response requires further evaluation of muscle weakness, poor balance, or blood pressure that drops. Multifactorial interventions should be employed such as reviewing medications to evaluate for side effects, teaching exercises to strengthen core muscles and improve balance, and evaluating the home for things that may trip the patient. Falls are as serious a health problem for older adults as heart attacks and strokes (Pighills et al., 2011).

Skin Assessment

Assessment of the aging patient's skin requires the same techniques a nurse would use in assessing any patient, including inspection of the scalp, head, neck, trunk, and limbs. The skin should be palpated to determine temperature, moisture, thickness, texture, and turgor. The amount of subcutaneous tissue present below the surface of the skin in the aging patient is decreased; thus, skin turgor may not be a reliable indicator for hydration status. Common skin changes in the aging patient include the presence of seborrheic or senile keratoses, senile lentigines also known as "liver spots," cherry angiomas, and development of skin tags. Assessment of the skin is discussed more in Chapter 58.

The most common skin disorders in older adults are skin cancers, which may be the result of many years of unprotected skin exposure to the sun. Many aging patients present with skin cancers, such as basal cell cancers, or precancerous lesions, such as actinic keratoses. Treatment includes surgical excision or removal via desiccation for precancerous lesions. Herpes zoster, which produces blistering lesions along a specific dermatome, also is more commonly found in the aging patient. The USPSTF recommends a yearly skin exam in individuals age 65 and older (AHRQ, 2009).

Dry skin is estimated to be present in approximately 75% of individuals 75 years and older (WebMD, 2010). It is worse during the winter when the air is drier, and develops when the skin loses water to the air. Keratosis and pruritus are chronic problems for many aging patients, fueling an industry that sells lotions, creams, and ointments to treat dry, itchy skin.

Neurological Assessment

Contrary to common myths regarding aging, it is not routine for older people to become senile or demented. However, by age 85, the risk of developing Alzheimer's disease, a type of dementia, is nearly 50% (Alzheimer's Association, 2010). Neurological assessment is covered in detail in Chapter 20. However, there are normal changes seen in the aging patient that must be taken into consideration. The brain atrophies with age, but there are no relationships between shrinkage and change in cognition. The sense of taste and smell decrease in the aging patient. Sometimes there is a lack of awareness that food has spoiled. This may predispose older individuals to nutritional problems. Changes in reflexes include decreased deep tendon reflexes in the legs and increased reflexes in the arms, with decreased vibratory sense.

There is some decrease in position sense as well. Many medical conditions are associated with pain in the older adult, but certain types of pain may be less severe than others. This may explain why a younger adult experiencing a myocardial infarction will report crushing chest pain, and the aging patient may report vague symptoms of discomfort, such as heartburn (Baseline, 2009).

Due to the changes just mentioned, neurological disease may be more difficult to assess in the older adult, since some "abnormal" neurological findings may in fact be "normal." Some disorders, such as normal pressure hydrocephalus (NPH) and dementia, may involve subtle changes in the patient's mental status. NPH is an abnormal increase of cerebrospinal fluid (CSF) in the brain's ventricles, which occurs when the normal flow of CSF throughout the brain and spinal cord is blocked. While this can occur in people of any age, it is most common in older adults. It may result from a subarachnoid hemorrhage, head trauma, infection, tumor, or complications of surgery. It also may occur when none of these factors is present; in these cases, the cause of the disorder is unknown. Symptoms of NPH include progressive mental impairment and dementia, problems with walking, and impaired bladder control, leading to urinary frequency and/or incontinence. The person also may have a general slowing of movements, with some complaining of feeling as though her feet are stuck. This abnormal state is hard to diagnose because the symptoms often resemble other neurological disorders, such as Alzheimer's disease, Parkinson's disease, and Creutzfeldt-Jakob disease (National Institute of Neurological Disorders and Stroke, 2007). Treatment for NPH involves surgical placement of a shunt in the brain to drain excess CSF into the abdomen where it can be absorbed. If not treated, the symptoms of NPH usually get worse over time. The success of treatment with shunts varies, but is generally favorable. Early diagnosis and treatment improves the chance of a normal recovery.

The term **dementia** is characterized by the loss of or decline in memory and other cognitive abilities. It is caused by various diseases and conditions that result in damaged brain cells. To be classified as dementia, it must meet certain criteria of memory loss involving cognitive abilities, recognition/identification of objects, and the ability to understand and process language in comprehension of a required task. The decline in cognitive abilities must be severe enough to interfere with daily life (Barnes et al., 2009) Presenting symptoms include:

- Asking the same questions repeatedly
- Becoming lost in familiar places
- Being unable to follow directions
- Getting disoriented about time, people, and places
- Neglecting personal safety, hygiene, and nutrition.

Dementia also may change a person's mood and personality. At first, memory loss and trouble thinking clearly may bother the person who has dementia. Later, disruptive behavior and other problems may start, but the person who has dementia may not be aware of these problems.

People with dementia lose their abilities at different rates. It is caused by many conditions; some are reversible and some are not. Reversible conditions can be caused by a high fever, dehydration, vitamin deficiency and poor nutrition, medication reactions, thyroid problems, or a minor head injury. Sometimes older people have emotional problems that can be mistaken for dementia. Feeling sad, lonely, worried, or bored may be common feelings for older people facing retirement or coping with the death of a spouse. Emotional problems and the medical problems previously noted should be professionally addressed. Family support also is critical to the care of people with dementia.

The two most common forms of dementia in older people are Alzheimer's disease (AD) and multiple-infarct dementia, sometimes referred to as vascular dementia. These types of dementia are irreversible. Alzheimer's disease is discussed in detail in Chapter 23 as a chronic neurological disease.

With multiple-infarct dementia, a series of strokes or changes in the brain's blood supply may result in the death of brain tissue. The location in the brain where the strokes occur and the severity of the strokes determine the seriousness of the problem and the symptoms that arise. Symptoms usually begin abruptly and progress in a stepwise fashion with repeated strokes. Strokes are fully discussed in Chapter 22.

Delirium is a sudden, fluctuating, and usually reversible cognitive disorder characterized by a disturbance in consciousness with decreased attention and a change in cognition or development of a perceptual disturbance that develops over a short period of time and tends to fluctuate throughout the day (Reuben et al., 2007). This change in cognition often manifests itself in disruptive behaviors in the hospital setting, such as disrobing, pulling out IV lines, striking out at caregivers, and resisting nursing care. Its incidence in the hospital setting is about 20%, with postoperative incidence up to 72%. It is an abnormal mental state, not a disease, and usually a sign of a newly developed disorder; it affects about one-third of hospitalized people age 70 or older.

Detection of delirium is difficult, but identification is critical. The Confusion Assessment Method (CAM) is a standardized tool developed in 1990 that is still widely used (Inouye et al., 1990). Any clinician can use this tool to identify delirium quickly and accurately. The short version consists of four features found to have the greatest ability to distinguish delirium from other types of cognitive impairment. The tool identifies the presence or absence of delirium, but does not assess the severity. The first two features that must be present for delirium to be diagnosed are difficulty focusing attention and evidence of an acute change in mental status from the patient's baseline or a fluctuation in behavior throughout the day. The presence of these features and either evidence of disorganized thinking, such as rambling or illogical conversation, or an altered level of consciousness must be present for diagnosis (Waszynski, 2007).

Once delirium is diagnosed, causative factors, such as infection or metabolic derangement, must be identified and treated. Urinary tract infections are the most common cause of delirium in older adults, and polypharmacy is the second most common cause (Voyer, McCusker, Cole, St-Jacques, & Khomenko, 2007). Metabolic disorders such as hypo- or hypernatremia must be corrected as well. Delirium is self-limiting; once the underlying problem has been corrected, it usually resolves after 5 days. In extreme cases, symptoms can last 3 to 6 months. If confusion and disorientation persist, other neurological disorders, such as dementia, must be considered. Dementia is diagnosed within 3 years in 60% of hospitalized patients with delirium (Voyer et al., 2007).

Weblink: Evidence-Based Geriatric Nursing Assessment Tools

Weblink: Key Facts About Seasonal Flu Vaccine

The USPSTF recommends cognitive impairment screening annually for the individual age 65 and older (AHRQ, 2009). The **Folstein Mini-Mental State Exam,** a classic, common screening tool used by clinicians to evaluate dementia, is easily administered after some training. The scoring ranges from 0 to 30 points, with 0 to 10 points typically scored for an individual with advanced dementia, 10 to 20 points for moderate dementia, and 21 to 26 points for mild dementia. A score of 27 to 30 is considered normal, with adjustments made for levels of education (Folstein, Folstein, & McHugh, 1975).

Within the last 10 years, there has been increasing recognition of older adults experiencing late-onset schizophrenia and bipolar disorders (Shawler, 2010). Late-onset schizophrenia tends to be attributed to organic factors and is often characterized by bizarre delusion and auditory hallucinations. Systematized delusions of physical or mental influence are seen in many of the patients, with grandiose, erotic, or somatic delusions occurring in some cases. Depressive symptoms also may be present. Psychoses may be a symptom of substance abuse, polypharmacy, delirium, or a mood disorder (Shawler, 2010).

Bipolar disorders in older adults are clinically heterogeneous and present with various courses, switching from recurrent depression to mania (Shawler, 2010). They can take on uncommon symptoms such as depressive or mixed behaviors, psychosis, mental confusion, or dementia. The prognosis of bipolar disorders in older adults is poor due to the high prevalence of recurrences, associated somatic disorders, reduced survival, and severe handicap. As with late-onset schizophrenia, there is an immediate need for collaboration between patients, families, and clinicians to provide health care services for this population.

Parkinson's disease is a neurodegenerative disorder associated with asymmetrical bradykinesia, hypokinesia, and rigidity. More information on this disorder is presented in Chapter 23. It is about 1.5 times more common in men, and has an average age of onset of 60 years. It currently is incurable; however, dopamine agonists are used to reduce dyskinesias and motor fluctuation, and levodopa is being used to improve motor function (Hauser, 2012).

Stroke, also discussed under multiple-infarct dementia, is one of the neurological disorders affecting older adults that can result in the greatest degree of disability. It is defined as loss of cerebral function lasting more than 24 hours or leading to death, with no apparent cause other than that of vascular origin. Ischemic stroke is caused by vascular insufficiency, often from a thromboembolism; hemorrhagic stroke is caused by a hemorrhage of a vessel. Strokes and their ramifications for nursing care are discussed in Chapter 22.

Resources are available that include collections of reliable assessment tools for the elder patient. One such website is from The Hartford Institute, www.consultgerirn.com.

Health Care Promotion and Preventive Care

The USPSTF is one of several groups that make recommendations for appropriate preventive services and screening exams in adults age 65 and older. As mentioned earlier, the USPSTF comprises an independent panel of experts in primary care and preventive care. The panel systematically reviews the evidence and effectiveness of clinical preventive services and develops recommendations (AHRQ, 2009). However, such recommendations do not specifically address the appropriateness of such testing in the frail aging patient with multiple medical problems, functional decline, and a limited life expectancy. When interpreting the guidelines, it is the responsibility of the aging patient and the health care provider to discuss which recommendations are appropriate, taking all of the previous factors and the individual's personal wishes into consideration.

Immunizations

Immunizations are one way the aging adult can proactively prevent potential debilitating illnesses. Hospitalization provides an opportunity for patients to update their immunizations. Vaccines in the aging adult are about 50% to 60% effective in preventing hospitalizations from pneumonia and 80% effective in preventing death (CDC, 2012). Pneumonia infections cause an estimated 50,000 deaths each year in the United States, more than any other vaccine-preventable bacterial disease (CDC, 2012). Influenza, which typically affects individuals during the winter months, has been associated with over 36,000 deaths per year with the majority being in the aging population (CMS, 2012).

Pneumococcal Vaccine

Streptococcus pneumonia is the organism responsible for pneumococcal pneumonia. All adults over 65 years old are candidates for initial vaccination, with a recommendation that those who may have received the vaccination at an earlier age due to chronic health conditions be revaccinated at age 65. The USPSTF recommends a pneumonia vaccination once at age 65, and suggests people in that age group consider repeating the vaccine every 6 to 7 years (CMS, 2012). The vaccine is administered intramuscularly in the deltoid muscle or subcutaneously. It can be given with the influenza vaccine via a separate injection in the other arm without an increase in the severity of reactions or by affecting antibody response.

Influenza Vaccine

Influenza vaccines have traditionally contained three virus strains: two type A and one type B. Following the increase in H1N1 influenza outbreaks in the United States, additional immunization against this variety was added to the CDC recommended list. During the influenza season, selected federal "sentinel reporters" who are health care providers submit nasal swabs of individuals who present to health care institutions with influenza-type symptoms. These data are used to develop the influenza vaccine for the upcoming year. In this way, the vaccine should represent the most common viruses to which individuals will likely be exposed in the upcoming influenza season. The influenza vaccine will not always prevent the aging patient from contracting the flu; in fact, although studies have shown the vaccine prevents severe illness, complications such as the development of pneumonia and death can occur (CDC, 2012). The USPSTF recommends annual influenza immunization in all individuals, especially those age 65 and older (AHRQ, 2009).

Safety Alert *The influenza vaccine is made from egg-grown viruses that are not infectious. Patients cannot get the flu from the vaccination; however, it is absolutely contraindicated in those who have a hypersensitivity to egg protein. CDC guidelines specify that the live attenuated influenza nasal vaccine should be administered only to persons age 2 to 49 years who are not pregnant.*

Tetanus Vaccine

Many older adults are not aware that they need a tetanus immunization, and others have poor recollection of their immunization history. Immunization against tetanus is recommended every 10 years in adults over 65 years of age (AHRQ, 2009). The vaccine is usually available in multiple-dose vials as tetanus-diphtheria toxoid (Td). The dosage for adults is 0.5 mL administered intramuscularly. The vaccine must be kept in the refrigerator to maintain its potency.

Herpes Zoster Vaccine

Herpes zoster virus vaccine is used to prevent herpes zoster virus, also known as shingles, in people over age 60. It contains live, attenuated varicella-zoster virus in a dose 14 times greater than the varicella (chickenpox) vaccine. This larger dose is needed to boost immunity against shingles in older persons. Herpes zoster virus vaccine decreases the occurrence of herpes zoster by about half; for those who do get herpes zoster, it reduces the severity and risk of developing postherpetic neuralgia. This is important because the pain that is associated with postherpetic neuralgia can be debilitating and persist long after the zoster rash has resolved.

About 50 million people are candidates to receive this vaccine. A single dose of zoster vaccine is recommended for adults age 60 or older whether or not they report a prior episode of herpes zoster (CMS, 2012).

Screening Exams

Addressing screening exams in the aging patient can be a challenge for several reasons. First, screening recommendations for seniors are not mandated, and they must take into account any comorbidities and the functional status of the individual. Second, when considering screening exams, the health care provider needs to know what will be done with the information obtained from the exam. If a patient indicates that he would not pursue treatment if cancer were found as a result of a screening test, ordering the test is most likely unnecessary. Finally, a factor that must be considered is whether the benefit of conducting the test outweighs the burden of administering the test itself. All of these decisions require the health care provider to fully discuss the screening exam with the patient in order to make informed decisions while taking the individual's wishes into account.

Vision

The USPSTF recommends visual screening and full eye exam on an annual basis for all individuals age 65 and older (AHRQ, 2009). Visual impairment is defined as visual acuity 20/40 or worse. Legal blindness is defined as 20/200 or less (National Federation of the Blind, 2012). Vision screening is important because some visual changes occur slowly over many years. Because of this, the aging patient may not be aware that his visual acuity has declined. Acuity testing and tonometry can identify refractive problems, cataracts, age-related macular degeneration, diabetic retinopathy, and glaucoma (Reuben et al., 2007). Mobile optometrists are available in some communities to travel to private homes, senior communities, and long-term care settings to evaluate individuals who are unable to travel to a traditional medical office. This is especially useful for evaluating individuals with dementia who may need eyeglasses, but who become agitated when moved from their familiar environment.

Hearing

Because hearing loss is the most common sensory impairment in the older adult, the USPSTF recommends hearing impairment screening on a yearly basis for all individuals age 65 and older (AHRQ, 2009). The canals must be free of cerumen for reliable testing. Evaluation consists of screening for hearing problems (medical history, questionnaire) and audiometry, which documents the decibel loss across frequencies along with the pattern of loss. Based on the findings, augmentation with hearing aids may be considered (Reuben et al., 2007). Hearing aids can cost up to $5,000 per pair. On admission, history relating to hearing should be collected as part of the initial assessment. As the nurse develops a plan of care relating to the patient's hearing deficits, directions for the management of the patient's hearing aids must be relayed to all care providers. Developing a plan of care is one of the components of the ANA standards of clinical gerontological nursing care.

Breast Exams/Breast Cancer Screening

The USPSTF recommends monthly breast self-exams and mammograms every 1 to 2 years up to the age of 70. For those over the age of 70, mammography should be continued for those who have a "reasonable life expectancy" (AHRQ, 2009), which is discussed in the Evidence-Based Practice feature.

Pap Smears

The USPSTF recommends a Pap smear at least every 3 years in women age 65 and older. However, Pap smears may be stopped after age 65 if there is one negative Pap smear at age 65 and the woman is low risk (USPSTF, 2012). A woman at low risk is one with an established sexual partner, history of consistent prior screening, and no history of abnormal Pap smears. Women without a cervix should not have Pap smears (Reuben et al., 2007; USPSTF, 2012).

Prostate Exam/Prostate Cancer Screening

Prostate cancer is the most common cancer, other than skin cancer, that affects men. About 1 in 6 men will be diagnosed with prostate cancer during their lifetime, but only 1 in 34 will die from it (American Cancer

EVIDENCE-BASED PRACTICE Mammogram Screenings in Older Adults

Clinical Problem

When considering health promotion and disease prevention, it is debatable as to which individuals over the age of 75 should receive screening mammograms. The recommendation for those over 75 is to only screen those with a "reasonable life expectancy," yet there is no definition of what "reasonable life expectancy" means. What criteria should be used when referring for a mammogram?

Research Findings

In the United States, breast cancer is the most frequently appearing, noncutaneous cancer that is diagnosed in women. More than 190,000 women are diagnosed yearly (Cibulka, 2011). In November 2009, the U.S. Preventive Services Task Force changed the age recommendations for mammography to state that women who are not at high risk for developing breast cancer can wait to begin screening until the age of 50. For those between the ages of 50 and 74, they recommend mammography screening every 2 years with the possibility of ending screening at age 75. The American Cancer Society recommends annual mammography beginning at age 40 to continue as long as the woman is in good health.

Implications for Nursing Practice

When addressing the need for a mammogram, the nurse must not just consider the exam itself, but also must consider the aging patient's overall condition. If the patient is bedbound or unable to participate due to an inability to remain still or follow instructions, a mammogram may not be appropriate. For patients with cognitive disorders or chronic illnesses, the nurse needs to ask this question: "If an abnormality were found, would the patient seek treatment?"

Critical Thinking Questions with answers can be found in the Osborn Student Resources at nursing.pearsonhighered.com.

Source: Cibulka, N. (2011). Update on breast cancer screening. *Journal for Nurse Practitioners, 7*(1).

Weblink: Key Statistics About Prostate Cancer
Weblink: Healthy People 2020

Society, 2010). The USPSTF recommends a yearly prostate surface antigen (PSA) test and a digital rectal exam (DRE) in males age 65 and older. However, it has been noted that men over the age of 75 with a negative DRE rarely die from prostate cancer, and the risks from treatment in this age group may outweigh the benefit (U.S. Preventive Services Task Force, 2008).

Prostate cancers tend to be slow growing in older patients, and for those with multiple comorbidities there is a greater chance death will occur from a disease process other than prostate cancer. Older men should discuss this subject with their primary care provider. PSA levels can be falsely elevated when obtained during hospitalization due to catheterization and infection; thus, they should not routinely be obtained during hospitalization.

Colon Cancer Screening

Colorectal cancer is the fourth most common cancer in the United States and the second leading cause of death from cancer (AHRQ, 2009). The USPSTF recommends colon cancer screening consisting of fecal occult blood testing (FOBT), sigmoidoscopy, and colonoscopy starting at age 50 for those at average risk for colorectal cancer. Those at high risk, such as individuals with a first-degree relative diagnosed with colon cancer before age 60, may consider screening at an earlier age. For those age 65 and older, FOBT is recommended yearly, sigmoidoscopy every 5 years, and colonoscopy every 10 years. The appropriate age to discontinue colorectal cancer screening is not known. Most screening studies have restricted enrollees to those less than 80 years of age. The burden of screening may outweigh potential benefits in patients with advanced age and comorbid conditions that limit life expectancy. Thus, the aging patient needs to discuss benefits and potential harms associated with each screening test with a health care provider before deciding on a screening strategy (AHRQ, 2009).

Healthy People 2020

Healthy People 2020 has added new objectives for the older adult. The new objectives are divided into two categories: Prevention and Long-Term Services and Supports. The short titles for the objectives are in Chart 10–4.

Pharmacology and the Aging Patient

A major emphasis in the health care community has been on appropriate medications for the aging patient, with a focus on prevention of complications from inappropriately prescribed medications (Moore, Cohen, & Furberg, 2007). This focus evolved from a 1991 publication identifying criteria of inappropriate medication use in the nursing home population (Beers, 1997). These criteria were initially developed to aid researchers in evaluating the quality of prescriptions, drug utilization systems, and educational efforts in the nursing home setting. Further updates have identified medications or medication classes that should generally be avoided in persons 65 or older for two reasons. First, there are medications that are either ineffective or pose unnecessarily high risks for older persons when safer alternatives are available. Second, certain medications should not be used in older persons known to have specific medical conditions. These criteria, now known as the *Beers criteria,* have been expanded to apply to older adults living in the community, because inappropriate prescribing by health care providers has been shown to occur in both inpatient and outpatient settings (Beers, 1997; Razzi, 2009). Older adults account for 34% of all prescriptions dispensed (Fitzsimmons, 2011). Often these medications may be unnecessary or inappropriately prescribed. The Evidence-Based Practice feature (p. 252) discusses these issues.

An **adverse drug reaction (ADR),** a noxious response to a drug when given at normal doses, or an **adverse drug event (ADE),** an

CHART 10–4 *Healthy People 2020* Objectives

Prevention

1. Use of Welcome to Medicare benefit, target 10% improvement.
   a. *Only 7.3% of older adults used the benefit in 2008.*
2. Older adults up to date on clinical preventive services, target 10% improvement.
   a. *Only 46.3% of males and 47.9% of females age 65 years or older were up to date on a core set of preventive services in 2008.*
3. Increase the proportion of older adults with one or more chronic health conditions who report confidence in managing their condition.
4. Receipt of diabetes Self-Management Benefits by older adults, target 10% improvement.
   a. *Only 2.2 percent of older adults received Diabetes Self-Management Benefits in 2008.*
5. Functional limitations in older adults, target to reduce by 10%.
   a. *In 2007, 28.3% of older adults had moderate to severe functional limitations.*
6. Leisure-time physical activities among older adults, target 10% increase.
   a. *Only 33.7% of older adults with reduced physical or cognitive function engaged in light, moderate, or vigorous leisure-time physical activities in 2008.*
7. Increase the proportion of the health care workforce with geriatric certification, target 10% improvement.
   a. *In 2004, 1.4% of registered nurses had geriatric certification.*

Long-Term Services and Supports

8. Reduce the proportion of noninstitutionalized older adults with disabilities who have an unmet need for long-term services and supports. Objective being developed.
9. Reduce the proportion of unpaid caregivers of older adults who report an unmet need for caregiver support services. Objective being developed.
10. Reduce the rate of pressure ulcer-related hospitalizations among older adults, target 10% improvement.
    a. *In 2007, there were 985.8 pressure ulcer-related hospitalizations per 100,000 persons age 65 years and over.*
11. Reduce the rate of emergency department visits due to falls among older adults, target 10% improvement.
    a. *In 2007, there were 5,235.1 emergency department visits per 100,000 persons due to falls among older adults.*
12. Increase the number of States, the District of Columbia, and Tribes that collect and make publicly available information on the characteristics of victims, perpetrators, and cases of elder abuse, neglect, and exploitation. Target 10% improvement.
    a. *In 2004, 3 states collected and made publicly available information on the characteristics of victims, perpetrators, and cases of elder abuse, neglect, and exploitation.*

Source: Healthy People 2020 (healthypeople.gov, 2010)

injury that results from taking the drug, can occur when a patient takes a medication that has been appropriately or inappropriately prescribed. Medications in general have the potential to cause adverse effects that can range from insignificant to life threatening. Many medications prescribed to older adults have narrow therapeutic windows; in other words, the levels required for clinical efficacy are very close to the toxic levels (Fitzsimmons, 2011).

Ethnic background also may place an individual at risk for ADEs. One meta-analysis of studies found this to be the case for cardiovascular medications in various ethnic groups. For example, Black patients taking angiotensin converting enzyme (ACE) inhibitors are five times more likely to experience angioedema compared with non-Black patients. Black patients have a higher risk of moderate or severe bleeding following thrombolytic therapy compared to non-Black patients. Antidysrhythmics and opioids are metabolized differently in Native American, African, and Asian patients. Thus, ethnic background must be considered in individuals experiencing ADEs (Adams & Koch, 2010).

Safety Alert *One method to ensure that patients are not re-prescribed medications that previously caused an adverse reaction is to enter those medications in the allergy section of the patient's chart or electronic health record, along with the reactions the patient experienced. Although not a true drug allergy, listing drug intolerances along with their corresponding adverse reaction as part of the medical record will direct providers to choose another medication for a particular condition when prescribing.*

Polypharmacy

Polypharmacy, one of the major medication issues affecting the aging patient, is defined as the administration of many drugs together, and/or the administration of excessive medications (Polypharmacy, 2007). However, the definition itself is controversial and varies from study to study, making application of research results in the clinical setting challenging. In the clinical setting, polypharmacy occurs when an individual is using more medications than is clinically indicated. This includes prescription medications, over-the-counter (OTC) medications, and nontraditional medications. Polypharmacy can occur in the acute care setting, in a structured care setting such as an assisted living facility, or at home.

A thorough nursing assessment on admission to the hospital provides an opportunity to identify and eliminate polypharmacy. Chart 10–5 outlines the information that should be collected on admission.

CHART 10–5 Assessment Criteria When Evaluating Polypharmacy

- Medical diagnoses and self-diagnosed health problems
- Known drug allergies
- History of previous adverse drug reactions
- All prescribed medications taken
- All OTC medications taken
- All nontraditional medications taken
- Length of time each medication has been taken
- Actual amounts of each medication taken and how often
- Reason for taking each medication, any adverse effects
- Any problems with taking the medication in its prescribed form

Medication Administration Principles for the Aging Patient

Medication administration principles for the aging patient go beyond practicing the "five rights" of medication administration (right patient, right drug, right dose, right route, right time). With regard to dosing, the adage to "start low, and go slow" should be followed. Often, when a patient needs a medication a nurse is given a range of doses to choose from. In the aging patient, the nurse should start with a lower dose than might be typically administered to a younger patient. The aging patient takes longer to metabolize and excrete medications due to decreased renal and hepatic function. Some medication reference guides list geriatric doses, which is helpful. For medications excreted through the renal system, the nurse can calculate the estimated creatinine clearance. Serum creatinine does not accurately reflect renal function in the aging patient due to decreased lean body mass. The Cockcroft-Gault formula is used to estimate creatinine clearance (CrCl):

$$\frac{\textit{Creatinine clearance} = (140 - \textit{age}) \times \textit{weight (kg)} \; (\times 0.85 \textit{ for women})}{\textit{Plasma creatinine (mg/dL)} \times 2.72}$$

For drugs excreted via the kidneys, dosage adjustments may be necessary if CrCl < 60 (Adams & Koch, 2010).

There is an increased risk that aging patients may have impaired swallowing or be unable to swallow medications in the traditional pill form due to altered cognition with agitation. These patients present a challenge for the nurse, who must be knowledgeable about other possible methods for medication administration. For example, a patient requiring long-term pain management who is unable to swallow or take pain medications on a consistent basis may be appropriate for medication delivery via a transdermal patch. A transdermal patch delivers a continuous amount of pain medication and only requires changing every 72 hours. This method of medication delivery also may reduce caregiver burden. Chart 10–6 lists some of the

CHART 10–6 Selected Medications with Potential Adverse Outcomes for the Aging Patient

Medication Class	Adverse Response
Antihistamines	Anticholinergic effects, sedation, confusion
Benzodiazepines	Anticholinergic effects, confusion, depression
Cimetidine	Depression, confusion
Digoxin	Reduced renal function can cause toxicity
Muscle relaxants	Anticholinergic effects, weakness, sedation
Nonsteroidal anti-inflammatory drugs	Fluid retention, nephrotoxicity, photosensitivity
Phenytoin	Confusion, slurred speech, double vision, ataxia
Ranitidine	Blood dyscrasias, liver dysfunction
Tricyclic antidepressants	Anticholinergic effects, confusion, hallucinations

Source: Adapted from Adams, M. P., & Koch, R. W. (2010). *Pharmacology: Connections to nursing practice.* Upper Saddle River, NJ: Pearson, 146–153.

EVIDENCE-BASED PRACTICE Medication Administration for Aging Patients

Clinical Problem

With all of the various mechanisms by which medications are metabolized in older adults, how is a nurse to know which ones are not appropriate in this population? Specifically, which medications should nurses tell their older adult patients to avoid?

Research Findings

The number of adverse drug reactions among older adults has increased 260% over the last few years. Approximately 90,000 serious events and 15,000 fatalities in older adults have been reported to the Food and Drug Administration (FDA) (Moore, Cohen, & Furberg, 2007). In 1991, the first research was published identifying inappropriate medication use in nursing home patients. From this original research, the Beers report update in 1997 became the accepted criteria for evaluating appropriate medication use in frail nursing home patients (Beers, 1997). By 1999, the criteria had been adopted by the Centers for Medicare & Medicaid Services for nursing home regulation. In 2003, the criteria were updated to generalize the criteria to older patients regardless of their residence. The Beers criteria identify medications or medication classes that should generally be avoided in persons 65 or older because (1) they are ineffective, (2) they pose unnecessarily high risk for this group, and (3) safer alternatives exist.

Implications for Nursing Practice

Any nurse caring for older adults needs to become familiar with the Beers criteria. In addition, most medication programs that can be installed on a personal digital assistant include a section on special considerations for the adults 65 or older. Any hospitalized aging patients who are exhibiting signs of delirium should have their medications reviewed to determine if adverse side effects of the medications are contributing to the delirium.

Critical Thinking Questions with answers can be found in the Osborn Student Resources at nursing.pearsonhighered.com.

Sources: Beers, M. H. (1997). Explicit criteria for determining potentially inappropriate medication use by the elderly. *Archives of Internal Medicine, 157,* 1531–1536; Moore, T. J., Cohen, M. R., & Furberg, C. D. (2007). Serious adverse drug events reported to the Food and Drug Administration, 1998–2005. *Archive of Internal Medicine, 167*(16), 1752–1759.

medications with potential adverse outcomes for the aging patient. The Evidence-Based Practice feature discusses the issues surrounding common medications and their effects on older adults.

Safety Alert *Medications with an enteric coating and sustained-release medications cannot be crushed. If the patient requires medications to be crushed or administered via nasogastric or gastrostomy tube, notify the physician or health care professional so that the equivalent short-acting medication may be ordered and crushed. Remember, if the medication is difficult to crush, there is a reason why!*

Resources for Caring for an Aging Population

When the aging patient can no longer live alone independently, all viable alternative resources should be explored. For example, 24-hour-a-day care may be needed, whether in a board and care facility, an assisted living facility, or a nursing home. Contrary to popular belief, Medicare does not cover private home care, board and care (a home that boards elders and cares for them), assisted living (apartments or condominiums where elders can live independently but have access to help if needed), or custodial nursing home care. Custodial care residents typically live in a nursing home for an extended period of time due to their need for 24-hour-a-day supervision, nursing care, and assistance with activities of daily living. ADLs include bathing, toileting, eating, and dressing. Generally, Medicare covers skilled nursing care when an individual has been hospitalized and requires a high level of nursing care or therapy at least daily. Examples of skilled nursing care include intravenous (IV) therapy, complicated wound care, and nutrition administered via a feeding tube. Examples of therapy include daily physical, occupational, or speech rehabilitation.

Board and care, assisted living, and many nursing homes cost between $4,000 and $7,000 per month depending on location and amenities offered. Individuals often exhaust their personal life savings paying for such care, and then rely on Medicaid to pay for their care for the remainder of their life. Some nursing homes will not accept Medicaid patients due to concerns that financial reimbursements for these patients have not kept pace with the cost of the care delivered. In fact, in many facilities, private-pay patients pay twice the amount per day that the state reimburses for Medicaid patients.

Medicare and Medicaid

A person's financial means directly affects his ability to pay for housing, food, and medical care. Medical care is of special interest as funding mechanisms have changed drastically in the past 50 years. Prior to the advent of Medicare, health care was primarily a fee-for-service industry. When an individual interacted with the health care system, the provider of care was paid directly for services provided. Medicare, a federally funded health care program for individuals over the age of 65, those under the age of 65 who are disabled, and those with end-stage renal disease, was signed into law in 1965 by President Johnson. Currently, Medicare pays for 54% of overall health care costs for its enrollees age 65 and over. Medicare Part A covers hospital stays, pints of blood for transfusions, home health services, hospice care, and some skilled nursing care (after a qualifying hospital stay). Most people or their spouses paid Medicare taxes while working, and they will automatically receive Medicare Part A coverage without having to pay a monthly premium. Medicare Part B covers medical services such as medical care by a doctor, nurse practitioner, or physician's assistant; outpatient care; and other medical services not covered by Part A. Enrollment in Part B is optional and there is a monthly premium to pay. The Part B deductible must be paid each year before Medicare begins to pay a share of Part B expenses. Some examples of services that fall under Medicare Part B are ambulance services, cardiovascular screenings, bone density measurements, mammogram screenings, and clinical laboratory services.

Individuals enrolled in Medicare can add drug coverage if they join a Medicare prescription drug plan. These plans are offered by private companies that work with Medicare to provide medication coverage. Premiums, copays, and yearly deductibles vary by plans. Each Medicare drug plan has a formulary, a list of covered drugs. The list must include at least two drugs in all classes of drugs commonly prescribed to individuals age 65 and older. For more details, review Chapter 2 of this text.

Some individuals choose to purchase a supplemental insurance policy to cover extra health care costs not covered by Medicare. This insurance, called a "Medigap" policy, is sold by private insurance companies to fill in the gaps in Medicare coverage. Typically, Medigap policies help pay a share of coinsurance, copayments, or deductibles related to the costs of Medicare-covered services. Usually when one buys Medigap insurance, both Part A and Part B are covered.

For those who are low income, Medicaid provides financial coverage for health care expenses. Medicaid is a federal program that was enacted in 1965 at the same time President Johnson enacted Medicare. It is administered individually by each state. Eligibility is based on income and assets. Medicaid covers 10% of overall health care costs for those age 65 and over. In 2006, new rules came into effect that required Americans to show proof of citizenship or risk losing their Medicaid benefits. This can be challenging for older adults who lack family support systems and suffer from dementia or mental illness (Centers for Medicare & Medicaid Services [CMS], n.d.). Most hospitals have patient advocates or other resources to help older adults submit the paperwork for Medicaid.

Some individuals enroll in Medicare advantage plans. With these plans, their Medicare is assigned to a preferred provider organization (PPO) or health maintenance organization (HMO), which is responsible for overseeing and coordinating care. Chapter 2 discusses these types of health plans in detail. Medicare advantage plans provide all of the coverage of Part A and Part B and must cover medically necessary services. Medicare pays an amount every month to these private health plans, whether or not services were used in that particular month. These organizations offer benefits greater than what Medicare alone covers, thus explaining their popularity in certain parts of the United States, such as California.

Legal and Ethical Issues of Aging

It is often difficult and challenging for the nurse to discuss legal and ethical concerns with a patient or family member. Many nurses have little experience in this area, and bringing up issues such as elder abuse or advance directives can feel awkward and unsettling. However, such difficult conversations become easier as a nurse gains experience and becomes knowledgeable about legal and ethical issues.

Elder mistreatment or *abuse* is a broad term that describes the outcome of abuse, neglect, exploitation, or abandonment of older adults. There are three categories of elder mistreatment: domestic, institutional, and self-neglect. Domestic mistreatment occurs in the older adult's home and involves significant others such as a child, spouse, or relatives. Institutional mistreatment occurs when an individual has a contractual agreement with a care facility, such as a nursing home, and is abused. Self-neglect occurs when an individual who is capable of making decisions and understanding consequences engages in behavior that threatens his safety or well-being. Chapter 6 discusses elder abuse in detail.

Advance directives provide a mechanism for individuals to state, in writing, their wishes regarding treatment should they become ill. Individuals typically execute such a document when they are well and able to think through the various scenarios they might experience as they age. Chapter 2 discusses advance directives in detail.

In the nursing home setting, a preferred intensity of care (PIC) or preferred intensity of treatment (PIT) form is used as an additional tool to enable patients or their designated representatives to clarify treatment wishes. Depending on the facility, such forms include yes/no boxes to check to address a number of medical interventions available in the nursing home, such as CPR, nasogastric or artificial feeding methods, IV antibiotics, and transfers to the hospital.

Care Options for the Aging Patient

For many aging patients, hospitalization represents a sentinel event, triggering a downward spiral of health and function (Fitzsimmons, 2011). Social issues as well as medical issues are brought to light when a frail patient is hospitalized. However, once the crisis of hospitalization has arrived, the nurse needs to look ahead toward discharge planning. Some discussion of post-hospitalization plans should even take place at the time of admission. When the subject of post-hospitalization discharge planning is broached, many older patients oppose returning to anywhere but home. Fortunately, a variety of housing and care options exist for the aging patient. These are outlined in the following subsections.

Independent Living

The older adult has many options for independent living beyond remaining at home. Life care communities or continuing care retirement centers offer an independent living option, with an opportunity to "age in place" if the individual requires more care as time progresses. Often, the independent living community offers apartment or town home living, with or without meals. Support such as housekeeping and social activities are available. Many facilities also offer assisted living and skilled nursing care so that residents can remain in the same community as their levels of need increase. The benefits of such communities are many. Most importantly, residents may move back and forth between levels of care as their health needs dictate, and couples with differing levels of health needs can be accommodated within one building.

Senior supported housing can vary from low-income apartment complexes for seniors that are subsidized by the government to privately paid apartments that provide some or all meals, housekeeping, and laundry services, in addition to social activities and transportation. Health plans and Medicare do not cover the expense of senior supported housing.

Adult Day Health Care and Adult Day Care

Adult day health care offers a program of health services, such as nursing care and therapy, meals, social and recreational activities, and social work services, in a structured daytime program. Individuals who require health services, social interaction, or supervision during the day can attend while continuing to live at home or in another care setting. Some programs offer transportation. A second type of adult day care, based on a social model, offers few or no health services. The emphasis of the social day care program is on fostering socialization among older adults. These programs aim to keep seniors as active and healthy as possible. These programs offer respite for families and caregivers who need some time away from the caregiver role.

Residential Care Facilities

A residential care facility is the formal name for the type of facility commonly referred to as "board and care" living. Their licensing oversight varies by state, falling under the department of health. These facilities provide on-site unlicensed caregivers 24 hours a day and assistance with ADLs such as bathing, dressing, and feeding. They provide three meals a day, social activities, housekeeping, laundry services, and limited transportation. Some facilities provide medication supervision by unlicensed personnel and are not medically focused. Many are operated by individual families.

Assisted Living Facilities

Assisted living facilities also are licensed as residential care facilities, but they tend to be larger in size, often with 50 to 200 residents, and many are part of a corporation that operates assisted living facilities

ETHICAL ISSUES Regarding Care of MS Patients with Urinary Retention Issues

Many patients with multiple sclerosis (MS) who are ambulatory and able to independently carry out most of their ADLs develop some degree of urinary retention due to their MS. Often, these individuals live in assisted living settings to maximize their independence. Most assisted living facilities will not accept residents with indwelling catheters. What should the nurse do when the individual develops moderate to significant urinary retention, resulting in multiple urinary tract infections and hospitalization for urosepsis?

Some options include:

- Discuss with the resident the risk/benefit of long-term catheter use; insist the resident consent to an indwelling catheter and move to a nursing home.
- Act as a patient advocate and discuss with the assisted living facility the possibility of obtaining a waiver to allow the individual with an indwelling catheter to remain living there.
- Discuss the risk/benefits of long-term urinary retention such as further damage to the bladder, antibiotic-resistant urinary tract infections, and the potential for urosepsis.
- Discuss treating the complications of urinary retention, such as urinary tract infections, when they occur.
- Discuss the goals of care with the patient given the progressive nature of the multiple sclerosis diagnosis, and determine whether the benefits of living in assisted living rather than a nursing home outweigh the risks of urinary retention and probable recurrent sepsis with hospitalization and death.

throughout the country. Most require individuals to be ambulatory, use a walker, or be able to propel their wheelchairs to a common dining area. Rarely are they able to accommodate special diets requiring modified food textures or special liquid consistencies. For example, rarely will an assisted living facility provide a puree diet with honey-thick liquid drinks. Some facilities will only accept an incontinent resident if that individual is able to manage her incontinence products independently. See the Ethical Issues box regarding care of patients with multiple sclerosis who have urinary retention issues.

These facilities cannot accommodate individuals who are bedbound. If an individual requires daily nursing care for problems such as pressure ulcers or an indwelling urinary catheter, the facility must apply for a special waiver to allow the person to remain in the facility. With such large variances in amenities, family members are encouraged to thoroughly examine what the assisted living facility will provide or allow in the way of services before placing a deposit. All types of residential care facilities are licensed by the department of health in the state where they are located.

Intermediate/Skilled Nursing Care

There are times when a frail aging patient has health needs that are beyond what can be provided in a home, board and care, or assisted living facility. In these situations, long-term care in an intermediate care or skilled nursing facility might be the best and, in some cases, only option. A skilled nursing facility may also be called a nursing facility, a nursing home, a convalescent home or hospital, or occasionally a rest home.

Intermediate care facilities (ICFs) and skilled nursing facilities (SNFs) are licensed by the department of health in the state where they are located. ICFs care for people who are moderately independent but require 24-hour-a-day supervision and assistance, as well as intermittent licensed nursing care. ICFs can provide special diets and moderate help with ADLs such as bathing and dressing. However, they cannot accept individuals who are nonambulatory, incontinent, or require skilled nursing care. ICFs tend to cost less than SNF care, reflecting a lower level of staffing and personal assistance.

Skilled nursing care is usually needed for a short period of time to recover from an acute illness or injury, often following hospitalization. Skilled nursing care is care that must be delivered by a licensed nurse, such as IV therapy, complicated wound care, or nasogastric or gastrostomy tube feedings. Individuals requiring daily physical, occupational, or speech therapy also would qualify for skilled therapy services. Health plans and Medicare cover skilled services and pay for nursing home days that meet established criteria.

Most residents in nursing homes receive custodial care. Custodial care residents live in a nursing home for an extended period of time, sometimes for the remainder of their lives. Some individuals recover enough to move to a less intensive level of care. For those who do not, custodial care provides a higher level of 24-hour-a-day supervision and assistance with ADLs. Licensed nursing staff are on site 24 hours a day to administer medications and deliver other nursing care. Residents who require walkers or wheelchairs for mobility and those who are bedbound or incontinent can be cared for in this setting. Some nursing homes are secured with perimeter fencing and a locked entrance/exit gate to enable those individuals with dementia who are prone to wandering to ambulate freely without becoming injured.

Medical management in the nursing home is handled on site by a physician and often a nurse practitioner who see residents at the facility. This nurse practitioner may be a **gerontological nurse practitioner (GNP),** a registered nurse with a master's degree from a nurse practitioner program specializing in the care of older adults. GNPs diagnose and manage acute and chronic diseases, using a holistic approach to address the medical, psychosocial, and functional needs of older adults.

Home Care

Older adults who choose to live independently in their homes for as long as possible can turn to supportive services, such as home care, to provide the needed assistance. Two types of home care are available: home health care and private duty care. The main difference between the two is who pays for the service.

Traditional hospital care involving IV therapy, tube feedings, some forms of dialysis, wound vacuums for pressure ulcer management, and oxygen therapy are now administered in the home. This is partially in response to individuals' preference for care in the home and, in some cases, in response to hospitals' efforts to rein in costs. Home health care may be covered by an individual's health plan, Medicare, or Medicaid if a physician determines the individual needs intermittent care by at least one professional, such as a registered nurse, physical therapist, occupational therapist, speech therapist, or social worker. A home health aide may be used if requested by the nurse or therapist coordinating the care.

The nurse's role as part of discharge planning during the patient's hospitalization is to determine if the patient, or a willing and able caregiver, is capable of administering such care in the home environment with support from the home health nurse. The ANA scope and standards of gerontological nursing practice, discussed in Chart 10–1 (p. 242), identify the nurse as the professional whose role it is to develop the discharge plan. The nurse should begin the teaching process before the individual leaves the hospital, with home health nurses providing specialized care and reinforcement of teaching. Home health nurses typically deliver intermittent care; they may visit daily, several times a week, or weekly, depending on the individual's needs. If an individual's care needs exceed what the family can provide or a home health nurse can accomplish in a home visit, the individual may need care in a skilled nursing facility setting.

Private duty or continuous care is rendered in the home by registered nurses or nursing assistants, homemakers, or companions with the goal to provide personal care and companionship. Caregivers are hired and paid privately by the individual receiving care or through an agency. Some long-term care insurance policies cover in-home private duty care.

Hospice

Hospice services are requested by patients and family members seeking expertise in end-of-life care. These services have been available in the home setting for a number of years. Hospice services also have been available in nursing homes for nearly 10 years. Once a patient is determined to be appropriate for hospice services in a nursing home, the expectations change from cure to acceptance that a decline is inevitable. At that time, the goals for the patient's care change to promoting comfort and quality for the remainder of the patient's life.

Palliative Care

Palliative care aims to relieve suffering and improve the quality of living and dying. It aims to address physical, psychological, social, spiritual, and practical expectations and needs of an individual with an acute or chronic life-threatening illness. Palliative care programs can provide transitions from symptom management to hospice care for the elderly as needed. See Chapter 11 for further discussion of the interaction between palliative care and hospice.

Innovations in Caring for the Aging Patient

Innovations in caring for the aging patient have been slow to evolve, primarily due to lack of funding and lack of mechanisms for reimbursement under traditional Medicare and Medicaid models. Innovations currently underway include team-based primary care in the home, the Program for All-Inclusive Care of the Elderly, and elder cohousing communities.

Team-Based Primary Care in the Home

The idea of health care professionals caring for an individual in the home is not new. Years ago, doctors made house calls to patients' homes. As communities grew, medical clinics emerged, mechanisms for funding health care changed with the advent of Medicare and Medicaid, and the days of house calls by a physician came to an end. The U.S. Department of Veterans Affairs (VA) has supported a program with home visits by a physician, a nurse practitioner, and an interdisciplinary team since its inception in 1972. The VA Home-Based Primary Care (HBPC) program provides comprehensive primary care in the homes of veterans with complex chronic disabling disease. Unlike home care that is focused on episodic, time-limited, and focused skilled care, HBPC provides comprehensive longitudinal care. However, most team-based care is only available for those with veterans benefits (Department of Veterans Affairs, 2007). There are community initiatives exploring home-based primary care such as the one in Durham, North Carolina, described at www.dukemagazine.duke.edu/issues/070810/depobs.html.

Weblink: Home-Based Primary Care in Durham, N.C.

Program of All-Inclusive Care for the Elderly

This government-sponsored program (Program of All-Inclusive Care for the Elderly, or PACE) was developed in the mid-1980s to provide all-inclusive care to the elderly through both national (Medicare) and state (Medicaid) government. An interdisciplinary team, consisting of professional and paraprofessional staff, assesses participants' needs, develops care plans, and delivers all services (including acute care services and, when necessary, nursing facility services), which are integrated for a seamless provision of total care. PACE programs provide social and medical services, primarily in an adult day health center, supplemented by in-home and referral services in accordance with the participant's needs. The PACE service package must include all Medicare- and Medicaid-covered services, as well as other services determined necessary by the interdisciplinary team for the care of the PACE participant.

PACE providers receive monthly Medicare and Medicaid capitation payments for each eligible enrollee. Medicare-eligible participants who are not eligible for Medicaid pay monthly premiums equal to the Medicaid capitation amount, but no deductibles, coinsurance, or other type of Medicare or Medicaid cost-sharing applies. PACE providers assume full financial risk for participants' care without limits on amount, duration, or scope of services (CMS, 2011).

Elder Cohousing

Another new and innovative housing option is elder cohousing. The concept is built on a Denmark-inspired, 30-year-old community planning model typically developed for intergenerational populations. In the past few years, it has become a focus for individuals over age 55. Cohousing communities exist in California, Virginia, and Colorado, and they exhibit similarities to a townhouse or condominium development run by a homeowners' association. The difference is that the residents are individuals who like living and doing things together. One community has 11 households, and all are represented on the board of directors. Members range in age from 55 to 75, with many professionals; some are retired, others are still working. Such communities are designed with the goal of encouraging aging in place through the use of universal design elements and an emphasis on home care (Nasser, 2009).

Innovations in Technology for the Aging Patient

Rapid advances in technology are beginning to have an impact on care of the aging patient in both traditional and nontraditional settings. With appropriate applications of technology, older adults who choose to remain at home or to live in board and care and assisted living during their aging years will be able to do so successfully. Challenges involving telephone communication, medication administration, and overall patient monitoring may be addressed using new technology.

Telephone Communication

The challenges for the older adult in using the telephone are numerous, due to hearing and vision difficulties. Traditional methods to address

RESEARCH OPPORTUNITIES Related to Technology

Research	Clinical Impact
How does body monitoring affect the health status of patients?	Constant body monitoring could identify changing homeostasis and would enhance early intervention.
Does the use of home dispensing machines decrease the frequency and adverse affects of medication error?	The dispensing, and remote adjustment, of medications in the home could prevent administration of the wrong medication, wrong administration time, and wrong dosage for patients who may be confused.
Does the use of technology increase the patient's quality of life?	Evaluate the patient's perception of quality of life with the use of technology and the ability to remain in her home.

such problems include phones with higher volume and text telephones (TTY) for those whose hearing renders them incapable of hearing speech over the phone. The TTY device allows an individual to type into a TTY keyboard, which generates tones that are converted into letters by another TTY device. Newer "smart" phones provide additional options for the aging patient to communicate. For example, many individuals are moving to the Voice over Internet Protocol (VOIP), which involves using the Internet rather than traditional phone lines to carry voices. The advantage is that an individual can communicate in several formats such as voice and text or through streaming video with multiple people at the same time. Also, videoconferencing is an ideal communication tool for the elderly. It is accessible to anyone with a computer, Internet service, and an attached camera and microphone, which many computers come with. The most commonly used videoconferencing application is Skype, which is free and easy to use (Berkenkamp, 2011).

Medication Administration Technology

Medication administration has advanced beyond the traditional pill reminder, divided up for time of day and days of the week in the home setting. Traditional methods such as pill reminders or alarm clocks that ring when a medication is due do not ensure the patient living at home is taking medications as prescribed. For those individuals, greater support may be needed to make sure they are taking their medication properly. Newer technologies offer devices that are the size of a small TV and serve as an "ATM for patient medications." Such devices are connected wirelessly to software that contains an individual's medication administration record, and they can be adjusted remotely by a pharmacist or health care provider. The device reminds patients when to take medications, selects the correct dose, and delivers it from the machine. (Medications are loaded via blister packs.) Such technology is beneficial for the home-dwelling patient who is forgetful, for someone with a complex drug regimen, and for someone who has difficulty understanding written directions (INRange Systems, 2011).

Continuous Body Monitoring Technology

Older adults who live at home alone may benefit from the use of technology involving continuous body monitoring. One device available is an armband, similar to a wristwatch in size, that is applied and collects continuous data on calories burned, duration and level of physical activity, and sleep–wake cycles. Using wireless transmission and software analysis, family members not living with the aging patient can be notified if, for example, the individual falls or fails to get out of bed. Those who might benefit most from this technology are individuals who live alone or have an inability to call for help. Such technology might be useful in collecting accurate data for those with chronic conditions to monitor overall health and physical status over time (Matthews, 2006). Future research regarding the use of technology and the older adult patient are presented in the Research Opportunities feature.

Summary

The older adult population will continue to grow and become the largest cohort of patients. In order to care for this cohort appropriately, the nurse must understand the physiologic changes that occur with aging and the most common challenges that the older adult will face during this time in his life.

NCLEX® PRACTICE

1. A nurse identifies the following when assessing an older patient. Which findings would the nurse evaluate as an expected age-related change? (select all that apply)

1. Shallow inspirations
2. Decreased taste sensation
3. Point of maximal impulse at the sixth left intercostal space, midclavicular line
4. Hyperactive bowel sounds
5. Presence of actinic keratosis on forearms

2. A 70-year-old patient asks which immunizations and screening are recommended for her. In compliance with the United States Preventative Services Task Force (USPSTF) for patients over 65 years of age, the nurse provides which information? (select all that apply)

1. Pneumococcal vaccine yearly
2. Tetanus vaccine every 4 years
3. Yearly vision screening
4. Fecal occult blood testing yearly
5. Influenza vaccine yearly

3. A nurse practitioner frequently refers to the Beers criteria when evaluating a patient's medications. What is the purpose of these criteria?
1. To list those medications that are illegal to use with older adults
2. To provide information on dosage changes necessary in older adults
3. To document the testing required when some medications are used in older adults
4. To identify medications that may be ineffective or harmful to older adults

4. An elderly patient presents from a nursing home, weeping and complaining of nausea. When placing the blood pressure cuff on the patient's arm, the nurse notices a large hand-shaped contusion on her bicep. What should the nurse do?
1. Confront the patient about what she did to deserve the injury
2. Ensure confidentiality and inquire directly about the contusion
3. Ignore the contusion because the patient is complaining of nausea
4. Call the local news to report the injury

5. A patient is being discharged from the hospital after recovering from a transient ischemic attack. The patient has no residual paralysis or parasthesias, is ambulatory with a cane, is continent, and is able to communicate. The patient will require assistance with medications. The patient and family want to consider a housing option that will meet the patient's needs and be covered by insurance. Which care option is most appropriate for this patient?
1. Skilled nursing care
2. Adult day care
3. Residential care facility
4. Senior supported housing

6. Which strategies, proposed by the nurse, would support the activity theory of aging for an 80-year-old patient? (select all that apply)
1. Joining a senior activity center
2. Offering to provide day care for a granddaughter's infant
3. Working crossword puzzles
4. Sharing quilting skills with a group of new quilters in her guild
5. Volunteering at a neighborhood library

Answers to NCLEX Practice questions can be found in Appendix D in the Osborn Student Resources at nursing.pearsonhighered.com. Practice additional NCLEX questions online at the Student Resources site.

Pearson Nursing Student Resources Find additional review materials at: **nursing.pearsonhighered.com**

REFERENCES

Adams, M. P., & Koch, R. W. (2010). *Pharmacology: Connections to nursing practice.* Upper Saddle River, NJ: Pearson.

Administration on Aging (AOA). (2009). A profile of older Americans: 2009. Retrieved from http://www.aoa.gov/AORoot/Aging_profile/2009

Agency for Healthcare Research and Quality (AHRQ). (2009). 2009 National healthcare quality & disparities reports. Retrieved from http://www.ahrq.gov/qual/grdr09.htm

Alexander, R. (Ed.). (2006). Avoiding fraud when buying long-term care insurance. Retrieved from http://www.consumerlawpage.com

Alzheimer's Association. (2010). Alzheimer's disease facts and figures. Retrieved from http://www.alz.org/alzheimers_facts_and_figures.asp

American Academy of Orthopaedic Surgeons. (2012). Bunions. Retrieved from http://orthoinfo.aaos.org/topic.cfm?topic=A00155

American Cancer Society. (2010). What are the key statistics about prostate cancer? Retrieved from http://www.cancer.org

American Nurses Association. (2010). *Scope and standards of gerontological nursing practice.* Silver Spring, MD: Nursebooks.org.

Barnes, D. E., Covinsky, K. E., Whitmer, R. A., Kuller, L. H., Lopez, O. L., & Yaffe, K. (2009). Predicting risk of dementia in older adults. *Neurology, 73*(3):173–179. doi: 10.1212/WNL.0b013e3181a81636

Baseline, R. W. (2009). Approach to geriatric patient. Retrieved from http://merckmanuals.com/professional/sec23/ch340b.html

Bauer, J. (2009). Green House concept combines best new thinking for elderly. *The Grand Rapids Press.* Retrieved from http://www.globalaging.org/elderrights/us/2009/green.htm

Beers, M. H. (1997). Explicit criteria for determining potentially inappropriate medication use by the elderly. *Archives of Internal Medicine, 157,* 1531–1536.

Berkenkamp, A. (2011). Skype—the ideal communication for the elderly. Retrieved from http://www.theelderlytechnologyandsocialmedia.blogspot.com

Centers for Disease Control and Prevention (CDC). (2012). Pneumonia can be prevented – vaccines can help. Retrieved from http://www.cdc.gov/Features/Pneumonia/

Centers for Medicare & Medicaid Services. (n.d.). Proof of citizenship. Retrieved from http://www.cms.hhs.gov/MedicaidEligibility/05_ProofofCitizenship.asp

Centers for Medicare & Medicaid Services (CMS). (2012). Immunizations. Retrieved from http://www.cms.gov/Medicare/Prevention/Immunizations/index.html?redirect=/immunizations

Centers for Medicare & Medicaid Services (CMS). (2011). PACE fact sheet. Retrieved from https://www.cms.gov/Medicare/Health-Plans/pace/downloads/PACEFactSheet.pdf

Cibulka, N. (2011). Update on breast cancer screening. *Journal for Nurse Practitioners, 7*(1):67–68.

Congdon, J. G., DeCamp, J., Fletcher, K., Henningson, B., Kaplan, K., & Resnick, B. (2001). *Scope and standards of gerontological nursing practice* (2nd ed.). Silver Spring, MD: American Nurses Association.

Department of Veterans Affairs. (2007). *Home-Based Primary Care Program: VHA handbook 11404.01.* Washington, DC: Veterans Health Administration.

Elzavy, B., & Higgins, K. E. (2011). The geriatric assessment. *American Family Physician, 83*(1): 48–56.

Falicov, C. J. (1998). *Latino families in therapy: A guide to multicultural practice.* New York: Guilford Press.

Fitzsimmons, S. (2011). Healthy aging. *Western Schools CE Express,* 67–118.

Folstein, M. F., Folstein, S. E., & McHugh, P. R. (1975). Mini-Mental State: A practical method for grading the cognitive state of patients for the clinician. *Journal of Psychiatric Research, 12*(3), 189–198.

Galanti, G. A. (2008). *Caring for patients from different cultures.* Philadelphia: University of Pennsylvania Press.

Harwood, J. (2007). *Understanding communication and aging.* Thousand Oaks: Sage.

Hauser, R. A. (2012). Parkinson disease treatment & management. Retrieved from http://www.emedicine.medscape.com/article/1831191-overview

HealthyPeople.gov. (2010). Healthy people 2020. Retrieved from http://www.healthypeople.gov/2020/topicsobjectives2020/default.aspx

Heron, M. P., & Smith, B. L. (2007). Deaths: Leading causes for 2003. *National Vital Statistic Report, 5*(10), 1–92.

Hobbs, F. B. (2011). The elderly population. Retrieved from http://www.census.gov/population/www/pop-profile/elderpop.html

Inouye, S., van Dyck, C., Alessi, C., Galkin, S., Siegal, A., & Horwitz, R. (1990). Clarifying confusion: The confusion assessment method. *Annals of Internal Medicine, 113*(12), 941–948.

InRange Systems. (2011). EMMA. Retrieved from http://www.inrangesystems.com/#1

Jaffe-Gill, de Benedictis, & Segal. (2008). Elder abuse and neglect. Retrieved from http://helpguide.org/mental/elder_abuse_physical_emotional_sexual_neglect.htm

Lipson, J. G., & Dibble, S. L. (Eds.). (2005). *Culture & critical care.* San Francisco: UCSF Nursing Press.

Ljubuncid, P., & Reznick, A. Z. (2009). The evolutionary theories of aging revisited—A mini-review. *Gerontology, 55,* 205–216. doi10.1159/000200772

Matthews, J. T. (2006). Existing and emerging healthcare devices for elders to use at home. *Generations, 30*(2), 13–19.

Mayo Clinic. (2007a). Colchicine (systemic). Retrieved from http://222.mayoclnica.cm/health/drug-information/DR202160

Mayo Clinic. (2007b). Probenecid and colchicine (oral route). Retrieved from http://www.mayoclici.com/health/drug-information/DR600297

Moore, T. J., Cohen, M. R., & Furberg, C. D. (2007). Serious adverse drug events reported to the Food and Drug Administration, 1998–2005. *Archive of Internal Medicine, 167*(16), 1752–1759.

Mui, A., & Shibusawa, T. (2008). *Asian American elders in the twenty-first century: Key indicators of well being.* New York: Columbia University Press.

Nasser, J. E. (2009). Seniors at home in co-housing. *USA Today.* Retrieved from http://www.usatoday.com/money/economy/housing/2009-05-03-co-housing_N.htm

National Center on Elder Abuse. (2007a). About NCEA. Retrieved from http://www.ncea.aoa.gov/ncearott/Main_Site/index.aspx

National Center on Elder Abuse. (2007b). Adult protective services. Retrieved from http://www.ncea.aoa.gov/ncearoot/main_site/find_help/APS/About_APS.aspx

National Center on Elder Abuse. (2007c). Major types of elder abuse. Retrieved from http://www.ncea.aoa.gov/ncearoot/Main_Site/FAQ/Basics/Types_of_abuse.aspx

National Federation of the Blind. (2012). Legally blind. Retrieved from http://www.nfb.org/legally-blind-definition

National Guideline Clearing House. (2007). Preventive services for adults. Retrieved from http://www.guideline.gov/summry/summary.aspx?doc_id=11699&nbr+0060046&string=P

National Institute of Neurological Disorders and Stroke. (2007). Normal pressure hydrocephalus information page. Retrieved from http://www.ninds.nih.gov/disorders/normal_pressure_hydrocephalus

National Osteoporosis Foundation. (2007). Fast facts on osteoporosis. Retrieved from http://www.nof.org/osteoporosis/diseasefacts.htm

Pighills, A. C., Torgerson, D. J., Sheldon, T. A., Drummond, A. E., & Bland, J. M. (2011). Environmental assessment and modification to prevent falls in older people. *Journal of the American Geriatrics Society, 59*(1):26–33.

Poh, C. H., Navarro-Rodriguez, T., & Fass, R. (2010). Review: Treatment of gastroesophageal reflux disease in the elderly. *American Journal of Medicine, 123*(6):496–501.

Polypharmacy. (2007). Retrieved from http://www.Mercksource.com/pp/us/cns_searchresults.jsp

Pool, I. (2007). Demographic dividends: Determinants of development or merely window of opportunity? *Aging Horizons, 7*, 28–35.

Porth, C. M., & Matfin, G. (2009). Pathophysiology: concepts of altered health states. (8th ed.). Philadelphia: Lippincott Williams & Wilkins.

Rantz, M. J., Phillips, L., aud, M., Popejoy, L., Marek, K. D., Hicks, L. L., et al. (2011). Evaluation of aging in place model with home care services and registered nurse care coordination in senior housing. *Nursing Outlook, 59*(1), 37–46.

Razzi, C. C. (2009). Incorporating the Beers criteria may reduce ED visits in elderly persons. *Journal of Emergency Nursing, 35*(5):453–454.

Red Horse, J. (1981). American Indian families. Paper presented at the Conference on American Indian Family Strengths and Stress. Elmsford, NY: Pergamon Press.

Reuben, D. B., Herr, K. A., Pacala, J. T., Pollock, B. G., Potter, J. F., & Semala, T. P. (2007). *Geriatrics at your fingertips: 2007–2008* (9th ed.). New York: American Geriatrics Society.

Roy, H., & Russell, C. (2005). *The encyclopedia of aging & the elderly.* MedRounds ebook. Retrieved from http://www.medrounds.org/encyclopedia-of-aging/2005/12/activity-theory.html

Shawler, C. (2010). Assessing and maintaining mental health in elderly individuals. *Nursing Clinics of North America,45*(4):635–650.

Tovey, D. (Ed.). (2007). *Clinical evidence handbook.* London: BMJ.

Urden, L. D., Stacy, K. M., & Lough, M. E. (2009). *Critical care nursing: Diagnosis and management* (6th ed.). St. Louis, Mosby.

U.S. Census Bureau (2011). *State & county quick facts.* Retrieved from http://quickfacts.census.gov/qfd/states/00000.html

U.S. Preventive Services Task Force. (2012) Screening for cervical cancer. Retrieved from http://www.uspreventiveservicestaskforce.org/uspstf/uspscerv.htm

U.S. Preventive Services Task Force. (2008). Screening for colorectal cancer. Retrieved from http://www.uspreventiveservicestaskforce.org/uspstf/uspscolo.htm

U.S. Preventive Services Task Force. (2008). Screening for prostate cancer: U.S. preventive services task force recommendation statement. *Annals of Internal Medicine, 149,* 185–191.

Voyer, P., McCusker, J., Cole, M. G., St-Jacques, S., & Khomenko, L. (2007). Factors associated with delirium severity among older patients. *Journal of Clinical Nursing, 16*(5), 819–831.

Waszynski, C. M. (2007). The confusion assessment method (CAM). *Try This: Best practices in nursing care to older adults, 13.* New York University College of Nursing: The Hartford Institute for Geriatric Nursing.

WebMD. (March 3, 2010). Elderly skin conditions. Retrieved from http://www.webmd.com/skin-problems-and-treatments/guide/elderly-skin-conditions

Caring for the Patient at End of Life

11 CHAPTER

Sally Brush
Cheryl Wraa

Outcome-Based Learning Objectives

After studying this chapter, the learner will be able to:

1. Differentiate ethical issues that influence decisions in end-of-life care.
2. Critique the nurse's role in the advance directives process during end-of-life care.
3. Compare and contrast pharmacological and nonpharmacological therapies used for relief of pain at end of life.
4. Compare and contrast the interdisciplinary team's roles in planning and delivering end-of-life care.
5. Generate a plan for providing hospice during end-of-life care.
6. Critique the principles of palliative care.

KEY TERMS

futile care p.263
hospice p.266
palliative care p.259
palliative care team p.261

PARTICIPATING IN THE CARE OF PATIENTS AT THE END OF LIFE can be an extremely difficult and complex situation for caregivers. This is particularly true in the acute care setting, because the critical nature of the patient's illness or injury is often sudden and unexpected. When a patient is injured or becomes ill suddenly, the health care team focuses on a curative model. As the patient progresses, however, it may become clear that further care may be futile. It can be difficult for both the health care team and the patient and family to change from a curative mindset to one of comfort care. Patient and family satisfaction depends largely on the information the family receives during this time and the way it is provided. After the patient has died, the family may not remember exactly what was done or said, but they will remember how they felt.

End of Life in the Acute Care Setting

Palliative care, comprehensive care focused on alleviating suffering and promoting the quality of a patient's remaining life when living with a chronic, life-threatening, or terminal illness, allows patients and families to guide treatment based on identified goals for care at the end of life (Morgan, 2011). Although palliative care is well defined for patients who are terminally ill, it has not been well defined for patients in the acute care setting who are critically ill.

For health care providers, several reasons exist why making the transition from providing "curative care" to "comfort care" can be difficult. First, ethical dilemmas may arise on a daily basis as to the choice of extending life versus postponing death. Second, nurses are influenced by their own values, culture, religion, education, and life experiences. Third, the nurse's role as a member of the health care team requires both the nurse and others to assist patients and families to make fully informed decisions with full knowledge of their options. It is critical that everyone involved with the patient's care communicate with one another and reach consensus prior to discussions with the family. This chapter discusses key nursing interventions that are important at all phases of patient care, but especially at the end of life. These key nursing interventions include:

- Recognition of autonomy
- Honesty
- Expert communication
- Presence
- Compassion
- Touch
- Assisting in transcendence or developing a sense of meaning and peace with death (Saunders, 2007).

Advances in technology, changes in managed care, and changes in social and family structures have also added to the complexity of end-of-life care (Wallace, Grossman, Campbell, Robert, Lange, & Shea, 2009). Advances in technology in critical care medicine have added therapeutic options never before available; these are discussed in the following text. Today, patients who were considered physiologically unstable, including those who are elderly or chronically ill, are receiving operations and complex procedures. Most will survive their operations and recover with few or no complications. Issues arise, however, when complications occur. In these cases, the patient continues to deteriorate and further care is often deemed futile.

EVIDENCE-BASED PRACTICE For End-of-Life Care

Clinical Problem

In the hospital setting, conflicts between families and health care providers regarding end-of-life decisions are common. Decisions should be a cooperative effort to achieve treatment goals. When discussions are perceived as conflicts, families often feel misunderstood or isolated, and may doubt the health care providers' commitment to the patient's well-being (Bjarnason, 2009).

Research Findings

Decisions made regarding a patient's care are often based solely on clinical data (Mahon, 2010). Within the acute care setting, patients and families may be confused and upset because of a new diagnosis or the exacerbation of a chronic illness. The psychological stress felt by the patient and family can be increased by the need to make decisions regarding patient care. Of all of the caregivers, nurses spend the most time with patients and families at the end of life (Wallace et al., 2009). For this reason, it is imperative that nurses communicate well and are able to assist the patient and family in understanding the plan of care and in making health care decisions.

Implications for Nursing Practice

Supportive communication involves active listening and letting the patient and family know that providers are present and are accepting of their strong emotions. For the family, knowing that caregivers listen to and understand what they are going through is therapeutic. A model developed by Jonsen, Siegler, and Winslade (2006) to guide the integration of ethics into patient care decision making is very applicable for the nurse to use in assisting the patient and family. The model's four dimensions are outlined in Chart 11–1.

Critical Thinking Questions with answers can be found in the Osborn Student Resources at nursing.pearsonhighered.com.

Source: Bjarnason, D. (2009). Nursing, religiosity, and end-of-life care: Interconnections and implications. *Nursing clinics of North America, 44,* 517–525; Jonsen, Siegler, & Winslade. (2006) *Clinical ethics: A practical approach to ethical decisions in clinical medicine* (6th ed.). New York: McGraw-Hill Companies; Mahon, M. M. (2010). Clinical decision making in palliative care and end-of-life care. *Nursing Clinics of North America, 45,* 345–362.

CHART 11–1 Integration of Ethics Into Patient Care Decision Making

Dimension	Example
Medical indications	The medical indication dictates the choice of therapies. For instance, the patient with a chronic illness may be treated with medications that allow her to live as well as possible. The patient's medical condition should be the first consideration in treatment options.
Patient preferences	Decisions should be made in terms of the patient's values, preferences, and goals of care. Before stating preferences, it is important that the patient and family understand the disease, injury, or other pathophysiologic considerations. They also need to understand the goals of treatment, the likelihood of achieving the goal, and the burden of the treatment. What will the patient's quality of life be if they agree to the treatment?
Quality of life	Quality of life is not only about what *quality* of life is acceptable to the patient, but also an understanding of what quality of life is realistic with the proposed treatment. Decisions should not be made solely on whether the patient will live or die, but also about how the patient lives.
Contextual factors	Contextual factors include relationships (family and social), the hospital, and financial and legal factors. They refer to identifying elements that affect the ability to implement the decision. For instance, a patient may wish to receive treatment at home, but his insurance may not cover home health and may require the patient to go to a skilled nursing facility instead.

Conversations regarding the option to continue to perform procedures may be a barrier to discussions with families when offering comfort care as opposed to curative care. For instance, although the patient may have a devastating traumatic brain injury, the health care team may tell the family that the patient has developed pneumonia and offer to start antibiotics. The team providing care may view the patient's failure to respond medically as a failure on the part of the medical system or team. The nurse working in this environment may need to address her feeling of defeat as well as to assist the family in approaching the medical team to begin discussions regarding end-of-life issues. See the Evidence-Based Practice feature for discussion surrounding decision making between families and health care providers.

End of Life in the Intensive Care Unit

Typically, patients who face life-threatening complications are placed in the intensive care unit (ICU) on varying degrees of life support. The ICU is one area where many technological innovations have been developed to prevent death; nonetheless, many patients die in this environment. Monitoring in the ICU provides an enormous amount of data regarding the patient's condition, including pulse, blood pressure, cardiac output, and oxygen saturation. The data may be confusing to the family, because one bit of information could bode well at the same time that another bodes poorly. Patients and families do not make an instant transition from hope of survival to acceptance of death and pursuit of comfort care.

Nurses spend most of their time at the bedside and are integral to relaying and reinforcing information to patients' families and other members of the health care team. Families in crisis often need information repeated or explained in a different way. It is essential that every member of the health care team, especially nurses because of their close and frequent contact with the patient and family, be included in discussions with the family and participate in the patient's plan of care. Nurses are instrumental in helping the family not feel abandoned at the end of life. A core nursing function at the end of life is to be present and bear witness during the dying process and to help the patient and family find meaning in the experience.

Families, when surveyed, revealed that not just communication but continuity of communication is an essential ingredient (Morgan, 2011). As the plan of care shifts from cure to comfort, it is important to repeatedly reassure the family through words and actions that neither they nor their loved one will be ignored or abandoned and that attentive palliative care will be provided.

Research has shown that nurses in the ICU can feel immense frustration and moral distress about the lack of consensus concerning end-of-life care in the critical care arena. In 2008, the Society of Critical Care Medicine updated recommendations published in 2001 for clinicians managing end-of-life care in the intensive care unit (Truog et al., 2008). One of the first steps addressed in this process is preparation of the clinical staff, as well as the patient and family, for what will follow as the patient care goals shift from cure to comfort. Although critical care clinicians often deal with death, planning for end of life is often done poorly. Involvement of end-of-life specialists, either as consultants or as caregivers who assume the care of the dying patient, should be considered. Inclusion of a **palliative care team,** physicians, nurse practitioners, and nurses that specialize in palliative care who provide consultation to the primary team members in interdisciplinary team meetings regarding individual patients may improve outcomes and educate clinicians regarding palliative care. Open communication among all members of the health care team will also assist them in dealing with the psychological and emotional stress incurred by ICU staff who are involved in palliating a dying patient, as discussed further in the Evidence-Based Practice box.

Nurses who do not care for patients who are terminally ill on a daily basis may not have a familiarity with end-of-life care. Research shows that there is a need to improve end-of-life care and to improve palliative care nursing education (Wallace et al., 2009). In the late 1990s, the American Association of Colleges of Nursing (AACN) and the City of Hope National Medical Center developed a core curriculum for end-of-life care called the ELNEC program. This was accomplished through grant funding by the Robert Woods Johnson Foundation. Information about the course and descriptions of the modules is available on the AACN website, www.aacn.nche.edu/ELNEC.

Ethical Issues at End of Life

The transition to end-of-life care in the acute care setting begins with the process of shared decision making to change the focus from care aimed at cure to care aimed at comfort and freedom from pain. When the health care team begins to discuss decisions regarding life-sustaining versus end-of-life interventions, ethical issues and dilemmas are inherent in the discussions. Ethical decision making involves a systematic appraisal of a situation using moral principles and ethical theories to justify the resolution (Monturo & Hook, 2009). All of the principles of ethics, reviewed in Chapter 2 of this textbook, are relevant to end-of-life care by nurses. These include privacy, autonomy, veracity, beneficence, nonmaleficence, and justice.

Advanced Care Planning

Patients must have the capacity to comprehend information in order to make informed consent. If the patient is unable to consent for himself, it is important to determine whether he has done any advanced care planning. Advance directives including *living wills* and *durable power of attorney* and are discussed in detail in Chapter 2.

Safety Alert *It is the nurse's responsibility to be aware of a patient's advance directive and to advocate for respecting the patient's wishes.*

Communication During End-of Life Care

Patients and their families have expressed that communication with caregivers is an extremely important factor during end-of-life care (Mahon, 2010). Even though health care providers feel overburdened with time constraints, it is important to take the time to sit with the patient and family and communicate with them in an open, genuine manner regarding the patient's illness.

Many clinicians have difficulty initiating a straightforward discussion about death with a patient and/or family because they have been trained to restore health. If the primary goal is to make patients well, then death is often viewed as failure. Adding to the conflict is the question of how certain the health care team is about the patient's prognosis. Complex disease processes often complicate prognosis. If the patient, family, and clinicians are always brought back to the goals of care for the patient, decision making becomes easier. For example, the goals of care for a young adult with traumatic injuries who was previously in good health will be considerably different than for an older adult with many preexisting health problems. Taking each new problem/complication at a time to reevaluate goals of care is one method of reducing the complexity of end-of-life decision making.

Caring for the acutely ill patient may require that decisions and interventions be made quickly, although the appropriateness of some of these decisions may become clearer as time passes and the illness takes its course (Morgan, 2011). If the patient is in a teaching hospital, the family may receive conflicting messages from the multiple teams of physicians caring for the patient. It is better to have a representative from each team present during a family meeting and to ask open-ended questions of the family to ascertain if they clearly understand what is discussed. Recommendations are to give information at a ninth-grade level with as little medical jargon as possible. Family members are under stress and their ability to understand large amounts of information is difficult. In addition, many clinicians do not feel comfortable with death and are not trained in good communication skills. This combination creates difficult situations for dying patients and their families. The ability to give compassionate, nurturing, end-of-life care is based on the caregiver's ability to be comfortable with death. Many resources are available to teach clinicians who are generalists in the care of patients about end-of-life and palliative care. One such organization is the End of Life/Palliative Care Resource Center (EPERC) available online at www.eperc.mcw.edu. In addition, the American Association of Colleges of Nursing has developed teaching materials for nurses, nurse educators, and others through the End-of-Life Nursing Education Consortium (ELNEC), including material developed by international nursing specialists in end-of-life care (www.elnec.com).

Weblink: End of Life/Palliative Care Resource Center

Weblink: End-of-Life Nursing Consortium

Ensuring the Patient's Comfort

The transition from curative care to comfort care can be inconsistent; some therapies may be aimed at comfort and some at cure instead of completely rewriting orders to only address the patient's comfort. In a study done by Heyland et al. (2006), patients and their families identified four issues that were considered extremely important in end-of-life care: (1) having trust and confidence in the physicians caring for them, (2) avoiding inappropriate prolonging of death, (3) communicating information about their illness in an honest manner, and (4) completing personal needs (getting papers in order, etc.) and preparing for life's end.

One suggestion for making the transition from curative to comfort care is to completely rewrite the patient's orders and review the plan of care as if the patient were just now being admitted. Each test or intervention should be reviewed for its need and how it will further the patient's wishes, improve symptom relief, and ameliorate emotional or spiritual concerns. The treatment orders should be organized by symptoms

Weblink: Southern California Cancer Pain Initiative

rather than by organ system or disease. The symptom list should include actual and potential symptoms, and each symptom should be managed separately.

Pain

Careful assessment of pain is a critical nursing function that is necessary at all disease stages to determine underlying causes and to make appropriate treatments. Pain at the end of a patient's life is not necessarily related to advanced disease. If the patient is unable to communicate, assessment of pain may rely on evaluation of physical signs, such as consciousness, breathing pattern, change in blood pressure and heart rate, and facial grimaces. Close attention to all body systems followed by thoughtful analysis of the cause of pain will lead to the most appropriate management of pain. Dr. Betty Ferrell (2010), a pioneer in end-of-life care, has outlined several key principles in the management of pain at end of life including the following:

- Vital role of pain assessment,
- Pharmacologic management of pain,
- Integration of complementary therapies,
- Attention to suffering, and
- Use of an interdisciplinary team for management of pain at end of life.

Ferrell (2010) contains excellent information regarding pain management at the end of life.

In dealing with pain at the end of life, it is important to always start with the simplest remedies first before advancing to higher level medications. Combining oral and parenteral pain medications allows for pain control at several sites. When changing from one route or agent to another, it is helpful to use equianalgesic dosing. The Southern California Cancer Pain Initiative (SCCPI) has developed a pocket reference card describing pain management guidelines, opioid side effect management, and equianalgesic dosing. The reference card is available on the SCCPI website (http://sccpi.coh.org) for duplication. The nurse must pay careful attention to all body systems in treating the patient for pain. Use of narcotics and sedatives can lead to reduced bowel motility and severe constipation, which the nurse must also address.

Environment also plays a factor in the patient's comfort. The hospital is rarely considered a peaceful environment, although measures can be taken to enhance the patient's comfort, such as reducing lighting and noise, eliminating unnecessary monitors and machines, removing restraints, and providing room for the patient's significant others. Cultural and spiritual factors such as prayer, ritual, and music can also increase the patient's comfort. See the Ethical Issues box regarding pain management at end of life.

Pharmacologic Therapies

The use of pharmacologic therapies, with consideration for the pharmacokinetics and pharmacodynamics of the drugs used, can ease many or all of the symptoms the dying patient may experience. The symptoms most often experienced by dying patients are pain, fatigue, dyspnea, excessive respiratory secretions, nausea and vomiting, constipation, and diarrhea (Saunders, 2007). In addition to the specifics discussed in the following subsections, the Pharmacology feature provides more information about the use of medications for a patient who is at the end of life.

ETHICAL ISSUES for Pain Management at End of Life

Management of pain at the end of life is the patient's right and the caregiver's duty. Many families state that their loved ones suffered from untreated pain at the end of their lives (Mularski et al., 2009). Failure to treat pain adequately can arise from the caregiver's fear of violating ethical and moral tenets in the administration of pain medication to the dying patient.

At the end of life, the use of opioids, benzodiazepines, and other medications in doses high enough to control the patient's symptoms may unintentionally hasten death. This is referred to as *double effect*, where an action may have two possible effects, one good and one bad. The action is not considered immoral if it is undertaken with the intention of achieving the good effect without intending the bad effect, even though the negative effect may be foreseen. At the end of life, failing to administer a drug to relieve symptoms because it may hasten death is viewed as causing the patient harm and increased suffering.

Opioids

Opioids are the most common class of drug used for the treatment of pain and suffering in the dying patient. Opioids instill analgesia, sedation, and euphoria by binding to receptor sites in the brain and spinal cord to prevent the release of neurotransmitters involved in pain transmission. The most frequently used opioids are morphine, hydromorphone, and fentanyl. Meperidine is not recommended because its metabolite, normeperidine, produces signs of central nervous system (CNS) excitation such as tremors; if not excreted, as in the patient with renal insufficiency, meperidine is toxic to the CNS and places the patient at risk for seizures (Mularski et al., 2009).

Most patients in the acute care setting are already receiving analgesics and may have already developed some tolerance to their effects. For this reason, there is no set dosage for opioids at the end of life. Analgesic drips should be titrated to effect and should not be limited by recommended maximum doses. As stated previously, increasing the titration of the opioid is intended to relieve pain and suffering, not to directly cause death (Tilden & Thompson, 2009).

Safety Alert *It is important to document clearly the indication for increasing the dose.*

It is also appropriate to use anticipatory dosing. For example, when withdrawing mechanical ventilation, increased dyspnea can be anticipated. It would not be sufficient to wait for the patient to experience distress before responding, so adequate medication should be given prior to withdrawing mechanical ventilation (Mahon, 2010).

Benzodiazepines

Benzodiazepines have a synergistic sedative effect with opioids, are anticonvulsants, and may help prevent the development of premorbid seizures (Adams & Koch, 2010). Midazolam, when administered intravenously, changes to a lipophilic (i.e., having an affinity for fat) compound that rapidly penetrates the CNS. The drug is short acting but has a sustained effect when given by continuous infusion. Starting doses for adult continuous infusion range from 1 to 5 mg/hr. Lorazepam is an intermediate-acting benzodiazepine that reaches a peak effect approximately 30 minutes after intravenous infusion. The starting dose for adult continuous infusion is 1 to 8 mg/hr. Further discussion about the use of opioids and benzodiazepines at the end of life is provided in the Ethical Issues box.

PHARMACOLOGY Summary of Drugs Used in End-of-Life Care

Medication Category and Action	Application/Indication	Nursing Responsibility
Opioid analgesics **Action:** Bind with and activate opioid receptors in brain and spinal cord to produce analgesia and euphoria	Treatment of pain and other symptoms associated with dying	Conduct regular, frequent assessment of pain and other symptoms (e.g., shortness of breath, anxiety). Ensure safe and timely reduction of pain and symptom levels. Address barriers to effective pain management, including inappropriate fears of risk of side effects, addiction, respiratory depressions, or hastening of death.
Benzodiazepines **Action:** Produce a calming effect and relax skeletal muscles by increasing the activity of gamma-aminobutyric acid, a major inhibitory neurotransmitter in the brain.	Synergistic sedative effect with opioids. May help prevent development of premorbid seizures.	Same as for opioids.

Neuroleptics

Neuroleptics, such as haloperidol, may be helpful for patients exhibiting delirium. It is important to try to distinguish between anxiety and delirium, an acute state of confusion. The distinction is important because the use of opioids or benzodiazepines can worsen the symptoms of delirium. Starting doses of haloperidol in adults range from 0.5 to 20 mg. Recommendations are to titrate additional doses at 30-minute intervals until symptoms are controlled. The use of restraints should be avoided when possible (Adams & Koch, 2010).

Dyspnea

Dyspnea, which is shortness of breath, can be extremely distressing and frightening. The neuropathways responsible for the sensation are poorly understood (Kuebler, Heidrich, & Esper, 2007). Many patients may be unable to report dyspnea due to their level of consciousness. Physical symptoms that should be considered signs of dyspnea are tachypnea, restlessness, accessory muscle use, grunting at the end of each breath, and nasal flaring. Nonpharmacologic techniques that may lessen the sensation of dyspnea are to (1) elevate the head of the bed to reduce choking sensations and promote expansion of the lungs, and (2) use fans to circulate the air. Cool air directed gently on the face may reduce the perception of breathlessness (Morgan, 2011). The use of oxygen may be effective if the patient is hypoxic, but the use of a face mask may increase the sensation of dyspnea if it makes the patient feel claustrophobic (Morgan, 2011). Opioids are highly effective in relieving dyspnea by depressing respiratory drive; causing vasodilation, which can reduce pulmonary vascular congestion; and producing sedation and euphoria. The use of opioids for relief of dyspnea in a patient who is near death is considered the standard treatment (Kuebler et al., 2007).

Dyspnea is reported in up to half of all dying patients. It is important to educate the family and the patient, if the patient is conscious, regarding the specific symptoms of dyspnea, as well as the ways to relieve the sensation and make the patient comfortable (Morgan, 2011).

Fever

Fevers and infections occur frequently in the acute care setting. For the dying patient, fever can be uncomfortable, and antipyretics should be given. Any measure that would cause the patient more discomfort, such as a cooling blanket or alcohol bath, should not be used.

Complementary and Alternative Therapies

Complementary therapies regarding spiritual aspects of death may be helpful to patients who are at the end of life, as discussed in the accompanying Complementary & Alternative Therapies box (p. 264).

Withdrawal of Life-Sustaining Treatments

The goal of palliative and end-of-life care is to achieve the best quality of life for the patient and her family, consistent with their goals and values, regardless of the patient's location. Palliative care should be offered, discussed, and incorporated into the plan of care at the time of diagnosis of a life-threatening illness. As the disease progresses, the patient or family may decide to forgo or withdraw life-sustaining treatments. When discussing with the family the decision not to initiate cardiopulmonary resuscitation, providing survival statistics to the family can facilitate decision making. Chances of survival to discharge for patients who have suffered an arrest in the hospital range from 6% to 15%, with 30% of survivors suffering a significant decrease in quality of life and the ability to be independent (Mularski et al., 2009). The debate will continue regarding whether futile care must be offered to a patient. **Futile care** can be defined as care that does not produce a benefit to the patient.

Terminal Wean of Mechanical Ventilation

Discontinuation of mechanical ventilation usually occurs when the burdens of continuing life-prolonging interventions outweigh their benefits. Withdrawal of mechanical ventilation should be planned carefully, ensuring the patient's comfort and allowing the family to be present at the bedside if they wish.

An advantage to terminal weaning is that the patient does not develop any signs of upper airway obstruction; with the proper administration of sedatives and analgesics, the patient does not even develop symptoms of acute air hunger. These advantages promote the patient's comfort and reduce the family's anxiety. The disadvantage of terminal weaning is that it may prolong the death by several days and some family members may perceive it as an attempt to have the patient successfully survive separation from the ventilator.

Nancy Yilk

AT THE CORE OF HOLISTIC HEALTH is the recognition of the wholeness of a person, including her human values and life experiences. Use of complementary health care embraces the possibility that there is a spiritual aspect to one's life and dying is holistic in nature.

A British study determined that one of the greatest fears for many Britons is to die alone. More than half the complaints received by the UK National Health Service (NHS) concern end-of-life care, with an emphasis on spiritual matters. The dying process appears to involve an instinctive need for spiritual connection and meaning, requiring compassionate understanding and respect from those who provide end-of-life care (Fenwick & Brayne, 2011).

Spirituality does not necessarily mean religious dogma, but rather an individual's philosophy, values, and understanding of the meaning of life. Nurses are intimately involved with patients and maintain a unique position of safeguarding the patient's wholeness and integrity (Chan, 2010).

In a study aimed to identify the spiritual needs and concerns of neuro-oncology patients from a patient perspective and how nurses currently support the patients, spiritual needs and concerns identified were: supportive family relationships, emotional support, loneliness, religious needs, need to talk, reassurance, anxiety, solitude, denial, plans for the future, thoughts about the meaning of life, end-of-life decisions, and discussion of beliefs (see Chart 11–2). The implications of the findings of this study are that nurses need to be aware and responsive to these spiritual needs (Nixon & Narayanasamy, 2010).

Utilizing a three-step process, the Spiritual Distress Assessment Tool (SDAT) was used in a study attempting to develop a clinically acceptable instrument to assess spiritual distress in hospitalized elderly patients.

Four dimensions of spirituality (Meaning, Transcendence, Values, and Psychosocial Identity) and their corresponding needs were defined (see Chart 11–3). These preliminary results suggest that the SDAT is an acceptable instrument to assess spiritual distress in hospitalized persons. The instrument provides a tool for communication between disciplines of health care providers and other caregivers such as chaplains and hospice workers. Using a shared vocabulary, SDAT provides a new basis for integrating spirituality into the patient's plan of care (Monod, Rochat, Büla, Jobin, Martin, & Spencer, 2010).

CHART 11–2 Examples of Statements Made by Patients Experiencing Unmet Needs

Need for Life Balance	"I know I've got to find a way to cope, but I just can't manage. I just don't have the strength any longer."
Need for Connection	"I think that God has abandoned me."
	"I am no longer able to paint, and it was the painting that kept me in touch with the force that kept me going."
Need for Values Acknowledgement	"I'm just a number here. The staff doesn't know who I am."
Need to Maintain Control	"I don't know what I'm doing here in the hospital. Why hasn't anyone given me any medicine?"
Need to Maintain Identity	"My friends don't come and visit me; my family has no idea of what I'm going through here; I just don't know myself any longer."

Source: Monod, S. M., Rochat, E., Büla, C. J., Jobin, G., Martin, E., & Spencer, B. (2010, December 13). The Spiritual Distress Assessment Tool: An instrument to assess spiritual distress in hospitalized elderly persons. *BMC Geriatrics, 10*, 88.

CHART 11–3 Spiritual Needs Model: Dimensions of Spirituality and Corresponding Needs in Hospitalized Patients

Dimension of Spirituality	Definition of Dimension	Needs Associated with Dimension
Meaning	The dimension that provides orientation to an individual's life and promotes his or her overall life balance.	The need for life balance: The need to rebuild a new life balance and the need to learn how to better cope with illness or disability.
Transcendence	An anchor point exterior to the person; the relationship with an external foundation that provides a sense of grounding. The group considered that everyone has an external foundation, even if different from God. For some people, this transcendence might be found in nature, beauty, or art.	The need for connection: The need for connection with her existential foundation and the need for beauty (aesthetic sense).
Values	The system of values that determines goodness and trueness for the person; it is made apparent in the person's actions and life choices.	*The need for values acknowledgement: The need that health professionals know and respect an individual's values.
		*The need to maintain control: The need to understand and to feel included in decision-making processes and to be associated with health professionals' decisions and actions.
Psychosocial Identity	The patient's environment; those elements, such as society, caregivers, family, and close relationships, that together make up the person's singular identity.	The need to maintain identity: The need to be loved, to be heard, to be recognized, to be in touch, to have a positive image of oneself and to feel forgiven.

*In the hospital setting, two different needs were clearly distinguished to translate the values dimension.

Source: Monod, S. M., Rochat, E., Büla, C. J., Jobin, G., Martin, E., & Spencer, B. (2010, December 13). The Spiritual Distress Assessment Tool: An instrument to assess spiritual distress in hospitalised elderly persons. *BMC Geriatrics, 10*, 88.

References

Chan, M. F. (2010). Factors affecting nursing staff in practicing spiritual care. *Journal of Clinical Nursing, 19*, 2128–2136. doi: 10.1111/j.1365-2702.2008.02690.x

Fenwick, P., & Brayne, S. (2011, February). End-of-life experiences: Reaching out for compassion, communication, and connection—meaning of deathbed visions and coincidences. *American Journal of Hospice and Palliative Care, 28*(1), 7–15. Epub 2010 Aug 27.

Monod, S. M., Rochat, E., Büla, C. J., Jobin, G., Martin, E., & Spencer, B. (2010, December 13). The Spiritual Distress Assessment Tool: An instrument to assess spiritual distress in hospitalised elderly persons. *BMC Geriatrics, 10*, 88.

Nixon, A., & Narayanasamy, A. (2010, August). The spiritual needs of neuro-oncology patients from patients' perspective. *Journal of Clinical Nursing, 19*(15-16), 2259–2370. Epub 2010 Jun 7.

Terminal Extubation

The obvious advantage to terminal extubation is that it does not prolong the dying process and it allows the patient to be free from an unnatural tube. It is important to anticipate the distress a patient may experience during terminal extubation. Therefore, the patient should receive anticipatory doses of analgesics and sedatives that are then titrated as necessary to the observed level of the patient's distress.

An issue may arise during both terminal weaning and terminal extubation with the patient who is receiving neuromuscular blocking agents. An effort should be made to allow restoration of neuromuscular function before withdrawing mechanical ventilation. Unfortunately, in some patients with multisystem organ failure, the clearance of the drug may become prolonged; if that happens, restoration of full neuromuscular function could take days or weeks. Therefore, it may be morally justified to withdraw mechanical ventilation from a patient who is still experiencing the effects of residual blocking agents that were started prior to the decision to forgo life-sustaining measures. This decision must be balanced between the reasons to wait for restoration of neuromuscular function versus the added suffering of continued use of life-sustaining interventions.

Environment

When a patient is dying, it is important to create an environment that facilitates family presence. Discussions with family members regarding end-of-life decisions should not be held in a hallway or in the busy ICU. Finding adequate space for all family members to wait without being in high traffic areas is important, as is scheduling a time and finding a quiet place where family members can listen and feel comfortable asking questions. Once the decision is made to provide only comfort care, the patient care area should facilitate comfort for the patient and her family and friends. If possible, the patient should be located in a room or area that is quiet and has space for family to be with their dying relative. In some hospitals, special areas are designated for patients who are actively dying. However, if the patient has been in one area of the hospital for a long time, moving to another area may be disruptive to both the patient and clinician. Rules regarding visiting hours and numbers of persons allowed in the room should be adjusted. The goal at this point is comfort and privacy for the patient and her family.

Cultural Considerations

The manner in which individuals handle death is influenced by their culture, religion, family traditions, and individual preferences (Kuebler et al., 2007). Increasing diversity in the United States contributes to a need for each nurse to identify and understand her patients' cultural issues. Culture can be defined as a system of shared views that link an individual to a group or others. There is variability within each group, and each culture is constantly evolving. Cultural practices bring security, integrity, and a sense of belonging to the individual. In many situations, religious beliefs may dictate the patient or family's response to death. Care of the body after death may be dictated by either culture, religion, or both. Rituals during dying or immediately after often carry significant meaning for the patient and family. Therefore, it is important to ask the family about their preferences and to facilitate any ritual that may be important or meaningful. Although it is not possible to know about all cultures, it is easy to find resource material regarding culturally appropriate care at the end of a patient's life. EPERC

CULTURAL CONSIDERATIONS
Resources for Cultural Considerations in End-of-Life Care

- Purnell, L. D. (2009). *Guide to culturally competent health care* (2nd ed.). Philadelphia, PA: F.A. Davis Company.
- Coakley, S., & Kaufman Shelemay, K. (2008). *Pain and its transformations: The interface of biology and culture.* Cambridge, MA: Harvard University Press.
- Robben, A. C. G. M. (2005). *Death, mourning, and burial: A cross cultural reader.* New York: John Wiley.
- End of Life/Palliative Education Resource Center (EPERC), Milwaukee, WI. Fast Facts and Concepts:
  - African Americans and End-of-Life Care
  - Asking About Cultural Beliefs in Palliative Care
  - Cultural Aspects of Pain Management

Available at http://eperc.mcw.ed

Weblink: End of Life/Palliative Care Resource Center

(www.eperc.mcw.edu) offers guidelines to specific cultural and religious practices at end of life.

Particular customs may come into play during communication with the patient and his family. Things to be aware of include conversational style and pace, eye contact, personal space, touch, and time orientation (Lipson & Dibble, 2007).

Grief and Loss

At the end of life, loss, grief, and bereavement can have a profound effect on the family and members of the health care team. Part of the nurse's role at the end of life includes facilitating the grieving process. What is important to understand is that an individual must experience the grief process to finally accept the reality of the loss. The patient and his family may suffer anticipatory grief when faced with a terminal diagnosis. Normal grief affects all aspects of a person's being—physical, emotional, cognitive, behavioral, and spiritual.

Interventions are designed to help an individual accept the reality of the loss. Interventions may include:

- Presence, active listening, touch
- Providing emotional support
- Encouraging verbalization
- Identifying support systems
- Normalizing the grief process and allowing for individual differences
- Identifying the need for additional assistance and making referrals.

To be effective caregivers at end of life, nurses must come to terms with their own views on death and dying. As with patients and their families, nurses' level of comfort with death is affected by their personality, culture, spiritual belief system, and life experiences. Encouraging nurses to verbalize their feelings and express emotions will help them to process grief and loss and provide quality care at the end of life. Refer back to Chapter 9 for more information on grief and loss.

End-of-Life Care for Patients Who are Terminally Ill

End-of-life care for patients who are terminally ill follows the same principles as those used for patients and families faced with an unexpected death. The main difference is that the patient with a terminal illness has the opportunity to participate in the planning for his death.

Hospice

Hospice is the provision of care at the end of life aimed at comfort instead of cure. It is based on a interdisciplinary model that is tailored to meet the values and goals of the patient and family. The care is aimed at relieving physical, psychosocial, and spiritual suffering for the patient and facilitating the grieving and coping strategies of families and caregivers.

Death is an inevitable aspect of the human condition; dying badly is not. As the aging of the population continues, more and more individuals will face decisions regarding their end-of-life care. The challenge of end-of-life care will grow during the next three decades because the population of seniors in the United States is projected to more than double during the next 30 years, rising from 34 million in 1997 to more than 69 million by 2030. Despite significant advances in preventive care and treatment modalities that prolong health and life, all but those who die suddenly and unexpectedly will have to make decisions about serious or life-threatening illness.

Nurses play a crucial role in assisting patients and families in increasing their knowledge of hospice care and dispelling myths and fears. Hospice care focuses on comfort care versus curative care. An interdisciplinary team of health care providers including physicians, nurses, social workers, spiritual counselors, dietitians, home health aides, and volunteers provide hospice. The care plan encompasses both the patient and family/caregiver as the unit of care, and the care plan is individualized to meet their values and goals. Patients receiving hospice care are generally defined as those patients who have a prognosis of 6 months or less if their terminal disease runs a normal course.

Hospice care is provided to the patient in various settings, although most often this is the patient's home or living facility. Hospice care is also provided in the inpatient setting. In fact, many hospice programs have beds or inpatient units dedicated to hospice care. Hospice care providers may also contract to provide hospice care within the general inpatient care areas of an acute care facility if that facility does not have its own inpatient unit. Inpatient care is generally provided for management of symptoms and periods of caregiver crisis.

Hospices also provide respite care. Respite is care given to a hospice patient by another caregiver so the usual caregiver can rest. Respite care is provided in a hospice facility, hospital, or a skilled nursing facility. Hospices may also provide short-term continuous nursing care in a patient's home to prevent a hospitalization during a period of medical crisis. This allows patients to remain in the comfort of their own home and attain symptom control.

In addition, hospice care encompasses bereavement services after the patient's death. These services are available for a minimum of 1 year after the patient's death and provide support for families and caregivers during the grieving process. Bereavement counseling is provided by telephone and in person, and on either an individual or group basis. Most hospice programs also have groups that are available to the community to deal with grief and coping issues such as going to a school after the unexpected death of a teacher or of some students.

The concept of comfort care versus curative care is important for nurses who are caring for patients with life-limiting disease to fully understand. Comfort care is aimed at improving the quality of life, but not necessarily aimed at prolonging the quantity of life. Effective symptom relief may not only improve the quality of life but occasionally will demonstrate some secondary gain in quantity of life. The key to understanding comfort care versus curative care is to ask "What is the primary intent of the treatment intervention?" There are instances where modalities such as chemotherapy and radiation are curative in nature. For example, providing radiotherapy to decrease tumor size may result in less pain. This is different from choosing these therapies in the setting of a more aggressive approach, with the goal being the final cure of the tumor.

Interdisciplinary care involves interdisciplinary teamwork, which is a hallmark of hospice care. Utilizing the knowledge and expertise of physicians, nurses, social workers, spiritual counselors, dietitians, aides, and volunteers, the care is designed to be comprehensive and constantly updated to meet the patient's and family's needs. Team meetings are held at regular intervals to discuss all aspects of a patient's care including symptom management, patient and family psychosocial needs, spiritual needs, and the ability to maintain or receive assistance in activities of daily living. All members of the team bring their individual perspectives to the care and have input into care decisions. The goal of hospice is to address all of these needs in an integrated and holistic manner.

Hospice care has expanded over the years to include serving patients other than just those with cancer diagnoses. Hospices now care for patients with other life-limiting, chronic illnesses such as heart disease, respiratory disease, and HIV/AIDS. In 2010, NHPCO reported that in 2009, only 40% of hospice patients had a cancer diagnosis. NHPCO reports the top noncancer causes of death include nonspecified disability, heart disease, dementia, lung disease, stroke, and end-stage renal disease.

NHPCO (2010) reported that, as of 2009, the racial/cultural makeup of hospice care recipients changed little: 94% of recipients were non-Hispanic; 5% claimed themselves to be Hispanic. Further breakdown revealed that 80% were Caucasian, 8.75% were multiracial, 8.7% were Black, 1.9% were Asian, and just 0.2% claimed Native American status. Identified differences between ethnic groups included age, cultural adaptation, high-risk behaviors, caregivers, and payment method. Hospice programs have begun to focus on increasing awareness of services within minority communities, including offering hospice educational material in multiple languages other than English and holding support groups within culturally diverse communities.

Sexual diversity applies to groups such as lesbians, gays, bisexuals, and transgendered individuals. These groups require special consideration in hospice care due to the fact that, despite advances, social stigmas still exist within certain groups and locales. This may discourage patient access to hospice care, especially if the terminal illness is associated with lifestyle choices.

The Role of Nursing in Hospice

The professional nurse plays a number of key roles in hospice care. The nurse is critical in not only directing the provision of high-quality, competent care, but also in promoting the hospice concept and advocating for patients and families. Most hospice programs identify the registered nurse as the case manager for a panel of hospice patients. The nurse is accountable for the interdisciplinary collaboration and oversight of the care of the patient and family.

The nurse can play a role in influencing physicians and other health care providers to consider the hospice option for their patients. The nurse can provide knowledge and information, correct myths and preconceptions, and influence the effort for earlier referrals to hospice. The nurse also plays a key role in educating patients and families about hospice, exploring their concerns and fears, and assisting them in navigating the numerous care options. The nurse is always the patient advocate, ensuring that whatever course is chosen is aligned with the patient's and family members' values and goals and done with their full knowledge about their options and the implications of their choices.

Hospice programs have grown tremendously during the past 10 years. NHPCO (2010) reported that in 1992 there were 1,935 hospice programs, growing to 3,650 in 2004 and now to over 5,000 in the United States. More patients and families are choosing hospice care, up from 246,000 in 1992 to 1,060,000 in 2004. Despite this growth, there are challenges. Access issues and barriers to care continue. Hospices are faced with an increasingly diverse population. These challenges exist in a health care system faced with an increasing number of aged Americans, issues of payer reimbursement, and complex regulations from payers, government agencies, and accrediting organizations. However, there is reason to be optimistic. The hospice movement and the palliative care movement collaborate to improve the overall quality of end-of-life care. Structured end-of-life education is being provided to physicians during training and later as continuing education. Hospice/Palliative Medicine is now a board specialty available as a post-graduate fellowship. Education in end-of-life care is being presented to nurses, and increasing numbers of hospice nurses are receiving certification in the specialty of hospice and palliative care. Professional organizations such as NHPCO and state hospice organizations are advocating legislative reforms to increase access to hospice programs; decrease barriers, especially with regard to eligibility; and promote increasing the lengths of stay in hospice programs. To provide the impetus for policy and practice changes that will increase access to hospice care, hospice must be re-envisioned as a concept of health care—a new way of thinking about the nature and goals of health care itself, rather than an end-stage form of care.

Palliative Care

Palliative care is a relatively new field in nursing. Nurses traditionally have contributed their resources to a health care system that has focused primarily on attempts at curing diseases. Yet many diseases carry significant potential to limit life and offer limited opportunity for cure. Diseases such as congestive heart failure (CHF), chronic obstructive pulmonary disease (COPD), some cancers, stroke, and dementias are common and carry a heavy symptom burden. The current medical treatment of these diseases relies heavily on a system of symptom management. Symptom management is at the heart of palliative care and may provide a greater quality of life when used in conjunction with the medical management of the disease.

Palliative care nurses serve patients with incurable illnesses, and their family members, by assisting in the management of their multifaceted symptoms, ultimately enabling them to live within the confines of their illnesses. Traditional disease-centered focus should be aligned with the caring model of nursing, one that focuses on the whole patient, embracing a model that includes the art of caring for ill patients, as well as the science.

Palliative care was recognized as its own field of medicine in 1987, with its roots stemming from hospice, being viewed as active care versus total care (Kuebler et al., 2007). In 1990, the WHO introduced its definition of palliative care as "the active total care of a patient whose disease is manageable but not curable." This includes interventions that:

1. Affirm life and regard dying as a normal process.
2. Neither hasten nor postpone death.
3. Provide relief from pain and other distressing symptoms.
4. Integrate the psychological and spiritual aspects of patient care.
5. Offer a support system to help patients live as actively as possible until death.
6. Offer a support system to help the family cope during the patient's illness and in their own bereavement.

Nurses should be familiar with how palliative care emerged and the types of programs and activities available to patients and their families. It is also important to recognize the barriers faced by those providing palliative care.

Emergence of Palliative Care

There is a rapidly growing national movement to improve end-of-life education and the delivery of palliative care. Forces behind the motivation to change include changes in the delivery of health care in the last century, results of research studies, and the development of programs and projects by renowned organizations.

Changes in the last century in medical science have led to unparalleled progress in the effective treatment of disease, which has, for many, led to prolonged periods of illness, decline, and suffering. Although surveys indicate that most people would prefer to die at home, greater than 50% of deaths occur in the hospital. Approximately 15% of patients in the ICU die in the unit (Mularski et al., 2009). Fear of the dying process is a very real emotion for many adults. Many fear the care they will receive during and before end of life, the loss of control they will experience, being attached to machines, dying away from home, and being separated from loved ones.

End-of-life education for health care professionals has been scarce at best. Since 2010, many changes have been made to medical education, including rotations at the undergraduate and resident level to include palliative/hospice care. An example of this education can be seen at Stanford University, which supplies web-based education for physicians from any discipline regarding end of life (End of Life Education for Medical Teachers, Stanford Faculty Development, 2010).

Several organizations are aspiring to improve the end-of-life care provided around the country. They are committed to the vision of ensuring a "good death" for patients and their families, where the period prior to death is dignified and comfortable. Among these organizations are the Last Acts Campaign of the Robert Wood Johnson (RWJ) Foundation, the Education for Physicians on End of Life Care of the American Medical Association, the Center to Advance Palliative Care, and Americans for Better Care of the Dying.

The End-of-Life Nursing Education Consortium of the American Association of Colleges of Nursing and the City of Hope National Medical Center is a program funded by the RWJ foundation. This 3-day course is designed to train nurses who provide continuing education courses and equip them with the resources to integrate end-of-life care into their courses. Renowned researchers, educators, authors, and leaders facilitate the training in the specialty of palliative care. Modules include nursing care at the end of life, pain and other symptom management, cultural issues, ethical/legal considerations, communication, bereavement, and care and preparation for death.

Provision of Palliative Care

As the specialty of palliative care is emerging, so is the evolution of the provision of care. Types of programs are varied, yet many of the activities are common.

A palliative care service may include either inpatient and/or outpatient consultations that range from comprehensive case management or care coordination to a one-time visit. Types of patients to be seen may

Weblink: WHO Definition of Palliative Care

Weblink: End-of-Life Care Online Curriculum

Weblink: Guidelines for Quality Palliative Care

include those with chronic illnesses that are incurable and decline over time, such as CHF, COPD, dementia, cancers, and strokes. No single health care provider can successfully meet all of the palliative care needs of patients who have incurable illnesses and the needs of their families. The interdisciplinary team approach is essential because it comprises a variety of disciplines that pool their data to reach a consensus about goal setting and the development of a comprehensive plan of care. Team members may include, but are not limited to, physicians, nurses, social workers, and chaplains. Other ancillary support may be needed depending on the patient's needs, including input from experts in the fields of mental health, physical therapy, nutrition, pharmacy, respiratory therapy, and ethics.

Nurses working in a palliative care program should understand that targeted interventions are common regardless of the program design. These include pain and symptom management, end-of-life care planning, and support that encompasses psychosocial and spiritual needs. The National Guidelines box discusses standards and guidelines for palliative care.

Another key function of the palliative care team is to assist the patient who has an incurable illness to develop a plan of care prior to advancement of his disease process. The plan should be rational and customized to the individual patient's goals and values. This can be accomplished in an interdisciplinary team setting and should include the patient and key people in his life. A systematic or methodical approach may be very beneficial. It would include a discussion regarding what the patient knows or wants to know about his disease state, as well as whether or not he is ready to engage in this type of discussion. The provider may then educate the patient regarding the potential trajectory of the illness, as well as the risk, benefit, and burden measure of each treatment option. Next, the patient is assisted to set goals of care based on the individual's values.

Paramount to providing good palliative care is the ability of the provider to be absolutely honest with the patient. The concept of truth-telling urges practitioners to overcome the tendency to avoid inaccurate disclosure when talking to dying patients so they may begin planning for their end-of-life journey (Saunders, 2007). Nurses build relationships with dying patients that allow for discussions centered on shifting the focus of care from curative to more of a palliative model. Often, nurses are successful in opening a window to alternatives to a curative model. Discussions of end-of-life options should be in congruence with the patient's medical, nursing, and social needs.

To be effective in providing palliative care for those with terminal illnesses, providers need to understand the various psychosocial needs of the patient and family. Nurses need to be able to recognize grief and assist with the appropriate interventions to cope, whether that is by nursing actions or consultation with the palliative care team for appropriate referral to psychiatrists, grief counselors, social services, or spiritual counselors. Patients facing incurable and life-threatening illnesses experience losses of function, control, independence, body image, dignity, and a future.

Spirituality is an inherent and pervasive dimension for persons, particularly those faced with the closure of their lives. Effective palliative care nurses must become comfortable and competent in performing a spiritual assessment. When the nurse queries a patient about spiritual issues, the patient is assisted to reflect on his own humanity. In doing so, the nurse is offering support for patients who naturally grapple with spiritual issues surrounding illness and impending end of life. Last, it is an opportunity for the nurse to be present and witness the sacredness of this life event. Nurses who assist patients may find this involvement in the intimate stories of patients' lives to be an honor, a gift, and a tremendous opportunity for growth as a person.

NATIONAL GUIDELINES for Quality Palliative Care

In 2002, the Hospice and Palliative Nurses Association and the American Nurses Association developed the *Scope and Standards of Hospice and Palliative Nursing Practice*.

Patients' symptoms will vary according to the disease state and should be monitored and controlled regardless of the proximity to end of life. For patients close to the end of life, symptoms experienced are often distressing and include pain, dyspnea, nausea, constipation, anxiety, restlessness, delirium, fatigue, dehydration, and gurgling from airway secretions. Palliative care nurses play a pivotal role in accurately assessing, reporting, and ensuring that symptoms are appropriately managed. A patient's quality of life is contingent on an astute, competent nurse who has received thorough education in pain and symptom management and who possesses the critical thinking and clinical judgment skills necessary to advocate for patients in an environment where the proper use of analgesics and adjunct medications is critical to maintaining patient comfort. For example, pain medication doses will need to be titrated and tailored to a level particular to the individual.

National Guidelines

In 2004, the National Consensus Project for Quality Palliative Care, the Center to Advance Palliative Care, and the Last Acts Partnership created the *Clinical Practice Guidelines for Quality Palliative Care;* these were subsequently updated in 2009 (National Consensus Project for Quality Palliative Care, 2009). More than 100 experts contributed to the evidence-based guidelines. The framework for the clinical practice guidelines include:

- Structure and processes of care
- Physical aspects of care
- Psychological and psychiatric aspects of care
- Social aspects of care
- Spiritual, religious, and existential aspects of care
- Cultural aspects of care
- Care of the imminently dying patient
- Ethical and legal aspects of care.

The guidelines are very comprehensive and can be accessed at www.nationalconsensusproject.org/guideline.pdf.

Source: National Consensus Project for Quality Palliative Care. (2009). *Clinical practice guidelines for quality palliative care* (2nd ed.). http://www.nationalconsensusproject.org.

Nursing Management

Variation in the delivery of care to patients is a leading cause of inadequate care. The number of patients who have died in the ICU following a decision to withdraw life support or limit therapy is increasing. Even so, evidence indicates that patients and families are dissatisfied with the care given during end of life (Mularski et al., 2009). Educating health care professionals in end-of-life care is an important aspect of improving their ability to properly care for dying patients and their families. The goal is to add life to the patient's time, not simply time to the patient's life. A detailed patient care plan for end-of-life care is provided in the Nursing Process box.

Collaborative Management

Achievement of a pain-free and meaningful death experience for the patient and family requires a multidisciplinary approach. In order to meet desired patient outcomes, it is essential that this interdisciplinary

NURSING PROCESS: Patient Care Plan for End-of-Life Care

Assessment of End-of-Life Status Using Gordon's Functional Health Patterns:

- Health Perception Health Management Pattern
- Nutrition Metabolic Pattern
- Activity Exercise Pattern
- Cognitive Perceptual Pattern
- Values and Belief Pattern

Subjective Data	Objective Data
Assessment of Therapeutic Regimen Are all members of the health care team clear on the plan of care, goals, and expected outcomes? What did the doctor tell you about your family member's prognosis? Do you know your family member's resuscitation wishes and are you in agreement? Is there a written advance directive?	**Assessment of Therapeutic Regimen** Family and significant others are able to verbalize an understanding of the treatment regimen. Health care team demonstrates understanding of the treatment plan.
Assessment of Grieving What is your past experience with loss? Do you have a support system? Are there any cultural or religious practices that I can assist you with?	**Assessment of Grieving** Observe family interaction with staff and significant others. Observe the family members' comfort level while in the patient's room. Observe the patient/family's ability to cope with the situation.
Assessment of Pain On a scale of 1–10, with 1 being a little pain and 10 being the worst pain you have ever felt, at what level is your pain? Do you routinely take pain medication at home? If yes, what is the name of the medication and why do you take it? Are you allergic to any medications? Where is your pain? Is it getting worse? Is the medication working? Have you tried other pain relief methods?	**Assessment of Pain** Facial grimacing Change in breathing pattern Change in blood pressure and/or pulse rate Diaphoresis Agitation
Assessment of Respiratory Distress Are you feeling short of breath? What helps relieve your shortness of breath?	**Assessment of Respiratory Distress** Observe nonintubated patient for: Tachypnea Restlessness Work of breathing Mentation Skin signs—pale to dusky, cool, clammy to diaphoretic Accessory muscle use Grunting at the end of each breath Nasal flaring
Assessment of Body Temperature Do you feel cold? Do you feel too warm? Do you feel like you have a fever or chills?	**Assessment of Body Temperature** Assess: Skin temperature Tachypnea Tachycardia Shivering

Outcomes and Evaluation Parameters	Planning and Interventions with *Rationales*
1. NURSING DIAGNOSIS: Ineffective Therapeutic Regimen Management ***related to the acceleration (expected or unexpected) of illness symptoms*** **(NANDA-I © 2012)**	
Outcome: The health care team has a clear understanding of the plan of care. ***Evaluation Parameters:*** All members of the health care team express understanding regarding: Disease process Rationale for treatment regimen Expectations of regimen Methods to monitor condition Signs or symptoms of complications Honoring the patient's wishes.	Request a multidisciplinary meeting with the health care team *to identify concerns and clarify goals and expected outcomes for the patient.* Facilitate multidisciplinary family conference. Be respectful of cultural conversational norms. Listen to identify concerns. Attempt to match expressed needs with services the nurse can provide or facilitate. Demonstrate honesty, consistency, and stability. Maintain pre-established contacts in person or by phone. *To build trust and strength.*

(*continued*)

NURSING PROCESS: Patient Care Plan for End-of-Life Care, *continued*

Outcomes and Evaluation Parameters	Planning and Interventions with *Rationales*
Outcome: The patient and/or family verbalize understanding of the seriousness of the patient's preferences and prognosis. ***Evaluation Parameters:*** The patient and/or family will verbalize an understanding of the seriousness of the patient's condition. The patient and/or family will be able to verbalize patient's preferences for quality-of-life issues.	Discuss with patient and/or family their understanding of the prognosis; perception of its seriousness; perceived level of anxiety; support system; emotional status; and cognitive ability *to identify factors that influence understanding.* Solicit expressions of feelings and questions. Identify if any advance directives were done and/or who will be responsible for care decisions. Encourage patient and family to seek information and make informed decisions. *To promote active participation of the patient and family.*
2. NURSING DIAGNOSIS: Grieving *related to anticipated loss of physiological well-being* (NANDA-I © 2012)	
Outcome: Patient/family will demonstrate the ability to make mutual decisions regarding the anticipated death. ***Evaluation Parameters:*** Expresses thoughts, feelings, and spiritual beliefs about the loss. Verbalizes fears/concerns regarding the impending death. Exhibits no somatic distress.	When assisting with family discussions use clear words, such as *death* or *died*, rather than euphemisms (i.e., *passed on*). Assist patient/family to verbalize fears/concerns regarding the impending loss, including its impact on the family unit. *To assist the patient/family to share mutual fears, plans, and concerns with each other.* Teach the patient/family about the normal events of the dying process. Encourage patient/family to implement cultural, religious, and social customs associated with death. Teach the patient/family characteristics of normal and abnormal grieving. *To help the patient and family move through the grieving process.* Arrange equipment and furniture in the patient's room to facilitate family presence and interaction with the patient. Remove as much monitoring equipment and intravenous lines from the patient as possible. Facilitate privacy for the family. Facilitate cultural/religious rituals. *To provide a peaceful, pain-free death for the patient and to create a supportive environment for the family.* Refer to appropriate resources: support groups, legal assistance, financial assistance, social services, and chaplain. *To assist the patient and family with putting the patient's legal affairs in order and to create an environment for emotional closure.*
3. NURSING DIAGNOSIS: Pain *related to disease process* (NANDA-I © 2012)	
Outcome: Pain level will be tolerable and the patient will not suffer. ***Evaluation Parameter:*** Patient will not exhibit symptoms of pain or suffering.	**Nonpharmacologic** Reduce lighting and noise, eliminate unnecessary monitors and machines, remove restraints, and provide room for the patient's significant others. Cultural and spiritual factors such as prayer, ritual, and music can also increase the patient's comfort. *Promotes relaxation and comfort.* **Pharmacologic** **Narcotics** Morphine drip: titrate for symptom relief. At end of life, there is no recommended maximal dose. *Titration is intended to relieve pain and suffering.* **Benzodiazepines** Midazolam drip: starting dose for adult continuous infusion: 1–5 mg/hr. Titrate for symptom relief. Lorazepam drip: starting dose for adult continuous infusion: 1–8 mg/hr. Titrate for symptom relief. *Benzodiazepines have a synergistic sedative effect with opioids, are anticonvulsants, and may help prevent the development of premorbid seizures.*

(*continued*)

NURSING PROCESS: Patient Care Plan for End-of-Life Care, *continued*

4. NURSING DIAGNOSIS: Ineffective Breathing Pattern *related to dying process* (NANDA-I © 2012)

Outcome: Breathing pattern will be effective.

Evaluation Parameter: Patient will not exhibit symptoms of respiratory distress.

Nonpharmacologic

Elevate the head of the bed.

Place a fan in the room that blows gently on the patient's face.

To promote comfort.

Pharmacologic

Morphine drip: titrate for symptom relief. At end of life there is no recommended maximal dose.

Titration is intended *to relieve pain and suffering.*

5. NURSING DIAGNOSIS: Imbalanced Body Temperature *related to disease process* (NANDA-I © 2012)

Outcome: The patient will not exhibit signs of physical discomfort from a fever.

Evaluation Parameters: Normal body temperature

Free from shivering

Pharmacologic

Administer an antipyretic *to decrease body temperature. Any measure that would cause the patient more discomfort, such as a cooling blanket, should not be used.*

Source: Adapted from Wilkinson, J. M., & Ahearn, N. R. (2009).

team communicate openly with one another in developing and evaluating care of the patient and family (IOM [Institute of Medicine], 2010). The nurse is in a pivotal role to bring together the members of the team necessary to achieve this objective. It is the nurse's responsibility to ensure that all members of the team are notified regarding the patient's and family's needs. Many services, as well as assistance from community collaboratives, are needed to optimally assist the patient and family with the dying process. Services that may be used include the hospital ethics committee, chaplain services, psychologists/psychiatrists, legal services, financial assistance, social services, hospice, and specific support groups for family members.

The ethics committee intervenes when there is conflict among the health care team and/or family regarding the prognosis and continuation of curative care for the patient. Once the decision is made to place the patient on palliative care, the family may need help regarding legal and financial assistance to ensure the patient's affairs are in order. The chaplain, social services, or a psychologist/psychiatrist assists the family to work through the grieving process and bring closure to the situation. If the patient is able to return home to die, hospice services aid the patient and family to facilitate this process in the home setting. Finally, specific support groups will help the family to work through the grieving process both before and after death.

Research

There is an abundance of literature and research regarding hospice care for the terminally ill. Unfortunately, little research has been done with regard to end-of-life care when the death is unexpected. See the Research Opportunities box for research topics in this area.

Many hospitals and organizations are working to improve end-of-life care and are committed to ensuring that all patients and families experience a "good death." Unfortunately, though, deciding who is "dying" in the acute care setting can be subjective or more of a matter of perspective. Caregivers feel comfortable when pursuing a cure, but once the decision is made that any further care would be futile, caregivers often feel uncomfortable because this is not the "norm." Today's health care system is tailored to handle emergencies and injuries, diagnostic tests, and the most technologically advanced care in the world. However, it is not designed to accommodate the diverse needs of patients who are dying. Education and care guidelines will help to alleviate the discomfort of caregivers when they end up doing something that is perceived as the opposite of their normal goals.

RESEARCH OPPORTUNITIES Related to End-of-Life Care

Research Area	Clinical Impact
What interventions will help to relieve the discomfort experienced by critical care nurses caring for end-of-life patients?	Developing interventions to relieve the discomfort surrounding end-of-life care will improve the care that nurses provide to patients at end of life.
Is there a way to measure quality of life as an end point of treatment?	A tool that could accurately measure quality of life would assist in decisions for the end point of treatment.
What interventions can be done to support culturally appropriate end-of-life care?	Take steps to promote cultural customs and rituals surrounding end-of-life care.
Compare the efficacy of terminal weaning versus terminal extubation during withdrawal of care.	This research could determine the best approach to withdrawal of ventilatory life support.

Summary

As a nurse, one of the most rewarding experiences is to allow natural death for a patient and to support him or her during this time. Helping the patient and significant others to meet their goals at end of life is challenging and rewarding. Preparing nurses both educationally and emotionally for the challenge of being with dying patients with presence and focused compassion is a vital task. Nurses must continue to advocate for patients, including those at the end of life.

NCLEX® PRACTICE

1. A family member states, "There are so many different people taking care of Mom now that she is in palliative care. Why are there so many?" How should the nurse respond to this statement?
   1. "Integrating the goals and expertise of many different disciplines encourages the development of the most comprehensive plan of care for your mom."
   2. "Increased numbers of health care teams can help to ensure continuity in communication with your mom and your siblings."
   3. "Using an interdisciplinary team approach decreases liability after new treatment decisions."
   4. "A multidisciplinary approach to end-of-life care guarantees that the latest in palliative care technology will guide patient care goals."
2. Which statement made by a novice nurse would indicate the need for further instruction regarding end-of-life care?
   1. "The focus of the plan of care should be changed from curative processes to comfort advances."
   2. "The rights of self-determination and confidentiality are essential for all palliative care patients."
   3. "The patient has the right to conclude what treatments or lack of treatments affect his own body."
   4. "The family usually finds it easier to withdraw life-sustaining treatments than to withhold them."
3. The nurse has just completed educating a patient about advance directives. Which statement made by the patient would indicate the need for further instruction?
   1. "Advance directives will guide the health care team as to my wishes regarding medical treatments should I become incapacitated."
   2. "By signing the advance directive, my appointed family member will have the ability to make health care decisions for me if I become ill."
   3. "The advance directive is supposed to help direct the decision-making process about my intentions for life-sustaining treatments."
   4. "My living will is a type of advance directive that describes what level of life-prolonging care I desire in the event I become incapacitated."
4. The patient is being admitted for inpatient hospice care. Which instructions should be provided to the patient and his or her family regarding pain control?
   1. "We will provide medication for pain before we do procedures."
   2. "We are going to limit family visits because the excess stimulation can be detrimental."
   3. "We are planning on reducing the amount of anxiety medication for fear of dependence."
   4. "We feel all the excess lights and noise will help the patient forget all about the pain."
5. A new nurse is being oriented to a hospice position in a culturally diverse area. Which statement made by this new employee would reflect a thorough understanding of cultural diversity as it relates to end-of-life care?
   1. "Many followers of Judaism believe that death is a private matter; therefore, the dying person should be left alone."
   2. "Some Russians may make their elderly family members a DNR so they will die comfortably and without life-sustaining treatments."
   3. "Believers in the Baha'i faith consider the body as just a shell, so cremations are common and organ donation is encouraged."
   4. "Persons from South Asia may remain positive and upbeat when around the health care team but then mourn in private."
6. A nurse is assisting a patient in making end-of-life decisions. Which nursing statements reflect a concern for the context of these decisions? (select all that apply)
   1. "You will live longer if you consent to this treatment."
   2. "The oncologist wants you to have this done."
   3. "How does your family feel about this procedure?"
   4. "Will your insurance pay for the procedure?"
   5. "Will you be alright with being hospitalized for a week after the procedure?"

Answers to NCLEX Practice questions can be found in Appendix D in the Osborn Student Resources at nursing.pearsonhighered.com. Practice additional NCLEX questions online at the Student Resources site.

Pearson Nursing Student Resources Find additional review materials at: **nursing.pearsonhighered.com**

REFERENCES

Adams, M. P., & Koch, R. W. (2010). *Pharmacology: Connections to nursing practice.* Upper Saddle River, NJ: Pearson.

Bjarnason, D. (2009). Nursing, religiosity, and end-of-life care: Interconnections and implications. *Nursing Clinics of North America, 44*(4), 517–525.

Chan, M. F. (2010). Factors affecting nursing staff in practicing spiritual care. *Journal of Clinical Nursing, 19*(15-16), 2128–2136. doi: 10.1111/j.1365-2702.2008.02690.x

Fenwick, P., & Brayne, S. (2011, February). End-of-life experiences: Reaching out for compassion, communication, and connection—meaning of deathbed visions and coincidences. *American Journal of Hospice and Palliative Care, 28*(1), 7–15. Epub 2010 Aug 27.

Ferrell, B. (2010). Pain management at end of life. Medscape Nurses. Retrieved from http://www.medscape.com/viewarticle/731405

Heyland, D. K., Dodek, P., Rocker, G., Groll, D., Gafni, A., Pichora, D., Shortt, S., Tranmer, J., Lazar, N., Kutsogiannis, J., & Lam, M. (2006). What matters most in end-of-life care: perceptions of seriously ill patients and their family members. *Canadian Medical Association Journal 174*(5): 627–633.

IOM (Institute of Medicine). (2010). *The future of nursing: Leading change, advancing health.* Washington, DC: The Academic Press.

Jonsen, A. R., Siegler, M., & Winslade, W. (2006). *Clinical ethics: A practical approach to ethical decisions in clinical medicine* (6th ed.). New York: McGraw-Hill Companies.

Kübler-Ross, E., & Kessler, D. (2007). *On grief & grieving: Finding the meaning of grief through the five stages of loss.* New York: Scribner.

Kuebler, K. K., Heidrich, D. E., & Esper, P. (Eds.). (2007). *Palliative and end of life care.* St. Louis, MO: Saunders.

Lipson, J., & Dibble, S. (Eds.). (2007). *Culture and clinical care.* San Francisco: UCSF Nursing Press.

Mahon, M. M. (2010). Clinical decision making in palliative care and end of life care. *Nursing Clinics of North America, 45,* 345–362.

Monod, S. M., Rochat, E., Büla, C. J., Jobin, G., Martin, E., & Spencer, B. (2010, December 13). The Spiritual Distress Assessment Tool: An instrument to assess spiritual distress in hospitalised elderly persons. *BMC Geriatrics, 10,* 88.

Monturo, C., & Hook, K. (2009). From means to ends: Artificial nutrition and hydration. *Nursing Clinics of North America, 44,* 505–515.

Morgan, D. Y. (2011). Improving quality of life for patients with life-limiting illnesses: The key role of nursing in palliative care. Retrieved from http://www.nursingconsult.com

Mularski, R., Puntillo, K., Varkey, B., Erstad, B. L., Grap, M. J., Gilbert, H. C., et al. (2009). Pain management within the palliative and end-of-life care experience in the ICU. *Chest, 135*(5), 1360–1369.

National Consensus Project for Quality Palliative Care. (2009). *Clinical practice guidelines for quality palliative care* (2nd ed.). Retrieved from http://www.nationalconsensusproject.org

National Hospice and Palliative Care Organization. (2010). Facts and figures. Retrieved from http://www.nhpco.org/files/public/Facts_Figures_for2004data.pdf

Nixon, A., & Narayanasamy, A. (2010, August). The spiritual needs of neuro-oncology patients from patients' perspective. *Journal of Clinical Nursing, 19*(15-16), 2259–2370. Epub 2010 Jun 7.

Saunders, C. A. (Ed.). (2007). *End of life: A nurse's guide to compassionate care.* Philadelphia, PA: Lippincott Williams & Wilkins.

Stanford Faculty Development Center for Medical Teachers (2010). End-of-life care online curriculum. Retrieved from http://sfdc.stanford.edu/previous_programs/

Tilden, V. P., & Thompson, S. (2009). Policy issues in end-of-life care. *Journal of Professional Nursing, 25*(6), 363–368.

Truog, R. D., Campbell, M. L., Curtis, J. R., Haas, C. E., Luce, J. M., Rubenfeld, G. D., Rushton, C. H., & Kaufman, D. C. (2008, May). Recommendations for end-of-life care in the intensive care unit: A consensus statement by the American College of Critical Care Medicine. *Critical Care Medicine, 36*(3), 1699–1715.

Wallace, M., Grossman, S., Campbell, S., Robert, T., Lange, J., & Shea, J. (2009). Integration of end-of-life care content in undergraduate nursing curricula: student knowledge and perceptions. *Journal of Professional Nursing, 25*(1), 50–56.

Wilkinson, J. M., & Ahearn, N. R. (2009). *Prentice Hall nursing diagnosis handbook* (9th ed.). Upper Saddle River, NJ: Prentice Hall.

World Health Organization. (2006). WHO definition of palliative care. Retrieved from http://www.who.int/cancer/palliative/definition/en

UNIT 3 Physiological Concepts Related to Nursing Practice

Content in Unit 3 that addresses the **Institute of Medicine (IOM)** competencies, **Nursing Core Competencies (NCC),** the **Quality and Safety Education for Nurses (QSEN)** competencies, and **Concepts** for concept-based learning is listed below.

Competencies	Feature or Text		Location
IOM, QSEN, NCC Providing patient-centered care	Pain as a Multidimensional Phenomenon Cultural Considerations Related to Patient Responses to Pain Management Management of Patients Who Are Substance Abusers Cultural Considerations Related to Refusal of Blood Products		Chapter 12, page 277 Chapter 12, page 279 Chapter 12, page 282 Chapter 13, page 304 Chapter 16, page 396
IOM, QSEN, NCC Working in teams	Collaborative Management, Pain Collaborative Management, Substance Abuse Collaborative Management, Infection Collaborative Management, Fluid and Electrolyte Balance Collaborative Management, Electrolyte Balance Collaborative Management, Acid-Base Balance Collaborative Management, Fluid Infusion Therapy		Chapter 12, page 292 Chapter 13, page 319 Chapter 14, page 341 Chapter 15, page 350 Chapter 15, page 359 Chapter 15, page 371 Chapter 16, page 393
IOM, QSEN, NCC Employing evidence-based practice	Evidence-Based Practice: Pain Management Evidence-Based Practice: Effects of Infection and Antibiotic-Resistant Bacteria on Wound Healing Evidence-Based Practice: Transfusion of Blood Products		Chapter 12, page 282 Chapter 14, page 341 Chapter 16, page 406
IOM, NCC Applying quality and safety improvement	Infection Prevention and Control Complications Associated with Infusion Therapy Blood Supply Safety		Chapter 14, page 332 Chapter 16, page 389 Chapter 16, page 395
IOM, QSEN, NCC Using informatics	Documentation of Pain Assessment Documentation for Insertion and Removal of VADs		Chapter 12, page 281 Chapter 16, page 388
NCC Applying ethical and legal responsibilities	Ethical Issues in Nonmalignant Pain Management Risks Associated with Transfusion Therapy		Chapter 12, page 276 Chapter 16, page 403
NCC Developing professionally	Impaired Health Care Professional Nursing Responsibilities Before, During, and After Transfusions		Chapter 13, page 319 Chapter 16, page 406
NCC Educating patients	Discharge Planning, Health Promotion, Pain Patient Teaching & Discharge Priorities for Pain Management Patient Teaching & Discharge Priorities for Substance Abuse Health Promotion, Acid–Base Balance		Chapter 12, page 293 Chapter 12, page 296 Chapter 13, page 318 Chapter 15, page 371
Concepts covered in Unit 3 include:	Acid-base balance Addiction behavior Aging Comfort	Fluids and electrolyte balance Immunity Pain	Stress and adaptation Thermoregulation Tissue perfusion

Pain Assessment and Management

CHAPTER 12

Gail Thurkauf
Annita Watson

Outcome-Based Learning Objectives

After studying this chapter, the learner will be able to:

1. Evaluate pain as a distinct and frequently encountered human problem in health care.
2. Distinguish among common pain assessment tools and strategies to elicit details of the multidimensional pain experience.
3. Differentiate between acute, chronic, and cancer-related pain.
4. Compare the basic pharmacodynamic and pharmacokinetic properties of commonly used pharmacologic therapies.
5. Examine the usefulness of nonpharmacologic interventions used to help alleviate pain in clinical practice.
6. Determine the role that nurses play in advocating for patients in pain.
7. Generate a plan of care for patients with acute, chronic, and cancer-related pain.

KEY TERMS

absorption p.283
acute pain p.277
adjuvant medications p.287
affective dimension of pain p.278
agonist p.285
agonist-antagonist p.285
antagonist p.287
balanced or multimodal analgesia p.283
behavioral dimension of pain p.279
biotransformation p.283
breakthrough pain p.277
Brief Pain Inventory (BPI) p.280
cancer pain p.277
chronic pain p.277
cognitive dimension of pain p.278
distribution p.283
elimination p.284
endorphins p.278
enkephalins p.278
equianalgesic dose p.285
hepatic first-pass metabolism p.284
McGill Pain Questionnaire (MPQ) p.280
neuropathic pain p.278
nociception p.277
nociceptive pain p.277
numeric rating scale (NRS) p.280
pain p.276
recurrent pain p.277
sensory dimension of pain p.278
simple verbal descriptive scale (SVDS) p.280
transduction p.277
transient pain p.277
visual analog scale (VAS) p.280

PAIN IS a symptom common to almost every illness, disease, or traumatic injury; it occurs without regard to age, gender, or socioeconomic status. All cultures recognize the experience of pain, although the ways they express and respond to it may differ. Pain alerts an individual to an injury and encourages guarding of the injury to prevent further damage. In most cases, pain is a transient and unpleasant experience that persists temporarily before becoming an annoyance and then a memory. For most people, the experience of pain leads to a diagnosis of the source of pain, successful treatment, and resolution of pain within a relatively short period of time. For others, pain becomes a complex experience that may not result in a diagnosis or successful treatment. For a few patients, pain is a disease. These patients may live with pain that persists for years, and possibly for the rest of their lives.

Pain is a health problem of epidemic proportions Institute of Medicine [IOM], 2011. Millions of patients are unable to find health care providers who are knowledgeable and willing to treat pain (American Academy of Pain Medicine, 2008; IOM, 2011). Pain management specialists are relatively few in number, clinics are generally located only in metropolitan areas, and health care coverage for pain treatment is often limited. Health care professionals, patients, and their family members are often misinformed, resulting in misconceptions and myths regarding pain and pain treatments that can create conflict as patients seek relief from their pain. In this challenging environment, patients are burdened with navigating an unfriendly health care system at a time when they are in pain, are unable to—or have a limited ability to—advocate for themselves, and are vulnerable to accepting whatever health care they

Weblink: Stanford Encyclopedia of Philosophy: Pain Weblink: Ethics and Pain Management in Hospitalized Patients

can access easily. When pain is chronic, patients are likely to experience personal distress from strained relationships, loss of independence, and depression. Patients in chronic pain often are unable to consistently participate in work-related activities, leading to loss of income and financial instability (Cowan, 2011; Jacques, 2010; Singh, 2012).

Epidemiology

A national health survey estimates that one-fourth (26%) of adults in the United States reported that in the past 30 days they had a problem with pain that persisted for more than 24 hours. One in 10 said that the pain lasted for a year or more (National Center for Health Statistics, 2009).

Pain is associated with significant personal, economic, and social distress. Research indicates that hospitalized patients suffering unrelieved pain are more likely to experience delayed wound healing, pneumonia, and other postoperative complications (Dunwoody, 2008). Pain also is associated with agitation, decreased mobility, sleep deprivation, and postoperative delirium (Pasero & McCaffery, 2010). In recent years, scientific studies have begun to uncover the connection between persistently unrelieved acute pain, subsequent hypersensitivity to pain, and the transition to chronic pain syndromes (Young, Casey, Greenberg, Nicassio, Harpin, & Hubbard, 2008; Polomano, Rathmell, Krenzoschek, & Dunwoody, 2008). These consequences of unrelieved pain are commonly associated with increased costs of providing health care (Cowan, 2011; Engebretson, 2012; Mayday Fund, 2009). They also create financial and personal burdens for patients and underscore the need to make every effort possible to relieve pain in the acute stages.

Pain management is associated with legal, ethical, and political concerns. In 2000, The Joint Commission released pain management standards that require accredited health care organizations to educate patients about their right to receive appropriate assessment and management of pain. As a result, patients are becoming better informed health care consumers who have expectations that their pain will be assessed and managed appropriately. Increased consumer awareness has improved patients' advocacy skills, resulting in increased legal liability for health care institutions, health care providers, and nurses (Dempski, 2009). More than ever before, nurses must be aware of the statutes and regulations that address the appropriate treatment of pain. Administering excessive amounts of pain medication can lead to sanctions and even criminal penalties for nurses. In addition, nurses who do not appropriately treat pain can be investigated and disciplined (Zalon, Constantino, & Andrew, 2008).

In addition to legal responsibilities, nurses have an ethical obligation to relieve pain. Nurses' ethical responsibilities when caring for patients are outlined in the American Nurses Association (ANA) *Code of Ethics* (ANA, 2001). Additionally, *The ICN Code of Ethics for Nurses* preamble states that nurses have the fundamental responsibility to alleviate suffering (International Council of Nurses [ICN], 2006). The use of placebos in the treatment of pain, treating the patient who has an addiction as well as pain, and treatment of pain at the end of life are examples of ethical challenges that nurses face in everyday practice. The American Society for Pain Management Nursing (ASPMN) (www.aspmn.org) has issued position statements that are useful guides for nurses when they are confronted with difficult ethical situations in the course of managing pain. The Ethical Issues box discusses additional ethical issues related to pain management.

In spite of positive strides, significant barriers prevent the provision of appropriate pain management for many patients. Patients and family members continue to be fearful that the use of opioids to treat pain will result in addiction. Health care professionals confuse physical dependence and tolerance to opioids as addiction, and consumers are bombarded with inaccurate data and information regarding opioid abuse and diversion. Health care provider, nursing, and pharmacy educational curricula lack evidence-based information regarding pain and pain management, and health care professionals enter their practice without adequate knowledge of pain management principles.

ETHICAL ISSUES in Nonmalignant Pain Management

Historically, the treatment of chronic nonmalignant pain has been controversial. This controversy is pervasive in those cases where the quality or state of the pain exceeds the expected norm for the diagnosis, as well as in cases where there is medical uncertainty regarding the etiology of the chronic pain (Vallerand & Nowak, 2010). These concerns are, in part, the reason that chronic pain is undertreated. In 2011, the American College of Physicians (ACP) established Clinical Practice Guidelines for the treatment of chronic pain, taking into account recent studies of patients' responses to chronic pain and patient satisfaction with pain assessment and management (Topolovec-Vranic et al., 2010). The Guidelines are directed toward the management of chronic pain precipitated by a variety of causes (e.g., low back pain, fibromylagia, osteoarthritis) and the ethical issues associated with treatment (ACP, 2012; Bolen, 2008). The guidelines can be seen on the following website: www.acponline.org/ckunucak_information/guidelines/guidelines/.

NATIONAL GUIDELINES for Pain Management

The National Institutes of Health provides a web page with a plan for comprehensive pain management that spans all age groups. Topics covered include:

- Diagnosis/symptoms
- Treatment
- Health check tools
- Alternative therapy
- Rehabilitation/recovery
- Coping
- Disease management
- Specific conditions
- Related issues.

Note: All of the information on this website is available in English and Spanish. In addition, a basic information sheet entitled "About Your Pain," which includes both the numeric and FACES pain scales, is available in many languages including Arabic, Chinese, Russian, and Tagalog.

Source: National Institutes of Health. (2008). Retrieved from http://medlineplus.nlm.nih.gov/medlineplus/pain.html#fromthenationalinstitutesofhealth.

Definitions of Pain

Discussion of pain is difficult without first defining the terms commonly used to describe pain. The lack of consistent language is confusing to patients and family members as well as health care providers. Is pain the same as suffering? What is the difference between acute pain and chronic pain? Improved understanding of the principles of pain management begins with learning the terms that are commonly used and then using consistent language in discussions with professional colleagues and when educating patients and families.

Pain is defined as an unpleasant sensory and emotional experience associated with actual or potential tissue damage, or described in terms of such damage (International Association for the Study of Pain [IASP], 2011). Pain is always a subjective experience (Aydede, 2010).

It is the subjective nature of pain that creates difficulty for the clinician who feels compelled to prove whether pain is present. Nurses must recognize that the physical assessment is *incomplete* without assessing patients' understanding of their illness including their pain. In 1968, Margo McCaffery's definition, "Pain is whatever the experiencing person says it is, existing whenever he says it does," described the need to appreciate that behaviors may not be consistent with the experience of pain and that the most reliable indicator of the presence of pain is the patient's report (McCaffery, 1968; National Institutes of Health [NIH], 1987).

Pain Descriptors

Acute pain is considered to be of relatively short duration and coincides with injury, surgery, or illness. When healing occurs, acute pain decreases and resolves within a relatively predictable period of time (Pasero & McCaffery, 2010). However, it is difficult to classify pain based only on duration. Acute pain may persist but still coincide with a high degree of pathology that does not meet the criteria expected for chronic pain. It may be appropriate to consider pain that is associated with high levels of pathology that can usually be linked to the injury, surgery, or illness as acute, regardless of its duration.

Recurrent pain is defined as acute pain episodes that are relatively short in duration and then completely resolve, leaving the patient pain free for a period of time before pain reoccurs. This type of pain is usually associated with a chronic disease process that is painless except for the episodes of acute pain (e.g., sickle cell disease, pancreatitis, or Crohn's disease). When resolution of pain does not occur within the expected time frame and is persistent beyond 3 to 6 months, it is considered to be **chronic pain.** Chronic pain is sometimes difficult to connect to an injury or illness and may persist for months, years, or even the patient's lifetime. Chronic pain is associated with low or absent levels of pathology that can be linked to injury, surgery, or illness. The intensity of pain perceived by the patient may appear to be inconsistent with the existing pathology (Borne et al., 2010). Common types of chronic pain complaints include headache, low back pain, arthritis pain, or pain resulting from damage to the peripheral nerves or to the central nervous system (CNS) itself. A less common example of chronic pain is pain that is not due to past disease or injury or any visible sign of damage inside or outside the nervous system (psychogenic pain) (National Institute of Neurological Disorders and Stroke [NINDS], 2007a). Untreated chronic pain is currently being recognized as a major health problem in the United States.

Transient pain is acute pain that is brief and then resolves completely, such as the pain associated with a needlestick for phlebotomy or an intramuscular injection. Transient pain is associated with minor tissue damage rather than disease or significant tissue damage (Porth, 2010).

Breakthrough pain is defined as intense increases in pain that occur with rapid onset even when pain-control medication is being used. Breakthrough pain can occur spontaneously or in relation to a specific activity (National Cancer Institute, 2010). It is referred to as breakthrough pain because the pain "breaks through" the patient's regular pain medication. Breakthrough pain is commonly associated with cancer pain, although it can occur with chronic pain as well. It may be easily confused with the pain caused by a painful procedure (acute pain) or the pain experienced as the effects of analgesic medications decline (end-of-dose failure).

Cancer pain is associated with malignancy and can be acute and chronic in nature. Acute cancer pain is generally caused by disease progression, surgery or procedures, and medications or therapies used in the treatment of cancer. Chronic cancer pain also can occur as a result of nerve injury leading to painful neuropathies (International Association for the Study of Pain [IASP], 2012). Cancer pain is discussed in detail in Chapter 57.

Weblink: Pain

Video: Chronic Pain

Pain as a Multidimensional Phenomenon

The currently accepted definition of pain and the evolving pain theories of the 21st century all support the rationale that pain is much more than the physical response to tissue damage. Pain is multidimensional and includes the patient's emotions, behaviors, and functionality, both physically and mentally, in response to the pain. A singular description of pain is not accurate: Consideration of all of the dimensions of pain is necessary to fully appreciate the individuality and complexity of the pain experience. The multiple dimensions of pain discussed in the following subsections are physiological, sensory, affective, cognitive, and behavioral.

Physiological Dimension

Both the peripheral and central nervous systems are involved in processing the perception of pain. Pain often is classified by its pathophysiology into two major types: nociceptive and neuropathic. **Nociceptive pain** involves normal neural processing of pain that occurs when free nerve endings are activated by tissue damage or inflammation. Neuropathic pain involves abnormal processing of stimuli from the peripheral or central nervous systems and is thought to serve no useful purpose (Pasero & McCaffery, 2010).

Nociceptive Pain

Nociception involves four processes: transduction, transmission, perception, and modulation. First, tissue damage releases chemical mediators such as prostaglandin, bradykinin, serotonin, substance P, and histamine. These substances activate nociceptors, which are nerve endings found in the skin, dental pulp, perisoteum, meninges, and some internal organs. Activation of the nociceptors results in **transduction,** which is the generation of an action potential (electrical impulse). In transmission, the second process, the action potential moves from the site of injury along afferent nerve fibers to nociceptors at the spinal cord. Release of substance P and other neurotransmitters carries the action potential across the cleft to the dorsal horn of the spinal cord. From there, the action potential ascends the spinothlamic tract to the thalamus and the midbrain. From the thalamus, fibers send the nociceptive message to the somatosensory cortex, parietal and frontal lobes, and finally to the limbic system, where the third process, perception, occurs (Cox & Karapas, 2010).

Perception, the conscious experience of pain, involves both sensory and affective components of pain. Recent clinical research has yielded an understanding of the role of the limbic system (which supports a variety of functions including emotion, behavior, long-term memory, and olfaction) and its role in the emotional response to pain. Modulation, the last nociceptive process, results from activation of the midbrain. Multiple types of neurons in this area that have a variety of neurotransmitters descend to lower areas in the central nervous system. These neurons stimulate the release of additional neurotransmitters that ultimately trigger the release of endogenous opioids and inhibit the transmission of the pain impulse at the dorsal horn (Wuhrman & Cooney, 2011).

Endorphins and **enkephalins** are endogenous morphine-like substances that reduce or suppress the pain perception in the descending pathways. These descending spinal pathways conduct inhibitory impulses by releasing serotonin, norepinephrine, and endorphins, which reduce nociceptive transmission in the CNS. This process modulates the pain, making it highly personal and individualized (Briggs et al. 2010; Porth & Marfin, 2009). Response to pain depends on the patient's past experience with pain, the cause of the pain, learned cultural responses, fear, anxiety, age, and individual beliefs.

Neuropathic Pain

The second type of pain, neuropathic pain, occurs when there is direct damage to the nerves (Porth & Marfin, 2009). **Neuropathic pain** is a result of injury or dysfunction in the peripheral nervous system. It can progress to the CNS, altering its function and resulting in a chronic, painful disease (NINDS, 2007a; Urch & Dickenson, 2008). Instead of loss of sensation, as would be expected with nerve damage, some injuries are associated with abnormal pain. Normal stimuli, such as light pressure, may result in significant pain; normal noxious stimulation, such as bumping the affected area, produces a supernormal pain response. Traumatic nerve injury, certain diseases (especially shingles and diabetes), and certain toxins (e.g., anticancer medications) can cause these painful neuropathies.

The type of injury or disease dictates the origin of the pain. Pain that originates in the skin and subcutaneous tissue is referred to as *superficial,* pain from muscles and bones is *somatic,* and pain originating in the organs is *visceral.* Somatic pain is typically described as dull or sharp, and aching. It is most commonly caused by a cut; heat, such as that from a burn injury; ischemia; or bone displacement. Visceral pain typically is described as dull or sharp, aching, and cramping. It is caused by distention, ischemia, spasms, and chemical irritants, such as medications or spicy food.

Physiological and Pathological Consequences of Unrelieved Pain

Undertreated pain can produce serious adverse physiological, psychological, and immunological effects. Inadequate pain control can stimulate a stress response that involves the cardiovascular, pulmonary, gastrointestinal, metabolic, and neuroendocrine systems (Dunwoody et al., 2008). Pain causes catabolism, which leads to poor wound healing, weakness, and muscle breakdown. Increased heart rate and blood pressure increases the risk of thromboembolic events due to stress hormone effects and decreased mobility. Chapter 9 describes the relationship of the stress response and pain. Pain can impair respiratory effort, increasing the risk of infection and hypoxemia. In addition, pain increases salt and water retention, resulting in fluid overload and hypokalemia. Pain also causes decreased gastrointestinal motility and increased blood pressure. Anxiety, depression, and sleep deprivation are commonly associated with pain. Immunologically, pain is associated with reduced natural killer cell counts indicating impaired immune response (Porth, 2010). Increasing evidence suggests that undertreated acute pain may predispose patients to chronic pain syndromes due to neuronal plasticity (Centers for Disease Control and Prevention, 2010).

Sensory Dimension

The **sensory dimension of pain** includes consideration of its location, intensity, quality, and temporal patterns. An understanding of these factors will influence the diagnosis and treatment. Many patients will experience pain in more than one location, and each location may be associated with a different intensity, quality, and pattern. Neuropathic pain, for example, is generally located along the anatomic distribution of the nerve or where the spinal cord is affected. Nociceptive pain may be localized to the injury and the immediate surrounding area. Pain intensity may be described in a variety of ways. Patients can be instructed to use numbers from a scale, select a drawing of a face that best illustrates their pain, or select descriptive words such as *mild* or *severe* (Chart 12–1). If encouraged to describe the quality of their pain, most patients can provide a fairly graphic description using one or two words without coaching. The temporal pattern of pain is generally described in terms of the onset and duration using terms such as *constant* or *steady*, *intermittent*, and *episodic* (Merck Manual of Diagnosis and Therapy, 2007b; Neuropathic Pain Management, 2011).

Affective Dimension

The **affective dimension of pain** describes the emotions patients assign to their pain, both positive and negative. For example, the patient recovering from surgery to remove a benign mass would possibly assign different emotions to his pain than would the patient with a malignant tumor. In addition to the patient's own emotions related to pain, the emotions and support of friends and family impact the pain experience. Feeling loved and supported by those who are meaningful in the patient's life can reduce the intensity of pain (Price, Riley, & Wade, 2010). Conversely, patients who do not have a good support system will report greater discomfort. Nurses have long noted that fear, frustration, anger, stress, and anxiety are all associated with increased pain intensity. Descriptive words such as *unbearable*, *punishing*, and *terrifying* convey a different meaning than do *annoying*, *tiring*, and *exhausting*. When negative emotions overwhelm the patient, the term *suffering* is used to describe the unpleasant physical and emotional components of pain. Hallmarks of suffering include feelings of uncontrollability, hopelessness, helplessness, and intolerability that undermine the patient's self-identity and integrity.

Cognitive and Cultural Dimensions

The **cognitive dimension of pain** includes the impact of personal beliefs, attitudes, and meanings attached to pain. Factors such as self-efficacy, self-control, and the locus of control can be beneficial or detrimental to the experience of pain. Patients who have a history of psychological problems generally report pain that is out of proportion to their physical disability and are prone to a greater degree of disability and depression when pain is chronic (Merck Manual of Diagnosis and Therapy, 2007b). Successful treatment of chronic pain often includes assisting the patient to convert unrealistic expectations into willingness to acknowledge and then accept pain as a part of his life. Acceptance enhances the patient's ability to cope and results in improved outcomes and satisfaction with the quality of life (Gordon et al., 2010; Mackintosh & Elson, 2008).

Nurses come to the patient's bedside carrying their own values and beliefs about pain and illness. It is important for nurses to recognize their own prejudices and values, and not to let them affect their perception of

CHART 12–1 Unidimensional Pain Intensity Measurement Tools

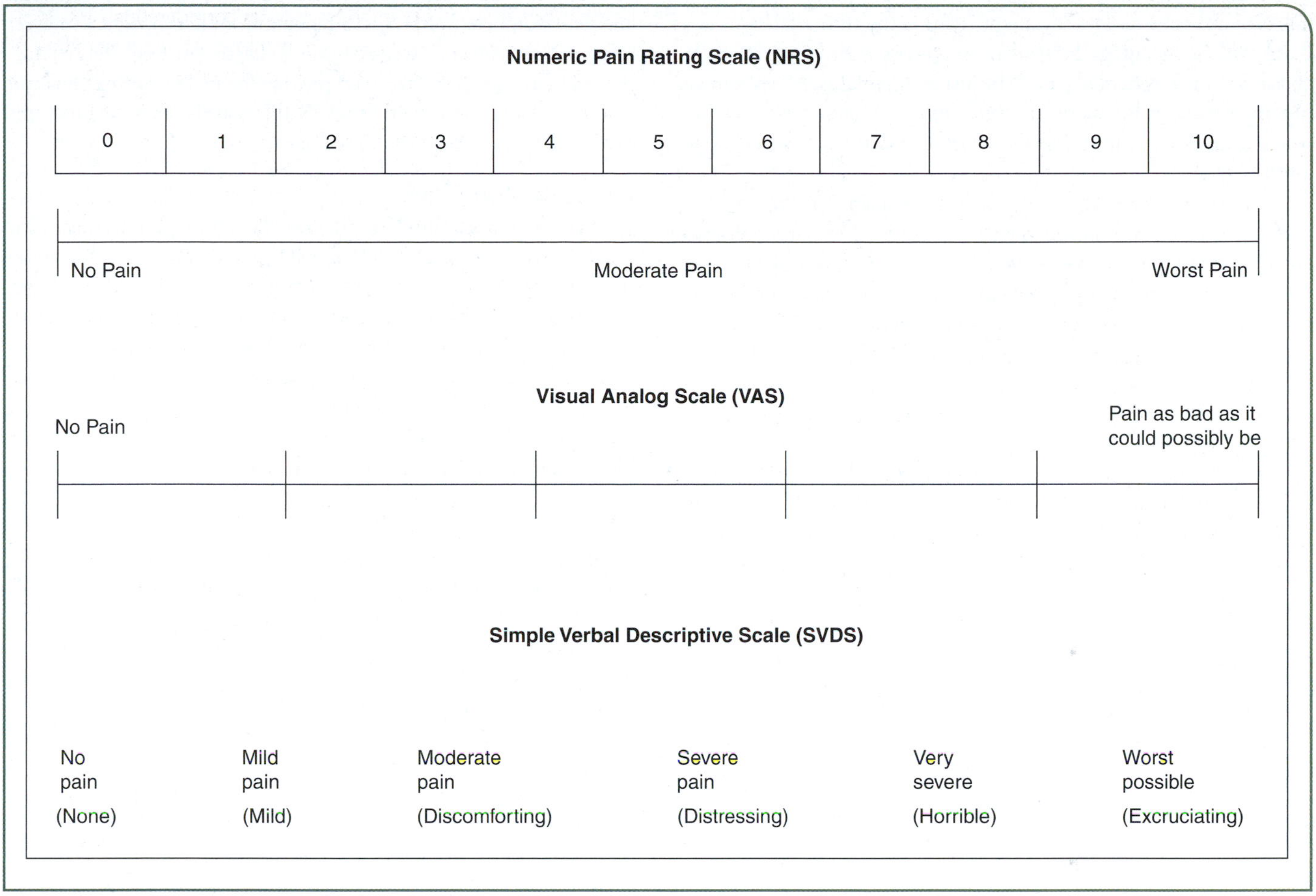

a patient's beliefs and pain concepts. Satisfaction with pain management is a nursing-sensitive outcome, yet many patients from different cultures may not be interested in pain management satisfaction. It is, therefore, imperative that nurses treat each patient as an individual and provide pain relief that best fits the patient's complaint (D'Arcy, 2009).

The Cultural Considerations box discusses how spiritual beliefs and culture affect patients' cognitive responses to pain.

Behavioral Dimension

The **behavioral dimension of pain** includes responses to pain that may be situational, developmental, or learned. Both nonverbal and verbal behaviors are commonly associated with the expression of pain. Grimacing, a furrowed brow, guarding, agitation, and avoiding required activities are examples of nonverbal expressions of pain. Verbal expressions of pain include crying, moaning, and screaming. It is appropriate to expect patients to demonstrate anxiety in situations that are not familiar to them, such as treatment in an emergency department or hospitalization. Patients who have developmental delays will demonstrate behaviors consistent with the situation and their developmental age. When pain is well controlled, pain behaviors alleviate or resolve; when this happens, patients appear more relaxed, are calmer, and are able to participate in both daily activities and required activities of recovery.

Failure to respond to a patient's report of pain may encourage the development of learned pain behaviors. Patients who think that their reports of pain will not be believed unless they appear to be uncomfortable may purposefully demonstrate behaviors consistent with pain when clinicians are present (Pasero & McCaffery, 2010).

CULTURAL CONSIDERATIONS
Related to Patient Responses to Pain

Spiritual beliefs, culture, and family affect patients' cognitive responses to pain. A child learns from an early age how to respond to and express pain from observations of family members. Acceptable responses vary among different cultures. Some cultures believe pain is a punishment for wrongdoing, whereas others feel it is a direct result of a past or future event. Spiritual rituals, such as prayer, may play an important comforting role in some cultures, whereas other cultures use food rituals to restore balance in the body. Patients may be stoic, remaining silent about their pain, or they may be verbally expressive and prone to pain behaviors such as moaning or crying. In some cultures, the patient may remain silent while the head of the family speaks for the patient. Each of these situations and responses plays an important role in the individual's cognitive responses to pain.

Pain Measurement and Assessment

Failure to measure and assess pain appropriately has long been recognized as a barrier to appropriate pain management. It is essential for nurses and all health care team members to understand the significance of assessing and providing effective pain management. To emphasize this point, the American Pain Society launched a campaign in the late 1990s to increase awareness of the importance of the pain intensity assessment. The statement "Pain is the fifth vital sign" was developed to encourage health care providers and organizations to consider the assessment of pain to be just as essential as the assessment of temperature, pulse, blood pressure, and respiratory rate. In other words, pain assessment should be incorporated into routine vital sign assessments.

Not only is it important to regularly assess pain, it is important to assess it correctly and thoroughly to create a pain management plan tailored to meet the patient's individual needs. The plan should be based on a unidimensional measurement of pain intensity and a complete assessment of the patient's multidimensional experience of pain.

Assessment and measurement tools have evolved over the past decades; multiple tools are now available to meet the specific needs of patients with different disease states, ages and developmental stages, and cognitive abilities. Depending on the patient's needs, any one of the tools may be appropriate in a given situation. Regardless of the tool selected, patients should be educated about its use. The same tool should be used consistently to encourage accurate trending of changes, to facilitate familiarity with the tool, and to ultimately increase the ease of use. Because these tools rely on the patient's ability to understand how to use them properly, patients who speak a language other than that of the health care team should be provided with a tool featuring numbers and descriptors written in their own language to prevent misunderstandings due to language barriers. Assessment tools should always be validated by research and found reliable in the patient population with which they are used (see the note in the National Guidelines box to learn how to obtain pain scales in many languages). Additionally, both the nurse and the patient are more likely to use and document tools that they can use easily (Gordon et al., 2011).

At times, nurses express frustration over their inability to verify the accuracy of the patient's report of pain intensity. Although most patients with pain will not attempt to lie or deceive, a few will. Although clinicians are required to accept the patient's report of pain, accepting does not require believing. When there is doubt regarding the truthfulness of a patient's response, it is important to recognize the potential for accepting a false report of pain, and that the possibility of providing an unnecessary intervention is offset by the importance of accepting the many reports of pain that are valid and truthful and that require appropriate interventions (Pasero & McCaffery, 2010). Nurses must value the fact that the patient is the only one who can identify the intensity of pain.

Unidimensional Measurement Tools

Unidimensional measurement tools are used to measure only one component of the pain. As a result, unidimensional measurement of pain is an incomplete assessment if the remaining multidimensional aspects of pain are not evaluated. In most cases, unidimensional tools are used to determine the patient's report of the intensity or severity of pain.

Numeric Rating Scale

The **numeric rating scale (NRS)** is a horizontal line with numbers from 0 to 10 ranging from left to right (see Chart 12–1, p. 279). Three interval descriptors of pain are located along the scale: "No Pain," "Moderate Pain," and "Worst Pain." Once a patient is instructed on how to use the scale, assessment can be completed within a few minutes, making it easy for both the patient and the clinician to use, document, and trend.

Simple Verbal Descriptive Scale

The **simple verbal descriptive scale (SVDS)** also uses a horizontal line with numbers from 0 to 10 ranging from left to right. However, interval descriptors of "No Pain," "Mild," "Discomforting," "Distressing," "Horrible," or "Excruciating" pain provide the patient with a few more descriptive options. As with the NRS, this scale is relatively quick and easy for both the patient and the clinician to use.

Visual Analog Scale

The **visual analog scale (VAS)** does not have numeric intervals; rather, it uses "No Pain" and "Pain as Bad as It Can Possibly Be" as descriptors at either end of a horizontal line measuring 10 centimeters in length. Each centimeter on the scale corresponds to a number from 0 to 10. The patient is instructed to draw a vertical line through the scale to indicate the intensity of pain. Although this scale is relatively easy for the patient to use, it requires measurement from the start of the scale to the point where the vertical line is drawn to determine the 0 to 10 score. This makes the scale less useful to a busy clinician.

Behavioral Assessment

When patients are unable to report their pain intensity (e.g., immediate postoperative patients, those with cognitivie impairment or who have dementia, those who are sedated, the critically ill, those who are unconscious), behavioral assessment tools can be used to guide observation for pain-related behaviors. This type of unidimensional tool, often validated for use with preverbal pediatric patients, should be used with caution in adults because pain-related behaviors may be inconsistent (either over- or underemphasized) with actual pain.

Patients who are critically ill represent a large population of nonverbal patients. These patients are at considerable risk for unrelieved pain. One of the primary reasons for inadequate pain relief is the lack of an appropriate pain relief assessment for nonverbal patients as previously described (Puntillo, 2007). Nursing researchers are currently studying ways to measure pain in this population (Gelinas, 2010; Gelinas, Fillion, & Puntillo, 2009; Pudas-Tähkä, Axelin, Aantas, & Salantera, 2009). To date, no valid standardized assessment tool exists for use in all populations of critically ill patients. However, the Critical-Care Pain Observation Tool (CPOT) has been researched and validated in nonverbal critically ill patients (Gelinas, 2010; Gelinas et al., 2009). This tool assesses four behavioral categories: (1) facial expressions, (2) body movements, (3) muscle tension, and (4) compliance with the ventilator for the patient on mechanical ventilation. Originally used in conjunction with research studies, this tool is being adopted by medical centers in North America (Gelinas, 2010).

Multidimensional Assessment and Measurement Tools

Multidimensional assessment and measurement tools such as the patient interview, the **McGill Pain Questionnaire (MPQ),** and the **Brief Pain Inventory (BPI)** assess more than one dimension of pain. The MPQ provides 20 sets of words patients can use to describe pain and scores their responses. Each set of words varies in intensity and measures either the sensory or affective dimension of pain. One set scores the intensity of pain. Patients also document the location of the pain on a body diagram provided as part of the questionnaire. In contrast, the BPI asks multiple questions regarding pain and its impact on patient function and addresses the multidimensionality of the pain experience.

Depending on the situation, these tools have advantages and disadvantages that may make them more useful or inappropriate. Most of these tools require the patient to have both the cognitive ability and the time to complete the tool. These two requirements make some of the tools difficult for both patients and busy nurses to use routinely. However, when pain management is complex, the time spent completing a multidimensional tool can be invaluable.

Patient Interview

The patient interview is the most commonly used multidimensional tool in nursing practice. The interviewer usually uses a unidimensional tool in addition to the interview questions to determine the patient's pain intensity. When appropriate, the patient interview can also be combined with any multidimensional tool. Prior to conducting an interview, the nurse should review the patient's medical history. Components of the patient's history that are specifically useful in the assessment of pain include:

- Previous experiences with pain, including trauma, surgery, or chronic pain
- Medications taken previously or currently to relieve pain
- Significant social history including drug, alcohol, or tobacco abuse
- Comorbid conditions, such as renal insufficiency, pulmonary disease, or hepatic dysfunction, which should be considered when administering analgesics.

During the patient interview, the nurse's demeanor should be supportive and interested. Allow sufficient time for the patient to answer the questions. Patients experiencing moderate to severe pain may have difficulty answering questions. Make every effort to make the patient as comfortable as possible before the interview takes place. Interview questions may include the following:

- Where are you having pain?
- Are you having pain anywhere else?
- How intense is the pain?
- What does the pain feel like?
- When did the pain begin?
- How long does the pain last?
- What makes the pain worse?
- Have you had this type of pain before?
- How does your pain affect your daily activities, sleep, mood, and relationships?
- What do you do to reduce the pain?
- On a scale of 1 to 10, what level of pain is acceptable to you?

Multidimensional Assessment of At-Risk Patients

Factors such as developmental delays, cognitive impairment, severe emotional disturbance, and critical illness may render patients incapable of providing an accurate report of pain intensity and preclude participation in the patient interview (Puntillo, 2007). Patients who are unable to report their pain intensity are at risk for undermanagement of pain (Chapman, 2008). Nurses should avoid erroneously concluding that a patient cannot provide a self-report. Studies have demonstrated that patients with mild to moderate cognitive impairment are able to report pain successfully using unidimensional measurement tools and short versions of some multidimensional assessment tools (Schofield, 2008). The PQRST method for pain assessment is a multidimensional approach to assessing a person's acute pain status. This mnemonic approach to pain assessment is shown in Chart 12–2.

CHART 12–2 PQRST Method for Pain Assessment

Provokes
- What causes pain?
- What makes it better?

Quality
- What does it feel like?
- Is it sharp?
- Dull?
- Stabbing?
- Burning?
- Crushing? (Try to let the patient describe her pain, as she sometimes says what she thinks the clinician would like to hear.)

Radiation/Region
- Where is it located?
- Does it go anywhere else?

Severity
- How severe is the pain on a scale of 1 to 10?

Time
- Time pain started?
- How long did it last?

Source: Adapted from Critical Care Nursing. (2010). PQRST method for pain assessment. Retrieved from http://micunursing.com/pain.htm.

Nurses should also evaluate other risk factors associated with the onset of persistent pain. Preoperative anxiety, being younger, being unmarried, having more invasive surgeries, and having greater preoperative emotional distress have been found to be predictors of long-term post-operative pain (Bruckenthal, 2008). Research indicates that persistent pain following common surgeries, such as hernia repair and breast and thoracic surgery, occurs in 10% to 50% of patients. Naturopathic pain is probably the most important cause of long-term postsurgical pain (Bruckenthal, 2008). Pasero and McCaffery (2010) suggest specific assessment approaches that will ensure that patients who are at risk of poor pain management are appropriately managed. Initially, make sure that the patient cannot report his own pain. Consider his pathological condition and individualized procedures that are known to be painful. Observe the patient for behaviors consistent with pain such as withdrawal, crying, and protective posture, or use a family member or caregiver to indicate the patient's perceived pain level.

The Evidence-Based Practice box describes patients' assessment of pain using three methods of measurement.

Documentation of Pain Assessment

As the health care team member most likely to spend the greatest amount of time with the patient and family, the nurse plays a pivotal role in the appropriate management of pain. Documentation of assessment findings is a vital part of the patient's medical record. Nursing documentation provides details that the multidisciplinary team members may not have had an opportunity to elicit. Because many team members will review the nursing documentation, it is important that details about the pain assessment, treatments, and the patient's response to treatments are accurately and completely documented on the medical record so that decisions regarding the plan of care are made with consideration of the information the nurse has compiled.

EVIDENCE-BASED PRACTICE Pain Management

Clinical Problem

Management of patients' pain is an ongoing nursing challenge. Due to patients' individual perceptions and responses, it can be difficult to quantify the pain. Typically, health care providers order a variety of medications and dosages that may be administered based on the level of pain. Therefore, it is essential that nurses make an accurate assessment of the pain in order to decide on the correct type and dose of medication. A number of pain intensity scales, as described earlier in this chapter, have been developed to assist nurses in standardizing pain levels and subsequent pain management, but the controversy continues about the best method to quantify pain.

Research Findings

McDonald, LaPorta, and Meadows-Oliver (2007) conducted a study to determine nurses' responses to patients' reports of pain. The study evaluated three different methods that patients used to describe their pain:

Personal description along with a numeric scale

Personal description only

Numeric scale only.

Nurses were randomly assigned to three groups; all were given a vignette about a trauma patient with moderate to severe pain. The vignettes were identical except for the patient's age and the three different methods used by the patients to describe their pain. The results showed that there was no difference in the nurses' responses to the pain management between the three modes. The authors further noted that a relatively small number of pain management strategies were identified by the sample nurses to respond to moderately severe pain.

Implications for Nursing Practice

Knowledge of effective pain management is still an evolving area of health care. It is a multifaceted area with issues of effective relief, addiction, and legal ramifications woven into the management decisions. Nurses are in a pivotal position and therefore must have knowledge of and an appreciation for these issues. Nurses' approach to pain management also requires sensitivity to individual responses to pain. When using the numeric scores, it is important to use the appropriate terminology and to inquire further about the reason for the score on the pain scale (Leleszi & Lewandowski, 2007). For example, some patients report a pain number and then state they are comfortable with a certain pain level as it relates to their diagnosis and do not require medication, whereas other patients report the same score and are not comfortable and therefore require treatment.

Prior use of both legal and illegal medications also may impact pain scores. Occasionally, patients with illicit drug histories demonstrate "drug-seeking" behaviors such as fabricating pain levels in order to receive medication. Nurses must come to understand patients' individual nuances to manage pain effectively. Use of both personal account and numeric scales provides the nurse with more data when making treatment decisions.

Critical Thinking Questions with answers can be found in the Osborn Student Resources at nursing.pearsonhighered.com.

References

Leleszi, J. P., & Lewandowski, J. G. (2007). Managing pain in patients at end of life. *Journal of the American Osteopathic Association, Supplement 4, 107*(6), E53–E59.

McDonald, D. D., Laporta, M., & Meadows-Oliver, M. (2007). Nurse's responses to pain communication from patients: A post-test experimental study. *International Journal of Nursing Studies, 44*(1), 29–35.

Whether recorded on a paper flow sheet, input into an electronic health record (EHR), or written in narrative, the nurse's documentation of pain assessment and measurement creates a baseline by which improvement or negative trends are measured. The Joint Commission's standards on pain management (2010) require that health care organizations have policies regarding the assessment and management of pain. These standards are reinforced in The Joint Commission's 2010 National Patient Safety Goals. The nurse must know and understand the contents of policies specific to the workplace, and the nursing documentation should reflect that nursing care was given according to institutional policy.

Safety Alert *Nursing documentation in the legal health record should reflect topics such as these:*

1. *Pain management that was delivered following institutional policy, with consideration of the patient assessment and responses to treatments, and in accordance with ordered interventions.*
2. *Responses to unrelieved pain, including administration of additional analgesic medications; use of nonmedication treatments; health care provider or licensed independent practitioner contact; and subsequent changes to the patient's pain management plan of care.*
3. *The avoidance of labels such as psychotic, whiner, drug seeker, or addict.*

Pain Management

In response to historical issues and more recent trends, the Agency for Healthcare Policy and Research and The Joint Commission have attempted to provide guidance to improve pain management. In the Joint Commission released the first standards addressing pain management in 1999. These standards, based on the same valid recommendations published in the AHCPR guidelines of 1992 and 1994, require health care organizations to implement a multidisciplinary team and create an institutional commitment to pain management (The Joint Commission, 2010). The current Joint Commission standards require hospitals to conduct a thorough pain assessment of every patient, and to conduct that assessment in a manner appropriate to the patient's age, condition and ability to understand. The Joint Commission also requires that the hospital treat the patient's pain or refer the patient for treatment, and to reassess pain according to established guidelines (The Joint Commission, 2010). The following sections outline therapeutic goals for pain management based on standards set by The Joint Commission and evidence-based practice.

Acute Pain Management Therapeutic Goals

Acute pain is often the result of surgical procedures, trauma, or burns. Acute pain problems are the most common reason why patients seek medical assistance. Nurses spend a significant portion of their time at the bedside providing pain-relieving treatments and medications (Coda & Bonica, 2009). The plan for pain management provides for organized and rational treatment appropriate to all phases of recovery including the critical or emergent phase, subsequent healing and recovery, and eventual rehabilitation.

Management of acute pain is focused on (1) reducing the sympathetic stress response, (2) safely optimizing comfort during treatment and recovery, (3) facilitating participation in recovery and rehabilitation activities, and (4) improving patient outcomes. Nurses educate patients and family members with the goal of improving their understanding of (1) the importance of pain management in the patient's recovery, (2) the role of medications and nonmedication treatment, and (3) the differences between physical dependence, tolerance, and addiction to opioid medications. Establishing comfort and function goals encourages the patient and health care team to work toward meeting a defined pain intensity score and a specific functional goal rather than an elusive or poorly defined therapeutic goal. For example, the patient with acute pain might select a pain intensity score of 3 from the 0–10 NRS with the goal of ambulating three times daily as a postoperative recovery activity.

Chronic Pain Management Therapeutic Goals

The long-term, persistent nature of chronic pain increases the likelihood that psychosocial and environmental factors will contribute to the emotional distress and physical disability that is frequently seen with pain that has limited ongoing pathology. Management of chronic pain is focused on (1) reducing the focus on pain; (2) safely optimizing comfort through appropriate use of analgesic treatments and complementary or alternative strategies; (3) increasing active participation in ADLs, work, and relationships; and (4) restoring joy and a sense of purpose despite persistent pain (Health Care Guidelines, 2011). Nurses educate patients and family members with the goal of improving understanding of (1) the role that anxiety, depression, and anger can have in escalation of pain; (2) the role of medications and complementary or alternative treatments in improving function; and (3) the differences between physical dependence, tolerance, and addiction to opioid medications.

When encouraging the patient with chronic pain to establish comfort and function goals, the process is the same as with acute pain, but the scores and functional goals are likely to be very different. Patients who experience moderate to severe pain on a daily basis may consider even a very small reduction in pain intensity as a success. Often functional goals are focused around achieving or maintaining independence in ADLs, work, or relationships and leisure activities. It may be necessary to encourage the patient to identify realistically achievable goals as an intermediate step to achieving ultimate goals in order to avoid discouragement.

Cancer Pain Management Therapeutic Goals

The management of cancer pain is a combination of the acute and chronic pain therapeutic goals mentioned previously. Given the dual nature of cancer pain, it is appropriate to have goals that address healing, recovery, and rehabilitation for the acute pain associated with surgery and cancer treatments. However, it also is appropriate to consider the role that a potentially lethal diagnosis has on increasing the likelihood of emotional distress and physical disability that are frequently seen with the pain of malignancy. Management of cancer pain is focused on (1) reducing the sympathetic stress response following surgeries or treatments; (2) safely optimizing comfort through appropriate use of analgesic treatments and complementary or alternative strategies; (3) facilitating participation in recovery and rehabilitation activities; (4) increasing active participation in ADLs, work, and relationships; and (5) preserving a sense of purpose despite a potentially lethal diagnosis. An in-depth discussion of the diagnosis and treatment of cancer is included in Chapter 57.

Pharmacologic Strategies for Managing Pain

In pain management pharmacology, the interdisciplinary team focuses on establishing a regimen that includes a balance of nonopioid, nonsteroidal anti-inflammatory, adjuvant, and opioid medications as necessary to optimize the quality of analgesia with minimal medication side effects. This method of managing pain is often referred to as **balanced or multimodal analgesia.** The pharmacologic pain management plan is accomplished through the combined efforts of multiple disciplines. The selection of medications requires that the health care provider consider the patient's medical history, including previous and current pain, and the findings of the patient interview and pain assessment as previously discussed. Treatment plans crafted in the absence of this information are often unsuccessful in relieving pain and may cause adverse effects that could potentially harm the patient.

Nurses are central to the effectiveness and safety of medication administration; they carry multiple responsibilities at every stage of the prescription process. Nurses must review prescriptions on the medical record and consider their appropriateness based on the patient assessment and relevant laboratory studies. If there are questions regarding the prescription, the nurse must contact the prescribing health care provider for clarification. When it is time to administer the medication, the nurse completes rigorous double checks to ensure the correct prescription is administered to the patient.

Pharmacologic Interventions

When discussing pharmacologic interventions, it is necessary to consider the patient's physiological status in relationship to the pharmacology of each medication selected. Considerations include how each medication is absorbed, distributed, metabolized, or biotransformed, and eventually excreted. The mechanism of action and the therapeutic and adverse effects of each medication should guide the selection and monitoring necessary to ensure patient safety.

Absorption describes the process by which the medication leaves the site of administration to cross membranes as it journeys to the site of action (Kee, Hayer, & McCuistian, 2009). For example, medications that are administered into the gastrointestinal system absorb from the stomach, small intestine, large intestine, colon, and even the rectum into the systemic circulation for distribution. In contrast, medications administered directly into the systemic circulation bypass the absorptive process and are immediately distributed.

Distribution refers to the process of moving the medication into the bloodstream, the extracellular and intracellular compartments, and the compartment that is the site of absorption and storage (Kee, Hayer, & McCuistian, 2009). Factors that affect the distribution of a medication are the size of the molecule, the degree to which it binds to protein, and the solubility of the medication. Large molecules and those that bind to protein usually stay in the bloodstream. Hydrophilic drugs, like morphine, are more slowly distributed in both the bloodstream and the extracellular compartments. Lipid-soluble medications, like fentanyl, are more rapidly absorbed and distributed throughout all three compartments (Miyoshi & Leckband, 2009).

Biotransformation or metabolism describes the process of changing a medication's structure in preparation for elimination (Kee, Hayer, & McCuistian, 2009). Metabolism occurs primarily in the liver, but also occurs in the kidneys and, to a very small degree, in other organ

Weblink: American Society for Pain Management in Nursing

Weblink: Tolerance, Physical Dependence, and Addiction

systems. Once a medication has metabolized, it is no longer the same and effectively discontinues its pharmacologic activity. **Hepatic first-pass metabolism** refers to the reduction of a medication's effect due to partial metabolism in the liver prior to distribution to the ultimate site of action. Medications may produce active metabolites that then exert a pharmacologic action of their own. This is of particular concern when the metabolite has significant adverse effects. For example, the morphine metabolite norpropoxyphene causes the following adverse effects: hypoglycemia, respiratory depression, and cardiac conduction abnormalities (Johnson, 2007).

Elimination is the process of excretion from the body that is generally accomplished in the renal system (Kee, Hayer, & McCuistian, 2009). A medication may be eliminated in its primary form or after it has metabolized. Alterations in the renal system that impair elimination prolong the effects of the primary medication and any metabolites that have been formed, potentially increasing the risks of adverse effects.

Classifying Analgesics

The three-step analgesic ladder designed by the World Health Organization (WHO) outlines recommendations for classes of analgesic medications that are appropriate for treating mild, moderate, and severe pain (World Health Organization, 2012). Figure 12–1◆ illustrates the WHO three-step analgesic ladder. This ladder provides a stepped approach based on pain severity. For example, step 1 analgesics include acetaminophen or a nonsteroidal anti-inflammatory drug (NSAID). If the pain persists or worsens despite appropriate dose increases of step 1 drugs, a change to a step 2 or step 3 analgesic is indicated. If the patient presents with moderate to severe pain, step 1 can be skipped (National Cancer Institute, 2007).

It is reasonable to choose the step that most closely describes the patient's pain intensity as a guide in determining a pain treatment plan that is likely to provide the best level of analgesia with the fewest potential adverse effects. The steps on the analgesic ladder are additive, meaning that as one progresses up the ladder, more medications are added to those already in use to achieve improved analgesia and a balanced or multimodal approach to pain management. It is important to recognize that when pain is severe, it is appropriate to begin at the top step of the analgesic ladder; movement through each step to reach the top is *not* necessary. This method of medication selection

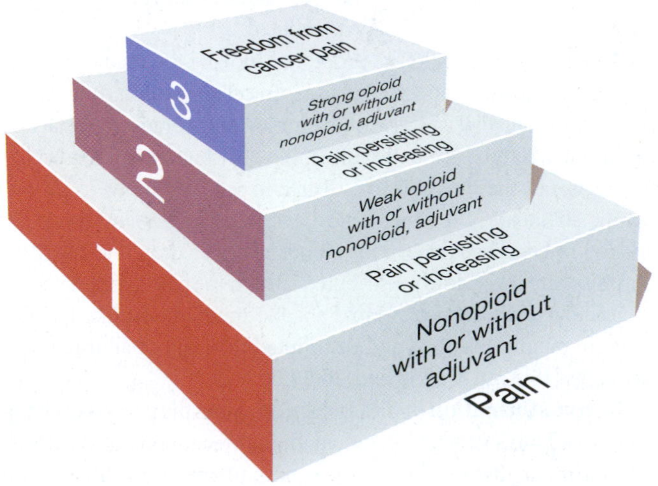

FIGURE 12–1 ◆ WHO three-step analgesic ladder.

has proven effective in acute, chronic, and cancer pain management. Nurses are vital to the medication administration and monitoring process and must understand the basic mechanism of action, pharmacology, and adverse effects of each group of medications to function effectively in their role.

Acetaminophen

Acetaminophen is one of the most widely used analgesic medications and is considered a first-line analgesic for treating mild acute and chronic pain (Miyoshi & Leckband, 2009). It is the first step in the WHO three-step approach to pain management. Its use also is important in steps 2 and 3. The Pharmacology feature includes an in-depth discussion of acetaminophen.

Safety Alert *Acetaminophen overdose is one of the most common poisonings worldwide. Patients, caregivers, and the public should be aware that acetaminophen is present in many combination cold and allergy medications such as Nyquil®, TheraFlu®, and Triaminic®. Additional doses of acetaminophen should not be taken along with these products. In 2011, the Food and Drug Administration (FDA) instructed manufacturers of prescription combination products containing acetaminophen to keep the upper limit of acetaminophen in each tablet or capsule to 325 milligrams. Manufacturers will also be required to ensure labels of all prescription combination acetaminophen products warn of the potential risk for severe liver injury.*

Nonsteroidal Anti-Inflammatory Drugs (NSAIDs)

NSAIDs effectively reduce inflammation, pain, and fever. More than 20 different NSAIDS are currently available in the United States; they are one of the most commonly used classes of drugs in the world. At equal doses, all NSAIDs are equally effective in relieving pain. However, there is an intrapatient variability in response that warrants a patient trying a different NSAID if the desired effect is not achieved by the patient's current NSAID at the maximum recommended dosage (APS, 2011). NSAIDs, along with acetaminophen, are the first step in the WHO analgesic ladder (see Figure 12–1) for mild to moderate pain. They should be used in conjunction with acetaminophen and opioids on the second and third steps for moderate to severe pain. The Pharmacology feature includes an in-depth discussion of NSAIDs.

Opioids

Opioids are morphine-like medications that play a major role in the management of moderate to severe pain for acute, cancer, and, in certain situations, chronic pain. As with all analgesic medications, opioids should only be initiated after an assessment of the patient's pain in conjunction with the significant findings of the medical history and physical exam (Chou et al., 2009).

Opioids should be added to nonopioids, NSAIDs, and adjuvants for pain that does not respond to these analgesics alone. Unlike acetaminophen and NSAIDs, opioids do not have a ceiling effect; unless combined with acetaminophen or an NSAID (e.g., Lortab, Percocet, Vicoprofen), an opioid dosage can be escalated as needed to relieve pain. The analgesia achieved by opioid administration is dose dependant, meaning that the effects of the drug change when the dose of the drug is changed. If the dosage is increased, the patient should experience less pain. With the appropriate dosing, opioids can usually relieve all intensities of pain (Miyoshi & Leckband, 2009). There is, however, a wide variation in the dosages required by individual patients to achieve pain relief. It is unrealistic to expect the same dose of opioid to be safe and effective for all patients. Therefore, opioid dosages should be increased or decreased incrementally to achieve the best level of pain relief with the lowest incidence of opioid-induced side effects. The type of opioid and the route of administration may need to be changed to achieve these desired results.

In clinical practice, it is often necessary to change either the route or the drug in the patient who is receiving opioid analgesics. Examples include (1) The patient has become NPO and must switch from oral to parenteral; (2) the patient is transitioning from postoperative parenteral to a different drug given orally; (3) high or escalating doses of one opioid are causing unacceptable side effects and must be changed. In doing so, it should be recognized that not all opioids are equally created. There are variations in metabolism, potency, available routes of administration, toxicity, side effect profile, and interaction with the opioid receptors in the body. These factors must be considered when changing the patient's medication in order to arrive at the proper dosage of the new medicaton. This determination is referred to as an **equianalgesic dose,** a new drug or route of administration that is approximately equal in ability to relieve pain as the original drug given. Equianalgesia tables are used when switching from one opiate to another, or when switching routes of administraton. This helps to minimize problems related to underdosing or overdosing (Arbuck, 2012).

Major barriers to the effective use of opioid medications are usually centered on misunderstandings regarding tolerance and physical dependence and on unfounded concerns that addiction is inevitable. Opioids require a prescription and are regulated by the Drug Enforcement Administration (DEA) to reduce the risk of abuse and diversion. The challenge of finding a balance between this risk and the need for appropriate management of pain with opioids is an additional barrier. It is of concern that the most significant barriers to effective pain relief using opioid analgesics are not complicated pharmacology or lack of good medications, but bias, regulatory scrutiny, and lack of education (Miyoshi & Leckband, 2009). Discussion of opioid tolerance, physical dependence, addiction, and pseudoaddiction is provided in Chart 12–3.

Opioids are available in two major groups, agonists and agonist-antagonists. **Agonist** opioids are often referred to as morphine-like, or mu, agonists because they bind to the mu, kappa, and delta receptors of the cell, which are located in the CNS, peripheral nervous system, and gastrointestinal tract. Agonist opioids include opioids such as morphine, codeine, meperidine, dihydromorphinone, and methadone. **Agonist-antagonist** opioids are kappa and mu receptor partial agonists and are generally considered to be less efficacious than the pure mu agonists. It should be noted that a ceiling effect on analgesia has been identified with this group of opioids (Miyoshi & Leckband, 2009). Agonist-antagonist opioids include opioids such as buprenorphine, butorphanol, pentazocine, nalbuphine, and dezocine.

CHART 12–3 Opioid Tolerance, Dependence, and Addiction

One of the most significant barriers to pain management is the concern that opioid analgesics will cause addiction. *Opiophobia* (Morgan, 1985) is the term frequently used to describe the fears that health care providers and patients share: that exposure to opioids will cause addictive disease.

When nurses have insufficient knowledge of the risks and realities of addictive disease, unethical clinical practices such as withholding opioids, administering subtherapeutic dosages when therapeutic dosages are prescribed, administering placebos, and withholding compassionate nursing care may become the hallmark of their professional practice. Nurses play a pivotal role in pain management and are recognized as patient advocates whose professional practice should be based on scientific understanding of addictive disease. Nurses must recognize the important role of opioid therapy in pain management and develop the skills necessary to provide appropriate nursing care and education to patients who have fears regarding opioids, who are recovering from opioid addiction, or who have active addictive disease.

Confusion regarding opioid tolerance, physical dependence, and addiction is common. Defining these conditions and then using these definitions consistently in professional as well as patient interactions is the first step.

- *Tolerance* is "a state of adaptation in which exposure to a drug induces changes that result in a diminution of one or more of the drug's effects over time" (American Academy of Pain Medicine [AAPM], American Pain Society [APS], & American Society of Addiction Medicine [ASAM], 2001).
- *Physical dependence* is "adaptation that is manifested by a drug class specific withdrawal syndrome that can be produced by abrupt cessation, rapid dose reduction, decreasing blood level of the drug, and/or administration of an antagonist" (AAPM/APS/ASAM, 2001).
- *Addiction* is "a primary, chronic, neurobiological disease with genetic, psychosocial, and environmental factors influencing its development and manifestations. It is characterized by behaviors that include one or more of the following: impaired control over drug use, compulsive use, continued use despite harm and craving" (AAPM/APS/ASAM, 2001).

Tolerance, physical dependence, and addiction are individual conditions that are often found in combination. *Pseudoaddiction* is a term used to describe the behaviors that can result from undertreatment of pain, such as watching the clock, requesting medications more frequently than allowed or in larger doses (drug seeking), and expressing anger or feelings of being unfairly judged. Pseudoaddiction is commonly mistaken for addiction; however, unlike addiction, its behaviors will resolve when pain is appropriately relieved (Weissman, 2008).

The following are suggestions for the nurse to consider when administering opioids for pain management:

- Assume the patient and family members have concerns regarding the risk of addiction and provide education based on scientific evidence to refute misconceptions.
- Manage pain appropriately and advocate for improvement when pain is unrelieved.
- Recognize that an opioid-tolerant patient will require higher dosages of opioid to achieve pain relief and that this need does not equal addiction.
- Respond promptly, with respect and compassion, to requests for pain medications for all patients including those with opioid tolerance, dependence, or addiction.
- Avoid personal biases, labeling of patients, or unethical practices.

Opioids that have modified release formulations to make them long acting are not appropriate for prn or "as needed" dosing (Adams & Koch, 2010). Prescribed medications with prn dosing are administered according to the judgment of the nurse or caregiver and at the patient's prerogative. (See discussion of prn dosing strategy on page 289.) Controlled-release or sustained-release opioids are designed to provide 12 to 24 hours of analgesia (up to 72 hours of analgesia in the case of transdermal fentanyl patches). Many of these opioids take as long as 4 hours to achieve peak effects and last much longer than short-acting opioids, increasing the risk of oversedation and respiratory depression with prn use. Controlled or sustained-release oral preparations must never be crushed or dissolved for administration through an orogastric or nasogastric tube because of the risk of overdose.

PHARMACOLOGY Summary of Medications Used for Pain Relief

Medication Category and Action	Application/Indication	Nursing Responsibility
Acetaminophen		
First-line analgesic for treating mild acute and chronic pain. Available over the counter in a variety of formulations including liquid, tablets, capsules, caplets, and rectal suppository. Found in combination with many medications, such as the opioids hydrocodone with acetaminophen (Lortab) and oxycodone (Percocet). An intravenous form of acetaminophen was approved for use by the FDA in November 2010. ***Action:*** Specific action is unclear; thought to be inhibition of the third isoform of the cyclooxygenase (COX-3) pathway only found in the CNS. Absorbed rapidly from the gastrointestinal tract, its low molecular weight permits easy penetration of the spinal tissues.	The first step in the WHO three-step analgesic ladder approach to pain management; included in steps 2 and 3 (see Figure 12–1, p. 284). Used in addition to anti-inflammatory medications, opioids, and adjuvants in the analgesic treatment plan unless contraindicated. The Food and Drug Administration (FDA) now requires acetaminophen to be labeled with warnings for the patient who consumes alcohol on a daily basis.	Use with caution in patients who have been fasting for prolonged periods of time or who drink more than three alcoholic beverages per day. Caution all patients to avoid exceeding eight tablets of 500 mg or a total of 4,000 mg total in 24 hours. Monitor liver function studies. Educate patients about potential side effects of overdose to prevent overdose and liver damage.
Nonsteroidal Anti-Inflammatory Drugs (NSAIDs)		
Aspirin Celecoxib Ibuprofen Indocin Ketoprofen Ketorolac (only injectable NSAID) Nabumetone Naproxen Piroxicam ***Action:*** Inhibit prostaglandin production, primarily the prostaglandin E series, via inhibition of the COX enzymes. Absorbed from the gastrointestinal tract and are, in general, highly protein bound.	First step in the WHO three-step analgesic ladder approach to pain (see Figure 12–1). Used alone for mild to moderate pain. Used in conjunction with acetaminophen and opioids on the second and third steps for moderate to severe pain. Aspirin inhibits platelet aggregation for the life of the platelet, making it useful for preventing thromboembolic events. When using NSAIDs in combination with opioids, frequently the dose of the opioid can be reduced (Chou et al., 2009). NSAIDs act as adjuvant drugs.	Assess character, duration, and intensity of pain prior to administration to determine baseline for effectiveness. Monitor for gastric pain, bleeding, and acute renal failure. Monitor BUN, ALT, AST, creatinine, and hemoglobin before and during continued use. Discontinue for several days to 1–2 weeks, if taking aspirin, before surgery or invasive procedures to reduce the risk of bleeding.
Opioids		
Codeine Dihydrocodeine Fentanyl Hydrocodone Hydromorphone Levorphanol Meperidine Methadone Morphine Oxycodone ***Action:*** A natural or synthetic morphine-like substance. Both pharmacologic effects and side effects are achieved by binding to opioid receptor cells throughout the CNS and peripheral tissues. There are three types of opioid receptors: mu, kappa, and delta. When the mu receptor is stimulated, analgesia, euphoria, reduced gastric motility, sedation, nausea, tolerance, and physical dependence occur.	Third step in the WHO three-step analgesic ladder (see Figure 12–1).Symptomatic control of moderate to severe pain and as preanesthetic medication.	Assess character, duration, and intensity of pain prior to administration to determine baseline for effectiveness. Monitor vital signs before and during treatment. Do not administer opioids if the respiratory rate is less than 12 per minute. Monitor level of consciousness and respiratory rate and depth after administration. Obtain allergy history and current and prior drug use. Monitor liver function tests. Document bowel movements. Administer antihistamines (pruritus) and antiemetics (nausea) as ordered. Have a narcotic antagonist (Narcan) readily available if respirations fall below 10 per minute. Monitor urinary output for urinary retention.

PHARMACOLOGY Summary of Medications Used for Pain Relief, *continued*

Medication Category and Action	Application/Indication	Nursing Responsibility
Anticonvulsants		
Carbamazepine Diazepam Gabapentin Phenytoin **Action:** Limit aberrant nerve firing, leading to neural membrane stabilization.	Neuropathic pain syndrome that is shooting or electrical in nature.	Assess character, duration, and intensity of pain prior to administration to determine baseline for effectiveness. Assess for alteration in vision, concentration, and coordination.
Antidepressants		
Amitriptyline Amoxapine Doxepin Imipramine Nortriptyline Trazodone Venlafaxine **Action:** Precise mechanism of analgesic effect unknown. Thought to inhibit the reuptake of serotonin and norepinephrine involved in the descending inhibitory pain pathway. Enhanced endorphin secretion, sodium channel blockade inhibition of substance P, a neuropeptide involved in both pain and depression. Doses for pain relief are lower than doses for depression.	Chronic pain, cancer pain, fibromyalgia, tension migraine headaches, postherpetic neuralgia, diabetic neuropathy, arthritis, low back pain. Most effective in treating burning neuropathic pain.	Assess character, duration, and intensity of pain prior to administration to determine baseline for effectiveness. Monitor for nausea and dry mouth. Gum will help with the dry mouth. Patient education includes time of onset (tricyclics take several weeks to achieve therapeutic effect). Monitor patient for oversedation and insomnia. Educate patient not to discontinue use abruptly. Monitor for orthostatic hypotension. Instruct patient not to rise suddenly from a lying position.
Glucocorticoids		
Betamethasone Cortisol Dexamethasone Methylprednisone Prednisone **Action:** Exert anti-inflammatory properties through inhibiting leukotriene and prostaglandin synthesis.	Nerve compression pain, chronic pain.	Assess character, duration, and intensity of pain prior to administration to determine baseline for effectiveness. Due to the impact on certain conditions, prior to therapy assess patient for infection, osteoporosis, diabetes, heart failure, hypertension, and renal disease. Instruct patient to take medication with food and water to prevent gastric irritation. Do not discontinue drug abruptly; therapy needs to be tapered off.

Sources: Adams, M. P., Josephson, D. L., & Holland, L. N. (2010). *Pharmacology for nurses: A pathophysiological approach* (3rd ed.). Upper Saddle River, NJ: Pearson Prentice Hall; Adams, M. P., & Koch, R. (2010). *Pharmacologic connections to nursing practice.* Upper Saddle River, NJ: Prentice Hall; American Pain Society (APS). (2012). *Principles of analgesic use in the treatment of acute pain and cancer pain* (6th ed.). Glenview, IL: APS; Deglin, J. H., & Valleran, A. H. (2009). *Davis's drug guide for nurses* (11th ed.). Philadelphia: FA Davis; Kee, J. L., Hayer, E. R., & McCuistian, L. E. (2009). *Pharmacology: A nursing process approach* (6th ed.). St. Louis, MO: Saunders; Pasero, C., & McCaffery, M. (2010). *Pain assessment & pharmacologic management.* St. Louis: Mosby.

Both agonist and agonist-antagonist effects are reversible with the administration of a pure antagonist such as naloxone. **Antagonists** displace and replace the opioid at the receptor, reversing the opioid's pharmacologic effect and side effects such as respiratory depression. The Pharmacology feature outlines essential information about opioids.

Adjuvant Medications

Adjuvant medications are pharmacological agents that help and enhance the effect of a drug or treatment. These medications are traditionally prescribed and administered for reasons other than pain relief; for example, they often are used in pharmacologic treatment plans for chronic and cancer pain. In addition, antidepressants and anticonvulsant medications may be used as adjuvant therapy with opiates. Although less commonly used in acute pain, these medications may be of benefit in cases of trauma, burns, and some complex acute pain situations. These medications may enhance the effects of the opioids or NSAIDs, provide analgesia on their own, or reduce the side effects of other analgesic medications (Knotkova & Pappagallo, 2007). Adjuvant medications, by definition, are not primarily indicated for treatment of pain (Kroenke, Krebs, & Bair, 2009), so the nurse must be aware of the rationale for the specific medication within the context of pain management. The nurse should also be prepared to offer education regarding the use of adjuvant medications to patients and family members to prevent confusion. Adjuvants may include tricyclic antidepressants, antiepileptic medications, local anesthetics, glucocorticoids, skeletal muscle relaxants, antispasmodic agents, antihistamines, benzodiazepines, caffeine, topical agents, and dextroamphetamines. Bisphosphonates and radionuclides also are useful in the treatment of metastatic bone pain (Haslbauer & Feigl, 2009).

Routes of Administration

Pain medications are available in a variety of formulations that can be administered via many different routes. The prescribing provider selects a route of medication administration based on the patient's individual needs given the specific situation. Routes of medication administration provide for a range of absorption times from rapid onset (e.g., transmucosal, intravenous) to delayed onset (e.g., transdermal). Each route of administration has advantages and disadvantages that should be considered. It is appropriate to deliver medications by the least invasive route possible.

Oral Route

The oral route of administration is generally preferred because it is the least invasive, most convenient, and often the most cost-effective route. Most analgesic medications come in tablets, capsules, or in liquid formulations that allow for ease of oral administration. The oral route of administration is preferred for the treatment of chronic and cancer pain because it reduces the need for frequent analgesic administration. The disadvantages of the oral route of administration are slower onset and delayed peak effect. The rate of gastric emptying and intestinal motility can increase or decrease medication absorption (Kee, Hayer, & McCuistian, 2009).

Oral Transmucosal Route

The oral cavity provides several locations for medication administration via the vascular mucosal membranes, including the sublingual, buccal, and gingival mucosa. When administering a medication sublingually, the medication is placed under the tongue and held there until it is completely dissolved and absorbed. Buccal administration requires the medication to be placed between the gums of the upper molars and the cheek. Gingival drugs are placed between the gums of the upper incisors and the upper lip (Kee, Hayer, & McCuistian, 2009).

The nurse should assess the patient's ability to hold the medication under the tongue until completely absorbed. Many patients are unable to either understand or tolerate sublingual administration and instead swallow the medication, resulting in gastric absorption and hepatic metabolism, which reduce the effectiveness of the medication dramatically.

Rectal Route

The rectal route of medication administration is generally reserved for use when nausea or vomiting precludes oral administration and in situations where the additional expertise of intravenous administration is not available or desirable. Most medications that can be taken orally may be given rectally with similar dissolution, absorption, and effectiveness. Relatively rapid systemic absorption and avoidance of hepatic metabolism are possible if the medication is inserted just past the rectal sphincter (Pasero & McCaffery, 2010). Medications that are formulated or coated so that absorption occurs in the intestine (e.g., enteric coated) are not effective when administered using the rectal route. The pH of the colon is alkaline and enteric-coated medications require the acidic environment of the intestines (Pasero & McCaffery, 2010).

Intravenous Route

Intravenous (IV) administration of medications allows for the most rapid onset of effect because medications are delivered directly into the systemic circulation. First-pass hepatic metabolism is avoided. When administering opioids to treat severe pain, IV boluses can be administered by titration (frequent administration of small doses) for rapid control of escalating pain (Miyoshi & Leckband, 2009; Pasero & McCaffery, 2010). Because of the rapid onset of effect, the IV route of administration is also associated with the highest level of toxicity. Care must be taken to administer medications slowly or in small doses in order to reduce adverse effects (Pasero & McCaffery, 2010).

The IV route of administration is commonly reserved for acute pain management. It is also used in cases of chronic and cancer pain where patients experience severe pain that requires rapid relief, as well as when patients are unable to take oral analgesics due to adverse effects or situations, such as a disease that impairs gastrointestinal function.

Intramuscular Route

Intramuscular (IM) injection of analgesics should be avoided. The IM route of administration has significant disadvantages. The IM absorption is unreliable with a 30- to 60-minute lag time to peak effect with a rapid falloff of action as compared with oral analgesic administration (Berman & Snyder, 2012; Kee, Hayer, & McCuistian, 2009). If the IM route of administration must be used, the deltoid muscles and vastus lateralis muscles have better perfusion and may absorb the medication more rapidly than the gluteal muscles.

Subcutaneous Route

The subcutaneous route of administration is similar to the IM route of administration but carries the disadvantages of painful injection and variability of absorption based on the location of injection. Hepatic first-pass metabolism is avoided. However, in situations where oral and IV routes of delivery are not available, the subcutaneous route offers an alternative for administering analgesics. If subcutaneous medications are delivered by continuous infusion, the volume of the medication should be limited to 2 or 3 mL/hour to optimize absorption. If higher infusion rates are necessary, the total volume to be infused can be split between two sites to prevent irritation, pain, necrosis, and sloughing at the site (Pasero & McCaffery, 2010).

Transdermal Route

Transdermal administration of analgesic medications relies on absorption of lipid-soluble medications through the barrier of the intact skin into the local tissues and the systemic circulation. These medications are generally formulated in transdermal patches or topical creams, ointments, or gels. Absorption of the medication can be unintentionally increased with the application of heat or by massaging the skin to increase the blood flow to the area, resulting in rapid absorption and potential overdose (Pasero & McCaffery, 2010). Fentanyl, lidocaine, and clonidine are examples of transdermal medications that are commonly used in pain management.

Spinal (Epidural and Intrathecal) Route

Epidural and intrathecal routes of administration are useful for acute pain management for post-operative pain, trauma pain, and specific cancer and chronic pain management situations. These routes of medication administration bypass metabolism in the liver and systemic circulation. For this reason, the dosage of medication used to achieve adequate analgesia is very small compared to the dosage necessary when administered by other routes.

The epidural space is separated from the spinal cord by the spinal meninges. When opioids, anesthetics, or other medications are administered by the epidural route, they must diffuse across the meninges, into the cerebrospinal fluid (CSF), and subsequently penetrate the spinal cord tissues. Medications injected directly into the intrathecal space have immediate access to the spinal cord tissues without diffusion across the meninges.

Both epidural and intrathecal administration of medications require access to the spinal tissues through an invasive procedure, either injection through a spinal needle alone or in combination with placement of an indwelling catheter. The epidural or intrathecal catheter is usually temporarily indwelling and can be a potential source of infection. If the intention is to use the epidural or intrathecal route for longer durations, either a permanent catheter is tunneled under the subcutaneous tissue to reduce the risk of infection or a fully implanted infusion pump with catheter is placed during a surgical procedure.

Regional Nerve Route

Injection of anesthetic medications into or near a nerve is commonly referred to as *regional anesthesia* or a *nerve block*. A variety of regional anesthetic blocks are performed to diagnose nerve pain, for use as a prognostic prior to a more invasive procedure, or to relieve chronic and cancer pain. When the anesthetic is injected, it is delivered directly to the nerve tissue. The anesthetic blocks the conduction of both afferent and efferent neural fibers (Buckley, 2009).

Continuous infusion of anesthetics to regional nerves is becoming a very popular option for acute pain management and in situations where it is desirable to reduce the amount of opioid a patient receives throughout the operative and postoperative course (e.g., multiple comorbidities). The nerve block generally is established prior to surgery as a single dose. In some cases, a catheter is placed to allow for continuous infusion of anesthetic so that the medication effects continue throughout the operative course and into the postoperative period, improving the quality of pain relief for the patient.

Methods of Medication Delivery

Clinical decisions regarding the dosing intervals for the various analgesic medications are based on multiple factors, including the type and intensity of the pain, the pharmacologic attributes of the medication, the patient's weight, and the clinical setting. Analgesics may be given as a single dose, in multiple intermittent doses, by continuous dosing, or at the patient's request. As with many aspects of pain management, the dosing schedule should be customized to meet the patient's individual needs to achieve the best results.

Single Dose

Single dosing of analgesic medications generally is used to treat pain caused by a painful procedure or, in some circumstances, injury. When used to premedicate a patient for a painful procedure, the analgesic should be administered so that the peak effects occur just prior to the start of the procedure. Single doses of analgesics are sometimes administered as a loading dose in order to rapidly achieve therapeutic blood levels before starting a continuous infusion. A loading dose is a higher amount of drug, often given only once or twice to prime the bloodstream with a level sufficient to induce a therapeutic response (Adams & Koch, 2010).

Pro re Nata (prn)

Pro re nata (prn), or "as needed," is a common dosing strategy that allows for flexibility in the dosing schedule when pain is intermittent and the analgesic medication is appropriate for intermittent dosing. It is most commonly used for acute pain when pain is not consistent or when pain is expected to decline rapidly as healing occurs. Disadvantages of the prn dosing schedule are evident when a patient waits too long between doses of medication, allowing the pain to become severe, or when continuous pain would be best managed with a continuous dosing pattern.

If continuous pain is managed with prn dosing, the patient can be taught to determine the duration of pain relief experienced with a dose of medication and to then schedule the prn doses at that frequency to be taken routinely. This is an effective strategy for severe acute pain and for chronic or cancer pain.

The use of prn dosing is appropriate when treating breakthrough pain episodes that occur in spite of well-controlled persistent pain. Breakthrough pain generally is unpredictable and severe, requiring the flexibility of a short- or rapid-acting analgesic that can be administered as soon as the breakthrough pain begins. For example, the patient is using a fentanyl transdermal patch once every 72 hours and treats breakthrough pain episodes two to three times daily with oral transmucosal fentanyl citrate (Actiq) units prn.

At times, the ordered interval for prn dosing is not frequent enough to allow dosing prior to the onset of pain, resulting in undertreated pain if the dosing schedule is followed. When this occurs, the nurse is responsible for informing the prescribing clinician and advocating for an appropriate dosing interval or an increase in dosage based on assessment findings. Likewise, if the prescribed dosing interval is too frequent to be realistically implemented, it is appropriate for the nurse to contact the prescribing clinician and advocate for an alternative dosing schedule or method.

Continuous

When pain is present consistently, analgesic medications should be administered continuously. This dosing strategy is most commonly used for severe pain to maintain a therapeutic level of the medication to provide optimal pain relief without adverse effects. To accomplish this goal, short-acting analgesics may be administered ATC as mentioned or infusion pumps can be used to deliver continuous IV analgesics. Continuous dosing of opioid analgesics should be used with extreme caution when patients are opioid naïve due to increased risk of adverse effects (Chou et al., 2009).

Patient-Controlled Analgesia

Patient-controlled analgesia (PCA) is a dosing strategy that allows patients to request a small dose of analgesic medication when they begin to feel pain. PCA infusion pumps are designed with a patient dose button that the patient can press to activate medication delivery. The dosage and dosing interval are programmed into the pump so that the patient receives the prescribed dosage no more often than allowed by prescription in spite of the possibility of more frequent button presses to request doses. The PCA can be used successfully to administer analgesic medications by a variety of routes including IV, subcutaneous, epidural, intrathecal, and peripheral nerve. The PCA may be used alone as a prn dose or in combination with a continuous infusion. PCA dosing is generally used in moderate to severe acute pain or in cases of chronic pain where alternate routes of analgesic administration are not available or effective.

The benefits of PCA include increased patient control and participation in pain management. PCA is very effective for acute pain management postoperatively or post-trauma when patients are unable to take oral analgesics and when the severity of pain requires an unrealistic frequency of IV medication administration given the nurse's other responsibilities. Reduced time waiting for the nurse to deliver a requested analgesic is a benefit that often makes patients reluctant to relinquish control even when they are able to transition to oral analgesics prn. As mentioned previously, use of continuous dosing of opioids should be used with extreme caution for opioid naïve patients. This is especially true when continuous dosing is combined with PCA dosing. A balanced analgesic medication treatment plan is the foundation of acute and cancer pain management. This is rapidly becoming the case in chronic pain management as well.

The nurse should have a basic understanding of common complementary therapies and include an assessment of the patient's use of complementary therapies in the overall assessment of pain. Patients may be reluctant to discuss their decision to use a complementary or alternative therapy for fear of ridicule or out of concern that the nurse will attempt to dissuade them from its use (Khatta, 2007). The following questions may be used to encourage discussion regarding complementary therapies the patient might be using or have a desire to learn more about:

- Do you do anything to treat your pain besides taking medications?
- Have you ever used music, massage, or meditation to distract you when you are in pain?

The Complementary & Alternative Therapies feature discusses the use of acupuncture in managing pain (p. 292).

Nursing Management

The nurse's knowledge of the many dimensions of pain management, effective assessment techniques, and common pharmacologic and complementary or alternative strategies provides the foundation necessary to deliver safe and appropriate nursing care. Consistent with the nursing process, data gathered from the pain assessment and from all other aspects of the physical assessment are analyzed and used to plan interventions.

Assessment

The assessment findings related to the physiological dimension should prompt the nurse to recognize the potential harm that unrelieved pain may cause to patients, especially those patients who are acutely or critically ill, are frail or debilitated, or have multiple disease states that would likely be impacted by a significant stress response.

Specific assessment data include:

- Type (sharp, dull, burning, pressure)
- Location (including transmission patterns)
- Duration
- What brings it on?
- What relieves it?
- When did it start?
- Is it getting worse or better?
- Intensity? (Using a pain scale, What level of pain is acceptable to the patient?)

Analysis of the data gathered regarding the sensory dimension of pain provides a baseline against which future data may be compared in order to determine if the treatment plan is resulting in a positive trend toward adequate pain relief. The quality of the pain will provide some direction in the selection of medications suited to nociceptive or neuropathic pain. The temporal pattern of the pain is important to the selection of formulations and timing of the administration of medications. Sustained-release, modified release, or continuous infusions of analgesics are particularly suited to pain that is constant and persistent, but they carry the potential to cause harm when administered for pain that is intermittent or transient. The sudden onset of severe breakthrough pain may require the use of a rapid-acting transmucosal or IV opioid.

Affective Assessment

The affective dimension of pain yields assessment data that have the potential to undermine even the most carefully planned treatments. It is essential to consider the patient's emotions and assignment of meaning to the pain when prioritizing time spent with the patient. Nurses must tailor education and emotional support to the specific needs of patients who are suffering or who have a negative perception of their pain. Involvement of a psychiatric specialist, psychologist, or social worker may be indicated by the analysis of the affective dimension findings. The nurse is in an excellent position to advocate for this on behalf of the patient who may not be able to recognize that this is a concern.

Consideration of assessment findings in the cognitive dimension assists the nurse in providing for the patient's specific religious and cultural needs. In addition, understanding culturally appropriate responses to pain helps the nurse in interpreting pain-related behaviors more accurately. For example, when a patient who is culturally inclined to be quite stoic in the expression of pain becomes more vocal, it should prompt the nurse to consider that pain might be severe in spite of the patient's subdued response. Patients who feel a loss of control might be comforted by having choices in their pain treatment whenever possible. For example, opioids that are ordered to be administered IV prn might be administered using a PCA infusion device, allowing postoperative patients significant control and increasing self-efficacy in their acute pain management.

Assessment of the behavioral dimension of pain is a necessary baseline to determine whether pain-related behaviors decrease following the implementation of the pain treatment plan. This is particularly important for patients who are unable to describe their pain. The nurse who finds that the patient has developed some unfortunate learned pain behaviors has the opportunity to reduce the use of these behaviors by establishing a trusting relationship; providing pain treatments before the patient begins to demonstrate pain-related behaviors rather than waiting for the behaviors to manifest; and reassuring the patient that the health care team is committed to relieving pain and will do everything possible to accomplish that goal. In addition, findings from behavioral assessments should prompt the nurse to consider encouraging and assisting patients to develop cognitive-behavioral coping strategies such as meditation, journaling, or redirecting thoughts into a more positive pattern.

Planning

The analysis of assessment findings and planning of interventions should be focused around the therapeutic goals described in this chapter. The baseline assessment of the patient's pain intensity and functional ability is matched, establishing comfort and function goals whose progress may be measured. Interventions are defined and initiated using the goals established in the planning phase. Evaluation will determine whether the goals and patient outcomes have been accomplished and redirect the plan if they have not.

Nursing Diagnoses

Nursing diagnoses that may apply to the patient experiencing pain include:

- *Pain, Acute*
- *Pain, Chronic*
- *Fatigue*
- *Coping, Ineffective*
- *Hopelessness*
- *Mobility, Impaired*
- *Powerlessness*

NANDA-I © 2012

Interventions and Rationales

Implementation of interventions, particularly pharmacologic interventions, is multifaceted and focused on patient safety as well as optimizing the potential efficacy of the treatment plan. The nurse uses the knowledge of pharmacologic interventions to review the medications that have been prescribed for the patient. Consider asking the following questions when reviewing patient medications:

- Could this medication or dosage cause the patient to experience adverse effects given her physiological status (e.g., allergies, other medical conditions)?
- Is the medication appropriate to treat this patient's source of pain (e.g., neuropathic, nociceptive)?
- Is it likely that this medication and dosage will be able to relieve the intensity of pain this patient is experiencing?
- Is this medication ordered with an appropriate frequency for administration?
- Is the formulation (long-acting, short-acting, etc.) and route of administration appropriate to treat this patient's pattern of pain?
- Does the patient understand how to use the medication to prevent harm through inadvertent misuse?
- Are there other medications that might be appropriate to add to this treatment plan to optimize the effectiveness and safety of pain relief for this patient?

The nurse is the "guardian of patient safety," ensuring that when medications are administered they do not cause harm (Campbell & Osborn, 2010). Safety is a quality indicator established by the Quality & Safety Education for Nurses (QSEN) project. It is imperative that nurses take this responsibility very seriously (QSEN, 2011). If there is any concern that the prescribed medication may not be appropriate or ordered in an appropriate dosage or frequency of administration, it is the nurse's responsibility to notify the prescribing clinician and request clarification of the order. The patient's physical condition must be considered when implementing pharmacologic strategies to avoid administration of a medication that has the potential to cause adverse effects that could result in patient harm. Because pain medications, particularly opioids, have the potential to cause serious adverse effects, this important nursing role cannot be stressed enough.

The patient's physical condition must be considered when selecting or implementing complementary or alternative strategies. Successful implementation of such interventions is based on the selection of a strategy that is embraced by the patient and family. Some interventions are less demanding of the patient's time and energy (e.g., music, massage), whereas others require the patient to be actively engaged (e.g., meditation, journaling). It is important to consider the selected strategies given the patient's specific needs and to consider alternative strategies if necessary.

Prior to initiating interventions, the nurse must educate the patient and family regarding the goals, rationale, expected outcomes, and potential adverse effects associated with each intervention. Some patients will only be able to understand or desire to learn the most basic concepts regarding their treatments. For these patients, a base of knowledge should be established and then built on through subsequent educational opportunities. Ensure that the patient does not have a cultural barrier to learning, such as speaking a different language or having a cognitive impairment (e.g., confusion, sedation). It is important to remember that the presence of severe pain is a barrier to learning and should be relieved as quickly as possible to facilitate the patient's participation in care. For patients who want detailed information, the nurse may need to provide education on multiple occasions to fully answer all of their questions. Educational tools such as diagrams, diaries, audiovisual programs, and demonstrations may provide another avenue of learning for patients who learn more effectively from visual instruction. The education provided must be tailored to meet the specific needs of each patient and their family members.

Management of Unrelieved Pain

As an advocate for change, it falls to the nurse to accurately and concisely communicate to the health care team the details of the pain assessment, interventions that have been implemented, and the evaluation of the patient's response.

Evaluation

Evaluation data are used to determine whether pain relief has been achieved. The nurse needs to evaluate each tenant of the plan to determine which interventions have been most effective. It may not always be realistic to achieve total relief, especially with chronic diseases such as arthritis. A more realistic goal may be a level of comfort that allows the patient to perform activities of daily living and maintain some quality of life. It is essential that the nurse helps the patient and family identify behaviors that increase pain and teach them how to avoid these activities.

Reassessment of pain and assessment of the patient's response to interventions are necessary to measure improvement in the quality of pain management as compared to baseline assessments. The reassessment of pain should follow the same pattern used at baseline, and use the same tools to reinforce the concepts taught during the assessment. Some minor alterations should be made to elicit the details needed to determine if there has been a change after intervention. For example:

- How would you rate your pain intensity on the 0 to 10 scale at rest? With activity? During ______________ (the patient's previously identified most painful time)?
- Is your pain in the same place?
- Do you have any new pain?
- Does your pain feel the same (e.g., aching, burning)?
- Do you feel like the pain treatments are helping to relieve your pain?
- Are you having any nausea, vomiting, itching, or constipation?
- Are you able to urinate (if opioid analgesics have been administered)?
- Do you feel alert and able to keep up with conversations around you when you are not resting?
- Are you able to do ______________ (the patient's previously identified goal for function)?

COMPLEMENTARY & ALTERNATIVE THERAPIES Acupuncture

Nancy Yilk

ACUPUNCTURE IS PRACTICED WORLDWIDE as a clinical mechanism to treat diseases and related pain disorders. Basically, it is used as a form of pain management. In a Chinese study, fMRI was used to reveal the central nervous system's (CNS) neuroimaging signatures of acupoint stimulation. The study sought to determine if acupuncture effects have two phases (i.e., the early acute effects, which involve the instant cerebral response to needling manipulation, and the delayed long-lasting effects). It was concluded that both the needling sensation and the following neural cascades may contribute to the overall effect of acupuncture through dynamic reconfiguration of complex neural networks (Qin et al., 2011).

In a Korean study, a prospective comparative design was used to examine the effect of an integrated care service which included a combination of oriental and Western care on health outcomes in elderly patients with degenerative arthritis (Lee & Sun, 2011). The study enrolled 85 elderly patients with degenerative arthritis in the lower extremities who were followed in a hospital outpatient department for 8 weeks. The participants were divided into two groups, the integrated care service group and the Western care group. The 36 patients assigned to the integrated care service group received a combination of physical therapy, acupuncture, Western medicines, or herbal medicines. The Western care group, consisting of 49 patients, only received physical therapy or Western medicines. Dependent variables consisting of functional independence, walking speed, rotation balance, pain intensity, service satisfaction, and total medical costs for the two groups were compared at 8 weeks.

Functional independence and walking speed improved significantly in the integrated care group while pain intensity improved significantly in the Western care group. The integrated care group reported higher scores for service satisfaction and higher medical costs than the Western care group. The results suggest the use of integrated care is effective in improving mobility and quality of life for seniors with degenerative arthritis (Lee & Sun, 2011).

Norrbrink and Lundeberg (2011) enrolled 30 Swedish participants in a study to explore the possibility of using acupuncture and massage therapy for relieving neuropathic pain following spinal cord injury (SCI). Participants were equally divided into two groups, those receiving either massage or acupuncture. Treatments were provided to both groups twice weekly for 6 weeks. Participants' responses to treatments were evaluated at the end of treatment and again after a 2-month follow-up. Researchers used an intention-to-treat analysis of data, meaning that an analysis was based on the initial treatment intent, not on the treatment eventually administered. Data analysis found a significant difference in ratings of present pain, general pain, pain unpleasantness, and coping at the end of treatment after acupuncture compared to baseline values. Pain interference as measured by the Multidimensional Pain Inventory improved following massage therapy. However, significant improvements were not noted on the 2-month follow-up evaluation. Comparisons of worst pain intensity at the end of treatment and unpleasantness and coping with pain between the two groups were found to be more favorable in those participants who received acupuncture versus massage therapy. Upon completing treatment, the majority of participants in both groups (15 who received acupuncture and 9 who received massage therapy) reported an improvement on the Patient Global Impression of Change Scale. This positive effect continued during the follow-up evaluation for 6 patients in the acupuncture group and 1 patient in the massage group. Few side effects were reported and neither group experienced dropout from the study due to unfavorable events. Those conducting the study concluded that both acupuncture and massage therapy may relieve SCI neuropathic pain. They noted that a larger randomized study was indicated for assessing the long-term effects of these treatments on pain management for those with SCI (Norrbrink & Lundeberg, 2011).

References

Lee, J., & Sun, Jr., E. (2011). Effect of an integral care system: A combination of oriental and Western care for older adults with degenerative arthritis. *Journal of Korean Academy of Nursing, 41*(1), 18–25. doi: 10.4040/jkan.2011.41.1.18

Norrbrink, C., & Lundeberg, T. (2011, April 6). Acupuncture and massage therapy for neuropathic pain following spinal cord injury: An exploratory study. *Acupuncture Medicine.*

Qin et al. (2011). The temporal-spatial encoding of acupuncture effects in the brain. *Molecular Pain, 7*, 19.

In addition to these assessment questions, the patient's vital signs should be checked with specific attention given to the patient's respiratory status including depth, quality, and rate of respirations when opioid analgesics have been administered.

If the analgesic treatment plan includes delivery of medications using infusion devices such as a PCA pump, analyzing the data from the device becomes an important component of the evaluation process. The nurse should review the pump settings to ensure appropriate programming will prevent errors or encourage rapid identification of an error should one occur. PCA pumps track the number of milligrams, micrograms, or milliliters of medication that is administered to the patient. The PCA pump also tracks the number of times the patient pushes the PCA button to request a dose and the number of times he actually receives a dose. Evaluation of these data can provide important trending information, providing a prompt to initiate a change when necessary.

The frequency of evaluation or reassessment is determined by institutional policies and procedures. However, it is the nurse's obligation to increase the frequency of reassessment if the patient's condition warrants. For example, if the nurse finds a patient who is not scheduled for reassement for 2 hours to be slightly drowsy with a marginal respiratory rate of 10 breaths per minute, the nurse should identify the potential for significant respiratory depression and reassess the patient more frequently until the patient's respiratory status is stable.

Collaborative Management

A successful pain management plan requires the focused attention of the interdisciplinary team. Because nurses are the team members most likely to spend significant amounts of time with the patient, they play a vital role in the coordination of the multidisciplinary team's care. In order to meet desired patient outcomes, it is essential that this interdisciplinary team communicate openly with one another in developing and evaluating care of the patient and family (IOM, 2010). It is the nurse's responsibility to assess the ongoing effects and intensity of pain, administer pharmacologic and nonpharmacologic treatments, communicate changes in the patient's condition to the other members of the team, and advocate for change. Members of the health care team depend on the knowledge and skill of the nurse to manage the patient's pain sufficiently in order to facilitate participation in necessary therapies and procedures and promote healing.

To meet the goals of pain management, the multidisciplinary team draws on the additional support of services such as pain management services, chaplain services, psychologists/psychiatrists, financial assistance, social services, and specific support groups for patients and family members. Pain management services provide expert assistance with complex pain management problems and are skilled in the management of high-technology modalities such as IV PCA, epidural or intrathecal infusion of opioids and anesthetics, and regional anesthetic techniques. Chaplain services, psychologists/psychiatrists, and social services assist with identification and management of concerns in the affective, cognitive, and behavioral dimensions of pain. Financial services assist the patient in meeting immediate needs, such as purchasing medications and obtaining specialty pain management care, and provide counseling regarding long-term needs if the patient is unable to return to gainful employment. Finally, specific support groups may be especially beneficial to patients with chronic and cancer pain. Meeting with others who are living with similar challenges allows the patient and family to openly discuss their concerns, exchange ideas, and receive encouragement.

Discharge Planning

Transitioning from one care setting to another can cause both patients and family members to feel anxious, frightened, confused, and frustrated as they try to understand their pain management plans and adapt to the new environments. Patients and family members should be prepared for discharge throughout the entire course of the admission through the coordinated efforts of all members of the multidisciplinary team. Nurses play a significant role in assessing the needs of the patient and family for discharge.

Initial Discharge Planning

Planning for the pain management regimen in the next care setting should begin with consideration of the patient's ability to use the medications and complementary or alternative strategies. Complex medication plans, although they may provide superior pain relief, may not be appropriate if the patient will not be able to manage the complexity of the plan independently after discharge. Likewise, patients are less likely to use nonpharmacologic strategies that are difficult to perform without expert skills.

Consideration of patient financial concerns, such as prescription drug coverage or ability to pay for prescription medications, will enhance the patient's willingness and ability to adhere to the medication regimen after discharge. Many patients do not have adequate health care insurance or prescription coverage; for these patients, the cost of pain medications may be a financial burden. When possible, medications should be selected based on the lowest appropriate cost that will meet the patient's needs. However, care must be taken to avoid selecting a less costly medication based on cost alone. A medication that causes side effects that must be treated with yet another medication will negate any cost savings to the patient.

Some patients have complex pain management needs and may require the care of a pain management specialist after discharge. In these cases, it is appropriate to begin the process of referral early to facilitate a smooth transition of care after discharge. If a pain management specialist is not available in the patient's community, appropriate follow up care may be available from another health care provider or licensed independent practitioner in the community. Time will be needed to select a provider and secure an appointment for follow up care.

Health Promotion

Patient teaching prior to discharge should be a review of the teaching that has been provided during the patient's stay. New information will be very difficult for the patient and family to incorporate this late in their care. Every effort should be made to ensure that the plan for pain management is to provide adequate relief of pain and optimal function with minimal side effects and to avoid last-minute changes when possible.

The nurse is the patient's final contact before discharge in most settings. Discharge responsibilities include presenting information in a calm and reassuring manner that will support the patient's confidence that he will be able to efficiently continue the plan independent of the health care team's support.

Determining when to take pain medications can be confusing and requires a thought process similar to that needed to manage diabetes with insulin injections. Patients must "measure" their pain and its impact on function to determine if and how much additional pain medication is needed. To facilitate optimal understanding, it is important to provide clear and accurate written discharge instructions. Supportive graphics to illustrate the use of each medication may be useful when discussing more complex pain management concepts such as persistent pain and breakthrough pain. Written instructions should include the times that medication was given to the patient while the patient was admitted, including when the last dose was taken and when the next dose is due. The nurse should explain how medication administration is recorded to reduce reliance on memory and the chance for errors. Encourage patients to use a similar system to track their own medications after discharge. Patients may find it helpful to use a notebook to document their pain scores, daily function, side effects, and when medications are taken. A written record may provide additional understanding of how much medication they are taking and the impact that pain has on their lives. Patients' and family members' perceptions regarding pain management are occasionally different; therefore, a written record may help each to gain an appreciation of the other's perspective. Strategies that may be used to clarify pain management instructions are shown in Chart 12–4, which stresses communicaton with low or limited literacy levels. The suggestions may be used with any patient or family that is having difficulty or variances in understanding pain management techniques.

If the patient participated in a complementary or alternative strategy as part of the pain management plan, the nurse should provide written instructions that include when the strategy was used and how it was most effectively executed (e.g., which music was most relaxing). The nurse should also provide appropriate referral information in cases where the strategy requires a specialist (e.g., acupuncture).

CHART 12–4 Strategies Used to Clarify Pain Management Instructions

- Create an environment conducive to exchanging information.
- Use audio tapes to convey the instructions.
- Use "plain language" materials; do not use medical or technical jargon.
- Use innovative multimedia.
- Use peer educators or patient advocates.
- Provide instruction materials comparable to level of health literacy.

Weblink: Chronic Pain In The Elderly Weblink: A Statistical Profile of Older Americans Aged 65+

The patient and family should be given the opportunity to voice any concerns or questions they may have prior to discharge. In addition, the nurse should review the following concepts:

- Pain management plays an important role in the recovery process.
- Several different pain medications may be prescribed together to relieve pain through different mechanisms.
- When pain is persistent, pain medications should be taken routinely.
- Physical dependence and tolerance to opioid pain medications are not addiction.

Many times patients and families are overwhelmed and are not sure what to ask. The nurse should provide the patient and family members with the name of their provider and the phone number to contact if they have questions after discharge. Discharge instructions are outlined in the Patient Teaching & Discharge Priorities box.

Ongoing Discharge Planning

Once a pain management plan is determined, it should be implemented and modified until the greatest level of pain relief and functionality are achieved with minimal side effects. When pain medications are administered, the nurse should instruct the patient and family members regarding expected onset of relief, side effects that may be experienced, and when additional medication will be provided or should be requested. The nurse should also review treatments of medication side effects with the patient and family. When assisting a patient with the use of a complementary or alternative strategy, it is imperative to provide the patient with adequate opportunity to practice the technique to facilitate the skillful use of the strategy after discharge. Repeated administration of medications and use of nonmedication strategies will allow the patient and family members the opportunity to hear instructions many times before discharge. This approach reduces the stress of having to learn everything on the day of discharge.

If the patient will be discharged on high doses of opiates or one of the stronger opiates, one of the health care providers (nurse, physician, case manager) should contact the patient's home pharmacy to ensure that they carry the drug and in sufficient quantities. The pharmacy may have to place a special order; this should be done prior to the patient's discharge to avoid any situation where the medication required to control the patient's pain is not available when needed.

Gerontological Considerations

Pain in the older patient (over 65 years of age) is often undertreated and misunderstood. By 2030, an estimated 20% of the population will be over age 65 (Administration on Aging, 2008). Today's older patients can expect to live longer and have a more active retirement lifestyle because of advances in medical science. If pain prohibits activity and limits functionality, it can lead to sleep disturbances, depression, anxiety, decreased social interactions, and increased health care utilization and costs (Bruckenthal & D'Arcy, 2007).

Pain is very common in patients over age 65. In a large sample of nursing home residents age ≥65 years, almost one-half reported persistent pain, yet one-fourth had received no pain medications within the preceding month and fewer than half of them had standing orders for analgesics (Herr, 2010; McDonald, 2009).

Undertreatment may be due to health care providers' age bias or knowledge deficits as well as to patient characteristics (D'Arcy, 2009). Health care providers may not prescribe opioid medications for pain in the older patient for fear of oversedation or other side effects. Patients may fear that they will become addicted to opioids; constipation is a common fear for older adults as well. One in five older patients reported taking pain medication only occasionally. Reluctance to take pain medications, financial constraints, and prescriber reluctance may contribute to a cycle of undertreatment (Bruckenthal & D'Arcy, 2007). In addition, many patients have fixed incomes and very minimal or no health care benefits. Financial concerns may cause them to delay seeking health care or to choose not to purchase prescribed medications. In addition to these and other age-specific barriers, many patients have multiple medical diagnoses and increased sensitivity to analgesic medications due to altered hepatic and renal function.

Consequences of Unrelieved Pain

The impact of undertreated pain in the older adult is costly on many levels. The consequences of untreated pain include sleep disturbances, malnutrition, declines in social and recreational activities, deterioration of physical functioning, falls, depression, anxiety, and impaired cognitive functioning. This combination of effects can result in decreased quality of life and increased health care utilization with its subsequent costs (Herr, 2010).

Pain Assessment and Measurement

In most cases, assessing and measuring the multiple dimensions of pain in the older adult can be accomplished in the same manner as with any adult patient. However, keep in mind that older persons may be reluctant to report pain for reasons such as:

- They think that pain is a normal part of aging.
- They react to perceived belief that they are unreliable pain reporters.
- They do not want to be a "nuisance" and/or perceived as a hypochondriac or addict.
- They fear that their intermittent confusion may limit their credibility.
- They do not like to take medications (e.g., tablets for pain relief).
- The expectation or concenrn that the clinician will give a low priority to pain in comparison to other medical problems.
- They fear the consequences of acknowledging pain, such as expensive testing or hospitalization.
- They fear that pain may indicate impending death (Bruckenthal & D'Arcy, 2007; Kumar & Allcock, 2008; Matteson, 2011).

Although some may require large print versions, most older adults can use the usual one-dimensional assessment scales such as the numeric rating scale, the visual analog scale, and the FACES pain rating scale. Older patients may need extra time to respond when asked about their pain rating.

Pain management of the older adult can be further complicated when the older patient is confused, cognitively impaired, or nonverbal. The American Society of Pain Management Nursing (ASPMN) has published practice guidelines to assess pain in the nonverbal patient with advanced dementia (Ferris, 2008). The first step is the same as for all patients—ask.

- **Step 1:** ***Ask the Patient About the Pain:*** Obtaining the older patient's report of pain is essential even if cognitive or functional deficits are present. Ask about the pain using words like "hurt" or "ache." Touch or point to the body part of concern while asking the patient to help clarify the pain's location (Ferris, 2008).

PATIENT TEACHING & DISCHARGE PRIORITIES for Pain Management

Need	Teaching
Prescription Management	Prescriptions for pain medications should be filled as soon as possible so that the next dosage can be taken on time. (It is advisable to contact your pharmacy prior to discharge to be sure that the medications will be available in case they need to be specially ordered.)
Patient/family	Secure prescription pain medications to prevent loss or theft.
	Avoid opening medication bottles over the sink or toilet.
	Follow your prescribed pain medication taper plan.
	• Contact your prescribing health care provider prior to taking extra doses of medication or if the dosage needs to be reduced.
	Report unrelieved or new pain to your health care provider.
	If an additional prescription is necessary, notify your prescribing health care provider 2 to 3 days before it is needed.
	Assess pain intensity and ability to perform necessary activities prior to taking pain medications.
	• Take routine medications on schedule without skipping dosages.
	• Take "as-needed" medications prior to the onset of severe pain.
	• Use a notebook or journal to record the pain score, activity at the time of medication, the time and dosage of medication, and notes describing your concerns.
	Assess for pain medication side effects.
	• Take pain medications with food to prevent nausea.
	• Take stool softeners and stimulating laxatives routinely if taking opioid pain medications to prevent constipation. Drink plenty of fluids to avoid becoming dehydrated, unless your doctor has advised you not to.
	• Contact your prescribing health care provider if your opioid pain medication causes excessive sleepiness or heavy snoring.
	Assess knowledge of pain medications and pain management plan.
Family/support system	• Assess knowledge of pain medication side effects and treatments.
	• Assess knowledge of physical dependence, tolerance, and addiction.
	• Assess financial needs and resources for prescription coverage.
	• Provide example of journal or notebook for patient use.
Setting	Assess discharge referral needs: Pain management specialist/clinic, psychiatrist or psychologist, primary care provider.
	Assess need for follow-up appointments.
Nonmedication Strategy Management	Nonmedication strategies that were helpful during admission should continue to be used in addition to pain medications.
Patient/family	Assess pain intensity and ability to perform necessary activities prior to performing nonmedication strategies.
	• Record the pain score, activity at the time of the nonmedication strategies, the time, and notes describing your feelings or concerns in the journal or notebook.
Family/support system	Assess knowledge of selected nonmedication strategies in the pain management plan.
Setting	Assess discharge referral needs: physical therapist, massage therapist, acupuncture practitioner.
	Assess for need for follow-up appointments.
Painful Procedure Management	Medications that are prescribed for use prior to painful procedures should be taken, allowing sufficient time for onset of pain relief prior to beginning the procedure.
Patient/family	Assess pain score prior to, during, and after procedure.
Family/support system	• Utilize nonmedication strategies to encourage relaxation or distraction.
Setting	• Report unrelieved pain during procedures to your prescribing health care provider.
	Assess understanding of the role of premedication in successful procedural pain management.
	Assess knowledge of pain medications and nonmedication strategies to be used prior to and during painful procedures.
	Assess for need for professional home health assistance with procedural pain management.

- Step 2: *Search for Potential Causes of Pain:*
  - Consider chronic conditions, especially musculoskeletal disorders or neuropathies.
  - When a patient has limited mobility, consider the need for repositioning.
  - Look for sources of discomfort such as skin irritation, constipation, recent falls.
- Step 3: ***Observe Behaviors:*** Observation of behavior is a valid approach to pain assessment for the patient who is unable to describe his own pain. It is important to remember, however, that behaviors do not necessarily reflect pain intensity (Heer, Coyne, & Key, 2006).
  - Behaviors that may be signs of pain include guarding a body part, reluctance to move or be moved, decreased mobility, and crying out or wincing when touched or with movement.
  - Nonspecific distress behaviors that may or may not be associated with pain include restlessness, irritability, and vocalizations.
- Step 4: ***Seek Surrogate Reports of Pain:*** If the patient cannot self-report pain, family, friends, and other caregivers can function as surrogates to help recognize a patient's pain. Family members may be able to describe patterns associated with pain such as changes in mood, affect, appetite, or activity (Ferris, 2008).
- Step 5: *Do an Empiric Analgesic Trial:*
  - If pain is identified or suspected because of diagnosis, behaviors, or surrogate reports, an empiric trial (one derived from experiment and observation rather than theory) of analgesics is indicated.
  - For pain thought to be mild to moderate, a trial of around-the-clock acetaminophen might be successful (Ferris, 2008). If pain behaviors subside, pain can be confirmed and analgesia continued.

Pharmacologic Considerations

When selecting analgesic medications for the treatment of pain in the older adult, the changes that occur with aging must be considered in order to reduce the risk of medication side effects. Changes in gastric pH, increased gastric emptying, and decreased intestinal blood flow are common changes that will slow the absorption of medications. When the older adult has decreased lean body mass, increased body fat, decreased body water, and increased plasma protein, the distribution of medications is altered (Arnstein, 2010). Medications are stored in the tissue longer, extending their effects. When hepatic changes such as decreased hepatic mass and blood flow are present, metabolism is impacted, increasing the half-life of medications and reducing clearance or elimination as a result. Older adults also may experience decreased clearance or elimination of medications as a result of decreased glomerular filtration rate, decreased creatinine clearance, and decreased renal blood flow (Hutchinson, 2010).

The physiological changes that occur with advancing age often result in a more potent effect and longer half-life of medications commonly used to treat pain. Generally, those adults who are older than 70 and who also have altered absorption, distribution, metabolism, and excretion should be started on 25% to 50% of the recommended adult starting doses (Ferris, 2008). Once the patient's response to the medication is determined, dosages should be slowly increased or decreased as indicated until the desired effects are achieved. Specific medication cautions for the older adult are listed in Chart 12–5.

CHART 12–5 Medication Cautions for the Older Adult

NSAIDs	Highly protein-bound NSAIDs, such as aspirin, diflunisal, ibuprofen, naproxen, indomethacin, meclofenamate, and piroxicam, are more likely to cause toxicities in older adults.
Meperidine (Demerol)	The active metabolite normeperidine can cause CNS irritability, leading to seizures. Delirium and agitation are more likely when used to treat the postoperative older adult. Metabolite accumulation and toxicity occur when renal function is impaired.
Pentazocine (Talwin)	More likely to cause seizures, cardiac arrhythmias, and agitation. Analgesia is similar to aspirin.
Tricyclic Antidepressants	Anticholinergic effects are often intolerable for older adults.
Sedatives, Hypnotics, and Antiemetics	Long duration of action and sedation side effects make the older adult more prone to delirium and unstable gait, both of which can lead to increased risk of falls. Can cause respiratory depression, especially when given with opioids.
Antihistamines	Anticholinergic effects are often intolerable. Use should be limited to less than 12 weeks, and in lower dosage ranges.

Sources: Hutchinson, L. C. (2010). *Fundamentals of geriatric pharmacotherapy: An evidence-based approach.* Bethesda, MD: American Society of Health-System Pharmacists; Jansen, M. (2008). *Managing pain in the older adult.* New York: Springer Publications.

Research

The science of pain management is expanding with astonishing speed due to the ongoing efforts of scientists, nurses, and other health care providers who have dedicated time and energy to discovery. The "Decade of Pain Research" provides an opportunity to accomplish even more. The Research Opportunities feature provides a list of both medical and nursing research topics still under investigation.

Summary

Pain is a physical and psychological phenomenon that most people experience in their lifetime. This chapter has defined pain from a theoretical perspective. The multiple dimensions of pain are explored as is the approach to pain management from a cultural viewpoint. Assessment and measurement tools for determining the intensity of pain are included and pharmacological strategies for managing pain are discussed. Nursing management of patients with pain is a central focus of the chapter and includes a collaborative approach to caring for patients experiencing pain. Gerontological considerations for assessing and managing pain are included in the chapter.

RESEARCH OPPORTUNITIES Related to Pain

Research Area	Clinical Impact
Assessment tools that are culturally sensitive for ethnic minorities who speak English dialects (with use of accent, grammar, and vocabulary from their native country) and have low literacy levels	Improved ability to assess pain in this at-risk population of patients
Assessment tools that are disease specific	Improved ability to capture the unique components of pain in diseases such as sickle cell, HIV, or cancer
Outcomes related to high-technology implanted modalities	Improved understanding of when high technology will improve outcomes to facilitate development of clinical guidelines outlining best practices
Neural remodeling as a mechanism of chronic pain	Identification of preventive, management, and restorative treatment possibilities
Use of opioids for the treatment of chronic pain	Improved understanding of the impact of opioids on long-term health to facilitate development of clinical guidelines and consensus on best practice
Gender differences in chronic pain	Improved understanding of gender-related factors and mechanisms that could lead to the development of new medications and management strategies
Clinical trials of complementary and alternative therapies	Establishment of a base of scientific evidence to validate the use of these therapies in specific pain states
Genes that are relevant to pain and inhibitory mechanisms	Development of gene therapy models targeting specific structures within the central nervous system
The role of sleep and circadian variations in perception and modulation of pain	Understand the differences in pain perception and modulation for patients who have unusual sleep/rest/activity needs (e.g., night-shift workers, people with insomnia)
Barriers to patient compliance with pain treatment plan	Development of assessments, tools, educational materials, or specific helps that are demonstrated to improve compliance

CLINICAL PREPARATION READ DOCUMENT APPLY

READ: **History of Present Illnesses** >> Laboratory Study Results >> Critical Thinking Questions

As the on-coming nurse on the orthopedic nursing unit in a major trauma hospital, you are reviewing a report from the night nurse about Walter Wyatt, a 27-year-old male who was admitted to the hospital following a motor vehicle collision in which he was the unrestrained driver. Mr. Wyatt was ejected from the vehicle, but did not lose consciousness. He was able to provide a brief medical history to paramedics at the scene. In the report, the night nurse states that the patient was now 24 hours post-op following stabilization of an open book pelvic fracture with external fixation. He has multiple lacerations over his arms and legs and a large laceration on his head that the plastic surgeon repaired during surgery.

Medical–Surgical History

Mr. Wyatt's past medical history includes asthma and multiple knee arthroscopies for sports-related injuries.

Social History

Mr. Wyatt is married and the father of two children ages 1 and 3. Mr. Wyatt's wife and parents are at his bedside. He denies medication allergies, alcohol, smoking, or drug abuse.

Physical Exam

Mr. Wyatt is alert and oriented, with no sedation. His respiratory status includes deep, even respirations at a rate of 14 breaths per minute. He is able to maintain oxygen saturations of 93% to 97% on room air. He has clear breath sounds.

Mr. Wyatt's pulse is regular and strong with an apical heart rate of 68 beats per minute with no extra heart sounds. He has 3+ peripheral pulses with capillary refill < 3 seconds in all extremities. Blood pressure is measured at 132/56.

Bowel sounds are present in all four quadrants of the abdomen and he denies nausea. He has passed flatus and his surgeon has prescribed advancement of diet as tolerated. He has not had a bowel movement since the surgery.

A urinary catheter has been placed and is draining approximately 30 mL of dark yellow-brown urine per hour.

Current Pain Assessment

Mr. Wyatt reports pain in his lower abdomen bilaterally, right groin, and right shoulder. He rates his pain intensity using the numeric rating scale of 0 to 10 as 7/10 in his abdomen, 9/10 in his right groin, and 5/10 in his right knee. Mr. Wyatt describes the pain in his abdomen and right groin as constant, sharp, and stabbing with occasional spasms; he describes the right knee pain as a constant, aching, throbbing pain. He reports his pain is unbearable when he is turned in bed to change the linens.

Mr. Wyatt expresses frustration and anger that his pain is unrelieved and that his life is ruined because of the injuries he has sustained. His wife expresses concern that he is not coping as he usually does when faced with difficult circumstances. The hospital chaplain has attempted to visit with Mr. Wyatt and his wife on two separate occasions, but each time Mr. Wyatt declines the visit, stating that he is in too much pain. When Mr. Wyatt's wife leaves the room he is calm and watches the sports channel on the TV.

CLINICAL PREPARATION, *continued*

Admitting Medical Orders

Admit to trauma service
Diagnosis: multiple lacerations over arms, legs, and head; rule out internal injuries; open book pelvic fracture
No known allergies
Vital signs every 4 hours
Bed rest
Sequential compression devices (SCD) to lower extremities
Sterile 0.9% saline to clean pin sites q12h
Foley catheter
Intake and output
IV: D51/2NS plus KCl 20 mEq at 125 hour
NPO
Incentive spirometer q1h while awake and q4h at night
Clean lacerations with normal saline q8h
Call house officer: Pulse 110/minute; BP 160 systolic; temperature $>$ 38.5; urine output 30/hour

Scheduled Medications

IV PCA morphine 1 mg/mL; no continuous infusion, 1 mg PCA demand dose, a 6-minute lockout time, and a 12-mg hourly limit; may bolus with 2 mg every hour prn severe pain

PRN Medications

Phenergan 25 mg IV q6h prn nausea
Ativan 0.5–2 mg IV q6–8h prn anxiety (not to exceed 10 mg/24 hours)
Tylenol 650 mg PR q4h for pain
Benadryl 25–50 mg IV qhs

Ordered Laboratory Studies

CBC q6h times 24 hours, then daily; basic metabolic panel daily, UA × 1 now

Ordered Diagnostic Studies

12-lead ECG
PA and lateral chest x-ray
X-ray of right knee and pelvis post-fixation

READ: History of Present Illnesses >> **Laboratory Study Results** >> Critical Thinking Questions

Test	Day 1	Day 2	Day 3
Potassium	4.4 mEq/L	3.8 mEq/L	3.7 mEq/L
Chloride	106 mEq/L	106 mEq/L	111 mEq/L
Sodium	142 mEq/L	141 mEq/L	144 mEq/L
Carbon dioxide (CO_2)	24 mEq/L	24 mEq/L	27 mEq/L
Anion gap	12.4 mEq/L	11.8 mEq/L	7.1 mEq/L
Glucose	97 mg/dL	99 mg/dL	119 mg/dL
Blood urea nitrogen (BUN)	22 mg/dL	22 mg/dL	20 mg/dL
Creatinine	0.8 mg/dL	0.8 mg/dL	1.4 mg/dL
Calcium	8.2 mg/dL	8.2 mg/dL	7.7 mg/dL
Hemoglobin	10/10.2/9.8/10/ 9.9/10.1 g/dL	10.1 g/dL	10.4 g/dL
Hematocrit	33/33.4/34/ 32.3/33/34/33/%	33.6 %	34%

Test	Day 1	Day 2	Day 3
Urinalysis			
Appearance and color	Dark amber and clear		
pH	6.2		
Protein	6 mg/dL		
Specific gravity	1.025		
Leukocytes, nitrates, ketones, and bilirubin	All negative		
Urobilinogen	0.02 units/mL		
Crystals and casts	None		
Glucose	None		
WBC and RBC	None		

Pearson Nursing Student Resources *Log on to* **nursing.pearsonhighered.com** *to download forms*

DOCUMENT:

>> Summary of Hospitalization
>> Pathophysiology Form
>> Laboratory Values
>> Laboratory Results Explanation

APPLY:

>> List of Potential Nursing Diagnosis
>> Concept Map
>> Critical Thinking Questions and Concept Map

APPLY: History of Present Illnesses >> Laboratory Study Results >> **Critical Thinking Questions**

1. Which dimensions of pain would you consider significant when reviewing your assessment of Mr. Wyatt's pain?
2. Which nursing intervention would be appropriate for the change in behavior when Mr. Wyatt's wife leaves the room?
3. What additional assessments would be important to consider prior to contacting the prescribing health care provider to advocate for changes to Mr. Wyatt's pain medications?

Answers to Critical Thinking Questions can be found in Appendix D in the Osborn Student Resources at nursing.pearsonhighered.com.

NCLEX® PRACTICE

1. Which information regarding pain should the nurse include when conducting an educational session for newly licensed nurses?
   1. Pain is a common symptom to most illnesses, disease processes, and traumatic injuries.
   2. There are few cultural differences in the recognition, expression, and response to pain.
   3. Today's health care system understands pain and is willing and able to manage it.
   4. Pain is rarely associated with significant personal, social, or economic distress.
2. A nurse is designing a basic plan of care for patients following the Clinical Practice Guidelines for chronic nonmalignant pain established by the American College of Physicians. Which concept should the nurse include in this plan of care?
   1. Expect that the pain experienced will be directly proportional to disease severity.
   2. Exclude the use of chronic opiates if the patient also requires treatment for concurrent psychiatric disorders.
   3. Recognize the fundamental responsibility of all nurses to help alleviate patient suffering and relieve pain.
   4. Acknowledge the potential for criminal penalties for patients receiving excessive amounts of opiates.
3. A patient has been diagnosed with chronic pain. The nurse is educating the patient about this condition. The nurse knows the patient has a clear understanding of chronic pain with verbalization of which statement?
   1. "My pain should be brief and then resolve completely."
   2. "The pain I am having is associated with my recent surgery."
   3. "This pain will not last long, but will come back soon."
   4. "My pain may last for months, years, or for my whole life."
4. Which tool should the nurse select to evaluate the multidimensional aspects of a patient's pain? (select all that apply)
   1. The patient's pain intensity self-report
   2. The McGill Pain Questionnaire
   3. The Numeric Rating Scale
   4. The Visual Analog Scale
   5. The Brief Pain Inventory
5. A physician in the pain control clinic has added a nonsteroidal anti-inflammatory drug (NSAID) to the opioid treatment already established for a patient with chronic back pain. The nurse can expect which action to follow this change?
   1. An increase in the opioid dosage
   2. No change in the opioid dosage
   3. A decrease in the opioid dosage
   4. A medical review since these two drugs are not used together
6. The nurse is planning to administer the first dose of an intravenous opioid to an opioid naïve patient. Which nursing actions are necessary? (select all that apply)
   1. Have Narcan available for administration.
   2. Observe the patient's respiratory status.
   3. Monitor the patient for pruritus.
   4. Monitor the patient's hemoglobin and hematocrit levels.
   5. Monitor the patient for nausea.

Answers to NCLEX Practice questions can be found in Appendix D in the Osborn Student Resources at nursing.pearsonhighered.com. Practice additional NCLEX questions online at the Student Resources site.

REFERENCES

Aaron, L. A., Turner, J.A., Mancl, L. A., Sawchuk, C. N., Huggins, K. H., & Truelove, E. L. (2006). Daily pain coping among patients with chronic temporomandibular disorder pain: an electronic diary study. *Journal of Orofacial Pain*, 20:125–137.

Adams, M. P., Josephson, D. L., & Holland, L. N. (2010). *Pharmacology for nurses: A pathophysiological approach* (3rd ed.). Upper Saddle River, NJ: Pearson Prentice Hall.

Adams, M. P., & Koch, R. (2010). *Pharmacologic connections to nursing practice*. Upper Saddle River, NJ: Prentice Hall.

Administration on Aging. (2008) *Snapshot: A statistical profile of older Americans aged 65+*. U.S. Department of Health & Human Services. Last updated February 6, 2008. Retrieved from http://www.aoa.gov

American Academy of Pain Medicine, American Pain Society, & American Society of Addiction Medicine. (2008). *Definitions related to the use of opioids for the treatment of pain.* Glenview, IL: American Pain Society.

American College of Physicians. (2012). ACP Clinical Practice Guidelines. Retrieved from http://www.acponline.org/clinical_information/guidelines/guidelines/

American Nurses Association. (2001). *Code for nurses with interpretive statements.* Kansas City, MO: Author.

American Pain Society. (2012). Principles of analgesic use in the treatment of acute pain and cancer pain (6th ed.). Glenview, Il: American Pain Society.

Arbuck, M. M. (2012). New views on opioid equivalency. *Pain-Topics.org News/Research Updates.* Retrieved from http://updates.pain-topics.org/2012/02/new-views-on-opiod-equivalency.html

Arnstein, P. (2010). Balancing analgesic efficacy with safety concerns in the older patient. *Pain Management Nursing, 11*(2), S11–S22.

Aydede, M. (2010). Pain. In E. N. Zalta (Ed.), *The Stanford encyclopedia of philosophy* (Spring 2010 Edition). Retrieved from http://plato.stanford.edu/archives/spr2010/entries/pain/

Barrett, K., Barman, S., & Boitano, S. (2009). *Ganong's review of medical physiology* (23rd ed.). New York: McGraw-Hill.

Berman, A. J., & Snyder, S. (2012). *Fundamentals of nursing* (9th ed.). Upper Saddle River, NJ: Pearson.

Bjorling, E. A. (2009). The momentary relationship between stress and headaches in adolescent girls. *Headache: The Journal of Head and Face Pain. 49*:1186–1197. doi: 10.1111/j.1526-4610.2009.01406.x

Bolen, J. (2008). Ethical issues in the treatment of chronic non-malignant pain: A focus on the legal side. *The Pain Practitioner, 18*(1), 3–8.

Borne, T., et al. (2010). Reducing patient barriers to pain and fatigue management. *Journal of Pain and Symptom Management, 39*(3), 486–501. DOI:10.1016/j.jpainsymman.2009.2008.007

Briggs, A. M., Jordan, J. E., Buchbinder, R., Burnett, A. F., O'Sullivan, P.B., Chua, J.Y., et al. (2010). Health literacy and beliefs among a community cohort with and without chronic low back pain. *Pain, 150*(2): 275-283.

Bruckenthal, P. (2008). Risk factors associated with the onset of persistent pain. Retrieved from http://www.medscape.org/viewarticle/576473

Bruckenthal, P., & D'Arcy, V. M. (2007). Assessment and management of pain in older adults: a review of the basics. *Topics in Advanced Practice Nursing.* Retrieved from http://www.medscape.com/viewarticle/556382_print

Buckley, P. F. (2009). Regional anesthesia with local anesthetics. In *Bonica's management of pain* (4th ed.). Ambler, PA: Lippincott Williams and Wilkins.

Campbell, C. E., & Osborn, K. (2010). Pain assessment and management. In K. S. Osborn, C. E. Wraa, & A. B. Watson (Eds.), *Medical surgical nursing: Preparation for practice* (1st ed., pp. 332–364). Upper Saddle River: NJ: Prentice Hall.

Centers for Disease Control and Prevention (CDC), National Center for Disease Prevention and Control. (2010). CDC's issue brief. Unintentional drug poisoning in the United States. Retrieved from http://www./cdc/gov/homeandRecreationalSafety/Poisoningbrief.htm.2010

Chapman, C. R. (2008). Progress in pain assessment: The cognitively compromised patient. *Current Opinion in Anesthesiology, 21*(4), 610–615.

Chen, L-M, Miaskowski, C., Dodd, M., & Pantilat, S. (2008). Concepts within the Chinese culture that influence the cancer pain experience. *Cancer Nursing, 31*(2), 103–108.

Chen, Y. L., & Francis, A. J. (2010). Relaxation and imagery for chronic, non-malignant pain: Effects on pain symptoms, quality of life and mental health. *Pain Management Nursing, 11*(3), 19–25, 159–168.

Chou, R., et al. (2009). Clinical guidelines for the use of chronic opioid therapy in chronic noncancer pain. *Journal of Pain, 10*(2), 103–130, e22.

Clark, H. L. (2010). Stress management: identifying your stressors. Retrieved from http://www.keepandshare.com/blog/2010/05/06/stress-management-identifying-your-stressors/

Coda, B. A., & Bonica, J. J. (2009). General considerations in acute pain. In J. C. Ballantyne & J. P. Rathmell (2009), *Bonica's management of pain* (4th ed.). Ambler, PA: Lippincott Williams and Wilkins.

Cowan, P. (2011). The financial costs of pain. *American Chronic Pain Association Chronical, 9*(1), 5. Retreived from http://www.iom.edu/Reports/2011/Relieving-Pain[in-American0A-BluepringOforTransforming-Prevention-Care-Education-Research.aspx

Cox, D. S., & Karapas, E. T. (2010). Taxonomy for pain management in nursing. In St. Marie, B. (Ed.), *Core curriculum for pain management nursing* (2nd ed.). Dubuque, IA: Kendall Hunt Publishing.

Critical Care Nursing. (2010). PQRST method for pain assessment. Retrieved from http://micunursing.com/pain.htm

D'Arcy, Y. (2008). Pain in the older adult. *The Nurse Practitioner, 33*(3), 18-24.

D'Arcy, Y. (2009). The effect of culture on pain. *Nursing Made Incredibly Easy! 7*(3), 5–7.

Deglin, J. H., & Valleran, A. H. (2009). *Davis's drug guide for nurses* (11th ed.). Philadelphia: FA Davis.

Dempski, K. (2009). Pain control. In S. J. Westrick & K. Dempski (Eds.), *Essentials of nursing law and ethics* (pp. 88–91). Sudbury, MA: Jones & Bartlett.

Dunwoody, C. J., Krenzischek, D. A., Pasero, C., Rathmell, J. P., & Polomano, R. C. (2008). Assessment, physiological monitoring, and consequences of inadequately treated acute pain. *Journal of Perianesthesia Nursing, 23* (suppl 1): S15-S27.

Engebretson, J. (2012). CDC report: Americans in pain. *Acupuncture, 8*(11). Retrieved from http://www.acupuncturetoday.com/mpacms/at/article.php?ed=31440

Ferrell, B., Levy, M. H., & Paice, J. (2008). Managing pain from advanced cancer in the palliative care setting. *Clinical Journal of Oncology Nursing, 12*(4), 575–581. doi: 10.1188/08.CJON.575-581

Ferris, M. (2008). Pain in the cognitively impaired elderly: Guidelines for clinicians. *Topics in Advanced Practice Nursing eJournal.* Posted May 15, 2008. Retrieved from http://www.medscape.com/viewarticle/573642

Gelinas, C. (2010). Nurses' evaluations of the feasibility and the clinical utility of the critical-care pain observation tool. *Pain Management Nursing, 11*(2), 115–125.

Gelinas, C., Fillion, L., & Puntillo, K. (2009). Item selection and content validity of the critical-care pain observation tool for non-verbal adults. *Journal of Advanced Nursing, 65*(1), 203–216.

Gmyrek, R., & Dahdah, M. (2009). Local and regional anesthetics. *E medicine from WebMD.* Retrieved from http://emedicine.medscape.com/article/1831870

Goebel et al. (2010, June). Addressing patients' concerns about pain management and addiction risks. *Pain Management Nursing, 11*(2), 92–98.

Gordon, D. B., Polomono, R., Pellino, T. A., Turk, D. C., McCracken, L., Sherwood, G., Farrar, J., Paice, J., Wallace, M., & Strassels, S. (2010). Psychometrics of the revised American Pain Society Patient Outcome Questionnaire/APS-POQ for quality improvement of acute and cancer pain management. *Journal of Pain, 11*(11), 1172–1186.

Haslbauer, F., & Feigl, M. (2009). Biphosphonates as adjuvant therapy in multimodal pain management. *MEMO: Magazine of European Medical Oncology, 2*(3), 161–165.

Herr, K. (2010). Pain in the older adult: An imperative across all healthcare settings. *Pain Management Nursing, 11*(2), S1N–S10.

Herr K., Coyne, P. J., Key, T., et al. (2006). Pain assessment in the nonverbal patient: Position statement with clinical practice recommendations. *Pain Management Nursing, 7,* 44–52.

Hutchinson, L. C. (2010). *Fundamentals of geriatric pharmacotherapy: An evidence-based approach.* Bethesda, MD: American Society of Health-System Pharmacists.

Im, E.-O., Guevara, E., & Chee, W. (2007). The pain experience of Hispanic patients with cancer in the U.S. *Oncology Nursing Forum, 34*(4), 861–868.

International Association for the Study of Pain. (1993). Outline curriculum on pain for schools of nursing. Retrieved from http://www.iasp-pain.org/nursing_toc.html

International Association for the Study of Pain. (2009). Coping with pain. Retrieved from http://www.iasp-pain.org/AM/AMTemplate.cfm?Section=Home&SECTION=Home&TEMPLATE=/CM/ContentDisplay.cfm&CONTENTID=15082

International Association for the Study of Pain. (2011). IASP taxonomy. Retrieved from http://www.iasp-pain.org/Content/NavigationMenu/GeneralResourceLinks/PainDefinitions/default.htm

International Association for the Study of Pain. (2012). Identification and treatment of neuropathic pain in patients with cancer. Pain Clinical Updates. 20(2). Retrieved from http://www.iasp-pain.org/AM/AMTemplate.cfm?Section=Home&CONTENTID=15349&TEMPLATE=/CM/ContentDisplay.cfm&SECTION=Home

International Council of Nurses. (2006). *The ICN code of ethics for nurses.* Geneva, Switzerland: Author.

Institute of Medicine (IOM). (2010). *The future of nursing: Leading change, advancing health.* Washington, DC: The Academic Press.

IOM (Institute of Medicine). 2011. *The Future of Nursing: Leading Change, Advancing Health.* Washington, DC: The National Academies Press.

Jacox, A., Carr, D. B., Payne, R., et al. (1994, March). *Management of cancer pain* (Clinical Practice Guideline No. 9, AHCPR Pub. No. 94-0592). Rockville, MD: Agency for Health Care Policy and Research.

Jacques, E. (2010). Living with chronic pain. *About.com. Chronic Pain.* Retrieved from http://pain.abouta.com/od/livingwithchronicpain/a/living_with_cp.htm

Johnson, S. J. (2007). Opioid safety in patients with renal or hepatic dysfunction. Pain Treatment Topics. Retrieved from www.Pain-Topics.org

Kee, J. L., Hayer, E. R., & McCuistian, L. E. (2009). *Pharmacology: A nursing process approach* (6th ed.). St. Louis, MO: Saunders.

Khatta, M. (2007). A complimentary approach to pain management. *Topics in Advanced Practice Nursing eJournal, 7*(1). Retrieved from http://www.medscape.com/viewarticle/556408

Knotkova, H., & Papopagallo, M. (2007). Adjuvant analgesics. *Medical Clinic of North America, 91*(1), 113-124. Retrieved from http://www.ncbi.nlm.nih.gov/pubmed/17164107

Kroenke, K., Krebs, E. E., & Bair, M. J. (2009). Pharmacotherapy of chronic pain: A syntheses of recommendations from systematic reviews. *General Hospital Psychiatry, 31*(3), 206–219.

Kumar, A., & Allcock, N. (2008). Pain in older people. *Help the Aged.* Retrieved from http://www.britishpainsociety.org/book_pain_in_older_age_ID7826.pdf

Lee, J., & Sun, Jr., E. (2011). Effect of an integral care system: A combination of oriental and Western care for older adults with degenerative arthritis. *Journal of Korean Academy of Nursing, 41*(1), 18–25. doi: 10.4040/jkan.2011.41.1.18

Leleszi, J. P., & Lewandowski, J. G. (2007). Managing pain in patients at end of life. *The Journal of the American Osteopathic Association (JAOA),* Supplement 4, *107*(6), E53–E59.

Mackintosh, C., & Elson, S. (2008). Chronic pain: Clinical features, assessment and treatment. *Nursing Standard, 23*(5), 48–56.

Matteson, M. (2011). Chronic pain in the elderly. Virginia Henderson International Nursing Library. Retrieved from http://www.nursinglibrary.org/vhl/handle/10755/177780

McCaffery, M. (1968). *Nursing practice theories related to cognition, bodily pain, and man–environment interactions.* Los Angeles: University of California at Los Angeles Students' Store.

McDonald, D. (2009). Older adult's pain descriptions. *Pain Management Nursing, 10*(3), 142–148.

McDonald, D. D., LaPorta, M., & Meadows-Oliver, M. (2007). Nurses' response to pain communication from patients: A post-test experimental study. *International Journal of Nursing Studies, 44*(1), 29–35.

Mayday Fund. (2009). A call to revolutionize chronic pain care in America: an opportunity in health care reform. Mayday Fund Pain Research, Education & Policy. Retrieved from sites.tufts.edu/prep/tag/mayday-fund/

Merck Manual of Diagnosis and Therapy. (2007a). Neurogenic pain. Retrieved from http://www.merckmanurals.com/professional/see16/ch209/ch209c.html

Merck Manual of Diagnosis and Therapy. (2007b). Types: Pain. In *The Merck Manual of Medical Information—Home Edition.*

Retrieved from http://www.merck.com/mmhe/sec06/ch078/ch078b.html?qt=types:%20pain&alt=sh

Miyoshi, H. R., & Leckband, S. G. (2009). Systemic opioid analgesics. In S. M. Fishman, J. C. Ballantyne, & J. P. Rathmell (Eds.), *Bonica's management of pain* (4th ed.). Ambler, PA: Lippincott Williams and Wilkins.

Morgan, J. P. (1985). American opiophobia: Customary underutilization of opioid analgesics. *Advances in Alcohol and Substance Abuse, 86*(5), 163–173.

National Cancer Institute. (2007). Pain PDQ: Pharmacologic management. Retrieved from http://www.cancer.gov/cancertopics/pdq/supportivecare/pain/HealthProfessional/Page3

National Cancer Institute. (2010). Dictionary of cancer terms. Retrieved from http://www.cancer.gov/dictionary

National Center for Health Statistics. (2009). *Public health report 2007, 122*(2), 268-269. Retrieved from http://www.ncbi.nlm.nih.gov/pmc/articles/PMC1820434/

National Institute of Health. (1987). The integrated approach to the management of pain. *Journal of Pain and Symptom Management, 2,* 35–44.

National Institute of Neurological Disorders and Stroke. (2007). Chronic pain information page. Retrieved from http://www.ninds.nih.gov/disorders/chronic_pain/chronic_pain.htm

National Institutes of Health. (2008). Fact sheets – Pain Management. Retrieved from http://medlineplus.nlm.nih.gov/medlineplus/pain.html#fromthenationalinstitutesofhealth

Neuropathic Pain Management. (2011). *WebMD.* Retrieved from http://www.webmd.com/pain-management/guide/neuropoathic-pain

Norrbrink, C., & Lundeberg, T. (2011). Acupuncture and massage therapy for neuropathic pain following spinal cord injury: An exploratory study. *Acupuncture Med.*29, 108-115. doi: 10.1136/aim.2010.003269

Pasero, C., & McCaffery, M. (2010). *Pain assessment & pharmacologic management.* St. Louis: Mosby.

Polomano, R. C., Rathmell, J. P., Krenzoschek, D. A., & Dunwoody, C. J. (2008). Emerging trends and new approaches to acute pain management. *Pain Management Nursing, 9*(1), S33–41.

Porth, C. M., & Matfin, M. (2009). *Essentials of pathophysiology: Concepts of altered health states* (72nd ed.). Philadelphia: Lippincott Williams & Wilkins.

Price, D. D., Riley, J. L., & Wade, J. B. (2010). Psychological approaches to measurement of the dimensions and stages of pain. In D. C. Turk & R. Melzack (Eds.), *Handbook of pain assessment* (3rd ed., pp. 53–75). New York: Guilford Press.

Pudas-Tähkä, S., Axelin, A., Aantaa, R., & Salanterä, S. (2009). Pain assessment tools for unconscious or sedated intensive care patients: A systematic review. *Journal of Advanced Nursing, 65*(5), 946–956.

Puntillo, K. A. (2007). Managing pain, delirium, and sedation. *Critical Care Nurse* (Suppl.), 8–10.

Qin et al. (2011). The temporal-spatial encoding of acupuncture effects in the brain. *Molecular Pain, 7*(19).

Quality and Safety Education for Nurses (QSEN). (2011). Retrieved from http://www.qsen.org/about_qsen.php

Schofield, P. (2008). Assessment and management of pain in older adults with dementia: A review of current practice and future directions. *Current Opinion in Supportive and Palliative Care, 2*(1), 128–132.

Singh, M. K. (2012). Chronic pain syndrome. Medscape Reference. Retrieved from http://emedicine.medscape/com/article/310834-overview

Sullivan, M., & Ferrell, B. (2005). Ethical challenges in the management of chronic nonmalignant pain: Negotiating through the cloud of doubt. Retrieved from http://www.ampainsoc.org/press/2005_jop/0105.html

The Joint Commission. (2009, October 5). The Joint Commission announces 2010 National Patient Safety Goals. *Accreditation Connection.* Retrieved from http://www.hepro.com/ACC-239979-851/The-Joint-Commission-announces-2010-National

The Joint Commission on Accreditation of Healthcare Organizations. (2010). *Comprehensive accreditation manual 2010.* Chicago, IL: The Joint Commission.

Topolovec-Vranic, J., Canzian, S., Innis, J, Pollmann-Mudryj, M. A., McFarlan, A.W., & Baker, A.J. (2010). Patient satisfaction and documentation of pain assessments and management after implementing the adult nonverbal pain scale. *American Journal of Critical Care, 19,* 345–354. doi:10.4037/ajcc2010247

Urch, C. E., & Dickenson, A. H. (2008). Neuropathic pain in cancer. *European Journal of Cancer, 44*(8), 1091–1096.

Vallerand, A., & Nowak, L. (2010). Chronic opioid therapy for nonmalignant pain: The patient's perspective. Part II—barriers to chronic opioid therapy. *Pain Management Nursing, 11*(2), 126–131.

Weissman, D. E. (2008). *Fast facts and concepts #69. End of Life/Palliative Education Resource Center (EPERC).* Milwaukee, WI: Medical College of Wisconsin.

World Health Organization. (2012). WHO's pain ladder. Retrieved from http://www.who.int/cancer/palliative/painladder/en/

Wuhrman, E., & Cooney, M. F. (2011). Acute pain: Assessment and treatment. *Topics in Advance Nursing Practice ejournal.* Posted: 1/3/2011. Retrieved from http://www.medscape.com/viewarticle/735034

Young Casey, C., Greenberg, M. A., Nicassio, P. M., Harpin, R. E., & Hubbard, D. (2008). Transition from acute to chronic pain and disability: a model including cognitive, affective, and trauma factors. *Pain, 134*(1-2), 69-79. Retrieved from http://www.ncbi.nlm.nih.gov/pubmed/17504729

Zalon, M. L., Constantino, R. E., & Andrew, K. L. (2008). The right to pain treatment: A reminder for nurses. *Dimensions of Critical Care Nursing, 27*(3), 93–101.

CHAPTER 13

Substance Abuse Assessment and Management

Gail Thurkauf
Annita Watson

Outcome-Based Learning Objectives

After studying this chapter, the learner will be able to:

1. Explain the major theories of substance-related disorders.
2. Analyze how the physical, psychological, and withdrawal effects of the major categories of substances manifest themselves.
3. Incorporate nursing assessment components to detect patients who have substance-related disorders.

KEY TERMS

delirium tremens (DTs) p.305
postacute withdrawal syndrome (PAWS) p.303
substance abuse p.303
substance dependence p.302
substance intoxication p.303
substance withdrawal p.303
substance withdrawal syndrome p.303
tolerance p.302
withdrawal p.302

SUBSTANCE ABUSE is the clinical term for the use or abuse of prescription or recreational substances in order to satisfy an urge, such as a need for relief, escape, relaxation, and/or feeling happy. The high incidence of substance abuse in society demands that nurses exhibit competence when treating patients with addictions. The American Nurses Association (ANA) Standards of Addictions Nursing Practice are the most current guidelines for validating the need for nurses to understand the implications of addiction (ANA, 2004). See the National Guidelines box for a list of the ANA standards (p. 303). The first step in gaining understanding and competence is becoming familiar with the terminology used to explain substance use and abuse; these terms are defined in the following sections. The major current theories of how substance abuse occurs are discussed later in this chapter, followed by management of care related to patients suffering from substance abuse.

Definitions and Terminology

Accurate nursing assessment and high-quality care of patients with substance abuse problems are based on an understanding of terms commonly used in the treatment of substance abuse. Patterns of behavior consistent with each definition are included in the following discussion.

Substance-Related Disorders

According to the *Diagnostic and Statistical Manual of Mental Disorders,* Fourth Edition, Text Revision (DSM-IV-TR) (American Psychiatric Association [APA], 2000), substance-related disorders are disorders that are (1) a consequence of abusing a drug (such as alcohol), (2) the side effects of a medication (antihistamines, for example), or (3) related to exposure to a toxin (fuel, paint, or other inhalants). Substance-related disorders are divided into two groups:

1. Substance-use disorders, which include substance dependence and substance abuse.
2. Substance-induced disorders, which include substance intoxication, substance withdrawal, substance-induced cognitive disorders, and substance-induced mood disorders.

This chapter focuses on substance abuse, including intoxication and withdrawal issues for some classes of substances that have traditionally been called psychoactive drugs.

Substance Dependence

Substance dependence is defined as a maladaptive pattern of substance use leading to clinically significant impairment or distress. The two main indicators of this pattern are tolerance and withdrawal:

- **Tolerance** is the need for increased amounts of a substance to achieve the desired effect.
- **Withdrawal** is the term used for the uncomfortable and maladaptive physiological and cognitive behavioral changes that are associated with lowered concentrations of a substance in the blood or tissue after an individual has been engaged in heavy use of the substance.

Characteristic behaviors during the pattern of tolerance and withdrawal include the following:

- Compulsive use, or not being able to sustain normal functioning without the use of the drug
- Need for increasing amounts of the drug to achieve the desired effect

NATIONAL GUIDELINES for ANA Standards of Addictions Nursing Practice

Standard 1: Assessment: The addictions nurse collects patient health data.

Standard 2: Diagnosis: The addictions nurse analyzes the assessment data in determining diagnoses.

Standard 3: Outcome Identification: The addictions nurse identifies expected outcomes individualized to the patient.

Standard 4: Planning: The addictions nurse develops an individualized plan of care that prescribes interventions to attain expected outcomes.

Standard 5: Implementation: The addictions nurse implements the interventions identified in the plan of care.

Standard 5a: Therapeutic Alliance: The addictions nurse uses the "therapeutic self" to establish a therapeutic alliance with the patient and to structure nursing interventions to promote development of insight, coping skills, and motivation for change in behavior that promotes health.

Standard 5b: Health Teaching: The addictions nurse, through health teaching, assists individuals, families, groups, and communities in achieving satisfying, productive, and healthy patterns of living.

Standard 5c: Self-Care and Self-Management: The addictions nurse uses the knowledge and philosophy of self-care and self-management to assist the patient in learning new ways to address stress, maintain self-control, accept personal responsibility, and integrate healthy coping behaviors into lifestyle choices.

Standard 5d: Pharmacologic, Biologic, and Complementary Therapies: The addictions nurse applies knowledge of pharmacologic, biologic, and complementary therapies and uses clinical skills to restore the patient's health and prevent consequences from addiction.

Standard 5e: Therapeutic Milieu: The addictions nurse structures, provides, and maintains a therapeutic environment in collaboration with the patient and other health care providers.

Standard 5f: Counseling: The addictions nurse uses counseling interventions to assist patients in promoting healthy coping abilities, preventing addiction, and addressing issues related to patterns of abuse and addiction.

Standard 6: Evaluation: The addictions nurse evaluates the patient's progress toward attainment of expected outcomes.

Source: Reprinted with permission from American Nurses Association and International Nurses Society on Addictions, Scope and Standards of Addictions Nursing Practice, © 2004 Nursesbooks.org, Silver Spring, MD.

- Unsuccessful attempts to cut down or regulate substance use
- Devotion of time trying to obtain the substance
- Using the substance or recovering from the effects of the substance
- Continued use of the substance despite the recognition of associated adverse effects and difficulties (Psych Central, 2011).

Substance Abuse

Substance abuse is characterized by a pattern of repeated consumption of substances that are used even though this use causes harm, such as the failure to fulfill major role obligations (such as parenting), using substances in physically hazardous situations (such as crack houses), and repeated social and relationship problems such as domestic violence.

Substance Intoxication

Substance intoxication refers to a reversible syndrome of maladaptive physiological and behavioral changes that are due to a substance's effects on a person's central nervous system (CNS). The syndrome includes disturbances of mood, the sleep–wake cycle, attention, thinking, judgment, perception of the current situation, and psychomotor and interpersonal behavior (Doweiko, 2011).

Substance Withdrawal

Substance withdrawal refers to the development of maladaptive physiological, behavioral, and cognitive changes that are due to reducing or stopping the heavy and regular use of a substance. The physical symptoms may include muscle aches, nausea, diarrhea, and increased blood pressure. **Substance withdrawal syndrome** is associated with distress and/or impairment in important areas of social functioning such as the ability to relate to people and/or unpredictable behavior.

Postacute Withdrawal Syndrome

Postacute withdrawal syndrome (PAWS) is a cluster of symptoms that occur in recovering addicts and alcoholics. PAWS symptoms usually begin to occur between 7 and 14 days after the acute period of withdrawal and usually peak 3 to 6 months after the start of abstinence (Battaglia, 2009). This phenomenon has been described as a "bio-psycho-social syndrome, that results from a combination of damage to the nervous system caused by alcohol or drugs and the psychosocial stress of coping with life without drugs or alcohol" (Battaglia, 2009, p. 1). The syndrome is manifested as the body attempts to repair residual physical remnants of neurotransmitter production and/or receptor site damage in the brain and other organs. Neurotransmitter production problems, either overproduction or underproduction, affect mood, interpersonal interactions, and cognitive skills. Receptor site damage means that naturally produced neurotransmitters cannot be normally recognized or absorbed or provide feedback. Therefore, normal functioning is impaired.

The symptoms of PAWS may be classified into six types: inability to think clearly, memory problems, emotional overreactions or numbness, sleep disturbances, physical coordination problems, and stress sensitivity (National Center for Alcohol and Drug Detox [NCADD], 2011). Evidence of PAWS is seen as unusual or flattened affect, disabilities in functioning in demanding zones such as personal finances and stressful situations, poor occupational/vocational functioning, and difficulties establishing and maintaining relationships. This creates social stressors in addition to the physiological and cognitive problems.

Etiology

The etiology of substance abuse describes how the problem of using substances came into being for a particular patient. It is important to determine where and why the problem started in order to develop interventions to address the source.

Biologic Theories

Substance abuse prior to conception and pregnancy in both males and females damages the child's genetic makeup. Research demonstrates that children of people who abuse alcohol have a fourfold risk

Weblink: The Genetics of Addiction.

of becoming alcohol abusers themselves (addictionsandrecovery.org, 2011). Even if different families adopt them at birth, there is more than a 60% chance that identical twins of alcoholic parents will both become alcoholics; for fraternal twins, the likelihood of both becoming alcoholics is just under 30% (Hasin, Hatzenbueler, & Waxman, 2010). Neurobiologic studies support the theory that biologic factors such as genetics shape vulnerability to substance-related disorders and also result from them (Erickson, 2007). Additional biologic foundations can be seen in the treatment of substance abuse. For example, the body's response to medications that have anxiolytic and antidepressant effects used in detoxification and relapse-prevention treatment further supports a biologic framework for substance abuse.

The biologic explanation of substance abuse has had a great deal of support from recent developments in technology. The use of magnetic resonance imaging (MRI) and positron emission tomography (PET) scans provides greater detail about the brain's function. These scans help explain substance abuse in terms of changes in the limbic area of the brain (Doweiko, 2011). Other studies have found biologic explanations of substance abuse and how genes affect the functioning of different biochemical systems, indicating a relationship with substance abuse problems, and the role of family genetics in the development of substance use disorders (Hasin et al., 2010).

Psychological Theories

Psychological theories about substance abuse suggest that the psychological underpinnings of experiences and behaviors come together to form the motivations for using substances in a destructive manner. People respond to environmental influences through their underlying neurobiologic system. The remarkable frequency of some disorders—such as bipolar disorder—co-occurring with substance abuse further suggests how psychological experiences and symptoms may affect subsequent maladaptive coping (Doweiko, 2011).

Dimensions of certain personality disorders can be detected in drug abusers. Routinely identified characteristics include inner dishonesty and self-centeredness, although self-centeredness could be related to the addiction itself. For example, when someone is addicted to a substance, nothing is as important as the substance and the acquiring of it. The addicted person's behaviors may reflect this preoccupation.

Sociocultural Theories

A sociocultural theoretical framework holds that both the social influences on an individual and the culture within which that social structure exists define what has happened to create substance abuse (Medeiros, 2011; Roy, 2008). Poverty and wealth can contribute to the stressors that influence some individuals to abuse substances, as can both youth and age. Some of the sociocultural reasons for substance use include the following:

- It was learned from the family and/or friends where the person thinks it is normal and usual.
- It results from a lack of alternative coping skills.
- It helps with anger.
- It helps deal with the side effects of medications.
- It makes the person feel better (smarter, interesting, creative, powerful, etc.).
- It helps the person cope with the difficulties of life.
- It numbs sexual, physical, and emotional trauma (Medeiros, 2011).

In a sociocultural framework, the roles that different family members play and the importance of family rituals contribute to the problem of substance abuse and its treatment. For example, the family of a person who abuses alcohol may see the annual family reunion as a time when excessive drinking is not only allowed but expected and part of the fun. Similarly, the family of a young man who is abusing a methamphetamine with cardiac implications may nurse him back to health with each setback; the role of caretaker may be more important to the family than any other role that the individual members may assume, such as parent or sibling (McCrady, 2010).

Management of Patients Who Are Substance Abusers

Competent medical and nursing management of patients who use substances involves an understanding of substance abuse and how to treat the problem most effectively. This chapter focuses on the most common substances of abuse.

Alcohol Abuse

Alcohol is a legal, liquid, recreational drug. Besides providing relaxation, alcohol can have a destructive power. Mood changes in those who abuse alcohol include euphoria, depression, and lability. Behavioral changes include outbursts, ataxia, slurred or incoherent speech, vomiting, and violence (Benton, 2011). The nurse needs to know how this drug affects the patient's physiology. The range of physiological impacts on a patient with blood alcohol levels ranging from 0.05 to 0.5 g/dL include disinhibition (behaviorally and sexually), memory and concentration degradation, decrease in reasoning abilities, blackouts, motor skill degradation, labored breathing, severe respiratory depression, drowsiness, stupor, unconsciousness, coma, and death (Dryden-Edwards, 2011a).

Alcoholism has been, and often still is, viewed as a sign of weakness by those who are unenlightened; however, clinical investigation has redefined alcoholism as a disease. As more people become aware of the biochemical aspects of alcoholism, the social stigma attached to alcoholism is decreasing and prompting more people to seek help (Alcohol Answers, 2009). Professionals, laypeople, students, alcoholics, and nonalcoholics are attending seminars and college courses on alcoholism. Recovery programs are reported widely in the popular media, and rehabilitation programs have become part of mainstream culture. Information about alcohol recovery programs is easily found on the Internet and in print materials.

Some of the effects of alcoholism include depression; loss of self-respect; alienation from family, friends, and coworkers; malnutrition; decreased competence in self-care; infections; and damaging physiological effects to most body systems. The patterns of alcohol use vary; an individual may regularly drink large amounts of alcohol every day, engage in regular heavy drinking limited to weekends, or experience long periods of sobriety interspersed with binges of heavy drinking that last for weeks or months. No matter what the pattern, it does not change the physiological effects or the designation "alcoholic."

Physiological Effects of Alcohol

A sedative anesthetic (CNS depressant), alcohol begins to be absorbed in the mouth, with absorption completed in the stomach and small intestine. Approximately 95% of alcohol is broken down by the liver; the rest is excreted through the lungs, kidneys, and skin.

Generally, a person can metabolize 30 mL of alcohol (1 oz of whiskey) every 90 minutes. The rate of absorption varies on the basis of weight, intake of food, liver function, and many other factors. If taken in exceedingly high doses, alcohol can depress respiration and cause death. Intoxication occurs when a person has a high blood alcohol level (BAL), also known as blood alcohol content (BAC). A BAL of 0.08% is the legal definition of inebriation in all 50 states, and the District of Columbia.

A short assessment tool frequently used in health care provider's offices and urgent care centers is the four-question T-ACE test; these four questions are (1) T: Does it Take more than three drinks to make you feel high? (2) A: Have you ever been Annoyed by people's criticism of your drinking? (3) C: Are you trying to Cut down on drinking? (4) E: Have you ever used alcohol as an Eye opener in the morning? A "yes" answer to two of the four questions on the T-ACE test is an indication of a possible alcohol abuse or dependence problem (National Institute on Alcohol Abuse and Alcoholism, 2012).

Another assessment aid for alcohol abuse is the World Health Organization's Alcohol Use Disorders Identification Test (AUDIT), which was developed in 1992. It is considered to be accurate 94% of the time, in addition to being accurate across ethnic and gender groups. The test contains 10 multiple choice questions that are scored on a point system. A score of more than 8 indicates an alcohol problem. Two disadvantages of the test are (1) it takes a long time to administer and (2) it is more difficult to score than are the shorter tests (Buddy, 2010). Complete information about the development and implementation of this test may be obtained from Babor, Higgins-Biddle, Saunders, and Monteiro (2001).

Other assessment tests that may be used to obtain an individual's propensity for alcohol abuse include the Five-Shot Questionnaire, the Rapid Alcohol Problems Screen (RAPS), the TWEAK test, the MAST test, the FAST test, the Paddington Alcohol Test, and the SAAST test. All of these tests have pros and cons in terms of their accuracy and predictability. They are not discussed in this chapter, but they may be located with full discussion on the Internet by searching on the keywords "alcohol screening tests" (Buddy, 2012).

Alcohol Withdrawal Syndrome

Alcohol withdrawal often includes the symptoms described in the following subsections and in Chart 13–1. Minor withdrawal symptoms can occur within 4 to 6 hours after the last alcohol ingestion by a person who is dependent on alcohol (MedlinePlus, 2011a).

The following can help to lessen the unpleasant and painful symptoms that can develop after drinking too much alcohol, commonly referred to as a "hangover" (Buddy, 2007b). Sugar and fluids help to overcome hypoglycemia and dehydration. Anti-inflammatory drugs can reduce headache. (However, note that aspirin may irritate the stomach and alcohol amplifies the toxic effects of acetaminophen on the liver.)

CHART 13–1 Alcohol Withdrawal Symptoms

Symptom	Occurrence Time Frame After Last Drink	Duration Time Frame
Slight at-rest tremors/ pronounced and irregular during activities	24 hours	1 week
Diaphoresis and thirst	24 hours	3–4 days
Nausea, vomiting, anorexia	24 hours	3–4 days
Gastritis	24 hours	3–4 days
Increased vital signs	24 hours	3–4 days
Agitation, restlessness, tremulousness, inner shakiness	24 hours	2 weeks
Insomnia, vivid nightmares	24 hours	At least 2 weeks
Fatigue	24 hours	2 weeks
Visual hallucinations (usually of disasters during everyday events)	24 hours	3 days
Auditory hallucinations, feeling persecuted, agitation, increased risk for lethality (self and others)	24 hours	3 days to 2 weeks
Delirium tremens (delirium, generalized seizures, disorientation for time and place, visual hallucinations, agitation, panic)	24–48 hours	3–5 days
Rum fits (generalized seizures)	24–48 hours	3–5 days

Sources: Alcohol Detox Centers. (2008). Alcohol withdrawal symptoms—alcohol detox withdrawal symptoms. Retrieved from http://www.alcohol-detox-centers.com/alcohol-withdrawal-symptoms/alcohol-withdrawal; MedlinePlus. (2011a). Alcohol withdrawal. U.S. National Library of Medicine and National Institutes of Health. Retrieved from http://www.nih.gov.medlineplus/ency/article/000764.htm.

Weblink: Alcohol Withdrawal   Weblink: Alcohol Detox Withdrawal Symptoms

Delirium Tremens

Delirium tremens (DTs) is the most severe form of alcohol withdrawal (MedlinePlus, 2011b). It is manifested by an altered mental status (overall confusion) and sympathetic overdrive (autonomic hyperactivity or heightened stimulation), which can progress to cardiovascular collapse (Burns, 2011). Protracted contact with alcohol results in inhibition of the inhibitory gamma-aminobutyric acid (GABA) A-type and NMDA-type glutamate receptors located in the CNS. Without the alcohol, greater CNS excitability develops, resulting in a condition of severe memory disturbance, agitation, fever, tachycardia, anorexia, and hallucinations. Generally, DTs begin a few days after drinking stops and persist for 5 to 7 days. They may, however, appear as late as the second week of abstinence from alcohol, especially when there is cross-addiction to other drugs (Burns, 2011; Mosby's Medical Dictionary, 2009).

With DTs, there are severe alterations in oxygen consumption and delivery, resulting in an increase in cardiac output (Gist, Sullivan, & Serianni, 2011). For example, hyperventilation resulting in respiratory alkalosis is common. Hypovolemia is also common, due to vomiting (Gist et al., 2011). Delirium tremens is still a fatal disease if it is not recognized and treated appropriately. In fact, 5% to 15% of alcoholics die of delirium tremens or its consequences (Burns, 2011; Gist et al., 2011). Early intervention, the use of benzodiazepines, and better intensive care have decreased the mortality rate, but it is still significant, especially if the patient has other alcohol-related diseases such as pancreatitis, cirrhosis, or pulmonary disease due to tobacco use.

Medical and Nursing Management

Medical treatment of alcoholism involves the management of withdrawal symptoms and the use of medication to deter the addicted individual from drinking.

Weblink: Clonidine

Alcohol withdrawal occurs after the individual stops drinking. This syndrome is composed of a constellation of physiological and behavioral symptoms that occur when the alcohol level drops; these were previously described in this chapter. Medical and nursing treatment for withdrawal includes the following:

1. Monitoring the patient's fluid status. Although some patients are overhydrated, many are dehydrated or have the potential to develop a fluid volume deficit. Fluids should be encouraged, up to 3,000 mL/day, if no condition exists to contraindicate this. Intravenous fluids are indicated if the patient is unable to take fluids by mouth.
2. Administering magnesium sulfate and thiamine, if appropriate.
3. Prescribing benzodiazepines, such as lorazepam (Ativan), diazepam (Valium), or chlordiazepoxide (Librium), to help prevent DTs.
4. Prescribing disulfiram (Antabuse, an agonist medication) and naltrexone (ReVia, Trexan). Developed in 1984 for treatment of heroin abuse, this drug was approved in January 1994 for blocking the craving for alcohol (see Pharmacology table, p. 307).
5. Monitoring the laborary data from tests used to detect alcohol (see the Laboratory and Diagnostic Tests box, p. 308).

Laboratory Tests

Findings from laboratory studies assist the health care provider in determining whether the patient has an alcohol abuse problem. Common laboratory tests in which elevated values are associated with excessive alcohol intake are listed in the Laboratory and Diagnostic Tests box. Abnormal laboratory findings are only one of the alerting factors for problem drinking. (The Laboratory and Diagnostic Tests box provides an overview of the rationale for these tests.) No single test or combination of tests alone is appropriate for clinical screening. Confirmation of the excessive use of alcohol in a sensitively conducted assessment interview remains the preferred assessment approach and is considered a prerequisite for successful intervention.

Nursing Management

Many patients who experience chronic alcoholism, especially patients experiencing an acute exacerbation of the disease or another major illness or trauma-related injury, are cared for in the acute care setting. They also are seen by nurses in an outpatient setting (e.g., community health setting), or in a chronic care rehabilitation setting such as an alcoholic recovery program. Assessment of the patient and implementing a plan of care are essential to the recovery of the patient. The care plan for a patient with chronic alcoholism (p. 309) details the nursing process used to treat these patients.

Amphetamine Abuse

Amphetamines, also known as "speed," belong to a group of compounds called the sympathomimetics. This group of compounds comprises synthetic drugs derived from ephedrine that stimulate the release of adrenaline and speed up someone's system, thus the common name.

Medical use of amphetamines began in the 1920s (Doweiko, 2011). In the 1950s and 1960s, amphetamines were heralded as wonder drugs for depression, management of obesity, and exhaustion. By the 1970s, their dangers became known, and today they are prescribed less frequently because alternative compounds are available to treat those symptoms effectively and safely. Amphetamines still are used to control appetite and to treat depression, narcolepsy, and minimal brain dysfunctions as well as attention deficit hyperactivity disorder in children. Common brand names of drugs that contain or metabolize into amphetamines include Adderall, Dexedrine, Dexostat, Desoxyn, ProCentra, and Vyvanse (Encyclopedia of Mental Disorders, 2011). Amphetamine abusers tend to be teenagers or young adults who are looking for a "good time" or who have a desire to improve their performance at school or work. The desire for alertness and improved performance through use of these substances can lure truck drivers working on long road trips, students during exams, and athletes, among others, into the "speed trap."

In small doses, amphetamines cause people to feel energetic, euphoric, and in touch with their surroundings. Users take these CNS stimulants to feel good. Women are more likely than men to seek weight loss by using methamphetamines (MAs); men report improved sexual performance as a motivator (Buxton & Dove, 2008). A growing number of people take amphetamines and barbiturates in a cyclic fashion, using amphetamines (the upper) to balance the effects of barbiturates (the downer). Amphetamines are dangerous because they alter judgment and obscure sensations. Taken in high doses or intravenously, amphetamines can have dangerous effects, such as abnormally high blood pressure; rapid and irregular heart rate and rhythm; seizures; damage to blood vessels in the brain; accumulation of excess fluid in the lungs, brain tissue, and skull; impaired regulation of heat loss; internal bleeding; and breakdown of muscle tissue leading to kidney failure (Buxton & Dove, 2008).

Amphetamines act by mimicking two of the brain's most important neurotransmitters, dopamine and norepinephrine. A drug must be able to act on a receptor site or on a number of receptor sites to have an impact. The body may not have a specific amphetamine or cocaine receptor site, so amphetamine and cocaine take what is called "illegal control" at the existing receptor sites (Doweiko, 2011). Dopamine and dopamine receptor sites are intricately involved in the effects of abused substances on the nervous systems of patients. Chronic use of methamphetamines changes the way a person thinks and behaves because the brain's cortex is no longer activated during decision making. This change in the brain's ability to transport dopamine to any significant degree creates clinical characteristics of severe psychiatric symptoms (Doweiko, 2011).

Tolerance develops rapidly, and chronic abusers may suffer a toxic psychosis presenting with the symptoms of paranoid schizophrenia. Argumentativeness, delusions, hallucinations, stereotypic compulsive behavior, increased libido, interpersonal sensitivity, panic, and violence may occur (The GoodDrugsGuide.com, 2012). Substance abuse with amphetamines means a craving for these drugs that requires higher and higher dosages to satisfy. Abusers are rowdy, paranoid, and irritable. A "crash" (depression), often with suicidal symptoms, may last for several weeks. This is so uncomfortable that the user ingests more of the drug in an attempt to feel better and develops a cyclical pattern of abuse and crashing.

Physiologically, the overuse of speed has been tied to stroke and death. Depression, anxiety, and increased stress symptoms are the most common psychological pitfalls in recovering from the use of

PHARMACOLOGY Summary of Medications to Treat Substance-Related Disorders

Medication Category and Action	Application/Indication	Nursing Responsibilities
Replacement Agent/Anticonvulsant		
Magnesium sulfate ***Action:*** Anticonvulsant activities produced by CNS depression; acts as a replacement for lost magnesium	Many people who abuse alcohol suffer from a magnesium deficiency due to malnutrition; administering magnesium decreases irritability caused by low magnesium levels and prevents seizures.	Monitor the patient for adverse effects: hypotension, hypothermia, stupor, respiratory depression. Observe the patient for signs of magnesium toxicity: cathartic effect, profound thirst, sedation, confusion, muscle weakness. Have calcium gluconate available as an antidote. Monitor the patient's ECG and vital signs when given IV. Monitor the patient's renal function, magnesium, calcium, and phosphorus levels.
Anxiolytic/Anticonvulsant		
Diazepam (Valium) Chlordiazepoxide (Librium) Lorazepam (Ativan) ***Action:*** Reduces withdrawal symptoms by action on limbic and subcortical levels of CNS	Symptoms of acute alcohol withdrawal, prophylaxis and treatment of seizures, delirium tremens.	Monitor the patient's CBC and liver function if used long term. Warn the patient not to abruptly stop the drug.
Antialcohol Agent		
Disulfiram (Antabuse) ***Action:*** Produces undesirable symptoms as a deterrent to alcohol ingestion by inhibiting acetaldehyde dehydrogenase, which normally detoxifies and metabolizes alcohol	Acetaldehyde is highly toxic, producing nausea and hypotension. Hypotension leads to shock and may be fatal. If the patient uses alcohol, a powerful disulfiram reaction may occur and last for up to 2 weeks. Alcohol cessation aid.	Monitor the patient's liver function, CBC. Do not administer unless the patient has been alcohol free for a minimum of 12 hours. Be aware of drug interactions (warfarin, phenytoin, barbiturate, and others). Warn the patient not to consume alcohol in any form including cough and cold preparations, mouthwash, sauces, etc. Warn the patient of potential severe reactions (myocardial infarction, convulsions, respiratory depression, sudden death) if alcohol is ingested (including alcohol-based cough syrups, cold remedies, or oral hygiene products) while on medication for up to 2 weeks following ingestion of the drug.
Opiate Antagonist		
Naltrexone (ReVia) ***Action:*** Reduces euphoria and drug craving by binding with opioid receptors	Adjunct to treatment of narcotic addiction and alcohol dependence. Blocks the craving for alcohol and the pleasure derived from it. Thus, it may help prevent relapse. It has had more success as an active treatment mode than disulfiram.	Give a naloxone challenge test before starting naltrexone. Monitor the patient for adverse effects: nausea, vomiting, abdominal cramps, muscle pain, insomnia, and anxiety. Monitor the patient's liver function. Warn the patient to check with a health care provider before using OTC drugs. Warn the patient of the risk of overdosing if opiates are used.
Vitamins	Because alcohol interferes with the absorption of B vitamins.	
Thiamine (vitamin B_1) ***Action:*** Necessary for conversion of carbohydrates to energy and maintaining proper functioning of the heart, nervous system, and muscles.	Used to treat malnutrition caused by alcohol or other drugs.	Obtain the patient's dietary history to determine need for thiamine replacement. Collaborate with a dietitian and family members to develop a dietary teaching plan that can be managed by the patient and ensures compliance. Assess for signs of thiamine toxicity: tachycardia, hypotension, and anaphylaxis like symptoms. Instruct the patient and family about dietary sources that are rich in thiamine. Advise the patient to take vitamin supplements exactly as prescribed.

Source: Adams, P. M., & Koch. R. W. (2010). *Pharmacology: Connections to nursing practice.* Upper Saddle River, NJ: Pearson.

LABORATORY AND DIAGNOSTIC TESTS for Substance Abuse

Tests with Description, Rationale, and Normal Values	Expected Abnormality
Liver Function Profiles	
Gamma-glutamyl transferase (GGT) *An enzyme found mainly in the liver that is sensitive for detecting liver disease. The serum level rises early in cell destruction and remains elevated as long as cellular damage persists. High levels of GGT occur after 12 to 24 hours of heavy alcoholic drinking and may remain increased for 2 to 3 weeks after cessation of alcohol intake* Normal values: Men: 4–23 international units/liter (IU/L) Women: 3–13 IU/L	Elevated
Alanine aminotransferase (ALT) *An enzyme primarily found in the liver cells that is effective in diagnosing hepatocellular destruction.* Normal value: 10–35 IU/L	Elevated
Aspartate aminotransferase (AST) *An enzyme found mainly in the heart muscle and liver that increases during an acute MI and when the liver is damaged.* Normal values: Men: 4–36 IU/L Women: Normal value may be slightly lower	Elevated
Lactate dehydrogenase *An intracellular enzyme present in nearly all metabolizing cells, the liver having one of the highest concentrations. Increased levels may represent liver damage.* Normal value: 100–190 IU/L	Elevated
Alkaline phosphatase *An enzyme produced mainly in the liver and bone that is useful for determining liver and bone disease.* Elevated ALP may be indicative of hepatocellular cirrhosis. Normal value: 42–136 IU/L	Elevated
Total bilirubin *Bilirubin is formed from the breakdown of hemoglobin by the reticuloendothelial system and is carried in the plasma to the liver where is conjugated to form diglucuronide and is excreted in the bile. Direct or conjugated bilirubin frequently is the result of obstructive jaundice. The conjugated bilirubin, which cannot escape in the bile through the intestine, thus backs up and is absorbed into the bloodstream. Damaged liver cells cause a blockage of the bile sinusoid (a distensible vascular channel), thereby increasing the serum level of direct bilirubin. Hepatitis and cirrhosis may cause bilirubin to be elevated.* Normal value: 0.1–1.2 milligrams/deciliter (mg/dL)	Elevated
Cholesterol *This is a blood lipid synthesized by the liver. It is used by the body to form bile salts for fat digestion and the formation of hormones. High serum cholesterol levels can be due to a biliary obstruction and can indicate liver disease as well as coronary artery disease.* Normal value: $<$200 mg/dL	Elevated, but may be decreased in the presence of severe malnutrition
Triglycerides *These blood lipids are processed from dietary fatty acids by the intestine and transported in the bloodstream. The liver also is responsible for manufacturing triglycerides. Persons who drink alcohol are at a high risk of elevated triglyceride levels. Increased levels may indicate alcoholic cirrhosis.* Normal value: $<$160 mg/dL	Elevated
Breathalyzer *Determines the blood alcohol level (BAL) following ingestion of an amount of alcohol.* Normal value: negative for evidence of alcohol intake.	Evidence of alcohol, and the amount of alcohol ingested

Source: Key, J. L. (2010). *Laboratory and diagnostic tests with nursing implications.* Upper Saddle River, NJ: Pearson.

NURSING PROCESS: Patient Care Plan for Chronic Alcoholism

Assessment of Coping Status Using Gordon's Functional Health Patterns:

- Sleep/Rest Pattern
- Nutrition Metabolic Pattern
- Coping-Stress Tolerance Pattern

Subjective Data

Assessment of Coping Style and Effectiveness

How much and what type of alcohol do you drink on a typical day?

How long have you been an alcoholic?

What do you consider stressful?

Does stress seem easier to manage when you drink?

How many hours do you sleep at night?

What do you do to promote sleep for yourself?

What do you usually eat throughout the day?

Objective Data

Assessment of Coping Style and Effectiveness

Inability to manage stress without resorting to substance use

Limited coping skills

Compromised liver function

Insomnia

Poor metabolic health

Malnutrition

Outcomes and Evaluation Parameters

Planning and Interventions with *Rationales*

1. NURSING DIAGNOSES: (a) Coping, Ineffective *related to alcohol abuse;* (b) Sleep Deprivation *related to alcohol abuse;* (c) Nutrition, Imbalanced: Less Than Body Requirements *related to alcohol abuse.* (NANDA-I © 2012)

Outcomes: Reduction of ineffective and self-destructive coping through alcohol abuse and regular use of more effective coping styles.

Sleeping a total of a reasonable number of hours/night indicates successful resolution of sleep deprivation.

Patient eats three meals every day plus snacks and takes multivitamin as recommended.

Evaluation Parameters: Has begun to substitute effective coping for alcohol use when stressed.

Uses sleep-inducing strategies nightly and reports satisfaction with quality of sleep.

Reestablishes a consistently healthy sleep routine.

Patient identifies and understands relationship between alcoholism and malnutrition.

Patient gains weight through a balanced diet.

Identify two effective coping mechanisms. *Patients need to have ready choices on how to cope with stress without their addictive substance.*

Inventory those situations that challenge patient's abilities to cope. *This prepares the patient for difficulties so rehearsal and skill building can take place.*

Rehearse various coping strategies to prepare and select two for regular use. *Rehearsal allows the patient to get familiar with the skill and to learn how to use it.*

Teach alternative, healthy coping mechanisms. *Revision of coping styles requires identification of the situations placing the patient at risk, typical problematic responses, and acknowledgment of a need to learn.*

Assess for cirrhosis of the liver. *Years of substance abuse may result in cirrhosis.*

Assess for depression and feelings of self-reproach and guilt for years of drinking and the effect on others. *Alcohol is a depressant and contributes to deepening existing depressions.*

Promote recognition of automatic mechanisms involved in habitually responding to stress with alcohol. *How to cope with stress in adaptive ways will be a new skill.*

Consider AA groups, psychiatric treatment, hospitalization, 28-day alcohol treatment programs. *These specialized interventions may be necessary to treat the acute problem.*

Evaluate suicide or violence potential. *Alcohol as a depressant certainly raises risk of lethality, plus abstinence may highlight the deep and various life problems the patient has where problem solving sober may seem too big a burden to bear.*

Assess for history of insomnia. *Alcohol initially causes somnolence, but chronic use causes insomnia.*

Assess current sleep pattern and effective strategies. *Teach and promote healthy sleep hygiene such as warm milk, reading, and other relaxation strategies that counteract ineffective sleep hygiene routines.*

Employ effective sleep strategies regularly. *To counteract the alcoholism-disturbed sleep pattern, retraining must take place.*

Assess malnourishment from chronic alcoholism. *Vitamins, especially vitamin B, are not metabolized well in an alcoholic's body.*

Long-term alcoholism interferes with self-care abilities such as proper nourishment. *Malnutrition from chronic alcoholism can be addressed with a comprehensive nutrition program.*

Monitor intake of meals and snacks *to ensure proper intake.*

Initiate dietary consult *to explore depth of nutrition problem and educate patient about healthy eating.*

Investigate dietary preferences *to maximize patient's abilities to expand intake appropriately. It is easier to reshape a patient's diet when preferences are incorporated.*

Educate patient regarding the impact of chronic alcohol ingestion on the digestive tract, metabolism, and overall health. *Alcohol impacts are not commonly known or understood.*

Offer frequent food and fluids throughout contacts *to reestablish proper electrolyte, protein, and carbohydrate levels.*

Sources: Adapted from Wilkinson, J. M., & Ahearn, N. R. (2009). *Prentice Hall nursing diagnosis handbook* (9th ed.). Upper Saddle River, NJ: Prentice Hall.

Weblink: Clonidine

speed. Changes in neurotransmitter activity increase the patient's sensitivity to stress and may contribute to the spontaneous recurrence of amphetamine and methamphetamine psychosis, called flashbacks. Recurrent flashbacks contribute to recurrent major mood disorders (Encyclopedia of Mental Disorders, 2011).

Methamphetamine

Recipes for the manufacture of methamphetamine (also known as crystal meth) in home drug labs using everyday ingredients (over-the-counter pseudoephedrine, starter fluids, and drain cleaner) are widely available and have affected how these products are sold (see the Combat Methamphetamine Epidemic Act of 2005). Lower quality MA is called "speed" or "crank"; higher-quality MA is sold in small chunks known as "glass" or "ice" because of its crystalline appearance. It is a maximum stimulant with maximum risks. The manufacture of this drug presents serious dangers due to the volatile chemicals, toxic by-products, and the potential for fires and explosions that cause injuries and burns (Wells, Noonan, Wells, Holian, & Wibbenmeyer, 2009).

Exposure to MA is neurotoxic, and long-term use leads to extensive neural damage. Physiological changes include cognitive impairments, MA-induced psychosis, inadequate perfusion, and ischemic lesions of the brain. People experiencing long-term use usually are unable to competently perform activities of daily living (brush teeth, wash face, etc.), have difficulty remembering or problem solving, and may persist with delusional accusations or react with strong emotional content to something they are experiencing (seeing, hearing, feeling). MA morphologically changes the corpus callosum (the bank of nerve fibers that divides the cerebrum into left and right hemispheres) and causes skin lesions, perinatal complications, and hypertension (Buxton & Dove, 2008; Wells et al., 2009). Each of these physiological changes has consequences that are far reaching for a person's health and functioning (e.g., motor movements, sensory perception, and cardiac irregularities) (Richards, 2011). Before-and-after photographs of people who use methamphetamines reveal a striking difference in their appearance due to weight loss, skin integrity problems, and a generally poor state of health.

Medical and Nursing Management

The treatment of methamphetamine dependence is challenging because of high rates of dropout and relapse and ongoing episodes of psychosis. If patients are experiencing hyperactivity or agitation, a dopamine-blocking agent such as haloperidol may be used. No medication has been demonstrated to be effective for the treatment of amphetamine abuse and dependence, so health care providers have to rely on behavioral and cognitive therapies, which have not shown to have long-term benefit (Buxton & Dove, 2008).

Cannabis Abuse

Marijuana is derived from an Indian hemp plant (*Cannabis sativa*) and contains a psychoactive substance, tetrahydrocannabinol (THC), which is found in the sticky yellow resin secreted by the tops and leaves of the ripe plants. THC is transformed into metabolites in the body. Unlike alcohol, which is water soluble and leaves the body through urine, breath, and perspiration, THC is stored in the fatty tissues (especially those of the brain and reproductive system). Consequently, it can be detected in the body for up to 6 weeks (Doweiko, 2011). The potency of marijuana has steadily increased over the years. Although marijuana contains more than 400 chemicals, the THC content determines the potency. With an increase in potency comes an increase in health problems. There is compelling evidence that underlying neurochemical mechanisms are at work reinforcing the reward and dependence features of this drug and contributing to addiction (Doweiko, 2011).

Researchers have found that marijuana produces a significant analgesic effect and is modestly effective against the nausea and vomiting associated with chemotherapy. Medicinal applications of both THC and cannabidiol (a nonpsychoactive cannabinoid of marijuana) for pain have been examined and show significant pain relief. Dronabinol is a synthetic delta-9-tetrahydrocannabinol or delta-9-THC that contains standardized THC content in an FDA-approved pharmaceutical. It is used mainly to treat the weight loss, nausea, and vomiting associated with a number of medical conditions (Bryson & Frost, 2011). Long-term marijuana smoking is associated with lung damage, increased risk of respiratory cancer, and poorer pregnancy outcomes.

Although marijuana was declared illegal in the United States in 1937 with adoption of the Marijuana Tax Act; it has been, and continues to be, fairly easy to obtain, and one of the most commonly used illicit drugs. Fourteen states have legalized the use of marijuana for medicinal purposes (Genen, 2011), but possession is still prohibited by federal law.

Cocaine Abuse

Cocaine is a stimulant drug that is extracted from the leaves of the coca plant found in Bolivia, Peru, and Colombia (Dryden-Edwards, 2011b). Cocaine is used as a local anesthetic in ear, nose, and throat surgery. When inhaled or injected, cocaine produces alertness and energy and makes users feel sociable and confident. The drug blocks appetite and erases fatigue, which makes it appear to be an ideal performance booster, although that is an illusion. Cocaine addicts develop a tolerance to the drug and eventually may use amounts that would have been lethal to them earlier (DeMaria & Weinkauf, 2011).

Cocaine—also referred to as coke, nose candy, or snow, or crystal or rock if in a solid form—is a highly addictive stimulant. Its effects are both behavioral and biochemical. Intravenous injection or smoking produces a euphoria that diminishes after approximately 5 to 10 minutes. Snorting results in slower absorption, lower plasma levels, and longer effects.

Cocaine initially increases dopamine (DA) neurotransmission, causing euphoria, but this is followed by DA depletion, resulting in the letdown, which lasts for 30 to 60 minutes, referred to as the "postcoke blues" or cocaine abstinence syndrome (DeMaria & Weinkauf, 2011). Anxiety, depression, and fatigue are part of this syndrome. The crash intensity appears to be related to the amount of cocaine used. Addicts often use other drugs, such as alcohol, marijuana, or sleeping pills, during the crash.

Ultimately, although cocaine no longer produces pleasure, not taking it makes the individual feel even worse. As the DA eventually becomes depleted, the user becomes chronically fatigued, irritable, and anxious. Psychiatric symptoms such as confusion and paranoia emerge. Suicide attempts, accidents, and overdoses are common (Dryden-Edwards, 2011b). The only effect of cocaine that increases as tolerance develops is its ability to induce a convulsion or seizure.

Cocaine causes significant cardiovascular effects primarily owing to the intense sympathetic stimulation. The acute effects include dysrhythmias, systemic and pulmonary hypertension, coronary vasoconstriction, and cardiac ischemia that can lead to myocardial infarction. Chronic changes include myocardial hypertrophy, hypertrophic cardiomyopathy, and accelerated atherosclerosis. Cocaine-induced ischemia has been successfully treated with oxygen, aspirin to prevent thrombus formation, nitroglycerin to reverse coronary vasoconstriction, and early management with intravenous benzodiazepines to reduce heart rate and blood pressure (Phillips, Luk, Soor, Abraham, Leong, & Butany, 2009). Research with cocaine users indicates that the drug bromocriptine mesylate (Parlodel), a DA receptor agonist, eliminates the craving that users feel after they stop using cocaine (Dryden-Edwards, 2011b).

Potential neurologic complications include stroke from cerebral arterial vasospasm, thrombosis, or cerebrovascular hemorrhage. Cocaine also can precipitate seizures in patients without a history of seizure disorder, and it lowers the seizure threshold in patients with epilepsy. Chronic cocaine use by inhaling/snorting can lead to ischemic necrosis of the midfacial structures. Reports of effects range from perforation of the nasal septum to destruction of the hard palate, the maxilla, and the orbital wall (DeMaria & Weinkauf, 2011).

According to the National Institute on Drug Abuse (2010a), an estimated 5.7 million Americans use cocaine habitually. A statistical review documented in Dryden-Edwards (2011b) indicates that more than 25 million people in the United States have used it at least once; 4.6 million people tend to use it once per month or less, and about 2.4 million people use the substance at least twice a week. "More than 5% of people who use cocaine just once go on to develop cocaine dependence within two years after the first use" (Dryden-Edwards, 2011b, p. 3). It is available to all cultural and socioeconomic groups and is used equally by women and men. The federal government considers cocaine use a widespread problem (Botvin, Griffin, & Gilchrist, 2011; United States Drug Enforcement Administration, 2010). The cocaine industry is a multibillion dollar illegal drug enterprise that affects every aspect of civilization (Kenney, 2010).

Crack and Freebase

Crack, or "rock," cocaine is a highly addictive potent form of hydrochloride cocaine that is mixed with baking soda and water, heated, allowed to harden, and then broken or "cracked" into little pieces and smoked in cigarettes or glass water pipes (Helmenstine, 2012). Smokable forms of cocaine have effects similar to those of the injectable drug. Crack is more insidious, addictive, and toxic than cocaine. It is not unusual for someone to become addicted after using crack twice.

A crack high has a rapid onset and is intensely euphoric, followed by a dramatic crash. Within seconds after the crash, users feel compelled to smoke more crack. Repeatedly smoking cocaine affects the central serotonergic and dopaminergic functions of the brain. The long-lasting and selective disruptions in serotonin pathways following chronic cocaine use may provide a neurochemical basis for the mood changes commonly reported during cocaine withdrawal (Doweiko, 2011).

Symptoms of crack use include irritability, paranoia, depression, and physical symptoms that go along with the smoking of a toxic chemical, such as wheezing, coughing blood, and black phlegm. Cardiac arrhythmias caused by crack use may lead to death.

Treatment for this addiction is very difficult. Many people seek help only when they can no longer support their habit. Because crack is cheap and easily acquired, that point is much farther along than it would be with a more expensive drug, so patients are very debilitated by the time they seek treatment and have usually been coerced by others to do so. It is an extremely problematic drug to stop using, with a high recidivism rate estimated to be more than 90% (Carvalho & Seible, 2009).

Freebase is a purified form of cocaine made by applying solvents to ordinary cocaine. Melting the cocaine with a small butane torch helps in the purifying and delivery process. This action alone is dangerous, owing to the hazard of the solvent exploding. Freebase cocaine is typically smoked, which releases a substance known as methylecgonidine, which has damaging effects on lung and liver tissue, making smoking of freebase particularly cardiotoxic (MedicineNet.com, 2011). The effects of the freebase are brief but intense, and the short euphoria (3 to 5 minutes) immediately becomes a restless desire for more "base."

Long-Term Effects of Cocaine and Crack Addiction

Drug addiction increases the risk of a number of negative life stressors and conditions. For example, cocaine abusers are at increased risk for domestic violence (Carvalho & Seible, 2009). They also have increased risks for medical crises, such as aortic dissection, heart attack, and hypertension.

Medical Management

The primary goals for treatment of cocaine and crack addiction symptoms are abstinence, relapse prevention, and rehabilitation. Detoxification for cocaine abusers is the first step in treatment. This process depends on the patient's symptoms but usually is performed in a hospital or other inpatient setting, where medications used to treat withdrawal symptoms and frequent medical monitoring can be provided. The detoxification process from cocaine is the most difficult part of coping with the physical symptoms of addiction and tends to last days. Medications that sometimes are used to help cocaine addicts abstain from drug use include propranolol (Inderal) and vigabatrin (Sabril). Propranolol decreases some of the physical symptoms associated with cocaine withdrawal, such as irritability, suppressed appetite, sleep problems, and craving the substance. Vigabatrin is use to treat seizures (Dryden-Edwards, 2011b).

The management of psychological addiction is often more challenging and time consuming than recovery from the physical aspects of cocaine addiction. Because the depression associated with cocaine detoxification is significant, Tofranil or other tricyclic antidepressants may be given for several weeks after the acute detoxification. Tricyclics build up existing levels of neurotransmitters and make them available for transmission. Some people with less severe addiction may be managed on an outpatient basis. However, individuals with a more severe addiction, those who have relapsed after participation in outpatient programs, or those who also suffer from a severe mental illness might need the higher level of organizational structure and support and more frequent medical monitoring of an inpatient or rehabilitation service. Following inpatient treatment, the patient may benefit from living in a sober-living community, such as a group home, with counselors available to provide abstinence support.

It is important in treating cocaine addiction patients to help the parents or other family members and friends learn how to refrain from supporting addictive behaviors. The family may establish codependency by providing financial support, making excuses, or failing to acknowledge the addict's addictive behaviors. Discouraging codependency in family members and significant others is a key component to the recovery of the affected individual.

Nursing Management

Assessment of the patient who is suspected of having an addiction to cocaine is critical to developing a plan of care. The main focus of the assessment is determining the subjective and objective indicators of the patient's coping style and effectiveness. It is important to determine from the patient's perspective what types of experiences trigger a need for the drug, whether these experiences were considered stressful, whether the stress seems easier to manage when the patient uses cocaine, and how the patient's relationships are affected by cocaine use. Objective assessment includes verification of the patient's inability to manage stress without resorting to substance abuse, coping skills employed, and poor social and occupational functioning.

Beginning with the assessment, the major focus of care continues to be on helping the patient develop effective coping. The desirable long-term patient outcome is that the patient completes a cocaine detoxification program and remains free of cocaine. Short-term outcomes that will help the patient to achieve that goal include the development and use of healthier coping skills, such as the replacement of destructive ways of coping with effective individual coping options.

Interventions by nurses and other members of the health care team are directed toward helping the patient achieve short- and long-term goals. Interventions may take the form of individual meetings in which the consequences of drug use in the work, home, social, and physical arenas are discussed; helping the patient recognize the automatic mechanisms involved in turning to cocaine; assisting the patient in developing or recognizing other coping strategies; and monitoring drug-seeking behaviors. When drug-seeking behaviors are detected, the nurse interacts with the patient about her feelings and assists the patient in identifying these behaviors.

While ineffective coping is a primary focus for these patients, other aspects of substance abuse also may be relevant. The Nursing Process: Patient Care Plan for Cocaine Intoxication depicts a complete approach to caring for these patients.

Hallucinogens Abuse

Hallucinogens are a diverse group of synthetic and natural drugs that cause an alteration in perception, thought, or mood. These drugs represent a heterogeneous group whose compounds have different chemical structures, different mechanisms of action, and different adverse effects (Parish, 2011). Despite their name, most hallucinogens do not cause hallucinations, which are defined as false sensations that have no basis in reality. They are more likely to cause changes in mood or in thought than actual hallucinations.

According to Parish (2011), 23 drugs are classified as hallucinogens. They are often grouped by structural criteria as lysergamides, phenylethylamines, piperidines, indolealkylamines, and cannabinols. Most are derived from plants that have an impact on the CNS.

People around the world continue to use many species of hallucinogenic plants to achieve distortions in their state of mind (Doweiko, 2011). Peyote, the active hallucinogen in cactus buttons, is still an integral part of religious rituals of Native Americans in the southwestern United States and Mexico. Psilocybin, the active hallucinogen in certain mushrooms, is most often ingested by eating the substance; recipes using psilocybin mushrooms encompass everyday foods, tea, and honey concoctions. There continues to be controversy around whether psilocybin-containing mushrooms can be smoked to produce a psychoactive effect.

LSD (an abbreviation of the German words for lysergic acid diethylamide), which was developed in 1938 for scientific research, is the drug that is most commonly identified with the term *hallucinogen.* It is the most widely used drug in this class and is considered to be the typical halllcinogen. Characteristics of its action and effects apply to other hallucinogens, including mescaline, and psilocybin.

Phenylcyclohexyl piperidine (PCP), also known as phencyclidine, was first introduced in 1957 as an experimental surgical anesthetic that was designed to be given intravenously. However, it was soon found to have serious side effects including agitation and a drug-induced delirium and/or psychotic reaction that lasted up to 10 days; therefore, its use in humans was quickly discontinued. By this time, illicit drug-abusers had discovered PCP. The first reports of PCP abuse began to appear in the late 1960s. PCP is distributed in widely varying purities and forms such as powder, liquid, tablets, leaf mixtures, and rock crystal. Its abuse has risen and fallen over the years, and it is not currently considered a popular drug of abuse (Doweiko, 2011). However, many drug users are exposed to PCP inadvertently because it is often used as an adulterant in marijuana, LSD, and methamphetamine to save on production costs of those other drugs (Brenner & Corden, 2009).

Recent studies reveal an increase in the use of hallucinogens, especially among the high school and college-age population. Hallucinogens are the third most frequently abused class of drugs among high school students, after alcohol and marijuana (Parish, 2011). Hallucinogen use is most common in Caucasians, although there also is a high lifetime rate of use among American Indians and Alaska Natives. Hallucinogens are most frequently abused by males, age 18 to 25 years (Parish, 2011).

Patients present in a wide variety of states from inebriated and calm to agitated and, in some cases, extremely violent. They also may show symptoms of anxiety, delusions, depression, hallucinations, panic attack, paranoia, restlessness, and seizures (Schueler, Beckett, & Gettings, 2010). An important diagnostic clue is nystagmus (involuntary eye movement), which is seen in a majority of patients. (Brenner & Corden, 2009). See Chapter 64 for more information on nystagmus.

The dangers of hallucinogens include "bad trips" and flashbacks. Users who experience bad trips may appear psychotic and extremely fearful. Reassuring the person and pointing out reality are helpful; occasionally, tranquilizers or antipsychotic drugs are given. These symptoms usually disappear within 12 hours but may persist for months.

Medical and Nursing Management

Different hallucinogens present with a variety of organ system effects. PCP has been known to cause muscle rigidity, seizures, rhabdomyolysis (the breakdown of muscle fibers, resulting in the release of muscle fiber contents into the bloodstream), and coma. Anticholinergics have been associated with delirium, supraventricular tachycardia, hypertension, and seizures. Other hallucinogens (e.g., LSD, peyote, marijuana, nutmeg) rarely cause significant physical complications. Therefore, treatment depends on the type of symptoms displayed. Medications may be prescribed for symptomatic relief of the observed or expected symptoms. Caution should be used in this population because of the obvious potential for misuse or diversion of any medications. Regimens for this type of care are supported primarily by anecdotal evidence (Benner, 2012). The most important approach to management of PCP intoxication is the implementation of the safe use of physical restraints and chemical sedation. Benzodiazepines usually are effective in managing aggressive behavior. Anxiety and agitation generally can be managed by decreasing external stimuli such as light, noise, and touch.

NURSING PROCESS: Patient Care Plan for Cocaine Intoxication

Assessment of Coping Status Using Gordon's Functional Health Patterns:

- Coping-Stress Tolerance Pattern

Subjective Data	Objective Data
Assessment of Coping Style and Effectiveness	**Assessment of Coping Style and Effectiveness**
What kinds of experiences lead you to want to use cocaine? What do you consider stressful? Does stress seem easier to manage when you use cocaine? How are your relationships affected by your cocaine use?	Inability to manage stress without resorting to substance use. Limited coping skills. Poor social and occupational functioning.

Outcomes and Evaluation Parameters	Planning and Interventions with *Rationales*
1. NURSING DIAGNOSIS: Ineffective Coping *related to cocaine abuse.* (NANDA-I © 2012)	
Outcome: Reduction of ineffective and self-destructive coping through cocaine abuse and regular use of more effective coping styles. ***Evaluation Parameters:*** Has begun to substitute effective coping for cocaine use when stressed. Patient will complete a cocaine detoxification program and will remain free of cocaine. "Clean" urine 72 hours after last use. Replacement of destructive coping with two effective individual coping options.	Conduct individual meetings with patient regarding consequences of drug use in work, home, social, and physical arenas. *Defense mechanisms solidly in place throughout the substance abuse period make recognition of self-imposed difficulties difficult.* Discuss prioritization of the work on problem areas. *Immediate medical–surgical concerns take priority over the longer term issues of substance abuse treatment and therapy.* There will be treatment offered for cocaine withdrawal. Arrange access to individual and group therapy. *Team discussions will shape the treatment for the problem in the forefront.* Observe every 1/2 hour. *Withdrawal from cocaine can be a difficult and dangerous time. Lethality risk exists.* Monitor drug-seeking behaviors as an inevitable aspect of this problem. *Long-standing interpersonal styles are not immediately resolved.* When drug-seeking behavior (DSB) commences, interact about patient's feelings and educate about cravings and time frames for resolution. *DSB may be out of patient's awareness and needs to be labeled and addressed.* Help patient recognize the automatic mechanisms involved in turning to cocaine. *Over time, the patient sees the connection between stress and demands and the urge to escape through cocaine use.* Identify two effective coping mechanisms. *Patients need to have ready choices on how to cope with stress without their substance.* Help patient rehearse various coping strategies to prepare and select two for regular use. *Revision of coping styles requires learning and practice. Options for coping are more effective and promote resiliency.* Patient begins to substitute effective coping for cocaine use. *Once substitution occurs, there is still the risk of returning to familiar, if maladaptive, responses to stress.* Improve patient's awareness of behaviors, reduce denial, and educate about the addiction. *This intervention serves to supply an educative process that was missing or ineffective before addiction was established.*

Source: Adapted from Wilkinson, J. M., & Ahearn, N. R. (2009). *Prentice Hall nursing diagnosis handbook* (9th ed.). Upper Saddle River, NJ: Prentice Hall.

Safety Alert *During acute presentation in emergency departments or elsewhere, PCP abusers may become violent or suicidal and should be considered a danger to themselves and others, including staff members. Because of the analgesic effects of PCP and the lack of a normal pain response, PCP-intoxicated patients have sometimes been described as having extraordinary strength. PCP-intoxicated patients have broken out of vinyl restraints and handcuffs and have fractured their own bones in the process (Brenner & Corden, 2009).*

Inhalants Abuse

Inhalants are a diverse group of volatile substances whose chemical vapors can be inhaled to produce psychoactive (mind-altering) effects (National Institute of Drug Abuse [NIDA], 2010b). While some other abused substances can be inhaled, the term *inhalants* is used to describe substances that are rarely, if ever, taken by any other route of administration, e.g., (1) volatile solvents—liquids that vaporize at room temperature; (2) aerosols—sprays that contain propellants and solvents; (3) gases—found in household or commercial products used in medical anesthetics; and (4) nitrites—a special class of inhalants that primarily are used for sexual enhancement (NIDA, 2010b). A variety of household and workplace items can be used as inhalants, including office supply solvents, glue, spray paint, paint thinner, hair spray, deodorant spray, fabric protector, butane lighter

Weblink: Inhalants Weblink: Inhalant-Related Psychiatric Disorders

CHART 13–2 Chemicals Contained in Inhalants with Example of Inhalant

Chemicals	Inhalants
Toluene	Spray paints, rubber cement, gasoline
Chlorinated hydrocarbons	Dry cleaning chemicals, correction fluids
Hexane	Glue, gasoline
Benzene	Gasoline
Methylene chloride	Varnish removers, paint thinners
Butane	Cigarette lighter refills, air fresheners
Nitrous oxide	Whipped cream dispensers, gas cylinders

Sources: Brannon, G. E. (2010). Inhalant-related psychiatric disorders. Medscape Reference. Retrieved from http://emedicine.medscape.com/article/290344-overview; National Institute of Drug Abuse (NIDA). (2010b). NIDA infofacts: Inhalants. Idea Connection Limited. Retrieved from http://www.nida.nih.gov/infofacts/inhalants.htm

fluid, propane, whipped cream from an aerosol dispenser, and medical anesthetics. Nitrites often are sold in small brown bottles labeled as "video head cleaner, room deodorizer, leather cleaner, or liquid aroma" (NIDA, 2010b). Most people do not think of these items as drugs because they were never intended to be used as such. Yet, when introduced into the human body, they alter normal brain function and induce euphoria (Doweiko, 2011). These various products contain a wide range of chemicals (as shown in Chart 13–2), and with abusive use can result in irreversible effects that may include hearing loss, peripheral neuropathies or limb spasms, brain or central nervous system damage, and bone marrow damage. High concentrations of inhalants may cause heart failure and death.

Inhalants are popular among teenagers and school-age children because they are inexpensive and, since they are typically household items, easy to obtain. Individuals tend to abuse different products at different ages (Substance Abuse and Mental Health Services Administration, 2007 & 2008). Among new users ages 12 to 15, the most commonly abused inhalants are glue, shoe polish, spray paints, gasoline, and lighter fluid. Among new users age 16 or 17, the most commonly abused products are nitrous oxide or whippets (nitrous oxide found in small metal canisters used in refillable whipped cream canisters). Nitrites are the class of inhalants most commonly abused by adults.

Inhalants are sniffed or inhaled (called "huffing") in a variety of ways. Huffing a rag soaked with the inhalant and placed in a plastic bag or inhaling the gas directly from a tank are the two most common behaviors. Amyl and butyl nitrite (called "poppers") can be easily concealed and passed around a classroom, and paint thinner can be concealed in a soft drink can. Use of these inhalants and solvents can cause ventricular fibrillation, decreased cardiac output, serious brain damage, and sudden death (Brannon, 2010).

Medical and Nursing Management

Although withdrawal from inhalants must be managed, as with the other substances covered in this chapter, careful assessment, early identification, detoxification, education, and prevention are particularly critical because so many inhalant abusers are children under the age of 12. The dangerous consequences of young children's abuse of inhalants cannot be understated. Health care providers and nurses must be aware of the programs and resources available for treatment and prevention so that they can serve as a resource to individuals and families of inhalant abusers.

Nicotine Abuse

Nicotine is the psychoactive stimulating substance found in tobacco. The behavioral and physiological effects of nicotine frequently lead to addiction, and access to this legal drug for adults endangers individuals who are under the legal smoking age. Populations with psychiatric conditions and substance abuse problems have higher rates of smoking and show a lack of responsiveness to smoking cessation treatments (Doweiko, 2011).

Nicotine, a highly addictive chemical stimulant present in tobacco products, gives people a "rush" within about 10 seconds of being inhaled (The GoodDrugsGuide.com, 2011a). This chemical acts in the central and peripheral nervous systems on cells that are normally acted on by the neurotransmitter acetylcholine. In the CNS, nicotine occupies the receptors for acetylcholine in both the dopamine and serotonin neural pathways. This causes the release of dopamine and norepinephrine. Nicotine initially increases alertness and cognitive ability and then has a depressant effect (Lande, 2012). Smoking rates in the general population and nicotine addiction are fully discussed in Chapter 6.

Opiates Abuse

Opiates, also referred to as narcotics, are powerful pain relievers whose use dates back to antiquity (Preda, 2011). Opiates are defined by their ability to bind to and influence opiate receptors on cell membranes and can be divided into three classes: naturally occurring opioids—opium and morphine semi-synthetic opioids—heroin, oxycodone, oxymorphone, hydrocodone, and synthetic opiates—buprenorphine, methadone, fentanyl, alfentanil, levorphanol, meperidine, codeine (Preda, 2011).

Opiates have analgesic qualities and often are prescribed after a surgical procedure or for chronic pain. Because they act by binding to opioid receptors on neurons distributed throughout the nervous and immune systems, they can have profound effects on many organ systems and bodily functions, including pain, stress, temperature, respiration, endocrine activity, gastrointestinal activity, mood, and motivation. More than 20 clinically available medications bind opioid receptors, resulting in the following effects: pain relief, mood alteration (often producing euphoria and decreased anxiety), respiratory depression (which can cause death in overdose), cough suppression, decreased gastrointestinal motility (can cause constipation), suppression of corticotrophin-releasing factor and adrenocorticotropic hormone, pinpoint pupils (miosis), and nausea, vomiting, and pruritus (DrugRehab, 2011; Preda, 2011).

Opiates are legally available by prescription only; however, they also have become "street drugs" that are easily accessed for use without a prescription. Heroin is the most commonly abused opiate and has been for a long time (Drugs Testing Book, 2011). Its use crosses geographical areas and sociocultural lines. A white or brownish powder that usually is dissolved in water and then injected, heroin is known by a variety of street names, such as smack, big H, hell dust, and nose drops. Prescription opiates typically are taken in pill form and often are referred to by the brand names under which they are marketed such as Vicodin, Percocet, or Hydrocodone (Treatment Solutions Network, 2011). People tend to think that they are safe using opioid medications that are prescribed by health care providers, but this may not be the case. Opioids are not only effective as an analgesic, but also highly addictive. Many prescription opiate users eventually become heroin users as well. Both heroin abuse and prescription opiate abuse are serious problems in the United States (Cohagan, 2011; Cohen, et al., 2008).

Use of opiates, including heroin, is widespread. The 2006 National Survey on Drug Use and Health (NSDUH), sponsored by the Substance Abuse and Mental Health Services Administration (SAMHSA), provides data that graphically illustrate the increase in prescription opioid abuse in the preceding decade (SAMHSA, 2007). The number of persons ages 12 and older illicitly using prescription pain relievers doubled from 2.6 to 5.2 million over a 10-year period, more than any other illicit drug (Preda, 2011). Illicit use of opioids usually begins in late adolescence or early adulthood, starting with experimentation with cigarettes and alcohol. The period of time from initial use to dependency is extremely variable, ranging from a few weeks to several years. Males tend to abuse opioids more frequently than females, the male-to-female ratio being approximately 3:1 for heroin and 1.5:1 for prescription opioids (Preda, 2011).

Medical and Nursing Management

Initially, the health care provider must recognize the signs and symptoms of opioid use: lethargy and drowsiness; constricted pupils and reduced vision; shallow breathing; needle or track marks on the inner arms or other parts of the body from injecting needles; redness and raw nostrils from sniffing heroin; excessive perspiration; shaking, vomiting, chills, or other withdrawal symptoms; use or possession of paraphernalia including syringes, bent spoons, bottle caps, eye droppers, rubber tubing, cotton and needles, euphoria, psychomotor retardation, slurred speech, and/or drowsiness. Any of these may indicate opiate intoxication.

Safety Alert *A heroin overdose, if identified quickly, can be treated with naloxone (Narcan). Naloxone is a fast-acting narcotic antagonist that counteracts respiratory depression. The dose is usually 0.4 to 0.8 mg IV repeated in 5 to 15 minutes.*

Opiates are physically addictive; therefore, withdrawal is a physiological threat. People who use high doses of a drug and who use the drug intravenously are at high risk for severe withdrawal symptoms. Withdrawal symptoms usually are evident within 12 hours after the last dose. The duration of withdrawal depends on the half-life of the opiate (Galanter & Kleber, 2008).

Early symptoms of withdrawal include anorexia, anxiety, fatigue, headache, irritability, lacrimation, perspiration, rhinorrhea, and an increased respiratory rate. Later symptoms include abdominal cramps, broken sleep, hot or cold flashes, increased pulse and blood pressure, low-grade fever, muscle and bone pain, muscle cramps, nausea, and vomiting. Abdominal cramps, rhinorrhea, and lacrimation may be treated with belladonna alkaloids or phenobarbital.

Clonidine has been useful in managing symptoms (Encyclopedia of Mental Disorders, 2011). Clonidine blocks the withdrawal symptoms, making the detoxification process less painful. Psychologically, the patient feels less anxious and depressed. Clonidine may be administered by mouth as a tablet or as a transdermal patch. The advantages of using the patch include (1) the patient does not have to take pills several times a day, (2) more even blood levels are achieved, and (3) the buildup of withdrawal symptoms during the night is prevented (Galanter & Kleber, 2008).

In 1964, methadone was introduced to treat opiate addiction (Narconon News, 2011). Methadone, a synthetic narcotic, was dispensed daily at clinics to narcotic addicts by prescribers with special licensure to do so, as methadone was a federally controlled drug. Although addictive, methadone did not produce the ecstatic feeling associated with heroin (Drugs.com, 2011); however, it did alleviate the addict's craving for narcotics. It was, therefore, expected to decrease the illicit drug trafficking, theft, prostitution, and crime necessary to obtain money for the drugs. Methadone as a treatment option for these patients has been successful to a certain extent but has had controversial aspects. The ethics of methadone treatment, as well as the economic aspects of the treatment, are viewed as public health concerns (Farnum, 2011).

Other federally controlled substances, including buprenorphine, are alternatives to methadone. Buprenorphine is an opioid mixed agonist and potent analgesic (Wang & Christo, 2009). As a potential treatment for opiate addiction, buprenorphine is administered under the tongue via a small syringe by specially licensed professionals. Patients do not swallow the medication but allow it to be absorbed through the mucous membranes that line the inside of the mouth. This medication is not a replacement for methadone therapy provided through special methadone treatment facilities, but will provide the office-based prescriber with an opportunity to treat patients for addiction to heroin or other opiates, including prescription painkillers. Other potential drugs available to the prescriber are methadone, naltrexone, and LAAM (Levo-alpha acetyl methadol) (Smith, 2007).

Sedatives, Hypnotics, and Anxiolytics Abuse

Sedatives, hypnotics, and anxiolytics (SHAs) are a heterogeneous class of drugs that include benzodiazepines, barbiturates, carbonate, and various hypnotics (DuPont, Greene, & Lydiard, 2007). A sedative lowers excitement and calms the awake patient, a hypnotic produces drowsiness and promotes sleep, and an anxiolytic reduces anxiety (Reed Group, 2010). All are widely used, and all have the propensity for abuse and addiction (Sola, 2011). SHAs are commonly used to treat anxiety, insomnia, muscle tension or spasticity, and seizures, as well as to aide in alcohol/drug withdrawal (Reed Group, 2010). Sometimes they are used to treat high blood pressure. Occasionally, an individual who is prescribed one of these medications abuses it or develops substance dependence. These medications also may be sold on the street and used for recreational purposes.

Sedative-hypnotics are the most commonly prescribed psychoactive drugs. Approximately 12.5% of the adult U.S. population uses a prescribed anxiolytic in a year's time, and about 2% of the population takes one every day (Sola, 2011). The use of these drugs in the United States has significantly increased over the past 10 years (Sola, 2011). Sedatives, hypnotics, and anxiolytics often are prescribed for people in their 60s and 70s; however, nonmedical use is highest in people ages 26 to 35 years (Sola, 2011).

Barbiturates are a derivative of barbituric acid. The scientific name for barbiturates is secobarbital (Partnership for Awareness, 2010). A number of barbiturates act as a sedative or hypnotic (Mosby's Medical Dictionary, 2009). Trade names include Amytal, Nembutal, Luminal, Seconal, and Tuinal. They all depress the central nervous system and are used to induce apathy and sleep; in high doses, they function as anesthetics. They vary in their sedative effects, in the duration of their effectiveness, and in their toxicity. They also are frequently prescribed to reduce anxiety, prevent or relieve pain, and induce sleep. Nonetheless, they have inherent dangers because of their ability to cause significant CNS depression and death if used to excess. Barbiturates are popular on the streets for recreational use without a prescription. Known as "Barbies," they give a pleasurable high and are an inexpensive, temporary substitute for more potent drugs (Bergeson, 2010).

Anxiolytic drugs, typically the benzodiazepines (BZDs) and nonbenzodiazepines, began to be widely used because of their ability to reduce anxiety without causing significant CNS depression. These drugs

Weblink: Treating Opiate Addiction with Replacement Therapy

are thought to modify anxiety by altering the balance of neurotransmitters, especially norepinephrine and GABA, in the brain's limbic system, which is involved in the regulation of emotion. BZDs include diazepam (Valium), clorazepate (Tranxene), lorazepam (Ativan), and alprazolam (Xanax). These and others are known to produce dependence and withdrawal syndromes. They have a high risk for abuse and physical dependence. When the drug stops working and tolerance develops, people tend to increase the dosage just "to cope." Even the nonbenzodiazepines such as zolpidem (Ambien) and zaleplon (Sonata) can be used to excess and have dependence issues associated with use.

The liver conducts a staged metabolism of barbiturates. Oral ingestion is followed by initial absorption and partial metabolism. The unmetabolized parts of the drug become active metabolites that are stored in the patient's fatty tissues. Use of these drugs over a period of time causes a cumulative effect, unsuspected dependence, and possible overdose. Death from barbiturate overdose commonly occurs when people take alcohol and barbiturates together (Bergeson, 2010). While judgment is impaired, they may take more pills, thereby unintentionally overdosing. Because alcohol and barbiturates are synergistic, an overdose can occur quickly. A deep sleep is followed by decreased respiration, coma, and sometimes death. Barbiturates often are used in suicide attempts.

Medical and Nursing Management

Definitive treatment for patients who abuse SHAs is a lengthy process, taking months or years. Patients with mild or moderate withdrawal symptoms may be treated in the outpatient setting; those with severe withdrawal symptoms and those who have comorbid medical or psychiatric problems are generally treated as inpatients. If they have been using high dosages of the drugs or have a history of seizures, they may be treated in an intensive care unit. The general principles for treatment of sedative-hypnotic, anxiolytic drugs include the following:

- Withdraw the addicting agent slowly to avoid convulsions; taper doses on a weekly basis.
- Determine the patient's approximate drug tolerance level, because patients often inaccurately estimate the amount of drug they may have taken. Direct observation works well for this and may be best accomplished in a supervised setting.
- The use of a long-acting barbiturate decreases the severity of withdrawal symptoms; phenobarbital often is used because it has a longer half-life (Sola, 2011).
- The use of anticonvulsant agents that do not demonstrate cross-dependence with the addicting drug also may ease withdrawal symptoms.

Patients who have overdosed on any SHA must be treated immediately. They usually are admitted via the emergency department, where all lifesaving measures are implemented. The nurse assists the health care provider in establishing an adequate airway and ventilation, stabilizes and maintains the patient's hemodynamic status, and, once the patient is stabilized, induces emesis and performs lavage using standardized procedures. Following the emergency situation, when the patient is stable, he is cared for as an inpatient. At that stage, all potential complications should be addressed, such as aspiration, pulmonary edema, and respiratory failure due to hypnotic-sedative overdose. If a suicide attempt is suspected, the patient is placed on suicide precaution, and a psychiatric evaluation is requested by the health care provider (Sola, 2011). Consultations with a neurologist may be indicated if the patient has seizures that are unresponsive to the usual treatment of the withdrawal symptoms or when there are neurological symptoms that are not explained by the usual symptoms of intoxication or withdrawal.

Some individuals respond to treatment and stay in remission; others experience periods of relapse, in which they begin to use SHA after a period of remission. Some individuals are never able to abstain from use and do not experience any periods of remission.

Nursing Management

Medical–surgical nurses must be prepared to manage patients who have a substance abuse problem. This may occur when patients are admitted to the hospital for another primary diagnosis, such as trauma, painful acute pancreatitis, or acute chest pain, or when the patient is admitted directly for substance abuse.

Assessment

The major approaches to assessing for substance abuse include interviews, questionnaires, and biologic measures of biochemical and hematological markers. Nurses must keep up with current trends in drug use to assess and treat patients who are substance abusers. The nurse must make an accurate assessment of the substances used and abused to anticipate potential toxic and withdrawal effects. Different substances require different modes of treatment. For example, a patient with chronic alcoholism and a patient who abuses cocaine will have different symptoms. Specific diagnoses will be made based on the assessment of these symptoms. Examples of such are shown in the Nursing Process: Patient Care Plan for the Patient with Chronic Alcoholism (p. 309).

The nurse should conduct a thorough, nonjudgmental substance use assessment. The interview questions in the following list will assist. The patient is most likely to give accurate responses to these questions when they are part of an admission interview that includes general lifestyle inquiries about cigarette smoking, coffee consumption, and exercise habits. Experts agree that skillful assessment interviewing of patients and their family members remains the best source of data (Fischer, Neale, Bloor, & Jenkins, 2008).

- How many packs of cigarettes do you smoke daily?
- Do you take any prescription drugs now?
- Do you drink alcohol each day? If yes, do you drink a pint or about a quart? (Let the patient correct an overstatement.)
- Do you drink a pint or quart of alcohol or more on occasion?
- When was your last drink?
- Do you have a drug habit?
- What drugs do you use?
- What is your daily cost of drugs?
- When did you last drink more than you wanted to?

In an emergency situation, the patient may be unable to answer key questions such as these: What did you take? How much did you take? When did you take it? What have you taken in the last 24 hours? In the last week? If the patient is unable to answer questions, the nurse must rely on family or friends as data sources and then corroborate what is learned with the patient once she is alert.

People who abuse alcohol and other drugs tend to deny that they have a problem or may minimize the problem to make it appear perfectly normal: "I drink/use every day, but it rarely interferes with my work." Rationalization and denial are common: "I know I shouldn't use, and I'll stop as soon as I get through this problem. It keeps me calm so

I can do what I need to do." A detailed assessment generally reveals that the problem is worse than the patient says.

Substance abusers manipulate people and situations to get drugs. The term *drug-seeking behaviors* refers to these manipulations (Grover, Close, Wiele, Villarreal, & Goldman, 2011). Examples include feigning illness or an injury to get a drug. For these abusers, it becomes more important to obtain the substance of choice than to function with honesty, love, or reliability.

An assessment of behavioral changes can alert the nurse to drug use. Less dramatic physical findings that aid in detection may include dry skin, hangnails, malnutrition, ascites, elevated blood pressure, and the smell of alcohol or an inhalant on the patient's breath. As alcoholism progresses, the nurse should be alert to signs and symptoms of liver cirrhosis, such as jaundice, fatigue, weakness, loss of appetite, itching, and easy bruising (Lee, 2011). Drug screens of blood and urine may be used to determine evidence of drug use.

Nursing Diagnoses

Nursing diagnoses are derived from the results of the assessment of patients with substance abuse. They may be specific to the type of substance abused; however, generic diagnoses pertinent for all types of substance abuse include the following:

- *Chronic Low Self-Esteem* related to vulnerability, social stigma, abuse, life choices, biochemical body changes.
- *Ineffective Coping* related to personal vulnerability, negative role modeling, inadequate support systems, and previous ineffective coping skills with drug substitution.
- *Self-Care Deficit* related to inability to function cognitively and physically, attitude of not caring.
- *Imbalanced Nutrition* related to insufficient dietary intake to meet metabolic need for psychological, physiological, or economic reasons.
- *Ineffective Denial* related to personal vulnerability, difficulty handling new situations. Learned responses.
- *Powerlessness* related to substance addiction, attempts at recovery, episodic compulsive indulgence, lifestyle of helplessness.
- *Sexual Dysfunction* related to altered body function, neurological damage, debilitating effects of drug use, especially alcohol and opiates.
- *Dysfunctional Family Processes* related to substance abuse, resistance to treatment, emotional isolation/loneliness, denial of problem, inability to maintain substance abuse.
- *Knowledge Deficit Regarding Condition, Prognosis, Treatment, Self-Care, and Discharge Needs* related to lack of information, misinterpretation of information, cognitive limitations such as lack of recall.

NANDA-I © 2012

Outcomes and Evaluation Parameters

In designing care for substance abusers, outcomes must be specifically stated. Although the outcome of total and permanent abstinence may be achievable for some patients with some abuse disorders, for others it may be an unattainable goal. Each situation must be assessed individually.

Outcome criteria for the previously identified nursing diagnoses include: *Establishes feelings of self-esteem, Identifies and demonstrates coping behaviors, Completes self-care, Maintains an Improved nutritional status, Verbalizes acceptance of health status, Acknowledges perceived control of situation, Acknowledges the consequences of substance abuse for sexual health,* and *Family coping verbalized and Acknowledges substance use control.*

It is important to note that the extent of counseling and behavioral therapy may be limited in a medical–surgical environment. The patient's reason for admission to the hospital may be the physical result of substance abuse, and the patient may or may not desire treatment for the substance abuse on the current hospital admission. The nurse must maintain a nonjudgmental attitude toward every patient to foster the nurse/patient trust relationship and should make use of available internal consultants. If the hospital has an inpatient behavioral health unit, the nurses and clinical specialists from that area can be an invaluable resource.

Other desired outcomes include risk reduction; improvement of work, family, and social relationships; and lifestyle changes that may include a growing sense of spirituality. No addiction or abuse situation is going to be easy to abandon as a lifestyle. Interventions promote more effectiveness in using new attitudes and behaviors. Although the risk of relapse is always present, over time the craving for chemicals diminishes, and the patient establishes a healthier lifestyle. See the Patient Teaching & Discharge Priorities box (p. 318) for general guidelines on planning the discharge for these patients.

Planning and Interventions

Treatment for substance abuse includes promoting adaptive mechanisms and healthy perspectives on self-care and addressing the psychodynamics of drug addiction. In general, planning care focuses on reducing the harmful use pattern. Key nursing priorities include the following:

- Providing support for the decision to stop substance use.
- Assisting the patient to strengthen her individual coping skill.
- Facilitating learning of new ways to reduce anxiety.
- Promoting family involvement in the rehabilitation program.
- Facilitating family growth/development.
- Providing information about the patient's condition, prognosis, and treatment needs.

Treatment Settings

Several types of treatment settings are available for someone who is chemically dependent, all of which allow for prescribed interventions.

Inpatient/Residential Treatment

Inpatient treatment usually consists of a minimum inpatient stay of at least 28 days and medical management of detoxification (National Institute on Drug Abuse, 2008). The individual receiving inpatient or residential treatment is removed from the availability of alcohol and other drugs and daily outside distractions. This setting gives individuals the needed time to focus on the task of understanding and accepting the disease of chemical dependency and working on recovery. Those who are suicidal or acutely ill with DTs, hepatic coma, respiratory depression, or cardiac arrhythmias need to be at the acute care hospital. Life-threatening physiological symptoms are prioritized. When the patient is out of danger, the alcoholism or drug addiction issues are addressed.

Specialized Care Unit

Specialized care is given in inpatient hospital units that are geared specifically for the treatment of substance abuse. The physical environment is modified to handle the particular needs of substance abusers.

PATIENT TEACHING & DISCHARGE PRIORITIES for Substance Abuse

Need	Teaching
Involvement in substance abuse treatment	Patient will initiate and continue involvement with substance abuse treatment framework.
Awareness of the substance abuse problem and the necessary treatment	Family members are able to list the signs of substance abuse evident in their relative and the appropriate interventions applicable to the situation.
Contact and linkage with the treatment venue associated with the substance of abuse	The setting of the substance abuse treatment varies depending on the drug of abuse. Alcoholism can be treated via inpatient programs such as a detoxification unit, in a 28-day program, in a halfway house, through self-help such as Alcoholics Anonymous (AA), or as an outpatient.
	Other substances offer a similar array of treatment choices, with heroin addiction having an extra component of the methadone clinic as a treatment avenue.

For example, rooms devoid of furniture and potentially harmful materials offer a quiet, nonstimulating environment that helps to prevent convulsions and decrease anxiety. A primary nurse may be assigned to decrease confusion and stimulation. Members of the staff are experts in detoxification, education, and treatment.

Residential Rehabilitation Facilities

This type of treatment offers inpatients expert care for substance abuse; however, in some facilities, staff members are not skilled in treating medical or psychiatric problems. Extended care facilities provide services for people with physical impairments and a home for recovering alcoholics or drug addicts who may have nowhere to go after discharge.

Outpatient Treatment

This type of treatment offers more flexibility and provides less disruption to the individual's everyday life than does inpatient treatment. Those receiving outpatient treatment are able to remain living in their home environment and may be able to continue to work. The individual receives treatment on a short-term basis at the health care provider's facility.

Extended Treatment

This type of treatment usually is recommended at the conclusion of an inpatient or residential treatment program. This option is very structured and can range in length from 2 months to 2 years. During the period of extended treatment and rehabilitation, the individual moves into a halfway type house and usually gains employment prior to completion of the program.

Continuing Care/Aftercare

This type of treatment is a vital extension of the primary treatment program and ranges in length from 6 months to 1 year. Continuing care typically involves weekly aftercare group meetings and may include individual counseling sessions with a health care provider.

Self-Help Groups

Self-help groups tailored for specific addictions have goals similar to those of other self-help groups: to be a source of mutual aid to individuals seeking support. Further goals of self-help groups may include serving as a resource to addicts and loved ones as well as increasing awareness of the addiction in the community and its treatment among clinical professionals.

Twelve-step groups, such as Alcoholics Anonymous (AA) and Narcotics Anonymous (NA), as well as other self-help recovery groups such as Rational Recovery, are an integral part of maintaining sobriety or drug abstention. Individuals tend to attend a minimum of at least two meetings per week throughout treatment and continuing care.

Relapse

Relapse is common among substance abusers, and it seriously complicates treatment regardless of the type of setting. Authorities in the field of alcoholism estimate that 60% to 75% of people who complete alcohol treatment programs drink again within the first 90 days. Data suggest that only 10% to 20% of alcoholics remain abstinent for 1 year following treatment and that only 35% of these are abstinent 5 years later. In fact, recidivism rates are notoriously high across the spectrum of addictive substances (Doweiko, 2011).

Complementary and Alternative Treatment Therapies

Interest in alternative and complementary treatments for substance abuse has increased. Use of these treatments for substance abuse takes on a different form than use for many other health problems in that an herbal substance or food supplement is not substituted for the pharmaceutical or illicit drug of abuse. There are a number of complementary and alternative substances that can be abused for their escapist and stimulating qualities, so suggesting those as a mode of treatment would be counterproductive. It is important for the nurse to consider the therapeutic impact of the treatment and the holistic functioning of the person when integrating these aspects of care.

For substance abuse, alternative treatments may include more ethnomedical treatments, medical treatments based on the cultural beliefs and practices of specific ethnic groups, or those discovered through research on cross-cultural styles rather than substituting a botanical substance for the abused drug. Interventions based on behaviors and beliefs would be alternative to the medical model of drug treatment. Treatments that attend to the cultural aspects of human existence include encouraging values that discourage deviant behaviors such as using drugs, inducing a relaxation response and thus providing a healthy coping mechanism, and using a non-drug reward for abstinence through the traditional operant behavior analysis style.

Using Group Intervention/ Confrontation Strategies

Interventions for substance abuse can occur as soon as the problem is identified. Group intervention is one strategy whose goal is to break down the substance abuser's denial (NIDA, 2011). Nurses with specialized training are often "intervention specialists" and leaders in this process (Miller, 2010).

Several family members, friends, employers, coworkers, and an alcohol/drug intervention specialist confront the substance abuser in a private meeting. They list the evidence by going around the group, one by one. The family, friends, employer, and so on, following the leader's cues, speak calmly and slowly with minimal emotion. They are presenting the facts, the objective evidence, to the alcoholic or drug abuser. Yelling, blaming, and haranguing are avoided because the alcoholic or drug abuser will inevitably respond by denying the behavior or making excuses. However, confrontation by several people who really care and who persistently present the facts can break through the denial.

Health Promotion

Education, a vital component of nursing interventions, is discussed in the section on nursing interventions (pp. 317–318). Videotapes and talks by recovered substance abusers or experts on the effects of substance abuse can be helpful. Education may take place in or out of the hospital, in one comprehensive session or in several sessions over time. Nurse-educators should focus on the types of abused substances and their physical, psychological, and social effects. Family members are often involved in these sessions because substance abuse is a family problem. The belief underlying such education is that knowledge and awareness may be useful in decreasing self-destructive behavior. Culturally sensitive and relevant educational resources should be used.

Collaborative Management

Treating substance abuse in an effective manner involves an interdisciplinary team of nurses, health care providers, rehabilitation therapists, and psychotherapists (such as clinical nurse specialists, psychologists, and psychiatrists), social workers, dietitians, and peer advocacy/support. In order to meet desired patient outcomes, it is essential that this interdisciplinary team communicate openly with one another in developing and evaluating care of the patient and family (Institute of Medicine [IOM], 2010). This disease process is a composite of genetic predisposition, a variety of underlying psychological dynamics, exposure and reactions to stress, and the physiological consequences of drug abusing behavior as a coping mechanism.

Each team member contributes, in a planned manner, to the patient's movement toward recovery from substance abuse. The psychologist or psychiatrist may provide psychological testing when there are questions about coexisting psychological problems and can provide psychotherapy (individual or group) for patients whose problems require multifaceted clinical interventions. The dietitian focuses on the patient's nutritional status, which has been compromised by malnutrition and the interference of alcohol and other substances in metabolizing necessary vitamins and nutrients. The peer support approach of AA/NA has had a significant impact on people addicted to alcohol and drugs. The self-help component of this contact is an important factor in the overall success and recovery of an alcoholic/drug addict. Participants or representatives from self-help groups or outside treatment programs may also become part of the health care team, as may the patient and family.

As with all substance abusers, there may be a need to consult with rehabilitation specialists in physical therapy and occupational therapy. For example, the patient may need physical therapy to restore muscle mass and increase mobility. The occupational therapist may assist the patient in developing ways to manage in the home setting or rehabilitation environment. A family counselor or social worker may assist the patient and family in identifying and resolving home and family issues, such as role identity, enabling behaviors, sexual problems, and adjustment to the home or rehabilitation setting. The collaborative team approach offers the best response to the treatment needs of a patient from the day of admission to the ongoing, sustained approach that will help a patient obtain discharge goals and develop and maintain a healthier lifestyle.

Impaired Health Care Professional

Alcohol and drug dependence does not discriminate. Addiction is as prevalent among health care professionals as it is in the general population (American Psychological Association, 2011). Though it is difficult to determine exact statistics of incidence, alcohol and drug abuse/dependence affect a significant number of health care professionals. Many are afraid to report their abuse for fear of disciplinary action or loss of their license to practice, and other people in their lives often fail to recognize the signs and symptoms. However, available literature on the subject estimates that 10% to 15% of health care professionals are afflicted with alcohol and drug dependence (Nebraska Department of Health and Human Services, 2010). Health care professionals are at particular risk for chemical abuse/dependency for a number of reasons. These professionals may prescribe, administer, and dispense medications every day to treat and help patients. Exposure and accessibility to mood-altering medications, pharmacologic knowledge of the drugs (which fosters a false sense of control), and tendency to self-treat or self-medicate are contributing factors. Health care workers, in general, work under a great deal of stress and may have physical injuries leading to pain syndromes. When they need relief from pain and emotional stress, they may find themselves self-prescribing or taking a medication from a patient or from the stock supply. They convince themselves that "it is only going to happen once"; however, if they do not suffer any negative consequences while self-medicating, they may start doing it on a regular basis (American Psychological Association, 2011).

Health care providers become substance abusers for the same reasons anyone becomes dependent on or addicted to a substance. And as with any addict, the substance becomes more important than anything else in that person's life. Such behavior is dangerous in a health care environment, is a violation of state practice acts and ethical standards of practice, and, depending on the drug and method of obtaining it, may be a criminal offense (McCue, 2010). Colleagues of chemically dependent health care workers need to be alert to behavior that suggests a substance abuse problem. They should assess the safety of attempting to talk with the professional who is having difficulty and, if appropriate, use the contact to clarify impressions and gather facts. Typical behaviors of impaired health care professionals include: frequent absenteeism (usually before or after scheduled days off); always working (in order to obtain supply): abrupt mood changes; inappropriate affect; sloppy patient care; on duty when drugs are missing; frequent "wasting" of drugs or inaccurate control of drug records; frequent disappearance from assigned work area; offering to give medication to patients not assigned to them; patients receiving medications from the health care provider complain of little or no pain relief; multiple physical complaints; unkempt appearance; personality and behavioral changes; emotional or mental crises; and lying (Nebraska Department of Health and Human Services [DHHS], 2010).

Though it is very common for colleagues to collude in covering up the addicted person's behavior, this does not help the affected individual. Concerns about a colleague should be reported to a supervisor. A co-worker relationship, a friendship, family ties, and feelings of guilt or fear are not good reasons to neglect the responsibility of protecting patients from exposure to an impaired health care provider.

Instead of addressing the colleague's addiction directly, peers often engage in enabling behavior, such as ignoring, covering for, trying to protect, making excuses for, and doing the job for the impaired health care professional (Nebraska Department of Health and Human Services, 2010).

Shielding such a health care provider, whatever the professional discipline, puts patients, the health care provider, and the profession at risk and violates professional practice, the code of ethics, and the law in many states (McCue, 2010).

Nurses need to understand that their chemically dependent colleagues have a disease, not a moral problem. This understanding empowers nurses to work together to help each other. The goal is to assist the chemically impaired nurse or health care provider to recover and to achieve a healthy state. Gallagher (2011) suggested the following steps to take in supporting a colleague who is in recovery:

- Do not be judgmental or condescending.
- Let your colleague know that you will be there for him and be supportive.
- Be available to step in when the colleague's recovery is in jeopardy.
- Be honest about mentioning troubling behaviors.
- Be ready to intervene if evidence of relapse appears.
- Promote collaboration, not an "us-against-you attitude."
- Step in and take a stand when others are intolerant.
- If intolerant behavior continues, report it to management.
- Ask questions about recovery, addiction, and relapse.
- Treat the colleague as you would want to be treated.

Most states have drug treatment or support groups affiliated with the state nurses' association to address the impaired nurse. Disciplinary action, mandated treatment, and determination of suitability to practice all work well in a holistic approach (McCue, 2010). A humane and rehabilitative approach to treatment returns competent nursing colleagues to the workforce.

Gerontological Considerations

Substance abuse among older adults is a major health concern because the way in which drugs affect individuals changes with age (Pathology Education, 2011). With aging, natural variability in physiologic differences becomes heightened. Pharmacodynamic responses are blunted, the ability to eliminate drugs is diminished, and sensitivity to the toxic effects of drugs is increased. The effects of disease affect the response to drugs. These changes account for the concentration of adverse drug events in older adults (Pathology Education, 2011).

The concern for drug use in older adults is heightened by the disproportionate use of drugs in this population. People over the age of 65 consume more prescription medications than all other age groups combined (Naegle, 2008). This alone puts this group at risk for deliberate or inadvertent prescription drug abuse. Misunderstandings about how exactly the medication should be taken combined with poor or slow responses may encourage inaccurate or abusive ingestion (Pathology Education, 2011). Additionally, the medical health of older adults usually is compromised, making overuse or abuse of prescription substances more dangerous. Older adults often have less-than-optimal liver functioning and other system frailties that can potentiate physiological consequences.

Several factors increase the risks associated with alcohol and drug use for older individuals. General risk factors that affect their health include changes in body composition such as decreased muscle mass, decreased organ efficiency (especially kidney and liver), and increased vulnerability of the central nervous system. Specific risk factors for substance abuse for the older individual include the following: family history of dependence on alcohol, tobacco, prescription or illicit drugs, co-occurrence of addiction with dependency or abuse of another substance, such as alcohol and tobacco, lifelong pattern of substance use, including heavy drinking, male gender, social isolation, recent and multiple losses, chronic pain, co-occurrence with depression, and unmarried or living alone (Naegle, 2008).

Alcohol is the drug of choice in the older patient population. A national epidemiological survey revealed that more than 1 in 5 adults age 65 and over had a substance abuse disorder, and more than 1 in 20 had such a disorder in the past 12 months, primarily involving alcohol or tobacco (Lin et al., 2011). In 1998, the prevalence of alcoholism, alcohol abuse, or problem drinking in persons age 60 or older was estimated at 5% to 10% in community studies (Naegle, 2008). Approximately 11% of men and 9% of women who were age 75 years and older reported heavy alcohol use. This caused them to be at risk for a range of problems.

Identifying late-life alcoholism either sustained from earlier years or as a new addiction requires the nurse to have a significant knowledge base about alcoholism and aging. Recognizing the effects of alcoholism on the body and developing evidence-based practice for treating those effects is vital.

The onset of substance abuse late in life may not be the norm. Frequently, lifelong substance abuse continues into the later years and is evident through chronic damage to body systems. Addiction to a substance throughout adult milestones may have affected the patient psychologically. Fighting an addiction is not easy at any stage in life; trying to conquer substance abuse after decades of use can be overwhelming.

In assessing and treating the older population for any form of substance abuse, the nurse should remember that this is a distinct group of individuals whose physiological support structures are altered. Receptor sensitivity and responsiveness is changed, usually reduced. The ability to mount a compensatory physiologic response is diminished. Normal homeostatic mechanisms are dulled and sometimes produce inappropriate responses (Pathology Education, 2011). Even healthy older adults have diminished capacities. Aging occurs on a continuum, and older adults are stratified by degree of age. Those who care for older adults must be cognizant of these facts and assist older patients to get better or enhance their health-related quality of life.

Research

Substance abuse is a serious, continuous, global problem. Researchers are conducting ongoing research regarding the effects of treatment, use and abuse patterns, methods of prevention, and identification of trends that will promote early detection, consequences of abuse, and treatment options. Research has been instrumental in answering some of the questions about substance abuse, but it has not been enough. As the number of people suffering from drug abuse continues to grow and diversify, additional research is needed. The advent of new drugs that can be used medicinally and recreationally underscores this need. As a result of the increasing severity of prescription drug abuse, the National Institute on Drug Abuse (NIDA) published the results of a study identifying the prevalence of such drug abuse (2011). The goals of the study included identifying the scope of the prescription drug abuse problem in the United States and the factors that are driving the abuse of prescription drugs. Data gained from this survey will be used to foster the development of educational programs and promote new research endeavors.

RESEARCH OPPORTUNITIES Related to Substance Abuse

Research Area	Clinical Impact
Research demonstrates that children of alcoholics are at higher risk of becoming alcoholics.	Research into addressing the environments vulnerable children are raised in could ultimately lower the risk factors associated with having genetic predispositions to substance abuse.
Alcoholism-centered clinical investigations have redefined alcoholism as a disease.	Further research into alcoholism would drive the stigma and lack of knowledge into retreat and provide a better venue for the definitions of the illness, effective treatment frameworks, and acceptance of people with alcoholism.
Researchers have found that marijuana produces a significant analgesic effect and is modestly effective against the nausea and vomiting associated with chemotherapy (American Cancer Society, 2012; Science Daily, 2008).	Examination of substances for their beneficial actions contributes to opportunities to capitalize on available treatment and encourage the development of additional compounds to treat clinical problems.
For years, researchers and clinicians have been searching for an objective biologic marker that will reflect problem drinking and make assessment less challenging.	Finding an objective biologic marker for alcoholism can be formulated as prevention as well as enhancing treatment.
Research indicates that participation in a 12-step program can help prevent relapse. These programs focus on the patient maintaining sobriety, as opposed to having recovered or being cured (Moos & Timko, 2008).	Science showed that the vast majority of alcoholics relapsed quickly with negative consequences if they drank alcohol. Continued research keeps treatment accurately focused.

Other very recent reports of research related to drug abuse and addiction include studies on the prevalence of drug use among teens and information about cocaine addiction. Ostrow (2011) found in a survey of 72,661 teens that American Indian youths had the highest level of drug or alcohol abuse. The data also revealed that Black and Asian teens are less likely to drink or use drugs than are White teens. Dr. Eric Kendel, with other researchers from Columbia University, found the first physiological evidence that smoking cigarettes primes an individual for cocaine addiction (Michael's House, 2011). This research paves the way for further research into the impact of other drugs, such as alcohol and marijuana, on addiction to other illicit drugs.

There is a great need for continued research into drug/alcohol abuse and addiction. Examples of research opportunities related to substance abuse are shown in the Research Opportunities Related to Substance Abuse feature.

Summary

Substance abuse knows no social boundaries. It is important for nurses to educate themselves and others about the effects of substance abuse. Through the understanding of addiction, the nurse will be able to observe the patient for behaviors or physical symptoms of abuse and report the patient to the health care team. Caring for patients who are substance abusers requires knowledgeable and skilled nursing to develop and implement effective multidisciplinary plans of care.

NCLEX® PRACTICE

1. A patient says, "I didn't drink while I was pregnant, but my husband has been an alcoholic for many years. Will my children be at risk for alcoholism?" How should the nurse respond?

1. "Since you abstained from alcohol during your pregnancies, your children are not at risk."
2. "As long as the children are not around your husband when he is drinking, there should be no effect."
3. "The children of alcoholic parents have a much higher risk of developing alcoholism."
4. "As long as there were no genetically linked birth defects, the risk is very low for them developing alcoholism."

2. The nurse identifies the patient with which personality traits to be most at risk for disruptive substance abuse? (select all that apply)

1. The patient is self-centered.
2. The patient is very independent.
3. The patient is dishonest with himself.
4. The patient has poor coping skills.
5. The patient has anger control issues.

3. The nurse is caring for a patient with a history of alcoholism who has been in the emergency department for 8 hours. The health care provider has ordered disulfiram (Antabuse). How should the nurse proceed with this treatment?

1. Have the patient use a mouthwash rinse to control the metallic taste associated with this medication.
2. Plan to monitor the patient for development of hypertension after giving the medication.
3. Advise the patient that the medication causes coughing that can be controlled with any over-the-counter cough syrup.
4. Wait a minimum of 4 additional hours before administering the medication.

4. The nurse caring for a patient in the emergency department who has been sniffing paint solvents places priority on monitoring the patient for which occurrence?

1. Cardiac arrhythmias
2. Suicidal tendencies
3. Outbursts of rage
4. Visual hallucinations

5. A patient admitted to the emergency department is displaying symptoms of PCP intoxication. The nurse prepares to administer which priority drug?

1. A narcotic antagonist
2. An antiemetic
3. A benzodiazepine
4. A tricyclic antidepressant

6. Amphetamine abusers can often easily obtain their drug of choice because amphetamines are used to treat a variety of common disorders. Which disorders are commonly treated with amphetamines? (select all that apply)

1. Depression
2. Hypertension
3. Cardiac dysrhythmia
4. Narcolepsy
5. Minimal brain dysfunction

Answers to NCLEX Practice questions can be found in Appendix D in the Osborn Student Resources at nursing.pearsonhighered.com. Practice additional NCLEX questions online at the Student Resources site.

REFERENCES

Adams, P. M., & Koch, R. W. (2010). *Pharmacology: Connections to nursing practice.* Upper Saddle River, NJ: Pearson.

Addictionsandrecovery.org. (2011). The genetics of addiction. Retrieved from http://www.addictionsandrecovery.org/is-addiction-a-disease.htm

Alcohol Answers. (2009). Social acceptance of alcohol. Retrieved from http://www.alcoholanswers.org/alcohol-education/social-acceptance-of-alcohol.cfm

American Cancer Society. (2012). Marijuana. Retrieved from http://www.cancer.org/Treatment/TreatmentsandSideEffects/ComplementaryandAlternativeMedicine/HerbsVitaminsandMinerals/marijuana

American Nurses Association. (2004). *Scope and standards of addictions nursing practice* (revised edition). American Nurses Association. Retrieved from http://Association/dp/155810

American Psychiatric Association. (2000). *Diagnostic and statistical manual of mental disorders* (4th ed., text revision). Washington, DC: American Psychiatric Publishing.

American Psychological Association. (2011). Practitioners working with older adults. Retrieved from http://www.apa.org/p/aging/resources/guides/practitioners-should-know.aspx

Babor, T. F., Higgins-Biddle, J. C., Saunders, J. B., & Monteiro, M. G. (2001). *AUDIT, the alcohol use disorders identification test* (2nd ed.). Geneva: World Health Organization, Department of Mental Health and Substance Dependence.

Battaglia, E. (2009). Post-acute withdrawal syndrome—what you need to know. *Drug and Alcohol Addiction Recovery Magazine.* Retrieved from http://www.drugalcoholaddictionrecovery.com/?p=37

Benner, S. (2012). PCP Toxicity. Medscape Reference. Retrieved from http://emedicine.medscape.com/article/1010821overview

Benton, S. A. (2011). The high-function alcoholic. *Psychology Today.* Retrieved from http://www.psychologytoday.com/blog/the-high-functioning-alcoholic/20090/characterlist

Bergeson, B. (2010). Side effects of barbiturates to the body organs. LIVESTRONG.COM. Retrieved from http://www.livestrong.com/article/1831810side-effects-of barbiturates-to-the-body-organs/

Botvin, G. J., Griffin, K. W., & Gilchrist, L. Z. (2011). Drugs and alcohol abuse— school, college. Retrieved from http://education.stateuniversity.com/pages/1923/Drug-Alcohol-Abuse.html

Brannon, G. E. (2010). Inhalant-related psychiatric disorders. Medscape Reference. Retrieved from http://emedicine.medscape.com/article/290344-overview

Brenner, S., & Corden, T. (2009). Toxicity, hallucinogens—PCP. Medscape Reference. Retrieved from http://emedicine.medscape.com/article/1010821

Bryson, E. O., & Frost, E. A. M. (2011). The perioperative implications of tobacco, marijuana, and other inhaled toxins. *International Anesthesiology Clinics, 49*(1), 103–118.

Buddy, T. (2007a). Alcoholism is a family disease. About.com. Retrieved from http://alcoholism.about.com/es/info2/a/aa030597.htm

Buddy, T. (2007b). What is a hangover? About.com. Retrieved from http://alcoholism.about.com/od/hangovers/a/hangover.htm

Buddy, T. (2010). How to prevent getting a hangover. About.com. Alcoholism. Retrieved from http://alcoholism.about.com/od/hangovers/a/prevention.htm

Buddy, T. (2012) Short alcohol tests ideal for healthcare screening. About.com.Alcoholism. Retrieved from http://alcoholism.about.com/od/tests/a/tests.htm

Burns, M. J. (2011). Delirium tremens. Medscape Reference. Retrieved from http://emedicine.medscape.com/article/166032-overview

Buxton, J., & Dove, N. (2008). The burden and management of crystal meth use. *Canadian Medical Association Journal, 178*(12), 1537–1539.

Cohagan, A. (2011). Alcohol and substance abuse evaluation. Medscape Reference. Retrieved from http://emedicine.medscape.com/article/805084-overview

Cohen, J. S. (2011). Alcohol intoxication. Emedicinehealth. Retrieved from http://www.emedicinehealth.com/alcohol_intoxification/article_me.htm

Carvalho, H. B., & Seible, S. D. (2009). Crack cocaine use and its relationship with violence and HIV. *Clinics* [online]. *64*(9), 857–866. Retrieved from http://www.ncbi.nlm.nih.gov/pubmed/19759879

DeMaria, S., & Weinkauf, J. L. (2011). Cocaine and other club drugs. *International Anesthesiology Clinics, 49*(1), 79–101.

Doweiko, H. F. (2011). *Concepts of chemical dependency* (8th ed.). Belmont, CA: Brooks/Cole, Cengage Learning.

DrugRehab. (2011). 3 signs of opiate abuse. Retrieved from http://www.edrugrehab.com/3-sings-of-opiate-abuse.html

Drugs.com. (2011). Methadone. Retrieved from http://www.drugs.com/pro/methadone.html?printable=1

Drugs Testing Book. (2011). Opiates. Retrieved from http://drugtestingbook.com/interpretation-of-workplace-drug-test-results-by-medical-review

Dryden-Edwards, R. (2011a). Alcoholism and alcohol abuse. MedicineNet, Inc. Retrieved from www.emedicinehealth.com/alcoholism/page12_em.htm

Dryden-Edwards, R. (2011b). Cocaine and crack abuse. MedicineNet.com. Retrieved from http://www.medicinenet.com/script/main/art.asp?articlekey=38069&pf=3&page=2

DuPont, R. L., Greene, W., & Lydiard, R. B. (2007). Sedatives and hypnotics: Clinical use and abuse. UpToDate, Inc. Retrieved from http://www.uptodate.com/contents/sedatives-and-hypnotics-clinical-use-and-abuse

Encyclopedia of Mental Disorders. (2011). Clonidine. Retrieved from http://www.mindisorders.com/Br-Del-Clonidine.html

Erickson, C. (2007). The science of addiction: From neurobiology to treatment. College of Pharmacy: University of Texas at Austin. Retrieved from www.utexas.edu/research/asrec

Farnum, S. (2011). Treating opiate addiction with replacement therapy. Home Box Office. Retrieved from http://www.hbo.com/addiction/treatment/343_treating_opiate_addiction.html

Fischer, J., Neale, J., Bloor, M., & Jenkins, N. (2008). Substance abuse treatment, prevention, and policy. *BioMed Central LTD.* Retrieved from http://www.substanceabusepolicy.com/content/3/1/21. doi10.1186/1747-597x-3-21

Galanter, M., & Kleber, H. D. (2008). *Textbook of substance abuse treatment* (4th ed.). New York: American Psychiatric Publishing.

Gallagher, A. (2011). Moral distress and moral courage in everyday nursing practice. *The Online Journal of Issues in Nursing.* Retrieved from http://www.nursingworld.org/MainMenuCategories/ANAMarketplace/ANAPeriodicals/O

Genen, L. (2011). Cannabis compound abuse. Medscape Reference. Retrieved from http://emedicine.medscape.com/article/2286661-overview

Gist, R. S., Sullivan, M., & Serianni, R. P. (2011). Management of substance abuse in the hospital setting. *International Anesthesia Clinics, 49*(1),15–30.

GoodDrugsGuide.com, (2012). What are amphetamines? Retrieved from http://www.thegooddrugsguide.com/amphetamines/index.htm

GoodDrugsGuide.com (2011a). Nicotine addiction. Retrieved from http://www.thegooddrugsguide.com/addiction-types/drug-addiction/nicotine.htm

GoodDrugsGuide.com. (2011b). Common opiate use. Retrieved from http//www.thegooddrugsguide.com/addiction-types;/drug=addiction/opiate.htm

Grover, C. A., Close, R. J., Wiele, E. D., Villarreal, K., & Goldman, L. M. (2012). Quantifying drug-seeking behavior: A case control study. *Journal of Emergency Medicine, 42*(1), 15–21. Epub 2011. PMID:21958455[pubMED – indexed for MEDLINE].

Hasin, D., Hatzenbueler, M., & Waxman, R. (2010). Genetics of substance abuse disorders. In K. Carroll & W. Miller (Eds.), *Rethinking substance abuse: What the science shows and what we should do about it.* New York: Guilford Press.

Helmenstine, A. M. (2012). Crack cocaine facts. About.com. Chemistry. Retrieved from http://chemistry.about.com/od/drugs/a/crackcocainefaq.htm

Institute of Medicine (IOM). (2010). *The future of nursing: Leading change, advancing health.* Washington, DC: The Academic Press.

Kenney, M. (2010). The resilience of Andean cocaine. *Globality Studies Journal.* Stony Brook, NY: Stony Brook University. Retrieved from http://globality.cc.stonybrook.edu/?p=152

Key, J. L. (2010). *Laboratory and diagnostic tests with nursing implications.* Upper Saddle River, NJ: Pearson.

Krebs, C. P. Lande, R. G. (2012). Nicotine addiction. Medscape Reference. Retrieved from http://emedicine.medscape.com/article/287555-overview

Lee, D. (2011). Cirrhosis of the liver. Retrieved from http://www.medicinenet.com/cirrhosis/article.htm

Lin, J. C., et al. (2011). Alcohol, tobacco and nonmedical drug use disorders in U.S. adults aged 65 years and older: Data from the 2001–2002 national epidemiological survey of alcohol and related conditions. *American Journal of Geriatric Psychiatry, 19*(3), 292–299.

McCrady, B. (2010). Family and other close relationships. In K. Carroll & W. Miller (Eds.), *Rethinking substance abuse: What the science shows and what we should do about it.* New York: Guilford Press.

McCue, C. (2010). Using the AACN framework to alleviate moral distress. *The Online Journal of Issues in Nursing.* Retrieved from http://www.nursingworld.org/MainMenuCategories/ANAMarketplace/ANAPeriodicals/OJ

MedicineNet.com. (2011). Cocaine and crack abuse. Retrieved from http://www.medicinenet.com/script/main/art.asp?articlekey=38069&pf+3&page=2

Medeiros, J. (2011). A theoretical perspective on substance abuse: A sociocultural approach. Associated Content. Retrieved from http://www.associatedcontent.com/shared/print.shml?content_type=article&content_type_

MedlinePlus. (2011a). Alcohol withdrawal. U.S. National Library of Medicine and National Institutes of Health. Retrieved from http://www.nih.gov.medlineplus/ency/article/000764.htm

MedlinePlus. (2011b). Delirium tremens. U.S. National Library of Medicine and National Institutes of Health. Retrieved from http://www.nlm.nih.gov/medlineplus/ency/article/000766.htm

Michael's House. (2011). Cigarettes shown to be a "gateway drug" for cocaine addiction. Retrieved from http://www.michaelshouse.com/blog/cigarettes-shown-to-be-a-%e3%80%98gateway-drug

Miller, C. (2010). How to confront someone with a drinking problem. Demand Media LIVESTRONG.com. Retrieved from http://www.livestrong.com/article/170285-how-to-confront-someone-with-a-drinking-pro

Moos, R. H., & Timko, C. (2008). Outcome research on 12-step and other self-help programs. In M. Galanter & H. D. Kleber (Eds.), *Textbook of substance abuse treatment* (4th ed., pp. 511–523). Washington, DC: American Psychiatric Press.

Mosby's medical dictionary (8th ed.). (2009). Philadelphia: Elsevier.

Naegle, M. (2008). Substance abuse: Nursing standard of practice protocol: Substance abuse in older adults. Hartford Institute for Geriatric Nursing. Retrieved from http://consultgerirn.org/topics/substance_abuse/want_to+know+more

Narconon News. (2011). The history of drug abuse and addiction treatment in America: Part 9. Retrieved from http://news.narconon.org/history-drug-abuse-treatment-america/

National Center for Alcohol and Drug Detox (NCADD). (2011). Retrieved from http://www.detoxalcoholdrug.org/

National Institute on Alcohol Abuse and Alcoholism. (2012). Retrieved from http://pubs.niaaa.nih.gov/publications/arh28-2/78-79.htm

National Institute on Drug Abuse (NIDA). (2008). Genetics of addiction. Retrieved from http://drugabuse.gov/tib/genetics.html

National Institute on Drug Abuse (NIDA). (2010a). NIDA infofacts: Cocaine. National Institutes of Health, U.S. Department of Health and Human Services. Retrieved from http://www.nida.nih.gov/infofacts/cocaine.html

National Institute on Drug Abuse (NIDA). (2010b). NIDA infofacts: Inhalants. Idea Connection Limited. Retrieved from http://www.nida.nih.gov/infofacts/inhalants.htm

National Institute on Drug Abuse (NIDA). (2011). Topics in brief: prescription drug abuse. Retrieved from http://www.drugabuse.gov/publications/topics-in-brief/prescription-drug-abuse

Nebraska Department of Health and Human Services (DHHS). (2010). *Chemical dependency and health care professionals resource guide.* Lincoln, NE: Division of Public Health–Licensure Unit.

Ostrow, N. (2011). Black and Asian teens have lowest rates of drug and alcohol use. *Businessweek.* Retrieved from http://www.businessweek.com/news/2011-11-08/black-and-asian-teens-have-lowest-rates-

Parish, B. S. (2011). Hallucinogens. Medscape Reference. Retrieved from http://emedicine.medscape.com/article/293752-overview

Partnership for Awareness. (2010). Barbiturates. Retrieved from http://sites.google.com/site/partnershipforawareness/resources/drug-information/barbiturates

Pathology Education. (2011). Drug use and principles of clinical care in geriatric patients. Retrieved from http://www.iaop2010org/drug-use-and-prnciples-of-clinical-care-in-geriatric-patients.htm

Phillips, K., Luk, A., Soor, G. S., Abraham, J. R., Leong, S., & Butany, J. (2009). Cocaine cardiotoxicity. *American Journal of Cardiovascular Drugs, 9*(3), 177–196.

Preda, A. (2011). Opioid abuse. Medscape Reference. Retrieved from http://emedicine.medscape.com/article/287790-overview

Psych Central. (2011). Identifying signs of addiction. Retrieved from http://psychcentralcom/lib/2011/identifying-signs-of-addiction/

Reed Group. (2010). Sedative, hypnotic or anxiolytic dependence. *MDGuidelines* ™ Retrieved from http://www.mdguidelines.com/sedative-hypnotic-or-anxiolytic-dependence/diagnosis

Richards, J. R. (2011). Methamphetamine toxicity. Medscape Reference. Retrieved from http://emedicine.medscape.com/article/820918-overview

Roy, N. (2008). Vygotsky's sociocultural theory. *South Florida Psychotherapy, Substance Abuse Counseling, Psychotherapy Research.* Retrieved from http://www.nickroy.com/2008/vygotskys-sociocultural-theory

Schueler, S. J., Beckett, J. H., & Gettings, S. (2010). Drug abuse: Hallucinogens. FreeMED. Retrieved from http://www.freemed.com/drug=abuse-symptoms-hallucinogens.htm

Science Daily. (2008). Marijuana may be effective for neuropathic pain. Retrieved from http://www.sciencedaily.com/releases/200806/080626150628.htm

Smith, J. K. (2007). Drugs for drugs: Medications to treat addictions. *For the Record, 19*(24), 21.

Sola, C. L. (2011). Sedative, hypnotic, anxiolytic use. Medscape Reference. Retrieved from http://emedicine.medscape.com/article/290585-overview

Substance Abuse and Mental Health Services Administration. (2008). *Results from the 2007 National Survey on Drug Use and Health: National Findings* (Office of Applied Studies, NSDUH Series H-34, DHHS Publication No. SMA 08-4343). Rockville, MD.

Substance Abuse and Mental Health Services Administration. (2008). The NSDUH Report: Inhalant use across the adolescent years. Office of Applied Studies, Department of Health and Human Services. Retrieved from http://www.samhsa.gov/data/2k8/inhalants/inhalanys.pdf

Treatment Solutions Network. (2011). Opiate addiciton treatment. Retrieved from http://www.treatmentsolutionsnetwork.com/opiate-addiction-treatment.html

Wells, S. M., Noonan, C., Wells, K. M., Holian, A., & Wibbenmeyer, L. A. (2009). Effects of toxic gases: Methamphetamine inhalation. *Journal of Burn Care & Research. 30*(1), 152–153.

Wilkinson, J. M., & Ahearn, N. R. (2009). *Prentice Hall nursing diagnosis handbook* (9th ed.). Upper Saddle River, NJ: Prentice Hall.

CHAPTER 14

Infectious Process and Prophylaxis

Gail Thurkauf
Annita Watson

Outcome-Based Learning Objectives

After studying this chapter, the learner will be able to:

1. Explain the infectious process and its effects on the body.
2. Construct the chain of infection to understand onset and progression of infections.
3. Analyze measures used to prevent and control infection.
4. Classify common pathogens that cause infection.
5. Demonstrate correct hand hygiene practices.
6. Generate a plan for assessing and determining nursing interventions for a patient with an infection.

KEY TERMS

active immunization p.335
antigen p.331
antigenicity p.328
carrier p.327
chain of infection p.327
community-acquired infection p.332
empiric therapy p.341
endotoxins p.328
exotoxins p.328
fever of unknown origin (FUO) p.336
health-care-associated infection (HAI) p.332
infectivity p.328
invasiveness p.328
mode of transmission p.327
notifiable disease p.340
passive immunization p.335
pathogenicity p.327
portal of entry p.327
portal of exit p.327
reservoir p.327
viability p.328
virulence p.328

Weblink: Preventing Transmission of Infectious Agents in Healthcare Settings

INFECTIOUS DISEASE is a major health problem around the world. Infection occurs when a harmful microorganism enters the body and is able to colonize and multiply, leading to an infection and subsequent immune response. A microorganism is a microscopic body such as a bacterium, virus, fungus, or parasite. Some microorganisms live on the human body normally and are beneficial. For example, certain microorganisms live in the intestines and produce enzymes that facilitate digestion. However, if the immune and inflammatory systems are compromised, as can occur when an individual has decreased immunity, organisms that usually benefit the body can leave their normal sites and travel to other areas of the body. When this happens, an infection may develop.

A microorganism that produces disease is called a pathogen. In contrast to beneficial microorganisms that may cause infection when the body's defenses are compromised, true pathogens are able to cause disease regardless of the body's normal defenses.

In spite of heightened diligence to prevent and treat infections many infectious organisms remain, and new varieties and strains are developing. Some of these strains are resistant to antibiotics, making treatment more difficult and increasing morbidity, mortality, and length of hospital stay. Antimicrobial resistance, primarily due to prolonged or inappropriate use of antibiotics, is becoming an increasingly concerning problem in health care (Hildreth, Burke, & Glass, 2009). Some bacteria may survive the use of antibiotics and, given this evolutionary advantage, are able to change their genetic makeup, making the antibiotic ineffective against this type of bacteria. Currently, the best-known resistant organisms are methicillin-resistant *Staphylococcus aureus* (MRSA), multidrug-resistant tuberculosis (MDR-TB), penicillin-resistant *Streptococcus pneumoniae* (PRSP), vancomycin-resistant enterococci (VRE), vancomycin intermediate-resistant *S. aureus* (VISA), and vancomycin-resistant *S. aureus* (VRSA) (CDC, 2007). Antimicrobial resistance has occurred for a variety of reasons, including but not limited to inappropriate prescribing practices, inconsistent infection control techniques, promotion of antibiotic use by pharmaceutical companies, lack of public knowledge about appropriate antibiotic use, availability of antibiotics without prescription in some parts of the world, and use of antibiotics in agriculture on crops and livestock. Chart 14–1 lists various nursing actions that can be taken to address this problem.

CHART 14–1 Actions to Address Antimicrobial Resistance

- Use standard, approved infection prevention and control measures. Proper hand hygiene, as outlined in Figures 14–1◆ and 14–2◆, is essential. Wear gloves when necessary, and follow standard precautions for all patients.
- Teach patients the importance of practicing infection prevention and control, the importance of taking the full course of an antibiotic even after symptoms have disappeared, and how to recognize when antibiotics are necessary and when they are not.

Hand Hygiene Technique with Soap and Water

Duration of the entire procedure: 40-60 seconds

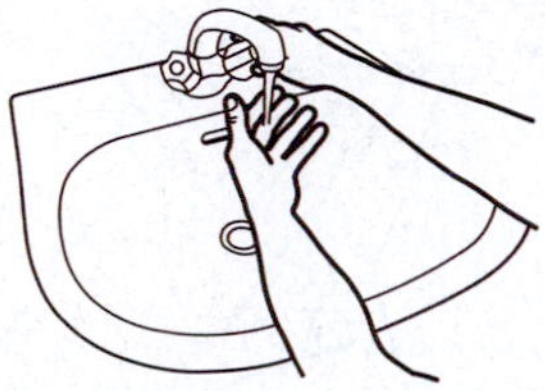

0 Wet hands with water;

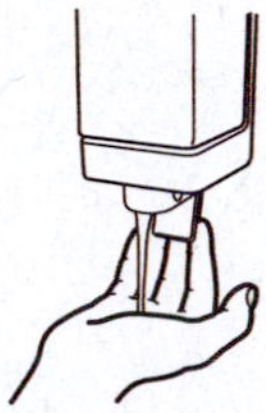

1 Apply enough soap to cover all hand surfaces;

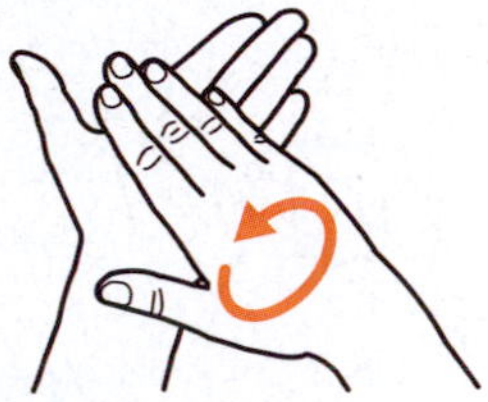

2 Rub hands palm to palm;

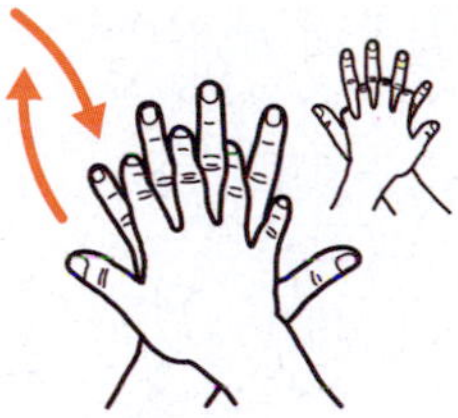

3 Right palm over left dorsum with interlaced fingers and vice versa;

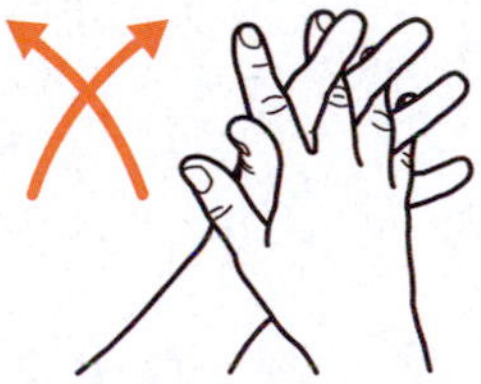

4 Palm to palm with fingers interlaced;

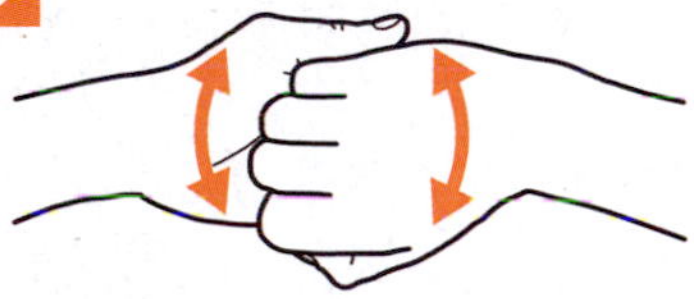

5 Backs of fingers to opposing palms with fingers interlocked;

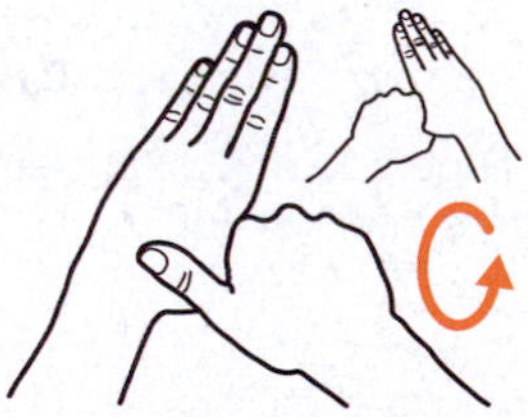

6 Rotational rubbing of left thumb clasped in right palm and vice versa;

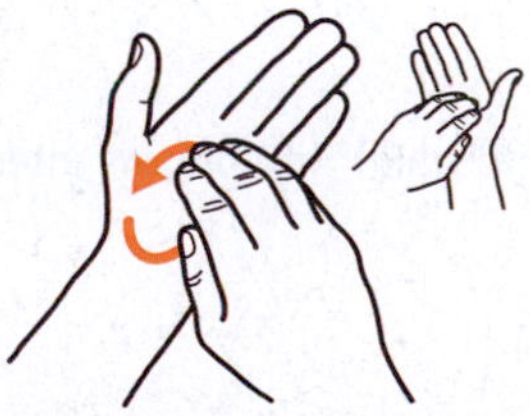

7 Rotational rubbing, backwards and forwards with clasped fingers of right hand in left palm and vice versa;

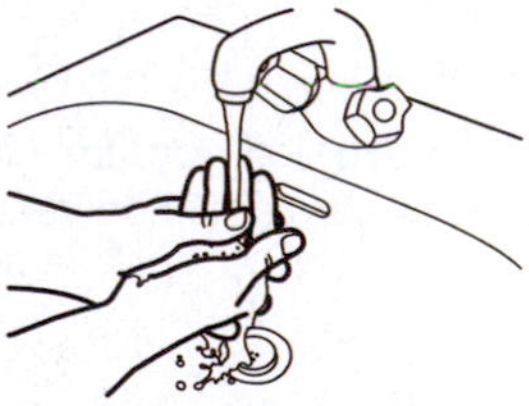

8 Rinse hands with water;

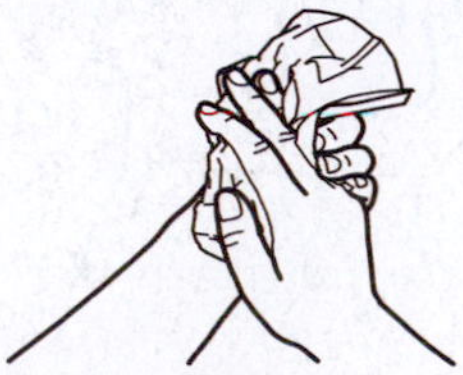

9 Dry hands thoroughly with a single use towel;

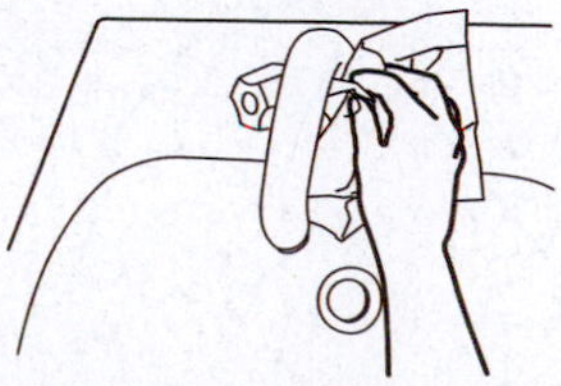

10 Use towel to turn off faucet;

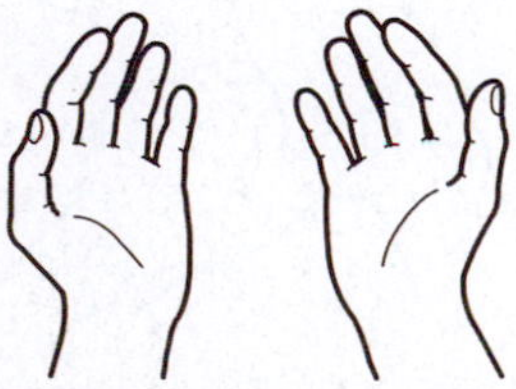

11 Your hands are now safe.

FIGURE 14–1 ◆ WHO hand hygiene technique with soap and water (used by permission).

Source: World Health Organization. (2009). *WHO guidelines on hand hygiene in health care.* Geneva, Switzerland: WHO Publications. Page 156. Retrieved from http://whqlibdoc.who.int/publications/2009/9789241597906_eng.pdf.

Video*: Hand Hygiene—Water with Cleanser **Weblink:** Hand Hygiene in Health Care

Hand Hygiene Technique with Alcohol-Based Formulation

Duration of the entire procedure: 20-30 seconds

1a 1b

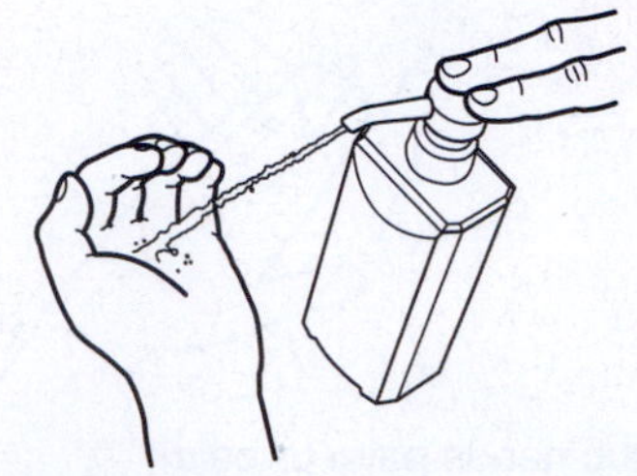

Apply a palmful of the product in a cupped hand, covering all surfaces;

2

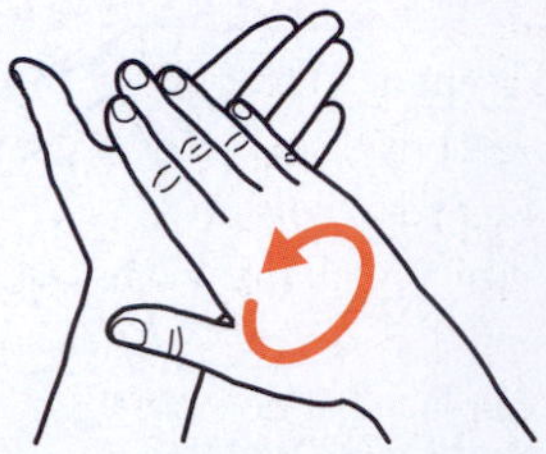

Rub hands palm to palm;

3

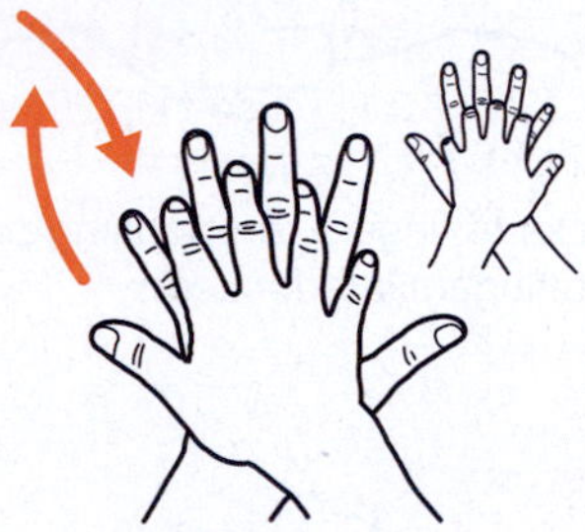

Right palm over left dorsum with interlaced fingers and vice versa;

4

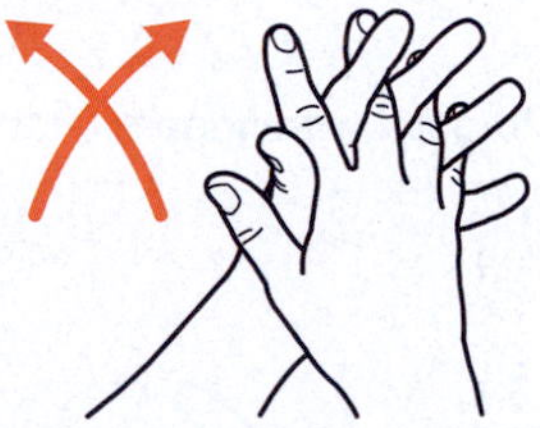

Palm to palm with fingers interlaced;

5

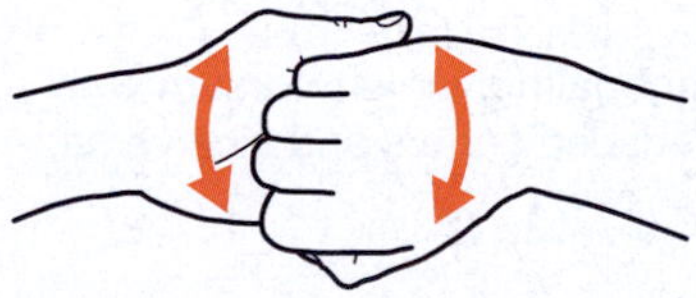

Backs of fingers to opposing palms with fingers interlocked;

6

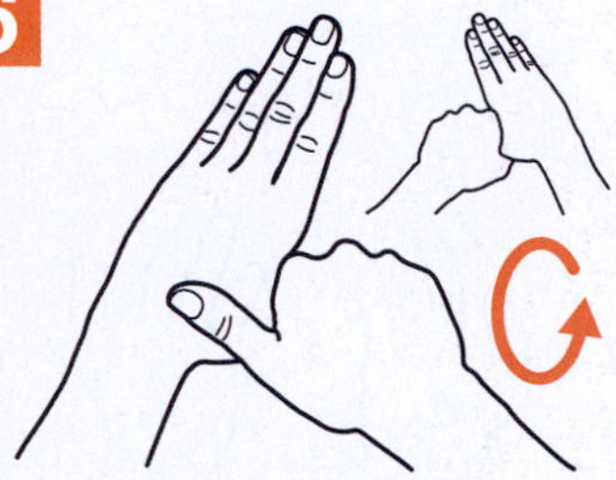

Rotational rubbing of left thumb clasped in right palm and vice versa;

7

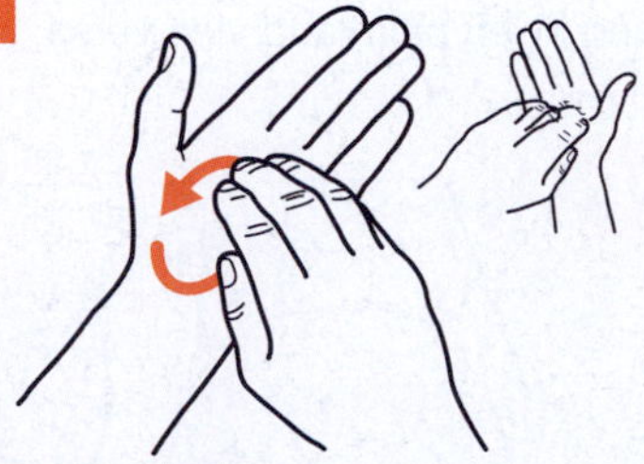

Rotational rubbing, backwards and forwards with clasped fingers of right hand in left palm and vice versa;

8

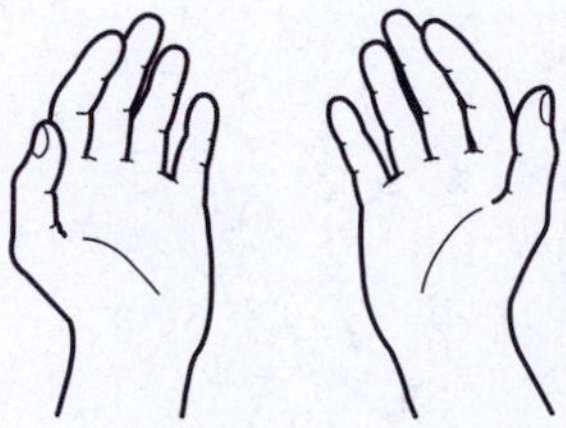

Once dry, your hands are safe.

FIGURE 14–2 ◆ WHO hand hygiene technique with alcohol-based formula (used by permission).

Source: World Health Organization. (2009). *WHO guidelines on hand hygiene in health care.* Geneva, Switzerland: WHO Publications. Page 155. Retrieved from http://whqlibdoc.who.int/publications/2009/9789241597906_eng.pdf.

Infectious Process

Infections can range from mild to debilitating to fatal. The severity of the infection depends on the **pathogenicity,** or disease-causing potential, of the microorganism; the number of invading microorganisms; and the host's defenses. The common sequence of events is known as the chain of infection. All links of the chain must be present for infection to occur. The **chain of infection** consists of a causative agent, a reservoir, a portal of exit, a mode of transmission, a portal of entry, and a susceptible host (Figure 14–3◆).

Chain of Infection

A causative agent or microorganism must exist for infection to occur. This can be any organism that is capable of causing disease. This organism must have a **reservoir,** that is, a place where it can survive and may or may not multiply. Humans can serve as reservoirs, as can inanimate objects such as soil, water, or equipment. Reservoirs can be **carriers** (people or animals that do not have symptoms of infection but carry an active pathogenic microorganism). These individuals can (1) be in a period of incubation or before the onset of symptoms, (2) have a subclinical infection, (3) be recovering from an infection, or (4) be chronic carriers of the pathogen.

There must be a **portal of exit,** or a path that allows the causative agent to escape from the reservoir. The portal of exit is usually associated with the site where the organism grows. Common human portals of exit include the respiratory system, the gastrointestinal system, the genitourinary system, and the skin and mucous membranes. Causative agents can be found in blood, sputum, emesis, stool, urine, wound drainage, and genital secretions. The portal of exit will vary depending on the microorganism.

To leave the reservoir, the organism needs a **mode of transmission,** which is the means by which it travels from the reservoir to a susceptible host. There are four modes of transmission: contact, airborne, vehicle, and vector-borne. *Contact transmission* can occur by direct contact, indirect contact, or droplets. Direct contact occurs when there is actual person-to-person or person-to-source physical contact, as occurs when a sexually transmitted infection is transmitted through sexual activity. Indirect contact involves the susceptible person being exposed to the organism through a contaminated object. An example of indirect contact is exposure to a contaminated dressing or surgical instrument. Droplet transmission occurs when the organism is expelled from its reservoir through the respiratory system in droplets, for instance, when someone sneezes or coughs. These large particles can travel up to 3 feet and can be inhaled by another susceptible person within a 3-foot radius around the person generating the droplets. They set up infection in a new susceptible host by being inhaled.

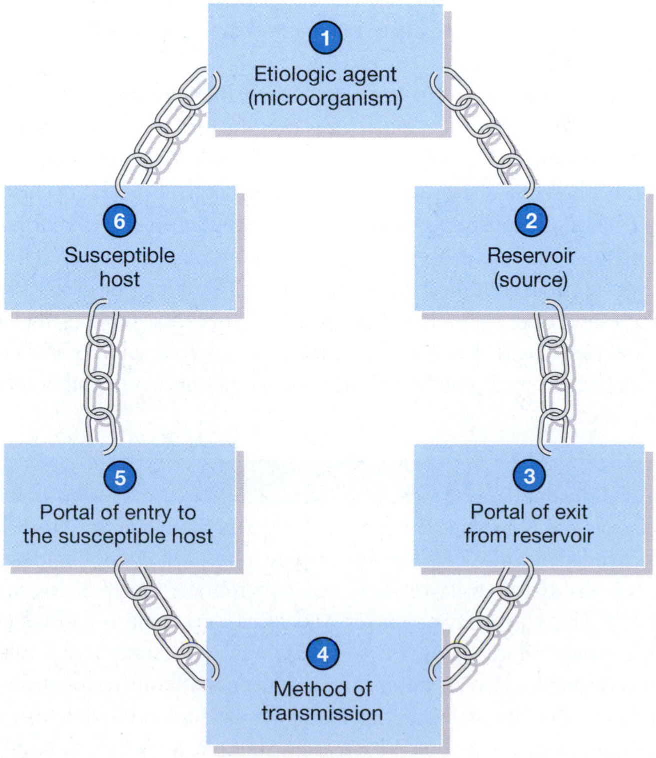

FIGURE 14–3 ◆ Chain of infection.

Airborne transmission occurs when the organism is expelled from the infected person and remains suspended in the air in tiny droplets no larger than 5 microns. These droplets are carried by air currents or on dust and inhaled by the susceptible host. They differ from droplet transmission in that these droplets are small enough to remain suspended in the air for prolonged periods of time. Tuberculosis (TB) is spread by airborne transmission.

Vehicle transmission occurs when the organism's life is maintained on something outside the reservoir until it is passed to the susceptible host. The vehicle is a nonliving object that is not normally harmful but acts as an intermediary for the infectious agent. Pathogenic organisms are contained in contaminated water or food, blood, or other items and transmitted to a susceptible host. This is the method of transmission for hepatitis B, which is transmitted through contaminated blood or blood products or through salmonella infection.

Vector-borne transmission occurs when a disease-producing organism is carried by a living intermediate host that transfers the organism to a susceptible host. Examples of vectors include mosquitoes that carry West Nile virus and ticks that carry Lyme disease.

A **portal of entry** is needed to continue the chain of infection. A portal of entry is the path by which the infective organism enters the new susceptible host. The sites of the portal of entry are usually the same as those for the portal of exit. Once the organism enters a host, the host must be susceptible to infection before an infection will occur. As long as the body's defenses against infection function normally, no infection will occur; however, if the body has weakened defenses and is at increased risk, infection can occur.

Stages of the Infectious Process

Once the organism enters the susceptible host, the infectious disease develops in four stages. The first stage is the incubation period. During the incubation period, the organism is establishing itself. It is replicating and spreading to other organs or tissues in the body but not yet causing symptoms. This stage can pass quickly or last for years; during this time, however, the infected person is contagious. The second stage is the prodromal stage. During the prodromal stage, the symptoms begin to appear. At this point, the symptoms are usually nonspecific, such as general malaise, fever, myalgia, and fatigue.

Acute illness occurs during the third stage. During this stage, the infective organism is growing and spreading rapidly in the body. The microorganisms produce toxins leading to cell lysis and death. An inflammatory response and an immune reaction occur, leading to tissue damage. Along with the vague symptoms, the patient develops more specific symptoms. These include the classic signs of inflammation: swelling, redness, pain, and warmth at the site of infection, along with tachycardia and tachypnea from increased metabolic demands. There are usually other, more specific symptoms related to the site of infection and the virulence of the pathogen. As the infection is contained and the pathogen is confined by the body's defenses, the individual enters the convalescent stage, the damaged tissues begin to heal and symptoms resolve.

An infection can be localized or generalized, and it can be acute or chronic. A localized infection affects the host in a small, focal area, such as an infected cut or laceration, an ear infection, or sinusitis. Proper care can control the spread of the infection and minimize the illness. Symptoms are localized and may include pain and tenderness at the wound site. A generalized or systemic infection indicates involvement of a large part of the body instead of a single organ or part, such as septecimia or bacteremia following a tooth extraction.

Infections are usually acute, which means that symptoms develop quickly and the body's response is temporary. However, infections can become chronic. In a chronic infection, the associated inflammation is covert, with the body trying to heal but the inflammation flaring up intermittently. It is almost like a battle without either the organism or the body's defenses ever gaining the upper hand. Sinusitis may vary between acute and chronic phases, as can hepatitis.

Pathogens That Cause Infectious Disease

Pathogens must be present in the right quantity in a susceptible host to cause infection. The number needed varies according to the pathogen and the host's susceptibility. The severity of the illness depends on the invading organism's pathogenicity. Several factors influence the pathogenicity of an organism, including the pathogen's infectivity or invasiveness, virulence, antigenicity, and viability:

- **Infectivity** or **invasiveness** is the pathogen's ability to enter the host and then live and grow. Some pathogens are capable of producing toxins or enzymes that help them to invade the host and increase their resistance to the host's defenses.
- **Virulence** is related to the severity of disease a pathogen is capable of causing. Virulence can vary depending on the host's ability to mount an immune response. It is expressed as the number of cases of infection that are serious or produce a disability in all those infected.
- **Antigenicity** is the pathogen's ability to elicit an immune defense in the host. It affects the host's ability to develop long-term immunity.
- **Viability** is the pathogen's ability to survive outside of the host. Most pathogens cannot live and grow outside the host.

Human pathogens are divided into different categories of disease-causing agents. These include bacteria, viruses, *Mycoplasma*, rickettsiae, fungi, and parasites.

Bacteria

Bacteria are single-celled microorganisms that have a cell membrane that can be penetrated by antibiotics. Cocci, bacteria that tend to form irregular colonies, can appear in pairs, called diplococci; or chains, such as streptococci; or in clusters, such as staphylococci. They can be rod-shaped bacilli, bacteria, spiral shaped as seen in spirochetes, or curved. Bacteria can be intracellular, such as *Neisseria gonorrhoeae,* or extracellular, such as *Staphylococcus.*

Bacteria can be classified according to their need for oxygen. Aerobic bacteria must have oxygen for survival; anaerobic bacteria, in contrast, can survive without oxygen. Bacteria are also classified according to their ability to be stained with crystal violet in a process known as Gram staining. Some bacteria have a substance in their outer cell wall that absorbs dye. Gram-positive bacteria stain blue when subjected to crystal violet stain; gram-negative bacteria remain colorless. Yet another classification for bacteria refers to their ability to form protective capsules and spores. See Chart 14–2 for classifications of common bacterial diseases.

Bacteria can cause disease in several ways. Gram-negative bacteria have **endotoxins** in their outer cell wall. These endotoxins are produced by live bacteria and are released when the bacteria are killed. Endotoxins stimulate the immune response, which can lead to changes in coagulation of blood and functions of vital body systems. Endotoxins can stimulate regulatory systems in humans, leading to inflammation, bleeding, hypotension, and fever. **Exotoxins** are proteins released by the bacterial cell during growth and have very specific actions. Exotoxins modify cell enzymes and functions, leading to cell death or dysfunction. They are usually named for the site they affect. For example, enterotoxins, toxins specific to the cells of the gastrointestinal mucosa, affect the gastrointestinal tract. Some toxins disrupt cell membranes, causing them to lyse, leading to cell death. Examples of bacteria include *Streptococcus, Staphylococcus, Neisseria gonorrhoeae, Enterococcus,* and *Pseudomonas aeruginosa.*

Viruses

Viruses are the smallest of human pathogens. They occupy the body intracellularly because they require the host cell's genetic material to replicate. Viruses contain a core made up of either RNA or DNA surrounded by a protein coat that helps the virus attach to the host cell. They cannot live and grow outside of a host cell. Viruses are classified according to the type of genetic material they incorporate (RNA or DNA), the type of disease they cause (e.g., hepatitis, herpes), and how they reproduce (e.g., retrovirus) or how they are transmitted (e.g., as an enterovirus or sexually).

Viruses attach to receptors on the host cell membrane and penetrate the cell. Once inside the cell, the virus uses the cell's genetic material to replicate itself. The virus then matures and exits the cell, ready to invade another host cell. The virus causes disease through the process of entering the cell and replicating, which leads to disruption of the cell's normal functions. The virus evokes an immune response against the host cell as it spreads from cell to cell. Most viruses are self-limiting, but viruses can also cause irreversible and lethal injury in a susceptible host. Examples of diseases caused by a virus include the common cold, acquired immunodeficiency syndrome (AIDS), hepatitis, mononucleosis, and herpes simplex.

Mycoplasma

Mycoplasma is a small pathogen that is neither bacteria nor virus. It lives independently and does not require a host cell. It does not have a cell wall but does have a lipid outer membrane (Porth & Matfin, 2009). This characteristic makes *Mycoplasma* resistant to antibiotics that usually attack cell walls. *Mycoplasma* has the ability to kill cells directly and leads to an autoimmune, antigen–antibody response and inflammation. It usually infects the respiratory tract and leads to many serious respiratory problems such as pneumonia. It also is responsible for pharyngitis, urethritis, and pelvic inflammatory disease (Porth & Matfin, 2009).

CHART 14–2 Common Classifications of Bacterial Disease

Organism	Area of the Body
Gram-Positive Cocci	
Staphylococcus aureus	Found in nasopharynx, skin, clothing. Common in subcutaneous and cutaneous abscesses, and foreign devices such as IVs. Frequent cause of osteomyelitis, pneumonia.
Staphylococcus epidermidis	Found commonly on the skin, nasopharynx, and lower genitourinary tract. Infection occurs with indwelling devices that are inserted through the skin, such as catheters. Can be a contaminant of cultures if area not properly disinfected prior to obtaining the culture.
Group A beta-hemolytic streptococci	Found in nose and throat, respiratory secretions, hands. Cause of acute pharyngitis, cutaneous impetigo, and systemic infection.
Gram-Positive Bacilli	
Corynebacterium diphtheriae	Present in nasopharyngeal secretions, respiratory infections, and skin infections. Transmitted by airborne droplets and direct contact with exudates from infected lesions.
Gram-Negative Diplococci	
Neisseria meningitidis	Found in the nasopharynx and transported through the respiratory tract. Causes meningitis.
Gram-Negative Bacilli	
Enterobacteriaceae	Important in nosocomial infections. Can be found in the intestinal tract. Causes lower respiratory tract infections, urinary tract infections, and traveler's diarrhea.
Pseudomonas	Found in the soil, water, raw fruits and vegetables, plants, animals, and man. Causes nosocomial infections. Can affect any body system but frequently seen in moist wounds and upper airways.
Anaerobic Bacteria	
Clostridium difficile	Occurs as an overgrowth in the gut of patients during or after antibiotic therapy. Also transmitted on the hands and unsterilized equipment and is a frequent colonizer of the hospital environment. It can live in the environment for long periods and is able to withstand normal cleaning procedures.

Rickettsiae

Rickettsiae are small, intracellular, gram-negative organisms. They have no cell wall and, therefore, require a host cell to live and multiply. Rickettsiae are transmitted through the bites of arthropods such as ticks, lice, fleas, or mites, or through exposure to the waste products of these organisms. Rickettsiae primarily attack vascular epithelial cells, causing vasculitis. Infections related to rickettsiae include Rocky Mountain spotted fever, typhus, and Q fever.

Fungi

Fungi have a nuclear membrane and a nucleus with several chromosomes. They can reproduce sexually or asexually. Fungi are classified as either molds or yeasts. Molds are organisms with hyphae that produce spores for reproduction. Yeasts are single-celled, oval-shaped organisms that reproduce by budding. Fungal disease is also known as mycosis.

Fungi are found almost everywhere on Earth. They can live in a wide variety of environments and do not necessarily need a host. Temperature is important to the survival of fungi. Some can grow only on cooler surfaces such as the skin; others require warmer core body temperatures. Cutaneous mycosis is caused by skin contact. Systemic mycosis is due to inhalation of the fungi, which are then spread through the lymphatic system. Examples of cutaneous mycosis include candidiasis, tinea pedis, and tinea capitis. Examples of systemic mycosis include cryptococcosis, histoplasmosis, and aspergillosis.

Parasites

Parasites are pathogens that infect and cause disease in other animals. Protozoa and helminths belong to this classification. Protozoa are small, single-celled animals that can be transmitted to the host by direct or indirect contact. They are mainly transmitted through ingested food or water or through an arthropod vector. They reproduce inside the host and are easily mobile in the body. Once inside, they stimulate an inflammatory response or cause disease by ingesting and/or invading human tissue.

Helminths are multicellular parasites. They require intermediate hosts and cannot reproduce inside the human host. Therefore, many exposures are required before a human can be infected. Helminths are transmitted by ingestion of eggs, breaks in the skin, or arthropod vectors. Like protozoa, helminths stimulate an inflammatory response. Infestation by helminths can lead to malnutrition and anemia in the host because they compete with the host for nutrients in the gastrointestinal tract.

Defense Mechanisms

Most human beings have defenses against infectious disease, including physical, chemical, and immune mechanisms. Whether or not an organism causes disease depends, in part, on the success or failure of these mechanisms. They include the skin, which acts as a protective barrier; enzymes that kill microorganisms; structures such as cilia that trap microorganisms and sweep them out of the bronchial tubes; membranes that secrete mucus to prevent the adherence of the organisms; chemical secretions such as hydrochloric acid in the stomach; and the immune system, which produces enzymes and uses other factors and cells to trap and kill microorganisms. Chart 14–3 lists human defenses against infection. Chapters 52 and 53 address immune assessment and immune response.

CHART 14–3 Defense Mechanisms Against Infection

Mechanism	Purpose
Skin	Offers a protective barrier of five to seven layers, with the top layer being shed constantly.
Mucous membranes	Lines orifices of body that are open to the environment; trap microorganisms; contain bacteriostatic agents; and secrete IgA, an immunoglobulin that fights infection by protecting mucous membranes from invading organisms. Help to wash out microorganisms and prevent them from adhering to mucosal surfaces.
Respiratory cilia	Traps microorganisms and sweeps them up and out of the respiratory tract.
Secretions of oil and moisture from glands	Inhibits penetration of pathogens; inhibits pathogen growth.
Normal flora	Flora that normally exists in the gastrointestinal tract and vagina and competes with pathogens for placement.
Chemical secretions	Gastric acid and acidic urine, which creates an atmosphere that is not conducive to the growth of microorganisms.

Inflammation

The body has physiological responses that eliminate invading organisms and protect against infection. The inflammatory response is a physiological process that attacks, confines, and kills invading organisms. It is a nonspecific response; the same steps occur no matter what the pathogen. It also allows for tissue repair after damage from an invading organism or from tissue injury and death. The steps in the inflammatory process, which involves a vasular phase and a cellular phase, are diagramed in Figure 14–4◆.

The vascular phase consists of the following processes, which occur almost simultaneously:

- temporary vasoconstriction to avoid blood loss after injury;
- vasodilation to increase blood supply to the area, leading to redness and increased warmth of the area;
- increased hydrostatic pressure related to the increase in blood flow;
- increased permeability of blood vessel walls caused by chemical mediators; and
- leakage of fluid and cells out of capillaries into interstitial spaces so that toxins are diluted.

This leakage of fluid and eventually protein leads to increased osmotic pressure in the interstitial spaces and edema.

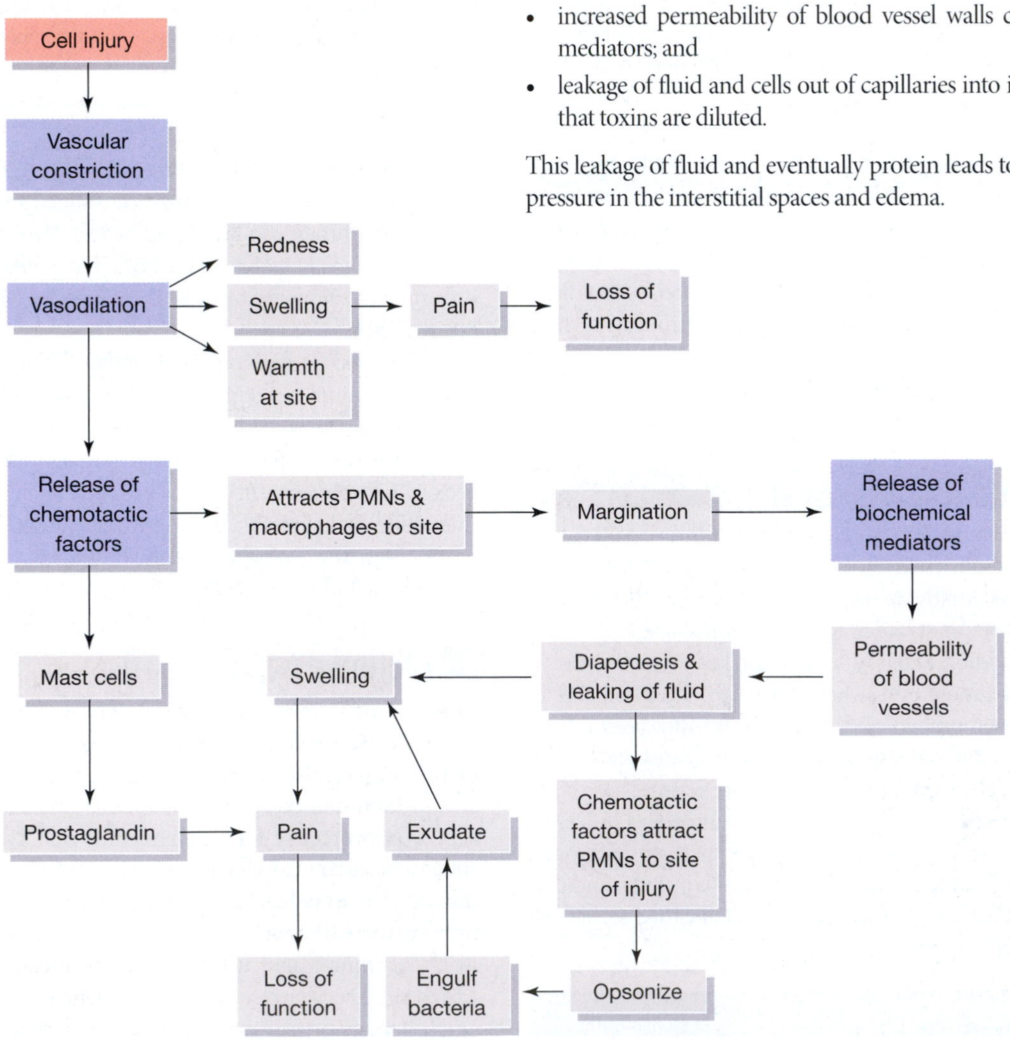

FIGURE 14–4 ◆ Steps in the inflammatory process.

The cellular phase involves the response of white blood cells (WBCs) to the cellular injury. It begins as chemotactic substances are released from the tissues by cellular injury and complement is activated. There are five types of WBCs: neutrophils, eosinophils, basophils, lymphocytes, and monocytes. Neutrophils are a form of granulocyte filled with tiny sacs of enzymes that help the cell to kill and digest microorganisms that have been engulfed or ingested by phagocytosis. They are the first type of WBC to arrive at the site of inflammation or infection to begin their job of ingesting bacteria. This process is described in Chapters 55 and 56. The inflammatory phase of wound healing is discussed in Chapter 60.

Manifestations of Inflammation

The signs and symptoms related to inflammation can be local and/or systemic depending on the location and severity of the inflammatory response. There are five cardinal local symptoms of inflammation: (1) redness from increased blood flow to the area, (2) heat due to increased blood flow to the area, (3) swelling due to the fluid exudates that form in the interstitial tissue, (4) pain caused by the pressure of the exudates and release of chemicals that irritate nerve endings, and (5) loss of function related to the pain and swelling.

The major systemic symptoms are fever and leukocytosis. Fever occurs because of the release of endogenous pyrogens, substances that induce fever, at the site of inflammation. These endogenous pyrogens consist of substances such as prostaglandins and leukotrienes from injured cells and WBCs that accumulate at the site. These substances are carried to the temperature-regulating center in the hypothalamus, where an increased temperature is stimulated. Fever is part of the body's defense mechanism and helps to fight infections.

Leukocytosis is a systemic sign of inflammation that is stimulated by the release of leukopoietins from damaged cells. Leukopoietins stimulate the increased production of WBCs and the release of mature neutrophils by the bone marrow. As inflammation continues, the bone marrow releases immature neutrophils known as bands to help meet the body's needs. An increase in the number of bands on a differential WBC count is known as a shift to the left and indicates an ongoing acute inflammation. WBC response to infection and inflammation is discussed further in Chapter 53.

Immune Responses

The immune responses are the body's specific reactions to being invaded by foreign materials. The immune responses are complex and not completely understood. However, it is known that they work to defend the body against agents that are able to produce infection.

The immune responses can be divided into two types: humoral immunity and cellular immunity. The humoral response involves the antigen–antibody reactions; the cellular response involves the reaction of the WBCs. Cellular and humoral defenses against infection also are discussed in Chapter 54.

Humoral Immunity

Foreign materials are called **antigens,** and the body responds to them by producing antibodies. These antigen–antibody responses are part of the humoral immune response. The humoral response is mediated by activated helper T cells that induce growth and differentiation of B lymphocytes. When B lymphocytes encounter an antigen, they are stimulated to differentiate into antibody-producing cells called plasma cells that secrete antigen-specific antibodies. These antibodies bind with the antigen-forming antigen–antibody complexes. The antibodies present the antigen to the T lymphocytes for identification and processing. These complexes serve to neutralize the bacterial toxins and viruses, lyse and destroy pathogens, and facilitate phagocytosis. Phagocytic cells can bind, engulf, and digest antigen–antibody complexes more effectively than is possible when the antigen is alone.

Cellular Immunity

The cellular immune response is a complex process involving an increase in the number of lymphocytes and macrophages in response to the invading organism. T cells mature in the thymus and in the process of growing become able to recognize specific antigens through the growth of antigen-specific receptors. After exposure to the antigens, the production of helper T cells is stimulated. This, in turn, increases the production of cytotoxic T cells and natural killer cells that enhance the engulfment and killing of the antigen directly by macrophages.

Increased Susceptibility to Infection

Some known factors make an individual more susceptible to infection. For instance, individuals who are very old or very young have an increased susceptibility to infection. For the very young, the immune system is not fully developed until about the age of 6 months. Susceptibility to childhood infections increases as children are exposed to pathogens at day care facilities and schools. In the older adult, the immune system weakens as a result of decreasing thymus gland function. Changes in lymphocytes may occur as people age, contributing to decreased defenses. It is known that some of the lymphocytes important to immunity become less responsive in the older adult, whereas others function normally.

Immunodeficiencies involve impaired functioning of one or more components of the immune response or inflammatory process. The failure of these defense mechanisms can be caused by a genetic abnormality or by an acquired abnormality such as cancer or human immunodeficiency virus (HIV). An immunodeficiency can lead to abnormal lymphocyte development, prevention of stem cell maturation into T or B cells, or a decrease in the production of a specific class of immunoglobulin. Regardless of the cause, a failure in the immune system will lead to a tendency to develop unusual or recurrent severe infections. Immunodeficiency should be considered when an individual has frequent severe, documented infections such as otitis media, pneumonia, candidiasis, or meningitis. It also should be suggested when the infections are unusual such as *Pneumocystis carinii*.

Defense mechanisms can be improved through lifestyle changes. Good hygiene is important in maintaining strong defense mechanisms. Skin that is unclean serves as a medium for bacterial growth and is more likely to allow invasion of microorganisms. Dust in the environment can serve as a reservoir for pathogens and helps with transportation of pathogens into the body. A balanced diet helps the body maintain an effective immune system by providing the nutrients needed for growth of new, healthy tissue. Protein is needed for the production of antibodies and the functioning of the immune system. Vitamins and minerals are also important to help the body digest and utilize nutrients so that cells can grow and remain strong. Individuals may develop a weakened immune system from chronic stress or chronic illness such as diabetes mellitus or chronic obstructive pulmonary disease.

People with known immunodeficiencies should be protected from infection. It may be unsafe or even fatal to administer certain types of immunizations or perform even simple procedures such as drawing blood on these individuals. Therefore, nurses should take care to avoid transmitting infectious organisms. An in-depth discussion of immunosuppression and immunodeficiency is included in Chapter 53.

Weblink: Guideline for Hand Hygiene in Health-Care Settings

Weblink: National Healthcare Safety Network Overview

Infection Prevention and Control

When an infection is acquired outside a health care facility, it is considered a **community-acquired infection.** When it occurs in a hospitalized patient, the infection is known as a **health-care-associated infection (HAI).** Health care facilities are prime reservoirs for the development and transfer of infectious organisms. HAIs, also referred to as nosocomial infections, are the cause of numerous complications in the hospitalized patient, leading to a cost of lives and health care dollars. Patients who develop HAIs often are critically ill with weakened defenses and an increased susceptibility to infection.

Many infections in the hospital are related to the use of invasive devices such as urinary catheters, intravenous catheters, surgical drains, nasogastric tubes, and endotracheal tubes. Because invasive devices increase susceptibility to infection, they should be used only when necessary for patient care and should be discontinued as quickly as possible. Clean or sterile technique should be used in caring for anyone with invasive devices in order to avoid infection. HAIs also may occur when broad-spectrum antibiotics are overused. These antibiotics alter the body's natural defenses and may lead to antibiotic resistance in harmful bacteria. Many of these infections are caused by multidrug-resistant organisms. The National Healthcare Safety Network (NHSN) system, a voluntary, hospital-based reporting system, was formed in 1970 by the Centers for Disease Control and Prevention (CDC) to create a national database of HAIs (CDC, 2010). The goals of NHSN are to: collect surveillance data, analyze and report surveillance data in order to identify trends, provide hospitals with data for comparison, assist hospitals in developing surveillance and analysis methods, and conduct collaborative research studies with NHSN hospitals. A complete description of these goals can be found on the NHSN website.

The NHSN's HAI database is used to (1) describe the epidemiology of HAIs, (2) describe antimicrobial resistance trends, and (3) produce HAI rates to use for comparison purposes. This information is used to help infection preventionists and hospital epidemiologists develop guidelines for prevention, timely recognition, and prompt intervention with appropriate infection prevention and control measures. The data show that urinary tract infections are the leading type of infection in hospitalized patients (Torrey, 2011). The respiratory tract, bloodstream, and surgical wounds are other common sites and are the most frequently monitored for the occurrence of infection. Although the rates of infection have decreased during the last 10 years, the prevention of infection in hospitalized patients remains part of the national health objectives for 2020 (U.S. Department of Health and Human Services [DHHS], 2010). Many actions can be taken to control and prevent infection. This is particularly relevant to health care facilities where HAI rates are as high as 30% in intensive care units (Teltsch, Hanley, Loo, Goldberg, Gurshaney, & Buckeridge, 2011).

Hand Hygiene

The single most important factor in the control and prevention of infection is good hand hygiene. Inadequate hand hygiene is considered the leading cause of HAIs and the spread of multidrug-resistant organisms. Hand hygiene is performed to remove dirt, organic material, and transient microorganisms and to prevent the spread of organisms leading to infection. The nurse's hands are contaminated daily simply through exposure to skin, patient gowns, bed linen, bedside furniture, and other objects in the patient's immediate environment that are contaminated with the patient's flora. Simple activities such as lifting a patient, taking a patient's pulse, or touching a hand or shoulder can result in contamination of the hands enough to spread infection to others. It is important to perform hand hygiene before and after patient contact. Other indications for hand hygiene include: following contact with body fluids and wound dressings, after removing gloves, before invasive procedures are performed, and when hands are moved from a contaminated body site to a clean body site during patient care.

The CDC has determined that alcohol-based products (70% ethanol) are more effective for hand antisepsis by health care workers (HCWs) than are soap and water or antimicrobial soaps (CDC, 2002). Alcohol-based products also have been shown to be less drying to skin with use over time.

The compliance of health care workers with hand hygiene recommendations is less than 50% (McGuckin, Waterman, & Govednik, 2009). The Joint Commission's National Patient Safety Goals (2010) include a requirement that hospitals implement a hand hygiene program that follows either the CDC guidelines or the guidelines of the World Health Organization (WHO). This program must include monitoring and improvement of compliance with hand hygiene based on established goals (The Joint Commission, 2010). Studies have shown that monitoring and publication of hand hygiene compliance rates do lead to improvement (Allegranzi & Pittet, 2009).

Health care workers often perform hand hygiene incorrectly and do not use it frequently enough. When using an alcohol-based product, the hands should be rubbed for 20 to 30 seconds. When using soap and water, the hands should be washed for at least 15 seconds, covering all surfaces of the hands and fingers so that nothing is missed. This allows time for the antimicrobial products to work. The area around and under the fingernails contains higher microbial counts and should be washed thoroughly. All debris should be removed from under the fingernails. (This is done by pursing all five fingers together, placing the fingertips in the palm of the other hand, and twisting back and forth, then repeating with the other hand.) The hands are then thoroughly rinsed to remove soap residue and then thoroughly dried. Microorganisms can be transferred more easily on wet hands than on hands that have been completely dried. Refer to Figures 14–1 and 14–2 to see the WHO recommended procedures for hand hygiene using soap and water and alcohol-based products.

Safety Alert *Alcohol-based preparations are not effective against* Clostridium difficile. *To prevent the spread of* C. difficile, *hand hygiene must be performed with antibacterial soap and water. For patients with this infection, most hospitals have adopted a symbol that accompanies the isolation sign outside the patient's door to indicate that soap and water must be used.*

Health care facilities have made alcohol-based hand rubs readily available by providing containers to be carried in the nurse's pocket for use at the patient's bedside or close to areas of patient care. Alcohol-based cleaners are not adequate, however, when there is visible dirt or contamination with protein-containing materials. Other antiseptic agents that are used for hand hygiene include chlorhexidine gluconate (CHG), hexachlorophene, and chloroxylenol. These agents work more slowly than alcohol but have effective residual effects. In addition, agents such as CHG have residual antimicrobial effects, unlike alcohol products.

The wearing of rings and artificial fingernails can contribute to the spread of infectious organisms (World Health Organization [WHO], 2009). Rings may increase the pathogen counts on the skin; the more rings that are worn, the greater the contamination. Therefore, rings should be avoided. Artificial nails are more likely to encourage the growth of microorganisms than are natural nails and should not be used when caring for patients at high risk for infection. Natural nails should be short enough to allow for thorough cleaning underneath the nail and to prevent tears in gloves. Microorganisms can be found in higher concentrations in subungual, under the nail, areas. Nail polish does not increase the microorganism count; however, chipped nail polish does support the growth of microorganisms on the hands. Most hospital dress codes now prohibit the wearing of artificial nails or nail extensions by any health care worker who has direct contact with patients.

Hand hygiene is important whether or not gloves are used. However, gloves do provide a protective barrier against the transmission of microbes and prevent heavy contamination of the hands. Some transmission can still occur because gloves may have small defects or be torn during use. The hands can also be contaminated during glove removal. Therefore, hand washing with soap and water or the use of an antiseptic hand rub is required after glove removal. Nurses should change their gloves between patients and between contaminated body sites. Single-use disposable gloves should not be reused.

Hand washing can lead to dermatitis from the frequent contact with water and cleansing agents. The cracked, dry skin associated with dermatitis is more readily colonized with pathogens. The tenderness of dry, cracked skin also can lead to the avoidance of hand washing. Therefore, it is important to prevent or correct hand dermatitis. Currently, the Occupational Safety and Health Administration (OSHA) recommends avoiding the use of petroleum-based moisturizers because they can cause latex gloves to deteriorate (OSHA, 2011). The use of an appropriate moisturizer that contains humectants, a substance used to help retain water, along with fats and oils can increase skin hydration, providing a protective skin barrier without interfering with gloves or antibacterial agents. The use of tepid water rather than hot water is also recommended to help prevent hand dermatitis and the spread of pathogens.

Patient Placement in the Hospital Setting

Proper placement of a patient with an infection in the hospital setting can be a significant factor in preventing the spread of infection. A private room is the best solution, especially if the infected patient has poor hygiene or cannot assist in implementing precautions to avoid transmission of the microorganisms. A recent study showed that when an ICU changed from a multibed arrangement to all private rooms, the acquisition of HAIs dropped by half (Teltsch, et al., 2011).

Protective Equipment

The use of personal protective equipment (PPE) such as gloves, gowns, and masks plays an important role in the prevention of the spread of pathogens. Protective gowns help prevent the contamination of clothing and protect the skin and clothing of wearers from exposure to blood and body fluids. Gowns can help prevent the transmission of pathogens from patients or equipment in the environment to other patients or equipment. The Healthcare Infection Control Practices Advisory Committee (HICPAC) of the CDC recommends the use of gowns and gloves to prevent HAIs. Nurses must wear gowns that are impervious to fluids when performing procedures that may involve fluids. Gowns should be tied at the neck and waist, not left hanging or drooping. They should always be removed before leaving the patient's room, and hand hygiene performed.

Health care personnel should wear masks, as well as face shields or eye shields, when performing procedures that are likely to cause splashing or spraying of blood or body fluids. These precautions protect the mucous membranes of the eyes, nose, and mouth from exposure to pathogens. When a patient with an infection that is spread by airborne organisms or droplets leaves her room, she should wear a surgical mask.

Housekeeping practices should be observed to decrease dust and environmental reservoirs of pathogens. Spills of blood and body fluids must be cleaned up immediately with hospital disinfectant or household bleach and water. Reusable equipment such as blood pressure cuffs and stethoscopes can also carry pathogens from patient to patient. Stethoscopes can be disinfected with isopropyl alcohol or other antimicrobial solution, or the health care provider can use disposable covers between patients. Before and after each shift and between patients, the bell, diaphragm, and earpieces of stethoscopes need to be wiped down with alcohol or another antibacterial solution. All equipment used in treating patients in isolation should be left in the room for use only with that patient. If not possible, any equipment that is removed from the room must be disinfected with hospital-grade disinfectant before being used with another patient.

Disposal of Soiled Equipment

Appropriate disposal of used and/or contaminated equipment is essential both to protect health care workers and to prevent the spread of disease. Linens should be changed in such a way that there is little contact between the dirty linens and the nurse's uniform. Linens are to be carried away from the nurse's body and placed in an appropriate hamper. Throwing dirty linen on the floor or laying it in a chair should be avoided because it could lead to further contamination of the environment. Linens should never be shaken in the air because that creates air currents that spread pathogens. Needles and syringes should be disposed of in a container specifically made for disposal of sharp objects. Inadvertent sticks with used sharps can lead to pathogen exposure.

Isolation Precautions

In 2007, the Healthcare Infection Control Practices Advisory Committee (HICPAC), updated their isolation precautions (Siegel, Rhinehart, Jackson, Chiarello, & HICPAC, 2007). HICPAC's guidelines follow a two-tiered program. The first tier involves standard precautions designed to reduce the risk of transmission of pathogens from blood and body fluids that contain blood. Patients with HIV or hepatitis B often have no apparent symptoms but can transmit the disease to others. Therefore, standard precautions apply to all hospitalized patients regardless of their diagnosis. The HICPAC guidelines are designed to control the spread of these diseases as well as other HAIs. The HICPAC guidelines should be used by all health care workers who have direct or indirect contact with patients or with their body fluids. This includes not only nurses and health care providers, but also the people who empty trash, change linens, or clean the room. Standard precautions apply to blood, body fluids and secretions, nonintact skin, and mucous membranes. The National Guidelines for Standard and

Weblink: Laboratory Safety: Latex Allergy
Weblink: The Hands Give It Away
Video*: PPE for Standard Precautions: Eyewear, Protective

Weblink: Healthcare-Associated Infections
Weblink: Preventing Transmission of Infectious Agents in Healthcare Setting
Video*: PPE for Standard Precautions: Gloves, Non-Sterile

NATIONAL GUIDELINES for Standard and Transmission-Based Precautions

Category	Precaution
Standard Precautions	
Hand hygiene	Perform hand hygiene after touching blood, body fluids, secretions, excretions, and contaminated items, whether or not gloves are worn.
Gloves	Wear clean, nonsterile gloves when touching blood, body fluids, secretions, excretions, and contaminated items. Put on clean gloves just before touching mucous membranes and nonintact skin.
Mask, eye protection, face shield	Wear a mask, eye protection, or face shield to protect mucous membranes of the eyes, nose, and mouth during procedures and patient care activities that generate splashes or sprays of blood, body fluids, secretions, or excretions.
Gown	Wear a clean, nonsterile gown to protect skin and prevent soiling of clothing during procedures and patient care activities that may generate splashes or sprays of blood, body fluids, secretions, or excretions. Gowns should be impervious to fluids.
Patient care equipment	Handle used patient care equipment that is soiled with blood, body fluids, secretions, or excretions in a manner that prevents exposure of skin and mucous membrane, contamination of clothing, and transfer of microorganisms to other patients and environments.
Environmental control	Adequate procedures should be in place for routine care, cleaning, and disinfection of environmental surfaces.
Linen	Handle soiled linen in a manner that prevents skin and mucous membrane exposure and contamination of clothing.
Occupational health and bloodborne pathogens	Prevent injuries when using and disposing of needles, scalpels, and other sharp instruments or devices. Never recap needles or use any technique that involves pointing the sharp end toward part of the body. Use mouthpieces, resuscitation bags, or other ventilation devices as an alternative to mouth-to-mouth resuscitation.
Patient placement	Place a patient who may contaminate the environment in a private room, if possible. If this is not possible, place patients with the same diagnosis in the same room.
Transmission-Based Precautions	
Airborne precautions	1. Place the patient in a private airborne infection isolation room (AIIR) with monitored negative air pressure, 6 to 12 air changes per hour, and appropriate discharge of air to the outdoors. Keep the room door closed and the patient in the room. 2. Wear a National Institute for Occupational Safety and Health (NIOSH)-approved N95 respirator mask that has been fit-tested by you when entering the room. 3. If leaving the room, the patient should wear a surgical mask. 4. Limit the movement and transport of the patient from the room.
Droplet precautions	1. Place the patient in a private room or in a room with cohort patients with the same disease. 2. Wear a mask when working within 3 feet of the patient. 3. If leaving the room, the patient should wear a mask. 4. Limit movement and transport of the patient from the room.
Contact precautions	1. Place the patient in a private room or with a very low-risk roommate. 2. Wear gloves when entering the room and remove gloves before leaving the room. Then perform hand hygiene. 3. Wear a gown when entering the room and remove the gown before leaving the room. 4. Limit the movement and transport of the patient from the room. 5. Dedicate the use of noncritical patient care equipment to a single patient.

Source: Siegel, J. D., Rhinehart, E., Jackson, M., Chiarello, L., & the Healthcare Infection Control Practices Advisory Committee. (2007, June). Guideline for isolation precautions: Preventing transmission of infectious agents in healthcare settings 2007. Retrieved from http://www.cdc.gov/ncidod/dhqp/pdf/guidelines/Isolation2007.pdf.

Transmission-Based Precautions box lists the HICPAC standard precautions (Siegel et al., 2007).

The second tier is the transmission-based precautions, also outlined in the National Guidelines box. These precautions are for patients "known or suspected to be infected by highly transmissible or epidemiologically important pathogens" (Siegel et al., 2007). They are used in addition to standard precautions and are classified into three types: airborne precautions, droplet precautions, and contact precautions (CDC, 2007). These precautions can be used either singly or in combination for diseases that have multiple routes of transmission.

Airborne precautions are designed to protect against infectious agents that are transmitted through particles that remain suspended in the air and can become inhaled or deposited on a host. These precautions require the use of special ventilation and air handling in an airborne infection isolation room (AIIR). This is a room with negative air pressure and an increased number of air changes, with the air discharged to the outside and no recirculation of the air in the room. If the air is recirculated, the return air must be filtered through a high-efficiency particulate air (HEPA) filter (CDC, 2007). Personal respiratory protection or a mask is indicated for anyone who enters the room when caring for the patient. Precautions include the use of a National Institute for Occupational Safety and Health (NIOSH)-approved N95 particulate respirator with qualitative fit testing of the respirator required. Use of these engineering controls is needed for TB, varicella (and disseminated varicella-zoster), measles, and smallpox.

Droplet precautions protect against the risk of transmission of infection through droplets in the air. Infected droplets can make contact with the conjunctivae or the mucous membranes of the nose or mouth. They are generated primarily during talking, coughing, or sneezing by someone who is infected with the organism. These droplets do not remain suspended in the air, and they travel only short distances (usually 3 feet or less); therefore, special air handling is not required. The wearing of masks is important when working closely with a patient during procedures such as suctioning, particularly with patients with meningitis or diphtheria.

Contact precautions reduce the risk of organism transmission by direct or indirect contact. Direct contact occurs when there is skin-to-skin contact such as might occur when turning or bathing a patient or even touching an infected patient's hand. Transmission could also occur from an infected patient to a susceptible patient if the patients shake hands or touch in some way. Indirect contact involves contact of a host with a contaminated intermediate object in the patient's environment. Contact precautions involve wearing gloves and gowns and dedicating the use of equipment to a single patient. This type of precaution would be necessary in caring for a patient with *C. difficile* infection or a major abscess.

Patients who are immunocompromised may be at high risk of developing infections, especially if they are severely neutropenic with an absolute neutrophil count of less than 500 cells/mm^3 (cubic millimeter) (Porth & Matfin, 2009). This may occur in patients who have had a transplant or have leukemia. These patients must be in a protective environment that minimizes exposures to pathogens. Of course, the standard isolation precautions are observed. The length of time this patient is outside the room for diagnostic procedures or other activities must be limited. If the patient must be outside the room, respiratory protection should be provided. The room should be kept very clean and without dust. All visitors and health care workers should perform hand hygiene carefully before entering the room or touching the patient. No one with any type of infection should be allowed to enter the room.

Immunization Programs

Prevention is the best approach to avoiding infection, and prevention can occur anywhere along the chain of infection. Efforts to prevent infection include anything from eradication of infectious agents to eliminating the reservoirs for infection to eliminating a vector that carries the disease. One method used to eliminate the risk for some infections is immunization. Active or passive immunization improves the host's defenses. **Active immunization** involves the introduction of a live, killed, or attenuated toxin of a disease organism into the body. The immune system responds by producing antibodies. Having produced the antibodies, the immune system will recognize the threat of another toxin attack. Active immunization provides long-term and possibly lifelong immunity, although some vaccines require boosters to maintain the immunity. Active immunizations include those for measles, mumps, hepatitis B, and hepatitis A.

Passive immunization provides immunity for a short period of time, usually around 6 to 12 weeks. This involves the injection of already formed antibodies into the body. The individual may still have the disease, but it will be a less severe case. An example of this type of immunity is immunoglobin injections given to people who have been exposed to hepatitis A. The recommendations regarding immunizations are based on scientific knowledge of the principles of active and passive immunization, the epidemiology and burden of disease, the safety of vaccines, and the cost analysis of preventive measures.

Certain benefits and risks are associated with immunizations. No vaccine is completely safe or 100% effective. Benefits include protection against the consequences of disease to the individual and to society as a whole. This protection includes not having to experience the symptoms of the illness, improved quality of life and productivity, and prevention of death. The risks of immunization include common, minor, and local adverse effects and rare, severe, and life-threatening conditions. The recommendations for immunizations represent a balance of the benefits for each person and society against the potential risks and problems associated with vaccinations. Vaccination schedules have been developed based on age-specific risks for disease, age-specific risks for complications, ability of an individual to respond to the vaccine, and potential interference with the immune response by passively transferred maternal antibodies. Studies have demonstrated that recommended ages and intervals between doses of multiple-dose antigens provide optimal protection or have the best evidence of efficacy. The immunization schedule for children is revised annually and published each year in January by the Centers for Disease Control and Prevention (CDC, 2011). The schedule for adolescents and adults is revised less frequently, except for influenza vaccine recommendations, which are published annually.

Although immunizations are relatively safe, there are some contraindications, and certain precautions should be followed. A contraindication is any condition that increases the risk for a serious adverse reaction. Most adverse reactions are temporary, and the vaccination can be given at a later time. The only true contraindication that is applicable to all vaccines is a history of a severe allergic reaction after a prior dose of vaccine or to a vaccine constituent. For example, a person who has an anaphylactic allergy to egg protein should not receive the influenza vaccine because the vaccine is grown on egg embryos and may contain a small amount of egg protein. If a recipient has a condition that might increase the risk for a serious adverse reaction or might compromise the vaccine's ability to produce immunity, precautions should be followed. For example, individuals with mild, acute illness such as diarrhea or upper respiratory tract infection can be safely vaccinated, while individuals with moderate or severe illness should be vaccinated as soon as possible after they have recovered from the acute illness.

All vaccines may cause adverse reactions that may be local, systemic, or allergic. Local reactions are the least severe and mainly involve redness or soreness at the site. Systemic reactions, fever, occur less frequently. Serious allergic reactions such as anaphylaxis are rare.

Nursing Management

Nursing management of a patient with an infection requires assessment of the patient and development of a specific plan to meet the individual patient's needs. Nursing care should be well planned and adapted as necessary so that the patient receives high-quality care, further infection is prevented, and infections are not transmitted to others. Nursing assessment is essential to identify potential complications and responses to treatment.

Assessment

When assessing the patient with an infection, the nurse should take into account the signs and symptoms of the infection, the site of the infection, the pathogenicity of the organism, and the body's immune response. A thorough assessment will help identify the infection and/or its complications so that appropriate therapy can be implemented.

Video*: PPE for Standard Precautions:Gown, Applying Non-Sterile

Weblink: 2012 Immunization Schedules

Fever

One feature common to most infections is a fever. Fever, defined as a body temperature of more than 38°C (100°F), indicates the severity of the inflammatory response in the patient who has an intact immune response. Fever is induced by mediators known as endogenous pyrogens that act directly on the hypothalamic regulating center that controls the body's temperature. Fever can be beneficial because some microorganisms are very sensitive to changes in temperature and cannot survive when temperatures go up. Fever can also be present when no infectious process is occurring, such as with malignancy or myocardial infarction. In these cases, the injured cells produce endogenous pyrogens, resulting in a fever.

Although a fever can have beneficial effects, a fever of 40°C (104°F) can be harmful. *Hyperpyrexia,* an elevated body temperature, leads to an increased metabolic rate, which increases the demand for oxygen and the need for calories. This is associated with tachycardia and tachypnea. These conditions put an increased workload on the heart and lungs and can lead to impaired function. In addition, the increased need for calories can lead to protein breakdown for energy. With the increase in temperature, diaphoresis increases; this can lead to dehydration.

The assessment of fever can provide information about the possible cause of the infection. The pattern of fever occurrence should be observed. Fever can be described as intermittent, remittent, sustained, or relapsing. An intermittent fever is defined as a fever that is cyclical; the temperature goes up and then returns to normal at least once in 24 hours. The remittent fever is one in which the fever stays elevated throughout the day but can vary a few degrees. Sustained fever is a continuous fever that has very little variation. A relapsing fever resolves but returns after a period of time during which the infection was thought to be resolved. A fever that lasts 2 weeks or more without identification of the cause is known as a **fever of unknown origin (FUO).**

Safety Alert *A fever of 40.5°C (105°F) can cause or worsen cardiac and pulmonary problems and also cause febrile seizures, although these are rare in adults. The health care provider should be alerted immediately if a fever this high develops, so appropriate interventions can be prescribed.*

Patient History

When assessing the patient, either for a risk of infection or the presence of an infection or fever, the first step is to take a history. A thorough history can help to identify the cause of the infection and can direct the focus for the physical examination and diagnostic tests. The first part of a patient history is the history of present illness. This section should provide an in-depth view of the patient's problem. One way to remember what should be included in the history of present illness is the mnemonic OLD CARTS (Chart 14–4). It is usually beneficial to begin with a general question such as "What brought you here?" Then direct the patient—without putting words in the patient's mouth—so that pertinent information is obtained.

CHART 14–4 History of Present Illness: OLD CARTS

The **OLD CARTS** mnemonic can be used to elicit information about a patient's current illness:

Onset	**C**haracter
Location	**A**ggravating/alleviating factors
Duration	**R**elieving factors
	Temporal factors
	Severity

Information pertaining to the patient's past medical history should include determining any previous infectious diseases such as hepatitis, sexually transmitted infections, or TB. History of childhood infections and vaccinations should be included in the inquiry. The patient should be asked about any preexisting conditions that might affect the immune system, such as steroid use, chemotherapy, transplants, or other chronic illnesses. The patient's travel history should also be included: Where has the patient traveled, how long, and what were the living circumstances? Hiking, camping, and caving can increase the risk of infection, as can travel to countries where sanitation is poor. It is important to note what foods the patient ate while traveling and whether the foods were cooked or raw.

Has the patient been exposed to any infected animals or rodents? If the patient has pets, how are the animal feces handled? Has the patient recently experienced any insect bites? Exposure to infected people is also important. The nurse should inquire about the patient's sexual history. It is important to know about all sexual partners and whether the patient engages in high-risk sexual activity. The nurse should also ask the patient about drug, tobacco, and alcohol use. Drugs and alcohol can lead to exposure to bloodborne pathogens via needles and sexual contact. Smoking increases the risk of respiratory infections due to the effects of smoke on cilia that normally protect the airway. Sharing tobacco products, drinks, lip balm, and so forth, has been implicated in the transmission of gram-negative diplococci *Neisseria meningitidis,* which may lead to meningococcal disease. The patient's diet history should be obtained related to what is eaten, as well as the sanitation of food, dining out, how food is cooked, and where it is obtained.

Physical Examination

Once the nurse completes the history, the physical examination should focus on the areas that were identified as potential sources of infection. A focused physical exam aimed at assessing for an infection should include the following:

- ***Vital Signs:*** Record the patient's height and weight, temperature, respiratory rate, pulse rate, and blood pressure.
- ***Skin and Mucous Membranes:*** Inspect the skin and mucous membranes for breaks in skin integrity, redness, warmth, rash, jaundice, signs of insect bites; check skin turgor and hydration status, as well as drainage from lesions or wounds. Inspect skinfolds for candidal skin infections and scabies.
- ***Head and Neck:*** Examine the eyes, nose, and ears for redness, drainage, or swelling. Assess the pharynx for redness, swelling, the presence of masses, and the presence of discharge or exudates. Inspect the oral mucosa for lesions and the teeth for caries, swelling of the gums, foul smell, or drainage. Palpate over the sinuses for pain or swelling.
- ***Lungs:*** Auscultate the lungs for abnormal breath sounds. Note decreases in breath sounds, as well as the presence of crackles, rhonchi, friction rubs, or wheezes. Note the presence of a cough. Note the color and consistency of sputum.
- ***Heart:*** Auscultate the heart to determine the rate and rhythm of the heart sounds. Note any abnormal sounds such as murmurs or friction rubs.
- ***Abdomen:*** Auscultate the abdomen for the presence of bowel sounds. Palpate for masses, tenderness, and enlarged liver or spleen. If diarrhea is present, note the amount, frequency, color, and

consistency. Note the presence of vomiting including the consistency, color, and amount.

- ***Genitourinary Tract:*** Assess the genitourinary tract for costovertebral angle (one of the two angles that identify a space over the kidneys), tenderness, suprapubic tenderness, and fullness over the bladder. Inspect the perineum for redness or drainage.
- ***Nervous System:*** Assess for changes in mental status. Note any changes in neurological signs such as weakness, tremors, seizures, or paresis.

Safety Alert *Areas where lines or tubes enter or leave the body need to be checked frequently for signs of infection, such as increasing redness or drainage around the tube. If found, the nurse should notify the health care provider immediately.*

Diagnostic Tests

Health care providers use diagnostic tests to confirm the diagnosis, to determine treatment or see the response to existing treatment, or to pinpoint the infection's location and severity. The Diagnostic Tests Related to Infection box summarizes the tests related to infection. One of the most important diagnostic tests is the complete blood count. The number and variety of white blood cells (WBCs) can give the nurse some insight into the presence and severity of an infection. The normal count is 4,500 to 10,000 WBC/mm^3. A WBC of more than 10,000 WBC/mm^3 usually indicates the presence of inflammation and/or infection. The higher the WBC count, the more serious the infection is thought to be. However, a viral infection can often cause the WBC count to decrease. The differential count of WBCs should also be assessed, including the percentages of neutrophils, eosinophils, basophils, lymphocytes, and monocytes.

Pathogen cultures also are very important in diagnosing and treating infections. The nurse often is responsible for collecting the specimen to be cultured. Each institution has its own policy for collecting specimens; however, it is very important to collect the specimen correctly so that the results of the culture are useful. The following guidelines should be followed:

- Collect sufficient material to ensure an accurate examination.
- Collect the specimen where the suspected organism is most likely to be found.
- Observe standard precautions when collecting the specimen.
- Culture only for a specific pathogen and not where there are areas of normal flora.
- Collect the specimen in a sterile container with a tight-fitting lid. Nurses who use polyester-tipped swabs in a collection system with a transport medium ensure the adequacy of the specimen for 72 hours.
- Place the specimen in a biohazard bag.
- Label the specimen correctly with patient information, the source of the specimen, and the time of collection.
- Make sure the specimen gets to the laboratory as soon as possible. Most specimens can be refrigerated for a few hours if necessary.

Safety Alert *It is imperative to collect specimens for culture before beginning treatment with an antibiotic. This gives a more accurate picture of the original infection, as antibiotic therapy that is started before the specimen collection could alter the results of the test.*

Emotional care of the patient is very important. Patients and their families may not know the origin of the infection and may therefore be apprehensive about the effectiveness of treatments. In addition, the use of standard precautions or transmission-based precautions makes visits with family and friends difficult. Hugs and touching are hindered by gloves and masks. The necessary use of protective masks, gloves, and gowns may make the patient feel isolated and rejected. Education about the necessity of isolation procedures is important for the patient and family. The nurse needs to allow the patient to verbalize feelings about the isolation and the concerns about being ostracized.

Health Promotion

Prevention and control of infection are the top priorities of health care no matter what the setting. The best way to address infection is to prevent it; this requires education of health care professionals and the general public. An educational program related to the prevention of infection has several facets. Everyone should be educated on the importance of proper hand hygiene. The public must understand the importance of immunization. Family members must be instructed to check all immunization records and keep them up to date. Community members should understand the disease they are being protected against, why the immunization is necessary, the relative safety of immunizations, and when booster doses are due.

It also is important to educate the public on the use of antibiotics. Antibiotics are not effective for all organisms; many infections will resolve completely without the use of antibiotics. Patients need to have an understanding of when antibiotics are effective and when alternatives may be appropriate. Health care providers must stress to patients that it is necessary to take all of the medication prescribed. If the full course of treatment is not completed, this may foster the development of resistant organisms. The Pharmacology Summary of Medications to Treat Infectious Disease box lists medications used to treat infectious diseases.

A healthy lifestyle is a deterrent to infection. An individual who practices good hygiene, eats a well-balanced diet, exercises regularly, and gets an adequate amount of sleep will have a strong immune system and be better able to resist infection. Although exposure will occur no matter how careful an individual is, it is important to prevent transmission of the organism. To decrease exposure, an individual should: avoid crowds and contact with susceptible persons, use disposable tissues when coughing or sneezing, use appropriate food-handling precautions, practice frequent hand hygiene, clean equipment and eating utensils, avoid contact with or sharing of body fluids through needles or razors; and use condoms during sexual activity.

Discharge Planning

With the movement toward decreasing the length of hospital stays, many patients are being cared for in their homes. In fact, many patients prefer receiving treatment there. Infection control has long been a concern of hospitals; with the trend toward home care, consideration should now be given to the home environment as well. The prevention of infection in the home is different than in the hospital. Patients who are being cared for at home are not exposed to other patients and do not encounter the reservoirs of pathogens that would be present in the hospital setting. In addition, home care patients are usually not as ill as hospitalized patients, so their ability to resist infections may be better. However, other environmental resources in the home, such as plumbing, sanitation, and ventilation, typically are more difficult to control than in an institution.

The basic principles of infection prevention and control still apply. The focus should not be on getting rid of household germs but on using good hygiene measures such as hand washing to prevent exposure to germs and cross infection. Families must be taught infection prevention and control principles so that they can develop their own

DIAGNOSTIC TESTS Related to Infection

Test with Description, Rationale, and Normal Values	Expected Abnormality
WBC Count	
WBC count increases in order to phagocytize or kill bacteria or cell debris.	Elevated in acute infections, tissue injury, and tissue necrosis.
4,500–10,000 cells/mm^3 is normal.	Decreased in viral infections, some bacterial infections, bone marrow depression.
Neutrophils	
Neutrophils are the first WBCs to arrive at the site of infection. They have a short life span and must be continually produced when needed. Therefore, the immature neutrophil or band will be elevated quickly.	Neutrophils and bands are elevated in acute infections.
50% to 70% of the total WBC count, normal; band, 0% to 5% normal.	
Basophils	
Involved in phagocytosis of antigen–antibody complexes.	Elevated with allergic and parasitic responses.
0.4% to 1.0% of total WBC count normal.	Do not respond to bacterial or viral infections.
Eosinophils	
Respond later in inflammation and help control the inflammatory process.	Elevated in allergic and parasitic reactions.
Phagocytic cells that perform like neutrophils but start later and stay longer in the bloodstream.	Elevated with infection, tuberculosis, bacterial endocarditis.
1% to 4% of total WBC count is normal.	
Lymphocytes	
Function to fight chronic bacterial infection and acute viral infections. Responsible for immune reactions.	Elevated with some bacterial diseases, infectious mononucleosis, leukemia, and some viral diseases.
25% to 35% of total WBC count is normal.	
Eosinophil Rate (ESR)	
Nonspecific test that measures the rapidity at which red blood cells (RBCs) clump together. This process occurs more rapidly when there is an alteration in blood proteins due to inflammation. Therefore, an elevation indicates the presence of an inflammatory process.	Elevated with acute and chronic infection, inflammation, cancer, tissue necrosis, rheumatoid, collagen diseases.
1% to 3% of total WBC count is normal.	
Culture and Sensitivity (C&S)	
If pathogens are present on the substance being tested, they will grow on a special culture medium and can be identified.	Positive if pathogens are present in the specimen. The culture will identify the organism and the sensitivity will identify what antibiotic will work best.
n = Organism is sensitive, or is intermediate or resistant to antibiotics.	
Gram Stain	
None with no organisms present	Differentiates between gram-negative and gram-positive organisms.
Useful for identifying the microorganisms so proper treatment can occur.	
Febrile Agglutinins	
A group of tests that helps identify the type of organism responsible for an infection based on antibodies.	Increased in infectious diseases such as rickettsial disease, salmonellosis, brucellosis, typhoid fever, and tularemia.
Normal ranges:	
Brucella: less than 1:20; less than 1:20 for individuals working with animals is normal.	
Tularemia: less than 1:40; less than 1:40 (nonvaccinated) is normal.	
Viral Antibody Tests	
Used to determine exposure to or existing viral infections that are difficult to culture. Includes several tests, each specific to an organism and antibody reaction. They must be specifically ordered.	This is a group of tests for specific viruses. They will be elevated with viral infections.
Negative culture result; no organisms present is normal.	
Fungal Antibody Tests	
Looks for the presence of antibodies related to fungal infections (or the presence of parasitic organisms) in serum and/or cerebrospinal fluid.	Elevated in the presence of a fungal-induced infection.
No antibodies present is normal.	

PHARMACOLOGY Summary of Medications to Treat Infectious Disease

Medication Category and Action	Application/Indication	Nursing Responsibility
Antibiotics		
Examples of Specific Types of Antibiotics		
Aminoglycosides • Amikacin • Gentamicin • Streptomycin • Tobramycin ***Action:*** Act as bactericidal agents by interrupting the bacteria's protein synthesis.	Used against gram-negative bacilli, aerobic gram-negative organisms, mycobacteria, and some protozoa. May be used to treat nosocomial infections, urinary tract infections, eye infections, and infections of the central nervous system.	Given intravenously because they are poorly absorbed through the GI tract. Assess kidney and hearing function. Check peak and trough levels so that blood levels are maintained in a narrow margin. Watch for drug interactions, drugs with other drugs.
Penicillins • Amoxicillin • Ampicillin • Carbenicillin • Nafcillin • Penicillin G • Piperacillin • Ticarcillin ***Action:*** Bactericidal action is through destruction of the cell wall of the bacteria.	Are broad spectrum and act against gram positive, gram-negative, and anaerobic organisms. Used for upper respiratory tract infections, syphilis, and endocarditis.	Assess for adverse reactions and interactions with other medications. Ensure adequate hydration of the patient. Provide small, frequent meals to minimize stomatitis and sore mouth. If the patient is female and of childbearing age, advise her to use a backup method of birth control.
Cephalosporins • Cefacetrile (cephacetrile) • Cefadroxil (cefadroxil) • Duricef • Cefaloglycin (cephaloglycin) • Cefazedone • Cefazolin (cephazolin; Ancef, Kefzol) ***Action:*** Inhibit bacterial cell-wall synthesis by binding to protein located on the cell membrane.	Act against gram-positive organisms and gram-negative organisms. Used for patients who are allergic to penicillin. Treat respiratory tract infections, skin infections, otitis media, urinary tract infections, septicemia, and endocarditis.	Take on an empty stomach. Refrain from drinking alcohol. Maintain adequate hydration.
Tetracyclines • Doxycycline • Minocycline ***Action:*** Bacteriostatic. Inhibit cell growth by inhibiting protein synthesis, leading to prevention of cell division.	Used for infections caused by rickettsia species, *Mycoplasma*, and *Chlamydia*. Treats Lyme disease, *Helicobacter pylori*, acne vulgaris, and skin infections.	Female patients must use an additional birth control method while taking. Absorption may be decreased if taken with some over-the-counter medications. Take on an empty stomach. Will cause increased sensitivity to the sun.
Macrolides • Erythromycin • Azithromycin • Clarithromycin ***Action:*** Can prevent the cell from dividing or can kill the bacterial cell. Act by inhibiting RNA-dependent protein synthesis.	More effective against gram-positive organisms than gram-negative organisms. Treats *Staphylococcus, Streptococcus, Chlamydia, Mycoplasma*. Used to treat urethral, endocervical, or rectal infections; bronchitis; pharyngitis; skin infections; respiratory infections; pharyngitis; and pneumonia.	Monitor the patient's hearing. Medication should be taken 1 hour before or 2 hours after meals.
Vancomycin ***Action:*** Has bacteriocidal activity that inhibits cell-wall synthesis by altering the cell's permeability.	Used to treat bacterial septicemia, endocarditis, bone and joint infections, and *Clostridium difficile* infections. Effective against streptococci and staphylococci.	Monitor hearing and renal function. Monitor fluid status. Assess peak and trough serum levels.
Carbapenems • Ertapenem • Imipenem • Meropenem ***Action:*** Bactericidal. Work by inhibiting cell-wall synthesis.	Have beta-lactam activity for use against anaerobes. Are broad spectrum and effective against gram-positive and gram-negative organisms. Frequently used for serious or life-threatening infections.	Give with caution in patients with head trauma or brain lesions because these medications can induce seizures.

(*continued*)

PHARMACOLOGY Summary of Medications to Treat Infectious Disease, *continued*

Medication Category and Action	Application/Indication	Nursing Responsibility
Monobactams • Aztreonam ***Action:*** Inhibits cell-wall synthesis, leading to cell death.	Effective against gram-negative aerobic organisms such as *Pseudomonas aeruginosa*. Also used to treat urinary tract infections, septicemia, skin, and lower respiratory tract infections.	Given intravenously or intramuscularly. Monitor for signs of thrombophlebitis at the insertion site.
Fluoroquinolones • Ciprofloxacin • Levofloxacin • Moxifloxacin • Ofloxacin ***Action:*** Interrupt DNA synthesis during bacterial replication, interfering with replication.	Used to treat urinary tract infections, respiratory tract infections, skin, bone and joint infections, pneumonia, gynecologic infections, and sexually transmitted infections.	Antacids will lead to decreased absorption. Avoid sunlight. Tendon rupture is a potential adverse event and should be assessed.
Oxazolidinone Linezolid (Zyvox) ***Action:*** Inhibits protein synthesis, interfering with replication	Used for gram-positive bacteria that are resistant to other antibiotics such as MSRA and VRE	Extremely expensive Long-term use (over 2 weeks) can lead to bone marrow suppression and low platelet counts
Sulfonamides • Sulfasalazine Sulfadiazine ***Action:*** Interferes with synthesis of folic acid needed for DNA synthesis. This prevents reproduction of the bacteria.	Treats urinary tract infections, lower respiratory tract infections, diarrhea, skin, bone and joint infections, and gynecologic infections.	Antacids will decrease absorption. Monitor folate deficiency. Monitor fluid intake. Photosensitivity can be a problem. Take on an empty stomach with a full glass of water. Monitor hematologic function.
Nitrofurantoin ***Action:*** Is bacteriostatic by inhibiting the energy production of the bacteria.	Is used only for urinary tract infections.	Monitor for peripheral neuropathy and pulmonary reactions.
Antivirals		
Used to treat viral infections Nucleoside analogues • Acyclovir • Famciclovir ***Action:*** Inhibits viral DNA polymerase, leading to disruption of viral growth.	Treat viral syndromes that occur in immunocompromised patients such as herpes simplex.	Monitor for adverse reactions. Monitor for nephrotoxicity. Is expensive, so consider referring patient to social services for financial help.
Influenza A and syncytial virus drugs • Amantadine • Oseltamivir (Tamiflu) • Rimantidine • Zanamivir ***Action:*** Appears to inhibit viral replication by blocking the uncoating of the virus particle and release of viral RNA into the host cell.	Used to treat influenza A infections and respiratory syncytial virus infections.	Should not be used with central nervous system stimulants such as alcohol.

approaches and make knowledgeable decisions related to reducing the chances of infection. Hand hygiene remains a very important part of preventing infection. Other procedures such as care of catheters and wounds can be adapted to the home. Equipment needs to be cleaned in the dishwasher if possible or with regular household cleaning products. Use of gowns, gloves, and masks is necessary only when family members need to be protected from the patient's infection.

There is a requirement that cases or suspected cases of certain diseases or conditions, called **notifiable diseases,** be reported to local, county, or state public health departments. This process helps with disease surveillance efforts so that the health of individuals and families can be protected and the diseases controlled or prevented. The list of diseases designated as reportable changes to reflect the needs of the public at any given time. Annual recommendations for what diseases should be on the list are made by the Council of State and Territorial Epidemiologists (CSTE) and the CDC. The infection preventionists in each hospital keep current with which diseases they need to report to the local and national health authorities. The reporting of a disease to a public health authority leads to an immediate response that includes case investigation, contact prophylaxis, and outbreak control. Analysis of the information supplied for the notifiable diseases allows for the establishment of public health priorities and the monitoring of trends.

EVIDENCE-BASED PRACTICE Effects of Infection and Antibiotic-Resistant Bacteria on Wound Healing

Clinical Problem

Antimicrobial resistance occurs when the antibiotics that are taken to stop the infection do not kill the bacteria that cause the infection. The bacteria resist the effects of the antibiotic, which allows them to continue to survive and grow, causing more harm. After repeated exposure to an antibiotic that does not kill them, microorganisms develop the ability to avoid the antimicrobial agent's inhibitory or lethal activity through several mechanisms. Research performed to increase understanding about how bacteria protect themselves shows that bacteria can become resistant by neutralizing the antibiotic, pumping the antibiotic out, or changing the antibiotic attack site so that the bacteria's function is not affected. Types of bacteria that were at one time killed by an antibiotic can become resistant through mutation of their genetic material or by acquiring pieces of DNA that code for the resistance properties from other bacteria. The transfer of one piece of DNA may allow the bacteria to become resistant to many antibiotics.

Several resistant pathogens are on the rise. These include penicillin-resistant *Streptococcus pneumoniae*, group A streptococci of enhanced virulence, and vancomycin-resistant enterococci. As long as bacteria are able to mutate, the battle against infection will be a struggle. One of the areas affected by infection and antibiotic-resistant bacteria is that of wound healing. The presence of bacteria in the wound leads to inflammation, delayed healing, and increased scarring. This becomes an issue of increasing importance as resistant strains of bacteria develop.

Research Findings

Ryan (2007) reviewed research on the effects of infection and antibiotic-resistant bacteria on wound healing. New mechanisms have been discovered by which bacteria protect themselves. For example, research has reported that bacteria use a biofilm cover; in addition, bacteria may mutate their genes and horizontally transfer them to other bacteria. Bacteria's ability to make adaptations like these causes concerns among those prescribing antibiotics. An understanding of these mechanisms help to identify other ways of attacking the bacteria.

Bacteria in wounds are initially gram-positive, but gram-negative bacteria also play a role in the delay of wound healing. For the right antibiotic to be prescribed, it is important for the health care provider to identify the right bacteria. Wounds are often contaminated with other materials or may grow different bacteria in different areas of the wound. A good understanding of how to take samples from the wound for culture is important.

The healing of the wound and signs of inflammation can be influenced by factors such as the presence of anemia and malnutrition, and medications that the patient may be taking, such as steroids or immunosuppressive agents, may delay wound healing and make the patient more susceptible to infection. Good nutrition with adequate amounts of vitamins A and C, iron, and zinc is necessary for wound healing. The traditional implementation of activities thought to be antibacterial is being questioned. Actions such as preoperative bathing and hair removal seem to have no effect on the rate of infection; however, research has shown proper hand hygiene, especially with alcohol-based cleaning products, to be effective in preventing infection.

Implications for Nursing Practice

This study demonstrates that nurses need to help prevent infections in wounds so that healing can occur. To do this, nurses need to perform hand hygiene before and after caring for the patient. Nurses should wear gloves when providing wound care. The patient's overall health should be enhanced through a well-balanced diet, proper hydration, good hygiene, and some exercise, if possible, to increase circulation. The proper use of antibiotics can help reduce the development of antibiotic resistance. Patients should be assessed for their response to antibiotic treatment to help health care providers decide if the antibiotic is effective. Patient education about the use of antibiotics is also supported in this research. Patients often want an antibiotic when one may not be indicated. Nurses can help the patient and the patient's family understand when the use of an antibiotic is needed and how to take the antibiotic properly.

Critical Thinking Questions with answers can be found in the Osborn Student Resources at nursing.pearsonhighered.com.

Source: Ryan, T. J. (2007). Infection following soft tissue injury: Its role in wound healing. *Current Opinion in Infectious Disease, 20*(2): 124–128.

Collaborative Management

The goals when caring for a patient with infection are to identify the site of the infection and the causative organism so that a cure can be achieved quickly and without complications. This requires a collaborative approach to care by an interdisciplinary team which may consist of nurses, health care providers, occupational therapists, physical therapists, nutritionists, psychologists, and pharmacists. In order to meet desired patient outcomes, it is essential that this interdisciplinary team communicate openly with one another in developing and evaluating care of the patient and family (Institute of Medicine, 2010). A thorough history and physical examination helps the team identify which body system is involved. The health care provider orders diagnostic tests to help narrow the focus and identify the site and causative agent. The nurse's responsibility is to continually assess the patient as the presenting signs and symptoms become more defined and to ensure that diagnostic tests are completed and specimens are collected correctly.

Once the infecting agent has been identified, therapy can be ordered that is narrowly focused on the patient's problem. A pharmacist will help identify the proper medications and educate the patient on their use and side effects. A viral infection will often resolve with only supportive care. If antibiotics are administered systemically, it is important to watch for any adverse effects caused by the drugs. The nurse also must protect the patient from contracting new infections and decrease the potential for spreading the infection to others.

The clinical and diagnostic evaluation is used to decide whether therapy should be instituted, as well as what type. If the severity of the infection merits, the health care provider may decide to begin therapy before the culture results are available. This is known as **empiric therapy,** in which the data used to decide on the medication of choice include the usual susceptibility of the suspected organism, the medication's capability to penetrate the site of infection, and patient factors such as other illnesses, medication allergies, immune status, and (in women of childbearing years) pregnancy status. Once culture results are available, the health care provider chooses the medication based on effectiveness against the identified organism with the least risk of toxicity and fewest adverse effects for the patient. Patient compliance, the cost, and the dosing schedule of the medication also is considered.

Nutritionists help the patient plan a well-balanced diet designed to keep the immune system strong. Physical and occupational therapists may be needed to maintain or regain physical functioning. Every member of the health care team, along with the patient and the patient's family, must be cognizant of the importance of proper hand hygiene and its huge role in the prevention of disease transmission.

Safety Alert *Always assess the patient for signs of an allergic reaction or side effects of the medication being given.*

The nurse serves as the patient advocate and liaison between the patient and other members of the health care team. In this role, the nurse coordinates and facilitates communication among all members of the health care team and the patient. In addition, the nurse is responsible for the patient's educational and emotional support needs.

Gerontological Considerations

Older people are at increased risk of acquiring an infection and typically have poorer outcomes (Wachter & Fretwell, 2007). The skin is more fragile and prone to breakdown or abrasion. Aspiration is more likely due to conditions such as dementia or stroke. Studies have shown that at least one-third of individuals over the age of 65 years have nutritional deficiencies that can adversely affect the immune system (Wachter & Fretwell, 2007). Factors that contribute to poor nutrition include altered sense of taste, social isolation, physical inability to prepare meals, altered nutritional absorption, and poverty. Also, older individuals are more likely to be on a large number of drugs for different conditions associated with aging, and these drugs may decrease the effectiveness of the immune system.

Because of age-related changes in the immune system, the older patient is at risk for acquiring urinary and respiratory tract infections, skin infections, and gastroenteritis such as *clostridium difficile*–related diarrhea. More deaths occur from infections in people over 65 years of age than any other group. The major host factor associated with community-acquired pneumonia is advanced age (Wachter & Fretwell, 2007). The same is true for influenza; 90% of deaths related to influenza occur in patients 65 years and over (Caterino, 2008). This is why it is so important for older people to receive both the pneumonia vaccine (pneumovax) and an annual influenza vaccination.

Studies have shown that in older hospitalized patients, the incidence of infection increases with the use of invasive devices such as central lines and urinary catheters. Early recognition of infection as well as restricted and shortest-term use of invasive devices can contribute significantly to decreasing the incidence of HAIs in older adults (Caterino, 2008).

The use of isolation for an infected older patient is also problematic. Being confined to a room decreases a patient's mobility; thereby hastening functional decline (Trowbridge, 2008). Deconditioning is a serious side effect of isolation and affects the patient's recovery. It also may be difficult to restrict the movement of patients who are physically able but cognitively impaired.

Isolation practices keep the patient from social interactions as well. Studies have shown that health care workers are half as likely to enter the rooms of patients on contact isolation compared to the rooms of nonisolated patients (Thames, 2011). If everyone entering the room is wearing PPE such as gowns, gloves, and perhaps face masks, the patient may feel confused and intimidated. The nursing care priorities for the older patient in isolation must include attention to physical mobility, social interaction, and emotional support.

Research

There are many research opportunities for nurses related to infection. The goals of research are to identify more effective means of caring for the patient with infection and to prevent infection from occurring. A list of research topics related to infection is provided in the Research Opportunities Related to Infection box.

Summary

The chain of infection is defined and explained in this chapter. Methods and mechanisms of developing an infection were discussed according to pathogen type: bacteria, viruses, mycoplasma, rickettsiae, fungi, and parasites. Infection prevention and control was emphasized, with differentiation made between hospital-acquired infections and community-based infections. The role of nurses in identifying and treating infections is emphasized throughout the chapter, including a summary of diagnostic tests used to identify the source of an infection and the drugs used to treat infections. The care of an older adult with an infection is incorporated, as is a section on future research opportunities. A case study provides the learner with an opportunity to apply critical thinking concepts in the development of a patient's plan of care.

RESEARCH OPPORTUNITIES Related to Infection

Research Area	Clinical Impact
Immunization	
Effects of nursing role on compliance with immunizations	Increases the number of people who are immunized so that the numbers exposed to infectious disease can be decreased.
Effects of laws on compliance with immunizations	
Adverse effects of vaccines on the outcomes of pregnancy or the unborn child	
Home Care	
Prevention techniques needed in the home	Little is known about the prevalence of infection in the home and the best techniques to prevent it.
The development of surveillance systems for infection in the home	
Prevention of Nosocomial or Hospital-Acquired Infections	
The degree and type of organisms related to environmental surface contamination	More information is needed about where the organisms come from and how to prevent their transmission.
Assessment of prevention strategies at specific sites such as ventilator-associated pneumonia	
Compliance of health care personnel with hand hygiene practices	
What agents are most effective for hand hygiene and what time intervals are needed	
What are the adverse effects of isolation on geriatric patients?	How can we prevent physical and mental decline?
Treatment	
Studies related to improved antibiotic usage and management of antibiotic resistance	Although much progress has been made in the treatment of infection, new problems are developing that need to be addressed.

READ: History of Present Illness >> Laboratory Study Results >> Critical Thinking Questions

Ralph Newman is a 68-year-old black male who was admitted with a diagnosis of "infection of right leg wound." Mr. Newman was struck in the right leg by a piece of wood while he was cutting up firewood. He finished cutting the wood, then went into the house and washed off his leg. However, three days later, the wound began to drain thick, greenish-yellow liquid and was painful. Mr. Newman visited his doctor, who cleaned the wound and put him on cephalexin. However, the wound continued to get worse, so Mr. Newman was admitted to the hospital. On the day of admission, he was taken to surgery for a cleaning and debridement of his leg wound.

READ: History of Present Illnesses >> **Physical Exam** >> Admitting Medical Records >> Laboratory Study Results

Medical–Surgical History

Insulin-dependent diabetes mellitus
Myocardial infarction 10 years ago but has been doing well since that time
Allergies: none known
Drug intolerance: none known

Social History

Retired and likes to work outside around his home
Smokes 1 pack of cigarettes per day
Lives with his wife in a rural area

Physical Exam

Weight: 200 lb; height: 5 ft 8 in.
BP 164/90; P 85; RR 20; T 101°F
HEENT: PERRLA, ears appear normal; pharynx pink with no exudates
Neck: no cervical lymphadenopathy; thyroid nonpalpable
Heart: regular rate and rhythm; no extra heart sounds
Lungs: clear to auscultation
Abdomen: bowel sounds present ×4 quadrants; soft and nondistended; no tenderness or masses; no hepatomegaly
Extremities: left leg 1+ pitting edema; brown discoloration from mid-calf down to ankle; toes slightly pink in color
Pedal pulses 1+ left foot
Pulses absent in right foot; toes on right foot pink and cool to touch
Right leg 2+ pitting edema
Open wound on anterior shin approximately 4 inches in diameter. Draining moderate amount of greenish-yellow, thick liquid. Necrotic tissue noted in wound bed. Skin around wound red and warm to touch
MS: moves all extremities; full ROM except right ankle due to pain; normal muscle strength
Neuro: sensation slightly diminished in both lower legs. DTRs 2+. CN ii-xii intact

Admitting Medical Orders

Admit to surgical service
Diagnosis: right leg wound infection; status post-incision and drainage of right leg
No known allergies
Vital signs with oxygen saturation q4h
Wet-to-dry dressing with Dakin's solution q4h
Up in chair
Bathroom privileges
1800 calorie ADA diet
Fingerstick blood glucose ac and HS
Sequential compression devices (SCD) to lower extremities
Incentive spirometry q hour while awake
IV: saline lock; NS flushes q8h
Intake and output
Call house officer: pulse < 60—greater than 110/minute; BP < 90—greater than 160 systolic; temperature greater than 38.5; urine output less than 30 mL/hr for 2 hours; respiratory rate greater than 30/minute: oxygen saturation less than 92%; blood sugar greater than 130

Scheduled Medications

Insulin 15 units SQ of 70/30 in a.m. and 10 units of 70/30 SQ at HS
Cefoxitin 1 g IV q8h
Aspirin 81 mg po daily
Lipitor 10 mg po daily

PRN Medications

Phenergan 25 mg IV q6h prn nausea
Mylanta 30 mL po q4–6h prn dyspepsia
Triazolam 0.25 mg po q noc, prn sleep
Ativan 0.5 mg IV q6h prn mild agitation
Milk of Magnesia 30 mL po daily, prn constipation
Tylenol 650 mg po/pr q4h
Vicodin 2 tabs po prn q6h for mild to moderate pain (Numerical rating 1–6)
Morphine sulfate 4 mg IV q4h prn severe pain (Numerical rating > 7)

Ordered Laboratory Studies

Wound culture
ESR × 1
Chemistry panel q a.m.
CBC q a.m.

Ordered Diagnostic Studies

Chest x-ray

CLINICAL PREPARATION, *continued*

READ: History of Present Illnesses >> **Laboratory Study Results** >> Critical Thinking Questions

Test	Day 1	Day 2	Day 3
Hemoglobin A_1C	9.1%		
Random glucose	160 mg/dL		
Fasting glucose	140 mg/dL	138 mg/dL	142 mg/dL
WBC	12,000/mm^3	15,000/mm^3	14,000/mm^3
Lymphocytes	11%	12%	11%
Monocytes	1%	2%	2%
Bands	12%	18%	17%
Neutrophils	78%	80%	79%

Test	Day 1	Day 2	Day 3
Basophils	10%	10%	9%
RBC	3.08/mm^3	3.10/mm^3	3.10/mm^3
Hemoglobin	9 gl/L	9.5 gl/L	9.7 gl/L
Hematocrit	27%	28%	28%
Wound culture	*Staph. aureus*		
ESR	48 mm/h		
Chest x-ray	Normal		

Pearson Nursing Student Resources *Log on to* ***nursing.pearsonhighered.com*** *to download forms*

DOCUMENT:

- >> Summary of Hospitalization
- >> Pathophysiology Form
- >> Laboratory Values
- >> Laboratory Results Explanation

APPLY:

- >> List of Potential Nursing Diagnoses
- >> Concept Map
- >> Critical Thinking Questions and Concept Map

APPLY: History of Present Illness >> Laboratory Study Results >> **Critical Thinking Questions**

1. When Mr. Newman is admitted to the unit, there are no private rooms available. The choices are as follows: room 110 with Mr. Jonas, who has a diagnosis of leukemia; room 115 with Mr. Smithson, who has a GI bleed; or room 122 with Mr. Kendrick, who was admitted for deep venous thrombosis. In which room should Mr. Newman be placed?
2. Should Mr. Newman be placed in isolation? If so, why?
3. What factors does Mr. Newman have that make him susceptible to infection?
4. What nursing diagnoses would be appropriate for Mr. Newman?

Answers to Critical Thinking Questions can be found in Appendix D. in the Osborn Student Resources at nursing.pearsonhighered.com.

NCLEX® PRACTICE

1. The nurse is caring for a patient with a wound infection. Which statement explains an increase in purulent exudate in the wound?
   1. Response of white blood cells to the cellular injury
   2. Temporary vasoconstriction to avoid blood loss after injury
   3. Vasodilation to increase blood supply to the area
   4. Leakage of fluid and cells out of capillaries into interstitial spaces
2. The nurse is assessing a patient with an infection. Which social history finding could be implicated in the development of this infection?
   1. The patient reports not having enough money to purchase nourishing foods.
   2. The patient has been treated for a personality disorder.
   3. The patient is age 45 and is employed in a bank.
   4. The patient lives in an urban apartment.
3. A patient is diagnosed with tuberculosis. The public health nurse would question the patient about which mode of transmission?
   1. Contact
   2. Airborne
   3. Vehicle
   4. Vector

4. While providing care to patients, the nurse realizes that preventing the spread of infection is a priority. Which action is an important part of hand hygiene?

1. Use water as hot as can be tolerated.
2. Clean under artificial nails prior to starting the shift.
3. Use a petroleum-based lotion to prevent skin dryness.
4. Rub hands for at least 20 to 30 seconds with an alcohol-based cleaner.

5. A patient is admitted with fever thought to be the result of rickettsia infection. Which assessment question should the nurse ask?

1. "Have you travelled out of the country in the last year?"
2. "Has anyone in your home or workplace been sick with cold or influenza symptoms?"
3. "Have you been bitten by a tick in the last year?"
4. "Have you had any dental work done in the last 6 months?"

6. A nurse conducting a public-health meeting about a new strain of influenza virus says, "This virus is especially virulent." How could the nurse have stated this fact in a way more understandable to the general public?

1. "This virus can stay alive on objects such as shopping cart handles and hand rails in the subway."
2. "This virus can make many people sick at one time."
3. "This virus can be killed with a very strong bleach and water solution."
4. "This virus can make a person very sick in a very short period of time."

Answers to NCLEX Practice questions can be found in Appendix D in the Osborn Student Resources at nursing.pearsonhighered.com. Practice additional NCLEX questions online at the Student Resources site.

Pearson Nursing Student Resources Find additional review materials at: **nursing.pearsonhighered.com**

REFERENCES

Allegranzi, B., & Pittet, D. (2009). Role of hand hygiene in healthcare-associated infection prevention. *Journal of Hospital Infection, 73* (4), 305–315.

Caterino, J. M. (2008). Evaluation and management of geriatric infections in the emergency department. *Emergency Medicine Clinics of North America, 26*(2), 319–343.

Centers for Disease Control and Prevention. (2002). Guideline for hand hygiene in health-care settings. *Morbidity and Mortality Weekly Report, 51*(16). Retrieved from http://www.cdc.gov/mmwr/preview/mmwrhtml/rr5116al.htm

Centers for Disease Control and Prevention. (2007). 2007 guideline for isolation precautions: Preventing transmission of infectious agents in healthcare settings. Retrieved from http://www.cdc.gov/hicpac/2007IP

Centers for Disease Control and Prevention. (2010). NHSN overview. Retrieved from http://www.cdc.gov/nhsn/PDFs/pscManual/1PSC_OverviewCurrent.pdf

Centers for Disease Control and Prevention. (2011). 2011 child & adolescent immunization schedules. Retrieved from http://www.cdc.gov/vaccines/recs/schedules/child-schedule.htm

Donskey, C. J., & Eckstein, B.C. (2009, January 15). The hands give it away. *New England Journal of Medicine, 360*(e3). Retrieved from http://www.nejm.org/doi/full/10.1056/NEJMicm0707259

Hildreth, C. J., Burke, A. E., & Glass, R. M. (2009). Inappropriate use of antibiotics. *Journal of the American Medical Association, 302*(7), 758.

IOM (Institute of Medicine). (2010). *The future of nursing: Leading change, advancing health.* Washington, DC: The Academic Press.

McGuckin, M., Waterman, R., & Govednik, J. (2009). Hand hygiene compliance rates in the United States—a one-year multicenter collaboration using product/volume usage measurement and feedback. *American Journal of Medical Quality, 24*(3), 205–213.

OSHA (Occupational Safety & Health) (2011). Laboratory safety: Latex allergy. Retrieved from http://www.osha.gov/Publications/laboratory/OSHAquickfacts-lab-safety-latex-allergy.pdf

Porth, C. M., & Matfin., G. (2009). *Essentials of pathophysiology: Concepts of altered health status* (2nd ed.). Philadelphia: Lippincott Williams & Wilkins.

Ryan, T. J. (2007). Infection following soft tissue injury: Its role in wound healing. *Current Opinion in Infectious Disease, 20*(2): 124–128.

Siegel, J. D., Rhinehart, E., Jackson, M., Chiarello, L., & the Healthcare Infection Control Practices Advisory Committee. (2007, June). Guideline for isolation precautions: Preventing transmission of infectious agents in healthcare settings 2007. Retrieved from http://www.cdc.gov/ncidod/dhqp/pdf/guidelines/Isolation2007.pdf

Teltsch, D. Y., Hanley, J., Loo, V., Goldberg, P., Gursahaney, A., & Buckeridge, D. (2011). Infection acquisition following intensive care unit room privatization. *Archives of Internal Medicine, 171*(1), 32–38.

Thames, D. (2011). Infection. In S. E. Meiner (ed.), *Gerontological nursing* (4th ed.). St. Louis: Mosby/Elsevier.

The Joint Commission. (2010). National patient safety goal #7. 2011 accreditation requirements for hospitals. Retrieved from http://www.jointcommission.org/standards_information/npsgs.aspx

Torrey, T. (2011). Another hospital infection to beware of: urinary tract infections (UTI). *About.com Health Patient Empowerment.* Retrieved from http://patients.about.com/od/atthehospital/a/hais.htm

Trowbridge, S. (2008). Hospital-acquired infections and infection control practices: What are the consequences to the elderly patient? *Perspectives (Gerontologic Nursing Association), 33*(1), 16–22.

U.S. Department of Health and Human Services. (2010). What's new for 2020. *Healthy People.* Retrieved from http://www.healthypeople.gov/2020/about/new2020.aspx

Wachter, T., & Fretwell, M. (2007). Practical guide to the care of the geriatric patient (3rd ed.). Philadelphia: Mosby/Elsevier.

World Health Organization. (2009). *WHO guidelines for hand hygiene in health care.* Geneva, Switzerland: WHO Publications.

CHAPTER 15

Fluids, Electrolytes, and Acid–Base Balance

Gail Thurkauf
Annita Watson

Outcome-Based Learning Objectives

After studying this chapter, the learner will be able to:

1. Evaluate the fluid status of an adult according to fluid and electrolyte values, and determine circumstances that might place the patient at risk for fluid and electrolyte imbalances.
2. Design nursing interventions to restore fluid and electrolyte balance in the body.
3. Critique the processes that produce respiratory and metabolic acids in the body and the processes by which they are eliminated.
4. Create a systematic stepwise process for the interpretation of the arterial blood gas values related to acid–base balance.
5. Explain the major causes, pathophysiology, signs, symptoms, consequences, and medical management for respiratory acidosis and alkalosis and metabolic acidosis and alkalosis.
6. Generate nursing assessment guides for the patient with fluid and electrolyte abnormalities and the patient with acid–base abnormalities.

KEY TERMS

acids p.360
aldosterone p.351
alkalis p.360
anion p.347
anion gap p.359
antidiuretic hormone p.351
atrial natriuretic peptide (ANP) p.351
base excess p.363
bases p.360
buffer p.360
calciphylaxis p.357
carbon dioxide p.360
carbonic acid p.360
cation p.347
compensation p.362
electromotive force p.351
electroneutrality p.359
hydrogen ion p.360
hydrostatic pressure p.348
hydroxyapatite p.356
hypercarbic drive p.362
hypertonic p.347
hyperventilation p.362
hypotonic p.347
hypoventilation p.362
hypoxic drive p.362
isotonic p.347
minute ventilation p.362
oncotic pressure p.348
osmolality p.347
osmosis p.347
sodium bicarbonate p.360
specific gravity (SG) p.348

FOR THE BODY TO MAINTAIN A HEALTHY STATE, it must maintain homeostasis, that is, a state of equilibrium. This is achieved through vital adaptive mechanisms that are inherent in the body system. Two of these adaptive mechanisms are the maintenance of fluid and electrolyte balance and the maintenance of acid–base balance. Imbalances of either of these critical mechanisms trigger a pathologic or disease-related response in the body. This chapter addresses both of these adaptive mechanisms.

Body fluid composition and function provide background information that can be used to determine normality and aberrations or imbalances from homeostasis. Patient symptoms, clinical manifestations, and the nursing management of fluid and electrolyte imbalances are discussed in this chapter, as are the systemic effects on body systems. Acid–base balance and its relationship to fluids and electrolytes are also defined and explained. Assessment data, including diagnostic studies, for both types of imbalances is included, as is the nursing management of patients with acid–base imbalances. The chapter also stresses the need for collaborative teamwork in caring for patients experiencing fluid, electrolyte, and acid–base imbalances and includes gerontological considerations and future research opportunities.

FLUID AND ELECTROLYTE BALANCE AND IMBALANCE

Fluids and electrolytes are the basic elements of life. All chemical reactions within the body take place in fluids. Electrolytes react because they have an electrical charge, negative or positive. The primary fluid of the body is water. It comprises 70% of living cells and 60% of an average adult's total body weight (Barrett, Barman, Boitano, & Brooks, 2010e). An average healthy person needs about 2 to 2.5 liters of water per day to meet the body's fluid requirements. This is based on the fact that healthy individuals need about 1 to 1.5 ounces of water per kilogram of body weight per day to dissolve and metabolize wastes (Rives, 2009). Fluids are continually lost through respiration, evacuation of urine and feces, and perspiration. Most adults produce about 1,500 mL of urine per day. Additional fluids may be lost during illness through *insensible fluid loss*, water that passes through the skin and from the respiratory tract and is lost by evaporation or with fever, wound drainage, vomitus, or diarrhea.

Body Fluid Composition and Function

There are two body fluid compartments: the intracellular fluid (ICF) compartment and the extracellular fluid (ECF) compartment. The ICF consists of fluids that exist within the cell cytoplasm and nucleus. The ECF consists of fluids that exist outside the cell, such as interstitial fluid between cells, fluid in the bloodstream (serum), cerebrospinal fluid (CSF) in the central nervous system, gastrointestinal (GI) secretions, sweat, and urine. Two-thirds of the body's water is in the ICF, and one-third is in the ECF (Felver, 2009). Only 5% of body fluid is normally in the blood (Johnson, 2011; Porth & Marfin, 2009).

Body fluids control or assist many bodily functions. For example, enzymes in saliva and mucus assist the passage of food into the gut and provide mechanisms for hydrolyzing food into elements the body can absorb. ECF in blood and CSF serve as a transport mechanism to deliver electrolytes, oxygen, nutrients, and hormones to tissues. Body fluids also carry immune system cells to injury sites for the body's defense. ECF eliminates the body's waste products through the kidneys, bowel, and perspiration. Body functions depend on fluids facilitating the movement of electrolytes from one body compartment to another, often multiple times per minute, to effect an electrochemical action (i.e., the heartbeat, secretion of a hormone, or a neuromuscular transmission). Another vital function of ECF is the regulation of body temperature through perspiration and capillary dilation to give off excess heat or conserve heat through the skin.

Osmolality

Osmolality is the number of molecules of solute per kilogram of water (Felver, 2009). The normal osmolality of blood is 275 to 295 milliosmoles per kilogram (mOsm/kg) of body weight. Fluids that have osmolalities within this range are known as **isotonic** fluids. Fluids with osmolalities above 295 mOsm/kg are known as **hypertonic** fluids, and those with osmolalities below 275 mOsm/kg are known as **hypotonic** fluids (Barrett et al., 2010d).

Electrolytes

Electrolytes are ionized minerals (sodium, potassium, calcium, magnesium, phosphorus, and chloride) that serve as energy transfer mechanisms to power normal bodily functions by attractions, repulsions, and combinations. Ions either have a positive charge (**cations**), such as sodium (Na^+), or a negative charge (**anions**), such as chloride (Cl^-). Because of their attraction forces, positively charged cations are always accompanied by negatively charged anions. The distribution of electrolytes between body compartments is influenced by their electrical change. However, one cation may be exchanged for another, provided it carries the same charge. For example, a positively charged H^+ ion may be exchanged for a positively charged K^+ ion. Ions do move from one body compartment to another via the fluids and cause movement of various body elements by electrochemical interactions. Fluids and electrolytes each have normal ranges in which the body functions well. When elements or fluids are outside normal ranges, dysfunction or decreased performance occurs.

Regulation of Body Fluid

Body fluids are regulated by osmosis, diffusion, and filtration. In **osmosis,** a solvent such as water moves through a semipermeable membrane from an area of lower particle concentration toward one of higher particle concentration, thus tending to equalize the concentration in the two areas (Figure 15–1◆). Osmosis is based on the relationship of the molecules of solute (i.e., electrolytes) to water molecules. Relationship refers to the presence or correlation of ions or electrolytes to water. In osmosis, the ions move from a dilute concentration to the heavily concentrated liquid of concentrated solution (light to heavy).

Diffusion occurs by movement of molecules (solutes) from an area of higher concentration to an area of lower concentration (Figure 15–2◆). Diffusion depends on the size of the molecules, electrical charges, and pressure gradients. An elevated pressure gradient resists the transfer of elements into the high-pressure area and filters ions from the high-pressure area into a lower-pressure area. An example of this process is the filtration provided by the kidneys (Barrett et al., 2010e). Pressure gradients are determined by conditions such as blood pressure within arterioles and the surrounding tissues. For example, the kidney juxtaglomerular apparatus exhibits higher pressure in the arterioles than in the renal collecting tubules, thus favoring movement of fluids and solutes into the renal collecting tubules. Molecules must be small enough to pass through semipermeable membranes. Thus, in the kidney, large protein molecules are not normally filtered. Electrical charges must balance negative and positive ions or move from an area of higher concentration to an area of lower concentration.

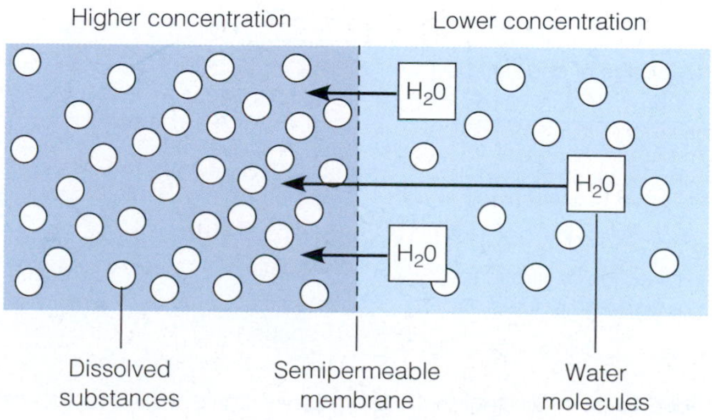

FIGURE 15–1 ◆ Osmosis: Water molecules move from the less concentrated area to the more concentrated area in an attempt to equalize the concentration of solutions on two sides of a membrane.

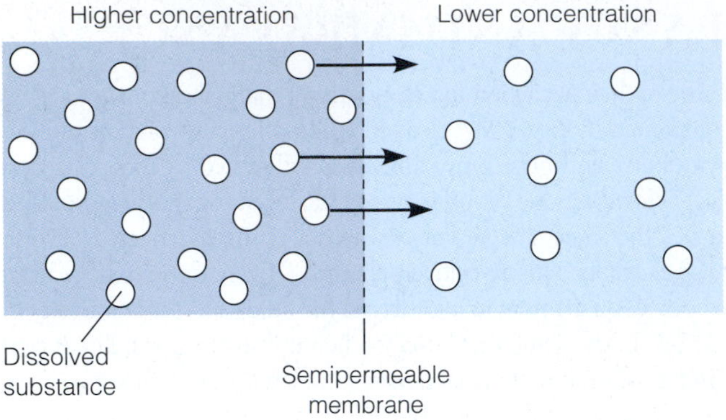

FIGURE 15–2 ◆ Diffusion: The movement of molecules through a semipermeable membrane from an area of higher concentration to an area of lower concentration.

Diffusion may be simple or facilitated. Simple diffusion is the passive movement of particles (atoms, ions, or molecules) from regions in which they are in higher concentration to regions of lower concentration. This process continues until the concentration of substances is uniform throughout. An example of simple diffusion occurs when lipid-soluble molecules pass through the phospholipid bilayers of cellular membranes and through protein channels for lipid-insoluble molecules (meaning that the lipids are fat-soluble but insoluble in water). Facilitated diffusion is the movement of specific molecules down a concentration gradient, passing through the membrane via a specific carrier protein. Each carrier protein has its own shape and only allows one molecule (or one group of closely related molecules) to pass through. Selection is by size, shape, and charge. Common molecules entering/leaving cells this way include glucose and amino acids. As an example, glucose is transported across erythrocyte membranes by a uniporter, which is a type of facilitated diffusion protein. This transport is passive and requires no energy from the cell (Porth & Matfin, 2009). The movement of an ion against an electrochemical gradient is called *active transport* because energy must be used to transfer the molecule (Bond, 2008).

Filtration takes place when molecules from an area of higher concentration move through permeable membranes to an area of lower concentration as a result of hydrostatic pressure (Figure 15–3◆) (Metheny, 2010). **Hydrostatic pressure** is the pressure exerted on the surrounding tissues because of the presence of water. Filtration occurs in the body because of hydrostatic pressure generated by the pumping action of the heart. On the arterial side of the capillary, the hydrostatic pressure is 32 millimeters of mercury (mmHg). On the venous side of the capillary, the hydrostatic pressure is about 15 mmHg. This favors movement of fluids from the bloodstream into the tissues on the arterial side of the capillary and back into the bloodstream on the venous side of the capillary after the fluids filter through the tissues and bathe the cells in interstitial fluid (Metheny, 2010).

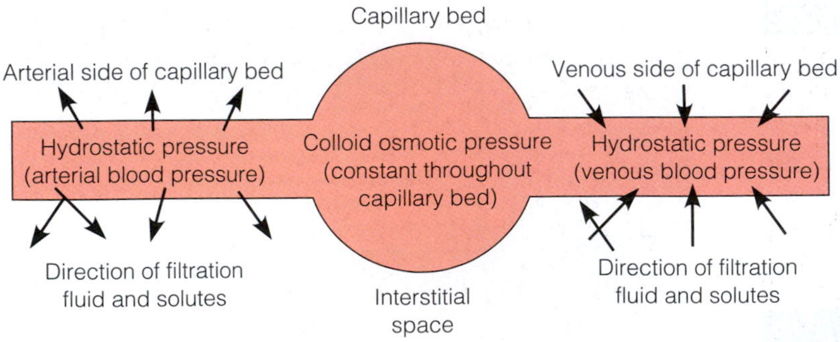

FIGURE 15–3 ◆ Schematic of filtration pressure change within a capillary bed. On the arterial side, arterial blood pressure exceeds colloid osmotic pressure, so that water and dissolved substances move out of the capillary into the interstitial space. On the venous side, venous blood pressure is less than colloid osmotic pressure, so that water and dissolved substances move into the capillary.

Filtration is directly opposed by the oncotic pressure of plasma proteins, especially albumin in the bloodstream (Metheny, 2010). **Oncotic pressure** is the result of the influence of plasma proteins on the movement of water into and out of the bloodstream based on the fact that plasma proteins maintain a negative ionic charge. Plasma oncotic pressure is about 22 mmHg. In a steady state, the ECF and ICF pressures are equal (Porth & Matfin, 2009). To maintain homeostasis, fluid loss must equal fluid intake.

Tests for Evaluating Fluid Status

Laboratories routinely test the osmolality of blood. The Diagnostic Tests box lists normal and low and high values for use in evaluating fluid status. The normal range is 275 to 295 mOsm/kg of water. Values above 295 indicate that there are too many molecules of solute per molecule of water, that is, there is a water deficit. Values below 275 indicate that there are too few molecules of solute per molecule of water, that is, there is a water excess. Both conditions can result in bodily dysfunction. Serum osmolality may be roughly calculated by doubling the serum sodium value (Barrett et al., 2010d).

Fluid (ECF) may accumulate in the interstitial space and ICF spaces (space within a cell, contains cytoplasm and nucleus). As a result, cellular edema occurs. Excess fluid between the cells will follow gravity and will be reflected by lower extremity edema in people who are upright and sacral edema (edema of the lower back over the sacral area) in people who are confined to bed. When cells are swollen with water, normal function is slowed or interrupted. Excess fluid volume is common in individuals with reduced renal sodium and water excretion and in patients with liver cirrhosis or congestive heart failure (Joy & Hladik, 2011).

Another test to evaluate hydration is the serum hematocrit measurement, which is the percentage of red blood cells in a given volume of blood. A normal value is ~ 40% to 50%, with males averaging 40% to 54% and females averaging 36% to 46%. If the serum is dilute (symbolic of overhydration), the hematocrit will be low with decreased values for sodium, chloride, potassium, and bicarbonate. If the serum is concentrated, the hematocrit, sodium, potassium, chloride, and bicarbonate values will be high. Normal laboratory values for measuring electrolyte and fluid balance are presented in the Diagnostic Tests box (p. 349). Serum concentration can be measured indirectly by measuring the osmolality (**specific gravity, or SG**) of urine. Normal SG is 1.015 to 1.024. SG will be low when the blood is dilute and high when the blood is concentrated (Barrett et al., 2010e) unless other physiological abnormalities are present.

Homeostatic Mechanisms

Serum osmolality is regulated by the osmoreceptors of the hypothalamus. When body water loss is 2% of normal body weight, the hypothalamus stimulates the posterior pituitary to secrete antidiuretic hormone (ADH). ADH signals the kidneys to conserve water by reabsorbing

DIAGNOSTIC TESTS for Evaluating Fluid Status (Adult Values)

Tests with Description, Rationale, and Normal Values	Expected Abnormality with Overhydration	Expected Abnormality with Dehydration
Urinalysis		
Specific gravity Normal = 1.005–1.030	<1.005	>1.030
Urine osmolality Normal = 50–1,200 mOsm/kg water	<50 mOsm/kg	>1,200 mOsm/kg
Urine Electrolytes		
Sodium Normal = 40–220 mEq/day	<40 mEq/d	>220 mEq/d
Potassium Normal = 25–120 mEq/day	<25 mEq/d	>120 mEq/d
Serum osmolality Normal = 280–300 mOsm/kg water	<280 mOsm/kg	>300 mOsm/kg
Hematocrit Normal = Male: 40–54% Normal = Female: 36–46%	Male: <40% Female: <36%	Male: >54% Female: >46%
Serum Electrolytes		
Sodium Normal = 135–145 mEq/L	<135 mEq/L	>145 mEq/L
Potassium Normal = 3.5–5.3 mEq/L	<3.5 mEq/L	>5.3 mEq/L
Chloride Normal = 95–105 mEq/L	<95 mEq/L	>105 mEq/L
Bicarbonate Normal = 24–28 mEq/L	<24 mEq/L	>28 mEq/L

Source: Kee, J. L. (2010). *Laboratory and diagnostic tests with nursing implications* (8th ed.). Upper Saddle River, NJ: Pearson Prentice Hall.

water from the distal renal tubules. Additionally, the perception of thirst is stimulated to promote drinking of water to restore normal serum osmolality (Barrett et al., 2010e).

In the presence of severe dehydration, such as that which results from vomiting, baroreceptors (pressure-sensitive cells) in the carotid artery sinuses and aorta stimulate the secretion of ADH. Baroreceptors in the afferent glomerular arterioles of the kidneys detect reduced perfusion and secrete renin. Renin causes the conversion of angiotensinogen to angiotensin I, which is converted to angiotensin II in the lungs by an angiotensin-converting enzyme. Angiotensin II stimulates aldosterone release from the adrenal glands, which promotes retention of sodium and, along with it, water (Barrett et al., 2010e). This mechanism becomes a problem in older adults. Atherosclerosis narrows the renal arteries as it does the coronary arteries. In response to decreased blood through the kidneys, renin is released, stimulating the cascade of sodium and fluid retention. Health care providers address this problem by prescribing angiotensin-converting enzyme inhibitors and angiotensin-receptor blocking medications.

Clinical Manifestations of Overhydration and Dehydration

The body normally does not have excess fluid in the absence of diseases such as renal failure, heart failure (HF), or syndrome of inappropriate antidiuretic hormone (SIADH). However, if the blood is dilute, water is redistributed by osmosis from the blood to the interstitial and ICF spaces, resulting in cellular edema. When cells are swollen with water, normal cell function is slowed or interrupted. Excess fluid volume is common in individuals with reduced renal sodium and water excretion and in patients with liver cirrhosis or HF (Joy & Hladik, 2011).

The most common cause of dehydration (pure water deficit) is the excessive loss of free water through urine, which occurs in people with diabetes insipidus (a condition in which antidiuretic hormone from the pituitary gland is lacking), hyperglycemia (serum glucose above 200 mg/dL and usually above 300 mg/dL), or diabetes mellitus; when diuretics are overused; or when the person fails to drink replacement fluids (as may happen in people with altered mental status) (Johnson, 2011).

Nursing Management

Assessing the hydration of patients is part of the initial and ongoing nursing assessments. Assessments, as defined in Chapter 6, include both the oral history and physical assessments. Many symptoms, such as headache, dizziness, or syncope (faintness), can be reduced with attention to adequate hydration. In the patient with heart failure, overhydration may lead to symptoms of dyspnea, shortness of

NURSING PROCESS: Patient Care Plan for Dehydration

Assessment of Fluid and Electrolyte Status Using Gordon's Functional Health Patterns:

- Nutrition Metabolic Pattern

Subjective Data	Objective Data
Assessment of Dehydration Are you feeling thirsty? Have you had difficulty drinking fluids or keeping them down? Have you had any nausea, vomiting, diarrhea, or fever lately? Have you experienced any dizziness on standing?	**Assessment of Dehydration** Weigh patient and compare weight to usual weight (loss of >2 lbs/day indicates dehydration). Measure temperature (>99°F or 37°C compatible with dehydration), pulse (greater than 100 beats/min), and blood pressure (lower than normal). Take pulse and blood pressure while patient is lying, sitting, and standing and observe for changes. Take respirations. Examine the mouth for cracked lips, dried tongue, and dry mucous membranes. Lift the skin on the back of the hands to assess for "tenting" (skin is slow to return to its normal position). Obtain urinalysis with specific gravity and serum electrolytes. Monitor urine output.

Outcomes and Evaluation Parameters	Planning and Interventions with *Rationales*
1. NURSING DIAGNOSIS: Risk for Imbalanced Fluid Volume ***related to excessive fluid loss/inability to take fluids as evidenced by low blood pressure, rapid pulse, increased body temperature, and dizziness on standing*** **(NANDA-I © 2012)**	
Outcome: Adequate fluid balance. ***Evaluation Parameters:*** Temperature, pulse, and blood pressure within normal limits. No evidence of dizziness on standing. Able to drink and retain 8 glasses of water per day.	Provide a source of fluids that the patient can retain (oral or parenteral). If nausea and vomiting are the source of dehydration, parenteral fluids will be needed. *Inadequate hydration requires restoration of normal circulating volume in order to maintain blood pressure and provide sufficient cardiac output to circulate nutrients to the body. When the fluids cannot be taken and retained orally, a parenteral source of fluids will be required to restore balance.*

Source: Adapted from Wilkinson, J. M., & Ahearn, N. R. (2009). *Prentice Hall nursing diagnosis handbook* (9th ed.). Upper Saddle River, NJ: Prentice Hall.

breath, and intolerance for walking and other activities of daily living (ADLs). Overhydration can lead to orthopnea (difficulty breathing when lying flat), which may necessitate propping the patient up in bed with several pillows or having the patient sit in a recliner chair to sleep (O'Gara & Braunwald, 2008). Sample hydration assessment questions are included in the Nursing Process: Patient Care Plan boxes for dehydration and overhydration. The care plans apply the nursing process to relevant nursing diagnoses and provide outcomes and interventions for patients with alterations in hydration.

Collaborative Management

To achieve the optimal balance of fluid and electrolytes, patients need a multidisciplinary health care team (Institute of Medicine [IOM], 2011). The team includes nurses, nursing assistants, health care providers, laboratory personnel, dietitians, and dietary assistants. In order to meet desired patient outcomes, it is essential that this interdisciplinary team communicate openly with one another in developing and evaluating care of the patient and family (IOM [Institute of Medicine], 2010). Nurses and health care providers assess the patient for alterations in fluids and electrolytes by conducting a thorough history and physical exam and by maintaining accurate intake and output (I&O) documentation. Nursing assistants often are responsible for maintaining I&O charts, particularly in inpatient settings. However, the nurse, as the supervisor for the nursing assistants, is responsible for the accuracy of the I&O data. Laboratory personnel assist by performing tests that provide more specific data about the fluid and electrolyte balances of patients. Dietitians and dietary assistants provide appropriate medical nutrition therapy for patients, including appropriate fluids in the right amounts.

Often, patients need to monitor their fluid status at home. Therefore, a plan for appropriate hydration (avoiding excesses and deficits) may be part of discharge planning. Daily weights may be part of the fluid assessment if patients have a tendency toward overhydration. For consistency, daily weights should be taken under the same conditions, on the same scale, at the same time of day, with the patient dressed in the same clothing (i.e., gown or pajamas). A weight gain of more than 5 pounds per day indicates that the health care provider should be notified because the retention of 1 pint of fluid results in a gain of 1 pound.

Electrolyte Balance

Electrolyte balance is the sum of electrolyte intake, absorption, distribution, and electrolyte loss through normal and abnormal routes. Intake is primarily oral but may include the rectal route if patients use enemas. Intravenous (IV) fluids are another source of electrolytes for patients (Felver, 2009). Once absorbed, electrolytes are distributed in different ways in the body. The reservoirs for calcium are the teeth and bones, the reservoir for potassium is in the intracellular compartment, whereas sodium and chloride are found primarily in the extracellular compartment. Most electrolytes are lost via the GI tract, urinary tract, and sweat.

NURSING PROCESS: Patient Care Plan for Overhydration

Assessment of Fluid and Electrolyte Status Using Gordon's Functional Health Patterns:

- Nutrition Metabolic Pattern

Subjective Data	Objective Data
Assessment of Overhydration Have you had any difficulty urinating lately? How much fluid have you ingested in the last 24 hours? Have you eaten a lot of salt or soy sauce? Have you experienced any shortness of breath with walking or exercise? Are you able to sleep lying flat? If not, how many pillows do you need for your head? Do you sleep sitting in a recliner chair?	**Assessment of Overhydration** Weigh the patient and compare weight to usual weight (an increase in weight greater than 2 lbs/day indicates fluid retention). Measure temperature, pulse, blood pressure (higher than normal), and respirations (will be more rapid than normal). Assess skin on the legs and ankles for dependent edema. If the patient is confined to bed, this will be in the sacral area. Obtain urinalysis and serum electrolytes.

Outcomes and Evaluation Parameters	Planning and Interventions with *Rationales*
1. NURSING DIAGNOSIS: Risk for Imbalanced Fluid Volume ***related to excessive fluid intake/decreased urination as evidenced by high blood pressure, rapid breathing, shortness of breath, and dependent edema*** **(NANDA-I © 2012)**	
Outcome: Adequate fluid balance. ***Evaluation Parameters:*** Temperature, pulse, and blood pressures within normal limits. No evidence of dependent edema. Voiding at least 240 mL/8 hr.	Reduce oral fluid and sodium intake as directed by health care provider or designee (about 1 L/day with most taken in the waking hours and <2,000 mg of sodium/day). A fluid-intake schedule is arranged and the patient instructed in fluid restriction. Administer diuretics as prescribed, monitoring serum potassium levels. *Overhydration requires restoration of normal circulating volume to decrease blood pressure and reduce the workload on the heart. When the fluids are excessive, fluids will cross the alveolar capillary barrier and pool fluids in the lungs (pulmonary edema), interfering with oxygen–carbon dioxide diffusion. This reduces blood oxygen levels. When dependent edema is present, it interferes with normal circulation in the tissues, resulting in lower tissue oxygen. The patient's cooperation is required to succeed at fluid restriction. Rapid diuresis will often result in low serum potassium. Serum potassium within the normal range is essential for normal cardiac function.* If the patient is not able to urinate due to renal failure, hemofiltration or dialysis may need to be arranged *to assist in restoration of normal fluid balance.* Potassium levels must be monitored *to ensure the patient is not retaining too much potassium.* Reposition patient every 2 hours *to decrease risk to skin.*

Source: Adapted from Wilkinson, J. M., & Ahearn, N. R. (2009). *Prentice Hall nursing diagnosis handbook* (9th ed.). Upper Saddle River, NJ: Prentice Hall.

Other sources of loss may be vomitus, nasogastric suction, wound drainage, or hemorrhage (Felver, 2009).

Electrolyte Imbalances

Because every bodily function depends on the **electromotive force** (the exchange of electrons between molecules), electrolyte imbalances decrease the body's ability to conduct normal activities. These activities include transmission of neural signals, contraction of muscles including the heart, secretion of hormones by secretory glands, and regulation of normal bodily functions, such as oxygenation and metabolization of wastes. The nature of the imbalance depends on which electrolyte is out of balance. Often, the complementary electrolyte with which the primary electrolyte combines also is affected. The following sections provide details about specific electrolyte imbalances.

Sodium

Sodium is the most abundant cation in the ECF. It maintains ECF volume through osmotic pressure, regulates acid–base balance by combining with chloride or bicarbonate ions, and conducts nerve impulses via the sodium channels of cells. Normal values for sodium are 135 to 145 milliequivalents/liter (mEq/L) (Coyle & Joy, 2011).

Three hormones are responsible for regulating the sodium level in the ECF: (1) **aldosterone,** a hormone secreted by the adrenal cortex; (2) **antidiuretic hormone (ADH),** secreted by the posterior pituitary gland; and (3) **atrial natriuretic peptide (ANP),** secreted by the atrium of the heart. Aldosterone is secreted in response to low ECF sodium levels, an increase in ICF potassium, low cardiac output, and stress. Aldosterone causes increased retrieval of sodium from the kidney filtrate. Water follows the osmotic attraction of sodium; thus, the volume of the ECF is increased. ADH is secreted in response to increased ECF osmolality detected by the osmoreceptors (receptors that detect the osmolality of the serum) in the hypothalamus and causes the reabsorption of water from the kidney distal tubules (Barrett et al., 2010d). When the atria are excessively stretched because of excessive ECF volume in the blood, ANP is secreted as an antagonist to aldosterone to cause increased sodium excretion through the kidneys. As a result, water also is lost into the urine, reducing blood volume and increasing water loss (Porth & Marfin, 2009).

Hypernatremia (Sodium Excess)

Hypernatremia (sodium above 145 mEq/L) represents a deficit of water in relation to the body's sodium levels. It occurs when there is an excess loss of body fluids that have a lower than normal concentration of sodium so that proportionately more water is lost than sodium. For example, Cushing's syndrome (aldosterone excess) causes excess sodium retention, and diabetes insipidus causes excessive fluid loss. Initially, fluid moves from the cells into the serum via osmosis to maintain osmolality within the normal parameters (below 300 mOsm/kg) and reduce serum sodium (to 145 mEq/L or below). Thirst increases because of the increase in serum sodium and osmolality (Verbalis & Berl, 2008).

Clinical symptoms resulting from hypernatremia caused by water loss are largely those of ECF fluid loss and cellular dehydration: thirst, low-grade fever, peripheral and pulmonary edema, and postural hypotension with excess fluid loss (Porth & Matfin, 2009). Laboratory values will show increased serum osmolality, elevated serum sodium, and a possible increase in urine specific gravity because of the water-conserving effect of ADH.

Pathophysiologic symptoms of hypernatremia are most likely to occur with sudden onset (Singer & Brenner, 2008). Neurologic symptoms resulting from hypernatremia may include altered mental status, neuromuscular irritability, and occasionally coma or seizures (Singer & Brenner, 2008). One cause of this type of hypernatremia is excess sweating without fluid replacement, such as in heat stroke. Mortality associated with serum sodium levels above 180 mEq/L is very high (Singer & Brenner, 2008).

The brain cells adjust to ECF hypertonicity after 24 hours by moving the excess ions into brain cells. The resulting hyperosmolality inside the cells results in increased hydration inside brain cells to correct cellular dehydration. A potential danger of administering IV fluids too aggressively to reduce the osmolality of the blood is that excess fluids will move into cerebral cells, resulting in cerebral edema. This can lead to cellular dysfunction in the brain and increased intracranial pressure. Seizures or permanent brain damage could result. Therefore, the water deficit should be replaced slowly over 48 to 72 hours, with oral fluids being the preferred route (Singer & Brenner, 2008).

Nursing Management

The nursing care of patients with hypernatremia, as outlined in the Nursing Process: Patient Care Plan for Hypernatremia, is very important because of the risk for cerebral edema if the serum sodium level is lowered too rapidly. The rate at which sodium is lowered should not exceed 0.5 to 1 mEq/hr (Porth & Matfin, 2009). To lower it more quickly risks brain dysfunction with neurological problems, such as seizures.

Hyponatremia (Low Serum Sodium)

Hyponatremia (serum values below 135 mEq/L) develops with excessive retention of water, inadequate sodium intake, or loss of sodium-rich fluids that are replaced with water. Diuretics, vomiting, diarrhea, GI suctioning, or loss of wound fluids from very large wounds (e.g., burn wounds) may cause sodium deficiency (Johnson, 2011). Excessive use of dextrose 5% IV fluid can result in hyponatremia owing to free water being created when glucose is metabolized. In fact, about 2.5% of hospitalized patients experience hyponatremia, largely caused by IV fluids (Verbalis & Berl, 2008). Diuretic-induced hyponatremia can result from the administration of thiazide diuretics by the blocking of sodium resorption in the distal tubules. Thus, water is retained in excess of sodium (Johnson, 2011).

Symptoms of sodium deficit are caused by the reduced ability of cells to depolarize and repolarize. Often patients are asymptomatic because both the relative sodium deficit and the rapidity of onset determines symptoms. As sodium levels drop below 120 mEq/L, neurological changes such as lethargy, headache, confusion, personality changes, apprehension, seizures, and even coma could result (Verbalis & Berl, 2008). These symptoms may reduce osmotic pressure in the blood to retain circulating fluid volume. Tissue edema may accompany dilutional hyponatremia caused by inappropriate IV fluids. In SIADH, the urine will be concentrated in spite of hyponatremia because of the lack of ADH. Permanent brain damage, such as central nervous system (CNS) demyelination, may occur if the serum sodium level drops below 115 mEq/L or is corrected too rapidly (Singer & Brenner, 2008). Symptoms of osmotic demyelination syndrome are flaccid paralysis, dysarthria, and dysphagia. Mortality is high with this syndrome, even in the hospital. The people who are most likely to suffer this syndrome are those with chronic hyponatremia (Singer & Brenner, 2008).

SIADH usually occurs as a result of brain trauma that causes increased secretion of ADH despite a normal fluid volume, or it may be caused as a side effect of lithium, diuretics, or anticancer drugs (Verbalis & Berl, 2008). Fluid overload and, hence, dilutional hyponatremia are the result. The serum sodium will be less than 135 mEq/L, and urine will be concentrated because of fluid retention. Symptoms are a bounding pulse, hypertension, pale dry skin, weight gain and edema, renal failure, weakness, confusion, and possible seizures. The cause must be identified and treated to restore fluid and sodium volumes to normal.

Nursing Management

The nursing care for a patient with hyponatremia is dependent on the cause. Therapeutic goals are to return the serum sodium level to near normal (135 mEq/L). Restriction of water intake to 1,000 mL/day is usually implemented to assist sodium increase and to prevent the sodium level from dropping further because of dilution. Foods that are high in sodium (e.g., highly processed foods, such as snack chips) will be given unless the patient is NPO (nothing by mouth). Correction of sodium levels may require adjusting other electrolytes to establish balance. Hypertonic saline IV fluids are used only in severe cases in which seizures have occurred (Johnson, 2011). Overly aggressive correction of chronic hyponatremia could result in permanent brain damage. When hypertonic saline IV fluid is given, only enough 3% sodium chloride is given to correct symptoms—not to return the sodium to 135 mEq/L (Porth & Marfin, 2009). The Nursing Process: Patient Care Plan for Hyponatremia (p. 354) provides further details on treating hyponatremia.

Potassium

Potassium (K^+) is an intracellular cation. In all, 98% of potassium is found within cells. In addition, small amounts are found in blood (3.5 to 5.3 mEq/L) and bone (Mount & Zandi-Nejad, 2008). The function of potassium is to maintain intracellular osmolality and participate in the sodium-potassium exchange that causes cellular depolarization and repolarization. The sodium-potassium-ATPase pump in cellular membranes uses active transport to move sodium out of the cell and potassium into the cell at a ratio of 3:2 to maintain the appropriate

NURSING PROCESS: Patient Care Plan for Hypernatremia (Sodium Excess)

Assessment of Fluid and Electrolyte Status Using Gordon's Functional Health Patterns:

- Nutrition Metabolic Pattern
- Cognitive Perceptual Pattern

Subjective Data	Objective Data
Assessment of Hypernatremia	**Assessment of Hypernatremia**
How thirsty have you been lately? Have you been able to drink water and keep it down? How much salt or soy sauce have you taken lately?	Excessive thirst Low-grade fever (99°F or 38°C) Peripheral edema Pulmonary edema (auscultation of S_3 heart sound at left apex and "crackles" in lungs) Postural hypotension (with large fluid loss) Cushing's syndrome Diabetes insipidus Decreased fluid intake or excessive sodium intake *Laboratory values:* increased serum osmolality, sodium, increased urine specific gravity
Assessment of Patient's/Family's Knowledge Regarding Cause of Hypernatremia	**Assessment of Patient's/Family's Knowledge Regarding Cause of Hypernatremia**
Do you understand how your/the patient's blood levels became out of balance? What will you be able to do in the future to keep this from happening again? Do you understand the risks involved with high salt in your blood?	Patient's/family's answers to previous questions and whether they reflect understanding Rehospitalization for similar conditions

Outcomes and Evaluation Parameters	Planning and Interventions with *Rationales*
1. NURSING DIAGNOSIS: Risk for Imbalanced Fluid Volume With Potential for Life-Threatening Cerebral Edema ***related to excess fluid loss or excess sodium retention as evidenced by serum sodium > 148 mEq/L*** **(NANDA-I © 2012)**	
Outcomes: Normal fluid and electrolyte balance Normal acid–base balance Adequate hydration ***Evaluation Parameters:*** Normal sensorium for patient Serum sodium 135–145 mEq/L Hematocrit: 37–47% for women, 40–50% for men Serum pH 7.35–7.45	Monitor fluids and electrolytes, acid–base balance, blood pressure, pulse, and temperature *to guide treatment decisions to ensure patient safety.* Administer IV *fluids to lower serum sodium slowly at a rate of 0.5–1.0 mEq/L until it reaches 147 mEq/L to avoid cerebral edema. Chloride follows sodium and chloride is involved in acid–base balance.* Assess level of consciousness every 4 hours. Observe for lethargy, headache, nausea, vomiting, increased blood pressure, or altered sensorium. Notify the health care provider or designee of changes. *To recognize the symptoms of cerebral edema early.*
2. NURSING DIAGNOSIS: Deficient Knowledge on Part of Patient and Family ***related to cause and treatment of hypernatremia*** **(NANDA-I © 2012)**	
Outcome: Appropriate knowledge of the definition, causes, and clinical manifestations of hypernatremia. ***Evaluation Parameters:*** Patient and family member verbalize understanding of causes and treatment of high serum sodium *to reduce likelihood of recurrence.* Patient adheres to treatment regimen *to reduce future threats to patient's health and need for hospitalization.*	Provide discharge instructions to patient and family member on causes and treatment of hypernatremia at an appropriate educational, cultural level *to inform patient/family why hypernatremia occurred, to promote adherence to treatment, and to prevent recurrence.* Provide reminders of adequate fluid intake and treatment adherence for Cushing's syndrome or diabetes insipidus *to prevent future occurrences of hypernatremia.*

Source: Adapted from Wilkinson, J. M., & Ahearn, N. R. (2009). *Prentice Hall nursing diagnosis handbook* (9th ed.). Upper Saddle River, NJ: Prentice Hall.

balance. About 70% of intracellular potassium is located in muscle. The remaining 30% is in the liver and red blood cells (Brophy & Gehr, 2011). Potassium is essential for cellular integrity, transmission of neuromuscular impulses, acid–base balance, conversion of carbohydrates into energy, and the formation of amino acids into proteins. Serum potassium affects the strength and rate of cardiac contraction. Both hypokalemia and hyperkalemia can result in potentially fatal cardiac dysrhythmias because of potassium's essential role in cardiac cell polarization and depolarization (Brophy & Gehr, 2011).

Potassium is gained by eating meat, potatoes, bananas, and other foods. (See Chapter 8 for information on nutrition.) Most people consume about 100 mmol/day. Because most foods contain some potassium, an increase in caloric intake leads to an increase in potassium intake. When the body is in an anabolic state (building new tissue), potassium is stored in the cells. Movement of potassium into the blood occurs (1) with tissue injury or catabolism, when cells are broken down for energy during starvation, or (2) during periods of acidosis, when excess hydrogen ions (cations) move into the cell, forcing potassium ions

NURSING PROCESS: Patient Care Plan for Hyponatremia (Sodium Deficit)

Assessment of Fluid and Electrolyte Status Using Gordon's Functional Health Patterns:

- Nutrition Metabolic Pattern
- Cognitive Perceptual Pattern

Subjective Data	Objective Data
Assessment of Sodium Deficit How thirsty have you been lately? Have much water have you been drinking? How much salt or soy sauce have you taken lately? Are you having any headaches? Are you having any difficulty thinking or remembering things?	**Assessment of Sodium Deficit** Is the patient receiving IV fluids? Does the patient have psychological problems leading to water intoxication? Is the patient taking diuretics that may have caused electrolyte imbalance? Does the patient exhibit neurological changes? *Laboratory values:* increased serum osmolality, sodium increased, decreased urine specific gravity.
Assessment of Patient's/Family's Knowledge Regarding Cause of Hyponatremia Do you understand how your/the patient's blood levels became out of balance? What will you do in the future to keep this from happening again? Do you understand the risks involved with low salt in your blood?	**Assessment of Patient's/Family's Knowledge Regarding Cause of Hyponatremia** Patient's/family's answers to previous questions reflect whether they understand. Rehospitalization for similar conditions.

Outcomes and Evaluation Parameters	Planning and Interventions with *Rationales*
1. NURSING DIAGNOSIS: Risk for Imbalanced Body Fluids With Potential for Life-Threatening Cerebral Edema ***related to excess fluid retention or sodium deficit as evidenced by serum sodium <135 mEq/L*** **(NANDA-I © 2012)**	
Outcomes: Fluid and electrolyte balance Acid–base balance Adequate hydration ***Evaluation Parameters:*** Patient free from injury with normal sensorium Serum sodium 135–145 mEq/L Hematocrit 38–47% (women), 40–50% (men) Serum pH 7.35–7.45	Monitor neurological status (orientation to person, place, time), fluid and electrolytes, and acid–base balance *to determine whether the patient's condition is worsening, improving, or staying constant.* Restrict fluids to <1,000 mL/day *to prevent further dilution of sodium.* Assess blood pressure, dizziness, and sensorium *to allow early intervention and maintain normal blood pressure.* Assist patient with ambulation. Maintain bed in lowest position with bed rails up and brakes on *to prevent falls and injury.* Explain to patient and family that disorientation is temporary *to decrease fear.* Use clocks, calendars, and familiar personal items *to reorient the patient and reduce confusion.* If seizures occur, administer hypertonic IV fluids (3% sodium) as ordered *to raise sodium to 135 mEq/L and prevent injury.*
2. NURSING DIAGNOSIS: Deficient Knowledge on the Part of the Patient and Family ***related to cause and treatment of hyponatremia*** **(NANDA-I © 2012)**	
Outcome: No future recurrence of low serum sodium ***Evaluation Parameters:*** Patient and family member identify the correct cause of the problem and identify proper treatment *to prevent recurrence*	Provide discharge instructions *to identify cause, to teach adherence to treatment, and to prevent future occurrences of hyponatremia.*

Source: Adapted from Wilkinson, J. M., & Ahearn, N. R. (2009). *Prentice Hall nursing diagnosis handbook* (9th ed.). Upper Saddle River, NJ: Prentice Hall.

(also positive ions) out of the cell and into the blood. Potassium is lost from the body via the kidneys, where it is exchanged for sodium, and via the GI tract, where it is used to buffer hydrochloric acid.

Hyperkalemia

Hyperkalemia (serum potassium greater than 5.0 mEq/L) may occur because of increased potassium intake, decreased urinary excretion, cellular damage that releases a lot of potassium into the blood (Mount & Zandi-Nejad, 2008), or inappropriate potassium supplementation in IV fluids during hospitalizations or potassium supplementation medication. Decreased potassium excretion, causing hyperkalemia, may be the result of acute or chronic renal failure (urine output less than 30 mL/hr) or use of potassium-sparing diuretics (amiloride, spironolactone, triamterene) (Brophy & Gehr, 2011). Severe acidosis may greatly increase serum potassium by movement of potassium out of the cells to allow the intracellular storage of hydrogen ion to the buffer blood pH. Cellular release of potassium can occur with surgery, fever, sepsis, or trauma. Decreases in the secretion of aldosterone can cause secretion of potassium in exchange for sodium and can increase serum potassium levels.

Clinical symptoms of hyperkalemia differ according to the degree of potassium elevation. Some common manifestations are muscular weakness and changes in the electrocardiogram (ECG) tracings with progressively widening PR and QRS intervals (Brophy & Gehr, 2011). Chapter 30 includes an in-depth discussion of ECG abnormalities.

Nursing Management

A thorough nursing assessment is essential to identify risks for and symptoms of hyperkalemia. Hyperkalemia is likely in cases of severe cellular injury such as crush injuries or burns, renal disease, insulin deficiency (diabetic ketoacidosis or hyperosmolar hyperglycemic nonketotic syndrome), Addison's disease (hypoaldosteronism), or the use of potassium supplements.

Assessment

Symptoms may include irregular pulse, irritability, abdominal distention, cramping, muscle weakness, paresthesia, and diarrhea (Mount & Zandi-Nejad, 2008). Arterial blood gases (ABGs) may show metabolic acidosis.

Outcomes and Evaluation Parameters

Nursing goals are to reduce cardiac risk within 6 hours of admission (Porth & Matfin, 2009). Positive results are a heart rate within the normal range of 60 to 120 beats/min and an ECG that is reflective of normal rhythm (contains a P wave, QRS is within 0.12 second with normal amplitude, ST segment is no longer depressed, and the T wave is less "tented" in its appearance). See Chapter 30 for more about ECGs.

Planning, Interventions, and Rationales

Treatment for hyperkalemia includes reducing oral or IV intake of potassium, treating the underlying cause of the hyperkalemia, and administering potassium-reducing agents. Kayexalate (sodium polystyrene sulfonate) enemas (retained for 30 minutes) are used to exchange potassium for sodium in the gut, or oral Kayexalate combined with sorbitol is used to rapidly remove potassium from the gut via diarrhea (Mount & Zandi-Nejad, 2008). Some drugs will temporarily reduce potassium to allow more time for correcting the underlying cause: (1) 1 ampule of 10% calcium gluconate is administered IV, (2) the concurrent administration of IV glucose (dextrose 50%) and IV insulin, (3) beta-adrenergic agonists such as albuterol, or (4) sodium bicarbonate (if the hyperkalemia is due to metabolic acidosis) (Brophy & Gehr, 2011). When correcting hyperkalemia, the nurse should observe for possible symptoms of hypokalemia due to overcorrection.

Safety Alert *In hyperkalemia, serum potassium levels greater than 6.0 mEq/L can be life threatening because of the heart's decreased ability to repolarize as evidenced by a "tented" T wave, loss of the P wave, and a wide, bizarre QRS with a depressed ST segment (Brophy & Gehr, 2011). Should this occur, the nurse should stop any potassium supplementation and take measures to reduce serum potassium before life-threatening dysrhythmias occur (Brophy & Gehr, 2011). The administration of IV glucose and insulin moves potassium into body cells temporarily, but it does not remove potassium from the body. It is a temporary measure. Emergent dialysis may be necessary if the patient has cardiac manifestations of excess potassium (Brophy & Gehr, 2011).*

Hypokalemia

Hypokalemia occurs when the serum potassium level is less than 3.5 mEq/L. Average daily losses of potassium are 5 to 10 mEq/L in feces, 0 to 20 mEq/L in sweat, and 40 to 120 mEq/L in urine. Lowered serum potassium may or may not reflect total body loss of potassium because potassium is primarily an intracellular cation. Generally, hypokalemia is not a problem unless people are receiving non–potassium-sparing diuretics, such as furosemide, bumetanide, or ethacrynic acid. Hypomagnesemia also is associated with hypokalemia. In fact, hypomagnesemia should be corrected before the potassium level is corrected because low magnesium promotes the loss of potassium from the kidneys (Brophy & Gehr, 2011).

Other common causes of low serum potassium are decreased potassium intake, GI and renal disorders, Cushing's disease, potassium-wasting diuretics, and elevated serum insulin. Diarrhea may increase excretion of potassium to 200 mEq/day. Vomiting or nasogastric suction can increase potassium loss due to GI fluid loss. Stress may predispose the body to hypokalemia because of increased aldosterone secretion in response to elevated ADH. This would result in increased sodium retention and increased potassium excretion in the urine. In acidosis, serum potassium moves out of the cell to allow hydrogen ions to move intracellular to buffer pH. Hypokalemia can occur when the potassium returns to the ICF and hydrogen ions return to the serum. During the temporary movement of potassium into the ECF to buffer hydrogen ions, potassium may have been lost in the urine, resulting in hypokalemia when the acidosis is corrected (Brophy & Gehr, 2011).

Nursing Management

Assessment

Clinical symptoms of hypokalemia are muscle weakness, cramps, nausea, vomiting, decreased bowel sounds with possible ileus (paralysis of the bowels), and paresthesias (Porth & Matfin, 2009). The cardiac manifestation of low serum potassium is a weak, irregular pulse. The ECG shows a flattened T wave followed by a U wave, which is an extra cardiac negative deflection that is not normally present. Ventricular ectopy may be common because of slow repolarization of the myocardium and could progress to dangerous dysrhythmias, such as ventricular tachycardia with hemodynamic changes (see Chapter 30) (Mount & Zandi-Nejad, 2008).

Planning, Interventions, and Rationales

Nursing interventions are directed at treating the underlying cause and replacing serum potassium as ordered without overcorrecting it (Brophy & Gehr, 2011). A diet containing about 50 to 100 mEq of potassium daily should be provided. Vegetables such as spinach, broccoli, carrots, green beans, tomato juice, acorn squash, and potatoes are good sources of potassium. Rapid correction of hypokalemia through oral supplementation is possible and may be faster than IV K^+ supplementation because of restrictions on how quickly IV supplements can be administered. Serum potassium can be increased by about 1–1.4 mmol/L in 60–90 minutes following an oral dose of 75 mmol of potassium. The oral dose is both effective and appropriate in patients with asymptomatic severe hypokalemia (Mount & Zandi-Nejad, 2008).

If the patient cannot tolerate oral potassium supplements or is experiencing life-threatening signs and symptoms of hypokalemia, the maximum possible IV infusion of K^+ should be administered for symptom control, followed by rapid oral supplementation (Mount & Zandi-Nejad, 2008). The usual dosage of IV potassium supplementation is 20 mEq potassium in 100 mL of normal saline administered over 1 hour. This is preferably administered through a large central vein to avoid venous pain, irritation, and sclerosis.

Safety Alert *Potassium must never be administered IV push. Too rapid administration of potassium can result in life-threatening dysrhythmias. If potassium is replaced too quickly, hyperkalemia may result (Brophy & Gehr, 2011).*

In cases of severe potassium depletion, patients may require as much as 300 to 400 mEq/day. It is common practice to dilute 40 to 60 mEq in 1,000 mL of 0.45% normal saline and infuse at a rate not exceeding 40 mEq/hour (Brophy & Gehr, 2011). Replacement of potassium at these rates requires continuous ECG monitoring.

Calcium

Calcium (Ca^{2+}) is important for neuromuscular transmission, contraction of muscles, blood clotting, bone and tooth construction, cellular membrane function, and energy conversion. Cellular membrane stability relies on calcium. It also exerts a sedative effect on nerves. Of all the calcium found in the body, 98% is found in the bones and teeth, whereas 2% is found in the blood serum (9 to 11 mg/dL, 50% ionized and 45% bound to albumin). Ionized calcium, 4.25 to 5.25 mg/dL, is responsible for the physiological actions of calcium, such as blood clotting and muscle contraction. Serum pH greatly affects the level of ionized calcium (Pollak, Yu, & Taylor, 2008). Metabolic acidosis decreases calcium binding to albumin, its carrier protein, and causes increased ionized calcium. Metabolic alkalosis has the opposite effect (Joy & Hladik, 2011). Tetany and muscle cramping occur. In the bone, calcium combines with phosphorus to form **hydroxyapatite,** the inorganic hexagonal matrix of bone (Pollak et al., 2008).

Regulation of calcium serum levels is controlled by vitamin D, calcitonin from the thyroid gland, and parathyroid hormone (PTH) from the parathyroid glands. PTH mobilizes calcium from the bones and causes increased reabsorption of calcium by the kidneys to increase serum calcium levels. Calcitonin inhibits calcium resorption, causes deposition of calcium in the bones and teeth, and increases renal excretion of calcium to lower serum calcium levels (Pollak et al., 2008). Vitamin D (cholecalciferol), a fat-soluble vitamin, is essential for the absorption of calcium and phosphorus from the gut. It may be consumed in the diet or manufactured in the skin by ultraviolet light. The kidneys must activate 1,25-dihydroxyvitamin D3 to vitamin D before it is physiologically active (Joy & Hladik, 2011).

Hypercalcemia

Hypercalcemia occurs when serum calcium is greater than 11 mg/dL or ionized calcium is greater than 5.25 mg/dL. Symptoms may occur with an increase in total calcium or an increase in ionized calcium because the ionized calcium is active. The latter may occur with acidosis (Pollak et al., 2008).

Three conditions account for 80% of hypercalcemia: primary hyperparathyroidism (dysfunction of the parathyroid gland), bone malignancy, and drug toxicity (from thiazide-related drugs; for example, thiazide diuretics, lithium carbonate, and vitamins A and D) (Guin, 2009). PTH mobilizes calcium from the bones and causes increased reabsorption of calcium by the kidneys, thus increasing serum calcium levels. Malignancy may involve bone metastasis, resulting in bone destruction and the liberation of calcium. Thiazide diuretics can cause renal tubule dysfunction and prevent the excretion of calcium. Vitamins A and D promote the absorption of calcium from the GI tract. Other causes of hypercalcemia are prolonged bed rest causing mobilization of bone calcium (bed rest equals decreased exercise, and a moderate amount of exercise is critical to preventing calcium loss), adrenal insufficiency, hyperthyroidism, and rhabdomyolysis (massive muscle destruction resulting in release of myoglobin into the blood with subsequent clogging of the renal glomeruli) (Guin, 2009).

Clinical symptoms of hypercalcemia affect most systems/organs of the body including the cardiovascular, nervous, renal, gastrointestinal, muscles, and the eyes.

Nursing Management

Treatment of hypercalcemia basically is treatment of the underlying cause such as partial parathyroidectomy for excess PTH, chemotherapy for malignancy, discontinuation of vitamins A and D and calcium supplementation with a low calcium diet, and discontinuation of thiazide diuretics.

Assessment

As with all electrolyte imbalances, assessment of the patient is critical. Key factors include monitoring the patient's intake and output to prevent fluid overload and ensure adequate kidney function. The patient should be turned carefully to avoid possible pathologic fractures secondary to calcium mobilization from the bones. The nurse also should auscultate breath sounds for crackles and rhonchi (see Chapter 25) and heart sounds for the development of an S_3 heart sound with vital signs to detect fluid overload at the earliest onset (see Chapter 29) (O'Gara & Braunwald, 2008). In the event that the patient is taking digitalis, digitalis toxicity must be considered.

Planning, Interventions, and Rationales

The treatment of chronic hypercalcemia depends on therapy aimed at the underlying cause. However, immediate therapy is required for patients with acute severe hypercalcemia or an acute worsening of chronic hypercalcemia. Some degree of volume depletion is almost always present with severe hypercalcemia (levels above 14 mg/dL) (Pollak et al., 2008). Normal saline is administered rapidly and concurrently with furosemide to dilute the blood and increase calcium secretion. Care must be taken during the administration of large amounts of saline and diuretic, particularly in hospitalized patients with concurrent cardiac or pulmonary disease.

Bisphosphonates are compounds with a high affinity for the hydroxyapatite bone matrix. They inhibit osteoclast (osteoclasts are rare cells that are responsible for bone reabsorption) function in areas of high bone turnover, promoting the retention of the bone matrix. These appear to be particularly effective in patients with breast cancer (Pollak et al., 2008). Glucocorticoids may be given to compete with vitamin D and decrease calcium absorption. They are most effective in hematologic malignancies such as multiple myeloma or Hodgkin's disease (Pollak et al., 2008). Calcitonin can be given to promote calcium deposition in the bone and increase calcium excretion. Gallium nitrate may be given to inhibit malignancy-related bone resorption.

Safety Alert *When treating hypercalcemia, if the patient is also receiving digitalis, the nurse should monitor for digitalis toxicity (visual green halo around objects, serum level >2 mg/mL) to avoid the occurrence of lethal dysrhythmias (Felver, 2009).*

Hypocalcemia

Hypocalcemia occurs when the serum calcium level is less than 9.0 mg/dL and ionized levels are less than 4.25 mg/dL. Because physiological effects depend on ionized calcium, symptoms of hypocalcemia may occur at higher serum levels, especially with a rise in serum pH (Pollak et al., 2008). Hypocalcemia can occur if the patient receives a large volume of citrated blood because the citrate combines with calcium, thus deactivating it.

Causes of hypocalcemia are reduced calcium intake or absorption (vitamin D deficiency or excessive phosphorus intake), decreased PTH, elevated serum phosphorus, decreased magnesium levels, hypoalbuminemia, and alkalosis. Often, the parathyroid glands are disrupted following thyroid surgery, and PTH is reduced. Unless the parathyroid glands were accidentally removed with the thyroid gland, this condition will be temporary. To monitor this condition, serum calcium concentrations should be checked every 6 hours for 1 to 2 days following thyroid surgery. On a worldwide basis, vitamin D deficiency is the most common cause of hypocalcemia; it also causes rickets and osteomalacia (Pai, Rohrscheib, & Joy, 2011).

Phosphorus and calcium combine in the GI tract under the influence of vitamin D and are exchanged for one another in the kidney. GI surgery, chronic pancreatitis, and small-bowel disease can result in decreased levels of vitamin D and, thus, decrease calcium and phosphorus absorption. Vitamin D supplementation may be needed by an IV route. Renal failure may decrease phosphorus excretion and result in excessive calcium loss. Large calcium losses may occur if the patient is taking loop diuretics (so named because they act on the nephron of the kidney at the site of the loop of Henle). Pancreatitis may cause decreased levels of ionized calcium because of free fatty acids binding calcium. Severe hypomagnesemia also may be associated with severe symptomatic hypocalcemia (Pai et al., 2011).

The faster the drop in serum calcium, the more acute the symptoms become. Symptoms of hypocalcemia include changes in the ECG showing prolonged QT intervals and cardiac contractility that may progress to congestive heart failure. Dysrhythmias, bradycardia, and hypotension also may occur. Patients with low calcium levels experience numbness and tingling of the hands and fingers, as explained later in the chapter, and around the mouth they may experience hyperactive reflexes, muscle cramps, laryngeal spasm, bronchospasm, muscle tetany, confusion, hallucinations, and possible tonic-clonic seizures (Mount & Zandi-Nejad, 2008). Mental changes can include anxiety, depression, or even psychosis. Pathologic fractures may occur because of calcium-poor bones.

Trousseau's sign (carpopedal spasm) or Chvostek's sign may be present. Trousseau's sign is induced by inflating a blood pressure cuff on the upper arm 20 mm above the systolic blood pressure and maintaining the inflation for 3 minutes, resulting in the patient's wrist and fingers contracting inward. Chvostek's sign is twitching of the facial muscles obtained by tapping the facial nerve just below the temple on the zygomatic arch. Laryngeal spasm can occur with severe hypocalcemia, resulting in asphyxiation (Pollak et al., 2008).

Nursing Management

Treatment of hypocalcemia includes oral or IV administration of calcium. Phosphorus levels should be checked to ensure that hyperphosphatemia is not the cause of the hypocalcemia. The elevated levels of calcium and phosphorus result in precipitation in the arteries, joints, soft tissues, and viscera and can result in tissue ischemia termed **calciphylaxis** (Pai et al., 2011). For tetany, 1 to 3 g of IV calcium gluconate is given over a period of 10 to 20 minutes, followed by a slow IV infusion (Pollak et al., 2008).

Too rapid administration of calcium can result in cardiac arrest or hypotension. Calcium gluconate is usually preferred over calcium chloride because calcium gluconate is less irritating to veins. Calcium should not be infused at a rate greater than 60 mg of elemental calcium per minute because severe cardiac dysfunction may result. IV calcium should be administered with caution in patients taking digitalis glycosides because cardiac dysrhythmias could result. Serum calcium concentrations should be monitored every 4 to 6 hours during the IV infusion (Pai et al., 2011).

For longer-term therapy, vitamin D should be administered to facilitate calcium absorption from the GI tract. Phosphate-binding antacids may be given to reduce phosphorus levels to promote calcium absorption. Oral calcium and vitamin D supplements will be prescribed for patients with chronic hypocalcemia. Discharge instructions include directions that oral calcium should be taken 30 minutes before meals or at bedtime for maximum absorption. Phosphorus-binding antacids should be taken with meals (Pai et al., 2011).

Magnesium

Magnesium (Mg^{2+}) is an intracellular cation. More than 50% of body magnesium is stored in muscle and bone; only 1% is in the blood (1.8 to 3.0 mg/dL). Two-thirds of serum magnesium exists in ionized form, and one-third is bound to plasma proteins. Of the magnesium in the body, 45% is intracellular; most of it is in the mitochondria, where it is a cofactor in enzymatic activities and contributes to neuromuscular interactions, neurotransmission, and cardiac contraction. Magnesium is involved in energy conversion of adenosine triphosphate, carbohydrate metabolism, protein synthesis, and muscular contraction (Pollak et al., 2008).

Magnesium is absorbed from food and excreted by the kidney. The body's requirement for magnesium is 4.5 mg/kg of body weight. In the average diet, 168 to 720 mg of magnesium are consumed each day. The proportion absorbed by the GI tract varies with the amount consumed. Sources of magnesium in the diet are green leafy vegetables, nuts, legumes, seafood, whole grains, bananas, oranges, and chocolate. Magnesium absorption decreases in kidney disease because vitamin D is not activated. Phytates, oxalates, and fat in the diet decrease magnesium absorption. In magnesium-depleted states, absorption of magnesium competes with calcium absorption. When calcium absorption goes up, magnesium absorption goes down. Average daily urinary excretion of magnesium is 100 mg/dL in men and 90 mg/dL in women. The kidney reabsorbs 20% to 30% of filtered magnesium. Excessive magnesium losses occur with diuresis. Alcohol ingestion decreases renal magnesium reabsorption. About 20% to 25% of alcoholics are frankly hypomagnesemic (Pollak et al., 2008).

Hypermagnesemia

Hypermagnesemia (serum levels greater than 3.0 mg/dL) may occur with renal failure. It can occur in people with adrenal insufficiency or in obstetrical settings where women receive IV magnesium to decrease symptoms of pregnancy-induced hypertension.

Clinical manifestations of hypermagnesemia are related to decreased neuromuscular activity, such as those seen in hyperkalemia. Cardiovascular symptoms are hypotension, bradycardia, flushing and sense of warmth, and possible respiratory or cardiac arrest. GI symptoms are nausea and vomiting; neurological symptoms are mental changes (drowsiness), respiratory depression, and decreased deep tendon reflex (Pollak et al., 2008). Deep tendon reflexes are usually lost at 8 mg/dL, and respiratory failure is likely if the serum level exceeds 10 mg/dL. Coma can occur at a level of 10 mg/dL, and cardiac arrest is possible at levels >15 mg/dL (Porth & Matfin, 2009).

Nursing Management

Nursing assessments should include tendon reflex as well as respiratory status. Both can be compromised with an increased magnesium serum level. Treatment for serious hypermagnesemia may involve immediate cessation of magnesium-containing products, IV push administration of 10 mL of 10% calcium gluconate, or dialysis. If the kidneys are intact, 0.45% normal saline may be given intravenously with diuretics to promote the renal excretion of magnesium (Brophy & Gehr, 2011).

Hypomagnesemia

Hypomagnesemia (serum magnesium of <1.8 mg/dL) occurs because of malnutrition (inadequate intake of magnesium-containing foods) or increased urinary excretion of magnesium due to alcoholism, osmotic diuresis in diabetes, and loop diuretics. It may occur by GI loss with vomiting, diarrhea, or malabsorption syndromes. The most common cause is a combination of factors. Because hypomagnesemia often is associated with an imbalance of other electrolytes such as K^+ and Ca^{2+}, many of the manifestations attributed to magnesium deficiency also may be explained by the frequent coexistence of hypokalemia and hypocalcemia in the same patient (Pollak et al., 2008).

Symptoms of hypomagnesemia are most common when the serum level is ≤1 mg/dL. Severe deficiency may cause confusion, lethargy, seizures, hyperreflexia of deep tendon reflexes, tetany, hallucinations, nausea and vomiting, hypertension, cardiac dysrhythmias, and death. Cardiac symptoms include supraventricular tachycardia, possible coronary artery spasms, and paresthesia (Pollak et al., 2008).

Nursing Management

Treatment for hypomagnesemia is parenteral and/or oral administration of magnesium supplements. Severe hypomagnesemia is treated with the IV route. The most common preparation is magnesium sulfate. In a patient who is seizing, 1 to 2 g may be administered intravenously over a 2- to 4-minute period. Otherwise, a slower rate of repletion is safer (Pollak et al., 2008). Magnesium must be administered carefully with close observation because of the possibility of developing hypermagnesemia due to overcorrection. Chronic, less severe hypomagnesemia is treated with oral magnesium salts, magnesium-containing antacids, and foods that are high in magnesium.

Phosphorus

In the human body, 85% of phosphorus is in a structural matrix with calcium and collagen, forming teeth and bones. The remainder is found intracellularly and in blood (2.5 to 4.5 mg/dL) (Pollak et al., 2008). Phosphorus is essential to carbohydrate, lipid, and protein metabolism and to nerve and muscle function. It is part of the body's basic energy units: adenosine triphosphate (ATP), adenosine diphosphate (ADP), and adenosine monophosphate (AMP). Phosphorus is in phospholipids, which make up the cellular and organelle membranes. It is also found in red blood cells in 2,3-diphosphoglycerate, which is a hormone that increases the amount of oxygen carried in red blood cells.

About 800 to 1,600 mg of phosphorus is consumed per day and absorbed with the help of vitamin D. Phosphate levels are regulated by calcitonin, parathyroid hormone, and vitamin D in conjunction with calcium regulation. PTH blocks the reabsorption of phosphorus. When calcium is reabsorbed from the kidney tubules, phosphate is excreted. However, under normal conditions, 80% to 90% of the phosphorus is reabsorbed. Plasma phosphorus levels vary with acid–base balance. The consumption of glucose, insulin, or sugar-containing foods temporarily shifts phosphorus into the cells.

Hyperphosphatemia

Phosphorus balance is regulated primarily by the kidneys. Hyperphosphatemia (serum levels greater than 4.5 mg/dL) is due chiefly to renal disease and decreased excretion of phosphorus. Other causes may be excessive phosphate replacement or the overuse of phosphate-based enemas. Acidosis may cause an extracellular shift of phosphorus because phosphate serves as a buffering anion in acidosis. Cellular destruction, which may occur with malignancy, chemotherapy, radiation therapy, or rhabdomyolysis, can release large amounts of phosphate, which is mostly an intracellular anion. As the serum phosphorus level increases, the serum calcium level decreases, which may result in hypocalcemia (Pai et al., 2011).

The most common complication of hyperphosphatemia is the deposition of calcium phosphate in soft tissues. This occurs when the product of the serum calcium level and serum phosphorus level exceeds 70 mg/dL. Deposition of calcium phosphate in the heart muscle could result in cardiac dysrhythmias. There are few symptoms directly due to hyperphosphatemia. Most adverse symptoms relate to the resulting hypocalcemia.

Nursing Management

Treatment for hyperphosphatemia is administration of phosphorus-binding antacids, such as calcium carbonate or calcium acetate. Phosphorus absorption is reduced, and excretion of phosphorus in the feces is increased. Calcium-based antacids are preferred in renal failure because of the potential for hypermagnesemia (Pollak et al., 2008). If hyperphosphatemia is accompanied by hypocalcemia, correcting the calcium level may reduce the phosphate level.

Hypophosphatemia

Hypophosphatemia occurs when the serum phosphate level is less than 2.5 mg/dL. Common causes are vitamin D deficiency (often seen in chronic alcoholism), bowel disorders that lead to malabsorption, excessive use of phosphate-binding antacids (aluminum hydroxide or magnesium hydroxide), alcoholism, or diabetic ketoacidosis. Prolonged respiratory alkalosis can contribute significantly to hypophosphatemia. In acidosis, such as diabetic ketoacidosis, phosphate is consumed as an acid buffer. The kidney may fail to reabsorb phosphorus in the presence of elevated PTH (Pollak et al., 2008).

Phosphate deficiency commonly impairs neurological function, which may be manifested by confusion, seizures, and coma. Peripheral neuropathy and ascending motor paralysis, similar to Guillain-Barré syndrome, may occur. Extrapontine myelinolysis (an osmotic demyelination syndrome that manifests as movement disorders, such as Parkinsonian movements) has been reported (Moore, 2010; National Institute of Neurological Disorders and Stroke, 2009).

Hematologic function also may be impaired. The hemolytic anemia associated with severe hypophosphatemia has been attributed to the inability of erythrocytes to maintain the integrity of cell membranes in the face of ATP depletion, leading to erythrocyte destruction in the spleen. Phosphate deficiency also compromises oxygen delivery to the tissues because of decreases in erythrocyte 2,3-diphosphoglycerate and the resulting leftward shift in the oxygen–hemoglobin dissociation curve, causing greater resistance of oxygen release to the tissues. Diminished oxygen delivery to the brain may be the cause of some of the neurologic manifestations mentioned earlier (Moore, 2010).

Nursing Management

Clinical symptoms of hypophosphatemia are due to decreased availability of ADP and reduced oxygen-carrying capacity of red blood cells as previously described, which leads to tissue hypoxia, cardiac dysrhythmias, and heart block (Moore, 2010). If the deficiency is severe, it can result in metabolic encephalopathy syndrome, in which the patient may be irritable and confused and may have seizures or chest pain. Respiratory failure is possible, owing to muscular weakness and diaphragmatic contractile dysfunction. Thus, the nurse should monitor phosphate serum levels for patients with respiratory weakness. Neurological symptoms may include apathy, delirium, hallucinations, and paranoia. Bones may be weakened because of resorption of the bone matrix to salvage phosphate. Bone pain and pathologic fractures may occur because of mobilization of phosphate to replace serum losses (Moore, 2010).

Treatment of hypophosphatemia is accomplished by treating the underlying cause and promoting a high phosphate diet, especially milk, if it is tolerated. Other foods that are high in phosphate are dried beans and peas, eggs, fish, organ meats (brain, liver, kidney), Brazil nuts and peanuts, poultry, seeds (pumpkin, sesame, sunflower), and whole grains (oats, barley, bran). Phosphate-binding antacids should be avoided. Mild hypophosphatemia may be corrected by oral supplements, such as Neutra-Phos liquid (sodium and potassium phosphate) or Phospho-Soda (sodium phosphate). IV phosphate salts are not commonly administered to correct hypophosphatemia because of the danger of hyperphosphatemia causing hypocalcemia followed by tetany (Pai et al., 2011). The IV route is reserved for cases of severe hypophosphatemia or in situations in which the bowel is not functioning (Moore, 2010). When IV hyperalimentation solutions are administered, 12 to 15 mmol/L of phosphorus should be added (Pai et al., 2011). Acidosis should be corrected, whether metabolic or respiratory.

Chloride

Chloride (Cl^-) is the primary anion in the ECF (blood level: 95 to 105 mEq/L). Chloride combines with sodium to create electrical neutrality in the body; therefore, it usually is found in combination with sodium. Chloride assists in the reabsorption of sodium in the kidneys. Another major function of chloride is to combine with hydrogen ion (H^+) to form hydrochloric acid for digestion and hydrolyzing nutrients for absorption in the GI tract. An ample amount of chloride ion is essential for reabsorbing hydrogen ion in the kidneys to buffer alkalosis. Bicarbonate is another major anion in the ECF, and chloride tends to vary inversely with the changes in bicarbonate. When carbon dioxide increases in the blood, chloride moves to the intracellular space to allow bicarbonate into the blood to buffer the carbonic acid. The range of variation of chloride in response to bicarbonate is 10 to 20 mEq/L (Barrett et al., 2010e).

Chloride is consumed with sodium in the diet in the form of salt, the recommended daily allowance being 750 mg/day. Normal excretion of acid by the kidneys includes the excretion of chloride. Chloride is lost through vomiting, through excessive sweating, and in the urine, especially with diuretics. Because the serum chloride level usually remains so stable, it is used to calculate the anion gap. The **anion gap** is based on the principle of **electroneutrality,** wherein the sum of all of the cation (positive) charges in the plasma must always be equal to the sum of all of the anion (negative) charges. It is calculated by adding the chloride and bicarbonate levels together and deducting the total from the sum of the sodium and potassium levels. A normal anion gap is 10 to 17. Anion gaps above 30 indicate excess organic acids, such as lactic acid or ketone acids (Kaslow, 2011). Further discussion of the anion gap is found on page 368 in the discussion of metabolic acidosis.

Hyperchloremia

Hyperchloremia (serum chloride $>$ 105 mEq/L) may result from metabolic acidosis (arterial pH $<$ 7.35). Common causes are hyperparathyroidism, dehydration, and respiratory alkalosis. Symptoms are increased depth and rate of respiration, lethargy, stupor, disorientation, and coma if the acidosis is not treated. Treatment is aimed at the underlying cause and includes the administration of saline solutions to repair volume losses and the administration of potassium (Agraharker, 2011).

Hypochloremia

Hypochloremia ($<$ 95 mEq/L) occurs because of a loss of gastric fluids in the form of hydrochloric acid with nasogastric suctioning and severe vomiting. The level of serum chloride will be reduced, and that of bicarbonate will be significantly elevated (30 to 40 mEq/L). One cause is stomach pyloric obstruction due to duodenal ulcer or prolonged vomiting, possibly caused by bowel obstruction. Diabetic ketoacidosis may result in chloride loss because of the osmotic diuresis and elevated bicarbonate. A rare condition is Bartter's syndrome, a congenital defect that prevents renal chloride reabsorption, resulting in decreased levels of chloride (Eaton & Pooler, 2009).

Hypochloremia may cause hypochloremic alkalosis (pH levels greater than 7.45). Bicarbonate will be excessively retained to maintain electrical neutrality and buffer acid–base imbalances. Symptoms of alkalosis are paresthesias of the face and extremities, muscle spasms and tetany, slow and shallow respirations, and dehydration. Initial management involves the administration of IV fluids, preferably normal (0.9%) saline (Ferry, 2009).

Collaborative Management

Care of the patient with electrolyte imbalances involves collaboration among members of a multidisciplinary team (IOM [Institute of Medicine], 2011). In order to meet desired patient outcomes, it is essential that this interdisciplinary team communicate openly with one another in developing and evaluating care of the patient and family (IOM [Institute of Medicine], 2010). The health care provider directs the patient's care and writes medication, fluid replacement, and laboratory test orders to ascertain the electrolyte status and the outcomes of directed therapies. Pharmacists ensure that the IV fluids and medications administered will bring about the desired change in the patient. Nurses are vigilant at the bedside to notify the health care provider of changes in the patient's clinical condition. Dietitians provide specified diets and nutritional teaching when patients are allowed to eat and are ready for discharge. The team collaboration aspect of care is reflected in the patient care plans that are provided in this chapter.

Gerontological Considerations

Older individuals have decreased perception of thirst due to aging and might not replace fluids appropriately. These older adults are particularly vulnerable to dehydration because many are taking prescription diuretics for high blood pressure. Other causes of fluid deficit may be nausea, vomiting, and diarrhea resulting from gastroenteritis (stomach flu) or food poisoning. Additionally, if the older adult has a fear of falling related to decreased mobility, he may choose not to walk to obtain fluids; this in turn may lead to dehydration.

Research

Opportunities for nursing research related to fluid and electrolyte imbalances are investigations into ways of promoting patient awareness of problems with electrolyte abnormalities and corrective actions to be taken. Because of its emphasis on prevention of osteoporosis, nutritional research might address overuse of antacids in combination with high milk ingestion or calcium-supplement therapy. The Research Opportunities box on this page outlines research topics on the area of fluid and electrolyte imbalances.

RESEARCH OPPORTUNITIES Related to Fluid and Electrolyte Imbalances

Research Area	Clinical Impact
Overuse of antacids in combination with high milk ingestion or calcium-supplement therapy	Prevention of osteoporosis
Low serum magnesium in diabetics due to the diuresis associated with hyperglycemia	Determining what role, if any, this electrolyte abnormality plays in cardiac symptoms in the diabetic population
Assessing the accuracy of bedside monitoring of intake and output reports	Improving the quality of data on patients' intakes and outputs of fluids

Weblink: An Acid—Base Tutorial

ACID–BASE BALANCE

Disorders of the balance between the acids and bases in the body are common clinical problems that result from or accompany a wide variety of pathologic conditions and diseases. A basic understanding of the effect of these imbalances on organ systems is important for nurses in assessing and caring for patients in all clinical settings.

Acid–Base Homeostasis

A **hydrogen ion** is a single charged particle (proton) that is not orbited by any electrons. The hydrogen ion (H^+) is the smallest ionic particle, and it is extremely reactive. Because of this reactivity, the hydrogen ion has a significant effect on physiological functions even though it is present in very low concentrations. The hydrogen ion combines with alkali/bases or other negatively charged ions at low concentrations. Proteins contain many negatively charged and positively charged groups within their structure. Therefore, even small changes in hydrogen ion concentration can alter protein and enzyme functioning. More extreme changes may totally disrupt the protein's structure, a process referred to as *denaturing* them. Disturbances in hydrogen ion concentration may result in abnormalities of function in many organs, such as the pulmonary, renal, or cardiac systems, and can also alter such processes as blood clotting and the metabolism of drugs (Schlichtig, 2011).

Plasma pH, an indicator of hydrogen ion concentration, is the negative logarithm of the hydrogen ion concentration measured in nanomoles per liter (nmol/L). A normal pH of 7.40 is equivalent to 40 nmol/L of hydrogen ion. In more commonly used terms, this would be equal to 0.0004 mEq/L. Contrast that with a normal serum potassium level of 4 mEq/L or a normal serum sodium level of 140 mEq/L. Because it is a *negative* log, as the hydrogen ion concentration increases, the pH decreases. Conversely, as the hydrogen ion concentration goes down, pH goes up. Homeostatic mechanisms work to keep pH within a relatively narrow range of 7.35 to 7.45 for optimal cell functioning. As the pH changes, either rising or falling, enzymes may stop functioning, nerve and muscle activity may weaken, and if the change is extreme, all metabolic activity may become deranged. The pH range that is usually considered compatible with life is 6.8 to 7.8.

Acids are compounds that form hydrogen ion in solution. Because of this, they are referred to as proton *donors*. As an example, hydrochloric acid (HCl) gives up H^+ when added to blood. Strong acids hold their hydrogen ion weakly, so the ion dissociates easily and can then act on other substances. Weak acids hold onto their hydrogen ion more tightly, so they do not contribute as much to the free hydrogen ion concentration. Because of this, the solution will have a higher (less acid) pH (Levitzky, 2007).

Bases or **alkalis** are compounds that combine with hydrogen ion in solution; they are proton *acceptors*. **Sodium bicarbonate** ($NaHCO_3^-$) removes hydrogen ion when added to the blood. Acids and bases constantly react with one another to neutralize changes in hydrogen ion concentration.

Carbon dioxide (CO_2) can be thought of as a potential acid. When it is dissolved in water, it becomes **carbonic acid:**

$$CO_2 + H_2O \rightarrow H_2CO_3 \text{ (carbonic acid)}$$

Carbonic acid then dissociates into hydrogen ion and bicarbonate:

$$H_2CO_3 \rightarrow H^+ + HCO_3^-$$

In plasma, under normal circumstances, there are 20 parts of bicarbonate to 1 part carbonic acid, a ratio of 20:1. If this 20:1 ratio is altered in either direction, the plasma pH will change (Schlichtig, 2011).

Body metabolism continually produces CO_2 (the respiratory acid) and other nonrespiratory acids, called metabolic acids. These acids are released into capillary blood, lowering the pH. Under normal conditions, this pH change is quite small. Blood arrives in the arterioles with a pH of 7.4 (which is equivalent to 40 nmol/L of hydrogen ion) and leaves the venules with a pH of 7.36 (equal to 44 nmol/L of hydrogen ion). Hydrogen ions have been added to the blood from the cell interior, which has a pH of about 7.0, equivalent to 100 nmol/L of hydrogen ion (Grogono, 2010).

The amount of respiratory acid produced is about 288 L/day (Grogono, 2010). This large amount is matched to the lung ventilation, which is how the respiratory acid is excreted from the body. By comparison, very little metabolic acid is produced on a daily basis, about 0.1 mol (100 mEq). The main metabolic acids are lactic acid, pyruvic acid, ketoacids seen in diabetic acidosis, acetoacetic acid, and beta-hydroxybutyric acid. These acids are eliminated by the kidneys or metabolized by the liver. The capacity for elimination of these metabolic acids from these organs is much lower than that of the lungs.

Abnormalities in the balance of acid to base can be grouped into four basic categories:

- ***Respiratory Acidosis:*** Excess of carbon dioxide leading to an acid pH
- ***Respiratory Alkalosis:*** Lower than normal level of carbon dioxide leading to an alkaline pH
- ***Metabolic Acidosis:*** Excess of hydrogen ion or a deficiency in bicarbonate leading to an acid pH
- ***Metabolic Alkalosis:*** Excess of bicarbonate leading to an alkaline pH.

Chart 15–1 provides a summary of acid–base terminology.

Maintaining Acid–Base Homeostasis

The body's response to changes in acid–base status has three components:

1. ***The First Defense:*** Buffering
2. ***The Second Defense:*** Changing the level of CO_2
3. ***The Third Defense:*** Changing the level of HCO_3^-.

Buffer Systems: The First Defense

A **buffer** is a compound that minimizes the change in hydrogen ion concentration and, thus, the change in pH when these ions are added

CHART 15–1 Acid and Base Terminology

Acidemia/Acidosis	Alkalemia/Alkalosis
Blood pH <7.40	Blood pH >7.40
Caused by loss of base/alkali; increase of acid	Caused by increase of base/alkali; loss of acid
Lowers the 20:1 bicarbonate-to-carbonic acid ratio	Raises the 20:1 bicarbonate-to-carbonic acid ratio
Less base/more acid	More base/less acid

or removed from solution. A buffer acts like a sponge: When there is an excess of hydrogen ion, the sponge soaks up the extra ions. When the level of hydrogen ion is decreased, the sponge can be squeezed out to release hydrogen ions back into the blood. Buffer systems act quickly to prevent excess changes in the pH.

There are buffers within body cells and in the ECF. The primary buffers of the extracellular system are carbonic acid and bicarbonate (Figure 15–4◆). The concentrations of these two substances are regulated by two independent systems. Carbonic acid is controlled by respiration via the lungs, and bicarbonate is controlled by excretion via the kidneys. Oxidative (aerobic) metabolism of amino acids and the anaerobic metabolism of glucose to lactate and pyruvic acid produce CO_2, which, again, can be thought of as a potential acid. Although CO_2 does not contain hydrogen ions, it reacts rapidly with water to form carbonic acid, which then dissociates into hydrogen and bicarbonate ions, as was noted previously. This reaction can be written:

$$CO_2 + H_2O \rightarrow H_2CO_3^- \leftrightarrow HCO_3^- + H^+$$

This reaction occurs throughout the body and, in certain circumstances, such as within red blood cells, can be sped up by the enzyme carbonic anhydrase.

Excess carbon dioxide is exhaled by the lungs as carbon dioxide gas. The concentration of bicarbonate ions is controlled by the kidneys. Under normal circumstances, the kidneys reabsorb and retain all of the bicarbonate presented to them by glomerular filtration. The kidneys also excrete small amounts of acid in the renal tubule. In alkalosis, either respiratory or metabolic, the kidneys retain hydrogen ion and excrete bicarbonate. In contrast, in respiratory acidosis and most cases of metabolic acidosis, the kidneys excrete hydrogen ion and conserve bicarbonate to correct the pH.

The intracellular buffer system is the phosphate buffer system. This system consists of dihydrogen phosphate ion (H_2PO_4) as the hydrogen ion donor (the acid) and hydrogen phosphate (HPO_4) as the hydrogen ion acceptor, the base. These two compounds are in equilibrium inside the cell. When there is excess hydrogen ion in blood plasma, the hydrogen ions cross the cell membrane, enter the intracellular fluid (ICF), and are consumed by reacting with HPO_4. If there is extra hydroxide, or base, these compounds enter the intracellular fluid, where they react with the H_2PO_4.

Protein buffers in the blood include plasma proteins and hemoglobin. Hemoglobin (Hgb) is the more important of these because it can bind to both CO_2 and H^+. Hemoglobin exists in two forms. It leaves the left side of the heart carrying its load of oxygen as oxyhemoglobin. After the hemoglobin has delivered the oxygen to the cell, its oxygen content is depleted and it has now become deoxygenated Hgb. Deoxygenated Hgb is a better buffer than oxygenated Hgb because it has a stronger affinity for both the CO_2 and the hydrogen ion. Oxygen unloading at the tissues increases the amount of deoxygenated Hgb, thus producing the superior buffer exactly where it is needed to buffer the additional hydrogen ion being produced by metabolism (Shlichtig, 2011).

At the tissue level, dissolved CO_2 enters the red blood cells (RBCs), where it combines with water to form carbonic acid. Carbonic anhydrase, present in the RBCs, is the enzyme that catalyzes this reaction. The carbonic acid then dissociates into bicarbonate and hydrogen ions. The hydrogen ions then bind to deoxygenated Hgb when they are soaked up by the buffer "sponge." Hemoglobin's buffering capacity is due to a chain within its structure, the imidazole chain. Imidazole can accept an extra proton, the hydrogen ion, or donate it back when the body pH is corrected (Levitzky, 2007). The bicarbonate ions that are formed by the dissociation pass through RBC membranes back into the plasma in exchange for chloride ions (Cl^-). This ensures that there is no gain or loss of negative ions within the RBCs.

When the RBCs reach the lungs, this process is reversed. Hydrogen ions that were bound to the hemoglobin recombine with the bicarbonate to form CO_2, which passes through the RBC membranes into the alveoli so it can be expired. The deoxygenated Hgb combines with oxygen to prepare to return to the tissues. This process is illustrated in Figure 15–5◆.

In addition to the buffer systems just described, bones also act as a buffer. The carbonate and phosphate salts in bone provide a long-term supply of buffer. They act as a reserve for alkalis. In acute metabolic acidosis, bone can take up hydrogen ion in exchange for calcium (Ca^{2+}), sodium (Na^+), and potassium (K^+). In chronic metabolic acidosis, calcium carbonate is released from bone as bone crystals dissolve. This situation can lead to the osteodystrophy (generalized defect in bone

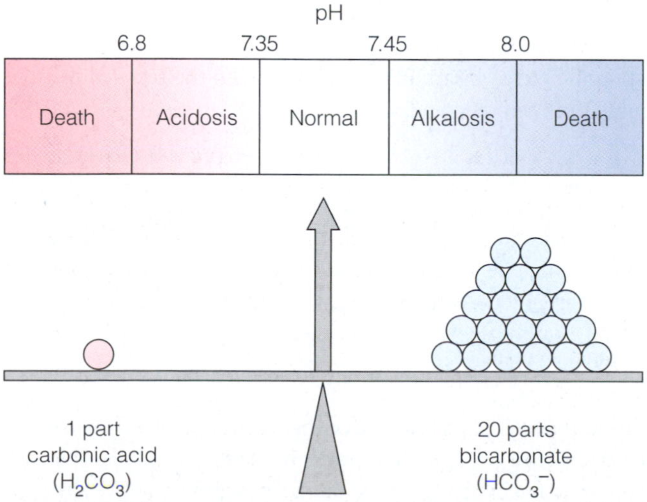

FIGURE 15–4 ◆ The normal ratio of bicarbonate to carbonic acid is 20:1. As long as this ratio is maintained, the pH remains within the normal range of 7.35–7.45.

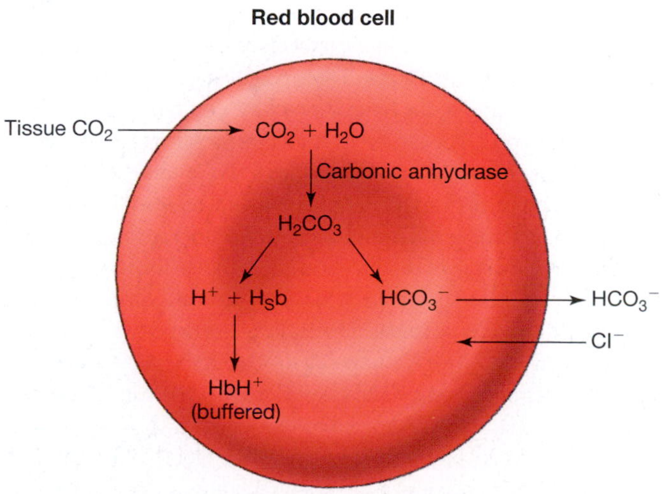

FIGURE 15–5 ◆ Oxygenation-deoxygenation cycle of erythrocytes.

development) that is often seen in chronic renal failure, which is a cause of chronic metabolic acidosis (DuBose, 2008).

Changing the Level of CO_2: The Second Defense

The lungs help to regulate plasma pH on a minute-to-minute basis by regulating the level of carbon dioxide, the respiratory acid. Carbon dioxide is measured as the partial pressure of carbon dioxide in arterial blood, denoted $PaCO_2$. This level is tightly controlled under normal conditions and kept within a narrow range of 35 to 45 mmHg at sea level. The lungs can either retain or excrete CO_2 by altering the rate and depth of ventilation. The amount of ventilation is generally quantified by how much air the lungs move in 1 minute, referred to as the **minute ventilation.** Minute ventilation is the product of respiratory *rate* and *depth*, referred to as the tidal volume (V_t). Normal resting respiratory rate is about 12 breaths per minute. Normal resting depth tidal volume is about 500 mL. This yields a normal minute ventilation of 6 L/min:

$$12 \text{ breaths/min} \times 500 \text{ mL } V_t = 6{,}000 \text{ mL or } 6 \text{ L}$$

This normal minute ventilation should yield a normal $PaCO_2$.

The respiratory center located in the medulla in the brainstem controls the rate and depth of ventilation in response to the $PaCO_2$. Chemoreceptors located on the surface of the medulla are in contact with cerebrospinal fluid (CSF). These receptors are termed "central" because they are located within the CNS. As the $PaCO_2$ rises, the arterial $PaCO_2$ reaches equilibrium with the CO_2 in the CSF. That CO_2 in the CSF combines with water to form carbonic acid, as previously described. The carbonic acid dissociates into hydrogen ion and bicarbonate. The CSF hydrogen ion diffuses into the medullary tissue and stimulates the chemoreceptors. They, in turn, stimulate the diaphragm and intercostal muscles to increase the rate and depth of ventilation. This increase in minute ventilation will "blow off" excess CO_2, returning it back toward normal, thereby correcting the pH.

The reverse happens when there are abnormally low levels of CO_2. In this state of hyperventilation, the medullary centers slow the rate and depth of ventilation to allow accumulation of CO_2 back toward normal, thereby correcting the pH.

The $PaCO_2$, acting on the central chemoreceptors by altering the pH of the CSF, is the most important single determinant of ventilation and is referred to as the **hypercarbic drive.** There are also peripheral chemoreceptors that are responsive to the level of oxygen in the blood and hydrogen ion, as well as the $PaCO_2$. These peripheral receptors are located in the carotid arteries at the bifurcation of the common carotid and in the arch of the aorta. The carotid receptors are sensitive to PaO_2, $PaCO_2$, and pH. The aortic receptors are sensitive to PaO_2 and $PaCO_2$ but not pH. Neural impulses from the carotid bodies increase as the PaO_2 falls below about 60 mmHg and stimulates the respiratory centers to increase both the rate and depth of ventilation in an attempt to increase the body's oxygen supply. This responsiveness to low oxygen tension, referred to as the **hypoxic drive,** is potentiated by acidosis and hypercapnia.

The hypercarbic drive is a response to acute respiratory acidosis. If a person suffers from chronic ventilatory failure, such as a patient with end-stage emphysema that leads to chronically high $PaCO_2$ levels (chronic respiratory acidosis), bicarbonate will cross the blood–brain barrier to buffer the CSF hydrogen ion changes. It takes hours to days for this adaptation to occur. Because of this increased bicarbonate on the brain side of the blood–brain barrier, the central chemoreceptors become less sensitive to changes in the level of CO_2, which results in a decrease in the strength of the ventilatory drive moderated by these central receptors. When this occurs, the only remaining drive to breathe is the stimulation of the peripheral receptors by a low PaO_2, known as the hypoxic drive.

In clinical practice, the terms *hyperventilation* and *hypoventilation* apply only to ventilation and its effect on the $PaCO_2$. A low $PaCO_2$, or hypocapnia, defines the state of **hyperventilation.** A high $PaCO_2$, or hypercapnia, defines the state of **hypoventilation.** There is a tendency to describe someone who is breathing rapidly and deeply as "hyperventilating," but whether this is actually the case cannot be determined without obtaining an arterial blood gas and looking at the $PaCO_2$.

In addition to the level of CO_2, an increase in the arterial hydrogen ion concentration will stimulate the central chemoreceptors of the respiratory control center, but to a lesser degree because hydrogen ions do not diffuse into the CSF as easily as the lipid-soluble CO_2; therefore, the response is slower. However, in a state of metabolic acidosis, such as that which exists during diabetic ketoacidosis, the medullary centers will stimulate the lungs to increase the minute ventilation to blow off CO_2, even if that level is normal. These rapid, deep respirations, referred to as Kussmaul respirations, are an attempt to correct the arterial pH by decreasing respiratory acid. This process is referred to as **compensation.**

Changing the Level of HCO_3^-: The Third Defense

The kidneys perform two basic functions to maintain acid–base balance: They secrete hydrogen ions, and they restore or reclaim bicarbonate ions. Bicarbonate ions are freely filtered in the kidneys by glomerular filtration. The level of bicarbonate in the renal tubular fluid is the same as that of plasma. To help make this clear, think of tubular fluid as being outside of the body. During glomerular filtration, plasma, water, and solutes are forced by hydrostatic pressure across the membrane of the glomerular capillaries into the lumen of the tubule. If substances remain in the tubular fluid or other substances are secreted into that fluid, they will eventually leave the body in urine. Secretion is the active process of moving substances, such as hydrogen ion, from the blood into the tubular fluid against the concentration gradient. If substances are reabsorbed from the tubular fluid back across the membrane and into the blood, they are being reclaimed back into the body.

The reabsorption of bicarbonate that has been filtered into the tubular fluid occurs primarily in the proximal convoluted tubule of the nephron. Filtered bicarbonate combines with the secreted hydrogen ions to form carbonic acid, which then dissociates into CO_2 and water:

$$HCO_3^- + H^+ \leftrightarrow H_2CO_3 \leftrightarrow CO_2 + H_2O$$

This reaction is catalyzed by carbonic anhydrase, the same enzyme that is contained in the red blood cells. The CO_2 crosses from the tubular fluid into the cells lining the tubule. Here, the CO_2 recombines with water to again form carbonic acid, which then dissociates to hydrogen ion and bicarbonate. This is the reverse of the preceding equation, or

$$CO_2 + H_2O \leftrightarrow H_2CO_3^- \ HCO_3^- + H^+$$

The bicarbonate passes from the cell back across the membrane into the blood while the hydrogen ion passes back into the tubular fluid. This hydrogen ion is exchanged for sodium ion, another positive ion.

In the face of a high load of metabolic acids, the kidneys also increase their production of the urinary buffer, ammonia (NH_4). Under normal circumstances, NH_4 excretion is about 30 mmol/day, or about 0.5 mmol/kg. This excretion can increase to about 280 mmol/day, but this response takes several days to be completed (DuBose, 2008).

In the event of respiratory acidosis, in which there is an excess of plasma CO_2, and in most cases of metabolic acidosis, the kidneys excrete hydrogen ion and conserve bicarbonate to help restore the acid–base balance and return the pH toward normal. In respiratory and metabolic alkalosis, the kidneys retain hydrogen ions and excrete bicarbonate ions. This metabolic compensation is slow in comparison to respiratory compensation; it can take hours to days to occur. Note that the average ventilation rate is about 6 liters per *minute*, whereas the renal excretion rate is only about 2 liters per *day* (Eaton & Pooler, 2009).

Assessment of Acid–Base Balance

ABG values are most often used to assess acid–base balance, although serum electrolytes will help fine-tune the analysis. The Diagnostic Tests box outlines the commonly assessed laboratory values.

Normal ABG values are:

$$pH = 7.40 \text{ (range: } 7.35-7.45)$$

$$PaCO_2 = 40 \text{ mEq/L (range: } 35-45)$$

$$HCO_3^- = 24-28 \text{ mEq/L}$$

Along with these values, most ABGs also report the **base excess.** This is a calculated value that is based on the bicarbonate level, the $PaCO_2$, and the hematocrit. The base excess refers to the number of milliequivalents of bicarbonate per liter of ECF of which there is too much (base excess) or too little (base deficit). As an example, suppose a patient has a base excess of +6. This indicates a metabolic alkalosis and quantifies it. Every liter of the patient's ECF has 6 mEq too much bicarbonate or other base. In an opposite example, suppose a patient has a base excess of −10. This indicates a metabolic acidosis, and every liter of ECF is deficient in bicarbonate by 10 mEq. This number can help guide clinicians who are considering how much bicarbonate to administer to a patient with severe metabolic acidosis. (*Note:* Although a positive number indicates a base excess and a negative number indicates a base deficit, in clinical practice, only the term *base excess* is commonly used.) A negative number is referred to as a "base excess of minus *x*." A normal base excess, then, is zero—not too little or too much bicarbonate. The normal range is usually considered to be ±2 mEq. Outlined here is the recommended stepwise approach for the interpretation of ABGs, which is also illustrated in Figure 15–6◆:

Step 1: ***Assess the pH:*** Is it normal, low, or high? This first step is crucial because it guides the approach to the rest of the values. If the pH is less than 7.35, there is an acidosis. If the pH is greater than 7.45, there is an alkalosis.

Step 2: ***Assess the Respiratory Component:*** Is the $PaCO_2$ normal, low, or high? If the cause of an abnormality is a respiratory problem, the $PaCO_2$ and the pH move in opposite directions. In ventilatory failure, the $PaCO_2$ rises and causes a lowered acid pH. If both the pH and the $PaCO_2$ have moved in the same direction (i.e., both are increased or both are decreased), then the cause of the abnormality is a metabolic one. Refer to the examples in Chart 15–2.

DIAGNOSTIC TESTS for Acid–Base Imbalances

Tests With Description, Rationale, and Normal Values	Expected Abnormality
pH *Plasma pH is an indicator of hydrogen ion concentration.* Normal range is 7.35–7.45.	↓'d < 7.35 in uncompensated respiratory or metabolic acidosis ↑'d > 7.45 in uncompensated respiratory or metabolic alkalosis
$PaCO_2$ *CO_2 is a respiratory acid. An excess will lead to acidosis; a deficiency will lead to alkalosis.* Normal range is 35–45 mmHg.	>45 mmHg in respiratory acidosis <35 mmHg in respiratory alkalosis
HCO_3^- *HCO_3^- is a base. A deficiency will lead to acidosis; an excess will lead to alkalosis.* Normal range is 24–28 mEq/L	<24 mEq/L in metabolic acidosis >28 mEq/L in metabolic alkalosis
Base Excess *Quantifies the milliequivalents of bicarbonate that are deficient/in excess per liter of ECF.* Normal range is +/− 2 mEq.	> −2 in metabolic acidosis > +2 in metabolic alkalosis
Serum Potassium *Excess hydrogen ion moves into cells and displaces K^+ out of the cell and into the serum.*	↑'d with acidosis
Ionized Calcium *Alkalosis ↑'s the binding of calcium to albumin, resulting in a decrease in free, ionized calcium in the serum.*	↓'d in alkalosis
Anion Gap *Indicates an increased anion load (lactic acidosis, ketoacidosis, ingestion of acids, rhabdomyolysis).*	↑'d above 10–17 in high anion gap acidosis
Loss of Bicarbonate (diarrhea, fistula, renal dysfunction) or ingestion of base.	Normal in nonanion gap metabolic acidosis

Source: Kee, J. L. (2010). Laboratory and diagnostic tests with nursing implications (8th ed.). Upper Saddle River, NJ: Pearson Prentice Hall.

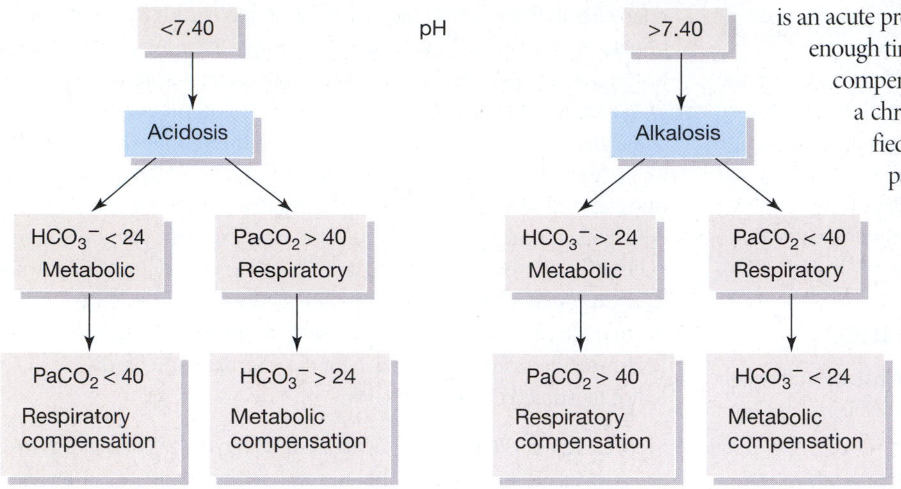

FIGURE 15–6 Stepwise approach to ABG interpretation.

CHART 15–2 Examples of Abnormalities of the Respiratory Component

Example 1: Mrs. A has a $PaCO_2 = 56$ and a $pH = 7.27$.

The $PaCO_2$ is increased (16 mmHg above normal). The pH is decreased by 0.13.

In respiratory acidosis, the $PaCO_2$ and the pH move in opposite directions, so: *Mrs. A has a respiratory acidosis.*

Example 2: Mr. B has a $PaCO_2 = 28$ and a $pH = 7.52$.

The $PaCO_2$ is decreased by 12 mmHg. The pH is increased by 0.12.

In respiratory alkalosis, the $PaCO_2$ and the pH move in opposite directions, so: *Mr. B has a respiratory alkalosis.*

Example 3: Ms. C has a $PaCO_2 = 52$ and a $pH = 7.48$.

The $PaCO_2$ is increased. The pH is also increased.

Because both the $PaCO_2$ and the pH are elevated (moving in the same direction), it cannot be a respiratory problem. If it isn't a respiratory problem, then it has to be a *metabolic derangement.* (This is known even though a value for bicarbonate hasn't been given.)

Step 3: ***Assess the Metabolic Component:*** Are the bicarbonate and the base excess normal, low, or high? In a metabolic abnormality, the pH and the bicarbonate move in the same direction. If the bicarbonate is increased, pH will be increased. If the bicarbonate is decreased, the pH will also be lower. Refer to the examples in Chart 15–3.

Steps 2 and 3 will identify the primary problem if there is one. Next, the nurse should evaluate compensation. Any change in the acid–base equilibrium will cause the system that is *not* the primary cause of the abnormality to respond to an attempt to restore the 20:1 ratio of bicarbonate-to-carbonic acid and bring the pH back toward normal. If the primary problem is a metabolic abnormality, the lungs will increase or decrease the total minute ventilation to attempt to bring the pH back toward normal. If the cause of the problem is respiratory, the kidneys will retain or secrete hydrogen ion and/or bicarbonate to restore balance.

Because renal/metabolic compensation is slower, taking hours to days, a health care provider can infer whether a respiratory abnormality is an acute problem or a chronic one. If the kidneys have not had enough time to compensate, the problem is acute. If metabolic compensation has taken place, the problem is likely to be a chronic one. Once the primary cause has been identified (CO_2 or HCO_3^-), look at the other value. If that parameter is abnormal but is moving in a direction that would bring the pH back toward normal, then compensation is occurring. If the pH is in the normal range, then complete compensation has occurred. If the pH is not within the normal range but is moving in the right direction, then partial compensation has occurred. See Chart 15–4 for a summary of the blood gas changes seen in respiratory and metabolic disturbances.

Complex Acid–Base Disorders

Sometimes patients will have combined disorders. For example, a critically ill patient who has recently suffered a cardiac arrest may have both respiratory acidosis and metabolic acidosis. It can be helpful, sometimes, to look at the magnitude of the change in the CO_2 or HCO_3^- and compare it to the expected change in the pH. A simple rule of thumb to use is this: For every 10 mmHg change in the $PaCO_2$, there should be a corresponding pH change of 0.08 to 0.1 in the opposite direction. Using the 0.1 is easiest to calculate:

$$\text{Normal } PaCO_2 = 40; \text{ normal pH} = 7.40$$

If the $PaCO_2$ increases to 50 (a change of 10 mmHg from normal), the pH should decrease by 0.10 to 7.30 if there is only a respiratory acidosis. Conversely, if the $PaCO_2$ decreases to 22 (a change of 18 mmHg from normal), the pH should increase to 7.58, a 0.18 increase, if there is only a respiratory alkalosis. However, if the $PaCO_2$ increases to 50 (a change of 10 mmHg), but the pH is 7.15 (a change of 0.25), this change in the pH is much greater than it would be if there was a respiratory acidosis alone. In this case, a concurrent metabolic acidosis must be causing the large drop in pH with a rather moderate increase in the $PaCO_2$.

CHART 15–3 Examples of Abnormalities of the Metabolic Component

Example 1: Mr. D has a HCO_3^- of 16 and a pH of 7.24. Base excess $= -6$.

The bicarbonate and the pH are both decreased. In a metabolic acidosis, the bicarbonate and the pH move in the same direction.

This is a metabolic acidosis. The base excess of –6 indicates that every liter of Mr. D's extracellular fluid needs 6 mEq of additional bicarbonate to normalize the pH.

Example 2: Mr. E has a HCO_3^- of 34 mEq and a pH of 7.50. Base excess $= +5$.

The bicarbonate and the pH are both elevated. In metabolic alkalosis, the bicarbonate and the pH move in the same direction.

This is a metabolic alkalosis. The base excess of +5 indicates that every liter of Mr. E's extracellular fluid has 5 mEq too much bicarbonate or other anion.

(A base excess is not as clinically helpful as a base deficit. A specific number of milliequivalents of bicarbonate cannot be dialyzed or otherwise removed, and acids are rarely administered to patients to correct a metabolic alkalosis.)

CHART 15–4 Blood Gas Changes in Acid–Base Imbalances

Acid–Base Disorder	pH Normal = 7.35–7.45	$PaCO_2$ Normal = 35–45 mmHg	HCO_3^- Normal = 24–28 mEq/L
Respiratory acidosis	↓	↑	Normal (↑'d if compensating)
Respiratory alkalosis	↑	↓	Normal (↓'d if compensating)
Metabolic acidosis	↓	Normal (↓ 'd if compensating)	↓
Metabolic alkalosis	↑	Normal (↑'d if compensating)	↑

Note: $PaCO_2$ and pH move in *opposite* directions; HCO_3^- and pH move in the *same* direction.

Acid–Base Imbalances

Imbalances between acids and bases almost always occur as a result of diseases, organ dysfunction, or other pathologic conditions. The following descriptions of the four imbalances describe them as distinct abnormalities, but the nurse must evaluate them in the context of the patient's underlying pathology when caring for patients in the clinical setting. Chart 15–5 summarizes the causes of acid–base imbalances.

Respiratory Acidosis

In respiratory acidosis, also referred to as primary hypercapnia, the primary derangement of acid–base balance is an excess of arterial CO_2 accompanied by a decrease in the pH. The CO_2 is regulated in part by the respiratory rate. When respirations increase, the CO_2 decreases and vice versa with a decreased respiratory rate, thereby increasing the CO_2.

Etiology and Pathophysiology

Whenever excretion of CO_2 via the lungs fails to keep up with the body's CO_2 production, respiratory acidosis will occur. This respiratory system failure may be *acute*, occurring rapidly because of a sudden event. In this situation, the elevation in the $PaCO_2$ results in acidemia and a low pH. Respiratory acidosis may also be *chronic*, when there has been a sustained increase in the $PaCO_2$ that leads to renal compensation and elevated serum bicarbonate. Causes of acute and chronic ventilatory failure are noted in Chart 15–6.

Most of these conditions impair the lung's ability to eliminate CO_2 by impairing ventilation. Conditions that cause alveolar hypoventilation can be categorized as being caused by a decreased respiratory drive (patients who "won't breathe") or a decrease in respiratory muscle or chest wall function (patients who "can't breathe"). Normally, an increase in the $PaCO_2$ leads to a marked increase in the ventilatory drive. If there is an abnormality of ventilatory control, there will be an inappropriately low to absent ventilatory drive despite elevations in the $PaCO_2$. This can occur with a neurological event such as cerebral anoxia or from depression of the respiratory centers by drugs such as narcotics.

Another influence on the respiratory drive is the level of CNS arousal. During non–rapid eye movement (NREM) sleep, the ventilatory response to $PaCO_2$ is blunted and the minute ventilation decreases, primarily secondary to a lower tidal volume. The $PaCO_2$ can increase by about 3 to 10 mmHg. This is not clinically a problem unless the person suffers from preexisting hypercapnia, in which case respiratory acidosis may worsen.

Chest wall or respiratory muscle abnormalities can be the result of CNS disorders, neuromuscular disorders, or restrictive lung conditions such as pulmonary fibrosis. These conditions can lead to acute or chronic hypoventilation. A condition worth noting in this category is obesity hypoventilation syndrome. Some people who are morbidly obese, which is defined as having a body mass index (BMI) > 40, have a syndrome that is characterized by chronic hypoventilation and chronic respiratory failure. Chronic respiratory failure develops over a longer period of time, allowing for renal compensation by the retention of bicarbonate. Chapter 28 discusses the diagnosis and treatment of respiratory failure. These patients have a decreased ventilatory drive and an increased work of breathing. This work of breathing increase is due to a reduction in lung compliance ("stretchiness") and abdominal influences. These individuals are prone to the development of obstructive sleep apnea, which causes both hypoventilation and hypoxemia.

In chronic obstructive pulmonary diseases such as emphysema or chronic bronchitis, elevations in $PaCO_2$ are thought to be a poor prognostic sign. With emphysema, there is decreased surface area for gas exchange; this leads first to a decrease in arterial oxygenation but, in the most severe cases, also leads to chronic hypercapnia. Trapping of air in the alveolar airspaces also leads to lung hyperinflation. This hyperinflation flattens out the diaphragm, which in the relaxed position is shaped like an upside-down bowl. When the lungs are permanently inflated, this flattened diaphragm impairs the person's ability to generate negative inspiratory pressure, which is needed to pull air into the lungs. This leads to impaired ventilation and greatly contributes to the sensation of breathlessness from which these patients suffer. (Try this yourself: Take a deep breath in and hold it. Now take in more air. Hard, isn't it? And very uncomfortable.)

In some conditions, the major problem is increased production of CO_2 rather than impaired elimination. These conditions include exercise, fever, burns, thyrotoxicosis (hyperthyroidism caused by the production of too much thyroid hormone), and catabolic states such as are seen with multiple-organ failure. In fever, for example, with every degree of temperature elevation, CO_2 production increases by about 13%. Thus, a patient with a fever of 40°C (104°F) must increase alveolar ventilation by about 40% to maintain a normal $PaCO_2$. Increased CO_2 production rarely leads to hypercapnia in otherwise healthy individuals because increased production leads to increased ventilation and subsequent CO_2 excretion. Patients with preexisting pulmonary diseases, however, may not be able to increase their ventilation enough to handle the excess CO_2, and their levels will rise.

In acute respiratory acidosis, cellular buffering occurs over minutes to hours. Renal compensation occurs over several days. The kidneys reabsorb bicarbonate and excrete acid. The plasma bicarbonate increases about 3.5 mEq/L for each increase of 10 mmHg in the $PaCO_2$. In acidemia, hydrogen ion moves into cells and displaces K^+ out of the cell into the serum, although respiratory acidosis does not usually cause clinically significant hyperkalemia.

Signs, Symptoms, and Consequences

Acute hypercapnia can be life threatening when it causes severe respiratory acidosis. This usually occurs in conjunction with hypoxemia. Carbon dioxide crosses cell membranes rapidly and leads to a low

CHART 15–5 Causes of Acid–Base Disorders

Acute Respiratory Acidosis	Metabolic Acidosis
CNS Depression	**Excess H^+ Production**
Drug overdose	Lactic acidosis due to tissue hypoxia
Head trauma	Ketoacidosis: diabetic, alcoholic, starvation
Encephalitis	**Ingestion of Acids**
Stroke	Poisoning with agents such as ethylene glycol (antifreeze) or aspirin
Neuromuscular Disease	**Inadequate Acid Excretion**
Guillain-Barré syndrome	Renal dysfunction
Myasthenic crisis	Endocrine disturbances (e.g., hypoaldosteronism)
Spinal cord injury	**Excessive Loss of Bicarbonate**
Airway Disease	Excessive diarrhea
Status asthmaticus	Acetazolamide
Upper airway obstruction	
Pleural or Chest Wall Abnormalities	
Pneumothorax	
Large pleural effusion	

Chronic Respiratory Acidosis	
Impaired Central Ventilatory Drive	
Central sleep apnea	Obesity hypoventilation
Neuromuscular Disease	
Amyotrophic lateral sclerosis	Multiple sclerosis
Muscular dystrophy	Spinal cord injury
Poliomyelitis	
Airway and Lung Parenchyma Disease	
Emphysema	Interstitial lung disease
Chronic bronchitis	
Other	
Kyphoscoliosis	Diaphragmatic paralysis

Respiratory Alkalosis	Metabolic Alkalosis
Central Nervous System	**Excessive Loss of H^+**
Pain	Protracted vomiting
Anxiety	Nasogastric suction
Psychosis	**Acid Shifts Into Cells**
Fever	Potassium deficiency
Stroke	**Excessive Reabsorption of Bicarbonate**
Meningitis, encephalitis	Hypochloremia
Tumor	Thiazide and loop diuretics
Trauma	
Hypoxemia	
Drugs	
Salicylates, nicotine, progesterone	
Pregnancy	
Sepsis	
Hepatic failure	
Iatrogenic on mechanical ventilation	

CHART 15–6 Causes of Hypercapnic Ventilatory Failure

Site of Disturbance	Acute	Chronic
Respiratory center	Drug overdose	Tumor
	Trauma	
	Stroke	
Neuromuscular disease	Guillain-Barré syndrome	Polio
	Myasthenia gravis	Spinal cord injury
		Amyotrophic lateral sclerosis
Chest wall	Trauma	Kyphoscoliosis
	Pleural effusion (large)	
	Pneumothorax	
Upper airway obstruction	Tumor	
	Laryngeal edema	
	Foreign body	
Peripheral airway obstruction	Asthma (severe)	Emphysema
		Chronic bronchitis
		Obesity
		Hypoventilation

intracellular pH, which can affect many body systems. CNS symptoms dominate, and their severity depends on the magnitude of the increase, the speed with which it occurs, and the accompanying degree of hypoxemia. Carbon dioxide rapidly crosses the blood–brain barrier and lowers CSF pH. The acute effects are cerebral vessel dilation, increased cerebral blood flow, and increased intracranial pressure. Clinical manifestations of these changes include anxiety, irritability, headache, confusion, disorientation, somnolence, and lethargy. Patients may complain of dyspnea. More serious alterations of consciousness such as stupor or coma are rare but are seen when the $PaCO_2$ is markedly elevated, typically more than 70 to 100 mmHg (Barrett et al., 2010b).

The other major body system that may be affected in respiratory acidosis is the cardiovascular system. Mild to moderate hypercapnia causes release of the catecholamines epinephrine and norepinephrine and peripheral vasodilation. Catecholamines usually cause peripheral vasoconstriction, but the elevated CO_2 has an inhibitory effect on vascular smooth muscle, which leads to vasodilation. These changes result in an increase in heart rate with normal or elevated blood pressure. Because of the peripheral vasodilation, the patient's skin is often warm, flushed, and diaphoretic.

In chronic hypercapnia, the effects are not as dramatic because organ systems have a chance to adapt and renal compensation has had time to occur. The cerebral blood flow returns to normal, and the only symptom may be a morning headache, mild irritability, and lethargy. It is important to remember that patients with chronic respiratory failure may develop acute respiratory failure as well. A patient with a chronically high level of CO_2 who presents with an acid pH is suffering from acute respiratory failure. See Chart 15–7 for examples.

Acid–base disturbances are rarely isolated conditions; they usually accompany other pathophysiologic processes. The main treatment for respiratory acidosis is correction of the underlying disorder that led to its development. This might include a reversal of a drug overdose to counteract respiratory depression, the use of inhaled bronchodilators

CHART 15–7 Acute Ventilatory Failure in the Patient Who Has Chronic Ventilatory Failure

Example 1: Mr. F has $PaCO_2 = 60$, pH = 7.37, $HCO_3^- = 35$ mEq/L.

Despite the elevated $PaCO_2$, the pH is normal because the kidneys have retained bicarbonate.

In this case, *Mr. F is at or near his baseline $PaCO_2$.*

Example 2: Ms. G has $PaCO_2 = 73$, pH = 7.28, $HCO_3^- = 35$ mEq/L.

The $PaCO_2$ is elevated, but the pH is acidic despite the elevated bicarbonate.

This $PaCO_2$ of 73 is higher than the patient's baseline. If it were her baseline, her pH would be at/close to the normal range.

This patient has an *acute respiratory failure superimposed on chronic respiratory failure.*

and steroids to treat the bronchospasm that accompanies acute asthma, or the use of antibiotics to treat pneumonia and improve ventilation, thus correcting the acidosis. Administration of sodium bicarbonate is almost never indicated in the treatment of respiratory acidosis because the bicarbonate will eventually be converted to CO_2. Thus, in the long run, it can actually worsen a respiratory acidosis, although its use may be considered in the situation of cardiac arrest with extremely low pH (< 7.0 to 7.1). In this situation, metabolic acidosis is usually combined with respiratory acidosis (Barrett et al., 2010c). The metabolic acidosis is a lactic acidosis that results from anaerobic metabolism that occurs because of the lack of tissue perfusion during cardiac arrest.

Treatment also is aimed at assisting or increasing ventilation. This can be accomplished invasively through endotracheal intubation and the use of mechanical ventilation or noninvasively through the use of nasal continuous positive airway pressure (CPAP) or nasal bilevel ventilation (BiPAP). Chapter 28 discusses CPAP and BiPAP.

Intubation

There are no absolute criteria for deciding when to intubate someone in respiratory distress, but the general rule is that intubation is indicated if the patient has a $PaCO_2$ in the 80- to 90-mmHg range and a pH of less than 7.10 to 7.25. It is often a clinical decision based on the medical team's estimation of whether the patient will be able to keep on or will approach exhaustion. Once the patient is on mechanical ventilation, the patient can be supported while health care clinicians work to correct the underlying pathology. After the problem has been treated, the patient can gradually be weaned off of the ventilatory support.

When patients with chronic hypercarbia are placed on mechanical ventilation, care must be taken to correct them slowly. Too efficient ventilation of the patient will correct the $PaCO_2$ too rapidly, and the patient will develop a metabolic alkalosis because of the excess retained bicarbonate. This can alkalinize the CSF and may cause seizures. Chapter 28 includes a discussion of the various modes of mechanical ventilation.

Supplemental Oxygen

Many patients with hypercapnia are also hypoxemic, so the use of supplemental oxygen may be indicated. Supplemental oxygen has been shown to decrease mortality and leads to better outcomes (Feller-Kopman & Schwartzstein, 2010). However, the use of supplemental oxygen in patients with chronic respiratory acidosis must be approached with caution. Because chronic hypercapnia blunts the central hypercarbic drive, these patients' main stimulus to ventilation is the peripheral hypoxic drive. These patients breathe because their level of PaO_2 goes down. High levels of supplemental oxygen may blunt this hypoxic drive, leading to a further decrease in ventilation and a worsening of hypercapnia. Oxygen should be administered carefully to keep the oxygen saturation level in the low 90% range with a PaO_2 of 60 to 65 mmHg.

Safety Alert *Patients with chronic obstructive pulmonary disease who have chronically elevated levels of $PaCO_2$ may have a blunted hypercarbic drive. Their main stimulus of ventilation is the hypoxic drive. If a person who is a chronic CO_2 retainer receives a high concentration of supplemental oxygen that raises her PaO_2 above the stimulus level, respirations may be depressed. This does not mean that these patients should not receive oxygen if they are hypoxemic. It means that clinicians have to be careful and monitor them more closely. (Note: This applies only to individuals who are chronic CO_2 retainers. Not all patients who have chronic lung disease retain CO_2.)*

Weblink: Use of Oxygen in Patients with Hypercapnia

Respiratory Alkalosis

Respiratory alkalosis is an acid–base derangement characterized by a lower-than-normal $PaCO_2$ accompanied by an elevated pH. Respiratory rate is a major determinant of the $PaCO_2$ level. Excessively fast or deep ventilation "blows off" the carbon dioxide, decreasing the level and increasing the pH, causing alkalosis.

Etiology and Pathophysiology

Respiratory alkalosis is an acid–base disturbance caused by alveolar overventilation. The overventilation leads to a decreased $PaCO_2$, altering the 20:1 bicarbonate-to-carbonic acid ratio and causing an increased pH. The lungs are removing carbon dioxide faster than the tissues are producing it. This can be an acute or chronic problem. In acute respiratory alkalosis, the pH will be higher than normal. In chronic respiratory alkalosis, the $PaCO_2$ is lower than normal, but the pH is within normal limits because the kidneys have had time to eliminate bicarbonate and normalize the pH. This is renal compensation and it takes about 2 to 4 days to be completed.

Under normal circumstances, a drop in the $PaCO_2$ has an inhibitory effect on the central respiratory centers, but certain disease processes or psychological conditions can stimulate ventilation and lead to hypocapnia. Acute respiratory alkalosis leads to changes in serum electrolytes. Hydrogen ions shift from the intracellular compartment to the plasma. The positively charged hydrogen ions move out of cells in exchange for other positively charged ions, specifically potassium and phosphate, which move into the cells, resulting in hypokalemia and hypophosphatemia. There is also a reduction in free serum calcium because, in alkalemia, there is increased binding of Ca^{2+} to serum albumin. Because the only calcium that is physiologically active is the free, nonionized calcium, the patient can develop symptoms of hypocalcemia.

Respiratory alkalosis is often caused by hypoxemia. When the PaO_2 drops, the peripheral chemoreceptors send impulses to the central respiratory control centers. They, in turn, increase ventilation in an attempt to raise the PaO_2. This increased ventilation, however, causes the patient to excrete (blow off) too much CO_2. This same process occurs in the presence of a metabolic acidosis; the lungs increase ventilation to eliminate CO_2 and normalize the pH.

Neurological conditions such as a stroke, meningitis, encephalitis, head trauma, or tumor can lead to excessive ventilation. Psychological conditions such as anxiety and panic or severe pain can also cause overventilation. During pregnancy, progesterone levels increase. This situation stimulates the respiratory center and can lead to respiratory alkalosis (Malish, Murdock, & Sassoon, 2010). It also can be an iatrogenic problem resulting from inappropriate machine settings when the patient is on mechanical ventilation.

Signs, Symptoms, and Consequences

The signs and symptoms of respiratory alkalosis are nonspecific and often vary according to the underlying illness or cause. Patients may appear anxious; tachycardia and tachypnea are common. CNS effects are caused by the cerebral vessel vasoconstriction that occurs with alkalosis. This vasoconstriction causes a significant decrease in cerebral blood flow. Vertigo, anxiety, clumsiness, and forgetfulness are often seen. The cardiovascular effects are nonspecific but may include tachycardia as well as atrial and/or ventricular dysrhythmias (Malish, Murdock, & Sassoon, 2010).

Alkalosis of any origin favors the binding of calcium to albumin. When there is increased binding of calcium, there is less free, ionized calcium in the blood. Because only free, ionized calcium is biologically active, any time there is less of it circulating, patients will exhibit signs and symptoms of hypocalcemia. Some of the symptoms that are seen with respiratory alkalosis may be the result of hypocalcemia and can include numbness and/or tingling around the mouth or in the hands and fingers. A positive Chvostek's sign or carpopedal spasm (Trousseau's sign) may be seen. Both Chvostek's sign and Trousseau's sign are discussed on page 357. Muscle cramps also may be experienced.

Medical Management

Treatment of respiratory alkalosis is directed primarily at correcting the underlying disorder. Respiratory alkalosis is rarely a life-threatening abnormality, and treatment is usually not indicated unless the pH is > 7.50 (Lambert-Drwiega, 2010). If the hypocapnia is secondary to hypoxemia, supplemental oxygen should be administered. If the patient is on mechanical ventilation, the tidal volume and/or respiratory rate settings should be adjusted to decrease the minute ventilation to the point where the $PaCO_2$ is in the normal range. Chapter 28 includes a discussion of ventilator settings and their impact on the acid–base balance.

Patients with psychological hyperventilation syndromes should benefit from reassurance and methods to decrease stress. During acute episodes, it may be necessary to have the patient breathe into a paper bag, which causes people to "rebreathe" their CO_2 and minimize loss through ventilation. The nurse plays an important role during this process by maintaining a calm, reassuring demeanor and explaining the reason for the rebreathing. Sedatives should be reserved for patients who do not respond to conservative treatment (Lambert-Drwiega, 2010).

Metabolic Acidosis

Metabolic acidosis is characterized by an increase in total body acid, leading to a decreased pH. Any disorder that alters metabolism in the body can contribute to the development of metabolic acidosis.

Etiology and Pathophysiology

Metabolic acidosis is a sign of some underlying disease process. It can be induced in two ways:

- An addition of hydrogen ions or an inability to excrete the H^+ load from dietary metabolism
- A primary decrease in plasma bicarbonate to $<$24 mEq/L.

The increased hydrogen ion load can come from numerous sources; lactic acidosis is believed to be the most common cause of metabolic acidosis in the hospitalized patient (Grogono, 2010). It represents an imbalance between lactate production and utilization. Tissue hypoxia is the most common cause of clinically significant lactic acidosis. The tissue hypoxia is the result of increased oxygen demand or decreased oxygen delivery to body tissues. Without oxygen, tissues resort to anaerobic metabolism. In the face of anaerobic metabolism, body tissues are unable to completely oxidize sugar to CO_2; instead, sugars are partially oxidized to lactic acid. This acid cannot be excreted via the lungs; therefore, it remains in the circulation and causes a metabolic acidosis.

Ketoacidosis from uncontrolled diabetes mellitus, alcoholism, or prolonged starvation can also cause an accumulation of the ketone bodies acetoacetic acid and beta-hydroxybutyric acid. Ingestion of toxins such as a salicylate (aspirin) overdose, methanol, and ethylene glycol (antifreeze) will also cause metabolic acidosis.

A certain amount of acid is produced when dietary proteins are metabolized. These proteins contain sulfate and phosphate groups that, after metabolism, form sulfuric and phosphoric acid. These acids normally amount to about 150 mEq/day, and they must be excreted through kidney filtration. If the kidneys fail, acidosis will occur in several days (Eaton & Pooler, 2009).

A failure to excrete the hydrogen ion load may be caused by renal damage at several sections of the nephron. The term *renal tubular acidosis* (RTA) refers to a group of renal pathologies that result in diminished hydrogen ion excretion or excess renal loss of bicarbonate. Type 1 RTA is referred to as classic RTA or distal RTA because the malfunction is at the level of the distal convoluted tubule. The problem here is an inability to maximally acidify urine. This results in a low acid secretion and continued excretion of bicarbonate at a time when it should be retained. There is also loss of sodium and potassium in the urine (Eaton & Pooler, 2009).

Type 2 RTA is also called proximal renal tubular acidosis because the site of damage is the proximal convoluted tubule. The pathology here results in impaired reabsorption of bicarbonate in the proximal tubule. The result is a high urinary bicarbonate loss, a systemic acidosis, and an inappropriately alkaline urine pH. There is accompanying renal loss of potassium that can lead to systemic hypokalemia.

Type 4 RTA is associated with a number of different conditions, but most patients with this pathology have renal failure that results in damage to the renal interstitium and tubules. Here, the defect causes impaired exchange of cations in the distal tubules. This results in reduced secretion of both hydrogen ion and potassium, which may result in hyperkalemia as well as acidosis (DuBose, 2008). (*Note:* There is a Type 3 RTA, but it is a rare variant of Type 1 RTA seen exclusively in children and not clinically relevant to the discussion here.)

Because not all ions are measured and reported by the laboratory, it may be necessary for the nurse who is assessing a patient with metabolic acidosis to calculate the anion gap. The primary cations that are measured in venous plasma are sodium and potassium; the main anions are chloride and bicarbonate or serum CO_2. Typically, there are more unmeasured anions than cations. Several other anions that are not normally measured include phosphates, sulfates, organic ions, and proteins (DuBose, 2008). Those anions make up the anion gap, which is calculated in one of two ways:

$$(Na^+ + K^+) - (Cl^- + HCO_3^-)$$

or

$$Na^+ - (Cl^- + HCO_3^-)$$

Because the value of potassium is so small (4 mEq/L), it is sometimes ignored in calculating the anion gap. A normal anion gap is 10 ± 4 when K^+ is not included in the equation, although different sources cite different values for this "normal":

$$(Na^+) - (Cl^- + HCO_3^-)$$

$$140 - (105 + 22) = 13$$

Figure 15–7◆ graphically depicts the anion gap.

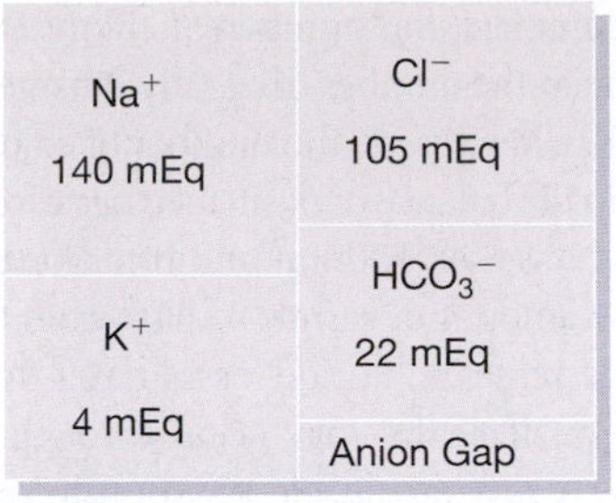

OR

Anions and Cations in Serum

The equivalents of cations in a solution always balances the equivalents of anions

Cations	Anions	
Sodium 140	Chloride 105	
Potassium 4.5	Bicarbonate 24	
Calcium 5	Other = 22	} Anion gap
Magnesium 1.5		
Total = 151	Total = 151	

FIGURE 15–7 ◆ Anion gap.

If the anion gap is abnormally large, there are more negative ions than can be explained by the usual unmeasured substances. These extra negative substances are often lactate or the ketone bodies seen with diabetic ketoacidosis: acetoacetic acid and/or beta-hydroxybutyric acid. In this situation, termed *high anion gap acidosis,* the acid dissociates into hydrogen ion and unmeasured anion. The hydrogen ion is buffered by bicarbonate while the unmeasured ion accumulates in the serum. For example:

$$pH = 7.1\ Na^+ = 145\ K^+ = 5\ Cl^- = 97\ HCO_3^- = 12$$

$$Gap = 145 - (97 + 12)$$

$$Gap = 36$$

This significant elevation indicates high anion gap acidosis. Sometimes, calculating the anion gap will help to identify a metabolic acidosis even when the pH is normal. High anion gap acidosis can also be caused by ingestion of salicylate, methanol, ethylene glycol (antifreeze), or other substances (DuBose, 2008).

If the patient has metabolic acidosis but the anion gap is within normal limits, the problem is likely to be a loss of bicarbonate rather than an excess of acid. This occurs with GI losses of bicarbonate such as that seen with extensive diarrhea or bowel fistulae that cause a high output of lower GI fluids. The intestinal fluids beyond the stomach, including pancreatic and biliary secretions, are alkaline and consist of both bicarbonate and other organic anions. When these fluids are absorbed through the intestine, they are converted to bicarbonate in normal metabolism. If these fluids are lost through diarrhea or fistula output, the bicarbonate cannot be reclaimed and pH falls. This scenario also is typically associated with an increase in plasma chloride concentrations. The chloride ions replace plasma bicarbonate. Urinary diversions, such as a ureterosigmoidostomy, can cause hyperchloremic metabolic acidosis in as many as 80% of patients. The colon has an anion exchanger that exchanges HCO_3^- for the high chloride usually found in urine. So when the urine is diverted to the colon, the urinary chloride is exchanged for bicarbonate, which is then lost in urine. In addition, the colon can directly absorb ammonia (NH_4), which is derived from urine and colonic bacteria. The absorbed NH_4 is converted into NH_3 and hydrogen ion in the liver, leading to hydrogen ion excess (Barrett et al., 2010a).

Signs, Symptoms, and Consequences

Patients with metabolic acidosis often complain of dyspnea because of the Kussmaul respirations that occur as the respiratory system tries to compensate. Tachypnea and hyperpnea (deeper than normal respirations) are usually prominent. If the acidosis is severe, with a pH < 7.10, patients may develop potentially serious or fatal cardiac dysrhythmias such as ventricular tachycardia. This abnormality may also reduce cardiac contractility and lead to hypotension and heart failure.

Neurological symptoms are nonspecific but may be manifestations of the underlying cause of the metabolic acidosis, particularly if it is associated with the ingestion of toxic substances such as ethylene glycol or methanol. Patients may complain of headache, visual changes, or mental confusion. GI symptoms include nausea and vomiting, abdominal pain, diarrhea, anorexia, and weight loss (Barrett et al., 2010c). Chronic metabolic acidosis such as that associated with uremia or RTA is associated with bone disease due to the buffering of calcium carbonate and increases the risk of fractures in adults.

Laboratory studies used in the evaluation of metabolic acidosis include an ABG, which shows a low pH and low HCO_3^- as well as a base deficit more negative than –2. (Remember that bicarbonate and pH move in the same direction.) If the lungs have increased their alveolar ventilation to attempt to compensate for the acidosis, the $PaCO_2$ may also be lower than normal.

A metabolic panel with electrolyte assay is required in assessing patients who have metabolic acidosis. The serum sodium, potassium, chloride, and bicarbonate levels are useful in calculating the anion gap. Hyperkalemia often complicates a metabolic acidosis. The excess hydrogen ions cross cell membranes and enter the intracellular space. They, in turn, "bump out" potassium ions, which are in high concentrations inside the cell. Glucose levels will be elevated in the presence of diabetic ketoacidosis; the blood urea nitrogen (BUN) and creatinine levels will be elevated in uremic acidosis.

Medical Management

Treatment of metabolic acidosis is directed at the correction or treatment of the underlying cause. The use of alkalinizing therapy is rarely indicated except in the most severe, life-threatening instances. In many cases, the treatment of the underlying cause and the restoration of intravascular volume and arterial oxygenation will be enough to allow for the metabolism of the organic acids (lactate and ketoacids) back to bicarbonate or for the kidney to regenerate new bicarbonate to replace the losses (Kraut & Madias, 2010).

The administration of sodium bicarbonate in acute metabolic acidosis is controversial. Recent studies have shown that giving bicarbonate is ineffective and may actually be detrimental to the patient's welfare (Kraut & Madias, 2010). The problem is that when exogenous bicarbonate is administered to a patient who is acidemic (increased acidity or low pH of the blood), the bicarbonate reacts with hydrogen ions to form carbonic acid. The carbonic acid then dissociates into CO_2 and water, so the $PaCO_2$ rises. When the CO_2 cannot be eliminated, the pH correction will be very slight, or the pH may become more acidotic (abnormal accumulation of acids in the blood and body tissues/fluids).

Metabolic Alkalosis

Metabolic alkalosis is characterized by a primary elevation in the plasma bicarbonate accompanied by an elevated pH. In metabolic imbalances, bicarbonate and pH move in the *same* direction. If bicarbonate is elevated, the pH will be elevated. If bicarbonate is decreased, the pH will decrease. The mortality rate of severe metabolic alkalosis is quite high: 45% in patients with an arterial pH of 7.55 and 80% when the pH is greater than 7.65 (DuBose, 2008).

Etiology and Pathophysiology

Metabolic alkalosis is caused by pathologic processes that lead to an accumulation of base or a loss of acid in the extracellular fluid. The increase in arterial pH usually causes a depression of the rate and depth of ventilation. This results in an increase in the $PaCO_2$ and a buffering of the alkalemia, which is the respiratory compensation component. Respiratory compensation for metabolic alkalosis is limited, however, because the respiratory center will not depress respiration to the point at which oxygenation begins to suffer.

Metabolic alkalosis is a relatively common disorder that is seen with diuretic use or the loss of gastric secretions due to excessive vomiting or nasogastric suction. It also can be caused by alkali administration, loss of hydrogen from extracellular fluid, or depletion of electrolytes such as chloride or potassium or from intravascular volume depletion.

In addition to the primary pathology, factors must be present that increase the reabsorption of bicarbonate from the kidneys. An excess of bicarbonate, or "base loading," is rarely a sole cause of significant persistent metabolic alkalosis because the normal kidney is very efficient at excreting bicarbonate (Dubose, 2008). Transient alkalosis may occur after a patient has received oral or IV $NaHCO_3^-$ or a basic/alkaline equivalent such as citrate. Citrate is used as the anticoagulant in transfused blood and fresh frozen plasma. When patients receive multiple blood or plasma transfusions, they receive a significant amount of citrate, and this can lead to metabolic alkalosis. Metabolic alkalosis also may occur temporarily in patients with a chronic respiratory acidosis who have been placed on mechanical ventilation and whose $PaCO_2$ has been corrected too rapidly, before their kidneys have had a chance to excrete the excess bicarbonate.

Loss of hydrogen can occur from the GI tract or in urine. Gastric contents have high concentrations of hydrochloric acid (HCl^-) and a smaller amount of potassium chloride (KCl^-). Gastric hydrogen secretion stimulates, and is matched by, pancreatic bicarbonate secretion. When the acid contents of the stomach pass through the pylorus into the duodenum, they stimulate the pancreas to secrete lytic enzymes and bicarbonate. This bicarbonate neutralizes the acidity of the stomach contents. If the patient suffers excessive vomiting or the gastric secretions are removed by nasogastric suction before they can pass into the duodenum, there is no stimulus to the secretion of bicarbonate, and it accumulates.

An excess loss of hydrogen in urine can be caused by a number of pathologic conditions or as a side effect of therapies. An increase in the secretion of the mineralocorticoid aldosterone causes an increased reabsorption of sodium from the kidney tubule back into the kidney interstitium. Certain classes of diuretics, the loop or thiazide diuretics, can cause an increased secretion of aldosterone and lead to increased urinary hydrogen secretion as well as decreased intravascular volume.

Chloride helps to maintain the balance of cations to anions in the extracellular fluid to maintain electroneutrality. It does this through its inverse relationship with bicarbonate. If excessive amounts of bicarbonate ions (anions) accumulate, the number of chloride ions (also anions) decreases to maintain the number of negative charges. If the number of sodium ions (cations) increases, the number of chloride ions increases as well, to maintain the balance of positive to negative charges. Chloride and sodium work together; sodium and bicarbonate have an inverse relationship. If the amount of serum sodium goes down, the amount of chloride also decreases. Chloride losses result in an increase in bicarbonate. Chloride depletion may occur through the loss of gastric secretions, which are rich in chloride ions, or through the kidneys with the loop or thiazide diuretics.

Hypokalemia participates in perpetuating metabolic alkalosis in several ways. When there is a decrease of K^+ in the extracellular fluid, hydrogen ions shift to the intracellular compartment to keep the electrical charge balanced. This makes the inside of the cells acidic. This intracellular acidosis stimulates reabsorption of bicarbonate from the collecting of the kidney. Hypokalemia stimulates an enzyme that promotes potassium ion reabsorption, but the potassium is exchanged for hydrogen ion, the loss of which leads to alkalosis (DuBose, 2008).

When a patient is hypovolemic and has lost relatively large volumes of bicarbonate-free fluid, this can lead to contraction alkalosis. The plasma bicarbonate concentration rises because there is a contraction of the extracellular volume around a relatively constant quantity of bicarbonate. This can occur when a loop diuretic is given to induce rapid fluid removal from a very edematous patient.

Signs, Symptoms, and Consequences

The symptoms of metabolic alkalosis are difficult to separate from the symptoms of the chloride volume or potassium depletion. The effect on the CNS is the same as with respiratory alkalosis. Cerebral vessels constrict and cerebral blood flow is decreased. This can lead to lethargy, confusion, and/or apathy. If the alkalemia is very severe, coma or seizures may result (Yaseen, 2009). The respiratory centers are depressed to attempt compensation, decreasing alveolar ventilation. This decrease in tidal volume can lead to problems with atelectasis and may contribute to the development of pulmonary infection in very ill or immunocompromised patients.

The increased binding of calcium to albumin described in the earlier section about respiratory alkalosis also occurs with metabolic alkalosis. This may lead to neuromuscular irritability, resulting in muscle twitching, muscle spasm, and tetany. Positive Chvostek's and Trousseau's signs (discussed previously) may also be present.

Metabolic alkalosis has effects on cardiac function. Myocardial contractility is depressed. Electrocardiogram (ECG) changes include prolongation of the QT interval as well as atrial and ventricular arrhythmias. Hypokalemia and hypomagnesemia often coexist with metabolic alkalosis, and these electrolyte imbalances may exacerbate the effect of the alkalosis on cardiac function and rhythm (Yaseen, 2009).

The cause of metabolic alkalosis is usually discerned from the patient's history. Episodic vomiting or the use of nasogastric suction or diuretic therapy is easily uncovered during a careful patient history. Sometimes, however, no obvious cause can be found. The metabolic alkalosis may be due to a patient's surreptitious use of diuretics or self-induced vomiting or to conditions that cause excess mineralocorticoids, usually aldosterone. With vomiting or diuretic use, intravascular volume depletion generally occurs; with hyperaldosteronism, mild volume expansion is usually present.

Medical Management

Once the origin of the metabolic alkalosis has been determined, the treatment is quite obvious. It is aimed at correcting the volume depletion, the potassium depletion, or the chloride depletion. In patients with low intravascular volume due to vomiting, gastric suction, or diuretic use, the administration of sodium chloride can correct the dehydration and replete the chloride. Any other electrolyte deficits should be corrected by replacing them. The administration of potassium chloride is important in the correction of metabolic alkalosis. This exogenous (from outside the body) potassium moves into body cells in exchange for hydrogen ion to maintain electroneutrality. This hydrogen ion buffers excess extracellular bicarbonate in the serum, bringing pH down toward normal. In addition, the correction of intracellular acidosis in renal tubular cells reduces the secretion of hydrogen ion and the reabsorption of bicarbonate (Yaseen, 2009).

If the primary cause is an excess of mineralocorticoid, steroids may be used to suppress hormone secretion, or the patient may be given the drug spironolactone. Spironolactone is a synthetic steroid with a structure much like that of aldosterone. It acts as a competitive antagonist at the aldosterone receptors in the kidney. This drug is administered until definitive therapy is undertaken to treat the primary disorder (Black, 2008). If the patient is on hemodialysis, the bath solution used for dialysis can be made more acidic. If the patient has posthypercapnic alkalosis, the administration of the drug acetazolamide can speed up the renal elimination of excess bicarbonate.

Nursing Management

Disorders of acid–base balance do not exist in a vacuum; they are a product of other underlying pathology. The nurse must be aware of whether a particular patient is at risk for acid–base disorders. The risk may be from the disorder itself or from a clinical manifestation such as fever, vomiting, diarrhea, age, or sepsis. The risk may be due to a treatment such as diuretics, mechanical ventilation, and total parental nutrition or enteral nutrition that is high in carbohydrates. Finally, the risk could be due to comorbid conditions such as respiratory or cardiac disorders or diabetes. The older adult may have multiple risk factors present from all three categories. The nursing care outlined in Nursing Process: Patient Care Plan for Acid–Base Imbalances (p. 372) must be incorporated into a larger plan of care that addresses the primary pathology or disorder. Caring for older patients who may have acid–base imbalances is discussed in the Gerontological Considerations section.

Collaborative Care

The care of a patient with a disorder that produces an imbalance of acid–base homeostasis involves nurses and health care providers but may also require respiratory therapy for assistance with bronchodilator therapy or assisted ventilation when treating respiratory causes of imbalance. Other nursing specialists such as dialysis nurses may also be called on for their expertise. Pharmacists may be brought in as consultants when electrolytes are being administered or when the absorption or action of medications may be altered in the presence of an abnormal pH. Case managers and discharge planners evaluate placement and discharge needs. They can provide assistance in the arrangement of home nursing and/or respiratory therapy and durable medical equipment such as nebulizers or CPAP or BiPAP machines. In order to meet desired patient outcomes, it is essential that this interdisciplinary team communicate openly with one another in developing and evaluating care of the patient and family (IOM [Institute of Medicine], 2010).

Health Promotion

Many patients with disturbances of acid–base balance suffer from chronic conditions that are the underlying causes of the imbalances. Nurses are in a unique position to promote healthy behaviors in the face of chronic illness. These interventions can decrease symptoms and improve quality of life. Several examples are presented here.

Patients with chronic ventilatory failure often experience disabling symptoms such as chronic dyspnea. This can lead to malnutrition because the patient is too short of breath to eat. The nurse can explore the patient's daily routines and make suggestions about switching to five or six small meals per day and limiting mealtime conversation to conserve energy. Dietitians can suggest the best types of foods to conserve energy while supplying adequate nutrition. Subjective feelings of breathlessness can be eased by keeping the environment relatively cool and using fans to create air movement. Positioning for optimal lung expansion may involve the use of a recliner for sleeping and supporting the arms on pillows. Patient and family education about the precautions to be taken when oxygen is in use in the home can help to decrease the risk of fire or excess oxygen administration. If the patient uses an oxygen concentrator, the patient and the nurse should formulate a plan about what to do in case of an emergency such as a power outage.

Patients with obstructive sleep apnea that leads to respiratory acidosis must be counseled about the dangers of excessive daytime sleepiness. When possible, patients should undergo an outpatient sleep study and evaluation for the use of nasal CPAP to decrease apneic arousal episodes at night and to promote better REM sleep. Patients are often reluctant to use home CPAP machines, and the nurse is in a position to provide encouragement about their use for patient safety. Patients who frequently fall asleep during the day should be counseled about the risks associated with driving because they are prone to accidents.

When patients with diabetes experience an episode of ketoacidosis, the nurse should explore with the patient and family what may have led to the episode. If it is a stressor such as infection, the nurse should begin or reinforce diabetic teaching. In addition, the patient should be counseled to have a "sick day" plan to decrease the chance that blood sugar levels will get out of control. To plan for a sick day is to plan ahead in the event that she becomes ill, to keep a garden variety flu from turning into something much worse (Diabetes Self-Management, 2012). In doing so, the patient should work with the health care team to discuss self-care management before she actually becomes sick. The plan for a diabetic patient includes ways of managing blood sugar, when to test for ketones, and when to seek medical help. Adequate diabetic supplies should always be kept on hand and stored properly. A friend, family member, or neighbor should be notified so they can check in on the patient. The underlying condition should be treated, and the health care provider should be kept informed. In essence, a plan is there for the patient to follow in the event that she becomes sick and experiences a sick day. If there is any suspicion that the patient is not following her diabetes management regimen adequately, the nurse will be able to explore the reasons for noncompliance. If the problem is a lack of knowledge, intensive diabetic teaching and reinforcement of previous teaching should be started in the inpatient setting and continued in the outpatient or home care setting.

Gerontological Considerations

The normal pH range of ECF is not affected by advanced age. Some changes in respiratory and renal function, however, may affect acid–base balance. However, these lung and kidney changes are more likely to affect the body's ability to respond to a physiological challenge.

NURSING PROCESS: Patient Care Plan for Acid–Base Imbalances

Assessment of Acid–Base Imbalances Using Gordon's Functional Health Patterns:

- Activity Exercise
- Nutritional-Metabolic

Subjective Data	Objective Data
Assessment of Respiratory Acidosis Do you have a history of shortness of breath or exercise-limiting symptoms? Do you have a cough? Is it productive? Sputum description? Do you have any history of sleep-disordered breathing? (Sleeping partner may be aware of excessive snoring.)	**Assessment of Respiratory Acidosis** Auscultate breath sounds; be alert for decreases in intensity, diffuse wheezing, stridor Respiratory rate Examine fingers for signs of clubbing Observe for presence of a barrel chest *Laboratory evaluation:* ABGs, complete blood count, serum electrolytes, drug screen (if there is suspicion of respiratory depression by drugs)
Assessment of Respiratory Alkalosis Do you have any shortness of breath, numbness around the mouth, or paresthesias? Do you have any history of anxiety or acute pain?	**Assessment of Respiratory Alkalosis** Assess respiratory rate *Laboratory evaluation:* ABGs, serum electrolytes, complete blood count
Assessment of Metabolic Acidosis Ask about symptoms that may help determine cause: history of diabetes, renal insufficiency/failure, diarrhea, or other loss of intestinal fluids. Ask about dyspnea; count respiratory rate. Observe for Kussmaul respirations.	**Assessment of Metabolic Acidosis** *Laboratory evaluation:* • ABGs; evaluate pH and HCO_3^-; also examine PaO_2 to evaluate for hypoxemia as a cause of lactic acidosis • Serum electrolytes; calculate anion gap • Urine electrolytes, osmolarity • Blood glucose (to evaluate for uncontrolled diabetes mellitus) • BUN and creatinine (to evaluate renal function) Evaluate for physical signs of malnutrition or dehydration
Assessment of Metabolic Alkalosis Ask about history that may help to identify a cause: vomiting, diarrhea, use of diuretics. Ask about symptoms of hypokalemia: weakness, muscle aches. Ask about symptoms of hypocalcemia: tingling around the mouth, muscles cramps.	**Assessment of Metabolic Alkalosis** Evaluate fluid volume status Evaluate for signs of hypocalcemia: tetany, Chvostek's sign *Laboratory evaluation:* ABGs; serum electrolytes and calcium, osmolarity; urine electrolytes

Outcomes and Evaluation Parameters	Planning and Interventions with *Rationales*
1. NURSING DIAGNOSIS: Impaired Gas Exchange ***related to ventilation perfusion imbalance, which is caused by hypoventilation and hypoxemia that may be a result of airway blockage*** **(NANDA-I © 2012)**	
Outcomes: Airway patency will be maintained. Gas exchange will be optimized. ***Evaluation Parameters:*** $PaCO_2$ will return to the patient's baseline with a pH in the normal range. Any dyspnea will be relieved as reported by the patient. Patient will return to baseline level of physical activity.	Position the patient sitting upright with arms supported on an over-bed table. (Positioning in a chair may be preferable to the bed.) *This position helps maximize lung inflation.* Administer any bronchodilators that are ordered. Ensure that the patient is using proper technique if self-administering. *Patients who self-administer metered-dose inhalers (MDI) at home often prefer to continue self-administration while in the hospital as a way to retain control. However, improper technique is a frequent problem in the use of MDI. Enlist the help of a respiratory therapist or pharmacist.* Encourage the use of an incentive spirometer. Use should be at least every 4 hours while awake. *This is one way to encourage the patient to take deep breaths to help prevent atelectasis.* Encourage early ambulation. Set increasing distance goals with the patient each time. *Helps the patient to avoid complications of immobility.*
2. NURSING DIAGNOSIS: Ineffective Breathing Pattern ***related to hyperventilation precipitated by anxiety, stress, and/or pain*** **(NANDA-I © 2012)**	
Outcomes: Gas exchange will be optimized. Any excess anxiety or pain will be relieved.	Encourage slow, deep respirations. In the acute stage, this may require the constant presence of the nurse. *A calm, reassuring nurse will help to promote relaxation in the patient.*

(continued)

NURSING PROCESS: Patient Care Plan for Acid–Base Imbalances, *continued*

Outcomes and Evaluation Parameters	Planning and Interventions with *Rationales*
Evaluation Parameters: $PaCO_2$ will return to the patient's baseline with a pH in the normal range. Respiratory rate and depth will be within normal parameters.	If that is difficult for the patient, the use of a rebreather mask or having the patient breathe into a simple paper bag may be required. *Promotes the rebreathing of exhaled CO_2 to help return levels to normal. Explain the reason for the rebreathing to the patient.* Evaluate for the presence of pain using objective criteria such as the visual analog scale. Medicate the patient to a level of pain that is acceptable to the patient. Reassess pain levels 30 minutes after IV medication and 1 hour after oral medication. *Pain can cause an increased respiratory rate. Relief of pain should help return the rate toward normal.* If the cause of the hyperventilation was anxiety or fear, help the patient to explore the cause to help identify strategies to avoid future episodes. *Patients may need guidance in stress relief or anticipatory guidance about how to avoid such stress in the future.*
3. NURSING DIAGNOSIS: Imbalanced Nutrition: More Than Metabolic Requirements *related to food intake that exceeds metabolic needs; high levels of carbohydrate can lead to metabolic acidosis, decreased pH and excess acidity.* Deficient Fluid Volume *related to dehydration caused by active fluid loss.* (NANDA-I © 2012)	
Outcomes: Acid–base balance will be restored. The underlying cause of the acidosis will be identified and treated. Recurrence will be avoided. ***Evaluation Parameters:*** Serum bicarbonate will return to normal levels with a pH within the normal range. Fluid balance will be optimized.	*Note:* Much of the nursing care will be directed by the underlying cause of the acidosis. Obtain a baseline weight, and weigh the patient frequently during rehydration, if applicable. *An accurate patient weight is a better parameter to measure than is the intake and output measurement. This is particularly true in cases in which the cause of any dehydration is excessive diarrhea or fistula output. The patient should be weighed with the same amount of clothing each time.* If the cause of the acidosis is an exacerbation of diabetes or renal failure, it is important to explore the reasons with the patient and family. The problem may be a failure to comply with recommended treatment or may be caused by a concurrent event such as an infection. *An assessment of the patient's knowledge of any underlying disease and its management may help to uncover causes of noncompliance or condition exacerbation. Extensive patient and family education or reeducation may be required to help prevent episodes in the future. This may be beyond the scope of the inpatient nurse when hospital stays continue to shorten. Referral to an outpatient facility or consultant such as a diabetes educator may be required.*
4. NURSING DIAGNOSIS: Deficient Fluid Volume *related to dehydration caused by active fluid loss.* (NANDA-I © 2012)	
Outcomes: Acid–base balance will be restored. The underlying cause of the alkalosis will be identified and treated. Recurrence will be avoided. ***Evaluation Parameters:*** Serum bicarbonate will return to normal levels with a pH within the normal range. Fluid balance will be optimized. Any excess vomiting or nasogastric suction will be corrected. Any chloride or potassium depletion will be corrected.	*Note:* Much of the nursing care will be directed by the underlying cause of the alkalosis. Obtain a baseline weight, and weigh the patient frequently during rehydration if applicable. *An accurate patient weight is a better parameter to measure than is the intake and output measurement. This is particularly true in cases in which the cause of any dehydration is excessive vomiting. The patient should be weighed with the same amount of clothing each time.* Control any vomiting with antiemetics. If the patient must be on continuous nasogastric suction, the use of a histamine-2 receptor blocker or a proton pump inhibitor may be indicated. *The goal is to stop the loss of hydrochloric acid from the stomach. The drugs decrease the secretion of acid into the stomach and, hence, stop its loss.* If the alkalemia is severe and the patient's respirations are depressed, encourage frequent deep breathing and the use of an incentive spirometer. *The decrease in tidal volume can lead to atelectasis and may contribute to the development of a pulmonary infection.* If there is no obvious cause for the alkalosis, a sensitive exploration into the possibility of self-induced vomiting or the use of diuretics may be required. *These may be attempts at weight loss or may be symptoms of a disorder such as bulimia.*

RESEARCH OPPORTUNITIES Related to Acid–Base Imbalances

Research Area	Clinical Impact
Patient Assessment	
• Assessing the severity of dyspnea	Establish a standard measure of dyspnea to measure severity and to gauge the effectiveness of interventions and relief strategies.
• Exploration of ethnic/cultural differences in the description of symptoms such as dyspnea	Enhance cultural sensitivity and ensure that symptoms are recognized and that strategies are undertaken to relieve symptoms.
• Assess accuracy of noninvasive methods of measuring $PaCO_2$	To promote noninvasive methods of assessing the adequacy of ventilation.
• Compare the accuracy of the recording of intake and output vs. accurate patient weight in the assessment of fluid loss/gain	Intake and output recording is time consuming and often inaccurate. Explore more accurate methods of assessment of fluid volume status.
Nursing Intervention Research	
• Effectiveness of interventions to relieve dyspnea • Enhancing quality of life in patients with chronic illness	Dyspnea is a strong, subjective experience of physiological distress. Relief of this symptom can enhance quality of life and improve end-of-life care.
• Examine the most effective methods of patient education during short hospital stays	Shorter inpatient hospitalization reduces the time available for patient and family education about disease processes and their management. Evaluation of the most effective methods that can be undertaken in a short time period has a goal of improving comprehension and retention of information.

In the lungs, there is uneven ventilation of the alveoli, which leads to an altered ventilation/perfusion balance. This causes a drop in arterial oxygen tension, but the $PaCO_2$ remains unchanged. This may be partly due to a drop in the production of CO_2 caused by a decrease in the basal metabolic rate that happens during the aging process (Hamer, Siera, & Thompson, 2010). The ability to hyperventilate in response to an acute metabolic acidosis may be blunted and lead to a persistent acidosis.

Renal tubular function is also affected by aging. The ability to conserve sodium and excrete hydrogen ion falls, so the aging kidney may be slower to respond to an acid load (either respiratory or metabolic), and blood pH may take longer to normalize. Dehydration is a particular problem because the aging kidney does not respond to fluid and sodium loss by its usual mechanism of increasing sodium retention, thus conserving water (Hamer et al., 2010). In addition, many drugs commonly used by older people, such as salicylates, diuretics, and laxatives, may precipitate acid–base disturbances.

Research

Current and future research needs to focus on control of symptoms with chronic conditions, such as dyspnea, and enhancing the quality of life of patients with chronic illnesses. Additionally, improved monitoring systems and treatment measures need to detect and treat symptoms before they progress to cause a debilitating state. The Research Opportunities box outlines research topics in the area of acid–base imbalances.

Summary

When the complexity of the body and of human nature is examined, it is easy to be amazed by the intricacies of balance that are required to keep bodily systems functioning in their normal condition. The human body has a complex internal environment that requires a balance of fluids and electrolytes, as well as acids and bases. The cations and anions of the electrolytes must balance in the proper fluid volume and space (ICF or ECF) to preserve life and prevent altered health states. Sodium, potassium, chloride, bicarbonate, calcium, magnesium, and phosphorus have separate roles and precise levels. Cellular life cannot exist outside these boundaries; cellular swelling or shrinkage is fatal. Proper maintenance of electrochemical and neuromuscular activity is dependent on each electrolyte being present in the proper ECF or ICF compartment when it is needed. Nurses can assist patients by educating them on electrolyte abnormalities that may occur as a result of disease processes and on how to avoid health problems.

Acid–base balance also is critical to maintaining health and averting disease. Thus, imbalances almost always occur in conjunction with the diseases or pathologic conditions that the nurse considers the primary focus when caring for the patient. A basic understanding of how these imbalances affect organ systems and blood chemistries will enable nurses to provide focused assessments of the patients in their care and plan nursing interventions accordingly.

NCLEX® PRACTICE

1. A patient is experiencing nausea with severe vomiting. The nurse realizes that this patient is at risk for which occurrence?

1. Interstitial fluid volume overload
2. Intracellular fluid volume deficit
3. Extracellular fluid volume deficit
4. Interstitial fluid volume deficit

2. The nurse has just received the following laboratory data report on a newly admitted patient. Which result causes the most concern to the nurse?

1. Na^+: 115 mEq/L
2. K^+: 4.0 mEq/L
3. Ca^+: 9 mg/dL
4. Mg^+: 1.8 mg/dL

3. The nurse is caring for a patient with severe vomiting and diarrhea and a nasogastric tube to low wall suction. The nurse includes monitoring for which electrolyte imbalance in this patient's plan of care?

1. Hypokalemia
2. Hypercalcemia
3. Hypermagnesemia
4. Hypophosphatemia

4. The nurse has admitted a patient in renal failure who has a serum potassium level of 7.1 mEq/L. Which admission order does the nurse recognize as the priority for this patient?

1. Neurological status checks every 15 minutes
2. Measure urine output hourly
3. Laboratory: Arterial blood gases
4. Obtain an electrocardiogram

5. The nurse is providing discharge instructions to a patient with hypokalemia. Which instruction should the nurse provide? (select all that apply)

1. Take oral Kayexalate as prescribed.
2. Limit the intake of spinach and carrots, as well as green, leafy vegetables.
3. Eat a balanced diet including tomato juice and potatoes.
4. Expect muscle cramps and weakness for at least 6 weeks.
5. Take oral potassium supplementation as prescribed.

6. A patient is admitted with the diagnosis of diabetic ketoacidosis. The nurse realizes that this patient's body will attempt to attain acid–base balance by which physiologic change?

1. Decreasing the respiratory rate.
2. Increasing the reabsorption of hydrogen ions.
3. Increasing the secretion of hydrogen ions.
4. Decreasing the reabsorption of bicarbonate.

Answers to NCLEX Practice questions can be found in Appendix D in the Osborn Student Resources at nursing.pearsonhighered.com. Practice additional NCLEX questions online at the Student Resources site.

Pearson Nursing Student Resources Find additional review materials at: **nursing.pearsonhighered.com**

REFERENCES

Agraharker, M. (2011). Hyperchloremic acidosis treatment & management. Emedicine. Retrieved from http://emedicine.medscape.com/article/240809

Barrett, K. E., Barman, S. M., Boitano, S., & Brooks, H. (2010a). Acidification of the urine & bicarbonate excretion. In K. E. Barrett, S. M. Barman, S. Boitano, & H. Brooks (Eds.), *Ganong's review of medical physiology* (23rd ed.). Section VIII, Chapter 40, 679–686. New York: McGraw-Hill Medical. Retrieved from http://www.accessmedicine.com/content.aspx?aID=5244356

Barrett, K. E., Barman, S. M., Boitano, S., & Brooks, H. (2010b). Gas transport & pH in the lung. In K. E. Barrett, S. M. Barman, S. Boitano, & H. Brooks (Eds.), *Ganong's review of medical physiology* (23rd ed.) Section VII, Chapter 36, 609-624. New York: McGraw-Hill Medical. Retrieved from http://www.accessmedicine.com/content.aspx?aID=5246110

Barrett, K. E., Barman, S. M., Boitano, S., & Brooks, H. (2010c). The regulation of acid–base status. In K. E. Barrett, S. M. Barman, S. Boitano, & H. Brooks (Eds.), *Ganong's review of medical physiology* (23rd ed.). New York: Mc Graw-Hill Medical. Retrieved from http://www.accessmedicine.com/content.aspx?aID=2774224

Barrett, K. E., Barman, S. M., Boitano, S., & Brooks, H. (2010d). Regulation of extracellular fluid composition & volume. In K. E. Barrett, S. M. Barman, S. Boitano, & H. Brooks (Eds.), *Ganong's review of medical physiology* (23rd ed.). Section VIII, Chapter 39, 665-678. New York: McGraw-Hill Medical. Retrieved from http://www.accessmedicine.com/content.aspx?aID=5244207

Barrett, K. E., Barman, S. M., Boitano, S., & Brooks, H. (2010e). Renal function and micturition. In K. E. Barrett, S. M. Barman, S. Boitano, & H. Brooks (Eds.), *Ganong's review of medical physiology* (23rd ed.). Section VIII, Chapter 38, 639-664. New York: McGraw-Hill Medical. Retrieved from http://www.accessmedicine.com/content.aspx?aID=5246287

Black, R. M. (2008). Metabolic acidosis and metabolic alkalosis. In R. Irwin & J. Rippe (Eds.), *Intensive care medicine* (6th ed., pp. 854–864). Philadelphia: Lippincott Williams & Wilkins.

Bond, E. F. (2008). Cardiac anatomy and physiology. In S. L. Woods, E. S. Sivarajan Froelicher, S. A. Underhill Motzer, & E. J. Bridges (Eds.), *Cardiac nursing* (6th ed.). Philadelphia: Lippincott Williams & Wilkins.

Brophy, D. F., & Gehr, T. W. B. (2011). Disorders of potassium and magnesium homeostasis. In J. T. DiPiro, R. L. Talbert, G. C. Yee, G. R. Matzke, B. G. Wells, & L. M. Posey (Eds.), *Pharmacotherapy: A pathophysiologic approach* (8th ed., pp. 877–888). New York: McGraw-Hill.

Coyle, J. D., & Joy, M. S. (2011). Disorders of sodium and water homeostasis. In J. T. DiPiro, R. L. Talbert, G. C. Yee, G. R. Matzke, B. G. Wells, & L. M. Posey (Eds.), *Pharmacotherapy: A pathophysiologic approach* (8th ed., pp. 845–860). New York: McGraw-Hill.

Diabetes Self-Management. (2012). Sick-day management. Retrieved from http://www.diabetesselfmanagment.com/Articles/High-Blood-Glucose/hyperglycemic_cris

DuBose, T. (2008). Acid–base disorders. In B. M. Brenner (Ed.), *The kidney* (8th ed.). Philadelphia: Saunders Elsevier.

Eaton, D. C., & Pooler, J. P. (2009). Control of sodium and water excretion: Regulation of plasma volume and plasma osmolality and renal control of systemic blood pressure. In D.C. Eaton & J. P. Pooler (Eds.), *Vander's renal physiology* (7th ed.). Chapter 7, 102-103. New York: McGraw-Hill Medical. Retrieved from http://www.acccessmedicine.com/content.aspx?aID=4528210

Feller-Kopman, D. G., & Schwartzstein, R. M. (2010). Use of oxygen in patients with hypercapnia. *UpToDate 19.2.* Retrieved from http://www.uptodate.com/contents/use-of-osygen-in-patients-with-hypercapnia

Felver, L. (2009). Fluids and electrolytes balance and imbalance. In S. L. Woods, E. S. Sivarajan Froelicher, S. A. Underhill Motzer, & E. J. Bridges (Eds.), *Cardiac nursing* (6th ed., pp. 53–157). Philadelphia: Lippincott Williams & Wilkins.

Ferry, R. J. (2009). Hypochloremic alkalosis treatment and management. EMedicine. Retrieved from http://emedicine.medscape.com/article/945263

Grogono, A. (2010). Acid–base tutorial. Retrieved from http://www.acid-base.com

Guin, P. R. (2009). Endocrine disorders. In *Lippincott manual of nursing practice* (9th ed., pp. 906–941). Philadelphia: Lippincott Williams & Wilkins.

Hamer, H. R., Sierra, F., & Thompson, L. V. (2010). Biology of aging. In H. M. Fillit, K. Rockwood, & K. Woodhouse (Eds.), *Brocklehurst's textbook of gerontology and clinical gerontology* (7th ed.). Philadelphia: Saunders Elsevier.

Institute of Medicine (IOM). (2010). *The future of nursing: Leading change, advancing health.* Washington, DC: The Academic Press.

Institute of Medicine. (2011). Leading health indicators for *Healthy People 2020.* Letter report. Retrieved from http://www.iom.edu/Reports/2011/Leading-Health-Indicators-for-Healthy-People-2020.aspx

Johnson, A. P. (2011). Sodium balance and imbalances. In M. A. Hogan & D. Wane (Eds.), *Fluids, electrolytes, and acid–base balance: Reviews and rationales* (2nd ed., pp. 37–59). Upper Saddle River, NJ: Pearson Prentice Hall.

Joy, M. S., & Hladik, G. A. (2011). Disorders of sodium, water, calcium and phosphate. In J. T. Dipiro, R. L. Talbert, G. C. Yee, G. R. Matzke, B. G. Wells, & L. M. Posey (Eds.), *Pharmacotherapy: A pathophysiologic approach* (6th ed.). New York: McGraw-Hill.

Kaslow, J. W. (2011). Anion gap. Retrieved from http://www.drkaslow.com/html/anion_gap.html

Kee, J. L. (2010). *Laboratory and diagnostic tests with nursing implications* (8th ed.). Upper Saddle River, NJ: Pearson Prentice Hall.

Kraut, J. A., & Madias, N. E. (2010). Metabolic acidosis: Pathophysiology, diagnosis and management. *Nature Reviews Nephrology, 6*(5), 274–285.

Lambert-Drwiega, A. (2010). Respiratory alkalosis treatment & management. Retrieved from http://emedicine.medscape.com/article/301680-treatment.

Levitzky, M. G. (2007). *Pulmonary physiology* (7th ed.). New York: McGraw-Hill.

Malish, S. L., Murdock, J. J., & Sassoon, C. S. (2010). Evaluation of respiratory alkalosis. Retrieved from https://online.epocrates.com/u/2911463.

Metheny, N. M. (2010). *Fluid and electrolyte balance* (5th ed.). Philadelphia: Lippincott Williams & Wilkins.

Moore, D. J. (2010). Hypophasphatemia in emergency medicine. Emedicine. Retrieved from http://emedicine.medscape.com/article/767855

Mount, D. B., & Zandi-Nejad, K. (2008). Disorders of potassium balance. In B. M. Brenner (Ed.), *Brenner & Rector's the kidney* (8th ed.). Section 2, Chapter 17, 640-688. Philadelphia: Saunders Elsevier.

National Institute of Neurological Disorders and Stroke. (2009). NINDS central pontine myelinolysis information page.

Retrieved from http://www.ninds.nih.gov/disorders/central_pontine/central_pontine__myelinolysis.htm

O'Gara, P. T., & Braunwald, E. (2008). Approach to a patient with a heart murmur. In E. Braunwald, A. S. Fauci, D. L. Kasper, S. L. Hauser, D. L. Longo, &, J. L. Jameson (Eds.), *Harrison's principles of internal medicine* (17th ed., pp. 207–210). New York: McGraw-Hill.

Pai, A. B., Rohrscheib, M., & Joy, M. S. (2011). Disorders of calcium and phosphate homeostasis. In J. T. DiPiro, R. L. Talbert, G. C. Yee, G. R. Matzke, B. G. Wells, & L. M. Posey (Eds.), *Pharmacotherapy: A pathophysiologic approach* (8th ed., pp. 861–870). New York: McGraw-Hill.

Pollak, M. R., Yu, A. S. L., & Taylor, E. N. (2008). Disorders of calcium, magnesium and phosphate imbalances. In B. M. Brenner (Ed.), *Brenner & Rector's the Kidney* (8th ed.). Chapter 16. Philadelphia: Saunders Elsevier.

Porth, C. M., & Marfin, M. (2009). *Essentials of pathophysiology: Concepts of altered health states* (8th ed.). Philadelphia: Lippincott Williams & Wilkins.

Rives, S. (2009). Healthy foods and eating. Retrieved from http://knol.google.com/k/health-foods-eating

Schlichtig, R. (2011). Acid–base balance. In *Textbook of critical care* (6th ed., pp. 829–838). Philadelphia: Saunders Elsevier.

Singer, G. G., & Brenner, B. M. (2008). Fluid and electrolyte disturbances. In E. Braunwald, A. S. Fauci, D. L. Kasper, S. L. Hauser, D. L. Longo, & J. L. Jameson (Eds.), *Harrison's principles of internal medicine* (17th ed., pp. 271–282). New York: McGraw-Hill.

Verbalis, J. G., & Berl, T. (2008). Disorders of water balance. In B. M. Brenner (Ed.), *Brenner & Rector's the kidney* (8th ed.). Chapter 13, 459-504. Philadelphia: Saunders Elsevier.

Yaseen, S. (2009). Metabolic alkalosis. Retrieved from http://emedicine.medscape.com/article1243160

Wilkinson, J. M., & Ahearn, N. R. (2009). *Prentice Hall nursing diagnosis handbook* (9th ed.). Upper Saddle River, NJ: Prentice Hall.

Fluid and Blood Replacement

16 CHAPTER

Gail Thurkauf
Annita Watson

Outcome-Based Learning Objectives

After studying this chapter, the learner will be able to:

1. Differentiate among the types of parenteral administration equipment and infusion devices according to intended use.
2. Critique all aspects of infusion nursing practice, including competencies, skill validation, and patient assessment, for consistency with standards of practice.
3. Generate a nursing plan of care to prevent infusion-related complications and create strategies to prevent complications for the patient receiving infusion therapy.
4. Critique the advantages of blood component therapy and the therapeutic use for each component.
5. Delineate the critical thinking and clinical judgment nursing skills necessary to appropriately treat adverse reactions to blood transfusions.

KEY TERMS

agglutinate p.396
albumin p.399
apheresis p.395
autologous transfusion p.401
blood transfusion p.395
blood type p.395
catheter embolism p.392
central vascular access device (CVAD) p.380
chelation p.405
cryoprecipitates p.399
drip factor p.386
electronic infusion device (EID) p.385
extravasation p.390
factor VIII p.399
flow control device p.383
flushing p.388
fresh frozen plasma p.399
frozen RBCs p.397
hemochromatosis p.405
homologous transfusion p.399
hypodermoclysis p.382
infiltration p.379
infusate p.378
intraosseous therapy p.382
intraspinal catheter p.382
intrathecal therapy p.382
leukocyte-reduced RBCs p.397
Luer-Lok p.384
metered-volume chambered sets p.383
needleless system p.393
Ommaya reservoir p.382
packed RBCs p.397
parenteral p.378
patient-controlled analgesia (PCA) pump p.386
perioperative blood salvage p.401
peripheral vascular access device p.378
phlebotomy p.405
platelets p.399
positive pressure infusion pump p.385
postoperative blood salvage p.402
Rh factor p.395
transfusion-related acute lung injury (TRALI) p.405
universal donor p.395
universal recipient p.395
vascular access device (VAD) p.378
vesicant p.380
volumetric pump p.385
washed RBCs p.397
whole blood p.397

FLUID AND BLOOD ADMINISTRATION are required when providing nursing care to patients in a variety of settings, both acute care and community-based. The parenteral administration of fluids and blood requires a competent level of skill development as defined by the Safety Standards of the Quality & Safety Education for Nursing (QSEN) report (QSEN, 2011) and in accordance with the policy and procedures of a given agency. Nurses must adhere to the standards established by the state nursing licensing act and demonstrate compliance with the standards established by the agency's accreditation and licensing bodies. This chapter discusses the rationale for and techniques of fluid and blood replacement. The nurse's roles and responsibilities as a member of the collaborative health care team that is managing infusion therapy also are discussed. The nurse's role as an educator and advocate for patients is emphasized within an ethical and legal framework and according to standards of practice.

FLUID INFUSION THERAPY

Infusion therapy involves the administration of medications and solutions through a needle or catheter. Today's research and technology have produced devices that are used for infusion therapy that can be easily inserted into vascular and nonvascular spaces and allowed to dwell (remain in place) for periods of several days to many months and sometimes years. These devices are used for delivery of prescribed **infusates** (solutions and medications) over a period of time for specific therapeutic indications or diagnostic evaluations. This method of delivery is referred to as the **parenteral** route, which means that medications and solutions are delivered by subcutaneous, vascular, intramuscular, or nonvascular routes. This chapter discusses these infusion therapies and focuses on the administration of infusates via the subcutaneous, vascular, and nonvascular routes.

Because infusion therapy requires that specific sterile compartments within the body be accessed, standard precautions and sterile technique must be practiced in doing all infusion-related procedures. More information about standard precautions is given in Chapter 14. Single-use catheters and infusion-specific products are used to promote safety for the patient and health care provider and to prevent and minimize development of infusion-related complications such as infections.

Hollow-bore needles, which are commonly used for obtaining blood samples, administering injections, or accessing vascular and nonvascular structures, are implicated in the transmission of bloodborne diseases because contaminated blood can become lodged within the internal space, or *lumen*, of the device. The pathogens associated with infusion therapy that pose the greatest health care risk are the hepatitis B and C viruses (HBV and HCV) and the human immunodeficiency virus (HIV).

Vascular Access Devices

A **vascular access device (VAD)** or catheter is a device that is introduced through the skin, into the vascular network, for the purpose of infusing parenteral solutions and medications (Navilyst Medical, 2011). The nurse must become proficient in insertion techniques, care and maintenance strategies for these devices, and patient assessment and monitoring practices.

Peripheral Vascular Access Devices

Peripheral vascular access devices, which are used primarily for infusion therapies administered via locations found on the upper extremities, or the peripheral vasculature, are addressed in the following sections. These devices are used with parenteral therapies administered in a variety of care settings (Easterlow, Hoddinott, & Harrison, 2010).

Peripheral-Short Catheters

Peripheral-short catheters are VADs that are less than 7.5 cm (3.0 inches) in length and are placed in the superficial peripheral vasculature of the adult's arms. Peripheral short catheters are manufactured in various configurations, lengths, and sizes. Certain materials such as Teflon (polytetrafluoroethylene) decrease the occurrence of catheter-related phlebitis and thrombogenesis. Another material, Vialon, is considered hemocompatible (compatible with blood without causing adverse reactions such as thrombosis or hemolysis) and becomes "slick" or smooth and slippery when moistened. It softens soon after insertion, which minimizes initial trauma and thrombus formation. Typically, the lengths of peripheral-short catheters vary from 1.5 to 7.5 cm (5/8 to 3.0 inches). Needles for peripheral-short catheters range in size, or gauge, from a 24-gauge needle, which is the smallest size, to 10- and 12-gauge needles, which are used for large-volume replacement and emergency and trauma care procedures.

During catheter insertion, the stylet is held stationary with the bevel up to prevent vein trauma and facilitate adequate blood flashback. The bevel is the slant or angle of the needle that facilitates puncture of the skin and cannulation of the vascular lumen. The *flashback chamber* is a small space in the hub of the stylet that allows for confirmation of the presence of blood and indicates access to the vascular lumen.

As a result of the Needlestick Safety and Prevention Act of 2000, manufacturers have made great strides in redesigning catheters to afford a measure of safety against accidental blood exposure and possible sharps-related injuries. One type of engineered safety mechanism is a self-sheathing stylet, which encases the needle in a protective chamber upon removal from the inserted catheter.

Dwell times (time left in the patient's vessel) for peripheral-short catheters usually range from 72 to 96 hours.

Removal or discontinuance of the catheter is accomplished by the nurse using standard precautions and aseptic technique. The nurse begins by removing the dressing from the catheter insertion site, then gently retracts the catheter from the vessel, followed by pressure until the bleeding stops. A dry sterile dressing is applied to the site. The nurse should also inspect the catheter for its condition upon removal to ensure that the catheter is intact. If a piece of catheter is left in the patient's vein, it could move centrally toward the heart or lungs, causing severe problems. If the catheter is not intact, the nurse must report this finding to the health care provider. The nurse must instruct the patient to keep the dressing in place and not lift heavy objects because the site could begin to bleed. The various types of peripheral-short catheters are discussed next. Figure 16–1◆ shows the most common veins used for intravenous infusions.

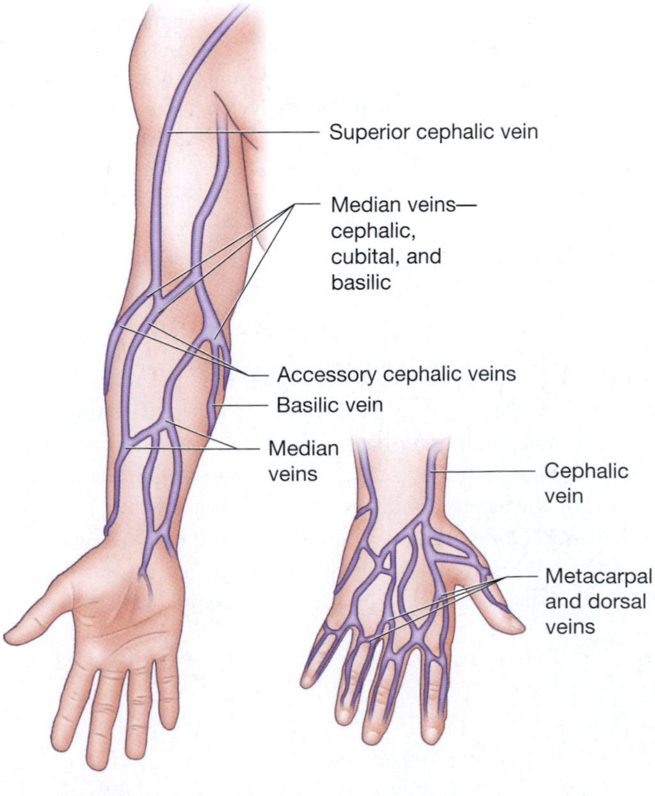

FIGURE 16–1 ◆ Common veins used for intravenous therapy.

Winged Steel Infusion Set

The winged steel infusion set is identified by its flexible plastic attachments, or "wings," that extend from either side of the steel needle to facilitate its insertion (Figure 16–2◆). Another common term for this type of device is a "butterfly." The needle of this device comes in several lengths, from approximately 3/8 to 1.5 inches. Needle gauges vary from 19 to 27. Steel needle gauges are often odd numbered, the lowest number being the largest lumen. Fastened to the winged attachments and needle is plastic tubing, which ranges in length to no more than 12 inches. Winged steel infusion sets are now manufactured with safety sheaths that the clinician must activate to prevent accidental needlesticks.

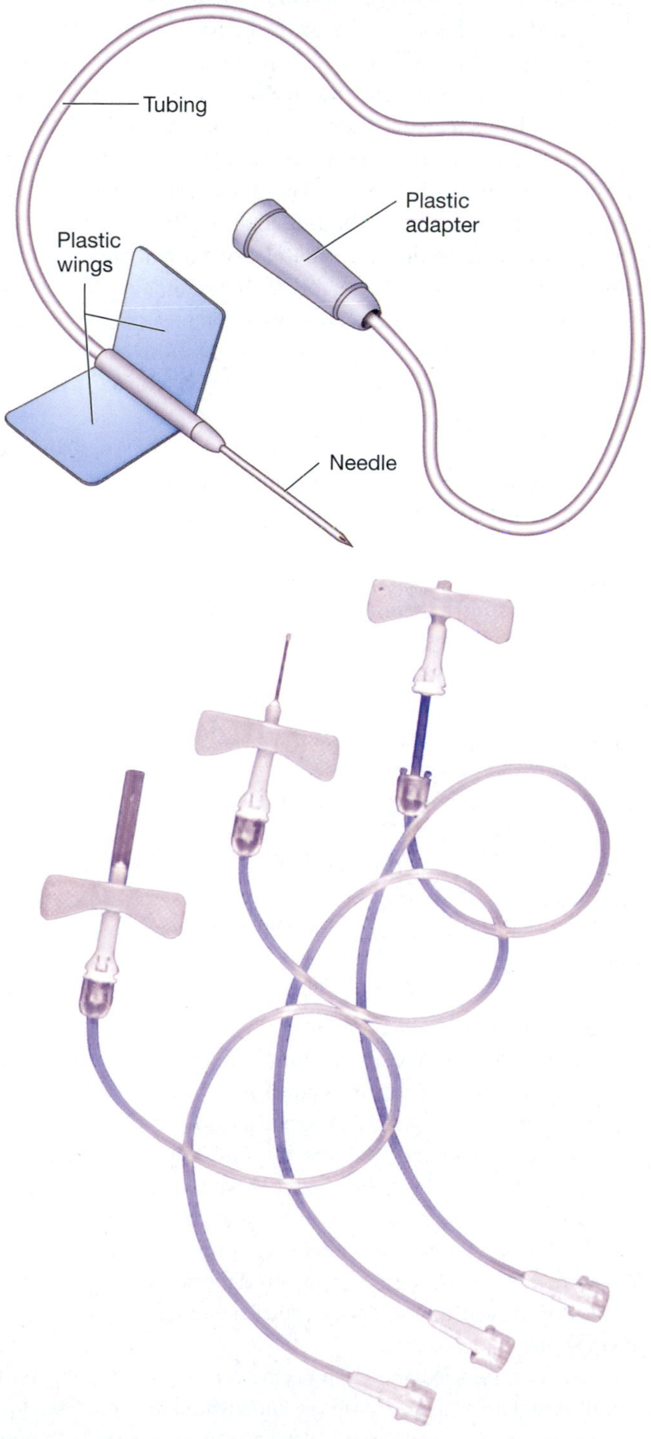

FIGURE 16–2 ◆ Winged steel infusion set.

Source: (bottom) Winged safety steel infusion set. Courtesy Exel International Inc., St. Petersburg, FL.

Because of the rigidity of the steel needle, development of complications is a potential; the needle is more apt to become dislodged, causing **infiltration** (the inadvertent administration of nonvesicant solutions or medications into surrounding tissues), or to pierce or erode the opposite wall of the vein, causing a clot to form within the vein or around the cannula (Rosenthal, 2007). Dwell times for winged steel infusion sets should be kept under 4 hours, and they should be relegated to single-dose therapies because of the increased incidence of complications such as associated with rigid devices. When the winged steel infusion set is used for continuous parenteral administration, the nurse needs to monitor the site frequently for signs of infiltration or bruising. Temporary supportive devices such as arm boards or splinting surfaces may be applied to assist in preservation of the infusion device's location during short-term therapy. The device is removed in the same manner as peripheral short catheters, described above.

Over-the-Needle Peripheral-Short Catheters

Over-the-needle peripheral-short catheters (Figure 16–3◆) are commonly used for short-term infusion therapies. They are 7.5 cm (3.0 in.) or less in length and made of radiopaque materials for ease of x-ray visualization. During the manufacturing process, a hollow-bore metal stylet needle is inserted through the lumen of the flexible catheter. This provides stability to the plastic catheter and facilitates penetration of the skin, as well as vascular or nonvascular structures, during device insertion. The presence of blood in the flashback chamber, situated on the posterior aspect of the catheter, indicates when the lumen of the vessel has been accessed. The stylet is then withdrawn as the catheter is moved forward into the vein. These devices are commonly referred to as angiocatheters.

Midline Catheters

Another example of a peripherally inserted VAD is the midline catheter. Made of materials similar to those of peripheral-short catheters, the midline (ML) catheter is approximately 7.5 to 20 cm (3.1 to 8.0 in.) in length. The recommended dwell periods of these devices is not to exceed 4 weeks. The catheter's insertion location is the antecubital fossa. The distal tip dwells in the basilic, cephalic, or brachial veins, and is level with the axilla. Because of the extended dwell time, insertion preparations are more extensive than those of the peripheral-short VADs in an effort to minimize development of complications. In most health care settings, midline catheters are inserted not by staff nurses, but by specially trained nurses such as those on an intravenous (IV) team.

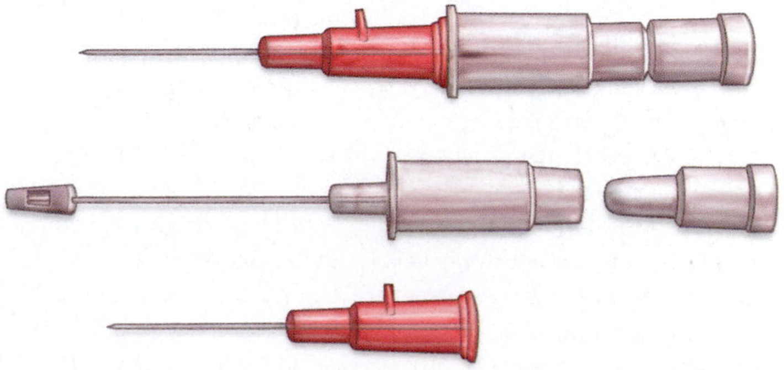

FIGURE 16–3 ◆ Introcan safety over-the-needle peripheral-short catheters.

A nurse may remove an ML catheter at the completion of therapy provided that the nurse is educated and skilled in ML catheter removal and is dependent on institutional policy. It is recommended that antiseptic ointment and an occlusive sterile dressing be applied to the exit wound after removal of the catheter. Because of the length of the device, the nurse must measure the catheter upon removal and compare the length to the pre-insertion catheter.

Midline catheters are useful for the administration of long-term antibiotic therapy and parenteral nutrition, provided that the fluid is appropriate for peripheral administration.

Central Vascular Access Devices

The **central vascular access device (CVAD or CVC),** a catheter inserted into a centrally located vein with the tip residing in the vena cava, was once relegated to emergent resuscitative procedures and therapies for critically ill patients. Today, use of this device has evolved to patients in multiple care settings, including those outside of the acute care setting (Encyclopedia of Nursing & Allied Health, 2011). After insertion but before initiation of therapy, the catheter tip location must be confirmed by radiologic examination.

Nontunneled and Noncuffed CVADs

Nontunneled and noncuffed CVADs are typically divided into three distinct categories for product identification and access configuration purposes. The nontunneled and noncuffed device (Figure 16–4◆) is inserted percutaneously via a direct skin puncture with passage of the catheter directly into the vasculature. A catheter inserted by using this method is generally not considered a long-term device because it is not tunneled under the skin. A percutaneous catheter may have a single lumen or multiple lumens. A common misnomer is to identify the catheter product by its vascular point of entry: "subclavian," "jugular," or "femoral," rather than by product name.

Typically, CVADs are inserted by health care providers or by advanced practice clinicians who are trained to perform the procedure. Once inserted, the device is usually sutured to prevent inadvertent dislodgement and loss of access. Insertion procedures require sterile technique and use of sterile gowns, gloves, and masks for health care personnel.

Removal of nontunneled and noncuffed devices may be done by a nurse who has been trained in the procedure. The patient is placed in a recumbent position and is instructed to perform the Valsalva maneuver, which is to take a deep breath, hold it, and bear down as if to defecate. When the patient bears down, air is prevented from entering the catheter wound and pathway, preventing an air embolism. While the patient is performing the maneuver, the nurse removes the catheter and applies pressure to the site. This is followed by immediate application of an antiseptic ointment and a sterile occlusive dressing to the site. Then the nurse instructs the patient to breathe normally and remain inactive and recumbent for approximately 30 minutes to achieve hemostasis. The nurse must inspect the integrity of the device, measure its length, and compare that length to the pre-insertion catheter length. This confirms whether or not the catheter has fractured, leaving a segment in the patient's circulation. Institutional policy will dictate whether staff nurses are authorized to remove CVCs.

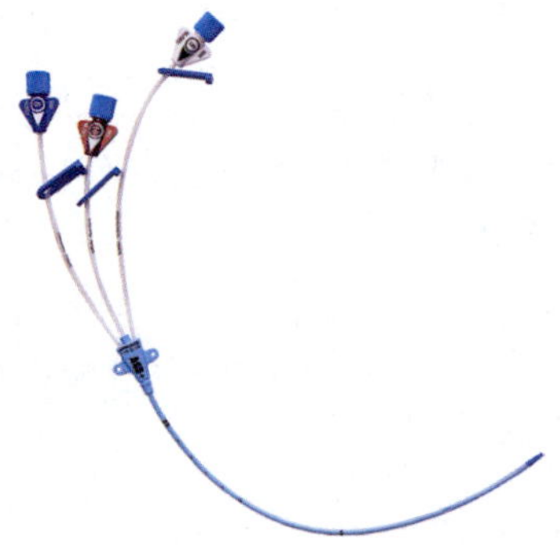

FIGURE 16–4 ◆ Triple-lumen noncuffed central catheters.
Source: Teleflex Incorporated

Another type of CVAD that falls into the category of percutaneously inserted nontunneled and noncuffed devices is the peripherally inserted central catheter (PICC). This is a long-term catheter that is typically inserted at the patient's bedside by a nurse who is educated and skilled in the procedure. A PICC is inserted in a peripheral vein, such as the basilic vein, or brachial vein and then advanced through increasingly larger veins, toward the heart until the tip rests in the distal superior vena cava. Therapies to be infused through a PICC include the following: those that require vascular access for several weeks to many months to as long as 1 year; those with extreme variations in solution pH (>5 and 600 mOsm/L) and including solutions that have irritant and **vesicant** (causes blistering) properties; and those commonly associated with CVADs such as parenteral nutrition and antineoplastic, anti-infective, and inotropic therapies.

Radiologic confirmation of the catheter tip location prior to therapy initiation is mandatory. Because of the insertion location in the antecubital region for most PICCs and ML catheters, the patient's ability to participate in self-care and self-administration practices makes these popular devices among both patients and health care providers.

The PICC also is less commonly associated with development of complications such as site infection, owing to the decreased bacterial ecosystem of the antecubital region, and air embolism, because the device does not externally penetrate the thorax. However, it does lend itself to other complications associated with VADs such as device fracture, tip malposition, device occlusion, infection, and thrombus formation. When removing a PICC, the educated and skilled nurse instructs the patient in the Valsalva maneuver, places the patient in a recumbent position, and performs the removal procedure following the same procedure indicated for removal of other CVADs. Documentation must include measurement of the PICC and comparison with the pre-insertion length.

Tunneled and Cuffed CVADs

A second category of CVAD is the tunneled and cuffed device (The Free Dictionary, 2011). The cuff is attached to the catheter in such a manner that the device is stabilized during its dwell time, and it reduces the risk of catheter-related infection by inhibiting the migration of microorganisms along the catheter track. Some cuffs are impregnated with antimicrobial agents such as a silver-impregnated collagen matrix. The catheter is configured with either single or multiple lumens. These CVADs often are identified by the name(s) of the health care provider(s) who developed such clinical devices, such as Broviac, Hickman, Raaf, and Groshong.

Insertion of tunneled and cuffed catheters is typically done in the surgical or radiology suite. Tunneling under the skin is the technique used to access the vasculature. An entrance wound is created at a point generally near a large vein, typically the subclavian vein. The catheter is inserted into the vena cava, and radiologic confirmation of tip placement is mandatory prior to initiation of therapy. After tip insertion, the catheter's remaining length is drawn through an exit wound located lower on the chest wall. By establishing mechanical barriers (the skin), this technique minimizes the potential for microorganisms to gain access to the body, and it enables the cuff to act as a securement device once the tissues heal from the procedure. These CVADs are intended for long-term infusion therapies, with the patient often participating in self-care in the home setting. They also may be used for blood sampling, thus avoiding numerous phlebotomy sticks. They are most commonly used in dialysis or with oncology patients.

Some tunneled catheters are open at the end, similar to a peripheral catheter. When not in use, they require the instillation of a small amount of heparinized saline to prevent clotting. Some, including the Groshong catheter, are closed at the tip but have a slit in the side of the catheter near its distal end. When infusions are running, the slit opens out. When the catheter is not in use, the slit closes so that no blood can enter the lumen of the catheter. This type of device requires only a flush with sterile normal saline, not heparin. When caring for a patient with a tunneled catheter, the nurse must know the type of catheter being used in order to provide optimal care to patients through demonstrating best practices and proper catheter management.

Implanted Ports

Implanted ports comprise the third category of central vascular access devices. Implanted ports are indicated for long-term or chronic therapies such as antineoplastic, inotropic, antimicrobial, and blood replacement therapies. An implanted port is a chambered device, containing either single or double reservoirs, with an attached silastic catheter (Figure 16–5◆). The catheter may be a single- or double-lumen catheter, depending on the configuration of the port. The catheter's tip is directed to dwell in a designated structure, which could be either vascular or nonvascular, depending on the intended infusion prescription.

Implanted ports are in their own category because of their unique physical structure, implantation procedures, clinical indications, and recommended lengths of dwell time. Typically, these devices are surgically placed either in the operating or radiology suite by health care providers or advanced practice clinicians. The device is considered long term because it can remain in place for several years. It is inserted, or implanted, under the skin in a surgically designed pocket of skin; the port or reservoir portion is usually placed over a bony surface to enhance port stability and facilitate access. When the port is not in use, it requires very little maintenance. However, most ports do require the instillation of heparinized saline to prevent clotting when the device is not in use (Drugs.com, 2012).

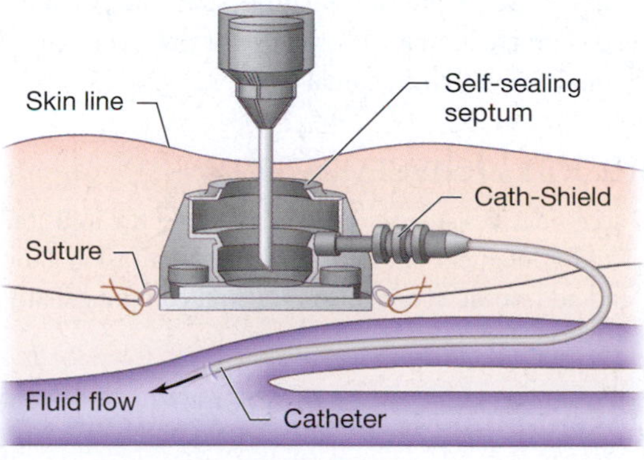

FIGURE 16–5 ◆ Implanted port.

Source: Courtesy of Infusion Nurses Society, PICC Education Module, 2003.

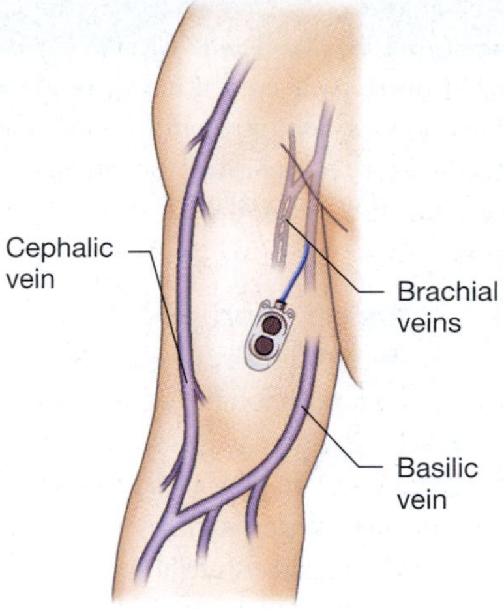

FIGURE 16–6 ◆ Double-lumen implanted ports.

Source: Courtesy of Bard Access Systems, Salt Lake City, UT.

The port chamber, or reservoir, will have one or two chambers leading to either a single- or double-lumen catheter with the catheter tip located in the vena cava (Figure 16–6◆). The port is usually less than 1 inch in height and diameter. There also are low-profile ports that are smaller, less than 1/2 inch in height and width, allowing for placement in the inner aspect of the adult's upper arm or ventral surface of the forearm.

The septum, a key factor for the port's optimal functioning, is the port's access point. If the septum becomes damaged in any way, the entire device must be surgically removed and replaced. The septum is designed to accommodate a noncoring needle. The bevel of the noncoring needle opens on the *side* of the needle at a gentle angle so that, when inserted, it makes a narrow "slice" in the septum as opposed to "coring" of the septum. This allows access to the port many more times before the septum is likely to leak. Damaging the septum would allow leakage of infusate from the septum, placing the patient at potential risk for infiltration and extravasation, air embolism, and infectious processes. It also would cause the patient to face another surgical procedure in order to replace the port. The needles used for implanted ports are usually bent at a 90° angle so that, once inserted, they lie parallel to the patient's chest, allowing easy stabilization of the needle. A special dressing, usually a clear film surrounded by a foam ring, is used to form an occlusive dressing that still allows visual inspection of the insertion site.

Implanted ports, once healed, are less prone to the development of infection because there is no break in the skin except when the device is in use and the access needle is in place. This makes them well suited for use in oncology patients who require intermittent chemotherapy, blood sampling, and blood transfusions.

The removal of tunneled and cuffed catheters and implanted ports and reservoirs is performed by the health care provider or by advanced practice clinicians.

In summary, CVADs are indicated for critical care and long-term therapies. These devices are used in all care settings such as hospitals; homes; long-term, rehabilitation, and subacute facilities; ambulatory infusion centers; and health care providers' offices. Certain properties of solutions and medications mandate the use of CVADs to avoid damaging the sensitive peripheral vascular structures. Additionally, CVADs are useful for medications, such as inotropics and antineoplastic therapies that are administered in cycles and over many months.

Nonvascular Access Devices

Infusion therapy can also be delivered by nonvascular routes such as the subcutaneous, intraosseous, and intraspinal routes. Although many of the prescribed therapies are complicated, the catheter products that are used in conjunction with these modalities are the same as those used with vascular access.

Subcutaneous Infusion Therapy

Subcutaneous infusion therapy involves the infusion of parenteral solutions and medications via absorption through the subcutaneous tissues (Gorski, 2009). The technique used to infuse a large amount of isotonic solutions in this manner is known as **hypodermoclysis** (Mei & Auerhahn, 2009). Infusing smaller volumes such as medications prescribed for pain control or diabetes mellitus is known as continuous subcutaneous infusions (CSI). The infusion devices are manufactured with extremely small gauge sizes (25 to 27 gauge) and are approximately 1/2 inch in length.

The needle may be positioned at a 90-degree angle and attached to an adhesive disk or may appear as a winged steel infusion set used for vascular access. The device is inserted over an area where there is adequate subcutaneous tissue and capillary beds to absorb the infusate. These areas, which include the abdomen, outer aspects of the thigh and upper arm, and subclavicular and subscapular regions, allow adequate visualization of the infusion site in addition to allowing the patient unfettered mobility.

Even though these are nonvascular insertion procedures, the nurse must prime the administration set and access device with the prescribed parenteral solution prior to initiation of therapy. The intended site is prepared with the appropriate antiseptic agent and allowed to dry before the device is inserted. The device must be aspirated with a syringe to confirm the absence of blood in the area of insertion. If no blood is found, the device is secured with sterile dressing material, and the infusion is started. If blood is obtained, the device is removed and another infusion site is selected and prepared. A new device is then readied and inserted, once again being aspirated to confirm the absence of blood at the insertion site.

Common complications associated with this type of treatment are localized skin irritation including erythema and itching, infection, and dislodgment of the access device. Systemic complications are associated with the medication or solution being infused. Ineffective dosing may require another infusion site or route to be secured. Site rotation usually occurs every 3 to 5 days, depending on the concentration and rate of the fluid or medication being administered.

Hypodermoclysis has been found to be an effective treatment for older patients who require short-term isotonic fluid resuscitation to treat dehydration. Additional criteria for this treatment modality include fluid needs of less than 3 liters per day, no evidence of existing coagulopathies, and intact skin sites.

Intraosseous Therapy

Intraosseous therapy is the insertion of a hollow-bore needle into the bone, with the device tip accessing the marrow space. The tip of the needle is protected by an obturator, which has screw-like threads that facilitate penetration of the bony structure. The sternum is usually the preferred site (Vizcarra & Clum, 2010). Patients with thermal injuries, trauma, cardiac arrest, or other life-threatening illnesses can be treated in this manner. Complications include bone fracture, infiltration, osteomyelitis, and cellulitis, in addition to occlusion of the obturator or needle and needle breakage. Emergent access of the bone core allows rapid infusion of large volumes of parenteral fluids and medications until vascular access can be obtained (Phillips et al., 2010).

Intraspinal Catheters

Intraspinal catheters are placed within the spinal spaces such as the epidural and intrathecal spaces. The intraspinal space has been used with great reliability for many procedures such as delivery of anesthesia, diagnostic testing, and infusions. Catheters used for the intraspinal route have 22- to 26-gauge lumens and vary from 10 to 30 inches in length. For temporary placement, the catheter is inserted percutaneously into the desired spinal space and secured externally. For more stable long-term placement and as an infection control measure, the catheter can be tunneled to an isolated exit site.

Implanted infusion ports also can be used for intraspinal access (Mosby's Medical Dictionary, 2009). These are usually reserved for patients with intractable pain who require lifelong pain control and have a life expectancy of months to a year (University Pain Centers, 2008). The device consists of a catheter whose tip is located in the epidural space, which is attached to an infusion pump that is often implanted under the skin, in the vicinity of the abdominal region or chest wall.

Infusates, drugs, and diluents must be preservative free because of the neurotoxic effects of preserving agents. The epidural space can usually accommodate an infusion rate no greater than 15 mL/min owing to limitations imposed by physical structures and restrictions of the epidural space. Medications and solutions given via this route have the ability to cross the dura mater, and have direct effects on the central nervous system (CNS). Surfactant-free filters on the administration system and alcohol-free skin antiseptic agents are used to prevent potential neurotoxic agents from entering the CNS.

Intrathecal Therapy

Intrathecal therapy involves the administration of medications directly into the cerebrospinal fluid (CSF) via an implanted reservoir system (Mosby's Medical Dictionary, 2009). The most common device, the **Ommaya reservoir,** allows delivery of medications directly into the CSF without relying on diffusion. The catheter attached to the reservoir terminates in the ventricular space of the cerebrum. The Ommaya reservoir is very effective for: delivering medications such as preservative-free opioids; administering selected antineoplastic agents such as methotrexate and cytarabine; measuring CSF pressures; draining excess CSF fluid; and obtaining CSF samples for laboratory assay. The reservoir is surgically placed via a burr hole in the skull, and the skin is secured over the device. Care and maintenance practices are dependent on the intended therapy, and standard precautions and sterile technique must be maintained. Complications with the use of this device are the same as those associated with intraspinal devices.

Infusion Delivery Systems

Vascular access devices are just one piece of the entire infusion delivery system. Fluid containers, administration sets, infusion flow control devices, and add-on devices also are integral components to effective therapy delivery.

Fluid Containers

Fluid containers in infusion delivery systems are made of either glass or plastic. In current practice, glass bottles are reserved for drugs that are incompatible with the polyvinylchloride in plastic IV bags. For example, amiodarone, nitroglycerin, and propofol must be administered in glass. Glass containers require a venting mechanism to be inserted into the container to facilitate solution delivery.

Plastic containers are the preferred type of container because of easy portability, easy storage, and reduced manufacturing costs. However, because of the flexibility of plastic containers, volume and dose administrations may be inaccurate. Plastic containers are highly amenable to fluctuations in temperature, which makes freezing of drugs after admixture advantageous for availability and storage.

Administration Sets

The *administration set* is the tubing that delivers the parenteral fluid from the infusate container to the catheter that is in the patient's vein. The administration set may be described as primary or secondary, depending on the function of the set. The *primary set* is the main tubing that extends from the infusate container to the access device. It permits fluid passage by using either gravity, or an electronic infusion device set, or a syringe pump-delivery system.

The *secondary set* is tubing that attaches to the primary set and permits additional infusion administrations. Typically, secondary sets are used to infuse medications and solutions that are administered on an intermittent basis (for example, every 4 hours). The secondary set is attached to a small bag of intravenous solution and is "piggybacked" into the primary set and hung up higher than the primary solution so that it infuses instead of the primary solution (Figure 16–7◆). When the bag is empty, the primary solution simply takes over again. The primary infusate and the secondary infusate must be compatible in order to prevent complications such as precipitate formation, which can result in occlusion of the fluid pathway.

Metered-volume chambered sets consist of an administration set topped with a metered, small-volume container that is attached to a fluid container (Figure 16–8◆, p. 384). Markings on the chamber vary from 1- to 5-mL increments. This administration set is often used for special patient populations, such as those in critical care units, and for older adults with fluid limitation needs requiring close observation and monitoring. Metered-volume chambered administration sets also are used for drugs and solutions that require significant control or intermittent delivery, and with titrated medications.

Clamping mechanisms are features of administration sets that regulate the prescribed infusion rates (Figure 16–9◆, p. 384). *Roller clamps*, generally found on primary infusion sets, allow the nurse to regulate the parenteral fluid by either opening or closing the clamp. *Slide and pinch* clamps are not volume controlling but instead provide an "on–off" feature to the set. These clamps are seen often on add-on equipment and secondary sets. *Screw* clamps may also be found on administration sets and offer "on–off" and flow regulation functions comparable to those of roller clamps.

Flow Control Device

The **flow control device,** an add-on device that can be used for regulation of fluid administration, is added to a gravity infusion system at the point closest to the patient and is used to regulate fluid flow instead of using the clamp provided on the set. Accuracy and consistency of infusion rates are affected by patient activity, height of the fluid container above the patient, and fluid composition and temperature. Once the flow rate is "dialed," or set, it is subject to wide variations in fluid delivery if the patient is ambulatory or the fluid container's height is adjusted. However, clamping mechanisms do not negate the need for close monitoring and fluid regulation by the nurse.

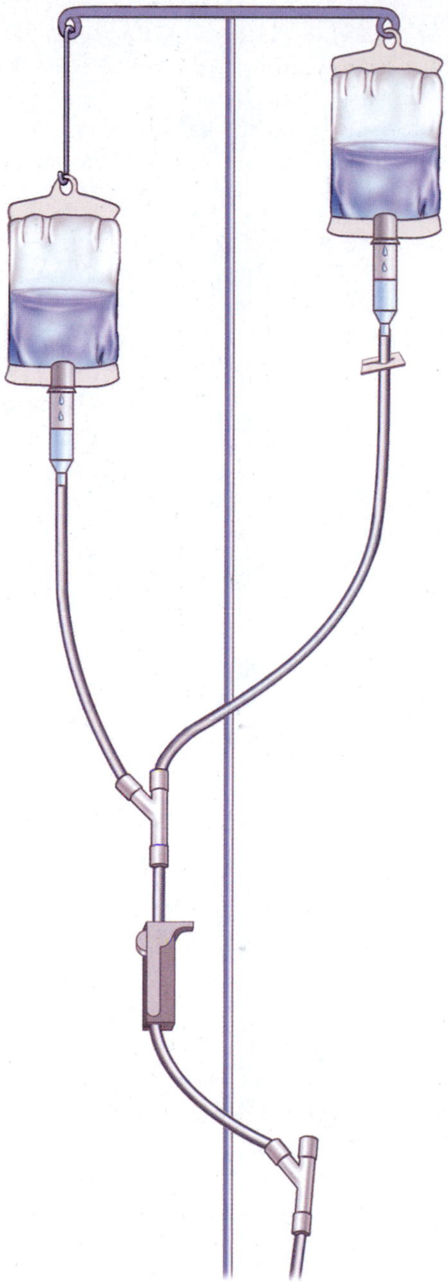

FIGURE 16–7 ◆ Piggyback system.

Some infusion products and medications, such as nitroglycerin, lipid emulsions, and blood products, have specific requirements associated with their delivery.

Specialized administration sets are manufactured with features that meet these requirements:

- Nitroglycerin is incompatible with standard PVC tubing. Hence, nitroglycerin administration sets are manufactured from non-PVC materials. Also, nitroglycerin comes in glass containers for medication delivery to minimize drug loss.
- Lipids are affected by containers and administration sets that contain DEHP (a plasticizer used in the manufacturing of articles made of polyvinyl chloride) (Alonge, 2010). Therefore, lipid emulsions are manufactured in glass containers.
- Blood infusion sets are designed to accommodate the specific properties of blood and its components. Blood administration

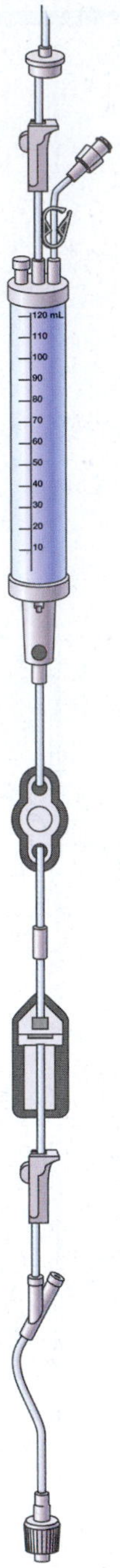

FIGURE 16–8 ◆ Metered-volume chambered set.

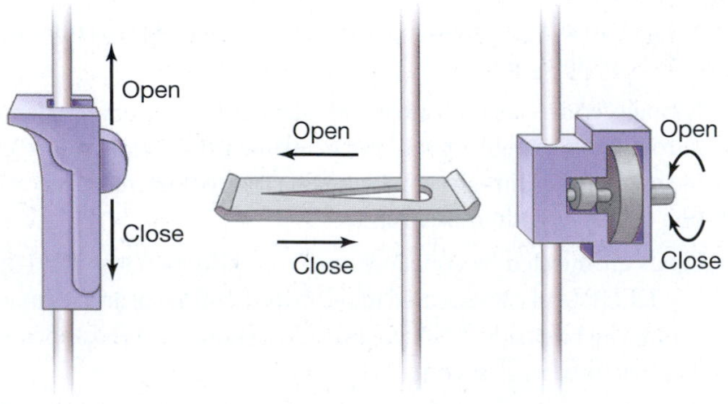

FIGURE 16–9 ◆ Administration set clamps.

sets may have Y-shaped tubing and will contain filter systems to remove debris and accumulated by-products that result from blood storage. Other systems require the nurse to attach a separate filter product to a standard administration set. The Y-tubing permits a container of 0.9% sodium chloride to be connected to one access spike of the set and the blood container to be connected to the second access spike. Some sets can be used for gravity infusion; others are compatible with electronic infusion devices. When rapid infusion is indicated, sets with in-line hand pump may be used, typically only in areas such as emergency departments, surgical suites, and intensive care units.

Add-On Devices

Add-on devices are pieces of equipment that extend the efficacy of the existing administration set. Devices are added to the administration set either proximally at the spike end or distally at the patient end. Devices can also be added at side ports along the administration set. Add-on devices are used to add length to the administration set, add filter infusates, and increase access to the patient's VAD. All connections to the catheter adapter and for add-on devices should be a **Luer-Lok** (a threaded mechanism that prevents inadvertent separation of equipment). The routine use of add-on devices is discouraged. Restricting their use will decrease occurrences of fluid contamination, accidental disconnection, and overall infusion supply costs. Here are some examples of add-on devices:

- ***Stopcock:*** A manually operated device that is used to direct the flow of an infusate. Stopcocks are used when multiple solutions are being infused. They have a three-way or four-way mechanism, permitting infusions to be connected at a common aperture, which is located at the VAD's hub. The stopcock requires the nurse to manually direct the infusion by turning the valve toward a specific infusion to initiate fluid flow.
- ***Extension Set:*** A device used to add length as well as additional side access ports to the existing administration set.
- ***Multiflow Adapter and Y Set:*** Devices used for administration of two or more infusates simultaneously. Access to the multiflow adapter is usually via a cap that maintains sterility of the fluid pathway. Each access of the adapter must be primed before attachment to the administration system and prior to attachment to the infusion catheter (Figure 16–10◆).
- ***Injection Port or Cap:*** A device used to gain access to the indwelling catheter. Manufactured with a resealable rubber cap, the device permits access with either needles or needleless safety infusion cannulas. Typically, the device is lightweight and varies in length from 1/2 inch to 2 inches (Figure 16–11◆).
- ***Filter:*** A filter is used to provide sterility to the infused parenteral medications or solutions. Filters remove particulate matter, eliminate air, and retain or capture microorganisms. Filters are not used when certain medications, such as amphotericin B or IV push medications are prescribed because the medication may become trapped on the filter bed and not reach the patient.

Infusion Delivery Devices

Several methods other than gravity are used to enhance effective delivery of prescribed parenteral solutions. These include mechanical infusion devices, electronic infusion devices, and positive pressure infusion pumps.

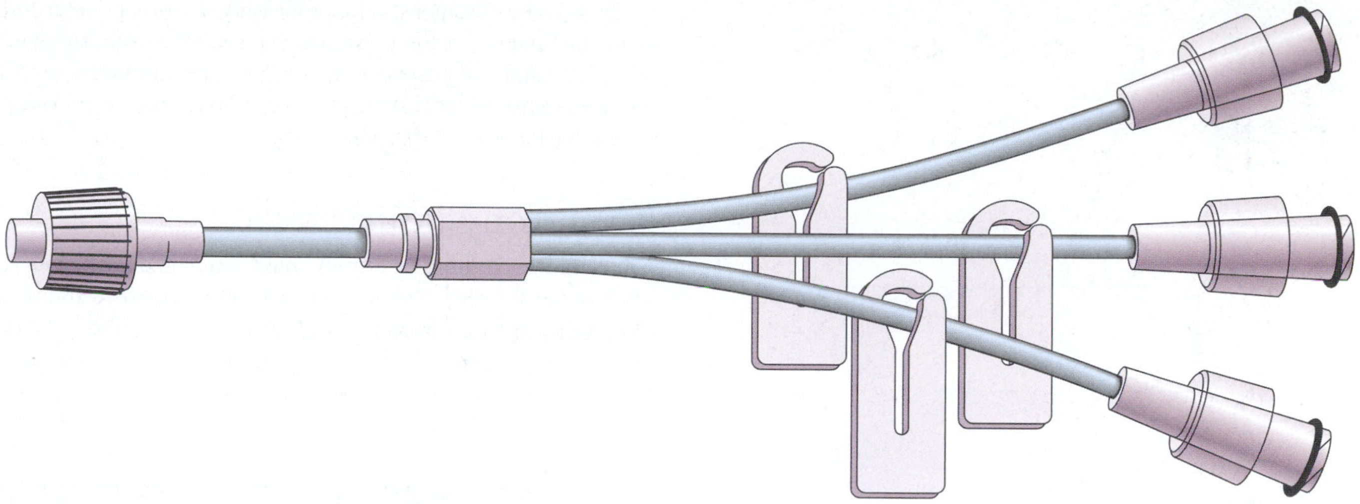

FIGURE 16–10 ◆ Three-lumen multiflow adapter.

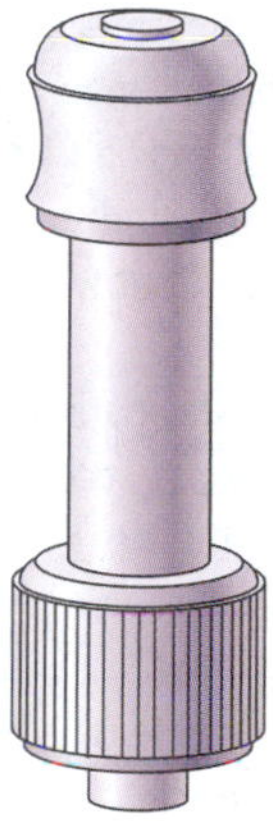

FIGURE 16–11 ◆ Injection cap.

Mechanical Infusion Devices

Mechanical infusion devices include these types:

- *Elastomeric balloons* are made of soft, expandable material contained within a transparent hard plastic casing. The prescribed medication is in the balloon-like container. Microbore tubing is attached to its outlet and, depending on its bore size, delivers the fluid at a corresponding rate over 30 minutes or more, depending on the volume of the fluid. The small size of the tubing impedes the flow, preventing undue pressure on the patient's catheter. These MIDs are usually reserved for home care situations and are a one-time use product.
- The *spring-coil syringe* acts by powering the plunger of a syringe and delivering the medication to the patient. Once the syringe is empty, a new syringe must be fitted into the locking mechanism. This type of delivery system is more bulky than elastomeric balloons, and its function is relegated to a specific syringe size.
- The *spring-coil container* is a combination of the spring coil and a collapsible disk. The mechanism is activated by applying pressure on the top and bottom disk, causing collapse of the container and allowing its contents to infuse with flow being controlled by microbore tubing. Both the spring-coil syringe and container are used for small-volume parenteral administrations and are seen in acute and home care settings.

Mechanical infusion devices (MIDs) are devices that do not require the use of an external power source to operate. MIDs are relatively easy to use and monitor, but the nurse should realize that these devices cannot detect flaws in the administration system such as air in the set, infiltration, or catheter occlusion.

Electronic Infusion Devices

Electronic infusion devices (EIDs) can be divided into two categories: pumps and controllers. The *pump* is a device that delivers its solutions via positive pressure; the *controller* is a device that relies on gravity to assist its action. A controller is often seen in general patient populations where uncomplicated therapies are used. Controllers usually do not contribute to infusion-related complications such as infiltration and vascular injury, so they are safe for special populations such as older adults and patients with most antineoplastic therapies. Most controllers use a drop sensor that attaches to the drip chamber of the administration set.

Positive Pressure Infusion Pump

The **positive pressure infusion pump** creates pressure to infuse the fluid and overcome vascular resistance (Figure 16–12◆, p. 386). Pumps have psi parameters somewhere in the vicinity of 10 psi. Positive pressure pumps are used in high acuity care areas such as critical care in which the therapies are complex. Depending on hospital policy, pumps may be used in the general medical–surgical areas or when medications are being delivered that requires strict monitoring, such as anticoagulation, parenteral nutrition, and inotropic therapies. The pump delivers infusate at an accurate prescribed rate and has an alarm system that detects infusion-related errors of delivery, such as free flow, air in the line, and changes in vascular resistance such as occlusion or infiltration.

A **volumetric pump** calculates the infusion volume delivered by the amount displaced in a reservoir. Drop sensors can also be included in this pump category. The sensor may be located internally in the pump where the fluid passes through a chamber, but it is usually found externally attached to the drip chamber. Syringe pumps are infusion specific and are limited to small-volume parenterals such as anti-infectives or pain medications. Syringe pumps are unable to detect "no flow" unless significant back pressure is generated from the distal set or indwelling catheter.

Alarms on infusion delivery devices indicate pending disruptions in fluid delivery. Not all devices have comparable alarms or a full array of similar controls. In effect, these systems serve to protect the patient by alerting the nurse when needed to evaluate the patient and the patient's infusion system. The following are some alarm features:

- ***Air in the Line:*** Detects the presence of air in the fluid pathway of the set.
- ***Occlusion:*** Infusion pumps detect disruption of flow above the catheter and resistance to flow occurring below the device.

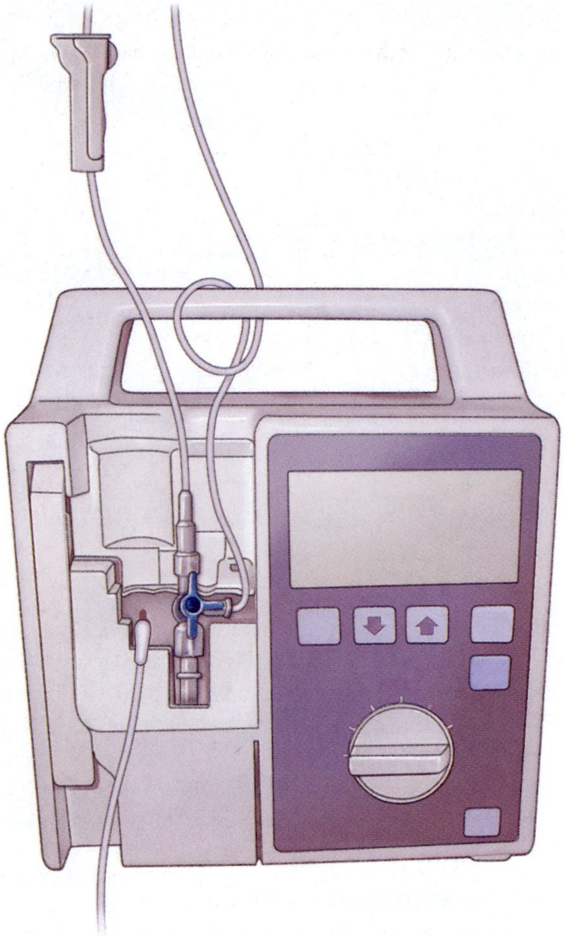

FIGURE 16–12 ◆ Positive pressure pump.

- ***Infusion Complete:*** This alarm sounds when a preset volume limit has been reached.
- ***Free Flow:*** This alarm is *essential* for preventing the inadvertent bolus dosing of fluid or medications. The administration set, upon its removal from the EID, must have a self-clamping mechanism that prevents free flow of infusate. The alarm detects rapid infusion of fluid as a result of partial disengagement of the pumping mechanism.

Ambulatory infusion pumps are lightweight and small enough to be easily carried. They may be used to administer continuous rate, automatic dose, demand dose, or a combination of these types of doses, and they may be used for administration of pain medications, insulin, and chemotherapy. Ambulatory pumps may be attached to the patient's belt, contained within a backpack, or placed on a table top. The power supply is usually a disposable battery. **Patient-controlled analgesia (PCA) pumps** are available in ambulatory, semiportable, or pole-mounted versions. The PCA pump is capable of delivering medication for pain management continuously or on patient demand. Multichannel and dual-channel pumps are contained in a single device. These channels can be operated independently of each other, so that different medications and solutions can be programmed for delivery at assigned times for predetermined doses via a single infusion pathway to the patient.

The infusion delivery device selection is essential. Specific controls and alarm systems are integral to the infusion delivery device as safety measures for the patient; they also ensure accurate administration of solutions and medications. Infusion delivery devices are never to be considered a substitute for nursing care; rather, they serve as an adjunct. Monitoring and evaluation of response to therapy, in addition to effective care and maintenance strategies for the infusion patient, provide the foundation for positive outcomes.

Infusion Nursing Practice

Nurses providing infusion therapy must have competency and skill validation in order to be proficient in its technical aspects, demonstrate competency in clinical judgment, and practice in accordance with their state's nurse practice act. Clinical competency validation are vital to health care organizations that participate in annual reviews (Infusion Nurses Society [INS], 2011).

Calculations

Infusion therapy is ordered by the health care provider or by a legally authorized prescriber. It is the nurse's responsibility to be knowledgeable of the drugs' and solutions' properties, intended outcomes, and potential side and adverse effects that may occur. Although many formulations are available for deriving correct dosing volumes and amounts, certain methods are relatively easy to use and are used consistently. These include calculation of the drip factor and the flow rate of the fluids being administered.

Keep in mind that certain patient conditions and patient populations (i.e., pediatric and older patients and patients receiving antineoplastic or antimicrobial therapies) have specific restrictions and requirements based on body surface area, weight, and age.

The drip factor referred to in administration sets can be described as macrodrip or microdrip, and the set may be classified as vented or nonvented. The **drip factor** is the number of drops that will equal 1 milliliter (mL) of infusate. Drip factor sizes vary from 10 to 60 drops/mL. A macrodrip calculation varies from 10 to 20 drops/mL, and a microdrip is 60 drops/mL, depending on the manufacturer. This information is critical in calculating the exact amount of solution to be infused. Several formulas are used for fluid delivery calculations; these are dependent on drip factors, prescribed drug, and infusate solutions, as well as other parameters such as body surface area and weight.

Flow rate determination is used to calculate the amount of fluid to be delivered over a specific time period. Flow rates can be ordered as milliliters per hour or minute, total volume over a set period such as multiple hours or a 24-hour period, or number of drops per minute. The nurse must be knowledgeable of the available drip factor of the administration sets on hand and select the most appropriate for the infusion prescription.

One simplified order conversion technique is to divide the milliliter rate per hour by a specific number associated with the drop factor. The formula and an example are given in Chart 16–1. Consistent use and knowledge of the variety of calculations associated with accurate dosing and therapy administration criteria will result in safe nursing practice for the clinician, fewer medication errors, increased patient safety, and positive infusion outcomes.

Infusion Nursing Standards of Practice

The goal of the *Infusion Nursing Standards (INS) of Practice* is to preserve the patient's right to safe, quality care, and protect the nurse who

CHART 16–1 Infusion Rate Calculation Formula

Example: The flow rate of therapy is ordered at 120 mL per hour via gravity. The administration set on hand has a drip factor of 15 gtts/mL. The following equation is used to calculate drops per minute:

$$\frac{120 \text{ (mL/hr)} \times 15 \text{ (gtt factor)}}{60 \text{ (time in minutes)}} = 30 \text{ drops per minute}$$

Typically, the 30 is divided by 4, and the nurse counts the number of drops in 15 seconds.

administers infusion therapy (INS, 2011). The INS standards define the criteria relative to nursing accountability in the delivery of infusion therapies. They provide a framework to use in evaluating patient outcomes and are used as a mechanism for evaluating the quality of patient care and the competency of the nurse delivering infusion therapy. The INS standards are applicable in all practice settings (e.g., hospitals, homes, long-term care facilities, and health care provider offices). Nurses are accountable for adherence to the standards regardless of the care setting.

National guidelines also are incorporated into infusion practice. An example related to infusion nursing is the *CDC Guidelines for the Prevention of Intravascular Catheter-Related Infections* (Centers for Disease Control and Prevention [CDC], 2011a). This publication provides recommendations that, when incorporated in practice, are designed to reduce infectious complications associated with infusion therapy (see the National Guidelines box).

Patient Assessment

Patient assessment is an ongoing process to determine the appropriateness of the therapy and ensure desired patient outcomes. The results of the initial assessment identify the baseline for the patient's care and treatment. Ongoing assessment chronicles the patient's response to treatment and provides data to measure outcomes. Pertinent information obtained during assessment and monitoring should be communicated to other health care professionals responsible for the patient's care.

Patient assessment should include the patient's past and present medical history, including diagnosis, medical and surgical histories, age, allergies, vascular access history, and patient preferences regarding VAD types and site locations. Prior to initiation, the prescribed therapy should be assessed for appropriate dose, route, and rate of infusion; potential incompatibilities among infusates, oral medications, and food; and appropriateness of the care setting.

NATIONAL GUIDELINES Prevention of Intravascular Catheter-Related Infections

The Centers for Disease Control and Prevention (CDC) guidelines for the prevention of intravascular catheter-related infections were developed for practitioners who insert catheters and for persons responsible for surveillance and control of infections in hospital, outpatient, and home health care settings. A complete copy of the guidelines can be found at http://www.cdc.gov/hicpac/pdf/guidelines/bsi-guidelines-2011.pdf.

Source: Centers for Disease Control and Prevention. (2011). CDC guidelines for the prevention of intravascular catheter-related infections. Retrieved from http://www.cdc.gov/hicpac/pdf/guidelines/bsi-guidelines-2011.pdf.

Because infusion therapy is directly related to the patient's fluid volume and electrolyte status, reviewing laboratory data is an important component of the assessment process. Necessary components of the process include, but are not limited to, the patient's electrolytes, serum proteins, blood chemistries, and renal function tests. Clinical assessment of the patient may include height and weight, body surface area, nutritional status, pain threshold, skin turgor, vital signs, intake and output, and vascular access integrity.

The type and frequency of patient monitoring will be determined by the prescribed therapy, access device, patient's condition and age, and care setting. In addition, the nurse must monitor the catheter–skin junction site and surrounding area, flow rate, clinical data, patient response, and side effects, as well as the patient's compliance with the prescribed therapy.

Site Selection

Vein selection for cannulation will need to accommodate the gauge and length of the catheter. Site selection is based on the patient's condition, age, and diagnosis; the vein condition, size, and location; the type and duration of prescribed therapy; and the patient's history. Veins that should be considered for peripheral cannulation are those found on the dorsal and ventral surfaces of the upper extremities, including the metacarpal, cephalic, and basilic veins (see Figure 16–1, p. 378). The nurse should avoid using the veins in the lower extremities of adults because of the risk of embolism and thrombophlebitis formation.

Site selection should be routinely initiated in the distal areas of the upper extremities with subsequent cannulations made proximal to previous cannulated sites. Areas of flexion should be avoided, except in placing a ML catheter or PICC. Veins in arms with compromised circulation, postmastectomy or postaxillary node dissection, or fistulated extremities should also be avoided.

The nurse should assess vascular access by applying a tourniquet 10 to 20 cm (4 to 8 in.) proximal to the intended venipuncture site. The nurse palpates the extremity to assess the vein's condition; an appropriate vein for venipuncture will feel soft and bouncy. In contrast, a hard, cordlike feeling indicates a sclerosed or compromised vein. Valves can be detected by a hard lump or "knot-like" feeling. Resilient veins that are easily depressed are required for successful venipuncture. Palpation also differentiates arteries from veins, because veins do not pulsate.

Site Preparation

While adhering to standard precautions during site preparation, the nurse disinfects the skin with an antiseptic solution before inserting the catheter. The agent should be applied by using friction and should be allowed to dry thoroughly before the venipuncture. Fanning, blowing, or blotting the prepared area is contraindicated. Agents recommended for skin preparation include 2% chlorhexidine-based solutions, 10% povidone-iodine, or 70% alcohol as single agents or in combination preparations. Agency policy should be consulted to determine the exact procedure nurses should follow for site preparation.

Dressings

Dressings are used to protect the catheter from external environmental contamination. Sterile dressings should be aseptically

Video*: Catheter Line Dressing Change

applied at the initiation of vascular access, when the integrity of the dressing is compromised, and at specified time intervals determined by organizational policy and procedure. Dressings should not be reinforced if they become damp, loose, or visibly soiled, but should instead be replaced with new dressing materials. Types of dressings include the following: gauze and tape dressings can be used to cover the venipuncture site, and changed according to agency pollicy; transparent semipermeable membrane (TSM) dressings which facilitate daily catheter–skin junction inspection without disruption of the therapy and allow direct observation of the insertion site. For peripheral-short catheter sites, a TSM dressing should be changed at the time of catheter site rotation and immediately if the integrity of the dressing is compromised. For other VADs, the TSM dressing should be changed per protocol or if the dressing has lost its integrity. Topical ointments should not be placed on the insertion site, because their efficacy at reducing infections has not been proven (CDC, 2011a).

Research on the choice of dressings is limited, and evidence does not support one choice over the other. The CDC recommends either a sterile gauze or a sterile, transparent, semipermeable dressing (CDC, 2011a). Antiseptic dressings, such as the chlorhexidine-impregnated foam dressing, are being used more frequently. A small, round disk or sponge is placed around the catheter at the exit site, covered with a transparent dressing. Studies have shown that these sponges can decrease infection rates and decrease the frequency of dressing changes (Timsit, et al., 2009).

Catheter Securement

Catheters must be stabilized so as not to interfere with assessment and monitoring of the site or impede delivery of the prescribed therapy. Devices used to secure and stabilize catheters include sterile tapes, sterile surgical strips, and sterile manufactured stabilization devices. Minimizing catheter movement helps to prevent mechanical irritation to the vein lining and reduces the risk of phlebitis formation. When feasible, using a manufactured stabilization device is preferred, as it prevents the catheter from telescoping within the vein or becoming dislodged (INS, 2011).

Flushing

Flushing, which is the infusion of a sterile solution, is performed to ensure and maintain patency of the VAD and to prevent mixing of incompatible medications and solutions. Routine flushing should be performed in the following situations:

- Administration of blood and blood components
- Sampling of blood
- Administration of incompatible medications or solutions
- Intermittent therapy
- Converting the VAD from continuous to intermittent therapies.

Patency flushing is performed at established intervals determined by organizational policy and procedure and the patient's condition. Acceptable flush solutions are saline (preservative-free 0.9% sodium chloride, injection) and heparin in the lowest concentration that will achieve patency while not affecting the patient's clotting factors. Many organizations flush intermittent peripheral devices with 0.9% sodium chloride solution only. The volume of the flush should be equal to two times the volume capacity of the catheter plus any add-on devices that are attached to the system.

An occluded or partially occluded catheter should never be forcibly flushed to restore patency because of the potential risk of embolizing the contents into the patient's circulation. The size of the syringe must be considered, because the smaller the syringe, the greater the pressure exerted on the catheter. Excessive pressure may cause the catheter or the vessel to rupture.

Compatibility flushing is accomplished by using 0.9% sodium chloride solution before and after medication administration. Flushing the catheter should prevent incompatible medications and solutions from forming precipitates that can occlude the device. When heparin is used to complete the flushing procedure, *SASH* criteria are used, as outlined in Chart 16–2 (AlternaCare Infusion Therapy, 2010).

Documentation

Accurate documentation in the patient's health record objectively describes the care rendered and the patient's response. It also allows for tracking patient outcomes and monitoring care. Chart 16–3 lists the pertinent information that should be documented when an infusion therapy-related procedure has been performed.

CHART 16–2 Intermittent VAD Flushing: The SASH Criteria

Saline
Administer medication/solution
Saline
Heparin (if necessary)

Source: AlternaCare. (2010). SASH technique. Infusion Pharmacy.

CHART 16–3 Documentation for Insertion and Removal of VADs

- Use of anesthetics for preprocedure medications
- Size, length, and type of catheter
- Location of insertion site
- Securement method and dressing
- Administration set, extension equipment, and access caps used
- Flush or infusate initiation
- Variations in the procedure such as patient sensitivity or allergy to preparatory agents, latex, or securement adhesives
- Patient's response to the procedure
- Name and title of the nurse

Similar documentation should occur when a VAD is removed including:

- Patient consent and education
- Size, length, and type of catheter, as well as its condition (e.g., whether the catheter was intact or fractured upon removal)
- Condition of the venipuncture site (evidence of erythema, drainage, bleeding, skin tears)
- Dressing materials applied
- Patient's response to the procedure
- Name and title of the nurse

Complications Associated with Infusion Therapy

Because of the invasive nature of infusion therapy, there is a risk for the development of complications that range from minor to severe. Complications increase hospital length of stay, length of therapy, cost of treatment, and can put the patient at risk for other medical problems. Most infusion-related complications are preventable, knowledge and understanding of the risks involved with infusion therapy and the use of measures to prevent their occurrence can eliminate many of the problems associated with this treatment (Nursing Made Incredibly Easy!, 2008).

Complications associated with infusion therapy are classified by their location. Local complications are generally seen at the site of venipuncture, whereas systemic complications are defined as those that occur within the vascular system distant from the venipuncture site. Although systemic complications are less common than local complications, they are often more difficult to treat. Timely recognition and nursing intervention can often prevent these complications from escalating into more serious occurrences.

Local Complications

Local complications are usually associated with traumatic injury to the vasculature and/or mechanical failure of the infusion system. Trauma to the vasculature may occur with unskilled venipuncture techniques, patient agitation, and noncompliance with infusion therapy. The injured vein will become edematous as a result, which can lead to interruption in the infusion prescription, tissue injury, phlebitis, thrombus formation, and possibly sepsis.

Mechanical Complications

Mechanical complications usually are the result of the infusion administration system's failure to deliver the prescribed therapy, as opposed to the venous access. They are typically the easiest complications to identify and correct. Areas to be evaluated in determining the causal factors include the patient and the cannulated extremity, the venipuncture site, the catheter, the administration set, and the infusate container and its contents.

The patient's extremity should be checked for constricting clothing, identification bands or bracelets, jewelry, tapes, physical positioning, and restraints. The catheter–skin junction at the venipuncture site and the immediate surrounding area should be assessed for swelling that can impede flow. Verification of catheter placement should be confirmed before initiation and periodically throughout the infusion period. A catheter that is inserted so that the tip is against a valve or venous bifurcation may impede the infusion by slowing or stopping the flow. The catheter may also become dislodged, bent, or kinked as a result of patient activity or inadequate device securement.

Placement of a catheter in an area of flexion may adversely affect the device's infusion rate and dwell time. If the flow rate slows or increases, the catheter can be stabilized by applying an arm board in accordance with the organization's policies.

Administration sets can easily be pinched, bent, kinked, or crimped. This will affect the infusion pathway and prohibit delivery of fluid from the infusion container to the patient. In-line filters or add-on equipment may become clogged owing to undissolved medications or precipitate formation from the introduction of incompatible medications into the administration system.

The infusate container and its contents need to be assessed as a contributing factor of mechanical failure. Inadequate height of the fluid container in relation to the patient and catheter insertion site can adversely affect gravity flow; an empty container can lead to diminished flow or cessation of flow. Rigid containers, such as those made from glass, should be checked for the presence of a venting mechanism. Soft, flexible plastic containers do not need to be vented. The entry port on a container must be completely penetrated in order for the solution to infuse into the patient. Refrigerated solutions need to be brought to room temperature prior to administration. Cold infusates not only cause discomfort for the patient but also may cause venospasm, resulting in vasoconstriction and decrease or cessation of flow.

Catheter-Related Complications

Complications related specifically to the vascular access device versus those related to the infusion system and infusate are readily identifiable. Addressing catheter-related complications should begin with the evaluation of the inserter's skill and technique.

Bruising

Bruising (skin discoloration due to infiltration of blood into the subcutaneous tissue) may be attributed to unskilled insertion technique, tourniquet placement (too tight), vigorous device securement and restraining techniques, or preexisting poor skin integrity. For example, patients who are prescribed long-term steroid or anticoagulant therapies are more susceptible to bruising.

Bruising may be particularly notable after multiple attempts at device insertion during a prescribed therapy period. These injuries adversely affect future visualization of intended venipuncture sites. Bruising may predispose the patient to development of cellulitis and other localized infections. The term *ecchymosis* is used to define generalized bleeding into the tissues, whereas *hematoma* describes uncontrolled bleeding at the venipuncture site that usually creates a hard painful lump.

Infiltration

Infiltration, as was mentioned earlier, is the inadvertent administration of nonvesicant solutions or medications into surrounding tissues. It is manifested by swelling either along the venous pathway or generally located around the venipuncture site (Figure 16–13◆). The patient may complain of "heaviness" or coldness in the extremity or may exhibit generalized swelling. The patient may realize that she cannot remove a ring or other piece of jewelry or cannot close her hand. The extremity will appear enlarged with the skin appearing stretched or shiny. The venipuncture site dressing may appear taut.

The amount of discomfort experienced by the patient is proportional to the type of infusate, rate of infusion, and infusion history. Isotonic solutions generally do not produce much discomfort when an infiltration occurs. Solutions with acidic or alkaline pH or those that are slightly more hypertonic are more irritating and usually cause discomfort (Rosenthal, 2007). If left undetected, infiltration may cause compression of pressure-sensitive tissues such as neurological and arterial structures.

A complete assessment of the patient, the venipuncture site and surrounding area, the involved extremity, and the infusion system may be necessary to determine whether an infiltration is present. The site around the tip of the catheter and the extremity should be inspected for swelling, blanching, stretched skin, firm tissues, and coolness. It may be helpful to compare the site with the same area on the opposite extremity. If both extremities appear edematous, the patient's medical status should be evaluated.

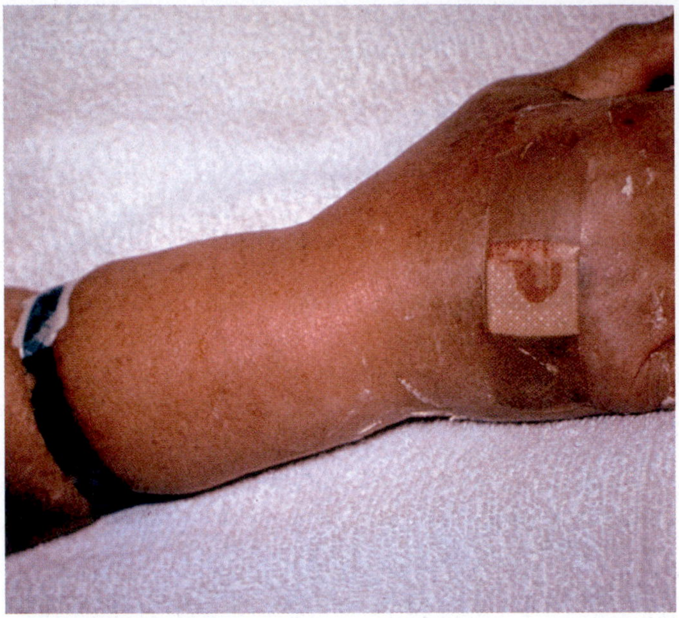

FIGURE 16–13 ◆ Infiltration.
Source: Johnson & Johnson

In determining the presence of an infiltration, pressure should be applied to the vein with a finger or tourniquet about 5 cm (2 in.) proximal to the insertion site. If the catheter is in the vein, manual pressure will slow or stop the infusion. If the infusion continues despite venous obstruction, an infiltration has occurred.

If infiltration is noted or suspected, the nurse needs to discontinue the infusion immediately and remove the catheter. Elevation of the affected extremity relieves patient discomfort and assists in absorption of excess fluids, leading to improved circulation.

Preventive measures can minimize the severity of the infiltration. When a VAD is being inserted, areas of flexion should be avoided if possible. The catheter should be secured adequately, and the site protected from excessive movement or pressure by use of an arm board.

Safety Alert *Be aware that despite the presence of a positive blood aspirate, an infiltration may have occurred. Remove the VAD immediately and restart it, preferably in the opposite extremity.*

Extravasation

Extravasation is the inadvertent administration of a solution or medication into the surrounding tissues. The solution produces tissue damage by causing blister-like formations with subsequent tissue sloughing. Initially, the patient may complain of pain or burning along the vein pathway or at the venipuncture site. Fluid can also seep into adjacent tissues as it passes through a previous proximal venipuncture site.

If the extravasated infusate was a vesicant, tissue sloughing may take several weeks to occur as the extravasation progresses from edema and erythema to necrosis. Necrosis not only may involve superficial skin layers but also may penetrate into basement supporting tissues, muscles, tendons, and bones. The severity of the injury is related to the type, concentration, and volume of the medication or solution infiltrated. This is an adverse condition that could result in loss of the extremity, prolonged hospitalization, protracted treatments involving surgery and rehabilitation, and potentially loss of life.

When an extravasation is suspected, the nurse should discontinue the infusion immediately and remove the catheter. The nurse then initiates treatment protocols established in written policies and procedures and establishes a new site, preferably in the opposite extremity or in a site above and away from the extravasated site.

Prevention is the key in minimizing extravasation episodes. Only qualified, skilled nurses who have demonstrated proficiency and knowledge in infusion therapy along with knowledge of medications that have the potential for causing injury should be allowed to administer vesicant medications. The venipuncture site must be observed for signs of pending extravasation prior to, during, and after the infusion treatment. Many organizations require that a new VAD be placed before the administration of vesicants to avoid questionable patency issues.

If a vesicant medication is delivered directly into a vein via a syringe, the nurse should ascertain the patency of the catheter throughout the infusion. The catheter should be appropriately secured so as to prevent movement in the vein, while simultaneously allowing for frequent visualization of the site and venous pathway throughout the administration procedure. Areas of flexion, bony prominences, and the hands should be avoided as access sites for vesicant therapies. Consideration should be given to the possibility of using a CVAD for vesicant therapies given the chronicity of many antimicrobial, inotropic, or antineoplastic therapies.

Phlebitis

Phlebitis is defined as an inflammation of the vein's tunica intima. It is a common catheter-related complication that is often associated with erythema along the venous pathway, discomfort and tenderness of varying intensities, and inflammation and warmth at the site. Causes of phlebitis include: inappropriate catheter length, gauge, or material; poor insertion technique, often caused by the nurse's inexperience; inappropriate site selection; prolonged dwell time for the catheter; infective device securement; chemical properties of the infusate(s); and the patient's age, infusion history, compliance, existing disease, or conditions.

Phlebitis can be classified by causative factors: chemical, mechanical, bacterial, and post-infusion phlebitis.

Chemical phlebitis is often associated with infusates with varying ranges of pH values or osmolarities. Improper admixing or dilution of some medications can result in incompatibilities that may cause irritation. Infusion rates also may cause irritation. For example, rapid fluid delivery can cause a higher concentration of medication within a localized area, resulting in poor or inadequate hemodilution, leading to inflammation. Particulate matter has been demonstrated to cause irritation of the vein wall.

Mechanical phlebitis is primarily associated with the catheter, its insertion, and the selected site. Using areas of flexion and too large a gauge size for the intended vein and prescribed therapy can result in the development of mechanical phlebitis. Poor device securement allows telescoping of the catheter within the vein. Patient noncompliance insofar as unrestricted physical activity will increase the risk of the development of phlebitis. In addition, the nurse's skill inserting the device may affect whether mechanical phlebitis develops.

Bacterial phlebitis is associated with infectious processes. It is a very serious condition because it may progress to a systemic infection that is potentially life threatening. Hand hygiene and the observance of aseptic techniques throughout the catheter insertion procedure are mandatory for the prevention of catheter- and infusion-related infections. All infusion-related equipment must be inspected prior to use to confirm product integrity and detect any presence of contaminants. Expiration dates, damaged packaging, particulate matter, and the presence of color or cloudiness are signs that may indicate compromised products. Appropriate site preparation reduces the opportunity for catheter-related infections. Shaving the intended venipuncture site is *not* recommended because of the potential to cause microabrasions that would allow for the entry of microorganisms into the circulation. If hair removal is necessary, the hair should be clipped.

Postinfusion phlebitis is commonly seen 2 to 4 days after the catheter has been removed. Occurrence is often attributed to the original insertion technique, patient condition, condition of the vein that was cannulated, the properties of the infusate that was delivered, size and length of the catheter, and the dwell time of the device. There are grades of phlebitis related to the severity. It can be a minimal erythema at the infusion site with or without pain, or as severe as being able to palpate the venous cord and/or show evidence of purulent drainage (INS, 2011).

The most effective treatment for phlebitis is prevention. Venipuncture sites should be assessed frequently. At the first signs of phlebitis, the nurse should remove and relocate the catheter. The venous pathway should be gently palpated at the tip of the catheter to ascertain tenderness while observing for warmth, edema, and induration. If an infection is suspected, the nurse should remove the catheter and obtain a health care provider's order to culture the catheter tip. The nurse also establishes a new venipuncture site, preferably in the opposite extremity. The nurse should document the degree of phlebitis in the patient's medical record and monitor the site frequently at specified intervals.

Thrombosis

Thrombosis is the formation of a blood clot within the vein. It is caused by an injury to the cells lining the vein, usually occurring at the junction where the catheter comes into contact with the tunica intima of the blood vessel. The causes of thrombus formation are similar to those of phlebitis, and include: poor insertion technique; multiple attempts at venipuncture; inappropriate catheter gauge and length for the patient and/or prescribed therapy; inadequate circulation; administration of incompatible medications and solutions, or those with extreme variations in pH and osmolarity; and the nature of the catheter material.

Thrombophlebitis is the combination of thrombus formation in association with inflammation of the vein. The inflammation may be first detected along the venous pathway, followed by edema, pain, and warmth. The vein will become markedly hardened as the thrombosis progresses.

The patient should be assessed for causative factors that may lead to the development of thrombosis and thrombophlebitis. Slowing or cessation of the infusion may be the first sign that complications are developing. Mechanical problems should be eliminated. If the infusion is being administered via an EID, occlusion alarms may offer an important clue. Patient complaints of discomfort and generalized swelling in the involved extremity are important clinical indications of this pending complication.

The degree of circulatory involvement should be monitored because deprivation of blood flow could seriously affect the functional use of the extremity. Thrombus formation has also been a precursor to systemic infections and embolic events. If thrombosis or thrombophlebitis is detected, the nurse should remove the catheter and establish a new venipuncture site in the opposite extremity, if possible.

To prevent these complications, the nurse needs skilled insertion techniques. Cannulation of veins in the lower extremities should be avoided, particularly in adults, because these veins are very small and allow pooling of blood with subsequent damage to the vein intima and clot formation. Appropriate catheter selection, avoidance of insertions over bony prominences and points of flexion, and proper catheter securement are nursing interventions that have proven to be effective preventive measures against thrombus formation.

Infection

Infection is considered a localized event when it occurs at the insertion site. Evidence of phlebitis may not be apparent. Typical signs of infection such as erythema, tenderness, and drainage will be detected at the catheter–skin junction. This type of infection is usually caused by a faulty insertion technique, such as nonadherence to aseptic technique during catheter insertion, site care, or device removal. The use of contaminated equipment, improper hand hygiene, or patient manipulation may also contribute to the development of an infection. There are instances when infection becomes apparent only after catheter removal.

If an infection is suspected, the nurse should remove the catheter immediately, apply a sterile dressing, obtain a health care provider's order to culture the catheter, and establish a new site. Antimicrobial infusions may be required, and surgical intervention may be necessary to treat the infection.

Occlusion

Occlusions are caused by thrombus formation, drug precipitates, or lipid deposits. Slowing or cessation of the flow from the solution container and an inability to flush the device are signs of occlusion. Catheters will become occluded if infusion containers are allowed to run dry or when incorrect flushing techniques are used. The administration of incompatible infusates may contribute to the development of occlusions.

When attempting to restore catheter patency, the nurse should never forcibly flush the catheter because catheter fracture or embolization of the catheter contents can occur. The occluded catheter must be removed, and another site must be located for continuation of the prescribed therapy. Containers of solution should be replaced when the contents are nearly empty, to avoid running dry. Frequent monitoring of the entire infusion system must occur at specified intervals. The nurse must establish compatibility of prescribed infusates prior to initiation and follow policies and procedures for flushing intermittent infusion devices.

Systemic Complications

Systemic complications are complications that occur in the circulation and have the potential to affect the entire body. Although these complications can occur in patients receiving peripheral infusion therapy, they are more frequently seen in those receiving therapies through a CVAD.

Air Embolism

The symptoms of an air embolism, which is caused by entry of air into the vascular system, include chest pain, shortness of breath, shoulder or low back pain, anxiety, cyanosis, hypotension, weak rapid pulse, and loss of consciousness. If an air embolism is left untreated, shock or cardiac arrest may result.

If the nurse suspects an air embolism, the nurse must identify the source of air intake and corrects the problem immediately. If the air embolism results from an open or leaking administration system, the nurse should change the administration set immediately and replace it with a new one flushed with solution. Measures need to be incorporated to prevent the occurrence of an air embolism. For example, administration sets should be clamped when they are being changed. Solution containers should be changed before they are completely empty. Luer-Lok connections should be used to prevent the accidental disconnection of infusion systems. Infusion systems need to be purged of air prior to the initiation of an infusion. Infusions using EIDs with "air-in-line" alarm systems should be used.

Safety Alert *Accidental disconnection of the administration set can lead to an air embolism. The nurse must be able to recognize symptoms of an air embolism and be prepared to administer resuscitative measures.*

Catheter Embolism

A **catheter embolism** occurs when a piece of catheter is fractured and enters the circulatory system. The catheter may block a major vein, causing loss of circulation, or may travel to the heart, causing cardiac irritability and cardiac arrest. Catheter fracture is commonly associated with poor insertion technique such as retracting a catheter back through an introducer, partially withdrawing a stylet from a catheter and then reinserting and advancing the now-torn catheter, or forcibly flushing an occluded catheter.

Signs that a peripheral catheter has broken are separation of the catheter and hub or a severed catheter on withdrawal from the venipuncture site. A rupture of a CVAD may not be noted until the device is used and the patient is symptomatic. If a catheter embolism is suspected, the nurse should observe the patient for signs of cyanosis, chest pain, hypotension, increased central venous pressure, tachycardia, fainting, and loss of consciousness.

For a peripheral catheter that has embolized, immediate interventions need to be initiated. The nurse secures a tourniquet on the patient's arm proximal to the venipuncture site and places the patient on bed rest to minimize the catheter's movement within the vascular system. If a central venous catheter embolism is suspected, the nurse places the patient on bed rest, notifies the health care provider, and monitors the patient for signs of shock. Radiographic studies will be ordered to detect the location of the catheter fragment. The extent of medical intervention will depend on the catheter location.

Pulmonary Edema

Pulmonary edema is caused by the presence of excess fluid volume in the circulatory system. If the condition persists, the patient can develop heart failure, shock, and cardiac arrest. This condition is frequently caused by too rapid infusion rates or too much volume infused within a given time period. The patients who are prone to developing pulmonary edema are pediatric and older patients and those patients with cardiac and renal disease. Pulmonary edema is discussed in detail in Chapter 28.

Before initiating infusion therapy, the nurse should assess the patient's cardiac and respiratory history, ability to tolerate fluid volume, and any previous problems associated with fluid volume while receiving infusion therapy. Patients receiving infusion therapy must be carefully monitored for tolerance of the amounts of fluids being administered. The nurse should maintain infusion rates as ordered and not increase rates for solutions that are behind schedule. The nurse should use volumetric devices and infusion controllers when accurate measurements are required or when the patient's condition warrants management to prevent fluid overload.

Septicemia

Septicemia is caused when pathogenic bacteria enter the bloodstream. Contributing factors placing the patient at risk for septicemia can lead to increases in the patient's susceptibility to infection and may allow microorganisms to enter the infusion system. Risk factors associated with septicemia are outlined in the Risk Factors box.

RISK FACTORS for the Development of Septicemia

- Patient susceptibility
- Alteration in host defenses
- Presence of other infectious processes
- Contaminated infusion equipment
- Inexperience of the nurse inserting the VAD
- Inadequate site preparation
- Dwell time of the device
- Manipulations of the administration delivery system
- Lack of hand hygiene or improper hand hygiene

Early symptoms of septicemia must be evaluated for possible causes. Fever in a patient with a CVAD should be attributed to the device until proven otherwise. Erythema at the insertion site could indicate an infectious process that could lead to sepsis. The health care provider should be notified and cultures of the catheter and the patient's blood may be ordered.

The most effective treatment for septicemia is prevention. Appropriate hand hygiene and strict adherence to aseptic technique should be used in initiating or manipulating an infusion system. All solutions and equipment should be inspected for intact packaging and product integrity. Venipuncture sites should be disinfected with approved antimicrobial agents. Catheter sites are to be rotated, dressings and administration sets changed, and sites monitored according to the *Infusion Nursing Standards of Practice* (INS, 2011) and organizational policy.

Allergic Reactions

An allergic reaction is a response to a medication or solution to which the patient is sensitive. The most common reactions are those seen as a result of administering antimicrobial, biologic, and blood products. The patient may experience chills, fever, urticaria, erythema, itching, shortness of breath, or wheezing. Patients should be assessed for a complete allergy history. Use of identification bracelets and special identifying labels on the patient's medical record serve to inform all health care providers about patient allergies.

If an allergic reaction is suspected, the infusion should be stopped immediately, the administration set and solution container should be changed, and vascular access should be maintained to allow for emergent treatment for possible anaphylactic shock. The health care provider should be notified, and the nurse should be prepared to administer resuscitative measures.

Needlestick Complications

Sharps-related injuries take place at an alarming rate. Estimates suggest more than 800,000 needlesticks occur annually among more than 5.6 million health care workers. Unfortunately, it is also estimated that at least one-half of these injuries go unreported. Additionally, of those injured, more than 1,000 reportedly contract a serious infection from the injury (Perry, Gomaa, & Jagger, 2009). Data collection for statistical information concentrates on four categories for risk of injury: injection devices, blood-drawing and vascular access devices, glass containers, and surgical instruments. Nurses report the most percutaneous injuries at 43.6% (Perry et al., 2009). The International Healthcare Worker Safety Center at the University of Virginia Health

System provides extensive resources on sharps safety and occupational exposure prevention: tools for conducting exposure surveillance, a list of safety-engineered sharps devices, and statistics (http://healthsystem.virginia.edu/internet/epinet).

The Needlestick Safety and Prevention Act of 2001 was introduced as a response to two issues: increased concern over inadvertent or accidental needlestick injuries in health care settings and advancements in technology to prevent health care professionals, patients, and caregivers from sharps-related injuries. The importance of using safety-engineered technologies in an effort to deliver safe infusion therapies is not diminished with the implementation of the act, because it also requires employers currently covered by the *Bloodborne Pathogens Standards* (2011) to continually evaluate and use devices that reduce the risk of injuries.

Needleless Infusion Systems

Needlestick injuries can occur as a result of unsafe products or improper use of a product. Factors that contribute to exposure to body fluids include equipment without adequate safety features, failure to observe standard precautions, and actively engaging in hazardous activities such as recapping needles. Needled syringes, winged steel infusion sets, vacuum blood collection tubes, and vascular access devices are often associated with high rates of injury (Tortorice, 2007).

Improper disposal of needles or other sharps puts many employees, patients, and visitors at risk. Used sharps should never be temporarily placed on food service trays or stuck into bed linens prior to disposal; those procedures greatly increase the risk of injury to others. Needles and syringes should be disposed of immediately after use. Drawing blood poses special risks to health care workers due to the heightened possibility of a "needlestick."

Other procedures can also pose a risk of exposure to blood or injury. Glass-based tubes may crack and break during phlebotomy procedures or during transport. Administration of infusates and medications presents special risks when piggybacking into primary infusion systems or when connecting to intermittent infusion devices. Injuries may occur when equipment is not properly attached and must be forced apart or when unfamiliar equipment is not used appropriately. Nurses who are not skilled at certain tasks, such as inserting infusion catheters or performing that type of procedure on specific patient populations, such as confused, combative, or older patients, are more susceptible to injury.

In response to these issues, manufacturers have devised engineered controls for sharps injury protection. Engineered safety products have demonstrated a reduction in needlestick injuries and subsequent exposure to bloodborne pathogens. Needleless systems are examples of engineering controls. A **needleless system** is a device that does not use needles for the collection of body fluids or withdrawal of such fluids after initial access has been established, for the administration of medications or fluids, or for any other procedure involving the potential for occupational exposure to pathogens due to percutaneous injuries from contaminated sharps.

The Food and Drug Administration (FDA) has approved more than 200 needleless products. Using prefilled syringes and other commercially prepared solutions and medications minimizes the occurrence of injuries during preparation. Needleless systems using vial adapters can prevent percutaneous injury. Vacuum tubes for laboratory analysis are now available in glass-free materials. Sharps disposal containers should be placed at eye level near the patient's bedside. They should also be emptied according to manufacturer's instructions, specifically when the container is three-quarters full.

Nursing Management

Infusion therapy is prescribed to deliver many types of solutions and medications to patients in all care settings via vascular and nonvascular routes. The nurse must possess a variety of skills and knowledge in order to safely manage patients receiving infusion therapies. These include the following:

- Knowledge of aseptic technique in order to prevent both local and systemic infections
- Skill in venipuncture
- Knowledge of care and maintenance procedures to preserve vascular access sites and devices
- Knowledge of the impact that solutions and infusion rates have on the body systems, especially in the presence of disease
- Ability to identify and treat catheter-related complications
- Critical thinking skills necessary to troubleshoot equipment problems when they occur
- Knowledge of the impact of medication administration via the intravenous route, including administering more than one medication simultaneously
- Ability to provide emotional support to the patient and family members.

The Nursing Process: Patient Care Plan for Infusion Therapy uses the nursing process to provide a comprehensive plan of care for patients receiving infusion therapy.

Collaborative Management

Members of the health care team involved in fluid infusion therapy include the primary health care provider, the nurse and members of the infusion team, the infection control practitioner, the pharmacist, and the case manager. With an emphasis on clinical care and performance competence, and in order to meet desired patient outcomes, it is essential that this interdisciplinary team communicate openly with one another in developing and evaluating care of the patient and family (IOM [Institute of Medicine], 2010). The team members will collaborate on specific issues such as appropriate VAD selection for the prescribed therapy and home-based infusion services and other indicated support systems as appropriate.

Once the health care provider has discussed the purpose of the treatment and ordered the patient's therapy, the nurse is responsible for the continued assessment of the patient's infusion needs. The nurse educates the patient about the treatment plan and, as the patient's advocate, determines the level of participation the patient can be engaged in. The patient's family or other caregiver also is included in the education process and taught the necessary skills, if needed, to assist the patient with the infusion care.

Others on the health care team who are involved with infusion therapy include infection control practitioners and pharmacists. The infection control specialist monitors sharps injuries, infection rates, and disseminated infection control practices. Pharmacists have knowledge of medication and solution concentrations, as well as compatibility issues. The case manager plays an integral role in the coordination of care for the patient within the care setting. Knowledge of the intricacies of insurance benefits, availability of health care providers and logistics coordination activities falls within the purview of the case manager.

Weblink: Safety-Engineered Sharps Devices and Statistics

NURSING PROCESS: Patient Care Plan for Infusion Therapy

Assessment of Infusion Delivery Status Using Gordon's Functional Health Patterns:

- Health Perception Health Management Pattern
- Cognitive Perceptual Pattern

Subjective Data

Assessment of Potential for Injury Secondary to Placement and Dwell Time of VAD and Disruption of the Infusion Delivery System

Do you know why you are having infusion therapy, and how long you expect to have it?

Have you ever had an intravenous catheter? If so, did you ever experience any problems with it?

Are you right handed or left handed?

Have you ever had a stroke (CVA) or surgery on your arm or chest, such as mastectomy, fracture, vascular surgery, AV fistula, or shunt?

Are you sensitive to tape or any antiseptic agents?

Do you use any ambulatory aids?

Assessment of Knowledge Deficit Related to Infection Control Measures Pertaining to Infusion-Specific Care and Maintenance Practices

Have you ever had an infection related to an earlier infusion?

Have you needed an infusion catheter replaced due to an occlusion or infiltration, infection, or catheter malposition?

Have you ever been assessed for a VAD reserved for long-term therapy such as a PICC or implanted port?

Objective Data

Assessment of Potential for Injury Secondary to Placement and Dwell Time of VAD and Disruption of the Infusion Delivery System

Does the patient have a preference for VAD location?

Does the patient have observable physical limitations or conditions that will impact site selection, site preparation, and dwell time of the VAD?

Assessment of Knowledge Deficit Related to Infection Control Measures Pertaining to Infusion-Specific Care and Maintenance Practices

Is the VAD dressing dry and intact?

Is there presence of erythema, swelling, or drainage along the vascular pathway or at the catheter–skin junction?

Is the patient complaining of discomfort or pain along the vascular pathway or at the catheter–skin junction?

Are the EID alarms going off frequently for "occlusion" or "no flow"?

Is there a lack of blood return?

Outcomes and Evaluation Parameters / Planning and Interventions with *Rationales*

1. NURSING DIAGNOSIS: Deficient Knowledge *related to therapeutic infusion management and maintenance practices* (NANDA-I © 2012)

Outcomes: Patient and/or caregiver will successfully demonstrate VAD care and maintenance practices.

Patient and/or caregiver will be educated in disease process and progression, signs and symptoms of distress, and indicated infusion-specific treatment regimen(s).

Evaluation Parameter: Verbalizes understanding of complications associated with infusion therapy.

Patient/caregiver will be able to:

Explain rationale for VAD placement.

Explain rationale for hand hygiene.

Describe appropriate condition of VAD location (i.e., intact dressing, clean securement device, intact skin integrity).

Describe symptoms of pending complications secondary to VAD dwell (i.e., infiltration, phlebitis, leaking of fluids [bloody drainage, exudates] from catheter–skin junction, pain, and erythema).

Describe signs and symptoms of potential infusion-related complications (i.e., air in the line, occlusion, empty infusion container, retrograde blood flow, nonflow of infusate, alarming of infusion assistive device).

Patient and/or caregiver will be able to identify signs and symptoms of possible catheter-related complications through education processes.

Patient/caregiver will be able to identify and seek emergency assistance as appropriate.

2. NURSING DIAGNOSIS: Infection, Risk for; Injury, *related to inadequate primary defenses, e.g., broken skin; increased exposure to environmental pathogens, and chemical exposure from IV fluids/medications* (NANDA-I © 2012)

Outcomes: The VAD will dwell according to established organizational policies and procedures.

The VAD will be asymptomatic for the length of dwell time.

The patient will achieve intended infusion-related outcomes.

Evaluation Parameters: The patient will be able to verbalize understanding of care and maintenance practices associated with the prescribed infusion therapy and mode of delivery to prevent catheter-related complications.

Patient/caregiver will be able to:

Explain rationale for hand hygiene.

Explain rationale for use of aseptic technique when changing infusion containers and administration sets.

Explain rationale for use of antiseptic agent(s) when preparing injection cap/access port for injection.

Patient and/or caregiver will be able to identify signs and symptoms of possible infusion-related complications through education processes.

Patient/caregiver will be able to identify and seek emergency assistance as appropriate.

Patient and/or caregiver will be able to identify sources for information and nursing support, and will be able to make informed decisions regarding infusion care.

Source: Adapted from Wilkinson, J. M., & Ahearn, N. R. (2009). *Prentice Hall nursing diagnosis handbook* (9th ed.). Upper Saddle River, NJ: Prentice Hall.

BLOOD INFUSION

Blood transfusion is defined as the infusion of blood products for the purpose of restoring circulating volume and increasing oxygen-carrying capacity. The benefit of a blood transfusion is that it reverses the tissue hypoxia caused by clinically significant anemia and/or blood loss. This reversal can be lifesaving.

Blood transfusions are given to approximately 5 million people in the United States annually (Dept. of Health & Human Services, 2007). Approximately 14 million units of blood are collected annually in the United States; of these, 12 million are transfused. About 60% of the U.S. population is eligible to donate blood; however, only 5% do (America's Blood Centers, 2011). As the population ages, the demand for blood products is expected to increase, perhaps exceeding the supply. The practice of transfusion medicine no longer consists only of storing and administering blood; it now also includes the management of blood resources to ensure that the right patients receive transfusions appropriately.

Blood may be administered as either whole blood or blood components. Blood is obtained from a donor, processed, and infused into a recipient. Whole blood contains red blood cells (RBCs), white blood cells (WBCs), and platelets, which are suspended in the plasma. Because patients seldom require all of the components of whole blood, blood component therapy has become the more frequently used method of transfusion. It is more appropriate and economical to separate blood into its component parts and use only the portion that the patient needs for a specific condition or disease. Two advantages of blood component therapy are that (1) blood resources are conserved, because one unit can be used for multiple recipients, and (2) the patient receives only the needed components, thereby decreasing volume overload and reducing side effects and complications.

Blood is fractioned into component parts by either a centrifuge or a cell separator. Each component is then processed and stored appropriately to maximize longevity and cell viability. (See the discussion about blood storage later in the chapter.)

Another type of transfusion is **apheresis,** a technique in which blood is withdrawn from a donor, a portion is separated out, and the remainder is returned to the donor. This is useful when a blood donor has been in a malaria-active area of the world, for example. The RBCs from such a donor cannot be used because they may carry the malaria virus, but the plasma portion of the blood can be used.

Blood Supply Safety

The Center for Biological Evaluation and Research (CBER) of the FDA, regulates the collection of blood and blood components, including manufactured pharmaceuticals derived from blood, such as clotting factors. Additionally, CBER develops and enforces quality standards, inspects blood donation centers, and monitors reports of errors, accidents, and adverse clinical events. This organization also works closely with the federal Public Health Service to identify and respond to potential threats to the blood supply and to develop safety and technical standards to ensure consistent monitoring of the blood supply. Once blood has been received from a donor, it is immediately tested for blood type and infectious diseases. A negative result for the disease testing is required before the blood is used, and each unit is labeled to certify the results.

ABO and Rh Factor Testing

Another element that is just as important as disease testing is accurate determination of **blood type.** Each individual has one of four types of blood: A, B, AB, or O. In a large percentage of the population, two related inherited antigens, A and B, occur on the surface of RBCs and form the basis for the ABO blood typing. Those individuals with A antigen have type A blood (41%), those with B antigen have type B blood (12%), and those with both A and B have type AB blood (3%). If neither A nor B antigens are present, the individual has type O blood (44%). Type O blood does not have the genetic information required to make any antigenic formation (Watson & Hearnshaw, 2010).

Antibodies develop in the serum of people who do not have the corresponding antigen, referred to as anti-A and anti-B. The person with blood type A has B antibodies, someone with type B has A antibodies, someone with type AB has no antibodies, and a person who has type O blood has both antibodies. Therefore, the person with type AB blood can receive any type of blood in an emergency situation and is referred to as the **universal recipient.** A person with the O blood type is considered a **universal donor** in an emergency situation. Chart 16–4 outlines each blood type, its antigens and antibodies, and what type of blood a person with each blood type can safely receive. Even if a person is a universal donor or recipient, unless there is an emergency, blood typing should be done to avoid transfusion reactions. ABO incompatibility may result in a fatal cause of transfusion reaction.

Safety Alert *In emergency hemorrhage situations, O negative blood can be lifesaving. It is referred to as "uncrossmatched blood," which means that the patient will not react to type O blood because there are no antigens or Rh factor. However, the number of units of O negative blood that can be given is still restricted because of the other antibodies in the blood that can be received via the transfusion. The use of uncrossmatched blood places the patient at high risk for transfusion reaction because of these other antibodies.*

The **Rh factor,** also called factor D, is made up of numerous complex antigens. When it is present on the surface of RBCs, the person is Rh positive (Rh^+); if it is not present, the person is Rh negative (Rh^-). Having a positive or negative Rh factor is influenced by race, with African Americans being approximately 95% Rh^+, Native Americans 100% Rh^+, and about 85% of Caucasians Rh^+ (Hall, 2011). An Rh^- person must receive only Rh^- blood to avoid antibody formation from Rh^+ blood. An Rh^+

CHART 16–4 Blood Types, Antigens and Antibodies, and Transfusion Types

Blood Type with Antigen	Antibody Produced	Type for Transfusion
Blood type A Antigen A	Antibody B	Can receive A or O blood
Blood type B Antigen B	Antibody A	Can receive B or O blood
Blood type AB Antigen AB	None	Can receive A, B, or O type blood Universal recipient
Blood type O No antigens	Antibodies A and B	Can receive O type blood only Universal donor

CHART 16–5 Blood Types and Crossmatch and Antigen Testing

Name of Test	Purpose of Test	Test Results
Blood type and crossmatch Mandatory test prior to blood transfusion (exception in extreme medical emergency/ hemorrhage)	Tests for antigens on the patient's RBCs: ABO antigens on RBCs determine blood type. Rh antigen determines negative or positive Rh factor.	Type A Type B Type AB Type O Rh^- Rh^+
Indirect Coombs' test Screening prior to blood transfusion	Tests for antibodies present in the patient's serum. Patient's serum is mixed with donor's RBCs. If the patient has antibodies to a specific antigen on the donor RBCs, an antigen–antibody complex is formed and agglutination (clumping) occurs. Blood is tested for more than 40 antibodies.	Normal results: no agglutination; negative for a specific antibody. Abnormal results: agglutination; positive for a specific antibody.
Direct Coombs' test Usually tested only if a transfusion reaction is suspected	Tests for antibodies on the patient's RBCs (not in the serum). Used to detect antibodies from the donor blood that are coating and destroying the patient's RBCs. Patient blood is mixed with Coombs' serum that contains various components of complement and antibodies to IgG to determine antigen–antibody reaction and agglutination.	Normal results: no agglutination; negative for antibodies. Abnormal results: agglutination; positive for antibodies.

Source: Plapp, F. V. (2008). *Essentials of transfusion medicine.* BookSurge Publishing.

person may receive either Rh^- or Rh^+ blood. The first time an Rh^- person receives Rh^+ blood, there is usually no reaction. However, antibodies will form during the next 2 to 4 weeks, and if the person receives another transfusion of Rh^+ blood, the antibodies will **agglutinate,** or clump, with the Rh antigens of the blood that are being transfused. Agglutination of cells causes obstruction of the capillaries and blockage of blood flow to the organs. Agglutination and antibody testing are done by using the direct Coombs' test (see Chart 16–5).

After the blood is taken from the donor, a series of procedures determines both donor and recipient ABO and Rh types. These procedures are referred to as "type and crossmatch" and are listed in Chart 16–5. Typing the blood determines the ABO and Rh factor, whereas crossmatching determines compatibility between donor and recipient blood. To determine blood compatibility, the donor's blood is mixed with the recipient's and observed for agglutination of the cells. If the cells do not agglutinate and the blood tests negative for diseases, then the blood is compatible and ready to transfuse into the recipient (Watson & Hearnshaw, 2010). The blood is stored in a blood bank until needed.

Disease Testing

The blood also is tested for the diseases outlined in Chart 16–6 before being released for patient use. A blood-screening test using nucleic acid technology (NAT) is able to detect minute amounts of the RNA and DNA of specific viruses in blood. Before NAT testing became available, blood could only be tested for antibodies to the virus. However, there is always a lag time between infection and production of antibodies during which the blood could test negative even though the virus is present. NAT testing markedly reduces this time period, thus making the blood supply safer. NAT testing has been approved by the FDA for hepatitis C, human immunodeficiency virus (HIV), and most recently West Nile virus.

Therapeutic Uses of Blood Products

The major therapeutic uses for blood are to restore circulating volume and to increase oxygen-carrying capacity. This makes blood transfusions useful for replacing blood volume during and after surgery and following trauma in which a person has lost a large amount of blood. Many surgeries could not be performed without blood transfusions.

Additional therapeutic uses for blood products are to replace platelets and other clotting factors, which is lifesaving for people with inherited clotting factor deficiencies such as hemophilia. Platelet replacement also is important for cancer patients receiving radiation and chemotherapy. Cancer treatments can cause bone marrow depression and platelet depletion. Blood also can provide protein and other nutrients in severely undernourished patients. Each unit of blood contains approximately 35 grams of protein in the form of plasma proteins, and further sources of protein are found in the cellular elements.

Cultural Considerations

Some individuals may refuse blood transfusions for cultural or religious reasons, as discussed in the Cultural Considerations box. Many people

CULTURAL CONSIDERATIONS
Related to Refusal of Blood Products

Certain religions ban the use of blood products. For example, Jehovah's Witnesses strictly prohibit receiving blood or agents in which blood is an ingredient in any form. This belief is based on scriptural references and precedents in the history of Christianity (Cutler, 2007). However, Jehovah's Witnesses do accept blood volume expanders and vigorously pursue blood alternative therapies as long as these do not contain any derivative of blood. Likewise, mechanical devices for circulating blood are acceptable as long as they have not been primed with blood.

Other religions' rules vary with regard to blood transfusion. For example, although the Christian Science Church does not forbid its members to use medicine or have surgery, most Christian Scientists do not believe in any type of medical interventions, though they will undergo those mandated by law such as immunizations. Thus, they do not accept or donate blood products. The Jewish religion prohibits the ingestion of blood (e.g., blood sausage, raw meats); however, this belief does not apply to receiving blood products. The following religions are among those that have no restrictions on the use of blood or blood products (New Mexico Donor Services, 2009): Protestant religions, Amish, Baha'i, Catholic, Hindu, Mennonite, Muslim, Seventh-day Adventist, Latter Day Saints, and Unitarian.

CHART 16–6 Transmission of Bloodborne Diseases

Disease	Test	Safety Margin
Hepatitis B	Core antibodies (anti-HBc) and surface antigen (HbsAG) are tested, not the virus itself. Research has just begun on the use of NAT (DNA) testing of blood products that will detect the virus itself.	There is still a window from the time an individual is infected to the time the antibodies are produced. Risk of transmission is 1 in 220,000. There is a 7- to 10-day window.
Hepatitis C	NAT testing for the DNA in the virus. Anti-HCV.	If the blood tests positive, it is sent out for confirmatory testing. If it is confirmed positive, it is not used. Risk of transmission is 1 in 1.6 million. There is a 7- to 10-day window.
HIV-1	NAT testing for the DNA in the virus. If the test comes out positive, the blood is sent for confirmatory testing.	This test reduces the period of time from infection to detecting the presence of antibodies from 12 weeks to 11 days. Risk of transmission is 1 in 1.8 million.
Human T-lymphocyte virus-1 (retrovirus present with leukemia)	Screened with enzyme immunoassays (EIA) for HTLV antibodies. If the test comes out positive, the blood is sent for confirmatory testing.	It is possible to have false positives and false negatives. If the blood tests positive, it is sent out for confirmatory testing. If it is confirmed positive, it is not used.
West Nile virus	NAT testing for the DNA in the virus.	If the blood tests positive, it is not used.
Syphilis	PK 7200 with RPR backup. PK 7200: Tests IgM and IgG antibodies for syphilis (*Treponema pallidum*). Immucor Captive CMV: Also tests for IgM and IgG antibodies. RPR test for reagent antibodies.	It is possible to have false positives and false negatives. If the blood tests positive, it is sent out for confirmatory testing. If it is confirmed positive, it is not used. If the test comes out positive, the blood is sent for confirmatory testing.
Malaria	If a donor has been in a malaria-active area of the world in the last 3 years, blood is not accepted.	The only exception is if an individual has taken prophylactic medication. Plasma apheresis (using the plasma portion of the blood only) is still possible because malaria is carried only on the RBCs.
Creutzfeldt-Jakob disease (mad cow disease)	If an individual has spent an extended period of time in Great Britain and Europe from 1980 to 1996, when there was increased incidence of this disease in those regions, the blood is refused.	If the blood tests positive, it is not used. No further testing is done. Diagnosis is usually made by autopsy, biopsy, or process of elimination.
Cytomegalovirus	PK 7200 and Immucor Captive CMV are performed as backup.	Transmission risk greater for premature newborns and immunocompromised recipients who are CMV negative. Leukocyte reduction helps reduce transmission of virus. CMV-negative blood is frequently specifically ordered.

Source: Plapp, F. V. (2008). *Essentials of transfusion medicine*. BookSurge Publishing; Seeber, P., & Shander, A. (2007). *Basics of blood management*. Massachusetts: Blackwell Publishing.

are frightened of disease transmission and therefore opt instead to replenish their blood supply with blood alternatives, iron supplements, and diet. Although slower, these treatments are effective unless there has been significant blood loss in a short period of time.

Types of Blood Products

Administering blood products has become more complex with the advent of blood component therapy. It is essential for the nurse to know the correct blood type and the specific rationale for administration, as well as any special considerations of a given blood product and patient. Chart 16–7 (p. 398) outlines the various types of blood products and their volume, storage, and uses. Chart 16–8 (p. 400) lists the information needed by the nurse to safely administer blood. In addition, the nurse must follow strict institutional guidelines and protocols to ensure safe administration with the fewest number of side effects. Each product has its own special consideration beginning with simple administration of whole blood.

Whole blood contains the normal constituents of blood. After it has been obtained from a donor, anticoagulants and preservatives are added, and the blood is ready for the recipient. Most of the platelets and WBCs are removed or destroyed during the processing of the blood. **Packed RBCs** have had the plasma portion of the blood removed by a centrifuge process. This is the most common blood product given in the hospital. **Washed RBCs** are indicated when previous transfusion reactions have occurred. The washing process increases the removal of immunoglobulins and proteins that cause reactions. **Frozen RBCs** are coated in glycerol before being frozen; after being thawed, they are washed to remove the glycerol prior to administration.

Leukocyte-reduced RBCs have had most of the WBCs removed as soon as the blood has been taken from the donor (prior

CHART 16–7 Types of Blood Product

Type of Blood Product	Amount	Action	Uses	Storage	Special Considerations
Whole blood	500 mL.	Increases RBCs to carry the oxygen (O_2) to the tissues. Increases plasma to augment intravascular volume as well as protein and clotting factors.	Shock, hemorrhage, low hemoglobin, hematocrit (volume of packed red blood cells found in 100 mL of blood, expressed as a percentage), and circulating volume.	For up to 35 days at 0–10°C. Warm for 20–30 minutes prior to administration.	Monitor for volume overload. Give slowly. Use fresh blood when possible to avoid increased amounts of potassium, ammonia, and cellular debris that accumulate in stored blood.
Packed RBCs	250–300 mL. 80% of plasma removed. Hematocrit 70%.	Increases RBCs, hematocrit. Increases O_2 carrying capacity.	Anemia associated with cancer, liver, and cardiac disease, renal disease, and for moderate blood loss. Useful when volume overload is a risk.	Same as whole blood.	More viscous than whole blood; slows transfusion. Most common blood product given.
Washed RBCs	250–300 mL. 80% of plasma removed. Hematocrit 70%.	Increases RBCs, hematocrit. Increases O_2 carrying capacity.	Same as packed RBCs, except previous transfusion reactions have occurred. Decreased fibrinogen coating.	Same as whole blood.	RBCs washed with sterile isotonic saline before transfusion. More viscous than whole blood; slows transfusion.
Frozen RBCs	250–300 mL. 80% of plasma removed. Hematocrit 70%.	Increases RBCs, hematocrit. Increases O_2 carrying capacity.	Storage of rare blood type or frequent transfusion reactions. Storage for autologous future use.	Frozen up to 3 years at −87°C (−188.6°F). Must be used within 24 hours of thawing. Storage in liquid state after 24 hr results in loss of clotting factors.	Relatively free of WBCs and microemboli. Expensive.
Leukocyte-reduced RBCs	200–325 mL. 80% of plasma removed. Hematocrit 70%.	Increases RBCs, hematocrit. Increases O_2 carrying capacity.	Previous sensitivity to WBC antigens from prior transfusions or pregnancy.	Same as whole blood.	Decreases transfusion reactions.
Fresh frozen plasma	200–250 mL.	Restores plasma volume in shock without increasing RBCs. Increases factors V, VII, VIII, IX, and X.	Bleeding due to liver disease and hemophilia, disseminated intravascular coagulation (DIC), hemorrhage, massive transfusion.	Frozen up to 1 year. Must be used within 24 hours after thawing to prevent deterioration of factors V and VIII.	Effective for rapid volume replacement. Give through a filter. No platelets in FFP.
Platelets	50–70 mL.	Increases platelets and maintains normal blood coagulability. Expected increase of 10,000 mm^3.	Bleeding due to thrombocytopenia (abnormally low amount of platelets) (<10,000 to 20,000 mm^3) and thrombocytopathy (a disorder of the blood coagulating mechanism that results from dysfunction of the platelets). Bone marrow depression and disseminated intravascular coagulation (DIC) (a disorder in which the proteins that control blood clotting become abnormally active, causing small blood clots to form in the blood vessels).	Five days at room temperature depending on type of collection and storage bag.	Can be made packed, washed, or leukocyte reduced. Bag needs to be agitated periodically. Failure to increase platelets after administration could be due to fever, sepsis, splenomegaly, and DIC.

(*continued*)

CHART 16–7 Types of Blood Product, *continued*

Type of Blood Product	Amount	Action	Uses	Storage	Special Considerations
Albumin (5% or 25% solution)	25-mL, 50-mL, and 100-mL bottles.	Increases plasma colloid osmotic pressure. Increases plasma volume.	Hypovolemic shock and chronic liver failure. Hypoalbuminemia. Burns. Pulmonary and peripheral edema and hypoproteinemia.	Up to 5 years. Check expiration date prior to administration.	No preservatives, so each bottle must be used at once. Rapid infusion can cause volume overload. Rate of infusion should not exceed 1 mL/min. Potential capillary leakage in shock due to increased permeability. Often administered with diuretic to prevent fluid overload.
Cryoprecipitate	5–20 mL/unit.	Increases factors VIII and XIII, von Willebrand's factor, and fibrinogen.	Hemophilia, congenital or acquired fibrinogen deficiency, von Willebrand's disease.	Frozen up to 1 year. When thawed, must be used within 6 hours.	Multiple units (8–15) typically given depending on reason for administration.
Factor VIIa	Number of units is stated on each vial.	Initiates coagulation independent of factors VIII and IX.	Acquired hemophilia A or B with inhibitors. Refractory postoperative bleeding conditions.	For intravenous bolus only. Keep at room temperature. Administer within 3 hours after reconstitution; do not freeze or store in syringes.	Effective in achieving rapid hemostasis. Thromboembolic complications may occur.
Factor VIII	Number of units is stated on each vial.	Increases factor VIII in the blood, adding to the total amount of factor VIII until a target amount is reached.	Hemophilia A.	Given either IV push or IV drip.	A factor VIII coagulant level of 30–50% is common end point therapy.
Factor IX	Number of units is stated on each vial.	Increases factor IX in the blood by replacing missing factor IX until the desired target level is reached.	Hemophilia B or Christmas disease, congenital factor VII or X deficiency.	IV push.	Factor IX levels need to be performed at intervals to determine response.

Source: Seeber, P., & Shander, A. (2007). *Basics of blood management.* Massachusetts: Blackwell Publishing.

to storage). The reduction is done before storage because the storage process causes necrosis of the WBCs, creating by-products that can cause serious adverse signs and symptoms for the blood's recipient. WBCs do not contribute to the efficacy of blood transfusions and are generally regarded as contaminants that potentially reduce transfusion safety. Until recently, the use of blood with fewer WBCs was reserved for patients who were considered a high risk for developing problems from the presence of WBCs; this group included immunocompromised individuals who have cancer or acquired immunodeficiency syndrome (AIDS) and transplant patients. Currently, the majority of the blood banks in the United States reduce the WBCs from every unit of blood.

Fresh frozen plasma (FFP) is prepared from whole blood by separating it from the cell portion and freezing it within 4 to 6 hours of taking it from the donor. **Platelets** are prepared from individual units of whole blood by a centrifuge process. Usually 6 to 10 units are given at one time, and the units are usually pooled into one bag for easier administration. **Albumin** is derived from the plasma portion of the blood. It is a commercially prepared product that has no risk of disease transmission and does not require ABO compatibility screening. **Cryoprecipitates** are collected by thawing FFP and collecting the white precipitate that remains (Seeber & Shander, 2007). This precipitate, which is rich in von Willebrand's factor, **factor VIII,** and fibrinogen are given to treat bleeding associated with hemophilia and disorders that cause a depletion of the clotting factors.

Safety Alert *The platelet count must be assessed within 1 hour following all types of platelet transfusions. This is the best way to accurately assess the therapeutic effect.*

Homologous Transfusion

A **homologous transfusion** is one in which blood is collected from a donor for transfusion into other individuals who are in need of blood. The blood may come from volunteers and/or designated donors.

CHART 16–8 Blood Administration Procedure

Equipment
- Y-type blood transfusion tubing (see Figure 16–14◆).
- 250- to 500-mL bag of normal saline (0.9% NaCl).
- Blood product from blood bank.
- Blood administration record for vital sign assessment.
- Nonsterile gloves.
- Alcohol wipes.
- Tape.
- 16- to 20-gauge IV catheter.
- IV pole.

Assessment Parameters
- Size of IV catheter (18 to 20 gauge).
- Health care provider's order for type, amount, and rate of blood administration.
- History of blood transfusion reactions.
- Religious or other personal objections to receiving blood products.
- Compatibility of blood product with recipient blood type.
- Circulatory and respiratory status.
- Vital signs before, during, and after transfusion.
- Presence of rash prior to transfusion.

Special Considerations
- No medications are to be piggybacked into a transfusion.
- The transfusion is never interrupted for medication administration.
- Only 0.9% NaCl is to be infused in the same line as the blood.

Planning for Blood Administration
- Obtain patient transfusion history (previous transfusions, transfusion reactions).
- Ensure the patient understands the need for blood administration and is willing to sign the informed consent. The blood is not given without the consent.
- Check the health care provider's order for type of blood product to be administered.
- Check size and insertion date of the IV catheter:
    - 18- or 20-gauge catheter, depending on the hospital protocol.

Nursing Implementation: Administration Protocol
- Wash hands and assemble appropriate equipment.
- Explain to patient/family the procedure and rationale, as well as length of transfusion, as appropriate. Assess understanding.
- Instruct the patient to report *any* unusual symptoms, such as might occur with a reaction.
- Follow hospital protocol for obtaining blood products from the laboratory.
- Close all three clamps on the Y-type blood tubing with filter and attach the 0.9% NaCl (NS) bag, open the clamp to the NS, and purge the Y-tubing (see Figure 16–4).
- Make sure the filter chamber is completely filled with saline.
- Using aseptic technique, connect tubing to the IV catheter or to the saline lock.
- Check the identification of the blood product with two (2) licensed staff nurses and the patient:
    - Two unique patient identifiers such as name and date of birth or medical record number.
    - Blood product type and unit number.
    - Blood ABO group and Rh factor of both donor blood and patient.
    - Expiration date of blood product (may be given up to midnight on expiration day).
    - Both nurses sign and date blood bank slip that is attached to the blood bag.
- Compare the above patient identification information with the patient's name band.
- Obtain baseline vital signs (TPR, BP) and document them on the chart.
- Prior to handling any blood products, put on nonsterile gloves and use standard precautions.
- Connect the blood bag to the free arm of the Y-tubing (see Figure 16–14) and open the roller clamp on the same arm of the Y.
    - Close the clamp on the NS side of the Y tubing before opening the clamp on the blood side of the Y tubing.
    - Begin infusion of blood product by adjusting the roller clamp closest to the patient's IV site.
    - The nurse must remain with the patient for this 15-minute period and observe the patient for transfusion reactions (Chart 16–9, p. 404). Blood products should be infused very slowly for the first 15 minutes of the transfusion.
    - Vital signs are taken after the first 15 minutes and at the frequency specified by institutional policy.
    - If there are no indications of a transfusion reaction, increase the infusion rate to the prescribed rate or the standard hospital infusion rate.
- Continue observation for transfusion reactions until the blood product has completely infused.
- Terminating the transfusion:
    - Flush the IV tubing with normal saline by closing the blood product roller clamp and opening the saline roller clamp.
    - Follow hospital protocol for discarding the blood product bag and tubing.
    - Flush the IV catheter after discontinuing blood tubing.

Documentation in Patient Record and Blood Administration Record (See Figure 16–15◆, p. 402)
- Date and time the infusion was started and completed.
- Volume of blood product and normal saline infused (intake and output record).
- Blood product and number.
- Signature of the two nurses who checked the blood product.
- Baseline and continuing patient assessment.

Special Equipment Used for Transfusion Therapy
- Blood warmers are used when blood is infused rapidly.
- Infusion pumps are used when blood needs to be given at a very specific rate to prevent fluid overload.

Nursing Evaluation
- Vital signs before, during, and after the transfusion.
- Lung assessment during and after the transfusion.
- Hemoglobin and hematocrit.
- Transfusion reaction.
- Changes in fatigue levels.
- Increased tissue perfusion.
- Clinical manifestations of anemia.

Source: Cheever, K. (2008). *IV therapy demystified: A self-teaching guide.* New York: McGraw-Hill.

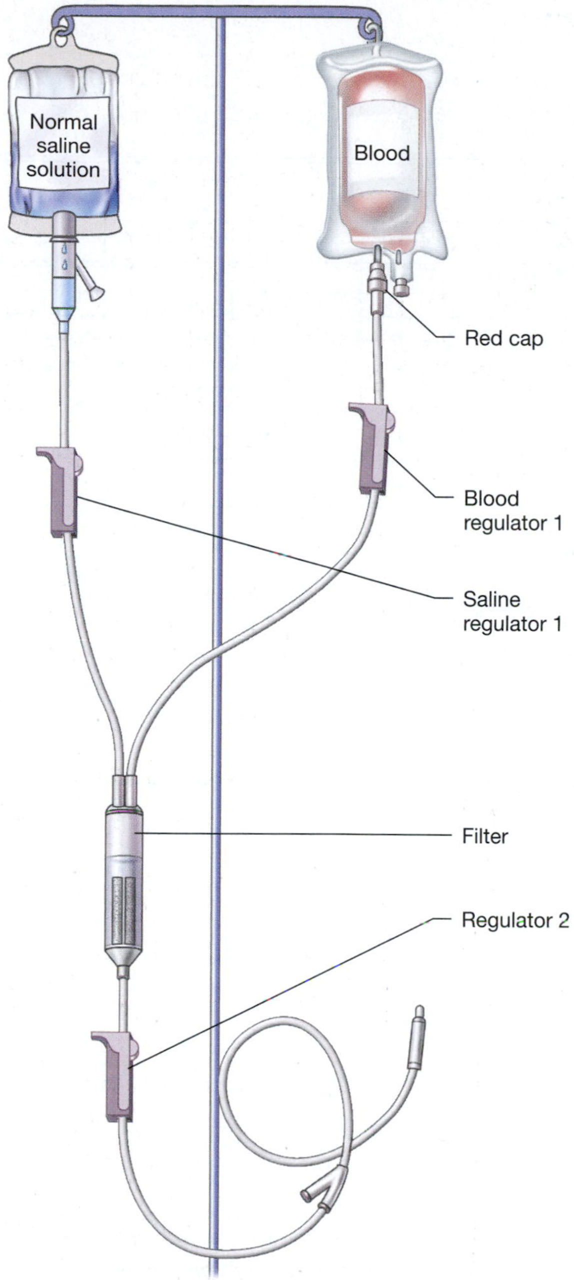

FIGURE 16–14 ◆ Y-type blood tubing.

Volunteer donors visit a blood bank periodically and donate a unit of blood to be used by an unspecified person. This blood is labeled "volunteer donor." Designated donors are individuals chosen by the intended recipient to donate blood. Regardless of which method is used to obtain the blood, it must be ABO and Rh typed and tested for all of the diseases outlined earlier in Chart 16–6 (p. 397).

Designated (Directed) Blood

Designated, or directed, blood is collected from a donor designated by the intended recipient. Compatibility testing is required, and the blood must meet all of the requirements of homologous blood including being free from transfusion-transmitted diseases. This method of blood donation is controversial because a donor whom the recipient knows might not disclose high-risk behaviors.

Autologous Transfusion

Autologous transfusion is the process of collecting and reinfusing the patient's own blood. There are three forms of autologous transfusion: (1) preoperative donation, (2) perioperative blood salvage, and (3) postoperative blood salvage. The advantages to this type of blood replacement are as follows:

- It eliminates infectious disease transmission.
- There is no risk of transfusion reaction.
- It provides a source of blood for individuals with a rare type or antibodies that make it difficult to find compatible donor blood.

Autologous blood products require special handling and labeling under strict guidelines by trained personnel before storage and reinfusion. Therefore, an autologous transfusion is more expensive than blood obtained from a volunteer donor (Seeber & Shander, 2007).

Preoperative Donation

In preoperative donation, the blood is collected from an individual who is preparing for surgery at a later date. This method is useful for healthy patients who are having elective surgery in which the potential need for transfusion is high (e.g., orthopedic surgery). Typically, the blood is collected 1 to 6 weeks prior to surgery and stored for reinfusion. The number of needed units varies depending on the surgical procedure. Individual units of blood components also can be collected and stored for future use. The American Red Cross (ARC) requires that blood collected for autologous use is given only to the donor. If the blood is not used for the surgery, it can be stored up to 10 years for future surgeries. It can never be placed in the general donor supply to be used by someone else.

Criteria for preoperative donation include a minimum hemoglobin of 11 g/dL, hematocrit of 33%, and no presence of infection. Individuals with unstable angina, acute cardiovascular and cerebrovascular disease, and hypertension may not donate. Cancer patients may donate provided that they meet the minimum criteria for donation (p. 387). Before the transfusion, the patient and blood are typed and crossmatched to confirm the ABO and Rh factors, and the patient is tested for diseases (see Chart 16–6, p. 397) to protect the people who will be handling the blood. The blood is processed and stored in designated blood banks until reinfusion.

Most patients take iron supplements (ferrous sulfate 325 mg three times per day or ferrous gluconate 325 mg five times daily) starting 1 week before donation and continuing until surgery. This helps to build up the number of RBCs. Occasionally, erythropoietin (Procrit, Epogen) is given to stimulate erythropoiesis (the process of forming new blood cells [erythrocytes] in the bone marrow) to maintain the required hematocrit. One unit of blood typically is collected each week.

Perioperative Blood Salvage

Perioperative blood salvage is the collection and reinfusion of blood lost during the intraoperative and early postoperative periods. This is a common procedure employed for major surgeries such as cardiovascular bypass, orthopedic, and vascular surgeries; splenectomy; organ transplantation; and trauma when major blood loss has occurred. The blood is collected under sterile conditions and may be reinfused back into the patient with a standard blood filter and gravity. Suction is used to salvage the blood but it does not traumatize the RBCs. The viability of recovered RBCs is comparable to that obtained with homologous transfusions. This salvage process has all the advantages of an autologous transfusion except that the blood has to be reinfused within 12 hours

Weblink: Blood Donation Eligibility Guidelines

Blood Administration Record

PATIENT PROGRESS RECORD

Date	Product	Unit#	Blood	Time		Pre-meds ?		Pre-Infusion				15 minutes				30 minutes				End of Infusion				Bld Wmr ?		S/S Reaction?		Signature
	Type		Type	Beg.	End	Y	N	T	HR	RR	BP	T	HR	RR	BP	T	HR	RR	BP	T	HR	RR	BP	Y	N	Y	N	

RECORD REACTION # IN THE "S/S REACTIONS?" COLUMN

Acute Reactions:
1 = fever
2 = temperature of > 1°C during or immediately following transfusion
3 = chills, mild itching or urticaria, sometimes confluent
4 = pain, sudden onset of dyspnea or complaints of inability to breathe
5 = hypotension
6 = sudden drop of systolic blood pressure 40 mmHg
7 = hemoglobinuria
8 = patient complaining of sense of impending doom (particularly for possible acute hemolytic reaction)
9 = abrupt change in urine color to a deep red/brown color or unexpected, sudden decrease in urine output
10 = unexplained bleeding or unexpected oozing from puncture/incision sites, chest pain, shock, pulminary edema

Delayed Reactions:
11 = unexplained onset of jaundice
12 = unexpected decrease in (or failure to increase) hemoglobin level occurring 5–13 days after transfusion
13 = unexpected elevations in liver function tests
14 = sudden and unexplained appearance of rash or diarrhea occuring 6–10 days

Transfusion Reaction Workup:

1. Send ASAP: 7mL clotted blood, and 10mL urine collected after reaction.
2. Six (6) hours post blood sample is required only for acute hemolytic transfusion reaction (HTR) or requested by Medical Director.
3. Send the remainder of the implicated unit(s) or empty blood bags, attached to administration set, all "Y" tubing with Transfusion Reaction investigation form to the Blood Bank.

FIGURE 16–15 ◆ Sample blood administration record.

after collection. The amount of blood recovered is usually about 50% of what is lost, so it often precludes the need for a transfusion.

Perioperative blood salvage has a number of disadvantages, however, the main one being a considerable loss of coagulation factors and platelets. Because of the risk of spreading infection, blood is not used if an infection is present or if intestinal contents have contaminated the sterile surgical field. Washing and filtering the blood does not eliminate bacteria from the salvaged blood. If malignancy is present, the blood is not used due to the risk of causing the cancer to metastasize to other organs.

Postoperative Blood Salvage

Postoperative blood salvage is used following major surgeries, typically cardiovascular, thoracic, and some orthopedic procedures. Blood is obtained from mediastinal and chest tubes and then reinfused. Even though the blood has been diluted with normal saline, it still has viable RBCs, making it useful for increasing tissue perfusion.

Therapeutic Apheresis

As was mentioned earlier, apheresis, a Greek word meaning to "separate," is a process in which blood is removed from the donor and passed through an automated cell separation device that removes specific components. The remaining blood is then returned to the donor. Apheresis platelets are collected from a single donor rather than multiple donors, and each unit contains 200 to 400 mL. This is equivalent to 6 to 8 units of platelets obtained from separate donors. Donors can have platelets apheresed about 24 times per year (American Red Cross, 2011a).

WBCs can be obtained in a similar manner, typically after the donor has received growth factors (G-CSF, GM-CSF) to stimulate WBC formation. Growth factors also release stem cells into the circulation that can be harvested over a period of several days and used for a peripheral blood stem cell transplant. Another use for apheresis is to remove specific components of the blood to treat certain diseases. For example, WBCs and platelets can be removed by a centrifuge process and the remaining blood given back to the patient. When platelets and WBCs are removed, the temporary reduction in the number of these cells decreases immunity, thus allowing time for chemotherapy to have a therapeutic effect. Finally, removal of plasma is typically done so that specific abnormal proteins can be transiently lowered until long-term therapy is initiated. This process is performed for many reasons, including autoimmune diseases such as Raynaud's phenomenon (Chapter 53), hematologic disorders such as sickle cell anemia (Chapter 56), and some neurological conditions including myasthenia gravis and multiple sclerosis (Chapter 23) (Linker & Gold, 2008).

Risks Associated with Transfusion Therapy

Transfusion therapy is associated with a variety of risk factors that need to be evaluated before the transfusion and monitored during the transfusion to ensure patient safety. Risks of transfusion therapy include disease transmission, bacterial contamination, acute or delayed transfusion reactions, and circulatory overload. Circulatory overload refers to an excess of fluid disrupting homeostasis, often caused by infusion at a rate greater than the patient's system is able to accommodate. Symptoms include dyspnea, cough, tachycardia, hypertension, widened pulse pressure, bounding pulse, and increased respiratory rate. Circulatory overload can lead to acute respiratory distress, congestive heart failure, and renal failure (Transfusion Medicine, 2012). When it is necessary to administer massive transfusions (replacement of greater than one blood volume in 24 hours), the risks include hypothermia, hemodilution, and platelet dysfunction (Seeber & Shander, 2007). Finally, there is a somewhat rare risk for the development of a pulmonary reaction to blood administration, referred to as *transfusion-related acute lung injury*, which is discussed in a later section. When the nurse is informing the recipient about the reason for the transfusion, it is important to explain the risks, the benefits, and what to expect during and after the transfusion. Patients must understand that the blood supply is not completely risk free. Each of the risks of transfusion therapy is discussed next. The nurse must be aware of how blood transfusions can affect older adults, as discussed in the Gerontological Considerations section.

Disease Transmission

The Food and Drug Administration (FDA) (2010b) states that the blood supply in the United States is not without risk of transmitting infectious disease, although the blood supply is safer than ever before. Currently, tests for the nine diseases outlined earlier in Chart 16–6 (p. 397) are conducted on each unit of blood (American Association of Blood Banks [AABB], 2012). It is a nursing responsibility to inform the patient that there are still some risks associated with blood transfusion therapy.

Bacterial Contamination

Bacterial contamination of blood products is very rare, but it may occur at any point from procurement to processing and during administration. A unit of contaminated blood product may appear normal, or it may have an abnormal color. The refrigeration process helps to prevent the growth of bacteria in the donated blood because most bacteria cannot survive the cold temperatures. Platelets are stored at room temperature as they do not tolerate refrigeration. When chilled, they are detected and rapidly removed from circulation. Because they are stored at room temperature, they are more susceptible to bacterial growth (Canellini, Waldvogel, Anderegg, & Tissot, 2010). Besides refrigeration, other measures that help prevent bacterial contamination and growth include meticulous care in the handling of blood products and following time guidelines when administering the blood. For example, whole blood and RBCs must be infused within 4 hours from the time of issue from the laboratory (refrigeration) because room temperature promotes bacterial growth.

The clinical manifestations of bacterial contamination might not occur until the transfusion is complete or in some instances several hours later, depending on the virulence of the infecting organism. Fever, chills, and hypotension are common initial symptoms. Endotoxic shock and even death will occur if the infection is left untreated (Seeber & Shander, 2007). Fluid replacement, antibiotics, and vasopressors (for blood pressure) are needed immediately to prevent irreversible shock and death.

Safety Alert *As soon as abnormal clinical manifestations occur when blood is being transfused, the nurse must stop the transfusion, notify the health care provider, and send the blood and tubing to the laboratory for testing and culturing. The nurse might not know the exact reason for the clinical manifestations; however, when they occur, the focus is on patient safety with the goal of preventing complications and, at times, death.*

Transfusion Reactions

With blood administration, there is always the risk of having a transfusion reaction occur. Therefore, it is essential for the nurse to know the signs and symptoms of each type of transfusion reaction and comprehend the importance of immediate treatment in order to prevent potentially fatal complications. During and after the transfusion, it is vital for the nurse to observe the patient for complications of transfusion therapy and know how to carry out the necessary interventions to reverse any reaction, if possible.

Transfusion reactions may be acute or delayed. Acute or immediate reactions can occur as soon as 5 minutes after starting the transfusion; delayed transfusion reactions may occur from 48 hours to 6 months later. There also may be a reaction when a patient receives multiple units of blood products due to preservatives used to store the blood. If possible before administering blood, the nurse should obtain a health history including allergies and reactions to previous transfusions. Patients with allergies potentially have a higher risk of transfusion reaction and need to be observed closely. Patients who have had previous transfusion reactions or have received multiple transfusions frequently are medicated with antipyretics and/or antihistamines prior to the transfusion because of the presence of antibodies. Chart 16–9 outlines the essential information related to transfusion reactions and the associated nursing care requirements. The Safety Alert discusses the essential nursing actions required during an acute transfusion reaction.

Safety Alert *When a transfusion reaction is occurring and it is necessary to stop the transfusion, it is essential for the nurse to keep the intravenous (IV) line patent. It may be needed to administer emergency medication to treat the presenting signs and symptoms. The line will need to be flushed with normal saline and/or the nurse must initiate a continuous infusion of fluid as soon as the blood transfusion is disconnected from the IV site.*

White Blood Cell Reduction

WBCs do not contribute to the efficacy of blood transfusions. They generally are regarded as contaminants that can reduce transfusion safety (American Red Cross, 2011b). As was mentioned earlier, until recently, reducing WBCs was reserved for patients who were considered to be at high risk for developing problems from the presence of WBCs, including immunocompromised patients. Recent advances in leukocyte reduction technology have contributed to the ease and effectiveness of removing leukocytes from blood and blood products, including whole blood and RBCs (Food and Drug Administration [FDA], 2010b). Most blood banks now reduce WBCs for every recipient. WBC reduction reduces the incidence of febrile transfusion reactions (see Chart 16–9) and the transmission of cytomegalovirus (American Red Cross, 2011b). The FDA concluded that adverse effects with leukocyte reduction had no significant adverse effects. All leukocyte-reduced blood products are specifically labeled "leukocyte reduced."

CHART 16–9 Transfusion Reactions

Class	Cause	Clinical Manifestations	Nursing Care
Allergic reaction	Recipient's sensitivity to foreign plasma proteins. Common in patients with allergies.	Itching, hives, flushing, and chills.	Slow the transfusion. Take vital signs. Notify the health care provider. May be necessary to medicate with antipyretic and/or antihistamine. Then resume the transfusion.
Febrile nonhemolytic reaction	Due to leukocyte or thrombocyte incompatibility (donor's WBCs or platelets react with recipient's antibodies). Usually occurs after multiple transfusions. Accounts for 90% of transfusion reactions. Fever begins about 2 hours after the transfusion. WBC-reduced blood helps prevent these reactions.	Increased pulse rate, temperature $> 1°C$, chills, headache, nausea and vomiting, anxiety, flushing, back pain, muscle aches.	Stop transfusion, but maintain IV site. Give antipyretics as prescribed. Take vital signs. Notify health care provider. Obtain urine and blood sample. Send blood bag, normal saline, and IV tubing to the laboratory. Consider using leukocyte-reduced blood.
Delayed hemolytic reaction	May occur up to 14 days after a transfusion when the level of the antibodies has increased to the extent that a reaction occurs.	Fever, anemia, increased bilirubin level, decreased or absent haptoglobin, and jaundice.	Generally not dangerous, but it is important to recognize the reaction because subsequent transfusions may cause a more severe hemolytic reaction. Typically not recognized or treated due to the mild nature of the reaction.
Acute hemolytic reaction	ABO incompatibility of the blood and recipient. May be due to a mistake in labeling by laboratory or blood bank or nursing error. Causes agglutination of cells, which causes obstruction of the capillaries and blockage of blood flow.	Bloody urine and decreased urine output. Petechiae, jaundice, decreased BP, chest tightness, low back pain, nausea, anxiety, and dyspnea. Hypotension, bronchospasm, and vascular collapse may occur. Hemoglobinemia, acute renal failure, shock, cardiac arrest, death. Symptoms typically occur within the first 15 minutes of the transfusion.	Emergent life-threatening situation. Stop transfusion, but maintain IV site and infuse IV colloid solutions to maintain BP. Give diuretics as prescribed to maintain urine flow. Insert urinary catheter to assess output and color. Obtain vital signs. Treat shock. Start CPR if necessary. Give epinephrine. Notify health care provider. Obtain urine and blood sample. Send blood bag, normal saline, and IV tubing to the laboratory.
Hemolytic or anaphylactic reaction	Reaction to donor plasma proteins. Specifically, infusion of IgA proteins to an IgA-deficient recipient who has an IgA antibody.	Wheezing, restlessness, anxiety; is progressing to cyanosis, shock, and possibly cardiac arrest.	Stop infusion, but maintain IV site. Give epinephrine per doctor's order. Initiate CPR if necessary. Notify health care provider. Obtain urine and blood sample. Send blood bag, normal saline, and IV tubing to the laboratory.

Source: Plapp, F. V. (2008). *Essentials of transfusion medicine.* BookSurge Publishing; Seeber, P., & Shander, A. (2007). *Basics of blood management.* Massachusetts: Blackwell Publishing.

Noninfectious Serious Hazards of Transfusion Therapy

According to the American Association of Blood Banks (AABB) (2001), there has been a 10,000-fold reduction in transfusion-transmitted infectious diseases in recent decades, but there has been very little progress in reducing the risk of noninfectious serious hazards from transfusions. As a result, patients are harmed from noninfectious hazards at a rate of 100-fold to an increase of 1,000-fold over a 10-year period (Hendrickson & Hillyer, 2009). The most common noninfectious transfusion-related problems include the following:

- Mistransfusion and ABO/Rh incompatible transfusion
- Cardiopulmonary toxicity/circulatory overload
- Transfusion-related graft versus host disease
- Transfusion-related acute lung injury

- Metabolic derangements in pediatric and massive transfusion
- Undertransfusion.

Mistransfusion and ABO/ Rh Incompatible Transfusion

Transfusion of incompatible blood (see Chart 16–9), known as mistransfusion, is the most common cause of serious morbidity and mortality associated with transfusions (AABB, 2001). Errors may occur at the time of sample collection, within the laboratory, when the blood is issued from the laboratory, or at the bedside. This type of transfusion reaction is typically fatal, and the incidence has not significantly decreased in the last 10 years (Callum, Lin, Lima, & Merkley, 2011; Clark, 2011).

Circulatory Overload

Circulatory overload can occur with transfusions when the blood is infused too rapidly or in too large a quantity, thus causing hypervolemia. The osmotic makeup of the blood causes fluid to be mobilized from the interstitial space, thereby increasing intravascular volume well beyond that given during the transfusion. High-risk patients include older adults and individuals who already have increased circulatory volume or who have a history of heart failure. Clinical manifestations of circulatory overload include dyspnea, tachycardia, distended neck veins, crackles in the lungs, and a rise in blood pressure. If the transfusion is not slowed down or stopped, pulmonary edema will result. A complete description of heart failure and a discussion of the impact of fluid volume are provided in Chapter 34.

If the blood is administered slowly, circulatory overload can usually be prevented. The only time blood is given rapidly is when a patient is hemorrhaging or is severely volume depleted. Packed RBCs are safer than whole blood for high-risk individuals because the plasma portion of the blood has been removed, which decreases the volume of the unit by approximately one-half. To decrease the circulating volume, diuretics are often administered between units or after transfusion to high-risk individuals. If pulmonary edema is present, oxygen, diuretics, morphine, and, in severe cases, mechanical ventilation may be necessary.

Transfusion-Related Graft Versus Host Disease

Graft versus host disease (GVHD) occurs in severely immunocompromised patients when transfused lymphocytes attack host lymphocytes or body tissues. Clinical manifestations include diarrhea, fever, diffuse red skin rash, nausea, vomiting, and hepatitis. The primary prevention measure is administration of leukocyte-reduced blood products. There is no effective therapy or cure for GVHD; therefore, nursing care focuses on managing the signs and symptoms. Mortality resulting from acute GVHD is directly related to severity, with overwhelming sepsis being the primary cause of death in patients with acute GVHD (Silvergleid, 2011).

Transfusion-Related Acute Lung Injury

Transfusion-related acute lung injury (TRALI) is a serious, life-threatening clinical syndrome that is a complication of blood transfusions. In fact, TRALI is the most commonly reported cause of transfusion-related deaths in the United States, surpassing those caused by ABO incompatibility and bacterial contamination (Clark, 2009). Because of the difficulty of specifically identifying the disorder, it is difficult to calculate the incidence. One group of investigators calculated that it occurs in approximately 1 in every 1,000 to 2,400 units of blood (Clark, 2009). No identifiable risk factors have been found.

The exact cause of this complication is not fully understood. One prevailing theory is that TRALI is thought to be caused by the presence of granulocyte antibodies and biologically active lipids in the donor plasma that the recipient reacts to. If antibodies are present in the donor's plasma, they stimulate the WBCs in the recipient's blood. Aggregates of WBCs form and occlude the microvasculature of the lungs (Kor & Gajic, 2010). Whatever the cause, the result is increased pulmonary vascular permeability leading to the clinical manifestations described next. Although all blood products can lead to this serious complication, high-plasma volume components such as FFP or platelets increase the risk 5 to 6 times compared to packed RBCs (Kor & Gajic, 2010).

Clinical manifestations include sudden onset of respiratory distress during or shortly after a transfusion. Hypoxemia, hypotension, severe pulmonary edema, cyanosis, and fever may also occur. Diffuse crackles and decreased breath sounds in the lungs are typically present. In its most severe form, TRALI is indistinguishable from adult respiratory distress syndrome (Chapter 28). It can occur during the transfusion and as late as 6 hours after a plasma-containing transfusion, but it most frequently occurs 1 to 2 hours after the transfusion. The severity of symptoms can range from mild to severe. The symptoms usually last about 96 hours and then begin to resolve. Treatment is supportive and related to the severity of symptoms. Frequently patients need ventilatory support, and diuretics are indicated if pulmonary edema is present (Clark, 2009). Once TRALI has occurred, the recipient should not receive any more transfusions from the same donor. Transfusion from other donors poses no increased risk.

See the Evidence-Based Practice: Transfusion of Blood Products box (p. 406).

Less Common Noninfectious Transfusion-Related Hazards

Other, less common noninfectious hazards of transfusion therapy include iron overload and the side effects of multiple and massive transfusions. Repeated exposure to blood transfusion not only carries an increased risk of the transmission of bloodborne diseases but also can cause iron overload.

Iron Overload

Iron overload, referred to as **hemochromatosis,** may occur in patients who have chronic transfusion requirements. One unit of RBCs contains 250 mg of iron. Patients who receive repeated transfusions acquire more iron than they need, and the excess builds up in the tissues. Over time, these deposits can cause organ damage, particularly to the pancreas, liver, heart, and testes. Laboratory tests conducted to diagnose hemochromatosis are the total iron binding capacity (TIBC), serum iron (SI), and serum ferritin (SF) tests. These values will all be elevated in iron overload.

The treatment goal is to induce a mild anemia and maintain it until the stored iron is greatly reduced. The SF test value is a measure of stored iron, and this number needs to come down to normal range. This is accomplished by bloodletting, that is, therapeutic phlebotomies. **Phlebotomy** is the removal of a full unit of blood from the patient, approximately 500 mL. This should be done in a medical setting. The schedule of this treatment should be twice a week or a minimum of once a week. **Chelation** therapy that is promptly initiated can prevent end-organ damage from iron toxicity.

Weblink: American Association of Blood Banks (AABB).

EVIDENCE-BASED PRACTICE Transfusion of Blood Products

Clinical Problem

Transfusing blood products is beneficial and often lifesaving, especially for critically ill individuals. Blood transfusions are not, however, without risk. Anemia is common among patients admitted to intensive care units (ICUs), and studies indicate that more than 40% of patients receive RBC transfusions while in the ICU (Napolitano, Kurek & Luchette, 2009). Two life-threatening risks are transfusion-related acute lung injury (TRALI) and fluid overload resulting in pulmonary edema. Nurses need to understand and apply evidence-based findings when administering blood in order to mitigate the occurrence of these complications.

Research Findings

Guangxi et al. (2010) conducted a study to assess the long-term survival and quality of life (QOL) of critically ill patients who had experienced TRALI and transfusion-associated circulatory overload (TACO) following blood transfusions. This study was based on continued reports of a high incidence of TRALI and TACO (Toy & Lowell, 2007) and failure of documented evidence of long-term effects on QOL. While prior outcome studies of TACO and TRALI have focused on short-term morbidity and mortality, long-term effects remain unknown (Guangxi et al., 2010). The researchers also were able to build on a prior prospective study of Gajic, Rana, Winters, et al. (2007), which identified those critically ill patients who had developed TRALI or TACO while being cared for in a medical intensive care unit of a tertiary hospital. For this study, TRALI was defined as "a syndrome of inflammation and increased pulmonary capillary permeability of inflammation and increased pulmonary capillary permeability that is associated with a constellation of clinical, radiologic, abnormalities of acute pulmonary edema that cannot be explained by left atrial hypertension" (Guangxi et al., 2010, p. 784).

Using a nested case-control study (a variation of a case-cohort study), the researchers compared the long-term survival and QOL between patients who developed TACO, TRALI, or possible TRALI after transfusion with transfused control patients matched by age ±10 years, sex, and admission diagnostic group. Patients who experienced possible TRALI were included in the study and identified as such. The QOL was assessed with the 36-item short-form health survey (SF-36) at 1 year after hospital discharge. The study subjects, 74 TRALI/possible TRALI and 51 TACO, with respective control groups, were followed for a median 825 days. The 1- and 2-year follow up rates were 98.5% and 97.6%, respectively. Baseline severity of illness was similar between cases and controls.

Results of the study revealed that the development of TRALI was associated with decreased long-term survival, with a statistical significance of $P = 0.006$. Additional poor prognostic indicators included older age, history of liver disease, and higher severity of illness. Compared with matched controls, TACO cases also had a reduced survival, but this difference was not statistically significant. Both TRALI and TACO were associated with prolonged ICU and hospital lengths of stay. QOL scores were lower than the age-adjusted population predictions but were not significantly different between responding survivors who did and did not develop transfusion-associated pulmonary complications.

Implications for Nursing Practice

The impact on nursing practice from the findings of this research is multidimensional and requires critical thinking skills. The nurse must be vigilant about the transfusion infusion rate for a given patient. The patient's age, medical history, current diagnosis, and hemodynamic stability all influence the infusion rate. Except in emergent situations in which acute blood loss affects hemodynamic stability, blood is transfused slowly in order to prevent fluid overload. Monitoring the patient's response to the transfusion also is of critical importance. Vital signs, lung sounds, and oxygen saturation are assessed during and after the transfusion in order to evaluate the patient's tolerance. It is essential for the nurse to report to the health care team any occurrence of abnormal lung sounds and/or a change in the rate and depth of respirations, as well as any decrease in oxygen saturation levels. The nurse needs to understand when ventilatory support is required and facilitate the plan to get it instituted.

The nurse also must be aware of the clinical manifestations of TRALI. Because this complication is often difficult to diagnose and can occur several hours after the transfusion, the nurse must continue ongoing monitoring of the patient subsequent to the transfusion. It is essential for the next shift of nurses to be told that the patient had a transfusion, especially if it was plasma, so that monitoring for side effects will be continued.

Critical Thinking Questions with answers can be found in the Osborn Student Resources at nursing.pearsonhighered.com.

References

Gajic, O., Rana, R., Winters, J. L., et al. (2007). Transfusion-related acute lung injury in the critically ill: Prospective nested case-control study. *American Journal of Respiratory Critical Care Medicine, 175*(9), 886–889.

Guangxi, L., et al. (2010). Long-term survival and quality of life after transfusión-associated pulmonary edema in critically ill medical patients. *Chest, 137*, 783–789. Publisher online October 16, 2009. doi:1378/chest.09-0841

Toy, P., & Lowell, C. (2007). TRALI—definition, mechanisms, incidence, and clinical relevance. *Best Practice & Research Clinical Anesthesiology, 27*(2), 183–193.

Multiple and Massive Transfusion Reactions

A massive transfusion is defined as the replacement by transfusion of more than 50% of a patient's blood volume in 12 to 24 hours. Patients who have repeated exposure to blood products and the preservatives used to store blood products have an increased risk of developing elevated blood ammonia titers, coagulation imbalances, hypocalcemia, acid–base imbalance, and hyperkalemia (Sihler & Napolitano, 2009). The ammonia level increases in stored blood due to decomposition of the blood products. Coagulation imbalance occurs because of dilutional thrombocytopenia and decreased platelets that are destroyed in stored blood. Depending on the age of the blood product, it may have few viable clotting factors; the longer the blood is stored, the more ineffective the clotting factors become. Therefore, an inability to clot normally may result from multiple transfusions. Replacement of clotting factors, plasma, and platelets is typically necessary (Sihler & Napolitano, 2009). The decrease in calcium is due to its binding with the citrate (the preservative), and hyperkalemia occurs when potassium leaks from the stored RBCs. Finally, hypothermia may occur with massive transfusions if refrigerated blood is rapidly transfused. This can be prevented by the use of a blood warming device. It is essential for the nurse to monitor for all of the potential side effects when a patient is receiving repeated transfusions.

Nursing Responsibilities Before, During, and After Transfusions

Nursing care of the patient receiving a blood transfusion requires the nurse to follow strict protocols set forth by the American Association of Blood Banks (AABB), state licensing boards, individual employers, the Infusion Nurses Society (INS), and the American Nurses Association nurse practice act. The nurse is responsible for all aspects of blood transfusion therapy and must continually assess the patient's response to the transfusion. Knowledge specific to blood transfusions includes blood types, blood component therapy, administration equipment, specific techniques for administering each component, and hazards of transfusion therapy. Critical thinking and clinical judgment skills are necessary because the clinical manifestations of a transfusion reaction are not always "textbook." The nurse is responsible for evaluating each situation and being knowledgeable about and able to respond with the appropriate care when problems occur.

Nursing Management

Blood transfusion therapy occurs most frequently in the acute care setting, although under certain circumstances patients will receive blood in other settings. Patients who need chronic transfusions may use freestanding infusion centers, ambulatory care settings, doctors' offices, and even private homes for their transfusions. Nurses must have the skill and knowledge to adapt to any of these settings when performing a blood transfusion. Use of the nursing process provides the template that enables the nurse to perform transfusion therapy in multiple settings.

Patients are required to sign a consent form prior to the transfusion. It is the health care provider's responsibility to explain why the transfusion is needed and what risks are associated with the procedure. The nurse's responsibility includes verifying that the patient understands the health care provider's explanation before signing the consent form. It is essential for the patient to understand that once the transfusion begins, any unusual signs or symptoms must be reported to the nurse.

Assessment

Before beginning a transfusion, the nurse should obtain a transfusion history from the patient. This includes information about previous transfusions, allergies, and any transfusion reaction. Information about the type of transfusion reaction, its manifestations, and treatment also is necessary and must be documented in the patient's record. This will alert the nurse to the patient's risk of transfusion reactions and possibly the need for premedication to prevent an allergic reaction.

The physical assessment includes vital signs prior to beginning the transfusion. This provides a baseline for vital sign assessment during the transfusion. An acute rise in the body temperature may indicate a transfusion reaction; therefore, it is essential to know the baseline temperature. Fluid overload causes changes in both pulse and blood pressure; obtaining baseline vital signs enables the nurse to monitor and assess significant changes. Additionally, lung sounds need a baseline assessment. The development of crackles may indicate fluid overload. Any concurrent health problems relating to cardiac, respiratory, or renal diseases need to be assessed.

Safety Alert *During a transfusion, it is essential for the nurse to assess the patient's vital signs and lung sounds. The heart rate and respiratory rate increase when fluid overload occurs and crackles can be heard in the lungs. Additionally, these patients tend to develop cardiac dysrhythmias. If these changes occur, the nurse should slow the transfusion and notify the health care provider.*

Planning

In addition to reviewing the patient's medical history, the nurse must plan for and prepare the equipment that will be used during blood administration.

Equipment Preparation

A 16- to 20-gauge catheter is required for RBCs to pass through without being damaged. Using a smaller gauge needle also may slow or stop the transfusion. Special Y-type blood tubing with an in-line filter is always used for the administration of blood products. Normal saline (0.9% NaCl) is attached to one of the Y sites and the tubing is primed with normal saline prior to blood administration.

Safety Alert *Only normal saline can be administered with blood. Dextrose solutions cause hemolysis of the cells. Calcium, which is present in lactated Ringer's solutions, can cause coagulation in citrated (preservative) blood. To increase the rate of the transfusion and decrease the viscosity of the blood, normal saline may run simultaneously to help thin the blood product.*

The purpose of an in-line filter is to trap clots and other debris from all blood components older than 5 days. Some institutions require additional in-line filters to be added to the blood tubing. These additional filters have two purposes: One type of filter augments the in-line filter in trapping clots and debris, and the other filter removes leukocytes for patients with a history of febrile reactions.

Other optional equipment used for transfusions includes electronic infusion pumps, pressure cuffs, and blood warmers. Electronic pumps regulate the rate or speed of the transfusion and are used when blood needs to be given very rapidly or very slowly. Special blood tubing can be inserted into infusion pumps, and the rate of administration is dialed into the pump. External cuffs may be applied to the outside of the blood bag and the cuffed bag is inflated, which pushes the blood in and therefore increases the rate of infusion. These bags are contraindicated unless large-bore catheters are used. The bag pressure should never exceed 300 mmHg. Blood warmers are used when rapid infusion of blood products is necessary and there is an increased risk of hypothermia. Cold blood may precipitate cardiac dysrhythmias and cardiac arrest associated with rapid, massive infusion of cold blood products. Blood warmers have a preset maximum temperature of 38°C (100.4°F) so as not to damage the RBCs. Blood should never be submerged under hot water or placed in a microwave oven for warming.

Outcome and Evaluation Parameters

The outcome of blood administration depends on the reason for the transfusion. For example, if blood is being administered because of a low RBC count, then the goal is to normalize the value. If the transfusion is needed because of low platelets resulting in bleeding, the goal is to normalize the platelet count and stop or prevent blood loss. Since blood administration is just part of a treatment plan, it is imperative that the reason for the abnormality be identified and corrected, if possible. Evaluation parameters include a normal RBC count, hemoglobin, hematocrit, platelet count, and clotting factors. Additionally, part of the evaluation would be relief from the clinical manifestations that resulted from the abnormality.

Interventions and Rationales

Once the blood has been taken from the blood bank, administration should begin within 30 minutes. Blood cannot be stored in the refrigerator on the nursing unit because the lack of temperature control may damage the blood. In administering a blood product, it is essential to follow institutional policy. The nurse must ensure positive patient identification, appropriateness of blood component, blood product inspection, verification of donor–recipient compatibility, and verification of the product's expiration date.

Additionally, the nurse must have knowledge of the appropriate rate at which to infuse the blood product. Occasionally, the health care provider will order a specific rate; otherwise, the institution will identify safe rates of infusion of various blood products in their blood administration policy and procedure. For example, a common infusion rate for a unit of whole blood is 4 hours. Chart 16–8 (p. 400) earlier in the chapter outlines the blood administration procedure.

Safety Alert *To protect both the patient and the nurse, strict hospital protocols must be followed when checking blood in order to prevent fatal transfusion reactions. It is the nurse's responsibility to know and follow the hospital protocol when checking blood. The protocols vary from institution to institution; however, most agencies require that two registered nurses (one of whom is the transfusionist) verify the correct unit, patient, blood type, and blood product.*

Weblink: Vein Identification and Structure

Evaluation

During and after the transfusion, the nurse evaluates the patient for response to the transfusion. The nurse must stay with the patient for the first 15 minutes of the transfusion to assess for any clinical manifestations of a transfusion reaction (see Chart 16–9, p. 404). If the patient begins to have clinical manifestations that indicate an abnormal response, the nurse must have knowledge of the appropriate interventions. It is a nursing responsibility to possess the necessary clinical judgment to evaluate a normal versus abnormal response during a blood transfusion. For example, vital signs are monitored at frequencies prescribed by the institution. Both immediate and delayed reactions are manifested by altered vital signs, which indicate an abnormal response to the blood. Additionally, the lungs are monitored during and after the transfusion to assess for signs of fluid overload.

The alteration in tissue perfusion that was occurring prior to the transfusion may be assessed by evaluating the hemoglobin and hematocrit. After administration of one unit of packed RBCs in a nonbleeding adult, the hemoglobin increases by 1 g/dL and the hematocrit by 3 percentage points (Department of Health and Human Services, 2007). The patient should have increased endurance and less fatigue after the transfusion due to the increased oxygen-carrying capacity.

Blood Alternatives

Because of the risks associated with blood transfusion, alternative treatments for replacement of hemoglobin are always being sought. For example, recombinant technology has provided a means to augment the production of blood cells within functioning bone marrow. Referred to as *blood modifier medications,* these drugs are being used in place of transfused blood in certain groups of patients. These medications have the same biologic activity as endogenous human erythropoietin. They induce erythropoiesis by stimulating the division and differentiation of cells in the bone marrow. Indications for their use are the same as those for blood transfusions: anemia associated with blood loss, HIV, cancer, and renal failure. These drugs are being used in place of a blood transfusion because they are a safe and effective way to improve oxygen uptake and therefore tissue perfusion (Cooperman & Allinson, 2011). In cases of massive hemorrhage, blood transfusion is still the treatment of choice due to the acute need for circulating volume and hemoglobin.

A second method used to minimize the use of blood products is recombinant factor VIIa. Clotting occurs with the administration of factor VIIa due to the activation of factor X, which causes additional generation of thrombin, resulting in the conversion of fibrinogen to fibrin. It is useful for a variety of clinical situations including the massive hemorrhage, thrombocytopenia, trauma, liver failure, oral anticoagulant toxicity, hemophilia, and surgical, intracranial, and obstetric hemorrhage (Seeber & Shander, 2007).

Administration of factor VIIa has resulted in cessation of bleeding, reduced blood product use, and an improved coagulation profile.

Gerontological Considerations

The nurse must possess critical thinking and clinical judgment skills in order to assess the patient's physical status and tolerance for all types of fluid replacement, including blood transfusion. The normal aging process causes many changes in the body, both psychological and physiological, and this has important implications for providing nursing care through infusion therapy to older adults. As the aging population grows, it is anticipated that most hospitalized older adults will receive some type of infusion therapy including blood transfusions (CDC, 2011b). It also is likely that the number of patients requiring IV therapy in assisted living or long-term care facilities will increase in tandem with the increase in the older population (CDC, 2011b), again accenting the need for specific nursing skills in administering fluids.

Treating dehydration with IV fluids and treating infections with IV antibiotics are the most common infusion therapies for older patients. Some will require blood transfusions. As individuals age, the nurse should be aware of localized changes in the skin and veins, which may obstruct or limit positive patient outcomes of infusion therapy. The skin loses its turgor, affecting insertion of the needle, and the veins undergo changes in each of its three layers (About.com, 2011). The innermost layer of the vein (tunica intima) is prone to scarring from caustic medications. Plaque from atherosclerosis may damage the semilunar values of this vein layer as well. The middle layer of the vein, the tunica media, is affected by changes in the body's temperatures. Older patients tend to be cold and often have cold skin, causing this layer to constrict, making it difficult to locate a vein. The outer layer of the vein, the tunica adventitia, is composed of supportive elastic tissue and collagen, which decreases with age, making this layer thin and no longer firm or supportive. This process, along with poor dietary intake, can cause veins to easily rupture, resulting in large bruises. Because older patients lack subcutaneous fat and muscle mass, their veins tend to "roll," making venipuncture difficult. Understanding these changes makes vein access and infusion therapies safer for this high-risk patient population.

With older adults, it is important to consider systemic reactions to fluid administration as well as the local considerations enumerated previously. For example, the nurse needs to be cognizant of the need to prevent fluid overload by administering the fluid or blood slowly unless the patient is acutely hemorrhaging or is significantly hypovolemic. The nurse needs to know the patient's medical history in order to be aware of the risk for this development. This is especially true for older patients with a history of heart failure or renal insufficiency or failure who would be more at risk than a young patient with a healthy heart. Frequent monitoring of high-risk patients will typically prevent complications. Often with older patients who have previous heart failure problems, the health care provider orders furosemide (a diuretic) to be given before or after a transfusion. In addition, if the patient is to receive more than one unit, furosemide is often ordered to be given between the two units. The nurse also must be alert to other possible systemic problems with infusions, such as respiratory difficulty and edema. This can be accomplished by monitoring fluid balance and electrolyte balance.

Research

Research within the specialty nursing field of infusion therapy, including blood infusion, is essential in order to advance the practice, but also to identify areas requiring specific data, supporting performance improvement indicators, and identifying concerns and considerations that affect anticipated outcomes and patient safety. Although ongoing assessment is critical for the patient receiving infusion prescriptions, post-therapy assessments and evaluation of indicators must also continue to suggest improved methods of infusion care, including transfusions. The goal of research is to identify areas in which current practice could improve and then evaluate and improve these areas. Advances in technologies affecting infusion care delivery will need to be addressed in all care settings. The Research Opportunities box provides a list of topics in promising areas of research still under investigation. Electronic databases also are a source for finding specific studies related to these topics.

RESEARCH OPPORTUNITIES Related to Infusion Therapy and Blood Infusion

Research Area	Clinical Impact
Infusion Therapy	
Evaluate the process of early patient assessment related to VAD selection.	Timely initiation of therapy Appropriate site and VAD selection to preserve sites and minimize the number of venipunctures Patient education to promote therapy compliance
Determine the efficacy of saline versus heparin flushes of CVADs in the home care patient.	Prevention of VAD occlusion Continuation of therapy without impacting patient's clotting mechanisms
Determine whether a 72- to 96-hour site rotation interval for peripheral-short catheters is appropriate.	Site preservation To minimize number of venipunctures To decrease risks associated with catheter-related complications
Blood Infusion	
Prevention of disease transmission.	To ensure a safe blood supply.
Development of a synthetic product that can be used to raise hemoglobin and replace volume quickly in emergent situations and for persons who refuse blood transfusions.	Would provide a safe method for volume and cell replacement when blood products are not available due to the type and crossmatch process. Will provide a safe, effective blood replacement for persons who refuse blood transfusions.
Development of a method to prevent ABO incompatibility errors.	To prevent the wrong blood from being given to a patient.
A storage process that prevents the loss of viable cells and clotting factors.	To increase the therapeutic effectiveness of blood products.
Evaluate the impact of infusion devices (IV pumps) on cell integrity.	To obtain evidence that supports or negates the use of infusion pumps.
The need for additional in-line blood filters to prevent the infusion of clots and other debris.	To obtain a safer blood product.

Summary

Infusion therapy will continue to be practiced in all care settings and administered to patient populations of all ages. Technologic advances affecting insertion, care and maintenance, and research-based practices will continue to shape this nursing specialty. Education and continued competence are necessary to keep nurses abreast of proper techniques and new technology that are essential components of the specialty practice of infusion therapy.

CLINICAL PREPARATION

READ DOCUMENT APPLY

READ: **History of Present Illness** >> Laboratory Study Results >> Critical Thinking Questions

Tom Ballou, an 86-year-old male, is admitted to the medical–surgical floor after being seen and evaluated in the emergency department (ED). His chief complaint is abdominal pain, nausea, and vomiting of moderate to large amounts of dark red liquid. Mr. Ballou has moderate to severe abdominal pain and nausea. He states he has been vomiting for 2 days and taken in very little food or water in 3 days. ED laboratory work: complete blood count (CBC), complete metabolic panel, UA, PTT, PT, and INR; liver function studies; troponin; type and crossmatch for 4 units packed cells. Vital signs in the ED were BP 90/60, HR 118, RR 28, T 37°C. On admission to the floor, the patient is awake and alert. He states he feels weak and light-headed. Two 500-mL fluid boluses of 0.9% NS were administered in the ED.

You are the nurse caring for Mr. Ballou on his second day of hospitalization. The night nurse reported that there had been no vomiting or bloody stools since his admission. He does continue to complain of abdominal tenderness. After morning report, you evaluate the patient's morning laboratory values. All laboratory work except the hemoglobin and hematocrit are normal. When you note that the hemoglobin is 8 g/dL and the hematocrit is 24%, you call the health care provider. Two units of packed RBCs are ordered to be given this a.m. followed by an Hgb & Hct and potassium. An endoscopy is scheduled for today.

READ: History of Present Illnesses >> **Physical Exam** >> Admitting Medical Records >> Laboratory Study Results

Medical–Surgical History

- Non-Q wave MI: 1998
- Osteoarthritis
- No known allergies
- Denies a history of syncope
- Denies history of gastric ulcers
- Denies fever, chills, and night sweats

Home Medications

- ASA 81 mg po daily
- Lipitor 50 mg po daily
- Lopressor 100 po mg bid
- Celebrex 200 mg po daily
- MVI po daily
- Surgeries: appendectomy in 1982

Social History

Mr. Ballou lives with his wife; he has three grown children who live in the local area

Physical Exam

Older male, mild discomfort due to abdominal pain
Oxygen sat 94% on RA
BP: 90/62 HR 118 RR 26
HEENT: normal
Neck: negative JVD, no bruits
Heart: NL S1, S2
Lungs: clear
Abdomen: mildly distended soft, tender, hyperactive bowel sounds
Pulses: present in all extremities; strong throughout; good cap refill
Normal neuro exam
No rash
Poor skin turgor
Osteoarthritis
12-lead ECG showed sinus tachycardia, low voltage, and nonspecific ST wave changes
Chest x-ray is within normal limits

Admitting Medical Orders

Medicine Service
Admit to Telemetry Unit
Admitting diagnosis: GI bleed of unknown etiology
No known allergies
Vital signs and oxygen saturation: q2h
Daily weight
Foley catheter
Strict I&O
NPO
Full code status
Call house officer: BP systolic <90 >150 & diastolic $>$ 90; HR >120 <60 & RR >30; <30 mL of urine per hour $\times$ 2 hours; oxygen saturation $<92\%$
NG: Salem sump lavage until clear and clamp; if vomiting occurs, apply low wall suction
Bed rest: out of bed to bedside commode with assist only
Incentive spirometer q2h
Sequential compression device (SCD) to lower extremities
IV: 0.9 normal saline with 20 mEq of KCl via infusion pump at 125 mL/hr
Keep 2 units of RBCs on hold at all times
GI consult ordered

Scheduled Medications

Protonix 40 mg IV once a day

PRN Medications

Morphine sulfate 2–4 mg IV push q2h prn for pain
Zofran 4 mg IV q8h prn nausea and vomiting

Ordered Laboratory Studies

Amylase and lipase now
Hgb & Hct now and q6h
Chem 7 panel now and in a.m.
Liver function studies now
PT, PTT, and INR in a.m.
Potassium after blood

Ordered Diagnostic Studies

Abdominal CT scan

READ: History of Present Illnesses >> **Laboratory Study Results** >> Critical Thinking Questions

Test	Pt. Values #1	Pt. Values #2	Pt. Values #3
Chemistry	Emergency department	Pre-blood	Post-blood
Sodium	148 mEq/L	143 mEq/L	
Potassium	3.5 mEq/L	3.7 mEq/L	4.2 mEq/L
Chloride	113 mEq/L	110 mEq/L	
Carbon dioxide (CO_2)	25 mEq/L	24 mEq/L	
Blood urea nitrogen (BUN)	40 mg/dL	9 mg/dL	
Creatinine	1.0 mg/dL	1.0 mg/dL	
Blood, glucose	150 mg/dL	136 mg/dL	
Calcium	8.1 mg/dL		
Amylase		60 units/L	
Lipase		82 units/L	
Magnesium	2.2 mEq/L		
Troponin I	0.2 ng/mL		
Albumin	3.9		
Alkaline phosphorus	100 units/L		

Test	Pt. Values #1	Pt. Values #2	Pt. Values #3
GGT (0–65)	56 units/L		
Total bilirubin	1 mg/dL		
CPK total	200 units/L		
CPK MB	2.5%		
LDH	166 units/L		
AST	42 units/L		
ALT	60 units/L		
Hematology			
WBC	8,000/mm^3	7,000/mm^3	7,000/mm^3
Hemoglobin	10.2 g/dL	8 g/dL	10 g/dL
Hematocrit	32%	24%	37.9%
RBC	5/mm^3		
Platelets	395/mm^3	325/mm^3	250/mm^3
PTT	24 seconds		
PT	16.4 seconds	12 seconds	
INR ($<$1.19)	1.5	1.19	
Urine analysis	Normal		

Pearson Nursing Student Resources *Log on to* **nursing.pearsonhighered.com** *to download forms*

DOCUMENT:

- >> Summary of Hospitalization
- >> Pathophysiology Form
- >> Laboratory Values
- >> Laboratory Results Explanation

APPLY:

- >> List of Potential Nursing Diagnoses
- >> Concept Map
- >> Critical Thinking Questions and Concept Map

APPLY: History of Present Illnesses >> Laboratory Study Results >> **Critical Thinking Questions**

1. What might be one cause of the gastric bleeding?
   1. Presence of a gastric ulcer
   2. Gastric irritation from daily use of ASA
   3. A tear in the gastrointestinal wall
   4. Esophageal varices
2. What are critical nursing assessments during blood administrations?
   1. Completion of a transfusion history (e.g., type, when, allergic reactions, if so, how treated)
   2. Baseline assessment of vital signs
   3. Signs and symptoms of fluid overload
   4. All of the above
3. For what might Mr. Ballou be at high risk during blood administration?
   1. Transmission of bloodborne diseases
   2. Hypothermia
   3. Development of transfusion-related acute lung disease
   4. Answers 1 and 3 only
4. Why is the health care provider ordering an amylase and lipase study?
   1. An elevation of amylase and lipase values may be indicative of damage to the pancreas, kidney failure, intestinal obstruction, and peptic ulcers.
   2. A decrease of amylase and lipase values may be indicative of damage to the pancreas, kidney failure, intestinal obstruction, and peptic ulcers.
   3. An elevation of amylase and lipase values may be indicative of blood clotting disorders.
   4. Answers 1 and 3 only.

Answers to Critical Thinking Questions can be found in Appendix D in the Osborn Student Resources at nursing.pearsonhighered.com.

NCLEX® PRACTICE

1. A patient, being discharged, will need to receive antibiotic therapy for an additional 3 weeks. Which peripheral vascular access device would be the best for this patient?
   1. A peripheral-short catheter
   2. A winged steel infusion set
   3. A midline catheter
   4. A PICC line
2. A patient receiving parenteral fluids is prescribed an intravenous medication to be infused every 6 hours. Which of the following infusion devices should the nurse use for this medication?
   1. Stopcock
   2. Extension set
   3. Elastomeric balloon
   4. Secondary administration set
3. The staff development department is planning an annual skills review day for the basics of intravenous therapy. If the *Infusion Nursing Standards of Practice* are being followed, what is the goal of this skills day?
   1. Ensure that all nurses follow standard precautions.
   2. Preserve the patient's right to safe, high-quality care and protect the nurse who administers infusion therapy.
   3. Ensure that the nurses are in compliance with all regulatory agencies.
   4. Ensure that the nurses' skill levels are adequate.
4. A patient is prescribed parenteral fluid therapy. What should be the nurse's first action?
   1. Wash hands.
   2. Gather the equipment to insert the peripheral access device.
   3. Prepare the flush to use once the peripheral access device is in place.
   4. Review the procedure with the patient and obtain consent.

5. A patient receiving parenteral fluid therapy complains of the arm "feeling cold" and says that the dressing "feels tight." The nurse suspects the intravenous infusion has infiltrated. What should the nurse do?

1. Check for a blood return in the catheter.
2. Stop the infusion and remove the catheter.
3. Turn off the infusion, reposition the catheter.
4. Change the dressing and observe the site for additional swelling.

6. A patient is to receive a transfusion of albumin. How should the nurse explain the purpose of this transfusion?

1. "Albumin pulls fluid into your vascular system from your tissues and helps to increase your plasma volume."
2. "Albumin is given to help your blood clot better."
3. "Albumin helps to give you more of the red blood cells that carry oxygen to your tissues."
4. "Albumin increases the number of white blood cells in your blood so that they can help you fight off the infection that you have."

Answers to NCLEX Practice questions can be found in Appendix D in the Osborn Student Resources at nursing.pearsonhighered.com. Practice additional NCLEX questions online at the Student Resources site.

Pearson Nursing Student Resources Find additional review materials at: **nursing.pearsonhighered.com**

REFERENCES

About.com. (2011). Vein. Biology. Retrieved from http://biology.about.com/od/anatomy/ss/vein2htm

Alonge, L. (2010). Could that plastic device harm your patient? The U.S. Food and Drug Administration—device safety alerts and notices. Retrieved from http://www.fda.gov/MedicalDevices/Safety/AlertsandNotices/TipsandArticlesonDeviceSafety/ucm228418.htm

AlternaCare. (2010). SASH technique. Olathe, KS: Infusion Pharmacy.

American Association of Blood Banks (AABB). (2001). Association bulletin #01-4. Retrieved from http://www.aabb.org/resources/publications/bulletins/Pages/ab01-4.aspx

American Association of Blood Banks (AABB). (2011). Testing of donor blood for infectious disease. Retrieved from http://www.aabb.org/Content/About_Blood/Facts_About_Blood_and_Blood_Banking/fabloodtesting.htm

American Red Cross. (2011a). Blood donation eligibility guidelines. Retrieved from http://www.redcross.org/services/

American Red Cross. (2011b). Leukocyte reduction Q&A. Retrieved from http://www.redcross.org/services/biomed/blood/supply/ulr/qanda.html

America's Blood Centers. (2011). 56 facts about blood. Retrieved from http://www.americasblood.org/go.cfm?do=Page.View&pid=12

Callum, J. U. L., Lin, Y., Lima, A., & Merkley, L. (2011). Transitioning from "blood" safety to "transfusion" safety: Addressing the single biggest risk of transfusion. doi: 10.1111/j.1751-2824.2011.01446.x Retrieved from http://onlinelibrary.wiley.com/doi/10.1111/J.1751-

Canellini, G., Waldvogel, S., Anderegg, K., & Tissot J. D. (2010). Bacterial contamination of platelet concentrates: perspectives for the future. Retrieved from http://labmed.ascpjournals.org/content/41/5/301.abstract

Centers for Disease Control and Prevention. (2011a). CDC guidelines for the prevention of intravascular catheter-related infections. Retrieved from http://www.cdc.gov/hicpac/pdf/guidelines/bsi-guidelines-2011.pdf

Centers for Disease Control and Prevention. (2011b). CDC's report: "The state of aging and health in America 2007." Retrieved from http://www.retirement-living.com/proaging-network/cdcs-report-the-s

Cheever, K. (2008). *IV therapy demystified: A self-teaching guide.* New York: McGraw-Hill.

Clark, C. T. (2009). Transfusion-related acute lung injury. *Journal of Infusion Nursing, 32*(3), 132–136.

Clark, C. T. (2011). Recent efforts and available technologies for safety in delivery of blood products. *Journal of Infusion Nursing, 34*(1), 23–26.

Code of Federal Regulations Title 21. (2008). Intravascular administration set. Retrieved from http://www.accessdata.fda.gov/SCRIPTs/cdrh/cfdocs/cfcfr/CFRSearch.cfm?fr=880.5440&SearchTerm=tubing

Cooperman, T., & Allinson, R. (2011). Specialty pharmaceuticals: Therapy class review: Blood modifiers. *Pharmacy Times. Online Edition January 13, 2011.* Retrieved from http://www.pharmacytimes.com/publications/issue/2011/January2011/Specialty-0111.

Cutler, C. (2007). Jehovah's Witnesses—position overview. Penn Medicine. Retrieved from http://www.pennmedicine.org/health_info/bloodless/026.html

Department of Health & Human Services. (2007). *The 2007 national blood collection and utilization survey report.* U.S. Department of Health and Human Services, American Association of Blood Banks. Retreived from dataprograms@aabb.org

Drugs.com. (2012). Implanted venous access ports. Retrieved from http://www.drugs.com/cg/implanted-venous-access-ports.html

Encyclopedia of Nursing & Allied Health. (2011). Central catheter maintenance. Retrieved from http://www.enotes.com/central-catheter-maintenance-reference/central-catheter-maintenance

Easterlow, D., Hoddinott, P., & Harrison, S. (2010). *Journal of Clinical Nursing, 19*(5-6), 721–727. Retrieved from http://www.ncbi.nlm.nih.gov/pubmed/20500315

Food and Drug Administration. (2010a). About CBER. Retrieved from http://www.fda.gov/cber/blood.htm

Food and Drug Administration. (2010b). Blood. Retrieved from http://www.fda.gov/cber/blood.htm

Gajic, O., Rana, R., Winters, J. L., et al. (2007). Transfusion-related acute lung injury in the critically ill: Prospective nested case-control study. *American Journal of Respiratory Critical Care Medicine, 175*(9), 886–889.

Gorski, L. A. (2009). Speaking of standards: Standard 64: Continuous subcutaneous access devices. *Journal of Infusion Nursing, 32*(4), 185–186.

Guangxi, L., Kojicic, M., Reriani, M. K., Fernández Pérez, E. R., Thakur, L., Kashyap, R., Van Buskirk, C. M., & Gajic, O. (2010). Long-term survival and quality of life after transfusion-associated pulmonary edema in critically ill medical patients. *Chest, 137*, 783–789. Publisher online October 16, 2009. doi:1378/chest.09-0841.

Hall, J. E. (2011). *Guyton and Hall textbook of medical physiology* (12th ed.). Philadelphia: Elsevier, Saunders.

Hendrickson, J. E., & Hillyer, C. D. (2009). Noninfectious serious hazards of transfusion. *International Anesthesia Research Society, 108*(3), 759–769.

Infusion Nurses Society. (2011). Infusion nursing standards of practice. *Journal of Infusion Nursing, 34* (Suppl.1), 1-43.

IOM (Institute of Medicine). (2010). *The future of nursing: Leading change, advancing health.* Washington, DC: The Academic Press.

Kor, D., & Gajic, O. (2010). Blood product transfusion in the critical care setting. *Current Opinion in Critical Care. 16*, 309–316.

Linker, R., & Gold, R. (2008). Use of intravenous immunoglobulin and plasma exchange in neurologic disease. *Current Opinion in Neurology, 21*, 358–365.

Mei, A., & Auerhahn, C. (2009). Hypodermoclysis: maintaining hydration in the frail older adult. Retrieved from http://www.annalsoflongtermcare.com/content/hypodermoclysis-maintaining-hydration-frail-older-adult

Mosby's Medical Dictionary. (8th Ed.). (2009). Philadelphia: Elsevier.

Napolitano, L. M., Kurek, S., & Luchette, F. A., et al. (2009). Clinical practice guideline: Red blood cell transfusion in adult trauma and critical care. *The Journal of Trauma, 67*(6), 1439–1442.

Navilyst Medical. (2011). Vascular access overview. Retrieved from http://www.navilystmedical.com/clinicians/index.cfm/11

New Mexico Donor Services. (2009). Religious views on organ, tissue and blood donation. Retrieved from http:www.donatelifenm.org/religiousviewsE.htm

Nursing Made Incredibly Easy! (2008). I.V. essentials: Complications of peripheral I.V. therapy. Lippincott's Nursing Center.. Retrieved from http://journals.lww.com/nursingmadeincrediblyeasy/Citation/2008/01000/Complications_of_peripheral_I_V__therapy.4.aspx

OSHA Fact Sheet. (2011). OSHA's bloodborne Pathogens standard. *OSHA Fact Sheet.* Retrieved from www.osha.gov/OshDoc/data_BloodborneFacts/bbfact01.pdf

Perry, J., Gomaa, A. E., & Jagger, J. (2009). Progress in preventing sharps injuries in the United States. In W. Charney (Ed.), *Handbook of modern hospital safety* (2nd ed.). Florence, KY: CRC Press, Inc.

Phillips, L., Brown, L., Campbell, T., Miller, J., Proehl. J., & Youngberg, B. (2010). Recommendations for the use of intraosseous vascular access for emergent and nonemergent situations in various healthcare settings: A consensus paper. *Journal of Infusion Nursing, 33*(6), 346–351.

Plapp, F. V. (2008). *Essentials of transfusion medicine.* BookSurge Publishing.

Quality and Safety Education for Nurses (QSEN). (2011). About QSEN. Retrieved from http://www.qsen.org/about_qsen.php

Rosenthal, K. (2007a). Infiltrations & extravasations. Resource Nurse. Retrieved from http://www.resourcenurse.com/feature_infiltration.html

Rosenthal, K. (2007b). Tonicity and IV fluids. Resource Nurse. Retrieved from http://www.resourcenurse.com/feature_toxicity_fluids.html

Seeber, P., & Shander, A. (2007). *Basics of blood management.* Massachusetts: Blackwell Publishing.

Sihler, K. C., & Napolitano, L. M. (2009). Massive transfusion: New insights. *Chest, 136,* 1654–1667.

Silvergleid, A. J. (2011). Transfusion-associated graft-vs-host disease. Up-to-date. Retrieved from http://www.uptodate.com/contents/transfusion-associated-graft-versus-host-disease

The Free Dictionary. (2011). Tunneled catheter. Retrieved from http://medical-dictionary.thefreedictionary.com/tunneled-catheter

The Joint Commission. (2011). Hospital: 2011 national patient safety goals. Retrieved from http://www.jointcommission.org/hap_2011_npsgs/

Toy, P., & Lowell, C. (2007). TRALI—definition, mechanisms, incidence, and clinical relevance. *Best Practice & Research Clinical Anesthesiology, 27*(2), 183–193.

Timsit, J. F., Schwebel C., Boudama, L., Geffroy, A., Garrouste-Orgeas, M., Pease, S., et al. (2009). Chlorhexidine-impregnated sponges and less frequent dressing changes for prevention of catheter-related infections in critically ill adults: a randomized controlled trial. *Journal of American Medical Association, 301*(12), 1231–41. Retrieved from http://www.ncbi.nlm.nih.gov/pubmed/19318651

Tortorice, J. (2007). Preventing needlestick injuries. *CEUFast.com.* Retrieved from http://www.ceufast.com/course/viewcourse.aspo?id=37

Transfusion Medicine. (2012). Circulatory overload. Canadian Blood Services. Retrieved from http://www.transfusion.medicine.ca/resources/books/vein-vein/complications-blood-transfus

University Pain Centers. (2008). Placement of spinal or epidural catheters. Retrieved from http://universitypaincenters.com/index.php?option-com.content&vi

Vizcarra, C., & Clum, S. (2010). Intraosseous route as alternative access for infusion. *Journal of Infusion Nursing, 33*(3), 162–174. Retrieved from http://www.nchi.nlm.nih.gov/pubmed/20442600

Watson, D., & Hearnshaw, K. (2010). Understanding blood groups and transfusion nursing practice. *Nursing Standard, 24*(10), 41–48.

Wilkinson, J. M., & Ahearn, N. R. (2009). *Prentice Hall nursing diagnosis handbook* (9th ed.). Upper Saddle River, NJ: Prentice Hall.

UNIT 4 Nursing Management of the Surgical Patient

Content in Unit 4 that addresses the **Institute of Medicine (IOM)** competencies, **Nursing Core Competencies (NCC)**, the **Quality and Safety Education for Nurses (QSEN)** competencies, and **Concepts** for concept-based learning is listed below.

Competencies	Feature or Text	Location
IOM, QSEN, NCC Providing patient-centered care	Nursing Assessment, Preoperative Nursing Physical and Functional Assessment Postanesthesia Care Unit Cultural Considerations for the Postoperative Patient	Chapter 17, page 416 Chapter 17, page 421 Chapter 18, page 450 Chapter 19, page 454
IOM, QSEN, NCC Working in teams	Collaborative Management, Preoperative Nursing Collaborative Management, Postoperative Nursing	Chapter 17, page 416 Chapter 19, page 453
IOM, QSEN, NCC Employing evidence-based practice	Evidence-Based Practice: The Benefit of Preoperative Patient Teaching for Pain Evidence-Based Practice: Prevention of Infection During Surgery Comparison of Postop Pain Management Using Two PCA Methods	Chapter 17, page 425 Chapter 18, page 444 Chapter 19, page 466
IOM NCC Applying quality and safety improvement	Surgical Safety Checklist Positioning the Patient to Prevent Injury Preventing the Retention of Foreign Objects Preventing Postoperative Complications	Chapter 18, page 448 Chapter 18, page 449 Chapter 18, page 449 Chapter 19, page 465
IOM, QSEN, NCC Using informatics	Preoperative Checklist Intraoperative Patient Record	Chapter 17, page 428 Chapter 18, page 448
NCC Applying ethical and legal responsibilities	Legal Preparation and Ethical Considerations, Preoperative Nursing	Chapter 17, page 428
NCC Developing professionally	Perioperative Nursing and Perioperative Nursing Practice Standards Guidance for Professional Practice	Chapter 17, page 416 Chapter 18, page 435
NCC Educating patients	Health Promotion, Preoperative Nursing Preoperative Teaching to Prevent Postoperative Complications Health Promotion, Intraoperative Nursing Ambulatory Surgery Discharge Patient Teaching & Discharge Priorities Following a Breast Biopsy Health Promotion, Postoperative Nursing Patient Teaching & Discharge Priorities for Postoperative Nursing	Chapter 17, page 425 Chapter 17, page 426 Chapter 18, page 437 Chapter 19, page 463 Chapter 19, page 463 Chapter 19, page 476 Chapter 19, page 478
Concepts covered in Unit 4 include:	Body image Grief Pain	Safety Skin integrity Thermoregulation Tissue integrity

Preoperative Nursing

17 CHAPTER

Leslie Flynn
Renée Holleran

Outcome-Based Learning Objectives

After studying this chapter, the learner will be able to:

1. Describe the components and significance of preoperative assessments.
2. Analyze critical preoperative assessment findings that require further intervention.
3. Discuss the elements of preoperative preparation.
4. Prioritize nursing interventions for the preoperative patient.
5. Generate a teaching plan for the preoperative patient.

KEY TERMS

cosmetic surgery p.415
curative procedures p.415
diagnostic procedures p.415
elective procedures p.416
emergent (emergency) surgery p.416
exploratory surgery p.415
holding area p.428
palliative procedures p.415
perioperative p.416
reconstructive surgery p.415
same-day admission p.415
urgent procedures p.416

ACCORDING TO data from the National Center for Health Statistics, approximately 45 million inpatient procedures were performed in 2007 (National Health Statistics Reports, 2010). Of these procedures, 15% were cardiovascular; of the remaining surgeries, those performed on the digestive tract, including endoscopy, colonoscopy, colectomy, appendectomy, and cholecystectomy, were the most common, followed by surgeries on the musculoskeletal system and the eyes. Surgeries are performed in hospital-based inpatient or outpatient settings or in freestanding surgical centers. **Same-day admission,** in which the patient reports from home directly to the reception area of the operating room, is becoming standard procedure for many surgeries, including complex cardiac procedures.

Categories of Surgery

Surgical procedures are categorized in a variety of ways, and any given procedure will fall into several categories. Each of the categorizations provides a small piece of information about the patient who is having surgery. For example, knowing the specific procedure to be performed allows the nurse to begin formulating plans for preoperative teaching. Knowing that a procedure needs to be done emergently gives information about patient acuity. Commonly, procedures are categorized according to the following:

- General anatomic location of the surgery (e.g., abdominal, gynecological)
- Specific procedure to be performed (e.g., colectomy, total hip replacement)
- Purpose of the surgery (e.g., diagnostic, cosmetic)
- Urgency of the surgery (e.g., elective, urgent, emergent)
- Degree of risk associated with the surgery (low, moderate, high).

Surgery may also be performed for diagnostic, curative, reconstructive, palliative, or cosmetic purposes. **Diagnostic procedures** are performed for the purpose of making or confirming a medical diagnosis. These procedures frequently require the removal of tissue or cells for analysis. Diagnostic surgeries include procedures such as breast biopsy, arthroscopy, and diagnostic laparotomy. In some cases, diagnostic surgery is referred to as **exploratory surgery** because the surgeon examines or explores the tissues and structures in order to decide what further procedures or treatments need to be done.

Curative procedures are done for the purpose of effecting a cure; for example, the successful treatment of a disease or condition. Many surgeries are done for this purpose, including cholecystectomy, hernia repair, and open reduction of a fracture.

Reconstructive surgery is done for the purpose of rebuilding tissues or body structures to achieve a more normal function and appearance. Examples include skin grafting and breast reconstruction following mastectomy.

Palliative procedures are done for the purpose of alleviating symptoms caused by disease or a condition. Palliative surgery does not effect a cure, but it frequently improves the patient's quality of life. Examples include debulking a tumor, performing a laminectomy to reduce spinal cord compression in a patient with metastatic cancer, and creating a colostomy in a patient with severe inflammatory bowel disease.

Cosmetic surgery is performed for the primary purpose of improving physical appearance. Examples include liposuction, rhinoplasty, and breast augmentation.

Weblink: National Health Statistics Report: National hospital discharge survey

Surgeries are also classified according to the urgency with which the procedure needs to be performed. **Elective procedures** are those that are scheduled in advance for a nonacute condition. Performing a procedure electively is always preferred because the patient will be in better health than he or she would be during an acute illness, and advance planning allows optimum physiological and psychological preparation of the patient. There also is a technical advantage to elective procedures because the tissues are not distorted by inflammation or infection. Knee replacement surgery is an example of a procedure that is most often elective.

Urgent procedures are performed for conditions that require prompt attention, within the next 48 hours, but that are not currently life threatening. An example might be an appendectomy performed for acute appendicitis. An **emergent** (or **emergency**) **surgery** is a procedure that must be performed immediately to prevent serious consequences. Failure to perform emergency surgery in a timely manner can result in a patient's death or disability. A fasciotomy performed to treat compartment syndrome in a fractured leg is an example of an emergent procedure.

Surgical procedures are accompanied by varying levels of risk. This risk is sometimes characterized by using the terms *minor* or *major surgery*. Minor surgery refers to procedures associated with minimal risks, for example, removal of warts or skin tags. These procedures are often done under local anesthetic and do not require hospitalization. Major surgery describes procedures accompanied by more significant risks. The surgical risk associated with particular procedures can also be described as low, moderate, or high. Low-risk surgeries (e.g., cataract removal) refer to those that have few complications; when complications do occur, they are not serious. High-risk surgery describes procedures that are associated with a larger number of complications and more serious complications. Carotid endarterectomy is an example of a high-risk surgery.

Common Surgical Suffixes

There is no standardization in the naming of surgical procedures. Consequently, any given surgical procedure may have several names that are used interchangeably. However, knowing the meaning of common surgical suffixes can help the nurse to understand what type of surgery is to be performed:

- ***Ectomy:*** Removal of, surgical excision to remove (e.g., colectomy)
- ***Ostomy:*** Surgical creation of a permanent opening (e.g., colostomy)
- ***Otomy:*** Surgical incision of or cutting into (e.g., thoracotomy)
- ***Plasty:*** Surgical repair or reconstruction of (e.g., rhinoplasty)
- ***Orraphy:*** Surgical repair or suture of (e.g., herniorrhaphy)
- ***Scopy:*** Use of a scope to view or look into an area (e.g., laparoscopy).

Perioperative Nursing and Perioperative Nursing Practice Standards

The term **perioperative** encompasses the entire surgical experience: preoperative, intraoperative, and postoperative (the prefix "peri" means "around"). The nurse's role in a perioperative setting includes preparing the patient for surgery, assisting and observing the patient during the operation, preventing and treating postoperative complications, and preparing the patient for discharge. Practice standards and practice guidelines are the basis for providing consistent, high-level care for the patient who is undergoing surgery. Practice standards developed by professional organizations set the expectations and responsibilities of professional nursing performance.

Standards are subject to ongoing evaluation and refinement so that they reflect current and best practices. The American Nurses Association's (ANA's) *Standards of Clinical Nursing Practice* and the *Code of Ethics for Nurses With Interpretive Statements* describe the roles and responsibilities of nurses regardless of practice setting. These standards are presented in Chapter 1. Specialty organizations in nursing use the ANA's conceptual framework for developing practice guidelines specific to the specialty. An example is the *Perioperative Standards and Recommended Practices for Inpatient and Ambulatory Settings* developed by the Association of Perioperative Registered Nurses (AORN, 2011). One part of the AORN standards, the *Standards of Perioperative Nursing Practice,* uses the nursing process (assessment, nursing diagnosis, outcome, planning, implementation, and evaluation) to describe how the perioperative nurse provides care to the surgical patient. Another part of the AORN standards, *Recommended Practices for Perioperative Nursing,* focuses on practices for perioperative nursing.

Several critical beliefs underlie AORN's standards. Among these is the belief that quality nursing care:

- Is a partnership between the nurse and the patient.
- Is individualized.
- Respects the patient's personal, cultural, and religious beliefs.
- Respects the patient's autonomy.
- Incorporates the patient's goals and preferences.
- Focuses on collaboration, education, and advocacy.

Another organization that is important to perioperative nurses is the American Society of PeriAnesthesia Nurses (ASPAN). This organization develops and publishes standards of practice for care of the patient during the preoperative and the postoperative phases. The postoperative period is divided into two phases. Phase 1 is immediately after surgery, when the patient is having the most physiological changes. Phase 2 occurs after respiratory and cardiac functions have returned to baseline and the patient is just gaining strength and cognition (ASPAN, 2010).

Perioperative nurses need to be familiar with standards developed by groups interested in promoting quality care. Such groups include the National Council of State Boards of Nursing (NCSBN), The Joint Commission, the Institute for Healthcare Improvement (IHI), and the Medicare Quality Improvement Community. Hospitals also develop policies and procedures for defining the quality of care. Hospital policies need to be rational, reasoned, current, and consistent with state and nationwide clinical and evidence-based practice (AORN, 2011). Practice guidelines and clinical pathways are used to promote high-quality care. Clinical pathways are evidence-based and reflect critical activities, interventions, time frames, and desired outcomes for specific surgeries or diseases. It is the responsibility of perioperative nurses to use standards, guidelines, pathways, and policies in conjunction with their expertise and judgment when delivering high-level nursing care.

Collaborative Management

A successful surgical experience includes all members of the health care team. In order to meet desired patient outcomes, it is essential that this interdisciplinary team communicate openly with one another in developing and evaluating care of the patient and family (IOM [Institute of Medicine], 2010). The surgeon, preoperative nurse, and anesthesia care provider assess the patient prior to surgery. Consults from specialty areas such as cardiology, endocrinology, or neurology may be required depending on the patient's past or current medical condition. Some surgeries, such as organ transplantation or the creation of an ostomy, will require the patient to learn a whole new set of health maintenance skills. In these situations, the health care team may include a nurse who works directly with the surgeon and specializes in health care teaching for those surgeries.

A preoperative health evaluation is done within 30 days of a planned operation and must be documented in the patient's medical record according to The Joint Commission requirements (American Society of Anesthesiologists [ASA], 2008). An internist, surgeon, or anesthesia provider performs the evaluation, which is frequently done as an outpatient examination. This evaluation is performed specifically to clear the patient for the planned surgical procedure. It provides data for confirming the overall appropriateness of performing the planned surgery (by answering questions such as "Is the patient healthy enough to have surgery?") and confirms the plan to perform the surgery on an outpatient, same-day admission, or inpatient basis. If abnormal findings are identified during this evaluation, further tests may be required before the patient is cleared to have the surgery. The preoperative evaluation includes a medical history; a focused review of issues pertinent to the planned anesthesia and surgical procedure; an abbreviated physical exam including height, weight, vital signs, and cardiac and pulmonary systems; and an assessment of the patient's overall functional ability (ASA, 2010). The preoperative health evaluation and any recommendations from the evaluation must be sent to the site where the surgery will be conducted. Although the history and physical exam can be completed 30 days prior to the surgery, many accrediting agencies, such as Medicare, require that this form be updated within 24 hours prior to surgery. This serves two purposes. It confirms that the surgery is still necessary (e.g., the patient may have already passed the kidney stone and no longer requires surgery), and it confirms that there has been no change in the patient's health since the initial evaluation.

The anesthesia provider conducts a separate preoperative history and physical exam. This preprocedure assessment includes a review of systems with a focus on issues that affect the choice and administration of anesthesia. The patient is asked about any family history of anesthetic problems and any history of motion sickness or anesthesia-related nausea and vomiting. The latter two are risk factors for postoperative nausea and vomiting. The anesthesia assessment includes an examination of the patient's airway, neck (for range of motion), and teeth. Permanent dental prostheses may be documented during the exam. The National Guidelines box lists the ASA guidelines for classifying a patient's physical status and operative risk. Patients are classified in one of six categories; lower classifications (e.g., I and II) represent patients who are healthy or have mild systemic disease and good operative risks, whereas higher classifications (V and VI) represent patients who have severe disease and are unlikely to survive surgery (ASA, 2008).

A newer approach to surgery, accelerated recovery programs, relies on a multidisciplinary team approach with an emphasis on collaboration. At the center of accelerated recovery programs, also referred to as fast-track surgery, is the view that patient outcomes are improved by expediting postoperative recovery. Key elements of accelerated programs include the following (Clifford, 2010; McCallin & Jones, 2011):

NATIONAL GUIDELINES for ASA Physical Status Classification

ASA I	A normal healthy patient
ASA II	A patient with mild systemic disease
ASA III	A patient with severe systemic disease that limits disease but is not incapacitating
ASA IV	A patient with severe systemic disease that is a constant threat to life
ASA V	A moribund patient who is not expected to survive 24 hours without the operation
ASA VI	A patient declared brain dead and whose organs are being removed for transplantation

Source: Adapted from American Society of Anesthesiologists. (2008). Classification of physical status. SAA Relative Value Guide. Retrieved from http://www.asahq.org/clinical/physicalstatus.htm.

- Preoperative education to prepare the patient to take an active part in recovery
- Use of anesthetics, analgesics, and surgical techniques that minimize surgical trauma and physiological stress, thereby allowing faster recovery
- Aggressive postoperative rehabilitation, including early feeding and intensive ambulation
- Selective and evidence-based use of traditional postoperative practices such as the use of drains, tubes, and monitoring.

In accelerated recovery programs, patient assessment and education are important collaborative roles for nurses working in preoperative care.

Nursing Management

Nursing management in the preoperative setting involves a cluster of activities (e.g., assessing, planning, teaching, and evaluating) performed by the nurse in anticipation of surgery. The purpose of preoperative care is to evaluate the patient's readiness for surgery, to identify potential risks and hazards of the surgery, to advise the patient about the surgical procedure, to prepare the patient for the postoperative experience, to plan for home care, and to provide emotional support.

Nursing Assessment

Assessment of the preoperative patient is a nursing responsibility identified in practice standards (AORN, 2011; ASPAN, 2010). A complete and thorough preoperative assessment serves several purposes. For example, the assessment identifies risk factors for intraoperative and postoperative problems. The risk level of surgery is influenced by several factors including the patient's age, health history, current cardiac and pulmonary status, functional ability, and the type of surgery planned (AORN, 2011). Once risk factors have been identified, the nurse takes steps to correct, minimize, or prevent potential problems. The assessment also provides the data necessary for developing preoperative and postoperative teaching plans. The preoperative assessment provides a baseline of physical and functional ability. Nurses caring for the patient postoperatively will use preoperative assessments in deciding whether a sign or symptom is a new finding; whether the patient is progressing as expected; and whether the patient needs specialized care, rehabilitation, or follow-up home services.

Weblink: ASA Physical Status Classification

Weblink: ASA Statement of Documentation of Anesthesia Care

The preoperative assessment may be done either in a separate appointment before the surgery or on the morning of the surgery. Many hospitals use their own forms for preoperative assessment to ensure completeness and simplicity. Most of these forms will represent an abbreviated version (e.g., using checklists) of the assessment. Preoperative assessment includes a patient history with physical examination and functional assessment. The patient history includes the following:

- Age
- Allergies
- Current health problem
- Type of surgery planned
- Plans for autologous blood donation
- Family history
- Past medical history
- Past surgical history and experiences with anesthesia
- Current medications
- Current herbal medications and nutritional supplements
- Alcohol, cigarette, and social drug use.

Each of these areas is discussed in more detail in the following subsections.

Age

Approximately one-third of all surgeries are performed on older adults. Age alone is not a contraindication for surgery; however, the risks of surgery increase with advancing age. (For more information, see the Gerontological Considerations section later in this chapter, p. 429.)

Allergies

Allergies and allergic reactions to medications, chemicals, and foods must always be identified and prominently displayed on the patient's wristband, in the medical record, and in the medication record. Patients with histories of allergic reactions have a greater risk of hypersensitivity to anesthesia, so the type of allergic reaction is very important. These patients also are much more likely to develop latex allergies. A special operating room setup is required for patients with latex allergy. Patients who are allergic to shellfish or iodine may also be allergic to povidone-iodine, a solution used for surgical preparation.

Safety Alert *Allergic responses to latex range from mild dermatitis to anaphylaxis. If latex allergy is suspected, the nurse needs to report it to the surgeon so that a blood or skin test can be performed to confirm the allergy. The nurse must create a latex-reduced environment for individuals who are allergic to latex.*

Current Health Problem

The patient's current health problem may influence various aspects of perioperative care, such as the type of anesthesia used, the type and amount of fluid replacement given, and the type of intraoperative monitoring performed. It may also determine priorities of postoperative care.

For women, anesthesia should be avoided during the first trimester of pregnancy. It is important for the health care provider to know the date of the patient's last menstrual period. If there is uncertainty about whether or not the patient is pregnant, she should perform a pregnancy test.

If a woman is lactating, the nurse should note this in the preoperative assessment. Certain medications may be avoided, and the patient will need to be instructed on when she can resume nursing and whether she needs to pump and discard the milk before she resumes nursing. This is done so the infant avoids exposure to any drugs that may have remained in the mother's milk.

Type of Surgery Planned

The surgical procedure that is planned influences every aspect of perioperative care including the preoperative assessment, preoperative teaching and preparation, the setup of the operating room, the type of anesthesia used, and the priorities of postoperative care. The preoperative assessment is a good time for the nurse to review the operative permit (e.g., consent), evaluate the patient's understanding of the surgical procedure to be performed, and clarify any matters about which the patient has questions.

Plans for Autologous Blood Donation

Patients who have scheduled elective surgery may make arrangements to donate their own blood in advance of the surgery. To be eligible for preoperative autologous donation, the patient must be in good health, be afebrile, have a hemoglobin level of 11 g/dL or higher, and have the approval of the health care provider or surgeon. Chapter 16 includes a complete description of autologous blood donation and its administration procedures and nursing interventions.

Family History

Family history is important to determine the presence of possible genetic predispositions. It is particularly important for the nurse to ask about any family history of diabetes, heart disease, sudden cardiac death, or malignant hyperthermia (MH). Malignant hyperthermia is a life-threatening condition of sustained muscle contraction precipitated by common agents of anesthesia such as inhalation agents and the muscle relaxant succinylcholine. Malignant hyperthermia (MH) is an autosomal dominant trait, so each child of a parent with MH has a 50% chance of inheriting the susceptibility. MH is discussed in detail in Chapter 18.

Past Medical History

In the medical history, the patient is asked about all previous diseases and conditions. Past medical problems can increase the risk associated with surgery as well as the possibility of postoperative complications. Preexisting disease influences many perioperative decisions, including whether or not to proceed with the operation, the type of anesthesia to be used, the need for additional testing or procedures prior to surgery, and the need for intraoperative and postoperative monitoring. The implications of specific conditions are discussed next.

Neurological conditions assessment includes asking about any history of stroke or transient ischemic attacks (TIAs). If a stroke is part of a patient's history, it is important to determine what, if any, deficits remain and whether or not the patient is receiving anticoagulation therapy. Deficits in cognitive functioning may affect the patient's ability to understand preoperative and postoperative instructions. Mobility deficits may place the patient at increased risk for postoperative atelectasis, pneumonia, abdominal distention, constipation, skin breakdown, and deep venous thrombosis. (Deep vein thrombosis is discussed in Chapter 35.) Patients who have neuromuscular disorders (e.g., myasthenia gravis, multiple sclerosis) or spinal cord injury also may be at a higher risk for postoperative complications associated with limited mobility. Patients who are experiencing transient ischemic attacks (TIA) may need to have a procedure to improve blood flow to the brain (carotid endarterectomy) prior to having any other surgical procedure in order to decrease the risk of a perioperative stroke. Seizure disorder also is a significant surgical factor because some anesthetic agents are known to lower the threshold for seizures.

The *cardiovascular disorders* assessment is important because surgery causes major stress to the heart as a result of the hemodynamic changes that occur with tissue injury and fluid loss. All anesthetic drugs have known cardiovascular affects. Disorders of the cardiovascular system are particularly important in establishing the patient's level of surgical risk. The highest risk is associated with acute myocardial infarction (AMI) (within 7 days preceding the operation), recent MI (occurred in the month prior to the operation), unstable angina, heart failure, significant dysrhythmia, and severe valvular disease (Babb, 2009). It is recommended that patients wait a minimum of 4 to 6 weeks after an MI to have elective surgery to prevent the likelihood of reinfarction. Patients with unstable angina may require stabilization with either medications or coronary revascularization prior to having any other surgical procedures. Patients with heart failure are at increased risk of postoperative pulmonary complications and of fluid and electrolyte imbalances (Babb, 2009). These patients will need to have their fluid status monitored closely during the intraoperative and postoperative periods. A chemical called brain natriuretic peptide (BNP) is released when the heart ventricle is stretched. Serum BNP is used preoperatively to screen or monitor for heart failure. Postoperatively, it is used to determine whether dyspnea is caused by heart failure or some other condition (Kee, 2010). Patients with valvular disorders may require antibiotic prophylaxis to reduce the risk of bacterial endocarditis (Chapter 33). These patients must also be monitored postoperatively for the development of worsening heart failure.

Patients with a history of dysrhythmias will require postoperative cardiac telemetry. Patients with pacemakers or implantable cardioverter defibrillators (ICDs) pose specific concerns during surgery. The presence of a pacemaker affects placement of the electrocautery grounding pad and choice of anesthetic agents. Electrocautery, used in the operating room to remove unwanted tissue or to seal blood vessels, can create an electromagnetic interference that may cause pacemaker dysfunction or damage (Rooke, 2007). The use of succinylcholine, a depolarizing muscle relaxant that is sometimes used during anesthesia, causes muscle fasciculations and postoperative shivering that can suppress pacemaker function (Rooke, 2007). Preoperative information that is required for patients with pacemakers includes identification of the underlying cardiac rhythm that necessitates the pacemaker and information about the pacemaker itself (e.g., type, device, lead system, availability of technical support). All patients with pacemakers need to have the unit interrogated (i.e., tested to check battery status and thresholds for sensing and pacing leads) within 3 months before scheduled surgery. Pacemaker interrogation after surgery is also recommended. Patients with ICDs also need to supply information about the device as well as evidence of unit interrogation prior to surgery. It is recommended that the tachyarrhythmia detection of the ICD unit be turned off prior to surgery (Rooke, 2007). Electromagnetic noise from electrocautery can mimic the signal for ventricular tachycardia or ventricular fibrillation, causing the ICD to deliver an unnecessary shock during surgery. A magnet is used to turn off the tachycardia detection feature on the morning of surgery. Postoperatively, the unit must be turned back on.

Patients undergoing cardiac surgery may have a beta-adrenergic blocking medication prescribed preoperatively to reduce the risk of developing atrial fibrillation postoperatively (Golembiewski, 2008). Generally, patients with hypertension will continue to receive antihypertensive medications throughout the perioperative period, especially patients with hard to control hypertension.

Patients with chronic respiratory conditions such as chronic obstructive pulmonary disease (COPD) and severe asthma, as well as older adults and people who smoke cigarettes, have an increased risk of postoperative atelectasis and pneumonia (Lauerman, 2008). Preoperative pulmonary function tests may need to be performed on patients with COPD, and surgery may be postponed for patients with an upper respiratory infection. Obstructive sleep apnea (OSA), a serious condition that is evaluated in the preoperative assessment, is associated with airway collapse, hypoventilation, and sensitivity to the respiratory depressant effects of medications such as anesthetics, narcotics, and sedatives (ASA, 2008).

Safety Alert *The nurse must notify the anesthesia care provider if the patient has suspected or documented OSA. It may be difficult to intubate this patient, and the patient will require continuous monitoring for hypoventilation and hypoxemia during surgery and postoperatively until he is stable.*

Patients with chronic renal failure (CRF) will require close monitoring of fluid and electrolyte balance and medication administration. The effectiveness of drugs may be altered because the kidney excretes most drugs. Patients with CRF are at a higher than expected risk of an intraoperative cardiac event (AORN, 2011). Preoperatively, it is important to ascertain when the patient was last dialyzed and confirm that labs have been drawn since the last dialysis treatment. Patients with benign prostatic hypertrophy (BPH) should be monitored postoperatively for problems with urinary retention.

Musculoskeletal conditions such as arthritis can have a major impact on the nurse's ability to properly position a patient intraoperatively and postoperatively. Therefore, the nurse must take care not to injure the patient's arthritic joints. Temporomandibular joint syndrome and limitations of neck mobility can interfere with intubation for general anesthesia. Myotonic dystrophy, a rare form of muscular dystrophy, increases the patient's sensitivity to anesthesia and narcotics.

Safety Alert *Patients with a history of certain neuromuscular disorders, such as myotonic dystrophy, may be highly sensitive to anesthesia and require special precautions in planning surgery. The patient should wear a medical alert bracelet, and all health care providers who work with the patient need to be aware of this condition. The use of narcotics should be monitored carefully.*

Several issues must be considered in caring for the surgical patient with an endocrine disorder such as diabetes. Type 1 diabetes is associated with an increased risk of perioperative cardiac morbidity (Ead, 2009). Poor glucose control is associated with higher rates of surgical site infections (Ead, 2009). Patients with diabetes also experience slower wound healing. The physiological stress of surgery changes the insulin requirement. Therefore, careful monitoring of blood sugar is needed to prevent hypoglycemia and ketosis.

Patients who are immunocompromised present a special surgical challenge. Examples of patients who are at high risk for immune system dysfunction include those with human immunodeficiency virus (HIV) or cancer; those who have undergone chemotherapy, splenectomy, or organ transplantation; those taking immunosuppressive drugs such as prednisone; and those who are malnourished, experience chronic pain, or abuse alcohol (Neil, 2007). Surgery depresses the normal immune system for up to a week, and this effect is heightened in patients who are already immunocompromised. Immunosuppression increases the surgical risks for hypothermia, infection, and hypoadrenal function. Preoperative assessment for immunosuppressed patients includes weight, blood pressure, a complete blood count, liver and renal function tests, and chest x-ray (Neil, 2007).

Other disorders that may affect surgery include anemia, bleeding or clotting disorders, cancer, and morbid obesity. Skin and tissues that have been irradiated as a treatment for cancer are more easily damaged and heal more slowly than other tissues. The effects of chemotherapy depend on the drugs given. Morbid obesity (a body mass index of 40 or greater) is associated with significant comorbidities including diabetes mellitus, hypertension, gastroesophageal reflux disease, and OSA (Reedy, 2009). Surgical procedures may also take longer, requiring a longer period of anesthesia (Reedy, 2009).

Past Surgical History and Experience with Anesthesia

A patient's previous experience with surgery and anesthesia will influence decisions about the current surgery. A complete surgical history should be obtained, focusing specifically on previous surgeries, dates they were performed, problems with anesthesia, and postoperative complications. Some problems are likely to repeat themselves. For example, if it was difficult to intubate the patient in a previous surgery, it will likely be difficult in the current surgery. Difficulty with intubation needs to be noted prominently in the medical record, and the patient should wear a colored wristband identifying the problem. Other problems with prior surgery might not reoccur because of changes in surgical techniques, improved technologies, better anesthetic agents, or new medications.

Safety Alert *The nurse needs to alert the anesthesia care provider if the patient reports a history of difficult intubation with a prior surgery. This patient needs an airway examination, and specialized airway equipment must be available.*

A preoperative risk assessment for postoperative nausea and vomiting (PONV) needs to be completed. Risk factors for PONV are outlined in the Risk Factors box. The preoperative risk assessment is used to plan for surgery and prophylaxis for postoperative nausea and vomiting. Patients with multiple risk factors may be given different anesthetics (e.g., total intravenous anesthesia or regional blocks) and preoperative medications (ASPAN, 2010). Patients with moderate to high risk of PONV need a multimodal approach to prevention. Some medications are given to the patient in the presurgical area; others, such as a transdermal scopolamine patch, are applied by the patient the night before surgery.

Current Medications

Patients are asked to provide a specific and detailed list of regularly taken medications, including over-the-counter (OTC) medications and herbal preparations. The list includes the name of the medication, as well as the amount, how often it is taken, and when the medication was last taken. Information regarding medications is used in numerous ways. For example, many medications have the potential to either increase or decrease the effect of anesthetic agents. Certain medications may necessitate specific preoperative tests. For example,

RISK FACTORS for Postoperative Nausea and Vomiting

Gender (women more than men)
History of nausea and vomiting with a previous surgery
History of motion sickness
Nonsmoker
Use of certain inhalation anesthetics (volatile anesthetic gases and nitrous oxide)
Use of opioid analgesics
Type of surgery (gynecologic, abdominal, and those on the ear or eye)
Longer surgeries.

Sources: American Society of PeriAnesthesia Nurses. (2006). ASPAN's evidence-based clinical practice guideline for the prevention and/or management of PONV/PDNV. *Journal of PeriAnesthesia Nursing, 21*(4), 230–250; Murphy, M., Hooper, V., Sullivan, E., Clifford, T., & Apfel, C. (2006). Identification of risk factors for postoperative nausea and vomiting in the perianesthesia adult patient. *Journal of PeriAnesthesia Nursing, 21*(6), 377–384.

patients taking digoxin or a diuretic (e.g., furosemide, hydrochlorothiazide) may need to have potassium levels tested prior to surgery.

Some medications, such as insulin, oral hypoglycemic agents, corticosteroids, and antihypertensive agents, require dose adjustments prior to surgery. In addition, medications that slow coagulation, such as aspirin, enoxaparin, heparin, vitamin E, and warfarin, are frequently discontinued prior to surgery.

It is important for the appropriate people to review the patient's medications and the problems that they may cause related to any surgery before surgery takes place. As a part of ensuring patient safety, the perianesthesia nurse needs to ensure that there is accurate communication about patient medications and their effects related to the surgical procedure that is going to be performed (Joy, 2009).

Current Herbal Medications and Nutritional Supplements

The use of herbal remedies and nutritional supplements is becoming increasingly common in the United States. Studies show that between 40% and 70% of patients do not tell their health care providers or pharmacists about their use of herbal remedies (Anastasi, Chang, & Capili, 2011; Somes & Donatelli, 2011).

Patients need to be asked specifically about the use of herbs and nutritional supplements in a preoperative assessment. Although many herbs are considered relatively safe, they do have pharmacologically active properties that can produce drug interactions or adverse effects. For example, several herbs are known to inhibit platelet function and delay clotting time (Anastasi, Chang, & Capili, 2011; Somes & Donatelli, 2011). In the United States, herbs are classified as diet supplements; they are not subject to federal regulation, and there is no standardization in herb potency. Consequently, it is difficult to know how much of a pharmacologic effect is exerted by any given herbal product.

The use of nutritional supplements can also affect surgery. Fish oil, a popular supplement that is thought to reduce the effects of atherosclerosis and prevent myocardial infarction and angina, may slow blood clotting. Patients should stop taking fish oil 2 to 3 weeks before surgery. Chart 17–1 lists some common herbs, their uses, and the implications for surgery.

CHART 17–1 Herbs, Uses, and Implications for Surgery

Herb	Uses	Implications for Surgery
Lutein	Energy and eye health	None recommended for eye surgery
Glucosamine	Joint health	None
Chondroitin	Joint health	None
Ginkgo biloba	Vertigo, tinnitus, intermittent claudication, Alzheimer's disease	Interferes with platelet aggregation and may lower seizure threshold
Lecithin	Heart health, decrease cholesterol	None

Source: Adapted from Rowe, D. J., & Baker, A. C. (2009). Perioperative risks and benefits of herbal supplements in aesthetic surgery. *Aesthetic Surgery Journal, 29*(2),150–157.

Alcohol, Cigarette, and Drug Use

A careful history of alcohol and illicit drug use is important because excessive and chronic use of these substances can interfere with anesthesia, increase the patient's tolerance to anesthesia, reduce the effectiveness of postoperative pain medication, and cause serious physiological issues such as drug or alcohol withdrawal syndromes. If surgery must be performed on patients who are addicted to alcohol or narcotics, then the careful titration of benzodiazepines (for alcohol) and methadone (for narcotics) may be used to prevent withdrawal symptoms.

Safety Alert *When the possibility of alcohol withdrawal exists, the nurse and surgical team need to monitor the patient closely. A standardized alcohol withdrawal rating scale, such as the Clinical Institute Withdrawal Assessment (CIWA) scale, helps in identifying serious withdrawal symptoms and in monitoring treatment for alcohol withdrawal syndrome.*

A lifetime history of cigarette smoking is described in pack-years, that is, the number of packs smoked per day multiplied by the number of years the person has smoked. Cigarette smoking increases surgical risk for several reasons. For example, smoking damages the mucociliary clearance system, resulting in increased secretions and a higher risk of postoperative atelectasis and pneumonia (Lauerman, 2008). Smoking also increases circulating carboxyhemoglobin, which reduces circulating oxygen, resulting in less oxygen delivery to body tissues. Smoking causes vasoconstriction, a serious concern for patients undergoing cardiac or vascular surgery. However, smoking cessation is thought to reduce sputum production, increase ciliary action and clearance of secretions, and improve small airway function. Patients are asked to stop smoking 6 to 8 weeks prior to surgery. For patients who are unable to quit before surgery, a nicotine patch can be applied postoperatively to prevent nicotine craving and withdrawal.

Physical and Functional Assessment

Although the assessment components remain the same regardless of the type of surgery being performed, the level of detail provided in certain categories may change by type of surgery. Patients who are admitted for neurosurgery will have a more thorough reporting of their neurological exam, whereas patients who are admitted for gastrointestinal surgery will need a more detailed abdominal and nutritional assessment. The patient's past medical history will also direct the nurse's attention toward specific categories of assessment.

Neurological Assessment

The neurological examination includes a baseline mental status examination as well as an assessment of motor and sensory function. An evaluation of mental status includes assessment of the patient's level of consciousness, judgment, ability to follow commands, appropriateness of behavior, speech, and the ability to express oneself and to understand what is being said. These data are especially helpful in designing preoperative and postoperative teaching plans. It is particularly important to document baseline performance for older patients because they are at higher risk than other adults of experiencing a surgery-related change in mental status. Evaluation of motor function includes evaluation of the patient's strength, movement, balance, and gait. Any physical limitations or impairments, such as difficulty with hearing, vision, speech, swallowing, or walking, should be noted, as well as any history of falls. The risk of falls is associated with many factors, but two factors are consistently identified across studies: (1) altered mental status and (2) impaired mobility (Braganza, 2009; Sly-Havey, 2009). During the evaluation, the nurse makes a determination about the patient's fall risk and begins developing a safety plan. A patient's neurological status may affect her ability to carry out activities of daily living (ADLs) independently such as bathing, dressing, toileting, feeding, walking, and transferring.

The nurse must ask the patient about issues of pain and pain tolerance. The nurse notes the location, description, and rating of preoperative pain and asks the patient about her successful strategies for dealing with the pain. This is a good time for the nurse to discuss postoperative pain, to teach about using a numeric pain rating scale, and to reassure the patient that pain control is a key concern for health care providers. Pain assessment and management are discussed in detail in Chapter 12.

Cardiovascular Assessment

Baseline vital signs are established for the preoperative patient. It is helpful to know baseline pulse and blood pressure because postoperative problems such as anxiety, pain, hypoxia, and dehydration can manifest via a change in vital signs. The nurse assesses heart rate and rhythm, blood pressure, and peripheral pulses in addition to observing the extremities for color, sensation, capillary refill, and the presence of edema. The nurse needs to notify the health care provider or surgeon of any cardiac-specific abnormalities that are present such as hypertension, chest pain, dyspnea, pedal edema, or heart rhythm irregularities.

Cardiac abnormalities may need further evaluation prior to surgery to prevent an intraoperative cardiac event (American Society of Anesthesiologists, 2011a). Additional evaluation may include an electrocardiogram, echocardiogram, cardiac stress test, and pacemaker or ICD interrogation. For patients with a history of cardiovascular disease, the health care provider investigates the disease's effect on the patient's ability to walk, exercise, and participate in ADLs. It is clearly important to document baseline activity levels for all patients.

Respiratory Assessment

Baseline findings of the preoperative respiratory assessment include respiratory rate and depth, quality of respiratory effort, lung sounds, and oxygen saturation level with room air and with oxygen to determine whether the patient requires oxygen. The nurse also asks the patient about any problems breathing; whether or not shortness of breath interferes with ADLs; and about the use of inhalers, oxygen, or continuous positive airway pressure (CPAP) devices at home. Baseline information is important because postoperative atelectasis is a common problem and the nurse is usually responsible for weaning patients off oxygen in the postoperative period.

Gastrointestinal Assessment

The preoperative physical exam includes palpation of the abdomen and auscultation of bowel sounds. Patients are asked about the usual pattern and consistency of bowel movements, the date of the last bowel movement, and what, if any, medications they take for their bowels. Abdominal distention and constipation can occur postoperatively as a result of factors such as anesthesia, limited physical mobility, and the use of narcotics for pain. A patient who has an ostomy is asked about any ostomy-specific issues such as skin care and regularity and about the supplies that will be needed during hospitalization. Some surgeries (such as bowel surgery) require a bowel prep prior to surgery. If a bowel prep was ordered, the preoperative nurse must ensure that it was completed and that the patient had good results.

Genitourinary Assessment

Patients are asked about their usual pattern of urinary elimination as well as urinary issues they may be having, such as difficulty starting a stream, difficulty controlling continence of urine, inability to completely empty the bladder, and dysuria (painful urination). Postoperatively, nurses monitor fluid balance by using urinary output. Urinary retention is a postoperative problem that is associated with certain surgeries, such as gynecologic and genitourinary procedures. It is also a problem for patients who have received a spinal anesthetic. Patients with chronic renal failure are asked whether they are anuric (no urine production) and their usual schedule for dialysis. If a patient is on dialysis, the arteriovenous (AV) fistula or graft, if present, is documented and palpated for the presence of a thrill and auscultated for a bruit, which indicates patency. Baseline data are important for interpreting postoperative findings and anticipating potential problems.

Musculoskeletal Assessment

Musculoskeletal assessment is concerned with patients' abilities to move themselves and their extremities. The nurse notes any problems with range of motion, arthritic joints, or mobility restrictions. These data are important to the proper positioning of the patient intraoperatively as well as postoperatively. If a patient uses a prosthetic device, electrocautery grounding pads, which are used in some types of surgery, should be placed away from the site of prosthesis to prevent potential injury to the tissue. Assistive devices (e.g., prostheses, crutches, a walker, a wheelchair) that the patient requires for mobilization need to be available to the patient postoperatively to facilitate early mobilization.

Endocrine Assessment

Patients with diabetes are asked about the frequency of glucose testing and use of oral hypoglycemic agents and insulin. Surgery and anesthesia can affect the regulation of glucose. The physiological and psychological stresses of surgery and illness tend to elevate serum glucose levels, whereas factors such as preoperative restriction of food and fluids tend to lower glucose levels. Therefore, the patient with diabetes should be scheduled for surgery early in the day to limit prolonged fasting. The patient will need frequent monitoring of serum glucose with insulin coverage using a sliding scale. Patients who ordinarily take oral hypoglycemic agents may need the temporary coverage of insulin during periods of stress and illness.

Nutritional Assessment

The nutritional assessment includes a baseline height and weight. The nurse asks specific questions about the patient's appetite, usual diet, food preferences, any recent weight loss or gain, and any problems with chewing or swallowing. The nurse notes signs of poor nutrition including brittle nails and dry, flaky skin. The patient's nutritional status has a profound effect on surgical outcomes. Surgery increases the basal metabolic rate and the need for proteins, vitamins, and calories. Patients who are malnourished with a negative nitrogen balance and deficits of vitamins A, C, and B complex are at risk for experiencing problems with their wound including infection, delayed healing, and dehiscence. A low serum albumin level (less than 3.5 mg/dL) and a low or declining prealbumin level are markers of poor nutrition and are associated with a higher risk of postoperative pulmonary complications (Freebody, 2010). Prealbumin or a transthyretin test is considered a more sensitive marker of nutrition than albumin and correlates with patient outcomes (Freebody, 2010). Postoperatively, a dropping prealbumin alerts the caregiver to a declining nutritional status.

Patients who are morbidly obese face a number of potential postoperative problems. For example, access to the operative site may be difficult, which may prolong the operation and length of time anesthesia is used. Anesthetic agents are absorbed by adipose tissue, prolonging the effects of anesthesia on all body systems in the obese patient. Research shows obesity to be a significant risk factor in the development of postoperative complications (Reedy, 2009). Wound approximation during surgical closure is difficult in obese patients, and decreased tissue vascularity contributes to slower healing. These factors and others such as insulin resistance increase the potential for wound infection, dehiscence, and evisceration in the obese patient.

Integumentary Assessment

The nurse asks the patient about skin sensitivities and problems; observes the condition of the skin for moisture, turgor, and color; and notes any area of injury or breakdown. The nurse should report to the surgeon any skin injury such as rashes, scrapes, or sores at or near the operative site. Because of the increased risk of infection, surgery may be cancelled if there is loss of skin integrity near the proposed surgical incision. The health care provider may also be concerned about the patient's likelihood of developing pressure ulcers during or after surgery. Therefore, many hospitals use a tool or scale to measure the patient's risk of pressure ulcer development. Refer to Chapter 60 for further information about the Braden Scale as well as other skin breakdown assessment data.

Maintaining skin integrity is a priority of care in the operating room. Surgical cleansing materials, surgical tape, electrodes, and other materials have the potential to cause allergic skin reactions. In addition, the grounding pad that is used with electrocautery can cause a burn if improperly placed. Pressure ulcers can develop within 2 to 3 hours of unrelieved pressure (Nicoladis, 2011). Preoperative risk factors for development of skin breakdown include older age; the presence of comorbidities such as diabetes, hypertension, and vascular disorders; poor nutritional status; and low hemoglobin and hematocrit levels (Allen, 2009). Chronic steroid use is also a risk factor for skin breakdown; therefore, paper tape may need to be used on these patients.

Psychosocial Assessment

Surgery is a stressful life event for patients and their significant others. Among the reported sources of anxiety are fears of the unknown, of death, of mutilation, of disability and loss of independence, of loss of sexuality, of waking up during the surgery, of pain, of separation from family, and of the financial impact. The nurse asks open-ended questions to elicit the patient's concerns about surgery and anesthesia. The nurse also assesses the patient for physiological indicators of stress and anxiety including crying, restlessness, tachycardia, tachypnea, diaphoresis, complaints of inability to sleep, stomach upset, nausea, and diarrhea. Numeric rating scales of anxiety, similar to those used to rate pain, are an effective, easy, and valid way to measure anxiety (Rosen, 2008). Patients' level of stress will influence their ability to listen and absorb perioperative instruction. It can also affect their response to anesthesia and pain medication and their ability to comply with postoperative care. Patients who are highly anxious about surgery may benefit from receiving preoperative medication with an antianxiety agent. A meta-analysis of 16 studies conducted in 2003 in which medication for anxiety was used preoperatively showed that using an antianxiety agent did not slow down the time frame for postoperative ambulation or discharge from the postanesthesia care unit (Walker, Smithy, & Pittaway, 2003).

The nurse asks about patients' support systems including family (traditional and nontraditional), friends, and other sources of support such as neighbors and religious affiliations. Patients are also asked whether there are spiritual or cultural rituals or traditions that they would like to maintain during their hospitalization. The nurse must be sensitive to the view that the hospital culture, such as its routines and food, may be alien to some patients. All cultures hold beliefs about health, illness, and healing. Culturally competent nurses support and build positive cultural health care practices. The Cultural Considerations box identifies cultural and ethnic concerns for the perioperative nurse.

Diagnostic Tests

Laboratory tests are not required for routine, non-high-risk surgical procedures unless there is a specific reason for performing the test (ICSI, 2010). Nevertheless, many patients have preoperative laboratory testing as part of a routine examination. Some hospitals require a complete blood count on all patients over a certain age, usually 55 years old. Generally, a hematocrit and hemoglobin, as well as a urine pregnancy test, are performed on all menstruating females. A patient may have a specific indication for performing a laboratory test. For example, a patient taking digoxin (Lanoxin) or a diuretic may need to have the potassium level checked. When laboratory tests are indicated, they should be performed within 30 days before the planned procedure; many surgeons prefer laboratory tests to be performed within the 1 to 2 weeks prior to surgery. If the health care provider anticipates the need for a blood transfusion, a blood type and crossmatch test of the patient's blood will be processed at the facility where the surgery will be performed.

Preoperative diagnostic studies depend on the patient and the surgery to be performed. These studies are determined by factors such as the reason the surgery is being done, the patient's overall health, the surgeon's preference, and any significant past medical history. In addition to any studies that are performed as part of the work-up of the patient's health problem, a chest x-ray, an electrocardiogram, and pulmonary function tests may be part of the preoperative tests for certain patients. A preoperative chest x-ray is not required for routine, low- to moderate-risk surgery but may be performed on patients who are older or who have a history of respiratory or cardiac disease. Similarly, pulmonary function tests are done preoperatively only if there is a specific indication, such as in a patient with severe asthma, a patient with chronic obstructive pulmonary disease, or a patient scheduled for removal of lung tissue (e.g., lobectomy, pneumonectomy). Electrocardiograms are recommended for all preoperative patients who are 55 years or older or in younger patients who have a specific indication (ICSI, 2010). Common preoperative diagnostic and laboratory tests and rationales are presented in the Diagnostic Tests box (p. 424).

CULTURAL CONSIDERATIONS
for Perioperative Nurses

If a patient does not speak English and the nurse does not speak the patient's primary language, the nurse should schedule an interpreter to assist with the assessment and teaching rather than relying on the patient's family member or significant other. The interpreter should be of the same gender as the patient, and the nurse should speak directly to the patient regardless of the interpreter's presence.

Certain culturally held beliefs will affect preparations for surgery. For example, in some cultures, an amulet may be worn to ward off evil or bad spirits. When possible, patients should be allowed to wear the amulet into the operating room. If the amulet needs to be removed, the nurse should remove it after induction of anesthesia and replace it as soon as the surgery is complete. In some cultures or religions (e.g., East Indian, Sikh), there are prohibitions against shaving body hair. In these situations, the nurse will need to work with the patient to determine an alternative method to prepare the surgical site.

Surgery and anesthesia may be viewed as harbingers of death in some cultures (e.g., Roma). The nurse should allow family members to stay with the patient as long as possible in the preoperative area and teach the patient and family about the surgical procedure to reduce anxiety.

The nurse should individualize the preoperative teaching. In some cultures, preoperative teaching is not a routine part of preoperative care and can actually increase the patient's anxiety level. The nurse should find out what kind of information and how much information the patient wants and tailor the teaching to meet the patient's needs.

Source: Adapted from Engebretson, J., Mahoney, J., & Carlson, E. D. (2008). Cultural competence in the era of evidence-based practice. *Journal of Professional Nursing, 24*(3), 172–178.

Nursing Management

Assessment

The nursing management of the perioperative patient involves patient education, assessing the patient's and the family's understanding of the operative procedure, and postoperative care. An important part of the preoperative assessment is the physical examination and functional assessment. During this assessment, the nurse documents the patient's baseline physical findings such as vital signs and mental status, as well as the patient's baseline functional ability. Components of this assessment include a neurological assessment, cardiovascular assessment, respiratory assessment, gastrointestinal assessment, genitourinary assessment, musculoskeletal assessment, endocrine assessment, nutritional assessment, integumentary assessment, and psychosocial assessment. Each of these components is discussed in depth in the Physical and Functional Assessment section of this chapter. Chapter 6 includes an in-depth health assessment.

Weblink: ICSI: Preoperative Evaluation

DIAGNOSTIC AND LABORATORY TESTS
Commonly Performed Preoperatively

Test, Normal Values, and Rationale for Abnormality	Expected Abnormality
Complete Blood Count	
Hemoglobin *Adult:* Male: 13.5–18 g/dL Female: 12–15 g/dL	Preoperative anemia could indicate blood loss and impair wound healing. A blood transfusion may be needed before surgery.
White blood cells total (WBC) *Adult:* 4,500–10,000 μL (mm^3) White blood cell differential Neutrophils *Adult:* 50–70 Segments: *Adult:* 50–65 Bands: *Adults:* 0–5	Provides information on the patient's immune status. Check for preoperative infection or inflammation. Preexisting infections, even those distant to the site of the operation, increase the risk of surgical site infection.
Platelet count *Adult:* 150,000–400,000 μL	Platelets promote coagulation. If the platelet count is low, the patient may be at risk for bleeding. Medications that affect platelets may need to be adjusted before surgery.
Serum electrolyte levels Sodium *Adult:* 135–145 mEq/L Potassium *Adult:* 3.5–5.3 mEq/L	Electrolyte imbalances, especially potassium, are corrected prior to surgery to prevent the potential for cardiac arrhythmias during the surgical procedure.
Glucose (Blood) *Adult:* 70–110 mg/dL	Low glucose can cause an altered level of consciousness and impair physiological processes. High glucose can impair wound healing.
Blood Urea Nitrogen (BUN): *Adult:* 5–25 mg/dL	Can be slightly higher in older adults.

Nursing Diagnoses

Nursing diagnoses will emerge from the preoperative assessment. Common diagnoses in the preoperative patient include the following:

- *Deficient Knowledge* related to the operative procedure
- *Anxiety* related to the operative process
- *Pain, Acute* related to the operative procedure and the recovery process
- *Risk for Perioperative Positioning Injury* related to the position in which the patient must be placed in order to perform the operative procedure
- *Ineffective Thermoregulation*
- *Impaired Home Maintenance* related to lack of knowledge about the effects of the operative procedure and the time needed to recover from surgery.

NANDA-I © 2012

Planning

Patient education decreases anxiety and increases the patient's participation in care. The patient should always be informed about what is going to happen before, during, and after the surgery. Before the procedure, the patient should be informed of the procedure's risks, its expected duration, and that repositioning may be required. Planning for interventions for the perioperative patient is multifaceted.

Outcomes and Evaluation Parameters

Outcomes for the perioperative patient include the following:

- The patient will demonstrate knowledge related to his surgery, preoperative preparation, and postoperative exercises such as coughing and deep breathing.
- The patient will verbalize decreased or tolerable levels of anxiety.
- The patient will report an acceptable level of pain.
- The patient will remain safe from perioperative injury.
- The patient will maintain a normal body temperature throughout surgery.
- The patient will demonstrate an understanding of discharge instructions.

Interventions and Rationales

Preoperative teaching is an important role of the perioperative nurse. The overall goal of preoperative teaching is to best prepare the patient for surgery, postoperative care, and discharge, as well as protect the patient's safety. Preoperative teaching has also been found to be important in pain management related to surgery. A study that identifies this is discussed in the Evidence-Based Practice box. Depending on where and how teaching is conducted, it serves the purposes of clarifying a patient's preoperative concerns, reducing the patient's anxiety about the perioperative experience, increasing the patient's compliance with perioperative care, decreasing patient-controlled risk factors of postoperative complications, and increasing the patient's satisfaction with nursing and with the surgical experience.

A preoperative patient needs information about the surgery and surgical routines, home preparation for the surgery, what to expect postoperatively, and preoperative exercises, such as coughing, deep breathing, and incentive spirometry, to prevent postoperative complications. Many operations are scheduled as a same-day procedure, so an easy way to start the teaching is to discuss some of the logistics that surround surgery. The nurse should provide the patient with information about transportation to the hospital, where to park a car, the cost of parking, what to wear, when to arrive at the hospital, where to report, where significant others may wait during the procedure, and how hospital personnel will communicate with significant others during and after the surgery. Many hospitals are instituting surgical liaison programs to facilitate ongoing communication and support for family members and significant others who are waiting for the patient during the surgical procedure. It has been shown that providing the family with updates on the patient's progress during surgery and early in the recovery period results in better coping and problem-solving skills and reduced anxiety in family members (Paull et al., 2010; Pritchard, 2011).

Similarly, there is a trend to allow, and even encourage, family members and significant others to visit the patient in the postanesthesia care unit (PACU), which can reduce anxiety for the family and provide comfort and support to the patient. Studies report that the presence of others during the perioperative period provides patients with a sense of comfort, safety, and control (DeWitt & Albert, 2010). Hospitals that have adopted PACU visitation often have an information sheet that instructs family and significant others about the experience (e.g., keep the visit short, no cell phones, respect the privacy of other patients, comply with requests to leave) (Dewitt & Albert, 2010). Patients who will be discharged home rather than admitted to the hospital are not

EVIDENCE-BASED PRACTICE The Benefit of Preoperative Patient Teaching for Pain

Clinical Problem

Patients who are about to undergo a surgical procedure have been found to be very concerned about pain and pain management (Kastanias, Denny, Robinson, Sabo, & Smith, 2009). At issue is what information patients want and whether nurses are providing this information as part of their preoperative teaching.

Research Findings

A study conducted by Kastanias et al. (2009) set out to identify what patients want to know about pain and pain management related to a surgical procedure. This study used a convenience sample of 150 patients who had undergone specific surgical procedures that would cause acute postoperative pain. The procedures included eye, knee, shoulder, wrist, and ankle arthroscopy, as well as hernia repair. The patients were surveyed by phone 72 hours after the procedure. There was a 74% response rate. The patients were asked to answer questions from the *Information Needs Questionnaire—Pain and Pain Management* tool. This tool consisted of 19 questions that were rated on a 10-point Likert scale. The weight of the answers ranged from 1 = not important to 10 = extremely important. The study found that many of the patients said that the preoperative teaching that they received did not provide adequate information about expectations of pain experience and severity, pain medication information, timing of the discharge instructions, anesthesia, functionality/activity, and the meaning of pain. Interestingly, many patients wanted more information about alternative methods of pain management.

Implications for Nursing Practice

These findings suggest that perioperative instructions related to pain management need to contain more information about the pathophysiology of pain or why pain occurs. Patients also want to know whether pain medications can cause addiction and whether there are other methods of managing pain besides medications. The research findings emphasize how important it is for the nurse to take the time to discuss pain and pain management with patients and their families. It also demonstrates the need to discuss other means to manage pain that may provide some pain relief but do not fully assist in the patient's recovery.

Critical Thinking Questions with answers can be found in the Osborn Student Resources at nursing.pearsonhighered.com.

Reference

Kastanias, P., Denny, K., Robinson, S., Sabo, K., & Snaith, K. (2009). What do adult surgical patients really want to know about pain management? *Pain Management Nursing, 10,* 22–31.

allowed to drive after the procedure and must be transported home by a responsible adult.

Preoperative education is shown to decrease preoperative anxiety, but it may also create worries, perhaps more so in individuals who feel healthy but are scheduled for major elective procedures. This highlights the need to individualize teaching. Preoperative education can improve patient outcomes (DeWitt & Albert, 2010; Paull et al., 2010; Pritchard, 2011; Swart & Houghton, 2010). A study conducted in 2003, which is still considered applicable, concluded that preoperative teaching and support can be categorized into five dimensions (Bernier, Sanares, Owen, & Newhouse, 2003):

- Situational and procedural information refers to teaching about the surgery and anesthesia.
- Sensation and discomfort information refers to teaching about what the patient can expect to see, hear, or feel.
- Patient role information refers to teaching patients how to participate in their own care.
- Skills training information refers to teaching about specific skills to be used postoperatively, such as how to get out of bed with less pain or how to use the incentive spirometer.
- Psychosocial support refers to interactions aimed at alleviating fears and anxieties.

Patient teaching is accomplished in several ways. Many hospitals schedule a preoperative appointment days or weeks before the surgery for the purpose of conducting preoperative assessment and patient education. It is increasingly common for patients to receive written instructions either at the time of the appointment or mailed to their home that reinforce important aspects of care. Some hospitals and surgical centers use videotapes or DVDs that explain the surgical procedure, as well as preoperative and postoperative care. Telephone interviews also are used for preoperative assessment, teaching, and follow up after discharge. Depending on the circumstances surrounding the surgery, preoperative teaching may be done at the patient's bedside the night before surgery if the patient is an inpatient or on the morning of the surgery if the patient is an outpatient.

Preoperative teaching is best accomplished in a calm, quiet, and private environment that facilitates discussion and questions and reduces the patient's anxiety or embarrassment. The nurse needs to be sensitive to the patient's level of anxiety, to the patient's ability to understand instructions and express herself, and to cultural issues. See the Cultural Considerations box on page 423.

Written instructions are important in reinforcing teaching and serving as a reference. When written instructions are given to patients, the instructions should not use medical jargon, should be written at a level that is easy to understand, and should be available in various languages. Before giving written instructions, the nurse must assess whether or not the patient is literate in English or in another language.

Health Promotion

Patients need to be prepared for how they will feel and how things will progress postoperatively. The patient should receive information about the surgery, including what will be done during the surgery, what the surgery will accomplish, where the incision(s) will be located, the anticipated length of the procedure, and the expected recovery trajectory. It is important that nurses give patients an honest, realistic view of the surgery without creating heightened anxiety. Patients need to know that their initial recovery from anesthesia occurs in a PACU where they will be monitored frequently until they are stable enough to be transferred to a surgical unit, or home in the case of outpatient procedures. If a patient is expected to go to an intensive care unit following the surgical procedure, the patient needs to know the routines of intensive care and the length of the anticipated stay.

It is important for the nurse to prepare the patient and family for any tubes, drains, devices, or attachments that may be present postoperatively. Some of these devices have alarms that can be frightening unless the patient is expecting them. In the PACU, the patient will have an intravenous catheter and intravenous fluid and will be attached to a cardiac monitor, blood pressure cuff, and pulse oximeter. Many patients will also have a urinary catheter to accurately measure postoperative urinary output and pneumatic compression boots or an alternative device to reduce the risk of deep venous thrombosis. Depending on the type of surgery performed, the patient may have a nasogastric tube for abdominal decompression, wound drains (e.g., Jackson-Pratt, Anderson sump, Hemovac), other drainage devices (e.g., chest tube, biliary tube, gastrostomy tube), or devices for pain control (e.g., PCA pump or epidural catheter).

Patients who are having orthopedic surgery may have equipment such as traction, continuous motion devices, or joint immobilizers. Patients should be prepared for postoperative routines so that they do not become excessively anxious with frequent assessments, measuring of vital signs, and observation and manipulation of the accompanying equipment and devices. Teaching is an important piece of health promotion and must be individualized for the patient and the surgery being performed.

Preoperative Teaching to Prevent Postoperative Complications

Fasting is implemented for patients who will have general anesthesia, regional anesthesia, or conscious sedation. Patients are instructed to abstain from food and fluids before the operation; the primary purpose of this restriction is to reduce the risk of pulmonary aspiration of stomach contents associated with anesthesia. Traditionally, patients were told to take nothing by mouth (NPO) after midnight on the night preceding surgery, but the American Society of Anesthesiologists' (ASA) 1999 guidelines loosened these requirements because the evidence showed that pulmonary aspiration rarely occurs with modern anesthesia (ASA, 2011b). Current guidelines recommend that patients abstain from solid food for 6 or more hours before procedures and from clear liquids for 2 or more hours. Clear liquids (nonparticulate fluids without fat) include water, fruit juices, carbonated drinks, broth, coffee, and tea (without cream or milk). No fried or fatty foods should be eaten for at least 8 hours before the procedure. The new standards allow individualization of fasting instructions so that a patient who is scheduled for an afternoon procedure need not fast excessively before the procedure. Patients with known delay in gastric emptying should be assessed on an individual basis and may require longer fasting periods (ASA, 2011b). On the day of surgery, patients are asked about the last time that they ate or drank. Surgery may need to be delayed or canceled if a patient has not complied with fasting requirements.

Patients may be given other instructions to follow at home prior to the surgery. For example, patients who smoke cigarettes are instructed to stop smoking 12 hours before surgery (Nagelhout & Plaus, 2010). Patients should also be advised to stop taking any herbal remedies 2 to 3 weeks before surgery because of the uncertain effect of herbs on anesthesia and, in some cases, on blood clotting. It is usually acceptable for patients to take their regular oral medications with a small amount of water, but not more than 150 mL, on the morning of surgery, but patients should check with the surgeon and the anesthesiologist.

Medications that interfere with blood clotting, such as heparin, enoxaparin, warfarin, clopidogrel, aspirin, and vitamin E, are usually stopped before surgery, although the time frame for stopping will vary according to the drug taken, the surgical procedure, the reason the drug is being taken, and laboratory tests. Some experts recommend stopping warfarin 5 to 6 days before surgery depending on the patient's INR (international normalized ratio), stopping enoxaparin 12 to 18 hours before procedures, and stopping heparin 6 to 8 hours before an operation. Some patients may need to be admitted to the hospital 2 to 3 days in advance to make a safe transition from warfarin to heparin in the preoperative period. Time frames for stopping anticoagulation are under investigation. A recent study of 80 patients taking enoxaparin found markedly elevated levels of anti-Xa heparin (a marker of anticoagulation activity) 14 hours after the last dose (O'Donnell et al., 2007). The finding suggests that stopping enoxaparin the evening before surgery might not allow enough time to minimize the risk of surgical bleeding.

Patients who take insulin need to check with their doctor about proper preoperative dosage. It has been recommended that short acting insulin not be used the morning of surgery. Oral hypoglycemic agents may require adjustment as well. The diabetic patient requires special and individualized care during surgery. The nurse needs to be aware of what each diabetic patient may require and prepare the patient appropriately in collaboration with the patient's surgeon and anesthesiology care provider (Ead, 2009).

Safety Alert *The nurse needs to document all diabetic medications taken in the 24 hours prior to surgery.*

Before the procedure, patients will receive surgery-specific instructions to follow at home. For example, patients who are scheduled for colorectal surgery may be asked to follow a special diet, take a laxative, and administer an enema on the night before and morning of surgery to empty the bowel of stool and reduce microorganisms (ASPAN, 2010). Patients who are scheduled for major surgery that reduces mobility and requires inpatient recovery should be taught breathing exercises, how to splint the incision, coughing (to help clear airways), leg exercises, and the importance of postoperative ambulation. The patient may also benefit from the use of an alternative therapy, such as the mind–body practice of eliciting the relaxation response, as discussed in the Complementary & Alternative Therapies box.

Breathing Exercises

Deep breathing is taught as an intervention to decrease the risk of the postoperative pulmonary complications of hypoxemia, atelectasis, and pneumonia. To perform deep breathing, the patient breathes out normally, then takes a deep breath through the nose or mouth, holds the inspiration to the count of three or longer, and slowly releases the breath. Postoperatively, the patient is asked to take 5 to 10 deep breaths every hour.

Deep breathing can also be used as a technique to reduce pain when moving. By encouraging the patient to focus on taking continuous deep breaths while moving or changing positions, the nurse may help to prevent the patient from tensing his muscles, which tends to worsen postoperative pain. One study found that patients who had received videotape instruction on how to use breathing and imagery while performing postoperative activities reported significantly less pain, more mobility, and more independent mobility than patients who had not received the instruction (Ong, 2009).

Incentive Spirometry

The use of incentive spirometry (IS) as a mechanism to encourage deep breathing is widespread. An incentive spirometer is a device that is activated by the patient's inspiratory effort. Incentive spirometers come in many different models, but there are two basic types: flow oriented and volume oriented. To operate the IS, the patient takes a deep breath, which causes a plate or a ball to rise upward in a calibrated cylinder. The cylinder displays either the inspired volume (a volume-oriented incentive spirometer) or the generated flow (a flow-oriented incentive spirometer). Currently, there is limited evidence to support the theory that IS reduces pulmonary complications in the postoperative patient. However, it is still widely used, and more research is needed before this common practice is stopped (Guimaraes, 2010).

COMPLEMENTARY & ALTERNATIVE THERAPIES Relaxation Response

Nancy Yilk

Description

MORE THAN 30% OF AMERICAN ADULTS use mind–body practices that elicit the relaxation response (RR). Although the mechanisms that mediate the RR remain unknown, it counteracts the effects of stress (Bailey, 2010; Halm, 2009). RR is an integrated psychophysiological response that originates in the hypothalamus and is the direct opposite of the stress response. It leads to a generalized decrease in central nervous system arousal. The RR is a hypometabolic state that can be useful in many situations. The patient who activates the RR can use the body's own innate mechanisms to calm and slow down. The RR can occur through the repetition of a word or short phrase. The patient can return to this gentle repetition whenever distracting thoughts occur. This technique triggers a series of physiological changes (slower breathing, heart rate, blood pressure, etc.) that reduce stress.

The pre- and perioperative areas are excellent settings in which to instruct the patient in various RR techniques, such as how to slow down, focus on breathing techniques, and repeat a simple relaxing phrase. The nurse can utilize this technique at the bedside or in the perioperative area prior to anesthesia. A good place for the nurse to begin is to instruct the patient to breathe in through the nose, out through the mouth, and "focus on my voice." The nurse should practice this technique often to help in its delivery. This technique is also used as a preliminary step in many other CAM therapies.

Research Support

Hart (2009) wrote a review paper that described the different types of methods that may be used to reduce discomfort and decrease stress for patients who are undergoing surgery. In this paper, Hart presents research that supports the use of guided imagery, music therapy, massage therapy, and hypnosis. Guided imagery was found to reduce pre- and postoperative anxiety, postoperative pain, and the need for additional opioid medication (Hart, 2009). Music, along with resting in bed after cardiac surgery, was found in one study to reduce stress. A group of 58 patients who had undergone coronary bypass surgery were evaluated for stress by measuring their serum cortisol level, heart rate, respiratory rate, mean arterial pressure, arterial oxygen tension and saturation, and subjective pain and anxiety level. The patients received 30 minutes of bed rest with uninterrupted music and then 30 minutes of bed rest or, alternatively, 60 minutes of bed rest. The patients who received 30 minutes of bed rest and 30 minutes of uninterrupted music demonstrated a decrease in cortisol levels (Nilsson, 2009). Bailey (2010) also wrote a review paper that identified multiple therapies to decrease anxiety in the perioperative patient. These therapies also included research that found music therapy reduced anxiety. Alternative therapies can provide methods to decrease anxiety for patients who are undergoing surgery.

References

Bailey, L. (2010). Strategies for decreasing patient anxiety in the perioperative setting. *AORN Journal, 92*, 445–460.

Halm, M. (2009). Relaxation: A self-care healing modality reduces harmful effects of anxiety. *American Journal of Critical Care, 18*, 169–172.

Hart, J. (2009). Complementary therapies before and after surgery. *Alternative and Complementary Therapies, 15*, 184–188.

Nilsson, U. (2009). The effect of music interventions in stress response to cardiac surgery in a randomized clinical trial. *Heart & Lung, 38*, 201–207.

Splinting the Incision

Patients with thoracic or abdominal incisions can be taught preoperatively how to splint the incision to prevent painful stress on the area. The patient can use a small flat pillow or a small folded blanket, sometimes referred to as a "cough pillow," to apply gentle, firm pressure over the incision when performing activities that tend to pull the incision, such as getting out of bed, getting up from a chair, or coughing. Splinting the incision is helpful in reducing pain.

Coughing

Postoperative patients have an increase in mucus production and a decreased ability to clear mucus from the airways as a result of anesthesia (Ong, 2009). Retained mucus places patients at risk for the development of atelectasis and pneumonia. Coughing can help to clear mucus from the airways and facilitate full expansion of the lungs because it requires an increase in intrathoracic pressure and a rapid expiratory flow (Ong, 2009). Coughing can be quite painful for some patients because of the stress it places on the suture line. Splinting the incision will help protect the suture and reduce some of the pain that occurs with movement of the incisional area. Coughing may be contraindicated after some surgeries because of the stress it puts on the incision (e.g., hernia) or because it increases intracranial pressure (e.g., craniotomy). Generally, a health care provider's order will be written to avoid coughing for surgical procedures for which it is contraindicated.

Leg Exercises

Guidelines on prevention of venous thromboembolism recommend that a risk assessment be performed on all surgical patients (Meguid, 2011; Recommended Practices, 2011). Most patients receive some form of prophylaxis against the development of deep vein thrombosis (i.e., venous blood clot in the leg) postoperatively. Leg exercises are a simple way of stimulating venous return in the patient with limited mobility. They are used in addition to other devices to prevent venous stasis. Deep vein thrombosis is discussed in detail in Chapter 35.

Several types of leg exercises can be performed. The exercises should be done on each leg and should be repeated several times before moving to the next exercise. Descriptions of various leg exercises follow:

- Alternate between flexing the foot and dorsiflexing the foot.
- Lift the foot off the bed and make circles with the ankle several times.
- Bend the knee and lift the leg off of the bed, holding the position for a few seconds.
- With the knees bent, push the ball of the foot into the bed or floor, contracting the calf and thigh muscles.

Ambulation and Mobility

Early ambulation is beneficial to the postoperative patient for a number of reasons. Ambulation increases the heart rate and cardiac output and stimulates circulation to all body systems. The increase in circulation helps to rid the body of the effects of anesthesia. Ambulation increases the respiratory rate and minute ventilation, and it helps to mobilize respiratory secretions. Increased circulation to the intestinal tract helps to stimulate peristalsis, and increased blood flow through the kidneys stimulates the production of urine. In addition, blood flow to the skin and muscles brings nutrients needed for wound healing. Ambulation stimulates calf muscles and increases venous return. Frequent ambulation, a minimum of three times per day, may help prevent some of the complications associated with immobility. Patients need to understand the importance of walking after an operation and be shown effective ways of getting out of bed postoperatively. If a patient cannot walk, alternative methods of mobility should be considered including dangling at the bedside or sitting up in a chair.

Weblink: Sample Informed Consent Forms **Weblink:** Preoperative Checklist

Legal Preparation and Ethical Considerations

Informed Consent

The patient must sign an informed consent form prior to surgery. The informed consent protects all parties involved: the patient, the surgeon, and the hospital. In order for the consent to be valid, there must be full disclosure of the treatment to be performed, the patient must sufficiently understand the information provided (i.e., must be competent), and the patient must voluntarily consent to the treatment. Full disclosure includes a description of the condition requiring surgery, the surgical procedure, the possible risks and benefits, alternative treatments, and prognosis. The surgeon is responsible for discussing the procedure with the patient and securing an informed consent. If a patient is unable to sign, an "X" is an acceptable substitute provided that there are two witnesses. Consent is voluntary and can be withdrawn at any time. The surgical consent form also may include additional consents such as consent for a blood transfusion and for the disposal of body tissues. The nurse's role in the process is to clarify information for the patient and advocate for the patient as needed.

If the patient is unable to participate in informed consent (e.g., an unconscious or incompetent patient), the consent is obtained from the person legally responsible for the patient. This person might be the patient's health care proxy, the next of kin, or a court-appointed legal guardian. In emergencies, telephone consent is acceptable. In cases of extreme emergency in which the legally responsible person is not available and delaying the operation might result in death or serious impairment, the medical emergency overrides the need for consent and the surgery proceeds without consent. In such circumstances, hospitals have set protocols for documenting in the patient's chart the gravity of the situation and the nature of the emergency.

Frequently, the consent for anesthesia is a separate process performed by the anesthesia care provider. The patient receives information about the type of anesthesia planned and the possible risks associated with it. Samples of informed consent forms can be seen at www.thedoctors.com. Chapter 2 provides a complete description of informed consent.

Resuscitation Orders

It is not unusual for a patient with a do-not-resuscitate (DNR) order to require surgery. Surgery might be done for palliative reasons (e.g., to decrease pain associated with tumor growth), to facilitate care (e.g., the insertion of a feeding tube), or to improve quality of life. Some older patients, even those who are in reasonably good health, may request a DNR order in case of an untoward event, even though the surgery to be performed is elective. In the past, DNR orders were suspended for the length of the surgery and early postoperative period.

Professional organizations of surgeons, anesthesiologists, and perioperative nurses have challenged the routine suspension of DNR orders (AORN, 2011; ASA, 2011a). The position of the AORN is that a patient's autonomy should be respected in the operating room and therefore DNR orders should not be routinely suspended for surgery. Instead, AORN recommends that there be a required reconsideration of the DNR order with the scheduling of surgery. The patient is given the opportunity to consider the consequences of withholding resuscitation efforts during surgery and what, if any, resuscitation efforts she might want performed. The decision whether to have a DNR order ultimately falls to the patient and must be clearly documented in the record. If the patient decides to suspend a DNR order intraoperatively, then the point at which the DNR is to be reinstituted needs to be clearly stated.

Common Routines and Medications

Preoperative care and routines are designed to protect the safety of patients and to minimize the likelihood of postoperative complications. Surgical preparation may include bowel preparation, skin preparation, and hair removal. Bowel preparation is usually ordered for major abdominal surgery of the colon or rectum. The goal of preoperative bowel cleansing is to clear the intestine of feces and to decrease intestinal bacteria. This preparation is thought to reduce the risk of contamination of the operative site with stool. Bowel preparation also may include the administration of oral antibiotics (e.g., neomycin and erythromycin or metronidazole). Bowel preparation is a time-consuming and exhausting process, and it can contribute to preoperative dehydration in older patients.

Skin preparation may require the patient to shower the night before surgery or the morning of surgery with an antiseptic solution (e.g., 2% chlorhexidine gluconate). Hair removal prior to surgery is a controversial practice. If hair is to be removed for an operation, the CDC recommends using sterile supplies, clipping rather than shaving, clipping in the direction of hair growth, and performing the procedure as close to the time of surgery as possible (Allen, 2009). Figure 17–1 ◆ shows the areas of skin preparation for common surgical sites.

Preoperative Medications

Preoperative medications refer to those that are given specifically in preparation for surgery. It is increasingly common for preoperative medications to be given in the **holding area** (a place where patients await surgery) of the surgical suite immediately prior to the operation.

Antianxiety agents are often given to relax the patient. Prophylactic antibiotics are given in many, but not all, surgical cases. Antibiotics are frequently given intravenously in the surgical holding area or at induction of anesthesia. Antibiotics should be administered on the basis of evidence and the institution's policy and procedure. Other preoperative medications that may be given include gastrointestinal stimulants, gastric acid blockers for gastric ulcer prophylaxis, and antiemetics to decrease nausea and vomiting. However, these medications are not recommended for the purpose of decreasing risk of pulmonary aspiration (ASA, 2011b). Beta-adrenergic blockers are given to patients prior to cardiac surgery to reduce the incidence of postoperative atrial fibrillation. Beta-adrenergic blocker therapy may also be given to high-risk cardiac patients or to those undergoing vascular procedures to reduce the risk of perioperative cardiovascular complications (ASPAN, 2010). Currently, it is recommended that beta-adrenergic blocker therapy be started days to weeks before elective surgery, although the ideal dose, drug, and timing have not been established.

Preoperative Checklist

Most hospitals use preoperative checklists to ensure and document the patient's readiness for surgery. A sample of a preoperative checklist can be seen at http://www.gwicu.com/Assets/Nursing%20Protocols/PreopNursingChecklist75-041.pdf. The admitting nurse completes the preoperative checklist for a patient who is having same-day admission surgery. If the patient is an inpatient, the clinical nurse caring for the patient completes the checklist. The patient scheduled for surgery is

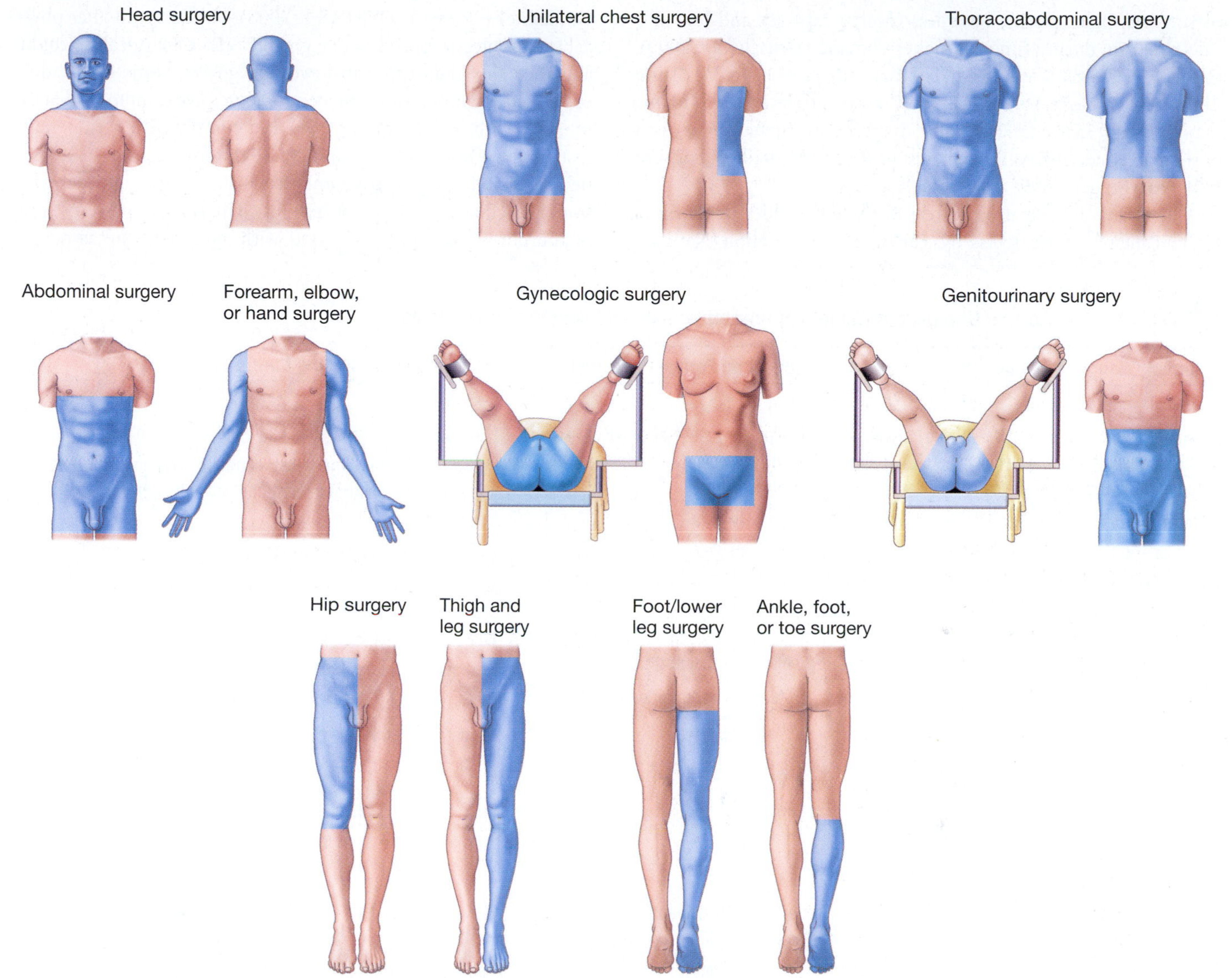

FIGURE 17–1 ◆ Skin preparation for common surgical sites.

identified by using two indicators (e.g., asking the patient his name and date of birth and also checking the wristband). The patient must have a hospital identification wristband in place and an allergy band if applicable. Before sending the patient to the operating room, the nurse ensures that a history and physical (H&P) performed within the past 30 days and signed surgical and anesthesia consents are on file. If the H&P, consent for surgery, or consent for anesthesia form is missing, the nurse contacts the appropriate health care provider. The nurse also checks that the medical record is complete, including recent laboratory tests, diagnostic tests, medication records, intake and output sheets, and vital sign graphic records. The nurse records the patient's physical assessment and a recent set of vital signs. The nurse then notes the medications, both routine and preoperative, that the patient took before surgery. The nurse also directs the patient to void before going to the operating room.

Cosmetics, including nail polish, are commonly removed preoperatively so that skin color and capillary filling can be observed. All jewelry is removed and locked up with other valuables according to the institution's policy. It is particularly important to note on the preoperative checklist where valuables are located to prevent loss. Most facilities allow the patient to wear a wedding band to the operating room if it is taped to the finger, but the patient may want to remove the ring if postoperative swelling is expected (e.g., in a mastectomy with lymph node dissection). Pierced earrings and other body piercings must be removed to prevent accidental burns from electrocautery (DeBoer, Seaver, Videa, Robinson, & Klepaccki, 2011).

All prosthetic devices, including dentures, removable bridges, and contact lenses, are removed prior to surgery. On occasion, the anesthesia care provider may prefer that the patient leave dentures in place to assist in airway maintenance. The presence of dentures in the mouth can assist in creating a tighter seal between the mouth and the oxygen mask. When dentures are removed, they must be labeled and stored safely to prevent loss. Patients may want to wear glasses or hearing aids to the holding area; this is acceptable, although they will be removed before the surgery. Patients are transported with their medical record, including the medication administration record, to the operating room via gurney.

Gerontological Considerations

Age is a major consideration in the nursing management of patients scheduled for surgery. Age-related changes to the body make it less able to respond and adapt to the physiological demands of surgery. Older people have less reserve capacity and less of a safety margin during times of higher demand (Doerflinger, 2009). Also, older people are more likely than others to have coexisting illnesses that increase surgical risk. Heart disease (e.g., angina, hypertension, heart failure, valve disease, and arrhythmias) is a particular concern because it is a significant predictor of surgical risk (Doerflinger, 2009).

Coexisting disease also is likely to place the older patient in a higher category of the ASA's Physical Status Classification (National Guidelines feature, p. 417) (ASA, 2008). Patients in higher physical status categories experience greater rates of surgical morbidity and mortality than those in lower categories. Some older adults experience memory impairment and depressive symptoms that can interfere with their ability to learn and comply with perioperative instruction. Other factors that increase the risk of surgery for older people include preoperative anemia, malnutrition, and dehydration, as well as limitations of mobility. Chart 17-2 presents some of the normal changes associated with aging and the associated

CHART 17–2 Normal Changes of Aging, Perioperative Risk, and Nursing Implications

Normal Changes of Aging	Impact on Perioperative Risk	Implications for Nursing Care
Overall		
Decreased reserve capacity of all body organs, which causes various systems to be overwhelmed during periods of physiological stress	Places the patient at a higher risk for many postoperative problems and complications	Minimize physiological stress as much as possible. Provide adequate oxygen, rest, nutrition, hydration, emotional support, and monitor and correct electrolyte imbalance.
Neurological		
Decreased reserve and increased sensitivity to physiological stressors such as fever and hypoxia Decreased ability to adjust to environmental changes and stimuli Slower reaction times Slower cognitive processes	Potential for acute confusion postoperatively that can take months to resolve Potential for sleep–wake disturbances while in the hospital Potential for knowledge deficit	Assess the patient's mental status every shift. Avoid using medications known to cause changes in mental status in older adults (CNS depressants, H2–receptor antagonists, lidocaine, phenytoin, anticholinergics). Provide for uninterrupted sleep. Avoid unnecessary room or unit changes. Encourage ambulation and participation in activities of daily living (ADLs). If acute confusion develops, look for and treat physiological stressors such as fever, hypoxemia, anemia, pain, and dehydration.
Cardiovascular		
Increased workload of the heart Increased arterial resistance Decreased cardiac output Reduction in the maximum attainable heart rate and cardiac output Decreased peripheral circulation Lowered ability to respond to demands for increased blood, oxygen, and nutrients	Potential for decreased cardiac output Potential for intraoperative cardiac complications Potential for activity intolerance postoperatively	Prevent or treat factors such as anemia that increase cardiac workload. Keep the patient warm to prevent shivering. Apply oxygen to keep oxygen saturation above 93%. Monitor fluid balance to prevent dehydration or fluid overload. Monitor BP, heart rate, oxygen saturation, fatigue, and dyspnea with activity.
Respiratory		
Decreased elasticity of lungs Loss of muscle mass, which weakens muscles of respiration Stiff chest wall, which reduces the ability to expand the lungs Less effective protective mechanisms such as coughing and mucociliary transport	Potential for postoperative pulmonary complications Potential for impaired gas exchange Potential for ineffective airway clearance	Encourage deep breathing postoperatively. Monitor for dyspnea as a sign of ventilatory dysfunction. Control pain but avoid overmedication with narcotics.
Gastrointestinal		
Decreased saliva Loss of teeth and changes in dentition More difficulty with swallowing Decreased peristalsis Decreased blood flow to internal organs	Risk of aspiration Potential for poor nutrition Potential for constipation	Follow aspiration precautions. Make sure dentures are in place when the patient is allowed to eat. Encourage mobility postoperatively to prevent abdominal distention and constipation.

(continued)

Weblink: National Center for Health Statistics

CHART 17–2 Normal Changes of Aging, Perioperative Risk, and Nursing Implications, *continued*

Normal Changes of Aging	Impact on Perioperative Risk	Implications for Nursing Care
Genitourinary		
Decreased renal blood flow Decreased renal function Decreased elasticity of bladder Decreased bladder capacity Enlarged prostate	Risk for impaired renal function postoperatively Risk of fluid and electrolyte imbalances	Monitor intake and output, BUN, and creatinine postoperatively. Ensure adequate hydration. Effects of drugs may be prolonged; choose drugs with short half-lives.
Musculoskeletal		
Loss of bone mass and height Changes in balance and gait Decreased range of motion in joints	Potential for falls	Perform a risk assessment for falls. Assist with ambulation. Use assistive devices as necessary. Perform a physical therapy consultation after surgery. Perform a home safety evaluation at discharge.
Sensory		
Decreased visual acuity and accommodation Decreased ability to adapt to changes in light Hearing loss and change in taste Atypical pain response	Potential for falls Potential for acute confusion Potential for alterations in communication	Make sure that glasses, hearing aids, and dentures are available postoperatively. Assess pain frequently.
Skin		
Slow replacement of epithelial cells Decreased elasticity of skin Loss of subcutaneous tissue Decreased circulation	Potential for tissue injury and pressure ulcers Potential for hypothermia Delayed wound healing and risk of infection	Document preoperative condition of the skin. Keep the patient warm postoperatively. Encourage adequate nutrition. Offer nutritional supplements as necessary.

potential perioperative problems. Chart 17–3 lists the most common surgeries performed on patients age 65 or older as reported by the CDC (2008).

Research

Research is important for improving the care of surgical patients. Advances in technology and changes in surgical technique create the need to research the effects of the change. For example, patients are sent home earlier after surgery than was typical in the past because surgical procedures have become less invasive. What effect does this have on the patient, the family, and the home health agency that now provides the care the patient once received in the hospital? Research is critical to nurses who want to know that the interventions they perform are based on scientific evidence. The Research Opportunities box (p. 432) lists some of the research problems that are important to the care of the preoperative patient. An example of a research study that could have a positive effect on perioperative nursing practice in regard to pain management is described in the Evidence-Based Practice box (p. 425).

CHART 17–3 Common Surgical Procedures in Older Patients

Gender	Common Procedures in Older Patients
Men	Prostatectomy
	Cardiac catheterization
	Coronary bypass
	Pacemaker insertion
	Repair of inguinal hernia
	Digestive system biopsies
	Cataract extraction
Women	Cardiac catheterization
	Reduction of fracture
	Pacemaker insertion
	Digestive system biopsies
	Cholecystectomy
	Cataract extraction

RESEARCH OPPORTUNITIES Related to Preoperative Care

Research Area	Clinical Impact
General Preoperative Teaching	
What is the effect of preoperative education on patients' self-care behaviors postoperatively?	A goal of preoperative education is to increase patients' self-care behaviors and participation in desired postoperative activities.
Is there a difference in knowledge outcomes of preoperative education presented in written versus oral versus video formats?	Provides data for selecting an appropriate format(s) for the presentation of preoperative information.
How does the availability of Internet information on surgical procedures change preoperative education provided by the nurse?	Increased use of the Internet by patients and family members may change the focus of preoperative teaching. It may also affect the type and amount of information desired.
Is there an optimal time for preoperative education?	Provides rationale for scheduling preoperative appointments and for providing written materials to the patient.
What factors (nurse, environment, patient) increase the effectiveness of preoperative education?	Provides background information necessary for understanding the educational process and for creating an effective teaching environment.
Does preoperative education improve patient outcomes postoperatively?	Provides a critical desired outcome of preoperative education programs.
Psychosocial Aspects of Preoperative Care	
How does the timing of preoperative teaching affect patient and family anxiety levels and coping strategies?	Provides information about an optimal time of psychological readiness for preoperative information.
Does family presence in the surgical holding area enhance the well-being of patients and family members?	Provides a rationale for designing a patient- and family-friendly environment for surgery.
How do the communication skills of novice nurses in the preoperative area compare to those of experienced nurses?	Provides a basis for understanding the development of therapeutic communication in nurses.
How does a nurse's skill in communication affect preoperative teaching?	Provides a basis for understanding how specific skills affect the teaching–learning process.
What is the effect of an emergency surgery on the informational needs of patients, families, and significant others?	Provides background information for prioritizing information in specific situations.
Culture	
What interventions can be done to support culturally appropriate care preoperatively?	Provides a rationale for developing a range of culture-specific interventions.
What are the differences across cultures regarding the type and amount of preoperative education desired by patients?	Provides information needed for designing culturally sensitive preoperative teaching plans.
Specific Preoperative Instructions	
What is the optimal time frame to quit smoking prior to surgery?	Provides important information about the time frame necessary to achieve positive outcomes.
Does a preoperative shower using antimicrobial soap decrease the risk of surgical-site infection?	Provides a rationale for a common preoperative instruction.
What are the physiological effects of a "good night's sleep" before surgery on the preoperative patient?	Provides important psychological and physiological information about the patient going into surgery.
Should gender, ethnicity, and body weight make a difference in the instructions for mechanical bowel preparation for surgery?	Provides information about differences in physiological responses that might support individualizing preoperative preparation.
Does the use of a preoperative risk assessment for venous thromboembolism correlate with reduced incidence of deep vein thrombosis postoperatively?	Provides the evidence for a current nursing practice recommendation.
Does specific information about deep vein thrombosis prophylaxis increase patients' compliance with leg exercises, ambulation, and use of intermittent pneumatic compression devices postoperatively?	Provides a rationale for preoperative teaching.

NCLEX® PRACTICE

1. A nurse asks a preoperative patient about the presence of allergies. What is the purpose of this information?

1. This knowledge helps to reduce adverse reactions to medications or to latex.
2. This information is essential in determining the type of anesthesia to be used.
3. The decision regarding the patient's postoperative care area depends upon preoperative assessment.
4. Allergy history is used to ensure correct blood products are available for the patient.

2. A nurse is assessing the cardiovascular status of a preoperative patient and learns of the patient's history of valve disease. Because of this finding, the nurse expects the addition of which intervention to this patient's preoperative care?

1. Addition of a normal saline bolus
2. Addition of intravenous potassium
3. Antibiotic prophylaxis
4. Placement of a temporary pacemaker

3. A 40-year-old patient who is scheduled for a total knee replacement reports using the herbal supplement ginkgo biloba to support memory. Which nursing instruction is correct?

1. "Since you are having memory problems, we will draw an arterial blood gas level preoperatively."
2. "It is recommended that patients stop using all herbal supplements 2 to 3 weeks before elective surgery."
3. "Ginkgo biloba affects blood glucose levels, so a hemoglobin $A1_C$ will be necessary a week prior to your surgery."
4. "You should avoid green leafy vegetables for at least one week prior to your surgery."

4. The nurse is planning preoperative care for an elderly patient. Which intervention is the priority to reduce the risk of pulmonary complications?

1. Encourage deep breathing and coughing.
2. Monitor oxygen saturation.
3. Monitor intake and output.
4. Elevate the head of the patient's bed.

5. During preoperative instruction, the patient states, "I don't want to be cauterized." How should the nurse respond to this statement?

1. "Everyone is cauterized during surgery."
2. "Can you explain to me what you mean by cauterized?"
3. "The surgeon will cauterize in the operating room if it's necessary."
4. "Who said anything about being cauterized?"

6. A preoperative patient tells the nurse that he researched the surgical procedure on the Internet and has no questions at this time. What is the best way for the nurse to respond to this statement?

1. Document that the patient studied the surgical procedure on the Internet.
2. Assess the patient's understanding of the procedure to supplement any areas not reviewed through the Internet.
3. End the preoperative teaching session.
4. Encourage the patient to use the call light in the event he decides he wants to discuss the procedure.

Answers to NCLEX Practice questions can be found in Appendix D in the Osborn Student Resources at nursing.pearsonhighered.com. Practice additional NCLEX questions online at the Student Resources site.

Pearson Nursing Student Resources Find additional review materials at: **nursing.pearsonhighered.com**

REFERENCES

Allen, G. (2009). Intraoperative risk factors for surgical site infection. *AORN Journal, 90*(6), 765–766.

American Society of Anesthesiologists (ASA). (2008). Statement of documentation of anesthesia care. Retrieved from http://www.asahq.org/For-Healthcare-Professionals/Standards-Guidelines-and-Statements.aspx

American Society of Anesthesiologists (ASA). (2010). Basic standards for preanesthesia care. Retrieved from http://www.asahq.org/For-Healthcare-Professionals/Standards-Guidelines-and-Statements.aspx

American Society of Anesthesiologists (ASA). (2011a). Practice advisory for the perioperative management of patients with cardiac implantable electronic devices: Pacemakers and implatable cardioverter-defibrillators. *Anesthesiology, VII4*, 247–261.

American Society of Anesthesiologists (ASA). (2011b). Practice guidelines for preoperative fasting and the use of pharmacologic agents to reduce the risk of pulmonary aspiration: Application to healthy patients undergoing elective procedures. *Anesthesiology, 114*, 495–511.

American Society of PeriAnesthesia Nurses. (2006). ASPAN's evidence-based clinical practice guideline for the prevention and/or management of PONV/PDNV. *Journal of PeriAnesthesia Nursing, 21*(4), 230–250.

American Society of PeriAnesthesia Nurses (ASPAN). (2010). *Standards of perianesthesia nursing practice.* New Jersey: Author.

Anastasi, J., Chang, M., & Capili, B. (2011). Herbal supplements: Talking with your patients. *Journal for Nurse Practitioners, 7*(1), 29–35.

Association of Perioperative Registered Nurses (AORN). (2011). *Perioperative standards and recommended practices 2011 edition.* Denver: Association of Perioperative Registered Nurses.

Babb, M. (2009). Clinical risk assessment: Identifying patients at high risk for heart failure. *Journal of AORN, 89*(2), 273–288.

Bailey, L. (2010). Strategies for decreasing patient anxiety in the perioperative setting. *AORN Journal, 92*(4), 445–460.

Bernier, M., Sanares, D., Owen, S., & Newhouse, P. (2003). Preoperative teaching received and valued in a day surgery setting. *AORN Journal, 77*, 563–582.

Braganza, V. (2009). Delirium in elderly patients with hip fractures. *Journal of Orthopaedic Nursing, 13*(4), 218–219.

Centers for Disease Control and Prevention. (2008). National Center for Health Statistics: Monitoring this nation's health. Retrieved from http://www.cdc.gov/nchs

Clifford, T. (2010). Reevaluation of the PACU patient before discharge. *Journal of Perianesthesia Nursing, 25*(6), 416–417.

DeBoer, S., Seaver, M., Videa, D., Robinson, B., & Klepaccki, J. (2011). Breasts, bellies, below and beyond: Body piercing jewelry and the transfer technique—When in doubt, don't necessarily take it out. *Journal of Emergency Nursing, 37*(6), 541–553.

Dewitt, L., & Albert, N. M. (2010). Preferences for visitation in the PACU. *Journal of Perianesthesia Nursing, 25*(6), 296–301.

Doerflinger, D. M. C. (2009). Older adult surgical patients: Presentation and challenges. *AORN Journal, 90*(2), 223–244.

Ead, H. (2009). Glycemic control and surgery: Optimizing outcomes for the patient with diabetes. *Journal of Perianesthesia Nursing, 24*(6), 384–395.

Engebretson, J., Mahoney, J., & Carlson, E. D. (2008). Cultural competence in the era of evidence-based practice. *Journal of Professional Nursing, 24*(3), 172–178.

Freebody, S. (2010). Implementation of a nutritional assessment tool for patients undergoing surgery. *International Journal of Orthopaedic Nursing, 14*(1), 25–31.

Golembiewski, J. (2008). Beta-blockers in the perioperative setting. *Journal of PeriAnesthesia Nursing, 23*(2),133–136.

Guimaraes, M. M. F. (2010). Incentive spirometry for prevention of postoperative complications in upper abdominal surgery. *Cochrane Database of Systematic Reviews, 4*(01-null-2010).

Halm, M. A. (2009). Relaxation: A self-care healing modality reduces harmful effects of anxiety. *American Journal of Critical Care, 18*(2), 169–172.

Hart, J. (2009). Complementary therapies before and after surgery. *Alternative and Complementary Therapies, 15*, 184–188.

Institute for Clinical Symptoms Improvement (ICSI). (2010). Preoperative evaluation. Retrieved from http://www.icsi.org/preoperative_evaluation/preoperative_evaluation_2328.html

IOM (Institute of Medicine). (2010). *The future of nursing: Leading change, advancing health.* Washington, DC: The Academic Press.

Joy, J. (2009). Nurses: The patient's first and perhaps last line of defense. *AORN Journal, 89*(6), 1133–1136.

Kastanias, P., Denny, K., Robinson, S., Sabo, K., & Snaith, K. (2009). What do adult surgical patients really want to know about pain management? *Pain Management Nursing, 10*(1), 22–31.

Kee, J. L. (2010). *Laboratory and diagnostic tests with nursing implications.* Upper Saddle River, NJ: Pearson.

Lauerman, C. J. (2008). Surgical patient education related to smoking. *AORN Journal, 87*(3), 599–605.

McCallin, A., & Jones, M. (2011). Older adults' recovery from hip fracture: A literature review. *International Journal of Orthopaedics and Trauma Nursing, 1*(7), 18–28.

Meguid, C. (2011). Best practice for deep vein thrombosis prophylaxis. *Journal for Nurse Practitioners, 7*, 582–587.

Murphy, M., Hooper, V., Sullivan, E., Clifford, T., & Apfel, C. (2006). Identification of risk factors for postoperative nausea and vomiting in the perianesthesia adult patient. *Journal of PeriAnesthesia Nursing, 21*(6), 377–384.

Nagelhout. J. J., & Plaus, K. L. (2010). *Nurse anesthesia* (4th ed.). St. Louis: Saunders Elsevier.

National Health Statistics Report. (2010). National hospital discharge survey: 2007 summary. Retrieved from http://www.cdc.gov/nchs/data/nhsr/nhsr029.pdf

Neil, J. (2007). Perioperative care of the immunocompromised patient. *AORN Journal, 85*(3), 544–565.

Nicoladis, C. (2011). A validated tool for the prediction of perioperative pressure ulcers. *Journal of Perianesthesia Nursing, 26*(1), 192.

Nilsson, U. (2009). The effect of music interventions in stress response to cardiac surgery in a randomized clinical trial. *Heart & Lung, 38*(3), 201–207.

O'Donnell, M., Kearon, C., Johnson, J., Robinson, R., Zondag, M., Turpie, I., et al. (2007). Preoperative anticoagulant activity after bridging low-molecular-weight heparin for temporary interruption of warfarin. *Annals of Internal Medicine, 146*(3), 184–187.

Ong, J. (2009). Effect of a preoperative instructional digital video disc on patient knowledge and preparedness for engaging in postoperative care activities. *Nursing Clinics of North America, 44*(1),103–115.

Paull, D. E., Mazzia, L. M., Wood, S. D., Theis, M. S., Robinson, L. D., Carney, B., et al. (2010). Briefing guide study: Perioperative briefing and postoperative debriefing checklists in the Veterans Health Administration medical team training program. *American Journal of Surgery, 5*(5), 620–623.

Pritchard, M. J. (2011). Using targeted information to meet the needs of surgical patients. *Nursing Standards, 25*, 35–39.

Recommended Practices (RP). (2011). RP summary: Recommended practices for prevention of deep vein thrombosis (DVT). *AORN Journal, 94*(5), 455–456.

Rooke, G. A. (2007). Pacemakers. Retrieved from http://www.vaanes.org/FORUMS/pacer.html

Reedy, S. (2009). An evidence-based review of obesity and bariatric surgery. *Journal for Nurse Practitioners, 5*(1), 22–29.

Rosen, S. (2008). Calm or not calm: The question of anxiety in the perianesthesia patient. *Journal of Perianesthesia Nursing, 23*(4), 237–246.

Rowe, D. J., & Baker, A. C. (2009). Perioperative risks and benefits of herbal supplements in aesthetic surgery. *Aesthetic Surgery Journal, 29*(2), 150–157.

Sly-Havey, M. (2009). Using the dementia quick screen to predict post-operative delirium in the total hip and knee replacement. *Journal of Orthopaedic Nursing, 13*(3), 141.

Somes, J., & Donatelli, N. (2011). Strange medication reactions. *Journal of Emergency Nursing, 37*(4), 388–390.

Swart, M., & Houghton, K. (2010). Preoperative preparation: Essential elements for delivered enhanced recovery pathway. *Current Anaesthesia & Critical Care, 21*(3), 142–147.

Walker, K., Smithy, A., & Pittaway, A. (2003). Premedication for anxiety in adult day surgery. *Cochrane Database of Systematic Reviews, 1*(CD002192).

Intraoperative Nursing

18 CHAPTER

Renée Holleran
Leslie Flynn

Outcome-Based Learning Objectives

After studying this chapter, the learner will be able to:

1. Discuss the sequence of events for the patient from the beginning of surgery to arrival in the postanesthesia care unit.
2. Differentiate the roles of the members of the surgical team.
3. Describe the interplay between the team members in bringing about a successful surgical intervention.
4. Prioritize nursing interventions to maximize patient safety in the operating room.
5. Evaluate effective nursing measures for patient advocacy in the operating room.
6. Prioritize the nursing care of patients experiencing selected intraoperative complications.
7. Differentiate the role of the certified nurse and that of the anesthesiologist for the anesthetized patient.

KEY TERMS

Bier block p.446
circulating nurse p.436
conscious sedation p.443
epidural anesthesia p.445
general anesthesia p.443
intraoperative p.437
intrathecal anesthesia p.445
malignant hyperthermia (MH) p.444
peripheral nerve block p.446
regional anesthesia p.445
scrub nurse p.436
spinal anesthesia p.445
surgical conscience p.448

THE GOAL OF PERIOPERATIVE OR INTRAOPERATIVE NURSING PRACTICE (nursing practice that occurs in, before, during, and after the operative procedure) is to assist patients and their families to achieve a level of wellness equal to or greater than the level they had before the procedure (Association of Perioperative Registered Nurses [AORN], Perioperative Nursing Data Set [PNDS-2007], 2011a). The nurse's most important role in this situation is to be a patient advocate. The essence of this advocacy is defined as protection, communication (giving a voice), doing, comfort, and caring.

Advocacy is described as an act of informing and supporting individuals so that they may make the best decisions possible for themselves. Advocacy also involves speaking up for someone who is unable to speak for himself. Advocacy is a critical issue for surgical patients who are unconscious or sedated and unable to make decisions related to their care. Protecting patients from harm is the essence of the nurse's advocacy role; it is a critical component for patients whose family members are not readily accessible and whose only possible advocate is the nurse. This is often the case for the patient having surgery. Advocacy in this situation may include helping patients who are uninformed or have not given adequate consent for surgical procedures, confronting an incompetent colleague, pressing for more analgesia for a patient who is in pain, or supporting the patient's view about prolonging life with extraordinary treatment or technology.

Safety Alert *Surgical patients can be compromised by stress, disease process, and sedation or general anesthesia, and they trust that a nurse will advocate in their best interest to ensure their privacy, dignity, rights, and safety.*

The nurse must accept accountability for nursing actions that safeguard the rights of the surgical patients. Nurses act as patient advocates by protecting them; therefore, they must be able to identify advocacy issues quickly and accurately and be ready to intervene on behalf of their patients (AORN, 2011b).

Guidance for Professional Practice

The term *perioperative* refers to the time around surgery. The practice of perioperative nursing is guided by professional organizations, including AORN, the Centers for Disease Control and Prevention (CDC), and The Joint Commission. AORN defines its mission as follows: "to promote safety and optimal outcomes for patients undergoing operative and other invasive procedures by providing practice support and professional development opportunities to perioperative nurses." AORN membership is composed of registered nurses in the United States and abroad who manage, teach, and practice perioperative nursing, who are enrolled in nursing education, and who are engaged in perioperative research (AORN, 2011a). This professional organization has developed a conceptual framework and vocabulary called the Perioperative Nursing Data Set (PNDS). The PNDS addresses the domains of safety, physiological responses, behavioral responses of the patient and family, and the environment of the perioperative setting within the health system.

The CDC's mission is to promote health and good quality of life by preventing and controlling disease, injury, and disability. It also influences perioperative practice. In 1999, the CDC issued guidelines for the prevention of surgical infection. Additionally, it reflected The Joint Commission's mission statement to continuously improve the safety and quality of care provided to the public through the provision of health care accreditation and related services that support performance improvement in health care organizations (The Joint Commission, 2011). In 2005, The Joint Commission developed The Joint Commission universal protocol to prevent wrong site, wrong procedure, and wrong patient surgeries (Conrardy, Brenek, & Myers, 2010). This protocol is presented later in the chapter. A complete discussion of The Joint Commission and the CDC is provided in Chapter 2.

Weblink: Association of periOperative Registered Nurses (AORN) Mission Statement

Video*: Perioperative: Sterile Field—Gloves, Sterile

Surgical Team

Successful surgery relies on the interplay of many individuals working as a team, complementing each other's skills and responsibilities. This multidisciplinary team includes the surgeon and assistants, the anesthesiologist and assistants, the nursing team, and support staff. Each of these professionals is responsible for specific functions and plays a role in supporting each of the other groups. This overlap of responsibilities ensures the safety of patients while they are in a most vulnerable situation and cannot give any personal input. The roles of each member are described next.

Surgeon and Surgical Team

The surgeon heads the surgical team and is responsible for performing the procedure, coordinating the team, and making decisions related to the surgical procedure. Depending on the procedure, an assistant might be required. This assistant could be another surgeon, a physician, a resident in a university teaching hospital, a physician's assistant, or a registered nurse first assistant (RNFA).

The role of RNFA is an expanded role for perioperative nurses. The RNFA collaborates with the surgeon and performs the role of first assistant during the operation. This role includes handling tissue, providing exposure, using instruments, suturing the wound, and providing hemostasis. The role of an RNFA is highly specialized and demanding. In 2008, with a revision in 2010, AORN approved a policy statement that defines the RNFA role, scope of practice, and qualifications (AORN, 2012). The RNFA must have a certification in perioperative nursing (CNOR); have completed a RFNA program that meets the AORN standards for RN first assistant education programs; and practice within all regulations, statutes, and institutional policies. The policies and scope of practice will vary from state to state (AORN, 2012).

Anesthesia Care Provider

The anesthesiologist is a health care provider who specializes in the administration of anesthetic agents and provides care to alleviate pain and promote relaxation. This professional is responsible for maintaining the airway; monitoring and ensuring gas exchanges, respiration, and circulation; estimating and replacing blood and fluid losses; administering medications to maintain hemodynamic stability; managing care in the event of a physiological crisis; and constantly communicating with the surgical and nursing team. The anesthesiologist heads the anesthesia team and might be assisted by a respiratory therapist, an anesthesia resident or fellow in a university teaching hospital, an anesthesia technologist, or a certified registered nurse anesthetist (CRNA).

The role of CRNA is an expanded role for perioperative nurses. As Chapter 1 discussed, the CRNA is an advance practice nurse who holds a master's degree from an accredited nurse anesthesia educational program. CRNAs administer anesthesia and anesthesia-related care in four general categories: (1) preanesthetic preparation and evaluation; (2) anesthesia induction, maintenance, and emergence; (3) postanesthesia care; and (4) perianesthetic and clinical support functions. The CRNA works under the supervision of the anesthesiologist.

Nurses

The perioperative nurse's primary role in the operating room (OR) is that of the circulating nurse. Most states have taken legislative measures to ensure that, for every surgical procedure in the OR, a registered nurse is present in the circulator role. The circulating nurse's duties are performed outside the sterile field and encompass responsibilities of nursing care management within the OR. The **circulating nurse** observes the surgical team from a broad perspective and assists the team to create and maintain a safe, comfortable environment for surgery. The circulating nurse communicates patient care needs to each member of the surgical team, facilitating a united effort while being the patient's advocate. In that role, the nurse is dedicated to ensuring that the patient's rights and wishes are respected and carried out.

The **scrub nurse** works directly with the surgeon within the sterile field (the area closely surrounding the OR table), passing instruments, sponges, and other items needed during the surgical procedure. Surgical team members who work within the sterile field perform a surgical scrub of their hands and arms with an antimicrobial solution and, in addition to the regular surgical attire, don a sterile gown and gloves. The role of scrub nurse can also be performed by personnel other than an RN, in which case the person is called a scrub technician. Other roles for RNs are team leader, assistant head nurse, head nurse or nurse manager, nurse educator, and clinical nurse specialist, as described in Chapter 1.

As with any specialty, the perioperative nursing assessment is the first step in providing individualized care for perioperative patients. The nursing process serves as a guide to make perioperative nursing assessments comprehensive and holistic in nature. The focus is aimed at promoting and maintaining wellness as well as identifying and preventing illness (Gillespie & Hamlin, 2009; Peterson & Kleiner, 2011). These assessments provide valuable information to the entire perioperative team. The nursing care plans that are developed on the basis of the assessment data are used to ensure continuity of care during each phase of the individual's perioperative experience. The assessment provides a baseline against which information about the individual's stability can be measured and monitored at any stage of the perioperative experience.

Perioperative Nursing Education

Given that most nursing programs offer limited or no operating room experience in their curricula, nurses initiating a career in the OR get their perioperative education either at the hiring institution or by enrolling in a postgraduate or fellowship perioperative program. Depending on the OR's activities, an estimated minimum of 3 to 6 months of instruction is required to adequately educate nurses with no previous OR experience (AORN, 2008a, 2011a). Topics of study in these programs may include the surgical environment, aseptic technique, perioperative assessment, anesthesia, positioning the surgical patient, sterilization and disinfection, surgical instruments, safety considerations, patient teaching, teamwork, scrubbing and circulating, and wound healing and hemostasis (AORN, 2008a, 2011c). In addition to didactic modules, nurses are often instructed through a cognitive apprenticeship model in the OR in which they take on increasingly complex responsibilities over time. Nurses may enhance their expertise in the surgical setting by becoming board certified operating room nurses (CNOR).

Health Promotion

Patient teaching for the **intraoperative** patient is usually done in a preadmission testing clinic or on the day before the surgery in a patient general surgical unit. Once in the preoperative area, the patient is often anxious and stressed and assumes a passive role as the recipient of technical care. The perioperative nurse performs the preoperative assessment of patients in the holding area. The perioperative nurse's responsibilities in this setting are to verify that the appropriate data have been obtained, assess the patient for readiness both physically and emotionally, and reinforce teaching as needed. This information is the basis for planning the patient's individualized perioperative care.

The use of the nursing process emphasizes a patient-centered approach. Health promotion in the perioperative arena has become more evident as perioperative nurses have gained great satisfaction from knowing that they are part of a team committed to an individual patient with an individualized outcome. This framework enables perioperative nurses to shift from a task-oriented role to that of providing a holistic view of the patient. Therefore, even if the nurse's main role is still to ensure patient safety throughout a patient's surgical experience, the nurse is now able to demonstrate the caring aspect of perioperative nursing by participating in a preoperative assessment of the patient.

Surgical Areas

Patients requiring surgery may have the surgical procedure performed in one of many settings:

1. ***Inpatient/Hospital Surgery:*** Complex surgical procedures, emergency surgical procedures, or less complicated surgical procedures on patients who have complex medical risks. Examples are major bowel, vascular, and orthopedic procedures.
2. ***Ambulatory/Standalone Surgery:*** Less complex surgery on patients with uncomplicated medical histories who are expected to go home the same day. Examples are cataract surgery, removal of skin lesions, and bunionectomy.
3. ***Specialty Clinics and Departments:*** Highly focused surgical procedure settings. Examples are cardiac catherization, labor and delivery and cesarean section.

Before being admitted to the surgical setting, the patient dons a gown and cap. Surgical-site skin preparation includes a baseline assessment, cleaning of the surgical site and surrounding area, hair removal, and application of an approved antiseptic agent, if required. Hair removal should be performed if the presence of hair could interfere with the procedure. If hair removal is indicated, care needs to be taken to maintain skin integrity and minimize injury. Ideally, the hair removal is done outside of the surgical suite as close to the surgery time as possible. Evidence suggests that shaving should be avoided immediately before a surgical procedure and hair should be removed instead by clipping (Anderson, 2011).

Presurgical or Preoperative Holding Area

The surgical area typically has a presurgical or preoperative holding area next to the operating rooms. The preoperative holding area, a *semi-restricted* area usually just inside of the surgical area, provides a quiet, calm transition area where the patient waits immediately before surgery. It provides a shield from the sights and sounds of the busy surgical suite and allows personnel to interview the patient and verify the documentation. Equipment should be readily available in the preoperative holding area for patient care and monitoring. This includes oxygen, suction, electrocardiogram machine, pulse oximetry, and a blood pressure cuff; an emergency medical cart and defibrillator also should be nearby.

In the holding area, the nurse must verify that all the relevant documents and studies (films, scans, etc.) are available before the start of the procedure, that they have been reviewed and are consistent with each other, and that they belong to this patient. Team consensus about the intended patient, procedure, and site (and implant, if applicable), is also needed. This verification should occur before the patient leaves the preoperative area and enters the surgical area.

When the operating room suite is ready to receive the patient, the patient is asked to empty her bladder to prevent incontinence or overdistention; an overly full bladder can hinder access to the surgical site and predispose the patient to inadvertent surgical bladder injury. The nurse accompanies the patient to the operating room, where the patient will be placed on the operating table and prepared for surgery.

Preoperative Operating Room Checklist

The preoperative checklist is a tool for continuing the patient assessment. On it, the nurse documents allergies as per facility policy. The nurse must accurately document the patient's height and weight to ensure proper dosage calculations of the anesthetic agents. The perioperative nurse goes through the checklist before the procedure begins and ensures that the results of all laboratory, radiographic, and diagnostic tests are on the patient's chart.

The nurse documents any abnormal results and reports them to the surgical team along with any special needs, concerns, or instructions, especially with regard to cultural or spiritual beliefs, physical impairments or limitations, and psychosocial conditions. For example, the perioperative nurse will advise the surgical team if the patient is a member of Jehovah's Witnesses and does not accept blood products or if the patient is hard of hearing and does not have his hearing aid (Gillespie & Hamlin, 2009). Showing respect for patients' spiritual beliefs, psychosocial conditions, and physical limitations facilitates rapport and trust. Experienced nurses understand the important role these factors play in how people cope with fear and anxiety related to their perceived perioperative experience.

The perioperative nurse also notes the medical diagnosis, previous surgical experience, patient's physical appearance, visual skin assessment, medical devices accompanying the patient or indwelling medical devices, and any prostheses, jewelry, dentures, and/or capped teeth. The nurse also ensures that the patient has taken any prescribed preoperative medications and that any medications that have been ordered to be given just prior to surgery, such as antibiotics, are documented on the chart accompanying the patient. The nurse also confirms the patient's NPO (*nil per os*, Latin for *nothing by mouth*) status to assess for any potential risk of aspiration. All relevant information is communicated to the surgical team.

Operating Room

Surgery may involve the removal, repair, drainage, replacement, or exploration of body tissue or organs. The operating room or operating suite is where the surgery will be performed. This room is a *restricted* area where the health care professionals wear attire that was donned in the surgery dressing room. This attire, commonly referred to as scrubs, includes a shirt, trousers, cap, shoe covers, and mask. The team members who are directly involved in the surgical procedure will have performed a surgical hand scrub and will be wearing sterile gowns and gloves when they enter the operating room.

Surgical hand preparation, previously known as a surgical scrub, is performed before participating in a surgical procedure to reduce the potential risk of surgical-site infections (SSI) by reducing the number of microorganisms on intact skin of the hands and forearms. Traditional scrub techniques involved the prolonged use of detergent, water, and brushes, which contribute to the deterioration of skin, sometimes leading to undesirable changes of hand skin flora and colonization. Hand preparation now includes the use of a broad-spectrum, fast-acting, nonirritating, FDA-approved antiseptic agent. Additionally, surgical facilities are examining ways to improve the use of physical resources and health care professionals' time. Compared to the traditional surgical scrub, waterless hand preparation boasts a reduction in microbial counts of hands, improved skin health, and reduced use of time and resources (Weight, 2010). The following list identifies recommended surgical hand preparation practices (AORN, 2008b, 2011c).

- Do not wear artificial fingernails.
- Keep the skin free from open lesions and breaks.
- Remove all jewelry from the hands and forearms before performing hand hygiene.
- Use only lotions that are approved by infection control staff; lotions must be compatible with the hand antiseptic and gloves and must be stored in disposable, hands-free dispensers.
- Use a standardized hand scrub procedure that follows the manufacturer's written guidelines and is approved by the health care facility.

Because of the rapid growth of surgical technologies and innovation during the past decade, many operating rooms have been renovated or reconstructed. This has been done in part to accommodate the abundance of equipment needed in today's operating rooms as well as for improved ergonomic design. Recent trends in surgery include the move toward less invasive techniques with shorter hospital stays and faster recovery periods.

One of the newest trends promising to transform surgery is the *intelligent OR*, which incorporates advanced robotic surgical systems. A speech recognition robot allows the surgeon to control the operating bed, lighting, video displays, and other devices with simple voice commands. A robotic endoscopic camera facilitates optimal views of the surgical field, and the robotic surgical assistant enables the surgeon to control precise technical movements of a robotic arm from a console station. Robotic systems are currently in use for certain cardiac procedures, and plans for expansion are on the horizon. Surgical robots make it likely that future surgeries could be performed at one facility with the surgeon operating the console from a distant facility. One of the nurse's roles in robotic surgery is to assist the surgeon at the patient's side during the operation.

Digital information is becoming the standard format for accessing patient information and images, for communicating with other areas of the hospital or consultants, and for conferring with other health care providers. The operating room requires convenient real-time access to these digital data and a way to manage the digital information acquired within the operating room. OR design may be categorized into three major areas: physical, information and communication systems, and management.

To accommodate an optimal workflow and facilitate observation of aseptic technique, certain physical considerations need to be taken into account, including the dimensions of the OR suite, positions of exits and entrances, and location of support services. In addition, integration systems are available that permit the control of medical devices, lighting, and the OR bed; access to images; and the routing of all this digital information to any particular monitor for display or to one or more recording devices for archiving. The information also may be sent to pathologists or radiologists via teleconferencing links. Control can be maintained from the surgical field by touch-screen or voice control interfaces, or from a nursing station (Figure 18–1◆).

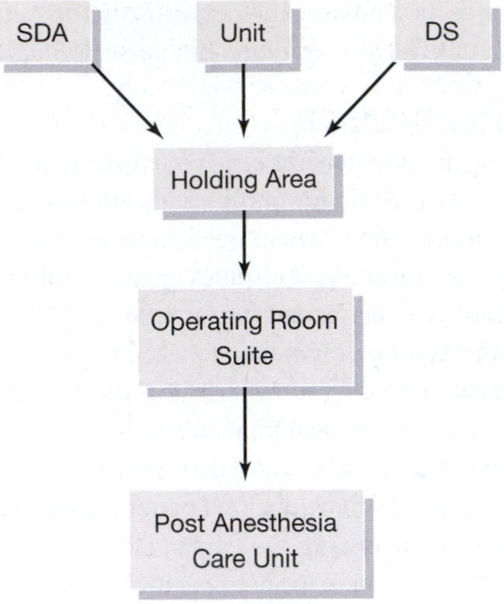

FIGURE 18–1 ◆ Layout of a typical surgical unit.
Note: (SDA = Same day surgery, DS = day surgery.)
Source: © J. Barabe/Custom Medical Stock Photo.

Intentional OR design considers the logistics of flow, maintains versatility, optimizes the use of resources, promotes communication, synchronizes services, and adopts technological advances while including all stakeholders in order to promote successful adoption. The ultimate goal of surgical technology adoption is to enhance patient care and improve patient outcomes.

The setup of the surgical table is specific to the procedure, facility, and surgeon preference. Scrub tables, however, are often standardized to facilitate efficiency and staff changeover. Instruments vary according to specialty and type of procedure.

Other perioperative nursing responsibilities include ensuring proper instrument functionality intraoperatively through cleaning and inspection. Inadvertent patient injury may occur because of an instrument malfunction, resulting in an undesirable effect such as tearing of tissue, loss of small instrument parts inside the patient, or improper reprocessing of instruments, leaving a residue of bioburden (bacteria or other contaminants) that can result in postoperative complications. The use of protocols, checklists, and detailed documentation of OR equipment is associated with a significant decrease in perioperative patient injury (Gillepsie & Chaboyer, 2010). Most surgical instruments are composed of high-grade stainless steel, although advances in surgery such as robotics and minimally invasive surgery have resulted in discoveries of innovative surgical materials and instruments. Surgical instruments are costly and require proper maintenance and care to preserve their longevity.

Patient Preparation

Once they enter the surgical suite, patients are cared for by the anesthetist, surgeons, and nurses. Members of the team take care to make the patient comfortable, apply monitoring devices, and insert additional lines as necessary. Every effort should be made to limit activity involving the patient until he has received a general anesthetic or been given a sedative, if warranted. For example, a patient should have his bladder catheterized after being given the general anesthetic whenever possible. Also, patients should be kept informed on an ongoing basis. This will prevent and limit anxieties created by the already stressful surgical experience. If regional anesthesia is being used, the patient will remain awake; therefore, a screen is placed in front of the patient's face so that the patient cannot see the procedure, which could be upsetting to watch. Sedatives, hypnotics, or tranquilizers are administered to decrease feelings of anxiety and provide sedation (i.e., a state of deep relaxation or sleep).

The perioperative nurse greets the patient on arrival and verifies the patient's identification by using at least two identifiers (e.g., name and date of birth). The nurse reviews the patient's medical record and preoperative checklist; ensures that the consent form has been signed; and verifies that all documentation, preoperative procedures, and orders have been completed. The nurse conducts the preanesthetic assessment by looking at the patient from a holistic viewpoint. This means recognizing the individual person as a dynamic entity made up of components that are continuously interacting. The perioperative nursing assessment is the first step in providing individualized care to the perioperative patient.

To harmonize care in all perioperative settings, the PNDS vocabulary can be used as part of the data collection tool. The PNDS describes the practice of perioperative nursing practice in four domains: safety, physiological responses, behavioral responses, and health care systems. The first three domains, which reflect phenomena of concern to perioperative nurses, are composed of nursing diagnoses, interventions, and outcomes that surgical patients and their families experience. The fourth domain, the health care system, comprises structural data elements and focuses on clinical processes and outcomes. The model is used to depict the relationship of nursing process components to the achievement of optimal patient outcomes (AORN, 2011b; Peterson & Kleiner, 2011).

Comprehensively written nursing care plans have been specifically adapted to the perioperative environment as clinical pathways. Because of the OR's fast-paced environment, patients' short lengths of hospital stay, and the many routines, some procedures and protocols can be documented on a flow sheet.

Surgical Approaches

Because of advances in technology, surgical approaches fall into the following major categories: direct visualization, endoscopic visualization, microscopic visualization, radiological guided visualization, or any combination of these approaches.

Direct visualization has classically been referred to as open surgery. Examples of direct visualization are open bowel surgery, orthopedic repair, and caesarean sections.

Endoscopic visualization is often referred to as minimally invasive surgery (MIS). Examples of endoscopic visualization are arthroscopy, laparoscopic cholecystectomy, cystoscopy assisted transurethral prostatectomy, and endoscopic nasal surgery. Advantages of MIS over open surgery include enhanced surgical visualization, less scarring, quicker recovery, shorter hospital stay, faster return to normal activities such as work, fewer problems with incisions, less pain, and less use of opioids, reducing the negative secondary effects associated with opioid use. Often patients who undergo MIS will be discharged the same day as surgery, whereas open surgery procedures can require 3 to 5 days of hospitalization. The intraoperative cost of MIS surgery is often higher but is offset by the lower costs involved in reduced hospital stay and quicker recovery (Dziedzic, 2010; Noblett & Horgan, 2007).

Microscopic visualization is utilized when the surgical structures are delicate or in confined spaces. Microscopic visualization is used in neurological surgery, eye surgery, micro hand surgery, and spine surgery.

Examples of radiologically guided surgery (surgery performed using an x-ray device as a guide) are cardiac stenting, percutaneous orthopedic repair of fractures, and ureteral stent placement in urology.

Anesthesia

Anesthesia is a pharmacologically induced and reversible state of amnesia, analgesia, loss of responsiveness, loss of skeletal muscle reflexes, decreased stress response, or all of these simultaneously. This state allows patients to undergo surgery and other procedures without the distress and pain they would otherwise experience. The anesthesia care provider considers the patient and selects the agent or a combination of agents that will produce the best anesthesia with the fewest negative effects for the patient (see Chart 18–1).

Anesthesia Pharmacology

To accomplish the level of anesthesia necessary to safely perform surgery, the anesthesia care provider will choose from a broad range of pharmacologic agents. Anesthesia agents may be delivered by inhalation, intravenous delivery, spinal or epidural block, regional block, and/or local injection.

Anesthesia needs to accomplish several things. It must produce sleep (hypnosis), lack of awareness and recall (amnesia), freedom from pain (analgesia), and muscle relaxation. A variety of anesthetic agents can produce these effects. The anesthesia care provider considers the patient and the procedure and selects the agent or combination of agents that will produce the best anesthesia with the fewest negative effects for that patient. Common agents are described in the following text and in the Pharmacology box on page 440.

CHART 18–1 Types of Anesthesia

Type of Anesthesia	Effect on Patient
Local anesthesia	The inhibition of sensory perception within a specific location on the body, such as a tooth, a finger or toe, or a small skin lesion.
Regional anesthesia	Renders a larger area of the body insensate by blocking transmission of nerve impulses between a part of the body and the spinal cord. Two frequently used types of regional anesthesia are spinal anesthesia and epidural anesthesia.
General anesthesia	The inhibition of sensory, motor, and sympathetic nerve transmission at the level of the brain, resulting in unconsciousness and lack of sensation.
Dissociative anesthesia	Dissociative anesthesia uses agents that inhibit transmission of nerve impulses between higher centers of the brain (such as the cerebral cortex) and the lower centers, such as those found within the limbic system.

PHARMACOLOGY Summary of Anesthetic Gases Used During Surgery

Agent	Action and Advantages	Disadvantages and Side Effects	Nursing Responsibility
Desflurane (Suprane)	Maintenance of anesthesia. Very rapid emergence. Good degree of muscle relaxation.	Must be heated to vaporize. Causes increase in heart rate and decrease in blood pressure. Has a strong odor, precluding its use for induction of anesthesia. May cause coughing if used for induction.	Monitor for hypotension.
Enflurane (Ethrane)	Maintenance of anesthesia. Good degree of muscle relaxation.	May lower the threshold for seizures. Increases heart rate and decreases blood pressure.	Monitor for hypotension. Contraindicated in patients with seizure disorders.
Halothane (Fluothane)	Maintenance of anesthesia. Rapid induction and emergence but less than that of isoflurane. Low incidence of postoperative nausea and vomiting.	Increases heart rate and triggers arrhythmias. Requires a higher degree of liver metabolization than other agents. Causes postoperative shivering.	Can cause hypotension. Monitor for premature ventricular contractions, ventricular tachycardia, and ventricular fibrillation with use of epinephrine. Provide warm blankets during recovery period.
Isoflurane (Forane)	Induction and maintenance of anesthesia. Faster induction and recovery than enflurane or halothane. Minimal metabolization by the liver.	Causes increase in heart rate and hypotension. Hypotension can be unpredictable and severe if concomitant use of antihypertensive agents. Weak stimulation of secretions.	Monitor for hypotension.
Nitrous oxide	Rapid induction and recovery of anesthesia. When used with other inhalants, it reduces the concentration of other agents.	Does not produce muscle relaxation.	
Sevoflurane (Ultane)	Induction and maintenance of anesthesia. Very rapid induction and recovery (3–4 minutes faster than Isoflurane). Minimal metabolization by the liver.		

Source: Adapted from Adams, M. P., & Koch, R. W. (2010). Anesthetics and anesthesia adjuncts. In M. P. Adams & R. W. Koch (Eds.), *Pharmacology: Connections to nursing practice.* Upper Saddle River, NJ: Pearson.

General Anesthesia

General anesthesia is achieved through combining medications, including inhalation and intravenous medications. When under anesthesia, the patient is completely dependent on the care of the surgical team, so it is critical that the nurse understand the pharmacology and potential complications that can occur with use of these medications.

Inhalation Agents

Inhalation agents are frequently used for anesthesia because they are fast acting and easily controlled. Anesthetic agents pass through a vaporizer and are mixed with oxygen. The patient inhales the vapors into the lungs. The gas crosses the alveolar membrane, dissolves in the blood, and is carried via circulation to body tissues, where it attaches to receptor sites on the cells to produce its effects, primarily depression of the central nervous system (CNS). Frequently, a mixture of gases is used to maintain anesthesia. Inhalation agents can cause respiratory and cardiovascular depression.

Intravenous Agents

A variety of intravenous (IV) agents are used to induce and maintain anesthesia. The Pharmacology box lists common intravenous medications that are used for anesthesia or as adjuncts to anesthesia. Induction of anesthesia may be accomplished by the administration of a sedative hypnotic or anxiolytic drug. Common drugs include barbiturates such as thiopental sodium (Pentothal) and sodium methohexital (Brevital). These drugs cause rapid, short-acting depression of the CNS (sedative hypnotic), but they have limited analgesic effects. A smaller test dose is initially given to make sure the patient tolerates the medication without reaction. These drugs quickly (within seconds) produce sedation and unconsciousness. Like inhalation agents, intravenous agents can cause respiratory and cardiovascular depression.

Nonbarbiturate drugs that depress the CNS may also be used to induce anesthesia. Etomidate (Amidate) produces rapid hypnosis but with less effect on the respiratory and cardiovascular systems than the barbiturate drugs have. This makes etomidate an attractive alternative for use with high-risk patients. However, etomidate suppresses cortisol secretion, causing hypotension. These effects are not significant in short procedures but can be an issue in longer surgeries. Etomidate is used primarily in short procedures. Ketamine hydrochloride (Ketalar) is a fast-acting CNS depressant that causes profound anesthesia but little skeletal muscle relaxation. It is associated with a difficult emergence phase that is characterized by hallucinations

PHARMACOLOGY Summary of Intravenous Anesthetic Agents and Other Adjuncts to Anesthesia Used During Surgery

Agent	Action and Advantages	Disadvantages and Side Effects	Nursing Responsibility
Intravenous Anesthetic			
Etomidate (Amidate)	CNS depressant used for induction and maintenance of anesthesia for short procedures. Hypnotic effect but no analgesia. Fewer respiratory and cardiovascular effects than other agents. Onset is 60 seconds with duration of 3–5 minutes.	Suppresses cortisol secretion. Postoperative nausea and vomiting. May cause transient skeletal muscle movements. Metabolized in the liver.	Good anesthetic for patients with asthma or cardiovascular disease. Used in neurosurgery because it causes a slight decrease in intracranial pressure. Monitor cortisol levels and blood pressure.
Diazepam (Valium)	Benzodiazepine with hypnotic and amnesiac properties. Used as adjunct drug in induction of anesthesia and as a preoperative medication to reduce anxiety.	May cause hypotension and tachycardia. Prolonged effect.	Monitor sedation postoperatively.
Ketamine (Ketalar)	CNS depressant used for induction of anesthesia. May supplement nitrous oxide anesthesia. Less postoperative nausea and vomiting than other agents.	Increases salivary secretions. Does not produce muscle relaxation. May increase heart rate and blood pressure. Depresses respirations and increases intracranial pressure. Associated with emergence reactions including hallucinations, dissociative feelings, and irrational behavior. Recovery can be prolonged.	Premedicate with anticholinergic agent to reduce secretions. Provide a quiet, calm, reassuring environment for recovery. Monitor heart rate and blood pressure. Monitor airway to prevent aspiration.
Midazolam (Versed)	Benzodiazepine with hypnotic, amnesiac, anxiolytic, and muscle relaxant properties. Used for induction of general anesthesia and for conscious sedation.	Slower induction than with barbiturates. May cause hypotension and tachycardia.	Prepare patient for amnesia. Monitor for respiratory depression.
Propofol (Diprivan)	CSN depressant used for induction and maintenance of anesthesia. Rapid onset with minimal excitation during induction.	Abnormal muscle movement. May cause hypotension.	Monitor blood pressure. Cautious use in patients with allergies to eggs.
Sodium methohexital (Brevital)	Barbiturate used for induction and maintenance of anesthesia. More potent and with a shorter onset and quicker recovery than thiopental.	May cause abnormal muscle movements, coughing, and laryngospasm. Hypotension occurs in some patients. Hiccups may persist postoperatively.	Patient should be recumbent during administration. Monitor blood pressure.
Thiopental sodium (Pentothal)	Barbiturate used for induction and maintenance of anesthesia. Depresses CNS, causing sedation and hypnosis. Ultrashort acting with onset in 10–20 seconds and duration of 20–30 minutes.	Depresses respiratory and circulatory function. Can cause anaphylaxis and laryngospasm. Metabolized by the liver.	Test dose given first.
Opioid Analgesics			
Alfentanil (Alfenta)	Narcotic used for induction, analgesia, and balanced anesthesia. Rapid onset and short duration make it a good choice for short surgical procedures.	Causes respiratory depression. Can cause bradycardia and hypotension. Bradycardia is more likely in patients who are taking a beta-blocking drug. Nausea and vomiting common.	Monitor vital signs. Report bradycardia.

(*continued*)

PHARMACOLOGY Summary of Intravenous Anesthetic Agents and Other Adjuncts to Anesthesia Used During Surgery, *continued*

Agent	Action and Advantages	Disadvantages and Side Effects	Nursing Responsibility
Fentanyl (Sublimaze)	Narcotic used as adjunct for induction to anesthesia and for analgesia supplement. The drug of choice for epidural analgesia. Short acting. Causes less nausea and vomiting than morphine.	Causes sedation and respiratory depression. May also cause bradycardia and hypotension.	Monitor vital signs. Watch for signs of respiratory depression.
Morphine sulfate	Narcotic used as premedication and for postoperative analgesia. Long-lasting effect.	Causes respiratory depression. Histamine release causes peripheral vasodilation and hypotension. Nausea and vomiting common.	Monitor vital signs.
Sufentanil (Sufenta)	Narcotic used for analgesic supplement in balanced anesthesia. More potent than fentanyl. Has a quicker onset and shorter recovery than fentanyl. Not associated with histamine release so there is less hypotensive effect.	Prolonged respiratory depression.	Monitor vital signs. Watch for signs of respiratory depression.
Depolarizing Muscle Relaxants			
Succinylcholine	Depolarizing neuroblocking agent with high affinity for acetylcholine receptor sites. Produces muscle relaxation and paralysis. Used to facilitate endotracheal intubation and to produce skeletal muscle relaxation for short surgical procedures. Short-acting agent with onset in 30–60 seconds and duration of several minutes.	Causes muscle fasciculations (twitching), bradycardia, and respiratory depression. Postoperative muscle soreness. May precipitate malignant hyperthermia in susceptible individuals.	Monitor vital signs. Maintain airway and clear secretions. Patient may complain of muscle soreness postoperatively. Comfort measures such as increased mobility may help to decrease the soreness.
Nondepolarizing Muscle Relaxants—Intermediate			
Mivacurium (Mivacron)	Intermediate, nondepolarizing muscle relaxant used for endotracheal intubation and to produce relaxation of skeletal muscles for surgery. Effect lasts 15–20 minutes.	Transient hypotension and bradycardia. Metabolized by plasma cholinesterase, potentially leading to paralysis.	Monitor vital signs.
Vecuronium (Norcuron)	Intermediate, nondepolarizing muscle relaxant used for endotracheal intubation and to produce relaxation of skeletal muscles for surgery. Effect lasts 20–40 minutes.	Metabolized by the liver. Causes respiratory depression. Minimal cardiovascular effects.	Monitor for delay of recovery postoperatively.
Nondepolarizing Muscle Relaxants—Long Acting			
Tubocurarine	Long-acting, nondepolarizing muscle relaxant used for maintenance of relaxation during surgery. Muscle relaxant effects last 30–40 minutes.	Causes histamine release with hypotension. Increases bronchial and salivary secretions.	Monitor blood pressure and airway until full recovery from drug. Observe for residual muscle weakness.
Metocurine (Metubine)	Long-acting, nondepolarizing muscle relaxant used for maintenance of relaxation during surgery. Muscle relaxant effects last 30–90 minutes.	Hypotension, increased salivary secretions, and respiratory depression.	Monitor blood pressure and airway until full recovery. May take several hours for complete neuromuscular recovery.

PHARMACOLOGY Summary of Intravenous Anesthetic Agents and Other Adjuncts to Anesthesia Used During Surgery, *continued*

Agent	Action and Advantages	Disadvantages and Side Effects	Nursing Responsibility
Pancuronium (Pavulon)	Long-acting, nondepolarizing muscle relaxant used for maintenance of relaxation during surgery. Muscle relaxant effects last 30–60 minutes.	Tachycardia, hypertension, and premature ventricular contractions.	Monitor vital signs.
Anticholinergics			
Atropine	Anticholinergic agent used to decrease salivary and respiratory secretions, to treat bradycardia and/or hypotension, and to reverse muscle relaxants.	Tachycardia, hypertension, urinary retention, and dry mouth. May cause cardiac arrhythmias.	Monitor heart rate and blood pressure. Heart rate is best indicator of response to the drug.
Glycopyrrolate (Robinul)	Anticholinergic agent used to decrease salivary and respiratory secretions and to reverse neuromuscular block.	Tachycardia, urinary retention, and dry mouth. Fewer problems with cardiac arrhythmias than atropine.	Monitor heart rate.

Source: Adapted from Adams, M. P., and Koch, R. W. (2010). Anesthetics and anesthesia adjuncts. In M. P. Adams & R. W. Koch (Eds.), *Pharmacology: Connections to nursing practice.* Upper Saddle River, NJ: Pearson.

and disassociative feelings (feeling separate from the environment). The patient who is recovering from ketamine will do better in a quiet, supportive environment. Propofol (Diprivan) is a rapid-acting hypnotic that causes minimal excitation effects during induction, thereby reducing the risk of the patient's vomiting or thrashing during induction. A test dose is initially given to test for allergy. Propofol is metabolized rapidly, so it does not accumulate in the blood when used to maintain anesthesia. Patients emerge from propofol quite quickly during the recovery period.

Muscle Relaxants

Muscle relaxants (neuromuscular blocking agents) primarily affect skeletal muscle. They are used in surgery to facilitate endotracheal intubation and to provide optimal operating conditions. A rapid-acting neuromuscular blocking agent is administered before intubation to paralyze the muscles of the jaw and vocal cords, making placement of the endotracheal tube easier. Muscle relaxation is used throughout the surgery to facilitate dissection of tissue. During surgery, the anesthesia care provider monitors the effects of muscle relaxant drugs with a peripheral nerve stimulator. Recovery from neuromuscular blocking agents after surgery is evidenced by the patient's ability to breathe on her own and hold her head upright, as well as the presence of a strong hand grasp. There are two types of neuromuscular blocking agents: depolarizing and nondepolarizing.

Succinylcholine is a depolarizing agent, the only one in clinical use. The drug has a strong affinity for acetylcholine receptor sites, and once it attaches to the site, it causes continuous depolarization of the motor end plate. Continuous muscle contractions and fasciculations are followed by flaccid paralysis of the muscles. The onset of paralysis is quick with intravenous administration, 30 to 60 seconds, and the effects last up to 10 minutes. Often succinylcholine is used for intubation because it works very quickly and wears off quickly, but the drug has disadvantages. The depolarization of muscle cells causes a transient increase in serum potassium that can produce cardiac dysrhythmia. Muscle fasciculation leads the patient to complain of muscle soreness postoperatively. Succinylcholine is known to trigger malignant hyperthermia (described later in this chapter) in susceptible individuals. The drug is broken down by the plasma enzyme cholinesterase. Prolonged paralysis occurs in individuals with insufficient amounts of cholinesterase, though this condition is rare.

Nondepolarizing agents work by blocking the depolarizing action of acetylcholine at the motor end plate of the neuromuscular junction, thereby producing muscle paralysis. Muscle fasciculations do not occur with these drugs, eliminating postoperative myalgia. Another advantage is that these agents can be antagonized or reversed with the administration of neostigmine, edrophonium, or pyridostigmine. Use of reversal agents reduces the risk of morbidity associated with anesthesia (Adams & Kock, 2010). Reversal drugs cause bradycardia, which is treated with atropine or glycopyrrolate. Nondepolarizing agents are divided into intermediate acting and long acting. Intermediate-acting agents have a quick onset, 60 seconds or less, and last 25 to 40 minutes. Examples of intermediate-acting nondepolarizing agents are vecuronium, atracurium, and mivacurium. Longer-acting nondepolarizing muscle relaxants also have a rapid onset but last 45 to 60 minutes. Examples are pancuronium, metocurine, and tubocurarine.

Other IV medications that are used in anesthesia include benzodiazepines and opioid analgesics. Examples of benzodiazepines are midazolam (Versed) and lorazepam (Ativan). The benzodiazepines are antianxiety agents that also have hypnotic, sedative, and muscle relaxant effects. Midazolam is sometimes used to induce anesthesia, but these drugs are more commonly used as premedication to reduce the patient's anxiety because they have an amnesic effect. Benzodiazepines are used in combination with other drugs to produce **conscious sedation** or as adjuncts to regional anesthesia to produce sedation and muscle relaxation. Opioids are used in anesthesia for their analgesic effect. Common medications include morphine sulfate, fentanyl citrate (Sublimaze), sufentanil, and alfentanil. Fentanyl is more potent than morphine and is the most commonly used analgesic in anesthesia. The opioid analgesics have good cardiovascular stability but cause respiratory depression.

Complications of General Anesthesia

The majority of patients experience **general anesthesia** without problems except for the complaint of a sore throat from the endotracheal tube. Other problems that may occur with intubation are damage to teeth or dental work and trauma to the vocal cords. Complications that arise from general anesthesia include hypoxia, hypotension,

EVIDENCE-BASED PRACTICE Prevention of Infection During Surgery

Clinical Problem

Mild perioperative hypothermia, which is common during major surgery, may promote surgical wound infection by triggering thermoregulatory vasoconstriction, which decreases subcutaneous oxygen tension. Reduced levels of oxygen in tissue impair oxidative killing by neutrophils and decrease the strength of the healing wound by reducing the deposition of collagen. Hypothermia also directly impairs immune function.

Research Findings

Research was done to test the hypothesis that hypothermia both increases susceptibility to surgical-wound infection and lengthens hospitalization. Maintaining normothermia (normal body temperature) intraoperatively is likely to decrease the incidence of infectious complications in patients undergoing colorectal resection and to shorten their hospitalizations (Anderson, 2011).

Other research was done on prewarming of patients' skin and its influence on core hypothermia (Lynch, Dixon, & Leary, 2010). Camus et al. (1995) found that a single hour of preoperative skin surface warming reduced the rate at which core hypothermia developed during the first hour of anesthesia.

Antibiotic Administration

Another measure to reduce infection in the operating room is proper timing of antibiotic administration. Antibiotic prophylaxis is being used in a variety of surgical procedures to reduce the incidence of surgical-site infections. Antibiotics should be chosen on the basis of their effectiveness against the pathogens that are most likely to be encountered. Skin floras (e.g., *Staphylococcus* organisms) are the usual target, so first-generation cephalosporins are most often chosen. Preoperative prophylactic antibiotics should be administered within 60 minutes before the initial incision is made to ensure that antimicrobial levels in the tissue are adequate and maintained for the duration of the procedure (Anderson, 2011; Wanzer, Goeckner, & Hicks, 2011; White & Schneider, 2007).

Implications for Nursing Practice

Evidence reported in the latest research results has generated changes of practice in the perioperative setting. In the preoperative area, nurses can use blankets and warming to maintain normothermia. For maintaining normothermia in the OR, policies and procedures can be implemented such as use of warming devices under the patient as well as the use of warm solutions. In addition, the temperature of the OR suite can be increased.

Nurses also can coordinate the timing of preoperative antibiotic administration. This will necessitate cooperation with both the surgeon and the OR staff to determine the optimal timing of antibiotic administration.

Critical Thinking Questions with answers can be found in the Osborn Student Resources at nursing.pearsonhighered.com.

References

Anderson, D. J. (2011). Surgical site infections. *Infectious Disease Clinics of North America, 25*(1), 135–153.

Camus, Y., Delva, E., Sessler, D., & Lienhart, A. (1995). Pre-induction skin surface warming minimizes intraoperative core hypothermia. *Journal of Clinical Anesthesia, 7*(5), 384–388.

Lynch, S., Dixon, J., & Leary, D. (2010). Reducing the risk of unplanned perioperative hypothermia. *AORN Journal, 92*, 553–565.

Wanzer, L., Goeckner, B., & Hicks, R. W. (2011). Perioperative pharmacology: Antibiotic administration. *AORN Journal, 93*(3), 340–351.

White, A., & Schneider, T. (2007). Improving compliance with prophylactic antibiotic administration guidelines. *AORN Journal, 85*(1), 173–180.

hypertension, cardiac dysrhythmia, residual muscle paralysis, hypothermia, and malignant hyperthermia. See the Evidence-Based Practice box for more information on hypothermia and wound infection.

Surgery

A drop in body temperature is common during surgery, as anesthesia interferes with the physiological mechanisms of thermoregulation. This effect, combined with environmental factors such as the ambient temperature in the OR, the exposure of body cavities, and the administration of cold solutions (e.g., blood products, IV fluids) or irrigants, leads to a reduction in core body temperature. Studies show that the most significant drop in body temperature occurs during the first hour of anesthesia (Hasankhani, Mohammadi, Moazzami, Mokhtari, & Naghgizadh, 2007; Lynch, Dixon, & Leary, 2010). Monitoring body temperature and using warming devices during surgery (e.g., blankets, thermal drapes, fluid warmers) are imperative (Hasankhani et al., 2007; Lynch, Dixon, & Leary, 2010). The American Society of PeriAnesthesia Nurses (ASPAN) has developed an evidence-based practice guideline that supports the use of forced-air warming blankets as the most effective method of preventing or treating hypothermia (Hooper et al., 2009). Some research suggests that using a forced-air warming blanket for 30 minutes prior to surgery helps to prevent intraoperative hypothermia and improves patient outcomes (Bitner, Hilde, Hall, & Duvendack, 2007; Burns, Wojnakowski, & Piotrowski, 2009).

Malignant Hyperthermia

Malignant hyperthermia (MH), which involves a sudden fast increase in body temperature and metabolism rate along with severe muscle contractions, is a rare but life-threatening complication of anesthesia. The predisposition for MH is genetically transmitted by an autosomal dominant trait. It is thought that MH is triggered by the medications or agents used in general anesthesia, the most common being succinylcholine or one of the inhalant anesthetics. Other factors such as stress, trauma, fatigue, or muscle injury also may play a role in increasing susceptibility to MH or in modifying the patient's response to the condition. Malignant hyperthermia occurs most commonly during induction of anesthesia, although it may present at any time during the surgery or early postoperative period.

MH is not well understood. In MH, calcium levels within skeletal muscle cells increase, although the reasons for this are not known. The elevation in intracellular calcium activates muscle rigidity and spasm and a hypermetabolic state. The increase in cellular metabolism leads to an increase in carbon dioxide production (hypercarbia) and a metabolic acidosis. As the process continues, the patient becomes hypoxic and hyperthermic and develops dysrhythmias and hypotension. Muscle breakdown with the release of myoglobins leads to myoglobinuria and an increased risk of renal failure. Damaged muscle cells then release intracellular potassium and creatinine phosphokinase into the circulation.

The presentation of MH is variable. Early signs are masseter spasm (contracture of jaw), sinus tachycardia, and an increase in expiratory carbon dioxide levels. The anesthesia provider first suspects MH because of a rise in the patient's expired carbon dioxide (CO_2), which is monitored throughout the surgery. An end-tidal CO_2 level that is two to three times normal is the earliest and most definitive sign of MH (Hernandez, Secrest, Hill, & McClarty, 2009; Martin, 2009). Other signs are rigor of muscles, hypoxemia evidenced by a drop in oxygen saturation, and tea-colored urine, indicating the presence of myoglobins. Laboratory blood test results show metabolic acidosis and increases in serum calcium, potassium, and creatinine phosphokinase. Hyperthermia is a late sign, and temperature elevations can be extreme, with increases of 1 to 2 degrees every few minutes. Other late signs are cardiac dysrhythmia and hypotension.

CHART 18–2 Management of the Patient with Malignant Hyperthermia

- Immediately discontinue the triggering agent.
- Stop surgery if possible. Otherwise, deepen anesthesia with opioids, sedatives, or nondepolarizing muscle relaxants.
- Ventilate with 100% oxygen.
- Change the anesthesia machine circuitry.
- Administer a bolus of dantrolene sodium (Dantrium) 2 to 3 mg/kg intravenously with additional bolus doses up to 10 mg/kg until decreased signs of hypercarbia.
- Administer cooling devices: Apply cooling blanket, use iced normal saline intravenously, or lavage open body cavities with iced saline.
- Hydrate with intravenous normal saline.
- Maintain a urine output greater than 2 mL/kg per hour. Administer diurectics if urine output is less than goal.
- Treat metabolic acidosis with intravenous sodium bicarbonate if it does not self-correct with treatment.
- Treat hyperkalemia with intravenous sodium bicarbonate, regular insulin with dextrose intravenously.
- Treat cardiac arrhythmia if it does not self-correct with treatment. Do not use calcium channel blockers.
- Continue to monitor vital signs, oxygen saturation, electrocardiogram, urine output, arterial blood gases, and blood chemistry.
- Transfer to the critical care unit for postoperative care.

Source: Reprinted from Redmond, M. (2001). Malignant hyperthermia: Perianesthesia recognition, treatment, and care. *Journal of Perianesthesia Nursing, 16,* 259–270. Copyright 2007, with permission from Elsevier. Retrieved from http://aspan.org/EdCeMalHyper.htm#head.

MH can be fatal. The key to treatment is early recognition of the syndrome, immediate discontinuation of the triggering agent, administration of dantrolene sodium to produce muscle relaxation, and provision of supportive care. Following emergency treatment, the patient is monitored in the intensive care unit for 24 hours or longer because a small percentage of patients experience a reoccurrence of MH (Hernandez, Secrest, Hill, & McClarty, 2009). Chart 18–2 summarizes the management of the patient with malignant hyperthermia (Martin, 2009).

Other Complications

Other adverse events or complications may occur in the operating room as a result of the surgical procedure. These include such things as excessive blood loss or inadvertent injury to surrounding organs or tissues. Intraoperative complication rates depend on the surgery, the type of anesthesia, and the patient's physical status.

Regional Anesthesia

Regional anesthesia is a general classification of anesthesia that includes spinal and epidural anesthesia, peripheral nerve blocks, Bier blocks, and local anesthesia. The common feature of all types of regional anesthesia is the local injection of a medication to block the transmission of sensory impulses from that area to the brain, thus effectively blocking the sensation of pain. Regional anesthesia has some advantages over general anesthesia. Usually, regional anesthesia does not depress respirations, so the patient is at lower risk of postoperative respiratory complications. This makes regional anesthesia a good choice for patients with severe cardiopulmonary disease. Patients who receive a regional anesthetic also usually experience less postoperative nausea and vomiting.

Regional anesthesia can be used for any number of surgeries. It is commonly used for repair of inguinal hernia, transurethral resection of the prostate, gynecologic procedures, and arthroscopies and other orthopedic surgeries, including repair of hip fractures in older adults. Typically, patients who are scheduled for regional anesthesia are premedicated in the holding area with an antianxiety agent to produce mild to moderate sedation. Opioid analgesics may be administered to reduce the pain associated with the insertion of needles and the administration of numbing agents.

Weblink: Malignant Hyperthermia

Spinal Anesthesia

Spinal anesthesia, also called **intrathecal anesthesia,** is the injection of a local anesthetic into the subarachnoid space and directly into the cerebrospinal fluid (CSF). The anesthetic blocks nerve fibers (i.e., sensory, motor, and sympathetic) at the level of the spinal cord. Spinal anesthesia effectively blocks motor and sensory nerves so that the patient cannot move the affected area (temporary paralysis) or feel pain, touch, temperature, or pressure. The spinal needle is inserted between the second and third lumbar vertebrae (L_2–L_3) or the third and fourth vertebrae (L_3–L_4). For insertion, the patient is placed in a sitting position or in a side-lying position with the head and knees flexed (i.e., fetal position). A spinal needle is inserted in the intervertebral space through the dura mater and into the subarachnoid space. Special spinal needles called *pencil point needles* enter the dura mater by separating the fibers rather than cutting them, reducing the risk of a CSF leak after the needle is removed.

Weblink: Malignant Hyperthermia

Commonly, spinal anesthesia includes the administration of local anesthetics such as lidocaine, bupivacaine (Marcaine), or chloroprocaine combined with an opioid analgesic such as fentanyl or preservative-free morphine. The medication may be mixed with a dextrose solution to create a hyperbaric solution (i.e., a solution that is heavier than CSF). Once a hyperbaric solution has been injected into the CSF, it travels by gravity. The anesthesiologist may have the patient sit for a few minutes to create a block in the lower extremities or place the patient supine with the head tilted slightly downward to create a higher block. After 10 to 15 minutes, the block sets and does not extend further.

Epidural Anesthesia

Epidural anesthesia is the injection of a local anesthetic into the epidural space. The epidural space is located adjacent to the dura mater and contains fat, tissue, and blood vessels. Anesthetic injected into the epidural space affects nerve roots as they leave the spinal cord, and some medication diffuses across the dura mater into the subarachnoid space and the CSF. The anesthetic spreads in both directions (i.e., cephalad and caudad) from the site of the injection, and positioning has less effect on movement of the medication than it does with spinal anesthesia.

The same medications that are used in spinal anesthesia are used in epidural anesthesia, but the concentration of the drugs in epidural anesthesia is greater because they must diffuse across several layers of tissue. The onset of epidural anesthesia is slower than that of spinal anesthesia. A test dose of lidocaine with epinephrine is injected to make sure that the needle is correctly placed in the epidural space and not in the subarachnoid space or in a vein. If the needle is mistakenly placed in a vein, the test dose produces transient tachycardia; if it is placed in the subarachnoid space, it produces mild numbness. Frequently, an epidural catheter remains in place after the operation to provide postoperative pain control. Caudal anesthesia is the administration of a local anesthetic into the epidural space, but the approach is through the caudal canal in the sacrum rather than through the lumbar vertebrae.

Complications of Spinal or Epidural Anesthesia

Spinal anesthesia may be complicated by the development of headache, hypotension, and meningitis. Spinal headache or post-dural puncture headache (PDPH) is a common postoperative complaint. PDPH is caused by the leaking of CSF through the hole in the dura (e.g., the puncture site). The loss of CSF causes irritation of meningeal nerves and vessels (Dale & Checketts, 2010). Because PDPH develops or worsens when the patient moves to an upright position, patients may be restricted to bed rest for the first 8 to 24 hours postoperatively to reduce the incidence of spinal headache. When headache develops, it is located in the occipital area and resolves in 1 to 3 days. Patients who develop a headache are treated with hydration and analgesics. The patient is placed on bed rest with the head of the bed maintained at less than 30 degrees to reduce CSF leak. PDPH that does not resolve quickly or that becomes intolerable may be treated with a "blood patch," which occurs when the anesthesiologist injects 5 to 10 mL of autologous blood into the epidural space at the site of puncture to seal the leak.

Whereas PDPH occurs postoperatively, hypotension is more likely to occur while anesthesia is still being administered. Hypotension is caused by vasodilation associated with the blocking of sympathetic nerves. When sympathetic nerves are blocked by anesthesia, arteries and veins lose muscle tone and the ability to constrict. This decreases venous return from the extremities and reduces cardiac output. Hypotension can occur with both spinal and epidural anesthesia. Hypotension is avoided with the administration of fluid volume, usually normal saline. Medications with strong alpha-adrenergic stimulation effects, such as ephedrine or phenylephrine, are used to prevent or treat hypotension.

Spinal anesthesia is associated with a low risk of aseptic meningitis. When it does occur, signs develop within the first 24 hours after surgery (Dale & Checketts, 2010). The patient presents with the typical signs of meningitis, fever, headache, nuchal rigidity, and photophobia.

Peripheral Nerve Block

A **peripheral nerve block** is the injection of a local anesthetic into or around a nerve plexus to produce anesthesia of a selected area. The major advantage of a nerve block is that anesthesia is confined to the area of the surgery and does not have a systemic effect. Long-acting local anesthetics used in the nerve block provide extended control of pain postoperatively. The local anesthetic blocks motor, sensory, and sympathetic nerves. Frequently, epinephrine is administered with the local anesthetic. Epinephrine causes vasoconstriction of the area and decreases vascular uptake of the medication, thus prolonging the effect of the local anesthetic. The duration of the block depends on the choice of anesthetic, the volume and concentration of the drug, and the site being injected. Frequently, nerve blocks are administered by anesthesia in the holding area because they may take anywhere from 5 to 30 minutes to take effect.

A nerve block can be performed at a number of different sites. For example, an interscalene or axillary block of the brachial plexus is done for surgeries on the shoulder, forearm, or elbow. Surgery on the lower leg may be accomplished by using a femoral or sciatic block. Peripheral nerve blocks are used alone or in combination with general anesthesia. When peripheral nerve blocks are used with general anesthesia, the amount of general anesthesia can be reduced. Complications that can occur with nerve blocks include hematoma at the site of the block, nerve damage, and toxicity from systemic absorption of local anesthetic. Other, specific complications depend on the site where the block is administered.

Peripheral nerve blocks may be performed as outpatient surgeries. Patients are taught that recovery of motor function occurs first, followed by recovery of sensation. Note that while the area is numb, the patient is at risk for inadvertently injuring the area.

A **Bier block** is a specific type of peripheral nerve block that is administered intravenously, but certain techniques are used to trap the anesthetic in the local area. Bier blocks may be used for surgeries on an extremity, usually the arm. An IV catheter is inserted in the extremity at the most distal site possible. A pneumatic tourniquet is applied proximal to the surgical site and inflated higher than the patient's systolic blood pressure. When the local anesthetic (lidocaine) is injected intravenously, the obstruction of blood by the tourniquet prevents the anesthetic from leaving the surgical area. At the completion of the surgery, the tourniquet is intermittently deflated so that the lidocaine enters the patient's general circulation slowly, preventing a toxic reaction to the anesthetic.

Nursing Management

The verification process consists of information gathering and verification, which begins with the determination to do the procedure and continues through all settings and interventions involved in the preoperative preparation of the patient, up to and including the time-out (discussed later) just before the start of the procedure.

Assessment

The nurse asks the patient to confirm the procedure to be completed, the surgical site, and the surgeon. The nurse verifies this information with the surgical consent form, a site verification form per organization policy, and the operating room schedule. In some cases, especially when the procedure involves a structure or body part on the left or right side, the correct area for surgery is marked on the patient. According to the AORN (2011d) position statement on preventing wrong patient, wrong site, wrong procedure events, a comprehensive approach is needed in each health care delivery system to prevent wrong site surgery. In 2003, AORN and the American College of Surgeons developed national guidelines that are to be used with every patient having surgery to eliminate inadvertently operating on the wrong surgical site (see the National Guidelines box).

Nursing Diagnoses

The actual and potential nursing diagnoses related to surgery include:

- *Stress, Overload*
- *Surgical Recovery Delayed*
- *Fear*
- *Infection, Risk for*
- *Pain, Acute.*

NANDA-I © 2012

Planning

To provide the safest and least stressful experience for the patient, planning is essential. Planning for the surgical experience typically begins with admission to the hospital. A comprehensive plan that organizes the care of the patient and family will facilitate the surgical process. The plan includes preoperative, intraoperative, and postoperative management and teaching. Communication is an essential part of executing the plan. Each hospital has specific forms that are used to guide the nurse through the process. Chapter 17 includes an example of a preoperative checklist.

Outcomes and Evaluation Parameters

The desired outcome for patients having surgery is that the patient transitions safely through the entire process. Evaluation parameters include the following: airway is maintained, oxygen levels are within

NATIONAL GUIDELINES Universal Protocol for Preventing Wrong Site, Wrong Procedure, and Wrong Person Surgery

The following guidelines are recommended by The Joint Commission and supported by both AORN and the American College of Surgeons.

1. Verify that the correct patient is being taken to the operating room. This verification can be made with the patient or the patient's designated representative if the patient is underage or unable to answer for him-/herself.
2. Verify that the correct procedure is on the operating room schedule.
3. Verify with the patient or the patient's designated representative the procedure that is expected to be performed, as well as the location of the operation.
4. Confirm the consent form with the patient or the patient's designated representative.
5. In the case of a bilateral organ, limb, or anatomic site (for example, hernia), the surgeon and patient should agree and the operating surgeon should mark the site prior to giving the patient narcotics, sedation, or anesthesia.
6. If the patient is scheduled for multiple procedures that will be performed by multiple surgeons, all the items on the checklist must be verified for each procedure that is planned to be performed.
7. Conduct a final verification process with members of the surgical team to confirm the correct patient, procedure, and surgical site.
8. Ensure that all relevant records and imaging studies are in the operating room.
9. If any verification process fails to identify the correct site, all activities should be halted until verification is accurate.
10. In the event of a life- or limb-threatening situation, not all of these steps may be followed.

Source: Reprinted from Carney, B. (2006). Evolution of wrong site surgery prevention strategies. *AORN, 83*(5), pp. 1115–1122. Copyright 2006 with permission from Elsevier.

Weblink: AORN Position Statement: Wrong Patient, Wrong Site, Wrong Procedure

normal limits, pain is managed, and any postoperative complications are effectively mitigated or controlled as much as possible.

Interventions and Rationales

The nurse must communicate pertinent information to the anesthesia team. Information may include allergies, lab/test results, skin condition, NPO status, sensory/mobility impairments, physical particularities, restrictions to jaw and neck range of motion, history of drug use including herbal medication, anticoagulants held for a specified number of days, implanted electronic devices, other implants, previous anesthesia/surgery history, artificial or loose teeth, previous surgery, comorbidities, particular patient requests, or any other information that the nurse deems crucial to intraoperative patient care. Although this verification takes place in the same-day admission unit or the surgical unit, many ORs have developed a presurgical checklist to ensure that all pertinent information is reviewed and communicated.

Patient Safety

Preventing Wrong Site Surgery

When a procedure involves a left/right distinction, one or more of multiple structures (such as fingers and toes), or one or more of multiple levels (such as spinal procedures), the intended site must be marked so that the mark will be visible after the patient has been prepped and draped. The purpose is to identify unambiguously the intended site of incision or insertion. The mark must be made by using a marker that is sufficiently permanent to remain visible after the skin preparation. The Joint Commission (2011) recommends that the method and the type of marking should be consistent throughout the organization and that the person doing the marking should be the one doing the procedure. Marking must take place with the patient involved and aware.

Safety Alert *Exemptions to the marking procedure may include single-organ cases (e.g., the heart or liver), interventional cases in which the point of insertion is not predetermined (such as cardiac catheterization), tooth extractions (although the involved tooth or teeth should be documented), and surgery on premature infants, for whom the mark may cause a permanent tattoo.*

As the patient's advocate, the perioperative nurse should communicate with all members of the surgical team to verify the correct surgical site. Individual facility policy should clearly delineate the role and responsibility of the health care provider and other team members in marking and verifying the correct surgical site. The 2006 statistics on sentinel events from The Joint Commission identify wrong site surgery as the second most reported sentinel event, accounting for 13% of reported sentinel events (AORN, 2011d). Although it is the surgeon's role to diagnose a patient's need for surgery and to delineate the surgical site, verifying the surgical site at the time of surgery is the responsibility of perioperative nurses and every member of the health care team (AORN, 2011d). To this effect, The Joint Commission has issued regulations and is endorsing the universal protocol as part of the 2007 National Patient Safety Goals (The Joint Commission, 2011).

Safety Alert *The goal of the universal protocol is to prevent wrong site, wrong procedure, and wrong person surgery. The Joint Commission's national guidelines to prevent wrong site surgery are based on the consensus of experts from the relevant clinical specialties and professional disciplines and is endorsed by more than 40 professional medical associations and organizations. The active involvement of the team and the patient or patient's representative and effective communication among all members of the operating room team are important for success.*

Surgical Time-Out

Safety initiatives that address communication issues such as the time-out are designed to promote correct site surgery. The time-out checklist, which has been adopted from the aviation industry model, requires surgical team members to cease all other activities to actively, verbally, and mutually verify information such as the correct patient, correct surgery, correct site/side, correct patient position, and possibly additional information such as prophylactic medications being administered at the appropriate time prior to surgery. Figure 18–2◆ shows a sample of a time-out checklist from the World Health Organization.

Wrong site surgery may be the result of operating on the wrong patient or performing the wrong procedure, but most commonly it is the result of operating on the wrong site or the wrong side; for example, the left hand is operated on instead of the right (The Joint Commission,

Weblink: WHO Surgical Safety Checklist

World Health Organization

SURGICAL SAFETY CHECKLIST (FIRST EDITION)

Before induction of anaesthesia ▸▸▸▸▸▸▸▸▸ Before skin incision ▸▸▸▸▸▸▸▸▸▸▸▸▸▸ Before patient leaves operating room

SIGN IN

☐ PATIENT HAS CONFIRMED
- IDENTITY
- SITE
- PROCEDURE
- CONSENT

☐ SITE MARKED/NOT APPLICABLE

☐ ANAESTHESIA SAFETY CHECK COMPLETED

☐ PULSE OXIMETER ON PATIENT AND FUNCTIONING

DOES PATIENT HAVE A:

KNOWN ALLERGY?
☐ NO
☐ YES

DIFFICULT AIRWAY/ASPIRATION RISK?
☐ NO
☐ YES, AND EQUIPMENT/ASSISTANCE AVAILABLE

RISK OF >500ML BLOOD LOSS (7ML/KG IN CHILDREN)?
☐ NO
☐ YES, AND ADEQUATE INTRAVENOUS ACCESS AND FLUIDS PLANNED

TIME OUT

☐ CONFIRM ALL TEAM MEMBERS HAVE INTRODUCED THEMSELVES BY NAME AND ROLE

☐ SURGEON, ANAESTHESIA PROFESSIONAL AND NURSE VERBALLY CONFIRM
- PATIENT
- SITE
- PROCEDURE

ANTICIPATED CRITICAL EVENTS

☐ SURGEON REVIEWS: WHAT ARE THE CRITICAL OR UNEXPECTED STEPS, OPERATIVE DURATION, ANTICIPATED BLOOD LOSS?

☐ ANAESTHESIA TEAM REVIEWS: ARE THERE ANY PATIENT-SPECIFIC CONCERNS?

☐ NURSING TEAM REVIEWS: HAS STERILITY (INCLUDING INDICATOR RESULTS) BEEN CONFIRMED? ARE THERE EQUIPMENT ISSUES OR ANY CONCERNS?

HAS ANTIBIOTIC PROPHYLAXIS BEEN GIVEN WITHIN THE LAST 60 MINUTES?
☐ YES
☐ NOT APPLICABLE

IS ESSENTIAL IMAGING DISPLAYED?
☐ YES
☐ NOT APPLICABLE

SIGN OUT

NURSE VERBALLY CONFIRMS WITH THE TEAM:

☐ THE NAME OF THE PROCEDURE RECORDED

☐ THAT INSTRUMENT, SPONGE AND NEEDLE COUNTS ARE CORRECT (OR NOT APPLICABLE)

☐ HOW THE SPECIMEN IS LABELLED (INCLUDING PATIENT NAME)

☐ WHETHER THERE ARE ANY EQUIPMENT PROBLEMS TO BE ADDRESSED

☐ SURGEON, ANAESTHESIA PROFESSIONAL AND NURSE REVIEW THE KEY CONCERNS FOR RECOVERY AND MANAGEMENT OF THIS PATIENT

THIS CHECKLIST IS NOT INTENDED TO BE COMPREHENSIVE. ADDITIONS AND MODIFICATIONS TO FIT LOCAL PRACTICE ARE ENCOURAGED.

FIGURE 18–2 ◆ WHO checklist.

Source: World Alliance for Patient Safety. (2008). WHO surgical safety checklist and implementation. Retrieved from http://www.who.int/patientsafety/safesurgery/ss_checklist/en/index.html.

2011). Although wrong site surgery is rare, the consequences can be devastating and warrant improved systems that promote effective communication such as the time-out initiative.

Intraoperative Patient Record

Most facilities have an intraoperative patient record that is used to record intraoperative information. In addition, perioperative nurses may chart information in the nurse's notes when warranted. For example, information may include personnel involved, length of surgery, position and accessories implemented, wound classification, anesthesia classification, and monitoring devices, to name a few.

Protecting the Patient from Infection

Surgical-site infections are the third most frequently reported type of iatrogenic (hospital-acquired) infection (Anderson, 2011; Wanzer, Goeckner, & Hicks, 2011). Preventing and minimizing associated risks of SSI are fundamental perioperative nursing responsibilities. It has been found that the most critical factor in postoperative infection is the sound judgment and proper practice of the surgical team in addition to the general health and disease state of the patient. For this reason, perioperative nurses have become quite expert in the areas of aseptic technique and surgical conscience (explained later in the chapter). Surgical aseptic practice or sterile conscience is based on the premise that most infections are caused by exogenous organisms, or organisms that come from outisde the body (Anderson, 2011; Nichols, 2001; Wanzer, Goeckner, & Hicks, 2011).

Asepsis is the absence of infectious organisms. In the OR, aseptic techniques are practices that minimize contamination due to microorganisms. Frequently, aseptic techniques and practices are criticized for being ritualistic in nature and lacking in scientific rigor; however, until empiric evidence demonstrates that a technique is unnecessary or ineffective, basic aseptic principles should be observed.

No sterilization processes completely eliminate all microorganisms. The best technologies available can only limit and reduce the presence of microbial life—such as bacteria, viruses, fungi, and spores—to an acceptable level. For this reason, nurses and surgical team members in the OR need to continually monitor the surgical field and develop strategies to minimize patient risk. An example may be inspecting sterile packaging, delivering items using proper aseptic technique, and ensuring that items have been appropriately sterilized.

SSIs may also be predicted on the basis of the surgical wound classification. The CDC publishes norms for SSI rates based on certain indicators, including wound classification (see the National Guidelines box). The CDC data provide benchmarks for health care professionals to evaluate their SSI rates so that they can investigate the problem and implement initiatives should the rates be unusually high.

Safety Alert *The purpose of surgical wound classification is to track and learn the cause of infections in order to prevent future incidence. This information is generally recorded on the patient's intraoperative record.*

Over time, surgical team members will develop a surgical conscience. A **surgical conscience** is defined as "An inner commitment to strictly adhere to aseptic practice, to report any break in aseptic

NATIONAL GUIDELINES for Surgical Wound Classification

Clean wounds	An uninfected operative wound in which no inflammation is encountered and the respiratory, alimentary, genital, or uninfected urinary tracts are not entered. In addition, clean wounds are primarily closed and, if necessary, drained with closed drainage. Operative incisional wounds that follow nonpenetrating (blunt) trauma should be included in this category if they meet the criteria.
Clean-contaminated wounds	Operative wounds in which the respiratory, alimentary, genital, or urinary tracts are entered under controlled conditions and without unusual contamination. Specifically, operations involving the biliary tract, appendix, vagina, and oropharynx are included in this category provided that no evidence of infection or major break in technique is encountered.
Contaminated wounds	Includes open, fresh, and accidental wounds. In addition, operations with major breaks in sterile technique (e.g., open cardiac massage) or gross spillage from the gastrointestinal tract, and incisions in which acute, nonpurulent inflammation is encountered, are included in this category.
Dirty or infected wounds	Includes old traumatic wounds with retained or devitalized tissue and those that involve existing clinical infection or perforated viscera. This definition suggests that the organisms causing postoperative infection were present in the operative field before the operation.

Source: Adapted from Giarrizzo-Wilson, S., Maxwell-Downing, D., & Chard, R. (2008). Wound classifications. *AORN Journal, 88*(1), 103–109.

technique, and to correct any violation whether or not anyone else is present or observes the violation. A surgical conscience mandates a commitment to aseptic practice at all times" (Spry, 2009). This allows personnel to function in a more efficient and safe manner.

One of the strategies employed to guard against SSIs is the creation of the sterile field. The sterile field begins at the surgical site (incision) and extends to the rest of the patient, the OR table, the surgical team, the scrub table, and a 1-foot parameter around the draped areas. This principle is applied to application of prepping solutions, patient draping, room setup, and so forth. It is commonly referred to as the *clean to dirty principle.*

Surgical attire, scrubbing, gowning, and gloving are all functions of OR aseptic technique. Figure 18–3 ◆ shows a nurse in proper OR attire and a surgical team member in scrub apparel.

Positioning the Patient to Prevent Injury

Patient positioning in the OR is chosen to accommodate surgical access, staff ergonomics, and view of the surgical site while maintaining the patient's skin integrity. This is why OR tables are narrow (ergonomic for surgeon) and firm (limits movement and allows for CPR). OR tables and accessories are designed to accommodate a wide range of positions to allow for the use of gravity to displace organs; to provide additional working space, surgical access, and enhanced ergonomics for the surgical team; and to prevent patient complications.

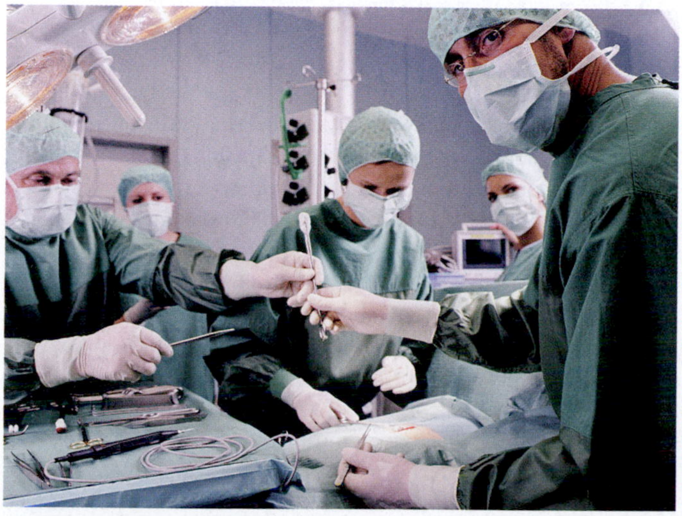

FIGURE 18–3 ◆ Correct surgical attire.

Source: Custom Medical Stock Photo, Inc.—Royalty Free

Complications secondary to positioning include compromised respiratory or circulatory responses, injury to nerves and muscles, and the development of pressure ulcers. Chart 18–3 lists common intraoperative positioning complications and potential causes. Nurses may review the patient's intraoperative position via the OR record and assess any relevant patient outcomes. Of these, pressure ulcers have received much attention as a preventable intraoperative complication. The incidence of pressure ulcers in surgical patients ranges from 4.6% to a high of 66% (Munro, 2010; Walton-Geer, 2009). Preoperative risk factors that are commonly cited across studies include age (e.g., higher risk for older patients); presence of comorbidities, particularly diabetes, hypertension, and vascular disorders; and poor nutritional status as measured by low serum albumin and anemia (Munro, 2010; Walton-Geer, 2009). Further research is needed to clarify intraoperative risk factors, but such factors probably include type of surgery (e.g., higher risk with vascular, cardiac, thoracic, and spinal surgery), length of operation (e.g., longer surgeries), care taken during perioperative skin preparation to reduce unnecessary moisture collection under the skin, hypotensive episodes during surgery reducing the blood available to tissues, and the type of anesthetic used. Perioperative nurses need adequate knowledge of anatomy and an understanding of the physiological effects of specific surgical positions. Appropriate positioning accessories and excellent communication between the anesthesia team that is monitoring physiological responses and the surgical team often requesting position changes is essential to prevent patient injury.

Safety Alert *The primary objective of patient positioning for surgery is to maximize exposure while ensuring patient safety. For example, proper positioning can help to maintain proper body alignment and access to intravenous and anesthesia support devices.*

Preventing the Retention of Foreign Objects

Surgical counts are the responsibility of perioperative nurses and are performed to prevent patient injury due to the high risk of retained foreign body, which can include gauzes, needles, or instruments. Retained foreign objects in patients have resulted in major injuries such as sepsis, bowel perforation, and death. Most facilities follow a legal counting procedure based on the AORN (2008b) recommended standards and practices. The desired patient outcome is a patient who is free from injury related to extraneous objects.

CHART 18–3 Intraoperative Positioning Complications

Potential Complications Secondary to Intraoperative Positioning	Potential Intervention
Decreased lung expansion due to supine position, resulting in compromised respiratory effects	Position bolsters correctly to minimize compression of thorax, facilitating full lung expansion.
Brachial plexus nerve injury	Position arm correctly to ensure proper arm alignment of less than 90 degrees, supinated, and adequately padded and protected.
Circulatory obstruction due to position, resulting in increased risk of postoperative deep vein thrombosis	Apply antiembolic stockings and sequential compression leggings. Use appropriate prophylactic anticoagulant medication administration.
Integumentary injury resulting in pressure ulcers, abrasion, and blistering	Use OR table equipment that will minimize pressure and maximize capillary refill. Appropriate equipment includes gel mattresses. Ensure proper lifting and securing of patient to prevent friction-related injuries.
Dislocation of acetabulum	Ensure proper placement of stirrups, and ensure that two health care professionals simultaneously lift, support, and place legs onto stirrups, observing correct alignment.

Estimating Blood Loss

The patient is monitored throughout the operation for blood loss. The calculation of blood loss is referred to as the estimation of blood loss (EBL). Blood in suction containers, wound drains, chest tubes, and nasogastric tubes is measured directly at frequent intervals during the surgery. If irrigating fluid is used, it is subtracted from the total amount of drainage to determine the amount of actual blood loss. Blood in sponges can be approximated from their weight with 1 gram of weight being equal to 1 mL of blood. Blood-soaked sponges are collected in a plastic bag and weighed. The weight of the dry sponge(s) and plastic container is subtracted from the total weight to determine blood loss.

Whether or not the patient needs a transfusion during surgery depends on blood loss as well as on factors such as age, general level of health prior to surgery, history of cardiovascular disease, how well the patient tolerates the blood loss, and the availability of autologous blood. Some religions, such as Christian Science and Jehovah's Witnesses, restrict the administration of blood products.

Adult patients who are generally healthy can tolerate surgical blood loss of up to 500 mL without the need for a transfusion. Blood loss is treated with the administration of packed red blood cells. Chapter 16 provides a complete description of blood administration indications and procedures.

Latex Allergy

There has been a significant increase in the number of people with latex allergy seen in the hospital, including the operating room. Some evidence suggests the increase correlates with the adoption of universal precautions and the increased use of latex gloves. Patients are asked preoperatively about the possibility of latex allergy. A latex sensitivity questionnaire can be used to identify patients who have a latex allergy or who are likely to develop the allergy. A high incidence of latex allergy is found in people with spina bifida, patients who have had multiple surgeries, those who work with latex products (health care workers, dental industry workers, rubber workers), and those with a genetic predisposition to allergies (atopy). Patients who report allergies to kiwis, bananas, and avocados are also at an increased risk of latex allergies, owing to the cross reactivity of the proteins present in these fruits and latex. Blood or skin tests can detect latex-specific IgE antibodies and are performed preoperatively when latex allergy is suspected.

It is virtually impossible to create a latex-free environment in the operating room—although it may become possible in the future as more products are being manufactured without latex. For patients with known latex allergy, a latex-reduced environment is created. Elements of a latex-reduced environment in the operating room include (1) scheduling elective cases as the first cases of the day to minimize contact with aerosolized allergen from latex gloves; (2) using vinyl gloves rather than latex gloves; (3) using powder-free gloves to limit the aerosolization of latex antigens; (4) avoiding latex on the sterile field; (5) using a plastic anesthesia mask; (6) using a stopcock rather than the rubber port for injection of intravenous drugs; (7) removing the rubber cap on medication vials rather than drawing a medication through the cap; (8) using nonlatex equipment such as a blood pressure cuff, stethoscope, and electrocardiogram leads; and (9) using nonlatex tape. Premedication of allergic patients with steroids or antihistamines is not recommended.

Allergic responses to latex can range from mild cases of contact dermatitis evidenced by a rash and urticaria to serious cases of anaphylaxis. When a latex allergy is suspected in the operating room, the source of latex in direct contact with the patient is immediately removed. Follow-up treatment includes the administration of 100% oxygen, intravenous fluids to support the blood pressure, and the administration of intravenous epinephrine. Diphenhydramine and steroids may also be given intravenously to attenuate the allergic response.

Postanesthesia Care Unit

Once the surgery is completed, the anesthetist and the nurse will accompany the patient to the postanesthesia care unit (PACU) for further monitoring. Concerns along this route will focus on safety, infection control, medication, communication, positioning, and equipment. The PACU is where the patient will recover from the anaesthetic he or she has received. This is an unrestricted area where the patient will no longer need to wear a head cover and the nurses wear regular uniforms. Visitors may be allowed in certain parts of the PACU under certain circumstances (e.g., if the patient is very anxious or may be dying).

Poor communication is one of the top contributing factors to medical errors. Therefore, nurses must strive to provide effective and consistent information during patient handoff to a transition unit such as the PACU or intensive care unit. It is important for the nurse to give any pertinent information to the unit members where the transfer of responsibility for the surgical patient is occurring and to provide interactive communication that is free of interruptions and includes a

CHART 18–4 Considerations for Older Patients Having Surgery

Physical Factors	Cognitive Factors	Sensorimotor Factors	Psychosocial Factors
Decreased tolerance to heat and cold Loss of skin tone Declining cardiac/renal function Atrophy of reproductive organs Increased incidence of preexisting health conditions	Decline dependent on pregeriatric state and general health and social involvement Decreased memory, inductive reasoning, and figural relations may occur Cognitive tasks may require more time to complete	Decreased visual acuity Diminished hearing Altered tactile sensation Changes in taste and smell Diminished response to stress and sensory stimuli Decreased mobility	Ego integrity important Stressors: end of life, changes in environment, increased cognitive demands Death of loved ones Concerns for general health increase

systematic process of verification. The Joint Commission recommends the mnemonic "I PASS the BATON" (The Joint Commission, 2008):

Introduction: Introduce yourself and your role/job (include patient)

Patient: Name, identifiers, age, sex, location

Assessment: Presenting chief complaint, vital signs and symptoms and diagnosis

Situation: Current status, medications, circumstances, including code status, level of (un)certainty, recent changes, response to treatment

Safety concers: Critical lab values/reports, socioeconomic factors, allergies, alerts (falls, isolation, etc.)

Background: Co-morbidities, previous episodes, past/home medications, family history

Actions: What actions were taken or are required AND provide brief rationale

Timing: Level of urgency and explicit timing, prioritization of actions

Ownership: Who is responsible (nurse/doctor/team) including patient/family responsibilities

Next: What will happen next? Anticipated changes? What is the plan? Contingency plans?

The PACU is discussed in detail in Chapter 19.

Gerontological Considerations

Individuals who are 65 years of age and older tend to require surgical interventions more often than younger people do because of age-related system changes and comorbid conditions. Degeneration of multiple systems, such as the musculoskeletal, nervous, cardiovascular, respiratory, genitourinary, endocrine, and hematopoietic systems, as well as hearing and vision, can influence intraoperative and postoperative outcomes. Changes in pharmacokinetics result in changes in drug absorption, distribution, metabolism, and excretion by the body. At this stage of life, both physical and cognitive abilities may vary greatly. Appropriate age-specific interventions should be considered for the older population, taking into consideration physical, cognitive, sensorimotor, and psychosocial factors. Chart 18–4 highlights the special considerations for the gerontological population.

The nurse will assess the older patient's history and general health status, in particular medications, previous surgeries, and comorbidities. Older patients might need the nurse to be attentive to making sure the patient is warm enough; if not, the nurse may use warming devices, if needed. The nurse should also assess the patient's range of motion before the patient is anesthetized in order to ensure that correct positioning accessories are available. Additional padding may be necessary owing to decreased adipose tissue and circulation, which will predispose the patient to the development of pressure ulcers. Efforts should be made to diminish the use of tapes that may lead to denuding of the older person's fragile thinner skin. The nurse must ensure that adequate time is available to communicate clearly and slowly, keeping in mind possible hearing impairment and the need for additional processing and response time.

Hyperglycemia is known to be associated with increased sepsis, so careful monitoring of glucose levels may be a way to reduce serious postoperative infections. Infections are a major concern for all hospitalized patients but are especially dangerous for older people. General risk factors for infection in older patients are known to include frailty, chronic undernutrition, reduced muscle mass, and poor dentition. More general factors that are common to all age groups are diabetes, aspiration, and the presence of an indwelling urinary catheter.

Patients with postoperative cognitive dysfunction (POCD) experience deterioration in cognitive function that may persist for years after the operation. POCD may be related to brain oxygenation during anesthesia, anesthetic agents, and the hospital environment (Prough, 2005).

NCLEX® PRACTICE

1. A preoperative patient is taken into the holding area. What nursing activities will occur in this area?
   1. Checking that surgical instruments are operational
   2. Sterilization of surgical dressings
   3. Interviewing the patient, verifying documentation
   4. Insertion of an indwelling urinary catheter, if necessary

2. A registered nurse first assistant (RNFA) is scheduled to assist a surgeon with a surgical procedure. What could be among this RNFA's responsibilities? (select all that apply)
   1. Administering anesthetic agents
   2. Serving as the patient advocate
   3. Providing the surgeon with instruments
   4. Suturing the wound closed
   5. Providing hemostasis

3. During the course of a surgical procedure, the patient's heart rate increases and the blood pressure drops. Which care provider would address these physiological changes?
1. Surgeon
2. Anesthesiologist
3. Registered nurse first assistant (RNFA)
4. Scrub nurse

4. While conducting a surgical time-out, the nurse says that the site of surgery is the right knee, whereas the left knee is marked as the site of the surgery. What action is indicated?
1. Operate on the right knee.
2. Operate on the left knee.
3. Ask a family member which knee is the site of surgery.
4. Stop all preparations until it can be verified which knee is the site of surgery.

5. While an anesthetized patient is being positioned on the operating room table, the patient's leg drops and hits the table. What is the best action of the nurse?
1. Continue with the positioning procedures.
2. Examine the leg for extent of injury and document the event.
3. Nothing, because this is considered an acceptable hazard of surgery.
4. Elevate the leg on a pillow.

6. During a surgical procedure, the patient begins to demonstrate signs of malignant hyperthermia. The nurse would expect to participate in which actions in the care of this patient? (select all that apply)
1. Administer calcium-channel blockers.
2. Apply a cooling blanket.
3. Notify the critical care unit of an impending admission.
4. Provide 21% oxygen.
5. Hydrate with intravenous normal saline.

Answers to NCLEX Practice questions can be found in Appendix D in the Osborn Student Resources at nursing.pearsonhighered.com. Practice additional NCLEX questions online at the Student Resources site.

Pearson Nursing Student Resources Find additional review materials at: **nursing.pearsonhighered.com**

REFERENCES

Adams, M. P., & Koch, R. W. (2010). Anesthetics and anesthesia adjuncts. In M. P. Adams & R.W. Koch (Eds.), *Pharmacology: Connections to nursing practice* (pp. 457–480). Upper Saddle River, NJ: Pearson.

Anderson, D. J. (2011). Surgical site infections. *Infectious Disease Clinics of North America, 25*(1), 135–153.

Association of Perioperative Registered Nurses. (2008a). AORN mission statement. Retrieved from http://www.aorn.org/AboutAORN

Association of Perioperative Registered Nurses. (2008b). RN first assistant. AORN. Retrieved from http://www.aorn.org/CareerCenter/CareerDevelopment/RNFirstAssistant/

Association of Perioperative Registered Nurses. (2011a). *AORN position statement: Orientation of the registered nurse and the certified surgical technologist to the perioperative setting.* Denver, CO: Author.

Association of Perioperative Registered Nurses. (2011b). Perioperative nursing data set model. Retrieved from http://www.aorn.org/PracticeResources/PNDSAndStandardizedPerioperativeRecord/PNDSModel/

Association of Perioperative Registered Nurses. (2011c). *Perioperative standards and recommended practices* (2011 edition). Denver, CO: Author.

Association of Perioperative Registered Nurses. (2011d). Position statement on preventing wrong patient, wrong site, wrong procedure events. Retrieved from http://www.aorn.org/PracticeResources/AORNPositionStatements/PositionCorrectSiteSurgery/

Association of Perioperative Registered Nurses. (2012). RN first assistants. Retrieved from http://www.aorn.org/Clinical_Practice/Position_Statements/Position_Statements.aspx

Bitner, J., Hilde, L., Hall, K., & Duvendack, T. (2007). A team approach to the prevention of unplanned postoperative hypothermia: Clinical report. *AORN Journal, 85*(5), 921–928.

Burns, S., Wojnakowski, M., & Piotrowski, K. (2009). Unintentional hypothermia: Implications for perianesthesia nurses. *Journal of PeriAnesthesia Nursing, 24*(3), 167–176.

Camus, Y., Delva, E., Sessler, D., & Lienhart, A. (1995). Pre-induction skin surface warming minimizes intraoperative core hypothermia. *Journal of Clinical Anesthesia, 7*(5), 384–388.

Carney, B. (2006). Evolution of wrong site surgery prevention strategies. *AORN, 83*(5), 1115–1122.

Conrardy, J. A., Brenek, B., & Myers, S. (2010). Determining the state of knowledge for implementing the universal protocol recommendations: A integrative review of the literature. *AORN Journal, 93*(1), 194–207.

Dale, M. C., & Checketts, M. R. (2010). Complications of regional anesthesia. *Aneaesthesia and Instensive Care, 11*, 85–88.

Dziedzic, M. E. (2010). Nursing challenges in the care of patients who undergo minimally invasive surgery—Are you prepared? *Clinical Updates.* Retrieved from http://www.nursingconsult.com/nursing/clinical-updates/full-text?clinical_update_id=198886

Giarrizzo-Wilson, S., Maxwell-Downing, D., & Chard, R. (2008). Wound classifications. *AORN Journal, 88*(1),103–109.

Gillespie, B. M., & Chaboyer, W. (2010). Enhancing communication in surgery through team training interventions: A systemic literature review. *AORN Journal, 92*(6), 642–657.

Gillespie, B. M., & Hamlin, L. (2009). A synthesis of the literature on "competence" as it applies to perioperative nursing. *AORN Journal, 90*(2), 245–258.

Hasankhani, H., Mohammadi, E., Moazzami, F., Mokhtari, M., & Naghgizadh, M. (2007). The effects of intravenous fluid temperature on perioperative hemodynamic situation, post-operative shivering, and recovery in orthopaedic surgery. *Canadian Operating Room Nursing Journal, 25*(1), 20–24, 26–27.

Hernandez, J. E., Secrest, J. A., Hill, L., & McClarty, S. J. (2009). Scientific advances in the genetic understanding and diagnosis of malignant hyperthermia. *Journal of PeriAnesthesia Nursing, 24*(1), 19–34.

Hooper, V. D., Chard, R., Clifford, T., Fetzer, S., Fossum, S., Godden, B., et al. (2009). ASPN's evidence-based clinical practice guideline for the promotion of perioperative normothermia. *Journal of PeriAnesthesia Nursing, 24*(5), 271–287.

Lynch, S., Dixon, J., & Leary, D. (2010). Reducing the risk of unplanned perioperative hypothermia. *AORN Journal, 92*(5), 553–565.

Martin, C. L. (2009). A practical guide for malignant hyperthermia management. *OR Nurse 2009, 3*, 20–26.

Munro, C. (2010). The development of a pressure ulcer risk assessment for perioperative patients. *AORN Journal, 92*(3), 272–287.

Nichols, R. L. (2001). Preventing surgical site infections: A surgeon's perspective. *Emerging Infectious Diseases, 7*(2), 220–224.

Noblett, S. E., & Horgan, A. F. (2007). A prospective case-matched comparison of clinical and financial outcomes of open versus laparoscopic colorectal resection. *Surgical Endoscopy, 21*(3), 404–408.

Peterson, C., & Kleiner, C. (2011). Evolution and revision of the perioperative nursing data set. *AORN Journal, 93*(1), 127–132.

Prough, D. S. (2005). Anesthetic pitfalls in the elderly patient. *Journal American College of Surgeons, 200*(5), 784–794.

Redmond, M. (2001). Malignant hyperthermia: Perianesthesia recognition, treatment, and care. *Journal of Perianesthesia Nursing, 16*(4), 259–270.

Spry, C. (2009). *Essentials of perioperative nursing* (3rd ed.). Sudbury, MA: Jones & Bartlett.

The Joint Commission. (2004). Procedures requiring surgical site marking. Retrieved from http://www.jointcommission.org/AccreditationPrograms/Hospitals/Standards/FAQs/Provsion[plus]of[plus]Care/Operative_HRP_Sed_Anesth/Surgical_Site_Marking.htm

The Joint Commission. (2008). National patient and safety goals. Retrieved from http://www.jointcommission.org/NR/rdonlyres/ACA4DBF6-90FD-4400-BE7E-4C6F881E5DCD/0/08_OBS_NPSG_Master.pdf. From the Department of Defense Safety Program

The Joint Commission. (2011). Wrong site surgery project. Retrieved from http://www.centerfortransforminghealthcare.org/projects/display.aspx?projectid=4

Walton-Geer, P. S. (2009). Prevention of pressure ulcers. *AORN Journal, 89*(3), 538–552.

Wanzer, L., Goeckner, B., & Hicks, R. W. (2011). Perioperative pharmacology: Antibiotic administration. *AORN Journal, 93*(3), 340–351.

Weight, C. J. (2010). Avagard hand antisepsis vs. traditional scrub in 3600 urologic procedures. *Urology, 76*(1), 15–17.

White, A., & Schneider, T. (2007). Improving compliance with prophylactic antibiotic administration guidelines. *AORN Journal, 85*(1), 173–180.

Postoperative Nursing

19 CHAPTER

Kimberly Yates
Renée Holleran

Outcome-Based Learning Objectives

After studying this chapter, the learner will be able to:

1. Prioritize nursing diagnoses and interventions for the patient in the postanesthesia care unit.
2. Discuss criteria for moving patients through the phases of postanesthesia recovery.
3. Discuss the assessment, prevention, and nursing management of common postoperative problems.
4. Generate a teaching plan for the discharge of a patient after surgery.
5. Identify and discuss areas of future research relevant to the care of the postoperative patient.

KEY TERMS

airway obstruction p.456
atelectasis p.465
dehiscence p.473
diuresis p.457
fast-tracking p.453
graduated compression stockings (GCSs) p.475
hematuria p.474
hemostasis p.456
hypothermia p.458
hypoxemia p.456
ileus p.459
intermittent pneumatic compression devices (IPCs) p.475
ischemia p.458
laryngospasm p.456
mydriasis p.460
normothermia p.459
piloerection p.458
postanesthesia care unit (PACU) p.453
postoperative nausea and vomiting (PONV) p.459
sanguineous p.457
serosanguineous p.457
surveillance p.454
third spacing p.457

THE POSTOPERATIVE PERIOD BEGINS with the completion of surgery and the patient's transfer to the **postanesthesia care unit (PACU),** where the patient recovers from the effects of anesthesia. The PACU, located close to the operating room, is designed to care for patients as they stabilize and recover from surgery and anesthesia. Important components of postanesthesia care include prevention of postoperative complications, wound healing and wound care, and postoperative pain management.

Entering the Postanesthesia Care Unit

Following surgery, the patient is transferred to the PACU, accompanied by the circulating nurse and a member of the anesthesia care team. In some circumstances, a surgical patient may be transferred directly to an intensive care unit (ICU) for recovery rather than to the PACU; however, most surgical patients stabilize in the PACU before discharge home or transfer to a clinical unit. After discharge from the PACU, postoperative care continues in the home for ambulatory surgical patients or in the hospital for patients who require a more monitored recovery.

Collaborative Management

The PACU nurse works in close collaboration with the anesthesia provider and surgeon. Nurse–health care provider collaboration is linked to better patient outcomes, including a reduction in mortality rates. In order to meet desired patient outcomes, it is essential that this interdisciplinary team communicate openly with one another in developing and evaluating care of the patient and family (IOM [Institute of Medicine], 2010). Generally, the anesthesia provider assumes responsibility for coordinating the patient's medical and surgical care in the PACU. The patient's condition in the PACU moves from instability to stability over the course of an hour to several hours. Chart 19–1 shows the typical trajectory of a postoperative patient.

Nursing Management

The nurse's assessment and intervention immediately after surgery focus on patient safety, hemodynamic stability, and the recognition and prevention of postoperative complications. Care in the PACU is organized around postanesthesia phases I and II. Phase I begins with the patient's arrival in the PACU and focuses on recovery of physiological homeostasis and protective mechanisms. During this phase, the patient requires intensive nursing observation and care.

Phase II begins when the patient becomes more alert and functional. In this phase, the patient requires less intensive nursing; if the patient will not be transferred to an inpatient unit, interventions focus on preparing the patient and significant others for the patient's discharge home. As such, phase II refers most specifically to ambulatory surgery. The term **fast-tracking** describes a situation in which the patient is transferred from the operating room to PACU phase II, bypassing PACU phase I. Fast-tracking is possible when surgical techniques are

Weblink: Nurse's Role in Immediate Postoperative Care

Weblink: ASA: Standards for Postanesthesia Care

CHART 19–1 Postanesthesia Patient Trajectory

Level of Consciousness

Unconscious → Semiconscious → Conscious

Airway

Unable to maintain airway → Rejects airway support → Supports own airway

Cardiovascular

Cardiovascular instability → Cardiovascular lability → Cardiovascular stable

Pain

No pain perception → Awareness of pain → Adequate pain control

Body Temperature

Hypothermia → Normothermia

Source: Adapted from Prowse, M., & Lyne, P. (2000). Clinical effectiveness in the post-anesthesia care unit: How nursing knowledge contributes to achieving intended patient outcomes. *Journal of Advanced Nursing, 31*(5), 1115–1124.

minimally invasive and anesthesia is of a short duration. Research continues to identify which patients are appropriate for fast-tracking, to standardize guidelines and develop protocols used in fast-tracking, and to follow patient outcomes (Kitching, 2009; Silbert, 2009).

Nurses in the PACU should be aware of certain specifics related to caring for postoperative patients from various cultures, as discussed in the Cultural Considerations box.

Assessment

The PACU nurse ensures patient safety during the transition from the operating room to the patient's home or to the clinical unit. The PACU nurse is an intensive care nurse who is prepared to identify and prevent the acute problems and complications associated with surgery and anesthesia. The nurse is skilled in the management of situations in which the patient's physiological condition is rapidly changing. The nurse is especially attentive to **surveillance** (the systematic and continuous assessment of the patient) and to the recognition and management of potentially catastrophic events (Lipke & Hyott, 2010, Anderson, 2011). The nurse also must be prepared to respond to patients' psychological reactions to surgery and anesthesia, providing reassurance and comfort. Care in the PACU is guided by the *Standards of PeriAnesthesia Nursing Practice* developed by the American Society of PeriAnesthesia Nurses (ASPAN), the professional organization for PACU nurses (ASPAN, 2010); the *Standards for Post Anesthesia Care* (ASA, 2009), hospital policies, and clinical guidelines. These care standards are found at www.asahq.org/Search.aspx?q=standards+postanesthesia+care.

The PACU nurse receives a report about the patient's condition from the anesthesia provider and the circulating OR nurse. The report provides a description of the patient's pertinent medical and surgical history, the condition that required surgery, the surgical procedure and any complications, the anesthesia, medications given during surgery, any difficulties with intubation, the estimated blood loss from surgery, the patient's fluid, any transfusions, and vital signs. Other pertinent information communicated to the nurse includes the type and location of incisions and drains; intravenous fluids; current medications and medications held prior to surgery; and impairments in skin integrity, swallowing, mobility, or communication. The PACU nurse is apprised of concerns the patient expressed preoperatively, any special requirements, and the presence of significant others waiting for the patient.

The nurse conducts a complete system assessment of the patient immediately on arrival at the PACU. The nurse uses the ABCs (i.e., airway–breathing–circulation) to prioritize the initial assessment of the surgical patient, starting with observation of the airway for patency. Unless contraindicated, recovering patients are placed in a lateral position to reduce the risk of aspiration. An artificial airway (oral or nasal) prevents the tongue from falling backward and occluding the airway. It may be used until the patient is able to support his

CULTURAL CONSIDERATIONS for the Postoperative Patient

- Modesty is extremely important in some cultures and in some religions (e.g., Hispanic, Arab, Muslim). The nurse should keep women modestly covered and expose only the body area necessary for examination or treatment. A cover for the head should be provided to female patients who desire it. It is best to provide same-gender caretakers when possible.
- Pain assessment may need to be modified for some patients. Numeric rating scales may not be appropriate for all cultures. In some situations, the FACES pain rating scale, which uses facial expressions to assess pain, may be more useful than numeric rating scales. Some patients may be reluctant to talk about their pain or to take pain medication.
- Pain expression is culturally influenced. In some cultures, pain may be openly expressed in words, sounds (e.g., moaning), and physical movement; in other cultures, patients are expected to be stoic about the presence of pain. Nurses need to be aware of and sensitive to cultural expressions of pain.
- The nurse should always consider cultural beliefs in the selection and use of pain medications. In some cultures, patients may be reluctant to talk about pain and to take pain medication for fear of addiction, dependence, or sedation. The nurse should explain to patients the importance of treating pain and be sensitive to alternative pain therapies.
- It is important to be aware of and sensitive to treatment restrictions. Some cultures or religions restrict or discourage the use of certain medical treatments such as blood transfusions or organ transplantation.
- The dietary practices of patients' cultures and religions should be recognized and supported. Many religions (e.g., Orthodox Jewish, Muslim, Seventh-Day Adventist, Catholic) have dietary requirements (such as vegetarianism or kosher food preparation) or dietary restrictions (such as avoidance of pork, shellfish, or caffeinated products). Hospital kitchens and health care providers need to accommodate these practices. The nurse should ask about and be sensitive to patients' special dietary needs. If family members wish to bring in specially prepared foods, the nurse should encourage them to do so.
- The nurse should ask about and support the use of alternative healing treatments when possible. Some alternative therapies, such as the use of prayer, anointment, healing touch, or communion, can be accommodated with little problem. Others, such as the use of herbal products to promote healing, may need to be evaluated for their effects on wound healing or medications. The nurse should talk with patients about what, if any, alternative treatments they believe are important to their recovery.
- Visitors should be encouraged. In some cultures, it is important for family members and extended family members to be present in the hospital with the patient. The nurse should consider ways to include family members in the patient's care.

Source: Hoke, M. M., & Robbins, L. K. (2011). Continuing the cultural competency through exploration of knowledge, attitudes, and skills with advanced practice psychiatric nursing students: An exemplar. *The Nursing Clinics of North America, 46*(2):201–205.

airway unassisted. Oxygen is provided via face mask and titrated to keep oxygenation saturation levels above 93% or at a level determined by the health care provider. The nurse assesses the patient's respiratory rate and depth, breath sounds, and oxygen saturation via a continuous pulse oximeter.

Some patients will remain intubated and on mechanical ventilation following the surgery. In such cases, the nurse performs the respiratory assessments described previously and, in addition, checks the endotracheal tube and ventilator settings. The nurse attaches a cardiac monitor and a blood pressure cuff to the patient. She also takes an apical pulse and blood pressure and notes the patient's heart rhythm. If the patient has a pulmonary artery catheter in place, pulmonary artery pressures and cardiac output are measured and recorded. The nurse assesses peripheral pulses and the patient's color as indices of the adequacy of circulation.

The patient's core body temperature is measured by using the monitoring device that is considered best according to agency policy and the nurse's judgment. The patient's temperature can fluctuate rapidly during recovery. Core body temperature can be measured in the tympanic membrane using a tympanic thermometer. Oral and axillary temperatures provide only an estimate of the core body temperature, and a rectal temperature is considered unreliable in hyperthermic crisis (ASPAN, 2010). A temporal scanner, which is a device that relies on an infrared scanner to detect the highest temperature of forehead skin, provides a rapid measurement of body temperature but may not be accurate in recording core body temperatures under some circumstances (Low et al., 2007).

The PACU nurse performs a systematic, head-to-toe assessment of the patient. The full PACU form can be found on the Osborn website. The following areas are assessed during the head-to-toe examination:

- ***Level of Consciousness (LOC):*** Is the patient unconscious, arousable, fully awake? LOC is documented every 15 minutes until the patient returns to baseline, then hourly thereafter. The nurse should describe pupil size and response. If awake, is the patient oriented to person, place, and time? Is the patient's speech clear? Intracranial pressure will be measured following selected cranial surgeries.
- ***Cardiovascular:*** The nurse records the patient's vital signs and cardiac rhythm. If applicable, the nurse measures and records cardiac output, pulmonary artery pressures, and central venous pressure. The extremities are examined for color, sensation, motion, and pulses. An ankle-brachial index may be measured in vascular procedures (Chapter 35).
- ***Respiratory:*** The nurse describes the patient's airway and need for artificial airway, respiratory rate, depth, breath sounds, oxygen saturation, cough, secretions, arterial blood gases, chest tubes, and need for suctioning, if applicable.
- ***Pain Management:*** The nurse describes the location, quality, and rating of pain. If a spinal or epidural pain management agent was used, the nurse should describe the sensory level of numbness and the motor ability of the extremities.
- ***Gastrointestinal:*** When the nurse does an abdominal assessment, is the abdomen flat and soft or firm and distended? Are bowel sounds present? If the patient is nauseated, is the nausea mild, moderate, or severe? Is the patient vomiting?
- ***Genitourinary:*** Does the patient have a urinary catheter? The nurse describes the amount and color of urine output. If there is no catheter, is the bladder distended? Has the patient voided? The nurse notes when the patient is due to void. If a gynecologic procedure was performed, the nurse describes any vaginal bleeding.
- ***Skin Integrity:*** The nurse describes the color and temperature of the patient's skin and any areas of bruising, redness, or ulceration.
- ***Temperature:*** The nurse records the patient's temperature on arrival at the PACU and after 30 minutes.
- ***Incision:*** The nurse describes the location and condition of the patient's incision. Any bleeding, wound drainage, or presence of a hematoma should also be described. If the suture line is not visible, the nurse should describe the condition of the dressing. If there are any wound drains, the nurse should describe the type and drainage.
- ***Activity/Movement:*** Is the patient able to hold her head up? Is the patient able to move all extremities? Are movements voluntary or on command? The nurse describes the strength of the extremities and notes whether or not it is equal on both sides. Does the patient have compression stockings, pneumatic compression boots, or another type of deep venous thrombosis (DVT) prophylaxis device in place?
- ***Psychosocial:*** If the patient is awake, the nurse describes the level of psychosocial comfort. Is the patient calm, relaxed, and sleeping or anxious and distressed?
- ***Intravenous Fluids:*** The nurse describes the location of intravenous catheters, the type of catheter, and the type and rate of intravenous fluid.
- ***Drains and Other Tubes:*** The nurse describes the type, location, and drainage of any tubes.
- ***Other Medical Devices:*** The nurse describes any other devices the patient may have, such as an arterial line, a pulmonary artery catheter, or traction.

The frequency of patient assessment in the PACU depends on the patient's stability. A patient's physiological status can change rapidly during recovery. In acute crisis, patients are continuously monitored (assessed every 1 to 5 minutes) until the situation no longer warrants such close observation. For patients who are stable, vital signs and patient assessment are performed on admission and every 15 minutes for the first hour (i.e., four assessments). This is followed by assessment every 30 minutes for the next 2 hours (i.e., four assessments), then every hour until discharge from the unit. Chart 19–2 (p. 456) lists abnormal findings on assessment that suggest the need for closer observation and consultation with the anesthesiologist.

Initially, patients are placed in a lateral position. As they become more awake, they are placed with the head of the bed elevated if this is not contraindicated by the surgery. Patients are repositioned every 1 to 2 hours or as needed. A patient who is experiencing nausea and vomiting may remain in a lateral position to prevent aspiration.

Nursing Diagnoses

The patient recovering from anesthesia and surgery is at risk for a number of problems. Some of these problems occur early in the course of recovery and are much more likely to be seen in the PACU than elsewhere. Others may occur both in the PACU and on the clinical unit. Some problems occur later in recovery and are more likely to be seen on the clinical unit or at home after discharge. Common nursing diagnoses with expected outcomes in the PACU are as follows:

- *Risk for Impaired Gas Exchange* (airway obstruction, laryngospasm, hypoxia)

CHART 19–2 Abnormal PACU Assessments That Are Reported to the Anesthesiologist

Neurological Findings
- Prolonged unresponsiveness
- Change in level of consciousness
- Abnormal responses such as slurred speech, asymmetrical smile, weak hand grasps, inability to move all extremities.

Cardiovascular Findings
- Heart rate >120 beats/min
- Hypotension (e.g., systolic blood pressure of less than 90 mmHg)
- New cardiac dysrhythmia
- Hypertension (e.g., systolic blood pressure 20% to 30% higher than baseline)
- Absence of peripheral pulses.

Respiratory Findings
- Oxygen saturation <93%
- Respiratory rate <10 breaths/min
- Indications of respiratory distress and/or hypoventilation such as stridor, retraction of intercostal muscles, minimal respiratory effort.

Other Findings
- Urine output <30 mL hour or <5 mL/kg per hour
- More than the expected amount of bleeding at the incision site
- Enlarging hematoma
- Loss of pulse(s) in a graft site
- Unexpected presence of blood in drainage tubes
- More than the expected amount of drainage from chest tubes or wound drains
- Vomiting associated with possible aspiration.

- *Risk for Imbalanced Fluid Volume* (bleeding, hypovolemia, fluid overload)
- *Risk for Decreased Cardiac Output* (dysrhythmia, hypotension, hypertension)
- *Risk for Imbalanced Body Temperature: Hypothermia*
- *Readiness for Enhanced Comfort: Nausea and Vomiting*
- *Readiness for Enhanced Comfort: Pain*
- *Anxiety.*

NANDA-I © 2012

Potential Complications in the Postoperative Patient

Most patients will arrive in the PACU with supplemental oxygen to prevent **hypoxemia** (insufficient oxygen content in the blood). Common causes of hypoxemia in the early postoperative period include airway obstruction, hypoventilation, and laryngospasm. Respiratory complications, especially the need for upper airway support, are the most frequent postoperative problems in the PACU (McAlister, Bertsch, Man, Bradley, & Jacka, 2005; Tarrac, 2006).

Airway obstruction occurs most often because medications used in anesthesia cause the muscles to relax. When the tongue relaxes, it can fall backward, blocking the airway. Signs of an obstructed airway include snoring, stridor, retraction of intercostal muscles, and a fall in oxygen saturation levels. To prevent airway obstruction, patients are positioned on their side and an artificial airway is inserted. An oral airway is effective with the patient who is minimally responsive; however, a patient who is more arousable may gag, choke, or spit out the airway. For these patients, a nasal airway may be more effective and comfortable. A patient who is experiencing an acute airway obstruction needs to be stimulated. If a patient is arousable, the problem can often be resolved by speaking to the patient, encouraging the patient to take deep breaths, and turning up the oxygen level, if necessary. Patients who are not arousable may need to have their airway opened. The nurse can perform the chin-tilt/jaw-thrust maneuver used in cardiopulmonary resuscitation to open the airway. An oral airway is inserted to maintain patency. Airway occlusion becomes less of a threat once the patient is more responsive and regains protective mechanisms.

In some patients, a delay in the excretion of neuromuscular blocking agents used in anesthesia can result in weakened respiratory muscles, causing *hypoventilation* (insufficient inspiratory and expiratory effort). Assessment should be focused on the complete respiratory function, including use of accessory muscles and depth and quality of respirations. Hypoventilation should be suspected in patients who are unable to sustain a head lift or have weak hand grasps, although this may be hard to evaluate in a patient who is obtunded. The prolonged effects of anesthetic agents also can produce a slow respiratory rate (i.e., less than 10 per minute) and shallow breathing. The continuous assessment of oxygen saturation helps to identify the patient who is becoming hypoxemic as a result of poor ventilatory effort. The nurse reports to the anesthesiologist a respiratory rate of less than 10 or oxygen saturation rate of less than 93% (or less than some other health care provider–prescribed value). Some patients experiencing hypoxemia may benefit from the application of continuous positive airway pressure (CPAP) to keep airways open (Brodsky & Margarson, 2011; Tallman, Ramachandran, Christensen, & O'Brien, 2011).

Laryngospasm occurs when the muscles of the larynx contract forcefully, causing a closure or partial closure of the airway. It can be caused by irritation from secretions, inhalants, or medications and is an emergency situation because the patient can quickly become hypoxic. Treatment may include opening the airway, suctioning secretions, administering oxygen, administering an aerosolized epinephrine solution, and, in severe cases, reintubation.

Postoperative Fluid Volume

The nurse monitors the patient postoperatively for evidence of bleeding, hypovolemia, and fluid overload. Bleeding is identified in several ways depending on the specific surgery performed. Bleeding can be seen on surgical wound dressings and in drainage tubes such as a nasogastric tube (NGT), a chest tube, a urinary catheter, or a wound drainage tube. The nurse examines the wound and dressing for signs of bleeding every hour, or more frequently if bleeding is found.

Often, the surgical wound is expected to ooze small to moderate amounts of blood or sanguineous drainage. The nurse does *not* take off the surgical dressing, because it aids in **hemostasis** (stopping bleeding). Instead, the nurse marks an area of drainage (e.g., circling it in pen) on the dressing, monitors it for enlargement, and reports any findings to the surgeon. The sheets under the patient are examined for evidence of bleeding because gravity may cause blood to leak from the dressing and pool underneath the patient. If blood soaks through a dressing, the nurse reinforces the dressing and reports the event to the surgeon. Drains are monitored when dressings are checked. The nurse reports the presence of blood or sudden increased amounts of drainage in a drain as a new finding to the surgeon. Certain tubes, such as chest tubes following a lung resection, an NGT following a gastrectomy, or wound drainage tubes, might be expected to drain blood initially, with the drainage gradually changing from **sanguineous** (blood in the drainage) to **serosanguineous** (blood and serum in the drainage) during the next several hours or days. The nurse needs to have a sense of the expected amount and type of drainage from a drainage tube in order to respond promptly to any increases in drainage. In addition, the surgeon must be notified of any increase or unexpected changes in the type of drainage.

Internal bleeding sometimes presents as distention of tissues or the formation of a bruise or hematoma. A hematoma forms in an area where blood is collecting and often causes increased pain. Generally, this will be in the area surrounding the wound; in some cases, however, a hematoma may form in what appears to be a distant site. Other signs of internal bleeding are seen when blood loss is large enough to produce a drop in blood pressure, an increase in heart rate, or a decrease in cardiac output (Neveleff & Kraiss, 2010). Initially, the heart rate increases in an attempt to maintain a normal cardiac output and blood pressure; thus, increased heart rate is an early sign of internal bleeding. Other indications include a change in the patient's level of consciousness (anxiety, agitation, and confusion), a decrease in blood pressure (hypotension) with an increase in heart rate (tachycardia) and respiratory rate (tachypnea), and a drop in oxygen saturation. The patient may appear pale, cold and clammy, or cyanotic. Urine output may decrease as a result of poor renal perfusion.

Significant postoperative bleeding is an emergency and is always reported immediately. An operation may be required to explore the surgical site, identify the source of the bleeding, control it, and stop it. If so, the patient is monitored continuously until arrangements for the operating room are complete. If an operation is needed to control the bleeding and the patient's condition does not contraindicate it, the patient is positioned with the head flat and the legs elevated or in the Trendelenburg position (head lowered and feet elevated) to increase venous return and raise the blood pressure. The patient is supported with supplemental oxygen to prevent hypoxemia and the administration of intravenous fluids, blood transfusions, and/or plasma expanders to replace blood volume. Chapter 54 provides a complete description of nursing care for the patient in shock.

Surgery has a significant effect on a patient's fluid balance, and it is unlikely that the patient will have a normal urinary output in the first 24 to 48 hours postoperatively (Young et al., 2009). In addition, the surgical patient is affected by factors that can lead to dehydration or fluid overload. Factors that contribute to fluid loss and dehydration in the surgical patient include preoperative fasting from foods and fluids, preoperative bowel preparation, hyperventilation from anxiety, blood loss intraoperatively, wound drains, nasogastric drainage, vomiting, evaporative water loss from exposed tissues during the operation, and decisions about intravenous (IV) fluid replacement. Some surgeons prefer a conservative approach to the administration of IV fluids in the operating room because research shows that these patients progress better postoperatively than patients who receive more liberal amounts of IV fluid (Young et al., 2009, Anderson & Comrie, 2009). Another factor in fluid balance is that tissue injury can cause a **third spacing** (fluids accumulating in the third space of tissues) of fluids that contributes to dehydration initially because the fluid is not in the intravascular space. Postoperatively, fever, hypermetabolism, and sweating can significantly increase insensible water losses from an average of 600 to 800 mL/day to as high as 1,500 mL/day (Young et al., 2009).

Alternatively, certain factors contribute to overhydration and *fluid overload*. The primary factor is the secretion of hormones that occurs with physiological stress. Stress, pain, and anxiety stimulate the release of epinephrine, aldosterone, and antidiuretic hormone (ADH). These hormones affect fluid balance by causing the retention of sodium and water. Fluid overload may also occur as a result of the administration of intravenous fluid. The replacement of fluids during surgery is a clinical approximation of fluid loss, and monitoring is needed to prevent fluid overload.

Although dehydration is more common than fluid overload postoperatively, patients are nonetheless monitored for signs of overhydration. The risk of overload is highest during the first 24 to 48 hours postoperatively when hormonal influences are at their peak. Most healthy patients can tolerate an overexpansion of fluid volume; however, the problem can be serious in those with altered physiological reserves. For those patients, the increased cardiac workload associated with fluid overload can precipitate heart failure or pulmonary edema. Patients who are at an increased risk of fluid overload are older patients and those with preexisting cardiac, pulmonary, or renal disease. Early indicators of fluid retention are heavy, swollen eyelids; edema in the hands and feet; weight gain; and fluid intake that is greater than output. The patient may complain of headache, apprehension, or dyspnea. Other signs are agitation, distended neck veins, crackles in the lungs, and a drop in urinary output. Vital sign changes include increases in heart rate, blood pressure, and respiratory rate. Treatment of fluid overload depends on the severity. Continuous close monitoring of weight, intake and output (I&O), and lung sounds is paramount, and the administration of IV fluids may be slowed or discontinued. In some cases, the patient may be given a diuretic, such as furosemide, intravenously to facilitate fluid excretion.

It is more common for a patient to be dehydrated after surgery than overhydrated (Young et al., 2009). Intake may exceed output for approximately 24 to 48 hours. Fluid balance begins to correct approximately 48 to 72 hours after surgery. At this time, fluid in the interstitial space begins to shift back into the vascular space and the effect of stress hormones decreases, producing **diuresis** (increased excretion of urine to decrease the amount of fluids in the third space).

Careful assessment of fluid balance is the key to maintaining adequate hydration and preventing fluid overload. Intravenous fluid is monitored closely. A number of formulas are available for calculating postoperative fluid replacement. As an example, approximately 2,500 mL/day (or 30 to 35 mL/kg body weight per day) is needed for routine fluid replacement with additional amounts, from 500 to 3,000 mL/day, for replacement of losses from third spaced fluid, drains, or other sources (Young et al., 2009). Isotonic solutions (normal saline, Ringer's lactate) are frequently used for routine IV fluid replacement.

In the PACU, urine output is measured hourly. A urine output that is less than 30 mL/hr or 0.5 mL/kg per hour is reported to the health care provider as a significant finding. Frequently, a low urine output in the postoperative patient is the result of depressed renal function from dehydration. Other indications of dehydration include dry mouth, dry tissues, poor skin turgor, and complaints of headache. Tachycardia occurs as a compensatory mechanism for dehydration, and the blood pressure tends to decrease as a result of too little blood volume.

A patient with low urine output or other signs of hypovolemia may be given a fluid bolus to expand blood volume and increase renal blood flow. A typical fluid bolus is 250 to 1,000 mL of 0.9% sodium chloride administered over 30 to 60 minutes. The nurse monitors urine output to determine the effectiveness of the fluid bolus. If it is effective, urine output increases. Vital signs may return to normal, although issues other than dehydration (e.g., anxiety, pain) affect vital signs. In some patients, particularly older adults, a fluid bolus can overwhelm the heart's pumping ability, resulting in heart failure and pulmonary edema. Older patients need to be monitored during a fluid bolus to ensure that they are able to tolerate the rapid administration of fluid. Crackles (i.e., rales) in the lungs, dyspnea, or a drop in oxygen saturation indicate that the patient is unable to tolerate the fluid.

Changes in Cardiac Output

Following surgery, patients may have problems with cardiac irregularities, hypotension, or hypertension. Abnormal cardiac rhythms are a frequent finding after surgery. Most abnormal rhythms are a result of expected postoperative issues such as pain or fluid and electrolyte imbalances, but an abnormal rhythm can also indicate a more serious problem such as cardiac **ischemia** (restriction of blood flow to the coronary arteries). Cardiac telemetry is used to monitor heart rhythms and abnormal beats in the PACU. Telemetry is normally discontinued when the patient is transferred to a clinical unit, but it will be continued for patients who have signs of myocardial ischemia or abnormal cardiac rhythms or for those who need monitoring for heart or blood pressure medications.

The apical pulse is a more reliable measure of heart rate and rhythm in the postoperative patient than is a peripheral pulse. The health care provider usually writes parameters that specify vital signs to report. The nurse relies on these parameters, as well as on clinical judgment, in reporting changes in the patient's condition. In addition to changes in heart rate, the nurse reports and investigates evidence of any new irregularity in the heart rhythm. Irregularity in the heart rhythm may indicate premature ventricular contractions or new-onset atrial fibrillation.

Sinus tachycardia (i.e., a heart rate greater than 100 beats/min) is the most common dysrhythmia; it is caused by fever, anxiety, pain, hypovolemia, anemia, and hypoxia, among other reasons. As a rule of thumb, a heart rate greater than 100 beats/min in a postoperative patient is investigated initially to determine the likely cause. If the patient is persistently tachycardic, the nurse must assess for other signs and symptoms (e.g., vertigo, syncope, hypotension, hypoxemia, chest pain) and report heart rates greater than 120 beats/minute. The goal is to treat the underlying cause (e.g., give pain medication, fluids, oxygen, or blood transfusion). Although many patients experience tachycardia in the postoperative period, it is important to remember that an increase in heart rate increases the heart's workload; therefore, in compromised patients, decompensation can occur rapidly.

Sinus bradycardia (i.e., a heart rate less than 60 beats/min) occurs postoperatively as a result of anesthetic medications or vagal stimulation. Patients with bradycardia are observed for its effect on cardiac output. If the patient is asymptomatic, further treatment is not usually necessary. However, bradycardia that produces hypotension, syncope, or other symptoms may need to be treated with medications such as atropine or with a pacemaker.

Premature ventricular contractions (PVCs) are not unusual after surgery. PVCs may be caused by anxiety, pain, hypoxia, hypovolemia, and electrolyte imbalances, particularly hypokalemia or hypomagnesia. Occasional PVCs are often benign and do not require treatment. The nurse reports an increase in the frequency of PVCs, the clustering of PVCs (i.e., couplets, triplets), and episodes of ventricular tachycardia (i.e., four or more PVCs in a row). Treatment is typically directed toward the underlying cause of the abnormal beats, but an antiarrhythmic drug such as amiodarone may be used to suppress episodes of ventricular tachycardia. It is important to remember that an antiarrhythmic drug given intravenously can also be proarrhythmic (i.e., it has the potential to trigger an abnormal rhythm); therefore, these drugs are used cautiously (Daniels, 2007). Chapter 30 includes a complete discussion of cardiac dysrhythmias.

Hypotension is a systolic blood pressure of less than 90 mmHg or a drop in the patient's systolic blood pressure of more than 20% from baseline. Hypotension can occur for a variety of reasons including bleeding, hypovolemia, depressed myocardial function, abnormal heart rhythm (e.g., atrial fibrillation), pulmonary emboli, and medications. Hypovolemia is the most likely cause of postoperative hypotension. The nurse reports hypotension and monitors the patient for other signs of decreased tissue perfusion. Interventions to treat hypotension depend on the underlying cause; they include placing the patient in the Trendelenburg position and administering IV fluids rapidly to increase blood volume.

Hypertension is a systolic blood pressure equal to or greater than 140 mmHg, a diastolic blood pressure equal to or greater than 90 mmHg, or an increase greater than 20% from baseline in the patient's blood pressure. There are many reasons for a postoperative patient to be hypertensive including pain, anxiety, hypothermia, fluid overload, and distention of the bladder. Interventions are focused on treating the cause. If the patient was on antihypertensive medications at home, these are restarted as soon as possible. Patients who are NPO are sometimes allowed to take medications with small sips of water, or they may be temporarily switched to an antihypertensive medication that can be given intravenously.

Hypothermia

Hypothermia is defined as a core body temperature of less than 36°C (96.8°F) or a condition, regardless of body temperature, in which a person experiences shivering, peripheral vasoconstriction, **piloerection** (elevation of hairs on the body to conserve heat, known as "goose bumps"), and feeling cold. Hypothermia is a common problem in the PACU, and it can have significant consequences for patients. Hypothermia is linked to patient discomfort, sympathetic stimulation, altered drug metabolism, increased intraoperative blood loss and the need for postoperative transfusions, impaired platelet function and clotting ability, slowed wound healing, increased susceptibility to infection, and untoward cardiac events such as angina (ASPAN, 2010; Lynch, Dixon, & Leary, 2010). Because of the slow drug metabolism associated with hypothermia, the hypothermic patient remains anesthetized longer than necessary.

Patients at risk for hypothermia include those with a history of vascular and endocrine diseases, those who are immunocompromised, those with open wounds, older patients, and persons who are malnourished and have low reserves of body fat. Relatively long surgeries (those lasting more than 1 hour) and the use of cold irrigation solution intraoperatively contribute to the development of postoperative hypothermia. On admission to the PACU, the nurse assesses the patient for evidence of hypothermia and takes the patient's core body temperature. Clinical guidelines for the prevention of hypothermia recommend maintaining an ambient room temperature between 20° and 24°C (68° and 75°F) and using passive insulation techniques such as applying warm cotton blankets, socks, and head coverings; limiting skin exposure; and using a circulating water mattress for all patients (ASPAN, 2010; Burns, 2009; Lynch, Dixon, & Leary, 2010). Hypothermic patients must be actively rewarmed using a forced-air warming system, which helps to raise body temperature by blowing warm air through a blanket that covers the patient. Other active warming techniques include warming IV fluids and applying warm, humidified oxygen (Hasankhani, Mohammadi, Moazzami, Mokhtari, & Naghgizadh, 2007; Lynch, Dixon, & Leary, 2010).

Patients who are hypothermic require more oxygen than they would if they had a normal temperature because shivering increases the oxygen demand of the tissues and workload of the heart. Achieving **normothermia** (i.e., a normal body temperature) reverses the immediate effects of hypothermia (e.g., shivering), but patients who experience perioperative hypothermia develop more cardiac events and wound infections postoperatively than patients who do not experience hypothermia (Burns, 2009; Lynch, Dixon, & Leary, 2010; Sedei, J., 2010). The nurse assesses the patient's temperature every 30 minutes until discharge. The patient must achieve a minimum core body temperature of 36°C (96.8°F) prior to PACU discharge.

Nausea and Vomiting

Postoperative nausea and vomiting (PONV) is a significant problem that can be more debilitating than the surgical procedure. Despite advances in anesthesia, a large number of patients are affected by nausea and vomiting. Nausea and vomiting contribute to the development of fluid and electrolyte imbalances, poor nutritional intake, and patient discomfort. Often, patients who experience nausea and vomiting are reluctant or unable to ambulate, increasing the likelihood of other postoperative complications. Predisposing factors for PONV include gender (women are more likely to experience it than men), type of surgery (there is a higher risk with gynecologic, abdominal, eye, and ear surgeries), length of surgery (increased risk with surgeries longer than 2 hours), use of opioid analgesics, use of inhalation agents during anesthesia, a history of motion sickness, a history of nausea and vomiting with previous surgery, and smoking status (ASPAN, 2006; Conway, 2009).

There are three types of PONV. Early PONV occurs quickly, within 2 to 6 hours after the surgery. Late PONV develops 6 to 24 hours after the surgery. Delayed PONV extends beyond the first 24 hours after surgery. The causes of nausea and vomiting are complex, and it may be that different types of PONV are caused by different factors and stimuli. PONV occurs as a result of stimulation of the vomiting center in the brain (Conway, 2009). The vomiting center is activated by pathways from (1) the chemoreceptor trigger zone (CTZ) in the brain, (2) the gastrointestinal (GI) tract and other viscera via the vagus nerve, (3) the vestibular apparatus in the ear, and (4) the cerebral cortex. The CTZ contains serotonin and dopamine receptors that, when stimulated by certain toxins, substances, and drugs, activate nausea and vomiting in the vomiting center. The GI tract also contains receptors—serotonin (5-HT3), dopamine (D2), and histamine (H1)—that, when stimulated, send messages to the brain via the vagus nerve to trigger nausea and vomiting. In addition, factors such as GI irritation, gastric distention, inflammation, or ischemia can cause nausea and vomiting. For the postoperative patient, anesthesia and medications, especially narcotics, are important triggers of nausea.

Most PONV occurs early in the course of recovery and improves over time. An important study done in 2000 involving 300 postoperative patients found that the highest incidence of nausea and vomiting occurred within 2 hours following surgery (Gunta, Lewis, & Nuccio, 2000). Interventions to reduce PONV begin in the preoperative or intraoperative period with the administration of antiemetic medication. Early administration of antiemetic drugs (i.e., administering the drug before emesis is triggered) is thought to be more effective than waiting until the patient experiences nausea and vomiting (Conway, 2009). When preventative therapy fails, experts recommend rescue therapy using an agent from a different antiemetic class (ASPAN, 2006). All patients with PONV need to be well hydrated with IV fluid.

The various antiemetic drugs have different modes of action, and the ideal drug or drug combination has yet to be found. In some cases, a combination of drugs may work more effectively than a single drug (Conway, 2009). Not all antiemetics are effective for the nausea and vomiting associated with anesthesia, and all of the drugs have limitations. The Pharmacology feature (p. 460) describes common antiemetics used for PONV.

Unfortunately, antiemetic medication does not work for everyone, and there are few effective alternatives to the use of drugs. Other methods that have been used to manage PONV include hydration, acupressure, oxygen, aromatherapy, and music therapy (Conway, 2009). The nurse provides comfort by allowing the patient periods of uninterrupted rest, offering empathy and support, and encouraging deep breathing. The nurse also offers application of a cool washcloth, frequent mouth care, and ice chips. Patients frequently report increased nausea with head elevation and movement. Slow position changes may help to prevent this trigger.

Pain

Achieving adequate pain control and comfort is a major goal of postoperative care. Studies continue to report the undermedication of pain in postoperative patients (Layzell, 2008; McMain, 2008, 2010; Rejeh & Vaismoradi, 2009).

The physiological effects of pain are well known; they include an increase in sympathetic stimulation with an increase in blood pressure, heart rate, respiratory rate, and cardiac workload. The body enters a catabolic state that uses up physiological reserves. From a psychological standpoint, pain contributes to loss of sleep, lack of appetite, depression, anxiety, anger, helplessness, and hopelessness. Postoperative pain is associated with delayed ambulation and diminished functional performance (Layzell, 2008; McMain, 2008, 2010; Rejeh & Vaismoradi, 2009). Pain control is necessary in promoting mobility and preventing complications such as atelectasis (described in the Preventing Postoperative Complications section later in this chapter), **ileus** (a hypoactive bowel with delay in peristalsis), DVT, and poor wound healing. The goal in postoperative pain control is to achieve a level of comfort without producing too much sedation or other side effects. Patients who are overly sedated will not be able to participate in postoperative breathing exercises or ambulation.

Incisional pain is expected to be highest in the first 24 to 48 hours postoperatively, followed by a gradual reduction in pain. However, the course of pain varies with the surgery and the individual. Activities and procedures can also alter the course of pain. Patients who have had cardiac surgery reported coughing as the most painful activity, followed by moving or turning in bed, getting out of bed, and using the incentive spirometer (Layzell, 2008; McMain, 2008, 2010; Rejeh & Vaismoradi, 2009).

Pain may come from sources other than the incision. Residual carbon dioxide, used to inflate the surgical area in laparoscopic procedures, can produce shoulder or back pain. The position used during surgery may cause specific muscle aches.

The PACU nurse continuously assesses the patient's level of comfort. The Agency for Health Care Policy and Research (AHCPR; now known as the Agency for Healthcare Research and Quality, AHRQ) developed guidelines for the management of acute pain in 1992. These guidelines recommend the use of a rating scale to measure the patient's report of pain. Most hospitals use a numeric rating system in which patients report their level of pain on a scale of 0 (no pain) to 10 (the worst pain imaginable) (ASPAN, 2010). Postoperative patients rate their pain at rest and with movement.

PHARMACOLOGY Summary of Common Drugs Used to Control Postoperative Nausea and Vomiting

Drug	Class and Action	Major Side Effects	Nursing Responsibility
Aprepitant	Neurokinin-1 (NK-1) receptor antagonist. Blocks NK-1 receptors in the central pathway of the vomiting center.	Headache, hypotension, bradycardia, pruritus, constipation.	Used only for prophylaxis of nausea and vomiting. Give as a single dose 3 hours before surgery.
Dexamethasone	Corticosteroid. Augments the antiemetic effect of 5-HT3 blockers. May also antagonize prostaglandins or release endorphins that increase mood and well-being.	Headache, gastrointestinal irritation, glucose elevation, retention of sodium and water.	Used in combination with other antiemetics. Watch for GI bleeding.
Diphenhydramine (Benadryl)	Blocks effects of histamine at H1 receptor sites.	Sedation, vertigo, hypotension.	Used most often for nausea associated with motion sickness or chemotherapy. Older adults may be very sensitive to the sedative effects of the drug.
Droperidol (Inapsine)	Blocks dopamine type 2 receptors in the chemoreceptor trigger zone in the brain to reduce nausea and vomiting.	Sedation, hypotension, tachycardia, extrapyramidal symptoms (dystonia, restlessness, tremor).	Low doses are used for postoperative nausea and vomiting. Watch for sedation and respiratory depression in patients receiving other CNS depressants. Monitor heart rate and blood pressure because it can cause QT prolongation or Torsade de pointes.
Metoclopramide (Reglan)	Increases gastric emptying and raises the threshold for triggering the chemoreceptor trigger zone.	Mild sedation, extrapyramidal symptoms (dystonia, restless, tremor).	Drug should be discontinued if extrapyramidal symptoms occur. Has not been shown to be effective in prophylactic management of PONV.
Ondansetron (Zofran)	Serotonin receptor antagonist.	Headache, diarrhea, or (more commonly) constipation.	Headache may be treated with Tylenol. Give stool softener or laxatives to prevent constipation.
Dolasetron Granisetron	Blocks 5-HT3 receptor sites in the CTZ and peripherally to reduce nausea and vomiting.	Headache, diarrhea, excessive tiredness, dizziness, pain, heartburn, chills, rash, fever, itching. Should not be used in patients with congenital long-QT syndrome. Hypokalemia and hypomagnesemia should be corrected before administering dolasetron.	To be administered 2 hours before surgery. Monitor for prolongation of QT interval.
Prochlorperazine (Compazine)	Phenothiazine that depresses CTZ in the brain.	Extrapyramidal symptoms, suppresses cough.	Be alert for development of extrapyramidal symptoms such as motor restlessness and parkinsonism.
Promethazine (Phenergan)	Long-acting phenothiazine derivative that depresses the chemoreceptor trigger zone.	Sedation, dizziness, dry mouth.	Monitor for increased sedation when administered with other CNS depressants. Monitor patient safety.
Scopolamine	Antagonizes muscarinic type 1 receptors in hypothalamus and vomiting center.	Visual disturbances, dry mouth, **mydriasis** (pupil dilation)	Used for prophylaxis of PONV, limited use in rescue because of delayed action.

Self-report is the best indicator of pain (AHCPR, 1992). Studies have affirmed that nurses and health care providers consistently underestimate patients' pain (Puntillo, Miaskowski, Kehrle, Stannard, Gleeson, & Nye, 1997; Sjostrom, Dahlgren, & Haljamae, 2000) or have difficulty distinguishing pain from anxiety except when they use a pain scale and listen to the patient's response (Layzell, 2008; McMain, 2008, 2010; Rejeh & Vaismoradi, 2009). Pain assessment in patients who cannot report its intensity is more complicated and relies on clinical judgment. If patients are unable to verbalize their pain, a behavioral pain scale must be used, such as the Checklist of Non-Verbal Indicators. Pain scales are available in Chapter 12. The nurse needs to consider the usual pain associated with a particular procedure or surgery and assess the patient for behavioral indicators of pain. Based on these factors, an analgesic is tried and evaluated for effectiveness (Layzell, 2008; McMain, 2008, 2010; Rejeh & Vaismoradi, 2009).

The American Society of PeriAnesthesia Nurses (ASPAN) published pain and comfort guidelines for postoperative patients in 2003 (ASPAN, 2003). Using these guidelines, the nurse documents the location and character of the pain. The patient is expected to feel pain at the area of the surgical incision; pain located in other areas requires further investigation. Pain in other sites may be caused by any number of factors and can be relatively benign. Examples include pain referred from the incision, pain as a result of positioning during the operation, or pain caused by the accumulation of carbon dioxide gas from a laparoscopic procedure. However, chest pain not related to an incision can be serious, indicating cardiac ischemia, and it requires further evaluation.

Postoperative pain should be well controlled with medications and other strategies. Early postoperative pain control is important for patient comfort, and it may play a role in reducing persistent postsurgical pain, a phenomenon in which pain continues long after the incision heals (Layzell, 2008; McMain, 2008, 2010; Rejeh & Vaismoradi, 2009). The nurse consults with the health care provider when the patient is not getting acceptable pain relief. Another situation requiring consultation is the report of increased pain when the pain was previously well controlled. This finding suggests the possibility of surgical complications, such as infection or hematoma formation, and requires prompt evaluation.

Safety Alert *Uncontrolled postoperative pain or a sudden increase in postoperative pain warrants an immediate investigation. These signs can signal a postoperative complication such as bleeding or leaking of the surgical anastomosis. Report findings to the health care provider immediately.*

Initially, most patients in the PACU receive small doses of intravenous narcotic analgesics for pain control. Common medications include morphine sulfate, hydromorphone, and fentanyl. A typical standing order may be written for morphine sulfate 1 to 5 mg IV every 5 minutes as needed to a maximum total dose of 0.3 mg/kg body weight. Fentanyl also is used in the PACU because it provides analgesia comparable to that of morphine but has a more rapid onset and excretion (Layzell, 2008; McMain, 2008, 2010; Rejeh & Vaismoradi, 2009). A typical standing order might read, "Fentanyl 25 mcg IV as needed to a maximum of 100 mcg." The nurse assesses the patient's responses to interventions every 15 to 30 minutes, or more frequently if appropriate. Patients are monitored for respiratory depression, and narcotics are withheld, or even reversed, if the respiratory rate falls to 10 per minute or less.

Safety Alert *Patients who require close neurological monitoring need an individualized regimen for pain control. Check with the anesthesiologist for special orders if the patient has major head trauma, has increased intracranial pressure, had a recent cerebrovascular accident, or had recent seizures.*

Patient-controlled analgesia (PCA) or patient-controlled epidural analgesia (PCEA) is commonly used to control postoperative pain. With PCA, a narcotic analgesic can be administered continuously at a basal rate, although continuous infusion is not standard because it increases the risk of adverse effects and opioid overdose (Beach, 2011; Eaden, Gilley, & Neff, 2009). More common is PCA in which a small bolus is administered when the patient pushes the control button. The PCA delivers a set amount of medication at specified intervals until a maximum amount of medication is reached. The computerized pump keeps a record of how often the patient attempts to access the medication and how many doses the patient receives. The nurse then uses this information to determine whether the patient is using the pump effectively. A typical PCA order for a postoperative patient might read, "PCA morphine sulfate 1 mg every 6 minutes with a lockout maximum of 10 mg/hour."

Patients receiving PCA are monitored for pain relief and for untoward effects of the narcotic, including a depressed respiratory rate, sedation, nausea, pruritus, and slowed GI function. In a review of studies comparing PCA with nurse-administered analgesics, researchers found consistent evidence that PCA provides better pain control and increased patient satisfaction with very few adverse effects (Hudcova, McNicol, Quah, Lau, & Carr, 2006).

PCEA delivers medication via a catheter to the epidural space. Like PCA, it can be set to deliver medication continuously, as a bolus, or both. PCEA is used to deliver a local anesthetic such as bupivacaine or ropivacaine alone or in combination with a narcotic. Fentanyl is frequently used as the narcotic of choice because it is lipid soluble and easily dissolves in epidural fat; however, preservative-free morphine also can be given as an epidural medication. Local anesthetics and opioids are thought to work synergistically to provide better pain relief in smaller doses.

The nurse checks the site of the epidural catheter for signs of infection and patency. Infection is uncommon, but since the catheter is taped, not sutured, displacement can occur. Catheter displacement is suspected when a patient who previously had good pain control with the epidural catheter complains of new pain. The nurse monitors the patient for overall pain control and notes the sensory level of the epidural (i.e., the area of the body where the patient reports diminished sensation). In the PACU, these assessments are made hourly; on the clinical unit, they are made every 4 hours unless the situation warrants more frequent assessments. It is also important to note any areas of motor deficit. The goal of epidural analgesia in the postoperative patient is to reduce sensation and pain without affecting motor ability. Morphine will give a broader coverage than fentanyl. If the epidural analgesia is affecting motor ability, the dose or timing will need to be adjusted downward so that the patient will be able to ambulate safely. Other possible side effects include nausea, pruritus, hypotension, and urinary retention. Some health care providers elect to leave a urinary catheter in place while a patient is receiving epidural medication to avoid urinary retention; others believe this practice to be unnecessary and that it may cause a urinary tract infection.

Safety Alert *If a patient with patient-controlled epidural analgesia is unable to lift his legs off of the bed or describes heaviness in the lower extremities, the health care provider should be consulted. These symptoms suggest that the dose of medication is too high, causing motor blockade.*

The use of PCA and PCEA is an important advance in control of postoperative pain. Many studies show that PCEA provides better pain control with fewer side effects and better functional outcomes than PCA (Carli et al., 2002; Cata, 2009; Mann et al., 2000; Nishimori, Ballantyne, & Low, 2006; Schumann, Shikora, Weiss, Wurm, Strassels, & Carr, 2003). Continuous epidural analgesia with local anesthetics for 24 to 72 hours postoperatively is associated with faster return of GI function, improved respiratory function, and a reduced stress response (Cata, 2009). As soon as appropriate, the patient is transitioned from intravenous or parenteral medications to oral medications.

Experts recommend a multimodal approach (e.g., using multiple agents with different modes of action) for postoperative pain management. When multiple medications are used, pain control can be achieved with smaller doses of narcotics and fewer adverse effects (Pasero & McCaffery, 2007). For example, infusions of local anesthetics may be used along with intravenous or oral opioids. A continuous wound infusion is the administration of a local anesthetic through a catheter implanted directly into the surgical site. An alternative is the use of continuous perineural infusion. In this type of infusion, a catheter is inserted near the peripheral nerves affected by surgery. An infusion of a short-acting local anesthetic in this area effectively blocks the pain from these nerves (Pasero & McCaffery, 2007).

Nonsteroidal anti-inflammatory drugs (NSAIDs) are used in conjunction with opioids for pain control except where contraindicated. Acetaminophen does not affect postoperative bleeding, so it can be added to most pain control regimens (Groudine & Fossum, 2011). Ketorolac (Toradol) is a particularly effective anti-inflammatory agent, but its use is often limited to 72 hours because of its deleterious effect on kidney function. The anticonvulsant agents pregabalin and gabapentin may be used postoperatively when there is a neuropathic component to pain as is frequently the case with orthopedic conditions (Pasero & McCaffery, 2007).

Other pain control techniques include the application of heat or cold (primarily cold for the postoperative patient) and elevation. Application of ice or a cold pack helps reduce tissue swelling, one factor that contributes to postoperative pain. Ice packs are applied for 20 minutes, then removed for 20 minutes and repeated as necessary. The application of cold is used with various orthopedic procedures as well as some plastic surgeries. Elevation of an affected area above the level of the heart also assists with pain control and reduces edema. Elevation is used most often with open reduction of an extremity fracture. Chapter 12 provides a complete description of pain management techniques.

Nurses use nonpharmacologic interventions to reduce pain, but these should complement medications, not replace them. Nonetheless, there is evidence that nonpharmacologic approaches can provide pain relief and give the patient comfort. Study patients have reported that the use of positioning, massage, distraction, therapeutic touch, and relaxation techniques have decreased their need for pain medications (Coakley & Duffy, 2010; Easter, DeBoer, Settlemyre, Staries, Marlowe, & Creech, 2010; Seers, Crichton, Tutton, Smith, & Saunders, 2008; Tracy, 2010). In a systematic review of relaxation interventions, researchers found these techniques effective in reducing pain in approximately half of the 15 studies they examined (Kwekkeboom & Gretarsdottir, 2006). Research needs to continue to explore the effectiveness of nonpharmacologic therapies for the management of postoperative pain.

Anxiety

For the postoperative patient, anxiety is an unpleasant emotional response that is associated with increased morbidity and mortality and longer, more complicated hospitalizations. Anxiety causes stimulation of the sympathetic nervous system, which can increase blood pressure by 30% to 40% and heart rate by 20% (Bailey, 2010). Anxiety depresses the immune system, delays wound healing, and alters blood coagulation. Other reported physiological responses to anxiety include increases in myocardial ischemia, cardiac dysrhythmias, and postoperative pain. The nurse assesses the patient for signs of anxiety, similar to the pain assessment. The best indicators of anxiety are patients' reports of how anxious they feel. Patients are encouraged to verbalize their fears and concerns.

Nurses play a critical role in reducing the anxiety of postoperative patients. The PACU nurse provides frequent reassurance to patients about their condition and how well they are progressing. Reassurance and caring are major factors in reducing anxiety. In one study of critically ill medical and surgical patients, subjects reported an overwhelming need to "feel safe" in their environment, and they identified nurses as the key to feeling safe or not feeling safe (Bailey, 2010). Whenever possible, the nurse should give patients choices regarding their care. Regaining a sense of control helps the patient to feel a sense of security (Susleck et al., 2007).

The nurse individualizes nursing interactions with patients and provides information consistent with the individual's personal coping style and preference for information. Some patients will want and need detailed information about their status; others may become more anxious if the nurse provides a great deal of information or explanations that are too explicit. The nurse should speak slowly and calmly and should maintain a quiet and restful environment. The trend toward allowing significant others to visit with the patient in the PACU is likely to be beneficial in reducing the anxiety of the patient and the significant other. Family and friends are an important source of support and comfort (Mayne & Bagaoisan, 2009; Susleck et al., 2007).

Other techniques that are helpful in reducing anxiety are sitting with the patient, touch, massage, distraction, meditation, guided imagery, relaxation exercises, and music. It may be very useful to incorporate music into a plan of care.

Despite the use of nonpharmacologic interventions, some patients may require antianxiety agents. A number of antianxiety agents are available. Lorazepam (Ativan) works quickly (1 to 5 minutes) when given intravenously but can also be administered as an intramuscular (IM) injection or given orally. The dose is titrated to produce desired effects so that oversedation is avoided (Cronrath et al., 2011). It is important for the nurse to follow up on the effectiveness of interventions to reduce anxiety.

Discharge from the Postanesthesia Care Unit

Patients are discharged from the PACU to home or to an inpatient unit. PACUs use written criteria and a numeric rating scale to determine the patient's readiness for move on to her next location. The Aldrete Post Anesthesia Discharge Score (PADS) (Figure 19–1◆) is one measure of a patient's readiness for discharge. The PADS assigns a

POST ANESTHETIC SCORE	
ACTIVITY	
Able to move 4 extremities voluntarily or on command	2
Able to move 2 extremities voluntarily or on command	1
Unable to move extremities voluntarily or on command	0
RESPIRATION	
Able to breathe deeply and cough freely	2
Dyspnea, limited breathing or tachypnea	1
Apneic or on mechanical ventilator	0
CIRCULATION	
BP plus or minus 20% of preoperative baseline	2
BP plus or minus 20%–40% of preanesthetic level	1
BP plus or minus 40% of preanesthetic level	0
CONSCIOUSNESS	
Fully awake	2
Arousable on calling	1
Not responding	0
O_2 Saturation	
Able to maintain O_2 saturation > 92% on room air	2
Needs O_2 inhalation to maintain O_2 saturation > 90%	1
O_2 saturation <90% even with O_2 supplement	0
TOTAL PAR SCORE	

FIGURE 19–1 ◆ Aldrete Post Anesthesia Discharge Score.
Source: Courtesy of Beth Israel Deaconess Nursing Department.

numerical rating of 0 to 2 for each of the following: vital signs, activity level, nausea and vomiting, pain, and surgical bleeding. Patients can be transferred to an inpatient unit with a PADS of between 8 and 10, but a score of 9 or better is required if the patient is being discharged home. If patients have a baseline PADS of less than 8 due to a preexisting condition, the anesthesia provider makes the decision to discharge on an individual basis.

Ambulatory Surgery Discharge

Ambulatory settings require a PADS of 9 or higher for discharge; however, other criteria also may need to be met before the patient is allowed to go home. Discharge criteria vary depending on the surgery, the patient, and the health care provider's preference. Additional discharge criteria may include the following:

- Stable vital signs for 1 hour
- Baseline level of consciousness
- Stable wound with minimal bleeding
- Able to take fluids orally (applicable to selected patients)
- Able to void (applicable to certain surgeries or selected patients)
- An acceptable level of pain
- Able to dress and ambulate with assistance
- Adult caretaker available to accompany the patient home.

Patients are no longer required to void or to take oral fluids prior to discharge. Evidence from research studies found that many patients can be safely discharged home without voiding or drinking fluids (Ead, 2006; Mulroy, Salinas, Larkin, & Polissar, 2002). Patients who are considered at low risk for urinary retention may be discharged home without voiding as long as their bladder is not distended. Patients are given explicit instructions to seek medical attention in the emergency department if they have not voided after 8 hours at home. Patients who do not void and who have bladder distention need an ultrasonic bladder scan and may require an intermittent catheterization before discharge. Patients at high risk of postoperative urinary retention are still required to void before discharge. Many patients will be able to drink fluids before discharge; however, in most cases, it is not necessary to delay discharge for those who do not tolerate oral fluids. Certain patients, such as those with diabetes, older adults, and frail individuals, remain under observation until they are able to drink fluids postoperatively.

Patients who are discharged home need complete and concise information about performing self-care. The information is presented verbally as well as in writing using simple language. When home care will involve performing a procedure, the nurse demonstrates the technique, then asks the patient to return the demonstration (Ross, 2007). The nurse reviews with the patient any new medications, including the purpose of the drug, the dose, the frequency of administration, and any significant side effects. Pain management is discussed, as well as wound care. The nurse reviews any restrictions on bathing, activity, and diet. Patients should be clear about how they are expected to feel after surgery and what symptoms require follow-up with their surgeon. Patients are then given instructions about how to contact their health care provider should a problem develop. Information about follow-up appointments is also given. The Patient Teaching & Discharge Priorities box provides examples of discharge priorities following ambulatory surgery for a breast biopsy.

Many ambulatory surgery centers contact the patient by telephone the day after surgery. The nurse performs the telephone follow-up and inquires about the patient's recovery. During this call, the nurse asks

PATIENT TEACHING & DISCHARGE PRIORITIES following a Breast Biopsy

Need	Teaching
Care of incision	Your incision is covered with Steri-Strips and a bandage. Leave the bandage in place tonight. Tomorrow, you may remove the bandage (but not the Steri-Strips) and shower. Gently wash the area and pat it dry. Leave the Steri-Strips in place until they fall off by themselves. If you have sutures, they will be removed during your follow-up appointment. It is not unusual to have mild bruising around the area of the incision.
Pain control	You should have very little pain after your biopsy. Your health care provider has given you a prescription for pain medication if you need it. Do not drive while taking the prescription medication. If your pain is mild, you may take acetaminophen (Tylenol) regular or extra strength every 4 to 6 hours as needed instead of the prescription medication. Do *not* take aspirin or ibuprofen because these medications may cause you to bleed.
	Ice will help to reduce swelling and discomfort. An ice pack wrapped in cloth can be inserted in the bra. Leave the ice pack in place until it gets warm, then remove and replace. Apply ice packs off and on for the remainder of today.
	You should wear a bra for the next 24 to 36 hours to support your breast. This means that you should sleep in the bra tonight. A soft, front-closing bra may be more comfortable for you than other types.
Activity level	Do not drive on the day of your surgery. You should rest and take it easy for the remainder of the day. You received medications during surgery that may make you feel tired. You may return to work when you feel able. For most people, this will be in 1 or 2 days after the procedure. You can begin performing normal activities tomorrow, but avoid strenuous exercise until the follow-up appointment with your health care provider.
Possible problems that require attention	You should watch for signs of infection. If your incision becomes red or painful or develops drainage, you should call your health care provider. You should also call if you develop a fever (>38°C [100.4°F]) or if you have pain that is not relieved by pain medication.
Follow up with the health care provider	The results of your biopsy will be available in 2 or 3 days. Your health care provider will call you at home with the results. If you have sutures, you should make a follow-up appointment for 7 to 10 days after the procedure. If you do not have sutures, you should make a follow-up appointment for 1 month after the procedure.

questions about pain, nausea and vomiting, voiding, and the surgical site, and gives the patient the opportunity to ask questions. Often, the surgeon or surgical assistant will also contact the patient at home to monitor her recovery. Follow-up phone calls help to ensure patient safety. They may also be helpful in reducing emotional stress and improving self-care abilities after surgery, although more research is needed in this area (Allard, 2007).

Transfer to an Inpatient Unit

The surgeon or anesthesiologist discharges patients from the PACU to an inpatient unit when the patient meets specific discharge criteria or an acceptable PADS. Other criteria for PACU discharge may require the patient to be normothermic, with pain and bleeding controlled, and all tubes, drains, catheters, and IV lines patent and functioning.

Postoperative orders are written before the patient's transfer to the nursing unit. The PACU nurse reports to the receiving nurse all pertinent information about the patient. The report includes relevant past history; a description of the surgery and type of anesthesia; any significant postoperative events; estimated blood loss from surgery; recent laboratory data; a summary of OR and PACU fluid status; recent vital signs; a description of the dressing, drains, pain medication, and antiemetics given; and any equipment required postoperatively.

Nursing Management

The nurse on the clinical unit admits the PACU patient and performs a head-to-toe assessment beginning with vital signs and an admitting weight. The elements of the assessment are similar to the PACU admission assessment described earlier. The nurse makes sure that all equipment is set up correctly and functioning well. The nurse assesses the patient's safety using a fall risk assessment tool. Patients at risk for falls need an individual plan to prevent a fall. Such plans often include simple strategies such as putting the call light within reach, placing the bed in the low position, monitoring the patient frequently, educating the patient and family about falls, and activating the bed alarm, if needed. Postoperative patients are assessed often because their condition can change rapidly. The usual routine on a surgical unit includes a full head-to-toe assessment at the beginning of a shift followed by frequent follow-up assessments as the day progresses. Vital signs with oxygen saturation are taken every 4 hours, although the timing of postoperative observations is based on tradition rather than on empirical evidence. Hospital policy or a health care provider's order may specify parameters for reporting changes in vital signs. Policies do not cover the range of events that can occur in the postoperative period.

The nurse uses clinical judgment in deciding which data require health care provider notification. Chart 19–3 describes findings that are usually reported to the health care provider. Initially, postoperative patients may run a low-grade fever as a result of tissue injury, inflammation, and mild dehydration. Mild temperature elevations are not cause for alarm (Nelson, 2011). The nurse reports a fever of 38°C (100.4°F) or higher unless otherwise directed by the health care provider. Atelectasis is often associated with the development of a fever in the first 24 to 48 hours after surgery, so the nurse assesses breath sounds and encourages deep breathing if fever is present.

Because of the risk of hypoxia, oxygen saturation is also an important postoperative measurement. Many patients arrive from the PACU with oxygen in place and orders to maintain oxygen saturation above 93%. If such a patient's oxygen saturation is acceptable, the nurse begins the process of titrating the oxygen downward.

CHART 19–3 Abnormal Postoperative Assessments that Need to be Reported to the Surgeon

Metabolic
- Temperature >38°C (100.4°F).

Neurological Findings
- Change in level of consciousness.

Cardiovascular Findings
- Heart rate 120 beats/min
- Hypotension (e.g., systolic blood pressure of less than 90 mmHg)
- New cardiac arrhythmia
- Hypertension (e.g., systolic blood pressure 20% to 30% higher than baseline)
- Chest pain
- Loss of pulses.

Respiratory Findings
- Oxygen saturation <93%
- Respiratory rate <10 breaths/minute
- Indications of respiratory distress such as dyspnea, crackles, wheezing.

Gastrointestinal
- Abdominal distention
- Vomiting uncontrolled by antiemetics.

Fluid Balance
- Urine output <30 mL/hr or <0.5 mL/kg per hour
- Unable to void in 6 to 8 hours.

Wound
- More than the expected amount of bleeding at the incision site.
- More than the expected amount of drainage from chest tubes or wound drains
- Incision with redness, purulent drainage, or opened areas.

Pain
- Pain not adequately controlled

Extremities
- Absence of peripheral pulses
- Swelling, redness, pain in calf.

Other
- Unexpected presence of blood in tubes

While performing the head-to-toe assessment, the nurse asks specific questions to assess the patient's level of consciousness, orientation, and cognition. The nurse also asks about the patient's ability to sleep in the hospital. A high rate of sleep disturbance exists in the hospital, and sleep is thought to have restorative functions (Windle, 2011). The nurse asks the patient to rate his pain and assesses the adequacy of the pain control measures that have been taken. If the patient is using PCA for pain control, the nurse checks the accuracy of the settings on the pump and reviews the history to see how frequently the patient is using the PCA. If the patient has an epidural catheter, the nurse assesses the insertion site on the patient's back for redness, swelling, leaking, or kinking of the tubing. The nurse also reviews the pump settings and evaluates the level of sensation and the patient's ability to move and use his extremities. The nurse listens to lung sounds, asks about sputum production, and evaluates the patient's ability to perform deep breathing exercises.

In addition, the nurse listens to bowel sounds, palpates the abdomen, and asks the patient about nausea, vomiting, passing flatus, and moving of the bowels. General anesthesia and narcotics slow peristalsis, but bowel function is expected to return within several hours after surgery unless the patient has had pelvic or abdominal surgery. In these surgeries, peristalsis may be delayed for 24 to 48 hours or longer. Patients are expected to void 6 to 8 hours after surgery, and urine output is measured and recorded with each void. If the patient has a urinary catheter in place, urine output is measured frequently. The nurse reports a urine output of less than 30 mL/hr or less than 0.5 mL/kg per hour to the health care provider.

The nurse examines the patient's wound dressing and notes the color and amount of any drainage. The nurse also checks the color, sensation, and motion of the extremities and the presence of pedal pulses. In addition, the nurse teaches the patient how to perform leg exercises and makes sure that any devices ordered to prevent DVT are in place and functioning properly.

At the conclusion of the assessment, the nurse works with the patient to establish goals for the day and a specific plan to accomplish the goals. One of the nurse's most important tasks is to assist the patient with rest and ambulation. It can be difficult to plan uninterrupted periods of rest, given frequent nursing assessments; health care provider visits; blood draws; consultations by physical therapists, nutritionists, case managers, and social workers, among others; visits with family and friends; and the noise level of the clinical unit. Despite these challenges, the nurse must create periods during which the patient can rest because rest is thought to be important in immune function, wound healing, and mental outlook (Neveleff, Kraiss, & Schulman, 2010).

Early ambulation is one of the most important interventions that can assist a patient in her recovery from anesthesia and surgery. Unless contraindicated, ambulation begins on the evening of surgery or on the first postoperative day. The nurse is present to assist patients with their first attempt at ambulation, as they may feel dizzy or nauseated when they first move to a sitting or standing position. Splinting the incision, deep breathing, moving slowly, and moving at the patient's pace may help to minimize pain, nausea, and vertigo. Patients should be allowed to sit on the side of the bed for a few minutes before moving to a standing position. Some patients may be inclined to hunch over to protect their incisions, but this posture creates muscle tension and distorts balance, so patients are encouraged to relax and assume the correct posture. If patients are only able to ambulate a short distance initially, the nurse should provide reassurance that the distance will gradually lengthen. Postoperative patients need to ambulate at least three times daily. Early ambulation and physical therapy are correlated with faster functional recovery after some surgeries (Ong, Miller, Appleby, Allegretto, & Gawlinski, 2011), particularly orthopedic procedures. Early and aggressive ambulation is an important element of accelerated recovery programs (Munro, 2009).

Collaborative Management

It is important for the nurse to work closely with the surgeon and other members of the health care team to facilitate the patient's rapid recovery from surgery and to prevent complications. Some hospitals are using a comanagement approach that teams the surgeon and nurse with a hospitalist in managing postoperative patients. In order to meet desired patient outcomes, it is essential that this interdisciplinary team communicate openly with one another in developing and evaluating care of the patient and family (IOM [Institute of Medicine], 2010).

Other members of the health care team are also closely involved in the patient's care. For example, clinical nurse specialists provide assistance in selected aspects of a patient's recovery such as wound care for more complicated wounds or teaching for a new ostomy or organ transplantation. Physical therapy and occupational therapy provide valuable information about postoperative exercises, ambulation, transfer, and use of assistive devices. A nutritionist may be consulted to make specific recommendations about diet or diet supplementation. Social workers are consulted to provide support and counseling for patients and their families. Case managers help provide a seamless transition from hospital to rehabilitation facility or to a patient's home with services. Many patients will be discharged home after surgery without the need for home services. Some postoperative patients, however, will require services at home such as physical therapy, speech therapy, intravenous antibiotics, wound and drain checks, or teaching. The nurse collaborates with home health agencies to make sure that the patient's discharge to home is a successful one.

Preventing Postoperative Complications

A significant role of the nurse on a surgical unit is to prevent postoperative complications when possible. Chart 19–4 (p. 466) lists postoperative problems that are common to many surgeries. Common problems that occur after surgery include atelectasis, pneumonia, abdominal distention, constipation, urinary retention, wound infection, and venous stasis. The Nursing Process: Patient Care Plan box (p. 468) is for a patient following general surgery. Examples of appropriate nursing diagnoses in the postoperative period are described in the care plan.

Atelectasis and Pneumonia

Atelectasis refers to the collapse of alveoli and the surrounding airways. When alveoli collapse, lung volume is reduced and mucus accumulates, causing localized airway obstructions from mucous plugs. If atelectasis remains untreated, it leads to fever and hypoxia. Although this has not been shown clearly by research so far, it is possible that the retention of secretions associated with atelectasis increases the risk of developing pneumonia (Atkinson, 2010). Pneumonia is the inflammation of lung parenchyma caused by a virus, bacteria, or other organism. The invasion of lung tissue by an organism causes an inflammatory response, and the alveoli fill with inflammatory exudates. These changes are seen on chest x-ray as new infiltrates. Signs of pneumonia include fever, dyspnea, crackles in the lung fields, purulent sputum, congested cough, hypoxia, and an elevation in the white blood cell count. The incidence of postoperative atelectasis varies according to the surgery performed.

Atelectasis and pneumonia are referred to collectively as postoperative pulmonary complications. Some researchers also include hypoxia in that description. It can be difficult to distinguish atelectasis from pneumonia initially, and the factors that predispose patients to atelectasis also predispose them to postoperative pneumonia. Older age, preexisting respiratory conditions, heart failure, decreased level of consciousness, poor functional ability, a history of cigarette smoking, and malnutrition predispose the patient to postoperative pulmonary complications. There is a higher risk of postoperative atelectasis and pneumonia with surgeries of the chest and abdomen because the incision is located close to the diaphragm, making it painful to take

EVIDENCE-BASED PRACTICE Comparison of Postoperative Pain Management Using Two Patient-Controlled Analgesia Methods

Clinical Problem

The effective management of postoperative pain is a significant challenge to nurses in the postoperative environment. Intravenous medication administration, including patient-controlled analgesia, takes time and may require additional nursing tasks to achieve pain management. This study evaluated patient-care tasks comparing the use of IV morphine with a fentanyl iontophoretic transdermal system (ITS). Iontrophoresis is basically an injection of medication without a needle, accomplished by application of an electric current to the skin. The patient population included patients who had total hip replacement surgery and abdominal/pelvic surgery.

Research Findings

In this study, patients who had undergone a surgical procedure were randomly assigned to receive fentanyl ITS or morphine IV PCA for up to 72 hours. The fentanyl dose was 40 µg over 10 minutes for up to 6 doses/hour for 24 hours or a maximum of 80 doses per system. After this, a new system was started. The PCA morphine dose was a 1-mg morphine bolus (with a 5- to 6-minute lockout interval between doses based on site-specific policies). The maximum was 10 doses/hour in 24 hours. The nurses who participated in the study were given a *Nurse Ease-of-Care Questionnaire* to evaluate the pain intervention. An important component in the questionnaire was *Satisfaction*. This was measured by two questions: *Pain control provided by the device* and *Overall satisfaction with the device*. Over 1,100 nurses participated in the study, which found that the fentanyl ITS appeared to be simpler, easier to use, and more satisfactory for nurses when providing postoperative pain management.

Implications for Nursing Practice

This study is significant because postoperative pain management is an important nursing intervention. Pain can cause significant physiological and psychological complications if not appropriately managed. In addition, pain medications can place a patient at risk of complications such as respiratory depression, leading to atelectasis and pneumonia; altered mental status, increasing the risk of falling; and hypotension, which could impede wound healing. The study found that patient movement was easier with the fentanyl ITS system than with the morphine PCA system. The ITS system was also much easier to set up and maintain. The researchers felt that this translated into better safety and comfort for patients having postoperative pain.

Critical Thinking Questions with answers can be found in the Osborn Student Resources at nursing.pearsonhighered.com.

References

Lindley, P., Pestano, C., & Gargiulo, K. (2009). Comparison of postoperative pain management using two patient-controlled analgesia methods: Nursing perspective. *Journal of Advanced Nursing, 65*, 1370–1380.

CHART 19–4 Common Postoperative Problems

Problem	Cause/High Risk	Goal	Assessment	Interventions
Pain	Cell injury, muscle spasm, inflammation from tissue manipulation, drains, anxiety.	Pain free, rate pain a 3 or less.	Pain rating scale 0–10. Increased heart rate, blood pressure, and respirations. Guarding, grimacing.	Narcotics: PCA or epidural. NSAIDs: Tylenol, Toradol. Comfort measures.
Fluid retention (overload)	Stress response, excess IV fluid, medical diagnosis such as heart failure.	Ensure adequate perfusion without causing overload. (Diuresis is expected by day 3 postop.)	Swelling in hands, feet, eyelids. Weight gain. Decreased urine output of <30 mL/hour or <0.5 mL/kg per hour. Crackles or rales.	Monitor urine output every 1–4 hours. Check breath sounds. Monitor IV fluid. Monitor vital sign trends for changes (i.e., increased heart and respiratory rate).
Fluid deficit (dehydration)	Excess fluid losses during surgery, from wound, drains; vomiting, fever.	Ensure adequate tissue perfusion.	Dry skin, mucous membranes. Decreased urine output of <30 mL/hour or <0.5 mL/kg per hour. HR >100, SBP <90 mmHg, narrow pulse pressure.	Fluid bolus: normal saline (NS) 250–500 mL over 1 hour per health care provider's order. Monitor urine output, heart rate, and BP.
Bleeding	High risk for surgery on vascular tissue or on patient with history of clotting disorder, use of anticoagulants, malnourished.	Hemodynamic stability.	Cool, clammy skin. HR >100, SBP <90 mmHg, narrow pulse pressure. Decreased Hct/Hgb. Decreased urine output of <30 mL/hr or <0.5 mL/kg per hour. Swelling or distention, oozing from wounds, hematoma, bloody drainage.	Fluid replacement: NS bolus. Transfusion with packed red blood cells (if active bleeding). Transfusion with fresh frozen plasma (if clotting factors need replacing).

CHART 19–4 Common Postoperative Problems, *continued*

Problem	Cause/High Risk	Goal	Assessment	Interventions
Atelectasis (risk of pneumonia)	Most common problem in first 48–72 hours postop. Primary cause is anesthesia. Risk increases with surgery on chest or abdomen, with uncontrolled pain, decreased mobility, obesity, smoker, chronic obstructive pulmonary disease, asthma.	Patient will demonstrate adequate oxygenation and will not develop postop pneumonia.	Fever is most common sign. Breath sounds diminished or crackles. Increased RR. Oxygen (O_2) saturation $<93\%$. Sputum: increased production and consistency.	Incentive spirometer or turn–cough–deep breathe 10 times per hour. Turn every 1–2 hours. Adequate pain relief. Splint incision during movement. Increase head of bed 30 degrees or higher. Ambulate 3 times per day. Titrate oxygen to maintain O_2 saturation $>93\%$.
Nausea and vomiting (N&V)	Most N&V peaks in 24–36 hours postop. Anesthesia, narcotics, antibiotics, retained gastric secretions.	Will not experience N&V or N&V will be relieved.	Nausea and vomiting. Nausea increases with movement. Abdominal distention.	IV fluid to maintain hydration. Medicate with antiemetic. (See Pharmacology feature, p. 460.) Maintain patency of nasogastric tube (NGT). Minimize use of opioids and increase use of nonopioids for pain. Advance diet slowly (ice chips—clear liquids—full liquids—regular diet).
Abdominal distention (postoperative ileus)	Following surgery on the bowel, it will take 3–5 days for return of GI function. Factors that decrease bowel function: anesthesia, surgical trauma, narcotics, decreased mobility.	Return of bowel peristalsis.	Abdomen is distended. No stool or flatus. Nausea and vomiting. No bowel sounds or hypoactive bowel sounds.	NPO until flatus; may be 3–5 days post-gastrointestinal (GI) surgery. NGT to suction for comfort if vomiting. Ambulate per health care provider orders. Advance diet slowly.
Syncope (orthostatic hypotension)	Anesthesia, immobility, dehydration, some medications.	Patient will not experience orthostatic hypotension.	Complaints of dizzy, light-headedness, diaphoresis. Increased symptoms with standing or sitting. Orthostatic (postural) vital sign changes: HR increases at least 10 beats/minute (from lying to standing); BP decreases by at least 10 mmHg (from lying to standing).	Get out of bed slowly; dangle legs before standing. If symptomatic, take orthostatic vital signs. If syncope is from dehydration, give patient a fluid bolus.
Urinary retention	Anesthesia, narcotics, anticholinergics, spasm of abdominal or pelvic muscles.	Patient will void (minimum 200 mL) after surgery or 6–8 hours after removal of Foley catheter.	No voiding or small, frequent voids. Fullness above symphysis pubis.	Ambulate. Avoid use of bedpan. Check intake and output. Offer fluids. Bladder scan. Catheterize (per order); if not, void in 8–12 hours.
Wound healing: risk of infection Dehiscence Evisceration	Infection usually not evident until 3–7 days after surgery. High risk with obesity, poor circulation, diabetes, malnourishment.	Wound well approximated and without drainage. Wound heals.	Local: redness, swelling, increased pain, edges not approximated, increased drainage from incision. Systemic: fever, elevated white blood cell count.	Adequate nutrition. Limit stress on wound. Prophylactic antibiotic for 24 hours only. Use sterile technique.
Deep venous thrombosis (DVT)	Occurs 5–7 days after surgery and is caused by venous stasis and pressure. DVT can dislodge and become a pulmonary embolus.	Adequate circulation without evidence of venous stasis.	Calf: red, painful, swollen. Positive Homans' sign.	Ambulate tid. Leg exercises. Antiembolism stockings or pneumatic compression boots. Antithrombotic medication. Avoid pressure under the knees.

NURSING PROCESS: Patient Care Plan for the Postoperative Patient Following General Surgery

Assessment of Postoperative Status Using Gordon's Functional Health Patterns:

- Health Perception Health Management Pattern
- Nutrition Metabolic Pattern
- Elimination Pattern
- Activity Exercise Pattern
- Cognitive Perceptual Pattern
- Activities and Exercise Pattern

Subjective Data

Assessment of Discomfort

Ask the patient to describe the pain, its location, and its intensity.

Ask the patient to rate the pain from 0–10 on the pain scale.

Assessment of Nausea and Vomiting

Ask patient about feeling nauseated.

Assessment of Fluid Volume—Deficient

Patient reports vertigo.

Are you thirsty?

Assessment of Fluid Volume—Excess

Patient reports dyspnea.

Assessment of Respiratory Status

Patient states it is painful to take deep breaths.

Assessment of Urinary Output

Patient states he cannot void or is only able to void small amounts.

Assessment of Activity Level

Patient states he has vertigo, fatigue, or dyspnea with activity.

Assessment of Wound

Patient states that incision feels painful and swollen.

Assessment of Blood Flow to the Extremities

Patient complains of pain in the calf.

Assessment of Knowledge Regarding Surgery and Postoperative Care

Patient states that she needs information on how to care for herself at home.

Objective Data

Assessment of Discomfort

Watch for physical signs of pain including guarding, grimacing, crying, increased blood pressure (BP), heart rate (HR), and respiratory rate (RR).

Assessment of Nausea and Vomiting

Patient vomits.

Abdomen is firm, distended with hypoactive bowel sounds.

Assessment of Fluid Volume—Deficient

Watch for signs of active bleeding including blood on dressing, hematoma, presence of blood in drainage tubes, and decreased hematocrit and hemoglobin.

Watch for signs of dehydration including heart rate (HR) $>$100, systolic blood pressure (SBP) $<$90, narrow pulse pressure, decreased urine output of $<$30 mL/hour or $<$0.5 mL/kg per hour.

Assessment of Fluid Volume—Excess

Swelling in hands, feet, and eyelids; weight gain; urine output $<$ 30 mL/hr or $<$0.5 mL/kg per hour; crackles in the lungs.

Assessment of Respiratory Status

Watch for fever, diminished breath sounds, crackles in the lungs, sputum production, increased respiratory rate, and decreased oxygen saturation.

Assessment of Urinary Output

Patient does not void or voids only small amounts.

Palpable fullness above symphysis pubis or a bladder scan showing a full bladder.

Assessment of Activity Level

Positive orthostatic vital signs with activity or an increased heart rate of $>$10 beats/minute, increased respiratory rate of $>$10 breaths/minute, decreased oxygen saturation, or labored breathing with activity.

Assessment of Wound

Incision is red, painful, or swollen. Wound edges are not approximated and the wound has increased drainage.

Elevated white blood cell (WBC) count and fever.

Assessment of Blood Flow to the Extremities

Calf is red, painful, and swollen. Patient reports a positive Homans' sign.

Assessment of Knowledge Regarding Surgery and Postoperative Care

Patient is being discharged home following a recent surgery.

Outcomes and Evaluation Parameters / Planning and Interventions with *Rationales*

1. NURSING DIAGNOSIS: Readiness for Enhanced Comfort ***related to surgical incision, muscle spasm, positioning in the operating room, the presence of drains, and anxiety*** **(NANDA-I © 2012)**

Outcome: The patient will be comfortable and rate the pain at or below the predetermined postoperative goal (if no predetermined goal was set, patient rates the pain at 3 or less).

Use pain scale (0–10) to assess pain every 2–4 hours. *Increases consistency in quantifying pain.*

Watch for physical signs of pain including guarding, grimacing, crying, increased BP, HR, and RR. *Some patients are reluctant to ask for pain medication. Different cultures respond to and express pain differently.*

NURSING PROCESS: Patient Care Plan for the Postoperative Patient Following General Surgery, *continued*

Evaluation Parameters: Patient is comfortable. Patient participates in postoperative activities and exercises without discomfort.	Administer pain medication, narcotics, and anti-inflammatory agents as prescribed. *Postoperative pain is highest in the first 48 hours after surgery.* Provide teaching about patient-controlled analgesia (PCA) or patient-controlled epidural analgesia (PCEA) if prescribed. Elevate affected area if *appropriate to decrease tissue swelling.* Apply ice to affected area if *appropriate to decrease tissue swelling.* Teach to splint the incision. *Provides stability to injured area.* Use nonpharmacologic interventions such as massage, distraction, and relaxation techniques. *These measures augment other pain control measures.*
2. NURSING DIAGNOSIS: Alteration in Nausea *related to anesthesia, narcotics, antibiotics, slowed peristalsis* (NANDA-I © 2012)	
Outcomes: Patient will get relief from nausea and vomiting. Patient will have a soft abdomen and pass flatus. Patient will have adequate intake of fluids. ***Evaluation Parameters:*** Abdomen soft. Appetite is present. Oral fluid intake is 1,500–2,500 mL in 24 hours. Passing flatus and stool.	Assess for nausea, vomiting, abdominal distention, and flatus. *Most nausea and vomiting peaks in 24 to 36 hours after surgery.* Maintain nasogastric tube (NGT) as prescribed for comfort. *An NGT decompresses the stomach and prevents vomiting.* Maintain NPO status until nausea recedes and bowel function returns. *Flatus and passing stool are the best indicators that bowel function has returned.* Advance diet slowly from ice chips to clear liquids to full liquids and regular diet. *Vomiting can occur when the diet is advanced too rapidly.* Medicate with antinausea medication as prescribed. *Early administration of medication is more effective than waiting until the patient experiences nausea and vomiting.* Encourage patient to change positions slowly. *Movement is a trigger for nausea and vomiting.* Provide comfort measures such as rest, a cool washcloth, mouth care, and deep breathing.
3. NURSING DIAGNOSIS: Deficient Fluid Volume *related to hemorrhage, blood loss with surgery, fluid loss, wound drains, vomiting, or fever* (NANDA-I © 2012)	
Outcome: Patient will have adequate hemostasis and normal intravascular volume. ***Evaluation Parameters:*** Normal vital signs. Urine output >0.5 mL/kg per hour. No evidence of active bleeding.	Assess for indications of bleeding and dehydration every 1–4 hours. *There is a higher risk of bleeding if surgery is performed on tissue that is vascular. The patient is most at risk for dehydration in the first 24–48 hours postop.* Report HR >120, systolic blood pressure (SBP) <90, urine output <30 mL/hour or <0.5 mL/kg per hour, or more drainage than expected on dressing or in tubes. *Indicators or risk of imbalanced fluid volume and possible postoperative bleeding.* Check dressing and circle any new drainage with pen *to monitor for bleeding.* Reinforce dressing as needed. *The surgeon changes the primary dressing.* Administer IV fluids as *ordered to replace fluids lost during surgery.* Administer normal saline fluid bolus if required. *Used to expand circulating blood volume and increase urine output.*
4. NURSING DIAGNOSIS: Risk for Imbalanced Fluid Volume *related to response to stress hormones, excess intravenous fluids, or preexisting medical condition such as congestive heart failure* (NANDA-I © 2012)	
Outcome: Patient will have adequate fluid volume without evidence of overload. ***Evaluation Parameters:*** Urine output is >30 mL/hr or >0.5 mL/kg per hour. Intake and output (I&O) is balanced. Clear breath sounds. Normal vital signs without tachycardia or tachypnea.	Assess for swelling, weight gain, urine output <30 mL/hr or <0.5 mL/kg per hour, crackles in lungs, and dyspnea every 1–4 hours. *The effect of stress hormones is greatest in the first 24–48 hours.* Monitor IV fluid administration carefully. *Fluid given too rapidly can exacerbate fluid overload.*
5. NURSING DIAGNOSIS: Ineffective Breathing Pattern *related to anesthesia, surgical pain, location of the surgery, limited mobility, a history of smoking, or preexisting medical condition* (NANDA-I © 2012)	
Outcome: Respiratory status will be stable and within normal limits. ***Evaluation Parameters:*** Afebrile. Clear lung sounds. Oxygen saturation >93%. Normal respiratory rate. Denies shortness of breath and air hunger.	Monitor respiratory rate, depth, breath sounds, and oxygen saturation every 4 hours *to assess for atelectasis.* Encourage deep breathing or use of incentive spirometry 10 times every hour *to increase maximal inspiration and stimulate surfactant.* Encourage patient to cough every hour. Splint incision if appropriate. *Coughing clears mucous secretions.* Elevate head of the bed 30 degrees or higher *to lower the diaphragm and facilitate lung expansion.*

(*continued*)

NURSING PROCESS: Patient Care Plan for the Postoperative Patient Following General Surgery, *continued*

Outcomes and Evaluation Parameters	Planning and Interventions with *Rationales*
	Provide adequate pain relief. *Patients consistently give high pain ratings to coughing and deep breathing.* Ambulate three times daily. *Increases RR, minute ventilation, and tidal volume.* Titrate oxygen (O_2) to maintain the O_2 saturation at or > 93%. *Oxygen dries the airways and reduces mucociliary clearance.*
6. NURSING DIAGNOSIS: Urinary Retention *related to anesthesia, narcotics, anticholinergic medications, or spasm of abdominal or pelvic muscles* (NANDA-I © 2012)	
Outcome: Patient voids >100–150 mL within 6–8 hours after surgery or after removal of indwelling urinary catheter. ***Evaluation Parameters:*** I&O is balanced. Voids adequate amounts without difficulty.	Monitor I&O *to determine adequacy of urine output.* Encourage oral fluids if appropriate. *Inability to void may be due to dehydration.* Ambulate frequently *to stimulate circulation and production of urine.* Perform measures to stimulate voiding reflex (i.e., use commode rather than bedpan; have male patients stand to use urinal; run water; run warm water over perineum; use spirits of peppermints). If patient is unable to void 8 hours after surgery or after indwelling urinary catheter is removed, perform a bladder scan and call the surgeon for an order to perform catheterization. *The patient should feel the urge to void when the bladder has 300 mL of urine.*
7. NURSING DIAGNOSIS: Activity Intolerance *related to anesthesia, narcotics, surgery, and limited mobility* (NANDA-I © 2012)	
Outcome: Patient will carry out postoperative activities and activities of daily living without signs of activity intolerance. ***Evaluation Parameters:*** Ambulates without experiencing symptoms. Completes activities of daily living without experiencing symptoms. Postactivity vital signs and oxygen saturation are within normal limits.	Encourage muscle strengthening activities every shift *to increase circulation.* Encourage use of slow changes in position. Dangle legs at bedside before attempting to ambulate. Assist with two people during first attempt at ambulation *to provide for patient safety.* If symptomatic, take orthostatic vital signs and notify surgeon. Anticipate administering a fluid bolus. *Positive orthostatic vital signs are an indication of dehydration.* Ambulate a minimum of three times daily.
8. NURSING DIAGNOSIS: Risk for Infection *related to altered skin integrity and high-risk factors (e.g., diabetes, obesity, diminished arterial circulation, malnutrition)* (NANDA-I © 2012)	
Outcomes: The patient will be free from infection. The wound will heal within appropriately 7–10 days. ***Evaluation Parameters:*** The patient is afebrile. The wound edges are well approximated without drainage, redness, or swelling.	Monitor temperature, WBC count, and serum glucose. *Infection causes a fever and increased WBC and glucose.* Change dressing every shift using sterile technique and monitor for signs of infection. *The inflammatory response in an infected wound will cause redness, pain, swelling, and drainage.* Encourage adequate nutrition that is high in protein and vitamins. *Protein, calories, calcium, iron, zinc, and vitamins A, B_6, B_{12}, and C are needed for wound healing.*
9. NURSING DIAGNOSIS: Ineffective Tissue Perfusion, Venous Stasis *related to immobility, surgical procedure, and high-risk factors (e.g., age, use of estrogen, cancer, history of previous deep vein thrombosis [DVT])* (NANDA-I © 2012)	
Outcome: The patient will have adequate peripheral circulation and no evidence of DVT. ***Evaluation Parameters:*** Palpable dorsal pedis and posterior tibialis pulses. Calf is pain free without evidence of redness or swelling.	Assess for signs of DVT. A red, warm, swollen, or painful calf alerts the nurse to the possibility of a venous clot. *Venous thrombosis is most likely to occur 5 to 7 days after surgery.* Administer anticoagulant medication as prescribed *to prevent clot formation.* Measure the circumference of the calf and thigh of each leg and compare them prn. *The leg will increase in size with DVT formation.* Any indication of a clot is reported immediately to the health care provider. *Early treatment will decrease the risk of further clot formation.* The patient is placed on bed rest until the possibility of a clot is evaluated. *There is an increased chance of clot migration with activity.* Encourage ambulation and leg exercises three times daily *to stimulate circulation.* Apply pneumatic compression boots, antiembolism stockings, or other antithrombotic devices as ordered *to increase venous return and prevent venous stasis.* Avoid pressure under the knees. *Venous compression contributes to the development of DVT.*

NURSING PROCESS: Patient Care Plan for the Postoperative Patient Following General Surgery, *continued*

10. NURSING DIAGNOSIS: Deficient Knowledge *related to postoperative care* (NANDA-I © 2012)

Outcomes: The patient will recover from surgery without complications.

The patient is knowledgeable about how to care for herself at home.

Evaluation Parameters: Demonstrates appropriate care of her wound and drains (if applicable).

Verbalizes an understanding of pain management.

Verbalizes an understanding of activity restrictions and other discharge instructions.

Verbalizes an understanding of danger signs and what to do about them.

The specific information taught depends on the surgery (refer to the appropriate disorder chapter in this text for specific information) and the preferences of the surgeon. General areas for teaching appear in the following list.

Teaching is done in the patient's native language, through an interpreter, if necessary.

- General information about recovery
- Wound care
- Activity
- Specific exercises to aid recovery
- Diet
- Medication
- Symptom management: pain, constipation, fatigue
- Recognition and prevention of complications
- Follow-up appointments
- Whom to call with questions

Source: Adapted from Wilkinson, J. M., & Ahearn, N. R. (2009). *Prentice Hall nursing diagnosis handbook* (9th ed.). Upper Saddle River, NJ: Prentice Hall.

deep breaths, turn, and ambulate. Studies show that vital capacity can decrease by as much as 60% in the first 24 hours following abdominal surgery (Wren, Martin, Yoon, & Bech, 2010). Immobility increases risk because the movement of the diaphragm and chest wall are restricted, resulting in diminished lung volumes (Atkinson, 2010). Surgeries that take more than 4 hours also increase the risk as a result of prolonged anesthesia (Wren et al., 2010). Other procedures associated with increased risk of postoperative pulmonary complications are neurosurgery, head and neck surgery, vascular surgery, and emergency surgery (Wren et al., 2010).

The nurse assesses the patient's respiratory rate, depth of respiration, lung sounds, and oxygen saturation at frequent intervals. Postoperative atelectasis most often occurs in the lower lobes of the lungs. Lung sounds may be diminished as a result of shallow respirations or crackles, which are most noticeable on inspiration and may be heard as collapsed alveoli are forced open. Crackles also occur with pneumonia as air is forced through mucus and fluid in the alveoli. The crackles with pneumonia may be present throughout the respiratory cycle. Atelectasis can clear with repeated deep breathing, so the nurse assesses lung sounds before and after deep breathing or use of the incentive spirometer. Fever can be present with either atelectasis or pneumonia and is caused by inflammatory mediators.

A number of interventions are designed to decrease postoperative pulmonary complications. Unless contraindicated, the patient is placed in a semi-Fowler's, Fowler's, or high-Fowler's position. By elevating the head of the bed 30 to 90 degrees, the patient's diaphragm is lowered, thus facilitating chest expansion.

The patient is encouraged to use lung expansion therapies, deep breathing, or incentive spirometry. Deep breathing reverses alveolar collapse by forcing and holding maximal inspiration. Techniques for deep breathing and incentive spirometry are discussed in Chapter 17. Deep breathing is most effective when maximal inspiration is held for 3 seconds or longer and when the exercises are performed frequently. Patients are encouraged to take 5 to 10 deep breaths every hour, although taking more is better. Nasal continuous positive airway pressure, a specially designed face mask and pump that forces air into the nasal passages at pressures high enough to keep the airway open, may be helpful to patients who are unable to perform deep breathing (Atkinson, 2010; Wren et al., 2010).

Forced coughing is used postoperatively to clear secretions. To have an effective cough, the patient must take a deep breath, increase intrathoracic pressure, and produce a high expiratory flow rate. Both volume and force of airflow are required to remove secretions. Coughing can be painful, and the incision should be splinted with a pillow or small rolled blanket held firmly across the incision to prevent undue stress. Coughing is usually performed with deep breathing exercises, but the practice is contraindicated in some situations (e.g., cranial surgery, eye surgery) because it can increase intracranial and intraocular pressures, and in other circumstances because it places too much stress on the incision (e.g., hernia surgery). Interventions to loosen and remove secretions such as percussion and postural drainage are recommended in specific situations, but they are not employed universally after surgery (Atkinson, 2010; Wren et al., 2010).

Ambulation is an important intervention to prevent postoperative pulmonary complications. Ambulation increases respiratory rate, minute ventilation, tidal volume, and inspiratory flow rates. Patients who walk more frequently and those who walk longer distances tend to recover more quickly and are discharged sooner than patients who are less mobile (Atkinson, 2010; Wren et al, 2010). There are no practice guidelines describing optimal postoperative ambulation. However, as soon as allowed by the surgeon, patients are encouraged to walk a minimum of three times daily. Patients are encouraged to walk with good posture and to take deep breaths with ambulation. More ambulation is likely to be better, provided that the patient does not overexert. Patients are monitored during ambulation for signs of activity intolerance. These include shortness of breath, tachypnea, hypoxia, tachycardia, chest pain, and fatigue. It is also beneficial for patients to get out of bed to a chair several times each day. Sitting facilitates excursion of the diaphragm, and it is associated with improved respirations and lung volumes (Atkinson, 2010; Wren et al., 2010).

Pain control is absolutely essential to getting patients to participate in pulmonary exercises and ambulation. Postoperative patients consistently give high pain ratings to turning, movement, coughing, and deep breathing. Higher pain scores are associated with reluctance to walk and to take deep breaths, as well as with higher rates of atelectasis and pneumonia (McMain, 2008, 2010; Pasero & McCaffery, 2007; Rejeh & Vaismoradi, 2009; Wood, 2010). Patients are given pain medication prior to periods of mobility; when possible, the nurse will ambulate patients when the effect of the pain medication is at its peak. Encouraging the use of nonpharmacologic interventions for pain control is also useful. In one study, the use of relaxation techniques 15 minutes before deep breathing exercises was associated with higher inspiratory volumes (Hoffman, Bohme, & Bigbee, 2008; McMain, 2008, 2010; Pasero & McCaffery, 2007; Rejeh & Vaismoradi, 2009; Wood, 2010).

The use of gastric tubes for patients with nausea and vomiting or symptomatic abdominal distention is shown to reduce the incidence of postoperative atelectasis and pneumonia. Conversely, quick removal of the gastric tube when it is no longer necessary may reduce microaspiration and bacterial colonization of the oropharyngeal area, both of which are risk factors for postoperative pneumonia (McMain, 2008, 2010; Pasero & McCaffery, 2007; Rejeh & Vaismoradi, 2009; Wood, 2010).

Other interventions may be helpful in reducing atelectasis and pneumonia, although the benefit has not been established through research. Titrating the patient off of oxygen may be helpful because supplemental oxygen can dry airways and reduce mucociliary clearance (McMain, 2008, 2010; Pasero & McCaffery, 2007; Rejeh & Vaismoradi, 2009; Wood, 2010). In 1997, the Centers for Disease Control and Prevention began recommending the use of sterile water to fill oxygen humidifiers and to rinse medication nebulizers to reduce the introduction of microorganisms to the respiratory tract (Centers for Disease Control and Prevention, 1997).

Poor nutrition correlates with postoperative pulmonary complications, but the routine use of enteral feedings using a gastrostomy tube, jejunostomy tube, or total parenteral nutrition is not recommended (Daniels, 2007). Dental plaque and poor oral care provide a site for bacterial growth and are thought to predispose patients to pneumonia. Good oral hygiene may stimulate salivary flow, reducing the growth of microorganisms in the mouth. Adequate hydration aids in mucous clearance (Daniels, 2007).

Safety Alert *A fever in the first 48 hours after surgery is commonly related to atelectasis. Encourage the patient to cough, deep breathe, and ambulate, if appropriate. If the fever is accompanied by crackles in the lungs, respiratory congestion, respiratory distress, or low oxygen saturations, contact the health care provider because these signs are consistent with pneumonia.*

Abdominal Distention, Ileus, and Risk for Constipation

As part of a routine gastrointestinal assessment, the nurse palpates the abdomen for firmness and tenderness and asks about the presence of nausea and vomiting, passing of flatus, and recent bowel movement. Multiple factors place postoperative patients at risk for abdominal distention, a bloated abdomen, and ileus. Surgical trauma, physiological stress, and the inflammatory process stimulate the release of catecholamines, neurotransmitters, and hormones that slow gastrointestinal motility. The inhibitory effects of anesthesia and opioids further reduce peristalsis. Despite these factors, most patients regain bowel function several hours after surgery except in abdominal procedures, after which the return of bowel function is delayed for several days.

A postoperative ileus (POI) occurs when peristalsis does not return as expected after surgery. An ileus is more likely to occur in patients who have had major abdominal surgery, particularly if inflammation or leakage of an abdominal organ was involved (e.g., appendix or gallbladder). Other factors such as postoperative fluid and electrolyte imbalance can cause POI. Minimally invasive surgical approaches (laparoscopy), epidural analgesia, and lower doses of opioids are associated with lower rates of POI (Miaskowski, 2009; Zeinali, 2009). Indications of an ileus include a hard, firm abdomen; hypoactive or absent bowel sounds; and no passing of flatus or stool. Patients with severe abdominal distention may also experience nausea, vomiting, pain, and hiccups caused by irritation of the diaphragm. Research efforts are focused on preventing postoperative ileus and on speeding the resolution of the ileus after abdominal surgery. Chart 19–5 lists some of the strategies used to prevent or correct postoperative ileus (Hocevar, Robinson, & Gray, 2010; Madsen, Magor, & Parker, 2010; Rasmussen, 2010).

Safety Alert *The nurse gives priority to performing an abdominal assessment early in the shift on patients who are recovering from abdominal surgery. A hard, distended, painful abdomen can indicate internal bleeding, and the surgeon must be notified as soon as possible.*

There are many approaches to the treatment of postoperative ileus, although not all treatments are evidence based. For example, POI may resolve with time alone or with the correction of dehydration or electrolyte imbalance. In some cases, an NGT or a longer intestinal tube is used to decompress the stomach and/or intestine. Studies done in 2006 showed that nasogastric intubation does not improve postoperative ileus (Saclarides, 2006), but it may provide comfort by reducing abdominal bloating, as well as nausea and vomiting. The NGT is attached to suction, and the nurse checks that the suction is functioning correctly. NGT drainage is measured every shift. If a disposable system is being used, the entire setup is replaced, rather than emptied, once a day or as often as needed. The NGT is taped firmly to the patient's nose to prevent dislodgement. Usually, an NGT can be flushed with 30 mL of normal saline to maintain patency except when contraindicated by the presence of internal sutures. The nurse does not flush an NGT if the patient has had esophageal or gastric surgery except by order of the health care provider because a strong flush could disrupt sutures and stimulate bleeding. Ambulation helps

CHART 19–5 Strategies Used to Reduce Postoperative Ileus

Strategies That Have Been Shown to Be Effective in Reducing POI	Strategies That Might Be Effective in Reducing POI
Use of minimally invasive surgical techniques	Use of epidural analgesia
NSAIDs for pain control	Opioid antagonists for pain control
Use of laxatives postoperatively	Chewing gum
Early feeding of patient postoperatively	Sham feeding: allowing patients to chew food without swallowing it
	Alternative therapies: guided imagery, mechanical massage, acupuncture

to stimulate peristalsis and return the bowel to normal function. Usually, it is acceptable to clamp an NGT temporarily for the purpose of ambulation or transfer to a chair.

The passing of flatus and stool marks the return of bowel motility and function. However, the presence of bowel sounds is not a good marker of the return of bowel function in the postoperative patient and is probably an unnecessary assessment (Zeinali, 2009). The trend in postoperative care is toward early feeding. Most patients (except those with abdominal surgery) will be started on clear fluids the evening of surgery. Traditionally, patients begin on clear liquids, and the diet is advanced if the patient tolerates clear liquids without nausea and vomiting.

Many postoperative patients experience constipation. Most patients receive a stool softener such as docusate sodium (Colace). Fluids, ambulation, and bulk laxatives such as Metamucil or MiraLax are also helpful to achieve postoperative bowel regularity. Patients who are unable to move their bowels may require a laxative or an enema, but health care provider approval is necessary in either case.

Urinary Retention

Many patients will have a urinary catheter for the first 12 to 24 hours after surgery. The nurse observes urine output frequently in patients with a urinary catheter. If urine output falls below 30 mL or 0.5 mL/kg per hour, the nurse notifies the health care provider. The catheter will be removed as soon as possible to avoid the possibility of a urinary tract infection (UTI). Once the catheter has been removed, however, the patient is often at risk for the development of urinary retention. Urinary retention occurs as a result of general anesthesia from relaxation of the detrusor muscle, spinal anesthesia from blocking parasympathetic fibers in the sacral region of the spine controlling micturition, certain preoperative medications, and narcotics. Urinary retention is also most likely to occur in surgeries of the lower abdomen, pelvis, and genitourinary tract, in which manipulation of tissues may cause swelling of or around the urethra.

Once the urinary catheter is discontinued, the patient must void within the next 6 to 8 hours. The time when the patient is due to void is noted on the intake and output (I&O) record and in the nursing note. The void must be substantial, a minimum of 100 to 150 mL, to be considered adequate. A patient who voids only small amounts may have urinary retention with overflow or a UTI.

When a patient is unable to void, the nurse palpates the bladder. A bladder scan can be used to estimate the amount of urine in the bladder and to determine the need for catheterization. The I&O record is also reviewed because dehydration may be partially to blame. Techniques to help patients void include running warm water over the perineum, allowing the patient to stand or use the bathroom rather than a bedpan, running water in the bathroom, and allowing the patient to smell spirits of peppermint. These techniques may help; however, their efficacy has not been demonstrated through research.

Patients who do not void within the specified time frame are usually straight catheterized to empty the bladder. However, the nurse needs a health care provider's order to perform urinary catheterization. Sometimes the catheter is left in place if more than 1,000 mL is drained during the catheterization. The patient is reassured and encouraged to continue to drink fluids. Urinary retention resolves over time, but it may take one or two straight catheterizations before the patient is able to void on his own.

Safety Alert *Urinary retention can place pressure on internal sutures in a patient recovering from some types of urological surgery. Contact the surgeon immediately if a patient is unable to void within the prescribed time period.*

Wound Care

Wound healing begins immediately after tissue injury. In the first stage (days 1 to 4), the inflammatory process is triggered, bringing blood, lymph, and fibrin to the area. Fibrin strands form along the area of injury, creating a blood clot that holds the wound edges together. Increased blood flow to the site brings white blood cells (WBCs), which remove damaged tissue and fight off microorganisms. In the second stage (days 5 to 14 or longer), epithelial cells migrate to the area and proliferate, forming a protective barrier at the wound site. While the process of epithelialization is occurring, collagen synthesis is taking place, filling in tissue gaps and giving the wound added strength. Collagen synthesis helps contract the wound, making it smaller than its original size.

Traditionally, the surgeon performs the first dressing change. Until then, the nurse monitors the surgical site for evidence of bleeding or drainage. Some amount of drainage is normal after surgery. As described earlier, small to moderate amounts of drainage are circled with a pen directly on the dressing. This allows the nurse to watch for an increase in the amount of drainage. The dressing can also be reinforced. Excessive amounts of bleeding or drainage are reported to the surgeon. After the first dressing change, the wound may be left open to the air or covered with a dry sterile dressing according to health care provider preference. Dressing changes are usually performed once or twice a shift using sterile technique. During the dressing change, the nurse notes the condition of the incision. It should be well approximated, slightly pink, and free of purulent drainage. Crusting along the incision is a normal finding. The nurse reports signs of wound infection, including pain and tenderness at the site, swelling, redness, purulent drainage, odor, or evidence of **dehiscence** (opening of the incision), to the surgeon. Systemic indicators of infection include fever (38°C [100.4°F] or higher), elevated WBC count, and elevated serum glucose. Wound care is discussed in detail in Chapter 60.

Prophylactic antibiotics may be necessary in situations in which an organ ruptured or leaked prior to surgery because these wounds are more likely to become infected (Steinberg et al., 2009). Other factors that may aid in wound healing include improving the patient's nutritional status. Protein, calories, calcium, iron, zinc, and vitamins A, B_6, B_{12}, and C are needed for wound healing. Chapter 8 provides a complete description of adequate nutrition. Chapter 60 discusses normal and abnormal wound healing.

Wound Drains

Drains are used for a variety of reasons. Wound drains are inserted through an intentional stab wound into an area close to the incision and site of the operation. The purpose of the drain is to remove inflammatory fluid (serum, blood, lymph) that might otherwise accumulate at the operative site, causing infection or abscess. The surgeon inserts a closed, suction-type drain such as a Jackson-Pratt or a Hemovac. Applying negative pressure in the drain reservoir creates suction in the drain and speeds the removal of fluid. The nurse empties the drain and records the color and amount of drainage every 8 hours or as often as necessary. The drainage may be sanguineous initially but progresses to serosanguineous and sometimes serous. The nurse reports an increase in the amount of drainage and any unexpected change in the type of drainage. Many patients are now discharged to home with wound drains in place. The nurse teaches these patients and their family members how to empty and measure the drainage so they will be able to continue the care at home. Chart 19–6 lists common tubes with their purpose and expected drainage. Chapter 60 further discusses drains and provides pictures.

Venous Thromboembolism

Deep venous thrombosis is the formation of a venous blood clot in a deep vein, usually in the lower leg or pelvis. It is a serious postoperative problem. Once the clot forms, there is a danger of detachment and the possibility of a pulmonary embolus (PE), a serious condition in which the clot obstructs an artery in the lungs. Venous thromboembolism (VTE) is the collective term for DVT and PE. It describes the process of

CHART 19–6 Common Tubes and Expected Drainage

Tube	Purpose	Drainage Amount	Drainage Color	Other
Urinary catheter (bladder).	Drains urine and decompresses the bladder.	1,500–2,500 mL in 24 hours or a minimum of 30 mL/hour.	Clear, yellow.	Report **hematuria** (blood in the urine) or cloudy urine. Report low urine output.
Three-way urinary (bladder). May have a 30-mL balloon rather than a 5- to 10-mL balloon.	Drains urine and is used for continuous bladder irrigation (CBI).	1,500–2,500 mL/24 hour and any irrigating fluid that is instilled.	If used for CBI, then expect urine to be pink.	Normal saline is used to irrigate. Regulate the CBI to keep the urine clear. Watch for bladder spasms and clots. Careful intake and output (I&O).
Suprapubic catheter (bladder).	Drains urine.	1,500–2,500 mL/24 hour or 30 mL/hour.	Clear, yellow.	Report no urine output. Report dislodgement.
Nephrostomy tube (kidney pelvis).	Drains urine from the kidney.	Amount depends on function of the kidney.	Clear, yellow.	Can be gently flushed with 5 to 10 mL of normal saline.
Nasogastric tube (NGT). Salem sump (stomach). Levine tube (stomach).	Decompress the stomach. Low, continuous, or intermittent suction is used; intermittent use needed if the tube does not have an air vent.	Depends on the situation; up to 1,500 mL/24 hour.	Usually pale, yellow-green.	Expect some blood in the drainage for 8 hours after gastrectomy. NGT can be flushed with 30 mL or more of saline except after gastric or esophageal surgeries.
Gastrostomy tube.	Drainage or feeding.	Varies.	Green to dark brown, bloody.	Flush with normal saline to keep patent.
Jejunostomy tube.	Drainage or feeding.	Varies.	Green to dark brown, bloody.	Flush with normal saline to keep patent.
Blakemore-Sengstaken tube (triple lumen; esophageal balloon, gastric balloon, drainage).	Drains stomach and compresses esophageal or stomach varices.	Varies.	Green to dark brown, bloody.	Measure pressure in esophageal balloon. Balloon is only inflated for a 48-hour period. Periodic release of balloon pressure.
Wound drains, such as Jackson-Pratt, Hemovac.	Drains inflammatory fluid from the area surrounding the incision.	Varies, but the need to empty the drain frequently (e.g., more than every 4 hours) should be cause for concern.	Sanguineous to serosanguineous. Drainage should become more serous over time.	Drains are usually removed when drainage is <30 mL in 24 hours.
Chest tube (pleural space).	Drains fluid or air from pleural space, restores negative intrapleural pressure. Re-expands the lung.	Not more than 100 mL/hour.	Drainage varies from sanguineous to serosanguineous to serous.	Must have a water seal. Record drainage at least every 8 hours. Clamp the chest tube *only* prior to changing the drainage system.
T-tube (common bile duct).	Drains bile if the common bile duct (CBD) is obstructed. Maintains patency of CBD after surgery on the bile duct.	Varies from 0 to 500 mL in 24 hours.	Green, yellow, or brown.	Normal bile production is 500–800 mL in 24 hours.

blood clot formation and travel through the veins. The overall incidence of DVT is around 9% to 10%, but the rate in some surgeries is much higher. For example, the incidence of DVT following general surgery has been reported at 20% to 30%, and the incidence of DVT following hip fracture may be as high as 50% (Autar, 2010; Dipaola, 2008). Nursing assessment, management, and prevention strategies are discussed in detail in Chapter 35.

DVT occurs as a result of vascular stasis (injury to the intimal layer of the vein) and hypercoagulability. The postoperative patient is at risk for DVT because anesthesia vasodilates vessels, leading to stasis and decreased venous return. Patients undergoing lengthy surgeries in which there is prolonged immobilization during the procedure have a higher risk of blood clot formation than patients with short surgeries. Reduced mobility after surgery also contributes to vascular stasis and DVT. Major orthopedic surgery, multiple trauma, and pelvic surgeries are associated with a higher risk of DVT than other procedures (Autar, 2010; Dipaola, 2008). Other risk factors include age (over age 60), obesity, prolonged immobilization, use of estrogen, cancer, and history of previous DVT (Maiocco, 2008).

Prevention of VTE is a goal for all postoperative patients, and the nurse should discuss prophylaxis with the health care provider if a postoperative patient arrives on the clinical unit without such orders (Dipaola, 2008). The American College of Chest Physicians (ACCP) in 2004 established guidelines for the prevention of DVT and PE at a consensus conference (Geerts et al., 2004). Several methods of DVT prophylaxis are recommended. The National Guidelines feature summarizes some of the recommendations for surgical patients.

Antithrombotic drug therapy is frequently used to prevent DVT. Low-dose unfractionated heparin (LDUH) or low-molecular-weight heparin (LMWH) is given subcutaneously in doses that are large enough to prevent clot formation but not large enough to produce systemic anticoagulation. LMWHs are better absorbed, have longer action, are more effective in producing anticoagulation, and cause bleeding less often than unfractionated heparin, but they are substantially more expensive (Adams & Koch, 2010). There are several types of LMWH; the most common are enoxaparin and dalteparin. An alternative to LMWH is fondaparinux, which inhibits Factor X and has a longer half-life, a more predictable response, and fewer adverse effects than does LMWH (Adams & Koch, 2010).

Oral medication, such as warfarin (Coumadin), can also be used for DVT prophylaxis in some situations, but the dose must be titrated to achieve a target INR of 2.5 (Adams & Koch, 2010; Geerts et al., 2004). Patients who are at higher risk for VTE may need to continue antithrombotic drug therapy for 2 to 4 weeks after hospital discharge. Examples of surgeries that involve higher risk for VTE and therefore require extended DVT prophylaxis include hip fracture repair, total hip or knee replacement surgeries, and major gynecologic surgeries.

Some patients should not receive either LDUH or LMWH, even in low doses, because if bleeding does occur it could be catastrophic. Patients who have had cranial surgery (which involves the risk of intracranial bleeding) or spinal surgery (which involves the risk of spinal cord compression from hematoma) might be better served by another form of prophylaxis.

Other ways to decrease the risk of DVT include intermittent pneumatic compression devices or graduated compression stockings. There are several manufacturers of **intermittent pneumatic compression devices (IPCs),** and all of these devices work on the basis of applying intermittent compression of the calf muscle, thereby increasing venous return. The pump is set to apply 45 mmHg of pressure with inflation. Pneumatic compression devices may be applied in the operating room and worn almost continuously (except when ambulating or bathing) for the next several days. Patients sometimes complain that the plastic leg sleeves are hot, cause sweating, or interrupt sleep. Some machines have a switch that cools the airflow through the sleeves. Experts suggest that pneumatic compression devices not be used on patients who are immobilized for 72 hours or more without prophylaxis. If a clot has formed, the device could dislodge it (Dipaola, 2008).

Graduated compression stockings (GCSs) are elastic stockings that apply varying degrees of pressure on the lower leg, with the greatest exertion of pressure at the ankle and the lowest pressure at the thigh (or knee in shorter stockings). GCSs increase venous return and velocity, thereby reducing venous wall distention and venous stasis (Dipaola, 2008). IPCs and GCSs may be used in conjunction with antithrombotic drug therapy, or they may be used as an alternative to it in patients who should not receive any type of anticoagulation.

Early ambulation is important in preventing DVT. Patients are encouraged to ambulate several times a day and to change positions in bed every 1 to 2 hours. Leg exercises can be done while the patient is in a chair or in bed. Chapter 35 contains a complete description of the causes and treatment of DVT.

NATIONAL GUIDELINES Summary of Recommendations for DVT Prophylaxis in the Surgical Patient

Level of Risk for Venous Thromboembolism	Recommendation
Low Risk	
Minor procedure, age <40 years, no other risks OR	Early and persistent ambulation
Gynecologic procedures lasting <30 minutes OR	
Low-risk urological procedures	
Moderate Risk	
Non-major general surgery, age 40 to 60 years	Low-dose unfractionated heparin (LDUH) 5,000 units bid OR
Gynecologic surgery (benign disease)	low-molecular-weight heparin (LMWH) <3,400 units daily
Higher Risk	
Nonmajor surgical procedure and age >60 years	LDUH 5,000 units tid OR
Extensive gynecologic surgery	LMWH > 3,400 units daily
Very High Risk	
Major surgery with multiple risk factors	LDUH tid OR
	LMWH (higher doses) daily AND
	Graduated compression stockings OR
	Intermittent pneumatic compression boots
High risk for bleeding	Intermittent pneumatic compression boots OR
	Graduated compression stockings

Source: Geerts, W., Pineo, G., Hit, J., Bergqvist, D., Lassen, M., Colwell, C., et al. (2004). Prevention of venous thromboembolism: The Seventh AACP Conference on Antithrombotic and Thrombolytic Therapy. *Chest, 126*(3 Suppl.), 338S–400S.

Gerontological Considerations

Care of the older adult after surgery is similar to care of younger adult patients with a few exceptions. Older adults have decreased physiological reserves, making them less able or slower to respond to the demands of surgery (Sullivan, 2011). For example, it may take older patients 48 hours or longer to fully recover from the effects of anesthesia (Stanton, 2010). Also, older adults tend to experience more postoperative complications than younger people because of preexisting illness, nutritional deficits, and alterations in how drugs are metabolized. When complications occur, older adults experience higher death rates (Stanton, 2010; Sullivan, 2011). The risk of postoperative complications varies depending on the surgery.

The assessment of older patients may show slight variations from the assessment of younger adult patients. For example, older adults tend to have slightly lower body temperatures and oxygen saturation levels (i.e., 93% to 95%) than younger patients, but the nurse needs to use the same parameters of concern for older adults that would be used for others. The nurse also uses the same priorities of postoperative care. The older adult may have special needs (e.g., replace hearing aids, dentures, and glasses as soon as possible) and problems. Major issues to address include pain management, postoperative delirium, medication management, restoration of functional ability, and discharge planning. Older patients also have a greater risk for falls even before any anesthesia admission and surgical procedure. Special attention needs to be paid to their safety.

Pain management is a challenge in older adults, and some studies report that their postoperative pain is undertreated (Stanton, 2010; Sullivan, 2011) or inappropriately treated. Teaching older patients about communicating their pain may improve pain treatment. The rule of thumb in treating pain in older patients is to start low and go slow (i.e., use the lowest doses first and slowly titrate medications upward). Opioids are used to control postoperative pain, but the concurrent use of NSAIDs can decrease the amount of narcotics required. All older patients receiving narcotics should also receive a stool softener to offset the constipating effect of the narcotic (Beach, 2011). Certain narcotics, such as meperidine (Demerol), are avoided in older adults because they produce toxic metabolites that can cause seizures or confusion.

Postoperative delirium, an acute change in cognitive function with decreased ability to focus or sustain attention and the presence of altered perceptions, is a serious problem for older adults. Postoperative delirium increases morbidity and mortality for those affected. The incidence of postoperative delirium ranges from 14% to as high as 56% in higher risk patients (DeCrane et al., 2011). Postoperative delirium can occur at any time during hospitalization, but it is more likely to occur shortly after surgery.

The development of postoperative delirium is multifactorial, with the most vulnerable and frail older adults being at highest risk. Risk factors include prior cognitive impairment, severity of illness on admission, depression, increased age, sensory deficits, impaired functional ability, and use of certain medications (DeCrane et al., 2011). Patients needing emergency surgery may be more likely to develop acute confusion than those admitted for elective procedures (Hudek, 2009).

Programs designed to prevent postoperative delirium have had some success in preventing delirium, reducing its severity, or shortening the course (Doerflinger, 2009). Such programs generally include identifying high-risk patients preoperatively, performing daily consultation with a geriatrician or advanced practice nurse specializing in geriatrics, reducing the use of unnecessary medications, training bedside nurses in the early recognition of acute confusion, and aggressively correcting factors that may be contributing to confusion (e.g., hypoxia, fluid and electrolyte imbalance, pain).

Older patients experience more adverse effects with medications than do younger patients. Aging causes changes in the absorption, distribution, protein binding, metabolism, and elimination of drugs (Doerflinger, 2009). These changes tend to increase the plasma concentration of some drugs and narrow the therapeutic range. In general, giving smaller doses of drugs or increasing the dosing interval may help reduce adverse effects. Certain drugs should be used sparingly or avoided altogether because of their propensity for causing sedation or confusion in older patients. Examples of these medications include meperidine, cimetidine, long-acting benzodiazepines (e.g., diazepam), and diphenhydramine (Doerflinger, 2009).

It is important to restore functional ability to the older surgical patient as soon as possible. A collaborative effort among health care providers, nurses, physical therapists, and others is required to optimize the older adult's recovery. Postoperative imbalances such as dehydration, electrolyte disturbances, or anemia should be corrected to preserve functional ability.

There are special concerns when discharging an older person home. The nurse needs to ask the patient about the availability of social support, the specifics of the home environment, and any surgery-related needs (Doerflinger, 2009). Specific concerns include the following:

- Is the patient able to perform self-care?
- Who is available to assist the patient in meeting her needs?
- Is the patient a primary caretaker for someone else?
- What is the condition of the home environment (e.g., stairs, location of bedrooms and bathrooms, availability of a telephone, presence of a lifeline)?
- Does the home environment need a safety evaluation?
- What supplies, medications, or other equipment (e.g., wheelchair, hold bars, chair-height toilet seat) does the patient need at home?
- How will the patient get to follow-up appointments?

Another concern for the nurse is the patient's psychological readiness for discharge. Patients need to feel that they will be safe at home. The sense of safety is related to patients' confidence in their ability to care for themselves and in the support they will have from others (Doerflinger, 2009). Nurses need to work closely with each patient so that the patient develops the confidence needed to feel safe and ready for discharge.

Health Promotion

Discharge teaching is critical now that the length of hospitalization is shorter. Surgeries that once required a 10-day hospital stay now require only a 3- to 4-day stay. Minimally invasive surgical techniques allow some patients to go home on the same day as surgery. It is not unusual to discharge patients home with dressings, drains, and even IV antibiotics or parenteral nutrition. Understandably, patients are concerned about how to care for themselves after discharge. Patients want information about wound care, medications, activities, diet, symptom management, and other aspects of self-care.

Teaching is provided to the patient as well as to others who will be involved in providing care for the patient. It is important to use language the individuals understand and to check their understanding of the information. Written or visual instructions are also critical. Research suggests that written or visual information fosters the patient's understanding and compliance with discharge instructions (Ong et al., 2011). Being able to call the nurse with questions may be especially important to patients in their adjustment after surgery (Ross, 2007). The teaching needs of the patient vary according to the surgery and other factors, but general areas to be covered in discharge teaching are discussed next.

Patients need to be advised about the trajectory of recovery. Postoperative recovery can be said to include four dimensions: physiological recovery, marked by a return of bodily functions; psychological recovery, a return of a sense of well-being; social recovery, a return to social activities and independence; and habitual recovery, a point at which the person returns to a full range of normal activities (Allvin, Berg, Idvall, & Nilsson, 2007). Patients need to be aware that recovery takes time. Uncomplicated surgery often takes 4 to 6 weeks, or even longer in older patients or patients with comorbid factors such as diabetes or obesity, for recovery. The effects from general anesthesia can linger, wound healing requires energy, it takes weeks to make sufficient red blood cells to replace those lost in surgery, and patients may experience pain or soreness until healing is well underway. Patients may lack their usual level of energy during recovery. Pain, fatigue, and depression are common symptoms during recovery from major surgery, but these symptoms will gradually resolve. Social support is important to the psychological well-being of patients as they recover from surgery.

Information on how to care for the wound following discharge is a common need for postsurgical patients. The nurse checks with the surgeon about any special requirements of wound care. Some patients will have a dressing in place that needs to be kept clean and dry until the follow-up appointment with the surgeon. In other situations, incisions are kept covered for the first 24 to 48 hours, and then the dressing is removed and the wound is left open to the air. These wounds are gently cleaned each day and the dressing replaced if there is risk of contamination. Staples and sutures are often removed 7 to 10 days after the surgery in a follow-up appointment with the nurse or health care provider. If Steri-Strips cover the wound, they are left in place until they fall off naturally. Wound drains are emptied as often as needed, and the amount and type of drainage are recorded. Any sudden increase in the amount of drainage or a change in the character or color of the drainage needs to be reported to the surgeon.

Information about activities that are allowed after surgery and those that are not allowed is especially important to provide. This information also is important because patients may judge their postoperative progress according to the activities they are able to perform. Examples of the types of questions that patients have are as follows:

- When can I bathe or shower?
- When can I exercise? Are there any restrictions on exercising?
- Can I do housework?
- When can I start driving?
- When can I resume sexual activity?
- How much rest should I get?
- When can I return to work?

Usually, patients are encouraged to bathe or shower daily. If a dressing is in place, it is to be kept clean and dry. After most surgeries, the patient is discouraged from lifting anything heavier than 10 to 15 pounds until the incision has healed in 4 to 6 weeks. Walking at a reasonable pace is encouraged and limited only by pain and fatigue, but heavier aerobic-type workouts are restricted until approved by the surgeon. Similarly, light housework is generally acceptable when the patient feels able, but heavier housework may be restricted. Most restrictions on driving are based on the need for road safety rather than potential injury to the wound. Often patients are allowed to drive when their ability to move is no longer restricted by pain or soreness. After some surgeries, driving is restricted for several days; after others, it may be several weeks. Once patients are able to drive, they are cautioned not to drive while taking narcotic analgesics. Except with certain gynecologic or genitourinary surgeries where sexual activity may cause pain because of the location and nature of the surgery, sexual activity after surgery is restricted as a result of pain. Most people will be able to resume sexual activity in 2 to 3 weeks. For patients who have had genitourinary or gynecological surgery, the time to return to sexual activity will be determined by the type of surgery that has been performed. These patients will need to use the counsel of their surgeons. The time frame for returning to work will depend on the surgery and the type of work performed. After less invasive procedures such as arthroscopy, patients can return to work in 2 to 4 days. Most patients will be out of work for 3 to 6 weeks following major surgery and up to 10 weeks for major abdominal or thoracic resections.

The postoperative diet for most patients emphasizes good nutrition for wound healing. Patients are encouraged to get adequate calories, proteins, and vitamins. Diet restrictions or recommended modifications are made for some surgeries, especially those involving the head and neck.

Research suggests that patients may not feel adequately prepared to manage their medication regimens at home (Cutilli, 2007). Discharge teaching includes a discussion of medications including purpose, how to take the medication, and key side effects. Most postoperative patients will be discharged with an oral narcotic for pain control, and some will have antibiotics prescribed. They need to know when to take pain medication, how much medication to take, alternative strategies for pain control such as elevation and ice applications, and how to prevent constipation, a common side effect of narcotics.

Early discharge puts the burden on the patient to recognize and respond to potential complications. Often, signs of wound infection take several days to develop and may not show up until after the patient is discharged home. Chart 19–7 lists some of the danger signs that patients should report to their health care provider. Discharge information includes contact phone numbers for emergencies. Most patients will have a follow-up appointment in 7 to 10 days after discharge.

The information needs of surgical patients are complex, and it is unrealistic to think that the needs of every patient can be met on discharge from the hospital. Nurses need to develop skills in evaluating patients for discharge. This includes carefully evaluating patients' ability to provide care for themselves at home and, when home assistance is required, making referrals to community services (e.g., visiting nurses

CHART 19–7 Danger Signs That Patients Should Report to Their Health Care Provider

- Temperature greater than 38°C (100.4°F)
- Fever with chills
- Pain that is increasing or that is not adequately controlled by medication
- Incision that is red, painful, or has drainage
- Difficulty voiding or unable to void
- Painful urination

association [VNA], physical therapy, hospice). Appropriate referrals not only improve patient care but also can prevent hospital readmission.

Surgical patients may need the services of a VNA or other home health agency to assist with their recovery. Services that may be appropriate, particularly for older adults, include home nursing care for dressing changes, wound checks, antibiotic administration, home safety evaluation, and the coordination of other services such as a home health aide to assist with meeting personal care needs, home physical therapy to assist with rehabilitation, and homemaker services for housekeeping and meal preparation.

Patients are discharged home when the health care provider and health care team determine that the patients no longer need the care and close attention of an acute care hospital and are safe to care for themselves at home. The nurse has an obligation to speak with the health care provider and advocate for patient safety if the nurse questions the patient's readiness for discharge. There are no set criteria for determining readiness for discharge; it is a clinical judgment, but the nurse can use indicators to assist in making this judgment. Indicators of stability and readiness for discharge are as follows:

- Stable vital signs; vital signs at patient's baseline
- Baseline level of consciousness
- Wound that is stable, without bleeding
- Able to take food and fluids orally without nausea and vomiting
- Able to void and move bowels
- Tolerates an acceptable level of pain
- Able to ambulate without assistance
- Able to perform ADLs independently or at baseline
- Home services are adequate to meet the patient's needs.

Discharge teaching for both the patient and the family/support system is outlined in the Patient Teaching & Discharge Priorities box.

Research

Research is changing the way nurses care for postoperative patients. Nurses are looking for evidence to support their practice. It is important to know whether or not nursing interventions are having the desired outcome. A culture of answering practice questions by using the best available research evidence or by designing a research study is evolving. The Research Opportunities box lists research problems that are important to the care of the postsurgical patient.

Research is also being used to design structures and nursing care delivery models to create healing environments. Single rooms in hospitals create space for privacy and personal control and provide a place for family members to stay overnight. Researchers are examining the effects of single rooms on outcomes such as infection control, pain management, and rest and recovery.

PATIENT TEACHING & DISCHARGE PRIORITIES for Postoperative Nursing

Need	Teaching
Incision and drain care	Assess for redness, warmth, swelling, increased pain, or drainage. Mild bruising around the wound is often normal.
	Keep wound dry for first 48 hours or as directed by the surgeon.
	After 48 hours, wash gently around the incision site(s) and pat dry.
	If Steri-Strips are in place, allow them to fall off by themselves.
	Sutures are usually removed in 7 to 10 days.
	If drains are in place, empty daily or as often as indicated. Note color and amount of drainage.
	Assess availability, knowledge, and comfort with treatment regimen.
	Report a fever >38°C (>100.4°F) or an incision that becomes red, painful, or swollen or has increased drainage.
	Assess respite needs and resources.
	Assess need for follow-up appointments.
	Assess need for wound checks by health professional.
Pain control	Take pain medication as prescribed.
	Do not drive while taking prescription pain medication.
	Increase fluids and take a stool softener to prevent constipation from prescription pain medication.
	Take acetaminophen (Tylenol) regular or extra strength for mild pain.
	Do *not* take aspirin or ibuprofen unless approved by your surgeon.
	Assess pain level and report any increase in pain.
	Assess environment for safety.
Activity	Expect that the effects of surgery, anesthesia, wound healing, and pain medication will make you feel more tired than usual.
	Fatigue may last several weeks. Plan rest periods, and pace your activities.
	Avoid strenuous exercise until the follow-up appointment with the surgeon.
	You will need to check with the health care provider about a time frame for returning to work and normal activities.
	Assess support systems for meal preparation, household chores, child care, or spousal care.
	Assess need for home care services.

RESEARCH OPPORTUNITIES Related to Care of the Surgical Patient

Research Area	Clinical Impact
Comparison of deep breathing exercises and incentive spirometry in reducing postoperative pulmonary complications.	Prevention of pulmonary complications in the postoperative period.
Effectiveness of alternative interventions (e.g., relaxation techniques) in reducing postoperative pulmonary complications.	Provides data to support or refute the use of innovative approaches to common postoperative problems.
Effectiveness of ambulation (distance and frequency) in reducing the incidence of postoperative complications (e.g., pneumonia, abdominal distention, urinary retention).	Improve postoperative management to produce more positive patient outcomes. Improve nursing interventions to promote safety and prevent complications.
Effectiveness of various interventions in treating postoperative urinary retention.	
Factors that increase wound healing postoperatively.	
Comparison of wound dressing technique, clean technique versus sterile technique, in the incidence of postoperative wound infection.	Earlier wound healing and prevention of infection.
Effectiveness of prewarming surgical patients to reduce surgical site infections.	
Effectiveness of interventions in the treatment of postoperative nausea and vomiting.	
Effectiveness of interventions to prevent postoperative confusion in older patients.	
Pain Management	
Effectiveness of nonpharmacologic interventions (e.g., splinting, elevation, application of ice, relaxation techniques) in reducing postoperative pain.	Increased patient comfort.
Evaluation of pain and discomfort associated with common postoperative interventions.	Improve interventions to decrease pain associated with the surgical experience.
Factors that influence the effectiveness of patient-controlled analgesia in the postoperative patient.	
Multimodal pain medication (fast and long-acting pain medication given at the same time)	Improve the pain scores immediately postop.
Factors that reduce persistent postoperative pain.	
Psychosocial Responses	
Predictors of anxiety in surgical patients.	Improve the psychological well-being of postoperative patients.
Factors that influence anxiety levels in the older surgical patient.	
Strategies to reduce anxiety in postoperative patients.	
Effect of family visits on postoperative anxiety.	
Description of the sleep and rest patterns in postoperative patients.	Understand the impact of sleep and rest on postoperative recovery.
Influence of sleep on postoperative recovery.	
Discharge	
Common problems experienced by the patient following discharge home.	Improve health care professionals' understanding of the issues that patients face following discharge.
Interventions used by patients to manage problems at home (e.g., fatigue, depression, constipation, pain, wound healing).	
Strategies to increase the patient's ability to manage symptoms at home.	Increase patients' competence in managing their own recovery.
Adjustment of discharge teaching to accommodate cultural differences.	

READ: **History of Present Illnesses** >> Laboratory Study Results >> Critical Thinking Questions

Ryan Landry is a 67-year-old man who is admitted to the surgical unit following a left hemicolectomy. Mr. Landry was in reasonably good health until 2 months ago when he began to experience cramping abdominal pain that he attributed to constipation and gas. When the abdominal cramping continued and he noticed that his stools were narrower than usual, he made an appointment with his primary health care provider. A routine exam uncovered occult blood in the stool, and Mr. Landry was referred for a colonoscopy.

Several polyps were removed during the colonoscopy, and biopsy results revealed adenocarcinoma of the colon. A left hemicolectomy without colostomy was performed. Once the results of lymph node biopsies taken during surgery are available, Mr. Landry will be referred to an oncologist for discussion of follow-up treatment, including possible chemotherapy. Currently Mr. Landry is second-day postoperative from the hemicolectomy.

Medical–Surgical History

Mr. Landry has hypertension and elevated cholesterol. He smokes 1 pack of cigarettes per day and has done so for the past 40 years. He has failed many times to quit smoking. His father died of colon cancer at the age of 70. His hypertension is treated with metoprolol 50 mg daily, and his elevated cholesterol levels are treated with atorvastatin 80 mg daily.

Social History

Mr. Landry lives with his wife and a grown son.

READ: History of Present Illnesses >> **Physical Exam** >> Admitting Medical Records >> Laboratory Study Results

Physical Exam

- Vital signs: T 101.4, HR 108, RR 20, BP 142/84
- Alert and oriented; reports feeling very anxious; asks frequent questions, often repeating them; looks worried and seems overly vigilant any time a health care worker comes into the room
- Reports a significant amount of pain, rating it as a 7 at rest and a 10 with movement
- Cardiac telemetry: sinus tachycardia with occasional premature ventricular contractions
- Taking shallow breaths; crackles in the lung bases bilaterally
- Oxygen saturation: 93% on 4 liters of oxygen via nasal cannula; using the incentive spirometer sporadically; weak cough
- Abdomen: slightly firm; distended with hypoactive bowel sounds and negative flatus
- Nasogastric tube attached to low intermittent suction; draining small amount of green fluid
- Complains of being thirsty and having a sore throat; slightly nauseated, especially with movement
- Foley catheter in place; draining concentrated urine
- Urine output in the last 2 hours: 42 mL
- Skin: warm and dry
- Abdominal incision covered by a primary dressing that is dry and intact
- 2+ pedal pulses bilaterally and no peripheral edema

Patient requires assistance with ambulation. He complains of severe pain and vertigo when standing. He ambulates a very short distance before requesting to go back to bed. Following activity, his respiratory rate was 32 and his heart rate was 118.

Admitting Medical Orders

- Surgical service
- Admit to Telemetry Unit
- No known allergies
- Vital signs every 4 hours
- Call house officer: pulse < 60 and > 110/minute; BP < 90 and > 160 systolic; temperature > 38.5; urine output < 30 mL/hr $\times$ 2 hours; RR > 30/minute; oxygen saturation $< 92\%$
- NPO
- Maintain nasogastric tube to low continuous suction
- Incentive spirometry 10 times every hour
- Foley to gravity drainage
- Monitor intake and output
- Sequential compression device (SCD) to lower extremities while in bed
- Ambulate three times daily
- Cardiac telemetry while receiving IV metoprolol
- IV: D5$^1/_2$NS with 20 mEq KCl at 125 mL/hr

Scheduled Medications

- Heparin 5,000 units subcutaneous twice a day
- Nicotine transdermal patch 15 mg daily
- PCA morphine sulfate 1 mg/mL incremental dose and lock out 6 minutes
- Metoprolol 5 mg IV every 6 hours while NPO

PRN Medications

- Phenergan 25 mg IV q6h prn nausea
- Mylanta 30 mL po/NG q4–6h prn dyspepsia
- Lorazepam 0.5 to 2 mg IV q6–8h prn anxiety
- Tylenol 650 mg po/pr q4h prn pain/fever
- Milk of magnesia 30 mL po/NG q4h prn constipation

Ordered Laboratory Studies

- Chemistry 20 and CEA on admission
- Chemistry 7 with magnesium, phosphorus, and calcium every 48 hours postoperatively
- CBC daily

READ: History of Present Illnesses >> **Laboratory Study Results** >> Critical Thinking Questions

Test	Day 1 (Preop)	Day 2 (Postop Day 1)	Day 3 (Postop Day 2)
Sodium	136 mEq/L		142 mEq/L
Potassium	4.1 mEq/L		3.9 mEq/L
Chloride	102 mEq/L		106 mEq/L
Bicarbonate	26 mEq/L		21 mEq/L
Blood urea nitrogen (BUN)	24 mg/dL		33 mg/dL
Creatinine	0.8 mg/dL		1.1 mg/dL
Glucose	113 mg/dL		153 mg/dL
Magnesium	2.2 mEq/L		2.4 mEq/L

Test	Day 1 (Preop)	Day 2 (Postop Day 1)	Day 3 (Postop Day 2)
Phosphorus	3.2 mg/dL		2.5 mg/dL
Calcium	9.3 mg/dL		10.1 mg/dL
White blood cell (WBC)	7,000/mm^3	11,000/mm^3	13,000/mm^3
Hematocrit	37%	32%	27%
Hemoglobin	13 g/dL	10.6 g/dL	9.2 g/dL
Carcinoembryonic antigen (CEA)	6.0 ng/mL		

Pearson Nursing Student Resources *Log on to* ***nursing.pearsonhighered.com*** *to download forms*

DOCUMENT:

- >> Summary of Hospitalization
- >> Pathophysiology Form
- >> Laboratory Values
- >> Laboratory Results Explanation

APPLY:

- >> List of Potential Nursing Diagnoses
- >> Concept Map
- >> Critical Thinking Questions and Concept Map

APPLY: History of Present Illnesses >> Laboratory Study Results >> **Critical Thinking Questions**

1. What five nursing diagnoses are of the highest priority for Mr. Landry today? Why?
2. Review Mr. Landry's current physical examination. What postoperative problems, if any, is Mr. Landry currently experiencing?
3. The following activities need to be performed with or for Mr. Landry: Change the syringe in the PCA pump, empty and record urine output, perform a.m. care, teach use of the incentive spirometer, and call the surgeon for an additional antiemetic order. In which order should the nurse perform these activities? Why?
4. Later in the day, Mr. Landry says to the nurse, "The surgeon told me he's pretty sure he got all of the cancer. I guess I won't need that appointment with the oncologist." What is the nurse's best response to this situation?

Answers to Critical Thinking Questions appear in Appendix D in the Osborn Student Resources at nursing.pearsonhighered.com.

NCLEX® PRACTICE

1. A postoperative patient in the PACU begins to demonstrate an increased heart rate. The nurse should assess for which finding first?
   1. Bleeding
   2. Anxiety
   3. Nausea
   4. Pain

2. A nurse is assessing a postoperative patient in the PACU. Which finding indicates the patient has entered stage II of postanesthesia and is approaching time for discharge to the inpatient unit?
   1. Breathing with an oral airway
   2. Easily arousable and moving all four extremities
   3. Urine output of 20 mL per hour
   4. Moderate amount of vomiting

3. A postoperative patient is demonstrating a distended abdomen with no bowel sounds. Which nursing intervention is indicated?

1. Advance to full diet.
2. Restrict fluids.
3. Ambulate three times a day.
4. Administer antiemetic medication.

4. The nurse is instructing a patient who had abdominal surgery under general anesthesia about care needed when at home. What should the nurse include in these instructions? (select all that apply)

1. "You will feel normal in the morning."
2. "Let these Steri-Strips fall off on their own."
3. "The health care provider will remove your staples at your 3-week checkup."
4. "Avoid lifting anything that weighs over 10 to 15 pounds for the next 4 to 6 weeks."
5. "You will need to take your narcotic pain medications prior to driving or walking very far."

5. The nurse would like to study how a nurse's critical thinking skills can be improved when working with a postoperative patient. Which research topic most clearly provides information on nurses' critical thinking skills?

1. Factors that influence anxiety levels in the older surgical patient
2. Strategies to increase the patient's ability to manage symptoms at home
3. Nurses' ability to manage postoperative pain
4. Adjustment of discharge teaching to accommodate cultural differences

6. A patient in the PACU is gagging and fighting the presence of the oral airway. The nurse removes the airway and the patient quiets; however, his oxygen saturation drops. What should the nurse do?

1. Replace the oral airway and place tape across it onto the patient's face.
2. Leave the airway out and stimulate the patient to breath every 5 seconds.
3. Insert a nasal airway into the most patent nare.
4. Call for endotracheal tube placement.

Answers to NCLEX Practice questions can be found in Appendix D in the Osborn Student Resources at nursing.pearsonhighered.com. Practice additional NCLEX questions online at the Student Resources site.

Pearson Nursing Student Resources Find additional review materials at: **nursing.pearsonhighered.com**

REFERENCES

Adams, M., & Koch, R. (2010). *Pharmacology: Connections to nursing practice.* Upper Saddle River, NJ: Pearson.

Agency for Health Care Policy and Research, Public Health Service, (AHCPR). U.S. Department of Health and Human Services. (1992). *Acute pain management: Operative or medical procedures and trauma—Clinical practice guideline* (AHCPR Publication No. 92-0032). Rockville, MD: Author.

Allard, N. (2007). Day surgery for breast cancer: Effects of a psychoeducational telephone intervention on functional status and emotional distress. *Oncology Nursing Forum, 34*(1), 133–141.

Allvin, R., Berg, K., Idvall, E., & Nilsson, U. (2007). Postoperative recovery: A concept analysis. *Journal of Advanced Nursing, 57*(5), 552–558.

American Society of Anesthesiologists. (2009). Standards for postanesthesia care. Retrieved from http://asahq.org/For-Healthcare-Professionals/Standards-Guidelines-and-Statements.aspx

American Society of PeriAnesthesia Nurses. (2003). ASPAN pain and comfort clinical guideline. *Journal of PeriAnesthesia Nursing, 18*(4), 232–236.

American Society of PeriAnesthesia Nurses. (2006). ASPAN's evidence-based clinical practice guideline for the prevention and/or management of PONV/PDNV. *Journal of PeriAnesthesia Nursing, 21*(4), 230–250.

American Society of PeriAnesthesia Nurses. (2010). *Standards of perianesthesia nursing practice.* Cherry Hill, NJ: Author.

Anderson, D. J. (2011). Surgical site infections. *Infectious Disease Clinics of North America, 2*(1), 135–153.

Anderson, M., & Comrie, R. (2009). Adopting preoperative fasting guidelines. *AORN Journal, 90*(1), 73–80.

Atkinson, M. C. (2010). Pneumonia. Evidenced-based nursing: Monographs. Mosby's Nursing Consult. Retrieved from http://www.nursingconsult.com/nursing/evidence-based-nursing/monograph?monograph_id=191486&filter=as&loe=&sortorder=title-a&pageno=1&parentpage=search&searchId=1203042496&searchTerm=Atelectasis+and+Pneumonia++AND+Postoperative+Nursing&search_type=allresults&page=&abstract=Pharm&bestBetId=BB_MNC_EBN_Pneumonia.bb&dropdown=EntireSite&area=EviNurse&bestbet=true

Autar, R. (2010). A review of venous thromboprophylaxis in patients undergoing hip fracture surgery. *International Journal of Orthopaedic & Trauma Nursing, 14,* 88–95.

Bailey, L. (2010). Strategies for decreasing patient anxiety in the perioperative setting. *AORN Journal, 92*(4), 445–460.

Beach, P. (2011). Acute pain: Evidence-based nursing: Monographs. Mosby's Nursing Monographs. Retrieved from http://www.nursingconsult.com/nursing/evidence-based-nursing/monograph?monograph_id=189121&filter=as&loe=&sortorder=title-a&pageno=1&parentpage=search&searchId=1202652581&searchTerm=PCA+&page=&bestBetId=&search_type=allresults

Brodsky, J. B., & Margarson, M. (2011). Weighing in on surgical safety. *AORN Journal, 93*(4) 518, continued on 432.

Burns, S. M. (2009). Unintentional hypothermia: Implications for perianesthesia nurses. *Journal of PeriAnesthesia, 24*(3), 167–176.

Carli, F., Mayo, N., Klubien, K., Schricker, T., Trudel, J., & Belliveau, P. (2002). Epidural analgesia enhances functional exercise capacity and health-related quality of life after colonic surgery: Results of a randomized trial. *Anesthesiology, 97*(3), 540–549.

Cata, J. P. (2009). Patient-controlled epidural analgesia (PCEA) for post-operative pain control after lumbar spine surgery. *Journal of Neurosurgical Anesthesiology, 20*(4), 256–260.

Centers for Disease Control and Prevention. (1997). Guidelines for the prevention of nosocomial pneumonia. *Morbidity and Mortality Weekly Report, 46*(RR-1), 1–79.

Coakley, A. B., & Duffy, M. E. (2010). The effect of therapeutic touch on postoperative patients. *Journal of Holistic Nursing, 28*(3), 193–200.

Conway, B. (2009). Prevention and management of postoperative nausea and vomiting in adults. *AORN Journal, 90*(2), 391–413.

Cronrath, P., Lynch, T., Gilson, L., Nishida, C., Sembar, M., Spencer, P., et al. (2011). PCA oversedation: Application of healthcare failure mode effect analysis. *Nursing Economics, 29*(2), 79–87.

Cutilli, C. (2007). Health literacy in geriatric patients: An integrative review of the literature. *Orthopedic Nursing, 26,* 43–48.

Daniels, S. M. (2007). Improving hospital care for surgical patients. *Nursing 2007, 8,* 36–41.

DeCrane, S. K., Sands, L., Ashland, M., Lim, E., Tsai, T., Pail, S., et al. (2011). Factors associated with recovery from early postoperative delirium. *Journal of Perianesthesia Nursing, 26*(4), 231–241.

Dipaola, C. (2008). Preventing deep vein thrombosis: A perioperative nursing imperative. *AORN Journal, 88*(2), 283–285.

Doerflinger, D. (2009). Older adult surgical patients: Presentation and challenges. *AORN Journal, 90*(2), 223–244.

Ead, H. (2006). From Aldrete to PADSs: Reviewing discharge criteria after ambulatory surgery. *Journal of PeriAnesthesia Nursing, 21*(4), 259–267.

Eaden, B., Gilley, B., & Neff, J. (2009). Implementation of evidence-based guidelines and PCA order sets for opioid naïve and opioid tolerant patients. *Pain Management Nursing, 10,* e2.

Easter, B., DeBoer, L., Settlemyre, L., Staries, C., Marlowe, V., & Creech, R. (2010). The impact of music on the PACU patient's perception of discomfort. *Journal of Perianesthesia Nursing, 26*(2), 79–87.

Geerts, W., Pineo, G., Hit, J., Bergqvist, D., Lassen, M., Colwell, C., et al. (2004). Prevention of venous thromboembolism: The Seventh AACP Conference on Antithrombotic and Thrombolytic Therapy. *Chest, 126*(3 Suppl.), 338S–400S.

Groudine, S., & Fossum, S. (2011). Use of intravenous acetaminophen in the treatment of postoperative pain. *Journal of Perianesthesia Nursing, 26*(2), 74–80.

Gunta, K., Lewis, C., & Nuccio, S. (2000). Prevention and management of postoperative nausea and vomiting. *Orthopaedic Nursing, 19*(2), 39–48.

Hasankhani, H., Mohammadi, E., Moazzami, F., Mokhtari, M., & Naghgizadh, M. (2007). The effects of intravenous fluids temperature on perioperative hemodynamic situation, postoperative shivering, and recovery in orthopaedic surgery. *Canadian Operating Room Nursing Journal, 25*(1), 20–24, 26–27.

Hocevar, B. J., Robinson, B., & Gray, M. (2010). Does chewing gum shorten the duration of postoperative ileus in patients undergoing abdominal surgery and creation of a stoma? *Journal of Wound, Ostomy & Incontinence Nursing, 37*(2), 140–146.

Hoffman, K. A., Bohme, M. A., & Bigbee, J. L. (2008). Nurse-directed early ambulation: A descriptive study. *Communicating Nursing Research, 41*, 430.

Hoke, M. M., & Robbins, L. K. (2011). Continuing the cultural competency through exploration of knowledge, attitudes, and skills with advanced practice psychiatric nursing students: An exemplar. *The Nursing Clinics of North America, 46*(2), 201–205.

Hudcova, J., McNicol, E., Quah, C., Lau, J., & Carr, D. (2006). Patient controlled opioid analgesia versus conventional opioid analgesia for postoperative pain. *Cochrane Library, 4* (CD003348).

Hudek, K. (2009). Emergence delirium: A nursing perspective. *AORN Journal, 89*(3), 509–520.

Institute of Medicine (IOM). (2010). *The future of nursing: Leading change, advancing health.* Washington, DC: The Academic Press.

Kitching, A. J. (2009). Fast-track surgery and anesthesia. *Continuing Education in Anaethesia, Critical Care and Pain, 9*, 39–43.

Kwekkeboom, K., & Gretarsdottir, E. (2006). Systematic review of relaxation interventions for pain. *Journal of Nursing Scholarship, 38*(3), 269–277.

Layzell, M. (2008). Current interventions and approaches to postoperative pain management. *British Journal of Nursing, 17*(7), 414–419.

Lindley, P., Pestano, C., & Gargiulo, K. (2009). Comparison of postoperative pain management using two patient-controlled analgesia methods: Nursing perspective. *Journal of Advanced Nursing, 65*(7), 1370–1380.

Lipke, V. L. & Hyott, A. S. (2010). Reducing surgical site infections by bundling multiple risk reduction strategies and active surveillance. *AORN Journal, 92*(3), 288–296.

Low, D., Vu, A., Brown, M., Davis, S., Keller, D., Levine, B., et al. (2007). Temporal thermometry fails to track body core temperature during heat stress. *Medicine & Science in Sports and Exercise, 39*(7), 1029–1035.

Lynch, S., Dixon, J., & Leary, D. (2010). Reducing the risk of unplanned perioperative hypothermia. *AORN Journal, 92*(5), 553–565.

Madsen, L., Magor, C., & Parker, B. A. (2010). Comparison of two bowel treatments to prevent constipation in post-surgical orthopedic patients. *International Journal of Orthopaedic & Trauma Nursing, 14*, 75–81.

Maiocco, G. (2008). DVT prevention for the obese patient: Evidenced-based nursing interventions. *Bariatric Nursing & Surgical Patient Care, 3*, 279–284.

Mann, C., Pouzeratte, Y., Boccara, G., Peccoux, C., Vergue, C., Brunat, G., et al. (2000). Comparison of intravenous or epidural patient-controlled analgesia in the elderly after major abdominal surgery. *Anesthesiology, 92*(2), 433–441.

Mayne, I., & Bagaoisan, C. (2009). Social support during anesthesia induction in an adult surgical population. *AORN Journal, 89*(2), 307–310.

McAlister, F., Bertsch, K., Man, J., Bradley, J., & Jacka, M. (2005). Pulmonary complications after noncardiac surgery. *American Journal of Respiratory and Critical Care Medicine, 171*(5), 514–517.

McMain, L. (2008). Principles of acute pain management. *Pain Management, 18*(11), 472–478.

McMain, L. (2010). Pain management in recovery. *Open Learning Zone, 20*(2), 59–65.

Miaskowski, C. (2009). A review of the incidence, causes, consequences, and management of gastrointestinal effects associated with postoperative opioid administration. *Journal of Perianesthesia Nursing, 24*(4), 222–228.

Mulroy, M., Salinas, F., Larkin, K., & Polissar, N. (2002). Ambulatory surgery patients may be discharged before voiding after short-acting spinal and epidural anesthesia. *Anesthesiology, 97*(2), 315–319.

Munro, C. A. (2009). The perioperative nurse's role in table-enhanced anterior total arthroplasty. *AORN Journal, 90*(1), 53–72.

Nelson, D. C. (2011). Perioperative care of the patient with rheumatoid arthritis. *AORN Journal, 94*(3), 290–300.

Neveleff, D. J., & Kraiss, L. W., & Schulman, C. S. (2010). Implementing methods to improve perioperative hemostasis in the surgical and trauma settings. *AORN Journal, 92*(5), S1–S15.

Nishimori, M., Ballantyne, J., & Low, J. (2006). Epidural pain relief versus systemic opioid-based pain relief for abdominal aortic surgery. *Cochrane Library, 4* (CD005059).

Ong, J., Miller, P., Appleby, R., Allegretto, R., & Gawlinski, A. (2011). Effects of a preoperative instructional digital video disc on patient knowledge and preparedness for engaging in postoperative care activities. *Nursing Clinics of North America, 44*(1), 103–115.

Pasero, C., & McCaffery, M. (2007). Orthopaedic postoperative pain management. *Journal of PeriAnesthesia Nursing, 22*(3), 160–174.

Prowse, M., & Lyne, P. (2000). Clinical effectiveness in the post-anaesthesia care unit: How nursing knowledge contributes to achieving intended patient outcomes. *Journal of Advanced Nursing, 31*(5), 1115–1124.

Puntillo, K., Miaskowski, C., Kehrle, K., Stannard, D., Gleeson, S., & Nye, P. (1997). The relationship between behavioral and physiological indicators of pain, critical care patients' self reports of pain and opioid administration. *Critical Care Medicine, 5*(7), 1159–1166.

Rasmussen, L. S. (2010). Constipation and defecation pattern the first 30 days after thoracic surgery. *Scandinavian Journal of Caring Sciences, 24*(2), 244–250.

Rejeh, N., & Vaismoradi, M. (2009). Perspectives and experiences of elective surgery patients regarding pain management. *Nursing and Health Sciences, 12*(1), 67–73.

Ross, J. (2007). Health literacy and its influence on patient safety. *Journal of PeriAnesthesia Nursing, 22*(3), 220–223.

Saclarides, T. (2006). Current choices—good or bad—for the proactive management of postoperative ileus: A surgeon's view. *Journal of PeriAnesthesia Nursing, 21*(2, Suppl. 1), S7–S15.

Schumann, R., Shikora, S., Weiss, J. M., Wurm, H., Strassels, S., & Carr, D. B. (2003). A comparison of multimodal perioperative analgesia to epidural pain management after gastric bypass surgery. *Anesthesia & Analgesia, 96*(2), 469–474.

Seers, K., Crichton, L., Tutton, L., Smith, L., & Saunders, T. (2008). Effectiveness of relaxation for postoperative pain and anxiety: Randomized controlled trial. *Journal of Advanced Nursing, 62*(2), 681–688.

Seidei, J. (2010). A preoperative forced-air warming protocol to maintain postoperative normothermia. ASPAN National Conference. *Journal of Perianesthesia, 25*, 193.

Silbert, B. S. (2009). Is fast-track cardiac anesthesia now the global standard of care? *Anesthesia and Analgesia, 108*(3), 689–691.

Sjostrom, B., Dahlgren, L., & Haljamae, H. (2000). Strategies used in post-operative pain assessment and their clinical accuracy. *Journal of Clinical Nursing, 9*(1), 111–118.

Stanton, C. (2010, September). Providing the right care to older adults. *AORN Connections.* Retreived from http://www.aorn.org/News/September2010News/OLDER/

Steinberg, J. P., et al. (2009). Trial to reduce antimicrobial prophylaxis errors (TRAPE) study group. Timing of antimicrobial prophylaxis and the risk of surgical site infections. *Annals of Surgery, 250*(1), 10–16.

Sullivan, J. M. (2011). Caring for older adults after surgery. *Nursing, 2011, 41*(4), 48–51.

Susleck, D., Willocks, A., Secrest, J., Norwood, B., Holweger, J., Davis, M., et al. (2007). The perianesthesia experience from the patient's perspective. *Journal of PeriAnesthesia Nursing, 22*(1), 10–20.

Tallman, K., Ramachandran, S., Christensen, R., & O'Brien, D. (2011). Cardiac arrest in the PACU: An analysis of evolving challenges for perianesthesia nursing. *Journal of Perianesthesia Nursing, 26*(1), 4–8.

Tarrac, S. (2006). A description of intraoperative and postanesthesia complication rates. *Journal of PeriAnesthesia Nursing, 21*(2), 88–96.

Tracy, S. M. (2010). Piloting tailored teaching on nonpharmacologic enhancements for postoperative pain management in older adults. *Pain Management Nursing, 11*(3), 148–158.

Wilkinson, J. M., & Ahearn, N. R. (2009). *Prentice Hall nursing diagnosis handbook* (9th ed.). Upper Saddle River, NJ: Prentice Hall.

Windle, P. (2011). Improving postoperative outcomes for patients with obstructive sleep apnea. *Journal of Perianesthesia Nursing, 26*, 188.

Wood, S. (2010). Post-operative pain 1: Understanding the factors affecting patients' experiences with pain. *Nursing Times, 106*(45), 16–22.

Wren, S. M., Martin, M., Yoon, J. K., & Bech, F. (2010). Postoperative pneumonia-prevention program for inpatient surgical ward. *Journal of the American College of Surgeons, 210*(4), 491–495.

Young, E., Sherrard-Jacob, A., Knapp, K., Craddock, T. S., Kemper, C., Falvo, R., et al. (2009). Perioperative fluid management. *AORN Journal, 89*(1), 167–182.

Zeinali, F. (2009). Pharmacological management of postoperative ileus. *Canadian Journal of Surgery, 52*(2), 153–157.

UNIT 5 Nursing Management of Patients with Neurological Disorders

Content in Unit 5 that addresses the **Institute of Medicine (IOM)** competencies, **Nursing Core Competencies (NCC),** the **Quality and Safety Education for Nurses (QSEN)** competencies, and **Concepts** for concept-based learning is listed below.

Competencies	Feature or Text	Location
IOM, QSEN, NCC Providing patient-centered care	Gerontological Considerations, Neurological Assessment Nursing Process: Patient Care Plans for Acute Brain Disorders Nursing Process: Patient Care Plan for Stroke Nursing Process: Patient Care Plans for Chronic and Degenerative Disorders Psychosocial Assessment and Intervention, Spinal Cord Injury Nursing Process: Patient Care Plan for Spinal Cord Injury	Chapter 20, page 500 Chapter 21, page 523 Chapter 22, page 564 Chapter 23, pages 606, 614, 617, 621, 625 Chapter 24, page 651 Chapter 24, page 654
IOM, QSEN, NCC Working in teams	Collaborative Management, pages 522, 534, 541, 545 Collaborative Management, page 580 Collaborative Management, page 628 Collaborative Management, page 657	Chapter 21 Chapter 22 Chapter 23 Chapter 24
IOM, QSEN, NCC Employing evidence-based practice	Evidence-Based Practice: Traumatic Brain Injury Evidence-Based Practice: Intracranial Hemorrhage Evidence-Based Practice: Family Caregiver Assistance Evidence-Based Practice: Respiratory Complications Related to SCI	Chapter 21, page 526 Chapter 22, page 569 Chapter 23, page 631 Chapter 24, page 646
IOM NCC Applying quality and safety improvement	Safety Alerts, pages 488, 490, 496, 497, 500 Safety Alerts, pages 511, 519, 528, 545 Safety Alerts, pages 552, 558, 574, 575 Safety Alerts, pages 610, 612 Safety Alert, page 644	Chapter 20 Chapter 21 Chapter 22 Chapter 23 Chapter 24
NCC Applying ethical and legal responsibilities	Ethical Issues Related to Brain Death Ethical Issues Regarding Huntington's Disease Genetic Testing	Chapter 21, page 522 Chapter 23, page 619
NCC Educating patients	Health Promotion for Acute Brain Disorders, pages 508, 541, 545 Patient Teaching & Discharge Priorities for Acute Brain Disorders, page 527 Health Promotion for Cerebral Vascular Disorders, pages 569, 579 Patient Teaching & Discharge Priorities for Stroke, page 583 Patient Teaching & Discharge Priorities for Chronic and Degenerative Neurological Disorders, pages 607, 616, 618, 622, 626, 629 Patient Teaching & Discharge Priorities for Spinal Cord Injury, page 658 Health Promotion, Spinal Cord Injury, page 658	Chapter 21 Chapter 21 Chapter 22 Chapter 22 Chapter 23 Chapter 24 Chapter 24

Concepts covered in Unit 5 include:

Body image	Fear	Mobility	
Cognition	Grief and loss	Perfusion	
Comfort	Intracranial regulation		

Nursing Assessment of the Patient with Neurological Disorders

20 CHAPTER

Christi DeLemos
Annita Watson

Outcome-Based Learning Objectives

After studying this chapter, the learner will be able to:

1. Correlate the anatomic and physiological aspects of the nervous system with the neurological examination.
2. Analyze the importance of history taking in the neurological assessment.
3. Associate the cranial nerves with common functional deficits seen in neurological disease.
4. Critique the rationale for and methods of measuring and documenting muscle stretch reflexes.
5. Organize assessment methods for identifying the presence of pathologic reflexes and the method of documentation.
6. Determine the normal age-related differences in the neurological examination of the older patient.

KEY TERMS

affect p.493
anisocoria p.496
anosmia p.494
apathetic p.493
aphasia p.493
Babinski reflex p.500
Battle's sign p.490
conjugate gaze p.495
decerebrate posturing p.497
decorticate posturing p.497
doll's eye reflex p.495
dysconjugate gaze p.495
dysphoria p.493
euphoria p.493
euthymia p.493
exophthalmos p.495
extinction phenomenon p.498
fasciculation p.497
graphesthesia p.498
Hamilton Depression Rating Scale (HDRS) p.500
hypotonia p.497
insight p.493
macrocephalic p.490
masked facies p.490
microcephalic p.490
muscle stretch reflexes p.498
muscle tone p.497
neuron p.485
nystagmus p.495
oculocephalic reflex p.495
oculovestibular reflex p.495
pathologic reflexes p.500
proprioception p.498
proptosis p.495
ptosis p.495
raccoon sign (eyes) p.490
superficial reflexes p.499
synapse p.485

THE COMPREHENSIVE NEUROLOGICAL ASSESSMENT provides essential information about the patient's current neurologic health and serves as an important tool in detecting disease and evaluating the patient's response to treatment. The initial neurological assessment becomes the baseline to which all further examinations are compared. Critical attention must be paid to providing an accurate assessment followed by documentation of findings. The documented assessment and reassessments are analyzed to identify any change in condition and direct the nursing plan of care.

This chapter presents guidelines for the assessment of the adult patient in a variety of clinical settings. The American Association for Neuroscience Nurses (2010) core curriculum for neuroscience nursing was used as a framework in determining neurological assessment guidelines.

Anatomy and Physiology of the Nervous System

Knowledge of normal neuroanatomy and physiology is essential to identify clinically significant abnormalities of the nervous system. Separated into three areas, the nervous system consists of the central nervous system (CNS), the peripheral nervous system (PNS), and the autonomic nervous system (ANS). Although the nervous system is complex, a basic understanding of its structure and function is critical so that the nurse can competently assess a patient.

The basic unit of the nervous system is the **neuron.** The primary function of the neuron is to receive information and subsequently transmit this information to other neurons. This information transmission takes place in the **synapse,** the channel between neurons, as shown

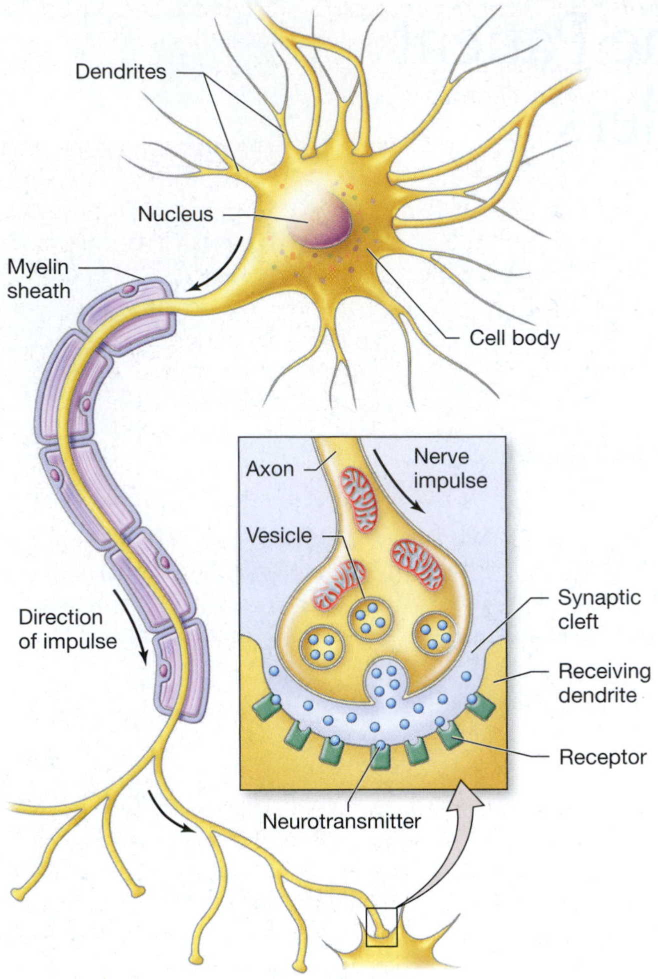

FIGURE 20–1 ◆ Two neurons with a synapse between.

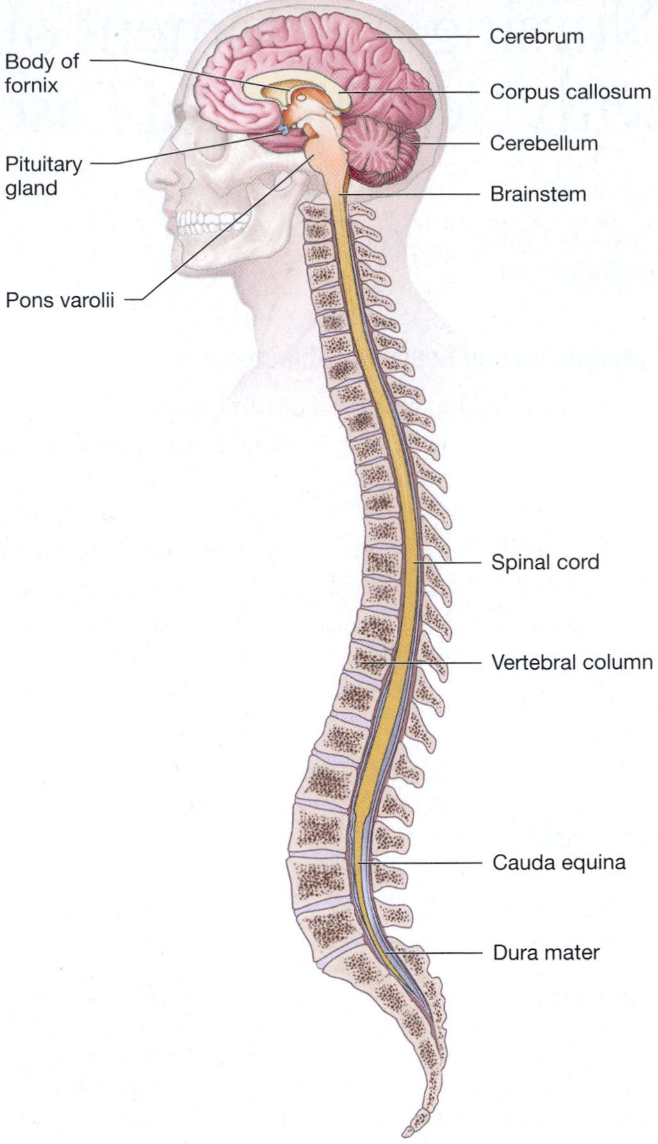

FIGURE 20–2 ◆ Brain and spinal cord.

in Figure 20–1◆. The size and shape of neurons are different based on their location in the nervous system, but conceptually all neurons are the same. Each neuron is a single cell body. From this body, several branches, or dendrites, extend. These branches communicate through the synapse to other dendrites.

A nerve fiber originating in the body, called the axon, can divide into several branches. Through these branches, impulses can be distributed to a number of destinations simultaneously. Information transmitted neuronally is dependent on cellular changes in electrical activity. When a neuron is stimulated, the electrical stimulus proceeds down the axon, stimulating vesicles containing chemicals called neurotransmitters. Neurotransmitters act in the synapse, stimulating the next neuron.

Neuroglias, the supporting cells of the nervous system, comprise the other major cellular component of the nervous system. Unlike neurons, neuroglias do not directly transmit information. There are five main types of neuroglias: oligodendrocytes, astrocytes, phagocytic microglial cells, ependymal cells, and Schwann cells. Oligodendrocytes form the myelin sheath that covers many neuronal axons. Astrocytes are a key component of the blood–brain barrier, and microglias have a role in removing cellular debris in nervous system damage. Ependymal cells are column-shaped cells that have microvilli and cilia that are thought to play an important role in cerebrospinal fluid (CSF) resorption. Schwann cells help to form the myelin sheath around axons and are found in the peripheral nervous system. Knowledge of the cellular components of the nervous system assists the nurse in understanding the etiology of disease states, such as multiple sclerosis or a primary neoplastic condition. Neurological disorders are discussed in Chapters 21 through 24.

Central Nervous System

The central nervous system consists of the brain and spinal cord, as shown in Figure 20–2◆. The CNS contains the majority of axons and synapses and is consistent in its apportionment of neurons. Areas with a high density of cell bodies are called gray matter; those primarily containing axons are referred to as white matter. Axons generally are myelinated, which results in a pale color; hence, the term *white matter*.

In general, CNS pathways conveying sensory information to the cerebral hemisphere cross over, or decussate, from one side of the CNS to the other. This holds true of descending pathways also. Therefore, each cerebral hemisphere generally perceives sensation from, and controls the movement of, the contralateral side of the body.

Three protective membranes called the meninges cover the brain and spinal cord. Specifically, these membranes are the dura mater, arachnoid mater, and the pia mater. The space between the arachnoid mater and the pia mater is known as the subarachnoid space. This is the space through which CSF flows. The CSF circulates through the brain in a series of open spaces called ventricles. The circulating CSF provides cushion to protect the brain and spinal cord from trauma. There are four ventricles, which are interconnected; they are named the right and left lateral ventricles, the third ventricle, and the fourth ventricle. The CSF flows through a series of holes or foramina (plural of *foramen*) that connect the spaces. CSF is produced by the choroid plexus and resorbed by the arachnoid villi (or granulations). Hydrocephalus, a condition in which there is too much CSF, can be caused by obstruction of flow through the ventricles or failure of the arachnoid villi to resorb CSF.

Blood is supplied to the brain through the internal carotid and vertebral arteries. When it enters the neck, the carotid artery bifurcates into the external carotid and the internal carotid. The internal carotid feeds the brain and divides into two main branches: the anterior cerebral artery and the middle cerebral artery. The vertebral system supplies the brainstem and cerebellum and is made up of the vertebral arteries, basilar artery, and cerebellar arteries. The venous drainage of the brain can be divided into deep and superficial sinus drainage systems. Superficial venous drainage runs along the surface of the brain and is organized into a complex linked system of sinuses including the superior sagittal sinus, straight sinus, transverse sinus, and cavernous sinus. The deep veins empty into the vein of Galen, which forms the straight sinus. The blood–brain barrier restricts substances that are circulating in the normal bloodstream from entering the brain. This prevents pathogens from entering the brain, but it also keeps most medications from reaching the brain. This poses important treatment challenges for patients with brain tumors that would benefit from chemotherapy.

Peripheral Nervous System

The peripheral nervous system is the link between the CNS and structures of the body. The CNS receives information (afferent pathway) and sends information to the skin, muscles, and tissues (efferent pathway). The PNS consists of two groups of nerves joined to the brain and spinal cord called the cranial nerves and spinal nerves. The spinal nerves are shown in Figure 20–2. The spinal nerves branch and combine in areas called plexuses and in groups of cell bodies in structures called ganglia.

The spinal cord lies in the hollow space of the vertebral column, which provides support and protection (Figure 20–2). Vertebrae are bones that are separated by intervertebral disks; these disks act as a cushion to the vertebrae and absorb stress. The spinal cord has 31 pairs of nerves corresponding to the vertebrae to which they are adjacent: 8 cervical, 12 thoracic, 5 lumbar, 5 sacral, and 1 coccygeal. Nerves C_1 through C_7 exit over their corresponding vertebrae, but thoracic nerve 1 (T_1) and the remainder of the nerves exit below their correspondingly numbered vertebrae. Cervical nerve 8 (C_8) exists in the space below C_7 and T_1. C_8 is unique in that there is no corresponding numbered vertebra. The spinal cord is shorter than the vertebral column, so the spinal roots extend downward. The spinal cord typically terminates between vertebral levels L_1 and L_2, but nerves L_2 through S_5 continue downward as the *cauda equina* ("horse's tail") (see Figure 20–2).

Safety Alert *Cauda equina syndrome is an injury or compression of the lumbosacral nerve roots within the spinal canal. This syndrome is often caused by acute disc herniation or injury. It is characterized by motor weakness of the lower extremities, saddle anesthesia (paresthesia or numbness and tingling in the crotch areas, sometimes interpreted as "unable to feel anything in the body areas that would sit on a saddle"), and new onset incontinence of bowel or bladder.* If *left untreated this syndrome can result in permanent neurological deficits.*

Autonomic Nervous System

Neurons that have the capacity to detect changes in, and control the activity of, the viscera are collectively called the autonomic nervous system (ANS). The components of the ANS are found in both the CNS and the PNS. The ANS innervates smooth muscle, cardiac muscle, and glands. The primary control of the ANS is the brain and spinal cord. The ANS is separated into two distinct divisions: the sympathetic and parasympathetic nervous systems. The sympathetic nervous system is used to mediate stress. The parasympathetic system, conversely, is associated with conserving and restoring energy. The nurse must have a thorough knowledge of the ANS when dealing with the spinal cord injury patient.

Safety Alert *Autonomic dysreflexia is a syndrome of unopposed sympathetic output that can follow spinal shock. It produces marked elevation in blood pressure and should be regarded as a medical emergency. It is commonly caused by bowel or bladder problems, irritation to the skin, and deep venous thrombosis. Care should be taken to immediately relieve suspected causes.*

History

In assessing the patient with neurological symptoms, a detailed history is vital for identifying possible causes of the symptoms (Cox, 2008). Special care must be taken to ensure that the history is comprehensive and accurate. The components of the history include the chief complaint, past medical history, past surgical history, family history, social history, environment, and cultural assessment (see Chapter 6).

The neurological assessment begins with the health care provider's first contact with the patient. The health care provider should assess the patient's general appearance, facial expression, distractibility, eye contact, and response to verbal stimuli. She also should note the patient's cognition, emotional expression, speech patterns, and ability to follow directions.

Biographic and Demographic Information

Biographic and demographic data consist of identifying facts such as age, sex, race, place of birth, current residence, marital status, and religion. These data points serve not only to establish who the patient is but also to give the nurse tentative suggestions as to what areas to explore further. Many neurological conditions occur in specific populations or age groups. Examples are the higher occurrence of Huntington disease in Western European populations and a lower incidence among Asians and Africans, a higher occurrence of Alzheimer's disease in older adults, and a higher occurrence of multiple sclerosis in the young adult. Ethnicity plays a role in cerebral vascular accidents; epidemiological studies indicate that minority populations are at higher risk (Centers for Disease Control and Prevention [CDC], 2007). The patient's current residence is an important piece of information that may prompt the health care provider to look at region-specific diseases such as West Nile virus or cysticercosis (CDC, 2007).

Chief Complaint

The chief complaint is the reason the individual is seeking care. It *is* best documented in the patient's own words, in quotations. Often, patients with neurological problems have a spouse, family member, or friend present at the time of initial assessment. This should be allowed, if possible, because it may provide both support and reassurance to the patient, as well as offer validation of the history. In the acute setting, the patient might not be capable of providing a health history because of age-related dementia or disease-related cognitive impairment. Confirmation of the health history by a relative or significant other can be critical in establishing the diagnosis and nursing plan of care.

History of the Present Illness

The history of the present illness can offer important clues to help establish the diagnosis and plan of care. The nurse should begin with the initial onset of the symptom and proceed to the present. Use of the mnemonic OLD CARTS is helpful in ensuring that all necessary information is obtained. This tool is shown in Chart 20–1 (Goldberg, 2008).

In gathering historical information, it is necessary to be very specific. An attempt should be made to clarify descriptors with as much detail as possible. For example, the term *dizziness* can be used to describe vertigo (a sensation that the environment is spinning around the patient or the patient is spinning in an immobile environment). Vertigo is commonly associated with disorders of the eighth cranial nerve or cerebellum. In contrast, light-headedness (a feeling of faintness) is commonly associated with cardiac dysfunction. The term *weakness* can be used to describe loss of muscle strength, lack of coordination, or a sensory disturbance. Chart 20–1 provides an example of taking the history of a patient who has presented with a headache.

Safety Alert *When evaluating a patient presenting with a headache in the ambulatory setting, difficulty with vision, large palpable temporal arteries, and temporal tenderness are the hallmark of temporal arteritis. This is a neurological emergency and will result in blindness if not treated.*

Safety Alert *A patient with the "worst headache of my life" with or without photophobia (sensitivity to light) and meningeal signs could have a subarachnoid hemorrhage. This is a neurological emergency and can result in death if not treated immediately.*

Past Medical History

The past medical history provides important information about the patient's overall health status and directs the examiner toward possible neurologic disorders that may be associated with the patient's current health problems or social habits. This includes a review of major illnesses, which encompass all hospitalizations, surgeries, ambulatory procedures, and illnesses, both acute and chronic. In addition, childhood diseases, immunizations, medications, and allergies are explored, as is the tendency to use one hand rather than the other, which is referred to as handedness, and tests muscle function and symmetry.

Medical and Surgical History

Several medical conditions are associated with neurological dysfunction. Some common health problems associated with neurologic disease are diabetes, hypertension, atrial fibrillation, neoplastic disease, and B_{12} dietary deficiency.

CHART 20–1 OLD CARTS Mnemonic for Assessment of Chief Complaint

Data Collected	Question	Headache (Example)
Onset of symptom:	When did the symptoms begin?	When did your headache first start?
Location of symptom:	Note the location of the manifestation.	What is the location of your headache (frontal, temporal, occipital, global)?
Duration of symptom:	How long has the manifestation been affecting you?	How long do the headaches last?
Characteristics:	Describe the characteristics of the manifestation in common language.	Describe your headache. Is it sharp pain? Is the pain throbbing (as with vascular or migraine headaches) or dull (as with chronic daily headaches or rebound headaches)? Are there any associated visual changes or nausea (as in migraine headaches)?
Aggravating/**A**ssociated factors:	What factors make the situation worse? What symptoms occur that are associated with the main symptom or manifestation?	What seems to make your headache worse? Do the symptoms change with position; for example, are they worse when sitting or standing, and improve with lying flat? (This can indicate increased intracranial pressure caused by, for example, a tumor, or low-pressure headaches, commonly seen with cerebral spinal fluid leakage.)
Relieving factors:	What factors alleviate the symptoms or make you feel better?	What seems to make your headache better? Do you take any medicines or herbal remedies for your headache? If so, what have you tried? (Record each medicine tried and the response to treatment.)
Temporal factors:	Is the onset of the manifestation gradual or sudden?	How often do the headaches occur? (if monthly, are they related to menses? daily?)
	When does it occur? How frequently does it occur?	Is the headache associated with any specific activity?
	Does it occur in specific settings or environments (e.g., usually after breakfast)?	
Severity of symptoms:	How severe is the problem? Rate on a scale of 1 to 10, with 10 being the most severe.	On a scale of 1 to 10, with 10 representing the most severe pain that you can imagine, how bad is your headache?

Source: Goldberg, C. (2008). *A practical guide to clinical medicine.* San Diego, CA: UCSD School of Medicine and VA Medical Center, San Diego, California 92093-0611. Retrieved from http://meded.ucsd.edu/clinicalmed/history.htm.

A history of any prior neurological illness is important, as this can affect baseline assessment performance. Key neurologic conditions include prior traumatic brain injury, seizures, stroke, cranial nerve problems, and neurodegenerative disorders. It also is important to review the history of surgical procedures. Cognitive impairment has been noted in up to three-quarters of all cardiac surgery patients (Newman, 2007).

Medications

The medication history should include all medications the patient is currently taking. In addition to prescribed medications, the history must list herbal medications, over-the-counter medications, home remedies, and supplements such as vitamins. It is important to specifically ask whether any of these nonprescription preparations are taken, because many people do not associate them with the term *medication.* This is especially important in minority and older populations.

Allergies

Many patients report that they have "allergies" to a medication, when in fact they have experienced an adverse drug reaction or a well-known side effect. The name of the medication and the specific reaction should be documented. The health care provider should specifically ask about iodine allergies, because many neurological conditions are best ruled in or out with a contrasted imaging study, which uses iodine. All patients should be questioned regarding an allergy to latex, as this has become a common allergy and latex materials are used in many medical settings (e.g., gloves).

Immunization History

The nurse should take a thorough inventory of all the patient's prior immunizations, his recent travels out of the country, and/or his exposure to disease. The nurse needs to ask about and record the patient's childhood diseases.

Family History

A thorough family history includes age, if living, and cause of death, if deceased, of all immediate biologic family members: parents, grandparents, siblings, and children. Some neurological disorders are familial. In others, a positive family history represents a risk factor. Refer to the Genetic Considerations Box to view the influence of genetics on the development of neurological disorders.

Social History

It is important to obtain the patient's social history in a nonjudgmental fashion. The social history begins with determining the highest level of education the patient has attained, as well as performance in school. Additional key elements include vocation, marital status, sexual orientation, and social habits such as tobacco, drug, and alcohol use.

GENETIC CONSIDERATIONS
for the Development of Neurological Disorders

In addition to the well-recognized inherited disorders such as Huntington disease or Friedreich's ataxia, research is under way to identify genetic links to stroke, amyotrophic lateral sclerosis (ALS), and multiple sclerosis (Alexander & Beach, 2008).

Environment

The home and workplace environment should be assessed for possible exposure to industrial toxins (lead, arsenic, asbestos, benzene, polyvinylchloride, and other carcinogens) as well as the use of any protective safety devices. The patient's potential for falls should be evaluated. Travel or exposure to contagious diseases also should be explored.

Cultural Considerations

Cultural components are present in all patients. Differences, both subtle and obvious, exist. The nurse must take care not to assume that any patient has a prescribed cultural behavior pattern, because this would constitute stereotyping. It is important to explore communication styles, nutrition, family relationships, health beliefs, and religion. This exploration can occur concurrently with the history portion of the assessment. The nurse should determine the patient's beliefs regarding the presenting problem. This exploration should include the patient's perceptions of what has caused the problem and treatments that have been tried. Being culturally aware is important to the nursing process, as discussed in the Cultural Considerations box.

Physical Examination

The physical examination of the patient with neurological symptoms is conceptually the same as any other system physical examination. Here, the findings of the physical exam are interpreted with the focus on the nervous system.

General Appearance

The patient's general appearance and grooming, facial expression, body habitus, skin color, symmetry of motor function, speech patterns, and general level of consciousness are observed. Many neurological disorders produce weakness or affect cognitive function, resulting in difficulty with self-care such as grooming.

Vital Signs

Vital signs should be taken by measuring the patient's height and weight and obtaining temperature, blood pressure, pulse rate, and respiratory rate. Many cardiovascular anomalies can result in neurological symptoms (see Chapters 30 to 35).

Skin

The nurse should take care to evaluate the skin for dryness, open areas, discoloration, or evidence of trauma. Some neurological diseases have hallmark skin findings, such as edema and temperature change (found in complex regional pain syndrome) or café au lait spots (which can be indicative of neurofibromatosis). *Café au lait* spots usually are oval, with the long axis situated along a cutaneous (skin) nerve tract. They are light to medium brown, as reflected by the name, which means "coffee with milk" in French. They usually are present at birth but may arise later, in the first few years of life. They are much more common in Black infants. To have a few such spots is totally normal. However, the nurse should take notice if there are more than six such spots greater than 1.5 mm in diameter in prepubertal children or greater than 5 mm in diameter in postpubertal children, because they are then essentially diagnostic of neurofibromatosis (although other features are required to make the diagnosis, and some individuals may have multiple spots without

CULTURAL CONSIDERATIONS
Related to the Health History

Maintaining cultural awareness indicates a nurse's recognition that patients' attitudes and reactions to illness are reflective of their beliefs as well as practices. Being aware of cultural beliefs and practices enables the nurse to more effectively evaluate and plan appropriate nursing interventions. Medication administration might need to be modified for various cultural groups to enhance communication and decrease misconceptions. For example, Hispanic, Chinese, and Asian patients often expect quick relief from symptoms, but they are cautious about American medicines and often initiate downward dosage adjustments to avoid even minor side effects. Chinese patients also consider American medicine to be quick and effective in removing symptoms but not in providing a permanent cure. Because they believe that traditional medicine can remove the cause of the illness, they tend to use American medicine for acute illness, surgery, and severe disease, but then rely on Chinese medicine for long-term treatment.

Cultural influences prevail in establishing interactions with health care providers. When patients of different ethnicities interact with health care providers, they often consider eye contact, body posture, and other forms of nonverbal communication significant, especially if a language barrier is present. Hispanic and Asian patients often are reluctant to speak up about their illness. Out of a misplaced deference for health care providers and a reluctance to share deeply personal information, they may minimize or conceal adverse events or might stop taking medications because of the side effects without telling the health care provider. They may agree with the plan of care out of this respect, although they may not intend to follow the medication instruction. This practice may have dangerous or life-threatening outcomes. Family involvement also is important in planning health care for Asian and Hispanic patients. In Hispanic families, the mother or grandmother (especially of the husband) usually makes the health care decisions. With Asians, the opinions of family members and the elderly are highly respected during illness. Egyptians are accustomed to the oral tradition of communication and thus may not keep reliable written records for medication schedules. A call from an Amish family is probably a true emergency because of their religious and cultural obligations to care for themselves first before seeking outside resources. Food rituals are important to the Appalachian, Jewish, Muslim, and Asian/Pacific Island people and must be incorporated into the plan of care if a prescription is to be followed.

Other cultural beliefs or rituals also need to be considered. In some other cultures, the practice of religious fasting can affect medication schedules or interfere with drug absorption. Self-medication and self-diagnosis are common among Asians. Hispanic patients tend to believe that the lack of symptoms means that they are cured. When symptoms abate, patients often stop taking their medications.

It is incumbent upon nurses to become knowledgeable of the customs and habits relevant to the patient populations for whom they are providing care (Grissinger, 2007). When patients are evaluated within the context of their cultural orientation and current health care beliefs, improved assessment and planning for interventions are more likely to occur. Chapter 1 contains a full discussion of cultural considerations and cultural competence.

having the disease—a trait that is itself inherited). The nurse also must pay special attention to the lower lumbar area at the base of the spine. A dimple, with or without a tuft of hair, in that area can signify spina bifida or meningocele (Vogel & Sturm, 2008).

Head, Neck, and Extremities

The nurse should observe the responsiveness of the patient's facial expression and look for asymmetry. Diseases such as Parkinson's disease can result in a poverty of facial expression, called **masked facies,** and facial asymmetry can be a subtle indication of dysfunction of the seventh cranial nerve. Inspection of the head should include observation for an abnormally large (**macrocephalic**) or small (**microcephalic**) head. The skin should be inspected for evidence of trauma and old incisions, and the skull should be palpated to detect deformities that may suggest previous surgery or fractures. Bruising immediately behind the ears, known as **Battle's sign,** and **raccoon sign** (or **eyes**), an ecchymosis around the periorbital area that generates the appearance of a raccoon, raise suspicion of basal skull fracture. The nurse should inspect the ear canal for evidence of clear fluid (otorrhea) caused by traumatic injury to the temporal bone producing a CSF leak. In addition, the nares should be inspected for evidence of clear fluid drainage (rhinorrhea) caused by traumatic injury or surgical opening of the frontal, ethmoid, or sphenoid bones. The temporal arteries should be palpated to note whether the patient experiences tenderness, which would signify temporal arteritis.

The nurse inspects and palpates the neck, looking for evidence of prior surgery, abnormal flexion (kyphosis) or extension of the neck, and adequate motor strength to keep the head in an erect position. If there is no evidence of trauma or cervical fracture, the nurse passively flexes the patient's neck to detect pain or limitation of movement, which suggests meningeal irritation.

Safety Alert *When examining the patient's neck, note whether the patient has pain on flexion or extension. Brudzinski sign is flexion of the hips when the neck is flexed from a supine position. This is consistent with meningitis and must be evaluated further.*

Cardiac

The cardiac system is intimately intertwined with functions of the central nervous system. The heart receives input from the medulla and vagus nerve for parasympathetic input, and the brain demands a constant flow of oxygen-rich blood for normal function. In states of low cardiac output, cerebral perfusion pressure is adversely affected. The nurse should auscultate heart sounds, noting the rate, rhythm, and tone and listening for murmurs. Blood pressure should be measured and trended over time, as abrupt increases or decreases in blood pressure can cause neurological injury. Blood pressure should be strictly controlled within the prescribed parameters.

Respiratory

The respiratory system relies on input from the brainstem to maintain a constant rate and oxygenation level. Three brainstem centers influence respiration: the apneustic and pneumotaxic centers, located in the pons, which governs tidal volume, and the medullary respiratory center, which controls muscles associated with breathing. The nurse should assess respiratory rate and pattern with an emphasis on observation for dyspnea, adequacy of air exchange, and ability to protect the airway. Several distinct patterns of breathing are associated with neurologic dysfunction. Detection of these patterns can provide important clues to the location of the injury. Common neurogenic patterns to recognize are summarized in Chart 20–2.

Neurological Examination

The neurological examination can be divided into six areas: mental status, cranial nerves, motor system, sensation, reflexes, and cerebellar function. Each element provides critical information about

CHART 20–2 Neurogenic Breathing Patterns

Breathing Pattern	Exam Findings	Location of Dysfunction/Injury
Apneustic breathing	Prolongation of the inspiratory phase followed by a pause and short expiratory phase	Pons
Ataxic breathing	Random irregular respiratory rate with periods of brief apnea and variable tidal volume	Medulla
Central neurogenic hyperventilation	Deep rapid regular respirations	Midbrain or upper pons
Cheyne-Stokes	Pattern of gradual increase in the rate and depth of respirations, followed by a similar decrease in the rate and depth of respirations with a short apnea phase and a repeating cycle	Bilateral hemispheric injury or injury to diencephalon
Cluster breathing	Cluster of breaths followed by a pause in a repeating pattern	Lower pons, high medullary

Source: Adapted from Barker, E. (2007). *Neuroscience nursing: a spectrum of care* (3rd ed.). Philadelphia. Mosby Elsevier. ISBN-10: 0323044018.

the primary functions of the brain. A comprehensive examination includes all variables and is performed in a systematic fashion aimed at detecting subtle changes in function.

Mental Status Examination

Mental status is defined as "the functional state of the mind as judged by the individual's behavior, appearance, and responsiveness to stimuli of all kinds, speech, memory, and judgment" (*Taber's Cyclopedic Dictionary of Medicine*, 2010). The mental status examination assesses the higher cortical functions of thinking and reasoning as well as the patient's level of consciousness, orientation, attention, memory, affect and insight, speech and language, fund of knowledge, and abstraction.

Level of Consciousness

Level of consciousness (LOC) is a critical component of the neurological assessment. Consciousness is a state of awareness and can be a sensitive indicator of cortical function. Arousal is a state of responsiveness to sensory stimulation governed by the reticular activating system. Arousal requires both hemispheres and the upper brainstem to be intact (Goldman & Ausiello, 2007). In documenting the patient's LOC, the nurse should include both the response and the stimulus that was required to produce the response. Evaluation of the LOC is most accurate when the patient is stimulated to a maximal state of arousal. Arousal refers to an individual's state of awareness of herself and her environment or her level of alertness; it is also known as response to stimuli. In determining level of consciousness, the nurse may stimulate the patient to respond to light stimuli such as normal voice tone, then progress to stronger stimuli such as a shout, light touch, and pain. If there is no response to voice or light touch, painful stimuli is needed. Central pain should be used first as a stimulant. Sternal rub, supraorbital (space above the orbit of the eye) pressure, or pinching the fleshy portion of the upper arm near the axilla are methods for introducing central pain.

The Glasgow Coma Scale (GCS) is the most widely recognized LOC assessment tool (Chart 20–3). The GCS was published in 1974 by Teasdale and Jennett and is commonly used in emergency departments, trauma units, and intensive care areas. This tool evaluates three areas: eye opening, verbal response, and best motor response. The highest score that can be attained is 15, and the lowest is 3. In general, a GCS score of 8 or lower indicates a coma. In completing the GCS, it is important to score the best response for each category.

CHART 20–3 Scoring for Glasgow Coma Scale

Eye Opening (E)	Verbal Response (V)	Motor Response (M)
4 = Spontaneous	5 = Normal conversation	6 = Normal
3 = To voice	4 = Disoriented conversation	5 = Localizes to pain
2 = To pain	3 = Words, but not coherent	4 = Withdraws to pain
1 = None	2 = No words; only sounds	3 = Decorticate posture
	1 = None	2 = Decerebrate
		1 = None

With the GCS, the examiner determines the best eye opening response, the best verbal response, and the best motor response. The score represents the sum of the numeric scores of each of the categories. Despite the limitations to its use, it is a practical evaluation tool to estimate level of consciousness and severity of injury at presentation in patients with neurological injury. When approaching the patient, the nurse should begin by observing for response in a normal speaking voice. If there is no response, the nurse should increase the stimuli in a stepwise fashion from a loud voice to gentle direct stimulation and finally to application of a painful stimulus to illicit a response. Central pain stimuli, as previously described, can be used if no limiting incisions or injuries are present. Speech content is scored on the basis of the best response to orientation questions. If the patient has an endotracheal tube in place, the patient is given an arbitrary score of T (intubated). For this reason, many examiners prefer to document the score by its individual components; therefore, a patient with a GCS score of 15 would be documented as follows: E4 V5 M6. An intubated patient would be scored as E4 VT (intubated) M6. Of these individual factors, the best motor response is probably the most significant.

Source: Wesley Medical Center. (2011). Trauma scoring-Glasgow coma scale (GCS) and revised trauma score (RTS). Retrieved from http://wesleymc.com/for-physicians/Glasgow-trauma-score.dot

Another validated tool that has been developed more recently than the GCS is the FOUR Score Consciousness Scale (Wolf, Wijdicks, Bamlet, & McClelland, 2007). This scale evaluates four components: eye, motor, brainstem, and respiration. Each component has a maximal score of 4. This scale provides greater neurological detail than the GCS does. In contrast to the GCS, verbal response is not a component of the FOUR Score Consciousness Scale, making it fully applicable to intubated patients. See Chart 20–4 for a description of the scale.

CHART 20–4 FOUR Score Consciousness Scale

Eye Response	Motor Response	Brainstem Reflexes	Respiration
4 = Eyelids open, tracking or blinking on command	4 = Thumbs up or fist to command	4 = Pupil and corneal reflex present	4 = Not intubated, regular breathing
3 = Eyelids open, not tracking	3 = Localizing to pain	3 = One pupil wide and fixed	3 = Not intubated, Cheyne-Stokes pattern
2 = Eyelids closed, but open to loud noise	2 = Flexion to pain	2 = Pupil **or** corneal reflex absent	2 = Not intubated, irregular pattern
1 = Eyelids closed, but open to pain	1 = Extensor posturing	1 = Pupil **and** corneal reflex absent	1 = Breathes above ventilator rate
0 = Eyelids closed with pain	0 = No response to pain or myoclonus status epilepticus	0 = Absent pupil, corneal, and cough reflex	0 = Breathes at ventilator rate or apnea

Source: Wolf, C. A., Wijdicks, E. F., Bamlet, W. R., & McClelland, R. L. (2007). Further validation of the FOUR score coma scale by intensive care nurses. *Mayo Clinic Proceedings, 82*(4), 435–438. PMID 17418071.

Orientation

The nurse should assess the patient for orientation to time, place, and person. Time orientation is assessed by evaluating the patient's awareness of the year, season, month, day of the week, and date. Place orientation is assessed via the patient's awareness of the name of the state he is in, followed by city, county, name of the current location (hospital or medical office), and floor the patient is currently on (or office number).

Time orientation often is the first sign of neurological change. In the hospitalized patient, this may be the result of a sleep disturbance and/or sensory overload. Impaired orientation to place may occur with moderate cerebral dysfunction (Dennis, 2007; Goldman & Ausiello, 2007). Orientation to person is generally the last parameter to be lost, and impaired orientation to person occurs with severe dysfunction such as delirium or dementia.

Confusion is defined as not being aware of, or oriented to, time, place, or self (*Dictionary of Cell and Molecular Biology*, 2008; *Taber's Cyclopedic Dictionary of Medicine*, 2010). Confusion may be acute or chronic. Etiologies include metabolic disorders, infections, changes in underlying neurological disorder, and drug or alcohol intoxication. A list of validated tools to assess cognition is shown in Chart 20–5.

Attention and Concentration

Attention is the ability to focus on a particular stimulus, task, or situation. Concentration is the ability to sustain attention. Alteration in attention and concentration can be early indicators of delirium (Snyderman, 2009; *Taber's Cyclopedic Dictionary of Medicine*, 2010). To evaluate attention and concentration, the nurse asks the patient to count backwards from 100 by 7 (93, 86, 79, 72, 65). If the patient is lacking in formal education, the nurse can ask the patient to say the days of the week or the months of the year backwards.

Memory

Memory is the ability to recover information about past events or knowledge. It can be subdivided into remote memory, intermediate memory, and recent memory. Most questions related to memory can be asked in the context of obtaining the history.

- ***Remote Memory:*** Remote memory can be evaluated by querying the patient about place of birth, where the patient went to high school, date of marriage, names and birthdates of the patient's children, or other details from the patient's past.
- ***Intermediate Memory:*** Intermediate memory can be evaluated by referring to personal and general events of the previous 5 years; for example, the patient could be asked to give a chronological

CHART 20–5 Cognitive Assessment Tools

Test Name	Evaluation	Scoring
Mini-Mental Status Examination (MMSE)	Evaluates orientation, language, memory, writing, ability to follow commands, calculations, and constructional abilities.	30-item examination scored by correct responses: Maximum score = 30 Average score = 27.6 Cognitive impairment = 25 or less.
Short Portable Mental Status Questionnaire (SPMSQ)	Evaluates orientation, language, personal history, awareness and remote memory, and calculation ability.	Ten-item instrument scored by errors. Score of 3 or greater indicates mild to severe impairment. Allow one more error if the person has only a grade school education. In this instance, a score of 4 or greater indicates mild to severe impairment. Allow one less error if subject has had education beyond high school, meaning that a score of 2 or more would indicate impairment. Allow one more error for Black subjects, using identical education criteria completed.
Cognitive Capacity Screening Examination (CCSE)	Evaluates orientation, memory, attention, calculation, and extracting abilities. Most reliable for distinguishing between delirium and dementia.	30-item instrument scored by correct responses. Most reliable for distinguishing between acute and chronic disorders. Maximum score = 30. Score of 20 or below indicates cognitive impairment.

CHART 20–6 Common Aphasias

Aphasia Type	Location	Exam Findings
Broca's aphasia	Damage to the dominant posterior frontal lobe.	Often able to comprehend but has difficulty with naming and expression of ideas; automatic speech may be preserved.
Conduction aphasia	Damage to the dominant posterior frontal and temporal/parietal regions.	Can produce speech and may be able to comprehend but is unable to repeat or write.
Global aphasia (a form of aphasia that involves both expressive and receptive aphasias)	Extensive damage to the dominant hemisphere. Lesions (extensive) of Broca's area, Wernicke's area, parietal-occipital area, and posterior frontal area.	Globally impaired speech production, verbal comprehension; difficulty with reading and writing.

account of the presenting illness, including dates. The nurse also could inquire about common events of the previous 5 years, such as presidential elections.

- ***Recent Memory:*** Recent memory can be tested in a variety of ways. Three-item recall is a common technique in which the nurse names three objects (i.e., apple, penny, table) and asks the patient to repeat them. The nurse then informs the patient that the nurse will be asking later for the patient to repeat the names of these objects. The nurse goes on to complete other aspects of the assessment and, after 5 minutes have passed, asks the patient to recall the three objects named previously. A person without cognitive deficit should be able to correctly recall the three objects.

Affect and Insight

Assessment of **affect,** or display of emotions, begins with observation. **Euthymia** refers to a normal state; that is, the patient is calm and appropriate. **Euphoria** is a state of being excessively or inappropriately cheerful. **Apathetic** is used to describe the patient who is flat or dull in affect. **Dysphoria** is a state of being depressed, despondent, or sad.

Insight refers to an individual's ability to assess and monitor her own cognitive, motor, or sensory function. Insight and reality orientation are frequently impaired in neurological diseases. The nurse can assess insight by asking the patient, "Why are you being seen today?" or "Why are you in the hospital?"

Speech and Language Fluency

Speech and language fluency refers to the spontaneity, articulation, hesitancy, and duration of the patient's response. Fluency of speech can be observed throughout the assessment. **Aphasia** is a disorder of speech and language caused by cerebral dysfunction. The three primary aphasic deficits are in comprehension of spoken language, expressive language, and naming. Aphasic deficits can be localized to the area of dysfunction. Approximately 90% of the U.S. population is right-handed and left hemisphere dominant for language. Among people who are left-handed, two-thirds are thought to have left hemisphere language dominance, while the others have varying degrees of mixed or right hemisphere dominance (Binder et al., 2011).

Most patients with neurological disorders have some communication function preserved. Carefully evaluating the patient's ability to communicate can aid the health care provider in localizing a lesion to a specific area of the brain. The various aphasias can be subdivided into categories and are listed in Chart 20–6 along with the respective areas of involvement.

- To assess comprehension, or the ability to understand the spoken word, the patient is first asked to follow a simple instruction, such as "Close your eyes." If the patient is able to do so, increasingly complex commands are given, such as "Touch your right ear with your left index finger." The ability to retain instructions and perform simple commands is a function of attention and, when abnormal, can be related to cortical dysfunction.
- To evaluate the ability to understand the written word, commands of increasing difficulty are written on cards that are shown to the patient, who is asked to follow the instructions. Examples include "Open your mouth," "Stick out your tongue," and "Point to your right ear."
- To assess the ability to express ideas verbally, the patient is asked to identify common objects, such as a pencil or a watch. The nurse then proceeds to ask open-ended questions, such as "Tell me about the kind of work you do" or "What types of activities do you enjoy in your free time?" or "Tell me about your illness."
- To test for naming, also called word finding difficulty, the patient is shown common objects, such as a pen and a watch, and is asked to name the object.
- If there is a question about the patient's ability to express himself in writing, the patient is given paper and pencil and asked to write his name and address. As with other aphasia evaluations, complexity is increased. After correctly writing his name and address, the patient could be asked to write an account of a current news event or to describe the weather.

Fund of Knowledge and Abstraction

The term *general fund of knowledge* refers to the patient's knowledge base—an understanding of her natural and social environment. This may be tested by asking age-appropriate questions related to historical and current events. The higher the number of correct answers, the better the patient's understanding and knowledge base, taking into consideration the individual's educational background and other training.

Abstraction is measured by assessing the patient's ability to determine similarities. For example, the nurse may ask the patient how two items, such as an apple and an orange or a car and an airplane, are alike. The answer to the first would be good if the patient said "fruit"; it would be poor if the patient said "round." The answer to the second would be good if the patient said, "modes of transportation." Proverbs can also be used to demonstrate intact abstract thinking.

Cranial Nerve Examination

Cranial nerves are part of the peripheral nervous system; they emerge from the cranium in pairs (Cox, 2008). The cranial nerves are numbered

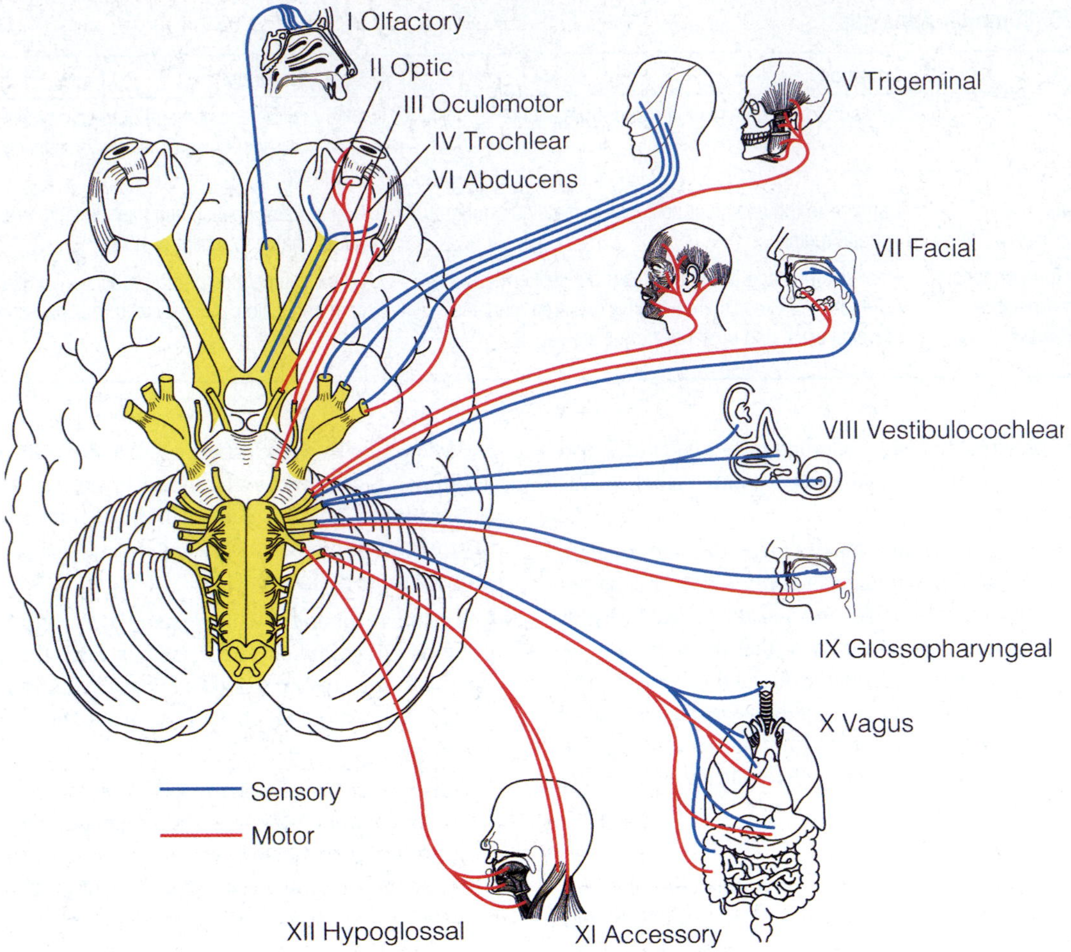

FIGURE 20–3 ◆ Dorsal aspect of brain with cranial nerves noted.

in Roman numerals I through XII and arise from the brainstem, as shown in Figure 20–3◆. They can have sensory or motor functions.

Olfactory Nerve (CN I)

CN I has sensory function only. The sense of smell is tested by occluding one nostril while testing the other. A common odoriferous substance is placed under the unobstructed nostril. Coffee, lemon oil, and peppermint are common substances used. **Anosmia** is the inability to smell. Common neurological causes of anosmia include tumors of the frontal lobe, fractures of the anterior fossa (basilar skull fracture), meningitis, hydrocephalus, and traumatic brain injury. Common nonneurological causes of anosmia include the common cold and inflammation of the nasal cavity. Recently, olfactory deficits have been described early in both Alzheimer's disease and Parkinson's disease (Luzzi, Snowden, Neary, Coccia, Provinciali, & Lambon, 2007). See Chapter 23 for a discussion of these diseases.

Optic Nerve (CN II)

CN II has sensory function only. Assessing the optic nerve involves inspecting the globe of the eye for abnormalities, foreign bodies, or other obvious deviations, as well as testing visual acuity and visual fields. A funduscopic examination, which may be performed by an advanced practice nurse or health care provider, can provide useful information in detecting increased intracranial pressure (see Chapter 64). To assess CN II, each eye is evaluated separately. Having the patient read from a newspaper can assess visual acuity; in the ambulatory setting, a Snellen chart is frequently used. A Snellen chart is an eye chart used by eye care professionals and others to measure visual acuity. Normal vision is 20/20, which means that the patient can read the Snellen chart from a distance of 20 feet. A reading of 20/30 means that the patient can read at 20 feet what the normal eye can read at 30 feet.

A visual field extends 60 degrees to the nasal side, 110 degrees to the temporal side, and 130 degrees vertically (Yanoff & Duker, 2008). Visual fields are assessed by using the confrontation test, whereby the patient and nurse face each other 2 feet apart. The patient is directed to cover one eye and look directly at the nurse. The nurse brings an object, such as a pencil, into each cardinal gaze, and the patient indicates when she first sees the object. The "cardinal positions" are six positions of gaze that allow comparisons of the horizontal, vertical, and diagonal ocular movements produced by the six extraocular muscles. The six cardinal positions are up/right, right, down/right, down/left, left, up/left. In each position of gaze, one muscle of each eye is the primary mover of that eye and is yoked to the primary mover of the other eye. Figure 20–4◆ shows each of the six cardinal positions of gaze. This test reveals only gross defects. Further testing would be indicated if it suggested any anomalies.

The funduscopic examination requires the use of an ophthalmoscope, a device with a special lens that is used to visualize the inside of

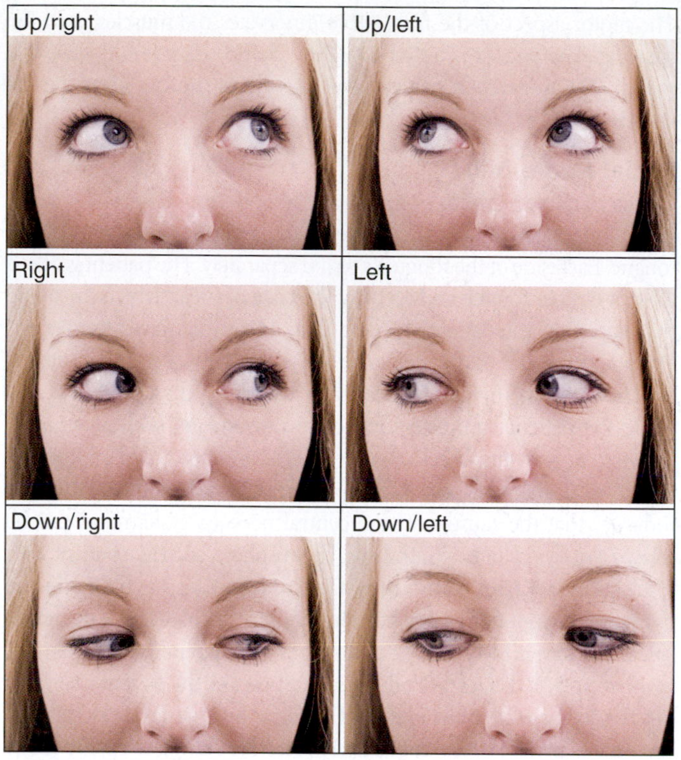

FIGURE 20–4 ◆ Six positions of cardinal gaze.

the eye by shining light directly into the eye. Alternatively, a penlight can be used to evaluate pupillary function. For best results, the room should be dimmed while this exam is performed.

The fundus includes the optic disc, macula, and blood vessels on the back wall of the eye. The funduscopic examination is perceived as a difficult task, and many nurses avoid performing it. However, it is essential for the assessment of papilledema, or optic disc swelling, which is a hallmark of increased intracranial pressure (see Chapter 64).

Oculomotor (CN III), Trochlear (CN IV), and Abducens (CN VI) Nerves

Cranial nerves III, IV, and VI are usually tested together because they supply the various muscles that move the eye, and because they have motor function only. These three nerves supply the extraocular muscles, pupils, and eyelids. The first step in assessing these nerve functions is to observe the eyes. Note the position of the eyeball within the head. Evaluate the eyes for symmetry. The abnormal protrusion of one or both eyeballs is called **proptosis** or **exophthalmos.** This commonly is seen in hyperthyroidism and less commonly in brain tumors that displace the globe. Next, note the position of the upper eyelid in relation to the pupil and iris in each eye, and compare them. **Ptosis** is the term for a drooping upper eyelid; it can be seen in injury to the third cranial nerve, Horner's syndrome, and myasthenia gravis.

Extraocular movements are evaluated by asking the patient to follow a finger or pencil through the six cardinal fields of gaze. In the patient without deficits, both eyes move at the same time in the same direction. This is referred to as **conjugate gaze.** If the eye movements are not the same, this is called **dysconjugate gaze.** Double vision may be present if the patient cannot move one eye in a particular direction. The loss of function of the muscles necessary for these movements may be caused by direct damage to the muscle or by injury of the cranial nerve. **Nystagmus** is an involuntary jerking or rotatory movement of the eyes that may be horizontal, vertical, or mixed in direction. There are multiple types of nystagmus; however, all involve a "jerky" movement of the eyes. Nystagmus can be a side effect of taking antiepileptic drugs for seizures.

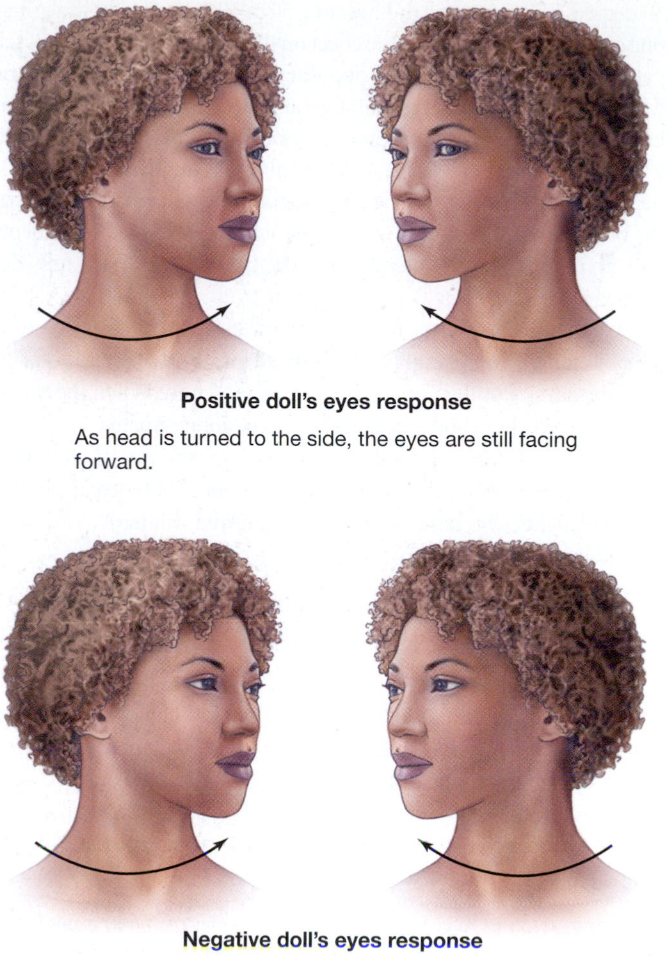

FIGURE 20–5 ◆ Doll's eyes reflex.

In assessing the unconscious patient, the oculocephalic reflex (doll's eye response) and the oculovestibular reflex (cold calorics) are evaluated for reflex movement of the eye. The **oculocephalic reflex,** or **doll's eyes reflex,** is one in which the eyes normally move in the opposite direction in which the head is turned, thus maintaining a more or less steady gaze (Figure 20–5◆). It is produced by moving the patient's head left to right or up and down. In a normal, alert person, this brainstem reflex is inhibited by gaze control mechanisms. The eyes go wherever the cortex wants them to go. In the comatose patient, this inhibition is lost, and the oculocephalic reflex becomes disinhibited and the patient's eyes remain stationary while the head is moved. In this response, the eyes stay focused on whatever they were looking at before the head was turned.

The **oculovestibular reflex,** or cold calorics, is a reflex movement that stabilizes images on the retina during head movement by producing an eye movement in the direction opposite to head movement. This can be produced by placing the patient's upper body and head at

Weblink: Aniscoria

30 degrees off horizontal and injecting 50 to 100 mL of cold water into one ear. The water has the same effect on the semicircular canal as if the patient's head was turned to the opposite side of the injection. Therefore, the patient's eyes will look toward the ear of injection. The eye deviation lasts for a sustained period of time. If the oculovestibular reflex is absent, a lesion of the pons, medulla, or, less commonly, the III, IV, VI, or VIII nerve is present. However, the presence of these reflexes indicates that the brainstem is intact. This test should only be performed on patients with an intact tympanic membrane. (The cold calorics test is fully described in Chapter 63.)

To assess the pupils, the nurse directs the patient to look at a stationary object in the room. Pupils are examined for size, shape, and equality. The normal size of the pupil ranges from 2 to 6 mm. When the pupils are compared, they should be equal; however, approximately 17% of the population has unequal pupil size without the presence of pathology (Eggenberger, 2010). This is called **anisocoria.** The normal pupil is round. Patients who have had cataracts removed will have a "keyhole" shaped pupil of the affected eye.

Safety Alert *An ovoid pupil indicates papillary dysfunction and is seen in early herniation. This is a neurological emergency and must be addressed immediately.*

The pupils are next tested for reaction to light. This is called the direct light reflex. A light is directed into each pupil and then withdrawn. When the light is shone into the eye, the pupil should constrict; conversely, when the light is withdrawn, it should dilate. Additionally, when the light is directed to the eye, the opposite eye should constrict slightly. This is called the consensual light reflex.

Safety Alert *A unilateral papillary dilation may represent excessive pressure and ultimately herniation of the medial temporal lobe. If this is seen, the nurse must communicate the assessment to the health care provider and observe the patient closely with serial assessments.*

The accommodation reflex is evaluated next. The patient is asked to focus on an object, such as the nurse's finger, that is positioned 2 or 3 feet directly in front of the patient and to follow it with his eyes. The finger is rapidly moved toward the patient's nose. The pupils should constrict when the patient is looking at the finger near his face.

In the unconscious patient, the maneuver to assess these nerves is called the doll's eyes maneuver, as previously discussed. To complete this maneuver, the nurse must first ensure that cervical injury has been ruled out. The nurse then holds the eyelids open and briskly turns the patient's head from side to side. Exam findings are observed as previously described.

Trigeminal Nerve (CN V)

The trigeminal nerve has both a sensory and a motor component. The sensory component is tested with the patient's eyes closed:

- The nurse places warm and cold objects on each side of the face randomly and asks the patient to identify the temperature.
- Using a piece of cotton or gauze, the nurse lightly touches each side of the face randomly and asks the patient to identify the sensation.
- The nurse uses a sharp object to lightly touch each side of the patient's face to test for pain.
- The nurse instills cool saline into the eye or lightly touches the cornea with cotton, resulting in the patient blinking the stimulated eye, to determine corneal reflex.

The motor aspect of the fifth nerve innervates the muscles used for chewing. The patient is asked to tightly clamp the jaw and close the mouth. The nurse then palpates the muscles of the jaw, checking for symmetry.

Facial Nerve (VII)

The facial nerve has both a sensory and a motor function. The seventh nerve innervates the sense of taste in the anterior two-thirds of the tongue. Each side of the tongue is tested separately. The patient is asked to stick out her tongue and identify the taste of sugar, which the nurse has placed on the patient's tongue. The nurse then gives the patient water to drink and then repeats the test with a salty or sour substance.

The motor component is tested by observing the face at rest and while the patient completes deliberate movements such as smiling, blowing air into the cheeks, wrinkling the forehead, and raising the eyebrows. Facial weakness with a pattern of weakness below the eyes indicates that the cause is in the central nervous system and can be related to a lesion in the contralateral hemisphere, such as a patient with a stroke. The patient with central facial weakness is unable to lift the corner of the mouth to smile but can wrinkle the forehead. If the entire side of the face is involved, the patient has a peripheral facial weakness, involving CN VII, such as Bell's palsy. In this case, the patient may have lost the ability to close the eyelids. The nurse must be aware of this and ensure that the eye is kept moist and protected. During sleep, the use of an eye moisture chamber is appropriate. These are clear plastic devices that allow moisture to remain yet protect the eye from trauma. Use of an eye patch or taping the lid closed while sleeping is appropriate as well.

Vestibulocochlear or Acoustic Nerve (CN VIII)

The acoustic nerve is a pure sensory nerve that is divided into two branches. The cochlear branch deals with hearing, and the vestibular branch is involved with balance. The vestibular branch is not routinely assessed. If the patient identifies symptoms of vertigo, tinnitus (noise or ringing in the ears), or disturbed balance, more specific testing can be done, generally by the neurologists. These symptoms are common in Ménière's disease and acoustic neuromas (see Chapter 63).

The cochlear branch is tested by the nurse whispering numbers and the patient repeating them or by the nurse asking the patient to close his eyes while the nurse rubs the thumb and first two fingers together, testing each ear separately and asking the patient to identify on which side he hears the noise. The Rinne Bone and Weber tests employ a tuning fork to distinguish between sensorineural and conductive hearing loss. Damage to this nerve can result in impaired hearing, tinnitus, vertigo, nystagmus, and unilateral or bilateral deafness.

Glossopharyngeal (CN IX) and Vagus (CN X) Nerves

The glossopharyngeal and vagus nerves are generally tested together because their innervation overlaps in the pharynx. They have both sensory and motor functions. The glossopharyngeal nerve supplies sensory function to the pharynx, tonsils, and posterior third of the tongue. The motor component elevates the pharynx. To test these nerves, the patient is directed to open the mouth and say "Aaah." The palate and uvula should move upward. The pharyngeal (gag) reflex is innervated by both the 9th and 10th nerves. To evaluate, the posterior pharynx is stimulated with a tongue blade. The pharynx should elevate and constrict, and the tongue should retract, or "gag." In the unconscious patient, the suction catheter can be used.

The vagus nerve controls swallowing and speaking by innervating the larynx and pharynx. When the patient has the mouth open and is saying "Aaah," the uvula should be midline. The quality of the patient's voice is assessed for hoarseness. The patient can be asked to repeat "No ifs, ands, or buts." Damage to the vagus nerve can result in impaired sensation, dysphasia, dysarthria, dysphonia, excessive drooling, and stridor (an abnormal, high-pitched, musical breathing sound caused by a blockage in the throat or voice box (larynx) (see Chapter 26).

Spinal Accessory Nerve (CN XI)

The spinal accessory nerve has motor function only. This nerve innervates the sternocleidomastoid and trapezius muscles. To assess function, the nurse first asks the patient to shrug the shoulders while the nurse uses resistance. The patient is then asked to turn the head to one side and push the chin against the nurse's hand. Damage to this nerve can result in impaired strength in lifting the shoulders or difficulty in turning the head to either side.

Hypoglossal Nerve (CN XII)

The patient is asked to open the mouth and stick out the tongue. The tongue is observed for deviation, atrophy, and **fasciculation,** a small, local involuntary muscle contracting or twitching visible under the skin. Next, the patient is asked to push the tongue against a tongue blade, to each side, to assess strength.

Motor Examination

The motor examination consists of assessing gait, muscle bulk, tone, and strength. The first aspect of the motor examination is the evaluation of the patient's gait. The patient is asked to walk naturally in the examination room. It is necessary to note posture, movement of body parts, and the type of steps taken. See Chart 20–7 for a description of gaits.

The nurse should inspect each of the muscles to be evaluated. Each side of the body is compared against the other. Palpating the muscles can assist with detecting atrophy. The nurse observes for fine or gross involuntary movements such as fasciculations, tremors, or myoclonic (quick involuntary) jerks. If muscles in an extremity appear asymmetric, the nurse should measure each limb. A difference of 1 cm or less is not significant. As a general rule, loss of muscle bulk may be due to a peripheral nerve dysfunction of the spinal roots or brachial plexus or Guillain-Barré syndrome.

Guillain-Barré syndrome is a disorder in which the body's immune system attacks part of the peripheral nervous system. It is characterized by an ascending paralysis that peaks in 3 to 21 days. The syndrome can result in variable motor dysfunction ranging from mild weakness to complete paralysis requiring ventilatory support. Involvement of the autonomic nervous system can result in life-threatening problems with blood pressure or heart rate—and is considered a medical emergency. This syndrome is fully discussed in Chapter 21.

Muscle tone represents muscle resistance to passive movements. Tone is assessed by passive range of motion. Slight resistance on movement is indicative of normal muscle tone. Each extremity should be assessed and should demonstrate smooth movement without change. Rigidity is a state of resistance that can be intermittent, such as cogwheel rigidity, when small regular jerks are felt. Flaccidity describes decreased muscle tone, or **hypotonia.** The muscle is weak and flabby.

In the unconscious patient, stimuli may elicit an abnormal motor response. Passive range of motion is done to assess muscle tone in these patients. Additionally, response to pain is evaluated. Pain is elicited by means of applying supraorbital pressure, squeezing the trapezius muscle, performing a sternal rub, or squeezing the Achilles tendon. Applying pressure to a nail bed should be avoided, as this can provoke a peripheral response rather than a central response to pain.

The nurse makes observations during the application of painful stimuli. Flexion of the arm, wrist, and fingers while adducting the upper extremity is known as **decorticate posturing** or abnormal flexion. The lower extremities are extended, internally rotated, and plantar flexed. **Decerebrate posturing** is an abnormal body posture that involves rigid extension of the arms and legs, downward pointing of the toes, and backward arching of the head; it is seen in the presence of noxious or painful stimuli. The patient clenches his teeth with arm extension in an adducted and hyperpronated fashion. Lower extremities are extended with plantar flexion. Because the lower extremities have similar positions in both motor responses, the upper extremities are used to identify the posturing. It is possible to demonstrate both abnormal responses simultaneously or each intermittently. Abnormal extension is believed to be the more grave of the two responses (Posner, Sapier, Schiff, & Plum, 2007).

Safety Alert *When caring for the unconscious patient, it is imperative for the nurse to contact the treating health care provider when a patient begins to demonstrate abnormal flexion or extension, as these indicate deterioration in the patient's neurological status.*

Muscle strength is evaluated in both the upper and lower extremities. Each muscle group is assessed by using passive range of motion against gravity, followed by active resistance positioned by the nurse and graded based on the ability to move against resistance. Chart 20–8 shows gradations of muscle strength.

To evaluate the upper extremities, the nurse begins by observing for symmetry of motor function. The nurse directs the patient to close her eyes and place the arms straight out in front with the palms up. The nurse then observes the patient for 20 to 30 seconds. If one arm lowers slowly, this is referred to as drift. If the hand pronates, this is noted as pronator drift. These are subtle signs of hemiparesis (muscle weakness

CHART 20–7 Descriptions of Gait

Gait	Description
Steppage	Associated with flaccidity of the leg and foot drop. Foot drop describes the inability to raise the front part of the foot due to weakness or paralysis of the muscles that lift the foot. As a result, individuals with foot drop scuff their toes along the ground or bend their knees to lift their foot higher than usual to avoid the scuffing, which causes what is called a "steppage" gait. Foot drop can be unilateral (affecting one foot) or bilateral (affecting both feet). The patient lifts the thigh and leg high, and the foot slaps against the floor. The patient looks as if she is walking up stairs.
Ataxic	Wide-based, staggering, and uncoordinated. The patient cannot stand with feet together.
Spastic	Leg extension. The patient shuffles with the legs stiff without lifting the feet.
Parkinsonian	In this gait, the hallmark is a slow, shuffling gait with loss of arm swing while walking. The head and body can be flexed forward, and the legs are rigid.

CHART 20–8 Muscle Strength

Muscle Function Level	Grade	Percentage of Normal
No evidence of contractility	0	0
Slight contractility, no movement	1	10
Muscle able to move with support against gravity	2	25
Muscle able to move without support against gravity	3	50
Muscle able to move without support against gravity with weakness to applied resistance	4	75

on one side of the body). The deltoid muscle is assessed by asking the patient to place her arms at her side with the elbows flexed and abducted to 90 degrees. Resistance is then applied. The biceps are tested by flexing the elbow; with the forearm supinated, the patient is directed to pull in against resistance. Then the patient is directed to push the arm away against resistance, which tests the triceps.

To evaluate the lower extremities, the patient is asked to sit on the examination table or on the edge of the hospital bed, with the legs dangling freely. The patient is asked to lift the knee up as if walking up stairs. Resistance is then applied, allowing the nurse to assess the iliopsoas muscle. The patient is then asked to pull the lower leg back toward the table, which tests the hamstring group. This is followed by directing the patient to push the lower leg out toward the nurse applying resistance, thereby testing the quadriceps.

Next, the feet are examined. The patient is directed to pull the toes up; this dorsiflexion tests the tibialis anterior. The patient then follows up with plantar flexion, which tests the gastrocnemius. These are important in assessing for foot drop. Chart 20–9 indicates major spinal cord segments with the corresponding functional ability and specific muscles to be tested.

Muscle strength assessment is a key factor in determining a diagnosis. Weakness or asymmetry can be seen in neuromuscular disorders such as myasthenia gravis, acute stroke, cranial space–occupying lesions, spinal cord lesions or compression, and many others.

Sensory Examination

In the evaluation of sensory function, the patient is tested with the eyes closed. As with muscle testing, the nurse compares each side of the body to the other. The examination is completed in a distal to proximal fashion. Areas for evaluation include the patient's hands, forearms, upper arms, trunk, thighs, legs, feet, and perineal and perirectal regions. Primary sensory modalities include light touch, superficial pain, temperature, position sense, and vibratory sense. A dermatome chart is helpful to use as a reference when assessing sensation and the patient's response to testing (Figure 20–6◆).

CHART 20–9 Muscle Innervations

Reflex	Spinal Level
Biceps	C_5–C_6
Triceps	C_6–C_7
Patellar	L_4

Light touch is tested by using a wisp of cotton as the stimulus. The patient is asked to identify when he feels something. The nurse lightly touches his skin with the cotton, beginning at the head and moving downward. Light touch can be preserved while other modalities are compromised in lesions of the spinal cord (see Chapter 24). Superficial pain is assessed in the same manner as light touch; however, the nurse uses a pin or other disposable sharp instrument for the stimulus. Temperature sensation is assessed in the same fashion as pain and touch. Test tubes filled with warm and cold water can be used. Others prefer to run warm and cold water over tuning forks, and then touch the skin with the tuning forks. The disparate temperature objects are used as the stimuli, and the patient is asked to identify warm versus cold on both sides of the body.

Vibratory sense is tested by using a tuning fork. The bony prominences are used, such as the great toe, malleolus, patella, elbow, and wrist. The vibrating tuning fork is placed on these areas, and the patient is asked to describe the feeling. Many patients will use the word "buzzing" to describe the sensation. The patient is then asked to tell the nurse when the feeling stops. Diminished distal vibratory sense is commonly seen in diabetic neuropathy, which may involve a single nerve (mononeuropathy) or occur in a stocking or glove distribution (Warren, 2010) (see Chapters 22 and 24).

To assess **proprioception,** the ability to determine spatial body position, the patient again is instructed to close the eyes. The nurse should grasp the patient's great toe by the side of the joint and move the toe in a forward-to-backward manner. This also may be done by using the thumb. Once the thumb or great toe is pointing in an upward or downward position, the patient is asked to state the direction in which the digit is pointing. This is repeated using both the upward and downward positions.

Two-point discrimination is tested by using a safety pin or paperclip. The nurse touches the patient, sometimes with one object and sometimes with two objects at the same time, and the patient reports whether she feels one or two touches. Stereognosis (recognition of form and shape of objects by touch) is assessed by placing common objects, such as a pencil or key, in the palm of the hand and asking the patient to identify the object. **Graphesthesia** (the sense by which a person recognizes figures or numbers written on the skin) is tested by tracing a number on the palm of the hand and asking the patient to identify the number. The **extinction phenomenon** is tested by lightly touching the patient in the same area simultaneously on both sides. The normal response is to feel both stimuli; an abnormal response is noted if the patient consistently feels only one of the stimuli. Abnormalities in these tests indicate cortical dysfunction.

Reflex Examination

Evaluating reflexes provides important information on the status of the central nervous system in both the conscious and unconscious patient. There are three categories of reflexes: muscle stretch reflexes, superficial reflexes, and pathologic reflexes. Abnormalities in reflex responses may be the earliest sign of CNS dysfunction.

Muscle Stretch Reflexes

Muscle stretch reflexes are also known as deep tendon reflexes. The nurse evaluates these reflexes first, using a percussion hammer at the muscle's point of insertion. The stimulus of the hammer causes the muscle to stretch. Sites commonly tested are the biceps, triceps, patella, and Achilles tendon.

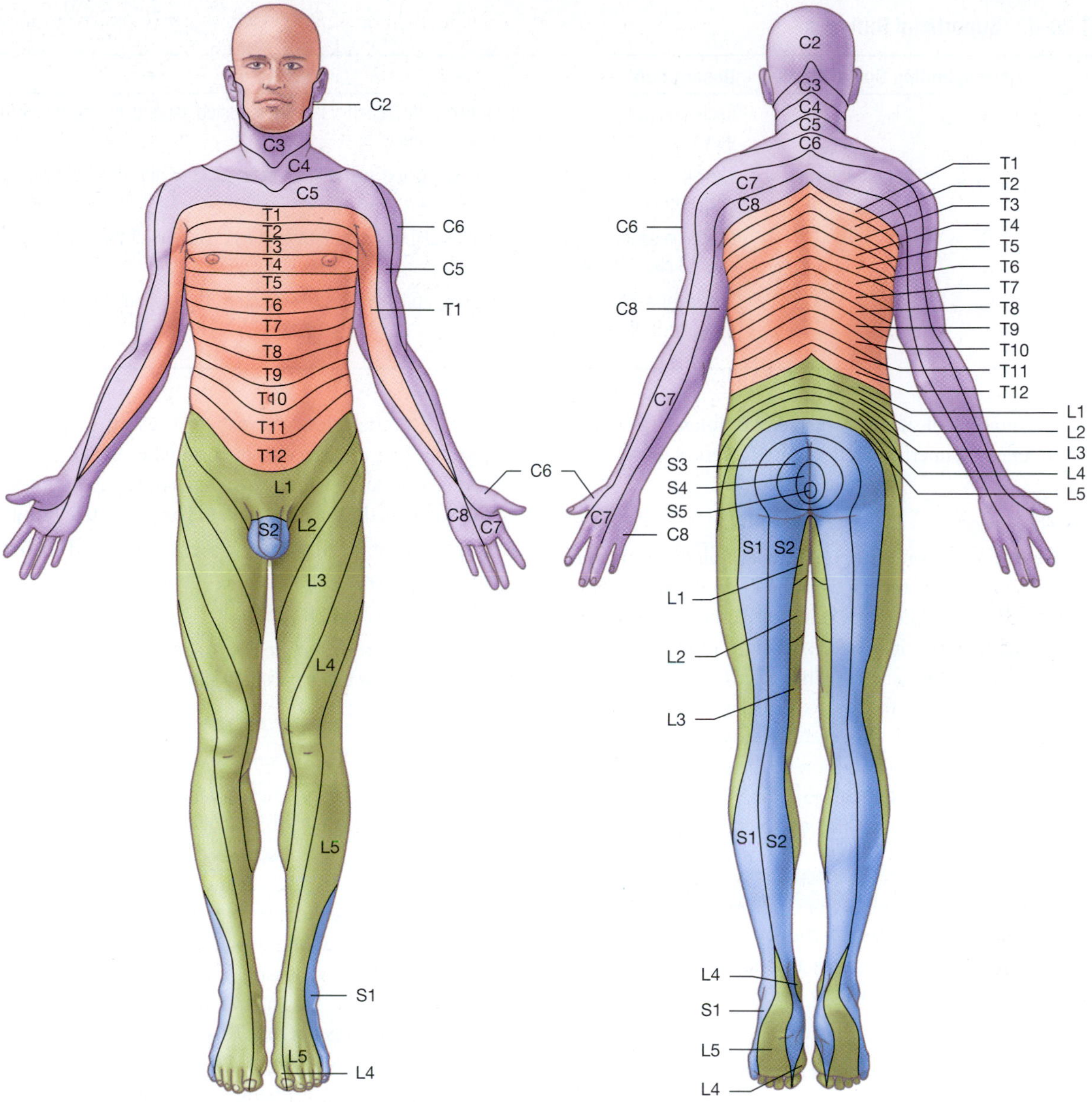

Levels of principal dermatomes

C5	Clavicles
C5, 6, 7	Lateral parts of upper limbs
C8, T1	Medial sides of upper limbs
C6	Thumb
C6, 7, 8	Hand
C8	Ring and little fingers
T4	Level of nipples
T10	Level of umbilicus
T12	Inguinal or groin regions
L1, 2, 3, 4	Anterior and inner surfaces of lower limbs
L4, 5, S1	Foot
L4	Medial side of great toe
S1, 2, L5	Posterior and outer surfaces of lower limbs
S1	Lateral margin of foot and little toe
S2, 3, 4	Perineum

FIGURE 20–6 ◆ Dermatome chart.

Forearm flexion is the normal response when the brachial tendon is tapped with the hammer. Forearm extension is the response to the triceps stimuli. Stimuli to the area just below the patella results in leg extension, and plantar flexion of the foot is seen when the Achilles tendon is tapped. Muscle stretch reflexes are graded based on the briskness of the response. The grade ranges from zero (no response) to four (hyperactive). Chart 20–10 illustrates muscle stretch reflexes.

Superficial Reflexes

Superficial reflexes are elicited by lightly stroking the skin or mucous membrane of the area tested. Chart 20–11 lists the most common

CHART 20–10 Muscle Stretch Reflexes and Scoring

Grade	Description
4+	Very brisk, hyperactive; muscle contracts multiple times, generally indicative of disease
3+	More brisk than 2+, can be normal for the individual
2+	Normal
1+	Diminished response
0	No response

Weblink: Neurological Disorders in the Elderly

CHART 20–11 Superficial Reflexes

Reflex	Corresponding Spinal Nerve	Description
Abdominal	$T_8, T_9, T_{10}, T_{11}, T_{12}$	Each side of the abdomen is stroked lightly. Each quadrant is tested separately. The umbilicus should move in the direction of the skin stimulated.
Anal	S_3, S_4, S_5	The skin at the side of the anus is scratched with a blunt instrument or pin. There should be puckering of the anus.
Bulbocavernous	S_3, S_4	Direct pressure is applied to the muscle behind the scrotum and pinching of the glans penis. The muscle should contract.
Cremasteric	L_1, L_2	The inner aspect of the thigh or lower abdomen is stroked lightly. There should be elevation of the opposite testicle, or both testicles.

reflexes tested. The grading of superficial reflexes is different from that of muscle stretch reflexes; superficial reflexes are scored as present (+) or absent (−).

Pathologic Reflexes

Pathologic reflexes are abnormal responses that result from an upper motor neuron lesion of the motor tracts in the brain or corticospinal tract. The most widely recognized is the extensor plantar response, also known as the **Babinski reflex.** It is tested by using a moderately sharp object, such as the handle of the percussion hammer, to stroke the lateral aspect of the sole of the foot from the heel to the ball of the foot, curving medially across the ball. The nurse observes the movement of the toes, which are normally in flexion. Dorsiflexion of the great toe with fanning of the other toes is seen. The Babinski reflex is normal in infants but abnormal after age 2 years. Figure 20–7 ◆ shows pathologic reflexes.

Weblink: The Hamilton Rating Scale for Depression

Cerebellar Examination

The cerebellar system is important in the coordination of movement. Various methods are used to assess balance and coordination. Following are some of the more commonly used methods:

- Starting with the arms outstretched, the patient is asked to touch her nose. Then the patient is asked to repeat the maneuver with her eyes closed.
- The nurse asks the patient to touch the nurse's index finger with her own index finger while the nurse is moving the finger, essentially asking the patient to touch a moving target.

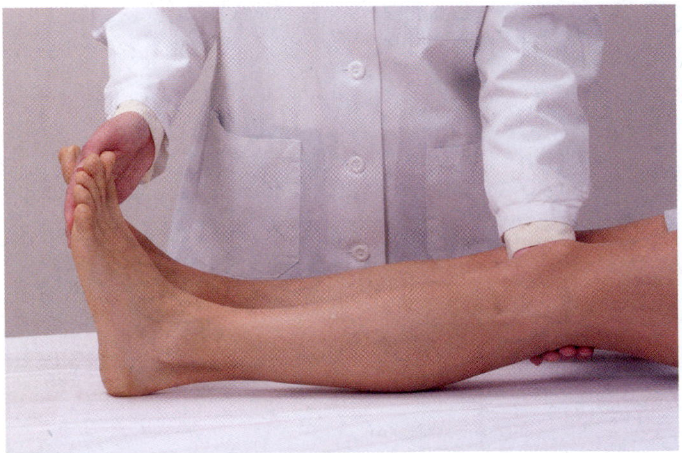

FIGURE 20–7 ◆ Procedure for testing pathologic reflexes.

- In the Romberg test, the patient is asked to stand with the feet together, first with the eyes open and then with the eyes closed. If the patient can stand with the eyes open but sways or loses balance with them closed, the patient is said to have a positive Romberg test.
- If the patient is supine, the patient is directed to run the heel of the foot down the shin of the opposite leg. The procedure is then repeated on the opposite leg.

Safety Alert *In performing the Romberg test, it is important for the nurse to stand close to the patient to prevent the patient from falling.*

Gerontological Considerations

Neurological disorders are the primary cause of disability in older adults. These disorders account for 50% of disability in those over 65 years of age and more than 90% of serious disabilities (Nadamuni, 2009,). The impact of neurological diseases and disorders on the older adult is significant. Whether the older adult is experiencing an acute neurological event or a chronic disabling condition, nurses are pivotal in assessment, treatment, and continuing care. The assessment guidelines are derived from the American Association of Neuroscience Nurses' (AANN) *Neurological Assessment of the Older Adult: A Guide for Nurses* (2007), a publication in AANN's Clinical Practice Guidelines Series.

When the nurse is assessing patients over 65 years of age, it is important to allow adequate time for processing the questions (Vance, 2009). If the patient uses adaptive devices, such as hearing aids, glasses, or a walker, the nurse should attempt to have them in place during the assessment (Armstrong & Mitchell, 2008).

Older patients generally have normal levels of consciousness and are alert. It is an abnormal finding if the patient is not oriented to situation, time, and place (Duthie, Katz, & Malone, 2007). Similarly, it is an abnormal finding if the patient has difficulty with calculations or impaired judgment. Remote and recent memory are normal; however, the processing speed and information retrieval capability are slowed (Duthie, Katz, & Malone, 2007). If the nurse notes that the patient has problems with speech and language, underlying pathology must be considered. Mood and affect should be evaluated. The **Hamilton Depression Rating Scale (HDRS)** is considered to be the gold standard in detecting depression, but a number of other validated tools also exist (Colasanti, Massimo Marianaetti, Miracchi, Amabilek, & Mina, 2010). The HDRS (Williams, 1988) is a standard test that measures the severity of depressive symptoms in individuals, including those who have already been diagnosed as having a depressive disorder. The HDRS is used to evaluate the outcomes or effectiveness of depression therapies and treatments, including the use of psychotropic medications. More information about the HDRS can be found at the following website: www.minddisorders.com/Flu-Inv/HamiltonDepression-Scale.html#ixzz1NOgLnHWS.

Cranial assessment of the older adult provides a basis for a functional assessment, which provides data regarding possible and potential impairments as well as the ability to provide self-care. Common cranial nerve changes include small pupils with reduced accommodation to light, hearing loss, and decreased taste discrimination.

Muscle tone can alter with age, with decreased tone being the most common state (Oommen, 2009). Bilateral strength is preserved except for a mild reduction in power proximally with advancing age; however, muscle atrophy may be noted (Duthie, Katz, & Malone, 2007).

The most common result of aging seen on the neurological examination is in the sensory evaluation. Impairment of loss of vibratory sense in the distal aspect of the lower extremities is a well-known finding. Conversely, proprioception is preserved. Decreases in two-point discrimination and stereognosis have been reported but are not well characterized (Sturnieks, St. George, & Lord, 2008).

Muscle stretch reflexes are generally preserved in the older adult, and absence or asymmetry generally indicates disease. Decrease in, or absence of, ankle jerks is common, but this is thought to be due to Achilles tendon inelasticity rather than true neurological change (Duthie, Katz, & Malone, 2007). Superficial reflexes may be diminished or absent due to musculoskeletal changes, e.g., relaxation of the abdominal muscles, possibly related to prior abdominal surgeries or previous pregnancies. The snout reflex, a pouting or puckering of the lips caused by light tapping of the closed lips near the midline, commonly seen in infants, may return; this is not considered pathologic in older adults. However, the suck and grasp reflex are indicative of frontal lobe disease.

Critical Thinking Related to Assessment Data

The purpose of neurological assessment is to detect disease and provide treatment early enough to prevent permanent neurologic injury or to arrest progress of the disease. Critical thinking skills are essential to correctly analyze assessment data and recognize abnormalities. On completion of the assessment, the nurse should be able to distinguish between normal and abnormal findings, recognize the need for a nursing intervention, and develop a customized nursing plan of care.

Health Promotion

Neurologic disorders often produce disability and result in dependence on others for activities of daily living and basic medical care. Efforts should be made to educate families regarding their risk factors for disease, management of symptoms of the disease, and their current medical regimen. Throughout the acute illness and recovery process, patients should be included in the plan of care to preserve independence and reduce loss of role. Rehabilitation services often are an essential element in achieving the optimum functional outcome.

Summary

The neurological assessment guides the nurse in determining the correct level of care and the need for intervention and protection. It also assists the nurse in identifying patients that would benefit from rehabilitation to maximize their functional outcome and prevent the development of self-help injuries (American Association of Colleges of Nursing, 2012). The examination consists of the evaluation of cognition, cranial nerves, motor function, sensation, and reflexes. The techniques described in this chapter will assist the nurse in incorporating the nursing process and developing a problem list of patient diagnoses, expected outcomes, and plan of care.

Weblink: Neurological History and Physical Examination

Weblink: Quality & Safety Education for Nurses (QSEN)

NCLEX® PRACTICE

1. The nurse is explaining to a patient's family the reason that a stroke on the left side of the brain affects function of the right side of the body. Included in this explanation should be that
   1. only the patient's dominant side will be affected by a stroke.
   2. physical limitations are highly dependent on the patient's physical fitness.
   3. pathways in the brain cross over, producing contralateral impairment when a stroke occurs.
   4. there is no predictability of where the physical limitations of a stroke will be experienced.
2. The nurse is assessing a patient who is demonstrating a neurological disorder. In which area of the health history would the nurse document information about the symptoms that the patient is demonstrating?
   1. Chief complaint
   2. History of present illness
   3. Medication history
   4. Past medical history
3. While assessing a patient's neurological status, the nurse notes that the patient is unable to move his head from left to right. This finding could indicate a disorder with which of the following cranial nerves?
   1. Vagus
   2. Hypoglossal
   3. Spinal accessory
   4. Facial
4. While assessing a patient's neurological status, the nurse uses the Glasgow Coma Scale. For which part of the mental status examination is this tool most likely used?
   1. Level of consciousness
   2. Language
   3. Memory
   4. Attention

5. After assessing a patient's patellar reflex, the nurse documents +2 on the patient's medical record. This document indicates that the patient's reflex is

1. indicative of disease.
2. more brisk.
3. normal.
4. diminished.

6. The nurse is going to assess for the presence of a Babinski reflex. Which of the following will the nurse use to assess this reflex?

1. Rubber triangle end of the reflex hammer
2. Handle of the reflex hammer
3. Safety pin
4. Cotton swab

Answers to NCLEX Practice questions can be found in Appendix D in the Osborn Student Resources at nursing.pearsonhighered.com. Practice additional NCLEX questions online at the Student Resources site.

Pearson Nursing Student Resources Find additional review materials at: **nursing.pearsonhighered.com**

REFERENCES

Alexander, S. A., & Beach, M. (2008). Genes and acute neurologic disease and injury: A primer for the neurologic intensive care nurse. *Critical Care Nursing Clinics of North America, 20*(2), 203–212. doi: 10.1016/j.ccell.2008.01.001

American Association of Colleges of Nursing. (2012). Quality & safety education for nurses (QSEN). American Association of Colleges of Nursing. Retrieved from http://www.acn.nche.edu/faculty/qsen

American Association of Neuroscience Nurses. (2007). *Neurological assessment of the older adult: A guide for nurses.* Glenview, IL: Author.

American Association of Neuroscience Nurses. (2010). *AANN core curriculum for neuroscience nursing* (Vol. 5 ed.). St. Louis, MO: Saunders Elsevier.

Armstrong, J., & Mitchell, E. (2008). Comprehensive nursing assessment in the care of older people. *Nursing Older People, 20*(1), 36–40.

Barker, E. (2007). *Neuroscience nursing.* (3rd ed.). Philadelphia: Mosby Elsevier. ISBN-10: 0323044018

Binder, J. R., Swanson, S. J., Hammeke, T. A., et al. (2011). Determination of language of dominance using functional MRI: A comparison with the Wada test. *Neurology, 76*(2), 1337. doi 10:1212/01.wnl.0000397065.05303.5d

Centers for Disease Control and Prevention. (2007). Prevalence of stroke—United States, 2005. *Morbidity and Mortality Weekly Report.* Retrieved from http://www.cdc.gov/MMWR/previdw/mmwrhtml/mm5619a2.htm

Colasanti, V., Marianetti, M., Micacchi, F., Amabile, G. A., & Mina, C. (2010). Tests for the evaluation of depression in the elderly: A systematic review. *Archives of Gerontology & Geriatrics, 50*(2), 227–230. doi: 10.1016/j.archger.2009.04.001

Cox, B. (2008). The principles of neurological assessment. *Practice Nurse, 36*(7), 45–50.

Dictionary of Cell and Molecular Biology. (2008). Confusion. Retrieved from http://cancerweb.ncl.ac.uk/cgi-bin/omd?confusion

Duthie, E., Katz, P., & Malone, M. (2007). *Practice of geriatrics* (4th ed.). Philadelphia: Saunders Elsevier.

Eggenberger, E. (2010). Aniscoria. Medscape reference. Retrieved from http://emedicine.medscape.com/article/1158571-overview

Goldberg, C. (2008). *A practical guide to clinical medicine.* San Diego, CA: UCSD School of Medicine and VA Medical Center. Retrieved from http://meded.ucsd.edu/clinicalmed/history.htm

Goldman, L., & Ausiello, D. (Ed.). (2007). *Cecil medicine* (23rd ed.). Philadelphia, PA: Saunders Elsevier.

Grissinger, M. (2007). Cultural diversity and medication safety. *Medication Errors, 22*(9). Retrieved from http://www.nipcweb.com/Medication_Errors.pdf

Luzzi, S., Snowden, J. S., Neary, D., Coccia, M., Provinciali, L., & Lambon, R. (2007). Distinct patterns of olfactory impairment in Alzheimer's disease, semantic dementia, front temporal dementia, and corticobasal degeneration. *Neuropsychologia, 45*(8), 1826–1831.

Nadamujni, S. (2009). 5 things you need to know about neurological disorders in the elderly. Livestrong.com. Retrieved from http://www.livestrong.com/article/9224-need-neurological-disorders-elderly/

Newman, M. F. (2007). Open heart surgery and cognitive decline. *Cleveland Clinic Journal of Medicine, 74*(1), 52–55.

Oommen, K. J. (2009). Neurological history and final examination. Medscape reference. Retrieved from http://emedicine.medscaape.com/article/1147993-overview

Posner, J. B., Sapier, C. B., Schiff, N., & Plum, F. (Eds.). (2007). *Plum & Posners diagnosis of stupor and coma.* Philadelphia: F. A. Davis.

Snyderman, D. R. B. (2009). Mental status exam in primary care: A review. *American Family Physician, 80*(8), 809. Retrieved from http://www.ncbi.nlm.nih.gov/pubmed/19835342

Sturnieks, D., St. George, R., & Lord, S. (2008). Balance disorders in the elderly. *Neurophysiologie Clinique/Clinical Neurophysiology, 38*(6), 467–478.

Taber's cyclopedic medical dictionary (21st ed.). (2010). Philadelphia, PA: F. A. Davis Company.

Teasdale, G., & Jennett, B. (1974). Assessment of coma and impaired consciousness: A practical scale. *Lancet, 2,* 81–84.

Vance, D. E. (2009, December 1). Speed of processing in older adults: A cognitive overview for nursing. The Free Library. Retrieved from http://www.thefreelibrary.com/Speed of processing in older adults: a cognitive overview for Nursing.-a0214101271

Vogel, L., & Sturm, P. (2008). Management of patients with developmental and hereditary spinal cord disorders. *Topics in Spinal Cord Injury Rehabilitation, 14*(2), 53–63.

Warren, E. (2010). Pain and diabetic neuropathy. *Practice Nurse, 39*(10), 25–27.

Wesley Medical Center. (2011). Trauma scoring-glasgow coma scale (GCS) and revised trauma score (RTS). Retrieved from http://wesleymc.com/for-physicians/Glasgow-trauma-score.do

Williams, J. B. W. (1988). A structured guide for the Hamilton Depression Rating Scale. *Archives of General Psychiatry, 455,* 742–747.

Wolf, C. A., Wijdicks, E. F., Bamlet, W. R., & McClelland, R. L. (2007). Further validation of the FOUR Score coma scale by intensive care nurses. *Mayo Clinic Proceedings, 82*(4), 435–438. PMID 17418071.

Yanoff, M., & Duker, J. (Eds.). (2008). *Ophthalmology* (3rd ed.). New York: Mosby, an imprint of Elsevier.

Caring for the Patient with Acute Brain or Cranial Nerve Disorder

21 CHAPTER

Joyce V. Colobong
Annita Watson

Outcome-Based Learning Objectives

After studying this chapter, the learner will be able to:

1. Generate a plan of care for patients experiencing the cranial nerve disorder trigeminal neuralgia.
2. Create a plan of care for the patient with increased cranial pressure (ICP), using the components of the nursing process.
3. Compare and contrast the various types and causes of head trauma according to level of injury.
4. Determine the differences between bacterial meningitis and viral meningitis, including causes, signs and symptoms, diagnostic evaluation, and treatment.
5. Differentiate among the major types of brain tumors—intra-axial, extra-axial, and metastatic—and explain the treatment options.
6. Analyze the causes and types of seizures as they relate to the development of nursing interventions.

KEY TERMS

acoustic neuromas p.538
aura p.506
autoregulation p.509
bacterial meningitis p.526
basal skull fracture p.516
Battle sign p.516
Bell's palsy p.505
brain abscess p.529
Brudzinski sign p.528
cerebral edema p.509
cerebral infarction p.515
cerebral ischemia p.515
cerebral perfusion pressure (CPP) p.509
cingulate herniation p.510
cluster headache p.507
comminuted skull fracture p.516
concussion p.520
contrecoup p.519
contusions p.519
coup p.519
Cushing's triad p.511
cytotoxic edema p.509
decerebrate (extensor) posturing p.511
decorticate (flexor) positioning p.511
depressed skull fracture p.516
diffuse axonal injury (DAI) p.521
encephalitis p.529
ependymomas p.537
epidural hematoma (EDH) p.517
extra-axial tumors p.537
gene mutations p.535
glioma p.536
Guillain-Barré syndrome (GBS) p.534
hemicrania continua p.507
herniation p.510
hydrocephalus p.542
intra-axial tumors p.536
intracranial pressure (ICP) p.508
ischemia cascade p.515
Kernig's sign p.528
linear skull fracture p.516
mass effect p.510
meningiomas p.537
meningismus p.528
migraine headache p.506
Monroe-Kellie doctrine p.508
otorrhea p.516
paroxysmal hemacronea p.507
persistent vegetative state p.522
postconcussion syndrome p.521
pupillometer p.511
rhinorrhea p.516
schwannomas p.538
second-impact syndrome p.520
seizure p.543
subdural hematoma (SDH) p.517
status epilepticus p.544
tension-type headache (TTH) p.506
transtentorial herniation p.510
traumatic brain injury (TBI) p.515
trigeminal autonomic cephalgias (TACs) p.507
trigeminal neuralgia (TN) p.504
uncal herniation p.510
vasodilatory cascade p.509
vasogenic edema p.509
viral meningitis p.527

ACUTE BRAIN and cranial nerve disorders include a wide range of conditions, such as cranial nerve disorders, headaches, traumatic injuries, brain tumors, and infectious diseases of the brain. Each of these disorders may affect not just the central nervous system, but every other system of the body as well. The symptoms of the disorders have a tremendous effect on the patient and on family, friends, and their community.

Cranial Nerve Disorders

There are 12 cranial nerves (CNI–CNXII) located within the cranial vault. Please refer back to the discussion of cranial nerves in Chapter 20. All 12 cranial nerves are subject to disorders caused by various types of injury or insult to the nerve. Many of the disorders resulting from trauma, infections, lesions, and surgery are discussed in other chapters throughout this book (e.g., spinal cord injury, chronic and degenerative neurological diseases, and visual disorders). Two specific disorders that affect the trigeminal nerve (CNV) and the facial nerve (CNVII) are addressed in this section of this chapter: trigeminal neuralgia and Bell's palsy. Guillain-Barré syndrome is discussed later in the chapter under Infectious Diseases, as it may occur following an onset of an infectious disease.

Trigeminal Neuralgia

Trigeminal neuralgia (TN), also referred to as *tic douloureux,* is a painful and chronic condition of the face characterized by episodes of intense, stabbing, shock-like paroxysmal pain. This pain radiates from the angle of the jaw to the branch of the trigeminal nerve (cranial nerve V [CNV]) (National Institute of Neurological Disorders and Stroke [NINDS], 2011f).

Etiology and Epidemiology

The exact etiology of TN has not been identified; however, a variety of associated factors have been recognized. One possible cause is the vascular compression of CNV causing irritation. TN may occur from focal demyelination of the trigeminal nerve or ganglia. Other possible causes are inflammation such as occurs with multiple sclerosis, infection, trauma, or compression on the trigeminal nerve from an aneurysm or tumor. It also is hypothesized that TN may be part of the normal aging process due to lengthening of the blood vessels. As they lengthen, they can come to rest and pulsate against a nerve (NINDS, 2011f).

TN occurs twice as often in females as in males. The disease begins after age 40 with a typical onset at 60 to 70 years in approximately 90% of patients. If it presents in patients ages 20 to 40, they are most likely to suffer from a demyelinating lesion in the pons secondary to multiple sclerosis. Symptomatic or secondary TN (that caused by a lesion) occurs in patients younger than the age of 20 (Singh, 2011). There also is some evidence that the disorder runs in families, perhaps due to an inherited pattern of blood vessel formation (NINDS, 2011f).

Pathophysiology and Clinical Manifestations

The trigeminal nerve, the fifth cranial nerve, is the largest of the cranial nerves and has both motor and sensory fibers. The nerve exits the pons and merges into the gasserian ganglion (a group of nerve cells of the sensory root of the trigeminal nerve; also known as semilunar ganglion), then separates into three major branches: the ophthalmic, maxillary, and mandibular branch (Figure 21–1◆). In many cases of symptomatic TN, degeneration of the gasserian ganglion and compression of the fifth nerve occur by anomalous blood vessels or tumors. The pain affects mainly the maxillary or mandibular branch of the nerve. This pain usually occurs abruptly and lasts for a few seconds to a few minutes. It is described as burning, stabbing, sharp, penetrating, or electric-shock-like and typically affects one side of the face (Buttaro, Trybulski, Baily, & Sandberg-Cook, 2008).

The majority of patients with TN can identify trigger zones, which usually are areas on the cheek, lip, gum, or forehead. These zones are sensitive to minimal stimulation such as touch, cold, pressure, or a blast of air, and may cause pain on stimulation.

Medical and Surgical Management

There are both medical and surgical interventions in the treatment for TN. Drug therapy usually is the first treatment attempted. Treatment begins with the administration of carbamazepine or phenytoin, which are both anticonvulsants. These drugs are believed to inhibit synaptic transmission in the spinal nucleus of the trigeminal nerve

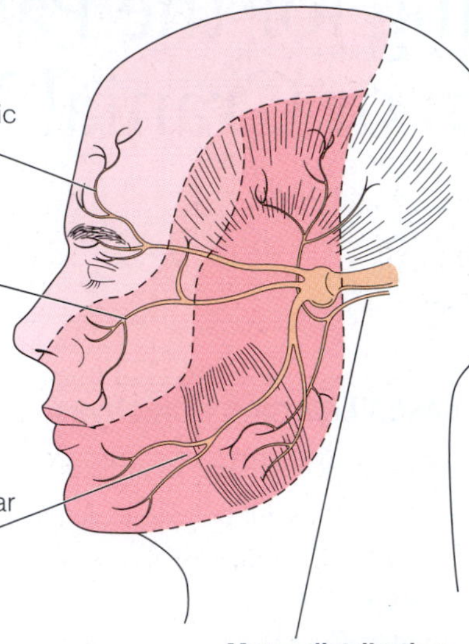

FIGURE 21–1 ◆ Trigeminal nerve.

(Barker, 2008). Other drug therapies include clonazepam or tricyclic antidepressants. At times, corticosteroids such as methylprednisolone may be useful. Patients with multiple sclerosis may be given long-acting prostaglandin E analog misoprostol.

Two-thirds of the patients with TN will initially respond to pharmacotherapy. Eventually, these patients are weaned from the drugs, and the maintenance dose of the drug is restarted only if attacks recur (Barker, 2008).

Surgical treatments are used for patients who do not respond to drug therapy. Gamma knife radiosurgery is an option for patients with either unilateral or bilateral TN. The surgeon uses highly targeted radiation of the trigeminal nerve, and pain relief usually occurs 4 to 6 weeks after treatment. Radiofrequency retrogasserian rhizotomy is another surgical treatment designed to produce a sensory defect in the affected division of the trigeminal nerve. This technique involves controlled thermal ablation of the trigeminal nerve fibers. Another surgical treatment is microvascular decompression. This is the most invasive of the surgical options, but it offers the highest probability that pain will not return (NINDS, 2011f). A posterior fossa craniectomy is performed, and any blood vessels that appear to be compressed by the trigeminal nerve are repositioned or padded away from the nerve. If there are no vessels that appear to be compressing the nerve, the trigeminal nerve may be partially dissected to provide pain relief, which causes some sensory loss to the face (Hickey, 2009).

Some patients choose to manage TN with complementary techniques that usually are combined with pharmacologic treatment. Complementary options include acupuncture, biofeedback, vitamin therapy, nutritional therapy, and electrical stimulation of the nerves (NINDS, 2011f).

Nursing Management

Patients with TN live with pain and multiple daily living challenges. Nursing management includes identifying triggers, assessing how frequently spasms occur, providing emotional support, and monitoring the effectiveness of medical or surgical treatment.

The pain triggered by chewing may cause the patient to avoid eating. A nutritional consultation with a registered dietitian may assist in determining daily caloric intake. In addition, strategies such as chewing on the unaffected side and staying away from foods and beverages at extreme temperatures may help the patient avoid pain. Eating small, frequent meals may increase caloric intake. The nurse may also need to encourage the patient to perform oral hygiene, as this is another activity that may trigger pain. The use of hot and/or cold packs on the face may reduce pain caused by brushing the teeth. Relaxation techniques such as listening to soothing music also may reduce or eliminate the onset of pain while patients engage in hygienic procedures. Other suggestions to offset the pain caused by TN include:

- Make a place to rest and relax in the home, a gentle place with quiet music that can be darkened easily, as light can make the pain worse. Make sure that this place is warm and cozy with a comfortable chair or bed and no drafts.
- Get enough sleep; exhaustion makes attacks much worse.
- Keep soft foods on hand for attacks.
- Keep teeth in good shape; get a good dentist who understands TN and can provide guidance in coping with the disease and its manifestations.
- Keep depression at bay by staying close to friends and family and doing enjoyable activities.
- Pain is exhausting, so learn what triggers the pain and pace life activities accordingly.

Teaching the patient and family to take prescribed medications at the time they are due may provide a steady blood level of the medications preventing pain. In addition, instructing patients to take analgesics at the first sign of pain will work more effectively than waiting to take them when the pain is becoming more severe. Providing individualized support and referral to national and local support organizations may be helpful to patients with TN.

Bell's Palsy

Bell's palsy is an acute and idiopathic disorder of cranial nerve VII, which is the facial nerve. It is characterized by an abrupt onset of unilateral facial weakness and sensory and parasympathetic function. This disorder is the most common cause of facial paralysis (NINDS, 2011d).

Etiology and Epidemiology

The annual incidence of Bell's palsy is approximately 23 cases per 100,000 persons, with the right side being affected 63% of the time. Bell's palsy can affect anyone but rarely affects people under the age of 15 or over the age of 60 (Mayo Clinic Staff, 2012). Men and women are affected equally; however, women within the ages of 10 to 19 years are more likely to be affected than men in the same age group (Taylor, 2011).

Bell's palsy accounts for approximately 60% to 75% of cases of unilateral facial paralysis. The disorder can also be recurrent, with a recurrence rate of 4% to 14%. This common disorder of the facial nerve mainly affects adults, people with diabetes, and pregnant women. In addition, people who are immunocompromised or women with preeclampsia are often affected (Taylor, 2011).

Bell's palsy is characterized by CNVII dysfunction involving all distal branches. Sudden occurrence of unilateral facial paralysis occurs, which peaks within 2 to 5 days and slowly resolves over 1 to 2 months (Hickey, 2009). The most common cause is believed to be herpes simplex virus; however, Bell's palsy has been seen with other conditions, such as Guillain-Barré syndrome or a stroke.

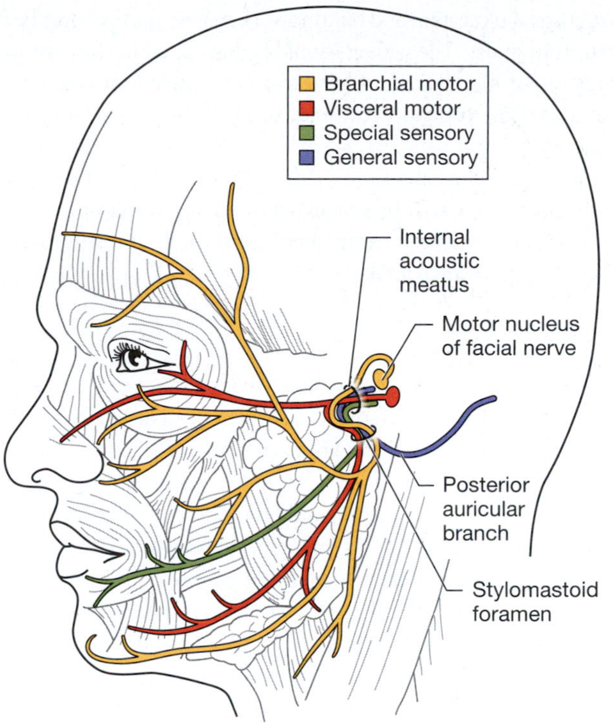

FIGURE 21–2 ◆ Facial nerve.

Pathophysiology and Clinical Manifestations

Cranial nerve VII is composed mainly of motor nerves that innervate the muscles of the face (Figure 21–2◆). Motor paralysis is characterized by complete loss of voluntary and autonomic expression over the affected side of the face, which remains motionless during attempts at expressions.

Characteristics of Bell's palsy include flattening of the nasolabial fold, sagging at the corner of the mouth, and displacement of the lips toward the unaffected side. In addition, the forehead flattens and the eyebrows are asymmetrical. The inability to blink occurs and results in the collection of tears in the lower lid. Pain around the jaws or in or behind the ear on the affected side also may be present. The patient may experience sensitivity to sound on the affected side, headache, and a decrease in the ability to taste (Mayo Clinic Staff, 2012). These symptoms are the result of demyelination of the facial nerve, which disrupts its function. In rare cases, Bell's palsy can affect the nerves on both sides of the face.

Medical Management

Treatment with a course of glucocorticoid therapy is generally believed to improve outcomes in people with Bell's palsy. Analgesics and possibly antiviral agents may further improve outcomes. Gentle massage, moistening of the head, and electrical stimulation of the nerve also may be used. Keeping the eye moist and protected from debris and injury is important. Physical therapy may be used to stimulate the facial nerve and help maintain muscle tone. If the patient does not respond to medical and/or physical therapy, surgery to decompress the facial nerve may be an option; however, this tactic is controversial (Taylor, 2011).

Nursing Management

Nursing care for the patient with Bell's palsy focuses on the prevention of complications and the need to provide psychological and emotional support to the patient. Eye care is essential because the patient cannot close the eyelid and is not able to blink; this results in dry eyes and may cause corneal ulceration and blindness. Therefore, the eye must be protected from injury. The patient should be instructed to close the eyelid manually. For lubrication, artificial tears are instilled into the eye four times a day. The patient's eyelid may be taped closed, or he may wear an eye patch.

Difficulty sipping through a straw, chewing, or controlling saliva on the affected side may be problematic and may result in weight loss. Instructing the patient to eat frequent small meals and soft food may increase her nutritional intake.

Headaches

Headaches are a common form of pain that is almost universally experienced. "More than 9 in 10 adults will experience a headache sometime in their life" (NINDS, 2011b). Headaches are classified as primary or secondary. A *primary headache* occurs independently and is not caused by another underlying medical condition. There are four main groups of primary headache disorders: migraine; tension-type; trigeminal autonomic cephalgias, which include cluster, paroxysmal hemicrania, and SUNCT (short-lasting, unilateral, neuralgiform headaches with conjunctival injection and tearing); and a miscellaneous group (NINDS, 2011b). *Secondary headaches* are symptoms of other health disorders that cause pain-sensitive nerve endings to be compressed or moved out of place (NINDS, 2011b). While many headaches are self-treated, a change in characteristics or intensity of a previous headache pattern may serve as an alarm, causing a person to seek medical attention. Careful questioning during the assessment process can assist the health care provider in determining whether the headache is considered to be primary or secondary. Diagnostic tests such as computerized tomography (CT) scans and magnetic resonance imaging (MRI) also may be useful in making this determination; however, they usually are not performed unless the presenting symptoms suggest that other neurologic processes are present.

Migraine Headaches

Etiology and Epidemiology

Migraine headaches are chronic disorders with episodic manifestations. These complex, recurring debilitating headaches are one form of vascular headache and are indicative of brain hyperexcitability, in which the threshold for headache attacks is lowered (National Headache Foundation, 2007). Migraines are one of the most common complaints of headache. More than 30 million people, or approximately 12% of the population, have one or more migraine headaches per year in the United States (NINDS, 2011b). In addition, 75% of all persons who experience migraines are women (Chawla, 2011). There is a genetic component to migraines, as approximately 70% of patients have a first-degree relative with a history of migraines (Chawla, 2011). A migraine without **aura** (a distinctive sensation or visual disturbance) is the most common. For people who have auras, focal neurological symptoms, such as light flashes or bright spots, either precede or accompany the headache. The pain is moderate to severe and is usually unilateral and throbbing. The headache may be accompanied by autonomic symptoms such as nausea, vomiting, diarrhea, light-headedness, photophobia, and sensitivity to sound or odor (Mayo Clinic Staff, 2011d). Migraines may be precipitated by stress, excessive or insufficient sleep, smoking, hormonal changes in women, food, sensory stimuli, medications such as vasodilators and oral contraceptives, or head trauma. Migraines occur more frequently in women than in men and can last 4 to 72 hours.

Nonpharmacologic treatments include control of risk factors and triggers, as well as behavioral interventions such as relaxation therapy and cognitive-behavioral therapy. Stress is a major component, and the health care providers should implement stress management interventions.

Medical Management

Acute treatment is directed toward stopping or preventing the progression of a headache or reversing a headache that has started. Preventative treatment aims to reduce the frequency and severity of the migraine attack, making acute attacks more responsive to acute treatment.

Nonsteroidal anti-inflammatory drugs are used for mild to moderate headaches. If the attack becomes severe, triptans and ergot alkaloids are very effective treatments that are best administered early. For patients who do not respond to pain relief measures and who go to the emergency department, IV metoclopramide or corticosteroids may be useful (NINDS, 2011b).

Tension-Type Headaches

Etiology and Epidemiology

Tension-type headache (TTH), commonly referred to as muscle contraction or tension headache, is the most common type of primary headache and accounts for 1% to 4% of all emergency department visits (Blanda, 2011). Its name signifies the role of stress and emotional or mental conflict in triggering the pain and contracting muscles in the neck, face, scalp, and jaw. TTHs, which typically are classified as episodic or chronic, affect women slightly more than they do men, and usually begin in adolescence, reaching peak activity in the 30s (NINDS, 2011b). Episodic TTHs tend to occur periodically, usually no more often than once or twice a month, and may occur when there is a stressful event. The intensity is moderate, self-limited, and usually responsive to nonprescription drugs. Episodic TTHs usually begin gradually and often occur in the middle of the day (Kunkel, 2011). Chronic TTHs are frequent and recur daily, usually occurring more than 15 days per month over a 3-month period. They are associated with contracted muscles of the neck and scalp, which precipitate bilateral and occipitofrontal headaches. The pain from chronic TTHs is more severe and disabling than that from episodic headache pain.

There is no single cause for TTHs (Kunkel, 2011). The TTH syndrome is not a trait that runs in families. For some people, a TTH may be caused by tightened neck and scalp muscles, which in turn may be caused by inadequate rest, sleep apnea, poor posture, jaw clenching, intense work, missed meals, and emotional or mental stress, including depression. For other people, tightened muscles are not part of tension headaches, and the precise cause is unknown. TTHs usually are triggered by some type of environmental or internal stress, which may be known (overt) or unknown (covert) to patients and their families. Common stressors include family, social relationships, friends, work, and school (e.g., losing a job, being overweight, competing in sports, and deadlines at work).

Medical Management

The pain of a TTH can have a throbbing quality with variable durations. The scalp may be sore to the point of causing pain when the person combs her hair. Episodic headaches often precede chronic TTHs. Treatment includes over-the-counter medications, relaxation techniques, regular exercise, sleep, and various modalities including hot or cold packs, ultrasound electrical stimulation, and stretching (Blanda, 2011).

Trigeminal Autonomic Cephalgias

Trigeminal autonomic cephalgias (TACs) are a special category of headaches caused by activation through the autonomic nervous system of the trigeminal nerve in the face (Headache Cooperative of New England [HCNE], 2011). These rare, short-lasting, and disabling headaches are characterized by severe pain in and around the eye on one side of the face and autonomic (involuntary) features on the same side (e.g., drooping eyelid, red and teary eye). These disorders differ in attack duration and frequency and have episodic and chronic forms (NINDS, 2011b). Episodic attacks occur on a daily or near-daily basis for weeks or months with pain-free remissions; chronic attacks occur on a daily or near-daily basis for a year or more with only brief remissions. TACs comprise cluster headache, paroxysmal hemicrania, and short-lasting unilateral neuralgiform headache attacks with conjunctival injection and tearing (SUNCT) (May & Goadsby, 2010), all of which are discussed in the following text. The medical treatment for TACs varies according to the specific type of headache within the category. For example, medical management for cluster headaches is different from the medical management of paroxysmal hemicrania headaches.

Cluster Headaches

Cluster headache, also known as histamine headache, is the most serious form of primary headache. It causes a severe, ipsilateral pain located in the orbital, supraorbital, or temporal area, or a mixture of these sites (Sheth, 2011). Cluster headaches are more common in men than women and are most common in adolescence and middle age. They tend to run in families and are more common in smokers than in nonsmokers. The attacks are usually severe and unilateral. Their duration is brief, lasting from a few moments to 2 hours, and they come in groups or "clusters." These headaches may occur one to eight times daily over a period of several weeks or months. They may awaken the person during the night and may be preceded by a migraine-like aura and nausea (NINDS, 2011b). The triggers for cluster headaches may include alcohol, smoking, histamine, or nitrogen. Research demonstrates a relationship between cluster headache and prior head trauma (NINDS, 2011b). An increased familial risk of these headaches suggests that there may be a genetic cause as well.

Treatment includes 100% oxygen inhaled using a face mask for 15 to 20 minutes. This may end the headache if used early. Drugs such as sumatriptan are used and have a rapid onset. Transitional treatment such as a short, tapered course of prednisone, ergotamine tartrate, or dihydroergotamine (DHE) is used for rapid suppression of the cluster attacks before preventive medications take effect.

Paroxysmal Hemicrania

Paroxysmal hemicrania is a rare form of primary headache that usually begins in adulthood with the same characteristics of pain, associated symptoms, and signs as cluster headache, but the attacks are shorter and more frequent. Attacks typically occur 5 to 40 times per day, with each attack lasting 2 to 45 minutes. Paroxysmal hemicrania occurs mostly in females without any familial pattern. It is described as severe throbbing, claw-like, or piercing pain on one side of the face in, around, or behind the eye and occasionally reaching to the back of the neck. At least one autonomic sign or symptom on the painful side is present, including conjunctival injection (redness of the sclera), tearing, or nasal congestion. Certain movements of the head or neck, external pressure to the neck, and alcohol use may trigger these headaches (NINDS, 2011b). The major diagnostic criterion is the absolute effectiveness of the nonsteroidal anti-inflammatory drug indomethacin (HCNE, 2011). Nonprescription analgesics and calcium-channel blockers can ease discomfort.

SUNCT

Short-lasting, unilateral neuralgiform headache attacks with conjunctival injection and tearing (SUNCT) is a rare type of headache that usually presents with a long clinical history of unilateral headache and eye pain, is side-locked (on the right or left side of head) with neuralgia pain of short duration (15 to 60 seconds), and occurs with high frequency (5 to 30 times per hour) (NINDS, 2011b). The cause is unknown. Symptoms include intense bloodshot eyes, watery eyes, stuffy or runny nose, sweaty forehead, puffy eyelids, increased pressure in the eye of the affected side of the head, and increased blood pressure (HCNE, 2011). Attacks of SUNCT may be precipitated by chewing, eating, or movements of the head and neck. It is very difficult to treat and is completely refractory to drug therapy, including indomethacin (HCNE, 2011). Anticonvulsants, anesthetics, and corticosteroid drugs may be used to relieve some of the symptoms and to treat the severe pain. Deep brain stimulation is being considered to reduce the frequency of attacks in severely affected individuals (NINDS, 2011b).

Miscellaneous Primary Headaches

The National Institute of Neurological Disorders and Stroke (NINDS) has established a category of headaches termed *miscellaneous primary headaches.* These include chronic daily headaches, primary stabbing headaches, primary exertional headaches, hypnic headaches, and ice cream headaches. Chronic daily headaches occur at least 15 days per month during a 3-month period. In addition to chronic tension-type headaches, chronic migraines, and medication overuse headaches, these headaches include **hemicrania continua,** a chronic form of headache marked by continuous pain that occurs on the same side of the face and head, and new daily persistent headaches. A *primary stabbing headache,* also known as an "ice-pick" or "jabs-and-jolts" headache, is characterized by intense piercing pain that strikes without warning and generally lasts 1 to 10 seconds (NINDS, 2011b). The stabbing pain usually occurs around the eye but may be felt in multiple sites along the trigeminal nerve. Onset occurs between 45 and 50 years of age, and most attacks are spontaneous. These headaches may be triggered by sudden movement, bright lights, or emotional stress. *Primary exertional headaches* are those that occur during bouts of coughing or sneezing, or during intense physical activity such as running, basketball, lifting weights, or sexual activity. The headache begins at the onset of the activity and typically lasts several minutes; on rare occasions, it may last up to 2 days. This type of headache tends to be consistent in individuals who have a family history of migraine. *Hypnic headache,* sometimes referred to as "alarm-clock" headache, mostly occurs at night in people who are 50 years of age or older. There is no known trigger. Mild to moderate throbbing pain usually lasts from 15 minutes to 3 hours after waking and usually is felt on both sides of the head. This disorder affects both men and women and may include other symptoms such as nausea or increased sensitivity to sound or light. Hypnic headaches tend to occur during dreaming. An *ice cream headache,* which sometimes is called "brain freeze," happens when cold materials such as cold drinks or ice cream hit the warm roof of the mouth. The local blood vessels constrict to reduce the loss of body heat, then relax to allow an increase in blood flow, resulting in a burst of pain that lasts for about 5 minutes. This type of headache is more apt to occur in individuals who have migraine headaches (NINDS, 2011b).

Pathophysiology of Headaches

The pathophysiology of migraine, cluster, and tension-type headaches is not well understood. It is believed that migraine and cluster headaches begin initially in the brain as a neurologic dysfunction, with subsequent involvement of the trigeminal nerve and cranial vessels. In cluster headache, which belongs to the trigeminal autonomic cephalgias classification of headache, most sufferers have overactivity of the parasympathetic nervous system (Kunkel, 2011). Tension-type headache is considered to be primarily a central neurologic disturbance similar to a migraine but may occur as a result of increased cervical and pericranial muscle activity (e.g., poor posture, anxiety with increased clenching or grinding of the teeth).

Migraine is an inherited disorder in which there seems to be an episodic instability of the neurovascular system. At times, the nuclei of the trigeminal nerve seem to become hyperactive and excitable. Efferent impulses travel over branches of the trigeminal nerve to the innervated cranial vessels, causing the release of substances that promote perivascular inflammation and vascular dilation (Kunkel, 2011). As the migraine attack progresses, the inflamed perivascular structures irritate nerve endings of the trigeminal nerve and cause afferent stimuli to travel back into the trigeminal neurons of the brain. The neurons become sensitized and continue to fire, demonstrating a cyclic process called central sensitization (Kunkel, 2011). As the cyclic process continues, the scalp becomes sore and tender to ordinary touch; this is called cutaneous allodynia. Dysfunction of other areas of the brainstem and hypothalamus account for the other symptoms of migraine, such as nausea and photophobia.

Medical Management and Laboratory and Diagnostic Testing

Diagnosis of any one of the primary headache syndromes is based on the condition and the presenting symptoms described by the patient. The health care provider generally will be able to identify the type of headache the patient is experiencing after talking with the patient. For some types of headaches, it is important to determine the cause of the headache and remove that cause as part of the treatment. This is particularly relevant in tension-type headaches. Examples of this type of cause are arthritis, obesity, and sleep apnea.

Abnormal physical or neurologic examination findings must be investigated. Laboratory studies may be useful in excluding metabolic or endocrine factors that might play a role. CT scans and MRIs are used to determine or rule out intracranial causes of headache and to identify or rule out lesions that cause neurologic or visual abnormalities associated with headache.

In most cases, medications are used to both treat and prevent headaches (NINDS, 2011b). Specific drug categories were previously discussed for each type of primary headache. In addition, oxygen therapy has been used as an effective treatment of cluster headaches and is considered a standard acute treatment. The patient inhales through a facial mask at a rate of 7 L/minute for 15 minutes several times daily. This treatment is used in combination with other acute therapies (Sun-Edelstein & Mauskop, 2011).

As part of the medical management of headaches, the nurse should discuss with the patient alternative therapies and lifestyle changes that can be used as a means of reducing pain. Some alternative therapies are biofeedback and relaxation training, acupuncture, meditation, physical therapy, and massage. Lifestyle changes include relaxation exercises; sleep patterns; diet; the use of herbs, vitamins, and minerals; and maintenance of a calm environment.

Nursing Management

Nursing management includes taking preventative measures and providing symptomatic relief. Patient education is very important. The patient, with the nurse's assistance, can identify headache triggers and learn how to avoid them. Identifying certain foods or scents as triggers can be accomplished by completing a headache diary. This also is true of daily activities and exercise. It is important to identify whether specific activities or specific events trigger a headache. Relaxation techniques such as massages or deep breathing may assist with headache relief. Lying in a quiet, dark room and getting additional sleep also may provide some pain relief. The patient will need to make lifestyle changes to avoid known triggers. A dietitian referral may be useful in providing guidance in making the dietary changes needed to prevent headaches.

Health Promotion

Headaches are a common occurrence. Most people experience at least one headache in their lifetime. However, the type of headache varies among people. The nurse must advise and educate the patient about the following factors regarding health promotion and the prevention of recurring headaches: identify the type of headache so that treatment can be prescribed accordingly and preventive measures unique to the type of headache can be implemented; identify signs and symptoms of impending headache; modify or eliminate activities or situations that tend to prompt a headache; modify lifestyle triggers, and identify treatments or remedies that help relieve the headache, which can be used if the same type of headache reoccurs.

Intracranial Pressure

An important and underlying physiological concept in the care of any patient with an acute neurological disorder is that of **intracranial pressure (ICP),** that is, pressure within the skull created by the brain, blood, and cerebrospinal fluid (CSF). Any disorder of the brain can cause an increase in intracranial pressure, which may have wide-reaching effects on the patient's neurological status and overall health.

Monroe-Kellie Doctrine

Once the sutures in the developing cranium become closed, the brain is sealed within a nonexpandable vault. The **Monroe-Kellie doctrine** acknowledges that the intracranial volume, which includes brain, blood, and CSF, is in a closed system in a nearly rigid skull. This theoretical model has formulated important principles that explain the mechanism of intracranial pressure. The Monroe-Kellie doctrine has two basic principles. The first principle is the relative incompressibility of the three intracranial contents: the brain tissue, blood, and CSF. The second principle is that changes in the volume of one component must cause reciprocal changes in the volumes of the other components (Hickey, 2009).

In some instances, brain volume actually decreases. This can occur, for instance, as part of the normal aging process, and it is detected on imaging studies of the brain as cerebral atrophy. However, the Monroe-Kellie doctrine holds true in this condition; the amount of CSF usually increases to offset the decreasing brain volume.

Pathophysiology of Intracranial Pressure

Due to the fixed nature of the skull, the volume of its contents—brain tissue, blood, and CSF—must remain constant. If the volume of one of these three components changes, the volumes of the other components also may change, thereby decreasing or increasing the ICP. A normal ICP ranges from 0 to 15 mmHg. Brain tissue itself, known as the parenchyma, is a relatively fixed mass. Thus, the presence of a space-occupying lesion, such as a hematoma, tumor, hydrocephalus, or edema, will ultimately cause compression and/or displacement of the two other components, the vasculature and CSF. The body has several compensatory mechanisms that it can access to adapt to changes.

Compensatory Mechanisms

For the brain to maintain a normal ICP, attempts are made to compensate for changes in any of the three components within the skull. Initial mechanisms may include changing the volume of CSF by decreasing production or altering absorption. A decrease in brain tissue may be accomplished by the compression of tissue. Alterations in blood volume may occur as a result of local changes in cerebral vasculature, cerebral perfusion pressure, and cerebral blood flow.

Cerebral Blood Flow

Cerebral blood flow (CBF) is the amount of blood that passes through 100 grams of brain tissue in 1 minute. Normal CBF is approximately 50 mL per minute per 100 grams of brain tissue. Because the brain has a high requirement for the oxygen and glucose found in blood, the maintenance of an adequate level is extremely important. The brain uses 20% of the body's oxygen and 25% of its glucose supply. However, the brain has the ability to alter its blood flow in response to its needs for oxygen and glucose, which is referred to as **autoregulation.** In a normal brain, autoregulation maintains adequate tissue perfusion by adjusting metabolic needs and by altering cerebral vasculature through either vasoconstriction or vasodilation. These adjustments are made to maintain normal ICPs.

Cerebral Perfusion Pressure

Cerebral perfusion pressure (CPP) is defined as the pressure gradient that drives cerebral blood flow and is the difference between the mean blood pressure and the opposing flow provided by the ICP. It is the amount of pressure needed to provide adequate blood flow to the brain. The purpose of autoregulation is to provide consistent CBF to ensure adequate CPP to meet the brain's metabolic needs. When the systemic arterial blood pressure is normal and ICP is normal, there is very little difference between the mean arterial blood pressure (MAP) and the CPP. In the brain, however, the compensatory mechanisms that usually preserve CPP are compromised (Noble, 2010). Initial mechanisms used by the components within the brain to maintain normal ICP begin to fail. Chart 21–1 shows the calculations that are used to determine CPP.

CHART 21–1 Calculation of Cerebral Perfusion Pressure

Cerebral perfusion pressure (CPP) = mean arterial blood pressure (MAP) − intracranial pressure (ICP)

MAP = diastolic blood pressure + 1/3 (systolic blood pressure)

Normal CPP = 70 to 100 mmHg

Normal ICP = 0 to 15 mmHg

When the CPP decreases, CBF also decreases, owing to the failure of autoregulation. As the CBF and CPP fall, neuronal ischemia (lack of oxygen to nerve cells) and death occur. CPP of 50 to 60 mmHg is necessary to adequately perfuse brain tissue. CPP of less than 30 is considered incompatible with neuronal life.

As previously noted, autoregulation maintains adequate tissue perfusion in a normal brain by adjusting metabolic needs and by altering cerebral vasculature through either vasoconstriction or vasodilation. These adjustments are made to maintain normal ICPs. When ICP is elevated, it is of utmost importance to maintain an adequate mean arterial pressure (MAP). Though CPP strives to maintain adequate tissue perfusion, this may not happen in all areas of the brain. The damaged brain may have areas of increased edema, causing a localized area of limited tissue perfusion, resulting in ischemia and further neurological compromise.

Increased Intracranial Pressure

Many conditions can cause an increase in ICP including intracranial tumors, stroke, traumatic brain injury, hematomas, subarachnoid hemorrhage, and abscesses. ICPs are considered elevated when sustained at greater than 20 mmHg. At approximately 20 mmHg, increased ICPs become evident by decreased CBF, decreased CPP, and distortion of brain tissue (Hickey, 2009). Increased ICPs are associated with increased mortality and morbidity. In the presence of increased ICP, many events take place to perpetuate the process. The **vasodilatory cascade** is a series of events triggered by hypoxia, the result being increased ICP. Common causes of hypoxia are decreased blood volume and decreased respiratory effort. Hypoxia, from any cause, is a potent vasodilator. The prevention of hypoxemia is crucial. Vasodilation stimulates increased CBF, increased ICP, and reduced cerebral perfusion pressure. In patients with acute brain injury, hypoxemia has been affiliated with considerable secondary brain injury (Barker, 2008).

Cerebral Edema

Several pathologic conditions affect the brain tissue. However, it is rare for these conditions to occur in the absence of an effect on the brain's other components, that is, the CSF and the vasculature. The most typical process capable of increasing brain tissue volume is cerebral edema. **Cerebral edema** is defined as an increase in the brain's water content. There are two separate forms of cerebral edema: cytotoxic and vasogenic.

Cytotoxic edema is the accumulation of damaged swollen cells with increasing intracellular water. This type of edema occurs as a result of a hypoxic or possibly toxic event that damages the cells' ability to pump water out of the intracellular space. Examples include anoxic events such as cardiac arrest or asphyxiation. Cytotoxic edema also is seen in severe water intoxication due to hyponatremia. This process may or may not be reversible (Quinn, 2008). **Vasogenic edema** represents an alteration in vascular permeability, with disruption of the blood–brain barrier resulting in increased extracellular space. Vasogenic edema precipitates an increase in brain water content, tissue swelling, and an increased ICP (Donkin & Vink, 2010). Vasogenic edema frequently is seen in neoplastic diseases, infection, and intracerebral hemorrhage. Treatments include corticosteroids and osmotic agents such as mannitol.

Cytotoxic edema and vasogenic edema may be seen together. An example of this is a malignant brain tumor in which vasogenic edema exists, causing increased ICP. This in turn decreases tissue perfusion, causing hypoxia to the brain, resulting in cytotoxic edema. Regardless of the process, an increase in brain mass causes the displacement of other components, which results in increasing ICPs.

Herniation Syndromes

When cerebral edema occurs as a result of a space-occupying lesion, such as a tumor or a hematoma, the pressure exerted on surrounding tissue causes compression of the veins and displacement of CSF, increasing the pressure within the skull (Kumar, Abbas, Fausto, & Aster, 2009). The result is a movement of brain mass from an area of high pressure to an area of lower pressure. This movement of brain tissue is referred to as **mass effect.** When a portion of the brain protrudes through an abnormal opening, the term is referred to as **herniation.** This can cause increased pressure on one compartment of the cranial vault, which causes uneven distribution among the other brain compartments. This pressure may cause compression and damage of the brain tissue, with possibly catastrophic results. Two categories of herniation are supratentorial and infratentorial herniation. The three most common forms of herniation are cingulate, transtentorial, and uncal, which are categories of supratentorial herniation (Barker, 2008). Herniation syndromes are shown in Figure 21–3◆.

Cingulate Herniation

Cingulate herniation, also referred to as falcine herniation, is caused by an expanding lesion located in one hemisphere that shifts toward the opposite hemisphere, forcing the cingulate gyrus under the falx cerebri and displacing it to the opposite side. This shift causes displacement and compression of the local blood supply, often that associated with the anterior cerebral artery. Cerebral edema, local cerebral tissue ischemia, and increased ICP follow. Cingulated herniation is common in head trauma and brain tumors; the signs and symptoms depend on the specific location affected.

Transtentorial Herniation

Transtentorial herniation, also referred to as central herniation, may cause a downward pressure from swelling or a unilateral space-occupying lesion in the frontal and parietal lobes toward the tentorial incisura on either side of the midbrain (Barker, 2008). The hemispheres, basal ganglia, diencephalon, or midbrain is displaced through the tentorial notch. Cerebral edema, ischemia, and possibly hemorrhage may occur. Signs and symptoms of transtentorial herniation may include constricted pupils, a loss of upward gaze, decreasing levels of consciousness, altered respiratory patterns, and contralateral motor weakness.

Uncal Herniation

The most common herniation syndrome is **uncal herniation,** also referred to as lateral transtentorial herniation. This type of herniation is a subset of descending transtentorial herniations. The uncus is displaced into the suprasellar cistern (Loh, 2011). Uncal herniation is caused by an expanding lesion, typically located in the temporal lobe. Pressure is exerted across the midline, pushing the medial edge of the uncus into the edge of the tentorium. Brainstem compression may occur in this process. The third cranial nerve (oculomotor nerve) may become compressed, causing ipsilateral pupillary abnormalities, such as a dilated pupil, a common early sign in uncal herniation (Loh, 2011).

Often, the first sign of impending uncal herniation is a sluggishly reactive pupil on the side ipsilateral to the lesion. This is an early sign and may be present before any other clinical symptoms. Later signs and symptoms of uncal herniation are contralateral hemiparesis and altered levels of consciousness, beginning with restlessness and progressing through sleepiness, obtundation, and coma. Late signs are altered respiratory patterns, such as Cheyne-Stokes, or pathologic positioning, such as decorticate or decerebrate positioning. Very late signs are dilated, fixed pupils (Barker, 2008).

Herniation into the foramen magnum occurs as the anterior spinal tracts in the ventral spinal cord become compressed against the bone of the posterior vertebral bodies. This complication of an uncal herniation can be clinically catastrophic as the brain extrudes through the foramen magnum. As with all herniation syndromes, this is a life-threatening neurological emergency that, if left untreated, can progress rapidly to death (Loh, 2011).

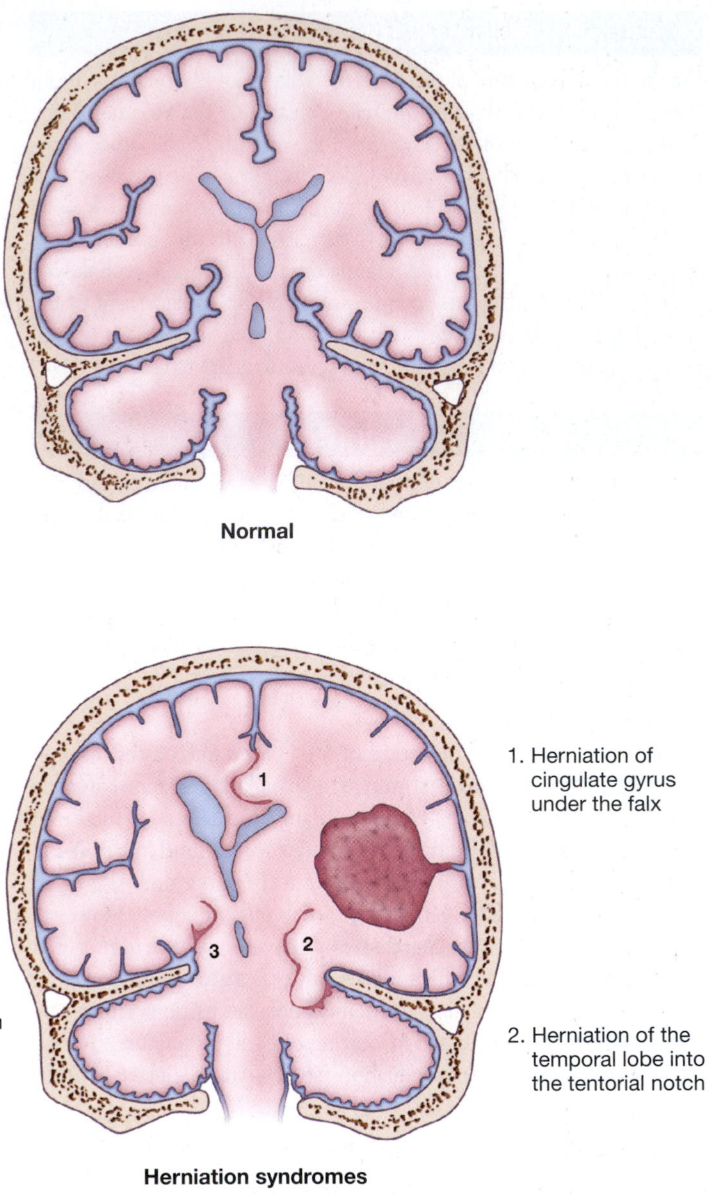

FIGURE 21–3 ◆ Herniation syndromes. (1) Herniation of cingulated gyrus under the falx. (2) Herniation of the temporal lobe into the tentorial notch. (3) Downward displacement of the brainstem through the notch.

Clinical Manifestations

The effect of increased ICP on the brain and the corresponding neurological exam depend on several common factors: the rate of the pressure increase and the location within the brain that is exerting the pressure.

Different parts of the brain, such as the brainstem, are less tolerant of pressure increases than others. The rate and location of pressure increase are reflected in the patient's neurological examination, as well as other body systems.

A complete neurological assessment, as described in Chapter 20, is essential to detecting increasing ICP. Alterations in the patient's level of consciousness (LOC) are usually the first sign of impending changes. These changes may be subtle, such as restlessness or slight confusion. They also may be catastrophic, presenting as coma or even death. The earlier the change is detected and treated, the better the prognosis.

Changes in the cranial nerve exam also may be an early sign of increased ICP that results in headache, vomiting, and papilledema/pupil changes. Edema and pressure on both the optic nerve and the oculomotor nerve (CNIII) by venous congestion resulting from ICP cause changes in the pupils; they may be unequal, dilated, pinpoint, sluggish, or nonreactive (Adoni & McNett, 2007). Decrease in motor function with presenting weakness in the extremities also may result, depending on the location of the pressure.

Safety Alert *New onset of restlessness, agitation, or confusion may be early signs of increased ICP and possible impending herniation. The nurse needs to perform hourly neurological assessment on patients diagnosed with neurological disorders and notify the health care provider of any changes in neurological status.*

Unrelieved increased ICPs may result in pathologic posturing of the body. These may be seen when a patient no longer is able to follow commands or display purposeful movements. **Decorticate (flexor) positioning** is manifested as flexion of the arms and wrists in an adduction posture when the patient is exposed to noxious stimuli, such as pain. The lower extremities are extended, internally rotated, and plantar flexed. See Figure 21–4◆. A more ominous sign is seen with **decerebrate (extensor) posturing,** which is an abnormal body posture that involves rigid extension of the arms and legs, downward pointing of the toes, and backward arching of the head. See Figure 21–5◆. This is seen in the presence of noxious or painful stimuli. The patient clenches his teeth with his arm extended in an adducted and hyperpronated fashion. His lower extremities are extended with plantar flexion. Because the lower extremities have similar positions in both motor responses, the upper extremities are used to identify the posturing. It is possible to demonstrate both abnormal responses simultaneously or each intermittently. Abnormal extension is believed to be the more grave of the two responses (Posner, Saper, Schiff, & Plum, 2007). Both of these postures indicate brainstem damage and also may indicate more serious conditions, such as herniation.

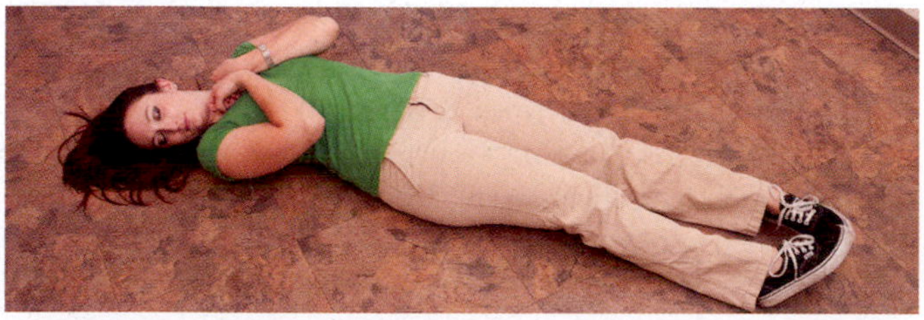

FIGURE 21–4 ◆ Decorticate positioning.

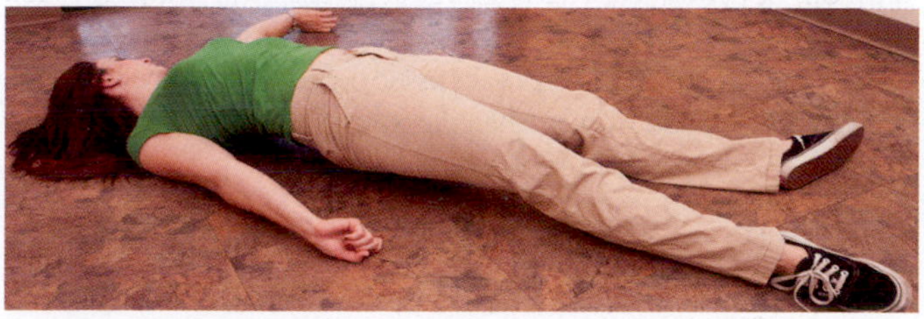

FIGURE 21–5 ◆ Decerebrate positioning.

Safety Alert *When caring for the unconscious patient, it is imperative for the nurse to contact the treating health care provider if a patient begins to demonstrate abnormal flexion or extension, as these indicate deterioration in the neurological status.*

Other signs, such as headache and vomiting, are less specific. Headaches generally are not a specific indication of ICP problems. However, headaches that are "different," such as more severe, unrelenting, and not responsive to modalities that are usually effective, may warrant notification of the health care provider. An example of a "different" headache is one that is "worse in the morning," which may be present with tumors in the posterior fossa. Projectile vomiting without prior nausea or warning may be an indication of increased ICP.

Changes in vital signs may be caused by pressure on the brainstem and/or the hypothalamus. They may be seen as increasing systolic pressure (widening pulse pressure), bradycardia, and/or irregular respiratory patterns. These are known as **Cushing's triad** and are a late indicator of increased ICP. Alterations in respiratory patterns may be a sign of impending neurological decline, especially when associated with a decrease in LOC and pupil changes, as previously discussed.

Medical and Surgical Management

The major goal of medical management of ICP is the prevention of secondary injury due to cerebral edema and increased ICP. The management of increased ICP requires an understanding of the various compensatory systems involved in the regulation of ICP. The goal is to monitor ICP dynamics, identify normal and abnormal values, and correct abnormal values. Blood pressure, ICP, volume status, and oxygenation must all be assessed to provide adequate management. Treatment may be medical or surgical.

Various modalities are available to determine, monitor, and treat abnormal ICP pressures. These vary by institution and by health care provider preference. Examples of these are external ventricular drains (EVDs), also called ventriculostomies; parenchymal bolts; a subdural monitor; or an epidural monitor. An EVD, considered the gold standard of ICP monitoring (Bader & Littlejohns, 2010), is a catheter placed into the ventricle and connected to a continuous monitoring device. The EVD allows the practitioner to monitor ICP at any given time, as well as assess trends based on the results. It also allows drainage of excess CSF if necessary to lower the ICP and to provide a sample for laboratory analysis (Nervous System Diseases, 2008).

Placement of ICP monitoring devices usually is done in an intensive care setting, emergency department, or operating room. Such devices are usually reserved for patients with decreased LOC or other manifestations of elevated ICPs.

One type of noninvasive monitoring device is the pupillometer. The standard subjective measurement of pupillary reaction has always been with a flashlight. The **pupillometer** is a small, handheld device that quantitatively assesses the changes in constriction and dilatation of the pupils to light. The basis of the pupillometer is the idea that patients with increased brain volume will have lower constriction velocities. At this time, the pupillometer is being used in some institutions as a supplemental monitoring device (Cecil, Chen, Callaway, Rowland, Adler, & Chen, 2010).

Another type of monitoring device is the brain tissue oxygen monitor, which may be used in conjunction with other methods of monitoring. The purpose is to recognize and treat ischemic injuries to the brain. Following an insult to the brain, compensatory mechanisms attempt to maintain autoregulation. The two most frequent causes of secondary injury are hypotension and hypoxia. Therefore, the measurement of oxygenation in brain tissue ($PbtO_2$) leads to valuable information regarding the supply of and demand for oxygen within the brain. Measurement of $PbtO_2$ is accomplished by the placement of an oxygen-sensitive probe into the brain tissue through an intracranial bolt or tunneled under the scalp from the site of a burr hole to exit at the desired location (the vascular area at risk for ischemia), which is approximately 6 cm from the burr hole (Deshaies, Jacobsen, Singla, Li, & Gorji, 2012). This probe is able to monitor both the level of oxygen and the temperature of the brain tissue. The oxygen sensor is positioned in the brain's white matter, preferably in the penumbra of the injured area. However, the most favorable location for normal brain measurements is in the uninjured brain. Lower levels of $PbtO_2$ correspond with lower levels of tissue oxygenation, translating to poor neurological outcome (Cecil et al., 2010).

A relatively new monitoring device is a directed CBF monitoring system. The brain depends on continuous blood flow to supply the body with glucose and oxygen. Regional CBF is an important monitoring parameter that can be used to evaluate tissue viability. This probe is able to measure CBF by calculating real-time tissue perfusion at the capillary level. The probe is placed through a burr hole into the white matter, optimally in the noninjured brain white matter or in the ischemic penumbra (Cecil et al., 2010).

Jugular bulb venous oxygenation saturation is another method of monitoring cerebral oxygenation. The internal jugular vein is cannulated via the catheter. The purpose is to obtain a continuous measurement of jugular venous oxygen saturation (SjO_2). This method provides a measurement of the oxygen saturation of venous blood leaving the brain. The goal of SjO_2 measurement is early identification of cerebral hypoxia. Saturation below 55% is indicative of global brain ischemia and needs immediate treatment (Barker, 2008).

The cerebral microdialysis system is used at the patient's bedside. This monitoring device identifies signals of cellular disturbances before clinical symptoms are manifested. Early identification may provide an opportunity for intervention and prevention of secondary injury. The microdialysis catheter allows frequent sampling of particular molecular substances within the interstitial fluid, including glucose, pyruvate, lactate, glycerol, and amino acids, such as aspartate and glutamate. An increase in these particular substances may be indicative of brain ischemia (Presciutti, Schmidt, & Alexander, 2009). A tiny microcatheter is threaded through a bolt or burr hole into the brain parenchyma. A microdialysis syringe filled with sterile perfusion fluid is then attached to the catheter. The ideal placement of the catheter is in the pericontusional penumbra of the injured brain. Through diffusion, the molecules related to the production of adenosine triphosphate are collected in the dialysate fluid and analyzed hourly. Changes in the cerebral metabolites indicate the presence of cerebral ischemia (Cecil et al., 2010).

Monitoring and maintaining the patient in a euglycemic (normal glucose content of the blood) state are critical to medical management. Brain trauma increases the release of glutamate, which increases cerebral metabolism. This, in turn, increases the metabolic breakdown of glucose, the major energy source for the brain. This process leads to tissue acidosis, ischemia, and a worsened neurological outcome due to secondary injury.

Normothermia (the normal body temperature) is another significant aspect of medical management. Fever occurs in up to 70% of neurologically injured patients and typically is a sustained response that may last up to 2 weeks following injury (Badjatia, 2009). Hyperthermia potentiates secondary injury and worsens neurological outcomes. The increased body temperature triggers pathophysiologic processes, increasing metabolic demand, CBF, cerebral blood volume, and ICP (Puccio, Fischer, Jankowitz, Yonas, Darby, & Okonkwo, 2009).

Various pharmacologic agents may be used in the management of refractory intracranial hypertension. Hyperosmotic fluids, such as mannitol or hypertonic saline solutions, can be used to decrease ICP. These solutions are effective because they move water from cerebral tissue into the circulation. Hemodilution of red blood cells occurs, reducing viscosity and allowing more blood flow to occur within smaller vessels. Vasoconstriction follows, which decreases ICP. It is important to closely monitor the patient's fluid status, including electrolytes and serum osmolality, to avoid negative fluid balance. Mannitol has been used more frequently for ICP control; however, mannitol also has been associated with severe diuresis, hyperkalemia, acute renal failure, hypotension, and rebound intracranial hypertension (Infanti, 2008).

Maintenance of adequate vascular volume is of utmost importance in the maintenance of adequate CPP. Central venous catheters and pulmonary artery catheters also may be used to adequately monitor volume status. These catheters are discussed in detail in Chapter 31. Also important in the management of CPP is close monitoring of arterial blood pressure with the use of an arterial line (Chapter 31). Vasopressor medications such as phenylephrine, norepinephrine, and dopamine may be necessary to elevate the systemic arterial blood pressure to support adequate CPP. The goal of treatment is based on the relationship of ICP and CPP, as previously discussed.

Patients who are at risk for neurological deterioration because of increased ICPs that are refractory to other methods of treatment may be placed in a barbiturate coma. A barbiturate such as pentobarbital is administered as a loading dose; then, a maintenance dose sustains the comatose state. This method is used to decrease LOC, thus decreasing cerebral metabolic needs. The negative aspect of barbiturate coma is that the neurological assessment—including the most basic reflexes, such as gag, swallow, and cough—is lost. It can also cause severe hypotension that requires the use of a vasopressor medication or an intravenous administration of fluids to expand the intravascular volume. The patient in pentobarbital coma must be mechanically ventilated (Chapter 28) (Bope, Kellerman, & Rakel, 2011).

Other, less aggressive means of sedation, such as the use of propofol, can be used to keep patients' pain and/or anxiety under control. The goal of sedation is to decrease ICP, CBF, and oxygen demand. Propofol has a short half-life, allowing practitioners to suspend infusion temporarily to accurately assess the patient's neurological status.

In some circumstances, the best method of treating increased ICP is surgical intervention. In cases of extreme cerebral edema, a hemicraniectomy may be performed. This is a surgical procedure in which a portion of the skull (bone flap) is removed. This method allows room for the swollen brain, lessening the risk for brain tissue damage. The bone flap often is replaced 2 to 4 months later when the patient's condition has stabilized.

Nursing Management

The nursing management of patients with elevated ICP is complex and requires constant vigilance in terms of the neurological exam and assessment of trends in the monitoring data. An increased ICP affects the brain's overall function and leads to dysfunction in many body systems, including the respiratory, cardiovascular, metabolic, and neurological systems. Therefore, nursing assessment of ICP must encompass all of these systems.

Assessment

Any patient with neurological compromise must be assessed for adequate respiratory function, since adequate oxygenation is essential to neurological function. Patients with a decreased LOC may have a decreased level of respiratory function. The patient's pulse oximetry also must be assessed. However, a health care provider's order is needed to administer supplemental oxygen to maintain oxygen saturations of 95% or greater, if required.

Ongoing assessment using the Glasgow Coma Scale (GCS) is an essential component of the neurological assessment. The GCS measures the LOC and is explained in detail in Chapter 20. Patients with a Glasgow Coma Scale score of 8 or less should be considered for intubation and mechanical ventilation. Assessment of the pupils also is critical to diagnosing increased ICP. Pupils should be examined for the following:

- ***Size and Equality:*** The normal size of the pupil is between 2 and 5 mm; the two pupils should be equal in size. A 1-mm discrepancy is considered a normal deviation. Pupil size should be assessed both before and after the pupil responds to direct light.
- ***Shape:*** The normal shape of the pupil is round. An irregular pupil may be the result of ophthalmological procedures, such as cataract surgery, and should be documented in the patient's record and confirmed with the patient and/or family. A pupil that is oval in shape may indicate the early compression of cranial nerve III due to increased ICP and therefore should be addressed immediately. If an oval pupil is detected, measures should be taken to decrease ICP. As ICP is reduced, the oval-shaped pupil should resolve. However, if ICP continues to rise or is not treated, the oval-shaped pupil will become further dilated and will eventually become nonreactive to light.
- ***Reactivity to Light:*** Pupil reactivity is reported as the response or reflex of each pupil to direct light. It is assessed by shining a low-beam flashlight inward from the outer canthus of each eye. Each eye should be checked separately. The light should not shine directly into the pupil because the glare or reflection may obscure visualization. The reaction that each pupil has to the light stimulus should be recorded as brisk, sluggish, or nonreactive. Normally, pupils should constrict briskly in response to light. A sluggish or slow pupillary response may indicate increased ICP, and nonreactive pupils are often associated with severe increases in ICP and/or severe brain damage.

A complete pupillary reactivity examination also includes assessment of the consensual pupillary response and accommodation. The consensual pupillary response is the constriction that normally occurs in a pupil when light is shone into the opposite eye. Because of this response, the trauma team should wait for several seconds after assessing the pupillary light reflex in one eye before assessing that in the second eye, as the second pupil may be temporarily constricted. Accommodation is the constriction of pupils that occurs when a conscious patient is focusing on a close object. Pupils should normally constrict bilaterally when an object is held within 4 to 6 inches of a patient's nose (Adoni & McNett, 2007).

Assessment of the patient's glycemic state also is important, as hyperglycemia with an ischemic brain has been shown to be an independent predictor of poor outcome. Hyperglycemia (a fasting blood glucose level higher than 140 mg/dL) disrupts the blood–brain barrier and promotes cerebral edema (Lab Tests Online, 2011). Glucose has been associated with brain tissue acidosis in patients who have experienced a major head injury (Moyer, 2009).

It is understood that fever in patients with neurological injury is associated with poor outcomes; therefore, monitoring of the patient's temperature is a key assessment factor (Puccio et al., 2009). The assessment of blood pressure also is essential. To prevent cerebral ischemia, adequate CBF is mandatory. Hypotension in the presence of brain trauma has a strong negative effect on outcome and may cause further brain injury.

Nursing Diagnoses

The following nursing diagnoses are applicable to patients with increased ICP:

- *Decreased Intracranial Adaptive Capacity* related to brain injury.
- *Ineffective Tissue Perfusion* related to increased intracranial pressure, cerebral edema, and decreased cerebral perfusion pressure.
- *Risk for Aspiration* related to reduced level of consciousness and depressed cough and gag reflexes.
- *Ineffective Thermoregulation* related to damage to the hypothalamus, dehydration, and infection.
- *Deficient Fluid Volume* related to fluid restriction.
- *Risk for Infection* related to ICP monitoring system (fiber-optic or intraventricular catheter).

NANDA-I © 2012

Outcomes and Evaluation Parameters

Outcomes and evaluation parameters consist of short-term goals with measurable determinants of achievement and are related to each nursing diagnosis cited in the previous list:

1. Patient will have intracranial pressure within normal range.

   ICP will remain less than 20.

   Glasgow Coma Scale score will be 13 or higher.
2. Patient will have a cerebral perfusion pressure (CPP) of at least 50, preferably 60.

   CPP = 60
3. Patient will not aspirate.

   Chest x-ray, lung sounds, and arterial blood gases normal or at patient's baseline.
4. Body temperature will remain within normal limits.
5. Patient will not have deficient fluid volume.

   Balanced fluid intake; normal laboratory values; moist mucous membranes, improved skin turgor.
6. Patient's risk for infection will be minimized.

   The patient will maintain normothermia and normal white blood cell count. Chest x-ray will be clear. Blood, urine, and sputum cultures will be negative.

Interventions and Rationales

Nursing interventions for patients with increased ICP require critical thinking and expert skill development. It is important for the nurse to be aware that activities such as turning, suctioning, and bathing tend to

CHART 21–2 Nursing Implications and Rationale for Actions for Patients with Increased ICP

Actual and Potential Problems	Nursing Action	Rationale for Action
Decreased intracranial adaptive capacity	Monitor neurological status, ICP, and vital signs at least every hour.	Maintenance of normal ICP is essential to prevent further brain injury.
	Notify health care provider and establish a protocol to respond to an ICP greater than 20.	Decreases resistance to venous return.
	Keep head of bed at 30°.	Prevents pulmonary complications.
	Maintain patient's head and neck in neutral position.	
	Monitor patient's temperature and maintain it within designated parameters.	
	Monitor patient's blood pressure and maintain it within designated parameters.	
	Monitor patient's blood gases and consult with health care provider to resolve hypercarbia (abnormally high level of carbon dioxide in the blood), hypocarbia (an abnormally low level of carbon dioxide in the blood), or hypoxia.	
	Monitor blood pressure and maintain within established parameters.	Maintains adequate perfusion to the brain. A CPP less than 50 should be avoided, since it is associated with loss of autoregulation of the brain.
	Calculate mean arterial pressure (MAP) and CPP. When CPP is decreased, institute methods to decrease ICP or increase MAP, contingent on the orders of the health care provider.	Positioning the patient with the head of the bed elevated has shown to be effective in reducing aspiration and pneumonia.
	Position the patient with the head of the bed elevated.	
	Provide mouth care per policy.	Mouth care may decrease the incidence of aspiration of bacteria.
	Ensure proper placement of a feeding tube and assess gastrointestinal functioning prior to and during feeding.	Proper tube placement limits the possibility of aspirating residuals.
Ineffective thermoregulation	Monitor body temperature.	Normothermia protects cerebral metabolic needs.
	Use cooling devices if necessary.	
	Administer appropriate antipyretics, if warranted.	
Deficient fluid volume	Maintain accurate record of intake and output.	Patients with severe brain injury should be kept normovolemic to maintain cerebral perfusion.
	Administer intravenous fluids as ordered.	
	Monitor patient for signs of "dryness" such as chapped lips, dry skin, diminished skin turgor, decreased urine output, dry mucous membranes, decreased blood pressure and pulse pressure, decreased venous filling, elevated hematocrit, increased body temperature, increased pulse rate, concentrated urine, and a change in mental status.	
Risk for infection	The ventricular system is a closed sterile system; therefore, it must be handled with sterile technique.	The nurse should prevent an infection from developing and causing additional physiological stress on the brain.
	Change the dressing at the insertion site according to agency protocol; keep it clean, dry, and occlusive. If the dressing becomes dampened with CSF, it should be changed and the health care provider should be notified.	
	Inspect the system once per shift or according to established policy.	
	Examine the site for signs and symptoms of infection.	
	Use sterile technique when the collection bag is changed (usually when it is three-quarters full). Clean technique can be used in repositioning the bag. If taking a CSF sample, complete a 3-minute scrub of the port.	
	Limit access into the drainage system.	
	Monitor the patient for signs of infection (e.g., elevated temperature), physical signs of a fever (e.g., flushed face, face feels warm to touch, fever blisters), and signs of dehydration.	

increase the ICP (Bell, 2009)). While most activities demonstrate only transient increases in ICP, the nurse needs to be aware of such tendencies for increasing ICP and administer these activities cautiously. Head injury patients are very vulnerable to random body positioning, which may cause changes in the ICP (Ledwith, Bloom, Maloney-Wilensky, Coyle, Polomano, & Le Roux, 2010). Chart 21–2 summarizes interventions related to each of the nursing diagnoses from the previous list.

Traumatic Brain Injury

Traumatic brain injury (TBI) is defined as a nondegenerative, noncongenital insult to the brain from an external mechanical force (Dawodu, 2011). Currently, injury to the brain accounts for 1.4 million reported injuries and 52,000 deaths each year in the United States (Cecil et al., 2010). The initial mechanical insult to the brain is called a primary injury. The brain's response to the initial injury is called a secondary injury.

Primary and Secondary Head Injuries

The *primary injury,* may be localized, such as occurs with a laceration, concussion, contusion, fracture, or diffuse axonal injury. The *secondary injury* is a progressive insult that evolves following the primary injury. When there is inadequate cerebral perfusion pressure, **cerebral ischemia** will occur, contributing to the risk of mortality and morbidity. This ischemia can then trigger the **ischemia cascade** (discussed in Chapter 22), which is a series of events that results in changes on the cellular level, which then results in **cerebral infarction** (Barker, 2008). It can be the result of a single event or a series of events. Secondary brain injury results from hypotension, hypoxia, anemia, and fever. Deficits in cellular metabolism in the brain can cause cell death, leading to death of brain tissue, compromised neurological function, and poor patient outcomes. Hypotension nearly doubles the mortality from head injury and may worsen the outcomes of the patients who survive (Marx et al., 2009).

Epidemiology and Etiology

TBI is a major health problem globally. In the United States, the Centers for Disease Control and Prevention (CDC) estimate that the incidence of patients with closed-head injuries admitted to hospitals is conservatively 1.5 million each year. Approximately 275,000 people with TBI are admitted to hospitals every year, with approximately 52,000 deaths (CDC, 2011). Although the causes of TBI differ by region, gender, and age group, most TBIs appear to be secondary to motor vehicle crashes, falls, and acts of violence, such as gunshot wounds and assault. Studies have shown that African American men have higher rates of brain injury than other groups (Arciniegas & McAllister, 2008). Penetrating head injuries represent approximately 10% of TBI; they are usually caused by firearms and are self-inflicted (Arciniegas & McAllister, 2008). Falls continue to be the leading cause of TBI in the United States. Motor vehicle crashes and traffic-related incidents are the second leading cause and resulted in the largest percentage of TBI-related deaths (Faul, Xu, Wald, & Coronado, 2010). For active duty military personnel in war zones, blasts are the leading cause of TBI (Champion, Holcomb, & Young, 2009). TBI rates are higher for males than for females in every age group (CDC, 2011). For some ethnic and socioeconomic groups, risk exposure for TBI is increased in various ways: increased exposure to physically demanding employment settings (such as construction and manual labor); increased exposure to personal violence; increased exposure to older homes and vehicles; and greater reliance on substandard housing (Mayo Clinic Staff, 2008). The Risk Factors box summarizes the risks for TBI.

Nearly 2% of the world population has a long-term or lifelong need for help in performing activities of daily living as a result of TBI (Oh & Seo, 2009). The impact on the lives of the patient, family, and community is beyond comprehension and impossible to calculate or predict. Acute head trauma occurs in varying degrees of severity and complexity. It can range from minor scalp lacerations requiring little to no treatment to severe TBIs resulting in prolonged hospitalization, permanent disabilities, or death.

RISK FACTORS for Traumatic Brain Injury

Age 18–25 or over age 70	High alcohol intake
Male (2:1 ratio)	Serving in the military
Participation in certain sports activities	

Source: Crippen, D. W. (2011). Head trauma. Retrieved from http://emedicine.medscape.com/article/433855-overview#a0102.

Superficial Injuries

Injuries to the scalp are relatively common. Although usually minor, they must be carefully assessed and treated diligently. The degree of subsequent treatment depends on the extent and depth of the injury. The scalp consists of five layers that cover the skull (Figure 21–6◆). The skin, or dermal, layer contains hair and protects the scalp. The subcutaneous fascia is a fatty, vascular layer containing blood vessels that may bleed profusely. The galea aponeurotica is a thick, flexible, and fibrous tissue. The subgaleal space is below the galea and is a potential space for blood to collect and form cephalohematomas, or "goose eggs." Below the subgaleal space is the periosteum, a thin layer of tissue covering the skull.

The most common and least severe scalp injury is a simple abrasion. An abrasion is a simple scraping of the skin that may bleed slightly. A contusion is a bruise of the skin. Treatments for both abrasions and contusions include a thorough cleansing of the wound with possible application of an antibiotic ointment.

Scalp lacerations account for a large number of emergency department visits. The scalp is extremely vascular, and exsanguination has been known to occur in extreme cases. This vascularity is what allows the scalp to heal well in most cases. With any scalp laceration, the possibility of an underlying skull fracture must be addressed. Therefore, an accurate history of the event surrounding the injury is very important. Depending on the mechanism of injury, if there is any reason to suspect a skull fracture, the health care provider should obtain a CT scan or,

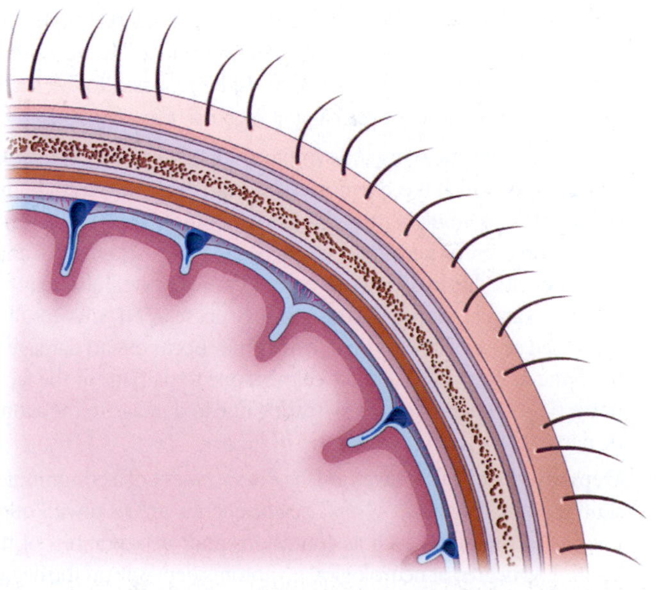

FIGURE 21–6 ◆ Scalp layers.

at the very least, a plain x-ray of the skull. Once the degree and extent of the scalp injury have been determined, the nurse should clean the wound with a standard skin-sterilizing solution, such as a povidone-iodine compound. The wound may require suturing. In addition to obtaining a history of the event, the nurse should assess the need for a tetanus toxoid and administer it, if appropriate.

Skull Fractures

The skull, or calvarium, is the bony structure that houses the brain. It is composed of the frontal, parietal, temporal, and occipital bones. It also includes the multiple facial bones that make up the facial structure. Of these facial bones, only the mandible is movable. The skull itself is asymmetrical and varies in thickness. The temporal bone is the thinnest; the occipital bone is the thickest. The floor of the skull, known as the skull base, is rough and uneven, contributing in an important way to brain injury. Skull fractures are categorized according to the type of break and severity of the fracture as follows:

- **Linear skull fractures** are the most common type of skull fracture. They are simple breaks in the continuity of bone, with no displacement, and most commonly are seen in low-velocity impact situations. Linear fractures of the temporal bone may result in a tear of the middle meningeal artery, resulting in more serious brain injury, such as an epidural hematoma.
- **Comminuted skull fractures** are fragmented interruptions of the skull resulting from multiple linear fractures. An area of bone depression at the point of impact is characteristic of a comminuted fracture.
- **Basal skull fractures** usually are an extension of a linear fracture into the skull base. The mechanism of injury generally is the same as that of linear skull fractures with a more serious result. The inner aspect of the skull is closely associated with the dura, the thin membrane that covers the brain. The skull base is rough and uneven, and its texture may cause tears to the delicate dura. Consequently, CSF may leak through the tear in the dura. This may result in CSF leaking from the nose or the ear. CSF leaking from the nose is called **rhinorrhea,** whereas CSF leaking from the ear is called **otorrhea.** Drainage of CSF may be visualized directly or may be seen on dressings or bed linens. It is distinguishable by its characteristic halo sign, which appears as blood with a yellow ring around it. The occurrence of CSF leak, while not unexpected, must be reported to the health care provider because the patient is at high risk for meningitis.

  Other characteristic signs and symptoms of basal skull fractures are **Battle sign,** which is ecchymosis (bruising) over the mastoid bone (Figure 21–7◆); bulging tympanic membranes; and the presence of raccoon eyes, or periorbital ecchymosis (Figure 21–8◆). Cranial nerve deficits, due to damage to various cranial nerves, also may occur. For example, damage to the olfactory nerve (CNI) may result in decreased sense of smell, visual deficits may occur due to damage to the optic nerve (CNII), facial weakness due to damage to the facial nerve (CNVII), and decreased hearing due to damage to the acoustic nerve (CNVIII).
- **Depressed skull fractures** are the displacement of a comminuted skull fracture (Figure 21–9◆). They frequently are seen with other injuries to the brain, such as contusions and/or lacerations of the brain. The degree of neurological symptoms depends on the degree and location of brain involvement. Hair, dirt, and other debris may be found within the wound and present risk for infection.

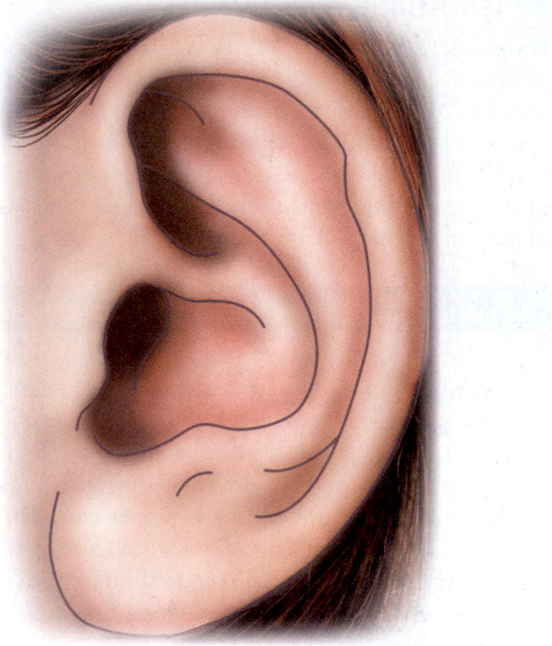

FIGURE 21–7 ◆ Battle sign.

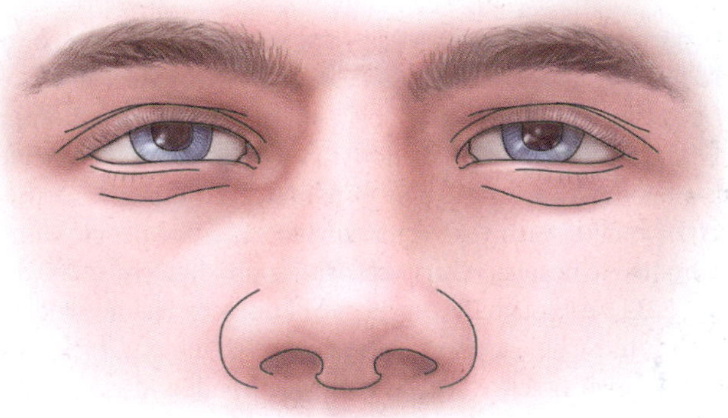

FIGURE 21–8 ◆ Racoon eyes/periorbital ecchymosis.

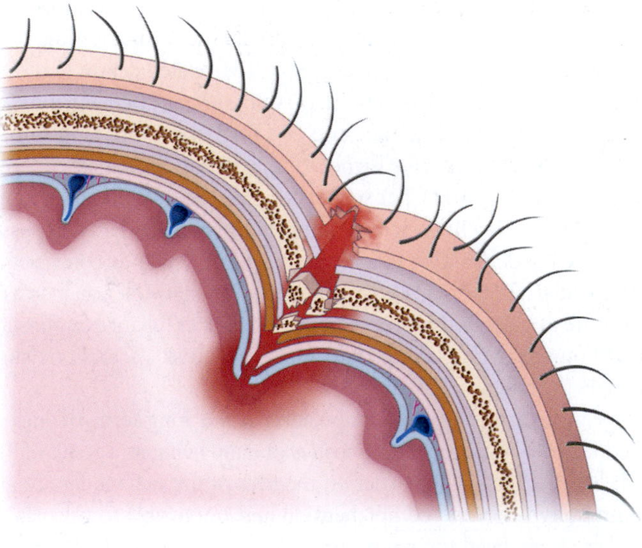

FIGURE 21–9 ◆ Depressed skull fracture.

Clinical Manifestations

Skull fractures alone do not cause neurological symptoms but frequently are seen in conjunction with other, more serious brain injuries, such as hematomas or contusions. In these cases, clinical manifestations are representative of the other brain injuries that may be present.

Laboratory and Diagnostic Procedures

A diagnosis of skull fracture can be made with plain skull x-rays. However, if a skull fracture is suspected on the basis of the health care provider's physical assessment and knowledge of the mechanism of injury, a CT scan of the patient's head should be obtained, because the question of underlying brain trauma must be addressed. Fractures of the facial bones and basal skull fractures may be seen best with a thin-cut CT scan. The Diagnostic Tests box provides more details about tests for skull fractures.

Medical Management

Treatment of a skull fracture depends on the type of fracture. Linear fractures usually do not require treatment other than close observation of the patient for neurological deterioration. Open or comminuted fractures should be considered contaminated, and careful wound debridement with surgical closure often is required. Depressed skull fractures may require elevation of the depressed bone as well as debridement of the wound. The possibility of infection must be considered, and antibiotics are started if considered appropriate.

Hematomas

Hematomas are collections of blood. Intracranial hematomas are defined by their location, either epidural or subdural. Chart 21–3 summarizes the types of hematomas, which are discussed in more detail in the following subsections.

Epidural Hematoma

An **epidural hematoma (EDH)** is caused by bleeding into the space between the skull and the dura, caused by the laceration of an artery or a vein (Figure 21–10◆). In the adult population, 90% of the patients with epidural hematomas have skull fractures, most commonly in the temporal bone, which lacerates the middle meningeal artery. Venous epidural bleeds may occur if the superior sagittal sinus tears (Bader & Littlejohns, 2010). As bleeding occurs, an enlarging hematoma develops as the dura is stripped away from the inner surface of the skull. The expanding lesion exerts pressure on the brain tissue, resulting in neurological compromise.

EDHs account for approximately 1% to 2% of all TBIs, and people in the age range of 20 to 40 are the most affected. The mortality rate is approximately 8%, which is the lowest rate of all the hematomas (Barker, 2008).

CHART 21–3 Types of Hematomas

Hematoma	Onset of Symptoms
Epidural	Immediate loss of consciousness, followed by lucid interval (considered "textbook presentation")
Subdural, acute	Up to 48 hours after injury
Subdural, subacute	48 hours to 3 weeks
Subdural, chronic	3 weeks to several months

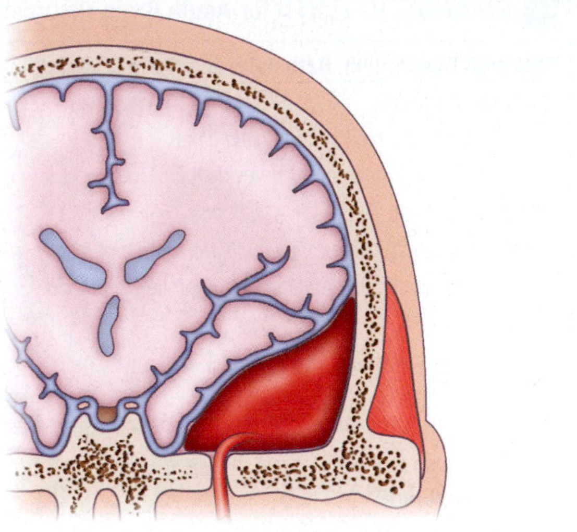

FIGURE 21–10 ◆ Epidural hematoma.

The classic clinical presentation of EDH is characterized by an immediate post-traumatic period of unconsciousness, followed by a lucid interval, which can last from minutes to hours. The "lucid interval" is considered a textbook presentation of EDH, and is seen in approximately 85% of patients with EDH. A rapid deterioration in LOC may follow, characterized by sleepiness, confusion, obtundation, coma, and possibly death. Neurological decline is caused by the rapidly increasing pressure, or mass effect, caused by the enlarging hematoma. Other possible signs and symptoms are an enlarging pupil on the same side of the injury (ipsilateral), increasing headache, seizures, motor weakness, and/or pathologic positioning (refer to Chapter 20 on assessment).

Subdural Hematoma

Subdural hematoma (SDH) is defined as bleeding between the dura and the arachnoid layer of the meninges (Figure 21–11◆). SDHs are the most common type of intracranial traumatic lesion, accounting for approximately 10% to 20% of lesions (Barker, 2008). They usually are caused by the tearing of bridging veins located over the surface of the brain. SDHs are divided into three categories based on the amount of

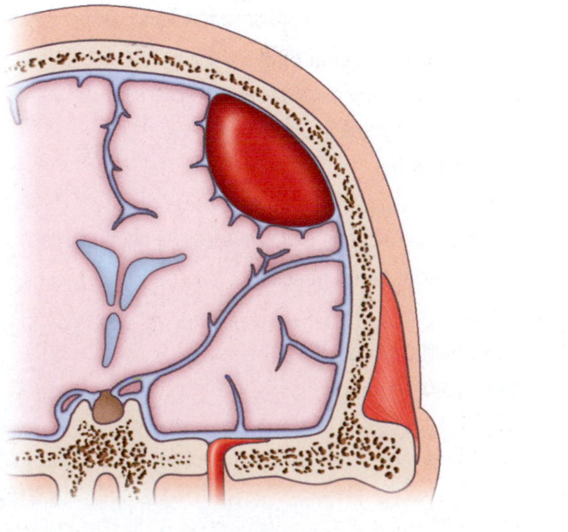

FIGURE 21–11 ◆ Subdural hematoma.

DIAGNOSTIC TESTS for Acute Brain Disorders

Test with Description, Rationale, and Normal Values	Expected Abnormality
Plain skull films *Skull fractures are best seen in plain films.* Normal findings should reveal no evidence of fractures.	Fracture lines, linear, basal, depressed, or comminuted
CT of head *CT scans are best suited to examining presence of blood, edema, CSF.* Normal findings should demonstrate no presence of blood or swelling.	Hematomas (SDH, EDH), contusions, hydrocephalus Test is time sensitive, as the presence of blood (in SDH) changes characteristics with time
MRI *MRI will demonstrate small lesions not seen on CT scan. Best suited to demonstrate heterogeneity of tumors.* Normal findings should not reveal tumors or lesions.	DAI (late) tumors
Lumbar puncture *Contraindicated until space-occupying lesions are ruled out because of the possibility of induced brain herniation.* Bacterial or viral pathogens affect glucose, protein, cell counts, red blood cells, and white blood cells.	Blood in CSF (subarachnoid blood) Abnormalities in fluid chemistry
Electroencephalogram (EEG) *Common in head trauma, brain tumors, and infectious process due to altered electrical activity in brain.* Normal findings reveal normal brain waveforms.	Seizure activity
Serum electrolytes: Sodium 135–145 mEq/L normal *Risk factor for increased cerebral edema.*	Hyponatremia (serum Na^+ less than 134 mEq/L) or hypernatremia (Na greater than 145)
Blood glucose 70–110 mg/dL normal *Indicative of steroid use (dexamethasone).*	May be elevated
Complete blood count (CBC) Normal: White blood cell count: 4,500–10,000 white blood cells per microliter **Hemoglobin:** Adult males: 13.5–18 gm/dL Adult women: 12–15 gm/dL **Hematocrit:** Adult males: 40–54% Adult women: 36–46% *Indicates infection.* *Also may be present with steroid use.* *Important for accurate hemodynamic monitoring, especially in patients at risk for vasospasm.*	Elevated white blood cell count Alteration in hemoglobin/hematocrit
Culture of cerebrospinal fluid *Indicated for suspicion of infectious CNS process.* No evidence of bacteria in culture.	Presence of pathogens
Tissue pathology *Indicated for suspicion of tumor or abscess.* Normal findings reveal no tumor, abscess, or abnormalities.	Presence of malignancy, pathogen
75–100 Arterial blood gases Normal: PO_2 75–100 mmHg PCO_2 35–45 mmHg *Depressed neurological state may also indicate depressed respiratory drive. Decreased levels of oxygen and increased levels of CO_2 are a concern for increasing ICPs.*	Hypoxia, hypercapnia

Source: Adapted from Kee, J. L. (2010). Laboratory and diagnostic tests with nursing implications. Upper Saddle River, NJ: Pearson.

time between the initial injury and the presentation of signs and symptoms: acute, subacute, and chronic.

Acute Subdural Hematoma

Acute SDH is characterized by the presentation of neurological signs and symptoms up to 48 hours after injury. The most common signs are severe headache with possible gradual deterioration of LOC, starting with drowsiness and progressing through confusion, obtundation, and coma. Pupillary signs also may be present, most commonly an ipsilateral dilation, and the person may exhibit sluggish reactivity. Hemiparesis of the contralateral arm and leg also may be present.

Subacute Subdural Hematoma

With subacute subdural hematoma, neurological signs and symptoms develop from 48 hours postinjury up to about 3 weeks. They are associated with less serious lesions, perhaps because the bleeding occurs at a much slower rate.

Chronic Subdural Hematoma

With chronic subdural hematoma, neurological signs and symptoms develop over 3 weeks to several months. These are associated with minor head injuries, possibly occurring weeks to months before the neurological signs become obvious. The SDH increases slowly in size, possibly from repeated small venous bleeds, until a significant mass effect develops and symptoms occur.

Chronic subdural hematomas are associated with older adults, since they may have an atrophic brain that provides more free space to bleed into. Another significant feature of the aging brain is the presence of bridging veins that are stretched as the brain atrophies. This stretching also may cause bleeding into the subdural space. Because there is more room for the clot to expand, the SDH may become quite large before symptoms occur. However, because chronic SDH may occur from repeated small episodes of subdural bleeding, it is not uncommon to have acute or chronic SDH, as evidenced by areas of varying density, demonstrated on a CT scan. Chronic SDHs usually do not present with the rapid and dramatic deterioration of neurological function that is seen with acute SDHs. The most common symptom of chronic SDH is increasing headache, slowing mentation, confusion, and drowsiness. Seizures also may be present.

Types of hematomas are summarized in Chart 21–3.

Safety Alert *Patients with a diagnosis of SDH are at risk for expanding hematoma. Therefore, the nurse must perform frequent neurological assessments (i.e., hourly until stable, then every 2 hours). A decrease in neurological function, such as increasing confusion or lethargy, increasing motor weakness, or an enlarging pupil, is a medical emergency. The nurse must notify the health care provider immediately.*

Diagnostic Procedures

A CT scan of the head remains the most accurate diagnostic tool, along with a thorough and accurate history of the event. EDH is characterized by a high-density elliptical-shaped mass adjacent to the skull. Mass effect also is seen with a shift of the brain from the side with the EDH to the opposite side. CT scan is highly diagnostic for SDH, as well as for the determination of the acute, subacute, or chronic type of hematoma.

Medical Management

The treatment for EDH is almost always surgical. The exception to surgical management is a small lesion that is causing little to no neurological impairment. The patient is hospitalized, possibly in the intensive care unit (ICU), with frequent neurological assessment. There, serial CT scans are taken to monitor the size of the hematoma. A decline in the patient's neurological assessment, with or without radiographic evidence of increased size, warrants emergent surgical evacuation of the hematoma.

The treatment for SDH depends on several factors. Observation with medical management may be appropriate for a small SDH with little to no neurological deterioration, because a small SDH may reabsorb with time. Because seizures are a common occurrence in SDH, the use of antiepileptic drugs (AEDs) may be warranted. A large SDH with significant neurological compromise requires immediate surgical evacuation. SDH is commonly associated with therapeutic anticoagulation, and correction of coagulopathy is a critical step in preparing the patient for operative care. It is possible to drain a small liquefied hematoma with twist drill burr holes. Burr holes are small holes made with a twist drill into the skull over the area of the hematoma. Commonly, a drain is left in to drain the hematoma over time. Larger acute, subacute, and chronic SDH may require an open craniotomy (surgical removal of a section of bone [bone flap from the skull]) for evacuation of the hematoma. Twist drill drainage of chronic SDH may not be possible, however, because the clotted blood is the consistency of motor oil and may be too gelatinous to be successfully evacuated with burr holes. The subdural evacuating port system (SEPS) is another treatment used for subacute or chronic subdural hematomas. It is a minimally invasive procedure in which a drain is placed into the SDH via a burr hole. This can be done quickly with local anesthesia, which makes this treatment ideal for older or very ill patients who may not tolerate general anesthesia (Kenning, Dalfino, German, Drazin, & Adamo, 2010). Postoperatively, the patient should remain in the ICU, with close monitoring of her neurological status. Use of intracranial monitoring is done with caution, because the monitoring system may cause the SDH to worsen. The patient may require hemodynamic monitoring to assess blood pressure and cardiac output (Chapter 31) and/or ventilatory assistance (Chapter 28), depending on the size and location of the lesion, as well as the presence of any accompanying injuries. The prophylactic use of antiepileptic drugs (AEDs) to prevent seizures is controversial, because they have many side effects and contraindications. If a patient has a seizure due to a lesion, the patient should be started on an AED such as phenytoin.

Cerebral Contusions

Contusions of the brain are defined as bruising of the brain tissue, often associated with other neurological injuries, such as skull fractures or hematomas. They may occur from blunt trauma, penetrating wounds, or acceleration/deceleration injuries. Causes may include motor vehicle crashes, falls, and assault. The injuries are referred to as **coup,** in which bruising occurs directly below the point of impact on the skull, or **contrecoup,** which occurs directly opposite the point of impact. Contrecoup contusions usually have a coup component, in which case they are referred to as coup-contrecoup contusions. Contrecoup contusions occur as a result of the brain moving with the skull and bruising itself against the skull during acceleration/deceleration movement (Figure 21–12◆).

Clinical Manifestations

The clinical presentation of cerebral contusion is highly dependent on the location, size, and amount of cerebral edema associated with the lesion. For example, a patient with temporal contusions, especially bilateral contusions, may have a significant decrease in LOC with motor and speech deficits. This patient is at high risk for cerebral edema and

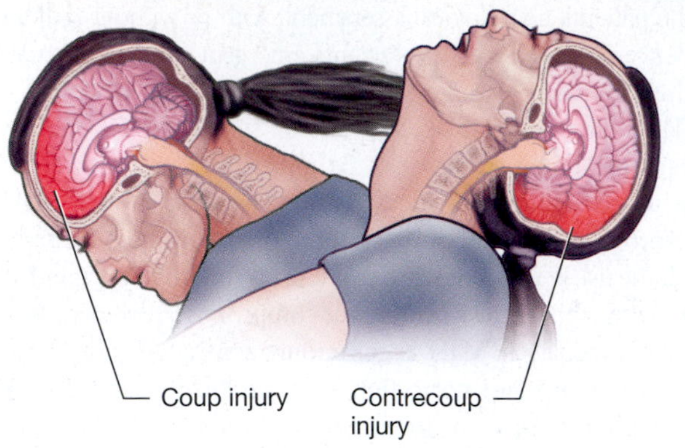

FIGURE 21–12 ◆ Coup and contrecoup injuries.

herniation. A patient with a frontal contusion may be alert, though possibly confused, and may be monitored in the hospital for a short period of time with no obvious consequences. However, the patient may experience more obvious neuropsychological deficits such as disinhibition in social situations; therefore, careful observation of the patient's cognitive status is warranted. For this reason, patients with neurocognitive deficits often require 24-hour care following discharge.

Diagnostic Procedures

As with all cerebral traumas, a thorough and accurate history is important. Diagnosis is made by radiographic detection on imaging studies to evaluate for the presence of contusion and possibly edema. Serial CT scans over several days may be warranted to assess the contusion's size as the brain heals. "Blossoming" or expansion of the contusion may occur at approximately 3 days.

Medical Management

Once the diagnosis of cerebral contusion is made, along with determination of the location and size of the contusion(s), treatment depends on the patient's neurological condition. Close monitoring of the patient's neurological assessment is important. Monitoring of the ICP (p. 508) may be necessary, since cerebral edema may be present.

Seizures may be a presenting sign; therefore, use of AEDs may be necessary. Prophylactic use of AEDs is controversial because of the potential risk of seizures, though some health care providers believe that their use is warranted for a limited time (usually 7 days) (Biros & Heegaard, 2009).

Hyponatremia is another common sequela to TBI. Hyponatremia results from dilution, osmotic therapies, inappropriate secretion of antidiuretic hormone, or cerebral salt wasting. Cerebral salt-wasting syndrome is defined as the development of extracellular volume depletion due to a renal sodium transport abnormality in patients with intracranial disease and normal adrenal and thyroid function" (Wedro, 2012). Management includes both salt supplementation and fluid restriction (Anderson, 2009).

Concussion

Concussion refers to a recognized collection of symptoms as a result of mild head injury. It is described as a temporary neurological dysfunction caused by an external force to the head. It is also described as a "shaking of the brain."

Clinical Manifestations

Concussion is associated with a myriad of symptoms, including confusion, possible brief loss of consciousness, headache, intellectual impairment, and memory loss. Concussion is characterized by a completely normal neurological exam with the inability to indicate a localizing process such as sensory changes, unilateral weakness, or difficulty ambulating The American Academy of Neurology grading scale is widely used to grade concussions (Rangel-Castilla 2011). This scale categorizes concussions according to three grades, with Grade 3 being the most severe and indicating a brief or prolonged loss of consciousness. However, some practitioners have abandoned the use of a grading scale and have chosen instead to use a symptom-oriented approach to determine the concussion's severity and its probability of being resolved. With perceived resolution of the concussion, the individual is able to resume all activities. This is particularly relevant to individuals who engage in sports activity and is referred to as a symptom-based approach to determining the concussion's severity (Halstead, Walter, & The Council on Sports Medicine and Fitness, 2010). Symptoms are evaluated in four categories: physical, cognitive, emotional, and sleep. The severity of the concussions and subsequent resumption of activity are determined according to the evidence of symptoms: physical performance, cognition (e.g., able to focus on school work), emotional response to the injury, and sleep pattern (whether the patient is able to sleep and, if so, whether the pattern is normal or abnormal) (Halstead, Walter, & The Council on Sports Medicine and Fitness, 2010).

Diagnostic Procedures

An accurate history of the event is essential, including questions regarding how long, if at all, the patient was unconscious; the presence of confusion; and the length of time until the symptoms subside. No radiographic findings are associated with concussions. However, if the patient has a focal neurological exam or an extended period of unconsciousness, the patient should be admitted to the hospital, and a CT of the head should be obtained to rule out other, more serious brain trauma.

Medical Management

The management of the concussion depends on the grade that has been determined. However, the treatment recommendations are merely guidelines. Each patient should be assessed individually, and the treatment should be planned according to the particular symptoms that are displayed, such as loss of consciousness, length of unconsciousness, inability to concentrate, headache, and vomiting.

Second-Impact Syndrome

Second-impact syndrome is characterized by a second concussion, within several weeks, that occurs before the brain can completely recover from the first concussion. The brain loses its ability to autoregulate intracranial and cerebral perfusion pressures, which then can lead to cerebral edema followed by brain herniation (Bey & Ostick, 2009). Because of poor brain compliance, persistent vascular congestion and increased ICP persist. This condition may persist for an indeterminate length of time. Because second-impact syndrome is the result of a second injury before the brain has recovered from the first injury, the result can be massive cerebral edema and possibly death. An example of this is the athlete who continues playing football after receiving one or more concussions and then collapses and dies on the sidelines after an apparent mild injury. The mortality rate is 50%, and the morbidity rate is 100% (Burns, Dunn, Brady, Starr, & Blosser, 2008). For this reason, patients should be counseled about the advisability of continuing risk-taking activities after receiving an initial concussion. Well-recognized return-to-play guidelines are now used that take a stepwise approach. The athlete has a period of rest and, when symptom free, may return to limited non-contact activity. The athlete progresses gradually each week toward full play if no symptoms such as headache or recurrent cognitive problems are experienced. However, the player must repeat the previous step if symptoms recur (Bey & Ostick, 2009).

Postconcussion Syndrome

Postconcussion syndrome is a condition that follows mild head injury and is characterized by one or more of the following symptoms: headaches (especially with exertion), dizziness, vertigo, tinnitus, hearing loss, blurred vision, light and/or noise sensitivity, alteration in smell, anxiety, depression, personality change, sleep disorders, decreased libido, decreased appetite, memory loss, alteration in cognitive function, personality changes, and physical or cognitive decline. The person should be evaluated by a CT and neuropsychiatric test prior to being allowed to return to play (DeLee, Drez, & Miller, 2009). Since there is an incomplete understanding of the etiology of symptoms after the event, the goal for postconcussive symptoms is to improve identified problems rather than affect a cure (Blyth & Bazarian, 2010). Counseling may be helpful to cope with personal and work-related problems.

Diffuse Axonal Injury

Diffuse axonal injury (DAI) is one of the most common and important pathologic features of TBI. DAI is defined as a diffuse injury to the white matter that results in tearing or shearing of axons and small blood vessels (Pangilinan, 2011). The main mechanical force that causes DAI is rotational acceleration of the brain, which results in unrestricted head movement. The shearing allows neurons to be pulled apart at the microscopic level; therefore, this tearing often it is not visible on imaging studies. However, magnetic resonance imaging (MRI) may detect small DAI lesions. Patients with DAI typically present in neurological compromise, such as coma, with decerebrate or decorticate posturing as described on page 511. Surgery is not indicated because the injury is diffuse. Treatment is determined by the patient's neurological presentation and usually is supportive. Support of respiratory and hemodynamic functions may be warranted. DAI is classified as mild, moderate, or severe. Patients with mild DAI may have only mild long-term cognitive disabilities, whereas severe DAI is associated with significant mortality and long-term disabilities.

Nursing Management

Nursing care of TBI patients has several goals. The first is protection of the patient's neurological function. This is accomplished by a thorough neurological assessment aimed at determining the patient's LOC and possible focal neurological deficits. Second, there is a need to prevent development of complications from the initial injury.

Assessment

A good neurological assessment is essential for communication between medical personnel as well as to establish a baseline for the nurse so she can detect changes. A tool such as the GCS is helpful in providing standardized information to other medical personnel. The GCS is a scoring system that is widely used in quantifying LOC following traumatic brain injury. The scale and its scoring mechanism are discussed in detail in Chapter 20. Any unfavorable change in a neurological exam, even the most subtle, may indicate deterioration in the patient's

NATIONAL GUIDELINES CDC Screening Instrument for Detection of Mild TBI

Questions

1. At the time of your trauma, did you experience any period of transient confusion, disorientation, or impaired consciousness?
2. At the time of your trauma, did you experience any dysfunction of memory?
3. Did you experience any of the following in relation to your trauma: seizures, headache, dizziness, irritability, fatigue, or poor concentration?
4. At the time of your trauma, did you experience any loss of consciousness lasting 30 minutes or less?

An answer of "yes" on any of these questions indicates mild TBI.

Source: Centers for Disease Control and Prevention. (2010b). Injury prevention & control. Retrieved from http://www.cdc.gov/TraumaticBrainInjury/index.html.

Weblink: Detection of Mild TBI

condition and is reportable. The National Guidelines box lists the questions used by the CDC to screen for detection of mild TBI.

TBI may be a mild head injury, such as a concussion or cerebral contusion, or it may be a severe, life-threatening situation. Other serious, life-threatening conditions also may be present. Patients with severe injury or potentially severe conditions are usually admitted to the ICU and monitored carefully. It is imperative to remember the ABCs of patient management with any trauma patient. Assessing and securing an adequate airway are always a primary consideration. Trauma victims frequently have respiratory compromise due to a number of factors, including other injuries. Whether a patient is severely injured and intubated or awake and talking, maintenance of an adequate airway is essential. Rate and quality of respirations should be assessed initially and then on an ongoing basis. A pulse oximeter may be of assistance in early determination of respiratory decline. This is especially important if the patient has an altered LOC. Any patient with a GCS score of 8 or less, with 15 being considered normal, should be considered for intubation. Maintenance of adequate oxygenation is an important tenet of ICP management.

Safety Alert *Patients with a decreased level of consciousness are at risk for aspiration and respiratory compromise. The nurse should monitor respiratory status carefully, suction as needed, and ensure airway protection.*

Assessment of adequate circulation is the last part of the ABCs of life support. Patients with TBI may exhibit alterations in circulatory function, such as bradycardia, hypotension, or hypertension. These patients also may be hemodynamically unstable due to blood loss secondary to trauma. Therefore, the initial nursing assessment must include a complete set of vital signs and a thorough assessment of the patient's circulatory status. After the initial ABCs of patient management, the most common concern for nurses caring for patients with TBI is that of increased ICP. Many patients with TBI require placement of a device to monitor ICP, previously described on page 511. The nursing management of patients with increased ICP was addressed earlier in this chapter. The Nursing Process: Patient Care Plan for Acute Brain Disorders (p. 523) includes nursing diagnoses, expected outcomes, and nursing interventions for patients with TBI.

TBI is almost always unexpected and usually comes at a time that finds both patients and their families unprepared. The early period of hospitalization requires critical thinking and astute assessment skills. It always requires understanding, empathy, and strong emotional support. Nurses may be equipped with the skills needed to care for TBI patients efficiently, but skills to appropriately care for families of patients with devastating, perhaps potentially fatal injuries are also extremely important. Families of severely injured patients are frequently overwhelmed, often angry, and commonly in denial. The nurse caring for their injured family member may be their only link for communication, support, and encouragement. It is important to keep the family as involved as they want to be in the care of their family member, as informed as possible, and given as much control as is possible. Experienced nurses often relate that the most frequent complaint heard from families is that they "don't know what is going on." It also is important to answer questions honestly, educating the family about the treatment plan and the expected rehabilitation process. Determining brain death in patients and working with patients' family members are discussed in the Ethical Issues box.

ETHICAL ISSUES Related to Brain Death

Brain death can be defined as damage to the brain that is irreversible and extensive to the point at which there is no potential for recovery. Criteria for the determination of brain death have been established in the United States by the Uniform Determination of Death Act adopted in 1980 (Uniform Law Commission, 2010). This Act recognizes cardiorespiratory and brain death in accordance with the criteria the medical profession universally accepts; however, the Act itself presents an ethical issue (Center for Bioethics, University of Minnesota, 2005; The Book of Doctrines and Opinions, 2011).

- While the Act allows for consistent criteria for determining death in all states, it also raises the question as to whether the Act's intention is to increase the number of organs available for transplant.
- The Act helps to reduce confusion and unnecessary delay for prompt retrieval of donated organs, but does it lead to misdiagnosis of brain death?
- The Act allows for accurate time of death declarations, but the use of the definition of brain death over and above cessation of heart and lung function remains debatable.
- The Act focuses on the human organism as a whole and recognizes the brain's role in the body's function as a complete organism, yet one may question whether irreversible loss of vital organ functioning (heart, lungs, brain) depends on whether or not a person can be revived. Revival may depend on the availability of CPR treatments and technologies, which can vary from location to location, and on the decision made by those present about whether to use these treatments and technologies.

It may be argued that the loss of brainstem function is an unnecessary requirement for brain death. A person dies when there is a loss of personhood, which comes from the functioning of the higher brain, the cerebrum and the cerebellum, and not the brainstem. Controversy remains over the definition and interpretation of brain death from bioethics, philosophical, and religious perspectives (The George Washington University Medical Center, 2008). Specific ethical issues to be considered when declaring brain death include the following:

- Who is making the decision to declare the individual brain dead? Is it the health care provider? Is there a conflict of interest related to a research study, an organ transplant option, or a personal religious or cultural philosophy?
- Are the religious and cultural values of the patient and the patient's family being considered?
- Is the patient really dead if the patient's body continues to maintain a degree of organ and tissue capacity, such as maintaining body temperature and eliminating wastes?
- Have the patient's rights to make decisions been violated? Who is authorized to make that decision? (Bagheri, 2007)

Persistent Vegetative State

The term **persistent vegetative state (PVS)** was proposed by Jennett and Plum (1972) to describe the state following coma in some patients who have experienced severe brain injury. In a PVS, the patient is in an awakened state without cognitive awareness. PVS patients have sleep–wake cycles, their eyes open spontaneously, and they maintain normal vital signs, including respiratory function. However, there is no attempt to follow commands or to communicate. In addition, there is no evidence of cognition.

Patients in a PVS may survive many years following a brain injury. This often presents a very difficult situation for the family. It is helpful if a living will is available and the patient and family have had discussions about the prolongation of life in a situation in which quality of life appears minimal at best.

Family conferences with health care providers, nurses, therapists, social workers, and clergy frequently are helpful in determining prognosis, including quality of life. Discussions involving discontinuance of medical treatment, including nutrition, are difficult and should be done with the patient's living will and/or advance directive. Assuring the family that such decisions are reflections of the patient's own wishes may be comforting and may assuage feelings of guilt or responsibility.

As the care plan for patients with acute brain disorders demonstrates, nursing interventions are both multifaceted and critical to the patient's treatment plan. The Evidence-Based Practice box addresses the multiplicity of nursing interventions and the manner in which they are performed.

Collaborative Management

The patient with TBI faces multifaceted challenges and requires an interdisciplinary focus. with active ollaboration among many specialists and ancillary services. In order to meet desired patient outcomes, it is essential that this interdisciplinary team communicate openly with one another in developing and evaluating care of the patient and family (IOM [Institute of Medicine], 2010). Medically, it is not uncommon for a TBI patient to be under the care of several health care providers, such as a pulmonologist to manage respiratory problems, a neurologist to manage seizures, an orthopedic surgeon and/or a trauma surgeon to manage coexisting injuries, and possibly a critical care specialist.

It also is important to have a dietitian involved in the TBI patient's care. Metabolic needs should be determined to ensure that the patient's caloric needs are met. TBI patients often require enteral feedings, and the type and amount are important to ensure that the patient receives the appropriate nutrition. Nutrition should be started as soon as it is medically possible (see Chapter 8).

Most TBI patients will, at some point in their hospital stay, require physical therapists, occupational therapists, and possibly recreational therapists. Speech pathologists also may be called on to assess the patient's swallow function as well as cognitive function. Sometimes a neuropsychologist will be consulted to assess higher cognitive function and to help determine the safety and feasibility of the patient either returning home or to a previous occupation. In some hospitals, a psychiatrist specializing in rehabilitation may be consulted to facilitate post-hospital therapies. Many TBI patients benefit from a post-hospital stay in a rehabilitation facility to prepare them for return to home and their previous lives.

NURSING PROCESS: Patient Care Plan for Acute Brain Disorders

Assessment of Neurologic Status Using Gordon's Functional Health Patterns:

- Nutrition Metabolic Pattern
- Activity Exercise Pattern
- Coping-Stress Tolerance Pattern
- Cognitive Perceptual Pattern

Subjective Data	Objective Data
Assessment of Altered Levels of Consciousness	**Assessment of Altered Levels of Consciousness**
Does the patient have any history of health problems, such as hypertension, heart disease, bleeding disorders, renal disease, or cancer? What were the patient's presenting symptoms/complaints? How long ago did the first symptoms present?	Neurological assessment, including mentation, cranial nerve examination, and motor and sensory examination. Imaging studies, including magnetic resonance imaging (MRI), computed tomography (CT) scan, and/or lumbar puncture. Laboratory data, including complete blood count (CBC), cerebral perfusion pressure (CPP), and drug levels.
Assessment of Airway and Gas Exchange	**Assessment of Airway and Gas Exchange**
Does the patient have any preexisting medical problems such as emphysema or asthma, or any cardiac diseases?	Respiratory rate (RR) Oxygen saturation (SpO_2) Arterial blood gases (ABGs) Vital signs Lung sounds Skin/nail bed/lip color
Assessment of Hemodynamic Status	**Assessment of Hemodynamic Status**
Does the patient have any preexisting cardiac or respiratory problems?	Vital signs, including heart rate (HR), blood pressure (BP), respiratory rate (RR), and central venous pressure (CVP), if available Oxygen saturation (SpO_2) Skin, lips, and nail bed color Lung sounds Cardiac rhythm strips or ECG
Assessment of Pain	**Assessment of Pain**
Does the patient complain of pain? Show negative facial expressions (i.e., grimacing)?	Increased heart rate (HR), blood pressure (BP), or respiratory rate (RR)?
Assessment of Coping	**Assessment of Coping**
What are the patient's complaints? What is the patient's understanding of the present condition or disease? What are the patient's concerns for the future?	What is the patient's level of education? What is the patient's occupation? What is the patient's family support system? Does the patient have a religious affiliation?

Outcomes and Evaluation Parameters	Planning and Interventions with *Rationales*
1a. NURSING DIAGNOSIS: Actual and Potential Alteration in Level of Consciousness ***related to traumatic brain injury (TBI), intracranial tumor, or infectious process*** **(NANDA-I © 2012)**	
Outcome: Improvement to optimum level of function. ***Evaluation Parameters:*** Stable neurological examination. Glasgow Coma Scale. Laboratory tests, including serum sodium and cultures of blood and cerebrospinal fluid (CSF), if suspicious for infection.	Monitor neurological examination hourly, or as directed. *Allows early recognition of pending neurological deterioration.* Monitor lab values, including serum sodium levels and cultures. *Early recognition and treatment of hyponatremia or infection.*
1b. NURSING DIAGNOSIS: Impaired Physical Mobility ***related to altered level of consciousness*** **(NANDA-I © 2012)**	
Outcome: Improvement to optimum level of motor function. ***Evaluation Parameters:*** Neurological motor and sensory examination. Level of participation in therapies and ADLs.	Monitor motor strengths and limitations. *Allows early recognition of neurological changes.* Initiate therapies, such as physical and occupational, unless contraindicated. *Early initiation of therapies helps to identify deficits and needed areas for improvement.* Initiate activity as tolerated, unless contraindicated. *Physical activity will increase strength and endurance, as well as decrease complications, such as pneumonia or blood clots.*

(continued)

NURSING PROCESS: Patient Care Plan for Acute Brain Disorders, *continued*

Outcomes and Evaluation Parameters	Planning and Interventions with *Rationales*
1c. NURSING DIAGNOSIS: Ineffective Tissue Perfusion *related to immobility* (NANDA-I © 2012)	
Outcome: Adequate tissue perfusion. ***Evaluation Parameters:*** Absence of deep vein thrombosis (DVTs) or pulmonary embolus.	Encourage activity as tolerated, unless contraindicated. *Physical activity will prevent immobility and the formation of blood clots.* Apply thigh-high elastic stockings and sequential compression stockings *to increase venous circulation.* Administer subcutaneous injections of low-molecular-weight heparin, if indicated *to discourage the formation of blood clots.* Monitor lower extremities frequently for signs/symptoms of DVT. *Early recognition and treatment of a DVT may prevent extension of the clot or pulmonary embolus.*
1d. NURSING DIAGNOSIS: Impaired Verbal Communication *related to anatomic defect* (NANDA-I © 2012)	
Outcome: Maximum level of communication. ***Evaluation Parameter:*** Ability to adequately communicate with others.	Assess type and degree of communication deficit *to determine patient needs and establish a baseline.* Arrange a speech therapy consult. *Early intervention and therapy optimize results.*
1e. NURSING DIAGNOSIS: Actual or Potential Alteration in Visual Perception *related to TBI or brain tumor* (NANDA-I © 2012)	
Outcome: Maximum level of vision/visual acuity. ***Evaluation Parameter:*** Formal and informal vision screening including visual fields.	Assess vision by informal testing (i.e., counting fingers, reading the clock) *to assess type and degree of visual deficit present.* Institute safety measures, such as placing call light within reach or orienting patient to surroundings, *to prevent accidents/falls.* Obtain occupational therapy evaluation if warranted. *Evaluation of visual deficits and education regarding coping mechanisms.*
1f. NURSING DIAGNOSIS: Ineffective Cerebral Tissue Perfusion *related to electrolyte imbalances in TBI, brain tumors, or infectious process* (NANDA-I © 2012)	
Outcome: Optimum neurological function. ***Evaluation Parameters:*** Stable neurological examination. Electrolyte levels, specifically sodium.	Monitor serum sodium as indicated, at least daily, *to assess for hyponatremia.* Conduct neurological assessments frequently *to assess for decreased level of consciousness.* Administer fluids as directed *to maintain adequate fluid balance.* Notify health care providers immediately of abnormal lab values or change in neurological examination. *Such changes may indicate hyponatremia.*
2a. NURSING DIAGNOSIS: Ineffective Airway Clearance *related to altered level of consciousness* (NANDA-I © 2012)	
Outcome: Adequate respiration status. ***Evaluation Parameters:*** Adequate arterial blood gases. Respiratory rate within normal limits. Normal oxygen saturation levels. Clear lung sounds. Mental status, such as confusion or agitation.	Monitor respiratory status (i.e., rate, rhythm, and quality). *Changes in respiratory rates or patterns may indicate pending respiratory failure. It may also indicate neurological change.* Monitor mental status. *Restlessness, agitation, or confusion may indicate hypoxia.* Monitor oxygen saturation *to assess adequacy of gas exchange.* Encourage deep breathing or use of an incentive spirometer *to promote adequate gas exchange.* Position with head in neutral position, head of bed elevated at 30 degrees, unless contraindicated *to promote adequate gas exchange.* Suction as necessary. *Patients with decreased neurological status may be unable to protect their airways.* Report changes in respiratory patterns to MD. *Such changes indicate possible risk for respiratory failure.* If patient not intubated, have necessary intubation equipment available. *Protecting the airway is the priority. Intubation may be necessary to protect airway.*
2b. NURSING DIAGNOSIS: Risk for Aspiration *related to altered level of consciousness* (NANDA-I © 2012)	
Outcome: No aspiration. ***Evaluation Parameters:*** Adequate oxygen saturation. Safe swallowing techniques.	Keep NPO until alert and/or swallow reflex is assessed and deemed safe. *Altered level of consciousness may depress the cough and/or swallow reflex.*

NURSING PROCESS: Patient Care Plan for Acute Brain Disorders, *continued*

Outcomes and Evaluation Parameters	Planning and Interventions with *Rationales*
3. NURSING DIAGNOSIS: Decreased intracranial adaptive capacity *related to increased intracranial pressure* (NANDA-I © 2012)	
Outcome: Hemodynamic stability. ***Evaluation Parameter:*** Adequate mean arterial blood pressure (MAP) to maintain central perfusion pressure (CPP). CPP = MAP – ICP. Stable vital signs, including central venous pressure (CVP), pulmonary arterial pressure (PAP), and intracranial pressure (ICP).	Monitor vital signs as directed *to establish a baseline and note changes in vital signs.* Administer fluids and medications as directed *to assist in maintaining blood pressure as ordered to maintain adequate CPP.* Monitor ECG rhythm *to assess for alterations in rhythm or rate.* Monitor intake and output *to assess fluid balance to maintain hemodynamic parameters.* Notify health care provider of hemodynamic changes. *Medical intervention may be necessary to prevent hemodynamic instability leading to neurological decline.* Monitor neurological assessments closely. *Hemodynamic stability is closely related to CPP and ICP changes in neurologically compromised patients.*
4. NURSING DIAGNOSIS: Readiness for Enhanced Comfort *related to brain tumor, head injury, meningitis, or surgical procedure* (NANDA-I © 2012)	
Outcome: Adequate pain control. ***Evaluation Parameters:*** Vital signs within normal limits. Patient verbalizes pain control.	Assess presence of pain or efficacy of pain control frequently *to ensure patient comfort.* Administer pain medications as ordered *to ensure patient comfort.*
5a. NURSING DIAGNOSIS: Ineffective Coping *related to knowledge deficit* (NANDA-I © 2012)	
Outcome: Patient and family will have information needed. ***Evaluation Parameter:*** Discussions with patient, with verbalization of condition and treatment.	Provide information as needed and answer questions honestly and completely. *Information and education are important to the patient.* Involve family as appropriate. *Family support is important for recovery.*
5b. NURSING DIAGNOSIS: Readiness for Enhanced Family Coping *related to neurological deficits* (NANDA-I © 2012)	
Outcome: Family will have improved coping with neurological disability. ***Evaluation Parameters:*** Discussions with patient and family with verbalization of concerns. Observation of family/patient interactions.	Reassure patient and family with honesty and compassion *to provide encouragement and information needed for coping.* Encourage family members to voice concerns *to help with assessment of family needs.* Provide family with support as needed, such as spiritual, therapies, or psychological. *Neurological disability affects the whole family and community.*

Source: Adapted from Wilkinson, J. M., & Ahearn, N. R. (2009). *Prentice Hall nursing diagnosis handbook* (9th ed.). Upper Saddle River, NJ: Prentice Hall.

Social services may be called on to assist in attaining resources the patient and family may need. Many patients and their families find TBI support groups to be helpful. This is especially important for the families of patients who need long-term rehabilitation or those experiencing significant changes in their jobs and/or lifestyles. Nursing support is important in providing and encouraging care for the caregiver in addition to providing and guiding care for the patient.

Health Promotion

The most important principle of TBI management is prevention. A vast number of programs in hospitals and communities nationwide are aimed at the prevention of TBI. Community education and public awareness programs are essential. Such programs include the promotion of helmets for bicycle and motorcycle riders and seat belt laws, which are known to have an effect on the severity of TBI due to motor vehicle collisions. Patient and public education on how to prevent a brain injury is critical. The following items should be covered:

- Wear a seat belt every time you drive or ride in a motor vehicle. The lap belt and shoulder belt should be secured across the pelvis and rib cage, respectively.
- Always buckle your child into a child safety seat, booster seat, or seat belt.
- Have children under the age of 13 ride in the back seat.
- Never drive under the influence of alcohol.
- Wear a helmet when riding a bicycle, motorcycle, or snowmobile; playing a contact sport; skating; riding a scooter; sledding; skiing or snowboarding; or horseback riding. The helmet needs to be fitted properly so it stays in place and does not limit visibility.
- When bicycling use protective clothing and to wear bright colors on reflective materials so they can be more easily seen.
- Avoid falls in the home by using a step stool to reach high objects, installing and using handrails on stairs, installing window guards to keep young children from falling out of open windows, and removing tripping hazards such as throw rugs and electrical cords.
- Use nonslip mats in the tub and shower.
- Place grab bars next to the toilet and in the tub or shower.
- Maintain a regular exercise program to improve strength, balance, and coordination.

Weblink: Hospital Admissions for TBI Weblink: Secondary Brain Injury

EVIDENCE-BASED PRACTICE Traumatic Brain Injury

Clinical Problem

TBI is a major health problem globally that occurs with varying degrees of severity and disability. Although it can affect people of all ages, the CDC (2010b) states that children ages 0 to 4, adolescents ages 15 to 19, and adults ages 65 years and older are most likely to sustain a TBI.

It is estimated that 71% of TBI hospitalizations are for patients with severe injuries necessitating critical care monitoring (Russo & Steiner, 2007). Neuroscience critical care nurses play an integral role in the care of the critically ill TBI patient, yet there is little evidence that documents specific interventions and clarifies the nurses' role on the interdisciplinary health care team. Evidence also is needed to analyze nursing judgments based on current standards of practice and existing therapies and to provide the foundation for determining how nurses impact patient and family recovery from TBI during the acute phase of injury (McNett & Gianakis, 2010).

Research Findings

Several descriptive reports have identified nursing interventions for critically ill TBI patients (Ladanyl & Elliot, 2008; Littlejohns & Bader, 2009). Reported responsibilities include monitoring patients' physiological parameters and ensuring hemodynamic stability, performing serial neurological examinations, preventing secondary injury, and providing emotional support for patients and families. With the advent of advanced technologies, additional responsibilities such as monitoring and maintenance of brain tissue oxygenation were added (Littlejohns & Bader, 2009). Collectively, a multifaceted role for nurses was described.

The presence of signs and symptoms also was determined to be an influencing factor in performing nursing interventions (McNett, Doheny, Sedlak, & Ludwick, 2010). For example, nursing judgments were influcenced by worsening values for oxygen saturation, ICP, and CPP (McNett, 2009). As values for oxygen saturation, ICP, and CPP fall farther from recommended parameters, nurses are quicker to consult with other members of the health care team before intervening.

Shift was also found to be a significant factor affecting nursing decsions (McNett, Doheny, Sedlak, & Ludwick, 2010). Nurses who work a day shift are more likely to rely solely on nursing interventions and less likely to consult with health care team members than are those working the night shift.

Prevention of complications was also evaluated by McNett, Doheny, Sedlak, and Ludwick (2010). These researchers found that when providing care to patients with subarachnoid hemorrhage, neuroscience critical care nurses were influenced by knowledge of current standards and therapies for fluid and hydration management.

In 2009, (McNett & Gianakis, 2010) conducted a study to determine which physiological and situational variables influence nursing judgments and actions regarding patients' risk for secondary brain injury. They also gathered data on whether patient management was dependent solely on nursing interventions or included consulting another member of the health care team. A multiple segment factorial anonymous survey design was administered to 67 nurses working in three ICUs at two Level I trauma centers who routinely cared for critically ill TBI patients. The survey consisted of three parts: (1) a series of questions about the last patient cared for, (2) a randomly generated case, and (3) demographic information about the nurse respondent. The registered nurse participants met three predetermined admission criteria: an active state license, employment as a clinical bedside nurse in an ICU that admits critically ill TBI patients, and employment in the current ICU for a minimum of 3 months.

Results of the study indicated that judgments about the risk for secondary brain injury were influenced by the patient's oxygen saturation, ICP, CPP, mechanism of injury, and primary diagnosis, as well as by nursing shift. The initial judgments made by nurses were the most significant variable predictive of follow-up judgments ($P < 0.001$). A significant difference also was found ($P < 0.001$) when the decision to consult another member of the health care team before making a nursing intervention was compared to making a solely independent nursing judgment (McNett et al., 2010). The four types of nursing interventions described—neurophysiological, psychosocial, injury prevention, and maintaining a therapeutic milieu—indicate that neuroscience ICU nurses must possess extensive knowledge of the pathophysiological processes associated with primary and secondary brain injury. They also must have the technical skills to manage these processes effectively and ensure neurological stability. Finally, excellent interpersonal skills are critical to communicating with family and other members of the health care team (McNett & Gianakis, 2010).

Implications for Nursing Practice

Nursing practice is increasingly influenced by evidence-based standards, and nurses are expected to be knowledgeable about research findings and clinical guidelines affecting their area of expertise. In the study by McNett et al. (2010), this would be neurological intensive care, specifically TBI. Findings from the study demonstrate how physiological and situational variables influenced ICU nurses' judgments about secondary brain injury. The findings highlight the need for standardized evidence-based content for ICU nurses regarding management of secondary brain injury. Information gained from this study may be used to guide nurses' educational initiatives and serve as a basis for future research on the educational interventions regarding the incidence of secondary brain injury and patient outcomes (McNett et al., 2010).

Critical Thinking Questions with answers can be found in the Osborn Student Resources at nursing.pearsonhighered.com.

References

Centers for Disease Control and Prevention (CDC). (2010b). Injury prevention & control. Retrieved from http://www.cdc.gov/TraumaticBrainInjury/index.html.

Ladanyl, S., & Elliot, D. (2008). Traumatic brain injury: An integrated clinical case presentation and literature review Part II: The continuum of care. *Australian Critical Care, 21*, 141–153.

Littlejohns, L., & Bader, M. K. (2009). *Monitoring technologies in critically ill neuroscience patients.* Sudbury, MA: Jones and Bartlett Publishers.

McNett, M. (2009). Intensive care unit nurse characteristics impacting judgments about secondary brain injury. *Dimensions of Critical Care Nursing, 28*, 182–188.

McNett, M., Doheny, M., Sedlak, C. A., & Ludwick, R.(2010). Judgments of critical care nurses about risk for secondary brain injury. *American Journal of Critical Care. 19*(3), 250-260. Retrieved from http://www.ncbi.nlm.nih.gov/pubmed/19542058.

McNett, M. M., & Gianakis, A. (2010). Nursing interventions for critically ill traumatic brain injury patients. *Journal of Neuroscience Nursing, 42*(2), 71–77.

Russo, C., & Steiner, C. (2007). *Hospital admissions for traumatic brain injuries, 2004* (HCUP Statistical Brief 27). Rockville, MD: Agency for Healthcare Research and Quality. Retrieved from http://www.hcupus.ahrg.gov/reports/statbriefs/sb27.pdf [Context Link].

- Have vision checked regularly to reduce the risk of falling.
- Keep firearms and bullets stored separately in a locked cabinet or safe when not in use (NHTSA, 2009).

In addition to preventive measures, health promotion related to brain injury includes factors directly related to helping the patient and family manage care at home. Specific instructions on how to control pain, avoid infections, achieve mobility, and gain emotional support for self and family are provided in the Patient Teaching & Discharge Priorities for Acute Brain Disorders box.

Infectious Diseases of the Central Nervous System

Meningitis, encephalitis, and cerebral abscesses are examples of infections of the central nervous system (CNS). These infections are caused by a number of pathogens including common bacteria, fungi, and viruses.

Meningitis

Meningitis is defined as an inflammation of the meninges. **Bacterial meningitis** is an inflammation of the meninges caused by a

PATIENT TEACHING & DISCHARGE PRIORITIES for Acute Brain Disorders

Need	Teaching
Wound infection: Patient/family support system	Assess surgical wound for signs/symptoms of infection, which include redness, tenderness, exudate and/or odor, swelling, and delayed healing. The presence of fever or any of the previous symptoms should be reported. Assess family knowledge and ability for wound management and provide support for needed assistance.
Mobility assistance: Patient/family support system Setting	Assess motor strengths and ability for ambulation. Obtain consults for physical and occupational therapy. Assess need for assistive devices, such as wheelchair, walker, or splints. Assess availability of family for support with mobility and activities of daily living (ADLs). Assess environment for risk factors.
Pain Management: Patient/family support system	Assess need for pain control. Is present medication regimen adequate? Is pain controlled sufficiently to allow patient to participate in ADLs? Assess need for family intervention in dispensing pain medication. Assess patient/family understanding of medication instructions.
Safety: Patient/family support system and setting	Assess patient cognitive status: Is patient at risk for falls? Assess safety awareness. Assess patient's understanding of medication schedule and needs. Assess patient's need for supervision. Conduct family teaching regarding need for supervision. Obtain consults for speech and cognitive evaluation. Obtain social service consult. Obtain home health consult. Assess family involvement in patient's recuperative period. Conduct family teaching regarding possible cognitive impairments. Assess environment for safety. May require home health or social service involvement.
Follow-up needs: Patient/family/support system and setting	Assess need for follow-up appointments for needed therapies or interventions: Outpatient therapies: physical, occupational, speech Health care provider appointments Laboratory visits for evaluation of drug levels or electrolytes Follow-up x-rays. Assess availability of resources for follow-up.

bacterial pathogen. **Viral meningitis** is an inflammation of the meninges caused by viral pathogens, such as herpes simplex virus, mumps, measles, or any other virus.

Epidemiology

Bacterial Meningitis

Despite the introduction and widespread use of antibiotics in addition to other advances in medical care, meningitis still has a high morbidity and mortality rate. Though the incidence of bacterial meningitis has fallen dramatically in the last 10 years, 31% from 1998 to 2007 (Thigpen, Whitney, Messonnier, et al., 2011), it remains a significant source of morbidity and mortality (Razonable, 2011a). The incidence of bacterial meningitis is about 0.6 to 4 cases per 100,000 population per year, with the greatest incidence in the pediatric population (Razonable, 2011a). Seppa (2011) estimates that 4,100 cases of bacterial meningitis occur annually in the United States. Risk factors for bacterial meningitis include the following: immunocompromised conditions due to immune system disorders such as HIV, organ transplantation, and radiation therapy; malnutrition: alcoholism; diabetes mellitus; and recent dental therapy (Bader & Littlejohns, 2010).

The patient's prognosis depends on multiple factors including age, presence of comorbidities, responsible pathogen, degree of severity at presentation, and degree of neurological impairment on admission (Mace, 2008; Razonable, 2011b).

Viral Meningitis

Viral meningitis is more common than bacterial meningitis but is less likely to be fatal unless the patient has a weakened immune system (Seppa, 2011). Viral meningitis accounts for approximately 26,000 to 42,000 hospitalizations each year in the United States, affecting mainly infants younger than 1 year of age and children 5 to 10 years of age, although it may affect older individuals as well (Di Pentima, 2012). The incidence of viral meningitis usually increases during the summer and fall. Epidemics of viral meningitis are uncommon (CDC, 2011; Wan, 2011).

Etiology and Pathophysiology

The most common cause of meningeal inflammation is irritation caused by bacterial or viral infections. Bacterial meningitis usually is characterized by an acute onset of meningeal symptoms and neutrophilic pleocytosis (an increase in the normal number of white blood cells in the CSF). Depending on the specific bacterial cause, this syndrome may be called haemophilus meningitis or Hib meningitis, staphylococcal meningitis, meningococcal meningitis, or tuberculous meningitis (Razonable, 2011a). Meningitis affects the layers of the meninges and the subarachnoid space. The brain is naturally protected from the body's immune system by a barrier that the meninges create between the bloodstream and the brain. However, with meningitis, the barrier becomes problematic. Once bacteria or other organisms have found their way to the brain, they are somewhat isolated from the immune system and can spread, triggering an inflammatory process. When the body tries to fight the infection, the problem can worsen; blood vessels become leaky and allow fluid, white blood cells (WBCs), and other infectious fighting materials to enter the meninges and brain. This, in turn, causes brain swelling and eventually results in decreased blood flow to the brain (Muller, 2011; Razonable, 2011a).

Bacteria can enter the meninges by various methods and structures. Bloodborne pathogens are the most common route for transporting bacteria to the meninges and subarachnoid space. Other routes include through the sinuses, the inner ear, dental procedures, or endocarditis. A dural tear caused by trauma or surgery can create a route for the introduction of pathogens via the CSF. Patients with skull fractures, for example, have a pathway to the CSF. If a route is available for CSF to leave the body, organisms have a route to enter the body. Unsterile technique during surgical procedures, including lumbar puncture, placement of an external ventricular drain (EVD), or collection of CSF from an EVD, is a method of introducing organisms into the CSF.

Viral meningitis typically is caused by enteroviruses, which account for more than 85% of all cases of viral meningitis (Wan, 2011). The majority of meningitis cases are caused by serotypes (distinct variations within a species of bacteria or viruses or among immune cells of different individuals) of coxsackieviruses and echoviruses. Enteroviruses usually enter the human host via the oral–fecal route but also can spread through the respiratory route. Arboviruses, which account for about 5 percent of viral meningitis cases in North America (Wan, 2011), consist of more than 500 viruses from different virus families; all are arthropod-borne diseases in which mosquitoes serve as transmitters. Some of the important arboviruses are West Nile, Japanese B, and the Colorado tick fever. Other causes of viral meningitis include mumps, herpesviruses, measles, and HIV.

Viral pathogens may gain access to the CNS via the hematogenous route (bloodstream) or the neural route. The actual mechanism of viral penetration into the CNS is not well understood. The virus may cross the blood–brain barrier (BBB) directly at the capillary endothelial level or through natural defects, such as the area postrema, a medullary structure lying at the base of the fourth ventricle, outside of the blood–brain barrier, and other sites lacking a blood–brain barrier. Some viruses may gain access to the CNS by retrograde transport along nerve roots (Wan, 2011).

Clinical Manifestations

The clinical triad of meningitis is fever, neck stiffness, and altered mental status. A common and early sign of bacterial and viral meningitis is that of meningeal irritation, or **meningismus.** Symptoms of meningismus include photophobia, nuchal rigidity (stiff neck), Kernig's sign, and Brudzinski sign. **Kernig's sign** is elicited by flexing the patient's hip to approximately 90 degrees, then straightening the leg at the knee. Pain in the hamstring area prevents the straightening of the leg. If present bilaterally, it is a positive Kernig's sign. **Brudzinski sign** is positive when flexion of the patient's neck elicits flexion of the hips and knees. The discomfort associated with meningismus is caused by inflammation of the meninges.

Headache is another common and early symptom of meningitis. They are usually described as severe and difficult to control. Fever also is common and usually is high. Altered levels of consciousness, such as lethargy, irritability, and confusion, may occur as the disease progresses. Seizures may be seen at the onset.

Laboratory and Diagnostic Procedures

To diagnose meningitis, blood tests are performed for markers of inflammation. These include C-reactive protein, complete blood count, and blood cultures. Once meningitis is suspected, lumbar puncture must be done to determine the presence and identity of organisms as well as other diagnostic criteria of CSF. Before a lumbar puncture can be done, however, a CT scan of the patient's head should be done to ascertain that no space-occupying lesion is present to cause the clinical manifestations. A lumbar puncture done in the presence of a space-occupying lesion could cause downward shifting of the brain and herniation through the foramen magnum, with neurologically devastating results.

Lumbar puncture can determine the presence of pathogens in the CSF. Also of benefit is examination of the fluid for other diagnostic factors. For example, the CSF may be turbid or cloudy in the presence of bacteria. The presence of protein and glucose in the CSF is diagnostic for bacterial meningitis. The amount of protein in the CSF is usually high, whereas the glucose level is low with bacterial meningitis (Razonable, 2011b). Viral meningitis differs in that the glucose count is usually normal, whereas the protein count remains elevated. The CSF appears clear. Intracranial pressure also may be measured via lumbar puncture.

Medical Management

A thorough and accurate history is very important, focusing on recent illnesses such as any "flu-like" illness. The presence of systemic viral infections is significant. A history of recent dental procedures, head trauma, and/or brain surgery also is pertinent.

Treatment for meningitis depends on the organism causing the infection, the patient's age, the extent of the infection, and the presence of other medical conditions or complications of meningitis. The treatment for bacterial meningitis is antibiotics. They are usually given intravenously but may be given intrathecally (through the theca of the spinal cord into the subarachnoid space). The type and route of antibiotics used are determined by identifying the pathogen from a CSF Gram stain and culture. Blood cultures also are obtained to assist with therapy determination. For an antibiotic to be effective in treating meningitis, it must have a bactericidal effect against the causative organism, and it must be able to penetrate the blood–brain barrier. It is important to note that some antibiotics interfere with the metabolism of other drugs, including phenytoin. This is significant because it generally decreases the blood levels of phenytoin, leaving the patient more susceptible to seizure activity.

Safety Alert *To protect the health care providers as well as family, droplet isolation (precautions used for patients infected with known or suspected illnesses transmitted by droplets, usually from coughing, sneezing, talking, or certain procedures such as suctioning or bronchoscopy) is usually maintained for 24 hours if there is a suspicion of meningitis. The antibiotic needs to be started within 30 minutes of clinical presentation because of the rapid progression of the disease (Barker, 2008).*

The prognosis appears to correlate with the causative agent; the patient's age; the degree of neurological impairment; the severity of the infection; the presence of underlying disease, such as diabetes; the patient's general health condition; and the timeliness of effective treatment. The mortality rate is between 5-40%, depending on the patient's age and etiology. There is a 10-30% rate of permanent neurologic deficits in survivors (Bope, Kellerman, & Rakel, 11).

Treatment of viral meningitis consists mainly of supportive measures; these include relief of symptoms, such as fever or pain. A more seriously ill patient may require respiratory and/or circulatory support.

Prognosis depends on variable factors, similar to those with the bacterial form of meningitis. Occasional neurological impairment has been reported, but full recovery usually occurs.

Encephalitis

Epidemiology and Etiology

Encephalitis is an acute infection and inflammation of the brain tissue. This rare disease may be caused by bacteria, viruses, fungi, or a parasite. Overall, viruses are the most common cause of encephalitis. Epidemiologic studies estimate the incidence of viral encephalitis at 3.5 to 7.4 cases per 100,000 persons per year (Gondim, 2011). The Centers for Disease Control and Prevention (CDC) estimates an incidence of approximately 20,000 new cases annually in the United States (Gondim, 2011). The two most common nonendemic causes of viral encephalitis in the United States are herpes simplex virus (HSV) and rabies virus. Other types of viruses include arthropod-borne, such as those carried by mosquitoes. Another cause of viral encephalitis is postviral disease from measles, mumps, or chickenpox. Typically, children and young adults are the groups most affected; however, severity usually is more pronounced in infants and older adults. Encephalitis tends to occur in warmer climates where mosquitoes are prevalent. This may be year-round or seasonal, depending on the location.

Pathophysiology

The mechanism by which a virus infects the brain varies with the type of virus. Viruses enter the CNS through the bloodstream and through retrograde neuronal dissemination. Retrograde neural dissemination is the main route of spread for rabies virus and may be a possible route for herpes simplex virus through the olfactory tracts. Humans are incidental terminal hosts of many viral infections. Viruses can be transmitted by an insect bite and then undergo local replication in the skin. Continuous replication leads to seeding of other sites, including the CNS. This results in structural damage to the brain. Effects include degenerative changes within the nerve cell, localized edema, hemorrhages, and areas of necrosis. Increased ICP may be present.

Clinical Manifestations

Clinical manifestations of encephalitis are usually more pronounced than those of meningitis. They also are dependent on the type of virus infecting the brain. Symptoms include severe headache, fever, nausea and vomiting, confusion, alterations in LOC such as lethargy, and focal deficits such as motor weakness. It is not unusual for patients to have seizures and bizarre behavior. If the virus is causing cerebral edema, the patient will have signs and symptoms of increased ICP, such as confusion or agitation, personality changes, seizures, loss of sensation in certain areas of the body, problems with speech or hearing, and loss of consciousness. Death or severe neurological deficits can occur if the condition is left untreated.

Laboratory and Diagnostic Procedures

Diagnosis of encephalitis is made primarily by examination of CSF. In encephalitis, glucose levels are low, protein levels are high, and WBCs are elevated. Brain imaging (MRI) often is the first test if symptoms and patient history suggest the possibility of encephalitis. The images may show swelling of the brain or another condition causing the symptoms. Early evidence of small localized hemorrhage lesions also may be revealed. Computerized tomography (CT) also may be used to gain an image of the brain. A lumbar puncture may be performed to extract and analyze the CSF fluid for the presence of a causative virus or other infectious agent.

A complete blood count (CBC) should be done to assess the systemic response to the disease. Specifically, the WBC count trends need to be tracked. Other laboratory tests that may be performed include analysis of blood and urine samples and analysis of excretions from the back of the throat to identify some of the viruses or other infectious agents that can cause encephalitis. An electroencephalogram (EEG) may be done to determine whether the brain pattern is normal or abnormal. A brain biopsy may be completed if symptoms are worsening, treatments are having no effect, and there is no working diagnosis; however, this is rarely done.

Medical Management

A thorough history is important to rule out other causes of the current illness. It is important to make a diagnosis as quickly as possible to initiate treatment, as a good prognosis often depends on early diagnosis and treatment. Treatment involves supportive management of symptoms, such as support of the respiratory system, management of increased ICP, nutritional support, and close evaluation of intake and output.

Antiviral agents, such as acyclovir or famciclovir, are the standard for treatment of HSV. They are given intravenously and must be started early in the disease process to be effective. Other important medications include dexamethasone to reduce cerebral edema, phenytoin for seizure management, and medication for pain and fever control. Medications used in the treatment of seizures are listed in the Pharmacology box. Neurological deficits such as cognitive impairment, nystagmus, motor weakness, seizure disorder, confusion, and personality changes are common adverse effects of antiepileptic drugs (Adams & Koch, 2010).

Brain Abscess

A **brain abscess** is a localized infection carried from other sites of the body into the cerebral tissue. There are several mechanisms by which an abscess can be introduced into the brain, such as infection, congenital abnormalities, or penetrating wounds.

Epidemiology and Etiology

Brain abscesses occur most often in the cerebellum but also can occur in the frontal, parietal, or occipital lobes. In addition, they can occur at any age. Because of improvements in the treatment of ear, sinus, and orofacial infections, brain abscesses are rare. Only 1,500 to 2,500 infections develop each year in the United States (Honda & Warren, 2009). An abscess may be caused by various agents, including bacteria, fungi, viruses, and parasites. The common primary causes have been sinusitis, otitis, and dental abscesses. Direct spread from a dental source proceeds from the abscess, which is often a molar, to the frontal lobe. Other sources include pulmonary infections, IV drug abuse, and liver infections. The initial focus for infection also may be head or facial trauma or a neurosurgical procedure. Finally, idiopathic brain abscess, in which no primary focus of infection can be identified, ranges from 10% to over 60% (Carey, 2010).

Pathophysiology

A brain abscess begins as an infectious organism that invades the brain from a nearby location, such as the sinuses, mastoid, or inner ear. Most often, brain abscesses originate in the white matter adjacent to the cortex, where increased vascular density may facilitate collagen deposits and promote capsule formation (Best Practice, 2012). A cerebral abscess develops in three stages. The first stage, early cerebritis, lasts approximately 3 days and is characterized by local inflammation, tissue necrosis, neutrophil infiltrate, and activation of microglia and astrocytes. The

PHARMACOLOGY Summary of Medications Used to Treat Acute Brain and Cranial Nerve Disorders

Medication Category and Action	Application/Indication	Nursing Responsibility
Analgesic		
Acetaminophen	Provides pain control and fever reduction.	Assess for pain relief and absence of fever. Monitor liver function tests periodically during prolonged and high-dose therapy. If overdose occurs, acetylcysteine is the antidote.
Tramadol (Ultram)	Provides pain relief.	Assess for pain relief. Assess for the adverse effects of vertigo, dizziness, headache, nausea, and symptoms of CNS stimulation. Also, be aware of the possibility of seizures.
Action: Acts centrally in the CNS by inhibiting COX. May exhibit the chemical mediators of pain, but its mechanism is unclear. The reduction of fever occurs by its direct action on the heat-regulating center of the hypothalamus to produce peripheral vasodilation, sweating, and dissipation of heat. Binds to the opioid mu receptor and inhibits norepinephrine and serotonin reuptake in spinal neurons, which inhibits the transmission of pain impulses.		
Antiemetic		
Metoclopramide (Reglan) Ondansetron (Zofran) Promethazine (Phenergan)	Reduces/prevents nausea when receiving chemotherapy. May also be used for migraines.	Assess for nausea, vomiting, and bowel sounds before and after administrations. Assess for extrapyramidal side effects such as pill rolling (a rhythmic tremor of the wrist and fingers), a mask-like face, shuffling gait, and muscle spasms throughout the course of therapy. Evaluate for signs or symptoms of dyskinesia such as uncontrolled rhythmic movement of the mouth, face, and extremities and lip smacking. Report these symptoms immediately since they may be irreversible. Life-threatening neuroleptic malignant syndrome may occur. Monitor for hyperthermia, muscle rigidity, altered consciousness, tachycardia, and diaphoresis.
Action: Stimulates motility of the upper gastrointestinal (GI) tract and accelerates gastric emptying. Blocks the effect of serotonin at receptor sites located in the vagal nerve terminals and chemoreceptor. Blocks the effects of histamine. Has inhibitory effect on the chemoreceptor trigger zone in the medulla, which results in antiemetic properties.		
Antiepileptic Drugs		
Clonazepam (Klonopin) Ethosuximide (Zarontin) Gabapentin (Neurontin) Lamotrigine (Lamictal) Phenobarbital Carbamazepine (Tegretol) Divalproex (Depakote) Phenytoin (Dilantin)	Prevents seizures. Can also be used to treat pain relief in trigeminal neuralgia. Used in the treatment of SUNCT, a type of headache. May also be used to treat pain relief in trigeminal neuralgia. Used in the treatment of seizures.	Observe and record the intensity, duration, and location of seizure activity. Evaluate for suicidal thoughts and behavioral changes. Evaluate for Stevens-Johnson syndrome, which may cause an increased frequency of tonic–clonic seizures. Monitor for suicidal thoughts, confusion, and depression. Assess for suicidal thoughts; observe skin for Stevens-Johnson syndrome. Monitor frequent vital signs. Resuscitative equipment should be readily available since it may cause respiratory depression. Monitor for thrombocytopenia and gingivitis. Monitor first given dose for allergic reactions.
Action: Causes sedative effects in the CNS by stimulating inhibitory GABA receptors. Antiepileptic drug: suppresses abnormal wave and spike activity of the brain associated with absence seizures. Mechanism of action is unknown. Thought to depress the CNS. Stabilizes neuronal membranes by inhibiting sodium transport. Depresses the sensory cortex, alters cerebellar function, and reduces motor activity by inhibiting transmission in the nervous system. Decreases seizure propagation by altering ion transportation.		
Benzodiazepines		
Diazepam (Valium) Lorazepam (Ativan) Clonazepam (Klonopin)	Treatment for seizure cessation, status epilepticus. Treatment for seizure cessation.	Conduct regular assessment for CNS depression. May increase drowsiness
Action: Depresses the CNS by potentiating GABA, which is an inhibitory neurotransmitter. Enhances the action of GABA in the brain, thus inhibiting the abnormal neuronal discharges characteristic of seizures.		

Medication Category and Action	Application/Indication	Nursing Responsibility
Calcium-Channel Blocker		
Verapamil ***Action:*** Inhibits the transport of calcium into vascular smooth muscles, causing vasodilation of peripheral arterioles, which lowers blood pressure.	Treatment for paroxysmal hemicrania headache.	Evaluate for arrhythmias, since it may cause prolonged PR intervals and CHF. Evaluate lungs, and monitor intake/output and daily weight.
Chemotherapy		
Temozolomide (Temodar) Procarbazine Cisplatin/carboplatin Vincristine Methotrexate ***Action:*** Death of rapidly replicating cells, resulting in regression or slowed tumor growth.	Treat malignant primary brain tumors.	Evaluate for seizures, fatigue, and headaches. Thrombocytopenia may occur; therefore, close observation of platelets is necessary.
Ergot Alkaloids		
Dihydroergotamine (DHE) ***Action:*** Vasoconstriction of dilated blood vessels.	Treatment of vascular headaches: migraines and cluster headaches	Evaluate for cardiac instability such as hypertension or angina. May cause myocardial infarction
Ergotamine		
Cafergot Ergotamine (Ergomar) ***Action:*** Causes constriction of peripheral and cranial blood vessels. Vasoconstriction of dilated blood vessels.	Used for cluster headaches Used for migraine headaches.	Evaluate for peripheral ischemia. Assess capillary refill. Monitor for chest pain or hypertension. May cause GI symptoms such as abdominal pain, nausea and vomiting.
H2-Blockers		
Famotidine (Pepcid) Ranitidine (Zantac) ***Action:*** Inhibits the action of histamine at the H2-receptor site, resulting in inhibition of gastric acid secretions.	Reduces acid in the stomach, which may be caused by other medications or dietary intake.	Thrombocytopenia.
Immunoglobulin		
Immune globulin ***Action:*** Contains gamma globulin antibodies.	Used in treatment of Guillain-Barré syndrome.	Monitor vital signs continuously during infusion and evaluate for anaphylaxis.
Muscle Relaxant		
Carisoprodol (Soma) Cyclobenzaprine (Flexeril) ***Action:*** Antispasmodics: skeletal muscle relaxation due to CNS depression. Decreases tonic somatic muscle activity at the level of the brainstem.	Muscle relaxant used to treat brain injuries.	Evaluate for oversedation or respiratory depression. Assess patient for dizziness, drowsiness, and confusion.
Nonsteroidal Anti-Inflammatory Drugs (NSAIDs)		
Ketorolac (Toradol) Indomethacin (Indocin) Ibuprofen (Motrin, Advil) Naproxen (Naprosyn) ***Action:*** Inhibits prostaglandin synthesis; therefore, decreases pain, inflammation, and fever.	Provides pain control and fever reduction.	Assess for signs and symptoms of GI bleeding such as tarry stools, hypotension, and light-headedness. Monitor renal and hepatic functions routinely.
Opioids		
Codeine Fentanyl (Sublimaze, Duragesic) Hydromorphone (Dilaudid) Hydrocodone (Lortab)	Provide pain control for moderate to severe pain. Provide pain control for mild to moderate pain.	Evaluate for respiratory depression, oversedation, constipation, and difficulty with urination. Administer bowel care as necessary. Respiratory depression, oversedation.

(*continued*)

PHARMACOLOGY Summary of Medications Used to Treat Acute Brain and Cranial Nerve Disorders, *continued*

Medication Category and Action	Application/Indication	Nursing Responsibility
Morphine Oxycodone (Percocet, Oxy-IR, OxyContin) ***Action:*** Binds to opiate receptors in the CNS. Inhibits reuptake of serotonin and norepinephrine in the CNS.		
Osmotic Diuretics		
Mannitol ***Action:*** Increases the osmotic pressure of the glomerular filtration; therefore, it inhibits reabsorption of water and electrolytes.	Reduce vasogenic edema.	The patient should be monitored in the intensive care unit. Monitor serum sodium and osmolality levels.
Prostaglandin Analogue		
Misoprostol ***Action:*** Decreases gastric acid secretions by direct action on the parietal cells through binding to prostaglandin receptor.	Treatment of trigeminal neuralgia.	Evaluate for abdominal pain or diarrhea. Evaluate whether the patient is pregnant, since misoprostol may cause miscarriages.
Proton Pump Inhibitor		
Omeprazole (Prilosec) ***Action:*** Decreases accumulation of acid in the gastric lumen; therefore, lessens gastroesophageal reflux.	Reduce acid in the stomach.	Assess routinely for abdominal pain. Monitor labs.
Reversal Agents		
Flumazenil (Romazicon) Naloxone (Narcan) ***Action:*** Antagonizes the CNS depressant effects of benzodiazepine compounds. Blocks the effect of opioids, producing any agonist effects.	Reverse benzodiazepine effects. Reverse opiate effects.	Monitor respiratory rate, rhythm, and depth. See above.
Sedative		
Propofol (Diprivan) ***Action:*** Short-acting. It is known to alter the structure of the brain's network and the way in which the brain transmits information (Ruskin, 2011). Exerts its sedative-hypnotic effects through a $GABA_A$ (gamma-aminobutyric) receptor interaction. This causes sedative actions (Drugs.com, 2011b; Propofol Mechanism of Action, 2011).	Provide sedation for patients with increased ICP, CBF, and oxygen demand.	Evaluate for oversedation. Monitor blood pressure and state of consciousness.
Steroids		
Dexamethasone Methylprednisolone Prednisolone ***Action:*** Suppresses inflammation and normal immune response.	Reduce vasogenic edema. Treatment of trigeminal neuralgia. Treatment of Bell's palsy, as well as migraine and cluster headaches. Also treatment for SUNCT.	Evaluate for psychosis, alteration in sleep, GI upset, leukocytosis, and hyperglycemia.
Tricyclic Antidepressants		
Amitriptyline (Elavil) Nortriptyline ***Action:*** Blocks the reuptake of norepinephrine and serotonin into presynaptic nerve terminals. This results in an increased action of both neurotransmitters in neurons.	Treatment of trigeminal neuralgia and migraines.	Assess for suicidal thoughts or arrhythmias.

References

Adapted from Adams, M. P. & Kochy, R. (2010). *Pharmacology connections to nursing practice.* Upper Saddle River, NJ: Pearson; Drugs.com. (2011a). *Propofol (systemic).* Retrieved from http://www.drugs.com/mns/propofol.html; MedicineNet.com. (2011a). *Gabapentin–neurontin.* Retrieved from http://www.medicinenet.com/gaabapentin-oral/article.htm; MedlinePlus. (2011b). Valparoic acid. U.S. *National Library of Medicine, NIH National Institutes of Health.* Retrieved from http://www.nllm.nnih.gov/medlineplus/druginfo/meds/a682412.html; Propofol mechanism of action. (2011). *AnesthesiaGeneral.com.* Retrieved from http://anesthesiageneral.com/proporol-mechanism-of-action/; Ruskin, K. (2010). *How do anesthetics work? Anesthesiology's Blog for Education & More.* Retrieved from http://page2anesthesiology.org/2011/how-do-anesthetics-work/; WebMD. (2011a). *Drugs & medications–depakote oral.* Retrieved from http://www.webmd.com/drugs/drug-1788-Depakote+Oral.aspx?drugid=1788&drugname; WebMD. (2011b). Meningitis–treatment overview. *Children's Vaccines Health Center.* Retrieved from http://chldren.webmd.com/vaccines/tc/meningitis-treatment-overview.

Weblink: How Do Anesthetics Work? **Weblink:** Depakote Oral **Weblink:** Proprofol Mechanism of Action **Weblink:** Valproic Acid **Weblink:** Gabapentin **Weblink:** Proprofol second stage, late cerebritis, occurs on days 4 to 9 and is represented by an organization in which lymphocytic and microglial infiltration is seen. During the last stage, a frank abscess forms; this is present after day 10 and is characterized by encapsulation and a suppurative collection.

Organisms may enter the brain through direct extension or spread through the blood. Increased permeability of the blood–brain barrier is present throughout the stages of abscess development. Direct extension may occur through necrotic areas of osteomyelitis in the posterior wall of the frontal sinus, as well as through the sphenoid and ethmoid sinuses. Frontal or ethmoid sinus infections generally spread to the frontal lobes. Odontogenic infections, those related to tooth development, can spread to the intracranial space via direct extension or through the bloodstream. Intracranial extension of the infection by the venous route is common in paranasal sinus disease. Chronic otitis media and mastoditis generally spread to the inferior temporal lobe and cerebellum, causing frontal or ethmoid sinus infection and dental infection of the frontal lobe. Trauma that causes an open skull fracture allows organisms to seed directly in the brain. Brain abscesses also can occur as a result of intracranial surgery and foreign bodies, such as a pencil tip, a lawn dart, a bullet, and shrapnel. Brain abscesses can occasionally develop after trauma to the face (Brook, 2011). The invading bacteria cause inflammation, cerebral edema, increased ICP, and necrosis.

Clinical Manifestations

Clinical symptoms of brain abscess may develop slowly over a period of several weeks, or they may develop suddenly. Initial symptoms are directly related to the location of the forming abscess. Headache is common, as are generalized malaise, fever, nausea and vomiting, and chills. Neurological deficits correspond to the location of the lesion and may include motor weakness, sensory deficits, cranial nerve weakness, speech disturbances, and alterations in LOC, such as confusion and lethargy. The patient also may experience seizures.

As the abscess develops, secondary symptoms caused by the expansion of the space-occupying lesion may occur. These symptoms which are dependent on the location of the lesion. may result in ataxia, nystagmus, or post-occipital headache (cerebellar); contralateral hemiplegia, aphasia, or personality changes (frontal area). Headaches may become more severe, and signs of increased ICP may occur. Herniation syndromes may occur if the abscess is left untreated.

Diagnostic Procedures

A diagnosis of brain abscess is made by history and by imaging studies such as a CT scan or MRI. Imaging studies show the encapsulated abscesses. A CT scan also is helpful in identifying hydrocephalus, mass effect, and cerebral edema. Occasionally, abscesses in the brain may appear to be cystic brain tumors. Diffusion-weighted MRI can be used to identify infectious brain lesions and to differentiate between cystic lesions and abscesses (Shetty, Moiyadi, Pantvaidya, & Arya, 2010).

Medical and Surgical Management

Medical management of a brain abscess consists of surgical drainage of the abscess, if possible, and administering the appropriate antibiotics, along with steroids. Recognition and treatment of symptoms, such as ICP management, and respiratory and cardiovascular systems are important. Management of fever and pain issues also is warranted. Prognosis is excellent if the abscess is treated early and aggressively. Another significant factor in determining prognosis is the number of abscesses noted. Patients with single lesions do considerably better than those with multiple lesions. Even though antibiotics, advanced neurodiagnostics, and surgical techniques have improved the mortality and morbidity statistics, reported mortality rates in cases of brain abscess are as high as 33% (Barker, 2008; Southwick, 2012).

Nursing Management

The single most important intervention on the part of the nurse and every hospital employee is prevention. The advent of universal precautions has been successful in educating employees in ways to prevent, or at least reduce, the occurrence of infections. The population of patients with neurological disorders, for example, appears to have an affinity for infections. One reason for this is the drugs that are often used to treat this patient population. Many patients are given steroids such as dexamethasone, which is an immunosuppressant. Radiation and chemotherapy also act as immunosuppressants. Additionally, many patients with neurological disorders have respiratory compromise, requiring intubation and possibly mechanical ventilation. These patients are at high risk for developing hospital-acquired infections.

Nutritional deficits also are predisposing factors for infection. Many patients enter the hospital in debilitated conditions, such as advanced stages of brain tumor or vegetative conditions. Finally, the widespread use of antibiotics for hospitalized patients plays a role in diminishing the normal flora of a person's immune system, leaving the patient vulnerable to hospital-acquired infection. Nursing plays a vital role in the prevention of these infections. The most obvious actions might be the observation of universal precautions, the practice of meticulous hand hygiene, and the monitoring of signs and symptoms of impending infection.

Assessment

Patients with infectious diseases of the brain such as meningitis, encephalitis, or brain abscess initially may appear to be neurologically intact but systemically ill. These patients and their families are usually frightened by the acuity of their illness. Often, the nurse identifies that the patient is becoming ill with symptoms such as fever or signs of nuchal rigidity and brings it to the health care provider's attention so that diagnostic testing can be done (see the Diagnostic Tests box, p. 518). The cardinal signs of a cerebral infection are those of any infection along with increased ICP. The patient's history may detail headache, stiff neck and back, malaise, photophobia, chill, and sometimes vomiting, twitching, and seizures. Therefore, obtaining the patient's history is critical to the assessment process. In taking the patient's history, the nurse should obtain information about prevailing symptoms such as irritability, loss of appetite, and headaches. There may be reports of a headache that become progressively worse, with accompanying vomiting, disorientation, or delirium. The patient also may note an increased sensitivity to light (photophobia), chills, fever, and seizure activity. Frequently, the patient and/or family describe a recent upper respiratory or other type of infection, such as ear, sinus, or lung infection.

Physical assessment of the patient includes checking for the following indicators of a cerebral infection:

- Opisthotonus, a spasm in which the back and extremities arch backward so that the body rests on the head and heels
- A petechial, purpuric, or ecchymotic rash on the lower part of the body.
- Positive Brudzinski and Kernig's signs (described on p. 528) and exaggerated and symmetrical deep tendon reflexes
- Altered LOC, ranging from confusion or delirium to deep stupor or coma
- Diplopia and other visual problems.

Nursing Diagnoses

Nursing diagnoses derived from assessment data may include the following:

- *Acute Pain* related to change in muscle tone, rigidity.
- *Altered Level of Consciousness* related to brain disorder.
- *Anxiety* related to fear of the unknown, anticipation of danger that causes apprehension.
- *Hyperthermia* related to fever, increased ICP, increased metabolic rate, decreased perspiration, dehydration, and medications.
- *Impaired Gas Exchange* related to ventilation perfusion imbalance.
- *Risk for Deficient Fluid Volume* related to dehydration and active fluid volume loss.
- *Risk for Impaired Skin Integrity* related to hyperthermia and physical immobilization, changes in fluid status, and nutritional status.

  NANDA-I © 2012

Outcomes and Evaluation Parameters

Outcomes and evaluation parameters related to the nursing diagnoses for patients with a cerebral infection are as follows:

- Patient will express feelings of comfort and relief of pain as evidenced by calm facial expression and demeanor, actual verbalization of relief.
- Patient will identify strategies to reduce anxiety.
- No evidence of hyperthermia; patient will exhibit normal temperature (normal temperature ranges are shown in Chart 21–3, p. 517); no evidence of dehydration.
- Patient will maintain adequate ventilation and oxygenation; no evidence of cyanosis, respiratory rate regular and within normal range, respirations even without evidence of gasping for air.
- Patient will maintain fluid volume within normal range; intake and output of fluid volume is balanced, no evidence of "dryness," such as diminished skin turgor, dry mouth, dry lips, decreased urine output, and mucous membranes.
- Skin integrity will remain intact; no evidence of reddened or broken skin.

Interventions and Rationales

Specific nursing interventions for patients with cerebral infections include the following:

- Pain management; alleviate pain or reduce pain to a level of comfort that is acceptable to the patient.
- Manage the patient's environment to promote optimum comfort; keep darkened if preferred, keep quiet and calm, allow visitors with the patient's permission.
- Assist in reducing anxiety by helping the patient identify ways to reduce it.
- Monitor temperature and vital signs.
- Assess respiratory status to ensure an adequate airway and adequate gas exchange.
- Administer oxygen, if ordered, and monitor its effectiveness to maintain adequate ventilation.
- Implement skin care precautions by monitoring pressure points, turning patient according to established protocol or as needed, and lubricating skin as needed to prevent pressure ulcers.

It is important to involve the patient and family in the decision-making process and keep them informed about the plan of care: treatments, medications, and consultations. Many patients and their family members are concerned because they do not understand the disease processes of meningitis, encephalitis, and brain abscess. This generates fear and concern as to whether these diseases are contagious. Therefore, their fears and questions must be recognized and answered by members of the health care team.

Collaborative Management

The health care team, the patient, and the patient's family all play a role in the patient's care. In order to meet desired patient outcomes, it is essential that this interdisciplinary team communicate openly with one another in developing and evaluating care of the patient and family (IOM [Institute of Medicine], 2010). Consultation with an infectious disease specialist may be indicated, if available. Commonly, the antibiotic course for cerebral abscess is 4 to 6 weeks in duration. Infectious disease health care providers specialize in the management of infections. Other health team members who might have a role in treating these patients include the respiratory therapist, who may assist the patient in maintaining adequate ventilation and air exchange; the physical therapist, who assists in developing a mobility plan; and the pharmacologist, who may consult with the team in prescribing medications and evaluating for effectiveness and drug interactions. The dietitian or nutrition consultant can help the patient achieve a balanced diet with adequate fluid intake. If the patient is having visual difficulties, an ophthalmologist may be consulted. A consultation with a social worker may be helpful in preparing the patient for discharge to the home environment.

Health promotion and discharge planning activities are the same as those for any patient experiencing a major cerebral disorder.

Guillain-Barré Syndrome

Guillain-Barré syndrome (GBS), an acute inflammatory polyneuropathy, is the most common cause of acute or subacute generalized paralysis (NINDS, 2011a). It is considered to be an autoimmune disorder that affects the peripheral nervous system, and it is characterized by varying degrees of motor weakness or paralysis. GBS primarily affects the motor component of the cranial and spinal nerves.

Epidemiology and Etiology

The annual incidence of GBS is 1.2 to 3 per 100,000 individuals; no racial preponderance exists (Andary, 2011). The rate of hospitalizations related to GBS in the United States increases with age. In North America, Western Europe, and Australia, most patients with GBS meet electrophysiological testing criteria for demyelinating polyneuropathy, a chronic relapsing polyneuropathy (Andary, 2011).

GBS has a male to female ratio of 1.5:1; male dominance is especially seen in older patients. In addition, GBS has been reported in all age groups, occurring at any time between infancy and old age. In the United States, the age distribution seems to peak in young adulthood, with a second, higher one in adults ages 50 to 75 years (Andary, 2011).

GBS is usually caused by an autoimmune response to a viral infection; typically, the patient gives a history of a recent acute infection such as a respiratory infection, gastrobacterial or intestinal infection, or viral pneumonia. In addition, vaccinations and other systemic illnesses have been associated with GBS.

Clinical Manifestations

GBS is characterized by motor weakness, areflexia (absence of reflexes), and flaccid paralysis. There usually is an ascending and symmetrical progression of weakness, with the lower limbs being involved prior to the upper limbs. Trunk, bulbar, and respiratory muscles may also be affected. Respiratory failure may occur due to the mechanical failure and fatigue of the intercostals and diaphragm. The facial nerve is most often affected if there is cranial nerve involvement. This is observed in 45% to 75% of patients with GBS (Davids, 2011). Physical presentation may include facial droop, diplopias, dysphagia, and pupillary disturbances.

Sensory changes may be present, causing paresthesia and pain. The paresthesia begins in the toes and fingertips, progressing upward; however, it does not extend beyond the wrists or ankles. Pain usually is located in the shoulder, back, buttocks, and thighs; frequently is described as aching or throbbing; and occurs with the slightest movements.

Autonomic changes include cardiac arrhythmias, orthostatic hypotension, paroxysmal hypertension, and urinary retention. These autonomic changes rarely persist in a patient with GBS (NINDS, 2011a). Respiratory involvement is the most immediate threat to life for patients with GBS. They may have dyspnea on exertion, shortness of breath, or difficulty swallowing. Ventilatory failure also may develop, requiring respiratory support.

Laboratory and Diagnostic Procedures

The diagnosis of GBS is based on clinical presentation in addition to diagnostic criteria. The criteria include progressive weakness of two or more limbs due to neuropathy, areflexia, disease course less than 4 weeks, and exclusion of other causes of the symptoms. A patient history of recent viral infection, elevated CSF protein levels via lumbar puncture, and a normal cell count are important to note (Hickey, 2009). Radiographic imaging such as a MRI or CT scan of the spine may be helpful in excluding other diagnoses (Miller, 2011).

Medical Management

There is no known cure for Guillain-Barré syndrome, but therapies can lessen the severity of the illness and accelerate the recovery in most patients. The most critical part of the treatment for GBS consists of keeping the patient's body functioning during recovery of the nervous system (NINDS, 2011a). Patients with GBS should be closely observed when admitted to the hospital. They require supportive therapy, including respiratory and cardiovascular monitoring as well as management. The need for this sophisticated machinery is one reason why patients with GBS are usually treated in hospitals, often in an intensive care unit. Approximately one-third of patients with GBS will require admission to the intensive care unit because of respiratory failure, which may require ventilator support (Davids, 2011). Frequent monitoring of vital capacity, tidal volume, or minute volume is essential. Immunotherapy such as immunoglobulin or plasmapheresis (therapeutic plasma exchange) is effective in most patients. The therapy usually is 4 to 5 days in duration and may require a second course of treatment because of relapse. Health care providers also look for and treat the many problems that can affect any paralyzed patient—complications such as pneumonia or bed sores (MedicineNet.com, 2012).

Nursing Management

Nursing management of the patient with GBS includes a comprehensive neurological and respiratory baseline assessment and ongoing monitoring for early recognition of changes. The patient's respiratory quality and rate as well as vital capacity should be assessed frequently. Insufficient breathing and oxygenation must be monitored with a pulse oximeter. If respiratory failure occurs, intubation will be necessary.

The nurse should assess the cranial nerves as well as motor and sensory function frequently to evaluate whether the GBS is developing further. Autonomic dysfunctions such as cardiac arrhythmias or vital sign changes must be monitored. Sleep cycles also may be altered by some of the autonomic changes and should be assessed on a regular basis (LoGuidice & Persin, 2011).

Pain and fear may be associated with GBS. The nurse will need to assess the patient's pain; IV narcotics and even IV continuous drips may be given for relief. Providing support for fearful patients is necessary. They may need continued reinforcement that their condition is reversible and that the prognosis is optimistic (Mayo Clinic Staff, 2011b). See the Nursing Process: Patient Care Plan for Acute Brain Disorders (p. 523) for a detailed description of nursing management.

Brain Tumors

The diagnosis of a brain tumor often brings feelings of fear and uncertainty to patients and their family members. Most patients have little understanding of the concept of brain tumors, and many harbor misconceptions about the cause, treatment, and prognosis of their disease.

Epidemiology

The American Cancer Society (ACS) estimated that approximately 22,340 people in the United States would be diagnosed with a malignant CNS tumor in 2011. In addition, approximately 13,110 people would die from brain, spinal cord, or other CNS malignancies (ACS, 2011). An estimated 64,530 new cases of primary nonmalignant and malignant brain and central nervous system tumors were expected to be diagnosed in the United States in 2011. In addition, the incidence rate of all primary nonmalignant and malignant brain and central nervous system tumors is 19.3 cases per 100,000 persons (Central Brain Tumor Registry of the United States, 2010). Glioblastomas are more common in men than in women, with a male-to-female ratio of 3:2 (Uddin, 2010). Meningiomas occur at an annual rate of 8.36 and 3.61 per 100,000 for females and males, respectively (Wiemels, Wrensch, & Claus, 2010). The chances of developing a malignant tumor of the brain or spinal cord is less than 1% (ACS, 2011).

Etiology

The cause of CNS tumors is not well understood. It is known that brain tumors, like other tumors, are caused by abnormal changes in the genes. DNA, found in all genes, is considered the "building block of life." Genes are inherited from parents, and they literally make people what they are. Abnormal genes are called **gene mutations** and also are inherited. Mutations can develop into diseases, including tumors. Cancer is believed to develop through an accumulation of genetic mutations or alterations, which allow the cells to grow out of control of normal regulatory mechanisms or to escape destruction by the immune system (see Chapter 53).

Some inherited diseases, such as neurofibromatosis, are associated with increased risk of developing CNS tumors. It also is known that some gene mutations are not inherited. Research into these mutations has led to experimental laboratory treatments for brain tumors, with further refinement expected in the future (ACS, 2011).

It is not known why some people have gene mutations that cause brain tumors. Much research has been done looking for causes for brain tumors, such as cell phone use or environmental factors. The overall evidence points toward an increased risk from cell phone use; however, the magnitude of the increase cannot be assessed at present because there is insufficient information on long-term use (Kundi, 2010).

Classification of Brain Tumors

The term *benign* can be misleading. It is used to refer to microscopic cells that are well differentiated and resemble normal cells but do not carry out the functions of normal cells. Instead, they form slow-growing, space-occupying tumors. Histologically, although a tumor may be benign, it is not resectable (capable of being surgically removed) if it is in a deep area of the brain that is not accessible surgically. A tumor that is not resectable can continue to grow, producing neurological symptoms and possibly death. Some benign tumors also may become malignant if left untreated. A patient whose benign tumors are surgically resected can be considered cured.

Malignant tumors are those with poorly differentiated cells. Malignant tumors tend to be both aggressive and invasive. Although surgical resection may reduce the tumor, it is typically not curative. The prognosis for malignant tumors usually is poor.

Brain tumors may be primary or metastatic. *Primary tumors* are those that originate in the brain. These tumors rarely, if ever, travel to other areas of the body. Metastatic tumors are those that originate in other areas of the body and metastasize to the brain. Metastatic tumors in the brain most commonly originate in the lung (35%), breast (20%), skin (10%), kidney (10%), and gastrointestinal tract (5%) (Bader & Littlejohns, 2010). Tumors within the brain are classified as *intra-axial, extra-axial,* or *metastatic.* Common brain tumors are summarized in Chart 21–4.

Intra-Axial Tumors

Intra-axial tumors, located in the cerebrum, the brainstem, and the cerebellum, arise from glial cells, astrocytes, primitive brain structures, and ependymal structures. Glial cells are the supportive or nourishing cells of the brain. Any tumor that arises from glial cells is referred to as a **glioma.** There are several types of gliomas: astrocytomas, oligodendrogliomas, and ependymomas. They are named for the type of cells they originate from and are graded for their degree of malignancy. Some tumors exist in a homogeneous form; others exhibit heterogeneous, or mixed, cell types.

Astrocytomas

Astrocytomas arise from the astrocyte cell. They have varying degrees of differentiation and are graded according to their degree of malignancy. Astrocytomas range from low grade (grades I and II) to anaplastic astrocytoma (grade III) to the most aggressive form of astrocytoma (grade IV), also known as glioblastoma multiforme. Low-grade astrocytomas, grade I or II, have well-differentiated cells. As the tissues become more malignant, cellularity increases, cell atypia increases, and mitotic activity increases. An astrocytoma with these cellular characteristics is termed an anaplastic astrocytoma and is considered to be more malignant.

CHART 21–4 Summary of Common Brain Tumors

Type and Age of Onset	Symptoms	Treatment	Prognosis
Meningioma Age 40–60s	Dependent on location and size Seizures Headaches	Surgery Radiation for residual or recurrence (gamma knife, cyberknife)	Excellent with resection
Astrocytoma Age: Variable	Dependent on location and size	Surgery Radiation for residual recurrence	3 to 7 years with treatment, dependent on grade and extent of resection
Glioblastoma multiforme (GBM) Age 50–60s	Dependent on location and size	Surgery Radiation Chemotherapy	12–18 months with treatment
Oligodendroglioma Age 40–50s	Dependent on location Seizures	Surgery Radiation Chemotherapy	5–10+ years with treatment
Ependymoma All ages (60% are children)	Signs and symptoms Increased ICP Hydrocephalus	Surgery Radiation Chemotherapy for recurrence May need shunt	7–8+ years with surgery, less with recurrence
Pituitary adenomas Age: Variable	Hormone abnormalities dependent on area of pituitary affected Visual disturbances Headaches	Medical Surgical possible Radiation possible	Excellent
Acoustic neuromas Age 40–50s	Hearing loss	Surgery Radiation for residual (gamma knife)	Excellent
Metastatic tumors Age: Variable	Dependent on location, size, single or multiple	Surgery if single metastasis or symptomatic Radiation (gamma knife) Chemotherapy	Usually poor, dependent on single or multiple and identification of primary disease

Astrocytomas are the most common type of malignant tumor. Approximately 75% of patients with this type of tumor will die within 5 years of diagnosis (Starkweather, Sherwood, Lyon, McCain, Bovbjerg, & Broaddus, 2011). They are seen most commonly in the 30- to 50-year-old population, though they do occur in all age groups. Though astrocytomas may spread into surrounding normal brain tissue, it is rare for them to spread outside the brain and CSF system. Some astrocytomas spread throughout the CNS via CSF pathways.

Survival rates depend on many factors, including grade of the astrocytoma, age of the patient, extent of surgical resection, and response to treatment. The strongest predictor of survival with low-grade gliomas is age. One study reported a mean survival time of 8.5 years for adults less than 40 years of age. This contrasts with 4.9 years for adults 40 years of age and older (Piepmeier, 1987). Though this study is over 20 years old, the age factor has remained a strong prognostic factor (Kennedy, 2011).

Anaplastic astrocytomas (grade III) are noted to be more aggressive than lower grade astrocytomas. The median survival time is 3 years from the time of diagnosis (Starkweather et al., 2011). Clinical manifestations depend on many factors, including the location and size of the lesion. The clinical manifestations may include a single seizure, behavior changes, headaches, or sensorimotor alterations.

Glioblastoma Multiforme

A grade IV astrocytoma is also referred to as a glioblastoma multiforme (GBM). These are the most malignant of the astrocytic tumors. Though they arise from astrocytes, as do all astrocytomas, they are characterized by much more aggressive and invasive cellularity. They are rapidly growing, sometimes doubling in size in as little as 10 days. The GBM is composed of heterogeneous cells, which demonstrate the transformation of cells within this tumor from a low-grade to a high-grade or more malignant tumor. They are characterized by the presence of necrosis and hemorrhage within the tumor.

GBMs occur more in men than in women, with peak incidence occurring between 45 to 70 years of age. Approximately 10% of glioblastomas occur in children (Ferri, 2011). The clinical history of GBM is relatively short. These tumors can exist for a time without clinical evidence of a lesion being present. They tend to present after a short clinical history, usually less than 3 months (Bruce, 2011). The most common presenting symptoms are seizure, focal symptoms such as motor weakness or aphasia, and nonfocal symptoms such as headache or personality changes. The most dangerous aspect of symptomatology is the potential for rapidly increasing ICP caused by the rapid proliferation of this tumor (Barker, 2008).

GBMs are the most malignant of all brain tumors. Despite improvements in surgical techniques and advances of adjunctive therapies such as radiation therapy, chemotherapy, and radiosurgery, the prognosis is grim. The median survival time varies from less than 1 year to 3 years after initial diagnosis (Starkweather et al., 2011). Although the prognosis is bleak, there is reason for hope in the treatment of high-grade gliomas. Research is ongoing, and new treatment protocols are being developed to treat this difficult and devastating disease.

Treatment is aimed at prolonging good quality of life and may include the following strategies: surgical resection, radiation therapy, stereotactic radiosurgery, chemotherapy, and Avastin. Avastin was approved by the FDA in 2009 (Hitti,, 2009) to treat glioblastoma multiforme that has not responded to other therapies. Avastin works by slowing the growth of new blood vessels, which are necessary for the growth of new cancer cells (Snowden, 2009). Despite what appears to be complete gross total resection, this group of tumors is thought to be highly invasive at a microscopic level. This accounts for tumor recurrence despite resection in most cases. Radiation therapy (RT) is considered adjunctive. The most common form of radiation is focal external beam RT or conformal RT. Gamma knife radiosurgery has been shown to increase survival time in some cases. Radiation is discussed in detail in Chapter 57.

In some institutions, the implantation of radioactive materials or a localized chemotherapeutic agent is used. This has met with mixed results; although it extends life by 4 to 10 weeks, it may be associated with seizures and craniotomy wound breakdown that requires additional hospital care. Chemotherapy also is a treatment option for GBMs. Most treatment decisions are made on the basis of the patient's life expectancy and personal goals. Some patients choose biopsy only and decide to spend their remaining time in their home with their family; others prefer to exhaust all treatment measures. Nursing support for the family during their difficult decision-making process is essential.

Oligodendrogliomas

Oligodendrogliomas are tumors that originate in the brain cells called oligodendrocytes. They grow and spread in much the same manner as astrocytomas. These slow-growing tumors can spread to the CSF pathways, but rarely spread outside of the brain or spinal cord. Presenting signs and symptoms of oligodendrogliomas depend on the tumor's size and location. Frequently, the initial presenting symptom is seizures. Oligodendrogliomas occur mostly in middle-age adults but are occasionally seen in children. Treatment is surgical resection and radiation therapy. Prognosis for survival is 9.8 years; 93% of patients survive 2 years, 73% survive 5 years, and 49% survive 10 years (Newton, Hickey, & Marrs, 2009).

Ependymomas

Ependymomas are tumors that originate in the ependymal cells lining the ventricles. They can be found in the brain or spinal cord. These tumors do not spread into normal brain tissue, but they may spread along the CSF pathways. Therefore, there is a much better chance for complete surgical resection of ependymomas, especially from the spinal cord. Because these tumors are found in and around the ventricles and the CSF pathways, they occasionally cause obstruction of CSF flow, in which case hydrocephalus may occur.

Signs and symptoms are related to the location of the lesion. Seizures, motor weakness, cranial nerve deficits, or alterations in LOC may be present, with symptoms of ICP if hydrocephalus is present,Treatment consists of surgical resection and placement of a shunt if hydrocephalus is present. Radiation also may be beneficial. Prognosis is excellent with surgical resection.

Extra-Axial Tumors

Extra-axial tumors are those that originate outside of the brain. The most common extra-axial tumors are meningiomas, schwannomas, and pituitary tumors.

Meningiomas

Meningiomas are the most common type of brain tumor, accounting for approximately 30% of all primary adult brain tumors; 90% of meningiomas are benign (Bohan & Glass-Macenka, 2009). They arise from the meninges, the layer of tissue covering the brain and spinal cord. These firm, encapsulated tumors are extremely slow growing. Because they grow so slowly, they can become quite large before they start causing symptoms. Meningiomas occur most commonly in middle-aged and older adults. The peak occurrence is in the 40- to 70-year-old age group.

Meningiomas occur twice as often in women as in men (Bohan & Glass-Macenka, 2009). Presenting signs and symptoms depend on the location and size of the lesion.

Treatment of meningiomas is surgical resection in most cases. Occasionally, a complete resection is not possible because of the size of the lesion and its proximity to vital structures within the brain. In this case, radiation and/or gamma knife radiosurgery may be necessary. It is important to follow these patients closely with yearly MRI scans to monitor the possible growth of the tumor. After total excision, the recurrence rates have been 0% to 20%. Patients with subtotal resection had a recurrence rate of 20% to 50% within 5 years (Ferri, 2011). In some cases, a lesion may be considered too small to warrant a surgical procedure. In these cases, monitoring of the lesion may be sufficient. Though meningiomas are considered benign, there is an atypical form and a malignant form of this disease, which may cause recurrence. It also is possible to have multiple meningiomas, which carry a high morbidity. Although the prognosis is extremely favorable with complete resection, it also is highly dependent on the degree of cell differentiation.

Schwannomas

Schwann cells are those that surround cranial nerves and other nerves. **Schwannomas** usually are benign tumors. The most common are schwannomas of the acoustic nerve (CNVIII), also referred to as **acoustic neuromas.** Acoustic neuromas usually are diagnosed when the patient experiences gradual hearing loss. Tinnitus and/or dizziness also may be noted. If left untreated, these lesions can become quite large, causing compression of the facial nerve (CNVII) or the trigeminal nerve (CNV).

For symptomatic lesions, gamma knife radiosurgery is the preferred treatment due to the ease of treatment, the excellent control of tumor growth, and reduction in unfavorable cranial nerve defects. Gamma knife treatment can also be planned to preserve hearing in those patients with acoustic neuromas who still have functional hearing.

Open surgery is more appropriate for lesions that exceed 3 cm (about 1 in.). Surgical resection of acoustic neuromas can cause damage to cranial nerves in proximity to the tumor. In some instances, hearing may be sacrificed in the attempt to remove the tumor. The proximity of the brainstem and cranial nerves may result in damage to these nerves. Acoustic neuromas are located in the cerebellopontine angle (CPA) with cranial nerves in proximity. Damage to the facial nerve (CNVII) may be present before surgery or as a result of surgery. Other cranial nerves also may be affected, specifically those involved with swallowing (CNIX, CNX, and CNXII). Therefore, a thorough cranial nerve assessment is important, both preoperatively and postoperatively.

If significant facial weakness is observed, special care should be taken to protect the eye that does not close adequately. It is important to protect the eye from dryness and even abrasions by keeping it well lubricated with eyedrops. Occasionally, complete resection is not possible owing to the size and location of the tumor. A residual tumor may be radiated and/or monitored with serial MRIs. Gamma knife radiosurgery also may be a beneficial adjunctive treatment.

Pituitary Adenomas

Tumors of the pituitary gland occur most frequently in the anterior lobe, but both lobes may show symptoms. Tumors are classified by the type of hormone secreted. Examples of these are prolactin, growth hormone, or ACTH secreting tumors. Pituitary tumors also are classified as functioning, hormone secreting, or nonfunctioning. Functioning pituitary adenomas produce endocrine symptoms, such as acromegaly, hyperprolactinemia, or Cushing's syndrome/disease (Cushings-Help.com, 2011). These disorders are fully discussed in Chapter 46. Nonfunctioning pituitary adenomas produce symptoms caused by pressure of the tumor on surrounding structures, such as the optic nerve. Frequently, visual loss is the presenting symptom; it may be in the form of decreased acuity, hemianopsia (loss of vision in one half of the visual field of one or both eyes), or scotomas (areas of depressed vision in the visual field, surrounded by areas of less depressed or normal vision), Headaches often accompany visual symptoms. Treatment may be medical and/or surgical. With treatment, prognosis is excellent. Chapter 64 discusses visual disorders. A complication of pituitary tumors is diabetes insipidus, although it is uncommon. Diabetes insipidus is characterized by hypernatremia and low urine specific gravity. Chapter 47 discusses diabetes insipidus.

Metastatic Tumors

Metastatic brain tumors usually originate in another part of the body from another type of cancer and metastasize to the brain. They are not considered to be cancer of the brain, but rather cancer from another source that has migrated to the brain.

Epidemiology and Etiology

Metastases to the brain come from many sources. The most common sites of primary disease are the lung, breast, and skin. Metastatic lesions are probably more common than primary brain lesions. The incidence of brain metastases depends on the specific primary tumor. For example, the chances of developing brain metastases is 1% in men with prostate cancer, whereas women with ovarian cancer have a 3% chance of developing brain metastases (Bradley, Daroff, Fenichel, & Jankovic, 2008). The method of spread of metastatic lesions varies by the type of primary disease. Lesions most commonly spread from their primary site via the arterial route. They also may spread via the meninges. Occasionally, direct extension of melanoma lesions of the head or neck may lead to melanoma in the brain.

Other characteristics of metastatic lesions vary by primary disease. The number and location of lesions also vary by primary disease. Single lesions are more common, but multiple lesions occur frequently in some types of primary disease, such as lung cancer. The cerebral cortex is the most common site of metastatic disease, with the cerebellum less so. Additional information on cancer and its treatment is found in Chapter 57.

Clinical Manifestations

Presenting symptoms of metastatic tumors depend on the location of the tumors. The most common symptoms are similar to those of primary tumors and include headache, motor weakness, alteration of mentation, and/or behavioral changes. Seizures are the presenting symptom in many cases.

Laboratory and Diagnostic Procedures

The actual diagnosis of a brain tumor is made by MRI of the suspected region. With this test, it is possible to determine the lesion's location, size, and characteristics, including heterogeneity and presence of necrosis or hemorrhage, calcification, cystic qualities, or enhancement. In addition, the MRI also shows ventricle size, which is important because hydrocephalus is a potentially dangerous side effect of the tumor's presence. The presence of edema and/or mass effect also can be determined. Although it is possible to diagnose a brain tumor with the aid of MRI, the MRI shows only the tumor's presence; it is not possible to determine the type of tumor. The only way to positively diagnose the tumor type is by obtaining tissue for pathology diagnosis.

Medical and Surgical Management

Diagnosis of brain tumors always begins with an accurate and thorough history and physical. Symptom analysis, including duration and frequency of symptoms, is a valuable tool for determining the presence and onset of symptoms. It also is important to have an accurate accounting of seizure events, including type and frequency. Once the diagnosis of brain tumor has been made, treatment options must be explored. Depending on the tumor type and stage, patients may choose to be treated with surgery, radiation therapy, or chemotherapy. Some patients may receive a combination of all three (UCSF Medical Center, 2011). Surgery is the most usual treatment for most brain tumors.

Surgical Excision

Surgical excision of a tumor will establish a positive diagnosis about the type of tumor type and grade, in order to establish the treatment plan. The second goal of surgery is to obtain the maximum tumor debulking possible while maintaining function. The success of the treatment and the prognosis are based on the amount of tumor resection. Craniotomy is the most common type of surgery to achieve these goals (Yale Medical Group, 2012).

Patients who have undergone surgical excision of a brain tumor require monitoring in an ICU setting initially. Some patients also may require ICP monitoring postoperatively. A postoperative MRI usually is done to assess the extent of resection and to assess the presence of hemorrhage, edema, and the status of the ventricles. The National Guidelines box provides the American Association of Neuroscience Nurses (AANN) national guidelines for the care of craniotomy patients.

Radiation Therapy

Once a pathologic diagnosis of brain tumor has been made, some patients will require a consultation with a radiation oncologist. Brain tumors that cannot be cured by surgery alone may be treated with radiation. Patients with recurrent, intermediate, or high-grade astrocytomas; metastatic tumors; incomplete or subtotal resections; or any other tumor deemed appropriate by the neurosurgeon or the neuro-oncologist may benefit from recommendations from a radiation oncologist. There are many types of radiation, and radiological treatment varies by pathologic diagnosis. Radiation is discussed in detail in Chapter 57.

Stereotactic Radiosurgery

Stereotactic radiosurgery is another treatment option. It is a form of radiation therapy that delivers a single, high dose of radiation directly at the tumor or tumor bed. Despite the terminology, it is not a surgical procedure. The goal of radiosurgery is to treat all tumor cells in its path. There are two main types of radiotherapy: external beam radiotherapy and internal beam or brachytherapy. The two types of external radiosurgery most commonly used for treatment of brain tumors are gamma knife and cyber knife radiosurgery.

NATIONAL GUIDELINES AANN Guidelines for the Care of Craniotomy Patients for Brain Tumor

Neurological
- Most complications occur within the first 6 hours postoperative
- ICU admission postoperative
- Frequent neurological assessments
  - Ask the neurosurgeon what complications or deficits are expected
- Incision care
  - Monitor the incision for drainage
  - Keep the incision dry
- Drains
  - Make sure the location of each drain is known; label clearly

Cardiovascular
- Cardiac arrhythmias
- Hypovolemic shock
- Monitor rate and rhythm
- Monitor blood pressure and maintain ordered parameters

Respiratory
- Related to decreased level of consciousness/inability to protect airway
- Especially relevant to surgery near brainstem
- Prevent atelectasis and pneumonia
- Maintain $SaO_2 > 94\%$
- Incentive spirometry unless contraindicated (transsphenoidal surgery)

Gastrointestinal
- Prevention of gastric ulceration (antacids, proton pump inhibitor, H2-blockers)
- Some drugs used in neurological treatment can contribute to gastric irritation (dexamethasone, phenytoin, some antibiotics)

Nutrition
- May require swallow evaluation
- May require enteral feedings

Serum Glucose
- Hyperglycemia may increase cerebral edema
- Hyperglycemia may result from steroid therapy
- Monitor blood glucose as ordered
- Maintain euglycemia

Serum Sodium
- Diabetes insipidus
  - Especially relevant to surgery involving or near the pituitary gland
  - Monitor intake/output and specific gravity
  - Notify health care provider for urine output > 200 mL/hr $\times$ 2 consecutive hours
- Syndrome of inappropriate antidiuretic hormone
  - Monitor sodium levels; treat as ordered

Activity
- Population at risk for deep vein thrombosis (DVT)
  - Early ambulation
  - DVT prophylaxis, such as low-molecular-weight heparin, when ordered
  - Therapy consults
- Pain control
  - Assess per hospital protocol
  - Administer pain medication as ordered
  - Offer other techniques for pain management, such as deep breathing or music

Source: Adapted from American Association of Neuroscience Nurses, AANN Reference Series for Clinical Practice. (2006). *Guide to the care of the patient with craniotomy post-brain tumor resection.* Glenview, IL: American Association of Neuroscience Nurses.

Gamma knife radiosurgery is a system that uses focused radiation in a single dose. The name is misleading because it is not really surgery and does not really use a knife. Rather, the radiation is used to irradiate very specific areas of the tumor, such as the tumor bed of a metastatic lesion. The ionizing radiation causes damage to cellular tissue. If the damage cannot be repaired, cell death occurs (Bader & Littlejohns, 2010). Gamma knife radiosurgery may be used to "shrink" the residual tumor when complete resection is not possible. It also may be beneficial in treating tumors that are considered inoperable or small enough that a surgical procedure is not necessary.

Cyber knife radiosurgery is a relatively new addition to the radiation arsenal. This radiosurgical system consists of a linear accelerator and a robotic arm. This system can locate tumors using image guidance and then deliver multiple beams of radiation directly to the tumor site. This system has some important advantages. It is a complete noninvasive procedure, and it offers flexibility in scheduling the treatment process and spreading the treatment over several sessions in cases of multiple lesions (Muacevic et al., 2010).

Brachytherapy is an internal radiation treatment given by placing radioactive material directly into a tumor or close to it. It is also called interstitial radiation therapy, intracavitary radiation therapy, intravascular radiation therapy, or seed implantation. This type of treatment prevents radiation exposure to other parts of the brain. In 2011, the U.S. Food and Drug Administration (FDA) approved a radiation therapy system for the delivery of brachytherapy in brain cancer patients. This system uses a dual balloon, comprised of an inner balloon that holds a liquid radioactive source and an outer balloon to provide safety in the event the inner portion is damaged (Waknine, 2011). This procedure is generally reserved for high-grade gliomas (Nader & Eden, 2011).

Chemotherapy

The purpose of chemotherapy is to destroy tumor cells, either by destroying the cells themselves or by destroying their capacity to reproduce. Chemotherapy uses anticancer drugs, which are given intravenously or orally. They also may be given intrathecally, usually into an implanted reservoir. The implantation of a wafer soaked in a chemotherapeutic agent is occasionally used in the treatment of GBMs. The types of drugs used, dosage, and route are determined by the tumor type. Special concerns when treating malignant brain tumors with chemotherapeutic agents include the following:

- The location of the tumor in the brain affects the choice of treatment.
- Cerebral edema affects drug entry into the brain.
- Brain tissue has a low capacity to remove dead tissue, cell debris, fluid, and drugs because there is no lymphatic drainage in the brain.
- Tumor cell resistance can occur (tumor cells are no longer susceptible to a particular drug).
- Malignant tumors (GBM) are composed of diverse (heterogeneous) cells, resulting in differences in the chemosensitivity of cells within the tumor.
- Many drugs cannot cross the blood–brain barrier.

Chapter 57 includes a complete discussion of chemotherapy drugs and their side effects.

Nursing Management

Nursing management of the patient with a brain tumor includes the opportunity to support patients and their families through one of the most difficult occurrences they will experience. The patient and family are presented with a life-altering diagnosis that will affect every facet of the patient's life and every member of the patient's family. Innumerable factors can affect the patient's needs, both emotional and physical. The response to the diagnosis by the family and the patient depends on many factors, including the type of tumor, location of the tumor, treatment plan, degree of neurological deficits, age of the patient, family dynamics, educational status of the patient and family, and other factors that may change as the disease course changes.

Assessment

The initial diagnosis of brain tumor may be made because of an event that brought the patient into the emergency department, such as a seizure. In this situation, the patient's respiratory status must be monitored carefully, especially if the patient is admitted with a decreased LOC. The ABCs of any emergency assessment (airway–breathing–circulation) are just as important in patients with neurological deterioration. Monitoring of respiratory rate, rhythm, and effort is paramount, with preparations made for emergency intubation should the patient's respiratory status decline.

Usually, however, the patient is not in medical distress or even particularly ill. The patient's first exposure to a hospital setting may be on admission for surgery to remove the brain tumor. The patient's level of knowledge regarding the diagnosis or plan may be unknown. An important nursing intervention is education, about both the surgical experience and what to expect postoperatively. The surgeon will review the planned surgery, surgical approach, projected length of hospital stay, and possible side effects with the patient and family. However, most patients and their families have many other questions that they might not ask the surgeon. Examples of these are: Will I have my head shaved? When will I be able to eat, or get out of bed, or go to the bathroom by myself? Will I be in pain? When can I go back to work? What's going to happen to me when I go home? It is not uncommon for the patient and family to depend on the nurse to provide them with the information that will affect their everyday lives.

Nursing Diagnoses

The following nursing diagnoses are applicable to patients with brain tumors:

- *Acute Pain* related to headaches due to tumor and increase in intracranial pressure.
- *Disturbed Body Image* related to upcoming hair loss and cranial incision.
- *Anxiety* related to unknown future and possible follow-up surgeries.

NANDA-I © 2012

Outcomes and Evaluation Parameters

Outcomes and evaluation parameters are related to each nursing diagnosis cited in the previous list:

1. The patient will have adequate pain control.
2. The patient will understand changes in physical appearance.
3. The patient will verbalize understanding of the disease, treatments, and prognosis.

A patient care plan for patients with acute brain disorders is discussed in the Nursing Process: Patient Care Plan for Acute Brain Disorders feature (p. 523).

Interventions and Rationales

There are usually additional nursing concerns related to patients with brain tumors. These patients usually are started on corticosteroids, such as dexamethasone (Decadron). Use of steroids usually increases blood glucose levels. Therefore, blood glucose levels need to be assessed regularly and might require treatment. Steroids also can increase WBC counts, thus limiting the use of WBC analysis when evaluating for infections. Steroids can cause significant alterations in behavior and may produce insomnia, elation, and even psychosis. Nursing care should include careful monitoring to detect behavioral changes. Refer to the Pharmacology box (p. 530) for more explanation of these medications.

Patients undergoing chemotherapy may experience many side effects, such as fatigue, nausea and vomiting, loss of appetite, rash, neuropathies, myelosuppression, constipation, and immunosuppression. Side effects differ with the agent and may range from mild to severe. Occasionally, the patient's treatment cannot be continued owing to the severity of the reaction. It is important for nurses to be aware of side effects specific to the treatment of each patient. The presence of severe side effects should be reported to the health care provider.

Although seizures may be seen with other acute brain disorders, they are closely associated with certain types of brain tumors. For example, they are the most common presenting symptom of patients with oligodendrogliomas. Seizures also are seen with other tumor types, especially those located in the temporal region, owing to the high intensity of seizure focus in that area. These seizures are treated with antiepileptic drugs such as phenytoin. The nursing implications of seizure treatment are discussed later in this chapter (p. 544).

Patients with newly diagnosed brain tumors may present with overwhelming emotional needs. Nursing interventions include education and support. An important discharge intervention may be acquainting patients and their families with available brain tumor support groups. Many patients and families feel that the diagnosis of brain tumor is one without hope. Providing them with education and support may be helpful in relieving the fear of the unknown.

Collaborative Management

The diagnosis, treatment, and management of patients with brain tumors require the expertise of multiple disciplines (IOM [Institute of Medicine], 2010). These interdisciplinary teams include, but are not limited to, nursing, neurosurgery, neuro-oncology, radiation oncology, physical therapy, speech and cognitive therapy, occupational therapy, pathology, rehabilitation specialists, neuropsychologists, research scientists and nurses, dietitians, and support groups. In order to meet desired patient outcomes, it is essential that this interdisciplinary team communicate openly with one another in developing and evaluating care of the patient and family (IOM [Institute of Medicine], 2010). Once the diagnosis of brain tumor has been made, the patient should be referred to a neurosurgeon. Postoperatively, the patient may require the services of various therapists, such as physical, occupational, and/or speech therapists. Therapies are important for evaluation, leading to treatment if necessary, and for discharge recommendations. Depending on the pathology of the tumor, consultations with neuro-oncology, medical-oncology, and/or radiation oncology may be warranted. These consultations may be for the purpose of recommendations, with or without treatment.

Upon discharge from the hospital, the patient may need further therapy in the form of outpatient therapies, home health therapy, or an acute inpatient rehabilitation stay. Determination of the patient's need for further therapy is usually made by specialists in rehabilitation medicine.

At the center of the brain tumor patient's plan of care is nursing. Newly diagnosed brain tumor patients are frequently in a state of confusion and emotional upheaval. Their lives are full of changes: physical, emotional, practical, and possibly financial. They may be facing the loss of a job and financial security, and there may be changes within their family structure (e.g., spouses becoming caregivers). It is important to supply patients with as much education and support as they require. If support groups are available, it is usually helpful to give this information to the patients and their families. Refer to the Patient Teaching & Discharge Priorities for Acute Brain Disorders box (p. 527) to assist patients with brain tumors in preparing to go home or to a rehabilitation unit.

Health Promotion

Management of patient care for patients who are recovering from brain tumor treatments begins when the patient is still in the hospital and continues postdischarge when the patient has returned home and to the community. Research has indicated that discharged patients are worried about matters such as a change in body image, their ability to resume work, their general health status, the availability of support, and their ability to control mood fluctuations (Schubart, Kinzie, & Farace, 2008). When interviewed, brain tumor patients indicated that the illness caused them to pause and reconsider their life values. When discharged, they wanted to walk out of the hospital themselves and to resume normal daily activities as soon as possible. They also were worried about the possible recurrence of the tumor (Bachuss, 2008). Some patients were shocked and dismayed by the resulting physical limitations (Schubart, Kinzie, & Farace, 2011). Paramount among patients' concerns was their ability to care for themselves or have sufficient caregiver assistance.

A patient education program needs to be developed to promote health and patient stability following discharge. The following factors should be addressed:

- ***Mobility:*** Patients should be referred to a physical therapist for an exercise program to help them regain strength and function. The nurse should advise the patient to maintain mobility by using supportive devices as necessary (e.g., walker, wheelchair, cane). The nurse should emphasize that if the patient is unstable on his feet, he should have assistance when walking. The patient and family should keep pathways clear of obstacles.
- ***Nutrition:*** The nurse should encourage the patient to eat a well-balanced diet. The diet needs to be tailored to the patient's ability to swallow. Maintaining adequate fiber intake helps to protect against both diarrhea and constipation, lowers elevated cholesterol and triglyceride levels, and assists in regulating blood sugar levels. The side effects of brain tumor treatment—fatigue, weakness, nausea, and reduced appetite—can sometimes hinder good intentions to eat well. The nurse should advise the patient to try eating smaller, more frequent meals; to chew thoroughly to maximize digestion; and to eat in a quiet, pleasant atmosphere to reduce stress (National Brain Tumor Society, 2011; Sidrah, 2011). It may be helpful for the patient to see a nutrition consultant.
- ***Pain Management:*** Some patients may still be experiencing pain. The nurse should advise them on how to take the medication prescribed for pain relief and to notify their health care provider if pain is not resolved with the medication. The nurse can encourage the patient to keep a journal of the frequency of medications taken and relief experienced.

- ***Infection:*** Patients who have had chemotherapy, radiation therapy, and/or corticosteroids are more susceptible to infection. The nurse should review with the patient ways to avoid risks for exposure to infection, such as caring for the scalp wound if postsurgery, maintaining hand hygiene, staying away from crowds, and avoiding contact with people who are ill. The nurse should encourage the patient to participate actively in immunization programs, with the health care provider's knowledge and concurrence.
- ***Body Image and Appearance:*** The nurse should allow the patient to discuss her concerns about appearance. If the patient's head was shaved, the nurse can assist in securing a wig or other types of covering. The nurse can also advise the patient on resources available in the community to assist with purchasing supplies.
- ***Fear of Tumor Occurrence:*** The nurse should allow the patient to verbalize any fears and recommend that the patient discuss them with the health care provider. The nurse should refer the patient to community resources for counseling, decision support, education, and emotional support. The patient may contact the Institute of Medicine's Cancer Care for the Whole Patient: Meeting Psychosocial Health Needs to secure resources (Bachuss, 2008).
- ***Financial, Housing, Transportation, and Caregiver Concerns:*** The nurse may refer the patient to the Brain Tumor Society for education, emotional support, and financial assistance. The nurse should also refer the patient to available community resources.

The nurse should provide the family and caregiver a copy of the resources given to the patient. Both the patient and the family or caregiver should be made aware of the symptoms of a developing brain tumor that were discussed earlier in this chapter, which could signal recurrence (p. 536).

Hydrocephalus

Hydrocephalus is broadly defined as a disturbance of formation, flow, or absorption of CSF that leads to an increase in volume occupied by this fluid in the CNS, specifically in the ventricles (NINDS, 2011c). A normal adult has approximately 125 to 150 mL of CSF at any one time. It is normally produced at a rate of approximately 25 mL per hour. Normally, the rate of absorption balances with the rate of production.

Epidemiology, Etiology, and Pathophysiology

Hydrocephalus may be caused by overproduction of CNS or inadequate drainage or absorption. This condition may be congenital or acquired. Congenital hydrocephalus may be caused by either events or influences that occur during fetal development or genetic abnormalities. Acquired hydrocephalus develops at the time of birth or at some point afterward. This type of hydrocephalus can affect individuals of all ages and may be caused by injury or disease.

The two types of hydrocephalus are communicating and noncommunicating. Communicating hydrocephalus occurs when the flow of CSF is blocked after it exits the ventricles. It is called communicating because the CSF can still flow between ventricles, which remain open. Noncommunicating hydrocephalus, also called obstructive hydrocephalus, occurs when the flow of CSF is blocked along one or more of the narrow passages connecting the ventricles. One of the most common causes of hydrocephalus is *aqueductal stenosis*, which results from a narrowing of the aqueduct of Sylvius, a small passage between the third and fourth ventricles in the middle of the brain.

Two other forms of hydrocephalus that primarily affect adults do not fit in the two categories previously mentioned (MedicineNet.com, 2011b). The first type, hydrocephalus ex-vacuo, occurs when stroke or traumatic injury causes damage to the brain. In these cases, the brain tissue may actually shrink. The second type is normal pressure hydrocephalus (NPH), which can occur at any age but is most common in older adults (MedicineNet.com, 2011b). It typically occurs following a subarachnoid hemorrhage, head trauma, infection, tumor, or complications from surgery. It also may be idiopathic.

The number of people who develop hydrocephalus or who are currently living with it is difficult to establish, as there is no national registry for such. However, experts estimate that 1 in every 500 children have hydrocephalus (NINDS, 2011c).

The causes of hydrocephalus are not well understood. It may result from inherited genetic abnormalities or the development of disorders associated with neural tube defects. Other possibilities include intraventricular hemorrhage, meningitis, tumors, TBI, or subarachnoid hemorrhage, all of which can block the exit of CSF from the ventricles (MedicineNet.com, 2011b). The most common cause of noncommunicating hydrocephalus is space-occupying lesions, such as tumors.

The most important concept for understanding hydrocephalus is that of resistance to the absorption of CSF, which can cause an increase of ICP. The most common cause of malabsorption of CSF is subarachnoid hemorrhage, in which protein from a blood product breakdown clogs the arachnoid granulations, hindering absorption of CSF. In the absence of a lymphatic drainage system in the CNS, open communication between the CSF and the interstitial fluid is necessary for maintenance of homeostasis (Urden, Stacy, & Lough, 2010).

In the presence of cerebral edema, there may be no increase in ventricular size, because of the pressure of the brain tissue (parenchyma) against the ventricular system. Ventricular size is a balance between brain tissue forces attempting to compress the ventricles and intraventricular pressure attempting to enlarge the ventricles. This concept of intracranial pressure was discussed earlier in the chapter (p. 508).

Clinical Manifestations

The presentation of increasing ventricular size in adults depends on the type of hydrocephalus. The symptoms are similar to those of increased ICP and include papilledema; headache; nausea and vomiting; incontinence; gait changes; difficulty with extraocular movements, particularly upgaze; and alterations in LOC.

Diagnostic Procedures

A CT scan of the head, without contrast, is the quickest and most definitive means of diagnosing hydrocephalus. MRI is also an effective diagnostic tool and may be a better choice for imaging when pathology such as a brain tumor is suspected. As always, close clinical correlation of the patient's history and presenting symptoms is recommended.

Medical Management

Hydrocephalus is a surgically treated condition. In emergency situations, removal of CSF by means of an external ventricular drain is a temporary solution. However, placement of a shunting device to remove extra CSF is the gold standard for treatment of hydrocephalus. There are several types of shunts; the most common are the ventriculoperitoneal shunt and the lumboperitoneal shunt. Other less commonly used shunts; the ventriculoatrial shunt, the ventriculopleural shunt, and the ventriculocyst shunt are used when the more common types of shunts are not successful or their use is not possible for some reason (Engelhard, 2010).

Disadvantages of shunts are obstruction of the proximal or distal end, infection, and failure due to disconnection. There also is the possibility of overshunting, that is, the drainage of too much CSF, resulting in headaches for the patient. In extreme cases, subdural hematoma (SDH), caused by tearing of bridging veins, may occur. Undershunting, or too little fluid removal, results in the ventricles remaining large and increase the ICP. A CT scan after placement of a shunt is recommended to document appropriate placement and to assess the efficiency of the shunt by checking for a decrease in ventricle size.

Nursing Management

Nursing management of patients with hydrocephalus consists primarily of accurate neurological assessment. Hydrocephalus can occur with virtually any neurological condition. Decrease in mental status can occur slowly, over days, or rapidly. Any change in neurological status is significant and should be reported. These changes include a change in LOC, decrease in ability to speak, decrease in ability to ambulate, and/or incontinence of bowel or bladder. Please refer to the Nursing Process: Patient Care Plan for Acute Brain Disorders box (p. 523) for the details of how to care for a patient with hydrocephalus.

Seizures

A **seizure** is described as a single, temporary event that consists of uncontrolled, electrical neuronal discharge in the brain that interrupts normal brain function. Seizures may occur as a result of most acute brain disorders: a brain tumor, brain trauma such as a hematoma or concussion, or in conjunction with an infectious process such as meningitis, encephalitis, or abscesses. They also may be seen with non-neurological disorders such as metabolic disorders, including severe dehydration and electrolyte imbalances, or in withdrawal from alcohol or drugs. Idiopathic seizures also may occur in the absence of underlying abnormalities. Epilepsy is a condition in which seizures occur spontaneously. They can recur owing to an underlying condition or without a known cause.

Epidemiology and Etiology

There are many causes of seizures. These causes are different depending on the patient's age at onset. Structural abnormalities, such as tumors, strokes, and trauma, are the most common cause in adults. Seizures may be caused by genetic predisposition or acquired brain damage (Stern, Rosenbaum, Fava, Biederman, & Rauch, 2008).

Clinical Manifestations

The clinical manifestations of seizures depend on the location of the electrical aberrancy, known as the seizure focus. Seizures are divided into two main divisions: generalized and partial.

Generalized Seizures

Generalized seizures affect the whole body; the most common type is the tonic–clonic seizure, formerly named the grand mal seizure (Hickey, 2009). The individual may exhibit alterations in mentation, behavior, sensation, and/or motor tonic–clonic activity. These seizures are characterized by bilateral, symmetric electrical discharges and are described as a stiffening of the body, with jerking of all extremities, ending in a limp state also known as the postictal phase (Hickey, 2009). The patient may become cyanotic, have excessive drooling, and bite the inside of her mouth and/or her tongue. Urinary incontinence is common with this type of seizure. The patient loses consciousness and is not communicative or interactive during the event. There may be pupillary changes, with a gaze deviation (away from the side of a structural abnormality, if present). However, the patient will have no memory of the seizure event. Chart 21–5 shows the characteristics of different types of seizures.

Video: Neurological: Seizures

Video: Neurological: Epilepsy—Etiology and Pathophysiology

CHART 21–5 Types of Seizures

Type of Seizure	Characteristics	Consciousness	Medications	Age Groups
Tonic–clonic Generalized Grand mal Absence	Bilateral Symmetric No warning Stiffening of the body Jerking Cyanosis Tongue-biting Incontinence Abnormal behavior Staring spells	Loss of consciousness for seconds to minutes	Phenytoin (Dilantin) Carbamazepine (Tegretol) Levetiracetam (Keppra) Lamotrigine (Lamictal) Phenobarbital Topiramate (Topamax) Valproic acid Divalproex (Depakote) Klonopin	All children
Partial, simple	Focal Motor and/or sensory May progress	No loss of consciousness	Same as above Pregabalin (Lyrica) Gabapentin (Neurontin) Oxcarbazepine (Trileptal)	All
Partial, complex	Focal Motor and/or sensory Automatisms	Altered state of consciousness Clouding or confusion Déjà vu	Same as above	All

Partial Seizures

Partial seizures, those that are focal or localized and affect only a part of the brain, are further divided into simple or complex, the differentiating factor being consciousness (MedlinePlus, 2011a). Simple partial seizures are described as seizures with specific motor or sensory abnormalities. These would include focal motor seizures or those with somatosensory components, such as the visualization of flashing lights or hearing noises that are not real. There is no loss of consciousness. Complex partial seizures may begin as a simple partial seizure. Although they may share many of the same features as simple partial seizures, consciousness is impaired. They also may progress to a generalized seizure.

Status Epilepticus

Status epilepticus is defined as 30 minutes of continuous seizure activity or two or more sequential seizures without full consciousness between seizures (Barker, 2008). Status epilepticus is a medical emergency, because continued seizure activity could result in severe neurological injury due to cerebral hypoxia. It also may result in respiratory and/or cardiovascular failure.

Diagnostic Procedures

The diagnosis of seizures depends on many factors. First, a detailed account of the event must be available. This includes clinical presentation, medications, and past medical history. A physical examination, with a focus on neurological assessment, is essential.

Diagnostic tests include, but are not limited to, imaging studies, such as MRI or CT scan, to rule out structural abnormality as a cause (see the Diagnostic Tests for Acute Brain Disorders box, p. 518). This does not address whether or not a seizure has occurred but rather is used to determine whether an underlying cause is present that could potentiate a seizure. EEGs record the brain's electrical potential. This is done by placing electrodes on the patient's scalp and recording tracings of the brain's electrical activity. Patients with epilepsy have abnormal electrical tracings. EEGs should be used in conjunction with other diagnostic tests, such as MRI, PET scans, or other tests that determine potential organic causes for seizures, such as a tumor. EEGs are very helpful in recording abnormal electrical activity if a seizure occurs during the tracing. However, these tracings can be normal in the interictal period (the period between seizure events). Other tests may be used to help determine the exact location of a seizure focus and the area and function of the brain affected. Wada tests, officially known as the intracarotid sodium amobarbital procedure (ISAP), are used to determine which side of the brain controls language function and how important each side of the brain is with regard to memory function. Functional MRIs also are very helpful to determine what areas in the brain are involved when the patient performs specific functions. For example, "when a patient with an arteriovenous malformation (AVM) lesion performs a left hand motor task, focal activation in the motor and sensory areas is seen in the right hemisphere, indicating a consolidated use of the cortex. When the same patient performs a right hand motor task, very weak activation in the left hemisphere is observed" (Northwestern Radiololgy, 2012, p. 2). Typically, the left hemisphere controls right-sided motor function. However, there is strong activation in the right hemisphere. The presence of the AVM may be disturbing the flow, making it difficult to detect activation around the AVM, and the right hemisphere activation may represent cortical remapping.

Medical Management

Medical treatment of seizures should begin immediately, although the type of treatment depends on the type of seizure. Antiepileptic drugs (AED) should be started immediately to prevent further seizures. Many antiepileptic drugs are available, and research is being done to determine the most efficacious according to seizure type. AEDs are described in the Pharmacology box (p. 530).

In some circumstances, surgical resection of an identifiable seizure focus is warranted. To determine suitability for resection, these patients may be evaluated extensively in a specialized monitoring unit (e.g., the epilepsy monitoring unit) equipped with 24-hour EEG and surveillance monitors to identify the seizure focus. Invasive EEG electrodes may be placed surgically. These data are reviewed along with continuous video surveillance of the patient and all possible seizure activity. This information, along with diagnostic imaging studies, gives useful information to specialists in seizures, called epileptologists. These specialized neurologists work closely with neurosurgeons to determine whether surgical resection of a seizure focus would be warranted. This surgery is referred to as a selective amygdalohippocampectomy (SAHC).

Management of status epilepticus has two important aspects. Termination of the seizure is of primary importance. This usually is accomplished with medications, such as short-acting benzodiazepines. Second are the ABCs of life support, such as assessment of the patient's respiratory status, with administration of oxygen by mask or nasal cannula and ventilatory support if necessary.

Nursing Management

One of the most important factors in the management of seizures is the reporting of the seizure event. Often, nurses are the ones who witness a seizure, and their assessment is critical to determining the seizure type and its management.

Assessment

Objective Data

Assessment of the patient experiencing a seizure should include the following objective observations:

- Was the seizure witnessed? If so, by whom?
- Were there precipitating events?
- Where did the seizure start? Did it progress to other areas?
- What type of movement of the extremities was observed?
- Were there pupillary changes?
- Was there gaze deviation? If so, in which direction?
- Was there incontinence of the bowel or bladder?
- What was the patient's mental status during the seizure (unconscious or awake and talking)?
- How long did the event last?
- After the seizure, what was the patient's mental status?
- Was there any motor weakness after the seizure?

Subjective Data

Subjective data are gathered through the following techniques:

- Inspection of the body for injuries
- Observation for safety hazards in the physical environment
- Observation for the presence of others.

Subjective assessment also may include asking the patient the following questions:

- Did anything happen to you just before you had the seizure; for example, were you upset about anything, or did some incident that was troubling for you occur before the seizure?
- What, if anything, do you remember about the seizure?
- Was anyone with you when you experienced the seizure?
- How did you feel after the procedure? Can you remember the date and time?
- How do your muscles feel? Are they strong or weak?
- Are you able to move your arms and legs? Do they feel weak?

Nursing Diagnoses

Nursing diagnoses for patients with seizures are derived from the assessment data.

- *Ineffective Airway Clearance* related to tonic–clonic muscle activity and tongue obstruction.
- *Anxiety* related to fear of the unknown and loss of control.
- *Deficient Knowledge* related to lack of understanding of seizures and unknown experiences.
- *Fear* related to threat of danger to self and unknown experience.
- *Risk for Injury* related to uncontrolled muscular coordination.

NANDA-I © 2012

Outcomes with Evaluation Parameters

Outcomes and evaluation parameters are based on patients' objectives, which guide the development of nursing interventions. These appear in the following list.

1. The patient's airway will be clear. *The patient is able to breathe comfortably; is free of mucus in the mouth and nose; has strong breath sounds, a normal respiratory rate, and normal respiratory rhythm; and has no evidence of cyanosis.*
2. The patient will have decreased anxiety. *The patient expresses feelings of decreased anxiety, uses available support systems, and develops coping skills.*
3. The patient understands his condition. *The patient communicates understanding of the condition and the treatment regimen.*
4. The patient acknowledges his fears and concerns. *The patient identifies fears and concerns and resumes active participation in social situations and activities.*
5. The patient remains free from injury. *The nurse finds no evidence of injuries to the patient's body and no evidence of falls.*

Interventions and Rationales

Nursing interventions for patients with seizures are as follows:

- Provide emotional support to patients and families *to assist patients in adjusting to their illnesses.*
- Encourage patient and family to express their fears and concerns. Suggest counseling to help them cope *and to assist the patient and family in developing coping mechanisms.*
- Maintain safety precautions for the patient to prevent injury (e.g., pad the bed rails), administer anti-seizure medications as ordered, and monitor the patient for side effects of medication (implement fall prevention protocol) *to maintain the patient's safety.*
- Do not leave the patient alone when she is having a *seizure in order to prevent the patient from injuring herself or choking, and assist the patient to protect herself by turning on her side.*
- Do not restrain the patient *as this may precipitate injury.*
- Monitor the patient for signs and symptoms of toxicity from medications, such as slurred speech, ataxia, lethargy, dizziness, drowsiness, nystagmus, irritability, nausea, and vomiting (Phenytoin, a commonly used anticonvulsive drug, may cause nausea, dizziness, gait and balance problems, gingival hyperplasia, and drug-induced fever), *in order to determine appropriateness of medication given to patient.* (See the Pharmacology box on p. 530.)
- If needed, prepare the patient for surgery to *keep the patient informed and prepared for upcoming treatment.*
- If necessary, provide preoperative and postoperative care appropriate for the types of surgery the patient is to undergo in *order to maintain patient safety and quality of care.*
- Protect the patient from secondary injury in the event that the patient stops breathing during a seizure. It also is important never to force anything into the patient's mouth, such as a "bite stick" (for example, a padded tongue blade) *to ensure patient safety.*
- Provide the patient and family with discharge and home health care guidelines *to assist the patient and family for the return to the home setting.*

The Nursing Process: Patient Care Plan for Acute Brain Disorders on page 523 may be used as an adjunct to the specific care plan for seizures.

Safety Alert *Confusion, lethargy, and/or seizure may be a sign of hyponatremia. The nurse should check recent serum Na^+ levels, check intake and output, and determine which intravenous fluids are infusing. The nurse needs to notify the health care provider of a Na^+ level less than 135 mEq/L. Patients with hyponatremia are at risk for seizures. In the presence of low sodium, the nurse institutes seizure precautions.*

Collaborative Management

Seizure management, specifically AED management, is a specialty area in some institutions. If an epileptologist (a neurologist specializing in seizure management) is available, a consult may be helpful, especially if management of the patient's seizures proves to be difficult. Other health care providers may also play a role in the patient's health. In order to meet desired patient outcomes, it is essential that this interdisciplinary team communicate openly with one another in developing and evaluating care of the patient and family (IOM [Institute of Medicine], 2010). Phenytoin dosing services are available in some institutions and are a welcome addition to management of this drug when dosing in accordance to laboratory drug levels. Pharmacists may be of assistance with the many drug interactions associated with AEDs. Many common drugs, as well as foods, can interact with and potentiate or diminish the effects of AEDs. It is important for the patient and family to be aware of these common foods and drugs and the effects they may have on seizure management. A nutritionist may be consulted to assist the patient and family in food management.

Health Promotion

Before discharge, it is imperative that the patient understands all medications, including the dosage, route, action, adverse effects, and need for routine laboratory monitoring of AEDs. The patient and family will probably need emotional support. This may be achieved by responding to their expressed concerns and answering any and all questions that they ask. Specific teaching points include the following:

- The nurse should explain to the patient and family the need for compliance with the prescribed drug schedule.
- The nurse should review medications with the patient: dosage, route, action, adverse effects, and the need for routine laboratory monitoring of drugs.
- The nurse should assure the patient that anticonvulsive drugs are safe when taken as prescribed.
- The nurse should instruct the patient to eat regular meals and consult with her health care provider before dieting. It is also important to explain that adequate glucose levels are needed to provide the necessary energy for the CNS to work normally.
- The nurse should teach the patient's family to avoid restraining the patient during a seizure as the patient may injure himself if he is thrashing against restraints.
- The nurse should advise the patient and family as to which social agencies in the community can help epileptic patients. The nurse may refer the patient to the Epilepsy Foundation for general information and to the state motor vehicle department for information about restrictions in obtaining a driver's license.

Gerontological Considerations

Acute brain disorders, such as TBI, brain tumors, or infectious diseases, can cause substantial injury to patients of any age. However, there are some specific considerations related to TBI in older adults. The incidence of TBI in older adults may be influenced by age-related changes, such as changes in vision, decreased mobility, decreased muscle and bone mass, and decreased physical agility. Fall risk of older adults is exacerbated by the fact that many of them live alone.

TBI in older adults carries a higher percentage of mortality and morbidity than in other age groups. Overall mortality of TBI in older adults is approximately 33.5%, with overall poor functional outcomes (Traumatic Brain Injury Services of California, 2011). Less favorable outcomes may be due to several factors, including chronic, preexisting comorbidities such as pulmonary or cardiovascular problems, thereby, increasing the risk of morbidity and mortality (Shiflett et al., 2010). Preexisting cognitive impairment is another factor that may influence outcome. Medications, specifically anticoagulation drugs, such as warfarin, also plays a significant role. These drugs and others taken for pre-exisiting conditions may be detrimental due to the increased risk of complications, such as bleeding.

According to Olson (2011), older patients with trauma to the head are at higher risk of developing a significant intracranial injury. This information supports the importance of recognizing the specific considerations of TBI in the gerontological population.

Research

It is important to work toward future advances in acute brain disorders that improve patients' lives. Therefore, investigation and continuing research are crucial. It is pertinent for the nurse to continue to monitor the epidemiological trends of CNS infections to understand infection dynamics and to develop appropriate health care interventions. Although the mortality rate for meningitis and encephalitis is still significant, it appears to be decreasing. One important trend is that the use of vaccines for meningococcal infections has decreased the incidence of *Streptococcus pneumonia* and Hib meningitis (Somand & Meurer, 2009).

A diagnosis of brain tumor is life altering at best. Even with more than 20 years of clinical trials and new technologies to combat this disease, few improvements in prognosis have been seen, especially in the treatment of high-grade tumors. There has been interest in an experimental drug called Cilengitide, an anti-angiogenesis agent that may cut off the tumor, which will prevent tumor growth. Clinical trials are underway using Cilengitide and GBMs (Stupp et al., 2010). The Radiation Therapy Oncology Group (RTOG) (2008) protocols also are important in identifying optimal RT programs for various tumor types. Radiosurgery has become and will continue to be important in the treatment of various tumor types. Information is being obtained and processed continually to determine the efficacy of various treatment plans.

Research into the genetics of brain tumors is dynamic. Genetic aberrations are being defined for the various glial tumors previously described. It is known that tumors can evolve by different pathways. Genetic aberrations differ from grade of malignancy and the type of tumor. Cataloguing of major genetic alterations in brain tumors is being followed, thus, allowing for development of novel pharmacologic therapies in the future (Rutka et al., 2009).

RESEARCH OPPORTUNITIES Related to Acute Brain Disorders

Research Area	Clinical Impact
Examine various treatment modalities for hyponatremia (i.e., hypertonic saline, salt tablets, fluid restriction, or other medications) and their impact on the treatment of hyponatremia in the presence of brain tumors.	Hyponatremia is relatively common in the patients with brain tumors and head injury, and it also is associated with cerebral edema. The appropriate treatment of hyponatremia may be significant to a positive patient outcome.
Examine the outcome of patients with TBI or brain tumor who are provided with rehabilitation services versus patients who receive no rehabilitation after discharge (retrospective study).	Define the benefits of therapies and rehabilitation to patients with brain injury due to TBI or tumor.
Examine different monitoring devices for the maintenance of adequate brain oxygenation.	Maintain adequate brain oxygenation, with the reduction of neurological injury.
Examine various administration routes (oral, enteral, IV) for the administration of phenytoin and any possible differences in the maintenance of adequate blood levels of the drug.	Maintain adequate blood levels of phenytoin, possibly reducing the risk of seizures.

READ: **History of Present Illness** >> Laboratory Study Results >> Critical Thinking Questions

As a nurse in the neuroscience ICU of a large metropolitan teaching hospital, you receive a phone call from the emergency department (ED), giving you a report on a new patient being admitted to your unit. The patient is a 32-year-old Hispanic male brought to the ED by his brother, who found him wandering outside their home, confused and disoriented. The patient's brother also noted that the patient had trouble opening the car door with his right hand. The brother stated that the patient had come home from his job stocking supplies in a grocery warehouse complaining of a headache. Coworkers told the brother that they had seen several boxes that had fallen but were unaware that any had actually struck the patient.

On admission to the ED, the patient received a CT scan, and the health care provider noted a moderate-sized subdural hematoma in the left temporal area, ruling out a skull fracture. The patient is now being admitted to the neuroscience ICU for close monitoring of his neurological status. A craniotomy for evacuation of the left temporal subdural hematoma is planned for early the following morning. The ED nurse tells you that the patient is on his way, and his family is accompanying him. His family consists of several siblings, his wife, his parents, and two small children. They are very concerned and do not speak English.

Medical–Surgical History

This history was obtained from multiple family members: On examination of the patient's records, you note that the patient, whose name is Jose Ramos, has no past medical history and has, in fact, never been in the hospital for any reason. He has no allergies and takes no medication. No illnesses are reported, with the exception of "usual" childhood illnesses, according to his parents.

Social History

Mr. Ramos has a wife, two small children, and multiple family members. His wife denies any drug or alcohol use; however, his brother relates moderate alcohol consumption "on the weekends." He works in a warehouse, stocking groceries and supplies. He has completed high school. He has lived in the United States for many years and is a citizen of this country. He has not traveled outside of the country since he was a young child.

READ: History of Present Illnesses >> **Physical Exam** >> Admitting Medical Records >> Laboratory Study Results

Physical Exam

His emergency department assessment and orders are as follows:

Young Hispanic male, resting quietly, appears in no distress
Vital signs: afebrile; HR 62 regular, RR 16, BP 134/74
HEENT: normocephalic, with small tender, bruised area near L temple
Heart: rhythm and rate regular, S_1S_2 heard, no abnormal murmurs, good capillary refill, pulses 2+ all extremities, no pitting edema
Lungs: clear to auscultation bilaterally
O_2 sat at 97% on room air
Abdomen: soft, nontender, bowel sounds heard all quadrants

Neurological Exam

GCS = E4 M6 V4 = 14; oriented to name only, confused to date and surroundings
Pleasant, cooperative, and attentive
Speech clear and fluent
Cranial nerves: CNII–CNXII intact bilaterally
Motor:
Right upper extremity 5/5
Right lower extremity 5/5
RUE pronator drift
Left upper extremity 5/5
Left lower extremity 5/5
Sensory: grossly intact to light touch bilaterally

Imaging Studies

Head CT scan done in the ED reveals an acute left-sided subdural hematoma
Chest x-ray: negative for abnormal pathology

Admitting Medical Orders

Admit to Neuroscience ICU
Diagnosis: acute left subdural hematoma
Condition: guarded
Allergies: none known
Vital signs and neuro assessment: q1h
Bed rest
Diet: NPO
Notify resident on call regarding any change in neurological status: increase in severity of headache or nausea, temperature >38°C, HR <60 or >120, systolic BP <100 or >160, RR <10 or >30, O_2 sat less than 92%, urine output <30 mL/hr × 2
Sequential compression devices (SCDs) to lower extremities prior to surgery
IV: 0.9% with 20meq KCL @ 75 mL/hr
Continuous ECG, pulse oximetry
Foley catheter
Intake and output q2h
Consent for craniotomy for evacuation of left subdural hematoma by Dr. Pramanik

Scheduled Medications

Pepcid 20 mg IV q12h

PRN Medications

Acetaminophen 650 mg po/PR q4h for pain or fever
Morphine sulfate 2–4 mg IV q2h for pain
Promethazine 12.5–25 mg po/IV/PR q4h for nausea

Ordered Laboratory Studies

ABG × 1 now
Serum and urine osmolality × 1 now
CBC now and q a.m.
PTT, INR. Chem 7 panel, magnesium, phosphorous, and ionized CA now and q12h
Urinalysis now

Ordered Diagnostic Studies

Preoperative ECG

After Mr. Ramos has been settled in your unit, you examine him. His vital signs and neurological assessment are unchanged from the admitting assessment. He is resting comfortably, is talking with the nursing staff, and is quite pleasant and cooperative.

CLINICAL PREPARATION, *continued*

He complains of a headache and is medicated with intravenous morphine. He has an IV line in place. He is denying nausea at this time but is not hungry. He is in the ICU for close monitoring. He is considered to be stable and safe to wait the few hours until morning to evacuate his hematoma.

About 2 hours after Mr. Ramos is admitted, he requests more pain medication because his headache is worse. Before you can bring his medication, he attempts to crawl over the side rails of his bed. He is clearly agitated, is worried about his family, and wants to go home. You convince him to return to bed. Within minutes, he has projectile emesis and now is clearly confused. He is unable to tell you his name or where he is. His vital signs are essentially unchanged, although his heart and respiratory rates are slightly elevated. His neurological examination is as follows: He is alert, restless, and agitated. He is clearly confused, unable to state his name or where he is. His pupils are equal, but his left pupil is slow to react. His right pronator drift is still present but does not appear to be any worse. The neurosurgical resident you call wants another CT scan but states that Mr. Ramos may go straight to surgery after his scan. As you are preparing to take him to radiology, you look up his labs and check his paperwork to make sure the surgical consent is in the medical record. While Mr. Ramos is receiving his scan, you go to the waiting room to speak to the family and keep them aware of the latest events.

READ: History of Present Illnesses >> **Laboratory Study Results** >> Critical Thinking Questions

Test	On Admission	6 Hours After Admission	Day 1 (AM Labs)
pH	7.36	7.40	7.39
$PaCO_2$	40 mmHg	40 mmHg	39 mmHg
PaO_2	80 mmHg	86 mmHg	82 mmHg
SO_2	96%	95%	95%
HCO_3	24 mEq/L	25 mEg/L	24 mEg/L
Sodium	140 mEq/L	139 mEq/L	138 mEg/L
Potassium	3.6 mEq/L	3.6 mEq/L	3.5 mEg/L
Chloride	92 mEq/L	92 mEq/L	91 mEg/L
Carbon dioxide	23 mEq/L	24 mEq/L	23 mEg/L
Blood urea nitrogen (BUN)	26 mg/dL	26 mg/dL	25 mg/dL
Creatinine	1.4 mg/dL	1.3 mg/dL	1.3 mg/dL
Blood glucose	93 mg/dL	90 mg/dL	92 mg/dL

Test	On Admission	6 Hours After Admission	Day 1 (AM Labs)
Blood alcohol	NA, 00.0%		
White blood cells	9,200/μL	9,000/uL	9,000/uL
Hemoglobin	14.2 g/dL	14 g/dL	14 g/dL
Hematocrit	39.8%	38 %	38%
Platelets	312,000 μL	310,000 uL	309,000 uL
Protime (PT)	11.8 seconds	11.7 seconds	11.6 seconds
International normalized ratio (INR)	0.9 INR	0.8 INR	0.8 INR
Partial thromboplastin time (PTT)	34 seconds	32 seconds	32 seconds
Serum osmolality	280 mOsm/kg	281 mOsm/kg	280 mOsm/kg
Urine osmolality	600 mOsm/kg H_2O	601 mOsm/kg H_2O	601 mOsm/kg H_2O

Pearson Nursing Student Resources *Log on to* ***nursing.pearsonhighered.com*** *to download forms*

DOCUMENT:

- >> Summary of Hospitalization
- >> Pathophysiology Form
- >> Laboratory Values
- >> Laboratory Results Explanation

APPLY:

- >> List of Potential Nursing Diagnoses
- >> Concept Map
- >> Critical Thinking Questions and Concept Map

APPLY: History of Present Illnesses >> Laboratory Study Results >> **Critical Thinking Questions**

1. What neurological findings might you expect in a patient with an injury to the left temporal area?
2. At what point did Mr. Ramos's neurological status change?
3. What is the significance of Mr. Ramos's change in mental status?
4. On the basis of the change in Mr. Ramos's condition, what might the nurse expect his CT scan to show?

Answers to Critical Thinking Questions appear in Appendix D. in the Osborn Student Resources at nursing.pearsonhighered.com.

NCLEX® PRACTICE

1. The nurse is monitoring a patient's intracranial pressure for a potential increase. The nurse is aware that the body may initially try to compensate for pressure changes in any of the components of the cranium by which of the following mechanisms?

1. Increasing production of CSF
2. Expansion of brain tissue
3. Blocking the autoregulation of cerebral blood flow
4. Increasing absorption of CSF

2. A patient is admitted with a gradual increase in intracranial pressure due to an enlarging tumor. Early signs of increased intracranial pressure may include which of the following?

1. Changes in the optic nerve (CNVIII) that may result in ringing in the ears
2. Decorticate movement observable in the arms
3. Complaints of a "different" headache and projectile vomiting
4. Cushing's triad

3. The nursing management for the patient with increased intracranial pressure involves assessment of respiratory, cardiovascular, metabolic, and neurological processes. Desired parameters to avoid complications include which of the following? (select all that apply)

1. Pulse oximetry should be used with supplemental oxygen to maintain saturations of 90% or greater
2. Normocapnia levels ($PaCO_2$ levels of 35 to 40 mmHg)
3. Euglycemic levels of 80 to 120 mg/dL
4. Normothermia and interventions for body temperatures >100.6°F rectally
5. Hypothermia with intervention to maintain temperature <95°F rectally

4. A 50-year-old patient is admitted to the ED with a scalp laceration that was bleeding profusely and was bandaged at the scene by emergency personnel. The patient is currently stable. The nurse is aware that before wound closure is initiated, which of the following activities is a priority?

1. A complete neurological assessment to rule out cerebral contusion
2. A CAT scan of the head to rule out skull fracture
3. A cerebral arteriogram to identify which vessel has been ruptured
4. A skull series to determine the presence of hematomas

5. A patient is being admitted for meningitis. The nurse is aware that the presenting signs and symptoms for bacterial and viral meningitis are the same, so the nurse must use laboratory data to differentiate between these acute processes. Which of the following is true concerning bacterial meningitis?

1. In the spinal fluid, protein levels will be high and glucose levels will be low.
2. In the spinal fluid, the color will be clear.
3. In the spinal fluid, the protein and glucose levels will be low.
4. The spinal fluid will be bloody.

6. A patient asks the nurse about the differences between a benign and malignant brain tumor. Which of the following statements reflects the characteristics of benign brain tumors that the nurse may include in her explanation?

1. These tumors are nonmalignant and are easily removed by surgery.
2. The tumors are self-limiting and do not influence the function of surrounding tissues.
3. Benign tumors may be surgically difficult to remove and may compress vital structures.
4. These tumors do not progress into malignant tumors.

Answers to NCLEX Practice questions can be found in Appendix D in the Osborn Student Resources at nursing.pearsonhighered.com. Practice additional NCLEX questions online at the Student Resources site.

Pearson Nursing Student Resources Find additional review materials at: **nursing.pearsonhighered.com**

REFERENCES

Adams, M. P. & Koch, R. (2010). Pharmacology: Connections to nursing practice. Upper Saddle River, NJ: Pearson.

Adoni, A., & McNett, M. (2007). The Pupillary Response in Traumatic Brain Injury. *The Journal of Trauma Nursing, 14*(4), 190–197.

American Association of Neuroscience Nurses, AANN Reference Series for Clinical Practice. (2006). *Guide to the care of the patient with craniotomy post-brain tumor resection.* Glenview, IL: American Association of Neuroscience Nurses.

American Cancer Society. (2011, June 20). What are the key statistics about brain and spinal cord tumors? Brain and spinal cord tumors in adults. Retrieved from http://www.cancer.org/Cancer/BrainCNSTumorsinAdults/DetailedGuide/brain-and-spinal-cord-tumors-in-adults-key-statistics

Andary, M. T. (2011). Guillain-Barré syndrome. Medscape reference. Retrieved from http://emedicine.medscape.com/article/315632=overview

Anderson, T. (2009). Current and evolving management of subarachnoid hemorrhage. *Critical Care Nursing Clinics of North America, 21*(4), 529–239.

Arciniegas, D., & McAllister, T. (2008). Neurobehavioral management of traumatic brain injury in the critical care setting. *Critical Care Medicine, 24*, 737–765.

Bachuss, C. A. (2008). Nursing management of glioblastoma multiforme. *Topics in Advanced Practice Nursing, Medscape.e-Journal, 8*(4). Retrieved from http://www.medscape.com/viewarticle/585174_print

Bader, M., & Littlejohns, L. (2010). *AANN core curriculum for neuroscience nursing* (5th ed.). Glenview, IL: American Association of Neuroscience Nurses.

Badjatia, N. (2009). Hyperthermia and fever control in brain injury. *Critical Care Medicine, 37*(7), S250–S257.

Bagheri, A. (2007). Individual choice in the definition of death. *Journal of Medical Ethics, 33*(3), 146–149.

Barker, E. (2008). *Neuroscience nursing* (3rd ed.). St. Louis: Mosby.

Bell, L. (2009). Nursing care and intracranial pressure. *American Journal of Critical Care, 18*(4), 338.

Best Practice. (2012). Brain abscess. Retrieved from http://bestpractice.bmj.com/best-practice/monograph/925/treatment/step-by-step.html

Bey, T., & Ostick, B. (2009). Second impact syndrome. *Western Journal of Emergency Medicine, 10*(1), 6–10.

Biros, M. H., Heegaard.,W. G. (2009). Head injury. In: Marx, J. A., Hockberger, R. S., Walls, R. M., et al., eds. *Rosen's Emergency Medicine: Concepts and Clinical Practice.* 7th ed. Chapter 38. Philadelphia, PA: Mosby Elsevier.

Blanda, M. (2011, September 16). Tension headaches. Retrieved from http://emedicine.medscape.com/article/792384-overview#a0199

Blyth, B., & Bazarian, J. (2010). Traumatic alterations in consciousness: Traumatic brain injury. *Emergency Medicine Clinics in Northern America, 28*, 571–594.

Bohan, E., & Glass-Macenka, D. (2009). It's not your "run of the mill" meningioma: Characteristics differentiating low-grade from high-grade meningeal tumors. *Journal of Neuroscience Nursing, 31*(3), 124–128.

Bope, E., Kellerman, R., & Rakel, R. (2011). *Conn's current therapy 2011* (1st ed.). Philadelphia: Elsevier.

Bradley, W., Daroff, R., Fenichel, G., & Jankovic, J. (2008). *Neurology in clinical practice* (5th ed.). Philadelphia: Elsevier.

Brook, I. (2011). Brain abscess. Medscape reference. Retrieved from http://emedicine.medscape.com/article/212946-overview

Bruce, J. N. (2011). Glioblastoma multiforme. Medscape reference. Retrieved from http://emedicine.medscape.com/article/283252-overview

Burns, C. E., Brady, M. A., Dunn, A. M., Starr, N. B., & Blosser, C. G. (2008*). Pediatric primary care* (4th ed.). Maryland Heights, MO: Saunders.

Buttaro, T. M., Trybulski, J., Baily, P., & Sandberg-Cook, J. (2008). *Primary care* (3rd ed.). St. Louis: Mosby Elsevier.

Carey, W. (2010). *Cleveland clinic: Current clinical medicine* (2nd ed.). Philadelphia: Saunders.

Castilla, L. (2011, June 14). Closed head injury. Retrieved from http://emedicine.medscape.com/article/251834-overview

Cecil, S., Chen, P., Callaway, S., Rowland, S., Adler, D., & Chen, J. (2010). Traumatic brain injury: Advanced multimodal neuromonitoring from theory to clinical practice. *Critical Care Nurse 31*(2), 25-26. doi: 10.4037/ccn2010226

Center for Bioethics, University of Minnesota. (2005). End of life care: An ethical overview. Retrieved from http://www.ahc.umn.edu/img/assets/26104/End_of_Life.pdf

Centers for Disease Control and Prevention (CDC). (2010a, March 18). *Facts for physicians booklet.* Retrieved from http://www.cdc.gov/concussion/headsup/pdf/Facts_for_Physicians_booklet-a.pdf

Centers for Disease Control and Prevention (CDC). (2010b). Injury prevention & control. Retrieved from http://www.cdc.gov/TraumaticBrainInjury/index.html

Centers for Disease Control and Prevention (CDC). (2010c). Meningitis questions & answers. Retrieved from http://www.cdc.gov.meningitis/about/faq.html

Centers for Disease Control and Prevention. (2011). Traumatic brain injury. Retrieved from http://www.cdc.gov/TraumaticBrainInjury

Central Brain Tumor Registry of the United States. (2010). Fact sheet of the Central Brain Tumor Registry of the United States. Retrieved from http://www.cbtrus.org/factsheet/factsheet.html

Champion, H., Holcomb, J., & Young, L. (2009). Injuries from explosions. *Journal of Trauma, 66*(5), 1468–1476.

Chawla, J. (2011, May 25). Migraine headache. Retrieved from http://emedicine.medscape.com/article/1142556-overview.

Crippen, D. W. (2011). Head trauma. Retrieved from http://emedicine.medscape.com/article/433855-overview#a0102

Cushing's-Help.com. (2011). Cushing's glossary. Retrieved from http://www.cushings-help.com/definitions.htm

Davids, H. (2011, Aug 26). Guillain-Barré syndrome. Retrieved from http://emedicine.medscape.com/article/315632-overview#aw2aab6b2b3

Dawodu, S. (2011). Traumatic brain injury (TBI)—definition, epidemiology, pathophysiology. Medscape reference. Retrieved from http://emedicine.medscape.com/article/326510

DeLee, J., Drez, D., & Miller, M. (2009). *DeLee and Drez's orthopaedic sports medicine* (3rd ed.). Philadelphia: Elsevier.

Deshaies, E.M., Jacobsen, W., Singla, A., Li, F., & Gorji, R. (2012). Brain tissue oxygen monitoring to assess reperfusion after intra-arterial treatment of aneurysmal subarachnoid hemorrhage-induced cerebral vasospasm: a retrospective study. *American Journal of Neuroradiology.* Published online on March 15, 2012. Retrieved from http://www.ajnr.org/content/early/2012/03/15/ajnr.A2971.full.pdf

Di Pentima, C. (2012). Viral meningitis: Epidemiology, pathogenesis, and etiology in children. Retrieved from http://www.uptodate.com/contents/viral-meningitis-epidemiology-pathogenesis-and-etiology-in-children

Donkin, J., & Vink, R. (2010). Mechanisms of cerebral edema in traumatic brain injury: Therapeutic developments. *Current Opinion in Neurology, 23*(3), 293–299.

Drugs.com. (2011a). Klonopin. Retrieved from http://www.drugs.com/klonopin.html

Drugs.com. (2011b). Propofol (systemic). Retrieved from http://www.drugs.com/mns/propofol.html

Engelhard, H. H. (2010, Feb. 23). Neurosurgery for hydrocephalus. Retrieved from http://emedicine.medscape.com/article/247387-overview

Faul, M., Xu, L., Wald M. M., & Coronado, V. G. (2010). *Traumatic brain injury in the United States: Emergency department visits, hospitalization, and deaths.* Atlanta, GA: Center for Disease Control and Prevention.

Ferri, F. (2011*). Ferri's clinical advisor* (1st ed.). Philadelphia: Elsevier.

Gondim, F. A. A. (2011). Viral encephalitis. Medscape reference. Retrieved from http://emedicine.medscape.com/article/1166498-overview

Halstead, M. E., Walter, K. D., & The Council on Sports Medicine and Fitness. (2010). Sports-related concussion in children and adolescents. *Official Journal of the American Academy of Pediatrics, 126*(3), 597–615.

Headache Cooperative of New England (HCNE). (2011). Trigeminal autonomic cephalalgias (2004). Retrieved from http://www.hacoop.org/p;rofessionals_6_2_html

Hickey, J. B. (2009). *The clinical practice of neurological and neurosurgical nursing* (6th ed.). Philadelphia: Lippincott.

Hitti, M. (2009). FDA OKs Avastin for glioblastoma. Retrieved from http://www.webmd.com/cancer/brain-cancer/news/20090506/fda-oks-avastin-for-glioblastoma

Honda, H., & Warren, D. (2009). Central nervous system infections: Meningitis and brain abscess. *Infectious Disease Clinics of North America, 23*(3), 609–623.

Infanti, J. (2008). Challenging the gold standard: Should mannitol remain our first-line defense against intracranial hypertension? *Journal of Neuroscience Nursing, 40*(6), 362–368.

IOM (Institute of Medicine). (2010). *The future of nursing: Leading change, advancing health.* Washington, DC: The Academic Press.

Jennett, B. & Plum, F. (1972). Persistent vegetative state after brain damage: a syndrome in search of a name. *Lancet.* I, 734–737.

Kee, J. L. (2010). Laboratory and diagnostic tests with nursing implications. Upper Saddle River, NJ: Pearson.

Kennedy, B. (2011). Astrocytoma. Medscape reference. Retrieved from http://emedicine.medscape.co/article/283453-overview

Kenning, T., Dalfino, J., German, J., Drazin, D., & Adamo, M. (2010). Analysis of the subdural evacuating port system for treatment of subacute and chronic subdural hematomas. *Journal of Neurosurgery, 113*(5), 1004–1010.

Klein, M. (2009, January 5). Post head injury endocrine complications: Clinical presentation. Retrieved from http://emedicine.medscape.com/article/326123-clinical

Kumar, V., Abbas, A., Fausto, N., & Aster, J. (2009). *Robbins and Cotran pathologic basis of disease* (8th ed.). Philadelphia: Elsevier.

Kundi, M. (2010). The controversy about a possible relationship between mobile phone use and cancer. *Ciencia & Saude Coletiva, 15*(5), 2415–2430.

Kunkel, R. S. (2011. Headache. Cleveland Clinic Center for Continuing Education. Retrieved from http://www.clevelandclinicmeded.com/medicalpubs/diseasemanagement/neurology/headache-syndromes/

Lab Tests Online. (2011). Glucose. Retrieved from http://labtestsonline.org/understanding/analytes/glucose/lab/test

Ladanyl, S., & Elliot, D. (2008). Traumatic brain injury: An integrated clinical case presentation and literature review Part II: The continuum of care. *Australian Critical Care, 21*(4), 141–153.

Ledwith, M., Bloom, S., Maloney-Wilensky, E., Coyle, B., Polomano, R., & Le Roux, P. (2010). Effects of body position on cerebral oxygenation and physiologic parameters in patients with acute neurological conditions. *Journal of Neuroscience Nursing, 42*(5), 280–287.

Littlejohns, L., & Bader, M. K. (2009). *Monitoring technologies in critically ill neuroscience patients.* Sudbury, MA: Jones and Bartlett Publishers.

LoGuidice, M. A., & Persin, M. (2011). Guillain-Barré syndrome. eMedicineHealth.com. Retrieved from http://www.emedicinehealth.com/guillain-bazrre_syndrome/article_em.htm

Loh, M. (2011). Brain herniation imaging. Medscape Reference. Retrieved from http://emedicine.medscape.com/article/337936-overview

Mace, S. (2008). Acute bacterial meningitis. *Emergency Medicine Clinics of North America, 26*(2), 281–317.

Marx, J., Hickberger, R., Walls., R., Adams, J., Barsan, W., Biros, M., et al. (2009). *Rosen's emergency medicine* (7th ed.). Philadelphia: Mosby Elsevier.

May, A. & Goadsby, P.J. (2010). Neuromodulatory approaches to the management of medically refractory cluster headache. *European Neurological Review* 5(1), 97–99. Retrieved from http://www.touchneurology.com/articles/neuromodulatory-approaches-management-medically-refractory-cluster-headache-0

Mayo Clinic Staff. (2008). Traumatic brain injury. Retrieved from http://www.mayoclinic.com/health/traumatic-brain-injury/DS00552/DSECTION=risk-fact

Mayo Clinic Staff. (2011a). Cluster headache. MayoClinic.com. Retrieved from http://www.mayoclinic.com/health/cluster-headache/DS00487/METHOD=print&DSECTI

Mayo Clinic Staff. (2011b). Encephalitis. MayoClinic.com. Retrieved from http://www.mayoclinic.com/health/encephalitis/DS00226/METHOD=print

Mayo Clinic Staff. (2011c). Guillain-Barré syndrome. MayoClinic.com reprints. Retrieved from http://www.mayoclinic.com/health/guillain-barre-syndrome/DS00413/METHOD=print

Mayo Clinic Staff. (2011d). Migraine. MayoClinic.com. Retrieved from http://www.mayoclinic.com/health/migraine-headache/DS00120/METHOD=print

Mayo Clinic Staff. (2012). Bell's palsy. MayoClinic.com. Retrieved from http://www.mayoclinic.com/health/bells-palsy/DS00168/METHOD=print

McNett, M. (2009). Intensive care unit nurse characteristics impacting judgments about secondary brain injury. *Dimensions of Critical Care Nursing, 28*(4), 182–188.

McNett, M., Doheny, M., Sedlak, C. A., & Ludwick R. (2010). Judgments of critical care nurses about risk for secondary brain injury. *American Journal of Critical Care, 19*(3): 250–260. Retrieved from http://www.ncbi.nlm.nih.gov/pubmed/19542058

McNett, M. M., & Gianakis, A. (2010). Nursing interventions for critically ill traumatic brain injury patients. *Journal of Neuroscience Nursing, 42*(2), 71–77. Retrieved from http://www.ncbi.nlm.nih.gov/pubmed/20422792

MedicineNet.com. (2011a). Gabapentin–neurontin. Retrieved from http://www.medicinenet.com/gaabapentin-oral/article.htm

MedicineNet.com. (2011b). Hydrocephalus. Retrieved from http://www.medicinenet.com/hydrocephalus/article.htm

MedicineNet.com. (2012). Guillain-Barré syndrome (cont.). Retrieved from http://www.medicinenet.com/guillain-bzarre_syndrome/pge3.htm

MedlinePlus. (2011a). Partial (focal) seizure. U.S. National Library of Medicine, National Institutes of Health. Retrieved from http://www.nlm.nih.gov/medlineplus/ency/article/000697.htm

MedlinePlus. (2011b). Valparoic acid. U.S. National Library of Medicine, National Institutes of Health. Retrieved from http://www.nllm.nnih.gov/medlineplus/druginfo/meds/a682412.html

Miller, A. C. (2011). Emergent management of Guillain-Barré syndrome. Medscape reference. Retrieved from http://emedicine.medscape.com/article/792008-overview

Moyer, M. (2009). Performance improvement measures in achieving glycemic control in the acute brain injury population. *Journal of Neuroscience Nursing, 41*(2), 72–82.

Muacevic, A., Kufeld, M., Wowra, B., Kreth, F., & Tonn, J. (2010). Feasibility, safety, and outcome of frameless image-guided robotic radiosurgery for brain metastases. *Journal of Neuro-Oncology,* 97(*2*), 267–274.

Muller, M. L. (2011). Pediatric bacterial meningitis. Medscape reference. Retrieved from http://emedicine.medscape.com/article/961497-overview

Nader, D., & Eden, B. (2011). HDR brachytherapy. Retrieved from http://www.cancercenter.com/conventional-cancer-tretment/radiation-therapy/hdr-brachty

National Brain Tumor Society. (2011). Brain tumor FAQ. *National Brain Tumor Society.* Retrieved from http://www.braintumor.org/patients-family-friends/about-brain-tumors-faq.html

National Headache Foundation. (2007). Migraine prevention summit proceedings: Advances in preventive therapies for migraine. Retrieved from http://www.headaches.org

National Highway Traffic Safety Administration (NHTSA). (2009). Traffic safety facts 2009 data. *U.S. Department of Transportation.* DDT HS B11 390. *NHTSA National Center for Statistics and Analysis.* Retrieved from www.nhtsa.gov/

National Institute of Neurological Disorders and Stroke. (2011a). Guillain-Barré syndrome fact sheet. Retrieved from http://www.ninds.nih.gov/disorders/gbs/detail_gbs.htm

National Institute of Neurological Disorders and Stroke. (2011b). Headache: Hope through research. Retrieved from http://www.ninds.nih.gov/disorders/headache/detail_headache.htm

National Institute of Neurological Disorders and Stroke. (2011c). Hydrocephalus fact sheet. Retrieved from http://www.ninds.nih.gov/disorders/hydrocephalus/detail_hydrocephalus.htm

National Institute of Neurological Disorders and Stroke. (2011d). NINDS Bell's palsy information page. Retrieved from http://ninds.nig.gov/disorders/bells/bells.htm

National Institute of Neurological Disorders and Stroke. (2011e). NINDS traumatic brain injury information page. Retrieved from http://www.ninds.nih.gov/disorders/tbi/tbi.htm

National Institute of Neurological Disorders and Stroke. (2011f). Trigeminal neuralgia fact sheet. Retrieved from http://www.ninds.nih.gov/disorders/trigeminal_neuralgia/detail_trigeminal_neuralgia.htm

Nervous System Diseases. (2008). Ventriculostomy: what is it? Retrieved from http://www.nervous-system-diseases.com/ventriculostomy.html

Newton, S., Hickey, M., & Marrs, J. (2009). *Mosby's oncology nursing advisor.* St. Louis: Mosby Elsevier.

Noble, K. (2010). Traumatic brain injury and increased intracranial pressure. *Journal of PeriAnesthesia Nursing, 25*(4), 242–250.

Northwestern Radiology. (2012). Clinical fMRI examples. Retrieved from http://www.radiology.northwestern,edu/reserach/brai/neuroimaging/clinical-fmri-examples

Oh, H., & Seo, W. (2009). Functional and cognitive recovery of patients with traumatic brain injury: Prediction tree model versus general model. *Critical Care Nurse, 29*(5), 12–22.

Olson, D. (2011, July 20). Head injury. Retrieved from http://emedicine.medscape.com/article/1163653-overview#showall

Pangilinan, P. H. (2011). Classification and complications of traumatic brain injury. Medscape reference. Retrieved from http://emedicine.medscape.com/article/3226643-overview

Piepmeier, J. M. (1987). Observations on the current treatment of low-grade astrocytic tumors of the cerebral hemispheres. *Journal of Neurosurgery, 67,* 177–181.

Posner, J. B., Saper, C. B., Schiff, N. D., & Plum, F. (2007). *Plum and Posner's diagnosis of stupor and coma.* (4th ed.). New York: Oxford University Press. Retrieved from http://www.nejm.org/doi/full/10.1056/NEJMbkrev58849

Presciutti, M., Schmidt, M., & Alexander, S. (2009). Neuromonitoring in intensive care: Focus on microdialysis and its nursing implication. *Journal of Neuroscience Nursing, 41*(3), 131–139.

Propofol mechanism of action. (2011). AnesthesiaGeneral.com. Retrieved from http://anesthesiageneral.com/proporol-mechanism-of-action/

Puccio, A., Fischer, M., Jankowitz, B., Yonas, H., Darby, J., & Okonkwo, D. (2009). Induced normothermia attenuates intracranial hypertension and reduces fever burden after severe traumatic brain injury. *Neurocritical Care, 11*(1), 82–87.

Quinn, E. (2008). Water intoxication—hyponatremia. Retrieved from http://sportsmedicine.about.com/od/hydrationandfluid/a/Hyponatremia.htm

Radiation Therapy Oncology Group (RTOG). (2008). Brain tumor protocols. Retrieved from http://www.rtog.org/summaries/brain.html

Rangel-Castilla, L. (2011). Closed head trauma. Medscape reference. Retrieved from http://medicine.medscape.com/araticle/251834-overview

Razonable, R. R. (2011a). Meningitis. Medscape reference. Retrieved from http://emedicine.medscape.com/article/232915-overview

Razonable, R. R. (2011b). Meningitis treatment & management. Medscape reference. Retrieved from http://emedicine.medscape.com/article/232915-treatment

Ruskin, K. (2011). How do anesthetics work? Anesthesiology's Blog for Education & More. Retrieved from http://page2anesthesiology.org/2011/how-do-anesthetics-work/

Russo, C., & Steiner, C. (2007). *Hospital admissions for traumatic brain injuries, 2004* (HCUP Statistical Brief 27). Rockville, MD: Agency for Healthcare Research and Quality. Retrieved from http://www.hcupus.ahrg.gov/reports/statbriefs/sb27.pdf

Rutka, J., Kongkham, P., Northcott, P., Carlotti, C., Guduk, M., Osawa, H., et al. (2009). The evolution and application of techniques in molecular biology to human brain tumors: A 25 year perspective. *Journal of Neuro-Oncology, 92*(3), 261–273.

Schubart, J. R., Kinzie, M. B., & Farace, E. F. (2008). Caring for the brain tumor patient: Family caregiver burden and unmet needs. *Neuro-Oncology, 10*(1), 61–72.

Seppa, N. (2011). Bacterial meningitis keeps falling. *Science News, 179*(13), 10.

Sheth, K. (2011). Cluster headache: all information. *University of Maryland Medical Center.* Retrieved frm http://www.umm.edu/ency/article200786all.htm

Shetty, P., Moiyadi, A., Pantvaidya, G., & Arya, S. (2010). Cystic metastasis versus brain abscess: Role of MR imaging in accurate diagnosis and implications on treatment. *Journal of Cancer Research and Therapeutics, 6*(3), 356–358.

Shiflett, V., Lorenzo, M., Mangram, A., Truitt, M., Amos, J., & Dunn, E. (2010). Should age be a factor to change from a level II to a level I trauma activation? *Journal of Trauma, 69*(1), 88–92.

Sidrah, S. (2011). Nutrition for brain cancer. LiveStrong.com. Retrieved from http://www.livestrong.com/article/368450-nutrition-for-brain-cancer-patients/

Singh, M. (2011, June 15). Trigeminal neuralgia. Retrieved from http://emedicine.medscape.com/article/1145144-overview#a0156

Snowden, R. V. (2009) Avastin apoproved for glioblastoma. *American Cancer Society.* Retrieved from http://www.cancer.org/Cancer/news/News/avastin-approved-for-glioblastoma

Somand, D., & Meurer, W. (2009). Central nervous system infections. *Emergency Medicine Clinics of North America, 27*(1), 89–100.

Southwick, F. (2012). Pathogenesis, clinical manifestations, and diagnosis of brain abscess. *UpToDate, Inc.* Retrieved from http://www.uptodate.com/contents/pathogenesis-clinical-manifestations-and-diagnosis-of-brain-abscess/contributors

Starkweather, A., Sherwood, P., Lyon, D., McCain, N., Bovbjerg, D., & Broaddus, W. (2011). A biobehavioral perspective on depressive symptoms in patients with cerebral astrocytoma. *Journal of Neuroscience Nurses, 43*(1), 17–28.

Stern, T., Rosenbaum, J., Fava, M., Biederman, J., & Rauch, S. (2008). *Massachusetts General Hospital comprehensive clinical psychiatry* (1st ed.). Philadelphia: Mosby.

Stupp, R., Hegi, M., Neynes, B., Goldbrunner, R., Schlegel, U., Clement, P., et al. (2010). Phase I/IIa study of cilengitide and temozolomide with concomitant radiotherapy followed by cilengitide and temozolomide maintenance therapy in patients with newly diagnosed glioblastoma. *Journal of Clinical Oncology, 28*(16), 2712–2718.

Sun-Edelstein, C., & Mauskop, A. (2011). Alternative headache treatments: Nutraceuticals, behavioral and physical treatments. *Headache, 51*(3), 469–483.

Taylor, D. C. (2011, March 29). Bell palsy. Retrieved from http://emedicine.medscape.com/article/1146903-overview

The Book of Doctrines and Opinions. (2011). Brain death—broader concerns. Retrieved from http://kaavvanan.wordpress.com/2011/01/15/brain-death-broader-concerns/

The George Washington Univeristy Medical Center. (2008). Diagnosing death: Why does it remain "well settled and persistently unresolved"? in *Rapid Public Health Policy Response Project, School of Public Health and Health Services.* Washington, DC: The George Washington University Medical Center.

Thigpen, M. C., Whitney, C. G., Messonnier, N. E., et al. (2011). Bacterial meningitis in the United States, 1998–2007. *New England Journal of Medicine, 364*, 2016–2025.

Thompson, H., Kirknes, C., & Mitchell, P. (2007). Fever management practices of neuroscience nurses, part II: Nurse, patient, and barriers. *Journal of Neuroscience Nursing, 39*(4), 196–201.

Traumatic Brain Injury Services of California. (2011). Traumatic brain injury (TBI) and elderly. Retrieved from http://www.tbisca.org/about-tbi/elderly.asp

UCSF Medical Center. (2011). Brain tumor. Retrieved from http://www.ucsf health.org/conditions/brain_tumor/

Uddin, A. S. (2010, April 19). Neurologic manifestations of glioblastoma multiforme. Retrieved from http://emedicine.medscape.com/article/1156220-overview

Uniform Law Commission. (2010). Determination of death act summary. Uniform Law Commission, The National Conference of Commissioners on Uniform State Laws. Retrieved from http://uniformlawls.org/ActSummary.aspx?title=Determination%20of%20Death%Act

Urden, L. D., Stacy, K., & Lough, M. (2010). *Critical care nursing* (6th ed). St. Louis: Mosby.

U.S. Bureau of the Census. (2010). United States Census 2010. Retrieved from http://www.census.gov/compendia/statab/2011/tables/11s0007.pdf

Waknine. Y. (2011). FDA clears brachytherapy system for brain cancer. Retrieved from http://www.medscape.com/viewarticle/749656

Wan, C. (2011). Viral meningitis. Medscape reference. Retrieved from http://emedicine.medscape.com/article/1168529-overview

WebMD. (2011a). Drugs & medications—Depakote oral. Retrieved from http://www.webmd.com/drugs/drug-1788-Depakote+Oral.aspx?drugid=1788&drugname

WebMD. (2011b). Meningitis—treatment overview. Children's vaccines health center. Retrieved from http://children.webmd.com/vaccines/tc/meningitis-treatment-overview

Wedro, B. (2012). Hyponatremia (low sodium). Retrieved from http://www.emedicinehealth.com/hyponatremia_low_sodium/article_em.htm

Wiemels, J., Wrensch, M., & Claus, E. (2010). Epidemiology and etiology of meningioma. *Journal of Neuro-oncology, 99*(3), 307–314.

Wilkinson, J. M., & Ahearn, N. R. (2009). *Prentice Hall nursing diagnosis handbook* (9th ed.). Upper Saddle River, NJ: Prentice Hall.

Yale Medical Group. (2012). Craniotomy. Yale School of Medicine. Retrieved from www.yalemedicalgroup.org/stw/Page.asp?PageID=STW029075

CHAPTER

22 Caring for the Patient with Cerebral Vascular Disorders

Christi DeLemos
Annita Watson

Outcome-Based Learning Objectives

After studying this chapter, the learner will be able to:

1. Differentiate the types of stroke and explain their impact on rehabilitation and recovery to a functional status.
2. Interpret treatment plans based on the basic pathophysiology of each type of identified stroke.
3. Analyze the events of the ischemic cascade as they relate to the pathophysiology of stroke.
4. Generate a nursing care plan for a patient with a ruptured aneurysm.
5. Integrate the nursing interventions associated with management of cerebral vasospasm into the total plan of care.

KEY TERMS

arteriovenous malformation (AVM) p.576
berry aneurysm p.571
brain herniation p.568
carotid endarterectomy p.558
cavernous malformation p.577
cerebral aneurysm p.571
cerebral salt wasting p.575
cerebral vasospasm p.574
coiling p.573
embolic strokes p.553
familial intracranial aneurysms p.571
Fisher grading scale p.573
fusiform aneurysms p.571
hemicraniectomy p.562
hemorrhagic stroke p.563
infarction p.552
ischemic strokes p.553
lacunar strokes p.553
lipohyalinosis p.554
nidus p.576
penumbra p.554
percutaneous angioplasty p.562
reperfusion injury p.554
Spetzler-Martin AVM grading scale p.576
stroke p.552
subarachnoid hemorrhage (SAH) p.571
thrombotic strokes p.553
transient ischemic attack (TIA) p.554
triple-H therapy p.575

CEREBRAL VASCULAR DISORDERS are a common cause of death and adult disability in the United States and abroad. More than 750,000 Americans suffer an acute stroke each year, but fewer than 30% seek emergency help immediately. This chapter will review essential information on the care of patients with stroke and vascular malformations. The prevalence, current modes of diagnosis and treatment, and nursing management of these disorders are discussed, as are the societal implications.

Stroke

Stroke is an interruption in the blood flow to the brain; it has been recently relabeled *brain attack*. This strong statement is indicative of the new emphasis on rapid identification of stroke symptoms and emergency care to restore blood flow. The more familiar term *stroke* is used throughout this chapter. The two subtypes of stroke are ischemic stroke and hemorrhagic stroke. With ischemic stroke, a blood vessel or artery is clogged or obstructed, which interrupts blood flow to a certain area of the brain. Hemorrhagic stroke is characterized by a sudden break in the vessel or artery, causing blood to spill out into the brain. This interrupts blood flow to a certain area of the brain. Both types of stroke cause ischemia, or lack of oxygen to the brain cells. Brain cells that are completely deprived of oxygen begin to die within minutes; this area of dead tissue is called an **infarction.**

As certain areas of the brain become damaged or infarcted, the control of various bodily functions may become affected. These functions include motor function, sensory function, speech, memory, and other cognitive mechanisms. The type and extent of neurological disabilities depend on the location of the stroke.

Safety Alert *The onset of neurological symptoms indicating stroke is a medical emergency. The nurse must notify the health care provider immediately if any new symptoms indicate the possibility of a stroke. Stroke protocols must be initiated immediately.*

Education has broadened public knowledge about stroke and clarified some misconceptions, changing the outlook for people who suffer strokes. Stroke is no longer viewed as a fatal or devastating disease. The term *cerebrovascular accident*, or *CVA*, once used to describe stroke, implies that stroke is an isolated event, somehow unexpected and random. For these reasons and others, this term has largely been abandoned.

Stroke is a vascular event that results from a disease of the blood vessels that may be mediated by the immune system (Mann, 2011).

Epidemiology of Stroke: Ischemic and Hemorrhagic

Stroke is a leading cause of death and disability in many developed nations. In the United States, it is the third leading cause of death, after heart disease and cancer. There are approximately 795,000 cases of stroke each year, of which 160,000 are fatal (American Heart Association [AHA], 2009).

Approximately 4 million people in the United States have survived a stroke and are living with the aftereffects, with an estimated 68.9 billion dollars spent in direct and indirect costs. Although stroke is considered a condition of older adults, it can happen to anyone—28% of stroke victims are under the age of 65 (AHA, 2009). Strokes in younger age groups are often related to cardiac comorbidities or abnormal coagulation states such as sickle cell disease (Munot, Crow, & Ganesan, 2011). The prevalence of stroke is almost twice as high among African Americans than Caucasians, and more men than women experience stroke. However, women account for approximately 60% of all stroke deaths (AHA, 2009). Stroke kills almost twice as many women as breast cancer (Martnez-Sanchez et al., 2011). See the Risk Factors for Stroke box and the Genetic Considerations Related to Stroke box for additional information.

Ischemic Stroke

Ischemic strokes are those that occur as a result of an obstruction within a blood vessel that supplies blood to the brain. They are the most common form of stroke, accounting for approximately 87% of all strokes (AHA, 2009).

Etiology and Classification

Ischemic strokes are further divided by mechanisms, which include embolic, thrombotic, and lacunar infarct. A small percentage of ischemic strokes are caused by other vascular conditions. Imaging studies often discriminate between ischemic and hemorrhagic subtypes of stroke.

Thrombotic Strokes

Thrombotic strokes occur most commonly in older individuals with underlying atherosclerosis (Cho, Lee, Kim, Moon, Ko, & Kim, 2011). Atherosclerosis is a condition characterized by a buildup of plaque (a mixture of cholesterol, lipids, and cellular debris), which narrows the lumen of the artery (National Heart Lung and Blood Institute, 2011). Narrowing of the arteries is referred to as stenosis. Blood clots may form on an atherosclerotic vessel, further narrowing the lumen of the artery and causing severe stenosis or acute occlusion. Large arteries, such as the internal carotid artery or the vertebral artery, can become stenotic, as can small, deep intracerebral vessels. Hypercoagulable states promote platelet aggregation, which increases clotting and the risk of acute occlusion.

RISK FACTORS for Stroke

Hypertension	Family history
Atrial fibrillation	Carotid stenosis
Hyperlipidemia	Diabetes mellitus
Stress	Excessive alcohol use
Sedentary lifestyle	Obesity
Smoking	Valvular disease
Coronary artery disease	

GENETIC CONSIDERATIONS Related to Stroke

Research has shown that the incidence of certain types of stroke is influenced by family history, gender, and race. Predisposition to stroke has been established within particular racial classifications. Black people have been found to have double the risk of first ischemic stroke when compared to Caucasians; this may be related to the higher incidence of hypertension in this population. The rate of hypertension in Blacks in the United States is higher than anywhere in the world and seems to be on the rise (Din Dzietham et al., 2007). Compared with Whites, Blacks developed hypertension earlier in life and had the highest rate of death from stroke (AHA, 2009). In addition, Black people with sickle cell disease or sickle cell trait have a higher incidence of stroke. Japanese people may develop multiple intracranial stenoses and are more likely to have a condition called Moyamoya disease; the name translates as "puff of smoke," and refers to the appearance (when viewed on x-rays) of the tangle of collateral blood vessels that develops to compensate for blocked vessels. Caucasians are predisposed to extracranial stenoses at the carotid bifurcation, requiring carotid endarterectomy. This is discussed later in the chapter (Cruz-Florres, 2011; Liebeskind, 2011).

The genetic association of intracranial aneurysm (aneurysms will be discussed starting on p. 570) with several connective tissue diseases is well established; these diseases include Ehlers-Danlos syndrome, Marfan syndrome, and polycystic kidney disease. In addition, a small percentage of patients will have familial aneurysm, in which more than two primary relatives have been diagnosed with intracranial aneurysm (Zacharia et al., 2010).

Familial type aneurysms tend to occur more frequently in women, as do other types of aneurysms. This is likely related to hypertension. As women age, they have a higher incidence of death from stroke. This is especially true of women who have experienced greater disabilities but survived a stroke.

Embolic Strokes

Embolic strokes result when a clot (embolism) breaks off and travels to an area of decreased circulation, interrupting blood flow. The tissue distal to the embolism becomes hypoxic, eventually infarcts, and ultimately dies. This embolism can be composed of plaque from within the arterial lumen or a blood clot that originates in the heart. Embolisms from cardiac sources are referred to as cardiogenic embolisms. The most common cause is atrial fibrillation, which accounts for almost 10% of all ischemic strokes irrespective of whether the atrial fibrillation is constant in nature or paroxysmal (AHA, 2009; Schirmer et al., 2010). Atrial fibrillation is discussed in detail in Chapter 31. Any condition that can cause a reduction in systemic blood flow can cause an ischemic event. Examples are shock, hypotension, and cardiac arrest. Extremely low rates of blood flow may be responsible for the lack of cerebral oxygenation, resulting in ischemia and infarction.

Lacunar Strokes

Lacunar strokes also are known as *small artery occlusive disease*. Although the terms *lacune*, *lacunar infarct*, and *lacunar stroke* often are used interchangeably, they are not the same thing (Wardlaw, 2008). The term *lacune* literally translates to "little lake." It is a descriptive term for the cerebrospinal fluid-filled cavities in the basal ganglia or white matter of the brain. *Lacunar stroke* describes a clinical stroke syndrome with the typical symptoms and signs referable to a small subcortical or brainstem lesion. *Lacunar infarct* should refer to a clinical stroke syndrome of lacunar type where the underlying lesion appears as an infarct on brain imaging. Lacunes characterize the brain's pathologic appearance as a result of infarcts in the deep brain tissue, such as the basal ganglia or the thalamus, which later fill with cerebrospinal fluid (CSF). This type of stroke is caused by thrombosis of a small penetrating artery that results in tissue death. While lacunes may appear small on imaging, they often occur in eloquent brain tissue that is rich with motor and sensory tracts. For these reasons, lacunar stroke is a significant source of morbidity. Lacunar syndromes can be further subdivided into four distinct types: pure motor syndrome, pure sensory syndrome, sensorimotor syndrome, and ataxic hemiparesis. Hypertension is the predominant risk factor.

Carotid Artery Disease

Carotid artery problems become more common as people age. The disease process that causes the buildup of plaque on the artery walls is called atherosclerosis, popularly known as "hardening of the arteries." The degree of stenosis usually is expressed as a percentage of the normal diameter of the blood vessel (The Internet Stroke Center, 2010a).

Transient Ischemic Attacks

Transient ischemic attacks (TIAs) are episodes of neurological deficit resulting from ischemia that is temporary and resolves in minutes to hours. This ischemia is a result of impaired blood flow to a defined vascular territory, and neurological deficits are directly related to the area with impaired perfusion. Examples of the signs and symptoms of focal neurological deficits are weakness or sensory loss to one side of the body, unilateral visual deficits, loss of speech, and/or facial droop. Global deficits, such as confusion or lethargy, are not indicative of TIAs.

TIAs are an important warning sign of cerebral vascular disease and may precede a large-vessel stroke. As in acute stroke, the onset of symptoms is sudden, but in a TIA, the deficits resolve in minutes to hours. Approximately 10% of people who experience a TIA will experience a major stroke within a year (Merwick & Kelly, 2011). The risk for stroke is greatest within the first 48 hours after a TIA (Ross & Nahab, 2009).

Pathophysiology

The pathophysiology of stroke varies on the basis of stroke subtype. Atherosclerosis is the strongest contributing factor to ischemic stroke. It begins with a fatty streak, located in the intimal layer of large arteries. Fatty streaks may be in existence for many years, possibly starting in the early adult years. The fatty streaks eventually form into fatty plaque, which grows and enlarges gradually over years. The patient often is asymptomatic until the plaque starts to invade the diameter of the artery and obstruct blood flow. The plaque eventually disrupts the integrity of the arterial lining, causing blood to enter the plaque, which in turn causes thrombus formation.

The blood flow to the anterior two-thirds of the brain is delivered by the carotid arteries. Carotid stenosis exceeding 60% decreases blood flow to critical structures of the brain and can be a precursor to thrombotic ischemic stroke.

Smaller arteries are probably affected by a different process. It is thought that they become coated with a lipid compound in a process called **lipohyalinosis.** Lipohyalinosis is indicative of a vascular abnormality due to hypertension (Ogata, Yamanishi, & Ishibashi-Ueda, 2011). This lipid coating causes the vessel walls to gradually become thicker until the lumen becomes extremely narrow and blood flow is obstructed. Lipohyalinosis is believed to be the mechanism behind lacunar strokes.

Regardless of the mechanism involved—plaque, embolus, or thrombus—the result is the same. As the vessel becomes obstructed, blood flow becomes inadequate to perfuse brain tissue, and ischemia results. Ischemia causes injury at the cellular level because of lack of blood flow. If this ischemia is left untreated, the tissue dies, which is referred to as cerebral infarction. The brain is extremely sensitive to lack of blood flow, and ischemic injury can occur within minutes. In cerebral infarction, an area of necrotic (dead) tissue exists at the core of the damage. Around the necrotic core, there exists an area referred to as the **penumbra.** The cells within the penumbra are hypoperfused but not destroyed, and they may be salvaged if blood flow is restored. The ischemic penumbra was described for the first time in 1970 as the hypoperfused zone surrounding an area of infarction. Clinically, this penumbra tissue is not functioning tissue, but it may be able to regain its function if promptly reperfused. Figure 22–1◆ depicts the time relationships among decreased cerebral blood flow (CBF), ischemia, and infarction.

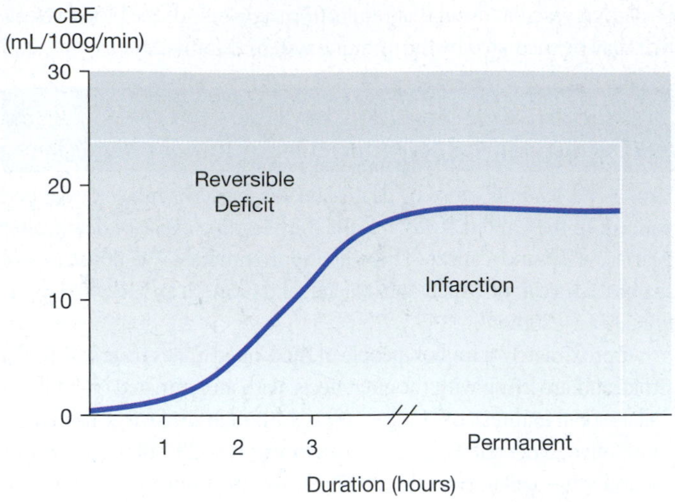

FIGURE 22–1 ◆ Time relationship among decreased CBF, reversible ischemia, and infarction.

Source: From Jones, T. H., Morawetz, R. B., Crowell, R. M., et al. (1981). Thresholds of focal cerebral ischemia in awake monkeys. *Journal of Neurosurgery, 54*, 773–782.

The ischemic penumbra that surrounds the infarcted core is composed of edematous, oxygen-starved brain cells. A process known as the ischemic cascade refers to a series of events that occur in response to cellular hypoxia. This process induces intracellular swelling, further propagating cerebral edema, cerebral ischemia, and, finally, cerebral infarction and cell death. This further extends the area of infarction, or the necrotic core. Chart 22–1 depicts the ischemic cascade. Note that the cells within the ischemic penumbra are viable and can be saved if blood flow is returned quickly; this important concept cannot be overstated. As the mantra goes, time *is* indeed brain. **Reperfusion injury** refers to an injury to cells due to release of oxygen free radicals that occurs after the blood supply has been re-established to the ischemic area. Reperfusion injury results in further injury to already damaged tissue that is compromised but viable, and it can present as a conversion to hemorrhagic stroke (Lieibeskind, 2010). Reperfusion injury is seen most often with thrombolytic therapy.

CHART 22–1 Ischemic Cascade

Hypoxic Ischemic Penumbra ⟶ Decreased Oxygen and Metabolites (i.e., Glucose) ⟶ Decreased Autoregulation ⟶ Decreased ATP Production ⟶ Failure of Na^+-K^+ Pump ⟶ Increased Membrane Permeability ⟶ Increased Intracellular Fluid ⟶ Increased Intracellular Edema ⟶ Increased Intracellular Death ⟶ Within Ischemic Penumbra ⟶ Increased Size of Necrotic Core.

Clinical Manifestations

The signs and symptoms of ischemic stroke vary widely and depend on the location of the vessel involved and the extent of the occlusion. Sudden weakness, numbness, difficulty talking, difficulty understanding, and a severe headache with no known cause are the hallmark symptoms of stroke. Examples of commonly occluded arteries and the signs and symptoms associated with occlusion in these arteries are found in Chart 22–2.

Diagnostic Procedures

Diagnosis of ischemic stroke is based on an accurate history of events, presenting symptoms, and physical examination findings. A noncontrast computerized tomography (CT) scan of the head should be obtained as soon as possible as the initial diagnostic imaging study to rule out hemorrhagic stroke. This is especially important if any condition exists that may predispose the patient to hemorrhage. Examples of these conditions are therapeutic anticoagulation, known bleeding disorders such as liver failure or hemophilia, known presence of lesions such as brain tumors, or a rapid deterioration of neurological status. It is important to rule out hemorrhage to provide the patient with the optimum treatment plan.

CT angiography is another test that uses imaging technologies. A contrast material is injected into a peripheral vein to produce detailed images of both blood vessels and tissues. The detailed view of the vasculature shows which artery is occluded and the extent of occlusion. Note that a CT scan does not immediately show infarcted tissue; the patient may have a normal CT scan, yet still have an occluded artery. Diagnostic tests are discussed in the Diagnostic Tests box (p. 556).

A variety of diagnostic imaging tools exist for the diagnosis of carotid stenosis including duplex sonography with Doppler imaging, CT angiography, and magnetic resonance angiography (MRA). Carotid ultrasound is the least expensive and most common tool used for the diagnosis of carotid stenosis, but its accuracy can be variable (UCSF Medical Center, 2011). When it is unclear whether the stenosis grade meets surgical criteria, patients often undergo CT or MR angiography to better define vascular flow and vessel patency.

CHART 22–2 Occluded/Affected Arteries with Accompanying Signs and Symptoms

Anterior Cerebral Artery	Contralateral paresis of lower extremity
	Sensory deficits in lower extremities
	Eye deviation to affected side
	Incontinence
	Personality changes
Internal Carotid Artery	Contralateral hemiparesis
	Visual field cuts
	Decreased visual acuity ipsilateral
	Cranial nerve deficits
	Aphasia if dominant hemisphere
	Eye deviation to the opposite side
Middle Cerebral Artery	Contralateral hemiparesis
	Eye deviation to opposite site
	Dysphagia if dominant hemisphere
	Aphasia if dominant hemisphere
	Contralateral sensory impairment
	Apraxia if nondominant hemisphere
Vertebral/Basilar Arteries (Posterior Circulation)	Visual field deficits
	Ataxia
	Cranial nerve deficits:
	Eye movement disorders
	Dysphagia
	Dysarthria
	Quadriparesis
	Vertigo
	Sensory deficits
	Mutism

Medical Management

Accurate diagnosis and treatment of stroke requires a review of predisposing risk factors, comorbidities, duration of symptoms, history of trauma, and age (Stanford School of Medicine, 2008). The term *neuroprotection* refers to therapies, both pharmacologic and nonpharmacologic, that are used to arrest the sequence of events that occur during the ischemic cascade (Pandya et al., 2011). During an ischemic stroke, the CBF decreases, causing ischemic tissue to become infarcted. It is important to restore blood flow by dissolving the clot. Currently, the only available treatment is tissue plasminogen activator (t-PA), which lyses the clot and restores blood flow (Adams & Koch, 2010). t-PA is an enzyme (serine protease) that has the property of fibrin-enhanced conversion of plasminogen to plasmin. It produces limited conversion of plasminogen in the absence of fibrin. When introduced into the systemic circulation at pharmacologic concentration, t-PA binds to fibrin in a thrombus and converts the entrapped plasminogen to plasmin; causing local fibrinolysis (clot breakdown).

The t-PA must be administered within 4.5 hours of onset of symptoms (Hacke et al., 2008). Administration of t-PA cannot restore function to the infarcted, necrotic core but may increase the blood supply to the penumbra, thereby limiting the extent of damage caused by ischemic stroke (National Institute of Neurological Disorders and Stroke t-PA Study Group, 1995). The protocol for use of t-PA as determined in the original 1995 trial continues to be used today (Cruz-Flores & Kulkarni, 2011).

The use of *permissive hypertension* also might be considered in the acute phase of the stroke as it helps maintain perfusion. It has been reported that allowing hypertension in a person who has had an ischemic stroke to at least 200 to 220 mmHg systolic may actually protect tissue that otherwise would be starved for oxygen (Darves, 2011; Jackson, 2009). This may not be applicable to patients who have been given t-PA, as their systolic blood pressure should be less than 185 mmHg (Darves, 2011). Also, it is not known how long permissive hypertension should last; typically, the blood pressure is reduced within 3 to 5 days and is accomplished before the patient is discharged. Vasopressors such as dopamine and dobutamine are used to induce and maintain the hypertension (see the Pharmacology box on p. 559).

Other medications used for the treatment of stroke include antiplatelet medications, which inhibit platelet adhesion and aggregation and are the cornerstone of therapy for vascular occlusive artery disease. Antiplatelet drugs such as aspirin, clopidogrel, and glycoprotein inhibitors work to block multiple platelet activation pathways, thus preventing clot formation and providing increased safety for patients with vascular disease (Pinto et al., 2009). Recently, clopidogrel (Plavix),

DIAGNOSTIC TESTS for Cerebrovascular Disorders

Test with Description, Rationale, and Normal Values	Expected Abnormality
Computed Tomography (CT) of the Head	
A CT scan of the head uses many x-rays to create detailed pictures of the face, skull bones, and brain. This exam is painless and takes less than 1 minute but delivers the highest amount of radiation of any scan. *CT scans are best suited to examine for the presence of blood, edema, and cerebral spinal fluid in the brain.* The normal exam would be negative for any abnormalities.	Detects ischemic stroke, evidence of a prior stroke, intracerebral hematomas, subarachnoid hemorrhage (SAH), hydrocephalus, subdural hematomas, calcifications of vascular malformations.
CT Angiogram	
A CT angiogram uses the same technology as a CT of the head, but contrast injection is used to define the vascular system of the brain. This provides a fast, reliable, detailed view of the arterial circulation for detection of aneurysm and cerebral vasospasm. The normal exam would reveal normal carotid and vertebral vascular structures, intact circle of Willis circulation with good visualization of distal vessels.	Detection of vascular abnormality, cerebral aneurysm, arteriovenous malformation, blockages of vascular flow, dissection.
Transcranial Doppler	
A transcranial doppler uses ultrasound waves through the skull to measure the velocity of blood flow through the brain's blood vessels. It is used to help in the diagnosis of stenosis or vasospasm from a subarachnoid hemorrhage (bleeding from a ruptured aneurysm), as well as other problems. The test requires skilled staff but is a relatively quick and inexpensive test. The normal exam would reveal no evidence of stenosis or vasospasm.	Detects cerebral vasospasm or stenosis in the setting of SAH.
Digital Subtraction Cerebral Angiogram	
Digital subtraction angiogram is the gold standard for visualization of the arterial system. A normal exam will reveal normal carotid and vertebral vascular structures, as well as intact Circle of Willis circulation with good visualization of distal vessels.	Detects vascular abnormalities, including cerebral aneurysms, arteriovenous malformations, blockages of a vessel, and dissection.
Magnetic Resonance Angiography (MRA)	
MRA employs a magnetic field and pulsed radio waves to form detailed pictures of the vascular structures. This can be accomplished with or without use of contrast injection. The pictures provide a detailed view of the vascular system, which works best when large aneurysms are present (>0.5 cm). A normal exam reveals normal vasculature with no evidence of aneurysm.	Detects vascular abnormalities including aneurysm >0.5 mm and arteriovenous malformation.
MRI, Including Diffusion-Weighted Images (DWI)	
Diffusion-weighted MRI is a specific magnetic resonance sequence that is particularly useful for detecting stroke. MRI will demonstrate early areas of infarction and small lesions not seen on a CT scan. Normal exam reveals intact brain parenchyma with no evidence of mass, ischemia, or prior infarct.	Detects ischemic abnormalities, cavernous malformations, and structural lesions such as tumors and traumatic injuries.
Lumbar Puncture	
A diagnostic procedure often performed in the emergency department to obtain information about the CSF. This test is valuable for detection of radiographically occult (hidden from imaging view) SAH. Lumbar puncture is contraindicated until space-occupying lesions are ruled out; the possibility exists of an induced brain herniation. The normal LP reveals clear, colorless CSF with normal cell counts and no bacteria.	Detects blood in the CSF (subarachnoid blood). Time-sensitive blood in the CSF presents as yellow with passage of time. Also may detect abnormal cell counts or bacteria to suggest meningitis.
Electroencephalogram (EEG)	
The EEG is an electrical recording of brain activity taken from scalp electrodes. The EEG is commonly used in head trauma, SAH, and vascular malformations to evaluate for seizures in patients with altered electrical activity in the brain. Normal EEG reveals no evidence of seizure or slowing.	Detects abnormal brain activity patterns including seizure activity.

DIAGNOSTIC TESTS for Cerebrovascular Disorders, *continued*

Test with Description, Rationale, and Normal Values	Expected Abnormality
Serum Electrolytes	
Serum electrolytes are a blood test collected from whole blood. This provides values for important electrolytes such as sodium, potassium, and magnesium. Several electrolytes are important when evaluating strokes. These include sodium, magnesium, and potassium. Common to SAH, low sodium levels are a risk factor for increased cerebral edema and altered level of consciousness. Hypomagnesemia lowers the seizure threshold. Abnormalities in potassium levels can alter cardiac function and predispose the patient to arrhythmia. Normal values are as follows: NA 135–145 mEq/L (goal > 140) Potassium 3.5–5.3 mEq/L (goal > 4.0) Magnesium 1.8–3.0 mg/dL (goal > 2.0)	Detects hyponatremia (serum Na^+ less than 134 mEq/L), hypomagnesemia, and abnormalities in potassium levels.
Blood Glucose	
Blood glucose is a test used to measure glucose levels in the blood. It is often performed as part of the emergency assessment as profound hypoglycemia or hyperglycemia can alter the patient's level of consciousness and mimic stroke. *Hyperglycemia can be associated with stress response, underlying diabetes, or steroid use.* *Hyperglycemia is also associated with worse stroke outcomes.* *Hypoglycemia can cause altered level of consciousness and often is seen in diabetes.* Normal blood sugar levels are 70–110 mg/dL.	Glucose levels may be elevated or decreased.
Complete Blood Count (CBC)	
The complete blood count is a blood test that provides comprehensive information regarding red blood cells, platelets, and white blood cells. High white blood cell counts are common and may indicate possible stress response, seizure, or infection. *Low platelet counts can be an important risk factor for bleeding. Severe anemia can also worsen the outcome in critical illness by depriving fragile tissue of oxygen needed for cellular repair. For these reasons, a hematocrit <30% in patients with any form of stroke is usually treated.* Normal cumulative blood count levels are as follows: Hemoglobin: 13.5–18 g/dL for men 12–15 g/dL for women Hematocrit: 40–54% for men and 36–46% for women White blood cell count: 4.5–10.0 cells per cubic millimeter Red blood cell count: 4.2–5.9 million cells per cubic millimeter Platelet count: 150–400 thousand cells per cubic millimeter	Detects anemia, leukocytosis, leucopenia, thrombocytopenia, or thrombocytosis.
Arterial Blood Gases	
Arterial blood gases measure the level of oxygen and carbon dioxide to determine how well the lungs are working. *A depressed neurological state may provoke a depressed respiratory drive and compromise oxygen supply to the brain.* Normal blood gas levels are as follows: pH: 7.35–7.45 PaO_2: 75–100 mmHg HcO_3: 24–28 mEq/L $PaCO_2$: 35–45 mmHg	Detects hypoxia, hypercapnia (an unusually high concentration of carbon dioxide in the blood), and acid–base balance of the blood.

a thienopyridine, has been added to the stroke arsenal for use in patients. Medications used to treat stroke are described in the Pharmacology box on page 559.

The medical management of stroke includes treatment of pain exhibited by the patient. One of the worst consequences that occur after a stroke is severe burning pain on the side of the body affected by the stroke. Poststroke pain, also referred to as thalamic pain, neurogenic pain, or central pain syndrome, occurs most frequently following strokes on the right side of the brain, which affect the left side of the body. Because the brain has been damaged, it interprets sensory input as pain when it should be interpreting it as a sensation that is not painful. The onset time for pain symptoms to develop is variable, ranging from days to months or years after the stroke. Though the exact cause of the pain is unknown, it is hypothesized that these sensations may be due to many factors, including damage to the sensory regions of the brain, stiff joints, or a disabled limb. An uncommon type of pain resulting from stroke is called central stroke pain or central pain syndrome (CPS). CPS results from damage to an area in the midbrain called the thalamus. The pain is a mixture of sensations, including heat and cold, burning, tingling, numbness, and sharp stabbing and underlying aching pain. The pain often is more severe in the extremities—the hands and feet—and is made worse by movement and temperature changes, especially cold temperatures (Cruz-Flores & Kulkarni, 2011).

Preventive medical treatment for ischemic stroke is aimed at addressing several modifiable risk factors that are outlined in the Risk Factors for Stroke box (p. 553). Hypertension is the most pervasive modifiable stroke risk factor. The lowering of blood pressure in the hypertensive patient has an undisputed effect on stroke. The recently published national guidelines for prevention of stroke recommend a systolic blood pressure less than 140 mmHg over a diastole of 90 mmHg (Goldstein et al., 2010). In a meta-analysis review, thiazide diuretics were found to be the most effective; they may be combined with ACE (angiotensin-converting enzyme) inhibitors, ARBs (angiotensive receptor blockade), or beta-blockers for refractory hypertension. The exception to this is patients with diabetes, for whom ACE inhibitors may be considered the preferred agent. Lipid-lowering drugs, such as the statins, are recommended for patients with dyslipidemia. These drugs also have a role in reducing risk factors of patients who are at risk for stroke or who have already had a stroke.

Medical management of patients with cardioembolic strokes due to atrial fibrillation is complex and requires careful evaluation of their health status. Selection of anticoagulation therapy is based on a number of clinical variables including age, functional status, and the presence of other risk factors. Warfarin has been the drug of choice for this group of patients. With warfarin administration, it is important for the nurse to monitor prothrombin time (PT) and INR (the international normalized ratio) to determine the patient's response to the warfarin and establish proper control. The nurse also should inspect the patient for bleeding gums, bruises on arms or legs, petechiae, nosebleeds, melena (black, tarry, foul-smelling stools caused by blood in the digestive tract), hematuria, and hematemesis (vomiting of blood). Patients also should be advised to avoid a high fat diet and consume only small amounts of foods rich in vitamin K, such as green tea, salad, and green vegetables (e.g., cabbage, cauliflower, broccoli, lettuce, and spinach), which can decrease the effectiveness of the warfarin. Cranberry juice and excessive alcohol also should be avoided, as they may increase warfarin's potency (Adams & Koch, 2010; Kee, 2010).

Safety Alert *Intracerebral hemorrhage is the most worrisome complication related to anticoagulation. The nurse needs to educate patients/families on dietary choices regarding foods rich in vitamin K, because variation in intake of vitamin K can interfere with the effects of the anticoagulants resulting in wide swings in INR. Supratherapeutic anticoagulation combined with minor trauma such as a fall can result in catastrophic bleeding. Patient education should include signs and symptoms of intracranial bleeding including decreased consciousness, headache, lethargy, seizures, and vomiting.*

Other drugs used in the treatment of strokes and other cerebrovascular disorders are listed in the Pharmacology box (p. 559).

Nearly 10% of patients with stroke affecting the middle cerebral artery will experience life-threatening malignant cerebral edema. This complication, which often manifests between day 1 and day 5 following stroke, can result in an 80% mortality rate (Cho, S.Y. et al., 2011). Hyperosmolar (a fluid of high osmolar concentration) treatment may be used to treat cerebral edema by reducing elevated intracranial pressure through two mechanisms: (1) plasma expansion with a resultant decrease in blood hematocrit, reduced blood viscosity, and decreased cerebral blood volume, and (2) the creation of an osmotic gradient that draws cerebral edema fluid from brain tissue into the circulation (Cruz-Flores & Kulkarni, 2011). The most common hyperosmolar treatments used are hypertonic saline and mannitol. Mannitol is a diuretic used to reduce cerebral volume and reduce intracranial pressure. Osmotic therapy requires that the serum osmolality be monitored closely (at a minimum every 8 to 12 hours), with a target serum osmolality of less than 320 mOsm/kg when using mannitol and less than 360 mOsm/kg when using hypertonic saline. If left untreated, the edema can result in increased infarction, herniation, and even death.

Surgical Management

Patients with atherosclerotic disease in selected vessels may be candidates for surgical intervention. The vast majority of such surgeries will be directed at restoration of the internal carotid artery or extracranial circulation. A minority of patients who suffer from intracranial stenosis are candidates for surgical revascularization. Endovascular procedures, discussed in the following sections, offer yet another alternative for restoration of blood flow. In acute stroke, thrombi that are occluding blood flow may also be retrieved from an artery endovascularly by using clot retrieval devices or mechanical thrombectomy (Nogueira et al., 2009). Surgical intervention may consist of a carotid endarterectomy or percutaneous angioplasty with or without intravascular stenting (p. 562). The goal of treatment is to prevent further strokes or TIAs.

Neurovascular procedures such as intra-arterial delivery of t-PA, clot retrieval or mechanical thrombectomy, carotid endarterectomy, stenting, and bypass procedures are highly specialized. The major risks common to all of the treatments are stroke and hemorrhage. The risks of percutaneous angioplasty with or without stenting are hemorrhage of the vessel, extravasation of contrast material, and stroke. However, these risks have decreased with the experience of the endovascular specialist and advances in medical devices. All surgical procedures carry risks of stroke, infection, and alteration in wound healing.

Carotid Endarterectomy

A **carotid endarterectomy** is a surgical procedure performed to correct carotid stenosis. In endarterectomy, the surgeon opens the artery and removes the fatty deposits called plaque. Surgical options depend on several variables: the location of the stenotic or occluded vessel, the extent of occlusion, and the accessibility of the appropriate facilities and surgical expertise. Carotid endarterectomy has been proven to be superior to medical treatment alone for the prevention of stroke by the North American Symptomatic Carotid Endarterectomy Trial (NASCET, 1991). Carotid endarterectomy continues to be used as a preferred treatment for atherosclerotic disease of the carotid artery.

Safety Alert *Patients who have had a carotid endarterectomy are at risk for hematoma at the incision, which increases the risk of airway patency. The nurse must monitor the incision at least every 2 hours for the first 24 hours. If hematoma occurs, the nurse notifies the health care provider immediately.*

PHARMACOLOGY Summary of Medications to Treat Cerebrovascular Disorders

Medication Category and Action	Application/Indication	Nursing Responsibility
Blood pressure medications:		
Labetalol hydralazine Metoprolol ***Action:*** Blocks beta-adrenergic pathways to provide a steady consistent drop in blood pressure without compromising cerebral blood flow. Because of nonselective beta-blocking properties, it should be avoided in severe reactive airway diseases and cardiogenic shock.	Reduce blood pressure. Blood pressure is gently lowered to maintain adequate perfusion of the ischemic penumbra.	Monitor blood pressure closely to maintain pressure within the ordered range (permissive hypertension may be ordered by the primary health care provider to limit infarct volume, in which case hypotensive drugs would not be given). Observe for signs of hypotension, bradycardia, or a decline in neurologic exam after administration of blood pressure-lowering agents, as this may require adjustment to the beta-adrenergic-blocker dose or other background medications. Report any episodes of hypotension to the health care provider to avoid neurological injury.
Nitroprusside (Nipride) ***Action:*** Dilates both arteries and veins, causing a hypotensive action due to direct relaxation of arteriolar smooth muscle and blood pooling in the veins. Tends to increase heart rate and decrease cardiac output.	Reduce blood pressure. Blood pressure is gently lowered to maintain adequate perfusion of the ischemic penumbra.	Monitor for increases in any raised ICP, as this is a known side effect. Monitor blood pressure closely to maintain pressure within the ordered range (permissive hypertension may limit infarct volume). Report any episodes of hypotension to the health care provider to avoid neurologic injury.
Nitroglycerine (NTG) Nitropaste ***Action:*** Forms nitric oxide in vascular smooth muscle, which is a potent vasodilator, causing relaxation of both arterial and venous smooth muscle. Dilation of veins reduces the amount of blood returning to the heart (preload) and reduces the risk of cerebral hyperemia. These agents should be avoided in patients suspected of having increased intracranial pressure (ICP) because they may cause intracerebral shunting of blood, which increases ICP.	Reduce blood pressure. Blood pressure is gently lowered to maintain adequate perfusion of the ischemic penumbra.	Monitor blood pressure regularly when drug is initiated and when dosage is titrated. Hold the drug and notify the health care provider if the systolic blood pressure is lower than the prescribed parameters. Monitor for headache. (While this is a known side effect of nitroglycerin, it can also be seen in hemorrhagic transformation or intracerebral hemorrhage, so any decline in neurologic condition should warrant discussion with the supervising provider.) Also monitor orthostatic hypotension.
ACE inhibitors: Enalapril Lisinopril ***Action:*** Works within the renin-angiotensin-aldosterone system (RAAS) to inhibit the vasoconstricting action of angiotensin II and the angiotensin-mediated secretion of aldosterone, thus causing blood vessels to dilate. This decreases systemic vascular resistance.	Reduce blood pressure. Blood pressure is gently lowered to maintain adequate perfusion of the ischemic penumbra. Secondary stroke is prevented by lowering blood pressure.	Monitor blood pressure closely to maintain pressure within the ordered range (permissive hypertension may limit infarct volume). Ensure that the patient is in a monitored unit if IV medications are used to control blood pressure. Report any episodes of hypotension to the health care provider to avoid neurologic injury. Monitor for ACE-inhibitor-induced cough, dizziness, hypotension, hyperkalemia, and worsening renal insufficiency.
Nimodipine (Nimotop) Nicardipine (Cardene) ***Action:*** Facilitates contraction in cardiac and smooth muscles. Calcium channel blockers selectively block channels in vascular smooth muscle, causing a decrease in the amount of intracellular calcium available for muscle contraction. Results in a fall in blood pressure and a diminished myocardial oxygen demand with preservation of cerebral perfusion pressure.	Reduce blood pressure. Reduce cerebral vasospasm. Blood pressure is gently lowered to maintain adequate perfusion of the ischemic penumbra. Administer nimodipine to patients with subarachnoid hemorrhage who are at risk for vasospasm.	Monitor blood pressure regularly when drug is initiated and when dosage is titrated. Hold the drug and notify the health care provider if the systolic blood pressure is less than the ordered range. Monitor for: Orthostatic hypotension Decline in neurological function If blood pressure is below the recommended range, discuss with the supervising provider cutting the dose in half and changing the nimodipine dosing schedule to every 2 hours instead of every 4 hours. Report any episodes of hypotension to the health care provider to avoid neurologic injury. Total fluid volume should be monitored with administration of Cardene, which can result in volume overload.

(continued)

PHARMACOLOGY Summary of Medications to Treat Cerebrovascular Disorders, *continued*

Medication Category and Action	Application/Indication	Nursing Responsibility
Dopamine Dobutamine ***Action:*** Acts as a vasopressor by stimulating dopaminergic receptors, especially in the kidneys, leading to vasodilation and increased blood flow, thereby increasing blood pressure. At high doses, it stimulates beta-1-adrenergic receptors, causing the heart to beat more forcefully and increase cardiac output. Also stimulates alpha-adrenergic receptors, thus causing vasoconstriction and raising blood pressure.	Increases blood pressure. Used as a medication to induce or maintain permissive hypertension when patients have experienced an ischemic stroke. May be given in small to large doses, dependent on the desired action of the drug. Administered as a continuous infusion only.	Continually monitor the patient for effects of the drug on the cardiovascular system and for signs of dysrhythmias and hypotension. Ensure patency of IV prior to beginning infusion. Observe the vein site diligently; dopamine is a vesicant drug that can cause severe, irreversible damage if the drug escapes from the vein into the tissue. Dopamine interacts with many other drugs (e.g., beta-blockers); therefore, the nurse should observe for onset of any ventricular arrhythmias.
Phenylephrine (Neo-synephrine) ***Action:*** Pure alpha-agonist that elevates the blood pressure without increasing the heart rate or contractility. Reflex bradycardia may result from the blood pressure increase.	Used to maintain blood pressure and prevent cerebral ischemia related to impaired cerebral perfusion pressure.	This medication should be administered through a central line in a monitored unit. Blood pressure must be monitored continuously with an arterial line to maintain the blood pressure within the prescribed parameter. Observe for bradycardia.
Anti-stroke medications:		
Clopidogrel (Plavix) Aspirin ***Action:*** Modifies coagulation in arteries by inhibiting ADP (adenosine diphosphate) receptors. Bleeding time is irreversibly reduced by reducing platelet aggregation.	Reduce the chance of thrombotic stroke. Can also be useful in lone atrial fibrillation for prevention of cardioembolic stroke.	Monitor closely for signs or symptoms of bleeding, including easy bruising, petechiae, coffee-ground emesis or frank bloody emesis, dark tarry stools, or frank blood in stools. Monitor for gastrointestinal (GI) side effects.
Dabigatran (Pradaxa) **Action:** Dabigatran is a direct inhibitor of thrombin. By inhibiting thrombin, it blocks the conversion of fibrinogen to fibrin and thus reduces clot formation.	Reduces the chance of cardioembolic stroke. Administer to patients with atrial fibrillation or mechanical valve. Unlike warfarin, it does not require laboratory monitoring or dietary restrictions to maintain a therapeutic effect.	Monitor closely for signs or symptoms of bleeding, including easy bruising, petechiae, coffee-ground emesis or frank bloody emesis, dark tarry stools, or frank blood in stools. Instruct the patient not to combine this medication with other medicines that may affect clotting time, such as aspirin, or other NSAIDs unless prescribed by the health care provider. Educate the patient that this medicine can interact with P-glycoprotein inhibitors.
Warfarin (Coumadin) ***Action:*** Anticoagulant which inhibits two enzymes that facilitate the formation of activated vitamin K, which is required for the synthesis of clotting factors II, VII, IX, and X. Inhibits the synthesis of new clotting factors but does not affect clotting factors that are already circulating in the blood.	Reduces the chance of cardioembolic stroke. Administer to patients with atrial fibrillation or mechanical valve.	Provide education about the risks of bleeding as previously detailed. Monitor lab tests such as PT/INR to ensure results are in the therapeutic range. Provide family teaching about the need to restrict dietary intake of vitamin K rich foods, which can alter INR levels. Instruct the patient not to combine this medication with other medicines that may affect clotting time such as aspirin or other NSAIDs unless prescribed by the health care provider. Educate the patient that this medicine can interact with P-glycoprotein inhibitors (amiodarone, verapamil, or quinidine and increasing levels of Pradaxa).
Heparin ***Action:*** Prolongs coagulation time by inhibiting excessive clotting within blood vessels. Activates the enzyme antithrombin III, which inhibits thrombin. High doses interfere with platelet aggregation.	Reduces the chance of venous thrombotic events. Administer to patients at risk for deep vein thrombosis including all patients who are non-ambulatory, have undergone a recent major surgical procedure, and have impaired mobility.	Provide education about the risks of bleeding as previously detailed in the aspirin example. Teach the patient and family about the importance of PTT (partial thromboplastin time) monitoring if fractionated heparin is prescribed. Provide family teaching for home care if heparin injections are prescribed.

PHARMACOLOGY Summary of Medications to Treat Cerebrovascular Disorders, *continued*

Medication Category and Action	Application/Indication	Nursing Responsibility
Alteplase (t-PA) Streptokinase ***Action:*** Promotes fibrinolysis by converting plasminogen to plasmin. Plasmin digests fibrin by breaking it into small soluble fragments, thereby accelerating the normal process of clot removal in the body.	Recanalize occluded arteries to restore oxygenation and cerebral blood flow. Administer to eligible patients who present with ischemic stroke within 4.5 hours.	Evaluate the patient carefully to determine whether the patient meets eligibility criteria. Inclusion criteria include onset of symptoms <4.5 hours ago, blood pressure <185/110 mmHg, no active bleeding, normal platelet count and INR. After IV infusion of t-PA, carefully monitor for bleeding or any decline in neurological status that could suggest intracranial bleeding or reperfusion injury. Ensure that the patient is in a monitored unit for the first 12–24 hours after administration of t-PA. Monitor blood pressure frequently and ensure that it is maintained <185/110 mmHg for the first 24 hours.
Anti-edema medications: Mannitol ***Action:*** Administered by IV route. Mannitol is filtered by the glomerulus of the kidney but is not capable of being reabsorbed by the renal tubule. This creates an osmotic gradient, resulting in decreased water and Na^+ reabsorption, and increased diuresis.	Reduce vasogenic edema. Control intracranial pressure, and correct hyponatremia. Administer to patients with cerebral edema and elevated intracranial pressure.	Carefully monitor blood pressure, intracranial pressure, and cerebral perfusion pressure. Monitor urine output hourly. Expect increases in urine output for up to 4 to 6 hours after mannitol administration. Measure serum osmolality every 8 hours to maintain less than 320 mOsm/kg.
Hypertonic saline ***Action:*** Reduces elevated intracranial pressure by expanding plasma with a resultant decrease in blood hematocrit, blood viscosity, and cerebral blood volume. Also creates an osmotic gradient that draws cerebral edema fluid from brain tissue into the circulation.	Reduce vasogenic edema. Control intracranial pressure, and correct hyponatremia. Hypertonic saline is indicated in patients with increased intracranial pressure (ICP > 20) and in patients with a serum sodium <135.	Monitor serum sodium levels every 6 hours if receiving continuous hypertonic saline. Monitor serum osmolality levels daily to maintain less than 360 mOsm/kg. Monitor ICP closely. Contact the supervising provider for elevated ICP refractory to external drainage of CSF and conservative measures to lower ICP (head of bed at 30 degrees, treat hyperthermia, control ventilation, provide sedation if indicated). Patients receiving hypertonic saline should be placed in a monitored unit.
Anticonvulsants: Phenytoin (Dilantin) Carbamazepine (Tegretol) Divalproex (Depakote) Gabapentin (Neurontin) Lamotrigine (Lamictal) Phenobarbital Clonazepam (Klonopin) Levetiracetam (Keppra) ***Action:*** Inhibits seizure activity by delaying the influx of sodium ions across neuronal membranes in the brain. Sodium ion movement is the major factor determining the initiation and propagation of neuron action potential. Abnormal discharges are slowed with antiseizure medications.	Prevent seizures. Administer to patients who have exhibited seizure activity or to patients at high risk for seizure.	Monitor closely for hypotension when giving loading dose intravenously. Carefully monitor for allergic reactions, which can include angioedema, hives, and anaphylaxis. As a class effect, anticonvulsants can cause drowsiness and difficulty with clarity of thought. Educate patients and families about the importance of routine lab testing including blood counts and liver function tests; if appropriate, drug levels should be drawn as ordered, as some agents can cause platelet abnormalities, abnormal liver function, and pancytopenia (abnormal depression of all the cellular elements of the blood). For patients taking phenytoin, gum side effects may occur, including bleeding and gum hyperplasia with long-term use. Educate patients and families about possible side effects affecting behavior, and encourage reporting any changes to the primary health care provider. These include aggressive behavior or new onset psychosis (Levetirazepam). Educate women of childbearing age about the risk of birth defects with anticonvulsants and review options for contraception. Review state-specific guidelines for patients with seizure disorders and advise no driving for patients who have not established seizure control.

(*continued*)

PHARMACOLOGY Summary of Medications to Treat Cerebrovascular Disorders, *continued*

Medication Category and Action	Application/Indication	Nursing Responsibility
Benzodiazepines: Diazepam (Valium) Lorazepam (Ativan) Midazolam (Versed) ***Action:*** Acts in the limbic, thalamic, and hypothalamic regions of the CNS to control seizures by enhancing the inhibitory action of (gamma-aminobutyric acid) GABA neurotransmitters, thus inhibiting the abnormal neuronal discharges characteristic of seizures.	Used as treatment for seizure cessation in status epilepticus.	Monitor for oversedation and review recommended dosing. Educate the patient and family about the risk of respiratory depression and recommend not combining this group of medications with any other sedative/hypnotic.
Opioid pain relievers: Codeine Hydrocodone Oxycodone Tramadol (Ultram) ***Action:*** Opioids act as analgesics by interacting with receptors in the CNS. The mu and kappa receptors are the most important in producing pain relief.	Control mild to moderate pain. Administer to patients with uncontrolled pain. Avoid excessive sedation that would interfere with neurological assessment.	Educate about the risk of addiction and dependence with long-term use. Recommend consideration of alternative nonnarcotic measures to control pain, such as nonnarcotic topical pain relievers, and biofeedback. Review the possible side effects with the patient/family including respiratory depression, constipation, and oversedation.
NSAIDs: Ketorolac (Toradol) Indomethacin (Indocin) Ibuprofen (Motrin, Advil) Naproxen (Naprosyn) Acetaminophen (Tylenol) ***Action:*** Nonsteroidal anti-inflammatory drugs act peripherally and inhibit the brain's ability to feel pain. They reduce the release of the enzyme cyclooxygenase (COX-1 and COX-2), leading to a reduction in the release of prostaglandin, thus, the pain message is reduced. It has a transient antiplatelet effect.	Control pain. Reduce fever. Administer to patients with pain or fever. Avoid in the setting of intracerebral hemorrhage as it has a transient antiplatelet effect.	Educate the patient about common treatment effects and side effects including GI upset and GI bleed. Advise the patient to take medication with food to minimize gastrointestinal side effects.

Source: Adams, M. P., & Koch, R. W. (2010). *Pharmacology connections to nursing practice.* Upper Saddle River, NJ: Pearson; Drugs.com. (2009). Torodol (ketorolac). Retrieved from http://www.drugs.com/toradol.html; Drugs.com. (2011). Pradaxa. Retrieved from http://www.drugs.com/pradaxa.html.

Endovascular Procedures

Endovascular procedures for the treatment of carotid stenosis to prevent stroke have largely been reserved for nonsurgical candidates. These interventional radiological procedures are performed by an endovascular neurosurgeon or neurointerventional radiologist. **Percutaneous angioplasty** is a form of catheterization with microcatheters. Vascular access is established by passing a catheter through the femoral or brachial artery and advancing it to the area of stenosis in the cerebrovascular circulation. The catheter then enters the stenosed vessel, and the atherosclerotic plaque is broken apart by inflation of a balloon within the catheter. The patency of the vessel may be preserved by the use of a *stent*, which is a tube of plastic or sprung metal mesh placed inside an artery to provide support to the vessel wall and widen the lumen. Neurointerventionalists can access the cerebral arteries to retrieve these clots or mechanically disrupt atherosclerotic thrombi to restore blood flow (Nogueira et al., 2009).

Hemicraniectomy

Hemicraniectomy is a surgical procedure to remove a large window of bone and sometimes necrotic tissue to give the salvageable brain room to swell. This reduces intracranial pressure and promotes improved blood flow to the brain. Hemicraniectomy is a valuable treatment option to relieve intracranial pressure in many other neurologic diseases such as traumatic brain injury, subdural hematoma, and cerebellar infarction (Kohrmann & Schwab, 2009; Staykov & Gupta, 2011).

Nursing Management

Nursing management of a patient who is experiencing an ischemic or hemorrhagic stroke demands good critical thinking and decision-making skills. Stroke is a life-threatening disorder that compromises brain function and requires immediate medical intervention. Warning signs of stroke include sudden numbness or weakness of the face, arm, or leg, especially on one side of the body; sudden confusion; trouble speaking or understanding; sudden trouble seeing in one or both eyes; sudden trouble walking, dizziness, loss of balance or coordination; and sudden severe headache with no known cause. The Nursing Process: Patient Care Plan that follows details the nursing management of care for the patient with stroke.

Hemorrhagic Stroke

Intracerebral hemorrhage is defined as bleeding into brain tissue. Also referred to as **hemorrhagic stroke,** it accounts for approximately 13% of all strokes. It is a potentially devastating type of stroke, associated with significant mortality and morbidity. The mortality rate in the first 30 days is approximately 35% to 50% (Lloyd-Jones et al., 2010). Though seen mostly in older adults, it can also affect people who are middle aged. The most common cause of intracerebral hemorrhage is uncontrolled hypertension, but it also can be caused by amyloid angiopathy (a disease most commonly seen in older adults, in which amyloid deposits form in the walls of the blood vessels of the central nervous system), antiplatelet/anticoagulation medications, illicit drug use, and underlying bleeding disorders. Hemorrhages can occur as a result of a broken blood vessel in the brain itself, known as an intracerebral or intraparenchymal hemorrhage. These differ from subarachnoid, subdural, and epidural hemorrhages, which are caused by a vessel rupture outside the brain.

Epidemiology

Intracerebral hemorrhage is more common in older patients, although it is seen in the younger population with certain high-risk factors. In younger age groups, trauma, such as motor vehicle crashes, assaults, and falls, contribute to intracerebral hemorrhage. When intracerebral hemorrhage is seen in a young adult and trauma is ruled out as the cause, drug use should be suspected, specifically cocaine or amphetamines.

Two types of hemorrhages are commonly associated with trauma. Subdural hematomas, described in the following section, occur in older populations, with a recent study citing a mean age of 80 (Miranda et al., 2011). Hemorrhages often are the result of falls and can be devastating when combined with oral anticoagulants. In contrast, epidural hematomas commonly occur in young people as a result of blunt trauma to the head.

Another type of hemorrhagic stroke is subarachnoid hemorrhage (SAH). The most common cause of SAH is rupture of an intracerebral aneurysm. SAH and cerebral aneurysms are discussed later in the chapter.

Etiology

The most common cause of intracerebral hemorrhage is hypertension (The Internet Stroke Center, 2010a; Liebeskind, 2011). Additional risk factors include smoking, anticoagulation with warfarin, excessive alcohol intake, and cocaine use (Rymer, 2011). Nonmodifiable risk factors include African American ethnicity, male gender, and older age (Staykov & Gupta, 2011).

Pathophysiology

The pathologic effects of hemorrhagic stroke are often produced by a combination of inadequate blood flow from a ruptured vessel and a space-occupying mass effect from the blood entering the brain (Liebeskind, 2011). The hemorrhagic stroke can produce increased intracranial pressure (ICP) related to acute hydrocephalus or from the volume of blood itself. Hydrocephalus is excessive accumulation of CSF in the brain, resulting in an abnormal widening of ventricles in the brain (National Institute of Neurological Disorders and Stroke [NINDS], 2011b). This event triggers a series of conditions, such as midline shift of intracranial contents, decreased CBF, and cerebral edema. It may further increase ICP and possibly lead to herniation. The events associated with hemorrhagic stroke are closely related to the pathophysiology of increased ICP and herniation syndromes (see Chapter 21 for a review of hydrocephalus and herniation syndromes).

The most common areas for hemorrhagic stroke are the putamen and the surrounding internal capsule. These very deep structures are the sites of approximately 50% of all hemorrhagic strokes due to hypertension (Lloyd-Jones et al., 2010). Other areas in which hemorrhages frequently are found are the thalamus, the cerebellum, the brainstem, and the white matter of the frontal, temporal, and parietal lobes.

Hemorrhagic stroke is most commonly caused by chronic uncontrolled hypertension (Liebeskind, 2011). The long-term strain caused by the force and excessive pressure of the blood on the vessel walls results in areas of weakness that later rupture under the stress of increased blood flow. The most common locations for vessel rupture are the small vessels of the brain including the lenticulostriate (branch of middle cerebral artery), thalamic vessels, and cerebellar vessels.

At the time of hemorrhage, the blood rushes into the brain, interrupting blood flow to the brain distal to the broken vessel, and causes local mass effect. Hemostasis is likely multifactorial, related to direct compression from local structures and activation of the clotting cascade. Hematomas often grow by as much as 30% over 24 hours, making correction of coagulopathy critical (Broderick et al., 2007). Coagulopathy is defined as abnormal function of the clotting system. This is normally measured by blood tests such as the platelet count, PTT, and INR. When there is bleeding in the brain, it is very important to restore normal clotting function to reduce the chance of continued bleeding. This is often accomplished by direct administration of medicines or blood products to normalize the PTT or INR. Common treatments include fresh frozen plasma, vitamin K, and factor VII. These treatments should be administered urgently to minimize growth of the hematoma, thus reducing the risk of morbidity and mortality.

Subdural hematomas occur as a result of tearing of the bridging veins in the subdural space, the potential space between the dura mater and the arachnoid membrane of the brain (refer to Chapter 21, Figure 21–11, p. 517). Because it is venous in nature, blood slowly fills the subdural space. The most common mechanism is a blunt head trauma or fall in the older adult. The blood accumulates over time and can result in a significant amount of blood, causing pressure on the brain. The size of the subdural hematoma is directly related to clinical symptoms. Subdural hematomas are discussed in detail in Chapter 21. In contrast, epidural hematomas result from tearing of an artery, most commonly the middle meningeal artery, and frequently are caused by blunt head trauma. Epidural hematomas are discussed in Chapter 21.

Clinical Manifestations

Like those of ischemic stroke, symptoms of intracerebral hemorrhage occur with no warning. Severe headache is often present and may help to distinguish it from ischemic stroke. The other signs and symptoms depend on the region of the brain affected and the size of the hemorrhage.

NURSING PROCESS: Patient Care Plan for Stroke

Assessment of Neurologic Status Using Gordon's Functional Health Patterns:

- Health Perception Health Management Pattern
- Nutrition Metabolic Pattern
- Activity Exercise Pattern
- Cognitive Perceptual Pattern
- Self-Perception Self-Concept Pattern
- Coping-Stress Tolerance Pattern

Subjective Data

Assessment for Level of Consciousness

Do you have any history of hypertension, heart disease, bleeding disorders, renal disease, or cancer?

What is your name?

What day is it?

Where are you?

How old are you?

Who is the president?

What was the last major holiday?

In your own words, tell me why you came to the hospital.

Assessment of Hemodynamic Status

Do you have any preexisting cardiac or respiratory problems?

Do you ever experience chest pain?

Do you have high blood pressure?

Are you taking any cardiac or blood pressure medications—if so, what are they?

Assessment of Motor, Sensory, and Cognitive Status

Can you move your arms and legs?

Where am I touching you?

Skin Assessment

Are you having pain on your skin in any area of your body?

Are you able to turn yourself in bed?

Are you able to get out of bed?

Nutrition Assessment

How is your appetite?

Do you have sores in your mouth?

What kinds of foods are you eating?

What kinds of foods do you like or dislike?

Are there any cultural practices that would influence your diet?

Does any type of food make you choke?

Have you noticed a change in your ability to swallow?

Assessment of Pain

Are you in pain? If so, where?

What makes the pain better or worse?

Does it radiate anywhere on your body?

Assessment of Communication Ability

Are you able to speak?

Has it become more difficult?

Objective Data

Assessment for Level of Consciousness

Glasgow Coma Scale (GCS) score (discussed in Chapter 20).

Neurological assessment, including pupil size and reactivity, mentation, cranial nerve examination, and motor and sensory function.

Imaging studies, including CT of head, magnetic resonance imaging (MRI), magnetic resonance angiography (MRA), and/or cerebral angiography.

Lumbar puncture (LP).

Laboratory data, including complete blood count (CBC), electrolytes, comprehensive metabolic panel (CMP), total cholesterol, HDL, LDL, and drug levels.

12-lead ECG results to detect dysrhythmias.

Observe response to voice, tactile stimuli, and ability to follow commands.

Assessment of Hemodynamic Status

Vital signs, including heart rate, cardiac rhythm, blood pressure, respiratory rate, and central venous pressure, if available.

Oxygen saturation.

Skin, lips, and nail bed color.

Lung sounds.

Cardiac rhythm strips or ECG.

Assessment of Motor, Sensory, and Cognitive Status

Motor and sensory function.

Pupil reactions.

Orientation.

Skin Assessment

Skin assessment for breakdown.

Patient's ability to move.

Patient's activity level.

Nutrition Assessment

Assess nutritional status.

Assess 24-hour food intake.

Assess for ability to swallow.

Assessment of Pain

Increased heart rate, blood pressure, or respiratory rate.

Facial expressions (i.e., grimacing).

Use pain scale (0–10) to quantify pain level.

Assess cultural or religious impact on the patient's response. Assess location, duration, and onset of pain.

Assessment of Communication Ability

Assess speech fluency and clarity.

Is there any slurring?

Does the mouth droop?

NURSING PROCESS: Patient Care Plan for Stroke, *continued*

Assessment of Coping

What are your complaints?

What is your understanding of the present condition or disease?

Have you noticed that you feel more emotional or depressed?

What are your concerns for the future?

Assessment of Coping

What is the patient's level of education?

What is the patient's occupation?

What is the patient's family support system?

Does the patient have a religious affiliation?

Facial expressions.

Mood.

Verbalization of fear regarding illness, impact on family, and future.

Assessment of Knowledge of Disease Condition

What do you understand about your illness?

Do you have questions about the treatment program?

What would you like me to tell you about your illness?

Assessment of Knowledge of Disease Condition

Patient/family verbalizes questions about the seriousness of illness and prognosis.

Outcomes and Evaluation Parameters	Planning and Interventions with *Rationales*
1. NURSING DIAGNOSIS: Altered Cerebral Perfusion Pressure ***related to decreased blood flow to the brain associated with (a) blockage of blood flow due to ischemic stroke; (b) cerebral hemorrhage resulting from the underlying disease process or loss of integrity of the ligated vessels; (c) compression of cerebral vessels as a result of cerebral edema; (d) spasm of the cerebral vessels from trauma or subarachnoid hemorrhage; (e) hypotension and decreased cerebral perfusion pressure due to hypovolemia or other causes*** **(NANDA-I © 2012)**	
Outcomes: Improvement to optimum level of neurological function. Improved level of consciousness. Intracranial pressure readings within normal limits. Normal or stable Glasgow Coma Scale score. ***Evaluation Parameters:*** Normal or stable Glasgow Coma Scale (GCS) score. Oriented to person, place, time, and event. Pupils equal, round, and reactive to light. Normal ICP waveform, a pressure-volume curve that demonstrates the effects of intracranial volume changes on ICP. (Normal ICP $<$ 20 mmHg) (Chapter 21). Normal serum sodium (Na^+), hemoglobin (Hgb), and hematocrit (Hct) levels. Vital signs, especially blood pressure (BP) and temperature, maintained per prescribed parameters (ischemic stroke may encourage permissive hypertension with blood pressures up to 220 mmHg systolic, while in hemorrhagic stroke blood pressure may be lowered to maintain a prescribed level).	Monitor neurological assessment using the Glasgow Coma Scale (GCS) at least hourly, or as ordered by the health care provider. *To assess changes in motor and sensory function, and orientation to person, place, time, and events.* Assess pupil size and reactivity. *To assess for increased intracranial pressure manifesting as pressure on the third cranial nerve.* Monitor ICP reading (the pressure inside the cranium composed of pressure from blood, brain tissue, and cerebrospinal fluid). *To assess changes in intracranial pressure that may be life threatening. To ascertain when medical intervention is necessary to decrease the pressure. To identify which interventions raise or lower the ICP.* Monitor lab values (serum Na^+). *To maintain a normal range to prevent fluid retention that would raise intracranial pressure.* Monitor vital signs, especially blood pressure and temperature, as ordered by the health care provider and report changes when values are outside ordered parameters. *To prevent a loss of cerebral perfusion pressure (CPP). To report any increase in temperature that may indicate an infection.*
2. NURSING DIAGNOSES: (a) Cardiac Output, Decreased ***related to arrhythmias, hemodynamic instability, and hypotension/hypertension;*** **(b) Actual or Risk for Ineffective Tissue Perfusion** ***related to decreased cardiac output*** **(NANDA-I © 2012)**	
Outcomes: Cardiac output within normal limits. Adequate tissue perfusion maintained. ***Evaluation Parameters:*** Stable rate and rhythm. Blood pressure maintenance within established parameters. Patient able to perform activities of daily living comfortably and independently.	Monitor ECG continuously. Notify health care provider of changes in rate or rhythm. Administer cardiac and hypertension medications as ordered and monitor for effectiveness. *To assess and treat cardiac dysrhythmias that affect cardiac output and detect rhythms such as atrial fibrillation that predispose to cardioembolic stroke.* Monitor vital signs and cardiac output. Cardiac output monitoring is described in Chapter 30 and atrial fibrillation in Chapter 31. Notify health care provider of changes in blood pressure. *To determine cardiac output, tissue perfusion, and embolic sources of stroke such as atrial fibrillation and evidence of heart failure.*
3. NURSING DIAGNOSES: (a) Self-Care Deficit ***related to altered motor and sensory function from neuro deficit;*** **(b) Actual or Risk for Impaired Physical Mobility** ***related to decreased strength and endurance;*** **(c) Risk for Injury** ***related to fall risk;*** **(d) Risk for Tissue Injury** ***related to immobility*** **(NANDA-I © 2012)**	
Outcomes: Patient will attain maximum motor function. Patient will be free from injury. Family/significant other available who is able to assist with care.	Monitor strengths and limitations. *Measure motor function through assessment of upper extremity and lower extremity muscle strength. Examination should include all of the major muscle groups and measurement of extremity drift to detect subtle changes in strength. Hand grip testing can be reflexive*

(continued)

NURSING PROCESS: Patient Care Plan for Stroke, *continued*

Outcomes and Evaluation Parameters	Planning and Interventions with *Rationales*
Adequate tissue perfusion. Patient will be safe from physical harm/injury. ***Evaluation Parameters*** Able to progress with ambulation and complete self-care. No deep vein thrombosis (DVT) or pulmonary embolism.	*and is not a good indicator of early weakness. Sensory function should be assessed though a systematic evaluation of detection of light touch and pain, comparing right to left. Evaluate cognitive functions that are necessary to complete sensory and motor rehabilitation activities. This may be done by questioning orientation to person, place, time, and situation. It is necessary to assess the patient's ability to follow directions by providing both single-step commands—"Close your eyes"—and multistep commands—"Take your left thumb and touch your right ear." The ability to follow instructions is important for patient safety in rehabilitation environments and can affect physical therapy treatment planning.* Initiate physical therapy consultation. Initiate activity as tolerated, unless contraindicated. Obtain an occupational therapy consult to assist with activities of daily living. *To regain and increase strength on the affected side and promote independence.* Encourage family involvement in patient care and mobility. *To promote family involvement and prepare for discharge.* Institute safety measures (i.e., place a call light within reach, ask the patient to call a nurse before getting out of bed). Apply restraints as ordered to prevent injury. Keep bed rails in high position at all times. *To promote safety and prevent falling.* Apply thigh-high elastic stockings or alternating leg pressure devices. Apply sequential compression stockings. Administer subcutaneous injections of heparin when ordered. Monitor lower extremities frequently for signs/symptoms of DVT, including unilateral swelling of a lower extremity, new pain in a lower extremity, pain behind the knee or calf, with dorsiflexion (Homans' sign). Notify health care provider for signs/symptoms of DVT. *To prevent, assess for, and treat deep vein thrombosis.*
4. NURSING DIAGNOSIS: Risk for Impaired Skin Integrity *related to immobility* (NANDA-I © 2012)	
Outcome: Skin intact and healthy, without evidence of breakdown. ***Evaluation Parameters:*** Patient will maintain skin integrity. Verbalizes importance of changing positions and is able to do it.	Turn and reposition every 2 hours, unless contraindicated. *To take the pressure off bony prominences and promote tissue perfusion.* Provide skin care frequently, keeping skin clean and dry. *To prevent breakdown.* Monitor skin for redness and possible skin breakdown. Do not position patient on areas of redness. *To detect areas that may be beginning to break down and treat them to prevent further deterioration.* Assess need for air mattress or other pressure relief bed. *To prevent breakdown.* Assess need for nutrition consult. *To provide the necessary nutrients to promote healing.* Monitor vital signs. *To assess for the presence of infection.*
5. NURSING DIAGNOSIS: Actual or Risk for Imbalanced Nutrition: Less Than Body Requirements *related to neurological deficit, impaired swallowing and intake of a chronic low protein diet, deficient in albumin* (NANDA-I © 2012)	
Outcomes: Stable weight. Adequate nutritional intake. ***Evaluation Parameters:*** No aspiration. Patient will maintain current body weight. Patient will maintain or improve albumin levels. Patient will tolerate diet or tube feedings.	Keep patient NPO until alert and/or swallow function is assessed and deemed safe. Conduct swallow evaluation *to assess safety.* Initiate aspiration precautions including head of bed position at 90 degrees for all oral intake with a chin tuck position. *To prevent aspiration and allow normal oral intake.* Monitor food intake. *Food intake needs to be adequate for healing.* Serve small amounts of high calorie, high protein food every 2 hours. *Patient is more likely to eat small amounts more frequently than large amounts less often.* *Monitor albumin levels daily; consult with dietitian to provide foods high in protein and calories, as protein contains albumin.* Provide a well-balanced diet with foods the patient likes. *Patient will be more likely to eat.*

NURSING PROCESS: Patient Care Plan for Stroke, *continued*

	Consult with a dietitian. Assess the need for parenteral or enteral feedings. *If the patient is unable to eat enough food orally to keep up with the body's demands, other avenues may need to be explored and utilized.* Keep calorie count. *To assess adequacy of intake.* Assess ability to swallow. Assess which foods make the patient choke—if any. *To prevent aspiration.*
6. NURSING DIAGNOSIS: Pain, Acute *related to impaired physical mobility and motor deficits* (NANDA-I © 2012)	
Outcome: Able to ambulate safely with little to no pain. ***Evaluation Parameters:*** Patient expresses pain control. Patient attains maximum motor function.	Administer pain medications as ordered. Use pain scale (0–10) to quantify pain level. *Quantifying pain increases consistency.* Instruct patient to inform nurse if pain is not relieved. *Indicates need to change pain management plan.* Assess cultural and religious impact on patient's responses. *Different cultures and religions respond differently to pain.* Correct misconceptions about risk of addiction and overdose. *To decrease anxiety related to medication addiction.* Explain, prepare, and medicate patient for painful procedures (physical therapy) and anticipated discomforts. *To control increased pain level related to procedure.* Provide a supportive environment where patient is able to express pain level. *Opens communication and facilitates pain management.* Use pain control measures before pain in extremities and muscles becomes intolerable to patient. *This increases comfort and decreases need for medication.* Teach nonpharmacologic method of control (i.e., guided imagery and massage) and breathing exercises. *These measures augment pain relief.* Plan diversional activities. *To augment pain relief measures.*
7. NURSING DIAGNOSIS: Actual or Risk for Impaired Verbal Communication *related to alteration of central nervous system and decreased circulation to the brain* (NANDA-I © 2012)	
Outcome: Patient is able to communicate needs and preferences verbally. ***Evaluation Parameters:*** Patient attains maximum communication. Speech skills begin to return.	Assess type and degree of communication deficit. *To identify the appropriate therapy.* Initiate speech therapy consultation. *To begin speech rehabilitation.* Provide communication board for intubated patient. *To facilitate communication.*
8. NURSING DIAGNOSES: (a) Ineffective Coping *related to sudden change in physiological status;* (b) Anxiety *related to apprehension regarding potential outcome* (NANDA-I © 2012)	
Outcome: Patient/family is coping with illness in a positive manner. Patient displays reduced anxiety. ***Evaluation Parameters:*** Manifests coping mechanisms with what is happening, verbally if possible, and by facial expression. Appears calm; discusses possible outcomes. Maintains self-composure when discussing the future. Verbalizes what relieves anxiety. Verbalizes absence of sensory perceptual disorders. Verbalizes absence of physical manifestations of anxiety.	Provide factual information concerning diagnosis, treatment, disfigurement, disabilities, and prognosis. *Truthful explanations increase trust, potentially decrease anxiety, and may increase coping.* Encourage family involvement. *To assist all members to learn to cope by decreasing fear.* Provide spiritual support as needed, if desired. Assess and document level of anxiety. *To track trends in anxiety levels.* Explore with the patient/family techniques to reduce anxiety. *This gives the patient a sense of control and opens communication about the subject.* Explain all procedures and allow time for mental preparation. *This decreases fear and anxiety of the unknown.* Explore with patient effective ways to minimize anxiety. *This gives the patient a sense of control.* Instruct patient on use of relaxation techniques. *To relieve anxiety.* Assess need for and administer antianxiety and pain medication. *If alternative measures are not effective, may need antianxiety agents.*

(*continued*)

NURSING PROCESS: Patient Care Plan for Stroke, *continued*

Outcomes and Evaluation Parameters	Planning and Interventions with *Rationales*
	Assist patient/family in setting realistic long-term goals for progress. *Indicates effectiveness of emotional adjustment.* Consider psychiatric counseling for patients/families who exhibit inability to accept situation or symptoms of depression. *Provide an ongoing plan and interventions to promote long-term relief of anxiety and depression.*
9. NURSING DIAGNOSIS: Deficient Knowledge *related to diagnosis* (NANDA-I © 2012)	
Outcome: Patient and family knowledgeable about condition and long-term ramifications. ***Evaluation Parameters:*** Patient and family or significant others verbalize understanding of condition and rehabilitative education provided.	Provide patient with information specific to their stroke subtype and anticipated plan of care. Educate patients and families about the disease process, treatments, and prevention strategies to reduce the risk of recurrent stroke. Provide support for smoking cessation in all tobacco users. Provide patient with resources as needed. *To increase their knowledge about all phases of illness and the necessary treatments.*

Source: Adapted from Wilkinson, J. M., & Ahearn, N. R. (2009). *Prentice Hall Nursing Diagnosis Handbook* (9th ed.). Upper Saddle River, NJ: Prentice Hall.

The most common clinical manifestations include severe headache, weakness or numbness on either side of the body, difficulty with speech or understanding speech, visual disturbances, and gait and balance problems. Patients with high volume intracerebral hemorrhage may present with loss of consciousness and severe neurological impairment. Hemorrhage volume is an independent predictor of outcome and can be used to predict survival (Broderick et al., 2007; Staykov & Gupta, 2011). High-volume hemorrhages cause rapid displacement of brain tissue and abrupt increases in intracranial pressure that may be nonrecoverable. The presenting signs and symptoms of hemorrhagic stroke may be focal signs associated with the specific location of the hemorrhage, but also may be those of increased ICP and herniation syndromes. Focal symptoms are localized and include weakness or paresis that may affect a single extremity, one-half of the body, or all four extremities; facial droop; monocular or binocular blindness; blurred vision or visual field deficits; dysarthria and trouble understanding speech; vertigo or ataxia; and aphasia. The neurologic deficits reflect the area of the brain typically involved. Increased intracranial pressure may be due to brain tissue swelling, blood or other fluid accumulating inside the skull, or a combination of these situations. The signs and symptoms that may indicate increased intracranial pressure are shown in Chart 22–3.

Brain herniation is a condition in which brain tissue, CSF, and blood vessels are moved or pressed away from their usual position inside the skull. This occurs when something else inside the skull produces pressure that moves brain tissues. Brain herniation can occur between areas inside the skull, as occurs with a hemorrhagic stroke, through the foramen magnum, or through an opening created during brain surgery. Signs and symptoms of brain herniation include hemodynamic instability, coma, lethargy, loss of all brainstem reflexes (blinking, gagging, pupils reacting to light), loss of consciousness, and respiratory arrest (MedlinePlus, 2010). Herniation and intracranial pressure (ICP) are fully discussed in Chapter 21.

CHART 22–3 Signs and Symptoms of Increased Intracranial Pressure

- Headache
- Nausea and/or vomiting
- Loss of consciousness (either current or recent unconsciousness)
- Dilated pupils that do not constrict when exposed to bright light (an early sign of serious head injury) or changes in pupil symmetry
- Lateral loss of motor nerve function in which one side of the body becomes paralyzed (may not occur immediately)
- Slow respiratory rate or change in respiratory pattern
- A steady rise in the systolic blood pressure (may not be present if there is significant bleeding elsewhere)
- A rise in the pulse pressure (systolic pressure minus diastolic pressure)
- Elevated body temperature
- Restlessness (indicates insufficient oxygenation of the brain)
- Slurred speech
- Convulsions or twitching
- Abnormal posturing

Source: MedlinePlus. (2010). *Brain herniation.* Retrieved from http://www.nlm.nih/gov/medlineplus/ency/article/001421.htm.

Medical Management

Treatment of hemorrhagic stroke depends on the location of the hemorrhage, the extent of the hemorrhage, and the neurological condition of the patient. Management usually is limited to medical management such as correction of coagulopathy and blood pressure control. Several studies have failed to show a benefit of surgical evacuation of deep hemorrhages (Adeoye & Broderick, 2010; Adeoye et al., 2010). As a result, surgical treatment is reserved for hemorrhage in the cerebellum or evacuation of subdural hematomas and epidural hematomas. Treatment of hemorrhagic stroke focuses on correction of coagulopathy, replacement of platelets if levels are abnormally low, and supportive nursing care to avoid secondary injury (Liebeskind, 2011). Treatments should be prioritized because bleeding in the brain often continues for hours after the initial event, leading to a worse outcome. This can be reduced by giving medicines or blood products to correct abnormal clotting.

In contrast, patients who present with subdural hematoma or epidural hematoma often require surgical evacuation. Clinical studies have shown that patients who have signs of shifting of the brain from the clot (transtentorial herniation) with normal coagulation will improve with surgical removal of the clot (Meagher & Lutsep, 2009).

After an initial neurological examination, the patient must be monitored closely in the intensive care unit (ICU), with frequent neurological

EVIDENCE-BASED PRACTICE Intracerebral Hemorrhage

Clinical Problem

Clinical manifestations of intracerebral hemorrhage (ICH) are usually sudden in onset with symptoms reflecting the vascular territory affected. The size of the hematoma is thought to be one of the most important factors in determining the outcome for patients with ICH. Hematomas may grow as much as 30% in the first 24 hours after onset of hemorrhage. For these reasons, strategies to stop bleeding would seem beneficial. Attempts to obtain hemostasis through reducing systemic blood pressure have also been interesting areas of clinical research.

Research Findings

Research has suggested that arresting expansion of the hematoma may improve the outcome for patients with ICH. A recent clinical trial (INTERACT 1) that focused on lowering blood pressure during the acute period has shown that hematoma volume can be reduced by lowering the blood pressure by as little as 12 mmHg (Anderson et al., 2010). The study evaluated 296 patients with intracerebral hemorrhage, elevated blood pressure (BP), and the ability to start an antihypertensive treatment within 6 hours of onset of intracerebral hemorrhage. Patients were randomly assigned to either normal treatment with a systolic <180 mmHg or intensive treatment with a blood pressure target of <140 mmHg for 7 days. Expansion of the hematoma and swelling were measured on serial CT scans. The investigators found that intensive blood pressure control reduced hematoma expansion by 20% to 30% (absolute value 2.8 mL). The study was not designed to detect functional clinical outcomes, and no obvious adverse effects were reported in the research results. This study is important because it is one of the first to demonstrate the safety and feasibility of aggressive BP reduction in the emergency department targeted at a systolic BP of 140 mmHg. It remains to be seen, however, whether intensive BP control can definitively reduce intracranial volume growth and improve outcome as a solo intervention (Mayer & Schwab, 2008).

The INTERACT 2 study, a replication of the INTERACT 1 study, was initiated in 2008, with ongoing enrollment at this time (The Internet Stroke Center, 2010b). The purpose of this second study is to investigate whether early intensive blood-pressure-lowering therapy can reduce death and disability from intracerebral hemorrhage compared to conservative management based on current stroke guidelines. This large-scale, randomized, controlled study employs the same blood pressure parameters as the original pilot study and intends to recruit 2,800 subjects from 140 sites across the world. Outcome measures include the effects of intensive lowering of blood pressure in the acute period with primary outcome measures for death and disability. Secondary outcomes of functional disability, cognitive function, quality of life, and mortality at 1 and 3 months also will be evaluated.

Preliminary findings of this study, with 633 participants, were reported in 2010. They indicated patient and clinical characteristics similar to those of INTERACT 1 (The Internet Stroke Center, 2010b). It also was reported that high levels of interest exist for INTERACT 2, and recruitment of study participants is on schedule to achieve the study goals. These data will advance understanding regarding the safety of acutely lowering blood pressure in the acute care setting of patients with ICH, and may lead to revision of stroke treatment protocols (Jeffrey & Nighiem, 2010).

Implications for Nursing Practice

Because intracerebral hemorrhage is complex, many health care professionals are involved in achieving the most favorable outcome. Nurses play a central role in the interdisciplinary team to coordinate care throughout the acute and subacute period (Miller et al., 2010). Blood pressure management and close monitoring of neurological status are major nursing responsibilities. Careful monitoring of blood pressure values to ensure that blood pressure stays within prescribed parameters is essential.

Hematoma expansion can be detected on clinical assessment. Any decline in the patient's neurological status could suggest a worsening condition. This possible decrease in neurological status warrants collaboration with the supervising health care provider to determine the need for urgent diagnostic imaging to assess for an increase in the size of the hematoma. Other important nursing responsibilities accompanying the monitoring of blood pressure include closely controlling the monitoring of blood glucose and other electrolytes, fever management, seizure management, and monitoring of physiological processes.

Critical Thinking Questions with answers can be found in the Osborn Student Resources at nursing.pearson.highered.com.

References

Anderson, C. S., Huang, Y., Wang, J. G., Arima, H., Neal, B., Peng, B., . . . Chalmers, J., for the INTERACT Investigators. (2008). Intensive blood pressure reduction in acute cerebral haemorrhage trial (INTERACT): A randomised pilot trial. *The Lancet Neurology, 7*(5), 391–399. doi: 10.1016/S1474-4422(08)70069-3

Jeffrey, S., & Nighiem, H. T. (2010). New AHA/ASA guidelines on management of intracerebral hemorrhage. Medscape reference. Retrieved from http://www.medscape.org/viewarticle/726269.

Mayer, S. A., & Schwab, S. (2008). Advances in stroke 2008. Stroke. doi: 10.1161/STROLEANA.108.544619

Miller, E. L., Murray, L., Richards, L., Zorowitz, R. D., Bakas, T., Clark, P., et al. (2010). Comprehensive overview of nursing and interdisciplinary rehabilitation care of the stroke patient: A scientific statement from the American Heart Association. *Stroke, 41*(10), 2402–2448. doi: 10.1161/STR.0b013e3181e7512b

The Internet Stroke Center. (2010b). Stroke trials INTERACT 2. Retrieved from http://www.strokecenter.org/trials/TrialDetail.aspx?tid+751.

assessment. Some patients will benefit from placement of an external ventricular drain (EVD) to monitor ICP and to treat elevation of ICP by drainage of CSF. The EVD is a small, soft tube that reduces the pressure on the brain by draining fluid from inside the brain to another place in the body where it drains naturally. Placement of the EVD and caring for the patient with a drain whose ICP is being monitored are discussed fully in Chapter 21. Medical support of blood pressure and respiratory effort also may be necessary. If the hemorrhage is large enough to cause a shift of brain tissue, a craniotomy may be done to evacuate the hematoma to relieve mass effect. The Evidence-Based Practice feature provides further information on intracranial hemorrhage.

Nursing Management

The nursing process provides the framework for managing the care of a patient who has had a hemorrhagic stroke. These patients require immediate assessment, diagnosis, and close monitoring of vital and neurologic signs. The Nursing Process: Patient Care Plan for Stroke on page 564 provides a complete approach to caring for patients with both ischemic and hemorrhagic stroke.

Health Promotion

The nurse plays an essential role in educating patients and families regarding ways to correct stroke risk factors and prevent secondary stroke. Hospital stays following stroke are often brief, challenging the bedside nurse to provide comprehensive education about stroke prevention, recognition of modifiable risk factors, and medication compliance within 48 to 72 hours.

Nursing management in the acute care setting is aimed at prevention of secondary injury and identification of modifiable risk factors. Nurses, as primary educators, should teach patients and/or their families regarding the administration, side effects, and drug interactions of their medications. If the patient has a new diagnosis of seizure, education regarding antiepileptic drugs is key to ensuring compliance and safety. Nurses also should be instructed if blood testing is required for evaluation of efficacy. Smoking cessation and avoidance of secondary smoke have been identified as important modifiable risks; nurses can assist the patient in identifying strategies to quit smoking or move away from secondhand smoke. Other modifiable risk factors include a low-fat diet, exercise, and a healthy

NATIONAL GUIDELINES National Stroke Association Prevention Advisory Board's 2010 Stroke Prevention Guidelines

Risk Factor	Guideline
1. Stage 1 hypertension. Systolic 140–159 mmHg Diastolic 90–99 mmHg Stage 2 hypertension Systolic > 160 mmHg Diastolic > 100 mmHg	Have your blood pressure checked annually. Lifestyle modification and drug therapy are recommended to treat HTN > 140 mmHg systolic and >90 mmHg diastolic. Thiazide-type diuretics are used for most. May consider ACEI, ARB, BB, CCB, or combination. Most patients will require two-drug therapy. Thiazide-type diuretic and one of the following: ACEI, ARB, BB, CCB, or combination. Compliance with antihypertensive medication is critical. A diet of low salt and low fat will help lower your blood pressure. Start and maintain an exercise program.
2. Atrial fibrillation	Be screened for atrial fibrillation if you are over the age of 65. Patients at high risk should have anticoagulation. Patients at low or moderate risk can be prescribed aspirin. In patients who are not candidates for anticoagulation but are at high risk for stroke, clopidigrel and aspirin given together offer more protection against stroke but have higher risks of bleeding.
3. Smoking	Stop smoking. Provide support, nicotine replacement, and formal programs to improve success rate. Cessation of smoking immediately decreases the chance for stroke. Smoking doubles the risk for stroke. Smoking is a completely preventable risk factor for stroke. Environmental secondhand smoke is also discouraged.
4. Alcohol use	Limit alcohol to no more than two drinks daily and no more than one drink per day in nonpregnant women. If you do not drink, do not start.
5. Hyperlipidemia	Use a statin drug to control lipid levels within national guidelines, LDL < 130. Fibric acid derivatives may be considered for patients with hypertriglyceridemia, but their efficacy in the prevention of ischemic stroke is not established. Niacin may be considered for patients with low HDL cholesterol or elevated lipoprotein(a), but its efficacy in prevention of ischemic stroke in patients with these conditions is not established. Treatment with other lipid-lowering therapies, such as fibric acid derivatives, bile acid sequestrants, niacin, and ezetimibe, may be considered in patients who do not achieve target LDL cholesterol with statins or cannot tolerate statins, but the effectiveness of these therapies in decreasing risk of stroke is not established.
6. Exercise	Get > 30 minutes of moderate to intense exercise per day to reduce the risk of stroke.
7. Diet and nutrition	Limit dietary sodium and increase dietary potassium to reduce blood pressure. A DASH-style (Chapter 8) diet, which emphasizes consumption of fruits, vegetables, and low-fat dairy products and is reduced in saturated fat, also lowers BP and is recommended. A diet that is rich in fruits and vegetables is beneficial and may lower risk of stroke.
8. Develop awareness of circulation problems.	See your health care provider if you experience circulatory symptoms, or if you have a history of anemia or sickle cell anemia.
9. Know the symptoms.	Know the signs and symptoms of stroke. Call 911 immediately if any of these occur.

lifestyle. Education of the patient and family is an invaluable service to help avoid future strokes.

Health promotion also may include helping the patients/families become involved in relevant community programs and services. The fact that stroke is the leading cause of death in the United States (AHA, 2009) has heightened public awareness of stroke and its risk factors. Both the public community and the professional community are becoming increasingly aware of the urgency in treating and/or preventing strokes. Stroke protocols are being set up in hospitals and in prehospital settings, saving precious time in the treatment of stroke. Community and post-hospitalization programs and services are readily available to assist people in modifying risk factors. These programs include nutritional counseling, smoking cessation clinics, stress reduction activities, and alternative medical therapies. Professional services also can assist individuals in determining whether they have genetic risk factors and, if so, how best to manage them on a daily basis.

The National Stroke Association's Prevention Advisory Board released its Stroke Prevention Guidelines, a set of recommendations on what the public can do to prevent stroke (Goldstein et al., 2010). The guidelines are presented in the accompanying National Guidelines box.

Vascular Malformations

Vascular malformations in the cerebral vasculature are relatively common; up to 15% of the general population harbors an abnormality in the cerebral circulation (Gloviczki et al., 2009). Most patients are asymptomatic. The most common problems associated with abnormalities in the cerebral blood vessels include headache, seizure, and intracranial bleeding. Treatment often is conservative with a watchful waiting approach unless the malformation is large enough to produce symptoms. In addition, the expected natural history given the size of the malformation may indicate that surgery should be considered.

Cerebral Aneurysms

The word *aneurysm* comes from the Greek word *aneurysma,* which means "widening." While aneurysms may occur in various parts of the

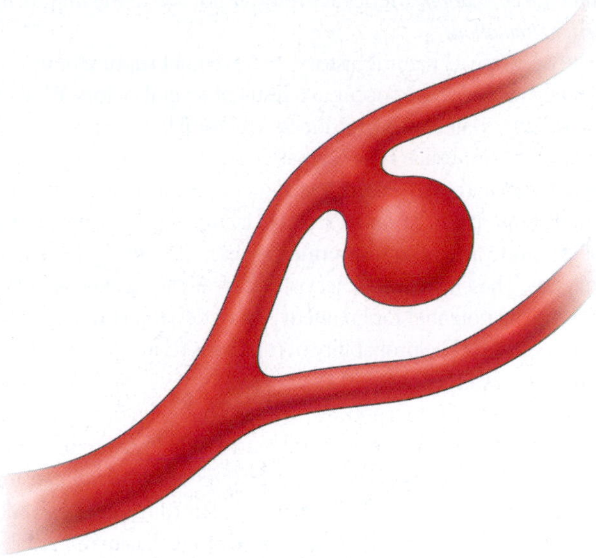

FIGURE 22–2 ◆ Cerebral aneurysm.
Source: Modified with permission from Barrow Neurological Institute

body, the following discussion focuses on cerebral aneurysm. A **cerebral aneurysm** is weakening of the wall of a blood vessel in the brain that results in ballooning or focal dilation, predisposing the weakened spot to rupture. Aneurysms may have a variety of shapes, but the saccular aneurysm, or **berry aneurysm,** a sac-like outpouching in a cerebral blood vessel that may seem berry-shaped, is by far the most common, accounting for approximately 85% to 95% of all intracerebral aneurysms (Figure 22–2◆). These aneurysms are generally located on a major artery at the site of maximum pressure of the blood moving through the vessel, and they have a neck as seen in Figure 22–2. Common locations are the middle cerebral artery, the anterior communicating artery, the anterior cerebral artery, and the internal carotid artery. Less common sites for saccular aneurysms are the posterior circulation on the vertebral or basilar arteries. Frequently seen in the posterior circulation are **fusiform aneurysms,** which are elliptical in shape. Intracerebral aneurysms may occur singularly or in multiples. **Familial intracranial aneurysms** are defined as two or more family members with documented cerebral aneurysms. The Genetic Considerations box discusses the familial tendency for aneurysms.

Rupture of an intracerebral aneurysm results in bleeding into the subarachnoid space, known as **subarachnoid hemorrhage (SAH).** Though SAH can occur from other causes, such as trauma, or can be idiopathic, it most often occurs from aneurysm rupture. This is referred to as *aneurysmal SAH*. Subarachnoid hemorrhage is discussed in detail in Chapter 21.

Epidemiology

Each year in the United States, there are approximately 30,000 new cases of aneurysmal SAHs (AHA, 2009). Autopsy studies demonstrate an incidence of approximately 5% of the population have this disorder. Despite vast improvements in medical technology and surgical techniques, outcomes of SAH are still poor, with a fatality rate of approximately 40% to 50% (Lloyd-Jones et al., 2010). Survivors of SAH may have significant neurological, physical, and/or cognitive deficits (Maud et al., 2009). The incidence of SAH increases with age, the mean age being approximately 50 years, and is higher in women than in men (Porras & Poussa, 2008).

GENETIC CONSIDERATIONS Related to Cerebral Aneurysms

Familial intracranial aneurysms often are defined as the presence of two or more family members among first- and second-degree relatives with proven aneurysms, either ruptured or incidental (asymptomatic), with recent research pointing to genetic linkages in addition to environmental exposure (Ruigrok & Rinkel, 2008). Multiple studies on familial aneurysms have determined that the incidence is between 7% and 20% (Zacharia et al., 2010). Because family members may have different risk factors and show no signs of other disorders that may predispose them to intracranial aneurysms, it is believed that there is a genetic component to familial intracranial aneurysms. Multiple aneurysms occur in approximately 10% to 20% of all patients with SAH (Inagawa, 2009).

Literature indicates that a number of nonmodifiable risk factors exist, including age, race, gender, and size and location of the aneurysm (Zacharia et al., 2010).

Etiology

The etiology of cerebral aneurysms is not clear. Genetic predisposition is one possibility. Genetic factors, combined with various intrinsic and extrinsic factors, may be an explanation. There are many intrinsic and extrinsic factors that affect the integrity of the vascular system; examples include hypertension and smoking. A genetic predisposition for weakened vasculature, coupled with hypertension and/or smoking that may exacerbate the weakened vessel, could cause rupture (see the Risk Factors for Aneurysms box).

The etiology of cerebral aneurysms remains an area of active research; however, the cause for some aneurysms is well understood. Some are caused by bacterial or fungal infections, resulting in mycotic aneurysms. Mycotic aneurysms are those that result from an infectious process involving the arterial wall. These aneurysms do not result in SAH.

Aneurysms also are classified by their size. Small aneurysms are the most common. Data from the International Study of Unruptured Intracranial Aneurysm (ISUIA) indicate that large aneurysms are more prone to rupture (NINDS, 2011a). Although giant aneurysms occasionally rupture, most often they cause patients to be symptomatic before they rupture, owing to compression on surrounding brain tissue.

Risk Factors for Subarachnoid Hemorrhage

Risk factors for SAH have been shown to include age, gender, and race, as described earlier. As with other types of stroke, smoking is a strong risk factor for SAH, especially in women, and is predictive of a poor outcome (Hashimoto, 2011). In the past, the use of oral contraceptives was felt to be a strong risk factor, but with the change in the estrogen composition of these drugs, the risk appears significant for thrombotic stroke but not SAH (Carwile, Wagner, Crago, & Alexander, 2009). Drug abuse has been associated with SAH, especially use of stimulants, such as cocaine and amphetamines. It appears that while the use of

RISK FACTORS for Aneurysms

Smoking	Hypertension
Previous aneurysms	Family history of aneurysms
Connective tissue disorder	Age greater than 40 years
Female	Blood vessel injury or dissection

cocaine or amphetamines may not actually cause a hemorrhage, the vasoactive properties of the drugs appear to worsen an already weakened vasculature. Smoking, drug use, and hypertension are all modifiable risk factors. Once an aneurysm ruptures, risk factors differ slightly. Factors such as the patient's initial clinical condition, the amount of subarachnoid blood, and the continued presence of hypertension are strong negative prognostic factors (Dupont, Wijdicks, Manno, Lanzino, & Rabinstein, 2009).

Pathophysiology

The saccular aneurysm, or berry aneurysm, is formed by a ballooning of the vessel at the weakened portion of the artery. In contrast, fusiform aneurysms look like "swollen" areas of the artery and are associated with fatty plaque buildup in the artery. Although fusiform aneurysms do not usually rupture, they may cause neurological compromise due to pressure exerted on the surrounding brain.

Aneurysms can be located along the course of four main arteries that enter the brain. The two internal carotid arteries enter in the front of the brain. Two vertebral arteries enter from the back. These four arteries form a ring that circles the underside of the brain, which is referred to as the *circle of Willis*. Many smaller arteries branch off from the larger arteries (Figure 22–3◆). Arteries at the top of the ring are in the *anterior circulation*; arteries at the lower portion of the ring are in the *posterior circulation*.

The occurrence, natural history, and eventual rupture of intracerebral aneurysms appear to occur as a result of several factors. Weakening of the vascular wall may occur due to structural limitations or weakening of the vessel's walls. Hemodynamic stressors caused by increased force of blood in the vessels further influence the formation and growth of aneurysms. Intrinsic and extrinsic factors, such as hypertension, smoking, and various autoimmune diseases, also affect the history of aneurysms. These risk factors act pathologically to weaken vessel walls, increasing the potential for an aneurysm to develop (Brain Aneurysm Resources, 2011). The probability of rupture is related to the tension on the aneurysm wall (Oman, 2011).

Once an aneurysm ruptures, the arterial pressure forces blood into the subarachnoid space, creating an SAH. Pressure of the brain tissue stops the bleeding. The blood irritates brain tissue, causing an inflammatory response, which may further cause cerebral edema. The circulating blood in the CSF is an irritant that may inhibit CSF absorption, causing hydrocephalus. The presence of SAH causes hemodynamic changes, with a resultant increase in intracranial pressure. The pathophysiology of increased intracranial pressure is discussed in Chapter 21.

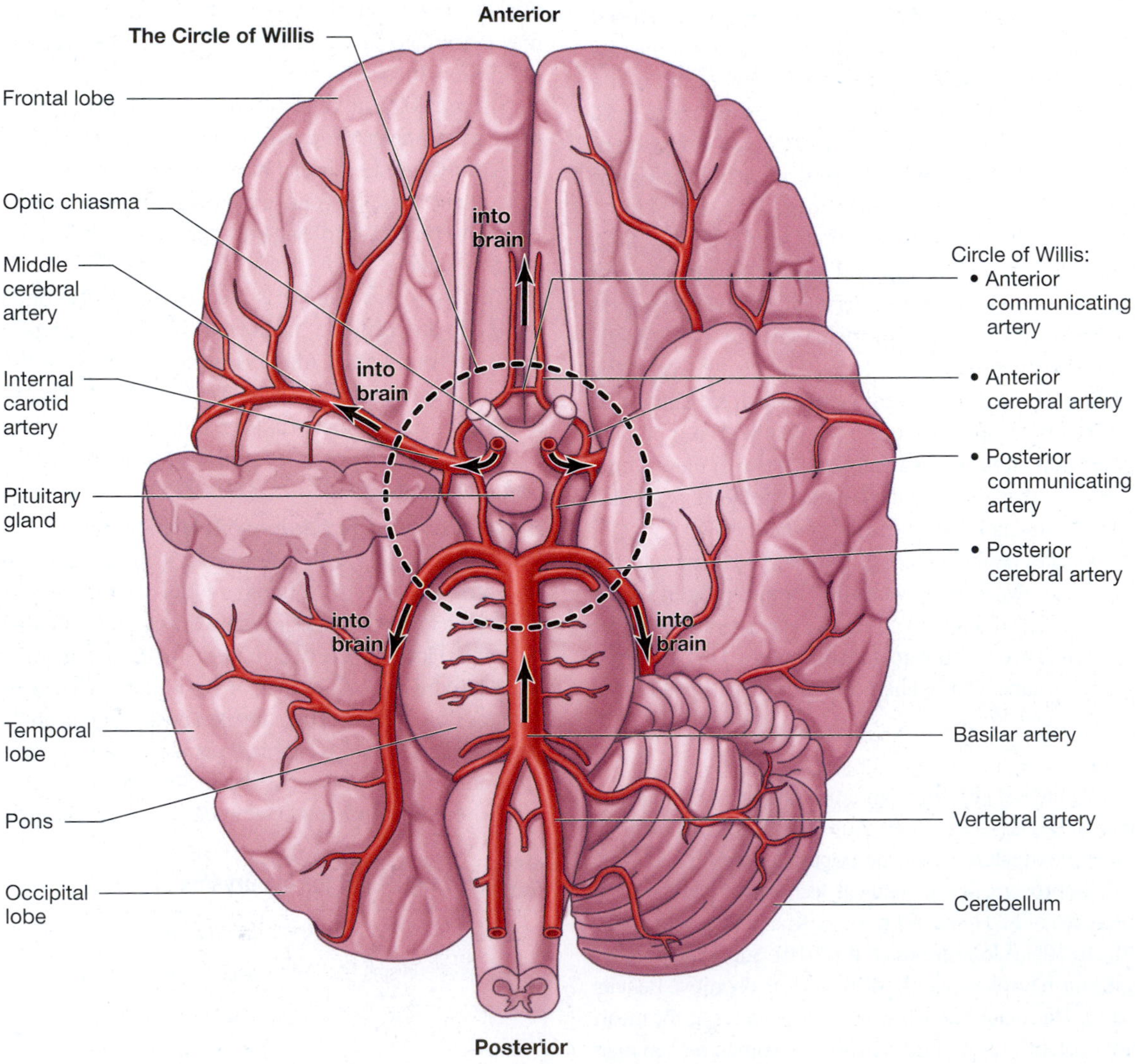

FIGURE 22–3 ◆ Circle of Willis.

Clinical Manifestations

The most common presenting symptom in aneurysmal SAH is the patient's complaint of the "worst headache of my life." Patients with aneurysms of the anterior circulation may have symptoms different from those of patients with aneurysms of the posterior circulation. Patients who experience SAH also have more severe neurological compromise than those without SAH. Clinical manifestations depend on the location and size of the hemorrhage. Certain differences exist between brain aneurysms of different sizes. Generally, small and large brain aneurysms behave similarly in that they tend to grow and rupture, whereas near-giant and giant brain aneurysms tend to cause symptoms related to compression or irritation of brain structures surrounding the aneurysms, such as seizures. The risks of death and disability associated with bigger brain aneurysms, particularly those in the back portion of the brain, are significantly higher than the risks with smaller aneurysms in the front part of the brain arteries (Brain Aneurysm Resources, 2011).

Ruptured Aneurysms

Neurological deterioration usually follows rupture of an aneurysm, with focal signs depending on the hemorrhage's location and size. Focal signs are disruptions of nerve, spinal cord, or brain function that affect a specific region of the body (e.g., weakness of the left leg). Seizures are not uncommon. Not infrequently, the presenting sign is death.

SAH in the posterior circulation also produces severe headaches. If the patient is conscious, extreme vertigo and nausea and vomiting usually are present. Neurological deterioration, manifesting as a decline in function, also may be present with posterior circulation aneurysms.

Unruptured Aneurysms

Although most patients with aneurysms are completely asymptomatic until rupture occurs, some aneurysms produce warning signs. However, these signs are frequently attributed to other causes and ignored. Occasionally, an aneurysm is found incidentally when the patient has imaging studies for another purpose. When an aneurysm becomes large enough to cause symptoms, the most frequent symptom appears to be localized headache and/or cranial nerve signs. The most common cranial nerve deficits are dilated pupil, decreased mobility of the eye, and ptosis (drooping of the eyelid), all due to pressure on cranial nerve III (oculomotor nerve). The aneurysm becomes a space-occupying lesion, causing symptoms that depend on the location and size of the aneurysm. Clinical manifestations of unruptured aneurysms of the posterior circulation are dizziness and balance difficulties. The symptoms are caused by the size of the aneurysm exhibiting mass effect.

Laboratory and Diagnostic Procedures

Initial diagnostic evaluation of a patient who presents with symptoms suggestive of SAH should always include a CT scan of the head with CT angiography (see the Diagnostic Tests box, p. 556). CT scan of the brain is a readily available test at most centers and is the most sensitive tool to detect blood in the brain parenchyma, ventricles, and subarachnoid space. The CT angiogram provides a detailed view of the arterial flow and can be invaluable in detection of cerebral aneurysms. Measurement of the volume and location of blood is important and provides critical information to predict the likelihood of complications such as hydrocephalus and cerebral vasospasm, a condition in which blood vessels spasm, leading to vasoconstriction. Based on the initial CT scan, the patient is assigned a grade based on the **Fisher grading scale** (Chart 22–4). This scale, which was designed to predict surgical outcomes, is used to communicate the amount of blood found on a CT scan. It also is used as a predictor for cerebral vasospasm. CT imaging and angiography have advanced to provide aneurysm diagnosis in less than 5 minutes. Lumbar puncture is less commonly performed but can be valuable in detection of radiographically occult SAH, one hidden from view on first imaging. The Diagnostic Tests box provides more information about tests used for determining whether an aneurysm or other cerebral vascular disorder exists.

CHART 22–4 Fisher Grading Scale

Group	Blood on CT Scan
1	No blood detected
2	Diffuse or vertical layers less than 1 mm thick
3	Localized clot and/or vertical layer greater than 1 mm thick
4	Intracerebral or intraventricular clot with diffuse or no SAH

Sources: Fisher, C., Kistler, J., and Davis, J. (1980). Relation of cerebral vasospasm to subarachnoid hemorrhage visualized by computerized tomographic scanning. *Neurosurgery, 6*(1): 1–9; Oman, J. S. (2011). Subarachnoid hemorrhage surgery. Medscape reference. Retrieved from http/emedicine.medscape.com/article/247090-overview.

Medical and Surgical Management

Care of the patient with a cerebral aneurysm depends on many factors. Key aneurysm characteristics that direct treatment include location, size, aneurysm shape, and evidence of rupture. The location of the aneurysm is important; aneurysms located outside the brain pose no risk of cerebral hemorrhage. The most important consideration is whether or not the aneurysm has ruptured. Patients with SAH due to ruptured aneurysm should be transported to facilities with the capabilities and training to appropriately treat patients with ruptured aneurysms.

The advent of endovascular procedures has presented nonsurgical options, such as coiling or stent-assisted coiling. The goal of any treatment is to prevent re-bleeding by eliminating blood flow to the aneurysm with either a surgical clip or a coil. **Coiling** consists of passing a thin plastic catheter into the femoral artery in the groin and navigating it through the vascular system into the brain arteries and into the aneurysm itself. Once the catheter is in the aneurysm, platinum coils are pushed into the aneurysm and released. These coils initiate a clotting or thrombotic reaction within the aneurysm that, if successful, will eliminate the aneurysm. In the case of broad-based aneurysms, a stent may be passed first into the parent artery to serve as a scaffold for the coils. Historically, the treatment of choice has been surgical intervention. Surgical clipping has been a standard in treating both ruptured and unruptured aneurysms (Figure 22–4◆). With clipping, the surgeon performs a craniotomy to attach a metal clip to the neck of the aneurysm where it connects to the blood vessel. This stops the hemorrhaging into the subarachnoid space and redirects the blood flow along its proper route. Functional outcomes have been optimized by advances in the technology of the clips themselves and by development of more efficient methods of approaching the aneurysm. Institutions that have a high volume of aneurysm clippings by experienced high volume surgeons are associated with more favorable patient outcomes.

With publication of the International Study Aneurysm Treatment (ISAT) study, which showed more favorable outcomes with endovascular coiling, most centers have reserved surgical treatment for complex aneurysms not amenable to coil-embolization techniques. These include aneurysms with complex anatomy in both the anterior and posterior circulation. Common anatomic reasons to avoid use of coil embolization include (1) the presence of an important vessel exiting the dome of the aneurysm, as occlusion would cause a stroke in the territory of the vessel, and (2) tortuous vessels that increase procedural risk of

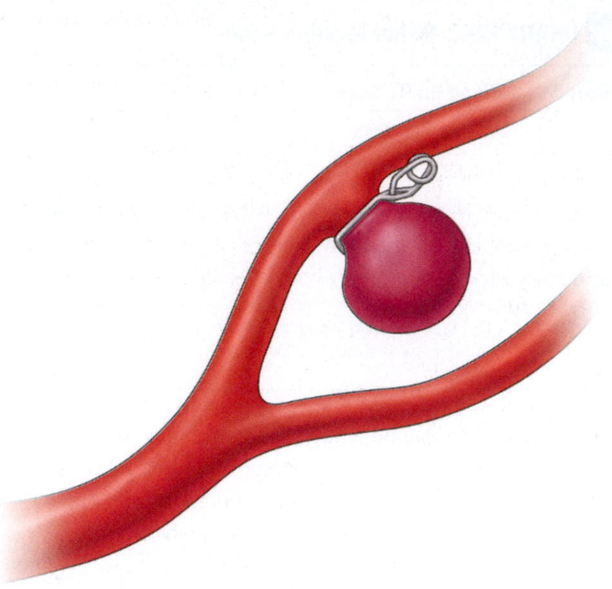

FIGURE 22–4 ◆ Aneurysm with clip applied.
Source: Modified with permission from Barrow Neurological Institute

vessel rupture or dissection. This challenge has led to the innovative use of localization aides that color the arterial circulation and techniques devised by cardiac surgeons to perform cardiac bypass surgeries. In a limited number of institutions, certain aneurysms are being clipped under cardiac standstill, a surgical procedure in which the patient's body is cooled and blood circulation is stopped. Large basilar artery aneurysms that are not amenable to coil embolization can be treated by surgeons skilled in this highly technical procedure.

Unruptured Aneurysms

In 1998, a group of researchers nationwide collaborated to study unruptured aneurysms to determine the most advantageous treatment plan. The International Study of Unruptured Intracranial Aneurysms (ISUIA) studied 1,449 patients with 1,937 unruptured aneurysms from 53 participating centers. In studies on clipping of unruptured aneurysms, the mortality rate was reported at 2.6% and the morbidity at 10.9%. The mortality rate for SAH was 66%. The high mortality rate associated with rupture of aneurysms suggests that preventive treatment for the obliteration of unruptured aneurysms is a good therapeutic option (Bedersen et al., 2009).

Ruptured Aneurysms

Patients with ruptured intracranial aneurysms should be treated as soon as possible after the hemorrhage. The purpose of treatment is to prevent re-bleeding. It also is important to aggressively manage medical complications associated with SAH, such as cerebral vasospasm, described in the following text. The choice of treatment—endovascular or surgical—is a source of ongoing debate. However, the choice of treatment should be based on a collaborative review of the angiographic features of the aneurysm by the neurosurgeon and neurointerventionalist.

The International Subarachnoid Aneurysm Trial (ISAT) Collaborative Group (2002) found that in patients with ruptured intracranial aneurysm for which both endovascular coiling and neurosurgical clipping are options, the outcome for survival free of disability at 1 year is significantly higher with endovascular coiling (Molyneux et al., 2002). Many years after the publication of this landmark trial, research continues to provide the most advanced devices for surgical treatment and coil embolization (NINDS, 2011b). These include coils that provide a stiffer structure for framing the inside of complex-shaped aneurysms, softer coils to fill the aneurysm, and stents to provide structural support across aneurysms lacking a neck. Bioactive coils have also been used to promote inflammation and reduce the complication of recanalization.

Complications of Subarachnoid Hemorrhage

The complications of aneurysmal SAH are varied and potentially life threatening. The major risks are re-bleeding, cerebral vasospasm, hyponatremia, seizures, and hydrocephalus.

Re-bleeding

The risk of re-bleeding is highest in the first 2 weeks after the initial bleed in unsecured aneurysms. Aneurysms re-bleed because the area of weakened vasculature is even weaker after it bleeds. Re-bleeding also is possible if risks, such as hypertension, remain. The increased force of the blood flow that exists with hypertension will continue to weaken the vessel, causing it to bleed again. The highest incidence of re-bleeding is in the first 24 to 48 hours. Re-bleeding is associated with a high mortality rate and remains the most worrisome complication until the aneurysm is secured (Dupont, Wijdicks, Lanzino, & Rabinstein, 2010). This underscores the importance of securing the aneurysm by either surgical clipping or coil embolization to prevent re-bleeding.

Cerebral Vasospasm

Cerebral vasospasm is a condition in which blood vessels spasm, leading to vasoconstriction. Cerebral vasospasm decreases CBF to the area supplied by the vessel, causing signs and symptoms of cerebral ischemia and leading to infarction if left untreated. Symptoms include: confusion, impaired level of consciousness, focal neurological impairment such as hemiplegia and aphasia, fever, and neck stiffness. This occurs in approximately 30% of all patients with SAH; the incidence is highest in patients with Fisher grade 3 aneurysm. The peak incidence of cerebral vasospasm is 3 to 14 days from the SAH, although it may occur up to 21 days after the bleed occurs.

Safety Alert *Patients with SAH are at significant risk for cerebral vasospasm. Monitor fluid intake and output carefully. IV fluid supplementation with a minimal goal of euvolemia (the presence of the proper amount of blood in the body) plays a critical role in the prevention of vasospasm. Check with the health care provider before discontinuing IV fluids. Monitor blood pressure at least hourly. Do not administer antihypertensive medications without parameters for administration.*

Diagnosis of cerebral vasospasm is made in several ways. The least invasive way is through transcranial Doppler studies (TCDs) (see the Diagnostic Tests box, p. 556). TCDs monitor the CBF using ultrasound to detect the velocity of flow in the major blood vessels of the brain. Using known normal values for CBF, high flow states can predict narrowing of a vessel. In contrast, cerebral angiography provides direct visualization of the artery to detect cerebral vasospasm as a narrowed vessel. CT angiography has become a valuable tool in detecting clinically symptomatic cerebral vasospasm. Digital subtraction cerebral angiograms are more invasive and take more time than TCDs, but are more definitive about the vessel itself and provide the access to treat the affected vessels intra-arterially. TCD studies can be performed at the bedside and may be ordered routinely on patients with SAH. The Diagnostic Tests box (p. 556) discusses these tests.

It is not uncommon for patients to demonstrate cerebral vasospasm by angiogram or TCD studies while being completely asymptomatic. Estimates indicate that up to 50% of patients with cerebral vasospasm are asymptomatic. Cerebral vasospasm can produce a focal ischemic zone that is characterized by a neurological decline distinguished by the specific territory supplied by the vessel in spasm. Patients may experience a decrease in the level of consciousness (LOC) and may exhibit motor weakness, aphasia, confusion, and/or cranial nerve deficits.

Treatment of cerebral vasospasm involves a medical triad of therapies referred to as triple-H therapy. **Triple-H therapy** consists of hypertension, hemodilution, and hypervolemia. The goal is to increase cerebral perfusion pressure and CBF, thereby reducing the risk for further neurological deficits.

Hypertension (the first H of triple-H therapy) is one form of therapy to treat cerebral vasospasm in the presence of a clipped or coiled aneurysm, as previously described. Hypertension can be therapeutic to augment CBF and reduce the chance of vasospasm. Systolic blood pressure should be kept at no less than 160 mmHg and may be kept as high as 180 to 200 mmHg in patients with cerebral vasospasm that does not respond to standard treatment. If necessary, hypertension may be induced with vasopressors, such as dopamine, phenylephrine, or dobutamine. Calcium channel blockers, such as nimodipine, have been shown to reduce ischemic neurological deficits after aneurysmal SAH (Tomassoni et al., 2008). It also has been shown to increase CBF. In many institutions, nimodipine is given routinely to patients with SAH. However, nimodipine has antihypertensive properties that might limit its effectiveness for some patients.

It also is common to use hypervolemia (the second H of triple-H therapy) as a method of maintaining blood pressure. Hypervolemia is achieved by administration of high volumes of isotonic fluids. This increases the central venous pressure and decreases the risk of vasospasm, although it may increase the risks of circulatory overload, pulmonary edema, and congestive heart failure. Patients must be in a monitored critical care unit, with a central venous catheter and a pulmonary artery catheter for hemodynamic monitoring (Chapter 31).

Hemodilution (the third H of triple-H therapy) increases CBF. The balance of viscosity and oxygen-carrying capability is maintained with a hematocrit of greater than 30% (Sheth et al., 2011). To maintain the hematocrit at this range, the infusion of volume expanders, such as albumin, may be used.

Cerebral vasospasm is a dangerous complication of SAH, often causing secondary neurological declines. Among patients with SAH, 13% die or have serious neurological impairments due to cerebral vasospasm (Zacharia et al., 2010). However, the treatment for cerebral vasospasm is not without risk. Patients with underlying pulmonary or heart disease are at risk for complications from triple-H therapy. Patients who develop neurologic changes associated with cerebral vasospasm may benefit from interventional treatment. Interventional treatment often involves direct angiography with intra-arterial injection of a calcium channel blocker into abnormal vessels to restore normal blood flow. Nurses play a critical role in the assessment and treatment of cerebral vasospasm. They must be aware of pulmonary compromise and congestive heart failure caused by catecholamine release and hypervolemic therapy in patients with preexisting pulmonary or heart conditions or those who are at risk due to age or other predisposing factors (Temes et al., 2010).

Hyponatremia

Hyponatremia is another common complication of SAH. Hyponatremia occurs in approximately one-third of all SAH cases (Dupont et al., 2010). Hyponatremia in SAH is most commonly caused by cerebral salt wasting. **Cerebral salt wasting,** a condition that causes excessive excretion of sodium, is thought to be centrally mediated by the brain due to injury or tumor. The primary symptoms include sodium levels less than 135 mg/dL with polydipsia (excessive urge to drink) and polyuria (excessive urination) in amounts up to 3 liters per day. Cerebral salt wasting can be distinguished from syndrome of inappropriate antidiuretic hormone (SIADH) because cerebral salt wasting results in hypovolemia. SIADH often produces normovolemia or hypervolemia because the body is saving water. Less commonly, patients with underlying pulmonary pathology can experience SIADH. The treatment for SIADH is fluid restriction, and the treatment for cerebral salt wasting is the addition of salt. This is an important clinical differentiation, because two of the risk factors for SAH are low volume and hyponatremia. Fluid restriction for patients with SAH can be catastrophic, contributing to increased cerebral vasospasm. Generally, the treatment for hyponatremia in SAH is hypertonic saline, with oral salt supplements, if possible. This is in addition to IV fluids, such as normal saline, administered at 100 to 150 mL/hour for the prevention of cerebral vasospasm. It is very important for the patient's serum sodium levels to be monitored frequently (e.g., every 6 hours if the patient is receiving hypertonic saline). It also is important for the patient's fluid intake and output to be carefully monitored. Hemodynamic monitoring also may be warranted. An important feature of hyponatremia in the presence of SAH is that it frequently accompanies cerebral vasospasm; thus, careful monitoring of this patient by the nurses is extremely important.

Safety Alert *Patients with SAH are at significant risk for hyponatremia. Monitor serum Na^+ levels at least daily. Levels at or below normal need to be reported to the health care provider. Standard treatment is the administration of salt, both as oral tablets and as IV hypertonic saline. Fluid restriction is absolutely contraindicated.*

The clinical picture of patients with hyponatremia usually is that of decreased LOC. This patient may become suddenly confused, restless, or lethargic. It is not uncommon for hyponatremia to become evident when the patient has a seizure. Patients with SAH should have sodium levels done at least daily, even if their levels are normal. Those with levels at baseline or slightly below should be treated to avoid worsening hyponatremia because these patients are very sensitive to cerebral vasospasm. The normal levels of serum sodium vary from hospital laboratories, and it is important to note the normal levels for any particular institution.

Seizures

Seizures also are not uncommon for patients with SAH. They can occur immediately after the bleed or may be delayed. The seizures may be generalized or focal, depending on the area involved. Treatment for seizures usually consists of phenytoin or levetiracetam (discussed in the Pharmacology box, p. 559) initially; other drugs may be added as needed. Prophylactic use of antiepileptic drugs is controversial.

Hydrocephalus

Hydrocephalus, an excessive accumulation of cerebral spinal fluid in the brain, is a common complication of SAH. As the blood products in the CSF break down, the high protein levels "clog" the absorption of CSF, causing communicating hydrocephalus. Symptoms of hydrocephalus include lethargy, confusion, and other focal neurological deficits. Hydrocephalus is diagnosed by a CT scan. Many patients have serial CT scans while hospitalized to monitor ventricle size. The treatment for hydrocephalus is placement of a shunt, usually a ventriculoperitoneal shunt. The ventriculoperitoneal shunt is a piece of small tubing that is placed inside the brain's ventricle and tunneled underneath the skin to the peritoneum. The peritoneum is a membrane that lines and protects the abdominal cavity and its contents (University of Maryland Medical Center, 2011). Hydrocephalus in SAH patients frequently occurs while the patient is still hospitalized, but it is not uncommon for delayed hydrocephalus to occur weeks after the initial bleed.

Nursing Management

Nursing management of the patient with a cerebral aneurysm follows guidelines of established stroke protocols (The Internet Stroke Center, 2010a). A cerebral aneurysm is a life-threatening condition wherein the patient may be asymptomatic initially if the aneurysm has not ruptured, or the patient may present with symptoms of a cerebral bleed. The diagnosis of cerebral aneurysm calls for nurses to act promptly and to take into account the major neurological deficits that the patient may be experiencing. Because these patients may be extremely ill with major neurological deficits, close observation of their neurological status is required. Monitoring the patient's status and helping to prevent complications to re-bleed and vasospasm are critical, as is helping the patient and family cope with the many problems associated with hospitalization.

Arteriovenous Malformation

Malformations of the cerebrovascular system are believed to be congenital anomalies that result from failure of the embryonic vasculature to develop properly (NINDS, 2011a). The two most common types of cerebrovascular malformations are arteriovenous malformations and cavernous malformations.

An **arteriovenous malformation (AVM)** is a tangled mass of abnormal blood vessels in which arterial blood flows directly into the venous system (Figure 22–5 ◆). AVMs contain blood vessels that are thin walled and do not have normal characteristics of blood vessels; therefore, bleeding is often the first symptom. AVMs may develop throughout the body; however, the focus in this chapter is on cerebral AVMs.

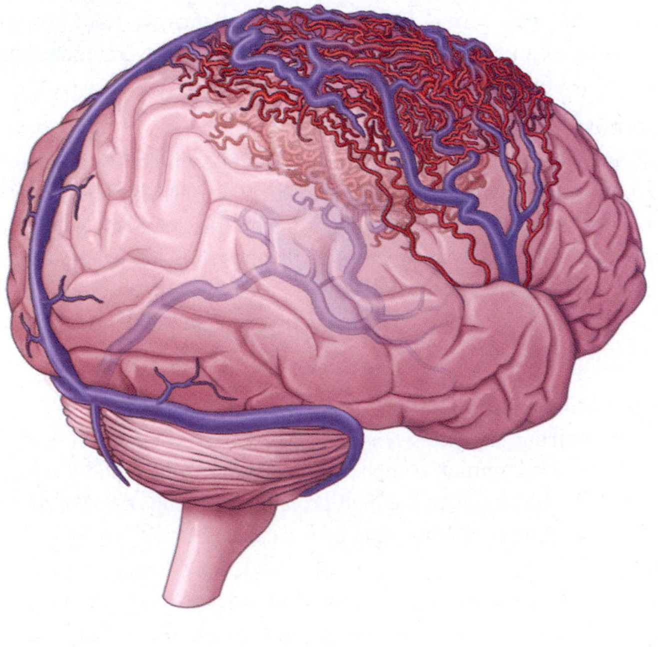

FIGURE 22–5 ◆ Arteriovenous malformation.

Source: Modified with permission from Barrow Neurological Institute

Epidemiology and Etiology of Cerebral Arteriovenous Malformations

AVMs account for approximately 8.6% of all SAH. The incidence is approximately 1 per 100,000 persons/year. There is a slight male prevalence, and the most common age at diagnosis is between 20 and 40 years old (NINDS, 2011a). About half of AVMs are diagnosed with hemorrhage as the presenting symptom. Since AVMs are congenital, there is a lifelong risk of hemorrhage (Sandalcioqlu et al., 2011).

Pathophysiology

An AVM is an abnormal direct connection between an artery and a vein without the benefit of a capillary bed to diffuse flow. The normal arterial function of delivery of oxygen is lost because the oxygenated blood is directly returned to the venous system with no nourishment of tissues. Since veins are not designed to accept high flow states, the veins dilate, resulting in a mass which displaces normal tissue as it grows. The presence of mass effect is possible, even in cases in which hemorrhage has not occurred. This means that there are symptoms related to a growing amount of substance (fluid or tissue) on the brain. A mass is formed that creates pressure on the brain. The largest concentration of abnormal vessels is located in the center of the AVM, referred to as the **nidus.** The nidus is composed of abnormal vessels that are a cross between veins and arteries. AVMs are supplied by one or more arteries and drained by one or more veins.

An AVM results in atypical shunting of arterial blood into the venous system (NINDS, 2011c). Elevated intravascular pressure predisposes the venous end to dilation, which increases the risk of rupture and hemorrhage of vessels. It also is possible for aneurysms to form on the artery that supplies the AVM. These aneurysms are prone to rupture due to high intravascular pressure. Approximately 6% to 7% of patients with AVMs have associated aneurysms (NINDS, 2011c). Neurological deterioration, such as new weakness, numbness, difficulty talking or understanding, or lapse in consciousness, may be rapid in the presence of hemorrhage. Diversion of arterial blood to the AVM may increase intravascular pressure, thus decreasing cerebral perfusion pressure. The brain tissue surrounding the AVM may become ischemic. Neurological deficits may progress slowly in the absence of hemorrhage. AVMs have three distinguishing characteristics: the size of the nidus, the eloquence of the surrounding tissue, and the presence/pattern of draining veins. The presence of aneurysms also is an important diagnostic factor. Nidus refers to the size of the AVM's focus. Eloquence refers to the location and to the "value" of identifiable neurological function. Eloquent areas are those in which speech, sensory and motor, and vision functions are located. The pattern of venous drainage refers to the characteristics of draining veins, whether they are superficial or located in deep subcortical tissue.

To assist in decision making regarding treatment of a lesion and to aid in consistency in referring to these lesions, a grading scale has been determined, and each AVM is given a grade based on a standardized scale. Spetzler and Martin (1986) devised a scale based on the degree of surgical difficulty in resecting these lesions. The **Spetzler-Martin AVM grading scale** rates AVMs by assigning points for size, eloquence, and the presence of draining veins (Chart 22–5). Lower-grade AVMs have a low morbidity and mortality rate with treatment; higher-grade AVMs have a high morbidity and mortality rate, and treatment is usually restricted to medical management and observation; thus, grades 4, 5, and 6 do not appear on the Spetzler-Martin grading scale (Lawton, Kim, McCulloch, Mikhak, & MPH Project, 2011).

CHART 22–5 Spetzler-Martin Grading Scale for Arteriovenous Malformations

Size of AVM*		Eloquence of Adjacent Brain†		Pattern of Venous Drainage‡	
Small (<3 cm)	1	Noneloquent	0	Superficial only	0
Medium (3–6 cm)	2	Eloquent	1	Deep component	1
Large (>6 cm)	3		. . .		. . .

*Measure the largest diameter of the nidus of the lesion on angiography.
†Eloquent areas include sensorimotor, language, visual, thalamus, hypothalamus, internal capsule, brainstem, cerebellar peduncles, and deep cerebellar nuclei.
‡The lesion is considered superficial only if all drainage is via the cortical drainage system.

Sources: Fisher, C., Kistler, J., & Davis, J. (1980). Relation of cerebral vasospasm to subarachnoid hemorrhage visualized by computerized tomographic scanning. *Neurosurgery, 6*(1): 1–9; Lawton, M. T., Kim, H., McCulloch, C. E., Mikhak, B., & MPH Project. (2011). A supplementary grading scale for selecting patients with brain arteriovenous malformations. *Neurosurgery, 66*(4), 702–713. Retrieved from http://www.ncbi.nlm.nih.gov/pmc/articles/PMC2847513/; Lindvall, P., Runnerstam, M., Birgander, R., & Koskinen, L. O. (2009). The Fisher grading correlated to outcome in patients with subarachnoid haemorrhage. *British Journal of Neurosurgery, 23*(2), 188–192.

Clinical Manifestations

Signs and symptoms of AVMs depend on several variables. The most important are size, location, and presence of hemorrhage. As the AVM grows, it can behave like a mass lesion, which is an abnormal growth of tissue resulting from uncontrolled, progressive multiplication of cells, causing pressure on other brain tissue. The symptoms exhibited by a patient with an unruptured AVM may be related to the location of the lesion and to the function of the brain it is displacing. This lesion is generally slow growing; neurological symptoms may progress slowly.

If the AVM has hemorrhaged, the symptoms may mimic hemorrhagic stroke with sudden onset of decreased LOC, weakness, numbness, or difficulty talking. For many patients with AVM rupture, severe neurological compromise, including coma or death, are the presenting symptoms. The severity of the neurological deficits depends on the size of hemorrhage and the eloquence of the brain affected. Because AVMs often affect cortical brain, seizures are common with AVM hemorrhage.

Diagnostic Procedures

Diagnosis of an AVM's presence, with or without hemorrhage, is usually done by CT scan or MRI. Once the diagnosis of AVM has been made, cerebral angiography is warranted to determine the involvement of cerebral vasculature, including the presence of associated aneurysms. (These tests are described in the Diagnostic Tests box, p. 556.)

Medical and Surgical Management

The treatment options for AVMs are surgical resection, endovascular embolization radiosurgery, or conservative treatment. Selection of the appropriate treatment is based on symptomatic control and presenting symptoms. The determination of a treatment plan for patients with cerebral AVMs is often influenced by the Spetzler-Martin grade given to the AVM.

Surgical Resection

Grades I and II have favorable results with surgical resection. Grade III may warrant surgical resection, depending on the individual analysis of the case. Grades IV and V usually call for other types of treatment, because surgical resection has high rates of morbidity and mortality even in the hands of the most experienced neurovascular surgeon.

Embolization

Higher-grade AVMs may benefit from endovascular treatment, such as embolization or coiling (p. 573). The use of specialized catheters has made navigation of the arterial system much safer and increased access to embolization for AVMs. In *embolization,* selected abnormal arteries, including aneurysms, may be obliterated by injecting glue into the vessel to seal it off or by placing a series of coils to block off an aneurysm or abnormal vessel.

The coiling of intra-AVM aneurysms with a Guglielmi detachable coil, such as those used in coiling of other intracerebral aneurysms, also has allowed some AVMs to be surgically resected that may otherwise not be amenable to surgical resection. The goal of embolization or coiling is to occlude aneurysms and other high-flow areas within the AVM. It is rarely used exclusively, since eliminating both arterial and venous flow is less likely with this technique. However, it is used commonly as adjunctive therapy before surgical resection or radiosurgery.

Radiosurgery

Gamma knife radiosurgery uses a beam of radiation given in a single session to obliterate an AVM. This treatment modality often is used to treat surgically inaccessible lesions or lesions that involve eloquent brain. It also is used to treat larger lesions in conjunction with other forms of treatment, usually surgical. Although gamma knife radiosurgery is delivered in a single session over a few hours, it takes 2 years or more for abnormal vascular tissue to be replaced with scar tissue (Mayo Clinic Staff, 2011). Over the 2-year period, the rate of hemorrhage remains unchanged, and patients can suffer symptoms associated with cerebral edema.

Conservative treatment usually is reserved for AVMs that are a higher grade (III through V) and are felt to be unsafe to treat. Patients with these AVMs should be monitored with serial magnetic resonance images (MRIs) and/or cerebral angiograms (see the Diagnostic Tests box, p. 556). Treatment consists of managing symptoms, such as headaches or seizures.

Weblink: Spetzler-Martin Grading Scale

Cavernous Malformations

Cavernous malformations also have been called cavernous angiomas, cavernous hemangiomas, capillary hemangiomas, and cavernomas (NINDS, 2011c). **Cavernous malformations** are composed of clusters of enlarged capillary channels, separated by dense fibrous tissue, with little to no intervening normal brain tissue. There are two types of cavernous malformations: sporadic and hereditary (or familial). Genetic considerations related to familial cavernous malformations are discussed in the Genetic Considerations box.

GENETIC CONSIDERATIONS
Related to Familial Cavernous Malformations

Genetics appears to play a part in the familial form of cavernous malformations. It has an autosomal dominant inheritance and is characterized by the presence of multiple lesions, often presenting with seizures (NINDS, 2011a). It appears to be more prevalent in Mexican American families (Labauge, Denier, Bergametti, & Tournier-Lasserve, 2007). Approximately 50% of documented cavernous malformations are believed to be familial (Smith & Scott, 2010). A gene contributing to cavernous malformations, both sporadic and hereditary, has been identified (Smith & Scott, 2010). It is important to ask the patient about any family history of cavernous malformations or family members with repeated unexplained intracranial hemorrhage.

Epidemiology and Etiology

Cavernous malformations are believed to affect approximately 0.5% of the population. They comprise approximately 5% to 10% of all cerebral vascular malformations (NINDS, 2011c). There is no gender bias, and they may be found in all age groups.

Pathophysiology

Cavernous malformations are clusters of enlarged capillary channels separated by dense fibrous tissue with little to no intervening brain tissue. These malformations increase in size as a result of recurrent bleeding and thrombosis. These lesions have a characteristic "grape-cluster" type of appearance (Figure 22–6◆). Gradual buildup of iron and other blood breakdown products occurs as a result of recurrent hemorrhages.

Clinical Manifestations

Clinical manifestations of cavernous malformations are dependent on several factors, including the location and size of the lesion and whether it has bled. A cavernous malformation may produce neurological symptoms because it is a space-occupying lesion. It is not uncommon for the patient to be unaware of the cavernous malformation until it bleeds, causing deficits based on its location. The most common presenting symptom of cavernous malformation is seizures. Other symptoms include headaches and/or focal neurological deficits, such as motor and/or sensory deficits or cranial nerve deficits. Repeated hemorrhages usually worsen the neurological deficits, especially if the lesion is in the brainstem (Duckworth, 2010). It is not uncommon for the patient to recover from neurological deficits, but rarely does the patient completely return to baseline.

Diagnostic Procedures

Because cavernous malformations are low-flow lesions, angiography is not diagnostic. Diagnosis is made via an MRI scan. A CT scan may be helpful to determine the presence of a lesion but will not identify the specific type of lesion. Furthermore, CT scans may be falsely negative in 30% to 50% of studies (see the Diagnostic Tests box, p. 556).

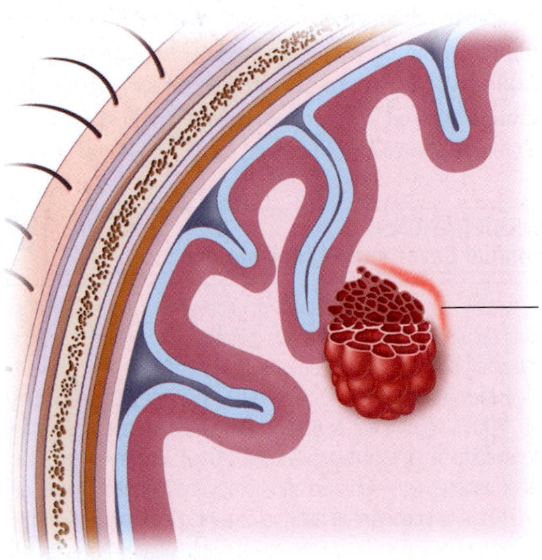

FIGURE 22–6 ◆ Cavernous malformation.

Medical and Surgical Management

Cavernous malformations usually are not diagnosed until they bleed, causing neurological deficits specific to the location of the lesion. These deficits may include weakness in the arms and legs as well as problems with vision, balance, memory, and attention. Treatment almost always is based on location, with surgical resection reserved for lesions that are in accessible areas. These lesions are curable if a complete resection is possible (Dukatz et al, 2011). Indications for surgery include refractory or worsening seizures, neurological deterioration due to repeated hemorrhages and/or mass effect, and neurological effects created by a mass that causes compression on the surrounding functional brain. Surgery may not be warranted if the lesion(s) are felt to be small and/or not threatening. These lesions are observed over time with serial MRIs.

As seizures are commonly seen with cavernous malformations, the use of antiepileptic drugs may be appropriate. (See the Pharmacology box, p. 559.)

Nursing Management

Nursing management of patients with a cerebral vascular abnormality focuses on observing trends in the neurologic exam to detect deterioration, preventing secondary injury by maintaining CBF and controlling intracranial pressure, and reinforcing strategies to maximize functional recovery. Patients who have experienced an ischemic or hemorrhagic stroke related to cerebrovascular malformations, aneurysms, AVMs, or cavernous malformations require careful attention to nursing care to limit further injury and expedite diagnostic tests to identify the abnormality and possible treatment options. Re-bleeding from vascular abnormalities can be fatal; this fact underscores the need for nurses to trend the patient's neurologic assessment and coordinate diagnostic tests to determine whether the abnormality would benefit from surgical or interventional treatment. Once the vascular abnormality has been secured by surgery or embolization, nursing care can be directed toward stabilization and rehabilitation.

Assessment

Initially, patients with hemorrhage related to cavernous malformations (cavernoma) present to the emergency department with symptoms of stroke of unknown type. It is imperative that nurses do complete and frequent neurological assessments aimed at detecting interval change and assessing the full extent of the deficits. Any change, regardless of how insignificant it may appear, should be reported. Initial evaluation should include assessment for the basic ABCs (airway, breathing, and circulation) followed by a comprehensive neurological examination that will serve as a baseline for future exams. This exam includes an evaluation of LOC, which is often captured in the Glasgow Coma Scale; a cognitive assessment; pupillary function exam; cranial nerve evaluation; a detailed motor and sensory assessment; and an evaluation of gait and balance as detailed in Chapter 20.

Repeated hemorrhage increases the risk of seizure and other neurological deficits. A thorough understanding of the patient's history will aid the nurse in developing a care plan for actual or potential patient problems. Ongoing assessment of any type of seizure activity is essential.

Nursing Diagnoses

Selection of appropriate nursing diagnoses is based on the examination, patient profile, and risk factors. These diagnoses include the *Risk for Altered Cerebral Tissue Perfusion* related to stroke. Additional common problems that should be included on the nursing care plan are related to the hemorrhage pattern, which may include the *Potential for Altered Nutrition* related to dysphagia, *Altered Mobility*, *Impaired Verbal*

Communication, Potential Aspiration and Aspiration Pneumonia, Fever related to lack of thermoregulation, *Altered Coping* related to threat and uncertainty of disease process, and *Knowledge Deficit* related to lack of understanding of the diagnosis, disease process, and secondary prevention strategies. The risk of future stroke is highest in patients who have just experienced a stroke or TIA (Lloyd-Jones et al., 2010). Identification of risk factors and appropriate medical management is essential for control of risk. In patients with cavernous malformations, appropriate nursing diagnoses may include *Knowledge Deficits* related to seizure, including seizure triggers, driving restrictions where applicable, and understanding of the need for compliance with antiepileptic agents or other newly instituted medical treatment.

NANDA-I © 2012.

Outcomes and Evaluation Parameters

Identification of expected outcomes from each nursing diagnosis provides the necessary structure to ensure preparation for a safe discharge to the community. The most worrisome problem is the potential for altered cerebral tissue perfusion, which can lead to further injury. An expected outcome would be stable neurological function as measured by the complete neurologic assessment. For patients with altered nutrition related to dysphagia, the expected outcome would be adequate dietary intake as measured by daily weight and percent of meals taken. If recurrent bleeding has produced weakness, altered mobility may be a problem. The expected outcome from nursing care would be optimal motor function and absence of injury related to impaired mobility. Seizures are a common problem faced by patients with recurrent cavernoma bleeding, placing the patient at risk for trauma related to large muscle control. Expected outcomes would include no injury to the patient during the observation period and an ability to verbalize activities and behaviors that reduce the chance of trauma related to seizure. Related to the patient/family's mental status, outcomes would be that the patient demonstrates understanding of his medical condition and expresses lack of fear or some degree of comfort with the diagnosis and plan of care. Outcomes also include the patient/family demonstrating preparation for rehabilitation and discharge to the home or community environment.

Planning and Interventions and Rationales

The plan of care includes ongoing assessment and treatment in order to identify any change in physiological findings, diagnostic tests, and exams. Efforts should be made to coordinate a rehabilitation plan to reduce disability. The nurse must perform routine neurologic assessments to detect any decline in neurologic function and prevent altered cerebral tissue perfusion. The nurse also should evaluate the patient and family's baseline understanding of cavernous malformations to identify knowledge deficits, form a plan for education, and coordinate efforts to ensure adequate rehabilitation and follow-up care.

The routine neurologic assessment is an important intervention for detection of altered cerebral tissue perfusion, seizure, and impaired verbal communication. Routine neurologic assessment generally includes a standardized measure of LOC exam such as the Glasgow Coma Scale, pupillary reaction, and cranial nerve, motor, and sensory function. Subtle changes such as new disorientation, a change in pupil size and reactivity, or new extremity drift may herald new problems such as worsening ischemia related to thrombosis, bleeding, or seizure. Changes that are apparent on examination may be sudden or may evolve over several hours; therefore, a comprehensive reproducible exam is needed that is trended over time. Nursing care of a patient with neurologic problems should also balance the need for any sedating medications with the importance of preserving the nurse's ability to conduct a neurologic assessment. Nursing interventions may also focus on integration of nursing care and rehabilitation services to optimize functional outcome in patients with altered mobility. A thorough understanding of normal brain anatomy and function can aid the nurse in predicting functional deficits based on the area of hemorrhage. Serial measurement of blood pressure and laboratory values help to establish modifiable stroke risk factors.

For patients who experience intracranial hemorrhage from an AV malformation, the management of blood pressure becomes a major nursing focus (UCSF, 2011). Blood pressure medications should be administered to keep blood pressure levels within the prescribed range. As patients transition to the outpatient setting, treatment goals are aimed at normotension and compliance with antihypertensive regimens, which should be emphasized to prevent re-bleeding or recurrent stroke.

Fever also is a possibility for patients with hemorrhage in thermoregulatory centers of the brain. In some cases, fever may be attributed to certain drugs, such as phenytoin. The presence of fever increases the brain's metabolic demands and may alter cerebral tissue perfusion; thus, every effort should be made to determine the cause of fever and to treat it aggressively. Interventions such as use of antipyretics (e.g., acetaminophen) and cooling devices are encouraged.

Patients with decreased LOC are prone to aspiration pneumonia because of their inability to protect the airway. However, this may not be readily apparent, predisposing the patient to experience "silent aspiration" with potentially serious consequences. Nursing interventions to prevent altered nutrition include coordination of a swallow evaluation by a speech therapist trained in dysphagia to determine whether a patient is able to swallow safely or whether alternative forms of nutrition are required, thus reducing the risk of inadvertent aspiration. If swallowing is preserved but impaired, strict aspiration precautions should be observed, including feeding with the head of the bed at a 90-degree angle, chin tuck positioning of the head, and repeated swallows after each bite with inspection of the oropharynx for pocketing of food.

Altered mobility can predispose patients to respiratory complications and deep vein thrombosis due to immobility. Appropriate nursing interventions are needed to prevent these potentially serious, even fatal, complications. These interventions include walking ambulatory patients a minimum of 150 feet per day and early mobilization for patients with weakness, combined with use of antiembolic stockings, alternating leg pressure devices, and use of anticoagulant medications where appropriate.

The nursing care of patients with cerebrovascular disorders is challenging but rewarding. Nursing care should address all affected body systems and reflect all actual and potential problems that were previously identified.

Health Promotion

Patients who have experienced an intracranial bleed from the rupture of vascular malformations and abnormalities need education from nurses and other members of the health care team on risk factors and methods of preventing a re-bleeding episode. It has been well documented that patient education and self-management are critical to the prevention of a re-bleeding occurrence (NINDS, 2011c).

Risk factors that should be discussed include high blood pressure, smoking, high alcohol intake, elevated cholesterol levels, diabetes, lack of exercise, a diet high in sodium and fat, and circulation problems. Instruction by the nurse on how to reduce or eliminate these risk factors is essential and may depend on lifestyle modifications by:

- Controlling one's blood pressure
- Quitting smoking

- Limiting alcohol intake
- Monitoring cholesterol levels
- Managing diabetes, if appropriate
- Developing an exercise program
- Eating foods low in sodium and fat
- Monitoring circulation problems with the help of the primary care provider (National Stroke Association, 2008).

Primary areas of patient instruction include knowledge of the disease process, modifiable risk factors, medications, functional impairments, dysphagia and nutrition, anticoagulation, and the emotional response of the patient/family to the diagnosis of stroke (National Stroke Association, 2008). These are discussed in the Patient Teaching & Discharge Priorities box. Additionally, patients should be instructed to find out whether they have atrial fibrillation (an irregular heartbeat, which allows blood to pool in the heart and may cause blood clots) (National Stroke Association, 2008). The Stroke Prevention Guidelines shown in the National Guidelines box on page 570 also are an excellent resource on risk factors and lifestyle modifications that can be used in patient education activities.

Health promotion may include helping the patients/families become involved in relevant community programs and services. The Stroke Prevention Guidelines shown in the National Guidelines box on page 570 also provide a strong educative tool for the public at large. A major preventative measure is community education as to what these cerebrovascular abnormalities are and what symptoms individuals should look for. Numerous community resources are available, including Internet education for the patient.

Collaborative Management

Patients who experience stroke—whether an ischemic stroke or an intracerebral hemorrhage due to a ruptured aneurysm, arteriovenous malformation, or a cavernous malformation—require a team of experienced professionals to manage the multisystem effects and to treat modifiable risk factors. Collaborative care, involving many disciplines, may be required to help each patient return to her optimum level of function. In order to meet desired patient outcomes, it is essential that this interdisciplinary team communicate openly with one another in developing and evaluating care of the patient and family (IOM [Institute of Medicine], 2010).

The patient with a cerebrovascular disorder usually experiences a complicated, multisystem disorder. These patients require the expertise of many health care professionals. Nursing care focused on detecting neurologic deterioration, preventing secondary complications, and ensuring the best functional recovery is a primary element of successful treatment.

Because the treatment goal for each patient is to optimize function, each team member plays a critical role to aid the patient in this endeavor. Once a patient has been admitted to the hospital with a diagnosis of a cerebral vascular disorder, the decision regarding treatment is made with the help of the appropriate specialists, usually neurologists, neurosurgeons, and/or endovascular surgeons.

During the patient's hospitalization, it is common to request the expertise of internal medicine or critical care health care providers to manage possible medical complications, such as respiratory failure, pneumonia, hypertension, electrolyte imbalances, and other preexisting conditions. After the initial treatment, the patient will require the entire team of nurses, specialists, and therapists to evaluate and assess for possible therapy needs. Patients with cerebral vascular disorders often benefit from physical therapy and occupational therapy to evaluate

COMPLEMENTARY & ALTERNATIVE THERAPIES Neurofeedback

Nancy Yilk

NEUROFEEDBACK IS TRAINING THE BRAIN to take advantage of the brain's own potential for neuroplasticity. Neurofeedback (NFB) has been used in the treatment of post-traumatic stress disorder, emotional and anxiety disorders, and depression, as well as the consequences of stroke and head trauma. It also has been used successfully in treatment of headaches, epilepsy, and chosen disturbances in cerebral palsy (Kubik & Przegl, 2010).

Using computer technology and electroencephalogram (EEG), it is now possible to monitor and "feedback" information to the brain about its activities. In a clinical setting, NFB begins with the placement of electrodes on the patient's head to measure her baseline brain waves. Placements are assessed for behavioral adaptation outcomes in the four following lobes: frontal lobe, affecting movement, speech, impulse control, emotional regulation, and short-term memory; parietal lobe, affecting social awareness, perception of touch, temperature, and pain; occipital lobe, affecting visual processing; and temporal lobe, affecting physiology stability, pattern recognition, auditory processing, and long-term memory

Determination is made as to the frequency to be used as "feedback" to either calm or activate the various lobes of the brain targeting clinical outcomes. In clinical studies, the use of reward tones heard by the patient is often utilized, while in clinical settings the use of video games that visually give reward clues are often preferred by clinicians and patients. The feedback to the patient and her participation begins the retraining of the brain, which moves it to a practiced way of neurological behavior. This is a skillful administration using modern technology that can, over time and repeated use, establish brain adaptation that offers measurable significance to patient cognitive health goals.

Surface ElectroMyoGraphy (SEMG) is a noninvasive technique of biofeedback for measuring muscle electrical activity that occurs during muscle contraction and relaxation cycles. To evaluate the efficacy of SMG's use in the treatment of stroke patients with chronic dysphagia, 11 consecutive patients with chronic dysphagia after stroke were analyzed. Patients were treated for dysphagia with SEMG as biofeedback, as an adjunct to normal exercises. All patients suffered from dysphagia after stroke. The average time after onset was 31.1 months. All patients had been previously treated by speech therapists without success. Functional swallowing was estimated using the Functional Oral Intake Scale (FOIS). At the start of the treatment, eight patients were tube dependent (FOIS $<$ or $=$ 4). Three patients were on an oral diet, but with restrictions (FOIS $>$ or $=$ 5). The patients were treated on average seven (7) times. The time between the first and last treatment session was on average 76.1 days (SD $+/-$ 44.0; range $=$ 29–168). Before treatment, the average FOIS was 2.6 (SD $+/-$ 2.3) and after treatment it was 5.6 (SD $+/-$ 1.6). The median scores improved from 1 to 6, showing a significant and clinically relevant improvement ($z = -2.820$: $p < 0.01$) in swallowing function. In six of the initial eight patients with percutaneous enteral gastrostomy tubes, the feeding tube could be removed after treatment. The use of SEMG as biofeedback in the treatment of chronic dysphagia after stroke could be an effective adjunct to standard therapy for swallowing disorders (Bogaardt, Grolman, & Fokkens, 2009).

Sources: Bogaardt, H. C., Grolman, W., & Fokkens, W. J. (2009, July). The use of biofeedback in the treatment of chronic dysphagia in stroke patients. *Folia Phoniatrica et Logopaedica, 61*(4), 200–205; Kubik, A., & Przegl, L. (2010). Neurofeedback and personal development, *67*(9), 716–720. Polish. PubMed PMID: 21387811.

and treat motor and functional deficits. It also is frequently beneficial for speech therapy to assess for cognitive deficits, some of which may not be readily apparent. Speech therapy also is of great benefit to assess and treat functional speech abnormalities, as well as swallow evaluations. Once the patient is medically stable, the need for further rehabilitation, frequently in an inpatient facility, may be addressed. See the Complementary & Alternative Therapies box for information on using neurofeedback for patient treatments.

Rehabilitation

Once a diagnosis has been made and treatment options have been explored and implemented, the promotion of optimum health centers on rehabilitation. Rehabilitation for patients with brain injury, whether it is a result of stroke, tumor, or trauma, is discussed in Chapter 21. The patient who has had a stroke as a result of a ruptured aneurysm, an intracerebral hemorrhage, or an ischemic infarction may have residual neurological deficits.

These deficits may affect cranial nerve, motor, sensory, or cognitive function. It is important that physical, occupational, and/or speech therapists be consulted and their recommendations initiated early in the patient's hospitalization. It also is important for nursing staff to be diligent in assessing the needs of stroke patients. The nurse is the first line in identifying and assessing deficits and in the education of the patient and family.

Several outcome measurement scales that are helpful in determining the type and degree of deficits are available. The scales also serve as a guide for how much nursing care and and professional assistance is required. One such scale from the National Institutes of Health (NIH) is shown in the National Guidelines box. Another, the Barthel Index (BI), is shown in Chart 22–6. The NIH scale is often used to quantify ischemic stroke severity and determine the need for thrombolytic therapy in patients who arrive at the hospital within 4.5 hours of stroke onset. A stroke scale score less than 6 indicates mild stroke from which the patient will likely recover without use of thrombolytic treatment. In contrast, patients with a stroke scale score more than 20 are unlikely to have a favorable outcome, have an increased risk of treatment-related complications with thrombolytics, and have an increased risk of death within the first 3 months following stroke. Both the NIH stroke scale and the BI provide valuable information about the severity of neurological deficits and allow the nurse to plan daily care and rehabilitation efforts. The BI is based on a rating scale that is completed by an observer. It covers personal toileting, feeding, mobility from bed to chair, transfers, bathing, walking, dressing, incontinence, and going upstairs. A total of 10 activities are scored, and the values are then added to give a total score ranging from 0 (totally dependent) to 100 (completely independent). Lower scores indicate greater dependency. Full credit is not given for an activity if the patient needs even minimal help or supervision (Stanford School of Medicine, 2011).

According to Sinoff and Ore (1997), total scoring on the BI can be interpreted as follows:

score of 80–100, independent
score of 60–79, needs minimal help with ADL
score of 40–59, partially dependent
score of 20–39, very dependent
score of < 20, totally dependent.

CHART 22–6 The Barthel Index

1. Feeding	10 = Independent; able to apply any necessary device; feeds in reasonable time
	5 = Needs help (i.e., for cutting food)
	0 = Inferior performance
2. Bathing	5 = Performs without assistance
	0 = Inferior performance
3. Personal grooming	5 = Washes face, combs hair, brushes teeth
	0 = Inferior performance
4. Dressing	10 = Independent; ties shoes, fastens fasteners, applies braces
	5 = Needs help but does at least half of the tasks within a reasonable time
	0 = Inferior performance
5. Bowel control	10 = No accidents
	5 = Occasional accidents
	0 = Inferior performance
6. Bladder control	10 = No accidents
	5 = Occasional accidents
	0 = Inferior performance
7. Toilet transfers	10 = Independent with toilet or bedpan
	5 = Needs help for balance, handling clothes, or toilet paper
	0 = Inferior performance
8. Chair/bed transfers	15 = Independent
	10 = Minimum assistance
	5 = Able to sit, but needs maximum assistance to transfer
	0 = Inferior performance
9. Ambulation	15 = Independent for 50 yards; may use assistive devices except for rolling walker
	10 = With help for 50 yards
	5 = Independent with wheelchair for 50 yards
	0 = Inferior performance
10. Stair climbing	10 = Independent
	5 = Needs help or supervision
	0 = Inferior performance

Sources: Adapted from Mahoney, G. K., & Barthel, D. (1965). Functional evaluation: The Barthel Index. *Maryland State Medical Journal, 15,* 56–61; Sinoff, G., & Ore, L. (1997). The Barthel Activities of Daily Living Index: Self-reporting versus actual performance in the old-old (>75 years). *Journal of the American Geriatrics Society, 45,* 832–836; Spinal Cord Injury Rehabilitation Evidence. (2010). The Barthel Index. Retrieved from http://www.scireproject.com/outcome-measures/barthel-index.

Weblink: The Barthel Index

NATIONAL GUIDELINES Outcome Grading Scales: The Modified National Institutes of Health Stroke Scale

Item	Name	Response
1A	Level of consciousness	0 = Alert 1 = Not alert, but arouses easily 2 = Not alert, obtunded 3 = Unresponsive
1B	Questions	0 = Answers both questions correctly 1 = Answers one correctly 2 = Answers neither correctly
1C	Commands	0 = Performs both tasks correctly 1 = Performs one task correctly 2 = Performs neither task correctly
2	Gaze	0 = Normal 1 = Partial gaze palsy 2 = Total gaze palsy
3	Visual fields	0 = No visual loss 1 = Partial hemianopsia 2 = Complete hemianopsia 3 = Bilateral hemianopsia
4	Facial palsy	0 = Normal 1 = Minor paralysis 2 = Partial paralysis 3 = Complete paralysis
5	Motor arm a. Left b. Right	0 = No drift 1 = Drift before 10 seconds 2 = Falls before 10 seconds 3 = No effort against gravity 4 = No movement
6	Motor leg a. Left b. Right	0 = No drift 1 = Drift before 5 seconds 2 = Falls before 5 seconds 3 = No effort against gravity 4 = No movement
7	Ataxia	0 = Absent 1 = One limb 2 = Two limbs
8	Sensory	0 = Normal 1 = Mild loss 2 = Severe loss
9	Language	0 = Normal 1 = Mild aphasia 2 = Severe aphasia 3 = Mute or global aphasia
10	Dysarthria	0 = Normal 1 = Mild 2 = Severe
11	Extinction	0 = Normal 1 = Mild 2 = Severe

It is in the patient's best interest for the nurse to facilitate a rehabilitation consult for either inpatient or outpatient therapy. It also is important to obtain information about the patient's home environment and the resources available at home. The availability of 24-hour supervision may make the difference between discharge to the home with family supervision and admission to a skilled nursing facility for therapies. Knowledge of a patient's occupation and level of responsibility on discharge also is important. It may be necessary for a patient to have neuropsychological testing prior to returning to the work environment.

It is important to teach the patient and family what to expect on discharge. Patients need to be told that there will be disappointments and setbacks as well as improvement. The nurse should encourage questions and give honest answers. It usually is helpful to evaluate the need for home health visits on discharge to support the family and patient and to answer any further questions or concerns they may have. It also is helpful to provide lists of resources for further support. The Patient Teaching & Discharge Priorities box lists some teaching suggestions for patients who have had strokes.

Gerontological Considerations

Age is an important factor in assessing stroke risk, as increased age is associated with a higher incidence of hypertension, atrial fibrillation, and hyperlipidemia. The prevalence of atrial fibrillation increases sharply with advanced age, predisposing older patients to cardioembolic stroke. More than 2.2 million people in the United States suffer from atrial fibrillation, with a median age of 75 (Schnabel, Sullivan, Levy, et al., 2009). Overall, atrial fibrillation accounts for more than 15% of all strokes in the United States, with one-quarter of the patients being over the age of 40 (Lip et al., 2010). The development of new anticoagulants that do not require laboratory monitoring and careful selection of patients may increase safety and use of anticoagulants in older patients (Maegdefessel, Spin, Azuma, & Tsao, 2010; Tulner et al., 2010). In the management of acute stroke, advanced age has been associated with poor outcome in large vessel occlusion. This may be related to declining neuroplasticity and aging body systems that are unable to tolerate additional insults. For these reasons, it is important to avoid secondary injury related to preventable complications. In the adult with advanced age, early mobilization is key to preventing DVT and potentially fatal pulmonary embolism. In addition, early control of hypertension is often not advised as this may increase the size of infarction and worsen neurologic injury (Cho, Oh et al., 2011).

Research

The nurse's role in the care of patients with cerebral vascular disorders presents exciting challenges for the future. Nurses have the responsibility and the challenge to explore opportunities to improve the care, and possibly the outcome, of patients experiencing cerebral vascular insult. There are many opportunities for nursing research, including the treatment of cerebral vasospasm, postoperative pain control, and the effect of nursing interventions on ICP (see the Research Opportunities box). Patients who have experienced stroke offer the nurse many opportunities to explore and research treatment modalities to improve patients' quality of life.

PATIENT TEACHING & DISCHARGE PRIORITIES for Stroke

Need	Teaching
Knowledge of disease process	Review the basic disease concepts with an emphasis on the signs and symptoms to recognize and key causes.
Disease prevention	Assess for the presence of modifiable risk factors for patients with cerebral vascular disease (lifestyle factors, exposure to tobacco smoke, smoking, hypertension, diabetes).
Medication teaching	Educate the patient and family regarding risk factors, and the appropriate interventions. Review the role of medication compliance in recurrent stroke prevention. Teach the medication, dose, route, side effects, and purpose of each medication. Assess for adequate primary care follow-up plan.
Knowledge of functional impairments and treatments to improve outcome	Encourage the patient/family to express understanding of the role of rehabilitation services including physical therapy, occupational therapy, and speech therapy. Explore available resources to avoid caregiver strain.
Dysphagia and nutrition	Educate the patient/family on swallowing techniques to prevent aspiration. Review the signs and symptoms of aspiration.
Anticoagulation	Assess the need for anticoagulation in cardioembolic stroke. Teach the signs and symptoms of deep vein thrombosis (DVT) and pulmonary emboli (PE). Reinforce the need for early mobilization to prevent DVT. Review the proper use of compression stockings and medications aimed at lowering risk of DVT. Assess risk factors concerning anticoagulation. Assess fall risk. Assess the family support and resources. Review the patient's dietary intake of vitamin K. Foods that are rich in vitamin K have been found to reverse warfarin, which can result in nontherapeutic INR levels and an increased risk of cardioembolic stroke. Common foods high in vitamin K include green leafy vegetables. Assess the patient's ability to comply with therapy and any needed laboratory tests.
Emotional adjustment related to loss of role	Assess the need for follow-up appointments for psychological therapy to manage emotional adjustment. Assess the patient for signs of depression or emotional lability. Teach the patient/family to report signs of depression to ensure identification and treatment.

RESEARCH OPPORTUNITIES Related to Cerebral Vascular Disorders

Research Area	Clinical Impact
Examine the various treatment modalities for hyponatremia, such as hypertonic saline, oral salt supplements, diet, or other medicines, and their impact on treating hyponatremia in the presence of subarachnoid hemorrhage.	Hyponatremia that occurs with subarachnoid hemorrhage is common. It is also associated with cerebral vasospasm. Evaluation of hyponatremia treatments may contribute to the successful treatment of cerebral vasospasm, thereby preventing further neurological compromise.
Examine the advantages of early ambulation and therapies in patients with stroke.	Earliest possible return to previous level of function.
Examine the impact of ruptured aneurysms in specific arterial locations and the potential for return to previous cognitive function. For example, study the rupture of anterior communicating aneurysms and the long-term cognitive impact.	Identifying cognitive risk factors associated with specific aneurysm locations may lead to early testing and intervention, resulting in improved cognitive function and quality of life.

CLINICAL PREPARATION READ DOCUMENT APPLY

READ: **History of Present Illness** >> Laboratory Study Results >> Critical Thinking Questions

Judith Myers is a 42-year-old woman admitted to the intensive care unit (ICU) in a major metropolitan hospital. She was brought into the emergency department (ED) by paramedics who responded to a frantic call from her husband. He reports that she has always been in perfect health until about 3 hours prior to admission. They were about to sit down to dinner with friends when she gasped, grabbed her forehead, and complained of the "worst headache of her life." She then lost consciousness and slid to the floor.

When paramedics arrived, they found Mrs. Myers moaning and localizing to pain with her left side. She had no obvious movement on her right side. Her respirations were labored, and her blood pressure was 192/110 mmHg. She was immediately transported to the hospital.

On arrival at the ED, her respirations became labored, and she required intubation to protect her airway. She was placed on a ventilator, and the health care provider requested a neurosurgical consult.

CLINICAL PREPARATION, *continued*

She was immediately sent for a CT scan of her head that revealed a subarachnoid hemorrhage (SAH). The neurosurgical resident immediately sent her for CT angiography, which revealed a ruptured aneurysm of the left middle cerebral artery. The surgeon and neurointerventional radiologist reviewed the angiographic findings and found that the aneurysm was suitable for coil embolization. The aneurysm neck was narrow, and the vasculature was nontortuous, suggesting the likelihood of success with coiling. The findings and recommended endovascular coil embolization were reviewed with Mrs. Myers's husband, and the radiologist obtained consent for treatment of the left middle cerebral artery aneurysm. While the endovascular team assembled, Mrs. Myers was admitted to the ICU.

READ: History of Present Illnesses >> **Physical Exam** >> Admitting Medical Records >> Laboratory Study Results

Medical–Surgical History

Obtained from husband
No known allergies
Medications: regular insulin, per sliding scale; occasional over-the-counter medications, such as acetaminophen
No past surgical history
No prior history of neurological illness

Social History

No tobacco use; rare social alcohol use; no history of recreational drug use
Married, with two daughters, ages 8 and 10
Works as a hotel manager

Physical Exam

Early-middle-aged woman appearing stated age, sedated, appears in no distress
Vital signs: temp 37.0°C rectally, heart rate 62, respiratory rate 12 (on intermittent mechanical ventilation), blood pressure 174/80
Cardiac: rhythm and rate regular, S_1S_2 heard, no abnormal murmurs, good capillary refill, pulses 2^+ all extremities, no pitting edema
Lungs: clear to auscultation bilaterally
Abdomen: soft, nontender; bowel sounds heard in all quadrants

Neurological Exam

GCS = E3 M4 VT1 = 8T (eyes open to speech only, withdraws her left side to pain, no verbal response, intubated)
Cranial nerves: CNII–CNXII intact bilaterally
Motor:
Left upper extremity: withdraws to pain
Left lower extremity: withdraws to pain
Right upper extremity: no response to pain
Right lower extremity: no response to pain
Sensory: unable to examine
Cerebellar: unable to examine

Imaging Studies

CT scan done in the ED reveals subarachnoid blood
Cerebral angiogram reveals the presence of a left middle cerebral aneurysm
Chest x-ray: no abnormal pathology
ECG: normal

Admitting Medical Orders

Admit to Neuroscience ICU
Diagnosis: subarachnoid hemorrhage; status postinsertion EVD
Condition: critical
Allergies: none known
Vital signs and neuro assessment q1h
Bed rest
NPO
NG tube to low intermittent suction
Foley catheter
Intake and output: q1h
Continuous ECG, arterial pressure, ICP monitoring
Keep EVD (external ventricular drain) at the level of the EAC (external auditory canal) open to drain for ICP > 20 until ICP is < 20; then resume monitoring
Call resident on call: any change in neurological status; any change in vital signs: HR < 60 or > 120; systolic blood pressure < 100 or > 140; RR < 12 or > 30; temperature > 38°C; O_2 saturation < 92%, ICP > 20; CPP < 70 or > 100; glucose < 70 or > 120 mg/dL
IV: NS with 20 mEq KCl @ 75 mL/hr
Ventilatory settings: FIO_2: 30%, TV: 500, IMV: 12
Consent for: craniotomy for coil embolization of left middle cerebral artery aneurysm by Dr. Johnson
Sequential compression stockings (SCDs) to lower extremities prior to surgery
Internal medicine consult for management of diabetes

Scheduled Medications

Sliding scale regular insulin, dosage to be determined by internist
Pepcid 20 mg IV bid
Nimotop 60 mg NG every 4 hours
Pravachol Hold

PRN Medications

Acetaminophen 650 mg rectal q4h prn fever
Morphine sulfate 2–6 mg IV q1h prn pain
Zofran 4 mg IV q8 prn nausea

Ordered Laboratory Studies

CBC, Chem 7 panel, PTT, PT, INR on admission and q a.m.
Accu-Chek q6h

Ordered Diagnostic Studies

Head CT scan in the morning postoperatively
Head CT scan stat prn if neuro signs change and notify health care provider
Transcranial Doppler study every other day

An external ventricular drain (EVD) is placed to monitor and assist clearance of blood products and to assist with controlling Mrs. Myers's ICP. Her opening pressure is 26, and her cerebrospinal fluid (CSF) is grossly bloody. A central line is placed to assist with hemodynamic monitoring. An arterial line is also being placed to assist with blood pressure monitoring. Laboratory tests, including coagulation studies done in the ED, are reviewed and are unremarkable. Mrs. Myers is sent to radiology for endovascular treatment.

Postoperatively, when Mrs. Myers returns to the ICU, she is still sedated but waking up. She opens her eyes and moves her left side purposefully. She does not move her right arm or leg. She remains intubated and ventilated with her EVD in place. A femoral sheath is in place from treatment. Pulses distal to the femoral sheath are intact.

Mrs. Myers is extubated on postop day 3. She is no longer sedated. Her neurological exam is as follows: GCS = E4 M6 V3. Her pupils are equal and reactive, and her gaze is conjugate. Her face shows some weakness on the right side. She follows commands by showing two fingers on the left side. She is unable to move her right arm or leg. Her speech consists of barely intelligible words. Her EVD is closed to drainage, and a follow-up CT scan the following morning shows no increase in ventricular size with the EVD closed, so it is removed.

Transcranial Doppler studies are being performed every other day to monitor blood flow in the affected arteries and to assess for cerebral vasospasm. Her laboratory values are stable, and her sodium level is 136 mEq/L. Medications include nimodipine 30 mg sublingual every 2 hours; Pepcid 20 mg orally bid; salt supplements, 2 grams three times a day with food; sliding scale insulin; and prn medications for pain, nausea, and fever. Her vital signs have been stable: afebrile, heart rate in the 70s, blood pressure 140/82–150/90, respirations stable at 16. She does not require supplemental oxygen. She is eating a pureed diet (due to impaired swallow reflex), and the nurses have been getting her out of bed to sit in a chair. Her IV is running at 100 mL/hr with a solution of NS.

She is transferred to general floor care on postop day 4. She has orders to increase her activity as tolerated and to attempt to eat solid foods. Her IV has been discontinued. Physical therapy and occupational therapy are ordered to assist with mobility and ambulation. Speech therapy is consulted to assist with the evaluation of her swallowing and to assist with her severe aphasia.

On postop day 5, the nurse notes that Mrs. Myers is slightly agitated. When she is questioned, the nurse notes that her speech has deteriorated to moans only. Her vital signs are unchanged with the exception of a blood pressure of 100/62 mm. The rest of her exam is unchanged. Laboratory values reveal a sodium level of 130 mg/L. The health care provider is called, and the patient is sent for a stat CT angiogram. The angiogram results show that Mrs. Myers has cerebral vasospasm of her left anterior and middle cerebral artery. She is placed on hypertonic saline for her hyponatremia. She is transferred back to the ICU, and her triple-H therapy is resumed.

READ: History of Present Illnesses >> **Laboratory Study Results** >> Critical Thinking Questions

Test	Day 1	Day 2	Day 3
Sodium	142 mEq/L	138 mEq/L	135 mEq/L
Potassium	3.8 mEq/L	3.5 mEq/L	3.6 mEq/L
Chloride	98 mEq/L	97 mEq/L	98 mEq/L
Carbon dioxide	22 mEq/L	22 mEq/L	23 mEq/L
Blood urea nitrogen (BUN)	22 mg/dL	21 mg/dL	22 mg/dL
Creatinine	1.2 mg/dL	1.2 mg/dL	1.2 mg/dL
Blood glucose	290 mg/dL	240 mg/dL	180 mg/dL
White blood cells	8,200 μL	8,100 μL	8,200 μL

Test	Day 1	Day 2	Day 3
Hemoglobin	12.3 g/dL	12.2 g/dL	12.4 g/dL
Hematocrit	35.4%	33%	34%
Platelets	210,000 μL	200,000 μL	205,000 μL
Protime (PT)	10.6 seconds	10.5 seconds	10.5 seconds
International Normalized Ratio (INR)	0.8 INR	0.8 INR	0.75 INR
Partial thromboplastin time (PTT)	33 seconds	34 seconds	32 seconds

Pearson Nursing Student Resources *Log on to* ***nursing.pearsonhighered.com*** *to download forms*

DOCUMENT:

>> Summary of Hospitalization
>> Pathophysiology Form
>> Laboratory Values
>> Laboratory Results Explanation

APPLY:

>> List of Potential Nursing Diagnoses
>> Concept Map
>> Critical Thinking Questions and Concept Map

APPLY: History of Present Illnesses >> Laboratory Study Results >> **Critical Thinking Questions**

1. What is the significance of Mrs. Myers complaining of "the worst headache of her life"?
2. What symptoms did Mrs. Myers experience that specified the location of the affected artery?
3. What symptoms of cerebral vasospasm did Mrs. Myers exhibit?
4. What interventions could be expected to treat cerebral vasospasm?

Answers to Critical Thinking Questions can be found in Appendix D in the Osborn Student Resources at nursing.pearsonhighered.com.

NCLEX® PRACTICE

1. The nurse is caring for a client with a diagnosis of ischemic stroke. Which of the following statements should the nurse include when discussing this patient's care with a student nurse assigned to the patient to enhance the student's understanding of the patient's diagnosis?

1. Ischemic strokes are hemorrhagic in nature.
2. The signs and symptoms of ischemic strokes resolve without permanent disability.
3. Ischemic strokes are commonly caused by atherosclerosis.
4. Patients experiencing ischemic strokes are usually younger.

2. The nurse is teaching a class in the community about stroke prevention and is planning to include information about the pathophysiology of a stroke. Which of the following would the nurse include as a process that can cause a stroke? (select all that apply)

1. Plaque formation that alters the internal diameter of a cerebral artery
2. Embolus that separates from a deep venous thrombosis in the left leg
3. Thrombus formation as a result of plaque formation
4. Lipohyalinosis, a vascular abnormality, caused by hypertension
5. Cardiac dysrhythmia such as atrial fibrillation

3. When describing the ischemic cascade to a group of students, the nurse educator uses which understanding when explaining the phenomenon?:

1. tissues that surround the necrotic area have themselves undergone anoxia.
2. ischemic cascade further extends the area of infarction.
3. this tissue may be reperfused, but its ability to function has been permanently impaired.
4. the penumbra of a stroke is the necrotic core.

4. The nurse is caring for a patient with cerebral vasospasm associated with subarachnoid hemorrhage who is being treated with triple-H therapy. The nurse must continuously assess for the complications by including?

1. Assessing renal output to detect the onset of cerebral salt wasting
2. Assessing lung and heart sounds to detect fluid overload
3. Detection of the nidus, which can warn of impending seizure onset
4. Monitoring for focal seizure onset, as this warns of a dire complication

5. The nurse is teaching the family of a patient with a ruptured cerebral aneurysm. When deciding about treatment options of endovascular coiling or neurosurgical clipping, the choice is based upon which of the following factors?

1. Endovascular coiling is associated with a longer length of hospital stay.
2. Neurosurgical clipping is associated with a higher survival and lower morbidity rate one year after the procedure.
3. Endovascular coiling is associated with improved outcomes with better potential that the patient may be able to return to their activities of normal living and work earlier than patients who had undergone neurosurgical clipping.
4. There is little difference in either treatment option other than the availability of an interventional neuroradiologist.

6. To assist a patient in reducing risk for stroke, the nurse may advise the patient to: (select all that apply)

1. keep blood pressure below 140/90.
2. investigate family history of stroke.
3. limit smoking to $<$ 1 pack per week.
4. limit alcohol intake.
5. engage in daily physical activity.

Answers to NCLEX Practice questions can be found in Appendix D in the Osborn Student Resources at nursing.pearsonhighered.com. Practice additional NCLEX questions online at the Student Resources site.

Pearson Nursing Student Resources Find additional review materials at: **nursing.pearsonhighered.com**

REFERENCES

Adams, M. P., & Koch, R. W. (2010). *Pharmacology connections to nursing practice.* Upper Saddle River, NJ: Pearson.

Adeoye, L., & Broderick, M. P. (2010). Advances in the management of intracerebral hemorrhage. Nature Publishing Group. Retrieved from http://www.medscape.org/viewarticle/729352_print

American Heart Association. (2009). *Heart disease and stroke statistics—2009 update.* Dallas, TX: Author.

Anderson, C. S., Huang, Y., Wang, J. G., Arima, H., Neal, B., Peng, B., et al. (2010). Intensive blood pressure reduction in acute cerebral haemorrhage trial (INTERACT): A randomised pilot trial. *The Lancet Neurology, 7*(5), 391–399. doi: 10.1016/S1474-4422(08)70069-3

Bederson, J. B., Connolly, E. S., Batjer, H. H., Dacey, R. G., Dion, J. E., Diringer, M. N., & Rosenwasser, R. H. (2009). Guidelines for the management of aneurysmal subarachnoid hemorrhage: A statement for healthcare professionals from a special writing group of the Stroke Council, American Heart Association. *Stroke, 40*(3), 994–1025. doi: 10.1161/strokeaha.108.191395

Bogaardt, H. C., Grolman, W., & Fokkens, W. J. (2009, July). The use of biofeedback in the treatment of chronic dysphagia in stroke patients. *Folia Phoniatrica et Logopaedica, 61*(4), 200–205.

Brain Aneurysm Resources. (2011). What is a brain aneurysm? American Society of Interventional and Therapeutic Neuroradiology. Retrieved from http://www.brainaneurysm.com/DisplayPage.aspx?pgID=MTA=

Broderick, J., Diringer, M., Hill, M., Brun, N., Mayer, S., Steiner, T., Skolnick, B., & Davis, S. (2007). Recombinant activated factor VII intracerebral hemorrhage trial investigators. Determinants of intracerebral hemorrhage growth: An exploratory analysis. *Stroke, 38*, 1072–1075.

Carwile, E., Wagner, A. K., Crago, E., & Alexander, S. A. (2009, February). Estrogen and stroke: A review of the current literature. *Journal of Neuroscience Nursing, 41*(1), 18–25; quiz 26-7.

Cho, H., Lee, J., Kim, Y., Moon, Y., Ko, S., & Kim, H. (2011). Comprehensive evaluation of coronary artery disease and aortic atherosclerosis in acute ischemic stroke patients: Usefulness based on Framingham risk score and stroke subtype. *Cerebrovascular Diseases, 31*, 592–600. doi: 10.1159/000326075

Cho, S. Y., Oh, C. W., Bae, H. J., Han, M., Park, H., & Seung-Bang, J. (2011). The prognostic factors that influence long-term survival in acute large cerebral infarction. *Journal of Korean Neurosurgical Society, 49*(2), 92–96.

Cohen, J., Itshayek, E., Moskovici, S., Gomori, J., Fraifeld, S., Eichel, R. & Leker, R. (2011, March). State-of-the-art reperfusion strategies for acute ischemic stroke. *Journal of Clinical Neuroscience, 18*(3), 319–323. Epub 2011 Jan 21.

Cruz-Flores, S., (2011). Ischemic stroke in emergency medicine treatment & management. Retrieved from http://emedicine.medscaape.com/article/1916852-treatment

Darves, B. (2011). Are you OK taking care of this patient? Today's Hospitalist.com. Retrieved from http://www.todayshospitalist.com/index.php?b=articles_read&cnt=930

Din-Dzietham, R., Liu, Y., Bielo, M., & Shamsa, F. (2007). High blood pressure trends in children and adolescents in national surveys, 1963 to 2002. *Circulation, 116*(13), 1488–1496.

Drugs.com. (2009). Torodol (ketorolac). Retrieved from http://www.drugs.com/toradol.html

Drugs.com. (2011). Pradaxa. Retrieved from http://www.drugs.com/pradaxa.html

Duckworth, E. A. (2010). Modern management of brainstem cavernous malformations. *Neurologic Clinics, 28*(4), 887–898.

Dukatz, T., Sarnhein, J., Sitter, H., Bozinov, O., Benes, L., & Sure, U. (2011, April 8). Quality of life following brainstem cavernoma in 71 patients. *Neurosurgery, 69*(3), 689–695.

Dupont, S. A., Wijdicks, E. F., Lanzino, G., & Rabinstein, A. (2010, November). Aneurysmal subarachnoid hemorrhage: An overview for the practicing neurologist. Seminars in Neurology, *30*(5), 545–554. Epub 2011 Jan 4.

Dupont, S. A., Wijdicks, E. F., Manno, E. M., Lanzino, G., & Rabinstein, A. A. (2009). Prediction of angiographic cerebral vasospasm after aneurysmal subarachnoid hemorrhage: Value of the hijdra sum scoring system. *Neurocritical Care, 11*(2), 172–176. Epub 2009 Jul 30.

Fisher, C., Kistler, J., & Davis, J. (1980). Relation of cerebral vasospasm to subarachnoid hemorrhage visualized by computerized tomographic scanning. *Neurosurgery, 6*(1), 1–9.

Gloviczki, P., et al. (2009, June). Vascular malformations: An update. *Perspectives in Vascular Surgery and Endovascular Surgery, 21*(2), 133–144.

Goldstein, L. B., Bushnell, C. D., Adams, R. J., Appel, L. J., Braun, L. T., Seemant, C., et al. (2010, December 6). Guidelines for the primary prevention of stroke. A guideline for healthcare professionals from the American Heart Association/American Stroke Association. *Stroke.* doi:10.1161/STR.0b013e3181fcb238

Hacke, W., Kaste, M., Bluhmki, E., Brozman, M., Dávalos, T., Guidetti, D., et al. (2008). Thrombolysis with Alteplase 3 to 4.5 hours after ischemic stroke. *New England Journal of Medicine, 359*(13), 1317–1329.

Hashimoto, Y. (2011). Smoking and stroke. *Brain Nerve, 63*(5), 483–490.

Inagawa, T. (2009). Incidence and risk factors for multiple intracranial saccular aneurysms in patients with subarachnoid hemorrhage in Izumo City, Japan. *Acta Neurochirurgica, 151*(12), 1623–1630. Epub 2009 Aug 11.

International Subarachnoid Aneurysm Trial Collaborative Group. (2002). International Subarachnoid Aneurysm Trial (ISAT) of neurosurgical clipping versus endovascular coiling in 2143 patients with ruptured intracranial aneurysms: A randomized trial. *Lancet, 360,* 1267–1274.

IOM (Institute of Medicine). (2010). *The future of nursing: Leading change, advancing health.* Washington, DC: The Academic Press.

Jackson, S. (2009). Today's big headlines in stroke care. Today's Hospitalist. Retrieved from http://www.todayshospitalist.com/index.php?b=articles_read&cnt=778

Jeffrey, S., & Nighiem, H. T. (2010, August 4). New AHA/ASA guidelines on management of intracerebral hemorrhage. Medscape reference. Retrieved from http://www.medscape.org/viewarticle/726269

Kallmunzer, B., & Kollmar, R. (2011). Temperature management in stroke—an unsolved, but important topic. *Cerebrovascular Diseases, 31*(6), 532–543. doi: 000324621 [pii]

Kee, J. L. (2010). *Laboratory and diagnostic test with nursing implications* (8th ed.). Upper Saddle River, NJ: Pearson.

Kohrmann, M., & Schwab, S. (2009). Hemicraniectomy for malignant middle cerebral artery infarction. *Current Opinion in Critical Care, 15*(2), 125–130. doi: 10.1097/MCC.0b013e328321826

Kubik, A., & Przegl, L. (2010). Neurofeedback and personal development. *Przegl Lek, 67*(9), 716–720.

Labauge, P., Denier, C., Bergametti, F., & Tournier-Lasserve, E. (2007). eneticcavernous iomas. *The Lancet Neurology, 6*(3), 237–244. doi: 10.1016/s1474-4422(07)70053-4

Lawton, M. T., Kim, H., McCulloch, C. E., Mikhak, B., & MPH Project. (2011). A supplementary grading scale for selecting patients with brain arteriovenous malformations. *Neurosurgery, 66*(4), 702–713. Retrieved from http://www.ncbi.nlm.nih.gov/pmc/articles/PMC2847513/

Liebeskind, D. S. (2010). Reperfusion for acute ischemic stroke: Arterial revascularization and collateral therapeutics. *Current Opinion in Neurology, 23*(1), 36–45. doi: 10.1097/WCO.0b013e328334da32

Liebeskind, D. S. (2011). Intracranial hemorrhage. *Medscape Reference.* Retrieved from http://emedicine.medscape.com/article/1163977-overview

Liebeskind, D. S. (2011). Hemorrhagic stroke in emergency medicine. Retrieved from http://emedicine.medscape.com/article/1916662-overview

Liebeskind, D. S., & Lutsep, H. (2010). Epidural hematoma. Retrieved from http://emedicine.medscape.com/article/1137065-overview

Lindvall, P., Runnerstam, M., Birgander, R., & Koskinen, L. O. (2009). The Fisher grading correlated to outcome in patients with subarachnoid haemorrhage. *British Journal of Neurosurgery, 23*(2), 188–192.

Lip, G. Y., Nieuwlaat, R., Pisters, R., Land, D. A., & Crijns, H. (2010). Refining clinical risk stratification for predicting stroke and thromboembolism in atrial fibrillation using a novel risk factor-based approach: The euro heart survey on atrial fibrillation. *Chest, 137*(2), 263–272.

Lloyd-Jones, D. et al. (2010). Heart disease and stroke statistics—2010 update: a report from the American Heart Association. Retrieved from http://www.ncbi.nlm.nih.gov/pubmed/20019324

Maegdefessel, L., Spin, J. M., Azuma, J., & Tsao, P. S. (2010). New options with dabigatran etexilate in anticoagulant therapy. *Vascular Health and Risk Management, 6,* 339–349. Dove Medical Press. Retrieved from http://www.pubmedcentral.nih.gov/articlerender.fcgi?artid=2879296&tool=pmcentrez&rendertype=abstract

Mahoney, G. K., & Barthel, D. (1965). Functional evaluation: The Barthel Index. *Maryland State Medical Journal, 15,* 56–61.

Mann, D. L. (2011). The emerging role of innate immunity in the heart and vascular system: For whom the cell tolls. *Circulation Research, 108*(9), 1133–1145.

Martnez-Sanchez, P., Fuentes, B., Fernndez-Domnguez, J., Ortega-Casarrubios, Mde. L., Aguilar-Amar, M. J., Abenza-Abildua, M. J., et al. (2011). Young women have poorer outcomes than men after stroke. *Cerebrovascular Diseases, 31*(5), 455–463.

Maud, A., Lakshminarayan, F. M., Suri, K., Vazquez, G., Lanzino, G., & Qureshi, A. (2009, May 11). Cost-effectiveness analysis of endovascular versus neurosurgical treatment for ruptured intracranial aneurysms in the United States. *Journal of Neurosurgery, 110*(5), 880–886. doi: 10.3171/2008.8.JNS0858

Mayer, S. A., & Schwab, S. (2008). Advances in stroke 2008. *Stroke.* doi: 10.1161/STROLEANA.108.544619

Meagher, R., & Lutsep, H. (2009). Subdural hematoma. Medscape reference. Retrieved from http://emedicine.medscape.com/article/1137207.

MedlinePlus. (2010). Brain herniation. Retrieved from http://www.nlm.nih/gov/medlineplus/ency/article/001421.htm

Merwick, Á., & Kelly, P. (2011, February). Transient ischaemic attack clinics and management of transient ischaemic attacks. *Current Opinion in Neurology, 24*(1), 50–58. doi: 10.1097/WCO.0b013e3283424c6b

Miller, E. L., Murray, L., Richards, L., Zorowitz, R. D., Bakas, T., Clark, P., et al. (2010). Comprehensive overview of nursing and interdisciplinary rehabilitation care of the stroke patient: A scientific statement from the American Heart Association. *Stroke, 41*(10), 2402–2448. doi: 10.1161/STR.0b013e3181e7512b

Miranda, L. B., Braxton, E., Hobbs, J., & Quigly, M. R. (2011). Chronic subdural hematoma in the elderly: Not a benign disease. *Journal of Neurosurgery, 114*(1), 72–76.

Molyneux, A., Kerr, R., Stratton, I., Sandercock, P., Clarke, M., Shrimpton, J., et al. (2002). International Subarachnoid Aneurysm Trial (ISAT) of neurosurgical clipping versus endovascular coiling in 2143 patients with ruptured intracranial aneurysms: A randomised trial. *Lancet, 360*(9342), 1267–1274.

Munot, P., Crow, Y. J., & Ganesan, V. (2011). Paediatric stroke: Genetic insights into disease mechanisms and treatment targets. *The Lancet Neurology, 10*(3), 264–274. doi: 10.1016/s1474-4422(10)70327-6

National Heart Lung and Blood Institute. (2011). What is a stroke? *People Science Health.* Retrieved from http://www.nhlbi.nih.gov/health/health-topics/topics/stroke/

National Institute of Neurological Disorders and Stroke (NINDS). (2011a). Arteriovenous malformations and other vascular lesions of the central nervous system fact sheet. Retrieved from http://www.ninds.nih.gov/disorders/avms/detail_avms.htm

National Institute of Neurological Disorders and Stroke (NINDS). (2011b). Hydrocephalus fact sheet. Retrieved from http://www.ninds.nig.gov/disorders/hydrocephalus/detail_hydrocephalus.htm

National Institute of Neurological Disorders and Stroke (NINDS). (2011c). NINDS arteriovenous malformation and other vascular disorders information page. Retrieved from http://www.ninds.nih.gov/disorders/avms/detail_avms.htm

National Institute of Neurological Disorders and Stroke (NINDS). (2011d). Stroke: Hope through research. Retrieved from http://www.ninds.nih.gov/disorders/stroke/detail_stroke.htm

National Institute of Neurological Disorders and Stroke t-PA Study Group. (1995). Tissue plasminogen activator for acute ischemic stroke. *New England Journal of Medicine, 333,* 1581–1587.

Nguyen, T. N., Babikian, V. L., Romero, R., Pikulam, A., Kase, C. S., Jovin, T. G., & Norbash, A. M. (2011). Intra-arterial treatment methods in acute stroke. *Frontiers in Endovascular and Interventional Neurology, 2,* 9. doi: 10.3389/fneur.2011.00009

Nogueira, R. G., Liebeskind, D. S., Sung, G., Duckwiler, G., Smith, W. S., MERCI, O. B. et al. (2009). Predictors of good clinical outcomes, mortality, and successful revascularization in patients with acute ischemic stroke undergoing thrombectomy: Pooled analysis of the mechanical embolus removal in cerebral ischemia (MERCI) and multi MERCI trials. *Stroke, 40*(12), 3777–3783. doi: 10.1161/strokeaha.109.561431

North American Symptomatic Carotid Endarterectomy Trial Collaborators. (1991). Beneficial effect of carotid endarterectomy in symptomatic patients with high-grade stenosis. *New England Journal of Medicine, 325*(7), 445–453.

Ogata, J., Yamanishi, H., & Ishibashi-Ueda, H. (2011). Review: Role of cerebral vessels in ischaemic injury of the brain. *Neuropathology and Applied Neurobiology, 37,* 40–55. doi: 10.1111/j.1365-2990.2010. cc. 01141.x

Oman, J. A. (2011). Subarachnoid hemorrhage surgery. Retrieved from http://emedicine.medscape.com/article/247090-overview

Pandya, R. S., Mao, L., Zhou, H., Zhou, S., Zeng, J., Popp, A. J., & Wang, X. (2011, April 27). Central nervous system agents for ischemic stroke: Neuroprotection mechanisms. *Central Nervous System Agents in Medicinal Chemistry, 11*(2), 81–07.

Pinto, A., Di Raimondo, D., Tuttolomono, A., Disciacco, R., Arnao, V., La Placa, S., et al. (2009). *Antiplatelet treatment in acute stroke treatment, 9*(14), 1298–1316.

Porras, J. S., & Poussa, K. (2008). Natural history of unruptured intracranial aneurysms: Probability of and risk factors for aneurysm rupture. *Journal of Neurosurgery, 108*(5), 1052–1080.

Ross, M., & Nahab, F. (2009, February). Management of transient ischemia attacks in the twenty-first century. *Emergency Medicine Clinics of North America, 27*(1), 51–69, viii.

Ruigrok, Y., & Rinkel, G. (2008, February 7). Genetics of aneurysm. *Stroke, 39,* 1049–1055. doi: 10.1161/STROKEAHA.107.497305

Rymer, M. (2011). Hemorrhagic stroke: Intracerebral hemorrhage. *Missouri Medicine, 108*(1), 50–54.

Sandalcioglu, I. E., Wanke, I., Zappala, V., Forsting, M., & Sure, U. (2011, March). The management of arteriovenous malformations. *Journal of Neurosurgical Sciences, 55*(1), 57–69.

Scaletta, T., & Kulkarni, R. (2011). Emergent management of acute subdural hematoma. Retrieved from http://emedicine.medscape.com/article/828005-overview

Schirmer, S. H., Baumhäkel, M., Neuberger, H.-R., Hohnloser, S. H., van Gelder, I. C., Lip, G. Y. H., & Böhm, M. (2010). Novel anticoagulants for stroke prevention in atrial fibrillation: Current clinical evidence and future developments. *Journal of the American College of Cardiology, 56*(25), 2067–2076. doi: 10.1016/j.jacc.2010.09.017

Schnabel, R. B., Sullivan, L. M., Levy, D., Pencina, M. J., Massaro, J. M., D'Agostino, R. B., & et al. (2009). Development of a risk score for atrial fibrillation (Framingham Heart Study): A community-based cohort study. *Lancet, 373*(9665), 739–745.

Schneck, M. J., & Origitano, T. C. (2006). Hemicraniectomy and durotomy for malignant middle cerebral artery infarction. *Neurologic Clinics, 24*(4), 715–727. doi: S0733-19(06)00069-7 [pii]10.1016/j.ncl.2006.06.011

Sheth, K. N., Gilson, A. J., Chang, Y., Kumar, M. A., Rahman, R. M., Rost, N. S., et al. (2011, February 8). Packed red cell transfusion and decreased mortality in intracerebral hemorrhage. *Neurosurgery.* [Epub ahead of print]

Sinoff, G., & Ore, L. (1997). The Barthel Activities of Daily Living Index: Self-reporting versus actual performance in the old-old (>75 years). *Journal of the American Geriatrics Society, 45*, 832–836.

Smith, E. R., & Scott, R. M. (2010). Cavernous malformations. *Neurosurgery Clinics of North America, 21*(3), 483–490.

Spetzler, R. F., & Martin, N. A. (1986). A grading system for arteriovenous malformations. *Journal of Neurosurgery, 65*, 476–483.

Spinal cord injury rehabilitation evidence. (2010). The Barthel Index. Retrieved from http://www.scireproject.com/outcome-measures/barthel-index

Stanford School of Medicine. (2008). Stroke prevention. Retrieved from http://strokecenter.stanford.edu/guide/prevention.html

Stanford School of Medicine. (2011). Barthel Index. Retrieved from http://strokecenter.stanford edu/scales/barthel.html

Staykov, D., & Gupta, R. (2011). Hemicraniectomy in malignant middle cerebral artery infarction. *Stroke, 42*(2), 513–516. doi: STROKEAHA.110.605642 [pii]

Temes, E., Tessitore, E. J., Schmidt, J., Naidech, A., Fernandez, A., Ostapkovich, N., et al. (2010, December). Left ventricular dysfunction and cerebral infarction from vasospasm after subarachnoid hemorrhage. *Neurocritical Care, 13*(3), 359–365.

The Internet Stroke Center. (2010a). About stroke. Retrieved from http://www.strokecenter.org/patients/ich.htm

The Internet Stroke Center. (2010b). Stroke trials INTERACT 2. Retrieved from http://www.strokecenter.org/trials/TrialDetail.aspx?tid+751

Tomassoni, D., Lanari, A., Silvestrelli, G.,Traini, E., & Amenta, F. (2008). Nimodipine and its use in cerebrovascular disease: Evidence from recent preclinical and controlled clinical studies. *Clinical and Experimental Hypertension, 30*(8), 744–766.

Tulner, L. R., Van Campen, J. P. C. M., Kuper, I., Gijsen, G., Koks, C., Mac Gillavry, M. R., & Brandjes, D. P. M. (2010). Reasons for undertreatment with oral anticoagulants in frail geriatric outpatients with atrial fibrillation: A prospective, descriptive study. *Drugs & Aging, 27*(1), 39–50. doi: 10.2165/11319540-000000000-00000000

UCSF Center for Cerebrovascular Research. (2011). What is an arteriovenous malformation (AVM)? American Stroke Association. Retrieved from http://avm.ucsf.edu/patient_info/WhatIsAnAVM/

UCSF Medical Center. (2011). Carotid artery disease. Retrieved from http://www.ucsfhealth.org/conditions/carotid_artery_disease/

University of Maryland Medical Center. (2011). Ventriculoperitoneal shunting–overview. Retrieved from http://www.umm.edu/ency/article/003019.htm

Wardlaw, J. M. (2008). What is a lacune? *Stroke, 39*,(11), 2921–2922. Retrieved from http://stroke.ahajournals.org/content/39/11/2921.full

Wilkinson, J. M., & Ahearn, N. R. (2009). *Prentice Hall Nursing Diagnosis Handbook* (9th ed.). Upper Saddle River, NJ: Prentice Hall.

Zacharia, B. E., Hickman, Z. L., Grobelny, B. T., DeRosa, P., Kotchetkov, I., Ducruet A. F., & Connolly, E. S. Jr. (2010, April). Epidemiology of aneurysmal subarachnoid hemorrhage. *Neurosurgery Clinics of North America, 21*(2), 221–233.

Zian, Y., Holloway, R. G., Chan, P. S., Noyes, K., Shah, M. N., Ting, H. H., et al. (2011). Association between stroke center hospitalization for acute ischemic stroke and mortality. *Journal of the American Medical Association, 305*(4), 373–380. Retrieved from http://www.ncbi.nlm.nih.gov/pubmed/21266684

Caring for the Patient with Chronic and Degenerative Neurological Disorders

23 CHAPTER

Joyce Colobong
Annita Watson

Outcome-Based Learning Objectives

After studying this chapter, the learner will be able to:

1. Differentiate among Alzheimer's disease, Parkinson's disease, amyotrophic lateral sclerosis, Huntington's disease, multiple sclerosis, and myasthenia gravis by describing the etiology and pathophysiology of each of these neurological disorders.
2. Analyze the presenting signs and symptoms for each of the neurodegenerative disorders discussed in the chapter by comparing similarities and differences.
3. Create a comprehensive plan of care for patients with each of the neurodegenerative disorders discussed.
4. Develop an inclusive discharge teaching plan for patients with each of the neurodegenerative disorders discussed.
5. Determine health promotion needs and gerontological implications for patients with each neurodegenerative disorder.

KEY TERMS

CARING FOR PATIENTS WITH THE NEURODEGENERATIVE DISORDERS of Alzheimer's disease, Parkinson's disease, amyotrophic lateral sclerosis, Huntington's disease, multiple sclerosis, and myasthenia gravis challenges the nurse's ability to manage diverse conditions. Characterized by neuronal loss in specific areas of the central nervous system (CNS), neurodegenerative disorders are chronic, progressive, and without cure. Although these disorders manifest with differing signs and distinctive symptoms, they share many aspects that contribute to the complexity of diagnosing and treating them.

In many cases, a diagnosis cannot be confirmed without autopsy. Clinically, neurodegenerative diseases often have a variable course. Patients and families face a future of uncertain prognosis—other than the knowledge that symptoms will worsen. Complicated treatment strategies compound the difficulty of these cases. As patients' mental and/or physical symptoms progress and the patients lose more and more of their ability to care for themselves, they begin to rely on a spouse, a close family member, or another lay caregiver. The ongoing and long-term care of a person with a degenerative disorder is labor intensive and can threaten the physical and mental well-being of the patient's family.

Nurses caring for patients with neurodegenerative disorders often find themselves in the dual role of caring for the patient and caring for the caregiver, and therefore often becoming a vital link among the patient, caregiver, and health care system in a variety of environments. Because of the prolonged, chronic nature of these diseases, the nurse commonly finds these patients in the home, outpatient clinic, or long-term care facility. Patients may be also hospitalized in the acute care setting during the initial diagnostic phase or for complications associated

Weblink: Alzheimer Disease
Weblink: Frontotemporal dementia

with their condition. The wide range of care for people with neurodegenerative disorders creates a unique opportunity for a nurse to have a profound impact on the patient's and family's response to a seemingly hopeless condition.

Degenerative Disorders

Alzheimer's Disease

Alzheimer's disease (AD) is an age-related, slowly progressive disease of the brain that develops over a period of years (National Institute of Neurological Disorders and Stroke [NINDS], 2011e). The most common form of dementia, it is characterized by impairment of memory and eventually by disturbances in reasoning, planning, language, and perception. Initially, people experience memory loss and confusion, which may be mistakenly identified as memory loss due to normal aging. However, the symptoms of AD gradually lead to behavior and personality changes, a decline in cognitive abilities such as decision-making and language skills, and problems recognizing family and friends. Ultimately, AD leads to a severe loss of mental function (NINDS, 2011e). Long-term care of AD patients is likely to take place in the home or in a nursing facility. Nurses who specialize in the treatment of neurological disorders most often provide ongoing clinical care in these settings; however, hospital nurses working in other specialties may see AD patients who have concurrent health issues.

Epidemiology and Etiology

Alzheimer's disease affects 8% to 15% of people over the age of 65 and is the sixth-leading cause of death in the United States (Alzheimer's Association, 2011b; Shawler, 2010). According to a 2010 report, AD affects approximately 5.3 million people in the United States (Anderson et al., 2011). A larger number of people have decreased cognitive function, a condition that frequently evolves into full-blown dementia. Researchers have calculated that by 2030, an estimated 7.7 million Americans ages 65 and older will have AD and that by 2050, that number will increase to more than 13 million (Anderson et al., 2011). AD affects both men and women; however, the risk of developing AD is significantly higher in women than in men. This may be due to women's longer life expectancy. AD and other dementias are more common in African Americans than in Caucasians. According to the Alzheimer's Association (2011b), in the population ages 71 and older, African Americans are almost 3 times as likely to have AD and dementias as Whites. In individuals age 65 and older, 7.8% of Caucasians, 18.8% of African Americans, and 20.8% of Hispanics have AD or other dementias. The prevalence of AD increases with age (Alzheimer's Association, 2011b).

Alzheimer's disease is the most common cause of dementia in people age 65 and older. **Dementia** itself is not a specific disease, but a group of symptoms that affect intellectual and social abilities severely enough to interfere with daily functioning. Dementia is caused by varying disorders and pathophysiological responses to disorders, including Creutzfeldt-Jakob disease (also known as "mad cow" disease), head trauma, HIV/AIDS, Huntington's disease, Lewy body disease, normal pressure hydrocephalus, and Parkinson's disease. However, Alzheimer's disease is the most common cause of a progressive dementia (Mayo Clinic Staff, 2011). This chapter focuses primarily on this most common form of dementia.

The causes of AD are not known; however, many scientists believe that it results from an increase in the production or accumulation of a specific protein (beta-amyloid protein) in the brain that leads to nerve cell death (Crystal, 2011). This is referred to as the amyloid cascade hypothesis and is discussed later in the chapter. Some researchers are investigating the hypothesis that individuals may inherit a gene that predisposes them to developing AD. A relatively common form of a gene located on chromosome 19 is associated with late-onset Alzheimer's disease. In the majority of AD cases, no specific genetic risks have yet been identified (Crystal, 2011). There are numerous risk factors for AD, which are summarized in Chart 23–1. Some of these risk factors are modifiable; others are not. Those that can be changed or individually modified are marked with an asterisk. The Risk Factors and Genetic Considerations boxes provide more information about Alzheimer's disease.

Pathophysiology

The pathology of AD is marked by the proliferation of amyloid plaques and neurofibrillary tangles, which form in the hippocampus and other parts of the brain critical to memory (Figure 23–1◆). The hallmarks of AD are the plaques and tangles in the brain. The third main feature is the gradual loss of connections between neurons in the brain, leading to diminished cell function and cell death (Crystal, 2011).

Neurofibrillary tangles were one of the discoveries that first described hallmark pathology in AD. The findings revealed a specialized protein known as **tau.** A key component of tangles, tau normally helps maintain the health of neurons. In patients with AD, mutations in tau cause it to distort and twist, creating tangled threads of the protein within neurons. The severity of Alzheimer's disease is determined by the number of neurofibrillary tangles (National Institute on Aging [NIA], 2011b; Querfurth & LaFerla, 2010). These neurofibrillary tangles eventually lead to cell death, neuronal degeneration, and the symptoms associated with AD (Anderson et al., 2011). Figure 23–2◆ depicts this process.

RISK FACTORS for Alzheimer's Disease

Increased age: the main risk factor

Genetic risk factors: 2% to 5% of patients develop the disease in the fourth or fifth decade of life; at least half of these early-onset patients have inherited gene mutations associated with the AD. Also, children of a patient with early-onset Alzheimer's disease who has some of these gene mutations have a 50% risk of developing AD. The genetic risk for late-onset cases is the gene located on chromosome 19 (Crystal, 2011).

Hypertension*	Alcohol use*
Coronary artery disease*	Family history
Obesity*	Smoking*
Insulin resistance	Diabetes
Elevated plasma homocysteine	Mild cognitive impairment (MCI)
Estrogen	General anesthetics
Lead	Possibly elevated blood cholesterol*
Inflammatory markers	Head injury

Completion of less than 8 years of education*

Down syndrome, patients develop the brain changes of AD by 40 years of age.

*Can be changed or individually modified.

Sources: Anderson, H., Brannon, G., Boswell, L., Feng, J., Haddock, J., & Schneider, R. (2011, June 9). Alzheimer disease. Retrieved from http://emedicine.medscape.com/article/1134817-overview#a0104; Crystal, H. (2011). Alzheimer's disease. Retrieved from http://www.medicinenet.com/alzheimers_disease_causes_stages_and_symptoms/article.htm. Mayo Clinic Staff. (2011). Frontootemporal dementia. MayoClinic.com. Retrieved from http://www.mayoclinic.com/health/frontemporal.

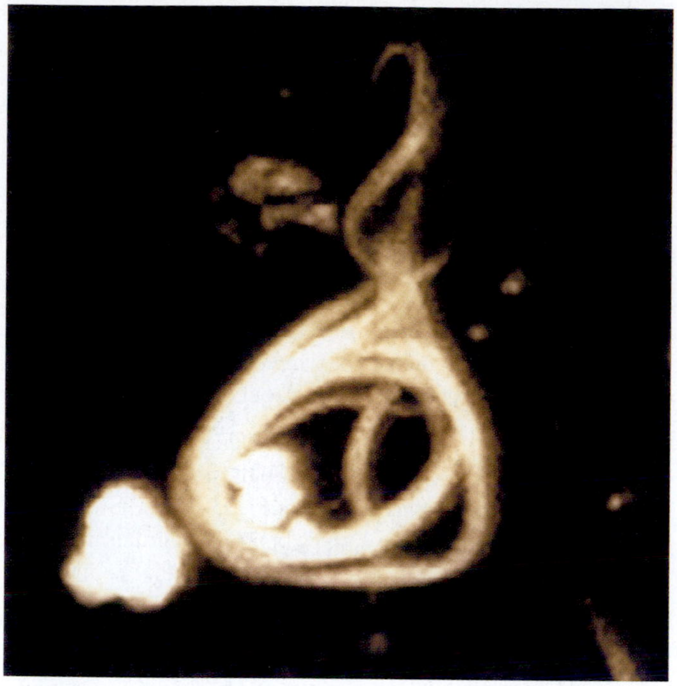

FIGURE 23–1 ◆ An AD neurofibrillary tangle.

Source: Photo from *Alzheimer's Disease: Unraveling the Mystery*, U.S. National Institute on Aging, 2002.

GENETIC CONSIDERATIONS
Related to Alzheimer's Disease

A genetic predisposition to AD can add to a person's susceptibility of developing the disease. In familial cases of early-onset AD (age 30s to 50s), gene mutations are known to produce abnormal amyloid precursor protein, the parent protein of beta-amyloid, and other abnormal proteins called presenilin-1 and presenilin-2. These mutations appear to increase the production of beta-amyloid, the protein found in the amyloid plaques that are characteristic of AD. While these findings help to delineate a genetic link to AD, familial early-onset cases are rare, and these gene mutations do not account for the more common occurrence of late-onset AD.

Also associated with the genetic risk of AD is the protein apolipoprotein E (ApoE), located on chromosome 19. The gene that produces ApoE has three alleles, e2, e3, and e4. The ApoE e4 allele has been linked to an increased risk of developing AD. This allele occurs in approximately 40% of late-onset cases whether or not there is a family history. A caveat to this discovery is that the presence of one or two ApoE e4 alleles does not predetermine the development of AD. Conversely, some people who develop AD show no ApoE e4 alleles. Thus, the ApoE e4 genotype represents an increased vulnerability for developing AD rather than being a causative factor. Another important factor in genetic investigation of AD is ethnicity. In one study, a significantly higher cumulative risk for dementia was noted among first degree relatives of African Americans with AD compared with those of Caucasians with AD.

Source:s Gies, C., & Lessick, M. (2009). Alzheimer disease in women. *Nursing for Women's Health, 13*(4), 314–324; National Institute on Aging, U.S. National Institutes of Health. (2011a). Genetics. Retrieved from http://www.nia.nih.gov/Alzheimers/Publications/ADProgress2008/LongWay/genetics.htm.

Most recently, researchers have focused on the impact amyloid plaques have on determining other pathologic characteristics of AD. Composed of the protein beta-amyloid and clipped from the larger amyloid precursor protein, these thick, insoluble plaques form around neurons, causing oxidative stress and inflammatory changes.

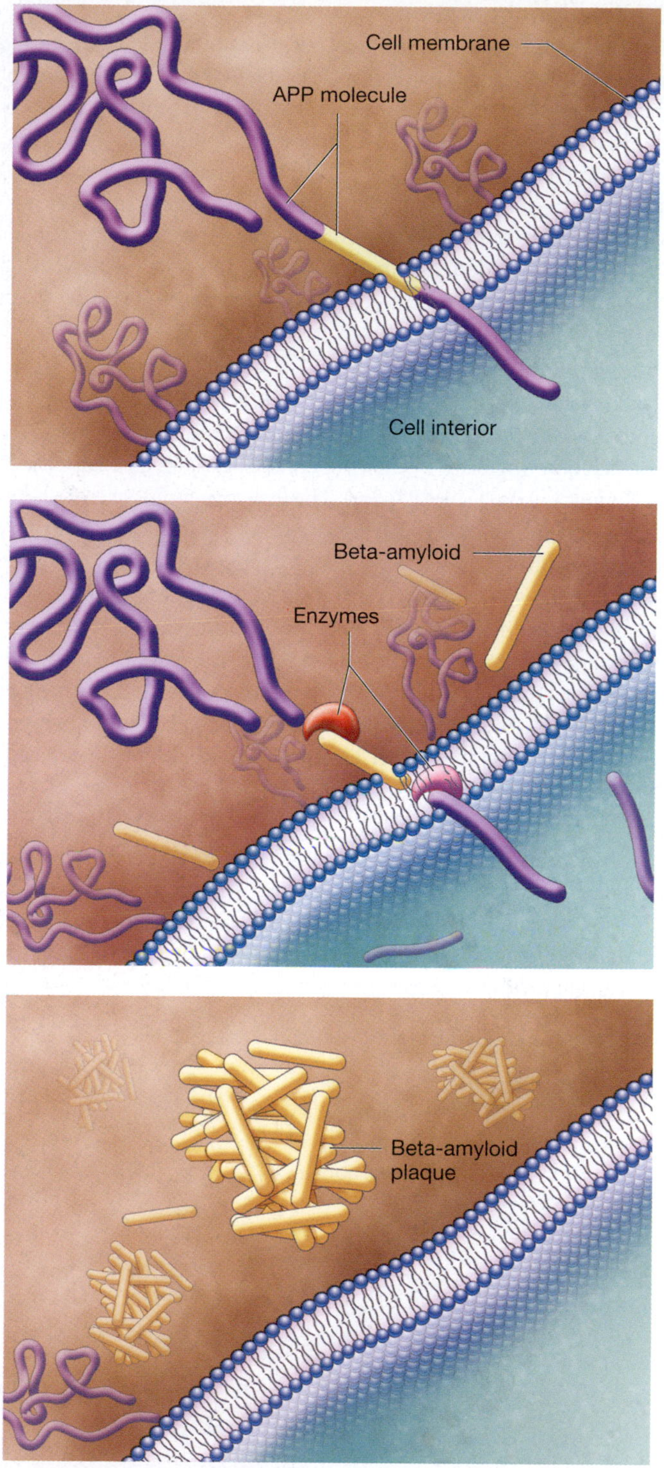

FIGURE 23–2 ◆ From amyloid precursor protein (APP) to beta-amyloid and formation of amyloid plaque.

A high serum cholesterol level may increase the risk of Alzheimer's disease. In recent studies, the administration of statins was shown to reduce the membrane pool of free cholesterol, thereby reducing risks (Querfurth & LaFerla, 2010). It is not known whether amyloid plaques cause AD or are a product of the disease process. Research continues to focus on oxidative stress, inflammation, and cholesterol and their relationship to the formation and presence of amyloid plaques in AD (NIA, 2011e).

Weblink: Signs and Symptoms of Alzheimer Disease

Weblink: Alzheimer's Disease Genetics Fact Sheet

Video: Alzheimer's Disease

Clinical Manifestations

The subtle onset of symptoms may occur over 1 to 25 years, with the average course being 8 to 10 years (Hickey, 2009). While the span of the disease varies in length and severity from patient to patient, its symptoms develop in stages that correspond to the area of the brain where degeneration is present (NIA, 2011e). Typically, neuronal degeneration starts in the hippocampus, an area of the brain that is critical to short- and long-term memory. From there, it spreads to other regions that control cognition, judgment, behavior, and physical movement. General descriptions of each of the four basic stages of AD are given next (NIA, 2011d).

Preclinical AD

Researchers suspect that the damaging effects of AD on the brain start 10 to 20 years before signs of the disease begin to show. Initially, the degeneration originates in the endocrinal cortex, an area adjacent to the hippocampus (Figure 23–3◆). The first symptom is likely to be an elusive, difficult-to-distinguish loss of memory. If the patient's memory loss appears to be greater than might be expected for his age while other functions of cognition remain intact, a diagnosis of *mild cognitive impairment* (MCI) may be rendered. In cases of MCI, the patient's experience of cognitive impairment may be uncorroborated by friends or family who do not notice the subtle behavior changes and memory anomalies of which the patient complains. The relationship between MCI and AD is not fully understood; however, MCI sometimes is considered a precursor to AD.

Mild AD

Once the degeneration of neurons spreads to the cerebral cortex (Figure 23–4◆), escalating problems with memory and cognitive function become obvious. Friends and family corroborate these difficulties, which may be considered warning signs of AD. Clinical testing will reveal the following signs of mild AD:

- Confusion about the location of familiar places
- Memory loss
- Slowness and difficulty in accomplishing simple tasks
- Misplacing things
- Difficulty handling money matters
- Poor or decreased judgment
- Problems with abstract thinking
- Loss of spontaneity and sense of initiative
- Mood swings and personality changes.

Moderate AD

At this stage of the disease, neuronal degeneration expands to areas that control language and reasoning. The symptoms worsen as atrophy continues to spread. The patient may have a bout of wandering and can be easily agitated by the routines of daily living. The following symptoms are indicators of moderate AD:

- Progressive memory loss and confusion
- Inability to recognize friends and family
- Language difficulties
- Difficulties with reading, writing, and simple math
- Problems learning new material, aligning thoughts, and thinking logically
- Hallucinations, delusions, and paranoia.

Severe AD

In the most advanced phase of AD, plaques and tangles have spread throughout the brain, causing generalized atrophy (Figure 23–5◆). The patient becomes completely dependent on others and cannot recognize loved ones. Other characteristics of advanced AD include the following: Inability to communicate, weight loss secondary to difficulty eating and swallowing, bowel and bladder incontinence, and increased sleeping. Death usually occurs as a result of aspiration pneumonia or from other concurrent health conditions.

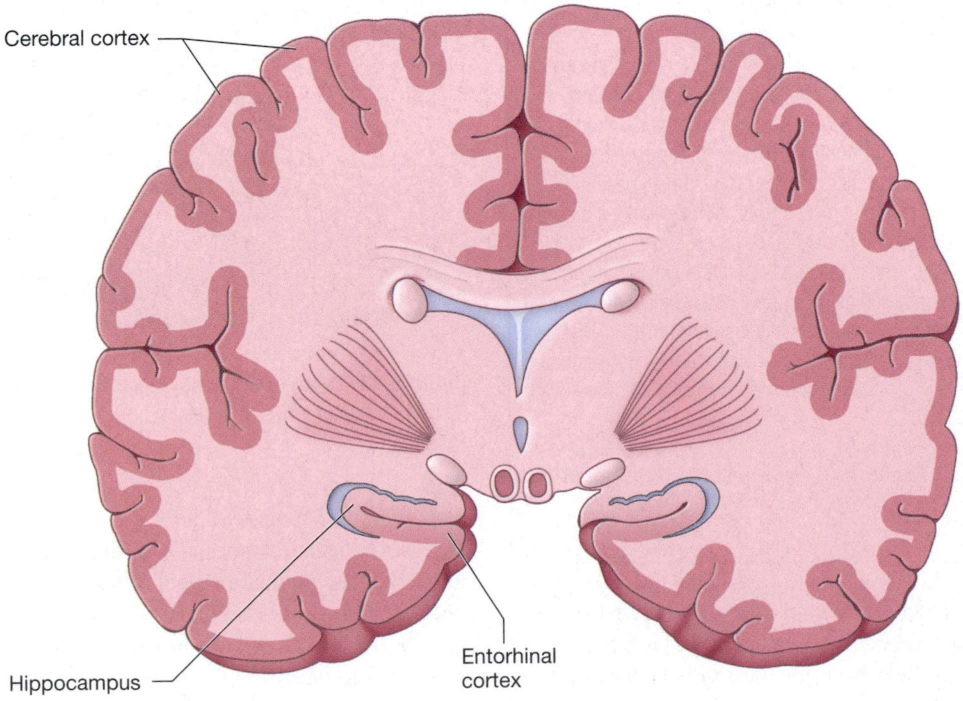

FIGURE 23–3 ◆ Preclinical AD.

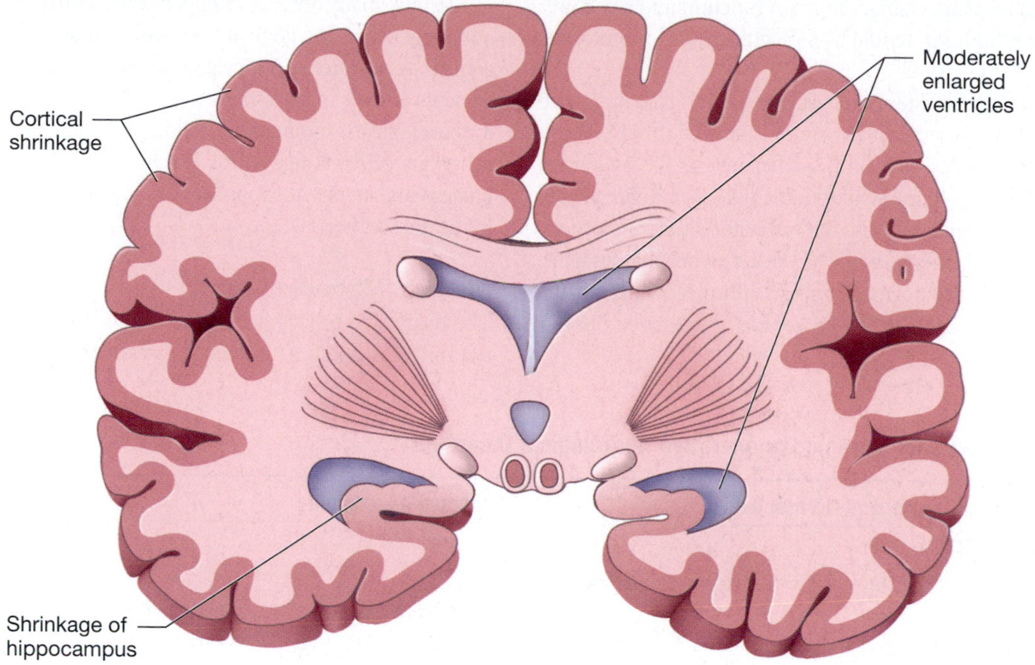

FIGURE 23–4 ◆ Mild AD.

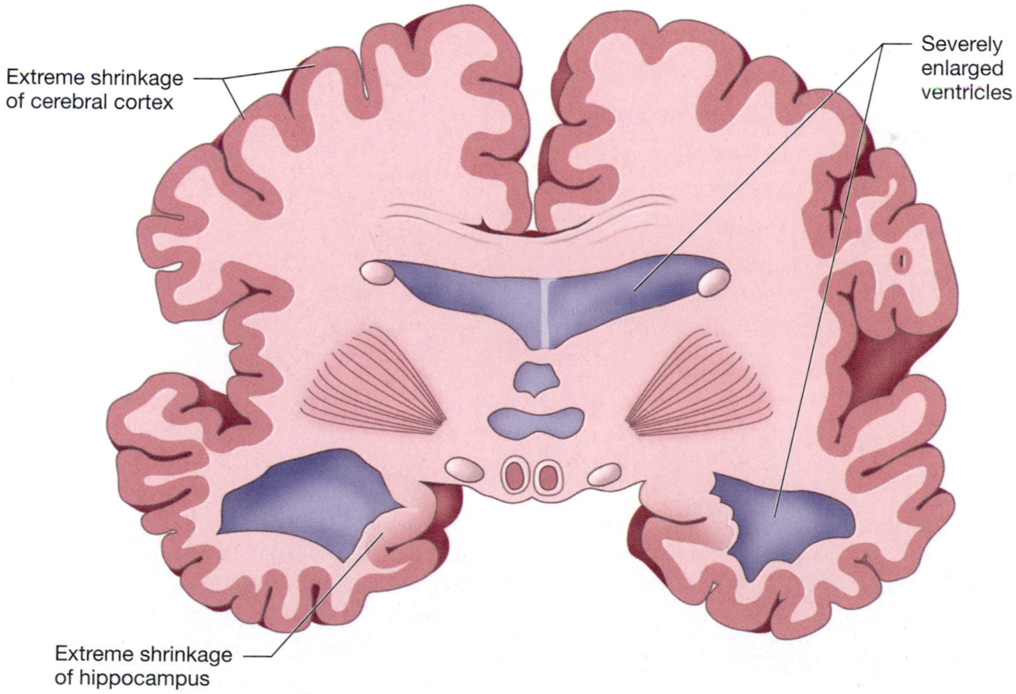

FIGURE 23–5 ◆ Severe AD.

Laboratory and Diagnostic Procedures

At the present time, there is no single diagnostic test that can detect whether a person has Alzheimer's disease. A definitive diagnosis of AD can be made only following a brain autopsy, which can determine the presence of the hallmark plaques and tangles. However, imaging technology designed to detect Alzheimer's plaques and tangles is becoming more precise and powerful. The newer positron emission tomography (PET) scans have confirmed the presence of beta-amyloid deposits in the brain (National Institute of Neurological Disorders and Stroke, 2011e). When AD is suspected, a magnetic resonance imaging (MRI) scan and the computerized tomography (CT) scan are performed, primarily to rule out other pathologic conditions such as normal pressure hydrocephalus or subdural hematoma. In advanced cases of AD, the MRI and CT scans, as well as the PET scans, may show diffuse cortical atrophy with disproportionate volume loss in the medial temporal lobe structures and atrophy in the hippocampal area (Meiner, 2010). However, only mild atrophy and normal age-related changes may be present early in the disease. Functional MRI (fMRI) is used primarily for research purposes to measure changes in brain function and structure, although it may have future potential as a diagnostic and monitoring tool (NIA, 2011b).

Routine laboratory and radiological tests are used to rule out other causes of dementia that present with symptoms similar to AD. These include metabolic imbalances, vitamin B_{12} deficiency, stroke, and brain tumor. Routine chemistry panels, blood counts, metabolic panels (e.g., TSH), spinal fluid analyses, and inflammatory markers are all within normal limits in patients with AD. Electroencephalographic (EEG) recordings usually are normal or show diffuse slowing in later states of AD (Tavee & Sweeney, 2011). These tests are described in the Diagnostic Tests box.

Because many other disorders can be confused with AD, laboratory and diagnostic tests alone are not sufficient to point to an ultimate diagnosis. A comprehensive evaluation is essential. The three major components of such an assessment are a thorough general medical workup; a neurological examination, including testing of memory and other functions of thinking; and a psychiatric evaluation to assess mood, anxiety, and clarity of thought. These assessment factors are discussed in the next section.

Medical Management

The diagnostic process includes a detailed medical history, a physical examination, and a neurological assessment. The health care provider

DIAGNOSTIC TESTS for Chronic Degenerative Neurological Disorders

Test with Description, Rationale, and Normal Values	Expected Abnormality
Complete Blood Count (CBC)	
Rule out metabolic abnormalities in the chronic neurodegenerative diseases discussed in the chapter. All values should be within normal limits. Complete blood count range of values: RBC—Red blood cells: 3.7–6.0 μL Hb/Hgb—Hemoglobin: 11.0–18.0 g/dL HCT—Hematocrit (Hct): 36.0–54.0 g/dL MCV—Mean corpuscular volume: 80–97 μm^3 MCH—Mean corpuscular hemoglobin: 27–34 MCHC—Mean corpuscular hemoglobin concentration: 28–36% RDW—Red cell distribution width: 11.5–14.5 Coulter S Platelets count ref. range: 140,000–390,000 (mm^3) MPV—Mean platelet volume: range 7.5–11.5 WBC—White blood cells (leukocytes): 5,000–10,000 μL Differential WBC count: Neutrophils: 35–45% Lymphocytes: 25–35% Monocytes: 4–10% Basophils: 0.5–1.0%	Values fall outside normal parameters with all diseases discussed: Alzheimer's disease (AD), Parkinson's disease (PD), amyotrophic lateral sclerosis (ALS), Huntington's disease (HD), multiple sclerosis (MS), and myasthenia gravis (MG).
Potassium and Sodium	
Potassium and sodium are evaluated as one method of ruling out neurodegenerative diseases as their symptoms of decreased or elevated values parrot many of the symptoms of the diseases AD, PD, ALS, HD, MS, and MG. *Potassium:* *Both hypokalemia and hyperkalemia cause symptoms similar to the neurodegenerative diseases.* Normal value: 3.5–5.3 mEq/L *Sodium:* *Both hyponatremia and hypernatremia cause symptoms similar to those of neurodegenerative diseases.* Normal value: 135–145 mEq/L	Hypokalemia may cause dizziness, hypotension, cardiac dysrhythmias, nausea, vomiting, diarrhea, abdominal distention, decreased peristalsis, muscle weakness, and leg cramps. Hyperkalemia may cause bradycardia, abdominal cramps, oliguria or anuria, tingling, and twitching or numbness of the extremities. Hyponatremia may produce symptoms of anxiety, muscular twitching, muscular weakness, and headaches. Hypernatremia may produce symptoms of restlessness; thirst; flushed skin; dry, sticky mucous membranes; and a rough, dry tongue. These are similar to symptoms characteristic of patients with AD, PD, ALS, HD, MS, and MG.
CPK (Creatine phosphokinase) Serum Level	
Indicates skeletal and myocardial breakdown of muscle tissue, which may occur with AD. This is a common phenomenon in skeletal muscle disease such as PD. Normal value = 5.25–5.35 mcg/mL in adults.	Value will be elevated with AD and PD.

DIAGNOSTIC TESTS for Chronic Degenerative Neurological Disorders, *continued*

Test with Description, Rationale, and Normal Values	Expected Abnormality
Cerebral Spinal Fluid (CSF) Studies *Uncovers signs of inflammation and myelin breakdown, a common phenomenon in MS.* Normal value: Normal CSF studies: values = 75–175 (mmH_2); 14–45 mg/dL protein, 119–132 chloride, and 40–80 mg/dL.	Elevated IgG index or synthesis rate in MS. Presence of oligoclonal bands in patients with MS.
Electromyogram (EMG) *Measures electrical activity of skeletal muscles at rest and during voluntary muscle contraction. May show signs of denervation, muscle wasting, and atrophy in ALS and MG.* Normal value: At rest, minimal electrical activity.	Fibrillations that are indicative of muscle disorders such as myasthenia gravis and amyotrophic lateral sclerosis are displayed.
MRI Brain and Spine *Rule out conditions that could mimic symptoms of AD and ALS, such as impaired mobility, confusion, language difficulties, paranoia, and weight loss.* Normal value: No evidence of abnormalities.	White matter lesion(s) identified, typical of MS. May show physical atrophy of different areas of the brain associated with later stages of Alzheimer's disease. Rule out other conditions, other than AD and MS (e.g., brain tumor, tumor, and hydrocephalus).
Electroencephalogram (EEG) *Measures the electrical impulses produced by brain cells; used to detect seizure disorder and identify a brain tumor, abscess, or intracranial hemorrhage.* Normal value: No abnormalities noted.	Abnormal tracing depicts seizures in patients with PD.
HIV Blood Test* *Rule out HIV as a cause of dementia.* Normal value: Negative.	Value will be positive in the presence of HIV; assists in determining cause of dementia.
Heavy Metals (e.g., arsenic, mercury, lead, aluminum, and zinc)* *Evaluate ingestion of metal, which causes changes in mental and central nervous system functions.* Normal value: Negative value for presence of heavy metals.	Long-term exposure causes slowly progressing muscular degenerative changes that mimic AD, PD, ALS, MG, and MS. There also is a potential link between the ingestion of heavy metals, leading to the formation of beta-amyloid plaques in the brain and possibly AD.
CT Scan *Rule out stroke, brain tumor, hydrocephalus, or other structural abnormalities.* Normal value: Within normal limits for age.	Will demonstrate stroke, brain tumor, hydrocephalus, or other structural abnormalities. In early stages of AD, mild atrophy may be present in hippocampal regions; in moderate to severe stages of AD, atrophy may be more generalized in areas of the brain.
Syphilis Serology* Normal value: Value within normal limit (WNL).	Rule out syphilis; symptomatic neurosyphilis can be confused with many similar neurological diseases or conditions, such as AD, ALS, and MG.
Thyroid-Stimulating Hormone (TSH) *Rule out hypothyroidism, as hypothyroidism often presents with symptoms similar to those with chronic, degenerative neurological disorders, such as AD and PD.* Result: WNL of 0.35–5.5 microinternational unit/mL (μIU/mL)	The level of TSH hormone will be decreased or elevated depending on the findings of hypothyroidism or hyperthyroidism. If elevated or decreased, it will rule out AD and PD.
Genetic Markers *Genetic markers consist of a gene or DNA sequence having a known location on a chromosome and associated with a particular gene or train. They are associated with certain diseases and can be detected in the blood. They are used to determine if an individual is at risk for developing a disease.* Normal value: No evidence of familial disease transmission genetic markers.	The presence of a genetic marker indicates a risk for development of AD, PD, ALS, HD, and MS. Families of individuals with early-onset familial AD may show an autosomal dominant pattern of inheritance. Currently, seven genes have been identified that form some kind of PD (National Human Genome Research Institute, 2011b).

(*continued*)

DIAGNOSTIC TESTS for Chronic Degenerative Neurological Disorders, *continued*

Test with Description, Rationale, and Normal Values	Expected Abnormality
	The familial form of ALS is caused by a specific genetic defect that leads to mutation of the enzyme known as superoxide dismulase 1. Other unidentified genetic causes may exist (National Institute of Neurological Disorders and Stroke [NINDS], 2011a).
The test analyzes DNA for the HD mutation by counting the number of CAG repeats in the Huntington gene. Normal value: Normal results are: Individuals who do not have HD usually have 28 or fewer CAG repeats (National Human Genome Research Institute, 2011a).	HD is a familial disease, passed from parent to child by a single abnormal gene (NINDS, 2010). The primary genetic risk factor of MS is the human leukocyte antigen (HLA)-DRB1*1501 allele (Briggs et al., 2010). Individuals with HD usually have 40 or more CAG repeats.
Inflammatory Markers *Inflammatory markers are biochemical substances the body sends out into the blood to signal to other cells how and where to act in response to a particular pathogen or injury. C-reactive protein is an inflammatory marker; the C-reactive protein test is the most well-known test used to measure general levels of inflammation in the body.* Normal value: Not usually present.	An elevated C-reactive protein signifies a chronic inflammation which occurs in AD. Chronic inflammation destroys brain cells.
VEP Visual Evoked Potentials *Identifies lesions in sensory pathway; may help identify lesion not easily visualized by MRI, for example, optic nerve.* Normal value: No lesions identified as would be expected with MS.	Will reveal slowed conduction of visual pathways with MS.
Vitamin B_{12} *Rule out vitamin B_{12} deficiency. Symptoms of vitamin B_{12} deficiency include symptoms similar to those found in neurological degenerative diseases: poor memory, apathy, mood swings, decreased cognitive function, low energy, fatigue, muscle weakness and soreness, and lack of coordination.* Normal value: Within normal limit of 200–900 pg/mL	Value may be low with MS.
Tensilon Test *The Tensilon test is an injection of edrophonium chloride and is used to diagnose myasthenia gravis (MG). The edrophonium blocks the action of acetylcholine esterase, thereby prolonging muscle stimulation and improving strength.* Normal value: No increase in strength of weakened muscles.	An obvious increase in the strength in weakened muscles strongly suggests the diagnosis of myasthenia gravis. The effect comes on rapidly and fades within minutes.
Acetylcholine Receptor (AchR) Antibody Assay *Used to determine the presence of AchR antibodies in patients with MG.* Normal value: Less than 0.02 to less than 0.03 nmol/L or negative	A positive result confirms the presence and autoimmune nature of MS.

*If history indicates.

References

Briggs, G. B., et al. (2010). Variation within DNA repair pathway genes and risk of multiple sclerosis. *American Journal of Epidemiology, 172*(92), 217–224. Kee, J. L. (2010). *Laboratory and diagnostic tests with nursing implications* (8th ed.). Upper Saddle River, NJ: Pearson. National Human Genome Research Institute. (2011a). Learning about Huntington's disease. National Institutes of Health. Retrieved from http://www.genome.gov/10001215. National Human Genome Research Institute. (2011b). Learning about Parkinson's disease. National Institutes of Health. Retrieved from http://www.genome.gov/1001217. National Institute of Neurological Disorders and Stroke. (2011a). ALS (amyotrophic lateral sclerosis) fact sheet. Retrieved from http://www.ninds.nih.gov/disorders/amyotrophiclateralsclerosis/detail_ALS.htm. National Institute of Neurological Disorders and Stroke. (2011b). NINDS dementia with Lewy bodies information page. Retrieved from http://www.ninds.nih.gov/disorders/dementiawithlewybodies/dementiawithlewybodies.htm. National Institute of Neurological Disorders and Stroke. (2011c). Multiple sclerosis: Hope through research. Retrieved from http://www.ninds.nih.gov/disorders/multiple_sclerosis/detail_multiple_sclerosis.htm. National Institute of Neurological Disorders and Stroke. (2011d). Myasthenia gravis fact sheet. Retrieved from http://www.ninds.nih.gov/disorders/myasthenia_gravis/detail_myasthenia_gravis.htm. National Institute of Neurological Disorders and Stroke. (2011e). NINDS amyotrophic lateral sclerosis information page. Retrieved from http://www.ninds.nih.gov/disorders/amyotrophiclateralsclerosis/detail_ALS.htm.

should pay particular attention to the duration and progression of the patient's memory loss. Complete and accurate charting of former and current medical conditions, medications, and behavioral symptoms are necessary considerations in prescribing treatments.

Whenever the patient has cognitive and memory difficulties, interviewing the primary caregiver and/or other family members can help to supplement the history. Cognitive status is often evaluated by using the Folstein Mini-Mental Status Exam (MMSE). The MMSE is an 11-question measure that tests five areas of cognitive function: orientation, registration, attention and calculation, recall, and language. The maximum score is 30. A score of 23 or lower indicates cognitive impairment. The MMSE takes only 5 to 10 minutes to administer and is, therefore, practical to use repeatedly and routinely. The MMSE is considered to be a national standard as a screening device to identify patients with cognitive impairment in both clinical practice and research (Kurlowicz & Wallace, 1999).

To establish the extent of AD and Alzheimer's, a three generation family history of the onset, duration, and progression of symptoms is needed to detect possible inherited patterns (Gies & Lessick, 2009). When MMSE results are monitored in cases of AD, scores drop at an average rate of 2 to 4 points per year (Barker, 2008).

The presence of depression can complicate the diagnosis of dementia or AD. Depression is thought to be present in 20% of older patients diagnosed with Alzheimer's type dementia. In hospitalized older adults with depression with psychotic features, AD has been estimated to be as high as 45%. Symptoms seen in both AD and depression include behavioral slowing, apathy, irritability, anxiety, and agitation (Geda et al., 2008). Depression can occur concurrently with AD; therefore, it is critical to separate the diagnoses of AD and depression before appropriate treatments can be implemented (Anderson et al., 2011).

Delirium also can manifest with symptoms similar to those of dementia; however, delirium is differentiated from dementia by the history. Delirium has a short onset within hours to a few weeks, while dementia is a chronic disturbance with a gradual onset. Delirium is a transient and potentially reversible condition, and the main objective in diagnosis is to identify treatable causes (Ferri, 2010). Common causes of delirium include renal or liver failure, vitamin B_{12} deficiencies, trauma such as hip fractures and head injuries, and medications.

The goals of pharmacologic treatment for AD are to preserve cognitive and functional abilities, minimize behavioral disturbances, and slow the progression of the disease (Hussey, 2011). With AD, levels of acetylcholine, a neurotransmitter that is critical in the process of memory formation, drops. The resulting decreases of acetylcholine and cholinergic activity in general are associated with memory impairment. Increasing available acetylcholine can potentially improve memory symptoms and help delay or prevent AD symptoms from exacerbating, mainly in the mild to moderate stages. The only medications approved by the Food and Drug Administration (FDA) for the treatment of mild to moderate AD are acetylcholinesterase inhibitors (AChEIs), which prevent the breakdown of acetylcholine, a brain chemical that is valuable for memory and thinking (Hussey, 2011). Three FDA-approved AChEIs—donepezil (Aricept), rivastigmine (Exelon), and galantamine (Reminyl)—are currently used in the treatment of AD. Late in 2003, the FDA approved the first *N*-methyl-D-aspartate (NMDA) receptor antagonist, memantine (Namenda), for the treatment of moderate to severe AD. See the Pharmacology feature for a description of these medications.

It is important for health care providers to treat or manage the challenging behaviors associated with AD. These patients do not tolerate changes in locations and routines well (Hussey, 2011). Nonpharmacologic approaches to managing behavioral symptoms center on reducing environmental stimuli, establishing predictable routines, simplifying tasks, and using distraction and redirection (Hussey, 2011). Restlessness, agitation, anger, anxiety, wandering, or psychotic symptoms may require treatment with psychotropic medications (Hickey, 2009). See the Pharmacology box (p. 598) for a list of drugs used to treat behavioral symptoms of AD.

Before implementing psychotropic medications, other conditions that may contribute to behavioral symptoms should be identified and eliminated, if possible. These include, but are not limited to, delirium, pain, infection, or other acute medical conditions (Geda et al., 2008).

The American College of Physicians and the American Academy of Family Physicians have established practice guidelines for the treatment of patients with dementia. These guidelines are published by the National Guideline Clearinghouse (2008). The major recommendations of the guidelines are shown in the National Guidelines box.

Nursing Management

Use of the nursing process facilitates a comprehensive approach to patient and caregiver support throughout the course of the disease (see the Nursing Process: Patient Care Plan for Alzheimer's Disease box, p. 606). Protecting the patient from injury, managing dysfunctional behaviors, and supporting the patient and caregiver in activities of daily living (ADLs) are the primary focus of nursing care. Cultural values and beliefs of patients and families with AD must be considered when establishing a therapeutic relationship with the patient and family. Elements to consider during the assessment process are found in the Cultural Considerations box, page 605.

The crippling effect of AD also comes with significant psychosocial ramifications. Often it will have an enormous impact on an older spouse or adult children who are called on to provide care and support. Research has demonstrated substantive implications of older adults caring for other older adults in terms of stress and the burden on an older caregiver's physical, mental, and financial well-being. Nurses must be prepared to assist family caregivers in dealing with denial, anger, guilt, grief, or clinical depression as the patient progresses, with the goal of helping the caregiver adjust and adapt to the changes associated with the progressive stages (Hussey, 2011; NIA, 2010) Referrals should be made to appropriate community resources, such as the state or local agency on aging or the local and national Association for Alzheimer's Disease.

Health Promotion

Health promotion is critical for the patient with AD as it is with the other diseases discussed in this chapter. Essential factors of health promotion include educational needs, dietary support, exercise and mobility, emotional and community support, and caregiver needs.

Education is paramount to helping patients remain as functional as possible and to preserve the quality of life over the course of the disease. Patients, their families, and caregivers need information and instruction on how to best take care of themselves and maintain activities of daily living in the home setting. These needs include maintaining a safe environment, taking medications, engaging in socialization, and in some instances maintaining occupational functions. Patients, families, and caregivers need to be apprised of resources on the health care team that are available to them, as well as community and organizational

NATIONAL GUIDELINES The American College of Physicians and the American Academy of Family Physicians Recommendations for Treatment of Dementia

Major Recommendations

Recommendation 1: Clinicians should base the decision to initiate a trial of therapy with a cholinesterase inhibitor or memantine on individualized assessment.

The decision to initiate therapy should be based on evaluation of benefits and risks for the individual patient. In particular, in cases of more advanced dementia, family members or other decision makers may not view stabilization or slowing of decline as a desirable goal if quality of life is judged to be poor. All of the drugs have known adverse events, and decisions made in managing the care of patients with dementia should balance harm against modest or even no benefit. Although the evidence shows statistically significant benefits of treatment with some cholinesterase inhibitors and memantine for all kinds of dementia, these benefits, on average, are not clinically significant for cognition and are modest for global assessments. However, limited evidence suggests, but does not demonstrate conclusively, that a subgroup of patients achieves clinically important improvements. Currently, there is no way to predict which patients might have a clinically important response. Therefore, the evidence does not support prescribing these medications for every patient with dementia. Evidence is insufficient to determine the optimal duration of therapy. A beneficial effect, if any, would generally be observed within 3 months on the basis of the duration of trials. This effect could be an improvement or stabilization. In addition, no evidence demonstrates when it is appropriate to stop the treatment if the patient becomes unresponsive or shows decline in various domains of dementia. However, if slowing decline is no longer a goal, treatment with memantine or a cholinesterase inhibitor is no longer appropriate.

Recommendation 2: Clinicians should base the choice of pharmacologic agents on tolerability, adverse effect profile, ease of use, and cost of medication. The evidence is insufficient to compare the effectiveness of different pharmacologic agents for the treatment of dementia. Because few trials compare one drug with another, evidence about their effectiveness is insufficient to support the choice of specific drugs for the treatment of dementia. Therefore, tolerability, adverse effect profile, ease of use, and cost of medication are reasonable criteria to help select a treatment. For example, when the benefits and harms related to a drug are being evaluated, the severe side effects associated with tacrine (an anticholinesterase medication that is sometimes prescribed in AD), especially as compared with the modest beneficial effects, make it an unreasonable choice.

Cholinesterase inhibitors are approved for treatment of mild to moderate dementia, and memantine is approved by the U.S. Food and Drug Administration (FDA) for the treatment of moderate to severe Alzheimer's disease. Patients with mild vascular dementia should benefit from memantine. However, memantine use in mild Alzheimer's disease has not been well studied. Major contraindications of cholinesterase inhibitors and memantine include, but are not limited to, uncontrolled asthma, angle-closure glaucoma (a type of eye disorder, discussed in Chapter 64), sick sinus syndrome and left bundle branch block (cardiac dysrhythmias, are discussed in Chapter 30).

Source: Adapted from American Psychiatric Association. (2000). *Diagnostic and statistical manual of mental disorders* (4th ed.). Washington, DC: Author.

PHARMACOLOGY Summary of Medications to Treat Patients with Chronic Degenerative Neurological Disorders

Medication Category and Action	Application/Indication	Nursing Responsibility
Acetylcholinesterase Inhibitors • Galantamine (Reminyl) • Rivastigmine (Exelon) • Donepezil (Aricept) **Action:** Increases acetylcholine levels in the brain; they are naturally degraded in the synaptic cleft by the enzyme cholinesterase; this allows elevation of acetylcholine (Ach), producing a more profound effect on Ach receptors.	Used to treat mild to moderate Alzheimer's disease (AD) by slowing memory loss and other progressive symptoms of dementia.	Monitor for positive response to medications, improved cognitive function and memory, decreased irritability and anxiety, and decreased signs of depression. Monitor for adverse effects of nausea, vomiting, diarrhea, and weight loss. Determine which symptoms of AD the patient is demonstrating, when they began, and whether there is anything that makes the symptoms worse or better. Evaluate the patient for improvement of symptoms after taking the medication. Determine the degree of depression, agitation, or anxiety that may be present. Obtain baseline laboratory tests, especially CBC, liver, and renal function tests; vital signs, weight, and vision checks. Determine whether safety issues are present, such as the inability to function independently, the inability to be left alone, or the inability to drive. Alert caregiver of any safety concerns.
N-Methyl-D-Aspartate (NMDA) Receptor Antagonist Memantine (Namenda) **Action:** Blocks action of glutamate, decreasing activation of NMDA receptors. It binds to the NMDA receptor, preventing glutamate from causing its excitatory actions and slowing nerve damage.	Used to treat moderate to severe AD.	Monitor for possible side effects of headache, constipation, confusion, and dizziness.

PHARMACOLOGY Summary of Medications to Treat Patients with Chronic Degenerative Neurological Disorders, *continued*

Medication Category and Action	Application/Indication	Nursing Responsibility
		Monitor patients' level of cognitive function, ability to self-administer medications, and ability to perform ADLs. Follow safety precautions as described with the use of the acetylcholinesterase inhibitors described previously.
Atypical Antipsychotics		
Olanzapine (Zyprexa) Quetiapine (Seroquel) Clozaril (Clozaaril) **Action:** Acts as antagonists of dopamine and serotonin by blocking the binding of dopamine to the receptors in various brain regions.	Used to treat delusions, hallucinations, agitation, and combativeness in patients with dementia and PD.	Monitor mental status and response to drug therapy. Monitor for orthostatic hypotension, somnolence, nausea, vomiting, and constipation.
Selective Serotonin-Reuptake Inhibitors		
Sertraline (Zoloft) Citalopram (Celexa) Fluoxetine (Prozac, Sarefem) **Action:** Inhibits uptake of the neurotransmitter serotonin in CNS, potentiating the effects of serotonin. Has little or no effect on other neurotransmitters.	Used to treat depression, irritability, and anxiety.	Monitor for mood changes, somnolence, and insomnia. Monitor for adverse effects: anxiety, drowsiness, headache, insomnia, sexual dysfunction, and tremors. Discontinue the use of MAO inhibitors 14 days prior to fluoxetine therapy. Combined therapy may result in serotonin syndrome: confusion, agitation, seizures, hyperpyrexia (an especially high fever), and hypertension. Monitor the CBC and differential white count periodically.
Carbidopa/Levodopa		
Immediate release Controlled release Carbidopa/levodopa/entacapone (Stalevo) **Action:** Levodopa is converted to dopamine in the basal ganglia, increasing dopamine concentration within the brain. Carbidopa blocks the peripheral decarboxylation of levodopa, making more levodopa available to the brain.	Symptomatic treatment of idiopathic Parkinson's disease; may be given alone or in combination with other anti-Parkinsonian drugs.	Monitor for nausea, hypotension, confusion, hallucinations, motor fluctuations, and dyskinesia. Monitor for impaired liver and kidney functions because metabolism and excretion of abnormalities could lead to toxic levels of the drug. Assess for symptoms associated with parkinsonism: tremors, muscle rigidity, bradykinesia, and postural instability. Obtain baseline and periodic blood tests, including a CBC and liver and renal function studies.
Dopamine Agonists		
Bromocriptine (Parlodel) Pergolide (Permax) Pramipexole (Mirapex) Ropinirole (Requip) Apomorphine hydrochloride (Apokyn) Rotigotine **Action:** Stimulates dopamine receptors in the brain at both presynaptic and postsynaptic sites in the striatum, thus helping to restore the balance of dopaminergic effects in the striatum.	May be given as initial treatment of Parkinson's disease (PD) or adjunctively with levodopa in advanced cases of PD.	Monitor for postural hypotension, nausea, confusion, and hallucinations. Evaluate all other medications taken by the patient for compatibility with dopamine agonists. Assess mental status, affect, mood, depression, and behavioral changes at regular intervals. Monitor for the presence of, reduction in, or increase of tardive dyskinesia (movements of the tongue, lips, face, trunk, and extremities), which is characterized by repetitive, involuntary, and purposeless movements.
Anticholinergics		
Benztropine (Cogentin) Trihexyphenidyl (Artane) **Action:** Acts by reducing the excess cholinergic effect associated with dopamine deficiency and restores neurotransmitter balance in the striatum.	Used to manage PD symptoms; reduces tremor and rigidity.	Monitor for symptom improvement (e.g., less tremors (shaking) and rigidity, better balance, and less muscle stiffness with improved range of motion). Monitor for side effects: dry mouth, constipation, urinary retention, blurred vision, hallucinations, and confusion. Monitor for symptoms of paralytic ileus, which is the only identified life-threatening effect.

(*continued*)

PHARMACOLOGY Summary of Medications to Treat Patients with Chronic Degenerative Neurological Disorders, *continued*

Medication Category and Action	Application/Indication	Nursing Responsibility
Antiviral		
Amantadine (Symmetrel) **Action:** Exact action is not clear; likely potentiates dopaminergic transmission in CNS. Possibly has the ability to release dopamine and norepinephrine from neuronal storage sites and prevent their reuptake.	Used to treat motor fluctuations and dyskinesia in PD patients.	Monitor for decreased extremity edema, unwanted effect of livedo reticularis (a cutaneous mottled reticulated vascular pattern that looks like a lacelike purplish discoloration on the extremities), urinary retention, and hallucinations. Assess for history of suicide attempts or substance abuse because this drug may exacerbate preexisting mental problems. Assess for CNS effects such as insomnia, light-headedness, nervousness, loss of concentration, and mental confusion. If present, report to the health care provider.
MAO-B Inhibitors		
Selegiline (Eldepryl) Rasagiline **Action:** Exact action not clear; believed to enhance dopaminergic activity in substantia nigra by blocking the enzyme MAO-B.	Sometimes given as monotherapy for initial treatment for PD; usually given adjunctively.	Observe for motor improvement in the early stages of PD, as well as a decrease in fluctuations in later stages of PD. Monitor for side effects: agitation, insomnia, vivid dreams, hallucinations, and orthostatic hypotension.
COMT Inhibitors		
Entacapone Tolcapone **Action:** Blocks COMT, an enzyme that metabolizes levodopa; enhances available dopamine.	Given adjunctively with levodopa/carbidopa for the treatment of PD.	Same as for levodopa.
Tricyclic Antidepressants		
Amitriptyline (Elavil) **Action:** Potentiates serotonin and norepinephrine in CNS.	Used to alleviate depression in patients with neurodegenerative disorders.	*Tricyclics:* Monitor for cognitive changes. May improve insomnia and drooling. Monitor for constipation.
Selective Serotonin Reuptake Inhibitors (SSRIs)		
Fluoxetine (Prozac) Sertraline (Zoloft) Paroxetine (Paxil) Citalopram (Celexa) **Action:** Inhibits uptake of neurotransmitter serotonin in CNS, potentiating the effects of serotonin. Has little or no effect on other neurotransmitters.		*SSRIs:* Monitor for restlessness or agitation. *All:* May take several weeks to reach therapeutic dose. Should not be discontinued suddenly. Assess suicide risk. Encourage concomitant counseling.
Glucocorticoid		
Fludrocortisone (Florinef) **Action:** Acts on distal renal tubule to promote sodium reabsorption and water retention.	Used to treat severe, chronic postural hypotension.	Assess medication regime for antihypertensives. Monitor blood pressure while sitting and standing. Monitor fluid balance and salt intake. Monitor for signs of fluid retention.
Vasopressor		
Midodrine (ProAmatine) **Action:** Stimulates alpha$_1$-adrenergic receptors, increasing total peripheral resistance, resulting in increased systolic and diastolic blood pressure.	Used to treat severe, chronic postural hypotension.	Assess medication regime for antihypertensives. Monitor blood pressure while sitting and standing. Monitor fluid balance and salt intake.
Genitourinary Antispasmodic		
Oxybutynin (Ditropan) Tolterodine tartrate (Detrol) **Action:** Exerts a direct spasmolytic (antispasmodic, disruption of spasm) action and an antimuscarinic action on smooth muscle, relaxing bladder smooth muscle.	Used to treat urinary symptoms of overactive bladder that may occur with PD.	Monitor for urinary frequency and urgency. Monitor fluid balance. Monitor for signs of urinary tract infection.

PHARMACOLOGY Summary of Medications to Treat Patients with Chronic Degenerative Neurological Disorders, *continued*

Medication Category and Action	Application/Indication	Nursing Responsibility
Pharmacotherapy of Amyotrophic Lateral Sclerosis (ALS)		
Riluzole (Rilutek) **Action:** Slows progression of ALS by protecting motor neurons through inhibition of glutamate production.	Only known drug with FDA approval for treating ALS.	Monitor for adverse effects: muscular weakness, dizziness, somnolence, nausea, diarrhea, and decreased lung function. Monitor liver function and blood count. Be aware of multiple drug interactions (theophylline, barbiturates, aminoglycosides, and others). Monitor riluzole plasma levels and observe for hepatotoxicity. Warn the patient that caffeine, cigarette smoking, high fat diet, and charcoal-broiled food may interfere with riluzole absorption. Give on an empty stomach.
Skeletal Muscle Relaxants		
Centrally Acting Diazepam (Valium) Baclofen (Kemstro, Lioresal) **Action:** Exact action is unknown; probably relaxes skeletal muscle by depressing afferent reflex activity at the level of the spinal cord.	Used to reduce spasticity and muscle spasms in ALS.	Monitor for adverse effects: drowsiness, dizziness, weakness, confusion, hypotension, nausea, and constipation. Monitor for psychiatric disturbances, especially in older adults. Monitor liver and kidney function, especially in older adults or if renal or hepatic disease is present. Warn the patient to avoid alcohol and other CNS depressants. Be aware that abruptly stopping the drug may result in adverse reactions. Monitor diabetics for hyperglycemia as drugs may increase blood glucose concentrations.
Peripherally Acting Muscle Relaxants		
Dantrolene (Dantrium) **Action:** Relaxes skeletal muscle by interfering with calcium ion release within the muscle.	Used to treat spasticity accompanying ALS.	Monitor for adverse effects: muscle weakness, slurred speech, fatigue, diarrhea, and constipation. Monitor blood count, as well as liver and renal function. Monitor for signs of pleural effusion and pericarditis in patients with cardiac disease, as well as respiratory depression in patients with pulmonary dysfunction. Warn the patient not to use alcohol, and to check with a health care provider before using OTC medications. Warn the patient about possible photosensitivity and the need for sunblock. Teach the patient the symptoms of hepatitis. Notify the health care provider, if present.
Antimalarial		
Quinine sulfate (Quinamm, Quiphile) **Action:** Reduces muscle cramping by direct action at the neuromuscular junction.	Used to reduce muscle cramping in ALS.	Monitor for adverse effects: headache, sweating, tinnitus, vertigo, visual disturbances, vomiting, diarrhea, abdominal pain, and cardiac arrhythmias. Be aware of multiple drug interactions; monitor for toxicity or decreased drug efficacy (digoxin, antacids, warfarin, anticonvulsants, and others). Give with food or milk.
Dopamine Receptor Blocking (Neuroleptics)		
Haloperidol (Halol) **Action:** Depresses the cerebral cortex, hypothalamus, and limbic system, which are parts of the brain controlling activity and aggression. Blocks neurotransmission to postsynaptic dopamine D_2 receptors and exhibits alpha, adrenergic blocking, and anticholinergic effects.	Used to suppress chorea (a type of movement disorder), agitation, and psychotic symptoms of Huntington's disease.	Monitor for adverse effects: blurred vision, dry eyes, constipation, dry mouth, hypotension, and neuroleptic malignant syndrome. Be aware of multiple drug interactions (nitrates, drugs with anticholinergic properties).

(*continued*)

PHARMACOLOGY Summary of Medications to Treat Patients with Chronic Degenerative Neurological Disorders, *continued*

Medication Category and Action	Application/Indication	Nursing Responsibility
		Observe for extrapyramidal side effects, which include tremor, slurred speech, akathisia (feeling of inner restlessness), dystonia, anxiety, distress, paranoia, and bradyphrenia (slowing of the thought processes). Monitor blood pressure and pulse frequently. May cause QT interval changes on ECG.
Risperidone **Action:** Exact action is not known. Believed to act by blocking the binding of dopamine to its receptors in various brain regions.	Used to decrease movement disorders such as those in Huntington's disease, as well as agitation.	Monitor for adverse effects: aggressive behavior, dizziness, headaches, cough, and constipation. Be aware of multiple drug interactions; may decrease the antiparkinsonian effects of levodopa, clozapine, and CNS depressants Monitor CBC and liver function tests frequently. Monitor for neuroleptic malignant syndrome and suicidal thoughts.
Dopamine-Depleting Agents		
Reserpine (Serpalan) **Action:** Depletes stores of catecholamines and 5-hydroxytryptamine in many organs, including the brain. The depression of sympathetic nerve function results in a decreased heart rate and lowering of arterial blood pressure, also producing a sedative and tranquilizing effect.	Used to decrease hyperkinesia or chorea in patients with Huntington's disease.	Monitor for adverse effects: hypotension, nasal congestion, nausea, vomiting, weight gain, and gastric intolerance. Obtain baseline ECG and vital signs including blood pressure. Assess neurological status and level of consciousness (LOC). Monitor for psychiatric disturbances: depression.
Tetrabenazine **Action:** Depletes presynaptic dopamine, norepinephrine, and serotonin storage, and antagonizes postsynaptic dopamine receptors. Its unintended action on serotonin and norepinephrine levels may account for tetrabenazine-associated depression.	Treat chorea in Huntington's disease.	Monitor for adverse reactions: extrapyramidal events, which include: tremor, slurred speech, akathisia or feeling of inner restlessness, dystonia, and anxiety, distress, paranoia, and bradyphreniad or slowing of thought processes, sedation, fatigue, depression, nausea, vomiting, dysphagia, upper respiratory infections, falls
Clonazepam **Action:** Enhances the action of gamma aminobutyric acid (GABA) neurotransmitters in the brain, thus inhibiting the abnormal neuronal discharge characteristic of seizures.	Reduces the potential of seizures and may be used to reduce anxiety or panic attacks in patients with Huntington's disease.	Monitor for adverse effects: sedation, drowsiness, palpitations, ataxia, and physical dependence. Monitor blood count and liver function tests. Monitor drug interactions: hormonal contraceptives, metoprolol, and phenytoin. For toxicity and overdose, Flumazenil may be given.
Lorazepam **Action:** Potentiates the actions of GABA, an inhibitory neurotransmitter in the CNS. Depresses the CNS to simple relaxation, to the induction of sleep, or to coma.	Used to manage excessive anxiety and agitation; may be used for those on mechanical ventilation or for treatment in neurologically compromised patients (e.g., Huntington's disease).	Monitor for adverse effects: dizziness, drowsiness, lethargy, apnea, and cardiac arrest. Monitor interactions with other medications: opioid analgesics, clozapine, valproate, and oral contraceptives. Monitor renal, hepatic, and hematologic functions.
Anticonvulsants		
Valproic acid **Action:** Increases levels of GABA and suppresses abnormal neuron discharges, leading to decreased seizure activity.	Stabilizes mood and used to treat behavioral agitation due to dementia, AD, or HD. Also used to treat absence seizures* and complex partial seizures. *Absence seizures are seizures where the abnormal discharges are coming from all over the brain at once.	Monitor for adverse effects: agitation, dizziness, headaches, depression, visual disturbances, abdominal pain, and tremors. Monitor for drug interactions with warfarin, aspirin, carbamazepine, and chlorpromazine. Monitor CBC, platelet count, and bleeding time. May cause leukopenia and thrombocytopenia. Also monitor hepatic function and serum ammonia.

PHARMACOLOGY Summary of Medications to Treat Patients with Chronic Degenerative Neurological Disorders, *continued*

Medication Category and Action	Application/Indication	Nursing Responsibility
Cholinesterase inhibitors		
Donepezil **Action:** Inhibits acetylcholinesterase, thus improving cholinergic function by making more acetylcholine available.	Improves cognition for those who are cognitively impaired, unable to perform ADL, and have behavioral problems, such as in chronic neurological disorders.	Observe for improved cognition, memory, and reasoning; ability to perform own ADL, and signs of less confusion, depression, or anxiety. Monitor for adverse reactions: headaches, diarrhea, and nausea. Monitor for drug interactions with succinylcholine, rifampin, dexamethasone, and phenytoin. Occasionally monitor heart rate due to possible bradycardia.
Immunomodulator/Interferons		
Interferon beta-1a (Avonex) Interferon beta-1b (Betaseron) Interferon beta-1a (Rebif) **Action:** Although action is not clear, thought to inhibit proliferation of leukocytes and antigens; modulate production of anti-inflammatory cytokines; and inhibit T-cell migration across blood–brain barrier.	Used to treat relapsing forms of MS.	Assess the frequency of exacerbations. Monitor hemoglobin, WBC, platelets, and blood chemistries. Instruct the patient on correct injection technique.
Immunomodulator		
Glatiramer acetate (Copaxone) **Action:** Although action is not clear, thought to modulate T cells to promote production of anti-inflammatory cytokines.	Used to treat relapsing-remitting forms of MS.	Assess frequency of exacerbations. After injection, assess for flushing, chest pain, palpitations, and dyspnea. Instruct the patient on correct injection technique.
Antineoplastic/Immunosuppressive		
Mitoxantrone (Novantrone) **Action:** Binds to DNA, causing strand splitting and inhibition of DNA synthesis. It is cell cycle nonspecific.	Used to treat rapidly worsening relapsing-remitting, progressive-relapsing, secondary-progressive MS.	Assess frequency of exacerbations. Monitor for cardiotoxicity, fatigue, nausea, and immunosuppression.
Monoclonal Antibody		
Natalizumab (Tysabri) **Action:** May hamper the movement of immune cells across the blood–brain barrier.	Used to treat relapsing forms of MS in patients who have inadequate response or who cannot tolerate other disease-modifying treatment.	Due to the risk of progressive multifocal leukoencephalopathy, a serious viral infection of the brain, this drug is available only at select authorized infusion sites requiring mandatory patient registration and follow-up.
Management of Selected Symptoms of Multiple Sclerosis		
CNS Stimulants		
Pemoline Modafinil **Action:** Produce CNS stimulation.	Used to offset/decrease fatigue.	Monitor for restlessness or sleep disturbances. Counsel the patient regarding the dosing schedule and titration.
Genitourinary Antispasmodics		
Oxybutynin (Ditropan) Tolterodine tartrate (Detrol) **Action:** Exerts a direct spasmolytic action and an antimuscarinic action on smooth muscle, relaxing bladder smooth muscle.	Used to correct bladder dysfunction.	Assess for urinary tract infection. Monitor for urinary retention. Monitor intake and output. Monitor overall elimination pattern.
Skeletal Muscle Relaxants		
Oral or intrathecal Baclofen **Action:** Acts at spinal cord level to decrease frequency and amplitude of muscle spasms.	Used to treat spasticity in patients with MS.	Time doses to maintain therapeutic blood levels. Titrate doses up. Monitor for sedation or cognitive symptoms. Intrathecal baclofen requires surgical insertion of a programmable pump; monitor closely during titration.

(*continued*)

PHARMACOLOGY Summary of Medications to Treat Patients with Chronic Degenerative Neurological Disorders, *continued*

Medication Category and Action	Application/Indication	Nursing Responsibility
Benzodiazepines		
Diazepam Clonazepam **Action:** Inhibits polysynaptic afferent pathways.	Used to treat spasticity in patients with MS.	Assess spasticity. Monitor vital signs during therapy. Assess risk of falls and implement fall prevention strategies. Monitor for psychological/physical dependence during long-term therapy.
Cholinesterase Inhibitors		
Neostigmine (Prostigmin) Pyridostigmine (Mestinon) Ambenonium (Mytelase) Edrophonium chloride (Tensilon) **Action:** Increases strength of muscle contraction by preventing the breakdown of acetylcholine at the neuromuscular junction.	Symptomatic treatment of myasthenia gravis, diagnosis of myasthenia gravis, and differentiation between cholinergic and myasthenic crises (not recommended for maintenance therapy due to short duration of action).	Monitor for adverse effects: abdominal cramping, nausea, vomiting, diarrhea, diaphoresis, blurred vision, bradycardia, hypotension, and bronchospasm. Monitor for cholinergic crisis. Assess vital signs, as well as respiratory and neuromuscular function. Have atropine and resuscitation equipment immediately available for treatment. Be aware of drug interactions (corticosteroids, aminoglycoside, antibiotics, and others).
Immunosuppressants		
Azathioprine (Imuran) Cyclosporine (Sandimmune, Neoral) **Action:** Suppresses immune response by inhibiting lymphocyte replication or disrupting helper T cells.	Used in treatment of myasthenia gravis.	Observe for improvement in symptoms 1 to 2 months after starting medication, such as increased muscle strength, improved control over eye movement, decreased ptosis or diplopia (double vision), and improved oropharyngeal muscle strength, thereby enabling the patient to chew, eat swallow, and talk better. Monitor for adverse effects: hirsutism (a condition in which women have excess dark coarse hair on the face), hypertension, nausea, vomiting, and infection. Observe for signs of toxicity: tremors, seizures, altered mental status, visual disturbances, and renal toxicity. Be aware of multiple drug interactions (digoxin, NSAIDs, erythromycin, verapamil, cimetidine, and others with cyclosporine; allopurinol, ACE inhibitors, warfarin, and others with azathioprine). Monitor for altered drug levels, nephrotoxicity, or leukopenia.
Corticosteroids		
Prednisone **Action:** Reduces acetylcholine receptor antibody levels; may enhance neuromuscular transmission.	Used with myasthenia gravis patients to initiate or maintain immunosuppression.	Observe for improvement in symptoms within the first weeks to months of starting prednisone, such as increased muscle strength. Strength may increase to total remission in the months that follow initial treatment. Some patients may experience increased weakness during the first 7 to 10 days of treatment; this lasts for approximately 6 days. Monitor for adverse effects: mood swings, anxiety, insomnia, nausea, vomiting, weight gain, acne, and delayed wound healing. Monitor the clinical response to guide incremental dosing. Observe for transient steroid-induced exacerbation of MG with initiation of drug. Be aware of drug interactions (theophylline, warfarin, and others). Monitor for toxicity or decreased efficacy. Warn the patient of the potential need for dose adjustment if ill or stress increases and to not abruptly stop the drug.

Sources: Adapted from Adams, M., & Koch, R. (2010). *Pharmacology: Connections to nursing practice.* Upper Saddle River, NJ: Prentice Hall.

CULTURAL CONSIDERATIONS for Care of the Patient/ Family with Alzheimer's Disease

There are three main elements of a cultural assessment within the clinical evaluation process for Alzheimer's disease. The health care provider:

- Needs to be sensitive to the preferred language of the patient and family, which may determine the service relationship with the health care provider. For example, in ethnically diverse populations, bilingual families may have quite different service engagement expectations and outcomes than monolinguals.
- Must be able to understand the patient's and family's customary ways of relating to others within their own group and with persons in authority, being aware that internal decision-making processes may vary both among and within different cultural groups. For example, the health care provider may be seen as the sole person in authority, with the expectation that he or she will be making detailed caregiving decisions. The health care providers must ascertain as early as possible in the assessment process how a family makes decisions and identify its primary decision maker, who may not be the person doing most of the "hands-on" caregiving.
- Needs to tap into underlying belief systems regarding Alzheimer's disease and other comorbid conditions. These underlying normative expectations are often expressed in terms of "folk understandings," which may influence the way in which people from diverse cultures receive and act on the information and directions provided by the health care provider. The health care provider should consult with the primary caregiver to identify beliefs about health and aging; learn about cultural taboos (e.g., direct eye contact); determine the language or dialect spoken by the patient and the patient's family; and use bilingual, bicultural health care providers as appropriate.

resources. Specific educational needs are addressed in the Patient Teaching & Discharge Priorities box (p. 607).

A dietitian or nutritionist who is familiar with dysphasia (impairment of speech and verbal comprehension), muscular weakness, swallowing abnormalities, and aspiration can be used to assess nutritional needs (see Chapter 8) and recommend adequate amounts of fluids and proper foods for such conditions. The nutritional goals for people who have mobility problems or impaired digestion include reducing constipation, improving fiber intake, providing adequate energy, preventing weight loss, maintaining hydration, and correcting vitamin D deficiency (Marcason, 2009). Good nutrition can aid in resistance to infection (Barker, 2008). A low-fat, high-fiber diet (see Chapter 8) is frequently recommended (National Muscular Sclerosis Society, 2008).

Patients should be encouraged to engage in a regular exercise program and practice healthy eating habits. Exercise may help manage fatigue, depression, muscle weakness, spasticity, and bowel and bladder problems, if present. Cardiovascular exercise, strength training, and muscle stretching routines can help combat loss of balance, dexterity, and normal movement. Exercise also will improve the strength, endurance, and compensatory qualities of the unaffected parts of the body (Hackney & Earhart, 2008; Vernon, 2009).

Physical and emotional stress can exacerbate the symptoms of many neurodegenerative diseases. Techniques to manage emotional stress should be emphasized. Patients are encouraged to remain active for as long as possible to reduce the stress accompanying all diseases. Referral for psychological and/or spiritual counseling may help the patient and family come to terms with the disease and its prognosis. Many patients and caregivers find support groups their most valuable asset in the struggle against the condition. Internet organizations also connect individuals who wish to communicate about the disease. Support organizations offer understanding and hope for both the patients and their families. Local and national support groups provide information, educational programs, and social activities tailored especially for people experiencing the patient's particular disease. Some patients may choose to participate in clinical research studies as a way of advancing science while managing their condition with the latest, most promising treatments.

The neurodegenerative diseases often are referred to as family diseases because the entire family is involved in and affected by the disease process. These diseases tend to have a devastating effect on all members of the family, leaving lasting and disturbing memories of loved ones. The genetic diseases, such as HD, carry the possibility that the disease has been or will be passed on to a loved one. AD, PD, MS, and MG also have possible genetic associations, thus causing additional family concerns. It is important, therefore, to refer the patient and family members for psychological and psychiatric support to assist them in dealing with the fear of developing the disease.

As with other degenerative neurological disorders, it is important to address the needs of the caregivers of patients with AD. They too will need instruction on how to best care for the patient and how to maintain their own health so they can continue to care for the patient. It is imperative that family members and caregivers be apprised of the resources available to them to assist in the actual care of the patient, in coping with the process of care and the patient's ultimate demise, and in dealing with their own concerns as caregivers.

Discharge Priorities

Discharge priorities focus on direct care of the patient in the home setting. Suggestions for both the patient and the family are included. Primary issues of protecting patient safety when performing self-care, taking medications, and resuming normal activities (as much as possible) are addressed. See the Patient Teaching & Discharge Priorities box for AD on page 607.

Other Forms of Dementia

Besides AD, other primary dementias include vascular dementia, Lewy body dementia, and frontotemporal dementia. While the diagnostic work-up for any form of dementia is the same, treatments for some types of dementia will make symptoms of other types worse; therefore, it is important to distinguish the type of dementia afflicting the patient. For example, antipsychotic drugs are used to treat frontotemporal dementia, but they may cause an adverse reaction in the patient with Lewy body dementia. Neuroleptic sensitivity could worsen the motor symptoms. The unique clinical and pathologic characteristics of and the treatment for various forms of dementia are summarized in Chart 23–1.

Parkinson's Disease

Parkinson's disease (PD) is second to Alzheimer's disease as the most common of the neurological degenerative disorders (Hauser et al., 2011). PD is a slowly progressive major disorder of the central nervous system that alters the brain centers that regulate movement (Barker, 2008).

Epidemiology and Etiology

PD is diagnosed in approximately 60,000 Americans each year, and an estimated 7 to 10 million people worldwide have the disease

NURSING PROCESS: Patient Care Plan for Alzheimer's Disease

Assessment of Neurologic Status Using Gordon's Functional Health Patterns:

- Health Perception Health Management Pattern
- Activity Exercise Pattern
- Cognitive Perceptual Pattern

Subjective Data

Assessment of Safety and Self-Care Ability

(Involve family members.)

Does the patient fall frequently?

Has the patient been hurt as a result of falling?

Does the patient wander?

Does the patient wear glasses or a hearing aid?

Does the patient use a walker?

Assessment of Cognition and Thought Processes

(Involve family members.)

Does the patient hear voices or see things that are not there?

Is the patient easily agitated?

Does the patient act impulsively?

Assessment of ADLs

(Involve family members.)

Does the patient bathe, groom, and dress independently?

Are these activities accomplished appropriately?

Does the patient become agitated during these activities?

Does the patient require assistance with self-care activities?

Do you have an established schedule for these activities?

Objective Data

Assessment of Safety and Self-Care Ability

Neurological status, including orientation, memory, sensory, gait judgment, and insight.

Wandering behavior.

Assessment of Cognition and Thought Processes

Neurological status, including orientation, memory, sensory, gait judgment, and insight.

Ability to follow instructions.

Agitation/restlessness.

Paranoia.

Assessment of ADLs

Neurological status, including orientation, memory, sensory, gait judgment, insight, apraxia, and agnosia.

Appearance.

Ability to draw bath or start shower, brush teeth, and select and put on clothing.

Ability to follow instructions.

Outcomes and Evaluation Parameters / Planning and Interventions with *Rationales*

1. NURSING DIAGNOSIS: High Risk for Injury *related to poor memory, insight, judgment, and self-control; unstable gait* (NANDA-I © 2012)

Outcome: Patient remains injury free.

Evaluation Parameters: Patient uses sensory aids and assistive devices.

Family identifies potential environmental hazards.

Patient does not fall.

Patient does not wander.

Encourage use of eyeglasses, hearing aids, and assistive devices such as a walker. *Optimal eyesight and hearing will help the patient with environmental awareness; assistive devices will stabilize gait.*

Remove potential hazards from the environment such as sharp objects and medications *to prevent patient from harming self.*

Ensure that the patient has an identification bracelet.

Encourage the family to register the patient with the Safe Return program of the Alzheimer's Association. *Patient may wander and cause harm to self or others.*

2. NURSING DIAGNOSIS: Disturbed Thought Processes (inappropriate reactions, dysfunctional behavior, delusions, and paranoia) *related to cognitive decline* (NANDA-I © 2012)

Outcome: Remains oriented to the extent possible given the stage of the disease.

Evaluation Parameter: Demonstrates fewer episodes of agitation, delusions, paranoia, or other dysfunctional behavior.

When communicating with the patient:

Approach the patient in a gentle, calm manner *to prevent the patient from being startled or frightened.*

Communicate using short, simple sentences and yes/no questions. *Negative feedback leads to increased confusion and agitation.*

Break directions down into short, simple steps. *Unable to follow complex directions; decreases frustration.*

Redirect conversation without contradicting or criticizing the patient's statements *to decrease anxiety, frustration.*

Maintain consistent daily schedule *to decrease anxiety; situational anxiety due to change can lead to agitation.*

Monitor for nonverbal behaviors such as grimacing or increased restlessness. *May indicate pain or discomfort, which may increase agitation.*

Create calming environment. Eliminate noise and clutter. *Sensory overload can contribute to disruptive behavior and agitation.*

NURSING PROCESS: Patient Care Plan for Alzheimer's Disease, *continued*

	Provide cues to orientation including verbal cues, clocks, and calendars. *Reorients patient to reality as much as possible.* Display pictures and mementos, and encourage reminiscence. *Can comfort patient and trigger memories.*
3. NURSING DIAGNOSIS: Self-Care Deficits (bathing, hygiene, dressing, grooming) *related to cognitive losses, impaired judgment* (NANDA-I © 2012)	
Outcome: Self-care needs are met. ***Evaluation Parameters:*** Performs self-care independently to the extent possible given the disease's progression. Daily routine of bathing, hygiene, dressing, and grooming is established with the patient and family. Staff and family assist with self-care needs.	Assist the patient to perform self-care activities such as bathing, dressing, and toileting *to obtain a baseline assessment of ability.* Keep instructions short, simple, and repeat frequently *to allow patient to perform activities; complicated directions can lead to frustration and agitation.* Avoid distractions during bathing, toileting, and dressing. *Sensory overload contributes to agitation and confusion.* Allow sufficient time to perform activities. *Rushing the patient may lead to agitation.* Provide privacy during self-care activities *to demonstrate respect for patient.* Maintain consistent schedule for bathing, dressing, and toileting. *Establishing routine may help decrease agitation during self-care tasks.* Provide care that patient is not able to do *to ensure that all care tasks are completed.*

Source: Adapted from Wilkinson, J. M., & Ahearn, N. R. (2009). *Prentice Hall nursing diagnosis handbook* (9th ed.). Upper Saddle River, NJ: Prentice Hall.

PATIENT TEACHING & DISCHARGE PRIORITIES for Alzheimer's Disease

Need	Teaching
Medication management: Patient/family	Adhere to medication schedule. Monitor response to medication. Monitor and report side effects.
Disease process: Patient/family	Describe diagnostic tests. Describe pathophysiology; cause not known. State signs, symptoms, and stages of disease progression. Describe possible treatments.
Activities of daily living: Family setting	Use wall calendar to mark events and activities to aid orientation and mark passage of time. Place clocks prominently around the house. Keep belongings consistently in one place. Use automatic dialing phone. Keep bathing and dressing routines consistent.
Safety: Family setting	Remove potential hazards. Cover the electrical outlets to prevent shock. Put locks on the cabinets that contain potentially hazardous materials such as medications, cleaning agents, kitchen appliances, knives, or razor blades. Store firearms in a locked area. Lower the water heater temperature to avoid burns. Remove furniture with sharp corners or pad the corners. Serve food on plastic plates to prevent breakage. Use professionally installed safety rails in the bathroom and stairway. Hide car keys if necessary. Use a signaling device if wandering is a problem. Enroll in the Alzheimer's Association's Safe Return program.
Managing wandering, aggression, agitation: Family	Reduce stressful situations. Establish daily routines. Simplify surroundings. Look for signs of pain or illness. Encourage light exercise, walking if possible.
Communication: Family	Listen and communicate patiently and in a calm, relaxed manner. Replace contradicting with listening and questioning in a caring manner. Use words or pictures to cue memories.

(*continued*)

Weblink: Fisher Center for Alzheimer's Research Foundation

Weblink: Common types of Dementia

Weblink: Alzheimer's Disease

PATIENT TEACHING & DISCHARGE PRIORITIES for Alzheimer's Disease, *continued*

Need	Teaching
Community resources: Family	Contact the Alzheimer's Association (1-800-272-3900) and its local chapter for information about the disease process, managing symptoms, and local support groups. Enroll in the Alzheimer's Association's Safe Return program if wandering is a problem. Contact a local area agency on aging for home care, respite, or adult day care referrals.
End-of-life issues: Patient/family	Establish an advance directive and/or living will. Explore the option of using hospice services.
Caregiver issues: Family	State the signs/symptoms of increasing stress and burnout. Get adequate rest. Eat balanced meals and nutritious foods. Exercise. Use relaxation techniques such as deep breathing or meditation. Use community resources for assistance and respite. Attend caregiver support groups.

Source: Fischer Center for Alzheimer's Research Foundation. (2011). *Alzheimer's disease cause, care, & cure.* Alzheimer's Research Foundation. Retrieved from http://www.alzinfo.org.

CHART 23–1 Overview of Other Common Types of Dementia

Type	Characteristics	Pathology	Treatment
Vascular dementia	Most common form of dementia after AD Abrupt onset with stepwise deterioration Focal neurological symptoms; signs or history of stroke Impaired learning, retention of new information, handling new tasks, and reasoning ability	Multiple infarcts on MRI	There is not yet a known cure for vascular dementia, so prevention is important. The best way to prevent vascular dementia is to lower the risk of stroke. This means getting high blood pressure under control, avoiding cigarettes, and controlling cholesterol levels and diabetes. Medications may be used to treat underlying symptoms such as hypertension, lipidemia, hyperglycemia, and blood clotting. Cholinesterase inhibitors and memantine (drugs used to treat Alzheimer's disease) also may be used to treat cognitive changes (e.g., judgment, planning, and memory).
Lewy body dementia (LBD)	Gradual onset Fluctuating cognitive deficits Noticeable variations in attention and alertness Parkinsonian symptoms (rigidity, bradykinesia) not responsive to levodopa Visual hallucinations Excessive daytime sleepiness and altered arousal	Lewy bodies (identified on brain autopsy) present in cytoplasm of cortical neurons	There is no cure for LBD. Treatments are aimed at controlling the cognitive, psychiatric, and motor symptoms of the disorder. Acetylcholinesterase inhibitors, such as donepezil and rivastigmine, are primarily used to treat the cognitive symptoms of LBD, but they may also be of some benefit in reducing the psychiatric and motor symptoms. Doctors tend to avoid prescribing antipsychotics for hallucinatory symptoms of LBD because of the risk that neuroleptic sensitivity could worsen the motor symptoms. Some individuals with LBD may benefit from the use of levodopa for their rigidity and loss of spontaneous movement.
Frontotemporal dementia (FTD)	Insidious onset Slowly progressive Psychiatric symptoms include uninhibited behavior, delusions, and social inappropriateness Neglect of hygiene/grooming Incontinence Change in eating patterns	Atrophy of frontal lobes and anterior temporal lobes Neuronal loss Tau tangles Gliosis	There's no cure for frontotemporal dementia and no effective way to slow its progression. Treatment relies on managing the symptoms. Antidepressants and antipsychotics may be used to control behavioral symptoms. Some types of antidepressants, such as trazodone (Desyrel, Oleptro), may reduce the behavioral problems associated with frontotemporal dementia. Selective serotonin reuptake inhibitors (SSRIs) have also been effective in some cases, although study results have been mixed. Antipsychotic drugs are sometimes used to combat the behavioral problems of frontotemporal dementia, side effects can include an increased risk of mortality in older people. Individuals with language difficulties may benefit from speech therapy.

Sources: Block, J., Smith, M., & Segal, J. (2012). Vascular dementia. *HELPGUIDE.org.* Retrieved from http://www.helpguide.org/elder/vascular_dementia.htm; Crystal, H. (2011). Alzheimer's disease. MedicineNet.com. Retrieved from http://www.medicinenet.com/alzheimers_disease_causes_stages_and_symptoms/article.htm; Halloran, L. (2011). Dementia: Forget about it! *The Journal for Nurse Practitioners, 7*(3), 242–243; Mayo Clinic Staff. (2011). Frontotemporal dementia. MayoClinic.com. Retrieved from http://www.mayoclinic.com/health/frontemporal-dementia/DS00874/DSECTION=treat; Meiner, S.E. (2011). *Gerontologic nursing* (4th ed.). St. Louis, MO: Mosby Inc.; National Institute of Neurological Disorders and Stroke, 2011e; Rakel, R., & Rakel, D. (2011). *Textbook of family medicine* (8th ed.). Philadelpha: Elsevier Saunders.

GENETIC CONSIDERATIONS
Related to Parkinson's Disease

Several recent studies confirm that PD is more common in relatives of PD patients than in people who have no relatives affected with PD. Studies of PD in twins have concluded that genetic factors do not play a significant role in those with onset commencing after age 50; however, genetic factors may be at work in earlier onset cases. While genetic research has linked mutations in the alpha-synuclein and parkin genes to PD, only about 1% of cases are clearly genetic (Schapira, 2009). However, recent studies have found that mutations in six genes have been unequivocally linked to PD (Klein & Djarmati, 2011). One such study found that "among 953 patients with the early-onset form of PD, approximately 17% harbored a mutation in one of these genes" (Klein & Djarmati, 2011, p. 1). These findings of possible genetic connections to PD raise important issues concerning genetic testing and genetic counseling for early-onset PD. These issues include consideration of the patient's rights versus the value of withholding information (e.g., Do people want to know if they are genetically predisposed to PD?). Is it appropriate to warn people of a possible fate of PD? How will this affect them now? Do they have appropriate coping mechanisms in place to handle this potential diagnosis? Is it a person's right to know if she may potentially develop this disease?

(Parkinson's Disease Foundation, 2011). The average age of onset is about 60 years, with occurrence in men more than in women (Bader & Littlejohns, 2010).

Although the cause of idiopathic PD is not known, both genetic and environmental factors have been implicated (Ferri, 2011). The consequential disease process appears to result from a complex interaction between genetic and environmental factors that differ from one individual to another (Hauser et al., 2011). (See the Genetic Considerations and Risk Factors boxes.)

Pathophysiology

Parkinson's disease is a disease of the basal ganglia, a structure deep in the brain that includes the corpus striatum and globus pallidus (Figures 23–6◆ and 23–7◆). These structures are critical to the system of connections that joins the cerebral cortex and the thalamus and allows for ease of movement. The origin of PD pathology lies in the **substantia nigra,** a structure located in the midbrain, beneath the basal ganglia. Neurons in the substantia nigra produce dopamine, a neurotransmitter that is necessary for smooth, voluntary movement. Through the connections of the nigrostriatal pathway, dopamine is transmitted from the substantia nigra to the striatum. This cycle allows for the smoothness and ease of normal, voluntary movement. In PD, the neurons of the substantia nigra inexplicably begin to degenerate and die. The resulting lack of dopamine production leads to difficulty with movement, tremor, rigidity, and difficulty maintaining posture.

When approximately 70% of the neurons in the substantia nigra have degenerated and/or died, the symptoms of PD begin to appear. Acetylcholine, another neurotransmitter, also is believed to be involved in the pathology. The lack of dopamine upsets the delicate balance between these two neurotransmitters. The defining pathologic feature of PD is the presence of Lewy bodies and neuronal loss in the substantia nigra (Schapira, 2009). Lewy bodies are detected only at brain autopsy, which is required for a definitive diagnosis of PD.

Several medications can cause parkinsonian symptoms, although they do not cause the idiopathic form of PD. These symptoms are often called drug-induced parkinsonism, or pseudo-parkinsonism. Drugs that can cause symptoms of PD include neuroleptics, such as haloperidol and risperidone, and antiemetics, such as prochlorpromazine and metoclopramide. Withdrawal from the offending agents will reverse the parkinsonian symptoms, although this can take weeks and possibly months. Since antipsychotic drugs can induce parkinsonism, older patients with a history of Parkinson's should be monitored closely when prescribed these medications. Antipsychotic drugs prescribed for behavior management should be used only for a short period of time. Atypical antipsychotic medications should be avoided in patients with dementia, if possible; if they are used, the patient must be monitored closely for the potential cerebrovascular or cardiovascular adverse effects and signs of infection (Lindsey, 2009).

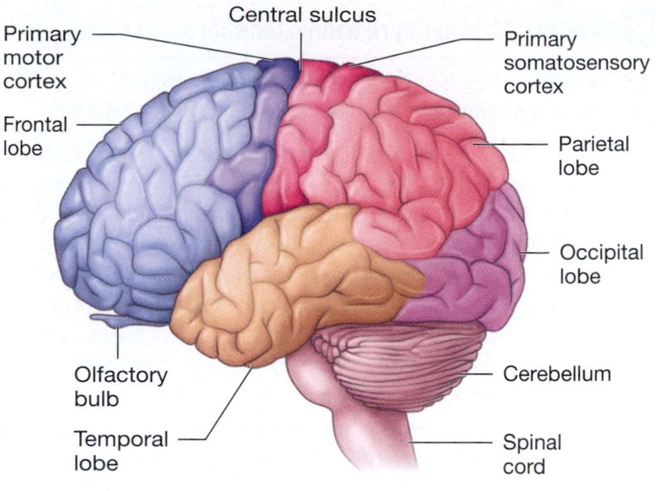

FIGURE 23–6 ◆ Cerebral hemispheres and brainstem.

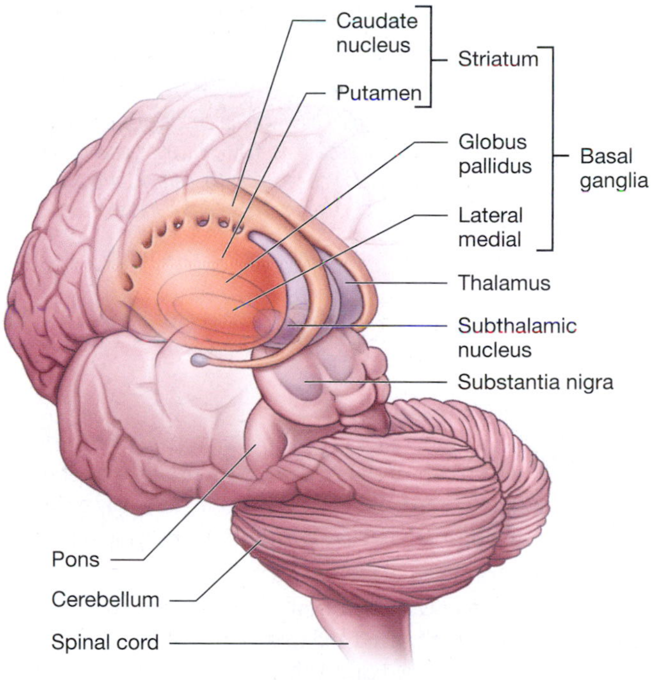

FIGURE 23–7 ◆ Main connections of the basal ganglia.

RISK FACTORS for Parkinson's Disease

Without a known cause, definitive risk factors for idiopathic PD are not clear. However, certain factors have been linked with PD, including the following:

Advancing Age. Although the disease occasionally develops in young adults, it most often manifests itself in the middle to late years of life. The risk continues to increase the older one gets. Some researchers assume that people with PD have neural damage from genetic or environmental factors that get worse as they age.

Sex. Males are more likely to get PD than females are. Possible reasons for this may be that males have greater exposure to other risk factors such as toxin exposure or head trauma. It has been theorized that estrogen may have neuroprotective effects. In the case of genetic predisposition, a gene that predisposes one to PD may be linked to the X chromosome.

Family History. Having one or more close relatives with PD increases the likelihood of getting it, though to a minimal degree. This lends support to the idea that there is a genetic link in developing Parkinson's.

Declining Estrogen Levels. Postmenopausal women who do not use hormone replacement therapy are at greater risk, as are women who have had hysterectomies.

Agricultural Work. Exposure to an environmental toxin such as a pesticide or herbicide puts one at greater risk. Some of these toxins inhibit dopamine production and promote free radical damage. Those who have been involved in farming and are therefore exposed to such toxins have a greater prevalence of Parkinson's symptoms.

Genetic Factors. An international study led by the Mayo Clinic Staff (2011) revealed that the gene alpha-synuclein may play a role in the likelihood of developing the disease. Studies showed that individuals with a more active alpha-synuclein gene had a 1.5 times greater risk of developing Parkinson's. These findings support the development of alpha-synuclein-suppressing therapies, which may in the long run slow or even halt the disease.

Low Levels of B Vitamin Folate. Researchers discovered that mice with a deficiency of this vitamin developed severe PD symptoms, while mice with normal levels did not.

Head Trauma. Recent research points to a link between damage to the head, neck, or upper cervical spine and PD. "A 2007 study of 60 patients showed that all of them showed evidence of trauma induced upper cervical damage. Some patients remembered a specific incident; others did not. In some cases, PD symptoms took decades to appear" (Parkinson's Disease Information, 2009).

Safety Alert *The nurse should be aware of common drugs that are contraindicated in Parkinson's disease as they can cause adverse and dangerous effects in the patient, such as tachycardia, cardiac arrest, laryngospasm, respiratory depression, and seizures. These drugs include:*

Antiemetics: *Prochlorperazine (Compazine) and metoclopramide (Reglan), and*

Neuroleptics: *Chlorpromazine (Thorazine) and haloperidol (Haldol)*

(Adams & Koch, 2010; Lindsey, 2009)

Clinical Manifestations

PD is characterized by four primary symptoms: resting tremor, rigidity, bradykinesia, and postural instability, which are all described in the following text. Secondary and autonomic symptoms also may be present. They often result from combinations of the primary symptoms.

Primary Symptoms

A parkinsonian tremor characteristically occurs at rest and manifests as involuntary shaking in the hand and wrist or feet while the muscles are relaxed. The tremor may decrease with activity. Lack of coordination is usually noted, and approximately 20% of patients first experience clumsiness in one hand (Hauser et al., 2011). The tremor usually is present only on one side of the body in the early stages of PD but may spread to the other side as the disease progresses. A "pill-rolling" action of the hand is classically seen in parkinsonian tremor (National Institute of Neurological Disorders and Strokes [NINDS], 2011f).

Rigidity, or muscle stiffness, may be felt throughout any given range of movement. Typically, parkinsonian rigidity is characterized as hypertonicity of muscles resulting in stiffness of motion and is often associated with aching and discomfort. Cogwheel rigidity is an abnormal rigor in muscles that are passively stretched; it often is likened to a ratcheting-link rhythm reminiscent of a circular jerking rigidity which continues throughout an entire range of movement and occurs mainly in the hands (Hickey, 2009).

Bradykinesia (slowness of movement), one of the more disabling symptoms of PD, is often the most prominent and disabling symptom. It also be particularly frustrating, since it is unpredictable (Goldenberg, 2008).

Postural disturbances comprise postural instability or flexed posture. Patients with PD have the tendency to have a stooped or flexed posture. In advanced stages of the disease, postural instability may occur with retropulsion (the inability to prevent oneself from going backwards) or propulsion (the inability to prevent oneself from forward motion) (Barker, 2008).

Secondary Symptoms

Secondary symptoms of PD usually are the result of the overarching, primary symptoms. For example, rigid facial muscles combined with bradykinesia lead to **hypomimia,** or decreased facial expression, resulting in the characteristic "masked" face of a PD patient. The decrease in facial expression often conveys lack of emotion or a depressed affect, which may or may not actually be what the person feels. Muscle rigidity, bradykinesia, and postural instability may combine to produce gait abnormalities, such as a shuffled walk, difficulty turning while walking, and stooped posture. Face and neck muscles used for talking may be affected as well (Goldenberg, 2008; Perlmutter, 2010). Voice changes associated with PD are known as **hypokinetic dysarthria.** They include **hypophonia,** or a soft, muffled speech. Similarly, the muscles used for swallowing become rigid, leading to dysphagia, or difficulty swallowing. **Micrographia,** or small, cramped handwriting, results from rigidity and bradykinesia in the hands (Barker, 2008; Ropper & Samuels, 2009).

Autonomic Symptoms

PD affects the autonomic nervous system, which can lead to symptoms not related to movement. Constipation is common; PD medications as well as inactivity, eating a poor diet, or drinking too little fluids may exacerbate it. Orthostatic hypotension, sexual dysfunction, excessive sweating, and urinary incontinence or difficulty urinating are other common symptoms (Barker, 2008; Goldenberg, 2008).

Neuropsychiatric Symptoms

The incidence of neuropsychiatric changes and cognitive impairments, including dementia, ranges from 20% to 40% with PD (Weintraub, Cornella, & Horn, 2008). Up to 50% of people with PD may suffer from depression. However, the depression may be underdiagnosed because some of the symptoms, particularly fatigue and insomnia, may be regarded as part of PD or aging (Vernon, 2009).

Disease Progression

As PD progresses, motor complications develop. **Dyskinesias**—involuntary, writhing motions that may involve the limbs, trunk, face, and neck—are a side effect of dopaminergic medications and result from overstimulation of dopamine receptors. Drug therapy regimes can create fluctuations in movement ability, known as **on–off phenomena.** When "on," the patient is experiencing a positive response to medication, but the effects may suddenly wear off, rendering the patient barely able to move, or "off." These reactions are related to building a tolerance to the medication or having an unpredictable response to it (Goldenberg, 2008). Dyskinesia and the associated motor fluctuations can cause a great diversity and range of physical capacity and disability during the course of an average day. The unpredictable nature of these fluctuations interferes greatly with the patient's ability to plan for and perform routine activities.

As motor function worsens, so can other PD symptoms. Dysphagia often worsens over time, and a feeding tube may be required to prevent the aspiration of food. In addition, worsening orthostatic hypotension and postural instability increase the risk of injuries resulting from a fall (Bader & Littlejohns, 2010). Although PD is not considered a fatal disease, the degrading effect it has on the patient's ability to carry out basic daily functions can cause susceptibility to more threatening conditions such as pneumonia or traumatic injury.

Laboratory and Diagnostic Procedures

There is no definitive laboratory or radiological test to diagnose PD. Diagnosis is based on a neurological exam and clinical history. In addition, laboratory tests and MRI are used to rule out other possible causes of the presenting symptoms. The positive response to dopaminergic medications reinforces the PD diagnosis.

Medical Management

Diagnostic criteria for PD include the following: bradykinesia and either resting tremor or rigidity; persistent asymmetry; clinical course lasting 10 years or more; positive response to levodopa; and other causes ruled out, such as drugs, stroke, or metabolic abnormalities. Definite diagnosis is made only by autopsy.

PD is commonly staged using the Hoehn and Yahr scale (1967):

- ***Stage I:*** Unilateral disease
- ***Stage II:*** Bilateral disease with preservation of postural reflexes
- ***Stage III:*** Bilateral disease with impaired postural reflexes; able to ambulate
- ***Stage IV:*** Severe disease requiring assistance
- ***Stage V:*** End-stage disease, confined to bed or chair (Barker, 2008; Meiner, 2010).

An effective treatment for protecting against the loss of dopamine-producing neurons remains to be discovered. Because PD involves the loss of dopamine-producing neurons and the subsequent diminished supply of dopamine in the striatum, dopaminergic drugs that can increase dopamine levels are the first line of treatment. Treatment of the secondary symptoms such as hypotension and constipation also is included in a broad approach to increase mobility, decrease symptoms, and improve quality of life, as the underlying disease progresses despite all treatments. There is no neuroprotective therapy that has shown any proven value. For example, nutritional supplementation does not cure or diminish the symptoms of PD.

Dopaminergic drugs enhance the levels of dopamine that are naturally produced in the brain. Levodopa was the first breakthrough in treatment for PD in the 1960s, and it is still considered the most effective drug for PD (Meiner, 2010; Poewe, 2009). Dopamine itself cannot cross the blood–brain barrier (Neuwelt et al., 2008), so the next best way to reduce symptoms is with levodopa, the amino acid precursor of dopamine, which can cross the blood–brain barrier. Once in the brain, levodopa is converted to dopamine (Neuwelt et al., 2008). However, a portion of levodopa is converted into dopamine by dopa-decarboxylase before the levodopa enters the brain, leaving dopamine in the circulating system and causing severe nausea and vomiting.

Levodopa is given with carbidopa, a dopa-decarboxylase inhibitor, which blocks premature conversion of levodopa into dopamine and minimizes nausea and vomiting (Vernon, 2009). A combination of carbidopa and levodopa is available in tablet form in various dosage combinations. For example, carbidopa/levodopa 25/100 tablets contain 25 mg of carbidopa and 100 mg of levodopa. The first number indicates milligrams of carbidopa; the second indicates milligrams of levodopa.

Although slightly less effective than levodopa, dopamine agonists are an alternative to levodopa for initial treatment of PD (Vernon, 2009). Dopamine agonists that have been approved for the treatment of PD include bromocriptine (Parlodel), pergolide (Permax), pramipexole (Mirapex), ropinirole (Requip), and apomorphine hydrochloride (Apokyn). Dopamine agonists act on dopamine receptors within the brain and essentially mimic the effect of dopamine. Dopamine agonists are prescribed initially in very low doses and slowly titrated upward to therapeutic amounts (Buttaro, Trybulski, Bailey, & Sandberg-Cook, 2008; Vernon, 2009).

Anticholinergics, the oldest class of medications used to treat PD, were commonly used before the discovery of levodopa. These medications are used primarily to treat tremor (Goldenberg, 2008). The most commonly prescribed medications in this category are trihexyphenidyl (Artane) and benztropine (Cogentin) (Hickey, 2009).

Catechol-O-methyltransferase (COMT) is an enzyme that metabolizes levodopa and dopamine. Inhibiting COMT abates the peripheral metabolism of levodopa, thereby prolonging the half-life of levodopa and providing more levodopa for transportation across the blood–brain barrier over a longer period of time (Hauser et al., 2011). Because they increase the effective duration of the levodopa dosage, COMT inhibitors are effective only when taken in conjunction with levodopa. They are used most often to counteract wearing-off responses (the effects of medication will start to wear off in between doses) (Barker, 2008). Approved COMT inhibitors are tolcapone (Tasmar) and entacapone (Comtan). Tolcapone is used less often because of the risk of liver toxicity. Stalevo combines both levodopa/carbidopa and entacapone into one tablet.

Amantadine, an antiviral drug, has proven to provide modest improvement for PD symptoms. It is particularly useful for treating dyskinesia (Barker, 2008). Inhibition of the enzyme monoamine oxidase type B (MAO-B) interferes with the metabolism of dopamine. Although the MAO-B inhibitor selegiline was thought to prevent degeneration of dopamine-producing neurons and delay the progression of PD, studies suggested that the effects may be more symptomatic than protective. Nonetheless, selegiline reduces the metabolism of dopamine, does improve PD symptoms, and slows the progression of PD symptoms by about 35% over 5 years (George et al, 2009; Vernon, 2009; Walsh et al., 2008). Other medications can be used to treat secondary symptoms of PD, including depression, cognitive changes, sleep problems, and genitourinary issues. The Pharmacology box (p. 598) provides more information about medications for Parkinson's disease.

Safety Alert *Meperidine, tricyclics, and selective serotonin reuptake inhibitors should not be given to patients taking selegiline because of the risk of fatal drug interaction (Walsh et al., 2008).*

Surgical Approaches

Neurosurgical intervention is an option reserved for certain carefully selected patients with advanced PD. Surgical treatments include ablative procedures, deep brain stimulation, and cell transplantation. Ablative procedures include thalamotomy and pallidotomy, which is the surgical placement of a permanent lesion in the thalamus or the globus pallidus, respectively. Ablative procedures are older procedures and rarely used today.

Deep brain stimulation (DBS) (Figure 23–8◆) has become the surgical option of choice for PD because it does not involve destruction of brain tissue and is reversible. In addition, bilateral procedures can be done without a significant increase in adverse events and the deep brain stimulation may be adjusted as the disease progresses. DBS involves surgically placing electrodes in targeted areas of the brain. As with ablative procedures, the most common targets are specific areas within the subthalamic nucleus or globus pallidus. The electrodes are attached to an external pacemaker-like device that is implanted underneath the collarbone. High-frequency stimulation provides effects similar to ablative surgery (Deiner & Hagen, 2009; Hauser et al., 2011). Like PD drug treatments, surgical interventions do not cure the disease but may alleviate symptoms.

Complementary and alternative therapies also may be used to treat PD. One such alternative exercise, is discussed in the Complementary & Alternative Therapies box.

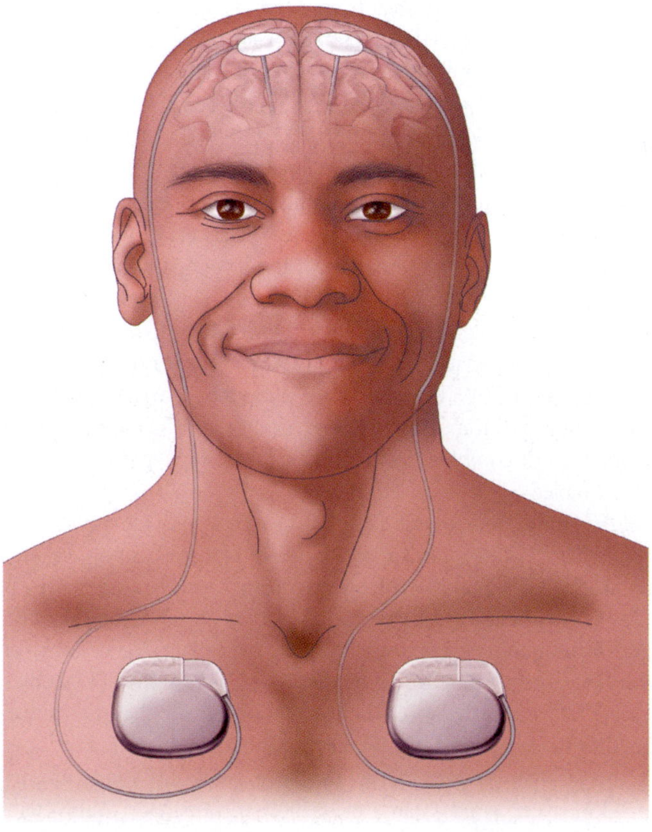

FIGURE 23–8 ◆ Parkinson's control therapy: deep brain stimulation.

Nursing Management

Application of the nursing process will facilitate a comprehensive approach to patient care for the patient with PD throughout the disease process. Many of the patient diagnoses and resultant care plans for patients with PD are the same as they are for patients with AD. However, with PD, there is more emphasis on maintaining independence and fostering the ability to communicate. See the Nursing Process: Patient Care Plan for Parkinson's Disease on page 614.

Health promotion and collaborative management are critical aspects of caring for patients with PD. The patient's health status often is compromised because PD is chronic and progressive. The patient's ability to care for self deteriorates and the patient becomes dependent on others to complete all self-care functions and to perform normal daily activities. The patient comes to rely on caretakers and a team of professional caregivers to maintain functionality. These topics are discussed on pages 628–630.

Discharge Priorities

Specific educational needs are addressed in the Patient Teaching & Discharge Priorities box (p. 616).

Amyotrophic Lateral Sclerosis

Amyotrophic lateral sclerosis (ALS) is a degenerative disease involving upper and lower motor neurons. Degeneration of motor neurons in the spinal cord, brainstem, and cerebral cortex leads to the characteristic symptoms of weakness, muscular atrophy, and spasticity. ALS, also known as Lou Gehrig's disease, is progressive, incurable, and fatal (Hickey, 2009).

Epidemiology and Etiology

Approximately 20,000 to 30,000 Americans have ALS. Another 5,000 diagnoses are made each year (NINDS, 2011a). In the 1930s, Lou Gehrig, a baseball player for the New York Yankees, was diagnosed with ALS; that is why the disease is identified by his name in the United States. His celebrity has brought recognition to this disease in terms of public awareness and research funding (Bradley, Daroff, Fenichel, & Jankovic, 2008).

The annual incidence rate of ALS is 0.4 to 1.74 per 100,000 population, and the disease affects nearly twice as many men as women. The onset of ALS typically occurs between 40 and 60 years of age; however, it can affect younger and older people (Ropper & Samuels, 2009).

The cause of ALS is unknown. The excitatory neurotransmitter glutamate is believed to have a part in motor neuron degeneration (Hickey, 2009). Other investigations have focused on autoimmune responses, environmental toxins, and infectious agents. Still, there is insufficient evidence to implicate any of these factors as causes of ALS (Bradley et al., 2008). A genetic link to ALS is possible, as discussed in the Genetic Considerations box.

Pathophysiology

In ALS, degenerative changes occur in the anterior horn cells of the spinal cord, the motor nuclei of the brainstem, and the corticospinal tracts. Upper motor neuron degeneration leads to spasticity and reduced muscle strength, while lower motor neuron degeneration causes flaccid muscles, paralysis, and atrophy. Cognition, sensory function, vision, and hearing are spared. Bowel and bladder functions are not affected until the later stages of the disease (Hickey, 2009).

Clinical Manifestations

Subtle at onset and slow in progression, the symptoms of ALS include painless muscle weakness and wasting, spasticity, cramping, fatigue,

COMPLEMENTARY & ALTERNATIVE THERAPIES Exercise to Treat Chronic Neurological Disorders

Nancy Yilk

AMONG THE FEARED EFFECTS OF AGING are loss of memory, cognitive decline, and loss of independence. Baby boomers have entered the "aged" group and are actively seeking ways to maintain strong bodies and minds. Clinical research suggests that keeping physically active and engaging in moderate to vigorous exercise may be vital to brain health. Exercise promotes neurogenesis, increased brain volume, and improved cognitive function; it also can help the aging brain to retain plasticity (Marks, Katz, & Smith, 2009).

There is a wealth of information suggesting that preventive strategies for neurodegenerative disorders may be more successful than treatments that exist today, primarily because of the fact that behavioral problems do not manifest until a majority of neurons are already dysfunctional or have undergone cell death, and general disease processes in the brain are already rampant (Granholm et al., 2008).

One of the mechanics of aging is the hippocampus shrinking in late adulthood, leading to impaired memory and increased risk for dementia. Studies have investigated whether the loss of volume of the hippocampus is inevitable, or if it could be reversed with exercise. To test this, 120 older adults without dementia were randomly assigned to an aerobic exercise group ($n = 60$) or to a stretching control group ($n = 60$), where they would exercise three times a week for a 1-year period. Magnetic resonance images were collected before the intervention, after 6 months, and again after the completion of the program. The groups did not differ at baseline in hippocampal volume or attendance rates.

Aerobic fitness (VO2 max) was assessed by graded maximal exercise testing on a motor-driven treadmill. The participants walked at a speed slightly faster than their normal walking pace, with increasing grade increments of 2% every 2 minutes. For the stretching and toning control, all sessions were led and monitored by trained exercise leaders. All classes started and ended with warm-up and cool-down stretching. During each class, participants engaged in four muscle-toning exercises using dumbbells or resistance bands, two exercises designed to improve balance, one yoga sequence, and one exercise of their choice. To maintain interest, a new group of exercises was introduced every 3 weeks. The results indicated that exercise training increased hippocampal volume by 2%, effectively reversing age-related loss in volume by 1 to 2 years. Correspondingly, results were consistent with the pattern of the hippocampal volume shrinking as we age, as the members of the stretching group experienced a 1.4% decline in volume over the 1-year interval (Erickson et al., 2011).

Other research investigated the effectiveness of exercise in improving the ability of a person with Alzheimer's disease (AD) to perform activities of daily living (ADLs) and physical performance. To research this, a study used 140 ambulatory patients with mild to severe AD from five participating nursing homes. Participants were randomly assigned into two groups of a collective exercise program. One group participated in 1-hour, twice-weekly, walking, strength, balance, and flexibility training; the control group did not. Both groups received routine medical care for 12 months. The ADL mean change from the baseline score for exercise program patients showed a slower decline than in patients receiving routine medical care without the exercise program (12-month mean treatment differences: $ADL = 0.39, P = 0.02$). A significant difference between the groups in favor of the exercise program was observed for 6-meter walking speed at 12 months. In the intervention group, adherence to the program sessions in exploratory analysis predicted change in the person's ability to perform ADLs. The results indicate that a simple exercise program, for 1 hour twice a week, led to a significantly slower decline in the ADL score (Rolland et al., 2007).

References

Erickson, K. I., Voss, M. W., Prakash, R. S., Basak, C., Szabo, A., Chaddock, L., et al. (2011, February 15). Exercise training increases size of hippocampus and improves memory. *The Proceedings of the National Academy of Sciences Online (U.S.), 108*(7), 3017–3022. Epub 2011 Jan 31.

Granholm, A. C., & Boger, H. (2008, July). Mood, memory and movement: An age-related neurodegenerative complex? *Current Aging Science, 1*(2), 133–139.

Marks, B. L., Katz, L. M., & Smith, J. K. (2009, April). Exercise and the aging mind: Buffing the baby boomer's body and brain. *Physician and Sportsmedicine, 37*(1), 119–125.

Ridgel, A. L., Vitek, J. L., & Alberts, J. L. (2009, July–August). Forced, not voluntary, exercise improves motor function in Parkinson's disease patients. *Neurorehabilitation and Neural Repair, 23*(6), 600–608. Epub 2009 Jan 8.

Rolland, Y., Pillard, F., Klapouszczak, A., Reynish, E., Thomas, D., Andrieu, S., et al. (2007, February). Exercise program for nursing home residents with Alzheimer's disease: A 1-year randomized, controlled trial. *Journal of the American Geriatrics Society, 55*(2), 158–165.

fasciculation (involuntary twitching) of the limb and tongue muscles, dysarthria, dysphagia, and dyspnea (Bradley et al., 2008; Hickey, 2009). Symptoms in an arm present first in roughly half of the cases; about 20% of occurrences first affect a leg. Initial complaints range from difficulty walking and problems with tripping and stumbling to trouble performing fine tasks such as buttoning clothing and writing. In 1% to 2% of people with ALS, the weakness starts in the respiratory muscles (Bradley et al., 2008; NINDS, 2011a).

As the disease progresses, weakness and atrophy extend throughout the muscles. The arms and legs become severely impaired. Muscles involved in speech and swallowing progressively deteriorate to the point of severe dysarthria and dysphagia (Barker, 2008; Bradley et al., 2008). Swallowing becomes difficult, so the risk of aspirating food or saliva into the airway increases. In addition, difficulties in eating lead to weight loss. Because cognitive functions remain intact, patients are highly aware of the disease and its progression. Anxiety or depression is likely to complicate the condition (NINDS, 2011a). In the final stage, speaking is nearly or completely impossible. Acute dyspnea sets in, and eventually a ventilator is required for breathing. Aspiration, infection, and respiratory failure are usually the ultimate causes of death. The average disease duration is 3 to 4 years (Barker, 2008; Bradley et al., 2008).

Laboratory and Diagnostic Procedures

As is the case for other neurodegenerative diseases, there is no definitive test that will confirm the presence of ALS. Diagnosis is based on medical history, neurological examination, symptoms, and laboratory tests that rule out other metabolic conditions (NINDS, 2011a). Electromyography (EMG) may distinguish characteristic fibrillations that result from denervation, muscle wasting, and atrophy (Barker, 2008). Brain and spinal MRI can detect structural lesions, herniated disks, or cervical spondylosis; this may help in eliminating other conditions that mimic ALS symptoms. In the same manner, nerve conduction velocity (NCV) tests can discount peripheral neuropathy and myopathy (NINDS, 2011a). Several different tests are commonly used to aid in the diagnosis of ALS, as presented in the Diagnostic Tests box on page 594.

Medical Management

Like other neurodegenerative diseases, ALS has no cure. Medical treatment focuses on slowing the disease progression and on symptom management. Riluzole (Rilutek), a benzothiazole, is the only drug known to slow the progression of ALS and the only drug approved by the FDA for the treatment of ALS (Barker, 2008). Riluzole is thought to protect motor neurons by inhibiting glutamate production. Patients who respond well to riluzole delay the need for ventilatory support and lengthen their life expectancies by an average of 3 months (Barker, 2008). While generally well tolerated, riluzole should be administered with strict monitoring of liver function. Dizziness, vertigo, and somnolence may result from taking the

NURSING PROCESS: Patient Care Plan for Parkinson's Disease

Assessment of Neurologic Status Using Gordon's Functional Health Patterns:

- Activity Exercise Pattern
- Cognitive Perceptual Pattern

Subjective Data

Assessment for Independent Activity

Do you have stiffness and slowness of movement?

Do these symptoms interfere with your daily activities?

Do you have trouble with balance?

Have you ever fallen?

Do you need assistance when you walk?

Do you use a cane or walker?

Does your medication regimen help your symptoms?

Do you have times during the day when you function better than at other times?

Assessment for Ability to Communicate

Do people ask you to repeat things?

Do you frequently feel misunderstood?

Do you get frustrated when trying to converse?

Assessment of Orientation to Time, Place, and Person

States name when asked.

Objective Data

Assessment for Independent Activity

Neurological status, including motor status (coordination, gait, balance, tremor, rigidity, bradykinesia).

Assessment for Ability to Communicate

Difficulty understanding patient

Lack of facial expression

Assessment of Orientation to Time, Place, and Person

Neurological status including level of consciousness, orientation, MMSE

Agitation

Visual hallucinations

Medication regimen

Signs of infection: fever

Hydration status, including intake and output

Laboratory studies including blood chemistry and CBCs

Outcomes and Evaluation Parameters / Planning and Interventions with *Rationales*

1. NURSING DIAGNOSIS: Impaired Physical Mobility *related to rigidity, bradykinesia, postural instability, altered gait* (NANDA-I © 2012)

Outcomes: Patient demonstrates maximum independent physical function.

Patient is free of immobility complications.

Evaluation Parameters: Patient maintains as much independent mobility as possible given the degree of disease progression.

Patient uses assistive devices to maximize mobility.

ADLs and therapy schedule coincide with medication peak effectiveness.

Planning and Interventions with *Rationales*

Assist the patient to ambulate and perform ADLs *to provide assessment of abilities.*

Consult with patient regarding medication schedule. *Medication schedule may be complex and may not fit traditional medication timelines.*

Schedule therapies and ADLs to coincide with optimum medication benefit. *Movement will be easier when medications are working at peak effectiveness.*

Instruct patient to stand as straight as possible and walk with a wide-based gait while swinging arms *to help maintain balance and momentum.*

Perform range of motion to all joints *to counteract the effects of rigidity.*

Encourage use of walker or other assistive device *to increase mobility by stabilizing gait.*

Use side rails or overhead trapeze on bed. *Both act as grab bars and assist with turning over in bed.*

Instruct the patient to use straight-back chairs with firm seats and arm rests when possible. *It is difficult for patients to get up from low, soft surfaces such as easy chairs or sofas.*

Consult with a physical therapist. *Can prescribe and tailor appropriate gait-assistive devices and also exercises to counteract stiffness and rigidity.*

Consult with occupational therapist. *Can assess need for adaptive aids for ADLs such as specialized eating utensils or button hook for dressing.*

NURSING PROCESS: Patient Care Plan for Parkinson's Disease, *continued*

Outcomes and Evaluation Parameters	Planning and Interventions with *Rationales*
2. NURSING DIAGNOSIS: Impaired Verbal Communication ***related to voice and speech changes and decreased facial expression*** **(NANDA-I © 2012)**	
Outcome: Patient is able to converse and communicate needs. ***Evaluation Parameters:*** Staff and family members are able to understand verbalizations. Patient and family members verbalize disease process and effect on speech and expression.	Assess and monitor for decreased voice volume, slurred or mumbled speech, and difficulties initiating speech. *Common symptoms of PD.* Observe the patient's ability to communicate needs and converse with family members. *Provides information about the impact of speech changes on family dynamics and assesses need for education.* Consult with speech-language pathologist. *Can evaluate speech difficulties and develop a treatment program, including assistive devices.* Eliminate background noise (TV, radio) while patient is speaking. *Decreases environmental interference when listening to the patient.* Allow ample time for the patient to speak and communicate. *Communicating takes longer for the patient; allowing ample time decreases stress and anxiety, which may improve speech.*
3. NURSING DIAGNOSIS: Disturbed Thought Processes (confusion, hallucinations, and delusions) ***related to cognitive changes, medication regimen, and/or infection*** **(NANDA-I © 2012)**	
Outcome: Patient remains oriented. ***Evaluation Parameters:*** Patient does not exhibit evidence of having delusions or hallucinations. Patient is oriented. Family remains calm in the event of visual hallucinations.	Assess and monitor the patient's level of cognitive functioning using a rating scale such as the MMSE. *Provides a basis of planning care.* Assess changes in the medication dosage and/or schedule and monitor for increased or decreased confusion or hallucinations and physical mobility. *Dopaminergic drugs can stimulate hallucinations or cause confusion and may need to be adjusted; these side effects may preclude a dosage high enough to improve mobility.* Assess for treatable causes of confusion such as infection, recent general anesthesia, and dehydration. *Can be sources of delirium or increased confusion.* Assess and monitor response to antipsychotic drugs. *May be prescribed to counteract hallucinations and delusions.* Reassure the patient and family during hallucinations. *Patient may or may not become frightened during hallucinations; hallucinations can be distressing to the family.* Minimize environmental hazards *to decrease the risk of injury due to confusion.*

Sources: Adapted from Ackley, B. J., & Ludwig, G. B. (Eds.). (2011). *Nursing diagnosis handbook: A guide to planning care* (9th ed.). St. Louis: Mosby; Gulanick, M., & Myers, J. L. (2011). *Nursing care plans: Diagnosis, interventions and outcomes* (7th ed.). St. Louis: Mosby; Meiner, S. (2010). *Gerontologic nursing.* St. Louis: Elsevier Mosby; Wilkinson, J. M., & Ahearn, N. R. (2009). *Prentice Hall nursing diagnosis handbook* (9th ed.). Upper Saddle River, NJ: Prentice Hall.

GENETIC CONSIDERATIONS
Related to Amyotrophic Lateral Sclerosis

Genetic research has discovered a defect occurring on the gene responsible for the production of the enzyme superoxide dismutase 1 (SODI1) that may be linked to ALS. SODI1 is a powerful antioxidant that protects against free radicals, which are thought to play a role in cell degeneration. The role of the SODI1 gene mutation in motor neuron degeneration is unclear. The theory is that the malfunctioning gene allows for an excessive accumulation of free radicals.

Between 90% and 95% of ALS cases are sporadic (appearing or happening at irregular intervals in time) while 5% to 10% are classified as familial (occurring or tending to occur in families). The SODI1 gene mutation accounts for approximately 20% of familial cases. Other familial forms involve mutations on the ALS2 gene, which also is implicated in the death of motor neurons (National Institute of Neurological Disorders and Stroke, 2011a).

drug. Other medications may be used for symptom management; these include diazepam or dantrolene for spasticity and quinine sulfate or baclofen for muscle cramping, as discussed in the Pharmacology box (p. 598).

Nursing Management

A home health care plan is critical for patients with ALS and their families. These people will be in particular need of ongoing support and assistance in coping with this progressive and fatal illness, as they will be faced with making difficult decisions regarding artificial feeding and ventilation. It is important that the choices be made before a crisis so that the patient's wishes, particularly those regarding end of life, are honored. Throughout this process, the nurse must respect cultural differences in the meaning of death and dying.

The nursing assessment, diagnoses, and expected or desired outcomes for patients with ALS are outlined in the Care Plan for ALS.

Collaborative management for ALS is discussed on pages 628–630. Many members of the interdisciplinary health care team will be included in the discharge plans for these patients.

Discharge Priorities

The Patient Teaching & Discharge Priorities box (p. 618) covers a wide range of topics that apply to the patient with ALS.

PATIENT TEACHING & DISCHARGE PRIORITIES for Parkinson's Disease

Need	Teaching
Disease process: Patient/family	Assess knowledge of disease process: PD is chronic and slowly progressive. No clear cause or cure is known. General progression through stages but progression varies from person to person. Treatment approaches.
Educational resources: Patient/family	National Parkinson Foundation (1-800-327-4545) Parkinson Disease Foundation (1-800-457-6676) American Parkinson's Disease Association (1-800-223-2732) Local support groups Internet resources
Dopaminergic medications: Patient and family	Side effects of dopaminergic medications: nausea/vomiting, light-headedness, drowsiness, confusion, and hallucinations. Take as directed, usually starting with low dose and titrating upward. Allow time to reach the dosage required for symptom improvement. Take carbidopa/levodopa 30 to 60 minutes before a meal or 1 to 2 hours after a meal for optimal absorption. Do not abruptly stop medications unless directed by health care provider. Use medication diary to track the schedule, dosage, and side effects. Need to work closely with the health care provider to arrive at optimal, individualized dosage.
Fall prevention: Family setting	Remove throw rugs. Move electrical cords out of walkways. Create clear, uncluttered walking paths. Rearrange furniture so that it is easy to get around. Install railings along hallways and on stairways. Minimize sharp edges or corners on furniture; minimize wet floors and hot surfaces. Install grab bars in the shower and next to the commode. Do not use towel racks as grab bars.
Nutrition: Patient/family	Hydration is important to counteract low blood pressure and constipation and for general health. Fiber helps to counteract constipation. Calcium is important for maintaining bone density and decreasing the risk of fracture from falls. Protein may interfere with levodopa absorption in a small percentage of patients. Take levodopa at least 30 minutes before eating or 1 hour after eating. Consult with dietitian for weight loss.
Exercise: Patient/family Setting (home/clinic)	Stress importance of the following in accordance with the patient's physical ability: • Resistance training to strengthen muscles and bones • Mild aerobic conditioning for cardiovascular health • Stretching to counteract stiffness and rigidity.
Constipation: Patient/family Setting (home/clinic/hospital)	Part of the disease process and worsened by medications. Avoid use of laxatives. May use stool softeners and bulking agents such as psyllium on a daily basis. Increase dietary fluid and fiber.
Urinary problems: Patient/family Setting (home/clinic/hospital)	Urinary frequency and/or urgency is common. Signs/symptoms of urinary tract infection (UTI): Foul-smelling urine and painful urination. Call health care provider if signs/symptoms of UTI develop.
Orthostatic hypotension: Patient/family Setting (home/clinic/hospital)	Signs of low blood pressure include light-headedness, dizziness, and fainting. Part of disease process; medications also contribute. Change the position slowly when rising from a lying or seated position. Increase fluids and salt if not contraindicated by other conditions. Use support stockings and elevate legs throughout the day. Remain seated for 20 to 30 minutes after a large meal or dose of medication. Sit down to use towel after hot bath or shower.

Sources: Bader, M. K., & Littlejohns, L. (2010). *AABN core curriculum for neuroscience nursing.* Glenview, IL: Elsevier; Hickey, J. V. (2009). *The clinical practice of neurological and neurosurgical nursing* (6th ed.). Philadelphia: Lippincott Williams & Wilkins; Meiner, S. (2010). *Gerontologic nursing.* St. Louis: Elsevier Mosby:

NURSING PROCESS: Patient Care Plan for Amyotrophic Lateral Sclerosis

Assessment of Neurologic Status Using Gordon's Functional Health Patterns:

- Activity Exercise Pattern
- Values and Belief Pattern

Subjective Data	Objective Data
Assessment for Comfort in Breathing	**Assessment for Comfort in Breathing**
Do you feel comfortable? Do you have a headache? Do you feel tired?	Neurological status including level of consciousness and cognition Vital signs Respiratory status, including respiration rate, pattern, lung sounds, accessory muscles, pulmonary function studies Skin and nail bed color Restlessness
Assessment for Ability to Swallow Foods and Liquids	**Assessment for Ability to Swallow Foods and Liquids**
Do you feel like you have trouble swallowing foods or liquids? Are you afraid of choking?	Neurological assessment including swallowing and gag reflex Vital signs Respiratory status including rate and lung sounds Choking on foods or liquids Tube feedings Swallowing studies
Assessment for Psychological and Spiritual Comfort	**Assessment for Psychological and Spiritual Comfort**
Do you have a spiritual counselor? Has your family ever experienced loss and/or death?	Patient/family interactions Patient/family cultural background and religious preferences Use of spiritual resources

Outcomes and Evaluation Parameters	Planning and Interventions with *Rationales*
1. NURSING DIAGNOSIS: Ineffective Breathing Pattern *related to neuromuscular dysfunction* (NANDA-I © 2012)	
Outcome: Patient receives ventilatory assistance to extent desired. ***Evaluation Parameter:*** Patient reports minimal respiratory discomfort.	Discuss wishes with the patient and family. Consult with spiritual care. Record advance directives/patient wishes for ventilatory assistance in the medical record. *Ensures that patient's wishes are met.* Assess respiratory rate and lung sounds q4h *to assess for respiratory distress.* Monitor pulmonary function studies and arterial blood gases as ordered *to assess adequacy of gas exchange.* Assess for morning headaches, restlessness, nightmares, or poor quality of sleep. *Indicates poor gas exchange with resultant brain hypoxia.* Assess skin and nail bed color. *Indicator of poor gas exchange with resultant tissue hypoxia.* Consult with respiratory therapist for noninvasive ventilatory device. *May be recommended if vital capacity is $<$ 70%.*
2. NURSING DIAGNOSIS: High Risk for Aspiration *related to impaired swallowing muscles* (NANDA-I © 2012)	
Outcome: Patient does not show signs of aspiration. ***Evaluation Parameters:*** Patient is able to swallow food without choking or aspirating. Patient does not aspirate oral secretions. Lung sounds are clear. No signs of infection.	Monitor for persistent coughing after swallowing liquids. *May indicate aspiration.* Consult with speech-language pathologist. *Can evaluate swallowing ability.* Consult with dietitian. *Can develop diet consistent with patient's swallowing abilities.* Administer and evaluate response to medications. *Medications may be given to dry oral secretions.* Discuss wishes regarding tube feedings with the patient and family. Consult with spiritual care if needed. Record advance directives/patient wishes for nutritional support in the medical record *to ensure that the patient's wishes are met.*

(*continued*)

Weblink: Amyotrophic Lateral Sclerosis
Weblink: Muscular Dystrophy Association
Weblink: ALS Association

NURSING PROCESS: Patient Care Plan for Amyotrophic Lateral Sclerosis, *continued*

Outcomes and Evaluation Parameters	Planning and Interventions with *Rationales*
3. NURSING DIAGNOSIS: Anticipatory Grieving, patient and family, *related to fatal illness* (NANDA-I © 2012)	
Outcome: Patient and family move through the grieving process and come to terms with the fatal illness.	Discuss cultural beliefs with the patient and family. *Provides knowledge of cultural beliefs that may influence the grieving process.*
Evaluation Parameters: Patient and family use culturally appropriate coping mechanisms to deal with their loss.	Provide the patient and family with an opportunity to verbalize feelings related to prognosis *to help facilitate acceptance.*
Patient and family utilize spiritual resources to cope with the pending death.	Encourage the patient/family to consult with a spiritual counselor consistent with the patient's culture and beliefs. *Can help facilitate acceptance and coping.*
Patient and family verbalize the grieving process and how it relates to their situation.	Encourage the patient and family to attend appropriate support groups. *Such groups provide a safe environment to express feelings.*
Patient and family express feelings related to the fatal illness.	Help the patient and family become familiar with the grieving process *to help facilitate acceptance and coping.*
Patient and family attend a support group.	
Patient and family formulate advance directives.	Encourage the patient and family to formulate advance directives. *Provides a sense of control and ensures that the patient's wishes are met.*

Sources: Adapted from Ackley, B. J., & Ludwig, G. B. (Eds.). (2011). *Nursing diagnosis handbook: A guide to planning care* (9th ed.). St. Louis: Mosby; Carpentino-Moyet, L. J. (2010). *Nursing diagnosis: Application to clinical practice.* Philadelphia: Lippincott; Gulanick, M., & Myers, J. L. (2011). *Nursing care plans: Diagnosis, interventions and outcomes* (7th ed.). St. Louis: Mosby; Wilkinson, J. M., & Ahearn, N. R. (2009). *Prentice Hall nursing diagnosis handbook* (9th ed.). Upper Saddle River, NJ: Prentice Hall.

PATIENT TEACHING & DISCHARGE PRIORITIES for Amyotrophic Lateral Sclerosis

Need	Teaching
Disease process:	Disease symptoms and progression; fatal illness.
Patient/family	Notify the health care professional of increasing weakness and/or difficulty swallowing.
	Contact the Muscular Dystrophy Association (1-800-572-1717; http://www.mdausa.org) or the ALS Association (1-800-782-4747; http://www.alsa.org) for educational materials.
Psychosocial:	Encourage consultation with the mental health professional.
Patient/family	Encourage participation in a support group.
Respiratory care:	Correct use of respiratory equipment such as oxygen therapy, noninvasive ventilatory devices, and suction equipment.
Patient/family	Guidelines for breathing: Don't lie down after eating, avoid eating large meals, and sleep with head elevated 15 to 30 degrees.
Communication:	Develop alternative methods to communicate, such as blinking, if not able to speak.
Patient/family	
Diet and oral care:	Clean corners of the mouth after eating.
Patient/family	Soft diet as tolerated.
	Pureed foods should be placed on the posterior tongue.
	Solid foods should be eaten slowly, in small pieces, and swallowed after every bite.
	Correct care of the feeding tube, if used.
Activity:	Balance activity with rest periods.
Patient/family	Mild low-impact aerobic exercise OK if able; do not exercise to exhaustion; stop if experiencing muscle cramping, heaviness in extremities, or prolonged shortness of breath.
	Correct use of braces, splints, or other orthotic devices.
	May enlist aid from the physical therapist.
	Correct positioning and transfer techniques.
End-of-life issues:	Need to make proactive decisions regarding mechanical ventilation, artificial hydration, and nutrition.
Patient/family	Hospice services can help ensure comfortable death at home in accordance with patient and family wishes.
	Encourage spiritual guidance in accordance with patient, family, and cultural beliefs.

Sources: Barker, E. (2008). *Neuroscience nursing* (3rd ed.). St. Louis: Mosby; Hickey, J. V. (2009). The clinical practice of neurological and neurosurgical nursing (6th ed.). Philadelphia: Lippincott Williams & Wilkins; Ward, R. L. (2009). End-of-life legal considerations. *The Journal for Nurse Practitioners, 5*(9), 668–672.

Genetic Disorders

Huntington's Disease

Huntington's disease (HD) is a devastating genetic and neurodegenerative disorder characterized by a gradual loss of motor coordination and mental function. This disorder was formerly called Huntington's chorea. **Chorea** (from the Greek word for "dance") is a motor phenomenon that involves nonrhythmic, rapid, irregular, brief, jerky movements. However, in Huntington's disease, chorea represents only a fraction of the total symptom burden (Barker, 2008).

Epidemiology and Etiology

Huntington's disease occurs in approximately 5 to 10 per 100,000 Caucasians and 0.9 to 6.37 per 100,000 African Americans in the United States. An estimated 30,000 individuals in the United States are affected, and more than 125,000 are believed to be at risk of inheriting HD (Barker, 2008). The mean age for onset of symptoms is 30 to 50 years. In some cases, symptoms may occur starting before the age of 20 years with behavior disturbances and difficulty learning at school (Bader & Littlejohns, 2010; Roos 2010).

Pathophysiology

HD passes within families from generation to generation due to an autosomal dominant gene. Offspring of an affected parent have a 50% chance of inheriting the gene. Everyone who carries this single faulty gene will develop the disease. Either sex can transmit and inherit it. This genetic mutation causes loss of neurons in the basal ganglia and frontal lobes of the cerebral cortex. Atrophy of these areas may be shown on an MRI or CT scan in advanced ages. Intracellular inclusions that contain aggregates of the abnormal *huntingtin* protein are observed in the degenerating regions of the brain. Current concepts suggest that the mutated huntingtin product cannot be cleared or degraded, causing buildup that appears to be toxic (Barker, 2008; Roos, 2010). The cell loss results in motor, cognitive, and emotional impairments. The manner in which this affects the development of Huntington's disease is discussed in the Genetic Considerations Related to Huntington's Disease box.

Clinical Manifestations

Symptoms of HD include intellectual decline and abnormal movements. Individuals may present with motor signs (about 60%), behavioral signs (approximately 15%), or both motor and behavioral signs (about 25%) (Bradley et al., 2008). The earliest sign of the disease is impairment in the ability to initiate saccadic or rapid eye movements (the term *saccadic* refers to rapid eye movements that bring an image from the periphery into the fovea). Other symptoms of forgetfulness and difficulty with speech, swallowing, coordination, and balance may occur. The combination of reported symptoms, serious clinical signs, and positive family history may be the basis of early diagnosis (Barker, 2008; Bradley et al., 2008). Behavioral changes such as irritability, anxiety, mood disturbances, and obsessive compulsive behaviors may occur in 98% of people with HD. In addition, 30% meet the criteria for major depressive disorder, which increases the risk of suicide as much as sixfold over that of the general population (Bradley et al., 2008).

Laboratory and Diagnostic Procedures

The HD genetic test makes it possible to identify carriers of the mutant gene long before they become symptomatic. These genetic markers evaluate the abnormal gene for HD containing 40 or more CAG repeats. The specificity and sensitivity are adequate, so this test is all that is needed to confirm the diagnosis (Bradley et al., 2008). Some people at risk might want to have this test; others might not. Some of the reasons for making a decision *not* to have the test are outlined in the Ethical Issues box (Health.com, 2012).

Computed tomography (CT) or magnetic resonance imaging (MRI) also may show evidence of gross wasting of the caudate nucleus and putamen. In mild-to-moderate HD, an MRI will demonstrate subcritical atrophy, which can be correlated with specific cognitive deficits. Single-photon emission computed tomography scanning shows a decrease in glucose metabolism and cerebral blood flow in the caudate nucleus greater than that of the putamen, consistent with the development of HD. In addition, positron emission tomography (PET) scanning has shown decreased glucose and oxygen metabolism with the caudate nuclei early in the course of HD. These findings lend support to the theory that disturbances in the metabolism of certain neurotransmitters and heightened sensitivity of particular neuroreceptors may contribute to the symptoms associated with HD.

GENETIC CONSIDERATIONS
Related to Huntington's Disease

The abnormal gene was localized on chromosome 4 in 1983. This gene contains a "triple repeat" mutation in which the DNA base sequence "C," "A," "G" is repeated several times. This CAG repetition produces longer polyglutamine segments, and evidence suggests that the expanded polyglutamine string is toxic to neurons. A person who inherits HD will usually have a gene with approximately the same number of repeats as that of the parent; this causes the offspring to have the same age of onset of the disease as the parent's. The CAG repeat sequences are usually longer in men with HD than in women; therefore, the first symptoms may occur much earlier in affected children of fathers with HD than in those of mothers with HD. This phenomenon is known as "genetic anticipation."

Sources: Barker. E. (2008). *Neuroscience nursing* (3rd ed.). St. Louis: Mosby; Bradley, W. G., Daroff, R. B., Fenichel, G. M., & Jankovic, J. (2008). *Bradley: Neurology in clinical practice* (5th ed.). Philadelphia: Butterworth Heinenmann Elsevier.

ETHICAL ISSUES
Regarding Huntington's Disease Genetic Testing

Reasons for wishing not to have the genetic test for Huntington's disease:

- News of a positive result might be devastating, and the affected individual might prefer to live without knowing that she might get Huntington's disease some day.
- The patient may feel that taking the test would destroy hope.
- The patient might be concerned about how the results will affect relationships. For example, if an individual does not have the disease gene, but a relative does, she may feel guilty. If the reverse is true, the individual may feel very angry and resentful toward her relatives.
- The test is expensive, and the individual has no way to pay for the test; insurance will not cover it.
- The patient is concerned about being discriminated against at work or with future health insurance if present insurance pays for the test. Many people worry that genetic information released to insurance companies may affect future employment.
- The patient may believe that there is no point in knowing now because there is nothing that can be done about it by changes in lifestyle or treatment to prevent the disease.

Medical Management

Currently, no neuroprotective or neurorestorative treatment is available for HD. The main medical management is supportive and symptomatic treatment. The use of particular medications may help to manage or alleviate certain neurobehavioral or movement abnormalities associated with HD. Certain antipsychotic agents, such as haloperidol, a dopamine antagonist, or benzodiazepines such as clonazepam may partially suppress choreic movements and help to control psychiatric abnormalities, including severe agitation, hallucinations, or psychotic delusions. These agents should be prescribed at the lowest possible dosages to decrease the risk of side effects. Monoamine-depleting agents may be used to alleviate chorea; however, they too may have serious side effects, such as depression, parkinsonism, and agranulocytosis (failure of the bone marrow to make enough white blood cells). Medical management also may include administration of certain agents to help alleviate depression, anxiety, or obsessive-compulsive behaviors associated with HD.

Late in the course of the disease, some patients with HD develop signs of parkinsonism. These patients may or may not respond to antiparkinsonism medications, such as levodopa. Medications are discussed in the Pharmacology box (p. 598).

The nurse may coordinate services with the health care provider to provide supportive management of individuals with HD. These services include speech therapy to help the patient maintain as much ability to communicate as possible as the disease progresses. Ensuring that the patient receives necessary nutrients and a sufficient intake of fluids is another supportive intervention. Ensuring that patients remain as physically fit as possible also may be helpful in improving overall quality of life.

There is no approved surgical intervention for HD; however, neural transplantation is being investigated. To replace lost neurons and/or to prevent the degeneration of neurons, fetal human striatal tissue is transplanted into the brain of the patient with HD. According to one study, positron emission tomography scans demonstrated increased metabolic activity as well as improvement in motor and cognitive functions with the implants (Sharon, Sharon, Wilkens, & Tulay, 2010).

Nursing Management

The primary goal of nursing management of the patient with HD is education of the patient and family. The nurse should present a concise description of HD, including symptoms, expected course of the disease, and future problems, and include counseling in the education. An overall assessment of the structure and function of the home environment may be planned to best accommodate the patient's declining health. Patients should be allowed to make their wishes clear regarding cardiopulmonary resuscitation and ventilation, and these wishes should be documented in the patient's medical record.

Families and patients should understand the autosomal dominant nature of HD and the risk of their children inheriting the disorder. HD affects the past, present, and future lives of all family members.

Since rates of depression and suicidal ideation are high in individuals with HD, risk of self-harm may be an issue. Psychiatric and psychological support is necessary for the patient, and counseling should be available for spouses and children to address caregiver burden. Genetic counseling should also be made available (Barker, 2008). The complete patient care plan for patients with HD is shown in the Nursing Process: Patient Care Plan for Huntington's Disease box on page 621.

Collaborative management for the patient with HD is discussed on pages 628–630.

Discharge Priorities

The Patient Teaching & Discharge Priorities box for Huntington's Disease (p. 622) covers a wide range of topics that apply to the care of patients with HD.

Autoimmune Disorders

Multiple Sclerosis

A chronic and progressive neuroimmunologic disease, **multiple sclerosis (MS)** is characterized by multiple areas of demyelization in the white matter of the brain and spinal cord. The demyelization leaves sclerotic areas, also known as plaques, and subsequent scarring that lead to a variety of neurological symptoms including weakness, spasticity, visual disturbances, and **paresthesia.**

Epidemiology and Etiology

There are almost 400,000 diagnosed cases of MS in the United States, according to the National Multiple Sclerosis Society. MS develops in early adulthood, with the onset of symptoms typically appearing at age 28 and diagnosed at age 33. Women are two times more likely to be diagnosed with MS than men (Litzinger & Litzinger, 2009). The risk for MS increases geographically from southern to northern latitudes, with MS occuring more often in people of northern European descent. "Rates of MS in these northern regions can be as much as 5 times higher" (Stachowiak, 2009, p. 1). Risk factors for developing multiple sclerosis are discussed in the Risk Factors box.

Pathophysiology

MS is a neuroimmunologic disease that attacks myelin, the protective sheath surrounding nerve fibers. Demyelinating lesions or plaques form along nerve fibers in the brain and spinal cord, producing symptoms that are related to the location of damage. The breakdown of myelin interferes with normal nerve conduction in the affected areas (Barker, 2008). Demyelination results from an inflammatory process that leads to irreversible axonal injury and permanent loss of nerve function (Buttaro et al., 2008; Tocco, 2008). Although viruses and environmental factors are suspected of having a role in MS, the cause is still unknown (see the Risk Factors box).

Clinical Manifestations

Because MS can damage different parts of the CNS, symptoms vary, not only from patient to patient, but also within the same patient over time. The most common initial signs include fatigue, nystagmus, vertigo, gait disturbances, sensory loss, lower extremity weakness, spasticity, bladder disturbance, and optic neuritis (inflammation of the optic nerve). Other symptoms that may present at any time during the course of the disease include cognitive changes such as euphoria or depression, and physical conditions such as muscle cramping and sexual dysfunction (Hickey, 2009; Ropper & Samuels, 2009).

Heat is a common aggravating factor in MS. With a one-degree elevation in body temperature, new symptoms may appear or old ones may re-appear. The elevation in temperature may be due to environmental heat, fever from an infection, or exercise.

The symptoms of MS are listed in four categories: sensory, motor, cerebellar, and miscellaneous. The symptoms correspond specifically with the area in the brain or spinal cord that is damaged. Sensory symptoms include numbness, paresthesia, loss of proprioception, and **L'Hermitte's sign** (a shock-like pain that results from flexion of the neck). Motor symptoms include weakness, particularly in the lower extremities, and spasticity. Cerebellar symptoms include **ataxia** (loss

NURSING PROCESS: Patient Care Plan for Huntington's Disease

Assessment of Neurologic Status Using Gordon's Functional Health Patterns:

- Nutrition Metabolic Pattern
- Activity Exercise Pattern

Subjective Data	Objective Data
Assessment for Limited Mobility	**Assessment for Limited Mobility**
Do you have difficulty walking? Do you have difficulty controlling your movements?	Neurological status including level of consciousness Vital signs Decrease reaction time Gait changes
Assessment for Adequate Nutrition	**Assessment for Adequate Nutrition**
Do you feel you are adequately eating your meals? Are you having difficulty swallowing?	Decrease subcutaneous fat and muscle mass Lack of interest in food Aversion to eating
Assessment for Comfort in Breathing	**Assessment for Comfort in Breathing**
Do you feel comfortable? Do you feel tired? Is it difficult to talk?	Neurological status including level of consciousness and cognition Vital signs Respiratory status, including respiration rate, pattern, lung sounds, accessory muscles, and pulmonary function studies Skin and nail bed color Restlessness

Outcomes and Evaluation Parameters	Planning and Interventions with *Rationales*
1. NURSING DIAGNOSIS: Impaired Physical Mobility *related to neuromuscular dysfunction* (NANDA-I © 2012)	
Outcome: Patient will be able to ambulate safely. ***Evaluation Parameter:*** Patient verbalizes feeling of increased ability to move and less fear of falling with physical activity.	Screen for mobility skills in various positions, including sitting and laying down, as well as transferring and walking activities. *Assessing mobility skills will evaluate the need for assistance.* Obtain any assistive devices needed for activity such as a walker, cane, or wheelchair. *Assistive devices can help increase mobility.* Before activity, observe for and treat for possible pain with massage, heat pack to affected area, or medication. *Pain limits mobility and is often exacerbated by movement.* Help the patient achieve mobility and start walking as soon as possible if not contraindicated. *Early mobilization improves function and prevents complications such as deep vein thrombosis.*
2. NURSING DIAGNOSIS: Imbalanced Nutrition: Less Than Body Requirements *related to neuromuscular dysfunction* (NANDA-I © 2012)	
Outcome: Patient will maintain weight or display weight gain toward the desired goal. ***Evaluation Parameter:*** Patient will gain weight toward the desired goal.	Assess the ability to chew, taste, and swallow. *Evaluation of swallowing ability is necessary to determine what texture of food would be adequate.* Weigh as indicated *to evaluate nutritional needs and adequacy of intact.* Prepare the patient for meals. *A pleasant environment helps promote intake.* If the patient lacks endurance, schedule rest periods prior to meals, open packages, and cut up food. *Nursing assistance will conserve the client's energy for eating.*
3. NURSING DIAGNOSIS: Ineffective Breathing Pattern *related to neuromuscular dysfunction* (NANDA-I © 2012)	
Outcome: Patient will maintain an effective respiratory pattern. ***Evaluation Parameter:*** Patient reports minimal respiratory discomfort.	Early discussion regarding the type of care should be discussed with the patient and family. Consult with spiritual care. Record advance directives/patient wishes. *Ensures that the patient's wishes are met.* Assess the respiratory rate and lung sounds q4h *to assess for respiratory distress.* Monitor pulmonary function studies and arterial blood gases as ordered *to assess adequacy of gas exchange.* Assess for morning headaches, restlessness, nightmares, or poor quality of sleep. *Indicates poor gas exchange with resultant brain hypoxia.* Assess skin and nail bed color. *Indicator of poor gas exchange with resultant tissue hypoxia.*

Sources: Adapted from Ackley, B. J., & Ludwig, G. B. (Eds.). (2011). *Nursing diagnosis handbook: A guide to planning care* (9th ed.). St. Louis: Mosby; Bader, M. K., & Littlejohns, L. (2010). *AABN core curriculum for neuroscience nursing.* Glenview, IL: Elsevier; Barker, E. (2008). *Neuroscience nursing* (3rd ed.). St. Louis: Mosby; Ralph, S., & Taylor, C. (2008). *Nursing diagnosis reference manual.* Philadelphia: Lippincott; Wilkinson, J. M., & Ahearn, N. R. (2009). *Prentice Hall nursing diagnosis handbook* (9th ed.). Upper Saddle River, NJ: Prentice Hall.

Weblink: Huntington Study Group
Weblink: Huntington Society of Canada
Weblink: Huntington's Disease Society of America

PATIENT TEACHING & DISCHARGE PRIORITIES for Huntington's Disease

Need	Teaching
Disease information: Patient/family	Contact the Huntington's Disease Society of America at www.hdsa.org.
	Huntington Society of Canada at www.hsc-ca.org.
	Huntington Study Group, an international consortium of academic research clinicians and basic scientists, at www.Huntington-Study-Group.org.
Speech and swallow: Patient/family	Dysphagia and dysarthria are common. The patient should sit upright in a sturdy chair with arms when eating, if possible; take small bites and clear the mouth prior to the next bite.
	Avoid or remove any distractions with eating such as watching TV.
	Physical and speech therapy may assist with increasing respiratory effort, volume, and articulation.
Loss of executive function: Patient/family	Inability to plan and initiate an activity.
	Diminished verbal fluency.
	Patient should be presented with two choices rather than open-ended questions.
	Activities and encouragement to begin with verbal prompting should be presented.
Falls: Patient/family	Patient may have clumsiness or a drunken gait as well as chorea.
	A walker may be provided to help maintain balance.
	Physical and occupational therapy may be necessary to provide home exercise programs.
	Remove rugs; in addition, provide grab bars in bathrooms and nonslip mats.
Genetics: Patient/family	HD is caused by an autosomal dominant gene.
	Provide genetic counseling. Notify the patient that he should realize that each of his children has a 50% chance of inheriting HD.
Suicidal Tendency: Patient/family	Patients with HD have a high incidence of depression and suicide attempts.
	Look for signs and symptoms of depression.
	Provide counseling to the family and patient as necessary.

Sources: Bader, M. K., & Littlejohns, L. (2010). *AABN core curriculum for neuroscience nursing.* Glenview, IL: Elsevier; Barker, E. (2008). *Neuroscience nursing* (3rd ed.). St. Louis: Mosby; Ralph, S., & Taylor, C. (2008). *Nursing diagnosis reference manual.* Philadelphia: Lippincott.

RISK FACTORS for Multiple Sclerosis

Research shows that people who spend their first 15 years in regions that are far from the equator (above 40 degrees latitude) are at higher risk of developing MS than those who spend that period of life in tropical regions (Stachowiak, 2009). A person who migrates from a high-risk region before the age of 15 takes on the lower risk. The highest incidence is across northern Europe, North America, and Australia and occurs mainly in Caucasians (Ascherio, 2008; Buttaro et al., 2008). Researchers are considering the possibility that puberty (hormones) and geography may somehow interact to increase MS risk (Stachowiak, 2009). Researchers also are considering the possibility that demyelization can be triggered by a virus or other environmental stimulus that activates T cells specific for the production of myelin basic protein (MBP). On the basis of indirect evidence, there has been support for the hypothesis that alterations in humoral and cell-mediated immunity to viral agents may be a precipitating factor (Ropper & Samuels, 2009).

There is evidence that a genetic link may influence an individual's susceptibility to MS. Generally, a person's chance of developing MS is about 0.1%; however, if there is a first-degree relative with MS, the risk jumps up to 3%. In identical twins, the chance that the second twin will develop MS if the first twin does is 30%; in fraternal twins, the risk is only 4%. Many researchers hypothesize that MS is not caused by a single gene, virus, or environmental factor but is the result of a combination of factors (NINDS, 2011b).

of balance and coordination) as well as speech difficulties including dysarthria or slurred and scanning speech (speech in which the normal "melody" or speech pattern is disrupted, with abnormally long pauses between words or individual syllables of words). Other symptoms such as fatigue and loss of vision associated with a central scotoma (a blind area in the field of vision) often are an early sign of the disease. Vertigo, sometimes accompanied by vomiting and nystagmus, affects some patients, while bowel and bladder problems beset others. Emotional disturbances and cognitive impairment may be present as well.

As with the wide range of symptoms, the course any particular case might take is varied. The four main types of MS are shown in Chart 23–2 (Bader & Littlejohns, 2010; Hickey, 2009; Ropper & Samuels, 2009).

Laboratory and Diagnostic Procedures

In addition to a comprehensive medical history and neurological exam, diagnostics for MS include MRI, cerebrospinal fluid (CSF) tests, and

CHART 23–2 Four Main Types of Multiple Sclerosis

- *Relapsing-remitting MS* is the most common type. It is known for its acute attacks followed by complete or partial remission. It makes up about 85% of initial diagnoses.
- *Primary-progressive MS* progresses without remission, although plateaus or minor improvements can happen. Approximately 10% to 15% of the diagnoses are for this form of the disease.
- *Secondary progressive MS* begins as relapsing-remitting, but then it develops into the primary-progressive course, which occurs in approximately 50% to 90% of patients with relapsing-remitting MS.
- *Progressive-relapsing MS* intersperses the progression of the disease with acute attacks.

Both age and duration of the disease have the greatest influence on the rate of relapse.

visual evoked potentials (VEP) (Buttaro et al., 2008; Ropper & Samuels, 2009). Lesions that represent inflammation or demyelization often are referred to as plaques and are easily detected with weighted and FLAIR MRI tests. FLAIR refers to fluid-attenuated inversion recovery, evoked potentials present in the MRI. FLAIR sequences suppress the signals generated by fluids in the body. Some MRI techniques cannot image lesions well, as bright fluid signals obscure them. FLAIR's suppression of fluid signals allows enhanced visualization of lesions (Multiple Sclerosis Foundation, 2009).

Cerebral spinal fluid (CSF) studies look for inflammatory proteins and oligoclonal bands (bands of immunoglobulins that are seen when a patient's blood serum is analyzed). The visual evoked potential (VEP) test is done to measure transmission of impulses across nerve fibers, which are slowed in areas of demyelization (BMJ Group Medical Reference, 2011; Ropper & Samuels, 2009). Other diagnostics are listed in the Diagnostic Tests box (p. 594).

Medical Management

Treatment of MS relies on drug therapy, relapse management, and symptom management. Disease-modifying drugs reduce the frequency of relapses and potentially delay progression of the disease. Interferon beta-1b (Betaseron) is used to treat ambulatory patients with relapsing-remitting MS and secondary-progressive MS. Interferon beta-1a (Avonex) helps relapsing forms of MS as well as the initial MS attack. Another interferon beta-1a (Rebif) treats relapsing forms of MS. These medications may produce side effects resembling flu symptoms, which may be reduced by administering nonsteroidal anti-inflammatory drugs pre- and post-treatment; in severe cases, prednisone may be given (Ropper & Samuels, 2009). Depression also is a possible side effect.

Glatiramer acetate (Copaxone) is not an interferon; nevertheless, it is a disease-modifying drug used to treat relapsing-remitting MS. Systemic reactions to this drug rarely occur; however, it may invoke tachycardia, sweating, anxiety, dyspnea, faintness, flushing, and nausea. Traditionally used as a treatment for cancer, mitoxantrone (Novantrone), an antineoplastic (controls or destroys neoplastic cells) drug, suppresses the activity of T cells, B cells, and macrophages. It is used to treat the secondary progressive, progressive-relapsing, and worsening relapsing-remitting forms of MS (Hickey, 2009; National Multiple Sclerosis Society [NMSS], 2008). Use of mitoxantrone for more than 2.5 years increases the risk of cardiac toxicity (Buttaro et al., 2008).

In 2006, the FDA approved natalizumab (Tysabri) for the treatment of relapsing MS. A laboratory-produced monoclonal antibody, this drug inhibits the movement of damaging immune cells across the blood–brain barrier and into the brain and spinal cord. This drug is available only through a restricted distribution program (Buttaro et al., 2008). The Pharmacology box (p. 598) provides more information about drugs used for the treatment of MS.

Relapse Management

A relapse is a new sign or a worsening of existing neurological symptoms with a duration that is greater than 24 hours. Recovery from relapse is variable. After the onset of neurological deterioration, symptoms plateau and patients recover over weeks or months. Symptoms gradually resolve, and patients recover fully or partially. Several conditions are known to precipitate symptoms or relapses. These include, but are not limited to, excessive exertion, extreme temperatures, infections, hot baths, fever, emotional stress, and pregnancy (Barker, 2008; Buttaro et al., 2008).

Relapses often are treated with an orally or intravenously administered glucocorticoid, such as methylprednisolone. Common side effects from the use of these types of drugs include weight gain, a metallic taste in the mouth, insomnia, hyperglycemia, and gastrointestinal ulceration and upset. Less common side effects include psychosis and blurred vision (Barker, 2008; Ropper & Samuels, 2009).

Detailing the history of relapse and the consequential symptoms becomes the basis of care and treatment of the MS patient. The record should show when the relapse began, the severity of symptoms, and the impact on the patient's daily activities. The patient care plan should address the patient's understanding of factors that can contribute to the worsening of symptoms, common diagnostic evaluations, and a review of common medical therapy.

Symptom Management

Fatigue, a common symptom in patients with MS, is the most disabling symptom (Barker, 2008; Buttaro et al., 2008; Johnson, 2008). MS fatigue may have sudden onset and interfere with normal functioning. The patient's sleep habits, current and former medications, experiences of depression, and applied coping strategies all need to be collectively, as well as individually, taken into consideration in managing fatigue. Patients should be instructed that a hot ambient temperature can trigger the onset of fatigue and symptoms. Countermeasures such as air conditioning, cool drinks, and ice packs can help to restore a patient's strength. In addition, occupational therapists can teach energy conservation strategies that can help the patient accomplish ADLs. The practices of light exercise, scheduling rest times between activities, and using labor-saving tools and appliances often become part of the therapy. Medications prescribed to combat fatigue include amantadine, pemoline, modafinil, and low-dose antidepressants (Frohman et al., 2011).

Muscle spasticity also is common in MS. Infection, disease relapse, incorrect body positioning, and a full bowel and/or bladder all can contribute to spasticity. The health care provider should obtain a detailed history of the time, place, and circumstances associated with spasticity. Treatment may include stretching and breathing exercises, cool-water therapy, and relaxation techniques. In some cases, orthotic devices are used to prevent contractures and maintain proper body posture and alignment. Medications used to treat spasticity include baclofen, tizanidine, clonazepam, gabapentin, and diazepam (Frohman et al., 2011). In some cases, injections of botulinum toxin or implantation of an intrathecal baclofen pump may be necessary (Frohman et al., 2011).

Bowel and bladder problems are common in MS. Bladder dysfunction can be classified as failure to store, failure to empty, or a combination of the two. Urinary tract infections, urinary urgency, incontinence, and dribbling are typical symptoms (Frohman et al., 2011). Medication management includes oxybutynin HCL (Ditropan), propantheline (Pro-Banthine), tolterodine (Detrol), and terazosin (Hytrin). The patient should be encouraged to avoid caffeine, alcohol, and other diuretics. The nurse may teach the Kegel technique of contracting and holding the pubococcygeal muscle and the Credé technique of applying pressure to the lower abdomen to express urine to help patients adjust to retention and elimination anomalies. In cases of urinary retention, intermittent catheterization may be necessary. The nurse should instruct the patient on correct straight catheterization technique and care. In some cases, a Foley or suprapubic catheter may be required (Barker, 2008). The management of constipation and bowel incontinence is best done with the help of a dietitian who is familiar with the needs of the MS patient. The nurse should stress the importance of a diet and hydration appropriate for the condition along with moderate exercise (Barker, 2008; Frohman et al., 2011).

About half of the people with MS suffer from some form of cognitive impairment as a result of the disease. Although the symptoms vary, they are most likely to manifest as short-term memory deficits and attention difficulties. At times, the person's mental condition may worsen when he is tired, stressed, or exposed to hot weather. Many patients turn to list making, calendar keeping, and tape recording to aid them with memory lapses (Frohman et al., 2011; Hunderfund & Bartleson, 2010). A neuropsychologist can help define the deficits and give recommendations (Buttaro et al., 2008).

Nursing Management

Application of the nursing process is important in caring for a patient with MS. Relevant nursing diagnoses, assessments, outcomes, and interventions are important parts of the nursing process. The Nursing Process box details the patient care plan for MS.

Collaborative management for patients with MS is discussed on pages 628–630.

Discharge Priorities

Discharge priorities for patients with MS focus on adaptive strategies for patients and their caregivers in the outpatient or home environment, as addressed in the Patient Teaching & Discharge Priorities box (p. 626).

Myasthenia Gravis

Myasthenia gravis (MG) is a chronic, autoimmune neuromuscular disorder in which acetylcholine receptors at the neuromuscular junction are destroyed. The two major clinical forms of MG are ocular and generalized (Ferri, 2011). The hallmark feature is fluctuating weakness and fatigability of voluntary muscles.

Epidemiology and Etiology

MG is a relatively uncommon disorder, with an annual incidence of 2 to 5 new cases per million people in the United States (Ferri, 2011). It can occur at any age, although the age of onset is commonly at 20 to 40 years for women and 60 to 80 years for men. Overall, the disorder is more common in women than in men, with a female-to-male ratio of 3:2 (Bope, Kellerman, & Rakel, 2011; Ferri, 2011).

Although the primary etiology of MG remains speculative, there is increasing evidence that the thymus plays an important role. Histological studies have shown prominent germinal centers (Barker, 2008). Epithelial myoid cells normally present in the thymus do resemble skeletal muscle cells and possess acetylcholine receptor (AChR) on their surface membrane; therefore, it is hypothesized that they may become antigenic and set free an autoimmune attack of the muscular endplate AChR by molecular mimicry. The majority of people affected by MG also have thymus gland abnormalities. A rare thymic tumor, thymoma, occurs in about 10% to 15% of patients with MG. It remains unclear why the disease predominantly affects the extraocular muscles.

Pathophysiology

Muscle weakness in MG is the result of dysfunction at the neuromuscular junction. Acetylcholine (ACh) is a neurotransmitter that is vital for the transmission of nerve impulses to skeletal muscles, and it is produced in motor nerve endings. In MG, antibodies generated by an autoimmune response bind to AChRs, blocking the transmission of nerve impulses. This inefficient neuromuscular transmission together with the normally present presynaptic rundown phenomenon results in a decremental amount of nerve fibers being activated by successive nerve fiber impulses. This accounts for the fatigability and characteristic muscular weakness of patients with MG (Barker, 2008; Bope et al., 2011).

Clinical Manifestations

Usually the initial complaint that leads to a diagnosis of MG is weakness in a specific muscle or set of muscles rather than generalized muscle weakness. The severity of the weakness typically fluctuates over hours, being least severe in the morning and worsening as the day progresses. It also varies over the course of weeks or months, with exacerbations and remissions. Exposure to sunlight, viral illness, surgery, immunization, emotional stress, menstruation, and physical factors might trigger or worsen exacerbations (Bope et al., 2011). As MG progresses, symptom-free periods decrease, and muscle weakness fluctuates from mild to severe (Hickey, 2009).

Symptoms may be classified as ophthalmic and nonophthalmic. A majority of the patients initially complain of ocular disturbance, mainly ptosis (drooping eye lid) and diplopia. Ptosis may be unilateral or bilateral, and it may shift from eye to eye. Eventually, 90% of patients with MG develop ocular symptoms. About 50% of patients present solely with ocular symptoms, and about 50% to 60% of these progress to develop generalized disease. Oropharyngeal muscle disturbances are the most common nonophthalmic symptoms, with approximately 5% to 10% of patients first experiencing difficulty in swallowing, talking, and chewing (Bope et al., 2011; Ropper & Samuels, 2009).

MG can affect any skeletal muscle group, with 10% of patients initially complaining of limb and trunk weakness. Weakness in the bulbar muscles produces dysarthria and dysphagia and a nasal quality to the voice. If facial muscles are involved, the patient may appear expressionless or have a snarling expression when attempting to smile. Involvement of respiratory muscles may lead to symptoms of respiratory insufficiency and even respiratory failure. Patients also demonstrate incremental weakness upon repeating the motor power test over and over.

Patients with MG are at risk for two life-threatening situations that have similar clinical pictures: myasthenic crisis and cholinergic crisis. In either case, the patient will present with extreme weakness and respiratory insufficiency. **Myasthenic crisis** is caused by undermedication (lack of acetylcholine) or by stressors such as infection, surgery, or incompatible medications. The less common **cholinergic crisis** results from overmedication (excess acetylcholine). Both conditions are medical emergencies because they require mechanical ventilation (Barker, 2008; Ropper & Samuels, 2009).

Laboratory and Diagnostic Procedures

Though not definitive, an electromyogram (EMG), which measures the electrical activity of muscles at rest and during contraction, may contribute to a diagnosis of MG. Repetitive nerve stimulation may be used to evaluate whether there is a decremental response in compound action potentials on EMG. In addition, a CT or MRI scan may be performed to evaluate the thymus gland and to rule out mass lesions compressing cranial nerves. Laboratory studies will include immunologic assays to detect AChR antibodies. Patients with MG have approximately 85% of the normal amount of circulating AChR antibodies (Barker, 2008; NINDS, 2011c). Thyroid function tests are indicated to rule out associated Graves' disease or hyperthyroidism. This is particularly essential in patients with ocular MG, in which the concomitant hyperthyroidism is most frequent.

NURSING PROCESS: Patient Care Plan for Multiple Sclerosis

Assessment of Neurologic Status Using Gordon's Functional Health Patterns:

- Health Perception Health Management Pattern
- Activity Exercise Pattern
- Elimination Pattern

Subjective Data

Assessment for Self-Care and Safety

Have you ever fallen?

Do you have double vision?

Do you have trouble sensing the temperature of water?

Assessment for Energy and Ability to Perform Own ADLs

How many hours per night do you sleep? Do you nap and, if so, how often? How many times do you get up during the night?

Are you or have you been feeling depressed?

Are you able to accomplish your usual activities during the course of a day?

Do you exercise?

Do you notice that you become very tired in hot temperatures?

Assessment for Ability to Void Normally

How many times per day do you void?

Do you feel like your bladder empties completely?

Are there times when you cannot make it to the bathroom in time?

Do you have sudden urges to void?

Do you dribble in-between voiding?

Is it hard to get started when voiding?

Do you have burning when you void?

Objective Data

Assessment for Self-Care and Safety

Neurological status including muscle tone, gait, balance, vision, and sensory perception

Assessment for Energy and Ability to Perform Own ADLs

Neurological status including gait, coordination, and spasticity

Nutritional status including appetite and weight

Activity level including exercise/therapy

Medications

Assessment for Ability to Void Normally

Intake and output

Voiding pattern

Bladder distention

Postvoid residual

Urine appearance/odor

Urinalysis, culture, sensitivity

Outcomes and Evaluation Parameters	Planning and Interventions with *Rationales*
1. NURSING DIAGNOSIS: Risk of Injury *related to muscle weakness, ataxia, decreased sensory perception* (NANDA-I © 2012)	
Outcome: Patient remains free of injury. ***Evaluation Parameters:*** Demonstrates correct use of mobility aids. Practices safety measures to compensate for sensory losses.	Ambulate patient *to evaluate gait, ataxia, and potential for falling.* Consult with physical therapist. *Can evaluate the need for mobility-assisting equipment.* Instruct on use of mobility aids such as a cane, walker, or wheelchair *to help prevent injury, provide security, and increase independent movement.* Consult with an occupational therapist. *Can provide instruction to compensate for sensory deficits while accomplishing ADLs.* Teach the patient and caregivers safety measures to compensate for sensory loss, such as the use of a thermometer to test water temperature or the wearing of an eye patch to alleviate visual disturbance such as double vision. *Impaired sensory perception increases the risk of injury.*
2. NURSING DIAGNOSIS: Fatigue *related to disease process* (NANDA-I © 2012)	
Outcomes: Patient verbalizes increased energy. Patient is able to accomplish daily routines. ***Evaluation Parameters:*** Patient verbalizes understanding that fatigue is part of the disease process. Patient practices prescribed energy conservation strategies. Patient uses prescribed assistive devices to accomplish ADLs. Patient verbalizes understanding that hot ambient temperatures worsen fatigue.	Discuss the relationship of fatigue and disease process with the patient and family; allow both to verbalize coping mechanisms. *Educates the patient and family and assesses their needs and coping strategies.* Provide rest periods between physical activity and activities of daily living *to minimize fatigue and conserve energy.* Teach the patient and caregivers to avoid prolonged exposure to hot ambient temperatures, hot baths, or showers. *Can trigger the onset of fatigue.* Consult an occupational therapist. *Can develop an energy conservation plan, and assess the need for and prescribe adaptive equipment to assist with ADLs, which helps to minimize fatigue.* Consult a physical therapist. *Can develop a light exercise regime, which may increase endurance and minimize fatigue.*

(*continued*)

NURSING PROCESS: Patient Care Plan for Multiple Sclerosis, *continued*

Outcomes and Evaluation Parameters	Planning and Interventions with *Rationales*
3. NURSING DIAGNOSIS: Impaired Urinary Elimination *related to spastic or flaccid bladder* (NANDA-I © 2012)	
Outcomes: Patient empties bladder completely by voiding and/or catheterizing. Patient remains free of urinary tract infection. ***Evaluation Parameters:*** Patient demonstrates correct techniques for bladder emptying. Patient is able to verbalize signs and symptoms of UTI.	Discuss voiding patterns with the patient. Encourage the patient to verbalize concerns. *Provides an opportunity for the patient to verbalize coping strategies and assesses voiding patterns.* Monitor voiding patterns *to establish baseline voiding patterns.* Assist the patient to use the bathroom *to assess patient mobility status and ability to get to and from bathroom.* Assess for signs of urine retention including bladder distention, urine overflow, and intake greater than output. *Signs of retention.* Assess for signs of urinary tract infection. *Urinary retention and catheterization increase risk of infection.* Teach the patient the Credé maneuver. *Fully expresses urine from the bladder for failure-to-empty difficulties, which decreases risk of infection.* Teach the patient Kegel exercises. *Contracting and holding pubococcygeal muscle strengthens it, which helps improve failure-to-store problems.* Teach correct technique for prescribed bladder elimination: intermittent catheterization and suprapubic or indwelling catheter care. *Decreases risk of infection and ensures emptying of bladder.* Monitor medications for therapeutic use and side effects *to aid in early detection of side effects or adverse reactions.*

Sources: Adapted from Ackley, B. J., & Ludwig, G. B. (Eds.). (2011). *Nursing diagnosis handbook: A guide to planning care* (9th ed.). St. Louis: Mosby; Wilkinson, J. M., & Ahearn, N. R. (2009). *Prentice Hall nursing diagnosis handbook* (9th ed.). Upper Saddle River, NJ: Prentice Hall.

PATIENT TEACHING & DISCHARGE PRIORITIES for Multiple Sclerosis

Need	Teaching
Disease information: Patient/family	Contact the National Multiple Sclerosis Society (1-800-FIGHTMS). Disease progression is variable; some patients never become incapacitated. MS is rarely the direct cause of death; expect a fairly normal life span.
Medication information: Patient/family	Explain the purpose, dosage, and administration schedule. Instruct on the correct technique for administering injectable medications. Administer on schedule.
Exacerbating factors: Patient/family Setting	Mild fever worsens symptoms; take prescribed medication promptly for any fever-associated illness. Prevent infections; use hand hygiene, avoid exposure to infection; get flu shot. Avoid emotional stress, undue fatigue, and exertion. Avoid exposure to heat, including home temperature, hot baths, or showers. Use air conditioning in warm months.
Bladder management: Patient/family	Teach correct technique for: • Catheterization, if warranted • Credé maneuver • Kegel exercises. Call the health care provider if signs/symptoms of UTI arise.
Relapse management: Patient/family	Report new or worsening symptoms to the health care provider.
Safety: Patient/family	Use thermometer to track water temperature for bathing.
Health promotion: Patient/family	Mild exercise is beneficial, but do not exercise to point of fatigue. Consume high-fiber, low-fat diet. Maintain adequate hydration.
Mobility: Patient/family Setting	Instruct how to correctly use mobility aids. Instruct methods of ambulation and transfer techniques. Complete home evaluation for adaptive equipment needs.

Sources: Bradley, W. G., Daroff, R. B., Fenichel, G. M., & Jankovic, J. (2008). *Bradley: Neurology in clinical practice* (5th ed.). Philadelphia: Butterworth Heinenmann Elsevier; Hickey, J. V. (2009). *The clinical practice of neurological and neurosurgical nursing* (6th ed.). Philadelphia: Lippincott Williams & Wilkins.

Medical Management

MG is initially diagnosed through a detailed history and physical assessment, including a neurological examination. The Tensilon test may be administered, in which 2 mg of edrophonium chloride (Tensilon), a cholinesterase inhibitor with rapid onset and short duration of action, is administered intravenously at 30- to 60-second intervals up to a total of 10 mg. Patients with MG will demonstrate a distinct increase in muscle strength within 30 to 60 seconds. However, administration of cholinergic drugs may precipitate a cholinergic crisis, which is a life-threatening situation. Symptoms of cholinergic crisis include muscle weakness, cramps, difficulty talking, difficulty swallowing, bradycardia, bronchospasm, excessive salivation, vomiting, diarrhea, and excessive sweating. A Tensilon test should not be administered without the ready availability of intravenous atropine, an antidote for edrophonium (Bope et al., 2011; Goldenberg, 2010).

Recently, the ice pack test (i.e., placing ice over the eyelid) has gained favor among ophthalmologists to assess improvement in ptosis and diplopia in ocular MG, the rationale being that cooling might improve neuromuscular transmission. This remains questionable, as some researchers (Chatzistefanou et al., 2009; Kearsey, Fernando, D'Costa, & Ferdinand, 2010; Roberts & Hedges, 2010) have demonstrated that patients with ocular MG actually improve on the ice, heat, and modified sleep tests. Hence, rest might be the cause of the improvement in ocular signs.

A wide range of treatments may be used for patients with MG. There is no consensus about which to start first or which ones to combine. Follow-up care of the patient with MS should be managed by the neurologist, who will orchestrate the treatment, and the ophthalmologist, who will follow up on the ophthalmic symptoms such as diplopia and ptosis (Awwad, Ma'luf, & Hamush, 2010). When ptosis becomes bothersome, it is best treated by using lid crutches. Lid crutches are spectacles which have been adapted to hold the upper lid up and away from covering the eye. Typically, a small wire or piece of metal is added to the top of the glasses, forming a ridge support that folds up into the eyelid. The eyelid closes over the support ridge, making it quite unnoticeable. Nose bridge pads are added to the glasses to prevent pressure. Each patient is individually fitted for this appliance. Surgery should be reserved for patients who are stable and refractory to other treatments. Diplopia is treated with the use of Fresnel prisms unless the deviation is large and variable, in which case an opaque lens over the affected eye is preferred (Yanoff & Duker, 2009).

Surgical treatment includes thymectomy (surgery to remove the thymus gland), strabismus surgery, and blepharoptosis (also referred to as ptosis; an abnormal condition of the eye in which one or both eyelids droop over the eye). Thymectomy may be performed in the absence of a thymoma. Approximately 85% of patients experience improvement, and 35% of these patients achieve drug-free remission. However, patients often experience some transient worsening of symptoms early in the postoperative period, and improvement usually is delayed for months or years. Strabismus surgery may be used for selected patients with a stable course of MG. If a patient has stable ptosis that has failed to respond to medical therapy, blepharoptosis may be performed.

Drug Therapy

The neurologist tends to coordinate the pharmacologic treatment. Cholinesterase inhibitors (neostigmine, pyridostigmine, or ambenonium) are used to treat the symptoms of MG by preventing the breakdown of acetylcholine at the neuromuscular junction. Pyridostigmine is the most commonly prescribed cholinesterase inhibitor, because it tends to have the least severe muscarinic side effects, including abdominal cramping, diarrhea, increased peristalsis, increased salivation, bradycardia, and blurred vision (Barker, 2008; Gold, Hohlfeld, & Toyka, 2008).

Patients with MG who remain symptomatic on cholinesterase inhibitors may require immunotherapy. Commonly prescribed immunotherapeutic drugs include corticosteroids, azathioprine, and cyclosporine (Gold et al., 2008). Although administration of corticosteroids leads to marked improvement in the majority of patients, there may be an initial worsening of symptoms. Transient glucocorticosteroids causing worsening of myasthenic weakness may occur in up to 10% of patients. For this reason, initiation of corticosteroids is reserved for hospitalized patients (Gold et al., 2008). The Pharmacology box (p. 598) lists other drug therapies for myasthenia gravis.

Plasmapheresis

Plasmapheresis may be used when a patient is in crisis or not adequately responding to other therapy. Circulating AChR antibodies are removed from the patient's circulation by removing whole blood, extracting the plasma from it, and returning the blood—along with fresh or frozen plasma—to the patient. The outpatient procedure is repeated three to four times over a period of 8 to 10 days (Barker, 2008; Ropper & Samuels, 2009).

Intravenous Immunoglobulin Therapy

Intravenous immunoglobulin (IVIG) therapy is an alternative to plasmapheresis for treating the patient with MG who is experiencing increasing weakness. It may be used as preoperative treatment before thymectomy. Monthly courses of IVIG may be administered until the slower immunotherapy approaches, such as corticosteroids, take effect. The mechanism of action for IVIG therapy is not certain (Barker, 2008; Ropper & Samuels, 2009).

Nursing Management

Application of the nursing process will facilitate a comprehensive approach to patient care throughout the disease process. Relevant nursing diagnoses, assessment, outcomes, and interventions are all part of the nursing process.

Assessment

Nursing diagnoses for the patient with MG will depend on the muscles that are affected in each individual. A thorough history of disease onset and progression should be reviewed. Baseline data for respiratory function, bulbar function, and fatigue should be established, including the following (Bader & Littlejohns, 2010; Hickey, 2009):

- Vital signs, with special attention given to respiratory rate
- Breath sounds and breathing pattern
- Lung vital capacity
- Integrity of gag/swallow reflex
- Ability to chew and swallow
- Ability to see correctly without diplopia, ocular motility disturbance, or ptosis
- Ability to perform self-care activities.

Nursing Diagnoses

Possible diagnoses include the following:

- *Ineffective Breathing Pattern* related to neuromuscular weakness.
- *Alteration in Vision Acuity* related to ocular muscle involvement and ptosis.

(NANDA-I © 2012)

- *Imbalanced Nutrition: Less Than Body Requirements* related to dysphagia, bulbar weakness.
- *Self-Care Deficit* related to weakness.
- *Deficient Knowledge* related to disease process, medications, and/or energy conservation (Carpentino-Moyet, 2010; Tocco, 2010).

NANDA-I © 2012

Planning

The overall goals of nursing care for the patient with MG are to minimize symptoms and to detect early signs of myasthenic or cholinergic crisis.

Outcomes and Evaluation Parameters

The outcomes and evaluation parameters are as follows (Barker, 2008; Carpentino-Moyet, 2010; Tocco, 2010):

- Respiratory rate of 16 to 20 breaths per minute
- Forced vital capacity >20 mL/kg
- Intact gag/cough reflex
- Able to read and establish visual field
- Heart rate of 60 to 100 beats per minute
- Weight maintained at baseline
- Patient and family members verbalize understanding of disease process, treatments, and signs of myasthenic or cholinergic crises.

In terms of evaluation parameters, the patient with MG will not show evidence of respiratory insufficiency. Weight will be at baseline. The patient will be able to complete ADLs independently and will verbalize an understanding of the disease process, treatment, and signs of myasthenic or cholinergic crisis.

Interventions and Rationales

The primary nursing concerns focus on the adequacy of the patient's airway and breathing. Because respiratory muscles are often affected, the patient with MG should be monitored closely for signs of respiratory insufficiency that could indicate impending myasthenic crisis or cholinergic crises. Myasthenic crisis is trigged by anything that worsens MG. Risk increases with a lung infection, fever, or being stressed. Characteristics of myasthenic crisis include worsening of muscle weakness, shortness of breath, difficulty swallowing or talking, and morning headaches. Cholinergic crisis is caused by an excess intake of acetylcholinesterase inhibitors. Symptoms may include an increase in perspiration, lacrimation, salivation and pulmonary secretions, nausea, vomiting, diarrhea, bradycardia, and fasciculations (involuntary muscle twitches) (Wendell & Levine, 2011).

MG often affects the bulbar muscles involved in chewing and swallowing, so the nurse should closely monitor the patient's ability to chew and swallow. Other nutritional parameters such as weight, intake and output, electrolytes, and serum albumin also should be monitored. The nurse should educate the patient on energy conservation techniques, such as taking frequent rests when completing ADLs. The patient might need assistance with bathing, dressing, cooking, shopping, and other ADLs.

If the patient is experiencing mobility issues, the nurse should address skin care as well as provide assistance with mobility, as well as assistive devices for mobility, if needed. Because MG affects the ocular muscles, the nurse should observe the patient for eye changes, in particular ptosis and double vision. Ptosis patches, which may be custom designed to fit the eye, may be used to keep the eyelid up off from the eye. If the patient is experiencing double vision, an eye patch may be used to assist the patient in seeing better. This eye patch may be rotated between the eyes.

Nursing interventions should always include providing emotional support for the patient and family who are experiencing this devastating disease. The nurse needs to help the patient recognize and address the fears and anxiety she is experiencing. Fear of respiratory failure or choking may be dominant. Other considerations the patient may have include fears about going home, taking care of herself, resuming work, and experiencing social economic decline.

Collaborative care for MG is discussed below.

Discharge Priorities

Discharge priorities for patients with MG are multifaceted and focus on the primary aspects of having myasthenia gravis. Knowing how and when to take medications is very important, as is an understanding of the potential respiratory complications caused by the disease. Nutritional counseling may be necessary if the patient cannot maintain his optimal weight. If the patient has difficulty swallowing or experiences aspiration, family members and/or caregivers need to understand what emergency measures to take. Infection also is a source of major concern, as a lung infection may lead to a myasthenic crisis. The patient should be taught measures to prevent respiratory infection and instructed to contact his health care provider immediately if signs or symptoms occur. The nurse should emphasize energy conservation strategies such as undertaking physical activities early in the day and alternating activity with frequent rest periods. It is critical for the patient and caregiver to know the signs and symptoms of myasthenic and cholinergic crises and to seek immediate help should they occur, as myasthenic crisis can lead to respiratory failure (Wendell & Levine, 2011). The patient should also wear a medical alert bracelet and carry a card stating the diagnosis, medication dose, and medication schedule (Barker, 2008; Carpentino-Moyet, 2010; Tocco, 2010). The Patient Teaching & Discharge Priorities for Myasthenia Gravis box provides specific patient and family instructions for care after discharge.

Collaborative Management

Collaborative management is imperative for all six types of chronic neurodegenerative disorders discussed in this chapter (IOM [Institute of Medicine], 2010). A multidisciplinary approach facilitates optimal disease management, thereby enabling the patient to achieve symptom relief, independence, dignity, and good quality of life within the confines of the disease. The interdisciplinary team develops a treatment plan intended to anticipate and manage patient care issues and concerns that evolve during the course of the disease. In order to meet desired patient outcomes, it is essential that this interdisciplinary team communicate openly with one another in developing and evaluating care of the patient and family (IOM [Institute of Medicine], 2010).

The treatment plan may include the following:

- Providing pertinent information, both written and verbal, about the disease
- Referring the patient and family to organizations for assistance with finding community resources, support groups, financial and legal advice, respite, and long-term care options
- Encouraging discussion about advance directives for management of advanced stages of the disease
- Assisting the primary caregiver in managing stress and developing coping mechanisms through psycho-educational interventions and individual and/or group therapy.

PATIENT TEACHING & DISCHARGE PRIORITIES for Myasthenia Gravis

Need	Teaching
Patient/family	Onset of symptoms is gradual, progressing over a period of 5 to 10 years. The severity of weakness and the muscles involved vary and may fluctuate within the hour or day. Weakness tends to worsen with use of the affected muscles and improves with rest.
Medication information:	Explain the purpose, dosage, and administration schedule.
Patient/family	Explain the side effects of medications.
	Advise to take medications on schedule, and to time the dose 1 hour before meals to obtain maximum relief when needed most (e.g., for best chewing and swallowing).
	Inform the patient of symptoms of overdosage and actions to take should a crisis occur.
	Encourage the patient to inform the dentist, ophthalmologist, and pharmacist of the myasthenic condition to avoid adverse drug interactions.
	Carry a card that has information regarding medications and the patient's primary health care provider.
Respiratory precautions:	If having difficulty breathing, assume emergency measures, and notify health care provider and hospital.
Physical activity and fatigue	Practice diaphragmatic breathing to strengthen muscles used to breathe.
	Be alert to choking and possible aspiration.
	Discuss emergency procedures to be used in the event of choking.
	Instruct the patient on the importance of rest and avoiding fatigue.
	Develop a plan to avoid fatigue when preparing and eating meals and when maintaining ADLs.
	To prevent muscle atrophy, instruct the patient on how to do active range-of-motion exercises or, if too weak, have the caregiver perform passive RPM.
	Wear sensible shoes to combat muscle fatigue and potential loss of balance.
	Encourage the patient to eat regular, balanced meals to prevent fatigue from lack of protein and to meet dietary requirements.
Impaired vision: Double vision or Ptosis:	Intersperse physical activities throughout the day with rest periods.
	Be alert to factors that can cause exacerbation.
	Instruct to call a health care provider if upper eyelid drooping occurs, as it could signify an exacerbation of symptoms.
	Suggest wearing an eye patch and rotating between the eyes.
Exacerbating factors	Infection (an annual flu shot is suggested); surgery, pregnancy, exposure to extreme temperatures, tonic and alcoholic drinks.
	Instruct the patient to avoid individuals with colds or respiratory infections.
Emergency measures:	Avoid extensive exposure to ultraviolet light.
Patient/family Setting	Teach patient signs of myasthenic and cholinergic crises. Myasthenic crisis is trigged by anything that worsens MG. Risk increases with a lung infection, fever, or being stressed. Characteristics of myasthenic crisis include worsening of muscle weakness, shortness of breath, difficulty swallowing or talking, and morning headaches. Cholinergic crisis is caused by an excess intake of acetylcholinesterase inhibitors.
	Symptoms may include an increase in perspiration, lacrimation, salivation and pulmonary secretions, nausea, vomiting, diarrhea, bradycardia, and fasciculations (involuntary muscle twitches) (Wendell & Levine, 2011).
	Prevent infections; use good hand hygiene, avoid exposure to infection.
	Avoid emotional stress, undue fatigue, and exertion.
	Avoid extreme temperatures.
	Use air conditioning in warm months.
Safety:	Instruct the patient to wear medical identification jewelry.
Patient/family	Suggest having an emergency code to alert family members if the patient is too weak to speak.
	Instruct the family about cardiopulmonary resuscitation techniques, how to perform the Heimlich maneuver, and how to contact the rescue squad, as well as how to explain the route to the hospital.
	Consult with vocational rehabilitation if home or work modification is needed (e.g., raised seat and handrail for toilet).
Health promotion:	Mild exercise is beneficial, but the patient should not exercise to the point of fatigue.
Patient/family	Consume high-fiber, low-fat diet.
	Maintain adequate hydration.
Mobility:	Instruct how to correctly use mobility aids.
Patient/family	Instruct patient regarding methods of ambulation and transfer techniques.
Setting	Complete home evaluation for adaptive equipment needs.

Sources: Barker, E. (2008). *Neuroscience nursing* (3rd ed.). St. Louis: Mosby; Carpentino-Moyet, L. J. (2010). *Nursing diagnosis: Application to clinical practice.* Philadelphia: Lippincott; Tocco, S. (2010, March 18). Myasthenia gravis. Retrieved from: Wendell, L. C., & Levine, J. M. (2011). Myasthenia crisis. *The Neurologist, 1*(1), 16–22. doi: 10.1177/1941875210382918.

Specific team members, by discipline, provide the following supportive services to the patient and family.

Neurologists and/or other health care providers often guide the development and implementation of the treatment plan. Neuropsychologists may play a critical role in the periodic evaluation of cognitive function. Psychiatrists may become involved either at the time of diagnosis or as behavioral symptoms increase.

Nurses are an integral part of the multidisciplinary team, providing a common link for all team members as well as providing education and support to the patient and family through all phases of treatment. Nurses maintain continuous contact with the patient in both inpatient and outpatient settings and are responsible for implementing the patient care plan.

Once patients have been stabilized, physical therapy evaluation and treatment are necessary to assist with optimization of function through range-of-motion exercises, strengthening exercises, and instructions regarding mobility and the use of adaptive equipment. As patients experience less mobility and perhaps become bed bound, physical therapy may be needed to counteract contractures. For patients who require rehabilitation, involvement of a physiatrist is needed to direct the rehabilitation efforts (Barker, 2008; Miller et al., 2009).

Respiratory therapists manage assistive ventilation based on periodic assessment of the patient's respiratory function. This may include using external inhalation devices, developing a respiratory exercise program, and/or consulting with the patient and family as to what, and when, respirations are inhibited. This is particularly relevant in the care of patients with ALS and MG, for whom the option of whether or not to apply mechanical ventilation will become a growing concern. Respiratory therapy can be applied as intermittent positive pressure ventilation (IPPV) or bilevel positive airway pressure (BiPAP). Both of these modes of ventilation are discssued in Chapter 28.

Occupational therapists assist the patient in maintaining self-sufficiency in daily routines such as eating and dressing for as long as possible. They are important in helping the patient develop energy conservation plans in order to avoid or alleviate fatigue. In addition, occupational therapists can provide assistive devices to improve functional abilities. They are instrumental in helping the patient return to a work enviorment or pursue former or new occupations.

Involvement of a social worker or mental health worker is required to assist with issues of depression and lifestyle changes as well as the scioeconomic impact of the disease. Patients will need help in identifying resources to assist them in transitoning back into the community. It is important that patients understand that they can continue to be active socially and recreationally despite their progressive disease process. Support groups, powers of attorney, living wills, financial assistance, and hospice services are areas where expertise in social services can help patients adjust to extremely difficult social issues. Spiritual counselors, if consistent with patient and family beliefs, can help the patient and family face the issue of inevitable death in the case of ALS and make plans as appropriate for them.

Dietitians and nutritionists can assess dietary needs and modify the patient's meals to maintain the desired nutritional status and prevent aspiration in patients who are at risk. For patients with ALS, as their condition deteriorates, the use of a gastrostomy tube may become an issue for both the patient and family. Nutritionists can assist in explaining to the patient and family the need for this device and the desired outcome of placing a tube in reponse to dietary needs.

Speech therapists may be able to help patients retain their speaking capabilities. This is particularly relevant for patients with PD, ALS, and MG. Speech therapists can teach adaptive strategies and techniques to cope with the effects of dysarthria. They may adapt a computer-based communication system to compensate for loss of speech. In addition, these therapists can evaluate and, more importantly, monitor the patient's ability to swallow. They may develop swallowing techniques that will prevent choking and enable patients to eat regular food (Parkinson's Disease Information, 2008).

Patients and caregivers are part of the interdisciplinary team and should participate in the planning and development of the treatment plan. Such participation enables patients to express their wishes regarding forms of treatment and assistive methods to help them move through the disease. Caregivers have opportunities to learn how to care for the patient in a home or community setting and opportunities to express concerns and limitations of providing care.

Gerontological Considerations

Many of the diseases discussed in this chapter affect older adults in particular. Therefore, gerontological considerations are a primary focus of health care for these patients. Because dementia primarily affects older adults, its signs are often misconstrued as naturally occurring senility common to old age. This misunderstanding could cause patients, family members, and caregivers to confuse the signs of dementia and AD with those of normal aging. This not only perpetuates fallacies of aging, but it also increases the risk of delaying early, accurate diagnosis and prompt treatment.

Because the highest prevalence rates of these disorders occur in the oldest segment of the population, nurses need to recognize the factors that influence an older person's response to drugs prescribed for AD. The aging patient is likely to have concurrent medical conditions that require multiple medications, raising the possibility of polypharmacy and presenting the potential for drug interactions and adverse effects (Hajjar, Cafiero, & Hanlon, 2007; Woodruff, 2010). Older adults may be taking too many medications, possibly prescribed by several different health care providers, as well as over-the-counter drugs such as vitamin and mineral supplements, analgesics, and herbal products. These medications may not be compatible with one another; they may even interact with one another, causing adverse reactions. The more drugs a person takes, the greater the risk of adverse reactions. Slowed renal clearance and hepatic metabolism also may influence medication tolerance. Drugs that cause sedation have an adverse effect on cognition. Nurses have a unique opportunity to identify patients who are at risk for inappropriate polypharmacy and to educate patients and families about risk reduction.

People with chronic degenerative neurological disorders encounter significant socioeconomic problems. The cost of medications for patients beyond their productive employment years can be particularly burdensome (Factor & Weiner, 2008). Housing, private care, and social interactions also may pose a problem.

Patients who have most of these neurodegenerative diseases can expect to live an average life span; however, patients with a severe progressive disability, such as MS and ALS, often have a shortened life span. To reduce complications and to increase longevity, a healthier lifestyle, cardiovascular health, and attention to bone density and diet are important (Barker, 2008).

EVIDENCE-BASED PRACTICE Family Caregiver Assistance

Clinical Problem

It is estimated that there are more than 44 million family caregivers in the United States who provide 83% of home care to chronically ill older adults (National Alliance for Caregiving, 2009; Wilkins, Bruce, & Sirey, 2009). Family caregivers may take on a multitude of tasks in the daily care of their loved ones, from assisting with ADLs to tasks requiring problem-solving skills and clinical judgment, such as managing symptoms and carrying out treatments as in medication regimes. In addition, family caregivers are often responsible for coordinating health care and social services (Wilkins et al., 2009). Decades of research has confirmed that providing care to an older, chronically ill family member is stressful and can negatively affect family caregivers' physical and mental health (Choi, Donahoe, Zullo, & Hoffman, 2011).

Studies have suggested that caregivers of individuals with other illnesses have similar negative physical and mental health outcomes. Nurses, particularly those who care for patients with neurodegenerative diseases, will encounter family caregivers in a variety of health care settings and are often the primary source for family caregivers to learn how to provide care (Hickman & Douglas, 2010).

Research Findings

MacNeil, Kosberg, Durkin, Dooley, DeCoster, and Williamson (2010) conducted a study to evaluate the caregiver's mental health and potentially harmful caregiving behaviors. Family members represent the front line of care for a growing number of ill, disabled, and demented older adults. Unfortunately, these informal caregivers may experience considerable stress and are at higher risk for poor mental and physical well-being than noncaregivers. In this study, 417 caregivers completed a face-to face interview. The results indicated anger was found to foster an intermediate emotion (or relation) between anxiety and potentially harmful behavior. In addition, increased anger positively correlated with increased scores on depression and resentment. The researchers summarized their discussion of the study by noting that decreasing depression in caregivers who report increased levels of anger may result in reduction of potentially harmful behaviors.

Implications for Nursing Practice

Although further research needs to be conducted regarding specific interventions to increase knowledge, skills, and self-care for caregivers, nurses should be aware that there may be common family caregiver needs and challenges across the span of neurodegenerative disorders. Specifically, family caregivers for individuals with neurological disorders identified high needs for information about the illness as well as the need for practical training on how to provide care. When providing education and support to individuals with these conditions, nurses need to identify and include the family caregiver. Furthermore, caregivers need information about self-care for their own health promotion, and encouragement to pursue activities to support their own health and well-being.

Critical Thinking Questions with answers can be found in the Osborn Student Resources at nursing.pearsonhighered.com.

RESEARCH OPPORTUNITIES Related to Neurodegenerative Diseases

Research Area	Clinical Impact
Quality-of-Life (QOL) Research	
Assessing domains of QOL.	Established domains of QOL.
Impact of disease progression on QOL.	Improved interventions that enhance QOL in the face of degenerative disease.
Factors that mediate QOL.	
Interventions that improve QOL.	
Cultural implications for QOL.	
Patient/Family Education Research	
Assessing the changing learning needs of the patient/family throughout the disease trajectory.	Proven interventions for effective patient/family education.
Efficacy of interventions to educate the patient/family throughout the disease trajectory.	
Factors influencing patient/family learning.	
Cultural implications for patient/family education.	
Caregiver Research	
Changing education and support needs throughout the disease trajectory.	Maintain family caregiver health.
Skill-building educational interventions.	
Factors influencing positive and negative caregiver experience.	
Barriers to accessing community resources.	
Cultural implications of family caregiving.	
Emotional and Psychological Research	
Sexuality and intimacy issues.	
Successful coping.	
Factors that influence patients/families to seek mental health services.	

The chronic and progressive nature of neuromuscular degenerative diseases can significantly affect older spousal caregivers, who may not have the physical strength to handle the weight of a patient with limited mobility. Caregivers often experience stress, diminished immune system, and impaired psychosocial functioning (Roland, Jenkins, & Johnson, 2010).

The nursing care needs of older patients are multifaceted and complex, encompassing both inpatient and outpatient care. Symptom management is a major area of focus, with nursing care concentrating on nonpharmacologic management, patient education, and support. Evidence-based practice asserts that family caregiver assistance is an issue and should be recognized for the health of the caregiver and chronically ill family member (see the Evidence-Based Practice box).

Research

Neurodegenerative conditions offer a plethora of opportunities for nursing research. Questions remain as to (1) what causes the diseases discussed in this chapter, (2) if treatments for these diseases can be improved, and (3) how caretakers of chronically ill patients cope with these situations. Research also is needed to explore the coping mechanisms used by patients/families and how they might be expanded, strengthened, or improved. New drug therapies are being explored; what is the nurse's role in this type of research? Genetics is discussed briefly in this chapter; increasing emphasis on the role of genetics also needs to be explored. Literature reveals little international research related to these chronic disorders. There is a great need to learn from each other to improve the overall care and treatment of chronic, degenerative neurological disorders. An example of research opportunities is shown on page 631.

CLINICAL PREPARATION

READ DOCUMENT APPLY

READ: History of Present Illness >> Laboratory Study Results >> Critical Thinking Questions

You are the on-coming nurse receiving the report on James Lee, a 65-year-old male admitted with a diagnosis of Parkinson's disease (PD). He underwent surgery today for unilateral deep brain stimulation (DBS) therapy. His surgery lasted approximately 5 hours. Mr. Lee was awake for the surgery, which involved placement of the DBS lead, so he did not have general anesthesia. There were no complications during surgery. The implantable pulse generator (also called the battery or pacemaker) will be placed in 1 week in outpatient surgery. Therefore, the leads are not yet generating electrical stimulation.

Medical–Surgical History

Mr. Lee was diagnosed with PD 10 years ago. His case of PD is currently staged as Hoehn and Yahr Stage III. He has had peak-dose dyskinesia for the past 3 years as well as unpredictable on–off fluctuations. His medical–surgical history is otherwise negative. His medications include ropinirole, carbidopa/levodopa LA 50/200, amantadine, citalopram, and apomorphine injections prn. His medical history is significant for an appendectomy at 21 years of age.

Social History

Mr. Lee is a retired bank manager. He is married and has two adult children.

Physical Exam

Mr. Lee is sleepy but easily aroused and oriented to person, place, and time. His pupils are equal, round, and reactive to light at 4 mm. His speech is low, muffled, and slightly slurred. He is able to move all four extremities equally, although movement is slow and stiff. He denies numbness and tingling in his extremities. He has pronounced tremor in his upper extremities. He denies nausea and has been sipping on clear liquids with assistance. His abdomen is soft, with bowel sounds present in four quadrants. His lungs are clear. He has voided in a urinal standing at the bedside. He has not had a bowel movement. He has a heparin lock in his right forearm. Mr. Lee has a 1-cm wound at the top of the cranium. He took his anti-PD medications last evening, but has not had any today. Mr. Lee needs assistance to sit at the bedside, and is able to turn himself over in bed.

READ: History of Present Illnesses >> **Physical Exam** >> Admitting Medical Records >> Laboratory Study Results

Admitting Medical Orders

Admit to Neurosurgical Floor, Neurosurgery Service
Diagnosis: Parkinson's disease, scheduled DBS surgery
Allergies: none noted
VS q4h
Neuro checks q1h × 4, then q2h × 2, then q4h
Ambulate with assistance
Bathroom privileges
I/O q shift
Diet: advance diet as tolerated
Call house officer: HR 120, systolic BP 160, temperature > 38.5°C, RR 30, change in neuro status, urinary output < 240 mL in 8 hours, O_2 saturation < 92%
Saline lock with NS flushes q8h
Wound care: dry sterile dressing to scalp wound daily and prn; if drainage is present, notify the health care provider

Scheduled Medications

Ropinirole 4 mg po tid
Carbidopa/levodopa CR 50/200 po tid
Amantadine 100 mg po bid
Citalopram 40 mg po daily

PRN Medications

Apomorphine 0.2–0.4 mL sq q4h prn for muscle stiffness or lack of muscle control
Lortab 1 tablet po q4-6h for pain, max 6 tabs/day

Ordered Laboratory Studies

CBC, Chem 7 panel, PT, PTT, and INR daily

Laboratory Findings

On admission, all lab values were WNL, including CBC, chemistry panel, and bleeding times.

READ: History of Present Illnesses >> **Laboratory Study Results** >> Critical Thinking Questions

Test	On Admission	Postop Day 1	Postop Day 2
Sodium	135 mEq/L	137 mEq/L	140 mEq/L
Potassium	3.5 mEq/L	3.7 mEq/L	3.7 mEq/L
Chloride	97 mEq/L	100 mEq/L	101 mEq/L
Carbon dioxide	22 mEq/L	23 mEq/L	24 mEq/L
Blood urea nitrogen (BUN)	22 mg/dL	23 mg/dL	25 mg/dL
Creatinine	1.3 mg/dL	1.3 mg/dL	1.2 mg/dL
Blood glucose	90 mg/dL	94 mg/dL	100 mg/dL
White blood cells	8,000 µL	8,200 µL	8,200 µL

Test	On Admission	Postop Day 1	Postop Day 2
Hemoglobin	14.0 g/dL	13.5 g/dL	13.6 g/dL
Hematocrit	50%	53%	50%
Platelets	200,000 µL	210,000 µL	220,000 µL
Protime (PT)	12 seconds	12 seconds	13 seconds
Partial thromboplastin time (PTT)	60 seconds	62 seconds	65 seconds
International Normalized Ratio (INR)	2.0 INR	2.0 INR	2.5 INR

Pearson Nursing Student Resources *Log on to* **nursing.pearsonhighered.com** *to download forms*

DOCUMENT:

>> Summary of Hospitalization
>> Pathophysiology Form
>> Laboratory Values
>> Laboratory Results Explanation

APPLY:

>> List of Potential Nursing Diagnosis
>> Concept Map
>> Critical Thinking Questions and Concept Map

APPLY: History of Present Illnesses >> Laboratory Study Results >> **Critical Thinking Questions**

1. What are potential postoperative complications for which you would want to carefully assess?
2. As Mr. Lee restarts his oral anti-PD meds postoperatively, what aspects of his neuro check would you carefully assess?
3. If Mr. Lee requests an injection of apomorphine, what would you assess before the injection?

Answers to Critical Thinking Questions can be found in Appendix D in the Osborn Student Resources at nursing.pearsonhighered.com.

NCLEX® PRACTICE

1. A patient is being seen in the neurology clinic and his wife reports that he has a recent history of being unable to identify common objects by name, such as keys and glasses. The nurse realizes this impairment is characteristic of which of the following disorders?
   1. Multiple sclerosis
   2. Alzheimer's disease
   3. Parkinson's disease
   4. Myasthenia gravis
2. A student nurse asks the nurse to explain a physician note that refers to the patient showing evidence of demyelinzation of nerve fibers and plaque formation. The nurse explains to the student that this patient is likely experiencing:
   1. Alzheimer's disease.
   2. myasthenia gravis.
   3. multiple sclerosis.
   4. Parkinson's disease.
3. The nurse is devising a plan of care for a patient with multiple sclerosis. Which of the following interventions should the nurse include to help reduce the incidence and frequency of fatigue?
   1. Discuss voiding patterns.
   2. Plan for a daily hot shower.
   3. Minimize the use of assistive devices.
   4. Instruct to avoid prolonged exposure to excessive heat.
4. The nurse is preparing a discharge plan of care for a patient with Parkinson's disease. Which of the following should be included to help the patient with constipation?
   1. Restrict fluids.
   2. Increase dietary fiber.
   3. Take a laxative every evening.
   4. Limit protein intake.

5. A patient with Alzheimer's disease is being cared for at home by her adult daughter. Which of the following should the nurse instruct the daughter to do to support her health promotion needs?
   1. Discuss advance directives for management of advanced stages of the disease.
   2. Encourage getting involved in clinical research studies.
   3. Instruct to avoid extreme temperatures and exposure to infections.
   4. Refer for psychological and spiritual counseling.

6. A patient with Parkinson's disease tells the nurse that she's worried about her 80-year-old husband's ability to care for her as she gets older. Which of the following would be an appropriate response for the nurse to make to this patient?
   1. "That's not something that you should be worried about."
   2. "You are so healthy now that I'm sure you won't be a burden to your husband."
   3. "Would you like to talk about things that can help you and your husband?"
   4. "I'll get the doctor for you so you can talk with him about your concerns."

Answers to NCLEX Practice questions can be found in Appendix D in the Osborn Student Resources at nursing.pearsonhighered.com. Practice additional NCLEX questions online at the Student Resources site.

Pearson Nursing Student Resources Find additional review materials at: **nursing.pearsonhighered.com**

REFERENCES

Ackley, B. J., & Ludwig, G. B. (Eds.). (2011). *Nursing diagnosis handbook: A guide to planning care* (9th ed.). St. Louis: Mosby.

Adams, M., & Koch, R. (2010). *Pharmacology: connections to nursing practice.* Upper Saddle River, NJ: Pearson.

Alzheimer's Association. (2007). FDA-approved treatment for Alzheimer's. Retrieved from http://www.alz.org/national/documents/topicsheet_treatments.pdf

Alzheimer's Association. (2011a). Alternative treatments. Retrieved from http://www.alz.org/alzheimers_disease_alternative_treatments.asp#ginkgo

Alzheimer's Association. (2011b). Alzheimer's disease facts and figures. *Alzheimer's & Dementia, 7*(2), 1–63.

American Psychiatric Association. (2000). *Diagnostic and statistical manual of mental disorders.* Washington, DC: American Psychiatric Association.

Anderson, H., Brannon, G., Boswell, L., Feng, J., Haddock., J., & Schneider, R. (2011, June 9). Alzheimer disease. Retrieved from http://emedicine.medscape.com/article/1134817-overview#a0104

Ascherio, A. (2008). Epidemiology of multiple sclerosis: From risk factors to prevention. *Seminars in Neurology, 28*(1), 17–28.

Awwad, S., Ma'luf, R., & Hamush, N. (2010, Feb. 18). Retrieved from http://emedicine.medscape.com/article/1216417-followup#a2645

Bader, M. K., & Littlejohns, L. (2010). *AABN core curriculum for neuroscience nursing.* Glenview, IL: Elsevier.

Barker, E. (2008). *Neuroscience nursing* (3rd ed.). St. Louis: Mosby.

Block, J., Smith, M., & Segal, J. (2012). Vascular dementia. HELPGUIDE.org. Retrieved from http://www.helpguide.org/elder/vascular_dementia.htm

Bope, E. T., Kellerman, R., & Rakel, R. E. (2011). *Conn's current therapy 2011.* Philadelphia: Saunders.

Bradley, W. G., Daroff, R. B., Fenichel, G. M., & Jankovic, J. (2008). *Bradley: Neurology in clinical practice* (5th ed.). Philadelphia: Butterworth-Heineman Elsevier.

Briggs, G. B., et al. (2010). Variation within DNA repair pathway genes and risk of multiple sclerosis. *American Journal of Epidemiology, 172*(92), 217–224.

Buttaro, T., Trybulski, J., Bailey, P., & Sandberg-Cook, J. (2008). *Primary care: A collaborative practice* (3rd ed.). St. Louis: Mosby.

Carpentino-Moyet, L. J. (2010). *Nursing diagnosis: Application to clinical practice.* Philadelphia: Lippincott.

Chatzistefanou, K. I., Kouris, T., Iliakis, E., Piaditis, G., Tagaris, G., Katsikeris, N., et al. (2009). The ice pack test in differential diagnosis of myasthenic diplopia. *Ophthalmology, 116*(11), 2236–2243.

Choi, J., Donahoe, M. P., Zullo, T. G., & Hoffman, L. A. (2011). Caregivers of the chronically critically ill after discharge from the intensive care unit: Six months' experience. *American Journal of Critical Care, 20*(1), 12–23.

Crystal, H. (2011). Alzheimer's disease. *MedicineNet.com.* Retrieved from http://www.medicinenet.com/alzheimers_disease_causes_stages_and_symptoms/article.htm

Deiner, S., & Hagen, J. (2009). Parkinson's disease and deep brain stimulator placement. *Anesthesiology Clinics, 27*(3), 391–415.

Erickson, K. I., Voss, M. W., Prakash, R. S., Basak, C., Szabo, A., Chaddock, L., et al. (2011, February 15). Exercise training increases size of hippocampus and improves memory. *The Proceedings of the National Academy of Sciences Online (U.S.), 108*(7), 3017–3022. Epub 2011 Jan 31.

Factor, S., & Weiner, W. (2008). *Parkinson's disease: Diagnosis and clinical management.* New York: Demos Medical Publishing.

Ferri, F. (2010). *Practical guide to the care of the medical patient* (8th ed.). St. Louis: Mosby.

Ferri, F. (2011). *Ferri's clinical advisor 2011* (1st ed.). Philadelphia: Mosby.

Fischer Center for Alzheimer's Research Foundation. (2011). Alzheimer's disease cause, care, & cure. Alzheimer's Research Foundation. Retrieved from http://www.alzinfo.org

Frohman, T. C., Castro, W., Shah, A., Courtney, A., Ortstadt, J., Davis, S., et al. (2011). Symptomatic therapy in multiple sclerosis. *Therapeutic Advances in Neurological Disorders, 4*(2), 83–98.

Geda, Y. E., Roberts, R. O., Knopman, D. S., Petersen, R. C., Christianson, T. J., Pankratz, V. S., et al. (2008). Prevalence of neuropsychiatric symptoms in mild cognitive impairment and normal cognitive aging: Population-based study. *Archives of General Psychiatry, 65*(10), 1193–1198.

George, J. L., Mok, S., Moses, D., Wilkins, S., Bush, A. I., Cherny, R. A., & Finkelstein, D. I. (2009). Targeting the progression of Parkinson's disease. *Current Neuropharmacology, 7*(1), 9–36.

Gies, C., & Lessick, M. (2009). Alzheimer disease in women. *Nursing for Women's Health, 13*(4), 314–324.

Gold, R., Hohlfeld, R., & Toyka, K. V. (2008). Review: Progress in the treatment in myasthenia gravis. *Therapeutic Advances in Neurological Disorders, 1*(2), 99–114.

Goldenberg, M. (2008). Medical management of Parkinson's disease. *Pharmacy & Therapeutics, 33*(10), 590–594.

Goldenberg, W. D. (2010, May 21). Myasthenia gravis in emergency medicine clinical presentation. Retrieved from http://emedicine.medscape.com/article/793136-clinical#a0217

Granholm, A. C., & Boger, H. (2008, July). Mood, memory and movement: An age-related neurodegenerative complex? *Current Aging Science, 1*(2), 133–139.

Hackney, M. E., & Earhart, G. M. (2008). Tai Chi improves balance and mobility in people with Parkinson disease. *Gait Posture, 28*(3), 456–460.

Hajjar, E. T., Cafiero, A. C., & Hanlon, G. T. (2007). Polypharmacy in elderly patients. *Amrican Journal of Geriatric Pharacotherapy, 5*(4), 345–351.

Halloran, L. (2011). Dementia: Forget about it! Differentiation and diagnosis of dementias. *The Journal for Nurse Practitioners, 7*(3), 242–243.

Hauser, R., Ahmed, I., Blackmer, J., Bloomfield, S., Campagnolo, D., Carroll, T., et al. (2011, June 20). Parkinson disease. Retrieved from http://emedicine.medscape.com/article/1831191-overview#showall

Health.com. (2012). Huntington's disease genetic test. Retrieved from http://www.health.com/health/library/topic/0,,uf6792a_uf6797m00.html

Hickey, J. V. (2009). *The clinical practice of neurological and neurosurgical nursing* (6th ed.). Philadelphia: Lippincott Williams and Wilkins.

Hickman, R. L., & Douglas, S. (2010). Impact of chronic critical illness on the psychological outcomes of family members. *AANN Advance Critical Care, 21*(1), 80–91.

Hoehn, M. M., and Yahr, M. D. (1967). Parkinsonism: onset, progression and mortality. *Neurology, 17*(5), 427–442.

Hunderfund, A. N., & Bartleson, J. D. (2010). Patient education in neurology. *Neurologic Clinics, 28*(2), 517–536.

Hussey, L. (2011, June 8). Tailoring nursing care to the special needs of Alzheimer's patients. Retrieved from http://www.nursingconsult.com/nursing/clinical-updates/full-text?clinical_update_id=200542&parentpage=topics&landingPageId=ALZHEIMERSDISEASE.lp

IOM (Institute of Medicine). (2010). *The future of nursing: Leading change, advancing health.* Washington, DC: The Academic Press.

Johnson, S. (2008). The concept of fatigue in multiple sclerosis. *Journal of Neuroscience* Nursing, *40*(2), 72–77.

Kearsey, C., Fernando, P., D'Costa, D., & Ferdinand, P. (2010). The use of ice pack test in myasthenia gravis. *Journal of the Royal Society of Medicine, 1*(1), 14.

Kee, J. L. (2010). Laboratory and diagnostic tests with nursing implications (8th ed.). Upper Saddle River, NJ: Pearson.

Klein, C., & Djarmati, A. (2011). Parkinson disease: genetic testing in Parkinson disease—who should be assessed? *National Review of Neurology, 7*(1), 7–9. Retrieved from http://www.nchi.nlm.nih.gov/pubmed/21221111

Kurlowicz, L., & Wallace, M. (1999). The mini mental state examination (MMSE). *Best Practices in Nursing Care to Older Adults, 3.*

Lindsey, P. (2009). Psychotropic medication use among older adults: What all nurses need to know. *Journal of Gerontological Nursing, 35*(9), 28–38. doi: 10.3928/00989134-20090731-01

Litzinger, M. H., & Litzinger, M. (2009). Multiple sclerosis: A therapeutic overview. *U.S. Pharmacist, 34*(1), HS3–HS9.

MacNeil, G., Kosberg, J., Durkin, D., Dooley, W., DeCoster, J., & Williamson, G. (2010). Caregiver mental health and potentially harmful caregiving behavior: The central role of caregiver anger. *Gerontologist, 50*(1), 76–86. doi: 10.1093/geront/gnp099

Marcason, W. (2009). What are the primary nutritional issues for a patient with Parkinson's disease? *Journal of the American Dietetic Association, 109*(7), 1316.

Marks, B. L., Katz, L. M., & Smith, J. K. (2009, April), Exercise and the aging mind: Buffing the baby boomer's body and brain. *Physician and Sportsmedicine, 37*(1), 119–125.

Mayo Clinic Staff. (2011). Frontotemporal dementia. MayoClinic.com. Retrieved from http://www.mayoclinic.com/health/frontemporal-dementia/DS00874/DSECTION=treat

Meiner, S.E. (2011). *Gerontologic nursing* (4th ed.). St. Louis, MO: Mosby Inc.

Miller, R. G., Jackson, C. E., Kasarskis, E. J., England, J. D., Forshew, D., Johnston, W., et al. (2009). Practice parameter update: The care of the patient with amyotrophic lateral sclerosis: Multidisciplinary care, symptom management, and cognitive/behavioral impairment (an evidence-based review). *American Academy of Neurology, 73*, 1227–1233.

Multiple Sclerosis Foundation. (2009). How is multiple sclerosis diagnosed? Retrieved from http://www.msfocus.org/diagnose-multiple-sclerosis.aspx

National Alliance for Caregiving. (2009). *Caregiving in the U.S.* Bethesda, MD: Author.

National Guideline Clearinghouse. (2008). *Guideline for Alzheimer's disease management.* Chicago, IL: Alzheimer's Association. Retrieved from http://www.guideline.gov/content.aspx?id=12691

National Human Genome Research Institute. (2011a). Learning about Huntington's disease. National Institutes of Health. Retrieved from http://www.genome.gov/10001215

National Human Genome Research Institute. (2011b). Learning about Parkinson's disease. National Institutes of Health. Retrieved from http://www.genome.gov/1001217

National Institute on Aging, U.S. National Institutes of Health. (2010). Caregiver guide. Retrieved from http://www.nia.nih.gov/Alzheimers/Publications/caregiverguide.htm

National Institute on Aging, U.S. National Institutes of Health. (2011a). Genetics. Retrieved from http://www.nia.nih.gov/Alzheimers/Publications/ADProgress2008/LongWay/genetics.htm

National Institute on Aging, U.S. National Institutes of Health. (2011b). Neuroimaging. Retrieved from. http://www.nia.nih.gov/sites/default/files/nia_2008_progressrpt_1.pdf

National Institute on Aging, U.S. National Institutes of Health. (2011c). Potential AD risk factors. Retrieved from http://www.nia.nih.gov/Alzheimers/Publications/ADProgress2009/Advances/Prevention/riskfactors.htm

National Institute on Aging, U.S. National Institutes of Health. (2011d). About Alzheimer's disease: Symptoms. Retrieved from http://www.nia.nih.gov/alzheimers/topics/symptoms

National Institute of Neurological Disorders and Stroke. (2010). Huntington's disease: Hope through research. Retrieved from http://www.ninds.nih.gov/disorders/huntington/detail_huntington.htm

National Institute of Neurological Disorders and Stroke. (2011a). ALS (amyotrophic lateral sclerosis) fact sheet. Retrieved from http://www.ninds.nih.gov/disorders/amyotrophiclateralsclerosis/detail_ALS.htm

National Institute of Neurological Disorders and Stroke. (2011b). Multiple sclerosis: Hope through research. Retrieved from http://www.ninds.nih.gov/disorders/multiple_sclerosis/detail_multiple_sclerosis.htm

National Institute of Neurological Disorders and Stroke. (2011c). Myasthenia gravis fact sheet. Retrieved from http://www.ninds.nih.gov/disorders/myasthenia_gravis/detail_myasthenia_gravis.htm

National Institute of Neurological Disorders and Stroke. (2011d). NINDS amyotrophic lateral sclerosis information page. Retrieved from http://www.ninds.nih.gov/disorders/amyotrophiclateralsclerosis/detail_ALS.htm

National Institute of Neurological Disorders and Stroke. (2011e). NINDS dementia with Lewy bodies information page. Retrieved from http://www.ninds.nih.gov/disorders/dementiawithlewybodies.htm

National Institute of Neurological Disorders and Stroke. (2011f). Tremor fact sheet. Retrieved from http://www.ninds.nih.gov/disorders/tremor/detail_tremor.htm

National Multiple Sclerosis Society. (2008). *Just the facts 2006–2007.* Washington, DC: Author.

Neuwelt, E., Abbott, N. J., Abrey, L., Banks, W. A., Blakley, B., Davis, T., et al. (2008). Strategies to advance translation research into brain barriers. *Lancet Neurology, 7*, 84–96.

Park, A., & Stacy, M. (2011). M. Dopamine-induced nonmotor symptoms of Parkinson's disease. *Parkinson's Disease,* 1–6. doi: 10.4061/2011/485063

Parkinson's Disease Foundation. (2011). Statistics on Parkinson's. Retrieved from http://www.pdf.org/en/parkinson_statistics

Parkinson's Disease Information. (2009). *Parkinson's Organization.* Retrieved from http://www.parkinsons.org/

Perlmutter, J. (2010). Assessment of Parkinson disease manifestations. *Current Protocols in Neuroscience, 14* doi: 10.1002/0471142301.ns1001s49\

Poewe, W. (2009). Treatment for Parkinson disease—past achievements and current clinical needs. *Neurology, 72* (7, suppl 2), S65–S73.

Poewe, W., Antonini, A., Zijlmans, J., Burkhard, P. R., & Vingerhoets, F. (2010). Levodopa in the treatment of Parkinson's disease: An old drug still going strong. *Clinical Interventions in Aging, 5*, 229–238.

Querfurth, H., & LaFerla, F. (2010). Alzheimer's disease. *The New England Journal of Medicine, 362,* 329–344.

Rakel, R., & Rakel, D. (2011). *Textbook of family medicine* (8th ed.). Philadelpha: Elsevier Saunders.

Ralph, S., & Taylor, C. (2008). *Nursing diagnosis reference manual.* Philadelphia: Lippincott.

Ridgel, A. L., Vitek, J. L., & Alberts, J. L. (2009, July–August). Forced, not voluntary, exercise improves motor function in Parkinson's disease patients. *Neurorehabilitation and Neural Repair, 23*(6), 600–608. Epub 2009 Jan 8.

Roberts, J. R., & Hedges, J. R. (2010). *Roberts: Clinical procedures in emergency medicine* (5th ed.). Philadelphia: Saunders Elsevier.

Roland, K., Jenkins, M. E., & Johnson, A. M. (2010). An exploration of the burden experienced by spousal caregivers of individuals with Parkinson's disease. *Movement Disorders, 25*(2), 189–193.

Rolland, Y., Pillard, F., Klapouszczak, A., Reynish, E., Thomas, D., Andrieu, S., et al. (2007, February). Exercise program for nursing home residents with Alzheimer's disease: A 1-year randomized, controlled trial. *Journal of the American Geriatrics Society, 55*(2), 158–165.

Roos, R. (2010). Huntington's disease: A clinical review. *Orphanet Journal of Rare Disease, 5*, 40. doi: 10.1186/1750-1172-5-40

Ropper, A., & Samuels, M. (2009). *Adams & Victor's principles of neurology* (9th ed.). Philadelphia: McGraw-Hill.

Schapira, A. (2009). Etiology and pathogenesis of Parkinson disease. *Neurologic Clinics, 27*(3), 58–603. doi: 10.1016/j.ncl.2009.04.004

Sharon, I., Sharon, R., Wilkens, J. P., & Tulay, E. (2010, Aug. 31). Huntington disease dementia. Retrieved from http://emedicine.medscape.com/article/289706-overview

Shawler, C. (2010). Assessing and maintaining mental health in elderly individuals. *Nursing Clinics of North America, 45*(4), 635–650.

Stachowiak, J. (2009). Multiple sclerosis. *About.com.* Retrieved from http://ms.about.com/bio/Julie-Stachowiak-Ph-D-25262.htm

Tavee, J., & Sweeney, P. (2011). Alzheimer's disease. The Cleveland Clinic Foundation. Retrieved from http://www.clevelandclinicmeded.com/medicalpubs/diseasemanagement/neurology/alzheimers-disease/

Tocco, S. (2008, March 14). Multiple sclerosis. Retrieved from http://www.nursingconsult.com/nursing/evidence-based-nursing/monograph?monograph_id=192906&filter=as&loe=&sortorder=title-a&pageno=1&parentpage=search&searchId=1180364398&searchTerm=multiple+sclerosis+demyelination&page=&bestBetId=BB_MNC_EBN_MultipleSclerosis.bb&search_type=allresults

Vernon, G. (2009). Parkinson disease and the nurse practitioner: Diagnostic and management challenges. *The Journal for Nurse Practitioners, 5*(3), 195–206.

Walsh, D., Caraceni, A., Fainsinger, R., Foley, K., Glare, P., Goh, C., et al. (2008). *Walsh: Palliative medicine* (1st ed.). Philadelphia: Saunders.

Ward, R. L. (2009). End-of-life legal considerations. *The Journal for Nurse Practitioners, 5*(9), 668–672.

Weintraub, D., Cornwella, C. L., & Horn, S. (2008). Parkinson's disease—part 3: Neuropsychiatric symptoms. *American Journal of Managed Care, 14*(2, suppl), S59–69.

Wendell, L. C., & Levine, J. M. (2011). Myasthenia crisis. *The Neurologist, 1*(1), 16–22. doi: 10.1177/1941875210382918

Wilkins, V. M., Bruce, M. L., & Sirey, J. (2009). Caregiving tasks and training interest of family caregivers of medically ill homebound older adults. *Journal of Aging and Health, 21*(3), 528–542.

Wilkinson, J. M., & Ahearn, N. R. (2009). *Prentice Hall nursing diagnosis handbook* (9th ed.). Upper Saddle River, NJ: Prentice Hall.

Woodruff, K. (2010). Preventing polypharmacy in older adults. *American Nurse Today, 5*(10). Health.Com Media. Retrieved from http://www.medscape.com/viewarticle/732131

Yanoff, M., & Duker, J. S. (2009). *Yanoff & Duker: Ophthalmology* (3rd ed.). St. Louis: Mosby.

CHAPTER 24

Caring for the Patient with Spinal Cord Injuries

Joyce Colobong
Christi DeLemos
Annita Watson

Outcome-Based Learning Objectives

After studying this chapter, the learner will be able to:

1. Compare and contrast the most common causes of acute spinal cord injury across the lifespan.
2. Differentiate between a complete and an incomplete spinal cord injury and determine the impact on patient care.
3. Incorporate the skills needed to assist families in coping with the psychosocial impact of spinal cord injury into the total plan of care.
4. Generate a patient care plan, using the nursing process, for a patient who has experienced a spinal cord injury.
5. Determine three complications of spinal cord injury and generate a patient care plan to prevent these complications.
6. Analyze rehabilitative needs and goals for discharge for the patient who has experienced a spinal cord injury.

KEY TERMS

areflexia p.643
atlas fractures p.643
autonomic hyperreflexia p.644
axis fractures p.643
complete spinal cord injury p.639
compression fractures p.643
compression injuries p.642
contusion p.642
hangman's fracture p.643
hyperextension injuries p.641
hyperflexion injuries p.641
hyperreflexia p.643
incomplete spinal cord injury p.639
neurogenic shock p.643
odontoid process p.648
paraplegia p.639
penetrating injuries p.642
proprioception p. 638
quadriplegia p.639
rotational injuries p.641
simple fractures p.643
spinal cord injury (SCI) p.636
spinal precautions p.646
spinal shock p.643
spondylitic disease p.639
teardrop fractures p.643
tetraplegia p.639
transection p.636

INJURY TO THE SPINAL CORD may be caused by trauma, neoplasm, hemorrhage, infection, or degenerative changes of the spine. Regardless of its etiology, spinal cord injury is a devastating event resulting in major morbidity and disability. Spinal cord injury and its associated complications present a significant and often permanent disability. People who have had a spinal cord injury not only experience the physical effects of this injury, but also face significant psychosocial impacts. Patients with spinal cord injury often are faced with major life changes including loss of prior lifestyle, decreased independence, economic uncertainty, and a negative body image.

Care of patients who have experienced a spinal cord injury poses significant challenges to nurses. The patient may have a profound physiological response to this injury, which can affect all major body systems. The patient's recovery from spinal cord injury can range from no discernible deficit to permanent, severe disability. Nurses caring for this population must have an understanding of the mechanisms of injury and subsequent sequelae, be able to perform an accurate neurological assessment, and institute appropriate interventions to optimize neurological function and avoid potential complications.

Spinal cord injury (SCI) is damage to any part of the spinal cord or nerves at the end of the spinal canal, causing a temporary or permanent loss of sensory, motor, or autonomic function below the level of injury. Although the spinal column serves as a protective structure shielding the delicate spinal tissue, vertebrae can be fractured or dislocated during trauma, resulting in compression, incomplete **transection** (severing), or complete transection of the spinal cord.

Epidemiology

It is estimated that more than 265,000 persons are living with an SCI in the United States, and approximately 12,000 new cases of SCI occur each year. Young adults are those primarily affected, and the majority of SCIs (approximately 80%) occur among males. The average age at injury, which is currently 40 years, has been gradually rising since the

1970s. This may be due to the increase of automobile crashes or sports incidents, though a definitive conclusion has not been reached (Centers for Disease Control and Prevention, 2010). The percentage of people over the age of 60 who have experienced an SCI has increased from approximately 5% of the total number of cases in 1980 to 12% in 2000 (National Spinal Cord Injury Statistical Center [NSCISC], 2012).

Nearly 40% of all spinal cord injuries will be high cervical injuries resulting in devastating loss of motor and sensory control below the level of the neck. More than 50% of all SCIs occur in the cervical spine. The thoracolumbar juncture is the second most common site for injury because of the relative mobility of the spine at this level (Hasler et al., 2011). The life expectancy for individuals who survive at least 1 year after injury depends on the person's age and the severity of injury, but is steadily increasing (NSCISC, 2011). Younger patients with less severe injuries have the best survival rate; older patients, those with severe injuries located high in the spinal cord, and those who are ventilator dependent have the least favorable survival rates (NSCISC, 2011).

Etiology

The majority of SCIs occur because of trauma to the spinal column. The vast majority of SCIs are the result of motor vehicle crashes and catastrophic falls (National Spinal Cord Injury Statistical Center [NSCISC], 2012). Over time, the incidence of SCI related to falls has increased in frequency to nearly 30% (related to an increase in the aging population who are subject to falls), followed by violent injury by gunshot at 15%. Sports- and recreation-related SCIs are more likely to occur in people under the age of 30, with nearly 40% of them being diving accidents associated with alcohol use (Vlok, Petersen, Dunn, & Stander, 2010). Other traumatic injuries also may be present and can influence outcomes after spinal cord injury. Morbidity and mortality after SCI generally is affected by the person's age at the time of injury and by the level and severity of the injury. Older adults and patients with severe injuries high in the spinal cord generally have higher mortality rates (van den Berg, Castellote, de Pedro-Cuesta, & Mahillo-Fernandez, 2010). Spinal cord injuries due to nontraumatic causes (those that result from chronic conditions, such as arthritis, cancer, inflammation or infections, or disk degeneration of the spine) are more likely to occur in people over 40 years of age (Mayo Clinic Staff, 2011b).

Fewer than 10% of SCIs are due to medical reasons such as neoplasm or hemorrhage from a vascular abnormality (Mayo Clinic Staff, 2011). Spinal tumors are broadly classified according to their location within the spine. They are divided into two broad anatomic categories: intradural/intramedullary and intradural/extramedullary. More specific tumor classifications are based on histology. Intramedullary lesions describe neoplasms that arise from within the spinal cord itself. These types of tumors can cause dilation and distortion of the central portion of the spinal cord, or they can infiltrate normal spinal cord tissue. The most common forms of intramedullary spinal cord tumors are infiltrative ependymoma in adults and astrocytoma in children. Ependymomas are most commonly seen in the conus medullaris and cauda equina and are surgically resectable. By contrast, gliomas such as astrocytomas are seen most frequently in the cervical and thoracic regions of the spinal cord and infiltrate the myelon, making surgical resection almost always incomplete (Grimm & Chamberlain, 2009).

Intradural/extramedullary lesions are neoplasms that occur between the dura and the spinal cord. These lesions tend to cause compression but do not invade the neural tissue. Schwannoma and meningioma are the most common intradural/extramedullary spinal tumors. Schwannomas can be found anywhere in the spine, but there is a slightly higher incidence in the thoracic spine. Meningiomas are seen most frequently in females after the age of 40 and have a higher incidence in the thoracic spine; they may be caused by arthritis, cancer, inflammation or infections, or disk degeneration of the spine.

Extradural lesions, or neoplasms that occur outside of the dural covering of the spinal cord, are the most common form of spinal tumors. Most of these tumors involve the bony structures of the spine, such as the vertebral bodies, and are metastatic in nature. These tumors cause destruction and weakening of the bone, resulting in spinal instability and collapse (Rose et al., 2009). Metastatic epidural spinal cord compression is a common problem associated with hematologic spread of cancer. The most common location of compression is the thoracic spine (60%), followed by the lumbar spine (25%) and cervical spine (15%) (Meyer, Singh, & Jenkins, 2010). Lung cancer is the most common origin of spinal metastatic lesion, followed by breast cancer (Hessler, Vettorazzi, Madert, Bokemeyer, & Panse, 2011). Other cancers that commonly metastasize to the spine include myeloma, prostate cancer, and lymphoma (Meyer et al., 2010).

Pathophysiology

To fully understand the pathophysiology associated with spinal cord injury, it is critical to understand the anatomy and physiology related to the spinal cord. The spinal cord extends from the first cervical vertebra to approximately the first lumbar vertebra in the adult. The spinal nerves exit the spinal cord in pairs. Each nerve has two roots, an anterior or ventral root and a posterior or dorsal root. The anterior root connects to the anterior portion of the spinal cord and contains *efferent* motor fibers, which carry motor information from the brain to the body. The posterior nerve root attaches to the posterior spinal cord and contains *afferent* sensory fibers, which carry sensory information from the body to the spinal cord (Figure 24–1◆). The spinal cord then transmits this information to the brain (Bader & Littlejohns, 2010).

The spinal cord is divided into segments according to regions and groups of nerves (Figure 24–2◆, p. 638). The segments are numbered according to the level of the vertebral column. For example, C_3 denotes the third cervical pair of nerves and the third cervical segment of the spinal column. The spinal cord tapers as it passes through the thoracic region and ends at the conus medullaris at approximately the first lumbar vertebra. Below this is the cauda equina. The cauda equina

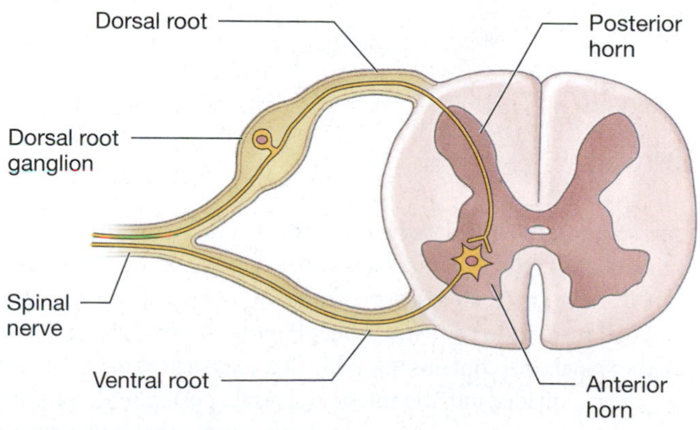

FIGURE 24–1 ◆ Ventral and dorsal nerve roots.

Source: Lindsay, K. W., & Bone, I. (2004). Localized neurological disease and its management: Peripheral nerves and muscles. In *Neurology and Neurosurgery Illustrated*, 4th edition.

Weblink: Spinal Cord Injury Fact Sheet
Weblink: Spinal Cord Injury
Weblink: Spinal Cord Injury Facts and Figures at a Glance
Video: Spinal Injuries—Etiology and Pathophysiology

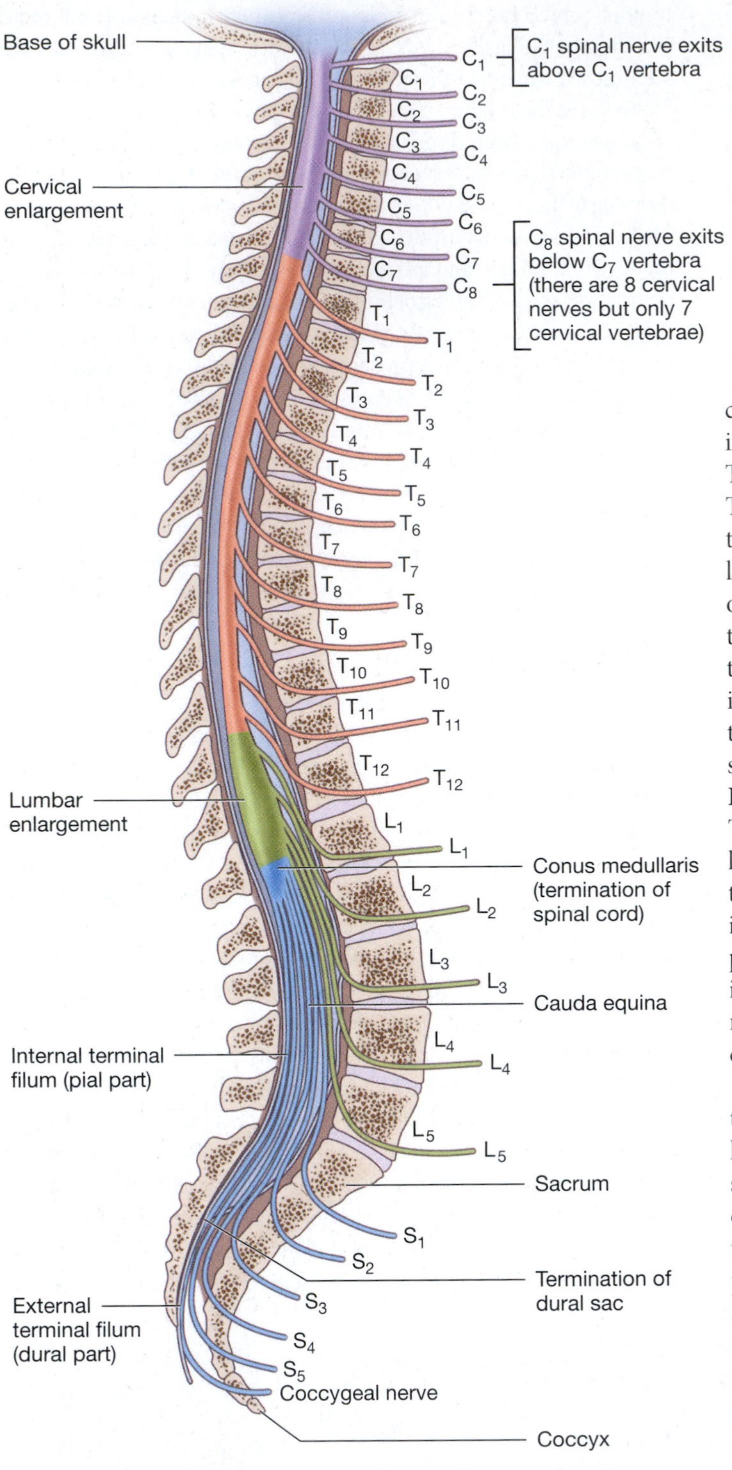

FIGURE 24–2 ◆ Spinal column.

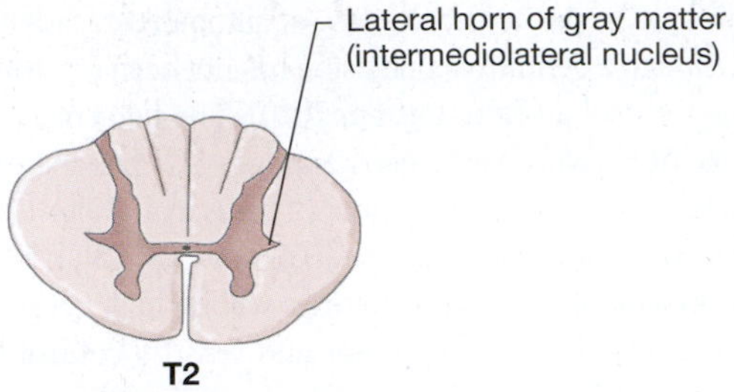

FIGURE 24–3 ◆ Cross section of the thoracic spinal cord.

comprises the lumbar and sacral nerve roots as they arise from the conus medullaris (Bader & Littlejohns, 2010). A cross section of the spinal cord reveals the gray matter, shaped like an "H" or butterfly, in the center of the cord, surrounded by white matter (Figure 24–3◆). The gray matter of the spinal cord contains unmyelinated cells such as the axons and dendrites. It is divided into the anterior (ventral), posterior (dorsal), and lateral columns or horns. The lateral columns of the gray matter extend only from T_1 to L_2 or L_3. The motor fibers of the anterior nerve roots originate in the ventral and lateral columns of the gray matter. The posterior columns of the gray matter receive sensory input from the dorsal nerve roots (Francisco de Assis Aquino Gondim, 2009).

The white matter serves to link the separate segments of the spinal cord and to link the spinal cord to the brain. It is composed of ascending and descending tracts that contain mostly myelinated nerve fibers. These tracts are organized into anterior, posterior, and lateral columns. The ascending tracts primarily contain sensory fibers; the descending tracts contain primarily motor fibers. The ascending tracts in the anterolateral columns of the white matter are responsible for the conveyance of pain and temperature sensations to the brain. Afferent impulses enter the spinal cord from the dorsal nerve roots. These impulses then cross the midline of the spinal cord to the contralateral side. From there, the impulses travel up the spinal cord to the thalamus. Injury involving the anterolateral columns will result in loss of pain and temperature sensation on the opposite side of the body below the level of the injury. **Proprioception** is defined as the sense of position and movement. The ascending tracts responsible for the conveyance of proprioception lie in the dorsal columns of the white matter. These tracts do not cross the spinal cord but ascend on the ipsilateral side to the medulla. Injury involving the ascending tracts in the dorsal column will result in loss of proprioception below the level of injury on the same side. The descending tracts are responsible for motor function and are located in the anterior columns of the white matter. These tracts do not cross in the spinal cord (Bader & Littlejohns, 2010).

The main vessels that provide the blood supply to the spinal cord are the anterior and posterior spinal arteries. These arteries run along the length of the spinal cord and have several vascular feeders. The anterior spinal artery arises from the vertebral arteries and lies along the midline of the spinal cord's anterior surface. This vessel perfuses the anterior two-thirds of the spinal cord, including the anterior and part of the posterior portions of the gray matter. It has a relatively poor collateral blood supply and is therefore susceptible to vascular disease or injury. The posterior spinal arteries are paired arteries that are located laterally on each side of the posterior aspect of the spinal cord. These arteries form a plexus on the posterior aspect of the spinal cord and have a rich collateral blood supply. As a result, the posterior aspect of the spinal cord is less susceptible to vascular disease or injury. The upper cervical spinal cord also is perfused by a plexus of vessels formed by the vertebral and subclavian vessels. The blood supply of the midthoracic region of the spinal cord is augmented by branches of the intercostal artery. The lower portion of the thoracic spinal cord and the conus medullaris receive additional perfusion from the artery of Adamkiewicz, which is the largest anterior segmental medullary artery. The sacral arteries supply perfusion to the sacrum and cauda equina (Barleben & Mills, 2010).

Classification

Spinal cord injuries are classified according to the degree of loss of motor and sensory function below the level of injury. Rehabilitation goals and degree of independence after recovery depend on the type of SCI.

Complete Spinal Cord Injury

A **complete spinal cord injury** is the complete loss of voluntary motor and sensory functions below the level of injury. Injuries involving the cervical spinal cord will result in **tetraplegia** (a Greek term; the Latin term is **quadriplegia**), or loss of motor and sensory function involving both the upper extremities, both the lower extremities, and bowel and bladder control. Injuries involving the thoracic or lumbar spinal cord will result in **paraplegia,** or loss of motor and sensory function in both of the lower extremities and loss of bowel and bladder control (Chart 24–1). In a complete SCI, the damage to the spinal cord is irreversible.

Incomplete Spinal Cord Injury

Patients who have experienced an **incomplete spinal cord injury** will have some preservation of sensory and/or motor function below the level of injury. In these patients, there is sparing of some of the spinal cord tracts, which allows neurotransmission to occur. Five main syndromes are associated with incomplete SCI, each classified according to the portion of the spinal cord damaged and the preservation of function below the level of injury (Figure 24–4◆) (Francisco de Assis Aquino Gondim, 2009).

Central Cord Syndrome

Central cord syndrome is the most common incomplete SCI. This injury can occur at any age but is seen most frequently in older patients who have degenerative bony changes in the cervical spine resulting in narrowing of the overall diameter of the spinal canal. It also may be caused by hemorrhage and intramedullary tumors such as central canal ependymoma (Francisco de Assis Aquino Gondim, 2009). It most often is caused by a hyperextension injury resulting in damage to the center of the spinal cord. The spinal tracts in the cervical spinal cord are arranged so that the fibers leading to the upper extremities are more centrally located, whereas the fibers leading to the lower extremities are located more laterally. Therefore, there is greater loss of motor and sensory function in the upper extremities than in the lower extremities. For these reasons, central cord syndrome is often referred to as "man in a barrel syndrome," since the arms are often weak but the patient maintains preservation of leg strength. The sensory loss often occurs in a dissociated cape-like pattern. The overall prognosis for recovery from this injury is generally favorable; however, a recent study found that older age, poor motor score on admission, and a larger amount of damage to the spinal cord on magnetic resonance imaging (MRI) were associated with poor outcome (Aarabi et al., 2010). The typical pattern of recovery is variable based on the pattern of injury but usually follows a return of lower extremity function first, followed by return of bladder function. Recovery of hand intrinsic function is variable and often the last to occur (Aarabi et al., 2010).

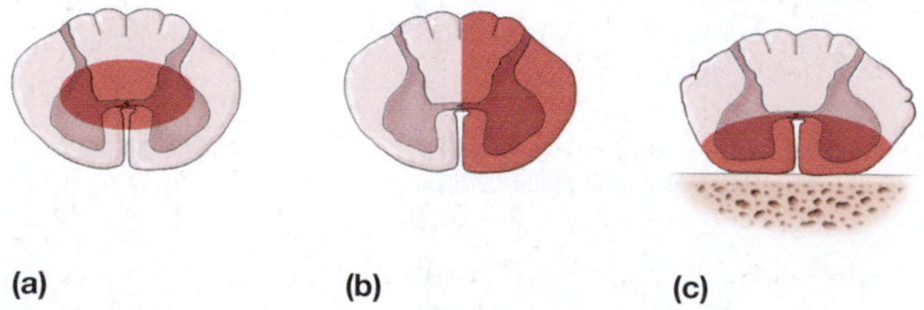

FIGURE 24–4 ◆ Incomplete spinal cord injury: (a) central cord syndrome, (b) anterior cord syndrome, (c) Brown-Séquard syndrome.

Source: Hickey, J. V. (2009). *The clinical practice of neurological and neurosurgical nursing* (6th ed.). Philadelphia, PA: Lippincott Williams & Wilkins.

Anterior Cord Syndrome

Anterior cord syndrome is caused by direct injury to the anterior portion of the spinal cord or disruption of the anterior spinal artery, resulting in ischemia and infarction of the anterior two-thirds of the spinal cord (Francisco de Assis Aquino Gondim, 2009). This often is due to compression from either an acute disk herniation or a hyperextension injury, resulting in fracture-dislocation of the vertebra. Paralysis and loss of pain and temperature sensation are evident below the level of injury. Light touch, vibration, and proprioception are preserved because these tracts are located in the dorsal columns of the spinal cord, which are perfused by the posterior spinal arteries. The prognosis for recovery from this injury is variable, though generally not favorable (McKinley, Santos, Meade, & Brooke, 2007).

Brown-Séquard Syndrome

Brown-Séquard syndrome usually occurs as a result of a penetrating injury causing transverse hemisection of the spinal cord. This injury accounts for fewer than 4% of all spinal cord injuries and is rarely seen in its pure form (Francisco de Assis Aquino Gondim, 2009; McKinley et al., 2007). Paralysis and loss of proprioception are seen on the ipsilateral side of the injury, and pain and temperature sensation are lost on the contralateral side. The spinal tracts responsible for motor and proprioception do not cross the spinal cord as they travel to the brain; however, the spinal tracts responsible for the conveyance of pain and temperature do cross to the opposite side of the cord. Functional recovery from this type of injury is the most favorable among the incomplete spinal cord syndromes (McKinley et al., 2007).

Cauda Equina Syndrome

Compression of the lumbar nerve roots below the level of L_1 can result in cauda equina syndrome. This is most commonly seen with large disk herniations at the L_4/L_5 level that cause mass effect (presence of additional tissue or fluid) on the nerve roots as they descend through the spinal canal. The deficits related to this syndrome are variable, depending on specific nerve root involvement, but can involve motor and sensory functions of the pelvic organs and lower extremities. Weakness, sensory deficits, loss of the Achilles reflex, and bowel and bladder dysfunction—including bowel incontinence, urinary retention, and overflow urinary incontinence—can be seen. Recovery is variable (Francisco de Assis Aquino Gondim, 2009).

Spinal Cord Injury without Radiographic Abnormality

Spinal cord injury without radiographic abnormality (SCIWORA) is defined as spinal cord injury following a traumatic event without signs of fracture, dislocation, or ligamentous injury on plain radiographs, computed tomography (CT), or myelography. This phenomenon was first described in older patients with spondylitic (related to spondylitis, which is inflammation of the vertebrae) changes of the cervical spine who developed central cord injury or acute myelopathy (any functional disturbance and/or pathologic change in the spinal cord), resulting in changes in sensory, motor, and reflex functions after experiencing a hyperextension injury. Although these patients had no evidence of radiographic spinal fracture or dislocation, they had significantly narrowed spinal canals because of the degenerative changes of the spinal column common in **spondylitic disease.**

CHART 24–1 Functional Loss After Complete Spinal Cord Injury

Level of Injury	Motor Function	Deep Tendon Reflexes	Sensory Function	Bowel and Bladder Function
C_1–C_4	Tetraplegia (quadriplegia) *Lost:* All motor function below the neck	All reflexes lost	*Lost:* All sensation from the neck down	Lost
C_5	Tetraplegia (quadriplegia) *Lost:* All function below the shoulders *Intact:* Sternocleidomastoid, cervical paraspinal muscles, trapezius, and diaphragm; may require ventilation	C_5, C_6 Biceps	*Lost:* Sensation below the clavicles Most of the arms, hands, chest, abdomen, and lower extremities *Intact:* Sensation to head, shoulders, deltoid, clavicle, lateral aspect of the forearm	Lost
C_6	Tetraplegia (quadriplegia) *Lost:* All function below the shoulders and upper arms *Intact:* Deltoid, biceps, rotator muscles of the shoulder	C_5, C_6 Brachioradialis	*Lost:* Sensation below the clavicles Chest, abdomen, lower extremities *Intact:* Sensation to the head, shoulders, arms, palms of hands, thumbs	Lost
C_7	Tetraplegia (quadriplegia) *Lost:* Function in portions of the hands and arms Possible loss of intercostal muscles *Intact:* Shoulder depressors, shoulder abductors, shoulder internal rotators, radial wrist extensors, and diaphragm	C_7, C_8 Triceps	*Lost:* Sensation below the clavicles Chest, abdomen, lower extremities *Intact:* Sensation to the head, shoulders, most of the arms and hands	Lost
C_8	Tetraplegia (quadriplegia) *Lost:* Function in portions of the hands and arms *Intact:* Elbow extensors, wrist, finger extensors and flexors; can breathe independently		*Lost:* Sensation below the chest and portions of the hands *Intact:* Sensation to the head, shoulders, part of the upper chest	Lost
T_1–T_6	Paraplegia *Lost:* Function below the midchest including the muscles of the trunk *Intact:* Shoulders, upper chest, arms, hands		*Lost:* Sensation below the midchest *Intact:* Everything above the midchest T_1, T_2 provide sensation to the inner arm T_4 provides sensation to the nipple area	Lost
T_6–T_{12}	Paraplegia *Lost:* Function below the waist *Intact:* Shoulders, arms, hands, long trunk muscles		*Lost:* Sensation below the waist *Intact:* Shoulders, arms, hands T_{10} provides sensation to the umbilicus T_{12} provides sensation to the groin	Lost
L_1–L_3	Paraplegia *Lost:* Most control of the legs and pelvis *Intact:* Shoulders, arms, hands, torso, and hip rotation	L_2–L_4 Knee jerk	*Lost:* Lower abdomen and legs *Intact:* Some sensation to the inner and anterior thigh and L_3 supplies the knee	Lost
L_3–L_4	Paraplegia *Lost:* Portions of the lower legs, ankles, feet *Intact:* Increased knee extension		*Lost:* Sensation to portions of the lower legs, ankles, feet *Intact:* Sensation to the upper legs	Lost
L_4–S_5	Incomplete paraplegia *L_4–S_1:* *Intact:* Abduction and internal rotation of the hip ankle dorsiflexion, and foot inversion *L_5–S_1:* *Intact:* Foot inversion *L_4–S_2:* *Intact:* Foot eversion *S_1–S_2:* *Intact:* Plantar flexion	S_1–S_2 Ankle jerk	*L_5:* *Intact:* Sensation to hip flexors: hip abductors; knee extension knee flexion; ankle dorsiflexion; and medial aspect of the foot *S_1:* *Intact:* Full leg, foot, and ankle control	Possibly spared *S_2–S_4:* Urinary control *S_3–S_5:* Bowel control

CHART 24–1 Functional Loss After Complete Spinal Cord Injury, *continued*

Level of Injury	Motor Function	Deep Tendon Reflexes	Sensory Function	Bowel and Bladder Function
	S_2–S_5: Bowel and bladder control, normal to impaired. Motor function of L_4 to S_5 spinal cord injury is limited as follows: Independent mobility with manual wheelchair; short distance to full ambulation with assistance; ambulate independently with or without assistance with S_1 to S_5 injury.		*S_2:* *Intact:* Full ankle control, posterior aspect of the thigh/calf *Lower* *Intact*: Innervation of perineal muscles for bowel, bladder, sexual function, and lower sacral nerves, and perineum.	

Sources: Adapted from Bader, M. K., & Littlejohns, L. (2010). *AABN core curriculum for neuroscience nursing.* Glenview, IL: Elsevier; Porth, C., & Matfin, G. (2009). *Pathophysiology: Concepts of altered health states.* Philadelphia: Wolters Kluwer/Lippincott Williams & Wilkins.

Magnetic resonance imaging (MRI) provides good imaging of the soft tissue structures of the spinal column, including the intervertebral disks, the ligaments, and the spinal cord itself. Patients who have experienced an SCIWORA often will demonstrate abnormality of the soft tissue structures or spinal cord on MRI that is not evident on standard radiography (Shah & Zollinger, 2011; Sharma et al., 2009).

Mechanisms of Injury

Regardless of the etiology of trauma-related SCI, there are five common primary mechanisms of injury to the spine: hyperflexion, hyperextension, rotation, compression, and penetrating injury. Each of these is related to the type of mechanical force that is applied to the spinal column. **Hyperflexion injuries** occur when there is a sudden deceleration in motion, such as can occur in a head-on motor vehicle collision or a diving accident. As a result of the deceleration, the head and neck are flexed forward in an exaggerated motion. This can result in fracture of the anterior portion of the vertebral body as well as fracture and dislocation of the facet joints in the posterior aspect of the spinal column. The posterior spinal ligament and the intervertebral disk also may be disrupted (Figure 24–5◆). The facet joints and the ligaments are important structures in maintaining the stability of the spine. If they are compromised, the spine will be unstable, and surgical stabilization of the spine may be required. The presence of fracture and dislocation of the facet joints increases the probability of injury to the spinal cord. These injuries often result in anterior compression and wedge deformities of the vertebral body.

Hyperextension injuries occur when the spine is extended backward, as can occur in rear-impact collisions when the head and neck are forcefully extended back, or in forward falls in which the chin or forehead is struck. The spinal cord can be stretched and degenerative changes of the spinal column, including the presence of bone spurs and hypertrophy of the ligaments, can cause excessive compression of the spinal cord, resulting in an SCI. Injury to the ligaments may not be evident, and dislocations are relatively uncommon. Fractures involving the posterior elements of the spinal column, including the spinous processes, may be present (Figure 24–6◆).

Rotational injuries occur when there is extreme lateral flexion or rotation and flexion of the spine (Figure 24–7◆, p. 642). This injury happens with sudden impact from a high-energy trauma, such as a car crash, a sports accident, or a fall from height. Rotational injuries occur most commonly in the neck because of the relative mobility of the spine in this region. The posterior ligaments may rupture, and fracture and dislocation of the facets may occur, resulting in spinal instability. If the facets on both sides of the spine are affected, the incidence of SCI is increased. The fracture and dislocation may need to be reduced with application of traction, and the spine will need to be surgically stabilized.

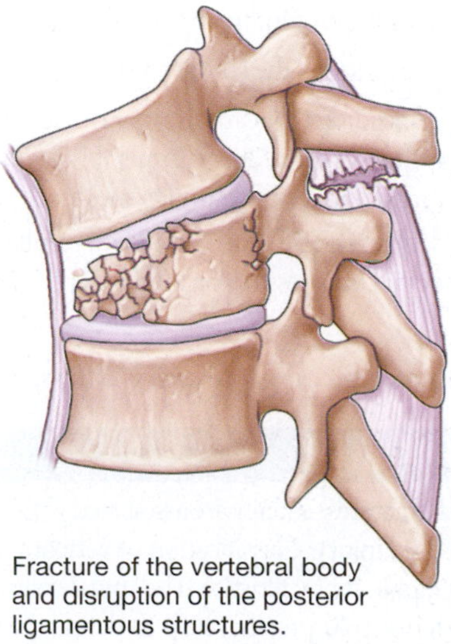

FIGURE 24–5 ◆ Flexion injury.

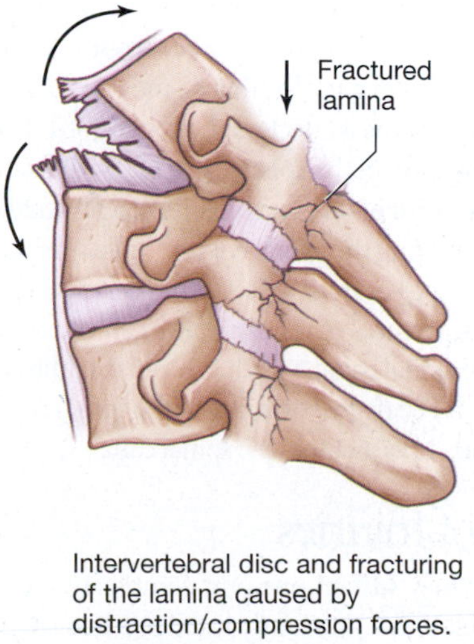

FIGURE 24–6 ◆ Hyperextension injury.

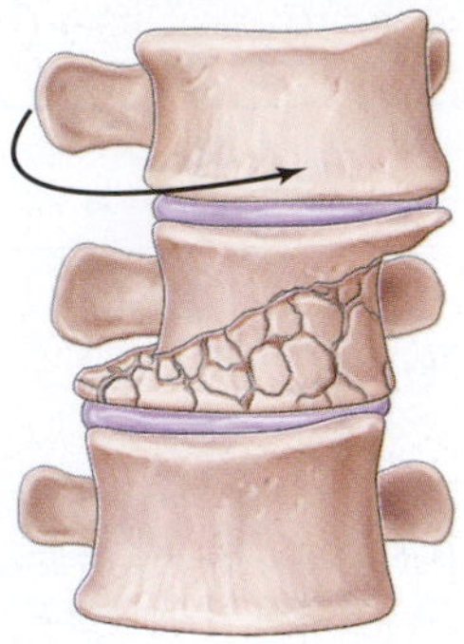

FIGURE 24–7 ◆ Rotational injury.

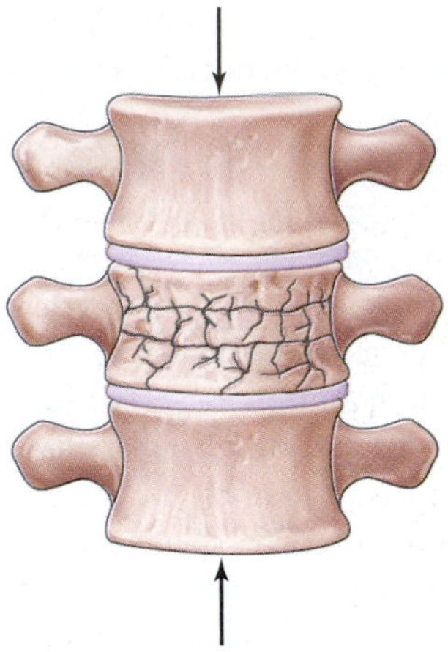

FIGURE 24–8 ◆ Compression fracture.

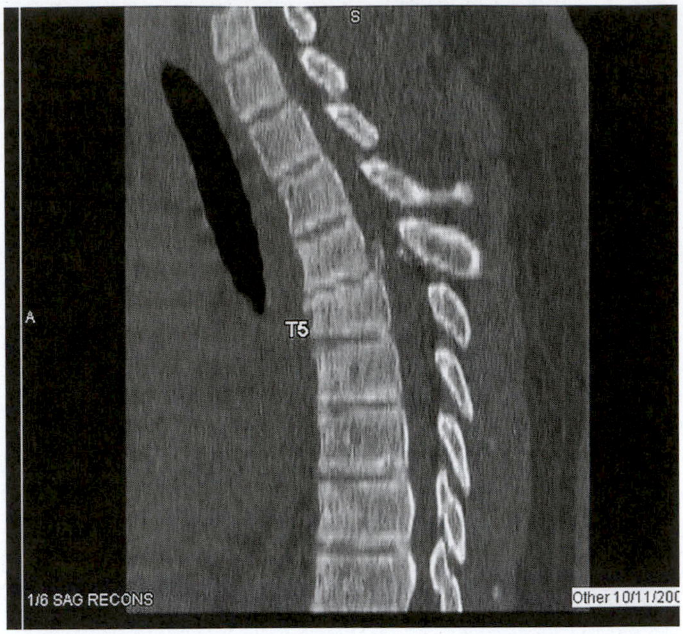

FIGURE 24–9 ◆ CT scan of a thoracic spine compression fracture.
Source: Laurie Baker.

Compression injuries occur because of axial pressure or loading of the spine. A vertical force is applied to the spine, causing fracture of the vertebral body (Figure 24–8◆). These injuries typically occur as a result of landing on the feet or buttocks after a fall from a significant height or from extreme flexion of the spine (Figure 24–9◆). A compression fracture also can occur because of weakening of the vertebral body due to infection, malignancy, or osteoporosis. Bone fragments from the fracture can *retropulse*, that is, move back into the canal and cause compression or mass effect on the spinal cord. These injuries may require decompression of the spinal canal and stabilization of the spine.

Penetrating injuries occur as a result of a projectile such as a bullet or sharp object entering the spinal column. The spinal cord can suffer a **contusion** (bruising) or even a partial or complete transection. Damage to the bony structures of the spine also can occur, resulting in bone fragments in the spinal canal, which can cause additional compression of the spinal cord. The degree of injury to the spinal cord is related to the velocity of the object as it enters the spinal canal.

Types of Injuries

The spinal cord may sustain one or a combination of several types of injuries as a result of the previously listed mechanisms of injury. Common spinal cord injuries are as follows (American Academy of Orthopedic Surgeons, 2010):

- ***Concussion:*** Usually occurs as a result of a blow to the spinal column. The spinal cord is jarred or shaken. A temporary loss of function can be seen for a period of hours or days.
- ***Contusion:*** Often caused by fracture, dislocation, or direct trauma to the spinal cord. The spinal cord is bruised, resulting in intramedullary hemorrhage and edema into the cord. Necrosis of spinal cord tissue may occur because of compression from bleeding or edema or because of direct damage of neural tissue. The degree of neurological dysfunction depends on the severity of the contusion.
- ***Compression:*** Occurs as a result of squeezing or pressure on the spinal cord. The pressure can last momentarily, as in a hyperextension injury, or can be prolonged because of structural damage to the spinal cord caused by the accumulation of bone fragments, a neoplasm, hemorrhage, or disk herniation (Figure 24–10◆).
- ***Laceration:*** A tear or cut in the spinal cord. Neurological deficits resulting from this type of injury are permanent.
- ***Transection:*** Severing of the spinal cord.
- ***Hemorrhage:*** Bleeding that can occur either within the spinal cord or the surrounding tissues. This can result in compression on the spinal cord or irritation to the neural tissues.
- ***Infarction:*** Ischemia of the spinal cord as a result of interruption of blood flow due to compression or injury to the vessels that perfuse the cord.

Vertebral fractures also can cause injury to the spinal cord.

Vertebral Injuries

Vertebral injuries (fractures) usually are associated with major trauma and can cause spinal cord injury. Classification of vertebral fractures is based largely on radiographic characteristics. The spinal column is divided into anterior and posterior columns that help to define the severity of injury and associated spinal stability (Reiter, 2012). Each vertebral region has unique anatomic and functional features that result in specific injuries.

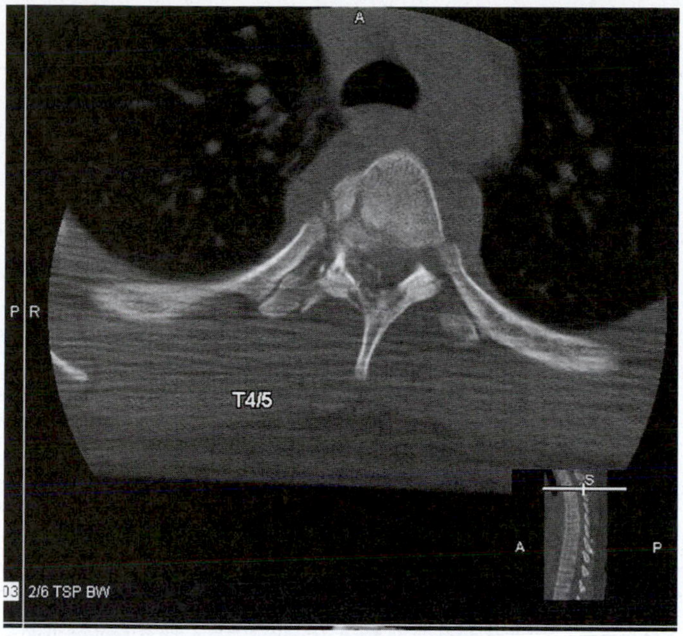

FIGURE 24–10 ◆ CT axial view of a thoracic spine fracture with bone fragments in the canal.
Source: Laurie Baker.

Simple fractures involve a single column injury that is easily visualized on plain films of the spine. Treatment generally is conservative, consisting of the use of pain medication and spinal bracing. **Compression fractures** commonly are related to osteoporosis or a fall causing flattening or wedging of the vertebral body. They generally are restricted to the anterior vertebral body and are easily visualized on plain x-rays. MRI of the spine may be useful to define fracture healing and determine the need for vertebroplasty to stabilize fracture fragments and reduce pain. **Teardrop fractures** often result from hyperflexion injury and are characterized by a chip off the anterior inferior edge of the vertebral body. This type of fracture may displace the bone laterally or posteriorly and typically is unstable. **Atlas fractures,** also known as *Jefferson fractures*, involve disruption of the anterior and posterior arch of C_1. MRI imaging is recommended to ensure that there is no disruption of the transverse ligaments. Atlas fractures found in isolation can be managed conservatively with an external orthopedic appliance that prevents or assists the movement of the spine or limbs (The Free Dictionary, 2011). **Axis fractures,** also known as odontoid fractures, are classified into three types based on radiographic findings. Type 1 odontoid fractures are characterized by a fracture of the tip of the dens (the odontoid process or peg is a projection of the axis [second cervical vertebrae], characterized by a neck where it joins the main vertebrae) and are considered stable. Type 2 odontoid fractures are considered unstable and involve a transverse oblique fracture through the body of the dens; they are routinely treated surgically with use of an odontoid screw. Type 3 odontoid fractures are fractures through the body of the axis and dens. Finally, **hangman's fracture** typically is caused by a hyperflexion injury of the neck. The radiographic findings include fracture through the bilateral pedicles of C_2 and separation of the C_2 and C_3 posterior elements.

Primary Injury

The initial insult to the spinal cord at the time of trauma is known as the primary injury. The spinal cord suffers physical damage as a result of this insult. The degree of damage to the spinal cord depends on the amount of force applied to the cord at the time of the initial injury and may range from mild cord concussion, resulting in a transient loss of function, to severe injury, resulting in complete and permanent loss of function. As a result of the initial trauma, the neural elements of the spinal cord, including nerve cells and the ascending and descending spinal tracts, will be disrupted at the level of the injury. The vasculature of the spinal cord also can be affected, resulting in hemorrhage and ischemia of the spinal cord (Martirosyan, Feuerstein, Theodore, Cavalcanti, Spetzler, & Preul, 2011).

Spinal shock is a state of **areflexia,** in which there is a loss of all motor, sensory, and reflex activity at the level of the injury and below. Spinal shock occurs as a result of the primary injury. The duration of spinal shock is quite variable, lasting as little as a few hours or as long as several weeks after injury. When the patient is in this state, it is impossible to determine the extent of the SCI. As spinal shock abates, signs of muscle spasticity and **hyperreflexia** (a reaction of the autonomic nervous system to overstimulation) become evident. The return of the bulbocavernosus reflexes usually occurs hours to weeks after injury (Bader & Littlejohns, 2010).

Secondary Injury

The initial or primary SCI sets forth a cascade of complex events that can worsen the extent of the injury by causing damage to the adjoining neural tissues. The exact mechanism of this injury is not entirely understood, but many of the current treatment strategies for SCI are directed at reducing the damage caused by this secondary process. The secondary process begins almost immediately after the initial trauma to the spinal cord. Ischemia within the spinal cord at the time of the primary injury leads to additional vascular changes, which worsen the disruption of the normal perfusion of the spinal cord (Martirosyan et al., 2011). As a result of these vascular changes, cell membrane permeability is affected owing to dysfunction of the cellular sodium-potassium pump (see Chapter 15). Intracellular potassium is depleted and sodium and calcium ions enter into the cell, resulting in cellular edema and subsequent cell death. The increased intracellular calcium triggers the release of enzymes and free radicals, which worsens cellular necrosis and leads to additional tissue damage. An inflammatory response is triggered, resulting in increased vascular permeability, edema, and macrophage activity, leading to additional tissue damage and glial scarring (Rodríguez-Zayas, Torrado, Rosas, Santiago, Figueroa, & Miranda, 2011).

Disruption of autonomic regulation occurs as a result of SCI and can lead to **neurogenic shock.** This phenomenon is most commonly seen in patients who have had an SCI at T_6 or above and should be differentiated from spinal shock. Spinal shock results in the loss of sensorimotor control and loss of the muscle stretch and cutaneous reflexes below the level of the injury. Neurogenic shock results in the disruption of the sympathetic nervous system. The sympathetic nervous system originates in the thoracolumbar region of the spinal cord and is responsible for elevations in heart rate and blood pressure and for vasoconstriction of the peripheral vascular system during stress situations. Neurogenic shock occurs when the normal impulses from the brainstem, which contribute to the reflexive control of heart rate and blood pressure, are disrupted, resulting in interruption of normal sympathetic outflow. Vagal tone is, therefore, left unopposed (Popa et al., 2010), leading to bradycardia, peripheral vasodilation below the level of injury (resulting in decreased systemic vascular resistance), hypotension, and decreased cardiac output. The resulting hypotension and diminished cardiac output are thought to further contribute to ischemia of the spinal cord at the site of injury.

Weblink: Autonomic Hyperreflexia

The trauma patient who is suspected of having an SCI also may experience hypovolemic shock. It is important to distinguish between neurogenic shock and hypovolemic shock to ensure that appropriate treatment strategies are implemented. Hypotension is a hallmark sign for both neurogenic shock and hypovolemic shock. The patient experiencing neurogenic shock will exhibit bradycardia with a heart rate of 50 to 70 beats per minute and will often require vasopressor support (drugs used to maintain mean arterial pressure of < 65 mmHg) for treatment; the patient's skin also will be warm and hyperemic. The patient in hypovolemic shock will exhibit tachycardia and will usually respond to volume replacement. Shock is discussed in detail in Chapter 54.

Safety Alert *It is easy to confuse neurogenic shock and hypovolemic shock in the trauma patient with SCI. The two conditions may both be present and will manifest with hypotension, but an important distinction is bradycardia. The nurse needs to assess patients for the symptoms of neurogenic shock and differentiate the symptoms from those of hypovolemia shock.*

Autonomic Hyperreflexia

Autonomic hyperreflexia occurs as a result of a noxious stimulus below the level of the SCI. Common causes include urinary tract abnormalities such as a distended bladder, abnormalities of the lower intestinal tract such as constipation or fecal impaction, and pressure ulcers. A sympathetic response is triggered by the noxious stimulus, resulting in vasoconstriction below the level of the SCI. Blood volume is shifted from the vasculature below the SCI to the vasculature above the injury, causing elevation of blood pressure. The baroreceptors in the carotid body and the aortic arch stimulate the vasomotor center of the medulla, which in turn triggers slowing of the heart and vasodilation. The vasculature above the level of injury responds, resulting in flushing of the skin, piloerection (the erection of hairs on the skin surface), and nasal congestion; however, these impulses are blocked at the level of the SCI, and vasoconstriction continues unchecked below the level of injury. This response will continue until the noxious stimulus is removed (Bader & Littlejohns, 2010). The National Guideline Clearinghouse publishes national guidelines for the acute management of autonomic hyperreflexia. These were last revised in 2006, and the summary was updated by the ECRE (Evidence-Based Care Rate) Institute in 2009. The guidelines currently in use are shown in the National Guidelines box.

Safety Alert *Autonomic hyperreflexia is a medical emergency that can lead to serious complications if left untreated. When the patient exhibits symptoms of autonomic hyperreflexia, it is important for the nurse to notify*

NATIONAL GUIDELINES for Acute Management of Autonomic Hyperreflexia

Guideline

Patients with SCI at or above T_6 are at risk for autonomic hyperreflexia.

Recognize the signs and symptoms of autonomic hyperreflexia:

Elevated blood pressure: a sudden, significant increase (20–40 mmHg) in both diastolic and systolic blood pressures above the patient's usual level

Pounding headache

Bradycardia: may be within normal range but relative slowing compared to the patient's normal heart rate

Profuse sweating above the level of the lesion, especially the face, neck, and shoulders

Piloerection above and possibly below the level of injury

Cardiac dysrhythmias including atrial fibrillation, premature ventricular contractions, and atrioventricular conduction abnormalities

Flushing of the skin above the level of injury, especially the face, neck, and shoulders

Patient complaint of visual disturbance such as blurred vision or spots in the visual field

Nasal congestion

Feelings of apprehension or anxiety

Symptoms may be absent or minimal despite significantly elevated blood pressure (silent autonomic hyperreflexia)

Treatment

- If the person is supine, immediately sit the patient up and lower the legs if possible. This allows the blood to pool in the lower extremities and may lower the blood pressure.
- Loosen any clothing or constricting devices.
- Monitor the blood pressure and pulse frequently. Blood pressure can fluctuate rapidly due to impaired autonomic regulation.
- Quickly assess the patient for the instigating cause and remove it as quickly as possible.
  - The most common cause of autonomic hyperreflexia is bladder distention:
    - Check indwelling catheter for patency and proper placement.
    - If the catheter is blocked, gently irrigate with 10 to 15 mL normal saline at body temperature.
    - Avoid compressing or tapping on the bladder.
    - If the catheter does not drain, remove and replace the catheter.
  - If no catheter is in place, catheterize the patient:
    - Instill 2% lidocaine jelly into the urethra and wait 2 minutes if time allows before inserting the catheter to decrease sensory input and relax the urinary sphincter.
  - The second most common cause of autonomic hyperreflexia is fecal impaction:
    - If systolic blood pressure is >150 mmHg, consider pharmacologic treatment to reduce blood pressure without causing hypotension prior to checking for fecal impaction.
    - If systolic blood pressure is <150 mmHg, check for fecal impaction:
      - Instill 2% lidocaine jelly into the rectum.
      - Wait 2 minutes.
      - Insert gloved, lubricated finger into the rectum and check for the presence of stool.
      - If stool is present, gently remove.
      - If autonomic hyperreflexia worsens, stop the manual evacuation, instill additional topical anesthetic, and recheck the rectum after approximately 20 minutes.
    - If urinary and fecal causes of autonomic hyperreflexia have been eliminated and symptoms persist, assess for other instigating causes and treat accordingly: pressure ulcerations, abdominal pathology, ingrown toenails, long bone fractures, and infection.

Education

Educate the patient and family about common causes of autonomic hyperreflexia and appropriate treatment strategies.

Source: National Guideline Clearinghouse. (2006). *Acute management of autonomic dysreflexia: Individuals with spinal cord injury presenting to a health-care facility.* Washington, DC: Consortium for Spinal Cord Medicine, Paralyzed Veterans of America. Retrieved from http://www.guideline.gov/summary/summary.aspx?doc_id=2964&nbr=002190&string=Autonomic+AND+dysreflexia. Reviewed in 2009.

the health care provider and to institute measures to treat the blood pressure and to identify and correct the cause.

Clinical Manifestations

The clinical manifestations of spinal cord injury are systemic in that the injury can affect the function of multiple organ systems depending on the level and severity of the injury. It is vital that nurses caring for this population understand the systemic effects of SCI so that appropriate assessment and interventions can be undertaken to avoid potential medical complications.

Cardiovascular

Cardiac dysfunction is the second most common cause of death among chronic SCI patients, affecting nearly one-quarter of survivors (Grigorean et al., 2009). Neurogenic shock resulting in cardiovascular compromise commonly occurs in the patient who has sustained an SCI at T_6 or above. Among patients with high cervical cord injury, 100% develop bradycardia and 16% develop cardiac arrest. Sympathetic innervation is lost, leaving vagal tone unopposed. Bradycardia, peripheral vasodilation below the level of injury, decreased systemic vascular resistance, and hypotension are seen. Cardiac preload and afterload subsequently are decreased, resulting in decreased cardiac output. The use of atropine to increase the heart rate and vasopressors such as norepinephrine, dopamine, or dobutamine may be required to increase the heart rate, promote vasoconstriction, and increase cardiac output (Grigorean et al., 2009).

Orthostatic hypotension also may be problematic for this patient population. The loss of sympathetic vascular tone results in blood pooling in the abdomen and lower extremities and a loss of arteriole vasomotor control. Prolonged immobility and decreased intravascular volume are contributing factors. The patient experiences a drop in blood pressure when placed in an upright position and may complain of dizziness, light-headedness, visual disturbance, or syncope because of diminished blood supply to the brain, a phenomenon referred to as orthostatic hypotension. If this phenomenon is left unchecked, cerebral ischemia is possible (Grigorean et al., 2009; Popa et al., 2010).

Pooling of blood in the peripheral vascular system, flaccidity of the extremities, and immobility predispose the patient with SCI to the development of deep venous thrombosis (DVT). This condition, if left untreated, could lead to the more serious complication of pulmonary embolus. The risk of development of DVT seems to be highest in the first 2 to 3 months after injury (Agarwal & Mathur, 2009). Patients may be asymptomatic initially unless they have some preservation of sensation. Signs of DVT include the presence of low-grade fever, edema in the affected limb, and change in temperature of the affected limb. Patients who have sensory sparing (preservation of sensation) may complain of pain and tenderness of the site. Diagnosis and treatment of DVT are discussed in detail in Chapter 35.

Pulmonary

Patients who have sustained an SCI above T_{12} have the potential for impairment of respiratory function. The degree of impairment depends on the level of injury. Generally, higher-level injuries mean more significant impairment (Chin, 2012). Atelectasis and pneumonia are common complications after SCI regardless of the involved spinal level and also can contribute to decompensation in respiratory function (Lieberman & Brown, 2011).

The diaphragm receives innervation from the phrenic nerve, which arises above C_5. The diaphragm is responsible for inspiration and deep breathing as well as the initiation of an effective cough. Injuries at C_4 or higher will cause paralysis of the diaphragm, necessitating intubation and ventilation (Bader & Littlejohns, 2010). Patients who have experienced injuries involving the lower cervical spine, thoracic spine, or lumbar spine usually will not require immediate intubation but warrant close monitoring for signs of respiratory decompensation because of loss of use of the respiratory accessory muscles. The intercostal and abdominal muscles that aid inspiration, forced expiration, and cough are innervated by the T_1–T_{12} nerves. Loss of use of these accessory muscles results in a decrease of about 70% of forced vital capacity and maximal inspiratory force in the acute period following SCI (Chin, 2012). Pulmonary embolus (PE) is a potentially life-threatening condition that may develop in spinal cord injury. A decline in oxygen saturation may be the only sign of PE; however, other symptoms may include chest pain or dyspnea. If any of these signs are evident and a PE is suspected, additional evaluation such as helical CT scan of the chest should be done immediately. Once PE has been diagnosed, treatment usually is supportive, involving the administration of oxygen therapy and anticoagulation medication (Bounameaux, 2010). PE is discussed in detail in Chapter 27.

Safety Alert *Pulmonary embolus is a life-threatening disorder that can result in death if not recognized and treated promptly. Common signs and symptoms include decrease in oxygen saturation, shortness of breath, and chest pain. If the patient exhibits any of these symptoms, the managing health care provider should be notified immediately.*

The Evidence-Based Practice box focuses on respiratory complications following spinal cord injury. The discussion explores the relationship of respiratory problems to aspiration and dysphasia in patients with a cervical spinal cord injury.

Weblink: Respiratory Complications **Weblink:** Kaun: Stress Ulcer Prophylaxis

Gastrointestinal

Gastrointestinal effects of spinal shock include gastroparesis, a loss of intestinal peristalsis, and ileus. This results in abdominal distention, which places the patient at risk for vomiting and aspiration and may interfere with respiratory function. Placement of a nasogastric or oral gastric tube often is necessary in the acute phase of SCI for decompression of the stomach and minimization of these risks (Coggrave, Norton, & Wilson-Barnett, 2008). A pharmacologic prophylactic medication regimen such as with antacids should be instituted in all SCI patients (Kaun, 2011).

Patients with SCI will experience abnormalities in both sensory and motor function of the bowel owing to disruption of the spinal tracts responsible for bowel control. Generally, patients with injury above T_{12} will experience decreased intestinal peristalsis, absent rectal sensation, and an increase in anal sphincter tone. Reflex activity may be preserved. These patients are prone to chronic constipation, tend to experience loss of tone throughout the colon and rectal sphincters, and are more likely to experience bowel incontinence (Fynne, Worsøe, Gregersen, Schlageter, Laurberg, & Krogh, 2011).

Genitourinary

The spinal tracts responsible for bladder control also are disrupted in SCI, resulting in loss of the normal bladder reflexes and loss of control of urination. As a result, the bladder becomes atonic, and the patient experiences urinary retention and bladder distention. Urinary incontinence

Weblink: Bedsores (Pressure Sores)

EVIDENCE-BASED PRACTICE Respiratory Complications Related to Spinal Cord Injury

Clinical Problem

Respiratory complications account for the most common cause of death in patients who have sustained a spinal cord injury. Serial examinations of the patient can assist in demonstrating signs of respiratory decompensation, fatigue, ascension of spinal cord lesion, or onset of pulmonary complications. Patients with injury in the cervical spine are at the highest risk for morbidity and mortality related to respiratory issues, owing in large part to disruption of innervation to the diaphragm and respiratory accessory muscles. However, aspiration also contributes to pulmonary-related complications (Bader & Littlejohns, 2010). Patients who have sustained a cervical spinal cord injury are at increased risk for aspiration not only because they cannot adequately protect their airways, owing to ineffective protective measures such as cough and to lack of control of chest and abdominal muscles, but also because these patients experience abnormality in swallowing (Barker, 2008).

Research Findings

Shin, Yoo, Lee, Goo, and Kim (2011) conducted a retrospective chart review of cervical spinal cord injury in patients who had undergone a video-fluoroscopic swallowing study (VFSS). The researchers evaluated the patients' swallow function and analyzed the features of dysphagia present in the study population. The sample size consisted of 121 cervical spinal cord injury patients. Ten patients showed evidence of aspiration on VFSS. Aspiration was statistically correlated with the patient's age and presence of tracheostomy, indicating dysphagia. They concluded that there is a possibility of silent aspiration, especially in patients with previous pneumonia, presence of a tracheostomy, or signs and symptoms indicating dysphagia.

A study performed by Shem, Castillo, Wong, and Chang (2011) showed that dysphagia following cervical SCI can increase the risk of pulmonary complications and delay the rehabilitation process. A bedside swallow evaluation (BSE) followed by a VFSS within 72 hours of the BSE was conducted on 29 patients within 31 days of injury. Dysphagia was diagnosed in 12 of the patients. Dysphagia was noted in 62% of patients with a tracheostomy.

Implications for Nursing Practice

As these studies show, patients with cervical spinal cord injury are at risk of aspiration due to swallowing abnormalities. Not only do these patients have abnormalities in the mechanics of swallow, but treatment modalities such as cervical bracing also contribute to swallowing dysfunction. It is important for nurses caring for this population to be aware of this risk so that appropriate assessment and prevention strategies can be instituted as part of the nursing plan of care. The patient and family also will need to be educated on the risk for aspiration as well as precautions to take to prevent it. If the patient exhibits signs of aspiration such as a wet quality to the voice, coughing with oral intake, or difficulty managing oral secretions, a referral for formal swallow evaluation is warranted. Aspiration prevention is a key strategy in decreasing the risk of pulmonary complications.

Critical Thinking Questions with answers can be found in the Osborn Student Resources at nursing.pearsonhighered.com.

References

Bader, M. K., & Littlejohns, L. (2010). *AANN core curriculum for neuroscience* nursing. Glenview, IL: Elsevier.

Barker, E. (2008). *Neuroscience nursing: A spectrum of care* (3rd ed.). St. Louis, MO: Mosby Elsevier.

Shem, K., Castillo, K., Wong, S., & Chang, J. (2011). Dysphagia in individuals with tetraplegia: Incidence and risk factors. *Journal of Spinal Cord Medicine, 34*(1), 85–92.

Shin, J. C., Yoo, J. H., Lee Y. S., Goo, H. R., & Kim, D. H. (2011). Dysphagia in cervical spinal cord injury. *Spinal Cord 41*(6), 347–353.

may occur as the result of overflow of urine from a distended bladder into the urethra. Over-distension of the bladder can cause complications such as autonomic dysreflexia (overactivity of the autonomic nervous system) and impairment of the blood supply to the bladder (David & Steward, 2010), thereby causing reflux of urine into the ureters and kidneys because of the increased bladder pressures. SCI patients are predisposed to complications such as urinary tract infection (UTI), hydronephrosis (distension of the pelvis and calyces of the kidney by urine that cannot flow past an obstruction in a ureter), decline in renal function, and the development of renal calculi. Chapter 34 discusses renal and urinary disorders. In some cases of incomplete SCI, bladder function may return after recovery from spinal shock. Post-void residuals should be assessed in these patients to ensure adequate bladder emptying (Bader & Littlejohns, 2010). Those with persistent post-void residuals greater than 150 mL may benefit from intermittent self-catheterization (Assis & e Faro, 2011).

Integumentary

Patients with SCI are at high risk for development of pressure ulcers because of impairment in sensory and motor functions as well as impairment of tissue perfusion due to hypotension and pooling of blood in the lower extremities. Risk factors for the development of pressure ulcers include patient age, completeness of injury, mobility, incontinence, and socioeconomic status (Henzel, Bogie, Guihan, & Ho, 2011). Additional factors that contribute to the development of pressure ulcers in this population include fever, infection, poor nutrition, and prolonged immobilization on the firm spinal board used to maintain optimal spinal alignment during transport to the hospital (Mayo Clinic Staff, 2011a). Once these wounds develop, they can be very difficult to heal and can increase the risk of infection.

General Evaluation and Management

Evaluation and management of SCI begin at the scene of the trauma and are continued throughout the acute care hospitalization and rehabilitation phases. Early assessment and management are vital for determining the extent of injury and minimizing secondary injury to the spinal cord. Acute care assessment and management are directed toward optimizing the patient's neurological function and avoiding early complications. Rehabilitative management and evaluation focus on adaptation and avoidance of long-term complications.

Prehospital Phase

Expert evaluation and management of the trauma victim at the scene can make a difference in the patient's ultimate neurological outcome. Improper mobilization of the trauma victim with an unrecognized, unstable spinal fracture can worsen or even cause injury to the spinal cord. Impairment of respiratory and circulatory function also can worsen SCI. First responders follow the general principles of trauma management, including rapid assessment of the victim, evaluation and management of the ABCs (airway, breathing, circulation), stabilization and control of life-threatening injuries, and rapid transport to an appropriate facility.

Spinal precautions are methods of immobilizing the spine and moving patients to prevent or avoid additional spinal injury. These precautions are initiated at the scene of the trauma and are carried out until spinal injury has been ruled out or appropriate treatment strategies have been implemented. Immobilization of the entire spine is necessary because an estimated 19% of patients with a spinal injury have injuries at more than one spinal level that are not contiguous (Miller, Brubacher, Biswas, Lawrence, Whang, & Grauer, 2011). Spinal precautions usually are implemented in any trauma patient; however, determination of the mechanism of injury at the scene can prove invaluable in helping to identify potential injuries. Victims of a traumatic event with a significant mechanism of injury are at greater risk for multiple organ injuries and neurological injuries. First responders should have a high suspicion of spinal injury in any victim with multiple injuries, complaint of spinal pain, spinal deformity, or abnormality on sensory and/or motor examination. Victims who are in a high-risk group; those with a head injury, loss of consciousness, an altered mental status, or complain of motor or sensory disturbance at the scene; and those who are under the influence of drugs or alcohol warrant more careful handling until a spinal injury can be ruled out (Saltzherr, Fung Kon Jin, Beenen, Vandertop, & Goslings, 2009).

Spinal precautions can be initiated with the patient in an upright position if necessary until extrication and movement to a long back board is possible. A rigid cervical collar is applied, and the patient is logrolled onto a back board in the supine position with the spine in a neutral position. Older patients may warrant special consideration with positioning owing to arthritic changes of the spine affecting spinal alignment. All trauma patients require vigilant monitoring of airway and respiratory function. Immobilization on a back board can contribute to respiratory impairment because forced vital capacity is decreased by approximately 20% (Chin, 2012).

Emergency Department

Once the patient arrives in the emergency department, a complete survey of injuries and continued stabilization of the patient will continue while spinal precautions are maintained. A baseline assessment of the patient's physical and neurological status as well as information pertaining to the trauma and the patient's past medical history will be obtained by the health care provider. Efforts should be made to expedite diagnostic testing to facilitate early identification of spinal cord compression or spinal instability so that appropriate surgical measures can be taken if needed or restrictive protective equipment can be removed if not required. After the initial assessment and diagnostic evaluation have been completed and the treatment plan has been established, the patient should be removed from the back board to avoid complications related to prolonged immobilization (Chin, 2012).

Evaluation of pulmonary and circulatory function takes precedence in treating the SCI patient. The patient is assessed and monitored for adequacy of respiratory efforts and ventilatory function by the nurse and other health care providers. All patients must have oxygenation monitored continuously with pulse oximetry, and a baseline arterial blood gas (ABG) must be obtained. Lung sounds are assessed on admission and repeated periodically. The patient with SCI may initially present with adequate respiratory function but can quickly deteriorate. Apnea; stridorous respirations; use of accessory muscles; rapid, shallow respirations; and decline of oxygen saturation are indicative of inadequate respiratory efforts (Chin, 2012). Ventilatory support should be considered if the patient exhibits signs of inadequate respiratory function. If intubation is necessary, care should be taken to ensure the spine remains in alignment and extension or flexion of the neck is avoided (Ahn et al., 2010).

Circulatory function including heart rate, rhythm, and blood pressure also is closely monitored. The patient with SCI may be bradycardic and hypotensive on presentation to the emergency department due to disruption in vagal tone due tp neurogenic shock. Blood pressure may be further compromised by hypovolemia. Central venous pressure monitoring is helpful in determining volume status and and identifying hypovolemic shock (Fehlings, Cadotte, & Fehlings, 2011).

Patients with SCI due to trauma also are at risk for other organ injuries. These patients may not be able to experience visceral pain because of the SCI. Therefore, it is vital that health care providers in the emergency department be vigilant in assessing for signs of other organ injury during the initial assessment.

A careful baseline neurological examination, including motor function, sensory evaluation, deep tendon reflexes, and perineal evaluation, is crucial in the initial assessment of the patient suspected of having a spinal injury. This assessment will be the basis for patient management as well as for determination of change in neurological status. The nurse should perform this assessment before the patient receives pain medication, sedatives, or paralytic medications, if possible, as these medications can interfere with the ability to obtain an accurate neurological assessment.

The overall level of consciousness should be assessed in all trauma patients using a Glasgow Coma Scale (GCS) score because there is a possibility of concomitant brain injury. The GCS score, as described in Chapter 20, is the sum of scores for the patient's best eye opening, verbal, and motor responses. This score provides a means for monitoring changes in the patient's mental status and predicting a prognosis from the time of injury in patients who have sustained a traumatic brain injury.

A detailed assessment by the nurse or health care provider of motor function of all major muscle groups in both the upper and lower extremities should be obtained as part of the initial assessment and repeated hourly as part of the routine monitoring of vital signs for the first 48 to 72 hours. The strength of each major muscle group is tested individually and compared with the corresponding muscle group on the contralateral side. The muscle strength is graded on a scale of 0 to 5 with 0 indicating no motor function and 5 indicating normal strength (Chart 24–2). Each muscle group is innervated by a corresponding spinal nerve (Chart 24–3, p. 648). Abnormalities in motor function can help with approximating the level of the SCI.

A sensory examination also is performed by the nurse or health care provider assessing the patient's response to pinprick in all dermatomes using a sequential side-to-side manner. Abnormalities in sensation are documented according to the corresponding dermatome. An anatomic dermatome chart is a helpful resource in determining the specific level of sensory abnormality (see Figure 20–6, p. 641, Chapter 20).

Evaluation of the deep tendon reflexes (DTRs) and rectal sphincter tone is included in the initial assessment by the nurse or health care provider. Each reflex is innervated by a corresponding spinal nerve (Chart 24–4). Reflex activity is lost below the level of injury when spinal shock is present. As spinal shock abates, reflexes will generally return. The DTRs usually are not tested on a routine basis after the initial assessment; however, the nurse can monitor sphincter tone and sensation during the routine bowel regimen (Chin, 2012).

In addition to the neurological assessment, the entire spine should be palpated as part of the initial evaluation. Bony deformity, alteration in alignment, pain, and focal tenderness should be noted because these signs may be indicative of spinal fracture or dislocation.

CHART 24–2 Grading of Muscle Strength

Grade	Strength
0	No contraction
1	Trace or flicker contraction
2	Movement with gravity eliminated
3	Movement against gravity
4	Movement against resistance
5	Normal strength

CHART 24–3 Major Muscle Group Innervation and Function

Spinal Nerve	Muscle	Function
C_5	Deltoid	Abduct arm
C_6	Biceps	Bend elbow
C_6, C_7	Extensor carpi radialis	Extend wrist
C_7	Triceps	Straighten elbow
C_8, T_1	Hand intrinsics	Spread fingers
L_1, L_2	Iliopsoas	Raise knee to chest
L_3, L_4	Quadriceps	Extend knee
L_5	Tibialis anterior	Dorsiflex the foot
S_1	Extensor hallucis longus	Extend the great toe
	Hamstring	Flex knee
	Gastrocnemius	Plantar flex the foot

CHART 24–4 Spinal Reflexes

Spinal Level	Reflex
C_5–C_6	Biceps
C_7	Triceps
L_4	Patellar
S_1	Achilles

Nursing Management

Nursing management in the emergency department setting requires rapid assessment and critical thinking to identify the primary injury as well as protect the spine from secondary injury. It is necessary to quickly obtain a report of the prehospital management and history of the injury event. The nurse will need to determine the circumstances of the injury, the patient's neurological status immediately after the injury, and treatment at the injury site (Hickey, 2009). It is necessary to query the patient and family as to what happened, when it happened, where it happened, and how it happened. All this information is necessary to assist the health care team in making a diagnosis as to the type of spinal cord injury and for planning appropriate emergency and ongoing care.

Immediate care consists of maintaining ventilation, establishing hemodynamic parameters that ensure optimal end-organ perfusion, evaluating motor and sensory functions, determining gastrointestinal status and possibly placing a gastric tube, stabilizing the injured portion of the spine, providing pain relief, and providing psychological support for the patient and family members. Treatment is discussed in the medical management section that follows.

Immobilization of the patient is critical in the emergency department and during transport to the next care unit. The patient who is diagnosed with a spinal cord injury is generally transferred to the intensive care unit for treatment. Nursing management of the patient in the acute care setting is discussed in the Nursing Process: Patient Care Plan on page 654.

Laboratory and Diagnostic Procedures

All patients who are suspected of having a spinal injury will undergo radiographic evaluation of the spine. Initially, plain x-rays are obtained of the entire spinal axis to assess spinal alignment and the integrity of the spinal elements. Anterior-posterior (AP) and lateral views are obtained. The **odontoid process,** the toothlike projection of C_2 that sits behind the anterior portion of C_1, is difficult to visualize on standard x-ray views; therefore, an x-ray through the patient's open mouth is used for visualization of the odontoid process and the C_1–C_2 junction.

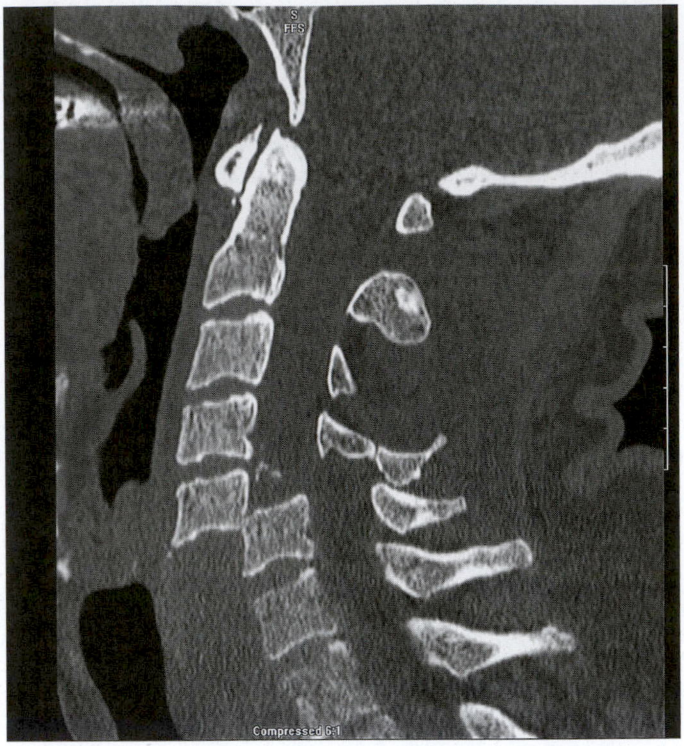

FIGURE 24–11 ◆ CT of C_5–C_6 fracture and subluxation.
Source: Laurie Baker.

The cervicothoracic junction also can be difficult to visualize with plain radiographs because of interference of the shoulder joint. Visualization of this area of the spine often requires pulling downward on the patient's shoulders or obtaining a lateral swimmer's view with the patient's arm fully abducted. However, this type of positioning may not be possible if the victim has sustained trauma to the upper extremities.

A computed tomography (CT) scan provides detailed imaging of the bony structures of the spine and is very helpful in identifying fractures that may be missed on plain radiographs (Figure 24–11 ◆). An MRI scan may be obtained to provide imaging of the soft tissue structures including the spinal cord, intervertebral disks, and ligaments; however, an MRI is not indicated for all patients (Figure 24–12 ◆) (Fehlings et al., 2011). See the Diagnostic Tests box for a listing of tests for acute SCI.

Medical Management

Decisions regarding treatment strategies for the patient with SCI are guided by the patient's presentation and the results of the imaging studies. The ultimate goals of treatment are to stabilize the spine at the level of injury, optimize neurological outcome, and prevent neurological deterioration. Early medical management of the patient with SCI is geared toward stabilization of the spine and lessening of the secondary injury processes.

If stability of the vertebral column or ligaments is in question, immobilization of the spine utilizing an orthotic device will be necessary. Most of these devices are noninvasive, and each device is designed to maintain alignment and stability of a particular spinal region. Rigid cervical collars are commonly used to provide stability to the cervical

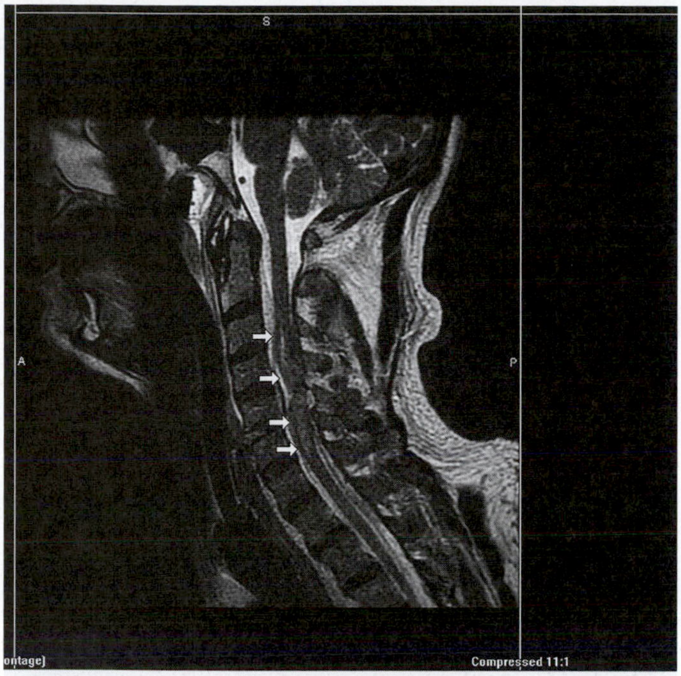

FIGURE 24–12 ◆ MRI of the cervical spine.
Source: Laurie Baker.

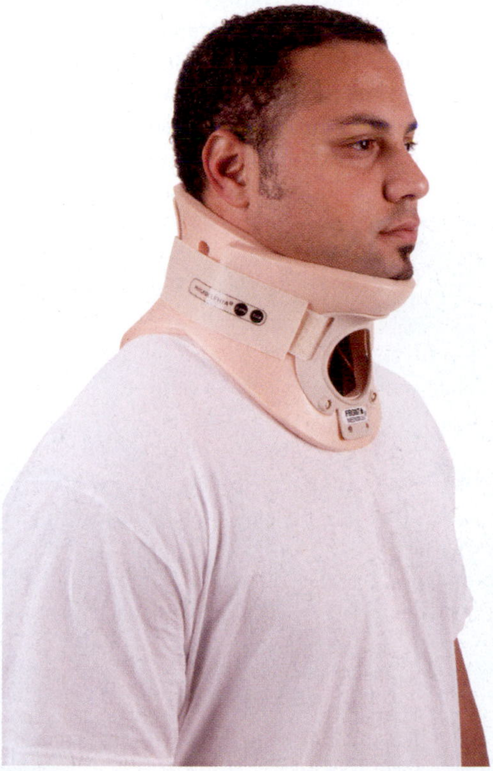

FIGURE 24–13 ◆ Philly collar.
Source: Courtesy of Ossur.

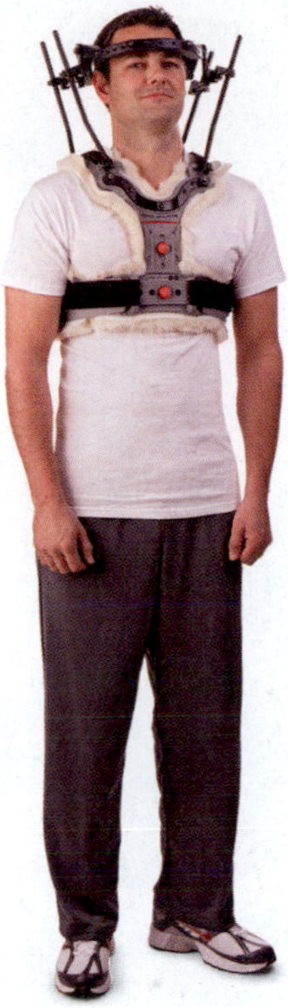

FIGURE 24–14 ◆ ReSolve Halo.
Source: Courtesy of Ossur.

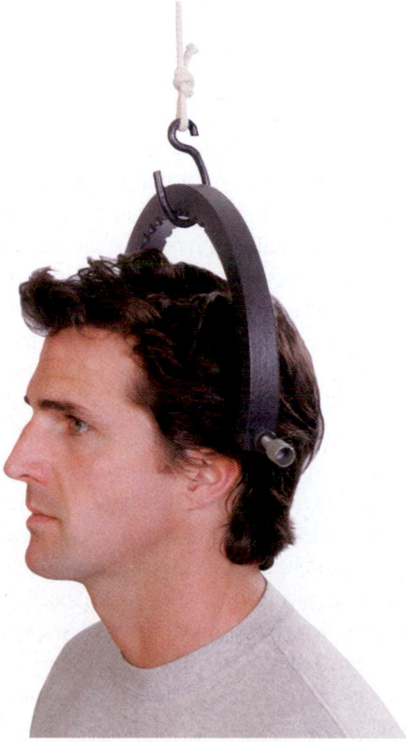

FIGURE 24–15 ◆ J tongs.
Source: Courtesy of Ossur.

spine (Figure 24–13◆). A halo brace also may be used to stabilize cervical fractures, especially if a collar does not provide adequate stability (Figure 24–14◆). The application of cervical traction with such devices as Gardner-Wells tongs (external tongs surgically inserted into the skull) may be necessary to reestablish alignment of the cervical spine or to reduce cervical fractures before surgical stabilization (Goodrich, 2010) (Figure 24–15◆).

Injuries in the cervicothoracic juncture or high thoracic spine require the use of a device that provides stabilization to both the lower cervical and upper thoracic regions such as a Sternal Occipital

Weblink: Bedsores (Pressure Sores)

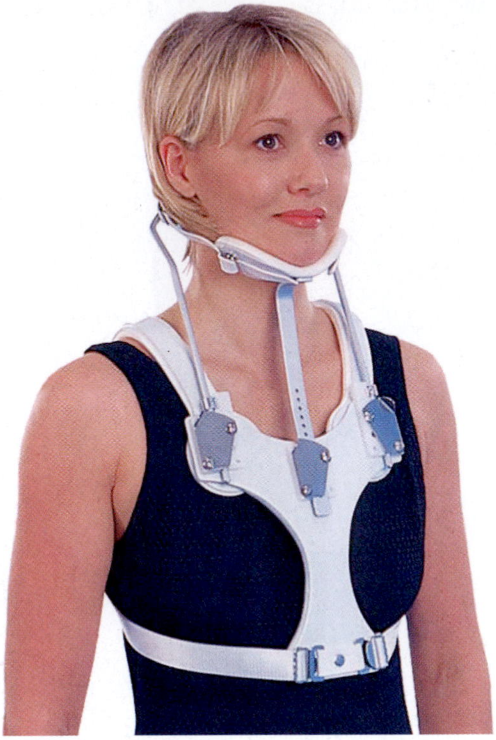

FIGURE 24–16 ◆ SOMI brace.
Source: Courtesy of Trulife.

Mandibular Immobilizer (SOMI) brace (Figure 24–16◆). A thoracolumbosacral orthosis (TLSO) will be required to stabilize the thoracic and lumbar regions. This orthotic device consists of a fiberglass or rigid plastic vest fitted specifically to the patient (Kulkarni, 2011).

The patient with a spinal cord injury may receive methylprednisolone (Medrol), a steroid, within the first 6 to 8 hours to reduce damage to nerve cells and decrease inflammation near the site of injury (Clinic Staff, 2011a). This medication does not cure spinal cord injury, but it may prevent further damage due to swelling. Methylprednisolone administration in acute SCI has become a standard of care in many treatment centers; however, there is much controversy in the literature regarding the effectiveness of this treatment strategy (Chin, 2012). Early studies indicated improvement of both motor and sensory function after administration of high-dose methylprednisolone; however, these results have not been duplicated in subsequent trials. Also, administration of high-dose steroids have associated risks, including sepsis, pneumonia, blood sugar elevation, and delayed wound healing. Despite the criticism in the literature, methylprednisolone remains a treatment option. The Pharmacology box lists this and other medications used for treatment of spinal cord injuries.

Current treatment strategies for medical management of acute SCI stress the importance of maintaining adequate oxygenation and blood pressure to ensure perfusion of the spinal cord. Hypotension is thought to be a contributor to aggravating spinal cord injury by worsening spinal cord ischemia. Systolic blood pressure should be maintained above 90 mmHg with mean arterial blood pressure targeted above 85 mmHg to ensure adequate spinal cord perfusion (Grigorean et al., 2009; Popa et al., 2010).

Surgical Management

Surgical management of spinal cord injuries is considered in patients who have fractures of the spinal column that are unstable and in those who have compression of the spinal cord as a result of bone fragments, disk herniation, tumor, or hematoma. Surgery to treat spinal cord injury may be performed immediately after the injury, within 24 hours, or at a later time. Urgent surgical intervention is more common in patients with incomplete SCI. There is some controversy among surgeons surrounding the optimal timing for surgical intervention, with some surgeons believing that early intervention may exacerbate coexisting clinical symptoms of the patient. Advocates for early surgical treatment point to the benefits of early decompression of the spinal cord. These benefits include improvement of spinal cord perfusion, resulting in preservation or possibly even improvement of spinal cord function by decreasing spinal cord ischemia, particularly in patients with incomplete injuries. Early stabilization of an unstable spinal column also will allow for earlier mobilization of the patient, resulting in improved pulmonary function and decreased risk of development of DVT and pressure ulcers (Carreon & Dimar, 2011).

Surgery for spinal cord injuries often consists of decompression of the spinal canal and/or fusion of the vertebrae to provide structural stability for spine fractures or dislocations. A laminectomy is the surgical procedure of choice for decompression of the spinal canal. This procedure is performed through a posterior approach and consists of removing the ligament and lamina from the back of the spinal column. Bone fragments, disc fragments, tumor, or hematoma resulting in compression of the spinal cord also will be removed when indicated. If the spine is unstable due to fracture, dislocation, or ligamentous injury, spinal instrumentation with fusion will be performed to restore spinal alignment and stability. Spinal fusion consists of placement of a combination of titanium screws, plates, wires, rods, or intervertebral cages and bone from either the bone bank or the patient's iliac crest to bridge fractured, unstable spinal segments with healthy, well-aligned bone. Fusion can be performed through either an anterior, posterior, or lateral approach to the spinal column (Figures 24–17◆ and 24–18◆).

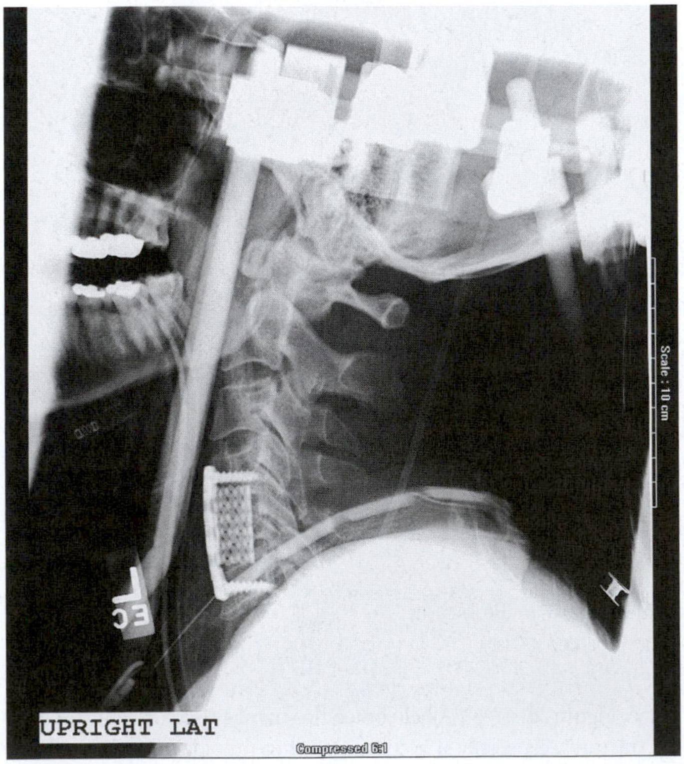

FIGURE 24–17 ◆ Lateral cervical spine x-ray of C_4–C_6 fusion.
Source: Laurie Baker.

DIAGNOSTIC TESTS for Acute Spinal Cord Injury

Test with Description, Rationale, and Normal Values	Expected Abnormality
Spine X-Rays	
Provides detailed images of the bones of the spine, and can be taken separately for the three main parts of the spine—cervical (neck), thoracic (middle back), and lumbar (lower back). *Common spinal x-ray views that aid in diagnosis of spinal problems include anterior/posterior (AP), lateral flexion, and extension views.* *Cervical spine x-rays should also include open-mouth views and swimmer's view.* Normal results: Normal spinal alignment. Bony elements of the spine are intact without evidence of fracture.	Subluxation of the vertebral bodies Compression or abnormal shape of the vertebral body Crush deformity of the vertebral body Widening or collapse of the intervertebral space
CT Scan of the Spine	
While some details of the soft tissue structures are seen, CT scans are best suited to identify problems with the bones of the spine. This exam is painless and takes less than 1 minute but delivers the highest amount of radiation of any scan. Normal results: The normal exam will reveal normal spinal alignment, normal configuration of the bony elements of the spine, no evidence of fracture, and no bone fragments within the canal.	Detects abnormal alignment of the spine (scoliosis, kyphosis); fracture of the bony elements of the spinal column; and bone fragments within the spinal canal
CT Myelogram	
Uses a contrast (a material that enhances the image of tissues) and x-rays to make the spinal canal visible. A myelogram can be done to find a tumor, an infection, problems with the spine (such as a herniated disc), or narrowing of the spinal canal caused by arthritis. *A dye is injected into the subarachnoid space. The dye moves through the subarachnoid space so the nerve roots and spinal cord can be seen more clearly. This test is used when a MRI is contraindicated or when existing spinal hardware makes MRI imaging difficult to interpret.* Normal results: No evidence of tumor, infection, or narrowing of the spinal canal.	Detects important problems such as cord compression by tumor or infection and determines whether it is outside the spinal cord (extradural) or part of the cord (intradural) Detects narrowing of the spinal canal (spinal stenosis) Also used to detect herniated discs and inflammation of the nerves called arachnoiditis
MRI of the Spine	
Uses a magnetic field and pulses of radio wave energy to make pictures of the spine. In many cases, an MRI gives different information than an x-ray, an ultrasound, or a CT scan. It often shows problems with soft tissue such as discs that cannot be seen with other imaging tests. MRI is indicated for patients with symptoms of degenerative disease, compressive lesions, or abnormal neurological exam suggesting spinal pathology. Normal results: Normal exam reveals spinal alignment that is maintained, with intervertebral disks intact. Spinal cord is surrounded by cerebrospinal fluid without evidence of compression or abnormality in signal intensity. Normal signal intensity given of the surrounding ligaments and tissue.	Abnormal alignment of the spine Protrusion of the intervertebral disk into the canal, causing compression of the spinal cord Narrowing of the spinal canal with compression of the spinal cord Hyperintensity within the spinal cord to suggest tumor or spinal cord abnormality Hyperintensity of the surrounding ligaments and tissues to suggest recent injury or pathology Hyperintensity of the exiting nerve roots to suggest nerve root avulsion or disease of the nerve root

Source: Kee, J. L. (2010). *Laboratory and diagnostic tests with nursing implications.* Upper Saddle River, NJ: Pearson.

Nursing Management

The focus of nursing care for the patient with an SCI is ongoing assessment of the patient and prevention of complications. Evaluation of the patient's physiological response to the injury and corresponding treatment and evaluation of the patient's emotional response to the injury are important aspects of the nursing assessment. All body systems should be included in the assessment and evaluation of patient care, since a secondary response to the injury may occur. The nursing assessment is vital in determining the treatment plan's effectiveness. It also aids in the prevention of potential complications and deterioration of the patient's status by allowing for early identification of problems and prompt intervention. The nursing plan of care will reflect the needs of the patient and family, and it will employ strategies to prevent complications and optimize the patient's functional status (see the Nursing Process: Patient Care Plan box, p. 654).

Psychosocial Assessment and Intervention

Patients who have experienced an SCI are faced not only with the physical challenges associated with this injury, but also with a significant psychosocial impact. These patients have changes related to altered body image, loss of independence, reduction or loss of control over their immediate environment, possible loss of economic security, and lifestyle changes. This injury also can place significant strain on existing relationships. The patient may exhibit a wide range of emotions including denial, grief, anger, hopelessness, and depression. The patient also may be at risk for suicidal thoughts (Bader & Littlejohns, 2010).

The nurse should monitor the patient for signs of inadequate coping, including withdrawal from social interactions, avoidance of eye contact, and refusal to participate in activities. The patient should be encouraged

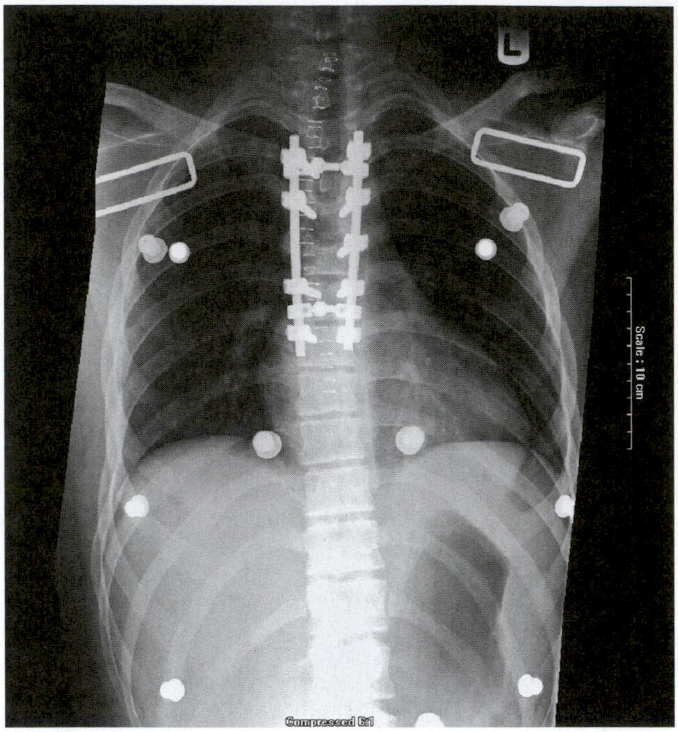

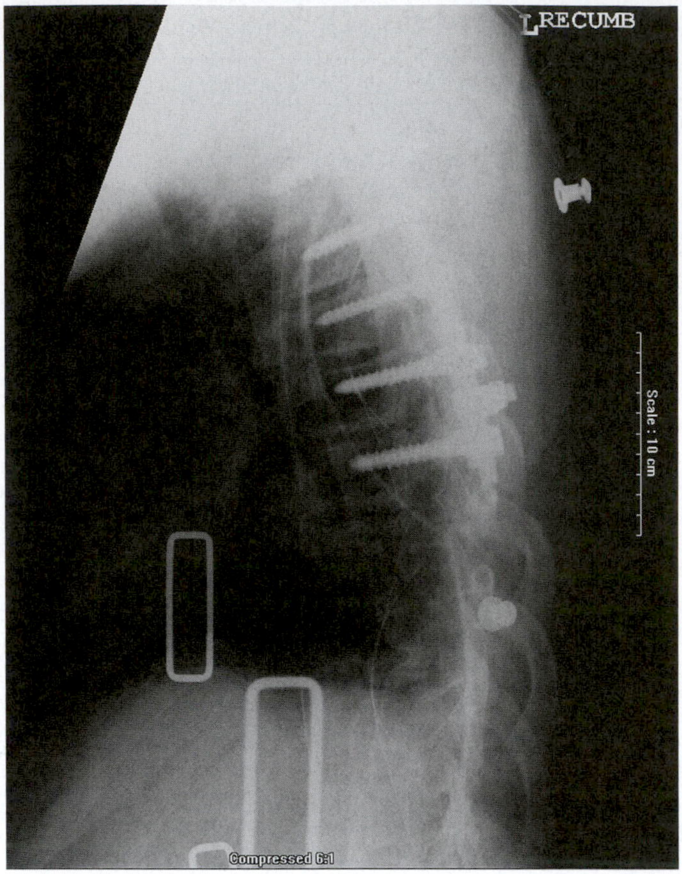

FIGURE 24–18 ◆ AP and lateral x-ray of posterior spinal fusion.
Source: Laurie Baker.

PHARMACOLOGY Summary of Medications Used in Early Spinal Cord Injury

Medication Category and Action	Application/Indication	Nursing Responsibility
Steroid		
Methylprednisolone ***Action:*** Stabilizes cell membrane permeability. Decreases immune response by blocking the actions of various chemical mediators in the inflammatory and allergic responses.	Decreases secondary injury due to inflammatory response.	Assess for side effects including mental status and mood changes. Monitor blood glucose levels. Monitor for symptoms of infection.
Cardiac		
Atropine Dopamine/dobutamine Norepinephrine ***Action:*** Inhibits action of acetylcholine or other cholinergic stimuli at postganglionic cholinergic receptors, including smooth muscles, secretory glands, and CNS sites. Alters autonomic activity of the heart, and acts to increase the heart rate. Blocks the parasympathetic activation by acetylcholine (Ach) and induces symptoms of the fight or flight response, increasing blood pressure and cardiac output.	Used to treat bradycardia and hypotension caused by neurogenic shock.	Monitor heart rate and rhythm. Monitor blood pressure. Titrate dosage to keep systolic BP > 90 mmHg and MAP > 85 mmHg.

PHARMACOLOGY Summary of Medications Used in Early Spinal Cord Injury, *continued*

Medication Category and Action	Application/Indication	Nursing Responsibility
Anticoagulant		
• Low-molecular-weight heparin • Warfarin sodium ***Action:*** Inhibits blood clot formation in the coagulation cascade. Activates the enzyme antithrombin III, which in turn inhibits thrombin production.	Prevention or treatment of DVT and PE.	Monitor patient for signs and symptoms of DVT formation. Monitor coagulation studies: PT, PTT, INR. Assess patient for signs of too much anticoagulation, such as excessive bleeding, bruising, or signs of gastrointestinal (GI) bleed.
Gastrointestinal		
Proton pump inhibitors: • Lansoprazole • Omeprazole • Pantoprazole ***Action:*** Inhibits gastric acid secretion by binding irreversibly to the enzyme H^+, K^+ -ATPase, thereby inhibiting the final pathway involved in acid secretion and effectively inhibiting the active proton pumps. *Stool softeners:* • Colace • Peri-Colace • Senokot ***Action:*** Promotes water retention in the stool, producing a laxative effect. *Bowel stimulants:* • Dulcolax suppository • Therevac *Osmotic laxative:* • MiraLax ***Action:*** Acts by irritating the mucosa in the colon and by altering intestinal and electrolyte absorption, thus maintaining water content of feces. Stimulates bowel activity.	Prevents gastric stress ulceration. Prevents constipation. Encourages regular emptying of the colon. Reduces anxiety related to hospitalization, injury, and loss of control over patient's own environment.	Monitor patient for development of stress ulcer: c/o abdominal pain, signs of GI bleeding. Monitor frequency and quality of bowel movements. Institute bowel program as soon as patient's medical condition warrants. Assess the patient's response to bowel stimulant medications, such as abdominal distention, cramping, and diarrhea.
Psychological		
Anxiolytics: • Diazepam • Alprazolam • Lorazepam ***Action:*** Potentiates the actions of GABA, an inhibitory neurotransmitter in the CNS, depressing the central nervous system and causing simple relaxation to the induction of sleep, to coma.	Mood stabilizers help the patient cope with the injury and focus on rehabilitative goals.	Assess for therapeutic effect, such as an alteration in mood. Assess patient needs for antianxiety drugs, including intensity and duration of symptoms, or factors that worsen anxiety or insomnia, such as physical symptoms, excessive drowsiness, or too little exercise or activity. Assess for signs and symptoms of overdose or abuse, such as somnolence, confusion, decreased reflexes, and coma.
Antidepressants: • Venlafaxine • Fluoxetine • Duloxetine • Sertraline • Paroxetine ***Action:*** Inhibits the reuptake of serotonin at the neuronal presynaptic membrane. This increases the amount of neurotransmitter available at the postsynaptic receptor sites, thus enhancing the actions of serotonin.	Used to treat depression.	Assess for depression before initiating therapy and reassess regularly. Obtain a comprehensive history of previous episodes of depression and factors leading to depression. Monitor for suicidal ideation. Encourage the patient to take drugs even if the immediate effects are not felt for several weeks. Assess for signs and symptoms of adverse reactions such as nausea, vomiting, insomnia, or restlessness. Evaluate for symptoms of a therapeutic response to medication.

Source: Adams, M. P., & Koch, R. W. (2010). *Pharmacology connections to nursing practice.* Upper Saddle River, NJ: Pearson.

NURSING PROCESS: Patient Care Plan for Spinal Cord Injury

Assessment of Neurologic Status Using Gordon's Functional Health Patterns:

- Health Perception Health Management Pattern
- Nutrition Metabolic Pattern
- Elimination Pattern
- Activity Exercise Pattern
- Cognitive Perceptual Pattern
- Coping-Stress Tolerance Pattern

Subjective Data	Objective Data
Assessment of Neurologic Status	**Assessment of Neurologic Status**
Are you able to move your arms, hand, legs, and feet? Do you have numbness or tingling anywhere?	Motor strength Sensory level Deep tendon reflexes Sphincter tone
Assessment of Pulmonary Function	**Assessment of Pulmonary Function**
Do you feel short of breath? Do you feel like you are unable to clear your secretions?	Lung sounds Monitor respiratory rate Use of accessory muscles for breathing Amount and character of secretions Adequacy of cough Monitor pulse oximetry Monitor arterial blood gases Change in mental status (i.e., anxiety, confusion, increased lethargy)
Assessment of Cardiovascular Status	**Assessment of Cardiovascular Status**
Are you dizzy or light-headed?	Heart rate and rhythm Blood pressure Urine output
Assessment of Tissue Perfusion	**Assessment of Tissue Perfusion**
Do you have any pain or pressure in your extremities? Have you noticed any abnormal swelling or redness in your extremities? Have you noticed a change in temperature in one or more extremity?	Peripheral pulses Temperature and color of the extremities Unilateral swelling in the extremities
Assessment of Gastrointestinal Function	**Assessment of Gastrointestinal Function**
Are you nauseous? Do you have any abdominal pain? When was your last bowel movement?	Abdominal pain Abdominal distention Bowel sounds Frequency of bowel movements Guaiac stools Hematocrit Dietary intake
Assessment of Urinary Elimination	**Assessment of Urinary Elimination**
Are you able to urinate? Do you feel like your bladder is full? Have you had any incontinence of urine?	Urinary output Bladder scans to assess for urinary retention
Assessment of Pain	**Assessment of Pain**
Are you having pain? Where do you hurt?	Facial grimacing Crying Increased spasticity Elevated blood pressure Elevated heart rate

NURSING PROCESS: Patient Care Plan for Spinal Cord Injury, *continued*

Assessment of Psychosocial State Are you feeling sad, depressed? How have you dealt with stress in the past? Who is your support person?	**Assessment of Psychosocial State** Refusal to communicate Refusal to participate in activities Avoidance of eye contact Anger Crying Expressing feelings of hopelessness
Assessment of Adaptation What are you able to do for yourself? What adaptive equipment do you have available and what will be needed?	**Assessment of Adaptation** Functional assessment based on preserved motor function Patient/caregiver knowledge of use of equipment Patient/caregiver knowledge of available resources

Outcomes and Evaluation Parameters	Planning and Interventions with *Rationales*
1. NURSING DIAGNOSIS: (a) Risk for Constipation *related to spinal cord injury;* (b) Disturbed Sensory Perception *related to spinal cord injury;* (c) Risk for Injury *due to spinal instability* (NANDA-I © 2012)	
Outcomes: Stabilization or improvement of neurological function. Maintenance of spinal alignment. ***Evaluation Parameters:*** Existing neurological function is preserved. Spine is immobilized with the appropriate orthotic device and mobility restrictions.	Spinal precautions maintained as ordered by the treating health care provider. *Measures to limit additional mechanical injury to the spinal cord.* Administer methylprednisolone per hospital protocol. *May limit inflammatory response and secondary injury to the spinal cord.* Maintain adequate oxygenation and mean arterial pressure (MAP) above 85 mmHg and systolic BP above 90 mmHg *to prevent secondary injury due to hypoxia and hypotension.* Monitor motor and sensory function *to assess for change in neurological function allowing for prompt medical attention if needed.*
2. NURSING DIAGNOSIS: (a) Ineffective Breathing Pattern *related to pulmonary complications of spinal cord injury;* (b) Ineffective Airway Clearance *related to the loss of spinal innervation of the respiratory muscles* (NANDA-I © 2012)	
Outcome: Adequate gas exchange. ***Evaluation Parameters:*** Adequate oxygenation is achieved as evidenced by normal blood gases and pulse oximetry. Patient is able to clear airway secretions. Patient is without complaint of dyspnea. Lung sounds remain clear. Patient remains alert and oriented without anxiety or restlessness.	Monitor respiratory status. *Evaluate for change indicative of declining respiratory function including increased use of accessory muscles, inability to clear secretions, drop in oxygen saturation, change in mental status, change in respiratory parameters (tidal volume, vital capacity, negative inspiratory force).* Institute pulmonary hygiene, including cough and deep breathing exercises, chest physiotherapy, assisted cough techniques, and suctioning *to promote gas exchange and airway clearance.* Administer humidified oxygen as ordered *to increase oxygenation.* Report decline in respiratory function to the medical team. *Medical management including mechanical ventilatory support may be necessary.*
3. NURSING DIAGNOSIS: Risk for Ineffective Tissue Perfusion *related to cardiovascular effects of neurogenic shock* (NANDA-I © 2012)	
Outcomes: Patient maintains hemodynamic stability. Patient is able to tolerate being in an upright position. ***Evaluation Parameters:*** MAP > 85 mmHg SBP > 90 mmHg HR > 50–60 Patient does not complain of dizziness or light-headedness.	Monitor hemodynamic status *to assess for change to allow for prompt medical intervention.* Administer vasoactive agents and atropine as ordered *to ensure adequate blood pressure, heart rate, and cardiac output.* Monitor intake and output and replace intravascular volume *to ensure adequate fluid status. Hypovolemia can contribute to hemodynamic instability.* Utilize abdominal binder and thigh-high compression stockings *to increase venous return to the heart and limit blood pooling in abdomen and lower extremities due to vasodilation.* Transition patient slowly into an upright position *to avoid orthostatic hypotension.*
4. NURSING DIAGNOSIS: Risk of Ineffective Peripheral Tissue Perfusion *related to deep venous thrombosis (DVT)* (NANDA-I © 2012)	
Outcome: Patient does not develop DVT. ***Evaluation Parameters:*** The patient does not exhibit signs of DVT: redness, edema, and change in temperature of extremity. Patient does not complain of pain or tenderness.	Utilize antiembolic hose and sequential compression boots *to limit blood pooling in the lower extremities.* Administer prophylactic dose of anticoagulant as ordered once cleared by the surgical team *to prevent formation of peripheral DVT.*

(*continued*)

NURSING PROCESS: Patient Care Plan for Spinal Cord Injury, *continued*

Outcomes and Evaluation Parameters	Planning and Interventions with *Rationales*
Peripheral pulses remain intact and adequate capillary refill.	Begin mobilization of patient including range-of-motion exercises as soon as cleared by the surgical team *to limit the effects of prolonged immobility.* Assess color, temperature, and size of extremities and check peripheral pulses. Report abnormalities to the medical team *to enable early detection and prompt treatment.*
5. NURSING DIAGNOSIS: (a) Risk for Constipation *related to impaired gastric motility due to spinal cord injury;* (b) Potential for Gastric Ulceration *related to stress of critical injury;* (c) Readiness for Enhanced Nutrition *related to increased metabolic need and inadequate caloric intake* (NANDA-I © 2012)	
Outcomes: Gastrointestinal function will be maintained. Patient will be without evidence of gastric stress ulceration. A regular pattern of bowel movements will be established. Patient will receive adequate nutrition to meet caloric requirements. ***Evaluation Parameters:*** Abdomen will remain soft, nontender, and nondistended. Patient will be without complaints of nausea, vomiting, constipation, or epigastric pain. Hematocrit will remain stable. Nutrition will be implemented.	Assess abdomen for tenderness and distention. Auscultate bowel sounds. *Evaluation of gastrointestinal function.* Monitor hematocrit and check stool for occult blood if drop in hematocrit noted without other explanation (i.e., surgery) *to assess for GI bleed due to gastric stress ulceration.* Use nasogastric tube if ileus is present *to provide for decompression of the stomach.* Administer stress ulcer prophylactic regimen as ordered by the medical team. Institute bowel regimen of stool softener, chemical stimulation such as a suppository, and mechanical (digital) stimulation *to establish a regular bowel elimination pattern.* Institute parenteral nutrition until patient is able to tolerate enteral feedings. Call for dietary consult *to determine patient's caloric needs.*
6. NURSING DIAGNOSIS: (a) Impaired Urinary Elimination *related to neurogenic bladder;* (b) Risk for Autonomic Dysreflexia *related to autonomic dysfunction as a result of spinal cord injury* (NANDA-I © 2012)	
Outcomes: The patient will establish a normal pattern of urinary elimination. The patient will be able to recognize the signs of autonomic hyperreflexia, identify potential causes, and describe treatment of hyperreflexia. ***Evaluation Parameters:*** The patient or caregiver is able to perform clean intermittent catherization (CIC). The patient and caregiver can verbalize common causes of hyperreflexia, common symptoms of hyperreflexia, and actions to take should hyperreflexia occur.	Use indwelling catheter during the acute period *to allow for complete bladder emptying and accurate measurement of urinary output.* Check post-void residuals by either intermittent catheterization or bladder scan *to assess for urinary retention.* Teach CIC to patient and caregiver *to encourage a consistent manner of bladder emptying.* Instruct patient and caregiver on common causes and signs of autonomic hyperreflexia and interventions to institute when these signs occur.
7. NURSING DIAGNOSIS: Readiness for Enhanced Comfort *related to injury and/or surgical procedure* (NANDA-I © 2012)	
Outcome: Effective control of pain. ***Evaluation Parameters:*** The patient will report improvement of pain. The patient is able to participate in therapies.	Assess pain utilizing a pain scale *to provide a method of measuring degree of pain and response to pain control measures.* Administer analgesics as ordered *to provide pharmacologic treatment of pain.* Utilize distraction and repositioning techniques *to augment pharmacologic treatment of pain.*
8. NURSING DIAGNOSIS: Ineffective Coping *related to loss of control over environment and uncertainty of the future* (NANDA-I © 2012)	
Outcomes: Patient will exhibit appropriate coping strategies. Patient will exhibit less anxiety. ***Evaluation Parameters:*** Patient reports improved mood. Patient participates in care. Patient is able to express feelings.	Encourage the patient to express her feelings *to provide for self-expression and identification of feelings.* Allow patient to participate in decisions *so the patient regains some control over self and the environment.* Request psychiatric consultation. *Assist with crisis counseling and to help the patient to identify appropriate coping strategies.* Administer anxiolytics and antidepressants as prescribed.
9. NURSING DIAGNOSIS: (a) Self-Care Deficit *related to spinal cord injury;* (b) Deficient Knowledge *related to adaptation strategies and resources* (NANDA-I © 2012)	
Outcome: Patient will implement self-care strategies utilizing the appropriate adaptive devices within the limitations of his injury. ***Evaluation Parameters:*** The patient participates in his own care. The patient will be able to identify available resources to help him to be independent within the limitations of his injury.	Schedule nursing care around PT/OT sessions *to ensure patient is able to participate in rehabilitative activities.* Have adaptive equipment readily available and encourage patient to use the equipment in self-care activities. *Encourages self-care strategies and reinforces education on the use of the equipment.* Assist the patient in identifying available community resources *to assist in independent living.*

Source: Adapted from Wilkinson, J. M., & Ahearn, N. R. (2009). *Prentice Hall nursing diagnosis handbook* (9th ed.). Upper Saddle River, NJ: Prentice Hall.

COMPLEMENTARY & ALTERNATIVE THERAPIES Healing Touch *Nancy Yilk*

EVERY HEALING INTENTION STARTS within the health care professional's intent to create a healing experience for the best patient outcome. Optimal healing environment (OHE) is a special focus on a patient's inner state and way of being in the world that can create a healing intention. The ability to create the patient's optimal sense of healing begins with the patient accepting a mindful and warm-hearted relationship with herself. In the mere nature of being human, the patient can only express what she has experienced as a reality for herself. The ability to develop congruence with core human desires such as present awareness in the moment, expressed love, and compassion allows a corresponding influence in the caregiver/patient relationship. Mindfulness is strongly related to compassion, and it is compassion that serves as a source for all healing intentionality. Compassion connects the patient's suffering with the healer's own suffering, and this emotional connection establishes a healing relationship through the power of empathy. This is the approach whereby a health care professional can elicit self-healing powers in patients through his inner attitudes (Leder & Krucoff, 2008).

Hands-on healing and energy-based interventions such as Reiki, Therapeutic Touch (TT), and Healing Touch (HT) have been found in cultures throughout history around the world. These complementary therapies are rooted in ancient Eastern healing practices. Reiki and HT are biofield therapies that arose in the nursing field in the late 1980s, and are used in a variety of settings (i.e., pain centers, surgical settings, and private practices) with reported benefits (i.e., decreased anxiety, pain, and depressive behaviors; increased relaxation; and a sense of well-being) (Anderson & Taylor, 2011).

Energy work with Reiki, TT, or HT is performed by the practitioner practicing mindfulness of the interconnectedness between himself and the patient, through the patient's etheric energy field. A practitioner of HT begins a session by recognizing the energy field between the patient and himself and proceeds by suspending his hands over the patient to direct the course of the disrupted energy, creating a peaceful and healing energy force. Bringing balance to energy disruption in the recipient's biofield allows a calm, soothing field for healing energy to promote itself uninhibited. The nursing diagnosis *"Energy Field, Disturbed"* is defined as a "disruption in the flow of energy surrounding a person's being." Nurses and nurse practitioners, as well as other health professionals (e.g., psychologists and health care providers), have integrated Esoteric Healing into their current practice (Settersten, 2011).

A randomized clinical trial involved 60 women who received HT along with their usual care or relaxation therapy immediately following their radiation treatment for cervical cancer. Healing Touch patients had a significantly minimal decrease in natural killer cell cytotoxicity (NKCC), which is an indicator of immune compromise, as compared to the other groups, which had a sharp decline. The Healing Touch group also showed greater decreases in depressed mood but there was no difference in quality of life, treatment delay, or clinically rated toxicities between groups. The researchers concluded that energy work with HT allows a compassionate connection through touch and presence between the provider and recipient with the intent to help or heal. The persistence of the metaphor "hands-on" to mean touch with intent to heal represents the essence of many of today's holistic nursing practices. Healing touch practices pervade nursing history, and the reemergence of holistic models, strengthened by societal demands, is suggestive of efforts to bring the heart back into the work of nursing (Lutgendorf et al., 2010).

References

Anderson, J. G., & Taylor, A. G. (2011, September). Effects of healing touch in clinical practice: A systematic review of randomized clinical trials. *Journal of Holistic Nursing, 29*(3), 221–228. Epub 2011 Jan 12.

Leder, D., & Krucoff, M. W. (2008, April). The touch that heals: The uses and meanings of touch in the clinical encounter. *Journal of Alternative and Complementary Medicine, 14*(3), 321–327.

Lutgendorf, S. K., Mullen-Houser, E., Russell, D., De Geest, K., Jacobson, G., Hart, L., et al. (2010). Preservation of immune function in cervical cancer patients during chemoradiation using a novel integrative approach. *Brain, Behavior and Immunity.* doi:20.2026/j.bbi.2010.06.014

Schmidt, S. (2004). Optimal Healing Environment (OHE): Mindfulness and healing intention: Concepts, practice, and research evaluation. *Journal of Alternative and Complementary Medicine, 10* (Suppl. 1), S7–14.

Settersten, L. (2011, June). What is esoteric healing? *Journal of Holistic Nursing, 29*(2), 132–139. Epub 2010 Oct 21.

to discuss his feelings and to participate in decision making whenever possible. The patient's family members also will need support and ongoing education to help them deal with the stress of having a critically ill loved one and the role changes associated with becoming a primary caregiver. In some cases, consultation with a chaplain, social worker, or psychiatrist may be necessary. Healing touch may also be helpful to patients with SCI, as discussed in the Complementary & Alternative Therapies box.

Once the patient is ready for discharge, the nurse should identify community resources that the patient and family may use for continued support and to assist the patient with reintegration into the home environment and community. Other patient teaching priorities are listed in the Patient Teaching & Discharge Priorities box.

Collaborative Management

The patient with an SCI will require a multidisciplinary team approach to treatment throughout the continuum of care. It is essential that this interdisciplinary team communicate openly with one another in developing and evaluating care of the patient and family (IOM [Institute of Medicine], 2010). The medical team often consists of members of the trauma team and surgical team until the patient's injuries are stabilized. In addition, health care providers specializing in critical care medicine are helpful in the management of cardiopulmonary issues in the acute phase after injury. A respiratory therapist assists with pulmonary management, including suctioning, coughing, and deep breathing strategies. Dietary consultation also is helpful to ensure that nutritional requirements are met.

Once the patient has been stabilized, physical and occupational therapy evaluation and treatment are necessary to assist with optimization of function through range-of-motion exercises, strengthening exercises, and instruction regarding mobility and use of adaptive equipment. Involvement of a social worker with expertise in SCI is vital to assist with issues related to lifestyle changes and loss of income as well as identification of resources to assist with the patient's transition into the community. The assistance of a mental health expert, such as a psychologist, may be helpful to assist with issues of depression and adjustment to lifestyle changes related to the injury. Once the acute care issues of hemodynamic and spinal stability have been addressed, the patient may need the involvement of a physiatrist to direct rehabilitation efforts. This is particularly relevant in the rehabilitation phase of recovery.

A social worker and a psychologist may work with patients and their families to assist with psychosocial issues related to lifestyle including sexuality and recreation. Patients will receive advice on maintaining an active lifestyle within the limitations of their injury. They also will receive instruction specific to sexual activity early in the acute rehabilitative period; this information will be frequently reinforced. It is important that patients with spinal cord injuries understand that they can continue to be active both sexually and recreationally despite their injury. It is even possible for them to have children in the future if they so desire. The ongoing support of a urologist or gynecologist after the patient's discharge from the rehabilitation facility will be important in maintaining her sexual health.

PATIENT TEACHING & DISCHARGE PRIORITIES for Spinal Cord Injury

Need	Teaching
Understanding of bowel/bladder regimen	The patient and family are taught how to perform placement of a continuous indwelling catheter (CIC) and how to perform bowel care including insertion of a suppository, digital stimulation of the bowel, and disimpaction of stool. The patient and family will understand the importance of maintaining a regular bowel and bladder regimen to avoid complications of UTI and bowel impaction.
Prevention of complications	The patient and family are taught strategies such as performing frequent position changes, routinely assessing the skin, and providing skin care to avoid the formation of pressure ulcers.
Safety	Proper instruction is given to the patient and family on the use of adaptive equipment and transfer strategies. The patient and family will be instructed on the signs and symptoms of autonomic hyperreflexia, common causes of hyperreflexia, and strategies to implement if autonomic hyperreflexia occurs.
Emotional adjustment of patient and family to psychosocial impact of SCI	The patient and family are encouraged to discuss their feelings openly. The patient and family will be able to identify supportive resources to help them cope with both the physical and psychosocial changes due to SCI.
Adaptation of environment	The patient and family will be provided with instructions on the neeeded adaptations to the home environment and resources to assist with completion of environmental changes required to accommodate the patient's deficits and adaptive equipment. If the patient cannot be discharged to a home environment, arrangements for an assisted living environment will be made.

Nurses are an integral part of the multidisciplinary team, serving as a common link for all team members as well as providing education and support to the patient and family through all phases of treatment.

Health Promotion

Health promotion focuses on prevention, education, and rehabilitation. All are critical elements in the patient's quest for optimum functionality. The majority of SCIs occur as a result of trauma, and many of these injuries are preventable. The key to reducing the incidence of these SCIs is to decrease high-risk behaviors such as driving while under the influence of drugs or alcohol, failing to use a seat belt, and diving into shallow water. Several educational programs geared to both adults and children have been designed to increase awareness of those high-risk behaviors as well as to educate the public on simple strategies to decrease the risk of sustaining an SCI. These programs have been implemented in schools, workplaces, and communities, often by a team of volunteers. This team often includes a person who has sustained a permanent SCI and an expert in health care in treating SCIs.

Rehabilitation after a spinal cord injury is essential to achieving the best possible clinical outcome and regaining functional independence. Recovery often occurs over months and combines skill-building activities and counseling for social and emotional support. Because mobility and communication are critical areas of function for independence, the initial efforts in rehabilitation are often directed toward restoring the patient's arm and leg function and communicating needs. For some patients, mobility will be possible only with the assistance of devices such as a walker, leg braces, or a wheelchair. For these reasons, the skills that are learned in the weeks to months after the person suffers an SCI have a significant impact on future health and independence. Once a therapy plan has been defined, patients and families can take an active role in recovery.

Achieving independence with management of bowel and bladder is an essential component of recovery and future health in SCI. Bladder and bowel management programs teach basic toileting routines, and patients also are taught self-grooming to take care of their basic hygienic needs. A bowel and bladder management program allows the patient to plan for bowel or bladder emptying in an acceptable manner when it is convenient for the patient. A bowel training program includes diet, medicines, and digital stimulation (touching inside the rectum to help the bowels move). Bowel training may take time, but can be successful. Spinal cord injury also may cause the messages between the bladder and brain to be changed. Normally, when the bladder gets full, nerves in the bladder send a message to the brain signaling a need to urinate. However, the message to the brain may be lost after spinal cord injury. Many different methods are available to assist in bowel and bladder training, such as daily bowel medications, intermittent catheterization, male condom catheters, and indwelling catheters. Each patient will choose a combination of methods or a single method that works best for him. Initially, with bladder training, a urinary (foley) catheter is placed to drain the bladder. When the indwelling (foley) catheter is removed, the nurse will check to determine when the bladder is full; when full, a straight catheter is used to drain the bladder. The patient or caretaker will be taught how to perform the straight catheterization, or the patient will wear an external catheter to collect the urine. Patients also acquire coping strategies for recurring episodes of spasticity, autonomic dysreflexia, and neurogenic pain.

Participation in vocational rehabilitation ensures that patients with SCI have the option of rejoining the workforce and continuing to be financially independent functional adults. Vocational rehabilitation begins with an assessment of the patient's basic work skills, current dexterity, and physical and cognitive capabilities to determine the likelihood for employment. Potential workplaces are identified by a vocational therapist who determines the type of assistive equipment that will be needed, and helps arrange for a user-friendly workplace. If disability prevents the patient from returning to the workplace, focus is placed on encouraging productivity through participation in activities that provide a sense of satisfaction and self-esteem, such as educational classes, hobbies, memberships in special interest groups, and participation in family and community events.

Surviving a spinal cord injury can be overwhelming, and every patient will experience it differently. Almost everyone feels frightened, anxious, or confused about what has happened. Acknowledging the patients' fear and providing time for therapeutic communication plays an important role in helping patients adjust to life after injury. It's important for patients to become engaged in outside activities that help them to reintegrate into normal daily life. Recreation therapy encourages patients to build on their abilities so that they can participate in recreational or athletic activities at their level of mobility. These activities help those with spinal cord injuries achieve a more balanced lifestyle and provide opportunities for socialization.

In summary, education is a key element in the health promotion efforts of SCI providers. Patients should be taught the importance of early detection and prompt treatment of problems such as alteration in skin integrity and UTIs in preventing more serious complications such as sepsis and osteomyelitis. The patient should understand the symptoms of complications and when to notify the health care provider. Patients should also be informed of the physical, psychosocial, and vocation potential commonly experienced by others in like situations.

Gerontological Considerations

The number of patients over the age of 60 who have sustained an SCI has gradually increased during the last decade and has risen by a factor of five in the past 20 years (Fassett et al., 2007). The number of older patients with spinal cord injuries is expected to increase as the older population increases. Particularly evident has been the increase in cervical spine injury. In the younger members of this age group (65 to 75 years of age), the main causes of cervical spine injuries are motor vehicle accidents (MVAs). In the older members (those over 75 years of age), falls from standing or high-seated positions, such as on a chair, bench, or stool, dominate (Walid & Zaytseva, 2009). Falls are particularly prevalent in community-dwelling for older adults, such as a board and care or extended care facility.

Older adults are at increased risk of injury to the spinal cord because of degenerative changes in the spinal column, including ossification and hypertrophy of the spinal ligaments and development of bone spurs within the spinal column, leading to narrowing of the spinal canal. Weakening of the bone due to osteoporosis and rheumatologic disease also increases the risk of spinal fracture in older adults. Management of acute SCI in this patient population is particularly challenging because of the high incidence of preexisting medical problems such as diabetes and heart disease as well as the normal effects of aging (Grimm & Mion, 2011).

Nursing management of the older adult with spinal cord injury is challenging. In addition to responding to other comorbid conditions that may be present, nurses must be aware of changes occurring in all the patient's body systems as a result of the aging process. Patients are likely to experience functional decline in areas such as recreation, independent activities of daily living (ADLs), and employment (Winkler, 2011). Services to limit or forestall patients' functional decline should be initiated to the extent possible. From a social and emotional perspective, patients may experience feelings of isolation, fear, and despair. Many older adults live alone or in some type of assisted living facility, have no family nearby, and have a limited cadre of friends to provide social and emotional support. It is essential that these patients' needs be recognized and addressed by the health care team.

Research

Current spinal cord injury research continues to focus on ways to improve outcomes for patients with SCI as well as improving functional ability (see the Research Opportunities box). Much of this research is focused on limiting the secondary effects of spinal cord injury as well as restoration of function. Research opportunities also focus on nursing care issues related to care of the patient/family with spinal cord injury.

RESEARCH OPPORTUNITIES Related to Spinal Cord Injuries

Research Area	Clinical Impact
Restorative therapy techniques.	Improvement and restoration of function.
Use of technology-assisted caregiving tasks on patients' sense of dignity. How do patients respond to the use of these devices—mobility aids, bathing aids, toileting aids?	Improvement of patient care, sense of comfort, dignity, and acceptance of technology-assisted caregiving tasks.
Use of technology-assisted caregiving aids by families in the home setting. Does the patient and family know how to access such devices? Are they educated in their use? (Kelly, 2011).	Improvement of patient care and reduction of caregiver stress by understanding how to use technology-assisted caregiving devices in the home postdischarge from the acute care or rehabilitative setting.
Assessment of emotional and social needs for an older patient with a spinal cord injury (SCI).	Improvement of patient care for the older patient. with an SCI by identifying emotional and social needs and intervening as appropriate.

READ: **History of Present Illness** >> Laboratory Study Results >> Critical Thinking Questions

You are the nurse assigned to Amit Patel, a 24-year-old male who sustained a spinal cord injury (SCI) 3 days ago. He dove into a pool from the roof of a friend's house while attending a party. When his friends noticed that he did not surface, they jumped into the pool and brought him out of the water. They estimated that he was submerged for 1 to 2 minutes. Once out of the water, Mr. Patel was noted to only shrug his shoulders. He was unable to move his arms or legs and complained of feeling "numb" and short of breath. His friends called 911, and Mr. Patel was transported to the hospital, where he was diagnosed with a compression fracture of C_6, spinal cord contusion at C_6, and a complete SCI. There was no evidence of continued spinal cord compression from bone fragments within the canal; thus, Mr. Patel was placed in a halo brace.

Medical–Surgical History

Mr. Patel denies significant past medical or surgical history.

Social History

Mr. Patel is single. He lives alone, and his parents live out of state. He smokes approximately 1.5 packs of cigarettes per day and drinks 24 to 48 cans of beer on the weekends. He denies recreational drug use.

Physical Exam

Mr. Patel has a halo brace in place, and the pin sites are clean. He has a triple-lumen, subclavian central line with normal saline infusing at 75 mL/hr in one port, and dopamine infusing at 15 mcg/kg/min into a second port to maintain a systolic blood pressure greater than 90 mmHg and O_2 saturation at 90%. He is receiving 50% oxygen via face mask. A nasogastric tube is in place, connected to low intermittent wall suction. An indwelling urinary catheter is draining yellow urine.

Mr. Patel is awake but does not open his eyes to answer questions or acknowledge staff. He is oriented to person, place, time, and current events. He denies complaint of pain but does report feeling short of breath. Cranial nerve testing is normal. Motor exam reveals 5/5 strength with shoulder shrug and deltoid function bilaterally. Bicep strength is graded as 4/5 bilaterally. He has 0/5 motor function in the triceps, wrist extension, and intrinsic hand muscles bilaterally. His lower extremities are flaccid.

He denies sensation to pinprick below the clavicle including the chest, abdomen, and lower extremities. He has intact sensation in the neck, shoulders, and palmar aspect of the hands. Deep tendon reflexes are 1+ in the biceps but otherwise absent. Rectal tone is absent. Lung sounds are diminished in the bases. The patient is tachypneic, and respirations are shallow. His abdomen is soft and nontender with hypoactive bowel sounds. He has not had a bowel movement since admission. His extremities are warm without erythema or edema. Peripheral pulses are intact.

Vital signs reveal a temperature of 37°C (98.6°F). Blood pressure is 90/46. Heart rate is 50 beats per minute, sinus bradycardia. Respiratory rate is 38 and shallow.

READ: History of Present Illnesses >> **Physical Exam** >> Admitting Medical Records >> Laboratory Study Results

Admitting Medical Orders

Service: Neurosurgical
Admit to Neurosurgical ICU
Diagnosis: compression fracture of C_6, spinal cord contusion at C_6, and complete SCI
Allergies: none reported
Vital signs: q1h
Bed rest
Diet: NPO
Nasogastric tube to low intermittent suction
Call house officer: HR < 50 or > 120, systolic blood pressure < 90 or > 160, RR < 12 or > 30, temperature > 38.5°C, urinary output less than 30 mL/hr × 2, O_2 saturation $< 92\%$
Respiratory care: incentive spirometer q1h when awake, IPPB respiratory treatment q4h
CVP monitoring q4h by obtaining reading from distal port of the central line, notify health care provider if < 8 or > 20
Foley catheter
Maintain I&O
Pin site care with 0.5% H_2O_2 and normal saline bid
IVs: normal saline at 75 mL/hr

Scheduled Medications

Famotidine 20 mg per NG bid
Senokot liquid 15 mL per NG bid
Dopamine titrated to keep the systolic BP above 90 mmHg

PRN Medications

Atropine 0.5 mg IV every 3–5 minutes (max 3 mg total) prn heart rate less than 45 beats per minute, and call health care provider

Ordered Laboratory Studies

Daily ABGs, Chem 7, CBC, and albumin weekly

READ: History of Present Illness >> **Laboratory Study Results** >> Critical Thinking Questions

Test	Day 1	Day 2	Day 3
ABGs			
PO_2	90 mmHg	88 mmHg	72 mmHg
PCO_2	36 mmHg	38 mmHg	48 mmHg
pH	7.35	7.34	7.31
Chemistry			
Sodium	141 mEq/L	145 mEq/L	142 mEq/L
Potassium	3.8 mEq/L	4.0 mEq/L	4.0 mEq/L
Chloride	95 mEq/L	102 mEq/L	103 mEq/L
CO_2	23 mEq/L	21 mEq/L	21 mEq/L

Test	Day 1	Day 2	Day 3
Glucose	134 mg/dL	121 mg/dL	118 mg/dL
Blood urea nitrogen (BUN)	8 mg/dL	12 mg/dL	16 mg/dL
Creatinine	0.8 mg/dL	1.1 mg/dL	1.0 mg/dL
CBC			
WBC	10.5 μ/L	11.3 μ/L	15.1 μ/L
Hgb	14.7 g/dL	13.8 g/dL	13.0 g/dL
Hct	40.6 mL/dL	39.6 mL/dL	39.8 mL/dL
Platelets	300,000 μL	350,000 μL	300,000 μL
Albumin	2.6 g/dL		

Pearson Nursing Student Resources

Log on to ***nursing.pearsonhighered.com*** *to download forms*

DOCUMENT:

- >> Summary of Hospitalization
- >> Pathophysiology Form
- >> Laboratory Values
- >> Laboratory Results Explanation

APPLY:

- >> List of Potential Nursing Diagnoses
- >> Concept Map
- >> Critical Thinking Questions and Concept Map

APPLY: History of Present Illness >> Laboratory Study Results >> **Critical Thinking Questions**

1. What are the indicators in the assessment that should alert the nurse to the potential for and/or actual decline in pulmonary status?
2. What measures should be instituted for DVT prophylaxis?
3. What are the indicators that Mr. Patel may be experiencing depression?
4. What are common signs for autonomic hyperreflexia and what are measures to take should this occur?

Answers to Critical Thinking Questions can be found in Appendix D in the Osborn Student Resources at nursing.pearsonhighered.com.

NCLEX® PRACTICE

1. The nurse is teaching a group of nursing students about the causes of spinal cord injury. Which of the following statements made by one of the students indicates a clear understanding of the topic?

1. "Forward falls in which the chin or forehead strikes the ground might produce compression spinal cord injuries."
2. "When axial pressure is loaded on the spine, the resultant rotational injuries might include fracture of the vertebral body."
3. "Hyperextension injuries can cause anterior vertebral body fractures and posterior spinal column facet fracture and dislocation."
4. "A sudden deceleration injury, such as a head-on motor vehicle collision, is frequently the cause of hyperflexion injuries."

2. The patient was involved in a motor vehicle collision with rear impact and is now experiencing severe neck pain and decreased upper extremity motor function, but there is normal motor function in the lower extremities. The patient complains of parasthesias in both the upper and lower extremities but greater in the arms. Based on these findings, the nurse suspects the patient may have which of the following types of injuries?

1. Anterior cord syndrome
2. Central cord syndrome
3. Cauda equina syndrome
4. Brown-Séquard syndrome

3. Which of the following statements would the nurse recognize as best describing appropriate prophylaxis for some of the most common complications that a patient may experience following spinal cord injury? (Select all that apply.)
   1. Use of an abdominal binder and compression stockings to decrease the peripheral venous pooling that can cause neurogenic shock
   2. Use of a Duplex Doppler ultrasound to dissolve deep vein thromboembolisms and reduce the likelihood of pulmonary embolus
   3. Use of a reclining wheelchair to gradually progress the patient into an upright position so as not to cause orthostatic hypotension
   4. Use of sound nutritional measures such as an increased caloric, protein, and micronutrient intake to promote bowel evacuation
   5. Learn the technique of straight catheterization to reduce the risk of urinary retention and decrease potential for urinary tract infections.
4. When planning educational opportunities for patients related to the psychosocial impact of spinal cord injury, the nurse understands that:
   1. the patient's family will need ongoing education to help deal with the stress of any role changes associated with the injury.
   2. the patient may exhibit any number of negative emotions about physical challenges, including elation and jubilation.
   3. the patient should be encouraged to discuss his feelings openly and to support the decisions made for him by the health care provider.
   4. the patient is usually so preoccupied with the physical challenges faced after a spinal cord injury that psychosocial problems rarely occur.
5. The nurse understands that the needs of the patient with a spinal cord injury (SCI) are unique. When planning the discharge of the patient with SCI, the nurse should include which of the following?
   1. Information regarding support systems that can help the patient and his family adjust to the changes in lifestyle and roles
   2. Referral to a rehabilitation program that uses a single, specialized discipline to help the patient adapt to his injury limitations
   3. Strategies such as infrequent position changes that avoid shearing and will help in the prevention of pressure ulcer formation
   4. Instruction on the importance of avoiding use of suppository medication or other bowel stimulation so as to prevent hyperreflexia
6. When planning care for the patient with spinal cord injury, which nursing diagnosis has the highest priority?
   1. *Risk for Imbalanced Nutrition Less Than Body Requirements* related to increased metabolic need and inadequate caloric intake
   2. *Anxiety* related to loss of independence, loss of control over environment, and uncertainty of the future
   3. *Risk for Ineffective Peripheral Tissue Perfusion* related to the formation of deep venous thrombosis
   4. *Ineffective Airway Clearance* related to the loss of spinal innervation of the respiratory and accessory muscles.

   NANDA-I © 2012

Answers to NCLEX Practice questions can be found in Appendix D in the Osborn Student Resources at nursing.pearsonhighered.com. Practice additional NCLEX questions online at the Student Resources site.

Pearson Nursing Student Resources Find additional review materials at: **nursing.pearsonhighered.com**

REFERENCES

Aarabi, B., Alexander, M., Mirvis, S. E., Shanmuganathan, K., Chesler, D., Maulucci, C., et al. (2010). Predictors of outcome in acute traumatic central cord syndrome due to spinal stenosis. *Journal of Neurosurgery: Spine, 14*(1), 122–130. doi: 10.3171/2010.9.spine09922

Adams, M. P., & Koch, R. W. (2010). *Pharmacology connections to nursing practice.* Upper Saddle River, NJ: Pearson.

Agarwal, N. K., & Mathur, N. (2009). Deep vein thrombosis in acute spinal cord injury. *Spinal Cord, 47*(10), 769–772.

Ahn, H., Singh, J., Nathens, A., Macdonald, R. D., Travers, A., Tallon, J., et al. (2010). Pre-hospital care management of a potential spinal cord injured patient: A systematic review of the literature and evidence-based guidelines. *Journal of Neurotrauma, 28*(8), 1341–1361. doi: 10.1089/neu.2009.1168

American Academy of Orthopaedic Surgeons. (2010). Fractures of the thoracic and lumbar spine. Retrieved from http://orthoinfo.aaos.org/topic.cfm?topic=a00368

Anderson, J. G., & Taylor, A. G. (2011, September). Effects of healing touch in clinical practice: A systematic review of randomized clinical trials. *Journal of Holistic Nursing, 29*(3), 221–228. Epub 2011 Jan 12.

Assis, G. M., & e Faro, A. C. (2011). [Clean intermittent self catheterization in spinal cord injury]. *Revista da Escola de Enfermagem da USP, 45*(1), 289–293. doi: S0080-62342011000100041 [pii]

Bader, M. K., & Littlejohns, L. (2010). *AABN core curriculum for neuroscience nursing.* Glenview, IL: Elsevier.

Barker, E. (2008). *Neuroscience nursing: A spectrum of care* (3rd ed.). St. Louis, MO: Mosby Elsevier.

Barleben, A., & Mills, S. (2010). Anorectal anatomy and physiology. *The Surgical Clinics of North America, 90*(1), 1–15.

Bounameaux, H. (2010). Contemporary management of pulmonary embolism: *Journal of Internal Medicine, 268*(3), 218–231. doi: 10.1111/j.1365-2796.2010.02254.x

Bradley, J. F., Jones, M. A., Farmer, E. A., Fann, S. A., & Bynoe, R. (2011). Swallowing dysfunction in trauma patients with cervical spine fractures treated with halo-vest fixation. *Journal of Trauma, 70*(1), 46–48.

Carreon, L. Y., & Dimar, J. R. (2011). Early versus late stabilization of spine injuries: A systematic review. *Spine, 36*(11), E727–E733. doi: 710.1097/BRS.1090b1013e3181fab1002f

Centers for Disease Control and Prevention. (2010). Spinal cord injury fact sheet. Retrieved from http://www.cdc.gov/TraumaticBrainInjury/

Chin, L. S. (2012). Spinal cord injuries treaatment & manaagement. *Medscape Reference.* Retrieved from http://emedicine.medscape.com/article/793582-treatment

Coggrave, M., Norton, C., & Wilson-Barnett, J. (2008). Management of neurogenic bowel dysfunction in the community after spinal cord injury: A postal survey in the United Kingdom. *Spinal Cord, 47*(4), 323–333.

David, B. T., & Steward, O. (2010). Deficits in bladder function following spinal cord injury vary depending on the level of the injury. *Experimental Neurology, 226*(1), 128–135. doi: 10.1016/j.expneurol.2010.08.014

Fassett, D. R., Harrop J. S., Maltenfort M., Jeyamohan S. B., Ratliff, J. D., Anderson, D. G. et al. (2007). Mortality rates in geriatric patients with spinal cord injuries. *Journal of Neurosurgery: Spine, 7*, 277–281.

Fehlings, M., Cadotte, D. W., & Fehlings, L. N. (2011). A series of systematic reviews on the treatment of acute spinal cord injury: A foundation for best medical practice. *Journal of Neurotrauma.* doi: 10.1089/neu.2011.1955

Francisco de Assis Aquino Gondim, M. (2009). Spinal cord, topographical and functional anatomy. Medscape reference.

Fynne, L., Worsøe, J., Gregersen, T., Schlageter, V., Laurberg, S., & Krogh, K. (2011). Gastric and small intestinal dysfunction in spinal cord injury patients. *Acta Neurologica Scandinavica, 125*(2). 123–128. doi: 10.1111/j.1600-0404.2011.01508.x

Goodrich, J. A. (2010). Lower cervical spine fractures and dislocations treatment & management. Medscape reference. Retrieved from http://emedicine.medscape.com/article/1264065-treatment

Grigorean, V. T., Sandu, A. M., Popescu, M., Iacobini, M. A., Stoian, R., Neascu, C., et al. (2009). Cardiac dysfunctions following spinal cord injury. *Journal of Medical Life, 2*(2), 133–145.

Grimm, D., & Mion, L. (2011). Falls resulting in traumatic injury among older adults. *AACN Advanced Critical Care, 22*(2), 161–168.

Grimm, S., & Chamberlain, M. C. (2009). Adult primary spinal cord tumors. *Expert Review of Neurotherapeutics, 9*(10), 1487–1495. doi: 10.1586/ern.09.101

Hardwick, M. E., Pulido, P. A., & Adelson, W. S. (2012, January–February). Nursing intervention using healing touch in bilateral total knee arthroplasty. *Orthopaedic Nursing, 31*(1), 5–11.

Hasler, R., Exadaktylos, A., Bouamra, O., Benneker, L., Clancy, M., Sieber, R., et al. (2011). Epidemiology and predictors of spinal injury in adult major trauma patients: European cohort study. *European Spine Journal, 20*(12), 2174–2180. doi: 10.1007/s00586-011-1866-7

Henzel, M. K., Bogie, K. M., Guihan, M., & Ho, C. H. (2011). Pressure ulcer management and research priorities for patients with spinal cord injury: Consensus opinion from SCI QUERI Expert Panel on Pressure Ulcer Research Implementation. *Journal of Rehabilitation Research and Development, 48*(3), xi–xxxii.

Hessler, C., Vettorazzi, E., Madert, J., Bokemeyer, C., & Panse, J. (2011). Actual and predicted survival time of patients with spinal metastases of lung cancer: Evaluation of the robustness of the tokuhashi score. *Spine (Phila Pa 1976), 36*(12), 983–989. doi: 10.1097/BRS.0b013e3181e8f7f8

Hickey, J. V. (2009). *The clinical practice of neurological and neurosurgical nursing* (6th ed.). Philadelphia, PA: Lippincott Williams & Wilkins.

IOM (Institute of Medicine). (2010). *The future of nursing: Leading change, advancing health.* Washington, DC: The Academic Press.

Kaun, L. E. (2011). Stress ulcer prophylaxis: The consequences of overuse and misuse. U.S.Pharmacist.om. Retrieved from http://www.uspharmacist.com/content/c/30500/

Kee, J. L. (2010). *Laboratory and diagnostic tests with nursing implications.* Upper Saddle River, NJ: Pearson.

Kelly, K. (2011). Family caregivers need access & training on assistive technologies. Family Caregiver Alliance, National Center on Caregiving. Retrieved from http://blog/govdelivery.com/usodep/2011/11/family-caregivers-need-access-training-on-a

Kulkarni, S. S. (2011). Spinal orthotics. Medscape reference. Retrieved from http://emedicine.medscape.com/article/314921-overview

Leder, D., & Krucoff, M. W. (2008, April). The touch that heals: The uses and meanings of touch in the clinical encounter. *Journal of Alternative and Complementary Medicine, 14*(3), 321–327.

Lieberman, S. L. & Brown, R. M. (2011). Respiratory complications of spinal cord injury. UpToDate, Inc. retrieved from http://www.uptodate.com/contents/respiratory-complications-of-spinal-cord-injury

Lutgendorf, S. K., Mullen-Houser, E., Russell, D., De Geest, K., Jacobson, G., Hart, L., et al. (2010). Preservation of immune function in cervical cancer patients during chemoradiation using a novel integrative approach. *Brain, Behavior and Immunity.* doi:20.2026/j.bbi.2010.06.014

Mayo Clinic Staff. (2011a). Bedsores (pressure sores). Retrieved from http://www.mayoclinic.com/health/bedsores/DS00570/METHOD=print&DSECTION=all

Mayo Clinic Staff. (2011b). Spinal cord injury. Retrieved from http://www.mayoclinic.com/health/spinal-cord-injury/DS00460/METHOD=print&DSEC

McKinley, W., Santos, K., Meade, M., & Brooke, K. (2007). Incidence and outcomes of spinal cord injury clinical syndromes. *Journal of Spinal Cord Medicine, 30*(3), 215–224.

Meyer, S. A., Singh, H., & Jenkins, A. L. (2010). Surgical treatment of metastatic spinal tumors. *Mount Sinai Journal of Medicine: A Journal of Translational and Personalized Medicine, 77*(1), 124–129. doi: 10.1002/msj.20162

Miller, C. P., Brubacher, J. W., Biswas, D., Lawrence, B. D., Whang, P. G., & Grauer, J. N. (2011). The incidence of noncontiguous spinal fractures and other traumatic injuries associated with cervical spine fractures: A ten year experience at an academic medical center. *Spine* (Publish Ahead of Print). doi: 10.1097/BRS.1090b1013e3181f1550a1096

National Guideline Clearinghouse. (2006). *Acute management of autonomic dysreflexia: Individuals with spinal cord injury presenting to a health-care facility.* Washington, DC: Consortium for Spinal Cord Medicine, Paralyzed Veterans of America. Retrieved from wiki.cns.org/wiki/index.php/Autonomic_Dysreflexia

National Spinal Cord Injury Statistics Center: Facts and figures. (2012). Birmingham, Alabama. Retrieved from https://www.nscisc.uab.edu/PublicDocuments/fact_figures_docs/Facts%202012%20Feb%20Final.pdf

Popa, C., Popa, F., Grigorean, V. T., Onose, G., Sandu, A. M., Popescu, M., et al. (2010). Vascular dysfunctions following spinal cord injury. *Journal of Medical Life, 3*(3), 275–285.

Porth, C., & Matfin, G. (2009). *Pathophysiology: Concepts of altered health states.* Philadelphia: Wolters Kluwer/Lippincott Williams & Wilkins.

Reiter, G.T. (2011). Vertebra fracture treatment & management. *Medscape Reference.* Retrieved from http://emedicine.medscape.com/article/248236-treatment

Rodríguez-Zayas, A., Torrado, A., Rosas, O., Santiago, J., Figueroa, J., & Miranda, J. (2011). Blockade of P2 nucleotide receptors after spinal cord injury reduced the gliotic response and spared tissue. *Journal of Molecular Neuroscience, 15*(3), 1–10. doi: 10.1007/s12031-011-9567-6

Rose, P. S., Laufer, I., Boland, P. J., Hanover, A., Bilsky, M. H., Yamada, J., et al. (2009). Risk of fracture after single fraction image-guided intensity-modulated radiation therapy to spinal metastases. *Journal of Clinical Oncology, 27*(30), 5075–5079. doi: JCO.2008.19.3508 [pii]

Saltzherr, T. P., Fung Kon Jin, P. H., Beenen, L. F., Vandertop, W. P., & Goslings, J. C. (2009). Diagnostic imaging of cervical spine injuries following blunt trauma: A review of the literature and practical guideline. *Injury, 40*(8), 795–800. doi: S0020-1383(09)00012-6 [pii]10.1016/j.injury.2009.01.015

Schmidt, S. (2004). Optimal Healing Environment (OHE): Mindfulness and healing intention: Concepts, practice, and research evaluation. *Journal of Alternative and Complementary Medicine, 10* (Suppl. 1), S7–14.

Settersten, L. (2011, June). What is esoteric healing? *Journal of Holistic Nursing, 29*(2), 132–139. Epub 2010 Oct 21.

Shah, L., & Zollinger, L. (2011). Congenital craniocervical anomalies pose a vulnerability to spinal cord injury without radiographic abnormality (SCIWORA). *Emergency Radiology, 9*(2), 144–148.doi: 10.1007/s10140-011-0936-9

Sharma, S., Singh, M., Wani, I. H., Wani, K. H., Sharma, S., Sharma, N., & Singh, D. (2009). Adult spinal cord injury without radiograpahic abnormalities (SCIWORA): Clinical and radiological correlations. *Journal of Clinical Medicine Research, 1*(3), 165–172. doi: 10.4021/jocmr2009.08.1256

Shem, K., Castillo, K., Wong, S., & Chang, J. (2011). Dysphagia in individuals with tetraplegia: Incidence and risk factors. *Journal of Spinal Cord Medicine, 34*(1), 85–92.

Shin, J. C., Yoo, J. H., Lee, Y. S., Goo, H. R., & Kim, D.H. (2011). Dysphagia in cervical spinal cord injury. *Spinal Cord, 41*(6), 347–353.

Suberviola, B., Gonzalez-Castro, A., Llorca, J., Ortiz-Melon, F., & Minambres, E. (2008). Early complications of high-dose methylprednisolone in acute spinal cord injury patients. *Injury, 39*(7), 748–752. doi: S0020-1383(07)00508-6 [pii]10.1016/j.injury.2007.12.005

The Free Dictionary. (2012). Spinal cord injury. Retrieved from http://medical-dictionary.thefreedictionary.com/spinal+cord+injury

van den Berg, M. E., Castellote, J. M., de Pedro-Cuesta, J., & Mahillo-Fernandez, I. (2010). Survival after spinal cord injury: A systematic review. *Journal of Neurotrauma, 27*(8), 1517–1528. doi: 10.1089/neu.2009.1138

Vlok, A. J., Petersen, J., Dunn, R. N., & Stander, J. (2010). Shallow-water spinal injuries—devastating but preventable. *South African Medical Journal, 100*(10), 682–684.

Walid, M. S., and Zaytseva, N. V. (2009). Upper cervical spine injuries in elderly patients. *Australian Family Physician, 38*(1/2), 43–45.

Williams, C. (2010). Ensuring a patient received appropriate bowel care following spinal cord injury. *Nursing Times, 106*(24), 40–41.

Winkler, T. (2011). Spinal cord injury and aging. Medscape reference. Retrieved from http://emedicine.medscape.com/article/322713-overview

UNIT 6 Nursing Management of Patients with Respiratory Disorders

Content in Unit 6 that addresses the **Institute of Medicine (IOM)** competencies, **Nursing Core Competencies (NCC)**, the **Quality and Safety Education for Nurses (QSEN)** competencies, and **Concepts** for concept-based learning is listed below.

Competencies	Feature or Text	Location
IOM, QSEN, NCC Providing patient-centered care	Nursing Process: Patient Care Plan for Head and Neck Cancer	Chapter 26, page 720
	Nursing Process: Patient Care Plan for Pulmonary Infection	Chapter 27, page 749
	Nursing Process: Patient Care Plan for Tuberculosis	Chapter 27, page 754
	Nursing Process: Patient Care Plan for COPD	Chapter 27, page 766
	Nursing Process: Patient Care Plan for Patient Receiving NPPV	Chapter 28, page 821
IOM, QSEN, NCC Working in teams	Collaborative Management, Upper Airway Disorders, pages 691, 707, 710, 719, 738	Chapter 26
	Collaborative Management, Lower Airway Disorders, pages 756, 760, 764, 771, 777, 779, 784	Chapter 27
	Collaborative Management, Complex Respiratory Disorders, pages 798, 805	Chapter 28
IOM, QSEN, NCC Employing evidence-based practice	Evidence-Based Practice: Sleep Apnea in Hospitalized Patients	Chapter 26, page 703
	Evidence-Based Practice: Multidisciplinary Health Care for Patients with COPD	Chapter 27, page 765
	Evidence-Based Practice: NPPV	Chapter 28, page 820
NCC Educating patients	Health Promotion, Respiratory Assessment	Chapter 25, page 681
	Patient Teaching & Discharge Priorities for Patients with Facial Fracture	Chapter 26, page 691
	Health Promotion, Upper Airway Disorders, pages 699, 710	Chapter 26
	Patient Teaching & Discharge Priorities for Patients with Head and Neck Cancer	Chapter 26, page 726
	Patient Teaching and Discharge Priorities for Asthma	Chapter 27, page 739
	Health Promotion, Lower Airway Disorders, pages 743, 753, 756, 761, 771, 774, 777, 779, 782, 784	Chapter 27
	Patient Teaching & Discharge Priorities for Pulmonary Hypertension	Chapter 27, page 777
	Health Promotion, Complex Respiratory Disorders, pages 798, 805	Chapter 28
	Patient Teaching & Discharge Priorities for a Patient with ARDS	Chapter 28, page 806
Concepts covered in Unit 6 include:	Gas exchange; Oxygenation; Perfusion; Acid–base balance	Infection; Thermoregulation

Nursing Assessment of the Patient with Respiratory Disorders

25 CHAPTER

Carol Rhoades
Cheryl Wraa

Outcome-Based Learning Objectives

After studying this chapter, the learner will be able to:

1. Describe the structure and function of the respiratory system.
2. Understand the importance of obtaining information on culture, nutrition, exercise, and recent travel as components of the patient history.
3. Use the data obtained from the review of a patient's social and occupational history to determine the patient's risk for pulmonary disease.
4. Differentiate normal breath sounds from adventitious breath sounds.
5. Generate an assessment plan using the essential components of a physical assessment of the pulmonary system.
6. Differentiate adjuncts used during physical assessment of the pulmonary system.

KEY TERMS

accessory muscles p.666
adventitious breath sounds p.677
bradypnea p.674
bronchial breath sounds p.677
bronchovesicular breath sounds p.677
capnography p.681
clubbing p.675
crackles p.677
crepitus p.676
deadspace ventilation p.667
dyspnea p.668
fremitus p.676
hemoptysis p.668
hemothorax p.671
hyperpnea p.674
hypoxemia p.666
pleural friction rubs p.678
pneumothorax p.671
resonance p.678
rhonchi p.677
shunt ventilation p.667
stridor p.678
subcutaneous emphysema p.676
tachypnea p.674
tracheal breath sounds p.677
vesicular breath sounds p.677
wheezes p.677

NURSES IN ALL HEALTH CARE SETTINGS need to understand the components of a comprehensive health history and physical assessment of the pulmonary system. This not only contributes to the health care team's efforts in making the differential diagnosis of respiratory complaints, but it also identifies potentially life-threatening events. The nursing history and physical examination can uncover clues to the origin of actual or potential problems that may limit the patient's ability to breathe effectively. Many pathologic conditions can interfere with the body's ability to exchange oxygen and carbon dioxide at both the pulmonary and cellular levels. Nursing assessment of a patient's respiratory status encompasses a focused patient interview, a thorough physical assessment, careful monitoring, and review of testing and laboratory results. Nurses should be familiar with normal assessment findings and recognize subtle deviations that signal deteriorating conditions. Early detection and intervention have the potential to improve patient outcomes and save lives.

Anatomy and Physiology of the Pulmonary System

The ability to correlate physical assessment findings and medical health history with alterations in ventilation and perfusion is contingent on a clear understanding of the anatomy and physiology of the pulmonary system as well as how other systems influence respiratory function. Even more so, a strong grasp of anatomic and physiologic processes will enable the nurse to have awareness of how these alterations can progress and deteriorate and therefore can guide the monitoring and prioritization of patient care.

Conducting Airways

Conducting airways are the airway structures from the nose to the terminal bronchioles that allow passage of air from the atmosphere

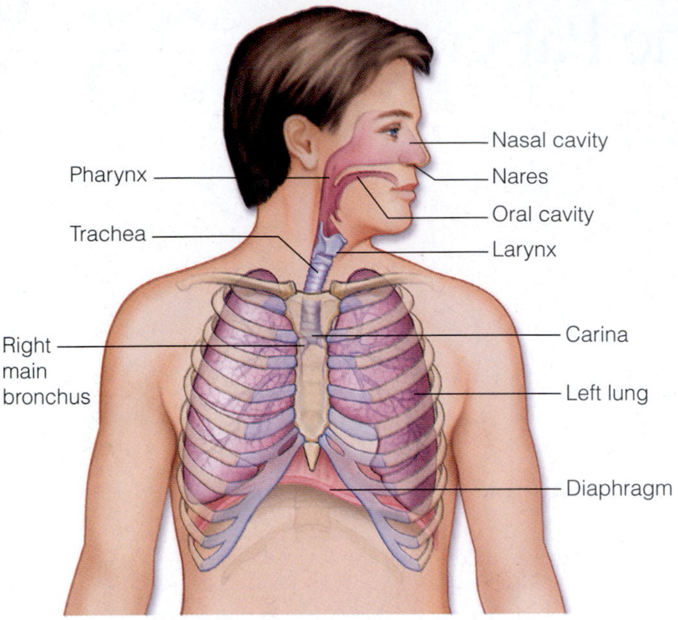

FIGURE 25–1 ◆ Anatomy of the respiratory system.

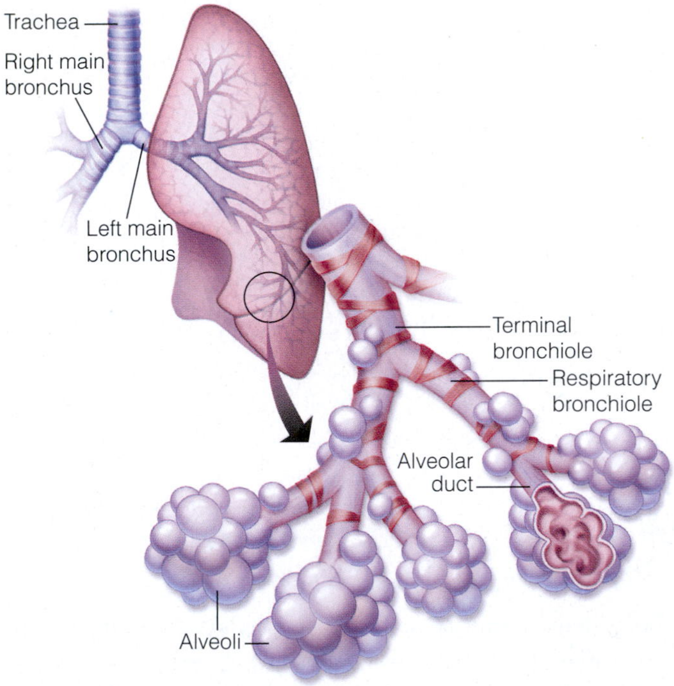

FIGURE 25–2 ◆ Respiratory bronchioles, alveolar ducts, and alveoli.

to the alveoli (see Figures 25–1◆ and 25–2◆). The trachea adds moisture to inspired air and warms or cools it to body temperature. The trachea also traps particulate matter such as dust, ozone, and bacteria to prevent it from reaching the alveolar membranes. Air flows through these passages, but they do not participate in gas exchange. Because of this, the conducting airways are referred to as the anatomic deadspace, which averages about 150 mL, varying with the patient's size and position. Obstructions in these conductive airways impair the adequate movement of air and oxygen to and from the alveoli for gas exchange.

Respiratory Muscles

The primary muscles that participate in respiration are the diaphragm and the external intercostals. Additional muscles, such as the internal intercostals, scalene (lateral neck), trapezius, abdominals, and sternocleidomastoids (anterior neck), can be recruited when additional work is needed to adequately ventilate. These are called **accessory muscles.**

Lungs

The lungs are the primary organs of the respiratory system. They are located in the thoracic cavity, bordered anteriorly at the apex (top) at the midclavicular line just above the clavicles and at the base at the sixth and eighth ribs at the midclavicular line and the midaxillary line, respectively (Figure 25–3◆). Posteriorly, the lung bases lie at the T10 spinous process and descend further on inspiration. The right lung is divided into the upper, middle, and lower lobes and is slightly larger than the left. The left lung is divided into an upper and lower lobe. The lungs house the right and left main bronchi, which branch into secondary, then tertiary, bronchi. The tertiary bronchi branch into progressively smaller bronchioles. When these bronchioles become microscopic, they are known as alveolar ducts (see Figure 25–2). These ducts enter the alveolar sacs, where diffusion of gases takes place in the alveoli. If the alveoli fill with fluid or collapse, gas exchange may be affected. However, the lungs have the capacity to shift blood flow away from areas that do not participate in gas exchange to areas that do, improving the oxygen-carrying capacity of the blood.

The lungs are covered by a membrane called the pleura. The pleura is composed of an inner layer, the visceral pleura, which lines the surface of the lungs, and an outer layer, the parietal pleura, which lines the thoracic cavity. The space in between the two layers, called the pleural space, contains a lubricating fluid that enables the lungs to expand fully and smoothly. If air or fluid enters the pleural space (e.g., in pneumothorax or pleural effusion), pressure is placed on the lungs, and this may affect the respiratory and cardiovascular status.

Ventilation

Ventilation is the movement of air between the atmosphere and the alveoli of the lungs. During inspiration, the diaphragm and intercostal muscles contract, dropping the diaphragm down and expanding the chest up and out, increasing the chest diameter, and reducing the pressures inside the lung. Pressures that are lower in the lung than in the atmosphere allow air to flow into the lung. The reverse happens with expiration. As the diaphragm and intercostals relax, chest size is reduced, increasing the pressure gradient and forcing air out.

Inspiration is an active process, and expiration is passive. The medulla oblongata, located in the lower half of the brainstem, is the primary respiratory regulator, either activating or deactivating inspiration via nerve innervation with the diaphragm and intercostal muscles. Stimulation of the medulla is influenced by chemoreceptors and receptor reflexes. Chemoreceptors located in the medulla respond to changes in blood pH. A decrease in blood pH (acidemia) will stimulate an increase in respiratory rate. Chemoreceptors in the aorta and carotid bodies are stimulated by a decrease of oxygen in the blood (**hypoxemia**), which also increases the rate and depth of ventilation. Stretch receptors in the bronchial wall respond to the stretch incurred during inspiration, stimulating the initiation of expiration. Receptors in the intercostal muscles influence the degree of respiratory muscle workload. The cerebral cortex allows individuals to have some conscious and voluntary

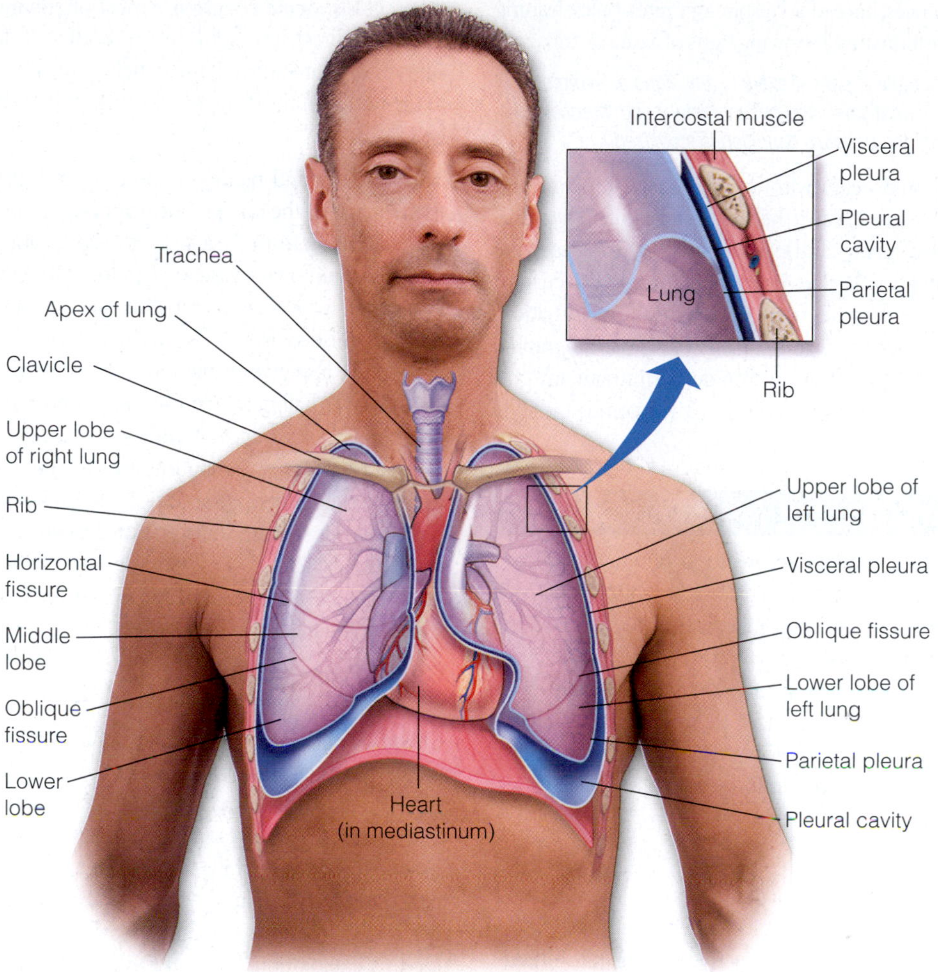

FIGURE 25–3 ◆ Anterior view of the thorax and lungs.

control over their ventilation. Expiration is predominantly passive and occurs through relaxation of the respiratory muscles and elastic recoil of the lungs. Diseases or injuries that affect the musculoskeletal system, brainstem, or nerve pathways may affect respiratory effort or efficiency.

Gas Exchange

Respiration involves the diffusion of oxygen from the alveoli into the pulmonary circulation and the release of carbon dioxide from the circulation into the alveoli. Carbon dioxide and oxygen exchange occurs at the alveolar level. Oxygen diffuses from the alveoli across the alveolar-capillary membrane and into the pulmonary vasculature. It attaches to the hemoglobin molecule for transport through the body for cellular consumption. Carbon dioxide is the by-product of cellular metabolism and is transported through the bloodstream back to the pulmonary vasculature, where it diffuses across the alveolar-capillary membrane into the alveoli and is expired through the conducting airways.

Ventilation/Perfusion

Adequate exchange of oxygen and carbon dioxide depends on ventilation of the alveoli and blood flow to the capillary membranes. In the healthy lung, ventilation and perfusion are nearly equal. If ventilation to the alveoli is compromised because of edema, secretions, or collapse, then ventilation/perfusion mismatch occurs. When blood flow (perfusion) to the alveoli is normal but ventilation is inadequate, not enough oxygen is delivered to the alveoli for diffusion, and blood flows past the alveoli without becoming oxygenated. This is termed **shunt ventilation.** If the lung cannot compensate, then the patient will exhibit signs and symptoms of hypoxia. Examples of shunt ventilation include atelectasis, pneumonia, pulmonary edema, and chronic obstructive pulmonary disease (COPD). All of these disorders are discussed in this unit.

Pulmonary perfusion is the blood flow through the pulmonary capillaries. When blood flow to normally ventilated alveoli is impaired, then **deadspace ventilation** exists. The classic example is pulmonary emboli. In addition, any condition that reduces cardiac output, such as shock, will also reduce the blood flow back to the lungs and subsequently pulmonary perfusion.

Pulmonary History

The patient's history includes both objective and subjective data. Because of this, the nurse needs effective interviewing skills to elicit pertinent data about the symptoms and the effect the symptoms have on the patient's ability to carry out daily activities. The interview should occur in a systematic format.

For acutely ill patients who display signs or symptoms of inadequate oxygenation or ventilation, the interview should be modified and shortened; the full history can wait until potentially life-threatening conditions have been attended to. Patients who appear anxious or fearful, are unable to speak in complete sentences, have rapid respiratory rates, or are leaning in a forward or braced position are all showing signs of acute distress.

Safety Alert *If an acutely ill patient exhibits any signs or symptoms of inadequate oxygenation or ventilation, the patient history and interview process should be curtailed until the patient's condition is stabilized.*

The health history should begin with the primary complaint that caused the patient to seek medical care (the chief complaint). The nurse should investigate what precipitates and exacerbates the symptoms. The past medical history may provide clues as to the nature of the current problem. The social history identifies support systems, home situation, occupational hazards, activity level, and sources of stress. Biographic and demographic data assist the interviewer in determining if any cultural or educational factors figure importantly into the manner and style of the interview process.

Chief Complaint

The chief complaint is the patient's interpretation of what prompted him to seek medical care. The nurse should record it in the patient's own words. Often, if the nurse asks what caused the patient to seek care, the patient will give information on both the symptoms and the impact the symptoms have had on his lifestyle and functional abilities. The chief complaint should direct a focused assessment of the patient's perception of the problem and the presenting symptoms. The most common presenting symptoms for patients with respiratory complaints are dyspnea, cough, sputum production, and chest pain.

Dyspnea

Dyspnea is the subjective feeling of shortness of breath or breathlessness. It is a common presenting symptom for patients with respiratory illness. Because dyspnea is considered a subjective finding, it is difficult to objectively quantify. The nurse should ask questions that provide further detail on the circumstances and causes of dyspnea. Because age, body size, and fitness level can influence shortness of breath, the nurse should attempt to determine how current symptoms have influenced changes in the patient's ability to perform daily activities. Anxiety can exacerbate or cause the symptoms and perceptions of shortness of breath. Patients may describe a feeling of being smothered; dyspnea can also be associated with a "pins-and-needles" sensation.

Patients might not be able to verbally complete the health history because of shortness of breath or difficulty breathing. Therefore, the nurse may need to obtain information from family members or the available medical record regarding the patient's basic history and to limit the history obtained from the patient to focused responses and information that is not available from other sources. The nurse may need to allow the patient to rest and limit all forms of exertion during the history. Asking yes and no questions or allowing the patient to write or use a communication board may be useful.

Cough

Coughing occurs when airways are irritated. It is a defense mechanism to rid the airways of mucus, pus, blood, foreign bodies, dust, or pollens, or to prevent inhalation of irritants, including very hot or cold air. Coughing may be caused by inflammation, tension in the airways, tumors, allergies, smoking, postnasal drip or esophageal reflux, and, less frequently, left-sided heart failure. The nurse must evaluate the symptom of coughing in relation to its timing, frequency, duration, and the nature of sputum produced. Cough should be described as chronic or acute. Chronic cough can be caused by asthma, reflux, smoking, or chronic bronchitis and is a classic warning sign of lung cancer and tuberculosis. Acute coughs are most often viral but are also caused by infections, bronchitis, and foreign bodies. If decongestants and cough suppressants are utilized, the cough may have a specific pattern related to the timing of the dosage. If so, this needs to be documented.

Sputum

The character and nature of sputum production give clues to the potential cause of the cough. **Hemoptysis,** coughing up blood or blood-stained sputum from the airway, is a significant finding that may indicate infection, pulmonary vasculitis, pulmonary emboli, pulmonary edema, bronchitis, lung abscess, tuberculosis, or cancer. Hemoptysis should be distinguished from hematemesis (vomiting blood). The color of the sputum also gives insight as to the causative organism. Pink, frothy sputum is the hallmark of pulmonary edema. In contrast, bronchitis and pneumonia are associated with yellow-, tan-, green-, or gray-colored mucus. The color of the sputum does not indicate a particular organism, nor should it influence the decision to obtain sputum cultures. Black or carbonaceous sputum may be related to burn trauma. A nonproductive cough may be related to angiotensin-converting enzyme (ACE) inhibitor use or irritation from dust or fumes. The amount of sputum production should be quantified as well.

Chest Pain

Cardiac causes should be investigated simultaneously with pulmonary causes of chest pain. Cardiac sources include myocardial ischemia or infarction, aortic dissection, and pericarditis. Refer to Chapter 29 on the assessment of patients with cardiovascular disorders for more information. Causes of pain associated with lung or chest wall disorders include bronchitis, pneumonia, pleuritis, trauma, asthma, and costochondritis (inflammation of the costal cartilage that connects the ribs to the sternum). The nurse may use any of a number of guidelines for this exploration. The OPQRST mnemonic in Chart 25–1 helps guide the patient to elaborate on the attributes of presenting symptoms and characteristics of pain (Bickley, 2009). The patient should be asked specifically when the symptoms began and the sequence in which they progressed. Aggravating and relieving factors must be explored, as well as the timing at which the symptoms occur.

Pain with respiration may cause patients to splint respirations (not take a deep breath), which will subsequently decrease inspired tidal

CHART 25–1 Symptom Characteristics Investigation: OPQRST

Onset	What was the patient doing when the symptom occurred? Are there environmental or emotional factors, specific activities, or other conditions that contribute to the symptoms? Was the onset sudden, gradual, or chronic?
Palliating/ Provoking Factors	Is there anything that will make the symptoms better or worse? Do the symptoms improve with rest?
Quality	What is the patient's description of symptoms? What is it like?
Radiation	Where in the body is the symptom? Does the pain or symptom extend to any other part of the body?
Severity	Scale of 0 to 10 with 0 being no pain and 10 being the worst pain possible.
Timing	When does it start? How long does it last? How often does it come?

volumes and promote atelectasis. Pain medication should be provided to patients so that they can participate in pulmonary rehabilitation activities and breathe deeply to prevent pneumonia and atelectasis. Cough suppressants should be used with caution because the cough's primary purpose is to remove secretions that block the airways.

Past History

The past history gives insight into the influence that prior illnesses and conditions may have on the presenting symptoms.

Childhood Diseases and Immunizations

Premature birth, childhood diseases, congenital pulmonary disease, and immunization (or lack thereof) are important to include in the history portion of the respiratory assessment. Current immunization status for influenza and pneumococcal pneumonia should also be assessed. Today, a number of adults present to health care systems with cystic fibrosis, often considered a childhood disease state. Asthma symptoms are frequently first seen during childhood. Cystic fibrosis and asthma are discussed in detail in Chapter 27. Finally, the nurse should ask the patient whether she had frequent colds, episodes of wheezing, or shortness of breath during childhood.

Patients who were born prematurely and were mechanically ventilated for long periods may suffer from primary or secondary pulmonary disease. Pulmonary disease in this population may be related to lung injury such as barotrauma (damage to alveoli from the extra-alveolar air during mechanical ventilation) from mechanical ventilation, prolonged use of high oxygen levels, or primary pulmonary disease such as pulmonary hypertension. It also may be related to primary congenital heart disease such as pulmonary atresia (a congenital heart defect where the pulmonary valve does not form properly) or valvular dysfunction. Neonatal respiratory distress syndrome is caused by a lack of surfactant in the immature lungs of premature babies. Although synthetic exogenous surfactant is available today to treat this complication of preterm birth, adults currently presenting with pulmonary problems might not have had treatment with the medication and are at risk for long-term or chronic complications.

The nurse should also ask the patient whether she suffered any childhood trauma. For example, swimming accidents during childhood could result in aspiration of water and resultant lung injury. Likewise, aspiration of foreign bodies in childhood may cause structural damage to airways.

Past Medical and Surgical History

The nurse should elicit from the patient the frequency of pulmonary infections, asthma exacerbations, infectious diseases, and associated hospitalizations. This will give insight into the potential severity of the patient's condition or the progression of the disease process. Treatment modalities, such as tracheostomy, chest tube insertion, intubation, and use of home oxygen, should also be elicited. Information about hospitalizations and illnesses not necessarily related to the pulmonary system is also important. Patients should be asked specifically whether any hospitalization was complicated by respiratory problems, including prolonged use of oxygen, intubation, or pulmonary embolus. For example, a patient who was hospitalized with a bowel obstruction may have suffered aspiration related to the reflux of gastric contents. Cardiac disease frequently has an adverse impact on the pulmonary system. Heart failure is a classic example of cardiac disease causing pulmonary symptoms and may result in residual pulmonary problems.

Treatment for thyroid disease may include local radiation therapy that could result in narrowing of the trachea due to goiter compression or tissue damage and edema from therapy. Patients who have been diagnosed with cancer may have metastases to the lung, or a treatment, such as radiation or chemotherapy, could have induced pulmonary injury. Thoracic trauma can cause lung lacerations, pulmonary contusions, hemothorax, pneumothorax, or pain. Liver failure associated with alpha$_1$-antitrypsin (AAT) deficiency is also associated with the development of emphysema and pulmonary disease.

The patient's response to hospitalization and previous illness gives the nurse information about the patient's prior experience with invasive and noninvasive testing and treatment. The analysis of previous illnesses and hospitalization also provides knowledge of comorbid conditions that may complicate diagnosis and care.

Medications

The patient should be encouraged to carry a list of all current medications. If possible, the medical record can also be explored for the prior use of medications. When discussing current medications with the patient, the nurse should inquire about dosage, frequency, and the last time the medication was taken. This is especially relevant if the patient is prescribed bronchodilators, anticholinergics, and steroids. Increased use of these medications may indicate that the patient's condition is worsening. Failure to take medications as directed also may increase pulmonary symptoms. The correct order in which to take inhaled medications is to take bronchodilators first to open the airways. Steroids should be taken after bronchodilators to improve absorption when the airways are dilated (open).

In listing the medications they take, patients may overlook over-the-counter (OTC) medications such as cough suppressants, expectorants, antihistamines, or herbal supplements. Because of this, the nurse should specifically ask about OTC medication use.

If the patient is currently prescribed medications to treat tuberculosis or antibiotics to treat pneumonia, the nurse should ensure that the patient is taking the medications as prescribed. Patients will frequently stop taking medications when they feel well. However, when patients fail to complete a course of antibiotic therapy, the pathogen may develop resistance, and the antibiotic will no longer be effective in its treatment. Use of medications other than those prescribed for pulmonary disease may cause pulmonary symptoms. For example, ACE inhibitors may cause cough, and amiodarone may cause pulmonary fibrosis. Respiratory medications are discussed in detail in Chapters 27 and 28.

Nurses need to request that the patients who use inhalers demonstrate their technique. If they are using metered-dose inhalers or spacers, the nurse should ensure that they are used correctly. For example, patients may assume that it is correct to use a spacer (described in Chapter 28) with all inhaled medications, when this is not true. For example, Advair, a combination inhaler, is not supposed to be taken with a spacer. Patients should be encouraged to bring all inhalers to their assessment. If patients bring inhalers that are no longer part of the prescribed regimen, the nurse should discard these inhalers to prevent the patient from potential overmedication.

Medications include the use of oxygen or ventilatory assist devices (BiPap, CPAP). Outpatient oxygen and ventilation therapy indicates that the patient has extensive or chronic pulmonary disease. Increased shortness of breath despite use of oxygen or ventilatory assistive devices or titrating up the support of these devices should send the nurse a warning about the potential for imminent decompensation. The nurse

Weblink: Cystic Fibrosis Foundation: Patient Registry Report

Weblink: Healthy People 2020 Objectives

should immediately assess the patient and determine whether the health care provider needs to be notified or the patient requires immediate intervention.

Allergies

Allergies frequently cause pulmonary symptoms ranging from simple congestion, coughing, and wheezing to anaphylactic reactions and airway obstruction. Patients should be instructed to report to the nurse allergies they have to plant products, foods, medications, dusts, molds, and animal sources. Knowledge of *all* allergies is important to the nurse because patients frequently do not realize that the contents of some medications or OTC supplements may contain allergens to which the patients are susceptible. For example, patients who are allergic to soy or nuts should not use Atrovent and Combivent (combination) inhalers. Patients may recognize that they are allergic to certain plants or pollens but not understand that most herbal supplements are made from plants and that they should carefully read the ingredients and understand the components of the supplements before taking them.

Family Health History

The family history seeks information on the age, health, and cause of death of the patient's grandparents, parents, and siblings. Respiratory infections, asthma, tuberculosis, hereditary disorders, and lung cancer may help in determining the cause of the patient's respiratory complaints as well as environmental and behavior-related risks for disease development. See the Genetic Considerations box for a discussion of cystic fibrosis, a genetic disorder.

In taking the family health history, the nurse should ask whether the patient has family members who smoke and whether any family members have had pulmonary disease, lung cancer, or cardiovascular disease. Lung cancer and cardiovascular disease tend to run in families. The familial risk of lung cancer is likely related to the presence of cigarette smoke in the household. The occurrence of childhood asthma and preterm birth is greater in instances where the mother smoked. Since cardiac disorders can present with respiratory symptoms, the cardiovascular health of family members should also be explored. The nurse also should inquire whether other family members are having similar respiratory complaints. See Chapter 29 for cardiovascular risk factors.

GENETIC CONSIDERATIONS Cystic Fibrosis

Cystic fibrosis is an autosomal recessive genetic disorder that causes the body to produce thick, sticky mucus in the lungs and digestive tract. The mucus builds up in the lungs and pancreas, leading to life-threatening infections and digestive problems. The thickness of the mucus is related to a defect in the cystic fibrosis transmembrane regulator (CFTR). CFTR affects the movement of sodium and water across epithelial tissues, producing thick mucus. Thick mucus is difficult to expectorate from the airways and promotes colonization of bacteria.

Most patients with cystic fibrosis are diagnosed in childhood. Pulmonary complications are the primary cause of death. In the 1980s, children born with cystic fibrosis had a median predicted survival age of 26 years. According to data collected by the Cystic Fibrosis Foundation, however, infants born in 2008 in the United States have a life expectancy of 37.4 years (Cystic Fibrosis Foundation, 2008). Refer to Chapter 27 for more information on cystic fibrosis.

Risk Factors

Cigarette smoking, inactivity, cardiovascular disease, obesity, substance abuse, and trauma are some of the more common risk factors that contribute to the development of respiratory disorders. The *Healthy People 2020* initiative cites physical activity, obesity, tobacco use, and substance abuse as leading health indicators. The goal in the area of respiratory diseases is to "promote respiratory health through better prevention, detection, treatment, and education efforts" (U.S. Department of Health and Human Services, 2010a).

Cigarette Smoking

Cigarette smoking remains the leading cause of premature preventable death in the United States (CDC, 2008). It damages the airways and alveoli of the lung, eventually leading to COPD. Smoking causes 85% of lung cancers as well as more than 90% of deaths from COPD (U.S. Department of Health and Human Services, 2010b). In addition, the CDC found that from 2000 to 2004, nearly 50,000 lung cancer and heart disease deaths were attributable to secondhand smoke. The three leading specific causes of smoking attributable to death are lung cancer, ischemic heart disease, and COPD. In the patient assessment interview, the nurse should ascertain the pack-year smoking history for patients who have been or currently are smokers. A patient's pack-year history is calculated by multiplying the number of packs per day smoked by the number of years the patient has smoked. For example, two packs per day for 10 years is a 20-pack-year history. In addition, nonsmokers should be asked whether they have a significant exposure to secondhand smoke. Smoking cessation techniques are discussed in Chapter 6.

Inactivity

Patients who are physically inactive are at higher risk for deep venous thrombosis (DVT) and pulmonary embolism. Immobility causes decreased venous return, venous stasis, and hypercoagulability. The longer the patient is inactive, the greater the risk for development of DVT. Patients with pulmonary disease may become short of breath with activity and become physically inactive so that they won't experience shortness of breath. This starts a cycle that further predisposes them to deconditioning, inactivity, and the potential for the development of thromboembolic disease.

Cardiovascular Disease

Patients with cardiovascular disease experience pulmonary complications related to the heart's inability to effectively pump blood to the lungs. Frequently, this results in a failure to adequately oxygenate or circulate oxygenated arterial blood to supply body tissues to meet metabolic demands. The result is activity intolerance, hypoxemia, and tachycardia, which further increase the myocardial oxygen demand and the potential for inadequate oxygen to supply these needs. A history of cardiovascular disease should alert the nurse to the potential for heart failure and pulmonary edema.

Obesity

Obesity has an impact on respiratory physiology, including increased airway resistance, altered gas exchange, increased work of breathing, and reduced lung volumes (Murugan & Sharma, 2008). These alterations are thought to be caused by excess weight on the chest and abdomen. There is increasing evidence that obesity is a risk factor for the development of several respiratory diseases, including obstructive sleep apnea (OSA), hypoventilation syndrome, and asthma.

OSA is commonly associated with obesity. Narrowing of the upper airway related to fat deposits in the neck and poor muscle tone in the upper airway cause intermittent partial and complete airway obstruction (Ferri, 2010). The inability of the pharyngeal muscles to maintain upper airway patency leads to intermittent upper airway collapse, which leads to apnea, hypoxia, hypercapnia, and increased respiratory effort. There is hypoventilation related to restriction of thoracic expansion by excess adipose tissue. In many obese patients, OSA interrupts effective sleep patterns.

Obesity-hypoventilation syndrome (OHS) is characterized by the combination of obesity, daytime hypoxemia, and daytime hypercapnia. Similar to sleep apnea, patients with OHS may complain of daytime sleepiness, fatigue, or morning headaches. The chronic hypoxemia and hypercapnia are associated with pulmonary hypertension and right-sided heart failure and, if left untreated, early mortality (Powers, 2009).

Substance Abuse

Patients who abuse intravenous (IV) medications are at risk for a multitude of complications affecting almost every organ system. IV drug abusers are at an increased risk for pneumonia, septic emboli, emphysema, pulmonary vascular disease, and increased incidence of fatal asthma (Karpel, 2009). Inhaled drugs may cause pulmonary injury or pulmonary hemorrhage. Central nervous system depression from alcohol or drugs can contribute to aspiration pneumonia, chemical pneumonitis, and respiratory arrest (Emergency Nurses Association, 2009).

Trauma

Thoracic and abdominal traumatic injuries predispose patients to the development of pneumonias, hypoventilation, and atelectasis. Fractures of long bones are most closely associated with fat emboli, although they also can occur with other invasive fat-related procedures such as liposuction and lipid infusions. Fat embolism syndrome generally manifests 24 to 72 hours post-injury. The classic triad of symptoms is hypoxemia, neurologic abnormalities, and petechial rash (broken capillaries in the skin that appear as red dots that do not blanche when pressure is applied) (Weinhouse, 2008). Early immobilization of fractures and surgical repair reduce the incidence of fat embolism.

Both blunt and penetrating trauma to the chest may cause pulmonary contusion, rib fractures, pneumothorax, and/or hemothorax. **Pneumothorax** is defined as air in the pleural space that prevents the lung from fully expanding and results in partial or complete collapse of the lung. If this pressure continues to build without intervention, it will develop into a tension pneumothorax in which the pressure pushes the airway and cardiovascular structures to the opposite side of the chest, causing cardiovascular collapse and, if untreated, death. In addition to blunt and penetrating trauma, pneumothoraces also may occur with medical procedures such as surgery or mechanical ventilation, Marfan syndrome, and pulmonary disease such as asthma and COPD. A **hemothorax** is defined as blood in the pleural cavity. It is most frequently caused by blunt or penetrating trauma. Hemodynamic compromise and shock will occur when there is significant blood loss. In addition, respiratory compromise develops when the lung is not able to fully expand because blood occupies space within the chest cavity.

Burn injury can occur in the pulmonary tree from inhalation of heated gases (see Chapter 61). The damaged lung tissue becomes edematous, and the patient develops acute respiratory distress. Edema of the airways can cause upper airway obstruction. Patients with signs of an airway burn should be aggressively considered for early intubation for airway protection. If clinicians wait until signs of airway distress and obstruction occur, the airway may be too edematous for placement of an endotracheal tube.

Trauma to the brain and spinal cord may also affect the respiratory system and assessment findings (see Chapters 21 and 24). The medulla and pons control respiratory rate and depth in response to changes in oxygen levels in the blood. Chemoreceptors relay information on blood pH to the cardiorespiratory centers in the brainstem. Spinal cord injuries above cervical level 4 will paralyze the muscles normally used in ventilation, including the diaphragm. Below cervical spine level 4, intercostal muscle paralysis may occur.

Personal and Social History

The personal and social history captures information relative to a patient's lifestyle, living conditions, work conditions, coping mechanisms, interests, and sources of support. It should include the patient's occupation, schooling, leisure activities, financial situation, home environment, and significant others. The nurse should also ascertain any sources of short- and long-term stresses that may affect the patient's ability to cope with illness. Determining the degree of connection with and assistance from family and friends is particularly important for older adults and disabled individuals.

Occupation

Many occupations are associated with exposure to airborne particles, vapors, and irritants. These occupational irritants can result in acute or chronic respiratory disease in susceptible individuals. The Occupational Safety and Health Administration (OSHA) sets and enforces standards in the U.S. work environment to ensure a safe work environment; however, it is impossible in many circumstances to prevent airborne or inhalation exposure, particularly in the outdoors. Farmers may be exposed to pesticides, and construction workers and masons may be exposed to cement dust. Even when personal protective equipment is available and recommended, it is each person's own decision to utilize precautions and protective equipment.

Asbestos inhalation is associated with the development of pleurisy and pleural effusion up to 20 years after exposure. Mesothelioma is a rare form of asbestos-related malignancy with a prolonged latency period in which symptoms might not appear for 40 years after exposure (Ferri, 2010). The use of asbestos was either reduced or banned in the 1960s. Patients at risk for asbestos-related pulmonary disease worked in naval shipyards, construction, mining, and insulation prior to the 1970s. Today, firemen and demolition workers are at risk of asbestos-related pulmonary disease because older buildings still contain significant amounts of asbestos. Asbestos is also present in vehicle brake linings, placing auto mechanics at risk.

Occupational asthma may occur in many settings. For example, people who work around animals are exposed to dander, hair, and allergens picked up from the environment. In the food industry, dust, proteins, and fumes may cause asthmatic reactions. Any occupation in which workers come into contact with fumes or vapors may provoke occupational asthma. This includes vapors from cleaning solvents that are utilized in work environments as well as the home. Symptoms associated with work-related asthma include wheezing, shortness of breath, and coughing when the worker is exposed to the allergen. The disease is progressive with each exposure. Initially, the person might have symptoms only while at work, but as the airways become more reactive, symptoms occur in any setting. Early recognition, diagnosis, and treatment of occupational asthma can prevent pulmonary complications.

Weblink: 2009 H1N1 Pandemic: Summary Highlights

CULTURAL CONSIDERATIONS
Cultural Practices Related to Respiratory Disorders

Cultural Practice	Nursing Considerations
Use of amulets (many cultures)	May interfere with diagnostic testing such as x-rays, MRI, and ultrasound. Suggest alternate placement of amulet for test duration or placement of amulet within eye contact.
Cupping (Southeast Asia, Greece)	May be mistaken for signs of abuse; may delay medical treatment. Burns or skin infections may occur and necessitate medical treatment.
Coining (Southeast Asia, Italy, and Russia)	May be mistaken for signs of abuse; may delay medical treatment. Burns or skin infections may occur and necessitate medical treatment.
Herbal remedies (used in many cultures)	Herbal remedies may be related to allergies because they are derived from plants that are associated with allergens. Herbal remedies may also interfere with the actions of medications and antibiotics or increase bleeding tendencies.

Culture

Culture plays an important role in the acceptance of diagnostic testing and treatment of respiratory symptoms (see the Cultural Considerations box). Cultural indoctrination may also influence the patient's responses to the nurse's attempts to obtain the patient's history and perform the physical examination. Therefore, the nurse needs to have an understanding of cultural considerations specific to the patient's frame of reference. For example, East Indian patients may feel that eye contact is rude. The nurse must make allowances for this conception and not conclude that the lack of eye contact indicates deception or abuse.

Cultural practices, such as the wearing of protective amulets, may interfere with planned diagnostic testing. Nonetheless, the nurse must respect the patient's belief and perhaps suggest an alternate placement of the amulet so that interference with diagnostic testing does not occur. For example, if a patient wears an amulet around the neck that would interfere with a chest x-ray, the nurse may suggest that the patient continue to wear the amulet but wrap it around the wrist during the diagnostic test.

Physical assessment of the patient may reveal cultural practices such as coining and cupping. Southeast Asian people may feel that respiratory illness is due to "wind illness" and traditionally treat the symptoms with "cupping." Cupping involves utilizing a cup applied to the skin to draw out the disease. This traditional therapy, which is also practiced by people in Greece, leaves circular marks on the skin. "Coining," which involves scraping the skin of the thorax with a coin or a spoon, is practiced in Southeast Asia, Italy, and Russia. Both coining and cupping may result in skin lesions or burns that may be mistaken as signs of abuse or cause complications that require medical treatment. Prior to coining or cupping, the skin may be treated with an herbal lotion or ointment (Spector, 2009).

If the patient is experiencing respiratory symptoms, some cultures feel that the patient should avoid water or bathing because these may contribute to illness. Many cultures have herbal remedies for respiratory illness. For example, a Native American herbal treatment for respiratory illness that is thought to boost the immune system is echinacea. Current research seems to vacillate regarding the effectiveness of this remedy. Among the Hmong (from Laos), opium is used as an analgesic. Smoking opium causes respiratory complications; however, the Hmong may consider lung disease an accepted part of life.

Environment

The nurse should explore the patient's home and work environment for potential allergens or contributing factors to the development of pulmonary symptoms. If the environment contains allergens, they should be removed. Patients with asthma should have allergy tests prior to receiving suggestions that specific allergens and triggers be removed from the home environment (such as pets). House dust mites are a common trigger for allergy and asthma symptoms. Weekly vacuuming and removal of stuffed products such as toys and pillows may help remove dust mites. Cockroach allergens may be removed by using commercial cockroach insecticides as well as preventive measures such as disposing of trash daily to an area outside of the home. Although little can be done regarding workplace allergen containment, the workplace should be reviewed regarding patient triggers, and accommodations should be made prior to specific activities such as painting, insecticide treatment, and use of specific cleansers. For individuals with reactive airway disease who work outdoors, environmental agents such as cement dust and specific fumes that affect the patient may be avoided with appropriate communication.

Habits

Cigarette smoking is the most specific habit that should be avoided. Even nonsmoking patients should be counseled to avoid situations in which cigarette smoking is present to prevent exposure to secondhand smoke. Personal hygiene habits should also be explored with the patient. Good oral hygiene can help prevent pulmonary disease. Oral infections can travel to the pulmonary tree to cause abscess formation or pneumonia. Hand hygiene is also important in the prevention and spread of disease. Patients should be counseled to wash their hands frequently and always before eating and drinking, as well as before preparing food.

Exercise

Exercise tolerance is often decreased in patients with pulmonary disease. The nurse should obtain specific information about the distance that the patient can walk on a flat surface as well as specific activities that cause shortness of breath. Frequently, the distance a patient can ambulate independently will affect the level of care necessary for the patient on discharge from the hospital. A specific plan for progressive exercise should be developed for each patient. Goals to be set for the patient on a daily basis require knowledge of the patient's baseline activity and exercise status.

Nutrition

Frequently, patients with shortness of breath have poor nutritional status. Shortness of breath can interfere with the patient's abilities to shop for, prepare, and consume food, activities that require energy. The nurse should also be aware that a typical body type is associated with certain pulmonary diseases. For example, the patient with chronic bronchitis or emphysema may be thin with muscle wasting. Inadequate nutrition places the patient at risk for infection. Nutrition is discussed in detail in Chapter 8.

Travel and Area of Residence

The patient's area of recent travel may become an important aspect of the history in diagnosing potential respiratory problems. The SARS (severe acute respiratory syndrome) and H1N1 (swine flu) outbreaks have demonstrated that some pulmonary diseases can be traced to a specific geographic location (Figure 25-4◆) (CDC, 2010). Therefore, recent travel and area of residence are important factors in the history

Weblink: Altitude Illness: Pulmonary Syndromes

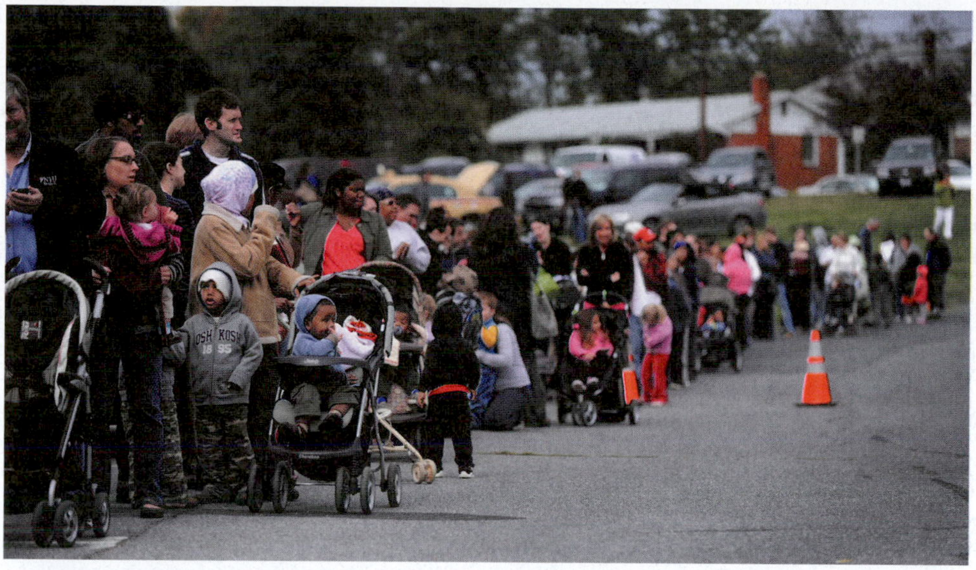

FIGURE 25–4 ◆ The H1N1 flu virus was first detected in California on April 15, 2009. By June 19, 2009, all 50 states reported cases of H1N1 infection. Hundreds of county residents waited in a long line for the H1N1 vaccination shot at a clinic held by the Montgomery County Health and Human Services on October 14, 2009, in Silver Spring, Maryland.

Source: Getty Images/Tim Sloan.

of respiratory symptoms, and the nurse should include questions about these in the interview process.

High-altitude illness refers to a group of syndromes associated with hypoxia at high elevation, generally greater than 5,000 feet. Pulmonary edema (HAPE) is a form of high-altitude illness marked by the accumulation of fluid in the lungs; it most often occurs at elevations greater than 6,500 feet, a common altitude of ski resorts. Some people appear to be predisposed to HAPE; however, anyone who travels to altitude is at risk regardless of age, medical condition, or fitness level (Harris & Nelson, 2008). Although HAPE is often associated with mountaineers, individuals with preexisting cardiovascular or pulmonary disease who have been managing adequately at or near sea level may develop symptoms of altitude illness when they travel to high altitude, such as flying from sea level to a ski resort. HAPE is discussed in detail in Chapter 28.

Biographic and Demographic Data

Assessment of biographic and demographic data includes information regarding age, race, gender, and culture that can influence the patient's understanding, preconceptions, and susceptibility to some pulmonary disorders. In some instances, knowledge of the patient's place of birth or current address may give clues to the origin of the current complaints. For example, if a patient with a productive cough and night sweats was born in or recently relocated from an area where tuberculosis (TB) is common, the nurse should suspect TB and initiate adequate precautions and testing. Places of residence may also include areas with poor air quality or the presence of allergens and irritants that affect the respiratory system.

Gender no longer appears to be a factor in the development of pulmonary disease. Lung cancer and COPD, which includes emphysema, occur only slightly more frequently in men than in women. Lymphangiomyomatosis is a disease affecting young women in their 20s and 30s that may have a genetic or hormonal component that causes changes in the smooth muscle tissue of the lung and cyst development. The symptoms and treatment of this disease are similar to those for emphysema. Normal aging may also play a part in activity-related shortness of breath. Therefore, the nurse must utilize knowledge of age-related changes in the pulmonary vessels and tissue when performing a respiratory assessment.

Physical Examination

The physical examination of the patient begins with first contact. It should proceed in an organized fashion utilizing the techniques of inspection, palpation, percussion, and auscultation. The nurse starts by taking visual cues of the patient's appearance and signs of distress. The nurse may also hear audible wheezes or stridor from a distance. When speaking with the patient, the nurse should note the number of words in each sentence and whether the patient's breath has a foul odor. The patient's general appearance, skin color, and presence of oxygen or assistive devices all provide data in the patient's assessment.

The patient's assessment should be systematic and proceed from noninvasive data collection to invasive data collection. The nurse should be aware of available resources and, when possible, review them before the interview. If the patient's medical records are available, they should be obtained and included in data collection. The patient's current physical status should be compared to findings in previous assessments. If findings indicate new symptoms or an increase in symptoms, the nurse must document these findings and take steps to ensure that the patient receives appropriate care. The nurse must pursue appropriate and complete evaluation of all physical findings and symptoms of respiratory dysfunction to assist in the determination of the cause and to prevent further compromise of the patient's ability to carry out activities essential to health and lifestyle satisfaction.

Inspection

Inspection is the nurse's initial visual survey of a patient. It involves observation of the patient's appearance, behavior, posture, speech, and motor activity. Some findings may identify potential health problems or characteristics that necessitate a more in-depth evaluation. Evaluation of the respiratory rate, pattern, and patient's ease of breathing should occur continually throughout the patient's assessment.

General Appearance

The nurse should evaluate the patient's general appearance. Does the patient appear to have the physical capability to take care of himself? Does the patient appear comfortable or assume a tripod position (see the following text) to facilitate breathing? Is the patient in obvious distress?

The patient's facial appearance may indicate that he is anxious or fearful, a symptom of hypoxia. Patients with COPD may exhibit facial flushing related to the effort of breathing. Pursed-lip breathing during exhalation prolongs the expiratory phase of respiration. This maintains the smaller airways in an open position, prevents alveolar collapse during expiration, and lengthens the time of gas exchange. It also helps to reduce trapped air in the alveoli for patients with COPD or asthma. Nasal flaring may also be evident in the patient with pulmonary disease. Nasal flaring indicates that the patient is making a voluntary effort to inhale through the nostrils, which is a sign of increased work in breathing.

Patients may assume a posture that eases the work of breathing. For example, the tripod position, in which the patient leans forward resting on both arms, allows expansion of the thorax and eases breathing. Sitting upright with the legs dependent may ease breathing in the patient with heart failure by decreasing venous return and the accumulation of fluid in the lungs.

Mentation

The brain relies on oxygen for function. Hypoxia causes changes in mental status, including agitation, poor judgment, poor memory, and attention deficits. Symptoms of elevated carbon dioxide in the blood include lethargy, headache, and decreased level of consciousness. The nurse must assess the patient for orientation to person, place, and time as part of the assessment process.

Safety Alert *The nurse should initially rule out hypoxia as the cause for anxiety or changes in mental status.*

Rate, Depth, and Rhythm of Respirations

The patient's respiratory rate should be counted for a full minute in patients with an irregular respiratory rhythm and for 30 seconds in patients with a regular rhythm. The normal respiratory rate for adults is 12 to 20 respirations per minute. **Tachypnea** is considered to be a respiratory rate greater than 20 breaths per minute. A respiratory rate greater than 24 indicates respiratory distress. **Bradypnea** is a respiratory rate less than 12 breaths per minute. Bradypnea may be related to neurological disease or oversedation. An increased respiratory rate may be seen with fever, anxiety, and exercise.

Hyperpnea refers to both increased rate and depth of respiration and is associated with metabolic acidosis. It is sometimes referred to as Kussmaul breathing. Cheyne–Stokes breathing is a pattern of breathing in which the patient breathes rapidly, then has a period of apnea. Shallow respirations may be seen with sedation, pneumonia, pain, or hypercalcemia. The respiratory pattern is normally rhythmic. Breathing patterns that are not rhythmic signal neurological dysfunction.

Thoracic Size and Shape

The size and shape of the thorax provide important clues about the risk for pulmonary disease. Structural abnormalities such as pectus excavatum (sternal depression) or pigeon chest (pectus carinatum), an outward bowing of the sternum, may indicate underlying structural abnormalities in the heart. Pectus excavatum may cause compression of the heart or great vessels. Barrel chest, an increased anterior-posterior diameter of the thorax, may indicate emphysema. Scoliosis and kyphoscoliosis (hunching and curvature of the spine) may prevent full expansion of the affected lung. These structural changes also prevent full lung expansion. Lung expansion is integral for oxygen and carbon dioxide exchange and for clearance of secretions. Cough may be ineffective to clear secretions in patients with structural deformities. This increases the risk of pneumonia.

Thoracic Expansion and Symmetry

During normal inspiration, the diaphragm flattens and the lower rib cage expands. During inspection of the thoracic cavity, the nurse should note the expansion and deflation of the chest wall with inspiration and expiration. The right and left chest should expand equally and simultaneously on inspiration as well as expiration. If expansion is unequal, it should be determined through observation whether one side is not expanding with inspiration, as with a flail chest, or whether one side is failing to deflate fully on expiration, as with a pneumothorax (See Chapter 27 on lower airway disorders for further discussion of these disorders). In some conditions, such as COPD, respirations are equilateral; however, excursion with inspiration is decreased. Normally, a 5- to 13-cm (2- to 5-in.) increase in chest diameter can be observed with COPD.

Use of Accessory Muscles

During normal inspiration, the diaphragm and intercostal muscles contract, expanding the thorax and moving it upward. These are the primary muscles of respiration. When extra effort is required to breathe adequately, secondary or accessory muscles may be recruited. Accessory muscles of inspiration include the trapezius (chest pectorals), sternomastoid (anterior neck), and scalenus (lateral neck). The use of these muscles may become pronounced in a patient with respiratory distress, fatigue, or diaphragmatic weakness, and may become progressively more prominent as the severity of symptoms increases. Abdominal muscles may also be used in patients with pulmonary disease to force expiration.

Color and Appearance of Skin and Extremities

The color and appearance of the patient's skin and extremities may give clues to the presence of hypoxia or anemia. Physical characteristics such as clubbing of the fingers may also indicate chronic hypoxia. Cardiovascular causes of pallor or skin changes must be explored as well. The nurse should corroborate findings of the physical examination with the patient to determine whether they are familial characteristics or changes related to disease progression.

Pallor

Pallor can be related to vasoconstriction from cold ambient temperatures, melanin deficiencies, and heredity. It may also indicate that the patient is anemic. The nurse should check the mucous membranes and conjunctiva if pallor is suspected due to anemia. Under normal conditions, 98% of the oxygen in the blood is bound to hemoglobin. In anemia, there is a decrease in hemoglobin and a resultant decrease in the oxygen-carrying capacity. Patients with anemia tend to compensate for the decrease in oxygen-carrying capacity by increasing the heart rate. Thus, the hemoglobin moves through the vascular tree more rapidly to the lungs to be oxygenated and then to the body, where it exchanges oxygen for carbon dioxide. Anemic patients are generally exercise intolerant because they cannot tolerate further increases in heart rate.

Cyanosis

Cyanosis is a bluish discoloration of the skin and mucous membranes. Central cyanosis refers to cyanosis present in the "central" part of the body, such as the lips, mouth, head, or torso. It is an abnormal sign that generally indicates lack of oxygenated arterial blood. This abnormality

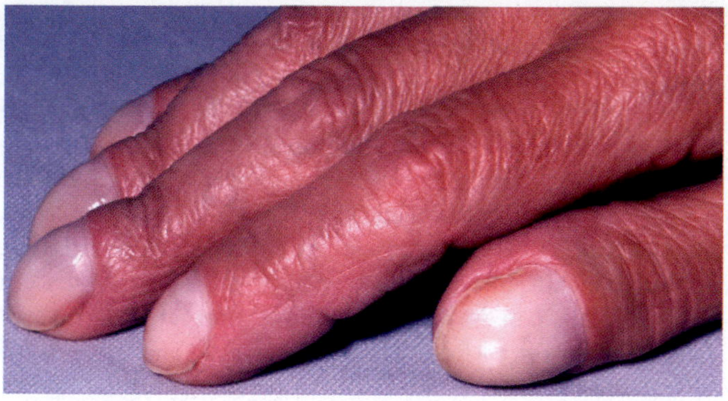

FIGURE 25–5 ◆ Clubbing of fingernails.

can be caused by a cardiac, pulmonary, or blood disorder. Peripheral cyanosis, a decrease in the oxygenated blood in the venous system, is most easily detectable in the hands and soles of the feet. It can be caused by exposure to cold temperatures, vasoconstriction, impaired blood flow, or a drop in cardiac output. When it occurs along with central cyanosis, it is most likely an indication of hypoxemia. Widening of the tips of the fingers and nail beds with loss of the normal angle may indicate chronic hypoxia. This finding is known as **clubbing** (Figure 25–5◆). Newborns may commonly exhibit peripheral cyanosis when cold or agitated; this is a normal reaction.

Cyanosis is a very nonspecific and somewhat subjective sign, subject to variation between clinician observations, room lighting, and natural skin pigmentation. As an indicator of hypoxemia, it can be unreliable. It takes approximately 5 g/dL of unoxygenated hemoglobin in the capillaries to produce the dark blue hue (Porth & Matfin, 2009). This relates to an arterial saturation of approximately 85% (PaO_2 of 50 mmHg) in patients with a normal hemoglobin level. In anemic patients, cyanosis is observed at lower saturation levels. For example, for a patient with reduced hemoglobin of 9 g/dL (the normal amount is 15 g/dL) cyanosis would not manifest until saturation reached about 73% (PaO_2 of 38 mmHg). Therefore, it is best not to rely on the absence of cyanosis to indicate adequate oxygenation.

Other less common causes of cyanosis are high concentrations of methemoglobin, which are seen mostly in drug reactions, particularly to nitrates (nitroglycerin). Some metals (silver, lead) or drugs (amiodarone, hydrochloride) can cause pseudocyanosis. To be certain, check saturations or arterial blood gas measurements.

Neck Inspection

The nurse should examine the patient's neck for tracheal deviation or the presence of goiter or lesions, which may cause upper airway obstruction and jugular venous distention. The trapezius, scalenus, and sternomastoid muscles may be enlarged in patients with COPD. Tracheal deviation occurs in pneumothorax and hemothorax. Deviation is contralateral to the affected lung. Neck vein distention (jugular venous distention) may be related to right heart failure, which decreases the flow of blood to the pulmonary tree for oxygenation. Jugular venous filling during expiration may be seen in COPD due to hyperinflation of the lungs.

Palpation

Palpation of the thorax and dependent extremities helps to determine whether changes are due to cardiac, vascular, or pulmonary causes. Edema of the lower extremities points to heart failure as the cause for edema. Palpation of the thorax may uncover subcutaneous emphysema, step-off defects (deformities) caused by rib fractures, and vibrations caused by respirations. Capillary refill time can indicate a cardiovascular cause for dyspnea.

Edema

Edema of the lower extremities is generally related to right heart failure or overall heart failure. Right heart failure and combined left- and right-sided failure are common in patients with COPD. Pulmonary hypertension causes right-sided failure. Chronic distention of the lower airways from high pressures makes forward blood flow more difficult. Over time, the right heart hypertrophies in an attempt to increase the force of blood through the pulmonary tree. Eventually, the right heart fails, and fluid that cannot be accommodated is sequestered in dependent interstitial spaces (usually the lower extremities and coccyx) and causes edema. Edema is classified as pitting or nonpitting and is graded according to depth. Using one finger, the nurse depresses the skin for 5 seconds and then releases it. If the nurse is able to depress the tissue up to 8 mm, the patient has 4+ edema; 6 mm, the patient has 3+ edema; 4 mm, 2+ edema; and 1+ edema measures 2 mm.

Skin Temperature and Moisture

The skin temperature and moisture status can give the nurse information about the patient's hydration, breathing effort, and temperature. Patients with COPD and asthma exacerbations may have very dry skin because of the loss of moisture through the respiratory tract. Shortness of breath with asthma and COPD exacerbations may prevent the patient from replacing fluids lost through rapid respiration, thus causing dehydration. Fever from pulmonary infections may increase skin temperature and moisture or cause cool, dry skin. Warm, moist skin may also be related to increased effort of breathing.

Clinical Reference Points

Although certain visible reference points, such as the trachea, nipple line, and sternum, are utilized in respiratory assessment, it is important to palpate and count ribs and intercostal spaces for accuracy (Figure 25–6◆). Landmarks that are utilized in the

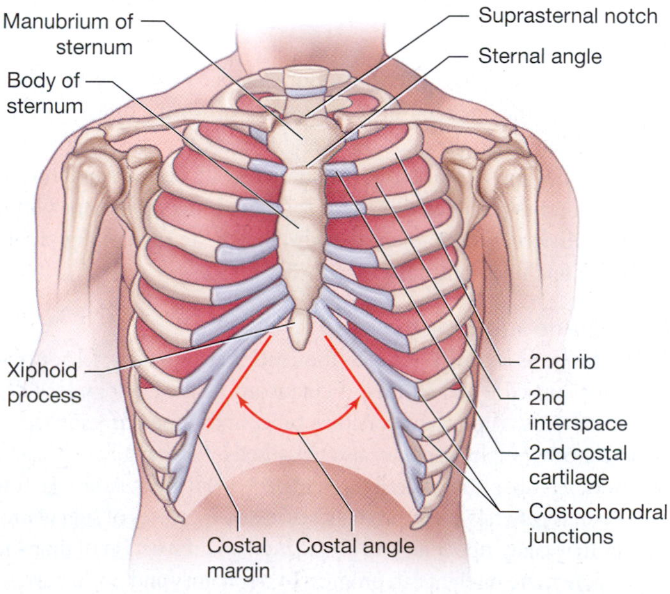

FIGURE 25–6 ◆ In a respiratory assessment, it is important to palpate and count ribs and interspaces to accurately record the location of lesions or adventitious breath sounds.

cardiorespiratory assessment include the anterior axillary line, the midaxillary line, and the midclavicular line. If a lesion is seen or adventitious breath sounds are heard along one of these lines, it is then described further by its vertical location as delineated by the rib number or intercostal space.

Chest Excursion

Chest excursion is measured by placing the hands on the patient's back, equidistant from the spine or the center of the back, at the level of the 10th rib. When the patient takes a deep breath, the nurse's hands should move an equal distance laterally. The normal chest excursion (i.e., the distance between the thumbs with inspiration) should be 5 to 10 cm (2 to 4 in.). Older adults may have decreased chest excursion as a normal finding. Patients with COPD may have decreased chest excursion due to anatomic flattening of the diaphragm from hyperinflation at the base of the lungs. Patients with rib fractures, pneumothorax, hemothorax, or pneumonia may also have decreased chest excursion.

Tactile Fremitus

Fremitus refers to the vibration transmitted through the lungs and chest wall and palpated on a patient's thorax during low frequency vocalization. Voice vibrations from the large airways are transmitted to the surface skin of the thorax. To assess the patient's fremitus, the nurse starts palpating with the ulnar side of the hand from the scapulae on the back or clavicles on the anterior chest and moves down bilaterally on each side of the thorax while the patient repeats the word "ninety-nine." The vibrations should be strongest over the large airways on the upper thorax and should decrease in strength as the nurse moves down the thorax, comparing each side for symmetry. Sound is transmitted better through solid, consolidated tissue than through air or fluid. Sound therefore increases when there is increased density of lung tissue. Examples of conditions in which there is increased fremitus include neoplasm, atelectasis, pneumonia, and fibrosis. Fremitus is decreased when there is fluid or air in the lung space. Examples of conditions in which there is a global decrease in fremitus include COPD and a muscular or obese chest wall. There is a unilateral decrease in pleural effusion, pneumothorax, bronchial obstruction, and neoplasm.

Tenderness

Point tenderness (pain when pressure is applied to a specific place on the body) may be seen in muscle strain or rib fracture. Excessive coughing may strain the intercostals and thoracic muscles. Pneumonia and consolidation may also cause tenderness with deep inspiration. To avoid tenderness from any of these conditions, the patient may limit chest excursion and breathe shallowly. Shallow respirations promote atelectasis and may contribute to hypoxia.

Subcutaneous Emphysema

Subcutaneous emphysema is the crackling sensation felt during palpation caused by air in the subcutaneous tissue. Etiology includes pneumothorax, ruptured bronchial tube, and ruptured esophagus. Subcutaneous emphysema can also be caused by gas gangrene. Because air rises, crepitus is not generally seen in dependent areas. Although this condition is generally asymptomatic, excessive increases of subcutaneous air may cause upper airway obstruction and restriction of thoracic expansion; more rarely, it can progress to respiratory and cardiac arrest. The term **crepitus** is often used interchangeably with *subcutaneous emphysema*; however, it more generally refers to the crackling or grating sound that is heard with subcutaneous air as well as when bone fragments rub together or when there are joint abnormalities.

Auscultation

Auscultation of breath sounds is performed in a systematic manner utilizing a stethoscope (Figures 25–7◆ and 25–8◆). The nurse should ensure as quiet an environment as possible when auscultating breath sounds and heart tones. The patient should be instructed to breathe normally through an open mouth. On the posterior and lateral chest, the auscultatory pattern should progress from the apices located above the scapula and then from left to right across the back and sides in a downward fashion to the lung bases. Auscultation across the anterior chest should follow a left-to-right pattern as well. The nurse should compare breath sounds bilaterally. The breath sounds on the left posterior chest are generally heard about 2.5 cm (1 in.) lower than those on the right side, owing to the location of the liver and increased height of the right diaphragm.

The nurse uses the diaphragm of the stethoscope to listen to breath sounds. Breath sounds are best auscultated with the patient in an upright position. The nurse should not listen to breath sounds over clothing or hospital gowns, since the movement of clothing causes rustling that will interfere with accurate auscultation of breath sounds. At least one full ventilatory cycle should be auscultated with each stethoscope position.

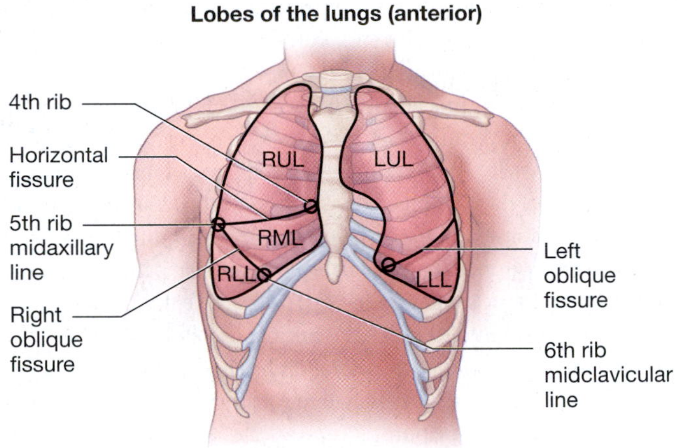

FIGURE 25–7 ◆ Lobes of the lung—anterior.

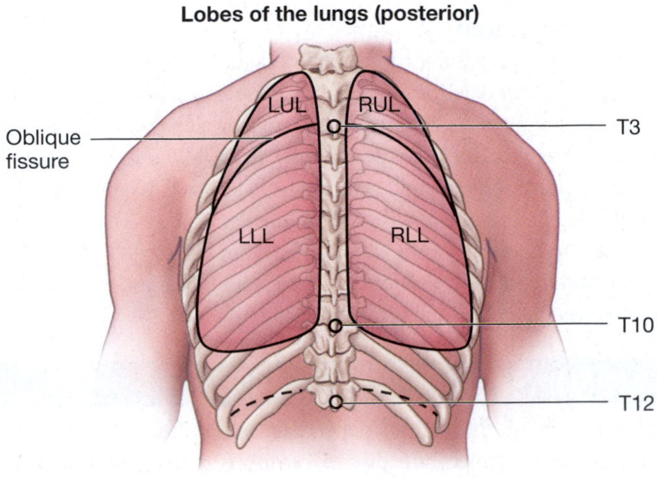

FIGURE 25–8 ◆ Lobes of the lung—posterior.

Normal Breath Sounds

When the nurse is auscultating the chest, the patient should be sitting upright so that the breath sounds can be auscultated bilaterally without interference and so that expansion is not restricted.

When the patient is obese, excess subcutaneous tissue can make it difficult to hear breath sounds because of the increased distance they must travel through the chest wall. Sometimes, having the patient stand so that gravity pulls subcutaneous tissue downward can aid in the auscultation of breath sounds in the obese person.

In the bed-bound patient, the dependent areas are restricted from fully expanding by the pressure of the mattress. If the patient must remain supine, it is best to listen to the dependent areas before the superior areas because fluid and exudates will migrate to dependent areas with gravity. When the patient is turned so that these areas are no longer dependent, evidence of consolidation or fluid may disappear.

Tracheal Breath Sounds

The loud, harsh, high-pitched breath sounds that are auscultated over the neck and trachea are called **tracheal breath sounds.** The sounds are caused by turbulent airflow through the trachea. Because this is the largest airway, these sounds are the loudest. As the airways become smaller, there is less turbulence and the sounds become softer and fainter. The duration of time that tracheal breath sounds are heard is equal during inspiration and expiration, with a short silence noted between the end of inspiration and start of expiration.

Bronchial Breath Sounds

Bronchial breath sounds are heard over the major airways (bronchi) in the chest, located at the manubrium. They can be auscultated over the anterior chest on either side of the sternum (over the right and left mainstem bronchus) from the second to fourth intercostal spaces. On the back, bronchial breath sounds are best heard lateral to the spine between the third and sixth intercostal spaces. They are loud and high pitched. They can be distinguished from tracheal sounds in that bronchial sounds are not as loud and expiration is longer than inspiration. As in tracheal sounds, a brief gap is heard between inspiration and expiration. They are abnormal if heard distal to the manubrium landmarks, in which case they suggest that fluid or solid tissue has replaced the normally air-filled space.

Bronchovesicular Breath Sounds

Bronchovesicular breath sounds represent air movement in the moderate airways between the main bronchi and smaller airways. They are best heard at the first and second intercostal spaces of the anterior chest and between the scapulae of the posterior chest. The duration of inspiration and that of expiration are equal, and no pause is heard between phases. They are of intermediate pitch and loudness between vesicular and bronchial breath sounds, and are abnormal if heard over the peripheral lung regions. It is an indication that the air in the lung is replaced by fluid, solid, or collapse, as in pneumonia or atelectasis.

Vesicular Breath Sounds

Vesicular breath sounds are the soft, low-pitched sounds heard over the majority of the lung fields. They are heard through inspiration and continue to expiration without a pause. The inspiratory phase is auscultated longer than the expiratory phase, even though expiration is twice the duration of inspiration, because the high-pitch sound over the final third of expiration is filtered out.

In summary, in a normal, healthy lung:

- Vesicular sounds are heard over most of the lung fields. Inspiration is longer than expiration, and there is no pause between inspiration and expiration.
- Bronchovesicular sounds are heard between the first and second intercostal spaces on the anterior chest. Inspiration and expiration are equal, and there is no pause between the phases.
- Bronchial sounds are heard over the body of the sternum. Expiration is longer than inspiration, and there is a gap between the phases.
- Tracheal sounds are heard over the trachea. Inspiration and expiration are equal, and there is a gap between phases.

Abnormal Breath Sounds

Abnormal breath sounds include decreased sound, absence of sound, or normal sounds in areas that they should not be heard, such as bronchial sounds over the peripheral airways. Diminished breath sounds may indicate atelectasis, shallow respirations, pneumothorax, or decreased respiratory effort. These findings should be correlated with the patient's clinical condition and diagnoses.

Adventitious breath sounds are extra, abnormal sounds that are not normally heard during auscultation of breath sounds (Chart 25–2). They represent pathologic conditions of the heart or lungs and indicate the presence of airway spasm, fluid, or secretions that disrupt airflow.

Safety Alert *Bronchial breath sounds over the large airways and diminished or absent breath sounds over smaller airways may indicate airway obstruction or pneumothorax.*

Crackles

Crackles, formerly termed *rales*, are sounds caused by either airways that collapse during expiration and "pop" open during inspiration or by air bubbles passing through fluid during respiration (Bickley, 2009). They are discontinuous, nonmusical, and of short duration. Crackles are described as wet or dry, coarse or fine, and inspiratory or expiratory. Fine crackles are soft, high-pitched, brief, and sound similar to rubbing a strand of hair between your fingers near your ear. They are usually associated with an interstitial disease process. Coarse rhonchi are louder and lower in pitch and have been described as sounding similar to opening a Velcro fastener. They are associated with chronic bronchiectasis (permanent dilation of the large airways caused by destruction of the muscle and elastic tissue) and asthma.

Wheezes and Rhonchi

Wheezes and **rhonchi** are continuous musical sounds caused by air flowing across airways that are narrowed or obstructed by constriction or swelling. They have been subdivided into sibilant and sonorous; however, many sources use the term *rhonchi* to describe sonorous sounds and *wheezes* to describe sibilant sounds. Sibilant rhonchi (wheezes) have a high-pitched musical or squeaky quality. They are most often caused by narrowing of the airways such as in asthma, allergic reactions, or reactive airways. They are usually heard during expiration but can also be heard during inspiration when the narrowing becomes more severe. Sonorous rhonchi have a lower pitched snoring or moaning quality caused by secretions in the larger airways, as in bronchitis and COPD. They are heard during inspiration and/or expiration, and may clear or partially clear with coughing.

Exercise-induced asthma, foreign-body obstruction, and tumors can also cause wheezing. The patient interview will help to discern possible causes.

Safety Alert *Absence of wheezing in a patient with asthma exacerbation indicates a lack of airflow and impending respiratory arrest. Notify the health care provider or arrange for emergency care (911) immediately.*

CHART 25–2 Characteristics of Adventitious Breath Sounds

Sound	Timing	Quality	Respiratory Cycle	Clearing	Cause
Crackles (Rales)	Discontinuous Brief	Nonmusical *Fine:* Soft, high pitched *Coarse:* louder, lower pitch	Predominantly inspiration	May clear with coughing	Popping open of collapsed airways or air bubbling through fluid in airway
Sibilant wheeze (Wheeze)	Continuous	Musical Relatively high pitched with hissing or shrill quality	Usually heard on expiration, but with increased severity also occurs during inspiration	Not usually cleared with coughing	Airway narrowing: Spasm, inflammation, secretions, or tumor
Sonorous wheeze (Rhonchi)	Continuous	Musical Relatively low pitched with snoring quality	Predominantly expiration	May clear with coughing	Loose secretions in larger airways
Stridor	Continuous	Harsh Crowing	Predominantly inspiration	Do not clear with coughing	Upper airway obstruction; croup
Pleural friction rub	Continuous	High-pitched grating/squeaking	Inspiration and expiration	Do not clear with coughing	Rubbing together of parietal and visceral pleural layers that cover the lung due to pleural inflammation

Stridor

Stridor is a high-pitched sound produced by turbulent airflow through partially obstructed upper airways (larynx to subglottic structures). The sounds that are produced are variable and can be described as harsh, crowing, musical, or breathy. Stridor can usually be detected without the aid of a stethoscope. Although it is audible during either phase of respiration, it is most commonly heard during inspiration. Because of their more anatomically narrowed airways, stridor is most commonly heard in infants and children with viral or bacterial infections, such as croup. Acute stridor occurs with foreign body obstruction or food aspiration. It is a potential medical emergency, and the underlying cause must be determined quickly. If stridor occurs, the nurse should notify the health care provider immediately. In turn, the health care provider should alert the nurse to the presence of airway obstruction and the need for interventions to relieve the mechanical obstruction. Bronchoscopy may be necessary to remove the obstruction.

Safety Alert *Moderate to severe respiratory stridor is a sign of airway obstruction and should be considered a medical emergency.*

Pleural Friction Rub

Pleural friction rubs are low-pitched creaking or squeaking sounds that occur when inflamed pleural surfaces rub together during respiration. They are most easily heard on inspiration. The pitch of the sound usually increases with chest expansion. To differentiate pleural friction rubs from pericardial friction rubs, the nurse should have the patient hold her breath. The pericardial friction rub will continue with each heartbeat, whereas the pleural friction rub will not occur when the patient is not actively breathing.

Percussion

Percussion helps to assess whether the underlying tissues are air filled, fluid filled, or solid. Sounds produced by percussion are described as flat, dull, resonant, hyperresonant, or tympanic. The lungs are approximately 99% air filled; therefore, percussion over the lungs produces resonance. Decreased sounds indicate a lack of air. Resonance should be heard throughout most lung fields during inspiration while they are air filled. **Resonance** is a low-pitched, clear sound that is heard over normal lung tissue.

Abnormal percussion sounds include hyperresonance and dullness. *Hyperresonance* is very loud, with a lower pitch and a longer sound than resonance. It indicates hyperinflation of the airways or an excess of air in the absence of lung tissue. Hyperinflation is seen and heard in COPD and asthma. Pneumothorax causes the collapse of lung tissue and excess air in the pleural space, thereby producing unilateral hyperresonance.

Dullness is a percussive tone that is heard over solid tissue. Dullness occurs over the lungs when air is absent. It is heard over the lower thorax during expiration, when consolidation is present (as in pneumonia), pleural effusion, hemothorax, or the presence of solid tumors. The sound that is elicited is a dull thumping sound without vibration.

Gerontological Considerations

Respiratory function decreases with advancing age for a variety of reasons. The capacity for exercise decreases. The chest wall becomes stiffer and harder to move, respiratory muscles weaken, and the lungs lose some elastic recoil (Bickley, 2009). Forced expiration diminishes, making coughing less effective. Skeletal changes from osteoporosis may cause stooped posture and decreased rib expansion. The rib cage becomes more rigid and the anterior-posterior diameter increases.

Older patients are at higher risk for pneumonia because of ineffective coughing related to these physiological changes and because older adults are more likely to have disease states that increase the risk for aspiration. Decreased subcutaneous fat may make the older patient more susceptible to cool room temperatures during respiratory physical assessment, so the nurse must take care to provide heat or warmed blankets or sheets to promote comfort during the examination.

Laboratory and Imaging

The decision to order laboratory and imaging studies is guided by the findings on the patient's history and clinical assessment. Some of the more common studies used in the differential diagnosis of lung disease or injury include chest radiography, sputum cultures, complete blood count (CBC), skin tests, pulmonary function tests (PFT), and arterial blood gases (ABGs). PFTs and ABGs are discussed in the monitoring section of this chapter.

A CBC includes a white blood count (WBC) with differential, red blood count (RBC), hemoglobin, hematocrit, and platelet count. A low RBC, hemoglobin, or hematocrit indicates anemia and therefore decreased oxygen-carrying capacity. A high RBC may indicate polycythemia and can indicate hypoxemia in advanced disease. An elevated WBC may indicate an infective or inflammatory process (pneumonia), cancer, stress, leukemia, or drug ingestion. The WBC differential targets specific types of white blood cells and can further identify the cause of elevation.

Sputum specimens are useful for diagnosing microorganisms causing respiratory infection and for detecting malignant cells in lung tissue (Kee, 2010). Studies performed on sputum associated with respiratory problems include culture and sensitivity (C&S), acid-fast bacilli (AFB), and cytology. Sputum cultures identify the presence of microorganisms causing a respiratory infection and the sensitivity to antimicrobials used to treat any identified pathogen. AFB is used to test sputum when tuberculosis is suspected. Cytology studies identify the presence of malignant cancer cells. Skin tests can be performed to diagnose or rule out tuberculosis and histoplasmosis.

Chest x-rays provide evidence of interstitial lung disease, trauma, pleural fluid or air, chest wall or spinal deformities, tuberculosis, and pulmonary lesions. High-resolution CT scanning is a more sensitive tool, but the expense and radiation dosage make it inappropriate in many situations. However, it is an important adjunct and should be used for patients who require further investigation after the initial chest x-ray and laboratory findings have been reviewed. CT angiography (CTA) is the current standard of care for detection of pulmonary embolus. In patients with a negative CTA, the likelihood of a subsequent thromboembolic event is extremely small (Ferri, 2010).

Bronchoscopy, mediastinoscopy, and thoracoscopy are diagnostic procedures that involve the exploration of airway structures for abnormalities, obtaining biopsy, or gathering a fluid sample.

Respiratory Monitoring

Respiratory monitoring involves observation, physical assessment, and the use of electronic monitoring devices. The nurse must be knowledgeable of the oxygen delivery method and the expected outcomes for the patient. For example, if a patient is receiving supplemental oxygen, the nurse should expect the patient to be able to maintain appropriate arterial oxygen levels. These are assessed by using ABGs, physical assessment, and pulse oximetry.

The standard of care for patients with cardiac and respiratory illnesses now includes continuous or intermittent observation of the patient's oxygen saturation. The peak flow is utilized to trend treatment effectiveness in patients with asthma.

Pulse Oximetry

Pulse oximeters provide a digital readout of the percentage of hemoglobin saturated with oxygen (Figure 25–9◆). Pulse oximeters use infrared light technology or reflectance photometry to reflect light off the hemoglobin molecules. The microprocessor in the pulse oximeter then measures and calculates the absorption of light by hemoglobin during pulsatile arterial waves.

Pulse oximetry has several limitations. The measurement is less accurate at lower values, and 70% has generally been considered the lowest accurate number; however, more recent studies suggest that the accuracy declines at 90% (Wilson, Cowan, Lord, Zuege, & Zygun, 2010). Decreased perfusion or blood flow will also affect oximeter readings. Since adequate arterial pulsation is required, any state that impairs perfusion to the site of probe placement will affect the measurement's accuracy. This includes hypotension, hypothermia, cardiac dysrhythmias, peripheral vascular disease, and heart failure. Sensors can be placed on the forehead or ear when distal circulation is decreased. Pulse oximetry probes should not be placed on extremities with automated blood pressure cuffs, hemodialysis fistulas, or arterial lines, because these interfere with blood flow.

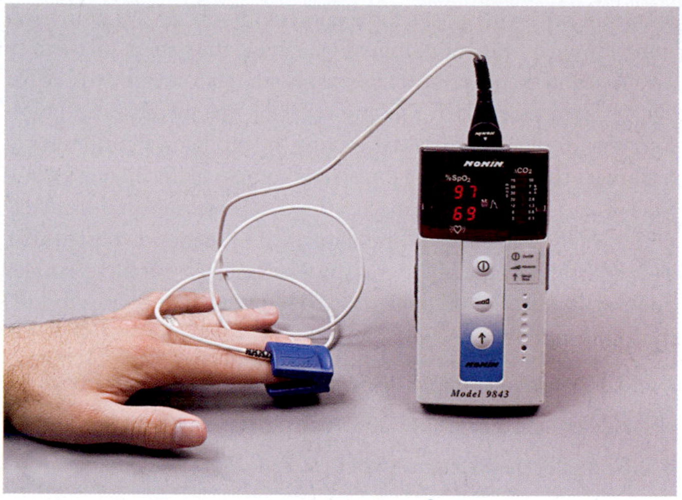

FIGURE 25–9 ◆ Pulse oximetry monitor.

Motion artifact, such as occurs with tremors, shivering, or seizures, can interfere with the oximeter's ability to detect the amount of light absorbed. The accuracy of the readout is suspect if the waveform does not match the patient's pulse rate. Manufacturers have recently developed new oximeters that claim "motion tolerance" and reportedly produce fewer artifact errors.

Some studies report that some nail polish colors, artificial nails, anemia, skin pigmentation, and ambient light may affect accuracy. Other studies have contradicted these results. Until definitive studies are completed, it would be prudent to remove artificial nails and fingernail polish from the sensor finger.

Pulse oximetry does not distinguish methemoglobin or carboxyhemoglobin from oxygen-saturated hemoglobin. The hemoglobin molecule has a much higher affinity to bind with carbon monoxide than to oxygen. This binding is referred to as carboxyhemoglobin. Even though pulse oximeters may read 100% saturations in patients with carbon monoxide toxicity, patients may in reality be profoundly hypoxic. Methemoglobin absorbs light at the same wavelength as oxyhemoglobin and therefore results in falsely high oximeter readings. Patients who have methemoglobinemia, as in suspected thiocyanate toxicity (prolonged use of sodium nitroprusside), or who have been exposed to carbon monoxide should have arterial blood gas monitoring to determine PaO_2.

Pulmonary Function Testing

Pulmonary function tests (PFTs) refer to a battery of standardized tools used to measure lung function. They include spirometry, lung volume measurement, diffusing capacity, and arterial blood gases.

A spirometer is the most simple and commonly used tool to measure pulmonary function. It involves having the patient take a deep breath in and then forcibly exhaling into the spirometer. Most of the devices used today have a microprocessor that measures and plots a graphic display of the data depicting the mechanical properties of the lungs. This includes the forced expiratory volume in one second (FEV_1) and forced vital capacity (FVC). These are used to determine whether the cause of pulmonary dysfunction is obstructive, such as asthma and emphysema, or whether it is restrictive, such as pulmonary fibrosis and neuromuscular disease. Other uses include the following:

- To diagnose and monitor respiratory symptoms and disease
- To determine the severity and progression of lung disease
- To monitor the effectiveness of treatment
- To identify preoperative risk
- As a tool for epidemiologic and other research studies.

A peak flow meter is a handheld over-the-counter device that measures peak expiratory flow rate, which is the amount of air a patient can exhale. It is used by patients with asthma to help keep their symptoms under control (Figure 25–10◆). The peak flow meter can reveal narrowing of the airways in advance of an asthma attack, alert patients when to seek medical care and when to stop or add medications (with health care provider direction), identify the effectiveness of treatment, and identify triggers of asthma attacks. Many peak flow meters utilize a red, yellow, and green zone to determine the severity of decrease in peak flow. Green is the "good zone," meaning that the patient meets at least 80% of normal. The yellow zone is a caution zone. Values in this area are below normal. The red zone means that the patient is in danger of respiratory complications and has a peak flow of less than 50% of the normal value. As a general rule, values of less than 400 L/min indicate poor airflow.

Arterial Blood Gas

ABG measurements are utilized to provide information on acid–base balance, arterial oxygenation, and carbon dioxide levels. The oxygen saturation, bicarbonate, and base excess are also calculated. The pH identifies acidemia or alkalemia of the blood. A pH of less than 7.35 is considered acidotic and greater than 7.45 alkalotic.

The carbon dioxide level is utilized as the major determinant for diagnosing adequacy of ventilation. Carbon dioxide combines with water to produce carbonic acid and lowers the pH of the blood. Any condition that produces hypoventilation and therefore accumulation of CO_2 will cause an acidotic state. Primary respiratory acidosis is defined as a pH < 7.35 with a $PaCO_2 > 45$ mmHg. High levels cause drowsiness and unconsciousness. Increased ventilation and treatment of cause will resolve acidosis. Intubation and mechanical ventilation may be required to achieve this goal. Causes of respiratory acidosis include the following:

- ***Airway Disorders:*** Bronchospasm (asthma), upper airway obstruction
- ***Lung Defects:*** Pulmonary edema, restrictive lung disease, exacerbation of COPD, acute respiratory distress syndrome
- ***Chest Wall Defects:*** Chest trauma (flail, hemothorax, contusion), pneumothorax, pain with respiration
- ***Central Respiratory Depression/CNS Dysfunction:*** Drug overdose, head trauma, high spinal cord injury, cerebral hypoxia
- ***Nerve and Muscle Disorders:*** Myopathies, Guillain-Barré syndrome, myasthenia gravis, toxins (organophosphates)
- ***Other:*** Inadequate mechanical ventilation, malignant hyperthermia (over-production of CO_2), rebreathing of CO_2

Primary respiratory alkalosis is caused by hyperventilation and blowing off of excess CO_2. It is defined as a pH > 7.45 and $CO_2 < 35$ mmHg. Symptoms are primarily nervous and cardiac system related. The patient may experience confusion, numbness, lightheadedness, and, at high pH levels, seizures. Cardiac symptoms include dysrhythmias and palpitations. Treatment involves correcting the underlying cause and monitoring for exhaustion and subsequent respiratory failure. Causes of respiratory alkalosis include anxiety, pain, increased metabolic demands (fever, sepsis), central nervous system lesions, and stimulants.

The PaO_2 is assessed for adequacy of oxygenation. A low oxygen level in the arterial blood is defined as hypoxemia. There are five primary causes of hypoxemia:

- ***Alveolar Hypoventilation:*** Decreased respiratory rate/depth or an increase in deadspace ventilation (ventilation to alveoli without blood flow in the adjacent pulmonary capillaries).
- ***Ventilation/Perfusion Mismatch:*** One of the most common causes of hypoxemia. In normal lungs, ventilation and perfusion are nearly equal. In diseased lungs, alveoli are perfused normally but insufficiently ventilated. As a result, blood passes through the pulmonary capillaries without achieving normal PaO_2 levels. This occurs in asthma and COPD.
- ***Low Inspired Oxygen:*** High altitude, low FiO_2.
- ***Right-to-Left Shunt:*** Conditions in which blood is transferred from the right side of the heart to the left without passing through the pulmonary arteries where oxygenation occurs. This may be seen in congenital abnormalities such as foramen ovale.
- ***Diffusion Defect:*** A clinically rare phenomenon in which there is a defect in the diffusion across the blood–gas membrane.

Chapter 15 includes a full discussion of all components of acid–base balance.

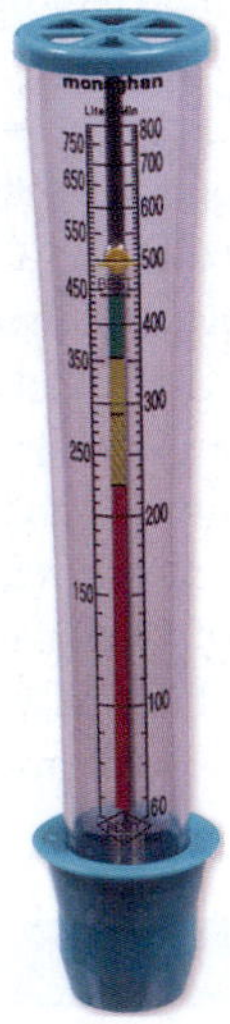

FIGURE 25–10 ◆ Peak flow meter.
Source: Courtesy of Monaghan Medical Corporation/True Zone.

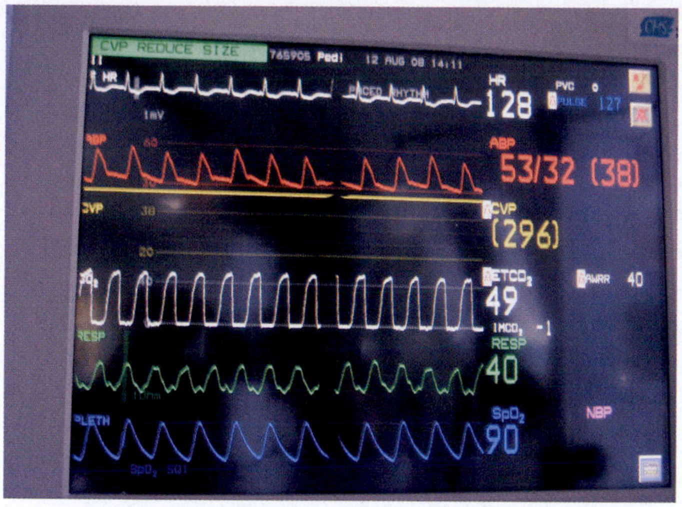

FIGURE 25–11 ◆ End-tidal CO_2 monitoring.
Source: Cheryl Wraa.

Capnography

Capnography is the measurement and graphic display of exhaled carbon dioxide, typically referred to as end-tidal CO_2 (Figure 25–11 ◆). A capnometer gives a digital readout of expired carbon dioxide without the graphic display. Small disposable capnometers, termed *calorimetric devices*, are used to test endotracheal tube placement by utilizing treated paper that changes color in the presence of an acid such as carbon dioxide.

Infrared spectrography is utilized in the majority of bedside or hand-held carbon dioxide monitors today. Carbon dioxide has a very specific infrared wavelength that is measured and analyzed as it is exhaled. Infrared spectrography is a useful tool in determining and monitoring endotracheal tube placement. It has been used to manage ventilation, assess adequacy of bronchodilator therapy, determine cardiac perfusion in cardiac arrest or shock states, and monitor for hypoventilation with procedural sedation. End-tidal monitoring has limitations. If the patient has carbonated beverages or re-breathed air from bag-mask ventilation in the stomach, the monitor may show CO_2 even if the endotracheal tube is not in the trachea, giving a false positive (Zwerneman, 2010). This CO_2 can be cleared from the stomach with several bag-valve-mask ventilations with 100% oxygen.

There are also limitations in using capnography to monitor ventilation. First, it should be recognized that the end-tidal CO_2 typically runs 2 to 5 mmHg less than the arterial CO_2. This is because of the variable rate of ventilation at the alveolar level. There are several conditions in which the end-tidal CO_2 is an unreliable indicator of arterial CO_2. In cases of hypoperfusion to the lungs (shock, cardiac arrest), end-tidal CO_2 is not reflective of arterial CO_2 levels. It is actually a better indicator of cardiac output than is arterial CO_2. As cardiac output falls, so does the end-tidal CO_2. The American Heart Association encourages clinicians to use capnography to identify CPR provider fatigue when the end-tidal CO_2 starts to fall. Hypoperfusion to the lungs can also be caused by deadspace ventilation in which alveoli are adequately ventilated but perfusion is decreased. The classic example of this is pulmonary emboli.

Finally, incomplete exhalation will render discrepancies between exhaled carbon dioxide and arterial CO_2. Even though ventilation and perfusion are normal, the respired air is not being completely exhaled and so is underestimated in the end-tidal CO_2 measurement. Examples of this state include asthma and COPD.

Health Promotion

Avoidance of cigarette smoking is a primary avenue to prevent the development of pulmonary disease. Adolescents and adults who do not smoke should not start; if they do smoke, they should stop. Nurses in all realms of practice should offer smoking cessation information and support for patients to stop smoking (Chapter 6).

Hand hygiene is recognized in health care settings as an important means to prevent the spread of infection. Frequent hand washing or the use of alcohol-based degermers in school settings and public places may prevent the spread of bacteria and decrease the spread of cold, flu, and pneumonia.

Flu vaccines and pneumococcal vaccines should be available to patients in high-risk populations. Adults who work in areas where they will be exposed to flu, such as health care workers, as well as older adults and patients with chronic conditions such as asthma and COPD should receive a yearly flu vaccination. Older adults and patients with chronic diseases should also receive pneumococcal vaccine to prevent pneumococcal pneumonia. Frequently, these frail patients are physically unable to go to local centers or wait in lines to obtain the vaccination. Communities need to develop and execute plans to get the vaccines to the patients instead of forcing these patients to come to the vaccine.

Governmental agencies have been active in promoting healthy and safe workplaces. Companies whose employees commonly encounter environmental irritants and allergens should provide education in the use of personal protective equipment on an ongoing basis. Although this equipment may be uncomfortable at first, the employer should consistently insist on its use. Construction workers have gotten used to hard hats; it is time for them to get used to respirator masks. Reduction of the effects of environmental allergens and irritants will prevent the development of chronic disease in this population.

Summary

The assessment of the respiratory system must include pertinent data regarding the patient's history and current complaints. Acute changes in respiratory status must be acted on quickly to prevent patient compromise. Patients with chronic pulmonary disease will have abnormal physical findings, but the patient's usual and customary status must be ascertained so that the patient's progression of symptoms and current status can be determined. This knowledge is also valuable in planning care for the patients. Data obtained from the respiratory assessment will determine whether the current plan of care is adequate for a patient's needs. Is the patient getting better or worse? Utilizing the objective data from the respiratory assessment, the nurse can advocate for the patient with the health care provider to ensure an appropriate plan of care. Early recognition of symptoms by the nurse is important to provide education in risk reduction and to assist in determining possible environmental irritants and allergens that can then be eliminated and thus prevent chronic disease.

NCLEX® PRACTICE

1. While auscultating a patient's lungs, the nurse hears intermittent popping sounds. How should the nurse document this finding?

1. Stridor
2. Crackles
3. Wheezes
4. Rhonchi

2. A patient tells the nurse that he just returned from visiting Asia and has had an upper respiratory infection for 2 weeks. Why is this information beneficial to aid in the care of this patient?

1. It will help determine the patient's socioeconomic status.
2. It will help determine the patient's occupation.
3. It might help to know whether there have been any recent outbreaks of pulmonary disorders in the area of travel.
4. It might help determine the patient's immunological status.

3. A patient comes into the clinic with symptoms of a respiratory disorder. Which questions should the nurse ask regarding this patient's social history while conducting the assessment? (select all that apply)

1. Do you have any heart problems?
2. Have you been to any activities or functions around other people with respiratory problems?
3. Is anyone in your family prone to respiratory infection?
4. Do you remember which immunizations you received as a child?
5. Do you use tobacco?

4. During the assessment of a patient with a respiratory disorder, the nurse observes 4+ edema over the lower leg. What is the priority reason this finding is important in this assessment?

1. It will indicate the patient's ability to ambulate.
2. Edema indicates the amount of fluid the patient can tolerate.
3. Edema may indicate heart failure, a common finding in a patient with COPD.
4. It aids in determining if the patient will need assistance with activities of daily living.

5. A patient is brought to the emergency department after being rescued from a structure fire. The patient's pulse oximetry reading is 90%. What nursing intervention is necessary?

1. Cover the probe to see if the reading is different.
2. Move the probe to another extremity.
3. Request arterial blood gas analysis.
4. Ask the patient not to move while the nurse takes another reading.

6. An emergency department nurse reports that the patient is using the sternocleidomastoid accessory muscles for breathing. Where would the admitting nurse observe to confirm this assessment?

1. Over the middle of the anterior chest wall
2. In the anterior neck
3. At the costal margins
4. In the abdomen, just below the diaphragm

Answers to NCLEX Practice questions can be found in Appendix D in the Osborn Student Resources at nursing.pearsonhighered.com. Practice additional NCLEX questions online at the Student Resources site.

Pearson Nursing Student Resources Find additional review materials at: **nursing.pearsonhighered.com**

REFERENCES

Bickley, L. (2009). *Bates' guide to physical examination and history taking* (10th ed.). Philadelphia: Lippincott Williams & Wilkins.

CDC. (2008). Smoking-attributable mortality, years of potential life lost, and productivity losses: United States, 2000–2004. *Morbidity and Mortality Weekly Review, 57*(45), 1226–1228.

CDC. (2010). The 2009 H1N1 Pandemic: Summary highlights, April 2009–April 2010. Retrieved from http://www.cdc.gov/h1n1flu/cdcresponse.htm

Cystic Fibrosis Foundation. (2008). Patient registry annual data report. Retrieved from http://www.cff.org/LivingWithCF/CareCenterNetwork/PatientRegistry/

Emergency Nurses Association. (2009). *Sheehy's emergency nursing* (6th ed.). St. Louis: Mosby.

Ferri, F. F. (2010). *Ferri's clinical advisor 2011* (1st ed.). St. Louis: Mosby.

Harris, N. S., & Nelson, S. (2008). Altitude illness: Pulmonary syndromes. Retrieved from http://emedicine.medscape.com/article/773065-overview

Karpel, J. (2009). Overview of pulmonary disease in injection drug users. In T. E. King (Ed.), UpToDate.

Kee, J. L. (2010). *Handbook of laboratory & diagnostic tests* (8th ed.). Upper Saddle River, NJ: Pearson Prentice Hall.

Murugan, A., & Sharma, G. (2008). Obesity and respiratory diseases. *Chronic Respiratory Disease, 5*(4) 233–242.

Powers, M. A. (2009). The obesity hypoventilation syndrome. *Respiratory Care, 53*(12), 1723–1730.

Porth, C., & Matfin, G. (2009). *Essentials of pathophysiology: Concepts of altered health states* (2nd ed.). Philadelphia: Lippincott Williams & Wilkins.

Spector, R. (2009). *Cultural diversity in health and illness* (7th ed.). Upper Saddle River, NJ: Pearson Prentice Hall.

U.S. Department of Health and Human Services. (2010a). *Healthy People 2020 objectives.* Retrieved from http://www.healthypeople.gov/2020/topicsobjectives2020/default.aspx

U.S. Department of Health and Human Services. (2010b). *How tobacco smoke causes disease: A report of the Surgeon General.* Washington, DC: Office of the Surgeon General.

Weinhouse, G. (2008). Fat emboli syndrome. In Polly Parsons (Ed.), UpToDate.

Wilson, B. J., Cowan, H. J., Lord, J. A., Zuege, D. J., & Zygun, D. A. (2010). The accuracy of pulse oximetry in emergency department patients with severe sepsis and septic shock: A retrospective cohort study. *BMC Emergency Medicine, 10*(9). doi:10.1186/1471-227X-10-9.

Zwerneman, K. (2010). End-tidal carbon dioxide monitoring: A vital sign worth watching. *Critical Care Nurse Clinics of North America, 18*(2), 217–225.

Caring for the Patient with Upper Airway Disorders

26 CHAPTER

Carol Rhoades
Cheryl Wraa

Outcome-Based Learning Objectives

After studying this chapter, the learner will be able to:

1. Compare and contrast nursing management of the most common facial fractures.
2. Generate a nursing plan of care for a patient with sinus disease.
3. Differentiate the essential components for developing a teaching plan for patients with infections of the upper airway.
4. Discuss the implications of the loss of the senses of smell, sight, and taste in patients with upper airway disorders and disfigurement.
5. Compare and contrast nursing management of patients with partial versus total airway obstruction.
6. Generate a plan of care for a patient with head and neck cancer including airway, wounds, pain, and nutrition.

KEY TERMS

anosmia p.697
aphonic p.706
chyle leak p.724
decannulation p.712
epiglottitis p.704
epistaxis p.685
hairy tongue p.702
hoarseness p.706
laryngeal spasm p.708
laryngectomy p.718
laryngitis p.707
laryngopharyngeal reflux disease p.710
Ludwig's angina p.704
mucormycosis p.698
myocutaneous flap p.719
nasal polyps p.697
otolaryngology (otorhinolaryngology) p.683
peritonsillar abscess p.704
pharyngitis p.704
rhinitis p.692
rhinosinusitis (sinusitis) p.696
sleep apnea p.699
stridor p.704
tonsillitis p.704
tracheostomy p.689
tracheotomy p.689

OTOLARYNGOLOGY, also called otorhinolaryngology, is the study of disorders of the head and neck, including the ears, nose, and throat. Disease and trauma that affect these structures affect a person's outlook on the world because they can change the way in which a person smells, tastes, breathes, sees, hears, and touches, as well as the person's body image. Any interference with facial appearance, basic human needs, or ability to communicate can be a devastating experience for the patient and family.

Disorders of the head and neck area not only can be physically disfiguring, but also can interfere with vital functions necessary to meet the patient's basic human needs, such as intake of air, fluids, and food. It is important for nurses to understand the physiological care needs of these patients and be sensitive to the impact on the patient's quality of life. Assisting and teaching patients how to cope with otolaryngologic illnesses and the subsequent life changes is an essential part of the healing process. Nurses must be aware of the immense impact of otolaryngology disordersand respond to their patients' needs accordingly.

Structural, Traumatic, and Deformity Disorders of the Nose and Facial Structures

The facial skeleton serves to protect the brain; house and protect the sense organs of smell, sight, and taste; and provide a frame for the soft tissues of the face. It also helps to facilitate eating, facial expression, breathing, and speech. The primary bones of the face are the nasal bones, mandible, maxilla, zygoma, temporal bone, and frontal bone. Numerous types of deformities affect the facial structures of the head and neck, many of which deal with fractures. Maxillofacial fractures are most often caused by motor vehicle crashes, domestic abuse, other types of assault, recreational vehicle crashes, industrial accidents, and sports activities.

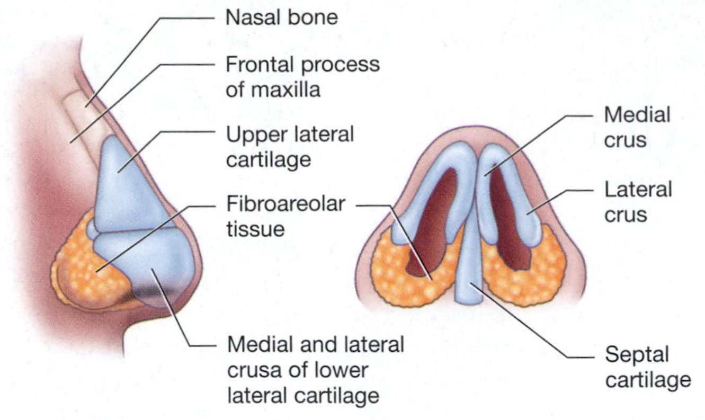

FIGURE 26–1 ◆ Anatomic relationship between nasal bones, cartilage, and septum.

Nasal Fractures

The skeletal structure of the nose is composed of paired nasal bones that form a framework to support the cartilaginous structures of the nose. The nasal bones rigidly support the upper portion of the nose between the eyes. The cartilages are flexible supports that maintain the shape of the lower portion of the nose. The septum divides the nostrils and is made of both cartilage and bone. Figure 26–1◆ shows the nose's anatomic structures. Within the framework of the nose are soft tissues, mucous glands, and nerves responsible for the nose's sensation and function. A nasal fracture may include bone, cartilage, nerves, skin, and/or mucosa (the nasal lining).

Epidemiology and Etiology

Nasal fractures are the third most common type of fracture in the body (behind clavicular and wrist fractures) and account for almost half of all facial fractures (Ross & Becker, 2009). Nasal fractures typically are caused by a traumatic injury to the bone or cartilage. With the increasing use of airbags in cars, the incidence of septal injuries without nasal bone fracture has increased. Fights, accidents, and sports account for approximately 85% of all nasal fractures in adults. Falls are the primary cause in the pediatric population (Ross & Becker, 2009). When nasal fractures are seen in children and women, physical abuse should be considered and appropriately ruled out.

Laboratory and Diagnostic Procedures

Nasal fractures may be diagnosed by facial x-rays (see the Diagnostic Tests box on page 690). The ethmoid bone lies posterior to the nasal bones at the base of the skull and can be damaged from direct trauma to the nose. If it is suspected that the ethmoid bone also is damaged because of its proximity to the nasal bones, neurological tests are indicated to assess cognition and response. A patient with this type of injury will have a profound headache and, owing to the close proximity to the brain, may have a cerebrospinal fluid (CSF) leak. Any clear fluid draining from the nose is highly suspect for CSF. A CSF leak is confirmed by allowing the fluid to drain onto a clean white dressing. If a halo of red-tinged fluid is demonstrated (halo test), then a CSF leak is present.

Clinical Manifestations

Patients with a nasal fracture usually present with some combination of deformity, tenderness, hemorrhage, edema, ecchymosis, instability, and airway passage obstruction. Nasal fractures can be displaced (i.e., the structures are moved) or nondisplaced (i.e., the structures are in alignment). Edema can mask underlying nasal bone displacement, which, if untreated, can result in both unfavorable appearance and function.

Air traveling through the nose normally is controlled by the position of the bones and cartilages; if these are displaced, obstruction of the nose can occur. Mucosal swelling and clotted blood also will limit airflow. An injured nose can bleed from lacerations of the skin or the mucosa inside the nose. These lacerations may need to be evaluated and repaired. A septal hematoma can injure or thicken the septal structures, impairing airflow through the nose. Bruises often migrate around the eyes and eventually down the cheeks. Repositioning or moving fractured bones and cartilage typically results in additional swelling.

Medical and Surgical Management

With an uncomplicated (nondisplaced) acute nasal fracture, no surgical treatment is indicated. To decrease pain and swelling, rest, cold compresses, pain medication, and elevation of the head are prescribed. Follow-up evaluation and management can safely be scheduled after the swelling resolves, usually within 3 to 5 days. If there is displacement of the nasal bones, reduction (realignment) should be accomplished between the 5th and 10th day after the injury, before the nasal bones start to fixate. In addition, septal hematomas should be drained if possible to prevent nasal obstruction.

Most acute nasal fractures can be reduced in a health care provider's office or hospital emergency department. A combination of medications inside the nose and injections around the nose lessens the discomfort of the reduction. However, for some fractures, surgical intervention under either local or general anesthesia is necessary to obtain proper alignment of the nasal bones. In some instances, the final aesthetic outcomes of closed-reduction techniques are less than optimal, and patients should be counseled that nasal reconstruction might eventually be necessary.

Nursing Management

Assessment is a key function of the nurse in caring for patients with a fractured nose. The nurse should evaluate the patient for type and severity of injury, bleeding, swelling, patency of airway, skin discoloration, and pain. The immediate goals are to control bleeding, reduce swelling with application of ice, and provide pain control. The nurse will need to assess for further injury by testing the patient for facial numbness or tingling. The presence of tingling needs to be reported to the health care provider as this may indicate pressure being exerted on a facial nerve. An isolated nasal fracture does not require hospitalization. Refer to Nursing Management of Facial Fractures on page 690 for more details.

Septal Deviation

The nasal septum is the wall that divides the nasal cavity into two halves; it is composed of a central supporting skeleton covered on each side by mucous membrane. The posterior portion is the ethmoid bone, and the front portion is a firm but bendable structure made of cartilage. The ideal nasal septum is exactly midline, separating the left and right sides of the nose into airway passageways of equal size. A septal deviation occurs when the septum is shifted away from the midline.

Etiology and Epidemiology

Deviations of the nasal septum may be congenital, caused by trauma, or due to surgical complications that further exaggerate the deviation.

Septal deviations are common; they typically cause no symptoms and require no treatment. The American Academy of Otolaryngology–Head and Neck Surgery (2007) reports that 80% of people have some degree of septal deviation.

The majority of symptomatic septal deviations (i.e., nasal obstruction) are caused by trauma to the nose. In some cases, the septal deviation may be severe enough to obstruct the passage of air through the nostrils. This obstruction predisposes the patient to sinusitis, infection, and epistaxis.

Clinical Manifestations

Although septal deviations are usually asymptomatic, they may cause one or more of the following: blockage of one or both nasal airways; nasal congestion; frequent nosebleeds; frequent sinus infections; at times, facial pain; headaches; postnasal drip; and noisy breathing during sleep.

In some cases, a person with a mildly deviated septum has symptoms only when she has an upper respiratory tract infection. In these individuals, the respiratory infection triggers nasal inflammation that temporarily amplifies any airflow problems related to the deviated septum. Once the infection resolves and the nasal inflammation subsides, symptoms of a deviated septum often also resolve.

Medical and Surgical Management

Treatment of a deviated septum can be either medical or surgical. A patient's complaint of an inability to breathe is the usual determinant of treatment. Decongestants, such as pseudoephedrine or phenylpropanolamine, will shrink the membranes and thereby enlarge the passages. Antihistamines, nasal cortisone spray, and other allergy treatments also may be temporarily beneficial. Normal saline drops and sprays are very helpful in loosening mucus in the obstructed side of the nasal cavity and preventing drying on the side receiving the majority of airflow. These therapies are useful in relieving symptoms but do not correct the problem.

If the patient complains of obstruction, a septoplasty, or surgical repositioning of the septum, may be performed with topical and/or local anesthetic and conscious sedation. Some surgeons insert nasal splints as a temporary structural support. A nasospecific procedure can be an alternative to surgery; in this procedure, a deflated balloon is inserted in the nare and inflated to a large enough degree to adjust the septal deviation. However, a practitioner trained in this procedure is necessary to successfully perform it.

Nursing Management

Nursing management focuses on maintaining a clear air passage, detecting signs of infection, and patient comfort. (See Diagnostic Tests for Facial Fractures on page 690.) The nurse is instrumental in teaching the patient how to instill nose drops and sprays and how to perform a saline lavage. In the event of a surgical repair, the nurse provides routine postoperative care and is alert for bleeding, swelling, and pain. Chapter 19 discusses postoperative patient management.

Epistaxis

Epistaxis, defined as any bleeding from the nostril, nasal cavity, or nasopharynx, is common because the linings of the nose are highly vascular. This condition can be caused by local or systemic problems. Air moving through the nose can dry and irritate the membranes lining the inside of the nose, forming crusts. These crusts bleed when irritated by rubbing, picking, or blowing the nose.

Etiology

Nosebleeds are very common. They tend to occur more frequently in the winter when viruses are common and heated indoor air dries out the nostrils. Common etiologies for epistaxis include injuries such as trauma; systemic problems, such as coagulation disorders or hypertension; environmental problems, such as dry air; irritation from nose picking; use of drugs and medications that irritate or dry the mucosa; or postoperative situations following any nasal or sinus surgery. A foreign object in the nose or direct impact to the nose also can cause a nosebleed. In addition, a deviated septum may make a person prone to nosebleeds.

Older adults are susceptible to nosebleeds for several reasons. As a person ages, the skin becomes more friable and retains less turgor. The same is true of the lining in the nose. Any mechanical irritation, such as nose picking or excessive rubbing, may cause a bleed. Individuals who use any type of inhaled drug also are at risk of damaging the nasal tissues and are highly prone to nosebleeds.

Pathophysiology

There are two areas within the nasal passage where a plexus of anastomotic vessels can be found. The anterior area is referred to as Kiesselbach's plexus (or Little's area), and the posterior area is known as Woodruff's plexus (Manes, 2010). These areas often are implicated in nosebleeds. Anterior bleeds from Kiesselbach's plexus are the most common, accounting for approximately 90% of nosebleeds (Manes, 2010). The bleeding erupts when the relatively thin nasal mucosa overlying a dilated septal vessel dries, scabs, and falls (or is picked) off. Posterior bleeds originating from Woodruff's plexus, which is located over the posterior middle turbinate, are less common. In these cases, the site of bleeding is higher and deeper within the nose and the blood flows primarily down the back of the throat. Identifying the anterior versus posterior origin of the bleed is an important factor in determining the appropriate therapy.

Only rarely is a nosebleed life threatening or actually fatal. In most cases of life-threatening nosebleeds, a systemic cause rather than a local one is implicated. Bleeding disorders such as hemophilia, VonWillebrand's disease, and thrombocytopenia can all lead to difficult-to-control epistaxis (Manes, 2010). Use of anticoagulant medication, aspirin, and non-steroidal anti-inflammatory drugs (NSAIDs) can affect the ability of the patient's blood to clot, leading to prolonged epistaxis. Garlic, ginseng, and ginkgo all inhibit platelet function and can contribute to epistaxis (Gifford & Orlandi, 2008). Hereditary hemorrhagic telangiectasia (also called HHT or Osler-Weber-Rendu syndrome, a disorder that causes development of multiple abnormalities in the blood vessels) may be evidenced by nosebleeds. This is a disorder involving a blood vessel growth similar to a birthmark in the back of the nose.

Clinical Manifestations

The clinical manifestation of epistaxis consists of bleeding from the nose. There may be slight or profuse bleeding dependent on the cause of the nosebleed. If the bleeding does not stop after 20 minutes, it is imperative that the patient seeks emergency care. If the nosebleed occurs after an injury to the head, this may indicate a skull fracture. It could also indicate a broken nose; therefore, x-rays should be taken no matter how trivial the blow seems to be at the time. Skull fractures are discussed in Chapter 21.

Laboratory and Diagnostic Procedures and Medical Management

Laboratory and diagnostic tests that may need to be performed (particularly if a systemic cause is suspected) include a complete blood

Weblink: Fact Sheet: Deviated Septum

Weblink: Facial Bone Anatomy

count (CBC), partial thromboplastin time (PTT) measurements, and prothrombin (PT) measurements. (Refer to the Diagnostic Tests box on page 690.) Nasal endoscopy (examination of the nose using a camera) also may be called for.

Anterior bleeds generally resolve on their own; this process can be helped along by pinching the nares together (not the nasal bones) and leaning forward for 15 minutes.

Safety Alert *The nurse should instruct the patient to lean forward or to the side to protect the airway and prevent swallowing of blood and subsequent emesis.*

Direct pressure is the primary method of stopping nosebleeds, but topical vasoconstrictors such as phenylephrine or oxymetazoline can also help stop the bleeding (Manes, 2010). In addition, chemical, electrical, or laser cautery or nasal packing may be used for bleeding that is resistant to pressure or vasoconstrictors (Figure 26–2◆).

Posterior packing is used for bleeding from a posterior origin. Patients with a posterior pack should be hospitalized and monitored closely for nasopulmonary reflex; in this situation, the nasal stimulation from the packing may cause hypoventilation or even apnea due to protective reflexes mediated by the trigeminal and vagal nerves. The process of this reflex is not well understood; however, changes in arterial oxygen tension can lead to hypoxia and subsequent myocardial infarction or cerebrovascular accident (Manes, 2010). If packing is ineffective, then the nurse should alert the healthcare team and recommend a consult with otolaryngology or interventional radiology for possible embolization or surgical intervention.

Nursing Management

Patients with epistaxis and packing may experience a feeling of airway obstruction. If this occurs, the nurse must take special note of the patients' concerns and provide reassurance as needed. For example, the nurse needs to elevate the head of the bed and provide a facemask for humidity. In the event of surgery, the nurse needs to follow routine postoperative care protocols (see Chapter 19) and provide pain medication as needed. Refer to Diagnostic Tests for Facial Fractures on page 690 for more detail.

Patients with posterior epistaxis, requiring posterior packing, should be observed closely in a monitored unit because of the possibility of hypoxia and hypoventilation. These patients are at risk for airway obstruction if the packs slip and for developing nasopulmonary reflex as previously described. Therefore, cardiac monitoring and pulse oximetry are mandatory.

The nurse should advise patients of risk factors for nosebleeds, which include a hot, dry climate; colds and allergies; a deviated septum; exposure to irritating chemicals; medical conditions; heavy alcohol use; and use of medications that interfere with blood clotting, such as aspirin. Patient education should include advice on preventive measures that can be taken. Instruction for any patient recovering from a nosebleed should include refraining from picking or blowing of the nose, not engaging in heavy lifting, and not straining for at least one week. Drying of the nasal cavity should be prevented by using gels, ointment, or a humidifier. Humidified tents rather than nasal cannula should be used for hospitalized patients.

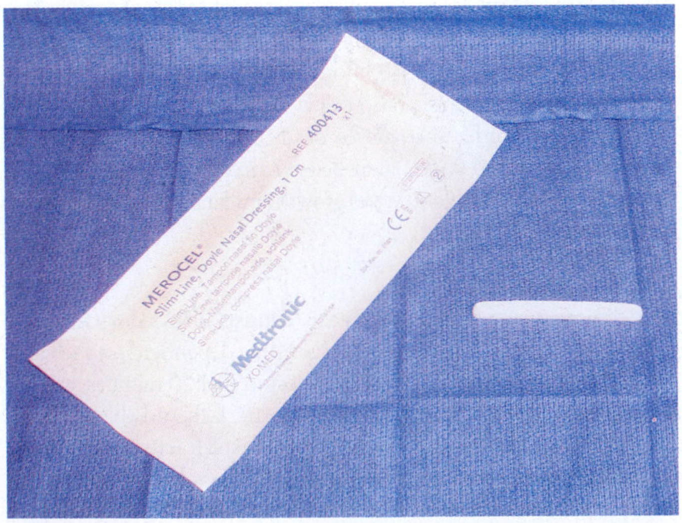

FIGURE 26–2 ◆ Nasal tampon for the treatment of anterior epistaxis. This is placed in the anterior nasal cavity, impregnated with normal saline, and left in place for at least 5 days. Most nasal packing is bilateral to provide pressure support on either side of the nasal septum.

Source: Ann E. F. Sievers, RN

Facial Fractures

Facial fractures are any injuries that result in a broken bone or bones of the face. Because nose fractures were discussed earlier, this discussion is restricted to the mandible, maxilla, zygoma, temporal bones, and the frontal bone. Multiple facial fractures may occur simultaneously, typically resulting from an injury to the face. When the nurse is caring for the patient with a facial facture, it is important to understand the characteristics and importance of each bone (see Figure 26–3◆ for an illustration of the facial bones).

Mandible Fracture

The mandible is a U-shaped bone; together with the maxilla, the mandible is the largest and strongest bone of the face. It forms the lower jaw and holds the lower teeth in place. The mandible consists of a curved, horizontal portion, referred to as the body that forms the chin and supports the lower teeth; two vertical portions, the rami, which unite with the ends of the body nearly at right angles; the alveolar process; the condyles that act as the ball of the ball and socket of the temporomandibular joint; the superior (upper) and posterior projection from the ramus, which forms the temporomandibular joint with the temporal bone; and the coronoid process, a projection from the ramus, which provides attachment to the temporalis muscle.

The inferior alveolar nerve, a branch of the mandibular division of the trigeminal (V) nerve, enters the mandibular foramen and runs forward in the mandibular canal, supplying sensation to the teeth. At the mental foramen, the nerve divides into two terminal branches: incisive and mental nerves. The incisive nerve runs forward in the mandible and supplies the anterior teeth. The mental nerve exits the mental foramen and supplies sensation to the lower lip (Babak & Blackwell, 2009). The mandible articulates with the two temporal bones at the temporomandibular joints. It is the only mobile bone of the facial skeleton, and, since it houses the lower teeth, its motion is essential for mastication.

Maxilla Fracture

The maxilla forms the largest component of the middle third of the facial skeleton and is a fusion of two bones along the palatal fissure that forms the upper jaw. The alveolar process of the maxilla holds the upper teeth and is referred to as the maxillary arch. The maxilla attaches laterally to the zygomatic bones (cheekbones) and assists in forming

Weblink: Temporal Bone Fractures

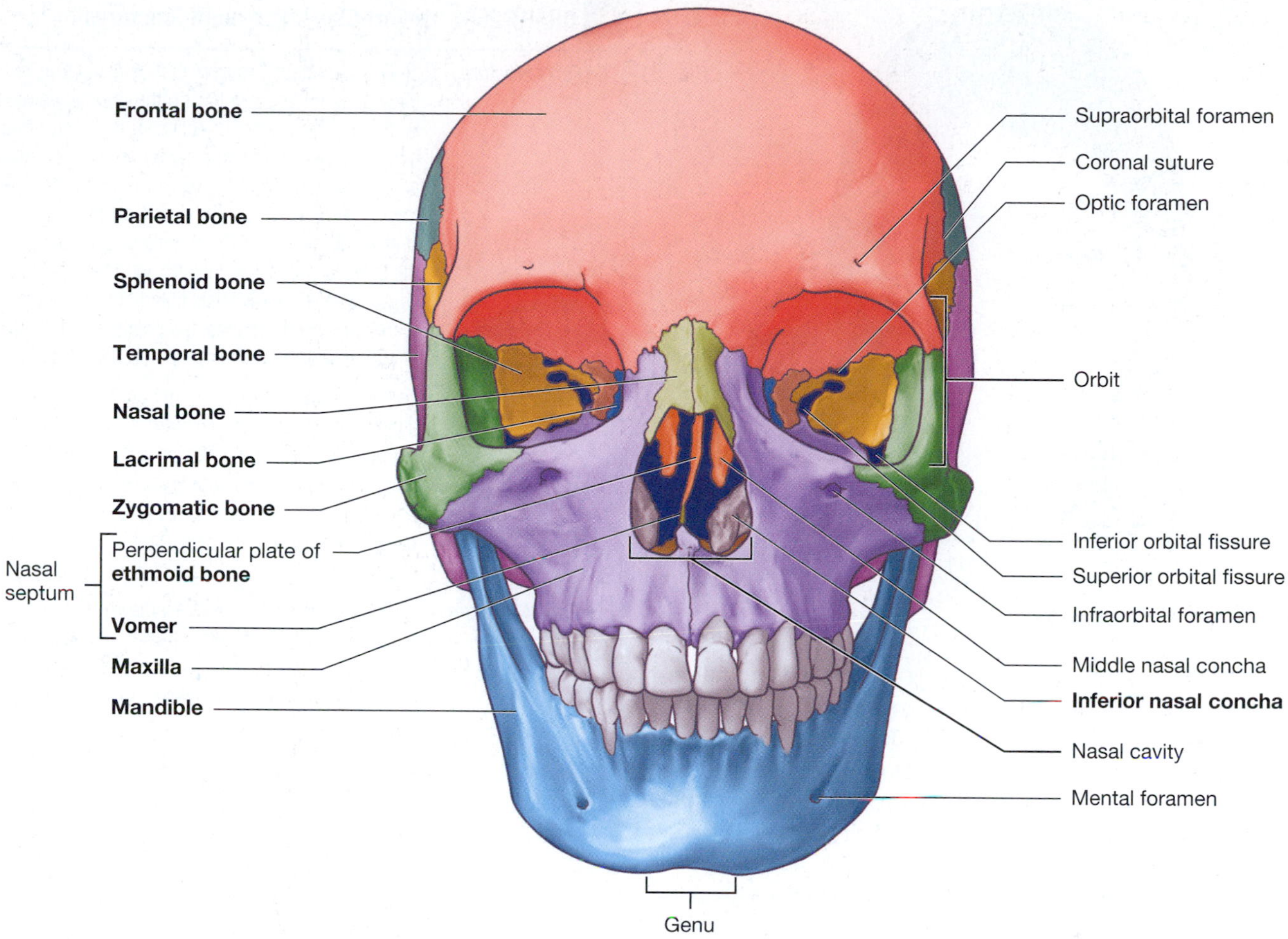

FIGURE 26–3 ◆ The facial bones.

the boundaries of three cavities: the roof of the mouth, the floor and lateral side of the nasal antrum, and the floor of the orbit. The maxilla articulates with nine bones: two of the cranium (frontal and ethmoid) and seven of the face (nasal, zygomatic, lacrimal, inferior nasal, concha, palatine, and vomer). The maxilla is a key bone in the midface that is closely associated with adjacent bones providing structural support.

Zygoma Fracture

The zygomatic bone (malar bone), a paired bone of the human skull, articulates with the maxilla, the temporal bone, the sphenoid bone, and the frontal bone. It forms the lateral portion of the interior orbital rim, as well as the lateral rim and lateral wall of the orbit. It is situated at the upper and lateral part of the face, forming the prominence of the cheekbone, part of the lateral wall and floor of the orbit, and parts of the temporal and infratemporal fossae. This bone presents a malar and a temporal surface; four processes—the frontosphenoidal, orbital, maxillary, and temporal; and four borders. Additionally, the zygoma forms the anterior zygomatic arch, which is made up of three bone components: the zygomatic bone, the bone coming off the zygomatic prominence of the maxilla, and the zygomatic process of the temporal bone.

Temporal Bone Fracture

The temporal bones are situated at the sides and base of the skull. The temporal bone is a thick, hard bone that is composed of multiple openings (foramina). These openings create an area of weakness that is susceptible to fractures (March, Connell, Belafsky, & Belafsky, 2010). The bone provides passage for many vital structures, including the ear canal; middle and inner ear structures; and portions of the facial nerve, carotid artery, and jugular vein.

Frontal Bone Fracture

The frontal bone is the large bone that makes up the forehead and the upper edge and roof of the orbit (eye socket). It forms the anterior portion of the cranium and articulates with a number of other bones including the parietal, nasal, ethmoid, maxillary, and zygomatic bones. The eyebrows and the buttress of the supraorbital rim demarcate the lower anterior border of the frontal sinus, which is a mucosa-lined, pyramid shaped, air-filled cavity that lies just above the orbit (see Figure 26–3). The sinus floor, which consists of membranous bone that is the thinnest of the sinus boundaries, is the nasal area most vulnerable to injury and forms two-thirds of the medial orbital roof. The primary purpose of the frontal sinus is to serve as a mechanical barrier to protect the brain from trauma. The frontal sinuses are positioned more anteriorly than the other paranasal sinuses and are situated to absorb anterior cranial facial trauma. Figure 26–4◆ shows the sinuses.

Maxillofacial Fracture Epidemiology and Etiology

Maxillofacial fractures usually occur as a result of blunt injury and less commonly from penetrating trauma. The most common etiologies of maxillofacial fracture are vehicular collisions, assault, falls, industrial accidents, and sports accidents. Because of increasing automobile safety standards, the number of injuries from crashes has trended

Weblink: Temporal Bone Fractures

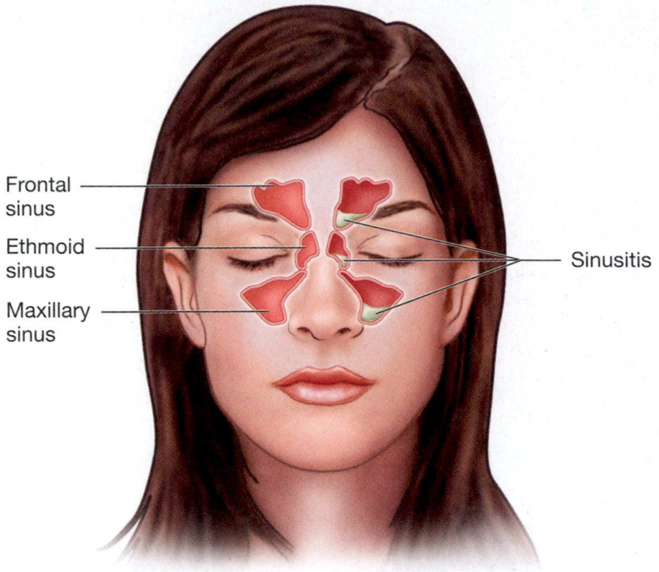

FIGURE 26–4 ◆ Sites of sinusitis.

CHART 26–1 Le Fort Classification of Fractures

Le Fort I Fracture	Le Fort I fractures (horizontal) may result from a force of injury directed low on the maxillary alveolar rim in a downward direction. The Le Fort I fracture, or transverse fracture, separates the alveolus as a mobile unit from the rest of the midface. The fracture extends through the base of the maxillary sinuses above the teeth, essentially separating the alveolar processes, palate, and pterygoid processes from the previously noted facial structures. With high-energy injuries, the palate may be split in the midline in addition to the Le Fort I fracture.
Le Fort II Fracture	Le Fort II fractures (pyramidal) may result from a blow to the lower or mid-maxilla. This fracture pattern begins laterally, similar to a Le Fort I, but medially diverges in a superior direction to include part of the medial orbit as well as the nose, separating the maxillary alveolus, the medial wall of the orbit and nose, from the rest of the facial bones.
Le Fort III Fracture	Le Fort III fractures (transverse) may result from impact to the nasal bridge or upper maxilla. A Le Fort III fracture, also referred to as a craniofacial disjunction, denotes a complete separation of the midface or facial bones from the cranium. This fracture transverses the zygomaticofrontal suture, continues through the floor of the orbit, and finally extends through the nasofrontal suture. The bones of the orbits are separated through the lateral wall, floor, and medial wall. It is unusual to have this fracture as a single segment of bone; more commonly, it connects with varying combinations of zygomatic, nasoethmoid, and orbital fractures. The fractures might not be symmetric on both sides, and minimal mobility may be present. Figure 26–5◆ shows the Le Fort fractures.

downward, while assault injuries, including domestic abuse, are on the rise (Zellweger, 2007). The etiology and incidence of maxillofacial trauma vary between and within countries depending on socioeconomic, cultural, and environmental factors. Alcohol consumption and being a young male (because of a greater propensity than females to engage in high-risk activities) are associated with a higher risk of facial injury (Zellweger, 2007).

A mandibular fracture generally is caused by trauma such as a direct blow or lateral blow to the face as a result of a motor vehicle crash, assault, fall, or contact sport. Mandibular fractures often are accompanied by a "twin fracture" on the contralateral (opposite) side. The mandible may be dislocated anteriorly (to the front) and inferiorly (downward) but very rarely posteriorly (backward). Like mandibular fractures, maxillary fractures are often the result of motor vehicle crashes. Fractures of the maxilla occur less frequently than those of the mandible or nose owing to the strong structural support of the maxilla. The midface consists of alternating thick and thin sections of bone that are capable of resisting significant force. This structurally strong bone provides protection for the globes and brain, protection of the midface, and support for occlusion (a person's bite). Reestablishing the continuity of these buttresses is the foundation on which maxillary fracture treatment is based. René Le Fort provided the earliest classification system of maxillary fractures in 1901. His model, which is still generally used, described "great lines of weakness in the face" using low-velocity impact forces directed against cadaver skulls. The categorization and assessment of Le Fort fractures are listed in Chart 26–1.

The bones that make up the zygomatic arch frequently are fractured in vehicular collisions and as a result of blunt trauma. These high-velocity injuries often produce fracture patterns that are not classified by the standard Le Fort system; they are described simply by the anatomic structure fractured and the degree of commination present.

Temporal bone injury is usually the result of blunt head trauma. Damage to the temporal bone typically requires the application of great force and may cause fracture, hemorrhage, nerve trauma, vascular damage, or disruption of the middle or inner ear structures. Temporal bone injuries reportedly occur in 14% to 22% of all skull fractures, with motor vehicle crashes causing approximately 31% of temporal bone fractures in the United States (March, Connell, Belafsky, & Belafsky, 2010). Temporal bone fractures are classified either as to the axis of the fracture—longitudinal (82%), transverse (11%), or mixed (7%)—or on the basis of the clinical relevance of the fracture: otic capsule-violating (OCV) or otic capsule-sparing (OCS) (Johnson, Semaan, & Megerian, 2008). Longitudinal fractures generally result from a temporoparietal impact, and transverse fractures result from a fronto-occipital impact. OCV fractures account for 2.5% to 5.6% of temporal bone injuries and have a high incidence of facial nerve injury, with subsequent facial paresis or paralysis, sensory and conductive hearing loss, balance disturbance, tinnitus, vertigo, cerebrospinal fluid (CSF) leak through the fractures, and underlying brain injury (Johnson, Semaan, & Megerian, 2008). Injuries to adjacent structures include vascular injury, cranial nerve palsies, and underlying brain injury.

Fractures involving the frontal region are some of the least common injuries that affect the facial skeleton. The incidence is 5% to 15% of all facial fractures (Piccolino, Vetrano, Mundula, Di Lella, Tedaldi, & Poladas, 2007). For purposes of initial evaluation, frontal sinus fractures should be regarded as head injuries. The majority of patients with such fractures are victims of automobile collisions with multiple injuries requiring a multiple-specialty team approach and complete evaluation.

Skull fractures are discussed in detail in Chapter 21.

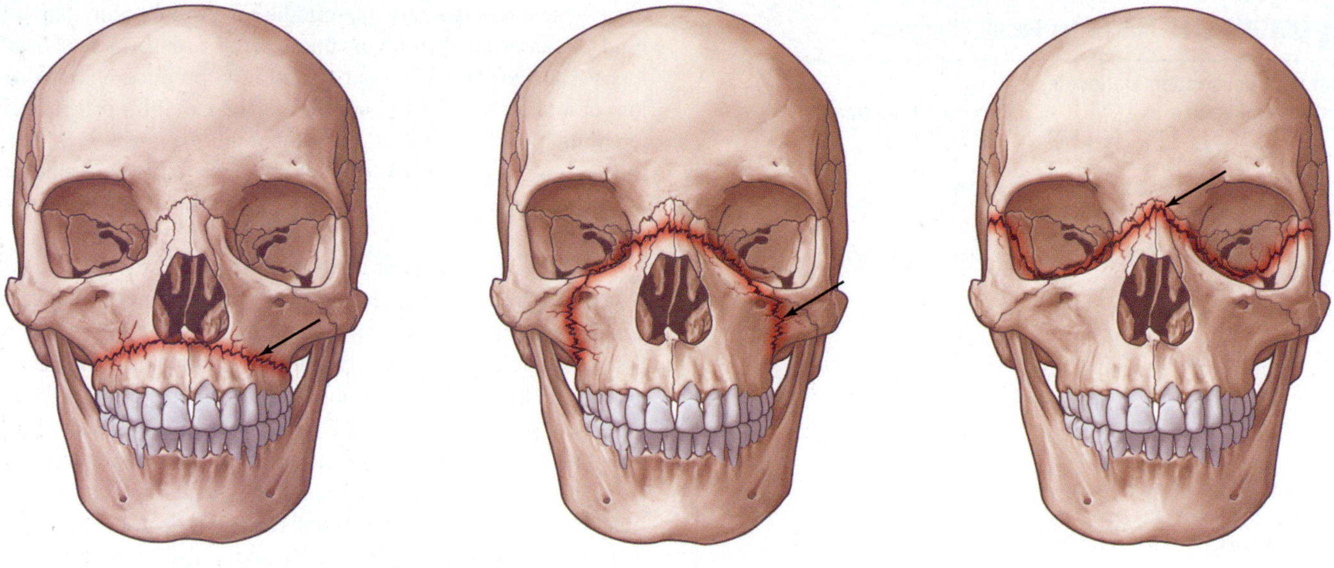

FIGURE 26–5 ◆ Le Fort fractures.

Laboratory and Diagnostic Procedures

In addition to the physical assessment, radiographs and CT scans aid in the identification of facial fractures. See the Diagnostic Test for Facial Fractures box.

Clinical Manifestations

With most facial bone fractures, there is some overt sign of the deformity, which may include bleeding, swelling, bruising, pain, or a change in the facial shape. With mandibular fractures, patients will have difficulty opening their mouths, talking, and chewing. Paresthesia and numbness also may be present on the affected side owing to swelling at the site of injury. With maxillary fractures, the face seems to be sunken; on palpation, irregularities and bony stepoffs (misalignments) demonstrate free movement. Because of considerable and extensive facial edema, the nurse might not fully appreciate the deformity until it is palpated. As with the mandibular fracture, patients will have pain, difficulty on opening the mouth and chewing, and sometimes difficulty talking. They also may have paresthesia or numbness or a sensation of "pins and needles" on the affected side owing to the proximity of the swelling to the trigeminal (CNV) and facial (CNVII) nerves. Of the three fracture types, the most extensive and life threatening is the Le Fort III. With this type of fracture, airway obstruction and severe bleeding are likely. The airway usually is supported with a temporary **tracheotomy,** or surgical airway created through the neck into the trachea. A **tracheostomy** is the opening created by the surgical procedure. The terms *tracheotomy* and *tracheostomy* are often used interchangeably.

In zygomatic and orbital fractures, the orbital contents can become entrapped by bony fragments from the floor of the orbit. The patient will experience pain, diplopia (double vision), difficulty with eye movement, and sometimes blindness. Global entrapment by the fracture must be surgically corrected very early on to prevent further visual damage. Swelling to the area may mask the fracture. Patients will have pain, difficulty on opening the mouth and chewing, and sometimes difficulty talking.

The two kinds of temporal bone fractures produce different findings. A longitudinal fracture runs vertically, usually causing injury to the tympanic membrane and ossicles of the inner ear. This produces conductive hearing loss, otorrhea, drainage from the ear of either blood or CSF, and, occasionally, facial nerve paralysis. Other findings include headache, nystagmus, or vertigo. Some temporal bone fractures are difficult to see on x-ray, and not all clinical findings may be present at the time of injury; some may develop later. Hearing impairment is discussed in detail in Chapter 63.

Medical and Surgical Management

Medical management of all facial fractures includes airway support, pain control, and closed reduction or surgical repair depending on the type and severity of the fracture. The patient's airway should be assessed for patency because hemorrhage or edema can cause airway obstruction. Surgical treatment generally consists of realigning the fractured pieces of bone with wires or repairing the break with metal plates and fine screws. If fragments of bone have pierced the skin or if teeth were lost or loosened, an antibiotic generally is ordered to reduce the risk of infection.

Maxillary fractures are treated by reduction and immobilization. Surgical repair of the fractures involves plating the bones together (surgically applying plates and screws to the bone to support the fractured site) to stabilize the bony facial structure (see Figure 26–3). The maxilla and mandible also may be wired together for further stabilization. Establishment of preinjury occlusion and midface buttress alignment provides the foundation for this treatment.

The goals of treatment of Le Fort fractures are to reestablish preinjury occlusion with normal height and projection of the face. To accomplish this, the structural buttress of the maxilla must be aligned and stabilized to provide the necessary support and contour to the midface. The proper occlusal relationship between the dental arches is established with intermaxillary fixation (IMF) or, as more appropriately termed, maxillomandibular fixation. IMF is established by securing arch bars to the upper and lower dental arches with individual wire ligatures around the teeth. The maxillary and mandibular arch bars are secured together. Early placement of the patient in IMF can eliminate some of the secondary deformities of the facial structure caused by Le Fort fractures. This is one of the simplest and most effective forms of treatment. However, IMF is

DIAGNOSTIC TESTS for Facial Fractures

Test with Description, Rationale, and Normal Values	Expected Abnormality
Plain Film X-Ray	
Normal facial bone anatomy without edema or foreign body identified *Plain films will identify bony fractures and foreign bodies, if present.*	Edema Foreign body Fracture of facial bone(s)
CT Scan	
Normal facial bone anatomy without edema or foreign body identified *CT scan quickly identifies detailed data on the integrity of the bony structures. Traumatic injuries can cause varying degrees of disruption and compromise.*	Facial bone fracture(s) Blood in the sinuses Foreign body
Hemoglobin and Hematocrit	
Hemoglobin: Male 13.5–18 g/dL Female 12–15 g/dL **Hematocrit:** Male 40–54% Female 36–46% *The hemoglobin and hematocrit should be obtained as a baseline to look for trends downward, signifying bleeding.*	Decreases or trends downward
Coagulation Studies	
International normalized ratio (INR): 2.0–3.0 in patients on anticoagulation Activated partial thromboplastin time (APTT): 20–35 secs Partial thromoplastin time (PTT): 60–70 seconds	May identify if the patient is on long-term anticoagulation at home. If the patient also has a traumatic brain injury, TBI causes the release of tissue thromboplastin, which increases INR.

more commonly used in conjunction with other immobilization and stabilization techniques.

Recent advances in the treatment of maxillary fractures include the use of extended open-reduction techniques with rigid plate and screw fixation (surgically exposing the fractured bone and applying plates and screws to support the fractured area) of the facial buttresses. Bone grafts have been used to replace missing or comminuted bone with early treatment of these injuries. This more aggressive surgical approach has dramatically improved the aesthetic results that are obtainable and allow for fewer secondary deformities.

Zygomatic and mandibular fractures are usually treated surgically. Fractures are reduced by using screws, bars, wires, and plates. Following open-reduction and internal fixation (ORIF) of the fractures, the jaws can be wired shut with or without plating of the fractures.

Management of temporal bone fractures generally is conservative. If the facial nerve (CNVII) is lacerated or impacted, the patient must undergo surgical facial nerve decompression. If a dural leak is suspected, systemic antibiotics are given to prevent meningitis. Transverse fractures across the middle ear produce pain, blood behind the eardrum (hemotympanum), and a sensorineural hearing loss. Facial nerve (CNVII) injury or paralysis produces a facial droop, loss of a blink reflex, and paresthesia. The care of a patient with a temporal bone fracture and/or a temporal bone resection is similar; the focus is on care of the eye after facial nerve resection, cable grafting, or repair. Eye protection and adding lubrication prevent corneal abrasions.

The long-range goals of treatment of frontal sinus fractures are cosmetic restoration and prevention of complications including acute and chronic sinusitis, mucocele (mucous cyst of the mucosa) formation, brain abscess, and osteomyelitis. The first step, however, is to evaluate and manage more serious life-threatening injuries. Thus, in the case of frontal fractures, the standard trauma protocol must be followed with an emphasis on ensuring an adequate airway, breathing, circulation, central nervous system (CNS) status, and cervical spine (refer to Chapter 67). Frontal sinus fractures do not require immediate surgical attention unless they are associated with a neurosurgical or ophthalmologic emergency. The choice of treatment usually is dictated by the site and extent of the damage (Piccolino et al., 2007).

Nursing Management

Nursing care of the patient with facial fractures involves assessment of airway, concomitant injury, pain, and nutrition.

Assessment

The nurse must assess and monitor the patient with a facial fracture for any airway compromise. Prevention of nausea and vomiting and intervention to prevent aspiration when necessary is of great importance. Careful initial and ongoing assessment of the cranial nerves' functions and the patient's ability to hear is necessary to determine entrapment/damage by the fracture or edema.

Nursing Diagnosis

Nursing diagnoses for the patient with a facial fracture may include the following:

- *Ineffective Airway Clearance* related to inflammation, blood, misalignment of bone
- *Risk for Aspiration* related to blood and misalignment of bone
- *Anxiety* related to wiring of mandible
- *Acute Pain* related to fracture
- *Risk for Infection* related to fracture
- *Imbalanced Nutrition: Less Than Body Requirements* related to misalignment of bone and pain

NANDA-I © 2012

Planning

The overall goals for the patient with facial fractures will be patency of the airway, control of pain, adequate nutritional intake, and prevention of infection.

Outcomes and Evaluation Parameters

The patient will have a patent airway as exhibited by normal respiratory effort, clear breath sounds, and adequate pulse oximetry. The patient's pain will be controlled as exhibited by the statement of his level of pain on a 1–10 scale. Nutritional intake will be adequate to maintain body weight and promote healing. The patient will be free from infection.

PATIENT TEACHING & DISCHARGE PRIORITIES for Patients with Facial Fracture

Need	Teaching
Airway protection	A patient with his mandible wired closed and his family must learn how to cut the wires so that he can open his mouth in case of vomiting or choking. The patient should always have wire cutters at hand.
Pain control	The patient and family will be instructed how and when to take pain medication, as well as given information on common side effects and safety precautions. The patient should report any increase in pain to his health care provider.
Avoiding epistaxis	The patient who is discharged with packing in place should be instructed to leave it in place until the health care provider removes it. The patient who does not have packing should be told the following: Do not blow your nose for 12 hours after a nosebleed. If bleeding occurs, sit up and bend forward, pinching the front half of the nose. Put petroleum jelly (e.g., Vaseline) inside the nares every morning. Use a humidifier in the home to make the air less dry. Do not take aspirin which may prolong bleeding. Try not to strain or lift heavy objects.

Interventions and Rationales

Effective oral care is essential for healthy healing and prevention of dental complications. Patient education includes use of the water pick for mouth and teeth cleaning and dietary requirements. A nutritional consult can assess the patient's nutrition and home requirements for enteral feeding or an oral soft or liquid diet. Chapter 8 includes a discussion of enteral feedings and their importance for maintaining nutritional balance.

Management of temporal bone fractures usually is conservative. The nurse must continually assess for nerve damage and hearing loss. It is essential to test for any otorrhea (discharge from the ears), which may indicate a CSF leak. The nurse needs to institute CSF leak precautions, which include the following:

- Keep the head of the patient's bed at 30 to 45 degrees at all times.
- Teach the patient not to bend over, strain, or lift heavy objects.
- Provide instruction about not straining during a bowel movement because this may prevent a CSF leak from healing or make it worse by increasing intracranial pressure.

A lumbar drain may be inserted to lessen the increased intracranial pressure at the site of injury and allow it to heal. If facial nerve injury is present, the nurse should provide eye care, including artificial tears every 2 hours, ointment at night, and use of an eye shield to protect the eye from drying and corneal abrasion.

Because of the amount of energy needed to fracture the frontal bone, patients who present with a frontal facial fracture have generally experienced other severe injuries as well. The nurse must be alert and assess for concomitant injury.

Safety Alert *Patients with mandibular wiring should be given postoperative antinausea medication to reduce the chances of vomiting. If, following surgery, the patient vomits and is unable to maintain her airway, the nurse (or family, if at home) should cut the wires to open the mouth to protect the airway. The patient must then have the wires re-secured to reestablish the fracture repair.*

Collaborative Management

The interdisciplinary team may consist of surgeons, dentists, speech therapists, and dietitians. In order to meet desired patient outcomes, it is essential that this interdisciplinary team communicate openly with one another in developing and evaluating care of the patient and family (IOM [Institute of Medicine], 2010). For example, patients with facial fractures that require immobilization will have difficulty meeting their nutritional needs. Therefore, involving nutritional services early to evaluate the patient and caloric intake is important. Dental follow-up is important during and after the 6-week healing process. The Patient Teaching & Discharge Priorities box discusses the long-term patient and family needs.

Inflammation, Infection, and Obstruction of the Nose and Paranasal Sinuses

Disorders affecting the nose and paranasal sinuses include inflammation, infection, and obstruction. The effects of these disorders lead individuals to feel ill, tired, and irritable. Common disorders that fall within these categories are discussed following a review of the anatomy and physiology of the paranasal sinuses.

Anatomy and Physiology of the Paranasal Sinuses

The paranasal sinuses are the eight cavities in the skull that connect with the nasal cavity. They are arranged bilaterally in four pairs: the maxillary sinuses in the maxillae, the frontal sinuses in the frontal bone, the sphenoid sinuses in the sphenoid bone behind the nasal cavity, and the ethmoid cells (sinuses) in the ethmoid bone behind and below the frontal sinuses. The exact function of the sinuses is not certain. They are believed to help the nose in circulating, warming, and moistening air as it is inhaled, thereby lessening the effect of cold, dry air to the lungs. The anatomy of the sinuses varies tremendously from person to person. In some individuals, anatomic differences may affect breathing and block the normal nasal drainage.

The mucous membrane in the nose and sinuses acts to condition inhaled air by warming, moisturizing, and filtering the air. The mucous membrane creates clear, wet, slightly sticky mucus that gathers dust, smoke, bacteria, or virus particles that may have been in the air. Tiny hairs along the membrane called cilia rotate to move the mucus along through the sinuses and out the nose. The mucous membrane is one of the body's frontline defense systems. Besides filtering out foreign particles, it releases chemicals that help to destroy bacteria and viruses. If a virus, bacteria, allergen, or other irritant is strong enough to prevent the mucous membrane and cilia from functioning, an infectious obstruction can occur in any of the pairs of sinus.

Rhinitis

Rhinitis is an inflammation of the linings of the nasal passages and sinuses that produces a full or partial combination of sneezing, rhinorrhea, nasal congestion, and nasal itching. Symptoms may extend to the eyes, ears, sinuses, or throat. It can be broadly categorized as allergic or non-allergic, with allergic being the most common cause. Although the symptoms of the two types of rhinitis may be similar, the etiology and treatment may vary.

Allergic rhinitis has traditionally been categorized as either seasonal-perennial or episodic-persistent. More recently, a version based on the severity and duration of symptoms, including intermittent (fewer than 4 days a week or 4 weeks a year), persistent (more than 4 days a week or 4 weeks a year), mild (if symptoms do not affect sleep or daily activities), and moderate to severe (if symptoms interfere with sleep or daily activities) has received support (Orban, Saleh, & Durham, 2008). Approximately 30% of adults and almost 40% of children are suspected of suffering from allergic rhinitis (Fletcher, 2011). About 70% of allergic rhinitis patients also suffer from allergic conjunctivitis marked by itchy, irritated, red eyes (Fletcher, 2011). The most common triggers are aeroallergins such as pollens, molds, and dust mites; however, rhinitis can also be triggered by food and occupational compounds.

Non-allergic rhinitis is distinguished by chronic symptoms that include nasal congestion, rhinorrhea, or postnasal drainage. Common triggers include tobacco smoke, motor vehicle exhaust fumes, temperature changes, strong fragrances, alcoholic beverages, and cleaning products (Fletcher, 2011).

Epidemiology and Etiology

Rhinitis is common among individuals and affects approximately 40 million people in the United States (Sheikh, 2007). This places a huge burden on society, with loss of school attendance and work productivity as well as a significant economic impact. Allergic rhinitis occurs in people of all races. However, the prevalence of allergic rhinitis seems to vary among different populations and cultures, which may be due to genetic differences, geographic factors, environmental differences, and/or other population-based factors. The prevalence of rhinitis is approximately equal between men and women in adulthood. The onset of rhinitis is common in childhood, adolescence, and early adulthood, with a mean age of onset of 8 to 11 years. However, allergic rhinitis may occur in people of any age, with 80% of cases developing by age 20. In older adults, rhinitis is less commonly allergic in nature (Sheikh, 2007).

Non-allergic rhinitis affects approximately 17 to 19 million Americans, accounting for close to half of the cases of chronic rhinitis (Joe & Patel, 2010). Non-allergic rhinitis is characterized by the presence of sneezing, rhinorrhea, nasal congestion, or postnasal drainage. It is difficult to distinguish from allergic rhinit is, although the presence of nasal and ocular itching, common in allergic rhinitis, is often absent in non-allergic rhinitis. Non-allergic rhinitis can be broadly categorized as inflammatory or non-inflammatory (Lieberman, 2011).

Non-allergic inflammatory rhinitis causes include the following:

- ***Infection:*** The most common causes are infections due to rhinovirus, coronavirus, adenovirus, parainfluenza virus, respiratory syncytial virus, or enterovirus.
- ***Drug Induced:*** Rhinitis may be caused by use of NSAIDs, antihypertensives, psychotropics, phosphodiesterase type 5 inhibitors, and cocaine. The symptoms are episodic and stop as soon as the drug has cleared the patient's system.
- ***Occupational:*** Occupational rhinitis causes patients to have symptoms only in the workplace. These symptoms usually are due to an inhaled irritant such as metal salts, animal dander, latex, wood dust, and chemicals.
- ***Sensitivity to Aspirin:***
- ***NARES (Non-Allergic Rhinitis Eosinophilic Syndrome):*** NARES is the most common type of inflammatory non-allergic rhinitis (Lieberman, 2011). The etiology of NARES is unknown, but there is some speculation that it is a precursor to aspirin-sensitive rhinitis (Orban, Saleh, & Durham, 2008). A distinguishing feature of NARES is the presence of eosinophils, usually 10% to 20% on nasal smears.

The causes of non-inflammatory rhinitis include the following:

- ***Emotional:*** Transient and rarely a problem.
- ***Idiopathic:*** All other possible causes have been excluded.
- ***Atrophic:*** Loss of secretory and humidifying function of the nose. This is often caused by bacteria, such as Klebsiella ozaenae.
- ***Gustatory:*** Occurs after eating, particularly hot and spicy foods. It is transient and rarely a problem. The end results are profuse watery rhinorrhea secondary to nasal vasodilation that is vagally mediated and generally occurs within a few hours of oral ingestion.
- ***Vasomotor:*** Believed to result from disturbed regulation of the parasympathetic and sympathetic systems in which the parasympathetic system dominates, resulting in vasodilatation and edema of the nasal vasculature. Causes include cold air, strong odors, stress, or inhaled irritants.
- ***Rebound Congestion:*** Associated with prolonged use of topical decongestant vasoconstrictor medications (rhinitis medicamentosa).
- ***Hormonal:*** Occurs during periods of hormonal imbalance including pregnancy, puberty, and menstruation.

Pathophysiology

An allergy is an inappropriate immune response to a substance in the environment that is normally harmless. When a person with an allergy to such a substance breathes in the allergen, histamine and other chemicals are released as part of the immune response, causing itching and swelling, mucus production, and, in serious cases, hives and rashes, as well as other symptoms.

Allergic rhinitis involves inflammation of the mucous membranes of the nose, eyes, eustachian tubes, middle ear, sinuses, and pharynx. It is a reaction that occurs when airborne irritants (allergens) trigger the release of immune mediators. The mediators that are immediately released include histamine, tryptase, chymase, kinins, and heparin. These mediators act via various interactions and ultimately lead to the symptoms of rhinorrhea. Mucous glands are stimulated, local vascular permeability is increased, and vasodilation occurs. This leads to an increase in secretions, plasma exudation, congestion, and pressure. Sensory nerves are stimulated, leading to sneezing and itching. Histamine causes inflammation and fluid production in the fragile linings of nasal passages, sinuses, and eyelids. All of these events can occur in minutes; hence, this reaction is called the early, or immediate, phase of the reaction.

Over 4 to 8 hours, these mediators, through a complex interplay of events, lead to the recruitment of other inflammatory cells to the mucosa, such as neutrophils, eosinophils, lymphocytes, and macrophages. This results in continued inflammation, termed the late-phase

CHART 26–2 Symptoms of Allergic Rhinitis

- Coughing
- Itching (nose, mouth, eyes, palate, throat)
- Impaired sense of smell
- Stuffy nose (nasal congestion)
- Tearing eyes
- Headache
- Runny nose
- Sneezing
- Sore throat
- Wheezing

response. The symptoms of the late-phase response are similar to those of the early phase, but usually with less sneezing and itching. In addition, more congestion and mucous production tend to occur. The late phase may persist for hours or days (Sheikh, 2007).

Non-allergic rhinitis follows the same path of symptom development as allergic rhinitis; however, autonomic stimuli have a greater effect on these patients than with those with allergic rhinitis. Autonomic imbalance favoring the parasympathetic system increases nasal blood flow, edema, and secretions, creating an overall presentation of rhinitis and nasal obstruction. Changes in body posture from erect to supine can increase nasal airway resistance. In the supine position, pressure is lower in the right nostril than in the left nostril when the patient lies on the right side. Temperature also can affect nasal blood flow and compliance, both of which decrease in cold environments (Ramakrishnan, 2010).

Clinical Manifestations

Clinical manifestations of non-allergic rhinitis mimic those of allergic rhinitis (Chart 26–2). Symptoms include an initial profuse, clear, watery rhinorrhea (which often turns cloudy later in the course of the illness), nasal obstruction, postnasal discharge, and fever. Obstruction of the sinuses and/or eustachian tube causes referred facial pain or ear fullness. Physical examination may demonstrate the "allergic shiner" (dark circles under the eyes that resemble bruises from a black eye) (Ramakrishnan, 2010). Many symptoms emanate from the edema of the mucosal membranes. Rhinitis usually causes self-limiting, but annoying, symptoms that resolve in 7 to 10 days.

Diagnostic Procedures

The most common diagnostic tests for allergic rhinitis are the percutaneous skin test and the allergen-specific immunoglobulin E (IgE) antibody test. Skin testing involves introducing controlled amounts of allergen and control substances into the skin to determine what the patient is allergic to. Allergic rhinitis can have an immediate or delayed response. Skin testing elicits both types of responses; however, the primary goal of skin testing is to detect the immediate allergic response caused by the release of mast cells or basophil IgE-specific mediators, which create the classic wheal and flare reaction after 15 minutes. The delayed response occurs 4 to 8 hours after exposure to the sensitizing allergen and is less useful in clinical diagnosis. Percutaneous testing is the most common type of skin testing because it is conventional, safe, and widely accepted. Occasionally, intradermal testing is used because it is more sensitive, but less specific than percutaneous testing. The Diagnostic Tests for Rhinitis box summarizes the tests.

Medical Management

Treatment options should be aimed primarily at resolving the underlying physiologic or causative problem. The health care provider must differentiate between acute and chronic rhinitis as well as allergic versus non-allergic rhinitis before a treatment method is chosen. Rhinitis is not a disease; it is simply a term used to describe the symptoms produced by nasal irritation or inflammation: a runny, itchy, or stuffy nose. If the rhinitis lasts less than 6 weeks, it is called acute rhinitis, which usually is caused by infections or chemical irritation and probably is classified as non-allergic rhinitis. If symptoms linger for longer than 6 weeks, the symptoms would be called chronic rhinitis. Chronic rhinitis may be caused by allergy or a variety of other factors. It often is difficult to differentiate among the types of rhinitis, but a thorough and comprehensive history usually suggests the correct diagnosis. Health care providers should focus on symptoms (i.e., duration, exposures, magnitude of reaction, patterns, and chronicity) and triggers. The symptoms of non-allergic rhinitis can be similar to those of allergic rhinitis but with a less prominent nasal itch and conjunctiva irritation. Symptoms also tend to be aligned with seasonal variation, environmental influences, allergies, medical history (e.g., trauma, family, and treatment histories), and current treatments. An acute onset of 1 week or less has a limited differential and usually suggests a viral etiology, an acute exacerbation of allergic rhinitis, or, less commonly, a foreign body, particularly when symptoms are unilateral with purulent discharge.

The treatment for allergic rhinitis involves avoidance of triggers, pharmacotherapy, and, when appropriate, allergen immunotherapy (Fletcher, 2011). It may be impossible to completely avoid all allergens that produce the sensitivity. In some cases, people outgrow an allergy as the immune system becomes less sensitive to the allergen. As a general rule, however, once a substance causes allergies for an individual, it can continue to affect the person over the long term. Trigger avoidance measures include the following:

- Reducing outdoor exposure during the season in which a particular type of pollen is present.
- Limiting outdoor exposure by keeping the windows and doors of the house and car closed as much as possible during the pollen season.

DIAGNOSTIC TESTS for Rhinitis

Test with Description, Rationale, and Normal Values	Expected Abnormality
Plain Film X-Ray	
Normal facial anatomy without edema or foreign body identified *Establishing possible structural abnormalities or for helping detect complications of comorbid conditions, such as sinusitis or adenoid hypertrophy.*	Edema Foreign body Structural abnormality
CT Scan	
Normal facial anatomy without edema or foreign body identified *Establishing possible structural abnormalities or for helping detect complications of comorbid conditions, such as sinusitis or adenoid hypertrophy.*	Structural abnormality Fluid/edema in the sinuses Foreign body
Rhinoscopy	
Normal facial anatomy without edema or foreign body identified *Use of a fiber-optic scope to visualize the nasal passages for structural abnormalities, edema, polyps, or foreign bodies.*	Structural abnormality Fluid/edema in the nares Foreign body

- Covering the mattress and pillow with impermeable covers to reduce exposure to dust mites, washing linens every 2 weeks, and treating carpets and rugs as appropriate.
- Reducing excessive humidity and removing standing water.
- Using environmental measures such as air purifiers, frequent vacuuming, and changing bed linens to control for dust mites and pet dander and to help reduce mold spores.
- Eliminating exposure to smoke, strong perfumes and scents, fumes, rapid changes in temperature, and outdoor pollution for patients with nonspecific triggers.
- For animal allergies, complete avoidance is the best option. Confining the animal to a noncarpeted room and keeping it entirely out of the bedroom can be of some benefit. For occupational allergens, as with animal allergens, avoidance is the best measure. When this is not possible, using a mask or respirator might be helpful.

Primary pharmacotherapy for allergic rhinitis uses intranasal glucocorticoids, oral and topical antihistamines, oral decongestants, cromolyn sodium, montelukast, and ipratropium bromide (refer to the Pharmacology box on page 700). Nasal decongestants and systemic glucocorticoids should not be routinely used in the treatment of allergic rhinitis (DeShazo & Kemp, 2011). Regular use of OTC decongestant nasal sprays can cause rebound nasal congestion, leading to accelerated use and dependency. Although effective, systemic glucocorticoids have significant side effects and should only be used in short courses in cases of severe rhinitis that do not respond to other medications. Topical intranasal glucocorticoids are currently the most beneficial treatment for allergic rhinitis and have few side effects. They have shown to provide better relief of nasal congestion, nasal drainage, sneezing, nasal itch, postnasal drip, and overall nasal symptoms than oral antihistamines (DeShazo & Kemp, 2011). Once-a-day preparations are available and convenient; they are most effective if taken in the evening. However, their effectiveness is reduced or negated if there is debris in the nose that prevents the drug from coating the nasal mucosa. Saline sprays can be used to clear the mucosa prior to applying the glucocorticoid.

First-generation antihistamines are available over the counter. They are effective in reducing the symptoms of rhinitis, although less so for nasal congestion. They do cross the blood-brain barrier and cause significant sedative effects that have been implicated in fatal motor vehicle collisions. Second-generation and third-generation antihistamines are longer-acting and have fewer CNS side effects. All generations are less effective than nasal steroids in relieving the symptoms of rhinitis. Second-generation antihistamines are often used for patients with mild or occasional symptoms. Topical antihistamine nasal sprays are also available by prescription. They have some effectiveness in reducing nasal congestion and anti-inflammatory effects. Antihistamines can also be combined with decongestants to deliver better symptom relief than antihistamine alone. Decongestants can cause hypertension, insomnia, and headaches. They should not be given to patients with hypertension and should be given with caution to patients with glaucoma, cardiovascular disease, or cerebrovascular disease (DeShazo & Kemp, 2011). Refer to the Pharmacology box on page 700 for more details.

Cromolyn sodium is a mast cell stabilizer that reduces allergic inflammation and inhibits histamine release. It is relatively free of side effects and is available OTC. It does require frequent dosing and is not as effective as other medications. Montelukast is an antileukotriene that is beneficial for patients with allergic conjunctivitis. These medications have been associated with anxiety, depression, and, rarely, suicide. Ipratropium bromide is available in a nasal spray to treat symptoms of rhinorrhea.

Immunotherapy involves administering an allergen in gradual, escalating doses in an attempt to modulate the abnormal immune response to trigger exposure. It is generally given in the form of subcutaneous injections. Immunotherapy is indicated in patients with significant allergic response to a known allergen, usually identified by skin testing, that is refractory to reduction in exposure and optimal medication regimen (Norman, 2011).

To prevent complications during allergy desensitization treatment, the health care provider should review a standard series of allergy questions with the patient prior to each injection. These questions include reactions to previous injections, any new medications, any changes in health status, any increase in allergy/asthma (seasonal response), and determining whether the patient has taken an antihistamine that day. Following the injection, the patient is monitored for reactions (Chart 26–3). After the injection is given, the patient is

CHART 26–3 Allergy Reactions and Treatments

Reaction	Symptoms	Treatment	Medications
Local reaction	Erythema arm swelling of 2–3 cm, itchy eyes, slight body itching, transient local itching	Ice elevation. Observe closely until reaction resolves. Fill out anaphylaxis treatment record in patient chart.	Antihistamines, steroids Claritin, Zyrtec, Benadryl
Systemic reaction, anaphylaxis	Conjunctivitis, urticaria, chest tightness, problems breathing, syncope, wheezing, difficulty swallowing, shortness of breath, dyspneic hives, decrease in blood pressure	Administer oxygen per health care provider's order. Place venous tourniquet above injection site. Check vital signs and peak flow using a peak flow meter (see Chapter 27), oxygen saturation every 5–10 min. Start two (14–16) IVs bolus 250–500 mL normal saline. Repeat fluid bolus as needed for BP stability. Continue to check vital signs every 5 min until reaction is resolved. Call 911 and transport to emergency department.	1:1,000 epinephrine up to 0.3–0.5 mL IM Chlorpheniramine 4 mg po or diphenhydramine 25–50 mg po or IM Albuterol 2.5 mg nebulizer or 8 puffs metered-dose inhaler if wheezing Prednisone 60 mg po or Solu-Medrol 125 mg IV Zantac 50 mg IV/Pepcid 20 mg IV Glucagon 1 mg (especially if on beta-blockers)

required to wait for 30 minutes. The risk for reaction is reduced by selecting low-risk patients and by educating patients about warning signs. Fatalities are rare, but they do occur.

Patients with chronic, non-allergic rhinitis generally do not respond as well to pharmacotherapy, although the topical intranasal glucocorticoids and the topical antihistamine azelastine have shown to be helpful (Lieberman, 2011). A combination of these two medications may be more effective in patients with moderate to severe disease. Ipratropium nasal spray can be added if the primary symptom is rhinorrhea. Patients with severe refractory disease may improve with laser turbinectomy (partial or complete removal of the posterior nasal turbinates). One alternative therapy that may be helpful to patients with upper respiratory mucus and swelling is the use of plant oils, as discussed in the Complementary & Alternative Therapies box.

Nursing Management

Nursing management of patients with rhinitis begins with the nurse taking a thorough history as described earlier. If allergy medications are to be administered, this is typically the nurse's responsibility. Before administering the medication, the nurse should advise the patient of the action, route, desired effect, and side effects of the medication. The nurse should stay with the patient after administration of the medication to determine any adverse effects. It also is incumbent on the nurse to advise the patient of warning signs of an allergic reaction and explain when and how to seek medical advice.

Another major component of the nurse's role is education, helping the patient identify the known allergen and how to avoid subsequent allergic reactions. During the target season, people should remain

COMPLEMENTARY & ALTERNATIVE THERAPIES Using Plant Oils for Healing Purposes

Nancy Yilk

ORAL TRANSLATION OF HUMAN USE of plant oils for healing purposes was first recorded in written form in the texts of the Egyptians, establishing the cultural use of essential oils as man's first medicine. Today, essential oils are used by complementary and alternative medicine practitioners as aromatherapy, having clinical uses in the areas of pain relief, relaxation and anxiety reduction, and enhanced energy. Essential oils have continuing use with midwives to help women cope with labor pain. Cancer patients have utilized eucalyptus oil (EO) to relieve the myelotoxicity of chemotherapy side effects (Kiecolt-Glaser et al., 2008). Studies have established the ability of oils to effectively lower systolic blood pressure and sympathetic nerve system activity in hypertensive patients (Cha, Lee, & Yoo, 2010).

To understand the mechanics of the effects essential oils have on the upper respiratory system, researchers used an animal study model utilizing pharmacologic magnetic resonance imaging (MRI). This study established inhalation of various oils measured from significantly increasing the surface fluid in the middle portion of the trachea at both 5 and 10 minutes after administration to moderate and negligible with other oils. The results helped develop a possible understanding of why the use of some oils is more beneficial than use of others in human respiratory illnesses (Nicolato, Boschi, Marzola, & Sbarbati, 2009).

There is a long history of home use of eucalyptus oil (EO) inhalation, steam dispensed by the traditional use of putting the oil drops in hot water in a large bowl and then using a towel or cloth tented over the head as a person places his face above the bowl to capture the airborne oil droplets as they rise, giving relief to congested airways. More recently, the biochemical details behind these effects have been further clarified. Although other plant oils may be more microbiologically active, the safety of moderate doses of EO and its broad-spectrum antimicrobial action make it an attractive alternative to pharmaceuticals. eucalyptus oil (EO) and its major component, 1, 8-cineole, have antimicrobial effects against many bacteria, including Mycobacterium tuberculosis and methicillin-resistant Staphylococcus aureus (MRSA), viruses, and fungi (including Candida). Surprisingly for an antimicrobial substance, there are also immune-stimulatory, anti-inflammatory, antioxidant, analgesic, and spasmolytic effects. Of the white blood cells, monocytes and macrophages are most affected, especially with increased phagocytic activity. Application by either vapor inhalation or oral route provides benefit for both purulent and nonpurulent respiratory problems, such as bronchitis, asthma, and chronic obstructive pulmonary disease (COPD) (Sadlon & Lamson, 2010).

Essential oil use as a topical agent can also afford benefits in critical care to lessen the patient's dependence on the benzodiazepines used for sedation during ventilation. Critically ill patients undergo prolonged painful interventions such as mechanical ventilation. To tolerate these unpleasant stimuli, infants and children in particular are sedated with continuous infusions of narcotics. Both insufficient and excessive use of sedatives can be harmful to patients. An 18-month-old previously healthy female was admitted with respiratory distress secondary to adenovirus pneumonia. Her pneumonia progressed to respiratory failure, requiring endotracheal intubation and mechanical ventilation within 48 hours of admission. She failed extubation on day eight of mechanical ventilation secondary to subglottic edema caused by thrashing from inadequate sedation. After reintubation, attempts to resume sedation at lower levels were not tolerated by the patient.

A bispectral index (BIS) monitor was placed to monitor the patient's level of sedation while receiving a continuous paralytic infusion. The BIS monitor is a processed, continuous electroencephalogram which objectively measures the depth of sedation and lack of recall. Bispectral index monitoring is used intraoperatively and in the intensive care unit when a patient is paralyzed and subjective measures of discomfort cannot be relied on to gauge discomfort. A goal BIS score of 40 to 60 was chosen to achieve minimal recall and adequate sedation. After 45 hours of sedation and paralysis on advancing doses of midazolam and morphine, the mean BIS score was 59 (40 to 77). The mother asked permission to massage her child while receiving mechanical ventilation. The massage oil consisted of a 7.5% total concentration of Roman chamomile (Anthemis nobilis), sandalwood (Santalum album), and galbanum (Ferula gummosa) in a base of jojoba oil (Simmondsia chinensis). The mother was instructed to apply 2.5 mL of the essential oil blend every 6 to 8 hours to her daughter's arms, legs, and chest. The child received two applications 9 hours apart. The second application was given when the child appeared agitated after a sponge bath. The BIS declined from 50 to 44 within 1 hour of the first application on the legs, reaching at nadir at 2 hours postapplication of 32. The midazolam infusion was reduced by 50% to 0.1 mg/kg/hour within 2 hours of the first application and remained at that level for the remainder of her mechanical ventilation. Mean BIS score postapplication was 41 for the remaining 16 hours before extubation despite the 50% reduction in midazolam infusion. She was discharged home 18 days after admission, 6 days after being successfully extubated (Hadayat 2008).

References

Cha, J. H., Lee, S. H., & Yoo, Y. S. (2010). Effects of aromatherapy on changes in the autonomic nervous system, aortic pulse wave velocity and aortic augmentation index in patients with essential hypertension. *Journal of Korean Academy of Nursing Korean, 40*(5), 705–713.

Hedayat, K. M. (2008). Reduction of benzodiazepine requirements during mechanical ventilation in a child by topical application of essential oils. *Explore (NY), 4*(2), 136–138.

Kiecolt-Glaser, J. K., Graham, J. E., Malarkey, W. B., Porter, K., Lemeshow, S., & Glaser, R. (2008). Olfactory influences on mood and autonomic, endocrine, and immune function. *Psychneuroendocrinology, 33*(2), 328–339.

Nicolato, E., Boschi, F., Marzola, P., & Sbarbati, A. J. (2009). Secretory response induced by essential oils on airway surface fluid: a pharmacological MRI study. *Ethnopharmacology, 124*(3), 630–634.

Sadlon, A. E., & Lamson, D. W. (2010). Immune-modifying and antimicrobial effects of eucalyptus oil and simple inhalation devices. *Alternative Medicine Review, 15*(1), 33–47.

Weblink: Acute Sinusitis

indoors in an air-conditioned atmosphere whenever possible. In many situations, this is difficult because patients are being asked to change their lifestyles or elements within their life that are very important to them (e.g., pets). In these instances, the nurse acts as a support person to the patient.

Sinusitis

Rhinosinusitis (sinusitis) is defined as the inflammation of the nasal cavity and the paranasal sinuses. It is traditionally subdivided into acute (symptoms lasting less than 4 weeks), subacute (symptoms lasting 4 to 12 weeks), and chronic (symptoms lasting more than 12 weeks) (Hwong & Getz, 2011). Recurrent acute rhinosinusitis is described as four or more intermittent episodes of rhinosinusitis annually.

Epidemiology and Etiology

More than 35 million people in the United States are estimated to have rhinosinusitis, with an estimated 1 out of 7 adults affected with the disease (Brook, 2011). Acute rhinosinusitis can be classified as viral rhinosinusitis (AVRS) or bacterial rhinosinusitis (ABRS). A viral infection associated with the common cold is the most frequent etiology. Chart 26–4 outlines the causes of rhinosinusitis.

Chronic rhinosinusitis (CRS) can be divided into different syndromes with significantly different causes, contributing factors, and medical management. They are CRS with nasal polyposis, many polyps (abnormal tissue growth from the mucous membrane), or overgrown tissue (20% to 33% of cases); CRS without nasal polyposis (60% to 65%); and allergic fungal rhinosinusitis (8% to 12%) (Hamilos, 2011). CRS with polyposis is associated with asthma and aspirin sensitivity (refer to the section on polyps on page 697). The polyps usually contain high levels of eosinophils, cytokines, and histamines. CRS without polyposis lacks nasal polyps or allergic mucin. It may include patients with anatomic abnormalities or immunodeficiency. Allergic fungal rhinosinusitis is identified by the presence of fungal colonization in the allergic mucin. These patients usually have polyposis and are immunocompetent (Benninger, 2010). Bacterial infections can further complicate all types of chronic rhinosinusitis.

Pathophysiology

The paranasal sinuses, which are part of the upper respiratory tract, are in direct communication with the nasopharynx. Because of the proximity to nasopharyngeal flora, obstruction can cause bacterial infection. When sinusitis is caused by a bacterial or viral infection, a person develops a sinus infection, which can result in a reduced ability of the paranasal sinuses to function normally. For example, if sinus and nasal polyps occur near the sinus openings (ostia), the sinuses can become obstructed. When the ostia are obstructed, the normal flow of air into the sinuses and mucus drainage out of the sinuses is impeded and the mucociliary transport system becomes impaired, leading to more stagnation of secretion and epithelial damage, with subsequent bacterial growth. The reduced flow of air and mucus allows mucus to become stagnant, which, in turn, contributes to the growth of bacteria and infection. Once a bacterial infection is present, it causes inflammation and swelling, which leads to an increase in mucus production. The cycle continues and ultimately leads to sinusitis.

CHART 26–4 Common Causes of Rhinosinusitis

Viral	Bacterial	Fungal
Rhinovirus	Streptococcus pneumoniae	Mucormycosis
Influenza	Haemophilus influenzae	Aspergillus
Parainfluenza	Moraxella catarrhalis	
Respiratory syncytial virus	Staphylococcus aureus	
Adenovirus		

Clinical Manifestations

Symptoms of sinusitis can include nasal congestion and obstruction, purulent nasal drainage, fever, weakness, maxillary tooth pain, facial pain that worsens when leaning forward, headache, fatigue, cough, and ear pressure (Hwang & Getz, 2011). Patients with high fevers and severe headache should seek immediate medical attention.

Chronic rhinosinusitis patients repeatedly present with at least two of the following complaints: purulent drainage, nasal obstruction, facial pain or pressure, and decreased sense of smell (Hamilos, 2011).

Laboratory and Diagnostic Procedures

Diagnosis of acute rhinosinusitis is made by clinical suspicion of presenting symptoms, particularly purulent rhinorrhea, nasal congestion, and/or face pain, although symptoms can be unreliable. Cultures lack accuracy, and radiographic studies are usually not necessary. Nasal endoscopy can be helpful in identifying patients with extensive disease marked by evidence of nasal polyps, deformation of the middle meatus, and nasal secretions (Leung & Katial, 2008). A CT scan also can be used to evaluate underlying disease and when medical management has been unsuccessful.

Medical and Surgical Management

Unlike a viral cold or an allergy, acute bacterial sinusitis requires antibiotic treatment to cure the infection. If sinus symptoms do not improve after 5 to 7 days, it becomes more likely that the infection is caused by bacteria and will respond to an antibiotic. However, about half of all bacterial sinus infections will resolve without antibiotics. Nasal corticosteroids may reduce inflamed nasal mucosa and, when used in conjunction with antibiotics, significantly relieve symptoms (refer to the Pharmacology box on page 700).

In general, treating chronic sinusitis is similar to treating acute sinusitis, which is done with administration of antibiotics if there is evidence of bacterial infection. When the cause is aspirin sensitivity, patients may benefit from aspirin desensitization. Leukotriene modifiers that block proinflammatory mediators can be helpful and have been shown to reduce polyp size (refer to the Pharmacology box on page 700). If patients are refractory to medical management, surgical intervention may be indicated. Functional endoscopic sinus surgery improves sinus ventilation and drainage. Because surgery does not treat the inflammatory disorder, it should always be followed with medical management to decrease inflammatory responses (Hamilos, 2011).

Nursing Management

Nursing care of the patient with rhinosinusitis relies heavily on assessment of signs and symptoms and obtaining a thorough patient history. The history must include the onset and duration of the symptoms, including site of pain or discomfort, redness of eyes, flushing of face across the nose, fever, weakness or fatigue, cough, congestion, sore throat, muscle ache, and sore teeth. It also is important to know whether any particular event or incident triggered the patient's symptoms.

If the patient requires surgical intervention, preoperative and postoperative care becomes important, as detailed in Chapters 17 and 19. Specific to the patient with rhinosinusitis would be airway management, pain control, and assessment for and prevention of infection. As these patients tend to have outpatient or short-stay surgeries, educating the patient about the signs and symptoms of potential complications contingent on the type of surgery is very important. For functional endoscopic sinus surgery, it is important to keep the nose free from build-up of crusts. This can be achieved by teaching the patient how to perform nasal douching with a neti pot. These are sold over the counter at most pharmacies and health food stores. Patient education also includes information about the cause of the rhinosinusitis and how to avoid its triggers: air pollution, diving, underwater swimming, and known allergens and irritants.

Nasal Obstruction

Nasal obstruction may be broadly described as any occurrence that blocks the flow of air in the nose. This feeling of blockage can result from many nasal disorders previously discussed in this chapter, such as those that cause a deformity of the cartilaginous or bony structures (e.g., fractures, a deviated nasal septum) and those that cause swelling and infections of the nasal lining and the turbinate bones (rhinitis and sinusitis). Two other common causes of nasal obstruction are nasal polyps and foreign bodies.

Nasal Polyps

Nasal polyps are small, saclike growths consisting of inflamed nasal mucosa and sinus linings. The nasal examination reveals a grayish, grapelike mass within the nasal cavity. Nasal polyps are smooth, pear-shaped growths of nasal mucosa that are gelatin-like, semitranslucent, and pale.

Polyps are usually benign, can occur on one or both sides of the nose, and are more commonly seen in adults than in children. The polyps may originate near the ethmoid sinuses (located at the top of the nose) and grow into the sinus cavities. Large polyps can obstruct this part of the upper airway. In adults, nasal polyps are most frequently associated with chronic sinusitis, asthma, and aspirin sensitivity (Wang, 2011). Almost one out of four patients with nasal polyps is intolerant to aspirin (Wang, 2011). In these individuals, ingestion of aspirin is followed by wheezing, excessive watery nasal discharge, and swelling of the throat, which can be fatal if not treated immediately.

The initial treatment of polyps usually is medical. Systemic corticosteroids, such as prednisolone, also reduce symptoms temporarily. Antibiotics are indicated if there is evidence of bacterial infection. Functional endoscopic sinus surgery for removal of the polyps is a standard of treatment and has shown to be efficacious, although complete eradication is uncommon (Bachert, Gevaert, & Cauwenberge, 2008). Most patients notice marked improvement in their breathing after removal of polyps, although they should be informed that polyps often recur. One way to prevent polyp regrowth is to continue to use topical steroid sprays for an extended period of time. Although most polyps are not cancerous, once removed, they should be sent for pathologic examination to ensure that no malignancy is present.

Nursing Management

Nurses assist in the examination of patients for polyps by assessing and documenting symptoms, including history, length of "stuffy nose" syndrome, and other related allergy symptoms. A major focus of nursing intervention and evaluation is patient education on the prevention of polyps. Patients can reduce their chances of developing or having nasal polyps recur after treatment through the following:

- Managing allergies and asthma by following the treatment plan
- Avoiding nasal irritants such as tobacco smoke, chemical fumes, and dust
- Practicing good hygiene by washing hands regularly to protect against bacteria and viruses that cause inflammation of the nasal passages and sinuses
- Using a humidifier at home if the air tends to be dry to improve mucus flow and prevent blockage and inflammation
- Using a nasal rinse or nasal lavage containing saltwater to improve mucus flow and remove allergens and other irritants.

It also is important for the nurse to complete a health history to determine allergic patterns and any signs of genetic implications.

Anosmia

Anosmia is the loss or impairment of the sense of smell. For most people, the ability to sense thousands of different odors is a normal occurrence. However, to a minority, this natural skill is lost due to a disorder of the olfactory system. Odors bring both enhancement and improvement of an individual's life, whether it is the smell of food, fragrances, or a scent associated with a particular event or person. Smell also has other functions. Taste is to a great extent determined by smell, so a loss of smell often leads to a loss of taste.

The loss of smell usually is the result of nasal congestion, a cold, or an obstruction, but sometimes it can indicate a neurological disorder. Loss of the sense of smell also may be idiopathic (without any identifiable cause). Some diminution of smell occurs normally with aging.

Temporary anosmia is common with colds and nasal allergies such as hay fever. It also may occur following a viral illness. In addition, the sense of smell is lost with disorders that prevent air from reaching the part of the nose where smell receptors are located (the cribriform plate located high in the nose). These disorders may include nasal polyps, nasal septal deformities, and nasal tumors. Other disorders that may cause anosmia include tumors of the head or brain, head trauma, endocrine and nutritional disorders, and neurological disorders.

Treatment of underlying disorders may correct the loss of sense of smell. This includes antihistamines (if the condition is related to allergy), surgical correction of physical blockages, treatment of other disorders, and changes in medication. If loss of the sense of smell is permanent, dietary counseling may include use of highly seasoned foods and stimulation of taste sensations that remain by eating foods that have that taste.

Nursing Management

Nurses are responsible for assessing the patient's symptoms, documenting and reporting them to the primary health care provider, and providing supportive care to the patient. Education as to the cause and alleviation of symptoms is a primary duty for the nurse. The nurse also plays a key role in assessing and evaluating the patient's response to treatment and communicating this to the primary care provider.

Nurses must educate the anosmic patient and her family about taking measures to ensure safety around the home. Electric appliances rather than gas appliances should be used, as should smoke detectors and technologies such as carbon monoxide alarms that detect the presence of gas fumes in the home.

Mucormycosis

Mucormycosis, also referred to as zygomycosis, is an opportunistic fungal infection that is capable of causing rhinal, orbital, cerebral, and pulmonary infections. This rare but often devastating disease typically develops in patients with weakened immune systems, diabetes, kidney failure, organ transplants, or those associated with chemotherapy. It also may develop in patients receiving an iron chelating drug called deferoxamine (Desferal) as treatment for acute iron poisoning.

Epidemiology and Etiology

The species of fungus responsible for human infection is generally acquired by inhaling the spores released into the air from decaying vegetation and soil. Since these agents are ubiquitous in the environment, potential for exposure is common. Spores can also be introduced through open skin lesions, such as those caused by trauma, or through the gastrointestinal route, although these routes of infection are less common (Kontoyiannis & Lewis, 2009). Most patients that develop mucormycosis have an underlying predisposing condition, most commonly diabetes (Kontoyiannis, 2011). Other risk factors include glucocorticoid treatment, burns, organ transplantation, traumatic injury, metabolic acidosis, cytotoxic chemotherapy, and chelation therapy with deferoxamine (see the Risk Factors for Mucormycosis box). Spores inhaled by immunocompetent persons are usually transported to the pharynx and then cleared by the gastrointestinal tract. Patients at risk tend to develop primary infection in the nasal turbinates and alveoli. Pulmonary mucormycosis most commonly occurs in patients with neutropenia or patients treated with corticosteroids, while rhino-orbital or rhinocerebral infections are more common in patients with diabetic ketoacidosis (Kontoyiannis, 2011).

RISK FACTORS for Mucormycosis

Diabetes mellitus	High glucose and acidic conditions stimulate growth, predisposing patients with ketoacidosis to increased susceptibility. Diabetes is the most common risk factor for mucormycosis.
Deferoxamine and iron overload	Iron enhances fungal growth and leads to increased host susceptibility. Deferoxamine, which is an antidote for iron or aluminum toxicity, increases iron uptake by the fungus. Patients with deferoxamine-related mucormycosis often have disseminated disease with high mortality rates. Newer iron-binding agents, such as deferasirox, do not increase susceptibility.
Prolonged neutropenia	The lowering of white blood cell count compromises immunity. Those who are immunosuppressed are more susceptible to the fungal infection. Leukemia, bone marrow or stem cell transplantation, and use of corticosteroids, cytotoxic agents, and broad-spectrum antibiotics that produce neutropenia are all recognized causes.
Hematologic malignancies	Etiology of mucormycosis in patients with hematologic malignancies is unclear. Proposed possibilities include use of voriconazole therapy (an independent risk factor), aggressive immunosuppressive agents, and reduction in mortality from aspergillosis in hematopoietic stem cell transplantation, allowing for the emergence of rare fungal infections.
Skin disruption	The most common transmission mode in immunocompetent patients. It can be due to burns, trauma, and intravenous drug use.

Pathophysiology and Clinical Manifestations

Mucormycosis is caused by fungi of several different species, including Mucor, Rhizopus, Absidia, and Rhizomucor. The fungus gains entry into the body through the nasopharynx. It can be inhaled into the lungs (pulmonary mucormycosis), or it can extend to the sinuses, orbit, and brain (rhino-orbital-cerebral). Upon gaining access to the mucous membranes of the patient's nose or lungs, the organisms multiply rapidly and invade the nearby blood vessels. The fungi destroy soft tissue and bone, as well as the walls of blood vessels. Regardless of the anatomic site involved, the organism causes tissue infarction and necrosis. The common sites include the following:

- Rhinocerebral mucormycosis involves the spread of spores into the orbit or brain following inhalation. The fungus destroys the tissue of the nasal passages, sinuses, or hard palate, producing a black or pus-filled discharge and visible patches of dying tissue. The overt symptoms of rhinocerebral mucormycosis include acute sinusitis, fever, eye swelling and protrusion of the orbit (proptosis), dark nasal eschar (scabbing), and redness progressing to ecchymosis of the overlying skin. General symptoms also may include headache, nausea, and lethargy. Visual loss secondary to thrombosis of the retinal artery or direct fungal invasion may occur. The fungus then invades the tissues around the eye socket and eventually the brain. At that point, the patient may have convulsions or paralysis on one side of the body.
- Pulmonary mucormycosis occurs when the fungus enters the patient's lungs, where it can cause airway obstruction, pulmonary vessel erosion, and potentially fatal pulmonary hemorrhage. It can travel across tissue planes and invade adjacent organs, including the diaphragm, chest wall, and pleura (Kontoyiannis, 2011). Early symptoms of pulmonary mucormycosis include fever, nonproductive cough, and progressive difficulty breathing. Vascular invasion can lead to massive hemoptysis (blood in the sputum).
- The symptoms of gastrointestinal mucormycosis are not unique to the disease; this may complicate diagnosis. Patients typically complain of pressure or pain in the abdomen and nausea and vomiting.

Safety Alert *When caring for a patient in diabetic ketoacidosis, if findings of orbital cellulitis and vision changes are present, the nurse must notify the healthcare team immediately to rule out mucormycosis. The progression of the disease occurs very quickly over a few hours, and the time lapse between recognizing the findings and instituting therapy is critical.*

Laboratory and Diagnostic Procedures

Diagnosis of mucormycosis usually is based on a combination of the patient's medical history and a visual examination of the nose, throat, and eyes. Once mucormycosis is suspected, obtaining tissue for culture is vital. Specimens should be obtained from areas such as suggestive skin lesions, necrotic areas found in the nasopharynx, and nasal discharge that may appear like clotted blood. A positive diagnosis is made when the tissue specimen reveals Mucor fungi and the species is oryzae. Other diagnostic procedures are listed in the Diagnostic Tests for Mucormycosis box.

Medical and Surgical Management

Treatment of mucormycosis involves managing the antifungal treatment and surgical debridement. Therapy should be initiated as soon as mucormycosis is suspected and not be delayed for culture

DIAGNOSTIC TESTS for Mucormycosis

Test with Description, Rationale, and Normal Values	Expected Abnormality
CT and/or MRI	
Normal facial anatomy without edema or foreign body identified *Serial CT and MRI scans are used to identify the extent of the disorder, as well as the destruction of soft tissue or bone in patients with advanced disease*	Edema Foreign body Structural abnormality
Chest X-Ray	
Normal chest and lung markings without fluid, blood, or collapse. *Chest x-rays sometimes reveal a cavity in the lung or an area filled with tissue fluid if the patient has pulmonary mucormycosis.*	Structural abnormality Fluid/edema/blood in the lung tissue

results. This is a rapidly progressive disease, and delay in early and aggressive treatment can be fatal. Effective antifungals include Amphotericin B, posaconazole, voriconazole, fluconazole, and flucytosine (refer to the Pharmacology box on page 700). Surgery is disfiguring for rhinocerebral mucormycosis because it may involve the removal of the palate and nasal and orbital structures. Reconstructive surgery is inevitable for those who have disfigurement due to severe rhinocerebral mucormycosis. Hyperbaric oxygenation, breathing 100% FiO_2 while under increased atmospheric pressure to hyperoxygenate the blood by dissolving oxygen in the plasma, may be indicated and has proven to be very helpful in conjunction with long-term therapy with antifungal drugs. In addition, underlying comorbidities such as hyperglycemia, acidosis in diabetic patients, nutritional problems, neutropenia, lymphopenia, and immunosuppression must be addressed.

Nursing Management

The nurse is responsible for assessing the patient for clinical manifestations of mucormycosis. Obtaining an accurate and complete patient history is essential. Following diagnosis and treatment, the nurse assumes preoperative and postoperative care of the patient. This includes administration of antibiotics, airway management, pain control, and preoperative and postoperative care as outlined in Chapters 17 and 19. During this phase, the nurse should be particularly sensitive to the fear and anxiety related to possible disfigurement and the high mortality rate of the disease. Postoperatively, the nurse should be careful to change occlusive dressings frequently and check the underlying skin for any signs of possible fungal infection.

Health Promotion

Follow-up care includes educating patients about the signs of recurrent mucormycosis, particularly facial swelling and a black discharge from the nose, and advising patients to see a health care provider at once if they notice these symptoms. Prevention also is critical for patients with mucormycosis. Patient and family education on protecting high-risk patients from contact with sugary foods that encourage fungal growth and avoiding inhalation of fungi from decaying plants, moldy bread, manure, and other breeding grounds for fungi is done during hospitalization and reinforced with discharge instructions.

Disorders of the Pharynx and Oral Cavity

The oral cavity, tongue, and pharynx are the anatomic conduits to the esophagus and airway. The pharynx assists in speech and swallowing and begins the division of the airway from the esophagus. The oral cavity, which includes the tongue, is responsible for ingestion, taste, and other sensory responses to food, chewing, swallowing, speech, and respiration. The tongue is an articulator for speech, a propulsion device for swallowing, and a sensor for taste. These organs are susceptible to disease, which may affect an individual's ability to communicate and take in nutrition. Disorders specific to the pharynx and oral cavity are discussed in the following sections.

Sleep Apnea

Sleep apnea is a disorder in which a person stops breathing for more than 10 seconds with at least five or more episodes per hour. Severe sleep apnea is defined as more than 30 apneic events per hour. The three main types of sleep apnea are central, obstructive, or a mix of both.

Etiology, Epidemiology, Pathophysiology, and Clinical Manifestations

The cause of central sleep apnea is impairment in the respiratory center drive such that the brain fails to send the appropriate signal to the breathing muscles to initiate respirations; thus, there is no respiratory effort. It is caused by an underlying factor that affects the brain, such as high altitude, or a disease process, such as renal failure. This is the less common form of sleep apnea. Obstructive sleep apnea (OSA) is caused by physical obstruction from tissues in the upper airway. Air cannot flow into or out of the person's mouth, despite continued efforts to breathe. This is evidenced by a paradoxical motion of the abdomen and rib cage with respiratory effort. The incidence of sleep apnea varies with how it is defined. It is estimated that 20% of the population have sleep apnea when defined as *five or more* apnea episodes per hour. Alternatively, 2% to 9% of the population has sleep apnea when defined as more than five apnea episodes per hour plus evidence of at least one clinical symptom such as daytime sleepiness and fatigue (Strohl, 2011).

Obesity is the single most important risk factor for OSA among middle-aged adults (see the Risk Factors box) (Pien & Pack, 2010). The greater the degree of obesity, the higher the prevalence of OSA. OSA is marked by nighttime symptoms as well as consequential symptoms during the day. Features of OSA that occur at night include loud

RISK FACTORS for Obstructive Sleep Apnea

Obesity
Upper airway or craniofacial anatomic abnormalities
Smoking (3 times more likely to have OSA)
Nasal congestion (regardless of cause)
$>$ 65 years of age
Male (2 to 3 times $>$ females)
Higher risk females include: postmenopausal

Source: Pien, G., & Pack, A. (2010). Sleep-disordered breathing. In R. Mason (Ed.), *Murray and Nadel's textbook of respiratory medicine* (5th ed.). Philadelphia: Saunders Elsevier.

Video: Sleep Apnea—Etiology and Pathophysiology

PHARMACOLOGY Summary of Medications Used to Treat Upper Airway Disorders

Medication Category and Action	Application/Indication	Nursing Responsibility
Decongestants		
Sympathomimetics: Pseudoephedrine Phenylephrine Phenylpropanolamine ***Action:*** Stimulates the sympathetic nerve endings including alpha-beta 1 and alpha-beta 2 receptors. Decreases nasal membrane edema by constricting nasal arterioles.	Common cold, sinusitis, allergic rhinitis, nasal congestion.	Monitor heart rate and blood pressure, especially in those with a history of cardiac disease. Patient teaching: Discontinue medication and consult healthcare provider if extreme restlessness or irregular heartbeats occur. Do not breast-feed while taking this medication.
Vasoconstrictors		
Oxymetazoline ***Action:*** Acts directly on alpha receptors of the sympathetic nervous system. Constricts smaller arterioles in nasal passages and has a prolonged decongestant effect.	Common cold, sinusitis, allergic rhinitis, nasal congestion.	Monitor use of nasal spray—if excessive use, discuss the possibility of rebound congestion. Patient teaching: Wash hands after handling spray; if rubbed into eyes, it may cause anisocoria (unequal pupil size) and blurred vision. Do not exceed recommended dosage. Do not breast-feed while taking this medication.
Antihistamines First Generation		
Diphenhydramine Chlorpheniramine Azelastine ***Action:*** H1-receptor antagonist and antihistamine with anticholinergic activity. Competes for H1-receptor sites on effector cells, thus blocking histamine release.	Temporary symptomatic relief of allergic reactions.	Monitor heart rate and blood pressure especially with pre-existing cardiovascular disease. Monitor for drowsiness and supervise ambulation. Older adults are especially prone to manifest dizziness, sedation, and hypotension. Patient teaching: Do not use alcohol or other depressants while using this drug. Do not drive or do other potentially hazardous activities. Increase fluid intake. Do not breast-feed.
Antihistamines Second Generation		
Loratadine Cetirizine ***Action:*** Long-acting antihistamine selectively blocks peripheral histamine H1-receptor activity.	Temporary symptomatic relief of allergic reactions.	Monitor heart rate and blood pressure. Report tachycardia or hypertension. Monitor for drowsiness and supervise ambulation. Patient teaching: May cause significant drowsiness in older adult patients and those with liver or kidney impairment. Do not drink alcohol or take other depressants. Do not breast-feed.
Antihistamines Third Generation		
Desloratadine Loratadine Levocetirizine ***Action:*** Long-acting, nonsedating antihistamine with selective H1 receptor antagonist properties. Reduces human mast cell release of the inflammatory cytokines exhibiting antiallergic effects.	Treatment of seasonal or perennial allergic rhinitis.	Monitor heart rate and blood pressure. Report tachycardia, palpitations, or change in BP. Monitor renal and liver function test. Patient teaching: May cause significant drowsiness in older adult patients and those with liver or kidney impairment. Do not use alcohol or other depressants. Do not take more often than every other day if a known renal impairment exists. Do not breast-feed.
Anticholinergic		
Ipratropium bromide ***Action:*** Produces local, site-specific effects on larger central airways including bronchodilation and prevention of bronchospasm.	Nasal spray—perennial rhinitis, colds. Nebulizer/inhalation—maintenance therapy for COPD.	Assess effectiveness—when given via nebulizer, assess breath sounds before and after; wheezes and tightness should decrease. Patient teaching: Medication is not an emergency agent—it has a delayed onset. For best results, allow 30 to 60 seconds between puffs. Rinse mouth after puffs to decrease bitter taste. Do not breast-feed.

Medication Category and Action	Application/Indication	Nursing Responsibility
Anti-infectives		
Fluoroquinolones/quinolones • Ciprofloxacin (Cipro) • Ofloxacin (Floxin) • Levofloxacin (Levaquin) • Moxifloxacin (Avelox) ***Action:*** Exerts bacteriocidal effect by disrupting synthesis of gram-negative and gram-positive bacterial DNA.	Acute exacerbation of chronic bronchitis, community-acquired pneumonia, sinusitis.	Monitor for effectiveness—decrease inflammation. Report any tendon inflammation or pain—the drug should be discontinued. Monitor urine output and pH—it should be less than 6.8 and patient should be well hydrated to prevent crystalluria. Administration with theophylline derivatives or caffeine can cause CNS stimulation. Patient teaching: Immediately report tendon pain. Fluid intake should be 2 to 3 L/day if not contraindicated. Restrict caffeine. Do not breast-feed.
Anti-infectives Tetracyclines		
• Doxycycline (Vibramycin) • Tetracycline (Sumycin) ***Action:*** Exerts bacteriostatic effect by inhibiting bacterial protein synthesis in gram-positive and gram-negative bacteria. May be bacteriocidal at higher doses.	Respiratory tract infections, Chlamydia, gonorrhea, tetanus, Helicobacter pylori, Lyme disease.	Monitor for effectiveness—decrease inflammation. Report sudden onset of painful or difficult swallowing—oral forms of medication are associated with esophagitis. Patient teaching: Take oral medication with a full glass of water to ensure passage into stomach and prevent esophageal ulceration. Avoid taking tablet within 1 hour of lying down. Avoid exposure to direct sunlight to reduce risk of phototoxic reaction (appears like an exaggerated sunburn). Do not breast-feed.
Antifungals		
• Amphotericin B • Posaconazole • Voriconazole • Fluconazole • Flucytosine ***Action:*** Causes fungal cell death by altering fungal cell membrane.	Progressive or potentially fatal systemic fungal or protozoal infections.	Monitor for effectiveness—decrease inflammation. *Note:* Drug may cause increase of ALT, AST, alkaline phosphatase, and bilirubin serum values. Monitor and report any elevation in BUN, serum creatinine, and liver function tests, as the drug can be hepatotoxic and effect renal function. Be aware of drug interactions and monitor for decreased efficacy or toxicity (oral hypoglycemics, Coumadin, phenytoin, theophylline, and others). Monitor for hypoglycemia in diabetic patients.
Corticosteroids Intra-Nasal		
Flunisolide Budesonide ***Action:*** Drug concentrations achieved at receptor sites in the nasal mucosa.	Allergic rhinitis.	Assess for effectiveness—decrease inflammation. Monitor nasal passages for dryness or crusting—provide lubricant. Patient teaching: Gently blow the nose to clear nostrils prior to using. If two sprays are prescribed, direct one toward the upper, and the other toward the lower, part of nostril. Wash the cap and nosepiece daily with warm water, dry thoroughly to prevent contamination with bacteria. Inhaled steroids do not provide immediate symptomatic relief.
Corticosteroid Oral		
Prednisolone tebutate ***Action:*** Analog of hydrocortisone with 3 to 5 times greater potency. Effective as an anti-inflammatory agent.	Anti-inflammatory.	Evaluate effectiveness—decreased inflammation. Give at mealtime to decrease gastric irritation. Be alert to masked infection and delayed healing—inspect oral cavity for Candida infection—white patches, black furry tongue, painful membranes and tongue. Patient teaching: Adhere to prescribed dose—do not increase, decrease, or omit doses or dose intervals. Report gastric distress or sign of an ulcer. Do not breast-feed.

snoring, apneic episodes, and snorting or choking sounds that may cause arousal. Common features of daytime symptoms include fatigue, sleepiness, and poor concentration. OSA occurs more frequently in the presence of systemic hypertension, pulmonary hypertension, cerebrovascular disease, cardiac arrhythmias, and ischemic stroke. If severe OSA is not treated, it can lead to heart failure and a three- to sixfold increase in mortality (Strohl, 2011).

Diagnostic Studies

A thorough history and a physical exam are important to differentiate OSA from other causes of daytime sleepiness. The standard of diagnosis of OSA is overnight polysomnography in a sleep laboratory. Sleep stages, respiratory effort, oronasal airflow, oxygen saturations, and electrocardiogram are monitored and measured. These measures are evaluated for frequency of occurrence and physiological effect. These tests are used both to diagnose sleep apnea and to determine its severity.

Medical Management

The treatment for central sleep apnea is to treat the underlying cause. For instance, if a patient experiences sleep apnea due to renal failure, nocturnal dialysis would optimize medical management and relieve the periods of apnea. If the patient has heart failure, use of CPAP (continuous positive airway pressure) by mask during sleep may relieve the periods of apnea (see the following text).

When evaluating for OSA, differential diagnosis includes restless leg syndrome, narcolepsy, insufficient sleep syndrome, medical conditions, depression, and side effects of medications. Treatment for OSA varies depending on the degree of sleep apnea and the patient's willingness and compliance. Behavioral changes such as weight loss are an important part of the treatment program. The individual should avoid the use of alcohol, tobacco, and sleeping pills. In some patients with mild sleep apnea, breathing pauses occur only when they sleep on their backs. In such cases, the use of pillows and other devices that help the person sleep in a side-lying position is often helpful. In cases of mild sleep apnea, some patients may obtain relief from the use of a dental device that moves the tongue or mandible forward.

Specific management strategies for OSA include positive airway pressure, an oral appliance, and surgical intervention. Patients with significant symptoms should be targeted for specific OSA therapy rather than waiting to see whether behavior modification is successful (Kryger, 2011). Positive pressure is a first-line therapy for severe OSA. The American Academy of Sleep Medicine recommends offering positive airway pressure therapy as an option to all patients diagnosed with OSA and recommends it for all patients with significant sequelae, such as daytime sleepiness or fatigue, desaturation, and/or greater than 15 apneic or hypopnea (overly shallow breathing or very low respiratory rate) episodes per hour.

Positive airway pressure is applied through a tight-fitting face or nasal mask and can be delivered as continuous positive airway pressure (CPAP), bilevel positive airway pressure (BPAP), or auto-titrating positive airway pressure (APAP). All forms force the airways open, preventing collapse and reducing apnea or hypopnea events. CPAP provides a continuous and constant level of airway pressure throughout the inspiratory and expiratory respiratory cycle. BPAP allows for the titration of inspiratory and expiratory pressures separately. APAP uses pressures that are more patient driven, depending on airflow, circuit pressure, or snoring. APAP tends to be better tolerated by patients, but clinically there is no proven benefit of one form of positive airway pressure over the others. CPAP and BPAP are discussed in detail in Chapter 28 (Care of the Patient with Complex Respiratory Disorders). Significant evidence demonstrates that positive airway pressure reduces nighttime events, reduces daytime symptoms, and improves quality of life (Kryger, 2011). Success in outcomes is related to compliance with therapy.

Oral appliances are devised to manipulate the mandible forward or retain the tongue in a forward position, preventing the soft tissues of the oropharynx from falling back and obstructing the airway. Surgical intervention is a successful option in patients with a surgically repairable obstructing lesion. In patients with severe, life-threatening apnea associated with serious cardiac dysrhythmias or frequent hypoxic events that do not respond to other therapies, a tracheostomy may be the only option.

Nursing Management

The nursing process guides the management of patients with sleep apnea. Nurses are in a unique position to assess sleeping patterns of hospitalized patients and refer the patients to experts if they display symptoms of sleep apnea (see the Evidence-Based Practice box). The outcome objective is to have normal airway function and relief of symptoms. Patients who undergo surgical intervention are placed on a pulse oximeter to monitor oxygen saturation level, and lung sounds are assessed for adventitious sounds. Patients who have had obstructive sleep apnea for an extended period of time develop higher pulmonary pressures due to the obstruction. Once the obstruction has been modified, the positive end-expiratory pulmonary (PEEP) pressures decrease. PEEP is the alveolar pressure above atmospheric pressure that exists at the end of expiration. This can result in a condition called flash pulmonary edema, which is potentially life threatening (see Chapter 28). This change can happen very quickly; therefore, the patient is monitored closely for shortness of breath, pink frothy sputum, and the inability to lie flat for the first 24 hours after surgery. The integrity of the surgical site in the posterior pharynx and tonsillar pillars is assessed by direct observation with a tongue blade and flashlight. As with most oropharyngeal surgery, use of straws is prohibited so as not to disrupt clot formation with higher intraoral pressures.

Oral Cavity Disorders

Disorders of the oral cavity involve the teeth, tongue, mouth, maxilla, and tonsils. These affect chewing, taste, nutrition, and speech articulation. *Healthy People 2020* identify oral health as central to a person's overall health and well-being. The stated 2020 goal is to prevent and control oral and craniofacial diseases, conditions, and injuries and improve access to preventive services and dental care (U.S. Department of Health and Human Services, 2010). See the National Guidelines box for additional information on oral health.

Hairy Tongue

Hairy tongue is a condition in which the tongue is covered with hair-like papillae and can appear black, brown, green, or white depending on the cause. Possible causes include poor hygiene, use of broad-spectrum antibiotics, or radiation treatment to head or neck. It is generally asymptomatic and can be treated by brushing the tongue with a toothbrush or a tongue scraper. A topical antifungal can be applied if Candida albicans develops.

Dental Caries

Dental caries are the result of the destruction of tooth enamel caused by dental plaque. Plaque, a substance formed by the interaction of saliva and food proteins, coats the teeth and breaks down tooth enamel. Deep crevasses in teeth, poor quality enamel, lack of fluoridated water, and

EVIDENCE-BASED PRACTICE Recognizing Obstructive Sleep Apnea in Hospitalized Patients

Clinical Problem

Although symptomatic obstructive sleep apnea (OSA) affects approximately 2% to 5% of the population, it is thought to be routinely underdiagnosed and consequently may go undiagnosed for many years. Since the problem occurs at night when patients are sleeping and is complicated by additional sleep pattern disturbances in hospitalized patients, OSA can be difficult to recognize and diagnose. It has been postulated that if nurses were aware of the risk factors for developing OSA, conducted focused sleep assessments, and monitored patients' sleep patterns, they could be influential in differentiating OSA from other sleep pattern disturbances of hospitalized patients. Early identification of OSA by nurses could lead to diagnosis, treatment, and improved patient outcomes.

Research Findings

Sheldon, Belan, Neill, and Rowland (2010) did a literature review of the risk factors associated with OSA as well as OSA screening tools in an effort to develop an evidence-based nursing assessment tool that would facilitate the recognition of OSA in hospitalized patients. They found several important risk factors and an applicable screening tool to support their goal. Risk factors include obesity, hypertension, and sleep position. The metabolic and anatomic changes that occur in the body with obesity dramatically increase the risk of OSA (Lavie, Vishnevsky, & Levie, 2007). Hallowell, Stelloato, Schuster, and colleagues (2007) found that approximately 90% of research participants with BMI >40 kg/m^2 had OSA and concluded that all persons with this index should be screened for OSA, whether or not they had other risk factors. In addition, Davidson and Patel (2008) found that a waist circumference >102 cm in both men and women, even in participants that were not obese, correlated strongly with OSA. They also found that the severity of OSA was greater in men than in women. Several studies have found that the incidence of OSA increased considerably in obese patients in the 40- to 65-year-old age range (Chung, Ward, Ho, Yuan, Kayumov, & Shapiro, 2007; Hwang et al., 2008; Martinez-Rivera, Abad, Fiz, Rios, & Morera, 2008; Okabayashi et al., 2007). Hypertension has also been associated with undiagnosed OSA (Davidson & Patel, 2008; Hwang et al., 2008). The correlation appears to be highest in persons with uncontrolled hypertension. Sleep position is a potential risk factor. Supine position has been shown to produce the greatest upper airway occlusion, with approximately 56% in patients with OSA that preferred the supine sleeping position, particularly so in younger patients (Richard, Kox, den Herder, Laman, van Tinteren, & de Vries, 2006). In regards to OSA screening tools, the Berlin Questionnaire (BQ) has shown the greatest statistical success in correlating high risk for OSA with confirmed diagnosis with polysomnography. The BQ consists of questions that focus on (a) snoring, (b) fatigue/sleepiness, and (c) hypertension/BMI. Patients are identified as high risk if they had significant risk in two of these three categories.

Implications for Nursing Practice

OSA can reduce quality of life and predispose patients to other medical problems that can increase morbidity and mortality. When patients with undiagnosed OSA are hospitalized, nurses are in a position to identify risk, monitor patients, detect apnea spells, and refer patients to experts for further work up. In addition, armed with the knowledge that the supine position predisposes a patient to airway occlusion and apnea episodes, nurses can advocate sleep positions that are not supine and that elevate the head of the bed by 30 degrees. Developing a tool for nurses that can help to identify the subjective and objective signs and symptoms of OSA risk and give nurses the autonomy to refer patients when criteria is met could have a direct impact on the quality of life and the morbidity and mortality of patients with OSA.

Critical Thinking Questions with answers can be found in the Osborn Student Resources at nursing.pearsonhighered.com.

References

Chung, F., Ward, B., Ho, J., Yuan, H., Kayumov, L., & Shapiro, C. (2007). Preoperative identification of sleep apnea risk in elective surgical patients, using the Berlin Questionnaire. *Journal of Clinical Anesthesia, 19*(2), 130–134.

Davidson, T. M., & Patel, M. R. (2008). Waist circumference and sleep disordered breathing. *Laryngoscope, 118*(2), 339–347.

Hallowell, P. T., Stelloato, T., Schuster, M., Graf, K., Robinson, A., Crouse, C., et al. (2007). Potentially life threatening sleep apnea is unrecognized without aggressive evaluation. *The American Journal of Surgery, 193*, 364–367.

Hwang, D., Shakir, N., Limann, B., Sison, D., Kalra, S., Shulman, L., et al. (2008). Association of sleep-disordered breathing with postoperative complications. *Chest: The Cardiopulmonary and Critical Care Journal, 130*(3), 1128–1134.

Lavie, L., Vishnevsky, A., & Levie, P. (2007). Oxidative stress and systemic inflammation in patients with sleep apnea: Role of obesity. *Sleep and Biological Rhythms, 5*(2) 100–110.

Martinez-Rivera, C., Abad, J., Fiz, J., Rios, J., & Morera, J. (2008). Usefulness of truncal obesity indices as predictive factors for obstructive sleep apnea syndrome. *Obesity, 16*(1), 113–118.

Okabayashi, K., Kasahara, E., Uchiyama, H., Yodota, K., Togashi, Y., Kono, C., et al. (2007). Obstructive sleep apnea-hypopnea syndrome patients with overweight and hypertension in a Japanese workplace. *Journal of Occupational Health, 49*(2), 117–124.

Richard, W., Kox, D., den Herder, C., Laman, M., van Tinteren, H., & de Vries, N. (2006). The role of sleep position in obstructive sleep apnea syndrome. *European Archives of Oto-Rhino-Laryngology, 263*(10), 946–950.

Sheldon, A., Belan, I., Neill, J., & Rowland, S. (2010). Nursing assessment of obstructive sleep apnea in hospitalized adults: A review of risk factors and screening tools. *Contemporary Nurse, 34*(1), 19–33.

NATIONAL GUIDELINES for Oral Health: *Healthy People 2020*

Risk Factor	Guideline Objective
Limited access to and availability of dental services: People who have the least access to preventative services and dental treatment have greater rates of oral disease. Education level, income, race, and ethnicity affect a person's ability to access oral health care.	Increase number of community health centers with an oral health component Increase the capacity of state dental health programs to provide preventive oral health services Increase the use of oral health care systems Increase the proportion of low-income children and children who receive preventative dental service Increase the proportion of school-based health centers with an oral health component
Increase in tooth decay in children 2 to 5 years old	Increase the proportion of children who have received dental sealants Increase the fluoridated water in community water systems
Health behaviors that lead to poor oral health and cancer include: • Tobacco smoke • Diabetes • Excessive alcohol use	Increase the oral and pharyngeal cancer screening Increase testing and referral for glycemic control

Source: Adopted from U.S. Department of Health and Human Services. (2010). *Healthy People 2020.* Retrieved from http://www.healthypeople.gov/2020/topicsobjectives2020/default.aspx.

poor dental hygiene also contribute to dental caries. If left untreated, dental caries can lead to a dental abscess and eventually loss of the affected tooth.

Ludwig's Angina

Ludwig's angina is an infection that arises from the floor of the mouth involving the sublingual and submaxillary spaces of the deep neck, usually seeded from an infected molar. The spread of a rapid growing and aggressive cellulitis develops that may lead to airway obstruction or aspiration pneumonia. Clinical presentation includes fever, chills, oral pain, drooling, and dysphagia. Dyspnea, stridor, and cyanosis may develop as the disease progresses. Diagnosis is usually made on the basis of imaging studies. Treatment includes airway management, broad-spectrum antibiotics, and surgery if any abscesses are identified, although this is uncommon. Intubation should occur prior to the onset of stridor; if this is not possible, an emergent tracheostomy should be performed.

Tonsillitis

The tonsils are masses of lymphoid tissue found in the root of the tongue (lingual tonsil), on both sides of the oropharynx (palatine tonsil), and on the superior wall of the nasopharynx (pharyngeal tonsil). **Tonsillitis** is an inflammation of the tonsils, most commonly caused by a virus, and occurs mainly in children. Symptoms are sore throat; red, swollen tonsils; dysphagia; odynophagia (painful swallowing); fever; and enlarged, tender lymph nodes in the neck. Tonsillitis usually is self-limiting and treated symptomatically. However, if a throat culture reveals the cause as group A beta-hemolytic streptococci, then an antibiotic will be prescribed. Complications such as sinusitis, mastoiditis, rheumatic fever, or peritonsillar abscess may occur with tonsillitis. Surgery to remove the tonsils (tonsillectomy) may be necessary for individuals with repeated infections.

Peritonsillar Abscess

Peritonsillar abscess, also known as Quinsy tonsillitis, is a rare complication of tonsillitis in which infection spreads to the tissue around the tonsillar capsule. Symptoms are severe throat pain, mouth breathing, drooling, and muffled voice. Physical examination reveals a large unilateral fullness of the affected tonsillar pillar and soft palate, and deviation of the uvula to the unaffected side. A peritonsillar abscess is treated with incision and drainage of the abscess, use of antibiotics, and supportive care such as pain management and hydration. A tonsillectomy may be necessary 4 to 6 weeks after recovery from a peritonsillar abscess. This prevents recurrent infection and removes scar tissue from the tonsillar area. Nursing care should focus on antibiotic therapy, pain control, hydration, nutrition, and airway protection during the acute episode.

Pharyngitis

Pharyngitis is an inflammation of the pharynx, which results in a sore throat. Upper respiratory infections such as the common cold or flu may lead to pharyngitis. It occurs most frequently in the winter months and usually resolves on its own. For symptomatic comfort the patient should increase fluid intake; take analgesics, such as NSAIDs; and gargle with warm saltwater. Pharyngitis from a Streptococcus infection requires antibiotics.

Epiglottitis

The epiglottis is a flap of tissue and cartilage that covers the opening of the trachea during swallowing. **Epiglottitis** is a life-threatening bacterial illness that may lead to airway obstruction. Epiglottitis is seen more frequently in children but also occurs in adults. The cause of the infection usually is Haemophilus influenzae group B. The incidence of epiglottitis has dramatically decreased since the H. influenzae vaccination was added to the regular immunization schedule in infants, although other strains of *H. influenzae*, streptococci, and *Staphylococcus aureus* can also lead to epiglottitis. The infection and inflammation affect the epiglottis and surrounding supraglottic structures. Symptoms are a cherry red epiglottis, drooling, inspiratory stridor, dyspnea, and high fever. **Stridor** is the raspy noise heard in the upper airway as the result of air attempting to move through a narrowed opening. Initial treatment focuses on maintaining a patent airway with conservative measures of oxygen, humidification, and inhaled respiratory therapy. An artificial airway, an endotracheal tube, or a tracheostomy should be considered early; waiting for signs of airway compromise is associated with increased mortality (Burns & Hendley, 2010). Antibiotic therapy, usually cefotaxime, ceftriaxone, or ampicillin, should be administered as initial therapy. Nebulized epinephrine and steroids have not proved to be effective in treating epiglottitis (Burns & Hendley, 2010). Rifampin prophylaxis is recommended for all household contacts.

Nursing Management

Nursing care of patients with oral cavity disorders should focus on administration of antibiotic therapy, pain control, hydration, nutrition, and airway protection.

Assessment

For all patients with oral cavity disorders, it is critical for the nurse to assess and monitor the patient for any airway compromise. Prevention of nausea and vomiting and intervention to prevent aspiration when necessary is of great importance.

Nursing Diagnosis

Nursing diagnoses for the patient with oral cavity disorders may include the following:

- *Ineffective Airway Clearance* related to inflammation
- *Risk for Aspiration* related to inflammation
- *Acute Pain* related to inflammation
- *Risk for Infection* related to untreated dental caries
- *Imbalanced Nutrition: Less Than Body Requirements* related to pain and difficulty swallowing

NANDA-I © 2012

Planning

The overall goals for the patient with oral cavity disorders will be patency of the airway, control of pain, adequate nutritional intake, and prevention of infection.

Outcomes and Evaluation Parameters

The patient will have a patent airway as exhibited by normal respiratory effort, clear breath sounds, and adequate pulse oximetry. The patient's pain will be controlled as exhibited by her statement of the level of pain on a 1 to 10 scale. Nutritional and fluid intake will be adequate to maintain body weight and promote healing.

Interventions and Rationales

Effective oral care is essential for healthy healing and prevention of complications. Patient education includes the importance for mouth and teeth cleaning and dietary requirements. A nutritional consult can assess the patient's nutrition and home requirements for enteral feeding or an oral soft or liquid diet. Chapter 8 includes a detailed discussion on nutrition.

Disorders Related to the Larynx and Trachea

Caring for a patient with a disorder of breathing requires that nurses have knowledge of airway anatomy and physiology. Nurses must advocate for these patients, who often are unable to speak and breathe without assistance. Specific disorders related to the larynx and trachea are discussed in the following text.

Anatomy and Physiology of the Larynx

The glottic structures include the larynx, the epiglottis, the arytenoids (small cartilages at the back of the larynx to which the vocal cords are attached), and the true and false vocal folds. The larynx and trachea are two major structures of the upper airway. The larynx, which connects the oropharynx to the trachea, is supported by firm cartilaginous structures that prevent collapse during inspiration. The larynx functions to protect the lungs from foreign substances and is needed for normal speech.

The epiglottis, which is located above the larynx, moves downward and acts like a sphincter during swallowing to cover the larynx, thus preventing food and fluid from entering the lungs. This same sphincter-type function is what allows for coughing, completion of a Valsalva maneuver (bearing down), and vocalization. Closing of the glottis (vocal folds) creates a brief increase in intrathoracic pressure and intra-abdominal pressure. Rapid opening of the glottic opening allows quick upward movement of the air and produces a cough or a bolus of air that can be transformed into speech.

The cavity of the larynx is divided into two pairs of folds: upper vestibular folds and lower vocal folds, also known as vocal cords. The vestibular folds function as protection. The folds and the space between the folds create the glottis. The vocal fold itself is composed of five layers: the epithelium, the superficial layer, the intermediate layer, the deep layers of the lamina propria, and the vocalis muscle (Figure 26–6◆). The larynx transmits air to and from the upper airway or the oropharynx and trachea and lungs. The vocal cords produce sound, and the oral cavity, palate, tongue, and lips function as articulators as the air passes through the oropharynx and mouth.

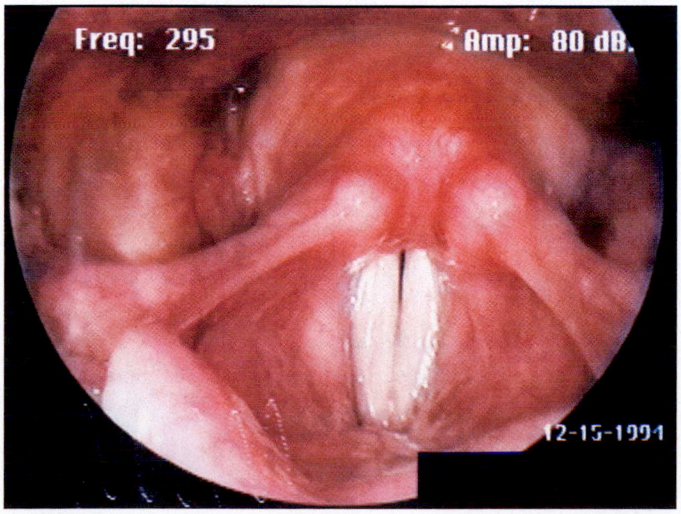

FIGURE 26–6 ◆ Normal vocal cords in resting position.
Source: Ann E. F. Sievers, RN

Two synovial joints in the larynx are of importance: the cricothyroid joint and the cricoarytenoid joint. The cricothyroid joint allows movement of the cords by changing the length of the vocal cords, thereby controlling vocal pitch. The cricoarytenoid joint allows for the adduction (movement toward the midline) and abduction (movement away from the midline) of the vocal cords during breathing, eating, and speaking. At the onset of inspiration, the laryngeal nerve is stimulated, which causes the vocal cords to abduct or open just before air is taken into the lungs.

These structures are vulnerable to trauma, disease, infection, inflammation, edema, and damage to the structures or to the nerves innervating these structures. This type of damage can result in respiratory, swallowing, and speaking disorders.

The 10th cranial nerve (vagus nerve) innervates the larynx. The superior laryngeal branch and the recurrent laryngeal branch are responsible for both motor function and sensation in the larynx. The location of these nerves makes them very vulnerable to damage by surgery or trauma to the neck and chest.

Safety Alert *Any patient who has undergone laryngeal or thyroid surgery or anterior chest or neck trauma must be observed for airway and voice changes. The implication is a temporary or permanent injury to the larynx. The nurse needs to observe the patient eating and drinking and assess for any difficulty with swallowing. This can include coughing, choking while eating, or experiencing a sensation as if something is caught in the throat. If noted, the nurse should alert the healthcare team and suggest a swallow study.*

Vocal Cord Paralysis

Vocal cord paralysis is a disorder that occurs when one or both of the vocal cords (vocal folds) do not open or close properly. This paralysis results in difficulty swallowing and coughing. Food or liquids slip into the trachea and lungs because the paralyzed cord or cords remain open, leaving the airway passage and the lungs unprotected.

Etiology, Epidemiology, and Pathophysiology

Vocal cord paralysis may occur at any age from birth to advanced age. It occurs equally in males and females from a variety of causes. It can be unilateral or bilateral and may occur as the result of an infectious process, trauma to the neck or chest area, neurological disorders, cancer, or surgical trauma. The most common cause of unilateral cord paralysis is surgical injury (thyroidectomy, carotid artery surgery, or transcervical procedures) (O'Handley, Tobin, & Shah, 2011). Cancer or tumors can also compress or invade the nerves, and must be ruled out. Etiologies of bilateral cord paralysis include cervical or thyroid surgery or CNS disorders. Bilateral cord paralysis can obstruct the glottis and cause significant respiratory distress. Because of the lengthy pathway of the vagus nerve to the recurrent laryngeal nerve, any surgery or injury involving the neck and chest area has the potential to lead to vocal cord paralysis. If the nerve is completely severed, there is little hope of regaining motion to the affected cord. However, if the nerve is stretched or bruised during the procedure, there may be a slow return of vocal cord function over a period of up to 12 months. Airway obstruction usually is not a problem with unilateral vocal cord paresis, but voice changes and possible aspiration remain a concern.

Clinical Manifestations

The primary clinical manifestation of vocal cord paralysis is a change in the voice. It may become hoarse (croaky or rough); breathy, as though the individual is exhaling excessive air when speaking; and weakened. Other clinical manifestations include the following:

- Shortness of breath
- Noisy breathing
- Choking or coughing while swallowing food, drink, or saliva
- The need to take frequent breaths while speaking
- Inability to speak loudly
- Inability to "bear down" (Valsalva)

If a patient indicates that he is breathing normally but is unable to speak—that is, the patient is **aphonic** (without a voice)—the nurse should suspect bilateral vocal cord paralysis. With bilateral cord paralysis, the patient will not be able to speak, produce an effective cough, or perform a Valsalva maneuver. If the patient has paralysis to only one of the vocal cords, the nurse can expect to hear a soft breathy or hoarse voice and minimal to no difficulty breathing. The severity of the patient's symptoms (breathy voice, ineffective cough, and dysphagia) depends on the position of the paralyzed cord, the degree of injury to the cord (paresis versus paralysis), and the ability of the opposite cord to compensate.

Damage to the vagus nerve and its branches can have a significant impact on the patient's quality of life. Because the vocal cords have an integral role in the protection of the airway from aspiration, damage here can affect the patient's ability to eat and drink. This damage also may alter the sensation of the larynx, making the individual unable to sense the insults of aspiration. Persistent aspiration can be significant enough that the patient will not be able to eat orally. The larynx and the vocal cords must be able to close completely to prevent food and fluids from entering the airway and to allow the patient to build up sufficient intrathoracic and intra-abdominal resistance to produce an effective cough. Additionally, the patient's ability to communicate is affected because this nerve is necessary to allow the opening, closing, and vibration of the vocal cords as air moves up from the lungs. Without this ability, the voice may be hoarse, weak, or nonexistent. Alteration in communication and method of eating are significant changes for any patient.

Diagnostic Procedures

Direct visualization of the vocal cord is done by flexible laryngoscopy. The scope is a thin flexible tube with a light and camera that can be passed down the patient's throat for direct visualization of the cords to determine whether one or both cords are affected. Additionally, laryngeal electromyography (EMG) is a test that assesses the spontaneous and voluntary activity of the laryngeal muscles, and is particularly helpful in identifying laryngeal nerve integrity (Woodson, Blitzer, Alexander, & Grant, 2010). This helps identify whether a neural lesion is the source of vocal cord paralysis. A CT scan is useful when a neoplasm (abnormal growth of tissue/tumor) is the cause of vocal cord paralysis. It helps to demonstrate the extent of the neoplasm on the vocal cords and surrounding structures.

Medical and Surgical Management

The treatment of unilateral paralysis is determined by the severity of **hoarseness,** an abnormal change in the quality of voice and aspiration risk. Speech and swallow therapy may help if the paralysis is mild. If aspiration or severe phonation difficulty is present, surgical intervention may be undertaken to protect the airway or to improve vocal ability. The procedure, termed medialization, brings the paralyzed cord into the adducted (closed) position so that the two cords can meet in the midline to allow for vocalization and prevent aspiration. The mobile cord still is able to move aside during breathing to allow adequate respiration. Medialization can be done either with the injection of a material such as a collagen derivative or with the placement of an implant.

The primary focus of bilateral cord paralysis is airway protection. If the cords are paralyzed in the adducted (closed) position, respiratory insufficiency and stridor exist. If they are paralyzed in the abducted (open) position, aspiration and severe phonation problems exist. Often, a tracheostomy is required to protect the airway. In the case of permanent cord paralysis, laser arytenoidectomy (removal of the arytenoid cartilage), cordotomy (freeing the vocal ligament and the vocal muscle from the vocal process of the arytenoids enlarging the airway), or vocal fold lateralization can be considered. These procedures are intended to improve the patient's ability to communicate and prevent aspiration.

Nursing Management

The nursing process guides the management of patients with vocal cord paralysis.

Assessment

Nursing assessment includes observation of the patient's ability to swallow thin liquids, voice changes (hoarseness or inability to speak loudly), and the inability to finish a sentence without taking multiple breaths. In addition, the nurse needs to monitor the patient's pronunciation of long -s sounds for signs of congestion and oxygen saturation. These parameters need to be assessed regularly and after each oral intake.

Nursing Diagnosis

Nursing diagnoses for the patient with vocal cord paralysis may include the following:

- *Ineffective Airway Clearance* related to cord paralysis and risk of aspiration
- *Risk of Aspiration* related to incomplete closing of the vocal cords
- *Risk of Infection* related to aspiration

NANDA-I © 2012

Outcomes and Evaluation Parameters

The expected outcome is prevention of aspiration. Evaluation parameters include the following:

- Lungs are clear to auscultation.
- Oxygen saturation is greater than 95% or within normal range.
- There is no increase in respiration or work of breathing.
- The patient denies feeling short of breath.
- Nutrition/swallowing
- Normal communication

Interventions and Rationales

Nursing interventions for the protection of the patient's airway include the following:

- Elevating the head of the bed to decrease pooling of secretions in the airway.
- Suctioning the oral cavity of excess secretions, and having suction available for the patient to use.
- Encouraging intake of fluids to keep the mucosa and the vocal folds hydrated to prevent irritation.

Nursing interventions to prevent aspiration include the following:

- Having the patient sit upright in a chair to eat and staying with the patient to observe for coughing or frequent throat clearing after swallowing. If the patient appears to be having significant problems with fluids or foods, the tray should be removed, and the patient's response to eating should be reported to the health care provider and documented.
- Having dietary services thicken any liquids to make them easier to swallow.
- Providing solid foods, thickened fluids, or foods with a custard-like consistency, which seem to be less of a problem because the patient has more control of the food bolus. This stimulates sensation when swallowing, thus decreasing the risk of aspiration.

Collaborative Management

A formal evaluation by a health care provider and a trained speech pathologist should be done, and a dynamic swallow study should be completed to determine the safest and most appropriate diet for the patient. In order to meet desired patient outcomes, it is essential that this interdisciplinary team communicate openly with one another in developing and evaluating care of the patient and family (IOM [Institute of Medicine], 2010). Patients with unilateral vocal cord paralysis are likely to have trouble with swallowing thin liquids safely and are prone to aspiration.

For some patients, their voice is their livelihood, and damage to their vocal cords can create psychological as well as physical changes. For example, singers, teachers, radio and television announcers, clergy, and politicians who depend on their voices may be unable to return to their chosen profession. Therefore, the patient should be observed for signs and symptoms of depression, and these should be discussed with the health care provider. Working with a speech therapist and learning how to maximize the remaining function of the vocal cords can help the patient physically by decreasing the risk of aspiration and mentally by improving the patient's communication skills.

Laryngeal Disorders

Hoarseness of the voice occurs because of the disruption of the normal vibration of the vocal cord. Hoarseness is defined as an abnormal change in the quality of voice. The voice may reflect altered pitch, breathiness, strained quality, weakness, or tremors. The causes of hoarseness include acute or chronic laryngitis, malignancy, benign vocal fold lesions, neurologic dysfunction, non-organic issues, or systemic causes. Hoarseness in older patients is discussed in the Gerontological Considerations section on page 725. Any patient with hoarseness that persists for longer than 2 weeks without the coexistence of an upper respiratory infection should be thoroughly evaluated, particularly if the patient is at risk of head and neck carcinoma (i.e., individuals who use tobacco and alcohol).

Acute Laryngitis

Laryngitis is an inflammation of the larynx and vocal cords or just the larynx. The most common cause of acute laryngitis is a viral upper respiratory tract infection or acute vocal strain. When laryngitis occurs as part of an upper respiratory infection, the patient also may experience coughing, rhinorrhea, and a mild sore throat. The infection causes edema and inflammation of the vocal cords, which prevents them from vibrating properly. Acute strain, often caused by loud yelling or protracted coughing, can lead to edema and hemorrhage to the vocal fold and cause laryngitis.

Acute laryngitis secondary to a viral infection usually is self-limiting and does not require medical treatment. Antibiotics rarely are necessary unless there is evidence of a coexistent bacterial infection. Humidification, hydration, and voice rest usually are sufficient to allow the edema to resolve and the voice to return to normal. Symptomatic relief of sore throat, fever, and cough is appropriate.

Chronic Laryngitis

Chronic laryngitis is a result of long-standing inflammation to the larynx and vocal folds. Examination of the larynx usually reveals redness of the true vocal cords and possibly edema. Causes include irritants that lead to injury over time, such as inhaled toxins (smoke, chemicals, and pollens), gastroesophageal reflux disease (GERD), chronic sinusitis, chronic alcohol use, or mechanical irritation from frequent coughing or throat clearing.

Chronic irritation can lead to a chronic inflammatory state that presents clinically as a hoarse voice and a barking cough. Individuals who overuse and abuse their voices, such as loud screaming sports fans or singers, teachers, preachers, and politicians who use their voice for long periods at a time day after day, may develop chronic irritation and inflammation to their vocal cords.

Medical Management

The health care provider should obtain a thorough medical history from any patient who presents with a hoarse voice. This includes observing specific qualities of the voice; exacerbating and ameliorating factors; pattern of onset; other head and neck symptoms; and a history of smoking, alcohol use, or GERD. In addition, the patient's troublesome or stridorous breathing should be assessed. It is essential to determine the use of any accessory muscles of respiration, because this indicates respiratory distress. The health care provider should assess risk factors such as a recent viral or bacterial illness, voice abuse or trauma, smoking and secondhand smoke exposure, and work environment for exposure to paint, chemicals, fertilizers, pets, or cleaning solutions. Chronic laryngitis is usually treated by the removal of the offending trigger. Resting the voice, hydration, humidification, and changes in voicing practices, such as how loudly a person speaks, may also be helpful.

Health Promotion

Instructions regarding voice rest must be reinforced for patients with laryngitis. The nurse should instruct patients that if they must speak, they should use a regular speaking voice and not a whisper. Whispering is more strenuous on the vocal cords than speaking in a normal voice and, thus, can exacerbate the problem. Patients should be instructed to carry a notepad and pen or a handheld communication device. If a patient is in the hospital for any condition that requires strict voice rest, the nurse needs to place a sign above the patient's bed indicating "Patient Is on Voice Rest."

Patients should be instructed to avoid inhaling irritants if this is the cause of the chronic inflammation. The nurse should stress the importance of smoking cessation and avoidance of secondhand smoke and should refer the patient to a smoking cessation program if needed. It may be necessary for the patient to wear a mask in the workplace if there are irritating substances in the environment. The nurse should encourage the patient to work with the occupational health nurse at the worksite and to find protective equipment to prevent further exposure to those substances.

Laryngeal Edema

Etiology and Clinical Manifestations

Laryngeal edema is defined as swelling in any region of the larynx. There are a variety of causes including anaphylactic allergic reactions, gastroesophageal reflux disease, laryngopharyngeal reflux disease, and endotracheal intubation. Allergic reaction is a common inflammatory response that can lead rapidly to airway obstruction. Laryngeal edema associated with anaphylaxis is usually of sudden onset and results from exposure to a specific allergen. Common precipitators are bee stings, foods, or medicines. The edema may be mild at first, causing hoarseness and a scratchy sensation in the throat. The reaction can progress rapidly to anaphylaxis, which involves airway obstruction and circulatory collapse if the patient is particularly sensitive to the allergen or has a significant exposure to a target food or medication. Anaphylaxis is a medical emergency and is discussed in detail in Chapter 53.

Nursing Management

The priority for nursing management of edema to the larynx is to summon medical assistance and support the patient's airway. While waiting for the healthcare provider's arrival, the nurse needs to elevate the head of the bed, monitor oxygen saturations, and provide supplemental oxygen. An intravenous (IV) line is inserted to administer medications to reverse the allergic response; these may include IV steroids and antihistamines. Epinephrine given subcutaneously or in aerosolized form via nebulizer treatments typically is effective. If the obstruction is severe and the patient does not respond rapidly enough to medications, a tracheotomy (p. 711) can establish an airway until the edema resolves. A tracheotomy is placed instead of an endotracheal tube because the swelling in the airway would make it impossible to view the landmarks needed to perform the intubation and the laryngeal edema would make it difficult to pass the endotracheal tube. Waiting until there is no air moving through the cords because of severe laryngeal edema can have fatal consequences. See the Nursing Management section on Airway Obstruction on page 711 for further details.

Vocal Cord Pathology

Vocal Cord Nodules

Vocal cord nodules, also called "singer's" or "screamer's" nodes, are a result of chronic microtrauma from vocal strain; they can be thought of as scars or calluses on the vocal cords (Figure 26–7◆). The nodules develop initially from submucosal hemorrhages resulting from an impact injury between the cords. The nodule may appear as a red edematous area on the cord, but with continued trauma to the area, it becomes thick and fibrosed. Vocal cord nodules typically occur in individuals who abuse their voices such as cheerleaders, singers, teachers, bartenders, coaches, and politicians. Smoking, allergies, and gastric reflux can exacerbate the situation and inhibit healing. These nodules, though painless, produce persistent hoarseness as they inhibit normal vibration and closure of the vocal cords. The patient will present with complaints of painless hoarseness, inability to sing in the higher ranges, inability to speak for a long period of time, or having a breathy voice. Typically the nodules will resolve with humidification, hydration, voice rest, and treatment by a speech therapist to teach the patient the correct way to use the voice and correct the underlying abuse issues. Some patients require surgical removal of the nodules.

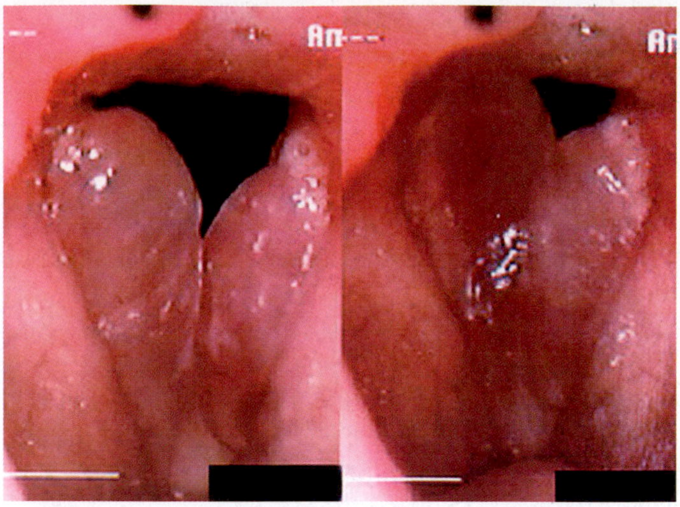

FIGURE 26–7 ◆ Vocal cord nodules/vocal hemorrhage/abuse.
Source: Ann E. F. Sievers, RN

Vocal Cord Polyps

A vocal cord polyp is a growth that typically occurs only on one side of the vocal cord, in a variety of shapes and sizes. Vocal cord polyps are a result of long-term vocal abuse or chronic irritation. The main irritants include tobacco, inhaled irritants, and gastric reflux. Some polyps can result from hemorrhagic trauma due to coughing. Hoarseness occurs because of the disruption of the vibration of the cord, and breathiness develops because of incomplete closure of the cords due to the polyp. Treatment for polyps is voice therapy, smoking cessation, treatment for GERD, and surgery with microlaryngoscopy to remove the polyp.

Because polyps may return after surgical removal if the same predisposing conditions exist, postoperative treatment must include treatment and education about the underlying etiologic factors to help prevent recurrence, as well as speech therapy to learn how to speak or sing without irritating the vocal cords. Smoking cessation is encouraged; the patient must be offered information on programs and support groups at the health care facility or in the community.

Laryngeal Papillomas

Laryngeal papillomas are benign laryngeal growths associated with the human papillomavirus (HPV). Although laryngeal papillomas can affect any age group, children seem to have the most aggressive form in terms of recurrence, spread, and requirements for frequent intervention. Laryngeal papillomas are thought to be acquired during vaginal delivery in mothers with HP.

The papillomas can be widespread, and patients present with hoarseness and, if severe, progressive respiratory distress. Treatment of this disorder involves carbon dioxide (CO_2) laser ablation of the papillomas during laryngoscopy. Despite frequent surgical interventions, the papillomas may recur or spread. It is important to keep them from becoming large enough to cause airway obstruction. Placing a tracheostomy tube in a patient with laryngeal papillomas should be avoided unless necessary to maintain a patent airway, as this puts the patient at risk for recurrence and spread into the lower airway.

Laryngeal Spasm

Laryngeal spasm is an abnormal reflexive response to a laryngeal insult. The laryngeal glottis reflexively closes in an attempt to prevent aspiration into the trachea. Laryngospasm is an abnormal response to this reflex. It may occur spontaneously or be triggered by vocal cord irritation, pain, GERD, or anesthesia. Laryngeal spasm is the most frequent cause of airway obstruction after the removal of an endotracheal tube (Hagberg, Georgi, & Krier, 2007). Patients will have stridor and retractions or use of accessory muscles. In most cases caused by irritants or GERD, the laryngospasm usually resolves spontaneously within a minute or two. However, if it is caused by extubation (removal of an endotracheal tube) or anesthesia, it can be life threatening and may require chemical paralysis and reintubation. Patients should have their airways suctioned prior to extubation to prevent saliva or blood from irritating the cords. Suctioning is discussed in Chapter 27.

Effective interventions include keeping the offending food or environmental stimulants (chemicals, cleaners, or perfumes) away from the patient in order to avoid triggering a spasm. If the laryngeal spasm occurs at night as a result of reflux, the nurse should educate the patient regarding diet, head elevations, and lifestyle changes, as discussed later in the section on laryngopharyngeal reflux disease (p. 710).

Laryngeal Injury

Etiology, Epidemiology, and Clinical Manifestations

There are two classifications of laryngeal injury: external and internal. External laryngeal injuries usually are the result of blunt trauma to the neck. The primary cause is motor vehicle collisions in which an unrestrained person or passenger using a lap-belt only is thrown forward and his hyperextended neck collides with the steering wheel. Other scenarios include clothesline injury (as when a motorcyclist impacts a fixed horizontal object), sports-related injuries, suicidal or homicidal strangulation, or penetrating trauma (knife or projectile) (Sandhu & Nouraei, 2010). Internal injury of the larynx can occur with caustic ingestion, thermal injury, and foreign body injury. Laryngeal injury after radiation treatment also can occur because radiation weakens the tissue and causes irritation; inflammation and stenosis also can occur as a result. The incidence of laryngeal trauma is rare, occurring in 1 in 137,000 persons annually (Sandhu & Nouraei, 2010). Laryngeal injury can also be caused by prolonged endotracheal intubation in patients in critical care units. The long-term complications associated with endotracheal intubation include laryngeal, subglottic, and tracheal stenosis as well as vocal cord paralysis. Irritation and inflammation to the subglottic (below the vocal cords) and upper tracheal mucosa most often are caused by the cuff on the ET tube. Before the advent of low-pressure endotracheal and tracheal cuffs, tracheal stenosis and tracheal esophageal fistulas were not uncommon in patients requiring long-term intubation. A fistula is a communication between two specific areas such as the oral cavity and the skin or between the trachea and the esophagus. Today, damage secondary to high cuff pressure is less of a problem than irritation and inflammation from the cuff on an improperly secured ET tube. This inflammation can cause subsequent scarring and subglottic stenosis. Endotracheal intubation is discussed in detail in Chapter 28.

Signs and symptoms of external laryngeal injury include hoarseness, dysphonia, dysphagia, anterior neck pain, dyspnea, and hemoptysis. Leaking of air into the tissues of the neck can be assessed by the presence of palpable crepitations. External landmarks, such as the thyroid cartilage (Adam's apple), may not be visible or appear abnormal. The neck should be examined for abrasions, hematomas, or lacerations. Stridor and respiratory difficulty are symptoms of bleeding or swelling that is invading the airway. Airway compromise can be immediate or delayed. If a cartilage fracture of the larynx penetrates into or obstructs the airway, or swelling occurs rapidly, the patient will immediately demonstrate signs of airway distress.

DIAGNOSTIC TESTS for Acute Laryngeal Injury

Test with Description, Rationale, and Normal Values	Expected Abnormality
Plain Film X-Ray Normal laryngeal anatomy without subcutaneous air, edema, or foreign body identified *To look for hematoma or swelling in the surrounding tissue*	Extraluminal air Edema Foreign body Fracture of laryngeal cartilage
Flexible Endoscopy Normal laryngeal anatomy *Endoscopy allows the healthcare provider to view the anatomic structures and how they are functioning.*	Laceration or hematoma in the larynx Alteration in vocal cord function Failure of vocal cords to meet on the same horizontal plane
CT Scan Normal airway structures *CT scan quickly identifies detailed data on the integrity of the larynx and surrounding structures. Traumatic injuries can cause varying degrees of disruption and compromise.*	Disrupted laryngeal or tracheal cartilage Hyoid fracture Internal or external laryngeal hematoma Dislocation of the cricothyroid or cricoarytenoid joints Decreased airway diameter

Diagnostic Procedures

The Diagnostic Tests for Acute Laryngeal Injury box outlines the tests needed to determine injury and function.

Medical and Surgical Management

Management of laryngeal injury depends on the extent of injury. Patients with minimal injury and good airway patency can be closely observed for at least 24 hours, placed on humidified oxygen, and given corticosteroids. Antibiotics should be given if there is a tear in the laryngeal mucosa. Patients with more significant injury often require surgical intervention. Hematomas, dislocated cricoarytenoid joints, and some lacerations can be repaired endoscopically (Sandhu & Nouraei, 2010). More severe disruption should be explored and repaired in an open surgical approach.

Airway assessment and stabilization is the top priority of laryngeal trauma. A patient who is stridorous and in respiratory distress should undergo an emergency tracheostomy immediately (Sandhu & Nouraei, 2010). However, endotracheal intubation is not the preferred method of stabilizing the airway. It has the potential to extend laryngeal injury or create a false passage. Care must also be taken to maintain cervical stabilization, as cervical injury is often associated with laryngeal injury. Once the airway has been secured, the larynx and surrounding structures can be explored.

Nursing management of laryngeal injury was previously covered in the section on laryngeal edema.

Safety Alert *Hoarseness and early respiratory distress are signs that must not be overlooked or discounted on initial exam. The nurse needs to assess patients with blunt neck trauma carefully for hoarseness, respiratory distress, hemoptysis (bloody sputum), and dysphagia because these symptoms indicate airway injury and respiratory compromise.*

Laryngopharyngeal Reflux Disease

Laryngopharyngeal reflux disease is the laryngopharyngeal manifestation of gastric content regurgitation. This may lead to pathologic conditions of the upper aerodigestive tract (the organs and tissues of the respiratory and upper part of the digestive tracts), including chronic laryngitis, otitis media, and chronic sinusitis (Ali Mel, 2008).

Etiology, Pathophysiology, and Clinical Manifestations

The etiology of laryngopharyngeal reflux (LPR) is retrograde reflux of gastric acid into the larynx. LPR differs from GERD in several areas. The clinical manifestations of GERD are heartburn and esophagitis because it is a problem with the lower esophageal sphincter and primarily occurs in the supine position. LPR, on the other hand, involves only a 40% incidence of heartburn complaints and only a 25% incidence of esophagitis. Rather, it is primarily a problem with the upper esophageal sphincter and occurs mostly in the upright position during physical exertion (Franco, 2011).

Patients with LPR most often seek medical care because of hoarseness and throat irritation rather than heartburn symptoms. Upon further questioning, the patient may say, "It feels like something is in my throat, and I seem to be clearing my throat a lot." Typical clinical manifestations include the following:

- Hoarseness/dysphonia
- Chronic (ongoing) cough
- Nonproductive throat clearing
- Pain or sensation of a lump in the throat.

LPR has also been associated with vocal fold granulomas, laryngospasm, vocal polyps, and subglottic stenosis (Franco, 2011).

Laboratory and Diagnostic Procedures

Usually the diagnosis of LPR is based on the patient's symptom history and examination of the larynx. Examination of the structures with a fiber-optic scope reveals laryngeal edema, vocal cord edema, and evidence of subglottic edema; however, these symptoms may also be present in patients without LPR. Twenty-four-hour pharyngoesophageal pH monitoring may be used in diagnosis, and some healthcare providers consider it the gold standard. However, this has been debated, and the literature is not convincing.

Medical and Surgical Management

The three major methods of treating LPR are (1) dietary changes, (2) behavior modification, and (3) medications. Foods and beverages that can weaken the esophageal sphincters include caffeine, alcohol, carbonated drinks, chocolate, peppermint, and low-acid or spicy foods (citrus, tomatoes, salad dressings, curry, hot peppers).

Behavior modification can limit LPR symptoms. For example, smoking stimulates acid production and should be curtailed. A full, distended stomach will force contents into the esophagus, so eating small meals and avoiding exercise for 2 hours after eating will reduce the incidence of LPR. Patients should not eat for 3 hours before bedtime.

When diet and lifestyle changes are ineffective or when the edema and irritation are significant on physical exam, medications that neutralize the gastric acid, increase gastric emptying, or decrease the secretion of gastric acids help lessen the exposure of caustic acids to the sensitive tissues of the larynx. Medical management for LPR is necessary for much longer than that for gastroesophageal reflux disease because the tissues of the larynx are much more sensitive to the gastric acid and, therefore, take longer to respond to therapy and heal completely.

A surgical option is available for patients whose LPR does not respond to dietary and lifestyle changes. Laparoscopic Nissen fundoplication tightens the esophageal sphincter, making it more difficult for the gastric acid to reflux into the esophagus and larynx.

Nursing Management

Nursing management of patients with laryngopharyngeal reflux disease depends on the severity of the disorder and the patient's general state of health. Assessment of the airway is the first priority and includes lung sounds, oxygen saturation levels, and respiratory rate and depth. Any difficulty with breathing and gas exchange must be addressed immediately.

Collaborative Management

The multidisciplinary team may include a gastrointestinal specialist, pulmonologist, respiratory therapist, and dietitian. In order to meet desired patient outcomes, it is essential that this interdisciplinary team communicate openly with one another in developing and evaluating care of the patient and family (IOM [Institute of Medicine], 2010).

Nutritional evaluation by the dietitian is especially important for the patient with LPR. Patients with severe dysphagia or unhealed esophageal burns and erosions will need nutritional supplementation through a gastrostomy tube to allow the damaged tissue to heal and the patient to receive adequate nutrition to aid the healing process.

Health Promotion

Patients with LPR may have a difficult time understanding how they can have irritation in the throat without experiencing irritation in the esophagus. The nurse should explain that the tissue of the larynx is much more sensitive to the acids from the stomach than the esophagus; therefore, it does not take as much exposure to create irritation in the throat as it does in the esophagus. It is important for the patient to understand the correlation between reflux disease and hoarseness. If the patient does not understand this connection, she may be reluctant to initiate the medication and dietary and lifestyle modifications required to treat this disease.

Upper Airway Obstruction

Upper airway obstruction is a potentially life-threatening event that requires immediate and aggressive intervention. If left untreated, complete obstruction will cause respiratory failure followed by respiratory arrest, cardiac arrest, and death within minutes. Intervention must be swift and appropriate. Partial airway obstruction may initially appear adequate; however, the condition may worsen quickly and convert to a complete obstruction with little warning. Prompt identification of precipitating cause and rapid initiation of treatment to prevent worsening of condition are necessary to reduce morbidity and mortality.

Etiology and Clinical Manifestations

Specific causes of acute obstruction include foreign bodies, viral and bacterial infections, fire or smoke inhalation, anaphylaxis, trauma, vocal cord dysfunction, angioedema (rapid swelling of the subcutaneous tissue, mucosa and submucosa), or an acute or chronic condition such as a tumor or cancer.

Patients with complete airway obstruction will have no lung sounds on auscultation, owing to no air movement, and the patient will not be able to speak or cough. There may, however, be some gagging or choking in an effort to clear the airway. If the patient can speak or the nurse can auscultate breath sounds, then the airway still has at least partial patency. Partial obstruction usually produces inspiratory stridor. Signs of worsening condition and imminent respiratory failure include ashen or central cyanosis, retractions, diminished air movement, decreased mental status, and either tachypnea or bradypnea.

Diagnosis and Medical and Surgical Management

Initial evaluation and assessment of airway obstruction should focus on the patency of the airway. Evidence of complete obstruction, or progressing partial airway obstruction, and/or respiratory failure calls for lifesaving management. The etiology of the airway obstruction needs to be considered in determining the appropriate intervention. If the patient is not in extreme distress as with a partial airway obstruction, the nurse should obtain a medical and surgical history from the patient or the family regarding the onset and progression of the respiratory difficulty. Questions should focus on recent symptoms of an infection (sore throat, runny nose, fever, cough, dysphagia, or odynophagia), head and neck trauma, new medications, foreign body ingestion, or recent dental extractions. The patient should also be asked whether he has recently been diagnosed and/or treated for a cancer of the head and neck, and the nurse should determine whether the patient has had any prior experience with respiratory difficulty. Often patients who present with partial obstruction secondary to a head or neck malignancy will relate recent weight loss, difficulty eating, coughing with meals, hoarseness, difficult or painful swallowing, or shortness of breath with minimal activity.

The nurse should note any surgical scars to the neck and ask the patient about those past surgeries. It is necessary to determine whether the patient had a thyroidectomy, carotid endarterectomy, goiter removal, tracheostomy, or cervical spine surgery with an anterior neck approach. This information can help the nurse focus on possible causes of the airway distress.

The nurse should place an IV line for medication and fluid administration. In addition, oxygen and humidification are indicated. The health care provider may order administration of IV steroids to decrease swelling in the airway. Even a small increase in the airway's diameter can make a significant improvement in the patient's symptoms. Antibiotic therapy is indicated if the cause is a bacterial infection.

Sudden onset of respiratory distress in a previously well person is likely due to foreign body obstruction or anaphylaxis. Anaphylaxis is reviewed in Chapter 53. If a foreign body is suspected in the presence of complete airway obstruction, the nurse should perform the Heimlich maneuver (abdominal thrusts for adults). If the obstruction cannot be removed, the nurse should perform direct laryngoscopic visualization and, if visible, remove the object with Magill forceps. If this is unsuccessful, the patient should receive advanced airway management such as intubation, cricothyroidotomy, or tracheostomy. Patients with complete airway obstruction require immediate cricothyroidotomy or tracheostomy to establish an airway. In the case of a full respiratory arrest secondary to airway obstruction, ventilating with a resuscitation bag will be futile. Therefore, it is critical to secure an emergency surgical airway.

Nursing Management

Nursing management of the patient with upper airway obstruction involves ongoing assessment and maintenance of the airway. Ongoing assessment includes the following:

- Presence of spontaneous breathing
- Rate, depth, and effort of respirations
- Presence of grunting or wheezing
- Use of accessory muscles of respiration
- Symmetry of chest expansion
- Vital signs
- Oxygen saturation level
- Quality of the voice, such as hoarse, raspy, weak, muffled, normal, or nonexistent
- Stridor or any type of noisy breathing
- Patient complaint of "not getting enough air"
- Air movement during auscultation.

Assessment also should include the patient's ability to handle oral secretions and whether the patient is having pain while speaking or swallowing. The nurse should note any frequent drooling or productive coughing to clear the airway. Drooling is an ominous sign that signifies an inability to swallow oral secretions, indicating near complete obstruction. It is essential to determine how long it has been since the patient has noticed voice or respiratory changes. Symptoms that have developed over a period of days may indicate a more slowly progressing airway problem.

The nurse should monitor the patient's orientation, mentation, and general demeanor on an ongoing basis. The patient may be cooperative and able to answer questions appropriately on presentation; however, as the obstruction increases, the patient may begin to appear anxious and agitated or confused. The patient who was cooperative initially may become disoriented and unable to follow directions. If the obstruction has been progressing gradually, the patient may not report as much discomfort when breathing as her appearance belies.

The nurse should place the patient in an upright position to straighten the airway and help alleviate the obstruction. Extending the patient's head and pulling the mandible forward to displace the tongue base away from the pharyngeal wall also may be helpful, particularly in patients with a decreased level of consciousness. This will straighten the airway and may improve air exchange until help arrives. Oxygen and an advanced airway are needed to relieve the obstruction.

Safety Alert *If the patient is having respiratory difficulty and the nurse suspects developing airway obstruction, the nurse should notify the healthcare team immediately. Airway obstruction is a medical emergency that requires immediate and aggressive treatment to prevent the potential of respiratory arrest leading to cardiac arrest and death.*

Tracheotomy

Patients with severe facial injuries, edema to the head and neck area, infection, surgery, large obstructive tumors, or neurological changes to the larynx may require an alternative airway. In these cases, a tracheotomy can be performed to provide an artificial airway.

Placement of a tracheostomy tube usually is temporary to support the patient through the initial period of obstructive swelling or to provide an airway in a patient with airway obstruction. Intubation is discussed in detail in Chapter 27. Most health care providers recommend a tracheotomy for patients whom they expect to be intubated for longer than 7 to 10 days. This decreases the risk of permanent injury to the vocal cords or tissues in the larynx or upper airway. Another indication for tracheotomy is for patients with severe obstructive sleep apnea who have failed conservative therapy and non-invasive positive airway pressure. Patients with short, thick necks and large tonsils or a large amount of soft tissue in the posterior pharynx may have their airways obstructed as they relax to sleep. The tracheotomy allows the patient to experience unobstructed breathing while sleeping.

The tracheotomy incision is below the prominent thyroid cartilage (Adam's apple) and below the cricoid cartilage, usually between the second and third or the third and fourth tracheal cartilages, and continues on through the anterior tracheal wall. The tracheostomy tube is placed into the tracheal stoma to keep the airway open. It is initially sutured into place to prevent inadvertent dislodgement. Ties are placed through the faceplate of the tracheostomy tube and around the neck to further secure the tube. The tube remains sutured in place until the tract from the anterior neck into the trachea becomes well established. The tracheostomy tubes are usually made of silicone, plastic, stainless steel, or silver. The tube consists of an outer tube and a removable inner cannula. The inner cannula serves as a safety device, in that it can be removed if it becomes obstructed with crusts or thick secretions. This helps reestablish a patent airway. The patient should always have an inner cannula in place except when it is being cleaned or when the tube is capped during weaning.

Tracheostomy tubes with a cuff are used for patients on mechanical ventilation to seal the airway around the tube (Figure 26–8◆). The cuff is not intended to hold the tube in place. At best, it keeps the tube centered in the airway. The trachea expands during inhalation, and secretions can fall from around the cuff into the mainstem bronchus. Sometimes special tubes must be used or customized to fit the patient appropriately. For example, for patients with thick necks, the regular length tube may not be long enough to reach into the trachea, so a tube with a longer shaft must be used (Figure 26–9◆).

Nursing Management

The nursing process is used to guide the care of the patient with a tracheostomy tube.

Assessment

Nursing assessment of the patient with a new tracheostomy tube includes auscultation of the lungs, monitoring of oxygen saturation, and assessment for any increase in the amounts of blood in the sputum, subcutaneous emphysema in the neck, respiratory distress, and patency of the tracheostomy tube itself.

Nursing Diagnosis

Nursing diagnoses for the patient undergoing tracheotomy may include the following:

- *Ineffective Airway Clearance* related to blood, thick secretions or malposition of the tube
- *Pain, Acute* related to the surgical site
- *Risk for Infection* related to surgical site and possible aspiration
- *Risk of Impaired Skin Integrity* related to pressure from tracheostomy tube cuff and plate

NANDA-I © 2012

Outcomes and Evaluation Parameters

Outcomes for the patient with an artificial airway include no complications and normal oxygenation as evidenced by adequate respiratory effort and oxygen saturations >95%. Airway complications can occur from a variety of causes including bleeding, tube obstruction or dislodgement, and displacement into the subcutaneous tissue of the neck. Most complications of tracheotomies can be avoided by securing the tube well.

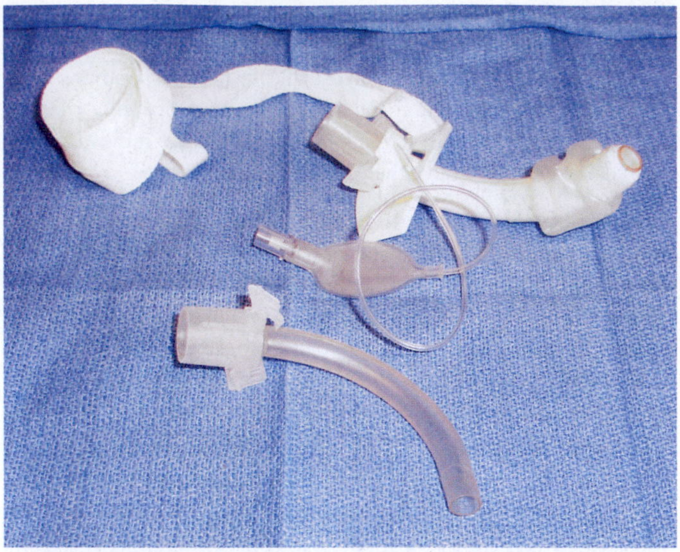

(A)

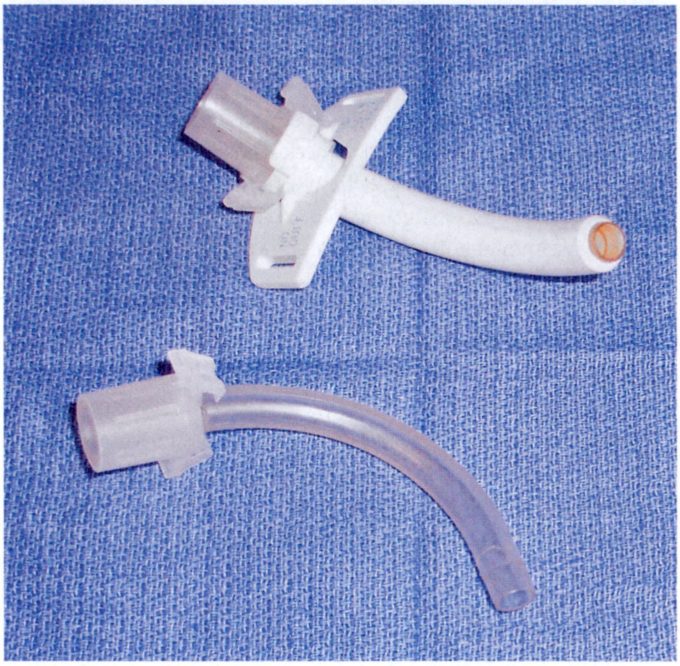

(B)

FIGURE 26–8 ◆ Shiley (A) cuffed and (B) uncuffed tracheotomy tube with disposable inner cannula.

Source: Ann E. F. Sievers, RN

Interventions and Rationales

A post-tracheostomy tray kept at the bedside or on the nursing unit contains instruments to help with reinsertion in the event of an early accidental **decannulation** (removal of the tube) or tube obstruction (Figure 26–10◆). The nurse should monitor the patient's oxygen and respiratory status and take note of changes in the patient's behavior. Increasing restlessness, agitation, or changes in mentation (decreasing level of consciousness or increasing confusion) could indicate that the patient is not well oxygenated. If these symptoms occur, the nurse should remove the inner cannula, make sure the tracheostomy tube is clear, then suction the patient (see Chart 26–5). If a suction catheter cannot be passed down the tracheostomy tube, the tube may have become dislodged. If the tube becomes displaced or dislodged, the nursing priority is to stay with the patient and to position the patient with the head up and slightly extended. A health care provider who is able to reinsert

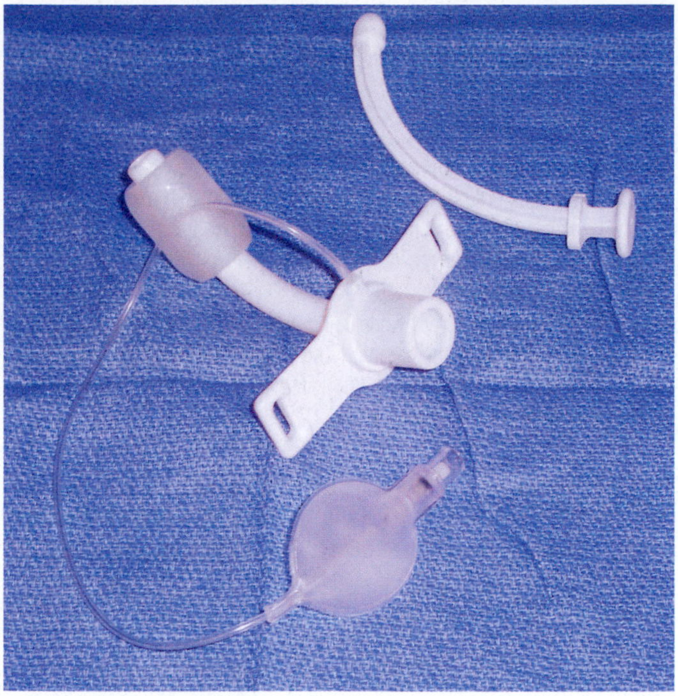

FIGURE 26–9 ◆ Shiley single-cannula tracheotomy tube used for patients who require an extra length to span the skin to trachea distance, or those who require a lower cuff placement. A single-cannula tube requires more aggressive nursing care to keep the single cannula free from lumen obstruction.
Source: Ann E. F. Sievers, RN

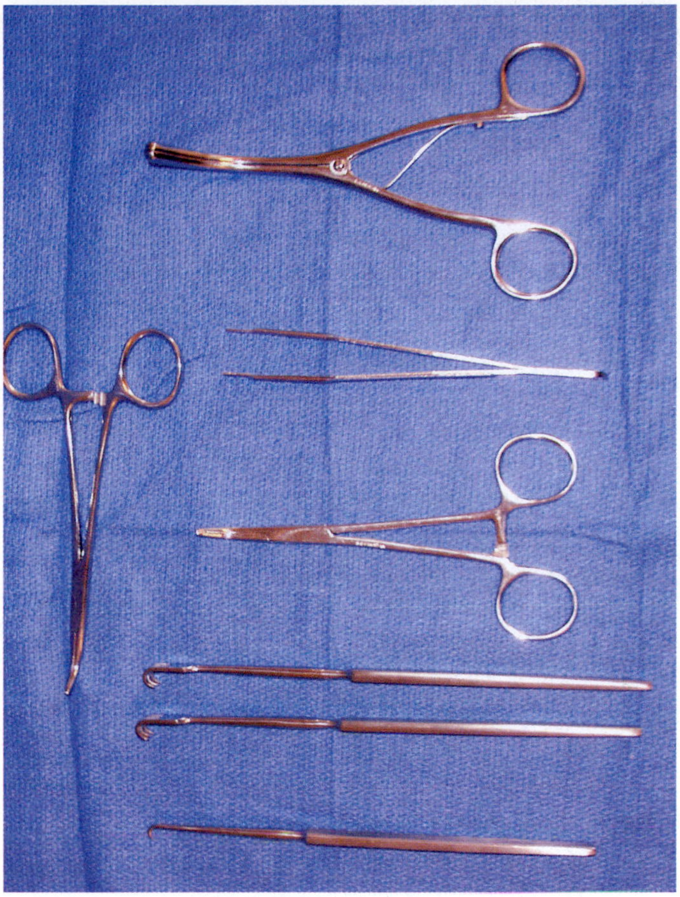

FIGURE 26–10 ◆ Post-tracheotomy tray instruments are kept near the new tracheotomy patient for surgical access in the event of accidental decannulation.
Source: Ann E. F. Sievers, RN

the airway tube needs to be summoned, and the patient needs reassurance that help is on the way. The patient might need to be ventilated with a resuscitation bag until the airway is replaced. Acute respiratory distress is very frightening for the patient; therefore, it is essential for the nurse to reassure the patient that everything is being done to rectify the situation. It is important to assemble the necessary equipment for reintubation or replacement of the tracheostomy tube. The obturator, which is used to guide the tracheostomy tube during insertion, should always be kept with the patient.

All patients who have an artificial airway require humidification to the airway because the normal upper airway passages that humidify sections are bypassed. This is done by tracheostomy cupola or collar. Many times in the early postoperative period, a patient is unable to clear secretions and may require bagging and deep suctioning. This procedure will mobilize mucus plugs, stimulate a cough, and clear the airway.

The patient should be encouraged to cough and to breathe deeply, and the nurse must suction as necessary to assist in clearing secretions if the patient does not have a strong enough cough or the secretions are very thick and difficult to expectorate. If the patient is able to take five to six deep breaths to maintain oxygenation, it is preferable to have the patient cough to clear secretions. The amount of tracheal suctioning should be limited, because excessive suctioning leads to irritation to the tracheal mucosa below the level of the tube. Suctioning of the artificial airway is discussed in Chart 26–5.

Safety Alert *In all cases of bleeding, the nurse must suction the tracheostomy tube to maintain patency of the patient's airway and inflate the cuff if one is present. The nurse must call for help, as this is an emergent situation.*

Ensuring that the inner cannula is changed routinely to prevent occlusion is an important component of the nursing care of a patient with a tracheostomy tube. Depending on secretions, the inner cannula can be changed every 8 to 24 hours. Care of the tracheotomy site itself involves cleaning around the tube with half-strength hydrogen peroxide on cotton swabs and rinsing with normal saline. Secretions under the tracheostomy plate can cause skin breakdown and can lead to infection if not cleaned regularly. Assess the area under the edges of the tracheostomy faceplate for signs of skin breakdown. Keep the faceplate flush with the skin of the neck. Check the ties frequently, and change them if they become wet or soiled. Cotton ties work well but do stretch as they become wet. The ties should be tied tightly enough so that only one finger can be placed between the skin and the ties.

Occasionally, owing to the patient's anatomy, the lower edge of the plate puts pressure on the skin and can lead to skin breakdown if not assessed and protected. A split gauze dressing provides some padding; alternatively, some form of manufactured skin barrier such as DuoDerm or a stoma wafer can be used to protect the skin. The nurse needs to assess frequently for secretions underneath the barrier and change the barrier as necessary.

The nurse should teach the patient to occlude the end of the tracheostomy tube with a finger in order to speak on exhalation. The patient should be instructed to inhale through the tube, cover the tube, and exhale through the natural airway. Regaining communication can be very rewarding for the patient.

Decannulation

Decannulation, or removal of the tube, occurs with the resolution of the airway problem. This process typically begins by downsizing the

CHART 26–5 Suctioning Procedure

Closed System Suctioning A suction catheter is in-line with the ventilator circuit so that the patient does not have to be disconnected from the ventilator to suction the airway. This method maintains PEEP (discussed earlier on page 702) and oxygen delivery and sterility of the suction catheter.

Open Suctioning Requires disconnection from the ventilator to suction using a sterile suction catheter.

Equipment and Supplies

Sterile suction catheter

Sterile gloves (open suction); clean gloves (closed suction)

Sterile normal saline for irrigation, when indicated, if the secretions are very thick and need thinning

Sterile disposable container

Suction source with calibrated, adjustable regulator

Pulse oximeter

Sterile sputum trap if specimen ordered

Stethoscope

Technique for Open Suctioning

1. Assemble the equipment, explain the procedure to the patient, adjust the bed to a comfortable working position, prepare the suction equipment, adjust the suction to between 80 to 110 mmHg, wash hands, and don gloves.
2. Preparation:
   - Select the suction catheter that does not exceed more that half the inner diameter of the artificial airway.
   - Place a pulse oximeter on the patient.
   - Monitor the patient's ECG as indicated based on her clinical condition.
   - Hyperoxygenate the patient with 100% oxygen for 30 to 60 seconds prior to suctioning either by adjusting the FiO_2 on the ventilator or using the temporary oxygen enrichment program available on most ventilators. Manual bag ventilation is not recommended because of the inconsistent oxygen delivery. If manual bag ventilation is the only alternative, then ensure that PEEP is maintained. Patients that are PEEP dependent (p.702) and cannot maintain open alveoli without the end expiratory pressure can decompensate their oxygenation status rapidly when PEEP is removed, and it can be difficult to oxygenate back to baseline. PEEP valve attachments are available for this purpose.
   - Check suction power by occluding the end of the suction tubing prior to attaching the catheter. The lowest pressure that will remove secretions should be used; in adults, this value should not exceed 110 mmHg.
3. Procedure:
   - Insert the suction catheter into the artificial airway without applying suction. Shallow suction (predetermined depth, usually the length of the artificial airway) is recommended to prevent trauma to the tracheal mucosa. Deep suctioning (advancing until resistance is met) is discouraged.
   - Withdraw the catheter slowly, applying intermittent suction. Each suctioning attempt should not exceed 15 seconds.
   - Monitor pulse oximetry and ECG during the procedure. Discontinue if there is evidence of dysrhythmia, bradycardia, or hypoxia.
4. Follow-up Care:
   - Hyperoxygenate for 1 minute as described earlier.
   - Patients should not be routinely hyperventilated.
   - Monitor for adverse reactions, including hypoxia, dysrhythmias, hypo-/hypertension, and bradycardia.
   - Clean suction tubing (open system).
   - Remove gloves and wash hands.

Source: Adapted from American Association of Respiratory Care (AARC) Clinical practice guidelines. (2010). Retrieved from http://www.rcjournal.com/cpgs/.

size of the tracheostomy tube and/or capping the tracheostomy tube to block air from moving through it and allowing the patient to breathe through the normal respiratory structures. A smaller tube allows enough air to pass around the tube and up into the natural larynx. This allows the patient to breathe in the normal physiological manner, taking in air through the nose and mouth and into the upper airway. Oxygen saturation is monitored continuously during and after this change. If the patient tolerates the downsizing, the tube is again downsized, and a cap is placed over the end of the tracheostomy tube (Figure 26–11◆).

Safety Alert *If at any time the patient experiences respiratory distress during weaning, the nurse must remove the cap and encourage the patient to cough. The nurse should suction if necessary and recap the tube if the patient is able to tolerate it.*

It also is critical for the nurse to teach the patient how to uncap or remove the cap of the tube. This can help allay fears that may be associated with capping or the process of decannulation. The nurse should cap the patient's tube and monitor saturations for an extended period, including a period while the patient is sleeping, before the tracheostomy is removed completely. If the patient tolerates the capping throughout the night without episodes of oxygen desaturation, the health care provider removes the tracheostomy tube and places a dry sterile occlusive dressing over the site. The nurse should explain to the patient the importance of putting pressure on the site when coughing or talking to prevent air from passing through the stoma. The more consistent the patient is in doing this, the sooner the stoma incision will close. The incision is never closed with sutures; it is allowed to heal from the inside out on its own. Closure of the skin edges before the tracheal incision itself closes can lead to subcutaneous emphysema in the neck. The dressing is changed as needed until there is no evidence of air passage through the incision and the skin edges are approximated. Wound care to the healing site is typically ordered twice a day and as needed, with half- or full-strength hydrogen peroxide and rinsing with normal saline before applying a dry dressing.

Oral communication is very important. If the patient cannot be decannulated for reasons such as vocal cord dysfunction, then the use of a speaking valve may help. These one-way valves allow the patient to breathe in through the valve; the valve then shuts and the patient breathes out through his natural airway (Figure 26–12◆). This flutter valve is very simple but very effective. Some types can be used in-line and assist ventilator-dependent patients to speak.

Discharge Priorities for Patients with a Tracheostomy

If a patient is to go home with a tracheostomy, the goal is for the patient to be safe at home, resume normal activities, and have an acceptable quality of life. Safety with an artificial airway is the priority for teaching. The patient and family must demonstrate safe care before discharge. This should include suctioning, saline instillation, wound care, inner

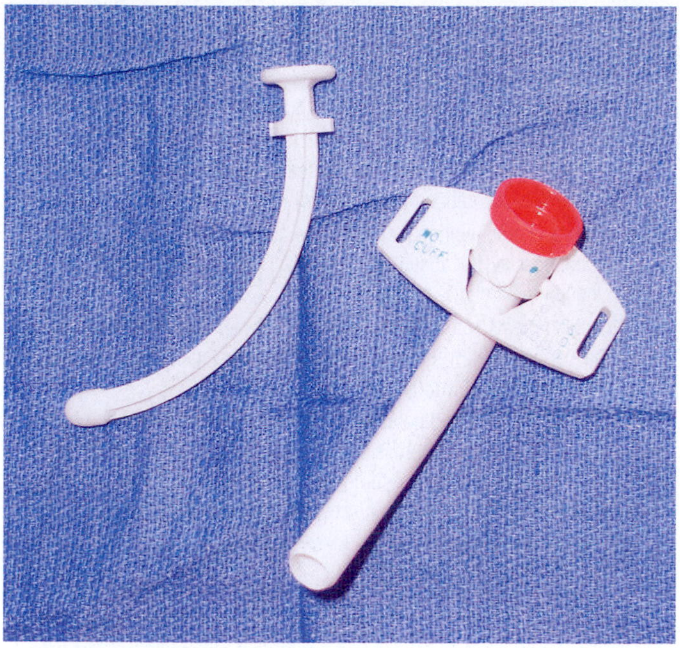

FIGURE 26–11 ◆ Shiley tracheotomy tube with red cap for weaning and eventual decannulation. If possible, the patient should be taught to uncap the tube if distress occurs. The nurse in the hospital must be vigilant for subtle and overt signs of distress during this process.
Source: Ann E. F. Sievers, RN

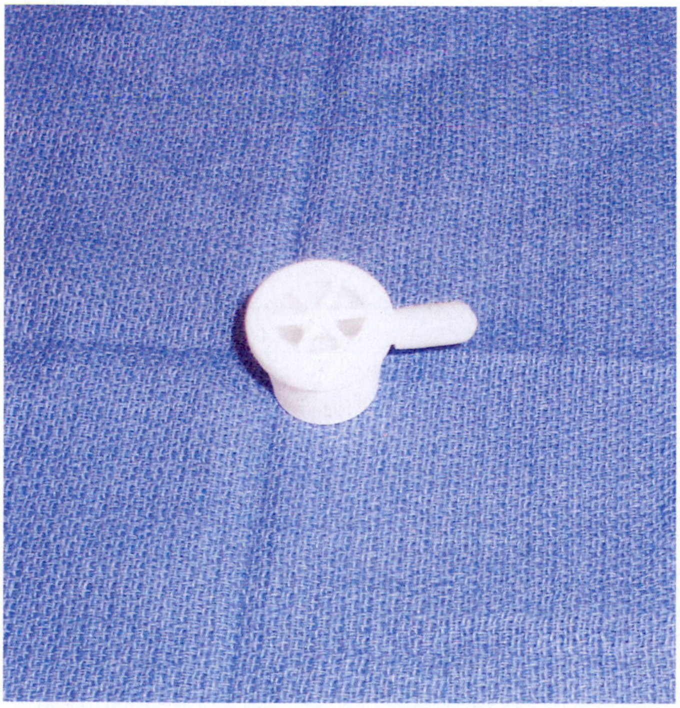

FIGURE 26–12 ◆ The Shiley speaking valve with oxygen port is a one-way valve that allows airflow on exhalation upward into the larynx, thereby supporting speech. These valves are fragile and any secretions interfere with their operation.
Source: Ann E. F. Sievers, RN

cannula care, tracheostomy change, and emergency measures. The nurse should encourage the patient and family to participate in care early in the hospitalization to increase their confidence.

Some individuals may not be able to write to communicate, which increases their frustration. The nurse should assess the patient's ability to read and write prior to surgery and establish a suitable form of communication.

Head and Neck Cancer

Head and neck cancer is a common form of cancer that presents intense and persistent challenges to the patient, family, and health care team during diagnosis, treatment, and recovery. Head and neck cancer may include tumors in the mouth, pharynx, larynx, nasal cavity and sinuses, thyroid, or salivary glands. Ablative surgery often is used to treat this type of cancer, leaving the patient with facial disfigurement and functional impairment. The use of an interdisciplinary team (early in diagnosis) will provide the patient with the clinical expertise that will optimize the patient's recovery potential and improve quality of life.

If detected early, head and neck cancer is treatable and curable. However, it is an insidious disease and may not present itself until the patient has a large tumor burden. Discussions with family and significant others often help to explain the consequences of head and neck cancer and its treatment. Unfortunately, if not treated, this type of cancer is very disfiguring and alters the normal functions of breathing, eating, smelling, tasting, and facial attributes and expressions. Decisions regarding treatment must be informed discussions that include the outcome with and without treatment and the implications, risks, and benefits of surgery and radiation therapy.

Epidemiology and Etiology

The worldwide prevalence of head and neck cancer is greater than half a million cases annually, making it the fifth-leading type of cancer in the world. The highest rates are in regions of the world where there is high tobacco use and alcohol consumption. It has been postulated that tobacco use and alcohol consumption account for almost 80% of head and neck cancers (Stenson & Brockstein, 2011). In the United States, head and neck cancer account for about 3% of malignancies. Because of the many different cell types in the head and neck region, the etiology of cancer is complex. Classification of tumors of the nasal cavity and paranasal sinuses alone encompasses over 50 different tumor types (Stenson & Brockstein, 2011). A variety of risk factors are associated with head and neck cancer, although some patients do not have any of the known risk factors. See the Risk Factors for Head and Neck Cancer box.

Pathophysiology

The predominant cell type in head and neck cancer is squamous cell cancer. Although there are many other types, they occur far less frequently. Squamous cells or epithelial cells line the aerodigestive tract and are irritated and altered by the environmental agents outlined earlier. Cells change from the normal division to altered cells that grow along tissue planes and into adjacent structures. Chapter 57 includes a complete discussion of the pathogenesis of cancer.

Diagnostic Procedures

Diagnostic tests used to diagnose cancer include CT scan, MRI, and positron emission tomography (PET) scans that are used to identify regional involvement of lymph nodes and metastasis. Esophagoscopy and bronchoscopy are used to visualize the tumor and to obtain biopsies. These tests aid in the classification and staging of carcinomas. See the Diagnostic Testsbox for some information on diagnostic tools used in identifying head and neck cancer. Further information on

RISK FACTORS for Head and Neck Cancer

Tobacco and Marijuana Use: Heavy tobacco and marijuana use increases the risk of head and neck cancer by 5- to 25-fold when compared to nonsmokers. The risk is correlated with the length and amount smoked or chewed. The risk declines after smoking cessation, with no increased risk after 20 years of not smoking. Smokeless tobacco (chew, snuff) increases the risk of oral and pharyngeal cancer. There has also been some suggestion that secondhand smoke may be a contributing factor.

Alcohol: Drinking alcohol can increase the risk of aerodigestive tract cancer. The combination of tobacco use and alcohol consumption increases the risk of head and neck cancer. The risk appears to be dose-dependent—the greater the amount, the greater the risk.

Viral Infection: Chronic viral infections may be associated with head and neck cancer. Epstein-Barr virus (EBV) and human papillomavirus (HPV) have the strongest correlation. EBV is associated with nasopharyngeal carcinoma, while HPV has been linked to invasive oral and oropharyngeal tumors.

Occupational Exposure: Occupational hazards linked to head and neck cancer include asbestos, pesticides, hydrocarbons, and dry cleaning agents. Workers at risk include textile workers, wood workers, cement workers, leather and paint workers, and farmers. Formaldehyde is associated with nasopharyngeal cancer.

Radiation: Radiation treatment for other diseases has been linked to salivary tumors, squamous cell cancers, and sarcomas.

Gender: Oral and oropharyngeal cancers are about twice as common in men as in women, possibly because men are more likely to use tobacco and alcohol, though this trend is changing.

Diet: Preserved meats with high levels of nitrates increases the risk of nasopharyngeal cancer when frequently consumed. Milk, vegetables, fruit, zinc, and green tea are thought to have protective factors.

Other: Poor oral hygiene and periodontal disease are associated with oral cavity carcinoma. Immunosuppression following cardiac and kidney transplant also show some correlation to developing cancers of the head and neck, particularly lip cancer in renal transplant patients.

Source: Stenson, K., & Brockstein, B. (2011). Overview of head and neck cancer. In M. Posner & M. Ross (Eds.), UpToDate, Waltham, MA: UpToDate.

diagnostic tests used in cancer diagnoses, as well as tumor classification and staging systems, can be found in Chapter 57.

Clinical Manifestations

Clinical manifestations of head and neck cancer vary with site involvement and include the following:

- ***Sinus Tumors:*** epistaxis and nasal obstruction (often unilateral)
- ***Nasopharyngeal:*** neck mass, hearing loss, pain, tinnitus, and cranial nerve abnormalities
- ***Oral Cavity:*** mouth ulcers that don't heal, weight loss, bleeding, loose teeth, difficult or painful swallowing, or poor fit in dentures. Tongue cancer is often painful and lip cancer presents with ulcerative lower lip lesions.
- ***Posterior Pharynx:*** often asymptomatic until there is advanced disease. Patients present with pain, bleeding, or neck mass.
- ***Larynx:*** hoarseness, difficulty swallowing, cough, hemoptysis, and stridor. Tumors may cause airway obstruction.

Medical and Surgical Management

Diagnosing head and neck cancer involves accurate assessment of the patient's health history, physical condition, social factors, and presence of support systems. When a patient presents to an otolaryngologist,

DIAGNOSTIC TESTS for Head and Neck Cancer

Test with Description, Rationale, and Normal Values	Expected Abnormality
Fine-Needle Biopsy Absence of carcinogenic cytology *Used to aspirate cells from the tissue in a neck mass for evaluation to make an initial diagnosis of cancer in patients suspected of head and neck cancer.*	Has a high degree of accuracy in identifying cancer in tissues of patients with head and neck cancer. However, a negative test is not reliable.
Fiber-Optic Laryngoscopy No evidence of tumor *Uses fiber-optic light bundle channel to transmit light.*	Used to look into the upper aerodigestive tract without using general anesthesia.
CT Scan and MRI No evidence of tumor *Used to define the extent of disease.*	CT scan identifies invasion of bone or soft tissue and evaluates cervical lymph nodes at risk of metastasis. The scan can be extended beyond the primary site if metastasis is suspected. MRI is superior to CT in soft-tissue definition and bone invasion. It is sometimes used when there is a suspicion of tumor extension into the orbit or brain. It is also the preferred method for oral and oropharynx tumor staging.
PET Scan (Positron Emission Tomography) No evidence of abnormality *Measures the metabolism of glucose in body tissues. Tumors have higher rates of glycolysis compared to healthy tissue. PET is used to identify primary head and neck tumors and metastasis to regional lymph nodes.*	Measures the biologic and metabolic changes associated with disease. Because the PET is limited in identifying the anatomic location of tumors/nodes, it is often integrated with CT imaging to improve localization.

Weblink: Oral Cancer

a thorough history is taken with emphasis on specific symptoms in the head and neck. The length of time each symptom has been present and sequence of symptom development also is documented. Treatment of head and neck cancer is complex because of the wide variety of tumors associated within this region as well as anatomic constraints. Preserving organ function is a primary concern. Patients with early stage disease are often managed with either primary surgery or radiation therapy and have a positive prognosis of 70% to 90% over five years (PubMed Health, 2011). Patients with tobacco- or alcohol-related cancers are at higher risk of developing a secondary malignancy over the following 5 years. Patients with more advanced disease generally receive a combination of surgery, radiation therapy, and/or chemotherapy. The 5-year survival rate is 30% to 60% (PubMed Health, 2011). Squamous cell cancer of the head or neck region often metastasizes to the cervical lymph nodes and is associated with a poor prognosis. In patients with distant metastatic disease, palliative chemotherapy and/or supportive care should be strongly considered. The patient should be informed of all aspects of therapy, including the pros and cons of each treatment. Chapter 57 includes a complete description of radiation and chemotherapy.

Surgical Resection

There are six general types of surgical resection: oral cavity resection, laryngectomy (partial or total), temporal bone resection, maxillary (with or without orbital removal) or bimaxillary resection, skull base resection, and the combination of each. Each surgery has its own subgroups based on the site of origin of the tumor. Each resection presents with unique requirements because of the location of the tumor. Essentially all of the surgical approaches have similar needs in relation to airway, wound care, nutrition, self-image, self-care education, and recovery.

Neck dissection may accompany tumor resections. Neck dissection includes lymph tissue, the jugular vein, the spinal accessory nerve, and the sternocleidomastoid muscle (SCM) and is necessary for metastatic disease in the lymph nodes of the neck or when there is a very high suspicion of tumor because of the behavior or tumor bulk at the primary site. Chart 26–6 outlines the various surgical approaches for head and neck cancer.

Collaborative Management

A multidisciplinary team of experts, including otolaryngologists, medical oncologists, radiation oncologists, social service providers, clinical nurse specialists, speech pathologists, nurses, and dentists or maxillofacial prosthodontists, enables a collaborative approach to providing care for patients with head and neck cancer. In order to meet desired patient outcomes, it is essential that this interdisciplinary team communicate openly with one another in developing and evaluating care of the patient and family (IOM [Institute of Medicine], 2010). This panel of experts reviews the patient's history, findings from the physical exam,

CHART 26–6 Otolaryngology Surgical Resections for Head and Neck Cancer

Type of Surgery	Major Areas Resected	Major Implications
Oral cavity resection	Tongue, buccal mucosa, mandible	Speech, articulation, chewing, swallowing, cosmetic changes
Oropharyngeal resections, bimaxillary resection	Tongue, base of tongue, tonsil, maxilla, mandible	Swallowing, speech, aspiration Facial cosmetic changes
Laryngectomy, partial (often called hemi or vertical hemi laryngectomy)	Larynx, partial	Speech, swallowing Aspiration (partial laryngectomy only) Cosmetic changes
Laryngectomy, total	Larynx, total	Speech, cosmetic changes Complete separation of airway and esophagus
Temporal bone resection	Temporal bone, parotid, maxilla, mandible	Hearing, balance Cosmetic changes Facial nerve impairment or paralysis Eye protection concerns
Maxillary, with or without orbital exenteration (surgical removal of all contents of the orbit)	Maxilla, orbit	Speech, swallowing, chewing, sight Cosmetic changes
Skull base resection (anterior, middle, posterior, or combination)	Skull base carotid artery	Cognition, speech, swallowing, balance Cosmetic changes
Neck dissection (radical, modified, paired with the above surgeries for lymph node involvement)	Lymph nodes, SCM, jugular vein, spinal accessory nerve CNXI	Impaired lymph drainage Trapezius muscle paralysis Facial edema (especially if bilateral neck dissections are performed at the same time) Cerebral edema with bilateral neck dissection
Combination of any of the previous surgical resections	Any anatomic combination as required by tumor invasion for oncologic purposes	All of the previous predicated on the location of the tumor and invasion

and results of radiologic studies. The team develops a consensus opinion for the best chance for cure and develops a plan of therapy. Then the plan is presented to the patient and family so they can make their decisions. The nursing role is to participate as a team member, to act as an advocate for the patient, and to help the patient and family interpret medical terms into lay terms.

The patient and family require assistance in understanding the choices and plan of care because many choices and decisions regarding treatment are available. Patients must understand that they may choose no treatment. Although this is unusual, some individuals elect no therapy as their option, with the ultimate outcome being death. When such a choice is made, alternatives in palliative and hospice care should be explored with the patient, family, and significant others. End-of-life care is discussed in detail in Chapter 11.

Total Laryngectomy

Removal of the larynx or **laryngectomy** necessitates a permanent tracheal artificial airway. This procedure is performed to manage malignant disease that does not, or cannot, preserve the larynx through other alternative medical or surgical interventions. A similar surgery called laryngotracheal separation is done for patients with severe aspiration that has resulted in repeated, frequent hospitalizations for aspiration pneumonia. In both surgeries, the trachea is transected, and the distal portion of the trachea is brought to the skin surface in the anterior neck and sewn into place. This surgery completely separates the trachea from the esophagus and thus prevents problems with aspiration. However, because air no longer passes through the structures of the larynx, such as the vocal cords, the patient will not be able to speak in the normal manner.

Losing the ability to communicate verbally can be very frightening for the patient. Few things are as disabling as the impairment resulting from total loss of laryngeal speech. The impact of the total removal of the larynx is so dramatic that it may affect the patient's decision regarding treatment. Much time and care must be taken with these patients and their families during the diagnostic and preoperative phases. It is important for the health care provider to explain to the patient and family all of the risks and benefits of each form of treatment. It is equally important that the patient feel support in whatever decision is made, even if it might not seem the best choice for complete removal of the disease. Some patients opt for other treatments first, such as radiation or a combination of radiation and chemotherapy, or may choose only a partial laryngectomy in order to preserve their voice. If cancer recurs or there is a significant problem with aspiration, then the patient may subsequently consent to a total laryngectomy.

Until the internal incision lines in the pharynx heal, the patient will not be able to eat orally. This typically takes 5 to 7 days post laryngectomy. For this reason, a nasogastric feeding tube is placed intraoperatively. Before the patient resumes an oral diet, a barium swallow is completed to evaluate the internal suture lines of the pharynx, thereby ensuring that the suture lines are intact and there is no leak of barium through the incisions, referred to as internal dehiscence. Aspiration is not a problem for these patients because the esophagus and airway are completely separated. However, there may be some swallowing issues initially as the patient learns to control food and fluids in the reconstructed esophagus.

As with the patient with a tracheotomy or someone on voice rest, it is important for the nurse to be patient with the new laryngectomy patient as he tries to communicate. This can be an extremely frustrating time for the patient and for the nurse if care is not taken to establish a workable form of communication. It is important to acknowledge the patient's frustration and to explain that writing and pantomiming, though tedious, are very effective communication tools. Some patients articulate well enough and use gestures so that writing may not be necessary all the time. For others, writing is the only way to communicate. Pen and paper or a dry erase board should be provided for this purpose.

It is important to determine whether the patient and spouse or other primary support person are able to read and write. Initially, this will be the most used form of communication for the patient to express his needs and concerns. The Cultural Considerations box addresses the needs of patients who may not understand English.

It is important for the patient with a laryngectomy to understand that various options are available for vocal restoration procedures. Meeting with a speech therapist preoperatively and discussing these options may help the patient realize that having a total laryngectomy does not necessarily mean the end of communication with some form of speech. It may be helpful to have someone who has had the same procedure and has been trained to work with patients visit with the patient to demonstrate how to speak after surgery and how the voice sounds.

Tracheoesophageal puncture (TEP) is a procedure that can be done at the time of the original surgery or at a later date when healing is completed. This procedure provides voice restoration to patients who have had a total laryngectomy. A puncture is made through the posterior wall of the trachea into the anterior wall of the esophagus. A feeding tube is threaded through this puncture and is used to help form a tract by acting as a stent. It also is used to feed the patient enterally while the surgical site heals. After the tract heals and matures, a one-way prosthetic valve is inserted into this tract for purposes of speech (Figure 26–13◆). The purpose of the valve is to allow the patient to shunt air from the trachea into the esophagus but not allow food and fluid from the esophagus to enter the trachea. The airflow through the one-way valve causes

CULTURAL CONSIDERATIONS
for Patients with Total Laryngectomy

For patients with a total laryngectomy who speak a language other than English, communication can be even more difficult. It is helpful to have the family assist by making signs with words both in English and in the patient's native language for things such as "pain," "bathroom," and "difficulty breathing." This allows the patient to just point to the appropriate sign. If no one in the family speaks English, typically hospitals have interpreting services available. If a staff member speaks the patient's native language, assign this person as one of the primary nurses. This can ease the patient's fears of not being understood.

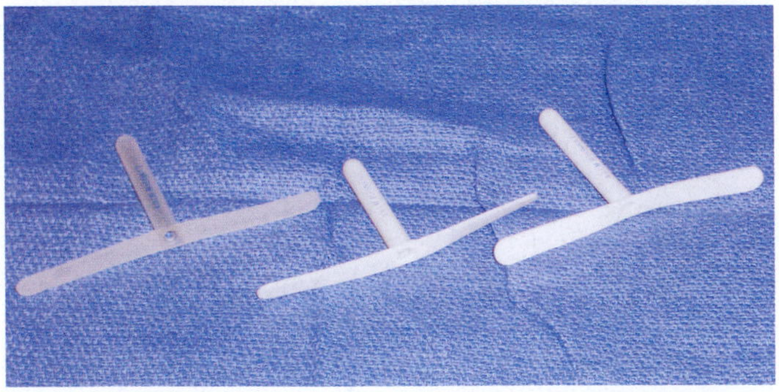

FIGURE 26–13 ◆ Bivona tracheoesophageal puncture speech prosthesis. This speech prosthesis is placed into the TEP to shunt air from the stoma (lungs) into the esophagus to produce speech after total laryngectomy.
Source: Ann E. F. Sievers, RN

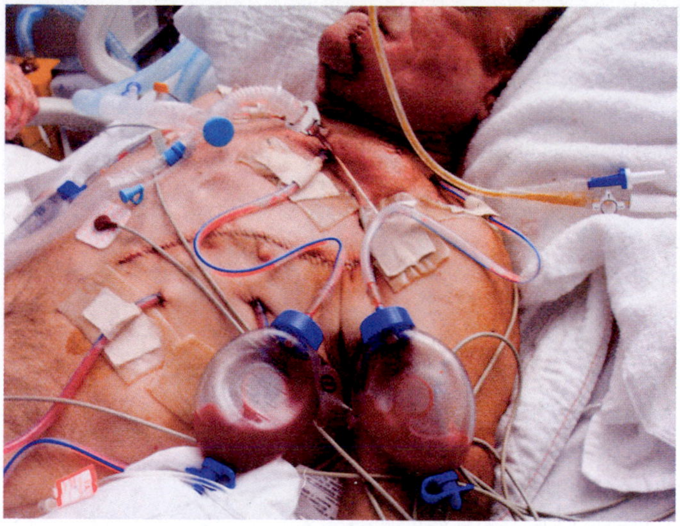

FIGURE 26–14 ◆ Pectoralis major myocutaneous reconstruction flap.
Source: Ann E. F. Sievers, RN

vibration in the upper esophagus when the stoma is occluded, and the mouth, tongue, and lips articulate the sound to produce speech.

Reconstruction Flaps and Grafts

In otolaryngology cancer surgery, after the tumor is resected, the goal is to reconstruct the patient for optimum function and cosmetics. The surgical site can be primarily closed or left open to granulate by secondary intention. Frequently, flaps and composite grafts of muscle, bone, and tissue are used for reconstruction. A **myocutaneous flap,** composed of muscle and skin, is used to reconstruct the defect caused by the tumor resection. A flap from the pectoralis major is commonly used for reconstruction. This rotation flap is supplied by its native blood supply, but rotated into the surgical defect. Free flaps that are harvested from a distant site also can be used for reconstruction. Common sites include the radial forearm, fibula, scapula, lateral arm, or lateral thigh. These flaps can include tissue, bone, and muscle, as well as the artery and vein for the microvascular anastomosis (Figure 26–14◆).

When the nurse assesses a reconstruction flap, myocutaneous or free, it should be pink and warm with brisk capillary refill (<2 seconds). A flap that is blue or cyanotic is a sign of venous congestion, white indicates no arterial supply, and deep red is a sign of partial venous congestion with a vigorous arterial supply. Tracheostomy and cupola ties (ties that secure the oxygen tracheostomy mask in place) should be positioned away from the graft to prevent pressure on the area, which may lead to impaired or decreased blood flow to the tissue and loss of the graft. The head position should be maintained straight or toward the operative side to prevent pressure or tension on the flap. The head of the bed is elevated to at least 30 degrees to facilitate drainage of fluid and to prevent edema of the head and neck area.

The free flap is assessed for a pulse by Doppler per the surgeon's order, typically every 2 hours (Figure 26–15◆). It also is important in the immediate postoperative period to maintain an adequate blood pressure with a mean arterial pressure (MAP) of at least 60 to ensure tissue perfusion to the graft. MAP is discussed in Chapter 31.

Nursing Management

Nursing care management priorities for patients with head and neck cancer are airway maintenance, pain management, nutrition, and wound healing. If surgery was performed, these patients have special

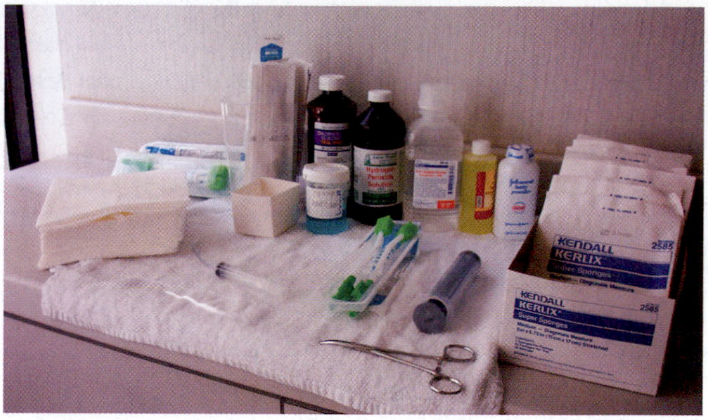

FIGURE 26–15 ◆ Nursing care equipment for Doppler monitoring for arterial patency following microvascular free flap reconstruction.
Source: Ann E. F. Sievers, RN

care needs including wound management, drain assessment and care, oral care, wound complications, and carotid artery exposure assessment and management. There are also special nursing management priorities related to reconstruction flaps. The Nursing Process: Patient Care Plan outlines the care for a patient who has had an orbital exenteration and maxillectomy.

Collaborative Management

Many patients with head and neck cancer present with inadequate nutrition caused by the tumor burden, cancer cachexia (weight loss, muscle atrophy, fatigue, loss of appetite, and weakness), or the mechanical difficulty of eating because of tumor impingement into the aerodigestive tract. Early recognition of nutritional inadequacy and nutritional intervention is critical to the healing process. Nutrition is discussed in detail in Chapter 8.

The inclusion of a nutritionist in the multidisciplinary team is mandatory. In order to meet desired patient outcomes, it is essential that this interdisciplinary team communicate openly with one another in developing and evaluating care of the patient and family (IOM [Institute of Medicine], 2010). Following cancer resection or during radiation therapy, nutrition consults are very helpful in targeting maintenance and replenishment goals. Replacement requirements need to be carefully calculated in order to ensure proper hydration as well as calories. The choice of feeding method, whether oral or enteral, depends on the patient's level of consciousness and ability to swallow. Feeding can proceed by an oral route, nasogastric route, gastrostomy, jejunostomy, or any combination thereof. Nutrition replacement must begin early and be continuous throughout the therapy for cancer. Most feeding can begin on postoperative day one and be advanced to goals as quickly as tolerated.

Dysphagia is a common issue that needs to be dealt with in patients with head and neck cancer. Swallowing is difficult because of tumor burden, invasion of the aerodigestive tract, and pain. Aspiration is a concern with patients who are unable to maintain their airway protection. See the Risk Factors for Aspiration box.

As the patient progresses through the hospital stay, it is important to include physical therapy in the plan of care. The patient who has had a neck dissection with the resection of cranial nerve XI will be unable to fully move the shoulder due to the enervation of the trapezius muscle. Physical therapy exercises help the patient to regain mobility, prevent a frozen shoulder, and improve general reconditioning. These exercises

NURSING PROCESS: Patient Care Plan for Head and Neck Cancer

Assessment of Respiratory Status Using Gordon's Functional Health Patterns:

- Health Perception Health Management Pattern
- Nutrition Metabolic Pattern
- Activity Exercise Pattern
- Cognitive Perceptual Pattern
- Self-Perception Self-Concept Pattern
- Values and Belief Pattern

Subjective Data	Objective Data
Assessment of Gas Exchange Do you feel like you are getting enough air? Are you short of breath? Do you have any preexisting health problems such as heart, lung, or kidney disease? Do you smoke? If so, for how long?	**Assessment of Gas Exchange** Oxygen saturation Work of breathing (e.g., gasping, increased rate, loudness) Heart rate Nail bed and skin color Use of accessory respiratory muscles Cough present, type of secretions Level of consciousness and orientation Lung sounds Arterial blood gases
Assessment of Knowledge Regarding Diagnosis and Treatment What do you understand about your diagnosis and treatment plan? Do you have questions about the treatment program? What would you like me to tell you about your diagnosis?	**Assessment of Knowledge Regarding Diagnosis and Treatment** Facial expressions Verbalization of questions by patient and family
Assessment of Cerebrospinal Fluid (CSF) Leak Related to Repair of Dural Defect Do you have a headache or blurred vision? Do you feel drowsy?	**Assessment of Cerebrospinal Fluid (CSF) Leak Related to Repair of Dural Defect** Nasal drainage for presence of CSF
Assessment of Perioperative Anxiety Related to Diagnosis, Hospitalization, and Surgery Tell me what you are feeling about your diagnosis and treatment plan. Who are the people in your life that are your support system? How have you handled fearful situations in the past?	**Assessment of Perioperative Anxiety Related to Diagnosis, Hospitalization, and Surgery** Facial expressions Mood Verbalization of fear regarding injury, impact on family, and future
Assessment of Impaired Skin Integrity Where are you hurting?	**Assessment of Impaired Skin Integrity** Color, blanching, odor, bleeding from graft donor and surgical site Size and depth of wound
Assessment for Infection Is your pain increasing in the surgical areas? Do you feel weaker?	**Assessment for Infection** Previously healed wounds are breaking down Open wounds not healing Partial-thickness injuries/donor sites converting to full-thickness injuries Increased odor and drainage from wound sites Wound cultures positive for organisms Fever Increased WBC
Assessment of Patient Safety Do you feel safe when up walking? How are you adapting to seeing out of only one eye? What adjustments have been necessary?	**Assessment of Patient Safety** Is the patient able to navigate safely? What assistive devices are necessary?
Assessment of Adjustment to Facial Disfigurement What impact does the change in your physical appearance have on your life? How do you plan to cope with these changes?	**Assessment of Adjustment to Facial Disfigurement** Does the patient look at the changes in the mirror? Does the patient ask questions about the wounds? Are the patient and family members willing to learn and participate in the required care after hospital discharge? Is the patient's perception realistic regarding body image changes?

NURSING PROCESS: Patient Care Plan for Head and Neck Cancer, *continued*

Assessment of Nutritional Intake Does your stomach feel full? Are you experiencing any nausea?	**Assessment of Nutritional Intake** Bowel sounds Lung sounds Residual volume
Assessment of Pain What is your pain level, using the 1 to 10 scale? (A 1 is very little pain; a 10 is the worst imaginable pain.) What is your experience with pain? Do you routinely take pain medications at home; if so, what for and what kind? Are you allergic to any pain medication? Do you have any cultural or religious beliefs that impact your pain control?	**Assessment of Pain** Grimacing upon movement Restlessness and irritability Taut facial expression
Outcomes and Evaluation Parameters	**Planning and Interventions with *Rationales***
1. NURSING DIAGNOSIS: Risk for Impaired Gas Exchange *related to potential for airway obstruction due to cancer or surgery* (NANDA-I © 2012)	
Outcome: Adequate gas exchange. ***Evaluation Parameters:*** Free of dyspnea: unlabored respirations < 24/min. Alert and oriented. Clear breath sounds. No restlessness, cyanosis, or fatigue. Oxygen saturation and ABGs are within normal limits.	Assess for adventitious or diminished breath sounds. Indicates decreased gas exchange. Note presence of cough and amount, color, and consistency of sputum to assess for inhalation injury. Monitor ABGs and oxygen saturation to assess adequacy of gas exchange and level of shock state. Monitor respiratory rate and depth to assess for respiratory distress. Monitor restlessness and confusion. Indicators of inadequate gas exchange with resultant brain hypoxia. Observe for cyanosis, especially in the mucous membranes. Indicators of inadequate gas exchange with resultant tissue hypoxia. Turn, cough, deep breathe, elevate head of bed, instruct on use of incentive spirometry. Measures to promote gas exchange. Administer humidified oxygen as prescribed *to loosen secretions and promote airway clearance.* Report respiratory distress to the health care provider. *Medical intervention may be indicated to prevent respiratory failure.* Assess need for suctioning and/or endotracheal intubation *to maintain adequate gas exchange.*
2. NURSING DIAGNOSIS: Deficient Knowledge *related to diagnosis and treatment* (NANDA-I © 2012)	
Outcome: Adequate knowledge of treatment regimen. ***Evaluation Parameter:*** Patient and family will verbalize understanding of treatments and care.	Assess patient/family's readiness and ability to learn and individual learning needs. The person must be psychologically ready to learn. Determine level of existing knowledge. Begin the teaching where existing knowledge ends. Instruct the patient and significant other about anatomic changes related to nasal and paranasal sinus surgery. Preoperative education empowers the patient and decreases anxiety. Provide factual information about diagnosis, treatments, and prognosis to increase knowledge and understanding. Explain all procedures in simple, concise language and allow for questions to increase understanding. Encourage questions. Keeps open communication and augments understanding. Provide ongoing education about the treatment plan and rationale. *Ongoing education is necessary as situations and conditions change.* Document response to teaching *to assist the health care team when implementing a teaching plan.*

(*continued*)

NURSING PROCESS: Patient Care Plan for Head and Neck Cancer, *continued*

Outcomes and Evaluation Parameters	Planning and Interventions with *Rationales*
3. NURSING DIAGNOSIS: Risk for Injury *related to CSF leak* (NANDA-I © 2012)	
Outcome: Orbital graft site will heal without complications. ***Evaluation Parameter:*** No evidence of CSF leak.	Observe all nasal drainage for CSF leak with a halo test. CSF on a clean dressing demonstrates as a halo of clear encircled with a red-tinged halo. Notify the surgeon when a leak occurs. This indicates an abnormal leak. Instruct the patient not to strain and to avoid excessive coughing to minimize increased intracranial pressure.
4. NURSING DIAGNOSIS: Anxiety *related to changes in health status/role functioning; situational crisis* (NANDA-I © 2012)	
Outcomes: Patient will verbalize fears and concerns. Accurate preoperative teaching will help decrease patient's fear of the unknown. ***Evaluation Parameter:*** Patient states she is comfortable with care and interventions.	Assess and document level of anxiety to track trends in anxiety levels. Explore with the patient/family techniques to reduce anxiety. This gives the patient a sense of control and opens communication about the subject. Provide factual information concerning diagnosis, treatment, disfigurement, disabilities, and prognosis. Truthful explanations increase trust and potentially decrease anxiety. Explain all procedures and allow time for mental preparation. This decreases fear and anxiety of the unknown. Explore with the patient effective ways to minimize anxiety. This gives the patient a sense of control. Instruct the patient on use of relaxation techniques *to relieve anxiety.* Assess the need to administer antianxiety and pain medication. *If alternative measures are not effective, the patient may need antianxiety agents.* Assist the patient/family in setting realistic goals for progress. *Indicates effectiveness of emotional adjustment.* Consider psychiatric counseling for patients/families who exhibit inability to accept the situation. *Provide an ongoing plan and interventions to promote long-term relief of anxiety.*
5. NURSING DIAGNOSIS: Impaired Skin Integrity *related to surgery* (NANDA-I © 2012)	
Outcome: Suture lines will heal normally, without complications. ***Evaluation Parameters:*** On inspection of the graft, no areas of dehiscence are seen. Continuous airway maintenance. Gas exchange within normal limits.	Assess wound and incisions. Cleanse incisions and initiate oral care per surgeon's order. Assess nutritional intake. No tracheostomy ties over reconstruction flaps or grafts. Preventing infection and promotion of wound healing. Provide orocutaneous, pharyngocutaneous care: • Wet-to-dry dressing that is packed carefully into the wound per surgeon's order. Protect the airway at all times to prevent infection and maintain airway. **Free Flap Care** • Do not change dressings. • Check neurovascular status. Radial forearm free flap: assess the fingers. Fibular free flap: assess the toes. Assessment of blood supply distal to the flap site. **Drain Care** Secure with Stomahesive and Elastoplast • Strip to prevent clots • Strict output recording • Call surgeon if sudden increase or decrease in output or air leaks from drains Pressure dressing 24 hours after drain removal. **Internal Carotid Artery** Exposed external or intraoral: • Wet to dry dressing to keep carotid in a wet and clean environment • Hespan at bedside

NURSING PROCESS: Patient Care Plan for Head and Neck Cancer, *continued*

	• Type and cross (or hold) two units of blood • Two large bore IV lines in place • Alert operating room that the patient is on precautions • If bleed occurs, apply DIRECT pressure—do not remove • Call surgeon and operating department emergently and prepare patient for transfer.
6. NURSING DIAGNOSIS: High Risk for Infection *related to loss of skin integrity and impaired healing* (NANDA-I © 2012)	
Outcome: Effective infection prevention. ***Evaluation Parameters:*** Surgical sites will not be colonized by organisms. Healing and re-epithelialization will occur as noted by wound closure. Skin integrity will be restored.	Cleanse wounds per protocol to prevent contamination. Assess for infection and document with each dressing change to prevent spread of infection. Assess for drainage: exudate, color, odor, and amount. These factors indicate infection. Assess for undermining or sinus tract formation. Indicates infection. Use strict aseptic technique to prevent infection. Notify health care provider of presence of infection or wound enlargement to facilitate medical intervention. Monitor serum WBC daily. Increased WBC indicates presence of infection. Maintain nutritional therapies. Malnutrition increases the risk of infection.
7. NURSING DIAGNOSIS: Risk for Falls *related to limited site and perception* (NANDA-I © 2012)	
Outcome: Patient will adapt safely to monocular vision. ***Evaluation Parameter:*** Patient is able to navigate safely in the hospital and home environment.	Explain the anatomic changes and discuss the implications for decreased vision. Discuss the implications of monocular vision and safety implications. Patient has knowledge of limitations. Encourage the patient to wear glasses as soon as possible. Helps improve vision. Arrange for home evaluation to make needed adjustments to ensure fall prevention. Improve the safety of the environment.
8. NURSING DIAGNOSES: (a) Disturbed Body Image *related to facial disfigurement and formation and functional loss;* (b) Anticipatory Grieving *related to body image change, risk of family role change, and possible occupational change* (NANDA-I © 2012)	
Outcomes: Acceptance of body image changes. Patient is safe and competent in wound care. Patient and family will cope with deficit. ***Evaluation Parameters:*** Patient will return to activities of daily living and social interactions. Patient verbalizes understanding of body changes.	Teaching will have begun preoperatively with patient education and informed consent. Teach the patient and family about the anatomy, reconstruction, and prosthetic rehabilitation. Begin teaching wound care, orbital packing, and obturator care as soon as possible after packing removal. To increase knowledge and potentially decrease anxiety of the unknown. Have the patient complete dressing with the nurse's support, instruction, and understanding of the visual implications of self-image changes. Begins the adjustment process and increases independence and autonomy. Use eye patch (flesh tones) until orbital prosthesis is made. More aesthetic and less visible.
9. NURSING DIAGNOSIS: Risk for Imbalanced Nutrition; Less Than Body Requirements *related to surgery* (NANDA-I © 2012)	
Outcomes: Patient will have sufficient nutrition to heal. Home nutritional care plan is instituted as needed. ***Evaluation Parameters:*** No weight loss. Nutritional parameters at normal levels. Intake and output within normal limits. Prealbumin levels normal. No aspiration.	Observe ability to orally nourish self safely without aspiration. Arrange for nutrition consult for calorie and protein requirements and intake. Measure intake and output with calorie counts. Nutrition is essential for wound healing. Institute enteral nutrition by nasogastric (NG) or gastrostomy (GT) tube feeding as necessary. • If chyle leak, feed only no-fat formula (Vivonex TEN or similar). • Do not move NG tube. • Secure with Stomahesive and tape to nares. • Do not remove nasal stitch. • Do not attempt to replace NG without health care provider order. • Aspirate NG/GT tube at regular intervals *to check residual volume. Hold tube feeding if greater than amount specified by health care provider.*

(*continued*)

NURSING PROCESS: Patient Care Plan for Head and Neck Cancer, *continued*

Outcomes and Evaluation Parameters	Planning and Interventions with *Rationales*
10. NURSING DIAGNOSIS: Pain *related to surgery* (NANDA-I © 2012)	
Outcome: Comfort level maintained. ***Evaluation Parameters:*** Able to communicate pain level and therapies that help alleviate it. Pain reduced and/or absent as evidenced by patient report and no pain behaviors (i.e., no grimacing). Nonpharmacologic method of control is effective as evidenced by patient report and no pain behaviors. Reports satisfaction with pain management program.	Use pain scale (0–10) to quantify pain level. Quantifying pain increases consistency. Instruct patient to inform nurse if pain is not relieved. Indicates need to change pain management plan. Assess cultural and religious impact on patient's responses. Different cultures and religions respond differently to pain. Correct misconceptions about risk of addiction and overdose to decrease anxiety related to medication addiction. Explain, prepare, and medicate patient for painful procedures (dressing change) and anticipated discomforts to control increased pain level related to procedure. Provide a supportive environment where patient is able to express pain level. Opens communication and facilitates pain management.

Sources: Adapted from Mulgrew, B., & Dropkin, M. J. (1991). Coping with craniofacial resection: A case study. *ORL–Head and Neck Nursing, 9*(3), 8–18; Wilkinson, J. M., & Ahearn, N. R. (2009). *Prentice Hall nursing diagnosis handbook* (9th ed.). Upper Saddle River, NJ: Prentice Hall.

RISK FACTORS for Aspiration

- Decreased level of consciousness (sedation, brain injury, drug overdose, alcohol intoxication, coma)
- Disorders of the aerodigestive tract (post head and neck cancer resection)
- Disorders of the esophagus
- Decreased or absent gag reflex
- Dysphagia
- Neuromuscular disease
- Endotracheal intubation
- Persistently high gastric residual volumes; delayed gastric emptying
- Need for prolonged supine position
- Presence of a nasoenteric tube
- Age
- Malpositioned feeding tube

should be continued after hospital discharge either in the home or on an outpatient basis. Written instructions with pictures are very helpful for the patient and family to follow. This also gives the home health nurse and outpatient physical therapist goals for home therapy.

Postoperative Complications

A number of postoperative complications can occur in the patient with head and neck cancer. Patients who have a history of radiation therapy or who have a poor nutritional status are at greater risk for alterations in wound healing and possible complications. Any type of excessive drainage may indicate a problem; if this is caught early, treatment will mitigate complications. For example, a large amount of milky colored fluid (possibly up to 1 liter in 24 hours) is referred to as a chyle leak. A **chyle leak** is a disruption in the lymph system that causes lymphatic fluid to leak from the thoracic duct on the left side and the lymphatic duct on the right side. The nurse should report this condition to the health care provider immediately because it can result in serious fluid and electrolyte imbalances. Shifts in potassium, sodium, calcium, and magnesium can be life threatening with serious cardiac manifestations. The affected drain is placed to gravity drainage, and a zero-fat diet is implemented. A decrease in fat in the diet will result in a decreased production of lymph. This is done with the hope that the leak will seal itself given the decrease in production of lymphatic fluid. The nurse must monitor fluid and electrolytes.

Bright red, excessive clots or large amounts of drainage indicate abnormal bleeding. Monitoring the patient's hematocrit (HCT) and hemoglobin (HGB) and carefully assessing vital signs are essential when bleeding occurs. The nurse must report any decrease in the HCT and HGB and/or any increase in the pulse rate and decrease in the blood pressure to the surgeon. Each drain is milked, or stripped, according to the surgeon's orders to ensure patency. Stripping will remove excess fluid, drainage, and clots from the surgical area, as well as tubing that may lead to problems of congestion, flap failure, and hematoma at the surgical site. The tube is stripped by first lubricating it with lotion or water-soluble jelly, then pinching the tube between two fingers and pulling down the length of the tubing, creating suction. Great care must be taken not to dislodge the tube from its position in the body. The nurse should report any suspected problems with drain function to the surgeon for immediate intervention.

Other possible postoperative complications include the accumulation of fluid (seroma) or blood (hematoma) in the bed of the surgical wound, infection, fistulas, carotid artery exposure, and flap failure. Fistulas are dehiscent wounds that traverse between two different tissue planes. In the head and neck, a fistula that occurs between the pharynx and the skin is termed a pharyngocutaneous fistula (Figure 26–16◆).

A serious, potentially life-threatening complication is carotid artery exposure and potential rupture. This can occur in the patient who has problems with wound healing, fistula formation, poor nutrition, and/or a history of radiation therapy to the area. A tumor that has been removed close to the carotid artery leaves the artery in jeopardy of rupture, and if the tumor recurs or a fistula forms, the risk further increases. If the primary closure of the surgical incision fails and the artery is exposed to air, it can lead to drying and weakening of the arterial wall. If this occurs, the nurse should place the patient on special alert for what is referred to as carotid blowout precautions. The patient should be in sight of a nurse at all times, and specific supplies are placed in the

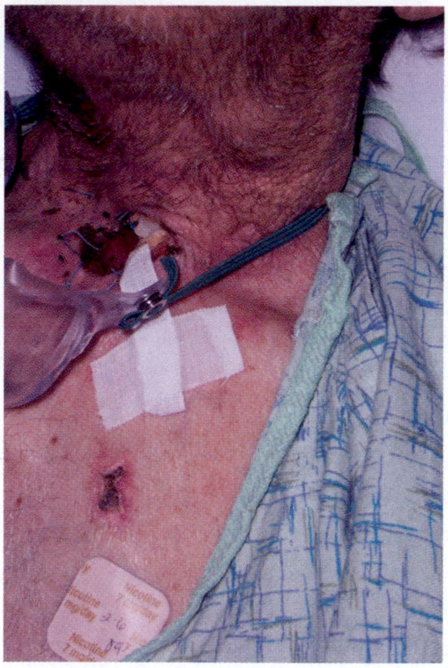

FIGURE 26–16 ◆ This post-laryngectomy patient developed a fistula on his left side just lateral to his laryngectomy stoma. Packing in place is changed four times a day to encourage healing and prevent saliva from entering his stoma.

Source: Ann E. F. Sievers, RN

CHART 26–7 Carotid Artery Precautions

1. Carotid tray at bedside
2. Four packages of fluffs at bedside
3. Dual-suction machines with large oral suction at bedside
4. Portable suction on unit for transport
5. One-liter lactated Ringer's solution at bedside with connecting tubing
6. Two large-bore IVs at all times
7. Blood administration set at bedside
8. Type and antibody screen every 48 hours (1 adult clot tube) or per hospital protocol
9. Two units Hespan (or similar) at bedside
10. Postoperative wound care: saline-soaked dressings (Wet to wet every 2 hours. When stable and healing, advance to every 2 hours while awake and every 4 hours at night, with wetting of the dressing with normal saline every 2 hours.)
11. Frequent observation of patient for "herald" bleed (prerupture bleed), dry or dark area of artery or aneurysm formation
12. Call the house officer or surgeon immediately if any of the above occur.
13. Assess for a higher level of care if other compounding problems are present such as infection.
14. Alert the OR and blood bank that patient is on carotid precautions.

patient's room that will be needed in the event of a rupture. A "herald" bleed (large bleed), or prerupture sign, indicating an imminent bleed, can occur 24 to 48 hours prior to a major carotid rupture. If a rupture occurs, direct digital pressure should be placed on the vessel and the airway maintained with suctioning and positioning. The patient is transported to the operating room immediately to undergo carotid resection. The nurse should never release direct pressure until surgical intervention has been secured. Chart 26–7 outlines typical health care provider orders for carotid artery precautions.

Discharge Priorities

Discharge priorities for patients with head and neck cancer are related to safety at home, airway maintenance, nutrition, wound care, follow-up therapy, compliance with the treatment regimen, and adaptation to illness (see the Patient Teaching & Discharge Priorities box). As these patients prepare for discharge, it is the nurse's responsibility to help the patient transition from hospital to home. All efforts of the clinical nurse specialist, dietitian, speech therapist, discharge planner, health care provider, physical therapist, and social services providers must be directed toward adaptation and safety. The most important part of the discharge process is to remember that discharge planning begins at the time of diagnosis.

Gerontological Considerations

In the older adult, hoarseness can be a result of changes in the texture or shape of the vocal cords from aging. It also can be the result of dehydration from poor nutritional intake and/or medications. Bowing of the vocal cords may occur, which does not allow the cords to meet fully in the middle. Stiffness may also decrease the normal vibratory action of the cords, resulting in a coarse and breathy voice. Arthritic changes in the cricoarytenoid joints can decrease the motion of the vocal cords. How the patient is affected by these changes depends on the severity of the decreased motion and how it manifests in the patient.

Other physical changes of aging that may affect the older patient's ability to heal from fractures and surgeries involving the upper airway include the following:

1. Declining cardiac/renal function
2. Diminished memory and inductive reasoning
3. Decreased visual acuity
4. Diminished hearing
5. Diminished response to stress and sensory stimuli
6. Decreased mobility.

Research

Improvement of patient care and outcomes is a constant goal in nursing. Through research nurses can achieve these improvements. The Research Opportunities box lists some areas of research related to upper airway disorders.

PATIENT TEACHING & DISCHARGE PRIORITIES for Patients with Head and Neck Cancer

Need	Teaching
Knowledge of home and self-care following surgery for head and neck cancer	Health care needs include verbal and written instructions for treatment plan and follow-up care. Assess patient and family understanding of disease process, surgical procedure performed, and health maintenance needs in the home setting.
Maintenance of airway	Patient and family are taught how to maintain an open airway by: • Providing verbal and written instructions on self-care needs, equipment usage, and indicators for emergency assistance. • Providing instructions on self-suctioning, wound care, change of tracheostomy tube, and safety precautions.
Nutrition	Patient and family are taught about nutritional needs by: • Instructing patient/family on nutritional needs, calories needed per day, and how to use enteral feedings. • Providing consultation from a dietitian as necessary.
Wound care	Ascertain the patient and family's ability to care for the wound using aseptic technique: • Instruct the patient and family on wound care and evaluate their ability to complete it by ensuring a return demonstration. • Provide all necessary supplies for wound care and ask the patient and family to keep track of the availability of necessary supplies.
Physical therapy	Determine the patient's ability to perform exercises as directed by demonstrating exercises.
Speech therapy	Establish means of communication; practice speech. Instruct the patient to keep track of therapy appointments and observe compliance to prescribed therapy.
Safety	Stress the importance of safety precautions by: • Instructing the patient and family to keep emergency numbers by the phone. • Instructing the patient to keep written instructions for self-care easily accessible. • Reinforcing instructions for airway maintenance.
Family/significant other support system	Assess the availability, knowledge, and compliance with treatment regimen. Assess for need for professional home health needs. Establish a plan for caretaker rest and support. Establish a plan for assurance of meeting the patient's rest needs. Discuss with the patient and family independence goals and establish markers for advancement toward independence.
Follow-up therapy	Assist the patient in establishing a calendar of appointments with the expected outcome that the patient will keep appointments.
Compliance	Evaluate the patient for knowledge of compliance needs in self-care including the patient maintaining ongoing appointments as scheduled.
Adaptation to illness	Assess the patient's and family's coping needs and methods of coping. Encourage open discussion of feelings and concerns. Provide psychological counseling as needed.

RESEARCH OPPORTUNITIES Related to Upper Airway Disorders

Research Area	Clinical Impact
Use of normal saline infusions by home health or the infusion center in the ambulatory patient with an artificial airway.	Better hydration and fluid replacement techniques. Decreased frequency of dehydration.
Quality of life for patients and caregivers of those with head and neck cancer.	Improved quality of life.
What is safe staffing for an otolaryngology unit or clinic given the fragility of patients with artificial and at-risk airways?	Ability to define the appropriate staffing mix for an ENT nursing unit or clinic based on nursing decisions, patient education, and interventions.

CLINICAL PREPARATION

READ DOCUMENT APPLY

READ: **History of Present Illnesses** >> Laboratory Study Results >> Critical Thinking Questions

Kara Cole, a 23-year-old female, was brought in by ambulance to the emergency department (ED). She was transported because of an injury to her anterior neck after being hit by a softball during practice. She was responsive, sitting in an upright forward position. She was initially evaluated by the ED health care provider. An otolaryngologist was urgently consulted because the patient's airway distress was increasing as her neck swelling increased. There was too much swelling to safely view the vocal cords for intubation. With fluid resuscitation and stabilization, the patient was taken to the operating room, where the health care provider performed a tracheotomy.

Following recovery from anesthesia, Ms. Cole was alert and cognitively intact and could write to the staff. After 2 days in the ICU to rule out any other injuries such as closed head injury, Ms. Cole was transferred to an acute care unit where you assumed care of her. Her tracheotomy was downsized from a cuffed #8 to an uncuffed #6 tracheostomy tube. She was taught to speak by covering the tube with finger occlusion. Her voice was very hoarse, and she coughed while drinking liquids. Aspiration precautions were initiated, and otolaryngology speech therapists were called in to assess Ms. Cole's voice and swallowing. Speech therapists continued to evaluate her hoarse, breathy voice and dysphagia. On fiber-optic examination, it was apparent that she was not able to medialize her right vocal cord and her larynx was insensate; this led to the hoarseness and inability to protect the airway during eating. Ms. Cole did not appear to be experiencing any further respiratory difficulties, and her vital signs and oxygen (O_2) saturations were all within normal limits.

A dynamic swallow study was done in the speech lab to further assess the degree of difficulty Ms. Cole had protecting her airway while eating and to evaluate her vocal cord status. The speech therapist worked with Ms. Cole with different types of food textures to determine which ones she could safely handle. It was determined that pureed food with thick liquids would be the safest diet for Ms. Cole.

Dietary services was notified of the change in diet, and a request was made to have the nurse deliver a food tray to Ms. Cole. That way, it was certain that she would be positioned properly in a chair or with the head of the bed at 90 degrees and that she would be observed for aspiration throughout the meal. Suction was available at the bedside for use as needed.

READ: History of Present Illnesses >> **Physical Exam** >> Admitting Medical Records >> Laboratory Study Results

Medical–Surgical History

Appendectomy and tonsillectomy as a child

Social History

Married, no children; attends graduate school
Travels frequently in the United States with her softball team

Physical Exam

Head: normocephalic, nontraumatic, no lacerations or bruising
Eyes: normal EOM bilaterally, PERL
Ears: WNL no hemotympanum or trauma
Nose: WNL
Mouth: WNL no evidences of trauma, tongue not swollen, occasional coughing of blood
Neck: Significant bruising was noted in the anterior of the neck; attributed to the direct injury of the softball
Cranial Nerves: CNI not tested; CNX impairment on the L side; others WNL

Admitting Medical Orders

Otolaryngology service
Admit to Medical–Surgical floor
Admitting diagnosis: 23-year-old woman admitted status postinjury to the neck by a softball; tracheotomy
Allergies: none known
Up ad lib with bathroom privileges
Head of bed at 90 degrees or up in chair for meals
Diet: pureed food with thick liquids
Vital signs and oxygen saturation q4h
Neuro assessment q4h
I&O
IV D51/2 NS at 75 mL/hr until tolerating fluids; then convert to saline lock: flush q8h with NS
Aspiration precautions
Routine tracheostomy care
Suction prn
O_2 per humidified trach collar to keep oxygen saturation >92%
Call house officer: pulse <60 and >130/minute; BP <90 and >160 systolic; temperature >38.5; urine output <30 mL/hr for 2 hours; respiratory rate >30/minute; oxygen saturation <92%
Sequential compression devices (SCDs) to lower extremities while in bed

Scheduled Medications

Morphine sulfate PCA: 1 mg incremental dose q10min. If pain not well controlled, give morphine sulfate bolus 1–5 mg IV × 1

PRN Medications

Temazepam 15–30 mg po qhs prn insomnia
Zofran 4 mg IV over 2 min as needed for nausea
Ativan 1 mg IV q6h prn anxiety
Milk of Magnesia 30 mL daily prn constipation
Tylenol 650 mg po/PR q4h prn for pain

Ordered Laboratory Studies

Chemistry 7 panel, CBC, ABGs, and magnesium daily
INR × 1

Ordered Diagnostic Studies

Flexible fiber-optic laryngoscopy
Videostroboscopy
Dynamic swallow study

READ: History of Present Illnesses >> **Laboratory Study Results** >> Critical Thinking Questions

Test	Day 1	Day 2	Day 3
Sodium	137 mEq/L	136 mEq/L	139 mEq/L
Potassium	3.8 mEq/L	3.8 mEq/L	3.7 mEq/L
Chloride	106 mEq/L	103 mEq/L	110 mEq/L
Blood urea nitrogen (BUN)	4 mg/dL	4 mg/dL	6 mg/dL
Creatinine	1.1 mg/dL	0.9 mg/dL	0.7 mg/dL
Blood glucose	143 mg/dL	120 mg/dL	98 mg/dL
Calcium	7.9 mEq/L	7.8 mEq/L	9.1 mEq/L
Total protein	6.3 g/dL	6.0 g/dL	5.8 g/dL
Magnesium	2.1 mEq/L	1.9 mEq/L	2.4 mEq/L
White blood count	12,600 µL	19.1 µL	13.4 µL

Test	Day 1	Day 2	Day 3
Hemoglobin	9.8 g/dL	10.6 g/dL	12.5 g/dL
Hematocrit	28.1%	29.6%	31.5%
Red blood cells	3.35 million/µL	3.26 million/µL	3.67 million/µL
Platelets	195,000 µL	189,000 µL	241,000 µL
INR	1.00 INR		
ABGs			
PaO_2	98 mmHg	112 mmHg	96 mmHg
O_2 sat	96%	99%	97
pH	7.44	7.46	7.56
$PaCO_2$	36 mmHg	35 mmHg	24 mmHg
HCO_3	25 mEq/L	25 mEq/L	20 mEq/L

Pearson Nursing Student Resources *Log on to* **nursing.pearsonhighered.com** *to download forms*

DOCUMENT:

>> Summary of Hospitalization

>> Pathophysiology Form

>> Laboratory Values

>> Laboratory Results Explanation

APPLY:

>> List of Potential Nursing Diagnoses

>> Concept Map

>> Critical Thinking Questions and Concept Map

READ: History of Present Illnesses >> Laboratory Study Results >> **Critical Thinking Questions**

1. Explain what the nurse's responsibility is to a patient who is unable to communicate by natural voice. What are the alternatives and what are the nurse's professional responsibilities?
2. Discuss the implications of nursing interventions used with a patient in airway obstruction following traumatic injury. How can the nurse help the patient adapt to a new airway?
3. Think of the quality-of-life implications for a 23-year-old athlete who has a tracheostomy and airway injury. Discuss the role of compassion and comportment in the nursing care of such a patient.

Answers to Critical Thinking Questions can be found in Appendix D in the Osborn Student Resources at nursing.pearsonhighered.com.

NCLEX® PRACTICE

1. The nurse is caring for a pediatric patient recovering from a fractured mandible. Which of the following should be included in this patient's plan of care?
   1. Provide system antibiotics to prevent meningitis.
   2. Once stable, instruct in the use of a water pick.
   3. Provide eye protection.
   4. Assess for facial droop every 2 hours.
2. What should the nurse include in self-care education for a patient with acute sinusitis?
   1. Drink no more than 1 liter of fluids each day.
   2. Take your antibiotics on time and finish the prescription.
   3. Stay on bedrest until your headache goes away.
   4. Make an appointment with your dentist for follow-up care.

3. The nurse is planning instruction for a patient with seasonal allergic rhinitis. What should be included in this instruction?
   1. Expect to have allergy injections for 6 months.
   2. Spend time outdoors to increase immunity to the allergen.
   3. Boil a pan of water on the stove every day to increase environmental humidity.
   4. Avoid exposure to strong perfumes, smoke, and rapid changes in temperature.
4. During an assessment, an older patient says, "I just don't smell things like I once did." What should the nurse ask this patient in regard to this statement? (select all that apply)
   1. "Do you have a smoke detector in your home?"
   2. "Can you move your neck as well as you once did?"
   3. "Has your appetite changed?"
   4. "Do you have any shortness of breath?"
   5. "What kind of cooking appliances do you use?"
5. A patient states, "I just can't stay awake in the afternoons. I don't think I sleep well at night." Which risk factors for the development of obstructive sleep apnea would the nurse look for in this patient's history? (select all that apply)
   1. The patient has a 24 pack-year smoking history.
   2. The patient is 10 pounds under desired weight.
   3. The patient is 41 years old.
   4. The patient is male.
   5. The patient was diagnosed with type 1 diabetes mellitus as a child.
6. A nurse is attending a picnic where a 9-year-old boy develops a nosebleed. What actions should the nurse take?
   1. Place pressure over the bridge of the child's nose.
   2. Have the child tilt his head back while someone applies ice to the back of his neck.
   3. Have the child pinch his nostrils together and lean forward.
   4. Stay with the child and have someone call 911.

Answers to NCLEX Practice questions can be found in Appendix D in the Osborn Student Resources at nursing.pearsonhighered.com. Practice additional NCLEX questions online at the Student Resources site.

Pearson Nursing Student Resources Find additional review materials at: **nursing.pearsonhighered.com**

REFERENCES

Ali Mel, S. (2008). Laryngopharyngeal reflux: Diagnosis and treatment of a controversial disease. *Current Opinion in Allergy and Clinical of Immunology, 8*(1), 28–33. doi: 10.1097/ACI.0b013e3282f3f44f

American Academy of Otolaryngology–Head and Neck Surgery. (2007). Fact sheet: Deviated septum. Retrieved from http://www.entnet.org/HealthInformation/deviatedSeptum.cfm

American Association of Respiratory Care (AARC). (2010). Clinical practice guildelines. Retrieved from http://www.rcjournal.com/cpgs/

Babak, J., & Blackwell, K. (2009). Facial bone anatomy. Retrieved from http://emedicine.medscape.com/article/835401-overview

Bachert, C., Gevaert, P., & Cauwenberge, P. (2008). Nasal polyps and rhinosinusitis. In F. Adkinson (Ed.), Middleton's allergy principles and practice (7th ed.). Philadelphia: Elsevier.

Becker, D., & Ross, A. (2009). Nasal and septal fractures. Retrieved from http://emedicine.medscape.com/article/878595-overview

Benninger, M. (2010). The pathogenesis of rhinosinusitis. In P. Flint (Ed.), *Cummings otolaryngology: Head & neck surgery* (5th ed.). Philadelphia: Mosby Elsevier.

Brook, I. (2011). Acute sinusitis. In B. Cunha (Ed.), Medscape reference. Retrieved from http://emedicine.medscape.com/article/232670-overview

Burns, J., & Hendley, J. (2010). Epiglottitis. In R. Mason (Ed.), *Murray and Nadel's textbook of respiratory medicine* (5th ed.). Philadelphia: Saunders Elsevier.

Cha, J. H., Lee, S. H., & Yoo, Y. S. (2010). Effects of aromatherapy on changes in the autonomic nervous system, aortic pulse wave velocity and aortic augmentation index in patients with essential hypertension. *Journal of Korean Academy of Nursing, 40*(5), 705–713.

Chung, F., Ward, B., Ho, J., Yuan, H., Kayumov, L., & Shapiro, C. (2007). Preoperative identification of sleep apnea risk in elective surgical patients, using the Berlin Questionnaire. *Journal of Clinical Anesthesia, 19*(2), 130–134.

Davidson, T. M., & Patel, M. R. (2008). Waist circumference and sleep disordered breathing. *Laryngoscope, 118*(2), 339–347.

DeShazo, R., & Kemp, S. (2011). Pharmacotherapy of allergic rhinitis. In J. Corren & A. Feldweg (Eds.), UpToDate. Waltham, MA: UpToDate.

Fletcher, R. (2011). An overview of rhinitis. In J. Corren & A. Feldweg (Eds.), UpToDate. Waltham, MA: UpToDate.

Franco, R. (2011). Laryngopharyngeal reflux. In D. Deschler & P. Eamranond (Eds.), UpToDate. Waltham, MA: UpToDate.

Gifford, T., & Orlandi, R. (2008). Epistaxis. *Otolarygologic Clinics of North America, 41*(3), 525–536.

Hagberg, C., Georgi, R., & Krier, C. (2007). Complications of managing the airway. In C. Hagberg (Ed.), Benumof's airway management (2nd ed.). Philadelphia, Mosby Elsevier.

Hallowell, P. T., Stelloato, T., Schuster, M., Graf, K., Robinson, A., Crouse, C., et al. (2007). Potentially life threatening sleep apnea is unrecognized without aggressive evaluation. *The American Journal of Surgery, 193*, 364–367.

Hamilos, D. (2011). Clinical manifestations, pathophysiology, and diagnosis of chronic rhinosinusitis. In J. Corren, D. Deschler, & A. Feidweg (Eds.), UpToDate. Waltham, MA: UpToDate.

Hedayat, K. M. (2008, March–April). Reduction of benzodiazepine requirements during mechanical ventilation in a child by topical application of essential oils. *Explore (NY), 4*(2), 136–138.

Hwang, D., Shakir, N., Limann, B., Sison, D., Kalra, S., Shulman, L., et al. (2008). Association of sleep-disordered breathing with postoperative complications. Chest: *The Cardiopulmonary and Critical Care Journal, 130*(3), 1128–1134.

Hwang, P., & Getz, A. (2011). Acute sinusitis and rhinosinusitis in adults. In D. Deschler, S. S. Calderwood, & N. Sokol (Eds.), UpToDate. Waltham, MA: UpToDate.

IOM (Institute of Medicine). (2010). The future of nursing: Leading change, advancing health. Washington, DC: The Academic Press.

Johnson, F., Semaan, M., & Megerian, C. (2008). Temporal bone fracture: Evaluation and management in the modern era. *Otolaryngolotic Clinic of North America, 41*(3), 597–618.

Joe, S., & Patel, S. (2010). Nonallergic rhinitis. In P. Flint (Ed.), Cummings otolaryngology: Head and necksurgery (5th ed.). Philadelphia: Mosby Elsevier.

Kiecolt-Glaser, J. K., Graham, J. E., Malarkey, W. B., Porter, K., Lemeshow, S., & Glaser, R. (2008). Olfactory influences on mood and autonomic, endocrine, and immune function. *Psychneuroendocrinology, 33*(2), 328–339.

Kontoyiannis, D. (2011). Mucormycosis. In L. Goldman & A. Schafer (Eds.), Goldman's Cecil medicine (24th ed.). Philadelphia, Elsevier Saunders.

Kontoyiannis, D., & Lewis, R. (2009). Agents of mucormycosis and entomophthoramycosis. In G. Mandell, J. Bennett, & R. Dolin (Eds.), Principles and practice of infectious diseases (7th ed.). Philadelphia: Churchill Livingstone.

Kryger, M. (2011). Management of obstructive sleep apnea. In R. Basner, M. Sanders, & K. Wilson (Eds.), UpToDate. Waltham, MA: UpToDate.

Lavie, L., Vishnevsky, A., & Levie, P. (2007). Oxidative stress and systemic inflammation in patients with sleep apnea: Role of obesity. *Sleep and Biological Rhythms, 5*(2), 100–110.

Leung, R., & Katial, R. (2008). The diagnosis and management of acute chronic sinusitis. *Primary Care: Clinics in Office Practice, 35*(1).doi: 10.1016/j.pop.2007.09.02

Lieberman, P. (2011). Chronic nonallergic rhinitis. In J. Corren & A. Feldweg (Eds.), UptoDate. Waltham, MA: UpToDate.

Manes, P. (2010). Evaluating and managing the patient with nose bleeds. *Medical Clinics of North America, 94*(5), 903–912.

March, A., Connell, S., Belafsky, P., & Belafsky, M. (2010). Temporal bone fractures. Retrieved from http://emedicine.medscape.com/article/857365-overview

Martinez-Rivera, C., Abad, J., Fiz, J., Rios, J., & Morera, J. (2008). Usefulness of truncal obesity indices as predictive factors for obstructive sleep apnea syndrome. *Obesity, 16*(1), 113–118.

Mulgrew, B., & Dropkin, M. J. (1991). Coping with craniofacial resection: A case study. *ORL–Head and Neck Nursing, 9*(3), 8–18.

Nicolato, E., Boschi, F., Marzola, P., & Sbarbati, A.J. (2009, July 30). Secretory response induced by essential oils on airway surface fluid: A pharmacological MRI study *Ethnopharmacol, 124*(3), 630–634. Epub 2009 May 5.

Norman, P. (2011). Subcutaneous immunotherapy for allergic disease: Indications and efficacy. In P. Creticos & A. Feldweg, UpToDate. Waltham: MA, UpToDate.

O'Handley, J., Tobin, E., & Shah, A. (2011). Otorhinolaryngology. In R. Rakel & D. Rakel (Eds.), Textbook of family medicine (8th ed.). Philadelphia: Elsevier Saunders.

Okabayashi, K., Kasahara, E., Uchiyama, H., Yodota, K., Togashi, Y., Kono, C., et al. (2007). Obstructive sleep apnea-hypopnea syndrome patients with overweight and hypertension in a Japanese workplace. *Journal of Occupational Health, 49*(2), 117–124.

Orban, N., Saleh, H., & Durham, S. (2008). Allergic and non-allergic rhinitis. In F. Adkinson (Ed.), Middleton's allergy principles and practice (7th ed.). Philadelphia: Elsevier.

Piccolino, P., Vetrano, S., Mundula, P., Di Lella, G., Tedaldi, M., & Poladas, G. (2007). Frontal bone fractures: A new technique of closed reduction. Technical strategies. *Journal of Craniofacial Surgery, 18*(3), 695–698.

Pien, G., & Pack, A. (2010). Sleep-disordered breathing. In R. Mason (Ed.), *Murray and Nadel's textbook of respiratory medicine* (5th ed.). Philadelphia: Saunders Elsevier.

PubMed Health. (2011). Oral cancer. Retrieved from http://www.ncbi.nlm.nih.gov/pubmedhealth/PMH0002030/#adam_001035.disease.prognosis

Ramakrishnan, V. (2010). Pharmacotherapy of nonallergic rhinitis. In A. Meyers (Ed.), Medscape reference. Retrieved from http://emedicine.medscape.com/article/874171-overview.

Richard, W., Kox, D., den Herder, C., Laman, M., van Tinteren, H., & de Vries, N. (2006). The role of sleep position in obstructive sleep apnea syndrome. *European Archives of Oto-Rhino-Laryngology, 263*(10), 946–950.

Sadlon, A. E., & Lamson, D. W. (2010, April). Immune-modifying and antimicrobial effects of Eucalyptus oil and simple inhalation devices. *Alternative Medicine Review, 15*(1), 33–47.

Sandhu, G., & Nouraei, S. (2010). Laryngeal and esophageal trauma. In P. Flint (Ed.), Cummings otolaryngology: Head and necksurgery (5th ed.). Philadelphia: Mosby Elsevier.

Sheikh, J. (2012). Allergic rhinitis. Retrieved from http://emedicine.medscape.com/article/134825-overview

Sheldon, A., Belan, I., Neill, J., & Rowland, S. (2010). Nursing assessment of obstructive sleep apnea in hospitalized adults: A review of risk factors and screening tools. *Contemporary Nurse, 34*(1), 19–33.

Stenson, K., & Brockstein, B. (2011). Overview of head and neck cancer. In M. Posner & M. Ross (Eds.), UpToDate. Waltham, MA: UpToDate.

Strohl, K. (2011). Overview of obstructive sleep apnea in adults. In R. Basner & M. Sanders (Eds.), UpToDate. Waltham, MA: UpToDate.

U.S. Department of Health and Human Services.(2010). *Healthy People 2020.* Retrieved from http://www.healthypeople.gov/2020/topicsobjectives2020/default.aspx

Wang, M. (2011). Etiologies of nasal symptoms: An overview. In J. Corren & A. Feldweg, UpToDate. Waltham, MA: UpToDate.

Wilkinson, J. M., & Ahearn, N. R. (2009). *Prentice Hall nursing diagnosis handbook* (9th ed.). Upper Saddle River, NJ: Prentice Hall.

Woodson, G., Blitzer, A., Alexander, R., & Grant, N. (2010). Neurologic evaluation of the larynx and pharynx. In P. Flint (Ed.), Cummings otolaryngology: Head and neck surgery (5th ed.). Philadelphia: Mosby Elsevier.

Zellweger, R. (2007). Maxillofacial fractures. *Australian and New Zealand Journal of Surgery, 77*(8), 613.

Caring for the Patient with Lower Airway Disorders

27 CHAPTER

Carol Rhoades
Cheryl Wraa

Outcome-Based Learning Objectives

After studying this chapter, the learner will be able to:

1. Differentiate between restrictive and obstructive lung diseases.
2. Compare and contrast the etiology, pathophysiology, clinical manifestations, nursing management, and prevention of the various pulmonary infections and inflammatory disorders.
3. Generate a nursing management plan for patients with COPD, chronic bronchitis, asthma, cystic fibrosis, pulmonary embolism, and cor pulmonale.
4. Evaluate the effectiveness of nursing interventions in the management of patients with lung cancer.
5. Create an education plan for prevention and health promotion for patients with pulmonary interstitial disease.

KEY TERMS

acute bronchitis p.731
asbestosis p.760
asthma p.732
atelectasis p.772
carbon monoxide p.782
chronic bronchitis p.761
chronic obstructive pulmonary disease (COPD) p.761
coal worker's pneumoconiosis p.760
cor pulmonale p.777
cystic fibrosis (CF) p.768
emphysema p.761
empyema p.752
hemoptysis p.752
influenza p.739
lung abscess p.755
metered-dose inhaler (MDI) p.737
near drowning p.781
pleural effusion p.779
pneumonia p.740
pneumothorax p.757
polycythemia vera p.763
pulmonary embolism (PE) p.771
silicosis p.759

A VARIETY OF PATHOLOGIES can affect the respiratory system. These respiratory alterations include infections; obstructive diseases; occupational diseases; restrictive disorders; and pleural, vascular, and malignant disruptions. This chapter discusses in depth the nursing management of the common respiratory diseases.

Infections and Inflammatory Disorders

Respiratory infections are common, and most individuals will experience symptoms of influenza at some point during their lifetime. However, infections of the respiratory tract can be potentially life threatening and are a significant cause of morbidity and mortality. The increasing number of resistant organisms heightens the complexity of treatment. The nurse's awareness of assessment, treatment, and prevention of respiratory infections is an important component of patient health and recovery.

Acute Bronchitis

Acute bronchitis is inflammation of the mid and large airways of the lung without evidence of pneumonia. Bronchitis can be acute or chronic. Acute bronchitis is one of the most common conditions treated by primary health care providers (File, 2011).

Etiology and Epidemiology

Acute bronchitis is most prevalent in children and older adults, and the incidence is highest in the winter. It tends to be brief and self-limiting. Individuals who are at increased risk include those with chronic respiratory or cardiac illnesses, smokers, young children and infants, and older adults (Blaivas, 2010). Acute bronchitis is most often caused by a viral infection, but the source can also be bacterial.

Pathophysiology

When airways are assaulted by chemical agents or microorganisms, the result is an inflammation of the lower bronchial mucous membranes. Acute bronchitis commonly follows a respiratory viral illness from the upper airway. The usual viral perpetrators vary by age and season. They include influenza A and B, rhinovirus, parainfluenza, and respiratory syncytial virus (RSV). There is no strong clinical evidence that bacterial infections that cause pneumonia (*Streptococcus pneumoniae, Haemophilus influenzae, Staphylococcus aureus*) also cause

Weblink: Acute Bronchitis

Video: Asthma—Etiology and Pathophysiology

acute bronchitis, unless an artificial airway is in place (Blaivas, 2010). Patients who smoke, have chronic respiratory conditions (COPD) (p. 761), or have impaired ability to clear their airway (e.g., cystic fibrosis) are at increased risk of developing acute bronchitis. Viruses that cause acute bronchitis do not affect gas exchange unless the bronchitis progresses to pneumonia or chronic bronchitis, which are discussed later in the chapter.

Clinical Manifestations

Acute bronchitisis characterized by cough, with or without sputum, which generally occurs with, or subsequent to, an upper respiratory infection (URI). Acute bronchitis may initially be difficult to distinguish from an URI. A persistent cough lasting more than 5 days is suggestive of acute bronchitis, and it generally lasts between 10 and 20 days (Blaivas, 2010). The cough is the last symptom to go away. About half of these patients will present with purulent sputum, which usually represents sloughing of cells from the tracheobronchial epithelium along with inflammatory cells and does not indicate bacterial infection (Blaivas, 2010). There is no correlation between sputum characteristics (clear, purulent) and etiology (viral vs. bacterial).

Laboratory and Diagnostic Tests

The majority of patients with acute bronchitis do not require diagnostic testing. Most are treated on the basis of their history and exam. If symptoms suggest pneumonia, such as labored or rapid breathing, reduced oxygen saturations, altered mental status, or abnormal breath sounds, then a chest x-ray (CXR) may be ordered to diagnose any lung involvement. Bacterial sputum cultures of patients with a negative CXR are not necessary, since bacteria is rarely the source of acute bronchitis (File, 2011). If there is a local outbreak of mycoplasma or chlamydophila or if pertussis is suspected, then culture collection is justified.

Medical Management

The airway inflammation caused by acute bronchitis is usually self-limiting. Treatment is generally targeted to symptomatic relief. These treatments include use of analgesics, anticholinergics (ipratropium), and nonsteroidal anti-inflammatories. Refer to the Pharmacology box on page 744. The literature shows limited support for antitussives (cough suppressants) and discourages antibiotic treatment. Antibiotics are often abused and overused in treating acute bronchitis and should not be routinely administered in otherwise healthy patients unless they are older adults, have comorbidities, or have pertussis. Cough suppressants should be reserved for cough-related sleeplessness. Inhaled corticosteroids may be ordered for persistent cough.

Nursing Management

The nursing process guides the care of patients with pulmonary infections. Diagnosis of acute bronchitis is based on symptom history.

Assessment

Assessment findings for acute bronchitis most commonly include a persistent cough, with or without sputum production, which lasts for more than 5 days. Patients frequently have significant bronchospasm with airway hyperreactivity. A mild fever may be present, but a high or prolonged fever is unusual and is suggestive of influenza or pneumonia (Bartlett, 2008).

Nursing Diagnoses

Priority nursing diagnoses for the patient with acute bronchitis include the following:

- *Airway Clearance, Ineffective* related to inflammation and bronchospasm
- *Gas Exchange, Impaired* related to inflammation
- *Activity Intolerance* related to inflammation and persistent cough

NANDA-I © 2012

Outcomes and Evaluation Parameters

The outcomes of nursing management include relief of the clinical manifestations and a return to the previous level of functioning. Evaluation parameters include whether cough has been suppressed and whether the patient has returned to her baseline activity level.

Interventions and Rationales

Nursing interventions for acute bronchitis focus on assisting patients with prescribed therapies. In addition to administering mild analgesics such as nonsteroidal anti-inflammatories or acetaminophen (Tylenol) for discomfort, the nurse encourages the patient to increase fluid intake to 2 to 3 liters per day for thinning secretions and to prevent dehydration. The nurse should advise the patient, and assist if necessary, to ambulate and cough; the nurse should also instruct the patient in deep breathing exercises to help mobilize secretions. Adequate rest and avoidance of known bronchial irritants, including smoking, will facilitate recovery. In addition, using a humidifier at night may help relieve a persistent dry cough. The patient should be instructed on prevention, such as hand washing and avoidance of risk factors. The nurse also should instruct the patient to recognize progression of symptoms such as persistent fever, increased sputum, and increased shortness of breath and ensure that the patient knows when to seek further medical care.

Asthma

Asthma, as defined by the National Heart, Lung, and Blood Institute (NHLBI, 2007), is a common chronic disorder of the airways that is characterized by variable and episodic symptoms, airflow obstruction, bronchial hyperresponsiveness, and airway inflammation. This inflammatory process causes wheezing, breathlessness, chest tightness, and coughing. These episodes are usually associated with airflow obstruction that is often reversible.

Epidemiology and Etiology

The prevalence of asthma has increased continuously since the 1970s, and the disorder now affects an estimated 4% to 7% of people worldwide (NHLBI, 2007). In the United States, more than 20 million people are affected by asthma, 6 million of whom are children, making it one of the most common chronic childhood diseases (Blair, Breit, & Peters, 2008). In approximately 75% of cases, asthma is diagnosed before the age of 7. Many adolescents will experience a remission during puberty, only to have the asthma recur several years later. Boys are more likely to acquire the disease before puberty and girls after puberty. Even though death rates have declined in recent years, mortality continues to be a significant problem. Worldwide, approximately 180,000 deaths per year are attributed to asthma; over 4,000 of these occur in the United States. The improvement in the mortality rates can at least partially be attributed to the use of inhaled corticosteroids, better access to medical care, recognition, and diagnosis. Death rates are higher among people over 65 years old, women, Puerto Ricans, and African Americans. Women have a 45% higher risk of dying than males. Puerto Ricans have the highest risk, at 3.6 times higher than the rate for Whites; the rate for African Americans is 2 times higher than that of Whites. This disparity might be explained

Weblink: Asthma

by factors such as access to health care, exposures to triggers in inner city areas, inaccessibility of medications, and health care inconsistencies (Lugogo, Que, Fertel, & Kraft, 2010).

The etiology of the increase in prevalence of asthma is unknown but is likely related to both environmental and individual factors, such as allergen exposure and obesity. The "hygiene hypothesis" is the speculation that exposure to endotoxins and bacterial and viral infections at a young age stimulates immune responses that help to develop tolerance. If exposure decreases, then tolerance is not developed. The lack of exposure in developed countries would at least partially explain why asthma prevalence is on the rise in countries where families are smaller, antibiotics are more readily available, living conditions are cleaner, and vaccinations are more prevalent.

Pathophysiology

In patients with asthma, inflammatory cells, particularly eosinophils (disease-fighting white blood cells), form an inflammatory infiltrate in the epithelium and smooth muscle of the airway. This initial inflammation is thought to result from an inappropriate immune response to an antigen in genetically predisposed individuals. This inflammation leads to structural changes (remodeling) in the airway and hypertrophy of the smooth muscle, narrowing of the airway, and increased reactivity to allergens, infections, parasympathetic stimulation, or other bronchoconstrictive triggers. (See the Risk Factors box.) Mucus plugging and peripheral blood eosinophilia are classic findings in asthma and may be a by-product of airway inflammation (Blair, Breit, & Peters, 2008). This process of inflammation, obstruction, and hyperreactivity is demonstrated in Figure 27–1◆. The degree of airway hyperreactivity generally correlates with the clinical severity of asthma.

The body's response to these triggers is reversible airway narrowing and uneven lung ventilation (Blair, Breit, & Peters, 2008). This alters the relatively equal ventilation-perfusion ratio in that vascular perfusion is now greater than alveolar ventilation. In the airways distal to bronchoconstriction, oxygen tension falls and carbon dioxide tension rises. This is usually compensated for by hyperventilating; however, in severe asthma, there is severe and diffuse bronchoconstriction/airflow obstruction that leads to air-trapping in the alveoli. The mechanics of respiration in these circumstances place a burden on the respiratory muscles, and the work of breathing increases. Oxygenation of the blood decreases and carbon dioxide levels rise, leading to respiratory and metabolic acidosis. If this condition is left untreated, respiratory and cardiac arrest will ensue.

RISK FACTORS Triggers for Asthma

Inhaled Allergens

- Dust mites (contained in house dust)
- Cockroaches
- Mold (indoor and outdoor)
- Pollen from trees and grass
- Animal dander (from the skin, hair, or feathers of animals)

Respiratory Irritants

- Tobacco smoke
- Air pollution
- Chlorine-based cleaning products
- Scented products such as perfumes
- Wood smoke from stoves or fireplaces
- Cold air or changes in weather
- Strong odors from painting or cooking
- Living in a large urban area
- Strong emotional expression (including excitement, anxiety, anger)

Comorbid Conditions

- COPD/emphysema
- Obesity
- Gastroesophageal reflux
- Depression/chronic stress
- Allergic bronchopulmonary aspergillosis
- Obstructive sleep apnea
- Rhinitis/sinusitis

Other

- Exercise
- Medications: Nonselective beta-blockers, aspirin, NSAIDs
- Sulfites in food (dried fruit) or beverages (wine)
- Complication of influenza
- Complications of pneumococcal infection
- Having one or both parents with asthma

Source: Fanta, C., & Fletcher, S. (2010). *An overview of asthma management.* In R. Wood & B. Bochner (Eds.), UpToDate. Waltham, MA: UpToDate.

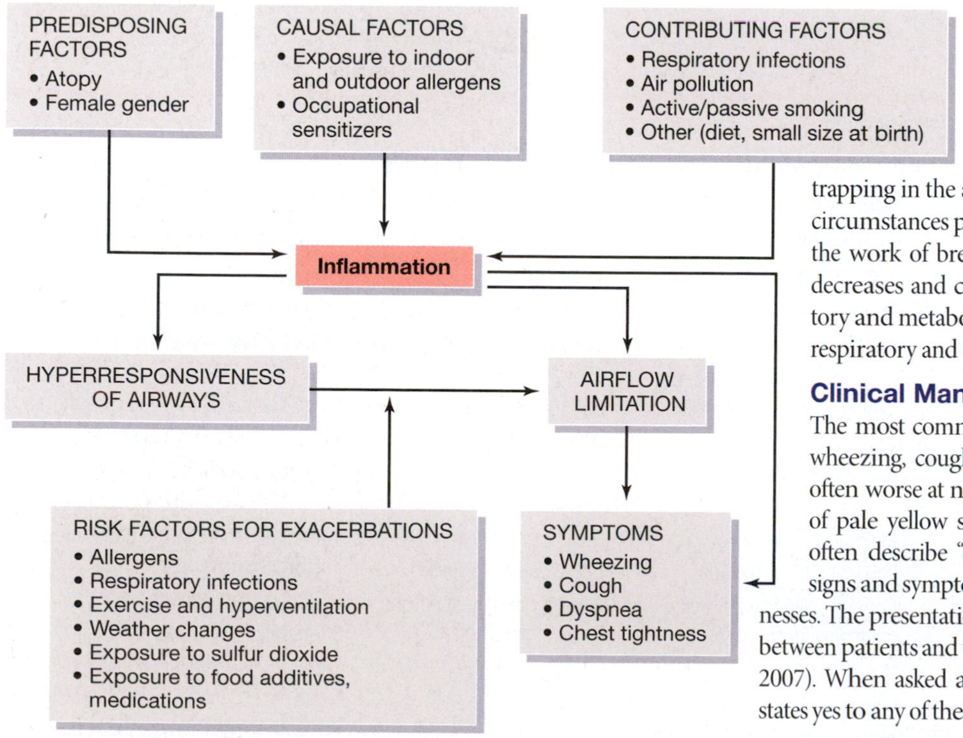

FIGURE 27–1 ◆ Pathophysiology of asthma.

Clinical Manifestations

The most common presentation in asthma is complaints of wheezing, coughing, and shortness of breath. The cough is often worse at night and can be nonproductive or productive of pale yellow sputum (discolored by eosinophils). Patients often describe "chest tightness" but rarely chest pain. These signs and symptoms are nonspecific and common in many illnesses. The presentation of symptoms and their triggers vary widely between patients and within patients over a period of time (NHLBI, 2007). When asked about the following symptoms, if the patient states yes to any of them, a diagnosis of asthma should be suspected:

- Sudden severe or recurrent episodes of coughing, wheezing, chest tightness, or shortness of breath

Weblink: Guidelines for Diagnosis and Management of Asthma

- "Chest colds" that take more than 10 days to resolve
- Coughing, shortness of breath, or wheezing that occurs at a particular time of the year
- Coughing, shortness of breath, or wheezing that occurs when exposed to certain things or certain places (refer to Trigger List).
- Symptoms that are relieved with OTC medications
- Symptoms that are worse at night
- Symptoms that occur with moderate exercise or activity.

The physical examination may or may not reveal findings that suggest asthma. Many patients do not show any airflow obstruction between attacks (by definition, asthma is episodic and variable). Wheezing or prolonged expiration may be signs of airflow obstruction. Use of accessory muscles, leaning forward, and hunched shoulders with the appearance of a hyperexpanded thorax is a position that asthmatics use to help force air out of their lungs. If the asthma is due to allergies, the nurse may note a rash on the skin.

As attacks become more severe, the individual may exhibit signs of using accessory muscles for breathing, distant breath sounds caused by air trapping, and loud wheezing. Fatigue develops as the attack progresses, with the skin becoming moist and anxiety and apprehension becoming obvious. Dyspnea may be severe, and often the person is able to speak only one or two words at a time before taking a breath. At the point at which airflow is markedly decreased, breath sounds become inaudible with diminished wheezing, and the cough becomes ineffective despite being repetitive and hacking (NHLBI, 2007; Porth & Matfin, 2009). Lack of breath sounds on auscultation is an ominous sign indicating that there is no airflow to the distal airways and respiratory and cardiac arrest is imminent.

The Global Initiative for Asthma (GINA) and the NHLBI Panel of Experts on Asthma classifies asthma as controlled, partly controlled, or not controlled. The components of severity are based on impairment and risk. They include frequency of daytime and nighttime symptoms, lung function (FEV_1 and FEV_1/FVC ratio), frequency of medication used to treat symptoms, and interference with daily activities (GINA, 2011) (See the National Guidelines for Asthma box).

Laboratory and Diagnostic Procedures

The NHLBI expert panel report on the diagnosis and management of asthma recommends that (1) diagnosis of asthma be based on episodic symptoms of airflow obstruction, (2) the airflow obstruction is at least partially reversible, and (3) other causes are ruled out (NHLBI, 2007). This can be accomplished through a medical history, physical examination, pulmonary function tests, and tests that exclude other causes. A patient history should inquire about symptoms, pattern of symptoms, precipitating or aggravating factors, family history, and social history (see Chapter 25 on Respiratory Assessment).

Once asthma is suspected, tests are performed to verify the presence of airflow obstruction. Pulmonary function tests diagnose not only airflow obstruction, but also the severity of the obstruction, which often does not correlate to physical findings (see Chart 27–1, Figure 27–2, and the Diagnostic Tests box on page 736). The patient also undergoes a detailed history to determine causes of airflow limitation in the environment as well as foods and stressful conditions.

Spirometry is the preferred method of testing for asthma (NHLBI, 2007). It measures FVC, which is the maximum volume of air forcibly exhaled after maximum inhalation. Spirometers also measure the FEV_1, which is the volume of air exhaled during the first second of testing the FVC. FEV_6 (volume expired in first 6 seconds) may be used instead of the FVC in patients who find the FVC too physically demanding. Obstruction is determined by a decrease in both FEV_1 and in the FEV_1/FVC ratio (or the FEV_1/FEV_6 ratio) using predictive chart references. Reversibility is determined by improvement in pulmonary testing after a short-acting bronchodilator is used. The

NATIONAL GUIDELINES Asthma Severity Classification

Classification of Asthma Control in Adults and Children ≥ 12 Years Old

	Characteristics	**Controlled**	**Not Well Controlled**	**Very Poorly Controlled**
Impairment	Daytime symptoms	≤2 days/wk	≥2 days/wk	Throughout the day
Normal FEV_1/FVC:	Nighttime symptoms/awakening	≤2x/month	1–3x/week	≥4x/week
8–19 yr 85%	Activity interference	None	Some	Extremely limited
20–39 yr 80%	Need for medication to relieve/ rescue symptoms	≤2 days/wk	≥2 days/wk but not >1x/day	Several times/day
40–59 yr 75%				
60–80 yr 70%	FEV_1 or peak flow	>80% predicted/personal best	60–80% predicted/ personal best	<60% predicted/personal best
	Exacerbations requiring corticosteroids	0–1 times/yr	≥2 times/yr	≥2 times/yr
	Recommended action	Maintain current action; Follow-up q1–6 months Consider step down if well controlled for ≥3 months	Step up 1 step Reevaluate in 2–6 wks Consider treatment options for adverse effects	Consider short course of systemic corticosteroids Step up 1 or 2 steps Reevaluate in 2 wks Consider treatment options for adverse effects

Source: Adapted from National Heart Lung and Blood Institute. (2007). *Expert panel report 3: Guidelines for the diagnosis and management of asthma* (NIH Publication No. 08-4051). Washington, DC: Author. Retrieved from http://www.nhlbi.nih.gov/guidelines/asthma/asthgdln.htm.

CHART 27–1 Pulmonary Function Tests

Pulmonary function tests (PFTs) are performed in a pulmonary function laboratory. After preparing the client, a nose clip is applied and the unsedated client breathes into a spirometer or body plethysmograph, a device for measuring and recording lung volume in liters versus time in seconds. The client is instructed how to breathe for specific tests: for example, to inhale as deeply as possible and then exhale to the maximal extent possible. Using measured lung volumes, respiratory capacities are calculated to assess pulmonary status. The specific values determined by PFT and illustrated in Figure 27–2◆ include the following:

- *Total lung capacity (TLC)* is the total volume of the lungs at their maximum inflation. Four values are used to calculate TLC.
  a. *Total volume (TV)*, the volume inhaled and exhaled with normal quiet breathing (also called tidal volume)
  b. *Inspiratory reserve volume (IRV)*, the maximum amount that can be inhaled over and above a normal inspiration
  c. *Expiratory reserve volume (ERV)*, the maximum amount that can be exhaled following a normal exhalation
  d. *Residual volume (RV)*, the amount of air remaining in the lungs after maximal exhalation.
- *Vital capacity (VC)* is the total amount of air that can be exhaled after a maximal inspiration. It is calculated by adding together the IRV, TV, and the ERV.
- *Inspiratory capacity* is the total amount of air that can be inhaled following a normal quiet exhalation. It is calculated by adding the TV and IRV.
- *Functional residual capacity (FRC)* is the volume of air left in the lungs after a normal exhalation. The ERV and RV are added to determine the FRC.
- *Forced expiratory volume (FEV_1)* is the amount of air that can be exhaled in 1 second.
- *Forced vital capacity (FVC)* is the amount of air that can be exhaled forcefully and rapidly after maximum air intake.
- *Minute volume (MV)* is the total amount or volume of air breathed in 1 minute.

In older clients, residual capacity is increased, and vital capacity is decreased. These age-related changes result from the following:

- Calcification of the costal cartilage and weakening of the intercostal muscles, which reduce movement of the chest wall
- Vertebral osteoporosis, which decreases spinal flexibility and increases the degree of kyphosis, further increasing the anterior-posterior diameter of the chest
- Diaphragmatic flattening and loss of elasticity.

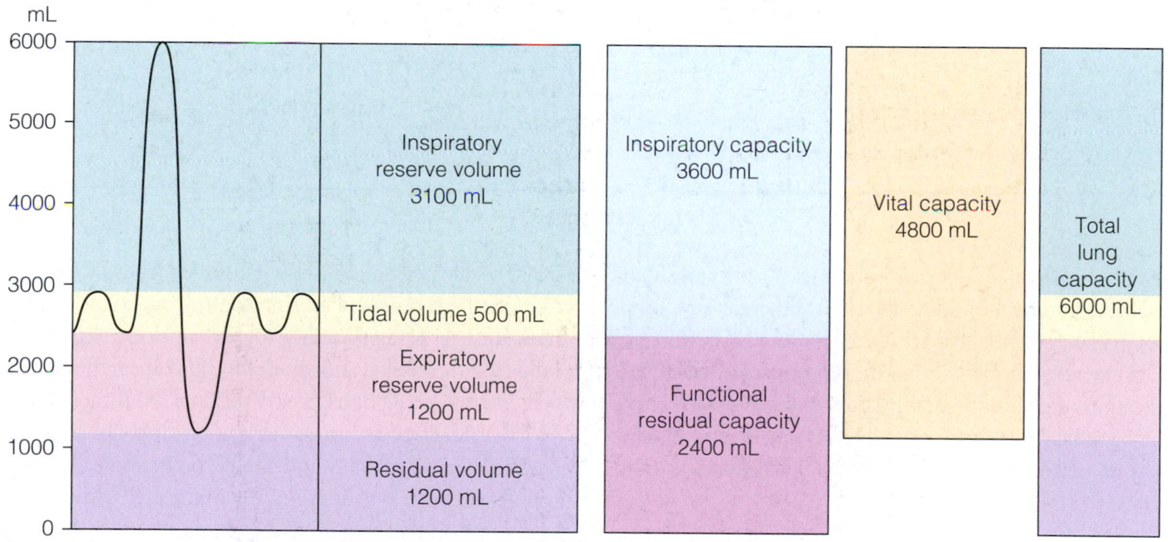

FIGURE 27–2 ◆ The relationship of lung volumes and capacities. Volumes (mL) shown are for an average adult male.

degree of reversibility correlates with the degree of airway inflammation (NHLBI, 2007).

Medical Management

The four essential components for the effective management of asthma, as outlined by the Expert Panel Report (NHLBI, 2007), are as follows:

1. Pharmacologic therapy
2. Control of environmental factors and comorbid conditions that affect asthma
3. Measures of assessment and monitoring to diagnose the severity, control, and responsiveness of asthma management
4. Education for a partnership in asthma care.

Pharmacologic Therapy

The method used in the pharmacotherapy of asthma management is to increase medications until asthma is controlled and then decrease them as soon as possible in an effort to minimize side effects. The NHLBI recommendations include a step-wise approach of adding medications based on severity of symptoms. The major classes of drugs used to treat asthma include bronchodilators (β_2-agonists, anticholinergics), corticosteroids, leukotriene modifiers, immunomodulators, and methylxanthines (Blair, Breit, & Peters, 2008). (Refer to the Pharmacology box on page 744.)

Trigger Control

Identification and avoidance of asthma triggers are important elements in the nonpharmacologic management of asthma. Successful avoidance

DIAGNOSTIC TESTS for Asthma

Test with Description, Rationale, and Normal Values	Expected Abnormality
Sputum Gram Stain and Culture	
Gram stains are done to identify the presence of eosinophils that are associated with antigen–antibody reactions that occur commonly in allergic reactions and asthma.	Eosinophils present in sputum.
Chest Radiography	
Used to rule out other potential causes with similar symptomatology. *Helpful in patients with difficult-to-control asthma for detection of comorbid conditions.*	Usually normal.
FEV_1 to FVC	
These spirometric results are expressed as an absolute volume and percent based on normal values for age, height, and weight (see National Guidelines box). *Refer to Figure 27–2 on page 735.*	With obstruction, the patient has difficulty exhaling from the lungs, reducing the FEV_1/FVC ratio to 70% or less.
White Blood Cell Count (WBC) with Differential	
4,500–10,000 μL *WBC will increase with infection and inflammation.* *Eosinophil is a type of white blood cell that responds to acute inflammation associated with allergies and asthma. It is identified on the differential.*	WBC count is likely to be elevated with infection and eosinophils elevated with allergic response.
Arterial Blood Gas (ABG)	
pH 7.35–7.45; $PaCO_2$ 35–45; PaO_2 75–100; HCO_3 24–28 *Arterial oxygen of less than 60 mmHg or an oxygen saturation of less than 90% on room air indicates respiratory failure. An arterial oxygen of less than 50 mmHg, arterial carbon dioxide of greater than 60 mmHg, and a pH of 7.30 or less indicates life-threatening illness.*	Shows hypoxemia or hypercarbia, acid–base abnormalities.
Allergy Testing	
Identifies triggers when allergic cause is suspected.	Reactivity in patients with allergy-induced asthma.

Source: Adapted from Kee, J. L. (2010). *Laboratory and diagnostic tests* (8th ed.). Upper Saddle River, NJ: Prentice Hall.

can reduce the need or frequency of medication use. Clinicians should perform a detailed assessment of domestic, environmental, and industrial exposures that are potential triggers (refer to the Risk Factors box on page 733) along with laboratory identification of sensitivities. Successful modification of environmental triggers requires a partnership between patient and health care personnel. Education in how to avoid triggers should be detailed, and assessment of the patient's learning should be verified.

Monitoring

The NHLBI panel of experts recommends periodic assessment of asthma control at 1- to 6-month intervals, depending on the adequacy of therapy until stabilization of symptoms occurs (NHLBI, 2007). Recommended measurements include signs and symptoms of asthma, pulmonary function, quality of life/functional status, asthma exacerbations, pharmacotherapy (adherence to treatment and potential side effects), patient-provider communication, and patient satisfaction. Assessment of the history of symptoms should include the frequency of daytime symptoms and nocturnal awakenings, use of SABAs for relief of symptoms, and impact of symptoms on the ability to perform daily activities and exercise. Pulmonary function should be measured frequently during the initiation and stabilization of asthma management and at least every 1 to 2 years thereafter. Patients who use a peak flow meter at home should have periodic assessment of its accuracy, particularly patients for whom use of the peak flow meter is known to be unreliable (older adults, very young, orthopedic or neuromuscular problems). The goal of asthma management should be not only to control symptoms, but also to improve the patient's quality of life. Assessing quality of life perceptions should include mental factors as well as physical ones. Perceptions of asthma control, quality of life, and depression may affect a patient's ability to participate in self-management and influence morbidity and mortality outcomes; therefore, the patient's perceptions should be assessed over time (NHLBI, 2007).

The history of asthma exacerbations that are either self-treated or require medical intervention should be periodically assessed. Exacerbations are described as episodes of increased symptoms and reduced lung function that require rescue medications, such as SABAs, to perform baseline activities. A history of exacerbations over a 1-year period is one of the strongest predictors of severe exacerbations that necessitate emergency department treatment and hospitalization (NHLBI, 2007). Clinicians should monitor the patient's compliance with the medical regime, pharmacology side effects, and inhaler technique. Patients who are having difficulty in controlling their asthma symptoms after 3 to 6 months of active therapy, have required hospital admission, are being considered for immunotherapy, or have comorbid complicating conditions should be referred to an asthma specialist for consultation.

Education

Open communication and partnership between the health care team and the patient are essential for a patient to successfully manage the asthma. The education plan should address identification and avoidance of triggers; correct use and timing of specific medication; proper use of inhalers, spacers, and metered-dose inhalers; exacerbation management; and instructions regarding when to seek medical help. The goals and treatment plan should be established collaboratively, documented, and reviewed with each visit.

Nursing Management

Nursing management of patients with asthma relies on a holistic approach to care. Immediate nursing care of a patient with asthma depends on the severity of the symptoms and whether the patient is being treated as an outpatient or inpatient. A major emphasis is education of the patient and family about the prevention of asthma attacks. Throughout the course of the illness, nurses also provide emotional support to the patient and family, who may be frightened and anxious because of the patient's dyspnea.

Assessment

Nursing responsibilities include a thorough assessment of the patient's symptoms and history of attacks and coordinating the plan of care as set forth by the health care provider. The nurse assesses the patient's respiratory status by monitoring the severity of symptoms, breath sounds, peak flow, pulse oximetry, and vital signs.

Nursing Diagnoses

Nursing diagnoses for the patient with asthma include the following:

- *Airway Clearance, Ineffective* related to inflammation and bronchospasm.
- *Gas Exchange, Impaired* related to inflammation.
- *Anxiety,* related to shortness of breath.
- *Fatigue* related to increased work of breathing.
- *Nutrition Imbalanced, Less Than Required* related to fatigue and shortness of breath.
- *Knowledge Deficit* related to self-care, treatment regimens, and discharge needs.

NANDA-I © 2012

Planning

The goal of nursing care is to promote an efficient breathing pattern and maintain effective airway clearance.

Outcomes and Evaluation Parameters

The patient with asthma will experience relief of chest tightness and dyspnea and will be able to exercise preventive strategies that alleviate frequency of symptoms. The patient will describe breathing as comfortable, lung sounds will be clear upon auscultation, use of accessory muscles for breathing will decrease, and the patient will show an improved flow rate (FEV_1). The patient will exhibit understanding of triggers and how to avoid them and the understanding of all medications and the treatment regime.

Interventions and Rationales

Administration of medications as ordered, having first obtained a history of any allergic responses to medications, is inherent in the nursing role. Patient education is paramount in ensuring that the patient will take medications as ordered. For example, regular use of anti-inflammatory medications via a **metered-dose inhaler (MDI)** controls the symptoms of asthma (see Figures 27–3◆ and 27–4◆).

A variety of respiratory medications are delivered through the aerosolized route using many different types of devices. Two of the most common devices are metered-dose inhalers (MDIs) with and without spacers and small-volume nebulizers (SVN). The nurse should be knowledgeable about the medication that is being administered and the important side effects. The nurse should understand how to use an MDI and how to teach patients to administer their medication appropriately.

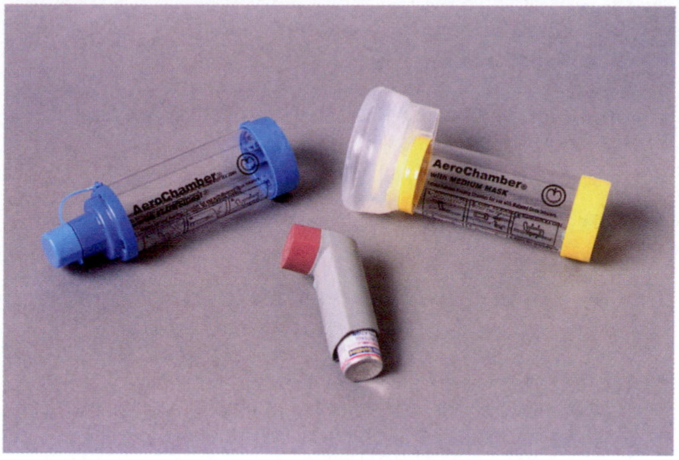

FIGURE 27–3 ◆ A variety of inhalers and their use.

Video*: Asthma—Using Inhaler

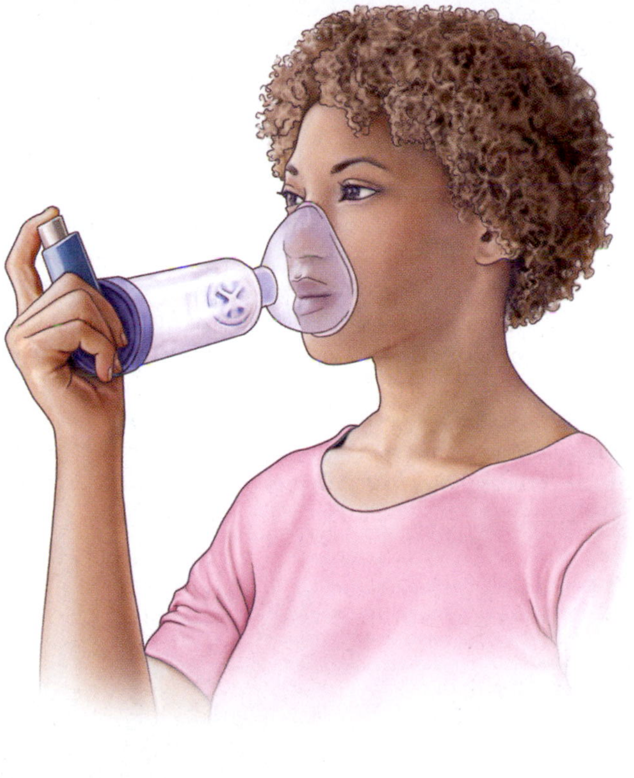

FIGURE 27–4 ◆ How to use a metered-dose inhaler.

Teaching patients about the proper use and side effects of medication is a basic nursing function. This is of particular importance when the patient has been prescribed respiratory medications. Improper timing and overuse of respiratory medications can prevent the medications from working properly and may, in a worst-case scenario, cause increasing symptoms and respiratory failure. For example, one of the most common devices used to deliver bronchodilators is the MDI. However, this device must be used correctly, and patients must be taught how to use it. One of the most effective methods of teaching patients about MDIs is for a member of the health care team to demonstrate use of the device and then to ask the patient to perform a return demonstration. This teaching can be accomplished in an acute care setting and usually takes less than 10 minutes. To teach the patient correctly, the nurse must follow the steps described in Chart 27–2.

CHART 27–2 Steps for Teaching a Patient How to Use a Metered-Dose Inhaler

The nurse should demonstrate this technique and then evaluate the patient's technique using the following checklist:

1. Removes cap from the MDI device.
2. Shakes the MDI.
3. Correctly inserts the MDI into the chamber.
4. Tilts head back and slowly exhales prior to actuation.
5. Places chamber into mouth and closes lips around chamber.
6. Slowly inhales through the mouth while pressing down on the inhaler one time to release the medication. If using a holding chamber, press down the inhaler first and then begin to slowly inhale.
7. Holds breath for more than 5–10 seconds after dose.
8. Waits at least 1 minute before administering next dose.

Source: Buddiga, P. (2011). Use of metered dose inhalers, spacers, and nebulizers. Retrieved from emedicine.medscape.com/article/1413366-overview.

When the patient is diagnosed with asthma, the nurse assists in preventing exacerbations by helping the patient and family develop a health maintenance routine that includes regular checkups, use of a peak flow meter, regular assessment of peak flow rates (Figure 27–5◆), and awareness of individual triggers that cause bronchospasm or exacerbations.

Corticosteroids are effective in improving symptoms and normalizing the FEV_1. The nurse will instruct the patient and family in the use of a spacer with this medication and instruct the patient to rinse his mouth afterwards to prevent thrush. A spacer is a device that is attached to the inhaler, allowing medication to accumulate as the patient inhales and preventing medication from escaping outside of the patient's mouth. These are particularly helpful for older patients and patients with poor dexterity.

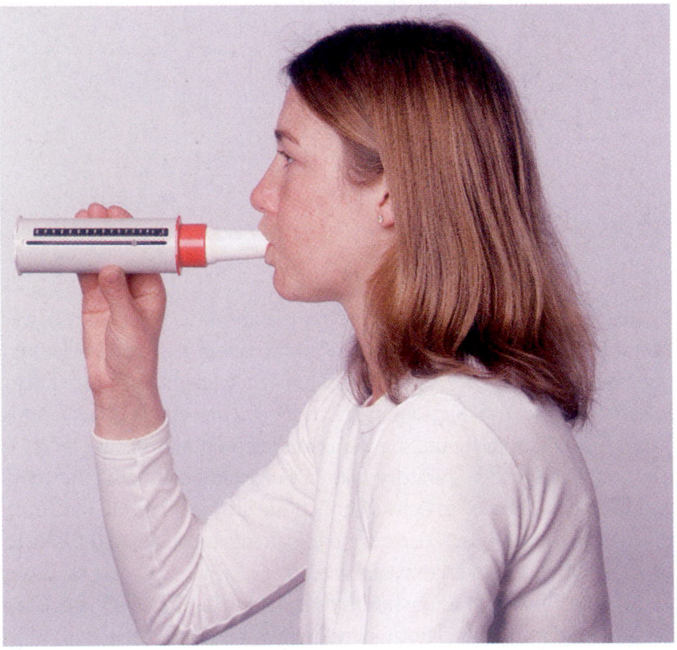

FIGURE 27–5 ◆ Use of a peak flow meter.
Source: © Dorling Kindersley.

Discharge Priorities

As part of the educational approach to care, the patient who has been diagnosed with asthma should be encouraged to keep a diary of her exposure and response to triggers. The nurse also should teach the patient to document home peak flow measurements in the diary. Tracking may also be done on internet-based home monitoring programs and mobile phones.

The importance of patient education cannot be overemphasized. The success of asthma management requires the patient's active engagement in collaboration with health care clinicians. The nurse should create an environment that invites open and honest communication of concerns and barriers to self-management. In addition, the nurse should tailor education to the patient's preference and verify understanding. Patients should be well informed of the causes, treatment goals, and pharmacotherapy of asthma management. Evidence supports that education in the self-management of asthma improves outcomes in chronic asthma (NHLBI, 2007). Refer to the Patient Teaching & Discharge Priorities for Patients with Asthma feature on page 739.

Collaborative Management

Comprehensive asthma management requires a multidisciplinary approach incorporating collaboration between medical health professionals, patients, family, and direct caregivers. In order to meet desired patient outcomes, it is essential that this interdisciplinary team communicate openly with one another in developing and evaluating care of the patient and family (IOM [Institute of Medicine], 2010). Contributions from health care providers, nurses, nurse practitioners, respiratory therapists, nutritionists, and occupational therapists may be involved depending on available resources and the disease's impact on the patient's functional status. If there are financial issues related to maintenance care and equipment, the social worker becomes involved. Referral to a home care nurse is instituted if the patient is not able to manage outpatient clinic or office visits. Any asthmatic patient who smokes should be referred to a smoking cessation clinic. Through integration of resources into the management of asthma, patients will have higher success in controlling symptoms, optimize functional status, increase participation, and reduce health care costs through stabilizing manifestations of the disease (Celli & ZuWallack, 2010).

Health Promotion

One of the objectives of *Healthy People 2020* (U.S. Department of Health and Human Services, 2010) is to "promote respiratory health through better prevention, detection, treatment, and education efforts." Asthma is one of the diseases specifically targeted in the objectives. Educating the public about the symptoms and dangers of asthma contributes to community well-being. This includes the role of environmental pollutants, smoking, allergens, chemicals, and inhalants. Effective asthma management will reduce hospitalization and emergency department visits, as well as allow patients to enjoy normal activities. Both health care providers and patients need to be educated on how to effectively assess and manage asthma. The National Asthma Education and Prevention Program (NAEPP) provides guidelines for asthma diagnosis and management that should be incorporated into professional health care academic curricula. *Healthy People 2020* identifies as a priority working with local community groups to promote and assemble community resources to develop a comprehensive, culturally and linguistically competent approach to controlling asthma among

PATIENT TEACHING & DISCHARGE PRIORITIES for Patients with Asthma

Need	Teaching
Knowledge of home medications	Health care needs include verbal and written instructions for treatment plan and follow-up care. Assess patient and family understanding of disease process, medications, and health maintenance needs in the home setting.
Maintenance of airway	When appropriate, patients are taught to do their own peak flow measurements and can discuss plans for possible emergencies at home or work and when to seek medical help. These include asthma attacks that are unresponsive to medication or require more medication than usual, peak flow measurements of 50% to 80% or personal baseline, drowsiness or confusion, severe chest pain, or severe shortness of breath at rest.
Knowledge of triggers	Assess patient's and family's understanding of asthma triggers and how to avoid exposure.

high-risk populations. It also encourages states to track occupational and environmental factors that cause or trigger asthma episodes and their impact on illness and disability.

Influenza

Influenza, also known as the flu, is a contagious respiratory disease that is caused by the influenza viruses. The stomach virus that many people call "flu" is not actually influenza but rather a form of gastroenteritis. Most people fully recover from influenza in 1 to 2 weeks, but some develop life-threatening complications such as pneumonia. At-risk patients include children younger than 4 years, adults older than 50 years, those with chronic medical conditions, the immunocompromised, women in the second or third trimester of pregnancy, those with impaired ability to handle airway secretions, and those with a body mass index (BMI) > 40 (Deriet, Sandrock, Nguyen, & Lawrence, 2011; Turner, 2009).

Safety Alert *Patients older than 50 years with a chronic disease or a respiratory disease or those who are immunocompromised should get an annual flu shot and should be inoculated with the pneumococcal vaccine. During admission assessment, the nurse should ask the patient whether she has received these vaccines. If not, the nurse should notify the health care team.*

Epidemiology and Etiology

Epidemics of influenza occur almost exclusively during winter months in the northern and southern hemispheres (and year round in the tropics). Influenza A and influenza B are the two types of influenza viruses that cause epidemic human disease. Influenza virus type C has not been classified and usually does not induce illness. Antigenic variations in influenza type A and B account for the yearly epidemics. These minor variations account for the yearly updating of vaccine strains.

Yearly epidemics of influenza begin abruptly and last 5 to 6 weeks. It generally occurs in two waves: first in schoolchildren and their household inhabitants and then in housebound or institutionalized people (Turner, 2009). Mortality is usually highest in older adults. In 2009, the H1N1 influenza A virus (swine flu) surfaced in Mexico and the United States, causing a pandemic. The population that experienced increased morbidity and mortality in this influenza was remarkable for the inclusion of previously healthy adults ages 24 to 29, the obese, and women who were pregnant or postpartum (CDC, 2009).

Pathophysiology

Transmission of influenza occurs by the transfer of respiratory secretions containing the influenza virus. It is generally transmitted by droplets and to a lesser extent as a small-particle aerosol (Lee & Treanor, 2010). This can happen when an infected person coughs or sneezes and droplets are propelled through the air and deposited on the mouth or nose of people nearby. Although a less frequent means of transmission, viruses also can be spread when a person touches respiratory droplets on another person or an object and then touches his own mouth or nose before washing his hands. The incubation period is 18 to 72 hours and is usually limited to the respiratory tract. Viral shedding is greatest at the onset of illness and continues for 5 to 7 days or longer in children. Pneumonia is the most common complication of influenza.

Clinical Manifestations

Typically, influenza has an abrupt onset and is characterized by fever, chills, headache, fatigue, dry mouth, cough, sore throat, nasal congestion, and myalgia. The cough may be associated with chest pain. The range of symptoms is widespread, but fever and a cough or sore throat is the most predictive (Lee & Treanor, 2010). However, older adults may present with fever, fatigue, and confusion and none of the respiratory symptoms. Fever usually persists for 3 to 4 days and occasionally 1 week, at which point systemic symptoms abate. Lung sounds are usually normal. The most common complication is pneumonia, which may be primary influenza pneumonia or a secondary bacterial pneumonia.

Laboratory and Diagnostic Procedures

During periods of outbreak, influenza can be diagnosed by clinical suspicion in patients with acute febrile respiratory illness. In cases of sporadic outbreak or in older patients, clinical criteria alone may not be enough to confirm or exclude the diagnosis of influenza (Dolin, 2011). Influenza diagnostic tests include immunofluorescence assays, rapid antigen immunoassays, and reverse transcriptase polymerase chain reaction tests. Patients should be tested if results will change the clinical management, such as initiating antiviral or antibacterial therapy for patients who are immunocompromised and hospitalized patients with acute febrile respiratory illness (Dolin, 2011).

Medical Management

Zanamivir and oseltamivir are two antiviral medications recommended for treatment of influenza. Two earlier medications, amantadine and rimantadine, are no longer recommended in the United States because of the high level of resistance against them (CDC, 2011). Providers should consult local health departments regarding the strain and sensitivities in their community. If taken within 2 days of getting sick, these drugs can reduce the symptoms of flu and shorten the time of illness by 1 or 2 days. Antiviral therapy is recommended for anyone requiring hospitalization, those who have severe progressive disease, and those who are at high risk for developing complications due to age or underlying medical condition (CDC, 2011). The best defense against acquiring influenza is annual vaccination and good hygiene techniques such as hand washing.

Nursing Management

The primary nursing care goals in treating influenza are relief of symptoms and prevention of secondary infection. The nurse advises the patient to rest, to drink plenty of fluids, to avoid using alcohol and tobacco, and to take aspirin or acetaminophen for symptom relief. (See the Nursing Process: Patient Care Plan for Pulmonary Infection feature on page 749.)

Pneumonia

Pneumonia is an acute inflammation of the lungs caused by infection. The cause, symptomatology, treatment, and prognosis depend on the source of infection, how it was acquired, and patient comorbidities. The infection can be categorized as either pneumonia acquired at an institution or pneumonia acquired in the community. Institutional-acquired pneumonia is further divided into hospital-acquired pneumonia, including ventilator-associated pneumonia, and health care-acquired pneumonia. Community-acquired pneumonia (CAP) is pneumonia that develops in a patient who has not been hospitalized within the last 90 days or has not received outpatient therapy, such as chemotherapy, wound care, or dialysis, in the previous 30 days and therefore was infected by the pneumonia in the community setting. Hospital-acquired pneumonia (HAP) is pneumonia that occurs more than 48 hours after hospital admission with no evidence of symptoms at the time of admission. Ventilator-associated pneumonia (VAP) is a type of HAP that develops 48 to 72 hours after endotracheal intubation. Health care-acquired pneumonia (HCAP) is pneumonia in a patient who has had substantial contact with health care agencies such as wound care, dialysis, chemotherapy, a long-term care facility, or intravenous therapy.

Epidemiology

Pneumonia is in the top eight leading causes of death in the United States for adults and children, the sixth-leading cause of death for people over age 65, and the number one cause of death from an infectious disease (CDC, 2010a; Donowitz, 2009). The incidence of CAP is likely grossly underreported. It is estimated that there are approximately 2 to 15 cases/1,000 people per year with a higher incidence in older adults (Donowitz, 2009). Risk factors for pneumonia include advanced age, a compromised immune system, underlying lung disease, alcoholism, altered level of consciousness, smoking, endotracheal intubation, malnutrition, and immobilization (see the Risk Factors for Pneumonia box).

Hospital-acquired (nosocomial) pneumonia is the leading cause of death among hospital-associated infections. Mortality estimates of patients with HAP range from 20% to 50%, although whether HAP specifically causes all these deaths is not clear (File, 2010a). Patients on mechanical ventilation are at high risk of developing HAP.

Etiology

Bacteria are the most common cause of pneumonia, although many pathogens can lead to pneumonia including viruses, fungi, and parasites.

Community-Acquired Pneumonia

Microaspiration of oropharyngeal secretions, usually during sleep, is the most common route of CAP. Gross aspiration is usually limited to patients with altered level of consciousness. This form of pneumonia can be caused by a large variety of microbial agents, making diagnosis and treatment decisions challenging. In patients requiring hospitalization, the most common identified pathogens are *Streptococcus pneumoniae, Mycoplasma pneumoniae, and Haemophilus influenzae* (Torres, Mendez, & Wunderink, 2010). A secondary route of infection for CAP is inhalation of aggressive microorganisms (e.g., Legionella, plague, anthrax) that have been aerosolized when an infected individual coughs, sneezes, or talks or from aerosolized water, such as infected respiratory equipment. Less commonly, it can seed in the lungs as a result of a bloodstream infection. The responsible pathogen is often staphylococcal sepsis as a result of intravenous drug use or gram-negative bacteremia in immunocompromised patients. Among patients with CAP who require admission to intensive care, the mortality rate averages between 13% and 36% (File, 2010b). This is related to predisposing factors that include general debility, malnutrition, endotracheal intubation, and contaminated respiratory therapy equipment.

Hospital-Acquired and Health Care-Acquired Pneumonia

Organisms responsible for HAP that develop during the first few days of hospitalization are usually similar to those that lead to CAP and tend to be susceptible to antibiotics. Those that present after 4 days of hospitalization are chiefly caused by methicillin-resistant *Staphylococcus aureus*, enteric gram-negative bacilli, or *Pseudomonas aeruginosa* (Torres, Mendez, & Wunderink, 2010). The highest risk for HAP is in patients on mechanical ventilation and is identified as ventilator-associated pneumonia (VAP). See the Risk Factors for Pneumonia box. Ventilator-associated pneumonia is discussed in detail in Chapter 28.

HCAP has an epidemiology more similar to that of HAP than to CAP. Mortality rates are higher, illness is more severe, and hospital length of stay is longer compared to CAP. Most likely pathogens are *S. aureus* and *P. aeruginosa*. See Chart 27–3 for common organisms responsible for CAP and HAP.

Pathophysiology

The lungs are constantly exposed to microbes and particulate matter from inspired air as well as organisms from oral airway secretions that

RISK FACTORS for Pneumonia

Community-Acquired Pneumonia	Hospital-Acquired Pneumonia
Advanced age	Mechanical ventilation
Immunocompromised state	Chronic lung disease
Underlying lung disease	Age > 70 years
Chronic disease	Depressed level of consciousness
Alcoholism	Aspiration
Smoking	Chest surgery
Immobility	H_2 blocker or antacid therapy
Malnutrition	Underlying illness
Crowded living conditions	Paralytic agents
Exposure to day care	

CHART 27–3 Microorganisms Associated with Pneumonia

Community Acquired	Hospital Acquired
Streptococcus pneumoniae	*Pseudomonas aeruginosa*
Mycoplasma pneumoniae	*Staphylococcus aureus*
Haemophilus influenzae	*Klebsiella pneumonia*
Oral anaerobic bacteria	**Health Care Acquired**
Influenza virus	*Staphylococcus aureus*
Legionella pneumophila	*Pseudomonas aeruginosa*
Chlamydial pneumonia	

COMPLEMENTARY & ALTERNATIVE THERAPIES Systemic Illnesses and Dental Health Care *Nancy Yilk*

INTEGRATIVE HEALTH CARE includes an acknowledgment of interdisciplinary congruence across medical practices that previously were considered to stand separate. Two of the areas that are developing a health concordance are the interrelationship of systemic illnesses and dental health care. Integrative dental medicine emphasizes an understanding of how dental disease and common chronic stress share underlying factors that affect outcomes globally in the body.

The medically complex patients require an improved understanding of the interplay between oral health and general health. For example, a heart transplant patient is instructed to have dental cleanings every 3 months to remove a biofilm found in dental plaque that has a corresponding influence on organ rejection complications. The 2007 American Heart Association guidelines for the prevention of infective endocarditis states, "Transient bacteria also occurs frequently during routine daily activities unrelated to a dental procedure, such as tooth brushing and flossing (20% to 68%), use of wooden toothpicks (20% to 40%), use of water irrigation devices (7% to 50%), and chewing food (7% to 51%)."

A biofilm is a complex, usually multispecies, highly communicative community of bacteria that is surrounded by a polymeric matrix. Treatment of these types of infections with traditional antibiotics alone is ineffective, and surgical removal of diseased tissue is still necessary (Ray & Triplett, 2011). Bacteria from the oral biofilms may be aspirated into the respiratory tract and contribute to the cause of initiation and progression of systemic infectious conditions such as pneumonia. Oral bacteria, poor oral hygiene, and periodontitis influence the incidence of pulmonary infections, especially nosocomial pneumonia episodes in high-risk subjects. Improved oral hygiene has been shown to reduce the occurrence of nosocomial pneumonia, both in mechanically ventilated hospital patients and nonventilated nursing home residents. It appears that oral colonization by potential respiratory pathogens possibly fostered by periodontitis, and possibly by bacteria specific to the oral cavity or to periodontal diseases, contributes to pulmonary infections.

The bacteria which cause hospital-acquired pneumonia (HAP) such as *Pseudomonas aeruginosa, Klebsiella pneumoniae,* and *Staphylococcus aureus* are thought to reside in the oropharynx before being aspirated into the lungs, causing pneumonia. These bacteria are more commonly found in the mouths of sick or institutionalized persons and are not considered part of the normal oral flora (Ewan et al., 2010). Additionally, studies have shown how oral biofilms serve as a reservoir for respiratory pathogens contributing to ventilator-associated pneumonia (VAP), one of the leading causes of morbidity and mortality in hospitalized patients in intensive care. Preventative care by dental intervention, such as oral irrigation, can influence treating biofilm buildup for treatment and prevention of lower respiratory disorders.

Pulsation and pressure are the critical mechanisms in the action of a dental water jet. The combination provides for phases of compression and decompression of the gingival tissue to remove supragingival plaque biofilm and expel subgingival bacteria and other debris as well as stimulating gingival tissue. A pulsating device is more effective than a continuous stream device because the pulsating action creates two zones of hydrokinetic activity: (1) the impact zone, where the solution initially contacts in the mouth at the gingival margin, and (2) the flushing zone, where the water or other irrigants reaches subgingivally.

In view of the emerging data suggesting inflammation's important role not only on periodontal diseases but also on the oral–systemic connection, the benefits of using the dental water jet may go beyond that of managing periodontal diseases, not only by reducing inflammation but also by affecting proinflammatory cytokines, which can affect the activities of a variety of body organs (Ciancio, 2009). It is suggested that positive clinical outcomes could be found in patients of all ages with reoccurring lower respiratory infections to introduce the use of oral irrigation into their health practices to address the possibility of oral biofilms influencing a successful outcome.

References

Ciancio, S. G. (2009, March). The dental water jet: A product ahead of its time. *Compendium of Continuing Education in Dentistry, 30* (Spec No 1), 7–13.

Ewan, V., Perry, J. D., Mawson, T., McCracken, G., Brown, A. N., Newton, J., & Walls, A. (2010, January). Detecting potential respiratory pathogens in the mouths of older people in hospital. *Age Ageing, 39*(1), 122–125. Epub 2009 Sep 11.

Ray, J. M., & Triplett, R. G. (2011, November). What is the role of biofilms in severe head and neck infections? *Oral Maxillofacial Surgical Clinics of North America, 23*(4), 497–505.

are aspirated during sleep. However, sterility of the lower airways is usually maintained by respiratory tract defense mechanisms. The defense mechanisms of the upper airways include nasal hair, mucociliary clearance, saliva, and cough. Host defenses of the conducting airways and lower respiratory tract include epiglottic reflexes, immunoglobulins, alveolar fluid, alveolar macrophages, neutrophil recruitment, and dendritic cells. It takes either a breakdown in these defenses, a particularly virulent organism, or the introduction of an overwhelming organism to infect the lungs. Microorganisms that reach the lower airways can then multiply and cause infection. The relationship between respiratory illness and dental health is of significance. Refer to the Complementary & Alternative Therapies feature above for a detailed discussion.

Clinical Manifestations

Symptoms suggestive of pneumonia include fever, chills, increased respiratory rates, bloody sputum, crackles, and x-ray abnormalities. Patients who are immunocompromised or hypothermic, as well as older adults, may not have a fever. In general, 20% of all patients presenting with pneumonia are afebrile. Nonrespiratory symptoms include headache, abdominal pain, nausea and vomiting, diarrhea, and muscle aches. Chart 27–4 summarizes the clinical manifestations of pneumonia.

CHART 27–4 Clinical Manifestations of Pneumonia

Fever, chills, or hypothermia	Respiratory rate greater than 20
Heart rate greater than 100	Crackles heard on auscultation
Chest discomfort	Dyspnea
Rusty-colored sputum	Cough
Fatigue, muscle aches, headache, nausea	

Laboratory and Diagnostic Procedures

Diagnosis of pneumonia is made primarily on the basis of clinical presentation. It can be supported with evidence of new or increasing pulmonary infiltrates on chest x-ray, positive sputum or blood cultures in bacterial infections, and leukocytosis. See the Diagnostic Tests for Pulmonary Infection box.

Medical Management

Antibiotics are the primary treatment for pneumonia and significantly improve survival when used appropriately. Selection of antibiotics should be based upon local and hospital pathogen and resistance data, risk factors for multidrug resistant (MDR) pathogens, recent antibiotic therapy (if any), the presence of underlying diseases, and available culture data (Fine, 2010b). Empiric broad-spectrum, multidrug therapy is recommended for patients with risk factors for MDR pathogens. Blood cultures should be drawn prior to administration of antibiotics; however, initiation of antibiotics should not wait for

DIAGNOSTIC TESTS for Pulmonary Infections

Test with Description, Rationale, and Normal Values	Expected Abnormality
Chest x-ray Clear *Helps to identify or rule out etiology of suspected infection.*	Evidence of pulmonary infiltrates, consolidation, cavitation, or abscess
Chest CT No abnormality *Used to identify lung pathology or degree of pathology when CXR provides insufficient data.*	Identification of pattern of injury caused by infection that suggests etiology of disease and the degree of pathology
Sputum Gram Stain and Culture No growth *Used to identify presence of microorganisms responsible for pulmonary infection.*	Presence of pathogen
Transtracheal Aspiration *An infrequently used method of obtaining sputum for culture that is not contaminated by oropharyngeal organisms in patients who cannot expectorate a sputum sample.*	Presence of specific pathogen
Bronchoalveolar Lavage (BAL) *A method of collecting sputum culture by passing a bronchoscope through the mouth or nose into the lungs, and squirting fluid into the small airways to collect a specimen for analysis. Used to diagnose infections and other pulmonary pathologies.*	Presence of a specific pathogen or abnormality
White Blood Cell Count (WBC) 4,500–10,000 μL *Leukocytosis (elevated WBC) is elevated when there is an infectious or inflammatory process.*	WBC $>$ 11,000
Serology *Laboratory examination of a blood or fluid sample that detects the presence of antibodies in the serum/fluid that are associated with specific microorganisms.*	Identification of microorganism
ABG Study pH 7.35–7.45; $PaCO_2$ 35–45; PaO_2 75–100; HCO_3 24–28 *Monitor for oxygenation or ventilation abnormalities that may be associated with pulmonary infection.*	Evidence of hypoxemia, hypercarbia, and/or acid–base abnormalities
Thoracentesis with Pleural Fluid Sample *Obtaining fluid from the pleural space for laboratory analysis allows for the differentiation between simple and complicated effusions. This is used to guide therapeutic intervention.*	Presence of abnormal cells and bacteria

culture results. Once results are available, therapy should be narrowed to antibiotics to which the identified pathogen is susceptible. The Pharmacology Summary of Medications Used to Treat Lower Airway Disorders box on page 744 lists the antibiotics used to treat pneumonia.

Nursing Management

Nursing management for patients with pneumonia is outlined in detail in the Nursing Process: Patient Care Plan for Pulmonary Infections box on page 749. In addition, the patient's oxygenation should be monitored so that the saturation is maintained at 93% (or the patient's baseline) unless otherwise specified by the health care provider. Pulse oximetry is the least invasive assessment tool, but arterial blood gas (ABG) studies should be done if the patient is suspected of being more severely hypoxemic. This may indicate that the patient should be given supplemental oxygen via a nasal cannula or mask (Figure 27–6◆). Chart 27–5 outlines the common oxygen delivery devices and percentage of oxygen that they deliver.

Priority nursing measures for the patient with pneumonia include management of airway clearance and patient comfort. The Nursing Process: Patient Care Plan feature on page 749 discusses the management of patients with pneumonia.

Discharge Priorities

Before discharging the patient recovering from pneumonia, the nurse emphasizes the importance of rest and a gradual increase in activity to avoid fatigue. Patients are instructed to maintain resistance to infection with proper nutrition, adequate rest, good hygiene, and an ample intake of fluids. They also are warned to avoid chilling and exposure to others with upper respiratory tract infections or viruses. They are instructed on the importance of taking medications as prescribed as well as other supportive treatments, such as home oxygen. Patients are informed of when they should call their health care provider for treatment. Symptoms that necessitate a call to their health care provider or a visit to the emergency department include worsening of cough, bloody sputum, difficulty or pain with breathing, light-headedness, persistent fever, or serious side effects with medications (rash, vomiting, or frequent diarrhea).

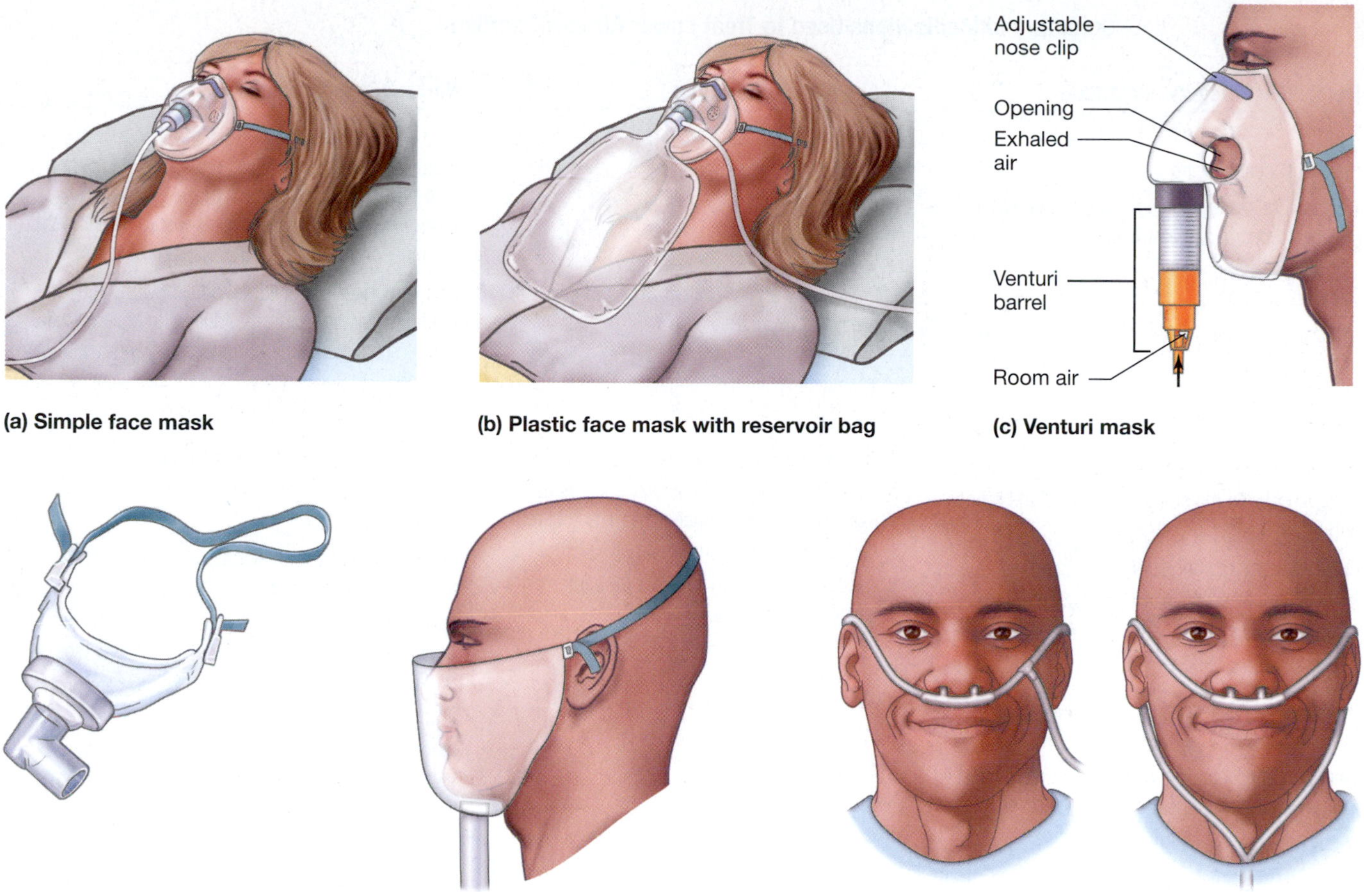

(a) Simple face mask (b) Plastic face mask with reservoir bag (c) Venturi mask

(d) Tracheostomy mask (e) Face tent (f) Standard nasal cannulas

FIGURE 27–6 ◆ Use of supplemental oxygen devices.

CHART 27–5 Common Oxygen Delivery Devices, FiO_2, and Flow Rates

Device	FiO_2 (%)	Flow Rate (L/min)
Nasal cannula	24	1
	28	2
	32	3
	36	4
	40	5
	44	6
Simple face mask	35 to 55	5 to 10
Venturi mask	24	3
	26	3
	28	6
	31	6
	35	9
	40	12
	50	15
Nonrebreather mask	60 to 80	10 to 15

Note: FiO_2 = fraction of inspired oxygen. These are only approximations, not absolute FiO_2 values, because the delivery is via a mask or cannula.

Health Promotion

Preventive measures can be taken to reduce the risk of acquiring pneumonia. These include annual influenza vaccinations, frequent hand washing, smoking cessation, and staying home when sick. Additional vaccines may be recommended for people at high risk of pneumonia, such as pneumococcal vaccine in older adults, the infirm, or those with chronic illness.

Pulmonary Fungal Infections

Fungi produce spores that are spread by wind, water, or contact. Fungal infections can be classified as opportunistic or primary infections (Chart 27–6). Opportunistic infections are those that generally do not

CHART 27–6 Fungal Infections of the Lung

Fungal Infections That Occur in Immune Competent Individuals	Fungal Infections That Occur in Immune Incompetent Individuals
Histoplasmosis	Aspergillosis
Coccidioidomycosis	Candidiasis
Blastomycosis	Mucormycosis
	Pneumocystis

PHARMACOLOGY Summary of Medications Used to Treat Lower Airway Disorders

Medication Category and Action	Application/Indication	Nursing Responsibility
Preventive		
Pneumococcal vaccine ***Action:*** Induces antibodies that enhance killing of *Streptococcus pneumoniae.*	Prophylaxis against pneumococcal infection.	Recommend for adults 65 years and older, people who have chronic illness, or those who live in environments with increased exposure, such as the immunocompromised and transplant patients.
Influenza vaccine ***Action:*** Induces formation of serum antibodies specific to the influenza virus strain.	Prophylaxis against influenza based on predicted exposure.	Recommended for children, adults over 50 years, the immunocompromised, adults and children with chronic conditions, pregnant women, and health care workers.
Asthma/COPD		
Bronchodilators ***Action:*** Relaxes the smooth muscle of the bronchi and bronchioles. Beta-2 adrenergic agonists: Short-acting beta-2 agonists (SABA): Albuterol (Proventil, Ventolin), Levalbuterol. levalbuterol (Xopenex), pirbuterol (Maxair) ***Action***: Selectively dilates the beta-2 receptors in the lungs. Rapid onset of action; short duration.	Bronchospasm caused by contraction of the smooth muscles of the airway such as asthma, exercise-induced bronchospasm, and chronic obstructive pulmonary disease (COPD). Used as a rescue medication for acute bronchospasm attacks.	Instruct the patient on proper techniques of inhalation devices (MDI, DPI [dry powder inhaler], nebulizer). Assess symptom relief. Instruct the patient to take as ordered, not to exceed the prescribed dosage. Inform the health care provider of all medications being taken, including OTC and herbal remedies. Instruct the patient to inform the health care provider if any worsening of symptoms occurs. Inhaled forms are faster acting, produce less systemic effects, and are preferred over oral forms. Tolerance may develop and require a dosage adjustment or addition of another medication. Check the medication record for drugs that may interact with beta-agonists, including MAOIs and beta-blockers. Monitor for nervousness, tachycardia, or hypertension as potential side effects.
Long-acting beta-2 agonists (LABA): formoterol fumarate (Foradil, Perforomist) salmeterol (Serevent). ***Action:*** Slower onset (10–25 minutes), longer duration (12 hours) They are often used in combination with short-acting beta- agonists to reduce symptoms and exacerbations. Anticholinergics (ipratropium, Atrovent; tiotropium - Spiriva) ***Action:*** Blocks the cholinergic receptors responsible for bronchial smooth muscle contraction. Methylxanthines (theophylline). ***Action:*** Relaxes bronchial smooth muscle and blocking bronchodilator and suppresses airway responsiveness to stimuli.	Used in combination with corticosteroids for bronchospasm prophylaxis and therapy in asthma and COPD. Because use of LABAs increases the risk of asthma-related death, they are prescribed only when short- or intermediate-acting drugs do not control symptoms. Never use as monotherapy. Often combined with a beta-2 agonist for an additive effect to improve relief of bronchospasm (e.g., Combivent). Is fast-acting and used to relieve acute attacks; tiotropium has a longer onset and is used for maintenance therapy. Due to extensive side effects and drug interactions, these are used primarily for long-term management of asthma that is unresponsive to other drug therapies.	LABAs: Due to long onset, they are NOT considered rescue medications, and patients should be well-educated not to use them for acute attacks. Side effects of inhaled anticholinergics are uncommon because there is very little systemic absorption. Assess patients for history of glaucoma (contraindicated). Instruct patients to rinse their mouths with water and spit after inhalation, to prevent swallowing and increased risk of systemic effects (GI distress, dry mouth, nausea). Assess for the presence of cardiac impairment, severe renal or liver disorders, and active peptic ulcer. Check the medication record for drugs that have known interactions. Monitor serum levels and report if results are toxic. Observe for common side effects: tachycardia, restlessness, insomnia, dizziness, headache, palpitations, and vomiting.
Anti-inflammatories		
Corticosteroids Inhaled (beclomethasone – Beconase AQ, budesonide - Pulmicort, flunisolide - Aerobid, fluticasone - Flovent).	Short courses of systemic corticosteroids are used to gain control of deteriorating symptoms or for long-term therapy for patients with severe disease.	Instruct patients on the proper technique of inhalation devices.

PHARMACOLOGY Summary of Medications Used to Treat Lower Airway Disorders, *continued*

Medication Category and Action	Application/Indication	Nursing Responsibility
Systemic (prednisone, methylprednisolone). ***Action:*** Decrease inflammation of the airways by inhibiting the synthesis and release of inflammatory mediators. These drugs suppress late phase inflammatory response to allergens and reduce inflammation of airways. They reduce asthma symptoms, improve lung function, and decrease inflammation of airways with greatly reduced side effects as compared to systemic corticosteroids.	Inhaled corticosteroids (ICS) are used for long-term asthma control. They are often combined with LABAs.	Assess for symptom relief.
Mast cell stabilizers: cromolyn, nedocromil sodium. ***Action:*** Prevent mast cell release of inflammatory substances, such as histamine.	Asthma. Allergic rhinitis COPD. May be combined with LABAs for long-term maintenance. Systemic: Rapid acting. Used in patients with severe disease unresponsive to other medications, or for short-term use in patients whose condition is rapidly deteriorating.	Assess symptom relief. Instruct the patient not to use these for acute attacks (except systemic corticosteroids). Monitor for adverse effects: headache, candidiasis, secondary hypocortisolism, osteoporosis, cataract, and Glaucoma. Monitor for masked signs of infection.
Leukotriene modifiers: montelukast (Singulair), zafirlukast (Accolate). ***Action:*** Leukotrienes are mediators of the inflammatory response. Modifiers either block leukotriene receptors or block synthesis.	Allergic rhinitis. Prophylaxis treatment of asthma and COPD.	Instruct patients not to use these for acute attacks. Monitor for side effects: nausea, vomiting, throat irritation. Observe for anaphylaxis, angioedema, and bronchospasm.
These drugs are chemicals released by inflammatory cells in tissues responding to allergic reactions and induce bronchoconstriction, mucus secretion, and airway edema.	Exercise-induced bronchospasm. Asthma. Allergic rhinitis. Used to control mild, persistent bronchospasm or as an adjunct to inhaled corticosteroids.	Instruct the patient not to use these medications for acute attacks. Observe for side effects: headache, nausea. Metabolized in the liver: Perform physical assessment for signs of hepatic impairment (jaundice, fatigue, dark urine). Monitor liver and coagulation lab tests. Monitor for signs of infections, particularly in patients over 55 years old. Instruct patients to take this drug on an empty stomach.
Immunomodulators: omalizumab (Xolair). ***Action:*** IgE is a naturally occurring substance in the body that binds to allergens, stimulating mucus secretion, bronchoconstriction, and inflammation.	Are useful for severe allergic rhinitis and asthmatics with high IgE levels. It relieves symptoms, decreasing exacerbations, and reducing corticosteroid requirements. Used in patients who have severe, persistent allergic asthma that cannot be controlled with other medications.	Monitor patients closely after omalizumab administration for signs of anaphylaxis, including bronchospasm, hypotension, syncope, and/or angioedema. Rare cases of anaphylaxis have occurred with administration of this medication, and clinicians should be prepared and equipped to treat this. Have lifesaving equipment immediately available. Observe for signs of respiratory infection and viral disease.
Pulmonary Infections		
Antiviral (zanamivir, oseltamivir) ***Action:*** Neuraminidase inhibitors that prevent the release of virions from the host cell. Shortens the duration of influenza symptoms and reduces the duration of viral shedding.	Treatment and prophylaxes of influenza A and B. Zanamivir: inhalation route (prophylaxis). Oseltamivir: oral route (prophylaxis and treatment).	Advise the patient that the drug is not a replacement for the annual influenza vaccine. Advise the patient to immediately report signs/symptoms of neuropsychiatric events (abnormal behavior, delirium, hallucinations). Patients should be advised not to reconstitute inhalation powder and not to use these in nebulizers. Advise patients of common adverse effects: diarrhea, nausea, sinusitis, cough, headache, dizziness.

(*continued*)

PHARMACOLOGY Summary of Medications Used to Treat Lower Airway Disorders, *continued*

Medication Category and Action	Application/Indication	Nursing Responsibility
Antibacterial ***Action:*** Inhibit cell wall synthesis (penicillins, cephalosporins, carbapenems, vancomycin). Inhibit metabolic pathways (sulfonamides). Inhibit nucleic acid synthesis (fluoroquinolones). Disrupt plasma membrane (azoles, polyene). Inhibit protein synthesis (aminoglycosides, tetracyclines, macrolides).	Treat bacterial infections of the lungs and airways. Antibacterial is selected depending on the identification of the causative pathogen as identified on culture and sensitivity (C&S) testing. Broad-spectrum antibiotics are often initiated for severe infections, or infections in immunocompromised patients until culture results are completed. Antibiotics may be administered to prevent infections in high-risk patients.	Instruct patients to: • Notify health care provider for worsening or persistent symptoms. • Take medication on schedule. • Take complete prescription, even if feeling better. • Avoid taking with certain foods if indicated. • Take medication with meal or on empty stomach, as prescribed. • Preventative measures: frequent hand washing; avoid sharing contaminated items/food. Monitor drug-specific adverse effects. Monitor labs, such as white blood cell count, and therapeutic antibiotic levels.
Antifungal • Amphotericin B • Azoles (fluconazole, ketoconazole) • Echinocandins (caspofungin) ***Action:*** Either slow the growth of the organism (fungistatic) or kill them (fungicidal) by altering the cell membrane, inhibiting cellular synthesis, or disrupting cellular mitosis.	Amphotericin B is used for the primary treatment of patients with progressive and serious fungal infections. Azoles: Used for less severe infections because of their safer profile or in combination with amphotericin B for severe fungal infections. Echinocandins: Used to treat candida and aspergillus species.	Initial treatment with amphotericin B can produce acute, infusion-related fever, chills, vomiting, anorexia, and headache, which can be reduced if premedicated with corticosteroids, antihistamines, aspirin, or antipyretics. Monitor cardiovascular and respiratory status during Amphotericin B infusion. Monitor BUN and creatinine for signs of nephrotoxicity. Monitor for ototoxicity and report any hearing loss. Advise patients of common side effects: nausea, vomiting, headache. Instruct the patient to report any skin rash.
Mycobacterium (TB and non-TB)	A minimum of 2 and as many as 7 antimycobacterial medications are administered concomitantly in the treatment of active TB due to the slow growth of mycobacteria and the incidence of multidrug resistance. Using a combination of drugs that kill mycobacterium by different mechanisms reduces the potential for resistance.	Monitor compliance with medication schedule for the entire prescribed period of 6 to 12 months. Monitor periodic sputum smears and cultures until at least two negative values are obtained. Monitor hepatic function tests and signs of hepatotoxicity (anorexia, fatigue, nausea, malaise).
Isoniazid (INH) ***Action:*** Thought to inhibit an essential cell wall component of mycobacteria.	Prophylaxis for prevention of tuberculosis to exposed or high-risk persons. Treatment of active tuberculosis. Treatment of atypical mycobacterial infections.	Severe and sometimes fatal hepatitis has been reported; advise patients not to drink alcohol owing to increased risk for hepatitis. Monitor for adverse effects: visual disturbances, neuropathy (burning, tingling, pain, or numbness to distal extremities), seizures. Monitor for hyperglycemia in the presence of diabetes.
Rifampin ***Action:*** Bactericidal: Inhibits bacterial RNA synthesis.	Active tuberculosis. Inactive tuberculosis. Prophylaxis against tuberculosis in high-risk patients (HIV). Always used in combination with other antimycobacterials.	Nephrotoxic: monitor renal functions. Monitor for side effects: influenza-like illness, nausea, loss of appetite. Advise patients that discoloration of urine, sweat, tears, and saliva is normal.
Pyrazinamide ***Action:*** Inhibits synthesis of essential cell wall components.	Used in combination with other antimycobacterials in the treatment of active TB.	Monitor uric acid levels and signs of gout or arthralgia due to hyperuricemia. Assess for signs/symptoms of gout or arthralgia.

PHARMACOLOGY Summary of Medications Used to Treat Lower Airway Disorders, *continued*

Medication Category and Action	Application/Indication	Nursing Responsibility
Ethambutol ***Action:*** Impairs cell metabolism of mycobacteria, causing cell death.	Treatment of active TB; always given in combination with other antimycobacterials. Treatment of some atypical mycobacterium.	Monitor visual acuity secondary to optic neuritis. Monitor uric acid levels and signs of gout or arthralgia due to hyperuricemia.
Cystic Fibrosis		
Bronchodilator ***Action:*** Refer to beta-2 adrenergic receptor agonists earlier in this table.	Improve airflow obstruction in patients with CF.	See earlier in this table for beta-2 adrenergic agonists.
Inhaled hypertonic saline. ***Action:*** Hydrates mucus in the airways of patients with CF.	Improve sputum clearance rate in patients with cystic fibrosis.	
Aerosolized DNase I (dornase alfa) ***Action:*** Cleaves long strands of DNA released from dying white blood cells into smaller pieces.	Decrease viscosity of purulent CF sputum and improve lung function.	Advise patients not to mix with other medications in the nebulizer. Advise patients of side effects: chest pain, conjunctivitis, laryngitis, pharyngitis.
Pulmonary Embolus		
Anticoagulants (low molecular weight heparin, unfractionated heparin) ***Action:*** Inhibit clotting factors in the coagulation cascade.	Used empirically in patients with high clinical suspicion of acute pulmonary embolism to prevent further clot formation.	Assess patient history for recent surgery, trauma, severe hypertension, bleeding disorders, or intracranial hemorrhage. Monitor for signs of bleeding. Keep heparin antidote (protamine) readily available. Monitor coagulation studies and report if out of therapeutic range. Maintain safe environment to reduce risk of trauma and subsequent bleeding.
Thrombolytics (streptokinase, urokinase, tPA) ***Action:*** Promote fibrinolysis by converting plasminogen to plasmin, accelerating the normal process of clot removal.	Used in patients with confirmed pulmonary emboli to accelerate clot lysis. Indications include persistent hypotension, severe hypoxemia, or patent foramen ovale.	Prior to administration, assess whether the patient has a history of recent trauma, severe hypertension, bleeding disorders, intracranial hemorrhage, or history of internal bleeding. Avoid invasive procedures. Assess frequently for signs of excess bleeding such as hematoma, bleeding gums, oozing at IV or catheter site, epistaxis. Assess neurologic status frequently while on medication and for 8 hours after infusion completed.
Pulmonary Hypertension		
Diuretics (hydrochlorothiazide, furosemide, spironolactone) ***Action:*** Increases excretion of water and sodium from the kidneys.	Used to treat fluid retention caused by pulmonary hypertension and right heart failure; reduces pulmonary congestion and thereby lowers pulmonary pressures.	Monitor for signs of dehydration: hypotension, dry mucous membranes, decreased urine output, poor skin turgor. Monitor potassium levels. Measure urine output to gauge response to drug.
Anticoagulants ***Action:*** See information under pulmonary emboli.	Prophylactic treatment in patients with pulmonary hypertension to reduce incidence of intrapulmonary thrombosis or embolism.	See anticoagulation under pulmonary emboli.
Digoxin ***Action:*** Positive inotrope: improves cardiac contractility.	Used in PH to control rapid heart rate associated with right heart dysfunction.	Instruct patient to report signs/symptoms of bradycardia. Advise patient against sudden discontinuation of therapy. Monitor for side effects: diarrhea, loss of appetite, nausea, vomiting, headache, visual disturbances. Assess therapeutic serum range and report subtherapeutic or toxic levels.

(*continued*)

PHARMACOLOGY Summary of Medications Used to Treat Lower Airway Disorders, *continued*

Medication Category and Action	Application/Indication	Nursing Responsibility
Calcium-channel blockers (rare): nifedipine, diltiazem, amlodipine ***Action:*** Blocks the influx of calcium into the arterial smooth muscle causing peripheral artery vasodilation and reduction of systemic vascular resistance.	May be trialed in patients with idiopathic pulmonary hypertension who have a positive vasoactive (affecting blood vessels with respect to constriction or dilation) test.	Monitor systemic blood pressure, heart rate, and oxygen saturations carefully during drug titration. Monitor for dysrhythmias. Observe for side effects: headache, dizziness, peripheral edema, nausea. Monitor for hepatotoxicity and congestive heart failure.
Prostanoids: epoprostenol (Flolan), treprostinil (Remodulin) ***Action:*** Stimulate vasodilation of pulmonary and systemic arterial vascular beds and inhibit platelet aggregation.	Used in patients with pulmonary arterial hypertension. Epoprostenol is delivered via a permanently implanted central venous catheter. Treprostinil can be given intravenously or subcutaneously.	Instruct patients that even brief interruptions in therapy may cause a rapid deterioration in condition. Advise patients to report IV pump alarms immediately. Monitor for side effects: diarrhea, arthralgia, flushing, headache. Instruct the patient to report signs/symptoms of pulmonary edema. Assess for bleeding. Assess for hepatic insufficiency.
Endothelin-receptor agonist (bosentan, ambrisentan) ***Action:*** Block the vasoconstrictor effects of endothelin-1, which is a potent vasoconstrictor produced by vascular endothelium.	Used in pulmonary arterial hypertension to improve exercise capacity, dyspnea, and hemodynamic measures.	Assess for hepatotoxicity. Advise patients with a history of congestive heart failure to report signs/symptoms of exacerbation caused by fluid retention. Assess for side effects: hypotension, palpitations, flushing, nausea, vomiting, headache.
Phosphodiesterase inhibitor: sildenafil (Viagra), tadalafil (Cialis) ***Action:*** Prolong the vasodilatory effect of nitric oxide; vasodilate the pulmonary vascular bed.	Used in pulmonary arterial hypertension to improve exercise capacity and hemodynamics.	Assess for epistaxis, headache, dyspnea, flushing, insomnia, and dyspnea. Instruct the patient to report sudden decrease or loss of hearing or vision. Assess for improvement in signs and symptoms of pulmonary hypertension.
Cor Pulmonale		
Diuretics (hydrochlorothiazide, furosemide, spironolactone) ***Action:*** Refer to diuretics under Pulmonary Hypertension.	Reduce peripheral edema, reduce pulmonary congestion, reduce blood volume, and lower blood pressure to reduce the workload of the heart.	Refer to information in the section on Pulmonary Hypertension. Patients with cor pulmonale are very dependent on preload (blood returning to the heart) and careful monitoring is necessary to prevent overdiuresis. Monitor blood pressure, heart rate, weigh loss, skin turgor, and dry mucous membranes.
Inotropes (dobutamine, milrinone) ***Action:*** Increase right ventricular contractility and decrease right ventricular afterload by inducing pulmonary vasodilation.	Rescue therapy for hemodynamically unstable patients due to cardiogenic shock associated with right heart failure. There are no oral inotropes that are safe for routine use in cor pulmonale.	These drugs are administered via continuous IV infusion and require continuous monitoring of vital signs. Monitor for hypotension and tachycardia: Hypotension is more likely at lower doses. Blood pressure should be stabilized with a vasopressor agent prior to initiation of these medications; patient should then be weaned off the vasopressor as blood pressure tolerates.

Sources: Adams, M. P., & Koch, R. W. (2010). *Pharmacology, connections to nursing practice.* Upper Saddle River, NJ: Prentice Hall; Wilson, B. A., Shannon, M. T., Shields, K. M., & Stang, C. L. (2007). *Nurse's drug guide 2007.* Upper Saddle River, NJ: Prentice Hall.

NURSING PROCESS: Patient Care Plan for Pulmonary Infection

Assessment of Respiratory Status Using Gordon's Functional Health Patterns:

- Activity Exercise Pattern
- Cognitive Perceptual Pattern

Subjective Data

Assessment for Pneumonia

Do you have a cough, chills, or chest pain?

Describe the sputum you are coughing, if any.

How are you treating the symptoms?

What seems to be most helpful?

Do you have any history of exposure to respiratory infections or pulmonary irritants?

Have you recently taken antibiotics?

Do you feel short of breath?

What triggers your discomfort?

Describe your sleeping pattern.

Assessment of Oxygen Status

Do you have a cough, chills, or chest pain?

Describe the sputum you are coughing, if any.

Do you have any history of exposure to respiratory infections or pulmonary irritants?

Have you recently taken antibiotics?

Do you feel short of breath?

Do you feel like you are getting enough air?

If not, what triggers your discomfort?

Assessment of Ability to Perform ADLs

Can you perform the normal activities of daily living (ADL)?

What activities lead to fatigue?

How much activity can you do before needing to stop and rest?

How is this different from your usual endurance?

Assessment of Patient/Family Knowledge

Tell me what you know about your health problems.

Do you have questions about your health care?

Objective Data

Assessment for Pneumonia

Lung sounds

Vital signs

Sputum cultures

Chest x-ray

Spirometry

ABGs

Oxygen saturation

Assessment of Oxygen Status

Lung sounds

Vital signs

Sputum cultures

Chest x-ray

Spirometry

ABGs

Oxygen saturation

Assessment of Ability to Perform ADLs

Exercise tolerance: How much activity can the patient tolerate before developing clinical manifestations?

Assessment of Patient/Family Knowledge

Verbalizes education needs.

Identifies mode of receiving educational material.

Participates in education discussion.

Outcomes and Evaluation Parameters

Planning and Interventions with *Rationales*

1. NURSING DIAGNOSIS: Ineffective Breathing Pattern *related to an infectious process in the lungs* (NANDA-I © 2012)

Outcomes: The patient demonstrates effective coughing and breathing techniques.

The patient drinks 3 liters of fluid per day.

Evaluation Parameters: The patient's vital signs and temperature are within normal range.

Upon auscultation, lung sounds in all fields are clear.

The health care team, patient, and significant other(s) report that the patient is drinking fluids as instructed.

Sputum is easily expectorated and liquefied.

Urine is clear light yellow.

Complete a physical assessment that includes vital signs, temperature, assessment of fever and/or chills, tachycardia, and tachypnea *to detect early signs of infection and/or exacerbation of infection.*

Inspect for accessory muscle retraction, cyanosis, grunting on expiration, and restricted chest movement. In addition, auscultate for bronchial breath sounds; inspiratory crackles; increased vocal fremitus due to pleural effusion, unless the bronchus is completely plugged, which decreases vocal fremitus; and egophony due to consolidation. *These clinical signs are associated with hypoxemia, atelectasis, and pulmonary congestion. A baseline assessment is performed to ascertain the degree of pulmonary congestion and hypoxemia.*

Assist the patient to perform controlled coughing and deep breathing, and place the patient in an upright position to do this. A small pillow used to splint the chest may facilitate coughing and increase comfort. When not sitting in a chair, the patient position should be changed frequently. *This assists with mobilizing secretions.*

(*continued*)

NURSING PROCESS: Patient Care Plan for Pulmonary Infection, *continued*

Outcomes and Evaluation Parameters	Planning and Interventions with *Rationales*
	Give mild analgesics for chest pain that the patient may experience *due to muscular fatigue as the result of frequent paroxysms of coughing. Coughing allows for expectoration of secretions and clearance of airways. A pillow supports the diaphragm and allows for deeper breaths.* Provide prescribed medications and teach the patient about the purpose of each. This may include the use of an MDI. Prior to discharge the patient should demonstrate accurate use of the MDI, inhalers, or other oxygen equipment, and state the purpose of each medication. In addition to bronchodilators, the patient may be placed on antibiotic therapy. The nurse reviews the therapy regime with the patient and ascertains that he is able to take the medications correctly at home. *The patient is placed on bronchodilator medications as well as antibiotics to open airways and clear secretions. Through providing teaching about medication and assessing the patient's ability, the health care provider ascertains that the patient will receive the prescribed dose at home.* Encourage fluids to 3 liters/day *to liquefy tenacious secretions and allow for easy expectoration.*
2. NURSING DIAGNOSIS: Impaired Gas Exchange *related to infectious process in the lungs* (NANDA-I © 2012)	
Outcome: The patient states she can breathe easily without distress. ***Evaluation Parameter:*** Pulse oximetry and/or blood gas results are within the normal range for the patient.	Assess the patient's dyspnea at rest, with exertion, and during sleep. Administer oxygen as ordered, usually via nasal cannula or mask, and position the patient in an upright position or with the head up at night. Explain the rationale for oxygen to the patient and family members. *Perfusion abnormalities related to pulmonary congestion cause hypoxemia and dyspnea. Supplemental oxygen with a nasal cannula or a mask provides relief. Ventilation is improved in the upright position because it allows for maximal expansion of the lungs. This is particularly important in the obese.*
3. NURSING DIAGNOSIS: Activity Intolerance *related to an infectious process in the lungs* (NANDA-I © 2012)	
Outcome: Patient is able to assist with ADLs and initiate short walks of one-quarter to one-half block without dyspnea. ***Evaluation Parameter:*** Patient's oxygen saturation remains normal during and after performance of ADLs and ambulation.	Assess the patient's ability to perform ADLs. Administering oxygen as necessary, encourage the patient to do partial completion of ADLs and assist to a chair position followed by ambulation at short distances until the goal is reached. *Dyspnea indicates increased work of breathing. In the hypoxemic patient, exercise should not be attempted without oxygen. Oxygen allows the patient to perform optimally by providing adequate oxygenation to the muscles and decreasing the work of breathing.*
4. NURSING DIAGNOSIS: Deficient Knowledge *related to disease process* (NANDA-I © 2012)	
Outcomes: Patient avoids risk factors related to pneumonia. Patient complies with follow-up care. ***Evaluation Parameter:*** Patient verbalizes understanding of health needs and importance of prevention.	Assess the patient's and family's learning needs, readiness to learn, and preferred method of education (verbal, written, audiovisual) to present information at a time and in a manner the patient and family can understand. The patient's understanding of the treatment measures decreases anxiety and promotes compliance. Instruct the patient to seek immediate medical attention for return of clinical manifestations *to promote seeking early medical treatment of a potential life-threatening illness.*

Source: Adapted from Wilkinson, J. M., & Ahearn, N. R. (2009). *Prentice Hall nursing diagnosis handbook* (9th ed.). Upper Saddle River, NJ: Prentice Hall.

cause illness unless the patient is immunocompromised, such as AIDS, diabetes mellitus, emphysema, tuberculosis, cancer, or those receiving corticosteroids or immunosuppressants. Primary fungal infections are those that are caused by inhalation of fungal spores that then lead to pulmonary infection.

Etiology and Epidemiology

North America is unusual among continents in that it is home to three native (endemic) fungi that can cause human infection (mycoses): histoplasmosis, blastomycosis, and coccidioidomycosis (Davies, Knox, & Sarosi, 2010). Fungal lung infections occur more frequently in areas where there are endemic fungi, which include the valleys of the Mississippi and Ohio rivers (histoplasmosis and blastomycosis), the southwestern United States, the San Joaquin Valley in California, and northern Mexico (coccidioidomycosis). Histoplasmosis is caused by the fungus *H. capsulatum,* which grows in soil enriched by bird droppings. It is widespread and common in endemic areas and is usually asymptomatic or mildly symptomatic and rarely diagnosed. Inhalation of the spores can occur either in enclosed spaces, such as chicken coops, or in open urban areas where the soil is disturbed by construction. The most severe forms of histoplasmosis occur in patients with acquired immunodeficiency syndrome (AIDS).

Blastomycosis is caused by the fungus *B. dermatitidis.* It resides in the soil and becomes airborne when disturbed. Outbreaks tend to arise around recreational waterways and increase when there is local excavation activity. It can disseminate to other organs including the skin and bones.

Coccidioidomycosis is caused by the fungus *C. immitis* or *Coccidioides posadasii,* which resides in soil in the southwestern United States and northern Mexico. It can be disturbed by the wind, and large outbreaks have been identified outside the endemic areas after large windstorms. Coccidioidomycosis is often asymptomatic, but it can also lead to fatal pulmonary or systemic disease. Patients with AIDS and coccidioidomycosis have a high mortality rate.

Fungi that affect immunosuppressed individuals include *Aspergillus* and *Candida,* as well as *Cryptococcus neoformans* and *Mucorales* (mucormycosis). In patients with limited defense mechanisms, these organisms can produce widespread systemic disease leading to death. A fungal etiology should be considered in immunosuppressed patients with radiologic abnormalities. *Pneumocystis jirovecii* is also an opportunistic infection; risk is highest in the first 6 months after organ transplant or during high levels of immunosuppression (Fishman, 2010).

Pathophysiology

Fungi can cause lung disease through direct infection of pulmonary tissue, through infection of pulmonary air spaces/lung cavities, or through the ability of fungi to trigger an immunologic reaction when the fungus is inhaled. Once in the lungs, the fungi elicit tissue responses ranging from acute local exudative reactions to a prolonged chronic course to dissemination to other organs causing systemic infections. Extrapulmonary complications include cavitation, pleural effusions, and bronchopleural fistulas.

Clinical Manifestations

Symptoms of pulmonary fungal infection can range from asymptomatic to overwhelming illness. Severe systemic disease is most often produced in those who are immunocompromised. Some fungal infections have characteristic manifestations of dissemination. For example, blastomycosis may develop skin lesions or involve the prostate. Histoplasmosis can involve the reticuloendothelial system of the liver, spleen, and bone marrow. Cryptococcosis can lead to chronic meningitis.

People infected with histoplasmosis are generally asymptomatic; when symptoms are present, they are similar to those of influenza: fever, chills, headache, myalgia, and nonproductive cough. The incubation period is 9 to 17 days. Blastomycosis can have acute or abrupt symptoms that resemble bacterial pneumonia and include fever, chills, and a productive, purulent cough (Davies, Knox, & Sarosi, 2010). Skin lesions may develop and vary widely in appearance. The incubation period for blastomycosis is 21 to 106 days. Approximately 60% of people infected are asymptomatic (Davies, Knox, & Sarosi, 2010). Common symptoms for coccidioidomycosis, when they are present, are fever, cough (usually nonproductive), headache, and chest pain. Most patients show pneumonitis on chest x-ray.

Laboratory and Diagnostic Procedures

Diagnosis is made by cultures, stains, occasionally serology tests, and more rarely biopsy. Other differential diagnoses that need to be ruled out are chronic pneumonia, tuberculosis, and tumors. Fungi are often identifiable on histology, but determining the specific fungus can be challenging. Serology tests may be useful in patients with systemic disease. A thorough patient history including area of travel is useful in identifying probable cause. See the Diagnostic Tests for Pulmonary Infection box.

Medical Management

Amphotericin B, the oral azoles (fluconazole, ketoconazole, etc.), and echinocandins are treatment options for most patients with fungal disease (Davies, Knox, & Sarosi, 2010). Amphotericin B is the drug most commonly used in treating serious systemic fungal infections. It is given intravenously and considered a toxic drug with many possible side effects, including renal toxicity, febrile reaction, chills, malaise, nausea and vomiting, and thrombophlebitis at the injection site. Recent advances in amphotericin B include the development of lipid formulations, which demonstrate reduced nephrotoxicity (Rose, 2010). Total treatment with the drug may last from 4 to 12 weeks. Many of the side effects can be avoided by premedication with steroids, an anti-inflammatory, and antihistamines. Renal function is monitored closely, and ensuring adequate hydration is essential. Fluconazole is effective in treating less serious fungal diseases or as a maintenance therapy in more ill patients that improved after a course of amphotericin B. The echinocandins are a newer class of antifungal agents that seem to be well tolerated. They are currently being used in combination with amphotericin B in seriously ill patients. More details on these agents are given in the Pharmacology box on page 744.

Nursing Management

For nursing management of pulmonary fungal infections, refer to the Nursing Process: Patient Care Plan for Pulmonary Infections.

Pulmonary Tuberculosis

Pulmonary tuberculosis (TB) is a chronic and contagious bacterial infection caused by *Mycobacterium tuberculosis (M. tuberculosis).* The lungs are the primary targets, but the disease can also spread to other organs. The disease can develop after inhaling droplets sprayed into the air from a cough or sneeze by someone infected with *M. tuberculosis.* The disease is characterized by the development of granulomas (granular tumors) in the infected tissues.

Epidemiology

In the 1900s, TB was the leading cause of death in the United States and Europe and killed an estimated 2 billion people worldwide. With the introduction of antituberculosis chemotherapy in the 1940s and the later addition of rifampin, isoniazid, ethambutol, and pyrazinamide, death rates have significantly declined in the developed world (Huang, 2010). The rates increased in the United States by 20% from 1984 to 1992 (partly due to HIV infections), but with increased funding and focused attention, the rates have continued a downward trend since 1993 (Huang, 2010). However, in developing countries, tuberculosis remains a problem of great magnitude. The World Health Organization (WHO) reports that, in 2007, there was an estimated 9.27 million new cases, of which 44% were highly infectious. Ninety-five percent of the persons with clinically active tuberculosis and 98% of those who die from it are from developing countries (WHO, 2009).

The most prominent risk factor for developing tuberculosis and rapid progression of the disease is HIV infection (Huang, 2010). This partially accounts for the rise in incidence of tuberculosis from 1984 to 1992. The introduction of antiretroviral therapy (for HIV) has substantially reduced the risk in the United States, and studies have shown that preventive treatment with isoniazid to the HIV population further reduces the incidence (Huang, 2010). Other risk factors include immunosuppressive diseases or therapies such as diabetes, steroids, or chemotherapy. Older adults have a higher risk primarily because of their exposure during years when the disease was more prominent; they are also more likely to have impaired immunity (Nardell, 2009).

Etiology

The organism *Mycobacterium tuberculosis* is a nonmotile, non-spore-forming, and acid-fast rod that secretes niacin. The tubercle bacillus is transmitted via aerosolization (airborne route). Individuals who are most commonly infected are those who have repeated close contact with an infected person who has not yet been diagnosed with TB.

The newest forms of TB are multidrug-resistant (MDR) TB and extensive drug-resistant (XDR) TB. They are resistant to two or more of the primary drugs used for the treatment of tuberculosis (MDR) and to the second-line drugs (XDR). Resistance occurs when bacteria develop the ability to withstand antibiotic attack. Noncompliance is a major cause of MDR and XDR TB. Tuberculosis patients who take their medications erratically or do not complete drug treatment increase the chance of proliferating resistant organisms. Multiple drugs are used in the treatment of tuberculosis so that organisms that are resistant to one drug will be eradicated by the others. If the regimen is not followed, MDR/XDR TB can occur, and the mutations then spread to other persons (Nardell, 2009). Although significantly controlled in the United States, MDR TB is increasing around the world. The cause is multifactorial and inflamed by inadequate drug supplies, HIV coinfection, weak treatment regimens, poor treatment supervision, institutional transmission, and inadequate laboratory facilities (Nardell, 2009).

Pathophysiology

TB is a highly communicable disease that is transmitted via aerosolization. The tubercle bacillus causes a primary infection that rarely leads to an acute illness. Approximately 95% of primary infections are asymptomatic and move to a dormant (latent) phase (Nardell, 2009). Primary infection occurs when an infected person laughs, sneezes, or sings. Droplet nuclei are produced and may be inhaled by others and dropped into the airspaces of the lower lung. Infection most often occurs at a solitary site. The bacilli are ingested by macrophages and can replicate inside of them and eventually kill them, causing an inflammatory response. Thus, a focal pneumonitis evolves. If the macrophages infected with bacilli migrate to lymph nodes, they can be spread to any other part of the body including long bones, kidneys, vertebral bodies, and meninges (Nardell, 2009). In most cases (95%), the immune system suppresses the replication of bacilli after about 3 weeks. The site of infection may develop into granulomas with necrotic centers. The bacilli can survive in granulomas for years. Whether the infection resolves, remains dormant, or becomes active depends on the person's resistance and the virulence of the microbe (Nardell, 2009). In the minority of cases, the primary site of infection progresses immediately, causing illness with pneumonia, pleural effusions, and lymph node enlargement.

A latent infection can turn into an active disease in approximately 10% of immunocompetent patients (Nardell, 2009). More than half of latent infections that activate occur in the first 1 to 2 years following infection; however, the infection can remain latent for decades. Reactivation most often occurs at the lungs; however, it can activate at any site where it seeded at the time of infection. Higher risks for activation include impaired immune system, use of some immunosuppressants such as corticosteroids, gastric surgery, stress, and diabetes. Through delayed-type hypersensitivity, granulomatous necrosis is produced, and lung lesions often appear cavitary (Nardell, 2009). Pleural effusions, **empyemas** (collection of pus in the pleural space), bronchopleural fistulas, and pneumothoraces may develop as a consequence of growth and/or rupture of the lesions.

Clinical Manifestations

Even in cases of moderate or severe tuberculosis, symptoms may be vague. Often symptoms do not develop until the disease is advanced. Common symptoms are cough, fever, and sweating. The cough progresses from nonproductive to productive of purulent and sometimes blood-streaked secretions. Breath sounds will progress from rales to coarse rhonchi as secretions build up. Occasionally there is frank **hemoptysis** (blood in the sputum). Sweats often occur during the evening and nighttime hours. Other signs and symptoms include fatigue, weight loss, chest pain, and shortness of breath. Tuberculosis that seats in other organs occurs about 15% of the time, more often in patients with HIV. Nonpulmonary sites include the lymphatic system, genitourinary system, gastrointestinal system, bone, central nervous system, and pericardium.

Laboratory and Diagnostic Procedures

The tuberculin skin test, chest x-ray, acid-fast bacillus smear, and sputum culture are used to diagnose TB. The skin test is falsely negative in 20% to 25% of adults, so clinicians should not rule out TB on the basis of a negative skin test alone. The chest x-ray is key in the diagnosis of TB. See the Diagnostic Tests for Tuberculosis box for details.

DIAGNOSTIC TESTS for Tuberculosis

Test with Description, Rationale, and Normal Values	Expected Results
Mantoux test for TB (PPD)	
An individual with a positive PPD test has been exposed to TB and has developed antibodies. This test will also be positive in individuals who have received the BCG vaccine used routinely in Europe and South America to provide resistance to TB (develops antibodies). Normal: no reaction.	A reaction at the injection site occurs 48 to 72 hours after injection of a small amount of intermediate-strength purified protein derivative (PPD) given intradermally into the forearm. A reaction includes induration (palpable raised hardened area) and erythema. The diameter of induration is measured at its widest part. An induration of 5 mm or greater may be significant for individuals at risk such as HIV patients. An induration of 10 mm or greater is significant in individuals with normal or mildly impaired immunity.
Chest X-Ray	
Used to visualize the extent of lung involvement but does not confirm diagnosis. Used to assess patients with a positive PPD. Normal: lung fields are clear.	Visualizes tuberculosis lesions, cavitation, and inflammation. In recent TB infections, lung abnormalities are seen in the middle and lower lobes; in reactivation TB, they are seen in the upper lobes. Cavitation appears in some cases of primary TB and is common in reactivation infection.
Sputum for Acid-Fast Bacilli	
Confirms TB diagnosis. Normal: negative smear.	Three sputum samples are positive on an acid-fast smear.

Medical Management

Most patients with tuberculosis are now treated on an outpatient basis and given instructions on how to prevent spreading the disease. Medical management for TB centers on drug therapy over a 6- to 9-month regimen (see the Pharmacology box on page 744). Multiple drugs are prescribed to reduce the likelihood that resistant strains will emerge. There are four drugs used in the initial treatment of drug-susceptible TB; isoniazid (INH), rifampin (RIF), pyrazinamide (PZA), and ethambutol (EMB). EMB is included in the initial treatment until drug susceptibility cultures are determined. If the strain is susceptible to the other three drugs, the EMB can be discontinued. Patients being treated outside the hospital should take preventive precautions for at least two weeks if they have drug-susceptible TB and longer if they have MDR TB, as the consequences of transmission are higher and drug responsiveness may be slower (Nardell, 2009). Sputum stains and cultures will be monitored regularly throughout the drug regimen to determine the success of medications and identify relapse. Because the medications can be toxic to the liver, hepatic enzymes will be monitored. TB diagnosis also is reported to the local health department, which follows up on patient progress through treatment and provides resources. If there is concern that the regimen is not being followed, the health department may decide to supervise medication administration throughout the course of therapy.

The hospitalized patient with active TB or suspected active TB is placed in a negative pressure room with respiratory airborne isolation and use of standard precautions. Negative pressure is effective in preventing the movement of airborne bacilli from the patient's room into the hospital's hallways and corridors. When entering the room, health care providers and visitors should wear an N-95 mask (or greater). The patient should remain in isolation until three consecutive sputum cultures have tested negative. Until the sputum cultures return negative, there is no certainty that an individual is not infectious.

Nursing Management

Nursing care for the patient with TB focuses on preventing the spread of the infection, assisting the patient and family to manage the environment, and monitoring prescribed pharmacotherapy. The nurse addresses patient anxiety related to the disease and issues such as poor nutrition, pain, and fatigue (see Nursing Process: Patient Care Plan for Tuberculosis).

Health Promotion

The main focus of TB management is prevention of the spread of infection. Most TB can be cured with drugs, but a patient must continually take the prescribed medication for the entire therapy regimen, usually for 9 months. Some patients require a year or more for successful treatment. If the drug is stopped before completion, the TB may return in a form that is more resilient than before. Surviving bacteria may become resistant to the drugs used to treat TB, causing MDR/XDR TB. Patients should be advised not to smoke and not to drink alcohol or take acetaminophen. The addition of alcohol and acetaminophen along with the hepatotoxicity of the antituberculin medications puts the liver at an additional risk of injury. Patients who have a positive PPD but no evidence of disease (latent infection) can be given INH for 9 months or rifampin for 4 months to greatly reduce the probability of the progression of latent to active TB later in life. Finally, all persons who live with or have been in close contact with the infected individual must be tested and then treated, if necessary.

Nontuberculosis (Atypical) Mycobacterium

Nontuberculosis mycobacterium (NTM) includes mycobacteria other than *Mycobacterium tuberculosis*. It is also referred to as atypical mycobacteria. NTM are commonly prevalent in soil, municipal and natural water sources, foodstuffs, and animals. More than 140 species have been identified (Griffith & Wallace, 2011). These include *Mycobacterium avium, M. intracellulare, M. kansasii, M. xenopi,* and *M. fortuitum*.

Epidemiology and Etiology

There is no required reporting for NTM infections, so the prevalence of the disease is uncertain. The majority of NTM infections in North America are caused by *Mycobacterium kansasii, Mycobacterium avium* complex (MAC), and *Mycobacterium abscessus*. MAC is the most common NTM worldwide. Disseminated disease usually occurs in the severely immunocompromised, particularly in patients with AIDS, although the incidence has greatly decreased since antiretroviral drugs became available. Because NTMs are so prevalent in the environment and contraction of the disease is relatively rare, it is likely that otherwise healthy individuals who fall ill have some form of susceptibility. There is no evidence of human-to-human transmission. Infection in the lungs caused by NTMs is the most common transmission route in the United States and is predisposed in persons with existing pulmonary disease such as COPD, bronchiectasis (condition that damages the airways, causing them to become flabby, scarred, and widen), or cystic fibrosis. MAC infections are known to predominate in two subgroups of patients. The first are middle aged to older men with a history of COPD, smoking, and alcoholism. The second group is women over 50 with no pulmonary or smoking history and who have reported several months of fatigue and cough.

Clinical Manifestations

NTM infections display a diverse set of symptoms. Most commonly, the onset is subtly progressive and includes one or more of the following symptoms: productive cough, fatigue, fever, weight loss, and/or hemoptysis (Nardell, 2009). Cavitary nodules similar to tuberculosis may present on chest x-ray. MAC infections can lead to disseminated disease in patients with advanced AIDS. Diagnosis is made by radiology studies that show pulmonary disease and mycobacteria identified in sputum cultures. Signs of disseminated disease are specific to organ involvement and may include neutropenia, hepatomegaly, elevated liver enzymes, or adenopathy.

Laboratory and Diagnostic Procedures

The American Thoracic Society and the Infectious Disease Society of America have provided guidance for the diagnosis of pulmonary disease caused by NTM. The key elements for diagnosis are exclusion of other diseases, microbiologic culture results, and radiologic evidence of disease consistent with NTM (Taiwo & Glassroth, 2010). It is recommended that positive cultures isolate the same NTM organism from multiple samples of secretions (sputum, bronchial lavage, biopsy). See the Diagnostic Tests for Pulmonary Infection box.

Medical Management

Medical management of NTM involves administration of prescribed multidrug therapy. Because NTMs are generally slow growing, the specific species should be identified before initiation of potentially toxic drug therapy. As in treating *M. tuberculosis*, a multidrug regimen is used to prevent the emergence of resistive strains of the bacteria. MAC infections are started with a macrolide, such as clarithromycin or

NURSING PROCESS: Patient Care Plan for Tuberculosis

Assessment of Respiratory Status Using Gordon's Functional Health Patterns:

- Activity Exercise Pattern
- Cognitive Perceptual Pattern

Subjective Data	Objective Data
Assessment of Airway and Gas Exchange	**Assessment of Airway and Gas Exchange**
Have you been exposed to TB? Have you had recent travels to foreign countries in which there is a high incidence of TB? Have you had any prior tests for TB? If so, what were they? Have you had the BCG vaccine? Have you had dyspnea, weight loss, cough, sputum production, sleep disturbances, night sweats, or fatigue?	Lung sounds Vital signs Sputum culture for acid-fast bacilli Chest x-ray Work of breathing Oxygen saturation
Assessment of Patient/Family Knowledge of Disease	**Assessment of Patient/Family Knowledge of Disease**
What is your understanding of TB? Do you know who you got it from? Do you know how it is spread? Can you list your medications and how to take them and what precautions are necessary? Do you understand the treatment of TB and how you can help clear your lungs?	Can you give examples of when you would call your health care provider? What are the best methods for preventing the spread of TB?
Assessment of Ability to Perform Activities of Daily Living (ADL)	**Assessment of Ability to Perform Activities of Daily Living (ADL)**
What daily activities can you accomplish without assistance? Describe your activity schedule. Describe any physical symptoms you have while exercising or performing ADLs.	Observation of physical status during exercise Oxygen saturation pre- and post-activity Lung sounds pre- and post-activity Vital signs pre- and post-activity

Outcomes and Evaluation Parameters	Planning and Interventions with *Rationales*
1. NURSING DIAGNOSIS: Ineffective Airway Clearance *related to tracheobronchial secretions as evidenced by copious sputum production* (NANDA-I © 2012)	
Outcome: Upon auscultation of lung fields by the nurse, breath sounds are clear or with fewer adventitious sounds. ***Evaluation Parameter:*** Upon assessment by the nurse, vital signs are within normal range and the patient is afebrile.	Instruct the patient on methods to facilitate airway clearance. Teach proper coughing, deep breathing, and postural drainage techniques. Encourage hydration with 2 to 3 liters of fluid daily. *Effective coughing and deep breathing techniques and good hydration promote liquefication of secretions and facilitate expectoration.* Assess respiratory status for changes, also observing for temperature spikes or recurrence of symptoms. The patient who is progressing well should show a remission of symptoms. *A temperature spike or changes in respiratory status may indicate a complication or drug resistance.*
2. NURSING DIAGNOSIS: Deficient Knowledge About Treatment Regimen and Preventive Health Measures *related to TB management as evidenced by inability to plan care without assistance* (NANDA-I © 2012)	
Outcomes: Patient demonstrates to the nurse accurate coughing and deep breathing techniques, positioning and postural drainage techniques, and proper use of humidification and hydration to facilitate airway clearance. ***Evaluation Parameters:*** Demonstrates an adequate level of knowledge with regard to the medication regime, side effects, and indications for contacting the health care provider. Describes methods for preventing the spread of TB. Describes methods for minimizing drug side effects such as regular checkups, laboratory evaluation, supplemental vitamins, and avoidance of alcohol and foods containing tyramine and histamine.	Review the necessary information regarding coughing and breathing techniques and drug therapy and provide written information and instructions. Information is repeated as needed, enlisting the support of family members. If the patient is not English speaking, an interpreter is sought as well as patient education materials in the appropriate language. The importance of scheduled laboratory evaluation of renal and liver function is stressed. Teach the patient that rifampin causes urine to become darker in color. In addition, rifampin can increase the metabolism of other medications, making them less effective. These include beta-blockers, oral anticoagulants, corticosteroids, digoxin, quinidine, oral hypoglycemic agents, oral contraceptives, theophylline,

NURSING PROCESS: Patient Care Plan for Tuberculosis, *continued*

Outcomes and Evaluation Parameters	Planning and Interventions with *Rationales*
	and verapamil. Patients taking isoniazid (also called isonicotinyl hydrazine or INH) are taught to avoid foods containing tyramine and histamine, such as tuna, aged cheese, red wine, soy sauce, and yeast extracts. Eating these foods while on INH causes headaches, flushing, hypotension, light-headedness, palpitations, and diaphoresis. Medications should be taken 1 hour before meals or on an empty stomach since food interferes with absorption. The patient is instructed to cover her mouth and nose when coughing and sneezing. The patient should alert the health care provider regarding any fever or recurrence of symptoms. She should avoid exposure to silicone or dust because these substances cause further lung damage. The patient also must understand that taking medications is the most effective method of preventing transmission. *The major reason treatment fails is that patients do not take medications regularly and for the prescribed duration. Adherence to the therapeutic regime is essential to recovery. Patients who are not compliant with medication regimes are likely to remain infectious, and also prone to developing resistant strains of TB that are much more difficult to treat.*
3. NURSING DIAGNOSIS: Activity Intolerance *related to fatigue as evidenced by inability to engage in normal activities without dyspnea or fatigue* (NANDA-I © 2012)	
Outcome: Maintains an activity schedule without fatigue or dyspnea. ***Evaluation Parameters:*** Walks one-half block without experiencing dyspnea or fatigue. Completes ADLs independently and without dyspnea. Oxygen saturation is within normal range at rest and after completion of ADLs.	Plan a gradual progression of activity to increase exercise tolerance and muscle strength.

Source: Adapted from Wilkinson, J. M., & Ahearn, N. R. (2009). *Prentice Hall nursing diagnosis handbook* (9th ed.). Upper Saddle River, NJ: Prentice Hall.

azithromycin, then ethambutol and rifampin for a 12-month period after cultures have converted to negative. If the patient experiences weight loss or wasting syndrome, the dietitian becomes involved with meal planning. Patients may require follow-up with a home care nurse, respiratory therapist, and dietitian upon discharge.

Nursing Management

Nursing care of the patient with atypical tuberculosis is similar to that of patients with pulmonary infections and tuberculosis (see Nursing Care Plans). This is not a transmissible disease; once diagnosis has been made, the nurse should ensure that the medication regime is understood and followed carefully. Refer to the Nursing Process: Patient Care Plan for the Patient with Pulmonary Infection on page 749.

Lung Abscess

A **lung abscess** is a pus-filled cavity located in the parenchyma of the lung. Traditionally considered bacterial in nature, a lung abscess can also be caused by fungal and parasitic infections. It may be referred to as *necrotizing pneumonia*, particularly in its more advanced state. It is distinguished from an empyema in that the pus collects in the parenchyma rather than the pleural space.

Epidemiology and Etiology

Most lung abscesses result from aspiration of an anaerobe species that generally resides in the mouth. Patients who present with this problem often have a predisposition to aspiration secondary to alterations in consciousness (drug abuse, alcoholism, seizure disorder, stroke, general anesthesia) or dysphagia (Bartlett, 2010). Periodontal disease, gingivitis, sinus infection, and bronchiectasis are sources of infections. Septic embolism is another cause of lung abscesses, most commonly occurring in IV drug abusers and usually producing multiple abscess sites rather than a singular one. Lung abscesses can be classified as (1) chronic or acute, (2) primary or secondary, or (3) by causative organism. Primary infections are infections that occur in otherwise healthy individuals, such as by aspiration. Secondary infections are from systemic causes such as an immunocompromised state, obstructive neoplasms, or surgical complications (Bartlett, 2010).

Clinical Manifestations

Clinical manifestations are often insidious and occur over several weeks. Typically, the patient experiences fever, night sweats, cough, purulent sputum, and pleuritic chest pain. The sputum has a putrid smell in about 50% of patients and an empyema is present in about one-third of patients (Lorber, 2009). Lung sounds may be diminished and there is dullness on percussion over the abscess. Depending on the size of the abscess, oxygen saturation may be decreased.

Laboratory and Diagnostic Procedures

A CT scan is used if there is a question of cavitation not clearly seen on chest x-ray and is also helpful in distinguishing a lung abscess from a malignancy. Pleural fluid and blood cultures may be obtained. If the health care provider is unable to obtain sputum, transtracheal aspiration via suction may be done to obtain a sample so that sputum can be cultured and the organism can be identified. The patient needs to be evaluated for signs of severe periodontal disease and infective endocarditis as a possible cause of the lung abscess. See the Diagnostic Tests for Pulmonary Infection box on page 742.

Medical Management

The type of organism isolated on sputum culture and the findings of the history, physical exam, and diagnostic work-up will determine the treatment required. The patient should be assessed for adequate cough and risk of aspiration. Some patients benefit from a percutaneous chest catheter placed for drainage of the abscess. Antimicrobial therapy is guided by Gram stain and probable source of infection, and then adjusted by culture and sensitivity. Clindamycin is the current drug of choice for anaerobic lung infections. Surgery for lung resection may be necessary for rapidly progressive disease. Immunocompromised patients may require more intensive antimicrobial therapy.

Nursing Management

The nursing management of patients with a lung abscess focuses on assessment, treatment, and evaluation. It is critical that the nurse assess the patient's recent past medical history and plan interventions based on the patient's knowledge base and understanding. The nurse also must take into consideration the patient's support system and ability to care for self.

It is important for the nurse to assess the patient's recent history of influenza, pneumonia, febrile illness, cough, and sputum production. Physical assessment of the patient often reveals a febrile patient who appears pale and fatigued. The patient may complain of pleuritic chest pain, which is stabbing in nature when taking a deep breath. Auscultation of breath sounds may reveal decreased sounds in the involved area of the lung. Bronchial breath sounds and fine crackles are heard over the site of the lesion. Refer to the Nursing Process: Patient Care Plan for Pulmonary Infections on page 749.

Collaborative Management for Pulmonary Infections

To optimize care of the patient with pulmonary infection, the nurse collaborates with the health care provider to monitor and adjust medications, treatments, patient education, and the overall plan of care. In addition, the pharmacist is consulted regarding medication effectiveness and side effects, and the respiratory therapist assists with administration of the pulmonary toilet, including breathing and coughing techniques that allow for clearing pulmonary secretions. In order to meet desired patient outcomes, it is essential that this interdisciplinary team communicate openly with one another in developing and evaluating care of the patient and family (IOM [Institute of Medicine], 2010).

The physical therapist may assist with ambulation and some physical rehabilitation if the patient is in a weakened state. The nurse provides adequate pain relief in advance of physical therapy. If anorexia is present, which is common with infections, especially TB, the nutritionist plans for small frequent meals and nutritional supplements as needed. The treatment of anorexia is discussed in Chapter 8. If monitoring is required after discharge, a social worker and home care nurse are enlisted. A community health nurse is likely to provide continuity of care.

Health Promotion for Pulmonary Infections

Patients should be taught principles of prevention. These include washing hands frequently, especially after using the bathroom, before meals, and after blowing the nose. Influenza vaccination is the primary method for preventing influenza and its severe complications. As indicated in a report from the Advisory Committee on Immunization Practices (ACIP) (CDC, 2011), an annual influenza vaccination is now recommended for all persons over 6 months old to prevent the spread of influenza.

Older adults and those with chronic diseases such as chronic obstructive pulmonary disease (COPD) and diabetes are at high risk for pneumonia and should avoid smoking. Exposure to environmental smoke, pollutants, and crowds also can be risk factors for these individuals. Those at risk should be inoculated with the influenza and pneumococcus vaccines. Individuals older than 65 years and younger patients who have chronic illnesses or are immunocompromised should receive the pneumococcal vaccine.

Interstitial Lung Diseases

Interstitial lung disease (ILD) is a broad category of over 100 diseases that have similarities in clinical presentation, chest x-ray characteristics, and physiologic traits. Chart 27–7 lists known causes of ILDs. Of the diseases that are considered ILDs, idiopathic pulmonary fibrosis and sarcoidosis of the lung are discussed in the following text. Others are covered in Chapters 51 and 53. The interstitium is the area between the alveoli and the capillaries and is important in the support and efficiency of gas exchange. Damage can occur from exposure (asbestos, mold), systemic tissue disease (rheumatoid), inflammation, or injury (Chapman, 2010). If the exposure continues or response to injury/inflammation

CHART 27–7 Causes of Interstitial Lung Disease

OCCUPATIONAL AND ENVIRONMENTAL

Long-term exposure to toxins may damage the lungs. These toxins include:

Asbestos fibers
Silica dust
Coal dust
Bird and animal droppings
Grain dust

RADIATION TREATMENTS

Patients who have had radiation treatment for lung or breast cancer may show signs of lung damage months or years after the initial radiation treatment. Severity depends on:

Amount of radiation received
Underlying lung disease
Amount of lung exposed
Use of adjunctive chemotherapy

MEDICATIONS

Many medications may cause lung damage. These include:

Chemotherapy
Medications to treat dysrhythmias such as amiodarone or propranolol
Some antibiotics such as sulfasalazine and nitrofurantoin

MEDICAL CONDITIONS

Rheumatoid arthritis
Systemic lupus erythematosus
Sarcoidosis
Scleroderma

is incomplete, the lung may be damaged permanently. The disease is not restricted to the interstitium and can include the alveoli and airway structures.

These diseases cause inflammation or scarring of the lung tissue or result in filling of the air spaces with exudate and debris (pneumonitis). The diseases can be characterized according to known and unknown (idiopathic) causes. Known causes include exposure, genetic, and systemic diseases (e.g., sarcoidosis, connective tissue disease).

Epidemiology and Etiology

The exposure-related etiologies include occupational exposure; drug, medication, and radiation exposure; hypersensitivity pneumonitis; and tobacco exposure. Occupational exposures are related to asbestosis, chronic silicosis, and coal worker's pneumoconiosis (described in the following text), all of which involve inhaling contaminants associated with the work environment (asbestos, silica, and coal dust). Many drugs and medications are known to cause ILD. There is no distinct physiologic, radiographic, or pathologic pattern associated with medication-induced ILD, and the diagnosis is usually made with respect to the timing of medication initiation and subsequent pulmonary problems (Chapman, 2010). Hypersensitive pneumonitis is an immune response to an inhaled antigen. Hypersensitivity can be caused by organic triggers (bacteria, fungi, animal proteins) or inorganic compounds (vaporized paints and plastics). Several forms of ILD have been associated with smoking.

ILD is a well-documented complication of sarcoidosis and connective tissue disease (CTD). The most common CTD-associated ILDs are scleroderma, rheumatoid arthritis, polymyositis, and lupus. The presentation is diverse. Sarcoidosis is an idiopathic multisystem inflammatory disorder, and sarcoidosis of the lung is the most common ILD in the United States (Chapman, 2010).

Of the idiopathic ILDs, idiopathic pulmonary fibrosis (IPF) is the most common. It is progressive and isolated to the lungs. The majority of patients who are diagnosed with IPF are over 60 years old, and it is rare in persons under 40. Most patients die within 4 years of diagnosis (Chapman, 2010).

Pathophysiology

Most ILDs, regardless of the cause, have a common pathogenesis. It is thought that these disorders are initiated by some type of pulmonary injury (exposure, systemic, idiopathic) followed by an attempted repair. If the exposure continues or the repair is imperfect, then diseased interstitial tissue replaces the normal capillaries, alveoli, and healthy interstitium of the lung. Gas exchange becomes impaired due to alteration in gas diffusion, ventilation-perfusion abnormalities, and alveolar shunting.

Clinical Manifestations

ILDs may be acute or insidious in onset, depending on the causes. The most common symptom is progressive dyspnea. A nonproductive cough and fatigue are also common. Hemoptysis may occur in patients with diffuse alveolar hemorrhage syndromes and vasculitis. Wheezing is an uncommon manifestation but can occur in patients with lymphangitic carcinomatosis (tumor spread through the lymphatics of the lung), chronic eosinophilic pneumonia, and respiratory bronchiolitis (inflammation and mucus buildup in the bronchioles). Chest pain also is uncommon, but pleuritic chest pain may occur in patients with rheumatoid arthritis, systemic lupus erythematosus, and some drug-induced disorders.

Many of the findings on physical exam, such as rales, rhonchi, or digital clubbing, are nonspecific. Some systemic findings may be associated with the causes of ILD, such as hepatosplenomegaly and lymphadenopathy associated with sarcoidosis.

Laboratory and Diagnostic Procedures

Although routine blood analysis only rarely leads to a diagnosis, the results can be helpful in identifying systemic disease.

Medical Management

Medical management depends on the specific diagnosis, which is based on findings from the clinical evaluation, imaging studies, and lung biopsy. When the cause is known, discontinuation of exposure to the inciting agent is essential. Corticosteroids, immunosuppressive agents, and cytotoxic agents are the mainstay of therapy for many of the interstitial lung diseases. Ancillary therapies include supplemental oxygen therapy, which alleviates exercise-induced hypoxemia and improves performance. Lung transplantation may be an option for advanced cases of fibrotic lungs; however, the mortality rate at one year (10% to 25%) and five years (50% to 60%) is high (Chapman, 2010). Many patients do not qualify due to age and comorbidities.

Idiopathic Pulmonary Fibrosis

Idiopathic pulmonary fibrosis (IPF) is a chronic, progressive, fibrosing interstitial lung disease of unknown etiology that usually affects adults over the age of 40 and is characterized by a poor prognosis and no proven effective treatment.

Epidemiology and Etiology

Approximately 80,000 cases of IPF have been identified in the United States, with an estimated 30,000 new cases developing each year. More males than females have been reported to have IPF. Patients with IPF are often middle aged, usually between 40 and 70 years of age. Approximately two-thirds of patients with IPF are over the age of 60 years at the time of presentation. IPF has no distinct geographic distribution. It is reported worldwide in both rural and urban settings with no predilection by race or ethnicity. Risk factors for developing IPF include exposure to smoke, hairdressing chemicals, farming dust, and metal dust (Budev & Wiedemann, 2010).

Typically, when detected, IPF is already at an advanced stage. The course of the disease is variable and unpredictable. Some patients exhibit a rapidly progressive fatal course over several months; others demonstrate deterioration in lung function over a longer period. The median survival is 3 to 5 years from the onset of symptoms.

Pathophysiology

The pathogenesis of IPF remains unknown. It is thought that some type of microinjury occurs to the alveolar epithelial cells that causes progressive scarring and fibrosis. This results in stiff lungs and loss of pulmonary function.

Clinical Manifestations

Clinical manifestations of IPF consist of progressive dyspnea upon exertion, nonproductive cough, interstitial infiltrates on chest radiographs, and abnormal pulmonary function tests indicating restrictive disease (Patel, 2008). Many patients have bibasilar (at the base of both lungs) inspiratory crackles and tachypnea. Symptoms depend on the extent of lung damage. Weight loss and fatigue are common. Pulmonary hypertension and right heart failure are seen as the disease progresses. Infection, **pneumothorax** (collection of air in the pleural space separating the lung from the pleural wall, causing partial or complete collapse of the lung), and pulmonary emboli are complications of the disease. Causes of death include respiratory failure, respiratory

DIAGNOSTIC TESTS for Interstitial Lung Disease

Test with Description, Rationale, and Normal Values	Expected Abnormality
Chest x-ray	
Clear *Helps to identify or rule out etiology of suspected disease.*	Demonstrates reduced lung volumes with reticular (network of lines) or reticulonodular (nodules at the intersection of the lines) opacities. IPF: almost all patients have findings of bilateral diffuse reticular or reticulonodular infiltrates at the periphery and the bases of the lungs. Sarcoidosis: enlarged lymph nodes and pulmonary parenchymal involvement is identified (Newman, 2009).
Chest CT	
No abnormality *Used to identify lung pathology or degree of pathology when CXR provides insufficient data.*	Defines the abnormalities that are particular for each disease. For example, interstitial pulmonary fibrosis often shows distortion of the lung anatomy and, in the later stages, a honeycomb appearance that represents multiple tiny cysts.
Serology	
Laboratory examination of a blood or fluid sample that detects the presence of antibodies in the serum/fluid that are associated with a specific microorganism.	Identification of microorganism.
ABG Study	
pH 7.35–7.45; $PaCO_2$ 35–45; PaO_2 75–100; HCO_3 24–28 *Monitor for oxygenation or ventilation abnormalities that may be associated with pulmonary disease.*	Evidence of hypoxemia. Decreased PaO_2.
Lung Biopsy	
Normal lung tissue *Obtaining tissue from the lung for laboratory analysis. This is used to guide therapeutic intervention.*	Presence of abnormal cells. May be necessary to definitively diagnose ILD. During the period of accelerated IPF, lung biopsy typically shows a combination of UIP with superimposed diffuse alveolar damage, characterized by fibroblast proliferation of the alveoli septa, hyperplasia of type 2 pneumocytes, and hyaline membrane remnants.

Source: Adapted from Kee, J. L. (2010). *Laboratory and diagnostic tests* (8th ed.). Upper Saddle River, NJ: Prentice Hall.

infection, or heart failure. The definitive diagnosis should be made only after clinical, radiologic, and pathologic evaluations of the patient and only after excluding other causes of interstitial lung disease.

Laboratory and Diagnostic Procedures

Blood test results are not specific for IPF; however, some abnormal values can be related to the pathophysiology of IPF. For example, an elevated hemoglobin value may reflect hypoxemia secondary to IPF. The erythrocyte sedimentation rate is elevated in many patients. Serologic test results are nonspecific; however, high titers should raise the possibility of connective-tissue disorders.

Pulmonary function tests are conducted with a typical finding of a restrictive ventilatory defect. The most common abnormality found in patients with IPF is a decreased diffusion capacity. Bronchoalveolar lavage, echocardiography, and bronchoscopy also may be done to isolate or confirm diagnosis. Refer to the Diagnostic Tests for Interstitial Lung Disease box above.

Medical Management

There is no proven treatment for IPF. Medical management is primarily supportive and focuses on preserving as much lung function as possible, thereby enabling the patient to engage in normal activities as long as possible. Oxygen therapy should be prescribed for patients with documented hypoxemia; this should improve exercise tolerance. A pulmonary specialist generally is consulted to manage the patient with corticosteroids and cytotoxic or antifibrotic agents, although these are considered experimental in the treatment of IPF. Patients with acute respiratory failure may require mechanical ventilation, with consultation from a critical care specialist.

Maintaining adequate nutritional intake and immunizations is important for quality of life. Participation in a pulmonary rehabilitation, where available, should be encouraged to maintain functionality and address psychosocial aspects of this disease. Lung transplantation also should be considered, and a referral to an appropriate transplantation center may be appropriate.

Sarcoidosis

Sarcoidosis of the lung, another form of ILD, is caused by an inflammatory immune system disorder that can affect any organ but most commonly attacks the lungs. Much evidence has suggested that the pathogenesis of the disease is an immune response, and it is widely believed that one or more antigens trigger a cascade of events in genetically predisposed individuals (Weinberger, 2007). However, no specific trigger or genetic factor has been found to occur in all patients with the disease.

Epidemiology, Etiology, and Pathophysiology

The identification of the prevalence and characteristics of sarcoidosis worldwide is problematic owing to lack of definition of the disease, precise diagnostic methods, and diagnostic bias. Sarcoidosis is relatively common in northern Europe (particularly Scandinavia), North America, and Japan. The lower reported incidence in areas such as China, Africa, and India may be due to undiagnosed or misdiagnosed disease (Weinberger, 2007). However, there does seem to be some geographic predilection, such as significantly higher incidence in northern vs. southern Italy, which suggests that climate may have a role in disease acquisition. In the United States, African Americans have a 3.8-fold higher incidence than Whites and present with more severe multisystem disease (Culver, 2010). Approximately 50% of people initially diagnosed with sarcoidosis are younger than 30 years old, and 75% are under 40. Women have a higher preponderance across ethnic backgrounds (Culver, 2010).

Evidence suggests that there is a genetic susceptibility that may be triggered when the person is exposed to a specific environmental antigen, although no single antigen or genetic factor has been identified (Weinberger, 2007). Both infectious and noninfectious causes have been suggested. A person-to-person transmission of infectious agents has some support in cases in which the diagnosed individuals share a common environment or infectious agent, such as fire fighters or nurses. Sarcoidosis has also been shown to develop in organ recipients from a donor with sarcoidosis. Although the exact cause of sarcoidosis is unknown, it is believed to occur when a person's immune system overreacts to an unknown toxin, drug, or pathogen that enters the body through the airways. Normally, a person's immune system helps protect the body from foreign substances and invading microorganisms, such as bacteria and viruses. But in sarcoidosis, T-helper lymphocytes—white blood cells that play a key role in the body's immune response—seem to respond too strongly to a perceived threat. This triggers small areas of inflammation called granulomas. As the disease progresses, granulomas and scarring (fibrosis) may occur in the tissue between the alveoli, stiffening the lungs and reducing the amount of air the lungs can hold.

Clinical Manifestations

Patients with symptoms of sarcoidosis most commonly present in winter and early spring, which suggests a possible environmental trigger. As many as 30% to 60% of these patients are asymptomatic and are diagnosed by review of a chest x-ray that was performed for unrelated reasons. Other symptoms include fever, night sweats, malaise, fatigue, weight loss, dry cough, wheezing, and dyspnea (American Lung Association, 2007).

Sometimes sarcoidosis develops gradually and produces signs and symptoms that last for years. Or it may appear suddenly and then disappear just as quickly. In either case, signs and symptoms can vary, depending on which organs are affected and how long the individual has had the disease (American Lung Association, 2007). Of these patients, 90% present with pulmonary involvement, and those who do not are likely to experience remission within 2 years or experience a milder disease presentation. Additional signs and symptoms of sarcoidosis that should be considered include small red bumps on the face, arms, or buttocks (a condition that is more common in African Americans than in Caucasians) and red, watery eyes.

Laboratory and Diagnostic Procedures

Diagnosis of sarcoidosis is usually made by radiography, biopsy, clinical assessment, and exclusion of other potential causes. Refer to the Diagnostic Tests for Interstitial Lung Disease box on page 758. The diagnosis can be confirmed with biopsy.

Medical Management

Approximately two-thirds of patients with sarcoidosis experience resolution of the disease within 2 years. Another 10% to 30% go on to have a chronic or progressive course (Weinberger, 2007). The disease is considered inactive once the symptoms fade. Medical management of sarcoidosis is individualized, with the need for medical therapy varying based on the symptoms and organ systems involved in each patient. When therapy is recommended, the main goal is to keep the lungs and other affected body organs functioning and to relieve symptoms. The decision to initiate drug therapy depends on the organ system that is involved and how far the inflammation has progressed. Patients who should receive therapy include those with progressive symptoms; markedly deteriorating or abnormal lung function; hypercalcemia; cavitation, fibrosis, or pulmonary hypertension on CXR; heart or nervous system involvement; renal or hepatic insufficiency; or disfiguring skin or joint disease (Newman, 2009).

Corticosteroids are the first-line treatment when aggressive systemic treatment is needed. They prevent granuloma formation and reverse immunologic abnormalities. Improvements in symptoms, chest radiographs, and lung function tests are typical; failure to respond within 2 to 3 months suggests the presence of steroid-refractory disease (Culver, 2010). The goal of corticosteroids is to relieve symptoms, improve the quality of life, and reduce morbidity and mortality related to organ damage. Other immunosuppressive medications, such as methotrexate, are used for patients who are refractory to corticosteroid therapy or who cannot tolerate the side effects. At present, there is no treatment to reverse the lung scarring (fibrosis) that might be present in advanced sarcoidosis. Frequent checkups are important so that the health care provider can monitor the illness and, if necessary, adjust the treatment.

Pneumoconiosis

Pneumoconiosis is a group of interstitial lung diseases associated with occupational exposures that cause interstitial lung fibrosis. They are usually caused by the inhalation of mineral or metallic dust. The exposure activates a cascade of inflammatory responses that ultimately lead to interstitial fibrosis. The two most common types of pneumoconiosis are silicosis and asbestosis. Other occupational-related lung diseases include coal worker's pneumoconiosis and COPD (caused by inhalation of coal dust), cobalt lung and asthma (caused by inhalation of hard metal dust), mesothelioma and bronchogenic cancer (caused by inhalation of asbestiform fibers), and lung cancer (caused by inhalation of silica).

Silicosis

Silicosis is a fibrosing interstitial lung disease caused by the inhalation of crystalline free silica dust, most commonly quartz. Because silica is a ubiquitous mineral, workers in a wide variety of industries are at exposure risk, including miners, foundry workers, and sandblasters. Types of silicosis include chronic, acute, and accelerated. Chronic silicosis develops over decades. Acute silicosis, in contrast, presents within several weeks or a few years after an intense exposure. Accelerated silicosis develops within 10 years of initial exposure and is associated with higher intensity exposures. Symptoms can range from asymptomatic for chronic silicosis to rapid progression of dyspnea, weight loss, and fatigue in acute silicosis. Diagnosis is made by a history of exposure, typical chest x-ray findings (nodular or ground glass appearance), and elimination of other possible causes. Fibrotic changes are believed to be irreversible, and medical management focuses on prevention of disease progression and complication development. Exposure to silicosis should be eliminated. Because of the interaction between silica exposure and smoking in the development of COPD, tuberculosis, and lung cancer, smoking cessation and exposure to secondhand smoke should be advised (Cowie, Murray, & Becklake, 2010). Management may include lung lavage, corticosteroids, and bronchodilators. Lung transplantation may be considered in young patients.

Coal Worker's Pneumoconiosis

Coal worker's pneumoconiosis (also called black lung or coal miner's lung) is caused by the inhalation of coal dust into the lung. The concentration of coal dust in the mine, the length of exposure over time, and the hardness of the coal all contribute to the risk of pneumoconiosis (Samet, 2007). When coal dust is inhaled, it causes an inflammatory lesion in the bronchioles and may extend into the alveoli. This may lead to fibrosis of the small airways and alveoli, and progress to larger nodules and extensive fibrosis. Nodular opacities of greater than 1 cm on radiography are considered progressive massive fibrosis. Patients with a simple form may be asymptomatic, although the chest radiography will demonstrate the typical nodular findings. Clinical presentation is usually productive cough, dyspnea, and altered pulmonary function. Progressive fibrosis is associated with pulmonary hypertension, dyspnea, or respiratory failure. No treatment is available for coal worker's pneumoconiosis, and medical management is supportive. As with silicosis, exposure should be eliminated, and smoking cessation should be advised.

Asbestosis

Asbestosis is pulmonary fibrosis caused by inhalation of asbestos fibers. Asbestos inhalation is also tied to mesothelioma, lung cancer, and laryngeal cancer (Samet, 2007). Asbestos has widespread industrial uses, particularly in construction and insulation. There is only low-level exposure to occupants of buildings in which asbestos fibers are used in construction and insulation; however, workers involved in removing or demolishing the buildings are at risk. Inhaled fibers cause an inflammatory response that ultimately leads to fibrosis. In advanced stages, it can destroy lung architecture, causing honeycombing (cavitations bordered by fibrosis), which makes lungs stiff and small. Patients are usually asymptomatic for 20 to 30 years after initial exposure (King, 2010). They initially present with progressive dyspnea on exertion. In advanced disease, patients may develop crackles, digital clubbing, and, in severe cases, cor pulmonale (discussed later in the chapter). Pulmonary function tests will be abnormal. Cigarette smoking worsens the disease. Chest CT is more sensitive than CXR in diagnosing asbestosis. Findings have a characteristic fibrotic pattern including honeycombing and linear densities. There is no treatment for asbestosis, and management is based on preventive measures, including smoking cessation, early detection, removal from exposure, prompt treatment of infections, and pneumococcal and influenza vaccinations (King, 2010).

Nursing Management of Patients with ILD

Nursing management of patients with ILD is based on the principles of caring for any patient with chronic lung or respiratory disorders. Supportive care plays a large part in this patient population.

Assessment

Nursing assessment of ILD includes identification of abnormal lung sounds, oxygen saturations, respiratory rate and effort, weight loss, change in activity tolerance, cough characteristics, digital clubbing, hepatosplenomegaly, or lymphadenopathy. Chronic hypoxia may also lead to cardiac involvement and the nurse should monitor for dysrhythmias and reduced cardiac output.

Nursing Diagnoses

Nursing diagnoses related to ILDs include the following:

- *Gas Exchange, Impaired* related to disease process.
- *Nutrition, Imbalanced Less Than Required* related to fatigue and shortness of breath.
- *Knowledge Deficit* related to disease process and plan of care.
- *Anxiety* related to shortness of breath.

NANDA-I © 2012

Planning

Because ILDs have a poor prognosis, much of the care is palliative. The main focus is on assisting the patient to remain functional and to maintain as much self-care and life management as possible.

Outcome and Evaluation Parameters

Desired outcomes for the patient with ILD include reduction or stabilization of dyspnea, cough, and exercise intolerance. The patient will verbalize understanding of disease management, including the importance of maintaining adequate nutrition, following the medication regimen, preventing pulmonary infection, and opting for smoking cessation.

Interventions and Rationales

The nurse caring for a patient with ILD provides supportive care and education to assist the patient and caregiver. Issues to be addressed are dyspnea, fatigue, and activity tolerance. Most patients with interstitial lung disease will require supplemental oxygen to facilitate maintaining activity levels and to possibly prevent or delay hypoxia-induced pulmonary hypertension. The nurse should provide education about the management of ILD. For patients with end-stage disease, the nurse should initiate a discussion of advanced directives. The nurse also should address emotional issues such as depression, anxiety, and anger as the patient's health deteriorates in the end stage.

Discharge Priorities

Discharge priorities for patients with ILDs include patient education regarding medication, criteria for contacting the health care provider, and actions to be taken in an emergency. Patients should contact a health care professional if they experience difficulty breathing, vision changes, or palpitations that may indicate progression of disease. Oxygen needs should be considered in making plans for transfer to home, and instructions should be given in writing. Referrals for home care and follow-up care are made if the patient and family require it.

Collaborative Management

The health care provider, nurse, respiratory therapist, physical therapist, and social worker are involved in the care of the patient with ILD. In order to meet desired patient outcomes, it is essential that this interdisciplinary team communicate openly with one another in developing and evaluating care of the patient and family (IOM [Institute of Medicine], 2010). Pulmonary rehabilitation referral may be helpful in some patients. Frequently, patients with sarcoidosis, because of their younger age, are able to return home and manage care independently; however, in the case of older patients and more extreme debilitation, referrals for physical therapy, respiratory therapy, and home care are required. If dyspnea is persistent, the health care provider may prescribe home oxygen and provide a referral to a home oxygen company.

Health Promotion

Since pulmonary infections can worsen an ILD, patients should be offered influenza and pneumococcal vaccination. Referral to smoking cessation classes should be emphasized for patients who smoke. Because both prednisone and methotrexate decrease the immune response, the patient is counseled to avoid crowds and children or persons with colds or infectious illnesses and to receive the flu and pneumococcal vaccines.

Workers who are exposed to the toxic agents that may cause ILDs must be fitted with appropriate safety equipment. In the industrial setting, the occupational health nurse advocates for the use of safety measures and reduced exposure to dust. The Occupational Safety and Health Administration (OSHA) issues regulations regarding dust control and ventilation that must be followed in the workplace. The nurse must be aware of these regulations to advocate for workers. Environmental checks must be initiated as required by OSHA. In addition, ongoing educational programs should be provided for workers so that they can be accountable for their own health. Refraining from smoking and receiving a yearly influenza vaccination contribute to good pulmonary health.

Chronic Obstructive Pulmonary Diseases

Chronic obstructive pulmonary disease (COPD) refers to a group of respiratory disorders characterized by chronic and recurrent obstruction of expiratory airflow in the pulmonary airways (Shapiro, Reilly, & Rennard, 2010). Several clinical pathologies fall within the definition of COPD; chronic bronchitis and emphysema are the two most prevalent forms. The Global Initiative for Chronic Obstructive Lung Disease (GOLD) consensus definition for COPD involves progressive and not fully reversible airflow limitation as well as an association with an abnormal inflammatory response of the lungs to noxious irritants. Chronic bronchitis is defined in clinical terms, and emphysema is defined in terms of anatomic pathology. Chronic bronchitis and emphysema are not usually seen as distinct clinical entities. Instead, they coexist in many patients, although one disease may predominate.

Chronic bronchitis is defined as the presence of a chronic productive cough that continues for 3 months of the year for at least 2 consecutive years when other causes of cough have been excluded. Symptoms are usually seen in the winter months. In chronic bronchitis infection, bronchial irritants contribute to increased secretions, edema, bronchospasm, and impaired mucociliary clearance. The mucous secretions are thicker and more tenacious than normal. Because of this, bacteria become embedded in the secretions where they reproduce rapidly.

Emphysema is identified by alteration of the lung architecture and destruction of alveolar walls. In this condition, lungs lose their elasticity. In addition, air spaces distal to the terminal bronchioles are abnormally enlarged or hyperinflated, causing limited airflow out of the lung.

Weblink: Bronchitis

Video: COPD—Etiology and Pathophysiology

Epidemiology and Etiology

Approximately 16 million people in the United States and more than 52 million worldwide have COPD (Juvelekian & Stoller, 2010). It is widely believed that these numbers underrepresent the actual disease prevalence, due to underdiagnosis and undertreatment. It is the fourth-leading cause of death in the United States, and mortality rates continue to rise. The incidence of chronic bronchitis is increased 20-fold in smokers and even more so in workers exposed to air pollution. COPD is particularly prevalent in the older population (McCance & Huether, 2007). The primary cause of COPD is exposure to tobacco smoke. Clinically significant COPD develops in 15% of cigarette smokers. Age of initiation, total pack-years, and current smoking status predict COPD mortality. Secondhand smoke or environmental tobacco smoke increases the risk of respiratory infections, augments asthma symptoms, and causes a measurable reduction in pulmonary function (Fayyaz, 2012). The rate of air pollution in the etiology of COPD is small when compared to cigarette smoking.

Alpha$_1$-antitrypsin (AAT) deficiency is the only known genetic risk factor for developing COPD, and it accounts for fewer than 1% of all cases in the United States (Fayyaz, 2012). Severe AAT deficiency leads to premature emphysema at the average age of 53 years for people who do not smoke and 40 years for people who do smoke.

Pathophysiology

With chronic bronchitis, diffuse airway obstruction occurs because of inflammatory changes in the bronchial walls that cause them to thicken and impinge on the airway diameter (Figure 27–7◆). Initially, chronic

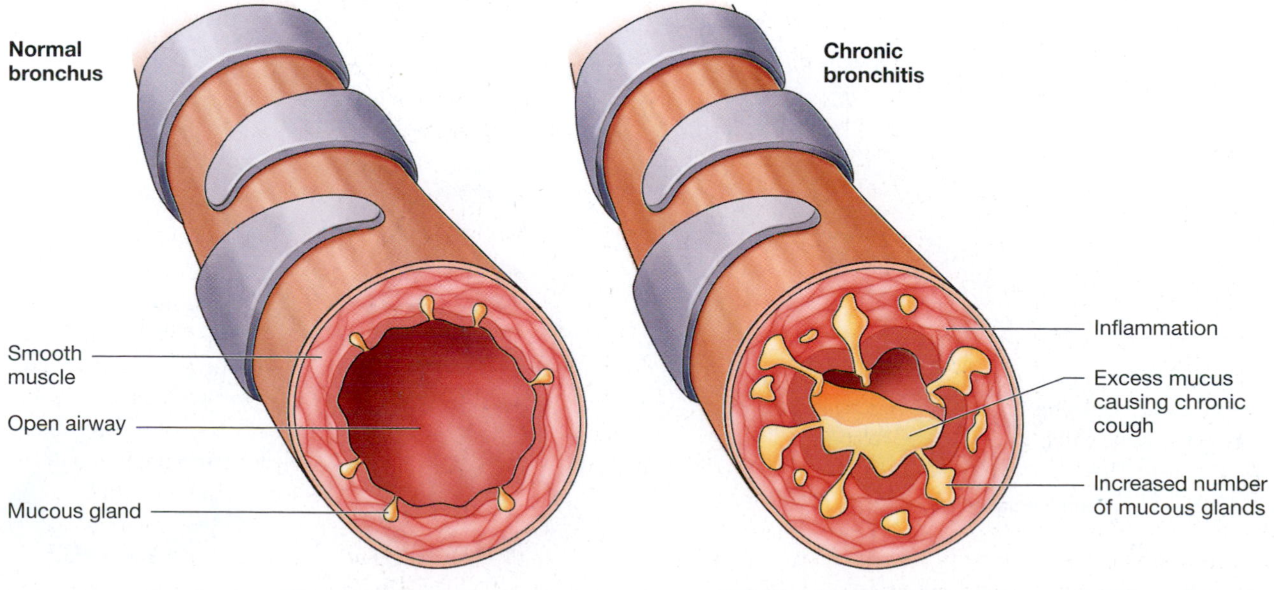

FIGURE 27–7 ◆ Bronchiolar changes as a result of chronic bronchitis.

bronchitis affects only the larger bronchi, but eventually it progresses to all airways. Obstructed airways are likely to close on expiration, causing air trapping in the distal portions of the lung. This leads to hypoventilation, increased arterial carbon dioxide levels, ventilation/perfusion abnormalities, and hypoxemia (McCance & Huether, 2007).

Chronic bronchitis is characterized by an increase in mucus production with inspired irritants and by an increase in the size and number of mucous glands and goblet cells in the airway epithelium (Figure 27–7). The mucus produced is thicker and more tenacious than normal. Because of this stickiness, bacteria become embedded in the airway secretions and reproduce there. Ciliary function is impaired, further reducing mucus clearance. The bronchial walls become inflamed and thickened from edema and the accumulation of inflammatory cells (McCance & Huether, 2007). Airway enlargement and loss of elastic recoil in the alveoli cause air trapping and limited airflow out of the lung.

In emphysema, there is enlargement of the distal airways (bronchioles and alveoli) caused by destruction of the walls of these airways (Figure 27–8 ◆). There are two types of emphysema: centrilobular and panacinar. Except in advanced disease, centrilobular emphysema affects primarily the bronchioles. It is mostly a disease of smokers. Panacinar emphysema involves both the alveoli and the bronchioles. One form of this is AAT protein deficiency, which leads to an imbalance of the neutrophil inflammatory response in the lungs as a response to smoking or other irritants. Without AAT, the neutrophils will digest lung tissue. In both forms, the result is collapse or narrowing of the small airways including bronchioles and the walls of small alveoli. Air becomes trapped in the alveoli, unable to expire through the restrictive airways causing hyperinflation. Hyperinflation of alveoli causes large air spaces (bullae) and air spaces adjacent to pleura (blebs) to develop.

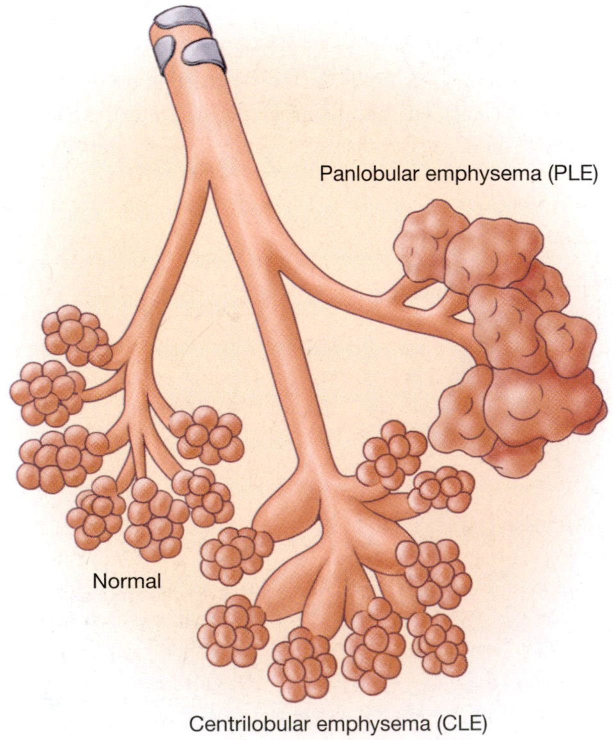

FIGURE 27–8 ◆ Changes in alveolar structure caused by various types of emphysema.

Clinical Manifestations

Patients with early stage COPD may present with only minor symptoms, but lead a very sedentary lifestyle. The health care provider may observe prolonged, forced expiration and note expiratory wheezes. As the disease progresses and airway obstruction increases, evidence of hyperinflation, basilar crackles, wheezing, and decreased breath sounds may occur. The diaphragm becomes depressed as hyperinflation increases and the anteroposterior diameter of the chest increases, often referred to as barrel chest (Figure 27–9 ◆). End-stage disease is indicated by use of accessory muscles, forced expiration through pursed lip breathing (Figure 27–10 ◆), and adopting a position of leaning forward with arms outstretched to help relieve shortness of breath (Figure 27–11 ◆). The patient may show cyanosis, tremors related to elevated carbon dioxide levels, and neck vein distention due to increased intrathoracic pressure and right heart failure.

Laboratory and Diagnostic Procedures

Laboratory assays are done initially to identify abnormalities of ventilation, oxygenation, and acid–base status. General laboratory tests are

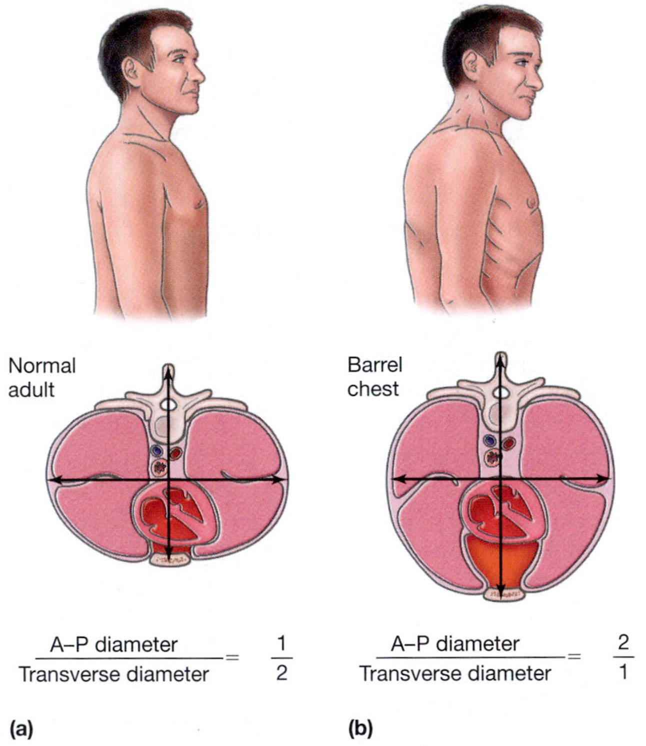

FIGURE 27–9 ◆ Barrel chest.

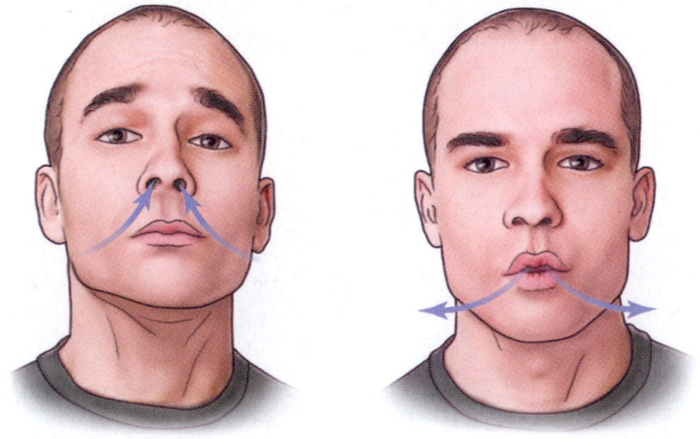

FIGURE 27–10 ◆ Pursed lip breathing.

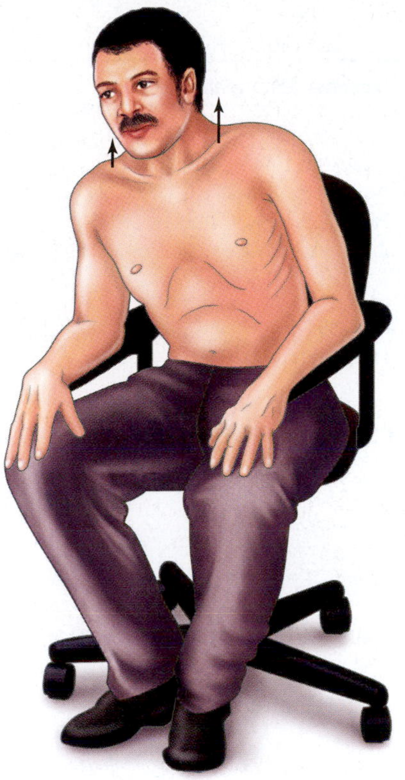

FIGURE 27–11 ◆ Typical posture of patient with COPD.

conducted to determine hematocrit levels, and tests to determine AAT levels are done in all patients younger than 40 years in whom COPD is suspected or those with a family history of emphysema at an early age. Pulmonary function tests are also indicated to determine restrictive or obstructive pulmonary abnormalities and degree of respiratory compromise. See the Diagnostic Tests for COPD box.

Medical Management

The goals of medical management of COPD include prevention of disease progression, symptom relief, improved exercise tolerance, improved health status, treatment and prevention of disease exacerbation, reduction of complications, and reduction in the risk of mortality (Shapiro, Reilly, & Rennard, 2010). Patient education and her active participation and involvement in the disease's medical management is paramount.

Smoking cessation, the most important therapeutic intervention, is the only treatment for COPD known to stop the progression of the disease. Smoking cessation in the early development of the disease can stop the progressive loss of lung function that characterizes COPD (Shapiro, Reilly, & Rennard, 2010). A smoking cessation plan involving behavioral and pharmacologic support is an essential part of a comprehensive management plan.

The pharmacologic therapy for COPD is directed at improvement of symptoms and prevention of exacerbations. The efficacy of the treatment should be weighed against the risks and side effects. Therapies are generally aimed at reducing both inflammation and smooth muscle tone. Inhaled bronchodilators relax smooth muscle and are useful in the symptomatic relief of COPD by decreasing dyspnea and increasing exercise tolerance. It is not acute bronchospasm, as in asthma, that causes dyspnea in COPD patients, but rather chronic obstruction combined with increased demands. Long-acting bronchodilators should therefore be used to help prevent symptoms rather than as a "rescue" medication (Shapiro, Reilly, & Rennard, 2010). The bronchodilators that are most commonly used in treating COPD are β_2 agonists, anticholinergics, a combination of the two, and methylxanthines. (Refer to the Pharmacology feature on page 744.)

The anti-inflammatory effects of inhaled corticosteroids (ICS) have shown airflow improvement and symptom relief in some patients when combined with bronchodilators. There is also evidence that ICS reduce the frequency and severity of COPD exacerbations (Shapiro, Reilly, & Rennard, 2010). It is reasonable to try using ICS on patients who have multiple exacerbations or who continue to have significant symptoms on bronchodilator therapy. The benefit may not be seen for several months. The practice of routinely prescribing oral and systemic corticosteroids is no longer recommended owing to significant side effects, and their use should be limited to the treatment of acute exacerbation.

Long-term oxygen therapy has been shown to prolong life in patients who are hypoxemic on room air ($PaO_2 < 55$ mmHg or saturation $<88\%$), and that 24 hours on oxygen is better than only 12 hours. Other benefits include reduced secondary polycythemia, improved exercise tolerance, and reduction in cor pulmonale (right-sided heart failure, discussed later in the chapter) (Hanania & Sharafkhaneh, 2010). **Polycythemia vera** is a condition that occurs when the hematocrit becomes elevated beyond the normal range as a compensatory mechanism of hypoxemia and the development of cor pulmonale. Cor pulmonale is an enlarged and weakened right ventricle that causes right-sided heart failure and is known to increase mortality in COPD. Oxygen therapy does not produce oxygen toxicity, and patients who have PaO_2 of < 55 mmHg while at rest should have oxygen prescribed. Oxygen therapy is also indicated for patients with a PaO_2 between 56 and 59 mmHg with hematocrit $> 55\%$ or evidence of right heart failure (Shapiro, Reilly, & Rennard, 2010). Oxygen may be considered to improve activity tolerance for patients who desaturate during exercise.

Although accumulation of mucus contributes to COPD symptoms, no mucolytics (agents that dissolve thick mucus) have been shown to demonstrate any clinical efficacy. Antibiotics are often required for acute exacerbations. About half of acute exacerbations of chronic bronchitis are related to bacterial infections, most commonly *H. influenzae, S. pneumoniae,* and *M. catarrhalis* (Shapiro, Reilly, & Rennard, 2010). Acute exacerbations must be distinguished from acute heart failure, pneumonia, pulmonary embolus, and pneumothorax. A chest x-ray and electrocardiogram are useful in the differentiation. Glucocorticoids and bronchodilators should be used aggressively in COPD exacerbation.

Safety Alert *Occasionally, large increases in carbon dioxide can lead to deterioration of mental status, causing the patient to become unresponsive. In such cases, decreasing oxygen delivery is the wrong action. The CO_2 narcosis inhibits respiratory drive to the point at which decreasing oxygen delivery leads to worsening of hypoxia. The correct action for the nurse is to notify the health care team and prepare for immediate intubation, oxygenation, and ventilation.*

Lung Transplantation

Lung transplantation has evolved as a viable alternative for patients with advanced end-stage pulmonary disease. The use of lung transplantation increased steadily from the early 1980s through the mid-1990s and has since leveled off. The biggest limitation to transplantation is a shortage of donors. There are four types of lung-associated transplantation: single-lung, bilateral lung, heart–lung, and living donor lobar transplantation. The most common indications for transplantation include COPD, idiopathic pulmonary fibrosis, α1-antitrypsin deficiency, cystic fibrosis, emphysema, and primary pulmonary hypertension. Selection of candidates for transplantation is guided by the prospective recipient's response to medical therapy, overall state of health, age, and nutritional status.

DIAGNOSTIC TESTS for COPD

Test with Description, Rationale, and Normal Values	Expected Abnormality
Chest X-Ray	
Overinflation results from air trapping and a flattened diaphragm are common clinical findings in chronic lung disease. Infiltrates are a common complication with infection and pneumonia.	Chest x-ray films of patients with COPD usually show marked overinflation, a flattened diaphragm (Figure 27–12◆), and decreased lung markings. Other abnormalities include infiltrates and pneumothorax.
Sputum Gram Stain and Culture	
Provides information about whether acute COPD exacerbation is caused by an infection. *Colonization with Haemophilus pneumonia, Streptococcus pneumoniae, and others is common.*	Identifies if there is a specific pathogen that is causing a respiratory infection.
Serum Theophylline Level	
Therapeutic range: 5 to 20 mcg/L *Theophylline is a weak bronchodilator with a narrow therapeutic window. It may be used in COPD patients for bronchodilation and to assist with increasing contractility of fatigued diaphragms. Dosing regimens should be individualized and serum levels checked regularly.*	Elevated levels or subtherapeutic levels may occur.
FEV_1 (Volume of Air that the Patient can Forcibly Exhale in 1 Second) to FVC (Forced Vital Capacity)	
COPD is classified from mild to severe and is diagnosed by pulmonary function tests or spirometry. This is used to evaluate airflow obstruction, which is determined by the FEV_1. With obstruction, the patient has difficulty exhaling or cannot forcibly exhale from the lungs, reducing the FEV_1.	Obstructive lung disease is defined as an FEV_1/FVC ratio of less than 70%.
WBC	
4,500–10,000 μL *Pulmonary infection commonly occurs related to copious mucus secretions and/or impaired airway clearance.*	WBC count is likely to be elevated with infection.
ABG	
pH 7.35–7.45; $PaCO_2$ 7.35–7.45; PaO_2 75–100; HCO_3 24–28 *Patients with arterial oxygenation of < 55 mmHg at rest will benefit from home oxygen therapy. A rising arterial carbon dioxide level and academia less than 7.30 is a sign of respiratory failure.*	Shows academia, hypoxemia or hypercarbia, and acid–base abnormalities.
Electrocardiogram	
Useful in differentiating acute COPD exacerbation from cardiac failure.	Should not indicate any cardiac ischemia or injury.

Source: Adapted from Kee, J. L. (2010). *Laboratory and diagnostic tests* (8th ed.). Upper Saddle River, NJ: Prentice Hall.

The primary postoperative concerns in transplantation include immunosuppression, infection, and rejection. Transplant patients are placed on a regimen of immunosuppressive agents after surgery. Infections are the leading causes of death in the postoperative period. Patients are at high risk of bacterial, viral, fungal, and protozoal infections (Reilly & Mentzer, 2010). Pneumonia is diagnosed in approximately 30% of patients in the first few weeks postoperatively. The risk of acute rejection is greatest in the first few months after transplantation. Symptoms of rejection include fever, chills, shortness of breath, elevated white blood count, desaturation with exertion, and declining pulmonary function tests per spirometry. These symptoms are similar to those of pneumonia, and bronchoscopy or biopsy is used for definitive diagnosis. High-dose corticosteroids are the first-line treatment for rejection. The body's response to organ transplant is discussed in detail in Chapter 53, and cardiac transplantation is discussed in Chapter 34.

Nursing Management

Nursing care goals for patients with COPD involve assessment of the patient for dyspnea, muscle fatigue, increased work of breathing, and worsening symptoms.

Nurses play a key role in teaching patients about recognizing and managing their symptoms. Education needs should be part of the initial assessment and should be reassessed regularly. Nurses will assist patients and families to manage their rest and activities, teach proper methods of using inhalants, educate patients and families about signs of worsening symptoms, and demonstrate good coughing techniques to clear mucus.

The nurse will instruct patients in how to perform pursed-lip breathing (Figure 27–10) and breathing while bending forward (Figure 27–11). Breathing training is geared toward selected patients with weak inspiratory muscle strength. Breathing retraining, use of postural drainage techniques, energy conservation, and physical reconditioning are the foci of education (Figure 27–12◆).

The Nursing Process: Patient Care Plan for Chronic Obstructive Pulmonary Disease depicts specific steps of the nursing process used in caring for the patient with COPD.

Collaborative Management

Any comprehensive management plan for individuals with COPD will involve collaborative efforts between nurses, respiratory therapists, physical therapists, social workers, pharmacists, and other

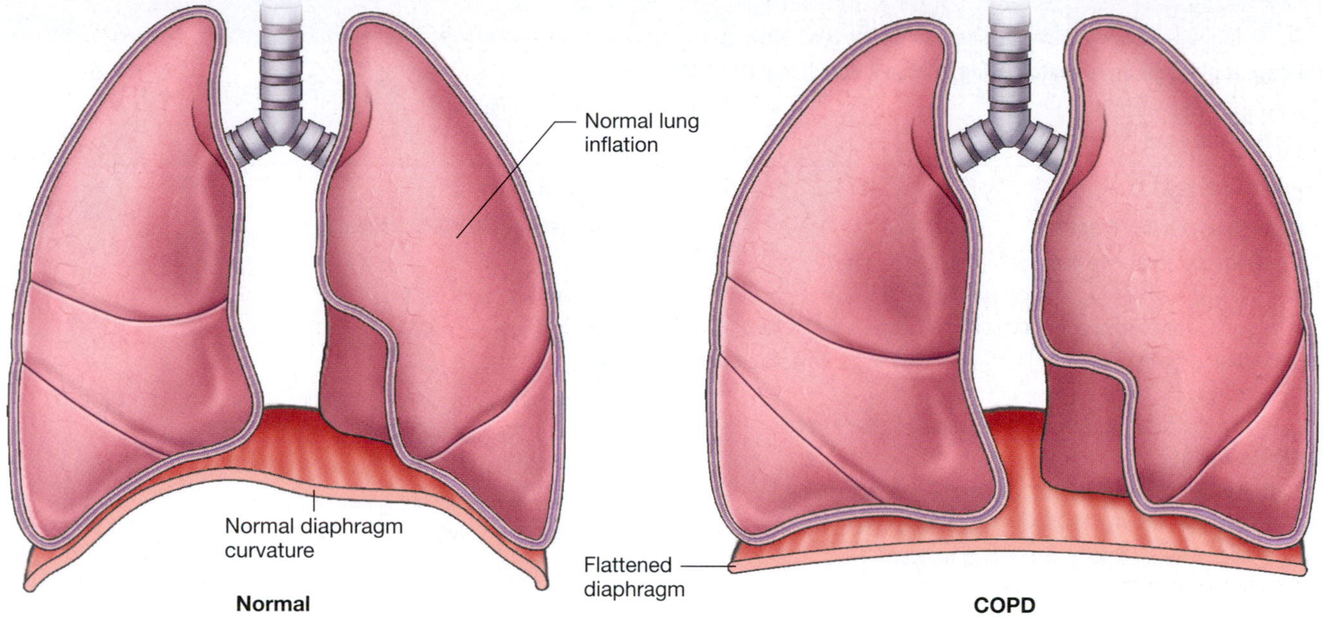

FIGURE 27–12 ◆ Overinflation and flattened diaphragm in COPD.

health care providers (see Evidence-Based Practice box). In order to meet desired patient outcomes, it is essential that this interdisciplinary team communicate openly with one another in developing and evaluating care of the patient and family (IOM [Institute of Medicine], 2010). Pulmonary rehabilitation has become an essential component in returning patients to the highest functional capacity possible and is on an equal plane with pharmacologic therapy. The benefits of rehabilitation include improved quality of life, decreased hospital days, improved independence, and better exercise tolerance (Saey, Bernard, & Gagnon, 2009).

Care of patients with COPD should be individualized and may include smoking-cessation counseling, healthy lifestyle education, exercise training, pharmacology optimization, exacerbation prevention strategy, education on early recognition of exacerbation, vaccinations, and discussion on advanced directives (Celli & ZuWallack, 2010). This approach focuses on an individualized care plan and comprehensive multidisciplinary assessment that stresses self-management and communication between the family, patient, and caregivers.

Health Promotion

Smoking cessation is the single most important factor in preventing COPD. The nurse refers the patient to a smoking-cessation program or assists in a personal plan. If a patient with COPD quits smoking, she is

EVIDENCE-BASED PRACTICE Multidisciplinary Health Care for Patients with COPD

Clinical Problem

Pulmonary rehabilitation is one of the recommended treatments for COPD patients and has demonstrated effectiveness in relieving dyspnea and fatigue, improving mental status, and augmenting patients' control over their disease. Unfortunately, pulmonary rehabilitation is not widely available because of cost and program capacity, so only a small proportion of patients with severe disease will benefit from this service.

Research Findings

Researchers asked the question of whether an integrated, multidisciplinary health care team available through primary care could have a similar impact on the health of COPD patients. They studied 106 COPD patients, 59 in the study group and 47 patients in the control group, over a 24-month period. The team members involved in patient management included a supervising primary health care provider, physiotherapists, a respiratory nurse, a physician assistant, a dietitian, a pharmacist, and a logistics manager. Some of the elements covered using a standardized written treatment protocol included personalized physical activity training, optimal medication prescribing and adherence monitoring, rapid action plans for exacerbations, and continuous self-management education. A validated health status assessment questionnaire and an international recommended 6-minute walking test were used to identify health status and functional capacity both at baseline and during the study period. At the end of the 24-month period, a considerable proportion of the patients in the study showed significant and clinically relevant improvements in health status and exercise tolerance. These results were similar to those found in the INTERCOM (Interdisciplinary Community-Based COPD Management Program) randomized controlled trial of COPD patients with moderate disease and exercise intolerance. The interventional group received exercise training, nutritional therapy, education, and smoking cessation counseling in a community-based multidisciplinary setting. Results proved favorable for exercise capacity, breathlessness, and quality of life for the study group versus the control group.

Implications for Nursing Practice

This study demonstrates how a planned, integrated approach to the care of COPD patients can improve health status over an extended period. In communities where pulmonary rehabilitation programs are not available or are limited, incorporating multidisciplinary teams in patient management may be a valuable alternative. Utilizing the knowledge and skill of a multidisciplinary team can have a favorable long-term impact on the health and quality of life in chronically ill patients. This also brings up the question as to whether this approach can be extended to additional chronic pulmonary diseases and is an area worthy of additional research.

Critical Thinking Questions with answers can be found in the Osborn Student Resources at nursing.pearsonhighered.com.

Source: Kruis, L. K., Adrichem, J., Erkelens, M. R., Scheepers, H., Veen, H., Muris, J. W., & Chavannes, N. H. (2010). Sustained effects of integrated COPD management on health status and exercise capacity in primary care patients. *International Journal of Chronic Obstructive Pulmonary Disease, 5*: 407–413 doi: 10.2147/COPD.S9654.

NURSING PROCESS: Patient Care Plan for Chronic Obstructive Pulmonary Disease

Assessment of Respiratory Status Using Gordon's Functional Health Patterns:

- Activity Exercise Pattern
- Cognitive Perceptual Pattern
- Self-Perception Self-Concept Pattern

Subjective Data

Assessment of the COPD Patient

Do you experience cough, shortness of breath, or wheezing?

Describe the type of cough you experience. Is it dry, hacking, productive, and/or triggered by smoking or other environmental, social, or emotional situations?

Is sputum clear or colored and how much would you say is expectorated per day?

Do you have any difficulty with sleeping and what position is most comfortable for you?

What are your current weight and eating habits? Has there been a change during the last month or year?

Do you or have you ever smoked any type of tobacco? If so, describe your smoking history.

Describe your medications and breathing treatments.

Do you use supplemental oxygen? If so, please describe.

Describe your activity tolerance. Has this changed during the last month or year?

If you experience wheezing or chest tightness, what situations seem to trigger this?

Assessment of Anxiety and Coping With Disease

How do you think you are coping with episodes of dyspnea or chest tightness?

What are triggers for increasing anxiety?

Assessment of Patient/Family Knowledge

Describe your disease history and the progression of symptoms. For example, has the shortness of breath worsened over time?

Objective Data

Assessment of the COPD Patient

Vital signs

Oxygen saturation with pulse oximetry

Spirometry results (FEV_1/FVC)

ABG results

Assessment of lung sounds and breathing pattern including use of accessory muscles

Presence or absence of clubbing

Presence or absence of barrel chest

Color of face, lips, and nail beds

Presence of cough

Color and amount of sputum production

Exercise tolerance

Oxygen requirements

Hemoglobin and hematocrit

Sputum culture and sensitivity results

Level of consciousness

Orientation

Note whether the patient responds with lucid answers and states them in complete sentences. Breathlessness may be so severe that the patient can only respond with one- or two-word answers.

Assessment of Anxiety and Coping With Disease

Facial expressions

Mood

Verbalization of fear regarding illness and its impact on family and the future.

Assessment of Patient/Family Knowledge

Able to verbalize prevention techniques.

Outcomes and Evaluation Parameters / Planning and Interventions with *Rationales*

1. NURSING DIAGNOSIS: Ineffective Airway Clearance *related to inadequate cough and excessive mucous production* (NANDA-I © 2012)

Outcome: Patient will demonstrate controlled cough.

Evaluation Parameters: After completion of pulmonary toilet, lung sounds are clear or significantly improved upon auscultation.

Oxygen saturation after pulmonary toilet is within normal range.

Patient expectorates secretions effectively upon assessment by the nurse.

Assess the patient's ability to mobilize secretions. If unable to do so, suction as necessary to remove secretions *to clear the airway.*

Teach chest physiotherapy or refer the patient to a respiratory therapist.

Note characteristics of sputum. *Secretions can obstruct airways and cause respiratory complications.*

Assess for presence of adventitious lung sounds every 4 to 8 hours. *Auscultation of lung sounds provides information on respiratory status.*

Observe the patient for drug effectiveness. *Airway dilation is the result of medications.*

Provide hydration of at least 2 L/day if not medically contraindicated.

Administer vaporization therapy and perform physical therapy as indicated. *Hydration and vaporization help to liquefy secretions.*

2. NURSING DIAGNOSIS: Anxiety *related to dyspneic episodes or asthmatic attacks* (NANDA-I © 2012)

Outcome: Patient is able to identify activities that tend to decrease anxious behaviors.

Evaluation Parameters: Demonstrates the ability to initiate purse-lipped breathing at the onset of dyspnea related to anxiety.

Ask the patient to identify in writing various factors that elicit an anxious response. *Clarifying thoughts gives the patient control and may decrease anxiety.*

NURSING PROCESS: Patient Care Plan for Chronic Obstructive Pulmonary Disease, *continued*

Verbalizes anxious feelings and thoughts. Anxiety is relieved by consistently demonstrating aggression and anxiety control, coping, impulse control, self-mutilation restraint, and substantially effective social interaction skills. Verbalizes absence of sensory perceptual disorders. Verbalizes absence of physical manifestations of anxiety. Behavioral manifestations of anxiety absent.	Help the patient formulate a plan for coping with dyspneic and/or wheezing episodes. *A plan allows the patient to prepare.* Encourage verbalization of feelings *to decrease anxiety.* Teach patient interventions for coping such as relaxation techniques and biofeedback. *These types of interventions decrease stress and anxiety.*
3. NURSING DIAGNOSIS: Deficient Knowledge *related to COPD* (NANDA-I © 2012)	
Outcome: Patient and significant others describe breathing exercises and energy conservation techniques prior to discharge. ***Evaluation Parameters:*** Patient demonstrates breathing exercises and energy conservation techniques prior to discharge. Patient and family members describe the treatment regime with rationale prior to discharge. Patient discuses emotional reactions to lifestyle changes prior to discharge. Prior to discharge, the patient and caregiver verbalize issues that constitute an emergency and what actions they should take. Patient and caregiver describe the appropriate contacts to make in the case of an emergency.	Instruct the patient on prevention of infection. Discuss stress with the patient: avoidance of crowded rooms or contact with known cases of colds or flu, avoidance of irritants such as tobacco smoke, importance of receiving pneumococcal and influenza vaccines, and importance of recognizing changes in sputum color and density. *These measures prevent complications of COPD.* The nurse, along with the respiratory therapist, physical therapist, and occupational therapist, teaches breathing techniques including breathing exercises and energy conservation strategies. Treadmills, weights, and bicycles may be used to improve muscle strength and endurance. Patients can incorporate use of portable oxygen systems into this exercise routine as needed. Inspiratory muscle training may be prescribed to strengthen muscles used in breathing. This requires that the patient breathe against resistance for 10 to 15 minutes a day, *thus conditioning muscles and increasing activity tolerance and ventilatory competence. Breathing exercises and physical reconditioning decrease the work of breathing and improve physical stamina.* Review the patient's treatment regime including medications, oxygen, breathing exercises, postural drainage, physical conditioning, and nutritional support. Attention to psychosocial issues is very important *since the patient with end-stage COPD is often discouraged because of immobility, and can easily become angry, depressed, and demanding. Making the necessary lifestyle changes requires that patients talk about the emotions associated with these changes.* Enlist family support and at the same time support caregivers who face these difficult issues daily. Attain resources for patient education from the American Lung Association, the American Association of Cardiovascular and Pulmonary Rehabilitation, the American Thoracic Society, and the American Association for Respiratory Therapy. The nurse plays a major role in educating the patient regarding the disease process and the medical regimen. *Enhancing the knowledge base of the patient and family is likely to facilitate health maintenance and prevention of complications.* Review what issues constitute an emergency and describe what actions patients should take in a simulated situation offered by the nurse. The health care team arranges for oxygen, if ordered, to be available in the home setting. Plans for transfer to home should be made in consideration of oxygen needs. Instructions should be given in writing. Arrangements are made with the home oxygen distributor to provide specific education regarding home oxygen and respiratory equipment. *Discharge is a time of transition and anxiety. Repetition of information and visual cues such as written information reinforce what has been taught.* Give contact numbers for nursing and other care providers to the patient and caregiver. The patient and caregiver are instructed to place these near the phone for easy access in case of an emergency.

Source: Adapted from Wilkinson, J. M., & Ahearn, N. R. (2009). *Prentice Hall nursing diagnosis handbook* (9th ed.). Upper Saddle River, NJ: Prentice Hall.

Weblink: Cystic Fibrosis Foundation

likely to prevent future complications. The nurse educates the patient about the hazards of smoking and provides counseling opportunities as needed. In addition, it is important to teach the patient some of the subtle changes that may occur, such as fatigue, dyspnea, and change in sputum color, consistency, or amount, which may indicate a respiratory infection.

To prevent infection, the nurse cautions patients to avoid extremes of temperature, exposure to crowds, poor air quality, or high pollen counts. Annual influenza vaccination can prevent influenza and decrease acute exacerbations by as much as 60% (Hanania & Sharafkhaneh, 2010). Pneumococcal vaccination should also be recommended to patients with more severe lung disease as well as older patients.

Genetic Disorders

Cystic Fibrosis

Cystic fibrosis (CF) is an autosomal recessive hereditary disease of the exocrine glands that primarily affects the respiratory and GI systems. In contrast to endocrine glands, which secrete their products into the bloodstream, exocrine glands secrete their products onto body surfaces either internally, such as the lungs, or externally, such as the skin. Some examples are mucus, sweat, tears, and digestive juices. CF leads to chronic airway obstruction, respiratory infections, exocrine pancreatic insufficiency, and gastrointestinal tract dysfunction, with consequential repercussions on nutrition, growth, and maturation (Boucher, Knowles, & Yankaskas, 2010). CF is the most common fatal recessive genetic disease among the Caucasian population.

Epidemiology and Etiology

Approximately 30,000 persons in the United States and 70,000 worldwide are afflicted with cystic fibrosis. The incidence in Whites is 1:2,500; in Blacks, 1:17,000. Cystic fibrosis is relatively rare in American Indians and Asian populations (Boucher, Knowles, & Yankaskas, 2010). It is estimated that 2% to 5% of the Caucasian population are carriers of the gene mutation but are completely asymptomatic. In 1970, fewer than 10% of those with CF survived into adulthood; however, with improvements in treatment, more than 45% of these patients are now over 18 years old, and the median age of survival is the mid-30s (Cystic Fibrosis Foundation, n.d.). More than 70% are diagnosed before 2 years of age.

Cystic fibrosis is caused by a mutation in a single recessive gene, the cystic fibrosis transmembrane conductive regulator (CFTR). This gene controls the production of a protein that regulates how salt and water are carried across the membranes that separate cells and affects nearly all exocrine glands. Disease manifestation requires that a person receive a CFTR defective gene from each parent.

Pathophysiology

The alteration in salt and water transport along the cell linings results in the accumulation of excessively thick and sticky mucus in the airways. The mucus clogs the airways and provides an environment that supports bacterial growth. White blood cells respond to the localized infection and release their sticky genetic material into the mucus, further aggravating the obstruction, inflammation, and infection. Cystic fibrosis patients frequently have ongoing and persistent infections that over time damage the lungs, leading to respiratory failure and eventually causing death. Thick secretions also clog pancreatic ducts, reducing digestive enzymes and causing malnutrition and slow growth and development. Abnormalities are also seen in the gastrointestinal tract, bile ducts, reproductive organs, and sweat ducts. The degree and presentation of CF vary between individuals partially owing to genetic mutations and environmental factors.

Clinical Manifestations

Clinical manifestations of CF usually occur in infancy, although milder forms of the disease may not be diagnosed until adulthood. Respiratory manifestations often start with intermittent cough and respiratory tract infections. The cough progresses in frequency, worsens at night, and becomes productive. Sputum is tenacious, purulent, and often green as bacterial infections seed. Wheezing may occur, but lung sounds are often normal. Chest radiography demonstrates lung hyperinflation. In the early stages of the disease, *Staphylococcus aureus* and *Haemophilus influenzae* are the predominant infections, followed by *Pseudomonas aeruginosa* (Strausbaugh & Davis, 2007). *P. aeruginosa* becomes the most common infection, affecting 80% of CF patients, and its acquisition is associated with deterioration of the disease, particularly the mucoid versions of the bacteria. Fungal infections are also common in CF patients, including *Candida,* aspergillus, and nontuberculous mycobacterium. Infections are very difficult, sometimes impossible, to eliminate. Hemoptysis is common as disease progresses and is associated with exacerbations. Exacerbations are characterized by tachypnea, increased shortness of breath, higher intensity cough, decreased activity threshold, loss of appetite, and weight loss. Additional physical signs of respiratory and other system abnormalities are shown in Chart 27–8.

Laboratory and Diagnostic Procedures

The diagnosis of CF is based on both clinical and laboratory assessment. The diagnostic standard for confirming suspected CF is the sweat test, which measures the amount of chloride in a person's perspiration. Patients who meet the clinical criteria and have a sweat chloride of

CHART 27–8 Clinical Manifestations of Cystic Fibrosis

Pulmonary Signs and Symptoms in Young Adults
- Persistent cough or wheeze
- *Pseudomonas aeruginosa* and/or *Staphylococcus aureus* in the sputum
- Hyperinflated lungs on chest x-ray
- Barrel chest and digital clubbing
- Chronic sinusitis
- Nasal polyps
- Recurrent episodes of pneumonia
- Chronic bronchitis

Gastrointestinal Manifestations
- Frequent loose and oily stools
- Pancreatic abnormalities
- Cramps and abdominal pain
- Rectal prolapse
- Malnutrition and weight loss

Endocrine Manifestations
- Glucose intolerance
- Polydipsia, polyuria, polyphasia

Reproductive
- Infertility in males
- High risk of complications with pregnancy
- Delayed sexual development

> 60 mEq/L are diagnosed with CF. Because of possible false-positive and false-negative results, the test is confirmed after two positive results. Clinical criteria used for confirmation include characteristic chronic pulmonary disease and GI abnormalities: chronic cough with sputum production, persistent respiratory infections with the characteristic pathogens, sinus disease/nasal polyps, chronic chest x-ray abnormalities, pancreatic insufficiency/recurrent pancreatitis, and meconium ileus (meconium material is found in the intestine of a newborn and is a common cause of intestinal obstruction in newborns). The diagnosis is often then confirmed by genetic verification of the CFTR mutation gene (Boucher, Knowles, & Yankaskas, 2010). Newborn screening now occurs in 48 of the U.S. states.

Other diagnostic studies used in diagnosing CF are chest x-ray, pulmonary function studies, fecal analysis for fat, pancreatic enzyme studies, liver function studies, and semen analysis to determine infertility in males (see Diagnostic Tests for Cystic Fibrosis box).

Medical Management

The goals of CF management are to control and prevent infections, clear mucus, improve nutrition, and provide psychosocial support. Early diagnosis and treatment are important in delaying the onset and severity of chronic illness in children with CF.

Prophylaxis against infections includes maintaining immunizations and obtaining an annual influenza vaccination. A neuraminidase inhibitor can be given for patients exposed to influenza (Rosenstein, 2008). Antibiotics should be initiated early when symptoms arise and ideally be based on pathogen identification. Antibiotic dosage is higher in CF patients than in non-CF patients due to clearance and distribution differences (Boucher, Knowles, & Yankaskas, 2010). Parenteral antibiotics are indicated for patients with severe exacerbation, particularly with *P. aeruginosa* infections.

Chest physical therapy is indicated as soon as pulmonary involvement is identified to facilitate clearance of retained mucus secretions.

DIAGNOSTIC TESTS for Cystic Fibrosis

Test with Description, Rationale, and Normal Values	Expected Abnormality
Sweat Chloride Test Normal: Adult < 60 mmol/L, Child: < 50 mmol/L 30 to 59 mmol/L = possible CF; > 60 mmol/L diagnosis of CF *The primary test of diagnosis of CF.* *Mucous plugging of the sweat duct causes malabsorption of sodium chloride.*	Chloride concentration in excess of 60 mEq/L.
Chest X-Ray *Used to identify extent of disease. Impaction of mucus, injury caused by persistent lung infections causes air-trapping in the alveoli.*	Early disease: hyperinflation. Bronchiectasis, focal atelectasis, peribronchial cuffing, pulmonary hypertension.
Fecal Fat *Pancreatic enzymes such as amylase, lipase, and trypsinogen do not reach the intestine to digest ingested nutrients. There is malabsorption of fat, protein, and fat-soluble vitamins. This results in steatorrhea (fatty stool).*	Fecal fat concentration is elevated.
Pancreatic Enzymes *Mucous plugging of the pancreatic duct results in fibrosis of the acinar glands of the pancreas. The exocrine function of the pancreas is altered and may be lost completely.*	Decreased.
Pulmonary Function Studies *Results are consistent with obstructive airway disease as disease progresses. Tidal volume, vital capacity, and other functions are below normal related to the disease process.*	Decreased forced expiratory flow. Decreased FVC and FEV_1.
Serum Glucose 70–110 mg/dL *Diabetes mellitus may occur because the islets of Langerhans become fibrotic. CF-related diabetes affects 15% of patients with CF.*	Elevated in some patients with CF.
Semen Analysis *Confirms infertility in males. CF causes maldevelopment of the vas deferens.*	Sperm count abnormally low.
DNA Analysis *Used to confirm diagnosis in patients with positive or intermediate sweat test results or in patients with strong clinical evidence despite negative sweat test.*	Two CF-related mutations; if only one mutation, an expanded test should be performed.
Liver Enzymes *Used to identify biliary cirrhosis involvement caused by mucous plugging late in the disease.*	Elevated.

Source: Adapted from Kee, J. L. (2010). *Laboratory and diagnostic tests* (8th ed.). Upper Saddle River, NJ: Prentice Hall.

Common techniques include postural drainage, percussion, vibration, and assisted cough. A variety of breathing and coughing techniques that don't require the aid of another person can be taught to older children and adults. No one method is identified as superior to another (Simon, 2010).

Bronchial plugging, inflammation, airway obstruction, and bronchial wall thickening may all contribute to airflow obstruction. Symptoms will be similar to those of asthma, such as wheezing, chest tightness, and cough (Simon, 2010). There is some evidence to suggest that bronchodilators are effective in patients who have milder disease. A guidelines committee for the Cystic Fibrosis Foundation recommends short-acting beta-agonists for patients before chest physiotherapy, exercise, or inhalation of medications to facilitate clearance of secretions and improve penetration and distribution of drugs within the airway. Anti-inflammatories may also be used. Ibuprofen in children < 13 years has shown an 8-fold slowing in the decline in lung function, but no benefit to older patients was identified (Boucher, Knowles, & Yankaskas, 2010).

Other medications that have been introduced to reduce mucus accumulation include inhaled hypertonic saline, aerosolized enzymes to lyse viscous DNA, and surface-rehydrating agents.

Removal of nasal polyps to relieve obstruction is the most common surgical procedure for patients with CF; although the incidence of recurrence is common, development of polyps tends to decrease over time. Lung lobectomy may be necessary in patients with massive hemoptysis who do not respond to artery embolization. More than 2,300 lung transplants have been performed worldwide in patients with CF. The survival rate is similar to that for lung transplants for other diseases. Although the transplanted lungs remain CF-free, they are subject to secondary infection (Boucher, Knowles, & Yankaskas, 2010). Live lobar transplant has shown similar success.

Careful attention should be paid to the social, emotional, and financial needs of the patient with CF and his family. Education in management of the disease should be ongoing, and counseling resources should be available to the patient and family. Active participation in the therapeutic regimen is essential for the well-being of persons with CF. Other issues for young adults include building self-esteem, self-confidence, and meaningful friendships and relationships. The decision to have children should be considered carefully. The nurse might suggest genetic counseling because men with CF are almost always sterile and women may have difficulty with pregnancy (some are infertile). Any children produced will either be carriers of or have the disease.

Nursing Management

Nursing management for the patient with CF focuses on assisting the patient to maintain adequate airway clearance, reducing risk factors associated with infections, preventing complications, assisting the patient to be able to perform ADLs, and involving the patient and family in planning and implementing the therapeutic regimen.

Assessment

Objective and subjective data should be obtained from the patient with CF and the family. Subjective data include obtaining a past health history of recurrent respiratory and sinus infection and persistent cough with excessive sputum production; use of and compliance with corticosteroids, bronchodilators, and antibiotics; functional health patterns, such as family history or diagnosis of cystic fibrosis in childhood; nutritional and metabolic needs and symptoms; elimination; activity patterns; cognitive perceptions of pain; and reproductive symptoms, such as menstrual irregularities.

Objective data include assessment of general impression, such as mood, anxiety, depression, restlessness, and failure to thrive; cyanosis of skin and nail beds; persistent runny nose, diminished breath sounds, and sputum characteristics; tachycardia; protuberant abdomen, abdominal distention, and foul and fatty stools; the possibility of abnormal ABGs and pulmonary function tests; and an abnormal sweat chloride test, chest x-ray, and fecal fat analysis. Determination of medications being used also is part of the assessment process.

Nursing Diagnoses

Nursing diagnoses related to CF may include the following:

- *Airway Clearance, Ineffective* related to thick and abundant mucus, weakness, and fatigue.
- *Breathing Pattern, Ineffective* related to bronchoconstriction, anxiety, and airway obstruction.
- *Infection, Risk for* related to chronic pulmonary disease.
- *Imbalanced Nutrition* related to dietary intolerances, intestinal gas, and altered pancreatic enzyme production.

NANDA-I © 2012

Planning

Planning goals for the patient with CF focus on the patient having adequate airway clearance, reduced risk factors associated with respiratory infections, the ability to perform ADLs, freedom from complications from CF, and active participation in planning and implementing a restorative regime.

Outcomes and Evaluation Parameters

Outcomes and evaluation parameters in treating CF include the following:

- The patient and family will demonstrate proficiency in providing pulmonary care, reducing pulmonary infection, and developing a plan for pulmonary care that fits the family's needs.
- The patient and family will demonstrate an understanding of a nutritional plan with adequate calories and pancreatic enzymes to support health and a plan of continuous evaluation of the patient's condition.

Interventions and Rationales

The goal of nursing interventions in CF is to assist the patient in gaining and maintaining independence by assuming responsibility for her own care. Active interventions include relief of bronchoconstriction, airway obstruction, and airflow limitation. The nurse is responsible for administering medications as ordered, providing oxygen therapy, and instructing the patient and family on nutrition and exercise. Home care instruction consists of postural drainage techniques, aerosol-nebulization therapy, and breathing retraining. The patient also should be taught controlled coughing techniques, deep breathing exercises, and progressive exercise conditioning.

Psychosocial support regarding the financial and emotional burden of the disease should be provided to the patient and family.

Discharge Priorities

Fatigue and weakness related to an exacerbation of cystic fibrosis may render a young adult who was formerly an active and independent participant in care incapable of performing the treatment regime independently. Therefore, the family should be included in all patient education and discharge planning. This includes instruction regarding the chest physical therapy regime, oral or IV medications, and aerosols and breathing treatments.

Collaborative Management

Comprehensive multidisciplinary CF treatment programs have led to a dramatic increase in the median age of survival for affected patients. Care is managed by a multidisciplinary team including the health care provider, nurse, social workers, respiratory therapist, physical therapist, and dietitian. In order to meet desired patient outcomes, it is essential that this interdisciplinary team communicate openly with one another in developing and evaluating care of the patient and family (IOM [Institute of Medicine], 2010).

The patient and family members work closely with the team to develop a successful regimen. Involvement of the patient is critical. Treatment depends on the severity of both the exacerbation and the underlying lung disease. The aim of interdisciplinary management of CF is to control symptoms, prevent complications, and improve perceptions of well-being.

Because of the pancreatic and gastrointestinal manifestations of cystic fibrosis, malnutrition is a serious complication. Good nutritional status is associated with long-term survival and a slower decline in pulmonary function, so prevention of malnutrition is an important goal (Welsh, 2007). A dietitian can work directly with the patient and family to assess nutritional status and identify caloric and nutritional needs. Approximately 7% of CF patients develop CF-related diabetes (Welsh, 2007) and may benefit from additional nutritional guidance. See Chapter 8 for details on nutritional management.

Health Promotion

Because the adult with CF is extremely vulnerable to infection, the nurse should emphasize to the patient and family that the environment be kept as free from infection as possible. The patient and family are encouraged to wash their hands before and after eating, after using the restroom, when coming home from school or work, or after being around ill persons. Hand washing is the most effective method of reducing infection. The nurse should emphasize the risk of exacerbations caused by smoking or exposure to secondhand smoke. Frequent oral hygiene is encouraged, especially after the chest physical therapy regime. Patients should avoid exposure to persons who are ill, especially those with upper respiratory infections. Patients with CF should be screened for *Mycobacterium tuberculosis* infection with yearly PPD skin tests and treated prophylactically with the same regimen used for non-CF patients. Vaccines and immunizations should be kept up to date.

Pulmonary Embolism

Pulmonary embolism (PE) is the obstruction of the pulmonary artery or one of its branches by material that originated elsewhere in the body (Thompson & Hales, 2010). Although the material can be due to thrombus, air, or fat, the most common cause is thrombotic and is the focus of this section. When a thrombus breaks loose from an attachment and blocks a branch of the pulmonary artery, it can produce widespread pulmonary vasoconstriction, impair ventilation and perfusion, and produce life-threatening hypoxemia and the potential for ischemia and pulmonary infarction.

Epidemiology

Statistics on the incidence of PE vary widely by report, but it is estimated that in the United States approximately 600,000 patients are diagnosed with PE every year, and nearly 100,000 deaths are attributed to PE (Thompson & Hales, 2010). The increase in incidence reported over the last 10 to 15 years is probably attributable to technologic advances that incorporate spiral CT scans into the identification of PE. At least 10% of diagnosed patients with PE die of its complications, and up to 30% of those with untreated PE will die (Thompson & Hales, 2010). More than 90% of PE originates from deep venous thrombosis (DVT) of the lower extremities. Both incidence and mortality are higher in Blacks than Whites, with mortality being about 50% higher. PE is relatively rare in Asians, American Indians, and children. PE is predominantly a disease of older individuals, and the highest incidence of recognized PE occurs in hospitalized patients. The incidence of venous thromboembolic events in older adults is more common among men than women. Among patients younger than 55 years, the incidence of PE is higher in females. Patients who survive an acute PE are at high risk for recurrent PE and the development of pulmonary hypertension or chronic cor pulmonale.

Etiology

The most common risk factors for PE are immobilization, surgery in the past 3 months, pregnancy, stroke, paresis/paralysis, chronic heart disease, history of venous thromboembolism, malignancy, and central venous instrumentation within the past 3 months (Thompson & Hales, 2010). Women have additional risk factors including obesity, heavy cigarette smoking, and hypertension. Additional factors that are associated with the development of DVT, which is most often the source of PE, include hypercoagulation disorders, trauma to the lower extremities, pregnancy/early postpartum, estrogen therapy, thrombophilia (a hereditary or acquired predisposition to develop blood clots), and CHF. Most emboli arise from thrombi in proximal deep veins. They also can originate from the pelvis, particularly in pregnant women and individuals with pelvic fractures.

Pathophysiology

A pulmonary occlusion occurs when a bloodborne substance occludes a branch of the pulmonary artery and obstructs blood flow to the area that the artery feeds. The source of embolism can be a thrombus, air accidentally injected through an IV catheter, fat from bone marrow after a fracture, or amniotic fluid that has entered the mother's bloodstream after rupture of the membranes at birth (Porth & Matfin, 2009). However, the most common origin is venous thromboembolism (VTE) from the lower extremities. After breaking off, the emboli travel through the venous system into the right side of the heart and lodge in one or more of the pulmonary arteries/vessels. The hemodynamic and pulmonary response to PE depends on the size of the occlusion, the number of emboli, the presence of any comorbidities, and the body's ability to dissolve the clot(s). Smaller obstructions may have no physiologic symptoms and resolve spontaneously, but large emboli, or even moderate obstructions in patients with previous cardiopulmonary disease, may produce hypotension. Recruitment and vasodilation of pulmonary vessels will compensate against the high pressures the right ventricle has to pump against due to obstructions. Compensatory mechanisms are lost once obstructions reach 50% to 60% and right arterial pressure rises sharply. Beyond this, right heart pressures rise, systemic hypoxia occurs, and hypotension occurs as blood to the left side of the heart falls and cardiac output decreases. In patients with previous cardiopulmonary disease, the degree of obstruction that produces hypotension is disproportionate, with moderate or mild obstruction generating hemodynamic instability (Morris & Fedullo, 2010).

Effects of PE on the pulmonary system include impaired gas exchange, alterations in ventilation/perfusion, and hypoxemia. Impaired gas exchange occurs when portions of the lung are not perfused and therefore diffusion of gases does not take place. The alveoli continue to be ventilated, but perfusion is reduced, leading to alteration in ventilation-perfusion, which is the primary cause of hypoxemia. Gas exchange abnormality is also related to the localized inflammatory response that leads to bronchoconstriction distal to the obstruction. If obstruction of blood flow persists, surfactant will become depleted, and **atelectasis** (collapsed alveoli) and edema will result. Pulmonary infarction occurs in fewer than 10% of patients with PE; the low rate is probably attributable to the presence of collateral blood flow in the pulmonary system (Morris & Fedullo, 2010).

Clinical Manifestations

The clinical manifestations of PE depend on its size, its location, and the amount of obstruction. Most PEs are small, asymptomatic, and physiologically inconsequential. Although small emboli may be asymptomatic initially, chronic small emboli gradually reduce the pulmonary bed, ultimately resulting in pulmonary hypertension. The Prospective Investigation of Pulmonary Embolism Diagnosis (PIOPED II) noted the signs and symptoms along with the frequency in which they occur out of nearly 800 patients in a multicenter study of patients with PE and with no preexisting cardiopulmonary disease (see Chart 27–9) (Stein et al., 2007).

Laboratory and Diagnostic Procedures

Because many of the signs and symptoms exhibited by patients with PE are also common in patients without PE, additional evaluation is required. Routine laboratory findings are nonspecific. The decision about which diagnostic modality to use should be based on what modalities are available at the institution (Thompson & Hales, 2010). See the Diagnostic Tests for Pulmonary Embolism box for details.

Medical Management

Management of PE depends on clinical severity and therefore will vary between patients. The initial focus of treatment will be to address any hemodynamic or respiratory compromise. Anticoagulation, fibrinolysis, inferior vena cava (IVC) filters, and embolectomy are other considerations in the treatment of PE.

Stabilization

The nurse should administer oxygen to any patient who is hypoxemic, and consider intubation and mechanical ventilation should be considered if the patient is in respiratory failure. Intravenous fluid administration is first-line therapy in patients presenting with hypotension. Since the right ventricle function may be deteriorating, fluid may cause further stress and ischemia. Boluses should be given in 500 to 1000 cc aliquots (Tapson, 2010). If hypotension persists after fluid resuscitation, vasopressor therapy should be initiated.

Anticoagulation

Since the mortality rate for patients with untreated PE can reach 30%, the nurse should initiate anticoagulation quickly, before definitive diagnosis with imaging studies, whenever there is a high clinical probability of PE and no potential bleeding contraindications. Anticoagulation reduces mortality and is the primary therapy for the treatment of PE (Tapson, 2010). Anticoagulants do not lyse or reduce the existing clot, but when therapeutic levels are reached within 24 hours, they reduce the risk of recurrence of clot formation. Recurrence of thromboemboli in patients who are untreated or are at nontherapeutic levels of treatment after 24 hours is approximately 25%. Low-molecular-weight heparin (LMWH) and unfractionated heparin are the drugs of choice for anticoagulation. LMWH is often preferred because it has more predictable dosing, has fewer side effects, doesn't require PTT monitoring, and allows subcutaneous dosing rather than IV infusion. Heparin therapy is usually required for 5 days, during which time the oral anticoagulant warfarin is started. This drug is continued and monitored for 3 to 6 months after discharge. Therapy duration is determined by the size and cause of the clot, risk factors, history of clot formation, and venous patency. See the Pharmacology table in Chapter 35 for a complete description of heparin.

Fibrinolysis

Thrombolytics reduce clot size and improve hemodynamic parameters. They also increase the risk of major hemorrhage, including intracerebral bleeding. Thrombolytics are generally reserved for patients with hemodynamic instability, and are considered in patients with oxygenation compromise, right ventricle dysfunction, or massive PE without instability. Heparin should be discontinued until the thrombolytic infusion is completed. The drugs that are currently available in the United States for the treatment of PE are streptokinase, urokinase, and recombinant tissue-type plasminogen activator (t-PA).

IVC Filters

IVC filters are placed into the inferior vena cava through the jugular or femoral vein. They allow blood to flow through while acting as a screen for large emboli to prevent them from reaching the lungs. Filters are indicated in patients who (1) have contraindications for anticoagulation, (2) have bleeding complications on anticoagulants, (3) have recurrent PE while on adequate anticoagulation, and (4) have massive PE in which any additional clot could be potentially fatal. IVC filters can be temporarily placed and removed within 2 weeks, and some newer models can be removed as late as 90 days after placement. Complications are uncommon and are associated with insertion problems and filter migration.

Embolectomy

Surgical or catheter embolectomy (clot removal) can be performed in hypotensive patients who are refractory to fluid and vasopressor therapy and have absolute contraindications to fibrinolytic or anticoagulant therapy. Catheter embolectomy is a technique that involves guiding a specialized catheter into the pulmonary artery to break up the clot. More research is needed in this field to compare outcomes of embolectomy with those of other modalities. Surgical embolectomy requires extracorporeal cardiopulmonary bypass and an experienced thoracic surgeon.

CHART 27–9 Signs and Symptoms of Pulmonary Embolism

Symptoms		Signs	
Dyspnea:	73%	Tachypnea:	54%
Pleuritic pain:	44%	Tachycardia:	24%
Leg pain:	44%	Rales:	18%
Leg swelling:	41%	Decreased breath sounds:	17%
Cough:	34%	Abnormal 2nd heart tone:	15%
Orthopnea:	28%	Jugular vein distention:	14%
Wheezing:	21%		

Circulatory collapse was found in only 8% of these patients.

Source: Stein, P., Beemath, A., Matta, F., Weg, J., Yusen, R., Hales, C., et al. (2007). Clinical characteristics of patients with acute pulmonary embolism: Data from PIOPED II. *American Journal of Medicine, 120*(10), 871–879.

DIAGNOSTIC TESTS for Pulmonary Embolism

Test With Description, Rationale, and Normal Values	Expected Abnormality
ABGs pH 7.35–7.45; $PaCO_2$ 35–45; PaO_2 75–100; HCO_3 24–28. *Used to identify altered gas exchange secondary to PE. Findings vary depending on the size and degree of obstructions and underlying co-morbidities.*	Often normal. Abnormal in some cases. May reveal hypoxemia, hypocapnia, or respiratory alkalosis. Massive PE with hypotension: hypercapnia, respiratory, and metabolic acidosis.
Pulse Oximetry $> 90\%$ *Used to detect early changes in oxygenation.*	Decreased in some cases, normal in most cases.
WBC 4,500–10,000 µL *Atelectasis and infiltrates occur, causing elevated white count.*	White blood cell count may be normal or elevated.
Troponin *Identifies right heart overload. Limited diagnostic usefulness, but elevated troponins are associated with adverse outcomes.*	Elevated in 30% to 50% of patients with large or moderate PE. Resolves in 2 days.
ECG *Identify right ventricular strain, cor pulmonale, and right ventricular dysfunction associated with pulmonary embolus.*	Nonspecific ST-segment and T-wave changes; atrial dysrhythmias, right bundle branch block, inferior Q-waves, and precordial T-wave inversion are associated with poor prognosis.
Chest X-Rays *Altered perfusion pattern not visible via chest x-ray. In patients with pulmonary complaints, this is useful. Major role of CXR is to rule out other diagnoses.*	Usually subtle/nonspecific. Atelectasis, pulmonary opacities, pleural effusion, cardiomegaly.
D-Dimer Test Negative Is < 250 ng/mL *The D-dimer test is a degradation product of cross-linked fibrin. This indicates activation of the fibrolytic pathway, meaning the body is trying to break down clots. Therefore, the D-dimer test will be elevated in any condition such as disseminated intravascular coagulation (DIC), PE, DVT, and myocardial infarction where clots are formed. Has good sensitivity and negative predictive value (normal level likely to indicate absence of PE). It has poor specificity and positive predictive value (an abnormal value is not predictive of PE).*	Abnormal (>250 ng/mL). Negative: PE unlikely. Positive: Further tests needed.
V/Q Scan *Perfusion pattern is altered by PE. If scan is of low or intermediate probability, other means of diagnosis should be pursued. V/Q has poor sensitivity, meaning that a positive V/Q probability score is not strongly associated with positive PE.*	Patients with high clinical probability and a high-probability V/Q score have a 95% likelihood of PE. Those with low clinical and V/Q probability have a 4% likelihood of PE. Combined low and high probabilities range from 15% to 86% likelihood.
Pulmonary Angiography *Gold standard for diagnosis of PE. Provides 100% certainty that an obstruction to pulmonary arterial blood flow does exist. A negative angiogram provides greater than 90% certainty in the exclusion of PE.*	Positive
Ultrasound *Detection of lower extremity DVT, which is treated similarly to a confirmed PE. However, many patients in whom a DVT is not detected on ultrasound may still be positive for PE.*	May detect presence of lower extremity DVT and suggest source of PE.
Spiral CT Scan (CT angiography = CTA) *CTA is being used increasingly in the diagnosis of PE. Diagnostic accuracy is similar to the V/Q scan. It is fast, available in most centers, and noninvasive. The PIOPED II study showed 96% specificity and 83% sensitivity. It is least accurate of emboli in smaller subsegmental vessels; therefore, a negative CTA does not necessarily rule out all PEs. CTA must be used with clinical probability scales.*	Low to high probability.

Nursing Management

The nursing process guides the nursing care for patients with a PE.

Assessment

Nursing assessment must include an evaluation of risk factors on admission and throughout the patient's hospital stay, including physical examination for evidence of DVT. Symptoms of PE are often nonspecific. There is usually a history of progressive shortness of breath over several days, a vague description of chest pain, tachypnea, and leg pain.

Nursing Diagnoses

Nursing diagnoses related to PE include the following:

- *Tissue Perfusion, Ineffective* related to a decrease in blood flow to the alveoli and systemic hypoxia.
- *Gas Exchange, Impaired* related to ventilation-perfusion mismatch.

NANDA-I © 2012

Other nursing diagnoses are directly related to the specific clinical manifestations described earlier that may or may not be present.

Outcomes and Evaluation Parameters

The expected outcomes for a patient with pulmonary embolus are (1) satisfactory ventilation, as evidenced by stable respiratory rate and ease of breathing, (2) decrease in shortness of breath, (3) adequate ABGs, and (4) improvement in hypoxia.

Interventions and Rationales

Nursing interventions for the patient with pulmonary embolus are aimed at assisting the patient to maintain the therapeutic regime during the acute period.

Safety Alert *Anticoagulant medication should be given on time and at the same time each day. The nurse monitors hemoglobin, hematocrit, platelet, INR levels, and other clotting studies as needed to assess the effectiveness of anticoagulants.*

The nurse should assess the patient's pulmonary status at least every hour to evaluate the severity of the PE and the effectiveness of interventions. Oxygen should be administered as prescribed by the health care team to prevent worsening hypoxia. The head of the bed should be elevated 30 to 45 degrees to promote respiratory excursion (movement of the diaphragm and chest wall) and reduce cardiopulmonary workload.

The nurse assesses the patient for symptoms of bleeding and heparin-induced thrombocytopenia (immune-mediated response to heparin that causes a decrease in platelet count and large-vessel venous or arterial thrombosis) and teaches the patient to do the same. Monitoring liver function is particularly important in older and critically ill patients receiving anticoagulants as heparin may cause elevations of AST and ALT and transient increases in serum LDH. The nurse has a major role in the prevention of DVT and PE. This is discussed further in the Health Promotion section that follows.

Discharge Priorities

Discharge priorities for the patient with PE include educating the patient and family about risk factors and treatment regimes and checking for understanding. Patients sent home on anticoagulants should avoid NSAIDs that may cause bleeding or ulcers. Since these patients will bleed more easily than usual while on these medications, the nurse should encourage them to wear rubber gloves or garden gloves for household or outdoor chores and advise them not to walk barefoot. Patients and families should also check the home environment for loose rugs or obstacles that could cause the patient to fall. This is particularly true of older adults, who have an increased incidence of cerebral hemorrhage from a ground level fall when on anticoagulation medications. Nurses should emphasize the importance of meeting outpatient appointments for laboratory tests such as INR, clotting studies, and liver function studies to monitor coagulation levels. Patients should watch for signs of swelling in their legs and wear elastic stockings when prescribed.

Health Promotion

Nurses should assess patients on admission for risk factors and throughout the hospital stay for signs and symptoms of PE and DVT. Patients who are at moderate to high risk for DVT, and thus PE, should be considered for prophylactic low-dose anticoagulation and intermittent pneumatic compression devices. Prevention of PE can be encouraged through regular exercise, not smoking, avoidance of constrictive clothing to the lower extremities, and drinking plenty of fluids unless restricted. Long-distance travel with prolonged inactivity can increase the risk of PE. Moving legs when sitting, getting up to walk every hour, and not sitting cross-legged can mitigate this.

Pleural Disorders

Pulmonary Hypertension

Pulmonary hypertension (PH) is a lung disorder characterized by increased pressures in the pulmonary artery and subsequent right ventricular overload and failure. PH develops when pulmonary vessels become constricted, hardened, blocked, or hypertrophied. It can be a life-threatening condition, and prognosis is poor if it is left untreated.

Epidemiology and Etiology

The initial classification of PH in 1973 was divided into primary or idiopathic (unknown cause) PH and secondary PH, depending on whether there was or wasn't any identifiable cause. Since that time, the categories have been changed to reflect groupings that are similar in pathologic and clinical features as well as therapeutic options (Simonneau et al., 2009). Chart 27–10 lists the current classification and associated diseases etiologies.

Idiopathic pulmonary arterial hypertension (IPAH) is rare, with an estimated prevalence of 6 per million people. Although IPAH has been reported in many patients over 70 years old, the mean age at diagnosis is 37 years, with a female to male ratio of 1.7:1 (McLaughlin et al., 2009). The association between appetite suppressants (e.g., fenfluramine, dexfenfluramine) and IPAH was well publicized in the 1980s when individuals who had been taking the drugs for as little as 3 months developed the disease. Other drugs that increase the risk of IPAH are rapeseed oil, amphetamines, L-tryptophan, and cocaine.

Pulmonary hypertension is a common complication of COPD, and the mortality rate is high among patients with significantly high pressures (>45 mmHg). Heart failure and dilated cardiomyopathy are also common causes of PH and are associated with a greater likelihood of death and hospitalization (Rubin & Hopkins, 2010).

Pathophysiology

Pulmonary hypertension is defined as a resting mean pulmonary artery pressure of > 25 mmHg (elevated) along with a pulmonary occlusion (wedge) pressure of < 16 mmHg (normal). These numbers indicate normal left heart function and elevated pulmonary pressures, the etiology of which would be lungs and/or right heart. The mean pulmonary

CHART 27–10 Classification and Conditions Associated with Pulmonary Hypertension

Group	Disorders

1
Pulmonary arterial hypertension
	• Idiopathic
	• Heritable
	• Drug-toxin induced
	• Specific disease associated
	  • Connective tissue disease
	  • HIV infection
	  • Portal hypertension
	  • Congenital hemolytic anemia
	• Persistent PH of newborn

2 PH owing to left heart disease	• Systolic dysfunction • Diastolic dysfunction • Valvular disease
3 PH owing to lung disease and/or hypoxia	• COPD • Interstitial lung disease • Sleep-disordered breathing • Alveolar hypoventilation disorders • Chronic exposure to high altitudes • Developmental abnormalities • Cor pulmonale

4
Chronic thrombo-embolic pulmonary hypertension (CTPH)
	• Pulmonary vessel obstructions
	  • Thromboemboli
	  • Tumors
	  • Foreign bodies

5 PH with unclear multifactorial mechanisms	• Hematologic disorders • Systemic disorders (sarcoidosis, pulmonary Langerhans cell histiocytosis, vasculitis, neurofibromatosis) • Metabolic disorders: thyroid disorders, glycogen storage disease • Other: chronic renal failure, tumoral obstruction

Source: Adapted from Simonneau, G., et al. (2009). Updated clinical classification of pulmonary hypertension. *Journal of the American College of Cardiology, 54*(1), S43–S53.

GENETIC CONSIDERATIONS
Related to Primary Pulmonary Hypertension

Abnormal bone morphogenetic protein receptor type II (BMPR2) seems to play an important role in the development of IPAH. Hereditary transmission of PAH has been reported in 6% to 10% of patients in Group 1 PAH (Chart 27–10). In the majority of these patients (50% to 90%), mutations in abnormal bone protein receptors (BMPR2) are identified (McLaughlin et al., 2009). BMPR2 has also been found in patients with IPAH and in 15% of PAH related to fenfluramine use. BMPR2 (IPAH1) appears to be transmitted as an autosomal dominant trait.

artery pressures are influenced by pulmonary flow (right ventricle cardiac output), pulmonary vascular resistance, and the mean pulmonary venous pressure. Increased resistance may be caused by conditions that occlude the vasculature of the pulmonary arteries and arterioles (IPAH, collagen vascular disease, HIV infection), decrease the vessel diameter (pulmonary emboli, interstitial lung disease), or cause hypoxic vasoconstriction (COPD) (Rubin & Hopkins, 2010). Increased flow is generally related to congenital heart defects with left-to-right shunt or liver cirrhosis. In addition, increased venous pressure may be caused by mitral valve disease, left ventricular dysfunction, or venous obstruction. Whatever the cause, the right ventricle will enlarge in response to the pressure and, if severe enough, will dilate, causing cardiac output to subsequently fall.

Clinical Manifestations

Symptoms of pulmonary hypertension may develop very gradually and often are nonspecific. Patients with mild or moderate PH may be asymptomatic. The clinical manifestations of PH frequently are masked by the underlying disease that leads to the PH. The most common presenting symptoms are as follows:

- Exertional dyspnea
- Fatigue and lethargy
- Angina
- Syncope
- Raynaud's disease (disorder of the blood vessels in the fingers and toes that causes the blood vessels to narrow)
- Peripheral edema.

On physical exam, heart murmurs, abnormal heart tones, and right bundle branch block develop as the right ventricle fails. Elevated jugular venous pressure, hepatomegaly, ascites, and pleural effusions are all signs of right ventricular failure that are associated with advanced PH disease.

Laboratory and Diagnostic Procedures

Several diagnostic studies are ordered in the differential diagnosis of the patient's presenting symptoms, starting with ECG and CXR. The ECG may be normal in some patients, but in many it suggests right ventricular hypertrophy. The degree of ECG change does not necessarily correlate with the severity of pulmonary hypertension. The CXR demonstrates an enlarged right ventricle, dilated pulmonary arteries, and reduced blood volume to the peripheral lung fields. An echocardiogram will rule out additional causes to these aberrations, estimate the pulmonary artery pressures, and assess right ventricle size and function. The echocardiogram will determine the likelihood of PH; heart catheterization can confirm the diagnosis and definitively determine hemodynamic and pulmonary compromise. Exercise testing is recommended to determine the functional severity of the disease (Rubin & Hopkins, 2010). Further tests are performed to identify the underlying cause of the pulmonary hypertension; these should be guided by the patient's history and physical exam. They include pulmonary function tests, ventilation-perfusion scans, overnight oximetry, and specific laboratory testing (HIV, liver function, and autoimmune serology).

Medical Management

The primary management of PH is directed at treating the underlying cause. Since advanced disease may be less responsive to interventions, therapy should be initiated as soon as PH is identified.

Several therapies can be applied to many patients with PH, regardless of the cause. These include diuretics, oxygen therapy, anticoagulation, digoxin, and exercise (Hopkins & Rubin, 2010). Diuretics are used to treat fluid retention that can occur with right heart failure by reducing hepatic congestion and peripheral edema. Care should be taken to avoid excess diuresis and reduction of cardiac output. Oxygen therapy should be considered in any patient with hypoxemia and is key in the treatment of Group 3 PH (Chart 27–10). Flow should be guided to maintain oxygen saturation above 90%. Patients with PH are at increased risk for intrapulmonary thrombosis or thromboembolism due to sluggish pulmonary blood flow, dilated right heart, venous stasis, and inactive lifestyle. Prophylactic anticoagulation should be considered, particularly in patients with Group 1 PAH, in which studies have demonstrated a reduction in mortality when treated with warfarin. Warfarin is the drug of choice unless contraindicated. Digoxin helps to control the heart rate in patients with right ventricular dysfunction and in some patients with COPD or left heart failure. Although exercise has not demonstrated any improvement in hemodynamic status, there has been some evidence that it improves patient functional status and is safe. Patients should avoid activities that lead to severe dyspnea, chest pain, or syncope or further exacerbate their symptoms (Hopkins & Rubin, 2010).

Additional therapies are targeted specifically at treating pulmonary hypertension rather than the underlying cause, particularly PAH (Group 1), and may be cautiously considered for other PH populations when primary therapy fails. These include calcium-channel blockers (rarely), prostanoids, endothelin-receptor antagonists, and phosphodiesterase inhibitors (Hopkins & Rubin, 2010). Experienced health care providers should administer these therapies.

Calcium-channel blocker studies have suggested prolonged survival and improved functional and hemodynamic status in some IPAH patients that had a positive vasoreactivity test. The studies at this point have been observational, and randomized trials are needed. Side effects are common and usually are associated with the vasodilatory effects (Hopkins & Rubin, 2010).

Prostanoids are an analog of prostacyclin, which is a naturally occurring substance in the body that induces vasodilation. A disruption in the prostacyclin pathways has been shown in patients with PAH and is thought to influence the vasoconstriction of pulmonary vessels. Medications in this class used to treat PH include epoprostenol, treprostinil, and iloprost. Epoprostenol is currently the first-line agent in patients with severe disease. It is delivered continuously through a portable infusion pump into an implanted central venous catheter. It has a short half-life, and interruption in the infusion can have life-threatening consequences. Treprostinil can be given IV, SQ, or more recently in an inhaled version. It has a longer half-life than epoprostenol and provides greater flexibility. Iloprost is an inhaled prostanoid. It has not been well studied, and its primary disadvantage is that it must be administered 6 to 9 times per day. Both treprostinil and iloprost have only been studied in small trials, and larger randomized trials are needed (Hopkins & Rubin, 2010).

Endothelin receptor antagonists mitigate the potent vasoconstrictor effects of endothelin-1. Studies have demonstrated improvements in exercise capacity, dyspnea, and hemodynamic measures. Drugs in this category include bosentan, ambrisentan, and sitaxsentan. The primary adverse effect is liver toxicity (Hopkins & Rubin, 2010).

Phosphodiesterase inhibitors prolong the vasodilatory effect of nitric oxide and are also used to treat erectile dysfunction. Sildenafil (Viagra, Revatio) and tadalafil (Cialis, Adcirca) both have shown some improvement in exercise tolerance and pulmonary hemodynamics. They are generally well tolerated.

Surgical Management

Bilateral lung or heart–lung transplantation has been performed on patients with severe, progressive IPAH that are refractory to medical therapy. The 3-year survival rate for transplantation for IPAH is approximately 50% (Hopkins & Rubin, 2010).

Nursing Management

Assessment

The nurse must be alert to the foremost signs and symptoms of pulmonary hypertension: exertional dyspnea, fatigue and lethargy, angina, syncope, Raynaud's disease, and edema of ankles and legs. The nurse also needs to be alert to progression of the disease that leads to right heart failure (refer to the Nursing Management section under the "Cor Pulmonale" heading).

Nursing Diagnoses

Nursing diagnoses related to pulmonary hypertension include the following:

- *Gas Exchange, Impaired* related to alterations in alveolar membrane structure and elevated pulmonary vascular resistance.
- *Fatigue* related to increased work of breathing.
- *Knowledge Deficit* related to disease process and plan of care.

NANDA-I © 2012

Planning

The primary goal of nursing management of pulmonary hypertension is to identify patients who are subject to or at high risk for this disorder. There are numerous conditions, but primary diseases include cystic fibrosis, COPD, hypoventilation syndromes, pulmonary fibrosis, congenital heart disease, pulmonary emboli, mitral valve disease, and connective tissue diseases. Management revolves around identifying, treating, and monitoring each of these disease entities.

Outcomes and Evaluation Parameters

The desired outcomes for the patient with pulmonary hypertension include maintaining oxygen saturation levels at greater than 90%. The patient will verbalize understanding of the medication regimen and will be able to remain active while minimizing overexertion, fatigue, and dyspnea.

Interventions and Rationales

Primary pulmonary hypertension often has limited treatment options, and care is supportive. This includes providing supplemental oxygen to reduce hypoxemia-related pulmonary vasoconstriction, administration of diuretics to reduce right heart volume and workload, and education of the patient and caregiver in managing the symptoms of the disease. Patients should be instructed in how to manage the activity and fatigue levels imposed by the disease, such as frequent rest intervals and identifying activities or diversions that minimize overexertion. Patients should be allowed to verbalize their concerns, identify support systems, and understand the disease progression. Conversations should include wishes for treatment and advanced directives.

Discharge Priorities

Discharge priorities for the patient with pulmonary hypertension are multifaceted and focus on self-care as well as education regarding medications and home equipment and emergency needs. Refer to the Patient Teaching & Discharge Priorities box. Fatigue and weakness related to the disease itself may render the patient dependent on others for daily care. Patients and families need to be advised about an activity regimen that the patient can safely assume. The physical environment also should be configured to provide easy and safe ambulatory or wheelchair navigation. The nurse should give the patient and family precise instructions as to how and when to take medications, and the patient should be instructed to keep the list in an easily accessible location along with emergency phone numbers. Family members should know the placement of these documents. If the patient is going to be on home oxygen therapy, instruction should be provided as to how to acquire and use the equipment.

PATIENT TEACHING & DISCHARGE PRIORITIES for Pulmonary Hypertension

Need	Teaching
Knowledge of disease process and prognosis	The patient should drink plenty of fluids unless restricted. The patient should eat a healthy diet, avoid obesity, and, if advised, eat a low sodium diet. The patient should stay physically active but avoid overexertion and heavy lifting. The patient or caregiver should contact the health care provider if: • The patient develops a fever. • New symptoms develop. • The patient's activity ability is reduced from baseline. The patient should seek emergency care if he develops chest pain or palpitations, increased swelling in the legs or abdomen, sudden shortness of breath, vomiting, or fainting spells.
Understanding of medications	The nurse gives the patient a list of medications and dosages to carry with him and advises him against taking any OTC medications, vitamins, herbs, or food supplements without discussion with the primary health care provider. The nurse teaches the patient the purpose, dose, and side effects of all medications. The nurse instructs the patient not to discontinue or reduce any medication without health care provider consent and to notify the health care provider if the medications are not helping. If patients are sent home on continuous infusion pumps of antipulmonary hypertensive medications, the nurse teaches the patient and family the sterile care of the catheter, the function and care of the infusion pump, and the dangerous consequences of stopping medications.
Psychosocial	The nurse allows verbalization of fears and provides realistic perceptions when patient seems ready. The patient's family or significant others should be included as appropriate in discharge teaching. The nurse provides information about support groups.
Health promotion	The nurse should advise the female patients against pregnancy as pulmonary hypertension carries a significant risk to the mother and fetus. Many medications given for pulmonary hypertension may cause birth defects. The patient should avoid strenuous activities and heavy lifting. The patient should avoid travel to high altitudes. The patient should stop smoking. The patient should receive the annual influenza and pneumococcal pneumonia vaccination.
Safety	The patient's home environment should be designed for easy ambulatory or wheelchair navigation. If medications produce drowsiness, the patient should not drive.

The patient and family's psychological adjustment to the patient's illness also must be considered. The diagnosis carries with it an uncertain and historically very bleak prognosis. Although new oral and chronic parenteral treatments have had a significant positive medical impact on the physical functioning of individuals with PH, patients often struggle with new short- and long-term psychosocial challenges (Wryobeck, Lippo, McLaughlin, Riba, & Rubenfire, 2007).

Collaborative Management

The health care provider, nurse, and social worker are involved in the care of the patient with pulmonary hypertension. They initiate the plan of care and assume responsibility for continuity. In order to meet desired patient outcomes, it is essential that this interdisciplinary team communicate openly with one another in developing and evaluating care of the patient and family (IOM [Institute of Medicine], 2010). Various diagnostic tests, as previously described, are performed. These are essential to determine the cause of pulmonary hypertension. Although there is no cure for PH, treatment as prescribed by the health care provider can relieve symptoms, improve the patient's quality of life, and prolong life. The nurse is responsible for implementing and evaluating the plan of care. The social worker, occupational therapist, and dietitian may be called on to assist the patient in making appropriate plans for discharge, physical set-up of the house that deters overexertion, self-care help, and dietary plans that reduce physiological stress. A consultation with a health care provider who specializes in the treatment of pulmonary hypertension should be considered to assist in managing the disease.

Health Promotion

Patients who are at risk for recurrent pulmonary embolism, which will increase PH, should be advised how to reduce their risk. This includes teaching patients how to minimize hypercoagulability, control obesity, and reduce venous stasis. Unless restricted, they should drink plenty of fluid. They should get exercise but avoid activities that exacerbate their symptoms. Stress can also lead to shortness of breath, and patients should be advised of stress reduction activities and programs such as yoga, meditation, and biofeedback. Patients with PH should not smoke; if they do, they should be referred to a smoking cessation program. Traveling to or living at high altitude can exacerbate PH. Women should not get pregnant and should not use oral contraceptives, which may cause blood clots. Because patients may be on a variety of medications, including anticoagulants, they should be advised to avoid situations that would put them at risk for experiencing side effects of the medications. They should not discontinue medications or take over-the-counter medications without consulting their health care provider. Counseling also is advised to help the patient cope with the serious and potentially life-threatening outcomes of their disease. Referral to a support group, locally or online, also may assist the patient in the coping process.

Cor Pulmonale

Etiology, Epidemiology, and Pathophysiology

Cor pulmonale is defined as an alteration in the structure and function of the right ventricle due to pulmonary hypertension caused by a disease that affects the lungs or its vasculature. This is listed in the pulmonary hypertension classification described previously in this chapter as Group 3: pulmonary hypertension owing to lung diseases and/or hypoxemia (Chart 27–10, page 775). Right ventricular disease caused by a primary abnormality of the left side of the heart or congenital heart disease (Group 2) is not considered cor pulmonale.

Cor pulmonale may develop from a variety of disease processes (Chart 27–11). The mechanisms associated with these diseases may include pulmonary vasoconstriction (hypoxemia, hypercapnia), increased blood viscosity (polycythemia, sickle cell), increased pulmonary blood flow, or anatomic reduction of the pulmonary vascular bed (pulmonary embolism, emphysema, COPD) (Wiedemann, 2011). The most frequent cause of cor pulmonale is chronic obstructive pulmonary disease (COPD). Most often, cor pulmonale is caused by a chronic process; however, patients may present with an acute, life-threatening condition when the right ventricle can no longer meet physiologic demand, either because the disease has progressed or due to another concurrent acute disease process (Wiedemann, 2011).

Laboratory and Diagnostic Procedures

Diagnosis of cor pulmonale is based on clinical suspicion and diagnostic tests. An echocardiogram is the most frequently used and accepted modality for the screening of pulmonary hypertension and right ventricular assessment. Although right-sided cardiac catheterization is the gold standard in diagnosing, quantifying, and characterizing pulmonary arterial hypertension, it is usually used only when an echocardiogram cannot provide adequate information. Diagnostic tests are summarized in the Diagnostic Tests box below.

CHART 27–11 Causes of Cor Pulmonale

Etiology	Disease Processes
Lung disease	• Chronic obstructive pulmonary disease • Cystic fibrosis • Interstitial lung disease
Disorders of the pulmonary circulation	• Pulmonary thromboembolism • Primary pulmonary hypertension • Tumor emboli • Sickle cell anemia • Schistosomiasis • Pulmonary veno-occlusive disease
Neuromuscular diseases	• Amyotrophic lateral sclerosis (ALS) • Myasthenia gravis • Poliomyelitis • Guillain-Barré syndrome • Spinal cord lesions • Bilateral diaphragmatic paralysis
Thoracic cage deformities	• Kyphoscoliosis
Disorders of ventilatory control	• Primary central hypoventilation • Sleep apnea syndromes

Source: Adapted from Wiedemann, H. (2011). *Cor pulmonale.* In J. Mandel & K. Wilson (Eds.), *UpToDate.* Waltham, MA: UpToDate.

DIAGNOSTIC TESTS for Cor Pulmonale

Test with Description, Rationale, and Normal Values	Expected Abnormality
Chest X-Ray *Used to identify changes in heart and pulmonary vessels caused by pulmonary hypertension.*	Enlargement of central pulmonary arteries; enlarged right heart.
Echocardiography *Identifies right ventricle hypertrophy or strain caused by chronic right ventricular overload. This causes increased thickness of the right ventricle and bulging of the septum during systole.*	Shows signs of chronic right ventricular pressure overload. Initially shows right ventricle hyperkinesis but progresses to hypokinesis as right atrium enlarges and tricuspid regurgitation manifests.
ECG *Identifies ECG changes secondary to right atrial enlargement and hypoxemia.*	Right axis deviation. Increased P-wave amplitude. Incomplete or complete right bundle branch block.
Cardiac Catheterization *Right heart catheterization is the gold standard for the diagnosis of pulmonary arterial hypertension that induces cor pulmonale. Used when echocardiography is inconclusive. Identifies chronic hypoxemia caused by pulmonary hypertension.*	Assesses degree of pulmonary hypertension and differentiates cor pulmonale from occult left ventricular dysfunction. Measures pulmonary artery pressures and vascular resistance.
Hematocrit Male: 40–54% Female: 36–46% *Polycythemia develops secondary to chronic hypoxemia.*	Abnormally elevated.
Serum Alpha 1-Antitrypsin 78–200 mg/dL *Deficiency of AAT causes COPD symptomatology and leads to cor pulmonale.*	Decreased.

Clinical Manifestations

Mild cor pulmonale is often asymptomatic and does not exhibit any significant radiographic alterations. Identification may be difficult because the signs are subtle and the nondescript symptoms are often confused and associated with those of the underlying disease process. Some of the more common symptoms associated with cor pulmonale are fatigue, exertional syncope, and lethargy. This is reflective of the disease's impact on the heart's ability to increase cardiac output in times of stress. The patients may also have some chest pain and, less commonly, cough and hemoptysis. Physical findings include changes in the second heart tone and/or murmur, peripheral edema, and enlarged and possibly pulsatile liver. Edema appears to occur primarily in patients with elevated serum carbon dioxide (hypercarbia).

Medical Management

Managing the underlying disease, when possible, will help to slow the development or progression of cor pulmonale. The treatment is focused on improving oxygenation, enhancing right ventricular contraction, and reducing pulmonary vasoconstriction. Oxygen therapy is a mainstay for patients with cor pulmonale and improves survival in hypoxemic patients with COPD (Wiedemann, 2011). This may be attributed to the reduction of pulmonary vasoconstriction and pulmonary vascular resistance that subsequently improves contraction of the right ventricle and cardiac output. Diuretics may improve cardiovascular function in patients with significant right ventricle overload by reducing the filling volume and dilation of the right ventricle. Diuretics should be used judiciously to prevent a drop in cardiac output and worsen cor pulmonale. Vasodilators and digoxin have been utilized to improve ventricular function and reduce pulmonary hypertension, respectively; however, these medications have not demonstrated any long-term benefit.

Nursing Management

Assessment

Because the physical assessment for identification of cor pulmonale is subtle and similar to assessment for the underlying disease, the nurse should hold a high level of suspicion of cor pulmonale in patients with chronic lung disease. The patient may appear acutely ill and complain of shortness of breath, and the nurse should ask how the current symptoms differ from the patient's baseline. Oxygen saturation levels should be immediately determined. The nurse should determine whether the patient has experienced any light-headedness with exertion, lethargy, chest pain, or fatigue. In addition, the nurse should examine the patient for the presence of peripheral edema, abnormal heart tones, murmur, or distended neck veins. The nurse also should assess the patient's blood pressure, pulse rate and rhythm, and breath sounds and determine whether the patient is complying with any home medications.

Nursing Diagnoses

Nursing diagnoses related to cor pulmonale include the following:

- *Decreased Cardiac Output* related to right heart pump failure.
- *Fluid Volume Excess* related to decreased myocardial contractility.
- *Activity Intolerance* related to hypoxia and increased work of breathing.
- *Knowledge Deficit* related to disease process and plan of care.

NANDA-I © 2012

Planning

Nursing management of cor pulmonale is directed at maintaining adequate oxygenation and cardiac output.

Outcomes and Evaluation Parameters

Desired outcomes for the patient with cor pulmonale include saturations > 90%, vital signs within acceptable limits, regular heart rate and rhythm (or baseline rhythm), urinary output > 30 mL/hr, maintenance of normal weight, and resolution of peripheral edema and shortness of breath.

Interventions and Rationales

In treating cor pulmonale, the nurse provides supplemental oxygen to maintain saturations > 90% to reduce pulmonary vasoconstriction. In addition, the nurse administers diuretics as prescribed to reduce overload to the right ventricle and monitors the patient for signs of adequate fluid balance such as absence or reduction of peripheral edema, maintenance of stable weight, and decrease in shortness of breath. The nurse provides education on any dietary restrictions such as low sodium intake, which can result in fluid retention and exacerbation of heart failure. The nurse should instruct the patient about managing stress and how anxiety can influence shortness of breath. Maintaining a calm, nonrushed approach can assist the patient in remaining calm.

Collaborative Management

A team approach should guide patients with cor pulmonale and their families in the use of prescribed medications, signs of respiratory infection, how to detect signs of fluid retention, and the importance of a low-sodium diet. In order to meet desired patient outcomes, it is essential that this interdisciplinary team communicate openly with one another in developing and evaluating care of the patient and family (IOM [Institute of Medicine], 2010).

The nurse should utilize a dietitian to review nutritional goals. Referrals to home health and pulmonary rehabilitation are usually needed to ensure safe care in the home setting. A plan for regular assessment of oxygen needs and medications should be in place before discharge.

Health Promotion

The single most important measure for preventing cor pulmonale is to encourage individuals to stop smoking and to avoid exposure to secondhand smoke and respiratory pollutants.

Pleural Effusion

A **pleural effusion** is the abnormal accumulation of fluid in the space between the parietal pleura, which covers the surface of the chest wall, and the visceral pleura, which covers the surface of the lungs (Figure 27–13◆). An estimated 50 different disorders can lead to pleural effusions (Lee, 2010) and are typically classified as either exudative (fluid that filters from the circulatory system) or transudative (caused by a change in oncotic pressure that is not inflammatory).

Epidemiology and Etiology

The etiology of pleural effusion can be either local or systemic. Pleural effusions are traditionally categorized as exudative or transudative. An exudate is a fluid high in protein and cellular debris that oozes from the blood because of inflammation or injury and is deposited into the tissue. Localized capillary permeability in the lung exudes fluid, protein, and cells into the lung tissue. There are many causes, including infection, malignancy, pulmonary embolism, gastrointestinal disease, collagen vascular diseases, drug interactions, trauma, asbestos exposure, and tuberculosis.

Transudate is fluid that is low in protein. It is usually the result of a decrease in oncotic pressure or an increase in capillary hydrostatic

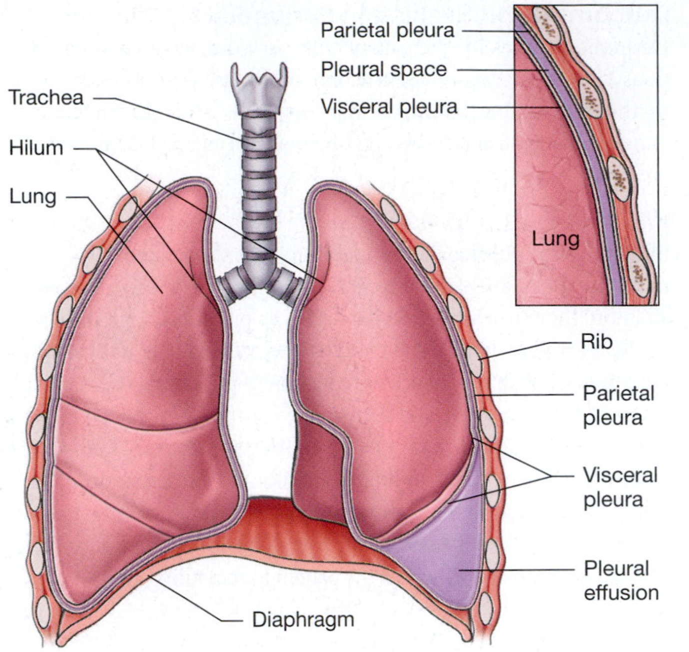

FIGURE 27–13 ◆ Pleural effusion.

pressure, which causes fluid to leak into the pleural space. The most common etiology is congestive heart failure (CHF), but transudate can also be caused by cirrhosis, central venous occlusion, renal disorders, peritoneal dialysis, pulmonary emboli, and myxedema (hypothyroidism). The top causes of pleural effusion in the United States are CHF, with an incidence of 500,000 per year; bacterial pneumonia, with an incidence of 300,000 per year; and malignant disease, with an incidence of 200,000 per year (Broaddus & Light, 2010).

Pathophysiology

The pleura is a thin, transparent, serous, permeable membrane that lines the thoracic cavity and encases the lungs. There are two layers. The parietal pleura lies adjacent to the chest wall, and the visceral pleura adheres to the outer surfaces of the lung. The small amount of serous fluid (10 to 20 mL) normally present between these two surfaces (pleural space) acts as a lubricant, allowing the chest wall and lung to glide across each other during inspiration and expiration. During the normal physiologic process, fluid enters the pleural space via capillaries and exits via stomas and lymphatics. A build-up of fluid occurs when too much fluid enters and/or too little fluid is removed. As this fluid occupies space in the thoracic cavity, the lungs are compressed, the diaphragm is depressed, and, in large effusions, the pressure on the heart may reduce filling pressures and potentially lead to cardiac tamponade. The effects of effusion on oxygenation are variable and usually depend on the function of the underlying lung (Broaddus & Light, 2010).

Clinical Manifestations

The symptoms of pleural effusion depend largely on the underlying disease and the size of the effusion. The patient may be asymptomatic even with large effusions. Inflammation of the pleura may cause the patient to complain of pleuritic chest pain, often described as sharp, unilateral, and worse with deep inspiration or cough. The pain may be referred to the shoulder, neck, or abdomen. A distortion of the lung may cause coughing. As the chest muscles stretch and the lung and diaphragm are displaced, the patient will experience dyspnea. Other clinical findings include decreased breath sounds and excursion on the affected side, dullness to percussion, absent tactile fremitus, and pleural friction rub.

Laboratory and Diagnostic Procedures

Accumulation of pleural fluid of 75 to 150 mL on lateral chest x-ray and 300 to 500 mL on an anterior/posterior upright chest radiograph can identify an effusion by the blunting of the costophrenic angles followed by diaphragmatic obscuration (diaphragm is difficult to distinguish). Effusions are more difficult to diagnose on supine films, as the fluid layers posteriorly. Massive effusions can completely opacify the hemithorax and cause a shift of mediastinal structures to the opposite side of the chest. Ultrasound and CT scans are helpful in identifying the extent of an effusion, lung tissue abnormalities, and masses. Imaging can identify the presence of an effusion, and clinical history may suggest the probable cause. However, most patients with large effusions should have a sampling of the fluid aspirated via thoracentesis, particularly when infection or malignancy is suspected. This analysis will first classify the sample as exudative (inflammatory fluid leaking from cells) or transudative (fluid produced from increased oncotic pressure without capillary injury). Additional cytology, cultures, and chemistry studies can further delineate the cause. For small or complicated effusions, the thoracentesis can be guided by ultrasound. Up to 25% of patients will not have a definitive diagnosis after pleural fluid testing and will require a further work-up (Lee, 2010).

Medical and Surgical Management

Asymptomatic pleural effusions generally do not require specific therapy, and treatment is directed at controlling the underlying cause. For patients who are symptomatic despite medical management, a thoracentesis is used to remove enough fluid to relieve dyspnea and other symptoms. Thoracentesis involves topical anesthesia and inserting a needle, tube, or catheter through the chest wall into the pleural space and aspirating fluid. In complex or small effusions, the procedure may be guided by ultrasound. Effusions may reaccumulate and the procedure may be repeated intermittently. If recurrences are frequent, other options include pleurodesis, indwelling pleural catheter with intermittent drainage, pleurectomy, or pleural-peritoneal shunt. A pleurodesis is a procedure that eliminates the pleural space by injecting a chemical irritant into the space that induces inflammation and fibrosis (Doelken, 2009). Success depends on full re-expansion of the lung so that the visceral and parietal layers have contact. Indwelling catheters are more often used in malignant effusions. Small catheters are tunneled into the pleura, and intermittent drainage can be performed at outpatient facilities. Pleurectomy (surgical removal of the pleura) is reserved for refractory effusions.

Nursing Management

The nurse caring for a patient with a pleural effusion will assess for signs and symptoms that indicate deterioration of ventilation and oxygenation status, including dyspnea, use of accessory muscles, tachypnea, abnormal breath sounds (crackles), decreasing saturations, and elevated carbon dioxide levels.

Nursing interventions can affect outcomes through the early detection of respiratory compromise. The nurse should monitor vital signs, respiratory pattern, and laboratory values to identify the patient's need for supplemental oxygen. Medications should be administered as prescribed, the patient should be encouraged to change positions frequently, and the head of the bed should be elevated to promote good lung expansion. Pain management is a priority, and the nurse assists the patient to assume positions of comfort and offers analgesics as needed.

Discharge Priorities

Patients with pleural effusions may be discharged with a pleural catheter for drainage. The nurse is responsible for educating the patient and family in the management and care of the catheter and drainage system. Otherwise, an effusion may become infected and turn into an empyema (abscess in the pleura) that requires additional therapy. The family should be familiar with signs of infection and know when to contact medical professionals. Another important issue for patient education is pain management. The patient and family should be given concrete instructions on medications to be taken for pain and what to do for breakthrough pain. Patients and families should be instructed to call the health care provider or health care team if dyspnea and discomfort are not relieved by the regimen suggested at discharge.

Environmental Injuries to the Lower Airway

Near Drowning

Although multiple definitions of drowning exist in the literature, **near drowning,** also known as submersion injury, is generally defined as the patient's survival, if only temporarily, after suffocation associated with submersion in a liquid medium (Chandy & Weinhouse, 2010).

Epidemiology and Etiology

Approximately 3,500 deaths per year are attributed to submersion injury, which is the second-leading cause of accidental death for children ages 1 to 14 years (CDC, 2010b). Men have a 3.7 times higher incidence of drowning than women, and African Americans have a 1.7 times higher incidence compared to Whites. Contributing or predisposing factors include inability to swim, risk-taking behavior, alcohol or drug use, inadequate adult supervision, hypothermia, concomitant trauma, and preexisting disorders (such as seizures). Alcohol use is estimated to account for up to 50% of submersion deaths in adolescents and adults. Drowning can occur in any body of water including the bathtub, artificial pools, swimming pools, buckets, toilets, freshwater sites, and saltwater.

The incidence of near drowning events is unclear, but they have an estimated incidence that is several hundred times greater than that of submersion deaths (Schoene, Nachat, Gravatt, & Newman, 2007). Many patients who have experienced near drowning require prolonged hospitalization and suffer lifelong neurologic disability.

Pathophysiology

The sequence of events that leads to drowning typically begins with panic, an abnormal breathing pattern, breath-holding, air hunger, and a struggle to stay above the water (Chandy & Weinhouse, 2010). Initial gasping leads to either aspiration or laryngospasm as water contacts the airways, followed by hypoxemia. Brain ischemia leads to unconsciousness and vomiting, and aspiration of gastric contents may ensue. Laryngospasm may be significant enough to cause hypoxemia without aspiration of water into the lungs. This is referred to as "dry" drowning.

Laboratory and Diagnostic Procedures

Diagnosis is made on the basis of the event's history. ABG analysis will identify the degree of oxygenation and ventilation compromise and will detect the presence of methemoglobinemia and carboxyhemoglobinemia (in those who lose consciousness by swimming close to the exhaust emissions from boats). Other tests to determine the effect of hypoxia on organ function include renal function tests (BUN, creatinine), liver enzymes, and cardiac troponin. Blood gases are obtained to determine the extent of hypoxemia and acidosis. A chest x-ray often does not adequately reflect pulmonary involvement but is indicated in symptomatic patients. A head CT to identify the presence of any cerebral edema or trauma is ordered if there is neurologic uncertainty. Cervical spine imaging is also indicated if there is suspected trauma.

Medical Management

Patients may be asymptomatic or in full cardiopulmonary arrest. Immediate resuscitation is the first priority. If hypothermia exists, pulses may be difficult to palpate, and the heart rate may be very low. Spinal precautions should be maintained until spinal trauma is ruled out. Unresponsive patients should be intubated, and supplemental oxygen should be applied to awake, spontaneously breathing patients. Wet clothing needs to be removed, and active (heating pads, forced warm air, etc.) or passive (blankets) rewarming is applied. Hypothermia has a neuroprotective effect, and there are reports of cold-water submersion patients recovering from cardiac arrest after prolonged resuscitation. Resuscitative efforts should continue until the core temperature reaches 32° to 35°C (90° to 95°F).

Hospital management is aimed at reducing secondary injuries due to ischemia, cerebral edema, acidosis, and fluid and electrolyte imbalances (Chandy & Weinhouse, 2010). Chapter 21 discusses the treatment of cerebral edema. Acidosis can lead to cardiac dysrhythmias and usually reverses with correction of hypoxemia, hypothermia, and hypovolemia. Patients who are alert and oriented are observed in the emergency department until the ABGs become normal and there is an absence of dysrhythmias. If hypoxemia or other complications do not resolve, patients are admitted for observation and treatment.

Nursing Management

Assessment

The nurse assesses the patient's respiratory rate and effort, breath sounds, oxygen saturation, mental status, and signs of pulmonary edema, such as frothy sputum. The nurse also obtains a history from the patient or family to determine the type of water the patient was submerged in, the temperature of the water, and the length of submersion.

Nursing Diagnoses

Nursing diagnoses related to near drowning include the following:

- *Impaired Gas Exchange* related to aspiration, pulmonary surfactant elimination, pulmonary capillary membrane damage, bronchospasm, and/or pulmonary edema.

NANDA-I © 2012

Planning

The goal of nursing care for the patient who has experienced near drowning is to maintain adequate oxygenation and ventilation.

Outcomes and Evaluation

For the patient who has experienced near drowning, the oxygen saturation will be ≥ 90%, and the respiratory rate will be within normal limits with easy, regular respiratory effort. The patient will be normothermic.

Interventions and Rationales

In treating the patient who has experienced near drowning, the nurse maintains an open airway and assists ventilations if needed with a bag-valve-mask device while maintaining cervical spine immobilization. Cervical spine injury is of particular concern in diving-related incidents. The nurse provides oxygen to maintain saturations ≥ 90% and is prepared to assist with intubation if the patient fails to respond or if the patient's level of consciousness does not provide airway protective mechanisms. Submersion injury can lead to pulmonary edema, hyaline membrane formation, and pulmonary capillary injury that may require mechanical ventilation to meet oxygenation and ventilatory requirements. If there is suspicion of child abuse, the nurse should coordinate the appropriate channels of reporting.

Carbon Monoxide Poisoning

Carbon monoxide is an odorless, tasteless, colorless gas that, when inhaled, causes cellular hypoxia. It is found in combustion fumes such as those produced by motor vehicle exhaust, small gasoline engines, stoves, burning charcoal and wood, and gas ranges and heating systems.

Epidemiology, Etiology, and Pathophysiology

Carbon monoxide (CO) toxicity is responsible for 5,000 to 6,000 deaths per year, making it one of the leading causes of poisoning death in the United States. The majority of deaths caused by CO poisoning are intentional suicide attempts (Clardy, Manaker, & Perry, 2010). Accidental CO poisoning causes approximately 500 deaths annually. Smoke inhalation is the primary cause of CO poisoning. Other causes include improper ventilation of fuel-burning devices (camp stoves, gas generators, kerosene heaters, charcoal grills) and running motor vehicles in poorly ventilated areas.

Normally, oxygen is carried to the tissues via the hemoglobin in red blood cells. Because carbon monoxide's affinity for hemoglobin is 200 to 240 times greater than that of oxygen, CO quickly binds with hemoglobin, replacing the oxygen molecule and reducing oxygen delivery to the tissues.

Clinical Manifestations

Diagnosis of CO poisoning is made from the history, clinical assessment, and carboxyhemoglobin blood levels. Signs and symptoms in general order of progression include nausea, headache, dizziness, difficulty concentrating, weakness, dyspnea, chest pain, confusion, syncope, seizures, obtundation (decreased level of consciousness), hypotension, coma, respiratory failure, and death.

Laboratory and Diagnostic Procedures

Carboxyhemoglobin is measured directly by arterial blood gas. Nonsmokers' typical levels are $< 3\%$, smokers' typical levels are 10% to 15%, and levels $> 15\%$ are consistent with CO poisoning (Clardy, Manaker, & Perry, 2010). Pulse oximetry is *not* valid because the hemoglobin is saturated by the carbon monoxide molecule, and oximeters cannot differentiate between carboxyhemoglobin and oxyhemoglobin.

Medical Management

The fundamental treatment for CO poisoning is removal of the patient from the source and administration of high-flow 100% oxygen via nonrebreather facemask or via intubation if the patient has a depressed level of consciousness or respiratory depression. CO is eliminated through the lungs, and its half-life is 3 to 4 hours. With administration of 100% oxygen, the half-life decreases to 30 to 90 minutes; hyperbaric oxygen reduces it to 15 to 23 minutes (Shochat, 2011). Many patients' symptoms resolve with high-flow oxygen therapy. Those who have high levels of carboxyhemoglobin or who continue to be symptomatic should be admitted to a hospital. In addition, transfer to a hyperbaric-capable facility should be considered. Hyperbaric oxygen (HBO) involves providing 100% oxygen at supra-atmospheric pressures. It is indicated for patients with high carboxyhemoglobin levels that do not respond to normal oxygen administration. HBO is most effective when initiated early. It reduces the half-life of CO and has the potential to decrease the neurocognitive sequelae associated with CO toxicity. This is accomplished by placing the patient in a chamber that allows manipulation of the atmospheric pressure. Increasing atmospheric pressure to 3 atm increases the amount of oxygen dissolved in the plasma and distributed to organ tissues. Chamber time is usually 90 to 120 minutes, and retreatment may be performed. Complications of HBO include decompression illness (release of dissolved nitrogen gas-forming bubbles in the body that may act as emboli and block circulation), barotrauma to the sinuses and middle ear, gas embolus, visual changes, and expansion of a pneumothorax.

Nursing Management

Having obtained the estimated exposure time from the patient, family, or EMS responders, the nurse will monitor the patient for confusion, headaches, vertigo, flu-like symptoms, visual disturbances, seizures, unresponsiveness, and respiratory failure. In monitoring arterial saturations, it is important not to rely on pulse oximetry saturations, which are unreliable as the CO attached to the hemoglobin will give a false reading. Instead, the nurse should monitor carboxyhemoglobin levels. The nurse should also assess for evidence of tissue and end-organ hypoxia including tachycardia, cardiac dysrhythmias/arrest, visual disturbances, hypotension, and acidosis.

The nurse provides 100% oxygen via nonrebreather mask at 15 liters. The patient's activity should be limited, as activity will increase the patient's oxygen demands. The nurse should be prepared to assist with intubation for patients with a decreased level of consciousness to protect the airway. A safe environment can be provided for patients with a decreased level of consciousness by placing the bed in a low position with the siderails up. In patients with CO poisoning due to smoke inhalation, the airway may become edematous and obstruct breathing. Since swelling can be occult, the nurse must monitor carefully and frequently for evidence of airway occlusion, including hoarseness, tachypnea, accessory muscle use, and stridor. The nurse will prepare the patient for transport to a facility with hyperbaric capabilities if ordered.

Health Promotion

Educating the public regarding the dangers of allowing exhaust fumes in small enclosed places, such as running cars in an enclosed garage, may reduce the incidence of CO poisoning. CO poisoning occurs more frequently in cold winter months when furnaces, portable heaters, and gas fireplaces are in use. To prevent accidental exposure, heaters and gas-burning appliances should be inspected regularly. Outdoor gas grills should not be used indoors. Carbon monoxide detectors should be installed in homes and offices to detect increased levels of CO within a closed space. In addition, nurses in home care and public health should make fire safety and the possibility of carbon monoxide escape a topic for environmental assessments. When unintentional carbon monoxide poisoning occurs, the nurse should contact the health department.

Lung Cancer

Lung cancer is a term used in reference to malignancies that originate in the airways or lung tissue. There are two main types of lung cancer: non-small-cell lung cancer (the most common) and small cell lung cancer (PubMed Health, 2011).

Epidemiology and Etiology

Lung cancer is the most common cause of cancer mortality in the world for both men and women, with an estimated 1.2 million deaths/year (Midthun, 2010). In the United States, the annual incidence of new cases is about 222,000 with deaths numbering approximately 157,000. Smoking accounts for almost 90% of all lung cancer deaths (Midthun, 2010). The extent of smoking and exposure to other carcinogens among smokers increase their risk. A 40-year pack-a-day smoker is 20 times more likely to develop lung cancer than a nonsmoker. Radiation therapy for other types of cancer can increase the patient's risk of secondary lung cancer. Environmental toxins, such as secondhand smoke or asbestos, are also risk factors. Other risk factors include pulmonary fibrosis, HIV infection, and genetics.

Pathophysiology

From a prognostic and therapeutic standpoint, lung cancers are separated into two major groups, small cell lung cancer (SCLC) and non-small cell lung cancer (NSCLC). In the United States, 85% of lung cancers are non-small cell lung cancer (NSCLC) and 15% are small cell lung cancer (SCLC) (Midthun, 2010).

SCLC almost always occurs in smokers. It is a highly aggressive, disseminated disease. At the time of diagnosis, it is often (60%) already widely disseminated. The stage of the disease at presentation is the most important prognostic indicator (Midthun, 2010). Staging is an important determinant, since therapeutic options are based on the extent of the disease. SCLC has two stages: limited and extensive. Limited SCLCs are confined to the regional lymph nodes and one lung. Extensive SCLCs extend beyond these confines. Patients who present with limited disease have a 5-year survival rate of 10% to 13%. If patients present with extended stage disease, the median survival time is 8 to 13 months with a 5-year survival rate of 1% to 2% (Midthun, 2010).

NSCLC consists of adenocarcinoma, squamous cell carcinoma, large cell carcinoma, and variants of these. Squamous cell tumors typically account for 20% to 25% of all lung cancers. These malignancies have a tendency to be slow growing, such that a visible mass may not be detected for 3 to 4 years.

Adenocarcinoma is now the most common form of lung cancer (40%) (Midthun, 2010). The rise in incidence is probably related to the rise in lung cancer in women; adenocarcinoma is the most common form of cancer in women. Progression is slow; however, adenocarcinoma invades the lymphatic and blood vessels early in the disease, resulting in a worse prognosis compared to that for SCLCs. There are seven levels of staging that are based on the combination and presence of tumor node metastasis, lymph node involvement, and distant metastasis. Common metastatic sites for all types of lung cancer include liver, bone, adrenal glands, and the brain. For a more detailed discussion of the pathophysiology of cancer, refer to Chapter 57.

Clinical Manifestations

Individuals with lung cancer tend to access the health care system once they start to experience multiple serious symptoms. Symptoms may relate to local, regional, or systemic effects depending on the spread of the disease. The most common symptoms are cough, hemoptysis, dyspnea, and chest pain. These symptoms need to be explored further so that their origin can be identified. Additional symptoms include hoarseness, pleural involvement (effusions), and superior vena cava syndrome. Superior vena cava syndrome occurs when a tumor obstructs or narrows the superior vena cava, reducing blood return to the heart, resulting in facial swelling; swelling of the hands, arms, and neck; distended neck veins; cyanosis of the upper torso; and dyspnea.

Laboratory and Diagnostic Procedures

Approximately 85% of patients with lung cancer are symptomatic at presentation; the other 15% are detected by radiographic evaluation exploring an unrelated problem (Mazzone, 2010). CXR and CT are performed for most patients when clinical signs and risk factors suggest lung cancer and abnormalities dictate further evaluation. Tissue samples will need to be collected to confirm lung cancer type and clinical stage. Depending on the location of the malignancy, flexible bronchoscopy, intrathoracic needle biopsy, and surgical approach can be used to sample tissue. Blood sampling for CBC, liver enzymes, and chemistries provides the clinician with information related to existing comorbidities, possible metastatic disease, and complications commonly found with lung cancer. An ECG and pulmonary function test may be ordered to determine baseline pulmonary and cardiac function, especially if radiation therapy will be part of the treatment plan.

Medical Management

The medical management of lung cancer differs on the basis of the cell type. Patients with limited stage SCLC will likely receive chemotherapy and radiation therapy. Those with extensive stage SCLC are treated with multidrug chemotherapy. Prophylactic radiation has demonstrated decreased incidence of brain metastases in patients with both limited and extensive stage SCLC. Surgical intervention is saved for patients with a rare subset of SCLCs. Patients with NSCLC may receive surgical resection, chemotherapy, and/or radiation therapy. For a better understanding of these three treatment options and the associated nursing responsibilities, refer to Chapter 57 on Caring for the Patient With Cancer.

Nursing Management

Nursing management of patients with lung cancer is challenging and complex. The nurse must possess an appreciation of the care required for patients who have undergone surgical resection, those who receive chemotherapeutic agents, and those who receive radiation therapy. Refer to Chapter 57, Caring for the Patient With Cancer, for a detailed description of nursing management of patients receiving chemotherapy and radiation therapy.

Assessment

Nurses should be alert for symptoms that are associated with lung cancer that need further exploration. These include cough, dyspnea, excessive sputum production, chest pain, and hemoptysis. The nurse will prepare the patient for further diagnostic tests including CXR, sputum and pleural fluid testing, biopsy, or pulmonary function tests.

Nursing Diagnoses

Nursing diagnoses related to lung cancer include the following:

- *Gas Exchange, Impaired* related to altered oxygen supply and surgical removal of lung tissue.
- *Ineffective Airway Clearance* related to increased secretions, restriction of chest movement, pain, fatigue, and weakness.
- *Knowledge Deficit* related to disease process and plan of care.
- *Fatigue* related to hypoxia and increased work of breathing.
- *Pain, Acute* related to cancer cell invasion of pleura and chest wall.
- *Anxiety and Fear* related to diagnosis, change in health status, and perceived threat of death.

NANDA-I © 2012

Outcomes and Evaluation Parameters

The patient treated for lung cancer should have a patent airway exhibited by clear breath sounds and oxygen saturations ≥ 90%. The patient will experience adequate pain control, and she and her family are able to verbalize understanding of medical management and plan of care.

Interventions and Rationales

The nurse will administer pain medications regularly to the patient with lung cancer to adequately control pain and discomfort. Oxygen is administered depending on the degree of dyspnea and to maintain oxygen saturations $\geq$ 90%. The nurse assesses for indications of retained secretions, such as rhonchi, wheezes, or audible respirations. The viscosity or amount of secretions, restricted chest movement, pain, fatigue, or weakness can affect the effectiveness of airway clearance. Therefore, the nurse instructs the patient on deep breathing, coughing, and splinting to assist with mobilization of secretions.

Collaborative Management

The multidisciplinary team for the patient with lung cancer may include health care providers, surgeons, nurses, nurse practitioners, respiratory therapists, radiation oncologists, nutritionists, and physical therapists, depending on available resources and the disease's impact on the patient's functional status. If there are financial issues related to maintenance care and equipment, the social worker becomes involved. In order to meet desired patient outcomes, it is essential that this interdisciplinary team communicate openly with one another in developing and evaluating care of the patient and family (IOM [Institute of Medicine], 2010). Referral to the home care nurse is instituted if the patient is not able to manage outpatient clinic or office visits. When the patient is near the end of life, a hospice nurse may be involved.

Health Promotion

Cigarette smoking is a major contributor to the development of lung cancer. The nurse is in a position to influence patients to begin smoking-cessation programs by educating them about the risks of smoking and being exposed to secondhand smoke.

Gerontological Considerations

Respiratory disorders and illness in older adults have significant consequences. One of the primary reasons older individuals seek medical care is the presence of respiratory symptoms (Hall & Ahmed, 2007). Additionally, chronic respiratory diseases contribute significantly to reduced pulmonary function, hospitalization, and higher mortality rates in older adults.

Pulmonary assessment in older individuals is complicated by comorbidities, patients' subjective perceptions, and physiologic changes associated with age. Studies suggest that older adults not only have a diminished recognition of the sensation of dyspnea, but also may not develop shortness of breath until a late stage of illness (Hall & Ahmed, 2007). Older adults often reduce their activity level when they do perceive shortness of breath, assuming that it is age-related. Assessment of older adults should always include questioning about changes in activity levels and taking complaints of shortness of breath seriously and investigating them thoroughly.

CHART 27–12 Pulmonary Manifestations and Disease Processes in Older Adults

- Decreased expiratory airflow may result in less effective cough and the development of hypoxemia.
- Decreased response to hypoxia and hypercarbia may lead to diminished or absent symptoms even with significant abnormality of arterial blood gases.
- Viral infections may precipitate new-onset asthma.
- Asthma development in older adults is common and often underdiagnosed.
- Gastroesophageal reflux that develops with age may lead to onset of asthma and wheezing.
- Older adults may not be able to participate with pulmonary testing due to cardiovascular or arthritic disease.
- Blunting of the immune system may mask respiratory disease symptoms, including failure to generate a fever with infection and lack of sputum production.
- COPD is more common in older adults and is associated with activity limitation and a patient's description of poor health. It is the fourth-leading cause of death in those over 65 years old.
- Pneumonia and influenza are the fifth-leading causes of death in older adults in the United States. Pneumococcal pneumonia and influenza vaccinations should be emphasized.
- Patients with unexplained pulmonary infiltrates should be evaluated for tuberculosis.
- Older adults are more prone to side effects of pharmacologic agents that may require the modification of standard guidelines.

Source: Adapted from Hall, W., & Ahmed, B. (2007). *Pulmonary disorders.* In E. Duthie, P. Katx, & M. Malone (Eds.), *Practice of geriatrics* (4th ed.). Philadelphia: Saunders Elsevier.

Older patients are at high risk for acquiring pulmonary infections and pneumonia because they often experience risk factors such as immobility and chronic disease. They are more likely to be malnourished or immunosuppressed. Pneumonia and influenza are the fourth- and fifth-most common causes of death for older adults in the United States. Although vaccines for influenza and pneumococcal pneumonia are safe and effective, they are generally underused (Hall & Ahmed, 2007).

Several considerations should be acknowledged with respect to pulmonary manifestations and disease processes in older adults. Refer to Chart 27–12.

Research

The treatment of lower airway disorders is aided by ongoing research on the topic, as outlined in the Research Opportunities box. The research opportunities enumerated here tend to focus on the use of complementary and alternative medicine, stimulation of positive health behaviors in older adults, enhancement of nursing knowledge, and student nursing learning gaps in caring for asthmatic patients.

RESEARCH OPPORTUNITIES Related to Lower Airway Disorders

Research Area	Clinical Impact
What complementary and alternative therapies are used by patients with chronic pulmonary disease, and are they effective?	A study by Lahmann et al. (2009) studied the effects of functional relaxation techniques on pulmonary parameters in asthmatic patients, showing a positive relationship. Singing, tai chi, yoga, laughing, and distractive auditory stimuli, among others, have also been researched for their benefits to patients with chronic pulmonary disorders, many with positive results. Specific data on these and other complementary and alternative therapies would add to the knowledge base about pulmonary disease treatment and could provide useful information for patient education. One research question might be: Which complementary and alternative modalities, such as homeopathy, herbal remedies, and acupuncture, as examples, have been most useful? Other research questions are: Do persons who use complementary and alternative therapies have fewer exacerbations? Is there a relationship between anxiety and use of complementary and alternative therapies?
Does reducing indoor triggers improve asthma control?	Takaro, Krieger, Song, & Sharify (2011) examined the benefits of moving low-income children with asthma into asthma-friendly homes. Asthma is the most common chronic condition in children, and the rate of asthma is disproportionally high in lower socioeconomic and racial/ethnic groups, partially owing to the levels of exposure to indoor allergens. Moving children into homes with moisture-reduction features and enhanced ventilation systems, as well as homes that were built with materials that minimized dust and off-gassing, resulted in large decreases in asthma morbidity. Research questions may include: What is the comparison of patient in-home asthma control education in patients who are and are not moved into a different environment? What is the feasibility of establishing building codes and construction practice modification to address environmental conditions that promote asthma triggers? Does the asthma-control benefit translate to other socioeconomic groups?
What is the validity of COPD severity index scales?	Jones et al. (2009) derived and validated a multicomponent assessment tool to identify COPD severity that is simple to use and applicable in all health care settings. The components include dyspnea, airflow obstruction, smoking, and exacerbation frequency (DOSE index). It covers a range of clinically relevant outcomes and is correlated with health status across varying national, disease status, and clinical settings. Research questions may include: How do interventions based on severity index scoring affect health status and lifestyle perceptions in patients with COPD? How can a severity index be used to manage patients with COPD? How can the DOSE index be combined with other multicomponent severity indices to provide additional management options?
Health promotion and attitudes on vaccination and flu prevention among university students	Wilson and Huttlinger (2010) looked at a university education strategy for flu prevention among university students living in dormitories. They found that despite education campaigns, approximately 25% of students were not aware of the virus and 60% did not believe that dormitory living posed a greater risk. Education was done primarily by posting flyers in prominent locations. Further studies that utilize social networking and electronic networking that are more consistent with mechanisms that students utilize are called for. Research questions may include: What types of education campaigns are most effective in improving knowledge and behaviors across age groups?
What is the effectiveness of various methods of smoking cessation?	Promotion of the most effective means of smoking cessation should aid patients in successful smoking cessation.
What is the effect of education on smoke avoidance in grade school on the rate of smoking in adolescence?	Early avoidance of primary and secondhand smoke should decrease the development of emphysema and COPD.

READ: **History of Present Illness** >> Laboratory Study Results >> Critical Thinking Questions

Glendon Hirsch is a 70-year-old man admitted to the emergency department with complaints of intermittent chest tightness and dyspnea, which he states have gotten progressively worse in the past week. He states that he is coughing up large amounts of thick, yellowish sputum and experiences muscle fatigue and dyspnea after bouts of coughing. Mr. Hirsch also indicates that he feels winded after a short walk to the bathroom of his apartment.

Mr. Hirsch is started on intravenous (IV) fluids at 125 cc/hr per day. He is started on Atrovent inhaler 2 inhalations four times a day, and he is continued on his captopril and glipizide orally. The nurse maintains a record of intake and output. A respiratory physical therapist assists Mr. Hirsch with postural drainage, as well as breathing and coughing exercises. He is maintained on 2 liters of nasal oxygen. The physical therapist and nursing staff ambulate him in the hallway four times a day with oxygen. He is placed on a 1,800-calorie diabetic diet, which he tolerates well.

Medical–Surgical History

Mr. Hirsch has a history of chronic bronchitis, hypertension, and colon cancer. He has had two to three hospital admissions per year for exacerbations of chronic bronchitis. Past surgical procedures include a hernia repair at age 50 and a colon resection for colon cancer at age 65. He underwent chemotherapy at that time and is currently in remission. He sees an oncologist every 6 months for follow-up. He is also a non–insulin-dependent diabetic. Current medications include glipizide and captopril.

Social History

Mr. Hirsch is married and lives with his wife. They have two children who live nearby in the same community. He has a history of smoking, but has quit within the last 5 years.

Physical Examination

Auscultation of lung sounds reveals crackles and a few expiratory wheezes throughout all lung fields. Mr. Hirsch's breath sounds are decreased in the bases. He uses his accessory sternocleidomastoid muscles for breathing. While at rest, his respiratory rate is 30. His vital signs are as follows: blood pressure 160/100, pulse 100 beats per minute, and temp 100.6°F orally. Auscultation of the heart reveals he is tachycardic with an S_3. He seems most comfortable sitting forward in a chair and appears to have a barrel chest.

READ: History of Present Illnesses >> **Physical Exam** >> Admitting Medical Records >> Laboratory Study Results

Admitting Medical Orders

Service: Medical floor
Diagnosis: dyspnea and shortness of breath
Allergies: none noted
Vital signs and O_2 saturations q4h
Ambulate in hall with assistance and with oxygen four times daily
Diet: 1,800-calorie diabetic diet
Call house officer: HR <60 >120, systolic blood pressure <100 >140, RR <12 >30, temperature >38°C, O_2 saturation $<92\%$, glucose <70 >150 mg/dL
IV fluids: 0.45 normal saline at 125 mL/hr
I&O q shift
Respiratory care: maintain on 2 liters of nasal oxygen; CPT and breathing and coughing exercises by physical therapist q4h

Scheduled Medications

Atrovent inhaler, 2 inhalations four times a day
Captopril 50 mg orally twice daily, 1 hour before meals
Glipizide 5 mg orally every day 30 minutes before breakfast
Day 2, Linezolid 600 mg IV every 12 hours

PRN Medications

Ibuprofen 400 mg orally every 4 hours as needed for discomfort

Ordered Laboratory Studies

CBC, and Chem 7 panel every morning
Sputum culture
Accu-Chek q ac and hs

Ordered Diagnostic Studies

Anterior/posterior and lateral chest x-ray

Nursing Care Day 2

On day 2, Mr. Hirsch is started on a broad-spectrum antibiotic given intravenously in addition to the other therapies. His dyspnea has eased and he is expectorating sputum more easily. Mr. Hirsch is tolerating ambulation and an increase in activity. His IV is changed to a saline lock through which he receives his antibiotic. His wife visits at his bedside regularly and is encouraged to assist with coughing and deep breathing exercises as well as a fluid intake of 8 glasses of water per day. Mr. Hirsch's vital signs are as follows: BP 130/70, HR 92, respiratory rate 24, and temperature 99.5°F.

READ: History of Present Illness >> **Laboratory Study Results** >> Critical Thinking Questions

Test	Day 1	Day 2	Day 3
O_2 saturation on room air	88%		
O_2 saturation on 2 L nasal O_2	92%	94%	94%
WBC	10,000 μL	10,000 μL	8,000 μL
Hct	54%	50%	49%
Hgb	17 g/100 mL	16 g/100 mL	15 g/100 mL
Platelets	200,000 μL	210,000 μL	225,000 μL

Test	Day 1	Day 2	Day 3
RBCs	4.6 ∞ 106/μL	5.0 ∞ 106/μL	5.2 ∞ 106/μL
Sodium	148 mEq/L	128 mEq/L	139 mEq/L
Potassium	4.0 mEq/L	4.2 mEq/L	4.5 mEq/L
Chloride	105 mEq/L	100 mEq/L	100 mEq/L
HCO_3-	35 mEq/L	35 mEq/L	32 mEq/L
Glucose	150 mg/dL	145 mg/dL	148 mg/dL
Sputum culture		*Staphylococcus aureus*	

Pearson Nursing Student Resources *Log on to* **nursing.pearsonhighered.com** *to download forms*

DOCUMENT:

- >> Summary of Hospitalization
- >> Pathophysiology Form
- >> Laboratory Values
- >> Laboratory Results Explanation

APPLY:

- >> List of Potential Nursing Diagnoses
- >> Concept Map
- >> Critical Thinking Questions and Concept Map

APPLY: History of Present Illness >> Laboratory Study Results >> **Critical Thinking Questions**

1. As the nurse on the unit where Mr. Hirsch is admitted, what further assessment data do you plan to collect?
2. Your initial impression is that Mr. Hirsch has a barrel chest. How do you verify this with objective data? What is the etiology of a barrel chest in the patient with COPD?
3. Mr. Hirsch is placed on Atrovent 2 puffs four times a day. How will this drug alleviate Mr. Hirsch's symptoms? What are some potential side effects?
4. After 3 days, Mr. Hirsch is to be discharged on 2 L nasal oxygen, which is to be administered continuously. His medications include glipizide, captopril, oral prednisone, an oral antibiotic to be taken for 3 more days, albuterol, and steroid inhalers to be taken three times a day. What patient education do you provide and what assessment do you want to make prior to discharge? Describe the patient education strategies and use of visual aids.
5. What are some nutritional considerations for Mr. Hirsch?
6. What benefits will continuous oxygen therapy afford Mr. Hirsch in terms of quality of life?

Answers to Critical Thinking Questions can be found in Appendix D in the Osborn Student Resources at nursing.pearsonhighered.com.

NCLEX® PRACTICE

1. A patient is seen in the emergency department with acute shortness of breath, coughing, wheezing, and chest tightness after cleaning her carpet at home. The nurse should continue assessment with which question?
   1. "Have you been exposed to the flu?"
   2. "Do you have asthma?"
   3. "Have you ever taken a pneumonia vaccine?"
   4. "Do you have cystic fibrosis?"
2. A client with community-acquired pneumonia is being discharged. What should the nurse include in this client's discharge plan of care?
   1. Take the prescribed antibiotics until the coughing stops.
   2. Limit fluid intake to reduce secretions.
   3. Avoid smoking or environments with smoke.
   4. Resume a normal activity level.
3. The clinic nurse is providing care to a client with chronic obstructive pulmonary disease. Which medication should the nurse anticipate that this client will receive?
   1. An inhaled long-acting bronchodilator
   2. Ibuprofen
   3. An oral corticosteroid
   4. An ACE inhibitor
4. The nurse has read the Mantoux test for TB (PPD) for the following clients. Which tests would the nurse document as positive? (select all that apply)
   1. The test that measures 9 mm of induration on the arm of a healthy 35-year-old female
   2. The test that measures 6 mm of induration on the arm of a client who has HIV
   3. The test that shows 3 mm of redness and no induration on the arm of a 12-year-old
   4. The test that measures 8 mm of induration on the arm of a client who has COPD
   5. The test that measures 12 mm of induration on the arm of a 28-year-old man

5. A client who has been diagnosed with idiopathic pulmonary fibrosis says, "I don't know what to expect. How will this disease affect my life?" Which nursing response is correct?

1. "As long as you stay on your medication, the disease should not have a serious impact on how you live your life."
2. "You will be pretty sick until you have surgery, but then you should feel well within 2 or 3 weeks."
3. "There really isn't a cure for this disease. You will have to work to manage symptoms as they arise."
4. "There is no treatment for this disease, but it will go away on its own in the next few months. Then you will feel much the same as you did before you got sick."

6. A nurse is providing disease management education to a 25-year-old client diagnosed with acute silicosis resulting from an industrial accident. Which information should the nurse provide? (select all that apply)

1. Bronchodilators are often prescribed to help manage symptoms.
2. Smoking cessation and avoidance of secondhand smoke are essential.
3. The fibrotic changes in the lungs will reverse.
4. Lung transplantation may be considered if the condition continues.
5. Exposure to silica dust should be strictly avoided.

Answers to NCLEX Practice questions can be found in Appendix D in the Osborn Student Resources at nursing.pearsonhighered.com. Practice additional NCLEX questions online at the Student Resources site.

Pearson Nursing Student Resources Find additional review materials at: **nursing.pearsonhighered.com**

REFERENCES

Adams, M. P., & Koch, R. W. (2010). *Pharmacology, connections to nursing practice.* Upper Saddle River, NJ: Prentice Hall.

American Lung Association. (2007). Sarcoidosis. Retrieved from http://www. lungusa.org/site/c.dvLUK9OOE/b.4061173/apps/s/content.asp?ct=5176723

Bartlett, J. (2008). Acute bronchitis. In R. Porter & J. Kaplan (Eds.), *The Merck manual online medical library.* Retrieved from www.merckmanuals.com/professional/pulmonary_disorders/acute_bronchitis/acute_bronchitis.html?qt=acutebronchitis&alt=sh

Bartlett, J. (2010). Lung abscess. In S. Calderwood & A. Thorner (Eds.), *UpToDate.* Waltham, MA: UpToDate.

Blair, R., Breit, J., & Peters, S. (2008). Asthma. In R. Porter & J. Kaplan (Eds.), *The Merck manual online medical library.* Retrieved from http://www.merckmanuals.com/professional/pulmonary_disorders/asthma_and_related_disorders/asthma.html?qt=asthma&alt=sh

Blaivas, A. (2010). Bronchitis. Medline Plus: National Library of Medicine. Retrieved from http://www.nlm.nih.gov/medlineplus/ency/article/001087.htm

Boucher, R., Knowles, M., & Yankaskas, J. (2010). In R. Mason (Ed.), *Murray and Nadel's textbook of respiratory medicine* (5th ed.). Philadelphia: Saunders Elsevier.

Broaddus, V., & Light, R. (2010). Pleural effusion. In R. Mason (Ed.), *Murray and Nadel's textbook of respiratory medicine* (5th ed.). Philadelphia: Saunders Elsevier.

Buddiga, P. (2011). Use of metered dose inhalers, spacers, and nebulizers. Retrieved from emedicine.medscape.com/article/1413366-overview

Budev, M., & Wiedemann, H. (2010). Exposure-related interstitial lung disease. In W. Carey & R. Dweik (Eds.), *Cleveland Clinic current clinical medicine* (2nd ed.). Cleveland, OH: Saunders Elsevier.

CDC (Centers for Disease Control and Prevention). (2009). 2009 H1N1 flu. Retrieved from http://www.cdc.gov/h1n1flu/qa.htm

CDC (Centers for Disease Control and Prevention). (2010a). Leading causes of death. Retrieved from http://www.cdc.gov

CDC (Centers for Disease Control and Prevention). (2010b). Unintentional drowning: Fact sheet. Retrieved from http://www.cdc.gov/injury/index.html

CDC (Centers for Disease Control and Prevention). (2011). Antiviral agents for the treatment of chemoprophylaxis of influenza: Recommendations of the advisory committee on immunizations practices. Retrieved from http://www.cdc.gov/mmwr

Celli, B., & ZuWallack, R. (2010). Pulmonary rehabilitation. In R. Mason (Ed.), *Murray and Nadel's textbook of respiratory medicine* (5th ed.). Philadelphia: Saunders Elsevier.

Chandy, D., & Weinhouse, G. (2010). Submersion injuries (near drowning). In D. Danzl & J. Grayzel (Eds.), *UpToDate.* Waltham, MA: UpToDate.

Chapman, J. (2010). Interstitial lung disease. In W. Carey & R. Dweik (Eds.), *Cleveland Clinic current clinical medicine* (2nd ed.). Cleveland, OH: Saunders Elsevier.

Ciancio, S. G. (2009, March). The dental water jet: A product ahead of its time. *Compendium of Continuing Education in Dentistry, 30* (Spec No. 1), 7–13.

Clardy, P., Manaker, S., & Perry, H. (2010). Carbon monoxide poisoning. In S. Traub, M. Ewald, & J. Grayzel (Eds.), *UpToDate.* Waltham, MA: UpToDate.

Cowie, R., Murray, J., & Becklake, M. (2010). Pneumoconioses and other mineral dust-related diseases. In R. Mason (Ed.), *Murray and Nadel's textbook of respiratory medicine* (5th ed.). Philadelphia: Saunders Elsevier.

Culver, D. (2010). Sarcoidosis. In W. Carey & R. Dweik (Eds.), *Cleveland Clinic current clinical medicine* (2nd ed.). Cleveland, OH: Saunders Elsevier.

Cystic Fibrosis Foundation. (n.d.). About cystic fibrosis. Retrieved from http://www.cff.org/index.cfm

Davies, S., Knox, K., & Sarosi, G. (2010). Fungal infections. In R. Mason (Ed.), *Murray and Nadel's textbook of respiratory medicine* (5th ed.). Philadelphia: Saunders Elsevier.

Deriet, R., Sandrock, C., Nguyen, H., & Lawrence, R. (2011). Influenza. Retrieved from http://emedicine.medscape.com/

Doelken, P. (2009). Management of refractory nonmalignant pleural effusions. In S. Sahn & H. Hollingsworth (Eds.), *UpToDate.* Waltham, MA: UpToDate.

Dolin, R. (2011). Diagnosis of seasonal influenza in adults. In M. Hirsch & A. Thorner (Eds.), *UpToDate.* Waltham, MA: UpToDate.

Donowitz, G. (2009). Acute pneumonia. In G. Mandell, R. Dolin, & J. Bennett (Eds.), *Mandell, Douglas, and Bennett's principles and practice of infectious disease* (7th ed.). Philadelphia: Churchill Livingston Elsevier.

Ewan, V., Perry, J. D., Mawson, T., McCracken, G., Brown, A. N., Newton, J., et al. (2010, January). Detecting potential respiratory pathogens in the mouths of older people in hospital. *Age Ageing, 39*(1), 122–125. Epub 2009 Sep 11.

Fanta, C., & Fletcher, S. (2010). Diagnosis of asthma in adolescents and adults. In P. Barnes & B. Bochner (Eds.), *UpToDate.* Waltham, MA: UpToDate.

Fayyaz, J. (2012). Bronchitis. eMedicine. Retrieved from http://www.emedicine.medscape.com/article/297108-overview

Fayyaz, J. (2012). Chronic bronchitis. eMedicine. Retrieved from http://www.emedicine.medscape.com/article/297108-overview

File, T. (2010a). Epidemiology, pathogenesis, microbiology, and diagnosis of hospital-acquired ventilator-associated, and healthcare-associated pneumonia in adult. In J. Bartless & A. Thorner (Eds.), *UpToDate.* Waltham, MA: UpToDate.

File, T. (2010b). Treatment of community-acquired pneumonia in adults in the outpatient setting. In J. Bartless & A. Thorner (Eds.), *UpToDate.* Waltham, MA: UpToDate.

File, T. (2011). Acute bronchitis in adults. In D. Sexton & H. N. Sokol (Eds.), *UpToDate.* Waltham, MA: UpToDate.

Fishman, J. (2010). Common infections in immunocompromised patients. In K. Marr & A. Thorner (Eds.), *UpToDate.* Waltham, MA: UpToDate.

Global Initiative for Asthma (GINA). (2011). Global strategy for asthma management and prevention. Retrieved from http://www.ginasthma.org/Guidelines/guidelines-resources.html

Griffith, D., & Wallace, R. (2011). Overview of unotuberculous mycobacterial infections in HIV-negative patients. In C. Fordham von Reyn & A. Thorner (Eds.), *UpToDate.* Waltham, MA: UpToDate.

Hall, W., & Ahmed, B. (2007). Pulmonary disorders. In E. Duthie, P. Katx, & M. Malone (Eds.), *Practice of geriatrics* (4th ed.). Philadelphia: Saunders Elsevier.

Hanania, N., & Sharafkhaneh, A. (2010). Chronic obstructive pulmonary disease. In E. Bope, R. Kellerman, & R. Rakel (Eds.), *Bope: Conn's current therapy 2011* (1st ed.). Philadelphia: Saunders Elsevier.

Hopkins, W., & Rubin, L. (2010). Treatment of pulmonary hypertension. In J. Mandel & K. Wilson (Eds.), *UpToDate.* Waltham, MA: UpToDate.

Huang, L. (2010). Tuberculosis. In R. Mason (Ed.), *Murray and Nadel's textbook of respiratory medicine* (5th ed.). Philadelphia: Saunders Elsevier.

IOM (Institute of Medicine). (2010). *The future of nursing: Leading change, advancing health.* Washington, DC: The Academic Press.

Jones, R., Donaldson, G., Chavannes, N., Kida, K., Dickson-Spillmann, M., Harding, S. et al. (2009). Derivation and validation of a composite index of severity in chronic obstructive pulmonary disease: The DOSE index. *American Journal of Respiratory Critical Care Medicine, 180*(12), 1189–1195.

Juvelekian, G., & Stoller, J. (2010). Chronic obstructive pulmonary disease. In W. Carey (Ed.), *Cleveland Clinic current clinical medicine* (2nd ed.). Philadelphia: Saunders.

Kee, J. L. (2010). *Laboratory and diagnostic tests* (8th ed.). Upper Saddle River, NJ: Prentice Hall.

King, T. (2010). Asbestos. In K. Flaherty & H. Hollingsworth (Eds.), *UpToDate.* Waltham, MA: UpToDate.

Kruis, L.K., Adrichem, J., Erkelens, M. R., Scheepers, H., Veen, H., Muris, J. W., & Chavannes, N. H. (2010). Sustained effects of integrated COPD management on health status and exercise capacity in primary care patients. *International Journal of Chronic Obstructive Pulmonary Disease, 5*: 407–413. doi: 10.2147/COPD.S9654.

Lahmann, C., Nickel, M., Schuster, T., & Sauer, N. (2009). Functional relaxation and guided imagery as complementary therapy in asthma: A randomized controlled clinical trial. *Psychotherapy and Psychosomatics, 78*, 233–239.

Lee, F., & Treanor, J. (2010). Viral infection. In R. Mason (Ed.), *Murray and Nadel's textbook of respiratory medicine* (5th ed.). Philadelphia: Saunders Elsevier.

Lee, G. (2010). Pleural effusion of unknown etiology. In S. Sahn & H. Hollingsworth (Eds.), *UpToDate.* Waltham, MA: UpToDate.

Lorber, B. (2009). Bacterial lung abscess. In G. Mandell, R. Dolin, & J. Bennett (Eds.), *Mandell, Douglas, and Bennett's principles and practice of infectious disease* (7th ed.). Philadelphia: Churchill Livingston Elsevier.

Lugogo, N., Que, L., Fertel, D., & Kraft, M. (2010). Asthma. In R. Mason (Ed.), *Murray and Nadel's textbook of respiratory medicine* (5th ed.). Philadelphia: Saunders Elsevier.

Mazzone, P. (2010). Lung cancer. In W. Carey (Ed.), *Cleveland Clinic current clinical medicine* (2nd ed.). Philadelphia: Saunders.

McCance, K., & Huether, S. (2007). *Pathophysiology: The biological basis for disease in adults and children* (5th ed.). St. Louis: Mosby.

McLaughlin, V., Archer, S., Badesch, D., Barst, R., et al. (2009). ACCF/AHA 2009 expert consensus document on pulmonary hypertension. *Journal of the American College of Cardiology Foundation, 53*, 1573–1619.

Midthun, D. (2010). Overview of the risk factors, pathology, and clinical manifestations of lung cancer. In J. Jett & M. Ross (Eds.), *UpToDate.* Waltham, MA: UpToDate.

Morris, T., & Fedullo, P. (2010). Pulmonary thromboembolism. In R. Mason (Ed.), *Murray and Nadel's textbook of respiratory medicine* (5th ed.). Philadelphia: Saunders Elsevier.

Nardell, E. (2009). Other mycobacterial infections resembling tuberculosis. In R. Porter & J. Kaplan (Eds.), *The Merck manual online medical library.* Retrieved from http://www.merckmanuals.com/professional/infectious_diseases/mycobacteria/other_mycobacterial_infections_resembling_tuberculosis.html?qt=mycobacterial infection&alt=sh

Nardell, E. (2010). Tuberculosis. In R. Porter & J. Kaplan (Eds.), *The Merck manual online medical library.* Retrieved from http://www.merckmanuals.com/professional/infectious_diseases/mycobacteria/tuberculosis_tb.html?qt=tuberculosis&alt=sh

National Heart Lung and Blood Institute. (2007). *Expert panel report 3: Guidelines for the diagnosis and management of asthma* (NIH Publication No. 08-4051). Washington, DC: Author. Retrieved from http://www.nhlbi.nih.gov/guidelines/asthma/asthgdln.htm

Newman, L. (2009). Sarcoidosis. In R. Porter & J. Kaplan (Eds.), *The Merck manual online medical library.* Retrieved from http://www.merckmanuals.com/professional/pulmonary_disorders/sarcoidosis/sarcoidosis.html?qt=sarcoidosis&alt=sh

Patel, R. J. (2008). Idiopathic pulmonary fibrosis. Retrieved from http://www.emedicine.com.med/topic1960.htm

Peters, S. (2010). Treatment of moderate persistent asthma in adolescents and adults. In B. Bochner (Ed.), *UpToDate.* Waltham, MA: UpToDate.

Porth, C. M., & Matfin, G. (2009). *Pathophysiology: Concepts of altered health states* (8th ed.). Philadelphia: Lippincott Williams & Wilkins.

PubMed Health. (2011). Lung cancer. Retrieved from http://www.ncbi.nlm.nih.gov/pubmedhealth/PMH0004529/

Ray, J. M., & Triplett, R. G. (2011, November). What is the role of biofilms in severe head and neck infections? *Oral and Maxillofacial Surgery Clinics of North America Journal, 23*(4), 497–505.

Reilly, J., & Mentzer, S. (2010). Surgical approach to lung disease. In R. Mason (Ed.), *Murray and Nadel's textbook of respiratory medicine* (5th ed.). Philadelphia: Saunders Elsevier.

Rose, B. (2010). Amphotericin B nephrotoxicity. In R. Sterns & T. Post (Eds.), *UpToDate.* Waltham, MA: UpToDate.

Rosenstein, B. (2008). Cystic fibrosis. In R. Porter & J. Kaplan (Eds.), *The Merck manual online medical library.* Retrieved from http://www.merckmanuals.com/professional/pediatrics/cystic_fibrosis_cf/cystic_fibrosis.html?qt=cystic fibrosis&alt=sh

Rubin, L., & Hopkins, W. (2010). Overview of pulmonary hypertension. In J. Mandel & K. Wilson (Eds.), *UpToDate.* Waltham, MA: UpToDate.

Saey, D., Bernard, S., & Gagnon, P. (2009). Pulmonary rehabilitation in chronic obstructive pulmonary disease. *Panminerva Med, 51*, 95–114.

Samet, J. (2007). Occupational pulmonary disorders. In L. Goldman & D. Ausiello (Eds.), *Cecil medicine* (23rd ed.). Philadelphia: Saunders Elsevier.

Schoene, R., Nachat, A., Gravatt, A., & Newman, A. (2007). Subscriptmersion incidents: Drowning and near-drowning. In P. Auerbach (Ed.), *Wilderness medicine* (5th ed.). Philadelphia: Mosby Elsevier.

Shapiro, S., Reilly, J., & Rennard, S. (2010). Chronic bronchitis and emphysema. In R. Mason (Ed.), *Murray and Nadel's textbook of respiratory medicine* (5th ed.). Philadelphia: Saunders Elsevier.

Shochat, G. N. (2011). Carbon monoxide toxicity in emergency medicine. Retrieved from http://emedicine.medscape.com/article/819987-overview#a0104

Simonneau, G., Robbins, I., Behgetti, M., Channick, R., Delcroix, M., Denton, C.P., et al. (2009). Updated clinical classification of pulmonary hypertension. *Journal of the American College of Cardiology, 54*(1), S43–S53.

Simon, R. (2010). Cystic fibrosis: Overview of treatment of lung disease. In G. Mallory & A. Hoppin (Eds.), *UpToDate.* Waltham, MA: UpToDate.

Stein, P., Beemath, A., Matta, F., Weg, J., Yusen, R., Hales, C., et al. (2007). Clinical characteristics of patients with acute pulmonary embolism: Data from PIOPED II. *American Journal of Medicine, 120*(10), 871–879.

Strausbaugh, S., & Davis, P. (2007). Cystic fibrosis: A review of epidemiology and pathobiology. *Clinics in Chest Medicine, 28*(2), 279–288.

Takaro, T., Krieger, J., Song, L., & Sharify, D. (2011). The breathe-easy home: The impact of asthma-friendly home construction on clinical outcomes and trigger exposure. *American Journal of Public Health, 101*(1), 55–62.

Taiwo, B., & Glassroth, J. (2010). Nontuberculous mycobacterial lung diseases. *Infectious Disease Clinics of North America, 24*(3), 769–789.

Tapson, V. (2010). Treatment of acute pulmonary embolism. In J. Mandel & K. Wilson (Eds.), *UpToDate.* Waltham, MA: UpToDate.

Thompson, B., & Hales, C. (2010). Overview of acute pulmonary embolism. Retrieved from http://www.uptodate.com/contents/overview-of-acute-pulmonary-embolism?source=search_result&search=overview+of+pulmonary+embolism&selectedTitle=1%7E150

Torres, A., Mendez, R., & Wunderink, R. (2010). Pyrogenic bacterial pneumonia and lung abscess. In R. Mason (Ed.), *Murray and Nadel's textbook of respiratory medicine* (5th ed.). Philadelphia: Saunders Elsevier.

Turner, R. (2009). Influenza. In R. Porter & J. Kaplan (Eds.), *The Merck manual online medical library.* Retrieved from http://www.merckmanuals.com/professional/infectious_diseases/respiratory_viruses/influenza.html?qt=influenza&alt=sh

U.S. Department of Health and Human Services. (2010). *Healthy People 2020* topics and objectives. Retrieved from http://www.healthypeople.gov/2020/topicsobjectives2020/default.aspx

Weinberger, S. (2007). Sarcoidosis. In L. Goldman & D. Ausiello (Eds.), *Cecil medicine* (23rd ed.). Philadelphia: Saunders Elsevier.

Welsh, M. (2007). Cystic fibrosis. In L. Goldman & D. Ausiello (Eds.), *Cecil medicine* (23rd ed.). Philadelphia: Saunders Elsevier.

Wiedemann, H. (2011). Cor pulmonale. In J. Mandel & K. Wilson (Eds.), *UpToDate.* Waltham, MA: UpToDate.

Wilkinson, J. M., & Ahearn, N. R. (2009). *Prentice Hall nursing diagnosis handbook* (9th ed.). Upper Saddle River, NJ: Prentice Hall.

Wilson, B. A., Shannon, M. T., Shields, K. M., & Stang, C. L. (2007). *Nurse's drug guide 2007.* Upper Saddle River, NJ: Prentice Hall.

Wilson, S., & Huttlinger, K. (2010). Pandemic flu knowledge among dormitory housed university students: A need for informal social support and social networking strategies. *Rural and Remote Health, 10*(4), 1526. Retrieved from http://www.rrh.org.au/articles/showarticlenew.asp?ArticleID=1526

World Health Organization (WHO). (2009). *Global tuberculosis control 2009: Epidemiology, strategy, financing.* Retrieved from http://www.who.int/tb/publications/en/

Wryobeck, J. M., Lippo, G., McLaughlin, V., Riba, M., & Rubenfire, M. (2007). Psychosocial aspects of pulmonary hypertension: A review. *Psychosomatics, 48*(6), 467–475.

CHAPTER

28 Caring for the Patient with Complex Respiratory Disorders

Carol Rhoades
Cheryl Wraa

Outcome-Based Learning Objectives

After studying this chapter, the learner will be able to:

1. Compare and contrast the etiology, incidence, and types of acute respiratory failure.
2. Define pulmonary edema and state three of the common etiologies of pulmonary edema.
3. Differentiate between noncardiogenic pulmonary edema and cardiogenic pulmonary edema in terms of patient symptomatology.
4. Determine the risk factors for ALI/ARDS.
5. Compare and contrast the common ventilator modes and important nursing implications for each mode.
6. Generate a plan of care for a ventilator-dependent patient.

KEY TERMS

acute lung injury (ALI) p.800
acute pulmonary edema p.794
acute respiratory distress syndrome (ARDS) p.800
acute respiratory failure (ARF) p.792
air-mask-bag unit (AMBU) p.804
alveolar ventilation (V_A) p.793
anatomic dead space p.793
barotrauma p.811
BiPAP p.818
cardiogenic pulmonary edema (CPE) p.794
continuous positive airway pressure (CPAP) p.810
dead space ventilation (V_D) p.792
endotracheal tube p.804
fraction of inspired oxygen (FiO_2) p.806
high-altitude pulmonary edema (HAPE) p.795
hypercapnia p.793
hypoventilation p.793
hypoxemia p.793
minute ventilation (V_E) p.801
negative pressure pulmonary edema (NPPE) p.795
neurogenic pulmonary edema (NPE) p.795
noncardiogenic pulmonary edema (NCPE) p.795
noninvasive positive pressure ventilation (NPPV) p.817
positive end-expiratory pressure (PEEP) p.810
perfusion (Q) p.792
shunt p.792
shunt ventilation p.792
surfactant p.791
ventilator-associated pneumonia (VAP) p.812
ventilation (V) p.792
ventilation/perfusion mismatching (V/Q) p.792
volutrauma p.811

PATIENTS WHO CAN'T BREATHE are one of the most challenging groups of patients for nurses. These patients can be agitated and confused or unconscious and apneic. They might require emergency arterial blood gases (ABGs) or an immediate lifesaving intervention such as intubation. They may need ventilator support and require immediate suctioning for a mucus plug or develop a tension pneumothorax that necessitates emergent placement of a chest tube.

This chapter addresses the different types of complex respiratory disorders that result in an alteration in oxygen perfusion to the tissues. It is important for the nurse to understand basic pulmonary physiology in order to care for patients with these complex respiratory disorders. The chapter discusses the relationship between oxygen and hemoglobin, how ventilation/perfusion mismatching produces hypoxemia, and the role of the alveolar–capillary membrane in respiratory failure. The reader is referred to other chapters to review such topics as interpretation of ABGs and other pertinent pulmonary physiology.

The heart and lungs are inextricably linked, and what affects one eventually affects the other. An appreciation of this association will aid the nurse in understanding complex disorders of the respiratory system. Respiratory complications are frequently a result of a primary disorder somewhere else in the body. Therefore, determining the primary organ system failure and focusing on the treatment of this pathology are the goals in treating many of the complex respiratory disorders. The nursing management of patients with complex respiratory disorders focuses on airway management and maintaining oxygen for tissue perfusion. A description of the complex respiratory disorders follows. The nursing management is similar for these disorders; therefore, nursing management is discussed after the descriptions of all the disorders, rather than with each one.

Respiratory Physiology

The acinus, the functional unit of gas exchange, is the terminal respiratory unit of the lung. It is composed of all structures from the respiratory

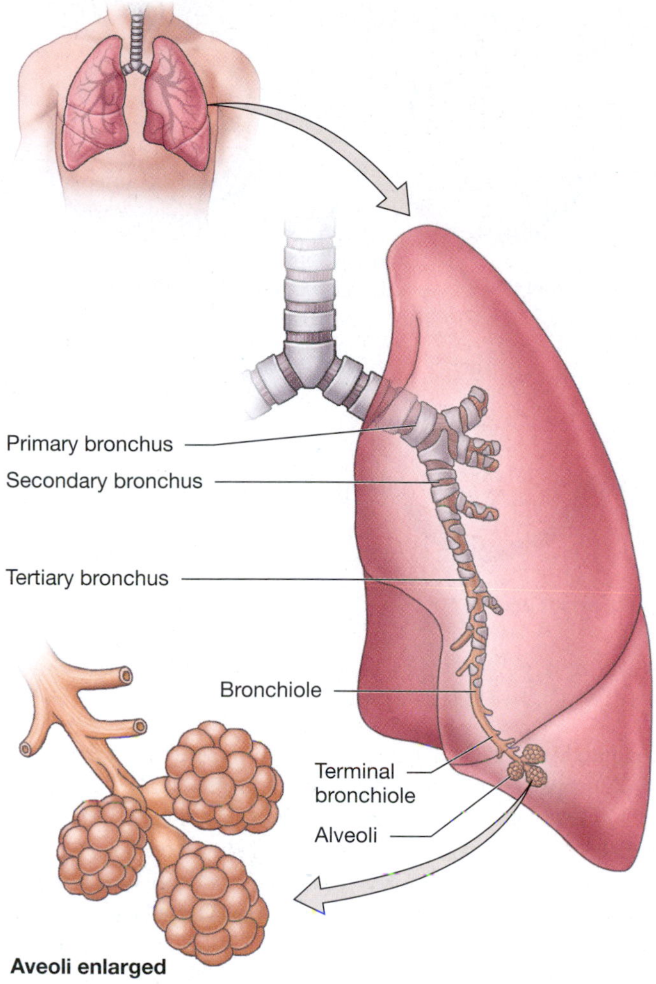

FIGURE 28–1 ◆ Alveoli with bronchioles.

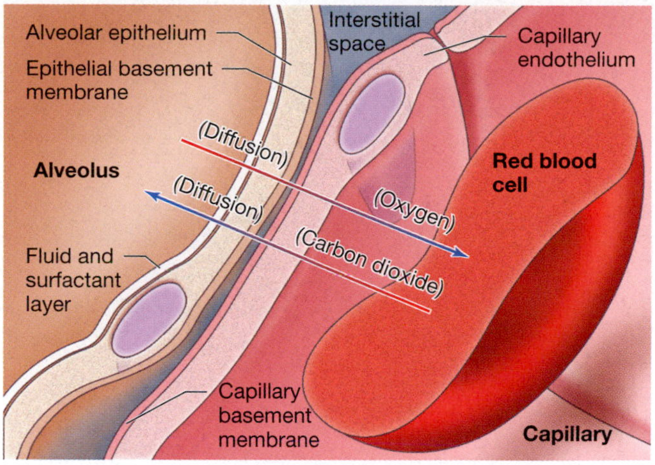

FIGURE 28–2 ◆ Alveolar-capillary membrane.

bronchiole to the alveolus, including alveolar ducts, alveolar sacs, and alveoli. These groups or acini permit 300 million alveoli to fit into the human thorax, providing a huge surface area for gas exchange and making the pulmonary organ system very efficient. Figure 28–1◆ represents a section of the lung showing many alveoli. The alveolar epithelium is coated with a thin fluid layer. An important component of this fluid layer is surfactant. **Surfactant** is a surface-active agent that promotes alveolar stability and reduces the likelihood of alveolar collapse. The type II alveolar cells that line the alveoli and the small bronchioles produce surfactant. The alveolus basement membrane provides structure for the alveolus. The next structure, in the middle of the membranes that separate the alveoli from the pulmonary capillary, is a potential space called the interstitial space (Figure 28–2◆).

The alveolar–capillary membrane (air–blood barrier) is the central component of gas exchange in the lungs. It is a very thin, strong barrier composed of surfactant, alveolar epithelium, capillary endothelium, and the basement membrane. The alveolar–capillary membrane (1) permits gas exchange between the alveoli and pulmonary capillary blood; (2) regulates the flux of fluid and solute between alveoli, interstitium, and blood; and (3) promotes fluid clearance from the alveolar lumen to the interstitial space. In the normal alveolar–capillary membrane, the interstitial space contains little or no fluid. In addition to the interstitial space, the pulmonary capillary is composed of a basement membrane and a capillary endothelium through which the gases diffuse. The oxygen diffuses into the red blood cells in the pulmonary capillary and attaches to the hemoglobin molecule. What is not shown in Figure 28–2 is the lymphatic system in the lungs, which allows transudated fluid to drain from the lungs into the lymph for removal. The pulmonary lymphatics prevent accumulation of fluid in the interstitial space. Normally, pressures exerted by water (hydrostatic pressure) and proteins (oncotic pressure) prevent fluid in the pulmonary capillaries and the lymphatics from entering the alveoli.

The alveoli are uniquely structured to prevent fluid from filling their air-filled spaces. The distance between the alveolus and the capillary is less than 0.3 micron (a micron is one millionth of a meter). Oxygen moves from the alveolus into the pulmonary capillary and carbon dioxide moves from the pulmonary capillary to the alveolus by simple passive diffusion, in which a substance moves from an area of higher concentration to one of lower concentration. The concentration (pressure) of CO_2 is higher in the pulmonary capillaries than it is in the alveoli, and the inverse is true for oxygen. This concentration gradient supports the diffusion of gases across the membrane.

Oxyhemoglobin Dissociation Curve

The oxyhemoglobin dissociation curve is a commonly used tool for understanding how blood carries and releases oxygen (Figure 28–3◆). Specifically, the oxyhemoglobin dissociation curve shows the percentage of oxygen saturation (SaO_2) at different oxygen pressures (PaO_2). This is determined by what is called hemoglobin's affinity for oxygen, that is, how readily hemoglobin acquires and releases oxygen molecules from its surrounding tissue. Oxygen saturation does not change significantly above a PaO_2 of 60 mmHg (flat portion of the curve). However, once a PaO_2 drops below 60 mmHg (steep portion of the curve), a very small change in PaO_2 causes a rapid decline in oxygen saturation. The curve can move to either the right or the left depending on the body's oxygen requirements. When the curve shifts to the right (lower saturations for a given PaO_2), the hemoglobin has less affinity for oxygen and O_2 is released easily to the cells. Increased carbon dioxide, decreased pH, and hyperthermia (heat, acidosis, and exercise) are three conditions in which the body requires increased access to oxygen so the hemoglobin more readily releases it. A shift to the left means that it is more difficult for hemoglobin to release oxygen to the tissues. Such a shift is caused by an increased pH, decreased carbon dioxide, and hypothermia. A clear understanding of the association between oxygen and hemoglobin is important to understand the respiratory system pathophysiology.

Weblink: Respiratory Failure

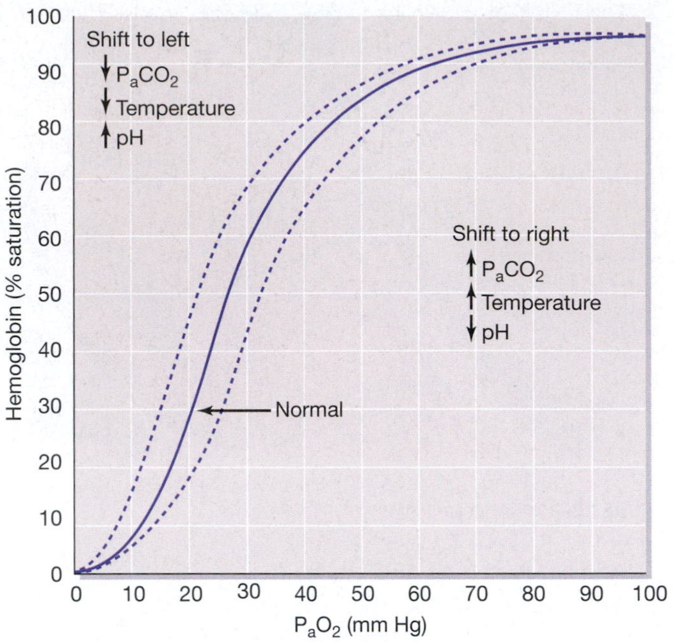

FIGURE 28–3 ◆ Oxyhemoglobin dissociation curve.

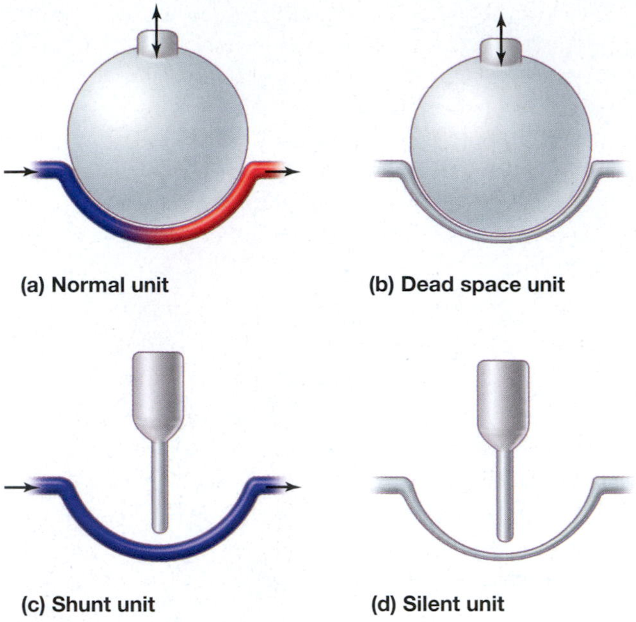

FIGURE 28–4 ◆ Ventilation/perfusion relationships: (A) normal unit; (B) dead space unit; (C) shunt unit; (D) silent unit.

Shunts and the Oxyhemoglobin Dissociation Curve

A **shunt** occurs when one thing bypasses another. In pulmonary physiology, a shunt can be anatomic or physiologic. An anatomic shunt occurs when blood bypasses the lungs, such as through an open channel between the right and left ventricles (ventricular septal defect) or a pulmonary anomaly in which blood flows directly from the pulmonary artery to a pulmonary vein. Increasing the fraction of inspired oxygen (FiO_2) will not improve oxygenation in these conditions. This is an important diagnostic clue that assists the health care professional in determining the cause of the hypoxemia. A physiological shunt occurs when blood goes through the regular pulmonary vasculature normally but does not come into contact with the air in the alveoli. This form of shunting is often seen in conditions such as pulmonary edema, pneumonia, and atelectasis (collapse of a segment of the lung) in which the alveoli are filled with fluid or collapsed. Low ventilation/perfusion states, discussed in the following text, are a form of physiologic shunt. Most patients with shunts do not have increased CO_2 levels in the blood because their respiratory center is responding to the hypoxemia by increasing the respiratory rate, thereby maintaining a near normal or slightly low level of CO_2.

Ventilation/Perfusion Mismatching

In pulmonary physiology, **ventilation (V)** refers to the inhaled *air* that reaches the alveoli and **perfusion (Q)** is the *blood* that reaches the alveoli. These are the primary determinants of blood oxygenation. The relationship between these two measurements is referred to as the V/Q ratio. Ideally, the amount of perfusion to the alveoli should equal the amount of ventilation to the alveoli, in which case the ratio would be close to 1.0. However, because different areas of the lung have varying degrees of ventilation and perfusion, the average value is actually closer to 0.8. When ventilation and perfusion are not matched or are only nearly matched, this state is referred to as **ventilation/perfusion mismatching (V/Q).** Figure 28–4A◆ shows an example of a unit in which the perfusion is normal and the ventilation is also normal; that is, V/Q is equal to 0.8. In Figure 28–4B, there is ventilation but no perfusion—note the air sac or alveoli without blood flow, hence no perfusion. This phenomenon is referred to as a **dead space ventilation (Vd),** or high V/Q, because there is normal ventilation and little if any perfusion. Examples of diseases in which there is a high V/Q ratio are pulmonary emboli and cardiogenic shock (decreased blood flow—perfusion—to the lungs). Figure 28–4C shows an example in which perfusion is normal but the alveoli are not adequately ventilated. This is referred to as **shunt ventilation** or low V/Q. In the example, there is perfusion but little or no ventilation—note that the air sac is collapsed. This occurs in atelectasis, pulmonary edema, pneumonia, asthma, and many other disorders that cause respiratory failure. Figure 28–4D demonstrates both abnormalities, in which neither ventilation nor perfusion occurs. Increasing the oxygen concentration can correct most types of hypoxemia caused by V/Q mismatch.

Acute Respiratory Failure

Acute respiratory failure (ARF) is a syndrome characterized by a failure of the lungs to oxygenate the blood and/or to remove carbon dioxide from the blood. The lungs no longer meet the body's physiological needs because of a failure of the heart, lungs, or both. The hallmark of ARF is respiratory difficulty with abnormal ABGs. Acute pulmonary edema, acute respiratory distress syndrome, and acute lung injury are common types of ARF that are discussed in more detail later in this chapter.

Etiology

The pulmonary system's purpose is to provide oxygen to the Body's cells and remove carbon dioxide and other waste products of metabolism. The respiratory system's inability to accomplish this function is termed *respiratory failure* and can have life-threatening consequences. Because respiratory failure is considered a syndrome, not a single disease process, its overall frequency is not well known (Kaynar, 2012).

Respiratory failure is classified as hypoxic (inadequate oxygenation) or hypercarbic (excessive carbon dioxide) respiratory failure. A failure of oxygenation produces **hypoxemia,** which is defined as an arterial oxygen tension or pressure (PaO_2) that is below normal range. The normal range of PaO_2 is between 80 and 100 mmHg. Therefore, a PaO_2 of less than 60 mmHg and an arterial saturation of oxygen (SaO_2) of less than 90% while breathing room air is representative of hypoxemic respiratory failure. This value of 60 mmHg is located on the steep part of the oxyhemoglobin dissociation curve (see Figure 28–3).

Safety Alert *The nurse should assess the patient carefully and notify the health care provider when $PaO_2 < 60$ mmHg from ABGs or $SpO_2 < 90\%$.*

The respiratory system's failure to ventilate produces the clinical sign of hypercapnia, also termed hypercarbia. **Hypercapnia** is a concentration of carbon dioxide ($PaCO_2$) in the blood above the normal range of between 35 and 45 mmHg. A $PaCO_2$ of greater than 45 mmHg represents hypercapnic respiratory failure and is associated with a pH of less than 7.35.

Acute respiratory failure happens quickly, over hours to days, and is not characterized by a gradual worsening of symptoms that would portray chronic respiratory failure. Chart 28–1 lists the major etiologies causing acute respiratory failure. This chart is divided into hypoxemic respiratory failure and hypercapnic respiratory failure.

Hypoventilation

With hypoventilation, the level of CO_2 in the blood rises because CO_2 is not exhaled adequately. Causes of hypoventilation include the following:

- Depressed central respiratory drive
- Obesity and obstructive sleep apnea
- COPD
- Chest wall deformity: trauma, kyphoscoliosis
- Neuromuscular disease: myasthenia gravis, Guillain-Barré syndrome, muscular dystrophy, amyotrophic lateral sclerosis.

CHART 28–1 Etiology of Acute Respiratory Failure

Type of Respiratory Failure	Diagnosis/Disease: Examples
Hypoxic respiratory failure	Acute lung injury
	Acute respiratory distress syndrome
	Pneumothorax
	Pneumonia
	Pulmonary thromboembolism
	Atelectasis
	Cardiogenic pulmonary edema
	Acute collagen vascular disease (Goodpasture's, lupus)
Hypercapnic respiratory failure	Medications causing respiratory depression
	Pulmonary diseases: COPD, asthma
	Neuromuscular
	Guillain-Barré syndrome
	Acute myasthenia gravis
	Spinal cord tumors
	Kyphoscoliosis
	Obesity

Although many patients with hypoventilation are also hypoxemic, oxygen therapy alone is inadequate in patients with hypercapnic respiratory failure. In some patients, such as those with COPD, oxygen therapy will widen the ventilation/perfusion mismatch and may worsen hypercapnia. Attention should focus on the cause of hypoventilation and making improvements in ventilation rather than oxygenation.

Hypoxemia

Hypoxic respiratory failure is usually caused by:

- Decreased fraction of inspired oxygen (FiO_2) at high altitude (less oxygen is available in the air)
- Ventilation/perfusion mismatch, which may occur in airway disease (asthma, COPD, bronchitis, pneumonia), interstitial lung disease, or disease of the pulmonary vasculature (pulmonary embolus, pulmonary hypertension)
- Anatomic shunt, which may occur in vascular disease (arteriovenous malformation), cardiac septal defects, or intrapulmonary alveolar disease (adult respiratory distress syndrome, atelectasis, pulmonary edema, pneumonia)
- Hypoventilation (see the previous text)
- Diffusion impairment caused by an interstitial lung disease.

Pathophysiology

As previously discussed, acute respiratory failure can be divided into two categories: hypoxic respiratory failure or hypercapnic respiratory failure. Hypercapnic respiratory failure is a result of alveolar hypoventilation. By definition, **hypoventilation** is decreased gas entering the alveoli per unit of time. **Alveolar ventilation (V_A)** is the cumulative gas exchange that takes place among all the alveoli. Although hypoventilation is a function of respiratory rate, the accurate measure of hypoventilation is the amount of gas exchanged at the alveolar level. It is not the quantity of gas that enters the large airways because the large airways, the trachea, and the bronchi down to the terminal bronchioles have no role in gas exchange. Their role is to transport ambient air beyond the terminal bronchioles where oxygen first meets the alveoli. These transporting airways compose the **anatomic dead space** because no gas exchange occurs. Ventilation of this anatomic region is defined as dead space ventilation (V_D).

Clinical Manifestations

Pulmonary symptoms, such as cough, sputum, and rales, are often related to the underlying cause of respiratory failure. The presenting symptom in acute respiratory failure regardless of cause is usually shortness of breath and tachypnea. Neurological function may deteriorate, and progressive failure may lead to fatigue and respiratory arrest. Chart 28–2 on page 794 compares the clinical manifestations of hypoxemic respiratory failure with those of hypercapnic respiratory failure.

The central cyanosis of hypoxemic respiratory failure and the muscle twitching caused by the acidosis in hypercapnic respiratory failure are unique for each condition. The patient with only hypoxemic respiratory failure will rarely become sleepy and usually will not have difficulty being aroused, but the patient who has high CO_2 levels commonly presents with somnolence and a decreased level of consciousness. It is important to understand that hypoventilation can lead to hypoxemia and that the symptoms can occur in tandem.

CHART 28–2 Clinical Manifestations of Acute Respiratory Failure

System	Signs/Symptoms	Hypoxemic Failure	Hypercapnic Failure
Respiratory	Dyspnea	✓	✓
	Tachypnea	✓	✓
Neurological	Anxiety	✓	
	Confusion	✓	
	Headache		✓
	Slurred speech		✓
	Lethargy/somnolence		✓
	Tremor		✓
	Asterixis (tremor of the wrist when extended)		✓
	Seizure	✓	
	Coma	✓	✓
Cardiac	Tachycardia	✓	
	Dysrhythmias (bradycardia, ventricular ectopy)	✓	
	Diaphoresis		✓
	Hypertension or hypotension	✓	

Laboratory and Diagnostic Procedures

ABGs are used to diagnose respiratory failure. The patient's history, physical assessment, and additional diagnostic tests, such as chest radiography, are used to identify the cause. See the Diagnostic Tests box for tests used in diagnosing acute respiratory failure.

Medical Management

The goals of medical management of acute respiratory failure are (1) correction of hypoxemia, (2) improving life-threatening acidosis, (3) maintaining or improving compromised cardiac output, (4) identifying and treating underlying cause, and (5) avoiding complications (Hudson & Slutsky, 2007). Hypercapnia is generally tolerated better than hypoxemia unless severe acidosis is present. Supplemental oxygen should be given until targeted treatment can reverse the hypoxemia.

Safety Alert *To treat life-threatening hypoxemia that does not respond to supplemental oxygen, endotracheal intubation is necessary. The nurse must have the knowledge and understanding to be able to assist with this procedure.*

Acute Respiratory Disorders

Acute Pulmonary Edema

Acute pulmonary edema is an abnormal accumulation of fluid in the lungs that can lead to acute respiratory failure. This fluid accumulates because of dysfunction of the lungs and/or the heart. The two categories of pulmonary edema are cardiogenic (generated by heart dysfunction) and noncardiogenic (having a noncardiac etiology). Acute pulmonary edema may be attributed to many different etiologies and types of pulmonary edema, which are discussed in the following text. These etiologies have different names, but all can be traced back to a failure of the heart, lungs, or both. Heart failure is discussed in detail in Chapter 34.

Epidemiology

Cardiogenic pulmonary edema (CPE) is a symptom of advanced heart failure. Heart failure is arguably the fastest-growing type of cardiac disease in the United States, with 2% of the population affected (Lloyd-Jones et al., 2009). Approximately 5% to 10% of patients with heart failure develop advanced stage disease typical of pulmonary edema. Cardiac disease is discussed in full detail in Unit VII.

Noncardiogenic pulmonary edema is a common medical problem with multiple etiologies. Adult respiratory distress syndrome (ARDS) and acute lung injury (ALI) are the most common causes. The prevalence of ALI is 86 per 100,000 people, and for ARDS is 64 per 100,000 people. As people age, the incidence increases for both; for those over 75 years, the incidence is 306 per 100,000 people (Siegel, 2011a).

Etiology

Whether pulmonary edema is acute or chronic depends on the time frame during which the fluid accumulation develops. In acute pulmonary edema, this occurs quickly, over minutes to hours. Some clinicians

DIAGNOSTIC TESTS for Acute Respiratory Failure

Test with Description, Rationale, and Normal Values	Expected Abnormalities
Arterial Blood Gases (ABGs)	
pH 7.35–7.45; $PaCO_2$ 35–45; PaO_2 75–100; HCO_3 24–28 *Measures the degree of hypoxemia and hypercarbia and determines hypoxic respiratory failure versus hypercapnic respiratory failure, or both. Identifies acid–base imbalance.*	pH $<$ 7.35 = academia PaO_2 $<$ 60 mmHg = hypoxemia $PaCO_2$ $>$ 45 mmHg = respiratory acidosis HCO_3 $<$ 24 = metabolic acidosis A low HCO_3 identifies a metabolic source of respiratory failure, such as sepsis. An elevated $PaCO_2$ identifies a respiratory cause of respiratory failure, such as COPD.
Chest Radiography (CXR, CT SCAN, MRI)	
Clear; no pathology *Used to identify possible etiology of respiratory failure such as pulmonary edema, ARDS, pneumonia, heart failure, COPD/asthma exacerbation, neoplasm.*	Consolidation (lung parenchyma is engorged with fluid), atelectasis, effusions, pneumothorax, cardiomegaly, and so on, that may contribute to respiratory failure.

use the term *flash pulmonary edema* to define pulmonary edema that occurs within minutes of a precipitating event. Reported causes of flash pulmonary edema include the classic cardiac pathologies of left ventricular dysfunction as a result of a massive myocardial infarction (MI) or valve dysfunction with or without papillary muscle rupture. When the pulmonary capillary pressure rises quickly and reaches two to three times the normal pressures in the pulmonary arteries, edema fluid floods the interstitial space. The pulmonary lymphatic system and other vessels have no time to compensate, so as the interstitial space quickly reaches its limit, fluid invades the alveoli. The etiology of pulmonary edema is divided into cardiogenic and noncardiogenic categories.

Cardiogenic Pulmonary Edema

Cardiogenic pulmonary edema (CPE) is pulmonary edema that results from left ventricular pump failure. Heart failure can be from cardiac muscle dysfunction or valvular problems. Dysrhythmias, especially tachydysrhythmias, such as supraventricular and ventricular tachycardias, can precipitate pulmonary edema.

Noncardiogenic Pulmonary Edema

Noncardiogenic pulmonary edema (NCPE) is pulmonary edema that is not caused by cardiac dysfunction. There are multiple etiologies that contribute to the development of NCPE (see Chart 28–3). Causes of NCPE include neurogenic injury, airway obstruction, high altitude, opiates, fluid overload, and toxin exposure.

One of the syndromes that is listed as a cause of NCPE is ARDS/ALI (acute respiratory distress syndrome/acute lung injury). Because of its prevalence and high mortality rate, this disease is discussed in more detail later in this chapter. Other forms of NCPE are listed in the following text.

Neurogenic Pulmonary Edema

Neurogenic pulmonary edema (NPE) is associated with direct insult to the central nervous system (CNS). It usually develops soon after the CNS injury. Seizures, cerebral hemorrhage, and traumatic brain injury are common precipitating factors in the development of NPE (Chapter 22). The pathophysiology of the edema formation is not clear, but it may be related to disruption in sympathetic tone related to increased venous pressure and hypertension. The most common symptom for these patients is dyspnea. Hemoptysis, tachypnea, tachycardia, and rales may also occur. Management of NPE includes treating the underlying events as well as supportive care. Most cases of NPE resolve within 48 to 72 hours (Mandel & Drislane, 2010).

Negative Pressure Pulmonary Edema

Negative pressure pulmonary edema (NPPE) is caused by attempting to breathe or ventilate against an airway obstruction. Postobstruction pulmonary edema and airway obstruction pulmonary edema are other names for the same disorder. This type of pulmonary edema occurs when negative intrathoracic pressure develops during forced inspiration against a closed glottis, such as with laryngospasm or airway obstruction (Johnson & Conde, 2010). As intrathoracic pressure becomes more negative, blood return to the right heart increases. This leads to pulmonary vessel dilation and an increase in the negative pressure in the interstitial space, causing a shift of fluid from the vasculature into the interstitium and the alveoli. This process will initiate a series of events that causes hypoxemia, catecholamine release, and systemic and pulmonary hypertension (Johnson & Conde, 2010). Patients who are at risk of NPPE include patients with obesity, a history of obstructive sleep apnea, a history of upper airway obstruction, and a history of ear, nose, or throat surgery. Pulmonary edema usually occurs immediately after the obstruction is relieved but can present several hours later. Treatment is primarily supportive with oxygen and diuresis. Bronchodilators and noninvasive positive airway pressure may prove beneficial.

High-Altitude Pulmonary Edema

High-altitude pulmonary edema (HAPE) is a form of noncardiogenic pulmonary edema precipitated by hypoxia due to low atmospheric pressures and low oxygen content at high altitudes. It is the most common cause of death related to high altitude. Any person who travels to high altitude is at risk, although some people seem to have a genetic predisposition to developing HAPE. HAPE generally develops within 2 to 4 days in persons who ascend to an altitude greater than 8,000 feet. Risk factors include genetic predisposition, degree of cold, altitude reached, rate of ascent, time spent at altitude, and underlying medical conditions (Gallagher & Hackett, 2011; Hackett & Roach, 2007).

The pathogenesis of the formation of pulmonary edema is unclear. The hypothesis is that diffuse pulmonary vasoconstriction occurs in response to environmental hypoxia, leading to pulmonary hypertension. This increases the pressure in the pulmonary capillaries, thus forcing fluid into the interstitial space and the alveoli. A direct injury

CHART 28–3 Common Causes of Acute Pulmonary Edema

Cause of Acute Pulmonary Edema	Disease/Condition
Increased pulmonary capillary pressure	Cardiogenic: left ventricular failure
	Noncardiogenic: pulmonary venous fibrosis, pulmonary occlusive disease
Increased pulmonary capillary permeability	Pneumonia: bacterial, viral, radiation-induced, aspiration
	ARDS/ALI
	Toxins
	Vasoactive substances, such as antihistamines
	Sepsis
	Immunologic reactions, such as transfusion reaction
	Immersion injury (near drowning)
	Smoke inhalation
	Uremia
Lymphatic insufficiency	Congenital or acquired
Decreased oncotic pressure	Hypoalbuminemia
	Malnutrition
	Protein loss
Increased negative	Upper airway obstruction (croup, epiglottitis, laryngospasm)
interstitial pressure	Re-expansion pulmonary edema
	Neurogenic
Mixed or unknown	High-altitude
etiology	Eclampsia (seizure in a pregnant woman that is not related to a preexisting brain condition)
	Pancreatitis
	Pulmonary embolism
	Heroin/narcotic

Source: Adapted from Mazor, R., & Green, T. (2011). Pulmonary edema. In R. Kliegman, B. Stanton, J. St. Geme III, N. Schor, & R. Behman (Eds.), *Nelson textbook of pediatrics* (19th ed.). Philadelphia: Elsevier-Saunders.

pattern from inflammatory mediators and oxygen free radicals also are believed to be responsible for some of the pulmonary capillary direct injury. Oxygen free radicals are components of oxygen that have an unpaired electron on an oxygen atom. These free radicals are believed to cause tissue injury at the cellular level. Symptoms of HAPE include nonproductive cough and exertional dyspnea. As the disease progresses, dyspnea becomes more severe and occurs at rest. Pink, frothy sputum or frank blood may be expectorated, and inspiratory crackles can be auscultated. Treatment of HAPE involves early recognition and immediate intervention. The most important treatment involves evacuation to lower altitude, supplemental oxygen, and limitation of cold exposure and physical exertion. This treatment is often effective. Hyperbaric therapy (see Chapter 27), noninvasive positive airway pressure, nifedipine, dexamethasone, and pulmonary vasodilators such as tadalafil and sildenafil have all been used in more severe cases (Hackett & Roach, 2007). Refer to the Pharmacology box on page 799.

Heroin-Induced Pulmonary Edema

Another type of noncardiogenic pulmonary edema, heroin-induced pulmonary edema (HIPE), develops within 24 hours of the administration of heroin, usually in the first several hours after injection. It can also occur with other opiates, including methadone and codeine. It is unknown why the injection of heroin induces pulmonary edema, but it is postulated that it causes either a direct injury or hypoxic injury to the alveolar–capillary membrane, leading to extravasation of fluid into the pulmonary interstitium (Maldonado & Limper, 2010). Treatment includes supplemental oxygen, mechanical ventilation using positive end-expiratory pressure (PEEP) (p. 810), and IV naloxone to reverse respiratory depression.

Excessive Intravenous Fluid Administration

Any patient who has a continuous intravenous infusion and receives a large amount of fluid over a short period of time can develop pulmonary edema. If the patient has any comorbidities such as cardiac, pulmonary, or renal disease, the risk of developing pulmonary edema increases. The pathophysiology of this type of pulmonary edema is very clear. Increased venous return of the excessive fluid contributes to increased pulmonary pressures that cause fluid to leak into interstitial spaces and then into the alveoli. Dialysis-dependent patients are at increased risk for this type of pulmonary edema. Fluid management for the patient who is in renal failure presents a challenge because under-resuscitation of hypotension can be as harmful as overresuscitation. Failure of the dialysis-dependent patient to follow dietary restrictions (e.g., salt intake) predisposes the patient to pulmonary edema.

Transfusion-Related Lung Injury

Patients who receive any type of transfusion are at risk for transfusion-related acute lung injury (TRALI), which can cause noncardiogenic pulmonary edema. Any blood product can precipitate TRALI, and whole blood, packed red blood cells, platelets, and fresh frozen plasma are the most commonly cited precipitators. This syndrome has also been reported following allogeneic stem cell transplantation. The classic symptoms of dyspnea, hypoxemia, and bilateral pulmonary edema occur within 4 to 6 hours of administration of blood products. A large percentage of the patients require support with either intubation or noninvasive ventilation. An impressive feature of this type of NCPE is the speed of development and onset of pulmonary edema. TRALI is discussed in detail in Chapter 16.

Toxin- and Drug-Related Pulmonary Edema

Toxin- and drug-related NCPE can be caused by inhalants or oral or parenteral toxins. Inhalants can cause direct injury to the lung, while orally or parenterally administered drugs and toxins can lead to NCPE by altering the clearance of fluid in the lungs or by targeting parenchymal or lung endothelium (Mullen, 2007). Most inhalants cause NCPE by causing lower airway irritation, and some may trigger a chemical reaction with lung tissue. In addition, some agents cause systemic toxicity and may add a cardiogenic component to the pulmonary edema. The more water-soluble an inhalant is, such as ammonia, the more likely it is to cause upper airway irritation rather than penetrating into lower airway and lung tissue. However, long exposure times can cause extensive lung injury. Phosgene, a highly toxic gas with a wide variety of industrial applications, is poorly water-soluble and may lead to cardiogenic pulmonary edema and cardiac anoxia. Other inhalants that are known to cause NCPE include acid fumes (hydrogen chloride, hydrogen fluoride, sulfur dioxide, sulfuric acid), bromine, chlorine, hydrogen sulfide, and fumigants.

In addition to heroin and methadone, discussed earlier, other known oral and parenteral agents that are toxic to the pulmonary system include opiate antagonists (naloxone), nonsteroidal anti-inflammatories (salicylate), thiazide diuretics, calcium-channel blockers, cytotoxins, and radiographic contrast agents (Mullen, 2007). Some bioterrorism agents, such as ricin and anthrax, also cause pulmonary injury and NCPE. More information on these types of agents is given in Chapter 65. Treatment of toxin exposure is largely supportive until the clinical manifestations subside.

Pathophysiology

The pathophysiology of acute pulmonary edema and the signs and symptoms of this dysfunction are related to the accumulation of fluid preventing adequate gas exchange across the alveolar–capillary membrane. This fluid accumulates in the interstitial space and floods the alveoli, thereby interfering with gas exchange.

Pathophysiology of Cardiogenic Pulmonary Edema

CPE results from left ventricular pump failure that leads to increased left ventricular filling pressures and consequently elevated pulmonary pressures. This can be caused by systolic dysfunction, diastolic dysfunction, valvular dysfunction, or pericardial tamponade. Refer to Chapter 34 for detailed descriptions of these disorders. Basically, the heart cannot sufficiently pump blood that is delivered to it, and this causes a backup, which increases the pressures in the pulmonary system. This pulmonary hypertension forces plasma to move from the pulmonary capillaries into the alveoli and pulmonary interstitium. The lymphatic system is responsible for removing excess fluid from the interstitium and may initially be effective; however, as drainage continues or increases, it may overwhelm the pulmonary lymphatic capacity. As fluid in the interstitium reaches capacity, fluid is forced into the alveoli. At this point, respiratory volumes and vital capacity are reduced, gas exchange is abnormal, and hypoxemia becomes severe. Eventually, if treatment is not instituted, more alveoli become flooded with fluid and collapse. Surfactant is washed out and deactivated. Lung compliance falls, and the work of breathing increases as more and more of the lung becomes unavailable for gas exchange. Chart 28–4 lists the stages of cardiogenic pulmonary edema. The pathophysiology of heart failure is discussed in detail in Chapter 34.

Pathophysiology of Noncardiogenic Pulmonary Edema

NCPE can be caused by increased capillary permeability, increased pulmonary capillary pressure, lymphatic insufficiency, decreased oncotic pressure, increased negative interstitial pressure, or unknown causes (see Chart 28–3). Regardless of the cause, the net result is fluid in the interstitium; if the pulmonary lymphatic capacity for fluid removal is reached, fluid will accumulate in the interstitium and alveoli.

CHART 28–4 Stages of Cardiogenic Pulmonary Edema

Stage	Physiological Abnormality
Stage I	Fluid and colloids move into the lungs' interstitial space from the pulmonary capillaries. The lymphatics are able to increase flow and remove the fluid. Blood gas exchange does not deteriorate, or it may even be slightly improved.
Stage II	The lymphatics become overwhelmed with fluid, and the efficient pump fails. The lung interstitial space becomes flooded. The interstitial space in the lungs is located around the bronchioles, arterioles, and venules in the dependent regions. The accumulation of liquid in the interstitium may compromise the small airways, leading to mild hypoxemia.
Stage III	Fluid continues to flow into the interstitial space. A large amount of fluid can be sequestered in this space in the lungs. With increasing fluid comes increasing pressure, and fluid flows across the alveolar epithelium into the alveoli, preventing gas exchange. The interstitial space can contain up to 500 mL of fluid. With further accumulations, the fluid crosses the alveolar epithelium into the alveoli, leading to alveolar flooding. This results in abnormalities in gas exchange and vital capacity, substantially reduced respiratory volumes, and more severe hypoxemia.

Source: Adapted from Sovari, A. A. (2008). Pulmonary edema: Cardiogenic. eMedicine. Retrieved from http://www.emedicine.com/med/topic1995.htm#.

Clinical Manifestations

Clinical manifestations of pulmonary edema vary with cause and severity. Initial symptoms include cough, dyspnea, tachypnea, and fatigue. As severity increases and fluid begins to invade the alveoli, patients will experience severe dyspnea, tachypnea, and frothy sputum production. Gas exchange is affected, and pulse oximetry will reflect decreased saturations. Crackles on auscultation may be audible in the bases of the lungs bilaterally as an early sign of pulmonary edema. The crackles could advance to fill the entire lung field. Other adventitious lung sounds, such as wheezes and rhonchi, also could be present. Central cyanosis and circumoral pallor (a bluish tinge to the lips and mucous membranes) reflect worsening respiratory conditions and are late signs of hypoxemia. Symptoms that occur rapidly are referred to as *flash edema* and are often related to capillary permeability causes of pulmonary edema (Matthay & Martin, 2010). Differentiating between NCPE and CPE can be challenging, but some symptoms may suggest cardiac failure as a source of pulmonary edema (Chart 28–5). In the cardiac assessment, some very subtle changes might assist the nurse in differentiating cardiogenic from noncardiogenic pulmonary edema.

Tachycardia with hypotension and cool diaphoretic skin would be prognostic of a cardiogenic pathology, whereas tachycardia with hypertension, bounding pulses and dry skin would be more predictive of a noncardiogenic cause of pulmonary edema such as sepsis. Jugular venous distention (JVD) occurs if there is right heart failure with a present hepatojugular reflex. JVD is a much more common finding in cardiogenic pulmonary edema than in noncardiogenic pulmonary edema. If a pulmonary artery catheter were placed, a pulmonary artery catheter wedge pressure (PCWP) or pulmonary artery occlusion pressure (PAOP) of greater than 18 mmHg would confirm a cardiogenic cause of the pulmonary edema. See Chapter 31 for a complete discussion of pulmonary artery catheters. Agitation and confusion are common symptoms of hypoxemia and sometimes are the first symptoms. The nurse should be sure not to discount these important symptoms when assessing a patient with any type of respiratory distress.

Laboratory and Diagnostic Procedures

Increased interstitial markings on a chest x-ray can be a diagnostic finding of pulmonary edema. The chest x-ray also may reveal an enlarged heart, particularly in CPE. Signs of increased pulmonary infiltrates will also be evident. In CPE, the infiltrates may start out centrally, referred to as a "bat wing" appearance, or have an even distribution through the lung fields. NPE has a diffuse and patchy infiltrate impression. Refer to Chart 28–5 for diagnostic findings used to differentiate CPE and NCPE.

Medical Management

Differentiation between NCPE and CPE is not always straightforward; however, it is an important distinction in establishing the treatment of pulmonary edema. The most important treatment in either case is to provide supplemental oxygen and, if necessary, intubation with

CHART 28–5 Differentiating CPE and NCPE

Signs and Symptoms	Cardiogenic Pulmonary Edema	Noncardiogenic Pulmonary Edema
History	Cardiac event (e.g., ischemic chest pain or hypertension)	Precipitating event (e.g., sepsis, aspiration, pneumonia, trauma, multiple transfusions)
PCWP (Pulmonary capillary wedge pressure): normal = 6–12 mmHg	>18 mmHg	<18 mmHg
New S3, S4 heart sounds	Associated with left heart failure	Not common
New or changed murmur		
Echocardiogram	Weak heart muscle or valvular abnormalities that would indicate heart failure	No cardiac muscle or valvular defects
Skin	Cool, diaphoretic	Warm (in sepsis)
Brain natriuretic peptide (BNP)	>500 pg/mL suggests heart failure	<100 pg/mL unlikely cardiac cause
Normal depends on age and gender. Should be < 100 pg/mL		
Chest x-ray	Enlarged heart, pleural effusions possible Even or central distribution of edema	Air bronchograms possible Diffuse bilateral patchy infiltrate pattern

mechanical ventilation to relieve the consequences of hypoxemia. Blood pressure support may also be necessary. Recently, noninvasive positive pressure ventilation (NPPV) using full or partial masks has been used to treat acute pulmonary edema. (Refer to page 817 for a discussion of NPPV.) This mode of treatment removes the risks of intubation. Supplemental oxygen should be titrated to increase the SpO_2 and relieve the patient's sensation of air hunger.

Medical Management of Cardiogenic Pulmonary Edema

After airway management, diuretics, vasodilators, and inotropes are the mainstay for treatment of cardiogenic pulmonary edema. Treatment should focus on aggressive preload and afterload reduction, not just diuretics. The administration of diuretics is not useful in hypotensive patients because poor renal perfusion reduces their effects. Morphine sulfate is a very helpful drug in the management of CPE because its vasodilatory effect reduces pulmonary capillary pressure without depressing myocardial contractility. This, along with the CNS sedative effect, reduces the heart's workload. Morphine should be titrated carefully to prevent hypotension or respiratory depression. See the Pharmacology box on page 799.

Continuous IV vasodilators, such as nitroglycerin or nitroprusside, are useful either in decreasing preload by redistributing blood peripherally or in decreasing afterload, allowing the heart to work more efficiently (Matthay & Martin, 2010). In acute pulmonary edema, the IV route is preferred because of its rapid onset of action and ability to relieve symptoms. The intravenous infusion can be discontinued, and the drug's effects are then quickly reversed. Other vasodilators include isosorbide and angiotensin-converting enzyme inhibitors. ACE inhibitors should not be given to patients having an acute MI. Intravenous (IV) furosemide is the diuretic of choice. Furosemide decreases venous return, reduces blood pressure, and decreases afterload. Diuresis should occur within 30 minutes of an intravenous dose.

Inotropes (drugs that increase cardiac contractility) are useful in CPE patients who have poor cardiac output and are hypotensive. Dopamine and dobutamine are the most common drugs used in the treatment of pulmonary edema. Dopamine when given at low doses will improve cardiac output, reduce systemic vascular resistance (afterload) and increase renal perfusion. Used in combination with a vasodilator, dopamine will balance the undesirable effect of venoconstriction that aggravates lung edema. Doses greater than 5 mcg/kg/min will increase heart rate and the incidence of dysrhythmias. Dobutamine, in contrast, does not cause vasoconstriction. It is an inotropic agent with some mild dilating effect that increases cardiac output and reduces afterload. It is useful in patients who are hypotensive due to poor ventricular contractility; however, it can precipitate or worsen hypotension in patients who have reduced intravascular volume. Chapter 34 includes a summary of the medications used for the treatment of pulmonary edema caused by heart failure.

Medical Management of Noncardiogenic Pulmonary Edema

Noncardiogenic pulmonary edema, which may result from a wide spectrum of diseases, is caused by either direct or indirect injury of the pulmonary capillary membrane that allows fluids to leak into the interstitial space and then into the alveoli. The treatment for NCPE is largely supportive and focuses on treating the underlying cause. Management strategies for acute lung injury are discussed in the next section.

Nursing Management

Assessment

The nurse should assess the patient with pulmonary edema for signs of hypoxia and progressive respiratory failure requiring ventilatory assistance. This includes dyspnea, restlessness, tachypnea, use of accessory muscles, increased respiratory effort, oxygen saturations, and cyanosis. The nurse also should auscultate all lung fields for crackles, which indicate fluid in the lungs. A patient history may elucidate the cause of pulmonary edema, including heroin or opioid use, toxin exposure, recent history of DVT or pulmonary embolus, list of current medications, and medical history.

Nursing Diagnoses

Nursing diagnoses for acute pulmonary edema include the following:

- *Gas Exchange, Impaired* related to fluid within the alveoli.
- *Fatigue,* related to increased work of breathing.

NANDA-I © 2012

Outcome and Evaluation Parameters

Adequate oxygenation as exhibited by normal respiratory rate and depth, relaxed respirations, absence of dyspnea, and arterial blood gas within patient's normal parameters.

Interventions and Rationales

The nurse should position the patient with head elevated at least 30 degrees to promote lung expansion and prevent aspiration. The nurse monitors oxygen saturations using continuous pulse oximetry and reviews arterial blood gas for arterial oxygen and carbon dioxide pressures. Oxygen levels are provided to maintain saturations $> 90\%$. The nurse should notify the health care provider of increasing oxygen requirements that may indicate a need for mechanical ventilatory support. The patient's energy level should be monitored for fatigue associated with breathing, which may render the patient incapable of sustaining the work of breathing. Therefore, the nurse must provide suctioning as needed to clear secretions that increase the work of breathing. The nurse closely monitors ABGs and reports any changes. Respiratory acidosis with an increasing carbon dioxide level indicates ventilatory failure, and a decreasing oxygen level despite escalation of inspired oxygen indicates hypoxic respiratory failure.

Collaborative Management

A team approach, including the nurse, respiratory therapist, health care provider, patient, and family, facilitates timely and accurate communication of the patient's fatigue level, oxygenation requirements, and assessment parameters that may indicate hypoxia. In order to meet desired patient outcomes, it is essential that the interdisciplinary team communicate openly with one another in developing and evaluating care of the patient and family (IOM [Institute of Medicine], 2010). If assessment indicates deterioration, intubation and mechanical ventilation should occur early rather than waiting for full decompensation. Preparation for intubation, the intubation process, the selection of ventilator settings, and the monitoring of adequacy of ventilation management require a team effort with clear and timely communication and the expert perspective of all bedside providers.

Health Promotion

To minimize exacerbation of heart disease that can progress to cardiac failure and cardiogenic pulmonary edema, the nurse should ensure that patients understand the importance of taking their medications on schedule as prescribed. Eating a healthy diet, limiting the amount of high fat and salty foods, and avoiding processed, canned, or fried foods will promote good health and well-being. The nurse should instruct patients on the signs of cardiac condition deterioration so that patients can seek medical attention early, before they become fully

PHARMACOLOGY Summary of Medications Used to Treat Complex Respiratory Disorders

Medication Category and Action	Application/Indication	Nursing Responsibilities
Diuretics		
Furosemide (Lasix) *Action:* Forces increased urine output by the kidney.	Increases water excretion. Used in cardiogenic pulmonary edema and noncardiogenic pulmonary edema to reduce pulmonary congestion, reduce systemic congestion, and decrease the workload to the heart.	Monitor for signs of dehydration: hypotension, dry mucous membranes, decreased urine output, and poor skin turgor. Overdiuresis will depress cardiac output and affect cellular perfusion. Monitor potassium levels. Measure urine output to gauge response to the drug.
Bronchodilators		
Short-acting beta-2 agonists (albuterol) Anticholinergics (Atrovent) *Action:* Relaxes smooth muscle of the bronchi and bronchioles.	Short-acting bronchodilators are fast-acting and used in acute respiratory failure associated with exacerbation of COPD, acute asthma attacks, or other diseases associated with bronchospasm.	Monitor signs and symptoms before and after treatment to identify presence of bronchospasm (wheezes) and response to therapy. Monitor for increased heart rate, palpitations, tremors, headache, nervousness, or dizziness that are associated with sympathomimetic stimulation. Obtain electrocardiogram in patients with chest pain or severe tachycardia. Beta-blockers may be ordered for symptomatic tachycardia or refractory hypotension unresponsive to fluid. Benzodiazepines may be administered for severe agitation or seizures.
Dexamethasone		
Action: A synthetic adrenocortical steroid. Has anti-inflammatory effects.	Prophylaxis of high altitude pulmonary edema. Mechanism of action is unknown.	Monitor for signs of infection. Corticosteroids decrease infection resistance and may mask signs of infection. Monitor for hypertension. Anaphylactic reactions have been reported; monitor vital signs after initial dosing.
Nifedipine		
Action: A nonspecific calcium-channel blocker that reduces pulmonary vascular resistance and pulmonary pressures; reduces systemic resistance and blood pressure.	Used in high altitude pulmonary edema when oxygen is unavailable and rapid descent is not possible.	Watch for hypotension. Have IV fluid available. Monitor for chest pain, especially in patients with severe obstructive coronary artery disease. May cause dizziness or headache. Patients should be advised to avoid activities that require coordination.
Phosphodiesterase Inhibitors		
Sildenafil Tadalafil *Action:* Inhibits PDE-5 in pulmonary vascular smooth muscle causing vasodilation and reduction in arterial hypertension.	Used in the prophylaxis and treatment of high altitude pulmonary edema (when oxygen and descent to a lower altitude are not options) to reduce hypoxic pulmonary vasoconstriction and pulmonary hypertension.	Assess for epistaxis, headache, dyspnea, flushing, insomnia, and dyspnea. Instruct the patient to report sudden decrease or loss of hearing or vision. Assess for improvement in signs and symptoms of pulmonary hypertension.
Naloxone (Narcan)		
Action: An opioid antagonist that competes with the opiate receptor sites in the central nervous system.	Reversal of opiate activity and respiratory depression.	Monitor blood pressure, heart rate, and respiratory rate. Monitor for withdrawal symptoms in patients with known or suspected opioid dependence. They will occur within minutes of naloxone administration and then subside in about 2 hours. Respiratory depression may then recur. Patients should be monitored for at least 2 hours after last dose.
Inotropes		
Dobutamine Milrinone Dopamine (at lower dosage) *Action:* Increase ventricular contractility and decrease ventricular afterload by inducing pulmonary and systemic vasodilation.	Helpful in patients with cardiogenic pulmonary edema associated with heart failure due to severe left ventricular dysfunction and low cardiac output. Unresponsive to diuretics or vasodilator therapy.	These drugs are administered via continuous IV infusion and require continuous monitoring of blood pressure and ECG. Monitor for hypotension and tachydysrhythmias. Blood pressure should be stabilized with a vasopressor, or dopamine should be used as the initial agent, prior to initiation of these medications, then wean the patient off the vasopressor as blood pressure tolerates.

(*continued*)

PHARMACOLOGY Summary of Medications Used to Treat Complex Respiratory Disorders, *continued*

Medication Category and Action	Application/Indication	Nursing Responsibilities
Vasodilators		
Nitroglycerin Nitroprusside ***Action:*** Veno- and/or vasodilators that reduce both the preload (blood returned to the heart measured as central venous pressure or pulmonary capillary pressure) and afterload (pressure the heart has to pump against measured by the systemic blood pressure).	Used in combination with diuretics in nonhypotensive patients for rapid symptom relief in patients with cardiogenic pulmonary edema. Reduces the heart's workload. Continuous IV infusions are recommended for patients to rapidly treat symptoms associated with acute pulmonary edema.	Frequent blood pressure monitoring and careful titration of continuous vasodilator infusions. Decrease drip rate or discontinue infusion for hypotension. Provide IV fluids if hypotension persists if not contraindicated by patient's condition. Do not use with phosphodiesterase inhibitors (sildenafil, tadalafil) as this may increase the risk of hypotension. Monitor for headaches and provide analgesia as ordered. Nitroprusside is associated with cyanide toxicity. Suspect in patients with prolonged infusions or renal insufficiency. Discontinue drip if encephalopathy, seizures, or coma develops. Treatment is hemodialysis.
Morphine		
Action: Induces peripheral vasodilation. Promotes respiratory depression by decreasing brainstem respiratory center's response to carbon dioxide tension and electrical stimulation. Promotes analgesia through interactions with opioid receptors in the brain.	Used in cardiogenic pulmonary edema to decrease the cardiac filling pressures through peripheral vasodilation.	Monitor for respiratory depression and worsening respiratory failure. Titrate dose in small increments and reassess respiratory and hemodynamic status.

decompensated. These signs and symptoms include weight gain of 3 or more pounds over 1 to 3 days, swollen ankles and feet, excessive coughing, increased shortness of breath or fatigue from baseline activity, and chest pain.

Acute Respiratory Distress Syndrome and Acute Lung Injury

Acute respiratory distress syndrome (ARDS) and **acute lung injury (ALI)** are types of ARF. ARDS is a syndrome of hypoxemic respiratory failure that leads to alveolar–capillary inflammation and damage. ALI is a less severe form of ARDS, differentiated by a lesser degree of abnormal oxygenation. In 1994, the North American–European Consensus Conference (AECC) on ARDS outlined criteria for ALI and ARDS. Chart 28–6 lists the criteria for both diseases, the only distinction between the two being the PaO_2/FiO_2 ratio. This ratio reflects the degree of hypoxemia; the lower the number, the worse the disease. The ratio requires ABGs to obtain the PaO_2, which is divided by the percent of oxygen the patient is breathing. For example, if a person's PaO_2 is 100 mmHg while breathing room air (21% or FiO_2 of 0.21), the ratio would be 476 (100/0.21). If the PaO_2 is 100 mmHg while breathing 100% oxygen (100/1.0), the ratio would be 100.

CHART 28–6 Criteria That Define Acute Lung Injury and Acute Respiratory Distress Syndrome

Type of Acute Lung Injury	Criteria
Acute lung injury	$PaO_2/FiO_2 < 300$ mmHg (regardless of PEEP level) Bilateral patchy infiltrates on chest x-ray PCWP < 18 mmHg if available or no evidence of left atrial hypertension
Acute respiratory distress syndrome	$PaO_2/FiO_2 < 200$ mmHg (regardless of PEEP level) Bilateral patchy infiltrates on chest x-ray PCWP < 18 mmHg if available or no evidence of left atrial hypertension

Source: Adapted from Lee, W., & Slutsky, A. (2010). Acute respiratory distress syndrome. In R. Mason (Ed.), *Murray and Nadel's textbook of respiratory medicine* (5th ed.). Philadelphia: Saunders Elsevier.

Epidemiology

Determining the incidence of ARDS and ALI has been challenging because many studies fail to use the AECC definitions and do not distinguish between ALI and ARDS. Current information suggests an incidence of 86 per 100,000 person-years for ALI and 64 per 100,000 person-years for ARDS. The incidence is highest among individuals older than 75 years (Siegel, 2011a). ARDS has a mortality rate of 30% to 50%, but the rate is highly variable depending on the severity of the disease. Patients usually die from multiple-organ failure, which results from the lack of oxygen to the cells rather than directly from the respiratory failure. The lower mortality usually is seen in centers that are accustomed to treating patients with ARDS and areas where the multidisciplinary team has a clear understanding of the goals of treatment and predicted outcomes. Some diseases and conditions increase the mortality of patients who acquire ARDS, as outlined in the Risk Factors box.

Etiology

ALI and ARDS are consequences of lung injury, either direct or indirect, that produces diffuse alveolar damage. Direct injury is caused by primary insult to the lung; causes include pneumonia, lung contusion, ventilator-associated injury (discussed later in this chapter), and aspiration. Indirect injuries that have nonpulmonary etiologies and lead to ALI/ARDS include sepsis, massive transfusions, and alcoholism or drug abuse. More than 60 potential causes of ALI/ARDS have been identified with more possibilities continuing to emerge (Siegel, 2011a). The most common disorders associated with ALI/ARDS are sepsis, gastric content aspiration, and massive transfusions; approximately 40% of all patients with sepsis develop ARDS (Lee & Slutsky, 2010). Sepsis is discussed in detail in Chapter 54. The Risk Factors box lists some of the more common causes of ALI. This list is not all-inclusive, and it is important to realize that almost any disease process that generates a large-scale inflammation and injury pattern in the human body can cause ALI and ARDS. Appreciation of this concept allows the nurse to recognize a worsening respiratory condition that may lead to ALI and initiate treatment quickly to prevent further hypoxemia and cellular damage.

Pathophysiology

ARDS and ALI are caused by injury to the alveolar–capillary membrane that allows fluids, proteins, and cell products to escape from the vascular space into the interstitium. As the lymphatic system becomes overwhelmed in removing excess fluid, the alveoli begin to fill with fluid and debris from injured cells. Surfactant is then lost which causes the alveoli to collapse. The fluid interferes with the exchange of oxygen and carbon dioxide across the alveolar capillary membrane. As alveoli collapse, the lungs become heavy, stiff, and difficult to ventilate. Hypoxemia, low lung compliance, and increased **minute ventilation (V_E)** (volume of gas ventilated in 1 minute) are the classic features of respiratory failure caused by ARDS. The initial injury to the alveolar–capillary membrane occurs when pro-inflammatory mediators, oxygen free radicals, and other cytokines are activated in response to injury. The complexity, interrelatedness, and mechanism of action of these host defense mediators are some reasons why no cure for ARDS has been found since the disease was first recognized as a syndrome.

Three overlapping and sequential phases have been described in ARDS: the acute exudative phase, the proliferative phase, and a final fibrotic stage. These are described next.

Acute Exudative Phase

The acute exudative phase occurs after initial injury and is marked by diffuse alveolar damage; it is thought to last 5 to 7 days. During this phase, the alveolar capillary membrane is damaged by the injury, as previously described, causing increased permeability and the leak of fluid and cellular debris. Neutrophils are activated and accumulate in the interstitium, and it is theorized that as the key cells in immunity generate a cascade of inflammatory responses and cytotoxic compounds then cause further destruction. As alveoli fill with fluid rather than air, the functional residual capacity (FRC), the amount of gas that remains in the lungs after normal expiration, is reduced.

RISK FACTORS That Cause or Predispose a Patient to ALI/ARDS

Sepsis	Bacteremia
Aspiration	Pneumonia
Severe trauma	Burns
Massive transfusion	Transfusion-related acute lung injury (TRALI)
Near drowning	Lung and hematopoietic stem cell transplantation
Drugs and alcohol	Pancreatitis
Fat embolism	Genetic determinants

Source: Adapted from TenHoor, T., Mannino, D. M., & Moss, M. (2001). Risk factors for ARDS in the United States: Analysis of the 1993 national mortality followback study. *Chest, 119*(4), 1179–1184.

Proliferative Phase

Some patients progress to the second, proliferative phase of lung injury. It is difficult to distinguish between disease progression and pathophysiological abnormalities that occur because of the high ventilator pressures and oxygen toxicity that must be used at times to treat ARDS at this stage of the disease. The air spaces that have been filled with fluid are now narrowed and filled with fibroblasts, specialized cells that attempt to restructure the alveoli. Type I alveolar cells have been replaced by type II cells in the alveolar epithelium. The alveolar–capillary membrane is thick and not efficient in gas exchange. This phase is marked by proliferation of these fibroblasts that are now present in the interstitial spaces and even in the air spaces that continue to collapse. The compliance of the lung is decreased now, and high pressures are needed to ventilate through narrowed air spaces and collapsed alveoli.

Fibrotic Phase

The final phase of ARDS occurs in some patients with persistent ARDS and is marked by pulmonary fibrosis. This phase can begin as early as 10 days after the initial insult. These stiff fibrotic structures can be seen on chest x-ray, and their "honeycombed" appearance is a classic finding. These structures are a result of the body's attempt to repair the damaged cells. These pathologic changes can be reversed if the patient's condition improves and the initial insult has been treated. Frequently, patients in this phase require long-term ventilator support until the lung injury is repaired. Because of these fibrotic changes in the lungs, increased CO_2 retention can be seen at this phase of the disease. CO_2 retention usually is not present until the disease reaches this final stage.

Clinical Manifestations

The patient with ARDS presents with all the symptoms of respiratory failure, usually after a precipitating event. An early sign of respiratory failure is hyperventilation with a corresponding respiratory alkalosis. At this stage of ARDS, the chest x-ray may appear normal; this rapid respiratory rate is the only clinical sign. As the hypoxemia increases, dyspnea, shortness of breath, and tachypnea with use of accessory muscles are frequent findings. The skin may appear cyanotic or mottled, and this does not improve with oxygen administration. Respirations are rapid and shallow with intercostal and suprasternal retractions on inspiration only (Kaplow & Hardin, 2007).

In auscultating the lung fields, the nurse may hear bilateral crackles in the bases or throughout the lung fields. Coarse rhonchi and wheezes, depending on the severity of the fluid that is flowing into the alveoli, also are heard. In some cases, the pink frothy sputum of classic pulmonary edema is seen. The hypoxemia quickly becomes refractory to standard oxygen therapies, and the patient requires intubation and mechanical ventilation to maintain oxygenation and ventilation (p. 805). The ABGs frequently demonstrate a respiratory alkalosis in the early stage and respiratory acidosis in the advanced stage. The chest x-ray exhibits the bilateral patchy infiltrates that are characteristic of ARDS. This "whiteout" can cover the entire lung field as the disease progresses. Late findings include hypotension and decreased cardiac output.

Laboratory and Diagnostic Procedures

ALI and ARDS are diagnosed primarily by exclusion, in which other possible causes of bilateral infiltrates, hypoxemia, and respiratory distress have been ruled out. Diseases that may mimic ARDS/ALI include cardiogenic pulmonary edema, pneumonias (cryptogenic, idiopathic eosinophilic, acute interstitial pneumonia), diffuse alveolar hemorrhage, and rapidly progressive cancer (Hansen-Flaschen & Siegel, 2010).

Cardiogenic pulmonary edema (CPE) is the most common disease to be confused with ARDS/ALI. Diagnostic tests that are used to exclude CPE include brain natriuretic peptide (BNP), echocardiography, and right heart catheterization. Refer to the Laboratory and Diagnostic Tests box. If clinical assessment, BNP, and echocardiogram are inconclusive, right heart catheterization (Swan-Ganz catheter) may be employed for definitive diagnosis. Swan-Ganz catheter indications and uses are discussed in Chapter 31. Once CPE has been ruled out, additional diagnostic tests such as bronchoscopy or lung biopsy may be used to rule out other etiologies.

Medical Management

Treatment of ARDS/ALI is primarily supportive and focuses on treating the underlying cause. Supportive treatment includes oxygenation/

LABORATORY AND DIAGNOSTIC TESTS for ARDS and ALI

Test with Description, Rationale, and Normal Values	Expected Abnormality
Brain Natriuretic Peptide (BNP)	
0–99 pg/mL	In patients with respiratory failure:
BNP is a hormone in the blood that is secreted from the ventricles of the heart in response to increased pressure that occurs with heart failure. The level is higher in women and increases with age. It is used to differentiate cardiac (congestive heart failure) versus pulmonary etiology (ARDS/ALI) of respiratory failure.	BNP < 100 pg/mL = ARDS/ALI etiology BNP > 500 pg/mL = cardiac etiology BNP 100–500 pg/mL = nondefinitive and requires further work-up.
Echocardiology	
Normal heart wall movement, and normal heart chambers and valve function. Ejection fraction 55% to 65%.	Normal or close to normal in patients with ARDS/ALI.
An echocardiogram uses sound waves to project images of the heart and determine the size of the heart, pump (ejection) strength, heart muscle motion, and heart valve function. It is used to identify heart function and differentiate cardiac versus pulmonary etiology of respiratory failure when BNP is inconclusive.	Compromised left ventricular function is suggestive of the cardiac etiology of respiratory failure.
Right Heart Catheterization	
Cardiac index: 2.8–4.2 L/min/body surface area Pulmonary systolic pressure: 17–32 mmHg Pulmonary mean pressure: 9–19 mmHg Pulmonary diastolic pressure: 4–13 mmHg Pulmonary capillary wedge pressure: 4–13 mmHg Right atrial pressure: 0–7 mmHg	Pulmonary wedge pressure >18 mmHg is associated with cardiac etiology of respiratory failure. Pulmonary wedge pressure < 18 mmHg is associated with pulmonary etiology of respiratory failure.
A Swan-Ganz catheter is inserted through a vein (usually subclavian or jugular) into the right side of the heart and threaded into the pulmonary artery. The pressures obtained indicate the pressures of the right heart, pulmonary vasculature, and left heart and identify and monitor cardiac function and blood flow, including cardiac output/index.Cardiac output/index is reduced and pulmonary wedge pressure increased in cardiac compromise. ARDS/ALI should demonstrate a normal wedge pressure.	
Arterial Blood Gases (ABGs)	
pH 7.35–7.45; $PaCO_2$ 35–45; PaO_2 75–100; HCO_3 24–28	pH < 7.35 = academia
Measures the degree of hypoxemia and hypercarbia	PaO_2 < 60 mmHg = hypoxemia
Identifies acid–base imbalance	$PaCO_2$ > 45 mmHg = respiratory acidosis HCO_3 < 24 = metabolic acidosis A low HCO_3 identifies the metabolic source of respiratory failure, such as sepsis. An elevated $PaCO_2$ identifies a respiratory cause of respiratory failure, such as COPD.
Chest Radiography	
Normal: clear, no trauma, good lung markings *Used to identify possible etiology of ARDS/ALI.*	Abnormalities in CXR can help to identify the source of respiratory failure. These may include pneumonia, pulmonary edema, pneumothorax, abscess, cancer, emphysema, or chest trauma. The progression of ARDS/ALI usually appears on the CXR as diffuse bilateral pulmonary infiltrates.
Sputum and Blood Cultures	
Normal: no growth *Used to identify the possible etiology of ARDS/ALI.*	May identify pathogens such as bacteria, fungus, or mycobacterium as a source of infection leading to respiratory failure.

ventilation management, hemodynamic management, and nutrition. The goals are to (1) reduce hypoxemia, (2) improve acidosis, (3) improve or maintain cardiac function, (4) treat the underlying cause, and (5) avoid complications. Ventilation and oxygenation therapies for the treatment of ARDS are discussed later in the mechanical ventilation section (p. 805).

Optimum fluid management in patients with ARDS is centered on conservative fluid administration in order to limit lung edema while also preventing overdiuresis, hypotension, and renal failure. If ARDS/ALI is induced by severe sepsis or septic shock, goal-directed therapy using the administration of crystalloid, blood, and vasoactive and inotropic agents should be followed for the first 6 to 8 hours (see Chapter 54 on severe sepsis).

Safety Alert *If the patient remains hypotensive after fluid resuscitation, the nurse must notify the health care provider, as vasopressor medications are indicated.*

To promote healing and prevent complications in patients who are seriously ill, adequate nutrition—either enterally or parenterally—is essential. If the patient can tolerate enteral feeding, this is the preferred route. Recent literature suggests that enteral nutrition is associated with fewer intravascular infections, less GI bleeding, and a decrease in bacterial translocation (Siegel, 2011b). There are no proven preferred enteral feeding formulas for the patient who has ARDS, and there is no benefit to overfeeding. Therefore, it is important to consult a nutritionist in order to calculate caloric goals for the patient and prevent overfeeding. See Chapter 8 for more information on nutrition.

Mechanical Ventilation

Life-threatening hypoxemia from respiratory failure is treated with intubation and institution of mechanical ventilation. Most patients who develop ARDS cannot be treated with supplemental oxygen alone. Therefore, mechanical ventilation should be initiated when saturations cannot be maintained at 90% with supplemental oxygen. Mechanical ventilation should be instituted early to prevent aspiration and reduce the patient's work of breathing, allowing the underlying initiating event to be treated and the lung to begin to heal.

The primary modes of positive pressure ventilation include volume-targeted and pressure-targeted ventilation. *Volume-targeted ventilation* uses a set inspiratory volume of gas (tidal volume) moving into the lungs with each breath. The inspiratory pressure will vary depending on the lung's compliance and resistance; the stiffer the lungs, the higher the pressure needed to deliver that volume. *Pressure-targeted ventilation* involves the delivery of a breath until a set inspiratory pressure is reached. The volume that is delivered to the lung will vary depending on the lung's compliance and resistance; the stiffer the lung, the less volume will be delivered before the set pressure is reached. There is no evidence that one mode has improved outcomes over the other. However, whichever mode is used, a lung-protective strategy should be employed to prevent ventilator-induced lung injury (VILI). A landmark study by the ARDS Network demonstrated that maintaining lower plateau pressures was associated with a statistically significant improvement in mortality as well as reduction in the number of days on the ventilator. These results are still affecting current practice (Acute Respiratory Distress Syndrome Network, 2000). Plateau pressure is the pressure applied to the small airways and alveoli during positive pressure ventilation and is measured during a portion of the inspiration phase on the ventilator.

Novel Medical Therapies

Although the mortality rate for ARDS/ALI has decreased since the 1990s, it remains over 40% (Zambon & Vincent, 2008). Many new and potentially exciting alternative therapies are being studied to determine whether they are efficacious for treating patients with ALI/ARDS. None of the following therapies have shown clear benefits in adults, partially because of the complex confounders in ARDS research. However, these alternatives continue to be explored and in time may show benefits. These therapies include extracorporeal gas exchange (ECMO), extracorporeal CO_2 removal (ECCO2R), high frequency ventilation (HFV), inhaled vasodilators, surfactant administration, liquid ventilation, and anti-inflammatory therapies (Siegel, 2011b).

Prone ventilation refers to positioning the patient in a prone position during mechanical ventilation. This process, which may be used for refractory hypoxemia in patients with ARDS/ALI, has improved oxygenation and reduced FiO_2 requirements in most patients with severe ARDS, although outcome studies are uncertain as of this writing (Alsaghir & Martin, 2008; Schwartz, Malhotra, & Kacmarek, 2010). Prone ventilation is usually used after conventional ventilation has failed to improve oxygenation above a PaO_2 of 60 mmHg. The duration of prone ventilation varies, and there is no evidence to suggest an ideal length of time for patients to be left in this position. This repositioning requires coordination between the nursing staff and respiratory therapists to ensure the stability of the endotracheal tube and IV access.

Nursing Management

The nursing process guides the care of patients who are experiencing ARF. Therefore, it is imperative that the nurse be knowledgeable about the pathophysiology of the disease that caused the ARF. The nurse also must recognize that the treatment for ARF is based on supporting the patient until the underlying disease can be resolved. Prevention of the complications of hypoxemia is a primary goal.

Assessment

The nursing assessment begins with the patient's airway and oxygenation status. This includes both subjective and objective findings. The patient must be questioned about whether he is feeling short of breath, fatigued, or anxious. Objective assessment includes the respiratory rate, the work of breathing, oxygen saturation, arterial blood gas results, mentation, breath sounds, sputum production, and tachycardia. The skin and nail beds need to be assessed for cyanosis and pallor. Patients often display anxiety when they feel short of breath, but anxiety is also a symptom of hypoxia. Therefore, saturations should be assessed immediately to rule out hypoxia as a cause of anxiety. Because respiratory status changes rapidly, it is imperative for the nurse to perform frequent and ongoing assessments.

Nursing Diagnoses

Nursing diagnoses that apply to patients with ARDS/ALI include the following:

- *Gas Exchange, Impaired* related to pulmonary shunt, interstitial edema, and alveolar edema.
- *Tissue Perfusion, Ineffective* related to hypoxia.
- *Coping, Ineffective* related to abrupt onset of life-threatening disease.
- *Nutrition, Less Than Required* related to patient's inability to take in nutrients due to intubation.
- *Infection, Risk for* related to disease process, invasive lines, and endotracheal intubation.
- *Skin Integrity, Risk for Impaired* related to immobility.

NANDA-I © 2012

Video: Set-Up and Assisting With Endotracheal Tube Intubation

Outcomes and Evaluation Parameters

Desired outcomes for the patient with ARDS/ALI include stable oxygen status and prevention of, or resolution of, respiratory failure. Evaluation parameters include vital signs and oxygen saturation within normal limits on room air. Lung sounds are clear and the patient denies shortness of breath or air hunger.

Interventions and Rationales

Nursing interventions for the patient with ARDS/ALI include encouraging the patient to engage in deep breathing and coughing exercises, having the patient use an incentive spirometer if ordered, and reporting to the health care provider when changes occur that may indicate a need for oxygen therapy and/or mechanical ventilation. Frequent turning and repositioning of patients has always been a standard component of the immobilized patient's nursing care to help mobilize secretions, facilitate comfort, and maintain skin integrity. Maintaining the head of the bed at least 30 degrees helps to prevent aspiration and the development of hospital-acquired pneumonia. The nurse should plan patient activity and rest periods to promote rest and recovery. In addition, the nurse will note any desaturation with activity and provide a short, temporary increase in FiO_2 to prevent hypoxia. Patients with ARDS frequently have little respiratory reserve and develop hypoxemia when turned, suctioned, or bathed. Sometimes this desaturation is related to turning on a certain side (related to unilateral lung disease) or occurs after an activity. The nurse can mitigate this hypoxemia by documenting the troublesome activity's effect so that it is not repeated.

Intubation and mechanical ventilation are two major medical interventions. Successful intubation is an important procedure that requires the nurse to know how to assist the health care provider, administer medications, demonstrate skill with suctioning and use of the **air-mask-bag unit (AMBU)** (a device used to deliver oxygen via a mask when a patient is not adequately ventilating or oxygenating), and document the event in the patient's record.

Nursing Priorities During Endotracheal Intubation

An indication for intubation is the respiratory system's inability to maintain oxygenation and/or ventilation. Other indications for intubation include airway protection and elective surgery. Assisting with intubation requires that the nurse know what equipment is necessary and its proper operation. It also requires that the nurse anticipate the needs of the health care professional who is performing the procedure.

Before the intubation procedure, the nurse should explain the process to the patient and her family. The patient is positioned on her back with a small blanket under the shoulder blades to hyperextend the neck and open the airway. The nurse confirms that the equipment is working properly and provides 100% oxygen via a nonrebreather mask (refer to Chart 27–3 in Chapter 27 for oxygen delivery systems) or AMBU. During the procedure, the nurse provides suction as necessary and monitors the patient's oxygen saturations by pulse oximetry, as well as the patient's heart rate and blood pressure.

Documentation of the intubation should include the size of the **endotracheal tube** (a tube used to deliver oxygen that is placed in the trachea) and where the tube is located in the airway. The nurse determines this by identifying the number of centimeters printed on the tube; this information is visible at the teeth or gum line. The nurse should also document medication administered and how the patient tolerated the procedure. Chart 28–7 includes a list of equipment necessary for intubation.

CHART 28–7 Equipment for Endotracheal Intubation

Personal protective equipment
Endotracheal tubes with intact cuff and 15-mm connectors
- Adult female: 7.0- to 8.0-mm tube
- Adult male: 8.0- to 9.0-mm tube

Laryngoscope handle with fresh batteries
Laryngoscope blades (straight or curved)
Spare bulbs for laryngoscope blades
Flexible stylet
Self-inflating resuscitation bag with mask connected to 100% oxygen
Oxygen source and connecting tubes
Nonsterile gloves
Luer-Lok 10-mL syringe for cuff inflation
Water-soluble lubricant
Rigid pharyngeal suction tip catheter (Yankauer)
Suction apparatus (wall or portable)
Suction catheters
Bite block or oropharyngeal airways
Endotracheal tube securing apparatus or tape
Stethoscope
Anesthetic spray or jelly (for nasal approach)
Sedating and/or paralyzing medication
Magill forceps
Monitor equipment for ECG, pulse oximetry, and end-tidal CO_2
Ventilator

Source: Adapted from Goodrich, C. (2010). Endotracheal intubation. In L. Wiegand (Ed.), AACN: Procedure manual for critical care (6th ed.). St. Louis, MO: Elsevier Saunders.

Nursing Priorities Post Endotracheal Intubation

Endotracheal intubation can be a lifesaving procedure. However, to prevent possible serious complications, the nurse must provide ongoing assessment with meticulous attention to detail. The placement of the tube is important. If it is too deep, it can be pushed down into the right main bronchus and not provide ventilation to the left lung, causing collapse of the left lung and hyperinflation damage to the right lung. If it is too shallow, it can dislodge above the vocal cords and out of the airway, and ventilation will be lost. The nurse should document and monitor tube position and ensure the tube is secured firmly in place (per institution protocol). Proper sedation may be necessary to prevent the patient from biting the tube or dislodging it either accidentally or purposefully, particularly the confused or head-injured patient. Securing straps can be loosened over time or with agitation, thereby displacing the tube. The nurse should keep the mouth and lips clean and dry for orally placed endotracheal tubes, and do the same for the nares for nasal endotracheal tubes. These areas must also be monitored for skin breakdown.

The cuff of the endotracheal tube occludes the space above the tip of the tube so that air does not escape out of the mouth when the patient is ventilated (Figure 28–5◆). The cuff also prevents most secretions from the oropharynx from being aspirated into the lungs. The cuff is situated just below the vocal cords. A pilot balloon is a small diameter tube that runs from the cuff and leads outside the mouth so that it can be inflated with a syringe after the tube is inserted. If too much air is added to the balloon, it can cause pressure and ischemic damage to the airway. If too little air is added, there is a poor seal and secretions leak down into the

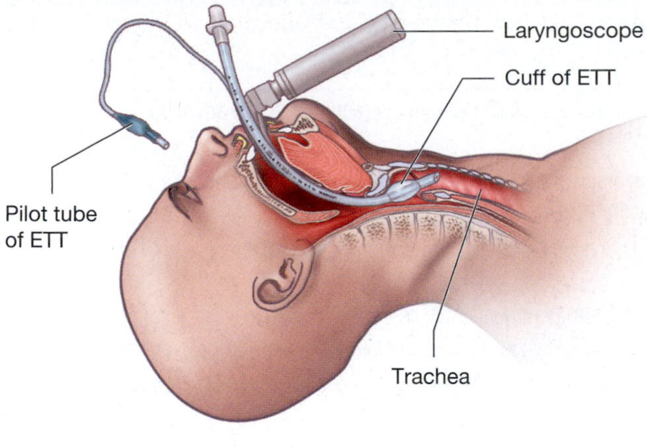

FIGURE 28–5 ◆ Using a laryngoscope to insert an endotracheal tube.

lungs, causing the tube to be more easily dislodged. Pressures should be set for minimal occlusion and should be monitored regularly. Some newer tubes have a separate port positioned above the cuff that allows for suctioning of secretions that may accumulate at the cuff, ideally preventing the possibility of microaspiration.

The nursing care of the ventilated patient involves not only understanding the purpose of mechanical ventilation, its basic operation, and common modes of ventilation, but also the complications of mechanical ventilation. Noninvasive positive pressure ventilation (NPPV) is being used to treat acute respiratory failure, especially with patients who have chronic obstructive pulmonary diseases and emphysema. NPPV is discussed in detail on page 817. Many of the complications of having an endotracheal tube in the airway are avoided with this type of ventilation. Because of technological advances in ventilator design as well as the positive results of controlled studies, this type of mechanical ventilation support is becoming more available to patients who previously were intubated.

Collaborative Management

The management of ARDS/ALI requires the collaboration of team members from many disciplines including nurses, health care providers (intensivist, pulmonologist, radiologist), infection control specialist, respiratory therapist, physical therapist, nutritional therapist or dietitian, and social worker. In order to meet desired patient outcomes, it is essential that this interdisciplinary team communicate openly with one another in developing and evaluating care of the patient and family (IOM [Institute of Medicine], 2010). Each discipline offers its own distinct contribution; together, these contributions provide the best possible care. Activity and care that need to be planned and coordinated include ventilation management, weaning from the ventilator, mobility, nutrition, sleep/rest cycles, management of underlying disease, family support, and possibly end-of-life decisions. Comorbidities add to the complexity of care and may require the addition of disease-specific specialists.

Health Promotion

It can be difficult to determine which people will develop ARDS/ALI. General preventive measures, such as good hand hygiene, not smoking, and having at-risk populations (older adults, immunocompromised individuals, patients with chronic illness) receive an annual influenza vaccine and pneumococcal vaccination, should be taken to prevent illnesses that may progress to ARDS/ALI. Patients with serious illness, infection, or trauma should seek treatment early to minimize the progression of disease.

Discharge Priorities for Patients with Respiratory Failure/ARDS

Quality-of-life research has helped to focus the discharge priorities for patients with ARDS and respiratory failure who spend weeks to months in hospitals receiving mechanical ventilation. Quality of life is an important but elusive (difficult to define and measure) outcome measure in many diseases, especially after critical illness. Quality of life means many different things to patients and has important implications for the nurses who care for patients as they recover from ARDS. It is important for the nurse who discharges these patients home or to a rehabilitation facility to understand how the quality-of-life issue affects these patients.

What is life like for the patient after surviving ARDS? Studies have suggested that quality of life after ARDS is diminished (Herridge et al., 2011). In a 5-year post ARDS survivor study, Herridge et al. identified some of the consequences of severe lung injury as exercise limitation, physical and psychological sequelae, decreased physical quality of life, and increased costs and use of health care service. A variety of contributors affect the lives of patients including depression, anxiety, and loss of cognitive ability. Recall of ICU events, including delusional memories, has precipitated post-traumatic stress syndrome. This has been described as overwhelming, and many patients have reported unpreparedness for its management (Cox et al., 2009). Caregivers of ARDS survivors are also affected by the long episodes of critical illness and recovery associated with the disease and may suffer from psychological dysfunction (Herridge et al., 2011).

Mechanical Ventilation

Indications for providing mechanical ventilation to the patient with acute respiratory failure include hypoxemia, hypercarbia, or both. Modern ventilators are termed positive pressure ventilators because they provide above atmospheric pressure on inspiration to the lungs. This is the most common type of ventilator used in the acute care setting. The high-frequency oscillator, a type of ventilator that uses a constant distending pressure with pressure variations oscillating at very high rates to create small tidal volumes, is used in pediatric and adult patients with decreased lung compliance. It produces an oscillating wave of pressures to deliver the gas.

Figure 28–6◆ displays the common components of a typical ventilator. The ventilator circuit is connected to the patient and consists of a single plastic tube that fits directly onto the endotracheal tube or tracheostomy. The circuit divides into an inspiratory circuit and an expiratory circuit that connect directly to the ventilator. An important component of this system is humidification. Oxygen delivered without humidification can cause drying of the airways and solidification of secretions. Humidification is discussed in more detail later in the chapter (p. 812).

The ventilator monitors rates, pressures, and volumes, and then delivers the set volumes or pressures (or a combination of the two) to the patient during the inspiratory cycle. The ventilator accomplishes this

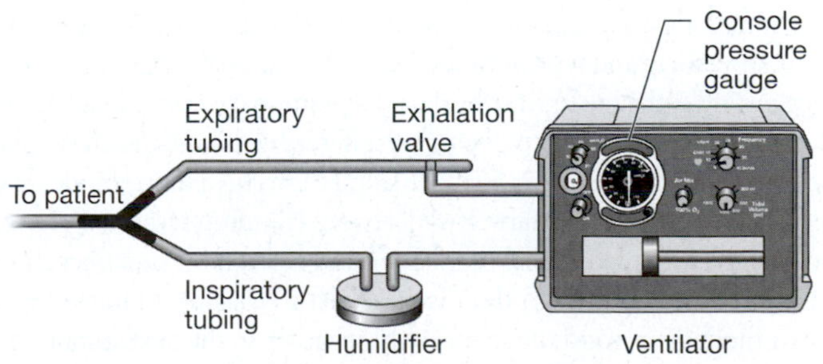

FIGURE 28–6 ◆ Model of volume-cycled ventilator.

PATIENT TEACHING & DISCHARGE PRIORITIES for a Patient with ARDS

Need	Teaching
Awareness of medications	• Teach the purpose and possible side effects of all medications and which side effects require medical attention. • Have the patient demonstrate proper use of an inhaler. • If home oxygen is ordered, teach proper use of oxygen therapy and safety measures in handling oxygen tanks. Provide information or coordinate through home health care to arrange for oxygen delivery.
Knowledge of continuing home care	• Explain the use of pulse oximetry if prescribed, as well as acceptable values and when to call a health care provider or seek emergency care. • Have the patient demonstrate proper use of an incentive spirometer and identify its frequency of use. • Have the patient demonstrate breathing exercises such as pursed-lip breathing or diaphragmatic breathing. • Provide written instructions of when to notify a health care provider or seek emergency care: fever, bloody sputum, increased shortness of breath, wheezing, or swelling in the legs, feet, or abdomen. • Describe the importance of keeping all follow-up appointments.
Understanding of disease recovery	• Stress that it may take 6 to 12 months or longer to regain normal lung function. • Explain that there may be some memory loss because of poor oxygen supply to the brain. • Anxiety, fear, and depression are normal feelings. Encourage the patient to talk to family, friends, or the health care provider about these feelings. • Inform the family or primary caregivers that they may also experience stress and depression. Encourage them to seek counseling if these feelings become overwhelming. • Encourage the patient to participate in an activity or exercise program under the guidance of the health care provider. • For patients who developed ARDS, provide information of ARDS support groups.
Promote ongoing health and disease prevention	Explain to the patient and family that they can reduce their chance of getting lung infections and other illnesses by doing the following: • Wash hands or use antimicrobial gel frequently. • Do not smoke. • Stay inside when air pollution or pollen count is high. • Stay inside during very cold or hot weather. • Avoid people with flu or cold. • Maintain a healthy diet.

monitoring and delivery of gas by using microprocessors to synchronize and detect when the patient inspires and expires to time the delivery of machine support. Another necessary component of the ventilator is the compressor. In hospitals that cannot provide compressed gas piped in from the wall, a compressor is attached to the ventilator. The compressor provides compressed air; this air is mixed with the required percent of oxygen to deliver the ordered FiO_2. Many ventilators are able to monitor respiratory waveforms, which allow the health care team to assess the lung mechanics by indicating pressure, flow, and volume over time. Analysis of the waveforms, which is done by a respiratory therapist, aids in deciding the mode of ventilation and fine-tuning settings.

Providing nursing care to the patient on a ventilator has become increasingly complicated for two reasons. First, the complexities of ventilators in use today have increased dramatically, and more and more of the functions have become automatic within user-defined limits. Second, the variety and type of ventilators that are available have increased. For example, the nurse who works on a pulmonary unit might have to learn the unique features of five or six different ventilators. Each ventilator manufacturer also uses many different terms to describe modes and ventilator operations. Chart 28–8 describes common respiratory terms associated with mechanical ventilation, and Chart 28–9 describes common ventilator settings. A discussion of all the available ventilators and their modes is beyond the scope of this chapter. In the next section, the most common ventilators and the modes they deliver are reviewed, as well as the implications for nursing care.

CHART 28–8 Common Respiratory Terms Associated with Mechanical Ventilation

Term	Definition
Fraction of inspired oxygen (FiO_2)	Amount of oxygen in the delivered gas; expressed as a percent or decimal
Minute ventilation (V_E)	Total ventilation per minute: Respiratory rate $\times$ V_T = V_E
Tidal volume (V_T)	Amount of gas inspired with each breath
Functional residual capacity (FRC)	Total amount of gas left in the lungs after a normal expiration
Residual volume (RV)	Amount of gas remaining in the lungs after a maximal expiration
Rapid shallow breathing index (RSBI)	Parameter used for determining weaning success: Respiratory rate/spontaneous tidal volume

The major resource for the nurse is the respiratory therapist who is responsible for the ventilator and for ensuring that the ventilator is meeting the patient's respiratory needs. The nurse is responsible for knowing how the ventilator functions and the meaning of different modes to ensure that the patient receives an integrative approach and

CHART 28–9 Common Ventilator Settings

Setting	Key Features	Nursing Implications
PEEP: Positive end-expiratory pressure	A pressure exerted on the airway throughout the respiratory cycle that prevents alveolar collapse. Used to improve oxygenation.	A PEEP of 5 cm H_2O is often used to compensate for endotracheal tube resistance. The ideal PEEP prevents atelectasis, but does not overdistend open alveoli. PEEP increases intrathoracic pressure and can cause hypotension at high levels.
FiO_2: Fraction of inspired oxygen	The percent of oxygen delivered to the patient. Prolonged $FiO_2 > 60\%$ can lead to lung injury.	Selected based on the clinical goal of PaO_2. PEEP can be added to improve oxygenation and reduced oxygen requirements.
V_T: Tidal volume	Volume of breaths delivered in volume-targeted ventilation modes. The ventilator will deliver a breath until the set volume is achieved.	Should be based on ideal body weight rather than actual body weight. The amount given is based on the health care provider's preference and the disease entity. Patients with ALI/ARDS have shown reduced morbidity and mortality with lower tidal volumes (6 mL/kg) and plateau pressures < 30 cm H_2O.
PIP: Peak inspiratory pressure/peak pressure	Pressure set in pressure-targeted ventilation modes. The ventilator will deliver a breath until the pressure limit is achieved.	Monitor for hypoventilation and hyperventilation by monitoring the minute ventilation.
VR: Ventilatory rate	Set rate delivered by the ventilator. Patients can breathe over the set rate; how that breath is supported depends on the ventilation mode.	The rate selected depends on age (pediatric, adult, newborn) and clinical goal. It usually is selected to meet a targeted pH. Increasing the rate will decrease the $PaCO_2$ and raise pH. Monitor for auto-PEEP and hyperventilation.

the best possible outcome. To ensure optimum care of a patient on a ventilator, the entire health care team must have a common goal: to liberate the patient from the ventilator. However, the respiratory therapist and the nurse have an added responsibility to work together in the care of the ventilated patient. The nurse and the therapist must ensure that they are communicating with each other about changes in modes, sedation levels, and daily plans for weaning.

The ventilator decreases the patient's work of breathing. If the ventilator does all the work of breathing, that breath is called a *mandatory breath*. The ventilator starts the breath, controls inspiratory gas delivery, and determines the end of inspiration. Assisted breaths are those breaths that the patient initiates, although the ventilator controls the inspiratory gas delivery and time. If the ventilator provides any type of support during inspiration or expiration, that breath is defined as an assisted breath. Spontaneous modes are breaths that are initiated, controlled, and terminated by the patient.

Basic Modes of Ventilation

There is no universal consensus on the classification of ventilation modes. However, as was discussed previously, the two primary methods of positive pressure ventilation are volume-targeted and pressure-targeted ventilation. Within these categories, ventilation modes can be broadly categorized on the basis of how a breath is initiated and controlled: mandatory, assisted, or spontaneous. CPAP (continuous positive airway pressure) is an example of the spontaneous ventilation mode since no rate, pressure, or volume is set on the ventilator, and the rate and volume of air inspired are driven by the patient. Chart 28–10 compares the modes, key features, and important nursing implications that are reviewed in this chapter.

The health care provider orders the mode that best meets the patient's needs. The mode is selected on the ventilator control panel. Figure 28–7◆ shows a ventilator that is commonly used in critical care units and an enlarged drawing of the control panel, demonstrating the complexity of today's ventilators.

Volume-Targeted Modes and Nursing Implications

Volume-targeted, also called volume-controlled, modes of ventilation have a selected set tidal volume that is delivered during the inspiratory phase of the ventilation cycle. When the tidal volume is reached, inspiration will stop and expiration will begin. The inspiratory pressure it takes to deliver the set tidal volume will vary depending on the compliance and resistance of the lungs. Resistant, noncompliant lungs will require higher inspiratory pressures to deliver the tidal volume.

Continuous Mandatory Ventilation

A breath that is initiated, controlled (volume of air delivered and time it takes to deliver it), and terminated by the ventilator is termed *continuous mandatory ventilation* (CMV). Patients can breathe at their own rate in between these mandatory breaths, but the patient-initiated breaths are essentially ignored by the ventilator. This mode of ventilation is uncomfortable for patients with a spontaneous respiratory drive and is usually reserved for patients who are heavily sedated or chemically paralyzed or who have no spontaneous effort.

Assist-Control Ventilation

In an assist-control (AC) mode, the patient initiates a breath, but it is controlled and ended by the ventilator. The health care provider orders a ventilatory rate and a tidal volume so that a minimum number of breaths are delivered. If the patient does not initiate the breath after a set time, the ventilator will initiate the breath. Regardless of how the breath is initiated, the preset volume is delivered to the patient each time a breath is initiated. This mode is often used in caring for the patient who requires ventilatory management because it gives the lungs a chance to rest and recover by allowing the ventilator to do much of the work of breathing.

Hyperventilation can occur in the AC mode of ventilation. The nurse should monitor minute ventilation (V_E) and ensure that alarm parameters are set appropriately. Minute ventilation is calculated by multiplying the respiratory rate (RR) by the tidal volume (V_T). Since the ventilator delivers a full tidal volume breath whenever the patient initiates a breath, the ventilator can precipitate hyperventilation for a

CHART 28–10 Common Ventilator Modes

Ventilator Mode/Setting	Key Features	Nursing Implications
Continuous mandatory ventilation (CMV)	Breaths are initiated, controlled, and terminated by the ventilator. The patient cannot initiate any breaths spontaneously.	Monitor for patient discomfort. Monitor for patient attempts to breathe beyond the set ventilated breaths. Consult with a respiratory therapist if the patient's effort to breathe is causing agitation or discomfort. Sedate the patient as needed.
Assist-control (AC)	Both the patient and the ventilator can initiate breaths. Each breath, whether patient or machine triggered, receives the full set tidal volume.	Monitor for hyperventilation. Ventilator alarms should include a high pressure limit. As the patient's lungs become less compliant, the pressure needed to deliver the tidal volume could rise to dangerous levels. Assess for patient-ventilator asynchrony. Monitor the inspiratory pressure, minute ventilation, and low inspiratory pressure alarms. Monitor PEEP (p. 810) levels to identify auto-PEEP and breath stacking (p. 810).
Synchronized mandatory ventilation (SIMV)	Both the patient and the ventilator can initiate breaths. Machine (preset rate) breaths receive a full set tidal volume. Spontaneous breaths are not assisted, and the patient sets the tidal volume.	Monitor for respiratory effort, as this mode places more work of breathing on the patient. If the patient becomes agitated, anxious, or appears to struggle to breathe, discuss the addition of pressure support with the respiratory therapist and/or health care provider.
Pressure control ventilation (PCV)	Both the patient and the ventilator can initiate breaths. Each breath, whether initiated by the ventilator or the patient, receives the full set inspiratory pressure.	Monitor tidal volume. With decreased lung compliance, the tidal volume delivered by the ventilator will decrease and may not meet respiratory demands.
Pressure support ventilation (PSV)	No set rate or volume. Each of the patient's spontaneous breaths receives support from the ventilator. The higher the set pressure support, the more the ventilator is doing the patient's work of breathing. This is used for weaning and may also be used in conjunction with SIMV.	Used for spontaneously breathing patients only. If the patient is too sedated and does not attempt to breathe, no support is received. Patient must have a reliable respiratory rate. Monitor for hypoventilation. Set the apnea alarm and a back-up rate if available.
Continuous positive airway pressure (CPAP)	Used in spontaneous ventilatory modes to maintain a positive pressure in the airway to reduce or prevent alveolar collapse.	Can be used in invasive and noninvasive modes of ventilation. Apnea alarms must be set. Assess for hypoventilation.
Noninvasive positive pressure ventilation (NPPV)	Ventilation is provided without the benefit of an endotracheal tube, using a tight-fitting mask.	Patient must be able to cooperate, must be alert and oriented, and must be able to clear secretions.

patient who is in pain or agitated, or who has an alteration in central breathing control. Additionally, to protect the lungs from injury due to high inspiratory pressures, limits should be set on the maximum inspiratory pressure. The nurse should be aware that if high-pressure limits are reached during the course of the tidal volume being delivered, the remaining tidal volume will be dumped and not delivered to the patient. For example, suppose the tidal volume is set at 400 mL and, after only 250 mL of it has been delivered, the patient breathes against the ventilator or coughs. This can drive the inspiratory pressure above the set limit. When the inspiratory pressure is reached, the ventilator will not deliver the rest of the tidal volume, thus delivering only 250 mL of the set tidal volume. If the problem causing this "patient–ventilator asynchrony" is not addressed, the patient will not be adequately ventilated and can become hypoxemic and/or hypercarbic. The nurse who is caring for this patient should be able to assess the situation and intervene to ensure that the patient and the ventilator are working together to prevent patient–ventilator asynchrony. Respiratory alkalosis is not uncommon with assist-control ventilation because of the patient's ability to increase minute ventilation (V_E).

Synchronized Intermittent Mandatory Ventilation

Synchronized intermittent mandatory ventilation (SIMV) is a mode of ventilation with a set rate during which the ventilator will deliver a set volume. This is the mandatory minimum rate. Otherwise, patients can breathe between the set rates and receive whatever tidal volume is determined by their effort. Pressure support, discussed in the following text, can be added to this mode to give some support to the spontaneous breaths. The synchronization means that the ventilator will wait for the patient to initiate a breath and then deliver the set mandatory breath in concert with the patient. If the patient does not inspire within the programmed time, the ventilator will initiate the breath.

SIMV is one of the most common modes used in the United States for patients on ventilators. Respiratory alkalosis is not much of a problem unless the set rate is too high. The nurse should record the set rate as well as the patient's rate to determine whether the patient is breathing over the ventilator. Most health care providers want the patient to breathe over the set rate in order to use their respiratory muscles. If the patient does not breathe over the set SIMV rate, the team should

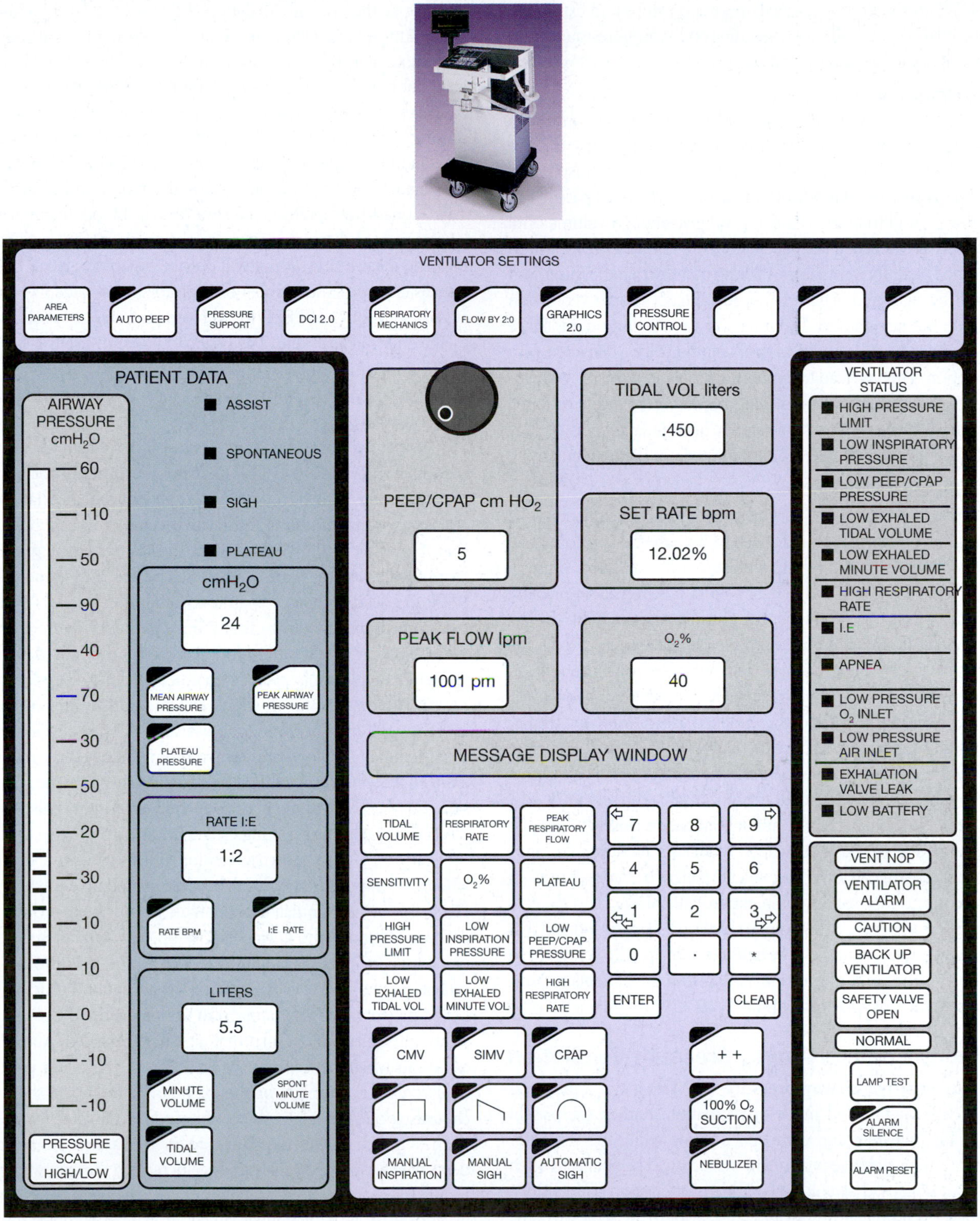

Third-generation control panel for the 7200 ventilator displays potential patient settings. If the mean airway pressure button is selected, the cmH_2O could be 24. In the next section the inspiratory to expiratory ratio is 1:2. If the rate in breaths/minute is selected that will be displayed in this window. The center panel illustrates 5 ventilator settings. In the example the PEEP is 5 cm H_2O, the tidal volumne is .450 liters, and the rate is 12 with a peak flow of 100 liters and an oxygen concentration of 40%.

FIGURE 28–7 ◆ Puritan-Bennett 7200 ventilator and control panel.
Source: Christielle Montichard/Nellcor Puritan Bennett LLC.

evaluate the levels of sedation and analgesia and consider decreasing them, as they may cause respiratory depression. Also, the set SIMV rate may be set too high. Decreasing the set rate will allow more opportunity for the patient to initiate a breath.

Pressure-Targeted Ventilation

Pressure-targeted, or pressure-controlled, modes of ventilation have a set inspiratory pressure. During the inspiration phase of the ventilatory cycle, an inspiratory breath is delivered until the inspiratory pressure setting is reached. When the limit is reached, inspiration stops and expiration begins. The tidal volume will vary depending on the lung's resistance and compliance. Resistive, noncompliant lungs will have a reduced volume.

Pressure-Control Ventilation

Pressure-control ventilation (PVC) is similar to AC ventilation except that, instead of a set volume being delivered, a set inspiratory pressure is targeted. The health care provider sets the rate and the inspiratory pressure. This is an assisted mode of ventilation in which the patient can initiate a breath, and then the ventilator will give enough volume until the set pressure is reached. If the patient does not initiate a breath within a programmed time, the ventilator will do so in order that the minimum set rate will be delivered. There is no guaranteed minute ventilation in this mode because the tidal volume will vary as lung compliance changes. As lungs become stiff, less tidal volume will be delivered with each inspiration. This can lead to hypoventilation and respiratory acidosis. Alternatively, as lungs heal, more tidal volume will be delivered to the set inspiratory pressure, which can lead to hyperventilation and respiratory alkalosis. The nurse should monitor minute ventilation regularly.

Pressure-Support Ventilation

Pressure-support ventilation (PSV) is an assisted form of ventilation. The patient must have a reliable respiratory effort because there is no set rate or set tidal volume delivered by the ventilator. If the ventilator senses a negative pressure, indicating a respiratory effort, it delivers a set pressure to assist with inspiration. The higher the pressure support is set, the less work the patient has to do. It is a common weaning mode in which the pressure support is gradually decreased, allowing the patient to take on more of the workload. If a patient requires high pressure support levels, the ventilator is taking on much of the workload of breathing, and the patient is not ready to be removed from the ventilator. A minimum pressure support level is used to overcome the resistance of the artificial airway, that is, an endotracheal tube or tracheostomy. Since there is no set rate or tidal volume, the nurse should monitor minute ventilation closely to identify hypoventilation and set the apnea alarm. Ventilators also allow the clinician to set a backup rate that will kick in if the patient becomes apneic.

PSV is commonly used in combination with SIMV. The patient's spontaneous breaths in the SIMV mode receive pressure support so that these potentially weak efforts will be assisted, allowing the ventilator to take on more of the work of breathing and giving the patient's respiratory muscles some rest and healing time.

Continuous Positive Airway Pressure Ventilation

Continuous positive airway pressure (CPAP) is not a pressure-targeted or volume-targeted mode of ventilation. Rather, the patient breathes at his own rate and own tidal volume while the ventilator places a continuous positive pressure in the airway. The goal is to open up or prevent collapsed alveoli. This mode is often used to identify a patient's ability to ventilate without assistance prior to the removal of the endotracheal tube. CPAP may also be used in patients who do not have a ventilation or oxygenation abnormality but have an artificial airway in place for airway protection, such as patients with a swollen upper airway that is at risk of obstruction. This mode should not be used in patients who are at risk of neurogenic or hemodynamic compromise in which spontaneous respirations are unreliable.

Positive End-Expiratory Pressure

Positive end-expiratory pressure (PEEP) is not a mode of ventilation but a ventilator setting. (See Chart 28–9 for other ventilator settings.) Normally, the pressure in the alveoli is equal to atmospheric pressure at the end of exhalation. PEEP exerts continuous pressure above atmospheric levels on the airways during both inspiration and expiration. This helps to prevent the cyclic opening of alveoli during inspiration and collapse during expiration. This action, referred to as *cyclic atelectasis,* may cause a local and systemic inflammatory response, causing further lung injury. Oxygenation status is affected by increasing FiO_2 and/or adding PEEP. The pressure exerted in the airway improves oxygenation by opening up collapsed airways and increasing FRC. This reduces intrapulmonary shunting of blood through collapsed lung regions and therefore improves ventilation/perfusion mismatching. The ideal PEEP setting will recruit collapsed alveoli but will not overdistend and injure functioning alveoli. Most patients benefit from at least 5 cm H_2O of PEEP to overcome the airway resistance exerted by the endotracheal tube. The goal should be to use the least amount of PEEP to achieve a PaO_2 of 55 to 60 mmHg with a FiO_2 of less than 60%. Prolonged FiO_2 above 60% can cause cytotoxic (producing a toxic effect on cells) injury.

There are negative consequences to PEEP, so it should be used with caution in some patients. PEEP increases the intrathoracic pressure and reduces venous return to the heart. If patients already have a reduced circulatory volume, adding PEEP can precipitate or aggravate hypotension. However, this hypotension can be mitigated or minimized by ensuring that volume status is addressed before PEEP is increased. High PEEP can lead to hemodynamic instability in patients with cardiac failure or compromise by further reducing cardiac output. PEEP should be increased gradually while blood pressure is monitored meticulously. As PEEP is applied in patients with unilateral lung disease, it will follow the path of least resistance, which will be to the healthy lung. This can lead to overdistention of the healthy alveoli, causing alveolar injury, and constriction of the vasculature surrounding the alveoli, leading to worsening of the shunt. If possible, it might help to position the patient on his side with the healthy lung in the dependent position. This will improve blood flow to the healthy lung via gravity and improve gas exchange.

Auto-PEEP (also known as residual PEEP or intrinsic PEEP) occurs when air is trapped in the alveoli because of incomplete exhalation. This can occur in nonventilated patients in whom there is obstruction or collapse of the airways during expiration, such as patients with COPD or asthma. Patients are taught to reduce auto-PEEP through exercises such as pursed-lip breathing, forcing the air out of the airways. In ventilated patients with expiratory flow abnormalities, PEEP may help by stenting the airways open so that air can be exhaled. Auto-PEEP also can occur when the respiratory rate set on the ventilator is too fast, the tidal volume is too high, or the expiratory time is too short. In these circumstances, the tidal volume cannot be completely exhaled before the next breath is delivered. This is referred to as breath stacking. In patients who are prone to air-trapping, increasing the expiratory time will facilitate alveolar emptying. The respiratory therapist can assess the level of auto-PEEP by a maneuver called an expiratory hold. Immediately before a breath, the expiratory port is closed for 2 seconds. As the flow ceases, the resistive pressure is eliminated and the resulting pressure demonstrates the alveolar pressure at the end of expiration. The consequences of auto-PEEP are serious. It increases the work of breathing, is uncomfortable for the patient, and can lead to patient–ventilatory asynchrony, which many nurses refer to as "bucking the ventilator." When this occurs, the patient is not being adequately ventilated. Sedation is not the answer to this problem, and every attempt should be made to assess the cause of the asynchrony before resorting to heavy sedation or paralysis. Auto-PEEP can also worsen gas exchange and induce hemodynamic compromise. PEEP increases intrathoracic pressure, reducing blood flow back to the heart. If severe and unrecognized, this can lead to cardiac arrest.

Finally, the clinician can cause auto-PEEP through the overaggressive use of bag-mask ventilation when the patient is removed from the ventilator for transport, CPR, or suctioning. Rapid bagging rates are used to ventilate the patient instead of the rate that was set on the ventilator. Treatment would involve disconnecting the patient from the bag-mask device or ventilator to allow the excess pressure to dissipate.

The ventilator panel in Figure 28–7 shows the modes that have been discussed. Note that the CMV mode on this particular ventilator is really AC. Some manufacturers use the term *CMV assist* or *CMV with trigger* to refer to AC ventilation. There is no standard classification of terms used by manufacturers of ventilators when describing modes. This can create confusion and is especially difficult when the novice is attempting to understand the different modes and their implications for patient care.

Complications of Mechanical Ventilation

As soon as a patient is intubated and mechanical ventilation is initiated, the nurse should immediately begin activating a plan to liberate the patient from the ventilator. The ventilator and endotracheal tube are necessary interventions to treat acute respiratory failure and other diseases in which the patient's own pulmonary or cardiovascular system cannot support exchange of oxygen and removal of carbon dioxide. However, ventilator support is not without some risk. For example, an endotracheal tube and positive pressure ventilation expose the patient to an increased risk of morbidity and mortality. One way in which the nurse can reduce this risk is to coordinate the care of the patient who is ventilated to ensure timely extubation. Another way is to recognize the possible complications that can occur and work diligently to prevent them if at all possible. The important complications of mechanical ventilation are presented next, organized by organ systems. This is not an exhaustive list, nor does it deal with some of the complications of long-term mechanical ventilation. Nursing implications and prevention strategies are also discussed.

Cardiovascular Complications

Cardiovascular complications of mechanical ventilation are variable and depend on the amount of pressure used to ventilate the lungs, the amount of PEEP, and the underlying heart and lung dynamics. The heart and lungs are a system, and what affects one component of that system will usually affect the other. In the setting of cardiac failure, mechanical ventilation can unload some of the stress exerted on the heart by decreasing the amount of blood coming into the heart (preload) and the amount of resistance encountered when the heart is attempting to pump blood into the circulation (afterload). This assistance by the ventilator remains invisible until the patient is weaned, and then chest pain and other symptoms of heart failure may develop.

One of the most common complications of mechanical ventilation is hypotension. This can occur immediately after intubation and initiation of positive pressure ventilation or anytime during the course of treatment. This hypotension is related to decreased cardiac output, hypovolemia, and positive pressure delivered by the ventilator. This positive pressure changes the pressure in the thorax. Positive pressure ventilation can reduce ventricular filling by decreasing the amount of blood that flows into the atria (preload) and therefore decreasing filling during ventricular diastole. This decreased preload produces the hypotension. Compression of the pulmonary vessels can reduce blood flow into the left atrium or impede the ejection of blood from the right heart. The increased pressure in the chest produced by mechanical ventilation also can affect the dispensability (ability to produce optimal fluid ejection) of the chambers of the heart, especially during diastole. The increased pleural pressure from the chest can be transmitted to the heart and prevent filling.

Assessing the patient for heart failure and intervening with appropriate treatment in the patient on the ventilator are the nurse's primary tasks in preventing cardiovascular complications. If hypotension is the presenting symptom without other indications of cardiac failure, fluid boluses can be administered that usually correct hypovolemia and reverse the hypotension. The nurse should be prepared to intervene, report to the health care provider, and institute treatment for this common complication. Recognizing the hypotension as potentially being related to the mechanical ventilation is important. The premedications used prior to intubation also can cause hypotension but will respond to increasing intravascular volume. In some situations, vasoactive medications such as dopamine might be required to support the blood pressure. Increased levels of PEEP, whether set PEEP or auto-PEEP, also can cause hypotension. It is important to decrease set PEEP levels if hypotension is a direct result of increased PEEP. Preventing auto-PEEP by allowing time for the patient to exhale or preventing stacking of breaths, discussed previously, by adequately sedating the patient or selecting the correct mode also can prevent hypotension. Decreased cardiac output and decreased pH can predispose some patients to cardiac dysrhythmias. Careful attention to fluid and electrolyte replacement can help prevent this complication from occurring. Chapter 30 includes a complete description of cardiac dysrhythmias.

Pulmonary Complications

Barotrauma is defined as damage to lung tissue that can lead to alveolar rupture caused by increased pressure resulting from high ventilation pressures. **Volutrauma** is similar, but the lung damage is caused by increased volume that causes overdistention and hyperinflation of alveoli. These lung injuries are termed ventilator-induced lung injury (VILI) or ventilated-associated lung injury (VALI). In patients with severe ALI/ARDS, lungs are stiff and have reduced compliance. The amount of pressure required to fully inflate the lungs can lead to high inspiratory pressures that can cause barotrauma and volutrauma. The ARDS Network's landmark study demonstrated that plateau pressures above 35 cm H_2O were associated with increased morbidity and mortality (Acute Respiratory Distress Syndrome Network, 2000). Plateau pressure, the true pressure that is transmitted to the alveoli, is obtained by a maneuver the respiratory therapist performs called an inspiratory hold (as described earlier in the chapter). The ARDS Network study determined that low tidal volumes (6 mL/kg) in patients with ALI/ARDS correlated with improved outcomes. Monitoring of plateau pressures can alert the team to increased risk of barotrauma and volutrauma. Besides the damage that these high pressures inflict on the alveoli, increased pressure can lead to pneumothorax (Chapter 27), pneumomediastinum, or subcutaneous emphysema (emphysema that is produced when small pockets of air are trapped under the skin). Atelectasis can occur because of a mucus plug that obstructs the airway.

Severe airway injury can occur with high pressures, long-term ventilation, or a predisposing abnormality. In addition, the endotracheal tube, the tape, or other devices used to secure the tube can cause nasopharyngeal injury. Ulcerations of the lips, nose, and mouth are common in patients who have endotracheal tubes but can be prevented in most instances. Sinusitis is a common infection produced by the increase in secretions and the inability of drainage because of the tube's location in the upper airway. Tracheal damage and tracheoesophageal fistulas have

Video: Tracheostomy: Sterile

become less common with the universal use of low-pressure, high-volume cuffed endotracheal tubes.

Oxygen toxicity is another complication of mechanical ventilation that can occur with prolonged high FiO_2 levels. In the treatment of life-threatening hypoxia, 100% oxygen should always be administered; however, excessive or inappropriate oxygen delivery can lead to lung injury. It is unclear what the duration of hyperoxia or the threshold of FiO_2 is that leads to oxygen toxicity. Therefore, it is generally recommended that FiO_2 should be titrated to the lowest concentration that produces a PaO_2 of 55 to 60 mmHg in patients with lung disease (Malhotra, Schwartz, & Schwartzstein, 2009). Hypoxia may not be tolerated as well in patients with cardiac disease and those with neurologic injury; these patients need to maintain a PaO_2 of at least 60 mmHg and saturation of greater than 90%. Strategies that can be used to reduce FiO_2 include diuresis, recruitment maneuvers/PEEP, prone positioning, and bronchopulmonary hygiene.

Prevention of soft-tissue injury of the lips, nares, and oral mucosa from the endotracheal tube and its attachment can be accomplished by paying careful attention to how the tube is secured. Many different types of tube holders are available besides the standard cloth tape used to secure the tube. Frequent changes of the device and assessment of underlying soft tissue are important. The nurse and the respiratory therapist working together can prevent the patient from acquiring an injury that is preventable.

Humidification of the entire ventilator circuit prevents excessive mucus plugging. There are many methods of humidification, such as a heat and moisture exchanger (HME) and heater-humidifiers. Providing humidification is an important intervention in using any type of artificial airway that bypasses the natural humidification provided by the nose and upper airway. If this is not done, mucus plugging is a common complication of mechanical ventilation.

Suctioning of the endotracheal tube to remove secretions is an integral part of endotracheal tube management. This is a sterile procedure, so a sealed system should be used to minimize nosocomial contamination. The frequency of suctioning depends on the quantity of secretions. Suctioning techniques are discussed in detail in Chapter 26.

A tracheostomy tube may be inserted in patients who require long-term ventilation management to prevent some of the complications of ulcerations, sinusitis, and pressure injury to the trachea. Other benefits include patient comfort, a secure airway, enabling of effective airway suctioning, decreased airway resistance and dead space, better patient mobility, increased opportunities for communication, and the ability to eat.

There is very little information regarding the optimum time to perform a tracheostomy on a mechanically ventilated patient. The ability to insert a tracheostomy tube at the bedside via percutaneous dilation eliminates the need to transport patients who are critically ill to the operating room. This method of tracheostomy placement involves blunt dissection and dilation with the placement of a tight fitting tracheostomy tube. It is associated with fewer bleeding complications; however, if the tube is accidentally displaced immediately postoperatively, the stoma may become occluded (Neacy, 2009). This tube is more stable and secure and has less dead space than an endotracheal tube. The care and management of patients with tracheostomy tubes are discussed in detail in Chapter 26.

Gastrointestinal Complications

Abdominal distention is a common complication of mechanical ventilation. Gastric distention as a result of swallowed air from pressure ventilation necessitates the routine use of a nasal or oral gastric tube to decompress the stomach. Stress ulcer prevention is another important intervention to prevent gastrointestinal bleeding. Gastric ulcer formation is discussed in Chapter 37.

Psychological Complications

Agitation, anxiety, and confusion are all complications of mechanical ventilation. It is very uncomfortable for a patient to be attached to a machine to breathe and unable to communicate simple wishes. Lack of adequate sleep and use of analgesics and sedatives also may contribute to this state. Providing periods of uninterrupted sleep is important in preventing agitation in the patient on a ventilator. Use of a speaking board, lip reading, or a special tracheostomy tube that forces air through the vocal cords can assist the patient in communicating. Sedating appropriately using a sedation scale and individualized sedation for each patient is key to providing good nursing care.

Ventilator-Associated Pneumonia

Ventilator-associated pneumonia (VAP) is defined as pneumonia that develops more than 48 hours after intubation. It is the most common form of infection among patients in the ICU who receive mechanical ventilation and is associated with a mortality rate of 20% to 50% (Chastre & Luyt, 2010). The rate of pneumonia for intubated patients is 3 to 10 times higher than that of patients who are not intubated. Endotracheal intubation interferes with the body's defenses, impairs mucociliary clearance, inhibits cough, and facilitates microaspiration of bacterial secretions that pool above the cuff of the tube (Bartlett, 2008). Most infections appear to originate from microaspiration of pathogens from the oropharynx, dental plaque, and nasal sinuses that pool and leak from around the cuff into the subglottic area. This pooling also generates the formation of a biofilm around the inner and outer surfaces of the endotracheal tube. The pathogens that are involved vary with the underlying disease and whether the VAP is of early or late onset. Gram-negative bacilli represent approximately 58% of identified organisms, including *P. aeruginosa* and *Acinetobacter baumannii*, as well as *Proteus mirabalis*, *Escherichia coli*, *Klebsiella pneumoniae*, and *H. influenzae*. Many VAP infections are caused by multiple pathogens (Chastre & Luyt, 2010).

The prevention of VAP depends on a multifactorial, multidisciplinary program. These programs are often referred to as "care bundles" and include evidence-based interventions that are consistently applied to every patient on a daily basis. Failure to fulfill one portion of the bundle results in a failure of the entire bundle. A culture of prevention depends on the attitude, motivation, and consistent practice of all health care workers.

Many evidence-based interventions have no or low cost. These include the following:

- Maintaining the endotracheal tube cuff pressure above 20 cm H_2O to prevent secretions from leaking into the respiratory tract
- Reintubating patients quickly if they do not tolerate extubation
- Keeping the head of the bead up 30° to 45°, particularly in patients who are receiving enteral feedings
- Providing oral care every 2 to 4 hours and prn
- Paying attention to conventional infection control measures such as hand washing and wearing gloves
- Removing condensation from ventilator tubing
- Avoiding the placement of endotracheal or gastric tubes through the nares, and
- Reducing the duration of mechanical ventilation (Chastre & Luyt, 2010).

NATIONAL GUIDELINES for the Prevention of Health Care–Associated Bacterial Pneumonia

Recommendations for Nursing Care

1. Wash hands after contact with mucous membranes, respiratory secretions, or objects contaminated with respiratory secretions. Wash hands before and after patient contact.
2. Educate health care workers about nosocomial bacterial pneumonias and infection control procedures used to prevent these pneumonias. Involve workers in implementing strategies for intervention.
3. Wear gloves when handling respiratory secretions or objects contaminated with respiratory secretions.
4. Provide subglottic suctioning before deflating the cuff of an endotracheal tube or before moving the tube.
5. Elevate the head of the bed to 30° to 45° if not contraindicated.
6. Develop and implement a comprehensive oral hygiene program to provide oropharyngeal cleaning and decontamination with or without an antiseptic agent.
7. Use chlorhexidine gluconate antiseptic rinse during the perioperative period in adult patients who undergo cardiac surgery.

Source: Adapted from Cason, C .L., Tyner, T., Saunders, S., & Broome L. (2007) Nurses' implementation of guidelines for VAP from the CDC. *American Journal of Critical Care, 16,* 2–37.

There is some evidence that supports VAP reduction by using endotracheal tubes that are coated both internally and externally with an antiseptic product such as silver, which has an antimicrobial effect in blocking the formation of biofilm on the tube surfaces (Chastre & Luyt, 2010). Recommendations by the CDC specific to nursing interventions are listed in the National Guidelines box.

The other important intervention is providing oral care to patients who cannot perform their own oral care. Decontamination of the oral cavity with either tooth brushing or use of other interventions may reduce VAP. The American Association of Critical Care Nurses (2010) recommends developing and implementing a comprehensive oral hygiene program for patients in critical care and acute care settings who are at high risk for health care–associated pneumonia. Interventions include the following:

- Brush teeth, gums, and tongue at least twice a day using a soft pediatric or adult toothbrush.
- Provide oral moisturizing to oral mucosa and lips every 2 to 4 hours.
- Use an oral chlorhexidine gluconate (0.12%) rinse twice a day during the perioperative period for adult patients who undergo cardiac surgery. Routine use in other populations is not recommended at this time.

The Complementary & Alternative Therapies box discusses cupping, a practice that patients may use at home when their pneumonia is not severe enough to warrant hospitalization.

Nursing Assessment and Care of the Ventilated Patient

Many of the interventions that are provided by nurses when caring for a patient on a ventilator determine the success of weaning and the prevention of complications. The attention to details and basic nursing care in this population affects the outcome of patients who require ventilators. Among the most important of these interventions is an accurate and detailed assessment. This section reviews the priorities of assessment and care of the patient on ventilation. It includes a discussion of suctioning and weaning.

COMPLEMENTARY & ALTERNATIVE THERAPIES Cupping

Nancy Yilk

CUPPING REFERS TO AN ANCIENT CHINESE PRACTICE in which cups are applied to the skin to suck out noxious materials. The therapy has been used in China for thousands of years. The technique involves the use of small glass cups, into which a small cloth saturated with alcohol or an herbal mixture is inserted and then ignited. The cup is then pressed against the skin to create a vacuum. The cups are placed on specific acupuncture points and remain for a period of time or are moved across the skin in a dragging motion to follow specific terrains. The cupping often results in a purpling to the skin in round circles mimicking the placement of the cups. There is typically no pain and the purple areas fade in a few days.

Cupping has been used historically for a wide range of health complaints. It was primarily a home remedy that was performed by midwives and family members for respiratory complaints, pain, and fevers. This therapy was used widely in the United States in the 18th and 19th centuries. In fact, as late as 1931 it was indicated in the treatment of bronchopneumonia and acute myelitis. Cupping was included in U.S. medical textbooks prior to 1940 and performed in sanatoriums for tuberculosis. In fact, the therapy is still used today in many cultures.

Cupping fell out of use in the medical field with the onset of newer applications of drugs and surgeries, but remained a mainstay in cultural teachings in Traditional Chinese Medicine (TCM). Currently there is an upsurge in its use within the United States from immigrating families from Pacific Rim countries where family members practice it as a natural medicine.

Between 1959 and 2008, 550 clinical studies were conducted regarding the practice of cupping, including 73 randomized controlled trials (RCTs), 22 clinical controlled trials, 373 case series, and 82 case reports. RCTs on cupping therapy appear to have improved during the past 50 years in China, and the majority of studies show potential benefits for pain conditions, herpes zoster, and other diseases, though increasing an unbiased approach to results will improve the understanding of cupping's benefits and risk (Huijuan et al., 2010).

Researchers explored various distinctions regarding techniques that were employed in cupping patients for the common cold at its early stages and the time duration that the cups were applied. In a randomized trial, 60 patients who were starting to experience colds were assigned to either an observational or control group. The technique of flash cupping, in which the cup is applied to the skin and suctioned in a quick pumping of the cupping tool, was applied to five acupoints historically used for colds. The therapeutic effects were compared after applying the treatments twice to the back. The total effect rate was 93.3% (28/30) in the experimental group, which was superior to the results of 66.7% (20/30) found in the control group ($P < 0.01$) (Ye, Zhang, & Pang, 2011).

The results demonstrated that, in the instances of the common cold, the longer applications were more beneficial. With such a simple treatment, even people who do not know the classic names of the application points can learn the techniques and use them in their families. However, the need still exists to define proper use of cup application and the correct location of cups among both practitioners and participants who want to learn the technique and don't benefit from the oral teachings of an elder in their community.

References

Adapted from Huijuan, C., Mei, H., Xun, L., Shangjuan, D., Yongmei, S., Qian, W., et al. (2010). Clinical research evidence of cupping therapy in China: A systematic literature review. *Complementary and Alternative Medicine, 10,* 70.

Ye, X. F., Zhang, H. F., & Pang, Z. W. (2011). Therapeutic effects of common cold of wind-cold type at early stage treated by different cupping duration. *Zhongguo Zhen Jiu, 31*(4), 357–359.

Inspection

Observing the patient and the patient–ventilator interactions is a highly underrated task. To observe the patient on a ventilator, the nurse stands at the foot of the bed and observes how the patient is breathing. The nurse should use a standardized method of observation, such as the head-to-toe method. In this option, the nurse starts at the patient's head and observes important structures in an organized manner. The nurse checks the endotracheal tube for its size and depth of insertion. The nurse also assesses the method of securing the tube, since a loose tube can cause pressure ulcers or, worse, accidental extubation. In addition, the nurse notes the presence of an oral airway. Oral airways usually are placed to prevent the patient from biting the tube; however, they can cause significant oral trauma and prevent mouth care. The nurse inspects the ventilator circuit to ensure that it is not pulling on the endotracheal tube or creating tension on the tube. The ventilator circuit should be free of fluid. If fluid is in the tubing, it can get into the airway and contaminate it.

The nurse notes the amount and color of secretions in the endotracheal tube and the patient's mouth and nose and assesses the position of the patient's head. Some patients develop torsion of the neck muscles because they always keep their heads turned toward the side of the bed where the ventilator is situated. The nurse also assesses the patient for agitation. Hypoxemia should be ruled out as a cause of agitation and restlessness, especially before administering medication for sedation and analgesia. Cyanosis present around the mouth and mucous membranes suggests central cyanosis and hypoxemia.

Observation of the patient's chest wall for an adequate and symmetrical breathing pattern is crucial in assessing the patient on a ventilator. The nurse assesses for asymmetry between the right and left sides of the chest and observes for unusual movements. A tension pneumothorax or pleural effusion can change the size of the affected lung, making it appear larger. In contrast, the side where an atelectatic segment is located can appear smaller. The right and left sides of the chest should be symmetrical and should rise equally with inspiration and fall with expiration. Paradoxical breathing can occur with trauma to the chest but also with muscle fatigue of the diaphragm. On inspiration, the chest rises and the abdomen is drawn in because the fatigued diaphragm cannot descend on inspiration, as it should.

The nurse looks for use of accessory muscles of ventilation. For example, is the patient's work of breathing increased because of the ventilator mode or size of the endotracheal tube? Phrenic nerve injury or paralysis can affect the diaphragm and can be present on only one side of the chest, producing asymmetry in inspiration or paradoxical movement of the diaphragm. The nurse notes whether the abdomen is distended and protruding into the chest, preventing adequate ventilation. It is important to observe whether the upper extremities are more swollen than the feet, since patients who have been on a ventilator for a significant period often accumulate peripheral edema in the upper extremities (more so than in the feet). Mottling of the extremities signifies vasoconstriction. If the patient is shivering, monitor her temperature and assess for signs of pulmonary infection such as increased sputum; change in color, consistency, or odor of sputum; and increased oxygen requirements. Any noise of escaping air heard on expiration could be caused by too low a volume in the endotracheal tube cuff. Other signs of loss of cuff volume include bubbling of oral secretions and the patient's ability to phonate.

Palpation

Deviation of the trachea is seen in defects such as tension pneumothorax or tension hemothorax. The nurse begins by palpating the trachea, checking for its position as well as mobility. The chest wall is next; the nurse feels for any abnormalities, bulging, or depressions. The point of maximal impulse (PMI) is palpated. Palpating for fremitus is another important component of the assessment. Pleural friction fremitus is a palpable vibration produced when the swollen, inflamed pleural surfaces come in contact with each other. Pleural friction fremitus can usually be felt during both expiration and inspiration but sometimes only during inspiration. Rhonchial fremitus is vibration produced when air is forced through thick secretions.

The nurse also checks the chest wall and extremities for subcutaneous emphysema, which is produced by air being forced into the tissue from a pneumothorax or other communication with the airway. Subcutaneous emphysema prompts the team to check for this apparent pathology but usually resolves without treatment.

Auscultation

Auscultation is the most significant component of the assessment of the patient who is ventilated. The frequency of assessment is patient specific and based on other assessment parameters. For example, if the pulse oximetry reading falls to 88% from 99%, the nurse should, after ensuring that the patient is receiving oxygen and ventilation from the ventilator, immediately assess lung sounds. Absent lung sounds on the left, for instance, could signal a pneumothorax. The endotracheal tube placed in the right main stem bronchus preventing air from entering the left lung also could cause the absence of lung sounds on the left.

The nurse should listen posteriorly as well as anteriorly, starting at the top of the thorax and moving down. When listening, the nurse should compare the right against the left lung and never listen through clothing or other material. The nurse should listen laterally in order to appreciate certain lung segments that can be heard in this position. For example, on the right side, by listening laterally, the nurse can auscultate the anterior basal segment of the right lower lobe. Assessing lung sounds in a ventilated patient can be assisted by performing manual breaths with the ventilator or by removing the patient from the ventilator and having someone bag the patient while the other practitioner listens. Normal lung sounds heard in abnormal locations can alert the nurse to certain abnormalities. For example, bronchial or bronchovesicular sounds heard over the periphery can indicate consolidation caused by pneumonia. This sound can also be a result of atelectasis.

The nurse assesses adventitious or abnormal sounds to ascertain the apparent cause of the abnormality. Crackles occur first in the bases; without listening posteriorly, the nurse cannot assess the majority of the lung fields. Inspiratory or expiratory wheezes could be the result of a constriction of the bronchi. Initiation of a bronchodilatory treatment administered as a nebulization through the ventilator circuit might be indicated. Gurgles or rhonchi are low-pitched continuous sounds that are heard over the large airways and sometimes are so loud that the sound is transmitted throughout the lung field. This sound should prompt the nurse to assess the need for suctioning the endotracheal tube. Diminished lung sounds in the ventilated patient can be indicative of pleural fluid accumulation, pneumothorax, or obesity. Chapters 6 and 27 include in-depth discussions of the lung sounds.

Usually, when abnormal or absent sounds are observed in the ventilated patient, a portable chest x-ray is ordered, particularly if the absence of normal sounds is associated with pulmonary compromise such as desaturation. The use of a chest x-ray should not preclude an excellent clinical exam, an important component of which is auscultation of the lungs. Depending on the facility, it can take many minutes to take a portable chest x-ray and even longer to produce the film. Some disorders such as tension pneumothorax can produce a fatal outcome in a few minutes. Tension pneumothorax is more common in patients who are receiving positive pressure ventilation. Air enters the pleural space through a defect in the lung parenchyma and is trapped in the pleural space. As the pressure in the pleural space increases from the trapped air, the lung collapses, causing the pressure to displace the trachea and great vessels to the opposite side. If the pressure is not relieved, the remaining lung collapses. This can occur very rapidly. Successful treatment is a needle thoracostomy followed by placement of a chest tube.

Safety Alert *Abnormal or absent lung sounds can indicate an emergency situation. The nurse at the bedside must be able to quickly assess the change in the lung exam and alert the health care provider.*

Nursing Management

Many patients who are mechanically ventilated have chest tubes; therefore, part of nursing management is ensuring that the chest drainage system is intact and functioning properly. There are two types of chest tubes: pleural tubes and mediastinal tubes. A pleural tube is inserted in the pleural space in order to evacuate the air or blood and allow the lung to reexpand. The pleural tube re-creates the normal negative pressure in the chest that has been violated by trauma or surgery. Indications for insertion of a pleural tube include all the conditions listed in Chart 28–11.

A mediastinal tube is placed in the mediastinum after this area has been opened during cardiac or thoracic surgery. Mediastinal tubes prevent fluid and blood from collecting in the mediastinum and exerting pressure on the heart. These tubes do not look any different from pleural tubes. Usually they are inserted in the subxiphoid area, but only the surgeon or the operative report can alert the nurse to the difference in the two types of chest tubes.

Assessment

Pleural tubes are connected to underwater seal drainage or to a one-way valve. Both of these devices allow air to exit the chest but prevent air from entering the chest. Pleural tubes exhibit a characteristic called tidaling, in which the fluid in the tube can be seen moving with respiration. If there is no fluid in the tube, many chest drainage systems have a fluid diagnostic chamber in which the tidaling can be seen. It is important to assess this fluid movement either in the tube or in the diagnostic fluid chamber to ensure that the chest tube is in the thoracic cavity and there is no blockage.

Mediastinal tubes exhibit no tidaling because they are located in the mediastinal space and not the pleural space. Mediastinal tubes usually drain blood or other fluid. An important intervention with these tubes is to ensure that they are patent and draining freely. Most chest tube systems include an autotransfusion unit attachment so that blood can be reinfused.

Initially, chest tubes are connected to suction to increase the drainage and to assist the lungs in reexpansion. The suction is most commonly set at 20 cm of water pressure. Though disconnecting the chest tube from suction is not recommended, this action does not allow air to enter the chest; rather, it only stops the suction. As the drainage diminishes and the lung reexpands, the health care provider will discontinue the suction for a few hours prior to the tube's removal.

No chest tube should ever be clamped except under direct observation prior to removal. Clamping a chest tube can allow a tension pneumothorax to develop. The risk of a tension pneumothorax is increased when a patient is receiving positive pressure ventilation.

Insertion of a Chest Tube

The equipment needed for insertion of a chest tube is listed in Chart 28–12. Pleural tubes commonly are inserted at the bedside, whereas mediastinal tubes are inserted in the operating room during surgery. The tube's location on the chest is related to the reason for the chest tube insertion. If a chest tube is inserted to decompress a pneumothorax, it usually is inserted anteriorly, whereas a chest tube that is inserted to drain fluid or blood from the chest is inserted in a more posterior location on the chest wall. Air rises to the anterior surface of the chest when a patient is supine; therefore, placement of a chest tube is anterior if insertion is required because of a pneumothorax. If there is blood in the pleural space, a chest tube will be placed posteriorly because the blood will settle in the posterior portion of the chest cavity. Many different types of chest tube drainage systems are commercially available. Figure 28–8 ◆ (p. 816) shows an illustration of a typical device.

Nutrition

Another important concern for the nurse providing care to the patient who is mechanically ventilated is preventing malnutrition while simultaneously not overfeeding and producing excess CO_2. Most patients who are enterally fed in critical care units do not have their nutritional needs met for multiple reasons such as excessive residuals, interrupted feedings because of procedures, and loss of access. The consequences of malnutrition include loss of respiratory muscle mass, strength, and function as well as compromised immunity. Malnutrition may lead to infection, failure to wean from the ventilator, and atelectasis.

CHART 28–11 Indications for Insertion of a Chest Tube

Indications for a Pleural Tube
- Hemothorax
- Pneumothorax
- Hemopneumothorax
- Pleural effusion
- Drainage of pus (empyema), bile (cholothorax), or chyle (chylothorax) from the pleural cavity
- Postoperative thoracostomy

Indications for a Mediastinal Tube
- Drainage of the mediastinal space after surgical procedure
- Cardiac surgery
- Pericardial window

CHART 28–12 Necessary Equipment for Insertion of a Chest Tube

Chest tube insertion tray	Scissors
Tube (size specified by health care provider)	Sutures
	Sterile gloves
Scalpel with size 11 blade	4 × 4 gauze
Kelly clamps or artery forceps	Suction setup
10-mL and 20-mL syringe	Suction tubing
One small-gauge needle (size 25)	Chest tube collection system
A needle driver	Vaseline gauze
Local anesthetic (Xylocaine)	Silk tape
Antiseptic scrub	

Source: Adapted from Lynn-McHale-D., & Carlson, K. (2001). *AACN Procedure Manual* (4th ed.). Philadelphia: W.B. Saunders. This article was published in the *AACN Procedure Manual,* 4th ed., p. 110. Lynn-McHale-D, & Carlson, K. Copyright W.B. Saunders, Philadelphia, 2001.

Enteral feeding via a nasogastric or oral gastric feeding tube is the preferred method. Small lumen feeding tubes are being used more often than larger bore feeding tubes because of increased patient comfort. Aspiration and other complications including malposition can be prevented by instituting standard protocols and by monitoring problems associated with these tubes at the unit level (Metheny, Meert, & Clouse, 2007). Careful assessment of abdominal distention and bowel frequency can decrease the risk of aspiration. Interventions to prevent aspiration include keeping the head of the bed elevated and administering medications to assist with gastric motility. Instillation of blue food coloring in the enteral feeding is not recommended because of possible contamination of the tube feeding. A complete description of enteral feedings is presented in Chapter 8.

Communication and Sleep

All patients need the ability to communicate their needs to the people who are caring for them. Since an inability to communicate because of mechanical ventilation is a concern for the patient, the nurse should recognize this need. Many devices are now available to help the patient communicate. Some are sophisticated, such as a speaking tracheostomy tube that allows a patient on a ventilator to communicate. This special tracheostomy tube has a port that can be connected directly to another oxygen source. The port exits near the vocal cords, and with some training the patient can learn to speak. A much simpler device that allows the patient to communicate is a message board with an alphabet or symbols to which the patient can point if he is unable to write.

Lack of sleep is another concern for the patients who are receiving mechanical ventilation. The nurse should arrange for periods of rest and uninterrupted sleep in the patient's plan of care. Hospitalized patients typically receive very little uninterrupted sleep, and patients who are in critical care units or in other specialty units receiving mechanical ventilation are more likely to be suffering from lack of sleep.

Weaning From Mechanical Ventilation

Delay in removing a patient from mechanical ventilation leads to longer ICU stays, increased cost, increased risk of infection, and prolonged subjection of patients to circuit pressures (MacIntyre, 2010). The benefits of early extubation must be weighed against the risk of premature removal, which include loss of a patent airway, aspiration, and respiratory muscle fatigue. Weaning is the process of gradually reducing ventilator support to the patient. Patients who have a stable lung injury, have adequate gas exchange on low PEEP and low FiO_2 requirements, are hemodynamically stable, and are able to breathe spontaneously should be considered candidates for ventilator weaning. Objective clinical criteria should be used to evaluate weaning readiness. A panel of experts

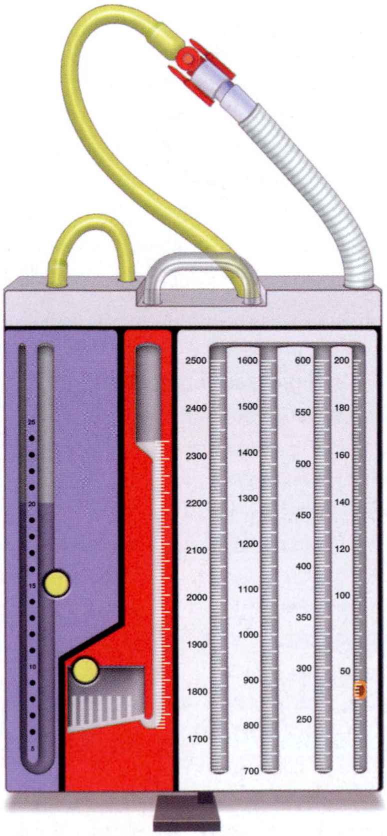

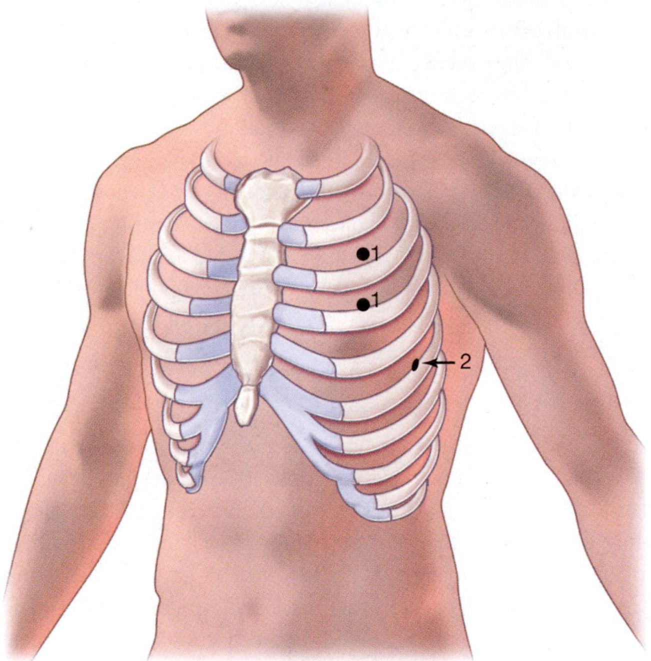

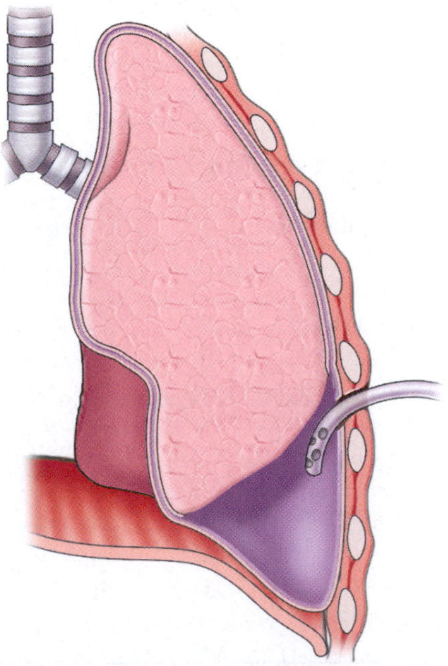

FIGURE 28–8 ◆ Chest tube drainage.

CHART 28–13 Clinical Criteria for Weaning Readiness

Required Criteria	Optional Criteria
Underlying cause of failure has improved.	Hemoglobin ≥ 8 to 10 mg/dL
$PaO_2/FiO_2 \geq 150$ or $SpO_2 \geq 90\%$ on $FiO_2 \leq 40\%$ and PEEP ≤ 5 cm H_2O	Core temperature ≤ 38° to 38.5°C
Hemodynamically stable (no or low dose vasopressors)	Awake and alert or easily arousable
Able to initiate inspiratory effort	

Source: Adapted from Epstein, S. (2010). Weaning from mechanical ventilation: Readiness testing. In P. Parsons & K. Wilson (Eds.), *UpToDate.* Waltham, MA: UpToDate.

CHART 28–14 Rapid Shallow Breathing Index

Definition	Clinical Example
f/V_T = RSBI Ratio of respiratory frequency (f) (breaths/minute) to tidal volume (V_T) (liters).	Calculate the RSBI for a patient whose respiratory rate is 28 breaths per minute and V_T is 250 mL or 0.25 liters: 28/0.25 = 112
If $f/V_T > 105$: probability that patient will fail to wean from the ventilator.	This patient is probably not ready to wean.

has proposed a set of required and optional criteria to identify patient readiness for weaning (Chart 28–13). Weaning predictor tests may also be used to support clinical criteria to determine whether patients can be successfully weaned. The process of weaning may involve an immediate change in full ventilatory support to unassisted breathing, called a *spontaneous breathing trial* (SBT). Alternatively, clinicians may choose a more gradual reduction in ventilator support (Epstein, 2010). One commonly used weaning predictor tool is the rapid shallow breathing index (RSBI) (Chart 28–14). The RSBI is the ratio of respiratory frequency to tidal volume. For example, a patient who has a respiratory rate of 30 breaths/minute and a tidal volume of 250 mL/breath will have a RSBI of 120 (30 bpm/0.25 L). Patients who cannot tolerate independent breathing will breathe fast and shallowly and therefore will have a high RSBI. Other more multidisciplinary screening tests, such as the Burns' Weaning Assessment Tool (Figure 28–9 ◆), have been developed that include other patient characteristics such as fever, strength, endurance, and other nonpulmonary system criteria.

Once the decision to wean the patient has been made, there are many different ways to attempt to wean. Methods that are commonly used for weaning include T-tube trials, intermittent mandatory ventilation, and pressure support. A T-tube is a tubing circuit connected to an oxygen source that attaches to the end of the endotracheal tube (it is not connected to the ventilator). This allows clinicians to observe the tolerance of spontaneous respirations without support. It is generally performed once per day for 2 hours or less; however, the literature suggests that a 30-minute T-tube trial is sufficient to determine readiness for extubation (Jubran & Tobin, 2009). Patients should be monitored for increased respiratory effort, tachypnea, dysrhythmias, desaturation, and onset of wheezing or crackles.

Weaning by the use of intermittent mandatory ventilation involves gradually allowing the patient to do more of the work of breathing and allowing the ventilator to do less. The rate is stair-stepped down gradually while the patient is monitored for distress. ABGs are done after approximately 30 minutes to verify that the pH is 7.30 or above. The rate can be further reduced as long as the pH does not decrease below 7.30.

Pressure support ventilation (PSV) weaning allows the patient to control the rate, depth, and flow of each spontaneous breath. The pressure support is decreased gradually so that the patient is taking on more of the workload of breathing. Maintaining a minimum of PSV compensates for the resistance of the endotracheal tube. Clinical trials have not been promising and have failed to identify the level of PSV necessary to overcome resistance and work of breathing (Jubran & Tobin, 2009).

When actively weaning the patient, the nurse should monitor the patient's SpO_2, respiratory rate, heart rate, respiratory effort, breath sounds, and blood pressure closely and be able to return the patient to the ventilator if the patient is in acute distress.

Safety Alert *During weaning, if the patient exhibits any adverse symptoms, the nurse should request that the patient be returned to the ventilator and that it be adjusted to the settings the patient was on before weaning. Symptoms that might prompt the nurse to terminate weaning include the following:*

Increase in respiratory rate and complaints of dyspnea

Increased work of breathing (nasal flaring, retractions, use of accessory muscles, and paradoxical chest motion with abdomen and chest)

Increase in blood pressure

Increase in heart rate and dysrhythmias

Decrease in SpO_2.

Other symptoms might include diaphoresis, nausea, and increased anxiety.

Successful weaning is important to ensure the patient's continued recovery from respiratory failure whatever the etiology. The nurse can assist with this process by being knowledgeable about the factors that are involved in weaning even though the best practice regarding weaning has not been fully clarified. The most important nursing action is assessment of the patient's tolerance to ventilator changes and ultimately being off mechanical ventilation. Vital signs, ABGs, and oxygen saturation levels are measured continuously. The patient may tire after being off the ventilator for an extended period of time and may therefore need to be placed back on the ventilator to rest. Typically, when the patient tires while off the ventilator, the heart and respiratory rate increase while the blood pressure and oxygen saturation decrease. It is essential for the nurse to intervene when changes occur in order to prevent complications such as a myocardial ischemia due to the physiological stress of trying to maintain oxygenation.

Noninvasive Positive Pressure Ventilation

Noninvasive positive pressure ventilation (NPPV) is the delivery of positive pressure ventilation through a noninvasive route, such as a face mask, nasal plugs, or nasal mask (Figure 28–10 ◆). The face mask appears to have the most success, probably because patients who are in respiratory distress tend to be mouth breathers. NPPV has been used for sleep apnea, obesity hypoventilation syndrome, neurologic disorders, chest wall disorders, post extubation failure, and acute respiratory failure (Bauman & Hyzy, 2011). It can also be used for patients who have "do not intubate" orders. NPPV, when successful, can reduce the work of breathing, bypass the complications of intubation, rest fatigued respiratory muscles, improve alveolar ventilation, and improve gas exchange (Rhoades & Linsler, 2010). In the case of acute respiratory failure, the strongest evidence for the support of NPPV is in patients with severe exacerbation of COPD complicated by hypercapnic acidosis and patients with cardiogenic pulmonary edema (Bauman & Hyzy, 2011). NPPV can be delivered by using the same modes as invasive ventilation; however, the most common modes are pressure support, AC, CPAP, and BiPAP. Pressure limited modes tend to be better tolerated. CPAP is

BURNS' WEAN ASSESSMENT PROGRAM (BWAP)
Copyright Burns 1990

Patient Name ____________________ Patient History Number ____________

Patient Weight ________________ kg

I. GENERAL ASSESSMENT

YES	NO	NOT ASSESSED	
___	___		1. Hemodynamically stable? (Pulse rate, cardiac output)
___	___		2. Free from factors that increase or decrease metabolic rate (seizures, temperature, sepsis, bacteremia, hypo/hyperthyroid)?
___	___		3. Hematocrit > 25% (or baseline)?
___	___		4. Systematically hydrated? (weight at or near baseline, balanced intake and output)?
___	___		5. Nourished? (albumin > 2.5, parenteral/enteral feedings maximized) If albumin is low and anasarca or third spacing is present, score for hydration should be "no."
___	___		6. Electrolytes within normal limits? (including Ca++, Mg+, PO_4). Correct Ca++ for albumin level.
___	___		7. Pain controlled? (subjective determination)
___	___		8. Adequate sleep/rest? (subjective determination)
___	___		9. Appropriate level of anxiety and nervousness? (subjective determination)
___	___		10. Absence of bowel problems (diarrhea, constipation, ileus)?
___	___		11. Improved general body strength/endurance? (i.e., out of bed in chair, progressive activity program)?
___	___		12. Chest x-ray improving or returned to baseline?

Figure 2. Burns Wean Assessment Program (BWAP), RR respiratory rate; ETT, endotracheal tube; ID, inner diameter; NIP, negative inspiratory pressure; PEP, positive expiratory pressure; STV, spontaneous tidal volume; VC, vital capacity: MV, mechanical ventilation.

FIGURE 28–9 ◆ Burns' Weaning Assessment Tool.

the delivery of positive pressure continuously and equally throughout inspiration and expiration. **BiPAP** is a pressure-limited mode in which the inspiratory pressure (IPAP) and the expiratory pressure (EPAP or PEEP) can be adjusted separately. Inspiratory pressures are usually set at 8 to 12 cm H_2O and are increased gradually as the patient tolerates. Expiratory pressure is usually started at 4 to 5 cm H_2O and increased to reduce hypoxemia. This is the preferred mode for COPD exacerbation (Bauman & Hyzy, 2011). Most modern day ventilators can provide NPPV. BiPAP is also the name of a portable ventilator designed to deliver BiPAP manufactured by Respironics, which should not be confused with BiPAP, the mode of ventilation. Figure 28–9 shows an example of a ventilator used for NPPV. Figure 28–11◆ illustrates one type of interface, an oronasal mask that is used to initiate NPPV.

The success of NPPV is associated with user expertise, familiarity with the equipment, and patient selection (Rhoades & Linsler, 2010). Patient populations associated with NPPV failure include those with pneumonia, ARDS, decreased level of consciousness, respiratory rate ≥ 30, severe illness, and pH < 7.25 (Reardon, Mason, & Clinton, 2009). Chart 28–15 outlines the contraindications for NPPV.

Nursing Management

NPPV is an intervention that can be successful in preventing intubation but only when a comprehensive approach to the patient is used. Patients receiving NPPV require many of the continuous monitoring devices that patients who are intubated require. The nurse should be aware that the most serious potentially fatal complication of NPPV is aspiration. Because the airway is not protected as in the patient who is intubated, patients receiving NPPV typically require more frequent assessments. Continuous heart rate, pulse oximetry (SpO_2), and especially trained nurses and respiratory therapists who are experienced with NPPV are essential for these patients. Two other common

II. RESPIRATORY ASSESSMENT

Gas Flow and Work of Breathing

YES NO NOT ASSESSED

____ ____ 13. Eupnic respiratory rate and pattern (spontaneous RR <25, without dyspnea, absence of accessory muscle use).
*This is assessed off the ventilator while measuring #20–23.
RR = _____

____ ____ 14. Absence of adventitious breath sounds? (rhonchi, rales, wheezing)

____ ____ 15. Secretions thin and minimal?

____ ____ 16. Absence of neuromuscular disease/deformity?

____ ____ 17. Absence of abdominal distention/obesity/ascites?

____ ____ 18. Oral ETT > #7.5 or trach > #6.0 (I.D.)

Airway Clearance

____ ____ 19. Cough and swallow reflexes adequate?

Strength

____ ____ 20. NIP <−20 (negative inspiratory pressure)
NIP = _____

____ ____ 21. PEP >+30 (positive expiratory pressure)
PEP = _____

Endurance

____ ____ 22. STV . 5 ml/kg (spontaneous tidal volume)?
Spont VNT = _____ STV/BW in kg =

____ ____ 23. VC > 10–15 ml/kg (vital capacity)?
VC =

ABCs

____ ____ 24. pH 7.30–7.45

____ ____ 25. $PaCO_2$ - 40 mmHg (or baseline) with M.V. <10 L/min
* This is evaluated while on ventilator.
$PaCO_2$ - _____ MV =

____ ____ 26. PaO_2 >60 on FiO_2 <40%

Figure 2. Continued.

FIGURE 28–9 ◆ Burns' Weaning Assessment Tool. *continued.* To score the BWAP: Divide the number of "yes" responses by 26.

Source: From Burns, S., Earven, S., Fisher, C., Lewis, R., Merrell, P., Schubart, J., Trawit, J., Bleck, T., University of Virginia Long Term Mechanical Ventilation Team. (2003). Implementation of an institutional program to improve clinical and financial outcomes of mechanically ventilated patients: One-year outcomes and lessons learned. *Critical Care Medicine, 31*(12), 2752–2763.

complications of NPPV are facial trauma related to the tight-fitting mask and abdominal distention.

Selection of patients who are good candidates for NPPV is discussed in the Evidence-Based Practice box. A comprehensive approach to the patient who is a candidate for NPPV is outlined in the Nursing Process: Patient Care Plan for the Patient Receiving Noninvasive Positive Pressure Ventilation box. This care plan applies the nursing process beginning with a diagnosis of altered respiratory status. Key interventions with rationales are listed for selection, initiation, and assessment of the patient on NPPV.

Health Promotion

Teaching the patient how to remove the ventilator mask and what the different alarms on the ventilator mean helps decrease patient anxiety. The nurse and therapist work closely together to accomplish this patient teaching. It is important to determine whether the patient and spouse or primary support person are knowledgeable about the reason for the mask and the limitations the patient will experience while wearing it.

After removal of the mask, the patient is reminded to continue deep breathing and coughing exercises at least every 2 hours. Before

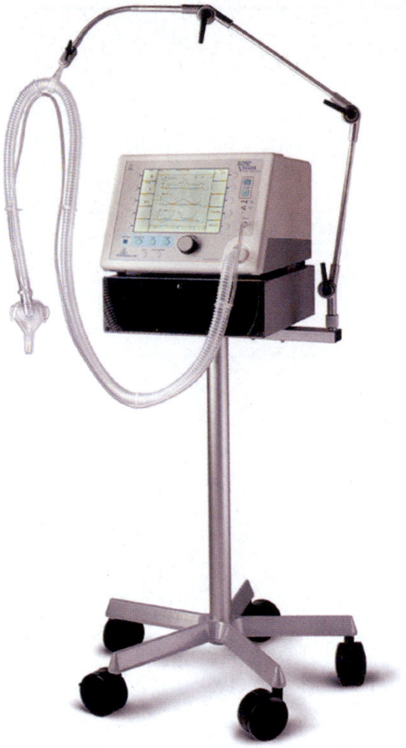

FIGURE 28–10 ◆ Example of NPPV: BiPAP.

Source: Courtesy of www.respironics.com.Photo Shari Urick.

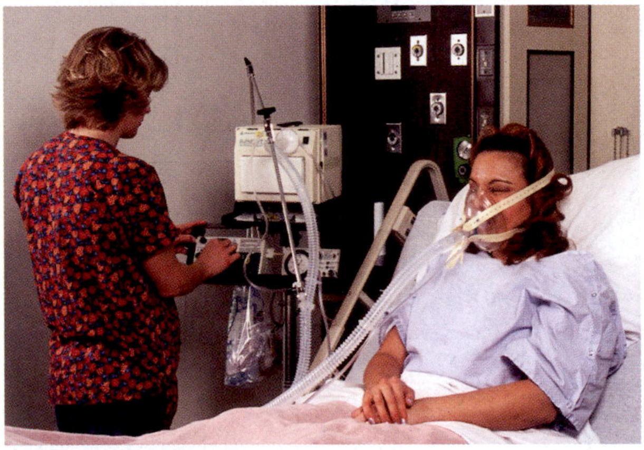

FIGURE 28–11 ◆ Oronasal mask.

CHART 28–15 Contraindications to Noninvasive Positive Pressure Ventilation

- Impending cardiac or respiratory arrest
- Inability to cooperate
- Inability to protect the airway
- Altered mental status
- Inability to clear respiratory secretions
- Hemodynamic instability
- Facial trauma, surgery, or deformity that limits placement of the NPPV mask
- Upper airway obstruction
- Severe gastrointestinal bleed/surgery (need for NG tube)
- High aspiration risk

Source: Adapted from Yeow, M., & Santanilla, J. (2008). Non-invasive positive pressure ventilation in the emergency room. *Emergency Medicine Clinics of North America, 26,* 835–847.

EVIDENCE-BASED PRACTICE Noninvasive Positive Pressure Ventilation

Clinical Problem

There are some patient characteristics and some absolutes with regards to patient selection. But how does the health care provider, nurse, or respiratory therapist decide who would be a good candidate for NPPV? It is difficult to predict which patients will tolerate NPPV. For example, some patients who are agitated and anxious when placed on NPPV become calm and relaxed; in these cases, the cause of the agitation is hypoxemia that is resolved by application of the NPPV. If the patient does have any potential contraindications to NPPV, attempting a trial of this therapy is probably the best course for deciding whether the patient will tolerate NPPV. However, there is some research that could assist the team in this regard.

Research Findings

The use of NPPV has long been accepted in patients with obesity hypoventilation syndrome and sleep apnea. In addition, over the past decade its use has become more popular in treating acute respiratory diseases in an attempt to prevent intubation with mechanical ventilation and its sequelae. A meta-analysis report demonstrated a consistent, positive effect on mortality, ICU days, and ventilator-associated pneumonia when using NPPV as a weaning strategy in patients with COPD (Burns, Adhikari, Keenan, & Meade, 2010). A large, multicenter randomized controlled study comparing traditional oxygen therapy against NPPV in patients presenting to the emergency department with acute cardiogenic pulmonary edema showed that NPPV provided earlier improvements in the resolution of breathlessness, reduction of respiratory distress, and reduced hypercarbia and acidosis when compared to the oxygen therapy group (Gray et al., 2009). Because of the complications of intubation in asthmatic patients, interest has been shown in using NPPV in patients with severe acute asthma. Scala (2010) reported on the review of the literature pertaining to NPPV in asthma. The available random controlled trials are few and the study groups small, leaving the application of NPPV in asthmatic patients unclear. This is an area where random controlled trials are clearly needed to identify efficacy in clearly defined patient parameters.

The use of NPPV in hypoxemic respiratory failure remains controversial. The cause of the hypoxemia appears to dictate its success. Agarwal, Aggarwal, and Gupta (2010) reviewed 13 studies (540 patients) on the efficacy of NPPV in patients with ALI/ARDS. They found an almost 50% NPPV failure rate and cautioned against its use in ALI/ARDS. They identified a need for a uniform NPPV protocol for use in patients with ALI/ARDS.

A case-controlled study involving 124 medical wards in 26 hospitals in Guangzhou and Hong Kong determined that the use of NPPV in SARS patients was an independent risk factor for spreading nosocomial outbreaks of SARS. NPPV has exhalation ports that allow exhaled air to escape. This may generate droplet nuclei and disperse infective aerosols, resulting in super spreading events (Tang, Eames, Chan, & Ridgway, 2007).

Implications for Nursing Practice

In the final analysis, if the patient does not meet any of the absolute contraindications and is cooperative, a trial of NPPV might be warranted if the clinical team feels that the patient might benefit from this therapy. The clinical judgment of health care providers, nurses, and respiratory therapists is a key element in ensuring a successful intervention. The research has provided evidence that patients with COPD exacerbation and those with cardiogenic pulmonary edema might benefit from this therapy.

Critical Thinking Questions with answers can be found in the Osborn Student Resources at nursing.pearsonhighered.com.

NURSING PROCESS: Patient Care Plan for Patient Receiving Noninvasive Positive Pressure Ventilation

Assessment of Ventilatory Status Using Gordon's Functional Health Patterns:

- Health Perception Health Management Pattern
- Nutrition Metabolic Pattern
- Activity Exercise Pattern
- Cognitive Perceptual Pattern
- Self-Perception Self-Concept Pattern

Subjective Data	Objective Data
Assessment for Selection, Initiation, and Assessment of Patient on NPPV	**Assessment for Selection, Initiation, and Assessment of Patient on NPPV**
Do you think you could attempt a trial of NPPV? Which interface would you prefer? Are you experiencing any episodes of nausea or vomiting? Have you ever had problems with claustrophobia?	Level of consciousness Hemodynamic stability Ventilation Work of breathing Oxygen saturation Abdominal and genitourinary assessment Vital signs ABGs
Assessment for Level of Consciousness, Patient's Ability to Communicate, and Procedural Tolerance	**Assessment for Level of Consciousness, Patient's Ability to Communicate, and Procedural Tolerance**
What is your name, where are you, what is the date, and why are you here?	Glasgow Coma Scale Follow commands
Assessment of Level of Comfort	**Assessment of Level of Comfort**
What is your pain level at, using the 1–10 scale? A 1 is very little pain and a 10 is the worst imaginable pain. What is your experience with pain? Do you routinely take pain medications at home; if so, what for and what kind? Are you allergic to any pain medication? Do you have any cultural or religious beliefs that impact your pain control? Does the pain get worse with deep inspiration? Describe the pain: burning, sharp, aching, or any other term that is descriptive of it.	Grimacing on movement Restlessness and irritability Taut facial expression
Assessment of Hemodynamic Stability	**Assessment of Hemodynamic Stability**
Do you become light-headed or pass out? Do palpitations or light-headedness occur at the same time? Do your feet swell and, if so, under what circumstances?	Vital signs: BP and HR Oxygen saturation Level of consciousness ECG Lab values: electrolytes and measures of acidosis Cardiac output Lung/cardiac Urine output
Assessment of Respiratory Effort	**Assessment of Respiratory Effort**
Do you feel short of breath? Is it becoming worse or better? How long have you been experiencing shortness of breath? Do you have it at rest or just with activities?	Oxygen saturation ABGs Skin color and temperature Respiratory rate Lung sounds

(*continued*)

NURSING PROCESS: Patient Care Plan for Patient Receiving Noninvasive Positive Pressure Ventilation, *continued*

Subjective Data	Objective Data
Assessment for Sufficient Oxygen Saturation Related to Altered Blood Gas	**Assessment for Sufficient Oxygen Saturation Related to Altered Blood Gas**
Do you have any preexisting health problems such as heart or lung disease?	Lung sounds Oxygen saturation Work of breathing (e.g., gasping, increased rate, loudness) Vital signs Skin and nail bed color ABGs Oxygen saturation
Assessment of Patient's Coping Abilities	**Assessment of Patient's Coping Abilities**
How are you feeling about your health and illness? Tell me what you are feeling about your illness and being on NPPV. Who are the people in your life that are your support system? How have you handled fearful situations in the past?	Facial expressions Mood Verbalization of fear regarding injury, impact on family, and future
Assessment of Soft-Tissue Injury of Skin, Nose, Mouth, and Nasopharynx	**Assessment of Soft-Tissue Injury of Skin, Nose, Mouth, and Nasopharynx**
Are you experiencing pain around, under, or near the mask?	Skin breakdown near and under the mask
Assessment of Abdominal Pain	**Assessment of Abdominal Pain**
Are you having any abdominal pain? Do you feel like you are swallowing air? Are you nauseated?	Abdominal girth Oxygen saturation Vomiting Bowel sounds
Assessment for Aspiration Related to Insecure Airway	**Assessment for Aspiration Related to Insecure Airway**
Are you feeling like you are getting enough air? Do you feel more short of breath?	Lung sounds Oxygen saturation Vital signs Increased work of breathing Bowel sounds Abdominal distention
Assessment of Knowledge Deficit	**Assessment of Knowledge Deficit**
What are your concerns about the diagnosis of respiratory disease in terms of prognosis, changes in lifestyle, and progression of disease? Do you understand how to take medications and their potential side effects? Do you understand what symptoms you might have, how to monitor them at home, and when to contact the health care provider?	Patients may be anxious, confused, and need repeated information.

Outcomes and Evaluation Parameters	Planning and Interventions with *Rationales*
1. NURSING DIAGNOSIS: Ineffective Breathing Pattern That Can Be Treated with Noninvasive Pulmonary Pressure Ventilation (NPPV) ***related to Impaired Gas Exchange, Ineffective Airway Clearance, and Ineffective Breathing Pattern*** **(NANDA-I © 2012)**	
Outcomes: Patient is candidate for NPPV. Improved gas exchange on NPPV. ***Evaluation Parameters:*** Arterial blood gases improved within 3 hours of NPPV. Decreased work of breathing as exhibited by the patient. Alert and oriented.	Assess level of consciousness and ability to follow commands and cooperate *to determine the presence of cerebral hypoxia.* Assess compliance with keeping the mask in place *to determine if the treatment is being tolerated.* Assess level of sedation *to determine if more or less is needed to keep the patient comfortable.*
2. NURSING DIAGNOSIS: Tissue Perfusion Ineffective: Cerebral ***related to decreased oxygenation and increased CO_2 levels*** **(NANDA-I © 2012)**	
Outcome: Tolerance of NPPV until it is not needed. ***Evaluation Parameters:*** Able to follow commands. Responds correctly to questions of time and place. *Glasgow Coma Scale (GCS) < 10 and/or inability to follow commands would disqualify patient from receiving NPPV.*	Assess neurological status frequently after initiating NPPV. Increasing confusion related to increased CO_2 levels would signify failure of NPPV.

NURSING PROCESS: Patient Care Plan for Patient Receiving Noninvasive Positive Pressure Ventilation, *continued*

3. NURSING DIAGNOSIS: Pain *related to ventilation or other preexisting conditions* (NANDA-I © 2012)

Outcomes: Pain controlled with analgesia. Level of sedation is adequate. ***Evaluation Parameters:*** Appears relaxed. Expresses relief of pain.	Assess pain and sedation level. *Increasing levels of pain would require increased analgesics that might decrease respiratory drive.* Provide adequate sedation. *Increasing anxiety would prevent patient from tolerating NPPV. Too much sedation could decrease respiratory rate and prevent the patient's ability to cooperate.*

4. NURSING DIAGNOSIS: Decreased Cardiac Output *related to heart failure and hypotension* (NANDA-I © 2012)

Outcome: Hemodynamically stable. ***Evaluation Parameters:*** Adequate blood pressure. Heart rate less than 100 beats per minute. Respiratory rate less than 18 breaths per minute while resting. Urine output minimum of 30 mL/hr. Lungs clear to auscultation. Intake and output within normal limits.	Monitor blood pressure and heart rate. *Hemodynamic instability, severe tachycardia, and/or hypotension (shock) would exclude patient. Uncontrolled ischemia or arrhythmias would also disqualify patient.* Auscultate heart sounds. Palpate pulses. Assess cardiac rhythm if patient is on monitor. Obtain 12-lead ECG to *further evaluate rhythm.* Administer antiarrhythmic and/or beta-blockers as prescribed. Assess extremities for edema. Assess fluid status and JVD. Weigh patient. Administer diuretics. Monitor intake and output. *Fluid overload can prevent adequate gas exchange.*

5. NURSING DIAGNOSIS: Ineffective Breathing Pattern, *related to lung constriction, lung collapse, low tidal volumes* (NANDA-I © 2012)

Outcome: Improved ventilation after application of NPPV. ***Evaluation Parameters:*** Decrease in respiratory rate, decreased use of accessory muscles, and decreased dyspnea. Oxygen saturation and ABGs within normal limits. Patient denies increased work of breathing.	Assess respiratory status for appropriateness of application of NPPV. *The following respiratory parameters would prompt the provider to not attempt NPPV:* *Inability to clear secretions* *Excessive secretions* *No cough or gag* *Impaired swallowing* *Respiratory arrest or unreliable respiratory drive.* Assess facial trauma or anatomic abnormalities that would prevent adequate mask fit. Assess breathing pattern, rate, and depth. Monitor respiratory rate and quality *to assess improvement in ventilation with NPPV.* Assess chest expansion. Note paradoxical respirations. Assess cough and ability to clear secretions. Assess use of accessory muscles during inspiration or prolonged expiratory phase. Assess nasal flaring or pursed-lip breathing.

6. NURSING DIAGNOSIS: Impaired Gas Exchange *related to pulmonary disease/infection* (NANDA-I © 2012)

Outcome: Improved oxygen saturation after application of NPPV. ***Evaluation Parameters:*** $SpO_2 > 92\%$ on room air. No increased work of breathing. Lung sounds clear.	Review ABGs and monitor SpO_2. *Ensure that initial ABG/SpO_2 value does not require immediate intervention such as endotracheal intubation.* Severe acidosis (pH < 7.2) and hypoxemia ($PaO_2 < 60$) would require invasive intubation. Auscultate breath sounds. Note any adventitious sounds such as wheezes or crackles in the bases. Assess pulse oximetry for absolute value as well as adequacy of waveform. *Waveform should always be monitored with SpO_2 to ensure that SpO_2 is accurate. Dampened waveform can reflect probe displacement.* Maintain $SpO_2 > 92\%$ *to provide appropriate level of oxygen therapy via mask.* Obtain chest x-ray as ordered. Compare film to previous studies *to assess lungs.* Administer bronchodilators if appropriate to increase ventilation.

(*continued*)

NURSING PROCESS: Patient Care Plan for Patient Receiving Noninvasive Positive Pressure Ventilation, *continued*

Outcomes and Evaluation Parameters	Planning and Interventions with *Rationales*
7 NURSING DIAGNOSIS: Anxiety *related to discomfort, inability to communicate, lack of adequate sleep, and use of analgesics and sedatives* (NANDA-I © 2012)	
Outcome: Reduced anxiety and confusion. ***Evaluation Parameters:*** Calm demeanor; acceptance of therapy. Patient can communicate and eat. Mask fits appropriately.	Provide constant observation and coaching of patient once NPPV therapy is instituted. *Explaining procedure to patient and coaching will decrease anxiety and promote acceptance of therapy.* Select appropriate mask for patient. Examine patient and note face size. Discuss interfaces and plan for initiation with patient and team (health care provider, respiratory therapist, and patient). *Use of an oronasal or full-face mask with gel mask improves compliance, is more efficient for gas exchange, and allows mouth breathing.* Transition to nasal mask if appropriate as patient improves.
8. NURSING DIAGNOSIS: Risk for Impaired Skin Integrity of Face and Nose *related to poor fitting mask* (NANDA-I © 2012)	
Outcome: Absence of soft-tissue injury. ***Evaluation Parameters:*** No tissue breakdown noted. Skin and soft tissue clear and intact.	Apply protective device on the bridge of the nose *to prevent skin breakdown.* Provide frequent oral care *to prevent mouth dryness and to prevent increase in plaque.* Keep dentures in place *to assist with mask fit.*
9. NURSING DIAGNOSIS: Risk for Injury and Abdominal Distention *related to high pressures, long-term ventilation, and predisposing abnormality* (NANDA-I © 2012)	
Outcome: No abnormal abdominal distention noted. ***Evaluation Parameters:*** Abdomen soft and nontender. Bowel sounds present. Patient free of nausea and vomiting.	Assess abdomen for distention, pain, or tenderness. Assess presence of bowel sounds in all four quadrants.*Persistent nausea and vomiting would be a contraindication to NPPV. Lack of bowel sounds and/or a distended abdomen might increase risk of aspiration with NPPV.* If abdomen is distended, consider obtaining order for placement of nasogastric tube *to decompress stomach.* Stop all feeding and oral intake until patient is stable on NPPV. Position patient with head of bed $>$ 30 degrees.
10. NURSING DIAGNOSIS: Risk for Aspiration *related to mask* (NANDA-I © 2012)	
Outcome: Free of aspiration. ***Evaluation Parameters:*** Clear lungs. Oxygen saturation within normal limits.	Instruct patient how to remove mask if vomiting occurs. *Aspiration is a significant risk for patients with NPPV.*
11. NURSING DIAGNOSIS: Deficient Knowledge *related to the diagnosis, treatments, and long-term management* (NANDA-I © 2012)	
Outcomes: Patient/family understand: The diagnosis of respiratory disease. Their prognosis and treatments. Lifestyle changes. Symptoms to monitor. ***Evaluation Parameters:*** Patient/family will: Ask appropriate questions. Follow appropriate medication regimen. Call when their symptoms worsen for urgent evaluation when needed.	Discuss with patient/family the cause and prevention of respiratory disease. *This will enhance their understanding of risk factors and prevention.* Discuss how the NPPV works and how to prevent complications. *This will provide the fundamental treatment strategies and should increase compliance.* Discuss the common symptoms of respiratory disease with the patient and family, describing shortness of breath, cough, fatigue, activity intolerance, weight gain/edema, palpitations, chest tightness, and poor concentration. *This will enable patients to recognize their symptoms and reinforce calling early when their symptoms worsen, so they can be seen and have adjustments made in their medications, preempting an urgent hospitalization.*

Source: Adapted from Wilkinson, J. M., & Ahearn, N. R. (2009). *Prentice Hall nursing diagnosis handbook* (9th ed.). Upper Saddle River, NJ: Prentice Hall.

discharging the patient, the nurse emphasizes the importance of rest and a gradual increase in activity to avoid fatigue. Patients are instructed to maintain resistance to infection with proper nutrition and adequate fluid intake. They also are warned to avoid exposure to others with upper respiratory tract infections or viruses and to obtain annual influenza and pneumococcal vaccine if advised by their health care provider.

Treating the underlying cause of respiratory failure is an important facet of reducing the need for NPPV. The nurse should inform the patient of the importance of taking all medications as prescribed on a set and regular schedule. Other regimens advised by the health care provider, such as weight loss and smoking cessation, should be followed. Nurses can provide written instructions for home medications and can refer the patient to smoking-cessation classes.

Collaborative Management

One of the primary examples of collaborative management is the multidisciplinary team of health care providers, nurses, and respiratory therapists who work together to successfully initiate NPPV for a patient. In order to meet desired patient outcomes, it is essential that this interdisciplinary team communicate openly with one another in developing and evaluating care of the patient and family (IOM [Institute of Medicine], 2010).

The health care provider's role is to assess the patient and make the decision that NPPV is an option for the patient. There are many contraindications for NPPV. Timing in initiation of NPPV is crucial. This therapy must be started before the patient is exhausted and unable to sustain a reliable respiratory effort. The respiratory therapist and nurse work together to select the appropriate interface or mask that will fit the patient and prevent large air leaks. The mask needs to be comfortable but tight enough to allow a flow of air to the patient. Coaching the patient and explaining the goal of NPPV is another important role of the nurse and the respiratory therapist.

Gerontological Considerations

As the population of older patients increases, the potential exists for an increase in the incidence of acute respiratory failure because there are some significant differences in the older adult's respiratory system that predispose these individuals to developing respiratory failure. These differences have to do with the physiological effects of aging. Chart 28–16 outlines the physiological effects of aging on the pulmonary system. Nurses who care for older adults must be aware of these important differences.

A decrease in the forced expiratory volume in 1 second (FEV_1) begins after age 30 and is further pronounced if the patient smokes. The other criteria listed in Chart 28–16 include many important physiological parameters that are accentuated as the person ages and the muscles become deconditioned. Outcome studies on the morbidity, mortality, and functional status of older adults who have been mechanically ventilated are contradictory; however, these studies suggest that age is an independent predictor of increased mortality in older adults (Barnato, Albert, Angus, Lave, & Degenholtz, 2010; Feng et al., 2009). Given the lower physiologic reserve and concomitant comorbidities of older adults, a careful and attentive approach toward intubation and mechanical ventilation is called for.

CHART 28–16 Physiological Effects of Aging on the Pulmonary System

- Decreased lung elasticity and increased ventilation/perfusion mismatch
- Reduced responsiveness to hypoxemia and hypercarbia
- Decreased FEV_1
- Decreased chest wall compliance and muscle strength
- Decreased cough effectiveness and mucociliary clearance
- Diminished cardiopulmonary reserve
- Changes in lung parenchyma that impair gas exchange and reduce PaO_2

Research

Research on complex respiratory disorders has led to tremendous advances in their diagnosis and treatment, ultimately saving lives and improving the quality of life. The treatments outlined earlier in the chapter represent evidence-based practice that resulted from ongoing research. There continue to be unanswered questions related to all aspects of complex respiratory disease. Therefore, research continues to strive to answer these questions in order to decrease the morbidity and mortality associated with these life-threatening disorders. The Research Opportunities box outlines future directions in research studies related to complex respiratory diseases.

RESEARCH OPPORTUNITIES Related to Complex Respiratory Disorders

Research Area	Clinical Impact
Effectiveness of prone ventilation in adults with ARDS	May improve promotion of alveoli and movement of secretions
Ventilator management for the treatment of ARDS:	Improving oxygenation and preventing further lung injury
Ventilator settings	
Mode selection	
Pressure versus volume	
High frequency oscillatory ventilation (HFOV)	
Liquid ventilation	
Extracorporeal membrane oxygenation (ECMO)	
Appropriate fluid management in ARDS	Effective support of cardiovascular status without increase in alveolar secretions
Ventilated-associated pneumonia (VAP)	Increased prevention of VAP
Role of mouth care in decreasing pathogenic organisms in the oral plaque biofilm	Decrease amount of pathogens from mouth to lungs
Other methods of preventing VAP:	
Patient positioning	Recruitment of alveoli
Use of subglottic endotracheal tube	Decrease amount of pathogens from oral cavity to lungs
Antibiotic-coated endotracheal tube	
Use of NPPV and weaning	Improving weaning
Incorporate this mode of ventilation into weaning strategies	
NPPV and indications for instituting this mode of ventilation in cardiac failure and respiratory failure	Wider use of NPPV for many types of cardiac and respiratory failure
NPPV interfaces (face mask, nasal mask, helmet, etc.)	Improved interfaces that will improve patient comfort and compliance

READ: **History of Present Illnesses** >> Laboratory Study Results >> Critical Thinking Questions

Philip Arnott is a 52-year-old man admitted to your unit with a diagnosis of pneumonia with increasing shortness of breath during the past several days. He is admitted from the emergency department receiving oxygen via nasal cannula at 6 L/min. Three days ago, Mr. Arnott stated that he "didn't feel right" and stayed home from work. He thought he had a cold and was congested and sneezing. He reported not being able to sleep lying flat. Last night he was awakened by an episode of severe shortness of breath. He called 911 and was transported to the hospital. On admission to the emergency department, he was febrile at 39.4°C (102.9°F) with a pulse oximeter of 88% on room air. Oxygen via nasal cannula was instituted, which increased the pulse oximetry reading to 92%. A portable chest x-ray demonstrated consolidation of the right middle and lower lobe. Blood, sputum, and urine cultures were obtained, and antibiotics were initiated. The patient was admitted to the special respiratory unit for further treatment. Continuous pulse oximetry, coughing and deep breathing encouragement, and Tylenol for fever are the nursing priorities for Mr. Arnott on admission. Careful attention to the timing of his antibiotic doses also is a priority.

Medical–Surgical History

Mr. Arnott has never been hospitalized before but has a history of hypertension that is being treated with the angiotensin-converting enzyme inhibitor irbesartan (Avapro), 150 mg, and hydrochlorothiazide, 12.5 mg, each once a day.

Social History

Mr. Arnott is a sedentary business executive who is 6 ft 3 inches (76 inches) tall and weighs 250 pounds. He lives by himself and has no close relatives locally.

Physical Examination

On physical exam, Mr. Arnott is alert and oriented but anxious. His cardiac exam reveals bounding pulses with normal heart sounds and no jugular venous distention. He denies any chest pain or any type of pain except discomfort related to breathing and shortness of breath. His respiratory rate is rapid, but his chest excursion is equal bilaterally. He is using accessory muscles for respiration and is sitting straight up in bed. On auscultation, he has decreased breath sounds on the right side with wet crackles heard posteriorly over the entire right lung field. His cough is productive for sputum that is thick, yellow, and tenacious. His blood pressure is 150/90; heart rate is 100 beats per minute with a respiratory rate of 34 to 36 per minute; and pulse oximetry fluctuating between 90% and 92% on 6 liters nasal cannula. His temperature is running 38° to 40°C (100.4° to 104°F). His abdomen is large but soft and nontender. He denies any problems with urination or defecation. His last bowel movement was yesterday. Skin is warm and dry with no areas of breakdown noted. An intravenous infusion is present in his left forearm with antibiotics infusing.

READ: History of Present Illnesses >> **Physical Exam** >> Admitting Medical Records >> Laboratory Study Results

Admitting Medical Orders

Admit to MIC
Service: MICU
Condition: guarded
Admitting diagnosis: pneumonia
Allergies: no known drug allergies
Vital signs and O_2 sats q1h
Activity: bed rest
Diet: regular
Daily weight
Continuous cardiac monitor
Continuous pulse oximetry
Call house officer: HR < 60 or >120, systolic blood pressure < 90 or >160, RR < 12 or > 30, temperature > 38.5°C, urinary output less than 30 mL/hr × 2, O_2 sat < 92%
IV: D5 1/2 NS @ 50 mL/hr
Strict I/O q1h
Oxygen: via 6 liters nasal cannula; maintain oxygen saturation > 92%
Respiratory care: incentive spirometer q1 hours when awake
Sequential compression stockings to lower extremities while in bed

Scheduled Medications

Irbesartan (Avapro) 150 mg PO once a day
Hydrochlorothiazide 12.5 mg PO once a day
Ceftazidime 2 grams every 8 hours IV

PRN Medications

Tylenol 650 mg po q4h for fever
Morphine 3 to 5 mg IV q4h prn pain
Temazepam 15 to 30 mg po at bedtime prn insomnia

Ordered Laboratory Studies

CPK-MB q8h ∞ 3
Chemistry panel, CBC, and magnesium daily
ABGs daily and prn for respiratory distress

Ordered Diagnostic Studies

Chest x-ray q a.m.

Nursing Priorities

Six hours later, the nurse is called to Mr. Arnott's room. His dinner tray is on his bedside stand. He is cyanotic with a pulse oximetry reading in the 70s. He is coughing sporadically with a respiratory rate in the high 40s. Lung sounds are decreased, but bronchial sounds are heard throughout the lung fields except for the right side, which is very decreased. The health care provider is called, and an emergency chest x-ray is ordered. Oxygen is changed to a face mask, 100% nonrebreather. Mr. Arnott's pulse oximetry increases to 85%. ABGs are obtained. (The ABGs are listed in the table with the laboratory results.)

The chest x-ray reveals a new infiltrate in the posterior segment of the left upper lobe and an increasing pattern of consolidation in the right lung. A presumptive diagnosis of worsening pneumonia with possible aspiration pneumonia is considered. On questioning, Mr. Arnott states that he had difficulty swallowing his dinner and remembers that after drinking some of the milk his coughing increased and he vomited. Soon he can barely talk because he is so short of breath and is increasingly anxious with nasal flaring. His respiratory rate has increased to 45 breaths/min, his heart rate has increased to the 120s, and his blood pressure is

150/100. Other laboratory tests are ordered with electrolytes and troponin to rule out any cardiac involvement.

Mr. Arnott's status is deteriorating. His respiratory rate is increasing, and he is complaining of becoming tired. A repeat ABG is drawn (see the following text) and shows increasing hypoxemia. The health care provider recommends a trial of noninvasive positive pressure ventilation (NPPV). Mr. Arnott is placed on an NPO regimen and fitted for a mask. The mode on the noninvasive ventilator is set for BiPAP (two levels of CPAP) with an inspiratory pressure (IPAP) of 15 cm H_2O and an expiratory pressure (EPAP) of 5 cm H_2O.

An hour after being placed on the NPPV, Mr. Arnott is less anxious. His respiratory rate is 24 to 26. An ABG examination demonstrates improvement in his hypoxemia. The nurse continues to monitor his progress.

READ: History of Present Illnesses >> **Laboratory Study Results** >> Critical Thinking Questions

Test	Day 1	Day 2	Day 3
Sodium	135 mEq/L	136 mEq/L	135 mEq/L
Potassium	4.1 mEq/L	4.0 mEq/L	4.0 mEq/L
Chloride	103 mEq/L	104 mEq/L	95 mEq/L
Carbon dioxide	26 mEq/L	25 mEq/L	25 mEq/L
Blood urea nitrogen (BUN)	16 mg/dL	15 mg/dL	14 mg/dL
Creatinine	1.2 mg/dL	1.3 mg/dL	1.2 mg/dL
Glucose	134 mg/dL	123 mg/dL	120 mg/dL
Phosphorus	2.2 mg/dL	3.4 mg/dL	3.8 mg/dL
Calcium	9.1 mg/dL	8.7 mg/dL	9.1 mg/dL
Albumin	3.7 g/dL	3.7 g/dL	3.5 g/dL
Alkaline phosphatase (ALP)	70 units/L	76 units/L	77 units/L
Bilirubin	0.8 mg/dL	1.0 mg/dL	1.0 mg/dL
Alanine transaminase (ALT)	15 units/L	20 units/L	30 units/L
Magnesium	2.0 mg/dL	1.9 mg/dL	1.9 mg/dL
Creatine kinase	64 units/L	67 units/L	62 units/L

Test	Day 1	Day 2	Day 3
CK-MB	0 ng/mL by immunoassay	0 ng/mL by immunoassay	0 ng/mL by immunoassay
Troponin I	0 mcg/mL	0.2 mcg/mL	0.1 mcg/mL
Troponin T	0 mcg/mL	0.1 mcg/mL	0.1 mcg/mL
WBC	4,500/µL	5,000/µL	8,000/µL
RBC	4.89 × 10_{12}/L	5.09 × 10_{12}/L	4.92 × 10_{12}/L
Hemoglobin	15.9 g/dL	16.5 g/dL	15.9 g/dL
Hematocrit	45.5%	47.8%	45.6%
Platelets	295,000/µL	256,000/µL	300,000/µL
ABGs	Admission	After aspiration	After NPPV
pH	7.35	7.30	7.35
PaO_2	70 mmHg	53 mmHg	76 mmHg
$PaCO_2$	47 mmHg	50 mmHg	39 mmHg
HCO_3	26 mmHg	25 mmHg	24 mmHg
SpO_2	93%	86%	92%
Oxygen delivery	6 liters nasal cannula	100% FiO_2 via nonrebreather mask	NPPV with BiPAP; IPAP of 15 and EPAP of 5

Pearson Nursing Student Resources *Log on to* ***nursing.pearsonhighered.com*** *to download forms*

DOCUMENT:

>> Summary of Hospitalization
>> Pathophysiology Form
>> Laboratory Values
>> Laboratory Results Explanation

APPLY:

>> List of Potential Nursing Diagnoses
>> Concept Map
>> Critical Thinking Questions and Concept Map

APPLY: History of Present Illnesses >> Laboratory Study Results >> **Critical Thinking Questions**

1. What are the risks of placing Mr. Arnott on NPPV versus intubating him and placing him on conventional ventilation?
2. What types of devices are available for administering NPPV and what are the benefits of each?
3. What are the nursing priorities involved with monitoring Mr. Arnott?

Answers to Critical Thinking Questions can be found in Appendix D in the Osborn Student Resources at nursing.pearsonhighered.com.

NCLEX® PRACTICE

1. Arterial blood gas results from a patient complaining of shortness of breath reveal a PaO_2 of 56 mmHg on room air. What is the most important action by the nurse?

1. Administer oxygen 2 liters nasal cannula and recheck the patient in 15 minutes.
2. Coach the patient to breath slowly and deeply along with the nurse.
3. Contact the patient's health care provider regarding these results.
4. Monitor the patient for development of cardiac dysrhythmia.

2. A patient presents to emergency department triage with a new onset of dyspnea, shortness of breath, tachypnea, and increased anxiety. The triage nurse notes increased crackles, coarse rhonchi, and pink frothy sputum. The nurse should notify the emergency department that they are about to receive a patient with which probable disorder?

1. Congestive heart failure
2. Aspiration pneumonia
3. Pulmonary edema
4. Haemophilus influenza A

3. The nurse is caring for a patient experiencing noncardiogenic pulmonary edema. The nurse should collaborate with the health care provider regarding which patient information? (select all that apply)

1. Heart rate has increased from 100 bpm to 120 bpm.
2. Brain natriuretic peptide result is 96 pg/mL.
3. The nurse auscultates a new S_4 heart sound.
4. PCWP is now 16 mmHg.
5. This morning's chest x-ray reveals cardiomegaly.

4. A patient, admitted with respiratory failure, has developed ARDS. Which assessment finding would alert the nurse that this patient will soon require intubation?

1. Chest x-ray is showing absence of infiltrates.
2. Oxygen saturation on oxygen therapy is 82% to 86%.
3. Arterial blood gas pH is 7.35.
4. Auscultation of lung fields reveals bilateral coarse crackles.

5. A nurse notes that the patient on a ventilator is experiencing acute distress with a decrease in oxygen saturation to 82%. What should be the nurse's initial intervention?

1. Call the respiratory therapist stat to assess the problem.
2. Remove the patient from the ventilator and use the AMBU bag with 100% oxygen.
3. Call the health care provider stat regarding the drop in oxygen saturation.
4. Administer a sedative per health care provider's orders to reduce the patient's anxiety.

6. A patient on a ventilator with 5 cm H_2O PEEP develops severe hypotension when disconnected from the ventilator. How should the nurse interpret this hypotension?

1. The patient should not be removed from the ventilator when PEEP is used.
2. The PEEP setting has resulted in the patient being hypovolemic.
3. The patient is anxious about being removed from the ventilator.
4. The AMBU rate being used is too aggressive.

Answers to NCLEX Practice questions can be found in Appendix D in the Osborn Student Resources at nursing.pearsonhighered.com. Practice additional NCLEX questions online at the Student Resources site.

Pearson Nursing Student Resources Find additional review materials at: **nursing.pearsonhighered.com**

REFERENCES

Acute Respiratory Distress Syndrome Network. (2000). Ventilation with lower tidal volumes as compared with traditional tidal volumes for acute lung injury and the acute respiratory distress syndrome. *New England Journal of Medicine, 342*(18), 1301–1308.

Agarwal, R., Aggarwal, A., & Gupta, D. (2010). Role of noninvasive ventilation in acute lung injury/acute respiratory distress syndrome: A proportion meta-analysis. *Respiratory Care, 55*(12), 1653–1660.

Alsaghir, A., & Martin, C. (2008). Effect of prone positioning in patients with acute respiratory distress syndrome: A meta-analysis. *Critical Care Medicine, 36*(2), 603–609.

American Association of Critical Care Nurses. (2010). Practice alert: Oral care in the critically ill. Retrieved from http://www.aacn.org/wd/practice/content/oral-care-practice-alert.pcms?menu=practice

Barnato, A., Albert, S., Angus, D., Lave, J., & Degenholtz, H. (2010). Disability among elderly survivors of mechanical ventilation. *American Journal of Respiratory and Critical Care Medicine, 183*(8), 1037–1042.

Bartlett, J. (2008). Hospital-acquired pneumonia. In R. Porter & J. Kaplan (Eds.), *Merck manual for health care professionals.* Whitehouse Station, NJ: Merck Sharp & Dohme Corporation.

Bauman, K., & Hyzy, R. (2011). Noninvasive positive pressure ventilation in acute respiratory failure in adults. In P. Parsons & K. Wilson (Eds.), *UpToDate.* Waltham, MA: UpToDate.

Burns, K., Adhikari, N., Keenan, S., & Meade, M. (2010). Noninvasive positive pressure ventilation as a weaning strategy for intubated adults with respiratory failure. *Cochrane Database Systematic Reviews*, Aug 4 (8), doi: 10.1002/14651858.CD004127.pub2

Cason, C. L., Tyner, T., Saunders, S., & Broome, L. (2007). Nurses' implementation of guidelines for VAP from the CDC. *American Journal of Critical Care, 16,* 2–37.

Chastre, J., & Luyt, C.-E. (2010). Ventilator-associated pneumonia. In R. Mason (Ed.), *Murray and Nadel's textbook of respiratory medicine* (5th ed.). Philadelphia: Saunders Elsevier.

Cox, C., Docherty, S., Brandon, D., Whaley, C., Attis, D., Clay, A., Dore, D., et al. (2009). Surviving critical illness: Acute respiratory distress syndrome as experienced by patients and their caregivers. *Critical Care Medicine, 37*(10), 2702–2708.

Epstein, S. (2010). Weaning from mechanical ventilation: Readiness testing. In P. Parsons & K. Wilson (Eds.), *UpToDate.* Waltham, MA: UpToDate.

Feng, Y., Amoateng-Adjepong, Y., Kaufman, D., Gheorghe, C., & Manthous, C. A. (2009). Age, duration of mechanical ventilation, and outcomes of patients who are critically ill. *Chest, 136*(3), 759–764.

Gallagher, S., & Hackett, P. (2011). High altitude pulmonary edema. In D. Danzl & J. Grayzel (Eds.), *UpToDate.* Waltham, MA: UpToDate.

Goodrich, C. (2010). Endotracheal intubation. In L. Wiegand (Ed.), *AACN: Procedure manual for critical care* (6th ed.). St. Louis, MO: Elsevier Saunders.

Gray, A., Goodacre, S., Newby, D., Masson, M., Sampson, F., Dixon, S., et al. (2009). A multicenter randomized controlled trial of the use of continuous positive airway pressure and non-invasive positive pressure ventilation in the early treatment of patients presenting to the emergency department with severe acute cardiogenic pulmonary edema: The 3CPO trial. *Health Technologic Assessment, 13*(33), 1–106.

Hackett, P., & Roach, R. (2007). High-altitude medicine. In P. Auerbach (Ed.), *Wilderness medicine.* Philadelphia: Mosby Elsevier.

Hansen-Flaschen, J., & Siegel, M. (2010). Acute respiratory distress syndrome: Definition; clinical features; and diagnosis. In P. Parsons & K. Wilson (Eds.), *UpToDate.* Waltham, MA: UpToDate.

Herridge, M., Tansey, C., Matte, A., Tomlinson, G., et al. (2011). Functional disability 5 years after acute respiratory distress syndrome. *New England Journal of Medicine, 364*(14), 1293–1304.

Hudson, L., & Slutsky, A. (2007). Acute respiratory failure. In L. Goldman & D. Ausiello (Eds.), *Cecil medicine* (23rd ed.). Philadelphia: Saunders Elsevier.

Huijuan, C., Mei, H., Xun, L., Shangjuan, D., Yongmei, S., Qian, W., et al. (2010). Clinical research evidence of cupping therapy in China: A systematic literature review. *Complementary and Alternative Medicine, 10*, 70.

IOM (Institute of Medicine). (2010). *The future of nursing: Leading change, advancing health.* Washington, DC: The Academic Press.

Johnson, M., & Conde, M. (2010). Overview of the management of postoperative pulmonary complications. In S. Manaker & K. Wilson (Eds.), *UpToDate.* Waltham, MA: UpToDate.

Jubran, A., & Tobin, M. (2009). Methods of weaning from mechanical ventilation. In P. Parsons & K. Wilson (Eds.), *UpToDate.* Waltham, MA: UpToDate.

Kaplow, R., & Hardin, S. R. (2007). *Critical care nursing: Synergy and optimal outcomes.* Boston: Jones & Bartlett.

Kaynar, A. M. (2012). Respiratory failure. Retrieved from http://www.emedicine.medscape.com/article/167981-overview

Lee, W., & Slutsky, A. (2010). Acute respiratory distress syndrome. In R. Mason (Ed.), *Murray and Nadel's textbook of respiratory medicine* (5th ed.). Philadelphia: Saunders Elsevier.

Lloyd-Jones, D., Adams, R., Camethon, M., De Simone, G., Ferguson, B., Flegal, K., et al. (2009). Heart disease and stroke statistics—2009 update: A report from the American Heart Association Statistics Committee and Stroke Statistics Subcommittee. *Circulation, 119*(3), 480–486.

Lynn-McHale, D., & Carlson, K. (2001). *AACN procedure manual* (4th ed.). Philadelphia: W.B. Saunders.

MacIntyre, N. (2010). Principles of mechanical ventilation. In R. Mason (Ed.), *Murray and Nadel's textbook of respiratory medicine* (5th ed.). Philadelphia: Saunders Elsevier.

Maldonado, F., & Limper, A. (2010). Drug-induced pulmonary disease. In R. Mason (Ed.), *Murray and Nadel's textbook of respiratory medicine* (5th ed.). Philadelphia: Saunders Elsevier.

Malhotra, A., Schwartz, D., & Schwartzstein, R. (2009). Oxygen toxicity. In S. Manaker & K. Wilson (Eds.), *UpToDate.* Waltham, MA: UpToDate.

Mandel, J., & Drislane, F. (2010). Neurogenic pulmonary edema. In P. Parsons & K. Wilson (Eds.), *UpToDate.* Waltham, MA: UpToDate.

Matthay, M., & Martin, T. (2010). Pulmonary edema and acute lung injury. In R. Mason (Ed.), *Murray and Nadel's textbook of respiratory medicine* (5th ed.). Philadelphia: Saunders Elsevier.

Mazor, R., & Green, T. (2011). Pulmonary edema. In R. Kliegman, B. Stanton, J. St. Geme III, N. Schor, & R. Behman (Eds.), *Nelson textbook of pediatrics* (19th ed.). Philadelphia: Elsevier Saunders.

Metheny, N. A., Meert, K. L., & Clouse, R. E. (2007). Complications related to feeding tube placement. *Current Opinions in Gastroenterology, 23*(2), 178–182.

Mullen, W. (2007). Toxin-related noncardiogenic pulmonary edema. Pulmonary, Critical Care, Sleep Update, 21. Retrieved from http://www.chestnet.org/accp/topics/PCCSU%20Volume%2021

Neacy, K. (2009). Tracheostomy care. In J. Roberts & J. Hedges (Eds.), *Clinical procedures in emergency medicine* (5th ed.). Philadelphia: Saunders Elsevier.

Reardon, R., Mason, P., & Clinton, J. (2009). Basic airway management and decision-making. In J. Roberts & J. Hedges (Eds.), *Clinical procedures in emergency medicine* (5th ed.). Philadelphia: Saunders Elsevier.

Rhoades, C., & Linsler, R. (2010). Mechanical ventilation. In R. Holleran (Ed.), *ASTNA: Patient transport principles and practice* (4th ed.). St. Louis, MO: Mosby Elsevier.

Scala, R. (2010). Noninvasive ventilation in severe acute asthma? Still far from the truth. *Respiratory Care, 55*(5), 630–637.

Schwartz, D., Malhotra, A., & Kacmarek, R. (2010). Prone ventilation. In P. Parsons & K. Wilson (Eds.), *UpToDate.* Waltham, MA: UpToDate.

Siegel, M. (2011a). Acute respiratory distress syndrome: Epidemiology, pathophysiology, pathology, and etiology. In P. Parsons & K. Wilson (Eds.), *UpToDate.* Waltham, MA: UpToDate.

Siegel, M. (2011b). Novel therapies for the acute respiratory distress syndrome. In P. Parsons & K. Wilson (Eds.), *UpToDate.* Waltham, MA: UpToDate.

Sovari, A. A. (2008). Pulmonary edema: Cardiogenic. eMedicine. Retrieved from http://www.emedicine.com/med/topic1995.htm#

Tang, J., Eames, I., Chan, P., & Ridgway, G. (2007). Factors involved in the aerosol transmission of infection and control of ventilation in health care premises. *Journal of Hospital Infections, 64*, 100–114.

TenHoor, T., Mannino, D. M., & Moss, M. (2001). Risk factors for ARDS in the United States: Analysis of the 1993 national mortality followback study. *Chest, 119*(4), 1179–1184.

Wilkinson, J. M., & Ahearn, N. R. (2009). *Prentice Hall nursing diagnosis handbook* (9th ed.). Upper Saddle River, NJ: Prentice Hall.

Ye, X.F., Zhang, H.F., & Pang, Z.W. (2011). Therapeutic effects of common cold of wind-cold type at early stage treated by different cupping duration. *Zhongguo Zhen Jiu, 31*(4), 357–359.

Yeow, M., & Santanilla, J. (2008). Non-invasive positive pressure ventilation in the emergency room. *Emergency Medicine Clinics of North America, 26:* 835–847.

Zambon, M., & Vincent, J. (2008). Mortality rates for patients with acute lung injury/ARDS have decreased over time. *Chest, 133* (5), 1120–1127.

UNIT 7 Nursing Management of Patients with Cardiovascular Disorders

Content in Unit 7 that addresses the **Institute of Medicine (IOM)** competencies, **Nursing Core Competencies (NCC),** the **Quality and Safety Education for Nurses (QSEN)** competencies, and **Concepts** for concept-based learning is listed below.

Competencies	Feature or Text	Location
IOM, QSEN, NCC Providing patient-centered care	Nursing Process: Patient Care Plan for Dysrhythmias Nursing Process: Patient Care Plan for Acute Coronary Syndromes Nursing Process: Patient Care Plan for CID, pages 980, 1002, 1010 Nursing Process: Patient Care Plan for Heart Failure Ethical Issues Related to Heart Failure Nursing Process: Patient Care Plan for PVD, pages 1074, 1087	Chapter 30, page 887 Chapter 32, page 961 Chapter 33, page 980 Chapter 34, page 1042 Chapter 34, page 1052 Chapter 35
IOM, QSEN, NCC Working in teams	Collaborative Management, pages 944, 960, 966 Collaborative Management, pages 991, 1004, 1019 Collaborative Management, page 1041 Collaborative Management, pages 1063, 1072, 1089	Chapter 32 Chapter 33 Chapter 34 Chapter 35
IOM, QSEN, NCC Employing evidence-based practice	Evidence-Based Practice: Genetic Considerations of Atrial Fibrillation Evidence-Based Practice: Gender Considerations in CAD Evidence-Based Practice: Antibiotic Prophylaxis Considerations Evidence-Based Practice: Use of Teach-Back Techniques Evidence-Based Practice: VTE Prophylaxis	Chapter 30, page 869 Chapter 32, page 938 Chapter 33, page 1005 Chapter 34, page 1036 Chapter 35, page 1084
IOM NCC Applying quality and safety improvement	Safety Alerts, pages 834, 835, 839 Safety Alerts, pages 852, 858, 859, 880, 884, 898 Safety Criteria When Using a Defibrillator Safety Alerts, pages 905, 906, 914 Safety Alerts, pages 924, 926, 927, 929, 932 937, 949, 959 Safety Alerts, pages 974, 984, 985, 987, 990, 995, 999, 1004 Safety Alerts, pages 1035, 1036 Safety Alerts, pages 1070, 1079, 1080, 1086	Chapter 29 Chapter 30 Chapter 30, page 890 Chapter 31 Chapter 32 Chapter 33 Chapter 34 Chapter 35
NCC Educating patients	Patient Teaching & Discharge Priorities for Cardiac Devices Patient Teaching & Discharge Priorities for CAD, pages 946, 963 Patient Teaching & Discharge Priorities for CID, pages 983, 1004, 1007 Patient Teaching & Discharge Priorities for Heart Failure Patient Teaching & Discharge Priorities for PVD, pages 1090, 1091	Chapter 30, page 898 Chapter 32 Chapter 33 Chapter 34, page 1047 Chapter 35
Concepts covered in Unit 7 include:	Perfusion Oxygenation	Inflammation Infection

Nursing Assessment of the Patient with Cardiovascular Disorders

29 CHAPTER

Brenda McCulloch
Kathleen Osborn

Outcome-Based Learning Objectives

After studying this chapter, the learner will be able to:

1. Critique the significance of cardiovascular assessment findings.
2. Differentiate the relationship between current health status and the presence of cardiac risk factors.
3. Compare and contrast the patient's physical manifestations to the data obtained from the review of the social history.
4. Implement a comprehensive cardiovascular physical assessment.

KEY TERMS

abdominojugular reflux p.839
auscultation p.840
bruits p.843
clinical reference points p.839
clubbing of the nail bed p.837
cyanosis p.837
dyspnea p.834
edema p.834
heaves p.840
innocent murmurs p.844
jugular venous distension (JVD) p.838
jugular venous pressure (JVP) p.839
murmurs p.842
nocturia p.834
orthopnea p.834
pallor p.837
palpitations p.834
pericardial friction rub p.842
point of maximal impulse p.840
S_1 p.841
S_2 p.841
S_3 p.842
S_4 p.842
skin turgor p.837
split heart sound p.842
summation gallops p.842
syncope p.834
thrill p.840

NURSES NEED in-depth knowledge and skills in order to rapidly assess the cardiovascular status of their patients. Although the cardiovascular system is complex, its purpose is simple: to deliver oxygen and nutrients to the body's tissues and cells. An understanding of cardiovascular anatomy and physiology is essential for cardiovascular assessment. Additionally, it is important to gather data about the patient's medical history, as well as the presenting symptoms, because they can provide clues to her cardiac status. The relationship between risk factors and the patient's susceptibility for disease is an important concept this chapter presents.

A thorough physical examination, including inspection, palpation, and auscultation, helps the nurse to evaluate an individual's ability to carry out the cardiovascular system's physiological function. Nurses must recognize normal assessment findings and, more importantly, identify subtle abnormalities or deviations from normal that might indicate worsening of the patient's condition. Accuracy in the monitoring and reporting of data is essential; therefore, nurses have access to a wide variety of noninvasive and invasive technological devices that assist in cardiovascular monitoring and assessment. These devices are discussed in subsequent chapters in this unit.

Anatomy of the Cardiovascular System

The heart is housed directly behind the central section of the thorax, an area referred to as the mediastinum, as seen in Figure 29–1◆ (p. 832). Two-thirds of the heart lies to the left of the midline. The apex lies just above the diaphragm and the base of the heart lies approximately at the level of the third rib. The exact size of the heart varies, but on the average it is approximately 5 inches long and about 3 inches wide, resembling the size of a closed fist.

The heart is a four-chambered muscular organ composed of two separate pumps, each having one atrium and one ventricle. The heart's upper chambers (atria) are separated by the interatrial septum, and the ventricles are separated by the interventricular septum. The two atria are located at the base or top of the heart, and the lower chambers are located at the bottom or apex of the heart. The upper chambers are thin walled and receive blood as it returns to the heart. The right atrium receives blood from the systemic venous circulation, while the left atrium receives blood from the pulmonary circulation. The lower chambers have thicker walls and pump blood out of the heart: The right ventricle pumps blood into the pulmonary circulation, while the left ventricle pumps blood into the systemic circulation. Although

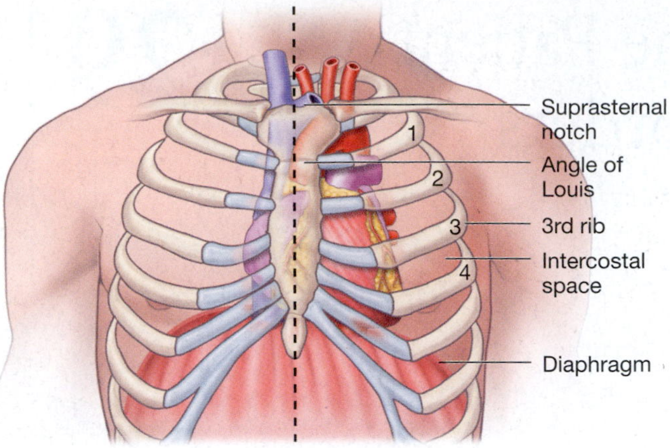

FIGURE 29–1 ◆ Diagram of the heart in the chest.

each ventricle pumps the same volume of blood, the left ventricle has a larger, stronger muscle. This increased strength is needed because the left ventricle has to pump blood into the systemic circulation, which has five times greater pressure than the pulmonic circulation.

The heart wall is composed of three layers: (1) the epicardium, the smooth outer serous layer; (2) the myocardium, the middle muscular layer, which is the thickest of the three layers and is responsible for the heart's ability to contract; and (3) the endocardium, the inner lining of the heart, which is composed of thin connective tissue. This smooth inner surface and the valves allow blood to flow more easily throughout the heart.

Cardiac Valves

There are four valves in the heart (Figure 29–2◆). The purpose of the valves is to ensure that blood travels in only one direction through the heart. The valves open to fill a chamber and then close when the pressure in the chamber builds, thereby allowing blood to continue to flow in one direction. The atrioventricular (AV) valves are located between the atria and the ventricles (see Figure 29–2). These valves are referred to as the tricuspid valve and the bicuspid or mitral valve. The tricuspid valve lies between the right atrium and the right ventricle and is so named because it has three cusps. In contrast the mitral or bicuspid valve has only two cusps and is located between the left atrium and the left ventricle. The cusps of both the mitral and the tricuspid valves extend into the ventricles where they attach to the chordae tendineae. Chordae tendineae are cords of dense connective tissue that attach to the papillary muscles (see Figure 29–2). The chordae tendineae and the papillary muscle work together to prevent the valve cusps from fluttering back into the atrium and interrupting forward blood flow. The semilunar valves are the pulmonic and the aortic valves. Each semilunar valve contains moon-shaped (semilunar) cusps. The pulmonic valve is located between the right ventricle and the pulmonary artery. The aortic valve is located between the left ventricle and the trunk of the aorta.

As blood is filling the ventricular chamber, pressure is rising. The ventricular muscle fibers respond to an increase in blood volume by stretching to allow more fluid into the chamber (Starling's law). As pressure in the ventricles increases, the ventricular muscles stretch. When the pressure in the right ventricle is greater than the pressure in the pulmonary system, and likewise, when the pressure in the left ventricle is greater than the pressure in the aorta, the AV valves (tricuspid and mitral) snap together to close as the semilunar valves (pulmonic and aortic) open. The ventricular muscles contract, and blood is ejected through the open pulmonic valve to the pulmonary artery and the pulmonary circuit, as well as through the open aortic valve to the aorta and the systemic circulation.

Surrounding the heart is a two-layered sac referred to as the pericardial sac (Figure 29–3◆). The outer layer, called the parietal pericardium, is in direct contact with the pleura (lung). This layer consists of a tough, nonelastic, fibrous connective tissue and serves to prevent overdistention of the heart. The thin, serous inner layer of the pericardium, called the visceral pericardium, lays directly on the epicardium or outer layer of the heart. There is a small amount of fluid between the heart wall and the pericardial sac (approximately 10 mL). This fluid acts as a lubricant to prevent friction during contractions.

Cardiac Circulatory System

The heart has its own circulatory system, which provides constant nourishment of blood to the cardiac muscle. The heart's circulatory system consists of coronary arteries and veins (Figure 29–4◆). The openings into the coronary arteries lie at the base of the aorta, just above

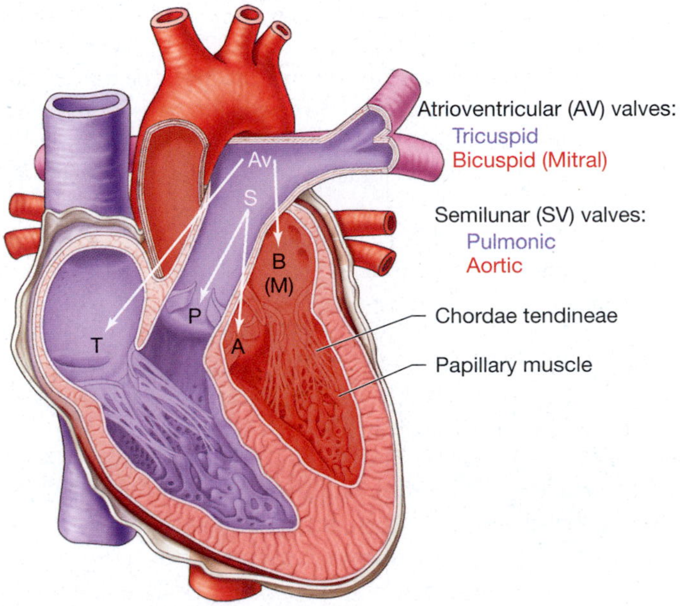

FIGURE 29–2 ◆ Cross section of the heart.

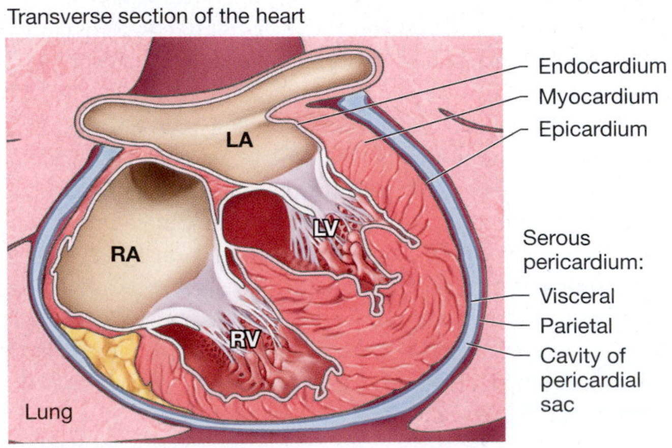

FIGURE 29–3 ◆ Layers of the heart.

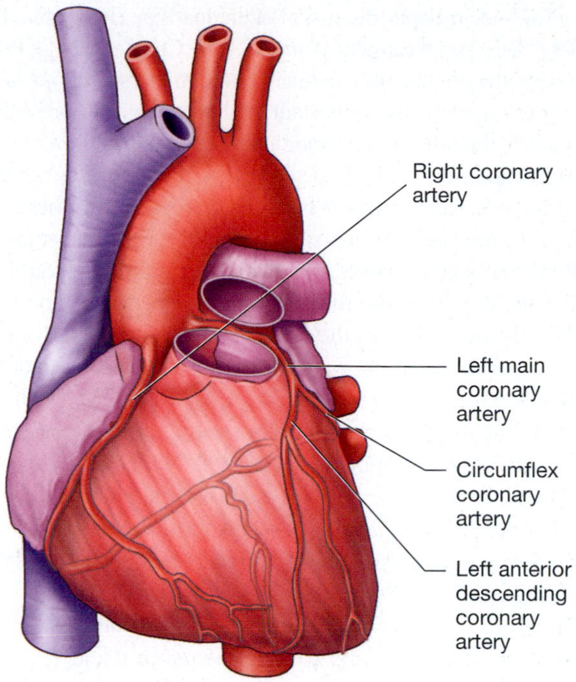

FIGURE 29–4 ◆ Coronary arteries.

the aortic valve. The two main coronary arteries are the right and left coronary arteries. The right coronary artery and its branches normally supply the right atrium and ventricle, as well as a portion of the inferior and posterior wall of the left ventricle. The left coronary artery branches into the left anterior descending (LAD) and the circumflex arteries, both of which feed the left atrium and the left ventricle. The left coronary artery carries 85% of the blood flow to the myocardium. The LAD artery feeds the anterior wall of the left ventricle and the interventricular septum. The circumflex artery feeds the lateral and posterior portions of the left ventricle. The veins of the heart return blood to the coronary sinus, which empties into the right atrium.

The pulmonary circulation consists of blood flow between the heart and lungs. Blood leaves the right ventricle, enters the pulmonary artery and lungs, picks up oxygen, and travels to the left side of the heart. The systemic circulation consists of a network of arteries, capillaries, and veins. Blood leaves the heart, travels through these vessels delivering oxygen and nutrients to the tissues, and then returns to the right side of the heart to pick up more oxygen.

Physiology of the Cardiovascular System

The right atrium is the central point in the body where unoxygenated blood from the systemic circulation returns. It then travels through the tricuspid valve to the right ventricle, through the pulmonic valve to the pulmonary arteries into the lungs, through the pulmonary alveolar–capillary network into the pulmonary veins, into the left atrium, through the mitral valve into the left ventricle, and finally out the aortic valve to the systemic circulation.

Freshly oxygenated blood, traveling through the aortic valve, also enters into the coronary arteries to supply the myocardium with oxygen. Normally the myocardium extracts 75% of the available oxygen from the coronary arteries. This is more than is extracted from any other tissue in the body; the rest of the body extracts about 40%. If oxygen needs are not met from this near maximal extraction, then blood flow must be increased. With a healthy heart, blood flow is increased in two ways. First, the arteries are able to dilate, thereby increasing their capacity. Second, the myocardial muscle increases the force of the contraction, pumping more blood into the arteries. These two mechanisms result in an increase in the cardiac output and blood flow to the myocardium.

Cardiac Cycle

The pumping action of the heart consists of contraction and relaxation of the myocardial layer of the heart's wall. Each contraction and relaxation is one cardiac cycle. During relaxation or diastole, blood flows into the ventricles; the contraction that follows, termed *systole*, propels blood out of the heart. The heart functions as a unit because both atria contract simultaneously, and then both ventricles contract. When both atria contract the ventricles are filled to capacity, and then the ventricles contract and blood is ejected into both the pulmonary and the systemic circulation. At the time of ventricular contraction, the mitral and tricuspid valves are closed by the pressure from the contraction while the pulmonic and aortic valves are opened. The cardiac cycle represents the actual time sequence between ventricular contraction and ventricular relaxation.

Autonomic Nervous System

The autonomic nervous system is a built-in control center for the body. Its purpose is to regulate functions of the body that are not under conscious control. There are two major divisions: the sympathetic and the parasympathetic nervous systems. Most of the organs of the body are innervated with both systems, although the blood vessels are innervated with only the sympathetic nervous system. The sympathetic nervous system (SNS) prepares the body for activity (flight or fight), whereas the parasympathetic nervous system (PSNS) regulates the calmer (rest and digest) functions. Because the SNS and the PSNS innervate the heart, neural impulses are not needed to maintain the cardiac cycle. In other words, the heart will beat in the absence of any nervous system connection. The SNS and the PSNS affect only the speed of the cardiac cycles and the diameter of the coronary arteries. It is said that these nervous systems only "fine-tune" the cardiac cycle.

Receptors and Neurotransmitters

The nerve endings of both the SNS and the PSNS secrete neurotransmitters. The SNS has two types of receptors at the nerve endings, the alpha- and the beta-receptors. These nerve endings are called adrenergic. The neurotransmitter for the SNS is norepinephrine, which causes an increase in heart rate and contractile force of the cardiac fibers. The PSNS nerve endings are known as cholinergic, and the neurotransmitter is acetylcholine, which causes the heart rate and blood pressure to go down.

Patient History

Obtaining a thorough patient history will help the nurse identify cardiovascular symptoms as well as current or potential problems that may affect cardiovascular function. Information learned from a history and physical exam could help prevent undesirable responses to current therapies and treatment plans and potentially prevent the progression of the cardiac disease. The essential assessment data included in the cardiovascular history are outlined in this section.

Biographic and Demographic Data

Assessment of biographic and demographic data includes information regarding age, race, gender, and ethnicity, which can impact the

Video*: Heart Sound: Irregular Weblink: Heart Diesease and stroke Statistics 2012

susceptibility to some cardiovascular disorders. For example, African Americans have a higher incidence of hypertension than Caucasians, and premenopausal women have a lower incidence of atherosclerotic coronary artery disease than men (American Heart Association, 2010b). Additionally, the presenting symptoms of cardiovascular diseases in women are often atypical, which may either delay diagnosis or make diagnosis more difficult. For example, women more frequently present with shortness of breath instead of the classic pain in the midsternal chest.

Chief Complaint

During the assessment process the nurse obtains a complete description of the present illness, paying particular attention to the chief complaint, or the reason the patient is seeking health care. The chief complaint focuses the history-taking process and prioritizes treatment regimens. For example, if the patient is complaining of chest pain, then the history should include information regarding the nature of the pain, associated symptoms, and exacerbating and alleviating factors, as well as radiation of the pain and intensity of the pain. It also is important to determine what brings the pain and what relieves it.

Presenting Symptoms

A review of symptoms helps define the current functional status of the patient. The nurse needs to ask questions about the date and mode of onset of the symptoms to find out when and how the symptoms first began. For example, has the shortness of breath been a problem for many weeks, or is it a new occurrence? Have the symptoms changed in intensity or duration? Additionally, questions about what causes the symptoms to worsen and alleviating factors are important.

Safety Alert *Nurses should be particularly aware of the following common cardiovascular symptoms: chest pain, palpitations, dyspnea, orthopnea, cough, and nocturia. The most severe symptoms should be assessed in greater depth and reported to the health care provider, if indicated.*

The most life-threatening symptoms should be addressed first. If the patient is complaining of **dyspnea** (shortness of breath), it needs to be assessed immediately. The presence of dyspnea may indicate an imbalance of arterial oxygen supply and demand. Airway management and oxygen status must be stabilized before the remainder of the assessment is completed. The management of the patient's airway is discussed in Unit VI. Other respiratory assessment findings may include **orthopnea,** which is the presence of dyspnea when the patient lies flat and is frequently a manifestation of cardiac disease. Often the degree of orthopnea is measured by the number of pillows (for example, 2- to 3-pillow orthopnea) the patient uses to breathe comfortably while sleeping. A cough may suggest pulmonary congestion resulting from fluid accumulation in the lungs due to either cardiac pump failure or fluid overload. Types of coughs related to pulmonary disease are discussed in Unit VI.

Next, ask the patient about the presence, site, and intensity of pain. The primary cardiovascular concern is pain associated with cardiac muscle ischemia, referred to as angina pectoris. The clinical manifestations of angina vary among patients; therefore, specific questions must be asked during the assessment in order to ascertain the cause of the pain. Pain may be described as indigestion, burning, numbness, tightness, or pressure in the midchest, or as epigastric or substernal pain, which can radiate to the shoulder, neck, arms, jaw, or back. It is essential that the nurse inquires about what brings the "pain on" and what makes it "go away." An in-depth discussion of angina-type chest pain, the assessment data, and treatment is included in Chapter 32. Patients might deny the presence of chest pain but admit to sensations of chest discomfort; therefore, it is important to allow patients to present their symptoms in their own words prior to analyzing their symptoms.

Palpitations are typically described by the patient as sensations of a racing heartbeat, irregular beats, or skipped beats. These sensations may be normal, or they may signify cardiac rhythm disturbances. **Nocturia,** the need to urinate often at night, may indicate heart failure, although there are other disorders that cause frequent urination, such as an enlarged prostate. During the day as a patient is up and moving, fluid shifts to extremities and extravascular spaces, which serves to decrease fluid workload on a decompensated heart. At night, however, when the patient lies flat, fluid is returned to the central intravascular column, thereby increasing the amount of fluid to the kidneys and the heart. Patients with heart failure may report paroxysmal nocturnal dyspnea, which is acute dyspnea that usually occurs within an hour or two after falling asleep, caused by lung congestion and edema that occurs due to the shifting fluids.

Edema, or fluid accumulation in the extravascular spaces of the body, may be due to decreases in venous return. Fluid retention is manifested by weight gain, a feeling of being bloated, or clothes or shoes that no longer fit comfortably. Changes in weight should be specifically addressed. Large, sudden weight gains correlate with fluid volume overload.

Dizziness, **syncope** (fainting), or light-headedness may be experienced with sudden changes of position, and all are related to a decreased cardiac output, which decreases blood to the brain. These clinical manifestations are exacerbated by sudden position changes.

Fatigue, a common complaint with cardiovascular patients, is due to a decreased supply of oxygen to the tissues. Metabolic demands are higher than normal in chronic cardiovascular conditions; however, due to a lowered cardiac output, demands are not met and the result is fatigue. The fatigue is usually progressive over time, and the patient may report a decreased ability to complete usual activities of daily living. Additionally, patients may report a lack of energy or the need for more rest than usual. Medications such as diuretics, beta-adrenergic blockers, calcium-channel blockers, digoxin, and antihypertensive drugs have long been thought to contribute to fatigue. For example, beta-adrenergic blockers block the response from the beta nerve receptors, which serves to slow down the heart rate and lower the blood pressure. This desired physiological change, which decreases the myocardial oxygen demand, also may cause an undesired side effect of fatigue. Therefore, the risks of adverse effects (fatigue) should be considered in context with the well-documented benefits of medications such as beta-adrenergic blockers.

Problems with the peripheral vascular system are frequently manifested with intermittent claudication. The patient reports pain in the muscles of the lower extremities associated with activity, which may be due to arterial insufficiency. Chapter 35 includes a complete discussion of both venous and arterial peripheral vascular disorders.

Past Medical History

Past medical history should be reviewed because many past illnesses or disorders of other systems of the body can affect the cardiovascular system directly or indirectly. Additionally, the clinical manifestations of other diseases may mistakenly be attributed to cardiovascular disorders. For example, it is important to determine the presence of respiratory disorders to assess a patient's complaint of dyspnea properly, or a history of rheumatic heart disease may have damaged the heart valves. Unit VI discusses respiratory management, and Chapter 33 discusses rheumatic fever and valve disorders.

Childhood Illnesses and Immunizations

Childhood illnesses, congenital heart diseases, history of murmurs, cyanosis, streptococcal infections, anemia, and rheumatic fever should all be assessed. They can either exacerbate current cardiovascular conditions or contribute to the development of additional cardiovascular problems and disease states. Nurses should question the status of immunizations.

Previous Illnesses and Hospitalizations

Heart failure, coronary artery disease (CAD), stroke, heart valve disease, mitral valve prolapse, previous myocardial infarction (MI), peripheral vascular disease, diabetes mellitus, hypertension, hyperlipidemia, dysrhythmias, murmurs, endocarditis, psychiatric illnesses, thrombophlebitis, deep vein thrombosis, and systemic or pulmonary emboli are all important components of or contributors to cardiovascular disease. Their presence, or a history of their presence, and the potential impact on the present health state must be assessed.

Diagnostic/Interventional Cardiac Procedures or Surgeries

Data from previous diagnostic tests, particularly for cardiovascular symptoms, should be obtained. The patient should be asked whether he had any cardiac studies or interventions in the past such as cardiac catheterizations, cardiac ultrasounds, electrocardiograms (ECGs), exercise tolerance tests (stress tests), or myocardial imaging. Previous chest x-rays or ECGs may be helpful to view for baseline data.

Past surgeries, treatments, or hospital admissions should be explored. Assess for a history of previous percutaneous coronary interventions, including balloon angioplasty or stent placement. See Chapters 30 to 35 for more information on diagnostic and interventional therapies for heart disease.

Medications

Review the patient's current and past medications, including over-the-counter (OTC) and prescription medications. The use of herbal remedies or dietary supplements should be specifically assessed because some cardiovascular complications have been linked to these substances. Consideration is made of other common medications and their potential side effects on cardiovascular status. Common medications that affect the cardiovascular system are discussed in the subsequent chapters in this unit as they relate to a specific disorder.

Allergies

Certain diagnostic tests to evaluate heart disease use contrast media and medications, so the presence of any allergies, especially to radiographic contrast agents or iodine, should be assessed. Drug interactions or intolerance should also be noted. Information as to the nature of allergic reactions, such as rash, anaphylaxis, or dyspnea, is essential.

Family History

The link between familial history of cardiovascular disease and the risk for similar events is well established (World Heart Federation, 2011). Specifically, the patient should be asked whether blood relatives have suffered from any of the following: CAD at or under age 55, myocardial infarction, hypertension, stroke, diabetes mellitus, and/or lipid disorders. Collagen vascular diseases such as lupus or scleroderma may be important, because they are linked to the development of cardiac disease or pericarditis. Additionally, a family health history of noncardiac conditions such as asthma, renal disease, and obesity is noted due to their impact on cardiovascular function.

Risk Factors

Several risk factors have been identified that can lead to cardiovascular disease. Risk factors are classified as either nonmodifiable or modifiable. Nonmodifiable risk factors include such things as age, gender, family history, and race. They cannot be changed, and they impact the development of cardiovascular diseases. Modifiable risk factors include cigarette smoking, hypertension, hypercholesterolemia, physical inactivity, diabetes, stress, and obesity. Modifiable risk factors can be treated with interventions to decrease their impact. Additionally, recent dental work or infection may put the patient at risk for development of cardiac complications such as endocarditis. Chapter 32 includes a complete description of cardiac risk factors.

Social History

An assessment of social history is important because of the relationship between social history and the development of, acceleration of, and response to cardiovascular diseases. While taking a social history, nurses gain valuable information from patients about the presence of risk factors. Nurses then have an important role in assisting patients to recognize unhealthy habits that require education in order to modify or change these habits to prevent the progression and complications associated with the development of cardiovascular disorders.

Occupation

Job stress is a common condition that promotes the occurrence of cardiovascular events. Therefore, previous and recent job-related stressors should be explored. Stress and tension regardless of their etiology cause vasoconstriction, which increases afterload, oxygen consumption, and release of catecholamines, which in turn can contribute to the development of cardiac symptoms. Another occupational hazard that should be considered is exposure to noxious or harmful substances, and the potential effect of them on the cardiovascular system.

Culture

Because nurses care for diverse populations, knowledge about the health practices of other cultures and religions is essential. Beliefs and values related to health, illness, and death, as well as daily habits, nutritional preferences, and health practices, are impacted by cultural norms and beliefs and may conflict with the health care standards or even the function of the cardiovascular status. Nurses need to inquire about cultural celebrations or rituals that may affect dietary patterns. For example, nurses should ask patients about the salt content in their food, because an increased amount may precipitate an episode of heart failure and/or high blood pressure. Health and well-being of a culturally diverse population can be promoted by incorporating the therapies that patients have traditionally used. During the assessment nurses must gather information on the use of all therapies, including complementary and nontraditional therapies.

Safety Alert *One of the most important complementary therapies that should be addressed during assessment is the use of herbal products. There is a known risk of interaction between herbal products and conventional medications.*

Environment

It is understood that heart disease develops as a result of complex interactions between genes and the environment in which we live. Additionally, environmental issues may be correlated with the risk for cardiovascular disease. Environmental conditions such as living

Weblink: Sodium Recommendations
Weblink: FAQs About Stress

NATIONAL GUIDELINES American Heart Association National Guidelines for Diet and Lifestyle Recommendations

Achieve an Overall Healthy Eating Pattern

- Choose an overall balanced diet with foods from all major food groups, emphasizing fruits, vegetables, and grains.
- Consume a variety of fruits, vegetables, and grain products.
- Eat at least 5 daily servings of fruits and vegetables.
- Eat at least 6 daily servings of grain products, including whole grains.
- Include fat-free and low-fat dairy products, fish, legumes, poultry, and lean meats.
- Eat at least 2 servings of fish per week.

Achieve a Healthy Body Weight

- Maintain a level of physical activity that achieves fitness and balances energy expenditure with caloric intake; for weight reduction, expenditure should exceed intake.
- Limit foods that are high in calories and/or low in nutritional quality, including those with a high amount of added sugar.

Achieve a Desirable Cholesterol Level

- Limit foods with a high content of saturated fat and cholesterol. Substitute with grains and unsaturated fat from vegetables, fish, legumes, and nuts.
- Limit cholesterol to 300 milligrams (mg) a day for the general population and 200 milligrams a day for those with heart disease or its risk factors.
- Limit *trans* fatty acids. Trans fatty acids are found in foods containing partially hydrogenated vegetable oils such as packaged cookies, crackers, and other baked goods; commercially prepared fried foods; and some margarines.

Achieve a Desirable Blood Pressure Level

- Limit salt intake to less than 1.5 grams (1,500 milligrams sodium) per day, slightly more than 1 teaspoon a day.
- If you drink, limit alcohol consumption to no more than one drink per day for women and two drinks per day for men.

Source: American Heart Association. (2010a). *Dietary guidelines: At-a-glance.* Retrieved from http://www.livestrong.com/article/425639-american-heart-association-sodium-recommendations/.

conditions and the presence of any cardiovascular toxins must be assessed. Environmental risk factors are not limited to the better known risk factors of smoking, poor diet, and lack of exercise, but also include exposure to chemicals and pollutants, such as air pollution.

Habits

Lifestyle habits and dietary habits such as the use of tea, coffee, alcohol, recreational drugs, OTC drugs, and smoking are assessed and documented. If the patient smokes, the number of pack-years of smoking (packs smoked per day multiplied by the years smoked) should be calculated. The patient's attitude about smoking and any attempts to stop smoking should be documented. The presence of secondhand smoke also must be assessed. Alcohol use, including type of beverages, amount, frequency, and any change in the reaction to it should be assessed. The use of habit-forming drugs and recreational drugs also should be noted.

Exercise

Physical activity has long been known to reduce the risk of cardiovascular events. Low levels of physical activity as well as consumption of excess calories, combined with inherited genes, cause obesity. Obesity, especially abdominal obesity, is a predisposing factor for the development of cardiovascular disease, as well as hypertension and type 2 diabetes mellitus. The physical activity patterns of a patient, including the type of exercise, the duration and frequency of the exercise, and the presence of any cardiovascular symptoms, should be documented. Any decrease in previous abilities or changes in the response to physical activity should be noted, because they may be indications of the advent or progression of heart disease.

Nutrition

It is important to assess the patient's weight and diet history. An assessment of weight in comparison to height and build must be completed. Being overweight or underweight may be related to certain cardiovascular disorders or may put the patient at risk for developing certain cardiac problems. Usual dietary intake including amounts of salt, saturated fats, triglycerides, and fluids should be determined. It may be important to identify which dietary habits are related to cultural preferences and which habits are the results of the environment or social situations. For example, an executive may consume many meals at restaurants with clients. In addition, the patient's attitudes and plans in relation to diet should be discussed. The American Heart Association's guidelines for healthy eating are outlined in the National Guidelines box. Nutrition as it relates to heart disease is discussed in this unit and in Chapter 8.

Personal Factors

Baseline cognitive functioning; recent life changes, especially within the last 12 months; sleep–rest patterns, and relationship issues should all be considered during the assessment. Emotional state, such as the evidence of psychological stress, anger, anxiety, or depression, causes the release of catecholamines, which results in vasoconstriction, thereby increasing cardiac workload and potentially resulting in a decreased cardiac output. Perception of illness and its meaning for the future should also be noted.

Personality type may also be a consideration for cardiovascular assessment. Type A personality behavior has been associated with increased incidence of cardiovascular disease (American Heart Association, 2011). Type A personality behavior may be a "trigger" that precipitates coronary events rather than affecting the process of atherosclerosis. The role of stress and the manner in which an individual deals with life stressors may also have an important role. Individuals with type A personality may respond to stress with hostility or aggression, which may exaggerate sympathetic and hemodynamic responses leading to greater cardiovascular reactivity.

Type D or *distressed* personality (Denollet, Schiffer, & Spek, 2010) is another personality type that has been linked to an increased risk for cardiovascular morbidity. Individuals with type D behavior have a tendency to experience negative emotions, but they inhibit these emotions and avoid social contacts. Both type D dimensions (negative affectivity and social inhibition) are associated with greater cortisol reactivity to stress, which increases the risk for coronary heart disease.

Physical Examination

A thorough physical examination is the foundation for accurate assessment of the cardiovascular system and encompasses skills of inspection, palpation, and auscultation. Percussion is not utilized for assessment of the cardiovascular system.

Inspection of Skin and Extremities

A great deal of information can be obtained about the status of the cardiovascular system by simply observing and touching the patient. By observation, the nurse is able to assess the patient's general appearance quickly, including facial expressions; body posture and mentation, as well as color and temperature; and clubbing of the nail beds. Then it is necessary to relate the findings to the patient's current cardiovascular status.

General Appearance

General appearance includes a brief visual inspection of a patient's physical appearance. Observations of a patient who looks unwell, lethargic, exhausted, or breathless are important findings and may indicate reduced cardiac output or heart failure. Observation of facial expression may indicate important findings, such as the assessment of apprehension, pain, or fear. Body posture may indicate the amount of effort it takes to breathe. For example, a patient in acute heart failure may need to sit upright, whereas a patient with pericarditis may lean forward in order to breathe comfortably (Lynn-McHale Wiegand, 2010). An obese person who has fat evenly distributed over the body is vulnerable for serious cardiovascular health consequences. Additionally, an accumulation of abdominal (visceral) fat, measured by waist circumference, is a known risk factor for cardiovascular and other diseases.

Normal neurological function indicates adequate cerebral perfusion. A quick and easy method to estimate baseline cognitive function is to assess the patient's orientation to person, place and time, and situation. Confusion could indicate hypotension or low cardiac output.

Color and Appearance of Skin and Extremities

The skin and mucous membranes are inspected for color and temperature. Extremities should be assessed bilaterally for equal temperature and appearance. The extremities are inspected for signs of peripheral arterial or venous vascular disorders. Chapter 35 includes an in-depth description of peripheral vascular disease.

Cyanosis is a bluish tinge to the skin due to deoxygenated hemoglobin in the blood vessels close to the skin surface; it can be either central or peripheral. Central cyanosis, which is noted on the lips or tongue, is often characteristic of impaired gas exchange. Central cyanosis may result from a cardiac right-to-left shunt due to septal defects, in which deoxygenated venous blood mixes with blood from the left heart and is ejected into the systemic circulation. In heart failure with significant pulmonary congestion, oxygenation of blood in the pulmonary vascular bed can be impaired, which leads to deoxygenated blood returning to the left heart and being pumped out into the systemic circulation. Peripheral cyanosis, which occurs in the extremities or under the nail beds, may indicate poor circulation. The room where the examination is taking place must have a comfortable temperature because nail beds can become cyanotic with cold temperatures.

Pallor suggests poor perfusion, which may be related to peripheral vascular disease; a release of catecholamines and subsequent vasoconstriction; or a low hemoglobin and hematocrit. All of these conditions should be thoroughly assessed. Additionally, temperature changes such as generalized warmth or coolness may indicate altered peripheral perfusion.

Clubbing of the nail bed is easily assessed and appears as swelling of the subcutaneous tissue over the base of the nail and absence of the normal angle between the nail and the nail base (Figure 29–5◆). The presence of clubbing indicates long-term oxygen deficiencies such as congenital heart defects or pulmonary diseases with hypoxemia.

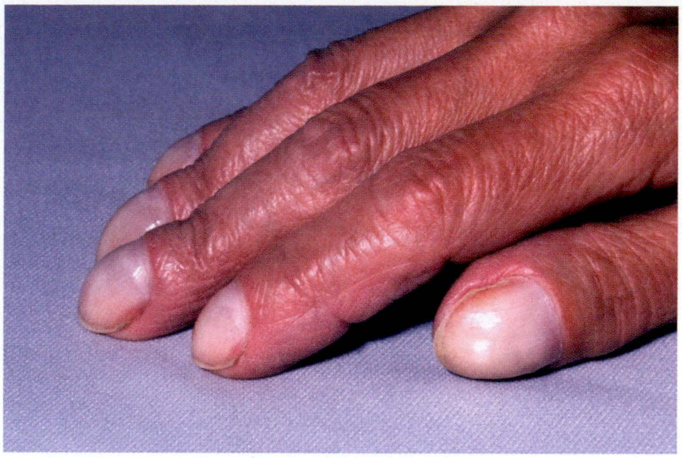

FIGURE 29–5 ◆ Clubbing of the nail beds.
Source: @Medical-on-line/Alamy.

Palpation of Skin and Extremities

Palpation of the skin and extremities during a cardiovascular assessment includes an assessment of edema, skin turgor, capillary refill, and the arterial pulses for abnormalities associated with cardiovascular disorders.

Edema is defined as an increase in interstitial fluid that is clinically evident. Although there are many types of edema, cardiovascular patients typically experience edema associated with the accumulation of fluid in the extracellular spaces, particularly the skin of the extremities, as discussed earlier. Edema of the skin can be painful, and it interferes with normal blood circulation. Edema is an important assessment finding because it is indicative of an underlying disease process and requires treatment.

Edema can be localized in one area of the body or can be generalized throughout. Dependent edema occurs when there is an increase in extracellular fluid volume in a dependent limb or area. Edema is assessed by firmly placing a thumb against a dependent area of the body (arms, hands, legs, feet, ankles). When the pressure is released, an indentation on the skin may be observed. When the indentation remains on the skin after releasing pressure, it is referred to as pitting edema. The degree of pitting edema can be rated on a 4-point scale (Chart 29–1).

Palpation for assessment of **skin turgor,** or elasticity, reflects the skin's state of hydration. A small section of the patient's skin (anterior chest, under clavicle, forearm, or abdomen) is pinched between the examiner's thumb and forefinger. As the skin is slowly released, the speed at which the skin returns to its original contour is observed. It should return to normal rapidly. If there is poor skin turgor, the skin returns to

CHART 29–1 Scale for Rating Edema

+0″ No pitting
+1 0″–1/4″ pitting (mild)
+2 1/4″–1/2″ pitting (moderate)
+3 1/2″–1″ pitting (severe)
+4 Greater than 1″ pitting (severe)

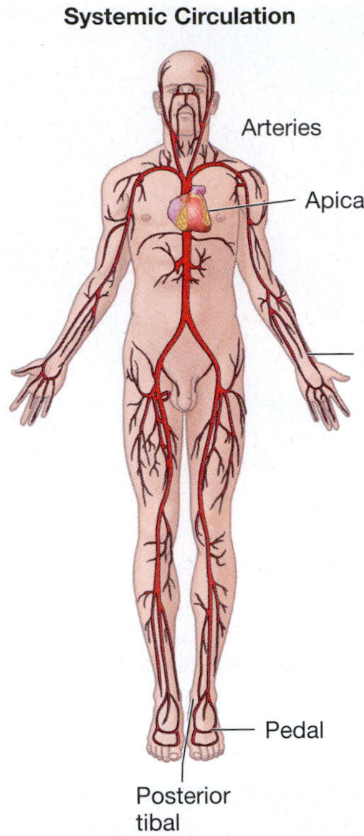

FIGURE 29–6 ◆ Arterial pulses.

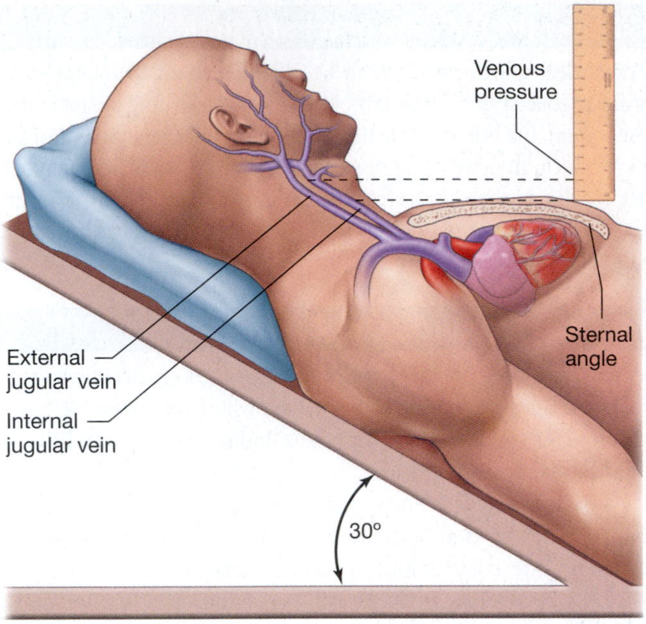

FIGURE 29–7 ◆ Jugular veins.

its original contour very slowly. Dehydration, scleroderma, or aging can decrease skin turgor.

Capillary refill, the rate at which blood refills empty capillaries, is a quick method of assessing blood flow to the peripheral microcirculation. The nurse compresses the tip of the patient's finger until blanching of the nail bed is noted. When pressure is released, a return of color should be noted within 2 to 3 seconds. A delayed return of color is a sign of vasoconstriction or poor peripheral perfusion. A delayed capillary refill may be observed in heart failure, peripheral vascular disease, or shock.

Palpation of the arterial pulses in the neck and extremities provides information about arterial blood flow, particularly volume and pressure within the vessels. Arterial pulses are palpated bilaterally to compare characteristics of the arteries on the right and left sides of the body (Figure 29–6◆). The volume of the pulsations is judged and recorded as normal, bounding, thready, or absent. Additionally, a common scale can be used for the documentation of pulses (see Chart 29–2). A normal pulse feels like a tap, whereas a vessel that is narrowed or bulging will vibrate. The rate and rhythm of arterial pulses are palpated. The nurse counts the number of pulsations in a minute to determine the heart rate. At the same time, the nurse judges the regularity of the pattern of pulses and the intervals between pulses. Pulses can be normal or abnormal. Abnormalities in the rate and rhythm of arterial pulses may indicate inadequate cardiac output or cardiac dysrhythmias.

CHART 29–2 Scale for Rating Arterial Pulses

0 Absent pulse.
+1 Pulse is present but is weak and thready.
+2 Pulse is present with normal amplitude.
+3 Full and bounding pulsation.

Jugular Venous Distention/ Jugular Venous Pressure

Jugular venous distention (JVD) and jugular venous pressure (JVP) or pulse are assessed using the right external and internal jugular veins (Figure 29–7◆). Although these terms are often used interchangeably, there is a physiological significance in distinguishing between JVD and JVP. Anatomically, the right jugular veins drain blood from the head into the right atrium of the heart. Both veins reflect activity on the right side of the heart. The internal jugular vein lies in a straight path to the right atrium; however, because it is buried beneath the sternomastoid muscle, it is difficult to visualize. The external jugular vein curves a few times before entering the right atrium, and because it is located closer to the skin it is easier to visualize. Findings from neck vein assessment are helpful in confirming suspicions of heart failure; however, the information must be put in context of the presenting clinical manifestations and current health status. The importance of volume status and its impact on cardiovascular function is an important hemodynamic concept. Chapter 34 includes an in-depth discussion of the significance of distended neck veins with heart failure.

Jugular venous distention (JVD) is assessed by visually observing the right external jugular (REJ) vein. Generally noting that this vein is full or overdistended is sufficient for the nursing assessment and provides useful information pertaining to the hemodynamic volume status of the cardiovascular system. The REJ vein is always distended when the patient is lying flat and is eliminated as the patient becomes more upright. From a flat position, slowly elevate the head of the bed and observe the right external jugular vein, noting the degree of elevation at which the distention is eliminated (30, 45, 60, or 90 degrees). The finding is reported by noting the highest height of the head of the bed (HOB) when JVD was appreciated; for example, "presence of JVD was noted with HOB elevated to 45 degrees" (Lynn-McHale Wiegand, 2010).

Safety Alert *The finding of JVD during inspection of the neck veins can contribute to diagnosis of right heart failure. Treatment to reduce volume, such as diuretics or vasodilators, may be needed. The finding of JVD may also help to explain other findings noted during the exam, such as shortness of breath (SOB), diaphoresis, or confusion. This finding needs to be reported for the health care provider.*

Jugular venous pressure (JVP) is measured using the right internal jugular (RIJ) vein. The RIJ lies deep in skin and soft tissues, and its pulsations are transmitted to the overlying tissues. These pulsations are produced by the right atrial and right ventricular activity (Lynn-McHale Wiegand, 2010). Changes in pulsations can be a diagnostic tool for the skilled practitioner. Assessment of RIJ for jugular venous pressure (JVP) provides valuable information as well, and it is a more reliable indicator of central venous pressure (CVP), or the pressure that exists in the central venous system, than is the right external vein assessment. To examine the JVP, stand on the patient's right side and turn the patient's head slightly to the left. The neck muscles should be relaxed. The head of the bed should be elevated high enough to visualize the top of the column of blood in the internal jugular vein. Observe the highest point of pulsation during exhalation. The vertical difference between this location and the sternal angle (see Figure 29–7) is measured in centimeters. The normal measurement should be 4 centimeters or less. A measurement of more than 4 centimeters suggests increased JVP, an increase in pressure in the right heart, and therefore an increased CVP. Because the distance between the sternal angle and the mid-right atrium is approximately 5 centimeters, to measure CVP, 5 centimeters is added to the measurement of JVP. The upper limit of normal is a CVP measurement of 9 centimeters (JVP of 4 plus 5 centimeters) (Woods, Sivarajan Frolicher, Motzer, & Bridges, 2010). An example of how this finding is reported is "JVP estimated at 9 centimeters with the head of the bed elevated to 45 degrees."

The **abdominojugular reflux** (sometimes called *hepatojugular reflux*) is a test to detect extra fluid volume in the abdomen. It can be assessed using a noninvasive technique. In heart failure, or volume overload, blood volume that normally is pumped proficiently by the heart begins to be displaced throughout the body as a mechanism to minimize cardiac workload. Volume may be displaced in the abdomen, particularly the hepatic system, which has a large capacity to hold fluid. The technique to observe abdominojugular reflux is done by compressing the right upper abdomen for 15 to 30 seconds. Observe for JVD before, during, and after abdominal compression. This pressure causes volume in the abdomen to be pushed back to the right atrium. The failing heart will not be able to accommodate this increase in volume, and the pressure will be reflected in the jugular veins. Sustained JVD (longer than 10 seconds) with abdominal compression is another indicator that aids the diagnosis of cardiac failure (Moser & Riegel, 2008).

Inspection and Palpation of the Precordium

Inspection and palpation of the bony structures of the thorax, including the sternoclavicular joints, the manubrium, and the upper part of the sternum, are performed using clinical reference points. The precordium is assessed for pulsations, heaves, and thrills, which are described in the following text. These conditions may indicate vessel abnormalities.

The normal **clinical reference points** or landmarks of the chest wall, as well as specific auscultatory areas, should be noted on every patient during cardiovascular assessment in a consistent manner. Experience enhances the ability to identify abnormalities and their significance to cardiovascular disorders (Figures 29–8◆ and 29–9◆).

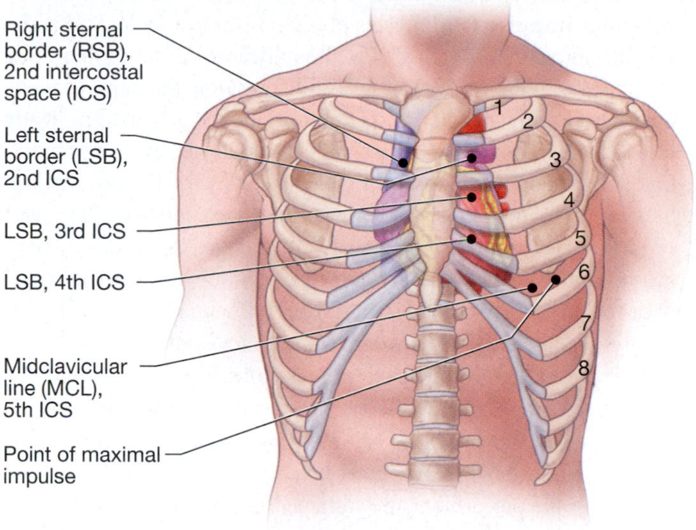

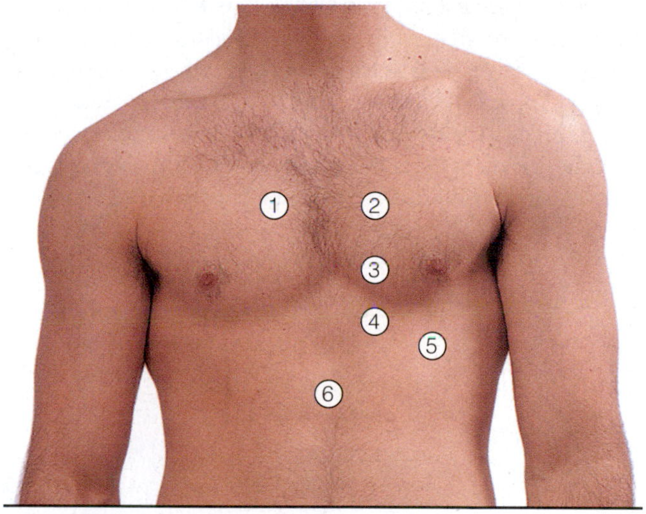

FIGURE 29–8 ◆ Clinical reference points for palpation.

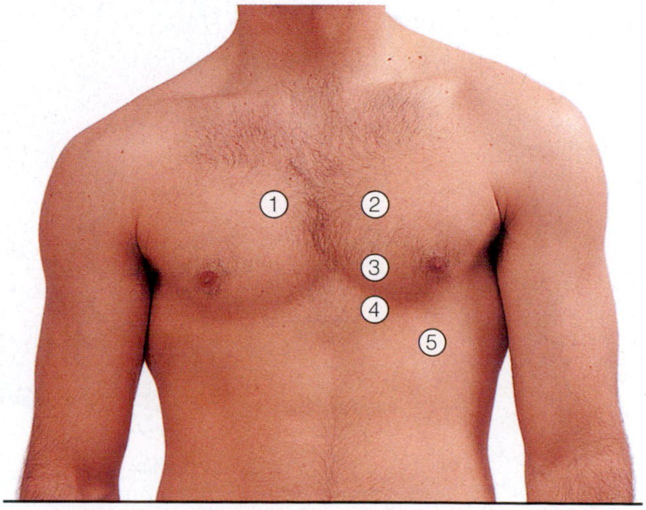

FIGURE 29–9 ◆ Auscultatory areas.

The mitral valve area of the thorax is palpated for the **point of maximal impulse (PMI).** This pulsation is normally located at the left fifth intercostal space (ICS) at the midclavicular line (MCL) (see Figure 29–8). With the patient in a sitting position, the nurse uses fingertips to identify the PMI. Sometimes having the patient lean slightly forward enhances the PMI. The PMI is normally felt as a single pulsation or light tap, and is 1 to 2 centimeters in diameter. The position and the diameter of the PMI should be recorded in relation to the MCL and ICSs. If the patient has cardiomegaly (an enlarged heart) due to heart failure, ventricular hypertrophy, or pregnancy, the PMI may be enlarged or displaced laterally and downward. The PMI may also be visualized as a pulsation on the chest in a patient with cardiovascular disease.

The precordium is inspected for pulsations, heaves, and thrills. Although rare, pulsations may be visualized on the chest wall, particularly in thin patients, and may be caused by pulmonary hypertension or a significant aneurysm. **Heaves** or lifts, which are normally not seen or felt over the precordium, are sustained lifts of the chest wall in the precordial area due to forceful cardiac contractions that cause a slight to vigorous movement of the sternum and ribs. Heaves may be caused by ventricular enlargement or hypertrophy. A **thrill** describes a palpable vibratory sensation from turbulent blood flow across cardiac valves. The sound a thrill makes is typically described as that of a purring cat.

Findings in various clinical reference points may indicate specific cardiac disorders. The respiratory system is observed simultaneously, because the purpose of the cardiovascular system is to deliver oxygen to the tissues that was received from the respiratory system. Alterations in rate and depth of respirations may indicate cardiovascular, respiratory, or neurological disorders.

Auscultation of the Precordium

Cardiac **auscultation** is an efficient, noninvasive manner to assess both normal and abnormal heart sounds. Although the technique is simply performed with only a stethoscope, a great deal of practice and expertise is required to appreciate and differentiate cardiac abnormalities associated with valvular alterations. The art of auscultation includes the ability to discriminate subtle differences in intensity, pitch, location, radiation, duration, timing, and intervals of heart sounds (Hurst, O'Rourke, Walsh, & Fuster, 2009). Generally, nurses should be able to perform the technique proficiently, be able to recognize normal auscultatory sounds, and most importantly be alert to variations from normal that can provide valuable clinical clues and may indicate a change or deterioration in cardiac status.

The skill of auscultation begins with good technique and a quiet environment. The stethoscope should have a bell, a diaphragm, and comfortable earpieces. The stethoscope is applied directly to the skin; listening over clothing will obscure the sound. The patient must be in a comfortable position and asked to lie still and not talk. Imagine the position of the heart and the cardiac valves under the chest wall (see Figure 29–1, p. 832). Find the angle of Louis, felt as a ridge just below the suprasternal notch. Feel the ribs on each side of this angle and the intercostal space below each rib. Using the bell and the diaphragm of the stethoscope, listen to heart sounds at each auscultatory area (see Figure 29–9, p. 839), first with the diaphragm for high-pitched sounds and then with the bell, using very light pressure for low-pitched sounds at each auscultatory site. Listen for the normal heart sounds (described in the following text) at each site, and note the intensity, the presence of split sounds, and the effect of the respiratory cycle on the regularity of the sounds. Also note the time between the regularity of the normal heart sounds. Listen for extra heart sounds and abnormal heart sounds at each site. If abnormal sounds are heard, note the timing, pitch, loudness, duration, and location on the chest wall. If a murmur is heard, note where it can be heard best and whether it is a low-, medium-, or high-pitched sound. The presence of any pericardial friction rubs should also be noted.

In order to become proficient at cardiac auscultation, nurses need to have knowledge of the physiology of the cardiac cycle, the normal landmarks of the chest (see Figure 29–8, p. 839), and the auscultatory sites on the chest wall that correspond to specific valve sounds (see Figure 29–9, p. 839). When listening to dynamic blood flow across cardiac valves, the sounds associated with the closure of the valves are not heard directly over that valve area, but rather in the direction of the flow of blood. It is helpful to imagine the physical position of the heart under the chest wall, as well as the path or direction of blood flow (Figure 29–10◆). Because sound is not transmitted through bone, the best auscultatory area of a particular valve is the area on the chest wall that is in line with

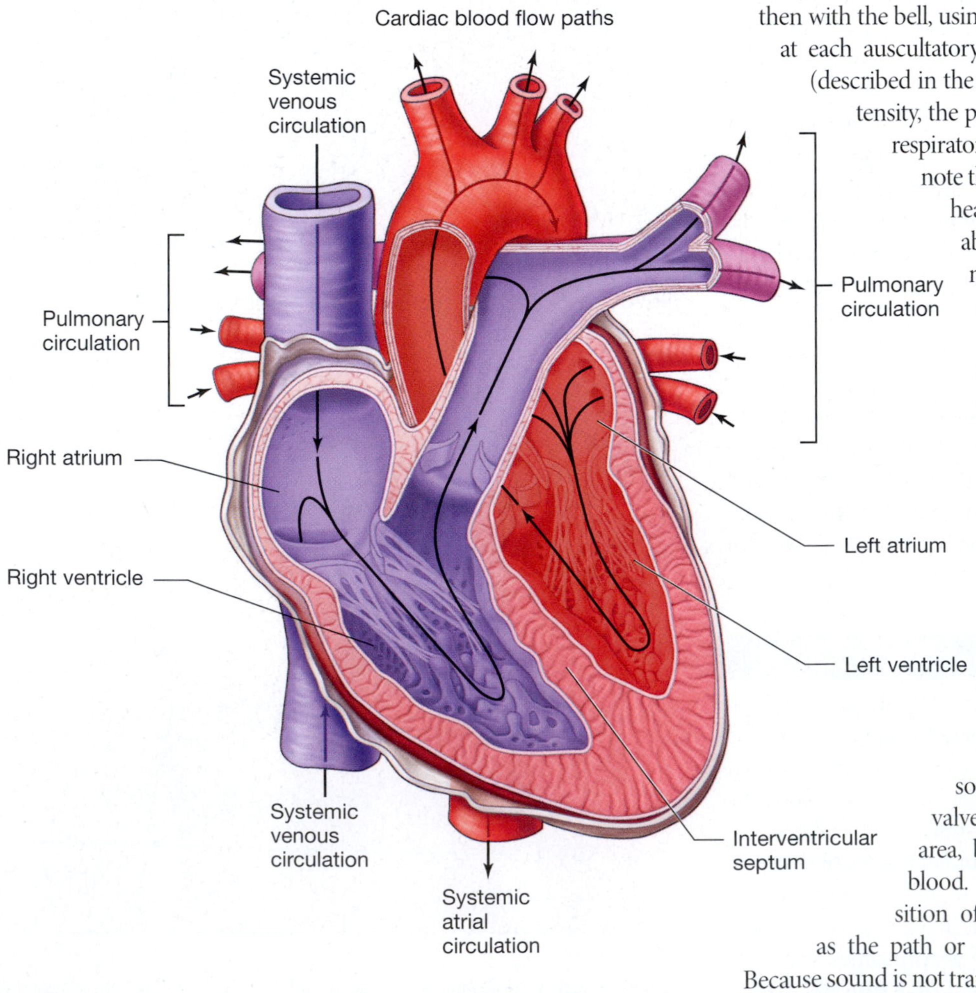

FIGURE 29–10 ◆ Cardiac blood flow path.

the path of blood flow. The key to a good auscultatory exam is to listen to one sound at a time in each auscultatory area. The nurse should be in the habit of listening to all the auscultatory areas with the diaphragm and then again with the bell.

Normal Heart Sounds: S_1 and S_2

Normal heart sounds are created by the turbulence of blood flow as the cardiac valves open and close during the cardiac cycle. As the valves move, some turbulence in blood flow is created. Two heart sounds can be heard with each cardiac cycle. The first heart sound is referred to as S_1 and the second heart sound, S_2. **S_1** is called a systolic sound because it signals the beginning of systole. When the pressures in the pulmonary artery, right ventricle, and left ventricle begin to equalize, systolic ejection tapers off and the AV valves, tricuspid and mitral, close to prevent regurgitation of blood back into the atria during ventricular contraction. The second heart sound, S_2, occurs at the end of systole and is the closing of the semilunar valves, pulmonic and aortic, which prevent regurgitation of blood back into the ventricles after ventricular

Video*: Heart Sounds: Normal

CHART 29–3 Summary of Heart Sounds

Heart Sounds		Cardiac Cycle Timing	Auscultation Site	Position	Pitch
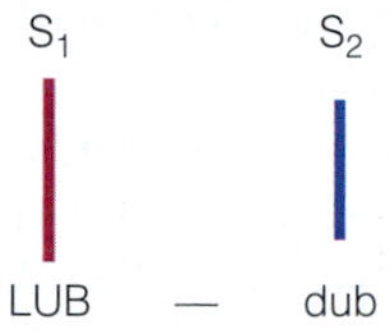	S_1	Start of systole	Best at apex with diaphragm	Position does not affect the sound	High
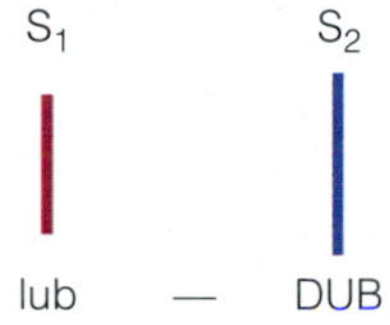	S_2	End of systole	Both at second intercostal space (ICS); pulmonary component best at left sternal border (LSB); aortic component best at RSB with diaphragm	Sitting or supine	High
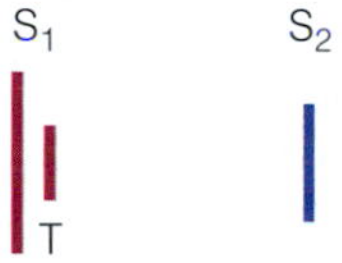	Split S_1	Beginning of systole	If normal, at second ICS; LSB abnormal if heard at apex	Better heard in the supine position	High
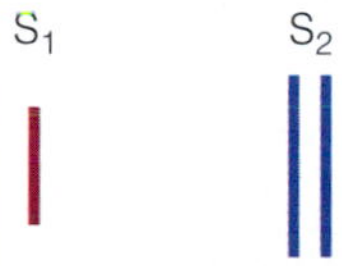	Fixed split S_2	End of systole	Both at second ICS: pulmonary component best at LSB; aortic component best at right sternal border (RSB) with diaphragm	Better heard in the supine position	High
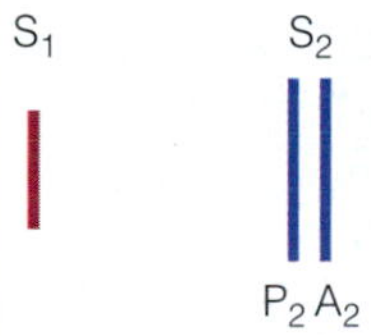	Paradoxical split S_2	End of systole	Both at second ICS; pulmonary component best at LSB; aortic component best at RSB with diaphragm	Better heard in the supine position	High
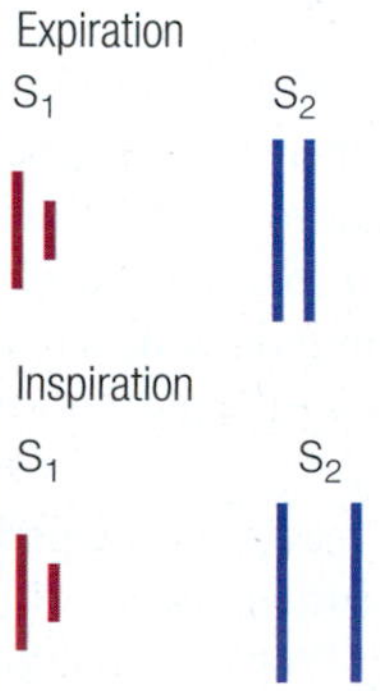	Wide split S_2	End of systole	Both at second ICS; pulmonary component best at LSB; aortic component best at RSB with diaphragm	Better heard in the supine position	High
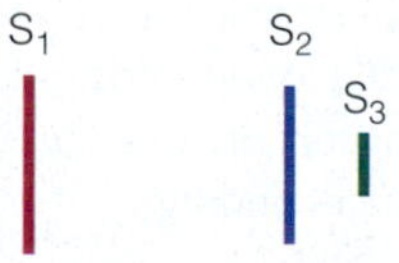	S_3	Early diastole right after S_2	Apex with the bell	Auscultated better in left lateral position or supine	Low
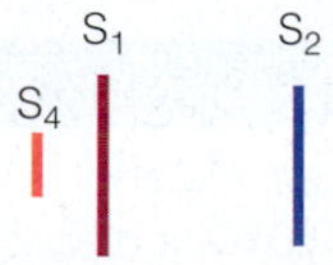	S_4	Late diastole right before S_1	Apex with the bell	Auscultated better in left lateral position or supine	Low

Video*: Heart Sounds: Split S2 Video*: Heart Sound: Irregular

contraction (Chart 29-3). The S_1 and the S_2 are both high-pitched sounds heard best with the diaphragm. The S_1 is normally loudest over the apex or mitral area, while the S_2 is best heard over the base of the heart, or the aortic area.

It is helpful during auscultation to differentiate the S_1 from the S_2. When there is an abnormality, it must be described as a systolic sound (occurring with or after the S_1) or a diastolic sound (occurring with or after the S_2). By determining where in the cardiac cycle the abnormality occurs, the listener can better estimate which cardiac valve is affected. For example, if the nurse hears an abnormality of the S_1 sound, she would know there is an alteration in either the mitral or the tricuspid valve. The S_1 and the S_2 sounds can be differentiated by three methods. The first is timing. During the cardiac cycle, the amount of time spent in diastole is longer than the amount of time spent in systole. Therefore, there should be a pause between the S_2 and the next S_1 (Chart 29–3, p. 841). Of course, this method is accurate only when the heart rate is slow enough to appreciate the diastolic pause. If, however, the heart rate is accelerated, the S_1 can be identified by palpating either the PMI (point of maximal impulse) or the carotid arterial pulsation. As the practitioner is listening with the stethoscope on the chest wall to the heart sound, she should be palpating these pulsation points. When the pulsation is felt, the S_1 is heard. Pulse points, further downstream, such as the radial artery should not be used to establish correlation, because they are too far away from the heart and are not likely to correspond with the S_1.

Split S_1 and Split S_2

Because the right and left heart are two separate pumps that function simultaneously, it is normal to hear the closure of two valves, the right and left AV valves, and the right and left semilunar valves, as one sound. Many conditions can alter the timing of the cardiac cycle on the right or left side of the heart, causing one valve to close slightly later than normal. When this happens, the sounds of S_1 (closure of the tricuspid and mitral valves) or the sounds of S_2 (closure of the pulmonic and aortic valves) are heard separately. This is referred to as a **split heart sound.**

The S_1 is normally heard as a single sound, although there might be a slight split between the mitral component (M_1) and the tricuspid component (T_1) of the S_1. The S_2 exhibits a normal split on inspiration. This is called a *physiological split*, because it is associated with a normal physiological pattern. This physiological split S_2, heard best over the pulmonic area, is a result of asymmetry with the closure of the aortic (A_2) and pulmonic (P_2) valve sounds that make up the S_2 (A_2P_2). On inspiration, there is an increase in intrathoracic pressure that causes an increase in venous return to the right heart. The increased volume causes a delay in ventricular emptying, and thus the pulmonic valve closure (P_2) is slightly delayed. This effect is removed, however, during expiration; the A_2 and P_2 should be closer in synchrony, and the two components of the second heart sound are heard as one. Numerous other conditions, such as ventricular septal defects (VSDs), bundle branch blocks, and ventricular failure, can cause abnormal splitting of S_2.

Extra Heart Sounds

Extra heart sounds are classified in relation to their timing in the cardiac cycle. Although the presence of an S_3 or S_4 can be normal, these extra heart sounds often signify cardiac disorders. Therefore, nurses must be knowledgeable about these sounds, as well as their significance in relation to heart disease, in order to detect and report their presence. Third and fourth heart sounds, if present, are both heard during diastole. S_3 and S_4 are low-frequency soft sounds, which are best heard by applying the stethoscope softly on the skin or just firmly enough to create a skin seal. It is easier to detect the S_3 or the S_4 by positioning the patient in the left lateral position, which brings the heart closer to the chest wall. S_3 sounds and S_4 sounds are not affected by respirations and are heard as single sounds.

S_3 is heard early in diastole just after the S_2 and is heard best in the apex (see Chart 29–3, p. 841). One cardiac cycle (S_1, S_2, S_3) sounds like lub-dub-DUB, similar to the cadence of the word "Kentucky." S_3 sounds, sometimes called ventricular gallops, are heard early in diastole because they are associated with abnormalities of ventricular filling. S_3 sounds are markers of systolic dysfunction. When there is ventricular systolic dysfunction, the ventricle is not able to empty sufficiently with each systolic contraction. During each consecutive diastolic filling period, turbulence occurs as the "new" load of blood attempts to enter when the previous load of blood has not completely left the ventricle.

An S_3 heard over the left ventricle in children and young adults is normal, although after ages 35 to 40 the presence of a third heart sound is usually abnormal and may indicate systolic dysfunction. An S_3 and the presence of increased JVD are regarded as specific signs of heart failure. The presence of an S_3 in an older person may be the only clue to abnormal left ventricular function (Hurst, O'Rourke, Walsh, & Fuster, 2009).

S_4 occurs late in diastole just before the S_1 and is heard best in the apex (Chart 29–3, p. 841). One cardiac cycle (S_4, S_1, S_2) sounds like LUB-lub-dub, similar to the cadence of the word "Tennessee." S_4 sounds, sometimes called atrial gallops, are heard late in diastole because they are associated with the atrial kick component of diastole. S_4 sounds are markers of diastolic dysfunction. An S_4 occurs when the atria attempt to pump blood into a stiff, noncompliant ventricle that is resistant to further volume expansion.

Diastolic dysfunction may occur with ventricular hypertrophy associated with hypertension, with aortic stenosis, or with altered ventricular compliance associated with ischemia. Normal fourth heart sounds are common in older adults and are associated with an age-related decrease in left ventricular compliance (Hurst, O'Rourke, Walsh, & Fuster, 2009). A fourth heart sound is almost always abnormal in children and may contribute to a decrease in ventricular compliance. An S_4 cannot be heard during atrial fibrillation, because S_4 sounds are associated with atrial contraction against a noncompliant ventricle.

Summation gallops occur when both an S_3 and an S_4 are heard (S_4, S_1, S_2, S_3) (Chart 29–3, p. 841); in other words, there is a combined ventricular and atrial gallop. A summation gallop is associated with advanced heart failure. The S_3 and S_4 may be heard as two distinct sounds in diastole or, in the case of tachycardia, as a single mid-diastolic sound. Summation gallops are sometimes described as galloping hooves (LUB-lub-dub-DUB).

Pericardial friction rubs are due to inflammation of the pericardial sac surrounding the heart in conditions such as pericarditis. Pericarditis is described in detail in Chapter 33. Pericardial friction rubs are a high-pitched sound heard best at the left sternal border. The sound that is produced is a squeaky, rubbing, muffled sound. Pericardial friction rubs are heard best with the patient leaning forward or lying on the left side. These rubs may be a transient assessment finding.

Murmurs

Murmurs are audible vibrations heard over the heart and great vessels. Murmurs are caused by turbulent blood flow across a diseased valve (stenosis or regurgitation), turbulence caused by increased blood

CHART 29–4 Classifications of Murmurs

Timing	Timing within the cardiac cycle. Systolic or diastolic (early, mid, late, continuous). Systolic murmurs are often benign. Diastolic murmurs are never benign.
Location	Auscultatory area the murmur is best heard. Aortic, pulmonic, mitral, tricuspid. Presence of murmurs at specific valve sites leads to the identification of the affected valve.
Frequency	High-pitched or low-pitched sound. Low-pitched murmurs are caused by a low velocity of blood flow. High-pitched murmurs are caused by a rapid velocity of blood flow.
Quality	Descriptive quality of the sound. Harsh, rumbling, musical, soft, blowing, gurgling. Quality may indicate regurgitation or stenosis.
Pattern	Configuration of sound if one was to draw it. Crescendo, decrescendo, diamond shaped.
Radiation	Sounds may be radiated to the neck, back, shoulders, sternal border, jaw, arm, or left axilla. Some murmurs radiate in the direction of the bloodstream, by which they are produced.
Intensity	Grading scale of loudness. I/VI Very soft, barely audible. II/VI Soft, but loud enough to be appreciated. III/VI Loud, easily heard, no thrills or vibrations. IV/VI Loud, soft palpable thrill. V/VI Loud, heard with stethoscope barely touching chest wall; palpable thrill. VI/VI Very loud, can be heard with stethoscope fully off chest wall, pronounced palpable thrill.

flow through normal structures, or blood flow into a dilated chamber (Chart 29–4). Whereas murmurs are auscultatory sounds caused by vibrations or turbulence in the heart and great vessels, **bruits** are auscultatory sounds associated with vibrations or turbulence in a blood vessel outside the heart.

Murmurs are caused by valve stenosis or regurgitation. A stenotic valve is one whose valve leaflets are hardened, calcified, or narrowed, thereby obstructing the flow of blood through a narrowed, stenotic valve orifice. Valve regurgitation occurs when the valve leaflets fail to close completely. This causes valve insufficiency, and a portion of the systolic blood volume is allowed to flow backward. Causes of abnormal valves are discussed in Chapter 33. As blood flows through these two different types of valve alterations, the sounds generated are very distinct. For example, blood flowing through a stenotic valve would sound very harsh because blood is being forced through a narrow opening, whereas blood flowing through a regurgitant valve would sound softer and have more of a gurgling quality. The sounds associated with particular valve disorders would be best heard at the corresponding valve's auscultatory site (Chart 29–5) and Figure 29–9 (p. 839). When a murmur is auscultated, the etiology can be suggested

CHART 29–5 Summary of Murmurs with the Associated Valve Disorder

Aortic Stenosis

1. Midsystolic, crescendo-decrescendo
2. Harsh
3. Usually heard best in the aortic area
4. Often heard widely over the chest
5. Often radiates to the carotid arteries
6. Loudness unrelated to severity

Aortic Regurgitation

1. Present in early diastole
2. Decrescendo configuration
3. High-pitched blowing
4. Heard best with the patient leaning forward; often faint
5. Loudness along left lower sternal border (LLSB)

Mitral Stenosis

1. Long, rumbling diastolic murmur
2. Low pitched
3. Heard best with bell
4. Localized to mitral area (apex)
5. Often accompanied by a diastolic thrill in the area
6. Crescendo occurs in late diastole

Mitral Regurgitation

1. Pansystolic
2. Loudest in mitral area (apex)
3. Radiates to left axilla
4. Usually blowing in quality
5. Systolic thrill usually present in mitral area

Innocent Murmur

1. Short, soft, systolic
2. Normal S_1 and S_2
3. Normal ECG and chest x-ray
4. Crescendo-decrescendo
5. Heard in primary aortic area

by understanding the physiology of the cardiac cycle and heart sounds. For example, during systole the aortic valve is open, allowing blood to flow from the left ventricle through the aortic valve to the aorta. At the same time, the mitral valve is closed, preventing blood from flowing back into the left atrium. If the aortic valve were stenotic, the sound would be a harsh murmur during systole over the aortic valve area. Likewise, if the mitral valve were regurgitant, one would typically hear a gurgling sound over the mitral valve area. During the assessment the nurse needs to evaluate the patient for head bobbing in an up-and-down manner in synchrony with the heartbeat, because this is characteristic of severe aortic regurgitation (D'Amico & Barbarito, 2009).

Systolic murmurs, heard during systole, include mitral regurgitation, tricuspid regurgitation, aortic stenosis, and pulmonic stenosis. Diastolic murmurs, heard during diastole, include mitral stenosis, tricuspid stenosis, aortic regurgitation, and pulmonic regurgitation.

Weblink: Heart Diesease and stroke Statistics 2012

Some murmurs may be classified as **innocent murmurs,** also known as *functional murmurs.* An innocent murmur is a sound made by the blood circulating in the heart chambers or valves, or through the blood vessels near the heart. Innocent murmurs are often soft and may vary or disappear with position changes, whereas pathologic murmurs are generally louder and seldom disappear with position changes. Innocent murmurs are harmless, asymptomatic, and are commonly heard in children. Further diagnostic tests may be performed to rule out other conditions.

When a murmur is heard, it is important to describe the sound properly. Murmurs should be described in terms of their timing in the cardiac cycle, the auscultatory location in which they are heard best, frequency, intensity, radiation, and quality. A summary of murmurs associated with valve disorders is presented in Chart 29–5 (p. 843).

Gender Implications/ Gender Differences

Before the 1980s, it was believed that cardiovascular disease (CVD) affected primarily men. This was due in large part to the fact that most research studies involved men. It is now well known that women respond uniquely to CVD as well as to other diseases. For example, women experience the signs and symptoms associated with CVD differently than men. In addition, more women than men have asymptomatic and undiagnosed CVD. It is difficult to apply preventive cardiovascular care to women who have not been identified as having CVD. Mortality rates of CVD, particularly from sudden death, are currently higher in women than in men (AHA, 2010b). This suggests that women previously deemed at intermediate risk for the development of CVD from standard available guidelines, but who have concerning features in their medical history such as a strong family history, may benefit from stress testing, which may provide further gender-specific prognostic information. However, further studies are needed to identify gender-specific predictors of cardiac disease, and more comprehensive approaches to CVD prevention and treatment are needed for women. Although many of the gender-specific differences in CVD are not well explained, it is well understood that postmenopausal women are at greater risk of developing CVD than are premenopausal women. This is due to the cardioprotective effect of estrogen in premenopausal women. Genetic predispositions to cardiovascular disease are discussed in the following sections.

Genetic Considerations

A great deal is known about the independent risk factors for the development of cardiovascular disease. Advances made in the area of genetics since the Human Genome Project in 1988 have helped scientists understand the genetic causes of cardiovascular disease. It has become clear that most cardiovascular diseases result from various genetic causes (Kumar & Elliott, 2010). Gene mutations and the interaction of genes and the environment are currently being examined. For example, polygenic disorders, such as hypertension, are caused by the combined effect of more than one mutated gene. Interestingly, the nature and severity of polygenic disorders vary significantly and are unpredictable in nature (Kumar & Elliott, 2010).

Coronary artery disease is an example of a multifactorial disorder. Multifactorial disorders may have a genetic component, but the presentation is largely affected by environmental factors. For example, multifactorial disorders may include an interaction of genetic factors (genetic abnormalities that result in lipid disorders, hypertension, and obesity) with nongenetic factors such as smoking, increasing age, and physical inactivity.

Through a thorough cardiovascular assessment, and potentially future genetic testing, inherited cardiovascular diseases or the susceptibility to diseases can be identified. The hope is that early detection and diagnosis will identify individuals at risk. Then prevention or modulation of the effects can be undertaken by the implementation of a treatment plan, education, and counseling. The goal of genetic testing would be to save lives through preventive treatment and therapeutic interventions. Nurses can complete family history assessments and initiate appropriate referrals for genetic counseling.

Gerontological Considerations

The number of elderly people over age 65 in the U.S. population has been steadily increasing; therefore, it is reasonable to assume that the number of elderly patients cared for in health care settings will also increase. The gerontological population has unique considerations that are important in cardiovascular assessment. Physiological changes associated with aging include myocardial hypertrophy; an increase in collagen and scarring; a decrease in elasticity; fibrotic and sclerotic changes of the atria and ventricles; calcification, sclerosis, or fibrosis of the cardiac valves; and rigidity and fibrosis of the vessels of the arterial system. These changes can lead to a drop in cardiac output, systolic or diastolic murmurs, increased frequency of dysrhythmias, and altered blood flow dynamics, all of which affect tissue perfusion. For example, elderly persons may have elevations in systolic or diastolic blood pressures. Additionally, in the response to injury or shock, the heart becomes less able to respond or initiate the stimulation of catecholamines needed to increase heart rate and contractility (Moser & Riegel, 2008). It is not uncommon to hear an S_4 in an elderly person due to decreased compliance of the left ventricle or a systolic murmur due to aortic or mitral valve abnormalities. Thickened myocardial fibers can also affect the heart's conduction system and cause cardiac irritability and dysrhythmias. Diseases affecting other body systems also can affect the heart and blood vessels. Diabetes mellitus is one example of a disease that can have damaging effects on the peripheral vasculature; another is chronic obstructive lung disease, which contributes to right-sided heart failure.

Normal physiological changes in the elderly can contribute to the significance of cardiovascular signs and symptoms. For example, loss of muscle mass is a normal physiological change but can contribute to symptoms of weakness or fatigue. It is essential to encourage a healthy diet and regular exercise program. The gerontological population is more susceptible to cognitive impairments that make them more vulnerable to the effects of cardiac diseases and their treatments (Moser & Riegel, 2008). Dementia and delerium are cognitive impairments found in the geriatric population. Cognitive losses of dementia affect an individual's overall ability to interact successfully with the environment. The way the individual responds to stimuli from touch or stimuli from the environment may vary among individuals and should be considered prior to the exam. The nurse needs to understand that there may be limitations in the patient's abilities to learn and apply new knowledge. It will be much more difficult for the individual who is cognitively impaired to manage the complexities of his cardiovascular disease and its treatment. Changes in cerebral perfusion due to atherosclerosis may also be present. When cognitive impairments such as dementia or delerium are suspected, the ability to provide accurate information for the health history will be altered.

Critical Thinking Related to Cardiovascular Assessment

Critical thinking is essential in order to prioritize the most significant clinical manifestations that need further investigation. Cardiovascular clinical manifestations can range from conditions as benign as an innocent murmur to life-threatening disorders such as heart failure. It is imperative that the nurse be able to distinguish normal from abnormal, benign from serious. The nurse must rely on critical thinking skills in interpreting the patient's symptoms and assessment findings to determine possible and potential patient diagnoses and to consider the appropriate actions to take. Analysis of these data allows the nurse to make a diagnosis and then follow up with an intervention. It is imperative that the nurse communicate and collaborate with other members of the health care team in developing and implementing a plan of care.

Because cardiac disease manifestations can mimic other abnormalities such as pulmonary disease, the nurse must question each symptom and then compare and contrast symptoms. For example, when the patient reports a sudden onset of chest pain, the nurse must possess knowledge of the difference in manifestations between the causes of cardiac versus pulmonary chest pain and assess the patient for each of them. Making an assumption that the pain is cardiac in nature would be inappropriate and shortsighted. Effective critical thinking skills include being curious and not making any assumptions. Regardless of the health problem, each symptom identified should be thoroughly described in order for the nurse to gain a full understanding. The nurse can say to the patient, "Tell me more about the problem," or "How did it start?" The patient usually proceeds with a discourse about the symptoms. The nurse then uses skillful interview techniques to explore and investigate each symptom further. Any symptom analysis would be incomplete without a thorough description of its characteristics.

Health Promotion

A good time to discuss the concept of health promotion with a patient is during a cardiovascular exam. Assessment can be a time to review current health status, examine problem areas, identify risk factors that need to be modified, identify possible health goals, discuss options, and potentially develop a plan of care. During a health assessment, nurses need to provide health education and supply the patient with educational materials. Nurses are in a unique position to help patients recognize health problems or potential health problems. When abnormalities or positive findings are discovered during the health history process, an opportunity exists to discuss the issue in greater detail. Nurses should also recognize their role in promoting healthy lifestyles and their abilities to empower a patient and her family to make needed changes in their lives. Be aware that certain health topics are very personal, and some nurses have difficulty discussing these sensitive issues with patients.

As the populations that are served in health care settings continue to change and nurses are caring for more diverse populations, they need to be knowledgeable about the health practices of other cultures. Integrating culturally competent care includes incorporation of complementary therapies into the plan of care that will ultimately help nurses accomplish the goal of health promotion for all patients.

Cardiovascular Monitoring

Cardiovascular monitoring is an integral part of nursing management and includes many technologies used to augment the physical exam. Monitoring devices range from simple noninvasive monitoring, including assessment of heart rate, blood pressure, and pulse oximetry, to more invasive monitoring, such as hemodynamic monitoring using indwelling pulmonary artery catheters and arterial catheters. Discussions of invasive hemodynamic monitoring are included with the cardiac disorders where monitoring is indicated in Chapter 31. The goal of cardiovascular monitoring is to obtain the data needed to complete the cardiovascular assessment in a timely fashion, in the safest, most cost-efficient manner.

Assessment of Heart Rate

Counting the number of pulsations of the heart per minute determines the heart rate. Assessment of the heart rate should be performed when the patient is at rest in a calm environment. Many factors can alter the heart rate. For example, exercise, pain, and anxiety can cause an increase in circulating catecholamines, which may elevate the patient's heart rate and blood pressure. Endocrine and metabolic conditions can also affect the heart rate. The heart normally beats 60 to 100 times per minute.

The regularity of the pulse should also be assessed. Irregularities suggest an alteration in cardiac conduction and should be further evaluated. Electrocardiogram (ECG) monitoring is a noninvasive method used to assess the heart rate and rhythm, and is commonly utilized in acute care settings. Interpretation and analysis of the ECG is discussed in Chapter 30.

Assessment of Blood Pressure

Arterial blood pressure (BP) is a measure of the pressure exerted by blood against the walls of the arterial system as it is ejected from the left ventricle. Blood pressure is a dynamic, multidimensional indicator of a person's cardiovascular state (Woods et al., 2010). Assessment of blood pressure reflects the events of the pulsatile cardiac cycle and is expressed as systolic/diastolic. The systolic blood pressure (SBP) is the peak pressure exerted against the arteries when the heart ventricles contract during systole. The diastolic blood pressure (DBP) is the residual pressure existing in the arterial system at the end of diastole when the ventricles are relaxed and are filling with blood from the atria.

The recording of blood pressure can provide important information about blood volume, cardiac output, and peripheral resistance. It is a critical component of vital signs and therefore is a basic parameter for nurses' physical assessments. When the systolic and diastolic blood pressures are elevated, so is the risk of developing the cardiovascular disorders discussed in this unit.

Blood pressure can be measured in several ways: (1) indirectly by use of auscultatory methods such as indirect sphygmomanometers, (2) by use of the electronic automatic blood pressure cuffs that produce a digital readout, or (3) directly by use of invasive monitoring devices. In many clinic and hospital settings the most common way to obtain blood pressure recordings is by auscultation with the use of an indirect sphygmomanometer. Measurement techniques for blood pressure are discussed in detail in Chapter 35.

It is important for nurses to understand that the blood pressure in an artery is a dynamic number and changes throughout the day. It is the lowest during sleep, rises on waking, and can rise with excitation, nervousness, or activity. Therefore, a single reading of high blood pressure is not used to make a diagnosis of hypertension. Diagnosis and treatment of hypertension is discussed in Chapter 35.

The term *prehypertension,* introduced in the JNC 7 report (National Heart, Lung, Blood Institute [NHLBI], 2010), describes those individuals with a blood pressure finding on two or more office visits of 120 to 139 mmHg systolic or 80 to 89 mmHg diastolic. These individuals are at twice the risk of developing hypertension as those with lower values. Prehypertension is the early phase when the relationship between the blood pressure measurement and the need for health education is the primary focus of care. The individual demonstrating prehypertension is at risk for development of stage 1 or stage 2 hypertension. The JNC 7 report emphasizes the need to reduce blood pressure levels and prevent the development of high blood pressure in the general population through the education of health care professionals.

Classification of Blood Pressure

Blood pressure readings are classified into four stages: normal tension, prehypertension, stage 1 hypertension, and stage 2 hypertension, as shown in the National Guidelines box. A severe form of hypertension, referred to as *malignant hypertension,* is a hypertensive urgency and emergency that reflects the patient's markedly elevated blood pressure and acute target organ damage requiring immediate hospitalization and parental drug therapy.

In addition, *white coat phenomenon* is an elevated blood pressure when the assessment of the blood pressure is done by a health care professional. If this phenomenon occurs frequently over time, the patient is responding to a perceived stressful situation and may need early hypertensive treatment. Often the health care provider will request the patient measure her blood pressure in the home setting. This process is used to determine if the patient is demonstrating white coat phenomenon.

Hypertension is further categorized by cause. There are two types: essential and secondary hypertension. *Essential hypertension* is defined as a chronic elevation in blood pressure that occurs without the evidence of disease. *Secondary hypertension* is high blood pressure that is a result of some other disorder such as kidney disease. Essential hypertension may be systolic, diastolic, or both systolic and diastolic.

Risk Factors

Certain identifiable contributing elements increase the risk of the development of high blood pressure. These risk factors are classified as modifiable factors and nonmodifiable factors (see the Risk Factors box). The modifiable factors are those that the patient can control, whereas nonmodifiable factors cannot be controlled by the patient.

A patient evaluation includes determining the risk factors, lifestyle, possible causes of hypertension, and target organs for damage including the heart (e.g., from coronary heart disease). A review of the multiple risk factors contributing to high blood pressure, as listed in the Risk Factors box, can be done while taking the patient and family history. The nurse needs to assess the patient for the presence or absence of each risk factor and causes of hypertension. Chart 29–6 outlines the causes of high blood pressure.

RISK FACTORS for Hypertension

Modifiable Factors

- High sodium dietary intake
- Excessive alcohol consumption
- Smoking
- Dyslipidemia
- Obesity (BMI > 30 kg/m^2)
- Low potassium intake
- Physical inactivity

Nonmodifiable Factors

- Age (older than 55 years for men and 65 years for women)
- Family history of premature cardiovascular disease (men under age 55/ women under age 65)
- Race
- Gender
- Diabetes mellitus
- Microalbuminuria or estimated GFR < 60 mL/min

Source: National Heart Lung Blood Institute. (2010). *The seventh report of the Joint National Committee on Prevention, Detection, Evaluation, and Treatment of High Blood Pressure (JNC 7).* Retrieved from http://www.nhlbi.nih.gov/guidelines/ hypertension/index.htm.

Culture, Environment, Race, Genetics, and History

The assessment of an individual's culture, environment, and race is obtained from the patient and family. The health care provider needs to be cognizant that African American individuals have twice as high a possibility of developing high blood pressure as do Caucasian Americans. If the patient lives in the southeastern portion of the United States as opposed to other parts of the country, the incidence of high blood pressure also is higher. In addition, environmental factors such as obesity, cigarette smoking, sedentary lifestyle, use of illegal drugs, and sodium intake have an impact on blood pressure.

The family may contribute medically historic information and report on any therapies the patient may have used. The interview may be both a teaching and learning opportunity, giving the nurse a further opportunity to gather data concerning the lifestyle of the patient and family. The Genetic Considerations box addresses how genetics might affect a patient's propensity for high blood pressure.

NATIONAL GUIDELINES Classification of Blood Pressure for Adults

BP Classification	SBP (mmHg)	DBP (mmHg)	Lifestyle Modification Encouraged
Normal	<120	and <90	
Prehypertension	120–139	Or 80–89	Yes
Stage 1 hypertension	140–159	Or 90–99	Yes
Stage 2 hypertension	>160	Or >100	Yes

Note: DBP, diastolic blood pressure; SBP, systolic blood pressure. Treatment determined by highest BP level.

Source: National Heart Lung Blood Institute. (2010). The seventh report of the Joint National Committee on Prevention, Detection, Evaluation, and Treatment of High Blood Pressure (JNC 7). Retrieved from http://www.nhlbi.nih.gov/guidelines/hypertension/index.htm.

CHART 29–6 Causes of Hypertension

- Sleep apnea
- Chronic kidney disease
- Renovascular disease
- Coarctation of the aorta
- Chronic steroid therapy and Cushing's syndrome
- Cause may be unknown
- Drug-induced or -related causes
- Primary aldosteronism
- Pheochromocytoma
- Thyroid or parathyroid disease

Sources: Lynn-McHale Wiegand, D. (2010). *AACN procedure manual for critical care.* Philadelphia: W. B. Saunders; Moser, D. K., & Riegel, B. (Eds.). (2008). *Cardiac nursing: A companion to Braunwald's heart disease.* Philadelphia: Saunders Elsevier; Porth, C., & Matfin, G. (2009). *Pathophysiology: Concepts of altered health states.* Philadelphia: Wolters Kluwer/Lippincott Williams & Wilkins.

GENETIC CONSIDERATIONS Related to Hypertension

The genetic profile may assist nurses by providing information about alterations in the genetic coding of angiotensinogen in the hypertensive population. Hypertension is seen most often with persons who have a family history of hypertension, thus implicating a genetic predisposition. If an individual has two or more family members with hypertension before the age of 55 years, he has a 3.8 times greater risk for the development of hypertension (Porth & Matfin, 2009). In addition, a family history of high blood pressure and heart disease may suggest a genetic predisposition for the development of these disorders.

Psychosocial Factors

When the nurse is obtaining a patient's psychosocial data, care must be used when listening to how the patient describes the meaning of the diagnosis of high blood pressure. Life stresses can make the patient's ability to participate in a partnership of care difficult. Areas of stress may be related to job stresses, economic position, losses and/or gains of any kind, and many other issues of life. When a patient experiences severe stress, the amount of catecholamine release is increased, which then increases the blood pressure.

Assessment of Oxygen Delivery

Pulse oximetry allows noninvasive estimation of hemoglobin oxygen saturation, or SpO_2, which is the amount of hemoglobin saturated with oxygen. Normal oxygen saturation values are 97% to 99% in a healthy individual, but a value of 95% is clinically acceptable in a patient with a normal hemoglobin level (Lynn-McHale Wiegand & Carlson, 2010). These devices are discussed in detail in Chapter 25.

Summary

A thorough and accurate cardiovascular assessment is an important nursing tool. Findings from cardiovascular assessments can lead to early identification of potentially life-threatening conditions and provide an opportunity for timely application of preventative measures and treatment modalities. Nurses may implement preventative strategies, initiate treatment plans, or provide education or counseling.

NCLEX® PRACTICE

1. A patient reports having difficulty sleeping at night secondary to becoming short of breath when lying down. In order to further assess the degree of orthopnea, the nurse should ask which question?
   1. "How often do you wake up at night?"
   2. "How many pillows do you sleep on?"
   3. "Do you experience palpitations that awaken you?"
   4. "How often do you get up to urinate during the night?"

2. The patient presents to the emergency department (ED) with complaints of chest pain. Which questions should the nurse ask? (select all that apply)
   1. "Are you short of breath?"
   2. "What exacerbates the pain?"
   3. "Have you been sick to your stomach?"
   4. "Have you had a temperature?"
   5. "When did your chest pain start?"

3. The nurse is reviewing the history of a patient who was admitted with complaints of chest pain. Which patient statements are significant to this complaint?
   1. "I lived in Alabama as a child."
   2. "When I was a child I had strep throat a lot."
   3. "My father was an alcoholic."
   4. "I played football in college."
   5. "I remember the day my grandfather had his heart attack."

4. The patient makes each of these statements during the health interview. Which statement should the nurse interpret as reflecting a "type D" personality?
   1. "Sorry I am late to my appointment; there were a lot of idiot drivers on the road today."
   2. "My life is pretty boring and I don't have many friends."
   3. "My sister and I are going shopping this afternoon."
   4. "Are you going to need a urine specimen? I need to go to the bathroom."

5. The clinic nurse notices that a 70-year-old patient seems more confused than at the previous visit. The nurse continues further assessment based upon which primary concern?
   1. The patient is likely becoming senile.
   2. The patient is probably not eating and drinking well.
   3. There may be a cardiac issue that is decreasing cerebral perfusion.
   4. It is likely that the patient is not taking prescribed medications correctly.

6. The nurse locates the patient's point of maximal impulse (PMI) at the sixth intercostal space (ICS), just medial to the left midaxillary line. How should the nurse interpret this information?
   1. The patient's right lung may be distended.
   2. The patient likely has a thinner than normal chest wall.
   3. The patient's heart is probably enlarged.
   4. The patient has a positive hepatojugular reflux response.

Answers to NCLEX Practice questions can be found in Appendix D in the Osborn Student Resources at nursing.pearsonhighered.com. Practice additional NCLEX questions online at the Student Resources site.

Pearson Nursing Student Resources Find additional review materials at: **nursing.pearsonhighered.com**

REFERENCES

American Heart Association. (2010a). Dietary guidelines: At-a-glance. Retrieved from http://www.livestrong.com/article/425639-american-heart-association-sodium-recommendations/

American Heart Association. (2010b). Heart disease and stroke statistics 2010 update: At-a-glance. Retrieved from http://www.americanheart.org/downloadable/heart/1265665152970DS-3241%20HeartStrokeUpdate_2010.pdf

American Heart Association. (2011). Frequently asked questions about stress. Retrieved from http://www.heart.org/HEARTORG/GettingHealthy/StressManagement/HowDoesStressAffectYou/FAQs-About-Stress_UCM_307982_Article.jsp

D'Amico, D., & Barbarito, C. (2009). *Health and physical assessment in nursing.* Upper Saddle River, NJ: Pearson Prentice Hall.

Denollet, J., Schiffer, A. A., & Spek, V. (2010). A general propensity to psychological distress affects cardiovascular outcomes: Evidence from research on the type D (distressed) personality profile. *Circulation, 3,* 546–557.

Kumar, D., & Elliott, P. (2010). *Principles and practice of clinical cardiovascular genetics.* New York: Oxford University Press.

Lynn-McHale Wiegand, D. (2010). *AACN procedure manual for critical care.* Philadelphia: W. B. Saunders.

Moser, D. K., & Riegel, B. (Eds.). (2008). *Cardiac nursing: A companion to Braunwald's heart disease.* Philadelphia: Saunders Elsevier.

National Heart Lung Blood Institute. (2010). *The seventh report of the Joint National Committee on Prevention, Detection, Evaluation, and Treatment of High Blood Pressure (JNC 7).* Retrieved from http://www.nhlbi.nih.gov/guidelines/hypertension/index.htm

O'Rourke, R., Walsh, R., & Fuster, V. (2009). *Hurst's the heart manual of cardiology* (12th ed.). New York: McGraw Hill.

Porth, C., & Matfin, G. (2009). *Pathophysiology: Concepts of altered health states.* Philadelphia: Wolters Kluwer/Lippincott Williams & Wilkins.

Thayer, M. S. (2010). *The only EKG book you'll ever need* (6th ed.). Philadelphia: Lippincott Williams & Wilkins.

Woods, S. L., Sivarajan Frolicher, E. S., Motzer, S. A., & Bridges, E. J. (Eds.). (2010). *Cardiac nursing* (6th ed.). Philadelphia, PA: Lippincott Williams & Wilkins.

World Heart Federation. (2011). Family history. Retrieved from http://www.world-heart-federation.org/cardiovascular-health/cardiovascular-disease-risk-factors/family-history/

Caring for the Patient with Disorders of the Cardiac Conduction System

CHAPTER 30

Brenda McCulloch
Kathleen Osborn

Outcome-Based Learning Objectives

After studying this chapter, the learner will be able to:

1. Differentiate intrinsic cardiac activity with ECG wave patterns.
2. Calculate heart rate, rhythm, PR interval, QRS complex, and QT interval from an ECG rhythm strip.
3. Compare and contrast the etiology and significant ECG features of the following dysrhythmia classifications: sinus, atrial, junctional, block, ventricular, and asystole.
4. Interpret the significance of each of the dysrhythmias and formulate nursing responsibilities for each dysrhythmia.

KEY TERMS

ablation p.891
absolute refractory period p.852
action potential p.852
anion p.851
artifact p.861
asystole p.885
atrial dysrhythmia p.865
atrial fibrillation p.868
atrial flutter p.867
atrial kick p.850
atrioventricular (AV) node p.850
automaticity p.851
automated external defibrillator p.890
AV dissociation p.878
Bachmann bundle p.850
bigeminy p.880
bipolar lead p.854
bundle branch block p.879
bundle of His p.851
bundles p.850
capture p.895
cardiac conduction system p.850
cardiac depolarization p.852
cardiac pacemaker p.891
cardiac repolarization p.852
cardiac resynchronization therapy (CRT) p.896
cation p.851
cardioversion p.886
conductivity p.851
contractility p.851
defibrillation p.890
dysrhythmia p.862
ECG waveform p.860
ectopic focus p.861
electrocardiogram (ECG) p.853
electrode p.856
electrophysiology study p.891
excitability p.851
fascicles p.851
fill time p.863
first-degree AV block p.875
graph paper p.859
implantable cardioverter defibrillator p.890
Holter monitoring p.856
intra-atrial pathways p.850
ion p.851
isoelectric line p.860
J point p.853
junctional dysrhythmia p.872
junctional escape rhythm p.872
junctional tachycardia p.873
lead axis p.857
millivolts p.852
Mobitz I/Wenckebach p.875
Mobitz II/second-degree block p.875
negative deflection p.857
nodes (bundles) p.850
normal sinus rhythm (NSR) p.861
P wave p.853
pacemaker cell p.851
pacemaker sensitivity p.896
permanent pacemaker p.894
positive deflection p.857
PR interval p.853
premature atrial contraction (PAC) p.865
premature junctional contraction (PJC) p.873
premature ventricular contraction (PVC) p.880
pulseless electrical activity (PEA) p.885
Purkinje network fibers p.851
QRS complex p.853
QT interval p.860
quadrigeminy p.880
refractory period p.852
relative refractory period p.852
resting membrane potential p.852
sick sinus syndrome (SSS) p.871
sinoatrial (SA) node p.850
sinus arrest p.863
sinus arrhythmia/dysrhythmia p.863
sinus bradycardia p.862
sinus tachycardia p.863
ST segment p.853
supraventricular tachycardia (SVT) p.868
T wave p.853
temporary transcutaneous pacing (TCP) p.894
temporary transvenous pacing p.892
third-degree AV block (complete heart block) p.876
threshold p.851
Torsade de pointes p.884
trigeminy p.880
12-lead ECG p.853
U wave p.853
unipolar lead p.854
ventricular dysrhythmia p.880
ventricular fibrillation (VF) p.884
ventricular tachycardia (VT) p.881
Wolff-Parkinson-White syndrome (WPW) p.871

THE ELECTROCARDIOGRAM (ECG) is the most important and definitive noninvasive diagnostic procedure that shows a graphic depiction of the electrical activity of the heart. It is used to assist the health care team in diagnosing and monitoring cardiac electrical system function. First used in the 1900s, initially the equipment was large and cumbersome and had limited use. As equipment improved, ECG bedside monitoring became possible in the 1960s. Today, due to increased patient acuity levels, the use of cardiac monitors is widespread, having moved outside the traditional critical and emergent care settings. This has greatly expanded the need for nurses to understand the ECG and dysrhythmia recognition. In order to orient the learner to the cardiac conduction system, this chapter provides a brief overview of the anatomy and electrophysiology of the heart. This review is followed by information on how to obtain the graphic representation of the electrical activity of the heart, the ECG (also referred to as the EKG). This chapter also describes the equipment and skills needed to obtain an ECG before guiding the learner in the necessary steps to interpret both normal and abnormal cardiac rhythms and describing appropriate nursing interventions and evaluation criteria.

Anatomy of the Heart

Recognition of common cardiac rhythms measured by an electrocardiogram requires a basic understanding of cardiac anatomy and physiology. A complete description of the cardiac anatomy is outlined in Chapter 29. Knowledge of the cardiac conduction system needed for ECG interpretation is presented in this chapter.

Cardiac Conduction System

The heart contains its own **cardiac conduction system** composed of specialized cell fibers called either **nodes** or **bundles.** These fibers enable the heart to generate and transmit action potentials (p. 852) without stimulation from the body's nervous system. The heart's conduction system is responsible for the electrical activity that controls each normal heartbeat. The fibers are located beneath the endocardium, or inner lining of the heart, in the cardiac conduction system. These are referred to as the sinoatrial (SA) node, the atrioventricular (AV) node, and the Purkinje network (Figure 30–1◆). Although the sympathetic nervous system (SNS) and the parasympathetic nervous system (PSNS) innervate the heart, these external neural impulses are not needed to maintain the cardiac cycle. The pacemaker cells are capable of initiating electrical activity automatically and act as a pacemaker; therefore, the heart will beat in the absence of any nervous system connection. The SNS and the PSNS affect only the speed of the cardiac cycles and the diameter of the coronary arteries. It is essential to understand the heart's electrical conduction system in order to be able to understand an ECG strip interpretation. Each component of the system follows.

Sinoatrial (SA) Node

The **sinoatrial (SA) node** is located in the upper posterior portion of the right atrial wall, near the opening of the superior vena cava. The node is made up of hundreds of cells that compose a knot of modified heart muscle. The SA node is capable of generating impulses that travel throughout the muscle fibers of both atria, resulting in atrial depolarization. The SA node is commonly referred to as the primary pacemaker of the heart because under normal conditions it depolarizes more consistently, frequently, and reliably than other normal pacemaker cells. The normal firing rate of the SA node is 60 to 100 beats per minute. Depolarization of the atria occurs as the impulse leaves the SA node and travels in a downward or waterfall fashion through the conduction pathways. If the SA node (pacemaker) fails to fire due to some abnormality, other pacemaker cells, such as the AV node or the Purkinje network, are able to take over. The emergence of a pacemaker that is lower in the heart and that sustains a heart rate when the SA node fails is referred to as an *escape* mechanism or rhythm. During an escape rhythm, the heart rate is slower than the dominant pacemaker. If the rhythm originates in the junctional tissue, it is referred to as a junctional escape rhythm. If the rhythm originates in the ventricle, it is referred to as a ventricular escape rhythm.

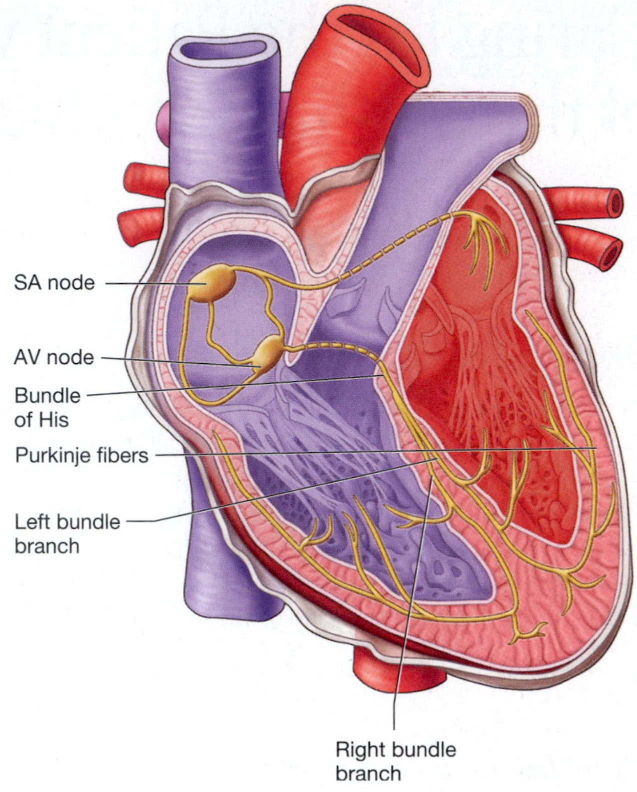

FIGURE 30–1 ◆ Electrical conduction system of the heart.

Intra-Atrial Pathways

The **intra-atrial pathways,** located in the atria, transport impulses from the SA node to the AV node. There are three pathways: the anterior, middle, and posterior intranodal or intra-atrial pathways. The **Bachmann bundle,** which is a part of the anterior pathway, is a group of fibers contained in the left atrium. All of the intranodal pathways and the Bachmann bundle receive electrical impulses as they exit the SA node, distribute these impulses throughout the atria, and transmit them to the AV node (Moser & Riegel, 2008).

Atrioventricular (AV) Node and AV Junction

The **atrioventricular (AV) node** is located on the floor of the right atrium just above the tricuspid valve. Electrical activity at the AV node is delayed approximately 0.05 second to allow for atrial contraction, which increases the amount of blood reaching the ventricles. Atrial contraction, commonly referred to as **atrial kick,** augments the blood supply going to the ventricles and, ultimately, cardiac output. This delay also serves to stop the transmission for a very rapid succession of impulses that can occur under abnormal conditions. These abnormalities, called atrial flutter/fibrillation, are discussed later in the chapter.

The AV junction contains fibers that can polarize spontaneously, forming an impulse that can spread through the heart chambers. This means that if the SA node fails or falls below its normal range, the AV node can take over and assume the role of a secondary pacemaker. Under normal conditions, the AV junction is the only pathway for the conduction of atrial impulses to the ventricles.

Bundle of His and Bundle Branches

The **bundle of His** lies on top of the interventricular septum, between the right and left ventricles. This area, also referred to as the common bundle, contains pacemaker cells that are able to self-initiate electrical activity at a rate of about 40 to 60 beats per minute. At the top of the interventricular septum, the bundle of His divides into two bundle branches, the right and left bundles. The right bundle, a long, thin structure that lies beneath the endocardium, runs down the right side of the interventricular septum and terminates at the papillary muscles in the right atrium. The left bundle is shorter than the right bundle and divides into pathways that spread from the left side of the interventricular septum throughout the left ventricle. The two pathways of the left bundle branch are called **fascicles,** one being anterior and the other posterior. The anterior fascicle carries electrical impulses to the anterior wall of the left ventricle. The posterior fascicle spreads electrical impulses to the posterior ventricular wall. The bundle branches continue to divide until they finally terminate in the Purkinje network fibers.

Purkinje Network Fibers

Purkinje network fibers consist of a network of fibers that carry impulses directly to the ventricles. The rapid spread of the electrical impulse through the left and right bundle branches, the Purkinje network fibers, and the ventricular muscle initiates ventricular contraction. Purkinje fibers also may be pacemaker cells; they fire at an intrinsic rate of 20 to 40 beats per minute.

Cardiac Cells

There are two basic cardiac cell groups: the myocardial working cells and the specialized pacemaker cells of the electrical conduction system. The atria and the ventricles are constructed of myocardial working cells, which have an abundance of contractile filaments needed to generate cardiac muscle contraction. Cardiac muscle contraction is what actually pumps the blood through and out of the heart into the pulmonic and the systemic circulation. The myocardial working cells have the ability to contract in response to chemical, electrical, or mechanical stimuli.

The second type of cardiac cell is the specialized **pacemaker cell,** whose primary function is to generate and conduct electrical impulses (stimuli). Found in the heart wall and septum (membrane dividing the right and left sides of the heart), these cells control the heart rate and rhythm by coordinating regular cardiac muscle depolarization (contraction) (see Figure 30–1). The myocardial contractions pump the blood through and out of the heart.

The term **threshold** refers to the point at which an electrical stimulus produces a cell response. When a stimulus is strong enough for cardiac cells to reach this threshold, all of the cells will respond to the stimulus and cause a muscle contraction. This is called the "all-or-none phenomenon"; in other words, either all the cells respond, or none of the cells respond. This principle allows for a coordinated muscle contraction and greater efficiency in pumping blood. Cardiac cells possess four primary characteristics: automaticity, excitability, conductivity, and contractility. These characteristics are described next.

Automaticity

Automaticity is the ability of the pacemaker cells to generate their own electrical impulses without depending on nervous system stimulation external to the heart. This spontaneous activity is what produces regular depolarization of the cardiac muscle. This characteristic is specific to only certain pacemaker cell sites within the conduction system: the sinoatrial (SA) node, the atrioventricular (AV) node, and the Purkinje network fibers.

Excitability

Excitability is the ability of the electrical cell to respond to a stimulus. Also referred to as irritability, this ability is shared by all electrical cardiac cells. When cardiac cells are highly irritable, a cell other than the normal pacemaker may cause a contraction. Cell irritability can be caused by a number of problems, including cardiac muscle ischemia due to hypoxia, or a lack of oxygen. Cell irritability is the most common cause of cardiac dysrhythmias, the abnormal rhythms of the heart.

Conductivity

Conductivity is the ability of the cardiac cell to accept and then transmit a stimulus to other cardiac cells. All cardiac cells share this characteristic, thereby portraying the all-or-none property of the heart muscle; the cardiac cells function as a unit.

Contractility

Contractility is the ability of the cardiac cells to shorten and cause the muscle to contract in response to an electrical stimulus. This ability also is referred to as rhythmicity. Contractility is the only mechanical function of the heart. Excitability, conductivity, and automaticity are electrical functions of the heart. Contractility may be thought of as the mechanical coordination of cardiac muscle contractions producing a heartbeat.

In addition to these cell characteristics, normal cardiac function depends on maintaining electrolyte concentrations inside and outside the cell membrane. Specific electrolytes and their relationship to cardiac function are described next.

Electrolytes Affecting Cardiac Function

An electrolyte is a substance or compound whose molecules dissociate into positively or negatively charged components, or **ions,** when placed in water. A positively charged ion is called a **cation.** A negatively charged ion is called an **anion.** Myocardial cells are bathed in electrolyte solutions; thus, both the mechanical and the electrical cardiac functions are influenced by electrolytes.

The major cations that affect cardiac function are potassium (K), sodium (Na), and calcium (Ca). Magnesium (Mg), although an important cation, is not as influential as K, Na, and Ca with regard to stimulating the action potential discussed here. Magnesium, potassium, and calcium are intracellular cations, meaning they reside within the cell; in contrast, Na is an extracellular cation, residing outside the cell. Chloride (Cl) is a major anion in electrocardiac function. Chloride provides electroneutrality in relation to Na. Transport of chloride is passive and follows the active transport of sodium (Na).

Abnormally high or low levels of electrolytes, especially K, can potentiate very serious, life-threatening ventricular dysrhythmias.

Therefore, monitoring and maintaining normal electrolyte values is essential. Nurses have a responsibility to report any significant abnormal values immediately to the health care provider.

Safety Alert *Assessing laboratory values is an essential nursing responsibility. Each time laboratory results are completed on a patient, the nurse needs to compare the new results with reference normal values and previous findings, if applicable, and report significant changes and/or trends.*

Cardiac Depolarization and Repolarization

When impulses travel through the myocardial muscle, they cause changes, referred to as depolarization and repolarization, in the muscle fibers. **Cardiac depolarization** refers to cardiac muscle contraction resulting from an electrolyte exchange in the cardiac cells that changes the electrical charge. As with all cells of the body, cardiac cells are electrically charged, with the inside of the cell more negative than the outside. To move Na and K across the cell membrane requires active transport by a mechanism referred to as the sodium-potassium adenosine triphosphatase (ATP) pump (Na-K pump). The Na-K pump is an energy-driven mechanism by which 3 Na ions are pumped out for every 2 K ions. Two enzymes, adenosine triphosphate (ATP) and adenosine triphosphatase (ATPase), are involved in the energy production for the pump (Porth, 2008).

Prior to depolarization the cells must be in a resting state, referred to as the **resting membrane potential.** In this state, the myocardial cell is negatively charged to –90 millivolts (mV). The cell maintains this negative state until depolarization occurs. When a muscle cell receives a stimulus due to the Na-K pump exchange, a rapid change occurs in the resting membrane potential, known as the **action potential,** which is measured in **millivolts** (a unit of electrical voltage or potential difference equal to one-thousandth of a volt). Once the action potential occurs, the cell moves toward a positive charge. The phases (0–4) of the action potential are shown in Figure 30–2◆. Phase 0 is rapid depolarization, phase 1 is rapid repolarization, phase 2 is the plateau, phase 3 is final repolarization, and phase 4 is the resting state. To generate this action potential and the resulting muscle depolarization, the threshold potential must be reached, which is phase 0. To initiate phase 0, Na enters the cell, causing a sharp positively charged rise of the intracellular ions. The cell moves from –90 millivolts (mV) in its resting state to a positive 15 to 30 millivolts, causing myocardial depolarization to occur. When the threshold is reached, the cell will continue to depolarize with no further stimulation; this phenomenon is referred to as automaticity. During phase 1, the depolarized stage, the interior of the cell has a net positive charge. In this effort to continue to make the inside of the cell more positive, calcium enters; this is phase 2, the plateau phase. During phase 3 the calcium channels close, and sodium (Na) is pulled from the cell by the Na-K pump. This returns the cell to its polarized negative resting membrane potential state (phase 4) (Figure 30–3◆). The first area of the cardiac muscle to be depolarized is the first area that is repolarized. For example, after the atria depolarize they repolarize while the ventricles are depolarizing. Thus, when the SA node fires again, the muscle will be ready to respond with a new action potential.

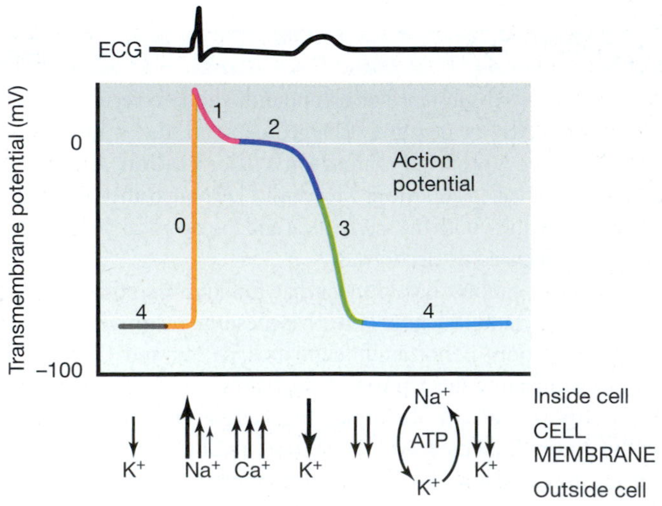

FIGURE 30–2 ◆ Action potential.

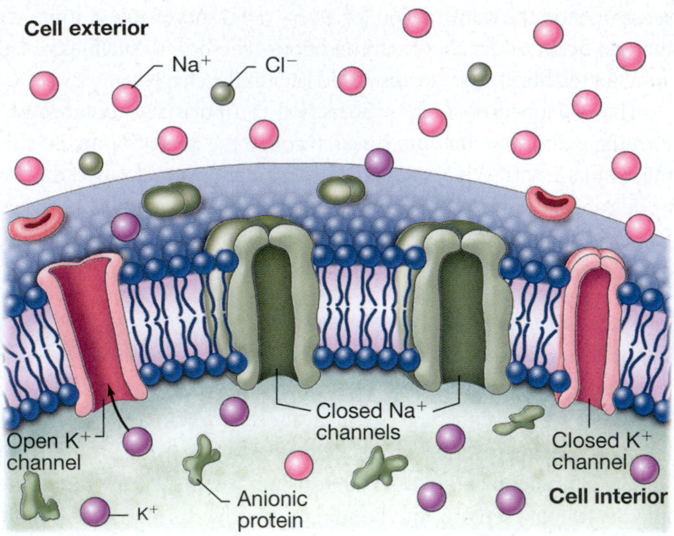

FIGURE 30–3 ◆ Electrolyte movement during an action potential.

Cardiac repolarization is the process whereby the depolarized cell is polarized, causing a return to the resting membrane potential (see Figure 30–2). Repolarization also is referred to as the recovery phase that every cardiac cell must go through in order to be ready to accept another stimulus. Repolarization is a slower process than depolarization. During repolarization, the muscle is *refractory* (resistant) to stimulation. This **refractory period** consists of two stages: the absolute and the relative refractory periods. During the **absolute refractory period,** which is the majority of time for repolarization, the cardiac cell is unable to respond to any stimulus and thus cannot spontaneously depolarize (see Figure 30–2).

The **relative refractory period** is a period when repolarization is almost complete (see Figure 30–2). This is the vulnerable period of cardiac cell repolarization. If a stimulus is strong enough, it can cause life-threatening depolarization. Depolarization during refractory periods is discussed later in this chapter. The refractory periods play a major role in either causing or preventing cardiac dysrhythmias. Further discussion of their role is presented regarding the various dysrhythmias and throughout the chapter.

Summary of the Cardiac Conduction System

The electrical impulse begins in the SA node located in the upper right atrium, causing atrial contraction. The impulse then travels through the atria along intra-atrial pathways to the AV node located near the center of the heart. After leaving the AV node, the impulse moves down into the bundle of His, through the right and left bundle branches, and into the Purkinje network fibers, causing ventricular contraction followed by repolarization (see Figure 30–1, p. 850). Then the cycle begins again.

Cardiac Waveform and Time Intervals Measured on ECG

When caring for patients with actual or potential cardiac conduction abnormalities, it is essential that the nurse understand how the cardiac conduction system is graphically depicted on an electrocardiogram. Recognizing and interpreting these electrical impulses and their relationship to heart disease is an essential nursing responsibility. A discussion of how the electrical conduction system is depicted in an ECG follows.

When the electrical impulse leaves the SA node, a graphical representation of the signal, referred to as a waveform, is produced and recorded with monitoring equipment. As the electrical impulse travels through the cardiac conduction system, waveforms characteristic of a given anatomical location are recorded. These waveforms are referred to as P, Q, R, S, and T. Time intervals, which represent the time it takes for the impulse to travel from one anatomical location in the heart to another, are also recorded. These time intervals are called PR, QRS, and QT. One complete cardiac cycle has five to six waveforms and time intervals. These are described here and depicted in Figure 30–4◆.

- *P Wave:* The **P wave** represents contraction or depolarization of the atria. Both the right and left atria depolarize at the same time.
- *PR Interval:* The **PR interval,** sometimes referred to as the PRI or PR segment, represents the time it takes for the impulse to travel from the SA node down the intra-atrial pathways to the ventricles. In other words, it represents the beginning of the atrial contraction to the beginning of the ventricular contraction.

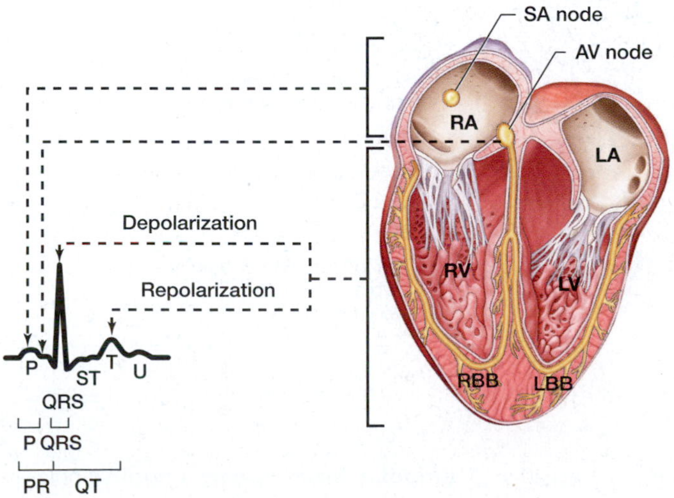

FIGURE 30–4 ◆ Waveform relationship to cardiac conduction system.

- *QRS Complex:* The **QRS complex** consists of the Q, R, and S waves, and represents the conduction of electrical impulses from the bundle of His near the AV junction to the Purkinje network fibers located in the ventricles.
- *J Point:* The **J point** is the point at which the QRS meets the ST segment is called the J point.
- *ST Segment:* The **ST segment** is a line extending from the S wave that gradually curves upward to the T wave, represented on the ECG as an almost isoelectric line. The ST segment signifies ventricular repolarization.
- *T Wave:* The **T wave** is ventricular recovery or repolarization. This is often referred to as the resting phase of the cardiac cycle. Both the absolute and the relative refractory periods are in place during the T wave.
- *U Wave:* The **U wave** is present only on some people's ECG. It follows the T wave. Its etiology is unknown, but it is frequently seen in exercise and in drug toxicity; it is seen most frequently with low potassium levels.

Changes in the configuration of the waveforms or lengthening and/or shortening of time intervals may indicate an abnormality in the heart. These abnormalities are discussed in detail in Chapters 32–35. The following sections discuss the method used to evaluate waveforms and time intervals.

Electrocardiogram

The **electrocardiogram (ECG)** is a body surface recording of the electrical activity of the heart introduced in 1902 by Willem Einthoven. The standard **12-lead ECG** derives its name from the 12 leads that provide 12 different "views" of the electrical activity as it traverses the myocardium (Chart 30–1). These views are derived from the four limb and six precordial (chest) electrodes attached to the patient (Figure 30–5◆). Think of the heart on a pedestal that one is able to move around while a camera takes pictures from various angles. Examining the electrical signals from the heart in different leads (views) provides the clinician with accurate information about a variety of cardiac conditions.

12-Lead Electrocardiogram (ECG)

Cardiac bedside continuous monitoring provides from 1 to 3 leads, whereas a 12-lead ECG provides 12 individual views or "snapshots" of the heart's electrical patterns. These added views provide a complete picture of the cardiac electrical system, both top to bottom and front to back. A 12-lead ECG is useful in evaluating not only the presence of damage but also the location in the heart where that damage

CHART 30–1 Myocardial Infarct Location by Lead

Infarct Location	Lead ST Elevation Found In
Anterior or Septal	V1, V2, V3, and V4
Posterior	V1 and V2
Inferior	II, III, and aVF
Low lateral	V5 and V6
High lateral	I and aVL

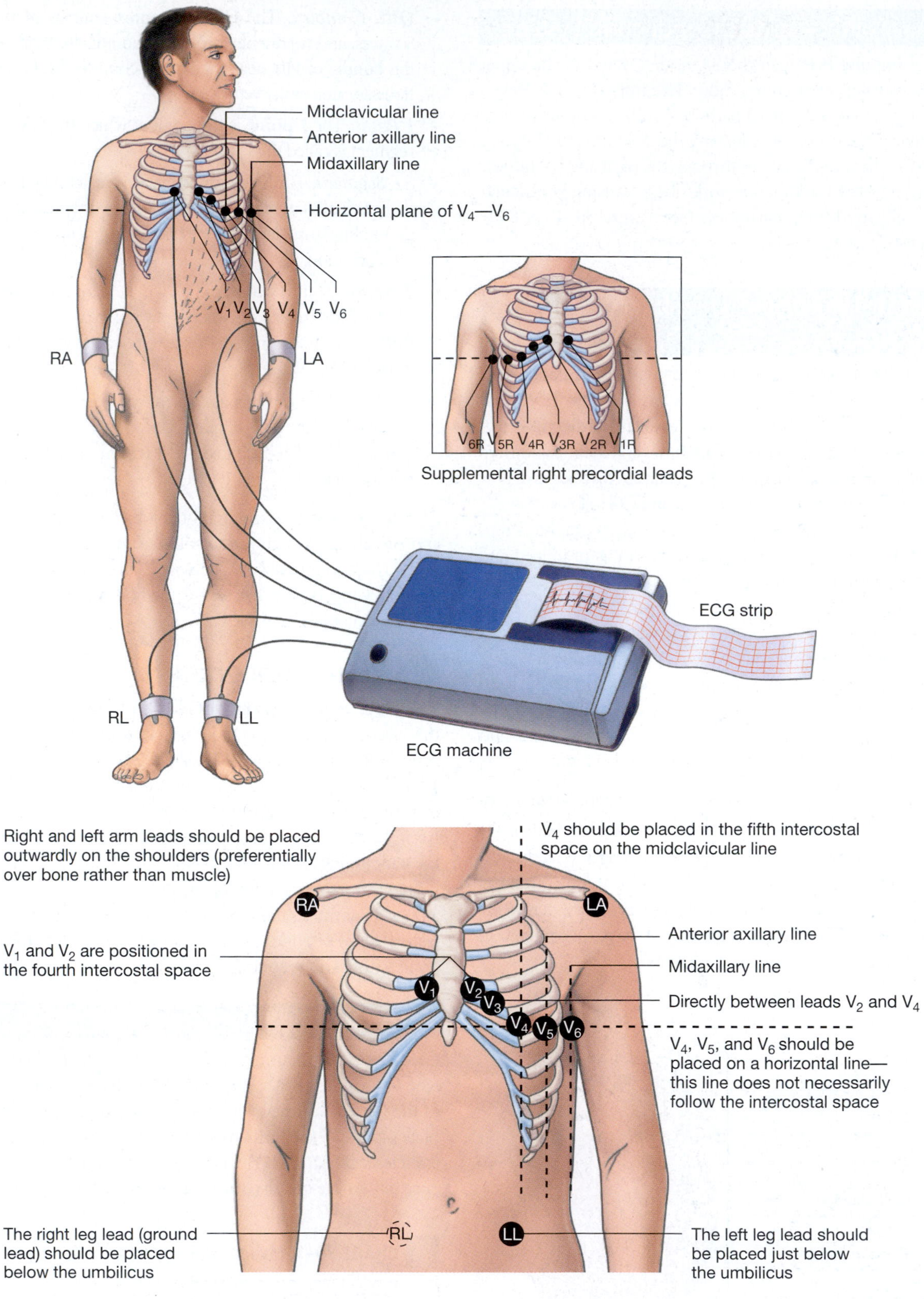

FIGURE 30–5 ◆ Position of the electrodes in the 12-lead electrocardiogram.

occurred. To assess damage accurately frequently requires viewing the area with more than one lead. Chart 30–2 provides the indications for a 12-lead ECG.

There are 3 bipolar and 9 unipolar leads in a 12-lead ECG. A **bipolar lead** has electrodes with opposite polarity, one positive and one negative. A **unipolar lead** has only a positive polarity (Baltazar, 2009). Both bipolar and unipolar leads provide information in one direction only—between two points. The two dimensions on the chest in which leads can be placed are the frontal plane (up and down) and the horizontal plane (around the chest).

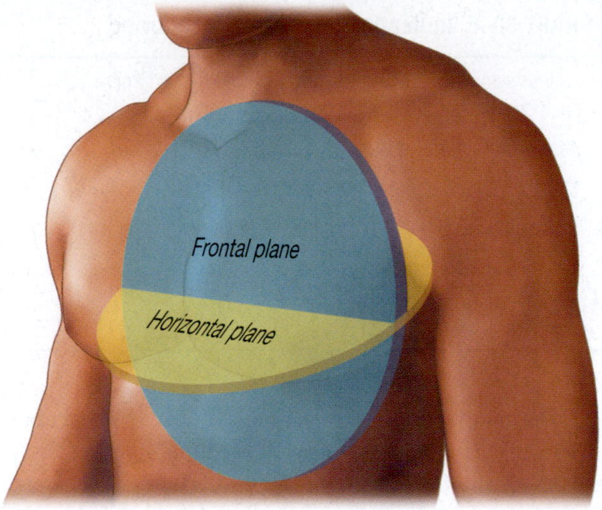

FIGURE 30–6 ◆ Horizontal and frontal planes.

CHART 30–2 Indications for a 12-Lead ECG

Evaluation of

- Axis deviation
- Cardiac valve disease
- Chamber dilation or hypertrophy
- Chest pain/angina
- Dysrhythmias
- Effect of cardiac drugs
- Electrolyte imbalance
- Hypothermia
- Myocardial ischemia
- Myocardial patterns of ischemia, necrosis, and infarction
- New versus old myocardial infarction
- Pericarditis
- Pulmonary embolism

Figure 30–6◆ shows the horizontal plane and the frontal plane views.

The axis of a lead is the imaginary line drawn between the positive and the negative electrode in a bipolar lead and between the positive electrode and the zero reference point in a unipolar lead. Thus, depending on where a given lead is placed, it provides a picture of the electrical activity from that vantage point within the heart. Electrical current flowing toward a positive electrode creates a positive deflection on the ECG paper, whereas electrical current flowing toward a negative electrode creates a negative deflection on the ECG paper (Baltazar, 2009).

The standard bipolar limb leads—I, II, III—are applied to the right arm (RA), left arm (LA), and left leg (LL). Each lead records the following electrical conduction pattern:

- Lead I records conduction from RA to LA.
- Lead II records conduction from RA to LL.
- Lead III records conduction from LA to LL.

The right leg electrode acts as a grounding electrode.

Three more frontal plane, unipolar augmented limb leads can be created by using a central terminal. Augmented leads are so named because they generate such small waveforms that the ECG machine must augment, or increase, their size so they will show up on the ECG paper (Baltazar, 2009). These leads are aVR, aVL, and aVF. Each lead records the following electrical conduction pattern:

- aVR: central terminal to right arm
- aVL: central terminal to left arm
- aVF: central terminal to left leg.

The standard bipolar leads and the augmented limb leads provide the 6 frontal plane leads of the 12-lead ECG, whereas the 6 chest (precordial) unipolar leads, V_1–V_6, evaluate the horizontal plane of the heart. The positive electrode is placed on 6 different sites across the chest as shown in the diagram in Figure 30–5 (p. 854). These chest leads provide the 6 horizontal leads of the 12-lead ECG. Chart 30–3 describes the procedure for obtaining a 12-lead ECG, and Chart 30–4 lists conditions detectable with a 12-lead ECG.

For example, lead V_1 evaluates the right ventricle; leads V_2 and V_3 span the interventricular septum; lead V_4 is over the cardiac apex; and leads V_5 and V_6 evaluate the lateral wall. The Q wave, T wave, and ST segment are used to evaluate the presence of damage, and the lead placement is used to identify the area of damage. Chapter 32 discusses the myocardial damage associated with changes in the Q wave, T wave, and ST segment.

CHART 30–3 12-Lead ECG Procedure

Electrode Placement	Bring the portable ECG machine to the patient's bedside in any type of patient care setting.
	Use 10 electrodes for the standard 12-lead ECG: 6 on the chest and 4 on the limbs. Figure 30–5 (p. 854) shows the correct placement of the electrodes.
	Place the limb electrodes away from bony prominences and areas of significant muscle movement to prevent interference of other muscle activity.
	Palpate the intercostal spaces along the sternal border, until the fourth one is reached, for placement of the first chest electrode.
Cable Connection and Machine Operation	Connect the cable that is attached to each of the electrodes to the ECG machine.
	Adjust the ECG machine to obtain a clear picture of the cardiac electrical activity.
	After completing the ECG, remove electrodes and clean the skin as necessary.
	Leave the electrodes in place if the patient is going to have serial ECGs to ensure consistency of multiple readings.
Patient Instructions	Explain the procedure and the rationale for the test prior to performing an ECG.
	Advise the patient to lie still, breathe normally, and refrain from speaking while obtaining the ECG.

CHART 30–4 Clinical Conditions Detectable from the 12-Lead Electrocardiogram

1. Myocardial ischemia, injury, and infarction
2. Cardiac dysrhythmias
3. Electrical conduction abnormalities
4. Cardiac hypertrophy
5. Medication effects (i.e., digitalis toxicity)
6. Electrolyte abnormalities

CHART 30–5 Indications for Holter Monitoring

1. Assess symptoms that may be related to a dysrhythmia, such as syncope or palpitations.
2. Assess therapy response such as cardiac medications.
3. Monitor the rate of atrial fibrillation.
4. Analyze pacemakers or implantable cardioverter defibrillators.
5. Detect silent myocardial ischemia.
6. Assess heart rate variability.

Nursing Management

When performing an ECG, the nurse must have knowledge of the lead placement for each of the 12 leads. Improper placement may result in inaccurate information and treatment. The electrodes must have firm, unbroken contact with the skin. The limb leads are placed on the flat surfaces just above the wrists and ankles. If there is an amputation, the lead is placed on the remaining stump. Chest hair may interfere with skin contact and, if so, should be cut as short as possible but not shaved. To improve the accuracy of the test, care must be taken to ensure correct positioning of the leads and firm contact with the skin. Patient factors that can negatively influence the quality of the tracing include motion artifact, morbid obesity, and chronic obstructive lung disease. Motion artifact distorts the baseline, introducing error into the interpretation. Morbid obesity and obstructive lung disease interfere with transmission of the electrical activity of the heart. Although the ECG alone gives the clinician much valuable information, the tracing must always be interpreted in the context of the patient's symptoms, laboratory values, and likely diagnosis.

The type and sophistication of ECG machines varies; some can record only one lead at a time, whereas others can record 3, 6, or all 12 leads simultaneously. Each ECG machine has its own method of identifying specific lead names (V_1, V_2, etc.) and a diagram of where to place them. To obtain an ECG tracing, specific equipment is needed, including an electrode, lead wire, and monitor or oscilloscope. An **electrode** is most commonly a round adhesive pad that is impregnated with conducting gel in the center and is attached to a lead wire. Electrodes are sensing devices that detect the electrical activity of the heart and conduct the electrical impulses from the skin surface back to the ECG machine, where they are converted into waveforms. An electrode is much like a camera in that it takes pictures of the electrical activity in the heart. The lead wire connects the electrode to the ECG machine.

When obtaining an ECG, the nurse must know which rhythms require immediate notification of the health care provider for emergent treatment. The significance and severity of the individual rhythms are presented under each rhythm discussed throughout the chapter.

Signal Averaged Electrocardiogram

Certain abnormal impulses are conducted during diastole, or when the heart is filling with blood, which is late into the QRS complex and ST segment. These impulses may be present in a patient who has survived an acute myocardial infarction and, if present, can result in ventricular tachycardia and sudden cardiac death. These signals, referred to as late potentials, are low-amplitude, high-frequency spikes that occur at the end of the QRS complex and extend into the ST segment. With the assistance of a computer, a signal-averaged ECG is able to distinguish low-level signals not detected by the traditional ECG. Therefore, the risk for lethal dysrhythmias can be assessed. A signal-averaged ECG also is used to evaluate bundle of His activity, presence of a left ventricular mass, effects of thrombolysis, and surgical repair of congenital heart disease.

Ambulatory Electrocardiogram Monitoring

Ambulatory ECG monitoring, also known as **Holter monitoring,** is often used in the outpatient setting to detect dysrhythmias. There are many indications for Holter monitoring; it is a valuable noninvasive tool with numerous clinical applications (Chart 30–5) (Thaler, 2010).

Current ambulatory ECG monitoring systems consist of leads placed on the chest that are connected to a small recording device that can be worn around the waist or on a strap over the patient's shoulder. Typically two or three leads of ECG data are recorded, either continuously for 24 to 48 hours or when activated by the patient during periods of symptoms such as palpitations or dizziness. In general, continuous recordings are indicated for assessment of frequent (at least once a day) symptoms that may be related to a dysrhythmia, syncope or near syncope, and unexplained palpitations (Kee, 2010). Ambulatory ECG monitoring is safe and relatively inexpensive. Because the electrodes must remain in place for 1 to 2 days, skin preparation is very important to ensure tracings free of artifact. Patients should be instructed not to pull at the electrodes and to go about their normal daily activities. Frequently they are asked to keep a diary to record their activities and the occurrence of any symptoms during monitoring.

If the symptoms occur very infrequently and other diagnostic tests have failed to provide a diagnosis, an implantable loop recorder can be utilized. Typically placed subcutaneously in the left subclavian or parasternal areas, this device can be left in place for months or even years, increasing the probability of capturing the ECG during the time of the clinical event (Heart Rhythm Society, 2011).

Bedside ECG Monitoring Equipment

Electrocardiography detects cardiac electrical impulses at various points on the surface of the body. The graphical depiction of these impulses, waveforms, and time intervals is obtained either with an electrocardiograph (ECG machine) or on a bedside cardiac monitor. The same type of equipment that is used for obtaining a 12-lead ECG is used for bedside monitoring. Instead of the electrodes and lead wires connecting to an ECG machine, they are connected to the bedside cardiac monitor. The lead wires are color coded according to machine manufacturer, and these colors assist the health care professional in attaching the lead wires to the appropriate electrode. The cardiac monitor records the electrical impulses and provides

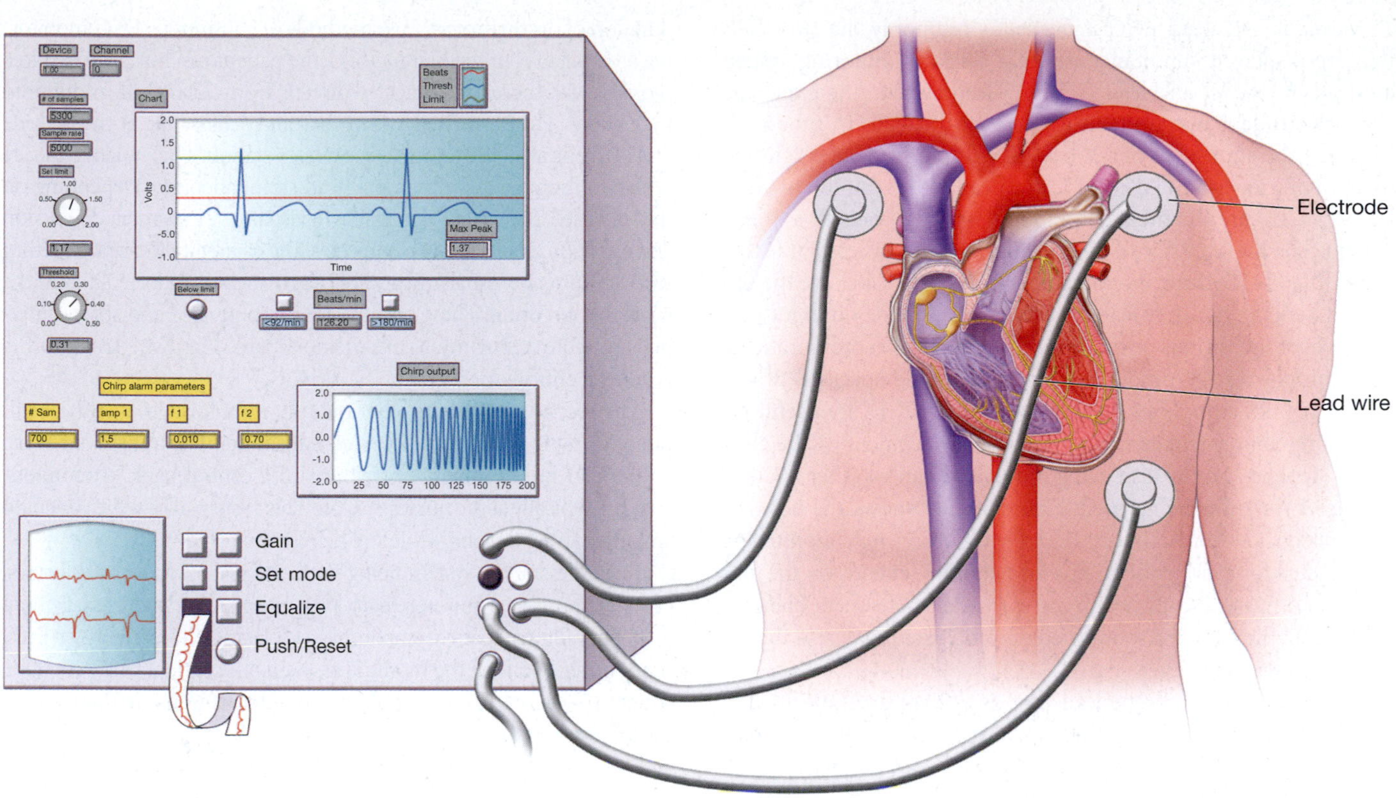

Video*: Electrocardiogram Placement of 3 Electrodes

FIGURE 30–7 ◆ Electrodes, lead wire, and cardiac monitor.

a real-time visual tracing of the waveforms on the screen and/or a printed version on specialized ECG graph paper, described next. The printed version is referred to as a rhythm strip or ECG strip. The rhythm strip gives the clinician information about where the pathological processes are occurring in the heart. Figure 30–7 ◆ shows the electrodes, lead wire, and cardiac monitor.

The term *lead* is used in different contexts when discussing ECGs. In addition to using the term as just described, as a connector from the electrode to the cardiac monitor, the term also is used when discussing a view or picture of the heart from a particular angle or vantage point. In this respect the lead can be thought of as the "eye of the camera."

Lead Placement

Body tissues and fluids surround the heart and conduct the electrical action potentials produced in the heart throughout the body. Therefore, the impulses, or action potentials, can be detected from any point in the body. In order to obtain a clear picture of the electrical impulses in the heart, electrodes must be placed on certain positions on the body. There also must always be a positive, a negative, and a ground electrode/lead. The ground lead minimizes outside electrical interference. Each electrode senses the flow of current in the heart in relation to the lead axis. The **lead axis** refers to the imaginary line drawn between the positive and negative electrodes. If the axis is directed toward the positive lead, there is an upward or **positive deflection** on the ECG tracing (above the isoelectric line). If the axis is directed toward the negative lead, there is a **negative deflection** on the ECG tracing (below the isoelectric line) (Figure 30–8 ◆). Multiple leads, as seen with a 12-lead ECG, view cardiac electrical conduction from different perspectives. Once again, think of the heart on a pedestal that is able to move around while a camera takes pictures from various angles. This gives the provider 12 different views of the cardiac electrical activity.

For bedside monitoring, it is not practical or necessary to have a 12-lead ECG or 12 continuous views of the heart. One or two leads are chosen for continuous bedside monitoring because they give a clear view of cardiac activity and abnormalities. To do this, a minimum of three electrodes is required: one positive, one negative, and one ground.

There are two types of bedside monitors: monitors with a 5-lead system and monitors with a 3-lead system. The 5-lead system has an exploring chest electrode that can be used to obtain the same

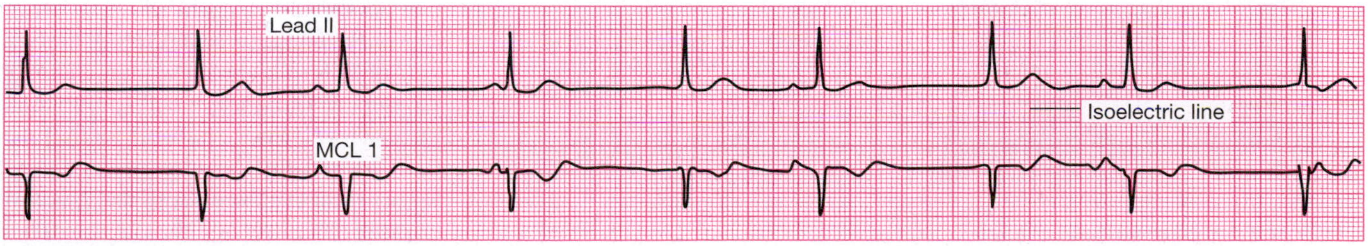

FIGURE 30–8 ◆ Lead II and MCL_1 ECG configurations.

12 views as a 12-lead ECG if needed. Commonly the two leads that are displayed simultaneously in a 5-lead monitoring system are leads V_1 or V_6 and lead II. In a 3-lead system, the exploring chest electrode is not available and one of the leads is "modified" to obtain the equivalent of a V lead. This modified lead is referred to as MCL_1 for modified chest $lead_1$. Lead II or a modified chest $lead_1$ (MCL_1) are the most commonly displayed leads in a 3-lead system. The MCL_1 is one of the V leads from the 12-lead ECG that is modified for bedside monitoring. It is important to have the option of viewing multiple leads because they provide different perspectives of the various normal and abnormal ECG configurations. For example, lead II produces easily identifiable upright P waves and clear QRS complexes. Leads V_1, V_6, and MCL_1 are useful for evaluating abnormalities in the ventricles. Placement of the electrodes depends on the lead being monitored and whether a 3-lead or 5-lead system is being used. Figure 30–9◆ shows the position of the electrodes for both lead II and MCL_1. No single monitoring lead is ideal for every patient. The lead chosen depends on the unit policy and nurse and/or health care provider preference. The specific dysrhythmia being monitored or anticipated may also dictate the type of lead chosen.

The color coding on the lead wire gives the nurse information about whether the lead is positive or negative. Typically the color black is negative, white is positive, and green is ground. In the 5-lead system red and brown colors also are used; their polarity changes depending on the lead being monitored.

Cardiac Monitoring Systems

The purpose of continuous ECG monitoring is to detect new and changing abnormal heart rhythms and to trend data relative to frequency and duration of dysrhythmias. Two methods of continuous ECG monitoring are available. In the first method, the patient can be hardwired to a monitor with the leads connected directly from the bedside monitor to the patient. The hardwired system has an oscilloscope at the bedside and in a central location such as the nurses' station. This system typically is able to monitor more than one lead simultaneously. Depending on the lead used, the system also is able to visualize ST segment depression and elevation. Hardwired systems have the capability to print a rhythm strip and provide visual and audible alarms when abnormalities in the heart rhythm occur. These systems are computerized and able to interpret and store dysrhythmias in a memory bank. Hardwired monitoring is done in critical care areas.

The second method for continuously monitoring patients is with radio waves from a battery-operated transmitter. The transmitter, worn by the patient, transmits the rhythms to a central bank of monitors, which is typically at the nurses' station. This system allows the patient to ambulate about the unit while still being monitored.

Regardless of the system being used, the patient must be informed of its purpose and any necessary precautions. Nursing management of the monitored patient encompasses placing the patient on ECG monitoring, checking the monitor, assessing the patient, and providing patient education. These critical nursing interventions are discussed in the following section.

Nursing Management

Prior to placing the patient on ECG monitoring, the nurse needs to explain the procedure and why it is necessary. It is essential that the patient understand that the heart is only being *monitored*, not controlled, by the equipment. Describe the electrodes, where they are placed, and how they are connected to the monitor. Skin preparation, electrode placement, and monitor connection are described in Chart 30–6.

The nurse needs to be knowledgeable about electrode placement for the lead that has been designated for monitoring the patient. Some manufacturers have the electrode and the lead wire attached, whereas others produce them separately. The electrode placement should be as comfortable as possible for the patient. Documentation of the lead used needs to be included in the patient's record.

Safety Alert *Precise lead placement is critical to accurate continuous cardiac monitoring. The nurse must verify correct lead placement at the beginning of each shift.*

All cardiac monitors have alarm systems to alert the nurse when abnormalities occur. Alarm systems have both a high and a low setting that alert the nurse when the heart rate goes above or below the set parameters. At the beginning of each shift, the nurse must ensure that the monitor alarms are on and set with the appropriate parameters established for the patient (see Chart 30–6). The nurse needs to explain to the patient that these alarms may go off with excessive movement or if the lead wire falls off. The nurse also needs to assure the patient and family that the nurse will respond to the alarm

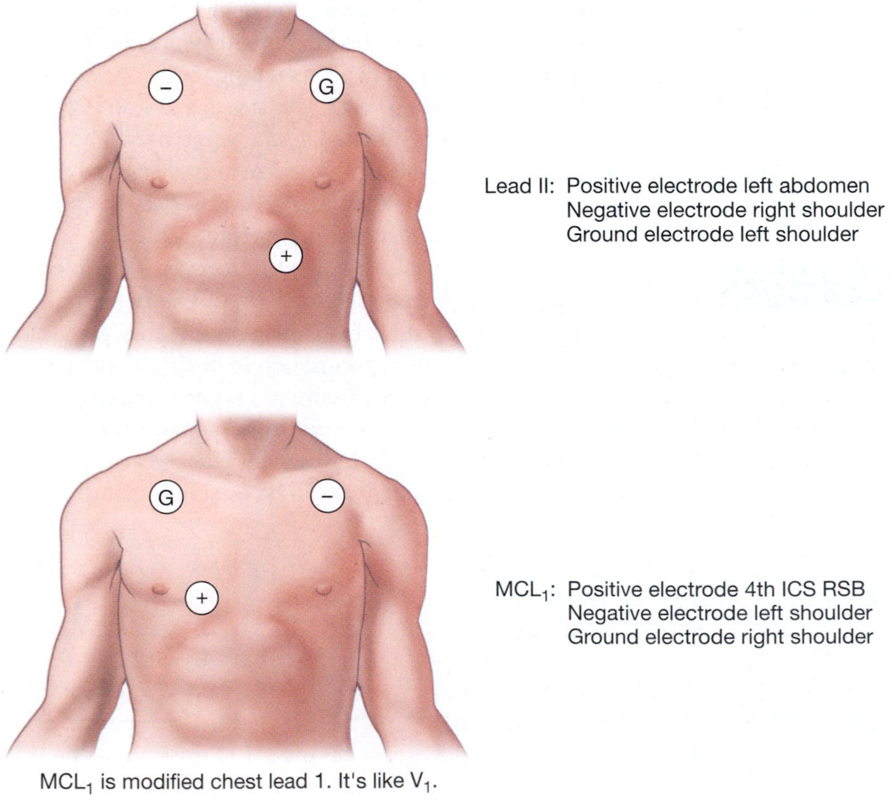

FIGURE 30–9 ◆ Electrode placement for bedside cardiac monitoring.

CHART 30–6 Procedure for Continuous ECG Monitoring

Electrode Attachment

- Choose an area to place the electrodes where there are no bony prominences, thick muscles, or skin folds, because these areas are prone to produce noncardiac waveforms and interference.
- Prepare the skin for electrode placement by making sure that it is clean, dry, and free of hair. It may be necessary to shave the chest area of male patients.
- Remove dead skin cells to improve electrical conductivity by rubbing the skin with the rough patch on the back of the electrode, a dry washcloth, or a gauze pad. The skin will become reddened with the rubbing; be careful not to cause skin breakdown.
- Wipe the skin, if it is oily, with an alcohol sponge or a moist wipe; allow it to air dry.
- Make sure that the electrode pads are moistened with conducting gel prior to placing them on the chest to increase electrical conductivity. A dry electrode is not effective for conducting the electrical activity. When the electrode becomes dry or loose, it needs to be replaced. If the skin around the electrode becomes irritated, the electrode must be removed and relocated.
- Position electrodes on the chest wall at prescribed locations depending on the lead or leads being monitored.
- Change electrodes when wet, poor contact exists, unclear tracing occurs, and/or every 48 hours to avoid skin irritation.
- Attach the opposite end of the lead wire to the cable. The cable has individual color-coded receptacles or holes for each lead wire.

Monitor Connection and Adjustment

- Attach the cable to the monitor.
- Adjust the monitor to increase the size of the PQRST complex for more accurate interpretation.
- Read the operating instructions for the specific brand of monitor prior to use.

Alarm Setting

- Always leave the alarm on.
- Recognize that the alarms have upper and lower heart rate limits.
- Set the alarm approximately 20 beats above and below the patient's resting intrinsic heart rate.
- Follow institutional policy, if present, to determine different alarm limits.
- Be aware that when the alarm sounds, the first nursing responsibility is to check the patient.
- Recognize that movement by the patient may cause the alarm to sound falsely.

Documentation

- Document lead used.
- Document PR interval, QRS width, QT interval, ectopic beats, and type of rhythm/dysrhythmia.
- Record ECG changes and patient's response to changes.

each time it sounds and that an alarm does not necessarily mean there is a problem with the heart. The nurse must stress that excessive movement will cause the alarm to sound frequently.

Safety Alert *When the monitor alarms go off, it is essential that the nurse evaluates the clinical status of the patient prior to any other activities in order to assess for the presence of cardiac abnormalities and the patient's clinical response to the abnormalities.*

Nursing responsibility for monitored patients includes knowing the patient's specific rhythm in order to assess for changes. The more familiar the nurse is with the patient and the monitoring system, the more quickly problems can be diagnosed and appropriate action taken. Assessment of patient tolerance of rhythm changes is the first nursing action, occurring prior to assessing for problems with the equipment.

Safety Alert *When abnormalities appear on a cardiac rhythm strip it is an essential nursing responsibility to assess the patient's tolerance of the rhythm, especially if it is a new abnormality. The nurse needs to know what changes must be reported to the health care provider. The rhythm needs to be documented on the patient's record.*

Tolerance to the rhythm is assessed by obtaining and evaluating vital signs; neurological status; and the presence of signs and symptoms of decreased cardiac output, such as angina. After determining patient status and stability, the nurse then troubleshoots the equipment for problems such as a dry electrode or a disconnected wire. The problem could be as simple as the patient's tapping the electrode, in which case no action would be necessary. It also is essential that the nurse know which cardiac disturbances are reportable and/or life threatening, such as ventricular tachycardia or fibrillation.

Communication with all personnel caring for the patient and observing the monitor is critical. They must be kept informed of when the patient needs to be off the monitor or of physical activities, such as bathing, that may sound the alarms. For example, if there is a monitor technician, that person must be informed if the patient will be leaving the floor and engaging in increased physical activities.

Because it may be stressful and frightening for a patient to have his heart monitored continuously, patient education is essential. In particular, the nurse should ensure that the patient understands that this system does not report clinical manifestations (e.g., angina, dyspnea, and weakness), and it is necessary for the patient to report these conditions as they occur. Providing clear information about how the monitoring system works and what the patient can expect during monitoring will help alleviate patient and family member anxiety.

ECG Graph Paper

ECG **graph paper** is specialized paper on which the ECG pattern is recorded. The paper is designed to allow the measurement of various calculations related to the electrical activity of the heart. It is standard nursing protocol to measure these calculations for the patient on a cardiac monitor. These measurements help determine whether the rhythm falls within the time limits of normal cardiac activity. Abnormal measurements may indicate a malfunction of the cardiac conduction system; these will be discussed later in conjunction with the various dysrhythmias.

The ECG graph paper is arranged as a series of horizontal and vertical lines. This paper is standardized to allow for consistency in ECG measurement and strip analysis. Both the amplitude and the voltage may be measured on the paper. The vertical axis measures the amplitude and is stated in millivolts (mV). Two large squares on this axis equal 1 millivolt. This measurement is rarely used because the size of the picture or millivolts can be adjusted at the monitoring station, thereby reducing the consistency of this measurement.

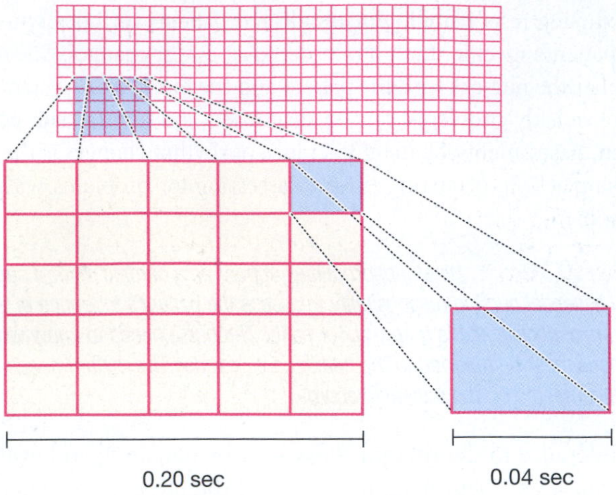

FIGURE 30–10 ◆ ECG graph paper.

The horizontal axis is divided into small squares. The squares on the ECG paper are used to measure the length of time required for the electrical impulse to traverse a specific part of the heart. Figure 30–10◆ shows an example of ECG graph paper.

These squares are used to measure time intervals as follows:

- The smallest square is 1 millimeter (mm) in length and represents 0.04 second in time.
- The large square is 5 mm in length and represents 0.20 second in time.
- The large square equals 5 small squares.
- Five large squares represent 1 second.

ECG Measurements

When assessing either a rhythm strip or a 12-lead ECG, the nurse must evaluate both the individual PQRST complexes and the relationship of each individual complex to the overall rhythm. The assessment of an ECG configuration includes the following:

- ***P Wave:*** There should be one P wave for every QRS complex.
- ***PR Interval:*** This is measured from the beginning of the P wave to the beginning of the QRS complex. The normal PR interval is from 0.12 to 0.20 second or 3 small boxes to 1 large box.
- ***QRS Complex:*** The QRS complex is measured from the beginning of the Q wave to the end of the S wave. The normal range is from 0.06 to 0.12 second or 1.5 boxes to 3 boxes. The shape of the QRS complex varies from individual to individual and also depends on the ECG lead being used. For example, QRS complexes are mostly positive in the lead II and mostly negative in the MCL_1 lead (see Figure 30–8, p. 857). Not everyone has a discernable Q wave.
- ***QT Interval:*** The **QT interval** is measured from the Q wave to the end of the T wave. The normal QT interval is 0.34 to 0.43 second or 8.5 to 11 boxes.
- ***Heart Rate:*** This is measured by using the very top of the ECG paper, which is marked off in 3-second intervals with tick marks. The tick mark is a small straight line or hash mark above the tracing. Count up the number of PQRST complexes that occur in 6 seconds and multiply that number by 10. This method provides a general estimate of the heart rate, which is most accurate when the heart rhythm is regular. A more accurate method for measuring heart rate is to count the number of large squares between two R waves and divide the total into 300. The normal HR is 60 to 100 beats per minute.
- ***Heart Rhythm:*** This is determined by measuring the distance between P waves for atrial rate and two R waves for ventricular rate and then measuring each subsequent R wave to ensure it is the same distance apart as the previous ones. With a regular rhythm, the distance between R waves is equal.

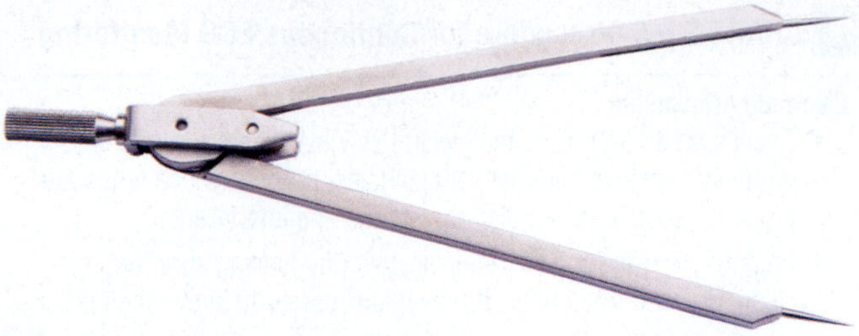

FIGURE 30–11 ◆ Calipers.

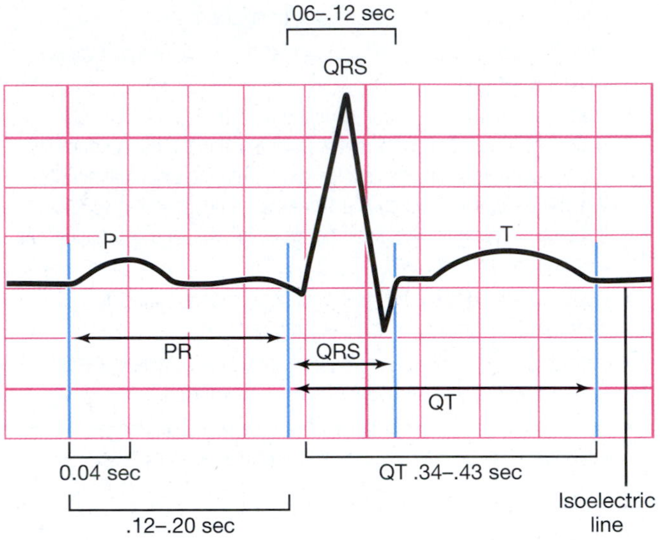

FIGURE 30–12 ◆ ECG measurement.

Calipers (Figure 30–11◆) are the instruments used to take all these measurements. Figure 30–12◆ demonstrates where each measurement begins and ends.

Isoelectric Line

The **isoelectric line** marks the beginning and ending point of all waves. When the SA node fires, the **ECG waveform** (the actual tracing on the graph paper) begins to move away from the isoelectric line. Any wave that has an upward deflection above the isoelectric line is referred to as a positive deflection; any waveform that goes below the line is referred to as a negative deflection. Depending on the lead, certain waves normally are positive and certain ones are negative. In a lead II, the normal P wave has a positive deflection, the PR interval is isoelectric, the Q wave is the first negative deflection, the R wave is positive, the S wave is negative, the ST segment is isoelectric, and the T wave is positive.

Artifact

Artifact is defined as a false and abnormal pattern on the ECG graph paper created by sources other than the heart. Any one of the following sources may cause this type of interference:

- Malfunction of electrodes, possibly due to dry conductive gel, clammy skin, or dense chest hair
- Patient movement, which precipitates a fluctuating isoelectric line that corrects itself when the patient lies still
- Improper grounding, which occurs when a patient is in contact with an outside source of electricity, such as poorly grounded beds and/or IV infusion pumps
- Equipment failures, such as broken wires or cables on the ECG equipment, which need to be exchanged for new equipment.

Because of this interference or artifact, the baseline or isoelectric line becomes fuzzy. When artifact is present, it is difficult to diagnose cardiac abnormalities, making it necessary to correct the cause of the artifact. Figure 30–13◆ depicts artifact.

Ectopic Focus

Ectopic focus is a heartbeat originating from a site other than the primary cardiac pacemaker tissue. Ectopic foci may affect cardiac output and must be assessed and documented carefully for their impact on the hemodynamic stability of the patient. The terms *dysrhythmia, arrhythmia,* and *ectopic focus* all mean the same thing and are used interchangeably.

ECG Rhythm Strip Evaluation and Documentation

When evaluating an ECG rhythm strip, using a simple stepwise process provides a consistent method for rhythm strip evaluation. This is shown in Chart 30–7. If the rhythm strip falls out of the normal parameters, then there is a high probability of an abnormality occurring in the conduction system. These abnormalities are discussed at length throughout the remainder of the chapter.

Normal Sinus Rhythm

Normal sinus rhythm (NSR) is a cardiac rhythm initiated from the SA or sinus node that has all the normal waveforms (PQRST) and normal time intervals (PR, QRS, QT) (Figure 30–14◆).

The following criteria must be present to be NSR:

- P wave has a normal and consistent shape and appears before every QRS complex.
- There is a 1:1 ratio of P wave to QRS complex.

CHART 30–7 Stepwise Process for ECG Interpretation

P Waves	Are the P waves regular?
	Is there one P wave for every QRS and one QRS for every P wave?
	Is the P wave in front of the QRS or behind it?
	Is the P wave normal and upright in lead II?
	Do all the P waves look alike?
	Are the abnormal P waves associated with ectopic beats?
PR Interval	Are all the PR intervals constant?
	Is the PR interval measurement within normal range (0.12 to 0.20 second)?
	If the PR interval varies, is there a pattern to the changing measurements?
QRS Complex	Are all the QRS complexes of equal duration?
	What is the measurement of the QRS complex size?
	Is the QRS complex measurement within normal limits (0.06 to 0.12 second)?
	Do all the QRS complexes look alike?
	Are the unusual QRS complexes associated with ectopic beats?
QT Interval	What is the length of the QT interval?
	Is it normal or prolonged?
	Is the patient on a treatment that prolongs the interval?
Rate	Atrial: how many P waves in 6 seconds times 10.
	Ventricular: how many R waves in 6 seconds times 10.
	A second method is to count the number of large boxes between two R waves and divide by 300. Both methods work best when the rhythm is normal.
	What is the heart rate?
Regularity (also called rhythm)	Is it regular?
	Is it irregular?
	Are there any patterns to the irregularity?
	Are there any ectopic beats; if so, are they early or late?
Ectopic Beats	Are they present?
	What are they?
	How is the patient tolerating them?
	Do they require treatment?

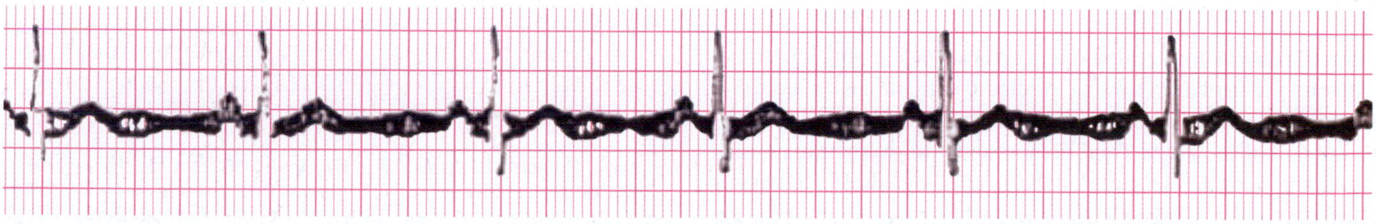

FIGURE 30–13 ◆ Artifact.

Video: Dysrhythmia—Etiology and Pathophysiology

Video: Dysrhythmia Animation

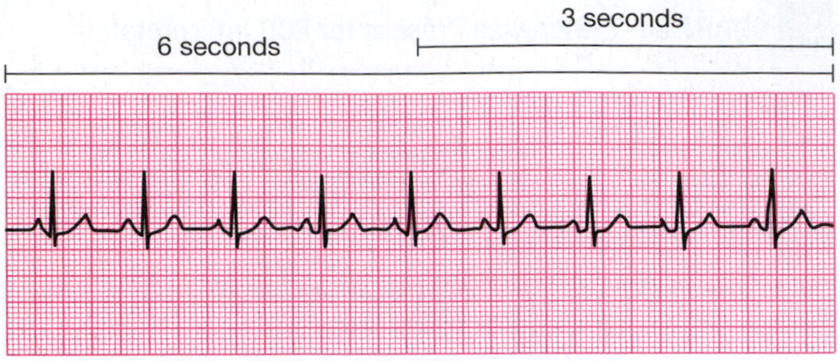

P Wave: Present 1 P wave/QRS complex; PR Interval: 0.18 second; QRS Complex: 0.06 second; QT Interval 0.36 second; Heart Rate: Atrial: 90 beats per minute (bpm); Ventricular: 90 bpm; Rhythm: Regular, Ectopic Beats: None.

FIGURE 30–14 ◆ Normal sinus rhythm.

- PR interval is between 0.12 and 0.20 second.
- QRS complex is between 0.06 and 0.12 second.
- QT interval is between 0.34 and 0.43 second.
- Atrial and ventricular rate is between 60 and 100 beats per minute (beats/minute).
- Atrial and ventricular rhythm is regular.

Nursing Management

When the patient is on a cardiac monitor, it is the nurse's responsibility to measure, assess, and document the patient's rhythm strip at least every shift and more frequently depending on the patient's condition and agency protocol. Whenever changes occur in the heart rhythm, the nurse must begin the same process again: measure, assess, and document the rhythm strip. The nurse must know when it is appropriate to report a change in the ECG to the health care provider.

Nursing Documentation

When documenting the heart rhythm in the patient's record, most institutions require that a rhythm strip be placed in the patient's record once every shift and/or when a change in the rhythm occurs. The patient's name, the date and time of rhythm strip collection, and the ECG lead used for the rhythm strip should be documented. The electrical features of the rhythm, including the presence of a P wave, the PR interval, the width of the QRS complex, the QT interval, the heart rate and rhythm (regular versus irregular), and the presence of ectopy (ectopic focus), should also be documented. Corresponding clinical manifestations associated with a given rhythm, such as a change in blood pressure, level of consciousness, and urine output, also need to be documented in the record.

Dysrhythmias

When the cardiac muscle does not receive enough blood, it becomes ischemic and irritable, causing cardiac dysrhythmias to occur. A **dysrhythmia** is an abnormal disturbance of the electrical conduction system of the heart. There are a number of dysrhythmias, each originating in different parts of the heart. This chapter addresses dysrhythmias according to location in the heart, beginning at the top with the atrial dysrhythmias. As the dysrhythmias occur anatomically lower in the heart, their severity increases due to their impact on cardiac output. Cardiac output decreases as the severity of the dysrhythmia increases.

Heart rhythms are categorized according to their site of origin, or the cardiac structure in which they begin. The most common dysrhythmias begin at the top of the heart with the SA node. These types of dysrhythmias are called sinus dysrhythmias due to their origin in the SA, or sinus, node. The next area in the heart where dysrhythmias may occur is in the intra-atrial pathways. Dysrhythmias that occur here are referred to as atrial dysrhythmias. Moving anatomically down to the next area of the conduction system, the AV node or junction is where junctional dysrhythmias occur. The final area of the heart where dysrhythmias may occur is in the ventricles. These ventricular dysrhythmias are considered to be the most dangerous because they precipitate the most profound decrease in cardiac output.

When observing, assessing, and treating dysrhythmias, it is critical for the nurse to remember to treat the patient, not the dysrhythmia. Treatment is always based on the hemodynamic impact of the dysrhythmia.

Sinus Dysrhythmias

The four common dysrhythmias associated with the sinus area of the heart are sinus bradycardia, sinus tachycardia, sinus arrhythmia/dysrhythmia, and sinus arrest.

Sinus Bradycardia

Sinus bradycardia, often called "sinus brady," occurs when the SA node is firing at a rate of less than 60 beats per minute. Sinus means the rhythm originated in the SA node; therefore, P waves are present. The only difference between sinus bradycardia and normal sinus rhythm (NSR) is the heart rate: Because of this variable, sinus bradycardia is not normal. Sinus bradycardia may result in decreased cardiac output because, while there is adequate time for the heart to fill up with blood, there are not enough contractions per minute to pump the amount of blood needed for normal cardiac output. Significant slowing of the heart rate predisposes the patient to an ectopic focus assuming the role of pacemaker in order to generate sufficient cardiac output. This condition may lead to serious dysrhythmias and warrants careful monitoring. An ECG strip showing sinus bradycardia is shown in Figure 30–15◆.

Significant ECG features of sinus bradycardia include:

- Both atrial and ventricular rates are less than 60 beats per minute.
- The QT interval tends to lengthen.

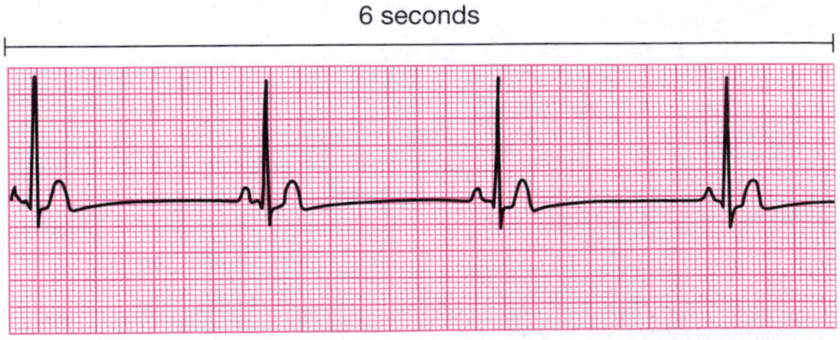

P Wave: Present, 1 P wave/QRS Complex; PR Interval: .16 second; QRS Complex: 0.08 second; QT Interval: 0.32 second; Heart Rate: Atrial: 40 bpm; Ventricular: 40 bpm; Rhythm: Regular; Ectopic Beats: None.

FIGURE 30–15 ◆ Sinus bradycardia.

The etiology, physical assessment findings, and treatment for sinus bradycardia are included in Chart 30–8.

Sinus Tachycardia

Sinus tachycardia is defined as a firing of the SA node at a rate greater than 100 beats per minute. It is called *sinus* tachycardia because there is a P wave present, although it may be related to an abnormality of the SA node itself. For example, an acute myocardial infarction (AMI) may cause a decrease in the blood supply to the SA node, resulting in an abnormal response such as tachycardia.

Sinus tachycardia results in increased oxygen consumption, increased workload of the heart, and decreased cardiac output. Whenever the heart rate increases, more oxygen is required to nourish the muscle, resulting in increased work of the heart and increased oxygen consumption. Whenever the heart rate increases, there is a loss of the time needed for blood to flow into the heart (**fill time**), which in turn decreases the amount of blood pumped out of the heart (cardiac output). An ECG strip showing sinus tachycardia is shown in Figure 30–16◆. Significant ECG features include:

- Atrial and ventricular heart rates are over 100 beats per minute.
- As the sinus rate accelerates, both the PR interval and the QT interval tend to shorten slightly.
- The rhythm may be slightly irregular as the rate begins to accelerate, but then becomes a rapid regular rhythm.

The etiology, physical assessment findings, and treatment for sinus tachycardia are outlined in Chart 30–8.

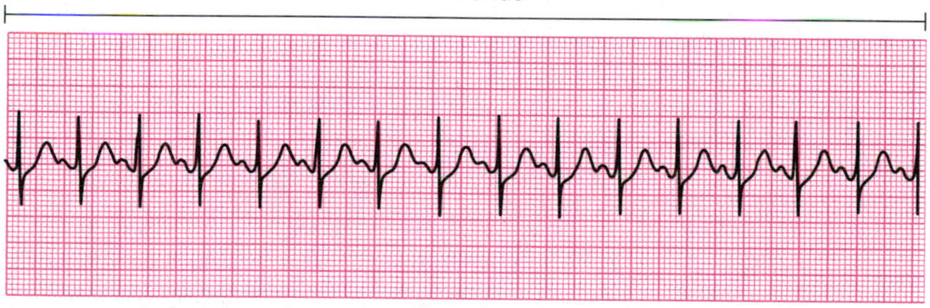

P Wave: Present, 1/QRS Complex; PR Interval: 0.14 second; QRS Complex: 0.08 second; QT Interval: 0.36 second; Heart Rate: Atrial: 140 bpm, Ventricular: 140 bpm; Rhythm: Regular; Ectopic Beats: None.

FIGURE 30–16 ◆ Sinus tachycardia.

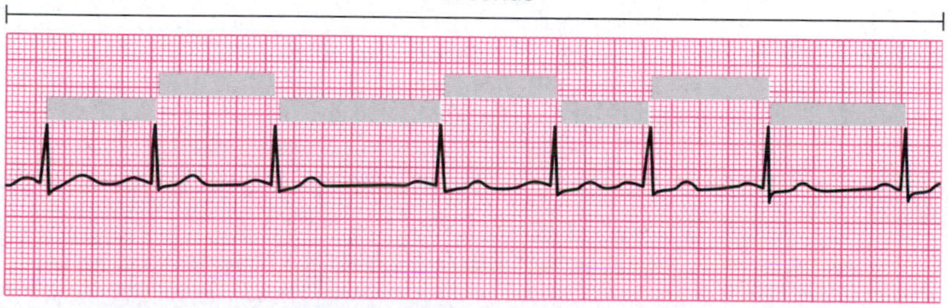

P Wave: Present 1/QRS Complex; PR Interval: 0.18 second; QRS Complex: 0.08 second; QT Interval: 0.40 second; Heart Rate: Atrial: 80 bpm, Ventricular: 80 bpm; Rhythm: Irregular; Ectopic Beats: None.

FIGURE 30–17 ◆ Sinus arrhythmia/dysrhythmia.

Sinus Arrhythmia/Dysrhythmia

Sinus arrhythmia/dysrhythmia resembles normal sinus rhythm, except for the slight irregularity in the heart rhythm. The rate of impulse formation and conduction varies with the respiratory cycle; thus, the P to P and R to R intervals change with respiration. The heart rate increases during inspiration and decreases with expiration. It tends to disappear when the heart rate increases (e.g., with exercise). Typically there is no clinical significance with this dysrhythmia; it is considered a variant of normal. However, the cyclic decreased heart rate may make the heart muscle more susceptible to other dysrhythmias. Figure 30–17◆ shows an ECG strip of sinus arrhythmia/dysrhythmia. Significant ECG features of sinus arrhythmia/dysrhythmia include:

- PR interval may change slightly as the heart rate changes.
- QT interval changes with the heart rate, becoming longer during the slow phase of the rhythm.
- Heart rate is 60 to 100 beats per minute; however, the slow phase may drop below 60 beats per minute.
- Heart rhythm is regularly irregular, with a variance of more than 0.08 second in the acceleration and deceleration phases.
- Ectopic beats may occur during the slow phase of the rhythm.

The etiology, physical assessment findings, and treatment for sinus arrhythmia/dysrhythmia are outlined in Chart 30–8.

Sinus Arrest

Sinus arrest is a momentary cessation of sinus impulse formation (SA node failure) that causes a pause in the cardiac rhythm followed by spontaneous resumption of electrical activity. Sinus arrest also is called sinus pause. With a sinus pause there is an absence of the PQRST complex on the ECG strip and a loss of cardiac output. Figure 30–18◆ shows an ECG strip of sinus arrest (pause). Significant ECG features of sinus arrest include:

- There is an absence of one entire PQRST complex.
- QT interval changes with the heart rate, becoming longer during the slow phase of the rhythm.
- There may be marked bradycardia due to long sinus pauses.
- Underlying heart rhythm is regular except when the pauses occur.

The etiology, physical assessment findings, and treatment for sinus arrest are outlined in Chart 30–8.

Nursing Management

The nurse should first evaluate the patient's response to and tolerance of any dysrhythmia. Depending on the type of dysrhythmia, the patient may or may not be symptomatic. However, if the abnormal rhythm results in a decreased cardiac output, it is important to assess for the changes outlined on Chart 30–9 (p. 865).

The nurse must also address the psychological impact of experiencing dysrhythmias. Most patients find the clinical manifestations of cardiac dysrhythmias, such as angina, dizziness, syncope, diaphoresis, and

CHART 30–8 Sinus Dysrhythmias: Etiology, Physical Assessment, and Treatment

Dysrhythmia	Etiology	Physical Assessment	Treatment
Sinus bradycardia	Decreased sympathetic tone, or anatomic changes Hypothermia Drugs, such as morphine, digoxin, verapamil, and some sedatives Toxins Vagal stimulation, as with vomiting or Valsalva maneuver Hypothyroidism Infectious diseases Acidosis Hypovolemia Hypo/hyperkalemia Hypoglycemia Cardiac tamponade Tension pneumothorax Thrombosis: Coronary and/or pulmonary Trauma Increased intracranial pressure Normal conditions: Sleeping and a well-conditioned athlete's heart	Pulse: Less than 60 beats per minute and typically regular. Blood pressure: Lower than usual if for pathological conditions. If cardiac output is decreased the clinical manifestations described in Chart 30–9 may occur.	Treat only if symptomatic. Treatment is typically instituted when syncope and/or alteration in consciousness occurs. If symptomatic, it means there is a significant drop in cardiac output. Attempt to identify and treat the cause. Assess for changes in vital signs. Observe for other dysrhythmias. With poor perfusion, typical treatment includes: • Oxygen • IV access • Drug therapy (atropine) • Epinephrine or dopamine • Pacemaker evaluation.
Sinus tachycardia	Exercise Smoking Alcohol Caffeine Cocaine Fever Blood loss/anemia Hypovolemia Early sepsis Hypermetabolic state (e.g., burn injury) Heart failure Allergic reactions Emotions Anxiety Pain Decreased PSNS Increased SNS stimulation Drug side effect of many over-the-counter cold drugs and drugs used to treat asthma and sinus conditions Compensatory response to a decreased cardiac output	Pulse: Greater than 100 beats per minute. BP: Lower than normal. If cardiac output is decreased the clinical manifestations described in Chart 30–9 may occur.	Treat only if symptomatic. Attempt to identify and treat the cause. Treatment may include: • Drug therapy, such as beta-adrenergic blockers, adenosine, diltiazem, and digoxin • Carotid massage/vagal maneuvers • Cardioversion • Anxiety medications • Fluid replacement. If causes are identified and managed, generally the rhythm converts back to NSR.
Sinus arrhythmia/ dysrhythmia	Common and normal finding, especially in children and young adults Pathological causes include underlying cardiac disease, such as sick sinus syndrome and myocardial infarction Digoxin Factors that cause heart rate variability including exercise, mental stress, and circadian rhythms	Pulse: Irregular.	Not treated unless the bradycardic phase causes clinical manifestations described under bradycardia. Atropine for bradycardia. Provide reassurance that this rhythm is not dangerous, but it needs to be evaluated to rule out more serious dysrhythmias.

(*continued*)

CHART 30–8 Sinus Dysrhythmias: Etiology, Physical Assessment, and Treatment, *continued*

Dysrhythmia	Etiology	Physical Assessment	Treatment
Sinus arrest	Hypoxemia Cardiac muscle ischemia Damage to the SA node Digoxin Aspirin Abnormal potassium levels Myocardial infarction Vagal dominance Hypersensitive carotid sinus reflex (e.g., tight shirt collar)	If cardiac output is decreased the clinical manifestations described in Chart 30–9 may occur.	Treat only if patient is symptomatic and/or condition is complicated by other dysrhythmias. Ascertain and treat cause, if possible. Typical treatment may include permanent or temporary artificial pacemaker for repeated episodes, depending on the prognosis, age, and presence of clinical manifestations.

Source: Adapted from Osborn & Watson, 2011.

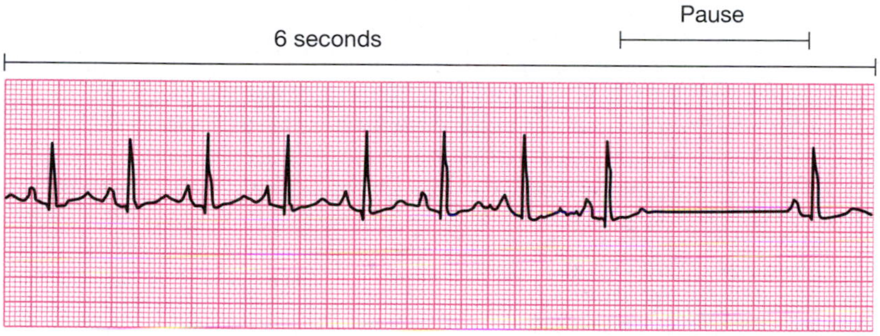

P Wave: Present 1/QRS Complex; PR Interval: 0.20 second; QRS Complex: 0.10 second; QT Interval: 0.40 second; Heart Rate: Atrial: 90 bpm, Ventricular: 90 bpm; Rhythm: Regular except for the pause; Ectopic Beats: None. Conclusion: Sinus arrest (pause).

FIGURE 30–18 ◆ Sinus arrest (pause).

disorientation, frightening. Patients need comfort measures and reassurance that all appropriate treatment is being provided. The nurse should ensure the patient has a quiet environment and provide treatments to alleviate clinical manifestations. The nurse should also provide support by actively listening to the patient's concerns and including family members in the plan of care.

The cause of the dysrhythmia, as outlined in Chart 30–10 (p. 866), must be evaluated and corrected, if possible. Typically the patient is treated only if he becomes symptomatic and/or the condition is complicated by other more serious dysrhythmias. When a dysrhythmia occurs, the nurse needs to do an in-depth assessment of the patient to determine the clinical manifestations. A dysrhythmia may not always occur due to an abnormality in the heart, but may be due to a variety of reasons not associated with a cardiac abnormality. For example, pain and anxiety are two noncardiac causes of tachycardia. Therefore, treatment may consist of pain medications or, for the anxious patient, supportive measures such as talking with the patient. If the patient is hemodynamically unstable, the health care provider should be notified. Chart 30–10 (p. 866) outlines the standard treatments for each of the sinus dysrhythmias.

CHART 30–9 Clinical Manifestations of Decreased Cardiac Output

Lower than usual blood pressure	Exercise intolerance	Altered mentation
Decreased or increased heart rate	Dizziness	Shortness of breath
Syncope	Alteration in consciousness	
Generalized weakness	Angina	

Note: Clinical manifestations depend on the degree of decreased cardiac output.

Atrial Dysrhythmias

Atrial dysrhythmias usually result from an irritable focus in the atria that initiates an electrical impulse before the SA node has fired in a normal fashion. Because the electrical impulse does not come from the SA node, the P wave configuration of the ECG is different. However, the QRS complex is normal because the electrical impulse travels down the normal pathway from the AV node through the ventricle. Six different atrial dysrhythmias are discussed next: premature atrial contraction, atrial flutter, atrial fibrillation, supraventricular tachycardia, Wolff-Parkinson-White syndrome, and sick sinus syndrome.

Premature Atrial Contraction

Premature atrial contraction (PAC) is an ectopic focus in the atria that occurs early, before the next expected SA node impulse, causing depolarization and contraction of the cardiac muscle. This electrical impulse originates outside the SA node. It frequently occurs when the underlying rhythm is normal sinus rhythm (NSR) and the only abnormality is the PAC. When there are more than 5 to 6 PACs per minute, they are termed frequent and have more clinical significance. Whenever beats are premature, there is a loss of the time needed for blood to flow into the heart (fill time), which in turn decreases the amount of blood pumped out of the heart (cardiac output). Therefore, if the beats occur frequently, cardiac output decreases. An increase in the frequency of the dysrhythmia also indicates irritability of the atrial muscle. This is a cause for concern because it tends to increase the risk for other dysrhythmias. Figure 30–19 ◆ shows premature atrial contractions. Significant ECG features include:

- P wave is present and is premature, and configuration (shape) may look different because electrical impulses do not come from the SA node.

CHART 30–10 Atrial Dysrhythmias: Etiology, Physical Assessment, and Treatment

Dysrhythmia	Etiology	Physical Assessment	Treatment
Premature atrial contraction	Mitral stenosis Mitral valve prolapse Cor pulmonale Underlying cardiovascular disease including ischemia and myocardial infarction Hypoxia Infectious diseases Electrolyte imbalance Increased sympathetic tone Stimulants Drug toxicity (e.g., digoxin) Stress Anxiety	Pulse: Irregular. BP: If frequent PACs, may be decreased. If cardiac output is decreased the clinical manifestations described in Chart 30–9 may occur.	Observe the frequency of the PACs, and observe for decreased cardiac output (Chart 30–9). Treat the underlying cause (e.g., stress, anxiety, electrolyte imbalance). Frequent PACs or those that cause sustained tachycardia may require treatment with drugs that prolong atrial refractoriness, such as digoxin, verapamil, or propranolol.
Atrial flutter	Coronary atherosclerosis Valvular disease Cor pulmonale Pulmonary edema Myocardial infarction SA node disease Pulmonary embolism Digitalis toxicity ETOH abuse Postsurgical complication: one of the common dysrhythmias following open heart surgery. On rare occasions it may occur with normal healthy hearts.	Pulse: May be regular or irregular. BP: Lower than normal if cardiac output is decreased. If cardiac output is decreased the clinical manifestations described in Chart 30–9 may occur.	Cardioversion is a common intervention. Drug therapy is used to reduce AV conduction: Digitalis, propranolol, and diltiazem. If this is a chronic situation, the patient may be placed on anticoagulants like warfarin.
Atrial fibrillation	Acute myocardial infarction Left atrial stretch due to mitral stenosis and mitral regurgitation May be a chronic rhythm associated with heart failure Transient after open-heart surgery Long-standing hypertension Digoxin toxicity Alcohol intake, chronic or acute, moderate to heavy Idiopathic	Pulse: Irregular (hallmark feature). BP: Lower than normal. If cardiac output is decreased the clinical manifestations described in Chart 30–9 may occur.	Control the ventricular response (i.e., heart rate). If a rapid ventricular response, control with drugs: Digoxin is still the drug of choice; beta-blockers (propranolol) and calcium channel blockers (verapamil, diltiazem) may also be used. Calcium channel blockers work the fastest, and are the drug of choice when patient is medically unstable. Prevent thromboembolic events with anticoagulant therapy (e.g., warfarin). Cardioversion: Is used if new onset, especially when hemodynamic instability is present. If successful, digoxin is used to prevent reoccurrence.
Supraventricular tachycardia includes paroxysmal atrial tachycardia Atrioventricular node reentry tachycardia AVNRT	Heart disease Rheumatic heart disease Coronary artery disease (CAD) Hypoxia May be precipitated by a premature atrial contraction (PAC)	Pulse: Very fast. BP: Decreased if drop in cardiac output. If cardiac output is decreased, the clinical manifestations described in Chart 30–9 may occur.	It is necessary to find and treat the cause (e.g., stress, hypokalemia). Vagal maneuvers (i.e., bearing down, coughing, and carotid artery massage). Specific treatment may include: Oxygen therapy and cardioversion.

CHART 30–10 Atrial Dysrhythmias: Etiology, Physical Assessment, and Treatment, *continued*

Dysrhythmia	Etiology	Physical Assessment	Treatment
	May occur in healthy adults from a variety of causes: Overexertion Stress Excessive use of stimulants Smoking Hypokalemia		Drug therapy: Adenosine is used to briefly terminate the rhythm for differential diagnosis. Verapamil is a calcium channel blocker; decreases heart rate. Cardioversion is performed if drug therapy and vagal maneuvers are unsuccessful.
Wolff-Parkinson-White (WPW) syndrome	Congenital in origin: Twice as common in males, and occurs in 0.1% to 0.3% of the general population	Pulse: Rapid. Frequent episodes of palpitations. If cardiac output is decreased the clinical manifestations described in Chart 30–9 may occur.	Same as that for supraventricular tachycardia. Radiofrequency ablation used to terminate the accessory pathway.
Sick sinus syndrome	Coronary artery disease Drugs: Cardiac glycoside, antihypertensive agents, calcium channel blockers Frequently intermittent and unpredictable, may occur in the absence of heart disease Myocardial infarction Inflammatory or degenerative processes	Pulse: Bradycardia that alternates with tachycardia, referred to as brady-tachy syndrome. BP: May decrease due to decreased cardiac output. If cardiac output is decreased, the clinical manifestations described in Chart 30–9 may occur.	Clinical manifestations and ECG findings determine treatment. Anticoagulants are used because of blood stasis if atrial flutter/fibrillation is present. The only definitive treatment is a permanent pacemaker to replace the SA node.

- PR interval may be shorter or longer than regular beats.
- PACs are premature, making the rhythm irregular.
- P wave after the PAC falls earlier than expected because of the early electrical discharge, which then resets the SA node rhythm, referred to as a noncompensatory pause.
- Heart rate and rhythm are typically within normal limits, except when the PAC occurs.

The etiology, physical assessment findings, and treatment of PACs are outlined in Chart 30–10.

Atrial Flutter

Atrial flutter is a rapid, regular, atrial rhythm with an *atrial* rate exceeding 350 beats per minute (Baltazar, 2009). There is loss of SA node dominance, which is the preferential pacemaker. Only a fraction of the atrial impulses is conducted through the AV node to the ventricle. Most of the atrial beats fall during the AV node refractory period when the cardiac cell is unable to respond to any stimulus. This makes the AV node the "gatekeeper" for the ventricles, because it prohibits all of the atrial impulses from reaching the ventricles, thereby limiting ventricular rate. Atrial flutter also causes a decreased cardiac output due to the loss of the atrial kick or normal atrial contraction. Atrial kick forces more blood into the ventricle, which augments cardiac output. With atrial flutter, the atria are just fluttering instead of contracting, resulting in a decreased cardiac output by as much as 30% (Moser & Riegel, 2008). The loss of the atrial contraction causes blood stasis and pooling to occur, leading to an increased incidence of clot formation, which in turn leads to stroke. Finally, due to the rapid atrial rate,

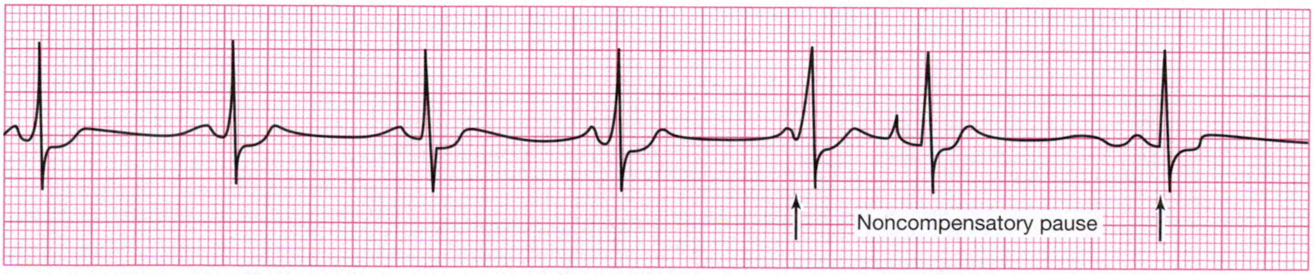

P Wave: Premature; PR Interval: 0.16 second; QRS Complex: 0.10 second; QT interval: 0.40 second; Heart Rate: Atrial: 70 bpm; Ventricular: 70 bpm; Rhythm: Regular except for premature beats. Ectopic Beat PAC. Conclusion: One premature atrial contraction.

FIGURE 30–19 ◆ Premature atrial contraction.

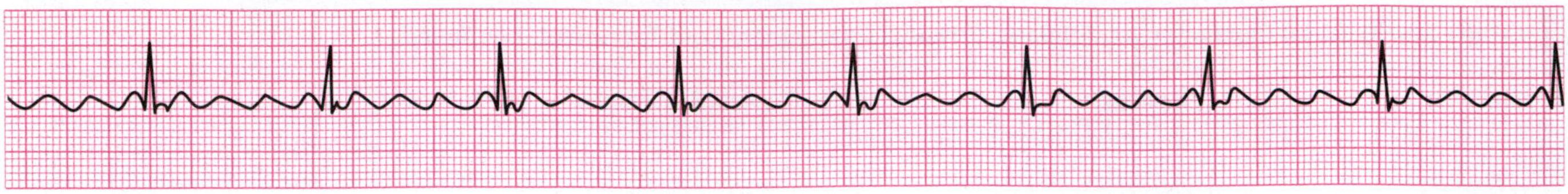

P Wave: None, flutter waves; PR interval: None; QRS Complex: 0.08 second; QT Interval: unable to obtain; Heart Rate: Atrial: about 300 bpm, Ventricular: 90 bpm; Rhythm: Regular; Ectopic Beats: Flutter waves.

FIGURE 30–20 ◆ Atrial flutter.

myocardial oxygen consumption increases. This eventually leads to the development of hypoxia of the myocardial muscle and predisposes left ventricular to fail. Figure 30–20◆ presents a rhythm strip showing atrial flutter. Significant ECG features of atrial flutter include:

- P waves are not identifiable; instead, there are flutter waves (F waves), creating a "sawtooth" baseline on the ECG strip.
- PR intervals are not measurable.
- QT interval is not measurable because the T waves are buried in the F waves.
- Atrial and ventricular rhythms typically are regular, but they may be irregular depending on how often the AV node allows impulses to travel to the ventricle.

The etiology, physical assessment findings, and treatment of atrial flutter are outlined in Chart 30–10.

Atrial Fibrillation

Atrial fibrillation, also referred to as "atrial fib" or "a-fib," is a common dysrhythmia. The Evidence-Based Practice box outlines the genetic considerations of atrial fibrillation.

Atrial fibrillation is characterized by a disorganized, very rapid, and irregular atrial rhythm resulting in an irregular ventricular rhythm, its hallmark feature. Rapid or slow ventricular heart rate, referred to as the ventricular response, depends on the rate at which the AV node allows impulses to be conducted to the ventricles. The cells in the atria have an increased irritability, typically due to cardiac muscle hypoxia, which causes many sites in the atria to become pacemakers and initiate electrical impulses. The firing of these multiple sites causes the atria simply to quiver instead of contracting effectively. Atrial fibrillation causes three significant clinical manifestations: (1) loss of SA node pacemaker dominance, which is the most reliable pacemaker; (2) decreased cardiac output due to loss of atrial kick; and (3) increased myocardial oxygen consumption.

The immediate concern for atrial fibrillation is the ventricular response because it determines cardiac output. A heart rate that is too slow or too fast could potentially decrease the cardiac output.

With the loss of the atrial kick, blood stasis and pooling occur, leading to an increased incidence of clot formation. Therefore, those individuals with atrial fibrillation are at high risk for a cardiovascular accident (CVA) and/or pulmonary emboli. The rapid atrial firing also increases the workload on the heart, eventually causing hypoxia of the myocardial muscle. Long-term hypoxia predisposes to left ventricular failure. Figure 30–21◆ presents a rhythm strip showing atrial fibrillation.

Significant ECG features of atrial fibrillation include:

- P waves are not identifiable due to the atrial quivering, referred to as "f" waves, occurring at 350 to 750 beats per minute.
- PR intervals are not measurable.
- QT interval is not obtainable because the T waves are buried in the f waves.
- Irregularly irregular rhythm occurs, meaning that there is no pattern to the irregularity.
- f waves are ectopic beats.

The etiology, physical assessment findings, and treatment of atrial fibrillation are outlined in Chart 30–10 (p. 866).

Supraventricular Tachycardia

Supraventricular tachycardia (SVT) is a tachycardia that is generated somewhere above the ventricles. This general term encompasses all fast (tachy) rhythms with normal QRS complexes and heart rates greater than 100 beats per minute. Rhythms included under the

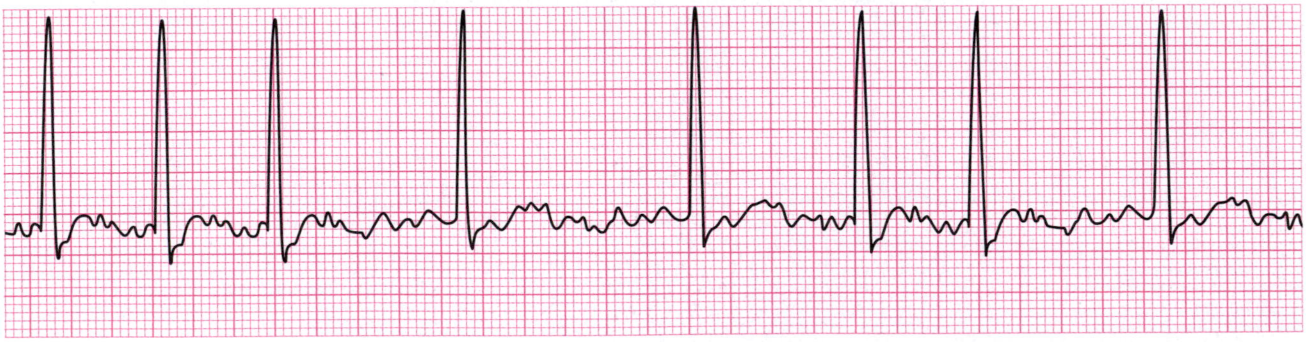

P Wave: None; PR Interval: None; QRS Complex: 0.10 second; QT Interval: unable to obtain; Heart Rate: Ventricular: 80 bpm; Rhythm: Irregular; Ectopic Beats: f waves.

FIGURE 30–21 ◆ Atrial fibrillation.

EVIDENCE-BASED PRACTICE Genetic Considerations of Atrial Fibrillation

Clinical Problem

More than 2 million people in the United States have atrial fibrillation (AF), the most common dysrhythmia reported. The incidence of AF increases with age; it is projected that by the year 2050, approximately 5 to 12 million Americans will have AF. There is significant morbidity and mortality related to AF, predominately because of the increased risk of thromboemoblic stroke and death. While AF is commonly associated with heart disease, such as valvular heart disease, research has demonstrated that "lone" atrial fibrillation has a substantial genetic basis and occurs with no underlying heart disease.

Research Findings

Since the completion of the Human Genome Study in the early 2000s, a number of genetic associations for AF have been evaluated. An early Mayo Clinic study in 2003 noted that up to 15% of lone AF could be attributed to genetic causes. In 2006, the Mayo Clinic reported that 40% of patients referred to their Arrhythmia Services had at least one relative with AF. In a Framingham Heart Study, patients were found to be twice as likely to develop AF if one of their parents had it. In a study done in Iceland in 2006, the authors reported that the risk of developing AF was almost doubled for those who were related to someone who also had AF. A 2009 meta-analysis by the National Heart Lung and Blood Institute assessed genome-wide association studies and found specific chromosome variants associated with AF. Extensive research is still needed to completely identify the genetic variants involved with AF to enhance early diagnosis and treatment.

Implications for Nursing Practice

Implications for nursing practice begin with nursing assessment. It is essential to specifically question the patient for a family history of AF. This is especially important if the patient is experiencing a new onset irregular pulse and clinical manifestations. The nurse must document any family history of AF in the patient's medical record. The nurse also must document the presence of other risk factors for the development of AF including:

Increasing age
Smoking
Caffeine
Excessive alcohol consumption
Extreme stress or fatigue
Heart failure, hypertension
Hyperthyroidism
Chronic lung disease, including emphysema, chronic obstructive pulmonary disease (COPD), asthma
Heart disease, including valvular heart disease, coronary artery disease, and cardiomyopathy

The patient and family need counseling about the increased risk for the development of AF, including instructions regarding the need for medical attention if additional symptoms occur. Patients with a family history need more frequent and diligent testing. Treatment for AF is outlined in Chart 30–10 (p. 866).

Critical Thinking Questions with answers can be found in the Osborn Student Resources at nursing.pearsonhighered.com.

Sources: American Heart Association (2011a); Campuzano & Brugada (2009); Lubitz, Yi, & Ellinor (2009); Mayo Clinic (2011).

Weblink: Atrial Fibrillation

Weblink: Hereditary Component of Atrial Fibrillation

SVT umbrella include sinus tachycardia, paroxysmal atrial tachycardia (PAT), and junctional tachycardia (JT). Clinicians use the term *supraventricular tachycardia* when it is impossible to identify the source of the tachycardia.

Usually this rhythm is benign and is self-limiting when the cause is removed. If sustained, loss of blood *fill time* (diastole) causes a drop in cardiac output. Prolonged episodes of supraventricular tachycardia increase myocardial oxygen demand and may result in a conversion to atrial flutter or fibrillation. Eventually, signs and symptoms of congestive heart failure will be present. Figure 30–22 ◆ presents a rhythm strip showing supraventricular tachycardia (SVT).

Significant ECG features of supraventricular tachycardia include:

- Heart rate is 100 to 250 beats per minute.
- P wave is not seen; it is buried in the QRS complex.
- PR interval is not discernable.
- QRS complex is within normal limits unless distorted by the buried P waves.
- QT interval is not obtainable because the T waves are buried.
- Heart rhythm may be regular or irregular due to varying conduction rates through the AV node.
- Ectopic beats may or may not be present, depending on the pacemaker site.

The etiology, physical assessment findings, and treatment of supraventricular tachycardia are outlined in Chart 30–10 (p. 866).

Atrioventricular Nodal Reentry Tachycardia

One phenomenon that can cause supraventricular tachycardia is atrioventricular nodal reentry tachycardia (AVNRT). Normally

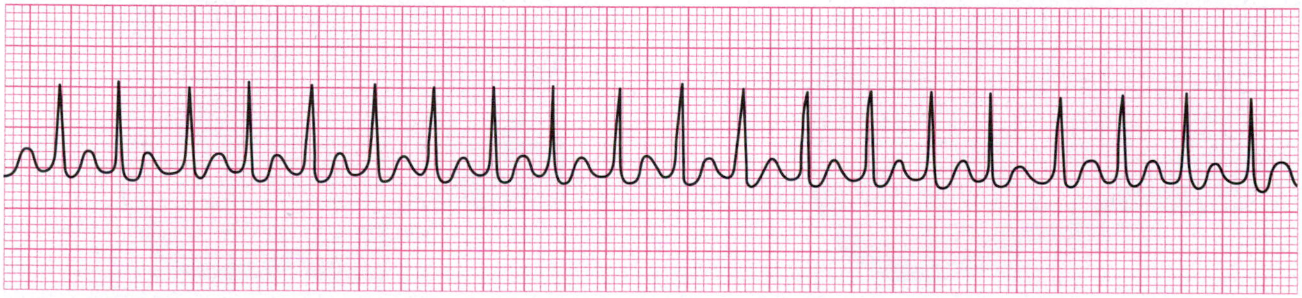

P Wave: None; PR Interval: None; QRS Complex: 0.10 second; QT Interval: unable to obtain; Heart Rate: ⟶ Atrial rate rapid, Ventricular: 200 bpm; Rhythm: Regular; Ectopic Beats: Depends on pacemaker site.

FIGURE 30–22 ◆ Supraventricular tachycardia (SVT).

people are born with only a single electrical pathway at the base of the right atrium where impulses travel to the AV node. However, some individuals are born with two separate electrical pathways leading to the AV node, each with its own respective properties. Each pathway has its own refractory period, one fast (beta) and one slow (alpha). The fast track has a long refractory period, and the slow track has a fast refractory period. Impulses travel the two separate pathways simultaneously. When the impulse begins down these two pathways, because of its speed, the one in the fast track stimulates the AV node and bundle of His, causing ventricular depolarization and a normal-width QRS complex. The fast track impulse also travels retrograde (backward transmission) back through the slow track, meeting the impulse coming down the slow track. When the two impulses meet, 99.9% of the time they cancel each other out and the rhythm is normal. If for any reason, such as the presence of a refractory period in the fast track, the fast track is unable to transmit the impulse, then the slow track transmits the impulse, causing depolarization of the ventricles. The QRS complex will still be within normal limits, but the PR interval will be longer than the ones coming from the fast track. This creates rhythm strips that have identical QRS complexes but two different PR interval lengths. These beats still are considered to be sinus complexes, as opposed to coming from another atrial ectopic focus. The PR interval length differences are a result of the conduction alternating intermittently between the two functioning tracks.

The AVNRT phenomenon occurs when a reentrant circuit or loop is created along the two pathways and the AV node (Figure 30–23◆). An early impulse, such as a PAC, hits the two pathways; the fast track is in refractory and therefore cannot accept the impulse, but the slow track can. The impulse travels from the slow track, to the AV node, and then retrograde up the fast track because this track has recovered, is no longer in a refractory state, and can accept the impulse. The impulses are now able to continue to cycle the circuit or loop and initiate ventricular depolarization at a fast rate; this is referred to as AVNRT (Baltazar, 2009).

It is estimated that AVNRT occurs in approximately several cases per thousand persons worldwide and in 60% of patients presenting with paroxysmal (sudden onset) SVT. Although more predominant in women, AVNRT may occur with individuals of any age and is common in young adults. Usually well tolerated, it often occurs in patients with no structural heart disease. Clinical manifestations are the same as with any tachy-dysrhythmia, although AVNRT may cause angina or myocardial infarction in patients with coronary artery disease. Prognosis for patients without heart disease is usually good (Baltazar, 2009). Treatment is aimed at breaking the reentrant cycle with the use

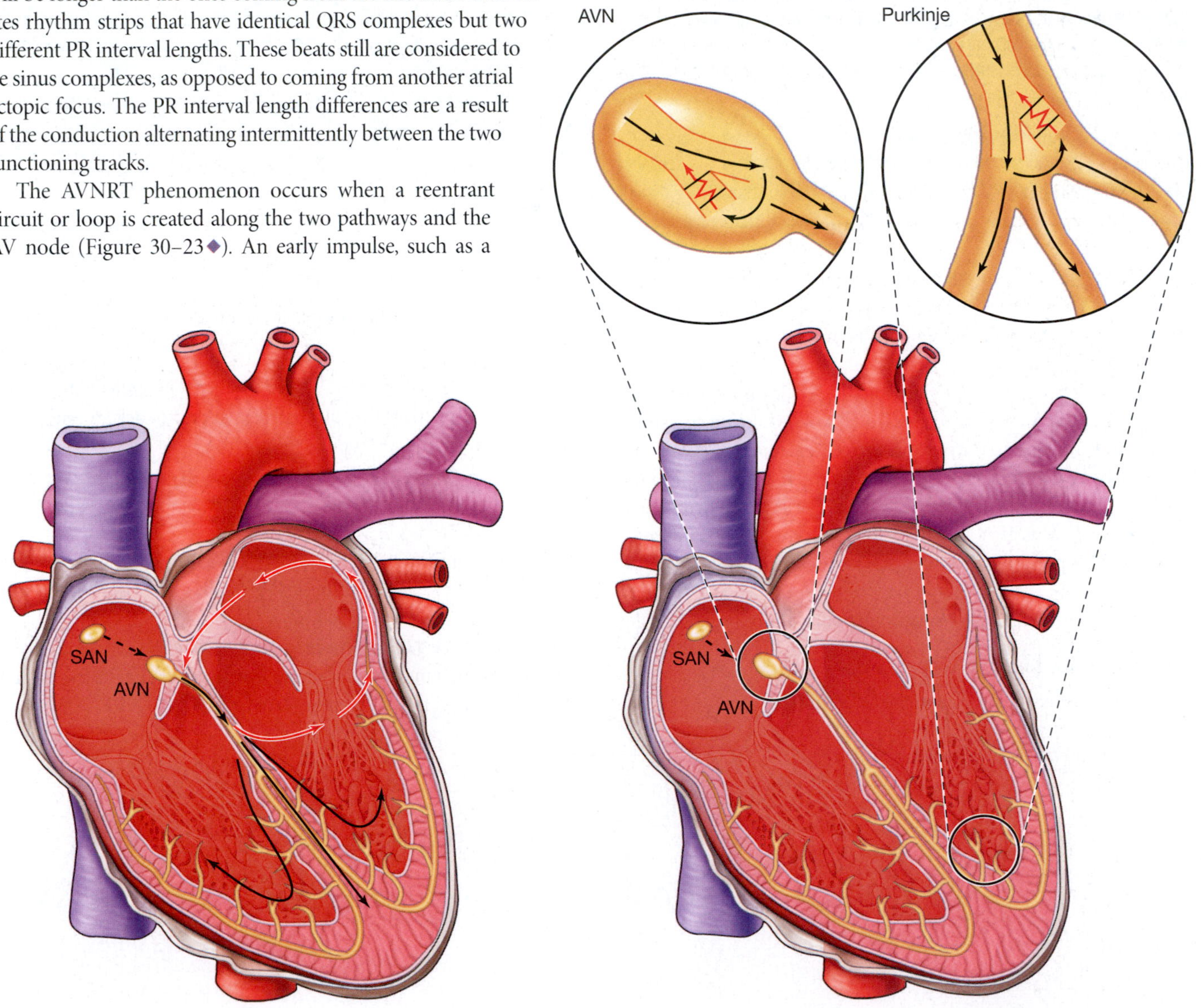

(a) Macro reentry circuit: antegrade through AV node and retrograde across an accessory pathway.

(b) Micro reentry at the cellular level in the AV node and Purkinje fibers.

FIGURE 30–23 ◆ Reentrant circuit.

of vagal maneuvers such as breath holding, stimulating gag reflex, and carotid sinus massage.

Wolff-Parkinson-White Syndrome

Wolff-Parkinson-White syndrome (WPW) is a genetic AV conduction disorder characterized by the presence of two AV conduction pathways, one normal and one abnormal. An impulse leaving the atrium may travel down one or the other pathway without any specific pattern. The abnormal pathway, called the Kent bundle, is composed of an extra muscle bundle made up of working myocardial tissue. This extra muscle bundle forms a connection between the atria and the ventricles outside the normal conduction system, referred to as an accessory pathway. This connection allows impulses coming from the atrium to bypass the normal AV connection. The hallmark feature on the ECG strip for the abnormal pathway is the presence of a delta wave, a slurred upstroke at the beginning of the QRS complex. The delta wave occurs when the impulse travels via the accessory pathway to the ventricles. Because the conduction is outside the normal conduction system, it takes longer for the impulse to travel through the ventricles, thus creating an abnormally wide, bizarre QRS complex (Baltazar, 2009).

Atrial flutter, atrial fibrillation, and supraventricular tachycardia that results in heart rates of greater than 250 beats per minute are common dysrhythmias in patients with WPW. The increased heart rate increases the workload and oxygen consumption of the heart, predisposing to heart failure, and therefore may cause sudden cardiac death. When the patient does not exhibit any dysrhythmias, but has the delta wave, this is called WPW pattern. When the patient becomes symptomatic or develops dysrhythmias, then the correct terminology is WPW syndrome. Significant ECG features of Wolff-Parkinson-White syndrome include:

- PR interval shortens to less than 0.12 second because the AV node is bypassed and delta waves appear just prior to the beginning of the R wave.
- QRS complex is greater than 0.12 second due to the delta waves.
- QT interval shortens if tachycardia occurs and lengthens with bradycardia.
- Heart rate is frequently tachycardic.
- Heart rhythm is regular, except during heart rate changes.

The etiology, physical assessment findings, and treatment of WPW syndrome are outlined in Chart 30–10 (p. 866).

Sick Sinus Syndrome

Sick sinus syndrome (SSS) encompasses a broad range of abnormalities, including disorders of impulse generation and conduction, failure of pacemakers, and a susceptibility to paroxysmal or chronic atrial tachycardia. This disorder also is referred to as sinoatrial disease. Sinoatrial dysfunction is caused by a severely depressed nonreliable SA node due to heart disease. Sick sinus syndrome can also be caused by certain cardiac drugs, such as cardiac glycosides, sympatholytic antihypertensive agents, beta-adrenergic blockers, calcium channel blockers, and membrane active antiarrhythmic agents. When the tachycardia occurs with SSS, increased oxygen consumption and workload for the myocardium result. Profound sinus bradycardia with SSS may progress to sinus pauses or arrest, thereby decreasing cardiac output. Figure 30–24◆ presents a rhythm strip showing sick sinus syndrome. Significant ECG features of sick sinus syndrome include:

- P waves may be present or absent depending on which dysrhythmia is occurring.
- PR interval varies due to changing P wave sites.
- QT interval varies due to rate changes.
- Heart rate may be rapid or slow, or a combination of both.
- Heart rhythm is irregular and highly variable.
- Ectopic beats may be present when a slow rate occurs.

The etiology, physical assessment findings, and treatment of sick sinus syndrome are outlined in Chart 30–10 (p. 866).

Nursing Management

When any dysrhythmia occurs, the nurse's responsibility is to assess the patient's response to the rhythm. This is especially true if it is a new onset dysrhythmia and/or if the dysrhythmia causes a drop in the cardiac output. The atrial dysrhythmias do not have the impact on cardiac output that the more serious ventricular dysrhythmias do, but any change in cardiac output may cause clinical manifestations and requires an in-depth assessment. The nurse evaluates the patient for the clinical manifestations of reduced cardiac output as outlined in Chart 30–9 (p. 865). The nurse needs to monitor vital signs and clinical manifestations frequently to assess tolerance of the rhythm, especially if it is sustained. The nurse must notify the health care provider, especially if this is a new rhythm, because medical intervention must be initiated to convert the rhythm back to normal sinus rhythm.

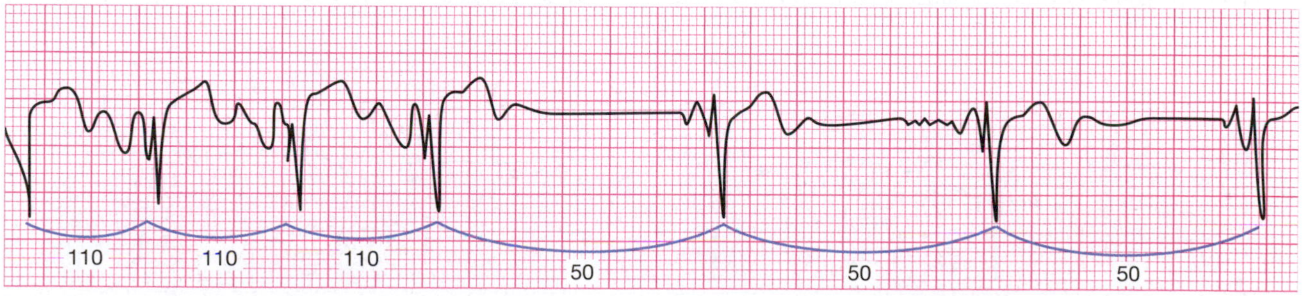

P Wave: Present, but variable configuration; PR Interval: 0.14 second; QRS Complex: 0.08 second; QT Interval: 0.40 second; Heart Rate: Atrial: 60 bpm, Ventricular: 60 bpm; Rhythm: Irregular; Ectopic Beats: May occur with slow rate.

FIGURE 30–24 ◆ Sick sinus syndrome.

Video: Dysrhythmia⊠Etiology and Pathophysiology
Video: Dysrhythmia Animation

Atrial flutter and fibrillation may occur as a transient dysrhythmia in healthy young individuals. If these conditions are chronic, they are typically associated with heart disease, including atrial muscle disease or atrial distention with disease of the sinus node. Atrial fibrillation also is seen in congenital heart disease. If the atrial flutter and/or atrial fibrillation are chronic conditions and normal sinus rhythm cannot be reestablished, the patient often is placed on an anticoagulant such as warfarin. This treatment is indicated because a fluttering/fibrillating atrium creates blood stasis, which increases the risk of clot formation. If these clots travel out of the atrium, they tend to lodge in the brain and, on rare occasions, in the lung, causing an alteration in normal function in these areas.

Treatment of atrial fibrillation/flutter may include cardioversion, which is the delivery of electrical voltage in order to stop unwanted electrical activity and allow the SA node to resume the heart's pacemaker. Cardioversion is discussed on page 886. This treatment increases the risk for myocardial infarction, cerebral vascular accident (CVA), and pulmonary embolus. The nurse needs to assess the patient post-cardioversion for clinical manifestations of these disorders. Myocardial infarction is discussed in detail in Chapter 32. Cardiovascular accident (CVA) is discussed in Chapter 22, and pulmonary embolus is discussed in Chapters 27 and 28.

Besides heart disease, there are other causes for atrial cardiac dysrhythmias that must be evaluated and treated (e.g., stress, pain, and anxiety). Appropriate treatments may include narcotics for pain relief or antianxiety medication to relieve stress and decrease anxiety. In some cases, the nurse may need only to sit and listen to the patient and provide emotional support.

Junctional Dysrhythmias

Junctional dysrhythmias, also referred to as nodal rhythms, result from an irritable focus in the junctional tissue that discharges before the SA node has had a chance to, or because the SA node has failed to fire; therefore, the junctional node becomes the secondary pacemaker. AV junctional dysrhythmias may occur if the impulse from the SA node is blocked as it exits the SA node or if it is not conducted through the atria. AV junctional dysrhythmias have a distinctive pattern on ECG tracings because the impulse is not initiated in the SA node. The impulse is initiated in the AV junctional tissue and must travel in a backward (retrograde) direction to activate the atria. Due to this retrograde conduction, the P wave is inverted or negatively deflected and may occur before, after, or buried in the QRS complex. Retrograde conduction means that the impulse originates in the AV junction so it stimulates the atria from the bottom up instead of the top down. The impulse simultaneously initiates both atrial and ventricular contractions. The location of the P wave, therefore, depends on the speed with which the impulses travel in both chambers. The QRS complex configuration is normal in appearance because the impulse travels the normal pathway from the AV junctional node through the ventricles. AV junctional dysrhythmias are not considered lethal or life threatening. As always, the most important indicator of the clinical significance of any dysrhythmia is the patient's response to or tolerance of the rhythm. The three AV junctional dysrhythmias discussed in this chapter are (1) junctional escape rhythm, (2) premature junctional contractions, and (3) junctional tachycardia.

Junctional Escape Rhythm

Junctional escape rhythm occurs when there is a problem with normal SA node function. The SA node either fails to produce an impulse, or the SA node's rate of firing falls below the intrinsic rate of the AV node. At this time the AV node will assume the role of the pacemaker. The ability of the AV node to assume this role is a safety measure in that it becomes the pacemaker for the heart when the SA node fails to do so. When an isolated beat from the AV junction occurs, it is called a junctional escape beat or complex; a series of beats is called a junctional rhythm. When a rhythm is generated from the junction, the rate is between 40 and 60 beats per minute. If the rate is greater than 60 but less than 100, it is referred to as an accelerated junctional rhythm. If the rate is greater than 100, typically it is called junctional tachycardia. Figures 30–25◆ and 30–26◆ are ECG rhythm strips that show junctional escape rhythm and accelerated junctional rhythm, respectively. Significant ECG features of junctional escape rhythms include:

- P wave is inverted, negatively deflected, due to retrograde conduction, and either occurs before, after, or buried in the QRS complex.
- PR interval is dependent on the location of the P wave; thus, the PR interval may or may not be present or normal.
- QRS complex is normal in duration and shape, unless distorted by a buried P wave.
- QT interval is within the normal range, unless impacted by the heart rate. It is prolonged with a slow heart rate or shortened with an increased heart rate.
- Heart rate is usually within the normal range for a rhythm generated from the AV junction and is 40 to 60 beats per minute. For an accelerated junctional rhythm, the rate is 60 to 100 beats per minute; for junctional tachycardia, the heart rate is greater than 100 beats per minute.

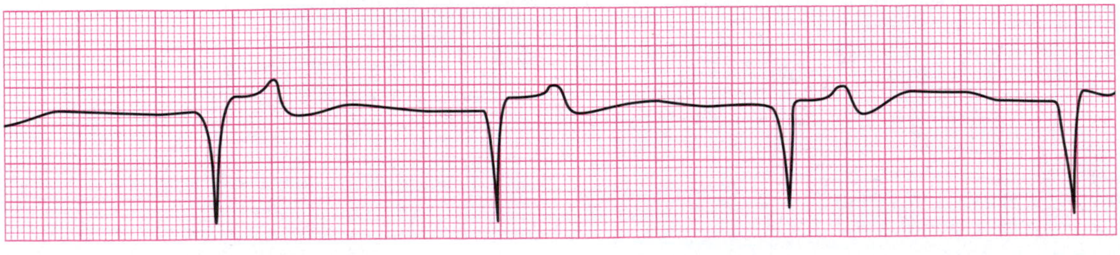

P Wave: None, or buried in QRS Complex; PR Interval: Not measurable; QRS Complex: 0.10 second; QT Interval: 0.40 second; Heart Rate: Atrial: Not measurable, Ventricular: 40 bpm; Rhythm: Regular; Ectopic Beats: None.

FIGURE 30–25 ◆ Junctional escape rhythm.

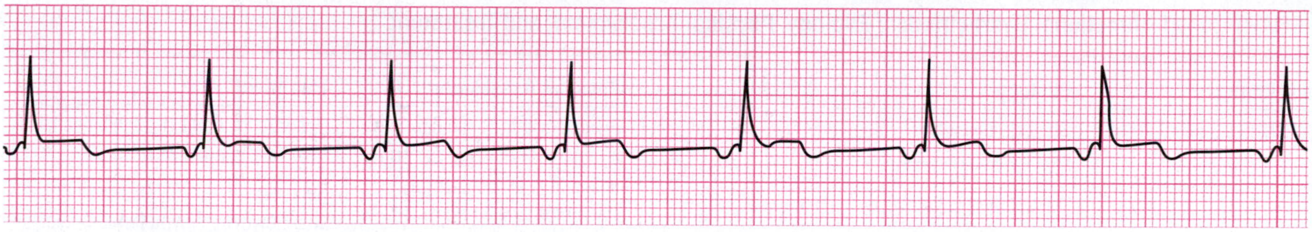

P Wave: Inverted and regular; PR Interval: 0.14–0.16 second; QRS Complex: 0.08 second: QT Interval: 0.44 second; Heart Rate: Atrial: 80 bpm, Ventricular: 80 bpm; Rhythm: Regular: Ectopic Beats: None.

FIGURE 30–26 ◆ Accelerated junctional rhythm.

- Heart rhythm is typically regular.
- Entire rhythm is composed of ectopic beats because they all come from the AV junction instead of the SA node. Other ectopic beats may occur with slow heart rate.

The etiology, physical assessment findings, and treatment of junctional escape rhythms are outlined in Chart 30–11.

Premature Junctional Contraction

A **premature junctional contraction (PJC)** originates as an ectopic beat that is initiated in the atrioventricular (AV) junction. It discharges before the next expected SA node impulse, causing simultaneous atrial and ventricular contraction to occur. This is not a dangerous dysrhythmia, although it does indicate that some degree of cardiac ischemia is occurring. Figure 30–27 ◆ presents a rhythm strip showing premature junctional contraction. Significant ECG features of premature junction contractions include:

- P wave is inverted and occurs before, after, or buried in the QRS complex.
- PR interval is dependent on the location of the P wave; thus, the PR interval may or may not be present or normal.
- QRS complex is normal in duration and shape, unless distorted by a buried P wave.
- QT interval also is normal unless impacted by the heart rate.
- Heart rate is that of the underlying rhythm.
- Heart rhythm is irregular when PJCs are present; or it may be described as regular with premature beats.
- Ectopic beat is the PJC.

The etiology, physical assessment findings, and treatment of PJCs are outlined in Chart 30–11.

Junctional Tachycardia

Junctional tachycardia is defined as an irritable focus in the AV junction that assumes the pacemaker role by discharging impulses more rapidly than the SA node. The term *junctional tachycardia* sometimes is used interchangeably with the term *accelerated junctional rhythm*. This rhythm produces a junctional rate of over 60 beats per minute. Significant ECG features of junctional tachycardia include:

- Heart rate is usually greater than 60 beats per minute.
- P wave is inverted and occurs before, after, or buried in the QRS complex.
- PR interval depends on the location of the P wave; thus, the PR interval may or may not be present or normal.
- QRS complex is normal in duration and shape, unless distorted by a buried P wave.
- QT interval shortens due to increased heart rate.
- Heart rhythm is essentially regular. It may become irregular as the rate increases.
- Entire rhythm is composed of ectopic beats because they all come from the AV junction instead of the SA node.

The etiology, physical assessment findings, and treatment of junctional tachycardia are outlined in Chart 30–11.

Nursing Management

Like atrial dysrhythmias, junctional dysrhythmias generally are not life threatening. However, the decreased and/or increased heart rate does have an impact on cardiac output. This is especially true in the presence of heart disease when the heart is unable to increase the

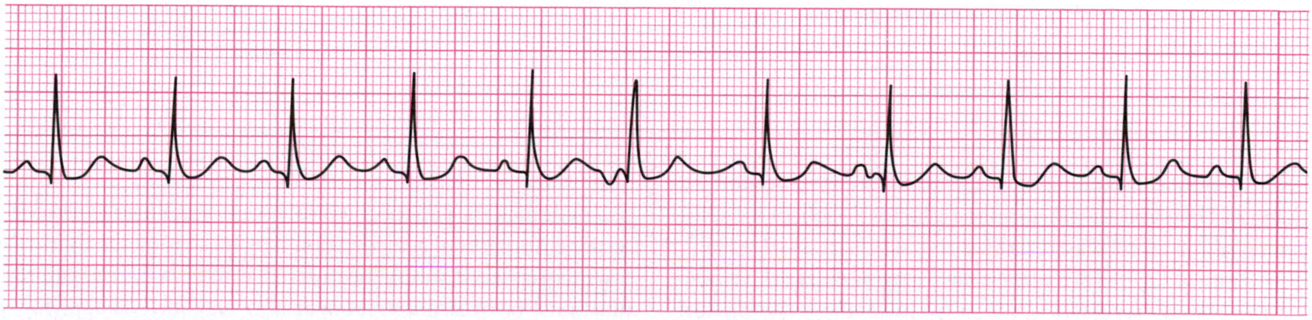

P Wave: Present and regular except for premature beat; PR Interval: 0.16 second; QRS Complex: 0.08 second; second; Heart Rate: Atrial: 110 bpm, Ventricular: 110 bpm; Rhythm: Regular except for premature beats: Ectopic Beats: None

FIGURE 30–27 ◆ Premature junctional contraction (PJC).

CHART 30–11 Junctional Dysrhythmias: Etiology, Physical Assessment, and Treatment

Dysrhythmia	Etiology	Physical Assessment	Treatment
Junctional escape rhythm	SA node disease Myocardial infarction Hypoxia and ischemia Heart failure Increased vagal tone Certain cardiac drugs (e.g., digoxin, beta-adrenergic blockers, and calcium channel blockers) Sinus bradycardia Digoxin toxicity Hyperkalemia Valve disease	Pulse: Rhythm is regular with a usual rate of 40 to 60 bpm unless it is an accelerated rhythm of > 100 bpm. If cardiac output is decreased, the clinical manifestations described in Chart 30–9 may occur.	Observe for other dysrhythmias if a slow rate is present. Generally this condition is asymptomatic; however, if symptomatic, typical treatment includes: Oxygen Drug therapy (atropine, dopamine) Pacemaker Cardioversion
Premature junctional contraction (PJC)	Irritability of the AV junctional tissue caused by: SA node disease Myocardial infarction Sinus bradycardia Mitral stenosis Mitral valve prolapse Cor pulmonale Hypoxia Ischemia Infectious diseases Increased vagal tone Increased sympathetic tone Electrolyte imbalances Digoxin Stimulants Stress Anxiety May precede AV block	Pulse: Irregular. BP: Normal unless PJCs occur frequently enough to decrease cardiac output.	Rarely causes symptoms, thus typically not treated. Find and treat the underlying cause, if possible. If it initiates a more serious dysrhythmia, such as tachycardia, therapy becomes more aggressive, contingent on the type of dysrhythmia. If occurring frequently, more than 5 times per minute, they can drop cardiac output, and predispose the patient to other dysrhythmias. Oxygen Drugs such as stimulants, sympathomimetics, and digitalis may be discontinued.
Paroxysmal junctional tachycardia	May occur at any age with no prior history of underlying heart disease Digoxin toxicity (common cause) Inferior wall myocardial infarction Myocarditis Ischemia Untoward response to open heart surgery Frequent ingestion of stimulants Anxiety Increased catecholamine secretion	Pulse: Rapid, with patient experiencing a fluttering sensation. BP: Lower than usual due to decreased cardiac output. If cardiac output is decreased, the clinical manifestations described in Chart 30–9 may occur.	Find and treat the cause, as junctional tachycardia may be a predisposition to lethal dysrhythmias, heart failure, and shock. Vagal maneuvers may be applied. Oxygen. Drug therapy initiated; includes amiodarone or beta-adrenergic blockers. Cardioversion may be initiated if necessary.

force of the muscle contraction sufficiently to compensate for the rate changes. Therefore, the nurse must evaluate the patient for clinical manifestations of decreased cardiac output (Chart 30–9, p. 865). When rhythm is slow, other ectopic foci may attempt to become the heart's pacemaker; therefore, the nurse must assess the rhythm for other aberrancies. The nurse needs to notify the health care provider to determine cause and treatment, especially if it is a new onset dysrhythmia. It is essential that the nurse assist the health care provider in determining the cause and treatment of dysrhythmias. Since some prescribed medications (e.g., digoxin) cause significant dysrhythmias, the patient's medical history should be reviewed to determine if a particular medication may be causing the dysrhythmia. Serum drug levels should be ordered as indicated. For symptomatic junctional tachycardia, treatment also may include applying vagal maneuvers, initiating drug therapy, and completing cardioversion if necessary. As always, the nurse needs to report any significant rhythm change or the appearance of new onset dysrhythmias to the health care provider.

Due to the clinical manifestations of these dysrhythmias, the patient and family may experience anxiety. The nurse must assess and treat patient and family anxiety with supportive measures, such as listening to the patient's concerns, offering reassurance, providing a calm environment, and medicating for anxiety and pain relief as appropriate.

Conduction Block Dysrhythmias

Cardiac conduction block dysrhythmias occur due to an interruption in the continuity of the cardiac electrical conduction system. This discontinuity is caused by a loss of blood supply to the conduction system as a result of ischemic heart disease or coronary artery disease. Heart blocks are classified according to the degree of the block, noting either partial or complete obstruction of the electrical conduction pathway. Conduction block dysrhythmias may be either permanent or transient, and minor or significant. The clinical significance of an AV block depends on the degree (severity) of the block, the rate of the escape pacemaker (junctional vs. ventricular), and the patient's response to that ventricular rate. Four types of heart block dysrhythmias are discussed next: first-degree AV block; Mobitz I/Wenckebach/Type I second-degree heart block; Mobitz II second-degree block; and third-degree AV block (complete).

First-Degree AV Block

First-degree AV block represents a conduction disturbance in which electrical impulses flow normally from the SA node through the atria but are delayed at the AV node. There is a prolongation or slowing of conduction rather than an actual block. Because of this consistent delay the PR interval is greater than 0.20 second, making it abnormal. First-degree AV block is not actually a dysrhythmia; rather, its presence indicates only a delay at the AV node, not a definite block. Figure 30–28 ◆ presents a rhythm strip showing first-degree AV block. Significant ECG features of first-degree AV block include:

- P waves are present and normal in size and shape.
- PR interval is prolonged, greater than 0.20 second, but constant.
- QRS duration usually is normal.
- QT interval is normal unless there is an abnormal rate.
- Heart rate is usually within the normal range.
- Heart rhythm is regular.

The etiology, physical assessment findings, and treatment of first-degree AV blocks are outlined in Chart 30–12 (p. 876).

Mobitz I/Wenckebach/Type I Second-Degree Heart Block

The terms *Mobitz I/Wenckebach/Type 1 second-degree heart block* are used interchangeably to refer to the same abnormality. This abnormality is depicted as a progressive prolongation of the electrical impulse delay in the AV node until there is a complete loss of the QRS complex, and therefore no ventricular contraction. This dysrhythmia is characterized by progressive lengthening of the PR interval until a QRS complex fails to appear after a P wave. **Mobitz I/Wenckebach** is one of the two types of second-degree block that occurs in the AV node. Figure 30–29 ◆ (p. 878) presents a rhythm strip showing Mobitz I/Wenckebach dysrhythmia. Significant ECG features of Mobitz I/Wenckebach dysrhythmia include:

- P waves are present and precede the QRS complexes.
- PR interval progressively prolongs until there is a dropped QRS complex, and then the progressive prolongation begins again.
- QRS complexes are normal in shape and duration.
- QT interval is within normal limits, unless no QRS complex occurs.
- Atrial heart rate is normal and regular; ventricular heart rate is less than that of the atrial rate.
- Atrial rhythm is regular; the ventricular rhythm is irregular.

The etiology, physical assessment findings, and treatment of Mobitz I/Wenckebach/Type I second-degree heart block are outlined in Chart 30–12 (p. 876).

Mobitz II Second-Degree Block

Mobitz II/second-degree block results from an intermittent block of the AV node, the bundle of His, or bundle branches. This dysrhythmia occurs when this block causes an intermittent interruption in the electrical conduction system near or below the AV node, which prevents the sinus or atrial impulses from getting to the ventricles. On the ECG strip, the P wave (atrial contraction) is present at regular intervals because the SA node is generating impulses in a normal manner. When the block occurs, however, the P wave is not followed by a QRS complex. An AV conduction ratio of 2 Ps for every 1 QRS; 3 Ps for every 1 QRS, or greater is common, with or without a bundle branch block. In other words there are 2, 3, or 4 P waves for every QRS complex, which may result in enough dropped QRSs to impact cardiac output significantly. Therefore, Mobitz II is a more serious dysrhythmia than either first-degree AV block or Mobitz I (Wenckebach/Type I second-degree heart block)

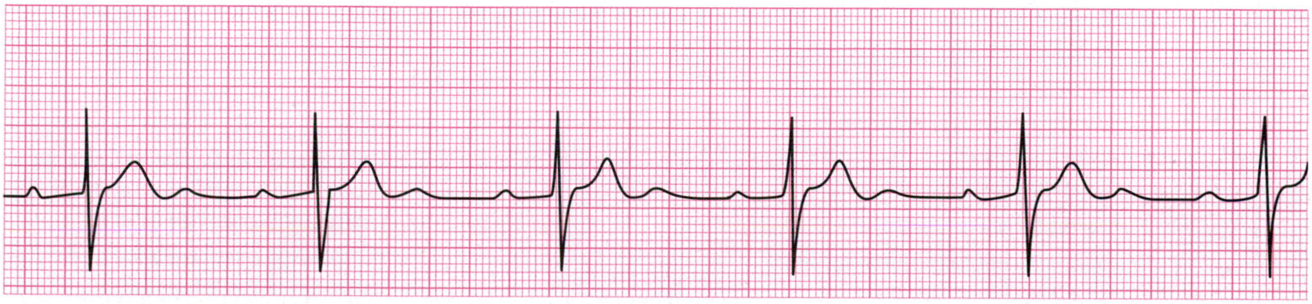

P Wave: Present and regular; PR Interval: 0.24 second; QRS Complex: 0.06 second; QT Interval: 0.40 second; Heart Rate: Atrial: 60 bpm, Ventricular: 60 bpm; Rhythm: Regular; Ectopic Beats: None.

FIGURE 30–28 ◆ First-degree AV block.

Video: Dysrhythmia—Etiology and Pathophysiology

Video: Dysrhythmia Animation

because of the impact on the cardiac output and an increased risk of progression to third-degree block or complete heart block. Figure 30–30◆ (p. 878) presents a rhythm strip showing Mobitz II/second-degree block. Significant ECG features of Mobitz II/second-degree block include:

- QRS complexes are intermittently absent and may be normal to prolonged when present. They are usually prolonged due to bundle branch block.
- P waves are present and regular.
- PR intervals are constant with conducted beats.
- QT intervals are within normal limits.
- Atrial heart rate is usually normal; ventricular heart rate is less than the atrial rate.
- Atrial rhythm is regular; ventricular rhythm may be regular or irregular. The ventricular rhythm is irregular when the AV block is intermittent.
- Ectopic beats may be present due to the slow heart rate.

The etiology, physical assessment findings, and treatment of Mobitz II heart block are outlined in Chart 30–12.

Third-Degree AV Block (Complete)

Third-degree AV block, or **complete heart block,** is the independent excitation and contraction of the atria and ventricles due to the inability of any atrial impulses to reach the ventricles. In other words, the top and bottom of the heart are not communicating: They are beating independently. This dysrhythmia also is referred to as

CHART 30–12 AV Block Dysrhythmias: Etiology, Physical Assessment, and Treatment

Dysrhythmia	Etiology	Physical Assessment	Treatment
First-degree AV block	May occur without any underlying heart disease May occur in athletes Occurs in about 13% of the population Drug reactions to digoxin, beta-blockers, and CA channel blockers Cardiac-related causes include: Ischemia Myocardial infarction Rheumatic heart disease Coronary artery disease	Pulse: Within normal limits. BP: Within normal limits.	This is not a dangerous rhythm in itself and usually is asymptomatic. May progress to a more advanced heart block, especially in the presence of a myocardial infarction. Observe closely and place on an ECG monitor to detect additional signs and symptoms.
Mobitz I/ Wenckebach/ Type I second-degree heart block	Conduction delay within the AV node Most commonly associated with AV nodal ischemia secondary to occlusion of the right coronary artery Other causes may be: Myocardial infarction Inferior/right ventricular structural heart disease or an anatomical abnormality Myocarditis Transient side effect of open heart surgery Increased vagal activity Drug toxicity (e.g., digoxin)	Pulse: Irregular. BP: May be decreased with frequently dropped beats due to decreased cardiac output. If cardiac output is decreased, the following clinical manifestations may occur: Angina Syncope Generalized weakness Dizziness Shortness of breath Altered mental state may be present, although rare.	This is often a transient rhythm and will revert to a normal rhythm without treatment. Usually asymptomatic because the ventricular rate often remains nearly normal and cardiac output is not significantly affected. If symptomatic, and is a result of medications, they should be withheld. If the heart rate is slow and serious, clinical manifestations such as low BP, angina, or shortness of breath occur, atropine or temporary pacing is considered. When occurs in conjunction with acute myocardial infarction, observe for increasing AV block.
Mobitz II second-degree AV block	Septal wall necrosis Acute inferior or right ventricular MI Myocarditis Advanced coronary artery disease (general ischemia) Electrolyte imbalance Digitalis toxicity Reaction to amiodarone, beta-blockers, or calcium channel blockers	Pulse: Slow and typically irregular, depending on ventricular response. BP: Decreased due to low cardiac output. If cardiac output is decreased, the following clinical manifestations may occur: Angina Syncope Generalized weakness Dizziness Shortness of breath Altered mental state may be present.	Often considered an emergent situation. The health care provider should be notified at once. May progress to a third-degree AV block and ventricular asystole; thus, a standby cardiac pacemaker is indicated for asymptomatic patients, and temporary cardiac pacing is required for symptomatic patients. For sustained permanent block, a permanent pacemaker is inserted.

(*continued*)

CHART 30–12 AV Block Dysrhythmias: Etiology, Physical Assessment, and Treatment, *continued*

Dysrhythmia	Etiology	Physical Assessment	Treatment
Third-degree AV block (complete)	Ischemic damage Septal wall necrosis Acute inferior or right ventricular MI due to the effect of vagal tone and ischemia on the AV node Acute anterior MI Myocarditis Coronary artery disease Cardiomyopathies Cardiac muscle diseases Rheumatic heart disease Drug toxicity, reaction to amiodarone, beta-blockers, or calcium channel blockers Electrolyte imbalance Rheumatic heart disease Congenital condition usually located at the level of the AV junction	Pulse: Slow and usually irregular. BP: Lower than usual. If cardiac output is decreased, the following clinical manifestations may occur: Angina Syncope Generalized weakness Dizziness Shortness of breath Altered mental state may be present.	Treatment is essential as third-degree block is potentially lethal. If an AV junctional or ventricular escape pacemaker does not take over following a sudden onset of third-degree AV block, asystole will occur. Clinical manifestations depend on the ventricular heart rate, especially for slow rates. If the QRS is narrow and the patient is symptomatic, initial management is atropine and/or transcutaneous pacing. If the QRS is wide and the patient is symptomatic, transcutaneous pacing is started. A temporary pacemaker is inserted, and may be followed by a permanent pacemaker.
Bundle branch block (BBB)	Causes vary depending on whether it is the right or left BBB Right BBB may be present in healthy individuals with apparently normal hearts without any apparent underlying cause Common pathological causes include: Coronary artery disease Cardiac tumors Cardiomyopathy Myocarditis Atrial septal defect Cardiac surgery Congenital RBBB Acute anterioseptal MI Acute pulmonary embolism or infarction Acute heart failure Unlike RBBB, LBBB always indicates a diseased heart and generally is more common in individuals with diseased hearts Common causes include: Hypertensive heart disease Cardiomyopathy Myocarditis Syphilitic, rheumatic, and congenital heart disease Cardiac tumors Idiopathic degenerative disease of the electrical conduction system Aberrant ventricular conduction associated with supraventricular premature contractions and tachycardia	Pulse: Within normal limits. BP: Within normal limits.	Specific treatment usually is not indicated if it is present alone and is not the result of an acute MI. Temporary cardiac pacing is indicated for the treatment of a right or left bundle branch block under the following conditions: Results from an acute MI, is complicated by a first- or second-degree AV block, or both, especially in the setting of an acute MI if the block progresses to a complete AV block.

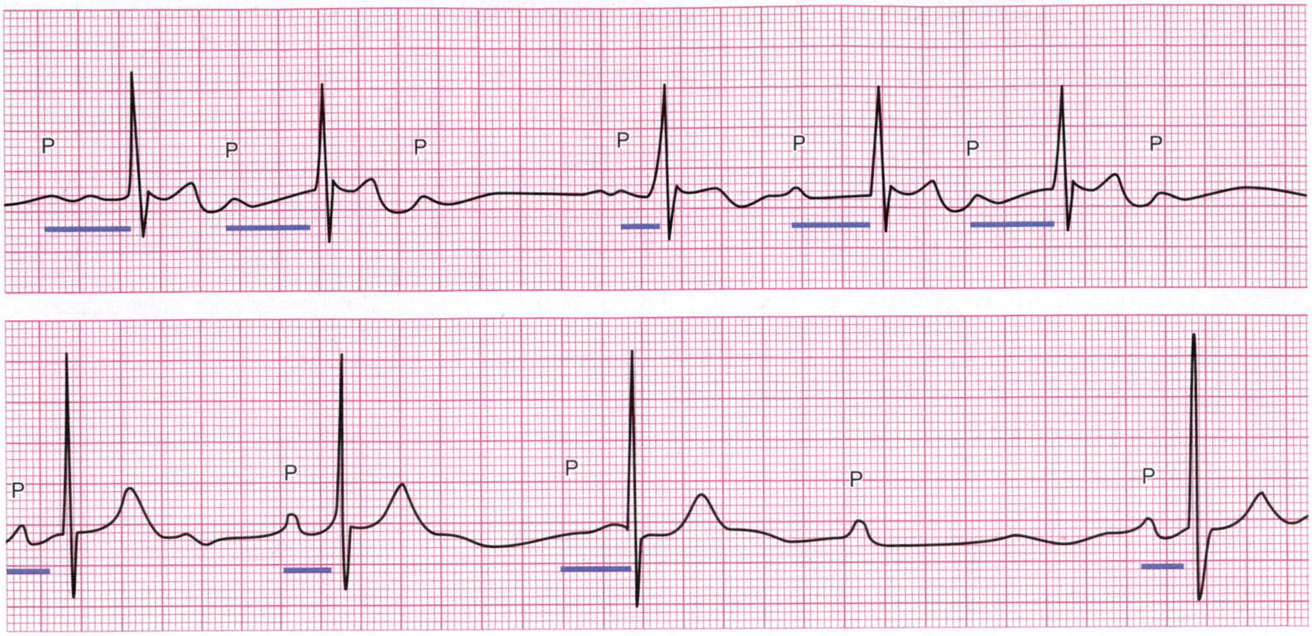

P Waves: Present and regular; PR Interval: Progressively prolonged until one P wave is not conducted and the sequence begins again; QRS Complex: 0.10 second; QT Interval: 0.42–0.60 second; Heart Rate: Atrial: 70 bpm, Ventricular 50 bpm; Rhythm: Atrial: Regular, Ventricular: Irregular due to dropped beat; Ectopic Beats: None. Conclusion: Mobitz I/Wenckeback Second-Degree Heart Block.

FIGURE 30–29 ◆ Mobitz I/Wenckebach/second-degree heart block.

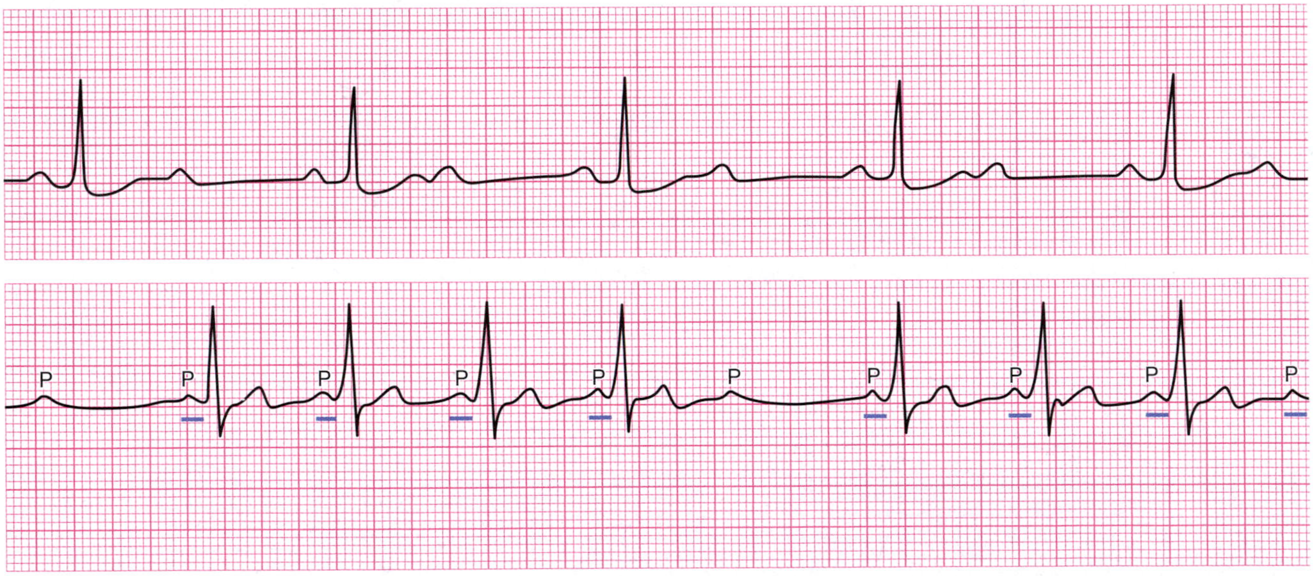

P Waves: Present and regular; PR Interval: 0.24 second; QRS Complex: 0.06 second; QT Interval: 0.48 second; Heart Rate: Atrial: 100 bpm, Ventricular 50 bpm; Rhythm: Atrial: Regular, Ventricular: Irregular due to dropped beat; Ectopic Beats: None.

FIGURE 30–30 ◆ Mobitz II/s econd-degree heart block.

AV dissociation because of the independent function of the atria and the ventricles. The SA node fires at regular intervals, producing P waves at a normal rate of 60 to 100 beats per minute, while the ventricles are paced by either a pacemaker site in the ventricles themselves or in the junctional tissue. If the QRS complex is narrow, the pacemaker is in the junctional tissue with a rate of 40 to 60 beats per minute. However, if the QRS complex is wide, the pacemaker is in the Purkinje network and the heart rate ranges from 20 to 40 beats per minute; this is referred to as an idioventricular rhythm. Complete AV block associated with an inferior myocardial infarction is thought to be a block in the bundle of His, and often occurs after progression from first-degree AV block or second-degree AV block, type I. Third-degree heart block is the most serious type of heart block because it may progress to asystole (a complete cessation of electrical activity), and the slow ventricular heart rate results in decreased cardiac output. Since the ventricular rhythm may not be able to sustain adequate cardiac output, third-degree heart block is referred to as a lethal dysrhythmia. Figure 30–31◆ presents a rhythm strip showing third-degree or complete heart block. Significant ECG features of third-degree heart block include the following:

- Atrial and ventricular rhythms are independent of one another (dissociated). Atrial rhythm usually is regular, depending on the underlying sinus, atrial, or junctional rhythm. Ventricular rhythm may be regular or irregular.
- P waves are present and regular, but there is no relationship to QRS complexes.
- PR interval is absent.
- QRS complex may be narrow with a junctional rhythm or wide with an idioventricular rhythm.
- QT interval may change with the rate change, but it is not directly affected.
- Atrial heart rate is regular, 60 to 100 beats per minute; nodal rate is 40 to 60 beats per minute; and ventricular rate is 20 to 40 beats per minute.
- Atrial and ventricular rhythms are independent of one another (dissociated). Atrial rhythm usually is regular, depending on underlying sinus, atrial, or junctional rhythm. Ventricular rhythm may be regular or irregular.
- Ectopic beats usually are present due to slow rate.

The etiology, physical assessment findings, and treatment of Mobitz II heart block are outlined in Chart 30–12 (p. 876).

Bundle Branch Block

Bundle branch block, also referred to as intraventricular conduction defect, is a discontinuity of conduction, complete or incomplete, in one branch of the bundle of His that affects normal transmission of the impulse through the ventricles. When one bundle is blocked, the ventricles depolarize asynchronously. Bundle branch block is characterized by a delay of excitation to one ventricle; therefore, an abnormal spread of electrical activity through the ventricles occurs. This delayed conduction causes a widening of the QRS complex to more than 0.12 second. When measuring the QRS complex, it is necessary to observe the axis of the complex to determine whether it is right or left bundle branch block. Figure 30–32 ◆ presents a rhythm strip showing a bundle branch block. Significant ECG features of bundle branch block include:

- QRS complex is more than 0.12 second if a complete bundle branch block is present. P waves are present and regular.
- PR interval is 0.12 to 0.20 second.
- QRS measuring 0.10 to 0.12 second is called an incomplete right or left bundle branch block.
- QT interval is within normal limits.
- Heart rate is 60 to 100 beats per minute.
- Heart rhythm is regular.

The etiology, physical assessment findings, and treatment of bundle branch block are outlined in Chart 30–12 (p. 876).

Nursing Management

The type of heart block determines the severity of the dysrhythmia and, therefore, nursing responsibilities. As with any dysrhythmia, the nurse must evaluate the patient's response to the new rhythm. Because first-degree heart block and bundle branch block in isolation do not impact cardiac output, patients are not symptomatic. With first-degree heart block, the nurse must observe the cardiac monitor for any changes in the rhythm that indicate a progression to a more severe type of heart block.

Mobitz I/Wenckebach often does not require treatment, but ECG monitoring and patient assessment are necessary because this type of block may lead to either a more serious Mobitz II or a complete heart block. The nurse must check the monitor frequently to identify potential changes. As with any new dysrhythmia, the nurse needs to report Mobitz I/Wenckebach to the health care provider.

The onset of Mobitz II and complete heart block are emergent situations that require immediate intervention. Mobitz II is described as a "treacherous and unpredictable" rhythm that can

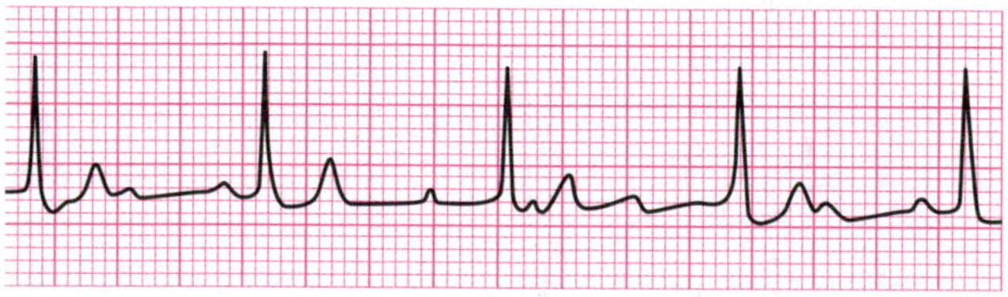

P Waves: Present and regular; PR Interval: None; QRS Complex: 0.12 second; QT Interval: 0.38 second; Heart Rate: Atrial: 90 bpm, Ventricular: 40–50 bpm; Rhythm: Regular; Ectopic Beats: None.

FIGURE 30–31 ◆ Third-degree (complete) heart block.

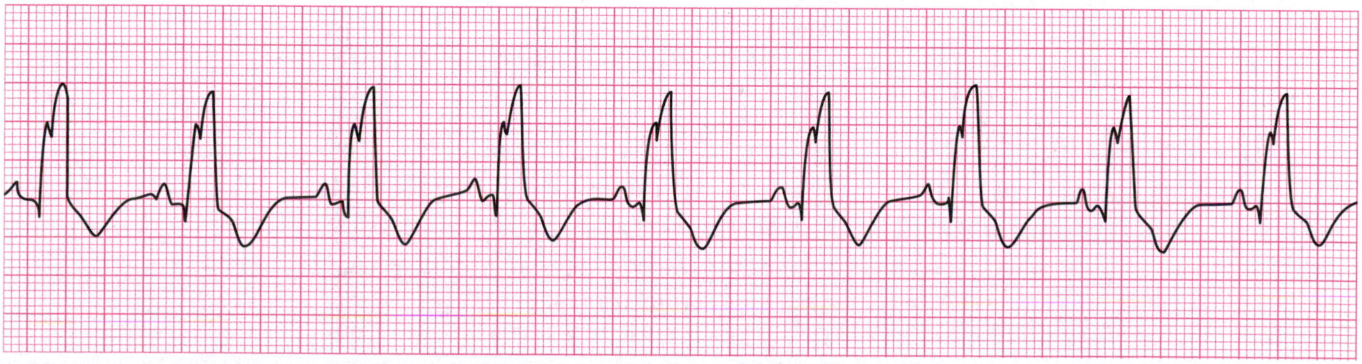

P Wave: Normal sinus rhythm; PR Interval: 0.16 second; QRS Complex: 0.20 second; QT Interval: 0.40 second. Heart Rate: Atrial: 90 bpm, Ventricular: 90 bpm; Rhythm: Atrial: Regular, Ventricular: Regular; Ectopic Beats: None.

FIGURE 30–32 ◆ Bundle branch block.

Video: Dysrhythmia Animation
Video: Dysrhythmia—Etiology and Pathophysiology

deteriorate to become a complete heart block. If untreated, these rhythms may progress to cardiac asystole and sudden death. At any indication of rhythm changes indicative of Mobitz II or complete heart block, the nurse should notify the health care provider at once. The nurse should prepare for a temporary pacemaker insertion (p. 892), which generally is indicated for these types of dysrhythmias. A permanent pacemaker may be necessary if the block persists. When working with monitored patients, it is the nurse's responsibility to be familiar with equipment location and operation.

Safety Alert *Signs and symptoms of third-degree AV block are the same as those in symptomatic sinus bradycardia. Third-degree AV block can appear more ominous on the ECG monitor, especially when associated with wide and bizarre QRS complexes. If an AV junctional or ventricular escape pacemaker rhythm does not take over the pacing of the heart following the sudden onset of third-degree AV block, ventricular asystole will occur. Temporary cardiac pacemaker is required immediately for treatment of symptomatic third-degree block with wide QRS complexes. The nurse must report this rhythm immediately to the health care provider in order to initiate treatment before a significant drop in cardiac output occurs.*

Ventricular Dysrhythmias

Ventricular dysrhythmias are caused by ectopic or irritable foci in the walls of the ventricles. The pacemaker cells in the ventricles may, in certain circumstances, serve as the heart's pacemaker. When the SA node fails or the impulse does not get through the AV node, the ventricles take over the pacing role. In this situation, an electrical impulse may be instigated from both the bundle of His and the Purkinje network. The intrinsic ventricular rate is only 20 to 40 beats per minute; therefore, cardiac output is severely compromised. Also, if the atrium is not contracting there is no atrial kick, causing further decrease in cardiac output. Because the rhythm originates in the ventricle, there is no P wave; because it is an abnormal conduction pathway, the QRS is wide and distorted. Ventricular dysrhythmias are considered to be very serious dysrhythmias mainly due to their impact on cardiac output. The various types of ventricular dysrhythmias are discussed next: premature ventricular contraction, ventricular tachycardia, Torsade de pointes, ventricular fibrillation, pulseless electrical activity, and asystole.

Premature Ventricular Contraction

A **premature ventricular contraction (PVC)** is caused by an irritable focus within the ventricle that discharges before the next sinus impulse, stimulating the ventricle directly and causing a contraction. PVCs are more likely to occur during bradycardia when there is more time for them to emerge. Premature ventricular contractions (PVCs) are individual beats—one ectopic beat, not a rhythm. PVCs have a wide and bizarre QRS complex that is more than 0.12 second in length. Because the activation begins outside the normal conduction system, it takes longer to travel the ventricular conduction pathways, thereby prolonging the QRS length. PVCs are followed by a full compensatory pause, meaning the SA node rate and rhythm are unaffected by the PVC. In other words, the rate prior to the PVC resumes, following the PVC. A compensatory pause is measured by:

- Measuring the two beats preceding the PVC
- Moving the calipers along, and marking where the next beat should have fallen
- Then placing the calipers on the spot where the beat should have occurred and measuring the distance to the next beat. There should not be a change in the cadence of the rhythm.

The full compensatory pause is one of the factors used when evaluating and diagnosing PVCs. To distinguish PVCs from atrial and junctional ectopic beats, the full compensatory pause must be present. Typically, atrial and junctional ectopic beats do not have a full compensatory pause; they are said to be noncompensatory or partially compensatory, meaning that there is a rhythm change following these dysrhythmias. Figure 30–33 ◆ presents a rhythm strip showing premature ventricular contractions (PVCs) with a full compensatory pause.

Unifocal and Multifocal PVCs

Premature ventricular contractions (PVCs) occur in various patterns. Each pattern differs in its severity and prognosis. First, if the PVC configuration (size and shape) remains the same consistently, the dysrhythmia is coming from one irritable focus in the ventricle. These are referred to as unifocal PVCs. If PVCs occur with every other beat, the rhythm is referred to as **bigeminy.** If PVCs occur every third beat, the rhythm is called **trigeminy;** occurrence every fourth beat is called **quadrigeminy.** The more often the PVC occurs, the greater the drop in cardiac output and, therefore, the more serious the

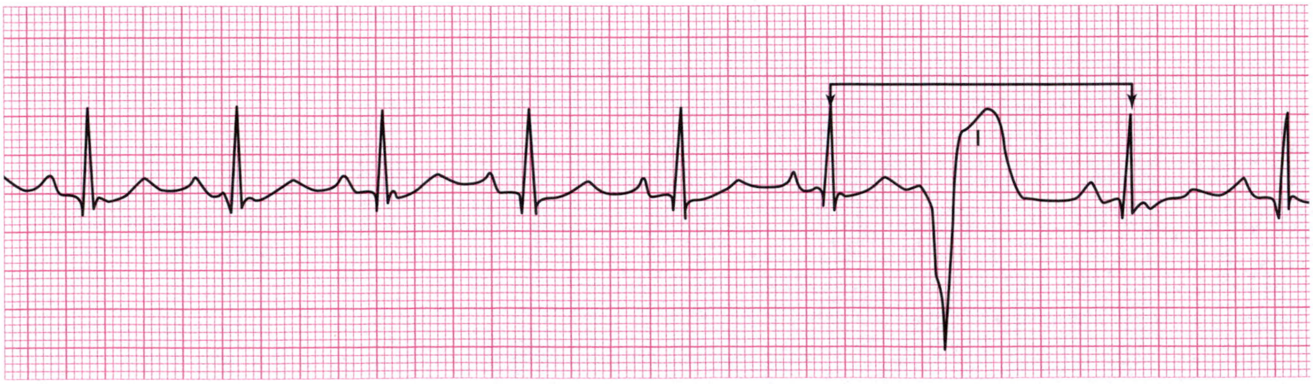

P Wave: Present and regular, except where absent (PVC); PR Interval: 0.20 second; QRS Complex: 0.08 second; QT Interval: 0.42 second; Heart Rate: Atrial: 70 bpm, Ventricular: 80 bpm; Rhythm: Atrial: Regular, Ventricular: Regular except for premature beat; Ectopic Beats: One PVC.

FIGURE 30–33 ◆ Premature ventricular contractions (PVCs).

dysrhythmia. The decrease in cardiac output is due to the premature occurrence of the rhythm, which does not allow for sufficient diastole or ventricle filling time. As cardiac muscle ischemia increases, the muscle becomes more irritable, causing PVCs to be initiated in more than one place in the ventricle. This is referred to as multifocal PVCs. When multifocal, the morphology (shape) of the QRSs varies. Multifocal PVCs are more serious than unifocal PVCs because they indicate that there is more ischemia occurring in the myocardium.

PVC Patterns

When PVCs occur for two or more consecutive beats, the pattern is referred to as paired salvos. When there are three or more consecutive PVCs salvos, it is defined as ventricular tachycardia. Ventricular tachycardia may be life threatening due to the severe drop in cardiac output.

The most serious or dangerous time for a PVC to occur is during the relative refractory period, which is the top of the T wave on the ECG. This is referred to as an R on T phenomenon, and this occurrence may precipitate a run of ventricular tachycardia. Significant ECG features with PVCs include:

- QRS complex is premature, 0.12 second or greater in width, and complexes are larger than the normal beats, with the T wave always occurring on the opposite side of the isoelectric line from the R wave.
- P waves are not present or are buried in the PVCs.
- PR interval—none.
- QT interval is prolonged for the ectopic beat only.
- PVC occurs prematurely.
- Heart rate usually is within the normal range, but depends on the underlying rhythm.
- Heart rhythm is irregular because the PVCs are premature.
- Ectopic beats are the PVCs.

The etiology, physical assessment findings, and treatment of premature ventricular contractions are outlined in Chart 30–13 (p. 882).

Ventricular Tachycardia

Ventricular tachycardia (VT), often referred to as v-tach, is a life-threatening ventricular rhythm arising from an excitable ventricular focus in the tissue distal to the bifurcation of the bundle of His. In general, ventricular tachycardia affects the diseased heart, although it has been described in patients with apparently normal hearts. It is a rhythm that discharges repetitively, acting as the dominant pacemaker. It is present when three or more PVCs occur in a row at a rate of greater than 100 beats per minute (Baltazar, 2009). This dysrhythmia frequently begins rapidly. It is initiated by a PVC, which then becomes the heart's pacemaker. A sustained ventricular tachycardia is a rhythm that lasts longer than 30 seconds and usually requires termination by antiarrhythmic drugs, antitachycardia pacing techniques, or electrical cardioversion. A nonsustained rhythm lasts less than 30 seconds, and terminates spontaneously. Ventricular tachycardia is an emergent situation, requiring urgent evaluation to assess cardiac output and the presence or absence of the pulse. Treatment is guided by published advanced cardiac life support (ACLS) guidelines and varies based on the presence of a pulse. When sustained but hemodynamically stable (with pulse), ventricular tachycardia is treated with pharmacologic agents such as lidocaine, procainamide, or amiodarone (Hazinski, 2010). Ventricular tachycardia that is hemodynamically unstable and pulseless is treated using the ACLS guidelines for pulseless cardiac arrest (Hazinski, 2010). These guidelines dictate that the nurse assess the patient for a pulse; if none is present, the nurse initiates cardiopulmonary resuscitation (CPR) and calls for help. The nurse administers oxygen and the patient is placed on a monitor/defibrillator when available. The nurse must be prepared to shock the patient per AHA guidelines. Vasopressors may be administered when intravenous access has been established. The nurse repeats CPR and defibrillation cycles per ACLS guidelines until a viable rhythm is established or death occurs. Figure 30–34 ◆. Significant ECG features of ventricular tachycardia and ventricular fibrillation include:

- QRS complexes are uniform in appearance, usually wide and bizarre, measuring 0.12 second or greater, with the T wave occurring on the opposite side of the isoelectric line from the R wave.
- P waves in rapid VT are usually not recognizable. At slower ventricular rates, P waves may be recognized and may represent normal sinus node depolarization at a rate slower than VT, but the electrical activities do not affect one another.
- PR interval is not discernable.
- QT interval is not measurable.
- Heart rate is greater than 100 beats per minute and usually not faster than 200 beats per minute.

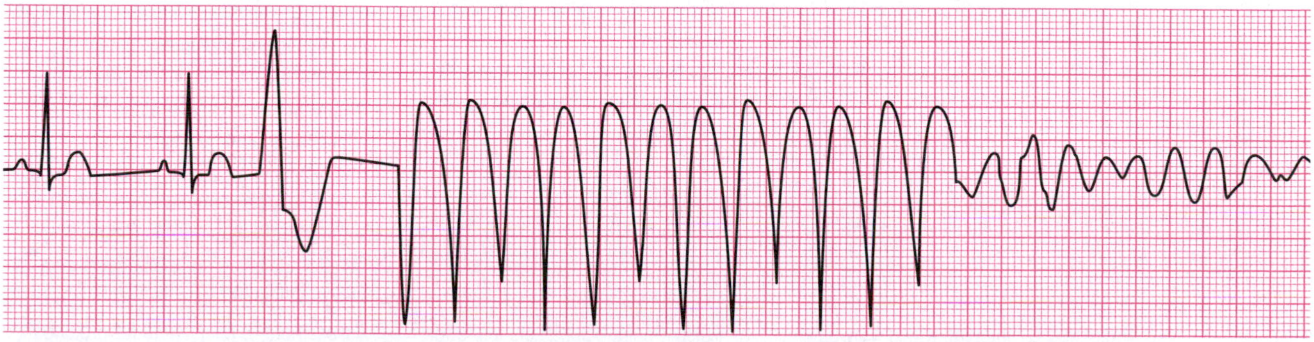

P Wave: Two normal P waves present; PR Interval: Not discernable during dysrhythmia; QRS Complex: Wide and distorted during dysrhythmia; QT Interval: Not discernable during dysrhythmia; Heart Rate: Atrial: Not discernable, Ventricular: Rapid; Rhythm: Both regular and irregular; Ectopic Beats: PVCs, ventricular tachycardia/fibrillation.

FIGURE 30–34 ◆ Ventricular tachycardia.

CHART 30–13 Ventricular Dysrhythmias: Etiology, Physical Assessment, and Treatment

Dysrhythmia	Etiology	Physical Assessment	Treatment
Premature ventricular contraction (PVC)	Organic heart disease Coronary artery disease Myocardial ischemia/irritability and infarction Cardiac valve disease Mitral valve prolapse Heart failure Primary electrical instability Fever Fluid volume deficit Electrolyte imbalance (e.g., hypokalemia, hypercalcemia, hypomagnesemia) Acid/base imbalance Drug excess (e.g., tricyclic antidepressants; digitalis, sympathomimetic amines, and antiarrhythmic agents) Moderate to excessive alcohol intake Increase in catecholamine release and sympathetic tone as in emotional stress Sarcoidosis Change in posture Exercise Emotional excitement Vagal stimulation Normal variation that increases with age	Pulse: May be irregular due to asynchronous firing of the ventricles. The corresponding QRS complex may be detected on the monitor while contractions are felt as a peripheral pulse. BP: Normal or lower than usual due to decreased cardiac output leading to decreased perfusion. Thumping sensation in chest/throat Palpitations If cardiac output is decreased, the following clinical manifestations may occur: Angina Syncope Generalized weakness Dizziness Shortness of breath Altered mental state may be present.	PVCs may be isolated when there is no underlying heart condition. Usually, then, they have no significance and require no treatment. Treatment depends on the cause and clinical manifestations. It is essential to identify and treat the underlying cause. When provoked by fast or slow heart rate, correcting the rate can abolish PVCs. Treatment usually is not required. Treatment is directed at uncovering the etiology and providing adequate oxygenation, pain relief, and rapid identification of causes. Antidysrhythmic drugs such as amiodarone and lidocaine should be administered as ordered per frequency of occurrence.
Ventricular tachycardia (VT)	Precipitated by the same conditions as premature ventricular contractions (see above)	Pulse: Rapid and weak. BP: Hypotensive. Cardiac output is decreased; therefore, the following clinical manifestations occur: Angina Syncope Generalized weakness Dizziness Shortness of breath Changes in mental status, starting with confusion and restlessness, leading to unconsciousness. Conscious sensation of ineffective cardiac activity often accompanied by anxiety. Presence and severity of the signs and symptoms depends on rhythm duration.	Initial treatment is based on the presence or absence of a palpable pulse. If hemodynamically stable, with a pulse, drug intervention is appropriate (e.g., procainamide, amiodarone, lidocaine). If hemodynamically unstable (pulseless), defibrillation and cardiopulmonary resuscitation (CPR) is indicated. After initial stabilization, other treatments which may be considered include: Implantable cardioverter defibrillator Electrophysiology Studies (EPS): Ventricles are stimulated to produce VT; then, antiarrhythmic drugs are administered, followed by a second attempt to produce the VT. If unable to reproduce the dysrhythmia, the drug is considered effective and continuous therapy is instituted. Drugs used include procainamide, amiodarone, and lidocaine. Radio-frequency ablation, burning the area or focus in the ventricle where the VT is coming from, may also be considered. Chapter 32 has a complete description of EPS and ablation.
Torsade de pointes (TdP)	Prolonged QT interval, which may be congenital or acquired Severe bradycardia	Pulse: Rapid, palpitations felt, often the first symptom. BP: Low due to decreased cardiac output.	Assessment of QT interval for prolongation. Magnesium is the treatment of choice to shorten the QT interval.

(continued)

CHART 30–13 Ventricular Dysrhythmias: Etiology, Physical Assessment, and Treatment, *continued*

Dysrhythmia	Etiology	Physical Assessment	Treatment
	Electrolyte imbalance (e.g., hypokalemia, hypomagnesemia) Central nervous system lesions Tricyclic antidepressants Antidysrhythmic drugs (e.g., quinidine, procainamide, amiodarone) Antihistamines (e.g., seldane) Antibiotics (e.g., erythromycin) Diuretics Liquid protein diets Starvation Or any combination of the above	If cardiac output is decreased the following clinical manifestations may occur: Angina Syncope Generalized weakness Dizziness Shortness of breath Changes in mental status, starting with confusion and restlessness, leading to unconsciousness. Seizures may be present with a prolonged rhythm. Clinical manifestations are related to the decreased cardiac output caused by the dysrhythmia.	If unsuccessful, overdrive ventricular pacing to keep the heart rate up and the QT interval within normal limits. Stress testing and Valsalva will prolong QT interval and can be used to diagnose congenital prolonged QT interval. All agents that cause Torsade de pointes are immediately discontinued. Administer potassium intravenously if QT interval is abnormal. Cardioversion and overdrive pacing are used to terminate Torsades, but may only be temporary. Drugs are modified or discontinued if QT interval is prolonged.
Ventricular fibrillation (VF)	Severe myocardial ischemia Coronary heart disease Myocardial infarction Advanced heart block Abnormal repolarization Vagal stimulation Drug toxicity (e.g., psychotropics, digoxin) Metabolic abnormalities (e.g., hypokalemia, hypomagnesemia) Hypoxia Trauma Terminal event in many disease states Electrical shock	Pulse: None palpable and heart sounds usually absent. BP: None. Unconscious Seizures Apnea Death, if untreated	Initiate CPR and defibrillation per ACLS guidelines.
Pulseless electrical activity	Profound hypovolemia Massive myocardial damage Excessive vagal tone due to loss of sympathetic tone Obstruction of blood flow to or from the heart (e.g., severe pulmonary embolism) Pericardial tamponade Myocardial rupture Massive cardiac trauma resulting in cardiac tamponade and/or tension pneumothorax Severe acidosis Hyperkalemia Hypothermia Drug overdose (e.g., tricyclics, beta-blockers, calcium channel blockers, digoxin)	Pulse: None palpable. BP: None. Unconscious Seizures may occur Death, if untreated	Assess for pulse and blood pressure; initiate CPR protocol per ACLS guidelines. Find cause and treat.
Asystole	Cardiac standstill from massive cardiac muscle damage	Pulse: None palpable. BP: None. Unconscious Death, if untreated	Check the rhythm in two leads in order to rule out the possibility of fine ventricular fibrillation. Also, check the lead placement to make sure it has not fallen off. Initiate CPR and ACLS protocols. Administer drugs per ACLS guidelines, agency protocol, or health care provider's orders.

- Heart rhythm is essentially regular but may be irregular.
- Entire rhythm is ectopic beats.

The etiology, physical assessment findings, and treatment of ventricular tachycardia are outlined in Chart 30–13 (p. 882).

Torsade de Pointes

Torsade de pointes, frequently referred to as "Torsades," is a form of ventricular tachycardia that is usually accompanied by prolongation of the QT interval. The QT interval usually is more than 0.50 second in the beats preceding the onset of the rhythm. Once the rhythm has occurred, the QRS complexes have varying shape and width (morphology) that usually begin after a pause in the rhythm or bradycardia. The name *Torsade de pointes* is derived from the French term that signifies the "twisting of the points." The name characterizes the rhythm in that it resembles a turning or twisting motion along the baseline or isoelectric line. This form of VT, which is rare, is due to age; gender; drug toxicity; or an idiosyncratic reaction to certain cardiac drugs such as quinidine, procainamide, disopyramide, or other agents that prolong the QT interval. Electrolyte imbalance, such as hypokalemia and hypomagnesemia, also can initiate Torsade de pointes (Baltazar, 2009).

In addition to being a life-threatening dysrhythmia, Torsade de pointes tends to recur repeatedly. It is, therefore, essential to find and treat the underlying cause. Figure 30–35◆ presents a rhythm strip showing Torsade de pointes. Significant ECG features of Torsade de pointes include:

- QRS complex height varies and undulates.
- P waves are not discernable.
- PR interval is not measurable.
- QT is not measurable.
- Heart rate varies; approximately 200 to 250 beats per minute.
- Heart rhythm may be regular or irregular.
- Entire rhythm is ectopy.

The etiology, physical assessment findings, and treatment of Torsade de pointes are outlined in Chart 30–13 (p. 882).

Ventricular Fibrillation

Ventricular fibrillation (VF), often referred to as v-fib, is a dysrhythmia marked by rapid, disorganized depolarization of the ventricles. There are no organized electrical impulses and, therefore, no coordinated atrial or ventricular contraction or palpable pulse. The myocardial cells appear to quiver rather than depolarize normally. With this dysrhythmia, multiple ventricular sites initiate electrical impulses that are not transmitted through the normal conduction pathway. There are no waveforms apparent on the ECG strip. The rhythm appears disorganized, rapid, and irregular with waves whose morphology varies greatly. Ventricular fibrillation may be classified further as coarse or fine, just like atrial fibrillation. Coarse waveforms are more easily visible and are greater than 3 mm; those that are less than 3 mm frequently are referred to as fine VF. Coarse VF responds better to treatment than does fine VF. Also, coarse VF typically progresses to fine VF unless treatment is initiated in a timely manner. Fine VF indicates that the rhythm has been present for an extended period of time. Figure 30–36◆ presents a rhythm strip showing ventricular fibrillation.

Safety Alert *Ventricular fibrillation (VF) is an ineffective quivering of the heart muscle that results in no blood delivery to tissues. VF must be treated immediately. Detection of VF on a monitor requires immediate patient evaluation by the nurse to begin prompt treatment and to rule out equipment malfunctions that mimic VF, such as ECG artifacts produced by loose or dry electrodes, broken ECG leads, or patient movements or muscle tremors.*

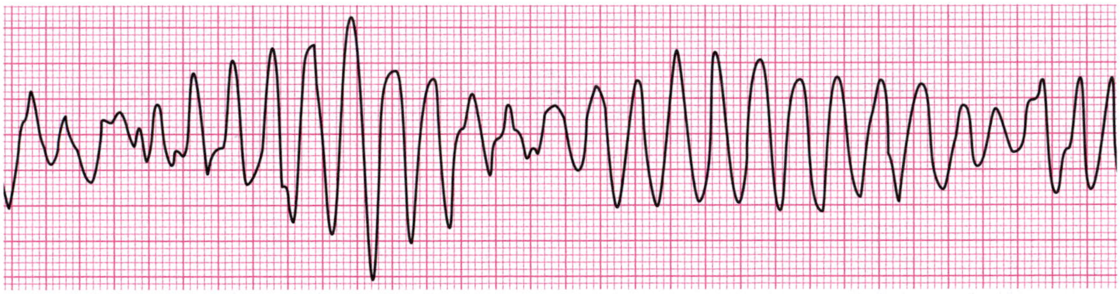

P Waves: Not discernable; PR Interval: Not discernable; QRS Complex: Wide, distorted, and varying heights; QT Interval: not discernable; Rate: Rapid; Rhythm: Both regular and irregular; Ectopic Beats: All.

FIGURE 30–35 ◆ Torsade de pointes.

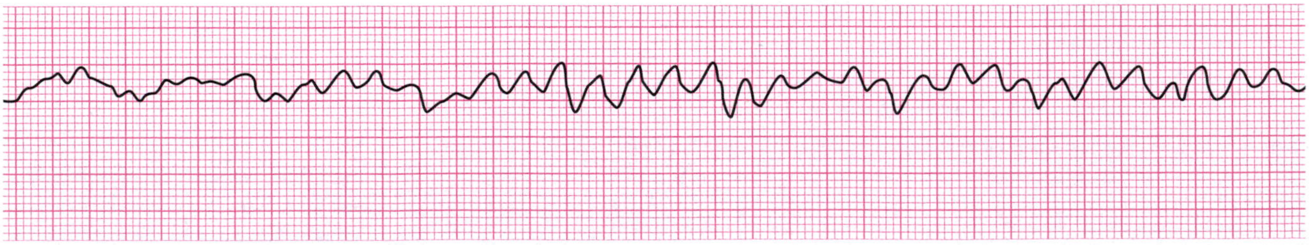

P Waves: Not discernable; PR Interval: Not discernable; QRS Complex: Wide, distorted, and varying heights; QT Interval not discernable; Heart Rate: Not discernable; Ectopic Beats: All.

FIGURE 30–36 ◆ Ventricular fibrillation.

Significant ECG features of ventricular fibrillation include:

- P waves, PR intervals, QRS complexes, and QT intervals are all absent.
- Heart rate is not discernable because there are no waves or complexes to measure.
- Heart rhythm is irregular.
- Entire rhythm is ectopy.

The etiology, physical assessment findings, and treatment of ventricular fibrillation are outlined in Chart 30–13 (p. 882).

Pulseless Electrical Activity

Pulseless electrical activity (PEA) is a clinical phenomenon that occurs when the heart muscle loses its ability to contract even though cardiac electrical activity is present. Although cardiac electrical activity is seen on the monitor, the patient has no detectable pulse or blood pressure. Though the electrical activity is represented as an organized rhythm (other than VT or VF) on the cardiac monitor (e.g., bradycardia, heart block), the heart muscle is unable to respond to electrical stimuli. Due to a variety of cardiac and noncardiac disorders such as acidosis, electrolyte imbalance, trauma, and cardiac rupture, the muscle is unable to respond to the stimuli, causing cardiac output and tissue perfusion to cease and clinical death to occur. When PEA occurs, biological death follows within minutes unless the cause is identified and treated (Hazinski, 2010). Formerly, pulseless electrical activity was called electromechanical dissociation (EMD). The clinical outcome usually is poor despite aggressive life support measures. Significant ECG features of pulseless electrical activity include:

- P waves may or may not be present dependent on rhythm.
- PR intervals may or may not have a relationship to QRS complexes.
- QRS complexes may be narrow or wide.
- QT interval is variable.
- Heart rate and rhythm are variable, usually bradycardia.
- Ectopic beats may be present.

The etiology, physical assessment findings, and treatment of pulseless electrical activity are outlined in Chart 30–13 (p. 882).

Asystole

Asystole is a complete termination of all cardiac electrical activity. Without an electrical impulse, the atria and ventricles do not contract, causing immediate loss of oxygen supply to the brain and tissues. In hospital settings, efforts are usually made to reestablish cardiac activity; these often are futile. Figure 30–37◆ presents a rhythm strip showing asystole. In asystole, no measurable electrical activity exists and the rhythm strip appears as a straight line on the ECG monitor. The etiology, physical assessment findings, and treatment of asystole are outlined in Chart 30–13 (p. 882).

Weblink: AHA Guidelines for CPR and ECC

Nursing Management

As with any dysrhythmia, the first nursing responsibility for ventricular dysrhythmias is to assess the patient's response to the specific abnormality. Nurses need to complete a health history to assess the risk factors related to the occurrence of ventricular dysrhythmias that are outlined in Chart 30–13 (p. 882). Cultural awareness of populations that are at increased risk for ventricular dysrhythmias is discussed in the Cultural Considerations box.

Ventricular dysrhythmias have the greatest impact on cardiac output and are, therefore, the most serious. Depending on the variation in configuration and the frequency of occurrence, ventricular dysrhythmias require a variety of interventions ranging from simple observation, to drug intervention, to advanced life support treatments. Generally, the health care providers provide protocols or some type of emergency orders for treating each type of ventricular dysrhythmia. The nurse must know the treatment regimens required for each of the ventricular dysrhythmias based on the standing orders, basic cardiac life support (BCLS), ACLS, and agency-specific protocols. When reporting ventricular dysrhythmias, the nurse needs to give the health care provider a detailed description of the dysrhythmia pattern and the patient's clinical response so that treatment may be tailored to the specific dysrhythmia. The seriousness and treatment of ventricular dysrhythmias depend on their duration and impact on hemodynamic stability (blood pressure and cardiac output).

If resuscitation efforts are initiated, it is imperative that family and significant others are kept informed and allowed to participate in the

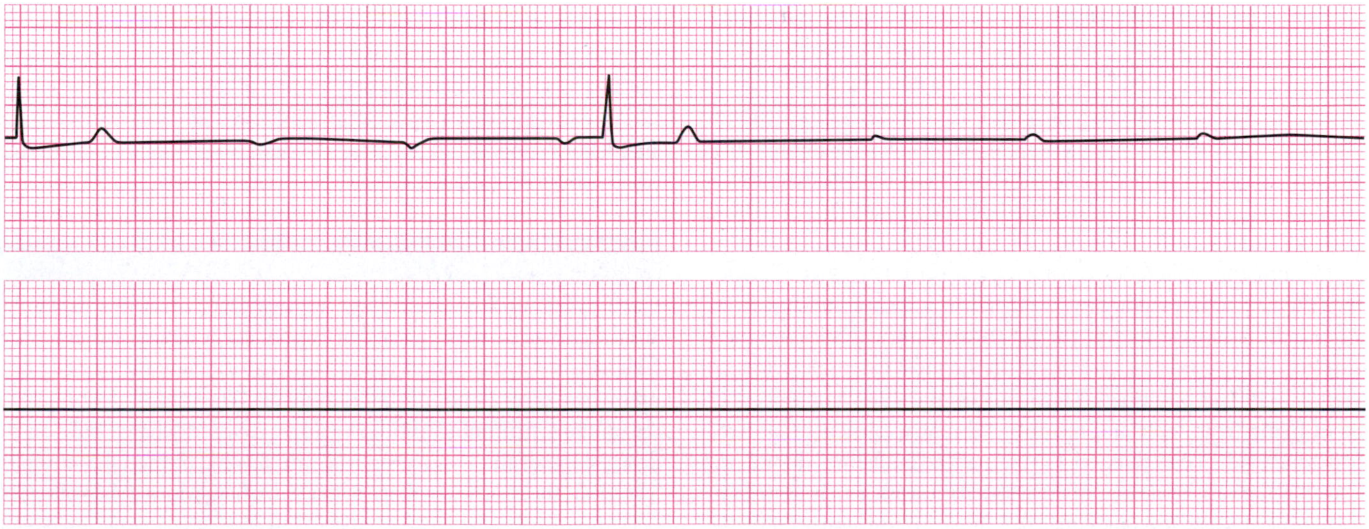

No measurable electrical activity.

FIGURE 30–37 ◆ Asystole.

Weblink: Brugada Syndrome Weblink: AHA Guidelines for CPR and ECC Weblink: International Liaison Committee on Resuscitation

CULTURAL CONSIDERATIONS Brugada Syndrome

The term *Brugada sign* is an abnormal finding on an electrocardiogram (ECG) that refers to a distance of at least 0.10 second from the onset of the QRS complex or the bottom of the S wave. Its presence may indicate Brugada syndrome, an abnormality in the heart's electrical system that causes life-threatening heart rhythm disturbances such as ventricular fibrillation. Brugada syndrome occurs in patients with a structurally normal heart, few or no coronary artery disease risk factors, and a family history of sudden cardiac death. It is possible to have a Brugada sign without having Brugada syndrome. This syndrome occurs most often in young adults. It also occurs with increased frequency in Asians. The cause is not clear, but it appears to be inherited in some cases.

Nursing implications are to assess young patients and patients of Asian descent with ventricular dysrhythmias and little to no risk of heart disease for a family history of sudden cardiac death. Those considered at risk have:

- A family history of sudden cardiac death in young relatives
- A personal history of serious heart rhythm problems
- A personal history of severe fainting spells.

Immediate treatment for ventricular fibrillation is outlined in the American Heart Association ACLS guidelines for 2010. Long-term treatment includes antidysrhythmic medication therapy and an implantable defibrillator.

Source: Adapted from: *Brugada Syndrome* (2005). MayoClinic.com. http://www.mayoclinic.com/health/brugada-syndrome/AN00551.

decision-making process. It is imperative that the health care team offers this opportunity and is sensitive to the family during this crisis period. If possible, it is optimal to have a health care team member be assigned to the family to answer questions, clarify information, and provide comfort (Hazinski, 2010). Since the nurse is at the bedside, it typically becomes a nursing responsibility to keep the family informed, act as a liaison, and advocate for the patient. Chapter 11 includes a complete description of end-of-life issues.

National Guidelines for Cardiopulmonary Resuscitation and Emergency Cardiovascular Care

Since 1974 the American Heart Association has been publishing guidelines for cardiopulmonary resuscitation and emergency cardiovascular care. The guidelines were most recently updated in 2010 and are based on evidenced evaluation from the 2010 International Consensus Conference on Cardiopulmonary Resuscitation and Emergency Cardiovascular Care with Treatment Recommendations (International Liaison Committee on Resuscitation, 2011). These guidelines supersede the published 2005 guidelines for cardiovascular resuscitation and emergency cardiovascular care. The current guidelines contain recommendations designed to improve survival from sudden cardiac arrest and acute life-threatening cardiopulmonary disorders. These guidelines are based on the most extensive evidence review of CPR yet published. They confirm the safety and effectiveness of many treatments and recommend new treatments that have undergone evidence evaluation. Given that the guidelines do not apply to all situations, the leader of the resuscitation attempt may need to adapt application of the guidelines to unique circumstances. Finally, the guidelines streamline the amount of information that rescuers need to learn and remember, and clarify the most important skills that rescuers need to perform. The National Guidelines box outlines the 2010 AHA national guidelines for selected CPR and emergency cardiovascular care.

NATIONAL GUIDELINES for Cardiopulmonary Resuscitation and Emergency Cardiovascular Care

- Adult basic life support
- Advanced cardiac life support
- Electrical therapies
- CPR techniques and devices
- Adjuncts for airway control and ventilation
- Management of cardiac arrest
- Management of symptomatic bradycardia and tachycardia
- Monitoring and medications
- Post-resuscitation support, including therapeutic hypothermia
- Stabilizing of the patient with acute coronary syndromes

Source: Adapted from Hazinksi, MF (Ed). (2010). Highlights of the 2010 American Heart Association Guidelines for CPR and ECC.

Nursing Management

Nursing responsibilities when caring for patients experiencing cardiac dysrhythmias are discussed throughout this chapter. To assist the learner, the patient care plan outlines a systematic approach to assessing and providing nursing care for these patients (see Nursing Process: Patient Care Plan for Dysrhythmias).

To assist the nurse in the comprehensive assessment and interpretation of cardiac dysrhythmias, Chart 30–14 (p. 888) summarizes the characteristics of each type of dysrhythmia.

Electrical Treatment of Cardiac Dysrhythmias

Cardioversion and defibrillation are common procedures used to treat cardiac dysrhythmias. Both of these procedures use a defibrillator that delivers a preset level of electrical voltage to the heart for the purpose of terminating an unwanted dysrhythmia. The electrical current depolarizes the myocardial cells; repolarization follows. During repolarization the sinus node usually is able to take over its role as the heart's natural pacemaker. Assessment of three major factors determines when to use cardioversion versus defibrillation: timing of the delivery of the electrical current, rationale for use, and amount of voltage used. Cardioversion and defibrillation are discussed next. Chart 30–15 outlines safety rules when using a defibrillator.

Cardioversion

Cardioversion is indicated for the treatment of tachyarrhythmias: atrial tachycardia, rapid atrial fibrillation, atrial flutter, and junctional tachycardia. Cardioversion typically is performed at the bedside on a unit where cardiac monitoring is available. The cardiac defibrillator is set on the synchronous mode, meaning it will discharge only on the down slope of the R wave or with the S wave of the QRS complex. Therefore, the electrical voltage will not discharge during the vulnerable period of ventricular repolarization (T wave), which could precipitate ventricular tachycardia and ventricular fibrillation (referred to as the R on T phenomenon). The nurse should instruct the patient not to eat or drink for at least 6 hours prior to the procedure and withhold digoxin

NURSING PROCESS: Patient Care Plan for Dysrhythmias

Assessment of Cardiovascular Status Using Gordon's Functional Health Patterns:

- Activity–Exercise Health Perception
- Coping/Stress Tolerance

Subjective Data

Assessment of Cardiac Output

- Do you feel palpitations in your chest?
- Do you ever feel your heart beat fast, beat irregularly, or skip beats?
- Do you get light-headed? If so, under what circumstances?
- Do you ever experience any of the following:
  - Syncope
  - Dizziness
  - Fatigue
  - Chest discomfort

Assessment of Activity Tolerance

- Are you able to complete your activities of daily living without fatigue or chest pain?
- Are you able to walk up a flight of stairs without getting short of breath or experiencing chest pain?
- Do you exercise on a regular basis?
- Are you able to walk in the hall without experiencing fatigue, SOB, chest pain, or dizziness?

Assessment of Patient/Family Knowledge of Disease and Treatment

- Tell me what you know about your problems with your heart.
- What medications are you on, when are you supposed to take them, and what are the side effects you should watch for?
- When are you supposed to see your doctor?
- Has anyone explained your health problems to you?
- Would you tell me what you know about cardiac dysrhythmias?
- Do you feel anxious about your health problems?
- Do you have family members or close friends who provide emotional support?
- Do you see your health care provider on a regular basis?
- Do you know what symptoms are important to report to your health care provider immediately?

Objective Data

Assessment of Cardiac Output

Health history and social habits that are high risk for the development of heart disease

- Smoking
- Alcohol intake
- Sedentary lifestyle
- Obesity
- Prescription and over-the-counter medications

Comorbid condition such as: diabetes

- Chronic obstructive pulmonary disease
- Kidney disease (electrolyte imbalance)

Assessment of Activity Tolerance

- Monitor vital signs (heart rate, blood pressure in both arms, mean arterial pressure, respiratory rate, oxygen saturation) before and after activity.
- Assess heart sounds.
- Assess lung sounds

Outcomes and Evaluation Parameters	Planning and Interventions with *Rationales*
1. NURSING DIAGNOSIS: Altered Cardiac Output and Alteration in Tissue Perfusion ***related to cardiac dysrhythmias*** **(NANDA-I © 2012)**	
Outcome: Maintain adequate cardiac output. Dysrhythmias controlled by effective treatment. ***Evaluation Parameters:*** Heart rate, blood pressure, and urine output within normal limits. No light-headedness, shortness of breath, or chest pain.	Monitoring and managing the dysrhythmia to prevent or mitigate clinical manifestations due to a drop in cardiac output. Finding the cause *to treat or prevent its occurrence if possible.* Reducing risk factors through patient teaching *to decrease incidence of heart disease that results in dysrhythmias.*
2. NURSING DIAGNOSIS: Anxiety and Knowledge deficit ***related to fear of the unknown about cardiac dysrhythmias*** **(NANDA-I © 2012)**	
Outcome: Reduced anxiety. ***Evaluation Parameters:*** Verbalizes understanding of disorder and treatments. Verbalizes prevention of heart disease.	Explain what causes the dysrhythmias and what treatment can prevent or control them. Explain when to call the health care provider and where the nearest hospital is located. Describe the cardiac risk factors and how to control/prevent them. *Increasing knowledge and minimizing anxiety to prevent dysrhythmias.* Promoting home and community-based care *to decrease progression of heart disease.*

Source: Adapted from Wilkinson & Ahearn (2009).

CHART 30–14 ECG Measurements for Cardiac Rhythms

ECG Rhythm	P Wave	PR Interval	QRS	QT Interval	Rate	Rhythm	Ectopic Beats
Normal sinus rhythm	Present and regular	0.12–0.21	0.06–0.12	0.34–0.43	60–100 bpm	Regular	None
Sinus bradycardia	Present and regular	Normal limits	Normal	Lengthens to greater than normal	40–60 bpm	Regular	None
Sinus tachycardia	Present and regular	As the sinus rate accelerates, the PR interval tends to shorten slightly.	Normal	Usually shortens	100–180 bpm	May be slightly irregular as rate accelerates; then becomes a rapid regular rate	None
Sinus arrhythmia	Present and irregular	Normal limits	Normal limits	Changes with the heart rate, becoming longer during the slow phase of the rhythm	60–100 bpm	Regularly irregular, with a variance of more than 0.08 seconds	May occur during the slow phase of the rhythm
Sinus arrest (pause)	Present and irregular	May be the same before and after sinus pauses	Normal limits	Changes with the heart rate, becoming longer during the slow phase of the rhythm	There may be marked bradycardia due to long sinus pauses	Underlying regular rhythm except where the sinus pauses occur	Possible during sinus pauses
Premature atrial contraction (PAC)	Present and irregular when PAC occurs.	Normal limits. May change with PAC only.	Normal limits	Normal if rate is normal	60–100 bpm	Regular except for premature PAC which may reset rhythm	PAC
Atrial flutter	No P wave f waves	None	Normal limits	Unable to obtain as T waves are buried in f waves	Depends on the AV conduction ratio; could be fast or slow	Atrial rate regular Ventricular rate may be regular or irregular	Flutter waves
Atrial fibrillation	No P wave f waves	None	Normal limits	Unable to obtain because the T waves are buried in the f waves	T waves are buried in the f waves	Irregular	Fibrillation waves
Supraventricular tachycardia (SVT)	Not seen—buried in QRS complex	Not discernable	Within normal limits, unless distorted by buried P waves	Unable to obtain as T waves are buried	100–250 bpm	Regular or irregular due to varying conduction through the AV node	Rapid ectopic focus takes over rhythm
Paroxysmal atrial tachycardia (PAT)	At onset of rhythm, shape of P waves different from sinus P waves	Varies with rhythm change	Within normal limits, unless distorted by buried P waves	T waves buried, so unable to obtain with fast rhythm	100–250 beats/minute dependent on reference source	Irregular due to varying heart rates	Ectopic focus at onset of rapid rhythm
Wolff-Parkinson-White syndrome	Present and regular	Less than 0.12 second because the AV node is bypassed and contains presence of delta wave	Greater than 0.10 second due to delta waves created by the abnormal conduction pathway	Shortens with tachycardia and lengthens with bradycardia	High incidence of tachydysrthrymias	Regular, except during heart rate changes	Delta waves: Occur just prior to R wave
Sick sinus syndrome	Present or absent depending on which dysrhythmia is occurring	Variable depending on the rhythm	Normal limits	Variable due to rate change	Bradycardia to tachycardia	Atrial: Irregular Ventricular: Irregular	May be present with slow rate
Junctional escape rhythm	May occur before, after, or buried in the QRS complex	Less than 0.12 second if the P wave occurs before the QRS complex	Normal unless distorted by P wave	Normal unless impacted by rate	Usually 40–60 (normal intrinsic rate for junctional tissue)	Regular	May occur with slow rates

(continued)

CHART 30–14 ECG Measurements for Cardiac Rhythms, *continued*

ECG Rhythm	P Wave	PR Interval	QRS	QT Interval	Rate	Rhythm	Ectopic Beats
Premature junctional contraction (PJC)	May occur before, after, or buried in the QRS complex	Less than 0.12 second if P wave occurs before QRS complex for the ectopic beat	Normal unless distorted by P wave for the ectopic beat All others normal	Normal	That of underlying rhythm	Regular except for the premature beat	PJC
Junctional tachycardia	May occur before, after, or buried in the QRS complex	Less than 0.12 second if P wave occurs before QRS complex for the ectopic beat	Normal unless distorted by P wave for the ectopic beat	No specific change unless it is heart rate related	Greater than 100 beats per minute	Appears regular, but may increase its rate	May occur due to muscle irritability
First-degree AV block	Present and regular	Greater than 0.20 second	Normal	Normal	Variable	Regular	None
Mobitz I/ Wenckebach	Sinus P waves	Progressively prolonged until one P wave is not conducted and the sequence begins	Within normal limits	Within normal limits	Atrial rate within normal limits; ventricular rate slower than atrial	Atrial rhythm is regular; ventricular rhythm is irregular	Usually none
Mobitz II/ second-degree block	Present Not always followed by QRS	Constant with conducted beats	Intermittently absent; may be normal (AV node) or prolonged when present	Within normal limits	Atrial rate is regular; ventricular rate irregular and bradycardic	Atrial is regular; ventricular is irregular	May occur due to slow rate
Third-degree (complete) heart block	Present and regular	P wave has no relationship to QRS complexes; therefore, no PR interval is present	May be narrow (junctional rhythm), or wide (idioventricular rhythm)	May be rate related, but not directly affected	Atrial rate is regular, 60–100 bpm; ventricular rate is 20–40 bpm	Atrial is regular; ventricular may be regular or irregular	May occur due to slow rate
Bundle branch block	Present and regular sinus P waves	0.12–0.20 second	Greater than 0.12 second	Within normal limits	60–100 beats/minute	Regular	None
Premature ventricular contraction (PVC)	None with PVC	None with PVC	Broad, premature, and has increased amplitude R and T waves opposite sides of isoelectric line	Prolonged with PVC	Underlying rate may be normal or abnormal	Irregular because PVCs are premature	PVC more likely to occur during bradycardia when there is more time to emerge
Ventricular tachycardia	None visible	Not discernible	Wide and bizarre, measuring $>$ 0.12 second R and T waves opposite sides of isoelectric line	Not discernible	100–250 beats/minute	Essentially regular	All waves are ectopy
Torsade de pointes	Not discernible	Not discernible	Height undulates	Usually $>$ 0.50 seconds in the beats preceding the onset of the rhythm	Rates vary 200–250 beats/minute	Typically regular	All waves are ectopy
Ventricular fibrillation	None	None	None	None	Atrial: Absent Ventricular: Absent	Irregular	All waves are ectopy
Pulseless electrical activity	May or may not be present	May or may not have a relationship to QRS complexes	May be narrow or wide complex	Variable	Variable, depends on rhythm; usually bradycardic	Variable, depends on rate	May be present but none of the beats perfuse
Asystole	None	None	None	None	None	None	None

Source: Megan Redeen, (2007). California State University, Sacramento.

Video: Automatic External Defibrillator Video: Cardiac Arrest—Defibrillation Weblink: AED Programs Q & A

CHART 30–15 Safety Criteria When Using a Defibrillator

- Use designated conductor pads or paddles.
- Use designated conductor medium: gel, pastes, sheet.
- Place pads or paddles so they are not in contact with the patient's clothes or bed linen, or placed near medication patches and monitor leads.
- Do not place pads or paddles near a direct oxygen source to prevent a fire hazard.
- For cardioversion, defibrillator must be set in a synchronous mode.
- For defibrillation, defibrillator must be set in an asynchronous mode.
- For cardioversion, make sure the monitor leads are attached to the patient.
- Do not charge the defibrillator until ready to shock, and keep fingers off discharge buttons until ready to discharge voltage.
- Exert enough pressure on the paddles to ensure adequate contact prior to discharging the voltage.
- Call for everyone to clear the area prior to discharging the defibrillator.
- Document the entire procedure and effectiveness of the intervention.
- Inspect the skin for burns after the procedure and report and treat per health care provider's orders.

for 48 hours prior to the procedure to ensure resumption of sinoatrial (SA) node activity and normal conduction to the atrioventricular (AV) node. The patient is sedated intravenously prior to the procedure and full resuscitation equipment is available, if necessary. The voltage on the defibrillator begins at 10 to 20 joules (J). If unsuccessful, it is increased to 50 joules and increased at intervals to a maximum of 360 joules. The lower the joules, the less the chance of complications such as cardiac necrosis. A successful outcome is conversion to normal sinus rhythm with adequate cardiac output.

Nursing responsibilities include recording the postcardioversion rhythm, cardiac output, and vital signs for 2 to 3 hours after the procedure. Other responsibilities include measuring vital signs, level of consciousness, and oxygen saturation until the patient recovers from the sedation. If the patient converts back to the unwanted rhythm, the nurse must report this to the health care provider immediately.

Defibrillation

Defibrillation is basically the same as cardioversion in that electrical voltage is delivered to the myocardium to terminate unwanted rhythms, except defibrillation is done in an emergency situation for life-threatening dysrhythmias. Defibrillation is indicated for patients in ventricular tachycardia and ventricular fibrillation when they have lost consciousness and cardiopulmonary resuscitation is in progress. Unless there are discernable T waves, the defibrillator is usually set in an asynchronous mode. The voltage on the defibrillator is set at 360 joules. After each defibrillation, the rhythm is evaluated and voltage delivery is repeated as necessary until there is a viable rhythm or resuscitation is stopped. Between each defibrillation, CPR is performed to maintain tissue oxygenation. Medications such as lidocaine, amiodarone, epinephrine, and vasopressin typically are administered during resuscitation to assist in conversion to normal sinus rhythm. During both cardioversion and defibrillation, paddles or conductor pads are applied to the patient's chest and attached to the defibrillator. Figure 30–38◆ demonstrates normal paddle placement using both the standard and anteroposterior placement. Whichever type of pad is used, it must have a conducting medium to prevent burning the patient's skin.

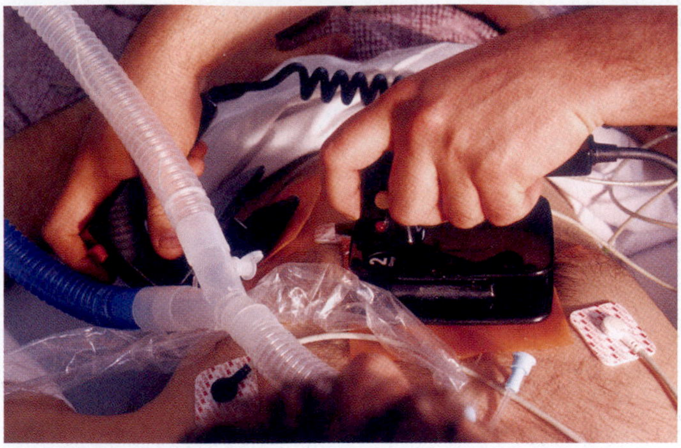

FIGURE 30–38 ◆ Defibrillator paddle.

Automated External Defibrillator

An **automated external defibrillator (AED)** is a small, lightweight device that can recognize and treat ventricular fibrillation (VF), also known as sudden cardiac death (SCD). The AED is designed for use by lay rescuers or "first responders." If SCD is present, an AED will talk the responder through the very simple steps to defibrillate. These devices have been shown to decrease mortality when used in conjunction with cardiopulmonary resuscitation (CPR) (American Heart Association, 2011b). Once the domain of only highly trained emergency professionals, these technologically advanced defibrillators are now available on board airlines, on cruise ships, and in other public places. These defibrillators are appropriate for use with infants and children as well as adults, as long as the appropriate pads are used. Typically, children over 55 pounds (25 kilograms) or 8 years of age are defibrillated as adults. Precautions when using AEDs include:

- Ensure pulseless criteria are met before AED is applied.
- Withhold unit analysis of the rhythm during cardiopulmonary resuscitation (CPR).
- Withhold unit analysis of the rhythm if the patient is seizing.
- Use caution with rhythm analysis in a moving vehicle.
- Stop frequently for rhythm analysis during transport.
- Place electrodes without shaving chest; not required for effective placement.
- Ensure skin is dry and free of nicks and cuts for effective electrode placement.
- Perform regular maintenance and battery placement according to manufacturer's recommendations.

Implantable Cardioverter Defibrillator

An **implantable cardioverter defibrillator (ICD)** is a device that can automatically terminate potentially lethal dysrhythmias of ventricular tachycardia and ventricular fibrillation. ICDs, like all pacemakers, are programmable and can combine a variety of therapies in one device, including:

- Tiered electrical therapy—the ability to deliver low-voltage cardioversion or high-voltage defibrillation

- Antitachycardia pacing—the ability to pace the heart at a faster rate than a tachycardia (supraventricular or ventricular), enabling the device to capture (control) the intrinsic heart rate and gradually slow it down to a normal heart rate
- Programmable ventricular or atrial pacing.

Current ICDs have effectively proven their lifesaving value for patients with repeated episodes of ventricluar tachycardia (p. 881).

ICD System

The ICD system is similar to traditional pacemakers in that it consists of a pulse generator and defibrillation leads for both dysrhythmia detection and delivery of therapy (Carlson, 2009). Unlike early devices that required open thoracotomy, current ICDs are usually implanted transvenously with generator placement under the chest wall. Depending on the programmed functions of the ICD, the patient may have one, two, or three leads. A single-chamber ICD requires only one lead in the right ventricle. The ventricular leads are similar to pacemaker leads in their ability to sense and pace the heart.

Complications

Potential complications of ICD include those related to traditional pacemaker therapy, such as lead dislodgment or fracture and infection. Long-term potential complications unique to ICD include electromagnetic interference (electrocautery during surgery, radiofrequency transmitters, high-powered electromagnetic fields, etc.) that can result in inappropriate shocks or inhibition of the device (Carlson, 2009).

If the patient requires external defibrillation, care must be taken not to position the paddles on or near the generator. In any event, the ICD must be thoroughly evaluated after any episode of external defibrillation.

Nursing Management

Nursing management of the patient immediately after ICD implantation is similar to care of the patient with a permanent pacemaker. Most patients and their families also need support in coping with the emotional response to ICD implantation (Carlson, 2009). Although the shock delivered by the ICD is lifesaving, it is unpredictable and painful: Patients typically equate a shock to being kicked in the chest or being slammed to the ground. If the shock is delivered when the patient is at work or out in public, she may report feeling embarrassed at her reaction to the shock and by her loss of control during the episode. In addition, anyone touching the patient during an ICD firing will also feel the shock. The result is not fatal but can be painful. Some patients report that a shock has been delivered when in fact the ICD has no record of delivering a shock; this phenomenon is called a "phantom shock." Providing emotional support for the ICD patient and her family before the device is implanted and during follow-up can promote acceptance of the technology and lead to improvement in quality of life.

Electrophysiology Study

The **electrophysiology study (EPS)** is an invasive procedure that involves placing multiple multipolar catheter electrodes into the venous and sometimes the arterial side of the heart. These electrodes are positioned at various locations inside of the heart and have two purposes: to record the electrical signal within the heart and to deliver an electrical stimulus at precisely timed intervals (programmed stimulation).

Currently EPS is the standard test for reproducing dysrhythmias in a controlled environment in order to diagnose and treat the disorder. During EPS, catheters with several electrodes are advanced percutaneously and positioned within the heart; the exact location depends on the source of the dysrhythmia. Detailed recordings of the electrical activity of the heart are obtained, including interval measurements (time for the electrical activity to travel from one area of the conduction system to another) as well as the direction of conduction. Programmed electrical stimulation involves using the catheters to deliver a programmed stimulus in order to initiate the dysrhythmia. A series of impulses is delivered to the myocardium in an attempt to cause a tachyarrhythmia. If successful, the dysrhythmia is termed inducible. Treatment is instituted and the same procedure is repeated; if the tachyarrhythmia cannot be induced, the treatment is successful. Medications to increase the heart rate, such as epinephrine or isoproterenol, also may be used to assess the conduction system (Woods, Froelicher, Adams (Underhill), and Bridges, 2010).

In addition, EPS can assess the function of SA and AV nodes and assess the effectiveness of specific antiarrhythmic medications. When assessing the cardiac conduction, the rate is turned up faster than the intrinsic rate, allowing the catheter to be the cardiac pacemaker. Then the stimulus is shut off and the time it takes for the SA node to take control is assessed. If the time is prolonged, the SA node is diseased.

Ablation of dysrhythmias, which has become a frequently performed procedure, refers to destruction of an area of the myocardium through localized delivery of chemicals or electrical energy to heat the myocardium in very specific locations, destroying the tissue responsible for dysrhythmia formation and propagation. Patient preparation for EPS is similar to that for cardiac catheterization, described in Chapter 32. The patient must be able to tolerate lying flat and relatively still for an extended period of time. Complications are very rare, but can include death (usually from intractable ventricular dysrhythmias), myocardial perforation (a risk any time catheters are introduced inside the heart), and thrombosis. The need for anticoagulation will depend on the length of the procedure and the position of the catheters. Procedural sedation or general anesthesia may be required for long procedures.

Nursing management postprocedure includes a complete cardiovascular assessment, with special emphasis on the ECG as well as the access site. Specific parameters will depend on the type of procedure. Patients are usually discharged the same day after a diagnostic EPS. Discharge instructions include care of the access site, bathing, driving, and return to work. Specific instructions regarding the results of the EPS will depend on the indication for the test.

Cardiac Pacemakers

A **cardiac pacemaker** is an electronic device that is capable of delivering an electrical stimulus to the heart. These devices are used to augment or replace the natural cardiac pacemaker when there is either a congenital abnormality or a disease of the cardiac conduction system. Pacemakers deliver impulses to multiple chambers of the heart in order to treat not only bradycardias, but also tachydysrhythmias (greater than 100 beats per minute) originating from either the atria or the ventricles. Pacemakers are able to vary the heart rate in accordance with a change in the patient's metabolic demand or activity level. Specialized pacemakers can also cardiovert and/or defibrillate (ICD) or improve cardiac output in patients with heart failure (chronic resynchronization therapy).

Pacemaker Components

A pacing system is composed of a generator and lead(s). The type of generator and the type and number of leads will depend on the reason for implementing pacemaker therapy. There are basically two types of pacemakers: temporary and permanent. Pacemakers may be single- or dual-chambered. Single-chambered devices pace a single chamber of the heart, such as the right ventricle. Dual-chambered pacemakers pace at least two chambers of the heart, such as the right atrium and the right ventricle, or both ventricles. A single-chambered right ventricular and a dual-chambered right atrium and right ventricular are shown in Figure 30–39◆. The *generator* contains the electronic circuitry and the power source, and is synonymous with the term *pacemaker* (Figure 30–40◆).

The pacemaker *lead* is the connection between the generator and the myocardium (Figure 30–40). Permanent pacemaker leads are placed inside the cardiac chambers (most common) or on the surface of the heart (epicardial leads). Leads contain tip electrodes, a conductor, and insulation (Figure 30–41◆). The tip electrode is embedded directly into the cardiac tissue. The lead conducts the electrical stimulus between the negative and positive electrodes (poles). Electrical current flows between two metal poles.

Temporary Pacemakers

Temporary pacing can be performed using transvenous, epicardial, or transcutaneous methods. The system used will depend on factors such as the clinical diagnosis and stability of the patient (elective or emergency situation). Temporary pacing is indicated in a variety of conditions (Chart 30–16). Generators for temporary pacing systems are connected to the pacemaker lead(s) but remain outside the body. They are powered by ordinary batteries and are manually programmed as needed (Figure 30–42◆, p. 894).

CHART 30–16 Indications for Temporary Pacemakers

- Symptomatic sick sinus syndrome
- Symptomatic second- or third-degree heart block
- Drug refractory dysrhythmias
- Prophylactic after cardiovascular surgery
- Prior to insertion of a permanent cardiac pacemaker
- Development of significant conduction disturbances after acute myocardial infarction
- Overdrive tachydysrhythmias
- During cardiac resuscitation
- Bradycardia unresponsive to atropine

Temporary Transvenous Pacing

Temporary transvenous pacing involves insertion of the lead through a major vein, such as the internal jugular, subclavian, or femoral. The pacing lead is threaded into the right side of the heart; the proximal end is sutured outside the body and connected to an external generator. If an epicardial lead is used, the lead is attached to the outside of the heart (typically during cardiac surgery) and is introduced through the chest wall. Temporary pacemakers can be either single-chambered (lead in the ventricle only) or dual-chambered (leads in both the atrium and the ventricle).

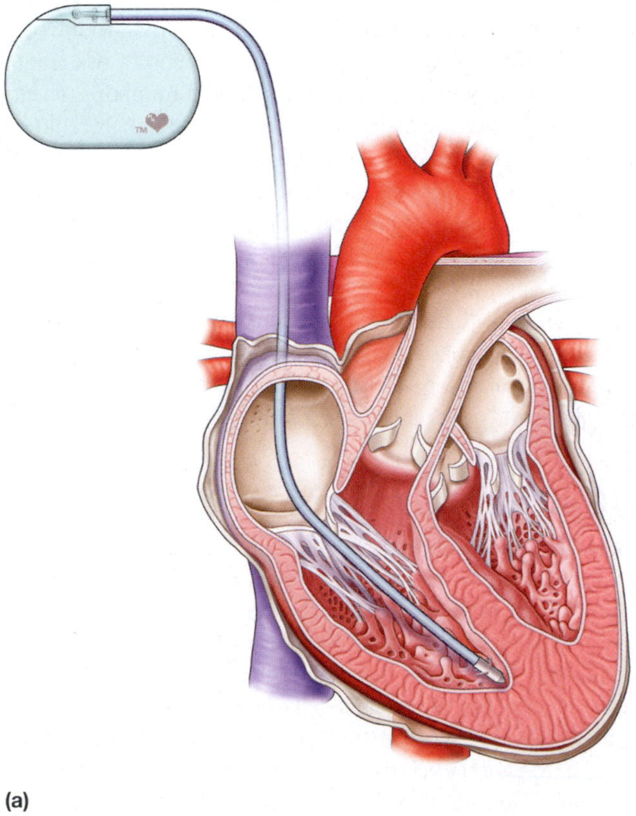

(a)

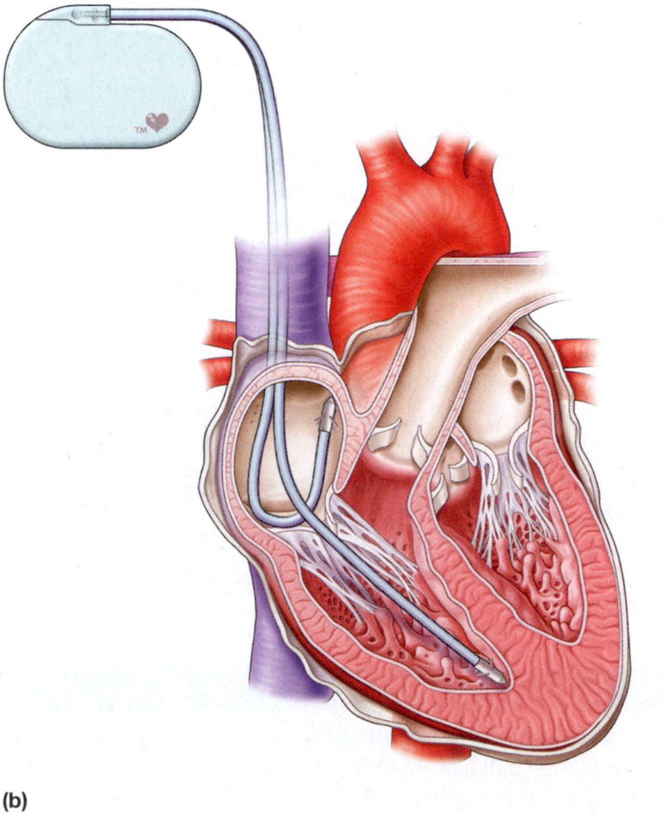

(b)

FIGURE 30–39 ◆ (A) Single- and (B) dual-chambered pacemakers.

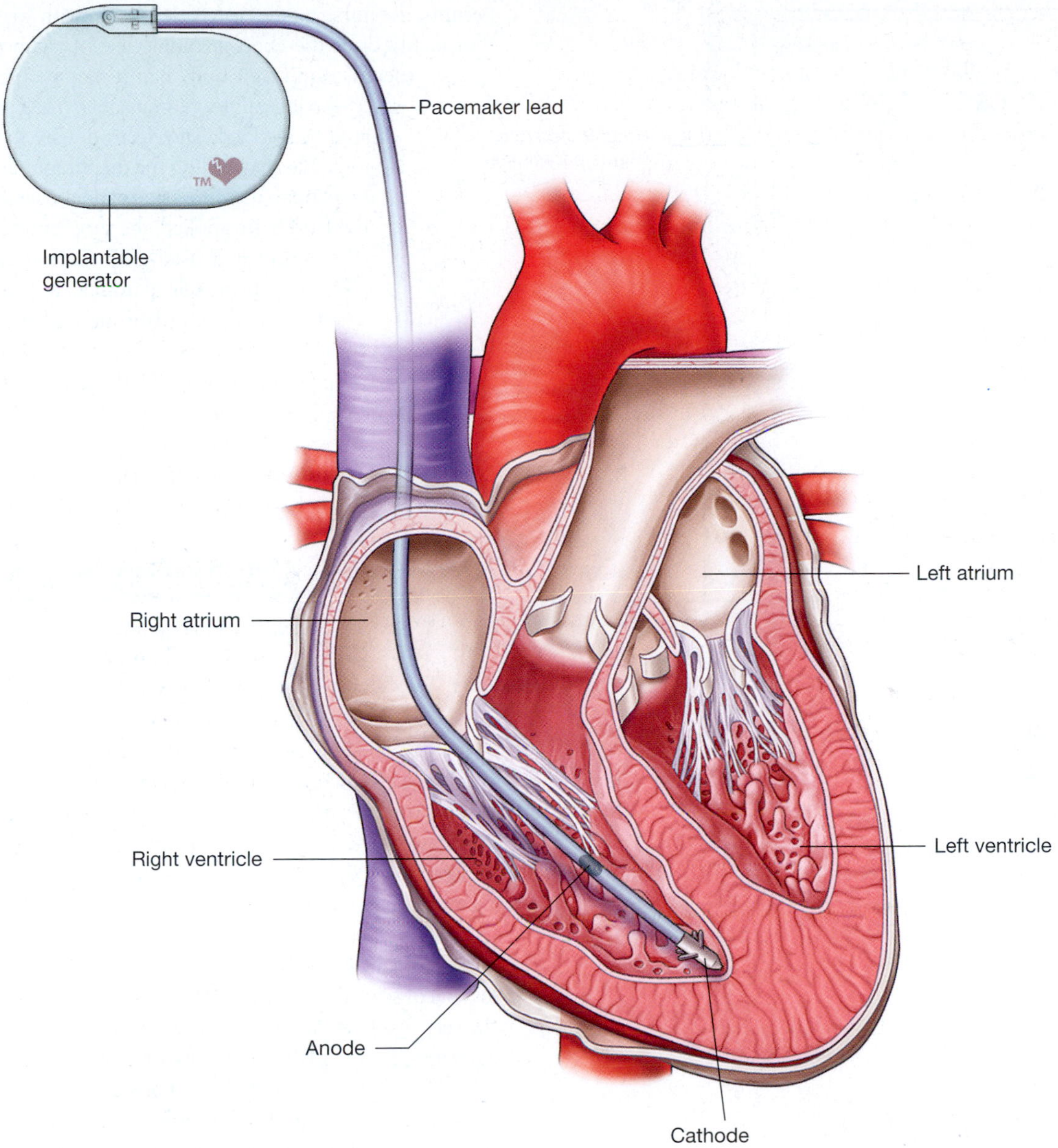

FIGURE 30–40 ◆ Pacemaker components.

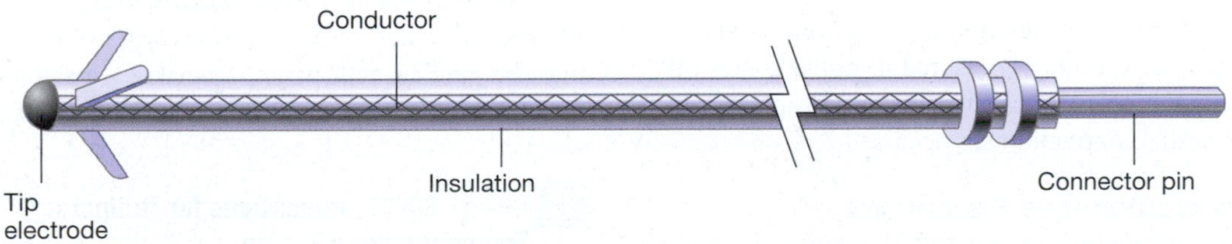

FIGURE 30–41 ◆ Pacemaker lead components.

Dual-chambered temporary pacemakers are not widely used at this time outside of the pediatric and adult cardiac surgery patient population.

Once the leads are connected to the generator, the system must be programmed. At a minimum, this consists of setting the rate at which the pacemaker will fire, the amount of energy delivered with each paced beat (output), and the sensitivity (Figure 30–42).

The programmed rate determines the patient's minimum heart rate. For example, a single-chamber temporary transvenous pacemaker (VVI) set at 60 beats per minute (beats/min) will deliver an electrical stimulus to the ventricle only when the patient's rate drops below 60. If the patient generates his own heartbeat faster than 60 beats per minute, the pacemaker will be inhibited (Figure 30–43◆). This is referred to as a *demand* pacemaker.

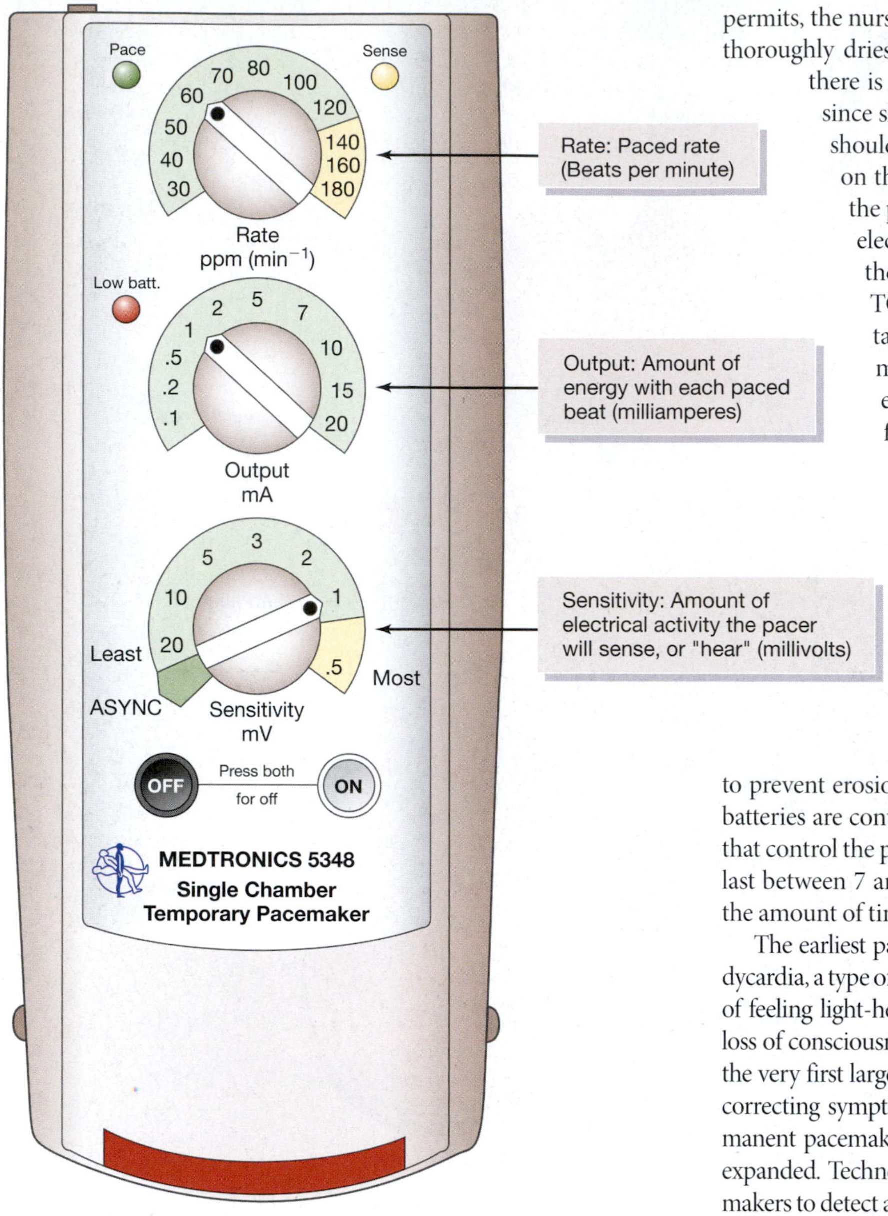

FIGURE 30–42 ◆ Temporary pacemaker generator.

The programmed output, the amount of energy delivered by the generator with each paced beat, is measured in milliamperes (ma). The amount of energy must be sufficient to cause capture, which means that a myocardial contraction has occurred.

Temporary Transcutaneous Pacemaker

Temporary transcutaneous pacing (TCP) is accomplished by delivering the electrical stimulus directly through the chest wall. A variety of devices is currently available; most portable defibrillators are now equipped with optional external pacing capabilities (Figure 30–44◆). Technological advances have resulted in TCP systems that are more reliable and safer to use, resulting in expanded indications for TCP (Chart 30–17).

Large-surface adhesive electrodes, similar to defibrillation electrodes, are placed on the anterior and posterior chest wall over the heart (Figure 30–45◆, p. 896). If this is not feasible, the pads may be placed on the anterior chest wall on the right shoulder and over the left apex. Skin preparation is critical to optimize capture. If time permits, the nurse washes the patient's skin with soap and water and thoroughly dries the chest, avoiding use of alcohol or benzoin. If there is significant body hair it may be trimmed carefully; since shaving can leave small cuts, making TCP painful, it should be avoided. The electrodes are then placed firmly on the chest, avoiding the diaphragm and any metal on the patient, including permanent pacemakers. After the electrodes are applied, the programmed rate is set and the output increased until there is *capture*. Because TCP results in skeletal muscle movement, it is important to verify capture through palpation of a pulse in a major vessel, preferably the femoral artery. Problems encountered with TCP include failure to capture, failure to sense, and painful stimulation of the chest wall. Patients may require sedation or analgesia during sustained TCP therapy. Newer systems have overcome many of these limitations.

Permanent Cardiac Pacemakers

Permanent pacemakers are small and usually implanted in the pectoral area. The generators of permanent pacemakers typically are composed of titanium and are hermetically (airtight) sealed to prevent erosion from contact with bodily fluids. Lithium-iodine batteries are contained within the generator, as are microprocessors that control the pacemaker's various functions. Implanted generators last between 7 and 10 years, depending on multiple factors such as the amount of time the heart is actually paced.

The earliest pacemakers were implanted to treat symptomatic bradycardia, a type of bradycardia that causes the patient to have symptoms of feeling light-headed, dizzy, confused, or even experience complete loss of consciousness. Figure 30–46◆ shows various pacemakers from the very first larger units to the current small, compact unit. Although correcting symptomatic bradycardia remains the cornerstone of permanent pacemaker therapy, indications for implantation have greatly expanded. Technological advances have expanded the ability of pacemakers to detect and treat a variety of dysrhythmias as well as structural abnormalities such as cardiomyopathy. Indications for a permanent pacemaker are outlined in Chart 30–18.

Permanent Pacemaker Vocabulary

In order to understand the various types of pacemakers, the nurse must be familiar with basic pacemaker terminology and functions. A standard pacemaker code system was originally developed in

CHART 30–17 Indications for Temporary Transcutaneous Pacing

1. Hemodynamically significant (resulting in symptoms such as dizziness or syncope) bradycardia unresponsive to atropine
2. Bradycardia with escape rhythms
3. Pacing for patients in cardiac arrest with profound bradycardia or pulseless electrical activity secondary to drug overdose, acidosis, or electrolyte imbalance
4. Standby pacing in anticipation of clinical deterioration, such as development of bifascicular block in acute myocardial infarction or transport of critically ill patients

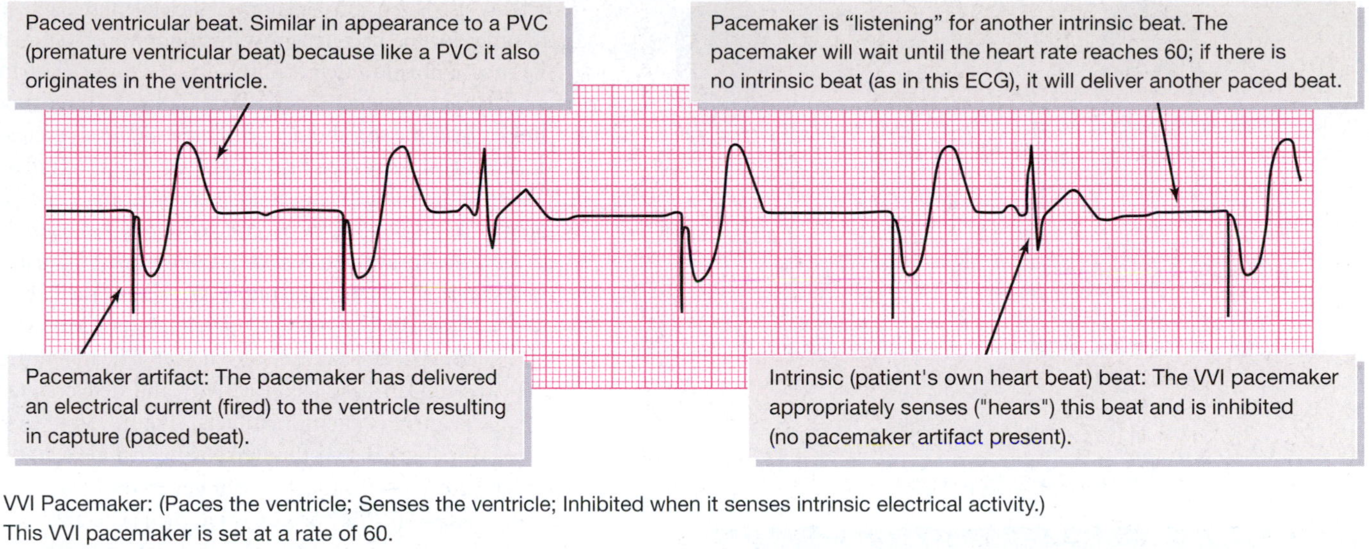

FIGURE 30–43 ◆ VVI pacemaker.

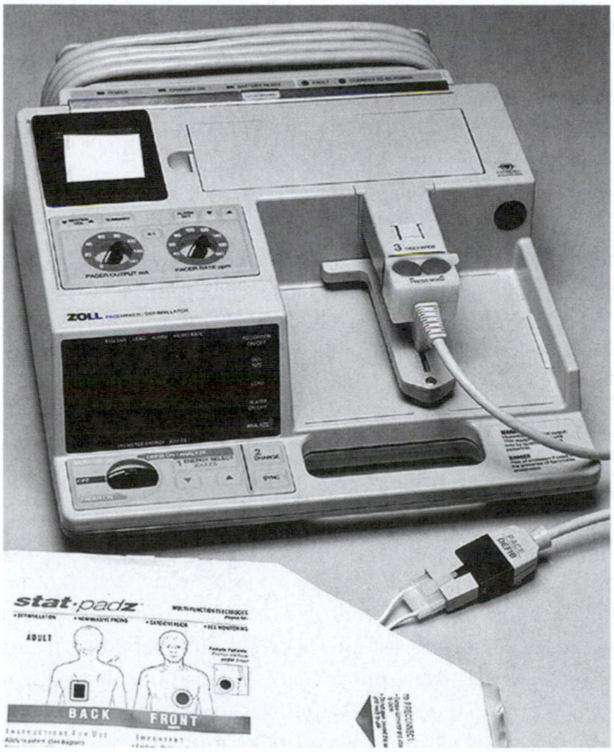

FIGURE 30–44 ◆ Temporary transcutaneous pacemaker.
Source: Courtesy of ZOLL Medical Corporation

1974 by the Inter-Society Commission for Heart Disease (ICHD) to describe the properties of any pacemaker. The original code contained three letters; however, with the advent of the more complex dual-chambered pacemakers, the code was expanded to five letters in 1987 (Chart 30–19, p. 896). It is not always necessary to use all five categories to identify clinically significant information. For example, two of the most commonly used pacing modes are VVI and DDD. The VVI pacemaker has the ability to pace the right ventricle (V), sense the intrinsic electrical activity in the right ventricle (V), and inhibit itself (not deliver an electrical stimulus) when sensing intrinsic activity (I). The DDD pacemaker (also referred to as a dual-chambered or physiological pacemaker) has leads in both the right atrium and the right ventricle. The first D (dual) in the code indicates that the pacemaker can deliver atrial or ventricular paced beats, or both, depending on the settings. The second D indicates the ability to sense intrinsic electrical activity in both the right atrium and right ventricle. The third D indicates the ability of the pacemaker to be either inhibited or trigger in response to a sensed activity. DDD pacemakers are commonly referred to as physiological pacemakers because of their ability to produce atrial contraction followed by ventricular contraction, which most closely mimics normal intrinsic cardiac activity. The fourth letter of the code indicates programmability and rate modulation. In the United States, the overwhelming majority of modern permanent pacemakers have rate modulation, the ability to adjust the pacing rate automatically in conjunction with the patient's activity level, as a programmable feature.

CHART 30–18 Indications for Permanent Cardiac Pacemaker

1. Acquired atrioventricular block in adults
2. Chronic bifascicular and trifascicular block
3. Atrioventricular block associated with acute myocardial infarction
4. Sinus node dysfunction
5. Prevention and termination of tachydysrhythmias
6. Hypersensitive carotid sinus and neurocardiogenic syncope
7. Patients with congenital heart disease
8. In certain conditions:
   a. Hypertrophic obstructive cardiomyopathy
   b. Idiopathic dilated cardiomyopathy
   c. Cardiac transplantation.

Pacemaker Capture

Capture is the depolarization of cardiac muscle response to a paced electrical stimulus that results in myocardial contraction (Figure 30–47A◆). Loss of capture is noted when pacing artifact is present without depolarization and is seen on the ECG as pacing

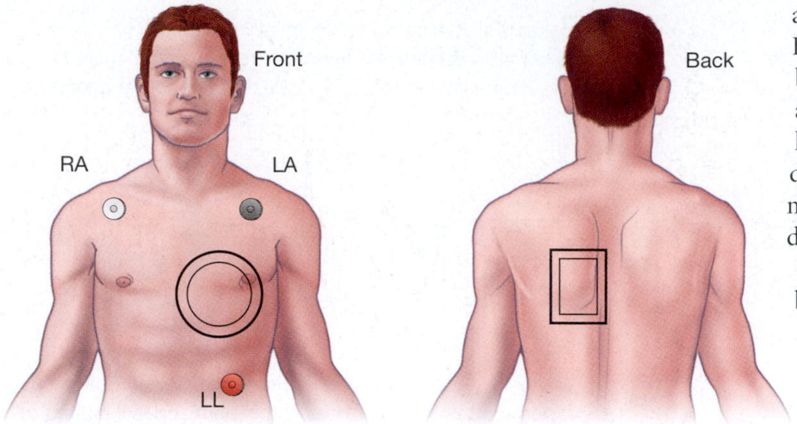

FIGURE 30–45 ◆ Transcutaneous conductor pad placement.

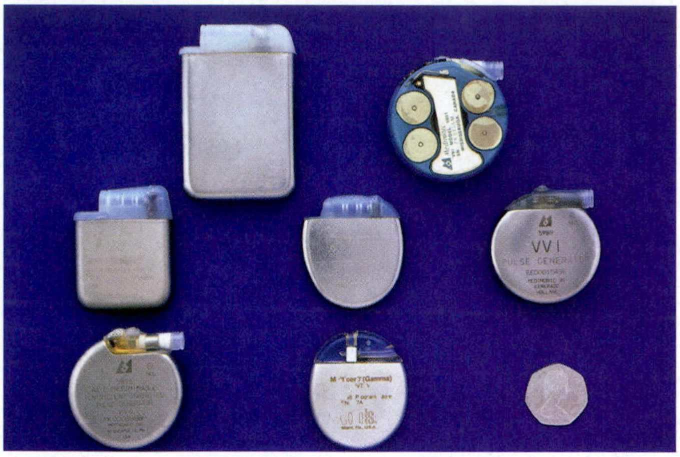

FIGURE 30–46 ◆ Permanent pacemakers.
Source: Reproduced with permission of Medtronic, Inc.

artifact with no paced beat (see Figure 30–47B). Loss of capture can be continuous or intermittent.

Once loss of capture is identified, it is important to assess the patient because loss of capture can result in profound drop in cardiac output and hypotension. Etiology for loss of capture in a temporary pacemaker includes lead dislodgment (most common), lead fracture, battery failure, altered pacemaker thresholds, perforation of the myocardium by the lead wire, and generator failure.

Pacemaker Sensitivity

Pacemaker sensitivity is the ability of the pacemaker to detect or "hear" intrinsic electrical activity and respond appropriately. Electrical activity also is generated by normal skeletal muscle activity. In order for the pacemaker to function properly, it must be programmed to detect only normal *cardiac* electrical activity. The sensitivity is usually set at two to three times higher than the threshold level. Threshold levels increase during the first few days after implantation due to inflammation at the tip site. Threshold levels are usually checked daily while the temporary pacemaker remains in place.

In order to evaluate sensing, there must be intrinsic beats on the ECG and the nurse must know the current pacemaker program. *Undersensing* occurs when the pacemaker fails to detect ("hear") intrinsic electrical cardiac activity and delivers inappropriate pacing artifacts (Figure 30–48A◆). Possible causes of undersensing include lead displacement or fracture, loose connections, or generator failure.

Oversensing (Figure 30–48B) occurs when the pacemaker is inhibited by inappropriate electrical artifact, such as extraneous muscle activity, or by the T wave on the ECG. Airport security systems are a common cause of oversensing. Patient education must include instructions not to go through airport security because the pacemaker will interpret the system's "electrical noise" as cardiac activity and inhibit itself. Depending on the length of exposure, the patient could experience a drop in cardiac output. Chart 30–20 outlines the nursing assessment of the patient who has a pacemaker.

Cardiac Resynchronization Therapy

Cardiac resynchronization therapy (CRT) refers to atrial-synchronized biventricular pacemakers. The three leads necessary for this system are a right atrial lead, a right ventricular lead, and a left ventricular lead. The right leads are positioned inside the cardiac chambers; the left ventricular lead is usually placed in a left lateral vein via the coronary sinus.

Normally the right and left ventricles are activated almost simultaneously, resulting in synchronous systole and diastole. In patients with systolic heart failure, approximately 30% have a prolonged QRS complex (>120 milliseconds). A prolonged QRS results in a significant delay in the electrical activation of the left ventricle, resulting in ventricular dyssynchrony (left ventricular systole occurs after right ventricular systole). This dyssynchrony between the right and left ventricles results in a paradoxical motion of the interventricular septum; that is, instead of contracting with the left ventricle, the septal wall moves toward the right ventricle. Ventricular dyssynchrony forces a mechanical disadvantage on an already failing heart and results in a further drop in cardiac output and heart failure.

CHART 30–19 Inter-Society Commission for Heart Disease Pacemaker Code

Chamber Paced	Chamber Sensed	Response of Sensing	Programmability	Antitachycardia Pacing Functions
0 = None	0 = None	0 = None	0 = None	0 = None
A = Atrium	A = Atrium	T = Triggered	P = Simple programmable	P = Antitachycardia pacing
V = Ventricle	V = Ventricle	I = Inhibited	M = Multiprogrammable	S = Shock
D = Dual (A and V)	D = A and V	D = Trigger and inhibited	C = Communicating	D = P and S
			R = Rate Modulation	

Sources: Code adapted from Parsonnet, Furman, Smyth, & NPD (1974). Bernstein et al. (1987).

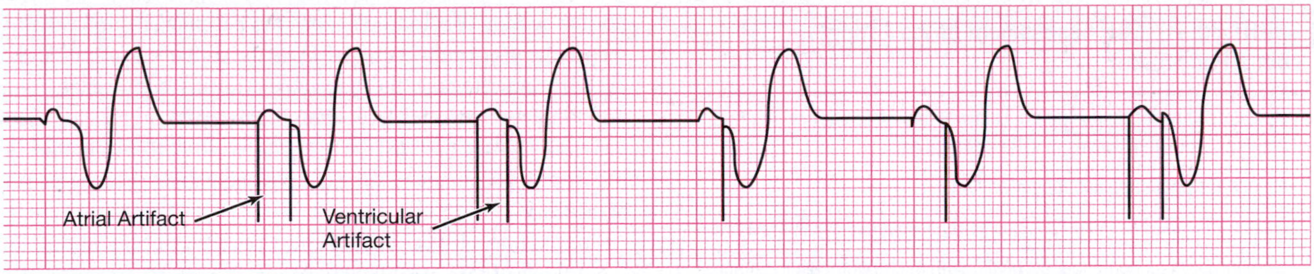

DDD (Dual: Paces both atria and ventricle, Dual: Senses both atria and ventricle: Dual: Can be programmed to be inhibited or triggered in response to intrinsic activity) pacemaker with evidence of 1:1 atrial and ventricular capture. Every pacing artifact is followed by depolarization. Note that pacemaker sensing can not be evaluated from this ECG because there is no intrinsic rhythm.

(a)

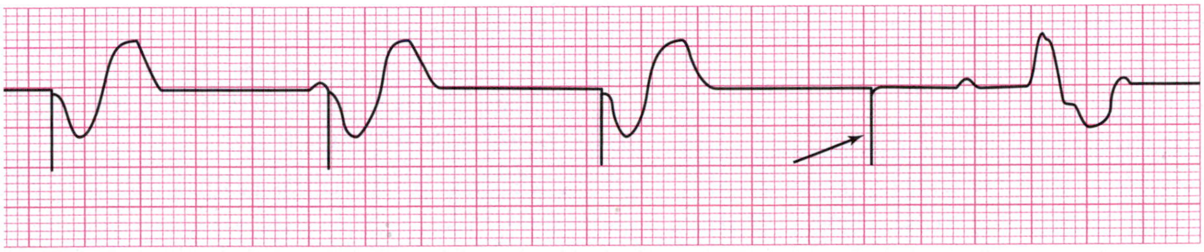

The first three beats exhibit 1:1 capture. After the 4th pacer artifact (arrow), there is no corresponding paced beat. The last QRS complex is an escape beat representing intrinsic ventricular activity.

(b)

FIGURE 30–47 ◆ Pacemaker capture: (A) and (B) loss of ventricular capture.

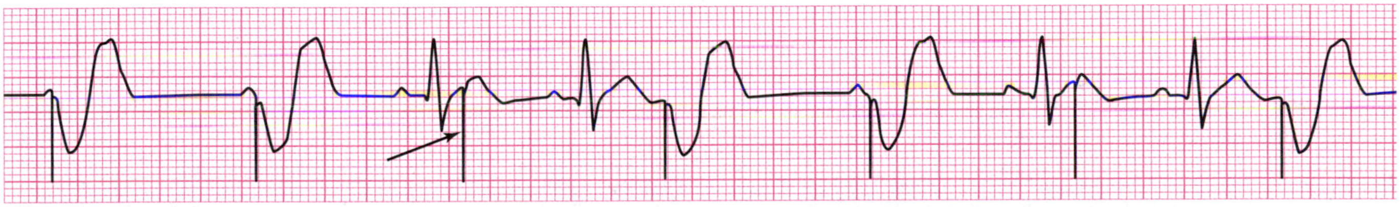

Undersensing. VVI pacemaker programmed at a rate of 60. Pacemaker fails to sense (hear) the intrinsic beat and delivers a pacing artifact into the ST segment of the intrinsic beat (arrow). Pacemaker artifact in this location has been noted to initiate a run of ventricular fibrillation (R on T phenomenon).

(a)

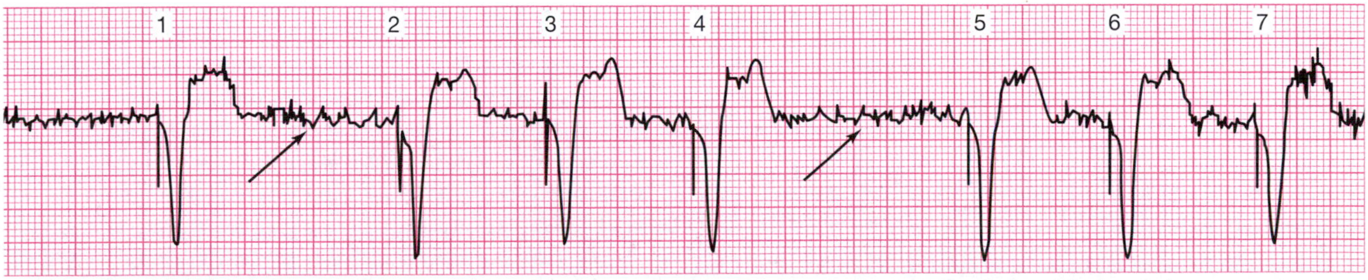

Oversensing. VVI pacemaker programmed at a rate of 60. Pacemaker is inhibited by extraneous electrical activity (arrows). When the pacemaker does fire, there is 1:1 capture.

Note: ECGs from Medtronics, Inc.

(b)

FIGURE 30–48 ◆ Pacemaker sensing: (A) undersensing and (B) oversensing.

Biventricular pacemakers were first implanted in the early 1990s. These devices are used for patients with severe systolic heart failure who have a prolonged QRS and remain symptomatic despite optimal medical management; these patients experience improved cardiac function with CRT. This therapy increases cardiac output and decreases ventricular filling pressures, which results in a decrease in heart failure symptoms and improved quality of life. The latest advances in CRT devices include combining cardioverter/defibrillation capabilities with biventricular pacing, eliminating the need for a separate ICD (discussed previously) in certain patients.

CHART 30–20 ECG Assessment of the Patient with a Pacemaker

1. Assess for any intrinsic electrical activity (the patient's own rhythm). Look for intrinsic P waves or QRS complexes.
2. Assess for pacing spikes (pacer artifact).
3. Examine the ECG in more than one lead for evidence of pacing activity.
4. Look for capture beats (paced beats) with each pacemaker artifact (1:1 capture).
5. Calculate the heart rate. What is the pacemaker's programmed rate?
6. Assess the patient's hemodynamic (Chart 30–9) tolerance of the current settings.

Nursing Management

Care of the patient with a pacemaker includes a complete cardiovascular assessment with special attention to the heart rate. The nurse needs to evaluate the rhythm strip to determine whether capture is occurring appropriately (Chart 30–20). If it is a single-chambered pacemaker, the nurse must determine if there is a QRS after each pacemaker spike; if it is a dual-chambered pacemaker, the nurse determines if there is a P wave after the atrial spike and a QRS after the ventricular spike (Figure 30–47, p. 897). Additionally, the nurse needs to assess for normal sensing. For example, does the pacemaker inhibit itself when there is intrinsic cardiac activity? Does the patient's heart rate and blood pressure indicate that the pacemaker rate is appropriate? Another important assessment is how often the pacemaker is pacing the heart. Frequency of pacing typically is expressed in percentages and usually is a close approximation; for example, the patient is being paced 50% of the time.

In addition, electrical safety practices are critically important, because the leads are capable of carrying electrical current directly into the heart.

Safety Alert

1. *Always wear gloves when handling the pacemaker leads or connecting cables to avoid microshocks.*
2. *Verify that all connections are securely fastened.*
3. *Verify that all equipment in the room is electrically grounded.*
4. *Do not touch any of the pacemaker components on first entering the patient's room to avoid static electricity.*

With the temporary pacemaker, the generator should be securely attached to the leads in order to avoid accidental dislodgment. Care of the surgical access site should incorporate standards of care for any vascular access site. Chapter 11 discusses care of vascular access sites.

The patient should be assessed frequently for signs and symptoms of inadequate cardiac output that could be related to the pacemaker, such as hypotension, dizziness, or sudden syncope.

PATIENT TEACHING & DISCHARGE PRIORITIES for Pacemaker/Implantable Cardioverter Defibrillator Devices

A nursing care plan made for patients after implantation of cardiac devices includes monitoring patient's post-implantation, teaching patients about the device, providing postoperative care, monitoring for adverse complications, and encouraging appropriate follow-up.

Need	Teaching
Patient/family • Provide patient education related to device and need for scheduled follow-up.	• Heart failure medical therapy will augment device therapy and will continue indefinitely. • Limit arm movement to affected side for 1 to 2 weeks (use of sling as needed). • No lifting with affected side for 3 to 4 weeks. • Assess site for signs and symptoms of infection/drainage/bleeding. • Call for abnormal sensation of chest wall muscle movement (indication of dislodged lead or diaphragmatic/pectoral pacing). • Follow-up will be in 1 week to assess site, at 1 month, and then every 6 months and as needed for device interrogation and battery life assessment.
Family/support system • Patients with an automatic implanted cardioverter defibrillator (AICD) may be shocked by the device.	• Family/supports need to understand this is the intended purpose, and that the patient will need follow-up with his cardiologist to assess appropriateness of device. • Patients may need support for anxiety due to the potential or real shocks from an implantable cardioverter defibrillator (ICD).
Setting • In hospital and at home: Assess postoperative pain. • In hospital and at home: Assess incision site.	• Have patient rate pain. • Provide pain medicines as ordered. • Continue to assess level of responsiveness and relief of pain. • Call cardiologist for unrelieved or new pain. • Assess for bleeding, other drainage. • Hematoma. • Call cardiologist for changes.

Source: Adapted from Woods et al., 2010.

Assessment of Pacemaker Function

In order to evaluate the pacemaker completely, information obtained from the ECG must be combined with knowledge of the specific type of pacemaker as well as a complete assessment of the patient. The nurse should review the reason for the pacemaker, the date of insertion, the program settings, and the patient's intrinsic rate, if present. The ECG should be examined in a systematic fashion regardless of the type of pacemaker (Chart 30–20).

Discharge Teaching

Discharge instructions include caring for the access site and providing the patient with the pacemaker information card provided by all pacemaker manufacturers. The patient should carry this information with her at all times. A letter from her health care provider and a medic alert bracelet will aid travel through airport security systems. Finally, even though current technology has rendered pacemakers relatively easy to implant and maintenance free, careful long-term follow-up is necessary to avoid potential problems. The complexity of modern pacemakers makes it difficult to evaluate pacemaker function fully with only the ECG. Pacemaker device questioning by a trained professional is necessary to evaluate pacemaker function and settings completely. This may occur in the office or by telephone. See the Patient Teaching & Discharge Priorities box.

Gerontological Considerations

The majority of patients who receive implantable devices such as pacemakers and ICDs are over the age of 65 (Baddour et al., 2010). Because elderly patients already are at increased risk for falls due to a variety of natural physiological changes, health care professionals must be aggressive in providing careful pacemaker follow-up in order to prevent potential complications in this vulnerable population. The timing of follow-up evaluation depends on several factors, including clinical status of the patient, age of the pacemaker, and geographic location of the patient to a health care facility. Family members may need to be enlisted to ensure that patients adhere to their appointments. Telephone follow-up may be an option if patients have difficulty traveling.

NCLEX® PRACTICE

1. After reviewing the patient's electrocardiogram, the nurse interprets the tracing as normal. Which findings were present on this ECG?
1. PR interval less than 0.8 second
2. QRS complex 0.10 second
3. Absent PR interval
4. QT interval greater than 0.50 second

2. The nurse is assessing the QRS complexes on a patient's electrocardiogram. The complex spans 3 small boxes on the ECG paper. The nurse would identify this patient's QRS complex to be how long?
1. 0.03 second
2. 0.06 second
3. 0.12 second
4. 0.15 second

3. The nurse identifies a small wave that appears after the T wave in a patient's ECG. Which test would the nurse anticipate related to this finding?
1. Repeat ECG in the morning
2. Potassium level
3. Fasting blood glucose
4. Blood urea nitrogen (BUN)

4. The patient's cardiac monitor reveals a regular ventricular rhythm with a rate of 110. The baseline appears to have a jagged saw-tooth configuration. How would the nurse document this rhythm?
1. Ventricular fibrillation
2. Sinus arrhythmia
3. Premature ventricular contractions (PVC)
4. Atrial flutter

5. The nurse identifies a single early beat in a patient's cardiac rhythm strip. The beat looks like the rest of the rhythm except that the P wave is inverted. How would the nurse document this rhythm?
1. Atrial fibrillation
2. Premature ventricular contraction (PVC)
3. Premature junctional contraction (PJC)
4. Sinus arrhythmia

6. The client's cardiac monitor strip has revealed sinus rhythm since admission. The nurse has just identified that the PR interval is 0.24 second. No other changes have occurred. How should the nurse interpret this rhythm?
1. Sinus arrhythmia
2. Atrial fibrillation
3. First-degree AV block
4. Ventricular tachycardia

Answers to NCLEX Practice questions can be found in Appendix D in the Osborn Student Resources at nursing.pearsonhighered.com. Practice additional NCLEX questions online at the Student Resources site.

Pearson Nursing Student Resources Find additional review materials at: **nursing.pearsonhighered.com**

REFERENCES

American Heart Association. (2011a). Risk Factors for Atrial Fibrillation. Retrieved from http://americanheart.org/presenter.jhtml?identifier=3032937

American Heart Association. (2011b). Automated External Defibrillation. Retrieved from http://www.heart.org/idc/groups/gwtg-public/@wcm/@private/@ecc/documents/downloadable/ucm_309676.pdf

Baddour, L. M., Epstein, A. E., Erickson, C. C., Knight, B. P., Levison, M. E., Lockhart, P. B., ... Taubert, K. A. (2010). Update on cardiovascular implantable electronic device infections and their management: a scientific statement from the American Heart Association. *Circulation, 121,* 458–477.

Baltazar, R. F. (2009). *Basic and bedside electrocardiography.* Philadelphia, PA: Lippincott Williams & Wilkins.

Bernstein, A. D., Camm, A. J., Fletcher, R., Gold, R. D., Rickards, A. F., Smyth, N. P. D., Spielman, S. R., & Sutton, R. (1987). The NASPE/BPEG: Pacemaker Code for antibradyarrhythmia and adaptive-rate pacing and antitachyarrhythmia devices. *PACE, 10,* 794–799.

Campuzano, O., & Brugada, R. (2009). Genetics of familial atrial fibrillation. *Europace, 11,* 1267–1271.

Carlson, K. K. (2009). *AACN advanced critical care nursing.* St. Louis: Saunders Elsevier.

Hazinksi, M. F. (Ed.) (2010). Highlights of the 2010 American Heart Association Guidelines for CPR and ECC. Retrieved from http://www.heart.org/idc/groups/heart-public/@wcm/@ecc/documents/downloadable/ucm_317350.pdf

Heart Rhythm Society. (2011). Available at HRS/EHRA Expert Consensus on the Monitoring of Cardiovascular Implantable Electronic Devices (CIEDs): Description of Techniques, Indications, Personnel, Frequency, and Ethical Considerations; accessed January 11, 2011.

International Liaison Committee on Resuscitation. (2011). Retrieved from http://www.ilcor.org/en/home/

Kee, J. L. (2010). *Laboratory and diagnostic tests with nursing implications.* Upper Saddle River, NJ: Pearson.

Lubitz, S. A., Yi, B. A., & Ellinor, P. T. (2009). Genetics of atrial fibrillation. *Cardiology Clinics, 27,* 25–33.

Mayo Clinic. (2010). Brugada syndrome. Retrieved from http://www.mayoclinic.com/health/brugada-syndrome/DS01142

Mayo Clinic. (2011). Hereditary component of atrial fibrillation revealed. Retrieved from http://www.mayoclinic.org/medicalprofs/atrial-fibrillation-hereditary-component.html

Moser, D. K., & Reigel, B. (2008). *Cardiac nursing: A companion to Braunwald's heart disease.* St. Louis: Saunders.

Osborn, K., & Watson, A. B. (2011). ECG: *The Art and Science of Interpretation.* Upper Saddle River, NJ: Pearson.

Parsonnet, V., Furman, S., & Smyth, N. P. D. (1974). Implantable cardiac pacemakers; Status report and resource guideline. Pacemaker Study Group, Inter-Society Commission for Heart Disease Resources (ICHD). *Circulation, 50,* A21–A35.

Porth, C. M. (2008). *Essentials of pathophysiology: Concepts of altered health states* (8th ed.). Philadelphia: Lippincott Williams & Wilkins.

Redeen, M. (2007). ECG Measurements for Cardiac Rhythms. California State University, Sacramento.

Thaler, M. S. (2010). *The only ECG book you'll ever need.* Philadelphia: Wolters Kluwer/Lippincott Williams & Wilkins.

Wilkinson, J., & Ahearn, N. (2009). Nursing Diagnoses Handbook. (9th ed.). Upper Saddle River, NJ: Pearson.

Woods, S. L., Froelicher, E. S. S., Adams (Underhill), S., & Bridges, E. J. (Eds.) (2010). *Cardiac nursing* (6th ed.). Philadelphia: Lippincott Williams & Wilkins.

Hemodynamic Monitoring

31 CHAPTER

Brenda McCulloch
Kathleen Osborn

Outcome-Based Learning Objectives

After studying this chapter, the learner will be able to:

1. Summarize the concept of hemodynamic monitoring.
2. Differentiate the components of a hemodynamic monitoring system.
3. Compare and contrast the types of data obtained from arterial, central venous, and pulmonary artery pressure monitoring.
4. Generate nursing management parameters for arterial lines, central venous catheters, and pulmonary artery catheters.
5. Critique how alterations in preload, afterload, and contractility affect cardiac output.

KEY TERMS

afterload p.903
Allen's test p.906
arterial line p.906
cardiac index (CI) p.902
cardiac output (CO) p.901
central venous pressure (CVP) p.903
contractility p.903
ejection fraction (EF) p.902
Frank-Starling law p.903
hemodynamic monitoring p.901
inotropic p.911
leveling p.904
mean arterial pressure (MAP) p.907
mixed venous oxygen saturation p.913
phlebostatic axis p.904
preload p.903
pulmonary artery catheter (PAC) p.911
pulmonary artery occlusion pressure (PAOP) p.912
stroke volume (SV) p.901
thermistor p.911
thoracic impedance p.917
transesophageal ultrasound p.916
zero referencing p.905

HEMODYNAMIC MONITORING is the monitoring of blood flow and pressures within the body. Current technology allows for the monitoring of both the cardiac and neurological systems. This chapter describes invasive and noninvasive hemodynamic monitoring techniques used for the cardiovascular system. The purposes of hemodynamic monitoring are to (1) aid in the diagnosis of various disorders, (2) assist in guiding therapies to minimize or correct dysfunction, and (3) evaluate the patient's response to therapy. For safe operation of hemodynamic monitoring devices, nurses must be familiar with the anatomy and physiology of the system being monitored. Moreover, nurses must be knowledgeable about therapeutic interventions and their rationales in order to achieve optimal, patient-specific outcomes. Nurses must be prepared to provide care based on the findings obtained from the hemodynamic monitoring, to institute interventions, and to report any changes to the health care provider.

Hemodynamic monitoring capability is not restricted to the intensive care unit (ICU). Patients who require hemodynamic assessment are also treated in emergency departments, postanesthesia care units, and intermediate care units. The level of intervention differs depending on the patient's diagnosis and hemodynamic stability. It may involve monitoring arterial blood pressure, central venous pressure, or intracardiac pressures, all of which are discussed in this chapter.

Hemodynamic Terminology

Invasive and noninvasive hemodynamic monitoring provide for close examination of cardiac function. This section explains the terms used in performing hemodynamic monitoring and provides examples to clarify their use. Chart 31–1 (p. 902) summarizes these terms.

Stroke Volume

Stroke volume (SV) is the amount of blood leaving the left ventricle with each contraction. For a healthy heart, the expected SV is 60 to 100 mL per beat. Stroke volume is sensitive to alterations in preload, afterload, and contractility, which are discussed later in this chapter.

Cardiac Output

Cardiac output (CO) is defined as the amount of blood leaving the left ventricle per minute. Cardiac output is calculated by multiplying heart rate (HR) by stroke volume (HR × SV). With a healthy ventricle, this amount is between 4 and 6 L/min. Adequate cardiac output is essential for circulation and tissue oxygenation. A drop in CO, which occurs when the heart is failing and cannot pump effectively, reduces the amount of oxygen and nutrients delivered to the tissues.

Weblink: Hemodynamic Monitoring

CHART 31–1 Hemodynamic Parameters

Parameters	Calculation	Expected Value
Cardiac Output (CO)		
Stroke volume (SV)	$\frac{CO \times 1000}{HR}$	60–180 mL per beat
Stroke volume index (SVI)	$\frac{SV}{BSA}$	33–47 mL/m^2 per beat
Cardiac index (CI)	$\frac{CO}{BSA}$	2.5–3 L min m^{-2}
Heart rate (HR)		60–100 beats/min
Cardiac output	$HR \times SV$	4–6 liters/min
Preload		
Central venous pressure (CVP)		2–6 mmHg
Right atrial pressure (RAP)		4–6 mmHg
Left atrial pressure (LAP)		4–12 mmHg
Pulmonary artery diastolic pressure (PAD)		5–12 mmHg
Pulmonary artery occlusion pressure (PAOP, PAWP, or PCWP)		5–12 mmHg
Right ventricular end-diastolic pressure (RVEDP)		0–8 mmHg
Left ventricular end-diastolic pressure (LVEDP)		5–12 mmHg
Afterload		
Mean arterial pressure (MAP)	$DBP + \frac{(SBP - DBP)}{3}$	
Systemic vascular resistance (SVR)	$\frac{MAP - CVP \text{ (or RAP)} \times 80}{CO}$	800–1,200 dyn sec cm^{-5}
Systemic vascular resistance index (SVRI)	$\frac{MAP - CVP \text{ (or RAP)} \times 80}{CI}$	1,500–2,400 dyn sec cm^{-5}
Pulmonary vascular resistance (PVR)	$\frac{PAM - PAOP \text{ (or PAWP)} \times 80}{CO}$	120–200 dyn sec cm^{-5}
Pulmonary vascular resistance index (PVRI)	$\frac{PAM - PAOP \text{ (or PAWP)} \times 80}{CI}$	255–285 dyn sec cm^{-5}
Contractility		
Ejection fraction (EF)	$\frac{LVEDV \times 100}{SV}$	55–75%
	$\frac{RVEDV \times 100}{SV}$	45–50%

Source: Adapted from Chulay, M., & Burns, S. (2010). *AACN essentials of critical care nursing* (2nd ed.). New York: McGraw-Hill; Woods, S. L., Froelicher, E. S. S., Adams (Underhill), S., & Bridges, E. J. (Eds.). (2009). *Cardiac nursing* (6th ed.). Philadelphia: Lippincott Williams & Wilkins.

Cardiac Index

Cardiac index (CI) is a more accurate measurement of circulation than cardiac output. The calculation for cardiac index incorporates the patient's body surface area (BSA). The cardiac index is the CO per square meter of the body. BSA can be calculated by using the DuBois scale, by using BSA calculation software in a personal digital assistant (PDA), or by computing it as follows:

$$BSA = (\text{weight in kg} \times 0.425) \times (\text{height in cm} \times 0.725) \times 0.007184$$

Whichever method is used to obtain a BSA, the BSA value is then divided into the cardiac output to obtain the cardiac index. An adequate CI is between 2.5 and 3 L/min. Most bedside monitors automatically calculate the BSA during a cardiac output measurement, provided that the patient's height and weight have been preprogrammed into the monitor. The CO and CI are hemodynamic parameters obtained with a pulmonary artery catheter, discussed later in this chapter.

Ejection Fraction

With each contraction, the left and right ventricles of the heart do not empty completely. The percentage of the total volume that is ejected with each beat is called the **ejection fraction (EF).** Ejection fraction is a calculation, expressed as a percentage, that compares the end-diastolic volume to the stroke volume. A normal EF is 55% to 70%, meaning that 55% to 70% of the blood in the left ventricle is ejected with each heartbeat under normal resting circumstances and 30% to 45% is left for periods of high demand.

The volume of blood remaining in the ventricle is considered a reserve. During periods of stress or exercise, this cardiac reserve, combined with a healthy ventricular contraction, assists in meeting the increased demand for adequate tissue oxygenation. Myocardium with abnormal contractile fibers is unable to pump as effectively as usual; thus, more blood remains in the ventricle with each beat, thereby decreasing the EF. Ejection fraction is an important parameter because a low EF value indicates ventricular dysfunction. An EF of less than 35% indicates serious ventricular failure.

Contractility

Contractility is the force generated by the contracting myocardium. The ability of the ventricles to contract or squeeze against resistance is determined by the contractile force of the ventricle. The force of contraction is related to the ability of the ventricular muscle fiber to lengthen or stretch. According to the **Frank-Starling law,** the muscle fibers in healthy ventricles will stretch to accommodate the venous return received during diastole. Generally, if the ventricle receives excess venous blood return during diastole, the ventricular contraction will be more forceful, resulting in an increased stroke volume. A filling pressure between 10 and 12 mmHg is considered optimal (Porth & Matfin, 2009). When the pressure exceeds 12 mmHg and the myocardial fibers are overstretched, the force of ventricular contraction will decrease, eventually resulting in heart failure.

Contractility is enhanced by circulating catecholamines, sympathetic nervous system stimulation, and medications such as digoxin, dopamine, or dobutamine that increase contractility. Contractility is depressed with acidosis, hypoxemia, and beta-adrenergic blocking medications.

Preload

Preload, the volume of blood in the ventricle at the end of diastole, is referred to as an end-diastolic pressure (EDP). Right ventricular preload is dependent on total blood volume returning to the heart, cardiac output, and venous vascular resistance (Porth & Matfin, 2009). **Central venous pressure (CVP)** and right atrial pressure (RAP) are measurements that reflect venous return to the right side of the heart. When assessment of preload must be more precise, a pulmonary artery catheter with a lumen in the right ventricle provides measurement of right ventricular volume using the previously described transducer system.

Afterload

Afterload is the pressure or resistance the ventricles must overcome to eject blood during systole. Vascular resistance is the major determinant of afterload. The right ventricle pumps blood into the pulmonary system through the pulmonic valve into the pulmonary artery. Afterload of the pulmonary system is termed *pulmonary vascular resistance* (PVR). The left ventricle pumps blood into systemic circulation through the aortic valve. Systemic afterload is termed *systemic vascular resistance* (SVR).

Equipment

Both noninvasive and invasive devices are available for hemodynamic monitoring. The required equipment depends on the parameter to be monitored. Noninvasive monitoring often involves a stethoscope and sphygmomanometer; however, technologies such as ultrasound and impedance cardiography are also considered noninvasive.

Invasive monitoring necessitates the insertion of a catheter into an artery or vein for direct and ongoing measurement of vascular pressures and volumes. Hemodynamic pressures are transmitted from the intravascular space via this specialized catheter into the monitoring system for the health care team to read and interpret.

Invasive monitoring requires knowledge about the safe use of equipment and techniques needed during the procedure. Assembling the equipment and maintaining the system are usually the nurse's responsibilities.

Components of the Monitoring Equipment

An invasive hemodynamic monitoring system has five basic components: the monitor, flush system, transducer, high-pressure tubing, and catheter (Figure 31–1◆). The system, referred to as a *transducer system*, is assembled in an identical fashion whether used for an artery or vein. Chart 31–2 describes the step-by-step process for setting up the hemodynamic monitoring system.

These systems require a constant flow of sterile solution in order to maintain patency and decrease the risk of clot formation. The most common solution used is 0.9% normal saline (NS). Because these catheters are placed into high-pressure systems in the body, a sleeve or pressure bag is placed over the NS bag and inflated to 300 millimeters of mercury (mmHg) to counteract the pressure in the vessel and allow the solution to flow into the patient. High-pressure tubing instead of flexible intravenous (IV) tubing is necessary to withstand the external pressure exerted by the sleeve and to decrease the distortion of the waveform (discussed later in the chapter).

After the transducer system has been assembled and attached to the catheter, the infusion rate is held constant by the transducer system and the pressure sleeve. The information on the transducer package insert

CHART 31–2 Setup of Pressure Transducer System

1. Obtain an intravenous (IV) flush solution of normal saline and a transducer system.
2. Wash hands.
3. Attach the transducer system to the IV flush solution and prime all tubing, ensuring that air bubbles are removed from the system.
4. Replace all vented caps with nonvented (dead-end) sterile caps.
5. Inflate the pressure bag to 300 mmHg.
6. Assist the patient to the supine position with the head of the bed elevated no more than 45 degrees.
7. Accurately measure and mark the patient's phlebostatic axis with an indelible marker.
8. Level the air–fluid interface to the phlebostatic axis.
9. Zero the system.
10. Set alarm limits.

Source: Adapted from Lynn-McHale Wiegand, D. J. (Ed.). (2010). *AACN procedure manual for critical care* (6th ed.). Philadelphia: Elsevier.

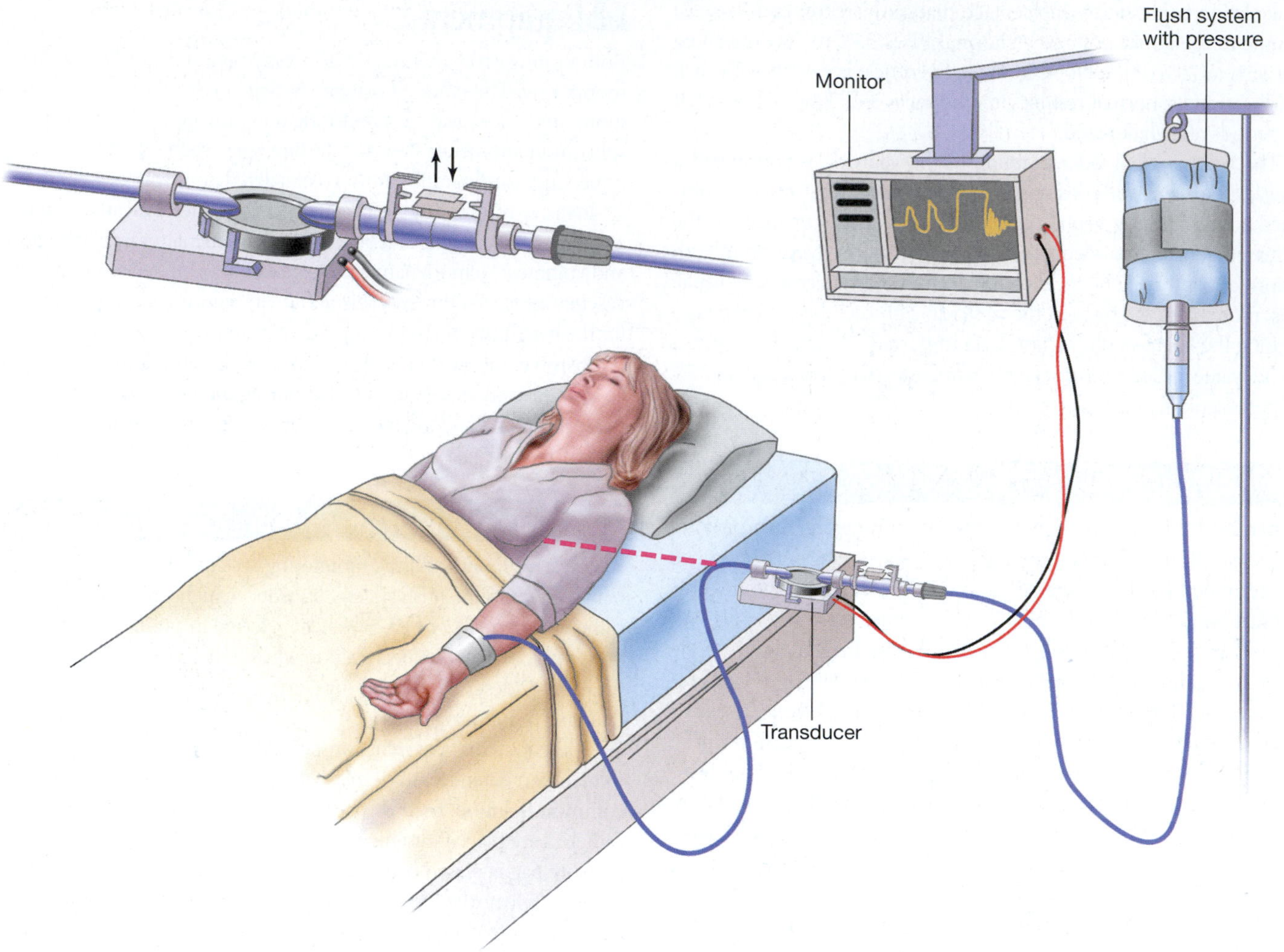

FIGURE 31–1 ◆ Components of the hemodynamic monitoring system.

will indicate the constant infusion rate, but 1 to 3 mL/hour is common (Lynn-McHale Wiegand, 2010). The transducer converts pressure detected at the catheter tip into an electrical signal, which is displayed as a waveform on a bedside or portable monitor.

Leveling the transducer and zero referencing are nursing responsibilities when patients have hemodynamic monitoring catheters in place. Variability in technique among clinicians conducting these operator-dependent procedures influences the accuracy of the hemodynamic data (Woods, Froelicher, Adams, & Bridges, 2009). Each of these variables is discussed next.

Leveling the Transducer

Leveling the transducer means placing the transducer at the same level as the tip of the catheter sitting in the patient. A reference point on the patient, referred to as the **phlebostatic axis,** is identified to use as a baseline for consistent transducer height placement. To locate the phlebostatic axis, a horizontal line is identified that is halfway between the anterior diameter and posterior diameter of the chest. This horizontal line intersects with a vertical line from the fourth intercostal space (Figure 31–2◆). Marking this reference point with an indelible marker permits ready identification by others. The transducer is typically mounted on an IV pole beside the bed. A yardstick with a carpenter level aids the nurse in aligning the transducer with the phlebostatic point. Figure 31–3◆ illustrates an adjustment of the reference point for

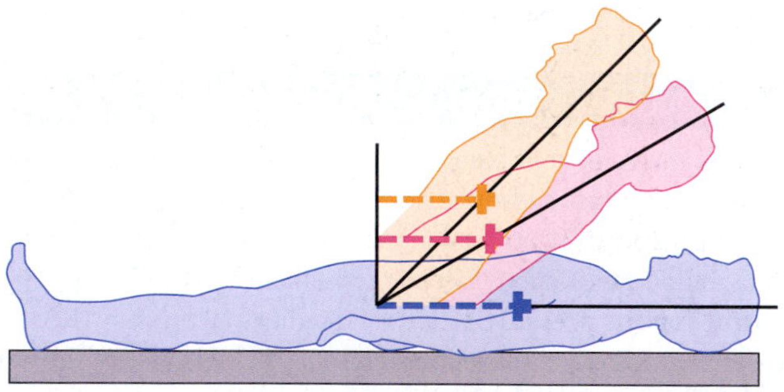

FIGURE 31–2 ◆ Phlebostatic axis.

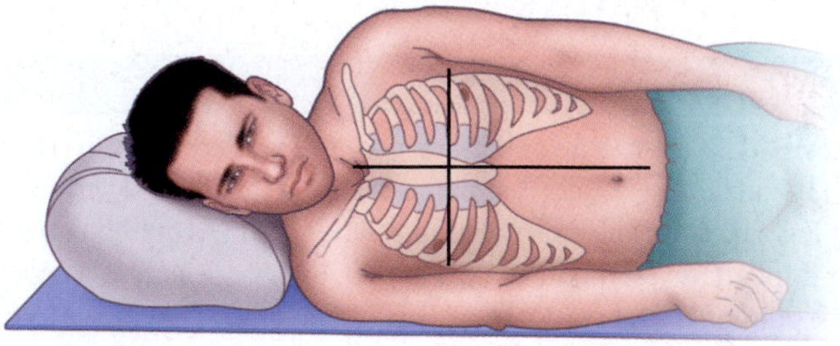

FIGURE 31–3 ◆ Identification of phlebostatic axis when patient is in the lateral position.

a patient in a lateral position. Research has shown that when the patient is supine, with the head of the bed elevated up to 45 degrees, the accuracy of pressure readings does not change (Woods et al., 2009).

The importance of using the same reference point cannot be overstated. Incorrect transducer placement results in invalid pressure readings. Positioning the transducer above the reference point will decrease the pressure reading, and lowering the transducer will increase the reading. This discrepancy can expose a patient to unnecessary or erroneous treatment.

Safety Alert *To ensure accurate pressure readings, it is imperative that when the patient is repositioned, including raising or lowering the head of the bed, the transducer must be zeroed out again at the phlebostatic point. When the transducer is pole mounted and the bed height is raised or lowered, the zeroing out process should be repeated.*

Zero Referencing the Transducer

Once the transducer is level with the reference point, the next step is to zero reference the system. Prior to performing this procedure, the nurse should ensure that the transducer system is intact, the tubing is without air bubbles, and connections are tight. **Zero referencing** the transducer calibrates the equipment to atmospheric pressure. Figure 31–4◆ illustrates the leveling and zero referencing. To zero the transducer, the nurse turns the stopcock closest to the patient to the off position. This turns the transducer off to the patient. The nurse then removes the cap from the transducer to allow for equilibration of the transducer with atmospheric pressure. The nurse initiates the zero function on the monitoring system, waits for the display to read zero, then turns the stopcock knob back to the neutral position.

The frequency of zeroing the transducer varies between institutions. However, zeroing should be done once per shift, after a patient is turned, and whenever pressure readings are questionable (Lynn-McHale Wiegand, 2010).

Normal Hemodynamic Pressures

Human physiology relies on a dynamic balance between blood flow, resistance, and pressure. Hemodynamic monitoring provides an overall assessment of this balance with individual components focusing on circulation, perfusion, and tissue oxygenation. This in-depth assessment of these interactions helps health care providers as they diagnose, guide, and evaluate therapies.

When an invasive catheter senses the cardiovascular system's pressures, they are displayed on a monitor as pressure waveforms. Pressure changes produce positive and negative deflections. The waveform correlates with the cardiac cycle; however, because the pressures are being transmitted through fluid-filled tubing, there is a slight delay. Simultaneous dual-channel recording of the electrocardiogram (ECG) and pressure waveforms improves the accuracy of the pressure waveforms (Figure 31–5◆) (Woods et al., 2009). Pressure waveforms are most accurate at the end of expiration when the effect of intrathoracic pressure is negligible.

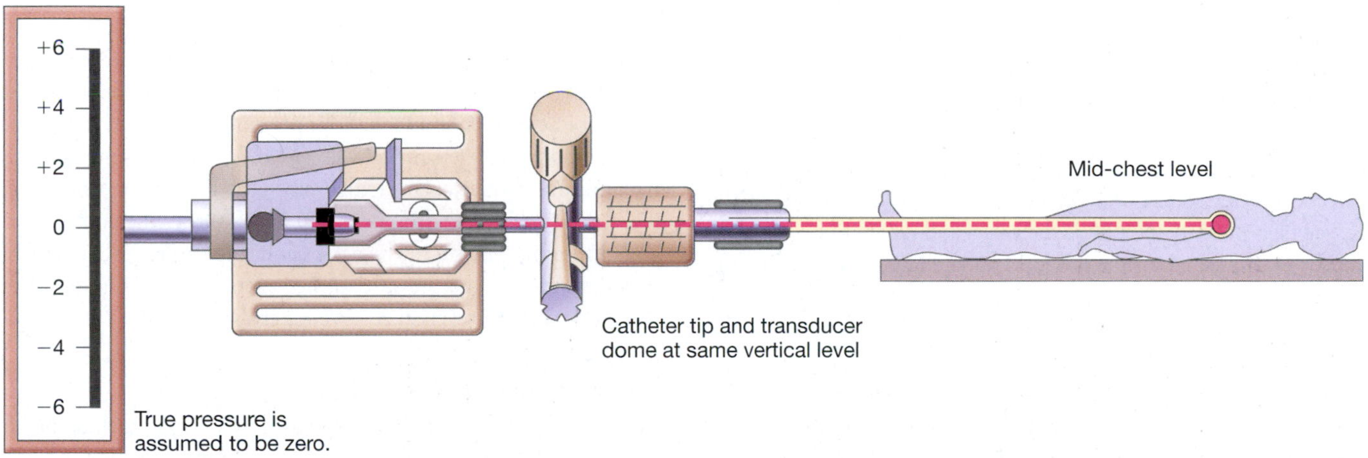

FIGURE 31–4 ◆ Leveling and zero referencing the transducer to the phlebostatic axis.

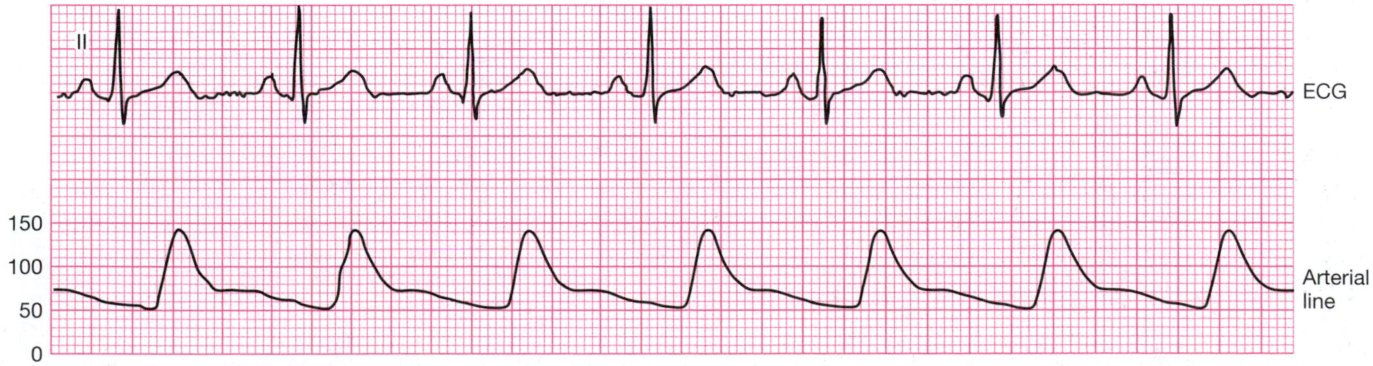

FIGURE 31–5 ◆ Single-lead ECG and arterial pressure waveform.

Invasive Pressure Monitoring

Invasive hemodynamic monitoring provides a method of direct measurement of vascular pressures. Medical therapies are based on the interpretation of the parameter being assessed. Systemic, central venous, and pulmonary artery monitoring devices are frequently used for this purpose. Each of these is discussed in this section along with information on complications and details about nursing management.

Intra-Arterial Catheters

An intra-arterial catheter, also known as an arterial catheter or **arterial line,** is an indwelling catheter inserted into an artery by a health care provider or an advanced practice nurse in order to monitor blood pressure (BP). Arterial catheters, which are inserted either percutaneously or by a surgical cutdown technique, are recommended for patients whose blood pressure is unstable and therefore requires frequent monitoring. These patients include those who are hypotensive, hypertensive, or receiving vasoactive medications that require titration and careful monitoring. Arterial lines also provide access for obtaining frequent blood specimens.

Safety Alert *An arterial line is* never *used for infusion of IV solutions or medications. Both IV solutions and medications are irritating to the vessel and may compromise tissue perfusion distal to the catheter.*

The radial artery is the most common site for arterial catheter placement. Other sites such as the brachial, axillary, femoral, dorsalis pedis, and posterior tibial are possible alternatives. To decrease the risk of infection, the femoral site should be avoided whenever possible. The radial artery is easily accessible because of its proximity to the skin surface, making it the preferred site.

An **Allen's test** is performed prior to insertion of the radial arterial catheter to assess ulnar circulation in the hand (Figure 31–6◆). To perform an Allen's test, the nurse raises the patient's hand above her head and asks the patient to make a tight fist. While the fist is tight, the nurse applies pressure to occlude the radial and ulnar arteries simultaneously. The nurse lowers the patient's hand and asks her to release the tight fist. The nurse then releases the pressure over the ulnar artery and observes the return of color to the hand. An Allen's test is positive if the color returns to the hand in 7 seconds or less after release of the ulnar artery. If the return time is greater than 7 seconds, the test is inconclusive; however, if it is greater than 15 seconds, the test is negative. If color does not return to the hand after the ulnar artery is released, the health care provider should be notified and arterial puncture should not be performed, because the superficial palmar arch is not intact. This may place the patient at risk for vascular thrombosis and arterial occlusion, which may lead to necrosis and, in severe cases, amputation of the hand. The nurse must always document that the Allen's test was performed, the results, and any action taken if the test is negative. Ongoing assessment of circulation distal to the insertion site is the nurse's responsibility.

Safety Alert *The Allen's test can be performed on an unconscious patient by holding the patient's arm above his head and clenching the patient's hand into a fist. Apply pressure to both the ulnar and radial arteries while the arm is overhead. Lower the arm, and release the pressure from the radial artery.*

Ensuring the integrity of the monitoring system, preventing infection, and assessing for thrombus formation are fundamental nursing responsibilities associated with arterial line placement (Woods et al., 2009). The arterial catheter can be sutured in place. Prior to applying the occlusive dressing, the nurse should check that the arterial catheter is tightly attached to the hub on the pressure tubing. The monitoring system has upper and lower limit alarming capabilities, and it is the nurse's responsibility to set, adjust, and ensure these alarms are engaged at all times.

Safety Alert *Always set the patient's alarms based on the patient's baseline hemodynamic pressures and the abnormality being monitored. Never turn the alarms off entirely. To allow alert patients to have periods of uninterrupted rest, the intensity or volume of the alarm can usually be adjusted on bedside monitors without affecting the alarm signal or message from the central station.*

Arterial Pressure Waveforms

When the pressure transducer system is attached to the arterial catheter, an identifiable arterial waveform appears on the monitor. This waveform represents systolic and diastolic pressures generated by the heart's mechanical activity (Figure 31–7◆). The systolic pressure represents maximum left ventricular systolic pressure. The dicrotic notch represents closure of the aortic valve and distinguishes the end of systole and beginning of diastole, which is a significant cardiac event. Diastolic pressure indicates the pressure in the ventricle at rest and is directly related to blood vessel elasticity (Woods et al., 2009).

Complications of Arterial Blood Pressure Monitoring

Complications of arterial blood pressure monitoring include hemorrhage, emboli, vascular occlusion or spasm, and infection. Bleeding

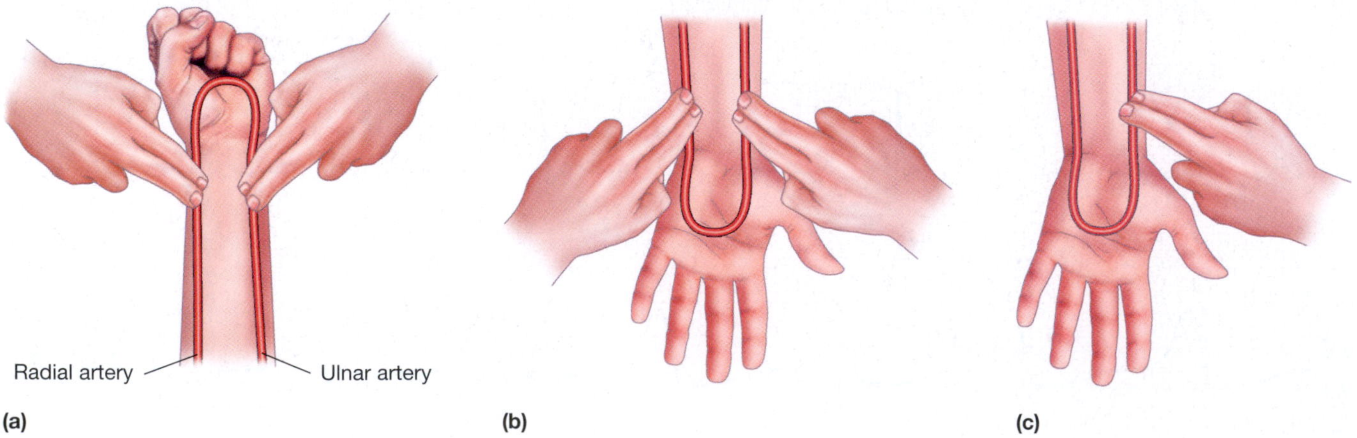

FIGURE 31–6 ◆ Performing the Allen's test.

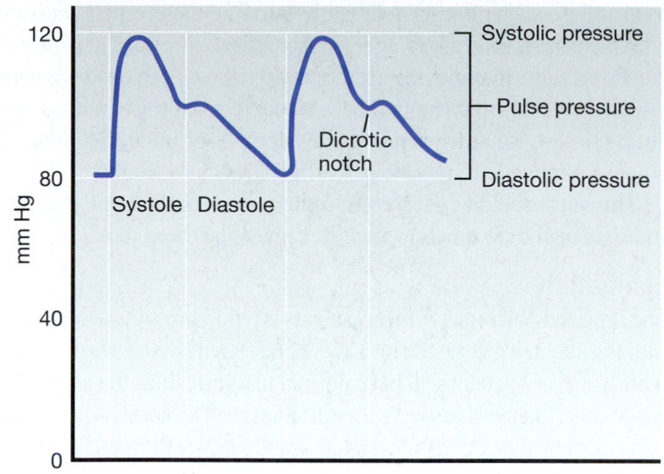

FIGURE 31–7 ◆ Analyzing an arterial pressure waveform.

may occur, particularly after a femoral artery catheter has been inserted. Signs of hypovolemia, lower abdominal firmness, or swelling or bruising at the site should alert the nurse to notify the health care provider immediately. Because of the high pressure in arteries, massive blood loss can occur if the catheter dislodges, if it is disconnected from the patient, or if the connections are loosened. Assessment of circulation distal to the insertion site, prior to insertion of the catheter, does not preclude the occurrence of vascular ischemia and necrosis. Arterial clots, fibrin, or air may cause emboli. Risk factors include multiple arterial punctures of the same limb or site, vasoconstriction, low cardiac output, severe peripheral vascular disease, prolonged duration of catheter, and an active infectious process (Woods et al., 2009). Vascular occlusion or spasm cannot be predicted, and risk factors for spasm are the same as those for embolic events. Aseptic technique is used for all dressings and sterility is maintained when obtaining blood specimens.

Factors Influencing Arterial Pressure

Alterations in the heart's conduction system influence arterial pressure. Patients who have irregular cardiac rhythms, such as atrial fibrillation or premature atrial contractions, demonstrate arterial waveforms with varying systolic pressures. These patients experience a decrease in systolic pressure as a result of the decrease in diastolic filling time. With less blood volume filling the heart, there is less volume to eject on the next systole, which results in the lower arterial systolic pressure. Figure 31–8 ◆ illustrates this phenomenon.

As the distance between the heart and the catheter site increases, the shape of the arterial waveform will change: The systolic pressure waveform becomes higher, and the diastolic pressure waveform becomes lower. The mean arterial pressure, however, remains constant irrespective of the arterial catheter site. **Mean arterial pressure (MAP)** is the average pressure in the arteries during one cardiac cycle. When vasoactive medications are to be administered, the MAP is usually specified as the titration parameter. Mean arterial pressure is used in the equation to calculate afterload or SVR.

Nursing Management

Explaining the procedure to the patient and family will assist in decreasing their anxiety and potentially elicit their cooperation. After an arterial line has been placed, a padded armboard is sometimes necessary to keep the wrist hyperflexed and to optimize the waveform. The nursing process serves as a guideline for nursing management of patients with arterial lines.

Assessment

An in-depth assessment can identify patients at risk so that actions can be taken to prevent complications from the arterial line. The nurse needs to assess the arterial line insertion site for redness, pain, and swelling, which are indications of infection. Assessment of the circulation also is essential to prevent ischemic changes due to compromised circulation. The nurse should regularly observe for changes in skin color and assess for motor and sensory changes in the extremity distal to the insertion site. Assessment of the BP is done on a continuous basis and documented according to health care provider orders or unit guidelines. The nurse must note the waveform; when changes occur, the patient should be reassessed, and troubleshooting should be done on the equipment.

Nursing Diagnosis

Nursing diagnoses related to arterial line placement include:

- *Risk for Infection* related to invasive procedures
- *Impaired Tissue Integrity* related to invasive procedures

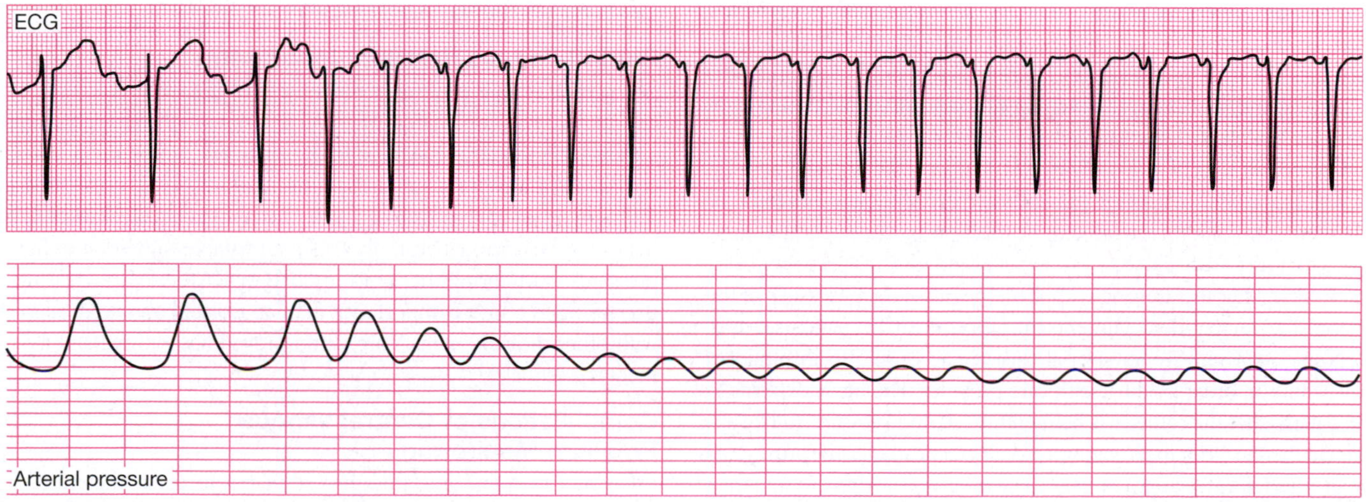

FIGURE 31–8 ◆ Effect of atrial tachycardia on arterial pressure.

- *Ineffective Tissue Perfusion risk for* related to catheter obstructing blood flow
- *Deficient Knowledge* related to hemodynamic monitoring equipment
- *Anxiety.*

NANDA-I © 2012

Planning

A collaborative and comprehensive approach to care of the arterial line is essential. Many hospitals have prescribed guidelines that dictate arterial line care protocols. Professionals who use the arterial line to either measure BP or obtain blood samples include health care providers, respiratory therapists, and nurses. All persons who access the arterial must follow the prescribed plan and must be responsible for prevention of complications, such as infection.

Outcomes and Evaluation Parameters

Outcomes for patients with arterial lines include the following:

- Stabilization of the blood pressure without vasoactive drugs
- No infection at the catheter site or in the bloodstream
- No bleeding from the arterial line site or catheter
- Having the arterial line discontinued due to blood pressure stabilization.

Interventions and Rationales

An arterial line can be inserted for the sole purpose of obtaining blood specimens. More commonly, however, it is placed so that blood pressure can be closely monitored. Nursing interventions include monitoring the blood pressure and assessing the effectiveness of vasoactive therapy, if administered. When a patient is receiving vasoactive medications, which either increase or decrease blood pressure, the nurse is responsible for medication titration to keep the blood pressure within the parameters ordered by the health care provider. Frequent assessment of blood pressure (usually at 5- to 10-minute intervals) and documentation of the amount of medication infusing are required. When the target blood pressure is achieved and maintained, then the institutional policy related to documentation is followed.

Each monitor has the ability to notify the nurse that the blood pressure is too high or too low. After the arterial line has been inserted, the nurse should set the high and low alarm limits. These alarms should never be turned off when the nurse leaves the room. When high or low alarms occur, the nurse assesses the patient for changes. If changes occur in the arterial waveform, the nurse *first* assesses the patient and takes a manual cuff pressure. If the cuff pressure varies from the arterial pressure, the nurse must troubleshoot the equipment by systematically inspecting and, if necessary, tightening all connections and tubing from the insertion site to the pressure bag.

Care of an arterial line site includes changing the dressing per unit protocol, as well as whenever the occlusive dressing becomes loose or when contamination is suspected. If infection is suspected, the nurse needs to notify the health care professional and institute preparation for a new line. After the dressing is applied, the nurse obtains a strip of the arterial line tracing and documents the procedure in the patient's record.

Nurses can remove an arterial catheter according to institutional policy and on order by the health care provider. The nurse explains to the patient that the catheter is being removed and pressure will be applied to the site. Prior to removing a radial artery catheter, the nurse dons goggles and nonsterile gloves. The nurse removes the dressing and then removes the suture, if present, with a suture removal kit. With one hand, the nurse gently removes the catheter and applies direct site pressure as soon as the catheter is removed. The nurse continues to apply pressure until hemostasis is achieved, then applies a sterile dressing. The procedure is the same in removing a femoral arterial catheter; however, with the large femoral artery, more time is required to achieve hemostasis by direct pressure. Routinely sending catheter tips for culture after removal is not recommended (Alexander, Corrigan, & Gorski, 2009).

The nurse should observe the catheter site regularly for bleeding and/or hematoma formation after the catheter has been removed.

Evaluation

The expected outcome for these patients is blood pressure stabilization with the intent of getting the invasive catheters removed as soon as possible. Not every patient will have normal readings; thus, the goal is for the discontinuance of vasoactive medications with a blood pressure that is tolerated by the patient. One gauge of tolerance is the patient's ability to perform activities of daily living.

Central Venous Catheters

Single- or multiple-lumen catheters are inserted for monitoring central venous pressure, which is the pressure in the right atrium. The subclavian, internal or external jugular, and femoral veins are potential insertion sites. Depending on the selected site and the length of the catheter, the tip transmits pressure from the right atrium, superior vena cava, or inferior vena cava. Specialized central venous catheters with a fiberoptic sensor allow for measurement of systemic central venous oxygen saturation ($ScvO_2$) (Woods et al., 2009).

Insertion of Central Venous Catheters

If the subclavian or a jugular vein site is selected and if tolerated, the patient may be placed in the Trendelenburg position. This position facilitates venous dilation of the central veins and reduces the risk of an air embolus. The patient may be asked to turn her head away from the insertion site to minimize contamination of the site. Patients should be informed of the necessity of maintaining a sterile barrier, which for upper torso sites involves temporarily covering the patient's face with sterile drapes. The health care provider and anyone assisting with catheter insertion must wear a cap, mask, sterile gown, and gloves.

When the catheter is secured, the sterile drapes are removed and a sterile dressing is placed over the insertion site. The catheter should not be accessed for intravenous infusions or monitoring until a chest x-ray confirms correct placement and a pneumothorax, or collapsed lung, is ruled out. A chest x-ray is not necessary for femoral lines.

Central Venous Pressure Monitoring

The central venous pressure reflects the pressure within the vena cava and the right atrium. When the central venous catheter is attached to a transducer system, a CVP or RAP waveform can be obtained. The CVP or RAP waveform should be continually displayed on the bedside monitor. A venous pressure of 2 to 6 mmHg is adequate; however, patients may be hemodynamically stable or unstable with lower or higher pressures. Monitoring the trend in CVP or RAP, either increasing or decreasing, is of more importance than an isolated observed value. As with other measurements, correlation of findings with patient assessment is essential.

Complications of Central Venous Pressure Monitoring

Infection can occur any time the catheter is in place; therefore, prevention of infection is an important nursing responsibility. When compared to arterial catheters and pulmonary artery catheters, central venous catheters have the highest rate of catheter-related infections. Almost 250,000 bloodstream infections occur in U.S. hospitals each year (CDC, 2010a). It is believed that a large proportion of these are associated with the presence of a central vascular catheter, though this is an area where more study is needed. These infections are termed *central line-associated bloodstream infections* (CLABSI). Bloodstream infections are usually serious infections that typically cause a prolongation of hospital stay and an increased cost and risk of mortality. Transmission of organisms is preventable when strict aseptic technique is maintained during catheter insertion and dressing changes. See the National Guidelines box for procedures to prevent CLABSI.

A pneumothorax is another risk associated with thoracic central line placement. It can occur when a needle or introducer penetrates the vessel wall, causing air to enter the pleural space. Assessment findings associated with a pneumothorax include those for an air embolus plus absence of breath sounds on the side of insertion. An air embolus is a rare complication that may occur during insertion or removal of a central catheter, if the IV disconnects from the catheter hub, or when obtaining blood specimens. Assessment findings that may indicate an air embolus include dyspnea, tachypnea, cyanosis, hypotension, and chest pain.

Nursing Management

Nursing management of central venous catheters focuses on preventing complications, starting with catheter insertion and ending with catheter removal. Further recommendations include replacing all central venous catheters if the patient is hemodynamically unstable and catheter-related bloodstream infection is suspected. In this instance, the nurse alerts the health care team to the need for catheter replacement and assists with placement of a new central line.

NATIONAL GUIDELINES Prevention of Intravascular Catheter-Related Infections

- Sterile full barrier precautions are necessary for all personnel assisting with central venous access insertion.
- A 2% chlorhexidine preparation is the preferred antiseptic before catheter insertion and during dressing changes.
- The antiseptic should remain on the insertion site and be allowed to air dry before catheter insertion.
- Inspect catheter sites visually or manually palpate on a regular basis. Remove the dressing to examine whether the site is tender to palpation.
- Regularly assess the need for the central venous line. Remove any vascular device that is no longer essential to patient care.
- Replace disposable transducers, tubing, and flush devices, and flush solution at 96-hour intervals.
- Replace administration sets, including secondary sets and add-on devices, no more frequently than at 72-hour intervals.
- To prevent infection, avoid routine replacement of central venous catheters. Avoid the use of the femoral site as much as possible.
- Vigorously clean the injection port ("scrub the hub") with 70% alcohol or iodophor for several seconds before accessing.
- Do not routinely culture catheter tips.

Source: Centers for Disease Control. (2010b). Overview of the patient safety component, device-associated module. Retrieved from http://www.cdc.gov/nhsn/wcOverviewNHSN.html.

Assessment

Nursing management of a central venous catheter involves patient education, assessing the site for infection and leakage, dressing changes, and monitoring of pressures. Prior to insertion of a central venous catheter, the nurse is responsible for assessing the patient for contraindications to the procedure. These include assessing the insertion site, assessing potential difficulties in positioning the patient, and obtaining a baseline physical assessment, including vital signs, pulse oximetry, and heart and breath sounds. Preassessment provides a point of reference for comparison when the procedure is complete. Ensure that external monitoring devices such as ECG wires and electrodes, noninvasive blood pressure cuffs, and pulse oximetry cables are clear of the insertion site.

Weblink: CLABSI Event Weblink: Patient Safety

Nursing Diagnosis

Nursing diagnoses related to arterial line placement include:

- *Risk for Infection* related to invasive procedure
- *Impaired Tissue Integrity* related to invasive procedure
- *Risk for Ineffective Tissue Perfusion* related to use of artery
- *Deficient Knowledge* related to arterial line placement
- *Anxiety.*

NANDA-I © 2012

Planning

Patient education decreases anxiety and increases patient participation in care. The patient should always be informed when routine dressing changes and close examination of the insertion site are to occur. Before the procedure, patients should be informed of the risks of the procedure, the expected duration of the procedure, and that repositioning may be required. Planning for interventions for care for the patient with invasive lines is multifaceted. Each institution has specific procedures for maintaining a sterile occlusive dressing over the line insertion site. The nurse must be knowledgeable of these procedures and carry them out within the required time frames.

Outcomes and Evaluation Parameters

Outcomes associated with central venous catheters include:

- Stabilization of the central venous pressure readings to within normal limits
- No infection at the catheter site or in the bloodstream
- No bleeding from the site or catheter
- Having the central venous catheter discontinued due to patient stabilization.

Interventions and Rationales

Once the central venous catheter is in place, the nurse is responsible for site care and dressing changes. Routine site inspection includes assessing the insertion site and the surrounding skin for signs of infection or leakage. Institutional policies vary as to the type of dressing applied; however, hand hygiene and nonsterile gloves are always used to remove the old dressing. The nurse who is using a prepackaged dressing kit should don the sterile gloves and clean the insertion site and catheter using the disinfectant provided. This disinfectant should be allowed to air dry. The nurse should not fan the area to speed the drying time because this may lead to site contamination. After the new dressing has been applied, the nurse should document the procedure, including patient education, date and time of procedure, description of the catheter site, and type of dressing. Some institutions require the date and time

Weblink: Factors That Influence Cardiac Preload

of dressing change plus the initials of the person changing the dressing to be placed on the dressing. After assisting with placement of a central venous line, the nurse should not access the line until a chest x-ray has confirmed correct placement.

Monitoring the CVP, interpreting the information, and correlating the data collected with the patient's condition are nursing responsibilities. Monitoring the CVP is accomplished with the previously described transducer system. By leveling and zero referencing the transducer, the nurse can help ensure that the CVP values are accurate.

The CVP reflects preload. Conditions that cause an increased CVP include venoconstriction, fluid volume overload, cardiac tamponade, pulmonary hypertension, and depressed cardiac function, especially right ventricular function. The nurse should corroborate elevations in CVP with physical assessment findings, which include dependent edema; tachypnea, dyspnea, or orthopnea; anxiety; crackles; and jugular vein distention. Central venous pressures below normal are indicative of venodilation or hypovolemia. Low pressures are frequently seen with major burn injuries, hemorrhage, and spinal cord injuries. Physical findings include postural hypotension, tachycardia, and decreased mean arterial pressure. If continuous monitoring of CVP is not routine, then institutional policy and the health care provider's orders dictate the frequency of obtaining readings. A single CVP value that is less than or more than normal is not as alarming as is a trend in values (up or down) coupled with a change in the physical assessment findings. The nurse should contact the health care provider when an abnormal CVP measurement correlates with assessment findings.

Removal of a central venous catheter is done in much the same manner as removal of an arterial catheter. However, in removing a central venous catheter from the subclavian or jugular site, the removal is timed with the inspiratory phase of the respiratory cycle. When the patient takes a deep breath, the intrathoracic pressure is increased. This maneuver decreases the potential for air embolus. At the peak of inspiration, the nurse gently removes the catheter and tells the patient to breathe normally. The nurse continues to hold pressure until hemostasis is achieved and then applies a sterile dressing.

Evaluation

Because of the risk of infection, the expected outcome for these patients is stabilization with the intent of getting the invasive catheters removed as soon as possible. Fluid balance as determined by heart rate, blood pressure, and urine output is the evaluation parameter. Not every patient will have normal readings; the goal is to achieve levels that are tolerated by the patient.

Measuring Cardiac Output

Variations in heart rate, preload, afterload, and/or contractility influence cardiac output. Healthy individuals maintain homeostatic balance through intact compensatory pathways. Athletes, for example, are frequently bradycardic (heart rate below 60 beats/min), but their CO is maintained with above-normal stroke volumes. Critically ill patients either lack reserves or have exhausted their compensatory responses. In other words, they are unable to significantly increase contractility to increase the stroke volume. The nurse must be knowledgeable about the components that influence cardiac output, because these factor into the evaluation of therapy.

Influence of Heart Rate on Cardiac Output

A slow or rapid heart rate affects cardiac output. Heart rates greater than 100 decrease diastolic filling time. For example, a heart rate of 150 beats/min and a reduced stroke volume to 20 mL is detrimental to CO:

$$HR\,(150) \times SV\,(20) = 3{,}000\ mL\ or\ 3.0\ L/minute$$

Dysrhythmias such as atrial fibrillation and atrial flutter cause not only a decreased diastolic filling time but also a loss of atrial kick, which is responsible for up to 25% of the total cardiac output (Chapter 30).

Bradycardia allows sufficient time for the ventricles to fill and usually is not detrimental to cardiac output because of compensatory mechanisms. However, when patients have lost their compensatory mechanisms, a bradycardic rhythm may not provide sufficient cardiac output. For example, a heart rate of 35 beats/min and a normal stroke volume of 60 mL/beat yield a CO of 2.1 L/min:

$$HR\,(35) \times SV\,(60) = 2{,}100\ mL\ or\ 2.1\ L/minute$$

Additionally, consider a patient with frequent premature ventricular contractions. If a patient has a heart rate of 80 but every other beat is a PVC, the heart rate is effectively reduced by one-half, due to little or no cardiac output with PVCs.

Influence of Preload on Cardiac Output

Reduced preload ($CVP < 2$, $RAP < 4$, $PAOP < 4$) signals vasodilation or volume loss. Exploration of cause is essential so that appropriate action can be taken. Treatment of hypovolemia is the administration of crystalloids, volume expanders, and/or blood products. Examples of obvious fluid losses are those that occur after trauma, during surgery, with diuretic therapy, in profuse sweating, or with excessive upper or lower gastrointestinal losses. Internal, nonvisible blood loss is an example of insidious hypovolemia and may go undetected unless considered as a suspected cause of preload reduction.

Vasodilation and loss of venous tone demonstrated in neurogenic or anaphylactic shock have a profound effect on preload. In neurogenic shock, the loss of vasomotor tone is secondary to the loss of neural output or spinal cord damage. This can result from general or spinal anesthesia or, in the case of spinal cord injury, from loss of sympathetic tone. In anaphylactic shock, the antigen–antibody response triggers the release of vasoactive chemicals in the body (histamine, bradykinin), which creates massive vasodilation. Shock is discussed in Chapter 54.

Excess preload ($CVP/RAP > 6$, $PAOP > 12$) may indicate hypervolemia or ventricular failure. Excessive circulating volume strains the heart and compromises adequate tissue oxygenation. Excess preload increases the heart's workload as well as myocardial oxygen demands. Diuretics and venodilators are ordered if the cause is hypervolemia. If patients do not respond to diuretic therapy or renal failure is diagnosed, then continuous renal replacement therapy utilizing ultrafiltration or dialysis may be considered. If ventricular failure is determined to be the cause, inotropic medications are prescribed.

Influence of Afterload on Cardiac Output

Reduced afterload ($PVR < 155$, $SVR < 900$) suggests vasodilation of the pulmonary and systemic vasculature. Decreased afterload lessens the workload on the heart and reduces myocardial oxygen requirements. With reduced resistance to ventricular ejection, an increase in stroke volume occurs as the ventricles empty. For example, patients with sepsis present with hypotension, fever, and vasodilatation, which reduce the SVR. The cardiac output of a patient with sepsis can elevate to as much as 10 L/min.

Excessive afterload (PVR > 255, SVR > 1,600) imposes great strain on the ventricles, increases the myocardial oxygen requirement, and decreases the stroke volume. Conditions that increase pulmonary resistance include hypoxia, acute respiratory distress syndrome, positive end-expiratory pressure, pulmonary embolism, chronic obstructive pulmonary disease (COPD), increased interstitial lung water, and pulmonary fibrosis (Woods et al., 2009). Left ventricular afterload is the resistance to ejection into the systemic circulation. Conditions that increase resistance include aortic valve stenosis, hypertension, and vasoconstriction of the peripheral vasculature.

Influence of Contractility on Cardiac Output

Contractility, the intrinsic ability of the myocardium to contract, occurs independent of changes in preload and afterload. Myocardial damage during an infarction or the presence of cardiomyopathy decreases contractility. Cardiomyopathy is discussed in detail in Chapter 33. Positive **inotropic** medications increase contractility and include drugs like dobutamine and epinephrine. These drugs also increase myocardial oxygen demand. In contrast, negative inotropic medications decrease contractility and are administered when myocardial work and oxygen consumption are detrimental, such as with a myocardial infarction. An example of this type of drug is a beta-adrenergic blocker.

Pulmonary Artery Catheters

A **pulmonary artery catheter (PAC)** is a flow-directed, balloon-tipped catheter. The brand name for this catheter is Swan-Ganz, so named for the inventors (Woods et al., 2009). Since the development of the PAC, it has evolved through multiple generations, although the basic technologies of the catheter remain identical. These catheters allow for assessment of cardiac function, calculation of vascular resistance, measurement of cardiac output, and infusion of IV fluids. The readings obtained with the PAC assist the health care team in diagnosing, treating, and estimating the prognoses of patients who are critically ill.

Ports and Lumens on a Pulmonary Artery Catheter

The pulmonary artery catheter is a multiple-lumen catheter, with each lumen having a specific purpose (Figure 31–9◆). The external ports of the catheter correspond to internal lumens that lie either in the right side of the heart or in the pulmonary artery. There are several types of PACs, some of which have more ports and lumens than others, depending on the catheter's intended purpose. Newer multifunction PACs with additional lumens are used to measure continuous mixed venous oxygen saturation (SvO_2), right ventricular volume, continuous cardiac output, or additional ports for insertion of transvenous pacing electrodes. Specialized pulmonary artery catheters are discussed later in the chapter.

The proximal port of the PAC sits in the right atrium and is used to infuse IV fluids and nonvasoactive medications. If a transducer is attached to this port, right atrial pressures (central venous pressures) can be obtained. The second port, which also sits in the right atrium, is the proximal injectate port, used for measuring cardiac output, which is discussed later. The distal port located at the end of the catheter is positioned in the pulmonary artery. The distal port is connected to the pressure transducer system with the flush solution and used for continuous monitoring of pulmonary artery pressures. The tip of the PAC also contains a thermometer, referred to as a **thermistor.** The thermistor permits measurement of the blood temperature in the pulmonary

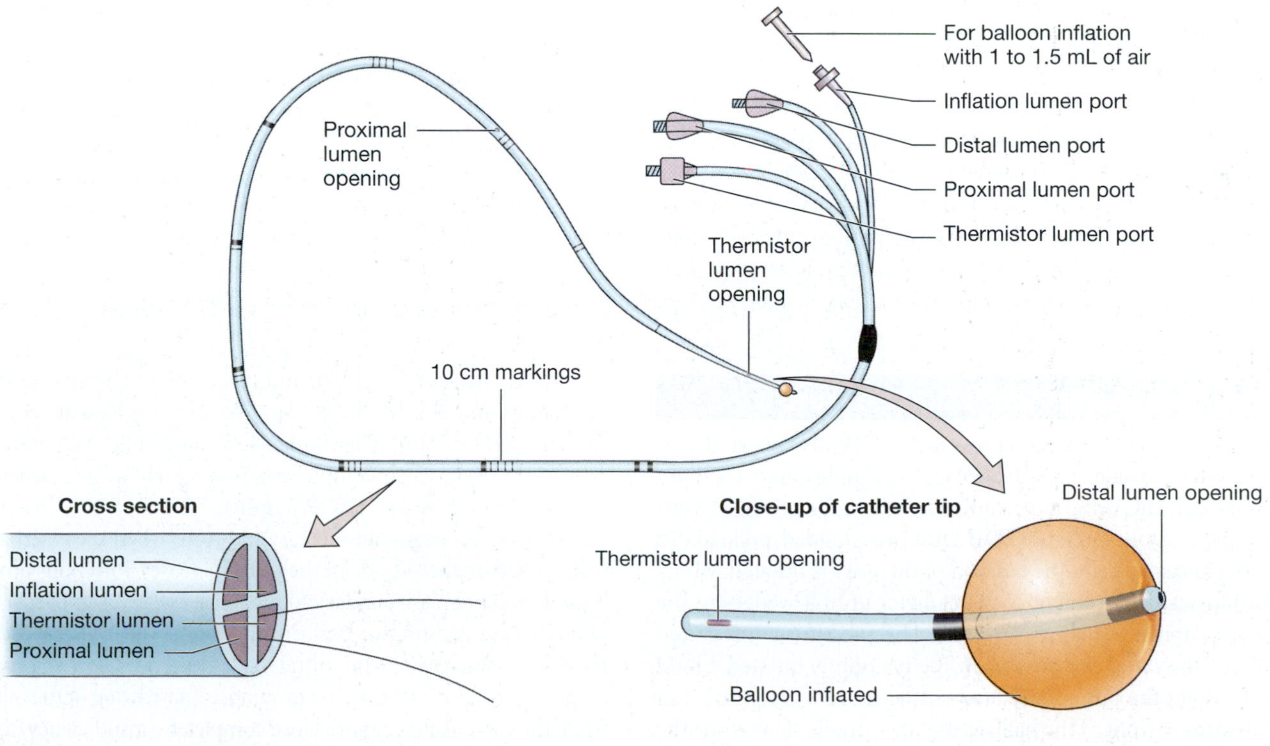

FIGURE 31–9 ◆ Ports and lumens of a pulmonary artery catheter.

artery, termed the *core temperature*. The external thermistor connector is attached to the cardiac output computer.

The final port is the balloon inflation port, which is used to inflate the balloon at the distal end of the catheter. The balloon is inflated during insertion to assist with "floating" the catheter through the heart. The balloon port is also used to obtain pulmonary capillary pressure or the **pulmonary artery occlusion pressure (PAOP).** The amount of air used to inflate the balloon is usually 1.5 mL; however, the balloon's capacity is limited by the catheter size. Manufacturers of PACs usually indicate the maximum balloon inflation volume on the catheter hub and provide a volume-limiting syringe to prevent accidental overinflation, which may cause rupture of the balloon or the pulmonary artery. Once insertion of the catheter is complete, the balloon *never* remains inflated but rather lies uninflated in the pulmonary artery until it is necessary to obtain the PAOP.

Insertion of the Pulmonary Artery Catheter

For PAC insertion, the patient is prepped and draped in a manner similar to that for any central venous access because strict sterile technique is required. An introducer is inserted in either the jugular, subclavian, or femoral vein. The PAC is passed through the introducer and advanced into the selected vessel to the right atrium. Once the catheter is in the right atrium, the balloon is inflated to allow it to flow with the blood through the heart chambers. This facilitates passage of the PAC through the tricuspid valve, right ventricle, pulmonic valve, and into the pulmonary artery. The balloon is then deflated and the introducer is sutured in place. Right atrial and right ventricular pressures are measured during the catheter's insertion.

Hemodynamic pressures and waveforms are generated by myocardial contraction (systole) and relaxation (diastole). When the PAC is advanced through the heart, each chamber has a characteristic waveform (Figure 31–10◆). As the catheter enters the right atrium, the waveform appears similar to a CVP waveform. The normal mean RAP is 4 to 6 mmHg. Normal systolic pressures in the right ventricle (RV) are between 20 and 30 mmHg, and diastolic pressures are between 0 and 8 mmHg (Lynn-McHale Wiegand, 2010).

As the catheter enters the pulmonary artery, the waveform resembles an arterial pressure waveform with not only systolic and diastolic pressures but also a dicrotic notch. The dicrotic notch represents closure of the pulmonic valve. The normal pulmonary artery systolic (PAS) pressure is 20 to 30 mmHg and the pulmonary artery diastolic (PAD) pressure is 5 to 15 mmHg. Notice that the normal right ventricular systolic pressure and the pulmonary artery systolic pressure are the same

Pulmonary Artery Occlusion Pressure

The pulmonary artery occlusion pressure (PAOP), also referred to as pulmonary artery wedge pressure (PAWP) and pulmonary capillary wedge pressure (PCWP), is an indirect measurement of left ventricular end-diastolic pressure (LVEDP), or left-sided preload. To obtain this measurement, the balloon of the PAC is inflated, which facilitates forward movement of the catheter until it wedges in the pulmonary capillary (Figure 31–11◆). The pressure is measured at the tip of the catheter; thus, when the balloon is inflated, blood flow in through the pulmonary artery is temporarily stopped, and only pressures in front of the balloon are measurable. Therefore, the PAOP is the most direct bedside measurement of left heart function. A normal PAOP reading is between 4 and 12 mmHg.

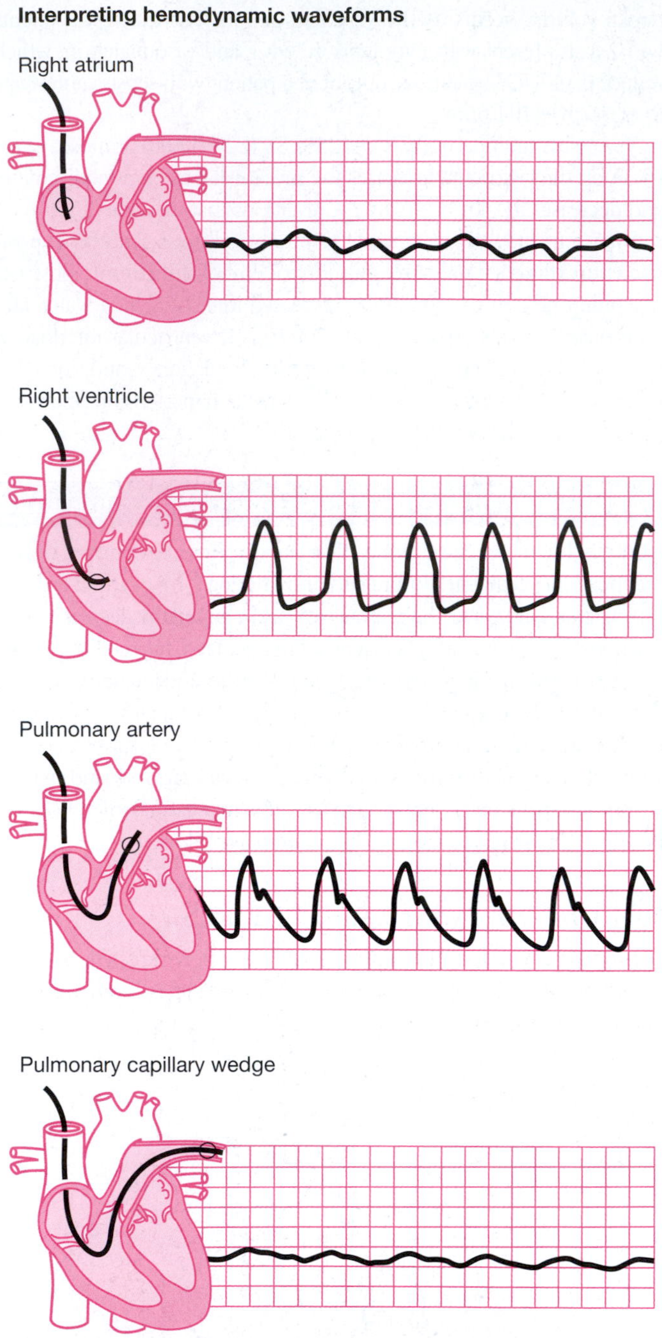

FIGURE 31–10 ◆ Cardiac pressures during PAC insertion.

Left ventricular (LV) failure and myocardial ischemia, constrictive pericarditis, mitral valve disease, and volume overload are conditions that elevate the PAOP. The diminished contractility and ensuing increase in left ventricular volume seen with LV failure and ischemia are reflected in an increased PAOP. Constrictive pericarditis, like pericardial tamponade, causes an increase in PAOP when the external pressure exerted on the left side of the heart increases. Infectious processes, trauma, and uremia secondary to renal disease are examples of conditions causing constrictive pericarditis. Mitral valve disease increases the PAOP either when the mitral valve does not allow for complete emptying of the left atrium due to stenosis (narrowing of the outlet) or when the valve leaflets cannot close completely (insufficiency), causing a reflux of blood into the left atrium during left ventricular contraction. The volume overload of the left heart is usually secondary to LV failure.

PAOPs decrease when patients are hypovolemic, in shock, or receiving vasodilating medications. Vasodilators decrease SVR, making it easier for left ventricular ejection and improvement in ejection fraction (Woods et al., 2009).

Thermodilution Cardiac Output

With the thermodilution method of obtaining a cardiac output reading, a specified amount of solution, typically 5 to 10 mL, is injected through the proximal lumen port of the PAC (see Figure 31–9, p. 911). This process is commonly referred to as "shooting" a cardiac output. The injectate is at room temperature (about 21°C [70°F]) when it enters the right atrium and mixes with blood (about 37°C [98.6°F]). The CO computer calculates the time required for the solution of a different temperature to reach the thermistor, located at the end of the catheter in the pulmonary artery. The change of temperature occurs over time to yield a CO curve, as shown in Figure 31–12 ◆. The area under the CO curve inversely corresponds to the cardiac output. When the area under the curve is large, the CO is low. Conversely, when the area under the curve is small, the CO is high.

Awareness of what constitutes a normal curve is important. Assessment of the shape of the cardiac output curve is necessary to determine whether the CO measurement should be accepted or rejected. A normal CO curve starts at the baseline and has a smooth incline and decline. Hesitation or starting and stopping during a CO injection would yield an invalid curve. The injectate should be injected smoothly and in less than 4 seconds. This prevents prolonged injection times that would yield a lower CO result. Additionally, injecting less than or greater than the recommended amount of injectate invalidates the measurement.

Cardiac output measurements are performed 1 to 2 minutes apart with an average of three measurements obtained. Also, the injectate should be timed to the end-expiratory phase of respiration. This will minimize the variation in intrathoracic pressure during respiration. Any CO that is questionable based on the curve or two CO measurements differing by 10% should be discarded (Lynn-McHale Wiegand, 2010).

Specialized Pulmonary Artery Catheters

The original PAC was a generic thermodilution catheter. As it developed, specialized models evolved. This section explains different PAC models and provides supplemental information. Although the PAC models are presented as separate entities in this discussion, in order to highlight their features, many PAC models combine several of these features.

Continuous Cardiac Output PAC

This catheter modifies the thermodilution PAC by adding a thermal filament that slightly warms the blood. The warmed blood is sensed at the thermistor in the catheter tip. The CO result is based on temperature changes at preset intervals, usually every minute (Woods et al., 2009). The updated calculation is then displayed on a CO monitor. The advantages to this system include recognition of CO as a dynamic, fluctuating parameter; the elimination of "shooting" cardiac outputs with the inherent risk of operator variability; plus the elimination of extra fluid a patient receives during that process.

Continuous Mixed Venous Oxygen Saturation

A **mixed venous oxygen saturation** (SvO_2) PAC provides information about the supply of oxygen to the tissues and demand for oxygen by the tissues (Woods et al., 2009). This catheter is positioned like a thermodilution catheter with the distal end in the pulmonary artery. These specialized catheters have fiber-optic fibers. One fiber emits a light wave to illuminate red blood cells (RBCs), and the

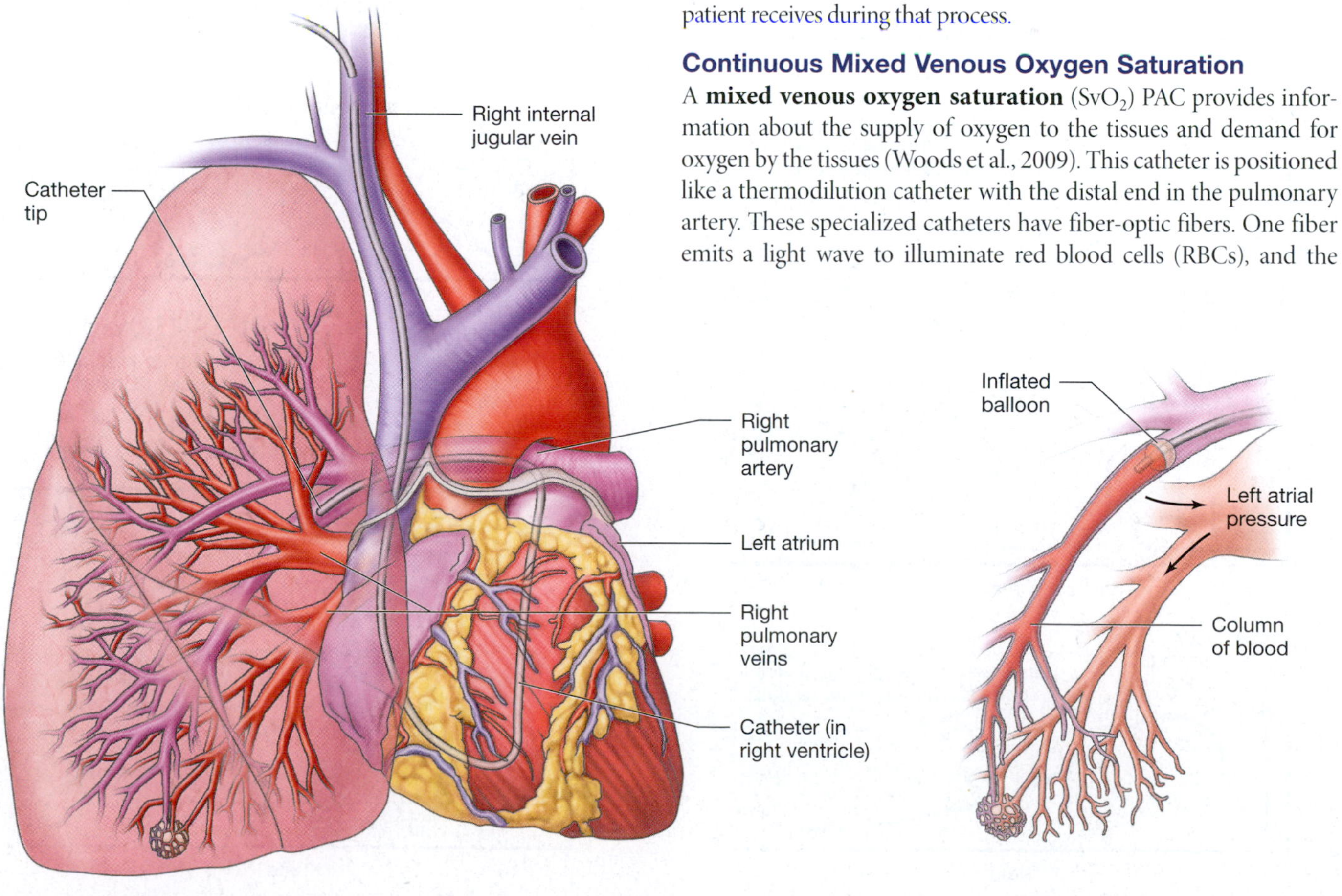

FIGURE 31–11 ◆ Position of pulmonary artery catheter during PAOP.

second fiber receives the reflected light signal. The amount of light reflected by the RBCs is determined by their hemoglobin saturation. Because this analysis occurs in the pulmonary artery, it reflects the saturation of all venous blood returned to the right side of the heart. This means that the SvO_2 reflects the consumption of oxygen at the tissue level. The numeric value displayed on the SvO_2 monitor reflects the saturation of mixed venous blood or the amount of deoxygenated blood that returns to the heart. The normal SvO_2 value is 60% to 80%.

Four factors affect mixed venous oxygen saturation: cardiac output, hemoglobin, arterial oxygen saturation, and oxygen consumption. Mixed venous oxygen saturation parallels cardiac output, hemoglobin concentration, and arterial oxygen saturation: A drop in cardiac output, hemoglobin, or oxygen saturation will cause a decrease in SvO_2; an increase in cardiac output, hemoglobin, or oxygen saturation will elevate SvO_2. High tissue extraction of oxygen (low SvO_2) occurs when patients are in pain (high oxygen demand) or when patients are experiencing respiratory failure (low oxygen supply). Low tissue extraction (high SvO_2) occurs when patients are sedated (low oxygen demand) or after blood transfusions (high oxygen supply). Nursing procedures such as patient repositioning and dressing or linen changes are oxygen-consuming activities for the patient and correspondingly lower the SvO_2.

Safety Alert *Use the information offered by the SvO_2 catheter to prioritize and plan nursing interventions. Patients who are compromised do not tolerate turning, suctioning, and dressing changes in a short time interval.*

Right Ventricular Ejection Fraction Volumetric Catheter

This catheter provides data on right ventricular systolic and diastolic volumes. Two sensors in the catheter, one in the right ventricle (RV) and one in the pulmonary artery, detect ventricular depolarization, heart rate, and temperature change. Using the information on systolic volume and diastolic volume, the ejection fraction is calculated. Accurate measurement of preload using the right ventricular end-diastolic volume instead of estimation of preload by CVP or PAOP is helpful in assessing the fluid requirement after right ventricular infarction and during high levels of positive end-expiratory pressure (PEEP) on mechanically ventilated patients (Woods et al., 2009). Accurate calculation of RV systolic and diastolic volumes relies on temperature consistency. Large-volume resuscitations with room temperature IV fluid or cool blood components diminish the accuracy of RV end-diastolic volumes and influence the calculation.

Transpulmonary Thermodilution with Pulse Contour Analysis

Using a special thermistor-tipped catheter inserted in the femoral or brachial artery and a regular central venous catheter, intermittent and continuous cardiac outputs can be evaluated. For an intermittent CO, a preset volume of cold injectate is injected into the central venous catheter. After completion of the vascular circuit, the temperature change is detected by the thermistor in the arterial catheter. As with the previously described thermodilution method, the calculation of CO is based on temperature change over time. For continuous cardiac

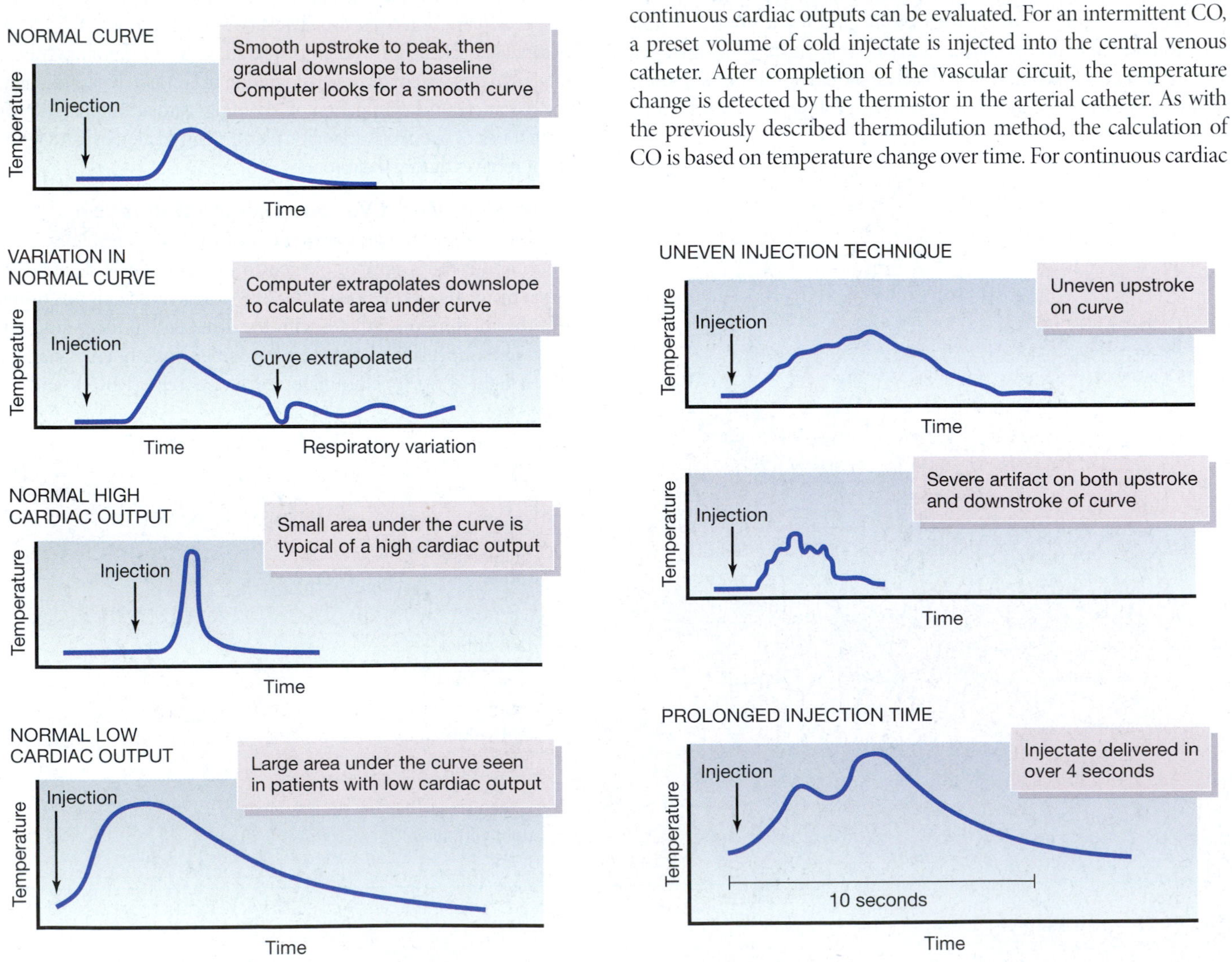

FIGURE 31–12 ◆ Normal and abnormal cardiac output curves.

output monitoring, the value obtained by an intermittent CO is used to calibrate the monitoring equipment. An internal algorithm combines this information with continual analysis of the arterial pressure wave contour to determine CO. Rather than measuring preload, afterload, and stroke volume, this device calculates intrathoracic volume and pulmonary volume by analysis of the CO distribution curve. End-diastolic volumes are automatically calculated. The advantage of measuring end-diastolic volume during fluid resuscitation without a PAC is useful.

Complications of a Pulmonary Artery Catheter

As with central venous catheters, complications from a pulmonary artery catheter include infection, air embolus, and pneumothorax (Woods et al., 2009). However, with a PAC there are additional risks of pulmonary artery rupture, pulmonary infarction, balloon rupture, catheter coiling or displacement, arrhythmias, and conduction defects. Pulmonary artery rupture is a life-threatening complication, and although it is rare, the mortality rate is high. Rupture of the pulmonary artery may occur when the balloon is overfilled or if the tip of the PAC migrates through the pulmonary artery intima. In most cases, hemoptysis is the presenting symptom (Woods et al., 2009). If a pulmonary artery rupture is suspected, the nurse should immediately place the patient with the affected side down, to prevent blood from leaking into the unaffected lung, and notify the health care provider.

Balloon rupture may cause air or balloon pieces to embolize the pulmonary vasculature. The likelihood of balloon rupture increases with catheter duration, because the balloon loses its elasticity over time. If blood is noted in the air inflation port or if no PAOP tracing appears with balloon inflation, then after placing the patient with the affected lung down, the nurse should notify the health care provider.

Pulmonary infarction can occur if the balloon accidentally remains inflated or if the PAC tip occludes a branch of the artery. Continuous monitoring of the PAC waveform, noting the contour of the wave and the corresponding numeric values, is an important nursing intervention to detect pulmonary infarcts. It is especially important to note the return of the normal pulmonary artery waveform after obtaining the PAOP. If the nurse suspects that the PAC is remaining wedged despite balloon deflation, then turning the patient from side to side or having the patient cough may unwedge the catheter. If these techniques are unsuccessful, the catheter may need repositioning by the health care provider or advanced practice nurse.

Safety Alert *After obtaining the PAOP, remove the syringe from the balloon inflation port and allow passive deflation of the balloon. Using the syringe to remove the air causes damage to the balloon and may lead to rupture.*

The PAC may coil on itself at any time. Usually the coiling occurs within the right atrium or right ventricle. An x-ray is necessary to detect this complication, and it requires an invasive procedure to correct. Dysrhythmias and conduction defects result when the PAC is touching the endocardium and septal wall. Conduction defects, especially right bundle branch blocks (RBBBs), can occur when the PAC is advanced through the right ventricle. In patients with a preexisting left bundle branch block (LBBB), a new RBBB places the patient at risk for developing a complete bundle branch block. For a patient with a preexisting LBBB, having transcutaneous pacing equipment available is advisable.

Nursing Management

Nursing management of patients needing pulmonary artery catheters requires critical thinking and clinical judgment. These patients are typically critically ill and hemodynamically compromised. Insertion of a PAC is an intervention that will provide the nurse with advanced assessment parameters as well as a central intravenous line to administer the necessary medications and fluid.

The nurse is responsible for management of the pulmonary artery catheter from preinsertion until removal. These responsibilities include patient and family education, assisting with insertion, site care, assessment and interpretation of hemodynamic waveforms and parameters, and titration of vasoactive medications. The nurse must provide the family with information about the PAC and how the measurements obtained will direct therapy. Use of the nursing process facilitates an organized approach for management of patients with invasive catheters.

Assessment

Prior to insertion of a PAC, the nurse is responsible for assessing the patient in the same manner as for a central venous catheter. Inform the health care provider or person inserting the catheter if the patient is coagulopathic, has an electrolyte imbalance (particularly magnesium, potassium, or calcium), or has an acid–base imbalance. Patients with a coagulopathy are more likely to have bleeding complications, and patients with electrolyte or acid–base imbalances are at increased risk for cardiac irritability that may lead to intractable arrhythmias. Ongoing assessment includes monitoring the insertion site for infection, monitoring of PA pressures, measuring PAOP and cardiac outputs, and monitoring the patient when changes occur.

Nursing Diagnosis

Nursing diagnoses related to hemodynamic monitoring include:

- *Anxiety* related to disease process and invasive monitoring
- *Risk for Imbalanced Fluid Volume* related to physiological need for catheter
- *Risk for Injury* related to invasive line
- *Deficient Knowledge* related to placement of PAC
- *Risk for Infection* related to invasive procedure.

NANDA-I © 2012

Planning

Planning for interventions for care for the patient with invasive lines is multifaceted. Each institution has specific procedures for maintaining a sterile occlusive dressing over the line insertion site. The nurse must know these procedures thoroughly and carry them out within the required time frames.

Outcomes and Evaluation Parameters

Outcomes and evaluation parameters associated with pulmonary artery catheters include:

- Stabilization of the pulmonary artery readings to within normal limits
- Normal or stable cardiac output
- No infection at the catheter site or in the bloodstream as evidenced by no fever and a negative blood culture
- No bleeding from the site or catheter
- Having the PAC discontinued due to patient stabilization.

Interventions and Rationales

The nurse prepares the transducer system as previously described and flushes all ports with normal saline to remove air from the lines. The normal saline flush syringe may remain attached to the lumen until after the procedure. The nurse attaches the distal end of the PAC to the transducer system, zero balances the system, and tests the balloon on the PA catheter by inflating the syringe with the appropriate amount of air.

The nurse assists with setup of the sterile field and opening of sterile kits. Sterile barriers identical to those used for central venous catheters are employed for insertion of PACs. Once the central venous access is obtained and the introducer inserted, the port end of the PAC is given to the nurse, who flushes all of the ports with normal saline to remove air from the lines. The nurse tests the balloon on the PAC by inflating the syringe with the appropriate amount of air. The nurse then attaches the distal end of the PAC to the transducer system and zero balances the system.

During catheter insertion, the nurse watches the monitor for waveform changes as the PAC passes through the chambers of the heart. When the catheter is in the right atrium, the nurse inflates the balloon. This facilitates passage of the catheter through the tricuspid valve. During this time, the nurse watches closely for ventricular ectopy.

The nurse notes the distance the catheter is inserted. The PAC has thin and wide black lines on the exterior. The thin line represents 10-cm increments, and the wide line signifies 50 cm. The nurse documents the number of centimeters. This will serve as a reference for others caring for the patient.

Ongoing appropriate nursing interventions include changing the occlusive dressing according to hospital protocol, as well as if the dressing is loosened, and inspecting the site for redness, swelling, and leakage. The nurse must also possess the knowledge required to operate and troubleshoot the catheter. The nurse must inspect the transducer system for kinks and air bubbles from site to pressure bag. After leveling, zero referencing, and checking the dynamic response, the nurse usually documents the pulmonary artery systolic, diastolic, and mean pressures hourly and after changes in therapies. PAOP and CO readings are obtained when changes occur in the patient's clinical status; with initiation, titration, or discontinuation of vasoactive medications; when significant changes occur in heart rate or rhythm; or when greater than 5 cm of PEEP is applied during mechanical ventilation. Increases in PEEP over 5 cm are associated with increased intrathoracic pressure, which may decrease cardiac output. PEEP is discussed in detail in Chapter 28.

Evaluation

After the catheter has been placed, the nurse secures the site with an occlusive dressing and reassesses the patient to determine his tolerance to the procedure. The nurse follows through with the health care provider on orders for a chest x-ray. Once the x-ray confirms proper placement and rules out a pneumothorax, the nurse connects the IV infusions to the remaining ports of the PAC and obtains PAOPs and cardiac output measurements, as discussed previously.

The expected outcome for these patients is hemodynamic stabilization with the intent of getting the invasive catheters removed as soon as possible. Not every patient will have normal readings; thus, the goal is for readings that are tolerated by the patient. One gauge of tolerance is the patient's ability to perform activities of daily living.

Alternative Methods of Determining Cardiac Output

Patients who are coagulopathic or immunosuppressed are at high risk of complications from invasive devices. Additionally, patients who may not tolerate positioning for a pulmonary artery catheter or are clinically unstable may be candidates for noninvasive determination of cardiac output. Minimally invasive and noninvasive monitoring devices estimate hemodynamic pressures in patients who are critically ill and are used in ICUs. Some devices are gaining acceptance in intermediate care units, emergency departments, and outpatient clinics to evaluate and treat patients with congestive heart failure and to optimize pacemaker settings. These devices, the supporting hardware, and monitoring systems are incompatible with the transducer systems used in invasive monitoring. Therefore, separate supporting hardware must be available.

Transesophageal Ultrasound

Transesophageal ultrasound is a minimally invasive method for continuous monitoring of cardiac function. An ultrasound probe is inserted into the esophagus in a manner similar to the insertion of a nasogastric tube. When the probe is properly positioned, the ultrasound waves detect red blood cells descending through the aorta. Figure 31–13◆ illustrates the probe's position behind the aorta. The blood flow and velocity are transmitted to a display monitor, where an internal algorithm converts blood flow, velocity, heart rate, and diameter of the aorta into estimations of cardiac output and stroke volume (Woods et al., 2009). Sedation is recommended before passage of the probe. Nurses assisting with this procedure must have knowledge of procedural sedation protocols.

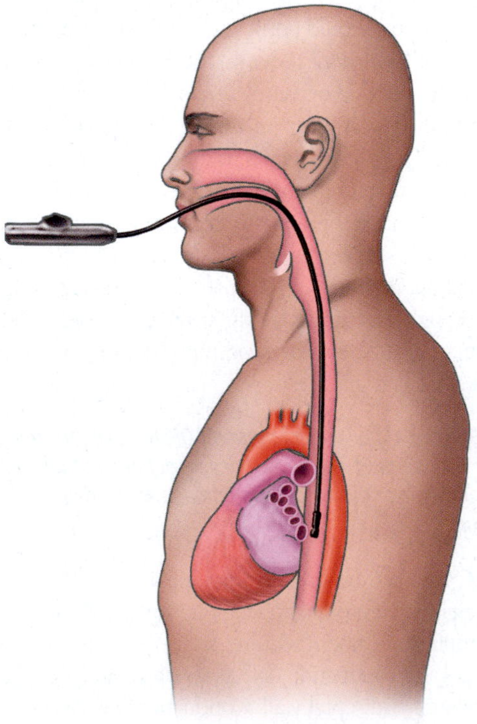

FIGURE 31–13 ◆ Transesophageal ultrasound.

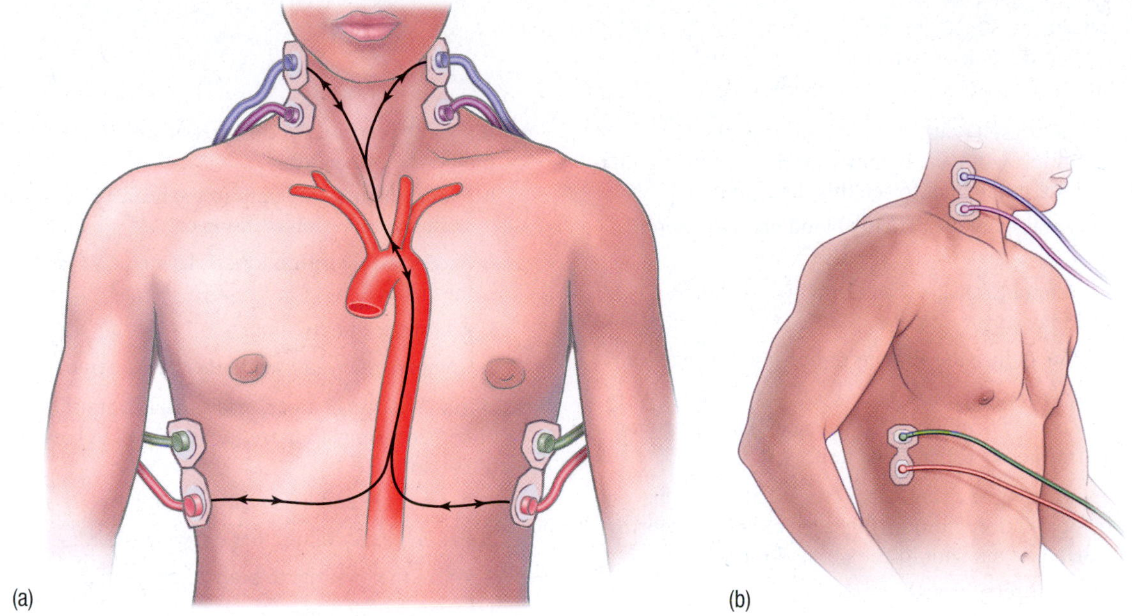

FIGURE 31–14 ◆ Electrode placement for thoracic impedance cardiography: (A) anterior view; (B) lateral view.

Thoracic Impedance

Thoracic impedance represents the resistance of electrical flow through the thoracic cavity (Calabrese & Thompson, 2010). Noninvasive thoracic impedance is done by placing special electrodes to the body, one set at the base of the neck and another set to both sides of the thorax (Figure 31–14◆), to measure the degree of resistance or impedance. Noninvasive thoracic impedance is a reliable indicator of increasing pulmonary congestion. However, this type of assessment is limited in that it must be done with the patient in the same position each time with the lead system continually in place. An invasive approach to measuring thoracic impedance involves placing a small device in the pectoral area and a coil within the right ventricle. Some pacemakers and implantable cardioverter defibrillators (ICDs) contain this technology.

Research

The evolution of hemodynamic monitoring does not preclude investigations of current technology. The nursing research discussed in this chapter needs replication, because study replication produces a body of knowledge that enhances nursing science and produces evidence-based practice. All nurses make a contribution in the research process, whether by collecting data or explaining in lay terms the research behind relocating a transducer after turning a patient. Nurses are prime candidates for identification of potential research projects, as outlined in the Research Opportunities box.

RESEARCH OPPORTUNITIES Related to Hemodynamic Monitoring

Research Area	Clinical Impact
Comparison of techniques used to secure arterial catheters	Results in fewer dislodged or accidentally removed arterial catheters, improved patient safety.
Techniques to decrease the infection rates associated with central venous catheters	Prevention of infections will decrease patient morbidity and mortality rates.
Continuous monitoring of left ventricular ejection fraction	Provides immediate information about cardiac function.
Noninvasive methods to accurately measure cardiac output	Decreases exposure to invasive catheters and the associated complications and risks.
Methods of facilitating family presence programs	Recognizes the impact of family systems on patient health and well-being.
The effect of prone positioning on hemodynamic pressures.	Provides for accurate hemodynamic assessment during therapeutic proning (face down on stomach).

NCLEX® PRACTICE

1. The nurse is glad to see that a patient who is in the ICU in critical condition will have hemodynamic monitoring initiated. Why is the nurse glad to see this development?

1. It will make measuring the patient's blood pressure more accurate.
2. Use of this technology helps with diagnosis, treatment, and evaluation of care.
3. These monitors reduce the amount of nursing time needed to provide care.
4. Information from this monitoring will be used to determine criteria for transfer to a step-down unit.

2. The nurse is assessing the waveform created after the placement of a hemodynamic monitoring device. The waveform appears distorted. What should the nurse do first?

1. Increase the flow rate through the device.
2. Reposition the catheter.
3. Check which type of tubing was used.
4. Begin interventions to improve hemodynamic stability.

3. During the placement of a pulmonary artery catheter (PAC), the patient demonstrates premature ventricular contractions on the cardiac monitor. Which intervention should the nurse anticipate?

1. Flushing the line with normal saline
2. Attaching the distal end of the PAC to the transducer
3. Zero balancing the system
4. Inflating the catheter balloon

4. A patient's central venous pressure is 10 mmHg. What should the nurse do?

1. Report the measurement to the health care provider and prepare for interventions.
2. Access the algorithm for an elevated CVP and begin the protocol.
3. Adjust the catheter tip.
4. Compare the result with other measurements.

5. While "shooting" a patient's cardiac output (CO), the nurse obtains readings that are inconsistent. What should the nurse do?

1. Begin again and inject the injectate over 10 seconds.
2. Eliminate any values that differ by 10%.
3. Warm the injectate to body temperature.
4. Use 45 mL of injectate.

6. A patient's central venous pressure (CVP) reading is 12 mmHg with a right atrial pressure (RAP) of 14 mmHg. The nurse plans care for this patient based on which interpretation of these values?

1. Fluid volume overload or ventricular failure
2. Hypotension
3. Vasodilation
4. Anaphylactic shock

Answers to NCLEX Practice questions can be found in Appendix D in the Osborn Student Resources at nursing.pearsonhighered.com. Practice additional NCLEX questions online at the Student Resources site.

Pearson Nursing Student Resources Find additional review materials at: **nursing.pearsonhighered.com**

REFERENCES

Alexander, M., Corrigan, A. N., & Gorski, L. (Eds.). (2009). *Infusion nursing: An evidence-based approach.* Philadelphia: Saunders.

Calabrese, M. S., & Thompson, M. J. (2010). Monitoring intrathoracic impedence in heart failure patients: Implications for use. *Dimensions in Critical Care Nurse, 29*(5), 203–210.

Centers for Disease Control. (2010a). Central-line associated bloodstream infection (CLABSI) event. Retrieved from http://www.cdc.gov/nhsn/PDFs/pscManual/4PSC_CLABScurrent.pdf

Centers for Disease Control. (2010b). Overview of the patient safety component, device-associated module. Retrieved from http://www.cdc.gov/nhsn/wcOverviewNHSN.html

Chulay, M., & Burns, S. (2010). *AACN essentials of critical care nursing* (2nd ed.). New York: McGraw-Hill.

Lynn-McHale Wiegand, D. J. (Ed.). (2010). *AACN procedure manual for critical care* (6th ed.). Philadelphia: Elsevier.

Porth, C., & Matfin, G. (2009). *Pathophysiology: Concepts of altered health states* (8th ed.). Philadelphia: Wolters Kluwer/Lippincott Williams & Wilkins.

Woods, S. L., Froelicher, E. S. S., Adams (Underhill), S., & Bridges, E. J. (Eds.). (2009). *Cardiac nursing* (6th ed.). Philadelphia: Lippincott Williams & Wilkins.

Caring for the Patient with Coronary Artery Disease

32 CHAPTER

Brenda McCulloch
Kathleen Osborn

Outcome-Based Learning Objectives

After studying this chapter, the learner will be able to:

1. Differentiate the epidemiological and risk factors that affect the development of coronary artery disease.
2. Implement a plan for nursing management of a patient experiencing angina pectoris.
3. Critique the pathogenesis of unstable angina (UA); a non Q wave, subendocardial, non–ST segment elevation myocardial infarction (NSTEMI); and a Q wave, transmural, and ST segment elevation myocardial infarction (STEMI).
4. Identify the complications of a myocardial infarction (MI) and discuss the variables that affect the patient's prognosis.
5. Summarize the major noninvasive and invasive diagnostic tests used to detect CAD and associated nursing management for a patient with progressive coronary artery disease.
6. Prioritize the nursing management for patients receiving percutaneous coronary interventional (PCI) procedures.
7. Identify three possible complications of coronary artery bypass graft surgery and implement nursing interventions that can potentially reduce the incidence of these complications.

KEY TERMS

acute coronary syndrome (ACS) p.945
akinesia p.945
angina pectoris p.932
arteriosclerosis p.920
arteriovenous (AV) fistula p.944
atheroma p.921
atherosclerosis p.920
cardiac catheterization p.940
cardiac risk factors p.924
cholesterol p.925
concentric p.922
coronary artery bypass grafting (CABG) p.964
coronary artery disease (CAD) p.919
creatine kinase (CK) p.950
dyskinesia p.945
eccentric p.922
fibrous cap p.922
high-density lipoprotein p.926
hypercholesterolemia p.925
hyperlipidemia p.924
hypokinesia p.945
ischemia p.920
low-density lipoprotein p.926
magnetic resonance imaging (MRI) p.940
metabolic syndrome p.930
MONA p.951
multislice helical CT p.939
myocardial hibernation p.924
myocardial infarction (MI) p.948
myocardial perfusion imaging (MPI) p.937
myocardial stunning p.924
myocardial viability p.940
myoglobin p.950
NSTEMI p.948
percutaneous coronary intervention (PCI) p.942
pseudoaneurysm p.944
remodeling p.958
restenosis p.943
stable angina p.933
STEMI p.948
stents p.942
sudden cardiac death (SCD) p.948
thrombus p.922
triglycerides p.927
troponin p.949
troponin I p.949
troponin T p.949
tunica adventitia p.920
tunica intima p.920
tunica media p.920
unstable angina (UA) p.945
variant, Prinzmetal, or vasospastic angina p.933

CORONARY ARTERY DISEASE (CAD) is defined as a progressive atherosclerotic disorder of the coronary arteries that results in narrowing or complete occlusion of the vessel lumen. The narrowing of the lumen decreases blood supply to the myocardium, resulting in a variety of clinical manifestations. This chapter discusses the clinical relevance to the prevalence, presentation, diagnostic work-up, and nursing care guidelines for patients with manifestations of CAD. Care providers, regardless of health care setting, are very likely to find themselves responsible for managing the care of a patient with CAD.

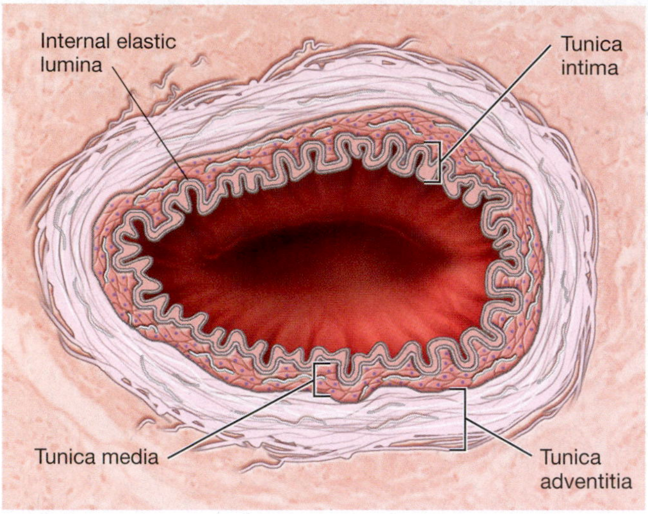

FIGURE 32–1 ◆ Normal artery layers.

Coronary Artery Anatomy

Coronary arteries comprise three concentric layers of differentiated cells separated by elastic membranes (Figure 32–1◆). The **tunica intima** is the inner layer, consisting of endothelial cells, connective tissue, and smooth muscle cells. The tunica intima was once considered simply a diffusing barrier between blood and the subintima; however, we now know that the endothelium regulates vasomotor tone, procoagulant and anticoagulant stimulation, mediation of inflammatory and growth factors, and the adhesion and entry of inflammatory cells and lipids into the vessel wall. Adjacent to the intima is the internal elastic membrane (internal elastic lumina), which is tissue that separates the intima from the medial layer.

The **tunica media** is the middle layer; it consists of multiple layers of smooth muscle cells and connective tissue made up of elastic fibers, collagen, and proteoglycans (Figure 32–1). The external elastic membrane (external elastic lumina) separates the medial layer from the adventitia. The external elastic membrane is composed of layers of elastin and is thinner than the internal elastic membrane.

The **tunica adventitia,** the outer layer of the artery, is a flexible stratum consisting of fibrous tissue made of collagen and elastic fibers surrounded by collagen bundles (Figure 32–1). The loose structure of the adventitia and adjoining collagen bundles facilitates coronary vessel diameter changes during vasodilation and constriction. The adventitia also contains nerve fibers and, in larger vessels, the vasa vasorum, which is a network of arteries and veins that provide blood to the vessel wall.

Epidemiology of Coronary Artery Disease

CAD is responsible for approximately 50% of cardiovascular events in both men and women under the age of 75. CAD causes about one out of every six deaths in the United States, making it the single largest killer of the American population. It is the leading cause of death in both males and females of White, African American, Hispanic, American Indian, and Asian Pacific Island ethnicities. The overall risk of CAD is greater in men than in women until menopause, when it becomes more equal (AHA, 2010b).

The economic impact of CAD is significant. According to the American Heart Association (2010b), CAD is the leading cause of early, permanent disability in the U.S. labor force. Medical costs are significant, with diagnostic testing of nearly 6 million patient visits to the emergency department (ED) annually for symptoms suspected of CAD and 1.7 million hospital discharges at an annual cost over $177 billion (AHA, 2010b). CAD is the leading cause of death, afflicts all ethnic groups and ages, and consumes the greatest portion of our national health dollars. The magnitude and pervasiveness of CAD provide sound rationale for allocating more funds for research targeted toward the prevention and treatment of CAD.

Etiology of Coronary Artery Disease

CAD is not an acute process but one that progresses over time and can begin as early in life as infancy. The rate of progression is related to risk factors such as genetic predisposition, gender, diet, sedentary lifestyle, and smoking. Atherosclerosis affects the arteries perfusing the heart, brain, and kidneys and the large arteries branching off the aorta. In general, men experience cardiac events when about 10 years younger than women for CAD and 20 years younger for serious events such as an acute myocardial infarction (AMI) or sudden cardiac death (SCD). Because women present with CAD at an older age, they have a greater risk of overall mortality and developing serious complications.

Pathophysiology of Coronary Artery Disease

CAD includes abnormal conditions such as arteriosclerosis, atherosclerosis, and arteritis (inflammation of the arterial wall, usually due to infection or auto-immune response) of the coronary arteries, all of which result in reduced flow of oxygen and nutrients to the myocardium. **Arteriosclerosis** is characterized by thickening, reduced elasticity, and calcification of the arterial wall. **Atherosclerosis,** a type of arteriosclerosis, is the most common etiologic process that causes reduced myocardial blood flow. Atherosclerosis is coronary artery luminal obstruction caused by buildup of plaque consisting of cholesterol, lipids, and cellular debris infiltrating the intimal lining of the arterial wall, causing a reduced blood flow to the myocardium. Reductions in myocardial blood supply, especially in times of increased demand, cause coronary syndromes, which include stable angina, unstable angina (UA), AMI, and SCD. These conditions depict a continuum of progressively worsening imbalances between the amount of oxygenated blood that is delivered and the amount that the myocardial tissues require.

Normally the myocardium extracts 75% of the available oxygen from the coronary arteries, which is more than is extracted from any other tissue in the body (the rest of the body extracts about 40% of available oxygen). If the oxygen needs are not met from this near maximal extraction, then myocardial blood flow must be increased. Normal coronary arteries are able to dilate and normal hearts are able to increase the force of contraction, resulting in increased blood being delivered to the cardiac muscle and increased cardiac output. With CAD the arteries are unable to dilate because of the plaque buildup and subsequent calcification. In addition, because of the decrease in blood supply, the heart muscle has significant difficulty increasing the force of the contraction in order to increase the cardiac output. The result of all of the unmet oxygen needs is the shift to anaerobic metabolism and myocardial tissue hypoxia, which results in angina. Myocardial **ischemia** or tissue hypoxia is a result of this oxygen imbalance.

Certain factors, whether experienced internally or environmentally, such as stress or physical activity, cause the heart to work harder,

CHART 32–1 Common Factors That Increase Oxygen Demand and Decrease Oxygen Supply

Increased Oxygen Demand	Rationale
Exercise	Increases the heart rate, which increases the heart's workload. Diseased coronary arteries are unable to deliver an increased amount of oxygen to the heart muscle.
Eating	During digestion after a heavy meal, the blood is diverted to the gastrointestinal system, causing low blood flow to the coronary arteries.
Emotions	Stimulate the sympathetic nervous system and increase the heart's workload by increasing heart rate and blood pressure.
Exposure to cold	Constricts blood vessels and increases metabolism, both of which put an extra workload on the heart.
Hypertension	Because the heart has to pump against greater pressure (afterload), it increases the workload and oxygen demands.
Sexual activity	Increases sympathetic nervous system stimulation, which increases the heart's workload.
Decreased Oxygen Supply	**Rationale**
Coronary artery spasm	Causes a decrease in the size of the lumen of the artery, which decreases blood flow to the tissues. When combined with CAD, it markedly decreases blood flow to the tissues.
CAD	Decreases vessel lumen, which decreases blood supply to the myocardium.
Hypotension	Decreases cardiac output.
Dysrhythmias	Decreases cardiac output if occurring in significant numbers and areas of the myocardium (ventricle).
Anemia	Decreases the oxygen-carrying capacity of the blood, which decreases oxygen to the myocardium.
Smoking	Causes vasoconstriction, which increases afterload and the heart's workload.

increasing the demand for oxygen. Whereas CAD decreases the blood supply to the myocardium, both abnormal demand and supply issues can cause angina to occur. Chart 32–1 outlines the most common factors that affect myocardial blood supply and demand.

The pathophysiology of plaque generation, development, composition, and injury provides the basis on which medical therapies for prevention of CAD and management of its sequelae have developed. The process of atherosclerotic development is described next.

Atherogenesis

An **atheroma** is an accumulation of plaque in the inner lining of an artery. The cause of plaque generation is still unclear to researchers. One theory proposes that plaque pathogenesis is a response to injury to the vessel wall. Potential causes of injury include mechanical, chemical, immunologic, viral, bacterial, and subendothelial stressors. Some of these stressors, as well as additional stressors, are included in Chart 32–2. Once the endothelial lining has been injured, it undergoes a number of structural and functional changes. There is a disruption in cell-to-cell contact or cell-to-underlying-connective-tissue contact, such that the once relatively impermeable endothelial monolayer can no longer protect or regulate the exposure of subendothelial constituents from elements in the circulating bloodstream. One effect of subendothelial cells coming into contact with blood is that there is a loss of endothelial vasodilatory control, as demonstrated by a decrease in focal endothelial-derived relaxing factor or nitric oxide synthesis and release and increased sensitivity to catecholamines. Thus, rather than stimulating compensatory vasodilation, ischemia causes vasoconstriction in areas of vessel disruption. Endothelial injury also causes stimulation of internal mechanisms that result in the smooth muscle extending into the inner layer of the vessel, thereby decreasing in the lumen of the artery and a loss of elasticity. Additionally, this process causes external recruitment of inflammatory and procoagulant cells (platelets and coagulation factors), causing them to aggregate and further decrease the size of the lumen.

CHART 32–2 Causes of Intimal Vessel Wall Injury

Stressor	Source and Effect
Mechanical	Sheer stress from blood flow at vessel branches/bifurcation due to hypertension (HTN); injury secondary to PCI procedures.
Chemical	Hypercholesterolemia; homocystinemia (abnormal accumulation of homocystein); hydrocarbons, nicotine, and carbon monoxide from cigarettes; free fatty acids, oxygen radicals, angiotensin, hormones; oxidized lipids; oxidant stress caused by cigarette smoking, HTN, and advanced glycation end products in diabetes mellitus; estrogen deficiency; vasoactive amines.
Immunologic	Exposure to antigen–antibody complexes; virally induced injuries; exposure to bacteria; activated macrophages; infectious microorganisms such as herpes viruses, *Chlamydia pneumoniae.*
Genetic	Alterations.
Biologic	Advancing age.

Stage I Lesion

Lesions in the coronary arteries develop in stages. In early atherosclerosis, grossly visible yellow lesions, known as fatty streaks, in the intimal layer are considered stage I lesions. This earliest form of plaque has been found in the aortas of newborns as well as in both young and old people. These streaks cause little or no obstruction to coronary blood flow. Early fatty streaks consist primarily of macrophages, foam cells, and T lymphocytes, suggesting that plaque genesis may be a response to inflammation. The lesion develops with the migration of smooth muscle cells and the accumulation of macrophages, T lymphocytes, lipids, and foam cells. In response to injury, circulating monocytes and platelets adhere to the damaged segment of endothelium. Activated platelets release their contents, and this release recruits and promotes adhesion of other platelets to the endothelium. This process then causes the release of growth factors, which inhibits cell proliferation and stimulates connective tissue formation, all of which cause a decrease in lumen size. Activated macrophages bind with lipoproteins to form foam cells. Macrophages and foam cells produce cytokines, growth factors, and other chemicals that induce and regulate the accumulation of lipids; the proliferation and migration of monocytes, T lymphocytes, possibly mast cells into the arterial wall, and smooth muscle cells from the media into the intima; and the synthesis of matrix components (Figure 32–2◆).

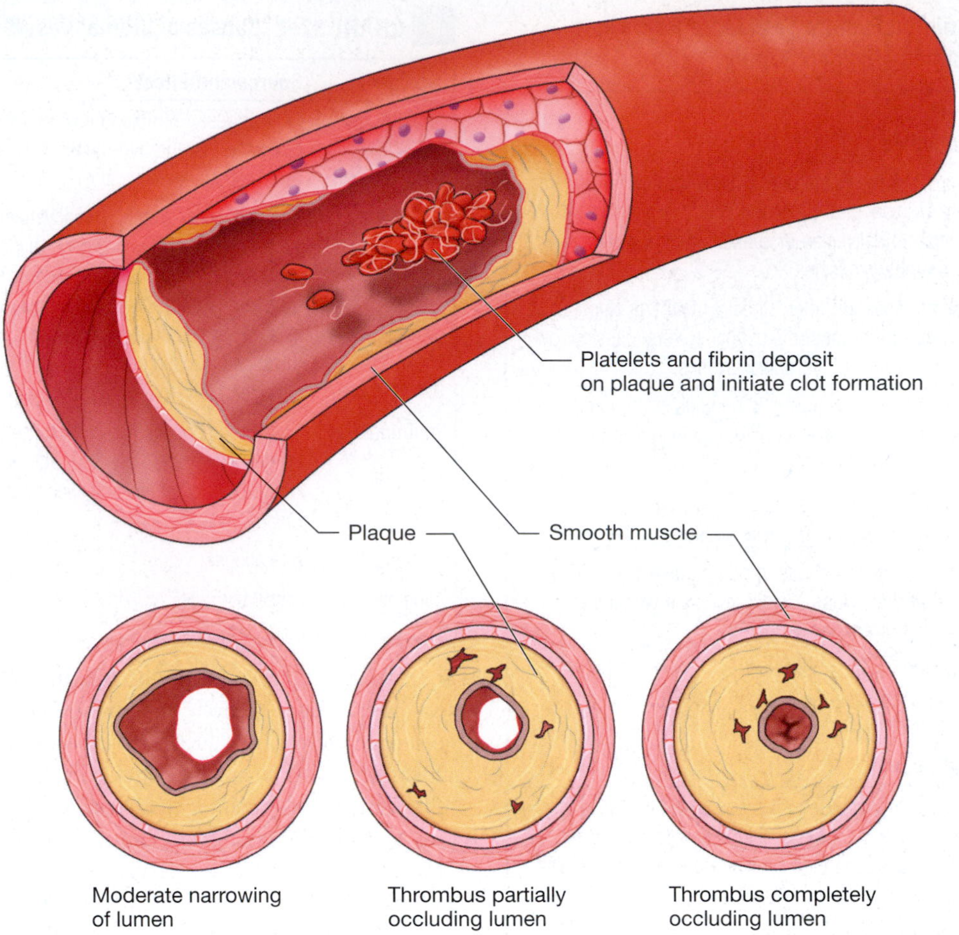

FIGURE 32–2 ◆ Stage of atheroma development in a coronary artery.

Stage II Lesion

Over time, perhaps as a result of repeated injury, plaque lesions may mature with the organization of a lipid core and the formation of a fibrous cap. This progression of the disease is referred to as a stage II lesion. During this stage, the medial smooth muscle cells invade the intimal lesion, leading to a further buildup of plaque that obstructs luminal blood flow. These lesions contain an accumulation of smooth muscle cells, macrophages, T lymphocytes, intracellular and extracellular lipids, foam cells, cellular debris from focal necrosis and foam cell apoptosis (cell death), and other blood components such as fibrin, fibrinogen, albumin, and white cells. The smooth muscle cells secrete collagen, elastin, and glycosaminoglycans, which form a dense connective tissue matrix called the **fibrous cap.** Stage II lesions are grossly white in appearance and most frequently develop where arteries bifurcate. Figure 32–3◆ shows the fibrous cap. Once arterial diameter is reduced by 70%, whether due to plaque size or thrombosis, the patient develops symptoms of CAD such as angina. Coronary artery stenosis is described as either **eccentric,** meaning that the lesion occupies part of the vessel wall circumference, or **concentric,** meaning that the lesion occupies the whole circumference.

Stage III Lesion

Advanced or stage III lesions consist of plaque with a well-established fibrous cap and lipid core. Further development and calcification of the fibrous matrix and lipid core, ulceration and hemorrhage of the fibrous cap and intimal surface, and increased risk of transluminal thrombosis characterize an advanced lesion.

In some lesions, the fibrous cap becomes vascularized and grows in size; other lesions calcify and become hardened; still others may be thin and poorly developed. Vessel segments with hardened fibrous caps are less responsive to ischemia-related vasodilatory compensatory mechanisms; the result is that the vessel does not dilate during periods of increased need for oxygen. In complicated lesions the lipid-rich core increases in size, may become calcified, and fills with necrotic cellular debris. As the atheroma enlarges, the intimal surface may develop fissures or cracks, referred to as plaque rupture, which exposes the subendothelial matrix and initiates the formation of a **thrombus** (a blood clot that forms in a blood vessel and remains at

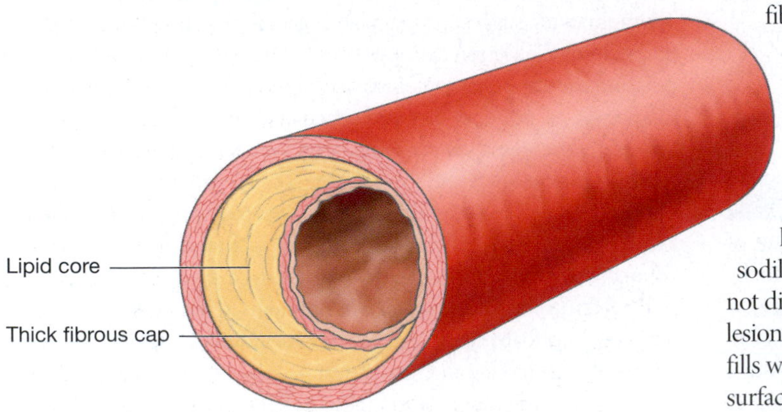

FIGURE 32–3 ◆ Fibrous cap.

the site of formation), depicted earlier (see Figure 32–2). When thrombus formation occurs in an already diseased coronary artery, it causes further obstruction to blood flow; if large enough, it may completely occlude the coronary artery. This may stop all blood flow to the tissues being fed by the artery, leading to tissue ischemia and, if sustained, apoptosis.

Plaque anatomy and defining plaque that is vulnerable to rupture have received a great deal of attention. Studies have identified certain characteristics that suggest plaque instability, which increases the risk for rupture (Moser & Riegel, 2008). Plaque that is prone to rupture is associated with the following factors:

- Positive remodeling
- A thin fibrous cap
- A core rich in lipids, calcium deposits, macrophages, T lymphocytes, and mast cells
- A paucity of collagen and smooth muscle cells
- Being large enough to cause mild to moderate luminal obstruction.

Acute Coronary Syndrome (ACS), which is discussed in detail later in the chapter, results when the plaque buildup in the artery becomes significant enough to cause ischemia that results in clinical manifestations.

When unstable plaque is conjoined with conditions of blood and myocardial maladies, the risk for ACS increases. Blood abnormalities include abnormal platelet function or structure, hypercoagulable states, and/or reduced anticoagulation factors. Having blood that is prone to coagulate because of one of these blood disorders increases the risk of thrombus formation when combined with plaque development or disruption. Myocardial maladies can be caused by dysrhythmias, reduced or abnormal ventricular function, and reduced myocardial perfusion. These patients are at higher risk of death from chronic and acute coronary artery occlusion.

In contrast, plaque that is more stable is associated with negative remodeling, a smooth surface with a predominant white color and no thrombi, a thick calcified fibrous cap with little smooth muscle cell or macrophage content, a smaller plaque core consisting of collagen, smooth muscle cells, and apoptotic necrosis (Moser & Riegel, 2008). Lesions of this type are less prone to plaque rupture.

Inflammation and Atherogenesis

The association between atherogenesis and the immune complex response has recently been described in the literature. Immune complex response is described in Chapter 52. At every stage of plaque development, leukocytes act as instigators and regulators of many processes that are associated with plaque development, such as endothelial dysfunction, procoagulant activity, subendothelial macrophage and smooth muscle cell activity, fibrous cap matrix formation and degradation, and enhanced lipoprotein transfer in the vessel wall. Research studies have suggested that certain infectious organisms may stimulate an immune response that results in plaque disruption, plaque growth, or thrombosis in areas of existing atheroma (Moser & Riegel, 2008; Woods, Froelicher, Adams [Underhill], & Bridges, 2010). Increased titers of antibodies to certain organisms such as cytomegalovirus, herpesvirus, *Chlamydia pneumoniae,* and *Helicobacter pylori* have been identified as possible predictors of elevated risk for coronary artery occlusions. It is unclear what effect these organisms have on the cells of the vessel lining; however, these organisms have been found in atheromatous lesions and organs either at autopsy or from atheroma samples. In addition, patients with ACS demonstrate elevated levels of serum markers of inflammation, activated leukocytosis, and their by-products of cytokine, growth factor, and smooth muscle cell activation, which indicate a heightened inflammatory response. These findings strongly suggest a role of inflammation in either propagating or promoting atherogenesis. Alternatively, inflammatory markers may be signs that plaque disruption is ongoing and thus are considered markers of increased risk for future sentinel cardiac events. Several serum markers of inflammation have been identified, including C-reactive protein (CRP). CRP levels that indicate CAD are included in Chart 32–3 (p. 926).

Pathophysiology of Myocardial Injury and Death

Myocardial injury from ischemia begins in the subendocardium and progresses to the epicardium (Figure 32–4◆). If blood flow is not restored within 20 minutes, apoptosis ensues, autodigestion of cells begins, and the inflammatory response is initiated. Rupture of the intracellular lysosomes is the final event signaling irreversible cell injury, apoptosis, and loss of muscle function. At this point, the intracellular enzymes are released into the bloodstream. The dead, nonfunctional tissue is referred to as the area of infarction, which has a central core composed of nonfunctional cells with disorganized structures. These are surrounded by peripheral cells with varying amounts of disruption (Figure 32–5◆, p. 925). Within hours, neutrophils infiltrate infarcted tissue, causing further endothelial damage, contraction of smooth muscles, and an increase in vascular permeability. Enzymes released by macrophages may lead to breakdown of connective tissue and cardiac muscle aneurysm formation or rupture, leaking of fluid into the pericardial space, and/or pericardial inflammation. Necrotic tissue is replaced by granulation tissue in 2 to 3 weeks, which can induce myocardial wall thinning and dilation. Fibroblasts eventually appear and synthesize a collagen matrix that provides the substrate for fibrous tissue and the formation of a mature scar in 2 to 3 months. Scarred or fibrotic myocardium becomes stiff and loses its ability to contract and relax, in other words, to function normally. Over time the myocardium may thin out. Muscle cells around scarred tissue enlarge or hypertrophy. Myocardial stiffening, thinning, and hypertrophy also can cause contraction abnormalities. In addition, myocardial scarring can cause abnormal conduction of cardiac impulses from the sinoatrial (SA) node to the ventricles (Porth, 2008). The cardiac conduction system is discussed in Chapter 30.

Surrounding the area of infarction is the zone of injury and the zone of ischemia (see Figure 32–5, p. 925). These zones are made of potentially viable tissues. The tissues can become necrotic and die or be reperfused with oxygen rich blood and remain functional. The goal of treatment for an AMI is to establish reperfusion as early as possible to prevent necrosis and salvage the myocardium.

Prevention of apoptosis, reversing cell injury, limiting infarct size or extension, and preventing myocardial remodeling (p. 958) are all dependent on a number of adaptive responses to acute and chronic ischemia. These include the timing of reperfusion, the presence of ischemic preconditioning, the extent of collateral circulation, myocardial stunning and hibernation, and apoptosis and oncosis (Porth, 2008). Reperfusion within 20 minutes will abort apoptosis (cell death). Fibrinolytic (clot-dissolving) agents (see the Pharmacology Summary of Medications to Treat Coronary Artery Disease box, p. 955) have a

Weblink: Strategies for Heart Disease and Stroke Risk Reduction

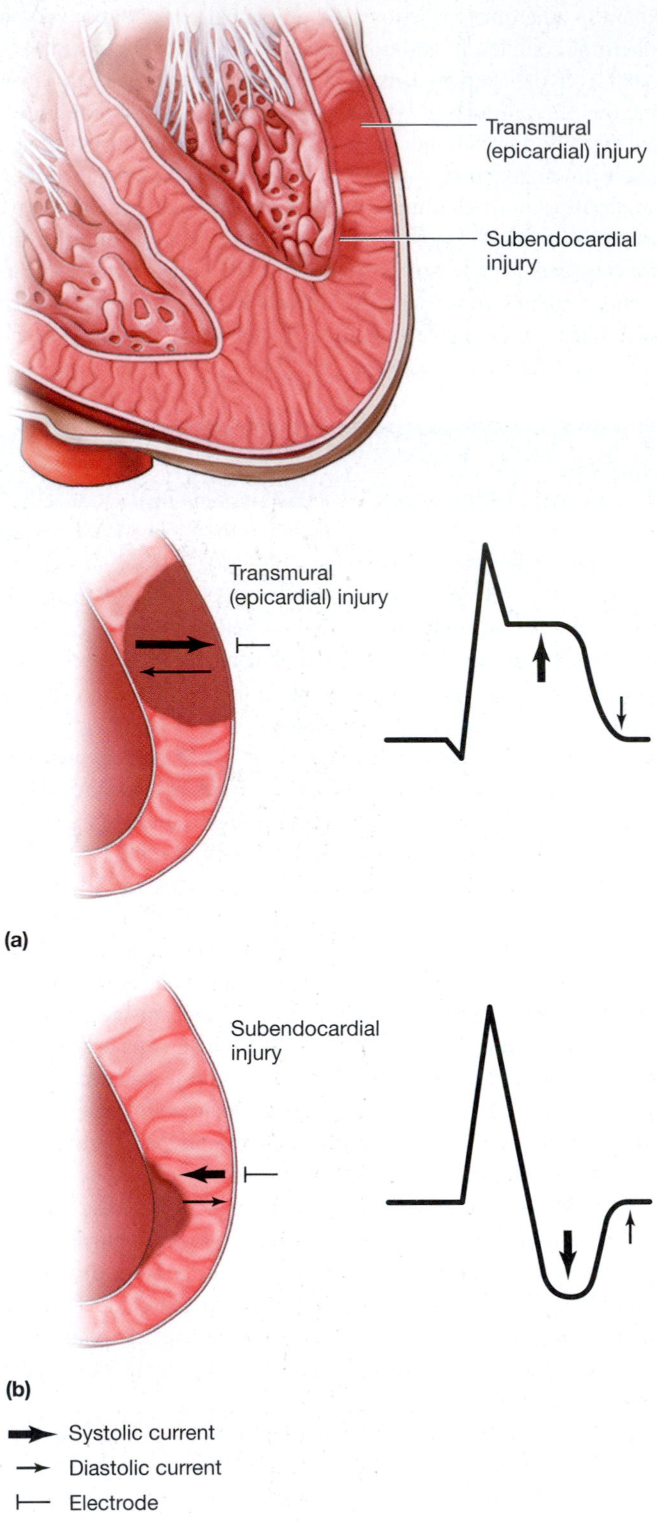

FIGURE 32–4 ◆ Subendocardial versus transmural damage.

window of less than 12 hours from symptom onset to achieve myocardial salvage. Vessels with chronic subacute thrombosis lasting a few minutes precondition the tissue for periods of longer ischemia, protecting it from infarction. Chronic, progressive coronary obstruction also stimulates the development of coronary collateral vessels. It is unclear whether these vessels are indigenous and simply recruited in times of coronary insufficiency or whether they represent neovascular development. Neovascular development can occur by angiogenesis, which is the growth of new microvessels budding from arteries in areas of healing infarcted tissue. Myocardial tissue stunning and hibernation are conditions of reversible muscle contractile dysfunction that are thought to be adaptive responses to chronic coronary occlusion. **Myocardial stunning** is a temporary dysfunction that occurs in response to artery occlusion of short duration or transient global hypoperfusion during a limited low flow state such as shock. The end result is that the myocardial muscle temporarily has a limited ability to contract, whereas with **myocardial hibernation** the tissue actually undergoes cellular structural changes and progressive apoptosis in response to prolonged occlusion. Hibernating tissue is thought to recover contractile function fully once perfusion is reestablished.

Cardiac Risk Factors

Since 1948 a longitudinal study has been conducted in Framingham, Massachusetts (Futterman & Lemberg, 2000). This study has been evaluating the lifestyles and habits of the city's inhabitants. The results have allowed researchers to identify factors that increase a person's risk for the development of CAD. The study is still going on and is now evaluating the third and fourth generation of subjects. It continues to provide important information about the development of heart disease. An abundance of other research also continues to refine and add to the body of knowledge about the development of CAD. **Cardiac risk factors** are habits, lifestyles, and/or genetic factors that predispose an individual to the development of CAD. Risk factors have various categories, which are typically referred to as modifiable versus nonmodifiable, as well as contributing factors. The risk factors for CAD disease are outlined in the Risk Factors box. Modifiable risk factors are ones over which an individual has some control, such as physical activity, stress, and cigarette smoking, whereas nonmodifiable risk factors are not controllable. Nonmodifiable risk factors include advancing age, male sex, and heredity. The AHA (2010e) recommends that all adults with or without established CAD be assessed for risk beginning at the age of 20. A review of lifestyle and predisposing factors at every annual physical evaluation or at least every 2 years should occur.

Research data from the last few decades have shown conclusively that it is possible to alter the natural history of atherosclerosis by either regression or stabilization of plaque with aggressive risk factor reduction (Moser & Riegel, 2008; Woods et al., 2010). Risk factor reduction efforts focus on factors that are modifiable, specifically lifestyle changes aimed at promoting smoking cessation, blood pressure control, exercise, weight reduction, low-fat diets, and pharmacologic therapies that control dyslipidemia. The Complementary & Alternative Therapies box discusses the impact of music on blood pressure and anxiety.

Modifiable Risk Factors

Identification of modifiable risk factors is important for both the assessment of risk and determining targets for intervention. The modifiable risk factors include hyperlipidemia, hypertension, tobacco smoke, diabetes, physical inactivity, and obesity/overweight.

Safety Alert *When educating patients about CAD, the nurse must stress that if the patient has nonmodifiable risk factors, it is essential to control the modifiable factors in order to prevent or slow the progression of CAD.*

Hyperlipidemia

Hyperlipidemia is defined as elevated cholesterol and/or triglyceride levels. Cholesterol and triglycerides are lipids that permeate the arterial wall, narrowing the lumen and ultimately decreasing blood

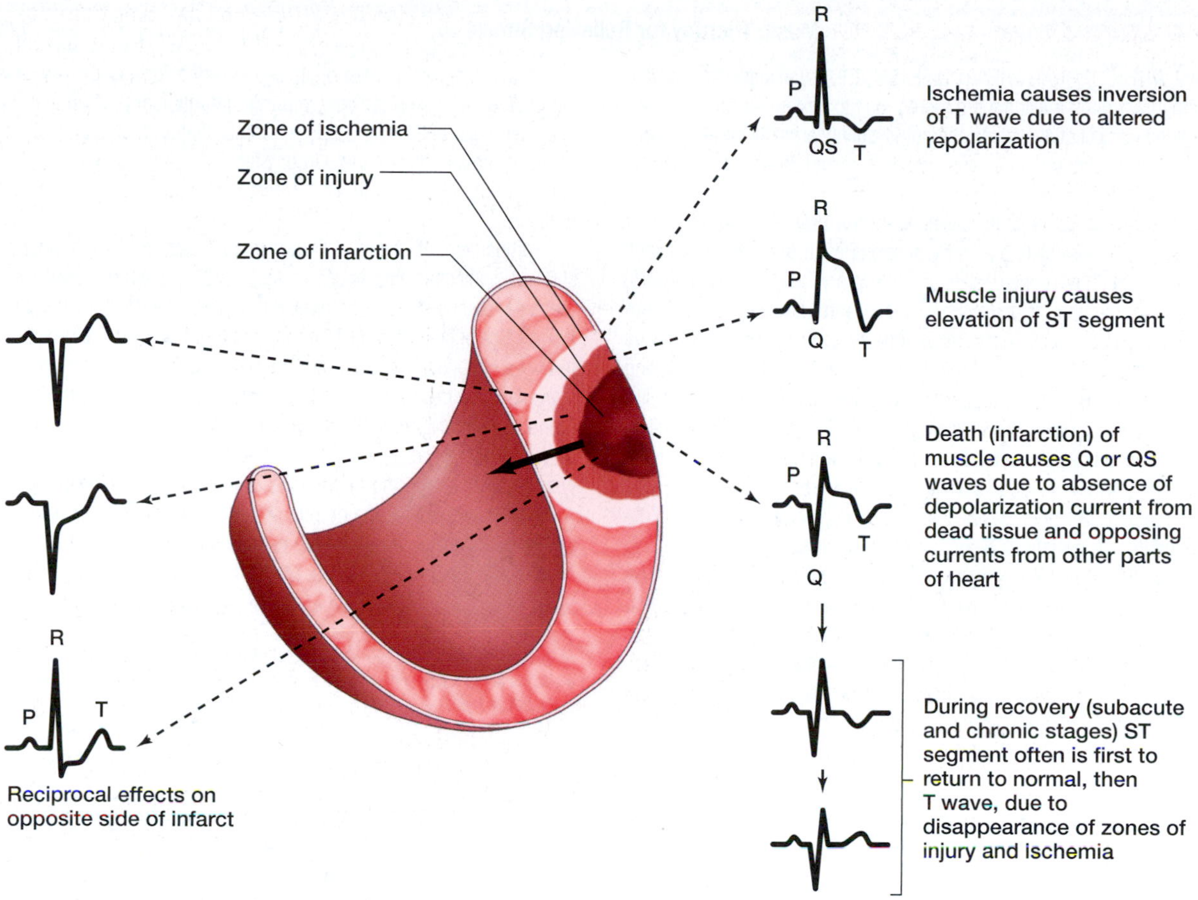

FIGURE 32–5 ◆ Zones of infarction and reciprocal ECG changes.

flow to the cardiac muscle. **Hypercholesterolemia** is defined as an increased cholesterol level in the blood. **Cholesterol** is a steroid molecule produced primarily by the liver that is essential for the formation and maintenance of cell membranes. The serum cholesterol level is a potent indicator of risk for CAD. Approximately 85% of cholesterol in the blood is produced by the body. The other 15% is consumed through the diet. For a person with no cardiac history or risk factors, a total cholesterol level less than 200 mg/dL is considered low risk for the development of CAD. A total cholesterol level of 200 to 250 mg/dL is considered moderate risk, and levels greater than 250 mg/dL are considered high risk. For patients with known CAD or risk factors, the desired serum levels are lower. Chart 32–3 outlines the desired goals for prevention of CAD.

Cholesterol levels tend to increase with age. Also, hypercholesterolemia may be inherited as a genetic defect that leads to excessive production of low-density lipoproteins or a decreased capacity for their removal. It also can be acquired through diet and lifestyle. Familial hypercholesterolemia is discussed in the Genetic Considerations box (p. 926). Cultural variations in cholesterol levels have been noted as well. The Cultural Considerations box (p. 927) discusses cultural groups that

RISK FACTORS for Coronary Artery Disease

Modifiable Factors	Nonmodifiable Factors	Contributing Factors
Elevated low-density lipoprotein cholesterol (LDL-C)	Increasing age	High-fat diet
Low high-density lipoprotein cholesterol (HDL-C)	Heredity	Alcohol consumption
Elevated Triglycerides	Male gender	Increased stress
Elevated total cholesterol		Increased homocysteine level
Hypertension		Increased C-reactive protein
Tobacco smoke		Hormone replacement therapy
Diabetes		
Physical inactivity		
Overweight and obesity*		

*Normal weight = 18.5 to 24.9 kg/m^2; overweight = 25 to 29 kg/m^2; obesity = > 30.0 kg/m^2; abdominal obesity is defined as waist circumference (men) > 102 centimeters (40 inches); (women) > 88 centimeters (35 inches).

COMPLEMENTARY & ALTERNATIVE THERAPIES Music Therapy for Relieving Stress

Nancy Yilk

INDIVIDUALS WITH CORONARY HEART DISEASE (CHD) often suffer from severe distress during treatment, making them more prone to anxiety, which puts them at greater risk for complications. Music therapy is a nonpharmacological intervention that has been used to reduce anxiety and distress and improve physiological functioning in patients.

An Italian study of 86 patients investigated the psychological effects of music, exploring the possibility that daily sessions of music-guided sessions with slow breathing may reduce 24-hour ambulatory blood pressure (ABP). Age-matched, sex-matched hypertensive patients were randomized into either the Intervention group, which used music-guided slow breathing exercises (4 to 6 breaths/min; 1:2 ratio of inspiration:expiration duration), comprising 29 subjects, or into two control groups that were told to relax while either listening to slow music (Control-26) or reading a book (Control-31). ABP monitoring was performed at baseline with follow-up at intervals of 1, 3, and 6 months.

Daily voluntary music-guided sessions with slow breathing demonstrated significantly reduced 24-hour systolic ABP and psychological factors. The average reduction of systolic 24-hour ABP at 6 months was 4.6 mmHg with confidence limits at 95% compared to control groups. Antihypertensive treatment was selected as a negative predictor of BP reduction. When antihypertensive treatment was inserted as a covariant, along with psychological factors assessed at baseline by the Mental Health Inventory questionnaire, the intervention of music was found to positively affect systolic blood pressure reduction at 6-month follow-up (Modesti et al., 2010).

Music intervention demonstrated positive effects on the physiological stress response and anxiety among mechanically ventilated patients in intensive care units in a study in China. Outcome measures included the Chinese version of the Spielberger State-Trait Anxiety Scale and physiological parameters (heart rate, respiratory rate, saturation of oxygen, and blood pressure).

Comparison of mean differences (pretest score and post-test score) showed significant differences in heart rate, respiratory rate, systolic blood pressure, and diastolic blood pressure as well as in the Spielberger State-Trait Anxiety Scale, but not in SaO_2 among the three groups; the greatest mean differences were found in the music listening group. A significant reduction in the physiological stress response (heart rate and respiratory rate) over time was found in the music listening group, and a significant increase in heart rate and respiratory rate over time was found in the control group, with no significant change over time in the headphone group. Using the Spielberger State-Trait Anxiety Scale, post-testing demonstrated a significant reduction in anxiety for the music listening group and the headphone group, but not the control group (Han, Li, Sit, Chung, Jiao, & Ma, 2010).

Sources: Han et al. (2010, April). Effects of music intervention on physiological stress response and anxiety level of mechanically ventilated patients in China: A randomized controlled trial. *Journal of Clinical Nursing, 19*(7–8), 978–987; Modesti et al. (2010, May). Psychological predictors of the antihypertensive effects of music-guided slow breathing. *Journal of Hypertension, 28*(5), 1097–1103.

CHART 32–3 Laboratory Test Parameters That Assess for CAD

Total cholesterol	<200 mg/dL	HDL-C	>40 mg/dL
LDL-C	<100 mg/dL	C-reactive protein	<0.175 mg/L
Triglycerides	<150 mg/dL	Homocysteine	<17

Source: Adapted from: Kee, J. L. (2010). *Laboratory and diagnostic tests with nursing implications.* Upper Saddle River, NJ: Pearson.

have a lower rate of CAD. Hypercholesterolemia has several alternative names, including type II hyperlipoproteinemia, hypercholesterolemic xanthomatosis, and low-density lipoprotein receptor mutation.

Cholesterol is carried in the blood via small proteins. When these carrier proteins join with cholesterol, they are called lipoproteins. The weight or density of lipoproteins depends on the amount of protein in the molecule. Total serum cholesterol is a composite value comprising all the types of cholesterol that carry lipoproteins. The lipoproteins that alter one's risk for CAD are the low-density lipoproteins, the high-density lipoproteins, and possibly lipoprotein A. The American Heart Association (2010e) recommends that total cholesterol levels be measured every 5 years. For men over 45 years, women over 55 years, and patients with elevated cholesterol, or low high-density lipoprotein cholesterol (HDL-C), cholesterol levels should be drawn more often.

Safety Alert *Patients need to be instructed that cholesterol and lipid panels should be drawn after fasting overnight, including no alcohol.*

Low-density lipoprotein cholesterol (LDL-C), often referred to as "bad cholesterol," is the major cholesterol carrier in the blood. When circulating LDL-C becomes oxidized, it is modified such that it attaches to and migrates through the cell membrane into the intimal lining of the vessel. Once inside the cell membrane, LDL-C attracts immune complexes from the blood into the intima. Smooth muscle cells from the medial layer of the vessel wall migrate into the intima, thus creating the surface for plaque development. Oxidized LDL-C also causes

GENETIC CONSIDERATIONS for Hypercholesterolemia

Familial hypercholesterolemia (FH) is an autosomal dominant inherited genetic disease that results in markedly elevated low-density lipoproteins (LDL), the bad cholesterol, beginning at birth. This leads to premature coronary atherosclerosis, which increases the risk of suffering an AMI or stroke at an early age. Men are more commonly affected, having rates of first AMI in their 40s to 50s, with 85% of them having an AMI by age 60. Women have an increased incidence of AMI, but it is delayed by 10 years.

An individual can inherit two genes for hypercholesterolemia, which magnifies the severity of the condition. In severely affected individuals, the cholesterol level may exceed 500 mg/dL, and waxy plaques (xanthomas) of cholesterol develop beneath the skin over elbows, knees, and buttocks; in tendons; and around the cornea of the eye. Atherosclerosis begins before puberty, and AMI and death may occur before age 30.

Patient teaching for individuals with a strong family history of hypercholesterolemia includes stressing the risk of early AMI. These patients should be evaluated with a lipid screen regularly. Proper diet, exercise, and the use of lipid-lowering drugs to bring the cholesterol down to safer levels are also recommended.

Source: Adapted from Moser, D. K., & Riegel, B. (2008). *Cardiac nursing: A companion to Braunwald's heart disease.* St. Louis: Saunders.

endothelial dysfunction by inhibiting the release of endothelial nitric oxide, a compound that not only prevents LDL-C oxidation but also is necessary for vasodilation. Thus, vessel segments damaged by plaque do not vasodilate in response to local hypoxia caused from vessel occlusion the way undamaged vessel segments do. The optimal target goal for LDL-C is less than 100 mg/dL. See Chart 32–4 for techniques to modify lipid panel results.

High-density lipoprotein cholesterol (HDL-C), sometimes called "good cholesterol," consists of heavier lipoproteins that bind to cholesterol, transporting it back to the liver, and may actually remove excess cholesterol from plaque in the arteries. High levels of HDL-C are thought to be cardioprotective. Levels greater than 40 mg/dL in men

CHART 32–4 Factors That Affect the Lipid Profile

HDL-C	Factors that ↑ HDL-C	Smoking cessation by 10%
		Exercise
		Weight reduction
	Factors that ↓ HDL-C	Smoking
		Trans fatty acids
		Sedentary
		Obesity
		Low-fat/high-carbohydrate diet
LDL-C	Factors that ↑ LDL-C	*Trans* fatty acids
		Saturated fats
		Cholesterol
	Factors that ↓ LDL-C	Polyunsaturated fatty acids
		Monounsaturated fatty acids
		Soluble fiber and soy protein
		Weight reduction
Triglycerides	Factors that ↑ triglycerides	Excess body weight
		Reduced physical activity
		Increased intake of sugar and refined carbohydrates, particularly with insulin resistance and glucose
		Increased alcohol intake intolerance
	Factors that ↓ triglycerides	Exercise
		Weight reduction
		Reduced carbohydrate consumption

and greater than 50 mg/dL in women with no CAD and no risk factors are desirable.

Safety Alert *When teaching patients about dietary control of cholesterol and lipids, it is important for the nurse to inquire about food preferences and cultural factors that may affect the patients' eating habits. The teaching needs to be tailored to include the patients' lifestyle and food preferences, as well as cultural considerations in order to increase compliance with the restrictions.*

Triglycerides are a form of fat derived and produced by the body from other sources such as carbohydrates. Elevated triglyceride levels are associated with high total cholesterol, high LDL-C, low HDL-C, heart disease, obesity, and diabetes (AHA, 2010f). Lowering levels to less than 150 mg/dL has become a part of risk prevention. Levels of 150 to 199 mg/dL are considered borderline high, levels of 200 to 499 mg/dL borderline high to high, and levels greater than 500 mg/dL very high.

CULTURAL CONSIDERATIONS for CAD Development

Not only is heart disease the leading cause of death in the United States, it is also the leading cause of death worldwide. Factors that have contributed to this include increasing longevity, smoking, an increase in high-fat diets, and increasing levels of inactivity (Libby, Bonow, Zipes, & Mann, 2008). As countries advance economically, there is a tendency for their citiziens to consume more calories. A key change has been an increase in the amount of saturated fats consumed accompanied by a decrease in the amount of plant-based foods. Cultural differences affect a patient's nutritional status, and it is important to have an understanding of the patient's typical diet. Some diets may be high in saturated fats (meats, dairy, coconut milk, condensed milk, oils), complex carbohydrates (rice, bread, pasta), or sodium (soy sauce, soups, casseroles, processed foods, food from fast-food restaurants). Such diets tend to promote heart disease.

Weblink: Diabetes

Weblink: Triglycerides

Lipid-Lowering Therapy

Multiple lipid-lowering drugs are now available. The Pharmacology box (p. 955) outlines these medications. Lipid-lowering agents are considered for patients with CAD and fewer than two risk factors if their LDL-C is ≥ 190 mg/dL, patients without CAD with two or more risk factors with an LDL-C ≥ 160 mg/dL, or patients with known CAD with an LDL-C ≥ 130 mg/dL. Drug therapy is delayed in men under age 35 and premenopausal women with LDL-C of 190 to 219 mg/dL, except in high-risk patient groups such as patients with diabetes or patients who are obese or with hypertension. However, patients with CAD and LDL-C between 100 and 129 mg/dL may still benefit from lipid-lowering therapy. Lipid-lowering therapy is also indicated for familial dyslipidemia.

Hypertension

Maintaining a blood pressure within the recommended normal range reduces the mortality from CAD. African Americans have the highest overall mortality rate from CAD of all ethnic groups in the United States, which is attributed to the higher prevalence of certain coronary risk factors, among them hypertension and type 2 diabetes (Moser & Riegel, 2008).

Tobacco Smoke

Cardiovascular adverse effects from smoking are attributed to carbon monoxide and nicotine. Carbon monoxide displaces oxygen on the hemoglobin molecule, thus reducing the blood's oxygen-carrying capacity. Carbon monoxide also may promote atherogenesis by causing endothelial damage. Nicotine increases myocardial oxygen demand by increasing blood pressure and heart rate and is thought to promote thrombogenesis through platelet aggregation. Nicotine also causes vasospasm and endothelial dysfunction. The risk of cardiovascular adverse events in male and female smokers who successfully quit dramatically decreases. In fact, within 2 to 3 years of smoking cessation, their risk level approaches that of nonsmokers. However, HDL-C levels increase after smoking cessation (Gepner, Piper, Johnson, Fiore, Baker, & Stein, 2011).

Diabetes

Various microvascular and macrovascular changes are thought to be responsible for the overall higher rate of cardiovascular morbidity and mortality found in patients with diabetes. Women have twice the risk of men of developing cardiovascular events associated with diabetes (AHA, 2010b). These vascular changes are thought to be mediated through intimal proliferation and other pathologies of endothelial function.

Reducing the risk of CAD for patients with diabetes goes beyond controlling known cardiac risk factors. Even without additional risk factors, people with diabetes are at greater risk for CAD (National Diabetes Information Clearinghouse [NDIC], 2010). Risk factor reduction focuses on aggressive treatment for diabetes including glycemic control (keeping blood sugar within a healthy range) and lifestyle changes. Moderate changes in diet, exercise, and weight reduction can decrease the development of diabetes. In addition, glycemic control has been shown to have an impact on decreasing overall CAD morbidity and mortality and reduces long-term mortality following an AMI.

Weblink: Physical Activity Weblink: Strategies for Heart Disease and Stroke Risk Reduction

NATIONAL GUIDELINES for Interventions to Promote Physical Activity and Dietary Lifestyle Changes for Cardiovascular Risk Factor Reduction

Cognitive-behavioral strategies can promote behavior change. These strategies focus on changing how individuals think about themselves, their behaviors, and surrounding circumstances and how to modify their lifestyle.

1. Assist the patient to set specific short-term goals for increased physical activity and/or dietary changes to reduce cardiovascular risk.
2. Provide feedback on the patient's progress toward her goals for cardiovascular risk reduction. Feedback helps patients to assess their progress and can improve their motivation and compliance with continued efforts toward risk reduction.
3. Provide strategies to help the patient self-monitor, such as logs for documenting weight, exercise, and/or food intake. Some patients may benefit from automated prompts, such as telephone messages or e-mail reminders.
4. Establish a plan for follow-up. Frequent contact helps patients to develop trust.
5. If patients are resistant, employ motivational interviewing strategies. Such strategies include:
   a. Asking for permission: "Do you mind if we talk about how you might increase your activity level?"
   b. Evoking change talk: "What would be good things that could come from changing your lifestyle?"
   c. Supporting the patient's ability to care for herself (self-efficacy): "If you did decide to change how you eat, what would need to happen first?"
   d. "Rolling with" resistance: "Help me to understand. You tell me that you want to live long enough to see your grandchildren graduate from high school, but you do not want to change your lifestyle so that you can do that."
   e. Develop discrepancies: "What do you think will happen if you don't change your lifestyle?"
   f. Reflective listening: Listen carefully to what the patient tells you has worked and not worked for her in the past.
6. Assist the patient with finding peer-based support groups. Patients are more likely to hear and personalize messages, leading to changes in attitude and behavior, if they believe the messenger is similar to them and faces the same concerns and pressures.

Source: Adapted from Artinian et al. (2010). Interventions to promote physical activity and dietary lifestyle changes for cardiovascular risk factor reduction in adults: A scientific statement from the American Heart Association. *Circulation, 122,* 406–441. Retrieved from http://www.ncbi.nlm.nih.gov/pubmed/20625115.

Physical Inactivity

Obesity, sedentary lifestyle, and lack of physical activity are mutually supporting cardiac risk factors. Regular exercise ($\geq$ 5 times/week lasting $\geq$ 30 minutes) of moderate intensity (such as brisk walking) decreases heart attack risk by 10% to 50% in both men and women. Cardioprotection from exercise is attributed to improved functional work capacity, decreased heart rate, decreased platelet adhesiveness, enhanced fibrinolysis, attenuation of the sympathetic stress response, weight loss, lowered triglyceride levels, and increased HDL-C levels. The AHA (2010d) recommends regular moderate-to-vigorous-intensity aerobic activity for at least 30 minutes on most days of the week. These 30-minute sessions can be broken down into two or three 10- to 15-minute periods of time and remain effective. See the National Guidelines box for ways of promoting physical activity.

Obesity and Overweight

Obesity is an increasing public health problem in the United States. Chronic obesity increases the risk of CAD in men and women. Obesity is attributed to increases in blood pressure, abnormal lipoprotein levels, insulin resistance, and platelet aggregation. The two units of measure associated with cardiovascular risk are body mass index (BMI) and abdominal circumference. BMI is a person's weight in kilograms divided by the square of one's height in meters, giving a measure of kilograms per square meter (kg/m^2). Abdominal obesity is defined as a waist circumference of > 40 inches in men and > 35 inches in women. Fat accumulation in the upper body, giving the body an appearance of an "apple," has been linked to a greater risk of CAD, as opposed to a "pear" shape with body fat accumulation in the gluteofemoral region. Abdominal obesity is associated with elevated levels of cholesterol and greater risk for CAD.

In counseling a patient in weight reduction, a multidisciplinary approach is typically most effective. To achieve lifetime changes in eating habits and adherence to an exercise program, the patient needs counseling from nutritionists, health care providers, nurses, physical therapists, and psychological counselors. Many cities have obesity clinics that provide these services.

Nonmodifiable Risk Factors

Nonmodifiable risk factors are those that cannot be modified through lifestyle and habit changes. Meticulous attention to controlling the modifiable risk factors is recommended to mitigate the effects of the nonmodifiable risk factors. The nonmodifiable risk factors include increasing age, heredity, and male gender.

Increasing Age

Cardiac aging results in stiffening of myofibrils, which cause a reduced ability of the muscle to relax, stretch, and contract. The number of myocytes decreases with age, cells enlarge or hypertrophy, the cells become less responsive to stimulation, and the rate of apoptosis or cell death increases. As was mentioned earlier, cholesterol and triglyceride levels increase with advanced age. Aging causes large arterial vessel walls to dilate and thicken and causes smooth muscle tone to increase; increased vessel stiffness increases as elastic and collagen are replaced with fibrotic tissue. The consequences of these changes are an elevated systolic blood pressure, arteriosclerosis, atherosclerosis, and a decrease in cardiac performance. Age is an independent risk factor for CAD and should be a part of every risk assessment.

Heredity

A familial history of CAD dramatically increases the risk that family members will have cardiac disease as well. Adult offspring of parents with a history of CAD also are more likely to have multiple risk factors for CAD and have a greater likelihood of an acute cardiac event, even after correcting for other disease risk factors. First-degree relatives (children, parents, and siblings); families with greater prevalence, meaning that more than one person in the family have CAD; and families with early onset CAD are at greater risk. Reasons for this familial connection are not known. Possible mediators may be environmental or social factors or genetic predisposition.

Health care personnel need to be mindful of the fact that family members are not always aware that others in their family have or are predisposed to heart disease, especially with regard to less obvious risk factors such as hypertension and hyperlipidemia.

Race is also included under the category of heredity. African Americans have a higher overall CAD prevalence and mortality rate than do Caucasians in the United States (U.S. Department of Health and Human Services, 2011). Additionally, African Americans present with a disproportionate number of CAD risk factors such as hypertension, type 2 diabetes, metabolic syndrome, abdominal obesity, stress, and inactivity. Reasons for these disparities are unclear but may include ethnic, cultural, and physiological differences. Studies have highlighted that African Americans (1) perceive cardiac pain differently and often ascribe symptoms to other noncardiac causes; (2) less often seek, ask for, or receive appropriate preventive, diagnostic, and interventional therapy for CAD and respond differently to it; (3) may be financially disenfranchised, which limits access to health care; (4) may experience psychosocial stress, racism, and frustration, leading to suboptimal interactions with the health care system; and (5) may have a genetic predisposition to vascular disease and atherosclerosis (Sirak, Chiadika, Daka, & Simon, 2008).

Male Gender

CAD prevalence and mortality rates are higher in men than in women, especially men 45 to 70 years of age, surpassed by women only in older age (AHA, 2010b). Even when women's death rate from heart disease increases after menopause, it is not as high as that of men. Men are more likely to seek and receive diagnostic and therapeutic interventions related to differences in pain perception, treatment bias, and social roles. Men also respond differently to therapy, often with separate prescription and guideline recommendations. As women achieve advanced financial and social status, there may be a change in CAD disease prevalence and mortality demographics.

Contributing Risk Factors

Contributing risk factors include those factors that an individual may have a tendency or likelihood to have because of genetics, gender, habits, or other related causes (see the Risk Factors box, p. 925). They are preventable risk factors that usually require self-discipline and motivation in order to avert. Contributing risk factors include a high-fat diet, alcohol consumption, stress, homocysteine level, C-reactive protein, and hormone replacement therapy, all of which are discussed next.

High-Fat Diet

The cornerstone of cardiac nutrition stresses a diet low in calories; low in total fat (saturated fats, *trans* fatty acids, and cholesterol); moderate in protein; and high in fruits, vegetables, and other complex carbohydrates. Limiting caloric intake aids in weight reduction and improves insulin resistance. Diets high in total fats are associated with excess body weight and elevated levels of circulating cholesterol and lipoproteins that are known to be atherogenic. Chapter 8 provides a complete description of heart-healthy diets.

Alcohol Consumption

Heavy use of alcohol also has been linked to CAD and related risk factors such as obesity, limited physical activity, diabetes, and malnutrition. Guidelines recommend limiting alcohol intake to no more than 2 drinks a day for men and 1 drink a day for women (AHA, 2010a). Alcohol in the form of red wine and dark beer may protect the heart in ways that have been recently discovered. Compounds known as flavonols that are found in red wine and dark beer, but are not as plentiful in white wine or other forms of alcohol, are thought to increase HDL-C, improve endothelial function, and reduce platelet aggregation (Heiss, Keen, & Kelm, 2010). However, drinking in excess of 1 glass of alcohol per day for women and 2 glasses for men, even red wine, is discouraged.

Weblink: Go Red for Women

Stress

Stress enhances autonomic stimulation. Sympathetic stimulation increases myocardial work, blood pressure, heart rate, and dysrhythmia generation and enhances platelet aggregation. Parasympathetic stimulation also predisposes one to dysrhythmias. Depression and lack of social support may affect autonomic impulses and may result in poor adherence to risk modification therapy. The association between psychosocial stressors and CAD is based only on epidemiologic studies thus far. People with greater spiritual awareness appear to display less distress, anxiety, and depression during times of personal turmoil, which may have a direct and indirect effect on cardiovascular risk. Spirituality includes a system of beliefs individuals have about the world and themselves. Chapter 9 contains a complete discussion of the impact of stress on maladaptive or disease processes.

Weblink: Alcohol and Cardiovascular Disease

Homocysteine Level

Homocysteine, an amino acid that has been found to be a predictor of CAD, promotes coagulation and endothelial injury. Smoking, aging, and chronic inflammation cause homocysteine levels to increase. Elevated levels of homocysteine (Hyc > 17 μmol/L) are associated with an increased risk of CAD, as well as peripheral vascular disease, stroke, and venous thrombosis. Vitamins B_6, B_{12}, and folic acid decrease the levels of homocysteine; either vitamin supplements or foods such as fruits, vegetables, cereals, and legumes are good sources of these nutrients (Moser & Riegel, 2008).

C-Reactive Protein Level

Inflammation is thought to contribute to ACS, and a marker of inflammation is C-reactive protein (CRP). CRP is produced and released by liver cells stimulated by activated macrophages. Elevated CRP is a predictor of increased risk for heart attacks, strokes, and peripheral vascular disease and is being used as a screening test for atherosclerosis for middle-aged and older people. Elevated levels (higher than 3.0 mg/L) are present in patients with unstable angina (UA) and acute MI and appear to be predictive of higher risk for short- and long-term cardiovascular morbidity and mortality (AHA, 2010c).

Hormone Replacement Therapy

Menopause is associated with significant elevations in serum dyslipidemias and a threefold increase in risk of CAD. This is thought to be related to a decrease in the level of estrogen. Current recommendations dissuade the use of hormone replacement therapy (HRT) as a CAD risk reduction strategy and suggest that women contact their health care provider to decide whether the therapeutic benefits of HRT outweigh the risks (Woods et al., 2010).

Safety Alert *The American Heart Association has created a free online toolkit designed to educate women about cardiovascular disease. It was developed as part of the association's "Go Red For Women" campaign, which calls attention to the devastating effects of heart disease in women. Access this and other campaign resources at http://www.goredforwomen.org/.*

Metabolic Syndrome

Metabolic syndrome is defined as having three out of the five following conditions: (1) elevated waist circumference, (2) elevated triglycerides, (3) reduced HDL-C, (4) elevated blood pressure, and (5) elevated fasting glucose ($\geq$100 mg/dL). This cluster of conditions correlates with a higher risk for CAD and type 2 diabetes onset (Alberti et al., 2009). Management of metabolic syndrome consists of targeting each abnormality with a modification of corresponding risk factors, especially weight reduction and increased physical activity, and use of direct therapeutic interventions to lower blood pressure, serum glucose, and serum lipids.

Clinical Manifestations of Coronary Artery Disease

CAD presents as clinical conditions of angina pectoris, UA, MI, and SCD. These conditions depict a continuum of progressively worsening imbalances between the amount of oxygen delivered to and required by myocardial tissues. The underlying pathophysiology of each disorder is the same: atherosclerosis, as described earlier. However, as vessel stenosis intensifies, distinctions in the manifestations of signs and symptoms occur that are important for appropriate disease management. The clinical manifestations of ischemia are described next. Chapter 30 discusses normal and abnormal electrocardiogram (ECG) rhythms.

Electrocardiogram Changes

When the heart muscle becomes ischemic, injured, or infarcted, depolarization and repolarization of cardiac cells are altered, causing changes in the ECG tracing. The ECG changes are manifested in three specific ways: ST segment elevation or depression, T wave extenuation or inversion, and QRS changes as in the development of pathologic Q waves. A bundle branch block and cardiac dysrhythmias also may occur. The ECG is useful (1) for identifying areas of injury or infarction, (2) for identifying the infarct-related artery, (3) for determining reperfusion following intervention, and (4) in monitoring for cardiac dysrhythmias associated with myocardial damage. The ECG should be completed within the first 10 minutes of admission to the emergency department.

ST Segment Changes

The ST segment begins at the end of the QRS complex and ends at the beginning of the T wave (see Figure 32–6◆). The point that marks the end of the QRS complex is referred to as the *J point* (see Figure 32–7◆). Normally isoelectric, the ST segment represents the time during which the ventricles have been completely depolarized and are beginning to repolarize. When cardiac tissue becomes ischemic, the ST segment becomes abnormal and indicates a total reduction in localized blood flow. When the muscle ischemia involves only a portion of the heart wall, it is referred to as subendocardial injury and results in ST segment depression (see Figure 32–8◆). When the ischemia traverses the entire width of the cardiac muscle, referred to as transmural ischemia, the ST segment becomes elevated (see Figure 32–7). Prolonged, persistent ST segment elevation indicates acute ischemia and injury or infarction and is associated with elevated cardiac blood markers (p. 949). The greater the displacement of the ST segment and the more leads that are involved on the 12-lead ECG, the greater the amount of tissue damage (Thaler, 2010). The morphology (shape) of ST segment elevation is dependent on the lead. Figure 32–7 depicts the various morphologies of ST segment elevation.

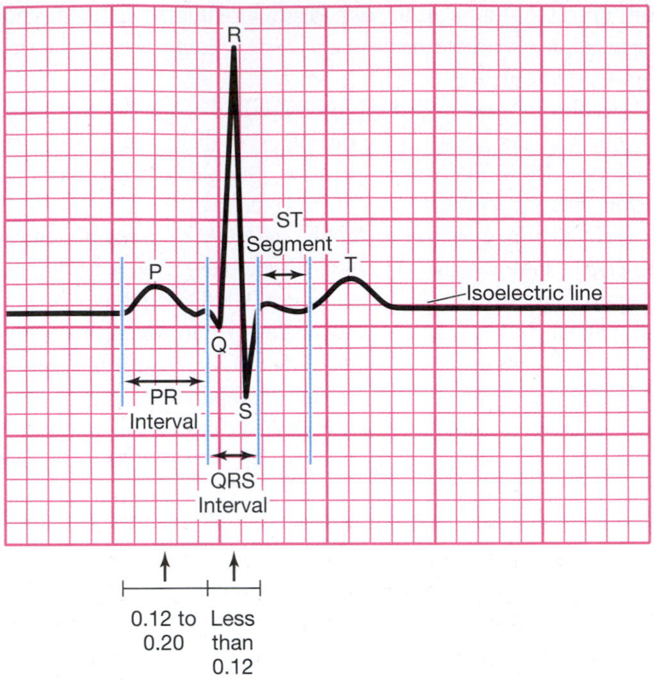

FIGURE 32–6 ◆ Normal ECG waveforms.

With transmural injury, the ST segment begins to rise almost immediately and can remain elevated for several hours to several days, as long as the ischemia continues. As the ischemia or injury subsides, the ST segment returns to the baseline. Once the ST segment has returned to the baseline, one of the main indicators of the acute MI is lost. Thus, obtaining a 12-lead ECG while the abnormality is present—in other words, while the patient is having chest pain—is essential for diagnosis and treatment of the cardiac event.

ST segment elevation greater than 1 millimeter, or 1 small box on the ECG graph paper, or ST segment depression greater than 0.5 millimeter, or one-half a small box, as determined on a 12-lead ECG, is considered a significant change. ST segment changes seen on continuous cardiac monitoring must be verified by obtaining a 12-lead ECG. The waveforms of continuous monitors are not calibrated and may be artificially enhanced by changes in the signal gain. Patients also may have a slight ST depression or elevation as a result of chronic cardiac disease, which can mimic an acute ECG change.

T Wave Changes

Normally, the T wave begins at the isoelectric line, gently slopes upward in a positive deflection, and represents ventricular repolarization (see Figure 32–6). Abnormal T wave changes occur with ischemia or injury, thus assisting with the diagnosis of ACS. When ischemia or injury occurs, the T wave inverts (flips over) in some leads and becomes tall or peaked in other leads. Marked T wave peaking and an increase in their width may be present in the very early stages of an acute MI. These are referred to as hyperacute T waves (see Figure 32–9◆). Even patients with unstable angina have marked T wave peaking and increased width. Peaked T waves, like ST segment elevations, are indicative of acute occlusion. If the occlusion is total and unrelieved, it will evolve into an AMI. Within 5 to 30 minutes of occlusion or ischemia, T wave inversion occurs (see Figure 32–9). The inverted T wave is symmetrical in shape, relatively narrow, and somewhat pointed. Unlike the ST segment, which returns to normal rather quickly, the T wave can stay inverted for weeks after the ischemic event.

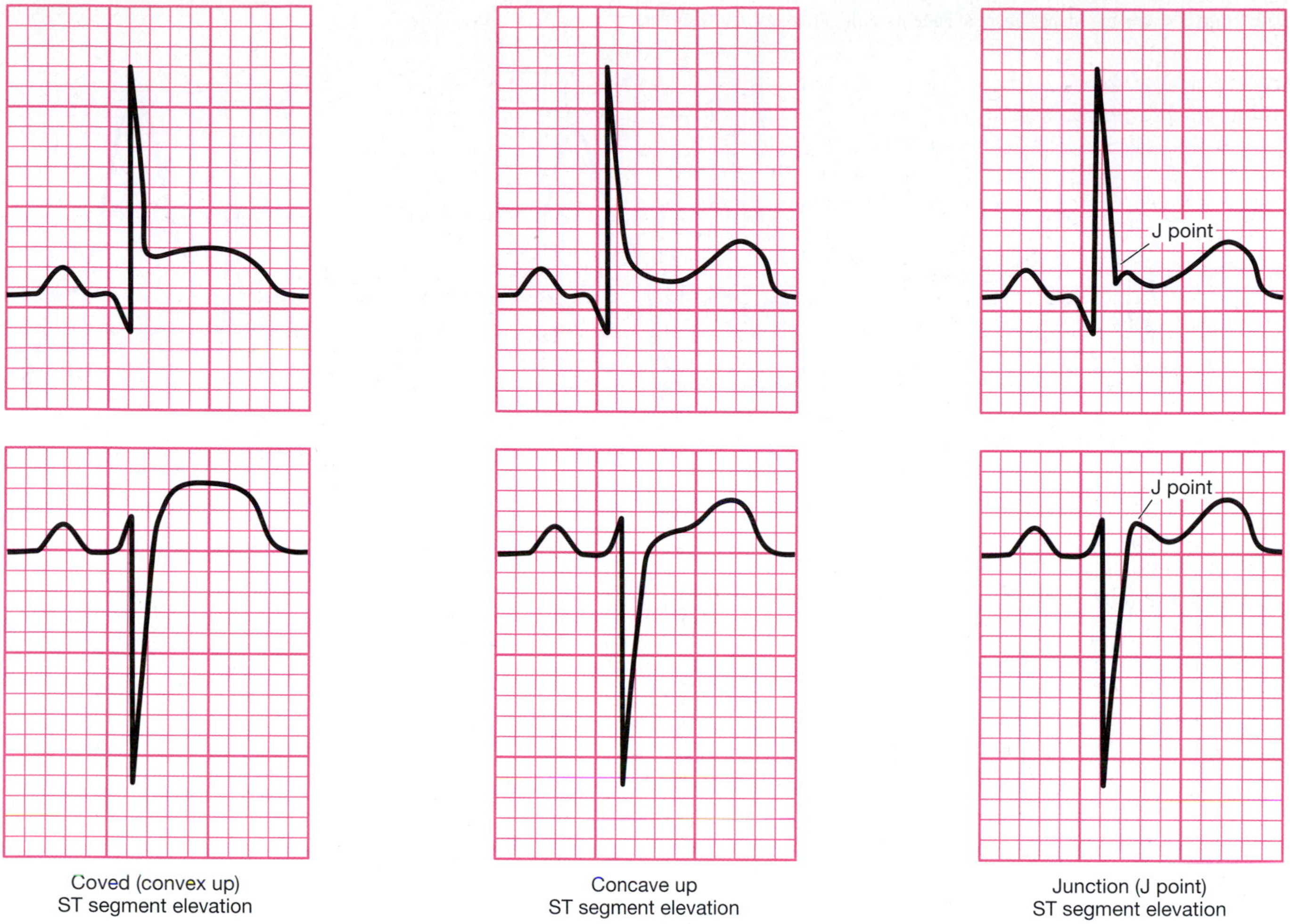

FIGURE 32–7 ◆ ST segment elevation morphology differences.

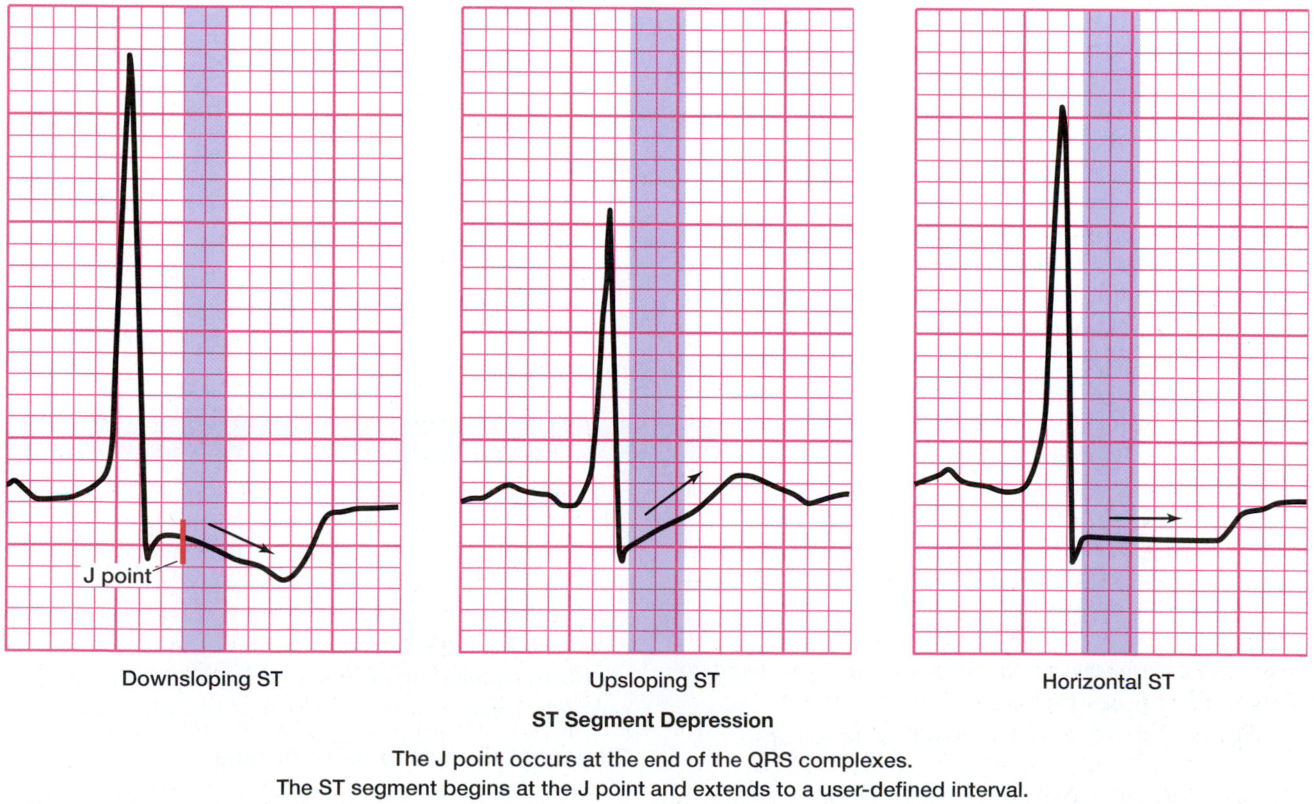

FIGURE 32–8 ◆ ST segment depression.

Video: Angina

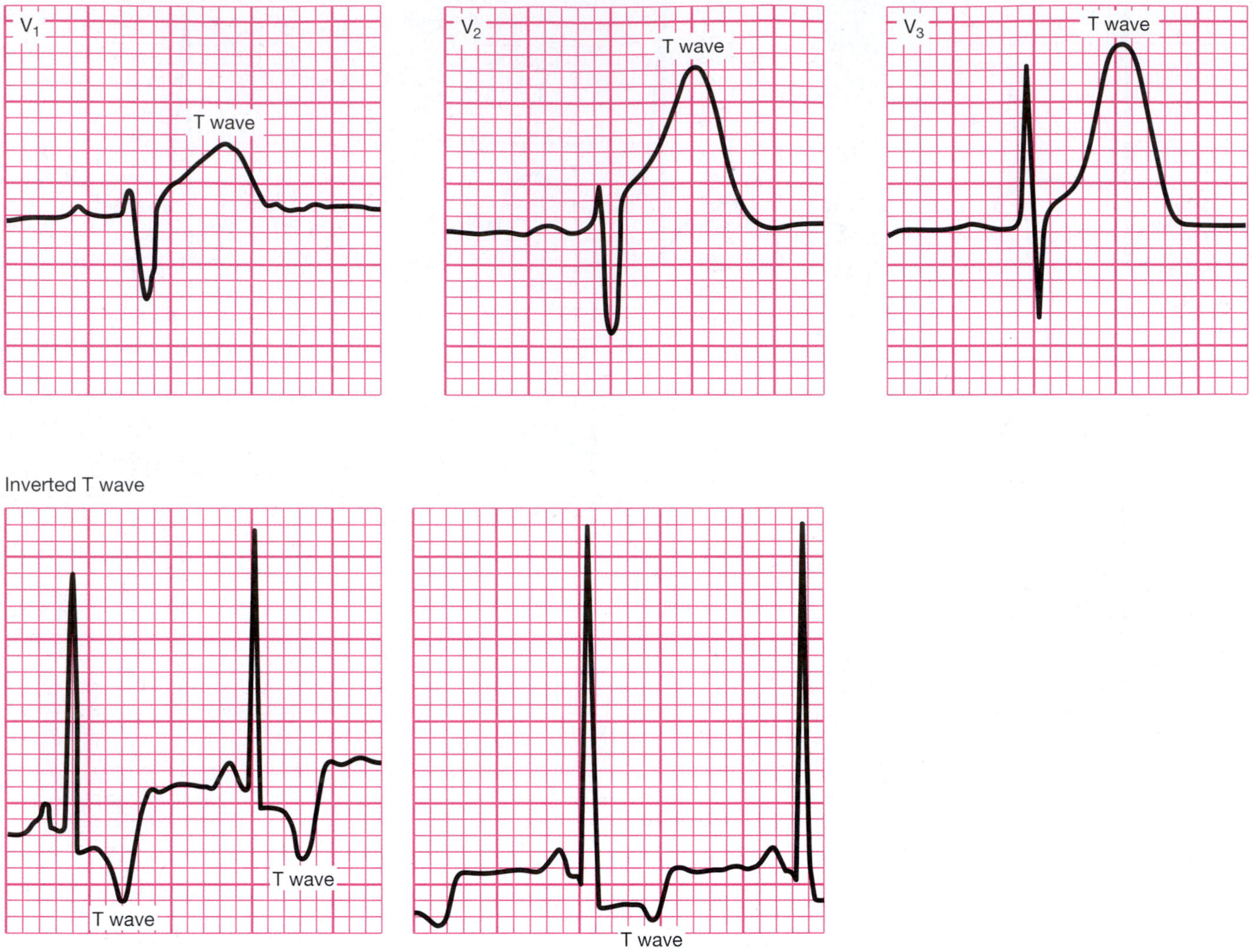

FIGURE 32–9 ◆ Abnormal hyperacute and inverted T wave.

Q Wave Changes

The Q wave is the first component of the ventricular complex, and under normal conditions it is a negatively deflected wave (below the isoelectric line). It is small in size, is less than 0.04 second in duration, and has less than 25% of the amplitude of the R wave (see Figure 32–10◆). The absence of Q waves is a normal variant of some people's ECG.

The development of an abnormal Q wave is a definitive diagnostic sign of myocardial necrosis. It appears later in time on the ECG than ischemia or injury evident by ST or T wave changes, because necrosis takes the longest to occur. During the first 24 to 48 hours after the AMI as the necrosis occurs, the Q wave becomes deeper and wider (see Figure 32–10).

Q waves will develop in the leads overlying the affected area. Abnormal Q waves are identified in three ways:

- An increase in duration of greater than 0.04 second
- Greater than 4 millimeters in depth or greater than one-fourth to one-third of the height of the R wave
- Appearance in leads where they have previously been absent.

The deep Q wave change seen on the ECG is due to necrosis, which is not reversible; therefore, Q wave changes on the ECGs are permanent, making previous MIs identifiable. The diagnosis of an "old" MI is made when there is a Q wave present in the absence of any ST segment elevation, patient symptoms, and positive blood markers. The ECG cannot determine how long ago the MI occurred.

Safety Alert *Because the dysrhythmias that accompany an MI are common and varied, it is essential that the nurse understand the impact of each on the patient's cardiac output and the necessary interventions to terminate the abnormal rhythm.*

Angina Pectoris

Angina pectoris is defined as transient chest pain due to myocardial ischemia caused by an inadequate supply of oxygen and nutrients for the myocardium. CAD is the most common cause of a decreased blood supply to the myocardium. Angina also can occur in people with normal coronary arteries without obstruction as a result of vasospasm, endothelial dysfunction, valvular heart disease, hypertrophic cardiomyopathy, uncontrolled hypertension, exacerbations of heart failure, and noncardiac conditions of the esophagus, chest wall, or lungs.

Clinical Manifestations of Angina

The clinical manifestations of angina pectoris include a sudden onset of discomfort in the chest, jaw, shoulder, back, or arm, aggravated by exertion or emotional stress and relieved with rest or nitroglycerin

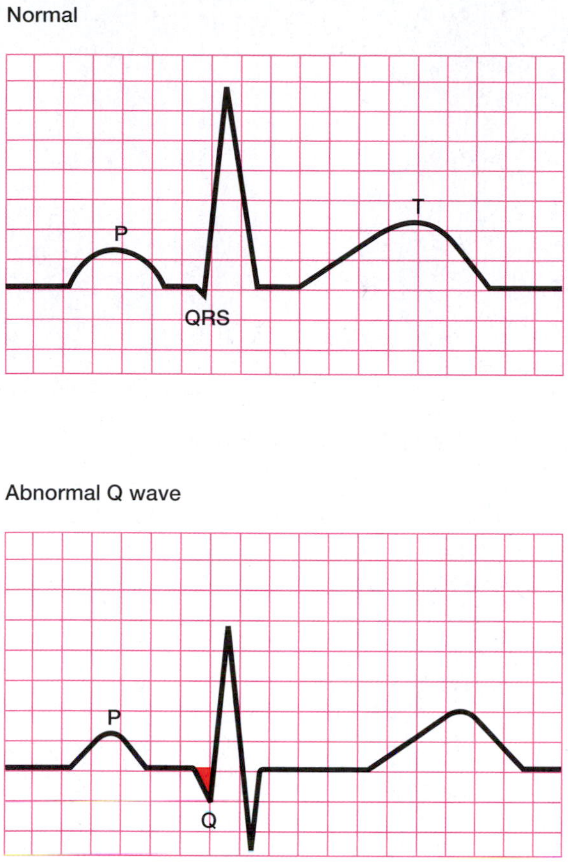

FIGURE 32–10 ◆ Normal and abnormal Q wave.

(Figure 32–11◆, p. 934). Terms such as *burning, crushing, suffocating,* and *pressure* are typical descriptors of chest pain from myocardial ischemia, often with pain radiating to other areas of the upper torso. Cardiac chest pain usually is described neither as sharp nor as localized to a defined spot.

Symptoms of chest pain alone are poor predictors of the presence of CAD and the severity of myocardial damage. In nearly one-third to one-half of individuals with myocardial ischemia, symptoms are not present at all. The clinician is faced with comparing data abstracted from the patient to a set of characteristics associated with diseases that have common presenting signs and symptoms. Charts 32–5 and 32–6 (p. 935) outline the presentation of patients with diseases that mimic chest pain associated with CAD.

Women, patients with diabetes, and older adults may not experience pain with myocardial ischemia. In addition, the way in which women characterize pain may be different from that of men; women tend to express pain in less severe terms, if at all, and often ascribe the pain to causes other than cardiac issues.

Types of Angina Pectoris

There are several accepted classifications for angina pectoris that are based on what triggers the occurrence, how long it lasts, when it occurs, what makes it go away, and its seriousness. Angina is classified as either typical or atypical, depending on signs and symptoms and/or by its severity. It also is assigned various terms that describe its timing, location, and position. Chart 32–7 outlines the classifications and descriptors of angina.

Two general categories or classifications are stable angina and unstable angina. **Stable angina,** the less serious type, is triggered by a predictable degree of exertion or emotions, and there is a pattern in what brings it on, its duration, its intensity of symptoms, and how to relieve it. Stable angina subsides by taking away the precipitating factors and using sublingual nitroglycerin. This condition is differentiated from unstable angina (UA) pathologically by the absence of plaque disruption and thrombus formation in the lumen of the artery. Unstable angina is discussed in the section of the chapter on acute coronary syndrome.

Variant, Prinzmetal, or vasospastic angina occurs when single or multiple sites in major coronary arteries and their large branches experience vasospasm. Most often, the right coronary artery is involved. Sites of vasospasm generally occur over eccentric lesions. Causes of vasospasm are unknown but may be related to an imbalance of vasoactive agents derived from damaged coronary endothelial tissue, vessel segment hypersensitivity to sympathetic stimulation, allergy, or hypomagnesemia. Symptoms are usually episodic, may last several minutes, are often associated with exercise, and can occur frequently at night.

Medical Management of Angina Pectoris

The majority of patients with stable angina achieve symptom control by medical management alone. When patients with symptoms of angina present to a clinician's office or an emergency department, they must be taken seriously and evaluated thoroughly by the health care team. Routine evaluations of patients who complain of chest pain include a review of their symptoms, their medical/social history for associated diseases and risk factors, an assessment for physical signs, and diagnostic tests. (See the Medical Management of Complications of Acute Myocardial Infarction section, p. 957.)

Predictors of higher risk for complications generally include angina that has increased in duration, in frequency, or at rest; associated ST segment or T wave changes on the ECG; and accompanying signs of heart failure such as new or worsening mitral regurgitation murmur; skin changes such as cool, pale, or clammy; pulmonary edema or presence of an S_3 or S_4 heart sound; tachycardia; and hypotension. Patients classified at lower risk are generally treated on an outpatient basis. Goals for outpatient management include treating conditions that exacerbate angina such as anemia, thyrotoxicosis, and dysrhythmias, as well as eliminating or suppressing symptoms through behavioral changes and prescribing antianginal agents.

Pharmacologic management for angina rests primarily on three classes of drugs: calcium-channel blockers, nitrates, and beta-adrenergic blocking agents. Symptom characteristics, exercise tolerance, and comorbid conditions dictate which antianginal agent to use. To date, no one drug category has proven more effective at improving the prognosis for patients treated for angina pectoris. Antianginal medications are outlined in the Pharmacology box (p. 955). In addition to antianginal agents, daily ASA is recommended.

Activity restriction and removing the precipitating factors also will help relieve angina because these methods decrease the oxygen demand on the heart. Supplemental oxygen is frequently ordered during periods of pain.

Nursing Management

Nursing management of a patient who is experiencing angina requires critical thinking and decision-making skills. Angina pectoris is a warning that the myocardium is not getting enough oxygen, and increased perfusion of oxygen and nutrients is needed to prevent permanent myocardial muscle damage.

Video: Angina

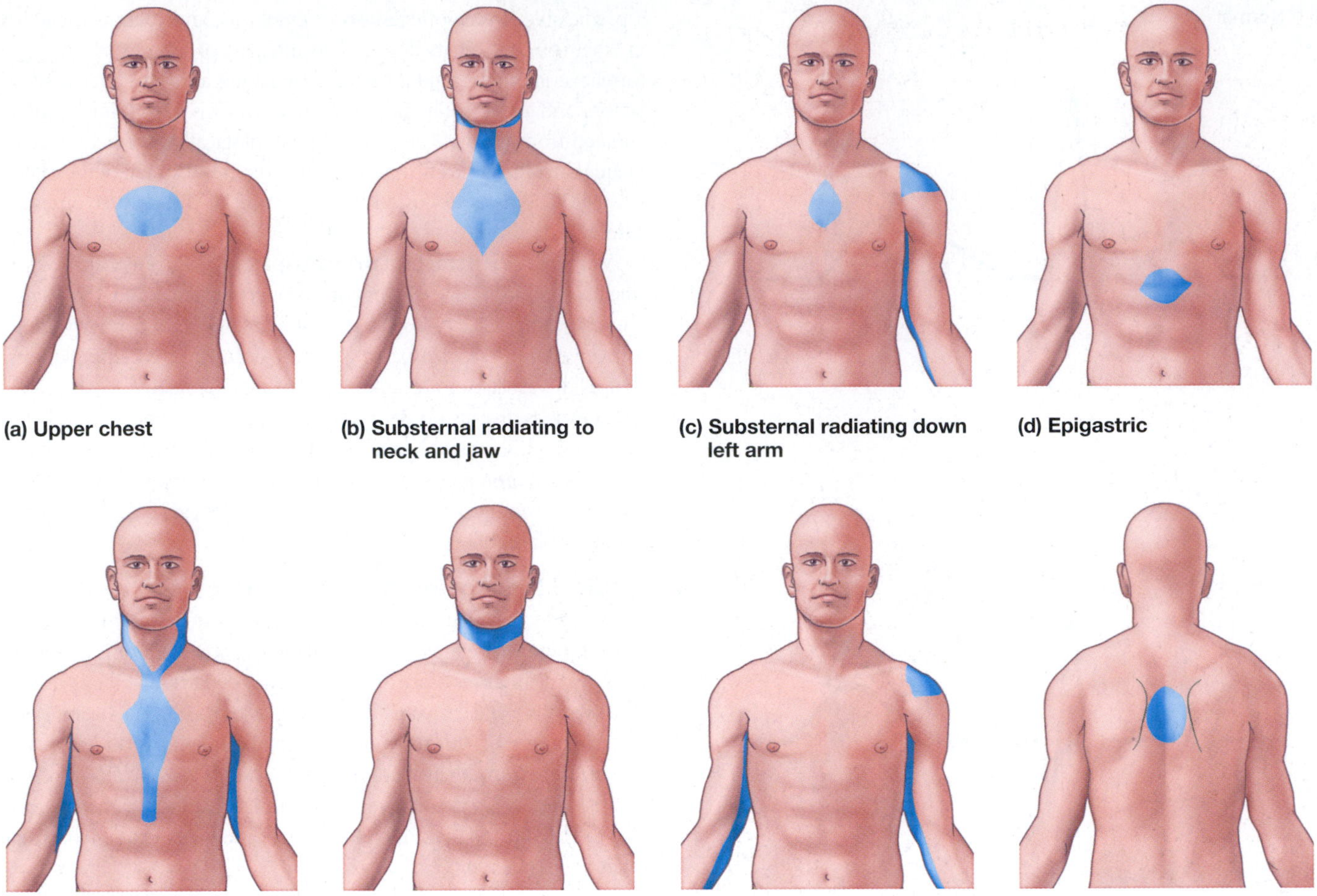

(a) Upper chest (b) Substernal radiating to neck and jaw (c) Substernal radiating down left arm (d) Epigastric

(e) Epigastric radiating to neck, jaw, and arms (f) Neck and jaw (g) Left shoulder and down both arms (h) Intrascapular

FIGURE 32–11 ◆ Location of anginal pain.

Assessment

The patient needs an in-depth nursing assessment of the pain, including the type of sensation, the location and transmission, the duration, what brings it on, and what makes it go away. The nurse must inquire whether this is new onset pain or whether there is a history of anginal chest pain. If this pain has occurred before, is there a change in the pattern or intensity? For example, stable angina is predictable in what causes it, what makes it go away, and its intensity, whereas unstable angina is more intense and less predictable in its pattern. The subjective and objective findings during an anginal attack may include tachycardia, increased or decreased blood pressure, cardiac dysrhythmias, apprehension/anxiety, diaphoresis, and pallor. The nurse must assess vital signs, the ECG monitor, and the associated clinical manifestations. Typically, the ECG is obtained during pain because the ischemic changes will resolve with treatment. It is also common to have cardiac dysrhythmias occur during angina, due to muscle irritability from the ischemia. Assessment for heart failure also is essential. Lung sounds, peripheral edema, increasing shortness of breath, and respiratory rate must be evaluated. Physical findings between periods of angina are usually normal and therefore not diagnostic.

Nursing Diagnosis

The nursing process serves as the platform to manage the patients experiencing angina pectoris.

Nursing diagnoses that pertain to the patient having angina include:

- *Pain, Acute* related to decreased blood supply
- *Anxiety* related to fear, pain, and knowledge deficit
- *Knowledge, Deficit* related to disease process
- *Tissue Perfusion, Ineffective* related to coronary artery disease

NANDA-I © 2012

Outcomes and Evaluation Parameters

The desired nursing outcome is to prevent the progression of ischemia to the myocardium, which would result in permanent cardiac muscle damage and worsening symptoms. The primary evaluation parameter is complete relief of the anginal pain, because this indicates that there is adequate blood supply to the myocardium. Associated outcome parameters include vital signs, cardiac output, activity tolerance, lungs, and mental orientation. The nurse must monitor the patient's vital signs both as the pain is beginning to subside and when it is totally relieved. The goal is for the heart rate and blood pressure to return to the patient's baseline. Normal ECG, absent or decreased dysrhythmias, and normal mentation also are outcomes that indicate an adequate blood supply to the myocardium. Absence of heart failure is an essential outcome because angina is a serious long-term complication. Finally, once the pain is relieved, the patient will verbalize less fear and anxiety.

Planning and Interventions With Rationales

Nursing interventions include administering prescribed antianginal medications. Whatever activity was occurring that precipitated the

CHART 32–5 Differential Diagnosis of Chest Pain: Common Etiologies

Pain Description	Associated Findings	History
Angina/Myocardial Infarction		

• Usually retrosternal
• Can originate or radiate at the back, anterior chest, epigastric area, jaw, shoulder, elbow, forearm, wrist
• May be relieved with rest, lasts < 30 minutes
	• Tachycardia
	• Tachypnea, dyspnea
	• Weak heart sounds
	• Rhonchi
	• Diaphoresis
	• Abnormal precordial impulses
	• Evidence of dysrhythmias
		• Cardiac risk factors
		  • Smoking
		  • Male gender
		  • African American
		  • Sedentary lifestyle
		  • Social stressors
		  • High-fat diet

• Heaviness, burning, tight pressure, aching, indigestion • Is not relieved with position change • May increase while supine • Is not aggravated by deep breathing	• Fever, elevated white blood cell (WBC) count, elevated sedimentation rate • Anxiety, sense of impending doom • Nausea/vomiting	• Cardiovascular disease • Heart failure • Dysrhythmias • PVD • Heart valve disease • Angina, unstable angina, MI cardiac interventions • Cardiac surgery • Catheter-based interventions
Pulmonary Embolism		
• Sudden onset • Sharp • Pleuritic • Lateral chest • Increases on deep inspiration	• Shock • Syncope • Dyspnea, shortness of breath (SOB), cyanosis • Tachycardia • Hemoptysis • Pleural friction rub • Expiratory wheeze • Fever	• Hypercoagulable state • Immobility • Surgery • Trauma • DVT
Gastrointestinal Disorders		
• Burning, squeezing, gripping • Retrosternal without radiation • Lasts many hours or days, constant in nature • Precipitated by bending over, drinking very hot/cold liquids, meals • Relieved with food or beverage	• Reflux • Dysphagia • Dyspepsia	• GERD • Esophageal motility disorders • Esophageal malignancy
Costochondritis		
• Usually superficial and localized • Described as tender, aching, sharp • Can be in any location • Duration variable • Aggravated/provoked by movement or touch	• Sudden movement • Tachypnea, shallow breathing • Tachycardia • Elevated blood pressure	• Falls or trauma • Immobility • Chest tubes newly removed
Acute Anxiety		
• Dull, stabbing	• Breathlessness, hyperventilation	• Acute stress, phobia • Inability to cope

Sources: Adapted from Moser, D. K., & Riegel, B. (2008). *Cardiac nursing: A companion to Braunwald's heart disease.* Philadelphia: Saunders; Woo, K., & Schneider, J. I. (2009). High-risk chief complaints I: Chest pain—The big three. *Emergency Medicine Clinics of North America, 27*(4), 685–712; Woods et al. (2010). *Cardiac nursing* (6th ed.). Philadelphia: Lippincott Williams & Wilkins.

pain must be stopped. The heart cannot meet the body's oxygen needs, and stopping the activity will decrease the need. The nurse may administer supplemental oxygen, according to health care provider orders, and observe vital signs and oxygen saturation levels. The nurse also assesses the effectiveness of these interventions continuously until the patient is pain free and the heart rate and blood pressure are within the normal range. If this is not achieved, it may indicate that there is a more serious problem; if so, the nurse must notify the health care provider to order further interventions and testing.

CHART 32–6 Differential Diagnosis of Chest Pain: Less Common Etiologies

Pain Description	Associated Findings	History
Pericarditis		
• Sudden, sharp • Dull, aching • Stabbing, knife-like • Retrosternal or precordial • Can radiate to neck, left shoulder and arm, back, epigastrium • Aggravated by deep inspiration, cough, rotation of the chest • Alleviated by sitting up and forward	• Pulsus paradoxus • Dyspnea • Low-grade erratic fever • Pericardial friction rub • Elevated neck veins • Tachycardia • Hiccups • Nausea/vomiting • Dizziness • Generalized malaise • Hoarseness • Abdominal pain	• AMI • Dressler's syndrome • Tamponade • Pericardial effusion • Constrictive pericarditis • Myocardial/pericardial injury • Connective tissue disease • Infection • Radiation therapy • Neoplasm
Dissecting Aortic Aneurysm		
• Acute sharp onset without warning • Tearing, ripping • In sync with heartbeat • Lasts for hours or days • Upper back, anterior chest, epigastric, shoulders, retrosternal • Radiates to hips, groin, lower extremity, neck, shoulders, costovertebral area, epigastric area, jaw • Settles in lower back	• Syncope • Diaphoresis • Tachycardia • Hyper/hypotension • Confusion • Fever • Blood pressure different in each arm • Absent or diminished pulses uni-/bilateral • Decreased level of consciousness • Melena, hematemesis, nausea, vomiting	• Hypertension • Congenital heart defects • Syphilitic aortitis • Blunt trauma • Males > 50 to 70 years • Third trimester of pregnancy
Spontaneous Pneumothorax		
• Sudden • Severe • Over lateral thorax	• Dyspnea • Tachycardia • Blood pressure difference in each arm • Hyperresonance and decreased breath sounds • Tracheal deviation toward affected side • Decreased respiratory excursion • Bulging intercostal muscles	• Severe underlying lung disease • Necrotizing pneumonia • ARDS • High airway pressures while on mechanical ventilation • Common ages 16 to 25 years • COPD • Cystic fibrosis • Blebs
Cholecystitis		
• Severe abdominal pain • Epigastric area • Tenderness in abdomen, right upper quadrant • May radiate to back and scapula	• Nausea/vomiting • Fever • Jaundice • Changes in bowel habit • Intolerance to fatty foods	
Pancreatitis		
• Extreme epigastric pain, alternating with dull aching sensation • Radiates to back, flank	• Hypotension • Fever • Change in bowel habit • Weight loss, malnutrition	

Sources: Adapted from Moser, D. K., & Riegel, B. (2008). *Cardiac nursing: A companion to Braunwald's heart disease.* Philadelphia: Saunders; Woo, K., & Schneider, J. I. (2009). High-risk chief complaints I: Chest pain—The big three. *Emergency Medicine Clinics of North America, 27*(4), 685–712; Woods et al. (2010). *Cardiac nursing* (6th ed.). Philadelphia: Lippincott Williams & Wilkins.

CHART 32–7 Angina Classifications and Descriptors

Term	Descriptor(s)/Definitions
Typical angina, three key characteristics	1. Central/substernal chest or left arm pain, discomfort, pressure, tightness, heaviness 2. Provoked by exertion or emotional stress 3. Relieved by nitroglycerin.
Atypical angina or ischemic equivalents, any two of the characteristics for typical angina	1. Jaw, neck, ear, arm, back 2. Weakness, dizziness, light-headedness, loss of consciousness, unexplained fatigue, diaphoresis 3. New or worsening dyspnea on exertion 4. Nausea/vomiting, unexplained indigestion, belching, epigastric pain or discomfort 5. Burning, aching, cramping.
Nocturnal angina	Occurs at night, usually during sleep. May be relieved by sitting upright. Commonly associated with left ventricular dysfunction.
Decubitus angina	Angina while lying down.
Preinfarction, postinfarction angina	Prior to or after infarction. Preinfarction angina may precondition the heart for episodes of subsequent infarction, resulting in a reduction in infarct size. Postinfarction angina denotes increased risk for death or recurrent MI.
Recurring/stuttering angina	Angina that comes and goes. Denotes instability, thrombus formation, and dissolution.

Sources: Adapted from Moser, D. K., & Riegel, B. (2008). *Cardiac nursing: A companion to Braunwald's heart disease.* St. Louis: Saunders. Woods et al. (2010). *Cardiac nursing* (6th ed.). Philadelphia: Lippincott Williams & Wilkins.

Safety Alert *The nurse must stay with the patient who is experiencing angina and continue an ongoing assessment until the pain is gone or until the nurse determines that the interventions are not effective and the health care provider needs to be notified.*

Health Promotion

Because angina pectoris is an indicator of decreased cardiac reserve, it is imperative that a comprehensive education program be initiated when the symptoms first occur. The best prevention program would be instituted before the clinical manifestations, but often the patient is not seen prior to admittance to an ED. The nurse is in an ideal position to begin education about lifestyle changes that will reduce or prevent progression of the disease. The education needs to include risk factor management (see the Risk Factors box, p. 925), medication instructions, and avoidance of precipitating factors. The nurse must assess the patient and family's ability to understand and be receptive to education. There may be language or cultural barriers, and/or the anxiety level may interfere with the patient's or family's ability to absorb the information. It is imperative that the teaching plan includes a review of medication regimens, side effects, symptoms of ischemia, and teaching about self-treatment and handling potentially emergent situations. Patients who receive beta-adrenergic blocking agents and calcium-channel blockers need to be taught how to count their pulse and what rate must be reported to the health care provider. If patients are taking nitrates, they should be taught about safe storage, handling, and side effects of different nitrate preparations, as well as how to take sublingual nitrates (see the Pharmacology box, p. 955). Patients must also receive coaching on their adaptation to and compliance with risk factor modification activities and be encouraged to seek assistance if therapy becomes a financial burden or creates conflicts within their support group. Families or significant others may need teaching about how to cope or help the patient deal with lifestyle and behavioral changes, or they may benefit from referral to community services to learn bystander cardiopulmonary resuscitation. The Evidence-Based Practice feature details some of the gender issues associated with CAD.

Evaluation of Coronary Artery Disease

Many types of stress testing are available to evaluate patients for CAD. Some require the patient to walk and/or run on a treadmill to increase the heart rate, and/or some require pharmacological stimulation (using adenosine, dipyridamole, or dobutamine) to increase the heart rate (Moser & Riegel, 2008). Some tests measure electrocardiographic changes only, while others use ultrasound or nuclear scanning to assess the heart's response to the elevated heart rate. Each of the tests will be discussed in the following text. See Chart 32–8 for indications and contraindications to stress testing.

Stress Testing

Treadmill or bicycle electrocardiogram testing is a commonly performed stress test that is often done in the outpatient setting. Patients exercise to increase their heart rate to a predetermined maximum predicted heart rate. Indications and contraindications for stress testing are outlined on Chart 32–8.

Radionuclide Imaging

Nuclear clinical cardiology techniques are used to establish the diagnosis, assess the severity of disease, calculate risk assessment, and evaluate outcomes of therapy in patients with acute and chronic coronary syndromes and heart failure (Kee, 2010). Exercise **myocardial perfusion imaging (MPI)** is the most common application of nuclear imaging techniques. In patients who do not have a normal baseline ECG or who for other reasons such as physical limitations are not suitable candidates for a standard exercise test, imaging techniques combined with a basic stress test improve the ability to detect significant CAD. In addition, imaging provides information regarding the location of ischemic myocardium, as well as an estimation of the amount of myocardium at risk. MPI is most useful in patients who have an intermediate risk of CAD.

During MPI a radioactive tracer is administered intravenously and given time to circulate in the bloodstream. The most commonly used radioisotopes are technetium-99m sestamibi and thallium-201.

EVIDENCE-BASED PRACTICE Gender Considerations in Coronary Artery Disease

Clinical Problem

Takotsubo cardiomyopathy (TC) is an unusual and infrequently seen disorder that mimics an acute MI (AMI). This disorder predominantly affects women. First described in 1990 by Japanese health care providers, it was named after the *takotsubo*, a fishing pot used to capture octopus, because the ballooning of the left ventricle that occurs with this disorder looks similar to the shape of the pot.

Takotsubo cardiomyopathy is characterized by the sudden onset of chest pain and/or shortness of breath and has accompanying ST-T wave changes on the electrocardiogram and moderately elevated troponin and CPK levels. Upon cardiac catheterization, little to no underlying CAD is found. More that 80% of the time, it is associated with stress of some type. Therefore, it is also referred to as *stress-induced cardiomyopathy* or *broken-heart cardiomyopathy*. Many potential triggers have been identified in the literature, including the following:

- Receiving notification of unexpected loss of spouse or child
- Witnessing or being in an accident
- Being the victim of a violent crime
- Fierce arguments
- Loss of large amounts of money/life savings
- Loss of employment
- Earthquakes, getting struck by lightning.

Takotsubo cardiomyopathy has also been noted to develop in association with other medical–surgical conditions such as acute pneumothorax, sepsis, severe hypoglycemia, seizures, and anesthesia/surgical procedures such as eye surgery, hip surgery, and cardiac surgery.

Takotsubo cardiomyopathy is 9 times more likely to occur in females than in males, and it is much more common in postmenopausal women (90% of all reported cases). Signs and symptoms mimic those of ACS, and about 20% of the patients may present to the hospital with severe heart failure due to marked left ventricular dysfunction. This ventricular dysfunction is reversible within 7 to 30 days. The long-term prognosis is good.

Research Findings

Since the first reports of TC in 1990, thousands of cases have been reported from all around the world. The exact mechanism of the disorder is unknown. The most widely accepted current theory for its onset is a neurohormonal cause leading to activation of the sympathetic nervous system. Many clinical studies have found that patients with TC have markedly elevated levels of catecholamines, such as epinephrine and norepinephrine, when compared to patients with AMI.

Implications for Nursing Practice

While TC accounts for fewer than 2% of patients who present to the emergency department with signs and symptoms of AMI, the initial medical treatment is different. Thrombolysis or percutaneous coronary intervention is the standard of care for AMI, especially ST segment elevation myocardial infarction. Patients with TC do not require either of those treatments. Early identification of the role of stress in the development of cardiac signs and symptoms may prevent a patient from unnecessarily receiving thrombolysis.

Patients with TC require regular nursing assessment of their cardiovascular system and monitoring for potential complications such as dysrhythmias and heart failure due to the left ventricular dysfunction. Dysrhythmias associated with TC include ventricular tachycardia, ventricular fibrillation, and AV nodal blocks. Prolonged QT intervals are also common, making these patients more susceptible to developing Torsades de pointes (Chapter 30). Because of heart failure, treatment with diuretics, beta-blockers, and/or ACE inhibitors may be indicated until the ventricle returns to normal. Some patients may initially have significant left ventricular dysfunction and require short-term support with intravenous inotropes and/or an intra-aortic balloon pump. Heart failure is discussed in detail in Chapter 34.

The need for patient and family counseling about TC and how it differs from AMI is important. Patients need to understand that this is a reversible disorder and that they will feel better within a short period of time. Recurrences of TC have been reported. It is important for these patients to better understand the impact of stress and how they manage stress in their lives.

Critical Thinking Questions with answers can be found in the Osborn Student Resources at nursing.pearsonhighered.com.

Sources: Adapted from Lindsay, J., Paixao, A., Chao, T., & Pichard, A. D. (2010). Pathogenesis of the takotsubo syndrome: A unifying hypothesis. *American Journal of Cardiology, 106*, 1360–1363; McCulloch, B. J. (2007). Transient left ventricular apical ballooning. *Critical Care Nurse, 27*(6), 20–28.

A gamma camera is placed over the precordium to record the amount of radioactive tracer emissions. Areas of the myocardium with normal coronary blood flow (normal perfusion) will absorb relatively large amounts of the tracer, whereas areas with compromised blood flow will absorb less. Because most significant coronary plaques are associated with normal blood flow at rest, it is necessary to image the heart during a period of maximal exercise. A perfusion defect that is imaged only during exercise, termed a *reversible defect*, denotes an area of viable (functioning) but ischemic myocardium. If a defect is present during both exercise and rest, it is termed a fixed defect and probably indicates an area of infarction (defect is not reversible). If the patient is unable to exercise to maximum capacity, pharmacologic agents such as dipyridamole or adenosine can be used to invoke a physiological response in coronary blood flow similar to that evoked by physical exercise. The results obtained with these methods appear to be as accurate as the results obtained with traditional stress tests (Moser & Riegel, 2008).

Exercise Thallium Perfusion Test

This test uses the radioisotope thallium 201 to assess myocardial perfusion during exercise. Thallium accumulates in the myocardial cells; when there is less blood flow to the myocardium, then less thallium accumulation is seen. This testing is useful in determining myocardial viability. This test is commonly performed in two phases: resting and stress. Many patients may benefit from having nuclear scanning (gated single-photon emission computed tomography [SPECT]) completed to assess for CAD.

Nuclear Persantine (Dipyridamole) Stress Test

This test is an alternative for patients who are unable to walk on a treadmill. Persantine is administered intravenously while nuclear scanning is done. Persantine dilates the coronary arteries and increases blood flow to the myocardium. The nuclear scanning is done with thallium or cardiolite as the isotope. Alternatively, adenosine can be administered to dilate the coronary arteries and increase myocardial blood flow (Moser & Riegel, 2008).

Nuclear Dobutamine Stress Test

This test is another alternative for patients who are unable to exercise. Dobutamine, a sympathomimetic drug, is given intravenously to increase heart rate, myocardial contractility, and blood pressure. The nuclear scanning is done with thallium or cardiolite as the isotope.

Electron Beam Computed Tomography

Electron beam computed tomography (EBCT) is a noninvasive test that quantifies CAD by identifying calcium inside the coronary arteries. Calcium deposits inside coronary arteries are part of the

CHART 32–8 Indications and Contraindications for Stress/Exercise Testing

Indications

1. To evaluate for CAD
2. To evaluate cardiac perfusion
3. To determine if ischemia is reversible
4. To assess for cardiac rehabilitation
5. To assess a patient's functional capacity
6. To evaluate efficacy of therapy

Contraindications

1. Myocardial infarction within 2 days
2. Unstable angina
3. Aortic stenosis
4. Uncontrolled dysrhythmias
5. Symptomatic heart failure
6. Active endocarditis
7. Uncontrolled hypertension
8. Any acute disorder that may affect exercise (infection, renal failure)
9. Inability to obtain informed consent

Source: Adapted from: Kee, J. L. (2010). *Laboratory and diagnostic tests with nursing implications.* Upper Saddle River NJ: Pearson.

development of atherosclerosis; these deposits are not found in normal coronary arteries. Thus, the ability to quantify the amount of intracoronary artery calcium may identify asymptomatic individuals at risk for coronary events.

The amount of calcium identified by EBCT is usually reported as a total calcium score. A calcium score of zero is normal. There is no currently accepted standard for a high score, but values over 100 are usually considered to indicate high risk for the presence of CAD. The higher the calcium score, the greater the extent of atherosclerosis. EBCT does not predict the need for percutaneous coronary intervention or coronary artery bypass surgery (Moser & Riegel, 2008).

Positron-Emission Tomography

Positron-emission tomography (PET) utilizes tracers that emit positrons (positively charged particles). The main advantage of PET scanning is the ability to label and image biologically active compounds such as glucose or drugs, which allows quantification of metabolic processes. PET scan is the current gold standard for assessment of myocardial viability.

Multislice Helical Computed Tomography

More recently, **multislice helical CT** has emerged as an exceptionally promising tool for visualization of general cardiac structures, the great vessels, and especially the coronary arteries (Figure 32–12◆). It is possible to scan the entire volume of the heart, the proximal great vessels, and the coronary arteries with a single 25-second breath hold (Figure 32–13◆). The spatial resolution of multislice helical CT is much higher than that of EBCT, allowing visualization of fine details of the coronary anatomy (Figure 32–14◆), such as small side branches and atherosclerotic plaques, including "noncalcified" plaques. In addition, multislice helical CT can also detect coronary calcification using a noncontrast, low-radiation-dose scan.

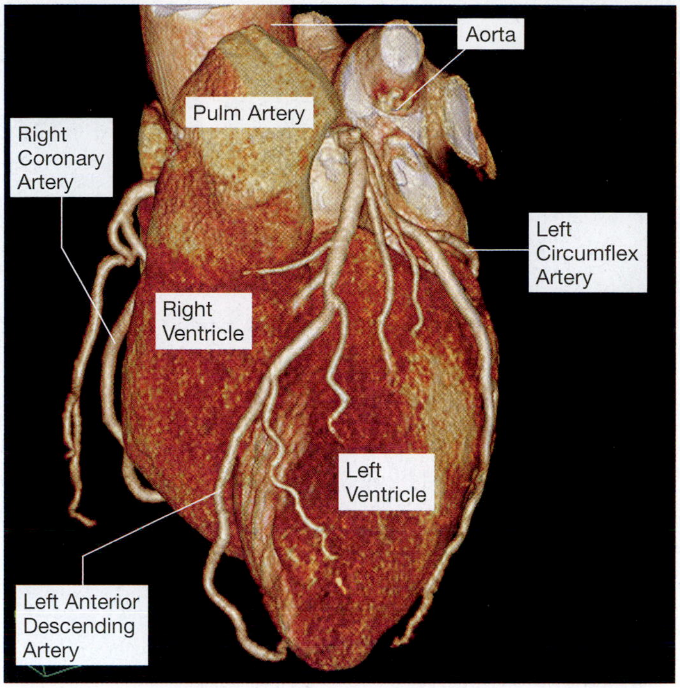

FIGURE 32–12 ◆ Multislice helical computed tomography (CT) image of the heart.

Source: Courtesy of Dr. Guy Weingold, Director of Cardiac CT, Washington Hospital Center, Washington, DC.

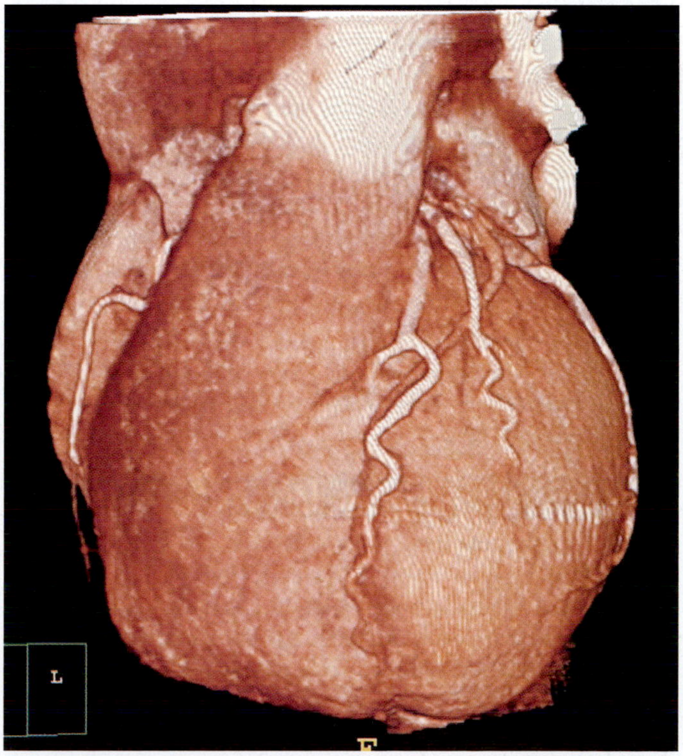

FIGURE 32–13 ◆ Multislice helical computed tomography (CT) image of the heart.

Source: Courtesy of Dr. Guy Weingold, Director of Cardiac CT, Washington Hospital Center, Washington, DC.

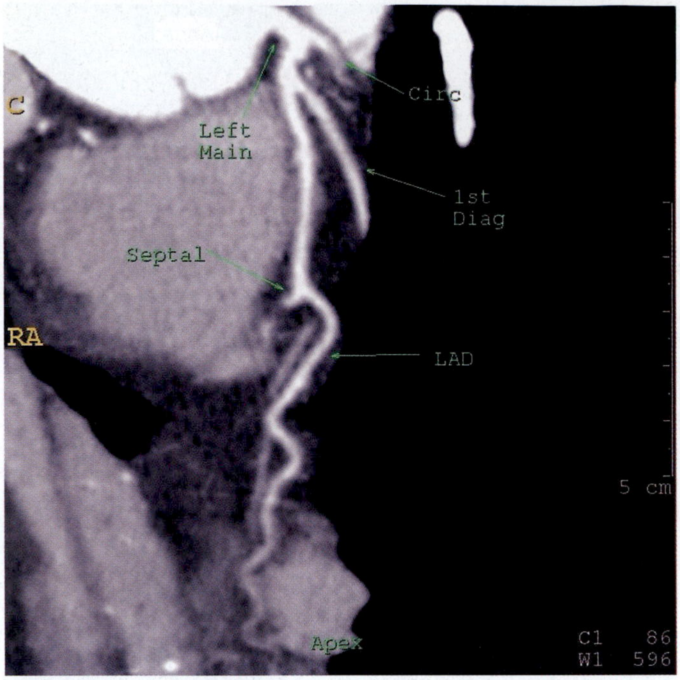

FIGURE 32–14 ◆ Multislice helical computed tomography (CT) image of coronary arteries.

Source: Courtesy of Dr. Guy Weingold, Director of Cardiac CT, Washington Hospital Center, Washington, DC.

The real advantage of multislice helical CT is its ability to visualize the lumen of the coronary artery with high detail, allowing the interpreter to measure the degree of luminal stenosis, something that EBCT cannot do.

Multi-Gated Acquisition Scan

Multi-gated acquisition (MUGA) scanning is a useful noninvasive tool for assessing the function of the heart, using a radioactive tracer. The moving images of the beating heart that can be obtained provide important information about the heart size, ventricular wall motion, and ejection fraction (Kee, 2010). If muscle damage has occurred, as with a myocardial infarction, the MUGA scan can localize the portion of the heart muscle that has sustained damage and can assess the degree of damage. But more important, the MUGA scan is able to measure the ejection fraction of the cardiac ventricles. The left ventricular ejection fraction (LVEF), which is the proportion of blood that is expelled from the ventricle with each heartbeat, is a commonly used measure of overall cardiac function.

Cardiac Magnetic Resonance Imaging

Magnetic resonance imaging (MRI) uses radiofrequency pulses from a large, powerful magnet to disrupt the normal spin of certain atoms within the body temporarily. MRI can be used to evaluate patients with presumed congenital heart diseases, such as coarctation of the aorta or atrial septal defects. It also is used to image heart structures such as the valves and the pericardium and to enable assessment of **myocardial viability.** This provides information about areas of the myocardium that appear to have normal functioning as well as areas that appear to be dysfunctional and may improve with revascularization (viable myocardium).

Introduced in the late 1970s, the term *hibernating myocardium* defines areas of the heart that initially appear dysfunctional but after restoration of blood flow (revascularization) are noted to have improved contractility. Similar improvements in function are noted in patients who have undergone successful thrombolytic therapy (p. 954). These areas are referred to as "stunned" myocardium because the contractile function of the heart is temporarily impaired by the sudden occlusion of the coronary artery during a myocardial infarction. The MRI is capable of identifying these areas of the heart.

Intravascular Ultrasound

Coronary angiography provides only a two-dimensional image of the coronary artery lumen and provides no information regarding the arterial wall. In contrast, ultrasound can be used to provide 360-degree cross-sectional images of the artery. The coronary lumen and the intima, media, and adventitia of the vessel wall can be assessed. Intravascular ultrasound is used as an adjunct in PCI to detect vessel wall pathology, to help determine the choice of PCI, and to evaluate the results of the intervention, especially intracoronary stenting. IVUS is safe, rapid, and reproducible (i.e., results are consistent when performed by different clinicians).

Cardiac Catheterization and Percutaneous Coronary Intervention

Cardiac catheterization, which includes right and left heart catheterization and coronary angiography, is a commonly performed procedure that is done in a special laboratory using x-ray. A catheter is inserted through a sheath and advanced into the left and/or right side of the heart to provide anatomic and hemodynamic information about the heart and great vessels. Cardiac catheterization provides information about:

- Hemodynamic pressures, which are used to evaluate cardiac and pulmonary function
- Heart chambers and the great vessels, which help determine structural abnormalities
- Pressure gradients across valves, which are used to evaluate the extent of stenosis or regurgitation
- The patency of coronary arteries, which is used to evaluate the extent of coronary artery disease.

Charts 32–9 and 32–10 outline the indications and relative contraindications for cardiac catheterization.

CHART 32–9 Indications for Cardiac Catheterization

- Identify coronary artery disease and assess its extent and severity.
- Determine the treatment strategy in patients with ACS.
- Assess the consequences of coronary artery disease (CAD):
  - Ischemic mitral regurgitation
  - Left ventricular dysfunction
  - Ventricular aneurysm.
- In patients with known CAD:
  - Correlate symptoms with extent of CAD.
  - Evaluate response to acute pharmacologic intervention.
  - Assess left ventricular dysfunction in cardiomyopathy.
- Evaluate and determine the treatment strategy in patients with congenital heart disease.
- Obtain hemodynamic information such as shunt size or pulmonary vascular resistance.

Right Heart Catheterization

To access the right side of the heart, a catheter is advanced through a major vein into the right heart (Figure 32–15A◆). Right heart catheterization allows for measurement and analysis of right heart pressures and oxygen saturations, measurement and analysis of pulmonary artery pressures including pulmonary capillary wedge pressures, screening for intracardiac shunts, and temporary ventricular pacing (Woods et al., 2010). Cardiac shunts, which are defects in which there is abnormal

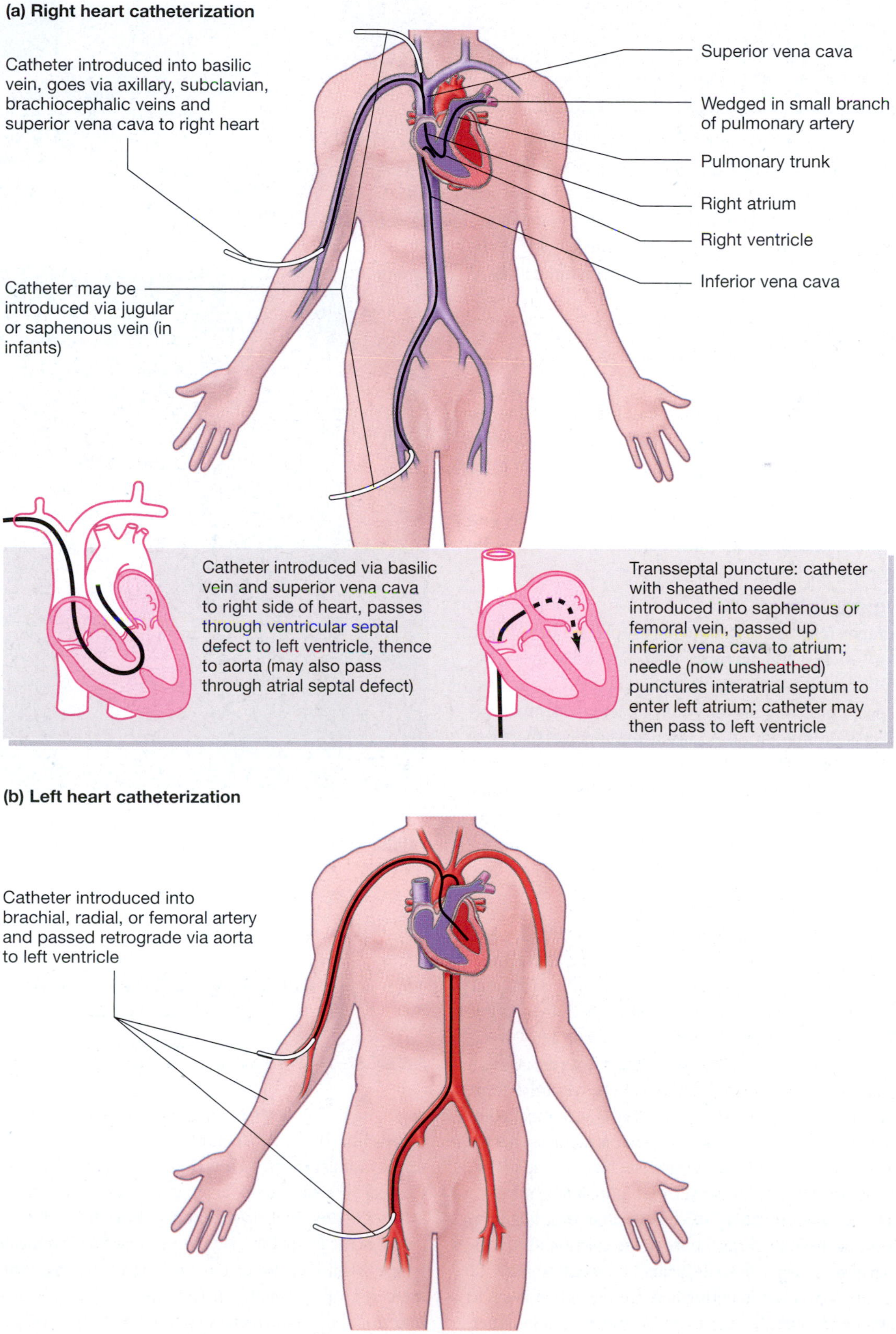

FIGURE 32–15 ◆ Heart catheterization. (A) Right catheterization and (B) left catheterization.

Source: All catheterization images courtesy of Boston Scientific.

CHART 32–10 Relative Contraindications for Cardiac Catheterization

- Severe congestive heart failure
- Severe electrolyte abnormalities
- Bleeding diathesis
- Serum creatinine ≥ 1.5 mg/dL
- Poor patient cooperation.

blood flow through an opening in the atrial or ventricular septum, can be detected by measuring oxygen saturation levels in the right heart. Clinically significant (needing closure) left ventricle-to-right ventricle shunts will be evident by a notable increase in the oxygen saturation levels in the right heart, as oxygenated blood from the left side of the heart crosses through the shunt and mixes with the desaturated blood in the right side.

Left Heart Catheterization

Left heart catheterization is usually performed by accessing the femoral artery, although the radial approach is gaining in popularity. The catheters are passed retrograde (in the direction opposite to blood flow) up the aorta to the openings of the coronary arteries, or they cross the aortic valve to enter the left ventricle (see Figure 32–15B). Left heart catheterization allows for the direct measurement of left heart pressures and pressures on both sides of the aortic valve, ventriculography to measure cardiac output, and evaluation of left ventricular function as well as the severity of any mitral or aortic valvular disease.

Coronary Angiography

Coronary angiography refers specifically to the use of contrast media to image the coronary arteries. It remains the gold standard to detect significant CAD. Both the left and the right coronary arteries are imaged, as well as any surgically placed saphenous vein or internal mammary artery grafts. Where plaque buildup has occurred, the lumen of the artery appears narrowed on the angiogram (Figure 32–16◆). In addition to evaluating the extent of CAD, angiography is used to define therapeutic options for treating CAD and to evaluate serial changes in the coronary artery lumen after revascularization or acute pharmacologic therapy (Woods et al., 2010).

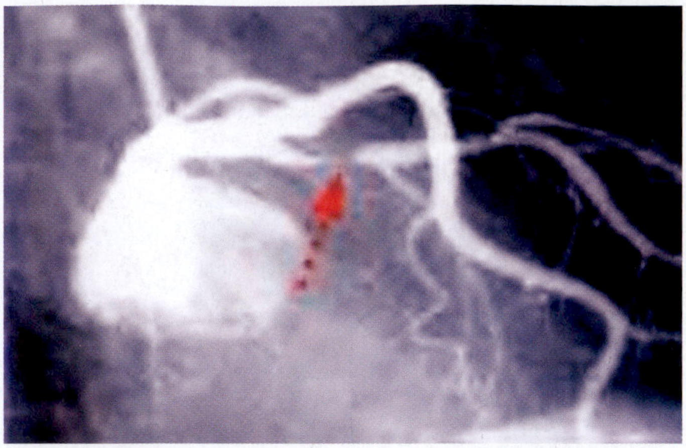

(A)

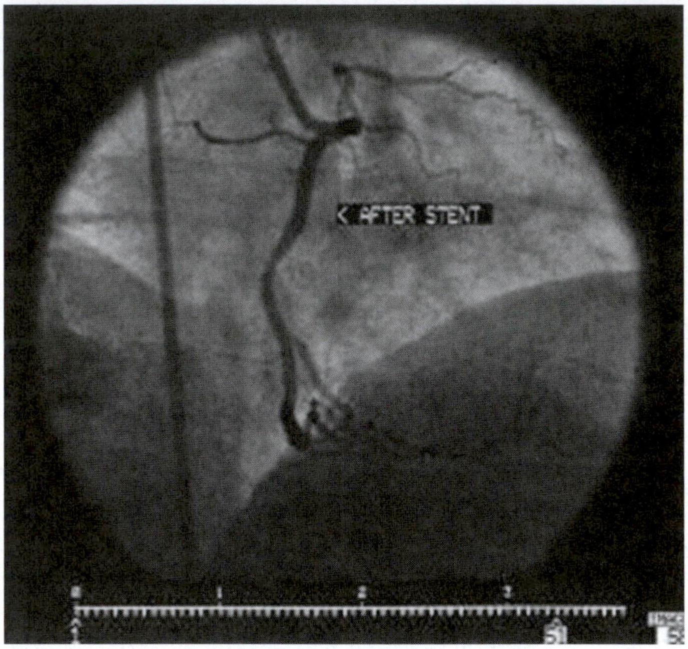

(B)

FIGURE 32–16 ◆ Coronary artery with contrast media: (A) before stent placement and (B) after stent placement.

Source: Courtesy of Dr. Walt Marquardt, Mercy Hospital

Percutaneous Coronary Intervention

Percutaneous coronary intervention (PCI) is a term that encompasses various catheter-based interventions available for the treatment of CAD. Balloon angioplasty uses expandable balloons to crack (tear or rupture) atherosclerotic plaque, enlarging the lumen of the artery (Figure 32–17◆). Other options include intracoronary lasers, which can be used to open totally occluded coronary arteries; atherectomy devices, which shave plaque and remove it; and thrombectomy devices, which extract clots. Coronary artery **stents,** the most commonly used PCI technique, are metallic mesh-like structures that are inserted permanently inside the coronary artery, compressing plaque and providing structural support of the vessel (Figure 32–18◆).

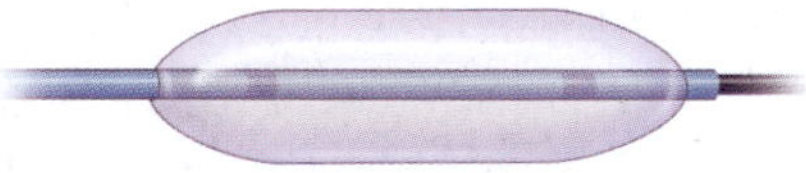

FIGURE 32–17 ◆ Balloon-tipped catheter for PCI.

PCI is indicated in a wide variety of clinical situations. Eligibility for PCI depends on the patient's clinical history, the extent of CAD, the presence of comorbidities, the left ventricular (LV) function, and the institution where the procedure is performed. Comorbidities such as diabetes, hyperlipidemia, renal failure, poor LV function, and hypertension are associated with higher morbidity and mortality rates during PCI. Outcomes are measured in terms of the success of the procedure and complications. A successful PCI procedure is usually defined as an angiographic success (minimal residual narrowing in the artery at the completion of the procedure) without any in-hospital major adverse cardiovascular event, such as death, emergency bypass surgery, or AMI. Clinical success includes angiographic and procedural success, as well as relief of any signs or symptoms of ischemia after the patient recovers from the procedure (short-term success) and ideally for more than 6 months after the procedure (long-term success). Although outcomes are constantly changing in response to new technologies, improved operator skills, and changes in adjunct pharmacology, the rate of PCI angiographic success is very high.

Restenosis is an accumulation of smooth muscle cells at the site of the original procedure that occurs because of the artery's response to

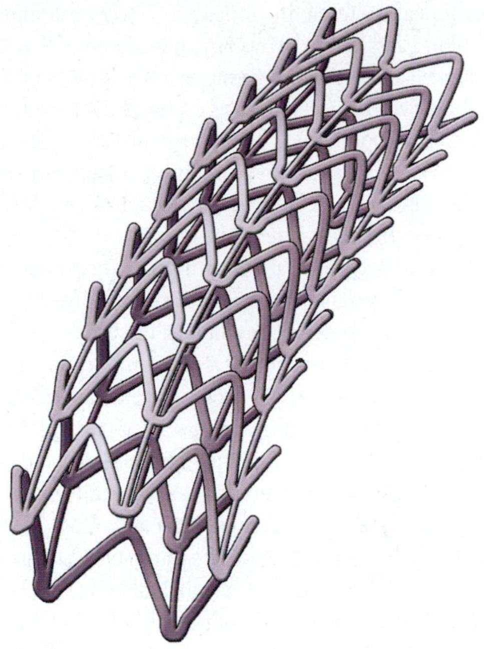

FIGURE 32–18 ◆ Intracoronary stent.

the injury from the PCI. Before stents were available, restenosis rates ranged from 30% to 50% within 6 to 12 months after the procedure, and patients again became symptomatic, requiring repeat procedures. The development of drug eluting stents (DES) has dramatically decreased the rate of restenosis following PCI. A DES is a metal stent that is coated with an immunosuppressive agent such as sirolimus or paclitaxel. The drug is emitted, or eluted, over a period of weeks to months to inhibit smooth muscle cell proliferation. Restenosis rates of less than 5% are common with current DES (Woods et al., 2010).

Nursing Management

Patients undergoing PCI range from the stable person having an elective first procedure to the patient with an acute MI who is hemodynamically unstable, requiring ventilatory and inotropic support during the procedure. The clinical status of the patient and the planned procedure will dictate the exact patient management.

Assessment

Before the procedure, the nurse should perform a complete patient assessment with special attention to the cardiovascular and peripheral vascular system. On the day of the procedure, the nurse should ask the patient and family about any medications taken that day, including warfarin, metformin, diuretics, or insulin. Warfarin, an oral anticoagulant, could lead to increased bleeding during and after the procedure. Metformin, an oral agent indicated in the treatment of non–insulin-dependent diabetes, has been associated with an increased risk of lactic acidosis after contrast administration. Diuretics in combination with the patient's NPO status can lead to hypovolemia during or after the procedure. Baseline laboratory values include serum chemistries, coagulation factors, and a complete blood count.

Following the PCI procedure, the patient is typically transferred to a specialized nursing care unit for continuing care. The patient is assessed for myocardial ischemia, hypotension, and bleeding complications. Patients are instructed to report any occurrence of chest pain, which can indicate acute thrombosis at the site of the PCI. The arterial access site and distal pulses are carefully and frequently assessed to observe for bleeding, hematoma, or loss of pulses.

Nursing Diagnoses

Nursing diagnoses that pertain to the patient undergoing PCI include:

- *Pain* related to *coronary artery disease*
- *Deficient Knowledge* related to disease process
- *Potential for Ineffective Tissue Perfusion* related to fluid balance
- *Bleeding, Risk for related PCI.*

NANDA-I © 2012

Outcomes and Evaluation Parameters

After the PCI procedure has been completed and the patient is returned to the nursing unit, the patient should remain hemodynamically stable and free of chest pain. The nurse assesses the ECG and evaluates the results for signs of abnormality. When the patient's anticoagulation status has normalized, the sheaths are removed from the femoral or radial artery. In many facilities, this is performed by the nurse. Hemostasis of the arterial access site can be obtained by using manual pressure or by using mechanical pressure through a device specifically designed for this use. The access site can then be covered with a small gauze pad or adhesive bandage. The use of pressure dressings and sandbags is not effective in preventing bleeding and hematoma development (Woods et al., 2010). Depending on the location and size of the sheath, the patient may need to be on bed rest for up to 4 to 6 hours following sheath removal. The nurse monitors the patient's vital signs, pain, pulses distal to the insertion site, and bleeding from the insertion site at frequent intervals per unit and health care provider protocols.

Planning and Interventions With Rationales

Before the planned procedure, the nurse must review the patient's and family's understanding of the procedure, including postprocedure care. Explaining the purpose of the vascular access devices and monitoring equipment will help to decrease anxiety for everyone during the procedure. Patients undergoing catheterization are told to have nothing to eat or drink for at least 6 hours before the test. Patients with preexisting renal failure and a history of anaphylactic reaction to contrast dye should be pretreated before the catheterization whenever possible. This pretreatment includes antihistamines and steroids (Woods et al., 2010). Patients with renal failure (serum creatinine $\geq$ 1.5 mg/dL) should receive intravenous normal saline for several hours before the procedure.

The length of the procedure will vary depending on the information needed; coronary angiography alone takes about 15 minutes. The patient should be warned that he may feel hot and flushed during the injection of any contrast medium; this will pass quickly. After the procedure, the patient will have to remain on bed rest for a few hours unless a vascular closure device has been inserted.

PCI is commonly done with procedural sedation to maintain the patient's comfort. The nurse's role during PCI usually includes close monitoring of the patient to ensure a safe environment for the procedure. The nurse must pay particular attention to the patient's airway and respiratory status during the administration of sedation agents such as midazolam. Continuous assessment of the cardiovascular system, including vital signs and ECG, is also necessary to avoid complications. ECG changes such as ST segment elevation (p. 930) indicating myocardial injury may occur before the patient experiences chest pain. The nurse must always be alert for signs and symptoms of any allergic reaction, such as hypotension or difficulty breathing. Rapid identification of any potential problems is necessary to initiate treatment and to provide optimal care for the patient.

Adjunctive pharmacology is required for patients undergoing PCI to maintain patency of the coronary artery. These drugs include oral antiplatelet agents, usually aspirin, and an adenosine diphosphate inhibitor (clopidogrel or prasugrel). Intravenous antiplatelet drugs, including the glycoprotein IIb/IIIa receptor inhibitors, such as abciximab, eptifibatide, or tirofiban, may also be used in some patients. Anticoagulant choices include unfractionated heparin, low molecular weight heparin, or direct thrombin inhibitors such as bivalirudin (Mehta et al., 2010). The drug, dose, and time of therapy will depend on the patient's exact clinical status. See the Pharmacology feature on page 955 for more information on these medications. In summary, the nursing management of patients with CAD who have undergone a PCI is challenging. The nurse must have an understanding of the procedure, including any complications that may arise and the typical medications that are crucial to optimum outcomes.

Complications of Percutaneous Coronary Intervention

During and after PCI, the patient can experience the complications associated with cardiac catheterization. Because of the larger sheaths and increased anticoagulation and antiplatelet medications used during PCI, patients can be at a higher risk of vascular complications, such as hematoma, pseudoaneurysm, and retroperitoneal hemorrhage, or bleeding into the retroperitoneal cavity.

Diagnosis of suspected arterial injuries is made through a careful physical assessment and confirmed through noninvasive vascular studies or arteriography. Physical examination of the femoral site is performed, assessing for the presence of localized tenderness, bruits, or a pulsatile mass. Hematomas are identified by swelling at the site of the arterial puncture. Large hematomas may need to be assessed by ultrasound to rule out the presence of pseudoaneurysms or arteriovenous fistulas.

A femoral **pseudoaneurysm** is an extravascular cavity communicating with the femoral artery by a channel or neck at the needle puncture site. Examination reveals localized tenderness and a palpable, pulsatile mass, often associated with a bruit. Although rare, large pseudoaneurysms can compress the adjacent nerves, causing significant discomfort for the patient. Diagnosis is confirmed through ultrasound with Doppler imaging that demonstrates a cavity communicating with the femoral artery as well as to-and-fro flow of blood through the neck of the pseudoaneurysm. Treatment depends on the size of the pseudoaneurysm and the clinical assessment of the patient. Asymptomatic patients with a well-defined pseudoaneurysm (lumen < 2 centimeters in diameter) can initially be managed conservatively. External compression guided by ultrasound is the standard of treatment for femoral artery pseudoaneurysms greater than 2 centimeters. Urgent operative repair should be considered for pseudoaneurysms associated with a rapidly expanding hematoma, because the expansion can lead to rupture of the pseudoaneurysm or compression neuropathy.

An **arteriovenous (AV) fistula** is a direct communication between the artery and vein, resulting in a high-velocity jet from the artery into the vein. Fistulae are identified by the presence of a bruit over the access site. Diagnosis is confirmed by Doppler ultrasound. An AV fistula that is detected in a clinically asymptomatic patient without evidence of expansion may be followed conservatively. If treatment is indicated, ultrasound-guided compression is usually attempted first. If this fails to close the fistula, or there is evidence of clinical deterioration, the patient is referred for surgical repair.

Retroperitoneal hemorrhage or hematomas are a rare but potentially fatal complication that accounts for significant morbidity. Bleeding into the retroperitoneal space can be difficult to detect until there has been significant blood loss. Early symptoms include abdominal, flank, or back pain, as well as nausea and vomiting, often associated with hypotension and bradycardia. Diagnosis is confirmed through abdominal CT scan. Small retroperitoneal hematomas in stable patients may be managed conservatively by discontinuing anticoagulation and administering volume and blood products. Surgical repair may be required in the patient whose condition deteriorates.

Infections at the access site are uncommon. Organisms are typically gram-positive cocci, usually *Staphylococcus aureus*. Treatment may require several weeks of appropriate antibiotic therapy.

Contrast-induced nephropathy is a rare complication after PCI but remains a major cause of hospital-acquired renal failure. Patients with preexisting renal dysfunction and diabetes are at particular risk (Moser & Riegel, 2008). Prevention and treatment options include hydration; discontinuing drugs such as diuretics, ACE inhibitors, and NSAIDs whenever possible; and administering intravenous fluids. Some patients may benefit from the administration of sodium bicarbonate infusions.

Discharge criteria vary but typically include stable vital signs, tolerating food and fluids, no evidence of complications at the access site, ability to ambulate without assistance, and voiding without difficulty. Discharge instructions to patients and family members should include management of the access site; when to shower, drive, and return to work; and what to do if the patient develops chest pain.

Collaborative Management

Care of patients with CAD undergoing urgent PCI requires a collaborative approach among all members of the health care team in different areas of the hospital, such as the emergency department, cardiac critical care unit, pharmacy, catheterization laboratory, cardiovascular operating room, and step-down units. In order to meet desired patient outcomes, it is essential that this interdisciplinary team communicate openly with one another in developing and evaluating care of the patient and family (IOM [Institute of Medicine], 2010). Staff in the emergency department must be aware of the need for urgent identification and treatment of any patient presenting with AMI. Appropriate medications need to be started as soon as the diagnosis is confirmed. Pharmacists can provide recommendations for dosing of thrombolytic, anticoagulation, and antiplatelet therapy based on the patient's weight and renal function. The patient needs to be transported to the appropriate area for treatment (catheterization laboratory, operating room, or nursing unit) without delay. Catheterization laboratory personnel, including invasive cardiovascular professionals, health care providers, and nurses, must be prepared to treat AMI patients quickly, whether it is during the middle of a busy day or in the middle of the night. All health care team members must cooperate in order to meet the goal of restoring blood flow to the occluded artery as quickly as possible.

Once the PCI is completed, the patient and family will require intensive education from the health care team regarding identification and management of all cardiac risk factors. For many patients, this procedure represents their first invasive cardiac procedure and usually requires significant changes in lifestyle. Many patients will benefit from a consultation with a dietitian to review needed dietary modifications. Because patients undergoing successful PCI may remain in the hospital for only a few days, this process should be started as soon as possible, because changes in lifestyle affect not only the patient but also the entire family. While most patients with CAD are discharged from the hospital quickly, patients who experienced extensive myocardial infarction and cardiogenic shock and have longer hospital stays may benefit from consultation and follow up with physical therapy for muscle strengthening.

Discharge Instructions for the PCI Patient and Family

Patients are able to leave the hospital 24 to 36 hours after an uncomplicated PCI. Serum laboratory values are checked before discharge to verify that hemoglobin, hematocrit, and creatinine levels are within an acceptable range and that there has been no abnormal elevation of cardiac enzymes. Physical examination includes a complete cardiovascular assessment, as well as auscultation and palpation of the vascular access site. If any tenderness, large hematoma, or bruit is noted, discharge must be postponed until the access site is stable.

Patients should be given written instructions regarding care of the access site and what to do if they experience chest pain or other symptoms of CAD. All medications should be reviewed, with emphasis on the importance of not stopping any medicine (especially antiplatelet and adenosine diphosphate inhibitor drugs) without first discussing this with the cardiologist. Finally, patients should be reminded of the need for careful follow-up with their health care provider. Comprehensive instructions are presented in the Patient Teaching & Discharge Priorities box (p. 946).

Medical Management of Coronary Artery Disease

Routine evaluation of patients who present with symptoms that may represent exacerbations of CAD includes a review of their symptoms, a review of their medical/social history for associated diseases and risk factors, an assessment for physical signs, and diagnostic tests. Tools used to determine the extent of myocardial perfusion depend on six indexes:

- The presence of physical signs and symptoms representative of tissue hypoxemia or heart failure
- Abnormal levels of blood serum markers indicating myocardial cell membrane damage
- ECG changes consistent with myocardial injury and muscle death
- The lack of uptake of substances by cardiac tissue
- Vessel patency as seen with angiography
- Assessments of global intracardiac structure and function.

Signs and symptoms, blood markers (p. 949), and ECG changes are completed expeditiously when a patient is admitted for suspected acute coronary ischemia. ECG testing is done either at rest, during an acute event such as the presence of angina, or during exercise to determine the extent of stress on the heart during work. Angiography, as previously discussed, is used to define or confirm areas of critical artery stenosis or obstruction, referred to as *culprit lesions*, as well as areas used for hemodynamic measurements. Viability studies employ the infusion of a radioactive indicator, typically technetium, that is taken up by tissue with good perfusion and is later "washed out" as perfusing blood dilutes the concentration of the isotope over time. Ventricular radiography done during coronary angiography identifies areas of abnormal heart contractility such as **dyskinesia** (impaired muscle movement), **akinesia** (severe loss or no muscle movement), and **hypokinesia** (hypoactive muscle movement) that can result from poor coronary perfusion. Echocardiography (Chapter 33) uses sonography to assess any damage to valve structure or chamber contractility at rest or during exercise that may result from chronic or acute myocardial ischemia. The Diagnostic Tests box (p. 947) summarizes the laboratory studies that are used to diagnose the presence and extent of CAD.

Physical findings associated with CAD also may be associated with other diseases such as systemic arterial hypertension, hyperlipidemia, valvular heart disease, heart failure, diabetes, or peripheral atherosclerosis. Thus, findings such as the following are not diagnostic for CAD specifically: elevated blood pressure; presence of an S_3, S_4, or paradoxically split S_2; diminished peripheral pulses; murmurs of aortic stenosis or mitral insufficiency; enlarged cardiac silhouette; changes in pulse cadence and rate because of ventricular or atrial ectopic beats; and presence of crackles. However, they may represent exacerbations of associated diseases that result in coronary insufficiency. The absence or presence of these findings also provides a baseline in the advent of complications, assists in excluding other conditions, and assists in stratifying risk for appropriate triage of patients who present with the clinical manifestations of CAD.

Pain is most effectively assessed by using a systematic approach to help ensure that all aspects are assessed, such as the following: aggravating and alleviating factors; timing related to frequency, duration, time of day, and relation to activity or rest; qualitative characteristics such as description, location, intensity, and radiation; and any other associated symptoms. Diagnostic tests for coronary artery disease are outlined in the feature box on page 947.

Acute Coronary Syndrome

Patients who present to the health care provider's office or the emergency department with a change in their previous pattern of angina or new onset angina are evaluated for the likelihood that their symptoms represent an **acute coronary syndrome (ACS)** secondary to CAD. They are evaluated for the presence of myocardial infarction, myocardial ischemia, and infarction-related complications, as well as a general state of hemodynamic stability. Disposition of patients to either outpatient management or admission to an inpatient unit, selection of therapy, and decisions about revascularization are based on these assessment data.

Categories of Acute Coronary Syndrome

Included under the umbrella of ACS are the diagnoses of unstable angina (UA), non–ST segment elevation myocardial infarction (NSTEMI), and ST segment elevation myocardial infarction (STEMI). Pathogenesis of ACS involves fibrous plaque disruption and thrombosis formation, and can result in either a partial or a total occlusion of the lumen of the coronary artery. This process will either markedly decrease or completely cut off blood flow to the myocardium.

Unstable Angina

Anginal symptoms controlled by rest or medical management are considered stable, as described earlier. **Unstable angina (UA)** depicts a transitory syndrome falling between stable angina and MI in which thrombus forms in an area of arterial stenosis but is subsequently fully or partially lysed, or dissolved, by endogenous antithrombotic mechanisms. Symptoms worsen such that the patient presents with the development of new onset exertion angina, angina present at rest for longer than 20 minutes, or symptoms that have accelerated in frequency, duration, or intensity (Moser & Riegel, 2008; Woods et al., 2010). When the vessels are assessed with cardiac angiography, these patients most often show the presence of stenotic eccentric lesions, collateral circulation, and the absence of a totally occluded coronary artery. Blood markers

PATIENT TEACHING & DISCHARGE PRIORITIES for Percutaneous Coronary Intervention and Heart Disease

Need	Teaching
Vascular Access Site	The patient should assess the site daily. Some amount of bruising and firmness/tenderness at the site is normal. The patient should call the health care provider if the area of firmness gets bigger instead of smaller. The bruising should resolve by 4 to 6 weeks. The patient should shower or bathe as usual. No special dressing is needed. The patient should take Tylenol for any discomfort at the site. If the access site was in the groin, the patient should avoid bending over or straining for the first 48 hours. The patient should avoid heavy lifting for the first week. If the patient experiences any of the following in the leg, toes, or foot, she should call the health care provider immediately: • Numbness • Tingling • Coolness. If the patient experiences bright-red bleeding from the site, she should lie down and have someone apply firm pressure just above the site for 20 minutes and then gently release the pressure. If the bleeding cannot be controlled, someone should call 911. If the access site was sealed using a special closure device, the patient will have received special instructions regarding the device. Usually no special care is required, but the patient needs to keep these instructions containing the name of the device in case the patient or the health care provider has questions or concerns about the site. The nurse should assess availability, knowledge, and compliance with the treatment regimen. The nurse should validate a follow-up appointment with the local health care provider. The nurse should assess the availability of emergency health care.
Activity	The patient should not resume or start an exercise program until she has been evaluated by the health care provider. The patient must notify the health care provider immediately if she experiences any of the following during exercise: • Chest pain, especially pain similar to typical angina • Nausea, vomiting, or cool, clammy skin • Extreme or persistent fatigue not relieved by a short rest period • Shortness of breath, especially if it makes talking difficult • A change in heart rhythm. The patient may be able to return to work quickly, depending on the type of work. This should be discussed with the health care provider. Following myocardial infarction, sexual activity can typically be resumed in 4 to 6 weeks after discussing the situation with the health care provider. The patient should notify the health care provider if any of the following occur during or after sexual activity: • Rapid heartbeat, palpitations, or shortness of breath persisting for 15 minutes • Chest pain • Extreme fatigue. It is critically important that the patient obtain regular follow-up from her health care provider. A heart-healthy lifestyle includes: • Weight control • Regular exercise • Smoking cessation • Diet high in fruits and vegetables and low in fat. Medications that may be prescribed include: • Aspirin therapy • Hypertensive control • Diabetes management • Lipid-lowering agent. Other medications may be indicated, depending on the health of the patient's heart. The nurse should assess availability, knowledge, and compliance with the treatment regimen. The nurse should assess the need for lifestyle modification for all family members. The nurse should assess the need for cardiac rehabilitation. The nurse should assess the patient's ability to obtain necessary medications after discharge.

DIAGNOSTIC TESTS for Coronary Artery Disease

Diagnostic Test, Normal Values, and Rationales	Expected Abnormality
ECG	
No ST segment elevation or depression.	ST segment elevation.
No T wave inversion.	ST segment depression.
No Q waves.	Q waves.
Identify ST segment or T wave abnormalities; the presence of pathologic Q waves indicates myocardial ischemia, injury, and necrosis, which assists in the diagnosis of an AMI.	
Stress Test (exercise treadmill or bicycle)	
Induces abnormal ECG changes, which occur when myocardial oxygen demand increases due to exercise.	ST segment or T wave changes during stress.
These changes occur only when the heart is stressed due to the heart's inability to increase cardiac output during periods of high demand.	
Nuclear Myocardial Perfusion Imaging	
Pharmacologic agent used to induce stress for those patients who cannot exercise.	ST segment or T wave changes during stress.
Identify both functional and nonfunctional myocardium when oxygen demand is increased.	
Dobutamine Stress Echocardiography	
Pharmacologic agent used to induce stress for those patients who cannot exercise.	ST segment or T wave changes during stress.
Identify both functional and nonfunctional myocardium when oxygen demand is increased.	Changes in ejection fraction.
Electron Beam Computed Tomography (EBCT)/Multislice CT	
Detect and quantify coronary artery calcification.	Calcium score is age dependent.
Coronary calcium is part of the development of atherosclerosis. It occurs exclusively in atherosclerotic arteries and is absent in the normal vessel wall. The presence of calcification in the coronary arteries indicates the presence of coronary atherosclerosis.	
MRI	
Identifies plaque size and composition.	Coronary artery stenosis.
Identifies area of plaque buildup from the presence and progression of CAD.	
Cardiac Catheterization	
Confirms patency of coronary arteries, determines blood flow in chambers and great vessels, and evaluates pressures across valves.	Coronary artery stenosis, valve damage, decreased ventricular function.
Identifies area of plaque buildup from the presence and progression of CAD.	
Intravascular Ultrasound	
Quantify plaque burden and composition from the presence and progression of CAD.	Coronary artery stenosis
Chest X-Ray (CXR)	
Evaluate heart size. Identify congestion or effusions. Identify tumors or masses.	Enlarged heart and lung congestion.
Determines heart failure, cardiomyopathy, and CAD.	Pulmonary edema, congestive heart failure.
	Presence of lung tumor or mass.
Echocardiogram, Transthoracic or Transesophageal (Chapter 33)	
Measures diameters of the cardiac chambers, evaluates structural abnormalities, and identifies valvular vegetation and pressure gradients.	Valvular damage; insufficiency, regurgitation, stenosis, or vegetation.
	Enlarged chamber size such as ventricular hypertrophy.
	Abnormal pressure gradients.
	Decreased ventricular function.
C-Reactive Protein	
<10 mg/L	Not usually present.
Acute phase reactant protein used to indicate an inflammatory process.	
Cardiac Enzymes	Chart 32–11 (p. 950)
Magnesium	
1.5–2.5 mg/dL	<1.5 mg/dL
Electrolyte balance; decreases ventricular irritability.	>2.5 mg/dL.
Potassium	
3.5–5.3 mEq/L	<3.5 mEq/L
Electrolyte balance; decreases ventricular irritability.	>5.3 mEq/L.

Source: Adapted from: Kee, J. L. (2010). *Laboratory and diagnostic tests with nursing implications.* Upper Saddle River, NJ: Pearson.

indicating myocardial damage are normal, and ECG changes, if present, are transitory and will return to normal. Based on the assessment and physical findings, patients are categorized as low, intermediate, or high risk and triaged and treated based on presenting symptoms.

Non–ST Segment Myocardial Infarction

The term **myocardial infarction (MI)** denotes a loss of myocytes or myocardial apoptosis as a result of prolonged muscle ischemia. Apoptosis results in a permanent loss of myocardial muscle function. Non–ST segment elevation myocardial infarction (**NSTEMI**) shares a common pathogenesis and clinical presentation with unstable angina. Both usually occur as a result of transient subtotal occlusion of a coronary artery with reduced coronary blood flow resulting from plaque disruption and ensuing pathophysiological processes. The presence of serum blood markers and persistent ECG changes distinguishes a more severe myocardial injury associated with NSTEMI and thus a higher risk of death and MI, versus no blood marker release and transitory or no ECG changes seen with UA. See Figure 32–6 (p. 930), which shows normal ECG waveforms, and compare it to Figure 32–8 (p. 931) and to Figure 32–19◆; the middle figure shows ECG changes associated with the partial obstruction seen with NSTEMI.

ST Segment Elevation Myocardial Infarction

ST segment elevation myocardial infarction (**STEMI**) refers to myocardial injury associated with ST segment elevation on the ECG (see Figure 32–7, p. 931). Besides the ST segment, STEMI compares differently to NSTEMI in a number of ways. The presence of ST segment elevation means that myocardial tissue is undergoing severe anoxia and cellular damage. In most cases this is a result of complete coronary artery blockage from thrombotic occlusion over an underlying plaque lesion (Libby et al., 2008). Unlike NSTEMI, the blockage is sustained. If blood flow is not reestablished in 20 minutes, apoptosis occurs. Ischemic damage traverses the myocardium vertically outward, starting with the subendocardial layer through to the epicardium (see Figure 32–4, p. 924). Before the current age of rapid revascularization therapies, ST segment elevation was usually associated with transmural MI and the appearance of Q waves on the ECG days later. The Q wave changes indicate apoptosis and permanent loss of muscle function in the affected area. If the occlusion is treated early, a patient presenting with STEMI may suffer only subendocardial cell damage without subsequent Q waves.

Silent Ischemia/Myocardial Infarction

Not all episodes of coronary artery ischemia cause chest pain. The presence of silent ischemia predicts greater risk of adverse outcomes in patients with stable and unstable angina and in patients following an AMI or revascularization therapy. Silent ischemia is more prevalent in older adults, women, patients with diabetes, and patients with three-vessel disease. The lack of symptoms has been attributed to altered pain regulation or perception, higher pain tolerance, higher levels of circulating endorphins, or altered senses secondary to pain pathway impairment (Libby et al., 2008).

Sudden Cardiac Death

Sudden cardiac death (SCD) is an unexpected cardiac arrest that results in death within an hour of symptom onset. The underlying causes of SCD include instability of the heart's electrical system, resulting in ventricular tachycardia and ventricular fibrillation. Bradycardia, asystole, and pulseless electrical activity can also occur. In some patients, SCD can be caused by vasospasm of one of the coronary arteries or congenital abnormalities of the coronary arteries. Cardiomyopathy can also be an underlying cause. About 75% of patients who experience SCD have underlying CAD (Moser & Riegel, 2008). Chapter 30 includes an in-depth discussion of these dysrhythmias.

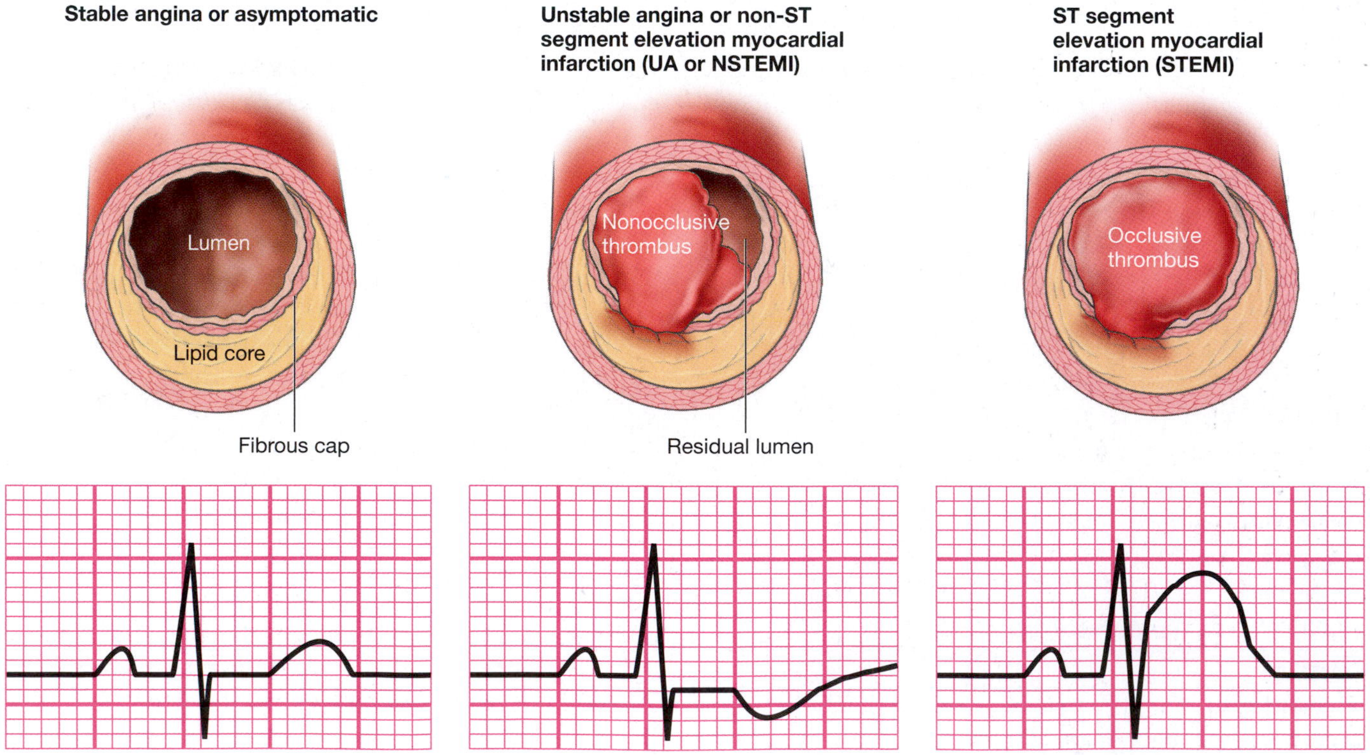

FIGURE 32–19 ◆ Clot formation and ST segment ECG changes associated with ACS.

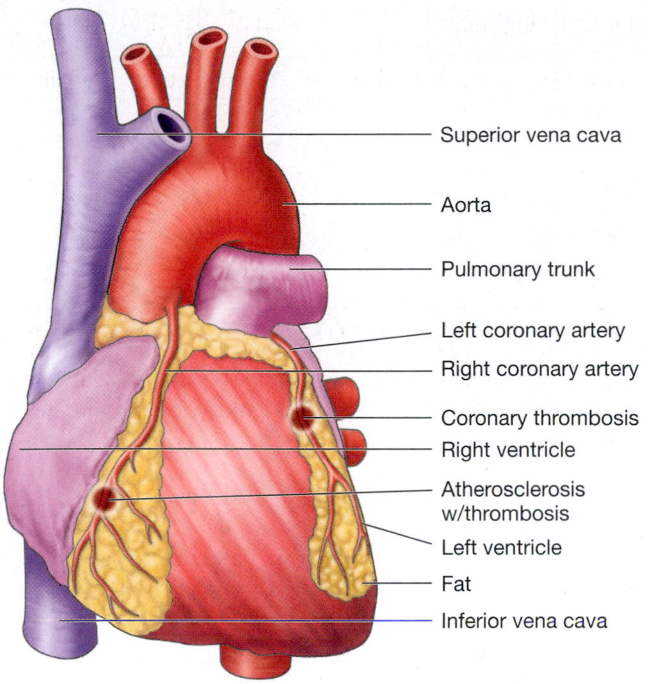

FIGURE 32–20 ◆ Thrombosis in a coronary artery.

Classifications of Myocardial Infarction

Both STEMI and NSTEMI are classified according to the coronary artery involved. Occlusion of the left anterior descending (LAD) artery is referred to as an anterior wall infarct. The LAD feeds the anterior left ventricle, anterior septum, papillary muscle, apex, bundle of His, and bundle branches. All or some of the function of these tissues is lost with an infarct to the LAD. Most infarcts affect the left ventricle.

Occlusion of the right coronary artery (RCA) results in an inferior wall MI. The RCA supplies the inferior left ventricle, inferior septum, papillary muscle, and right ventricle (the SA node in 60% of the population and the AV node in 90%). Occlusion of the circumflex artery results in a lateral wall infarct because it supplies the lateral wall of the left ventricle (the SA node in 40% of the population and the AV node in 10%).

Occlusion of the left main coronary artery results in a massive MI because it supplies blood to over 70% of the left ventricle. MIs involving the left main, often referred to as "widow makers," typically are associated with complications such as heart failure. Figure 32–20◆ shows a thrombosis in the coronary arteries.

Clinical Manifestations of Acute Coronary Syndrome

Presenting signs and symptoms of ACS vary greatly from person to person. Typical symptoms include chest pain, diaphoresis, shortness of breath, and generalized weakness. Patients describe the pain from an acute MI in the same terms as the pain from angina pectoris except that it is usually more intense and longer in duration. If the chest pain lasts longer than 20 minutes, cardiac damage may occur. The pain from an AMI is not relieved by rest and requires treatment with medications or interventions to open the occluded coronary artery.

Most frequently, patients report that the anginal pain occurs in the mid to lower sternal areas of the chest. It also may radiate to the left arm, right arm, neck, jaw, and back. Atypical angina occurs in the stomach and back. Owing to the close proximity to the epigastric region, many people mistake the pain for indigestion. Other frequent signs and symptoms associated with AMI include nausea, vomiting, dyspnea, syncope, anxiety, and a feeling of impending doom. Approximately one-third of the patients experiencing an AMI do not experience chest pain and initially exhibit other symptoms of decreased cardiac output such as shortness of breath and changes in sensorium or syncope.

Women having an MI have different signs and symptoms than men. Men having an MI report mid to lower sternal chest pain more often than women. Women, in contrast, are more likely to have an atypical presentation. Pain may be more generalized, it may come and go, or it may be described as indigestion. They may have nausea and vomiting. Women are more likely to experience pain in the neck, jaw, throat, shoulder, or back instead of the chest. In addition, women are more likely to have complaints of overwhelming fatigue, weakness, and sleep disturbances (Miracle, 2010; Moseley, Allen, & Martel, 2010). Figure 32–11 (p. 934) outlines the locations where angina occurs.

Safety Alert *Some patients are able to sense when a major cardiac event is occurring. Therefore, it is essential that the nurse pay close attention to patients who report impending doom.*

The physical assessment findings in a patient experiencing ACS are also variable. The blood pressure may be low because of decreased cardiac output, or it may be elevated owing to catecholamine release, fear, and anxiety. The heart rate may be bradycardic or tachycardic, depending on where in the heart the damage is occurring and the patient's anxiety level. There may be an S_3 or S_4 present and new systolic murmurs. Chapter 29 includes a description of heart sounds. The lung sounds may be clear unless there is associated heart failure, in which case rales or crackles and/or wheezes may be heard with an associated decrease in arterial oxygen saturation. Heart failure is described in Chapter 34.

Laboratory and Diagnostic Procedures to Diagnose Acute Coronary Syndrome

The clinical manifestations of CAD typically bring the patient to the emergency department or health care provider's office. The second indicators of acute coronary insufficiency are the laboratory tests and ECG changes that indicate the presence and extent of myocardial damage. As soon as the patient is admitted to the emergency department, laboratory tests are done to assist in determining the diagnosis. Many of the laboratory values are time sensitive, so it is essential that the blood is drawn immediately after admission. The initial laboratory and diagnostic workup includes blood serum markers and a 12-lead ECG.

Blood (Serum) Markers of Myocardial Ischemia

Laboratory tests commonly ordered include troponin (T or I), creatine kinase (CK total, CK-MB), and myoglobin. A rise in cardiac blood markers occurs when the myocardial cells become damaged from a lack of blood supply that occurs with myocardial injury and death. The cell membrane loses its integrity, and intracellular enzymes are released. The extent of enzyme release is relative to the amount of tissue damage and, thus, the size of the infarct. Therefore, blood marker levels are useful to help confirm the diagnosis and the extent of tissue injury.

Troponin

Troponins are biochemical markers for cardiac disease, especially acute MI. **Troponin T** and **troponin I** are found in cardiac muscle;

CHART 32–11 Cardiac Markers' Pattern Consistent with Acute Myocardial Infarction

Laboratory Test	Normal Values	Time to Elevation	Mean Time to Peak Elevation	Time to Return to Normal
Troponin I	0.1–0.5 ng/mL	1–3 hours	24 hours	5–9 days
Troponin T	Less than 0.2 ng/mL	1–3 hours	12 hours–2 days	10–14 days
CPK	5–35 mcg/mL	4–6 hours	18–24 hours	3–4 days
Myoglobin	12–90 ng/mL	2–6 hours	8–12 hours	12–18 hours

Source: Adapted from: Kee, J. L. (2010). *Laboratory and diagnostic tests with nursing implications.* Upper Saddle River, NJ: Pearson.

during periods of cardiac ischemia, intracellular troponin will leak from the inside of the cell because of changes in myocardial cell membrane permeability. Troponin levels can be detected soon after an ischemic event. Normal and abnormal cardiac markers are outlined in Chart 32–11.

Creatine Kinase

Creatine kinase (CK) is an enzyme found in high concentrations in the heart and skeletal muscle and in smaller concentrations in the brain. Laboratory studies are able to subdivide and analyze the total CK level into its three isoforms: CK-MM from damaged skeletal muscle, CK-BB from damaged brain tissue, and CK-MB from damaged cardiac tissue. Of the isoforms, only CK-MB, along with the CK total and percentage of CK-MB in the CK total, is relevant for determining cardiac ischemia and infarction.

Myoglobin

Myoglobin is a heme-containing, oxygen-binding protein that is exclusive to striated and nonstriated muscle. Because of its very small molecular weight, myoglobin is released into the interstitial fluid as early as 2 hours following damage to muscle tissue. Unlike CK-MB, the presence of an elevated myoglobin level is not a specific indicator of just heart damage. Rather, it is a sensitive indicator that muscle damage has occurred. For example, if a patient falls or has any type of muscle injury, the myoglobin level will rise. In other words, a patient who has had an acute cardiac event will have an elevated myoglobin; however, the diagnosis cannot be made on the myoglobin level alone because of its lack of specificity.

ECG Changes

12-Lead ECG Changes with Acute Myocardial Infarction

The 12-lead ECG provides 12 different views of the electrical activity in the heart. In evaluating a 12-lead ECG, the Q wave, T wave, and ST segment are used to determine the presence of damage. Descriptions of these waves are on page 930. Changes in specific leads reflect the specific location in the heart where the damage has occurred and which vessel(s) contain the culprit lesions (Chart 32–12). As the ischemia and injury evolve, so do the ECG changes. Figure 32–19 (p. 948) demonstrates the ECG changes that occur with a transmural AMI.

The ST segment is the major focus in evaluating ischemic injury to the myocardium. As was discussed earlier, the location of the AMI is identified by the involved coronary artery. Abnormal changes on the ECG correlate with the area in the myocardium where damage has occurred and thus identify the artery involved. For ST segment and T wave changes to be considered diagnostic, they must appear in two or more contiguous leads. This means that changes must be present in two or more leads that correspond to a given area of myocardium damage. For example, in order for the ECG criteria to be met for an inferior wall MI, a patient would have to have an ST segment elevation of 1 millimeter or greater in two of these three leads: II, III, and aVF.

Reciprocal ST Segment Abnormalities

When ST segment changes occur during an AMI, they are present in the leads on the 12-lead ECG that face the damaged myocardium and/or infarction and are referred to as the indicative leads. Reciprocal (electrically opposite) leads are distant from the injury and reflect in an upside-down mirror image the changes or damage seen in the indicative leads. Reciprocal ST segment changes present as horizontal or down-sloping of the ST segment. Other reciprocal changes include the absence of a Q wave, an increased height of the R wave in the QRS complex, and a tall, upright T wave. The presence of reciprocal changes is generally thought to indicate more extensive damage and a worse prognosis. When looking at a 12-lead ECG for indicative and reciprocal changes, the nurse should keep in mind that ST segment depression interpreted as reciprocal changes may in fact reflect injury rising from a culprit lesion in another vessel (Woods et al., 2010).

Bundle Branch Block

Bundle branch block (BBB) is defined as a discontinuity of conduction (complete or incomplete) in one branch of the bundle of His, which affects normal transmission of the impulse through the ventricles and causes the QRS to be wider than the normal 0.12 second. When one bundle is blocked, the ventricles depolarize asynchronously, which is characterized by a delay of excitation to one ventricle; therefore, an abnormal spread of electrical activity through the ventricles occurs. A spontaneous left BBB or right ventricular pacing-induced left bundle branch pattern obscures the electrocardiographic diagnosis of an AMI.

ECG Signs of Reperfusion

The goal for the management of AMI is rapid restoration of blood flow to the affected coronary artery. The lack of reperfusion is an important predictor of cardiac morbidity and mortality following AMI. The amount of time to restoration of blood flow directly correlates to the morbidity and mortality associated with AMI. For the therapy to be considered successful, the resolution of ST segment deviation should occur within 90 minutes following revascularization. Other markers of reperfusion include newly acquired T wave inversion within 4 hours after AMI, accelerated idioventricular rhythms of rates between 60 and 120 beats per minute, isolated premature ventricular contractions, and nonsustained asymptomatic runs of ventricular tachycardia. The development of sustained ventricular tachycardia or ventricular fibrillation often represents reocclusion of the coronary artery. Chapter 30 has a complete description of dysrhythmias.

CHART 32–12 ECG Changes During an MI, Correlated with Coronary Anatomy

Artery	Areas and Structures Supplied	Type of MI and Leads Involved	Associated Symptoms and Complications
Right Coronary Artery (RCA)	SA node (55%), AV node (90%) Bundle of His Right atrium and ventricle Inferior surface of left ventricle Posterior one-third of septum Left bundle branch Posterior/inferior division of right bundle branch	**Inferior MI (RCA)** II, III, aVF Reciprocal changes in I, aVL	Vagal symptoms: nausea and bradycardia AV blocks: most common = first degree and second degree type I (Wenckebach); third degree possible Usually transient; treat only if symptomatic
Left Anterior Descending (LAD)	Anterior wall of left ventricle Anterior two-thirds of septum Right bundle branch Anterior/superior division of left bundle branch	**Anterior MI (LAD)** $V_1 - V_4$ Reciprocal changes in II, III, aVF **Anterolateral (LAD/CIRC)** V_1–V_4 I, aVL, V_5, V_6 Reciprocal changes in II, III, aVF	Often associated with loss of large muscle mass If large myocardial infarction (MI), prone to develop diminished left ventricular branch function, signs and symptoms of heart failure, cardiogenic shock Rhythm disturbances: atrial and ventricular dysrhythmias, bundle branch blocks, AV blocks with second degree type II most common; may progress to third-degree block (complete heart block)
Left Circumflex Artery (CIRC, CX)	SA node (45%), AV node (10%) Inferior surface of left ventricle Lateral wall of left ventricle Left atrium Posterior/inferior division of left bundle branch	**Lateral MI (CIRC/LAD)** I, aVL, V_5, V_6 Reciprocal changes in V_1, V_3 **Anterolateral MI (LAD/CX)** I, aVL, V_5, V_6 V_1–V_4 Reciprocal changes in II, III, aVF **Posterior MI (RCA, CIRC)** Reciprocal changes only in V_1, V_2 unless 18-lead ECG is done	Frequently seen with large anterior MIs Occasionally seen with inferior MIs Least likely to alter hemodynamics or cause dysrhythmias Uncommon; involves both right coronary artery (RCA) and circumflex (CIRC) Hard to diagnose on traditional 12-lead; researchers developing 18-lead ECG Bradycardia with possible AV block; usually transient

Cardiac Dysrhythmias Associated with Acute Myocardial Infarction

Premature atrial and ventricular contractions, conduction abnormalities, tachycardia, and bradycardia can all be seen with myocardial ischemia and infarction. Premature beats and tachycardias occur because of acute tissue hypoxemia and irritability and derangement of electrical membrane potentials. Tachycardia also is a by-product of elevated levels of circulating catecholamines due to the stress response. Atrial fibrillation may result from MI because of enhanced vagal tone, increased atrial pressure, atrial infarction, or pericarditis. Conduction delays and bradycardia relate to the location of the infarct and the mass of involved myocardium.

Although a significant number of patients do not have ECG changes indicative of AMI on admission, these changes are still considered an important diagnostic indicator when used in conjunction with the patient's history, presenting signs and symptoms, and blood markers indicative of cardiac ischemia.

Medical Management of Acute Coronary Syndrome

Patients with unstable symptoms are at a greater risk and therefore warrant hospital admission for diagnostic work-up and treatment. An estimated 5 million or more adults present each year to the emergency department with a primary complaint of chest pain (Libby et al., 2008).

Patients with suspected cardiac ischemia but with nondefinitive results from the cardiac workup may be triaged to a cardiac observation unit located as part of an emergency department or inpatient unit. Observation units, also referred to as chest pain units, provide space for ischemia to be ruled out in patients by using specific protocols. These protocols involve serial ECGs, cardiac blood marker determinations, and possibly stress testing, echocardiography (Chapter 33), or perfusion tests. These patients are not admitted to the hospital unless ischemia is ruled in or still suspected after 24 hours.

Patients with ACS should be evaluated in an environment where aggressive therapy can be initiated quickly, such as a hospital emergency department, which has advanced life support backup and personnel to provide continuous monitoring. On admission to the emergency department or critical care unit, patients are made NPO, put on bed rest, given supplemental oxygen, and undergo continuous cardiac and oxygen saturation monitoring. Blood chemistries including cardiac markers are drawn, a 12-lead ECG is obtained, and the patient is placed on a cardiac monitor.

The mnemonic **MONA,** cited in the Advanced Cardiac Life Support (ACLS) guidelines, describes a protocol for treatment of patients with suspected MI. The mnemonic stands for morphine, oxygen, nitroglycerin, and aspirin. The platelet-inhibiting action of chewable aspirin in doses of 81 to 325 milligrams decreases platelet aggregation, and supplemental oxygen treatments are intended to increase oxygen supply to ischemic tissue. Nitroglycerin (NTG) dilates the large coronary arteries, thus increasing the blood supply to ischemic tissue. Initially, it is administered sublingually, as spray or tablets, although with persistent symptoms it may be given intravenously. Intravenous morphine sulfate, a potent analgesic, is used to relieve angina, although it is also effective in reducing anxiety. Morphine, along with nitroglycerin, can cause the veins to dilate, resulting in a decrease in the amount of blood returning to the heart (preload). This reduced preload (Chapter 31) helps to decrease myocardial oxygen demand.

Short-acting nitroglycerin and morphine can precipitate hypotension, especially in patients with a right ventricular infarction. Therefore, both drugs must be titrated cautiously to relieve pain without causing hypotension. For persistent symptoms of ischemia, IV or oral beta-adrenergic-blockers and heparin will be administered. Glycoprotein (GP) IIb/IIIa inhibitors may be added for unrelenting symptoms. A thrombolytic agent (see Pharmacology feature, p. 955) may be administered, or the patient is prepared for emergent percutaneous coronary intervention (PCI) (p. 940) as soon as the ECG and/or cardiac markers indicate the presence of an ST segment elevation MI (STEMI). Thrombolytic medications are contraindicated in patients with unstable angina (UA) and non–ST segment elevation MI (NSTEMI), because studies demonstrate a higher risk of bleeding and lower beneficial results compared to patients with STEMI (Libby et al., 2008).

Thrombolytic drug therapy is recommended for patients suspected of AMI who are younger than 75 years old, at low risk for bleeding, with symptoms lasting less than 12 hours. PCI is indicated when thrombolytic therapy is contraindicated or in patients with cardiogenic shock. PCI is recommended as an alternative first-choice therapy only if intervention can be performed within 60 to 90 minutes by skilled clinicians (those who have performed 75 procedures/year) in high-volume centers (>200 PCI cases/year) with demonstrated acceptable PCI success rates. Coronary artery bypass graft surgery (CABG) (p. 964) is recommended for patients with persistent pain or hemodynamic instability when treatment with PCI is unsuccessful or if medical management including thrombolytic therapy fails.

Once medically stable (without recurrent ischemia, electrical instability as shown by ECG, signs of heart failure, or other serious complications), patients with UA can be transferred to a non–critical care environment where oral nitrates, β-adrenergic blockers or calcium-channel blockers, and antiplatelet therapy will be initiated or adjusted to maintain symptom control and hemodynamic stability. For recurrent chest pain, the patient should receive an immediate 12-lead ECG to document ischemia during pain, followed by sublingual NTG and IV NTG if pain persists. Patients with unrelieved chest pain and ECG changes, pulmonary edema, hypotension, or new mitral regurgitation indicate a need for ICU monitoring. However, if minimal or no episodes of angina occur while the patient is being transitioned off oxygen and to a normal activity level, discharge can be expected in 1 to 3 days.

Noninvasive stress testing, perfusion scans, and/or cardiac catheterization may be scheduled to occur while in the hospital or as a follow-up procedure postdischarge. Discharge preparation includes teaching about cardiac risk factors, signs and symptoms of myocardial ischemia, how and when to access emergency medical services, and medication regimens. Improving the outcomes of patients following AMI is now one of the major goals of many institutions.

Nonpharmacologic and Pharmacologic Treatment of Acute Coronary Syndrome

Efforts aimed at increasing oxygen supply to ischemic myocardium revolve around five strategies: (1) Raise the amount of oxygenated blood delivered to the tissues with supplemental oxygen and blood transfusions; (2) relieve coronary smooth muscle vasoconstriction or spasm with vasodilators; (3) reperfuse ischemic tissue by dissolving thrombus with thrombolytic agents; (4) prevent thrombus formation with anticoagulant therapy; and (5) reestablish blood flow through invasive revascularization procedures such as CABG and PCI.

Activity Progression

Activity for patients with ACS is dictated by the emergence of anginal symptoms. Patients are advised to avoid certain activities, to refrain from sudden exertion, and to stop what they are doing if symptoms occur. Activity prescriptions, based on ischemic thresholds determined during exercise testing (p. 937), are recommended to maintain or enhance exercise tolerance, strengthen ventricular wall motion, or reduce ischemic episodes.

AMI patients without clinical signs of ischemia or depressed ventricular function are able to get out of bed after a 24-hour pain-free period. Certain self-care activities are allowed, such as toileting, feeding, bathing, weighing, transferring, and positioning, which require minimal energy expenditure and do not cause undue strain on the recovering heart. For elimination needs, during the first 24 hours, patients may use either a bedpan or a bedside commode, as they are equivalent in energy expenditure. Barring other limitations, patients admitted with UA can advance their activity after symptoms are controlled and hemodynamic stability has been achieved for 8 hours. After 24 hours, AMI patients should be up in a chair, during which time an assessment for orthostatic changes should be done. A drop in systolic pressure of 20 mmHg or more, or a heart rate increase of 20 beats per minute or more, represents a positive orthostatic change indicating that the patient is deconditioned. Muscle deconditioning, as it relates to cardiac function, refers to the delayed or inadequate response of the leg muscles to contract reflexively to increase return of peripheral blood volume as the patient progresses from a lying to a standing position. When a patient is deconditioned, blood pools in the legs, dropping systemic blood pressure and causing syncope or dizziness, risk of falls, and possible recurrence of ischemia. Orthostatic blood pressure and heart rate changes can be ameliorated by timing activity apart from administration times of vasodilating and diuretic medications and having the patient warm up with in-bed isotonic exercises, such as extending and flexing the feet, prior to rising.

Reducing Autonomic Stress Responses

Norepinephrine and epinephrine levels are elevated during the first few hours after an AMI. These catecholamines increase heart rate and systemic vascular resistance (SVR), both resulting in increases in myocardial oxygen demand. To lessen the cardiovascular impact of autonomic system overstimulation, interventions for patients with angina and AMI are aimed at identifying and eliminating triggers of autonomic nervous system stimulation. Following an acute event, patients are monitored for signs of excessive sympathetic nervous stimulation such as dysrhythmias, diaphoresis, cool/clammy skin, and elevations in hemodynamic parameters such as pulmonary artery wedge pressure (PAWP) (Chapter 31), afterload, heart rate, and blood pressure. Conditions that may cause or potentiate excessive catecholamine release such as abnormal electrolyte levels, hypoxemia, acidosis, hyper/hypotension, tachycardia/bradycardia, fever, anemia, volume depletion, immobility, discomfort, pain, or emotional stress are avoided or treated quickly. Pain is treated with intravenous (IV) morphine sulfate. Besides being a powerful pain reliever, morphine sulfate has the added benefit of being a vasodilator, thereby reducing both preload and afterload. Anxiety is treated with oral or IV benzodiazepine such as lorazepam (Ativan) or midazolam (Versed), although morphine sulfate also will help decrease anxiety. Family interaction is either liberal or restricted depending on patient preference; tolerance, defined in terms of cardiac signs and symptoms, is scheduled around adequate rest periods for the patient. Sleep is promoted by maintaining a quiet environment, keeping the lights off or low during the night, minimizing interactions with the patient during sleep periods, and utilizing pharmacologic sleeping aids. Dietary modifications that reduce sympathetic stimulation include avoidance of caffeinated beverages and beverages of extreme hot or cold temperature.

Overstimulation of the parasympathetic nervous system can be equally deleterious to recovery in an ischemic heart. Valsalva maneuvers such as bearing down, pain, or heightened emotional responses may stimulate the vagus nerve, causing a decrease in heart rate and electrical conduction through the heart. In contrast to healthy hearts, myocardium scarred from ischemia with a concomitant reduced blood supply cannot compensate for a drop in heart rate and cardiac output. Pain from procedures such as chest tube insertion or sheath pulling from angiography can cause local excitation of the vagus nerve, resulting in bradycardia and hypotension, called a vasovagal reaction. Precautionary treatments to avoid overstimulation of the parasympathetic nervous system include small frequent feedings, stool softeners and laxatives, analgesics prior to painful procedures, and avoidance of Valsalva maneuvers.

Pharmacologic Management of Coronary Artery Disease

Beta- (β-) Adrenergic Blocking (β-blockers) Agents

Inhibiting adrenergic stimulation by competitively binding sympathetic receptors with β-adrenergic blocking agents has been shown to reduce myocardial ventilation oxygen consumption (MVO_2). β-adrenergic blockers reduce heart rate at rest, attenuate heart rate with exercise, decrease myocardial fiber stretch and contractility, oppose platelet aggregation, and stabilize myocardial cellular membranes, thus, reducing dysrhythmia occurrence. These actions slow the heart rate and decrease the oxygen demand. Whether administered intravenously (IV) or orally, early β-adrenergic blocker therapy in the setting of AMI reduces infarct size, malignant ventricular dysrhythmia occurrence, chest pain, risk of cardiac arrest, and mortality without a greater incidence of heart failure or heart block. Because the risk of mortality is highest during the first year, therapy should begin soon after the first IV dose and continue for at least a year. When β-adrenergic blocker therapy is discontinued, the drug should be weaned down with decreasing doses.

Contraindications and reasons for discontinuing therapy include hypotension, sinus bradycardia, bronchial asthma, AV nodal dysfunction, claudication (pain in legs from peripheral arterial disease), and hyperglycemia from diabetes. Patients should be advised against abruptly discontinuing β-adrenergic blocking agents. Long-term therapy results in an increase in the number, affinity, and sensitivity of β-receptors. When no longer blocked, unopposed sympathetic stimulation is heightened, producing rebound tachycardia, hypertension, exacerbation of angina, ventricular ectopy, and greater risk of MI.

Angiotensin-Converting Enzyme Inhibitors

Low-dose angiotensin-converting enzyme inhibitors (ACEIs) that are started within 24 hours and continued indefinitely are part of the recommended therapy for patients suffering from an AMI because they reduce mortality and the incidence of left ventricular dysfunction and reinfarction. ACEIs are thought to be beneficial through a number of mechanisms: (1) increased production of superoxides by decreasing angiotensin II; (2) increasing endogenous nitric oxide, which increases vasodilation; and (3) positive influence on hemodynamic load, vascular function, myocardial remodeling (p. 958), and neurohumoral regulation. Side effects include hypotension, angioedema, persistent cough, and reduced creatinine clearance.

Angiotensin II Receptor Blockers in Myocardial Infarction

Angiotensin II receptor blockers (ARBs) have not been shown to be superior to ACEI alone or synergistic when added to ACEI, but they are recommended for patients who are intolerant of ACEI therapy.

Nitrate Therapy

Nitrate therapy is a staple in drug management of occlusive coronary syndromes, regardless of the underlying mechanism triggering ischemia. Administration of nitrates causes the vascular smooth muscles to relax, resulting in dilation of venous, coronary, and, to a lesser degree, peripheral arterial vessels. Nitroglycerin dilates areas of arterial stenosis, especially in eccentric lesions, and can relieve spontaneous coronary vasospasm directly or possibly through the release of prostacyclin, another potent vasodilator, which improves collateral flow to ischemic areas. Nitroglycerin also has been shown to inhibit platelet aggregation, inhibit platelet adhesion, and cause disbursement of formed platelet clumps.

Nitrates are used alone or in combination with beta-adrenergic blockers or calcium-channel blockers to reduce the frequency and duration of angina symptoms, incidence of silent ischemia/MI, and to improve exercise tolerance. Short-term benefits of IV nitroglycerin with UA and AMI are improved hemodynamics, decreased frequency and duration of symptoms, reduced infarct size, better patency rates following reperfusion therapy, greater residual left ventricular function, and decreased mortality. Long-term benefits of nitrate therapy on mortality and incidence of AMI in patients with symptomatic and asymptomatic ischemia have not been determined. Long-acting nitrates such as oral, ointment, or patch preparations are used to treat patients with symptomatic CAD prophylactically. Faster acting nitrates such as sublingual tablets or spray-on nitroglycerin are used as needed to alleviate breakthrough angina. Patients are instructed to take up to 3 sublingual tablets or sprays spaced 5 minutes apart to relieve anginal attacks, which can be repeated in 30 minutes if symptoms return. If symptoms do not abate or symptoms return despite rest and/or treatment, patients are instructed to call 911. Nitrates cannot be used within 24 hours after ingesting sildenafil citrate (Viagra) or like products because of the risk of severe vasodilation and death.

Other potential side effects of nitrate administration include reflex tachycardia, hypotension, headache, facial flushing, syncope, and cerebral ischemia. Over-the-counter analgesics usually relieve nitroglycerin-induced headaches. Patients should be cautioned about the potential for hypotension and reflex tachycardia when changing position from lying to standing.

Vasodilator Therapy to Relieve Vasoconstriction or Vasospasm

Nitroglycerin is the drug of choice for relief of coronary vasoconstriction during chronic and acute myocardial ischemic syndromes. Sodium nitroprusside also produces coronary artery vasodilation. Unlike nitroglycerin, which is selective for venous and larger arterial beds, sodium nitroprusside affects only arterial vessels. Sodium nitroprusside is recommended as a second-line vasodilator if satisfactory blood pressure control is not obtained with nitroglycerin and as the first-line therapy in the setting of AMI complicated with hypertension or acute heart failure.

Calcium-channel blockers, such as diltiazem hydrochloride (Cardizem), are used in combination with nitrates in patients with Prinzmetal, or variant, angina to produce smooth muscle relaxation.

Thrombolytic Agents

Fibrinolytic therapy (treatment with thrombolytics) has been shown to successfully establish reperfusion to the infarct-related artery in a timely fashion. This has allowed myocardial muscle salvage, which has decreased the overall mortality rate for patients with an AMI. Important general principles that guide the administration of thrombolytics are (1) contraindications, (2) timing of medication to time of event, and (3) monitoring for adverse reactions. Certain patient characteristics must be considered before administering thrombolytics. Essentially, patients who are at risk for bleeding because of recent use of blood thinners, who have a history of recent bleeding complications, or who are hemodynamically unstable may be considered ineligible for thrombolytic therapy.

An important aspect of administration of fibrinolytic therapy is the delay from symptom onset to treatment. Every hour past symptom onset decreases the survival benefit of thrombolytic therapy. Past 12 hours, thrombolytic administration is associated with a greater risk of complications.

Adverse reactions primarily include anaphylactic reactions, bleeding, and hemodynamic instability. Nurses must watch for signs and symptoms of an allergic reaction, which include rash, wheezing, shortness of breath, flushing, and hypotension. Patients should be monitored for signs of bleeding not only from obvious sites such as IV catheter sites but also from mucous membranes of the oral pharynx, gums, nose, lungs, and rectum. Neurological and vital sign checks should be performed according to institution protocol, monitoring for signs of intracranial hemorrhage and hemodynamic instability.

Anticoagulation Therapy

Anticoagulation therapies counteract thrombus formation in one or more of the following ways: deactivation of platelets, blocking of protein expression necessary for activation of the clotting cascade, and neutralization of thrombin generation or activity.

Antiplatelet agents deactivate platelets by either interfering with the production, release, or function of platelet-derived stimulants or the binding of GP IIb/IIIa receptors. Acetylsalicylic acid (aspirin), clopidogrel bisulfate (Plavix), prasugrel (Effient), and GP IIb/IIIa inhibitors form the constellation of antiplatelet agents currently used to treat ACS. Aspirin has proven to be the most cost effective and least adverse antiplatelet agent used to date. It is effective in risk reduction with MIs and sudden death in patients with angina; reduced recurrence of ischemic symptoms in patients with UA; and reduced infarct size, rates of reinfarction, and mortality in patients with MI. Although commonly used alone as prophylaxis against thrombus formation in patients with stable CAD, aspirin is frequently used in combination with other antiplatelet agents in circumstances in which there is a definite risk of plaque rupture.

Clopidrogrel bisulfate (Plavix) and prasugrel (Effient) are thienopyridines that inhibit the platelet-stimulating effects of ADP. They may be more effective than ASA in preventing thrombus formation following endothelial injury in that they inhibit both platelet adhesion and intimal proliferation. Clopidrogrel in combination with ASA has been shown to reduce recurrent coronary events in the ACS population, although the response to clopidogrel varies among patients and clopidogrel resistance has been observed (Kushner et al., 2009).

Adhesion of platelets to one another is dependent on fibrinogen contact with GP IIb/IIIa. Three intravenous GP IIb/IIIa antagonists are used in clinical practice: abciximab (ReoPro), eptifibatide (Integrilin), and tirofiban hydrochloride (Aggrastat). Abciximab is different from the others in that it is a monoclonal antibody that binds irreversibly to the GP IIb/IIIa receptor. Once given, the antiplatelet effects of abciximab cannot be reversed despite administration of new platelets. Abciximab only lasts the 7- to 10-day life cycle of the platelet. Eptifibatide and tirofiban are synthetic nonpeptide antagonists that compete with fibrinogen to bind with GP IIb/IIIa receptors. Unlike abciximab, the antiplatelet effects of eptifibatide and tirofiban can be reversed by withholding administration for 2 to 4 hours. Bleeding is the major complication; prevention of bleeding requires close monitoring and patient education. One major disadvantage of the GP IIb/IIIa blocking agents is that there is currently no simple, inexpensive method to monitor the extent of receptor blockade, which would allow dose titration and possibly reduce side effects.

Intravenous heparin is a combination of heparins with various densities and weights. Using heparin doses adjusted according to patient weight and level of anticoagulation as measured by activated partial thromboplastin time (aPTT) produces better results with less bleeding complications. Most sources suggest a therapeutic aPTT range of 1.5 to 2 times control, which is reported in seconds. The aPTT should be drawn every 4 to 6 hours until therapeutic range is achieved. Standardized nomograms, or dosing scales, which prescribe how and when to adjust heparin infusions based on aPTT values are beneficial to nurses responsible for heparin titration.

In summary, pharmacologic and nonpharmacologic measures to decrease oxygen demand and increase supply form the mainstay of initial management guidelines for patients with presenting signs of CAD, with resulting clinical manifestations of angina and ACS. See the Pharmacology Summary of Medications Used to Treat Coronary Disease box.

Intra-Aortic Balloon Pump

An intra-aortic balloon pump (IABP) may be used as an adjunct treatment for patients with ongoing ischemia, for those with complications related to AMI, and in high-risk patients who require prophylactic protection against ischemia before or during diagnostic, interventional, or surgical procedures. The IABP employs a large catheter with a balloon, which is inserted into the aorta between the left subclavian artery and the renal arteries' take-off branches. The balloon is inflated during the diastolic phase of the cardiac cycle and deflated right before systolic ejection. Inflating the balloon during diastole creates an elevated perfusion pressure back to the coronary artery located off the aortic route (McCulloch, 2010). This elevated perfusion pressure increases coronary blood flow, thereby enhancing oxygen delivery. The balloon is deflated during the contraction phase of the cardiac cycle so that ventricular pressure opens the aortic valve and blood is ejected out into the aorta.

PHARMACOLOGY Summary of Medications Used to Treat Coronary Artery Disease

Animation: Propranolol

Medication Category and Action	Application/Indication	Nursing Responsibility
Dihydropyridine calcium-channel blockers: Amlodipine (Norvasc) Felodipine (Plendil) Nicardipine (Cardene) Nifedipine (Procardia) ***Action:*** Dihydropyridines bind reversibly to closed type calcium channels to make them unresponsive to depolarization. **Nondihydropyridine calcium-channel blockers:** Diltiazem (Cardizem, Dilacor) Verapamil (Calan) ***Action:*** Nondihydropyridines are chemically different from the dihydropyridines as they bind to open type calcium channel blockers and slow repolarization.	Hypertension Chronic stable angina Vasospastic angina Hypertension Chronic stable angina Vasospastic angina Unstable angina	Monitor blood pressure regularly when drug is initiated and when dosage is titrated. Hold the drug and notify the health care provider if the systolic blood pressure is less than 90 mmHg. Monitor for: Elevated blood glucose Gingival hyperplasia Palpitations, weight gain, peripheral edema, skin rashes. Teach the patient to avoid grapefruit and grapefruit juice because of potential drug–food interaction.
Nitrates: Nitroglycerin (NTG) Isosorbide dinitrate (Iso-Bid, Isordil) Isosorbide mononitrate (Imdur, Nitro-Bid) ***Action:*** Potent vasodilator, leading to relaxation of both arterial and venous smooth muscle. Reduces preload to the heart. Lowers myocardial oxygen demand. Dilates coronary arteries.	Angina Hypertension Heart failure Acute pulmonary edema Acute myocardial infarction	Monitor blood pressure regularly when drug is initiated and when dosage is titrated. Hold the drug and notify the health care provider if the systolic blood pressure is less than 90 mmHg. Monitor for: Headache Orthostatic hypotension. Teach the patient to avoid sildenafil and other sildenafil-type drugs because of the risk of profound hypotension.
Beta-Adrenegic Blockers: Nonselective beta-adrenergic blockers: Nadolol (Corgard) Pindolol (Visken) Propranolol (Inderal) Sotalol (Betapace) Timolol (Blocadren) ***Action:*** Nonselective: Causes a decrease in blood pressure through a mixture of beta-blocking effects but does not cause reflex tachycardia or decreased heart rate. **Selective beta-adrenergic blockers:** Acebutolol (Sectral) Atenolol (Tenormin) Bisoprolol (Zebeta) Esmolol (Brevibloc) Metoprolol (Lopressor) ***Action:*** Selective: Completely blocks beta-1 receptor stimulation in cardiac smooth muscle.	Hypertension Dysrhythmias Angina pectoris Hypertension Heart failure Stable angina Myocardial infarction	Monitor blood pressure and heart rate regularly when drug is initiated and when dosage is titrated. Hold the drug and notify the health care provider if the systolic blood pressure is less than 90 mmHg and/or the heart rate is less than 60 per minute. Monitor for: Bradycardia Elevated blood glucose. Teach the patient to avoid abruptly stopping beta-adrenergic blocker agents.
Angiotensin-converting enzyme (ACE) inhibitors: Benazepril (Lotensin) Captopril (Capoten) Enalapril (Vasotec) Fosinopril (Monopril) Lisinopril (Prinivil, Zestril) Quinapril (Accupril) Ramipril (Altace) ***Action:*** Inhibits the conversion of angiotensin I to angiotensin II; suppresses renin-angiotensin-aldosterone system.	Hypertension Heart failure Acute myocardial infarction	Monitor blood pressure regularly when drug is initiated and when dosage is titrated. Hold the drug and notify the health care provider if the systolic blood pressure is less than 90 mmHg. Monitor for: Orthostatic hypotension Elevated serum sodium, potassium, and/or creatinine Angioedema of the extremities, face, lips, tongue, glottis, and larynx Drug-induced neutropenia. Teach the patient to avoid over-the-counter NSAIDs, as they can reduce the effectiveness of ACE inhibitors.

(continued)

Animation: Nifedipine

PHARMACOLOGY Summary of Medications Used to Treat Coronary Artery Disease, *continued*

Medication Category and Action	Application/Indication	Nursing Responsibility
Angiotensin II receptor blockers (ARBs): Candesartan (Atacand) Eprosartan (Teveten) Irbesartan (Avapro) Losartan (Cozaar) Valsartan (Diovan) ***Action:*** Blocks the vasoconstrictor and aldosterone-secreting effects of angiotensin.	Hypertension Heart failure	Monitor blood pressure regularly when drug is initiated and when dosage is titrated. Hold the drug and notify the health care provider if the systolic blood pressure is less than 90 mmHg. Monitor for: Orthostatic hypotension Elevated serum sodium, potassium and creatinine.
Lipid-Lowering Therapy		
HMG-CoA reductase inhibitors (statins): Atorvastatin (Lipitor) Lovastatin (Mevacor) Simvastatin (Zocor) Pravastatin (Pravachol) Fluvastatin (Lescol) Rosuvastatin (Crestor) ***Action:*** Inhibits HMG-CoA reductase enzyme, thereby preventing the formation of cholesterol in the liver. Statins lower total cholesterol, low-density lipoproteins–cholesterol (LDL-C), and triglycerides while increasing high-density lipoprotein–cholesterol (HDL-C). Statins have also been connected with stabilizing *rupture-prone* atherosclerotic plaque, thereby improving vasomotor tone, decreasing levels of proinflammatory proteins, decreasing factors that contribute to thrombosis, and improving myocardial perfusion.	Hyperlipidemia	Monitor for: Muscle pain, tenderness, or weakness Jaundice of the skin and eyes Abdominal pain, nausea, vomiting, anorexia, skin rash or hives Elevated CK levels, liver function tests (LFTs). Teach the patient to take statins in the evening because cholesterol biosynthesis is higher at night. Teach the patient to avoid grapefruit and grapefruit juice to avoid drug–food interaction.
Resins, or bile acid sequestrants: Cholestyramine (Questran) Colestipol (Colestid) Colesevelam (WelChol) ***Action:*** Binds with cholesterol-containing bile acids in the intestines and are then eliminated via stool.	Hyperlipidemia	Monitor for: Gastric distress, nausea, vomiting, increased bruising, tarry stools, or abnormal bleeding.
Fibrates: Gemfibrozil (Lopid) Fenofibrate (Tricor) ***Action:*** Lowers triglycerides and can increase HDL-C levels.	Hyperlipidemia	Monitor for: Increased bruising, epistaxis, hematuria Jaundice of the skin and eyes Upper abdominal pain, nausea, vomiting.
Antihyperlipidemics: Ezetimibe (Zetia) Ezetimibe/Simvastatin (Zetia and Zocor) Combination drugs: Ezetimibe and simvastatin (Vytorin) Work best when given with statin ***Action:*** Ezetimibe: Reduces blood cholesterol by inhibiting the absorption of cholesterol at the small intestine. This will decrease the level of cholesterol delivered to the liver. Simvastatin: Inhibits HMG-CoA reductase enzyme, thereby decreasing cholesterol production; increases HDL-C and decreases VLDL and triglycerides.	Hyperlipidemia	Monitor for: Abdominal pain, diarrhea, arthralgia. Instruct the patient not to take concurrently with bile acid sequestrants.

PHARMACOLOGY Summary of Medications Used to Treat Coronary Artery Disease, *continued*

Medication Category and Action	Application/Indication	Nursing Responsibility
Niacin: B vitamin ***Action:*** In high doses, lowers triglycerides and LDL-C levels, and increases HDL-C.		Monitor for: Flushing, nausea, pruritis, and bloating. Teach patient that taking one ASA 30 minutes prior to taking niacin can reduce uncomfortable flushing.
Fibrinolytic (thrombolytic) Therapy		
Tenecteplase (TNKase) Alteplase (Activase, tPA) Reteplase (Retavase) ***Action:*** Modified human tissue plasminogen activator that binds to fibrin and converts plasminogen to plasmin. It is fibrin specific, thus decreasing the systemic activation of plasminogen.	Acute ST segment elevation myocardial infarction (STEMI)	Monitor for: Excessive bleeding Hematoma Other bleeding, such as gum bleeding, epistaxis, oozing from puncture sites.
Antiplatelet Agents		
Acetylsalicylic acid aspirin (ASA) ***Action:*** Impairs hepatic synthesis of blood coagulation factors VII, IX, and X and possible inhibiting action of vitamin K.	Acute myocardial infarction (AMI) Prevention of AMI recurrence	Monitor for bleeding and increased bruising. Chewable aspirin is better absorbed and suppositories can be safely used if nausea, vomiting, or known upper-gastrointestinal disorders are present.
ADP receptor blockers: Clopidogrel (Plavix) Prasugrel (Effient) ***Action:*** Inhibits platelet aggregation by selectively preventing the binding of adenosine diphosphate to its platelet receptor.	Secondary prevention of MI Reduction in thrombosis formation after coronary artery stent placement	Monitor for: Bleeding, increased bruising, and gastrointestinal distress.
Glycoprotein IIb/IIIa blockers: Eptifibatide (Integrilin) Abciximab (ReoPro) Tirofiban (Aggrastat) ***Action:*** Binds the IIb/IIIa receptor sites on platelets, preventing fibrinogen and von Willebrand factor from adhering to the platelet.	Unstable angina Acute myocardial infarction Percutaneous coronary intervention	Monitor for bleeding and thrombocytopenia. Stop infusion if bleeding occurs and notify health care provider.

Sources: Adams, M. P., & Koch, R. W. (2010). *Pharmacology: Connections to nursing practice.* Upper Saddle River, NJ: Pearson; Bhatt, D. (2009). Prasugrel in clinical practice. *New England Journal of Medicine, 361*(10), 940–942.

The deflation of the balloon just before systole creates a suction effect within the vessel that helps pull more blood from the left ventricle and decreases the resistance the blood encounters when leaving the heart (afterload). A lowered afterload resistance decreases the heart's workload and enhances forward ejection of blood. The goal in using an intra-aortic balloon pump is to increase the supply of oxygen to the myocardium and decrease the demand (Figure 32–21◆).

Medical Management of Complications of Acute Myocardial Infarction

When myocardial blood flow is cut off for longer than 20 to 40 minutes, a dynamic process of apoptosis is initiated that extends over several hours. Cell necrosis produces a loss of cell membrane integrity and degradation of connection tissue, which in turn causes cell swelling, protein leakage, and changes in cellular structure and function. In response, systemic catecholamine stimulation raises MVO_2 and taxes nonischemic tissue. With reestablishment of flow, initially cell necrosis continues and cell disruption and death ensue. After apoptosis, myocardial tissue undergoes remodeling characterized by the deposition of collagen in place of normal myocytes, muscle thinning, and dilation. These pathologic changes result in a myriad of complications that include recurrent angina, ventricular failure, dysrhythmias, and mechanical defects.

Recurrent Chest Pain from Ischemia

Chest pain that reemerges 12 hours to 6 days after an AMI, waxes and wanes, and is sometimes called stuttering or recurrent chest pain may represent infarct extension. Recurrence of angina during recovery from AMI may depict coronary flow instability within the infarct-related artery. Pain, the most sensitive indicator of infarct extension, may be accompanied by ECG changes, myocardial serum marker elevation (CK-MB, troponin I, and troponin T), hemodynamic instability, dysrhythmias, or worsening heart failure. Medical management for recurrent ischemic pain includes IV nitroglycerin, beta-adrenergic blockers, and calcium-channel blockers. Continuing ischemic symptoms that are not controlled by medical management necessitate angiography to discern whether coronary occlusion is the cause and determine the appropriateness of repeat reperfusion therapy.

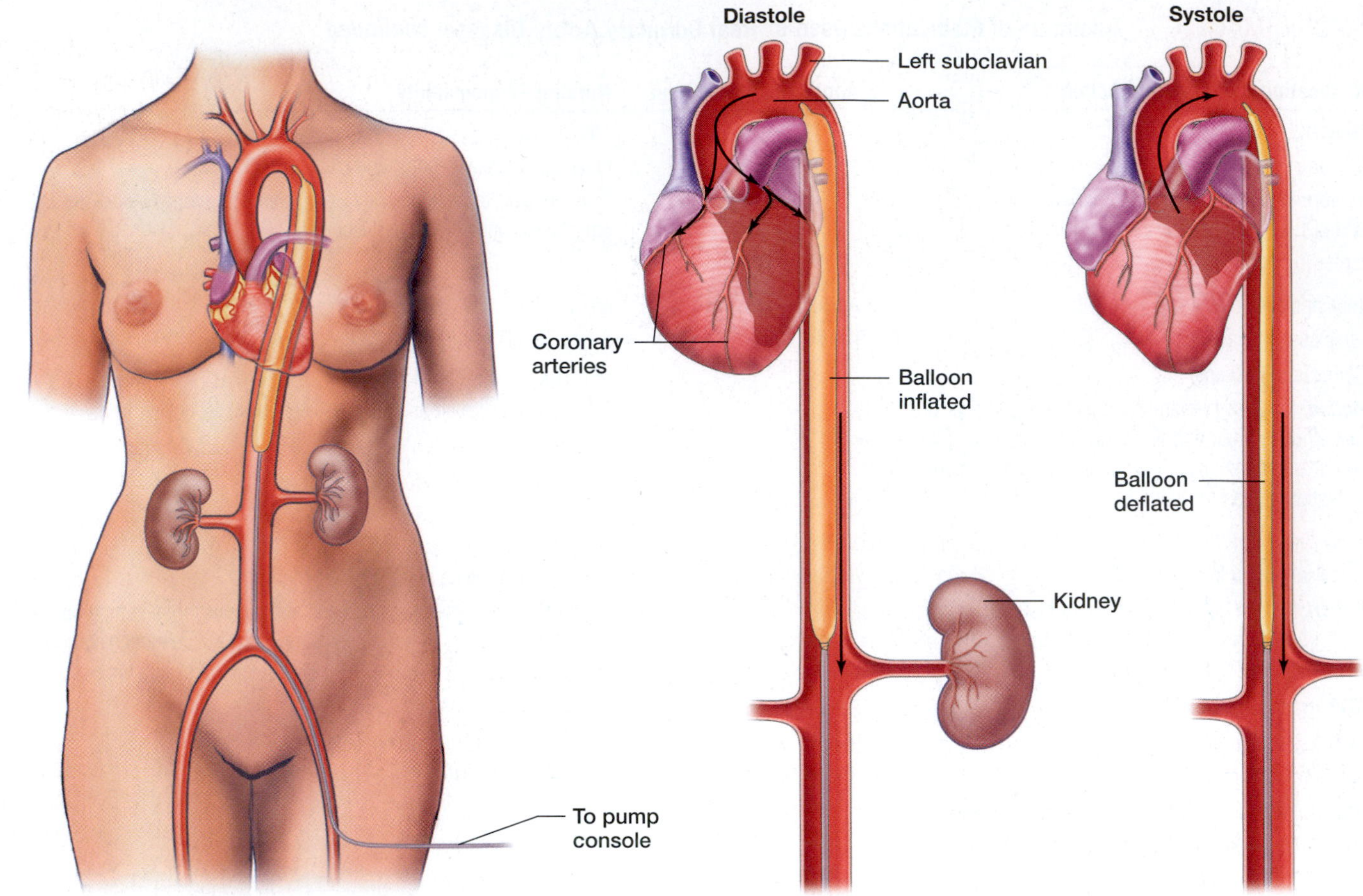

FIGURE 32–21 ◆ Intra-aortic balloon pump catheter.

Pericarditis

Extension of myocardial wall necrosis through to the epicardium causes pericardial inflammation in some post-MI patients. It can occur early or later in AMI. Early or acute pericarditis occurs 48 to 72 hours after an AMI and is associated with larger infarcts and lower ejection fractions. Dressler's syndrome (post-MI syndrome) connotes pericarditis that occurs 2 to 12 weeks after MI; it is thought to be an autoimmune or immunologic response to antimyocardial antibodies produced by myocardial necrosis (Moser & Riegel, 2008; Woods et al., 2010). Pericarditis often presents with pain accompanied by pericardial friction rub, pericardial effusion, dyspnea, fever, elevated erythrocyte sedimentation rate (ESR), leukocytosis, and ECG changes of J point elevation with concave upward ST segment elevation in all leads except aVR and V_1, persistently elevated T waves, or inverted T wave reversal. Absence of elevated CK-MB levels, symptom qualities, and ECG characteristics help to differentiate pericarditis from ischemic pain. Pericarditis is discussed in detail in Chapter 33.

Cardiogenic Shock

The incidence of cardiogenic shock following an AMI is 7% and occurs when more than 40% of the left ventricle is infarcted, usually with severe three-vessel disease (Woods et al., 2010). Despite available treatment, mortality remains high. Cardiogenic shock is discussed in Chapter 54.

Infarct Expansion, Ventricular Remodeling

Infarct expansion is the process of ventricular wall thinning and elongation of the infarct zone, which produces ventricular dyskinesia. Ischemia causes cellular inflammation, edema, and cell slippage, resulting in myocardial fibril changes. Ischemia also causes myocardial cell fibers to become soft and distensible and to rearrange in a wavy pattern, which results in a paradoxical fiber lengthening and wall bulging during systole and shortening during diastole. Eventually fibroblast proliferation causes collagen deposition and scar formation. Myofibrils are stretched and elongated and new fibrils are added, resulting in ventricular hypertrophy. The two processes of infarct expansion and ventricular hypertrophy cause ventricular remodeling, which can lead to development of heart failure and/or left ventricular rupture (Moser & Riegel, 2008; Woods et al., 2010). Myocardial **remodeling** is the process of replacing nonviable heart muscle tissue with nonelastic fibrinous collagen, which causes cardiac wall thinning, dilation, and subsequently an impaired ability for the ventricles to function normally. Myocardial remodeling begins in the early stages of infarction and can continue for months and years. It is a predictor of increased mortality.

Limiting infarct size and maintaining patency of the infarct-related artery with reperfusion therapies are two primary strategies for preventing ventricular remodeling. Clinicians should avoid the administration of drugs that inhibit healing and scar formation, such as steroids, indomethacin, and ibuprofen. Reducing ventricular wall stress by decreasing preload with NTG and afterload with an intra-aortic balloon pump (p. 954) and angiotensin-converting enzyme (ACE) inhibition medications is another means of limiting the extent of ventricular remodeling. Reduction in afterload and preload limits myocardial wall stress and subsequent infarct expansion and ventricular hypertrophy.

Left Ventricular Aneurysm and Thrombus Formation

Left ventricular aneurysm is a potential consequence of infarct expansion and remodeling. Aneurysm formation is associated with a greater risk of death, heart failure, angina, ventricular dysrhythmias, and embolization. Symptomatic patients may require temporary medical measures such as inotropic- and afterload-reducing agents, followed by surgical resection and/or endoventricular patching of the aneurysm, provided that their remaining myocardial function is normal.

Mitral Valve Disruption

Papillary muscle ischemia can cause valve leaflet regurgitation or complete rupture, which accounts for 5% of deaths from MI (Moser & Riegel, 2008; Woods et al., 2010). The posterior medial papillary muscle is affected more frequently because it receives its blood supply only from the posterior descending artery (Figure 32–22◆). Rupture can be complete, in which case rapid partial or total hemodynamic collapse ensues. Diagnosis of mitral valve disruption is made by two-dimensional echocardiography (Chapter 33) or cardiac catheterization (p. 940) with ventriculography. Afterload reduction with vasodilation therapy and intra-aortic balloon therapy (p. 954), preload reduction using nitrates and diuretics, and inotropic support may be necessary to stabilize the patient medically. Severe mitral valve disruption is treated with mitral valve repair or complete valve replacement. The diagnosis and treatment of valve disease are discussed in Chapter 33.

Ventricular Free Wall Rupture

Often fatal, rupture of the myocardial wall can be a result of an acute tear or a slow, incomplete rupture. It occurs in 1% to 3% of AMI patients and accounts for 10% of deaths from MI (Moser & Riegel, 2008; Woods et al., 2010). Administration of thrombolytic therapy and intravenous β-adrenergic blockers has been linked to a decreased incidence of myocardial rupture following a MI. Surgical repair is the only definitive treatment.

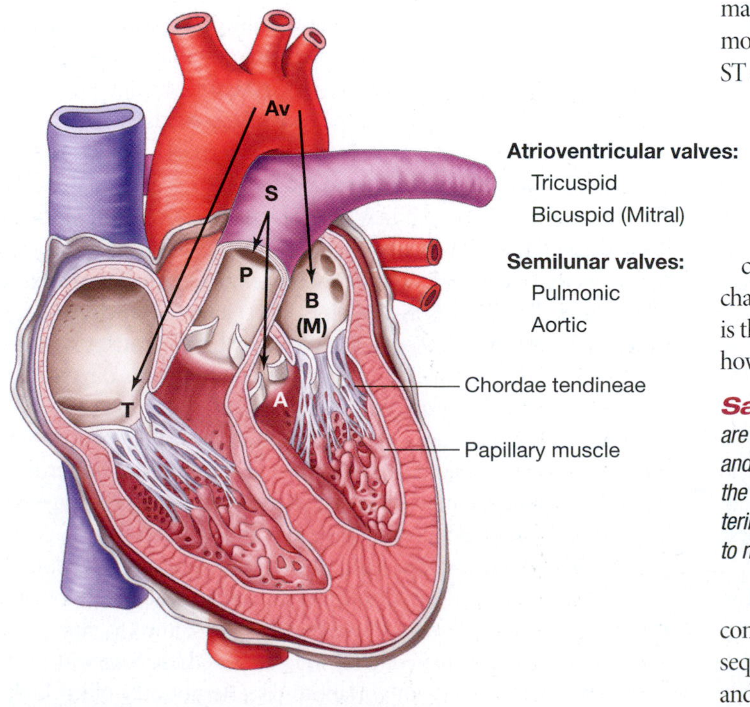

FIGURE 32–22 ◆ Structures supporting the valves.

Ventricular Septal Defect

Rupture of the ventricular septum results in a left-to-right shunting of the blood with symptoms of chest pain, syncope, and hypotension. Patients can quickly develop pulmonary edema and cardiogenic shock. Medical treatment includes the use of diuretics, vasodilators, inotropic agents, and intra-aortic balloon therapy aimed at decreasing the amount of blood shunted from left to right and increasing forward flow. Emergency surgical repair involves debridement of infarcted tissue and suture of a tissue or Dacron patch to healthy septal tissue.

Nursing Management

Nurses caring for AMI patients must understand when and how to intervene to decrease the heart's workload by increasing oxygen supply and decreasing oxygen demand. Nursing management of patients admitted to an intensive care unit (ICU) depends on which method was used to reestablish coronary blood flow.

For patients treated medically, care is aimed at reducing myocardial oxygen demand, monitoring for signs indicative of adequate myocardial oxygen supply, administering and titrating medications to balance oxygen demand and supply, monitoring for and managing complications, and teaching patients. Hemodynamic monitoring with a pulmonary artery catheter and intra-arterial pressure line (both discussed in Chapter 29) is warranted for patients presenting with severe or progressive heart failure or pulmonary edema, cardiogenic shock or progressive hypotension, or suspected mechanical/structural complications, as well as those who are being treated with vasoactive agents that affect blood pressure and therefore require medication titration. Continuous cardiac monitoring in leads that will show ischemia or dysrhythmias is required.

Intra-aortic balloon pump therapy may be needed to reduce myocardial oxygen demand in the presence of heart failure, cardiogenic shock, or complications following an AMI. The nurse will assess laboratory tests such as complete blood count, chemistry panels, and coagulation profiles to prevent complications and monitor the patient's response to treatments. The nurse also will evaluate serial ECGs and serum cardiac markers. Patients who have received thrombolytic therapy should be monitored for clinical signs of reperfusion including chest pain and ST segment elevation (p. 930).

Patients should be encouraged to inform the nurse of any new onset of chest pain or symptoms that were the same as those that occurred with the AMI. Anginal-type pain such as burning and pressure must be communicated between care providers. In many instances, health care providers supply the nursing staff with contingency orders to be followed if certain complications such as a change in blood pressure, chest pain, or cardiac dysrhythmias occur. It is the nurse's responsibility to understand when to use these orders and how to assess the patient for effectiveness of the treatment.

Safety Alert *A health care provider may give contingency orders that are to be implemented for a given clinical manifestation. An example is NTG and 12-lead ECG orders for the occurrence of chest pain. It is important that the nurse understands the importance of obtaining the ECG prior to administering the NTG because the medication will cause the ST segment to return to normal, thus losing important diagnostic information.*

Patients are categorized as having either high or low potential for complications, as well as either actual presence or absence of adverse sequelae. These categories determine the degree and duration of care and the aggressiveness of the required treatment. For example, patients with no complications are low risk and can be fast-tracked within 24 to

48 hours to a lower level of care and may be discharged early. Patients with secondary complications and active comorbid diseases are at higher risk and will require longer hospital stays in areas with cardiac and hemodynamic monitoring capabilities.

No empiric data define the level of care the patient should receive once discharged from an area of intensive monitoring. Given that the risk of sudden death is highest during the first 48 hours post-AMI and that intrahospital transfers can precipitate dysrhythmias, continuous cardiac monitoring for the first 48 hours of the hospital stay and/or the first 24 hours after discharge from the ICU is warranted. Other care needs during convalescence on a step-down, telemetry, or intermediate unit for the AMI patient are the same as those outlined for patients with UA, with the exception of added attention to monitoring the response to progressive activity in AMI patients.

The assessment data, which include sample questions specific to ACS, are found in the Nursing Process: Patient Care Plan for Acute Coronary Syndrome box. Nursing diagnoses are developed from the assessment data and follow the assessment in the first column of the Nursing Process: Patient Care Plan box. This provides a comprehensive care plan for a patient with ACS in the acute period. Documentation of patient conditions is essential in order to assess normal progress following an AMI.

Collaborative Management

Patients who have experienced an AMI often recover best when a multidisciplinary approach is put into place. These patients benefit from several subspecialties such as physical therapy, respiratory therapy, dietitians, social workers, and, of course, the cardiologist and nurse. In order to meet desired patient outcomes, it is essential that this interdisciplinary team communicate openly with one another in developing and evaluating care of the patient and family (IOM [Institute of Medicine], 2010).

A patient who has suffered a large MI can spend several days to a few weeks in the hospital. When this happens, the patient becomes weak from being in bed for such a long period of time and because the heart cannot function at its previous level. Physical therapists can help bridge this gap and get the patient ambulating and performing activities of daily living before discharge so that she may function at home. Furthermore, they can help transition the patient into a cardiac rehabilitation program. Associated with prolonged bed rest comes the high risk of developing a respiratory infection. The respiratory therapist plays a key role in daily pulmonary toileting to prevent any nosocomial respiratory infections. The dietitian focuses on proper in-hospital nutritional support as well as educating the patient and family about dietary changes at home. The dietitian emphasizes the need for a cardiac diet that is low in fat, cholesterol, and sodium. The social worker and discharge planner cannot go unnoticed in this collaborative approach. Often, the MI patient has a type A or D behavior pattern (see Chapter 29), is in denial, and is suffering from depression. Although the cardiologist can order some pharmacologic intervention, it is the social worker who can work best with these patients to help them understand their situation and learn more effective coping mechanisms. They can assist these patients with behavior modification.

The constant and consistent care provided by the nurse is the main link to these other disciplines. Only the nurse can provide an ongoing assessment of the patient and the patient's response to these interventions. It is important that nurses recognize that they are the link and help collaborate all of these services.

Health Promotion

The nurse is in a unique position to help in early treatment of the patient with a MI in a number of ways. First, nurses can collaborate with the community and establish educational programs that bring community awareness around the subject of timely treatment. Included in this is early recognition of symptoms and prompt initiation of emergency medical services. Nurses also can participate by teaching cardiopulmonary resuscitation so that, when an individual is experiencing life-threatening cardiac events, measures are being taken to increase the chance of survival.

Once the patient enters the hospital system, the nurse plays a key role in ensuring timely treatment. The nurse can advocate on behalf of the patient to the health care provider. The nurse's physical assessment, as well as her interpretation of the ECG and laboratory tests, is vital in deciding the appropriate reperfusion strategy for the patient. Once the patient is discharged, the nurse plays a vital role in educating the patient and family in the recovery process. It is often the cardiac rehabilitation nurse who "walks" patients through lifestyle changes, behavior modification, and an exercise program to promote a full recovery. The nurse in this role teaches classes to small groups to educate them on topics such as nutrition, exercise, stress reduction, and even some new alternative therapies such as yoga, herbal medicines, and even acupuncture. It is important to include the family or another support system the patient has in this process so that others also can support optimal recovery. The Patient Teaching & Discharge Priorities box (p. 963) presents the discharge needs for patients who have experienced a cardiac event.

Gerontological Considerations

Older adults make up the fastest growing portion of the American population. As a person ages, his heart undergoes physiological changes. These changes include stiffer ventricles due to the muscle's losing the ability to relax completely, decreased pumping function, decreased response to adrenaline, and decreased elasticity of the arteries. These changes can occur even in the absence of CAD but can be magnified in the presence of CAD.

Coronary artery disease is the leading cause of death in older adults. Although men usually have a higher rate of CAD than women during most of their lifetime, women have an equal, if not higher, rate after menopause. This may be due to the decrease in estrogen production. When an older individual experiences a heart attack, it may result in more complications and a longer hospital stay. Recovery is slower and presents many challenges. It may involve multiple systems in the body beyond just the cardiovascular system. This is often seen in patients with diabetes. Older adults also have a higher incidence of heart failure and rhythm disturbances as a result of CAD alone or in conjunction with an AMI. For this reason, it is imperative that the patient is monitored via a cardiac monitor, and nursing management is directed appropriately to any changes.

Silent heart attacks are not uncommon in older adults; this is attributed to their decreased sensation of pain. This is especially true in the diabetic population, where heart attacks can occur at any age but increase in the older population. Instead of the typical "I feel like an elephant is sitting on my chest" symptoms, these patients may experience atypical symptoms such as heartburn or gastrointestinal discomfort and shortness of breath. Older individuals grow accustomed to illness and discomfort and therefore frequently will overlook these otherwise overt symptoms. It is especially important to educate not only older adults about these symptoms but also the people who help with their daily

NURSING PROCESS: Patient Care Plan for Acute Coronary Syndrome

Assessment of Cardiac Status Using Gordon's Functional Health Patterns:

- Activity Exercise Pattern
- Cognitive Perceptual Pattern
- Nutritional Metabolic Pattern
- Coping–Stress Tolerance Pattern

Subjective Data

Assessment of Cardiac Output

Do you ever feel your heart beat fast, beat irregularly, or skip beats?

Do you ever feel light-headed?

Do you get short of breath when you walk distances?

Assessment of Fluid Status

Are you short of breath?

Do you monitor your weight?

Do you eat a lot of salt?

Do your feet swell, if so, when and under what circumstances?

Assessment of Pain

Do you have chest pain?

Does your jaw hurt or throat hurt?

Does it radiate anywhere else on your body?

Does it go away with a deep breath?

What makes the pain better or worse?

Assessment of Activity Tolerance

Are you able to complete your activities of daily living without fatigue or chest pain?

Are you able to walk up a flight of stairs without getting short of breath or experiencing chest pain?

Do you exercise on a regular basis?

Are you able to walk in the hall without experiencing fatigue, SOB, chest pain, or dizziness?

Assessment of Patient Ability to Cope

How are you feeling about your heart attack?

What are your thoughts about your future health?

Assessment of Patient/Family Knowledge of Disease and Treatment

Tell me what you know about your problems with your heart.

Tell me what you are doing about your risk factors.

Tell me about your dietary intake and your exercise program.

When do you develop chest pain and what makes it go away?

What medications are you on, when are you supposed to take them, and what are the side effects you should watch for?

When are you supposed to see your doctor?

Are you consistently participating in a cardiac rehabilitation program?

Has anyone explained your health problems to you?

Would you tell me what you know about your disease?

Objective Data

Assessment of Cardiac Output

Assess heart rate and rhythm for abnormalities.

Compare monitor to central and peripheral pulses.

Note quality of pulse (weak, bounding) at the radial site.

Monitor medications given and evaluate the patient's response, especially those given for tachycardia, bradycardia, or any dysrhythmias.

Monitor blood pressure.

Monitor respirations and SpO_2.

Assessment of Fluid Status

Assess lung sounds for rales or crackles.

Monitor blood pressure, jugular venous distention (JVD), vital signs, urine output, daily weight, and peripheral edema.

Assessment of Pain

Use a pain scale (0–10) to quantify pain level.

Assess the cultural or religious impact on the patient's response.

Assess the location, duration, and onset of pain and what provokes and relieves it.

Assessment of Activity Tolerance

Monitor vital signs (heart rate, blood pressure in both arms, mean arterial pressure, respiratory rate, oxygen saturation) before and after activity.

Assess heart sounds.

Assess lung sounds

Assessment of Patient Ability to Cope

Evaluate the patient's response to written and verbal teaching materials about the patient's heart attack.

Evaluate the patient's response to discussion about current and future health concerns.

Observe for manifestations of anxiety: restlessness, apprehension, withdrawal.

Assessment of Patient/Family Knowledge of Disease and Treatment

Patient/family may be anxious, confused, and need repeated information.

Note mistakes being made with treatment plan.

Self-care deficit due to clinical manifestations.

(*continued*)

NURSING PROCESS: Patient Care Plan for Acute Coronary Syndrome, *continued*

Subjective Data	Objective Data
How does this disease affect your daily life? Do you feel anxious about your health problems? Do you have family members or close friends who provide emotional support? Do you see your health care provider on a regular basis? Do you know what symptoms are important to report to your health care provider immediately?	

Outcomes and Evaluation Parameters	Planning and Interventions with *Rationales*
1. NURSING DIAGNOSIS: Decreased Cardiac Output ***related to dysrhythmias secondary to acute myocardial ischemia and infarction*** **(NANDA-I © 2012)**	
Outcomes: Patient maintains normal and regular heart rate and rhythm. Patient verbalizes less fear and anxiety. ***Evaluation Parameters:*** Vital signs within normal limits. Exercise endurance increases. No anginal-type chest pain. Cardiac output within normal limits. No clinical manifestations of heart failure. Alert and oriented. Lungs clear.	Monitor heart rate and rhythm. Treat symptomatic dysrhythmias as ordered by health care provider. Teach patient about antidysrhythmic medications ordered by health care provider, *to ensure proper dosages, time intervals, and evaluation of side effects.* Provide comfort measures to patient and assurance *to decrease fear and anxiety.*
2. NURSING DIAGNOSIS: Excess Fluid Volume ***related to fluid retention secondary to impaired myocardial contractility*** **(NANDA-I © 2012)**	
Outcome: Patient's body weight is within normal range; electrolytes will be maintained in normal range. ***Evaluation Parameters:*** Weight. Electrolyte values daily until stable. Lungs clear. No peripheral edema. Neck vein distention not present. Cardiac index and ejection fraction within normal limits.	Administer diuretics as ordered and teach the patient the rationale and side effects of medication. Weigh the patient daily and stress to the patient the importance of daily weights. Instruct the patient to notify the health care provider with greater than 2- to 3-pound gain. *This will allow the patient to identify weight gain from fluid.* Maintain fluid restriction and low-sodium diet as ordered in order *to decrease excess fluid accumulation.*
3. NURSING DIAGNOSIS: Acute Pain ***related to cardiac ischemia*** **(NANDA-I © 2012)**	
Outcome: Pain free or controlled with medication. ***Evaluation Parameters:*** Patient notifies nurse immediately on experiencing pain. Patient's ECG is normal and pain is relieved with sublingual NTG. Patient is able to verbalize how to take sublingual NTG and its side effects.	Instruct the patient to notify the nurse immediately of chest pain. Implement the health care provider's orders (i.e., ECG, sublingual NTG, morphine, oxygen). Teach the patient how to take sublingual nitroglycerin and note its side effects. *This encourages the patient to participate in his own care and teaches one of the most important interventions for patients with CAD.*
4. NURSING DIAGNOSIS: Activity Intolerance ***related to insufficient oxygenation secondary to decreased cardiac output*** **(NANDA-I © 2012)**	
Outcome: Patient enrolls in cardiac rehabilitation program and attends post-MI lectures. ***Evaluation Parameters:*** Patient regularly uses exercise log to record distances walked and symptoms experienced. Patient is able to monitor vital signs and adjust activity accordingly.	Encourage participation in the cardiac rehabilitation program. Teach the patient to use an exercise log to monitor distances walked and symptoms. Teach the patient how to monitor his heart rate, blood pressure, and respirations as a response to activity. *To increase endurance and strength and prevent weight gain.*
5. NURSING DIAGNOSIS: Ineffective Coping ***secondary to denial related to decreased physical status after MI*** **(NANDA-I © 2012)**	
Outcome: Patient verbalizes a decrease in problems and concerns. ***Evaluation Parameters:*** Vital signs within normal limits. Denies apprehension. Able to state an understanding of the disease process.	Determine degree of denial; do not directly confront patient's denial; support patient's behavior. Provide active listening *to assure patient you are working with her, not against her.*

NURSING PROCESS: Patient Care Plan for Acute Coronary Syndrome, *continued*

6. NURSING DIAGNOSIS: Deficient Knowledge *related to disease and treatment plan* (NANDA-I © 2012)

Outcome: Patient/family have an understanding of and comply with the treatment plan. ***Evaluation Parameters:*** Patient and family understand the treatment plan and safely become compliant. Patient and family understand the importance of risk factor control in preventing a progression of the disease. Patient and family participate in a cardiac rehabilitation program.	Describe the required diet, medications, activity, and limitations *to increase knowledge of the disease and treatment.* Describe what clinical manifestations need to be reported to the health care provider and when to access the emergency medical system *to ensure immediate care when necessary.* Have the patient/family repeat instructions *to assess understanding.* Provide information about the type, setting, cost, and location of a cardiac rehabilitation program, and assist with contacting the program *to decrease anxiety about the process.*

Source: Adapted from Wilkinson, J. M., & Ahearn, N. R. (2009). *Prentice Hall nursing diagnosis handbook* (9th ed.). Upper Saddle River, NJ: Prentice Hall.

PATIENT TEACHING & DISCHARGE PRIORITIES for Coronary Artery Disease/Acute Coronary Syndrome

Need	Teaching
Knowledge of disease process and prognosis	Provide written and verbal instructions for: • Specific diagnosis/treatment (i.e., heart catheterization procedures, PCI, stent, heart attack, heart failure, CAD) • Follow-up laboratory tests, health care provider appointments • Medications • Diet • Activity These instructions will reinforce the need to comply with therapy.
Understanding of medications	Teach the patient and family the purposes of the medications, their side effects, and their timing. These instructions will reinforce medication compliance and prevent over- or underdosing.
Safety	Stress the importance of wearing an identification bracelet to identify a heart problem to health care workers. Carry a stent identification card in a wallet to identify implant information to health care workers.
Disease prevention	Teach about dietary consumption. Stress the importance of a low-fat, low-cholesterol, low-salt diet. Teach about an exercise program. Stress the importance of exercise to prevent further CAD and keep current CAD from progressing. Offer cardiac rehabilitation program resources. Teach about behavior modification; decrease stress environment. Stress the importance of smoking cessation and offer resources for community programs.
Reportable clinical manifestations	Teach the patient to report chest pain or the anginal equivalent. Stress how to take sublingual nitroglycerin should the patient experience angina. Stress the importance of using the 911 emergency response system instead of driving self to the hospital. Teach about fatigue and shortness of breath, which may be indicators of an unstable plaque or valve problem exacerbating. Teach about dental prophylaxis if the patient was diagnosed with a valve problem or had an invasive coronary procedure.
Family/support system	Assess availability, knowledge, and compliance with the treatment regimen. Assess discharge needs (i.e., home placement, medications, driving). Involve discharge planning if specific needs are not met to offer community resources.
Emotional adjustment of patient/family	Answer questions honestly. Encourage verbalization of frustrations and anger. Encourage positive reinforcement from the family. Provide active listening. Provide additional hospital and community resources, as necessary.

care. Simple knowledge of this may prevent untoward outcomes among the older population.

Treatment options for older adults often present challenges. Different considerations are given to older adults in deciding on treatment options. For example, a patient who presents with a MI who might otherwise meet the criteria for thrombolytics may in fact *not* meet the criteria simply based on age. For example, a patient who is 75 years or older is at a higher risk for an intracranial hemorrhage than is a 50-year-old patient. The health care provider critically assesses the risk–benefit ratio in this instance, and the patient may or may not receive fibrinolytic therapy. The 50-year-old patient usually would receive fibrinolytic therapy because intracranial hemorrhage is not as great a concern in this age group. Another example that demonstrates the differences in treating older adults is a patient who presents with a ventricular dysrhythmia that might be treated with prophylactic lidocaine. Lidocaine can cause confusion and other side effects in older patients, thus negating its use in this patient population.

The management of older patients may also be different because they may be willing to accept a decrease in their quality of life. In addition, they may choose to refuse further invasive testing such as coronary angiography or bypass surgery. Instead, they may accept some degree of limitation and just be managed through medications.

Should patients choose a more invasive treatment strategy, they must be willing to accept longer hospitalizations and more complicated recovery patterns. Older patients often have other medical problems besides CAD. They also may have multiple cardiac problems as well that include hypertension, atherosclerosis, calcified valves, and rhythm disturbances. These patients may have a more complicated recovery from procedures or surgery due to renal impairment, mobility limitations, mental status changes, and poor nutrition. All of this must be considered in helping these patients to decide the pathway of care.

Lifestyle changes must not go unrecognized in older adults. Risk factor modification such as smoking cessation, weight reduction, and proper diet can have a dramatic impact on their quality of life. The American Heart Association has suggested age-appropriate measures to help promote a healthy lifestyle (AHA, 2010e). For example, physical inactivity is a modifiable risk factor for developing CAD. Lack of exercise also contributes to obesity, high blood pressure, a low level of HDL ("good") cholesterol, and diabetes. Even modest levels of physical activity are beneficial. The AHA states that a moderate amount of physical activity, preferably daily, is recommended for older adults. Healthy moderate activity for older adults includes:

- Longer sessions of moderately intense activities such as walking or swimming
- Shorter sessions of more vigorous activities such as fast walking or stair-climbing.

Surgical Management of Coronary Artery Disease

For more than three decades, **coronary artery bypass grafting (CABG)** has been a mainstay for the treatment of CAD. During this time, great advances have occurred in both technique and technology, leading to reduced rates of morbidity, mortality, and graft occlusion. Widely accepted indications for CABG include two-vessel disease with proximal LAD involvement, three-vessel disease, and left main disease, either isolated or in conjunction with other CAD. Before the decision is made to send a patient for CABG, the following factors must be carefully considered by the medical team (Patel, Dehmer, Hirshfeld, Smith, & Spertus, 2009):

- The patient's clinical presentation (stable angina, acute coronary syndrome)
- The severity of the patient's angina
- The extent of ischemia validated by noninvasive testing
- The presence of other prognostic factors such as heart failure, diabetes, or reduced LV function
- The extent of current medical therapies
- The extent of anatomical disease

Standard Operative Techniques

Standard coronary artery bypass surgery is done via a median sternotomy using cardiopulmonary bypass (CPB), cold cardioplegia solution to stop the heart, and systemic hypothermia (28° to 32°C). Cardiopulmonary bypass is a means to divert blood away from the heart and return it to the arterial system. The CPB machine temporarily performs the functions of the heart (circulation of blood) and lungs (gas exchange). This is accomplished by drainage of systemic venous blood directly to the CPB machine, through a cannula placed in the right atrium. The venous blood is then processed by the CPB machine. This entails a heat exchanger, which regulates the temperature of the blood; a filter, which does not permit air or emboli (air, thrombus, or cholesterol) to pass; and finally an oxygenator. Once the blood is oxygenated, it is returned to the body via the arterial cannula, which usually is placed in the aorta. Further protection of the heart is achieved by cooling the heart with a cardioplegic solution. Infusions of cardioplegia allow surgeons to interrupt coronary flow safely for up to 20 minutes.

Once the patient is on CPB, anastomosis, or connection, of the conduits will be done (Figure 32–23 ◆). The number of grafts usually varies from two to six. With the heart stopped, the surgeon can identify the obstructed artery. An end-to-side anastomosis is then carried out with the chosen conduit. The proximal end of the graft is then anastomosed to the aorta using a similar technique.

Some surgeons perform coronary artery bypass without using CPB. This is generally referred to as beating heart bypass. Because CPB is not used, the heart does not stop beating. Instead, mechanical stabilizers are placed on the area of the heart being bypassed to reduce motion. The advantage of this technique is the reduction of complications that can occur from CPB. The disadvantage is that the bypasses are more difficult to place accurately on a moving heart, which may lower the graft patency rate.

The left internal mammary artery (IMA) is the graft of choice due to its resistance to atherosclerosis and the ability to graft it as an *in situ* pedicle graft. This means that the artery remains connected proximally to the native subclavian artery. The 10-year patency rate for the IMA has been cited as 85% to 95% (Woods et al., 2010). Because of the success of the IMA graft and its superiority over vein grafts, some surgeons are now performing bilateral IMA grafting in nondiabetic patients. It is still too early to tell whether this will become common practice.

Vein grafts are typically the conduits used for the remaining bypasses. In most cases, the greater saphenous vein is harvested from the leg. If the greater saphenous vein is not of good quality, the lesser saphenous vein and cephalic vein can be used. Up until just recently, a patient who required multiple bypasses would require an incision that extended over the entire length of the leg. A new technique wherein the vein is retrieved using an endoscope with one to three incisions is now being used in most large medical centers. The use of this technique has great advantages, including a decrease in incidence of leg wound infections and less pain.

Because of the success of IMA grafts, surgeons are exploring the use of other arteries as conduits. The most common arterial conduit other than the IMA is the radial artery. Before using the radial artery, however, Doppler studies must be done to ensure that adequate flow to the hand will resume with the radial artery gone. There is a greater incidence of spasm in radial artery grafts. The use of radial arteries has not replaced the use of vein grafts because many surgeons are waiting for more

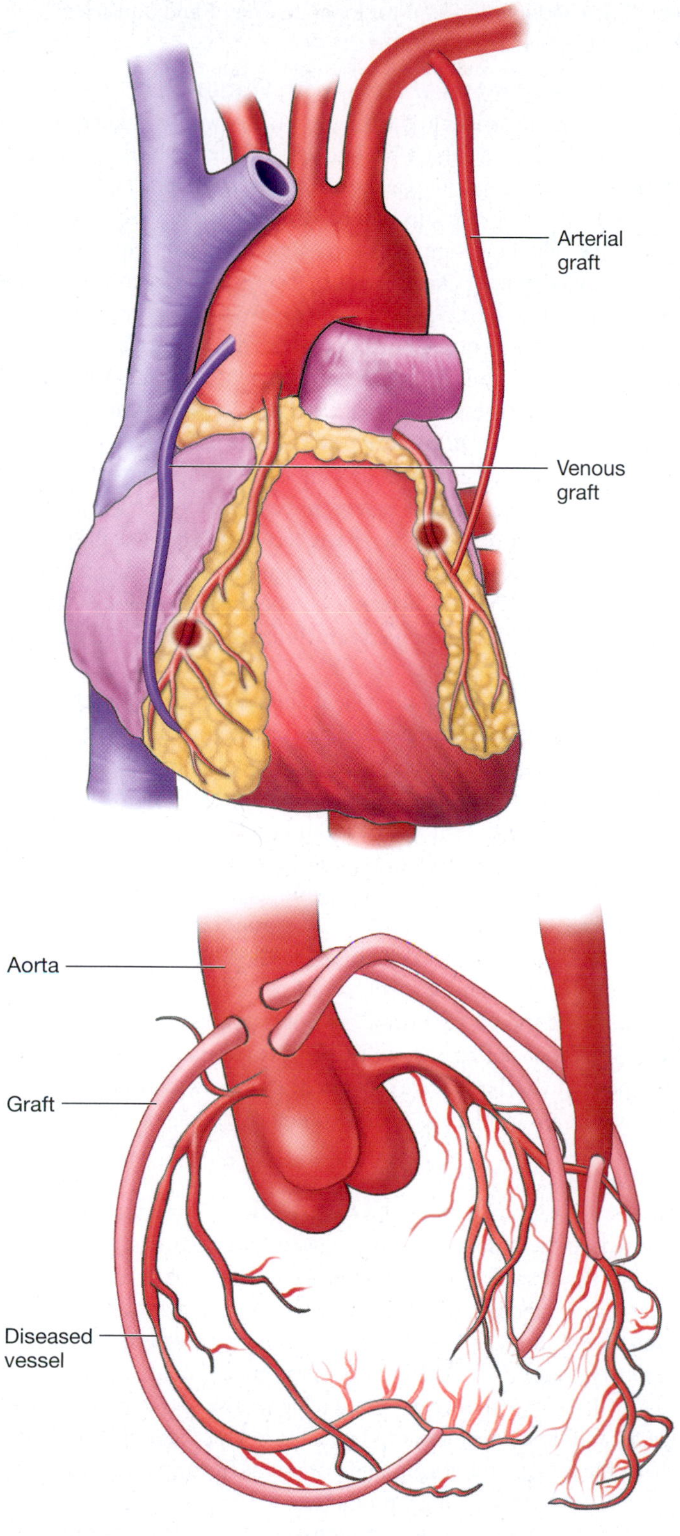

FIGURE 32–23 ◆ Heart surgery grafts.

long-term data. Other arterial conduits that are being experimented with are the right gastroepiploic artery and the inferior epigastric artery. Use of these will require more research before determining whether they can be used as alternatives to vein grafts.

New Surgical Techniques

Advances in cardiac surgery have introduced new techniques. Although their use is not widespread, initial results seem to be encouraging. Minimally invasive direct coronary artery bypass surgery (MIDCAB) was first done in Europe but quickly spread to the United States. MIDCAB is done via only a small left anterior thoracotomy incision. With the use of a thoracoscope and mechanical stabilizers, the left internal thoracic artery can be directly harvested and anastomosed. Similar to beating heart bypass, this procedure is done off CPB, so the heart remains beating. Medications are used to slow the heart, and stabilizers are used to reduce motion. The advantage of this approach is that it will reduce recovery time and potential postoperative complications such as CPB-related complications and wound infections. As with beating heart bypass, the disadvantage is that the bypasses are more difficult to place accurately on a moving heart, which may lower the graft patency rate. This technique is also usually limited to one or two types of bypasses.

The latest development in cardiac surgery is called port-access technique. This procedure combines a minimally invasive approach with an endovascular cardiopulmonary bypass–cardioplegic arrest system. This technique uses peripheral CPB via femoral vessels with an endaortic occlusion device. The heart can then be bypassed and stopped without opening the chest. This allows for more accurate anastomosis as well as use of multiple grafts. This technique has also been used on patients with mitral valve disease for valve repair or replacement (Chapter 33).

Postoperative Considerations

The overall rate of mortality for CABG is less than 3%, with the risk increasing according to the number of risk factors a patient may have (Society of Thoracic Surgeons, 2010). As with any surgical procedure, complications can occur. Chapter 19 includes an in-depth discussion of common postoperative complications. Serious complications of CABG include stroke, MI, and bleeding. Stroke can be a devastating complication that greatly affects recovery. Stroke is usually caused by an embolus from the ascending aorta or aortic arch. Surgeons use intraoperative echo to help detect irregularities within the aorta and avoid them while cannulating or clamping the aorta. Other postoperative complications include tamponade, renal failure, respiratory failure, dysrhythmias, wound infection, and both pericardial and pleural effusions.

A patient with a completely uncomplicated postoperative period can be discharged as soon as 4 days following surgery. Most patients, however, will leave the hospital within 6 days. Once home, patients will gradually increase their activity levels and should be able to resume regular activity after 6 to 12 weeks. The amount of time is individualized and is dependent on a patient's age and other health problems. Risk factor modification continues to be extremely important, and all patients should be counseled on diet, exercise, weight control, and smoking cessation. Patients with hypertension, diabetes, and hyperlipidemia need aggressive management of these conditions.

Nursing Management

Skilled postoperative nursing management for the CABG patient is crucial for a successful recovery and prevention of complications. In the immediate postoperative period, patients are typically taken directly from the operating room to a specialized ICU staffed by nurses who are trained in postcardiac surgery care. Depending on the institution and the patient's condition, some patients are extubated (the endotracheal tube is removed) prior to leaving the operating room. On arrival at the

ICU, it is imperative for the nurse to receive a report from the operating room on the patient, which should include the following:

- A summary of the surgery performed
- Amount of time the patient was "on pump" (cardiopulmonary bypass)
- Any intravenous drips that are running
- Recent laboratory values including arterial blood gases (ABG)
- Any problems that occurred in surgery
- Any coexisting illnesses that are pertinent.

Knowing the type of surgery that was performed and the amount of time a patient was on CPB is crucial to a patient's care. Prolonged bypass induces cytokine activation and an inflammatory response that results in red cell damage and hemoglobinuria, thrombocytopenia, clotting abnormalities, reduced pulmonary gas exchange, and cerebrovascular accidents.

Assessment

Nursing assessment includes close monitoring of the patient's hemodynamic status. Continuous monitoring of cardiac output, cardiac index, pulmonary artery pressure, central venous pressure, and blood pressure is done, and the results are assessed at regular intervals. Close observation of the patient's heart rhythm, blood pressure, and oxygen saturation can detect new imbalances or hypoxia. Serum electrolytes and complete blood counts are assessed at regular intervals to allow intervention before complications occur. For example, an abnormal potassium or magnesium level can precipitate life-threatening cardiac dysrhythmias, and a low hemoglobin and hematocrit can decrease the blood's oxygen-carrying capacity. Additionally, ventilator settings, chest tube drainage, and urine output are all assessed regularly.

Nursing Diagnoses

Nursing diagnoses that pertain to the CABG patient include:

- *Pain, Acute* related to surgical procedure
- *Airway Clearance, Ineffective risk for* related to anesthesia
- *Decreased Cardiac Output, Risk for* related to surgery and heart disease
- *Fluid Volume, Risk for Impaired* related to heart disease
- *Potential for Bleeding* related to surgery and anticoagulant medications
- *Infection, Risk for* related to loss of skin integrity
- *Knowledge, Deficit* related to *post-operative* needs
- *Mobility, Impaired* related to surgery
- *Sleep Deprivation* related to environment and care needs

NANDA-I © 2012

Outcomes and Evaluation Parameters

Extubation is an early outcome, and most hospitals will have protocols to wean the patient from ventilation as soon as possible. As a patient begins to wake up, it is important to prevent the patient from removing the endotracheal tube herself. Once a patient has been extubated and hemodynamic parameters are stable, the next outcome is to get the patient weaned off all intravenous drips and converted to oral medications. The nurse removes the pulmonary artery catheter on postoperative day 1 if the patient is stable. Neurological status is an essential evaluation parameter to establish; once a patient begins to awaken, the nurse must ask the patient to move each extremity and respond to simple questions. Early mobilization is important to reduce postoperative complications. It is standard for a patient to be out of bed and in a chair on postoperative day 1 and transferred out of the ICU if stable.

Planning and Interventions with Rationales

When the patient arrives in the ICU, laboratory work including chemistries, CBC, ABGs, a chest x-ray, and an ECG should be done as soon as possible so that a baseline can be established. Titration of intravenous drips is done to maintain adequate hemodynamic status such as cardiac output and blood pressure. The nurse should immediately report any abnormal change in a patient's status to the surgeon. Depending on the institution and surgeon, a patient will have two to four chest tubes. The nurse should document chest tube output hourly. Any increase in output of greater than 100 mL per hour should be reported, and serial CBCs should be done to assess for internal bleeding because it occurs most frequently in the early postoperative period. Some patients will have temporary pacemaker wires placed, and the nurse should connect and test the temporary pacemaker to ensure proper function (Chapter 30). These will be removed later when it has been established that the patient will not need them. It is common for patients to develop dysrhythmias such as atrial fibrillation (Chapter 30) on postoperative days 2 through 5. Should a patient develop a dysrhythmia, the nurse should perform an ECG and notify the surgeon.

Once out of the ICU, the patient should remain on a telemetry floor to continue monitoring of the heart rhythm. While the patient is on telemetry, aggressive mobilization and physical therapy must be a focus. Adequate pain control management is important to encourage ambulation as well as deep breathing and coughing. Common postoperative complications include pneumonia, deep vein thrombosis, and pulmonary embolism. Each of these complications can be minimized or prevented by ambulation and deep breathing exercises. As a patient's chest tube output begins to decrease, the chest tubes will be removed and the amount of pain a patient has will also decrease.

The nurse should perform a close observation of wounds for any signs of infection during each shift. Changes in wounds and fever need to be reported to the health care provider. Poor glucose control will greatly increase the risk of infection, so it is important to monitor glucose levels.

Health Promotion

Discussing risk factors and employing secondary prevention measures will reduce the number of patients who have recurrent events after CABG. Patients will usually take medications such as cholesterol drugs, aspirin, beta-blockers, and ACE inhibitors long term. In addition, daily exercise and adequate weight control will help reduce the risk of further coronary disease. If the patient smokes, the nurse should encourage him to stop. Patients with diabetes are at a higher risk for recurrent cardiac events and should be monitored for this closely. The nurse should instruct the patient on the signs and symptoms of angina and advise the patient to report any changes promptly.

Most patients will require repetitive counseling to change risk factors that have taken a lifetime to develop. Therefore, frequent follow-up with their primary health care provider and cardiologist is important to review risk factors and to monitor blood pressure, blood sugar, and cholesterol levels. Cardiac rehabilitative programs can assist the patient and family with the necessary lifestyle changes. The nurse can help to motivate the patient to take these important steps.

Collaborative Management

A multidisciplinary team approach, including health care providers; advance practice nurses, such as nurse practitioners and/or clinical nurse specialists; staff nurses; pharmacists; physical therapists; wound specialists; and dietitians; is important in the management of the patient undergoing CABG. In order to meet desired patient outcomes, it is essential that this interdisciplinary team communicate openly with one another in developing and evaluating care of the patient and family (IOM [Institute of Medicine], 2010). Health care providers oversee the patient's plan of care by determining what medical or surgical therapies are needed, including diagnostic testing, surgical procedures, and pharmacologic and nonpharmacologic interventions. Nurses implement the plan of care and are responsible for ongoing monitoring, assessment, and evaluation of interventions. Pharmacists oversee the patient's pharmacologic profile, assessing for appropriateness of dosing, drug-to-drug interactions, and potential adverse reactions of medications. Physical therapists are essential in assisting patients in gaining and maintaining strength and mobility, especially after extensive surgical interventions.

An assessment by a dietitian can provide helpful insight into the patient's nutrition and hydration status. For example, the dietitian can offer recommendations for foods or supplements that may promote healing. Patients following CABG are dealing with pain, anxiety, and altered body image and may benefit from interactions with social workers and hospital chaplains. A referral to a cardiac rehabilitation program can assist the patient with risk factor modification and building exercise tolerance.

Discharge Priorities

Thorough patient teaching is needed for the patient following CABG. Discharge medications most always include aspirin, beta-adrenergic blockers, cholesterol-lowering medications, and ACE inhibitors, described earlier. Detailed discharge instructions include medication management, signs and symptoms of infection and bleeding, risk factor management, and progression of activity levels. Patients with median sternotomy are taught sternal precautions, which include no heavy lifting, no extended reaching or twisting of the upper body, and no driving for 4 to 6 weeks. These discharge instructions can be the deciding factor in whether a patient will succeed as an outpatient and should be reviewed thoroughly with the patient and his family.

Research

Research is essential to improve the care, quality of life, and survival of patients with CAD. The goal of research is to identify areas where practice could improve and evaluate and test methods for these improvements. The research topics related to CAD are included in the Research Opportunities box. The list provides both medical and nursing research topics still under investigation. Electronic databases are a source for finding specific studies related to these topics.

RESEARCH OPPORTUNITIES Related to Coronary Artery Disease

Research Area	Clinical Impact
Physiological Research	
Stem cell injection after acute MI.	Stimulate new growth of myocardial cells and increase myocardial viability.
Gene therapy for chronic CAD patients who have no other alternatives.	Stimulate angiogenesis, thereby decreasing symptoms and increasing quality of life.
Facilitated PCI for acute MI.	Conjoined mechanical and pharmacologic interventions for AMI will decrease mortality and increase myocardial salvage.
Establish heart-healthy food supplements.	Decrease hyperlipidemia, thereby providing risk factor modification for some predisposed risk factors.
Identify predictors of vulnerable plaque and their impact.	Provide the ability to manage plaque and prevent plaque rupture, thus preventing future coronary events.
Establish standard of providing fibrinolytic therapy in the field.	Increase survival for acute MI patient.
Effect of community awareness programs on patients with ACS, emphasizing early symptom recognition and treatment.	Decrease adverse cardiovascular events and increase survival from out-of-hospital events.
Effect of immediately triaging women with ACS-like symptoms to chest pain unit.	Increase survival in the female population and bring awareness because their symptoms are often missed.
Long-term impact of drug-eluting stents on restenosis.	Restenosis is the major cause of repeat revascularization procedures.
Vascular management techniques.	Potential to reduce the patient's length of stay and improve patient comfort and safety after PCI.
Length of time to continue antiplatelet agents after PCI.	Reduce complications associated with these medications.
Risk factor modification.	Reduce incidence of CAD, as well as improve outcomes after PCI.
Effective teaching methods for discharge instructions.	Knowledge alone does not improve patient/family compliance.
Emotional and Psychological Research	
Denial of signs and symptoms of acute myocardial infarction.	Delaying treatment results in increased morbidity and mortality.
Risk factor modification.	Reduce incidence of CAD, as well as improve outcomes after PCI.
Use of alternative therapies such as guided imagery to reduce anxiety during PCI.	Lower stress during PCI while reducing need for sedatives/analgesics.
Effective teaching methods for discharge instructions.	Knowledge alone does not improve patient/family compliance.
Behavior modification techniques and their effect on CAD and its events.	Lower all modifiable risk factors, thereby decreasing cardiovascular events in a high-risk population.

CLINICAL PREPARATION READ DOCUMENT APPLY

READ: History of Present Illness >> Laboratory Study Results >> Critical Thinking Questions

You are a nurse in the coronary care unit (CCU) and have been notified that you will be receiving a patient from the cardiac catheterization lab with the diagnosis of STEMI. You receive the following report from the nurse in the catheterization lab: Daniel Ray is a 43-year-old male with a history of hypertension, hypercholesterolemia, gastroesophageal reflux disease (GERD), and hepatitis C. He developed substernal chest pain while doing some yard work at approximately 1:00 p.m. today. His pain radiated to his left arm and was accompanied by shortness of breath, nausea, and vomiting. He rated his pain as a 10/10 in severity. He presented to the emergency department, and his first ECG showed ST elevation in the anterolateral leads. He was initially treated with aspirin, nitroglycerin paste, morphine, oxygen 2 liters, and intravenous unfractionated heparin. He was then emergently taken to the cardiac catheterization lab.

Mr. Ray's cardiac catheterization showed a 100% thrombotic occlusion of his proximal left anterior descending artery. A drug-eluting stent was placed, and the patient was placed on an abciximab infusion.

On arrival at the CCU, Mr. Ray is awake and alert and denies any chest pain or shortness of breath. He denies any previous cardiac history. He is a pleasant man who appears to be in no acute distress.

READ: History of Present Illnesses >> **Physical Exam** >> Admitting Medical Records >> Laboratory Study Results

Medical–Surgical History

No known allergies
Medications: none
Hypertension
GERD
Hepatitis C
Surgeries: knee and hip had "pins" placed

Social History

Family history: no premature heart disease; parents both alive and in good health
Last used tobacco 20 years ago and denies any ethanol use. He did use intravenous drugs approximately 15 years ago. He is employed as a landscaper.

Physical Exam

Temp: 97.6, BP 120/83, HR 80, RR: 14
Caucasian man with multiple tattoos, in no apparent distress
HEENT: sclera anicteric, oropharynx clear
Neck: supple, no lymphadenopathy
Lungs: clear to auscultation bilaterally
Cardiovascular: JVP not elevated; normal S_1 and S_2; regular rate and rhythm, no significant murmur, rub, or gallop; carotids 2+ without bruits
Abdomen: soft, nontender, nondistended, normoactive bowel sounds
Extremities: no edema
Neurological: normal, alert, and oriented × 3
CXR: normal
ECG: see history of present illness

Admitting Medical Orders

Admit to cardiology, coronary care unit
Condition guarded
Admitting diagnosis: ACS
Diagnosis: acute anterolateral STEMI
Vital signs and oxygen saturation q1h
Bed rest
Call health care professional: pulse > 100/minute; BP ≥ 160 systolic; temperature > 38.5; urine output 30 mL/hr; oxygen saturation < 92%
Sequential compression devices to lower extremities
Diet: cardiac
Daily weight
Continuous cardiac monitor
Foley to gravity
Strict in/out
Oxygen per nasal cannula to maintain oxygen sat > 92%
IV: D5 1/2NS @ 50 mL/hr

Scheduled Medications

ASA 325 mg po daily
Pantoprazole 40 mg po daily
Metoprolol 25 mg po bid
Lisinopril 20 mg po daily
Clopidogrel 75 mg po daily
Abciximab infusion @ 0.125 mcg/kg/min for 12 hours
Atorvastatin 20 mg po daily

PRN Medications

Morphine 3–5 mg IV q3–5 min, max 15 mg q3h prn pain
Temazepam 15–30 mg po qhs prn insomnia
Ondansetron (Zofran) 4 mg IV every 6 hours—may repeat x 1 if needed.
Reglan (Metaclopromide) 10 mg IV every 6 hours (reduce to 5 mg IV if estimated CrCl < 30 mL/min) if Zofran not effective.

Ordered Laboratory Studies

Troponin I q8h × 3
CPK–MB q8h × 3
Basic chemistry panel q a.m.
CBC q a.m.
Magnesium q a.m.
Lipid panel in a.m.

Ordered Diagnostic Studies

ECG q a.m.
Echocardiogram in a.m.

READ: History of Present Illnesses >> **Laboratory Study Results** >> Critical Thinking Questions

Test	Day 1	Day 2	Day 3
Sodium	135 mEq/L	136 mEq/L	137 mEq/L
Potassium	4.1 mEq/L	4.0 mEq/L	4.0 mEq/L
Chloride	103 mEq/L	104 mEq/L	103 mEq/L
Carbon dioxide (CO_2)	26 mEq/L	25 mEq/L	25 mEq/L
Blood urea nitrogen (BUN)	16 mg/dL	15 mg/dL	14 mg/dL
Creatinine	1.2 mg/dL	1.3 mg/dL	1.2 mg/dL
Glucose	85 mg/dL	96 mg/dL	89 mg/dL
Phosphorus	2.2 mg/dL	3.4 mg/dL	3.8 mg/dL
Calcium	9.1 mg/dL	8.7 mg/dL	9.1 mg/dL
Albumin	3.7 g/dL	3.7 g/dL	3.5 g/dL
Alkaline phosphorus	70 units/L	76 units/L	77 units/L
Aspartate amino-transferase (AST)	70 units/L	76 units/L	77 units/L
Bilirubin	1.8 mg/dL	1.4 mg/dL	1.2 mg/dL
Alanine amino-transferase (ALT)	87 units/L	67 units/L	54 units/L
Magnesium	2.0 mEq/L	1.9 mEq/L	1.9 mEq/L

Test	Day 1	Day 2	Day 3
Creatine kinase	4,368 units/L	2,812 units/L	2,000 units/L
Relative index	>6.9%	>10.7%	>9.4%
CK-MB	>300.00%	>300.00%	259.7%
Troponin I	>100 ng/mL	82.86 ng/mL	52.00 ng/mL
WBC	11.5/mm^3	10.9/mm^3	9.3/mm^3
RBC	4.89/mm^3	5.09/mm^3	4.92/mm^3
Hemoglobin	15.9 g/dL	16.5 g/dL	15.9 g/dL
Hematocrit	45.5%	47.8%	45.6%
Platelets	295/mm^3	256/mm^3	300/mm^3
Cholesterol	280 mg/dL		
High-density lipoproteins (HDL)	22 mg/dL		
Low-density lipoproteins (LDL)	198 mg/dL		
Very low-density lipoproteins (VLDL)	68%		
Apolipoproteins	162 mg/dL		
Triglycerides	210 mg/dL		

Pearson Nursing Student Resources *Log on to* ***nursing.pearsonhighered.com*** *to download forms*

DOCUMENT:

- >> Summary of Hospitalization
- >> Pathophysiology Form
- >> Laboratory Values
- >> Laboratory Results Explanation

APPLY:

- >> List of Potential Nursing Diagnosis
- >> Concept Map
- >> Critical Thinking Questions and Concept Map

APPLY: History of Present Illnesses >> Laboratory Study Results >> **Critical Thinking Questions**

1. What factors in Mr. Ray's history would increase his risk for the development of coronary artery disease?
2. Why were cardiac markers ordered?
3. What is the purpose of abciximab in this patient?
4. When you review the ECG, what leads can you expect to be elevated with an acute anterolateral MI?
5. If, during the next couple of days, Mr. Ray complains of chest pain that mimics the pain that he had before, what steps would you take and anticipate?

Answers to Critical Thinking Questions can be found in Appendix D in the Osborn Student Resources at nursing.pearsonhighered.com.

NCLEX® PRACTICE

1. Which patient statement would the nurse evaluate as indicating a risk factor for the development of coronary heart disease that the patient cannot change?

1. "I am trying to quit smoking, but it is difficult."
2. "My blood sugars sometimes run a little high."
3. "I walk at least one mile every day."
4. "My father died of a heart attack at age 70."

2. A patient reports a history of having substernal chest pain. Which patient statement would help the nurse establish a diagnosis of stable angina?

1. "The pain usually lasts about 10 minutes."
2. "The pain has started waking me up at night."
3. "This last bout of pain was the worst yet."
4. "I'm having the pains more often than I used to."

3. A patient seen in the clinic reports having episodes of left arm pain and chest tightness that started after having an argument. The nurse concludes the pain was most likely typical angina pain when the patient also reports which occurrence?

1. Experiencing pain relief by taking nitroglycerin
2. Having just eaten a large meal prior to having the pain
3. Feeling very anxious when having the pain
4. Experiencing weakness and dizziness

4. The electrocardiogram (ECG) of a patient admitted with acute coronary syndrome (ACS) shows new ST segment elevation. The nurse plans this patient's immediate care based on which concern?

1. This patient is experiencing mild cardiac ischemia.
2. It is likely that this patient has experienced an MI in the past.
3. Severe damage to the patient's heart is inevitable.
4. Transmural ischemia may be occurring.

5. A patient admitted with complaints of epigastric pain since yesterday is evaluated for an MI. Blood markers are negative but the electrocardiogram (ECG) shows deep Q wave changes without ST segment elevation. The nurse plans the immediate care of this patient based on which concern?

1. The patient has suffered an MI some time ago.
2. The patient likely suffered an MI yesterday.
3. The patient's natural pacemaker is failing.
4. The patient has ventricular hypertrophy.

6. The patient presents to the emergency department (ED) with a history of substernal chest pain and shortness of breath that occurred 4 days ago. The nurse anticipates that blood work will be drawn to measure which indicator of myocardial infarction?

1. Troponin I levels
2. Myoglobin levels
3. C-reactive protein
4. CK-MB

Answers to NCLEX Practice questions can be found in Appendix D in the Osborn Student Resources at nursing.pearsonhighered.com. Practice additional NCLEX questions online at the Student Resources site.

Pearson Nursing Student Resources Find additional review materials at: **nursing.pearsonhighered.com**

REFERENCES

Adams, M. P., & Koch, R.W. (2010). *Pharmacology: Connections to nursing practice.* Upper Saddle River, NJ: Pearson.

Alberti, K. G. M. M., Eckel, R. H., Grundy, S. M., Zimmet, P. Z., Cleeman, J. I., Donato, K. A., et al. (2009). Harmonizing the metabolic syndrome: A joint interim statement of the International Diabetes Federation Task Force on Epidemiology and Prevention; National Heart, Lung, and Blood Institute; American Heart Association; World Heart Federation; International Atherosclerosis Society; and International Association for the Study of Obesity. *Circulation, 120,* 1640–1645.

American Heart Association. (2010a). Alcohol and cardiovascular disease. Retrieved from http://www.heart.org/HEARTORG/Conditions/HeartAttack/UnderstandYourRiskofHeartAttack/Alcohol-and-Cardiovascular-Disease_UCM_305173_Article.jsp

American Heart Association. (2010b). *Heart disease and stroke statistics—2010 update.* Dallas, TX: American Heart Association.

American Heart Association. (2010c). Inflammation, heart disease and stroke: The role of C-reactive protein. Retrieved from http://www.americanheart.org/presenter.jhtml?identifier=4648

American Heart Association. (2010d). Physical activity. Retrieved from http://www.americanheart.org/presenter.jhtml?identifier=4563

American Heart Association. (2010e). Primary prevention in the adult. Retrieved from http://www.americanheart.org/presenter.jhtml?identifier=4704

American Heart Association. (2010f). Triglycerides. Retrieved from http://www.americanheart.org/presenter.jhtml?identifier=4778

Artinian, N. T., Fletcher, G. F., Mozaffarian, D., Kris-Etherton, P., Van Horn, L., Lichtenstein, A. H., et al. (2010). Interventions to promote physical activity and dietary lifestyle changes for cardiovascular risk factor reduction in adults: A scientific statement from the American Heart Association. *Circulation, 122,* 406–441. Retrieved from http://www.ncbi.nlm.nih.gov/pubmed/20625115

Bhatt, D. (2009). Prasugrel in clinical practice. *New England Journal of Medicine, 361,* 940–942.

Futterman, L. G., & Lemberg, L. (2000). The Framingham heart study: A pivotal legacy of the last millennium. *American Journal of Critical Care, 9*(2), 147–152.

Gepner, A. D., Piper, M. E., Johnson, H. M., Fiore, M. C., Baker, T. B., & Stein, J. H. (2011). Effects of smoking and smoking cessation on lipids and lipoproteins: Outcomes from a randomized trial. *American Heart Journal, 161*(1), 145–151.

Han, L., Li, J. P., Sit, J. W., Chung, L., Jiao, Z. Y., & Ma, W. G. (2010, April). Effects of music intervention on physiological stress response and anxiety level of mechanically ventilated patients in China: A randomized controlled trial. *Journal of Clinical Nursing, 19*(7-8), 978–987.

Heiss, C., Keen, C. L., & Kelm, M. (2010). Flavanols and cardiovascular disease prevention. Retrieved from http://eurheartj.oxfordjournals.org/content/early/2010/09/18/eurheartj.ehq332.abstract

IOM (Institute of Medicine). (2010). *The future of nursing: Leading change, advancing health.* Washington, DC: The Academic Press.

Kee, J. L. (2010). *Laboratory and diagnostic tests with nursing implications.* Upper Saddle River, NJ: Pearson.

Kushner, F. G., Hand, M., Smith, S. C., Jr., King, S. B., 3rd, Anderson, J. L., Antman, E. M., et al. (2009). Focused updates: ACC/AHA guidelines for the management of patients with ST-elevation myocardial infarction (updating the 2004 guideline and 2007 focused update) and ACC/AHA/SCAI guidelines on percutaneous coronary intervention (updating the 2005 guideline and 2007 focused update): A report of the American College of Cardiology Foundation/American Heart Association Task Force on Practice Guidelines. *Circulation, 54*(23), 2271–2306.

Libby, P., Bonow, R. O., Zipes, D. P., & Mann, D. L. (2008). *Braunwald's heart disease: A textbook of cardiovascular medicine* (8th ed.). St. Louis: Elsevier.

Lindsay, J., Paixao, A., Chao, T., & Pichard, A. D. (2010). Pathogenesis of the takotsubo syndrome: A unifying hypothesis. *American Journal of Cardiology, 106,* 1360–1363.

McCulloch, B. J. (2007). Transient left ventricular apical ballooning. *Critical Care Nurse, 27*(6), 20–28.

McCulloch, B. J. (2010). Intra-aortic balloon pump and other cardiac devices. In S. Watson and K. A. Gorski (Eds.), *Invasive cardiology: A manual for cath lab personnel.* Sudbury, MA: Jones and Bartlett.

Mehta, S., Alfonso, C. E., Oliveros, E., Shamshad, F., Flores, A. I., Cohen, S., et al. (2010). Adjunct therapy in STEMI intervention. *Cardiology Clinics, 28*(1), 107–125.

Miracle, V. (2010). Coronary artery disease in women: The myth still exists unfortunately. *Dimensions of Critical Care Nursing, 29*(5), 215–221.

Modesti, P. A., Ferrari, A., Bazzini, C., Costanzo, G., Simonetti, I., Taddei, S., et al. (2010). Psychological predictors of the antihypertensive effects of music-guided slow breathing. *Journal of Hypertension, 28*(5), 1097–1103.

Moseley, M. J., Allen, D., & Martel, M. (2010). Electrocardiogram lead selection using critical thinking. *Dimensions of Critical Care Nursing, 29*(6), 253–258.

Moser, D. K., & Riegel, B. (2008). *Cardiac nursing: A companion to Braunwald's heart disease.* St. Louis: Saunders.

National Diabetes Information Clearinghouse (NDIC). (2010). Diabetes, heart disease, and stroke. Retrieved from http://diabetes.niddk.nih.gov/dm/pubs/stroke/

Patel, M. R., Dehmer, G. J., Hirshfeld, J. W., Smith, P. K., & Spertus, J. A. (2009). CCF/SCAI/STS/AATS/AHA/ASNC 2009 appropriateness criteria for coronary revascularization: A report of the American College of Cardiology Foundation Appropriateness Criteria Task Force, Society for Cardiovascular Angiography and Interventions, Society of Thoracic Surgeons, American Association for Thoracic Surgery, American Heart Association, and the American Society of Nuclear Cardiology. *Circulation, 119,* 1330–1352.

Porth, C. (2008). *Essentials of pathophysiology: Concepts of altered health states* (3rd ed.). Lippincott Williams & Wilkins.

Schneider, J. I. (2009). High-risk chief complaints I: Chest pain—The big three. *Emergency Medicine Clinics of North America, 27*(4), 685–712.

Sirak, T., Chiadika, S., Daka, M., & Simon, C. (2008). *Acute coronary syndrome in African Americans and Hispanic Americans.* New York: Springer Publishing.

Society of Thoracic Surgeons. (2010). Adult cardiac surgery database. Retrieved from http://www.sts.org/documents/pdf/ndb2010/1stHarvestExecutiveSummary%5B1%5D.pdf

Thaler, M. S. (2010). *The only EKG book you'll ever need.* Philadelphia: Lippincott Williams & Wilkins.

U.S. Department of Health and Human Services. (2011). Heart disease and African Americans. Retrieved from http://Kuminorityhealth.hhs.gov/templates/content.aspx?ID=3018

Wilkinson, J. M., & Ahearn, N. R. (2009). *Prentice Hall nursing diagnosis handbook* (9th ed.). Upper Saddle River, NJ: Prentice Hall.

Woods, S. L., Froelicher, E. S. S., Adams (Underhill), S., & Bridges, E. J. (Eds.). (2010). *Cardiac nursing* (6th ed.). Philadelphia: Lippincott Williams & Wilkins.

CHAPTER

33 Caring for the Patient with Cardiac Inflammatory Disorders

Brenda McCulloch
Kathleen Osborn

Outcome-Based Learning Objectives

After studying this chapter, the learner will be able to:

1. Compare and contrast the etiology, pathophysiology, and clinical manifestations of the four inflammatory disorders that affect the heart and the medical and nursing management for these disorders.
2. Integrate the etiology, pathophysiology, clinical manifestations, and treatment for valve stenosis, regurgitation, and mitral valve prolapse.
3. Explain the rationale and type of preventive therapy necessary for patients with valve disease.
4. Develop a plan of care for the patient undergoing valve repair or replacement in terms of patient care and education needs.
5. Compare and contrast the four types of cardiomyopathy in terms of etiology, pathophysiology, clinical manifestations, and medical and nursing management.
6. Apply nursing diagnoses and the nursing process to the care of the patient with inflammatory or structural heart disease.

KEY TERMS

allograft valve p.1001
annuloplasty p.999
annulus p.999
aortic valve regurgitation p.993
aortic valve stenosis p.994
arrhythmogenic right ventricular cardiomyopathy (ARVC) p.1016
autograft valve p.1002
Beck's triad p.984
biologic valve p.1000
cardiac tamponade p.983
cardiomyopathies (CMPs) p.1005
commissure p.999
commissurotomy p.999
constrictive pericarditis p.982
dilated cardiomyopathy (DCM) p.1006
Dressler's syndrome p.979
effusion p.974
echocardiography p.1019
homograft valve p.1001
hypertrophic cardiomyopathy (HCM) p.1009
infective endocarditis (IE) p.987
mechanical valve p.1000
mitral valve regurgitation p.993
mitral valve stenosis p.993
mitral valve prolapse (MVP) p.994
myocarditis p.986
pancarditis p.973
pericardial effusion p.983
pericardial friction rub p.983
pericardial window p.985
pericardiectomy p.985
pericarditis p.979
pulmonic regurgitation (PR) p.997
pulmonic stenosis (PS) p.995
pulsus paradoxus p.984
restrictive cardiomyopathy (RCM) p.1015
rheumatic fever p.973
rheumatic heart disease p.973
stress echocardiography p.1020
transesophageal echocardiography (TEE) p.1020
tricuspid regurgitation (TR) p.995
tricuspid stenosis (TS) p.995
valvular regurgitation p.992
valvular stenosis p.992
valvuloplasty p.999

CARDIAC DISORDERS may be caused by inflammation or by structural changes and abnormalities. Because they alter myocardial pumping ability, these disorders result in abnormal blood flow through the heart, thus affecting tissue perfusion. All three layers of the heart—the pericardium, myocardium, and endocardium—can be subject to inflammation and structural abnormalities. The manifestations differ depending on which layer is involved in the pathologic process. An in-depth discussion of disorders affecting each layer of the heart is presented in this chapter.

In recent years, the incidence of cardiac structural disorders has increased, due in part to advancements in the prevention and treatment of coronary artery disease (CAD). People are living long enough to develop the structural changes that are often associated with advanced age. This chapter presents the treatments for patients with these disorders and how the nursing process is applied for these patients.

Inflammatory Disorders

The heart is susceptible to bacteria and microbes that may be infecting other organs of the body. These infections cause an inflammatory response that can affect the heart's ability to maintain a normal cardiac output. In the acute stages, these infections are serious and potentially lethal. Additionally, long-term and potentially disabling damage can be done to the heart during the infectious process. The inflammatory conditions that affect the heart—rheumatic heart disease, pericarditis, myocarditis, and endocarditis—are discussed next.

Rheumatic Heart Disease

Rheumatic heart disease is a complication of rheumatic fever. The pathologic process of **rheumatic fever** begins with a pharyngeal infection caused by Lancefield group A beta-hemolytic streptococcus (strep). If left untreated, a small number of these pharyngeal infections result in rheumatic fever. The resulting rheumatic heart disease is thought to be caused by an abnormal autoimmune response to the original infection, but the exact pathogenesis remains unclear (Gerber et al., 2009). The primary long-term damage is scarring and malfunction of the heart valves.

Epidemiology and Etiology

Rheumatic fever was the leading cause of death 100 years ago in the United States in people 5 to 20 years of age. Antibiotics and early treatment have made rheumatic fever rare in developed countries, although it continues to be a challenge because of its high prevalence in the developing world. Rheumatic fever was thought to have been nearly eradicated from developed countries, but in recent years it has made a comeback in poor inner-city neighborhoods.

Rheumatic fever occurs most frequently in children from 5 to 15 years of age and tends to affect connective tissues, especially those of the heart, brain, skin, and joints. The risk factors associated with the development and spread of streptococcal infections are outlined in the Risk Factors box.

Worldwide, rheumatic fever and rheumatic heart disease affect 20 million people and are leading causes of death in people younger than 50 years of age (Gerber et al., 2009). Once a person has had rheumatic fever, she is more susceptible to recurrent infections. With each infection, more damage to the heart valve occurs.

Pathophysiology

As was previously mentioned, rheumatic fever develops following pharyngitis from Lancefield group A beta-hemolytic streptococcus. The infecting organisms attach to the epithelial cells in the upper respiratory tract and produce enzymes that damage and invade other tissues of the body. These organisms elicit an acute inflammatory response after an incubation period of 2 to 4 days. Several weeks after the initial infection resolves, rheumatic fever results. Only infections of the pharynx initiate and reactivate rheumatic fever. Patients remain infected for weeks after the resolution of symptoms and may serve as a reservoir for infecting others.

An abnormal autoimmune response is thought to occur in more than half of the cases of rheumatic fever. It is theorized that the invading organism produces toxins that precipitate an antigen–antibody response. The antibodies appear to cross-react with connective tissues and bind to receptor sites on the heart, joints, skin, brain, and subcutaneous tissue, causing an acute inflammatory response. In the heart, all three layers—the endocardium, myocardium, and pericardium—become inflamed, giving rise to the term **pancarditis** (meaning "inflammation involving all three layers of the heart"). Microscopic lesions, referred to as Aschoff nodules and composed of a collection of lymphocytes and histocytes, are found in the fibrinous interstitial septa of the myocardium. Additionally, wart-like raised fibrinous lesions develop on the closure lines of the valve cusps. As Aschoff nodules age, they become more fibrinous scar tissue, contributing to the transient heart failure that is associated with rheumatic fever. As the inflammation subsides, there is typically no long-term damage to the myocardium and pericardium. The long-term sequela of the inflammation is to the heart valves.

The inflammatory process causes swelling of the valves, and small bacterial vegetations form on the valve surface (Figure 33–1◆). The result is fibrous thickening and fusion of the valve leaflets, which cause valve dysfunction. Damaged valves either do not completely open (stenosis) or do not completely close (regurgitation). The severity of the symptoms depends on the valve that is involved and the degree of dysfunction. Valvular stenosis and regurgitation, described later in this chapter, cause an increase in the heart's workload. The symptoms typically become worse over time, and the most advanced condition leads to heart failure.

RISK FACTORS for Rheumatic Fever

Poor inner-city neighborhoods	Damp weather
Crowded living conditions	Malnutrition
Immunocompromised state	Poor access to health care.

Clinical Manifestations

Clinical manifestations of rheumatic fever typically begin about 1 to 6 weeks after a bout of strep throat (pharyngitis), although in some cases the infection may have been too mild to be recognized. The diagnosis of rheumatic fever and rheumatic heart disease is based on a cluster of clinical manifestations and laboratory findings. Clinical manifestations

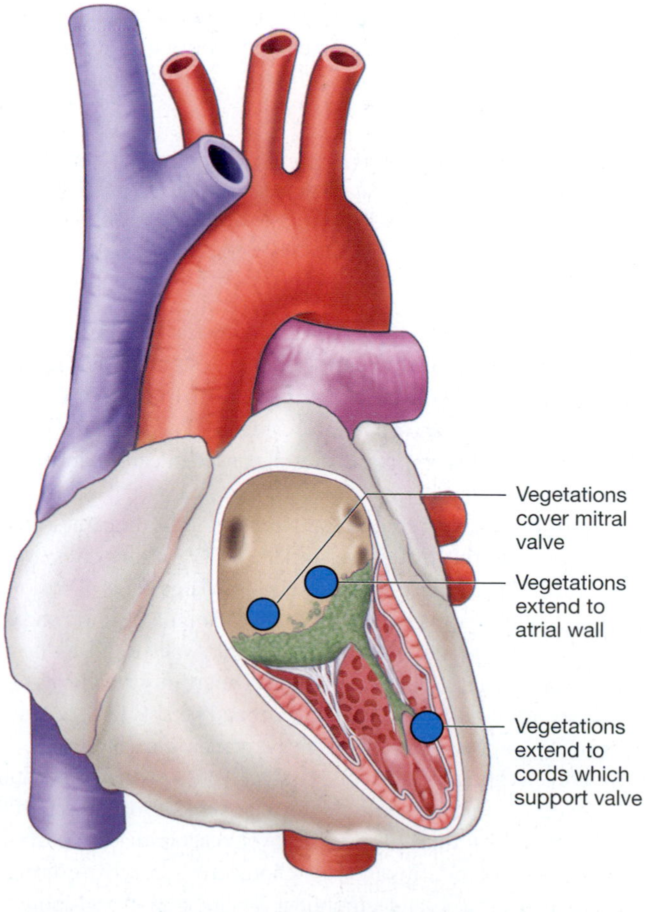

FIGURE 33–1 ◆ Vegetative growth on a heart valve.

Weblink: Rheumatic Fever

CHART 33–1 Clinical Manifestations of Acute Rheumatic Fever and Rheumatic Heart Disease

Acute Rheumatic Fever	Rheumatic Heart Disease
Fever	Chest pain
Malaise	Development of a new murmur or change in an existing murmur
Headache	Tachycardia and cardiac dysrhythmias
Erythema marginatum: red, raised, lattice-like rash, usually on the chest, back, and abdomen	Electrocardiogram (ECG) changes: prolonged PR interval
Swollen tender joints with small bony protuberances with or without the presence of subcutaneous nodules	Pericardial friction rub
May have weakness and shortness of breath	Symptoms of heart failure
Sydenham chorea: sudden, irregular, aimless involuntary movements that are self-limiting with no permanent damage	Cardiomegaly
Elevated white blood count (WBC)	Mitral and aortic stenosis

of acute rheumatic fever and rheumatic heart disease are outlined in Chart 33–1.

In addition to evaluating the clinical manifestations, the diagnosis of rheumatic fever and rheumatic heart disease is made by analysis of laboratory and diagnostic tests. Carditis is the most significant manifestation of rheumatic fever. New or changing murmurs are one of the major signs of cardiac involvement. The murmur is caused by valve insufficiency or regurgitation. Murmurs typically found with acute rheumatic fever are (1) the apical pansystolic, high-pitched murmur, which has a blowing quality that radiates to the left axilla, indicating mitral regurgitation; (2) the apical diastolic murmur, which is low pitched and rumbling, is present with active carditis, and accompanies severe mitral insufficiency; and (3) the basal diastolic murmur, a high-pitched, blowing, decrescendo murmur associated with aortic regurgitation (Hurst, O'Rourke, Walsh, & Fuster, 2009). A complete classification of murmurs is outlined in Chapter 29.

Safety Alert *If the nurse detects a new murmur during assessment of a patient with rheumatic fever, it needs to be reported to the health care provider. It may indicate the onset of rheumatic heart disease and requires further diagnostic testing. Where the murmur is heard depends on the valve that is involved.*

Heart failure may develop secondary to myocarditis or valve insufficiency. Another manifestation of cardiac involvement during rheumatic heart fever is pericarditis. A pericardial friction rub, distant muffled heart sounds, chest pain, and evidence of pericardial **effusion** (abnormal accumulation of fluid) are all consistent clinical manifestations of pericarditis.

Polyarthritis is the most common symptom and is the earliest manifestation of acute rheumatic fever in 70% to 75% of the cases (Mayo Clinic, 2010b). The arthritis typically begins in large joints of the lower extremities, and then migrates to other large joints of the lower and upper extremities. The affected joints are painful, swollen, and erythematous and have decreased range of motion. The arthritis reaches its most intense severity 12 to 24 hours after onset and persists for 2 to 6 days. Polyarthritis is not associated with any permanent disability.

Sydenham chorea is the major central nervous system manifestation and may occur in patients with rheumatic fever (Mayo Clinic, 2010b). It is characterized by difficulty writing, involuntary grimacing, purposeless movements of the arms and legs (choreiform), speech impairment, generalized weakness, and emotional lability. Sydenham chorea is slightly more common in females under age 18 than in males.

Laboratory and Diagnostic Procedures

When evaluating the patient with suspected rheumatic heart disease, the nurse must obtain a complete history and physical in order to evaluate the risk factors and the extent of the disease process. In addition to the clinical findings, a number of laboratory tests are useful in making the diagnosis. The Diagnostic Tests box describes the laboratory and diagnostic tests and the associated abnormalities that would be expected with rheumatic fever and rheumatic heart disease.

Medical Management

Prevention is the primary goal in the management of rheumatic heart disease. Early treatment of the streptococcal infection with antibiotics will usually prevent the development of rheumatic fever. People who have had previous attacks of rheumatic fever are more susceptible to future episodes, and each attack increases the amount of heart damage.

An antibiotic, typically penicillin, is used in the treatment of rheumatic fever. Oral penicillin V is the drug of choice. Following the acute stage, prophylactic antibiotics are indicated to prevent further damage to the valves. The recommendation in the United States is that after the initial course of antibiotics, an intramuscular injection of penicillin G be given every 4 weeks. This schedule is usually continued indefinitely for high-risk patients or for recurrent infections.

Aspirin and nonsteroidal anti-inflammatory drugs (NSAIDs) are used to treat joint pain and fever. If symptoms of moderate to severe carditis are present as evidenced by cardiomegaly (enlarged heart) and heart failure, steroid administration is typically added to the therapy and continued for 2 to 4 weeks (Mayo Clinic, 2010b).

If heart failure with left ventricular dysfunction (ejection fraction less than 40%) occurs as a consequence of rheumatic fever, treatment is needed. See Chapter 34 for the management of heart failure. See the Pharmacology feature (p. 976) for medications to treat inflammatory heart disease.

Bed rest is prescribed to reduce the cardiac workload, especially during the acute phase. Once the carditis subsides, the patient may begin a gradual schedule of increasing activity. Activity levels are dictated by the presence or absence of symptoms.

Nursing Management

Nursing management of the patient with rheumatic heart disease begins with an in-depth assessment of the clinical manifestations outlined in Chart 33–1. Further subjective and objective data related to clinical manifestations are outlined in the Nursing

DIAGNOSTIC TESTS for Cardiac Inflammatory Disorders

Diagnostic Test, Normal Values, and *Rationales*	Expected Abnormality
White Blood Cells (WBC) 4,500–10,000/mm^3 *Elevated levels are associated with inflammation and infection.*	Elevated with rheumatic fever, pericarditis, and myocarditis. Mild elevation with infective endocarditis (IE).
Red Blood Cells (RBC) Male: 4.6–6.0 mm^3 Female: 4.0–5.0 mm^3 *Occurs due to the inflammatory inhibition of erythropoiesis.*	Mild to moderate decrease with rheumatic fever.
Erythrocyte Sedimentation Rate Male: up to 15 mm/hour Female: up to 20 mm/hour *The test measures inflammation. Chronic inflammation and infection cause an elevation.*	Elevated rheumatic fever, pericarditis, IE, and myocarditis.
C-Reactive Protein Normally not present *Acute-phase reactant protein used to indicate an inflammatory illness.*	Elevated rheumatic fever, pericarditis, IE, and myocarditis.
Antistreptolysin O Titer (ASO) $<$100 international units/mL *Streptococcal antibody test used to determine whether a previous streptococcal infection has caused a poststreptococcal infection such as rheumatic fever.*	250 unit/mL with rheumatic fever.
Cardiac Marker: Creatinine Kinase MB (CK–MB), Troponin T, and Troponin I CPK–MB $<$6% Troponin T: $<$ 0.2 ng/mL Troponin I: $<$ 0.5 ng/mL *May be transiently elevated during the acute stages of myocardial cell damage.*	Elevated if carditis is present with all of the inflammatory disorders.
BNP $<$100 pg/mL or $<$ 100 ng/L *Marker of ventricular systolic and diastolic dysfunction. Useful to determine the presence of heart failure.*	Elevated with ventricular hypertrophy, severe hypertension, and heart failure.
Throat Culture Negative or normal flora *Quantifies and differentiates bacterial from viral throat infections.*	Positive for A beta-hemolytic streptococci with rheumatic fever.
ECG Normal conduction time intervals (see Chapter 30) *Conduction delays may be present with inflammation.* *ST segment changes may be present when myocardial ischemia is occurring.*	Prolonged PR interval with rheumatic fever. Diffuse ST segment abnormalities, T wave changes, dysrhythmias, and heart block with myocarditis. ST segment changes associated with myocardial ischemia and the conduction delays typical of IE.
Chest X-Ray Clear lungs and normal heart size *Cardiac enlargement occurs with inflammation, heart failure, and pericardial effusion.* *Congestion occurs with heart failure.*	Enlarged heart and lung congestion with pancarditis and heart failure. May show cardiac enlargement if a pericardial effusion is present. Diagnoses of heart failure and in right-sided IE may show evidence of septic pulmonary emboli.
Echocardiogram (ultrasound) Normal chamber size and normal cardiac structures *The inflammation causes structural changes in cardiac chambers and function.*	Valve damage and dilated chamber size, abnormal pressure gradients, decreased ventricular function, and/or pericardial effusion with structurally abnormal valves. Depressed systolic function, dilated chambers, and mild to no pericardial effusion may occur with myocarditis.

(*continued*)

DIAGNOSTIC TESTS for Cardiac Inflammatory Disorders, *continued*

Diagnostic Test, Normal Values, and *Rationales*	Expected Abnormality
	Determines the presence of pericardial fluid, motion of the heart walls, and the presence of restriction with pericarditis. Presence of thickening and calcification of the pericardium for IE.
Cardiac Catheterization	
Normal coronary arteries, chambers, and valve pressures *Inflammation causes changes in chamber size and valve function.* *Valve regurgitation causes a backflow of blood into the previous chamber. Valve stenosis disrupts blood flow causing enlarged chamber size.*	Valve damage, enlarged chamber size, decreased ventricular activity and/or function with rheumatic fever. Valvular and ventricular function abnormalities; test assists in evaluating need for valve replacement surgery.
Blood Cultures	
Negative for organisms *Organisms enter the bloodstream, adhere to the valve surface, and multiply.*	Positive and organism specific in 90–95% of cases with IE and therefore guide antibiotic therapy.
Viral Titers	
Negative *Viral titers are present for 8 to 10 days after onset of illness.*	Elevated.
Endomyocardial Biopsy	
Normal tissue *Often done within 6 weeks of acute illness while lymphocytic infiltration and myocyte damage is present.*	Presence of patchy cell necrosis and inflammatory changes confirm the diagnosis.
Autoimmune Serum Markers	
Negative *Intracellular adhesion molecules on cardiac myocytes is specific to autoimmune myocarditis.*	Presence of intracellular adhesion molecules on cardiac myocytes.

Source: Adapted from Kee, J. L. (2010). *Laboratory and diagnostic tests with nursing implications.* Upper Saddle River, NJ: Pearson.

PHARMACOLOGY Summary of Medications Used to Treat Cardiac Inflammatory Disorders

Medication Category and Action	Application/Indication	Nursing Responsibility
Antibiotics		
Penicillin Erythromycin Specific antibiotic depends on infecting organism ***Action:*** Inhibits cell wall synthesis. Inhibits protein synthesis. Disrupts plasma membrane. Inhibits nucleic acid synthesis.	Rheumatic fever Infective endocarditis Sepsis	Obtain and assess culture and sensitivity tests (blood, urine, sputum, wound, or other body fluids) before starting antibiotic therapy. Monitor for hypersensitivity reaction, and immediately report signs of allergy including rash, difficulty breathing, or swelling of the face, lips, or throat to the health care provider. Monitor for severe or persistent diarrhea. Instruct patients who are discharged home on antibiotics to take the antibiotic as prescribed until the prescription is completed.
Nonsteroidal Anti-Inflammatory Agents (NSAIDs)		
Acetylsalicylic acid aspirin (ASA) Acetaminophen (Tylenol) Indomethacin (Indocin) Ibuprofen (Motrin) Ketorolac (Toradol) ***Action:*** Aspirin and the ibuprofen-like NSAIDs block the synthesis of prostaglandins by inhibiting cyclo-oxygenase (COX-1 and COX-2).	Pain, discomfort Fever Rheumatic fever Infective endocarditis Pericarditis	Monitor for urticaria, prolonged bleeding time, abdominal distress, GI bleeding, elevated liver function tests, elevated BUN/creatinine.
Steroids		
Dexamethasone (Decadron) Hydrocortisone (Solu-Cortef) Methylprednisolone (Solu-Medrol)	Rheumatic fever Pericarditis	Monitor for elevated blood glucose levels, elevated lipid levels, and hypernatremia. Monitor level of immunosuppression and increased susceptibility to infection.

PHARMACOLOGY Summary of Medications Used to Treat Cardiac Inflammatory Disorders, *continued*

Medication Category and Action	Application/Indication	Nursing Responsibility
Prednisone ***Action:*** Reduce cell reproduction. Reduce inflammation. Suppress allergic response. Suppress immune response.	Prophylaxis of transplant rejection	Monitor for development of peptic ulcers. Monitor for changes in mood and behavior, nervousness, and hallucinations. Instruct the patient to take the medication as prescribed. Do not stop abruptly, doses need to be tapered.
Diuretics		
Bumetanide (Bumex) Ethacrynic Acid (Edecrin) Furosemide (Lasix) Torsemide (Demadex) ***Action:*** Increase the excretion of water. Block reabsorption of sodium in the loop of Henle.	Hypertension Heart failure Pulmonary edema Peripheral edema	Monitor intake and output. Monitor for excess fluid loss, hypokalemia, dysrhythmias, orthostatic hypotension. If patient is diabetic, monitor blood glucose levels, which may be affected by some loop diuretics.
Anticoagulant Therapy		
Heparin Low molecular weight heparin (Lovenox, Fragmin) Dabigatran (Pradaxa) Warfarin (Coumadin) ***Action:*** Inhibits specific factors in the clotting cascade and decreases the risk of thrombus formation.	Dysrhythmias, especially atrial fibrillation Venous thromboembolism prophylaxis	Monitor for bleeding from the gums, bleeding from puncture sites; hemoptysis, hematuria. Monitor laboratory values that assess coagulation: PT/INR, PTT. Monitor for thrombocytopenia. For patients on warfarin (Coumadin), provide detailed discharge instructions regarding PTT/INR follow-up and the potential impact of alcohol, food, and various other medications, including OTC and herbal preparations.
Anti-Anxiety Agents		
Alprazolam (Xanax) Chlordiazepoxide (Librium) Diazepam (Valium) Lorazepam (Ativan) ***Action:*** Central nervous system depression. Produces relaxation, calmness.	Anxiety	Monitor for drowsiness, ataxia, or dizziness. As appropriate, instruct the patient about nonpharmacologic techniques for relaxation; for example, deep breathing, massage, guided imagery.
Dihydropyridine Calcium-Channel Blockers:		
Amlodipine (Norvasc) Felodipine (Plendil) Nicardipine (Cardene) Nifedipine (Procardia) ***Action:*** Dihydropyridines bind reversibly to closed-type calcium channels to make them unresponsive to depolarization.	Hypertension Dysrhythmias	Monitor blood pressure regularly when drug is initiated and when dosage is titrated. Hold the drug and notify the health care provider if the systolic blood pressure is less than 90 mmHg. Monitor for: Elevated blood glucose Gingival hyperplasia Palpitations, weight gain, peripheral edema, skin rashes. Teach the patient to avoid grapefruit/grapefruit juice because of potential drug–food interaction.
Nondihydropyridine Calcium-Channel Blockers		
Diltiazem (Cardizem, Dilacor) Verapamil (Calan) ***Action:*** Nondihydropyridines are chemically different from the above as they bind to open-type calcium-channel blockers and slow repolarization.		

(*continued*)

PHARMACOLOGY Summary of Medications Used to Treat Cardiac Inflammatory Disorders, *continued*

Medication Category and Action	Application/Indication	Nursing Responsibility
Nitrates		
Nitroglycerin (NTG) Isosorbide dinitrate (Iso-Bid, Isordil) Isosorbide mononitrate (Imdur, Nitro-Bid) ***Action:*** Potent vasodilator, leading to relaxation of both arterial and venous smooth muscle. Reduces preload to the heart. Lowers myocardial oxygen demand. Dilates coronary arteries.	Hypertension Heart failure Acute pulmonary edema	Monitor blood pressure regularly when drug is initiated and when dosage is titrated. Hold the drug and notify the health care provider if the systolic blood pressure is less than 90 mmHg. Monitor for: Headache Orthostatic hypotension.
Beta-Adrenergic Blockers: Nonselective Beta-Adrenergic Blockers		
Nadolol (Corgard) Pindolol (Visken) Propranolol (Inderal) Sotolol (Betapace) Timolol (Blocadren) ***Action:*** Nonselective: Causes a decrease in blood pressure through a mixture of beta-blocking effects but does not cause reflex tachycardia or decreased heart rate.	Dysrhythmias Hypertension Heart failure	Monitor blood pressure and heart rate regularly when drug is initiated and when dosage is titrated. Hold the drug and notify the health care provider if the systolic blood pressure is less than 90 mmHg and/or the heart rate is less than 60 per minute. Monitor for: Bradycardia Elevated blood glucose. Teach the patient to avoid abruptly stopping beta-adrenergic blocker agents.
Selective Beta-Adrenergic Blockers		
Acebutolol (Sectral) Atenolol (Tenormin) Bisoprolol (Zebeta) Esmolol (Brevibloc) Metoprolol (Lopressor) ***Action:*** Selective: Completely blocks beta-1 receptor stimulation in cardiac smooth muscle.		
Angiotensin-Converting Enzyme (ACE) Inhibitors		
Benazepril (Lotensin) Captopril (Capoten) Enalapril (Vasotec) Fosinopril (Monopril) Lisinopril (Prinivil, Zestril) Quinipril (Accupril) Ramipril (Altace) ***Action:*** Inhibits the conversion of angiotensin I to angiotensin II; suppresses renin-angiotensin-aldosterone system.	Hypertension Heart failure	Monitor blood pressure regularly when drug is initiated and when dosage is titrated. Hold the drug and notify the health care provider if the systolic blood pressure is less than 90 mmHg. Monitor for: Orthostatic hypotension Elevated serum sodium, potassium, and/or creatinine Angioedema of the extremities, face, lips, tongue, glottis, and larynx Drug-induced neutropenia. Teach the patient to avoid over-the-counter NSAIDs as they can reduce the effectiveness of ACE inhibitors.
Angiotensin II Receptor Blockers (ARBs)		
Candesartan (Atacand) Eprosartan (Teveten) Irbesartan (Avapro) Losartan (Cozaar) Valsartan (Diovan) ***Action:*** Blocks the vasoconstrictor and aldosterone-secreting effects of angiotensin.	Hypertension Heart failure	Monitor blood pressure regularly when drug is initiated and when dosage is titrated. Hold the drug and notify the health care provider if the systolic blood pressure is less than 90 mmHg. Monitor for: Orthostatic hypotension Elevated serum sodium, potassium, and creatinine.

Sources: Adapted from Adams, M. P., & Koch, R. W. (2010). *Pharmacology: Connections to nursing practice.* Upper Saddle River, NJ: Pearson. Connolly, S. J., Ezekowitz, M. D., Yusef, Y., Eikelboom, J., Oldgren, J., Parekh, A., et al. (2009). Dabigatraban versus warfarin in atrial fibrillation. *New England Journal of Medicine, 36*(12), 1139–1151.

Process: Patient Care Plan for Inflammatory Heart Disease box (p. 980). The nurse must specifically note and report to the health care provider any progression of the clinical manifestations related to heart failure. In addition, any change in the loudness of the murmur must be documented and reported because this may indicate a progression of cardiac valve disorders.

The desired outcome for the patient with rheumatic fever is to make a full recovery with no residual cardiac pathology. Nursing management focuses on resting the heart, pain relief, eradication of the infecting organism, and emotional support. Nursing interventions require critical thinking and sound clinical judgment because patients do not all present with the same manifestations. It is essential to stress the importance of decreasing myocardial oxygen demand and cardiac workload. Strict bed rest is typically ordered, especially in the acute stages of these illnesses. The nurse must explain the importance of bed rest and activity restriction to the patient and family. Spacing care and activities to allow for periods of rest will decrease oxygen demand and, thus, cardiac workload.

Health Promotion

Prevention of a recurrence of the disease requires patient and family education about the need for vigilant hygiene, good nutrition, and rest. The patient needs to be instructed to avoid individuals with upper respiratory infections to minimize exposure. The nurse should stress the risk for recurrence if a streptococcal infection occurs. A list of clinical manifestations that would indicate a need to seek medical help must be provided. The nurse should stress that cardiac valve disease could develop and will require medical intervention. The Patient Teaching & Discharge Priorities box (p. 983) outlines specific discharge priorities.

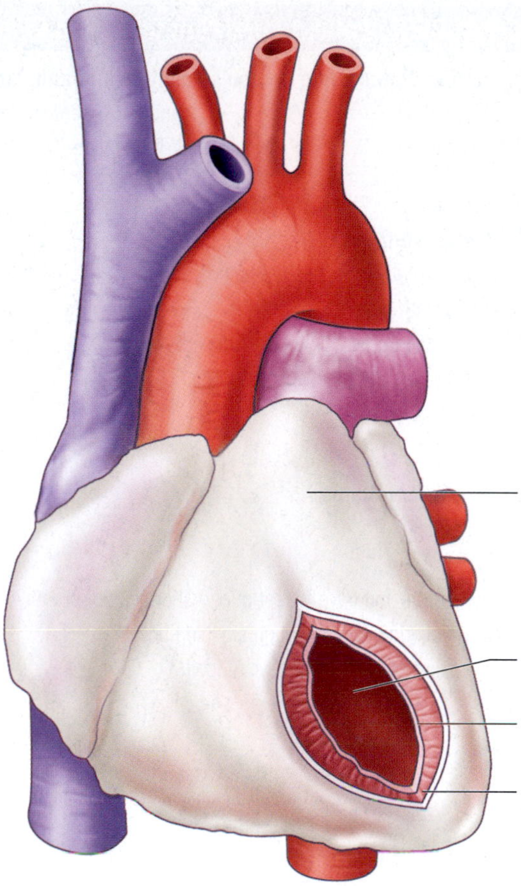

FIGURE 33–2 ◆ Layers of the heart wall.

Pericarditis

Pericarditis, an inflammation of the pericardial sac, is the most common pathologic process affecting the pericardium. The pericardium or pericardial sac is a double-walled membranous sac that encloses the heart and the roots of the great vessels. The purpose of the pericardial sac is to prevent excessive dilation during diastole, to act as a barrier from infections in adjacent tissues, and to prevent displacement of the myocardium and great vessels. The inner serous layer of the pericardium is the visceral pericardium or epicardium, and the outer layer is the parietal pericardium (Figure 33–2◆). The space between these two layers, referred to as the pericardial space, normally contains approximately 50 mL of fluid. The fluid serves to lubricate and decrease friction between the layers while the heart is moving during systole and diastole. Due to the inflammatory process, the two layers of the pericardium become inflamed and roughened, and the amount of fluid in the pericardial sac increases. Pericarditis can be acute and/or chronic constrictive (recurrent) and has several causes.

Epidemiology and Etiology

Pericarditis has three general causes: infectious, noninfectious, and hypersensitive or autoimmune. These causes are listed in the Risk Factors box (p. 984). If the cause is infectious, the infection often starts in some other organ in the body, usually the lungs and upper respiratory tract. The most common cause of pericarditis is infection with the coxsackie virus B, which is referred to as Bornholm disease. People in their 20s and 30s who have had a recent upper respiratory infection and men ages 20 to 50 years are most likely to be affected. Frequently, the cause of pericarditis is idiopathic. Noninfectious causes include uremia, which affects 6% to 10% of patients with advanced renal failure before initiation of dialysis. When patients with large effusions are studied, uremia may account for up to 20% of cases in some series. The widespread availability of dialysis has reduced the incidence of uremic pericarditis (Gowda, 2010). Noninfectious pericarditis also occurs after acute myocardial infarction (AMI) and following open heart surgery (postcardiotomy).

Hypersensitive or autoimmune responses are the third category of causes of pericarditis. This category includes connective tissue disorders, drug reactions, and rheumatoid diseases that affect the heart. **Dressler's syndrome,** also referred to as late pericarditis, occurs in 5% to 15% of the patients typically 1 to 4 weeks after an AMI. It is characterized by fever, pericarditis, chest pain, and pericardial friction rub and pleural effusions. Dressler's syndrome may persist for weeks or even months after an AMI (Mayo Clinic, 2010a). Because it is thought to be an inflammatory process, treatment focuses on decreasing inflammation and treating the pain. NSAIDs such as aspirin treat the inflammation, and opioids are used to treat the pain.

Pathophysiology

With the infectious form of pericarditis, microbes causing the infection form an exudate of fibrin, white blood cells (WBCs), and endothelial cells. This exudate covers the pericardium, causing further inflammation of the surrounding tissues. Acute pericarditis can be either dry or exudative. If exudative, the pericardial sac fills with the serofibrinous exudate. Anywhere from 100 to 3,000 mL of fluid or exudate has been known to accumulate in the pericardial sac. This excess fluid accumulation restricts cardiac filling and emptying, thereby decreasing cardiac

NURSING PROCESS: Patient Care Plan for Inflammatory Heart Disease

Assessment of Cardiac Status Using Gordon's Functional Health Patterns:

- Nutrition Metabolic Pattern
- Activity Exercise Pattern
- Cognitive Perceptual Pattern
- Self-Perception–Self-Concept Pattern

Subjective Data	Objective Data
Assessment of Cardiac Output	**Assessment of Cardiac Output**
Do you become short of breath at rest or with activity? Has your shortness of breath become worse? Do your legs become swollen at any time during the day? Have you noticed a blue tinge in your nail beds?	Determine heart rate and rhythm. Blood pressure. Lung sounds. Urine output. Capillary refill. Right-sided heart failure (JVD, hepatomegaly, peripheral edema).
Assessment of Respiratory Status	**Assessment of Respiratory Status**
Do you feel short of breath? When does it occur? How far can you walk before you have to rest due to shortness of breath? Do you have a cough and, if so, do you cough anything up? Do you become more short of breath when lying down?	Acid–base balance. Lung sounds. Respiratory rate. Assess for adventitious or diminished breath sounds. Note presence of cough, and amount and color of sputum. Monitor ABGs and oxygen saturation. Monitor respiratory rate and depth. Monitor restlessness and confusion. Observe for cyanosis, especially in the mucous membranes.
Assessment of Tissue Perfusion	**Assessment of Tissue Perfusion**
Do you have any pain in either leg? Have you noticed any swelling or hard reddened areas? Have you had any sudden chest pain that becomes worse when you take a deep breath? Have you had any headaches, loss of consciousness, or dizzy spells?	Lung congestion. Urine output and color. Abdominal pain. Neurological function. Skin and eyes. Nail beds. Calf deep vein thrombosis (DVT). Glasgow Coma Scale.
Assessment of Pain	**Assessment of Pain**
Do you have problems with pain? Where is the pain (joints, chest)? What brings the pain on; what makes it go away? What do you use to relieve it and is it effective? Is the pain getting worse? Describe the type of pain (i.e., sharp. dull, ache, pressure).	Use pain scale (0–10) to quantify pain level. Assess cultural and religious impact on patient's responses. Assess the onset of increased pain to evaluate the presence of disease progression and/or an embolic event.
Assessment of Activity Tolerance	**Assessment of Activity Tolerance**
What type of activity fatigues you? Has it been getting progressively worse? Does activity increase joint tenderness and swelling? Are you able to complete your ADLs without fatigue or shortness of breath?	Assess for joint tenderness, swelling, and decreased range of motion. Monitor vital signs during activity.
Assessment of Anxiety Related to Inflammatory Heart Disease	**Assessment of Anxiety Related to Inflammatory Heart Disease**
Has anyone explained your health problems to you? Would you tell me what you know about your disease? How does this disease affect your daily life? Do you feel anxious about your health problems? Do you have family members or close friends who provide emotional support?	Observe for manifestations of anxiety: restlessness, apprehension, and/or withdrawal.

NURSING PROCESS: Patient Care Plan for Inflammatory Heart Disease, *continued*

Assessment of Fever Do you feel hotter than normal? If so, how long have you been feeling that way? Have you had the chills?	**Assessment of Fever** Monitor temperature and WBC count.
Assessment of Knowledge of Health Problems What have you been told about your health problems? Tell me what you know about your health problems. What do you do when symptoms occur? Do you see your health care provider on a regular basis? Do you know what symptoms are important to report to your health care provider immediately?	**Assessment of Knowledge of Health Problems** Assess knowledge of need to rest the heart and decrease the oxygen needs. Explore the patient's understanding of the purpose of preventive antibiotic therapy.
Outcomes and Evaluation Parameters	**Planning and Interventions with *Rationales***
1. NURSING DIAGNOSIS: Decreased Cardiac Output and Ineffective Tissue Perfusion *related to infection, incompetent valves, and heart failure* (NANDA-I © 2012)	
Outcome: Sufficient cardiac output to perfuse organs. ***Evaluation Parameters:*** Minimal valve damage that decreases cardiac output. Stable vital signs, denies shortness of breath. Oxygen saturation levels within normal limits.	Auscultate heart sounds for murmur and S_3, S_4 *to evaluate valve function and onset of heart failure.* Provide oxygen per order *to increase oxygen to the heart and peripheral tissues.* Administer diuretics, inotropics, and a low sodium diet *to treat heart failure.* Plan rest period *to reduce cardiac workload.*
2. NURSING DIAGNOSIS: Impaired Gas Exchange *related to heart failure* (NANDA-I © 2012)	
Outcome: Adequate gas exchange is achieved. ***Evaluation Parameters:*** Normal arterial blood gases. No dyspnea: unlabored respirations < 24/minute. No ischemic ECG changes such as ST segment changes and dysrhythmias. Alert and oriented. Clear breath sounds. No restlessness, cyanosis, or fatigue. Oxygen saturation is within normal limits.	Monitor: ABGs, oxygen saturation, respiratory rate, lung sounds, and ECG. Turn, cough, deep breathe, elevate head of bed. Instruct on use of incentive spirometry. *Measures to promote gas exchange.* Administer humidified oxygen as prescribed *to increase oxygen levels.* Report respiratory distress to the health care provider. *Medical intervention may be indicated to prevent respiratory failure.* Assess need for suctioning and/or endotracheal intubation *to maintain adequate gas exchange.* Monitor fluid status *to assess heart failure.*
3. NURSING DIAGNOSIS: Ineffective Tissue Perfusion *related to dislodging of vegetative growths and immobility-related thrombophlebitis* (NANDA-I © 2012)	
Outcome: Occurrence of emboli diagnosed early and treatment instituted. ***Evaluation Parameter:*** Effective prevention of DVT.	Apply elastic compression stocking *to provide venous support.* Teach leg exercises *to promote venous return and decrease risk of DVT.* Report any new abnormal clinical manifestations to the health care provider. Monitor for therapeutic levels of anticoagulant therapy. Monitor for bleeding. *To prevent or mitigate side effects of anticoagulant medication.*
4. NURSING DIAGNOSIS: Pain, Acute *related to fluid buildup and inflammatory response* (NANDA-I © 2012)	
Outcome: Comfort level maintained. ***Evaluation Parameters:*** Patient is able to communicate pain level and therapies that help alleviate it. Pain is reduced and/or absent as evidenced by patient report and no pain behaviors: grimacing. Nonpharmacologic method of control is effective as evidenced by patient report and no pain behaviors. Patient reports satisfaction with pain management program.	Instruct the patient to inform the nurse if pain is not relieved. *Indicates need to change the pain management plan.* Obtain a clear description of the source of discomfort. *This will assist in developing a pain management plan.* Correct misconceptions about the risk of addiction and overdose *to decrease anxiety related to medication addiction.* Provide a supportive environment where the patient is able to express her pain level. *Opens communication and facilitates pain management.* Use pain control measures before pain becomes severe. *This increases comfort and decreases need for medication.* Teach nonpharmacologic method of control (e.g. guided imagery and massage) and breathing exercises. *These measures augment pain relief.* Teach the patient/family the correct dosage and time intervals for medication administration *to increase compliance and prevent complications.*

(*continued*)

NURSING PROCESS: Patient Care Plan for Inflammatory Heart Disease, *continued*

Outcomes and Evaluation Parameters	Planning and Interventions with *Rationales*
5. NURSING DIAGNOSIS: Activity Intolerance *related to decreased cardiac output, fatigue, and inflammation* (NANDA-I © 2012)	
Outcome: Able to complete ADLs without fatigue. ***Evaluation Parameter:*** Able to increase activity level with resolution of clinical manifestations.	Take 30- to 60-minute rest periods between all activities *to decrease cardiac workload.* Perform only essential activities until endurance improves *to decrease cardiac workload during the healing process.*
6. NURSING DIAGNOSIS: Fear and Anxiety *related to inflammatory heart disease* (NANDA-I © 2012)	
Outcome: Anxiety level is minimized and manageable. ***Evaluation Parameters:*** Verbalizes anxious feelings. Verbalizes what relieves anxiety. Verbalizes absence of sensory perceptual disorders. Verbalizes absence of physical manifestations of anxiety. Behavioral manifestations of anxiety absent.	Provide factual information concerning diagnosis, treatment, disfigurement, disabilities, and prognosis. *Truthful explanations increase trust and potentially decrease anxiety.* Explain all procedures and allow time for mental preparation. *This decreases fear and anxiety of the unknown.* Allow time and encourage verbalization of fears related to illness *to assist in relieving anxiety.* Explore with the patient/family techniques to reduce anxiety. *This gives the patient a sense of control and opens communication about the subject.* Explore with the patient effective ways to minimize anxiety. *This gives the patient a sense of control.* Instruct the patient on the use of relaxation techniques *to relieve anxiety.* Assess the need for and administer antianxiety and pain medication. *If alternative measures are not effective, the patient may need antianxiety agents.*
7. NURSING DIAGNOSIS: Hyperthermia *related to the infection* (NANDA-I © 2012)	
Outcomes: Normal temperature. Absence of chills. ***Evaluation Parameters:*** Effective antibiotic treatment. Resolution of infection.	Administer antipyretics *to decrease temperature.* Administer antibiotics *to treat the causative organism.* Cover the patient *to prevent shivering and subsequent temperature elevation.*
8. NURSING DIAGNOSIS: Deficient Knowledge *related to disease process and prognosis* (NANDA-I © 2012)	
Outcome: Verbalizes understanding of prevention. ***Evaluation Parameters:*** Reports regular dental appointments and follow-up visits. Verbalizes adherence and compliance to therapy.	See Patient Teaching & Discharge Priorities feature for home care and remainder of teaching needs.

Source: Adapted from Wilkinson, J. M., & Ahearn, N. R. (2009). *Prentice Hall nursing diagnosis handbook* (9th ed.). Upper Saddle River, NJ: Prentice Hall.

output and tissue perfusion. Without prompt treatment, shock and death will occur.

A number of causes of noninfectious pericarditis are listed in the accompanying Risk Factors box (p. 984). For example, blunt trauma to the chest and heart surgery cause inflammation of the cardiac tissues. Small blood vessels may leak due to trauma, and the inflammation caused by tissue injury causes fluid to accumulate in the pericardial sac.

Chronic **constrictive pericarditis** occurs when the pericardial layers adhere to each other as a result of fibrosis of the pericardial sac. This usually occurs as a result of tuberculosis, typically found in the immigrant and prison populations and in people with acquired immunodeficiency syndrome (AIDS). Constrictive pericarditis also may develop secondary to surgery, uremia, or radiation. The fibrosis causes scarring and thickening of the pericardium, which decrease cardiac filling and contracting, leading to decreased cardiac output and heart failure.

Clinical Manifestations

Pain from pericarditis varies among patients, with symptoms ranging from mild to severe. The pain usually comes on suddenly, often on the left side of the chest, and radiates to the left shoulder, neck, and back. Some patients describe the pain in the same terms as anginal-type chest pain; others describe it as a sharp pleuritic-type pain. One way to differentiate the pain of pericarditis from angina is that it becomes worse with inspiration, coughing, movement of the trunk, and deep breathing. It also typically is worse when the patient is lying flat and tends to decrease when the patient is sitting up and leaning forward, a position that moves the heart away from the diaphragmatic side of the lung pleura. This is often the key to the diagnosis. The chest pain often causes the patient to have dyspnea. Other causes of dyspnea include compression of the bronchioles from the inflamed heart and fever.

The onset of bacterial pericarditis is associated with high fever (39.4°C [103°F]), chills, leukocytosis (increased white blood cells), malaise, joint pain, and a rise in the erythrocyte sedimentation rate. Anorexia, weight loss, and nausea also accompany the acute stages of the disease.

Electrocardiogram (ECG) changes also occur with pericarditis. ECG changes may include transient PR interval depression, tachycardia, bradycardia, and atrial fibrillation. Concurrent with the onset of chest pain, ST segment elevation in leads I, II, aVF, V_4, and V_6 occurs, followed by T wave inversion without Q wave changes. The T wave remains inverted for weeks to months. ECG changes evolve over a period

PATIENT TEACHING & DISCHARGE PRIORITIES for Inflammatory Heart Disease

Need	Teaching
Knowledge of disease process and prognosis	Home care needs include verbal and written instructions for: • Treatment plan • Follow-up care • Activity restriction. These instructions will reinforce the need to comply with therapy.
Understanding of medications	Teach the patient and family to administer the antibiotics and to care for the infusion site using aseptic technique. Teach the purpose, dose, and possible side effects of all medications to increase compliance and prevent over/underdosing. Emphasize the need for regular laboratory testing to monitor therapeutic levels.
Oral hygiene	Emphasize the importance of good dental hygiene and regular checkups to decrease the risk of pathogen entry via the mouth.
Disease prevention	Explain the need for antibiotic prophylaxis before invasive procedures to prevent reoccurrence. Encourage avoidance of people with upper respiratory infections to prevent an increased risk of infection. Avoid intravenous (IV) drug use.
Safety	Stress the importance of a medic alert bracelet to identify a heart problem to health care workers.
Reportable clinical manifestations	Instruct the patient and family to report: • Change of exercise tolerance • New onset chest pain and fever • Clinical manifestations of heart failure • Spontaneous or unusual bleeding.
Family/support system	Assess availability, knowledge, and compliance with treatment regimen. Assess respite needs and resources. Assess discharge placement needs: • Home • Rehabilitation facility • Extended care facility. Assess the home environment for the need for assistive devices. Assess for the need for professional home health needs. Assess for the need for follow-up appointments.
Emotional adjustment of patient/family due to the chronic nature of the disease	Answer questions honestly. Encourage verbalization of frustrations and anger. Encourage positive reinforcement from the family. Stress that it is not uncommon to feel let down or depressed after discharge.

of weeks to months and are thought to be caused by superficial myocardial inflammation or epicardial injury. See Chapter 30 for a complete description of these ECG changes. Finally, the overall amplitude of the QRS complexes is typically decreased.

A **pericardial friction rub** is a key factor in the diagnostic assessment of a patient being evaluated for pericarditis. Friction rubs are described as a grating, scraping, squeaking, or crunching sound that is the result of friction between the roughened, inflamed layers of the pericardium. These sounds are best heard over the left sternal border in the second, third, or fourth intercostal space with the diaphragm of the stethoscope. The sounds become louder when the patient is sitting up and leaning forward. One way to distinguish it from a pleural friction rub is to ask the patient to momentarily hold her breath; if the rub persists, it is cardiac rather than respiratory in nature. Pericardial friction rubs are often transient and may vary in intensity from hour to hour (Hurst et al., 2009).

Pericardial effusion, an excess of pericardial fluid, is a threat to normal cardiac function. The fluid buildup in the pericardial sac is a result of an accumulation of infectious exudates or toxins and/or blood. The clinical manifestations depend on the rate and amount of fluid collecting in the area. If the buildup is gradual, the pericardial sac will stretch and accommodate 1 to 2 liters of fluid without causing cardiac compression. Conversely, a rapid buildup of fluid does not allow the pericardial sac to stretch, and cardiac compression will occur with only 80 to 200 mL of fluid. If a pleural effusion is present, heart sounds are typically muffled and may be difficult to auscultate. Large effusions compress adjoining structures in the pleural cavity (e.g., pulmonary compression causes coughing, dyspnea, and tachypnea). Compression of the laryngeal nerve causes hoarseness, and compression of the phrenic nerve may induce hiccups (Hurst et al., 2009).

Cardiac tamponade occurs when there is a rapid and large accumulation of fluid in the pericardial space. This is a medical emergency that is caused most frequently by bleeding, from either postoperative complications (thoracic surgery) or trauma. It also can be caused by an accumulation of pus or air and may be present with any type of pericarditis. This large collection of fluid raises the pressure in the pericardial sac, compressing the cardiac chambers, and prevents blood from entering the heart. Blood backs up into the venous system, raising venous

Weblink: Sudden Cardiac Death

RISK FACTORS for Pericarditis

Infectious	Bacterial: tuberculosis, streptococcus, staphylococcus, meningococcus, syphilis, pneumococcus, Lyme disease
	Viral: coxsackie virus B, echoviruses, endoviruses, adenoviruses, HIV, hepatitis
	Fungal
	Parasitic
Noninfectious	Chest trauma or injury
	Cardiac surgery
	Uremia
	Radiation therapy
	Cancer that has metastasized to the pericardium
	Acute myocardial infarction (AMI) (48–72 hr)
	Dissecting aortic aneurysm
Hypersensitive or Autoimmune	Systemic lupus erythematosus
	Rheumatoid arthritis
	Scleroderma
	Polyarteritis nodosa
	Ankylosing spondylitis
	Myxedema
	Post myocardial infarction syndrome or Dressler's syndrome (Chapter 32)
	Drug reactions: procainamide, hydralazine, minoxidil

Source: American Heart Association. (2010). *Sudden cardiac death.* Retrieved from http://www.americanheart.org/presenter.jhtml?identifier=4741.

pressure, while cardiac output and blood pressure (BP) fall because of a lack of blood filling the heart (decreased preload; see Chapter 31 for a complete explanation of preload). The drop in cardiac output and subsequent loss of tissue perfusion make this a life-threatening situation. It is essential that the nurse knows and understands the significance of the clinical manifestations of cardiac tamponade and how to intervene to prevent shock and death.

Clinical manifestations associated with tamponade are related to the decreased cardiac output and increased systemic venous congestion. A narrowing of the pulse pressure (systolic minus diastolic blood pressure to less than 30 mmHg) and tachycardia are hallmark signs of cardiac tamponade. The heart is attempting to compensate for the drop in cardiac output by increasing the rate. Without adequate preload, the increased rate cannot maintain a normal cardiac output, and the increased cardiac workload will lead to failure. Classic assessment findings for the patient with cardiac tamponade are referred to as **Beck's triad,** consisting of decreased blood pressure, muffled heart sounds, and jugular venous distention. Additionally, weak peripheral pulses and pulsus paradoxus are also present. A **pulsus paradoxus** is a greater than 10-mmHg drop in systolic blood pressure during inspiration. The blood pressure normally decreases during inspiration but does so by less than 10 mmHg. A drop of greater than 10 mmHg occurs when there is increased thoracic pressure as a result of pericardial swelling. This is an important diagnostic clue that is most frequently picked up by the nurse. The patient typically becomes restless and may have a decreased level of consciousness as the fluid accumulates and the cardiac output drops. Finally, the amplitude of the QRS complex of the ECG is low.

Safety Alert *The sudden onset of pulsus paradoxus is an indication that cardiac tamponade is occurring. The patient needs to be assessed for other signs of tamponade: tachycardia, diminished heart sounds, narrowed pulse pressure, and distended neck veins. The nurse should notify the health care provider immediately to institute diagnosis and treatment. Cardiac tamponade is a life-threatening complication of pericardial effusion.*

Laboratory and Diagnostic Procedures

The patient's clinical manifestations and diagnostic and laboratory tests are used to confirm the diagnosis of pericarditis. There are no specific laboratory tests to diagnose pericarditis, but tests are performed to rule out other possible causes of the symptoms. The earlier box titled Diagnostic Tests for Cardiac Inflammatory Disorders (p. 975) outlines the typical tests that are done to assist in confirming the diagnosis. In addition to the tests listed in that box, antibody titers, blood urea nitrogen (BUN), and tuberculosis testing are used to help determine the cause. An ECG, serial troponin, and cardiac isoenzymes are done to rule out a myocardial infarction. Computed tomography (CT) scans and magnetic resonance imaging (MRI) also are used to identify pericardial effusions and/or the pericardial thickening characteristics of constrictive pericarditis (Chapter 32).

Hemodynamic monitoring is used with acute pericarditis to assess pulmonary artery pressures and cardiac output. Elevated central venous pressures and pulmonary artery pressures are seen due to inflammation. Cardiac output is decreased especially in the presence of cardiac tamponade.

A pericardiocentesis, the removal of fluid from the pericardial sac, is both diagnostic and therapeutic when effusion is present. The procedure is performed under sterile conditions with ECG and hemodynamic monitoring capabilities. A health care provider inserts an 8-inch, 16- to 18-gauge needle into the pericardial sac, and the fluid is aspirated (Figure 33–3◆). Echocardiography (p. 1019) may also be used to provide ultrasound assistance during needle insertion. The needle is attached to an ECG monitor to guide the depth of needle insertion. Once the needle touches the epicardial surface, ECG changes occur. The health care provider and the nurse observe the ECG monitor for ST segment and T wave changes that indicate the epicardial surface has

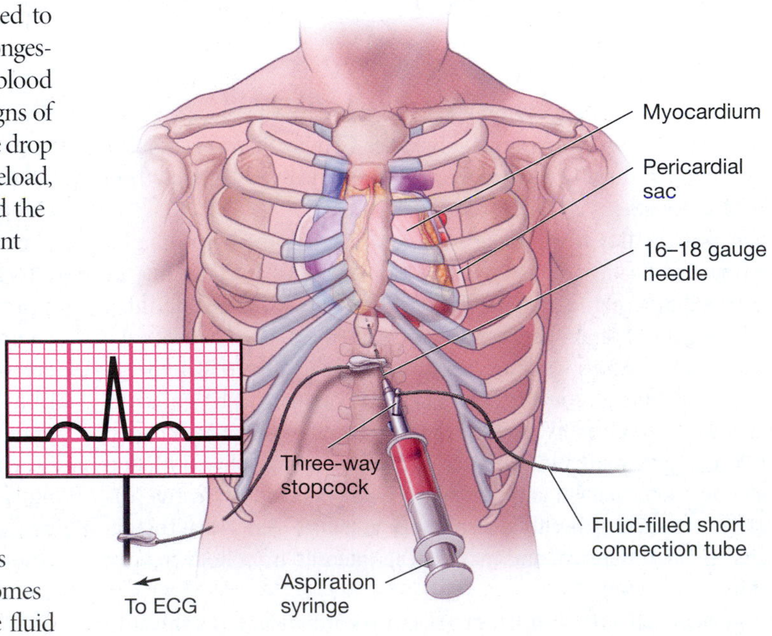

FIGURE 33–3 ◆ Pericardiocentesis.

been reached; when that occurs, the needle is withdrawn slightly. When the needle is in the proper position, a catheter is placed and the pericardial fluid is withdrawn. As the fluid drains, the pressures decrease and the clinical manifestations of tamponade begin to resolve. To assist in determining the cause of the pericardial effusion, the pericardial fluid is sent to the laboratory for culture and sensitivity analysis and cytology. If fluid buildup persists, the health care provider may choose to leave a catheter in the pericardium attached to a bag to allow for continuous draining of the fluid.

Medical Management

Medical management of pericarditis is directed toward finding the cause and instituting treatment to prevent complications. Because treatment is specific to the cause, it is essential that the cause of the pericarditis be determined. The diagnostic studies and clinical manifestations outlined previously assist in determining the cause.

Antibiotic treatment is indicated if the cause is a bacterial infection, and steroids are used when the pericarditis is secondary to systemic lupus erythematosus (SLE), a myocardial infarction (MI), or other immune system conditions. There is no specific curative treatment for viral pericarditis. It typically clears in 2 weeks to 3 months, and treatments are aimed at controlling symptoms. For example, drugs that are known to treat tuberculosis are indicated if that is the cause of the pericarditis. If renal failure is the cause, more frequent and intense dialysis treatments are needed.

Pain must be assessed to differentiate pericarditis from MI, because treatment for MI requires antiplatelet and anticoagulation therapies, which are contraindicated with pericarditis. Pain control is managed with NSAIDs such as indomethacin (Indocin), ibuprofen, and aspirin in large doses. In addition to their analgesic properties, these medications reduce swelling. See the Pharmacology feature (p. 976) for a list of medications used to treat inflammatory heart disease.

Activity restriction is necessary until the swelling begins to subside and the pain is effectively managed. Bed rest is indicated with the head of the bed elevated to reduce cardiac workload. Symptoms and activity tolerance will dictate when increased activity is appropriate. Oxygen may be needed in the acute stages or in the presence of pericardial effusion. ECG monitoring is necessary to monitor for cardiac dysrhythmias and myocardial injury.

Because cardiac tamponade is a life-threatening complication of pericarditis, assessing for it is critical to patient survival. A pericardiocentesis is done to relieve the constricting effects of cardiac tamponade and is indicated when the patient's blood pressure has decreased by 30 mmHg. Hemodynamic and ECG monitoring are necessary during and after the procedure to assess the patient's hemodynamic status. The amount of fluid that is removed is recorded on the output record in the patient's medical record. Fluid replacement after pericardiocentesis is needed to increase cardiac output and tissue perfusion. Complications from pericardiocentesis include dysrhythmias, pneumothorax, myocardial laceration, cardiac tamponade, and gastric fistula.

If recurrent effusions and tamponade occur or if there are adhesions from chronic constrictive pericarditis, the pericardium may have to be partially or completely removed surgically (**pericardiectomy, pericardial window**) to allow fluid to drain into the pleural space. This will relieve the compression on the heart and allow for adequate ventricular filling and cardiac output. Surgical resection of the pericardium is recommended in the early stages of constrictive pericarditis. Patients with advanced constrictive pericarditis have up to a 12% risk of mortality (Schwefer, Aschenbach, Heidemann, Mey, & Lapp, 2009).

Nursing Management

The goals of nursing management for the patient with pericarditis includes: pain and anxiety management, cardiac monitoring, treating, and reporting significant ECG changes; and evaluating the patient for the development of cardiac tamponade.

Assessment

The nurse must assess the patient's pain to distinguish it from anginal-type chest pain as described earlier. It is important to assess the pain for the amount, quality, and location to differentiate it from the pain of an acute MI. The ECG is monitored during pain because ST segment changes seen with an acute MI are seen only in certain leads depending on the location of the infarction, whereas ST segment changes seen with pericarditis are present in all leads except aVR and V_1 (Chapter 30). Additionally, the patient is assessed for the clinical manifestations of cardiac tamponade, including decreased blood pressure, muffled heart sounds, jugular venous distention, weak peripheral pulses, and pulsus paradoxus.

Nursing Diagnoses

Actual and potential nursing diagnoses related to pericarditis include:

- *Decreased Cardiac Output* related to *the pericarditis*
- *Ineffective Tissue Perfusion related to decreased cardiac output*
- *Anxiety related to the fear of pericarditis*
- *Activity Intolerance related surgery and heart disease*
- *Acute Pain related to surgery.*

NANDA-I © 2012

Outcomes and Evaluation Parameters

The desired outcomes for the patient with pericarditis include absence of pain and normal cardiac output. Finding and treating the cause will result in a relief of symptoms. Medical intervention with pericardiocentesis, as described earlier, may be a lifesaving measure. Evaluation parameters include normal heart rate and blood pressure as well as a balanced intake and urine output. There should be no unusual fatigue or shortness of breath.

Planning, Interventions, and Rationales

Administration of the anti-inflammatory analgesics is essential, and helping the patient find a position of comfort also helps to relieve the pain. Typically, the most comfortable position is sitting up and leaning forward on a bedside table to give the heart more room in the pleural cavity. A warm heating pad or hot water bottle also may help relieve the pain. Pain relief measures include elevating the head of the bed and administering anti-inflammatory agents as ordered.

Safety Alert *When a patient complains of chest pain, it is essential that an assessment be done to determine whether the pain is anginal-type pain associated with myocardial ischemia or is due to pericarditis. Anginal pain is typically described as a burning, pressure-type pain that is not associated with position change or deep breathing. It is relieved by nitroglycerin and rest. The chest pain that is associated with pericarditis is often described as sharp and gets worse with deep breathing. It is relieved by sitting up and taking anti-inflammatory drugs.*

The nurse needs to assess the ECG for ST segment changes associated with both types of pain. If the pain is unrelieved, the nurse needs to notify the health care provider for further orders.

Nursing management of the patient during and after a pericardiocentesis includes monitoring the patient's response to the procedure. The nurse monitors the pulmonary artery, the right atrial pressure or central venous pressure (CVP), pulmonary wedge pressures if invasive monitoring lines are in place (Chapter 31), and the ECG during and after the procedure. As the effusion is relieved, the CVP and pulmonary artery wedge pressure will decrease and the blood pressure will increase. The amplitude of the QRS complex also increases as the pressure is relieved. Vital signs and urine output provide information about cardiac output and typically are monitored every 15 to 30 minutes for the first hour, then every 30 minutes for another hour, and then every hour for the remainder of the first 24 hours. The amount of fluid removed is recorded on the output record and, if ordered, a specimen is sent to the laboratory for analysis. It is essential that the patient be monitored closely for a recurrence of tamponade. If the clinical manifestations prior to the pericardiocentesis return, a recurrence is suspected, and the nurse should notify the health care provider immediately. The patient's anxiety is typically reduced when he is informed of what to expect in terms of clinical manifestations and treatment. The patient may require an antianxiety agent.

Health Promotion

Health teaching for patients with pericarditis focuses on prevention. Teaching about the clinical manifestations and when to seek medical help is essential. Identifying risk factors specifically related to the cause and outlining how to mitigate them will also help with disease prevention. The Patient Teaching & Discharge Priorities for Inflammatory Heart Disease box outlines specific patient teaching and discharge priorities (p. 983).

Myocarditis

Myocarditis, a focal or diffuse inflammation of the myocardium or heart muscle, is an uncommon disorder that is frequently associated with pericarditis. The myocardium is the middle muscular layer of the heart. Its function is to provide the pumping action that propels the blood through the heart and into the peripheral circulation. Cardiac muscle contraction, referred to as systole, occurs when the blood is pumped out of the heart. Systole is followed by muscle relaxation, or diastole, when blood flows into the cardiac chambers. Myocardial dysfunction can be systolic, diastolic, or both. Myocarditis affects the heart's ability to pump blood normally, thereby affecting cardiac output. Most cases of myocarditis originate from a viral infection and often remain undiagnosed, due to the general lack of initial symptoms. In some cases, the disease presents as an acute catastrophic illness requiring immediate attention. Myocarditis may be mistaken for ischemic, valvular, or hypertensive heart disease and can be both acute and chronic.

Epidemiology and Etiology

The incidence of myocarditis in the United States is estimated to be 1 to 10 per 100,000 people. It can occur at any age and is more common in men than women. Viral infections are the most common cause of myocarditis, followed by bacterial and fungal infections. Approximately 1% to 5% of patients with acute viral infections have myocardial involvement (Howes, 2008). Whether there is a genetic predisposition for myocarditis is under investigation. Immunosuppressed patients are at higher risk. Approximately 10% of patients with HIV develop myocarditis because the virus infiltrates the myocardium. The Risk Factors box outlines the infectious and noninfectious risk factors and causes of myocarditis.

Pathophysiology

Myocarditis is an inflammatory disorder resulting from the causes outlined in the Risk Factors and Causes of Myocarditis box that typically occurs several weeks after the initial infection. The inflammatory process causes an infiltrate to build up in the cardiac myocytes, resulting in injury to the myocardial cells. Infectious agents infiltrate myocardial tissues, forming abscesses, and an autoimmune injury may occur when the immune system destroys both the invading organism and myocardial cells. The extent of damage determines the long-term effect on heart function. The majority of infections are self-limiting and often subclinical, although severe or repeated infections may cause progressive deterioration in cardiac function. The most severe cases develop into cardiomyopathy, described later in this chapter.

RISK FACTORS and Causes of Myocarditis

Risk Factors	Autoimmune and connective tissue diseases	
	Drug hypersensitivity or toxicity	
	Sarcoidosis	
	Hypersensitive immune reactions such as rheumatic fever	
	Postcardiotomy syndrome	
	Toxins	
	Chemicals	
	Alcohol use	
	Nosocomial infections	
	Large doses of radiation to the chest for treatment of malignancy	
Causes		
Viral Infection	Coxsackie B virus accounts for 50% of the cases	
	Coxsackie A virus	Adenovirus
	Echovirus	Mumps
	Rubella	Influenza A and B
	Epstein-Barr	Hepatitis
	HIV	Hepatitis C
	Poliovirus	
Bacterial Infection	Diphtheria	Typhoid fever
	Staphylococcus	Pneumococcus
	Tuberculosis	Tetanus
Fungal Infection	Chagas disease (South and Central America)	
	Toxoplasmosis	

Clinical Manifestations

The clinical manifestations of myocarditis vary, ranging from no overt clinical symptoms to severe heart involvement. Mild signs and symptoms include fatigue, malaise, shortness of breath, fever, gastrointestinal upset, and aching joints—very similar to flu symptoms. In contrast, myocarditis may appear suddenly with manifestations of heart failure or sudden cardiac death without prior symptoms. Symptoms of heart failure are discussed more thoroughly in Chapter 34. When myocarditis and pericarditis occur simultaneously, manifestations may include a pericardial friction rub, chest pain, and a pericardial effusion. Blood clots on the heart wall (mural thrombi) may develop if blood stasis is present. Early cardiac symptoms typically appear 7 to 10 days after the initial infection.

Laboratory and Diagnostic Procedures

Several laboratory tests are done to diagnose both the cause of myocarditis and the extent of the disease process. An evaluation of presenting symptoms followed by a thorough history and physical examination will determine the need for diagnostic and laboratory studies. The tests that assist in determining a definitive diagnosis are discussed in the Diagnostic Tests for Cardiac Inflammatory Disorders box (p. 975). WBCs must be monitored for elevations in diagnosing the disorder as well as periodically if symptoms reappear or worsen. Mild to moderate leukocytosis with atypical lymphocytes is common.

Medical Management

The primary aim of medical management for myocarditis is early diagnosis and treatment to mitigate the damage to the myocardial cells. Finding the cause and instituting timely and appropriate treatment make up the cornerstone of the medical management for the patient with myocarditis. A complete history and physical including an assessment of the risk factors is indicated, along with the previously described diagnostic studies. Bed rest, a quiet environment, and a semi-Fowler's position are measures that decrease metabolic demand and reduce myocardial workload. Activity restrictions of varying levels, depending on clinical manifestations, may continue for up to 6 months. Oxygen may be needed when heart failure symptoms are present in the setting of hypoxemia. Medications for treating myocarditis include the following:

- Immunosuppressive therapy includes the use of steroids to prevent cardiac damage when the cause is autoimmune myocarditis.
- Antimicrobial medications are used when the myocarditis is caused by a bacterial infection.
- ACE inhibitors (or angiotensin receptor blockers), beta-adrenergic blockers, digoxin, and diuretics are used if heart failure with left ventricular dysfunction occurs. See the Safety Alert regarding the use of digoxin with myocarditis.
- Antidysrhythmic medications are indicated to treat the dysrhythmias.
- Anticoagulants are used to prevent thromboembolism from mural wall blood clots.
- Antianxiety agents may be necessary for patients who are anxious because of the sudden onset of heart disease and its impact on the quality of their life.

Safety Alert

- Digoxin. *Patients with myocarditis are sensitive to the effects of digoxin. Digoxin increases the force of cardiac contractions, thus increasing the workload and oxygen demand of the heart muscle. These patients must be monitored closely for heart failure. Vital signs, lung sounds, increasing shortness of breath, and peripheral edema need to be monitored on a frequent and ongoing basis.*
- NSAIDs. *The use of NSAIDs with myocarditis is contraindicated because they appear to increase cardiac damage.*

See the Pharmacology Summary of Medications Used to Treat Cardiac Inflammatory Disorders (p. 976).

The prognosis for myocarditis caused by viral infections is excellent. Scarring and permanent myocardial damage from myocarditis vary from none to severe heart failure leading to death or requiring a heart transplant.

Nursing Management

The aim of nursing management for myocarditis is to rest the heart as much as possible. These patients are placed on strict bed rest and allowed minimal activities until the cause has been identified and treatment instituted. Increasing the level of activity can only progress when the symptoms subside with successful treatment.

Assessment and Nursing Diagnosis

Nursing assessment focuses on the clinical manifestations of heart failure. *Alteration in Cardiac Output* and *Altered Tissue Perfusion* are the two most important nursing diagnoses for these patients.

NANDA-I © 2012

The majority of patients who experience myocarditis make a complete recovery without residual complications. Note, however, that cardiomyopathy can be a long-term complication of myocarditis. Nursing management and patient education are pivotal in preventing complications.

Outcomes and Evaluation Parameters

The desired outcomes for the patient with myocarditis include absence of pain and normal cardiac output. Finding and treating the cause will result in relief of symptoms. Evaluation parameters include normal heart rate and blood pressure as well as a balanced intake and urine output. There should be no unusual fatigue and shortness of breath.

Planning, Interventions, and Rationales

With myocarditis, as with other cardiac inflammatory diseases, resting the heart by spacing activities and by providing pain relief, emotional support, and a quiet environment will promote healing and assist in preventing complications. As the patient's condition allows, active and passive range-of-motion exercises will help the patient to regain strength and joint motion and should be performed regularly until activity levels increase. The nurse must teach the patient to avoid excessive fatigue and stop all activities immediately when light-headedness, dyspnea, or faintness occurs. Changes in activity restrictions are based on the patient's tolerance and the occurrence of clinical manifestations.

The remainder of the nursing management is outlined in the Nursing Process: Patient Care Plan for Inflammatory Heart Disease box (p. 980).

Health Promotion

Teaching goals for the patient with myocarditis focus on having the patient make a full recovery and prevention of long-term complications. Gradually increasing the patient's activity levels promotes good muscle tone and strength. However, the patient must be taught to stop activity and revise the plan if clinical manifestations recur. It is essential for the nurse to outline the specific manifestations of heart failure and reinforce that the patient must seek medical care if they occur. Discharge medications need to be discussed, and the nurse must assess the patient's understanding of the regimen. Specific discharge planning is outlined in the Patient Teaching & Discharge Priorities for Inflammatory Heart Disease box (p. 983).

Endocarditis

The endocardium is the inner lining of the heart and is contiguous with the heart valves. Thus, an infection or inflammation of the endocardium affects the heart valve function. Figure 33–2 (p. 979) identifies the endocardium. **Infective endocarditis (IE),** previously known as *bacterial endocarditis,* is an infection of the endocardial layer of the heart that may involve one or more heart valves, the mural endocardium, and/or a septal defect. Infective endocarditis is a life-threatening disease that occurs most often in individuals who have structural abnormalities of the heart or great vessels, but it also can occur with normal hearts.

There are two types of IE: acute and subacute. With acute IE, the onset of symptoms is rapid, often in individuals with normal heart valves;

if untreated, it can lead to death within days to weeks. Acute IE is usually caused by a virulent organism and is more likely to follow infections of the respiratory, gastrointestinal, and/or genitourinary tracts and following open heart surgery.

Subacute IE is the more common form and is usually caused by organisms of low virulence that have a limited ability to infect other organs. It is present in an inactive state for long periods of time in people with preexisting valve disease. It often becomes symptomatic after dental work or with an invasive procedure, but it usually responds well to treatment.

Infective endocarditis is classified according to the causative organism, hemolytic streptococci being the most common. Other causes and predisposing factors are outlined later in the Risk Factors box. The increasing use of contaminated needles by individuals using illegal intravenous (IV) drugs has increased the number of cases of IE in recent years. These individuals have a high risk of bacteremia due to the insertion of a contaminated needle into the venous blood. The tricuspid valve is the most frequently affected valve with IV drug use, especially cocaine use.

RISK FACTORS for Infective Endocarditis

Recent dental surgery	Bleeding gums
Illegal intravenous drug use	Long-term central line placement
Weakened cardiac valves	Prosthetic heart valve
Previous history of endocarditis	Complex cyanotic congenital heart disease
Pneumonia	Cellulitis
Narrowed valve orifice	Rheumatic fever
Mitral valve prolapse with murmur	Marfan's syndrome
Degenerative valvular lesions	Aortic valve leaflet abnormalities
Nosocomial infections	Human immunodeficiency virus (HIV)

Chest trauma

Asymmetric septal hypertrophy (hypertrophic cardiomyopathy)

Invasive procedures: oral surgery, gynecologic procedures, implantation of a cardioverter–defibrillator, hemodynamic catheters, insertion of an indwelling urinary catheter, or renal shunts

Urinary tract infection.

CHART 33–2 Etiologic Organisms That Cause Infective Endocarditis

Staphylococci (*Staphylococcus aureus, S. epidermidis*)
Streptococci (hemolytic streptococci, enterococci, *Streptococcus bovis, S. pneumoniae*)
Gram-negative bacteria (*Escherichia coli, Klebsiella, Pseudomonas*)

Haemophilus	*Actinobacillus*
Cardiobacterium	*Eikenella*
Kingella	*Aspergillus fumigatus*
Candida albicans	

Epidemiology and Etiology

The incidence of IE continues to rise, with 15,000 to 20,000 new cases reported annually. Infective endocarditis is now the fourth-leading cause of life-threatening infectious disease syndromes (after urosepsis, pneumonia, and intra-abdominal sepsis) (Nishamura et al., 2008). Internationally, the incidence of the disease is similar throughout the developed countries. The greatest risk factor for the development of IE is preexisting heart damage. Infective endocarditis affects males twice as often as females and is distributed throughout all age groups. Infective endocarditis can develop in anyone, and the most frequent bacteria that cause IE are usually found in the mouth, intestinal tract, or urinary system. Nosocomial infections occur most often in patients who are debilitated and have long-term urinary and IV catheters. Patients who are immunosuppressed or who are receiving immunosuppressive therapy are at a higher risk for developing yeast or fungal IE. This population would include cancer patients, people with human immunodeficiency virus, and IV drug users.

Prosthetic heart valve IE, which may develop in the early postoperative period (60 days or less) or later on (greater than 60 days), accounts for 10% to 20% of the cases. Common infecting organisms for early IE development are staphylococcus, gram-negative bacilli, and *Candida albicans*. *Staphylococcus epidermidis*, streptococci, and enterococci cause the later infections (Woods, Froelicher, Adams, & Bridges, 2009). Infective endocarditis most frequently affects males over 60 years old and occurs most often with mitral valve replacements. Early prosthetic valve IE, usually due to a contaminated valve or preexisting bacteremia, has a rapid onset and high mortality rate. Late prosthetic valve IE follows the course of subacute IE. The Risk Factors box outlines the risk factors, and Chart 33–2 lists the organisms that cause IE.

Increased mortality is associated with increased age, infection of the aortic valve, development of heart failure, central nervous system complications, and other underlying diseases. Mortality rates also vary with infecting organism.

Pathophysiology

Several mechanisms are thought to contribute to the development of endocarditis. First, bacteremia (infection in the blood) occurs, usually as a complication of an infection originating somewhere in the body (e.g., urinary tract infection, pneumonia, cellulitis). Surgical procedures, dental work, and invasive diagnostics such as a colonoscopy also may allow bacteria to enter the bloodstream. Second, the narrowed orifice of a damaged valve reduces the movement of blood from the atria to the ventricle, allowing time for bacteria to grow and multiply. This increases the risk of bloodborne bacteria lodging on the endocardial valve surface, forming vegetative growths that adhere to the valve surface. These vegetative growths consist of fibrin, leukocytes, platelets, and the infecting microbe.

The infection spreads and becomes imbedded in the valve matrix, producing thinning and destruction of the valve and its supporting structures and ultimately causing valve dysfunction. Mechanical complications may occur, including rupture of chordae tendineae (Figure 33–4◆), development of valve stenosis due to overgrowth of large vegetations, and perforation of a valve leaflet. The organisms then spread from the valve to the myocardium, culminating in myocardial dysfunction and heart failure.

The infection can be on either the right or the left side of the heart or, in severe cases, both sides. Left-sided IE, which affects the mitral valve most often, is more common with bacterial infections and patients with underlying heart disease. Right-sided IE, which affects the tricuspid valve, is primarily a result of IV drug use and most often is caused by *Staphylococcus aureus*.

The friable vegetative growths on the valves may break off into the circulation, causing embolization. Left-sided emboli travel to the systemic circulation, affecting the brain, kidneys, and spleen and causing limb infarction. Right-sided emboli travel to the lungs, causing pulmonary complications. When the emboli become trapped in the organ,

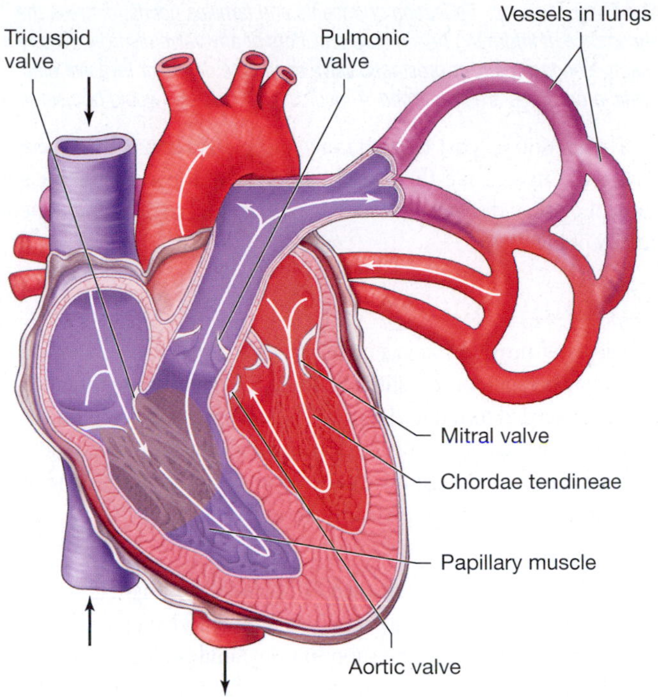

FIGURE 33–4 ◆ Cardiac valves, chordae tendineae, and papillary muscle.

abscesses may form, further spreading the infection and affecting organ function.

Clinical Manifestations

Endocarditis may mimic almost any systemic disease depending on the infecting organism and the associated complications. The signs and symptoms of IE can be nonspecific but may involve many organs, often making it difficult to differentially diagnose. Fever occurs in about 90% of the patients and is typically accompanied by tachycardia, fatigue, malaise, anorexia, weight loss, headache, and chills (Moser & Riegel, 2008; Woods et al., 2009).

Bacterial IE is associated with high fevers, shaking chills, and night sweats. Arthralgias, myalgias, back pain, abdominal discomfort, headache, clubbing of fingers, anorexia and weight loss, and a low-grade fever often accompany subacute IE.

The cardiac assessment reveals a heart murmur, usually on the aortic or mitral valve. The mitral murmur is typically a midsystolic regurgitant type, whereas the aortic murmur may be early diastolic. Murmurs are uncommon with right-sided IE because the pressures on the right side are too low to transmit the sound. (See Chapter 29 for a complete description of murmurs.) Dyspnea, cough, and chest pain are common complaints, especially if heart failure and decreased cardiac output have occurred. The accumulation of serous, purulent, and/or hemorrhagic fluid in the pericardial sac causes a pericardial effusion and possibly tamponade. Tamponade causes a decrease in cardiac output, leading to shock, heart failure, and death. Heart failure occurs in approximately 50% of patients with IE. ECG changes may include conduction delays (first-, second-, and third-degree heart blocks), diffuse ST segment changes, and PR interval depression. (Chapter 30 describes these and other ECG abnormalities.)

Vascular changes also may occur with IE, including the following:

- Splinter hemorrhages are black longitudinal streaks on the nail beds.
- Petechiae on the lips, buccal mucosa, palate, ankles, feet, antecubital space, and popliteal areas occur as a result of microembolization of vegetative lesions in these areas.
- Painful, red or purple, pea-size lesions, referred to as Osler's nodes, may be present on the fingertips or toes.
- Janeway's lesions, which are flat, painless, small, red spots, are found on the palms of the hand and soles of the feet.
- Roth's spots, which are round white spots surrounded by hemorrhage, may appear on the retina.

Finally, tiny emboli often break off of the heart valve and travel to distant organs, causing clinical manifestations associated with the specific organ: brain, heart, lungs, kidney, and/or spleen. Emboli also may travel to the limbs, interrupting peripheral perfusion.

Laboratory and Diagnostic Procedures

The diagnosis of IE is typically based on a constellation of clinical findings. The history of clinical manifestations is variable, often with vague symptoms, making it difficult to diagnose. The Diagnostic Tests for Cardiac Inflammatory Disorders box (p. 975) includes the tests used to diagnose IE. In addition to the standard tests described in that box, a positive rheumatoid factor and proteinuria are evaluated because they are present in some cases of IE. The echocardiogram evaluates the presence of thickening and calcification of the pericardium that occur most commonly with bacterial and fungal IE. Transesophageal echocardiography (TEE) is more sensitive than the traditional transthoracic echocardiogram, particularly for detecting small vegetative growths and extension of the infection into the myocardial tissue and for assessing prosthetic valve function. A description of the TEE procedure is discussed on page 1020. If right-sided IE is suspected, a ventilation/perfusion (V/Q) scan may be useful to evaluate pulmonary function. A CT scan also is useful for localizing the area of the abscess.

Medical Management

Due to the complex nature of IE and its ability to mimic other diseases, diagnosing it is often difficult. Underdiagnosis can lead to clinical catastrophe and death, while overdiagnosis may result in weeks of unnecessary antimicrobial therapy with excessive costs and potentially avoidable drug-related side effects. It is imperative to make a definitive diagnosis and begin a treatment plan in a timely manner. Clinical management is both curative and supportive in nature. The priorities for management of IE are finding the cause and starting treatment to eradicate the infecting organism, minimize valve damage, and prevent heart failure. A thorough health history is required to evaluate risk factors including recent high-risk procedures (see the Risk Factors box on p. 988) that may have precipitated an episode of IE. Most clinicians agree that patients who present with symptoms that are compatible with IE should be evaluated by using the following criteria:

- When symptoms appear, blood cultures obtained from separate sites are repeated two or three times over a 24-hour period and may be kept for up to 3 weeks to determine whether the causative organism is slow growing. The cultures may be negative if the patient is currently on antibiotic therapy.
- TEE confirms a mass, abscess, or prosthetic valve damage.
- Clinical manifestations as previously outlined include evidence of endocardial involvement.

Hospitalization is usually required for IE so that the patient can be given intravenous antibiotics and to administer supportive treatments for the clinical manifestations. Following the blood cultures, antibiotic therapy is initiated with drugs that are known to be specific to the organisms based on the laboratory sensitivity reports. Various classifications of antibiotics are used, including the penicillins, the cephalosporins, the aminoglycosides, and the antitubercular medications. If the cause is fungal, antifungal agents are used. Often a combination of these drugs is necessary to completely eradicate the organism.

Intravenous antibiotics are continued for 2 to 8 weeks depending on the organism, the blood culture, and the resolution of symptoms. The fibrin that covers the vegetative growths protects the colonies from antibiotic therapy; therefore, an extended course of multiple antibiotics is typically required. Prosthetic heart valve IE usually requires a combination antibiotic treatment for 6 to 8 weeks. Changes in antibiotic therapy may be necessary if allergic drug-related reactions occur and/or resistance to the medication develops. Resistance is measured by repeating the blood culture and sensitivity. The sensitivity portion of the test provides information about the medications' ability to kill the organism. Peak and trough drug levels also are measured to ensure that therapeutic levels of the drug are being given. Periodic blood cultures are done throughout the course of the illness. If the cultures remain positive, this indicates inappropriate therapy. Medications used to treat inflammatory heart disease are outlined in the Pharmacology box (p. 976).

Surgical intervention is required for the following reasons: (1) to repair valvular regurgitation, which causes heart failure and is the most common reason for surgery; (2) to remove large vegetative growths that are at risk for embolization; (3) to treat fungal infections; (4) to replace a severely damaged valve; and (5) to remove a valve (native or prosthetic) that is a continuing source of infection and does not respond to antibiotic treatment. No response after 7 to 10 days of antibiotics is an indication that valve replacement is necessary.

Home care is appropriate once the symptoms are under control and the patient has adequate support systems at home. Intravenous antibiotic therapy can be continued at home once the patient and family have been taught the skills. However, outpatient management is not advised for IV drug users because of issues with noncompliance. Patients with prosthetic valves typically stay in the hospital until the infection has resolved.

Prophylactic treatment for all individuals who have the medical indications outlined in Chart 33–3 is critical to preventing an episode of IE. Moreover, other behaviors such as IV drug use need to be discussed with a patient who is at high risk for the development of IE. The use of a medical alert bracelet would be helpful if an emergency situation occurred in which the patient was unable to speak for himself.

Safety Alert *Education of patients and families needs to stress the importance of informing health care providers of any valve disorder, history of infective endocarditis, or prosthetic valve each time dental or invasive diagnostic procedures are performed. A medical alert bracelet would be useful.*

The emotional cost to the family and patient cannot be overemphasized. This is a life-threatening illness with the potential for permanent cardiac damage that has a significant impact on the patient's quality of life.

Nursing Management

The goals of nursing management for a patient with IE include rest, pain management, and instituting the pharmacologic treatment and measures needed to reduce fever and other associated symptoms such as tachycardia, fatigue, malaise, anorexia, weight loss, headache, and chills. Patients with IE require a comprehensive plan of care. The nursing process serves as a template to develop the plan.

Assessment

Nursing care for the patient with IE includes an ongoing, in-depth physical assessment focusing on the patient's hemodynamic status, level of comfort, coping ability, and support from family or significant others. Nursing assessment is essential to prevent life-threatening complications. Frequent monitoring and assessment of trend changes in the vital signs and clinical manifestations will provide the most reliable information about the progress of these diseases. Careful monitoring of cardiac output and oxygenation also is necessary.

Nursing assessments specific to IE include murmurs, embolic events, and skin manifestations. Assessment for new and changing murmurs is essential because such changes indicate valve malfunction. The nurse should report any new or changed murmur to the health care provider. Heart sounds are assessed every 8 hours, or more frequently if ordered by the health care provider. Assessing for embolic events also is essential because they may be life threatening or cause serious organ damage. Embolization of the spleen is manifested in localized abdominal tenderness and rigidity, sharp upper left quadrant pain, and splenomegaly. Emboli to the kidneys often cause flank pain, hematuria, and azotemia. Small peripheral blood vessels also may be affected by emboli, causing gangrene. Neurological deficits occur when emboli lodge in the brain. Finally, pulmonary emboli are common with right-sided IE. Skin assessment includes evaluating for splinter hemorrhages on the nail beds; petechiae on the lips, buccal mucosa, palate, ankles, feet, antecubital space, and popliteal areas; Osler's nodes; and Janeway's lesions (which are a late finding).

CHART 33–3 Indications for Prophylactic Antibiotic Therapy with Infective Endocarditis

Medical Indications	Procedural Indications
Prosthetic heart valve	Dental procedures in which manipulation of gingival tissue, the periapical (root) area of the tooth, or perforation of the oral mucosa is likely, including periodontal procedures/dental implants
Previous episodes of IE	Bronchoscopy and/or pulmonary biopsy
Rheumatic heart disease	Cystoscopy/colonoscopy
Hypertrophic cardiomyopathy	Urinary catheterization when infection is present
Mitral valve prolapse with regurgitation and murmur	Incision and drainage of infective tissue, especially soft tissue
Sclerotic aortic valve	Vaginal delivery if infection is present
Most congenital heart malformations	Most surgeries
Surgically constructed systemic-pulmonary shunts or conduits	

Source: Gerber et al. (2009). Prevention of rheumatic fever and diagnosis and treatment of acute streptococcal pharyngitis. *Circulation, 119,* 1541–1551.

Nursing Diagnoses

Nursing diagnoses that apply to patients with IE include the following:

- *Acute Pain related to infectious process and impact on cardiac output*
- *Fatigue related to decreased cardiac output and infection*
- *Altered Cardiac Output related to impact of infection on cardiac function*
- *Hyperthermia related to infection*
- *Ineffective Tissue Perfusion related to impact of infection on cardiac function*
- *Anxiety related to fear about the infection and cardiac function*
- *Fear related to cardiac disorder.*

NANDA-I © 2012

Outcomes and Evaluation Parameters

The desired outcomes for the patient with IE include absence of pain and normal cardiac output. Finding and treating the cause will result in relief of symptoms. Evaluation parameters include normal heart rate and blood pressure, as well as a balanced fluid intake and urine output. There should be no unusual fatigue and fever. Education about prevention of a reoccurrence is critical. The patient and family need to understand the importance of the preventive measures discussed next.

Planning, Interventions, and Rationales

The focus of nursing management is to provide an environment that supports decreasing myocardial oxygen demand and cardiac workload. The patient is encouraged to eat nutritious meals, drink lots of fluid, and rest both mentally and physically. Strict bed rest is indicated only with heart failure, but restricted activity is necessary to decrease cardiac workload, especially if there is valve incompetence. It is essential that the nurse explain to the patient and family the importance of bed rest and activity restriction. Additionally, the nurse teaches the patient to avoid excessive fatigue and stop all activities immediately when chest pain, light-headedness, dyspnea, or faintness occurs. Changes in activity restrictions are based on the patient's tolerance and the occurrence of clinical manifestations. Fever, which typically persists for several days, is treated with antipyretics, forced fluids, cooling measures, and rest. Intravenous antibiotics and fluids are administered; as the antibiotics treat the infection, the patient's discomfort level will decrease.

Emotional support is essential for patients with IE. The patient needs to be given an opportunity to verbalize fears and concerns about a potentially life-threatening cardiac disorder that may cause permanent damage to the heart. Education about the clinical manifestations of heart failure and when it is necessary to seek medical attention also is essential. The Nursing Process: Patient Care Plan for Inflammatory Heart Disease box (p. 980) includes an in-depth care plan for patients with IE.

Health Promotion

Patient education includes information on how to avoid infection and making sure the patient knows that health care providers need to be informed that prophylactic antibiotics are necessary prior to the procedures outlined in Chart 33–3 (p. 990). Patients are taught to use a soft toothbrush and to floss regularly to protect the gums from bleeding. Overall good hygiene will help to prevent the reoccurrence of IE in high-risk patients. The patient must be taught the importance of seeking medical help if there is a return of clinical manifestations. In addition, it is important to stress seeking medical assistance if neurological or pulmonary symptoms occur, because these may indicate a serious complication. The specific education needed for management of the patient at home is outlined in the Patient Teaching & Discharge Priorities for Inflammatory Heart Disease box (p. 983).

Collaborative Management

A collaborative care approach is optimal for management of patients with inflammatory heart disease. These conditions tend to be chronic, with recurring remissions and exacerbations, therefore requiring lifelong management. A multidisciplinary team approach, including health care providers, nurses, physical and occupational therapists, psychologists/psychiatrists, and pharmacists, will facilitate the best possible quality of life for the patient and family. In order to meet desired patient outcomes, it is essential that the members of this interdisciplinary team communicate openly with one another in developing and evaluating care of the patient and family (IOM [Institute of Medicine], 2010). In addition to the role of the cardiologist and surgeon, the patient may need psychiatric counseling to assist in lifestyle adjustments necessitated by a chronic disease. The occupational therapist helps to facilitate realistic occupational goals, while the physical therapist assists in the maintenance of optimum conditioning given the activity restrictions. Because much of the treatment for inflammatory cardiac disorders centers on medication, the pharmacist's role is essential in educating the patient about how to manage the medications and their side effects. In addition to the nursing care described previously, the nurse plays a pivotal role in coordinating the efforts of the health care team. In the inpatient setting, the nurse facilitates communication between the members of the team and the patient and family. The nurse may also want to explore alternative therapies with the patient, such as music therapy, as discussed in Chapter 32.

Cardiac Valvular Disorders

Abnormalities in the physical structure of the heart impair blood flow and cardiac pumping ability. Therefore, these abnormalities result in decreased cardiac output and tissue perfusion. Structural abnormalities that affect the cardiac valves are discussed next, and structural abnormalities of the heart muscle itself, cardiomyopathy, are discussed in the following section.

The heart has four valves: two semilunar valves (the aortic and the pulmonic) and two atrioventricular valves (the tricuspid and the mitral) (Figure 33–5◆). Each valve is located in a strategic position to provide unidirectional blood flow through the heart (Figure 33–4, p. 989). Although the incidence of rheumatic heart disease, a common causative

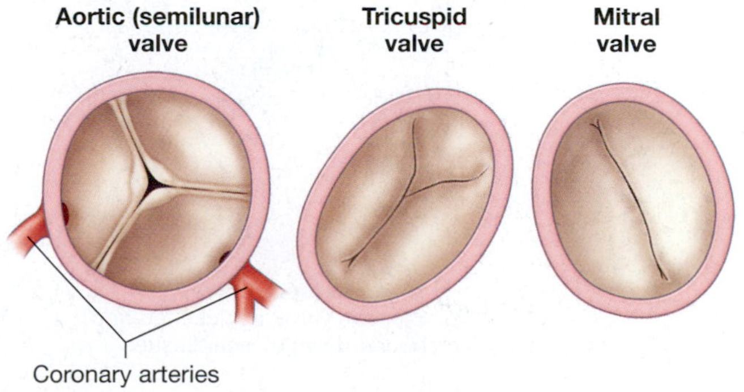

FIGURE 33–5 ◆ Normal cardiac valve shapes.

factor in valve disease, has declined, valvular heart disease remains common. Three factors influence this lack of change: (1) improvement in the assessment of valvular disorders, (2) an increased number of older adults, and (3) a larger number of recognized cases owing to improvements in diagnostic testing technology.

Valvular heart disease is classified according to the valve involved and the functional alterations, which include stenosis and regurgitation. A regurgitant valve is one that is unable to close normally, causing a backward flow of blood; a stenotic valve is unable to open normally, causing an impedance of blood flow. Valve regurgitation also is referred to as insufficiency or incompetence. When the valve is only mildly regurgitant or stenotic, the heart is initially able to adapt and maintain. In time, however, chamber dilation and myocardial muscle hypertrophy occur, causing decreased contractility, reduced cardiac output, and finally heart failure.

Valvular heart disease can be congenital or acquired, and it affects people of all ages. Most congenital valve repairs are performed immediately after birth or during early childhood. Significant advances have been made in the assessment and treatment of both congenital and acquired valve disease in the last several decades. Innovative diagnostic tools, pharmacologic developments, and improved invasive and surgical procedures have enhanced the quality of life for patients with valvular heart disease. The focus of medical and surgical intervention is to prevent heart failure and serious cardiac muscle damage.

Valvular Stenosis

Valvular stenosis is defined as a fibrotic thickening of the heart valve that causes fusion and calcification of the valve leaflet, resulting in a decrease in the size of the valve orifice (Figure 33–6◆). The thickened leaflets interfere with the valve's ability to open completely, thus obstructing blood flow through the valve orifice and decreasing cardiac output. Valvular stenosis can occur in the mitral, aortic, and tricuspid valves. The degree of stenosis will determine the reduction in cardiac output and the presence and severity of clinical manifestations. Patients with mild to moderate stenosis are able to maintain cardiac output at rest but become symptomatic with exercise because the heart is unable to respond to the increased need for oxygen.

Valvular Regurgitation

Valvular regurgitation is defined as the valve's inability to close completely during systole, resulting in a backflow of blood through the incompetent valve orifice into the previous chamber. In response to this, both chambers dilate, and hypertrophy results, due to the extra

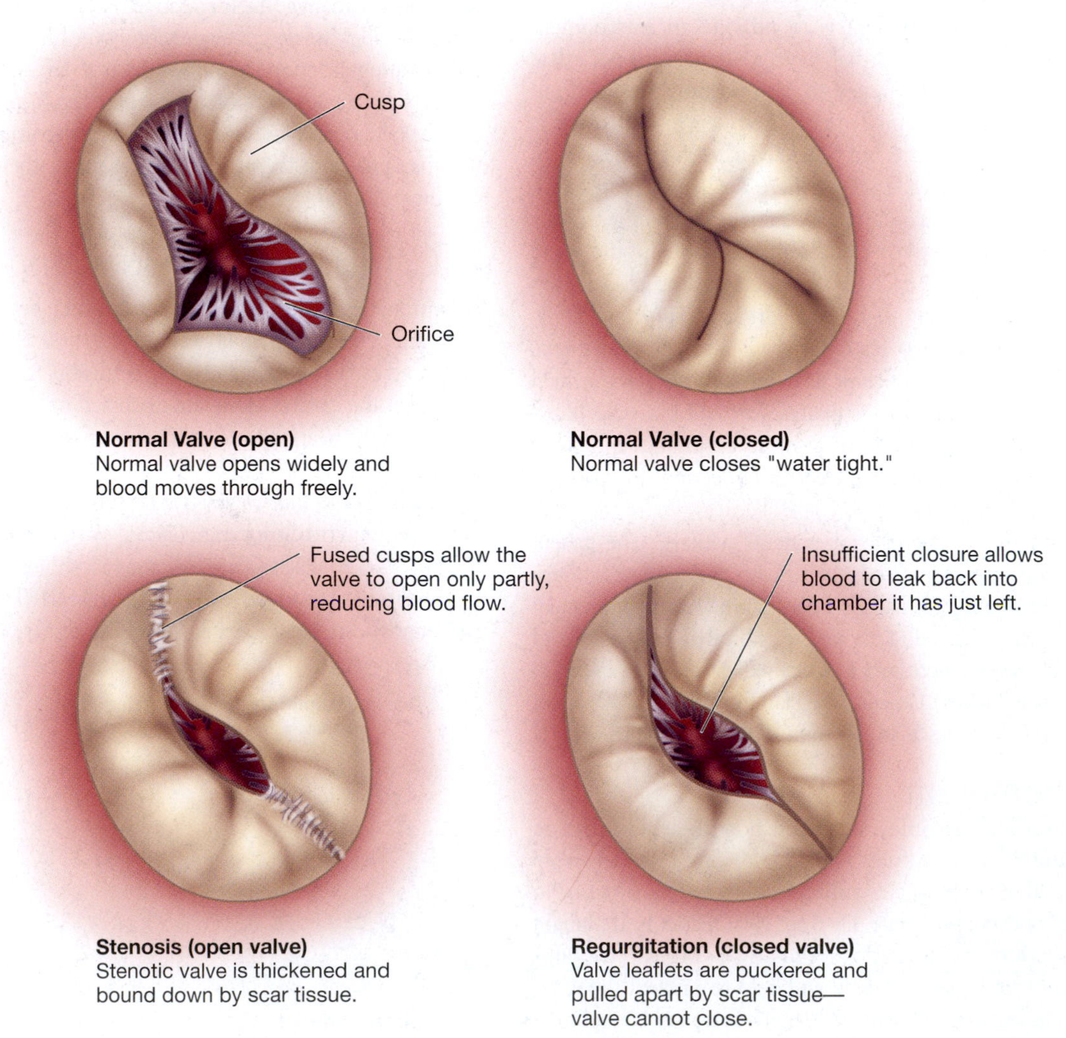

FIGURE 33–6 ◆ Normal versus abnormal stenosed valve.

workload and hypoxemia. This leads to progressive chamber failure and decreased cardiac output. Heart failure develops slowly but is the eventual outcome. Valve competence depends on normal leaflets, chordae tendineae, papillary muscles, and the valve annulus. A malfunction in any one of these structures will cause valvular regurgitation. Valvular regurgitation primarily affects the aortic and mitral valves and, on rare occasions, the tricuspid and pulmonic valves.

Mitral Valve Disease

The mitral valve, which lies between the left atrium and the left ventricle, controls blood flow between these two structures. Three diseases affect the mitral valve: stenosis, regurgitation, and prolapse. These disorders are discussed next.

Mitral Valve Stenosis

Mitral valve stenosis, a common disorder of the mitral valve, is a progressive and chronic disease. The mitral valve assumes an abnormal funnel shape due to thickening and shortening of the valve structures as a result of calcification. Contractures develop between the junctions or commissures (leaflets) of the valve (see Figure 33–6). The stenosis narrows the opening of the valve, which obstructs blood flow from the left atrium to the left ventricle. The obstruction may be mild or severe. The normal orifice of a mitral valve is 4 to 6 cm; with stenosis, it can become less than 1 cm.

Epidemiology, Etiology, and Pathophysiology

Among people with rheumatic heart disease, 40% develop mitral stenosis, making rheumatic heart disease the most common cause of this disorder. Less common causes include infectious endocarditis, congenital mitral stenosis, rheumatoid arthritis, thrombus formation, calcification of the annulus, atrial myxoma (tumor), and SLE. Mitral stenosis is more common in women (66%) than in men (Woods et al., 2009).

The inflammatory process caused by the infection results in fibrinous changes in the valve leaflet and chordae tendineae. The chordae tendineae shorten, causing narrowing of the outflow tract. The valve leaflets become fused and immobile and are unable to open completely. The narrowed opening causes an obstruction to blood flow from the left atrium to the left ventricle during diastole, creating a pressure gradient. The obstruction causes the volume of blood, and therefore the pressure, to build up in the atrium, eventually backing up into the pulmonary system and causing increased pressure in the pulmonary vasculature. Consequently, it takes more pressure to pump blood and thus the workload of the heart increases. Eventually, the prolonged rise in pressure and increased cardiac workload cause dilation and hypertrophy of the left atrium. Initially, the heart is able to compensate, but eventually pulmonary capillary congestion occurs, causing pulmonary hypertension and subsequent backup into the right side of the heart. The increased pressure in the pulmonary vasculature causes fluid leakage across the alveolar membrane, leading to pulmonary edema. Finally, the increased pressure causes dilation and hypertrophy of the right ventricle. If untreated, mitral stenosis will lead to heart failure.

Clinical Manifestations

The size of the opening of the valve orifice determines the acuity of symptoms, and clinical manifestations depend on cardiac output and pulmonary vascular pressures. The most frequent complaint with mitral stenosis is dyspnea, which results from the pulmonary involvement.

Symptoms typically appear gradually over the course of a 20- to 30-year period and typically begin late in the fifth decade of life. In some cases, if rapid progression occurs, it usually takes 2 to 5 years for symptoms to appear. The symptoms appear with exercise in the early stages and with rest in the later stages. Specific clinical manifestations of mitral stenosis are outlined in Chart 33–4 (p. 996).

Mitral Valve Regurgitation

Mitral valve regurgitation (MVR) or mitral insufficiency is defined as the mitral valve's inability to close due to an abnormality in the valve's structure and function. Fibrotic changes and calcification of the valve result in an inability to close completely during systole (see Figure 33–6). There are two types of MVR: chronic and acute. In chronic MVR, the left atrium, left ventricle, and pulmonary vasculature dilate to accommodate the chronic volume overload. With acute MVR, there is no chamber or vessel dilation, so pressures rise in both the left atrium and the left ventricle, ultimately backing up into the pulmonary system, causing pulmonary edema.

Epidemiology, Etiology, and Pathophysiology

Rheumatic heart disease is the primary cause of MR, and since rheumatic heart disease is on the decline, thanks to early and effective antibiotic treatment, the incidence of MVR also is declining. MVR from rheumatic heart disease is more common in women than men; MVR from nonrheumatic causes is more common in men. Mitral valve regurgitation is often present with mitral valve stenosis. Other causes of MVR include connective tissue disorders (Marfan's syndrome), congenital valve malformation, CAD, endocarditis, dilated cardiomyopathy, mitral valve prolapse, amyloidosis, ankylosing spondylitis, and MI.

With MVR, there is an abnormality of one or more of the valve structures: leaflets, annulus (the valve ring that attaches to the leaflets), chordae tendineae, or papillary muscle. Valve leaflets and the chordae tendineae may shorten or tear, and the annulus may be stretched by heart enlargement to dilation and hypertrophy. Ventricular dilation and scarring from a myocardial infarction cause the papillary muscle to rupture, stretch, or be pulled out of position.

Because the mitral valve is unable to close, there is a backward flow of blood into the left atrium during systole. During diastole, both the regurgitant blood and the normal blood flow into the ventricle, causing the left ventricle to become overfilled and dilated. This backward movement also increases the pressure in the left atrium and the pulmonary vasculature, resulting in varying degrees of chamber and vessel dilation and hypertrophy. The degree of involvement of these structures is determined by the etiology, severity, and duration of the MVR. For example, the acute MVR that occurs with myocardial infarction causes rupture of the papillary muscle and a sudden increase in left atrial distention and pressure. This increased pressure is transmitted to the pulmonary vasculature, resulting in rapid pulmonary edema and shock. In addition, cardiac output drops, thereby affecting organ and peripheral tissue perfusion. Conversely, in chronic MR, the volume overload on the left ventricle, left atrium, and pulmonary vasculature allows for dilation and hypertrophy of these structures. Patients typically remain symptom free for several years until the development of left ventricular failure.

Clinical Manifestations

The clinical manifestations of mitral regurgitation depend on the cause and the degree of incompetence. In acute regurgitation, the left atrium has not had time to dilate; therefore, the symptoms of pulmonary edema and shock appear quickly. The clinical manifestations of chronic MR often take years to appear. Atrial fibrillation is a common and potentially deadly dysrhythmia associated with MR. The remainder of the clinical manifestations for both acute and chronic MR are outlined in Chart 33–4 (p. 996).

Mitral Valve Prolapse

Mitral valve prolapse (MVP) (also referred to as Barlow's syndrome and floppy valve syndrome) is the most common form of heart valve disease in the United States. Mitral valve prolapse occurs when one or more of the valve leaflets bulge or prolapse into the left atrium during systole (Figure 33–7◆). This prolapse of the valve essentially results in valvular regurgitation. Varying degrees of valvular incompetence occur depending on the extent of the disorder. In many patients, the disease is benign, and they remain asymptomatic and undiagnosed; in other patients, serious complications result.

Epidemiology, Etiology, and Pathophysiology

Mitral valve prolapse affects approximately 2% to 6% of the population, is much more common in women than in men, and may be genetically inherited as a dominant trait (Verma & Mesana, 2009). Genetic predispositions to MVP are discussed in the Genetic Considerations box. Other causes of MVP include endocarditis, CAD, myocarditis, connective tissue disorders, cardiomyopathy, hyperthyroidism, and cardiac trauma. The cause also can be idiopathic.

Mitral valve prolapse can result from abnormalities of the valve leaflets, chordae tendineae, papillary muscles, and left ventricular dysfunction. With MVP, the leaflets of the valve are displaced upward into the left atrium during systole when the valve needs to be sealed shut to prevent a backflow of blood (see Figure 33–7). The blood then regurgitates into the left atrium, as is seen with mitral regurgitation. Severe mitral regurgitation is a complication of MVP. If progressive worsening of the regurgitation occurs, it can lead to heart failure.

Clinical Manifestations

Most patients with MVP remain asymptomatic for years. Often, the onset of symptoms is due to a major physiological stressor such as childbirth or emotional situations such as divorce or the death of a family member. The chest pain that accompanies MVP, which is described as sharp, is not due to inadequate blood flow to the heart muscle; instead, it may be due to stretching of the chordae tendineae and papillary muscle during prolapse. The chest pain can last for hours or days and is not brought on by exertion. Many patients experience panic attacks and a feeling of intense anxiety, and some feel an overwhelming sense of impending doom. The cause of these symptoms is unknown, but some clinicians believe that the anxiety felt during palpitations makes the body more sensitive to stress hormones, which in turn increases palpitations and the release of more stress hormones (Verma & Mesana, 2009; Woods et al., 2009). These symptoms can last from a few seconds to a few minutes.

If mitral regurgitation is present, the patient will present with the associated symptoms. Patients with MVP have no activity restrictions except those necessitated by the clinical manifestations (see Chart 33–4, p. 996).

GENETIC CONSIDERATIONS for Mitral Valve Prolapse

There is a genetic predisposition with some forms of MVP. It is associated with Marfan's syndrome, a disorder that is present from birth; Graves' disease; and connective tissue disorders (Verma & Mesana, 2009).

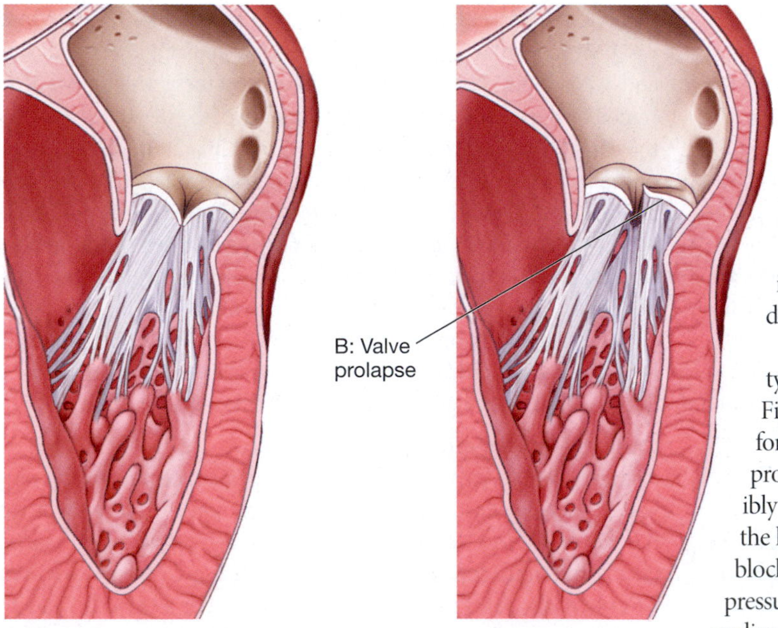

FIGURE 33–7 ◆ Mitral valve prolapse.

Aortic Valve Disease

The aortic valve lies at the root of the aorta in the left ventricle. It controls blood flow from the left ventricle through the aortic outflow tract into the systemic circulation. Diseases of the aortic valve include stenosis and regurgitation, which are discussed next.

Aortic Valve Stenosis

Aortic valve stenosis (AVS) is similar to mitral stenosis in that there is a narrowing of the aortic valve orifice (see Figure 33–6, p. 992). This stenosis results in an obstruction to blood flow from the left ventricle to the aorta during systole. Aortic valve stenosis is a progressive, chronic disease; if left untreated, it has a poor prognosis, leading to end-stage heart failure.

Epidemiology, Etiology, and Pathophysiology

Causes of AS include congenital leaflet malformation, rheumatic endocarditis, and degenerative changes associated with the aging process. It may also be idiopathic. Idiopathic AS is typically mild and does not decrease cardiac output. Aortic valve stenosis is more common in males than in females (Woods et al., 2009). In patients younger than 30 years old, AS is typically caused by a congenital malformation of the aortic valve. When AS is caused by rheumatic heart disease, typically the mitral valve also is involved and the AS occurs in individuals between the ages of 30 and 70 years. Rheumatic heart disease destroys both valve leaflets with calcification and fibrosis, causing them to become scarred and rigid. In people older than 70 years of age, in the absence of rheumatic heart disease, atherosclerosis and degenerative calcification are the primary causes of AS.

With AS, there is progressive narrowing of the valve orifice, typically over a period of several years or even decades (see Figure 33–6, p. 992). The narrowed orifice makes it more difficult for the left ventricle to eject its load of blood. As the valve stenosis progresses, the left ventricle contracts more slowly and less forcibly in an attempt to maintain normal cardiac output. Even though the left ventricle attempts to increase blood flow, the stenotic valve blocks it, producing a fixed cardiac output. Prolonged increased pressure in the left ventricle causes hypertrophy, which is another cardiac muscle compensatory mechanism to maintain cardiac output. The increased cardiac workload results in increased cardiac oxygen consumption. Additionally, due to the decreased cardiac output, coronary artery blood flow is decreased. Thus, both the increased oxygen need and the decreased cardiac output result in myocardial ischemia. As ventricular end-diastolic pressure rises, the left atrial pressure increases and, over time, backs up into the pulmonary vasculature. Pulmonary vascular congestion and pulmonary edema eventually occur. If AS is untreated, pulmonary hypertension and right ventricular failure eventually develop. With fixed cardiac output, the heart is unable to meet the body's oxygen demands during periods of increased activity, and clinical manifestations begin to appear.

Clinical Manifestations

As AVS progresses, usually over several years, compensation fails, and symptoms begin to appear. Typically, the clinical manifestations begin to appear between the ages of 50 and 70 years and are a result of increased narrowing of the valve orifice and the onset of left ventricular failure. Symptoms generally develop when the valve orifice becomes one-third its normal size. As in mitral stenosis, dyspnea is the most frequent complaint, usually accompanied by angina and exertional syncope. The clinical manifestations of aortic stenosis are shown in Chart 33–4 (p. 996).

Aortic Valve Regurgitation

Aortic valve regurgitation (AVR), also called aortic insufficiency, is similar to mitral regurgitation in that the blood regurgitates back into the left ventricle through a valve that is unable to close completely. This valve incompetence may be due to abnormal valve cusps or aortic root. The increased blood in the left ventricle causes dilation, hypertrophy, and eventually left ventricular dysfunction. Aortic valve regurgitation can be either chronic or acute.

Epidemiology, Etiology, and Pathophysiology

The common causes of chronic AR are rheumatic heart disease, congenital valve malformation, and cardiomyopathy (Woods et al., 2009). Less common causes of chronic AVR include connective tissue disorders (Marfan's syndrome), rheumatoid arthritis, ankylosing spondylitis, chronic hypertension, and syphilitic aortitis. Abrupt dilation of the aortic root, most commonly caused by a descending dissecting aortic aneurysm, causes acute AVR. Other causes of acute AVR are blunt chest trauma and endocarditis. Except in cases caused by rheumatic heart disease, AVR is more common in men than in women. In women, it is commonly associated with coexisting mitral valve disease.

With AVR, the left ventricle receives blood from the left atrium and the regurgitant blood coming back from the aorta, causing the left ventricular end-diastolic volume to gradually increase. The regurgitant blood flow is caused by an inability of the aortic valve to close to inflammation, scarring, and calcification of the valve leaflets from the causes listed earlier. With chronic AVR, as a compensatory mechanism, the left ventricle increases stroke volume in an attempt to increase cardiac output. The increased pressure causes ventricular dilation and hypertrophy (to increase muscle strength). As the condition progresses over time, the left ventricle loses its ability to compensate for the increased workload and cardiac output falls. The clinical manifestations of left ventricular heart failure begin to appear. If left untreated, AVR will lead to increased left atrial pressures and dilation, pulmonary hypertension and congestion, and finally right-sided heart failure.

Much as in acute mitral valve regurgitation, in acute AVR the left ventricle has not had time to develop compensatory mechanisms. Therefore, with the extra blood volume, the dramatic increase in cardiac workload results in a rapid decline in hemodynamic status, and patients develop fulminant pulmonary edema. If heart failure occurs rapidly, these patients often require emergent lifesaving measures.

Clinical Manifestations

Patients with chronic AR may remain asymptomatic for as long as 20 years. The first complaints are typically an uncomfortable awareness of a heartbeat or palpitation. This bounding heartbeat is due to the large ventricular stroke volume and rapid diastolic runoff. The hallmark clinical manifestation of AR is a diastolic murmur that is heard best at the second right intercostal space (aortic area) and radiating to the left sternal border. The remainder of the clinical manifestations for AR are listed in Chart 33–4 (p. 996).

Tricuspid Valve Disease

Tricuspid valve stenosis (TVS), which obstructs blood flow between the right atrium and the right ventricle, is an extremely rare and uncommon disorder (see Figure 33–6, p. 992). **Tricuspid valve regurgitation** is usually the result of pulmonary hypertension that increases right ventricular volume, causing the ventricle to dilate and stretch. This stretching distorts the leaflets, chordae tendineae, and papillary muscle, preventing complete closure of the valve. The low pressure on the right side of the heart decreases the risk of inflammatory changes and calcification associated with high-pressure areas of the heart (left side).

Etiology, Epidemiology, and Pathophysiology

Tricuspid valve stenosis (TVS) occurs with rheumatic heart disease, IV drug use, and concurrently with mitral stenosis. Like aortic and mitral stenosis, the scarred and fibrosed valve leaflets are unable to completely open, creating the obstruction to blood flow. Right ventricular filling is decreased and right atrial pressure is increased due to the obstruction to blood flow. The right atrium enlarges and increased right atrial pressure is reflected backward into the systemic circulation, causing congestion and clinical manifestations of right-sided heart failure. The decreased volume in the right ventricle reduces the blood flow to the lungs and left heart, resulting in a decreased cardiac output and tissue perfusion.

As with aortic and mitral valve regurgitation, with tricuspid valve regurgitation the valve is unable to close completely during systole. The valve and its supporting structures become damaged by rheumatic heart disease, inferior myocardial infarction, blunt chest trauma, and infective endocarditis. Volume overload occurs in both the right atrium and the right ventricle, causing decreased cardiac output and right-sided heart failure (Chapter 34).

Clinical Manifestations

Tricuspid stenosis increases the pressure in the right atrium, backing blood up into the venous circulation and resulting in right-sided heart failure. Atrial fibrillation (Chapter 30) is common owing to the stretching of the atrium. If tricuspid stenosis is present, the patient is at a high risk for thrombus formation. The murmurs that are heard with both stenosis and regurgitation become more intense with inspiration.

Safety Alert *Atrial fibrillation decreases cardiac output by 20% to 25%. If new-onset atrial fibrillation occurs, the nurse needs to assess tissue perfusion in the presence of a decreased cardiac output. Blood pressure, heart rate, respiratory rate, and presence of cyanosis need to be monitored frequently. The nurse must notify the health care provider so that measures can be instituted to terminate the abnormal rhythm.*

Pulmonic Valve Disease

Like aortic and mitral stenosis, **pulmonic valve stenosis (PVS)** restricts blood flow due to an inability of the valve to completely open (see Figure 33–6, p. 992). The blood from the right ventricle is obstructed

CHART 33–4 Clinical Manifestations of Cardiac Valve Disorders

Valve/Disorder	Clinical Manifestation
Mitral valve stenosis	Atrial fibrillation, when present, causes an irregular, often weak pulse and a drop in cardiac output and blood pressure. Dyspnea, dyspnea on exertion, orthopnea are all due to pulmonary hypertension. Low-pitched rumbling crescendo–decrescendo diastolic murmur heard best with the bell of the stethoscope. Mural thrombi and stagnate blood found with atrial fibrillation, causing embolization. Loud first heart sound heard (S_1). An opening snap occurs, reflecting high atrial pressures. Sound is best heard with the diaphragm of the stethoscope at the apex of the heart. Dry cough, dysphasia, and bronchitis due to bronchial irritation from the left atrial enlargement. Fatigue and weakness due to decreased cardiac output. Clinical manifestations of right-sided heart failure (Chapter 34). Palpitations and angina. Crackles in the lung bases. Hemoptysis.
Mitral valve regurgitation, acute	Sudden onset of dyspnea, thready peripheral pulses, and cool clammy skin. Pulmonary crackles. Decreased cardiac output. Atrial fibrillation with thrombus formation (occurs 75% of the time). Blowing high-pitched, systolic murmur. Left- and right-sided heart failure (Chapter 34).
Mitral valve regurgitation, chronic	Gradual onset of dyspnea, weakness, and fatigue, gradually progressing to orthopnea, paroxysmal nocturnal dyspnea, and peripheral edema. S_3 and pansystolic (both systole and diastole) murmur at the apex radiating to the left axilla. Cough, pulmonary crackles. Atrial fibrillation with thrombus formation (occurs 75% of the time).
Mitral valve prolapse (MVP)	Palpitations and irregular heartbeat. Sharp stabbing chest pain, especially during periods of stress. Paroxysmal atrial tachycardia, premature ventricular contractions, and ventricular tachycardia, precipitated by stress, caffeine, alcohol, and over-the-counter stimulants. Sharp stabbing chest pain that usually occurs at rest but may occur with exercise. Panic attacks, anxiety, and impending doom. Fatigue, weakness, and dyspnea. Chronically cold hands and feet and paresthesia (numbness and tingling) of arms and legs. Pansystolic murmur. Midsystolic to late-systolic click heard between S_1 and S_2. Light-headedness; dizziness, especially with position change; and low blood pressure.
Aortic valve stenosis	Dyspnea, angina, fatigue, and syncope, which increase with exertion and are due to the fixed cardiac output. Harsh crescendo–decrescendo systolic murmur heard best in the second intercostal space on the right sternal border; the sound radiates to the carotid arteries. Palpable thrill is present. Increased pulmonary artery pressure and decreased cardiac output. Prominent S_4. Lung congestion. Left- and right-sided heart failure (Chapter 34). Palpitations.
Aortic valve regurgitation	High-pitched blowing, crescendo–decrescendo diastolic murmur. Decreased diastolic pressure and a widening of the pulse pressure. Pistol-shot pulse auscultated over the femoral arteries. Some patients have head bobbing with each heartbeat (Musset's sign). Palpitations and exaggerated carotid artery pulsations. Sudden sharp pulse followed by a swift collapse of the diastolic pulse (waterhammer pulse). Exertional dyspnea, orthopnea, and paroxysmal nocturnal dyspnea.

CHART 33–4 Clinical Manifestations of Cardiac Valve Disorders, *continued*

Valve/Disorder	Clinical Manifestation
	Nocturnal angina with diaphoresis. Bounding atrial pulse. Apical pulse is displaced to the left. Widened pulse pressure with an increased systolic pressure and a decreased diastolic pressure. Dizziness and exercise intolerance. Angina that occurs mostly at night and may not respond to conventional therapy. Left- and right-sided heart failure (Chapter 34).
Tricuspid vlave stenosis and regurgitation	TR: high-pitched blowing systolic murmur heard over the xiphoid area. TS: low-pitched rumbling diastolic murmur heard best in the fourth intercostal space of the left sternal border. Right-sided heart failure (Chapter 34). Low cardiac output. Fatigue and weakness. Atrial fibrillation. Prominent waves in the neck veins due to vigorous atrial contraction. If in normal sinus rhythm, there are tall P waves.
Pulmonic valve stenosis and regurgitation	Dyspnea and fatigue. PR: high-pitched diastolic blowing murmur along the left sternal border. PS: systolic crescendo–decrescendo murmur heard in the second left intercostal space (pulmonic area). Right-sided heart failure (Chapter 34). PS: ECG has tall peaked T waves from atrial hypertrophy. Atrial fibrillation is common.

from flowing into the pulmonary vasculature during systole. With **pulmonic valve regurgitation (PVR),** the valve is unable to close completely, causing blood to regurgitate back into the right ventricle. As in tricuspid disorders, the pulmonic valve is on the low-pressure right side of the heart; therefore, it is at a lower risk for developing the inflammatory changes and calcification associated with the high-pressure areas of the left side of the heart.

Epidemiology, Etiology, and Pathophysiology

Disorders of the pulmonic valve are rare and are usually caused by a congenital valvular malformation, although endocarditis, tumors, and rheumatic heart disease also have been implicated as causes. Pulmonic valve regurgitation is slightly more common than pulmonic stenosis and is typically caused by infective endocarditis, pulmonary artery aneurysm, syphilis, and pulmonary hypertension. The pulmonary hypertension dilates the pulmonary orifice, preventing complete valve closure.

With PS, the blood backs up into the right ventricle because of obstruction to blood flow through the narrowed valve orifice. Pulmonic valve regurgitation allows the blood in the pulmonary artery to regurgitate back into the right ventricle due to an inability to close completely. Therefore, both PVS and PVR prevent the blood from reaching the left side of the heart, thereby decreasing cardiac output. The increased blood volume in the right ventricle caused by both disorders increases ventricular volume and pressure, causing dilation and eventually hypertrophy. The final consequence of both disorders is right-sided heart failure (see Chapter 34).

Clinical Manifestations

Pulmonic valve disease is frequently associated with diseases of other valves. Therefore, the clinical manifestations may be complicated by multiple valve involvement. The clinical manifestations that are specifically associated with pulmonic valve disease are listed in Chart 33–4.

Laboratory and Diagnostic Procedures for Cardiac Valve Disease

A heart murmur is usually the first indication of valve disease. Once valve disease has been identified by auscultation, diagnostic studies are done to determine the specific valve or valves involved and to confirm the progression of the disease. The most sensitive diagnostic test for valve disease is the echocardiogram (p. 1019) because it provides information about the structure and function of the heart valves and enlargement of the chambers that is often a result of malfunctioning valves. An echocardiogram can identify thickened valve leaflets, vegetative growths, thrombus, myocardial function, and chamber size. In addition, it is able to measure pressure gradients across valves, and allows pulmonary artery pressures to be estimated. Transesophageal echocardiography (p. 1020) is particularly useful not only for diagnosing but also for tracking the progression of the disease. A list of additional diagnostic tests for cardiac valve disease is included in the Diagnostic Tests for Cardiac Valve Disease box (p. 998).

Medical Management of Valve Disorders

Despite differences in pathophysiology among the valve disorders, the clinical management of patients with these diseases is similar. As always, the first priority is to find and treat the cause of the disorder with a goal of preventing complications and ultimately death. Treatment is based on the involved valve and the severity of the clinical manifestations and disease. Specifically, treatment focuses on preventing recurrent infective endocarditis, heart failure, and thromboembolism. Initially, the patient is treated medically; however, as the clinical manifestations become more disabling, surgical intervention is considered.

DIAGNOSTIC TESTS for Cardiac Valve Disease

Diagnostic Test, Normal Values, and Rationales	Expected Abnormality
Echocardiogram and Transesophageal Echocardiography (TEE)	
Echocardiogram (ultrasound): Normal chamber size and normal cardiac structures. *Vegetative growths and infection cause a thinning of valve leaflets, leading to abnormal function.*	Abnormal structure and function of heart valves, able to identify thickened valve leaflets, vegetative growths, myocardial function, and chamber size. TEE is particularly useful not only for diagnosing but also for tracking the progression of the disease.
Chest X-Ray	
Clear lungs and normal heart size *Abnormal valve function causes a change in blood flow, leading to changes in chamber size and valve structure.*	Pulmonary congestion, cardiac hypertrophy, chamber and great vessel enlargement, and calcification of the valves.
Cardiac Catheterization	
Normal coronary artery blood flow, chamber size, and valve function *Abnormal valve structure causes changes in openings, leading to increased pressures in the cardiac chambers and decreased cardiac output.*	The size of the valve opening and pressure gradients across valve surfaces are abnormal. Pressure in the heart chambers and pulmonary system is increased. Cardiac output typically is decreased.
Electrocardiogram (ECG)	
Normal conduction time intervals. *Changes occur due to diminished blood flow to the myocardium due to decreased cardiac output caused by abnormal valvular function.*	Conduction delays, atrial and ventricular dysrhythmias, and the presence of cardiac ischemia. Useful in detecting increased ischemia and the presence of life-threatening dysrhythmias.
Cardiac MRI	
Normal heart valve function *Abnormal valve structure causes changes in openings, leading to increased pressures in the cardiac chambers and decreased cardiac output.*	Valve size and competence.

Medical management begins with an in-depth history and physical examination. It is important to remember that a patient with valve disease may become ill suddenly or may develop the symptoms slowly over several years. The history needs to include information about the patient's health history, genetic factors, and social habits, such as IV drug use, that would increase the risk for developing valve disease. Specific questions need to be asked about a history of rheumatic fever and infective endocarditis. Each episode of these infections further increases valve dysfunction. The patient's fatigue level and ability to perform activities of daily living (ADLs) as well as the other clinical manifestations of valve disease need assessment during the physical exam.

After the cause of the disease has been identified and treatment has begun, the medical management focuses on maintaining cardiac output, evaluating activity tolerance, and preventing complications. The treatment plan includes rest and medication. Pharmacologic management depends on the clinical manifestations and the progression of the disease. If heart failure is present with left ventricular dysfunction, ACE inhibitors (or angiotensin receptor blockers), digoxin, diuretics, and fluid and sodium restrictions are typically prescribed. See Chapter 34 for a complete description of the management of heart failure. The Pharmacology box (p. 976) includes medications to treat cardiac valve disease.

Antidysrhythmic medications are used to manage the dysrhythmias that are common with valve disease. If atrial fibrillation occurs, every effort is made to terminate the dysrhythmia because it decreases cardiac output further in patients who may already have a compromised cardiac output due to their valve disease. Conversion to normal sinus rhythm is done with either drug therapy (calcium-channel blockers) or, if that is unsuccessful, synchronized cardioversion. After conversion, an antidysrhythmic agent is typically prescribed to prevent further episodes of atrial fibrillation and control the heart rate. Chapter 30 describes atrial fibrillation and cardioversion. If atrial fibrillation persists, the blood stagnates in the quivering atrium, and the patient is at a high risk for thrombus formation. Anticoagulant therapy is necessary to prevent strokes, pulmonary emboli, and deep venous thrombosis. Oral nitrates are prescribed for patients with aortic valve disease to increase peripheral dilation and decrease preload. This will decrease the pressure gradient in the left ventricle, thereby allowing it to pump more effectively and decreasing myocardial oxygen demand. Additionally, nitrates dilate the coronary arteries to increase perfusion to the myocardium.

The fixed and/or decreased cardiac output associated with valve disease limits physical activity. As the disease progresses, the need for surgical intervention is in part determined by the patient's ability to perform ADLs. Patients with asymptomatic AVS are instructed to get an echocardiogram every 6 months (Woods et al., 2009). The echocardiogram serves as a guide for appropriate surgical intervention. Medical management of patients with AVR includes vasodilators to decrease ventricular afterload, and an echocardiogram every 6 months (Woods et al., 2009).

Invasive Management of Valve Disorders

When medical management is no longer effective and the patient's hemodynamic status becomes unstable, invasive intervention is necessary to cure the problem or at least relieve symptoms. The need for intervention is determined in part by the impact of the clinical manifestations on the quality of life, the type and severity of valvular damage, and the patient's ability to tolerate the procedure. Options include either valve repair (annuloplasty, valvuloplasty, or commissurotomy) or valve replacement with a prosthesis. The reparative procedures do not result

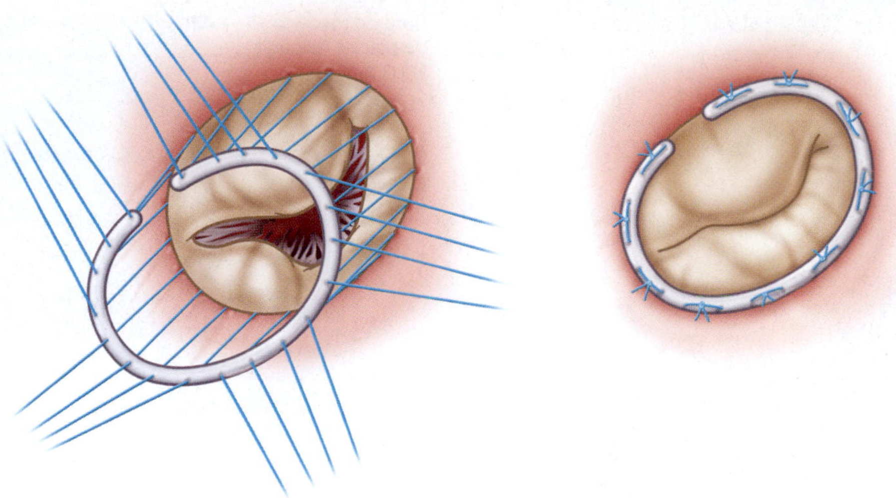

FIGURE 33–8 ◆ Annuloplasty.

in a normal valve leaflet but are associated with fewer side effects than valve replacement. The repaired valve functions more normally, and cardiac output is improved, therefore buying the patient more time.

Safety Alert *The nurse should instruct the patient to report to the health care provider when it is becoming too difficult to perform ADLs. This is one important indicator of the need for valve repair or replacement surgery.*

Annuloplasty

An **annuloplasty** corrects valve regurgitation by repairing the enlarged **annulus,** which is the fibrous ring at the junction of the valve leaflets and the muscular wall. This procedure is done when the valve leaflets are normal but the valve fails to close owing to this enlargement. The surgical procedure involves tightening the annulus with a prosthetic ring sutured in place, which reduces the size of the annulus (Figure 33–8◆). An annuloplasty requires open heart surgery and cardiopulmonary bypass.

Valvuloplasty

Repair of the valve leaflet, rather than replacement, is referred to as a **valvuloplasty.** The torn or damaged leaflet, chordae tendineae, or papillary muscle is surgically repaired under general anesthesia and cardiopulmonary bypass. This procedure is primarily performed to treat mitral and aortic stenosis, although it has been used to treat tricuspid and pulmonic stenosis.

The most common valvuloplasty is a **commissurotomy.** The objective of this procedure is to separate fused valve leaflets. The site where leaflets meet is referred to as a **commissure.** With stenosis, these commissures are abnormally fused either congenitally or due to calcification and scarring from inflammatory heart disease. A closed commissurotomy requires general anesthesia but not cardiopulmonary bypass. After a midsternal incision is made, a small hole is cut into the heart, after which the surgeon's finger or a dilator is used to break open the commissure. This procedure is useful for mitral, aortic, tricuspid, and pulmonic valve stenosis.

An open commissurotomy is performed with general anesthesia and cardiopulmonary bypass. This gives the surgeon direct visualization of the valve and has the added advantages of allowing any thrombi to be removed and the degree of valve calcification to be identified. Additionally, if necessary, the chordae tendineae and papillary muscle can be repaired. The goals of this procedure are to improve leaflet mobility and to increase the size of the valve orifice. The procedure is most effective when the valve leaflets are thin and pliable (Woods et al., 2009).

Percutaneous Transluminal Balloon Valvuloplasty

Percutaneous transluminal balloon valvuloplasty is an invasive, nonsurgical commissurotomy that is used to dilate stenosed mitral and aortic valves (Figure 33–9◆). In the cardiac catheterization laboratory with the patient under local anesthesia, a balloon-dilating catheter is inserted and positioned across the valve. To reach the mitral valve, the catheter is advanced through the femoral vein into the right atrium through the atrial septum and into the left atrium and across the mitral valve. The balloon is repeatedly inflated and deflated with dilute angiographic solution to dilate the stenosis. The valve is not completely occluded during inflation, thereby allowing some blood to flow to the left ventricle. The most common approach to treating aortic stenosis is to feed the catheter retrograde to blood flow in the femoral artery into the aorta until the valve is reached. To reach the tricuspid and pulmonic valves, a right-sided venous approach is used. This procedure is useful to relieve symptoms in patients who are too high a surgical risk (Woods et al., 2009). Some degree of mitral regurgitation is present after the procedure. Other complications include emboli and, rarely, a left-to-right arterial shunt through the opening created by the catheter.

Prosthetic Heart Valves

Patients with cardiac valve disease must be monitored regularly by a cardiologist to determine the best time for valve replacement surgery. The general clinical state of the patient is usually appraised by using the New York Heart Association classification system for functional disability (see Chapter 34). The goal is to replace the valve before permanent left ventricular damage occurs. Valve replacement is indicated when leaflets are calcified and immobile and when the clinical manifestations impact the patient's ability to perform ADLs.

Newer valves and improved surgical techniques have made valve replacement surgery safer. The goal for a valve is to be nonthrombogenic and durable, and to create the least amount of stenosis. The type of valve that is used for a given patient is determined by the anatomic suitability, ease of insertion, the patient's age, contraindications to anticoagulant therapy (e.g., pregnancy), and patient preference. Valve replacement surgery is done under general anesthesia using cardiopulmonary

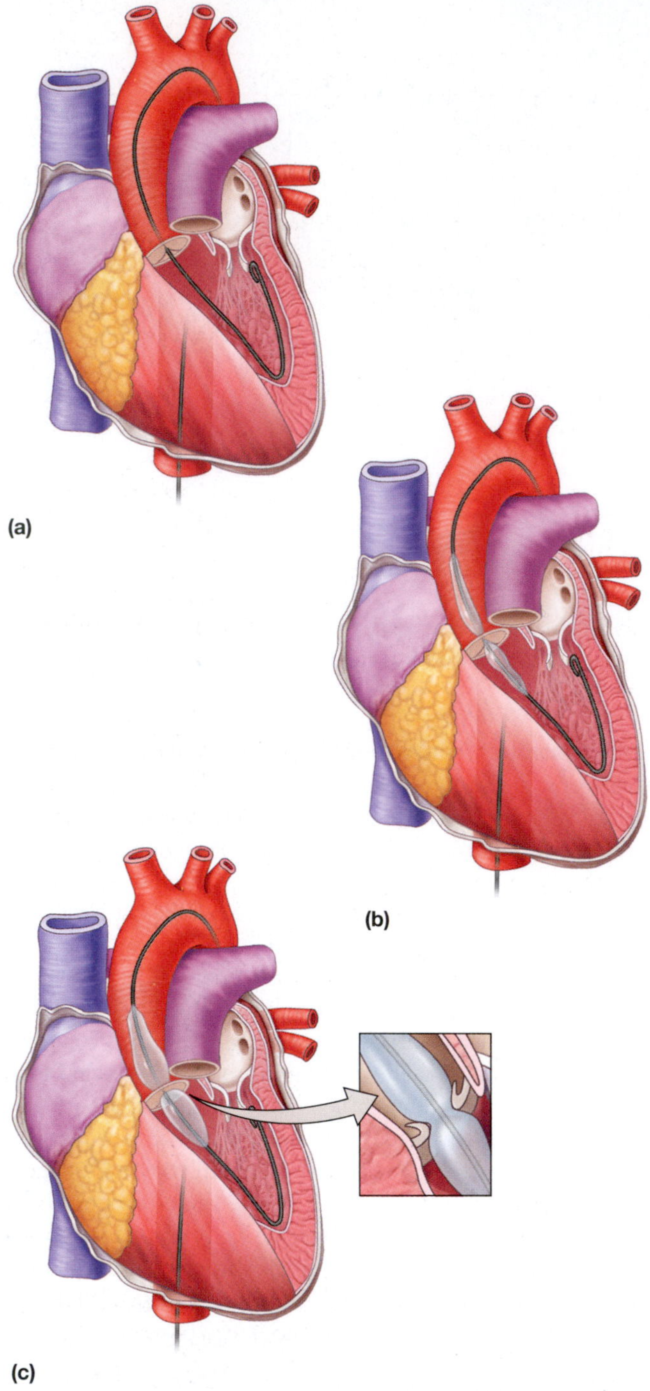

FIGURE 33–9 ◆ Valvuloplasty.

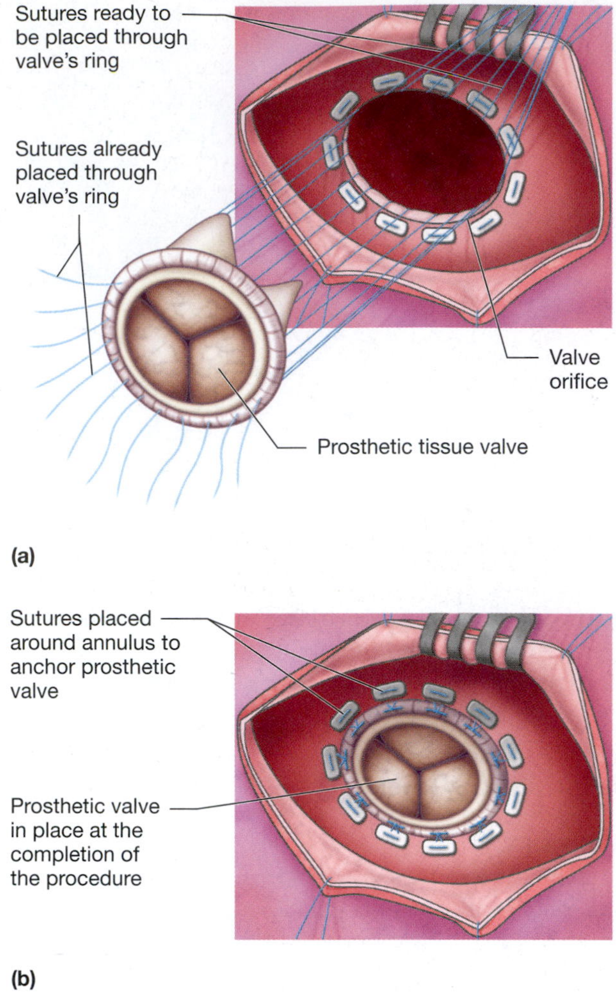

FIGURE 33–10 ◆ Valve replacement surgery.

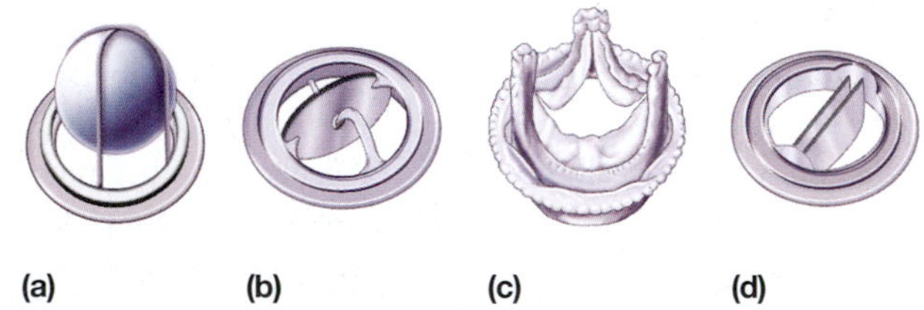

FIGURE 33–11 ◆ Valve types: (A) caged-ball valve, (B) & (D) tilting-disc valve, and (C) porcine heterograph valve.

bypass. After removal of the diseased valve, the new valve is sutured into the site of the native valve (Figure 33–10◆). There are two different types of valves: mechanical and biologic (Figure 33–11◆).

Mechanical Valves

Mechanical valves are commercially manufactured valves. With the caged-ball valve, the ball floats up and occludes the valve opening when the pressure from the blood rises (Figure 33–11A). The tilting disk valve operates on the same principle except that the disk closes when the pressure from the blood rises (see Figure 33–11B and D). There are two types of disk valves: single disk and double disk. The valve must have good hemodynamic design with the least amount of blood turbulence possible. The most frequently cited complications of mechanical valves are thromboembolism and anticoagulation-related problems (Woods et al., 2009). Conversely, structural failure is relatively rare with mechanical valves in comparison to biologic valves. Most mechanical valves are expected to last 20 to 30 years (Moser & Riegel, 2008; Woods et al., 2009). Descriptions of the specific valves, along with their advantages and disadvantages, are provided in Chart 33–5.

Biologic Valves

Biologic valves most commonly come from pigs (porcine valves; see Figure 33–11C), although cow valves (bovine) and human valves also are used. Because they have a lower incidence of clot formation compared to mechanical valves, long-term anticoagulation therapy is

CHART 33–5 Types of Prosthetic Heart Valves

Valve Type	Types	Description	Advantages	Disadvantages
Mechanical valve	Caged-ball: Starr-Edwards Smeloff-Cutter MaGovern-Cromie	Metal cage with struts mounted on a ring, with a ball on the inside of the cage (Figure 33–11A).	Occupies less space in the ventricle. Requires less force to move the ball. Long-term durability up to 20 years. Hemodynamically efficient.	Lifetime anticoagulation. Audible click. Risk of thromboembolism. Infections harder to treat. Risk of hemorrhage from anticoagulants. Very large size.
	Tilting disc: Bjork-Shiley Lillehei-Kaster Medtronic Hall	Mobile disk attached to a circular ring by two struts (Figure 33–11B and D).	Produces central blood flow through orifice, like native valves. Long-term durability. Hemodynamically efficient.	Lifetime anticoagulation. Audible click. Risk of thromboembolism under pivoting points as a result of blood stasis. Infections harder to treat. Risk of hemorrhage from anticoagulants.
	Bileaflet valve: St. Jude Medical Duromedics	Two pivoting disks that open, centrally attached to a ring.	Compact size, useful for children and patients with small aortic roots. Long-term durability. Hemodynamically efficient.	Lifetime anticoagulation. Audible click. Risk of thromboembolism. Infections harder to treat. Risk of hemorrhage from anticoagulants.
Biologic tissue valve	Xenograft, porcine (pig): Hancock Carpenter-Edwards Medtronic	Harvested aortic valve from pig that is mounted on a sewing ring (Figure 33–11C).	Low incidence of thromboembolism. Need anticoagulation for only 3 months. Hemodynamically efficient. Quiet. Easier to treat infections.	Prone to deterioration. Frequent replacement required (5–7 years). Cumbersome structural design.
	Xenograft, bovine (cow): Ionescu-Shiley Carpenter-Edwards	Three leaflets composed of the pericardium of a 16- to 18-month-old calf that is mounted on a Dacron-covered frame.	Less resistant to blood flow. Useful for patients with small aortic roots. Low incidence of thromboembolism. Need short-term anticoagulation. Hemodynamically efficient. Quiet. Easier to treat infections.	Limited durability.
	Homograft/allograft: Cadaver	Harvested aortic valve from human cadaver that is sewn in place with special mounting material.	Low incidence of thromboembolism. Only rare need for anticoagulation. Excellent hemodynamics.	Limited durability. Not useful for mitral or tricuspid valve replacement. Not readily available. Very expensive.
Autograft valve	Autologous	Excised pulmonic valve and portion of pulmonary artery from patient.	Lasts 20 years. Nonthrombogenic, anticoagulation is unnecessary. Will grow with child. Useful for women in childbearing years, young adults, and for those who cannot tolerate anticoagulation.	Possible only if the aortic valve is normal. May require double valve replacement.

not necessary with biologic valves. Biologic valves do tend to wear out faster (7 to 10 years), especially in the younger populations, who have increased amounts of calcium in the blood that break down the valve. Note, however, that biologic valves are useful for women of childbearing age because long-term anticoagulation therapy is not feasible for them; biologic valves will prevent bleeding complications associated with menses, pregnancy, and childbirth. Biologic valves also are used for older adults (greater than 70 years of age) and for patients with a history of peptic ulcer disease when anticoagulants are contraindicated.

There are two major types of biologic valves: homograft valves and autograft valves. **Homograft** or **allograft valves** come from human cadaver donations and are used primarily to replace the aortic and pulmonic valves. The valves are harvested from a cadaver and stored cryogenically, although they are not readily available and are very expensive.

Autograft valves or autologous valves are obtained from the patient's own pulmonic valve and pulmonary artery. The pulmonic valve replaces the diseased aortic valve, and then the pulmonic valve is either replaced with a homograft or left without a valve. If the pulmonary pressures are normal, the surgeon may elect not to replace the valve.

Nursing Management

Nursing care of the patient with valve disease is aimed at assessing the clinical manifestations and progression of the disease and conserving energy. The physical assessment begins with an in-depth history and an assessment of risk factors. Any episodes of rheumatic fever or endocarditis or habits that increase the risk of valve disease are evaluated. The physical assessment includes vital signs, dysrhythmias, fluid status, anxiety, lung sounds, and the clinical manifestations of right- and left-sided heart failure, as described in Chapter 34.

Nursing care focuses on conserving energy to maintain normal cardiac output and prevent the manifestations of heart failure and pulmonary congestion. Activity intolerance is a significant factor; therefore, the nurse spaces activities and visitors to allow for periods of rest. Because valve disease is a chronic debilitating disorder, it is important for the nurse to assess the patient's support systems. The Nursing Process: Patient Care Plan for Valve Disease provides a comprehensive plan of care for a patient with valve disease. The Patient Teaching & Discharge Priorities for Cardiac Valve Disease box (p. 1004) outlines the patient teaching and discharge needs for a patient with valve disease.

The chronicity of valve disease and its atmosphere of uncertainty may produce anxiety, fear, and depression for the patient and family or significant others. A nursing assessment of the patient's ability to handle the situation and its impact on the patient's quality of life is essential. The assessment findings are necessary in order to develop a comprehensive

NURSING PROCESS: Patient Care Plan for Valve Disease

Assessment of Cardiac Status Using Gordon's Functional Health Patterns:

- Health Perception Health Management Pattern
- Activity Exercise Pattern
- Cognitive-Perceptional Pattern
- Self-Perception–Self-Concept Pattern

Subjective Data	Objective Data
Assessment of Tissue Perfusion	**Assessment of Tissue Perfusion**
Do you become short of breath? What causes it to occur? How far can you walk before becoming short of breath? Do you experience leg pain? Do your hands and feet feel cold on a warm day?	Acid–base balance. The presence of and/or change in a murmur. Lung sounds. Respiratory rate. ECG. Peripheral pulses. Capillary refill.
Assessment of Activity Tolerance	**Assessment of Activity Tolerance**
What level of activity fatigues you? Have you been becoming more fatigued with less activity recently? Are you able to complete your ADLs without fatigue?	Monitor tolerance to activities while on bed rest in order to obtain a baseline to plan activities. Monitor for changes in symptoms and vital signs (VS) during activity. Determine if heart rate (HR), respirations, and blood pressure (BP) return to normal within 3 minutes after stopping activity.
Assessment of Anxiety and Fear Related to Cardiac Valve Disease	**Assessment of Anxiety and Fear Related to Cardiac Valve Disease**
What do you know about your disease process? How do your health-related issues impact your daily life? Do you feel anxious about your health? Do you have family members or close friends who provide emotional support?	Observe for manifestations of anxiety: restlessness, apprehension, withdrawal.
Assessment of Pain	**Assessment of Pain**
Do you have problems with pain? Where is the pain? What brings the pain on; what makes it go away? What do you use to relieve it and is it effective? Describe the type of pain (i.e., sharp, dull, ache, pressure)	Use pain scale (0–10) to quantify the pain level. Assess the cultural and religious impact on the patient's responses.
Assessment of Infection	**Assessment of Infection**
Do you have fever or chills? Do you have any pain or drainage at your surgical site?	Monitor for signs and symptoms of infection (e.g., temperature, heart rate, drainage, appearance of surgical incision, secretions, appearance of urine). Monitor lab values (e.g., CBC, differential results, cultures).

NURSING PROCESS: Patient Care Plan for Valve Disease, *continued*

Outcomes and Evaluation Parameters	Planning and Interventions with *Rationales*
1. NURSING DIAGNOSIS: Ineffective Tissue Perfusion *related to decreased cardiac output as a result of valve disease* (NANDA-I © 2012)	
Outcomes: Maintenance of cardiac output. Adequate tissue perfusion. ***Evaluation Parameter:*** Absence of heart failure. Absence of atrial fibrillation and/or successful conversion to normal sinus rhythm.	Assess for adventitious or diminished breath sounds. *Indicates decreased gas exchange and heart failure.* Note presence of cough and amount and color of sputum. *Assessing for heart failure.* Monitor ABGs and oxygen saturation *to assess the adequacy of gas exchange.* Monitor respiratory rate and depth *to assess for respiratory distress.* Monitor fluid status *to assess heart failure.* Monitor ECG for dysrhythmias, especially atrial fibrillation *to determine impact on cardiac output and risk for sudden death.* Monitor restlessness and confusion. *Indicators of inadequate gas exchange with resultant brain hypoxia.*
2. NURSING DIAGNOSIS: Fatigue and Activity Intolerance *related to decreased or fixed cardiac output* (NANDA-I © 2012)	
Outcome: Energy conservation. ***Evaluation Parameters:*** Endurance maintained. Balanced diet. Reports increased energy levels. Absence of clinical manifestations at rest.	Identify activities that increase fatigue *to avoid increasing cardiac workload.* Discontinue activity if chest pain, dyspnea, cyanosis, dizziness, hypotension, sustained tachycardia, or dysrhythmias develop *to aid in evaluating tolerance to activities.* Explore sedentary activities that the patient may enjoy *to provide a diversion that does not place a demand on the heart.* Maintain balanced nutrition to ensure adequate calories *to increase energy.*
3. NURSING DIAGNOSIS: Anxiety and Fear *related to chronic disease process.* Deficit Knowledge *related to disease process* (NANDA-I © 2012)	
Outcome: Anxiety level minimized and manageable. ***Evaluation Parameters:*** Verbalizes anxious feelings. Verbalizes what relieves anxiety. Demonstrates relief from anxiety through consistent aggression control, impulsiveness control, and self-mutilation restraint; and by improving coping and social interaction skills. Verbalizes absence of sensory perceptual disorders. Verbalizes absence of physical manifestations of anxiety. Behavioral manifestations of anxiety absent.	Provide factual information concerning diagnosis, treatment, disfigurement, disabilities, and prognosis. *Truthful explanations increase trust and potentially decrease anxiety.* Explain all procedures and allow time for mental preparation. *This decreases fear and anxiety of the unknown.* Allow time and encourage verbalization of fears related to illness *to assist in relieving anxiety.* Explore with the patient/family techniques to reduce anxiety. *This gives the patient a sense of control and opens communication about the subject.* Explore effective ways to minimize anxiety. *This gives the patient a sense of control.* Instruct the patient in the use of relaxation techniques *to relieve anxiety.* Assess need for and administer antianxiety and pain medication. *If alternative measures are not effective, may need antianxiety agents.*
4. NURSING DIAGNOSIS: Acute Pain *related to surgical procedure* (NANDA-I © 2012)	
Outcome: Comfort level maintained. ***Evaluation Parameters:*** Patient's comfort level is regularly assessed. The patient's comfort level is controlled and patient reports decreasing levels of pain.	Ongoing assessment of pain level is done to better control the patient's discomfort. Administer analgesics as ordered. Monitor vital signs, respiratory rate, and level of consciousness to assess comfort and monitor for side effects of narcotics such as respiratory depression. Reposition the patient, assist to a position of comfort as needed.
5. NURSING DIAGNOSIS: Potential for Infection *related to surgical procedure* (NANDA-I © 2012)	
Outcome: Patient remains free of infection. ***Evaluation Parameters:*** Normal body temperature, normal heart rate, normal white blood cell count, no drainage/discharge from surgical incisions.	Elevate head of bed to decrease the risk of ventilator-associated pneumonia when intubated. Encourage turning, coughing, and deep breathing and use of incentive spirometer to prevent postoperative atelectasis. Change dressings using aseptic technique.

Source: Adapted from Wilkinson, J. M., & Ahearn, N. R. (2009). *Prentice Hall nursing diagnosis handbook* (9th ed.). Upper Saddle River, NJ: Prentice Hall.

PATIENT TEACHING & DISCHARGE PRIORITIES for Cardiac Valve Disease

Need	Teaching
Knowledge of disease and progression of clinical manifestations	Detailed teaching materials about the disease process, medical regimen, and possible complications to increase knowledge and compliance.
Prevention	Antibiotics for dental work to prevent valve infection and repeated endocarditis.
Assess need for valve surgery	Seek medical help when unable to perform ADLs.
Safety	Medication dosages, frequency, side effects, and special considerations need to be explained to both the family and patient.
Postoperative learning needs to prevent complications	Anticoagulant therapy teaching needs to include: • Drug and dosage • Monthly INR to determine correct dosage. PT also may be used to monitor anticoagulants (1.2 to 2 times greater than normal). Report bruising, bleeding, epistaxis, and hemoptysis. Avoid large amounts of yellow and dark green vegetables and fatty foods, which increase the absorption of vitamin K (clots blood). Avoid alcohol, aspirin, and NSAIDs. Inform health care providers of anticoagulant therapy. Test stools and vomitus for blood. Use a soft-bristled toothbrush and an electric razor. Maintain an adequate level of anticoagulation without side effects.
Follow-up care	Medical follow-up continues for about a year to assess for complications, valve function, and compliance to therapy.

Sources: Adapted from Adams, M. P., & Koch, R. W. (2010). *Pharmacology: Connections to nursing practice.* Upper Saddle River, NJ: Pearson; Gerber et al. (2009). Prevention of rheumatic fever and diagnosis and treatment of acute streptococcal pharyngitis. *Circulation, 119,* 1541–1551.

plan and help with the adjustment to the disease. The patient needs to be given an opportunity to express concerns and fears in a nonthreatening environment. Explanation of the medical regimen with rationales often decreases fear and frustration in patients.

The postoperative nursing care of the valve surgery patient includes monitoring for the usual complications such as hemorrhage, wound infection, and pulmonary complications. Additionally, the hemodynamic status and cardiac output must be closely monitored. For the first 24 to 48 hours after surgery, the patient is admitted to the critical care area, where the ECG, cardiac output, and pulmonary artery pressures can be monitored and ventilatory support can be provided if necessary.

Following repair or replacement of the valve, the heart requires time to adjust to the improved hemodynamic function. Vasoactive agents may be necessary in the immediate postoperative period to optimize cardiac output. Inotropic agents may be necessary to improve cardiac contractility, and vasodilators may be needed to decrease afterload. Continuous monitoring for cardiac dysrhythmias is essential because the mitral and aortic valves lie close to the conduction pathway. Transient or permanent heart blocks may occur due to edema, ischemia, or damage to the conduction pathway. A temporary or permanent pacemaker may be required. Additionally, atrial dysrhythmias are a common complication of cardiac surgery and are even more common after valve surgery (Moser & Riegel, 2008; Woods et al., 2009).

If indicated on the basis of valve type, anticoagulant therapy is started within 48 hours of valve surgery.

Safety Alert *The nurse should report to the health care provider a PT (prothrombin time)/INR (International Normalized Ratio) that is either too low or too high. If the values are too low, there is increased risk of clot formation. If the values are too high, there is an increased risk of excessive bleeding. The nurse should also monitor hemoglobin and hematocrit and report any decreases, since these may indicate bleeding. If the platelet count is less than 50,000/mm³, there also is an increased risk of bleeding.*

Health Promotion

Because of the progressive nature of valve disease, health promotion begins as soon as the patient is diagnosed with a valve abnormality. Patient and family education focuses on controlling the clinical manifestations, reducing physical activity, and preventing reoccurrences of an infection in the valve. Education includes information on medications, lifestyle choices, and preventive care. The patient needs to be given specific instructions about when to seek medical advice for surgical intervention. When the patient can no longer perform ADLs, surgical intervention is usually discussed.

Once surgical intervention has occurred, formulating a teaching plan for the postoperative valve surgery also is an essential nursing function. The plan needs to include information about medications, activity, and the signs and symptoms that need to be reported to the health care provider.

Safety Alert *Following valve replacement surgery, the nurse teaches the patient that if fever, increased heart rate, fatigue, malaise, anorexia, weight loss, headache, chills, or night sweats occur, the patient needs to notify the health care provider. The clinical manifestations are a sign of postoperative infective endocarditis, which requires immediate medical attention.*

Collaborative Management

Because of the chronic and progressive nature of cardiac valve disease, a collaborative care approach is optimal for management. A multidisciplinary team approach, including health care providers, nurses, physical and occupational therapists, psychologists/psychiatrists, dietitians, and pharmacists, will facilitate the best possible quality of life for the patient and family. In order to meet desired patient outcomes, it is essential that this interdisciplinary team communicate openly with one another in developing and evaluating care of the patient and family (IOM [Institute of Medicine], 2010). It is essential that the health care provider monitor the progress of the valve disease and determine when surgical intervention is necessary. Psychiatric counseling may assist in lifestyle adjustments necessitated by a chronic disease process. The occupational therapist helps to facilitate realistic occupational goals, while the physical therapist assists in the maintenance of optimum conditioning given the activity restrictions.

Because medication is an essential part of the management of valve disorders, the pharmacist has a crucial role in educating the patient about how to manage the medications and their side effects. When cardiac valve disease is complicated by the presence of congestion, a symptom of heart failure, diet and fluid restriction counseling are necessary. The dietitian can educate the patient and family about salt restrictions and help them learn about satisfying meals that do not increase the risk of fluid retention. In addition to the nursing care described earlier, the nurse plays a pivotal role in coordinating the efforts of the health care team. In the inpatient setting, the nurse facilitates communication between the members of the team and the patient and family. The nurse also must include in the patient teaching the coordination of care after discharge (see the Patient Teaching & Discharge Priorities box on p. 1004).

Cardiomyopathy

Cardiomyopathies (CMPs) are defined as diseases of the myocardial muscle fibers. These diseases result in progressive structural and functional abnormalities of the myocardium. Cardiomyopathies are classified as primary and secondary. The etiology of the primary CMPs is unknown, and the only abnormality is in the heart muscle itself. Secondary CMPs are caused by other disease processes such as ischemia, viral infections, alcohol intake and drug abuse, inherited disorders, and pregnancy. Four types of CMPs will be reviewed in this chapter: dilated, hypertrophic, restrictive, and arrhythmogenic. Each type has its own pathology, clinical manifestations, and treatment. All types of cardiomyopathy can lead to cardiomegaly and heart failure.

EVIDENCE-BASED PRACTICE Antibiotic Prophylaxis Considerations in Valvular Heart Disease

Clinical Problem

Infective endocarditis can be a devastating illness that carries a poor prognosis and a high mortality rate. Patients who develop IE usually have underlying heart disease, such as valvular heart disease, a prosthetic cardiac valve in place, or congenital heart disease. Infective endocarditis also can be seen in patients with implanted cardiac devices, such as pacemakers, or in patients with hypertrophic cardiomyopathy. It also can occur in patients without underlying cardiac disease who are IV drug abusers.

Research Findings

For decades, prominent medical associations promoted the routine administration of antibiotics before invasive procedures in patients with known valvular heart disease or congenital heart disease. In 2008, the American College of Cardiology (ACC) and the American Heart Association (AHA) issued joint recommendations for the prevention of infective endocarditis in patients with valvular heart disease. This 2008 guideline abruptly reversed previous guidelines and the historical recommendations around antibiotic prophylaxis. Further guidelines, endorsed by the European Society of Cardiology, that were published in 2009 are consistent with the ACC/AHA recommendations.

The panels that were convened to develop these guidelines found no conclusive evidence linking dental, gastrointestinal (GI) tract, or genitourinary (GU) tract procedures with the development of IE. The panels also concluded that IE is much more likely to result from frequent exposure to random bacteremias associated with daily activities than from bacteremia caused by a dental, GI, or GU tract procedure. The guidelines stress the importance of thorough oral hygiene that includes frequent tooth-brushing and flossing and regular dental examinations.

Implications for Nursing Practice

Current thinking is that antibiotic prophylaxis prevents only a very small number of IE cases and that the risk of antibiotic therapy outweighs the benefit. There is controversy in the medical community regarding these guidelines, and their content has not been completely incorporated into clinical practice. Some health care providers will continue to provide routine antibiotic prophylaxis before all invasive procedures in patients with valvular heart disease. Ongoing medical research is needed to fully understand the role of IE prevention and to better delineate the high-risk patient groups.

As outlined in the 2008 and 2009 guidelines, the routine use of antibiotic prophylaxis is no longer recommended for routine dental cleanings. It is recommended for the high-risk patients who are at the most risk of poor outcomes if they develop IE, including the following groups:

- Patients with a prosthetic cardiac valve or in whom prosthetic material was used for cardiac valve repair
- Patients who previously had endocarditis
- Patients with congenital heart disease who meet these conditions:
  - Unrepaired cyanotic congenital heart disease, including palliative shunts and conduits
  - Completely repaired congenital heart defect with prosthetic material or a prosthetic device, whether placed by surgery or by catheter intervention, during the first 6 months after the procedure
  - Repaired congenital heart disease with residual defects (persisting leaks or abnormal flow) at the site or adjacent to the site of a prosthetic patch or prosthetic device (which inhibit endothelialization)
- Cardiac transplantation recipients who develop cardiac valve abnormalities.

Antibiotic prophylaxis is recommended in high-risk patients only for dental procedures that involve manipulation of either gingival tissue or the periapical region of the teeth (around the root) or perforation of oral mucosa. Antibiotic prophylaxis is no longer recommended for procedures involving the respiratory tract unless the patient is a high-risk patient and the procedure involves an incision into the respiratory tract mucosa. Antibiotic prophylaxis also is no longer recommended prior to gastrointestinal or genitourinary procedures unless an associated infection is suspected.

Patients who are at risk of IE should be taught the signs and symptoms, which include new onset fever, chills, fatigue, and shortness of breath. Some patients may develop stroke-like symptoms caused by emboli from diseased valves. The patient should be taught to contact her health care provider quickly if these symptoms develop.

Critical Thinking Questions with answers can be found in the Osborn Student Resources at nursing.pearsonhighered.com.

Sources: American Heart Association. (2011). Infective endocarditis. Available at http://www.heart.org/HEARTORG/Conditions/CongenitalHeartDefects/TheImpactofCongenitalHeartDefects/Infective-Endocarditis_UCM_307108_Article.jsp; Habib, G., et al. (2009). Guidelines on the prevention, diagnosis, and treatment of infective endocarditis. *European Heart Journal, 30*(19), 2369–2413. Nishimura, R. A., et al. (2008). ACC/AHA 2008 guideline update on valvular heart disease: Focused update on infective endocarditis. *Journal of the American College of Cardiology, 52*, 676–685.

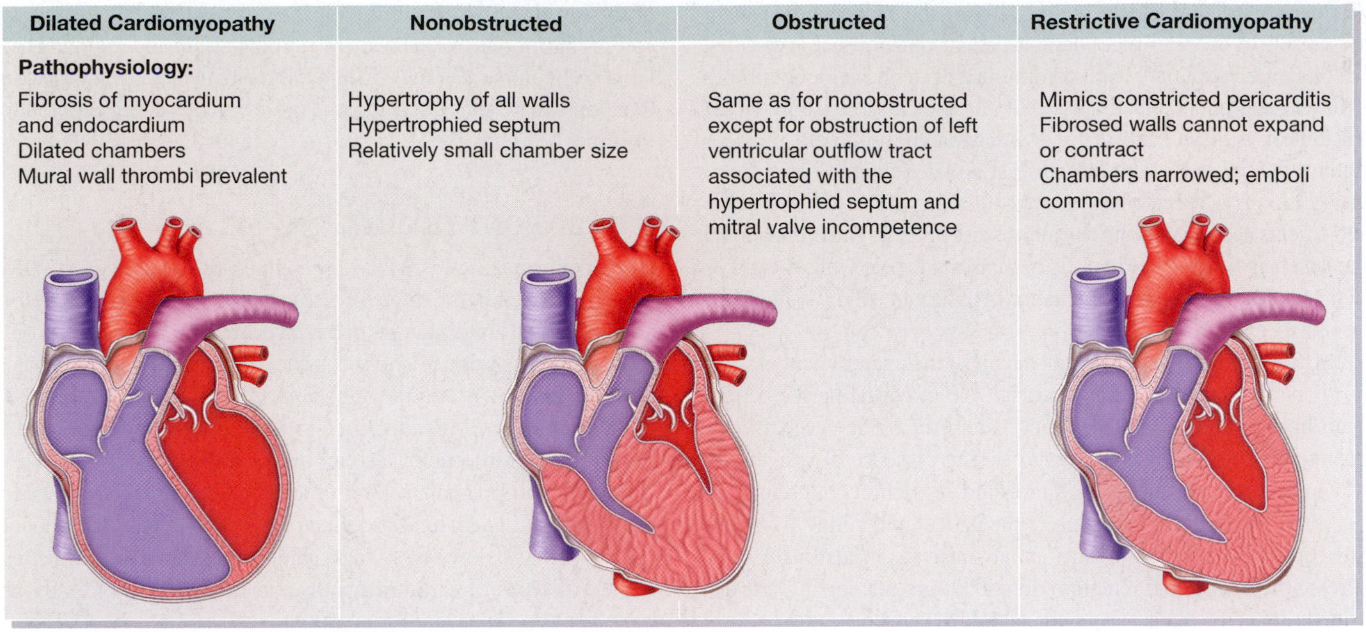

FIGURE 33–12 ◆ Types of cardiomyopathy.

Dilated Cardiomyopathy

Dilated cardiomyopathy (DCM), the most common form of cardiomyopathy, is a disorder of the myocardium characterized by dilation and impaired contraction of one or more ventricles. When dilation becomes severe, it may be accompanied by heart wall hypertrophy, which is an increase in myocardial wall thickness. Figure 33–12◆ compares the ventricle sizes for the different types of cardiomyopathy.

Epidemiology and Etiology

Dilated or congestive cardiomyopathy accounts for approximately 87% of all cardiomyopathies and is distributed throughout all age groups, with the majority in older adults (Porth & Matfin, 2009). The risk factors for development of DCM are listed in the Risk Factors box, although for 50% of cases, no cause can be identified. CAD is the most common cause of DCM in the United States (Woods et al., 2009). This type of cardiomyopathy most frequently develops following a myocardial infarction and ventricular tissue remodeling. Prolonged ischemia causes a loss of myocytes that are replaced by noncontractile scar tissue, thereby leading to heart failure. These changes lead to irreversible myocardial dysfunction.

After initial diagnosis and onset of clinical manifestations, 50% of patients with DCM are alive in 5 years, and 25% are alive in 10 years. Mortality rates from DCM are highest in older adults, males, and members of the Black race (Moser & Riegel, 2008; Woods et al., 2009).

Pathophysiology

Some forms of DCM are idiopathic but with a genetic cause. Known risk factors for development of DCM are outlined in the Risk Factors box. These factors cause the myocardial fibers to degenerate, become necrotic, and eventually be replaced by fibrotic tissue; this process is referred to as *tissue remodeling*. Dilation of the cardiac chambers

RISK FACTORS for Cardiomyopathy

- Long-term uncontrolled hypertension
- Coronary artery disease
- Viral myocarditis
- Cocaine
- Calcium overload
- Hyperlipidemia
- Obesity
- Diabetes mellitus
- Idiopathic
- Chemotherapeutic agents
- Alcohol abuse
- Genetic predisposition
- Neuromuscular disorders (Duchenne's muscular dystrophy)
- Endocrine disorders (diabetes, Cushing's disease)
- Electrolyte abnormalities (hypocalcemia, hypophosphatemia, uremia)
- Antiviral medications (zidovudine, didanosine)
- Cardiac valve disease
- Congenital heart disease
- Sleep apnea
- Radiation therapy
- Amyloidosis and sarcoidosis
- Smoking
- Familial cardiomyopathies
- Cardiac surgery
- Bacterial/parasitic infections
- Stress and/or sedentary lifestyle
- Toxins (lead, mercury, carbon monoxide, arsenic)
- Pregnancy and postpartum period
- Connective tissue disorders (SLE, scleroderma, giant cell arthritis)
- Nutritional deficiency (decreased thiamine, selenium, carnitine).

Source: Adapted from Porth & Matfin (2009). *Essentials of pathophysiology: Concepts of altered health states* (8th ed.). Lippincott Williams & Wilkins.

NATIONAL GUIDELINES for Two Controllable Causes of Dilated Cardiomyopathy

Risk Factor	Guideline
Alcohol intake	Moderate alcohol intake is defined as no more than 1 drink per day for women and no more than 2 drinks per day for men. However, some people should not drink any alcohol, including those who are: • Pregnant or trying to become pregnant • Taking prescription or over-the-counter medications that may cause harmful reactions when mixed with alcohol • Under the age of 21 • Recovering from alcoholism or are unable to control the amount they drink • Suffering from a medical condition that may be worsened by alcohol • Driving, planning to drive, or participating in other activities requiring skill, coordination, and alertness. Over time, excessive alcohol use can lead to the development of chronic diseases, neurological impairments, and social problems. These include cardiomyopathy.
Substance abuse	Expand research to identify and locate any genetic components that would predispose individuals to the risk of alcoholism and drug addiction. Encourage middle/junior high and senior high schools to use science classes to instruct students about the deleterious effects of alcohol and drug abuse on the body. Adopt strategies to counter and prevent substance abuse in young people that recognize various risky behaviors on their part as making up a complex whole, to which integrated and congruent approaches are required. Ensure that parents are integrated into national strategies against substance abuse by young people as partners on an equal footing with schools, communities, and other concerned elements of society. Support studies to determine the long-term biologic consequences for children who are born to mothers addicted to drugs or alcohol. Urge all agencies and individuals involved in acting to control substance abuse to begin interventions as soon as possible after the first offense, when success in preventing recurrence is more likely. Direct studies toward establishing whether youth exposure to advertisements for alcoholic beverages is altering attitudes about underage drinking and whether this in turn increases underage alcohol use. Increase research to explicate the nature and persistence of biologic and electrophysiologic changes in the brains of adolescent and adult abusers of alcohol and drugs.

Source: Healthy People 2020. Retrieved from http://www.healthypeople.gov/2020/default.aspx.

occurs because of the constant stress from overfilling. The stretching of the myocardial fibers increases the compliance of the ventricles but results in hypocontractility, reduced stroke volume, ejection fraction, and ultimately decreased cardiac output. Blood flows more slowly through the enlarged heart, causing mural thrombi (blood clots on the heart wall) to form, increasing the risk of atrial and ventricular emboli formation. Additionally, the extra blood that stays in the chambers after each contraction eventually backs up into the pulmonary system, causing heart failure symptoms and ultimately reducing blood flow to the tissues.

Cardiomyopathy that develops during pregnancy or after pregnancy, referred to as peripartum cardiomyopathy (PPCM), is thought to be caused by an interaction of pericardium physiology with infectious agents, leading to myocarditis, or by inflammatory, genetic, hormonal, or metabolic factors (Porth & Matfin, 2009). The diagnosis of PPCM is based on (1) the patient's having no other identifiable causes of heart failure, (2) heart failure within 5 months of delivery, (3) absence of heart disease before the last month of pregnancy, and (4) ECG revealing abnormal left ventricular systolic function. Most cases of PPCM occur in the postpartum period, with up to 50% of the related deaths occurring within 3 months after delivery (Woods et al., 2009).

Clinical Manifestations

The clinical manifestations of DCM have an insidious onset. Findings depend on the area and the degree of structural dysfunction. Initial complaints typically include a complaint of increasing fatigue, dyspnea, and activity intolerance, classic symptoms of heart failure. The failing heart may include one or both sides of the heart, manifesting both left- and right-sided heart failure clinical manifestations (see Chapter 34 for more information). Right-sided heart failure occurs later and is associated with a poor prognosis. Mitral and/or tricuspid insufficiency may develop because of ventricular dilation, preventing complete valve closure.

Some patients may be asymptomatic for months or even years and are diagnosed by laboratory findings; others have pronounced symptoms at the onset of the disease. Sudden death can occur at any stage of the disease.

Laboratory and Diagnostic Procedures

The diagnosis of DCM is made on the basis of an in-depth history and physical and ruling out other causes of the presenting clinical manifestations. (See Chapter 34 for the diagnostic evaluation of heart failure.) Etiologic predisposing risk factors listed in the Risk Factors box need to be evaluated. Additionally, other diseases need to be ruled out; for example, if the patient is complaining of chest pain, a MI evaluation is indicated (see Chapter 32). The Diagnostic Tests box outlines the tests that are usually done to evaluate DCM (p. 1008). Because DCM is a progressive disease, frequent and ongoing monitoring is necessary. Clinical manifestations typically dictate the need for further testing and evaluation.

Medical Management

Because DCM is a chronic, noncurable disease, management focuses on control of the disease, identifying precipitating factors, and controlling clinical manifestations. Interventions are aimed at controlling the progression of structural dysfunction that leads to heart failure, when possible. Treatment aims are more palliative than curative and focus on decreasing cardiac workload.

DIAGNOSTIC TESTS for Dilated Cardiomyopathy

Diagnostic Test, Normal Values, and *Rationales*	Expected Abnormality
Chest X-Ray	
Clear lungs and normal heart size *Cardiomyopathy causes an increase in heart size and predisposes heart failure.*	DCM: Cardiomegaly and enlargement of the heart. Lung fields have pulmonary congestion and edema.
Electrocardiogram (ECG)	
Normal conduction time intervals (see Chapter 30) *Stretching of the myocardium may also cause conduction disturbances.* *Heart failure causes abnormal axis deviation.* *Ischemia associated with heart failure causes the dysrhythmias and ST segment changes.*	Dysrhythmias. Axis deviation. Left bundle branch block. ST segment changes. Sinus tachycardia.
Echocardiogram (ultrasound) (p. 1019)	
Normal chamber size and normal cardiac structures *The disease causes enlargement of the chamber, which results in sluggish wall motion and decreased systolic and diastolic function.*	Enlarged chamber size, ventricular wall, and septum thickness. Sluggish wall motion. Decreased systolic and diastolic function.
Cardiac Catheterization	
(Chapter 32) to Rule Out CAD, Assess Hemodynamic Status, and Determine Chamber Size and Function: Normal coronary arteries, chambers, and valve pressures *The disease causes enlargement of the chamber, which results in a decreased force of muscle contraction, leading to decreased cardiac output.*	Enlarged chambers and decreased cardiac output.
Endomyocardial Biopsy Occasionally Done to Rule Out Other Causes of the Clinical Manifestations	
Normal myocardial tissue *Changes due to disease process.*	Myocardial cells positive for pathologic evidence of infiltration, fibrosis, or inflammation.
Radionuclide Study (Chapter 32)	
Normal chamber volumes and blood perfusion to cardiac muscle *The disease causes enlargement of the chamber, which results in a decreased force of muscle contractions leading to an increase in blood being left in the chambers and thereby decreasing myocardial perfusion.*	Abnormally increased ventricular volume and deficits in myocardial muscle perfusion.

The overall goals of medical management are to find the cause, improve contractile efficiency, and manage the symptoms and complications. If the cause can be identified and terminated, such as use of illicit drugs or alcohol, stopping the use of these substances will help to control and possibly reverse the progression of the heart disease. The multifaceted treatment program includes medications along with activity and dietary restrictions. Medication therapy includes anticoagulants for the blood stasis problems and diuretics and fluid/sodium-restricted diets to decrease fluid overload and pulmonary congestion. Cardiac devices may be indicated for significant left ventricular dysfunction or for bradycardia or heart block, as described in Chapter 30.

If heart failure with left ventricular dysfunction is present, then medical therapy with ACE inhibitors or angiotensin receptor blockers, beta-adrenergic blockers, and aldosterone blockers are the standard of care (Woods et al., 2009). Chapter 34 provides a complete review of pharmacologic management for left ventricular dysfunction. Beta-adrenergic blockers and ACE inhibitors together may be able to slow, stop, or even reverse the tissue remodeling that occurs with cardiomyopathy and heart failure (Woods et al., 2009). Antidysrhythmic medications help to control atrial and ventricular irritability, decreasing dysrhythmias. Finally, diuretics are prescribed to control congestion, and digoxin is used for continued symptoms of heart failure.

If left ventricular dysfunction is present with an ejection fraction of less than 35%, despite optimizing medications, an implantable cardioverter defibrillator (ICD) may be placed (Chapter 30). A pacemaker with a lead in both ventricles (Chapter 30), referred to as a biventricular pacemaker (or cardiac resynchronization therapy), is being used to treat heart failure when the ejection fraction is less than 35%, the QRS duration is greater than 120 milliseconds, and patients remain symptomatic despite optimal heart failure medicines. The pacemaker is able to synchronize cardiac contraction, beginning with atrial depolarization and ending with left ventricular depolarization. This produces significantly improved left ventricular performance, which results in an improved ejection fraction and cardiac output. The result is an improved heart failure status. See the Pharmacology Summary of Medications to Treat Cardiac Inflammatory Disorders (p. 976).

Activity restriction is essential during the acute illness. Over time, however, the nurse should encourage the patient to resume activities that increase strength and endurance. Early in the disease process, patients may find the activity restrictions difficult to accept. Thus, patient and family education needs to stress that physical and emotional stress exacerbate the disease. As the disease progresses, most patients experience severe clinical manifestations that limit activity. Alcohol is discouraged for patients with DCM because it depresses myocardial contractility and further decreases cardiac output. End-stage therapies for patients who have progressive and refractory disease include heart transplantation or permanent mechanical assist devices. These therapies are described in Chapter 34.

Nursing Management

Nursing management begins with a detailed history and in-depth physical assessment. The nurse must inquire about possible risk factors and other diseases that may mimic DCM. Continuous monitoring of assessment parameters of the patient for changes in systemic perfusion include mental status, heart rate and rhythm, peripheral perfusion, oxygenation, fluid status, and vital signs. Since this is a progressive disease, an ongoing assessment is necessary to note significant trends. See the Nursing Process: Patient Care Plan for Cardiomyopathy on page 1010.

Hypertrophic Obstructive Cardiomyopathy

Hypertrophic cardiomyopathy (HCM) is a disorder of the sarcomere, the contractile element of the cardiac muscle that is characterized by left ventricular and occasionally right ventricular hypertrophy, with greater hypertrophy occurring in the septum. This disorder has also historically been referred to as idiopathic hypertrophic subaortic stenosis (IHSS) and hypertrophic obstructive cardiomyopathy (HOCM). The rationale for the variation in names is described in the following text. Figure 33–13◆ demonstrates the difference between a normal ventricular wall and a hypertrophied wall.

Epidemiology and Etiology

Hypertrophic cardiomyopathy occurs in about 1 in 500 people in the general population, and it is the most common cause of sudden death in young people. In more than 50% of the cases, HCM is a genetic disorder, manifested by a defect in cardiac muscle development (Moser & Riegel, 2008). Close blood relatives (parents, children, or siblings) of someone with HCM often also have enlarged ventricular septums. In the majority of patients, HCM is transmitted as an autosomal dominant trait.

GENETIC CONSIDERATIONS for Hypertrophic Cardiomyopathy

Because of the genetic link of hypertrophic cardiomyopathy, the health care provider needs to test close family members for the disease. Echocardiographic screening is recommended for immediate family members of patients with hypertrophic cardiomyopathy.

Hypertrophic cardiomyopathy, which is frequently idiopathic, also can be caused by hypertension or hypoparathyroidism. Although HCM is most commonly found in young adults, it can also occur in the very young and in the aged population. Men and the Black population are affected more than other groups by HCM. It is usually diagnosed in young adulthood in more active athletic individuals (Moser & Riegel, 2008).

Hypertrophic obstructive cardiomyopathy has the same etiology as HCM, although patients with HOCM have the additional problem of having the left ventricular aortic outflow tract obstructed.

Pathophysiology

With HCM, the walls of the ventricle hypertrophy, or remodel, without an increase in the chamber size. Fibrotic infiltrates in the myocardium produce left ventricular stiffness and add to the hypertrophy of the wall and septum. One unique feature of HCM is that the cardiac muscle might not hypertrophy equally. The interventricular septum, especially the upper portion, tends to have a greater increase in size than the free wall of the left ventricle. These changes result in a decreased ventricular chamber size and cause the ventricles to take a longer period of time to relax. The result is diastolic dysfunction because the loss of ventricular compliance decreases the amount of blood that will flow into the ventricle during

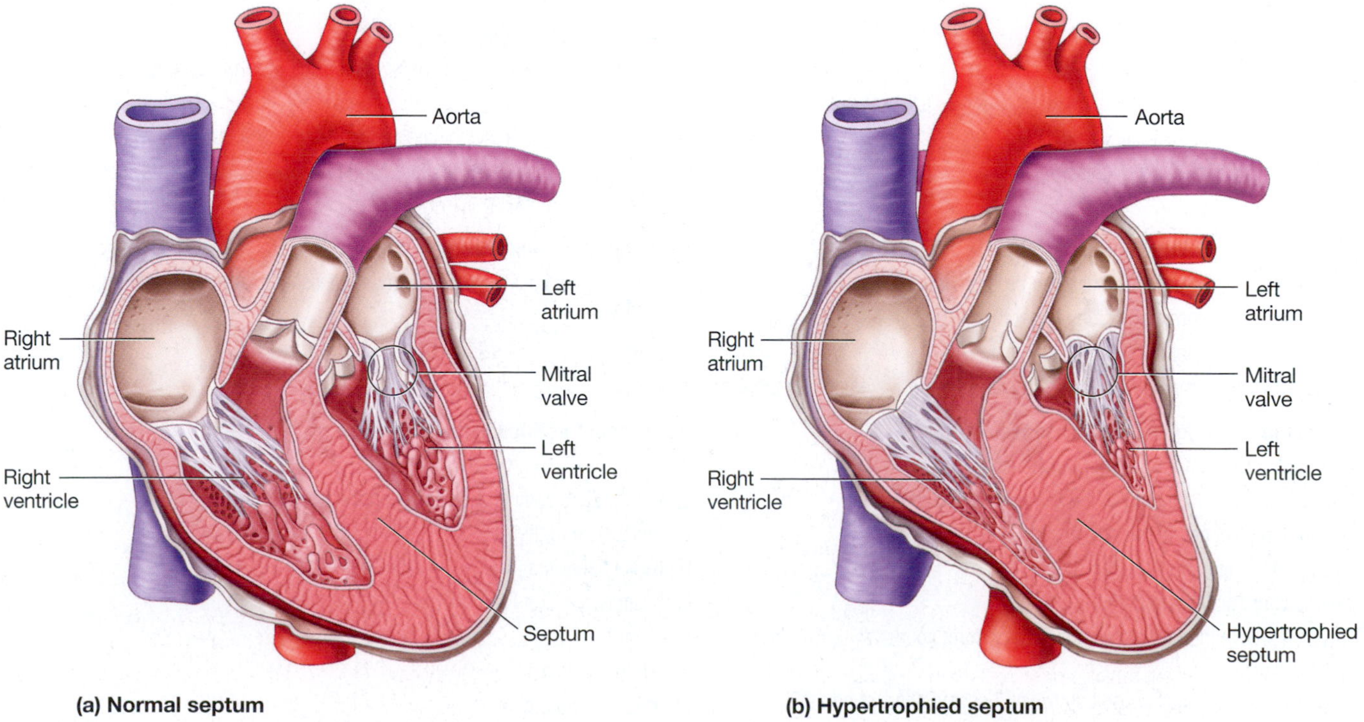

FIGURE 33–13 ◆ (A) Normal heart wall and (B) hypertrophied heart wall.

NURSING PROCESS: Patient Care Plan for Cardiomyopathy

Assessment of Cardiac Status Using Gordon's Functional Health Patterns:

- Health Perception Health Management Pattern
- Activity Exercise Pattern
- Cognitive Perceptual Pattern
- Self-Perception Self-Concept Pattern

Subjective Data	Objective Data
Assessment of Cardiac Output Do you feel weak or light-headed with activity? Do you become short of breath? If so, what causes it to occur? Is the shortness of breath getting worse?	**Assessment of Cardiac Output** Vital signs. Lung sounds. Weight: Is there recent significant gain? Cardiac output, cardiac index, and ejection fraction. Fluid intake and output.
Assessment of Tissue Perfusion Do you become short of breath? If so, what causes it to occur? How far can you walk before becoming short of breath? Do you experience leg pain? If so, what brings it on and is it getting worse? Do your hands and feet feel cold on a warm day?	**Assessment of Tissue Perfusion** Acid–base balance. Lung sounds. Respiratory rate. Cyanosis. Edema. Skin temperature. Capillary refill.
Assessment of Heart Failure How much activity are you able to do before becoming short of breath? Do you have a cough? If so, is it productive? Do your feet swell? If so, how much?	**Assessment of Heart Failure** Vital signs. Lung sounds. Jugular venous distention. Dyspnea. Confusion. Decreased urine output. Orthopnea. Pink frothy sputum. Skin temperature. Peripheral edema.
Assessment of Fatigue What level of activity fatigues you? Have you been becoming more fatigued with less activity recently? Are you able to complete your ADLs without fatigue?	**Assessment of Fatigue** Monitor tolerance to activities while on bed rest in order to obtain a baseline to plan activities. Monitor for changes in symptoms and vital signs (VS) during activity. Determine if heart rate, respirations, and blood pressure return to normal within 3 minutes after stopping activity.
Assessment of Anxiety What do you know about your disease process? How do your health-related issues impact your daily life? Do you feel anxious about your health? Do you have family members or close friends who provide emotional support?	**Assessment of Anxiety** Observe for manifestations of anxiety: restlessness, apprehension, and withdrawal.
Assessment of Knowledge of Disease What have you been told about your health? What is your understanding of the treatments you are on? Do you drink alcohol or use any recreational drugs? Do you take rest periods during the day? What is your level of activity? Do you feel any change in your ability to perform your activities of daily living (ADLs)? How much activity can you do before you become short of breath? What symptoms need to be reported to your health care provider?	**Assessment of Knowledge of Disease** Assess: Level of understanding of disease and treatment. Compliance with therapy. High-risk behaviors. Lung sounds. Vital signs. Peripheral edema. Shortness of breath. Cough—type of sputum.

NURSING PROCESS: Patient Care Plan for Cardiomyopathy, *continued*

Assessment of Compliance with Treatment Regimen What do you understand about your treatment plan? Are you able to comply with the restrictions necessary to prevent further progression of your disease? What can the health care team do to help you with treatment compliance?	**Assessment of Compliance With Treatment Regimen** Assess motivation and willingness to comply with therapy. Assess where the health care team can assist with barriers to compliance.
Assessment of Ability to Function in Usual Role What is your role in your family? Are you able to perform that role? Who takes over your role function when you are not able to? How do you feel about your inability to function in your role? Do you worry about your and/or your family's finances related to your illness?	**Assessment of Ability to Function in Usual Role** Determine knowledge of health status (see *Deficient Knowledge* nursing diagnosis). Assess level of functioning. Assess alternatives or alterations in role function.
Outcomes and Evaluation Parameters	**Planning and Interventions with *Rationales***
1. NURSING DIAGNOSIS: Decreased Cardiac Output *related to hypercontractility and obstruction to outflow* (NANDA-I © 2012)	
Outcomes: Patient is able to tolerate decreased cardiac output. Stabilization of cardiac output occurs. ***Evaluation Parameters:*** Clear lung sounds. No dyspnea. Normal vital signs. Skin warm and dry. Normal heart rate and rhythm. No abnormal heart sounds (S_3 and S_4). No jugular venous distention, peripheral edema, or ascites. Normal urine output.	Monitor vital signs, lung sounds, skin, heart rate and rhythm, edema, JVD, and ascites *in order to monitor response and tolerance of altered cardiac output (CO).* Administer negative inotropic medications as ordered *to decrease the hypercontractility.* Avoid a valsalva maneuver *because it impedes venous return (preload).*
2. NURSING DIAGNOSIS: Ineffective Tissue Perfusion *related to decreased cardiac output* (NANDA-I © 2012)	
Outcome: Adequate gas exchange. ***Evaluation Parameters:*** Normal ABGs. No dyspnea: unlabored respirations <24/minute. Alert and oriented. Clear breath sounds. No restlessness, cyanosis, or fatigue. Oxygen saturation is within normal limits.	Assess for adventitious or diminished breath sounds. *Indicates decreased gas exchange and heart failure.* Note presence of cough and amount and color of sputum. *Assessing for heart failure.* Monitor ABGs and oxygen saturation *to assess adequacy of gas exchange.* Monitor respiratory rate and depth *to assess for respiratory distress.* Monitor fluid status *to assess heart failure.* Monitor restlessness and confusion. *Indicators of inadequate gas exchange with resultant brain hypoxia.* Assess need for suctioning and/or endotracheal intubation *to maintain adequate gas exchange.* Observe for cyanosis, especially in the mucous membranes. *Indicators of inadequate gas exchange with resultant tissue hypoxia.* Turn, cough, deep breathe, elevate head of bed, and instruct on use of incentive spirometry. *Measures to promote gas exchange.* Administer humidified oxygen as prescribed *to increase oxygen levels.* Report respiratory distress to the health care provider. *Medical intervention may be indicated to prevent respiratory failure.*
3. NURSING DIAGNOSIS: Tissue Perfusion Ineffective *related to hypercontractility and aortic outflow obstruction* (NANDA-I © 2012)	
Outcome: Prevention of heart failure. ***Evaluation Parameters:*** Lungs clear. Patient denies shortness of breath. Patient verbalizes understanding and willingness to adhere to treatment plan.	Monitor BUN, creatinine, liver enzymes, and bilirubin *to assess blood supply to the liver and kidneys.* Monitor fluid balance and record as prescribed *to assess fluid retention that would exacerbate the symptoms of heart failure.* Report significant imbalances to the health care provider *to obtain the necessary intervention(s) to correct the imbalance.*

(*continued*)

NURSING PROCESS: Patient Care Plan for Cardiomyopathy, *continued*

Outcomes and Evaluation Parameters	Planning and Interventions with *Rationales*
4. NURSING DIAGNOSIS: Fatigue and Activity Intolerance *related to decreased cardiac output* (NANDA-I © 2012)	
Outcomes: No increase in fatigue. No decrease in activity levels. ***Evaluation Parameters:*** Absence of or no progression of peripheral edema, congested lungs, decreased CO, dyspnea, pink frothy sputum, diaphoresis, or decreased renal and liver perfusion.	Identify activities that increase fatigue *to avoid increasing cardiac workload.* Discontinue activity if chest pain, dyspnea, cyanosis, dizziness, hypotension, sustained tachycardia, or dysrhythmias develop *to aid in evaluating tolerance of activities.* Explore sedentary activities the patient may enjoy *to provide diversion that does not place a demand on the heart.*
5. NURSING DIAGNOSIS: Fear and Anxiety *related to disease process and sudden cardiac death* (NANDA-I © 2012)	
Outcome: Anxiety level minimized and manageable. ***Evaluation Parameters:*** Verbalizes anxious feelings. Verbalizes what relieves anxiety. Demonstrates anxiety relief by consistently controlling aggression, impulsiveness, and self-mutilation, and by improving coping and social interaction skills. Verbalizes absence of sensory perceptual disorders. Verbalizes absence of physical manifestations of anxiety. Behavioral manifestations of anxiety absent.	Allow time and encourage verbalization of fears related to illness *to assist in relieving anxiety.* Explore with the patient/family techniques to reduce anxiety. *This gives the patient a sense of control and opens communication about the subject.* Provide factual information concerning diagnosis, treatment, disfigurement, disabilities, and prognosis. *Truthful explanations increase trust and potentially decrease anxiety.* Explain all procedures and allow time for mental preparation. *This decreases fear and anxiety of the unknown.* Explore effective ways to minimize anxiety. *This gives the patient a sense of control.* Instruct the patient on use of relaxation techniques *to relieve anxiety.* Assess the need for and administer antianxiety and pain medication. *If alternative measures are not effective, the patient may need antianxiety agents.*
6. NURSING DIAGNOSIS: Deficient Knowledge *related to disease process, care needs, and complications* (NANDA-I © 2012)	
Outcomes: Understanding of disease process, care needs, and importance of compliance with treatment. ***Evaluation Parameters:*** Compliance with treatment plan. Activity level appropriate for cardiac workload.	Avoid high-risk behaviors (alcohol, cocaine). Report any increases in clinical manifestations to your health care provider *to retard the progression of the disease.* Comply with therapy *to prevent progression of the disease.* Activity restriction *to decrease cardiac workload.*
7. NURSING DIAGNOSIS: Noncompliance with Medication and Activity Restrictions *related to chronic progressive illness* (NANDA-I © 2012)	
Outcome: Shows willingness to comply with therapy. ***Evaluation Parameter:*** Accepts imposed restrictions and complies with treatment plan.	Suggest alternative solutions to barriers *to determine interventions that will increase compliance.* Monitor and evaluate compliance with therapy *to determine patient's ability to sustain treatment.*
8. NURSING DIAGNOSIS: Powerlessness Over Altered Role Function *related to chronic progressive illness* (NANDA-I © 2012)	
Outcomes: Verbalizes a realistic perception of control. Verbalizes realistic perception of abilities to perform. ***Evaluation Parameters:*** Identifies health outcome priorities. Verbalizes powerlessness. Identifies actions that are within her control and demonstrates ability to perform those actions. Reports adequate support from staff and family.	Discuss realistic options for self-care. *Gives patient hope and realistic view of limitations.* Reinforce personal strengths. *Decreases sense of powerlessness.* Encourage verbalization of feeling of powerlessness. *Opens communication.* Assist patient to increase independence when realistic. *Decreases powerlessness.* Allow control over surroundings and schedule when possible. *Decreases powerlessness.* Keep items within reach. *Decreases powerlessness.* Set short-term realistic goals. *Decreases powerlessness.* Explore patient's support mechanisms: family, church, and friends. *Needed as a source of support.*

Source: Adapted from Wilkinson, J. M., & Ahearn, N. R. (2009). *Prentice Hall nursing diagnosis handbook* (9th ed.). Upper Saddle River, NJ: Prentice Hall.

diastole. This has a direct negative effect on cardiac output and, thus, tissue perfusion. Another characteristic of HCM is hypercontractility of the muscle, rather than hypocontractility as seen in dilated cardiomyopathy. The hypercontractility occurs, particularly in the intraventricular system.

A third characteristic of HCM is obstruction to the outflow tract of the left ventricle (LV) leading into the aorta. The site and extent of hypertrophy dictates the degree of obstruction. The hypertrophy distorts the septum; in some patients, the anterior leaflet of the mitral valve is distorted, causing it to meet the septum, thus narrowing the left

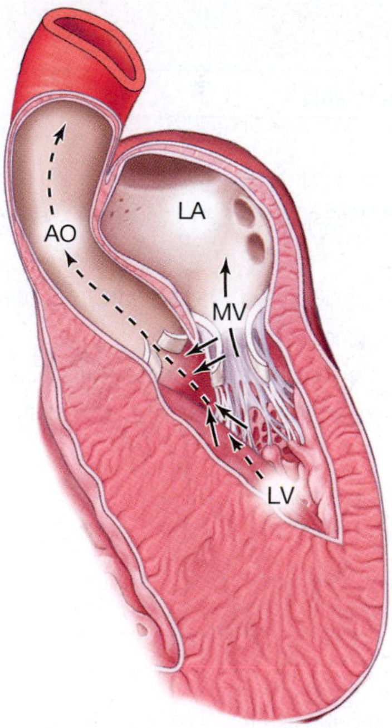

FIGURE 33–14 ◆ Hypertrophic obstructive cardiomyopathy.

ventricular outflow tract during systole (Moser & Riegel, 2008; Woods et al., 2009). This occurs because of the septum's inward movement during systole, which narrows the LV outflow and increases blood velocity. This increased velocity then pulls the mitral leaflet toward the septum (the Venturi effect). Figures 33–13 and 33–14◆ demonstrate how the septum and the anterior leaflet narrow the left ventricular outflow tract into the aorta.

Significant LV outflow obstruction is present in some patients at rest, while in others it is evident only during increased activity such as exercise. Reduced preload decreases chamber size and increased heart rate will increase LV outflow obstruction. Dehydration and suddenly sitting upright (which may cause orthostatic hypotension) are two examples of factors that will decrease preload; fever and exercise are two factors that increase heart rate. The result is a reduction in cardiac output that may range from minimal to severe and may lead to syncope, serious cardiac dysrhythmias (ventricular tachycardia), and sudden death. Heart failure is the eventual outcome as the disease progresses. Not all individuals with HCM have obstruction to outflow, but if obstruction is present, HCM is further classified as hypertrophic obstructive cardiomyopathy. If the obstructive process is present, the disorder is also referred to as idiopathic hypertrophic subaortic stenosis (see Figure 33–14).

Clinical Manifestations

Clinical manifestations most commonly begin in late adolescence or early adulthood but may appear at any age. Many of the clinical manifestations of HCM are similar to those of dilated cardiomyopathy. The most frequently reported manifestation is dyspnea, which is due to high pulmonary pressures created by the backup of blood from the restricted left ventricle. This type of cardiomyopathy also may occur without symptoms, although other frequently reported symptoms include chest pain, dizziness, presyncope or syncope, fatigue, orthopnea and paroxysmal nocturnal dyspnea, and palpitations. The symptoms appear gradually, progress over time, and are associated with deterioration of LV function. Exercise tends to precipitate the symptoms and increases the risk of sudden death. In some individuals, however, sudden death or severe heart failure is the first clinical manifestation of the disease. Right- and left-sided heart failure may be present. The risk of sudden death, which appears most often in young adults, can be decreased by avoiding strenuous exercise. Sudden death is the most common cause of death for individuals with HCM.

Both supraventricular (primarily atrial fibrillation) and ventricular (tachycardia and fibrillation) dysrhythmias occur with HCM, along with sudden death (Chapter 30). Additionally, it is common to have an abnormally forceful LV apical pulse, S_4, and a harsh crescendo–decrescendo systolic murmur of varying intensity that is heard best at the left lower sternal border and the apex. A systolic thrill may be palpated at the apex or lower left sternal border.

In severe cases of HOCM, pulmonary artery pressures are elevated because of increased backward pressure due to an inability of the left ventricle to empty. This eventually increases right ventricular pressure, causing the interventricular septum to shift to the left. The leftward shift causes further obstruction to the ventricular outflow tract (Moser & Riegel, 2008; Woods et al., 2009).

Laboratory and Diagnostic Procedures

The echocardiogram (p. 1019) is the most useful tool in diagnosing both HCM and HOCM. It allows visualization of the LV hypertrophy and will also reveal wall motion abnormalities and diastolic dysfunction. Because of the progressive nature of the disease, bedside hemodynamic studies are done to monitor the pressures in cardiac chambers and the pulmonary system as well as providing ongoing cardiac output readings. The other tests are described in the Diagnostic Tests box (p. 1014).

Medical Management

Preventing heart failure and sudden cardiac death is the primary treatment goal for patients with HCM. Improving the cardiac output is achieved by reducing ventricular contractility and relieving LV outflow obstruction. These measures improve ventricular filling and ultimately cardiac output and the quality of life. It is often difficult for young adults, in particular, to adhere to a regimen of decreased activity. Emotional support and education by both the nurses and the health care providers are essential to help the individual understand and comply with the reduced activity levels.

If possible, finding and treating the underlying cause is the first priority of medical management. The remainder of medical care is directed toward controlling clinical manifestations, preventing progression of the disease, and improving the individual's quality of life. The treatment plan, described in the following text, consists of medications, activity restriction, fluid stabilization, surgical interventions, and possibly implanting electronic devices. Genetic testing for HCM is discussed in the Genetic Considerations box (p. 1009).

Negative inotropic medications, such as beta-adrenergic blocking agents and calcium antagonists, provide the mainstay of medical therapy and are used to decrease the hypercontractility and outflow obstruction. These medications also decrease the heart rate, which decreases the cardiac workload and oxygen consumption. If the patient is in atrial fibrillation, anticoagulant medications are prescribed to assist in the prevention of clot formation. Antidysrhythmic medications are used to prevent life-threatening dysrhythmias and improve cardiac output. Likewise, ICDs are used to prevent sudden cardiac death (Chapter 30).

Dehydration needs to be avoided because it will decrease preload and cardiac output. Patient and family education must stress the importance of consistent normal hydration. Activities, foods, and drinks (alcohol) that cause dehydration must be avoided. Surgical management

DIAGNOSTIC TESTS for Hypertrophic Obstructive Cardiomyopathy

Diagnostic Test, Normal Values, and *Rationales*	Expected Abnormality
Chest X-Ray	
Clear lungs and normal heart size	Cardiac enlargement (cardiomegaly), specifically left atrial enlargement.
Due to progression of the disease process.	If heart failure is present, pulmonary congestion and edema exists.
Resting and Ambulatory ECG	
Normal conduction time intervals (see Chapter 30)	*Resting:* Increased voltage and duration of the QRS complex.
Due to the ventricular hypertrophy and myocardial ischemia.	Both atrial and ventricular dysrhythmias.
	Ambulatory: ST segment changes that occur with increased activity.
	Increased hypercontractility that increases with activity.
Echocardiogram (p. 1019) (ultrasound)	
Normal chamber size and normal cardiac structures	Left ventricular hypertrophy.
The disease causes enlargement of the chamber and septum and hypercontractility, which results in abnormal valve function and cardiac output.	Hypercontractility.
	Asymmetrical wall size.
	Diastolic dysfunction.
Cardiac Catheterization to Rule Out CAD, Assess Hemodynamic Status, and Determine Chamber Size and Function (Chapter 32)	
Normal coronary arteries, chambers, and valve pressures	Increased chamber size and may see changes in valve function and cardiac output.
Tissue hypertrophy and hypercontractility cause abnormal valve motion, resulting in obstruction of the aortic outflow tract.	
Radionuclide Study (Chapter 32)	
Normal chamber volumes and blood perfusion to cardiac muscle	Increased left ventricular and septal wall size.
Tissue hypertrophy and hypercontractility related to disease process.	Asymmetrical hypertrophy.
	Hypercontractility.
Cardiac Biopsy May Be Performed to Analyze Myocardial Tissue	
Normal cellular size and function	Tissue positive for infiltrations and fibrosis.
Changes due to disease process.	

is indicated for HCM if the patient has not responded positively to medical therapy and if marked obstruction to the aortic outflow tract is present due to the mitral valve meeting the enlarged septum. The surgical procedure, which is termed a ventriculomyotomy, involves excising some of the hypertrophied septal muscle. This widens the LV outflow tract, improves cardiac output, and relieves symptoms. Clinical manifestations and exercise tolerance are improved after this surgery in most patients (Moser & Riegel, 2008; Woods et al., 2009). A second surgical procedure that is sometimes used to decrease obstruction is the removal of the mitral valve, the chordae tendineae, and the papillary muscle (see Figure 33–4, p. 989). The mitral valve is then replaced by an artificial valve. This procedure substantially reduces the space taken up by the mitral valve and supporting structures, allowing blood to move more easily around the enlarged septum. In addition to surgical complications, a common problem is transient dysrhythmias caused by edema from surgery and shifts in electrolytes.

A nonsurgical treatment for HCM is an alcohol septal ablation, which involves injection of alcohol down the septal perforator branches of the left anterior descending artery, which provides blood flow to the area of hypertrophied muscle in the septum. The alcohol destroys the extra cardiac muscle without the need to surgically remove it, in effect causing an intentional myocardial infarction (Moser & Riegel, 2008).

An implantable cardioverter defibrillator (ICD) (Chapter 30) is useful for patients with HCM to treat ventricular tachycardia or ventricular fibrillation and to avert sudden death. If left ventricular dysfunction and an ejection fraction of less than 35% are present, a cardiac resynchronization therapy (biventricular pacemaker; see Chapter 30) may help to increase cardiac output (Moser & Riegel, 2008).

Nursing Management

The primary goals of nursing care are to assess and monitor progress of the disease and to provide patient education and emotional support for individuals with this chronic progressive disease. The nursing process provides a framework for the care of these patients. A complete plan of care for HCM is outlined in the Nursing Process: Patient Care Plan for Cardiomyopathy (p. 1010).

Assessment

Nurses must monitor and report changes in the assessment that indicate complications and progression of the disease. Specific nursing assessment data, interventions, rationales, and outcomes are outlined in the Nursing Process: Patient Care Plan for Cardiomyopathy (p. 1010).

Monitoring the patient's hemodynamic status is essential as the disease progresses. Increases in pulmonary artery pressure indicate the onset of heart failure, which increases the risk of further ventricular outflow obstruction. Moreover, the cardiac output needs ongoing monitoring to evaluate oxygenation and adequate tissue perfusion. The nurse needs to space activities for the hospitalized patient in order to allow for periods of rest.

Nursing Diagnoses

The nursing diagnoses that apply to HCM include the following:

- *Risk for Activity Intolerance* related to *decreased cardiac output*
- *Ineffective Tissue Perfusion related to decreased cardiac output*
- *Decreased Cardiac Output related to decreased cardiomyopathy*
- *Coping related to chronic disease state*
- *Fatigue related to decreased cardiac output.*

NANDA-I © 2012

Outcomes and Evaluation Parameters

Because of the risk of cardiac sudden death, both HCM and HOCM have a grave prognosis. However, end-stage therapies such as cardiac transplantation may be viable options. All options must be presented to the patient and family, and the nurse must assess their understanding of the situation. Evaluation parameters would include a verbalization of the options, including the lifestyle changes that organ transplantation would require.

Planning, Interventions, and Rationales

Providing emotional support for the patient with HCM is essential in planning the management of these patients, since this is a progressive chronic disease that could cause sudden death at any time. Identifying perceived stressors for both the patient and the family and assisting them in alleviating these stressors will decrease the emotional stress. The patient and family need to feel free to verbalize fears and concerns and need reassurance that these concerns are legitimate and that resources are available to provide assistance. Providing realistic hope helps to reduce anxiety and increase self-esteem; the patient needs to be encouraged to accomplish a goal no matter how small. If the patient is facing imminent death or waiting for a donor heart, the nurse must create an environment in which the patient and family can openly express concerns and acknowledge fears. Encouragement, a caring touch, and a listening ear will improve the quality of life for patients and families dealing with HCM.

See the Nursing Process: Patient Care Plan for Cardiomyopathy (p. 1010) for a complete nursing care plan to guide the care of patients with HCM and HOCM.

Safety Alert *Patients with hypertrophic cardiomyopathy have an increased risk of sudden cardiac death due to ventricular dysrhythmias such as ventricular tachycardia or ventricular fibrillation. Families of patients with HCM and HOCM should be encouraged to learn CPR and to find out how to access emergency care near their home.*

Restrictive Cardiomyopathy

Restrictive cardiomyopathy (RCM) is the least common type of cardiomyopathy found in the United States. This disorder is characterized by endocardial scarring that usually affects one or both ventricles and restricts filling of blood, resulting in systolic dysfunction. The ventricle has normal wall thickness, but the walls are rigid, producing elevated filling pressures and dilated atria. Involvement of the valve is common, but the outflow tract is spared (see Figure 33–14 , p. 1013).

Epidemiology and Etiology

The causes of RCM are divided into two classifications: primary and secondary. The cause of primary RCM is idiopathic, whereas secondary RCM is thought to be caused by a number of pathologic processes that are outlined in the following text. Idiopathic restrictive cardiomyopathy can present at any age, but its incidence is increased in older adults and is more common in women than men (Mogensen & Arbustini, 2009).

The incidence of cocaine-related RCM is on the rise. Cocaine causes both coronary artery constriction and peripheral vasoconstriction as well as high levels of circulating catecholamines. The combined effect causes an increased workload for the myocardium and a decreased supply of oxygen, leading to myocardial ischemia and infarction. The cells of the myocardium become damaged, leading to cardiomyopathy. These patients typically have a poor prognosis.

Pathophysiology

Secondary RCM may be caused by amyloidosis, endomyocardial fibrosis, disorders in glycogen storage, hemochromatosis, and sarcoidosis, or it may be idiopathic. With amyloidosis, a deposition of eosinophilic fibrinous protein buildup occurs in the heart, causing it to lose the ability to stretch. Idiopathic RCM is a poorly recognized entity of unknown cause characterized by nondilated, nonhypertrophied ventricles with diastolic dysfunction, resulting in dilated atria, with or without systolic dysfunction (Mogensen & Arbustini, 2009). Contractility is unaffected by restrictive cardiomyopathy.

Microscopically, the endometrial changes that occur with RCM include nonspecific patchy endocardial and interstitial fibrosis with increased collagen deposition and molecular hypertrophy. These changes result in the ventricle losing its ability to stretch, thereby decreasing compliance. It also results in an inability to fill and a drop in cardiac output. As intraventricular pressures increase and cardiac output decreases, manifestations of heart failure begin to appear. These manifestations typically progress rapidly, resulting in high mortality.

Clinical Manifestations

Patients with RCM have signs of pulmonary and systemic congestion. The most common symptom is dyspnea. In addition, patients complain of palpitations, fatigue, syncope, angina, generalized weakness, and exercise intolerance. In the advanced stages, clinical manifestations of either or both right- or left-sided heart failure are present. An S_3 is frequently present, and a systolic murmur from mitral and tricuspid regurgitation is common.

Laboratory and Diagnostic Procedures

As with all of the cardiomyopathies, the echocardiogram (p. 1018) is the most useful diagnostic test for the diagnosis of RCM. It reveals a thickened cardiac wall, a small ventricular chamber size, and dilated atria, as well as diastolic filling changes as the disease progresses. The echocardiogram also is useful in distinguishing restrictive cardiomyopathy from constrictive pericarditis, the major disorder that mimics restrictive cardiomyopathy. Hemodynamic studies identify elevated left atrial and left ventricular pressures. The Diagnostic Tests box describes the remainder of the diagnostic tests for RCM.

Medical Management

Currently, there is no specific treatment or cure for RCM. Therapy is aimed at controlling symptoms to improve the patient's quality of life. Like patients with HCM, those with RCM are taught to avoid situations that impair venous filling, causing a further drop in cardiac output. The patient and family need to have a clear understanding that activity such as strenuous exercise, as well as any situation that causes dehydration, needs to be avoided.

Medical management is aimed at reducing pulmonary and systemic congestion and reducing the heart's workload to diminish heart failure. There is no medical cure for this disease, although treatment of the underlying cause of secondary restrictive cardiomyopathy may be beneficial.

The cornerstone of the medical treatment for RCM is drug therapy. Antidysrhythmic medications are prescribed, depending on the specific

Weblink: Cardiomyopathy Association

DIAGNOSTIC TESTS for Restrictive Cardiomyopathy

Diagnostic Test, Normal Values, and *Rationales*	Expected Abnormality
Chest X-Ray	
Clear lungs and normal heart size *Restriction of blood flow leading to pulmonary venous backup of blood and resulting in cardiac enlargement heart failure.*	Cardiomegaly, specifically atrial enlargement. Pulmonary venous congestion. Pleural effusions may be present with heart failure.
Electrocardiogram (ECG)	
Normal conduction time intervals (see Chapter 30) *Distortion of the cardiac conduction system due to cardiomegaly. Cardiac ischemia causes dysrhythmias.*	Atrial fibrillation. Complex serious ventricular dysrhythmias. Tachycardia.
Echocardiogram	
Normal chamber size and normal cardiac structures *Restrictive nature of disease increases wall thickness and prevents myocardial fiber stretch to accommodate blood volumes. Blood backs up in atria, causing it to dilate.*	Thickened cardiac wall. Small ventricular chamber size. Dilated atria. Decreased diastolic filling as disease progresses.
Radionuclide Study (Chapter 32)	
Normal chamber volumes and blood perfusion to cardiac muscle *Restrictive nature of disease prevents myocardial fiber stretch to accommodate blood volumes, causing decreased cardiac output and tissue perfusion.*	Increased ventricular volume mass, decreasing chamber size. Areas of decreased perfusion.
Endomyocardial Biopsy	
Normal myocardial tissue *Changes occur due to disease process.*	Presence of amyloidosis and/or sarcoidosis.

dysrhythmia. Diuretics are used to decrease pulmonary congestion, although the patient has to be monitored closely to prevent dehydration. Calcium-channel blockers and beta-adrenergic blockers will decrease the heart rate, which then increases ventricular filling time. Anticoagulants are indicated for patients in atrial fibrillation to prevent thromboembolism. A low-sodium diet will decrease fluid retention and pulmonary congestion. As with dilated cardiomyopathy, the heart failure from RCM may be treated with a biventricular pacemaker. In addition, an ICD may be indicated to prevent sudden cardiac death (Chapter 30).

Both primary and secondary restrictive cardiomyopathies have a poor prognosis. Death is most frequently due to heart failure, sudden cardiac death, dysrhythmias, or stroke. Strategies for treating end-stage heart failure are more fully discussed in Chapter 34.

Nursing Management

Nursing management of restrictive cardiomyopathy focuses on decreasing the workload of the heart and conserving energy. Nursing care is similar to the care of the patient with the other types of cardiomyopathy. The Nursing Process: Patient Care Plan for Cardiomyopathy (p. 1010) outlines the care for all types of cardiomyopathy. The discharge priorities are presented in the Patient Teaching & Discharge Priorities box.

Arrhythmogenic Right Ventricular Cardiomyopathy

Arrhythmogenic right ventricular cardiomyopathy (ARVC), a rare inherited heart muscle disease, is defined as an electrical disturbance that develops when the muscle tissue in the right ventricle is replaced with fibrous scar and fatty tissues. In approximately 30% of patients, the left ventricle also is involved (Basso, Corrado, Marcus, Nava, & Theine, 2009). It is also known as arrhythmogenic right ventricular dysplasia/cardiomyopathy (ARVD/C) and arrhythmogenic right ventricular dysplasia (ARVD).

Epidemiology and Etiology

The precise cause of ARVC is unknown, although it has a possible familial link in some patients. The onset of the disease typically is between the late teens to early 20s. It is rare for ARVC to develop in early childhood or after age 40. It appears that men and women of any ethnic origin can be affected. When more than one member of the family is affected, the mode of inheritance appears to be an autosomal dominant gene (Basso et al., 2009).

Because little is known about the disease, it is difficult to estimate how many people are affected. However, it is reasonable to estimate in the light of current knowledge that approximately 1 in 3,000 to 1 in 10,000 people are affected (Cardiomyopathy Association, 2010).

Pathophysiology

Patchy areas of fat and fibrous tissues develop primarily in the right ventricle between the epicardial and endocardial layers, replacing functional cardiac muscle. The specific reason for this occurrence is under investigation. One theory suggests that an abnormal gene or genes leads to heart muscle cell damage and loss. The fibrous and fatty tissues are thought to replace these heart muscle cells as an attempt by the body to repair the damage. Once the muscle has been replaced, the areas become hypokinetic. Given the patchy nature of ARVC, abnormal areas may be surrounded by normal ones. Right ventricular thickening occurs early in the disease; as the disease progresses, it may involve the left ventricle. The patchy disorganized structure of the myocardium areas of the right ventricle may lead to one or more sites of abnormal electrical activity, accounting for abnormal ECG rhythm disturbances and abnormal contractile ability.

Weblink: Cardiomyopathy Association

PATIENT TEACHING & DISCHARGE PRIORITIES for Cardiomyopathy

Need	Teaching
Prevention of disease progression	Teach the importance of following a treatment plan that includes medications (that slow disease progression) and lifestyle changes. Teaching includes the following: • Add timed rest periods between activities. • Space activities to prevent dyspnea. • Avoid alcohol and drug use (cocaine). • Restrict sodium and fluid intake to prevent fluid overload.
Compliance with therapy	Teach the importance of complying with the treatment plan in order to slow the progress of the disease and prevent sudden death. Determine motivation factors for individual patients and create a plan that utilizes these factors. Comply with follow-up health care provider visits.
Prevent exacerbation of heart failure	Explain to the patient/family what clinical manifestations to monitor and report to the health care worker: • Sudden increase in weight in a short period of time (i.e., greater than 2–3 lb in a few days) • Shortness of breath at rest, possibly with chest pressure • Increased shortness of breath with activities • Persistent productive cough • Swelling ankles, feet, or abdomen • Waking breathless at night. Diet therapy: limit sodium to 2–3 g and 2 liters of fluid daily. Eat small, frequent meals. Plan rest periods between activities.
Reportable clinical manifestations	Consider clinical manifestations of heart failure (Chapter 34). Consider clinical manifestations of infective endocarditis. Consider new onset chest pain.

Clinical Manifestations

The degree and type of clinical manifestations and the risk of complications vary greatly among individuals with ARVC. Many patients report little or no difficulties or manifestations, whereas others have life-threatening problems. Typically, patients seek help for palpitations, light-headedness, and fatigue. More serious symptoms include syncope and symptoms of heart failure. The ECG exhibits complete or incomplete right bundle branch block. A signal-averaged ECG is abnormal. Patients may present with ventricular tachycardia that generally has a left bundle branch block contour, with T waves inverted over the right precordial leads. The ventricular tachycardia may be due to reentry. Supraventricular dysrhythmias also can occur, and exercise can induce the ventricular tachycardia in some patients. Chapter 30 provides an in-depth description of these dysrhythmias and tests. Sudden cardiac death is the most serious complication of ARVC and, at times, the very first sign of the disease.

Heart failure is a less common complication of ARVC and appears to occur later in the disease. Typically, right heart failure is more common than left heart failure and is manifested by prominent visible veins in the neck; distention of the liver, which may lead to a sensation of fullness or discomfort in the upper abdomen; and swollen legs or ankles. Left heart failure occurs late when the disease is in the advanced stages and is manifested by fatigue and shortness of breath (see Chapter 34).

Laboratory and Diagnostic Procedures

Research is showing that an MRI (Chapter 32) is a useful noninvasive test for diagnosis detection of right ventricular myocardial fibro-fatty changes in ARVD/C (Cardiomyopathy Association, 2010). The MRI has the unique ability to characterize tissue, specifically by differentiating fat from muscle. The echocardiogram also is a useful tool to assist in the diagnosis because it allows for visualization of the right ventricle and assessment of wall motion abnormalities. Because of the cardiac conduction changes that are associated with ARVC, serial ECGs are indicated to detect rhythm changes and serious life-threatening dysrhythmias. The remainder of the tests are described in the Diagnostic Tests box (p. 1018).

Medical Management

Other than heart transplant, there is no cure for ARVC. Medical management is aimed at controlling clinical manifestations and progression of the disease. Because of the familial nature of ARVC, medical management begins with an in-depth medical and family history. The heath care provider needs to assess any personal or family history of palpitations, light-headed sensation, or collapse.

Because the clinical manifestations and risk of sudden cardiac death vary with ARVC, there are no precise guidelines to determine which patients need to be treated, and there is not one best management approach. Established therapeutic options include beta-adrenergic blockers, antiarrhythmic drugs, catheter ablation, and an ICD. Pharmacologic therapy is the first choice of treatment for patients with well-tolerated and non–life-threatening ventricular dysrhythmias. Treatment includes beta-adrenergic blockers and class I and III antidysrhythmic drugs (sotalol or amiodarone) alone or in combination with beta-adrenergic blockers. If heart failure is present, the patient is treated with diuretics and vasodilators. Typically, medication efficacy is based on symptom improvement, although a more reliable approach is the use of 24-hour Holter monitoring or

DIAGNOSTIC TESTS for Arrhythmogenic Right Ventricular Cardiomyopathy

Diagnostic Test, Normal Values, and *Rationales*	Expected Abnormality
Electrocardiogram (ECG) Holter monitor: ambulatory recording of the ECG over 24 to 48 hours Exercise ECG: Normal conduction time intervals (see Chapter 30) *Dysrhythmias occur because of changes in the structure of the myocardial tissue causing abnormal conduction patterns.* *To detect exercise-induced ventricular dysrhythmias and assess functional capacity.*	Repolarization and depolarization abnormalities. Intraventricular conduction delay. Complete or incomplete right bundle branch block. Lethal ventricular dysrhythmias.
Cardiac Catheterization and Electrophysiological Study (EPS) (Chapter 32) *Determines the presence of other causes for the clinical manifestations.* *Fatty infiltration changes to myocardium cause ventricular dilation.* *Determines which drug will control the dysrhythmias.*	Able to rule out CAD. Right ventricular dilation and dysfunction. *EPS:* able to induce the dysrhythmias. (Chapter 30 discusses these tests.)
Endomyocardial Biopsy Normal cardiac tissue *Due to disease process.*	Fibrous scars and fatty infiltration changes to right ventricular myocardium.
Echocardiogram Normal chamber size and normal cardiac structures *Due to fibrous scarring and fatty infiltrations to the myocardium.*	Dilated right and left ventricles with diminished contractility.
Magnetic Resonance Imaging (MRI) (Chapter 32) Normal cardiac tissue and chamber size *Due to fibrous scarring and fatty infiltrations to the myocardium.*	Right ventricular myocardial fibro-fatty change.
Exercise Radionuclide Study Normal chamber volumes and blood perfusion to cardiac muscle. *Detects changes that occur only with exercise.*	To detect exercise-induced ventricular dysrhythmias and assess functional capacity.
Chest X-Ray Clear lungs and normal heart size *Due to fibrous scarring and fatty infiltrations to the myocardium.*	Cardiomegaly.

Source: Adapted from Kee, J. L. (2010). *Laboratory and diagnostic tests with nursing implications.* Upper Saddle River, NJ: Pearson.

stress testing to determine the effect of life activities and stress on dysrhythmic events. Chapter 30 discusses Holter monitoring.

Due to the risk for sudden cardiac death in patients with sustained ventricular tachycardia and/or ventricular fibrillation, antiarrhythmic drug treatment is indicated. Additionally, the need for an electrophysiology study (EPS) and guided drug testing must be evaluated. Currently, EPS is the standard test for reproducing dysrhythmias in a controlled environment in order to diagnose and treat the dysrhythmias. EPS is further described in Chapter 30.

Catheter ablation of cardiac tissue with radiofrequency may be done for patients with life-threatening ventricular dysrhythmias in whom drug treatment is (1) ineffective, (2) not applicable because of the inability to induce the clinical ventricular dysrhythmias during EPS, or (3) associated with serious side effects. Catheter ablation is a procedure done in the cardiac catheterization laboratory in which areas in the myocardium that initiate dysrhythmias are identified and destroyed with electrical energy or cold temperature (cryotherapy). The goal is to eliminate sites in the myocardium that initiate the dysrhythmia, thereby eliminating the dysrhythmia. When all medical options have been exhausted, ARVC patients may be candidates for heart transplantation (see Chapter 34) (Woods et al., 2009).

Nursing Management

As with all types of cardiomyopathy, nursing management of arrhythmic right ventricular cardiomyopathy focuses on decreasing the heart's workload and conserving energy. Additionally, these patients need to be monitored carefully for cardiac dysrhythmias. Nursing care is similar to the care of the patient with the other types of cardiomyopathy. The Nursing Process: Patient Care Plan for Cardiomyopathy box (p. 1010) outlines the care of all four types of cardiomyopathy. The discharge priorities are presented in the earlier Patient Teaching & Discharge Priorities box (p. 1017).

Health Promotion

The chronicity of a cardiomyopathy has an impact on the patient's quality of life, as well as that for the family and significant others. The nurse needs to evaluate the disease's impact on the patient's role in the family and community. Additionally, the nurse needs to involve the family in the treatment plan and educational program. It is essential to identify stressors and attempt to work with the patient and family to relieve them.

Providing appropriate explanations of all treatments and interventions will increase compliance by both the patient and family. Home health nurses can provide the patient and family with an ongoing assessment of the effectiveness of the treatment plan and facilitate changes when necessary. The goal of therapy is to keep the patient functional and out of the hospital, and home health nurses are essential in the accomplishment of that goal.

When educating patients, nurses must be knowledgeable about cultural factors that can affect the development of cardiomyopathy. The dietary customs and social habits of some cultures increase the risk for the development and progression of the disease. For example, excessive alcohol intake, which is a risk factor for the development and progression of dilated cardiomyopathy, is common in certain cultures. When developing a teaching plan, the nurse needs to evaluate the need for education related to alcohol intake and its impact on DCM.

For HCM and ARVC, patient education includes information on the importance of avoiding strenuous exercise in preventing symptoms, dehydration, and possibly lethal complications. Compliance with activity restriction is often difficult for the young adult with these disorders. Education also is necessary for increasing compliance with the medication regimen and dietary sodium restrictions. Patient compliance will help to prevent the progression of the disease process and can greatly improve the quality of life for the chronic disease. The Patient Teaching & Discharge Priorities box (p. 1017) discussed the discharge priorities and learning needs for patients with cardiomyopathy. Because HCM and ARVC have a genetic predisposition, family members need to be educated about having themselves tested for the disease.

Collaborative Management

Because of the chronic and progressive nature of cardiomyopathy, a collaborative care approach is optimal for management. Utilizing a multidisciplinary team approach, including health care providers, nurses, physical and occupational therapists, psychologists/psychiatrists, dietitians, and pharmacists, will facilitate the best possible quality of life for the patient and the family. In order to meet desired patient outcomes, it is essential that this interdisciplinary team communicate openly with one another in developing and evaluating care of the patient and family (IOM [Institute of Medicine], 2010). It is essential that the health care provider monitor the progression of the cardiomyopathy to determine the treatment plan. Psychiatric counseling may be necessary to assist in lifestyle adjustments necessitated by a chronic disease process. The occupational therapist helps to facilitate realistic occupational goals, while the physical therapist assists in the maintenance of optimum conditioning given the activity restrictions.

Because medication is an essential part of the management of cardiomyopathy, the pharmacist's role is crucial in educating the patient about how to manage the medications and their side effects. Given that heart failure is a common result of cardiomyopathy, the patient and family need to consult with the dietitian about dietary changes needed to control congestion that is exacerbated by excess salt and fluid intake. In addition to the nursing care described previously and in the Patient Teaching & Discharge Priorities for Cardiomyopathy box (p. 1017), the nurse plays a pivotal role in coordinating the efforts of the health care team. In the inpatient setting, the nurse facilitates communication between the members of the team and the patient and family.

End-of-Life Issues with Cardiomyopathy

Due to the severity and progressive nature of the disease, the risk of sudden cardiac death increases as the disease progresses. Therefore, the nurse should encourage family members and significant others to learn CPR and to determine how to access emergency care near their home. When patients reach the end stage and are refractory to available therapies, they should be considered for advanced therapies such as cardiac transplantation or permanent mechanical assist devices, or for palliative care and hospice. These options are discussed in Chapter 34. Finally, the nurse should ask the patient about end-of-life wishes, and the patient should sign an advance directive in advance of a sentinel life-threatening event.

Gerontological Considerations

The effects of rheumatic fever and episodes of infective endocarditis often do not become obvious until later in life. If valve stenosis or regurgitation occurs as a result of these infective processes, symptoms typically follow a slow, stable course. In developed countries, there is a latent period of 20 to 40 years from the occurrence of rheumatic fever to the onset of symptoms. Then it is usually another decade before symptoms become disabling. Once significant limiting symptoms appear, however, survival rates drop to less than 3 years. This progression of the disease tends to place the manifestations and need for treatment in the late decades of life. A decreased immune response and the existence of other debilitating diseases increase the risk for both medical and surgical complications in the older population. The stress of the illness and the normal physiological changes of aging put this group at risk for functional decline during hospitalization. Changes in cardiovascular, respiratory, and renal systems and the prevalence of comorbidities have been cited as possible causes (Moser & Riegel, 2008; Woods et al., 2009).

Dilated cardiomyopathy is also a disease of older adults. With the increasing geriatric population, more attention is being given to understanding diastolic failure induced by uncontrolled hypertension and cardiomyopathies. Researchers have demonstrated that the compensatory mechanisms associated with left ventricular diastolic dysfunction lead to elevated right heart pressures and eventually to right heart failure. When heart failure is present, the patient needs to be evaluated to differentiate between ventricular systolic and ventricular diastolic origins of the disease process. This is done to both understand the origins of the heart failure and to guide clinical management. Treatment goals must be directed toward controlling both systolic and diastolic pressures in order to achieve optimum outcomes. End-stage cardiomyopathy patients benefit from hospice support (see Chapter 34). Chapter 11 includes a complete description of services provided by hospice.

Echocardiography

If the ECG is the most frequently performed diagnostic test, the echocardiogram (echo) is a close second. This is not surprising because the echo exam provides a rapid, safe, and relatively inexpensive detailed examination of the heart. **Echocardiography** refers to the noninvasive assessment of the structures and function of the heart and great vessels utilizing high-frequency (ultrasound) sound waves (Kee, 2010). These waves are emitted from a transducer placed in standard positions on the chest wall. As the waves encounter an interface between solid (muscle) and liquid (blood), a portion of the ultrasound waves are bounced back to the transducer. Interfaces perpendicular to the ultrasound beam reflect echoes much more effectively than those that are not perpendicular. Because the speed of sound traveling in the body is known, the time it takes for the echo to return to the transducer allows the health care provider to determine the depth of the structure. The fast rate of travel of the ultrasound waves allows for almost instantaneous or real-time recording of the cardiac structures in motion.

The three noninvasive types of echocardiography are M-mode, two-dimensional, and Doppler ultrasound. M-mode (motion) echocardiography was the earliest form of clinical ultrasound. Images are transmitted from a single narrow line of ultrasound and recorded as moving lines that do not resemble cardiac structures. These can be difficult to interpret. M-mode provides information about the distance of each object (valve leaflet, pericardium, etc.) from the transducer and can be used to assess valvular motion and chamber wall thickness and motion. Two-dimensional (2D) echocardiography came into use in the 1970s. It provides an anatomically recognizable image of the heart by sending out pulsed ultrasound waves in a fan or arc-shaped configuration. Doppler ultrasound relies on analysis of frequency shifts as the beam encounters moving targets. In the heart, sound waves are reflected off moving red blood cells. The Doppler effect shifts the sound frequency as the cells move toward or away from the transducer; these shifts are viewed as color changes. Together they provide the clinician with detailed information about the structure and function of the heart and great vessels (Chart 33–6) (Kee, 2010). Currently, a complete echocardiography exam incorporates all three modalities: M-mode, 2D, and Doppler.

This ability to measure blood flow through the heart and great vessels provides hemodynamic data to supplement the anatomic information obtained from M-mode and 2D echo. Hemodynamic data include the amount and speed of blood flow through the valves, enabling the noninvasive detection and follow-up of stenotic or regurgitant heart valves, and measurement of intracardiac pressures, which can be used to detect abnormal flow states such as shunts across the atrial or ventricular septum.

The echocardiogram can also assess the pumping action of the cardiac muscle. This measure is known as an ejection fraction (EF). A normal EF is around 55% to 65%. Numbers below 45% usually represent some decrease in the heart's pumping strength; numbers below 30% to 35% are representative of an important decrease.

In certain populations, the standard transthoracic examination (TTE) has limitations that require the use of further tests to establish the diagnosis or determine the therapeutic course of action. Because ultrasound waves cannot travel through air, echocardiography performed on patients who have chronic obstructive lung disease or who are on mechanical ventilators may result in suboptimal or even inadequate images. Likewise, ultrasound cannot image through bone or heavily calcified structures. In the adult, this limits the transducer placement to the intercostal and subxiphoid positions. Finally, excess adipose tissue can make visualization of the borders of the heart difficult.

CHART 33–6 Indications for Echocardiography

Assessment of the Heart and Great Vessels

1. Size of the cardiac chambers
2. Size of the cardiac walls
3. Structure and function of the valves
4. Location and quantification of cardiac shunts (i.e., patent foramen ovale or a ventricular septal defect)
5. Cardiac tumors
6. Estimates of left ventricular functioning

Establishment of Clinical Diagnoses

1. Aortic dissection
2. Location and quantification of pericardial effusions
3. Cardiac tamponade
4. Endocarditis
5. Murmurs
6. Stroke: identification of intracardiac sources of embolization

Timing of Therapeutic Interventions

1. When to repair/replace defective cardiac valves
2. Rule out intra-atrial thrombus before cardioversion for atrial fibrillation
3. Intraoperative TEE guidance
4. Ischemic heart disease

Transesophageal Echocardiography

Transesophageal echocardiography (TEE) can overcome some of the limitations of TTE (Kee, 2010). During TEE, the miniaturized transducer is advanced down the esophagus. Because the esophagus passes directly behind the posterior surface of the heart, it affords excellent views of the posterior structures of the heart and great vessels. Because TEE is minimally invasive and usually performed under procedural sedation, it is associated with a slight risk (<0.02%) of complications such as trauma to the structures of the mouth or throat or adverse reactions to the procedural sedation (Kee, 2010). TEE is frequently used to detect and assess endocarditis, aortic dissection, intracardiac masses such as thrombi or tumors, pericardial effusions, valvular pathology, and congenital disorders in both children and adults. TEE also is helpful in critically ill patients requiring ventilator support because the posterior images are not distorted by the constant motion of the lungs as the ventilator cycles. The role of TEE intraoperatively is expanding as evidence mounts that TEE guidance during procedures such as valvular repair improves clinical outcomes in cardiac surgery procedures.

Stress Echocardiography

Stress echocardiography refers to the use of echocardiography to detect coronary artery disease (Kee, 2010). Although exercise electrocardiography is the standard noninvasive method of detecting CAD, in some settings this test is of limited value because of incomplete data or difficulty in interpreting the test results. These instances include patients who have baseline ECG abnormalities or who are unable or unwilling to exercise to their peak heart rate. In these instances, stress echocardiography can be used to make the diagnosis because the test results are based on echo images and not on ECG changes. Stress echocardiography is also used to evaluate patients with known coronary or valvular heart disease, populations who often cannot exercise to their peak heart rate and/or have baseline ECG abnormalities (Kee, 2010).

Stress echocardiography can be performed by using standard forms of exercise (treadmill or bicycle), or a pharmacologic agent such as

RESEARCH OPPORTUNITIES Related to Cardiac Inflammatory Disorders

Research Area	Clinical Impact
Effect of immunosuppressive treatment on myocarditis.	Improvement in left ventricular ejection fraction and evidence of healed myocarditis.
Identify predictors of embolic risk among the clinical and laboratory data obtained on hospital admission in patients diagnosed as having definite infective endocarditis (IE).	To identify high-risk individuals for embolic events associated with IE.
Lyme carditis and the incidence of myocarditis and/or pericarditis.	Diagnostic and complication guidelines.
Identify link between teeth brushing and infective endocarditis.	Identification of safer methods of teeth cleaning for patients with IE.
Herbal and complementary medicine to treat heart disease.	Lowers cholesterol, saturated fats, low-density lipoproteins, triglycerides, and blood pressure.
Heart valves that are durable and nonthrombogenic, with a low incidence of endocarditis.	Decreases need for multiple valve replacement and decreases complications of valve replacement surgery.
Septal ablation for hypertrophic obstructive cardiomyopathy.	Decreases obstruction of blood flow from the left ventricle to the aorta.
Prevention of sudden cardiac death with hypertrophic cardiomyopathy.	Increases survival of patients with HCM.
Stem cell homing and tissue regeneration in ischemic cardiomyopathy.	Repair of damaged tissue from ischemia.
Alcohol consumption's impact on heart failure.	Determine amount that is cardioprotective.
Use of beta-andrenergic blockers in the treatment of heart failure.	Slow the progression of heart failure and reduce mortality, including sudden cardiac death.
Thiamin status, diuretic medications, and the management of heart failure.	
Relationship of heart failure severity, left ventricular loading conditions, and repolarization length in advanced heart failure secondary to ischemic or idiopathic dilated cardiomyopathy.	
Nonsustained ventricular tachycardia in hypertrophic cardiomyopathy: an independent marker of sudden death risk in young patients.	Determine predictors of sudden death risk to institute preventive therapy, such as implantation of an ICD.
Improvement in hypertrophic cardiomyopathy after significant weight loss.	Associated with striking improvement in cardiac functional indices, which could have profound implications for long-term cardiovascular risk.

dobutamine, to increase the heart rate. The normal response to exercise is an increase in heart rate and contractility. The development of a new myocardial wall motion abnormality (failure to contract normally in one or more segments of the heart) or failure of the heart to increase strength of contraction during the test is a positive indication of reversible ischemia.

Contrast agents have been explored as a method of improving visualization of the left ventricle during echocardiography (Kee, 2010). Agitated saline, created by forcefully mixing normal saline with air, is the simplest contrast agent and is commonly used to detect intracardiac shunts. The visualization of bubbles in the left side of the heart after intravenous injection is considered positive proof of a cardiac shunt (abnormal opening in the atrial or ventricular septum).

Finally, the development of three-dimensional echocardiography (3D) allows the clinician to view the structures and valves of the heart in a three-dimensional view noninvasively. This technology, combined with other advances in echocardiography, is bringing diagnostic cardiology closer to having an all-inclusive noninvasive assessment of the anatomy and physiology of the heart.

Research

Research is essential to improve the care, quality of life, and survival of patients with inflammatory and structural heart diseases. The goal of research is to identify areas in which practice could improve and evaluate and test methods in these areas. The research topics related to the inflammatory and structural heart diseases are listed in the Research Opportunities box . The list includes both medical and nursing research topics under investigation. Electronic databases are a source for finding specific studies related to these topics.

CLINICAL PREPARATION READ DOCUMENT APPLY

READ: **History of Present Illness** >> Laboratory Study Results >> Critical Thinking Questions

You are the nurse on the telemetry floor, and you have been notified that you will be receiving a new patient from the emergency department (ED). The ED nurse calls the following report: Matthew Hollis is a 26-year-old male brought in by ambulance who was found unconscious in the driveway of his home. He is initially seen by ED health care providers and the trauma team. Initial work-up included normal head CT, chest x-ray showing no pneumothorax, C-spine x-ray with no fractures, complete blood count (CBC), chemistry 7 panel, INR, UA; all were normal. ECG showed sinus tachycardia, low voltage, and nonspecific ST wave changes. Drug toxicology is still pending. A medicine consult was requested by the trauma service for persistent shortness of breath (SOB) and an abnormal ECG.

At present, Mr. Hollis is awake and alert. He feels weak and is short of breath. He denies assault. He denies a history of syncope and chest pain. He denies abdominal pain but has mild nausea. He denies fever, chills, and night sweats. He states that he has a poor appetite but thinks he has gained weight due to swelling in his legs. He denies smoking cigarettes and admits to using crack/cocaine. He states that he drinks socially.

Of note, when the family is interviewed, Mr. Hollis's mother states that he is in good health and lives a very clean life. He is single, is unemployed, and lives above her garage. She states that he has no chronic health problems but was told in his youth that he had a heart murmur. To her knowledge, Mr. Hollis does not use any illegal drugs but does occasionally drink alcohol. Mr. Hollis's sister reports a very different story; she states that the patient drinks at least six beers per day and frequently uses cocaine.

READ: History of Present Illnesses >> Physical Exam >> **Admitting Medical Records** >> Laboratory Study Results

Medical–Surgical History

- No known allergies
- Medications: none
- Illness: diagnosis of heart murmur some years previously reported by mother, no clinical problems
- Surgeries: none

Social History

- Family history: Mother and father healthy. The mother states that the patient does not use any illegal drugs but does drink occasional alcohol. The patient's sister reports that the patient drinks at least six beers per day and frequently uses cocaine.

Physical Exam

- Young male, overweight, mild discomfort due to SOB
- Oxygen sat 90% on RA
- BP 160/90 HR 115 RR 26
- HEENT: normal but poor dentition
- Neck: +JVD, no bruits
- Heart: NL S_1, S_2, soft systolic murmur heard at PMI, S_3 present
- Lungs: mild bibasilar rales
- Abdomen: obese, soft, nontender
- 1+ lower extremity edema
- Strong pulses throughout, good cap refill
- Normal neuro exam
- No rash
- Chest x-ray: cardiomegaly, mild interstitial edema
- ECG: in history of present illness

Admitting Medical Orders

- Admit to Cardiology–Telemetry Floor
- Condition guarded
- No known allergies
- Admitting diagnosis: syncope unknown etiology: R/0 dysrhythmia, ischemia, valvular disease; R/0 CHF and cardiomyopathy related to admitted use of cocaine and alcohol
- Final diagnosis: cardiomyopathy and heart failure due to cocaine and alcohol abuse
- Oxygen at 2–3 liters nasal cannula, keep oxygen saturation > 92%
- Bed rest with bathroom privileges
- Vital signs q2h with continuous ECG monitoring
- Sequential compression device (SCD) to lower extremities
- Incentive spirometry q hour while awake
- Daily weight
- Strict in/out
- IV: saline lock; flush with NS q8h
- Fluid restrict 1,500 mL/day
- Low Na diet
- Call house officer: Pulse < 60–110/minute; BP 90–160 systolic; temperature > 38.5; urine output < 30 mL/hr for 2 hours; respiratory rate > 30/minute; chest pain

Scheduled Medications

- Lasix 40 mg IV every 12 hours for 2 days, then once a day
- Nitropaste 1 inch q6h to chest wall topically
- KCl 20 mEq po now and 20 mEq in 3 hours
- Lisinopril 12.5 mg po daily
- Lovenox 30 mg SQ bid
- Magnesium sulfate 3 g IV dilute in 100 mL and give over 1 hour for a Mg level of less than 1.5 mEq/L × 1 now

PRN Medications

- Phenergan 25 mg IV q6h prn nausea
- Mylanta 30 mL q4–6h po prn dyspepsia
- Triazolam 0.125–0.25 mg po q noc, prn sleep
- Ativan 0.5–2 mg IV q6–8h prn anxiety (not to exceed 10 mg /24 hours)
- Milk of Magnesia 30 mL daily, po prn constipation
- Tylenol 650 mg po/pr q4h prn for pain

Ordered Laboratory Studies

- Troponin I q3h × 3 days
- Myoglobin q3h × 3 days
- CPK–MB q8h × 3 days
- Chemistry 20 and PO_4 on admission and Chemistry 7 q12h for first 2 days then daily
- CBC q a.m.
- Mg^{2+} q a.m.
- Serum and urine drug toxicity screen

Ordered Diagnostic Studies

- Chest x-ray on admission and with adverse changes in O_2 saturation, increased shortness of breath, and/or increasing rales
- Echocardiogram
- Cardiac catheterization
- 12-lead ECG daily

READ: History of Present Illness >> **Laboratory Study Results** >> Critical Thinking Questions

Test	Day 1	Day 2	Day 3
Sodium	132 mEq/L	137 mEq/L	140 mEq/L
Potassium	3.0 mEq/L	4.0 mEq/L	3.8 mEq/L
Chloride	90 mEq/L	92 mEq/L	95 mEq/L
Calcium	8.6 mg/dL		
Venous carbon dioxide	25 mEq/L	24 mEq/L	26 mEq/L
Blood urea nitrogen (BUN)	28 mg/dL	25 mg/dL	22 mg/dL
Creatinine	2.0 mg/dL	1.7 mg/dL	1.2 mg/dL
Blood glucose	150 mg/dL	138 mg/dL	112 mg/dL
Total proteins	5.2		
Magnesium	1.0 mEq/L	2.0 mEq/L	2.0 mEq/L
Phosphorus	3.2 mg/dL		
Troponin I	0.26/0.23/0.28 ng/mL		
Myoglobin	110 µg/L		
Albumin	3.5 g/dL		
GGT	48 units/L		
T. bilirubin	1.1 mg/dL		
CPK total	212 units/L		

Test	Day 1	Day 2	Day 3
CPK MB	1.8%		
LDH	166 units/L		
AST	38 units/L		
ALT	28 units/L		
WBC	14,000/mm^3	12,000/mm^3	11,000/mm^3
Hemoglobin	10.2 g/dL	12.2 g/dL	13.8 g/dL
Hematocrit	32%	37%	40%
RBC	5/mm^3		
Platelets	395/mm^3	325/mm^3	250/mm^3
ABGs			
PO_2	70 mmHg	78 mmHg	80 mmHg
O_2 saturation	90%	91%	93%
Ph	7.30	7.34	7.38
PCO_2	50 mmHg	48 mmHg	43 mmHg
HCO_3	24 mEq/L	26 mEq/L	24 mEq/L

Cocaine metabolite screen, urine: positive

Cocaine metabolite screen, blood: positive

Blood alcohol level: negative

Pearson Nursing Student Resources

Log on to **nursing.pearsonhighered.com** *to download forms*

DOCUMENT:

>> Summary of Hospitalization

>> Pathophysiology Form

>> Laboratory Values

>> Laboratory Results Explanation

APPLY:

>> List of Potential Nursing Diagnoses

>> Concept Map

>> Critical Thinking Questions and Concept Map

APPLY: History of Present Illness >> Laboratory Study Results >> **Critical Thinking Questions**

1. What is the purpose of the echocardiography for this patient?
2. Why did the doctor order cardiac marker laboratory tests?
3. Why was a cardiac catheterization done?
4. What is the importance of assessing the potassium level frequently?
5. The teaching plan for this patient needs to include specific information about lifestyle changes that will not cause worsening of the heart disease. What information does this patient need to know and what referrals would be appropriate?
6. What is the goal of medical therapy for this patient? This answer drives much of the patient teaching and helps the nurse anticipate complications and potential problems with the patient as well as additional orders.

Answers to Critical Thinking Questions can be found in Appendix D in the Osborn Student Resources at nursing.pearsonhighered.com.

NCLEX® PRACTICE

1. A patient's history indicates a past history of rheumatic fever. The nurse plans to assess the patient for signs of which disorder?
   1. Pericarditis
   2. Endocarditis
   3. Mitral stenosis
   4. Pulmonary fibrosis
2. The mother of a 6-year-old who has a history of rheumatic fever brings the child and a 3-year-old sibling to the clinic because of fever and sore throat. Which statement, made by the nurse, is appropriate in the care of this child?
   1. "Since your child has had rheumatic fever, we must treat strep throat aggressively."
   2. "Because your child has already experienced rheumatic fever, no antibiotics are necessary."
   3. "At least your 3-year-old is not at risk for developing rheumatic fever."
   4. "All of the damage to your child's heart valves has probably already occurred."
3. The nurse is developing a teaching plan for a patient diagnosed with mitral valve prolapse. Which information should be included in this plan?
   1. Avoid having any dental work until the valve is replaced.
   2. Plan for rest periods throughout the day.
   3. Take your oral temperature every morning.
   4. Keep a diary of all the high-fat foods you eat.
4. A patient is scheduled for open surgical valvuloplasty of the mitral valve with thrombus removal. When preparing the patient for surgery, the nurse should include which information?
   1. Cardiopulmonary bypass will not be required for this procedure.
   2. Anticoagulation therapy will not be necessary in the postoperative period.
   3. The valve will be repaired, but not replaced.
   4. This procedure will prevent the need for future valve surgeries.
5. A patient is diagnosed with restrictive cardiomyopathy secondary to cocaine abuse. The nurse plans nursing care, recognizing treatment for this type of cardiomyopathy usually involves which procedure?
   1. Alcohol septal ablation
   2. Insertion of an implantable automatic defibrillator (ICD)
   3. Aortic valve repair
   4. Supportive therapy with medications
6. The nurse suspects a patient having frequent episodes of chest pain has pericarditis. To help confirm the suspicion, the nurse should ask which question?
   1. "Is the pain relieved by lying flat?"
   2. "Do you only experience the pain during the night?"
   3. "Does the pain become worse if you take a deep breath?"
   4. "Is the pain preceded by an episode of heart palpitations?"

Answers to NCLEX Practice questions can be found in Appendix D in the Osborn Student Resources at nursing.pearsonhighered.com. Practice additional NCLEX questions online at the Student Resources site.

Pearson Nursing Student Resources Find additional review materials at: **nursing.pearsonhighered.com**

REFERENCES

Adams, M. P., & Koch, R. W. (2010). *Pharmacology: Connections to nursing practice.* Upper Saddle River, NJ: Pearson.

American Heart Association. (2010). Sudden cardiac death. Retrieved from http://www.americanheart.org/presenter.jhtml?identifier=4741

American Heart Association. (2011). Infective endocarditis. Retrieved from http://www.heart.org/HEARTORG/Conditions/CongenitalHeartDefects/TheImpactofCongenitalHeartDefects/Infective-Endocarditis_UCM_307108_Article.jsp

Basso, C., Corrado, D., Marcus, F. I., Nava, A., & Theine, G. (2009). Arrhythmogenic right ventricular cardiomyopathy. *Lancet, 373*(9671), 1289–1300.

Cardiomyopathy Association. (2010). Retrieved from http://www.cardiomyopathy.org/

Connolly, S. J., Ezekowitz, M. D., Yusef, Y., Eikelboom, J., Oldgren, J., Parekh, A., et al. (2009). Dabigatraban versus warfarin in atrial fibrillation. *New England Journal of Medicine, 36*(12), 1139–1151.

Gerber, M. A., Baltimore, R. S., Eaton, C. B., Gewitz, M., Rowley, A. H., Shulman, S. T., et al. (2009). Prevention of rheumatic fever and diagnosis and treatment of acute streptococcal pharyngitis. *Circulation, 119*, 1541–1551.

Gowda, A. (2010). Pericarditis, uremic. eMedicine Web MD. Retrieved from http://www.emedicine.com/med/byname/pericarditis-uremic.htm

Habib, G., et al. (2009). Guidelines on the prevention, diagnosis, and treatment of infective endocarditis. *European Heart Journal, 30*(19), 2369–2413.

Healthy People 2020. Retrieved from http://www.healthypeople.gov/2020/default.aspx

Howes, D. S. (2008). Myocarditis. eMedicine. Retrieved from http://www.emedicine.com/emerg/TOPIC326.HTM

IOM (Institute of Medicine). (2010). *The future of nursing: Leading change, advancing health.* Washington, DC: The Academic Press.

Kee, J. L. (2010). *Laboratory and diagnostic tests with nursing implications.* Upper Saddle River, NJ: Pearson.

Mayo Clinic. (2010a). Dressler's syndrome. Retrieved from http://www.mayoclinic.com/health/dresslers-syndrome/DS00666

Mayo Clinic. (2010b). Rheumatic fever. Retrieved from http://www.mayoclinic.com/health/rheumatic-fever/DS00250/DSECTION=symptoms

Mogensen, J., & Arbustini, E. (2009). Restrictive cardiomyopathy. *Current Opinion in Cardiology, 24*(3), 214–220.

Moser, D. K., & Riegel, B. (2008). *Cardiac nursing: A companion to Braunwald's heart disease.* St. Louis: Saunders Elsevier.

Nishimura, R. A., Carabello, B. A., Faxon, D. P., Freed, M. D., Lytle, B. W., O'Gara, P. T., et al. (2008). ACC/AHA 2008 guideline update on valvular heart disease: Focused update on infective endocarditis: A report of the American College of Cardiology/American Heart Association Task Force on Practice Guidelines. *Journal of the American College of Cardiology, 52*, 676–685.

O'Rourke, R., Walsh, R., & Fuster, V. (2009). *Hurst's the heart manual of cardiology* (12th ed.). New York: McGraw-Hill.

Porth, C. M., & Matfin, G. (2009). *Pathophysiology: Concepts of altered health states* (8th ed.). Philadelphia: Lippincott Williams & Wilkins.

Schwefer, M., Aschenbach, R., Heidemann, J., Mey, C., & Lapp, H. (2009). Constrictive pericarditis, still a diagnostic challenge: Comprehensive review of clinical management. *European Journal of Cardio-thoracic Surgery, 36*(3), 502–510.

Verma, S., & Mesana, T. (2009). Mitral valve repair for mitral valve prolapse. *New England Journal of Medicine, 361*, 2261–2269.

Woods, S. L., Froelicher, E. S. S., Adams (Underhill), S., & Bridges, E. J. (Eds.). (2009). *Cardiac nursing* (6th ed.). Philadelphia: Lippincott Williams & Wilkins.

Wilkinson, J. M., & Ahearn, N. R. (2009). *Prentice Hall nursing diagnosis handbook* (9th ed.). Upper Saddle River, NJ: Prentice Hall.

Caring for the Patient with Heart Failure

34 CHAPTER

Brenda McCulloch
Kathleen Osborn

Outcome-Based Learning Objectives

After studying this chapter, the learner will be able to:

1. Evaluate the etiology, incidence, and prevalence of heart failure.
2. Distinguish between systolic and diastolic dysfunction.
3. Describe the pathophysiology of heart failure and the compensatory neurohormonal responses that occur.
4. Compare and contrast right-sided and left-sided symptoms of heart failure.
5. Evaluate the diagnostic work-up that is used to determine the presence of heart failure.
6. Describe a comprehensive treatment plan, including the medical, device, and surgical components of treatment, using the multidisciplinary team approach.
7. Describe the self-management concepts applicable to patients with heart failure.
8. Compare and contrast potential comorbidities associated with heart failure.
9. Describe components of end-of-life care for end-stage heart failure.

KEY TERMS

ascites p.1032
biventricular heart failure p.1028
cardiomegaly p.1030
crackles p.1032
diastolic dysfunction p.1028
euvolemia p.1036
heart failure p.1025
hepatojugular reflux p.1032
hypertrophy p.1029
left-sided heart failure p.1027
left ventricular ejection fraction (LVEF) p.1027
New York Heart Association (NYHA) classification system p.1030
pitting p.1032
right-sided heart failure p.1027
S_3 (abnormal third heart sound in the cardiac cycle) p.1032
S_4 (abnormal fourth heart sound in the cardiac cycle) p.1032
systolic dysfunction p.1026
tachypnea p.1032

HEART FAILURE is best defined as a complex and debilitating clinical syndrome caused by cardiac dysfunction, resulting in left ventricular dilation, hypertrophy, or both. If left untreated, the disease will progress, resulting in worsening symptoms, more frequent hospitalizations, and possibly death. Heart failure is a common, chronic condition that has a significant impact, not only on patients living with the disease but also on care delivery systems. Leaders in heart failure care, such as the Heart Failure Society of America and the American Heart Association with the American College of Cardiology, have updated guidelines to help providers with delivering appropriate, evidence-based care. These guidelines will be presented later in the chapter, after a complete discussion of heart failure.

Heart Failure

Current understanding of heart failure has matured from viewing it as a hemodynamic condition to recognizing it as a state in which complex neurohormonal changes result in an impairment of cardiac filling and/or ejection of blood. Treatments for heart failure have expanded significantly and are often able to improve symptoms and reduce morbidity, mortality, and hospitalizations. Heart failure is treated with therapies of increasing complexity: medications, cardiac devices, and surgical/interventional approaches. Special attention to controlling comorbid conditions and volume status is paramount. Medical therapy is aimed at reducing the detrimental neurohormonal response, discussed in the following text. Cardiac devices (p. 1039) play an expanding role in preventing sudden cardiac death, resynchronizing dyssynchronous ventricles, and even aiding in the assessment of fluid status. End-stage therapies may offer the opportunity to extend life with modalities such as cardiac transplantation or mechanical assist devices for eligible patients. Palliative care and hospice will be essential for patients whose prognosis is poor.

Multidisciplinary teams that use established disease management strategies to provide care improve outcomes. Nurses have been pivotal in patient care by providing self-management instruction, telephone management, and more (Steckler et al., 2010). The future of heart failure treatments will involve understanding genetic implications and integrating clinical research into practice. Genetic implications are discussed in the Genetic Considerations box (p. 1053).

Epidemiology

Heart failure is a major public health problem affecting nearly 6 million Americans (American Heart Association [AHA], 2010b). With over 550,000 new cases diagnosed each year in the United States, heart failure is reaching epidemic proportions. Contributing to the rising incidence of heart failure are the aging U.S. population and increased survival rates among patients with hypertension and coronary artery disease (CAD). Older adults are more likely to suffer from impaired heart function, and individuals who would have succumbed to an acute cardiac event in the past are now more likely to survive, albeit with impaired cardiac function (AHA, 2010b). Furthermore, the increase in conditions such as diabetes, obesity, and metabolic syndrome have significantly increased the risk of developing heart failure (Hunt et al., 2009).

Mortality

Despite advances in heart failure treatments, the mortality rate from heart failure remains high. Nearly 290,000 people die annually of heart failure in the United States. In addition, people with heart failure are six to nine times more likely than the general population to suffer from sudden death. The majority of patients diagnosed with heart failure die within 8 years (AHA, 2010b).

Etiology

The leading etiologies of heart failure are hypertension, CAD, and dilated cardiomyopathies. Other factors that contribute to developing heart failure include well-established risk factors for cardiovascular disease and exposure to substances that are toxic to the cardiac muscle. Risk factors that may lead to heart failure are summarized in the Risk Factors box.

RISK FACTORS for Heart Failure

Modifiable Risk Factors	Nonmodifiable Risk Factors
Atherosclerosis	Age
Cardiotoxic drug use (alcohol, illicit drugs, anthracyclines)	Positive family history of CAD
Diabetes	Gender
Hyperlipidemia	Genetics
Hypertension	
Metabolic syndrome	
Obesity	
Sedentary lifestyle	
Smoker	
Valvular abnormalities	

Sources: Adapted from Lindenfeld, J., Albert, N. M., Boehmer, J. P., Collins, S. P., Ezekowitz, J. A., Givertz, M. M., et al. (2010). Executive summary: HFSA 2010 comprehensive heart failure practice guideline. *Journal of Cardiac Failure, 16* (6), 475–539; Schocken, D. D., Benjamin, E. J., Fonarow, G. C., Krumholz, H. M., Levy, D., Mensah, G. A., et al. (2008). Prevention of heart failure. *Circulation, 117*, 2544–2565.

Pathophysiology

The dysfunction in heart failure can be systolic, diastolic, or mixed, and it leads to neurohormonal and circulatory abnormalities. Symptoms can vary but generally include fluid retention, shortness of breath, and fatigue, especially with exertion.

Two very different pathologic processes, commonly referred to as systolic and diastolic dysfunction, may lead to heart failure as a result of a wide range of left ventricular functional abnormalities. Systolic dysfunction and diastolic dysfunction usually result in the same set of symptoms and may occur simultaneously. Chart 34–1 outlines the etiologies of systolic and diastolic dysfunction leading to heart failure.

Systolic Dysfunction

Systolic dysfunction, also referred to as left ventricular systolic dysfunction (LVSD), is characterized by impaired ventricular function, which results in volume overload and decreased contractility. In the

CHART 34–1 Etiologies of Heart Failure

Heart failure is a syndrome of symptoms that occurs from two pathologic processes: systolic dysfunction (when the heart is unable to contract normally) and diastolic dysfunction (when the heart is unable to relax normally). The etiologies leading to either process are noted here.

Systolic Dysfunction	Diastolic Dysfunction
Hypertension	Hypertrophic or restrictive cardiomyopathy
Coronary artery disease (CAD)	Coronary artery disease (CAD)
Myocardial infarction	Systemic hypertension with hypertrophy
Ischemia (hibernating myocardium, stunned myocardium)	Infiltrative cardiomyopathy such as sarcoidosis
Diabetes	Hypertrophic or restrictive cardiomyopathy
Peripartum cardiomyopathy	Alcoholic cardiomyopathy
Drug-induced cardiomyopathy	Valvular cardiomyopathy
	Idiopathic cardiomyopathy

Sources: Adapted from Hunt, S. A., Abraham, W. T., Chin, M. H., Feldman, A. M., Francis, G. S., Ganiats, T. G., et al. (2009). Focused update incorporated into the ACC/AHA 2005 guidelines for the diagnosis and management of heart failure in adults: A report of the American College of Cardiology Foundation/American Heart Association Task Force on Practice Guidelines. *Circulation, 119*, e391–e479; Lindenfeld, J., Albert, N. M., Boehmer, J. P., Collins, S. P., Ezekowitz, J. A., Givertz, M. M., et al. (2010). Executive summary: HFSA 2010 comprehensive heart failure practice guideline. *Journal of Cardiac Failure, 16* (6), 475–539.

COMPLEMENTARY & ALTERNATIVE THERAPIES Coenzyme Q10 Supplementation *Nancy Yilk*

COENZYME Q10 (CoQ10 in humans) has been known for a number of years for its key role in mitochondrial bioenergetics; studies have demonstrated its presence in other subcellular fractions and in plasma. It has also been extensively investigated for its antioxidant role. These two functions constitute the basis on which research supporting the clinical use of CoQ10 is founded (Littarru & Tiano, 2007). Cardiovascular disease is still the main field of study, and the latest findings confirm that CoQ10 has a role in improving endothelial function. Furthermore, in cardiac patients, the plasma CoQ10 level was found to be an independent predictor of mortality (Littarru & Tiano, 2010).

In a New Zealand cohort study, 236 patients, with an average age of 77 years, who had been admitted to the hospital with heart failure were followed for a median of 2.69 years to investigate the relationship between plasma coenzyme Q10 and survival in patients with chronic heart failure. Patients with heart failure have low plasma concentrations of CoQ10, an essential cofactor for mitochondrial electron transport and myocardial energy supply. It was demonstrated that plasma levels of CoQ10 are an independent predictor of patient survival. This remains consistent with previous studies, which have shown myocardial CoQ10 depletion in heart failure, correlated with the severity of the underlying disorder. Several interventional studies have been undertaken with CoQ10 in heart failure, including randomized controlled trials with mostly positive outcomes in relation to improvement in plasma levels of CoQ10. A meta-analysis showed that CoQ10 resulted in an improvement in ejection fraction of 3.7% and a mean increase in cardiac output. In a subgroup analysis, studies with patients not taking ACE inhibitors found a 6.7% increase in ejection fraction (Molyneux, Florkowski, Richards, Lever, Young, & George, 2009).

Antioxidant supplementations have the potential to alleviate the atherosclerotic damage caused by excessive production of reactive oxygen species. To evaluate the effects of prolonged antioxidant treatment on arterial elasticity, as well as inflammatory and metabolic measures in patients with multiple cardiovascular risk factors, study participants were randomly assigned to two groups. Group 1 received oral supplementation with two capsules per day of 60 mg coenzyme Q10, vitamin C (500 mg), vitamin E (200 iu), and selenium (100 mcg). Group 2 received a matching placebo for 6 months. Patients were evaluated for lipid profile, HbA1C, insulin, C-peptide, hs-CRP, endothelin, aldosterone, plasma renin activity, and homeostasis model assessment insulin resistance. Arterial elasticity was evaluated by using pulse wave contour analysis. Results demonstrated that the antioxidant-treated group exhibited significant increases in large arterial elasticity index as well as small arterial elasticity index. A significant decline was found in HbA1C, along with a significant increase in HDL-cholesterol in this group. Metabolic measures were not observed in the placebo group. Antioxidant supplementation significantly increased large and small artery elasticity in patients with multiple cardiovascular risk factors (Shargorodsky, Debby, Matas, & Zimlichman, 2010).

Commercial CoQ10 formulations often show poor intestinal absorption. National Institutes of Health-funded clinical trials have shown the relative bioavailability of CoQ10 to be increased by its delivery system (Liu & Artmann, 2009). The high molecular weight of CoQ10 makes it poorly water soluble and consequently leads to low systemic availability. Several advances have been made to enhance the bioavailability of CoQ10 using various approaches such as size reduction, solubility enhancement, and use of novel drug carriers such as liposomes, microspheres, nanoparticles, nanoemulsions, and self-emulsifying systems. These methods should be assessed to determine the utility of complementary supplementation of CoQ10 as an adjutant therapy (Beg, Javed, & Kohli, 2010).

Sources: Adapted from Beg, S., Javed, S., & Kohli, K. (2010). Bioavailability enhancement of coenzyme Q10: An extensive review of patents. *Recent Patents on Drug Delivery and Formulations, 4*(3), 245–255; Littarru, G. P., & Tiano, L. (2007). Bioenergetic and antioxidant properties of coenzyme Q10: Recent developments. *Molecular Biotechnology, 37*(1), 31–37; Littarru, G. P., & Tiano, L. (2010). Clinical aspects of coenzyme Q10: An update. *Nutrition, 26*(3), 250–254; Liu, Z. X., & Artmann, C. (2009). Relative bioavailability comparison of different coenzyme Q10 formulations with a novel delivery system. *Alternative Therapies in Health and Medicine, 15*(2), 42–46; Molyneux, S. L., Florkowski, C. M., Richards, A. M., Lever, M., Young, J. M., & George, P. M. (2009). Coenzyme Q10: An adjunctive therapy for congestive heart failure? *New Zealand Medical Journal, 122*(1305), 74–79; Shargorodsky, M., Debby, O., Matas, Z., & Zimlichman, R. (2010). Effect of long-term treatment with antioxidants (vitamin C, vitamin E, coenzyme Q10 and selenium) on arterial compliance, humoral factors and inflammatory markers in patients with multiple cardiovascular risk factors. *Nutrition & Metabolism (London), 7*, 55. Published online 2010 July 6. doi: 10.1186/1743-7075-7-55

United States, the most common cause of LVSD is coronary artery disease (CAD), followed by hypertension (McMurray, 2010). In an era of improved therapies to treat CAD and acute myocardial infarction, people now survive such events, but many are left with a dysfunctional ventricle. This may lead to the syndrome of heart failure. Other causes of systolic dysfunction include idiopathic, valvular, and hypertrophic causes, as well as cardiotoxic substance use, such as chronic alcohol abuse. LVSD is diagnosed when the **left ventricular ejection fraction (LVEF),** or the proportion of blood ejected during each ventricular contraction compared with the total ventricular filling volume, is below 40%. The normal LVEF is 55% to 70% (Porth & Matfin, 2009).

Once LVSD occurs, progressive adverse structural and neurohormonal changes occur within the heart, leading to deteriorating cardiac function and symptoms of low cardiac output and congestion. Neurohormones such as norepinephrine, endothelin, and cytokines are released, leading to an adverse condition called cardiac remodeling. This detrimental effect on the myocardium results from volume overload or cardiac injury, which causes myocytes to revert to a fetal-type expression and ultimately changes the myocyte geometry from elliptical to spherical. These changes result in molecular, cellular, and interstitial changes of the cardiac muscle that are manifested clinically as changes in size, shape, and function of the heart, which leads to a reduction in ventricular function. Regardless of the etiology, once systolic dysfunction occurs, the heart is unable to pump enough blood to sustain the body's metabolic demands. Right, left, and/or biventricular (affecting both ventricles) heart failure can occur, depending on the extent and anatomy of the damage (Figure 34–1◆, p. 1028). Tissue remodeling is described in detail in Chapter 32. See the Complementary & Alternative Therapies box for a type of nontraditional therapy that affects the ejection fraction.

Left-sided heart failure, as the name suggests, is an abnormal cardiac condition characterized by impairment of the pumping ability of the left side of the heart, which eventually backs the blood up into the pulmonary circulation. Elevated pressure and congestion in the pulmonary veins and capillaries result as the disease progresses. Symptoms that eventually follow impaired left ventricular function include fatigue, activity intolerance, shortness of breath, and cough. Often, *orthopnea* (an abnormal condition in which a person must sit or stand to breathe deeply or comfortably) and paroxysmal nocturnal dyspnea (a disorder characterized by sudden attacks of respiratory distress that awakens the person, usually after several hours of sleep in a reclining position) will occur (Moser & Reigel, 2008).

Right-sided heart failure is an abnormal cardiac condition characterized by impairment of the pumping ability on the right side of the heart, leading to a backup of blood, followed by congestion and elevated pressure in the systemic veins and capillaries. The most common cause of right-sided dysfunction is left-sided dysfunction (Moser & Reigel, 2008). Right-sided heart failure may also be caused by a pathologic process in the lungs whereby blood cannot flow into the pulmonary vasculature or result from an isolated right ventricular myocardial infarction.

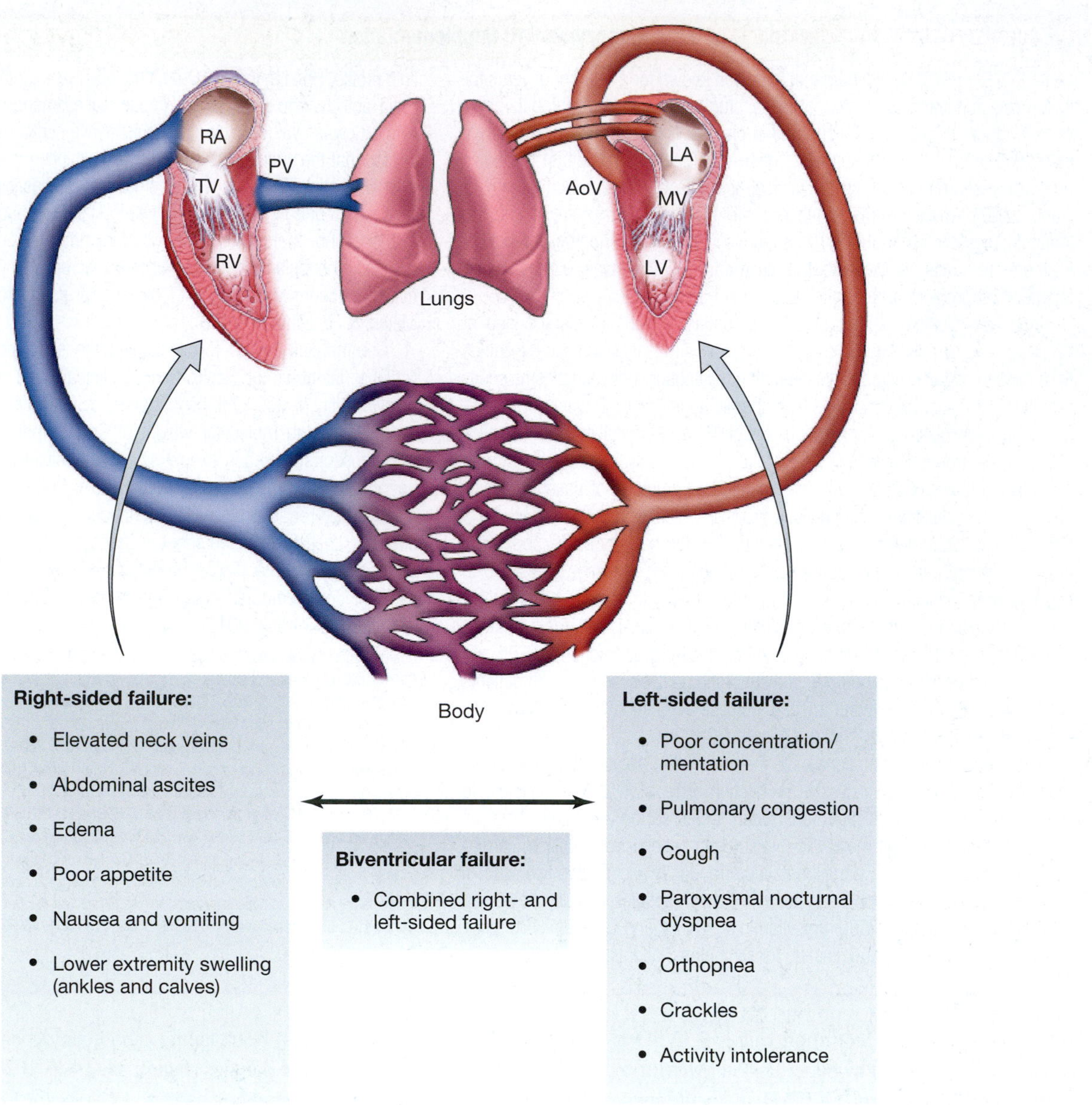

FIGURE 34–1 ◆ Right, left, and biventricular failure.

Symptoms of right heart failure result from volume overload leading to ascites and edema. Patients may complain of abdominal bloating and discomfort, often with a poor appetite and sometimes nausea and vomiting. Lower extremity edema is common, but the absence of edema does not exclude volume overload in patients with heart failure.

Biventricular heart failure refers to a global inability of both ventricles of the heart to pump blood effectively. Forward blood flow is compromised, leading to right and left heart failure symptoms. Symptoms are typically a combination of those from both right and left heart failure. Generalized malaise, activity intolerance, and even poor concentration are common as the disease progresses.

Diastolic Dysfunction

Diastolic dysfunction, also known as heart failure with preserved LVEF, is diagnosed when ventricular relaxation is slowed. In this condition, elevated filling pressures are found in the setting of normal ventricular volume and contraction (Hunt et al., 2009). Diastolic dysfunction is usually diagnosed when the clinical symptoms of heart failure are present with a normal LVEF. Patients with diastolic dysfunction are primarily older women, frequently with hypertension, diabetes, obesity, and atrial fibrillation (Lindenfeld et al., 2010). Diastolic dysfunction seems to be related to a stiff, noncompliant heart with prolonged relaxation. The result is decreased filling, increased left ventricular end diastolic pressure, and reduced stroke volume at rest or during exercise. Some causes of diastolic dysfunction include restrictive, obstructive, nonobstructive, hypertrophic, and infiltrative cardiomyopathies (see Chart 34–1, p. 1026). Cardiomyopathies are described in detail in Chapter 33. Principles of treatment focus on controlling hypertension, ischemia, and the ventricular rate when atrial fibrillation is present and on minimizing congestion (Lindenfeld et al., 2010). Given the robust data on systolic dysfunction and the lack of a standardized approach to treating diastolic dysfunction, this chapter focuses primarily on systolic dysfunction.

Neurohormonal Response

A series of compensatory mechanisms are triggered when the heart's pumping action is compromised. Regardless of the etiology of LVSD, the initial response to decreased cardiac output (the volume of blood expelled by the heart's ventricles equal to the amount of blood ejected at each beat multiplied by the heart rate per minute) is activation of the sympathetic nervous system (SNS) and the renin-angiotensin-aldosterone system (RAAS). Substances that are released with eventual detrimental cardiac effects include norepinephrine, angiotensin II, aldosterone, endothelin, vasopressin, and cytokines. Circulating levels play an important role in vasoconstriction, sodium retention, and toxic effects on the architecture of the heart described earlier (Hunt et al., 2009). In the early stages of heart failure, SNS and RAAS activation augments preload (the volume of blood being returned to the heart, causing the stretch of myocardial fibers at end diastole), ventricular contractility, and heart rate, thereby maintaining cardiac output, especially during exercise. But as cardiac function progressively worsens, these compensatory mechanisms can no longer maintain cardiac output, and ventricular function is further compromised. Unless this cycle is halted, it will result in ventricular remodeling, a process in which detrimental effects occur on the cardiac myocyte level.

Sympathetic Nervous System Activation

Increased SNS activity leads to elevated levels of norepinephrine. Norepinephrine causes vasoconstriction in the pulmonary and systemic vasculature and enhances venous tone, causing vasoconstriction. This initially maintains blood pressure and increases ventricular preload. Norepinephrine also causes renal vasoconstriction that allows for the glomerular filtration rate to remain stable despite decreased perfusion of renal blood flow. Circulating norepinephrine also increases sodium absorption, leading to fluid retention that initially increases intravascular volume with subsequent temporary improvements in cardiac output and blood pressure. In addition, myocardial contractility and heart rate are stimulated and therefore increase cardiac output. These neurohormonal effects provide short-term, necessary support to maintain cardiac output. In the long term, however, these effects are deleterious, causing increased cardiac wall stress, **hypertrophy** (an increase in the size of an organ caused by an increase in the size of the cells rather than an increase in the number of cells), chamber dilation, increased myocardial oxygen consumption, worsening myocardial ischemia (a decreased supply of oxygenated blood to a body organ or part), and pulmonary and systemic congestion (Lee & Tkacs, 2008).

Renin-Angiotensin-Aldosterone System Activation

Decreased renal perfusion triggers activation of the renin-angiotensin-aldosterone system (RAAS). Renin is released from the kidneys, causing a conversion of inactive angiotensin I into active angiotensin II. Angiotensin II is a potent vasoconstrictor that enhances venous tone and increases afterload (the load or resistance against which the left ventricle must eject its volume of blood during contraction). Angiotensin II also stimulates the secretion of aldosterone, causing sodium and fluid retention. In the short term, preload, cardiac output, and blood pressure are increased. However, long-term effects include increased cardiac workload, pulmonary and systemic congestion, and chamber dilation. Abnormal cell growth manifested by myocardial hypertrophy and adverse remodeling is also triggered by angiotensin II (Lee & Tkacs, 2008).

Course of Heart Failure

Heart failure progresses according to a predictable course (Figure 34–2◆). Formal diagnosis usually occurs when symptoms develop and functional status is compromised. Treatment of patients with heart failure, regardless of their course, involves providing supportive care for presenting symptoms and addressing needs for patients with chronic disease. Once standard heart failure therapies, including medications and/or devices, have been initiated, the patient's functional status usually improves for a period of time. As the disease progresses, after a period of stability of unknown duration, many patients experience episodes of exacerbation followed by periods of stabilization. Often, patients are unable to regain their prior level of functional ability. Exacerbations become increasingly frequent, and stabilization becomes more difficult. The disease progression eventually leads to death unless the patient is a candidate for end-stage therapies.

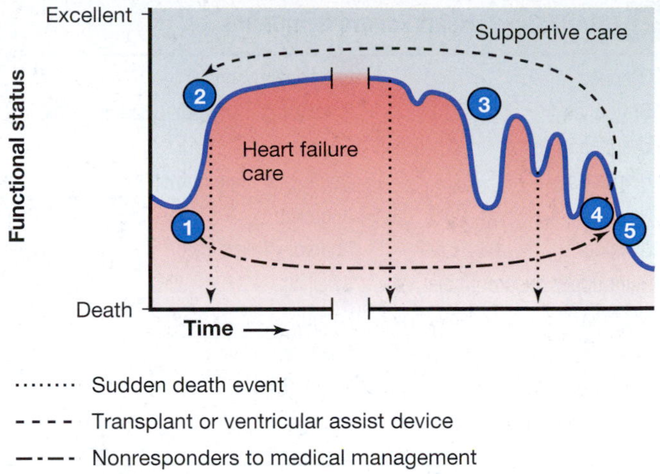

FIGURE 34–2 ◆ Course of heart failure.

Understanding the course of heart failure can help to guide not only therapeutic decisions, but also discussions with patients and families about a comprehensive approach to care. Even patients who respond to medical or device therapies with improvement of cardiac function may eventually decompensate, and only a select few may be eligible for advanced therapies such as cardiac transplantation or mechanical circulatory support. End-of-life care is essential for patients with a poor prognosis, who in general are not candidates for advanced therapies. Therefore, both patients and health care providers can better anticipate treatment options and the trajectory of the disease when they understand the course of heart failure. End-of-life management is discussed in Chapter 11. End-of-life planning for patients with heart failure is discussed later in this chapter.

Chronic Heart Failure

The onset of heart failure can be either insidious or acute. Patients with chronic heart failure tend to have a mixture of good and bad days, with ongoing dyspnea, fatigue, and activity intolerance. Patients typically complain of weight gain (despite a decreased appetite), nausea, vomiting, and slow changes in their ability to perform activities of daily living (ADLs). Patients may also complain of irritability, restlessness, or profound fatigue, causing them to have low energy levels. Increased urinary frequency and nighttime urination also are common. These symptoms will wax and wane in the majority of patients. Heart failure is a chronic condition and, with suboptimal or lack of treatment, will lead to progressive cardiac dysfunction, increasing symptoms, and eventually death (Chart 34–2).

Stages of Heart Failure

The American College of Cardiology (ACC) and the AHA (Figure 34–3◆) (Hunt et al., 2009) has designated four stages of heart failure. This system has better defined the evolution and progression of heart failure, thus helping to direct treatment strategies to assist in

CHART 34–2 Heart Failure Symptoms

Dyspnea	Exertional dyspnea
Orthopnea	Paroxysmal nocturnal dyspnea (PND)
Dyspnea at rest	Cough
Hemoptysis	Decreased urine output
Nausea	Anorexia
Bloating	Abdominal distention
Right upper quadrant pain	Swelling
Nocturia	Fatigue
Restlessness	Agitation
Weight gain or loss	Poor energy
Poor exercise tolerance	

halting disease progression. Criteria were set for Stages A through D to (1) identify risk factors for developing heart failure, (2) detect the presence or absence of structural disease, and (3) treat on the basis of well-proven strategies throughout the stages. The stages are described next.

Stage A

People who are in Stage A are at risk for developing the disease but have no structural abnormalities and no symptoms (Hunt et al., 2009). Risk factors for developing heart failure are similar to those for CAD: advancing age, diabetes, hypertension, hyperlipidemia, sedentary lifestyle, obesity, smoking, and excessive alcohol use (Hunt et al., 2009). Risk factors for the development of CAD are described in detail in Chapter 32. Interventions for individuals who are in Stage A aim at reducing the risk of developing CAD and may very well prevent heart failure.

Stage B

The people who are at Stage B are asymptomatic individuals who have structural heart disease. This is a difficult group to identify because symptoms are usually what will lead to the diagnosis of heart failure. Screening for heart failure indiscriminately is generally not recommended (Hunt et al., 2009), but screening could be undertaken selectively if risk factors were present. Individuals with a prior myocardial infarction or significant CAD or valvular disease are at particular risk in this stage. Evidence of structural disease can be detected on certain diagnostic tests including a 12-lead ECG (showing left ventricular hypertrophy); a chest x-ray showing **cardiomegaly** (enlargement of the heart); or an echocardiogram, chest CT, or MRI (showing ventricular hypertrophy or valvular dysfunction).

Evaluating the level of *B-type natriuretic peptide* (BNP) could be considered if there were clinical suspicions of heart failure; however, an abnormally elevated value alone is not sufficient to diagnose heart failure. B-type natriuretic peptide is a 32-amino-acid polypeptide secreted by the heart's ventricles in response to excessive stretching of myocytes in the ventricles. Levels of BNP are elevated in patients with left ventricular dysfunction, and levels correlate with both the severity of symptoms and the prognosis in congestive heart failure. The BNP level may also be elevated with acute myocardial infarction, acute pulmonary embolus, and renal failure; age alone may also cause elevation of the BNP level in some individuals. Valuation of BNP is most useful in its ability to exclude heart failure as a diagnosis if the value is normal. Elevations in BNP values have correlated with significant heart failure symptoms and increased risk of mortality. Reducing BNP has been shown to improve clinical status, yet the role of serial BNP measurements to guide therapy remains unclear (Hunt et al., 2009).

Treatments for Stage B patients include angiotensin-converting enzyme (ACE) inhibitors, angiotensin receptor blockers (ARB), and beta-blockers (as well as aspirin and a statin if CAD is present). Such treatments prevent further damage of the myocardium and delay progression to symptomatic disease. Treatments at Stage B should be coupled with the recommended preventive measures of Stage A (Hunt et al., 2009).

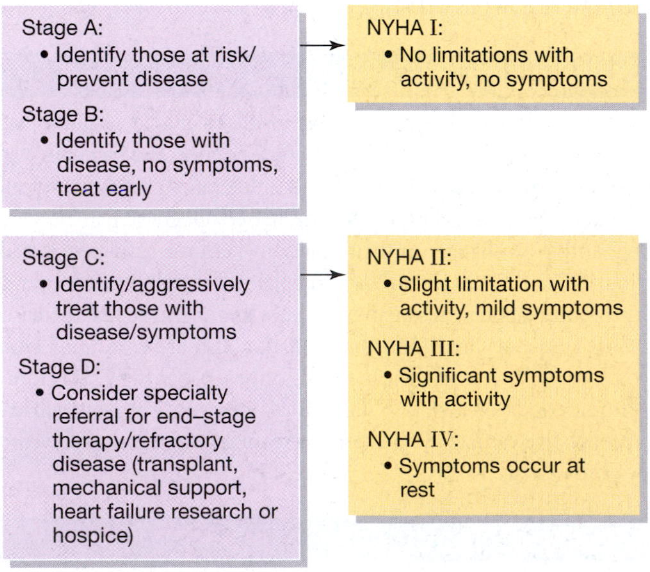

FIGURE 34–3 ◆ The American College of Cardiology/American Heart Association (ACC/AHA) stages of heart failure vs. the New York Heart Association (NYHA) classes.

Stage C

Patients who are at Stage C have symptomatic, structural heart disease. Recommended therapies include ACE inhibitors, angiotensin receptor blockers, beta-blockers, and digoxin. See the Pharmacologic Management section (p. 1033) for more detail. Diuretics are used to relieve congestive symptoms, and aldosterone blockade is added for persistent symptoms. Cardiac devices, such as internal cardioverter defibrillators and biventricular pacemakers, are used in appropriate candidates to reduce the incidence of sudden cardiac death, to improve the synchronous contraction in the ventricles, or do both. Chapter 30 discusses the pacemakers used for patients with heart failure.

Stage D

Stage D refers to end-stage heart failure. When little hope of recovery exists, advanced interventions including heart transplantation (p. 1040), implantation of mechanical circulatory devices (p. 1039), enrollment in heart failure research studies, or hospice may be warranted.

New York Heart Association Classification System

One measure used to quantify the degree of limitation and clinical symptoms of heart failure that are present in patients is the **New York Heart Association (NYHA) classification system.** This functional classification system categorizes a patient's subjective degree of symptoms into NYHA classes I through IV (McMurray, 2010). This system places patients in one of four classes depending largely on the degree of dyspnea present when the patient performs activities (AHA, 2010a).

Class I. Patient has no symptoms.

Class II. Patient has symptoms with ordinary exertion.

Class III. Patient has symptoms with less than ordinary exertion.

Class IV. Patient has symptoms at rest.

Diagnosing Heart Failure

Heart failure is a complex clinical syndrome for which no stand-alone test can establish the diagnosis (Hunt et al., 2009; Lindenfeld et al., 2010). Obtaining a full history, physical examination, and laboratory and diagnostic testing will help the clinician better understand the etiology, assess the severity of symptoms, and project the patient's prognosis.

A careful history of the onset, severity, and nature of symptoms will be critical in the initial evaluation when heart failure is suspected. The nurse should determine the patient's baseline ability to complete ADLs and the patient's NYHA class. A patient with heart failure tends to present with symptoms of volume overload and low cardiac output (Chart 34–3).

Dyspnea continues to be the most common presenting symptom, which patients largely identify as the key factor limiting their ADLs (Lindenfeld et al., 2010). The medical history should include questions about potential comorbid conditions, such as CAD and the use of cardiotoxic substances (Chart 34–4, p. 1032). The nurse should also get a thorough family history to identify possible familial tendencies (Chart 34–5, p. 1032).

Clinical Manifestations

The physical examination focuses largely on identifying signs of volume overload and decreased peripheral perfusion. As cardiac output deteriorates, specific physical manifestations become evident (Chart 34–6, p. 1032). General assessment may reveal that the patient is confused or disoriented, owing to low cardiac output and poor oxygen perfusion to the brain; more commonly, however, patients complain of forgetfulness and loss of concentration. Patients with chronic heart failure may appear to have cardiac cachexia (general ill health and malnutrition marked by weakness and emaciation usually associated with severe disease). Evaluation of the neck may reveal jugular venous distention (JVD) (bulging of the jugular vein that may be caused by increased blood volume in the jugular vein, reflecting increases in volume and

CHART 34–3 Symptoms of Congestion Versus Symptoms of Low Cardiac Output

Heart failure symptoms typically fall into two categories: those of congestion, or excess fluid retention, and those of poor perfusion, resulting from diminished cardiac output. These symptoms can be categorized by body system or function.

Organ System of Symptoms	Symptoms of Congestion	Symptoms of Low Cardiac Output
Pulmonary	Dyspnea, rest or exertional	
	Paroxysmal nocturnal dyspnea	
	Orthopnea	
	Cough	
Cardiac	Chest pain/tightness/discomfort	Chest pain/tightness/discomfort
		Decreased urination
Abdominal	Epigastric distention	Nausea or anorexia
	General discomfort	
	Discomfort with bending	
	Abdominal distention	
	Nausea or anorexia	
	Early satiety	
Extremities	Swelling; pedal, leg, sacral, scrotal/vulvar	Weakness, instability with ambulation
Cognitive	Fatigue	Impaired memory or concentration
		Confusion
Sleep	Sleep disturbance; air hunger, anxiety during sleep, need to sleep with head of bed elevated or in upright position	Sleep disturbance
		Daytime sleepiness
General	Fatigue	Lack of energy
	Lack of energy	Easy fatigability
	Malaise	Weight loss
		Malaise
		Decreased exercise tolerance
		Decreased urination

Source: Porth, C.M. & Matfin, G. (2009). *Pathophysiology: Concepts of altered health status* (8th ed.). Philadelphia: Lippincott Williams & Wilkins.

CHART 34–4 Past Medical History

Coronary artery disease	Prior myocardial infarctions
Hypertension	Diabetes
Hyperlipidemia	Valvular disease
Peripheral vascular disease	Rheumatic fever
Chest irradiation	Cardiotoxic agents
Alcohol consumption	Tobacco use
Obesity	Diabetes mellitus
Illicit drug use	Collagen vascular disease
Bacterial or parasitic infection	Thyroid disease
Pheochromocytoma	

CHART 34–5 Family History

Coronary artery disease	Hypertension
Diabetes	Hypercholesterolemia
Sudden cardiac death	Cardiomyopathies
Valvular disease	Peripheral vascular disease
Conduction system disease	Skeletal myopathies
Collagen vascular disease	

CHART 34–6 Clinical Manifestations of Heart Failure

Hypotension	Jugular venous distention
Rales	Crackles
Pleural effusion	Wheezing
Tachypnea	Tachycardia
Third and fourth heart sound	Ascites
Engorged liver	Positive hepatojugular reflux
Splenomegaly (enlarged)	Cyanosis
Cool extremities	Cachexia
Confusion	Disorientation
Pitting edema	

Source: Adapted from: Porth, C. M. & Matfin, G. (2009). *Pathophysiology: Concepts of altered health status* (9th ed.). Philadelphia: Lippincott Williams & Wilkins.

pressure of venous blood [Chapter 29]). Upon auscultation of the lungs, **crackles** (a common abnormal sound heard on auscultation of the lungs from the movement of fluid or exudate) may or may not be present in patients with chronic heart failure. In addition, a cough may be present due to an elevation in pulmonary venous pressure. A cough may or may not be productive; however, if pink frothy sputum is present, pulmonary edema should be suspected as a potential cause. Dull breath sounds may be heard in the presence of a pleural effusion.

Nursing Management

Due to the evolving course of heart failure, nursing management of this condition requires critical thinking and good clinical judgment skills. For example, an older patient may fall asleep during the physical assessment. The nurse should question whether this happened because of poor perfusion due to early heart failure or some neurological disorder. Therefore, it is essential to assess the patient for subtle symptoms of heart failure, which include the following:

- Crackles are absent in over 80% of people with elevated filling pressures.
- Edema in older adults is often unrelated to filling pressures.
- The easiest vital sign used to assess perfusion is blood pressure.
- Patients who fall asleep while interviewed may have poor perfusion.
- Cool forearms and legs may be more indicative of low cardiac output than are cold hands and feet.

A patient's clinical manifestations can change rapidly, owing to the progression of the heart failure. If there is an abrupt decline in cardiac output, the following signs and symptoms can occur:

- Narrow pulse pressure
- cool extremities
- altered mentation
- hypotension
- Cheyne–Stokes respiration
- resting tachycardia
- rise in BUN/creatinine
- oliguria (no urine output).

Patients may also have **tachypnea** (an abnormally rapid rate of breathing, more than 20 breaths per minute) while being examined. Palpation of the chest may reveal that the apical pulse is displaced laterally due to left ventricular hypertrophy. As part of the assessment and treatment of tachypneic patients, the nurse should do the following:

- Obtain the patient's oxygen saturation.
- Assess the patient's extremities for temperature and appearance of cyanosis.
- Assess the patient's neurological status.
- Obtain an order from the health care provider for oxygen, and place the patient on the oxygen.
- If the patient is currently on oxygen, assess these connections; if all are correct, increase the oxygen level and notify the health care provider.

On auscultation, an **S_3 (abnormal third heart sound in the cardiac cycle)** may be present with volume overload. An **S_4 (abnormal fourth heart sound in the cardiac cycle)** may be heard when patients have significant hypertension. Both S_3 and S_4 are discussed in Chapter 29. With increasing sympathetic stimulation, tachycardia (a condition in which the myocardium contracts at a rate greater than 100 beats per minute) may be present. Abdominal examination may reveal **ascites** (an abnormal intraperitoneal accumulation of fluid containing large amounts of protein and electrolytes) and an engorged liver and spleen. A positive **hepatojugular reflux** (an increase in jugular venous pressure when pressure is applied over the abdomen, which is suggestive of right-sided heart failure) may also be present if volume overload is found in the periphery. The extremities may exhibit edema measured by the degree of **pitting** (an indentation that remains for a short time after edematous skin is pressed with the finger). Cyanosis (bluish discoloration of the skin and mucous membranes caused by an excess of deoxygenated hemoglobin in the blood) and cooling of the extremities with a poor capillary refill can occur with shunting of blood to vital organs (Porth & Matfin, 2009).

Chapter 29 discusses cardiac assessment. The remainder of the nursing management of heart failure is discussed in the Nursing Process: Patient Care Plan, page 1042.

Laboratory and Diagnostic Procedures

Laboratory tests are done to evaluate for underlying diseases or conditions that can cause or exacerbate heart failure. Other specific laboratory tests should be done to help the health care provider understand the etiology of heart failure, precipitating factors, and/or the degree of organ compromise when heart failure is present. Applicable tests are shown in the Diagnostic Tests box (p. 1034). Recommended blood work may give clues about the etiology and/or comorbidities of heart failure using a complete blood count, ferritin, troponin, lipid panel, and thyroid function tests. Other laboratory values may give an indication of the severity of the disease by assessing liver function tests, BNP, and renal function (Hunt et al., 2009; Lindenfeld et al., 2010).

Various cardiac imaging techniques are employed to identify structural abnormalities of the heart (see the Diagnostic Tests box, p. 1034). An echocardiogram, a 12-lead electrocardiogram, and a chest x-ray are indicated for all patients undergoing an evaluation for heart failure (Hunt et al., 2009; Lindenfeld et al., 2010). These are the least expensive and most accessible tests in many institutions. Further cardiac testing will provide information on the etiology of heart failure, extent of disease, measure of cardiac function, ejection fraction (EF), cardiac anatomy, and hemodynamics. Other means to assess ventricular function may be used, such as cardiac magnetic imaging. Patients with angina should have an angiogram, but noninvasive imaging to detect myocardial ischemia may be used for patients for whom the diagnosis is less clear. Patients should also be screened for sleep-disordered breathing, because this has increasingly become recognized as a common contributing factor in heart failure (Lindenfeld et al., 2010).

Medical Management

Treatment goals for chronic heart failure include the following:

- Alleviate symptoms of congestion.
- Improve perfusion.
- Increase activity tolerance.
- Improve quality of life.
- Decrease hospitalizations.
- Reduce readmissions.
- Slow or reverse progression of cardiac dysfunction.
- Improve survival.
- Minimize risk factors.
- Provide palliative care.
- Decrease heart failure-related costs.
- Track outcomes.

Treatment options for heart failure have evolved tremendously. The rapid growth of heart failure treatment in the 21st century has led to the use of a combination of pharmacologic measures, cardiac devices, and surgical approaches. Medications, such as ACE inhibitors and beta-adrenergic blockers, have become the current standard of care for their role in not only decreasing morbidity and mortality but also decreasing heart failure hospitalizations.

Additionally, heart failure device therapies such as biventricular pacemakers and implantable-cardioverter defibrillators have a significant role, because they address the impact of sudden cardiac death and cardiac dyssynchrony (Chapter 30). Self-management and health promotion strategies will complete the heart failure treatment plan. Although a number of treatments have been shown to improve outcomes in patients with heart failure, the prognosis of these patients remains poor, resulting in frequent readmission to the hospital. Research is looking at the efficacy of using multidisciplinary strategies to improve outcomes for heart failure patients. This research is discussed in the Evidence-Based Practice box (p. 1036).

Pharmacologic Management

Although heart failure has no cure, effective pharmacologic treatments have shown clear benefits in improving the quality and length of life in patients with acute or chronic heart failure. Optimal pharmacologic management for patients with LVSD includes a combination of ACE inhibitors or angiotensin receptor blockers, beta-adrenergic blockers, diuretics, digoxin, and aldosterone antagonists. Despite advances in heart failure management, compliance with these proven therapies remains poor (Hunt et al., 2009; Lindenfeld et al., 2010). Strategies to keep patients on lifesaving medications are paramount, such as providing medication assistance programs to those in need, educating patients about the role of medical therapy, and addressing side effects that may limit quality of life.

The primary targets of pharmacologic therapies in chronic heart failure focus largely on inhibiting the neurohormonal response invoked by left ventricular dysfunction in addition to relieving the symptoms of congestion. In acute heart failure, primary pharmacologic therapy is based on a rapid and thorough assessment of volume status, the extent of peripheral and organ perfusion, and the presence of precipitating and life-threatening conditions. Treatment goals are usually aggressive for acute heart failure and are aimed at the following:

- Relieving symptoms
- Stabilizing hemodynamic parameters
- Improving organ function
- Eliminating precipitating or exacerbating causes (Hunt et al., 2009; Lindenfeld et al., 2010).

Angiotensin-Converting Enzyme (ACE) Inhibitors

All patients with left ventricular dysfunction who show evidence of an ejection fraction of less than 40% should be placed on an ACE inhibitor unless they have a known contraindication (Lindenfeld et al., 2010). This class of medication has shown improved survival, delayed progression of heart failure, and improved exercise tolerance (McMurray, 2010). Adverse effects from ACE inhibitors include cough, angioedema, renal insufficiency, and hyperkalemia. As doses are increased, hypotension may occur, and the nurse should monitor for it (Adams & Koch, 2010b).

Angiotensin II Receptor Blockers (ARB)

The RAAS system is only partially suppressed by the use of ACE inhibitors because angiotensin II is also produced by other pathways. ARBs cause inhibition by blocking RAAS activation at the angiotensin II receptor site. Angiotensin receptor blockers have been found to have clinical effects similar to those of ACE inhibitors with regard to the interference with the RAAS, yet they have not demonstrated results superior to those of ACE inhibitors in clinical trials (Hunt et al., 2009; Lindenfeld et al., 2010).

Beta-Adrenergic Blockers

Beta-adrenergic blockers, commonly referred to as beta-blockers, act primarily by blocking the SNS in patients with heart failure and have been a major advance in heart failure treatment (Hunt et al., 2009).

LABORATORY AND DIAGNOSTIC TESTS for Heart Failure

Test, Normal Values, and Rationale	Expected Abnormality
Blood Count	
Hemoglobin:	Anemia
Males: 13.5–18 g/dL	Infection
Females: 12–15 g/dL	
Hematocrit:	
Males: 40–54%	
Females: 36–46%	
White blood count: 5,000–10,000 μL	
Can determine whether anemia or infection is present, which can exacerbate heart failure symptoms. Anemia affects the blood's oxygen-carrying capacity, which could result in tissue hypoxia.	
Serum Electrolytes and Creatinine	
Sodium: 134–145 mEq/L	Renal insufficiency
Potassium: 3.5–5.3 mEq/L	Electrolyte deficiencies
Magnesium: 1.5–2.5 mEq/L	
BUN: 5–25 mg/dL	
Creatinine: 0.5–1.5 mg/dL	
Can determine whether there is underlying renal disease. Can determine whether electrolyte deficiencies are present and can obtain baseline measurements prior to the initiation of diuretic therapy.	
Liver Function Tests	
Bilirubin:	Hepatic congestion
Indirect unconjugated: 0.1–1.0 mg/dL	
Direct conjugated: 0.1–0.3 mg/dL	
Total: 0.1–1.2 mg/dL	
ALT or SGPT: 10–35 U/L	
LD/LDH: 100–190 IU/L	
GGT/GGTP:	
Males: 4–23 IU/L	
Females: 3–13 IU/L	
Alkaline phosphatase: 42–136 WI	
Can determine the impact of heart failure on the liver function.	
Urinalysis	
Thyroid function tests:	Renal dysfunction
TSH: 0.35–5.5 microinternational unit/mL	Hypothyroidism/hyperthyroidism
Serum thyroxine (T_4): 4.5–11.5 mcg/dL	
Serum triiodothyronine (T_3): 80–200 ng/dL	
Can determine whether the etiology or the exacerbation of heart failure is related to hypothyroidism or hyperthyroidism.	
Serum Ferritin	
Male: 15–445 ng/mL	Hemochromatosis
Female: 10–235 ng/mL	
Determines whether the etiology of heart failure is related to iron overload.	
Lipid Panel	
Cholesterol: 150–240 mg/dL	Hypercholesterolemia
Triglycerides: 10–190 mg/dL	Hyperlipidemia
Phospholipids: 150–380 mg/dL	
LDL: 60–160 mg/dL	
HDL: 29–77 mg/dL	
May indicate the presence of CAD.	

LABORATORY AND DIAGNOSTIC TESTS for Heart Failure, *continued*

Test, Normal Values, and Rationale	Expected Abnormality
BNP	
Less than 100 pg/mL	Elevated with left ventricular dysfunction
Abnormal levels correlate with both the severity of symptoms and the prognosis of heart failure.	
Digoxin Level	
0.5–2 ng/mL therapeutic range	Must be monitored until therapeutic range is stabilized
Determines need for dosage adjustment.	
Arterial Blood Gases	
PO_2	Low oxygen blood levels and acidosis/alkalosis
pH: 7.35–7.45	
$PaCO_2$: 35–45 mmHg	
HCO_3: 24–28 mEq/L	
Base excess: +/− 2 mEq/L	
Determines oxygen levels and acid–base balance	
DIAGNOSTIC TEST	
Chest X-Ray	
Can determine the presence of cardiac or great vessel enlargement, abnormal thoracic calcification, and pulmonary congestion.	Pleural effusion Cardiomegaly
Electrocardiogram (Chapter 30)	
Can determine the presence of dysrhythmias, left ventricular hypertrophy, and myocardial ischemia or insult.	Left ventricular hypertrophy Left bundle branch block Pathologic Q waves
Echocardiogram (Chapter 33)	
Can determine the size and function of atria and ventricles, segmental wall motion abnormalities, wall thickness, and valvular structure and function.	Left ventricular dysfunction Myocardial infarction Diastolic dysfunction
Cardiac Catheterization: Right Heart Catheterization (Chapter 32)	
Can determine the presence of volume overload or pulmonary hypertension.	Increased filling pressures, pulmonary artery pressures, cardiac output, and mixed venous blood gas
Cardiac Catheterization; Left Heart Catheterization and Selective Coronary Angiography (Chapter 32)	
Can determine whether CAD is present and whether intervention is possible.	Evaluation of coronary arteries and assessment of ventricular function
Cardiac Magnetic Imaging (Chapter 32)	
Useful in perfusion imaging to assess the viability of the myocardium.	Evaluation of the heart and the coronary arteries
Can determine the patency of coronary arteries.	

Source: Adapted from: Kee, J. L. (2010). *Laboratory and diagnostic tests with nursing implications.* Upper Saddle River, NJ: Pearson.

Patients placed on beta-blockers who have had a myocardial infarction and/or LVEF < 40% in addition to standard therapy of an ACE inhibitor, digitalis, and a diuretic have an improved survival rate and reduced symptoms (Lindenfeld et al., 2010). Other benefits include improved clinical status, decreased risk of sudden death, and improved overall exercise tolerance. Beta-blockers have been found to be effective in all classes of heart failure, including patients with severe but stable heart failure.

Safety Alert *Symptoms requiring adjustment of beta-blocker dose include worsening shortness of breath, weight gain, fatigue, hypotension, or light-headedness or syncope. If patients develop these symptoms, the nurse must notify the health care provider.*

Diuretics

The most effective method to relieve heart failure symptoms is to remove excess fluid with loop diuretics (Lindenfeld et al., 2010). Patients with advanced heart failure who need enhanced diuresis may require a thiazide-like diuretic, such as metolazone, to be added to loop diuretics. Hospitalized patients or those who are refractory to oral diuretics may require intravenous diuretics for rapid relief of congestive symptoms. Most diuretic agents work within the renal tubules to prevent sodium reabsorption and thereby cause natriuresis. Primary management when using a diuretic will require the nurse to evaluate laboratory work for close monitoring of serum electrolytes (because hypokalemia is common), to assess volume status (by evaluating symptomatology),

Weblink: Educating Patients

Weblink: Health Literacy Toolkit

EVIDENCE-BASED PRACTICE Use of Teach-Back Techniques in Patients with Heart Failure

Clinical Problem

Over 6 million Americans have heart failure, and its prevalence is increasing as treatments for acute cardiovascular diseases improve and the population ages. Heart failure is one of the most costly cardiovascular disorders, and much of the cost is due to hospital admission and re-admission for care of symptoms of decompensation because patients do not understand how to manage their disease.

Research Findings

The treatment of heart failure is complex and can be challenging for patients to manage. Patients who have a clear understanding of their after-hospital care instructions, including how to take their medicines and when to make follow up appointments, are 30% less likely to be readmitted or visit the emergency department than are patients who do not know this information (AHRQ, 2009). Many readmissions to hospitals for treatment of heart failure could be avoided by increasing patients' understanding. Some of the factors that contribute to re-admission are inadequate discharge instructions, non-adherence to medication regimen and dietary restrictions, and failure to follow up with health care providers (Manning, 2011). The American College of Cardiology and American Heart Association have identified six key areas of instruction for the heart failure patient: diet, activity, discharge medications, weight monitoring, treatment plan for worsening symptoms, and follow up appointments. Compliance with these recommendations is poor and ranges from 20% to 54% (Manning, 2011). A strategy that is being used successfully to educate patients with heart failure is the use of "teach back," in which patients relay back to the nurse what they have learned using their own words. It helps to confirm that the teaching has been done in a manner that the patient understands (AHRQ, 2010).

Implications for Nursing Practice

Nurses play a pivotal role in educating patients in ways that will help them be successful in managing their heart failure. When teaching patients about heart failure, the nurse should use simple language, avoid the use of medical jargon, and not speak too quickly. In addition, the nurse should focus on two or three key concepts (AHRQ, 2010) such as taking medications correctly, avoiding high-sodium foods, and weighing themselves regularly. Assess the patient's level of understanding by using the teach-back format rather than yes or no questions.

Critical Thinking Questions with answers can be found in the Osborn Student Resources at nursing.pearsonhighered.com.

Sources: Adapted from Agency for Healthcare Research and Quality (AHRQ). (2009). Educating patients before hospital discharge reduces readmissions, emergency department visits, and saves money. Retrieved from http://www.ahrq.gov/research/mar09/0309RA1.htm; Agency for Healthcare Research and Quality (AHRQ). (2010). Health care literacy universal precautions toolkit. Retrieved from http://www.ahrq.gov/qual/literacy/healthliteracytoolkit.pdf; Manning, S. (2011). Bridging the gap between hospital and home: A new model of care for reducing readmission rates in chronic heart failure. *Journal of Cardiovascular Nursing.*

to observe for excessive volume depletion (to ensure hypovolemia is prevented), and to monitor the response to diuretics (urine output and weight loss). Excessive volume depletion can also activate the RAAS system, negating the effect of the ACE inhibitor and ARB.

If patient compliance with sodium and fluid restriction is poor, escalation of diuretic doses may be needed to maintain **euvolemia** (when the body is in a state of equal fluid balance, without fluid retention). Patients who are placed on a diuretic will need nursing education regarding the mechanism of diuretic function and the importance of maintaining a euvolemic or "dry" weight (McMurray, 2010).

Digitalis

Digitalis is a weak, positive inotropic drug that increases the contractility of the weakened heart muscle, thus improving the volume of cardiac output. It is effective in improving symptoms and exercise tolerance in patients with heart failure. Although no mortality benefit has been identified with this medication, there has been a decrease in hospitalizations with the greatest benefit in patients with NYHA class III and IV symptoms (Hunt et al., 2009; Adams & Koch, 2010b). Adverse effects of digitalis use are largely related to toxic serum concentrations; therefore, patients should be placed on a low dose and be monitored to maintain a target therapeutic level < 1.0 ng/mL (Lindenfeld et al., 2010).

Aldosterone Antagonists

Aldosterone antagonists are recommended for patients with heart failure and/or postmyocardial infarction with continued NYHA class III or IV symptoms treated with a standard therapy of ACE inhibitors, beta-adrenergic blockers, and diuretics. Aldosterone antagonists provide a more complete blockade of the RAAS and reduce aldosterone release, resulting in a mortality benefit and a reduced hospitalizations (Lindenfeld et al., 2010).

Dysrhythmic Agents

Dysrhythmic agents should not be used routinely to treat heart failure; however, they may be used for recurrent atrial fibrillation or symptomatic ventricular dysrhythmias (Hunt et al., 2009; Lindenfeld et al., 2010).

Anticoagulant Agents

In patients with severe left ventricular dysfunction and an ejection fraction $\leq 35\%$, there is a potential for stasis within the ventricles that could lead to the development of thrombi. It may be reasonable to treat such patients with an anticoagulant such as warfarin (Hunt et al., 2009; Lindenfield et al., 2010). Patients with atrial fibrillation, mechanical heart valves, some mechanical assist devices, pulmonary embolism, transient ischemic attacks or cerebral vascular accidents, or other deep venous thrombosis also are candidates for anticoagulation therapy.

Safety Alert *Older adults with heart failure frequently void at night and therefore are at risk for falling if they rise from bed suddenly. Caution the patient about fall risks, including the use of regular toileting, a bedside commode, or a call light for assistance (for patients in the hospital) and home health and home needs assessment for those at home.*

Inotropic, Vasopressor, and Vasodilator Therapeutic Agents

In patients with acute decompensated heart failure and critical hypoperfusion, intravenous diuretics, inotropes, vasopressors, or vasodilator agents have been found to be beneficial in improving hemodynamics, including stroke volume and cardiac output, and thereby improving blood pressure and perfusion to organs and tissues (Hunt et al., 2009; Lindenfeld et al., 2010).

Medications for Select Patients

Hydralazine/nitrates were used in combination until ACE inhibitors showed superior results in patients with heart failure (Adams & Koch, 2010b). Now, this combination is recognized as a reasonable alternative for patients who are unable to take an ACE inhibitor, ARBs, and/or beta-adrenergic blockers for whatever reason (Lindenfeld et al., 2010). African American patients with continued NYHA class III or IV symptoms despite standard medical management with an ACE inhibitor or ARB and beta-adrenergic blockers have improved outcomes with hydralazine/nitrates, which should be added if blood pressure allows. The Pharmacology feature reviews all of the medications used to treat heart failure.

PHARMACOLOGY Summary of Medications Used to Treat Heart Failure

Medication Category and Action	Application/Indication	Nursing Responsibility
Angiotensin-converting enzyme (ACE) inhibitors: Captopril (Capoten) Enalapril (Vasotec) Fosinopril (Monopril) Lisinopril (Prinivil, Zestril) Quinapril (Accupril) Ramipril (Altace) ***Action:*** Works within the renin-angiotensin-aldosterone system (RAAS) to inhibit the vasoconstricting action of angiotensin II and the angiotensin-mediated secretion of aldosterone, thus causing blood vessels to dilate and decreasing systemic vascular resistance. Results in decreased afterload, decreased sodium resorption, and increased contractility.	Heart failure. Use in all patients with reduced ventricular function; left ventricular ejection fraction (LVEF) $< 40\%$. Heart failure patients on ACE inhibitors have improved survival and delayed progression of heart failure due to the favorable blockade of the RAAS.	Monitor blood pressure regularly when drug is initiated and when dosage is titrated. Hold the drug and notify the health care provider if the systolic blood pressure is less than 90 mmHg. Monitor for ACE inhibitor-induced cough, dizziness, hypotension, hyperkalemia, and worsening renal insufficiency. Angioedema may also occur in rare settings. Angioedema indicates an allergic reaction, and immediate intervention may be needed, depending on the patient's symptoms. Monitor for orthostatic hypotension, elevated serum sodium, potassium, and/or creatinine, and drug-induced neutropenia. Teach the patient to avoid over-the-counter NSAIDs as they can reduce the effectiveness of ACE inhibitors.
Angiotensin II receptor blockers (ARBs): Candesartan (Atacand) Eprosartan (Teveten) Irbesartan (Avapro) Losartan (Cozaar) Telmisartan (Micardis) Valsartan (Diovan) ***Action:*** Causes inhibition by blocking RAAS activation at the angiotensin II receptor site. They decrease afterload, decrease sodium resorption, and increase contractility.	Heart failure in patients who are intolerant to ACE inhibitors with an LVEF $< 40\%$. Heart failure patients on ARBs have improved survival and delayed progression of heart failure.	Monitor blood pressure regularly when drug is initiated and when dosage is titrated. Hold the drug and notify the health care provider if the systolic blood pressure is less than 90 mmHg. Monitor for dizziness, orthostatic hypotension, and elevated serum sodium, potassium creatinine Monitor for worsening renal insufficiency.
Beta-adrenergic blockers: Carvedilol (Coreg) Metoprolol succinate (Toprol) ***Action:*** Acts primarily by blocking the sympathetic nervous system (SNS), resulting in improved coronary blood flow and less ischemia. There also is a decreased workload on the heart and less myocyte hypertrophy resulting in decreased myocardial ischemia and hypertrophy.	Use in heart failure patients with LVEF $< 40\%$ or postmyocardial infarction. Heart failure patients on beta-blockers have been found to have improved survival, improvement in symptoms, a decrease in the risk of sudden death, and improved overall exercise tolerance.	Observe for signs of hypotension or bradycardia, as either condition may require adjustment of the dose. Patient education is imperative about the side effects of fatigue, dizziness, fluid retention, and worsening heart failure. It is also imperative that nurses instruct patients on how to monitor their pulse and blood pressure and to help them recognize when they should notify their provider. Beta-adrenergic blockers can worsen bronchospasm in patients with reactive airway disease and therefore should be monitored.
Cardiac glycoside: Digoxin (Lanoxin) ***Action:*** A weak, positive inotrope that increases the contractility of the weakened heart muscle, thus improving the volume of cardiac output. (It has also been found to have an impact on suppression of renin secretion from the RAAS.)	Use in heart failure patients with NYHA class III or IV symptoms. This medication has been found to decrease hospitalizations and to improve symptoms, quality of life, and exercise tolerance.	Nursing assessment for patients includes monitoring for toxic drug levels that can cause bradycardia and/or cardiac dysrhythmias, as well as conduction disturbances, gastrointestinal symptoms, and neurological complaints. Patients are taught to take their pulse daily before taking their digoxin. If their heart rate is below 60, they should hold the digoxin and contact their health care provider for further instructions.
Hydralazine and isosorbide dinitrate (BiDil) ***Action:*** This combination of vasodilators that act on both arteries and veins.	Heart failure patients on ACE inhibitors or ARBs, and beta-blockers may benefit when this combination is added. This combination has shown improved survival, reduced hospitalizations, and improved quality of life.	Monitor for headache, hypotension, and gastrointestinal complaints. This should not be used in patients that have not had a trial of ACE inhibitors or ARBs. Patient/family education must stress compliance owing to the multidose schedule required.

(continued)

PHARMACOLOGY Summary of Medications Used to Treat Heart Failure, *continued*

Medication Category and Action	Application/Indication	Nursing Responsibility
Nitrates: Nitroglycerin (NTG) Isosorbide dinitrate (Iso-Bid, Isordil) Isosorbide mononitrate (Imdur, Nitro-Bid) ***Action:*** Potent vasodilator, leading to relaxation of both arterial and venous smooth muscle. Reduces preload to the heart. Lowers myocardial oxygen demand. Dilates coronary arteries.	Indications include heart failure, acute pulmonary edema, and hypertension.	Monitor blood pressure regularly when the drug is initiated and when the dosage is titrated. Hold the drug and notify the health care provider if the systolic blood pressure is less than 90 mmHg. Monitor for headache and orthostatic hypotension.
Antidysrhythmics: Amiodarone (Cordarone) Dofetilide (Tikosyn) Ibutilide (Corvert) Sotalol (Betapace) ***Action:*** Class III antiarrhythmic agents have sympatholytic (or antiadrenergic) effects on the heart and atrioventricular nodal-blocking properties.	Used to treat dysrhythmias. May be used for rate and rhythm control for patients in atrial fibrillation, and to suppress significant ventricular dysrhythmias.	Possible side effects include pulmonary toxicities, skin discoloration, hepatic and/or thyroid derangements, corneal deposits, optic neuropathy, and interactions with warfarin and digoxin. May be proarrhythmic; monitor cardiac rhythm.
Diuretics		
Loop diuretics: Bumetanide (Bumex) Ethacrynic acid (Edecrin) Furosemide (Lasix) Torsemide (Demadex) Metolazone (Zaroxolyn) **Thiazide diuretics:** Hydrochlorothiazide (Hydrodiuril) ***Action:*** Increase the excretion of water. Block sodium and chloride reabsorption in the loop of Henle.	Use in heart failure patients exhibiting signs and symptoms of fluid overload. Diuretics increase urinary sodium excretion and decrease physical signs of fluid retention. Pulmonary edema. Peripheral edema. Hypertension.	Monitor intake and output. Monitor for excess fluid loss, hypokalemia, dysrhythmias, orthostatic hypotension. If the patient is diabetic, monitor blood glucose levels, as they may be affected by some loop diuretics. Monitor for hyperkalemia in patients who are also taking potassium-sparing diuretics, such as eplerenone or spironolactone. The nurse must provide the patient education regarding daily weights, sodium and fluid restrictions, and instructions to contact the health care provider when congestion/edema worsen.
Aldosterone antagonists: Eplerenone (Inspra) Spironolactone (Aldactone) ***Action:*** Blocks the release of aldosterone hormone secreted by the adrenal glands that, when activated in heart failure, causes sodium and fluid retention. By blocking the actions of aldosterone, these drugs enhance the excretion of sodium and the retention of potassium.	Use in heart failure patients with continued symptoms, despite therapies listed previously. Found to have a favorable mortality benefit and has been shown to decrease hospitalizations. These benefits are greatest in those patients with NYHA class IV symptoms.	Monitor for signs of hyperkalemia and renal dysfunction. A side effect of some aldosterone antagonists is gynecomastia (enlargement of breast tissue in males), which may require a change in antagonist used. Nursing instruction should include a discussion of the avoidance of high-potassium-containing foods. Nonsteroidal anti-inflammatory drugs and COX-2 inhibitors should be avoided, which can worsen hyperkalemia and renal dysfunction.
Phosphodiesterase inhibitors: Milrinone (Primacor) Inamrinone (Inocor) ***Action:*** Positive inotropic agents and vasodilators. Block the enzyme phosphodiesterase III in cardiac and smooth muscle, leading to increased amounts of calcium available for myocardial contraction.	Indications include heart failure and acute decompensated heart failure.	Place on a cardiac monitor for the duration of administration. Therapy is generally restricted to short-term intravenous infusion for 2 to 3 days. Monitor for ventricular dysrhythmias. Monitor blood pressure frequently due to vasodilatation. Monitor for thrombocytopenia (low platelet count) and headache.

Weblink: Dabigatran (Pradaxa)

PHARMACOLOGY Summary of Medications Used to Treat Heart Failure, *continued*

Medication Category and Action	Application/Indication	Nursing Responsibility
Nesiritide (Natrecor) ***Action:*** Structurally identical to endogenous beta-type natriuretic peptide (hBNP) which increases the excretion of sodium and water in response to increased stretch of the ventricular walls.	Indications include acute decompensated heart failure.	Place on a cardiac monitor for the duration of administration. Therapy is generally restricted to short-term intravenous infusion. Use is limited due to severe hypotension associated with its use and can persist after the infusion is discontinued.
Anticoagulant therapy: Heparin Low molecular weight heparin (Lovenox, Fragmin) Dabigatran (Pradaxa) Warfarin (Coumadin) ***Action:*** Inhibit specific factors in the clotting cascade and decrease the risk of thrombus formation.	Indications include dysrhythmias, especially atrial fibrillation, and venous thromboembolism prophylaxis and treatment.	Monitor for bleeding from the gums and puncture sites; hemoptysis, and hematuria. Monitor laboratory values that assess coagulation: PT/INR, PTT. Monitor for thrombocytopenia. For patients on Pradaxa, ongoing laboratory follow up is generally not indicated and there are no known food–drug interactions. For patients on Coumadin, instruct them to have PTT/INR follow-up and the potential impact of alcohol, foods containing vitamin K.
Anti-anxiety agents: Alprazolam (Xanax) Chlordiazepoxide (Librium) Diazepam (Valium) Lorazepam (Ativan) ***Action:*** Central nervous system depression. Produces relaxation, calmness.	Indications include anxiety.	Monitor for drowsiness, ataxia, or dizziness. Instruct the patient about relaxation, for example, deep breathing, massage, and guided imagery.

Source: Adams, M. P., & Koch, R. W. (2010a). Dapigatraban etexilate prescribing information. Retrieved from http://www.pradaxa.com/?sc=PRDACQWEBGGLWKT1006111.

In summary, multiple medications are used in the management of heart failure, with different indications and side effects. The entire health care team must share the responsibility of emphasizing the importance of medical therapy to patients, their families, and their caregivers. The complexity of the heart failure medication regimen increases the risk of noncompliance and medication errors.

Device Therapies for Heart Failure

Cardiac devices have a well-established role in the management of systolic dysfunction. These revolutionary devices have improved both the length and quality of life when added to medical therapy for people with heart failure. Cardiac pacemakers and the expanded use of implantable cardioverter defibrillators (ICDs) have become the standard of care for select patients. Internal cardioverter defibrillators have shown superiority over medical therapy alone in reducing sudden cardiac death. Cardiac pacemakers and ICDs are discussed in detail in Chapter 30.

Cardiac Resynchronization Therapy

Cardiac resynchronization therapy (CRT), also known as biventricular pacing, is useful in the treatment of heart failure in certain patients. The CRT device paces both ventricles simultaneously, restoring a synchronized contraction that had been lost because of conduction abnormalities and dyssynchrony, which occur in many heart failure patients. CRT is most effective for patients with moderate to severe symptoms, despite optimal heart failure medication, with a LVEF less than 35% and a QRS complex greater than 120 milliseconds (Hunt et al., 2009). Heart failure patients with myocardial damage often have conduction abnormalities such as a bundle branch block, in which there is a delay in the transmission of the electrical impulse down one or the other bundle branch, causing a wide QRS complex on the ECG. Chapter 30 discusses the width of the QRS complex. This intraventricular conduction delay results in dyssynchronous movements between the ventricles, abnormal septal wall motion, suboptimal filling during diastole, poorly coordinated ventricular contraction, decreased left ventricular ejection fraction (LVEF), and even impaired mitral valve function. Clinically, patients with a bundle branch block experience limited exercise tolerance, impaired quality of life, and poor functional capacity.

CRT implantation is similar to pacemaker insertion, except that a total of three leads are used, rather than one or two. One lead is placed in the right atrium, one in the right ventricle, and the third through the coronary sinus to a vein that is near the left ventricle. The potential complications, nursing management, and patient education for pacemakers are discussed in more detail in Chapter 30.

Ultrafiltration in Heart Failure

Ultrafiltration, also referred to as aquapheresis, is the mechanical removal of water and sodium from patients with fluid overload from heart failure. It is generally reserved for patients with declining renal function when diuretics cannot be used as safely. Blood is withdrawn from the patient, via a central line or peripheral venous line, and is filtered through a dialysis machine, removing the excess water and sodium while returning the blood to the patient (Kamath, 2011).

Surgical Treatments for Systolic Heart Failure

Specific surgical procedures are utilized if they are likely to improve left ventricular function, clinical manifestations, and survival and the patient is an appropriate surgical candidate. However, surgery places chronically ill heart failure patients with significant comorbidities of renal, lung, and other vascular disease at a higher risk of surgical morbidity and mortality. Some patients with mitral valve disease may benefit from mitral valve repair or replacement (Chapter 33) to relieve or control their heart failure symptoms (McMurray, 2010). Surgical reconstruction of the left ventricle has not been found to provide a clinical benefit to patients.

Cardiac Transplantation

Heart transplantation is a successful treatment for some patients with heart failure. Even though it remains the best long-term surgical treatment for heart failure, its use is extremely limited by the availability of donor hearts. Fewer than 3,000 heart transplantations are performed annually in the United States (AHA, 2010c).

Patients who may benefit from heart transplantation are those with ischemic cardiomyopathy, non-ischemic cardiomyopathy, and severe congenital defects or valvular heart disease (Carlson, 2009). Patients who have a history of psychosocial challenges such as psychiatric issues, substance abuse, and poor social support may not be able to comply with the complex post-transplant medical regimen that is required.

Patients who may be candidates for transplant are thoroughly examined and evaluated by a multidisciplinary team that includes health care providers, surgeons, nurses, social workers, dietitians, physical and occupational therapists, and insurance advisors. Testing includes a complete cardiac work-up including cardiac catheterization, thorough antibody and antigen testing, and screening for tuberculosis, hepatitis, HIV, and toxoplasmosis. Age criteria may also be considered; it is unusual for patients older than 65 years to receive a heart transplant. The average time between being listed and receiving a transplant is 2 or more years (Carlson, 2009).

When an appropriate donor heart is found, the patient is taken to surgery. In the most common approach to transplant, the patient's heart is removed or "explanted" except for sections of the left atria (orthotopic). The donor heart is then implanted and the surgical anastamoses are completed. In some patients, the patient's own heart is not removed, and the donor heart is placed alongside it (heterotopic procedure). This may be done when the patient's own heart can be used in conjunction with the donor heart (e.g., when the donor heart is small or when there is some chance of recovery of the patient's own heart).

The donor heart is denervated during harvesting, the process of surgical removal from the donor. Because of this, there can be abnormalities of cardiac rhythm and contractility once the heart is implanted into the recipient. The denervated heart does not respond to stimulation from the vagus nerve. Because sensory fibers are also severed during explanation, patients with transplanted hearts might not be aware of myocardial ischemia if it occurs.

Following surgery, in addition to the standard care of the open heart surgery patient, care is focused on monitoring the patient for rejection of the transplanted heart and managing immunosuppression. Signs of rejection include fever; signs of heart failure include fatigue, shortness of breath, dysrhythmias, edema, and decreased left ventricular function. Adequate immunosuppression is essential in the heart transplant patient to prevent acute and chronic rejection. Some of the agents that are used for this purpose are cyclosporine, tacrolimus, sirolimus, mycophenolate, methylprednisone, and prednisone. Patients receiving these drugs are at risk for infection. Regular, lifelong follow up care is essential for the patient after heart transplantation and includes regular clinic visits, frequent echocardiography, and intermittent heart biopsy to assess for early rejection. Immunosuppression is discussed in Chapter 53.

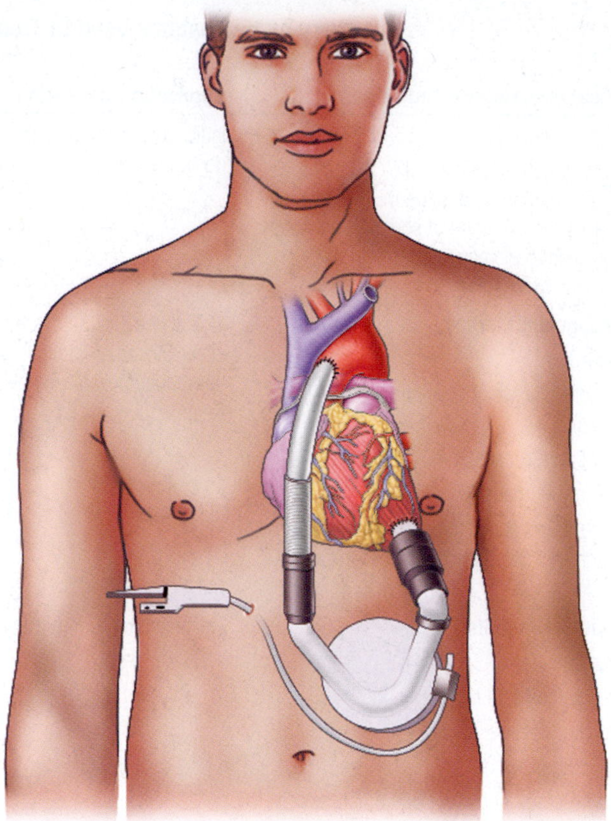

FIGURE 34–4 ◆ Ventricular assist device.

Mechanical Assist Devices

A growing field for patients with severe heart failure is circulatory support. This includes short-term devices such as the intra-aortic balloon pump and percutaneous ventricular assist devices (VAD) such as the TandemHeart and the Impella 2.5 and 5.0 (McCulloch, 2010). Longer term extracorporeal surgical devices are available that can support the patient's recovery after cardiac surgery. Implantable VADs are an option for some patients with end-stage heart failure (Figure 34–4◆). Patients with such devices are able to return to their home setting and live with a significant improvement in their length and quality of life. The devices were designed for patients who need a bridge to heart transplantation or as a bridge to myocardial recovery (McMurray, 2010). The future and success of this technology will be based on appropriate patient selection, improved device durability, and coordinated teams who can provide long-term management to this specific population.

Acute Decompensated Heart Failure

Acute heart failure, the source of considerable expense to health care systems because of the need for frequent hospitalizations, has become a leading public health issue (Hunt et al., 2009; Lindenfeld et al., 2010). Acute presentations of heart failure are manifestations of elevated ventricular filling pressures causing sudden congestion in the pulmonary vasculature and periphery, decreased cardiac output leading to poor perfusion of the periphery and kidneys, and increased systemic vascular resistance causing increased work for the heart (see Chart 34–1, p. 1026, for causes of heart failure). Severe dyspnea is the leading symptom resulting in hospitalizations for heart failure, and its relief is usually a treatment priority. Paroxysmal nocturnal dyspnea, orthopnea, productive

CHART 34–7 Precipitating or Exacerbating Factors for Developing Acute Heart Failure

Noncompliance	Silent or overt ischemia
Dietary indiscretion	Fluid indiscretion
Untreated hypertension	Acute or chronic infection
Uncontrolled hyperglycemia	Thyroid dysfunction
Inadequate follow up	Atrial fibrillation, new or rapid
Other dysrhythmias	Renal or hepatic insufficiency
Pulmonary embolism	Substance abuse
Worsening valvular or cardiac function	Over-the-counter supplementation
Iatrogenic factors	
Anemia	Pregnancy

Factors that may precipitate or exacerbate heart failure are numerous and may be related to new or poorly controlled comorbid conditions, noncompliance, iatrogenic causes, or lack of adequate follow-up.

Sources: Adapted from Hunt, S. A., et al. (2009). Focused update incorporated into the ACC/AHA 2005 guidelines for the diagnosis and management of heart failure in adults: A report of the American College of Cardiology Foundation/American Heart Association Task Force on Practice Guidelines. *Circulation, 119*, e391– e479; Schocken, D. D., et al. (2008). Prevention of heart failure. *Circulation, 117*, 2544–2565.

or nonproductive cough, bloating, right upper quadrant pain due to hepatic congestion, and palpitations due to excess volume in the atria may also present in the acute setting (Lindenfeld et al., 2010).

Acute decompensated heart failure can be precipitated by many conditions and situations (Chart 34–7). Cardiac decompensation generally can be attributed to issues with compliance, new or worsening comorbid conditions, and/or progressive disease. Compliance issues that contribute to decompensated heart failure relate to failing to take medications or taking them inappropriately, excess sodium and fluid intake, inadequate outpatient treatment, or inadequate follow up. If acute decompensated heart failure is not treated, cardiogenic shock, multiorgan failure, and death may result.

Goals for the treatment of acute decompensated heart failure include the following:

- To determine the reason for the decompensated state
- To relieve congestive symptoms
- To reverse hemodynamic compromise
- To treat dysrhythmias
- To assess for exacerbating comorbid conditions
- To use prognosis-altering medications
- To assess for their candidacy for cardiac devices or end-stage therapies
- To provide self-management education
- To document that appropriate heart failure care was provided as mandated by regulatory entities.

In preparing patients with heart failure for life outside the hospital, the nurse should consider which patients might benefit from the organized structure of a heart failure disease management program. On presentation, the patient can be classified on the basis of degree of perfusion and volume status: well perfused and either hypervolemic or hypovolemic, or poorly perfused and either hypervolemic or hypovolemic (Figure 34–5◆).

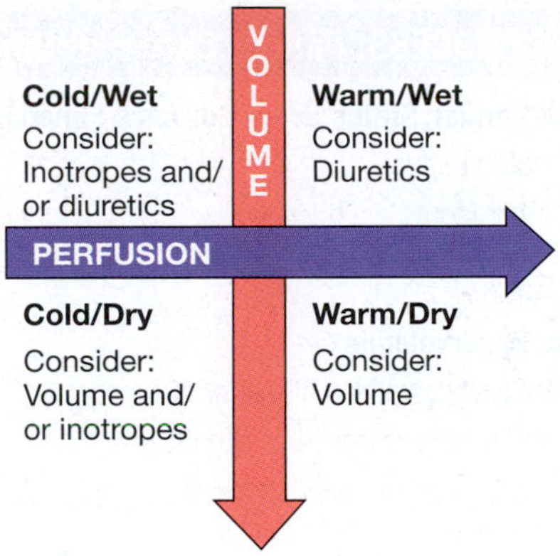

FIGURE 34–5 ◆ Volume versus perfusion.

Nursing Management

The nursing care of a patient with heart failure is directed at treating congestion and monitoring the patient's response to therapy. Fluid retention is the primary reason most patients with heart failure are admitted or readmitted to the hospital. Nursing goals of treatment for acute decompensated heart failure include assessing response to diuresis, monitoring intake/output and daily weights, assessing cardiac output, monitoring for dysrhythmias, encouraging increased levels of activity, performing ADLs, and enhancing patient knowledge of the disease process. Application of the nursing process will facilitate a comprehensive approach to patient assessment and care. The Nursing Process: Patient Care Plan for Heart Failure box applies the nursing process to the relevant nursing diagnosis of congestion and provides a comprehensive care plan for a patient with heart failure during hospitalization. The Patient Teaching & Discharge Priorities box outlines discharge care for patients with heart failure. It is also essential that cultural considerations be addressed because they potentially impact the patient's ability to prevent progression of the disease. The Cultural Considerations box (p. 1052) presents necessary considerations related to African American patients.

Collaborative Management

Patients with heart failure need a multidisciplinary team approach to achieve optimal recovery and return to society. Nurses at all levels collaborate with health care providers, health care provider assistants, dietitians, pharmacists, social workers, and cardiac rehabilitation specialists across various care settings. Close scrutiny by the team is required to provide optimal, evidence-based care. In order to meet desired patient outcomes, it is essential that the members of this multidisciplinary team communicate openly with one another in developing and evaluating care of the patient and family (IOM [Institute of Medicine], 2010). Nursing assessment of subjective and objective measures of adequate diuresis will allow for prompt notification of the health care provider if adjustments to the medical plan are needed. Nursing staff also can focus on the essential aspects of patient self-management, including instruction on medications, activity, daily weights, dietary guidance, and symptom management. A comprehensive nutritional plan should include helping patients follow a restricted salt and liquid diet. Dietitians provide patients and families with a greater understanding of appropriate food and fluid guidelines. When hypervolemia is present, patients generally have a decline in physical activity, with dyspnea being their primary source of limitation in activity. Cardiac rehabilitation specialists help mobilize patients with monitored physical activity during their

NURSING PROCESS: Patient Care Plan for Heart Failure

Assessment of Cardiac Status Using Gordon's Functional Health Patterns:

- Nutrition Metabolic Pattern
- Activity Exercise Pattern
- Cognitive Perceptual Pattern

Subjective Data

Assessment of Hypervolemia

Are you having difficulty breathing at rest or with activity?

How long have you had shortness of breath (SOB)?

Do you need to sleep with your head propped up, or do you awaken in the middle of the night feeling short of breath?

Do you have a cough?

Do you have abdominal bloating or lower extremity swelling?

Have you had recent weight increase over a short period of time (2 to 3 days)?

Assessment of Cardiac Output

How is your energy level?

Are symptoms limiting your level of activity?

Are you light-headed?

Are you having memory problems or trouble concentrating?

Are you making the same amount of urine as usual?

Objective Data

Assessment of Hypervolemia

Vital signs: weight, blood pressure, heart rate (HR).

Oxygen saturation.

Dyspnea with exertion.

Lethargy.

Anxiety.

Lung sounds: crackles/wheezes.

Restlessness.

Distended neck veins.

Ascites and/or lower extremity edema.

Daily weight.

Hemodynamic parameters:

1. Right atrial pressure (RAP) or central venous pressure (CVP)
2. Pulmonary artery pressure (PAP systolic [PAS], diastolic [PAD], and mean)
3. Pulmonary artery occlusion pressure (PAOP)
4. Cardiac output (CO) and cardiac index (CI).

Peripheral circulation:

1. Peripheral pulses.
2. Presence of edema using the edema scale.
3. Color and temperature.
4. Capillary refill time.

Intake and output:

1. Assess volume of fluid intake by any route (e.g., oral, intravenous).
2. Assess volume of fluid expelled by any route (e.g., urinary, nasogastric [NG], drainage, blood).

Evaluate laboratory/diagnostic findings associated with hypervolemia:

1. Serum sodium (may be decreased, normal, or elevated based on cause of hypervolemia).
2. BUN (may be abnormal).
3. Urine specific gravity (may be abnormal).
4. Hematocrit (may be decreased).
5. Chest x-ray (may show pulmonary congestion or cardiomegaly).
6. Right heart catheterization (may indicate elevated filling pressures).

Assessment of Cardiac Output

Cardiovascular system:

1. Heart rate
2. Heart rhythm
3. Blood pressure
4. Peripheral pulses
5. Presence of edema using the edema scale
6. Color and temperature
7. Capillary refill time.

Heart sounds: murmurs, clicks, rubs, splitting.

Pulmonary status.

Oxygen saturation.

NURSING PROCESS: Patient Care Plan for Heart Failure, *continued*

Hemodynamic parameters (as applicable) (Chapter 31):

1. Right atrial pressure (RAP) or central venous pressure (CVP)
2. Pulmonary artery pressure (PAP systolic [PAS], diastolic [PAD], and mean)
3. Pulmonary artery occlusion pressure (PAOP)
4. Cardiac output (CO) and cardiac index (CI).

Intake and output:

1. Assess the volume of fluid intake by any route (e.g., oral, intravenous).
2. Assess the volume of fluid expelled by any route (e.g., urinary, NG, drainage, blood).

ECG waveform (rhythm and intervals) as ordered (including cardiac rhythm, PR interval, QRS interval, QT/QTc interval, dysrhythmias) (Chapter 30).

Obtain weight.

Evaluate laboratory/diagnostic findings associated with decreased cardiac output:

1. Serum BUN and creatinine (may be elevated)
2. Serum hematocrit, hemoglobin (may be decreased)
3. Echocardiogram (may show depressed ventricular function, pericardial effusion)
4. 12-lead ECG (may show dysrhythmias, myocardial infarction, heart block, tachycardia, or bradycardia)
5. Blood gases (may show acidosis, hypoxemia) (Chapter 15)
6. Arterial–mixed venous blood gases may show an increased SaO_2/SvO_2 ratio.

Assessment of Activity Tolerance

How much activity are you able to do (i.e., walk for 5, 10, 30+ minutes, or not at all)?

Are you more or less active now than 1, 3, and 6 months ago?

Are you able to walk up 1 or 2 flights of stairs without stopping?

Do you have symptoms during exercise (chest pain, shortness of breath, palpitations, and light-headedness)?

Assessment of Activity Tolerance

Vital signs: blood pressure (BP) and heart rate (HR).

Oxygen saturation.

NYHA classification for heart failure assessment (p. 1030).

Pain scale.

6-minute walk.

Assessment of Dysrhythmias

Do you experience palpitations or feel that your heart races?

Do you become light-headed or pass out?

Do palpitations or light-headedness occur at the same time?

Assessment of Dysrhythmias

Vital signs: blood pressure, heart rate, and heart rhythm.

Oxygen saturation.

Level of consciousness.

ECG.

Laboratory values: electrolytes and measures of acidosis.

Lung/cardiac.

Abdomen.

Integument.

Urine output.

Cardiac devices (if present).

Assessment of Knowledge Deficit

Patient/family express concerns about the diagnosis of heart failure, in terms of prognosis, changes in lifestyle, and progression of disease.

Patient/family exhibits a lack of understanding of the therapies for treatment of heart failure.

Patient/family express concerns about how to take medications and their potential side effects.

Patient/family express concerns about what symptoms they might have and how to monitor them at home.

Patient/family express concerns about continuing a sexual relationship.

Patient/family express concerns about treatment options if medicines fail.

Patient/family express concerns about the mode of death.

Assessment of Knowledge Deficit

Patients may be anxious, confused, and may need repeated information.

(*continued*)

NURSING PROCESS: Patient Care Plan for Heart Failure, *continued*

Outcomes and Evaluation Parameters	Planning and Interventions with *Rationales*
1. NURSING DIAGNOSIS: Fluid Volume Excess *related to ventricular dysfunction and sodium/water retention* (NANDA-I © 2012)	
Outcome: Diuresis: improved volume status (i.e., euvolemia) and improved symptoms. ***Evaluation Parameters:*** Blood pressure target: 120/80 mmHg. Heart rate target: 60–100 beats/min. Improved New York Heart Association (NYHA) class (p. 1030). No signs of pulmonary congestion: airway patent; respiratory rate $<$ 20 breaths/minute; pattern regular and unlabored; lungs clear to auscultation all lobes bilaterally. Oxygen saturation $>$ 90% in patients breathing room air. Hemodynamic parameters (normal levels) (Chapter 31): 1. RAP 1–7 mmHg or CVP 2–8 cm H_2O 2. PAP 15–25/6–12 mmHg (mean 10–20 mmHg) 3. PAOP 6–12 mmHg 4. CO 3.5–5.5 L/min or CI 2.0–3.2 L/min/m^2. Peripheral circulation: 1. Pulse 2–3+ on pulse grading scale 2. No edema 3. Skin warm, natural color 4. Capillary refill time less than 3 seconds. Intake and output: 1. Intake/output difference greater than 1,000 mL/24 hours or as defined for diuresis per provider 2. Urinary output average of greater than or equal to 30 mL/hr. Daily morning weight less than the day prior. Abdomen soft, nondistended; no ascites. The following laboratory/diagnostic studies are within normal limits: Serum sodium Blood urea nitrogen (BUN) Urine specific gravity Hematocrit (laboratory and diagnostic studies, p. 1034).	Insert intravenous catheter *to facilitate intravenous medication administration.* Administer and titrate intravenous (IV) medications *to facilitate diuresis.* Record amount of intravenous (IV) fluid infused *to monitor intake.* Assess vital signs and urine output regularly (every hour or more frequently) *to assess adequacy of diuresis.* Monitor central venous pressure (CVP) and pulmonary artery occlusion pressure (PAOP), if possible (Chapter 31) *to assess the response to diuresis.* Obtain and track daily morning weight *to monitor the adequacy of diuresis.* Monitor serum electrolytes, hematocrit, serum creatinine, and report critical abnormalities to the provider *to monitor hematological changes associated with hypervolemia, possibly hypovolemia, electrolyte changes, and diuresis.* Instruct patient on fluid and sodium restrictions *to prevent excess oral intake, which would negate the effect of diuresis.*
2. NURSING DIAGNOSIS: Decreased Cardiac Output *related to ventricular dysfunction* (NANDA-I © 2012)	
Outcome: Adequate cardiac output as seen by improved organ, tissue, and cerebral perfusion related to improved cardiac output. ***Evaluation Parameters:*** Cardiovascular system: 1. Heart rate: 60–100 beats/min 2. Regular rhythm or patient's normal asymptomatic rhythm 3. BP: 120/80 mmHg 4. Pulses 2–3+ on pulse grading scale 5. No edema 6. Skin warm and normal color, no cyanosis noted 7. Capillary refill time less than or equal to 3 seconds. Heart sounds: normal S_1 and S_2. Airway patent; respiratory rate $<$ 20 per minute, pattern regular and unlabored; lungs clear to auscultation all lobes bilaterally. Oxygen saturation $>$ 90% in patients breathing room air. Hemodynamic parameters: 1. RAP 1–7 mmHg or CVP 2–8 cm H_2O 2. PAP 15–25/6–12 mmHg (mean 10–20 mmHg) 3. PAOP 6–12 mmHg 4. CO 3.5–5.5 L/min or CI 2.0–3.2 L/min/m^2.	Insert intravenous catheter *to facilitate intravenous medication administration.* Administer and titrate IV medications *to facilitate diuresis and inotropic support.* Record amount of IV fluid infused *to monitor intake.* Assess vital signs and urine output regularly (every hour or less) *to assess adequacy of diuresis and inotropic support.* Monitor hourly urine output *to assess adequacy of diuresis.* Monitor central venous pressure (CVP) and pulmonary artery occlusion pressures (PAOP, CO/CI), if possible *to assess adequacy of diuresis and inotropic support of cardiac output.* Monitor integument and neurological status *to assess for adequacy of tissue and cerebral perfusion.* Administer oxygen *to ensure proper oxygenation and tissue perfusion.* Administration of medications *to improve cardiac output, tissue perfusion, and diuresis.*

NURSING PROCESS: Patient Care Plan for Heart Failure, *continued*

Intake and output:

1. Intake/output difference greater than 1,000 mL/24 hours or as defined for diuresis per provider
2. Urinary output average of greater than or equal to 30 mL/hr.

ECG is stable, with regular rhythm or patient's normal asymptomatic rhythm, without evidence of ischemia, myocardial infarction, tachycardia/bradycardia, or heart block.

Cardiac intervals are within normal limits (Chapter 30):

- PR interval: 0.12–0.20 second
- QRS interval: < 0.10 second
- QTc interval: 0.37–0.047 second.

Daily morning weight less than the day prior.

The following laboratory/diagnostic studies are within normal limits: serum sodium, blood urea nitrogen (BUN), urine specific gravity, hematocrit, and ABGs (laboratory and diagnostic studies, p. 1034).

3 NURSING DIAGNOSIS: Risk for Activity Intolerance *related to impaired cardiac function secondary to chronic heart failure* (NANDA-I © 2012)

Outcome: Activity tolerance stabilizes or improves as seen by improved NYHA classification for heart failure, as well as decreased symptoms.

Evaluation Parameters: Normal vital signs.

Oxygen levels are within normal range: oxygen saturation ≥ 90%.

Patient has clear plan for activity, with reasonable goals.

Symptoms during activity are minimal.

Patients have action plan for symptoms that occur.

NYHA classification for heart failure has improved.

Pain scale improves.

Strength and balance improve.

Nutrition improves.

Weight reduction occurs (if needed).

Stress is reduced.

Smoking cessation is successful.

Monitor vital signs at rest, with activity, and 3 minutes after activity (heart rate, BP, respiratory rate) *to obtain a baseline for comparison.*

Monitor oxygenation before, during, and after activity *to obtain a baseline for comparison.*

Assess baseline activity level (including strength and balance) and tolerance to activity *to use as a basis for an individualized plan.*

Assess symptoms at rest and with activity *to use as a baseline for comparison.*

Patients understand the symptoms to monitor during activity: increased shortness of breath, chest pain, palpitations, light-headedness.

Monitor level of pain.

Assess degree of symptoms (NYHA class) *to use as a baseline for comparison.*

Assess the patient's perception of her quality of life (QOL) using a standardized tool such as SF-36. This information can be used as *a baseline for comparison during treatment.*

Promote activity: Start with a reasonable daily plan, increase slowly, set reachable goals, plan around periods of rest, and reassure that small improvements will lead to physical, emotional, and psychosocial benefits. *An individualized plan of care will promote change.*

Promote exercise prescription: type, activity, duration, intensity. Monitor level of strength *to individualize each patient's plan.*

Teach an appropriate diet to accompany an activity plan. Assess the body mass index (BMI). Monitor the current level of nutrition and calorie content *to enhance balanced nutrition and promote weight loss as needed.*

Teach strengthening exercises *to promote muscular strength to improve balance.*

Discuss level of stress and anxiety.

Teach stress reduction techniques *to facilitate well-being and foster an activity plan.* (More information is available in Chapter 9.)

Stress smoking cessation. *Smoking decreases oxygenation to muscles during activity.*

Teach heart failure symptoms to monitor and which need to be reported to the health care provider: shortness of breath, chest pain, light-headedness, passing out, and palpitations *to obtain a baseline for comparison and need for further treatment.*

(continued)

NURSING PROCESS: Patient Care Plan for Heart Failure, *continued*

4. NURSING DIAGNOSIS: Cardiac Output Decreased Due to Dysrhythmias Related to Impaired Cardiac Function *related to secondary ischemia, acidosis, hypoxemia, electrolyte abnormalities, structural/conduction abnormalities, or device implantation* (NANDA-I © 2012)

Outcomes and Evaluation Parameters

Outcome: Absence of hemodynamically significant dysrhythmias.

Evaluation Parameters: Heart rate is within normal range (60–80, or not > 100 beats per minute).

Breath sounds are normal and clear, without respiratory distress.

Oxygen levels are within normal range: Oxygen saturation ≥ 90%.

Patient has no altered level of consciousness (LOC) or anxiety.

ECG is stable, with regular rhythm or patient's normal asymptomatic rhythm, without evidence of ischemia, myocardial infarction, tachycardia/bradycardia, or heart block.

Cardiac intervals are within normal limits (Chapter 30).

Laboratory values are within normal limits:

Potassium, magnesium, digoxin level optimal, arterial blood gases within normal limits or normal enough that the patient is asymptomatic.

Abdomen is soft, without pain, ascites, and organomegaly.

Urine output remains normal.

Integument is dry, warm, and well perfused.

Cardiac device interrogation: shows properly functioning device with settings optimized and optimal battery life with leads intact.

Planning and Interventions with *Rationales*

Assess cardiovascular status: heart rate, regularity of rhythm (pattern), and blood pressure *to assess baseline and monitor for changes and response to therapy.*

Assess lung sounds *to assess for the presence of lung fluid from increased dysrhythmias, causing a drop in cardiac output.*

Assess oxygenation saturation *to monitor baseline for changes with dysrhythmias and response to therapy.*

Assess level of consciousness (LOC) *to assess for tissue perfusion.*

Assess ECG and waveforms (rhythm, PR, QRS, and QTc intervals, dysrhythmias) *to establish a baseline and determine the degree of abnormality and response to therapies.*

Assess lab and blood gas values (potassium, magnesium, calcium, digoxin level, presence of acidosis) *to establish a baseline and determine the degree of abnormality and response to therapies.*

Assess the abdomen *to assess for ascites, abdominal pain, presence of bowel sounds, and organomegaly.*

Assess urine output *to assess for decreases that may occur with dysrhythmias.*

Assess integument *to assess for cyanosis, pallor, or diaphoresis.*

Assess cardiac device if present (i.e., pacemaker, cardiac defibrillator) *to assess proper position of leads and for appropriate device function.*

5. NURSING DIAGNOSIS: Deficient Knowledge *related to the diagnosis of heart failure* (NANDA-I © 2012)

Outcomes and Evaluation Parameters

Outcomes: Patient/family understand:

The diagnosis of heart failure.

Their prognosis.

Treatments for heart failure.

Lifestyle changes.

Progression of the disease.

Symptoms to monitor.

Sexuality.

End-stage treatment options.

Mode of death.

Evaluation Parameters: Patient/family will:

- Ask appropriate questions about the course of heart failure.
- Follow appropriate medication adjustments, and consider recommendations for surgical procedures and devices.
- Come in with a completed self-care diary, following instructions between visits.
- Call when their symptoms worsen for urgent evaluation when needed.
- Express successful maintenance of a sexual relationship.
- Understand which end-stage therapies are available and for which they qualify.
- Understand the usual mode of death of heart failure, make appropriate plans with their health care team and family regarding their wishes, and complete advanced directives and power of attorney.

Planning and Interventions with *Rationales*

Discuss with the patient/family the course of heart failure using the diagram. *This will enhance their understanding of the chronic and progressive nature of the disease, which usually presents with periods of exacerbation and stabilization.*

Discuss how heart failure is treated with the patient and family. *This will provide the fundamental treatment strategies for heart failure including medications, surgical strategies, and devices.*

Discuss with patients/family self-management support (see Figure 34–6, p. 1048). *This will teach the basic concepts that will help them to understand their medications, about activity, the importance of daily weights, their diet, and what to do when their symptoms worsen.*

Discuss the common symptoms of heart failure with the patient and family, describing shortness of breath, cough, fatigue, activity intolerance, weight gain/edema, palpitations, chest tightness, and poor concentration. *This will enable the patient to recognize her symptoms and reinforce calling early when her symptoms worsen, so she can be seen and have adjustments made in her medications, preempting an urgent hospitalization.*

Discuss ways for the patient and significant other to maintain a sexual relationship. Patients will understand that having sexual intercourse is about the amount of effort involved in climbing two flights of stairs. If they are able to complete this activity without significant symptoms, then sexual intercourse will likely be safe. *Patients will understand other means of sexual intimacy and will understand what to do if symptoms worsen during sexual activities.*

Describe end-stage treatment options to the patient and family. Those who fail standard therapy might be considered for cardiac transplantation, mechanical assist devices, and heart failure research studies, or for hospice care. *The patient and family will understand which of the preceding end-stage therapies they might be considered for and why they might not be a candidate for others.*

Describe the mode of death for patients with heart failure. *Most patients with heart failure die either by a sudden dysrhythmia (caused by ventricular tachycardia or fibrillation) or by progressive deterioration of the cardiac muscle and its function. Dying suddenly will be a fast, typically painless, way to die. Dying of progressive disease is typically associated with more symptoms that will require an individualized plan for symptom relief by medicines such as narcotics, anxiolytics, nitrates, diuretics, and oxygen.*

Source: Adapted from Wilkinson, J. M., & Ahearn, N. R. (2009). *Prentice Hall nursing diagnosis handbook* (9th ed.). Upper Saddle River, NJ: Prentice Hall.

PATIENT TEACHING & DISCHARGE PRIORITIES for Heart Failure

Patients discharged from the hospital have multiple needs. Teaching strategies should be based on these needs, with the goals of preventing readmissions, slowing disease progression, and improving quality of life.

Several criteria must be met prior to discharge. For example, the patient must have stable blood pressure and renal function on oral medications. In the 24 hours prior to discharge, it is essential that the patient remain stable. The nurse must assess fluid status for euvolemia, vital signs must remain within normal limits for this patient, the patient must be able to walk without dyspnea or light-headedness, and the cardiac rhythm must be stable.

Once the patient is ready for discharge, it is essential that the nurse implement a teaching plan that will help prevent a recurrence of the patient's heart failure. A practical approach, tailored to individual patients, will be needed to help patients integrate self-management strategies at home.

Need	Teaching
Patient/family	Teach the patient about medications, activity, weights, diet, and symptoms.
• Prevent recurrent symptoms of congestion.	
• Optimize medical therapy for heart failure and comorbid conditions.	Provide a list of current medications to patients with dose and schedule, along with clear instructions on changes from prehospitalization. Instruct the patient about the purpose of medications; the need to refill prescriptions before running out; not doubling up for missed doses; and the importance of calling the health care provider if the patient experiences adverse effects.
• Increase activity tolerance.	Instruct the patient to increase activity as tolerated, monitoring for symptoms; to become active most days; and to call the health care provider if the patient experiences new or worsened symptoms or diminishing ability to perform ADLs.
• Minimize risk factors.	Review health maintenance strategies: smoking cessation, limited alcohol intake, regular exercise, stress reduction, eating a balanced diet, and optimally treating comorbid conditions.
• Provide palliative care.	Discuss the chronic nature of the disease; encourage a multidisciplinary team meeting that includes the patient and their caregiver(s) regarding overall plans for care. Have family members or a person living with the patient learn CPR if the patient wishes to be resuscitated.
Family/support system • Assess resources to assist with chronic illness in the home setting.	Provide resources based on the individual's needs: home health, hospice, and family/friends/neighbors to help with home care, meals, and transportation.
Setting • Assess home needs.	Assess safety from falls for patients who are weak and at risk for falling; use occupational therapy to assess home safety and for home aids for debilitated patients.

hospitalization and may provide a plan to follow after discharge. Social workers can evaluate and instruct patients on the psychosocial aspects of this diagnosis and address any financial concerns.

Since 2001, The Joint Commission (TJC) has mandated that patients admitted to the hospital with heart failure must have documentation of their care related to the following: (1) ventricular function is measured (most commonly by echocardiography); (2) patients with an LVEF less than 40% receive an ACE inhibitor (or ARB) unless contraindicated; (3) patients receive self-management instruction before discharge; and (4) smoking-cessation counseling is provided to smokers (TJC, 2010). Plans for optimal outpatient management should focus on ways to prevent readmissions for heart failure, to improve the prognosis, to decrease mortality, to foster adherence, and to restore the patient's functional capacity. Educating patients with heart failure about standardized self-management techniques has led to reductions in mortality and should be a focus prior to discharge.

Health Promotion

Heart failure management would be incomplete without the vital step of providing patients with self-management instruction and education from nurses and other members of the health care team. Research supports the importance self-management has on indexes such as quality of life, readmission rates, and functional status (Steckler et al., 2010). Not only have heart failure medications altered patients' prognoses, but evidence shows that the addition of self-management education can reduce mortality as well. Essential principles that focus on living with heart failure couple medications with nonpharmacologic therapies. Nonpharmacologic management strategies include appropriate diet and nutrition, health maintenance, and psychosocial lifestyle changes.

The key concepts that patients must learn to incorporate into their daily lives include medications, activity, weight, diet, and symptoms, as depicted in Figure 34–6◆ (p. 1048). If these concepts are followed, reductions in readmissions and costs associated with heart failure may occur (Steckler et al., 2010). A good self-management plan includes the following:

- Educating the patient and family about medications, activity, daily weight, low-sodium diet, fluid restriction, and changes in symptoms.
- Ensuring that the patient understands when to call the health care provider about worsening symptoms.
- Scheduling of a follow up appointment.

Medications

Patients need instruction about how their medications act to improve symptoms, prevent hospitalizations, and prevent death. The typical patient with heart failure is on a complicated medical regimen for the heart condition along with therapy for comorbid conditions. The more medications a person takes in a day, the more he is at risk for noncompliance or mistakes with the regimen. Patients need to understand the names of the medications, the times of the day they should be taken, their purpose, and what to do in case of missed doses and/or adverse

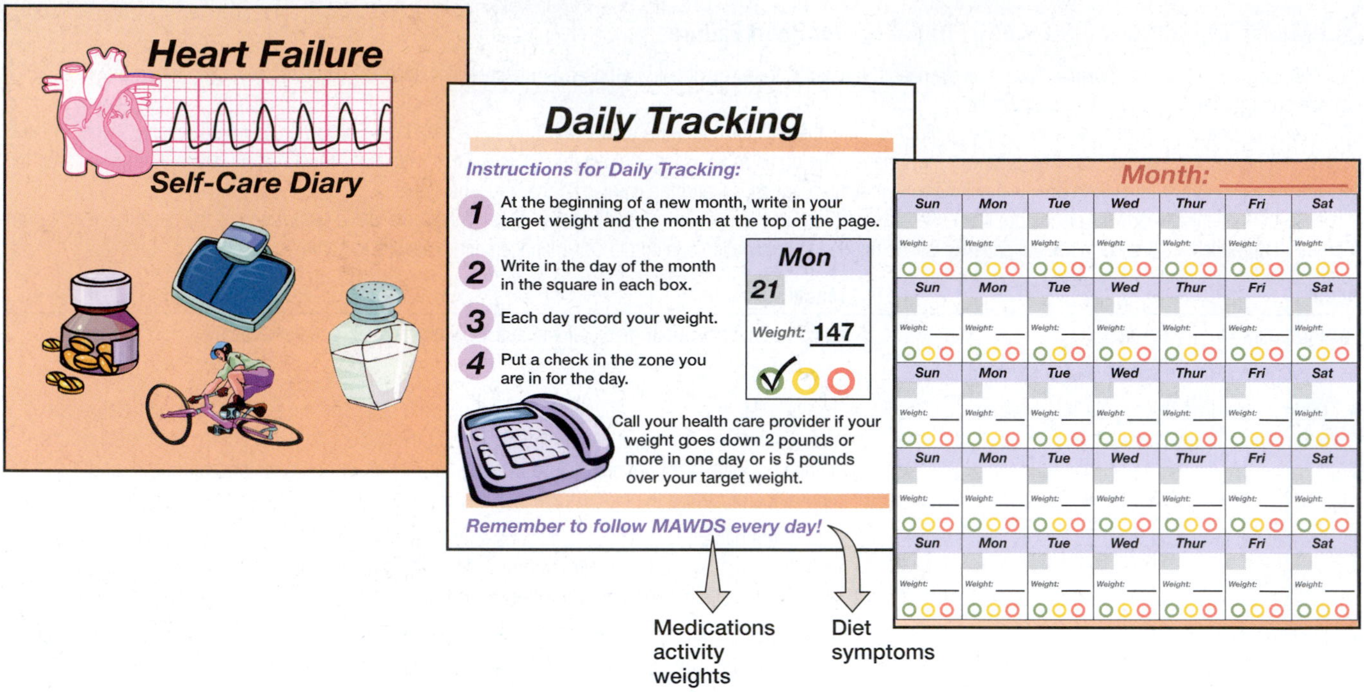

FIGURE 34–6 ◆ Heart failure self-care diary.

reactions. The nurse must plan strategies aimed to increase long-term compliance and access to medications for those with limited resources.

Activity

Exercise can have significant benefits for patients with heart failure. Hemodynamic parameters, quality-of-life indexes, functional status, and depression scores are all improved when people with heart failure exercise on a consistent basis (Lindenfeld et al., 2010). The reality of living with heart failure, however, is that the syndrome involves a cycle of inactivity that leads to further deconditioning. The challenge is, therefore, to encourage a reasonable exercise program that will lead to clinical benefits. Cardiac rehabilitation may be started during a hospitalization in stable patients. An exercise prescription given to patients must include the type, frequency, duration, and intensity of exercise (Chart 34–8). Working with patients to set reasonable goals is critical so that success with an exercise prescription may be achieved. Assessing behavioral and motivational issues is important for patients who have struggled with maintaining an active lifestyle.

Weight

One of the most important aspects of self-management for patients to understand is that they must record their weight daily and know what to

CHART 34–8 Exercise Prescription

Patients with heart failure usually fall into a cycle of inactivity leading to further deconditioning. Exercise is usually limited by symptoms of congestion or poor perfusion. It is important to provide thorough instructions to patients on how to exercise safely as they live with heart failure.

Exercise Prescription	Recommendation to Patients	Caution to Patients
Type of exercise	Walk, run, bike, swim, or hike. Factors such as personal preference, location, orthopedic challenges, and so on, will help plan the type of exercise. Choosing a type of exercise the patient will enjoy should help the patient to be motivated to continue this activity over the long term.	Do not pursue an activity known to exacerbate certain conditions patients may have (e.g., walking downhill, which causes more knee pain).
Intensity of exercise	Discuss in terms of being able to maintain a conversation while exerting, yet having a high enough amount of energy expenditure.	Having significant symptoms of dyspnea, chest pain, or light-headedness means that the patient should reduce or stop the activity.
Duration of exercise	Will depend on the baseline level of fitness. Start slowly and increase the duration of activity over time.	Reduce the duration and intensity of exercise if the patient is too tired to perform activities of daily living (ADLs) the day following an activity.
Frequency of exercise	Be active most days of the week.	The patient should not worry if he needs to skip a day occasionally. The patient should simply try being active most days.

Source: Adapted from Hunt et al. (2009). Focused update incorporated into the ACC/AHA 2005 guidelines for the diagnosis and management of heart failure in adults: A report of the American College of Cardiology Foundation/American Heart Association Task Force on Practice Guidelines. *Circulation, 119*, e391– e479.

do when it deviates from a dry weight. The ultimate goal is to maintain a state of euvolemia, in which the patient is not retaining fluid. This means less congestion and fewer symptoms (McMurray, 2010). As easy as this concept sounds, it can be quite a challenge to health care providers to work out a plan with patients related to their weight. Some terms used to describe a "goal" weight when there is an absence of congestion are *optivolemic* and *euvolemic*. This weight needs to be determined in conjunction with the health care provider and may change over time with weight gain or loss from causes other than fluid retention. Patients feel better when they are not congested and also are more likely stay out of the hospital.

Patients should be instructed to call their health care provider when their weight increases 2 or more pounds overnight or increases to more than 5 pounds from their "goal" weight. Conversely, patients who lose too much weight are at risk of dehydration and possibly syncope. A 5-pound or greater drop below their goal weight should prompt a call to their health care team. Patients should have an individualized plan for self-adjusted diuretic dosing regimens to achieve relief of congestion and limit the chance of readmission.

Diet

Patients need instruction to help them understand that treating congestion with diuretics offers the best result when coupled with limiting dietary sodium (Lindenfeld et al., 2010). Patients who have heart failure with congestive symptoms should be counseled to ingest less than 1.5 grams of sodium daily (AHA, 2011). Those with persistent evidence of volume overload should also ingest less than 2 quarts (or liters) of all fluids per day. Following a low-sodium diet is challenging, because the American diet usually consists of much more than 2 grams of sodium daily. In fact, most Americans complain about food lacking in flavor when they change to the reduced sodium preparation; herbs and spices should be encouraged, as they add flavor to foods without increasing sodium. See Chart 34–9 for a list of foods that are commonly known to be high in sodium content, along with recommended lower-sodium alternatives. Patients often need help to understand how to read food labels, how to calculate their sodium intake, and how to make wise food selections when eating out. Meeting with a dietitian and with other patients to share shopping and food preparation tips will likely heighten success and compliance. Chapter 8 includes a specific discussion of low-sodium diets.

Weblink: Dietary Sodium Recommendations

Weblink: Sodium

Many patients with heart failure complain of "thirst." This mechanism is a neurohormonal response that tries to trick the body into seeking and retaining more fluids so that blood volume will increase, leading to increased flow to the renal system. Unfortunately, in heart failure, the heart is unable to keep up with the body's demands, and backward flow results in "volume-overloaded" patients and worsened symptoms. Low sodium intake coupled with fluid restriction will assist patients in maintaining their goal weight and often lead to reductions in diuretic dosing.

Symptoms

It is vital that patients understand the typical symptoms of heart failure including exertional dyspnea, orthopnea, paroxysmal nocturnal dyspnea, cough, edema, fatigue, and activity intolerance. Symptoms of heart failure lead to a poorer quality of life and result in frequent hospitalizations (Hunt et al., 2009; Lindenfeld et al., 2010). Each patient should receive clear instruction on how to track her own symptoms and when to call if symptoms worsen. If a patient calls early enough, the issue may be managed on an outpatient basis, preventing an emergency department visit or hospitalization. Patients with heart failure need to understand that their symptoms will wax and wane, resulting in a combination of good and bad days. It is critical that patients listen to their bodies and keep track of objective information (such as weight, blood pressure, and heart rate) that should be reported. See Figure 34–6 for an example of a tool used to help patients monitor and

CHART 34–9 Dietary Sodium Recommendations

The sodium-restricted diet (1.5 g/day) is a well-known part of the heart failure patient's self-management. It is important that the patient understand this diet and the need to comply with it.

Food Group	High-Sodium Choice	Lower-Sodium Alternative
Meats/fish/poultry	Cured meats (bacon, ham) Processed meats: jerky, salami, sausage Stews, casseroles, anchovies, pickled herring, crab, canned meat/fish/poultry	Fresh lean meat seasoned with herbs/spices, roasted, baked, boiled, or poached
Vegetables	Canned soups or vegetables; canned vegetable juices; those in sauce or au gratin; canned beans including: refried beans, pork and beans, kidney beans	Any vegetables; stewed, steamed, fresh, or boiled, plain or seasoned with herbs/spices
Carbohydrates	Pretzels, potato chips, peanuts, popcorn, bagels, croissants, English muffins, oyster crackers, pita pockets, pancakes, stuffing, packaged puddings, pastries, cream pies, ice cream, creamed potatoes, noodles in cream sauce, fried rice	Fresh fruit, angel food cake, sherbet, frozen/nonfat yogurt, ice milk, gelatin, hard or soft rolls, plain bread or toast, unsalted crackers, breadsticks, mashed/baked/steamed/boiled potatoes, boiled or steamed rice, boiled noodles
Dairy/fats	Cottage cheese, Parmesan cheese, other hard and/or processed cheeses	Mozzarella cheese
Condiments	Canned gravies, salad dressings, canned sauces, soy sauce, ketchup, mustard, olives, pickles, bouillon	Homemade low-sodium gravy, other herbs/spices, oil and vinegar dressing, low-salt dressings
Fast foods	Hamburgers, cheeseburgers, fried chicken, pizza, onion rings, fish sandwiches, burritos	Salad bars, baked potatoes without toppings, broiled chicken sandwich without sauce, fresh fruits/vegetables, sandwiches with low-salt meat and cheese options and limited spreads
Other	Frozen foods, milkshakes, chocolate or whole milk, cocoa, alcoholic drinks	Fruit juices, skim milk, soft drinks, tea, or coffee

Source: Adapted from Mayo Clinic. (2012). Sodium: How to tame the salt habit. Retrieved from http://www.mayoclinic.com/health/sodium/NU00284.

record their weights. This tool also can be used to communicate with the health care team about changes that occur outside predetermined parameters of weight and symptoms.

Family/Significant Other Support

Heart failure, like other chronic diseases, requires support from family, significant others, and members of the community. Heart failure can pose both emotional and physical challenges to patients and those surrounding them. When patients are initially diagnosed, during times of exacerbations, and as they approach the end-of-life stage, patients with heart failure may need a significant amount of emotional and physical support. Patients and their loved ones need to understand the chronicity of the disease with which they live so they can make foreseeable adjustments to their daily activities to ensure an acceptable quality of life. This may include adjustments in all family-related activities such as family meal preparation and home maintenance. Meals should be planned that adhere to the patient's sodium and fluid restrictions. Available Internet resources, such as those found through the American Association of Heart Failure Nurses, can help both patients and families better understand how to live with this common condition.

Lifestyles and Habits

Promoting healthy lifestyles is critical for all patients, including patients with heart failure. General health promotion strategies, which should be age and gender focused, include the following:

- Smoking cessation
- Regular physical activity and weight control
- Limited alcohol use and discouraged illicit drug use
- Dental care
- Vaccination for influenza and pneumonia
- Stress reduction techniques
- Discontinuance of nonsteroidal anti-inflammatory drugs (NSAIDs)
- Regular health care follow up.

It is essential that patients with heart failure follow additional disease prevention strategies for infection, CAD, hypertension, diabetes, hyperlipidemia, obesity, and malnutrition. Infection prevention includes recommendations for an annual influenza vaccination and a current pneumococcal vaccination. For patients with valvular heart disease, endocarditis prophylaxis should be followed for dental and other invasive procedures (see Chapter 33). Primary prevention strategies for CAD include smoking cessation, regular exercise, and maintaining a healthy body weight. Additionally, CAD secondary prevention strategies focus on tight control of comorbid conditions that may influence the development or worsening of heart failure including diabetes, hypertension, hyperlipidemia, and obesity.

Hypertension and hyperlipidemia screening and treatment not only may prevent the development of CAD but also may prevent systolic dysfunction. Lifestyle changes including more exercise and better dietary choices will also help reduce hypertension and hyperlipidemia. Aggressively treating diabetes, targeting an optimal hemoglobin A_{1C}, and preventing target organ damage will limit the risk of developing CAD and subsequent systolic dysfunction. Regular exercise and an improved diet will also prevent obesity and malnutrition.

Heart Failure Resources for Patients and Families

Many resources are available to help the nurse educate the patient. It is also vital for nurses to instruct patients on how to access educational materials. In this multimedia era, numerous resource options are available to patients with heart failure. Web-based sites for heart failure represent many different entities providing information: organizations specific to heart failure and cardiology, hospital systems providing heart failure care, governmental agencies with guidelines for treatment, drug and device companies with product information and patient education, patients with their own websites, studies done on heart failure, and more. The nurse can help patients by providing tips about some of the more credible Internet sites, which are those ending in .edu, .gov, and .org. Well-established organizations that provide valuable resources include the Heart Failure Society of America, the American Association of Heart Failure Nurses, and the American Heart Association.

Other resources on heart failure can be obtained through books from hospital, university, or public libraries. Many companies have produced videos for patients to help them better understand heart failure. In addition, drug and device companies and hospital systems often produce tools that focus on patient and family education. Community-based resources include health care fairs, community lecture series, the local health department, the local chapter of the American Heart Association, and hospitals and care providers in the community. Patients with heart failure need resources that are sensitive to various cultures, presented in multiple languages, and developed at appropriate levels of literacy.

Patients with heart failure commonly have comorbid conditions that require thoughtful and optimal treatment. The need to evaluate other comorbidities in the progression of heart failure has become increasingly evident. Depression, anemia, renal insufficiency, diabetes, CAD, hypertension, and sleep apnea have all been found not only to worsen the patient's prognosis and increase morbidity and mortality rates, but also to confound heart failure treatment (Hunt et al., 2009).

Gerontological Considerations

Heart failure is generally a condition of older adults, and the aging baby boomers are contributing to the rise in its incidence. Heart failure is the major reason for hospitalization among older adults. There is little guidance provided in the literature on heart failure in older adults, yet as the baby boomers continue to age and improvements are made in the treatment of CAD, the number of people over age 65 living with heart failure will continue to grow. In fact, the incidence of heart failure is expected to double by 2030 partly because people are living longer (Schocken et al., 2008).

Due to the incidence of CAD and hypertension in older adults, they are more likely to have heart failure with preserved systolic function. Diastolic dysfunction is particularly common in obese older women (Hunt et al., 2009). Whether the cause of heart failure is systolic dysfunction or diastolic dysfunction, the prognosis is poor once the patient is hospitalized. Chart 34–10 summarizes prognostic predictors of increased mortality for older patients with systolic dysfunction.

The common symptoms of heart failure are similar at any age: dyspnea (especially with exertion), cough, orthopnea, and dependent edema. Older adults, however, may present with less common or less overt symptoms, such as fatigue, poor concentration, disorientation, and failure to thrive. Often, their symptoms may be confused with other disease processes or other comorbidities such as CAD, infection, or depression. A normal part of age-related changes of cardiac function

NATIONAL GUIDELINES Heart Failure Society of America: Guidelines for Nonpharmacologic Care for Chronic Heart Failure

- Dietary instruction regarding sodium intake is recommended in all patients. Dietary sodium restriction (2 to 3 g daily) is recommended.
- Restriction of daily fluid intake to less than 2 L is recommended in patients with severe hyponatremia (serum sodium less than 130 mEq/L). Fluid restriction should also be considered for patients who demonstrate fluid retention that is difficult to control despite sodium restriction and high doses of diuretic.
- Attention to nutritional management of the patient in chronic heart failure is essential. Measurement of nitrogen balance, caloric intake, and prealbumin may be useful in determining appropriate nutritional supplementation. Caloric supplementation is recommended. However, anabolic steroids are not recommended for cachexic patients.
- Patients on diuretic therapy and restricted diets should be considered for daily multivitamin-mineral supplementation to ensure adequate intake of the recommended daily value of essential nutrients.
- Documentation of the type and dose of nutritional or herbal products used by patients is recommended. Patients should be instructed to avoid using natural or synthetic products containing ephedra (ma huang), ephedrine, or its metabolites because of an increased risk of mortality and morbidity. Patients should be taught to avoid products that may have significant drug interactions with digoxin, vasodilators, beta-blockers, antidysrhythmic drugs, and anticoagulants. For example, large doses of garlic have been found to increase the risk of bleeding in patients on Coumadin, antiplatelet agents such as clopidogrel, and nonsteroidal anti-inflammatory agents (Kowalsky, 2011).
- Continuous positive airway pressure to improve the patient's functional capacity and quality of life is recommended in patients with documented obstructive sleep apnea.
- Supplemental oxygen, either at night or during exertion, is not recommended for patients unless there is underlying pulmonary disease. Patients with resting hypoxemia or oxygen desaturation during exercise should be evaluated for residual fluid overload or concomitant pulmonary disease.
- The identification of treatable conditions, such as sleep-disordered breathing, urologic abnormalities, restless leg syndrome, and depression, should be considered in patients who complain of chronic insomnia. Pharmacologic aids to sleep induction may be necessary.
- Patients should be routinely screened for depression upon diagnosis and periodically throughout the course of treatment. Pharmacologic management with selective serotonin reuptake inhibitors may be useful for some patients.
- Stress reduction strategies may be helpful in reducing anxiety for some patients.
- Treatment options for sexual dysfunction should be discussed openly with both male and female patients. The use of phosphodiesterase-5 inhibitors may be appropriate for some patients.

Sources: Adapted from Heart Failure Society of America (HFSA). (2010). Comprehensive heart failure practice guidelines. Retrieved from http://www.hfsa.org/hf_guidelines.asp; Lindenfeld, J., et al. (2010). Executive summary: HFSA 2010 comprehensive heart failure practice guideline. *Journal of Cardiac Failure, 16* (6), 475–539.

Weblink: Heart Failure Practice Guidelines

CHART 34–10 Considerations for Poor Prognosis in Older Adults with Systolic Dysfunction

Heart failure is a chronic disease that leads to death in 50% of patients within 5 years of diagnosis. Although difficulties remain with assessing prognosis, the indicators listed here, if present, provide objective evidence that suggests the patient's prognosis is poor.

High NYHA class	Low exercise capacity
Very low ejection fraction (EF)	Severely dilated left ventricle
Ischemic etiology	Renal failure
Hyponatremia	Ventricular dysrhythmias
Abnormal liver function tests	Shortened filling time of mitral filling pattern
Conduction system delays (left bundle branch block)	

Sources: Adapted from Schocken, D. D., et al. (2008). Prevention of heart failure. *Circulation, 117*, 2544–2565.

may include modest decreases in systolic function and decreases in cardiovascular response with increased workload. As a result, stressors in older adults may precipitate heart failure symptoms that might not present themselves in the younger population. These stressors include infection, hypothyroidism, hyperthyroidism, anemia, cardiac ischemia, hypoxia, hypothermia, hyperthermia, renal failure, nonadherence to drug or diet regimens, and potentially the use of certain drugs (nonsteroidal anti-inflammatories, beta-blockers, and some calcium-channel blockers).

Given the limited available data in the literature related to treating diastolic dysfunction, most of the therapies should be aimed at treating CAD, hypertension, and volume overload (Hunt et al., 2009; Lindenfeld et al., 2010). Because older adults are at risk of hypotension in the setting of volume depletion, cautious use of antihypertensive agents that have vasodilatory properties is recommended when diuretics are being use. Toxicities to medications may occur in older adults who have renal insufficiency. Digoxin should be started at low doses for those over the age of 70 years. Health care providers, however, must carefully monitor these levels because patients may be prone to toxicity due to reduced renal clearance (Adams & Koch, 2010b).

Coping with Heart Failure and End-of-Life Planning

People who have been diagnosed with heart failure face many challenges. There is the uncertainty about the prognosis, expectations related to their response to medications, and possible loss of earning potential for those in the workforce. As with many chronic conditions, the impact of depression on heart failure is significant. People diagnosed with heart failure need family or loved ones who participate actively in their life for the physical, psychological, and emotional support that is needed.

Despite medicine's best treatment options, individuals with heart failure will likely die from this disease process, as displayed in the course of heart failure (see Figure 34–2, p. 1029). As usage rates of medications that can alter the prognosis of heart failure improve, internal cardioverter defibrillators offer corresponding reductions in mortality. Using medications such as beta-adrenergic blockers can lead to a 5% to 15% increase in ejection fraction or even its normalization, which improves the patient's prognosis. Many factors contribute to the unpredictability of a given patient's course, such as his response to prognosis-altering medications, compliance, and timing and level of care.

When heart failure reaches a terminal stage and treatment options are limited, patient care needs to be geared toward comfort measures and reducing symptoms, which are typically manifested as respiratory distress and pain. Palliative care is treatment done to reduce symptoms and suffering in end-of-life planning and can be helpful for the patient with end-stage heart failure (Goodlin, 2009). Optimally, palliative care should be included in the management of heart failure from the time of diagnosis, designed as part of comprehensive care across the continuum. Discussions about the level of care need to be planned ahead of time, not during times of crisis. Advance directives, hospice care, resuscitation wishes, living wills, formalizing estate planning, and discussing wishes with family and health care providers must be completed. Chapter 11 discusses end-of-life care.

Care providers have struggled with how to predict when death is near for patients with heart failure. It has become clear that patients with hypotension who require dose reductions of ACE inhibitors (or ARBs) and beta-adrenergic blockers, as well as those with increasing creatinine and anemia, face a poor prognosis.

Patients and loved ones deserve an honest discussion related to caring for those who are near the end of life. Patients with heart failure will likely die of a sudden dysrhythmic event (if an ICD has not been implanted or has been deactivated) or the slower, progressive cardiac pump dysfunction. Clear decisions must be made regarding symptom management (often done with narcotics, diuretics, nitrates, and anxiolytics), and it is important to plan ahead so that medications are ready for use when needed (Goodlin, 2009). Engaging home care, family and loved ones, community resources, and hospice can assist with facilitating the patient's individual preferences. Discussing plans for turning off mechanical devices (pacemakers, defibrillators, ventricular assist devices) that may prolong life when little hope is present is often difficult but will be necessary as the use of these devices becomes increasingly common in treating heart failure. Planning for the end of life must take into account the patient's spiritual, psychological, physical, social, and cultural needs. Ethical issues regarding heart failure care that must be considered thoughtfully are outlined in the Ethical Issues box.

ETHICAL ISSUES Related to Heart Failure

Specific ethical issues for heart failure patients and their families include:

- Quality of life after the initial onset of left ventricle (LV) dysfunction
- Employability after clinical stabilization
- When to withhold or withdraw care
- Dignified and comfortable death
- Psychological adjustment
- Considerations of futility
- Financial costs of end-stage therapies (i.e., transplant, mechanical circulatory support, intravenous medications)
- Turning off an implantable cardioverter defibrillator (ICD) device in chronic, severe, refractory heart failure patients
- Pregnancy in female heart failure patients
- Therapeutic potential of embryonic stem cells in heart failure
- Differences of care between male and female heart failure patients.

CULTURAL CONSIDERATIONS for Risk Factors of Heart Failure

- Heart failure is more common in African Americans than other races and tends to be worse in severity than is the case for other ethnic groups. It occurs at an earlier age, and hypertension, obesity, and systolic dysfunction rather than myocardial ischemia contribute to its development. African Americans experience a higher incidence of hospitalization for heart failure issues (Bibbins-Domingo et al., 2009; Franciosa, Ferdinand, & Yancy, 2010).
- The African-American Heart Failure Trial (A-HeFT) results suggest that African Americans have improved outcomes when isosorbide dinitrate and hydralazine are added to standard heart failure medications (McMurray, 2010). Additional studies have suggested that treatment with hydralazine–isosorbide dinitrate, when added to an ACE inhibitor, a beta-blocker, and, in some cases, an aldosterone antagonist, resulted in a reduced rate of hospitalization for heart failure, improved quality of life, and increased survival.
- Salt sensitivity has been identified in some African Americans and can make the treatment of hypertension and resultant heart failure more challenging (Franciosa, Ferdinand, & Yancy, 2010).

Sources: Adapted from Bibbins-Domingo, K. (2009). Racial differences in incident heart failure among young adults. *New England Journal of Medicine, 360*, 1179–1190; Franciosa, J. A., Ferdinand, K. C., & Yancy, C. W. (2010). Treatment of heart failure in African Americans: A consensus statement. *Congestive Heart Failure, 16*(1), 27–38; McMurray, J. J. V. (2010). Systolic heart failure. *New England Journal of Medicine, 362*, 228–238.

Research

Cardiovascular research has led to tremendous advances in diagnosis and treatment. The Framingham Heart Study continues to be one of the research landmarks providing epidemiologic data on which studies of heart disease and treatment are based. Studies performed in the past 30 years on all the forms of heart failure treatment mentioned in this chapter have led to treatment guidelines for care. There has been an explosion of heart failure studies striving to find new treatments in hopes of finding methods to reduce mortality, to improve quality and length of life, and to reduce the treatment cost. Understanding heart failure management will include a sensitivity and awareness of cultural aspects of the patient's life (see the Cultural Considerations box).

Comprehensive disease management strategies have been shown to improve outcomes associated with chronic heart failure. Such strategies include telephone follow up with decision support software and protocol-driven pharmacologic management with close telephone nurse follow up (Steckler et al., 2010). Future directions for heart failure research studies can be found in the Research Opportunities box.

Genetic Considerations

Understanding genetic mechanisms of heart failure will broaden treatment approaches. Studies are needed that will evaluate genetic risk factors, therapies, legal implications, counseling, and screening issues. The Genetic Considerations box provides a more thorough review of genetic implications.

RESEARCH OPPORTUNITIES Related to Heart Failure Care

Research Area	Clinical Impact
Depression and anxiety in patients with mechanical cardiac devices	Patients with heart failure are increasingly having cardiac devices implanted to prevent cardiac death, to improve contractility, or to do both. Understanding optimal treatment for anxiety or depression will be critical given the growing use of device therapy.
Caregiver support for end-stage heart failure	Heart failure is increasing in incidence and prevalence; thus, learning how to support the caregiver will be imperative.
Cost-effectiveness of heart failure therapies	Given the increasing evidence to support the use of cardiac devices, such as ICDs, pacemakers, and left ventricular assist devices (LVADs), continual cost analysis of these therapies is essential.
Respiratory support for sleep-disordered breathing	Patients with heart failure frequently experience abnormal respiratory patterns. Treatment or prevention of these abnormal respiratory patterns may lead to a reduction in the incidence of heart failure.
External counterpulsation	This involves the use of a device that inflates and deflates around a patient's legs. This therapy has been shown to decrease the frequency of ischemic attacks in CAD patients. Larger trials are underway to determine its routine use in heart failure care.
Implantable hemodynamic monitors	Implantable monitors are able to monitor ventricular filling pressures. This form of technology may be able to prevent heart failure exacerbations prior to their occurrence.
Cardiac support devices	Several surgical devices are currently in design stages to assist in the reduction of physical stresses on the left ventricle.
Myocardial regeneration by activation of stem cells	The possibility of reconstituting dead myocardium by activation of stem cells is a promising area of research.
Understanding the knowledge deficits of patients with heart failure	Patient understanding of the course of heart failure and self-management strategies is essential. Identifying the most significant barriers to patient understanding of the disease and self-management is likely to improve outcomes.
Self-management strategies in heart failure	Identifying what improves patient compliance with self-management strategies may lead to improved outcomes.
The role of culture in patients with advanced heart failure	Identifying cultural barriers in providing patient care can help providers in formulating a comprehensive treatment plan.
Anthracycline-induced cardiomyopathy	Anthracyclines used to treat malignancies have been known to cause left ventricular dysfunction. More study is needed to learn how to prevent this, and to monitor and optimally treat this patient population.

GENETIC CONSIDERATIONS for Heart Failure

Risk Factors	Family history of early CAD, idiopathic or hypertrophic cardiomyopathy, sudden cardiac death.
	Virus exposure.
	African American race.
	Potential for thromboembolic events: atrial fibrillation, pulmonary embolism, intracardiac thrombi, or deep vein thrombosis.
Research	Familial Dilated Cardiomyopathy Research Project.[a]
	Viral genome; studying parvovirus B19, cause of Fifth Disease as a risk factor for myocarditis and heart failure.
	A-HeFT: African-American Heart Failure Trial: showed increased response to hydralazine and nitrates in addition to standard heart failure therapy.
	Genetic testing to assess low or high response warfarin dosing.
Counseling/ Screening	Counsel patients that genetic factors that led to their condition might also put their first-degree relatives at risk.
	Appropriate screening would be recommended, then starting treatment if left ventricular dysfunction is found.
	To screen those with risk factors or a family history suggests simple screening of first-degree family members with a limited history, physical examination, 12-lead ECG, and echocardiogram.
	Genetic screening by blood testing is not yet well understood but may guide future treatment.

Source: Adapted from Hunt, S. A. (2009). Focused update incorporated into the ACC/AHA 2005 guidelines for the diagnosis and management of heart failure in adults: A report of the American College of Cardiology Foundation/American Heart Association Task Force on Practice Guidelines. *Circulation, 119*, e391–e479.

READ: **History of Present Illnesses** >> Laboratory Study Results >> Critical Thinking Questions

As the on-coming nurse on a telemetry cardiovascular care unit, you receive report about Glen Craver, who was admitted with a diagnosis of heart failure 48 hours ago. He is a 56-year-old male who presented to his primary care provider with a 2-month history of worsening symptoms of dyspnea on exertion, a nonproductive cough, general fatigue, and decreased activity tolerance. Initially, the patient thought he had the flu; however, when the symptoms persisted longer than expected, he sought medical attention. At the office, Mr. Craver was found to have profound jugular venous distention, rhonchi in his lungs, and lower extremity swelling. After admission, he had an echocardiogram, and his serum BNP was found to be 1,560 pg/mL. Coronary angiography, which was performed to provide a definitive diagnosis, revealed no evidence of CAD. Echocardiogram shows moderate concentric hypertrophy of the ventricles, moderate left ventricular dysfunction, ejection fraction 33%, and mild to moderate mitral regurgitation. Angiogram: normal coronary arteries, ejection fraction 33%, confirmed reduction in ventricular function with a ventriculogram.

READ: History of Present Illnesses >> **Physical Exam** >> Admitting Medical Records >> Laboratory Study Results

Medical–Surgical History

- Hyperlipidemia: diagnosed 3 years ago
- Hypertension: diagnosed this past year
- Type 2 diabetes: diagnosed this past year
- Obesity: over 20 years
- Hypothyroidism: diagnosed 12 years ago
- Tonsillectomy: 40 years ago
- Cholecystectomy: 4 years ago

Current Medications

- Simvastatin 20 mg po qhs
- Levothyroxine 0.125 mg po daily
- Glipizide 15 mg po daily
- Hydrochlorothiazide 25 mg po daily

Physical Exam

- Vital signs: HR: 84 beats per minute; BP: 146/84 mmHg; temperature: 36.8°C; oxygen sat: 94% on 2 liters of oxygen.
- He is a well-nourished male with appropriate affect and no apparent distress.
- All extremities have palpable pulses, are warm to touch, and have a capillary refill of less than 3 seconds.
- 31 pitting edema is present in his lower ankles bilaterally, which extends to his midcalf; his lungs have bibasilar crackles without wheezing or retractions; he also has a nonproductive cough.
- Normal S_1 and S_2 are present. S_3, and the point of maximal impulse, is displaced laterally into the anterior axillary line of his chest.
- Positive hepatojugular reflux.
- Bowel sounds present and palpation is nontender.

Admitting Medical Orders

- Cardiology Service
- Diagnosis: acute heart failure
- Telemetry floor
- Condition guarded
- No known allergies
- Full code
- Bed rest with bathroom privileges
- Call house officer: pulse < 60 > 100/minute; BP < 0 >160 systolic; temperature > 38.5; urine output 30/minute; oxygen saturation < 92%; blood sugar < 60 >120
- Continuous cardiac monitor
- Oxygen per nasal cannula to maintain oxygen sat > 92%
- Vital signs and oxygen saturation q4hours
- Daily a.m. weights
- IV: saline lock-flush with NS q8h
- Blood sugars ac and hs
- Cardiac rehab evaluation and management
- Low-sodium (<2,000 mg/day), fluid-restricted (<2 L/day) diet
- Strict I&O
- Sequential compression devices (SCD) to lower extremities when in bed
- Incentive spirometry 2 hours while awake and q4 at night

Scheduled Medications

- Simvastatin 20 mg po qhs
- Levothyroxine 0.125 mg po daily
- Glipizide 15 mg po daily
- Furosemide 80 mg IV bid
- Potassium 40 mEq po bid
- Lisinopril 2.5 mg po daily

PRN Medications

- Morphine 3–5 mg IV q3–5min, max 15 mg q3h prn chest pain
- Temazepam 15–30 mg PO qhs prn insomnia
- Droperidol 1.25–2.5 mg IV q 6 hours prn nausea

Ordered Laboratory Studies

- Chemistry 7 panel daily
- CBC now
- BNP daily × 3
- Lipid panel

Ordered Diagnostic Studies

- Chest x-ray in a.m.
- Echocardiogram
- Angiogram

READ: History of Present Illnesses >> **Laboratory Study Results** >> Critical Thinking Questions

Test	Day 1 Admission	Day 1 Evening	Day 2 Morning
Potassium	4.8 mEq/L	3.5 mEq/L	3.8 mEq/L
Sodium	136 mEq/L	138 mEq/L	137 mEq/L
Chloride	103 mEq/L	104 mEq/L	103 mEq/L
Carbon dioxide (CO_2)	26 mEq/L	25 mEq/L	25 mEq/L
Calcium	8.8 mg/dL	8.7 mg/dL	9.1 mg/dL
Creatinine	1.8 mg/dL	1.4 mg/dL	1.2 mg/dL
BUN	30 mg/dL	24 mg/dL	18 mg/dL
Glucose	110 mg/dL	108 mg/dL	102 mg/dL
Hematocrit	40%	39%	44%
Hemoglobin	13.9 g/dL	13.5 g/dL	14.9 g/dL
Platelets	285/mm^3	266/mm^3	289/mm^3

Test	Day 1 Admission	Day 1 Evening	Day 2 Morning
WBC	8.5/mm^3	7.9/mm^3	8.3/mm^3
RBC	4.89/mm^3	5.02/mm^3	4.96/mm^3
BNP	1,560 pg/mL	662 pg/mL	422 pg/mL
Cholesterol	260 mg/dL		
High-density lipoproteins (HDL)	36 mg/dL		
Low-density lipoproteins (LDL)	187 mg/dL		
Very-low-density lipoproteins (VLDL)	70%		
Apolipoproteins	160 mg/dL		
Triglycerides	196 mg/dL		

Pearson Nursing Student Resources

Log on to ***nursing.pearsonhighered.com*** *to download forms*

DOCUMENT:

>> Summary of Hospitalization

>> Pathophysiology Form

>> Laboratory Values

>> Laboratory Results Explanation

APPLY:

>> List of Potential Nursing Diagnosis

>> Concept Map

>> Critical Thinking Questions and Concept Map

APPLY: History of Present Illnesses >> Laboratory Study Results >> **Critical Thinking Questions**

1. You are reviewing Mr. Craver's orders when coming on shift. List them in order of priority.
2. Why would Mr. Craver receive daily a.m. weights?
3. Which laboratory values may require notification to the ordering provider?
4. What should you monitor for after giving lisinopril 2.5 mg po daily?
5. Why is a beta-adrenergic blocker not listed on the ordered medications?

Answers to Critical Thinking Questions can be found in Appendix D in the Osborn Student Resources at nursing.pearsonhighered.com.

NCLEX® PRACTICE

1. The nurse identifies the following conditions in the medical history of a patient admitted with symptoms of heart failure. Which condition is most likely related to the heart failure the patient is currently experiencing?
   1. A recent episode of acute pancreatitis
   2. Chronic fatigue syndrome
   3. Aortic stenosis
   4. Pleural effusion
2. When caring for a patient with systolic dysfunction, the nurse anticipates the patient will most likely exhibit symptoms related to which cardiac condition?
   1. Decreased cardiac output
   2. Pain in the upper right abdomen
   3. Peripheral edema
   4. Bradycardia

3. The nurse is planning the care of a patient with heart failure who has experienced a decrease in cardiac output. Which neurohormonal response should the nurse consider when planning this care?

1. Activation of the sympathetic nervous system (SNS)
2. Activation of the parasympathetic nervous system (PNS)
3. Inactivation of the renin angiotensin system (RAS)
4. Suppression of cytokine release

4. The patient has been diagnosed with left-sided heart failure. Which common finding of this condition should the nurse consider when planning care?

1. Weight gain
2. Anorexia
3. Dyspnea
4. Peripheral edema

5. The nurse reviews the brain natriuretic peptide (BNP) levels of a patient admitted with dyspnea and activity intolerance. Because the levels are normal, the nurse draws which conclusion?

1. A diagnosis of heart failure can be excluded.
2. The patient has long-standing heart failure.
3. The patient is most likely experiencing cardiac ischemia.
4. The symptoms are related to pulmonary tissue damage.

6. The nurse should anticipate that the treatment of a patient with stage B heart failure will include which interventions?

1. Administration of ACE inhibitors and beta-blockers
2. Use of diuretics only
3. Insertion of an implantable cardiac defibrillator
4. Possible referral to hospice

Answers to NCLEX Practice questions can be found in Appendix D in the Osborn Student Resources at nursing.pearsonhighered.com. Practice additional NCLEX questions online at the Student Resources site.

REFERENCES

Adams, M. P., & Koch, R. W. (2010a). Dapigatraban etexilate prescribing information. Retrieved from http://www.pradaxa.com/?sc=PRDACQWEBGGLWKT1006111

Adams, M. P., & Koch, R. W. (2010b). *Pharmacology: Connections to nursing practice.* Upper Saddle River, NJ: Pearson.

Agency for Healthcare Research and Quality (AHRQ). (2009). Educating patients before hospital discharge reduces readmissions, emergency department visits, and saves money. Retrieved from http://www.ahrq.gov/research/mar09/0309RA1.htm

Agency for Healthcare Research and Quality (AHRQ). (2010). Health care literacy universal precautions toolkit. Retrieved from http://www.ahrq.gov/qual/literacy/healthliteracytoolkit.pdf

American Heart Association. (2010a). Classification of functional capacity and objective assessment. Retrieved from http://www.americanheart.org/presenter.jhtml?identifier=4569

American Heart Association. (2010b). Heart disease and stroke statistics: 2010 update at a glance. Retrieved from http://www.americanheart.org/downloadable/heart/1265665152970DS-3241%20HeartStrokeUpdate_2010.pdf

American Heart Association. (2010c). Organ donation. Retrieved from http://www.americanheart.org/presenter.jhtml?identifier=4697

American Heart Association. (2011). Sodium (salt or sodium chloride). Retrieved from http://www.heart.org/HEARTORG/GettingHealthy/NutritionCenter/HealthyDietGoals/Sodium-Salt-or-Sodium-Chloride_UCM_303290_Article.jsp#.Txw85W_OV2A

Beg, S., Javed, S., & Kohli, K. (2010). Bioavailability enhancement of coenzyme Q10: An extensive review of patents. *Recent Patents on Drug Delivery and Formulations, 4*(3), 245–255.

Bibbins-Domingo, K., Pletcher, M. J., Lin, F., Vittinghoff, E., Gardin, J. M., Arychyn, A., et al. (2009). Racial differences in incident heart failure among young adults. *New England Journal of Medicine, 360*, 1179–1190.

Carlson, K. K. (2009). *AACN advanced critical care.* St. Louis: Saunders Elsevier.

Franciosa, J. A., Ferdinand, K. C., & Yancy, C. W. (2010). Treatment of heart failure in African Americans: A consensus statement. *Congestive Heart Failure, 16*(1), 27–38.

Goodlin, S. J. (2009). Palliative care in congestive heart failure. *Journal of the American College of Cardiology, 54*; 386–396.

Heart Failure Society of America (HFSA). (2010). Comprehensive heart failure practice guidelines. Retreived from http://www.hfsa.org/hf_guidelines.asp

Hunt, S. A., Abraham, W. T., Chin, M. H., Feldman, A. M., Francis, G. S., Ganiats, T. G., et al. (2009). Focused update incorporated into the ACC/AHA 2005 guidelines for the diagnosis and management of heart failure in adults: A report of the American College of Cardiology Foundation/American Heart Association Task Force on Practice Guidelines. *Circulation,119*, e391– e479.

IOM (Institute of Medicine). (2010). *The future of nursing: Leading change, advancing health.* Washington, DC: The Academic Press.

Kamath, S. A. (2011). The role of ultrafiltration in patients with decompensated heart failure. *International Journal of Nephrology*, 2011(Article ID 190230).

Kee, J. L. (2010). *Laboratory and diagnostic tests with nursing implications.* Upper Saddle River, NJ: Pearson.

Kowalsky, P. E. (2011). Common interactions with herbal supplements and prescription drugs. *AACN Advanced Critical Care, 22*(2), 101–106.

Lee, C. S., & Tkacs, N. C. (2008). Current concepts of neurohormonal activation in heart failure: Mediators and mechanisms. *AACN Advanced Critical Care, 19*(4), 364–385.

Lindenfeld, J., Albert, N. M., Boehmer, J. P., Collins, S. P., Ezekowitz, J. A., Givertz, M. M., et al. (2010). Executive summary: HFSA 2010 comprehensive heart failure practice guideline. *Journal of Cardiac Failure, 16* (6), 475–539.

Littarru, G. P., & Tiano, L. (2007). Bioenergetic and antioxidant properties of coenzyme Q10: Recent developments. *Molecular Biotechnology, 37*(1), 31–37.

Littarru, G. P., & Tiano, L. (2010). Clinical aspects of coenzyme Q10: An update. *Nutrition, 26*(3), 250–254.

Liu, Z. X., & Artmann, C. (2009). Relative bioavailability comparison of different coenzyme Q10 formulations with a novel delivery system. *Alternative Therapies in Health and Medicine, 15*(2), 42–46.

Manning, S. (2011). Bridging the gap between hospital and home: A new model of care for reducing readmission rates in chronic heart failure. *Journal of Cardiovascular Nursing.*

Mayo Clinic. (2012). Sodium: How to tame the salt habit. Retrieved from http://www.mayoclinic.com/health/sodium/NU00284

McCulloch, B. J. (2010). Intra-aortic balloon pump and other cardiac assist devices. In S. Watson & K. A. Gorski (Eds.), *Invasive cardiology: A manual for cath lab personnel.* Sudbury, MA: Jones and Bartlett.

McMurray, J. J. V. (2010). Systolic heart failure. *New England Journal of Medicine, 362*, 228–238.

Molyneux, S. L., Florkowski, C. M., Richards, A. M., Lever, M., Young, J. M., & George, P. M. (2009). Coenzyme Q10: An adjunctive therapy for congestive heart failure? *New Zealand Medical Journal, 122*(1305), 74–79.

Moser, D. K., & Reigel, B. (2008). *Cardiac nursing: A companion to Braunwald's heart disease.* St. Louis: Saunders.

Porth, C. M. & Matfin, G. (2009). *Essentials of pathophysiology: Concepts of altered health states* (9th ed.). Philadelphia: Lippincott Williams & Wilkins.

Porth, C., & Matfin, G. (2009). *Pathophysiology: Concepts of altered health states.* (8th ed.). Philadelphia: Wolters Kluwer/Lippincott Williams & Wilkins.

Schocken, D. D., Benjamin, E. J., Fonarow, G. C., Krumholz, H. M., Levy, D., Mensah, G. A., et al. (2008). Prevention of heart failure. *Circulation, 117*, 2544–2565.

Shargorodsky, M., Debby, O., Matas, Z., & Zimlichman, R. (2010). Effect of long-term treatment with antioxidants (vitamin C, vitamin E, coenzyme Q10 and selenium) on arterial compliance, humoral factors and inflammatory markers in patients with multiple cardiovascular risk factors. *Nutrition & Metabolism (London), 7*, 55. Published online 2010 July 6. doi: 10.1186/1743-7075-7-55

Steckler, A. E., Bishu, K., Wassif, H., Sigurdsson, G., Wagner, J., Jaenicke, C., et al. (2010). Telephone titration of heart failure medications. *Journal of Cardiovascular Nursing, 26*(1), 29–36.

The Joint Commission. (2010). Heart failure. Retrieved from http://www.jointcommission.org/heart_failure/

Wilkinson, J. M., & Ahearn, N. R. (2009). *Prentice Hall nursing diagnosis handbook* (9th ed.). Upper Saddle River, NJ: Prentice Hall.

Caring for the Patient with Peripheral Vascular Disorders

35 CHAPTER

Brenda McCulloch
Kathleen Osborn

Outcome-Based Learning Objectives

After studying this chapter, the learner will be able to:

1. Critique the differences between prehypertension, stage 1 hypertension, and stage 2 hypertension.
2. Implement a plan of care and discharge instructions for a patient with hypertension.
3. Analyze the risk factors and clinical findings to develop a nursing care plan for patients with peripheral arterial disease, deep vein thrombosis, aortic aneurysm, Raynaud's disease, and aortic dissection.
4. Differentiate the clinical manifestations of potential complications of endovascular repair and surgical repair of diseased blood vessels and identify appropriate nursing interventions.
5. Generate a nursing plan of care for patients on anticoagulants and antiplatelet agents for the treatment of peripheral arterial disease.

KEY TERMS

aneurysm p.1078
ankle–brachial index (ABI) p.1070
aortic dissection (AD) p.1080
blood pressure (BP) p.1058
DASH diet p.1062
deep venous thrombosis (DVT) p.1081
diastolic blood pressure p.1059
embolectomy p.1076
endoleaks p.1079
hypertension p.1060
hypertensive crisis p.1069
hypertensive encephalopathy p.1069
intermittent claudication (IC) p.1069
lymphangitis p.1089
lymphedema p.1082
paresthesia p.1069
peripheral arterial disease (PAD) p.1069
peripheral vascular resistance p.1059
prehypertension p.1060
pulmonary embolism (PE) p.1082
pulse pressure p.1059
Raynaud's disease (RD) p.1076
stage 1 hypertension p.1060
stage 2 hypertension p.1060
sympathectomy p.1076
systolic blood pressure p.1058
thoracic outlet syndrome (TOS) p.1077
Unna's boot p.1088
varicose veins p.1082
venous thromboembolism (VTE) p.1082
Virchow's triad p.1083

VASCULAR DISORDERS include disorders of the body's arterial, venous, and lymphatic systems. Peripheral arterial disease includes occlusive, aneurysmal (dilated), and vasospastic disorders affecting the arterial system of the neck, abdomen, and extremities. Peripheral venous disease predominantly involves the legs and is usually due to thrombosis or insufficiency of the veins. Lymphatic disease leads to abnormal fluid collection, edema, and fibrosis. These peripheral vascular diseases may cause serious complications such as loss of limb or even loss of life.

Anatomy and Physiology Review

The peripheral vascular system is a network of branching blood vessels carrying oxygenated blood from the heart to the body's tissues and returning deoxygenated blood to the lungs. The peripheral vascular system is made up of arteries, veins, and capillaries. The lymphatics, also considered part of the peripheral vascular system, help maintain adequate blood volume by returning tissue fluid to the bloodstream.

Arteries consist of three distinct layers: the tunica intima, the tunica media, and the tunica adventitia. The innermost lining of the tunica intima consists of the endothelium, which provides a smooth surface for flowing blood. The middle layer, or the tunica media, is made up of smooth muscle cells, collagen, and elastin, providing elasticity and strength to the vessel. The tunica adventitia, the outermost layer of the artery, consists of connective tissue and anchors the vessel in the surrounding tissue.

The largest artery in the body, the aorta, ascends from the aortic root of the heart, passes through the chest, and descends into the abdomen, where it bifurcates about the level of the umbilicus. It branches off to various vital organs along the way. The major arteries are shown in Figure 35–1◆ (p. 1058). Arteries branch sequentially from large to

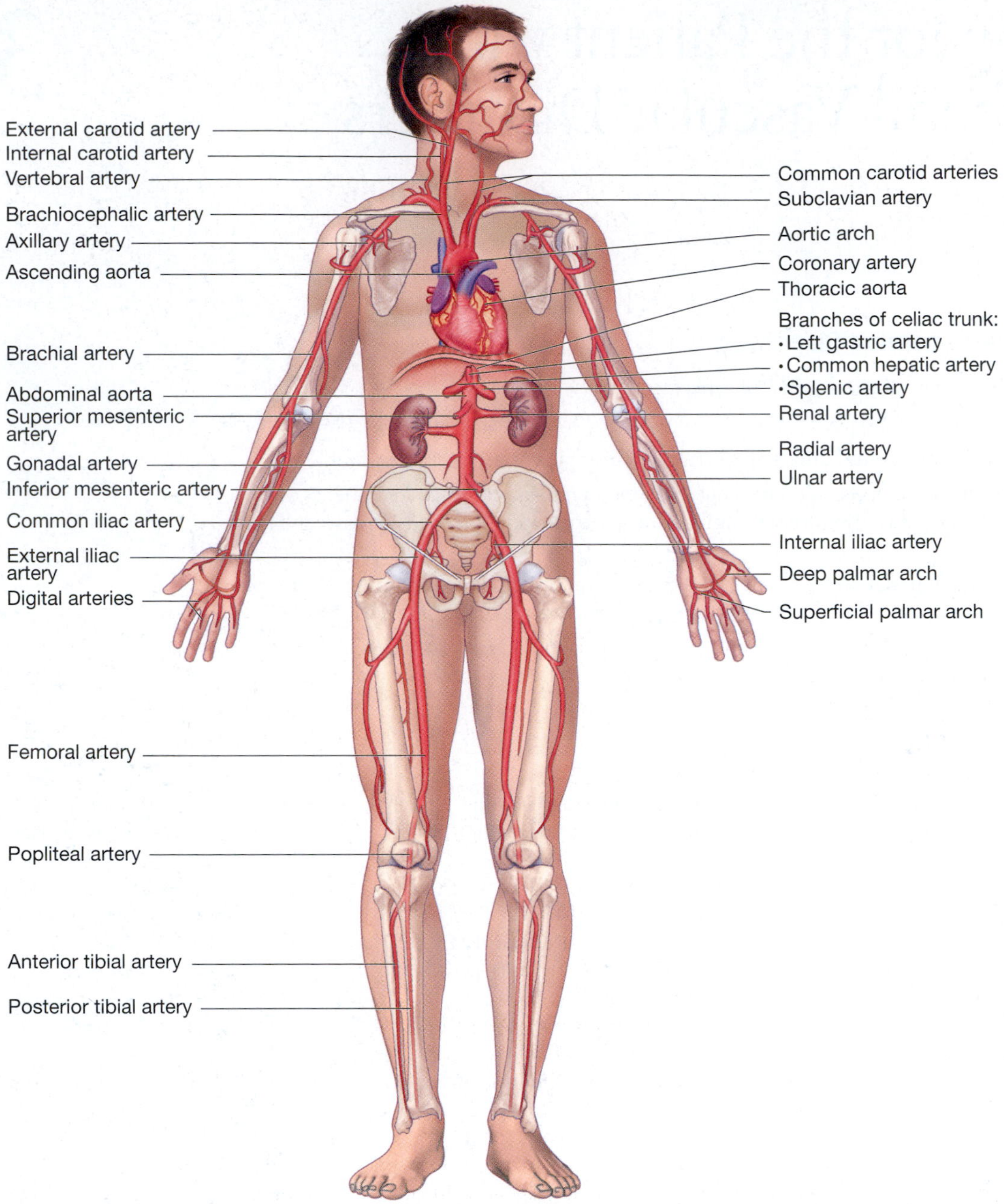

FIGURE 35–1 ◆ Major arteries of the body.

medium to the smallest arteries, called arterioles, before eventually reaching the capillary bed.

Capillaries, thin-walled structures consisting of a single layer of endothelial cells, help facilitate rapid nutrient and waste product transport and removal. Venules are formed when several capillaries join together. Small venules form progressively larger veins and return blood from the periphery to the right atrium. The major veins are shown in Figure 35–2◆. Veins are thin-walled structures in comparison to arteries, and the venous system is comparably low pressure as compared to the arterial system.

The lymphatic system is a network of vessels that transports lymph—a clear fluid that comes from the blood and bathes the tissues. Lymph contains water, protein, minerals, and white blood cells. Functions of the lymphatic system include the absorption of excess fluid and its return to the bloodstream, the absorption of fat, and an immune system function. The lymphatic system is shown in Figure 35–3◆.

Vascular Disorders

Hypertension

Hypertension is a significant risk factor in the development of all peripheral vascular disorders. Before discussing these disorders, we will review blood pressure regulation and hypertension. **Blood pressure (BP)** is defined as the pressure created by the circulating blood through the arteries, veins, and the chambers of the heart. Blood pressure readings are classified into four stages: normal tension, prehypertension, stage 1 hypertension, and stage 2 hypertension (National Heart, Lung, and Blood Institute [NHLB], 2011).

Regulation of the Blood Pressure

Because of the pulsating blood flow created by the heart's contraction and relaxation, there are two readings associated with blood pressure: systolic and diastolic. The **systolic blood pressure** is the maximum

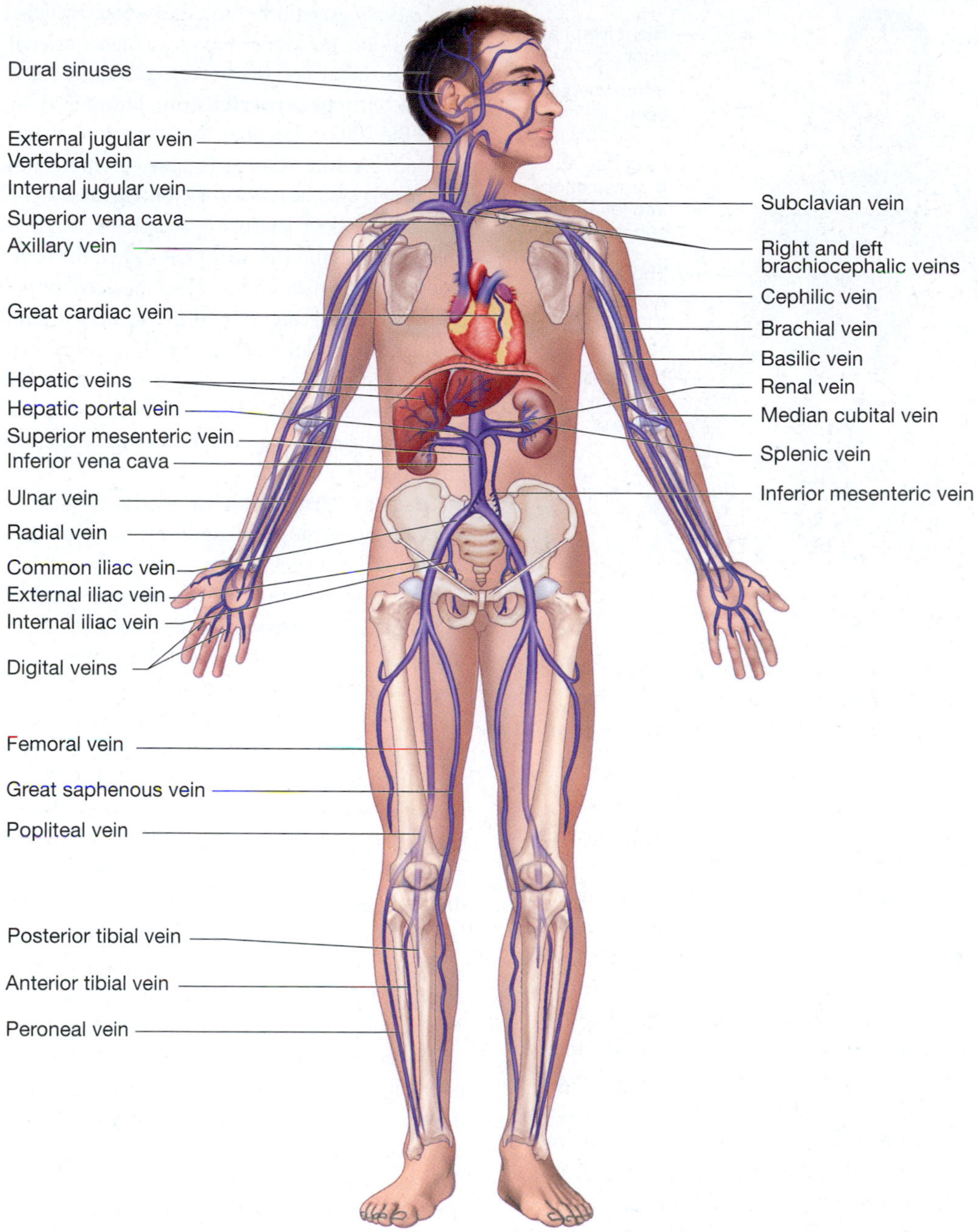

FIGURE 35–2 ◆ Major veins of the body.

pressure in the aorta and major arteries. It occurs when the left ventricle contracts and ejects blood into the central vascular system. The **diastolic blood pressure** reflects cardiac relaxation; thus, it is the minimum pressure in the arteries, which occurs just prior to the next cycle of ventricular ejection of blood. The difference between the systolic pressure and the diastolic pressure is called the **pulse pressure.**

Blood pressure is the product of cardiac output (the amount of blood pumped by the heart each minute) and systemic **peripheral vascular resistance** (the resistance to the flow of blood as determined by the vascular musculature and the diameter of the blood vessels, as well as influences on the cardiovascular system's ability to adapt). The homeostatic systems that influence blood pressure changes in accordance with body needs are neural regulation, arterial baroreceptors and chemoreceptors, regulation of fluid volume, and humoral regulation (Porth & Matfin, 2009).

Many body systems play a role in the regulation of normal blood pressure. For example, beginning in the brain, the pons and medulla are the neural control centers for blood pressure regulation. In these areas, the autonomic nervous system is integrated and modulated. It's also where the vasomotor control center and cardiovascular control center are located. In the periphery, baroreceptors located in the walls of blood vessels are pressure-sensitive receptors that respond to changes in the stretch of the blood vessels by sending impulses to the brain and heart to adjust the heart rate and smooth muscle tone. These stretch receptors are located in various large vessels throughout the body, such as the carotid sinus and the wall of the left ventricle. They respond to changes in arterial pressure (high or low) and signal the central nervous system (CNS). Signals are then transmitted back through baroreceptors to counteract the abnormal changes in the arterial pressure. A third mechanism that plays a role in blood pressure regulation is the body's

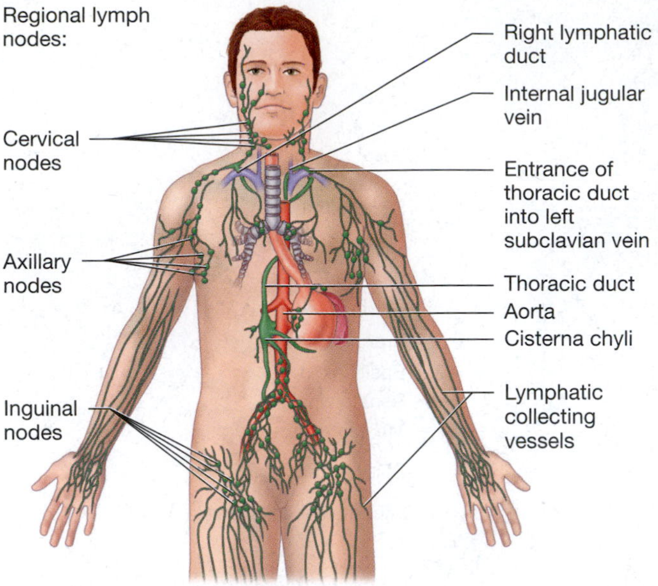

FIGURE 35–3 ◆ The lymphatic system.

intrinsic hormones. These include the renin-angiotensin-aldosterone mechanism, vasopressin, and epinephrine and norepinephrine. These hormones are essential in maintaining normal blood pressure on an ongoing basis.

Etiology and Epidemiology

Over 74.5 million American adults have hypertension (AHA, 2011). Nearly one-third of all adults 18 years and older are hypertensive with systolic blood pressure readings greater than 140/90 or are taking medications to control their blood pressure. The prevalence of hypertension is nearly equal between men and women. With the aging population, the prevalence of all cardiovascular diseases is projected to increase. People older than 65 years of age (especially older than 80 years of age) have a higher prevalence for all cardiovascular diseases, and this population segment will grow significantly in the next two decades. This will translate to an additional 27 million people with hypertension. Increasing body mass index has contributed to more than 50% of the increase in hypertension. Reversing the obesity epidemic will play a pivotal role in favorably impacting the projected hypertension trends. Hypertension accounts for 18% of cardiovascular deaths in Western countries and is a major risk factor for stroke, heart disease, and heart failure (Heidenreich et al., 2011). Because it has a higher prevalence than other cardiovascular conditions, hypertension is the most expensive component of cardiovascular disease.

Pathophysiology

Hypertension is defined as an average blood pressure that is higher than the accepted norm over a period of time consisting of two or more consecutive office visits. The May 2003 JNC 7 report (NHLBI, 2003) included revised guidelines for what constitutes hypertension and divided these parameters into three separate classifications for adults over the age of 18 years.

Multiple body systems interact to cause long-term elevation in blood pressure. These include hemodynamic, neural, humoral, and renal mechanisms. All forms of hypertension involve an increase in cardiac output, an increase in peripheral vascular resistance, or both. The sympathetic nervous system controls vascular resistance by releasing vasoconstrictor substances. The kidney also is a key player in causing hypertension. When the blood pressure rises normally, the kidney increases its excretion of salt and water. Evidence suggests that with hypertension, the kidney requires a higher arterial pressure to regulate the release of salt and water (Porth & Matfin, 2009).

The term **prehypertension,** introduced in the JNC 7 report (NHLBI, 2003), describes the condition of those individuals with a blood pressure finding on two or more office visits of 120 to 139 mmHg systolic or 80 to 89 mmHg diastolic. These individuals are at twice the risk of developing hypertension as those with lower values. Prehypertension is the early phase when the relationship between the blood pressure measurement and the need for health education is the primary focus of care. The individual demonstrating prehypertension is at risk for development of stage 1 or stage 2 hypertension. The JNC 7 report emphasizes increasing the awareness of the need to reduce blood pressure levels and prevent the development of high blood pressure in the general population through the education of health care professionals.

Stage 1 hypertension is a blood pressure of 140 to 159 mmHg systolic or 90 to 99 mmHg diastolic measured during multiple office visits following the guidelines for accurate blood pressure measurement. Lifestyle changes as well as medications are part of the therapeutic plan.

Stage 2 hypertension is a systolic blood pressure measured on multiple occasions during an office visit of greater than 160 mmHg or a diastolic pressure of greater than 100 mmHg. The measurement of the blood pressure follows the guidelines for accuracy. Both medications and lifestyle changes are part of the therapeutic plan.

White coat phenomenon is an elevated blood pressure that occurs when the blood pressure assessment is done by a physician or another health care professional. Often, the health care provider will ask the patient to measure his blood pressure in the home setting and record the findings in order to diagnosis high blood pressure. This process is used to determine whether the patient is demonstrating white coat phenomenon. If white coat phenomenon occurs frequently over time, the patient is responding to a perceived stressful situation and may need early hypertensive treatment.

Hypertension is further categorized by cause. There are two types: essential and secondary hypertension. *Essential hypertension* is defined as a chronic elevation in blood pressure that occurs without the evidence of disease. *Secondary hypertension* is high blood pressure that results from some other disorder such as kidney disease. Essential hypertension may be systolic, diastolic, or both systolic and diastolic.

Clinical Manifestations

High blood pressure is asymptomatic in the initial period. The patient with high blood pressure may be of any age ranging from early childhood to older adulthood. High blood pressure may be present in some individuals for many years prior to discovery. During this time, the major organs may be slowly damaged. Clinical signs and symptoms the patient describes may be nonspecific, such as a headache or dizziness, sleepiness, nausea and vomiting, irritability, and visual disturbances. More serious complications may occur when a patient remains undiagnosed for years. Myocardial infarction, heart failure, cerebral vascular accidents, and renal failure may all be the result of untreated hypertension.

Diagnostic Tests

There are no specific diagnostic tests for hypertension except the tracking of serial blood pressures. When any stage of hypertension is diagnosed, a complete work-up needs to be completed to determine the current state of target organs. This provides a baseline from which to assess future changes. The Diagnostic Tests box outlines tests that can

DIAGNOSTIC TESTS for Hypertension

Test with Normal Values	Expected Abnormality
Urinalysis	
Color: Clear	Urinalysis can be useful in the diagnosis of renal disease.
Appearance: Clear	Specific gravity can be low in renal disease because of the inability to concentrate urine.
Glucose: Negative	Protein in the urine is a sensitive indicator of renal dysfunction.
Ketones: Negative	
Blood: Negative	
Microscopic Examination	
RBC: 1 to 2 per low power field	
WBC: 3 to 4	
Casts: Occasional hyaline	
Blood Urea Nitrogen (BUN)	
Adult: 5 to 25 mg/dL *Can be slightly higher in older adults.*	Urea is formed as an end product of protein metabolism and is excreted by the kidneys. An elevated BUN can indicate prerenal failure, renal failure, or dehydration.
BUN/Creatinine Ratio	
Adult: 10:1 to 20:1	A decreased ratio is seen in acute tubular necrosis and low protein intake. An increased ratio is seen in reduced renal perfusion, glomerular disease, obstructive uropathy, or high protein intake.
Creatinine (blood)	
Adult: 0.5 to 1.5 mg/dL. Females may have slightly lower values because of their lesser muscle mass.	Creatinine is a more specific indicator of renal disease than BUN as it is not influenced by diet or fluid status. It is very useful in evaluation of glomerular function. Creatinine is increased in acute and chronic renal failure, shock, essential hypertension, diabetic nephropathy, and chronic heart failure.
Aldosterone (blood)	
Supine: Less than 16 ng/dL (fasting)	An increased serum aldosterone level is associated with hypertension and hypokalemia.
Upright (sitting for at least 2 hours): 4 to 40 ng/dL	Abnormally high levels of aldosterone cause the kidneys to retain salt and excrete potassium, causing the retention of water. This increases blood volume, leading to increased blood pressure.
Aldosterone (urine)	
6 to 25 mcg/24 hours	A 24-hour urine aldosterone test decreases the fluctuation seen in blood draws. Both urine and serum aldosterone levels will be increased in hyponatremia, low-salt diet, and hyperkalemia. Urine and serum aldosterone levels will be decreased in hypernatremia.
Renin (plasma)	
Adult: Normal sodium diet: Supine: 0.2 to 2.3 ng/mL Upright: 1.6 to 4.3 ng/mL Adult: Restricted sodium diet: Upright 4.1 to 10.8 ng/mL	Renin is an enzyme that is secreted by the kidneys that activates the renin-angiotensin system, leading to vasoconstriction and the release of aldosterone. This can lead to hypertension. Increased renin levels can occur in hypovolemia, malignant hypertension, renovascular hypertension, hyperaldosteronism, cancer of the kidney, acute renal failure, and Addison's disease. Decreased renin levels can be seen in essential hypertension, Cushing's syndrome, diabetes, hypothyroidism, and a high sodium diet.
Glucose (blood)	
Adult: 70 to 110 mg/dL	May be elevated in patients who are nonfasting or who have glucose intolerance or diabetes. Some medications (for example, steroids, thiazide diuretics, and loop diuretics) may cause elevated blood glucose.
Sodium (blood)	
135 to 145 mEq/L	Increased sodium levels increase fluid retention, which increases blood pressure. It is increased in dehydration, severe vomiting and diarrhea, heart failure, Cushing's disease, and a high-salt diet. Some medications (for example, thiazide and loop diuretics) can increase the sodium level.

Source: Adapted from Kee, J. L. (2010). *Laboratory and diagnostic tests* (8th ed.). Upper Saddle River, NJ: Pearson; http://www.nhlbi.nih.gov/guidelines/hypertension/index.htm.

Weblink: Adult Obesity

be used during the initial work-up of a newly diagnosed hypertensive patient.

Medical Management

The purpose of the therapeutic plan is to effectively lower and maintain the systemic blood pressure at a normal level. This plan needs to be individualized for each patient. The following factors should be considered when tailoring a plan for a given patient:

- Cultural food preferences
- Age
- Risk factors
- Degree of blood pressure elevation
- Coexisting diseases
- Cost of prescribed pharmacologic agents
- Family/social support
- Amount and type of follow-up care needed.

A comprehensive plan includes addressing all factors that influence the occurrence of hypertension. This includes dietary restrictions, weight reduction where appropriate, medication regimen, exercise program, and stress reduction. Additionally, an evaluation needs to be made to determine whether the patient is able to follow through with sustaining the lifestyle changes, monitoring her blood pressure, and maintaining contact with the health care team.

Diet

The Dietary Approaches to Stop Hypertension diet, known as the **DASH diet,** is low in sodium, saturated fat, cholesterol, and total fat. The diet focuses on fruits, vegetables, nuts, and low-fat dairy products. This plan is rich in potassium and calcium. Although lowering total and saturated fats has no direct effect on controlling blood pressure, it will lower cholesterol and have an effect on the development of coronary artery disease. Therefore, it is an important adjunct to the dietary plan. The DASH diet is described in detail in Chapter 8.

The patient with stage 1 or stage 2 high blood pressure should be encouraged to make the following lifestyle changes: Eat a low-sodium diet (DASH meal plan), reduced-calorie diet (weight reduction diet), or low-cholesterol diet; decrease the intake of saturated fats; limit the use of alcohol; and stop smoking. The DASH diet plan is considered to be equivalent to a single-drug therapy (NHLBI, 2011). Chapter 8 provides an overall description of healthy sensible eating plans, using the Food Guide Pyramid and a description of the DASH diet.

Exercise

Regular physical activities assist in the promotion of cardiovascular fitness and beneficial changes: They lower blood pressure and raise a person's high-density lipoproteins (the good cholesterol). It is essential to have an organized aerobic exercise program, approved by a health care provider, which is completed on a regular basis for 30 to 45 minutes three to five times per week. This plan is begun slowly and stopped if the patient develops shortness of breath, fainting, or chest pain. Physical conditioning has a positive impact on both lowering and maintaining normal blood pressure. Chapter 32 includes an in-depth discussion of the lipids and the benefits of exercise on the heart.

Light weight training is recommended to lower blood pressure; however, heavy lifting is known to raise blood pressure due to the vasovagal response that occurs with intense isometric exercise. Thus, heavy lifting should be avoided in hypertensive individuals. See the Complementary & Alternative Therapies box for a discussion of research related to exercise and patients with perivascular disease.

Weight Control

According to the Centers for Disease Control and Prevention (2010), there has been a dramatic increase in obesity in the last twenty years and rates continue to rise. A standard measurement for expressing the relationship (or ratio) of weight-to-height is the body mass index (BMI). Obesity and BMI measurements are discussed in depth in Chapter 32 (p. 928). A second risk factor for the development of high blood pressure is the presence of excess fat accumulated in the torso that is out of proportion to the rest of the body fat distribution. Men with a waist circumference of 40 inches or more and women with a waist circumference of 35 inches or more are at risk for developing high blood pressure (National Heart, Lung, and Blood Institute, 2011).

For individuals who are 10% or greater above ideal body weight, a reduction in weight by as little as 10 pounds will lower the blood pressure. Additionally, antihypertensive medication effectiveness is enhanced with weight reduction. During the weight reduction process, the blood pressure needs to be assessed regularly and medications adjusted appropriately.

Stress Reduction

A priority for the nurse is discussing the issue of stress with both the patient and family. Often, individuals are not fully aware of the impact stress has on their blood pressure. Individuals may also feel helpless about controlling their stress levels. It is important for the nurse to explain clearly the impact of stress on the development of high blood pressure. Teaching the patient stress reduction techniques is an essential part of the plan for controlling high blood pressure. Exercise, the use of support systems, and some alternative therapies have all been identified as stress reduction techniques. Stress and its impact on the body are discussed in Chapter 9.

Alcohol Consumption

Research indicates that regular consumption of three or more drinks per day increases the risk of hypertension. The systolic blood pressure is more affected by alcohol than is the diastolic blood pressure. The exact mechanism by which alcohol exerts it effect on blood pressure is unclear, but elevated blood pressure may improve and return to normal when alcohol consumption ceases. Since patients tend to understate the amount of alcohol they consume, the nurse needs to realize that the amount may be more and tailor his teaching to the possibility of greater consumption.

Pharmacologic Agents Used to Treat Hypertension

Care of the patient with high blood pressure may include the use of pharmacologic agents. These agents have reduced the morbidity and mortality associated with high blood pressure as well as the incidence of cerebrovascular accidents. The Pharmacology feature (p. 1064) outlines the medications used to treat high blood pressure.

Nursing Management

A partnership of care with the hypertensive patient involves the process of devising a role for each patient, family member, and the nurse. The nurse is the coordinator of care and provider of information concerning risk reduction, health promotion, disease prevention, and the nursing care plan. The nurse's tasks in caring for the individual with prehypertension or stage 1 or stage 2 hypertension focus on educating the patient about lifestyle changes and implementing the therapeutic regimen. One consideration in planning for patient education is the patient's culture,

COMPLEMENTARY & ALTERNATIVE THERAPIES Exercise in Peripheral Arterial Disease *Nancy Yilk*

Description

AN ACTIVE EXERCISE PROGRAM can improve symptoms in patients with early peripheral arterial disease (PAD). By performing a variety of exercises, such as the use of treadmills and elliptical machines, walking, and organized exercise classes, patients can improve peripheral vascular circulation.

Overwhelming evidence garnered from a number of sources, including epidemiological, prospective cohort, and intervention studies, suggests that cardiovascular disease is largely associated with physical inactivity. Exercise also alters vascular remodeling, which involves two forms of vessel growth: angiogenesis and arteriogenesis. Even modest increases in exercise intensity and frequency have hypotensive effects in sedentary hypertensive patients (Yung, Laher, Yao, Chen, Huang, & Leung, 2009).

Research Support

To determine whether supervised treadmill exercise or lower extremity resistance training improves functional performance, 156 patients with PAD were randomly assigned to one of three groups: (1) treadmill exercise, (2) lower extremity resistance training, or (3) a control group at an urban academic medical center.

The participants were supervised by an exercise physiologist. Treadmill exercise intervention consisted of treadmill exercise 3 times a week for 24 weeks. Participants began with 15 minutes of exercise per session and increased to 40 minutes per session by week 8. The initial treadmill walking speed was set at 2.0 mph, or lower if the participant was unable to keep that pace. Between weeks 8 and 24, researchers attempted to increase exercise intensity at least weekly either by increasing treadmill speed or by increasing the treadmill grade. Participants with leg symptoms were encouraged to exercise to near maximal level. Asymptomatic participants were encouraged to exercise to a level of 12 to 14 (moderately hard) based on the Borg rating of perceived exertion scale. The participants also completed the Walking Impairment Questionnaire and completed a 36-Item Short Form Health Survey physical functioning (SF-36 PF) score.

Participants in the lower extremity resistance training group exercised 3 times a week for 24 weeks with a certified trainer. Participants performed 3 sets of 8 repetitions of knee extension, leg press, and leg curl exercises using standard equipment. For each exercise, the 1 repetition maximum (1 rm) was measured at baseline and then subsequently every 4 weeks. Participants began exercising at 50% of their 1 rm. Weights were then increased over the first 5 weeks until participants were lifting 80% of their 1 rm. After that point, weights were used as needed to achieve an exercise intensity.

Those in the control group participated in 11 nutritional information sessions over 6 months. The 1-hour sessions were intended to provide regular contact with participants in the control group. Session topics included nutritional supplements, healthful restaurant eating, and increasing fruit and vegetable consumption. Sessions were led by registered dietitians but were not designed to change behavior.

The 6-month supervised treadmill exercise intervention findings noted increased walking endurance, measured by the 6-minute walk and treadmill walking performance, in patients with PAD both with and without classic intermittent claudication symptoms. Supervised treadmill exercise also increased brachial and arterial flow-mediated dilation and improved quality of life. However, a 6-month lower extremity resistance training intervention did not improve 6-minute walk distance in PAD participants. Resistance training did, however, improve maximal treadmill walking time and quality-of-life measures, particularly stair climbing ability.

Based on the findings reported in this trial, health care providers should recommend supervised treadmill exercise programs for PAD patients, regardless of whether they have classic symptoms of intermittent claudication (McDermott et al., 2009).

A Japanese retrospective cohort study, with a maximum of 13 years of follow-up, demonstrated that undergoing a 12-week supervised exercise training program reduced overall cardiovascular mortality by 52% and morbidity by 30%. In the study, 118 PAD patients were enrolled in a 12-week supervised exercise program. The long-term outcomes of the 64 patients who completed the training were compared with the outcomes of the 54 patients who did not. The primary endpoint was cardiovascular mortality, with the secondary endpoint being cardiovascular morbidity. The cardiovascular death-free rate was higher in patients who completed the training program than in those who did not. Multivariate analysis showed that independent predictors of cardiovascular death were age, the presence of diabetes mellitus, maximum walking distance, history of coronary revascularization, and completion of the training program. The cardiovascular event-free rate was also higher in patients who completed the training program.

Documentation shows that exercise training provides a significant reduction in the cardiovascular mortality and morbidity of patients with PAD. With self-reported physical activity improved by 62%, this suggests that patients were the ones who identified this functional improvement (Sakamoto, Yokoyama, Tamori, Akutsu, Hashimoto, & Takeshita, 2009).

Sources: Adapted from McDermott, M. M., Ades, P., Guralnik, J. M., Dyer, A., Ferrucci, L., Liu, K., et al. (2009). Treadmill exercise and resistance training in patients with peripheral arterial disease with and without intermittent claudication: A randomized controlled trial. *Journal of the American Medical Association, 301*(2): 165–174; Sakamoto, S., Yokoyama, N., Tamori, Y., Akutsu, K., Hashimoto, H., & Takeshita, S. (2009). Patients with peripheral artery disease who complete 12-week supervised exercise training program show reduced cardiovascular mortality and morbidity. *Circulation Journal, 73:* 167–173; Yung, L. M., Laher, I., Yao, X., Chen, Z. Y., Huang, Y., & Leung, F. P. (2009). Exercise, vascular wall and cardiovascular diseases: an update (part 2*). Sports Medicine, 39*(1): 45–63.

including ethnicity. The Cultural Considerations box discusses African Americans' susceptibility to high blood pressure.

Health Promotion

Health care providers are beginning to place more responsibility with the individual for healthy lifestyle choices across the life span because a healthy lifestyle assists in controlling high blood pressure. A healthy lifestyle includes eating three balanced meals per day, maintaining a healthy weight, exercising, limiting the use of alcohol, no smoking, getting adequate sleep (7 to 8 hours per night), and reducing stress. The individual and family need to be familiar with the individual's current blood pressure measurements. If the findings are higher than 120/80 mmHg, the nondiabetic individual needs to seek medical advice. In an individual who has diabetes, blood pressure higher than 130/80 mmHg should signal a need to seek medical advice because of the increased risk of cardiovascular disease in these patients.

Collaborative Management

The goal of therapy for high blood pressure is to reduce the risks of cardiovascular, cerebral vascular, and renal morbidity and mortality through achieving a systolic blood pressure of < 120 mmHg and a diastolic blood pressure of < 80 mmHg. If the patient has diabetes mellitus, the systolic blood pressure should not be greater than 130 mmHg and the diastolic blood pressure should be less than 80 mmHg.

Care of the patient with high blood pressure requires a multidisciplinary approach that will help the patient and family in making lifestyle changes. In order to meet desired patient outcomes, it is essential that this interdisciplinary team communicate openly with one another in developing and evaluating care of the patient and family (IOM [Institute of Medicine], 2010). The nurse and the primary health care provider are the coordinators of care, accessing the other health team members to facilitate the ongoing care of the patient and family. Multiple resources

PHARMACOLOGY Summary of Medications Used to Treat Peripheral Vascular Disease

Medication Category and Action	Application/Indication	Nursing Responsibility
Hypertension		
Thiazide diuretics: Chlorothiazide (Diuril) Chlorthalidone (Hygroton) Hydrochlorothiazide (Hydrodiuril, HCTZ) ***Action:*** Reduces blood volume through increased excretion of water and sodium. Reduced blood volume decreases peripheral resistance and lowers blood pressure.	Initial drug of choice for hypertension. Reduces hypertension-related morbidity and mortality. Frequently prescribed with other antihypertensive medications.	Teach the patient to take this medication at the same time daily. Monitor for hypokalemia, elevated blood glucose, and elevated uric acid levels. Encourage the intake of foods high in potassium such as bananas and orange juice. Review the frequency of prescription renewal as a measure of compliance.
Potassium-sparing diuretics: Amiloride (Midamor) Eplerenone (Inspra) Spironolactone (Aldactone) Triamterene (Dyrenium) ***Action:*** Reduces blood volume through a modest dieresis. Does not cause potassium depletion.	Hypertension.	Monitor for hyperkalemia, especially in patients with diabetes. Monitor for dysrhythmias. Teach patients to avoid excessive amounts of potassium in their diets: avoid salt substitutes, and take no oral potassium supplements unless prescribed by their health care provider. When given concurrently with ACE inhibitors or ARBs, there is an increased risk of hyperkalemia.
Loop diuretics: Bumetanide (Bumex) Ethacrynic acid (Edecrin) Furosemide (Lasix) Torsemide (Demadex) ***Action:*** Reduces blood volume through diuresis. Can cause a more significant drop in blood pressure than thiazide diuretics.	Hypertension.	Monitor for hypokalemia, dehydration, and orthostatic hypotension. Can cause ototoxicity (damage to the inner ear, potentially causing hearing loss).
Angiotensin-converting enzyme (ACE) inhibitors: Captopril (Capoten) Enalapril (Vasotec) Fosinopril (Monopril) Lisinopril (Prinivil, Zestril) Quinapril (Accupril) Ramipril (Altace) ***Action:*** Works within the renin-angiotensin-aldosterone system (RAAS) to inhibit the vasconstricting action of angiotensin II and the angiotensin-mediated secretion of aldosterone, decreasing blood pressure. Enhance the effects of thiazide diuretics.	Hypertension. Heart failure. Use in all patients with reduced ventricular function; left ventricular ejection fraction (LVEF) $< 40\%$.	Monitor blood pressure regularly when drug is initiated and when dosage is titrated. Hold the drug and notify the health care provider if the systolic blood pressure is less than 90 mmHg. Monitor for ACE inhibitor-induced cough, dizziness, hypotension, hyperkalemia, and worsening renal insufficiency. Angioedema may also occur in rare settings. Angioedema indicates an allergic reaction and immediate intervention may be needed, depending on the patient's symptoms. Monitor for: Orthostatic hypotension Elevated serum sodium, potassium, and/or creatinine Drug-induced neutropenia Teach the patient to avoid over-the-counter NSAIDs as they can reduce the effectiveness of ACE inhibitors.
Angiotensin II receptor blockers (ARBs): Candesartan cilexetil Eprosartan mesylate Irbesartan Losartan (Cozaar) Telmisartan Valsartan ***Action:*** Causes inhibition by blocking RAAS activation at the angiotensin II receptor site. Angiotensin receptor blockers have been found to have similar clinical effects as ACE inhibitors with regard to the interference with the RAAS. They decrease afterload, decrease sodium resorption, and increase contractility.	Hypertension. Heart failure in patients who are intolerant to ACE inhibitors with an LVEF $< 40\%$.	Monitor blood pressure regularly when drug is initiated and when dosage is titrated. Hold the drug and notify the health care provider if the systolic blood pressure is less than 90 mmHg. Monitor for: Dizziness, orthostatic hypotension Elevated serum sodium, potassium creatinine Monitor for worsening renal insufficiency.

PHARMACOLOGY Summary of Medications Used to Treat Peripheral Vascular Disease, *continued*

Medication Category and Action	Application/Indication	Nursing Responsibility
Dihydropyridine calcium-channel blockers: Amlodipine (Norvasc) Felodipine (Plendil) Nicardipine (Cardene) Nifedipine (Procardia) Nondihydropyridine calcium-channel blockers: Diltiazem (Cardizem, Dilacor) Verapamil (Calan) ***Action:*** Relax arterial smooth wall muscle leading to decreased peripheral resistance and lowered blood pressure. Usually not used as only therapy for hypertension.	Hypertension, especially as an additional agent in older and African American patients.	Monitor blood pressure regularly when drug is initiated and when dosage is titrated. Hold the drug and notify the health care provider if the systolic blood pressure is less than 90 mmHg. Monitor for: Reflex tachycardia Elevated blood glucose Gingival hyperplasia Palpitations, weight gain, peripheral edema, skin rashes Teach the patient to avoid grapefruit/grapefruit juice because of potential drug–food interactions.
Beta-adrenergic blockers: Non-selective beta-adrenergic blockers: Nadolol (Corgard) Pindolol (Visken) Propranolol (Inderal) Sotalol (Betapace) Timolol (Blocadren) ***Action:*** Nonselective: causes a decrease in blood pressure through a mixture of beta-blocking effects but does not cause reflex tachycardia or decreased heart rate. Selective beta-adrenergic blockers: Acebutolol (Sectral) Atenolol (Tenormin) Bisoprolol (Zebeta) Esmolol (Brevibloc) Metoprolol (Lopressor) ***Action:*** Selective: completely blocks beta-1 receptor stimulation in cardiac smooth muscle.	Hypertension. Dysrhythmias. Angina pectoris. Hypertension. Heart failure. Stable angina. Myocardial infarction.	Monitor blood pressure and heart rate regularly when the drug is initiated and when the dosage is titrated. Hold the drug and notify the health care provider if the systolic blood pressure is less than 90 mmHg and/or the heart rate is less than 60 per minute. Monitor for: Bradycardia Elevated blood glucose Teach the patient to avoid abruptly stopping beta-adrenergic blocker agents.
Alpha adrenergic antagonists: Doxazosin (Cardura) Prazosin (Minipress) Terazosin (Hytrin) ***Action:*** Lowers blood pressure directly by blocking sympathetic receptors in the arterioles, causing arterial dilation. Used concurrently with other classes of antihypertensive agents.	Hypertension.	May cause significant orthostatic hypotension, especially when first initiated. Older patients may have more orthostatic hypotension. Monitor for dizziness, light-headedness, and syncope. Monitor for headache, nausea, and vomiting. May contribute to decreased libido and erectile dysfunction.
Alpha agonists: Methyldopa (Aldomet) Clonidine (Catapres) ***Action:*** Inhibits the sympathetic nervous system. Lowers peripheral resistance leading to lower blood pressure.	Hypertension that has not responded to other antihypertensive agents. Tolerance can develop after a few months of therapy, requiring increased dosing. Hypertension.	Monitor for CNS effects, which are most prominent when initially started or when dosage is increased: drowsiness, depression, headache, sedation, bizarre dreams. Monitor for hepatotoxicity and hemolytic anemia. May contribute to decreased libido, inability to ejaculate, menstrual cycle irregularities, or gynecomastia. Interacts with many drugs, including alcohol, lithium, tricyclic antidepressants, and NSAIDs. Monitor for adverse CNS effects as previously noted, including dry mouth.

(*continued*)

PHARMACOLOGY Summary of Medications Used to Treat Peripheral Vascular Disease, *continued*

Medication Category and Action	Application/Indication	Nursing Responsibility
		When administered via transdermal patch, it can cause skin irritation and itching. Teach the patient the importance of continuing medication as prescribed. Abruptly stopping the drug can cause rebound hypertension, agitation, nervousness, and anxiety.
Vasodilators: Hydralazine (Apresoline) Diazoxide (Hyperstat) Fenoldopam (Corlopam) Nitroprusside (Nipride) Nitroglycerin (Tridil) ***Action:*** Lowers blood pressure rapidly by relaxing the smooth muscle tone of the blood vessel, thus reducing the peripheral resistance.	Treatment of acute hypertension in the hospital setting. Hypertensive crisis.	Monitor the blood pressure frequently after initiating therapy or dosage adjustment. Monitor for hypotension, dizziness, or flushing. Prolonged administration of nitroprusside can lead to thiocyanate toxicity. Monitor for lethargy, blurred vision, metabolic acidosis, or altered level of consciousness.
Direct renin inhibitor: Aliskiren (Tekturna) ***Action:*** Inhibits the production of renin, leading to lowered blood pressure.	Hypertension.	Monitor for diarrhea, cough, flu-like symptoms, and rash.
Anticoagulants		
Unfractionated heparin ***Action:*** Prevents clot formation by indirectly inhibiting thrombin. It binds to antithrombin III (AT-III), preventing the formation of fibrin clots.	Prevention of clot formation and extension in venous thrombosis and pulmonary embolism; prevention of postoperative deep venous thrombosis (DVT); treatment of disseminate intravascular coagulation (DIC) (Chapter 56); maintenance of venous access device patency.	Reponses to heparin vary considerably between patients. Monitor for bleeding from the gums and/or bleeding from puncture sites; hemoptysis; and hematuria. Monitor activated partial thromboplastin time (aPTT), blood count, and platelet count. Assess the patient for the presence of beef or pork allergy, history of heparin-induced thrombocytopenia (HIT), or active bleeding (contraindicated in these patients).
Low molecular weight heparin (LMWH): Enoxaparin (Lovenox) Dalteparin (Fragmin) Tinzaparin (Innohep)	Treatment of pulmonary embolism; treatment of DVT; prevention of venous thromboembolism.	Monitor for adverse effects, such as bleeding. Monitor for increased risk of bleeding in the presence of reduced creatinine clearance. Contraindicated in patients who have or will receive epidural or spinal anesthesia or puncture.
Warfarin (Coumadin) ***Action:*** Inhibits two enzymes required in the formation of activated vitamin K. Inhibits the synthesis of new clotting factors but does not affect clotting factors that are already circulating.	Long-term prophylaxis for thrombus formation (e.g., mitral valve replacement, atrial fibrillation, hypercoagulability disorders).	Monitor for adverse effects: bleeding, nausea, and vomiting. Monitor serum PT/INR. Assess current drug regimen prior to initiating warfarin. Assess for potential of drug interaction: NSAIDs, acetaminophen, phenytoin, barbiturates, and many others. For patients on warfarin (Coumadin), provide detailed discharge instructions regarding PT/INR follow-up and potential impact of alcohol, food, and various other medications, including over-the-counter and herbal preparations.
Antiplatelet		
Aspirin (acetylsalicylic acid, ASA) ***Action:*** Inhibits platelet aggregation.	Prevention of recurrent thromboembolism in MI, stroke.	Monitor for adverse effects: dyspepsia, nausea, heartburn, abdominal pain, and gastrointestinal bleeding. Monitor for signs of toxicity (tinnitus, altered hearing). Increase blood sugar monitoring in the presence of diabetes. Give with food. Warn the patient to avoid alcohol and other drugs containing salicylates.

PHARMACOLOGY Summary of Medications Used to Treat Peripheral Vascular Disease, *continued*

Medication Category and Action	Application/Indication	Nursing Responsibility
Clopidogrel (Plavix) Ticlopidine[a] (Ticlid) Cilostazol[b] (Pletal) ***Action:*** Inhibits adenosine diphosphate (ADP)-induced platelet aggregation. Promotes vasodilation.	Prevention of recurrent thromboembolism in MI and stroke.	Monitor for adverse effects: bleeding, abdominal pain, diarrhea, nausea, and headache. Monitor blood count, bleeding time, and platelet function. Check neutrophil count if an infection develops. Be aware of drug interactions (NSAIDs, diltiazem, vitamin A, anticoagulants, and others). Monitor for altered drug efficacy. Give with food. [a]Monitor for hematologic adverse reactions: agranulocytosis, aplastic anemia, thrombotic thrombocytopenic purpura. [b]Warn patient to avoid grapefruit and grapefruit juice.
Hemorheologic		
Pentoxifylline (Trental) ***Action:*** Prevents thrombus formation by decreasing red blood cell viscosity and improves microcirculation by decreasing platelet aggregation.	Intermittent claudication.	Monitor for adverse effects: dyspepsia, nausea, vomiting, tremors, dizziness, and headache. Monitor for toxicity in presence of impaired renal function. Be aware of drug interactions (cimetidine, insulin, and theophylline). Monitor for drug toxicity or reduced efficacy. Give with food.
Antidepressants		
Nontricyclic: Bupropion (Zyban, Wellbutrin) ***Action:*** Antidepressant neurochemical effect unknown.	Smoking cessation (off-label use for addiction to smokeless tobacco), depression.	Monitor for adverse effects: dry mouth, insomnia, sweating, blurred vision, weakness, vomiting, constipation, weight loss, or gain. Monitor for increased seizure potential if increasing dose, dose > 300 mg/day, or in presence of seizure disorder; head trauma history. Monitor for treatment-induced hypertension. Warn patient to avoid alcohol (increases seizure risk) and not to stop drug abruptly.
Tricyclic: Nortriptyline (Pamelor) ***Action:*** Antidepressant effect may be due to inhibition of norepinephrine reuptake.	Depression, smoking cessation (off-label use).	Monitor for adverse effects: orthostatic hypotension, urinary retention, constipation, dry mouth, dizziness, blurred vision or tachycardia. Monitor vital signs when initiating drug. Withhold and notify health care provider for systolic blood pressure decrease > 20 mmHg or sudden increase in pulse. Be aware of drug interactions (alcohol, antihypertensives, hypnotics, and others). Monitor for adverse reactions. Contraindicated in patients during or within 14 days of treatment with monoamine oxidase inhibitor (MAOI).
Anti-anxiety		
Alprazolam (Xanax) Chlordiazepoxide (Librium) Diazepam (Valium) Lorazepam (Ativan) ***Action:*** Central nervous system depression. Produces relaxation, calmness.	Anxiety disorders; short-term relief from anxiety symptoms.	Monitor for drowsiness, ataxia, or dizziness. As appropriate, instruct the patient about nonpharmacologic techniques for relaxation (e.g., deep breathing, massage, guided imagery).
Smoking Deterrents		
Nicotine: Gum (Nicorette) Transdermal patch (Habitrol, NicoDerm) Nasal spray (Nicotrol NS) ***Action:*** Replaces nicotine.	Symptom reduction of nicotine-dependent smoker during cigarette withdrawal.	Monitor for adverse effects: headache, dizziness, and nausea. Monitor for route-specific adverse effects: gum, tongue, mouth, throat irritation; jaw pain; patch: skin irritation; nasal spray: nasal, throat irritation, or rhinorrhea. Be aware of drug interactions with, for example, theophylline, insulin, and acetaminophen. Warn patient against smoking cigarettes or using smokeless tobacco while on replacement therapy.
Varenicline (Chantix) ***Action:*** Provides some nicotine effects through nicotine receptor agonist activity; blocks pleasurable effects of nicotine.	Nicotine withdrawal symptoms.	Monitor for adverse effects: nausea, vomiting, diarrhea, anxiety, headache, sleep disturbance, joint pain, and lethargy. Monitor for mood disturbances (depression, suicidal ideation).

Source: Adams, M. P., & Koch, R. W. (2010). *Pharmacology: Connections to nursing practice.* Upper Saddle River, NJ: Pearson.

CULTURAL CONSIDERATIONS
African Americans and Hypertension

African Americans are particularly likely to have hypertension, which is a major contributor to cardiovascular morbidity and mortality in this population. African Americans have disproportionately higher rates of fatal stroke, death from heart disease, heart failure, and hypertension-related end-stage kidney disease than Whites. Barriers to optimal care for many African Americans with hypertension have been identified as patient level barriers, health care provider level barriers, and systems level barriers. Patient level barriers include poor medication compliance, poor knowledge level about hypertension, and reluctance to adhere to lifestyle changes, such as weight loss, smoking cessation, and blood pressure monitoring. Health care provider level barriers include poor adherence to evidence-based and consensus guidelines that have been developed. An example of this is suboptimal pharmacologic management of systolic hypertension. Systems level barriers that can affect these patients may include lack of access to health care providers, high cost of medications, and lack of medical insurance.

Sources: Adapted from American Heart Association. (2011). High blood pressure. Retrieved from http://www.americanheart.org/presenter.jhtml?identifier=4623; Ogedegbe, G., Tobin, J. N., Fernandez, S., Gerwin, W., Diaz-Gloster, M., Cassells, A. N., et al. (2009). Counseling African Americans to Control Hypertension (CAATCH) Trial: A multi-level intervention to improve blood pressure control in hypertensive Blacks. *Circulation: Cardiovascular Quality and Outcomes, 2*, 249–256.

may be needed to support the patient and family during the management of this chronic illness. The roles of resource individuals for the patient are as follows:

- ***Clinical Dietitians:*** The patient and family will be making a number of lifestyle changes, including the selection of food and the amount to be eaten. The patient needs the clinical expertise of a therapeutic dietitian to assist in the modification of diet and recipes, as well as menu planning. This can be a major lifestyle change with many cultural consequences.
- ***Fitness/Exercise Leader:*** The fitness/exercise leader is employed by a recognized, organized health care system. The leader is able to assess, follow a health care provider's prescription, and modify the types and kind of activities for the individual with hypertension.
- ***Pharmacist:*** The pharmacist provides information about the action of the antihypertensive medications as well as precautions and side effects.

Complications of High Blood Pressure

The impact of uncontrolled high blood pressure on organs occurs insidiously over an extended period of time throughout the body. The JNC 7 report (NHLBI, 2011) referred to certain complications of hypertension as target organ damage, with the heart, kidney, brain, peripheral vasculature, and retina considered to be target organs. Prolonged untreated hypertension causes both large and small blood vessels to become sclerotic, tortuous, and weak. These changes cause narrowing of the artery lumen, decreased blood flow to organs, and increased blood pressure. Additionally, the weakened arteries are more prone to rupture. Large arteries tend to occlude or rupture, causing a loss of the blood supply to organs and tissues. Small arteries that are damaged decrease the blood supply to organs, resulting in structural changes. An increased diastolic blood pressure causes injury to the intimal wall of the arteries, resulting in plaque buildup and local inflammation, which in turn result in plaque rupture, platelet aggregation, and subsequent vessel occlusion. The result is a decreased blood supply to organs, leading to progressive loss of function. The organs that are most affected by these changes are the heart, brain, kidney, and retina. Chart 35–1 outlines the target organs that are most prone to damage.

CHART 35–1 Target Organ Damage

Left ventricular hypertrophy	Retinopathy
Angina or prior myocardial infarction	Prior coronary revascularization
Heart failure	Renal failure
Stroke or transient ischemic attack	Chronic kidney disease
Peripheral arterial disease	Peripheral ischemia
Vision changes leading to blindness	

Source: Adapted from National Heart Lung and Blood Institute (NHLBI). (2011). The Seventh Report of the Joint National Committee on Prevention, Detection, Evaluation, and Treatment of High Blood Pressure (JNC 7). Retrieved from http://www.nhlbi.nih.gov/guidelines/hypertension/index.htm.

Ischemic heart disease is the most common site of target organ damage associated with high blood pressure (NHLBI, 2011). As a result of prolonged hypertension, the coronary arteries are unable to deliver enough blood to the myocardium. This causes the heart muscle to lose its ability to contract sufficiently, resulting in decreased cardiac output. The shearing force of blood flowing with increased pressure over time causes irregularities in the intima of the lumen of the arteries. This causes an increased buildup of plaque, ultimately narrowing the lumen of the artery and decreasing blood flow to the myocardium, resulting in ischemic heart disease.

Heart failure occurs because of the increased cardiac workload due to pumping against an increased afterload, which is the increased pressure created by the narrowed lumen of diseased blood vessels, as the heart attempts to eject its blood supply. Eventually, the left ventricle hypertrophies to compensate for increased pressure. Left ventricular hypertrophy increases with age and is more prevalent in patients with higher systolic and diastolic pressures (Porth & Matfin, 2009). Heart failure is a systolic or diastolic ventricular impairment, which can be caused by both ischemic heart disease and long-standing uncontrolled high blood pressure. Chapter 34 has an in-depth discussion of systolic and diastolic heart failure.

Hypertension leads to nephrosclerosis, which is a common cause of renal insufficiency. This condition is caused by diseased blood vessels that are no longer able to deliver enough blood to the kidneys, resulting in decreased renal function. Additionally, high blood pressure accelerates other types of kidney diseases, particularly diabetes. The American Diabetic Association recommends that diabetics maintain a blood pressure of less than 130/80 mmHg (ADA, 2011). Chapter 39 includes a complete discussion of renal disease.

The patient with diabetes may have high levels of circulating cholesterol and other lipids, which affects the development of atherosclerosis, arteriosclerosis, and severe coronary heart disease, as well as multiple microcirculatory lesions. Due to the complications of diabetes, atherosclerosis increases the probability of developing hypertension, diabetic retinopathy, cataracts, and chronic renal disease.

Metabolic syndrome is being diagnosed more frequently in the adult obese population. In fact, it is estimated that one-fourth of the U.S. population has this syndrome. The characteristics are insulin resistance, hypertension, dyslipidemia, high triglyceride levels, diabetes mellitus, low HDL cholesterol level, and a tendency for the patient to form blood clots (NHLBI, 2011). Metabolic syndrome is discussed in detail in Chapter 32.

Cerebral vascular disease is caused by arteriosclerotic plaques that occur in the feeder arteries to the brain. When these arteries are damaged by prolonged hypertension, plaque forms and becomes vulnerable to rupture away from the wall of the artery. Ruptured plaque activates the clotting mechanism, and platelets aggregate, causing a clot to form and block the artery, leading to an acute loss of brain function in the local area (Porth & Matfin, 2009). High blood pressure may cause the vessel to rupture. Hemorrhage follows, compressing the local brain tissue. Subsequent clotting of the blood vessel leads to blood vessel blockage. Cerebral vascular disorders are discussed in Chapter 22.

Hypertensive eye disease affects the retinal arterioles, retinal parenchyma, choroids, and optic nerve. High blood pressure can be detected in the eye by the presence of diffuse arteriolar narrowing, bleeding, cotton wool patches, hard exudates, microaneurysms, zones of nonperfusion, and flame-shaped bleeding at or near the retina (NHLBI, 2011). All of these conditions are visible through an ophthalmoscope. The patient's level of visual acuity is dependent on the degree of pathology. Eye disorders are discussed in Chapter 64.

Hypertensive Emergencies

If left untreated, high blood pressure can lead to life-threatening emergencies. Approximately 90% of the cases of untreated hypertension will lead to death from myocardial infarction, stroke, renal failure, or aortic dissection. The most common emergencies are discussed next.

Hypertensive Crisis

Hypertensive crisis is rare and sometimes has a fatal occurrence characterized by the sudden onset of a diastolic blood pressure between 120 and 130 mmHg, the clinical manifestation of target organ vascular damage, and the presence of retinal exudates and hemorrhage. A diastolic blood pressure greater than 120 mmHg causes acute vascular damage, and structural organ changes begin to occur. Catecholamines are released and the renin-angiotensin mechanism is activated, raising the blood pressure even further. The symptoms may include unstable angina, pulmonary edema, myocardial infarction, eclampsia, stroke, life-threatening arterial bleeding, aortic dissection, morning headache, blurred vision, dyspnea, and renal failure.

The causes of a hypertensive crisis include acute and chronic renal failure, exacerbation of chronic hypertension, sudden withdrawal of antihypertensive medications, and vasculitis. The management of a hypertensive crisis includes immediate hospitalization in a critical care area such as a critical care unit. The goal of management is to bring the blood pressure down within 1 hour of the crisis without allowing it to drop too low. Decreasing the blood pressure too severely can cause cerebral and/or myocardial infarcts and renal failure. Short-acting or titratable intravenous medications, such as labetelol, nicardipine, nitroglycerin, or nitroprusside, can be useful (Adams & Koch, 2010).

Safety Alert *Hypertensive crisis is a medical emergency. It involves the rapid onset of a systolic blood pressure greater than 240 mmHg and/or a diastolic blood pressure greater than 130 mmHg. The nurse must notify the health care provider immediately of marked elevations in blood pressure.*

Hypertensive Encephalopathy

Hypertensive encephalopathy is a very dangerous state of multifocal cerebral ischemia due to a severely acute or subacute elevated blood pressure. The pathogenesis of hypertensive encephalopathy is the detrimental effect of high blood pressure on the brain's arterioles. The patient with this diagnosis needs urgent and immediate treatment. The decreasing incidence of hypertensive encephalopathy is due in part to the use of effective antihypertensive drugs.

Peripheral Arterial Disease

The American College of Cardiology and the American Heart Association (AHA) define **peripheral arterial disease (PAD)** as "vascular disease caused primarily by atherosclerosis and thromboembolic pathophysiological processes that alter the normal structure of the aorta, its visceral arterial branches, and the arteries of the lower extremities" (AHA, 2008). This chronic and progressive disorder is a largely underrecognized and underdiagnosed disease affecting millions of Americans. Atherosclerosis has been defined as the process of fatty substances, cholesterol, cellular waste products, calcium, and fibrin building up in the inner lining of an artery, resulting in plaque buildup and a narrowing of the lumen of the artery (AHA, 2008). Peripheral arterial disease is defined as the development of this atherosclerotic process at various levels in the aortic bifurcation, the iliac arteries, and the lower extremities, including the femoral, popliteal, peroneal, and tibial arteries. Atherosclerosis is further discussed in Chapter 32.

Etiology and Epidemiology

The incidence of PAD increases with age, and approximately 5% of people age 55 and older and 20% of those age 70 and older have signs and symptoms. The incidence in men is slightly higher than that in women; in addition, PAD is more common in the African American population. The risk factors, similar to those of heart disease and stroke, include cigarette smoking, diabetes, hyperlipidemia, hypertension, elevated C-reactive protein, and elevated homocystein levels (Muir, 2009). Screening for PAD is recommended for patients with exertional leg pain, patients over age 50 who have associated risk factors such as smoking and diabetes, patients who have had diabetes for more than 20 years, and all patients over the age of 70 (Christman, 2009).

Pathophysiology

Peripheral arterial disease is atherosclerosis of the peripheral arteries, including the aorta and the arteries that supply the arms and legs. Atherosclerosis is a disease process that occurs over many years, usually beginning in childhood. Lipids (fats) collect under the inner lining of damaged artery walls, eventually narrowing or blocking the artery and obstructing blood flow. Over time, this fatty tissue can erode the wall of the artery, diminish its elasticity, and interfere with blood flow. Plaque deposits also can rupture, causing debris to migrate downstream within an artery. Clots also can form around the plaque deposits, further interfering with blood flow and posing added danger if they break off.

Clinical Manifestations

Signs and symptoms of PAD may include intermittent claudication, weakness of muscles or limbs with use, absent or diminished pulses, poor hair growth, cool skin, resting limb pain, **paresthesia** (an abnormal physical sensation such as prickling, tingling, or numbness), and poor healing of sores or ulcers.

Intermittent claudication (IC), or exercise-induced leg pain, is the most common symptom of PAD. Patients may describe their pain as aching, cramping, tiredness, and/or fatigue. This pain can occur in the buttocks, hip, thigh, or calf, depending on the portion of the arterial tree affected by atherosclerotic disease. The muscle group distal to a stenotic (narrowed) or occluded (completely blocked) artery is affected by the decreased circulation. For example, more proximal lesions, such as aortoiliac lesions, will produce the pain of IC in the hip, buttocks, or thigh, whereas lesions lower in the femoral or popliteal arteries produce calf pain. When a muscle is at rest, the metabolic needs are minimal, and even diseased arteries can provide enough blood to maintain perfusion. With exercise, such as walking, metabolic demands are increased, and the diseased arteries cannot deliver the needed oxygen to the muscles or dispose of the metabolic by-product lactic acid. The buildup of lactic acid causes pain in the affected muscle group of the leg. When the walking ceases, or shortly afterward, the pain resolves and exercise may resume.

Intermittent claudication can remain stable for years, and walking can improve muscle endurance, especially if the patient stops smoking tobacco. The atherosclerotic process can, however, progress to a point at which the patient experiences pain in the foot at rest. Rest pain is a sign of severe ischemia or lack of sufficient oxygen supply to the tissues. It is characterized by pain in the forefoot and toes, usually worse at night when lying flat in bed, and can either awaken a person from sleep or prevent sleep altogether. Patients will usually be more comfortable with the leg in a dependent position, such as dangling over the edge of the bed or chair, because gravity can enhance arterial circulation. Narcotic pain medicines, such as opiates, are indicated but may not control the pain well due to the severe nature of the ischemic rest pain.

Ulceration (skin breakdown) can occur as a result of poor blood supply, pressure, or trauma to an ischemic limb. A nonhealing area of tissue injury is prone to necrosis or gangrene and infection. Arterial ulceration accounts for about 20% of all leg ulcers and is most likely to occur at the distal-most point of arterial flow. The toes are a common site for arterial ulceration. In arterial ulcerations, the base is pale, gray, or yellowish in color with little drainage and regular borders. Wounds are described in detail in Chapter 60. The foot pulses are diminished or absent, and the skin is pale and cool to touch. The patient typically complains of a burning, throbbing pain, unless the patient has peripheral neuropathy, most commonly seen in long-standing diabetes. Pain management can be challenging, requiring narcotics for relief (Christman, 2009).

Safety Alert *Ongoing and regular nursing assessment of ulcerations and wounds in the patient with peripheral vascular disorders is essential so that early signs and symptoms of infection can be detected and treated. Assessment finding in early localized infection can include low-grade temperature, warmth, tenderness, pain, edema, erythema, and new or increased drainage that may have a foul odor. If the patient develops mental status changes, hyperventilation, tachycardia, fever, chills, elevated white blood count, fatigue, or malaise, systemic infection (sepsis) may be occurring. The nurse needs to report these changes to the health care practitioner.*

Laboratory and Diagnostic Procedures

The diagnosis of peripheral arterial disease is typically based on the patient's history; physical examination findings; and resting **ankle–brachial index (ABI)** results, which is a simple-to-perform, noninvasive test that detects peripheral arterial disease of the legs (Figure 35–4◆). Patients who should have an ABI done include those patients with exertional leg pain or unhealed ulcers who are age 65 or more, or those patients with diabetes who smoke and are over 50 years of age (Rooke et al., 2011). To determine the ABI, the nurse checks the blood pressure of both arms with a Doppler and takes the higher reading. Using a Doppler over the posterior tibial and dorsalis pedis pulses, the nurse determines the blood pressure in the foot and takes the higher of the two. The ABI is the ratio of the highest ankle systolic pressure to the highest arm systolic pressure. An ABI ≥ 1.0 is considered normal, whereas a finding of ≤ 0.90 indicates peripheral arterial disease. A result less than 0.4 indicates severe arterial ischemia (Gardner & Afaq, 2008). The Diagnostic Tests box outlines the remainder of the diagnostic tests performed for peripheral arterial disease.

Medical Management

Patients with PAD should receive lifelong antiplatelet therapy with aspirin. Aspirin has antithrombotic effects and inhibits platelet aggregation.

$$\text{Right ABI} = \frac{\text{Average right ankle pressure}}{\text{Average brachial artery pressure}}$$

$$\text{Left ABI} = \frac{\text{Average left ankle pressure}}{\text{Average brachial artery pressure}}$$

Interpretation of ABI	
>1.30	Noncompressible
0.91–1.30	Normal
0.41–0.90	Mild-to-moderate peripheral arterial disease
0.00–0.40	Severe peripheral arterial disease

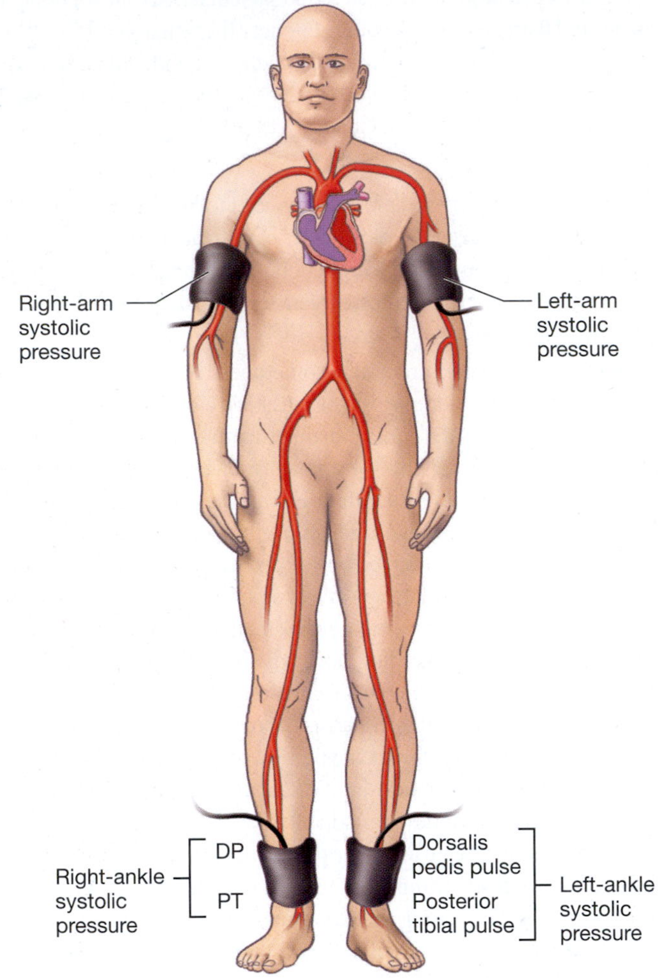

FIGURE 35–4 ◆ Ankle–brachial index chart.

Ticlopidine (Ticlid), clopidogrel (Plavix), and cilostazol (Pletal) or pentoxifylline (Trental) also may be indicated for some patients. Ticlopidine and clopidogrel, which are thienopyridine derivatives, inhibit adenosine diphosphate (ADP)-induced platelet aggregation. Cilostazol inhibits phosphodiesterase III, but its exact mechanism of action is not fully understood. It suppresses platelet aggregation and is a direct arterial vasodilator. Pentoxifylline has weak antithrombotic effects and lowers blood viscosity (Adams & Koch, 2010). Cardiovascular risk reduction strategies are also important for the patient with PAD and include the use of beta-adrenergic blockers, angiotensin receptor blockers, and lipid-lowering agents. Additional information about these therapies can be found in Chapter 32.

Endovascular repair is the treatment of vascular disease from inside the blood vessel (endoluminal) and includes angioplasty, stenting, and radiation therapy. Percutaneous transluminal angioplasty (PTA) is indicated for those patients who are limited by their pain when

DIAGNOSTIC TESTS for Peripheral Arterial Disease

Test	Expected Abnormality
Ankle–brachial index (ABI) Normal: 0.95 to 1.1	≤0.9 Indicative of PAD. ≤0.4 advanced ischemic disease with impending loss of tissue. Segmental arterial pressures and ankle–brachial indexes (ABIs) can be falsely elevated if the patient has calcified, noncompressible arteries. May be unreliable in patients with diabetes or patients with heavily calcified vessels. Suspect calcified arteries if the ABI is > 1.3 and/or if the ankle pressure is > 300 mmHg.
Treadmill exercise arterial studies	A decrease in the ABI following exercise indicates arterial insufficiency. Patients with intermittent claudication (IC) will demonstrate 20 mmHg or more decrease in ABI within 1 minute following exercise.
Duplex ultrasound	Uses sound waves to identify areas of stenosis in arterial vessels and defines severity of the stenosis. Identifies areas of turbulent flow and abnormal flow patterns.
Segmental arterial pressures	This procedure assesses the femoral, popliteal, dorsalis pedis, and posterior tibial arteries. A decrease in pressure of 20 to 30 mmHg from one segment to the adjacent, more distal segment implies a significant arterial obstruction in the vessels between the cuffs.
Angiography	Visualizes anatomy, areas of stenosis, and/or occlusion.
Computed tomography (CT)	Visualizes anatomy, areas of stenosis, and/or occlusion.
Magnetic resonance imaging (MRI) and magnetic resonance angiography (MRA)	Visualizes anatomy, areas of stenosis, and/or occlusion. Provides excellent anatomic detail. Arteries treated with stents may show artifact and be inaccurate.

there is a reasonable likelihood of improvement with intervention. Percutaneous transluminal angioplasty is an invasive percutaneous procedure that can be done using local anesthesia with sedation. It is performed in the interventional radiology suite or in the cardiac catheterization laboratory by vascular surgeons, interventional radiologists, and/or cardiologists. A balloon-tipped catheter is inserted into the arterial vasculature, usually the femoral artery, and positioned at the area of obstruction. The balloon is then inflated, disrupting the plaque and stretching the media of the artery, thereby enlarging the lumen and enhancing blood flow. Stents—tubular metal devices made of stainless steel, nitinol (nickel titanium), or titanium—are inserted to act as a mechanical scaffolding to hold a vessel open in the diseased area. Stents and other interventional devices are further discussed in Chapter 32.

Percutaneous transluminal angioplasty is indicated for the treatment of some arterial occlusive disease. It is most successful when performed for shorter lesions that are < 5 cm (2 in.) in the iliac artery and < 10 cm (4 in.) in the superficial femoral artery. Percutaneous transluminal angioplasty of lesions longer than these is more likely to restenose. Percutaneous transluminal angioplasty also may be done in the smaller tibial vessels if the lesion is < 2 cm (<1 in.) (Gardner & Afaq, 2008). The long-term results of PTA for these lesions are less than optimal, but performing this procedure may allow enough improved blood flow to permit wound healing and/or limb salvage and to prevent or delay amputation.

Complications of PTA are uncommon; they include bleeding and hematoma at the access site, distal embolization, arterial dissection, and occlusion at the dilation site. Other complications can include contrast allergy and contrast-induced renal failure. Following PTA, patients are discharged on aspirin and/or clopidogrel. Although the long-term results of this procedure are unknown at this time, PTA is rapidly becoming the initial intervention for revascularization of the lower extremities. The PTA technique is further discussed in Chapter 32 under percutaneous coronary interventions. Other adjunctive interventional techniques such as the use of lasers, cutting balloons, atherectomy devices, and thermal devices can be useful in treating the iliac, femoral, popliteal, and tibial arteries.

Surgical Management

Arterial bypass is the surgical revascularization procedure performed for debilitating peripheral arterial disease. Surgery is done when a patient has disabling claudication and/or limb-threatening ischemia due to blocked arteries in the lower extremities. These reconstructive procedures, which are performed by a vascular surgeon, involve bypassing areas of occlusion with the patient's own vein (autogenous) or a synthetic graft. Numerous types of surgical procedures are available for the treatment of peripheral arterial disease, depending on the level of the disease within the aorta and distal leg arteries. These include aortoiliac bypass; aortobifemoral bypass; iliac endarterectomy, or iliofemoral bypass; axillofemoral bypass; and femoropopliteal bypass, the most commonly performed arterial bypass (Figures 35–5◆ through 35–9◆, p.1073). Following arterial bypass surgeries, frequent and careful assessment of circulation to the leg and foot is essential (Figure 35–10◆). Pulselessness distal to the graft site indicates decreased or no blood flow.

Amputation may be indicated for uncontrolled infection, uncontrolled pain, and extensive tissue loss and in cases in which adequate revascularization cannot be accomplished. Chapter 50 discusses amputation.

Nursing Management

Peripheral arterial disease is a systemic process, and the majority of patients with PAD also have coronary artery disease (Gardner & Afaq, 2008). When assessing patients for PAD, the nurse needs to obtain subjective information from the patient about the present illness and symptoms, as well as the medical history, especially previous cardiac

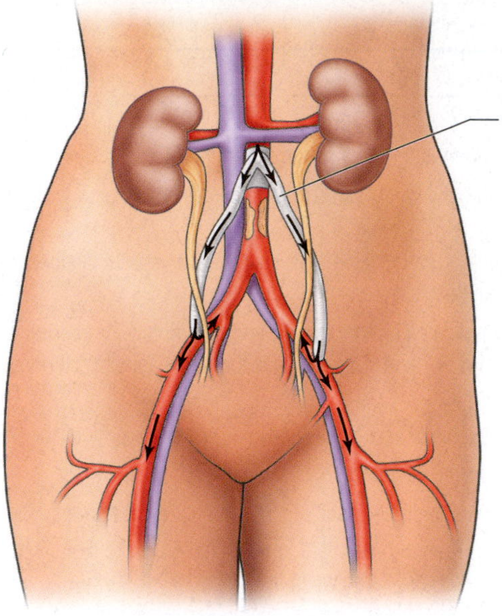

FIGURE 35–5 ◆ Aortoiliac bypass.

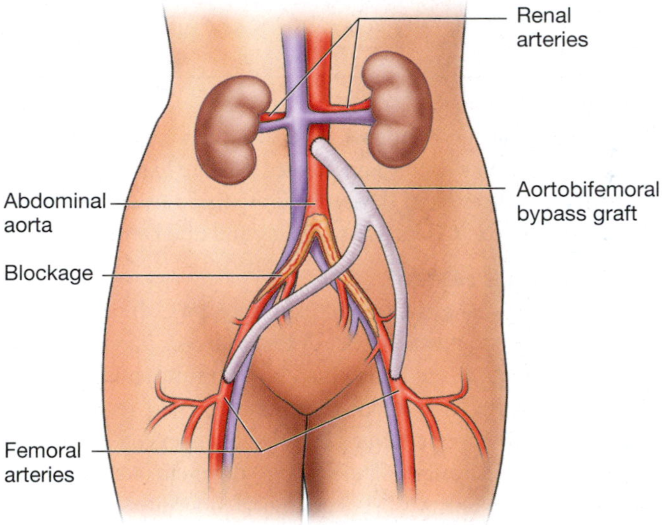

FIGURE 35–6 ◆ Aortobifemoral bypass.

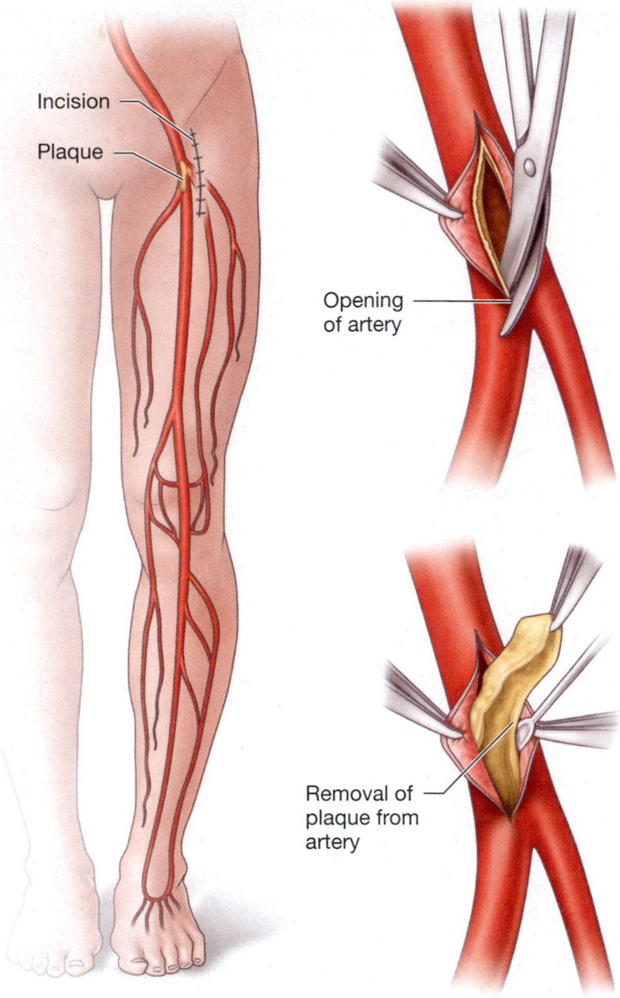

FIGURE 35–7 ◆ Iliac endarterectomy.

diagnoses such as myocardial infarction, hypertension, heart failure, and stroke. Obtaining information about the patient's history of smoking, hyperlipidemia, diabetes, family history, and activity level is important for planning necessary patient teaching about risk reductions.

Occlusive arterial disease can impair blood flow and obliterate pulses in the affected extremity. Skin color should be examined carefully and with the patient in various positions. If arterial disease is present, pallor may be present when the legs are elevated. When patients hang their legs over the side of the exam table or bed, the legs become a deep red in color (dependent rubor) because blood is pooling in the arterioles. Hyperpigmentation of the skin is associated with venous, rather than arterial, disease. Additional physical findings may include decreased capillary refill, increased venous filling time, skin discoloration, decreased warmth, muscle or limb weakness with use, and poor healing.

Peripheral arterial disease is a lifelong disease. The more information the patient is given, the better equipped she is to manage this chronic disorder. The nurse must be certain that the patient understands the basic pathophysiology of PAD, contributing risk factors and how best to manage them, prescribed medications and exercise programs, and signs and symptoms to report to the health care provider. The applicable nursing diagnoses and nursing interventions are further described in the Nursing Process: Patient Care Plan for Peripheral Arterial Disease box.

Collaborative Management

A multidisciplinary team approach—including health care providers; advance practice nurses, such as nurse practitioners and/or clinical nurse specialists; staff nurses; pharmacists; physical therapists; wound specialists; and dietitians—is important in the management of patients with PAD. In order to meet desired patient outcomes, it is essential that this interdisciplinary team communicate openly with one another in developing and evaluating care of the patient and family (IOM [Institute of Medicine], 2010). Health care providers oversee the patient's plan of care by determining what medical or surgical therapies are needed, including diagnostic testing, surgical procedures, and pharmacologic and nonpharmacologic interventions. Nurses implement the plan of care and are responsible for ongoing monitoring, assessment, and evaluation of interventions. Pharmacists oversee the patient's pharmacologic profile, assessing for appropriateness of dosing, drug-to-drug interactions, and potential adverse reactions of medications. Physical therapists are

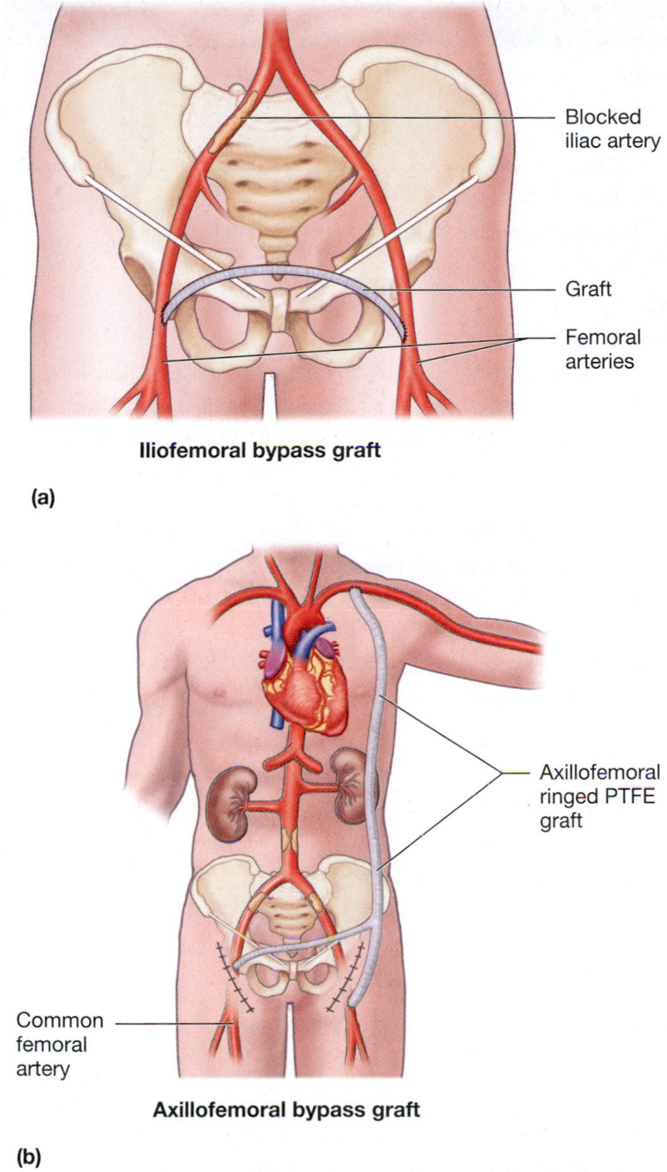

FIGURE 35–8 ◆ Femorofemoral bypass types: (A) iliofemoral bypass graft and (B) axillofemoral bypass graft.

essential in assisting patients in gaining and maintaining strength and mobility, especially after surgical interventions.

Wound specialists are a helpful resource for those patients who have sustained injury or infection and have wounds on their extremities. The wound care specialist assists with specialized treatments and dressings that promote healing. Whenever a patient has skin breakdown or wounds, a nutritional assessment by a dietitian can provide helpful insight into the patient's nutrition and hydration status. The dietitian can offer recommendations for foods or supplements that may promote healing. Patients with advanced PAD, who are dealing with pain, altered mobility, and/or potential amputation, may also benefit from interactions with social workers and hospital chaplains.

Health Promotion

Patient and family education is important in managing the patient with PAD. The nurse should begin by educating the patient and family about pathophysiology, IC, the mechanism by which the pain sensation occurs with walking, and the important and ongoing need for risk factor

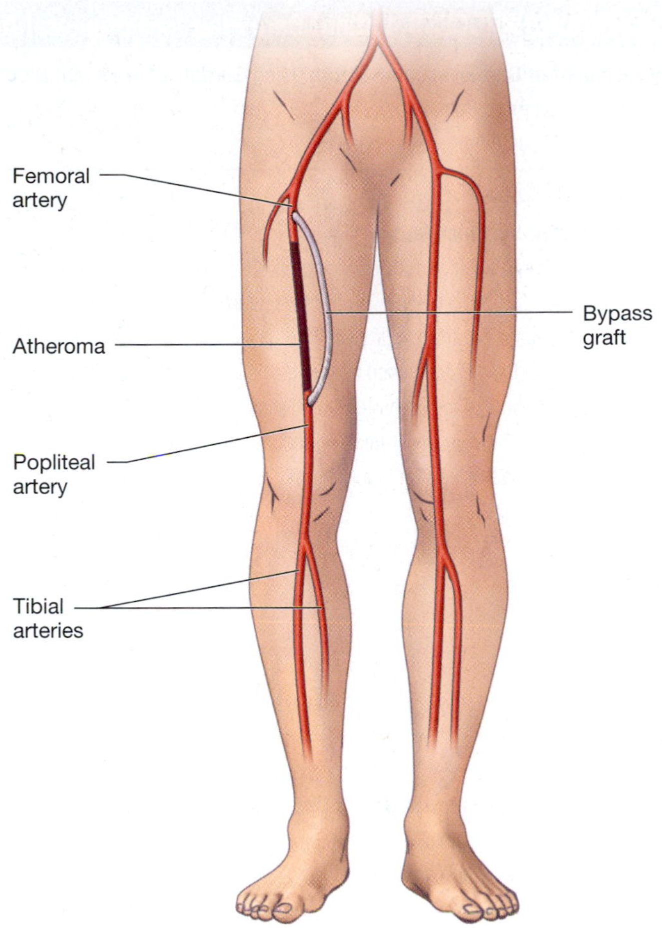

FIGURE 35–9 ◆ Femoropopliteal bypass.

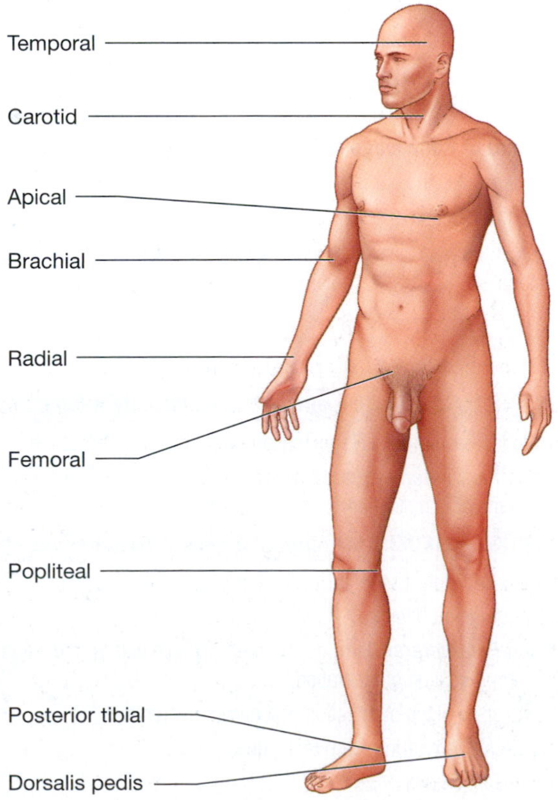

FIGURE 35–10 ◆ Peripheral pulses.

NURSING PROCESS: Patient Care Plan for Peripheral Arterial Disease

Assessment of Cardiovascular Status Using Gordon's Functional Health Patterns:

- Nutrition Metabolic Pattern
- Activity Exercise Pattern
- Cognitive Perceptual Pattern

Subjective Data	Objective Data
Assessment of Vascular Status	**Assessment of Vascular Status**
How far can you walk without experiencing pain? Does leg discomfort or pain keep you from sleeping? Does the pain wake you from your sleep? Do you use an aid for walking such as a cane, walker, or wheelchair? Do you need assistance to do your daily activities? How many blocks (stairs) does it take to produce your pain? Is the pain worse with elevation? Worse with cool temperatures?	Assess bilateral blood pressure. Assess capillary refill. Assess for carotid bruit. Assess the need for assistance with ambulation and activities of daily living. Assess peripheral pulses, including the brachial, radial, femoral, popliteal, dorsalis pedis, and posterior tibial, for presence, rate, equality, regularity, and strength of pulses. Assess and record as absent, diminished, normal, or bounding. Palpate abdomen for pulsatile mass. Inspect the lower extremities for pallor, cyanosis, or trophic changes—which include hair loss; thin, smooth, shiny skin; thick, brittle nails with or without fungal infection; tapering of toes or fingers. Assess peripheral pulses, temperature, and color of extremities. Assess for signs of ulceration, skin breakdown, impaired healing, and trauma. Assess walking distance.
Assessment of Peripheral Vascular Perfusion and Skin Integrity	**Assessment of Peripheral Vascular Perfusion and Skin Integrity**
Do your extremities feel cold? Do you have pain in your extremities? Do you have any areas of sores or ulcerations?	Assess extremities for perfusion: warmth, color, bilateral pulses, and edema. Assess extent of wounds, if applicable.
Assessment of Discomfort	**Assessment of Discomfort**
Do you have problems with pain when you are at rest? Do you have problems with pain during activity, or when in a cold environment? Where is the pain, what brings it on, and what makes it go away? Is the pain getting worse?	Use a pain scale (0–10) to quantify pain. If pain is increased, evaluate for disease progression or acute arterial obstruction.
Assessment of Knowledge of Self-Care Needs	**Assessment of Knowledge of Self-Care Needs**
Has anyone explained your health problems to you? How does this disease affect your daily life? Are you able to care for yourself independently? If not, how much assistance do you need?	Assess knowledge of disease process and progression, risk factors, and impact of smoking cessation. Assess patient's understanding of treatment plan, including medications and wound care, if indicated. Assess need for assistance.

Outcomes and Evaluation Parameters	Planning and Interventions with *Rationales*
1. NURSING DIAGNOSIS: Impaired Physical Mobility *related to disease and pain* (NANDA-I © 2012)	
Outcome: Increased mobility; decreased symptoms of claudication. ***Evaluation Parameter:*** Increased walking distance; decreased signs and symptoms of claudication.	Teach the patient the importance of regular and structured ambulation (30 minutes three times a week) *to promote collateral development and enhance existing circulation to decrease pain.*
2. NURSING DIAGNOSIS: Ineffective Peripheral Tissue Perfusion *and* Impaired Skin Integrity *related to diseased arteries* (NANDA-I © 2012)	
Outcomes: Sufficient tissue perfusion to perfuse extremities. Skin intact or ulcers healing. ***Evaluation Parameters:*** Warm extremities, palpable pulses, reduction in pain, and prevention of ulceration. No wounds or no signs of infection of the lower extremities. Demonstrates effective foot care techniques. Eats well-balanced diet. Does not smoke or use smokeless tobacco.	Notify the health care provider immediately if any of the six Ps of arterial ischemia occur abruptly: pain, pallor, pulselessness, poikilothermia (coldness), paresthesia, and paralysis of the affected extremity *to prevent tissue damage and loss.* Encourage the patient to keep his legs in the dependent position *to enhance arterial perfusion.* Encourage the patient to walk regularly and progressively *to promote conditioning and blood flow.*

NURSING PROCESS: Patient Care Plan for Peripheral Arterial Disease, *continued*

	Teach the patient the importance of smoking cessation *to reduce the adverse vasospastic effects of nicotine.* Teach the patient risk factor modification *to prevent worsening of the atherosclerotic process.* Initiate wound care as directed *to promote healing and prevent infection and further tissue loss.* Teach the patient to avoid trauma, heat, and sunburn to feet/legs *to prevent wounds and infection.* Teach the patient about foot care: Keep feet and toes clean, mild soap only; dry well between toes; use lanolin emollient; inspect feet daily; clip toenails straight; wear proper fitting shoes; avoid walking barefoot. Avoid extremes in temperature to the extremities (hot baths, heating pads, cold water) *because sensation may be diminished and therefore could cause skin breakdown.* Teach the patient signs and symptoms of infection such as fever, redness, tenderness, and drainage from a wound or incision. Teach the patient about good nutrition (Chapter 8) *to promote healing and prevent skin breakdown.*
3. NURSING DIAGNOSIS: Readiness for Enhanced Comfort *related to tissue ischemia* (NANDA-I © 2012)	
Outcome: Comfort level maintained. ***Evaluation Parameter:*** Patient states adequate pain control has been acheived.	Assess the pain so appropriate pain interventions can be initiated. Encourage periods of rest when walking *for pain relief.* Provide an environment where the patient is able to express his pain level *so that he feels supported.* Instruct the patient to inform the nurse if pain is not relieved *so that additional pain management strategies can be considered.* Use pain control measures before the pain becomes severe *to intervene early and with less medication.* Teach nonpharmacologic methods of pain control; that is, guided imagery and breathing exercises *to augment other treatments.*
4. NURSING DIAGNOSIS: Deficient Knowledge *of self-care needs and treatment plan related to tobacco use* (NANDA-I © 2012)	
Outcomes: Adequate knowledge level about underlying disease process, treatment plan, medications, and risk factor modification, such as smoking cessation. ***Evaluation Parameters:*** Patient/family are able to discuss disease process, risk factors, and current treatment plan. Patient verbalizes understanding of treatment plan. Information is provided where deficiency exists. Patient/family verbalize understanding of disease, management, and prevention.	Provide factual information about the diagnosis, treatment, risk factor modification, medications, and treatment plan *to enhance understanding.* Explain all procedures and allow the patient to ask questions *to promote his understanding.* Provide information about care assistance *to ensure adequate help to provide a safe environment.*

Source: Adapted from Wilkinson, J. M., & Ahearn, N. R. (2009). *Prentice Hall nursing diagnosis handbook* (9th ed.). Upper Saddle River, NJ: Prentice Hall.

modification. Patient compliance with the treatment plan is essential to help prevent possible complications such as ulceration, gangrene, amputation, and myocardial infarction.

It is vital that the patient understand the risk factors that worsen PAD. Cigarette smoking is the single most important risk factor; smoking cessation decreases the progression of PAD and improves the patient's functional status (Moser & Riegel, 2008). Smoking cessation is fundamental because of the detrimental effects of tobacco on the arterial system. Smoking and its impact on the body are discussed in detail in Chapter 6. Medications to assist patients with smoking cessation are included in the Pharmacology feature on page 1064.

For patients with diabetes, control of blood glucose is recommended. While there is no evidence that tight glycemic control (defined as a level of glycosylated hemoglobin < 7%) decreases IC or critical limb ischemia, tight control of blood sugar levels has been demonstrated to decrease microvascular complications and the risk of myocardial infarction (Christman, 2009).

For PAD patients with hypertension, blood pressure control should be consistent with the evidence-based 7th Report of the Joint National Committee on Prevention, Detection, Evaluation, and Treatment of High Blood Pressure recommendations of systolic blood pressure < 130 mmHg and diastolic blood pressure < 90 mmHg. Good blood pressure management has been found to decrease the risk of stroke, coronary artery disease, and mortality.

Patients also need to be taught to avoid trauma, heat, and/or sunburn to their legs and feet to prevent the development of wounds and possible infection. Foot care information essential for patients with PAD is discussed in the Nursing Process: Patient Care Plan.

Clinical trials have demonstrated the benefit of lipid-lowering agents for patients who have PAD and coexisting cardiovascular and/or cerebrovascular disease. Normalizing lipid levels has been shown to reduce disease progression and the severity of intermittent claudication. According to the evidence-based National Cholesterol and Education Program III, PAD patients should be managed in the same way as patients with coronary artery disease; the primary goal is to lower the LDL-C levels to below 100 mg/dL (AHA, 2010). Coronary artery disease and dyslipidemia are discussed in Chapter 32.

Complications of Peripheral Arterial Disease

Acute arterial ischemia occurs when trauma, thrombosis, or embolism abruptly stops arterial flow or greatly diminishes it. The most common cause of acute arterial ischemia is thromboembolism from the atrial appendage that occurs in patients with chronic atrial fibrillation or from the left ventricle in the patient following acute myocardial infarction or chronic heart failure due to clot formation from stagnant blood.

Safety Alert *Acute arterial ischemia is an emergency. Assessment findings in acute arterial ischemia include the "six Ps": pain, pallor, pulselessness, poikilothermia (coldness), paresthesia, and paralysis of the affected extremity. The nurse would notify the health care provider immediately if the patient develops any of these symptoms of arterial ischemia.*

Immediate contrast angiography may be performed to determine the cause of the ischemia accurately. Management of the patient depends on the cause of the ischemia. If it is caused by trauma, such as fractures or penetrating injuries, surgical repair is often required. Ischemia due to thrombosis or embolism is generally treated by immediate heparin therapy to stop the propagation of new clots and remove the clot, either pharmacologically with catheter-based thrombolysis (streptokinase, tenecteplase, alteplase, reteplase) or mechanically with **embolectomy,** the mechanical removal of the clot.

Raynaud's Disease

Raynaud's disease (RD) is an arterial vasospastic disorder caused by emotional distress or cold.

Etiology and Epidemiology

The fingers and hands are most commonly affected, but the toes and feet also can be involved. Individuals can have RD without any underlying disease associated with it, in which case it is called Raynaud's disease or primary Raynaud's. It also can be part of another disease, in which case it may be referred to as Raynaud's phenomenon or secondary Raynaud's. Raynaud's disease is more prevalent in women than men, and the typical onset is before age 30 (Saigal, Kansal, Mittal, Singh, & Ram, 2010).

Pathophysiology

The precise pathophysiology of RD is unclear. The symptoms are caused by a transient spasm of the small cutaneous and subcutaneous arteries and arterioles, which results in decreased blood flow to the affected extremity. Abnormalities of the endothelium may be responsible for initiating the vasospasm. Raynaud's disease is classified as primary or secondary. Primary or idiopathic RD has no known cause. In contrast, secondary RD is associated with many diseases, including connective tissue diseases, such as rheumatoid arthritis, scleroderma, and systemic lupus erythematosus (SLE), and myeloproliferative diseases, such as leukemia and polycythemia rubra vera. Occupational and environmental conditions are also associated with RD, particularly cold exposure, repetitive trauma, and vibration injury (e.g., from using chain saws, pneumatic drills).

Clinical Manifestations

The diagnosis of RD is made on the basis of the patient's clinical manifestations. Usually during times of high stress, strong emotions, or exposure to the cold, patients develop vasoconstriction of the arterial blood vessels, causing cooling of the temperature of fingers, toes, and earlobes. As the temperature decreases, the skin color of the affected parts changes. Three color changes occur with RD: (1) pallor (whiteness) in response to the vasospasms, (2) cyanosis (blue) due to the reduction of oxygenation of the blood, and (3) rubor (redness) when the vasospasms stop and the arterial blood returns (Saigal et al., 2010). Other factors that may trigger ischemia include smoking, caffeine intake, and use of alcohol, cocaine, or amphetamines. The vascular changes also cause paresthesia to the affected parts. The episode ends when the arterial spasm relaxes and perfusion normalizes. Digits appear normal between attacks.

Diagnosis

A cold stimulation challenge may be administered to induce symptoms of RD. In this challenge, the patient is exposed to cold temperatures by placing her hands in a basin of cold water. Patients with RD will quickly develop pallor and possibly cyanosis. When the hands are warmed, the patients experience redness and pain in their hands.

Nail-fold capillaroscopy can be performed to distinguish between primary and secondary RD (Saigal et al., 2010). The nail bed is examined by using a stereoscopic microscope or handheld ophthalmoscope to assess for the presence of enlarged, distorted, or deformed capillaries that may be associated with secondary RD.

Medical and Surgical Management

It is critical for the health care provider to obtain a complete medical history to find out whether the patient has other connective tissue disorders, such as SLE and scleroderma. The signs and symptoms are vague and consist of (1) malaise, (2) light sensitivity, (3) joint pain, and (4) skin lesions. Because the symptoms are vague, RD is difficult to diagnose. Treatment is based on the signs and symptoms presented. Nonpharmacologic management of RD is directed toward avoiding known stressors (cold, emotional stress); controlling exposure to extremes in climate; dressing warmly in cold weather; and limiting tobacco, caffeine, and alcohol intake. Some patients may benefit from learning relaxation techniques. Regular physical exercise is important because it improves circulation and warms the body temperature. If pharmacologic treatment is needed to manage symptoms, the dihydropyridine calcium-channel blocking agents, such as nifedipine, isradipine, amlodipine, and nicardipine, are used. Other agents that have been used to treat RD include prazosin (Minipress), fluoxetine (Prozac), losartan (Cozaar), pentoxifylline, captopril, and topical nitroglycerin.

Surgical **sympathectomy,** removal of the sympathetic ganglia, has been performed for patients with severe symptoms of RD. This interrupts sympathetic nervous system stimulation to the affected vessels, decreasing vasoconstriction and vasospasm. Following this procedure, patients may experience relief of pain, decreased tissue loss, and improved wound healing. There is no cure for RD.

Complications of Raynaud's Disease

Complications of RD are not common. Digital ulcers may occur as a result of the disorder. Most digital ulcers will heal over several weeks to months with conservative therapy, provided that the patient cares for his hands and/or feet carefully and seeks prompt treatment for signs and symptoms of infection. Surgery may be required when there is the threat of loss of a digit because of a nonhealing ulceration or gangrene.

Nursing Management

Careful history taking is important when assessing the patient with RD. The nurse should determine the patient's particular stressors and characteristics of attacks such as pain, numbness, color changes of the extremities, and frequency of attacks. The skin of the hands and toes should be assessed for the presence of ulcers and gangrene. It is important to obtain a detailed list of medications that the patient takes, since some medications, such as beta-adrenergic blockers, ergot alkaloids, and hormones, can precipitate episodes of vasospasm.

Because the treatment of RD is supportive and there is no cure, patient and family teaching is very important to assist the patient in preventing and managing vasospastic episodes. It is important that the patient clearly understands the disease process to avoid aggravating and alleviating events, such as cold environments and emotional stress. Smoking cessation counseling is essential. The patient may benefit from referrals for stress management class or relaxation techniques.

Health Promotion

Most patients with RD have only mild to moderate symptoms and can manage sufficiently by avoiding exposure to cold and tobacco. The nurse should teach the patient to wear warm clothes and gloves, mittens, and/or hand warmers when required to be in cold environments. Exposure to cigarette smoke also can cause symptoms. In addition, patients with RD should avoid oral contraceptives, beta-adrenergic blockers, and ergot preparations because they have been known to exacerbate the symptoms of RD. Behavioral modification therapy may be helpful for some patients because RD has such a strong emotional component.

Thoracic Outlet Syndrome

The thoracic outlet is a space between the thorax and the clavicle through which the main blood vessels and nerves pass from the neck and thorax into the arm. **Thoracic outlet syndrome (TOS)** is a rare disorder, more common in females than males, in which there is compression of the arm's nerves and arteries in the thoracic outlet. It may be due to an extra first rib or an old fracture of the clavicle, which reduces the space of the outlet. Compression may occur with repetitive activities that require the arms to be held overhead.

Clinical manifestations of TOS include pain, paresthesia, muscular weakness and fatigue or swelling, and coldness in the arm and hand. The symptoms can be confused with those of other conditions, such as a herniated disk in the neck, carpal tunnel syndrome, and even bursitis of the shoulder.

The diagnosis of TOS is usually based on patient history and physical examination. Many patients will have a history of an accident or trauma. To diagnose TOS, the elevated arm stress test (EAST) may be conducted. This is done by having the patient place both arms in 90 degrees of abduction and external rotation, then opening and closing the hands for 3 minutes. A positive EAST study occurs when there is reproduction of symptoms (Chang, 2008). Other noninvasive testing that may be useful in diagnosing TOS includes cervical and chest x-rays to assess skeletal abnormality, color flow duplex scanning, MRI, and ulnar nerve conduction or electromyography. Invasive testing that may be performed includes an arteriogram and venography.

Treatment of TOS is initially directed toward nonsurgical interventions, including physical therapy and pain management strategies. Physical therapy involves specific exercises aimed at strengthening the supporting muscles of the thoracic outlet structures. Muscle relaxants, nonsteroidal anti-inflammatory drugs such as aspirin or ibuprofen, moist heat, massage, analgesics, and short courses of steroids may be recommended. Surgical decompression of the thoracic outlet to remove the point of compression is indicated for patients with severe symptoms that limit their lifestyle.

Renovascular Disease

Renovascular diseases are disorders of the arteries of the kidneys, which result in systemic hypertension and kidney dysfunction.

Etiology and Epidemiology

Two disorders primarily affect the renal arteries: atherosclerotic renal artery stenosis (AS-RAS) and fibromuscular dysplasia (FMD). Fibromuscular dysplasia is more common in girls and women between the ages of 15 and 50 and frequently involves the main renal artery and its branches (McCulloch, 2010).

The atherosclerotic disease process accounts for approximately 70% to 90% of renovascular disease. It is the cause of 1% to 2% of all cases of hypertension, making it the most common cause of secondary hypertension (Porth & Matfin, 2009). The prevalence of AS-RAS increases with age, particularly in patients with diabetes, aortoiliac occlusive disease, coronary artery disease, or hypertension. However, many cases are never detected because hypertension or kidney failure does not develop (McCulloch, 2010).

Pathophysiology

Patients with AS-RAS have progressive abnormal narrowing of the renal artery, which occurs in about half of all patients within 5 years after the initial diagnosis has been made. Anywhere from 3% to 16% of the arteries eventually become totally blocked, and shrinkage of the kidney occurs in approximately 20% of patients. The resulting hypertension is caused by reduced renal blood flow and activation of the RAAS. The diminished blood flow to the kidney causes a release of excessive amounts of renin, which increases the circulating levels of angiotensin II. Angiotensin II vasoconstricts the peripheral vessels and acts as a stimulus to increase aldosterone levels and sodium retention. The result of all of these changes is systemic hypertension. One or both kidneys may be affected (Porth & Matfin, 2009).

Fibromuscular dysplasia is a noninflammatory, nonatherosclerotic disease that also can affect the renal arteries, causing alterations in the intimal and/or medial layer, leading to obstruction of blood flow. Fibromuscular dysplasia accounts for 10% to 25% of renovascular disease, and is seen almost exclusively in women (McCulloch, 2010). Unlike AS-RAS, FMD rarely leads to total renal artery blockage. The cause of FMD is unknown; however, theories have identified a genetic predisposition, smoking, hormonal factors, and disorders of the blood supply to the renal artery itself as some of the possible causes of the disease.

Clinical Manifestations

Patients with renovascular disease present with significantly elevated blood pressure that is difficult to control, although it is not readily distinguishable from other forms of hypertension. Certain classic features such as lack of family history of hypertension, recent onset of hypertension, or onset of hypertension before age 50 are more suggestive of renovascular hypertension than of other forms of high blood pressure. It is frequently higher than 180/100 mmHg and may be resistant to two or more medications.

Diagnosis

The goal of diagnostic studies is to assess perfusion to the kidneys and the RAAS. Duplex ultrasonography is recommended as the screening test to establish the presence of renal artery stenosis. CT angiography and magnetic resonance angiography (MRA) may also be used as screening tests. For example, contrast angiography may be performed to assess the renal–arterial vasculature. Angiographic findings of fibromuscular dysplasia demonstrate a very characteristic "string of beads" appearance in the lumen of the artery (McCulloch, 2010).

Medical and Surgical Management

Medical therapy of atherosclerotic renal artery disease is directed toward careful blood pressure control, antiplatelet therapy, lipid management, smoking cessation, and weight reduction. Angiotensin-converting enzyme (ACE) inhibitors may be indicated in the presence of renal stenosis (Porth & Matfin, 2009).

Endovascular therapy may be an option for select patients. Patients with fibromuscular dysplasia have good outcomes with renal angioplasty, which leads to improvements or a cure in over 90% of patients. Percutaneous ballooning and stenting of renal artery atherosclerotic lesions have success rates of near 100% when performed by an experienced health care provider (McCulloch, 2010). Complications of renal artery angioplasty and stenting may include cholesterol embolization, vessel rupture, renal infarction, temporary deterioration in renal function, retroperitoneal hemorrhage, and access site vascular complications such as bleeding and hematoma (McCulloch, 2010).

Surgical management for renovascular disease is limited to those patients who present with severe therapy-resistant hypertension and ischemic nephropathy. Procedures that may be performed include aortorenal bypass, the most common surgery performed for patients with renovascular disease, and renal artery thromboendarterectomy or renal artery reimplantation. Complications of untreated renovascular disease can include severely elevated blood pressure, stroke, renal insufficiency and failure, heart failure, retinopathy, and death.

Nursing Management

Caring for the patient who has undergone renal artery stenting is similar to the care of the patient who has undergone other types of peripheral angioplasty. Monitoring of blood pressure and urinary output is essential. Because renal stenting is performed by percutaneous arterial access, careful monitoring of the access site is needed, along with regular assessment of distal pulses. Follow-up laboratory testing of blood urea nitrogen (BUN) and creatinine levels is important to assess renal function.

Patients who have undergone surgical treatment of their renovascular disease, such as reconstruction of the renal arteries or aortorenal bypass, may require intensive care monitoring for several hours postoperatively. Postoperative monitoring includes frequent and ongoing assessment of the blood pressure. Postoperative nursing management is discussed in more detail in Chapter 19.

Health Promotion

Patients need to be instructed on the importance of regular and continuing medical follow-up. Close monitoring of blood pressure is required. Changes to the antihypertensive medication regime will likely be needed following stenting or surgical repair. Patients also must be monitored for progression of renovascular disease and decline in renal function.

Aortic Aneurysm

An **aneurysm** is a diseased segment of an artery that becomes thin and dilated because of degenerative changes in the tunica media layer.

Etiology and Epidemiology

Arterial aneurysms can occur throughout the body. Aortic aneurysms can be saccular (extending over only part of the vessel circumference), projecting from one side of the aorta only, or fusiform (involving the entire circumference), which is symmetrical involvement of the aorta. The prevalence of aortic aneurysm in the United States varies with advancing age, family history, gender, and tobacco use. The condition is more common in men, especially between ages 50 and 70. The incidence increases with age and develops more frequently in smokers. Additionally, aortic aneurysms tend to have familial tendencies. The most common causes of aortic aneurysms are atherosclerosis and degeneration of the vessel media (Porth & Matfin, 2009).

Pathophysiology

Aortic aneurysms can occur anywhere in the aorta, although the majority of them occur below the level of the renal arteries (infrarenal). These are referred to as abdominal aortic aneurysms (AAA). Thoracic aneurysms account for only 10% of the occurrences. The pathogenesis of an aortic aneurysm is not well understood. An aneurysm is a localized area of the aorta that is weakened because of decreased elastin in the medial layer, causing loss of medial smooth muscle cells with thinning of the vessel wall. Inflammatory changes may also play a part. Causes include congenital weakness, trauma, and disease. Once the aneurysm is initiated, it will grow larger as the tension on the vessel wall increases. The aneurysm may increase to the point at which it is putting pressure on the adjacent organs and interrupting blood flow. If a growing aneurysm is left untreated, it may rupture due to the increased tension (Porth & Matfin, 2009).

Clinical Manifestations

The clinical manifestations of an aortic aneurysm depend on its size and location. Aneurysms of the thoracic area present with substernal, back, and neck pain. Patients also may have dyspnea, stridor, and brassy cough due to pressure on the trachea. If the laryngeal nerve is compressed, hoarseness may occur (Porth & Matfin, 2009). AAAs are typically asymptomatic. Frequently, an unknown aortic aneurysm is discovered during abdominal imaging performed for some other reason or during routine physical exam. Visual inspection may reveal a pulsatile abdominal mass near the umbilicus in the lean patient. Auscultation of this mass reveals a bruit (see Chapter 29), caused by the turbulent flow in the widened area of the aorta.

Diagnosis

Diagnostic testing performed for aortic aneurysms includes abdominal ultrasound, CT scan, abdominal angiography, and MRA. These tests are described in Chapter 32. The aortic aneurysm is followed by serial diagnostic tests to evaluate the growth and impedance of surrounding organs. To be considered an AAA, the size must exceed 3 centimeters in diameter.

Medical Management

Medical management of the stable AAA includes ongoing surveillance with abdominal ultrasound performed every 6 months to assess the amount of aneurysmal growth, as well as smoking cessation, maintaining optimal blood pressure control, monitoring, and controlling fasting lipid values and discontinuance of steroids, if possible.

An endovascular stent graft covered with a thin layer of Dacron may be an option for some patients with an AAA. In endovascular repair of an AAA, the graft is placed into the aorta via access from the femoral artery. This procedure is performed in the operating room or in the cardiac catheterization laboratory using general, regional, or local anesthesia with sedation. Several endovascular stent graft systems are currently available (Figure 35–11◆). Advantages for the patient include no long abdominal incisions, faster recovery time, and shorter length of stay. This approach may be an option for the patient who is at very high

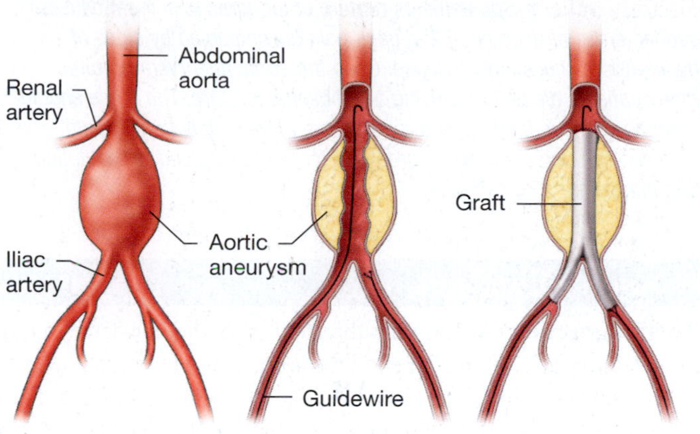

FIGURE 35–11 ◆ Endovascular stent graft.

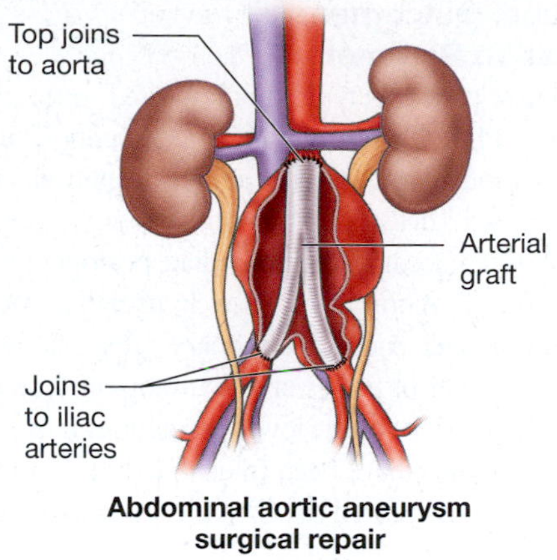

FIGURE 35–12 ◆ Repair of abdominal aneurysm.

risk for open-heart surgery because of extensive comorbidities, such as cardiac and/or pulmonary disease. Complications of endovascular stent graft repair of an AAA include **endoleaks** (continued leaking of blood into the aneurysmal sac), arterial trauma, occlusion of the renal or hypogastric arteries, renal impairment due to contrast administration, device migration, structural failure, and/or infection. The long-term durability of these stent grafts is not known; lifelong follow-up is needed for these patients. The early mortality rate for endograft repair generally has been less than 3% (Christman, 2009).

Surgical Management

Options for treating AAA are open surgical repair and endovascular repair, described previously. Surgical intervention for AAA has been performed for over 50 years. Patients with infrarenal AAAs measuring 5.5 centimeters or larger should undergo repair to eliminate the risk of rupture (Christman, 2009). Elective AAA repair is a major surgical procedure with mortality rates reported between 2% and 6% and post-operative complication rates up to 30%. Cardiac complications are most common. The perioperative administration of beta-adrenergic blockers, if not contraindicated, reduces the risk of adverse cardiac events and mortality in patients with coronary artery disease undergoing repair of atherosclerotic aortic aneurysms (Christman, 2009).

The surgical approach is dependent on the location of the aneurysm; however, the traditional approach is a midline or transverse incision with retroperitoneal dissection of the aneurysm. The aneurysm is then resected (removed) and replaced with Dacron graft material, with the aneurysm wall usually left in place to cover the Dacron graft. Aneurysms that extend above the renal arteries and into the thoracic aorta are more difficult to repair. If the ascending aorta is involved, cardiopulmonary bypass is required. Chapter 32 discusses cardiopulmonary bypass surgery. Figure 35–12 ◆ shows the repair approach for AAA.

Immediate surgical repair is indicated for the patient who presents with expanding aneurysm or rupture. The mortality rate for emergency surgery for ruptured AAA is as high as 40% (Christman, 2009).

Complications

Complications that can occur from AAA include rupture, thrombosis, and embolization. The risk of rupture is related to the size of the aneurysm and is very high if the aneurysm is larger than 5.5 centimeters. Factors that can increase the risk of rupture include hypertension, smoking, and family history of ruptured AAAs. Embolization from the aneurysm can decrease perfusion to the lower extremities, a condition that is referred to as "blue toe syndrome." This syndrome, caused by emboli, is an indication for surgical repair of the AAA.

Complications that can occur following open AAA repair include hemodynamic instability due to postoperative bleeding, hypothermia, myocardial ischemia and/or infarction, hypoxia due to atelectasis, fluid and electrolyte disturbances due to renal insufficiency, massive transfusions, inadequate hydration, ileus and abdominal distention due to ischemia or surgical manipulation of the bowel, and spinal cord ischemia due to interrupted blood flow during cross-clamping.

Nursing Management

The care of the patient undergoing endovascular or surgical repair of an AAA is complex. Depending on the extent of the procedure, the patient spends some time in the critical care setting prior to transferring to a lower level of care before discharge.

Assessment

A careful in-depth nursing assessment is essential for the patient undergoing surgical or endovascular repair of an AAA. Prior to repair, the nurse needs to monitor the patient closely for signs and symptoms of impending rupture: restlessness, abdominal pain and tenderness, hypotension, and shock. Any of these symptoms should be reported immediately to the health care provider/surgeon and the patient should be prepared for emergent surgery.

Safety Alert *The unstable patient who has experienced rupture of an AAA requires immediate nursing intervention. The nurse will administer intravenous immediate fluid and blood resuscitation as well as drugs to lower the patient's blood pressure, such as propranolol (Inderal) or nitroprusside (Nipride). The nurse will adminster analgesics for pain management and prepare the patient for emergency surgery.*

Nursing Diagnoses

The nursing process guides the postoperative care of the patient immediately following the open AAA surgery. Nursing diagnoses that pertain to these patients include:

- *Tissue Perfusion, ineffective risk for,* related to aneurysm.
- *Risk for Deficient Volumeand Gas Excahnge* related to anesthesia, possible fluid overload, and blood transfusions.
- *Readiness for Enhanced Comfort* related to surgical pain, immobility, and fear and anxiety.
- *Risk for Infection* related to the surgery.
- *Deficient Knowledge of Postoperative Care and Discharge Needs.* NANDA-I © 2012

Interventions, Outcomes, and Evaluation Parameters

The postoperative patient is typically monitored in the intensive care setting for 6 to 24 hours. Priority nursing interventions include blood pressure and hemodynamic support, aggressive pulmonary toilet, and prevention and early detection of surgical complications. Hemodynamic instability can occur in the immediate postoperative phase, and patients are generally monitored invasively using an arterial line and central venous catheter and/or pulmonary artery catheter. Frequent and careful assessment of pulses and neurological function (bilateral movement and sensation) in the lower extremities is essential because normal blood flow may have been interrupted during surgery. Urine output also must be monitored closely if the aneurysm occurred above the renal arteries.

Postoperative complications can be caused by bleeding, hypovolemia, and third spacing of fluid; myocardial ischemia or infarction; hypertension; and hypothermia. Vasoactive drugs may be required in the immediate postoperative phase to support and control the blood pressure and other hemodynamic parameters. Patients are placed on bedside ECG monitors to assess cardiac dysfunction and the presence of dysrhythmias (Chapter 30). The nurse should compare the postoperative cardiac rhythm to the preoperative ECG to assess for new changes that may indicate myocardial ischemia or infarction, such as ST segment depression or elevation. Hypothermia causes an increase in the systemic vascular resistance. Patients should be rewarmed 1 degree per hour until the core body temperature exceeds 36°C. Rewarming can be accomplished by using forced warm air blankets, administering warmed IV fluids or blood, warming the inspired ventilator air, and covering the patient's head with warm blankets.

Patients who have undergone open AAA repair require frequent assessment of pulmonary status, including signs of poor oxygenation and ventilation as evidenced by abnormal arterial blood gases, cyanosis, sluggish capillary refill, use of accessory muscles to breathe, nasal flaring, abnormally low oxygen saturation, and decreased level of consciousness. Regular assessment of the patient's airway is essential. Adequate pain management, frequent repositioning, and the regular use of incentive spirometry are essential to promote oxygenation and ventilation and prevent atelectasis.

Impaired renal function can occur due to decreased blood flow to the kidneys during surgery and with episodes of hypotension and hypovolemia. The nurse should monitor the urine output, BUN, and serum creatinine closely. Gastrointestinal disturbances can occur postoperatively because of ischemia and/or manipulation of the bowel during surgery. The nurse should assess for nausea, vomiting, abdominal pain/tenderness, distention, presence/absence of bowel sounds, blood in stools, and diarrhea. Spinal cord ischemia can occur because of an interruption of blood supply during cross-clamping of the aorta and cause sensory and motor deficits.

Health Promotion

Prior to surgery, the nurse should teach patients the importance of blood pressure control and compliance with their medication regime. Risk factor reduction is important. For example, patients should be counseled to stop smoking. Following surgery, risk factor modification teaching is reinforced. Additionally, the nurse teaches patients wound care, activity restrictions, the medication regime, and reportable symptoms, such as changes in sensation to the legs, which may indicate thrombosis of the graft, or gastrointestinal bleeding, which may indicate erosion of the graft into the duodenum.

Safety Alert *Spontaneous rupture of an aortic aneurysm causes sudden onset of abdominal and back pain accompanied by signs of hypotension, shock, and collapse. Once the aortic aneurysm ruptures, many patients die before arriving at a hospital for care. The nurse should monitor for these findings and report them immediately to the health care provider. The nurse should be prepared for fluid and blood resuscitation and immediate surgical repair.*

Aortic Dissection

Aortic dissection (AD) is a life-threatening condition whereby a tear in the intimal layer of the lumen of the aorta allows blood to flow into the medial layer. The flow creates a passageway, referred to as a "false lumen," that may block or diminish flow through the true lumen. This diminishes the blood supply distal to the area of dissection.

Etiology and Epidemiology

A dissection can occur anywhere in the aorta, although two-thirds of the dissections occur in the ascending aorta. As the dissection increases in size, pressure is placed on the surrounding organs, which may affect organ function. Risks for the development of AD include hypertension, degeneration of the medial layer of the vessel wall, trauma, Marfan's syndrome, and iatrogenic (treatment-induced) dissection caused by catheter-based interventions and aortic clamping during surgery. It occurs most frequently in people ages 40 to 60 and is more prevalent in males than females (Porth & Matfin, 2009).

Pathophysiology

The exact cause of AD is unknown. However, chronic stress from hypertension may play a significant role in the deterioration of the aortic wall. An aortic dissection begins with a tear in the intima, which allows blood to enter the aortic wall, stripping the intima from the adventitia of the aorta. Aortic dissection is classified according to its location. Dissection that involves the ascending aorta is the most common, and this type requires immediate surgical repair. Dissections that involve only the descending aorta generally require immediate surgery and are stabilized medically.

Clinical Manifestations

Most patients with AD present with sudden, sharp, shifting chest or back pain that can mimic acute myocardial infarction, pulmonary embolus, or ruptured AAA. The patient may describe it as "ripping" or "tearing." The pain is not affected by position changes, and it may wax and wane. These patients also may have syncope or altered level of consciousness. About 25% of patients with AD present with signs of ischemia from blood flow obliterated by the dissection, such as stroke, anuria (no urine output), and mesenteric and/or extremity ischemia that occurs because of the altered blood flow to the brain, kidneys, intestine, and legs (Porth & Matfin, 2009).

Safety Alert *Rapid identification of aortic dissection is key in preventing death. Signs and symptoms of aortic dissection (AD) can mimic other disorders such as acute myocardial infarction and pulmonary embolus, making the diagnosis difficult. The most classic symptom of AD is the abrupt onset of severe, tearing chest pain that may radiate to the back. Patients may also present with sudden onset aortic insufficiency, neurological changes, and cardiac tamponade. The nurse must monitor for these symptoms and notify the health care provider immediately if they occur.*

Diagnosis

The diagnosis of aortic dissection begins with taking the patient's history and doing a physical examination. An assessment of risk factors

DIAGNOSTIC TESTS for Aortic Dissection

Test with Normal Values	Expected Abnormality
ECG	
Normal conduction intervals. No ST segment elevation or depression.	May have ST segment elevation or depression if coronary arteries are affected by the ascending aortic dissection.
Chest X-Ray	
Normal findings. No mediastinal widening.	Widened mediastinum may be seen.
Transesophageal Echocardiogram (TEE)	
Normal valve function. No pericardial effusion; no signs of cardiac tamponade.	Detects cardiac tamponade, involvement of coronary arteries, and damage to aortic valve.
CT Scan	
Normal findings. No aortic tear or dissection.	Quickly confirms the location and extent of the dissection.
Angiography	
No false lumen. No dissection or tear in the coronary arteries.	Visualization of true and false lumen possible. Identification of coronary artery anatomy.
MRI/MRA	
No dissection or tear of the aorta or coronary arteries. No involvement of the aortic valve.	Shows intimal tear, type and extent of dissection, and involvement of aortic valve.

is essential. Because aortic dissection is a life-threatening situation, prompt and careful assessment of the clinical manifestations also is essential. Diagnostic tests that will assist with the diagnosis include aortic angiography, transesophageal echocardiography, CT scan, and MRI studies. The Diagnostic Tests box outlines the diagnostic tests used to evaluate AD.

Medical Management

Medical therapy is recommended for type B dissections or those that are in the descending aorta, although surgery may be required when there is poor blood pressure control, inadequate pain relief, and/or progression of the dissection. Control of hypertension is essential for the patient with AD. Aggressive control of blood pressure is managed using beta-adrenergic blockers such as esmolol (Brevibloc), labetalol (Normodyne, Trandate), propranolol (Inderal), metoprolol (Lopressor) (beta-adrenergic antagonist), and nitroglycerine or nitroprusside (Nipride) (vasodilator).

Endovascular repair of AD may also be an option for select patients. Because these procedures are less invasive than surgical repair, the patients have a shorter recovery period and a shorter length of stay. Complications, such as endoleaks, are similar to those seen in endovascular repair of AAA. Endovascular procedures are typically done with local anesthesia and procedural sedation.

Surgical Management

Surgical intervention is indicated for type A dissections, which are those that involve the ascending aorta when the patient develops ischemic complications and/or when medical management fails. If the proximal aorta is involved, the aortic valve may need to be replaced and the coronary arteries may need to be reimplanted. Surgical complications may include myocardial ischemia or infarction, arrhythmias, pulmonary atelectasis, renal failure, ischemic bowel, prolonged ileus, and leg ischemia.

Complications of Aortic Dissection

Disruption of the aorta can cause life-threatening complications or death if not rapidly recognized and treated. Abnormal blood flow into the false lumen of the aorta results in occlusion of the branches of the aorta. If the dissection occurs proximally in the aorta, there is a risk of shearing of the aortic valve and the coronary arteries, causing serious complications including myocardial infarction, acute aortic insufficiency, and pericardial tamponade. If the dissection moves distally in the aorta, there is a risk of damage to the arteries that supply the kidneys, spine, abdomen, and legs.

Nursing Management

The nursing care of the patient following open AD repair is complex and very similar to the nursing care of the patient who has had open AAA repair. Patients spend the first 1 to 2 days in the intensive care unit for careful monitoring. Goals of therapy are directed toward airway and blood pressure management, as well as pain control. Care of the postoperative patient is discussed in detail in Chapter 19.

Health Promotion

Patients must be instructed to control their blood pressure carefully for the rest of their lives. Compliance with their medication regime is essential to help prevent further damage to the aorta. Regular, ongoing monitoring of blood pressure and follow-up visits with the health care provider are important.

Venous Disorders

Venous disease is more likely to affect the lower extremities. The patient may experience intermittent swelling, tightness, and discomfort in one or both lower extremities due to a venous disorder. Unilateral extremity swelling may be associated with **deep venous thrombosis (DVT),** a clot that forms in the deep veins. Bilateral or diffuse edema may indicate that the patient has heart failure, valvular venous incompetence, or **lymphedema,** which is swelling due to obstruction of the lymphatic system.

The venous system of the lower extremities has two components: the superficial and deep systems. Perforation of communicating veins transports blood from the skin and subcutaneous tissues from the superficial system to the deeper venous channels, where it is then transported to the heart. The veins contain valves, which prevent retrograde flow, thereby maintaining normal flow of blood back to the heart. Muscle function also assists in moving the blood back to the heart. There are more venous valves located in the lower legs than in the upper legs. Loss of valve function causes venous insufficiency, after which venous hypertension can occur.

Varicose Veins

Varicose veins are dilated, tortuous veins that occur in the lower extremities as a result of the incompetence of valves of the deep and superficial venous system, which leads to valve reflux.

Etiology and Epidemiology

Risk factors for the development of varicose veins include older age, family history, female gender, occupations that require standing, obesity, and history of phlebitis or clots. Other potential risk factors include constipation/low-fiber diet, smoking, hypertension, pregnancy, and injury. Varicose veins are subcutaneous veins that remain dilated when the patient is standing or sitting. Figure 35–13◆ shows a normal venous structure and a varicose venous structure. In the general population, the incidence of varicose veins is between 5% and 30%, with a higher incidence in females (Leopardi, Hoggan, Fitridge, Woodruff, & Maddern, 2009).

Clinical Manifestations

Some patients with varicose veins may have no symptoms; other patients experience sensations of heaviness, tiredness, itching, burning, or aching in their leg(s). Symptoms may intensify by the end of the day, especially after the patient has been standing for long periods of time.

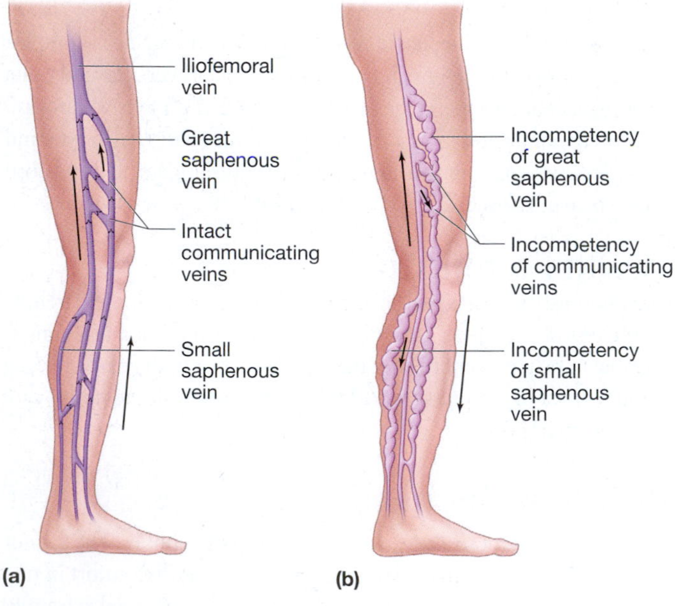

FIGURE 35–13 ◆ (A) Normal venous structure and (B) varicose veins.

Varicose veins may be more visible and more painful during pregnancy or menstruation.

Diagnosis, Medical, and Surgical Management

Diagnosis is made by physical examination and the patient's report of clinical manifestations. A frequent site of varicose veins is the greater saphenous vein. Doppler ultrasound may be used to assess blood flow in the large vessels, and angiography is used to assess valve function. Treatment may be required for patients with extensive varicose veins or those who are severely symptomatic. Interventional therapy, or nonsurgical alternatives to treatment for varicose veins, such as sclerotherapy, is performed less frequently because of the high incidence of reoccurrence. In sclerotherapy, generally reserved for small varicose veins and spider veins, the vein is injected with an irritating chemical, causing fibrosis and occluding the vessel lumen. This results in reduction of the varicose vein.

Surgical therapy for varicose veins may include ligation, stripping, laser therapy, or radiofrequency ablation of the vein, usually the saphenous vein (Leopardi et al., 2009). This is performed in the outpatient setting, and the patient's recovery generally takes a few days to 3 weeks at the most. Following venous sclerotherapy or surgery, patients must wear compression stockings to help prevent further varicosities. Complications of surgical repair of varicose veins may include hemorrhage, thrombophlebitis, edema, and infection.

Complications

Complications of untreated varicose veins can include increased risk of DVT and chronic venous insufficiency (CVI) leading to hyperpigmentation and ulceration of the feet and legs. This can increase the patient's susceptibility to injury and infection.

Nursing Management

Repair of varicose veins is generally scheduled as outpatient surgery in either a hospital or a surgical clinic. Bed rest is suggested for the first 24 hours, with the foot of the bed elevated; the patient is then encouraged to walk short distances every 2 hours. Compression stockings are usually worn for several days following surgery. Surgical incisions should be inspected daily for signs of infection such as redness, tenderness, warmth, and drainage. Patients should avoid showering or bathing the legs for the first 24 hours and should avoid the use of lotions and creams on the legs until the incisions are fully healed.

Health Promotion

Prior to discharge, the nurse should teach the patient to avoid activities that cause venous pooling, such as sitting for long periods of time and standing in one position for long periods of time. The nurse needs to explain the proper method for applying and wearing compression stockings. In addition, the patient should be encouraged to develop a walking program and to lose weight, if needed.

Venous Thromboembolism

Venous thromboembolism (VTE) consists of two conditions: deep venous thrombosis and pulmonary embolism. Venous thromboembolism is a common cardiovascular disorder affecting over 2 million people in the United States each year; an estimated 200,000 deaths in this country alone result from VTE (Stevens & Douketis, 2010). Multiple risk factors for the development of VTE are outlined in the Risk Factors box (p. 1083). **Pulmonary embolism (PE)** in this context is defined as the presence of a thrombus or blood clot in the pulmonary vessels that obstructs blood flow and impedes gas exchange. The diagnosis and treatment of PE are discussed in detail in Chapter 27. Deep venous thrombosis (DVT) will be covered here.

Etiology and Epidemiology

A deep venous thrombosis usually forms in one of the deep veins of the lower extremities and pelvis, although these clots can also occur in the upper extremities. Factors that contribute to the development of DVT include venous stasis, hypercoagulablity, immobility, and thrombus formations. Figure 35–14◆ shows common locations for DVT occurrence. Risk factors for DVT are outlined in the Risk Factors for Venous Thromboembolism box.

Pathophysiology of Deep Vein Thrombosis

The venous system is a low pressure system that relies on skeletal muscle action, as well as changes in abdominal and intrathoracic pressure, to return the blood to the heart and lungs. The venous system also is equipped with valves that help propel the blood back to the heart and prevent retrograde flow (Porth & Matfin, 2009).

In 1864, Virchow described the triad that is associated with the formation of DVTs. **Virchow's triad** includes venous stasis, damage of the endothelium, and hypercoagulability. This theory is still used to explain the thrombus formation of DVT. Blood stasis occurs with immobility, such as occurs when a patient is in surgery or on continuous bed rest. Vessel endothelial damage can occur from trauma, surgery, infection, and inflammation. Hypercoagulability can occur with deficiencies in antithrombin III and protein C and S that normally inhibit clot

RISK FACTORS for Venous Thromboembolism

- Spinal cord injuries; paresis
- Fracture of the pelvis, hip, or long bones
- Multiple trauma; burns
- Malignancy
- Myocardial infarction, heart failure, respiratory failure, sepsis, ulcerative colitis
- Intensive care unit admission
- Previous DVT or PE
- Age > 40 years
- Obesity
- Prolonged immobility of 3 days or more
- Varicose veins
- Pregnancy/postpartum
- Oral contraceptive use
- Acquired and inherited disorders of coagulation
- Presence of central venous catheters
- Major abdominal, thoracic, gynecologic, and/or urologic surgeries
- Major orthopedic surgeries such as total hip or total knee procedures.

Source: Adapted from Brotman, D. J., & Jaffer, A. K. (2008). Prevention of venous thromboembolism in the geriatric patient. *Cardiology Clinics, 26*(2), 221–234; Stevens, S. M., & Douketis, J. D. (2010). Deep vein thrombosis prophylaxis in hospitalized medical patients: Current recommendations, general rates of implementation, and initiatives for improvement. *Clinics in Chest Medicine, 31*(4), 675–689; Worel, J. N. (2009). Venous thromboembolism: What is preventing achievement of performance measures and consensus guidelines? *Journal of Cardiovascular Nursing, 24*(6), S14–S19.

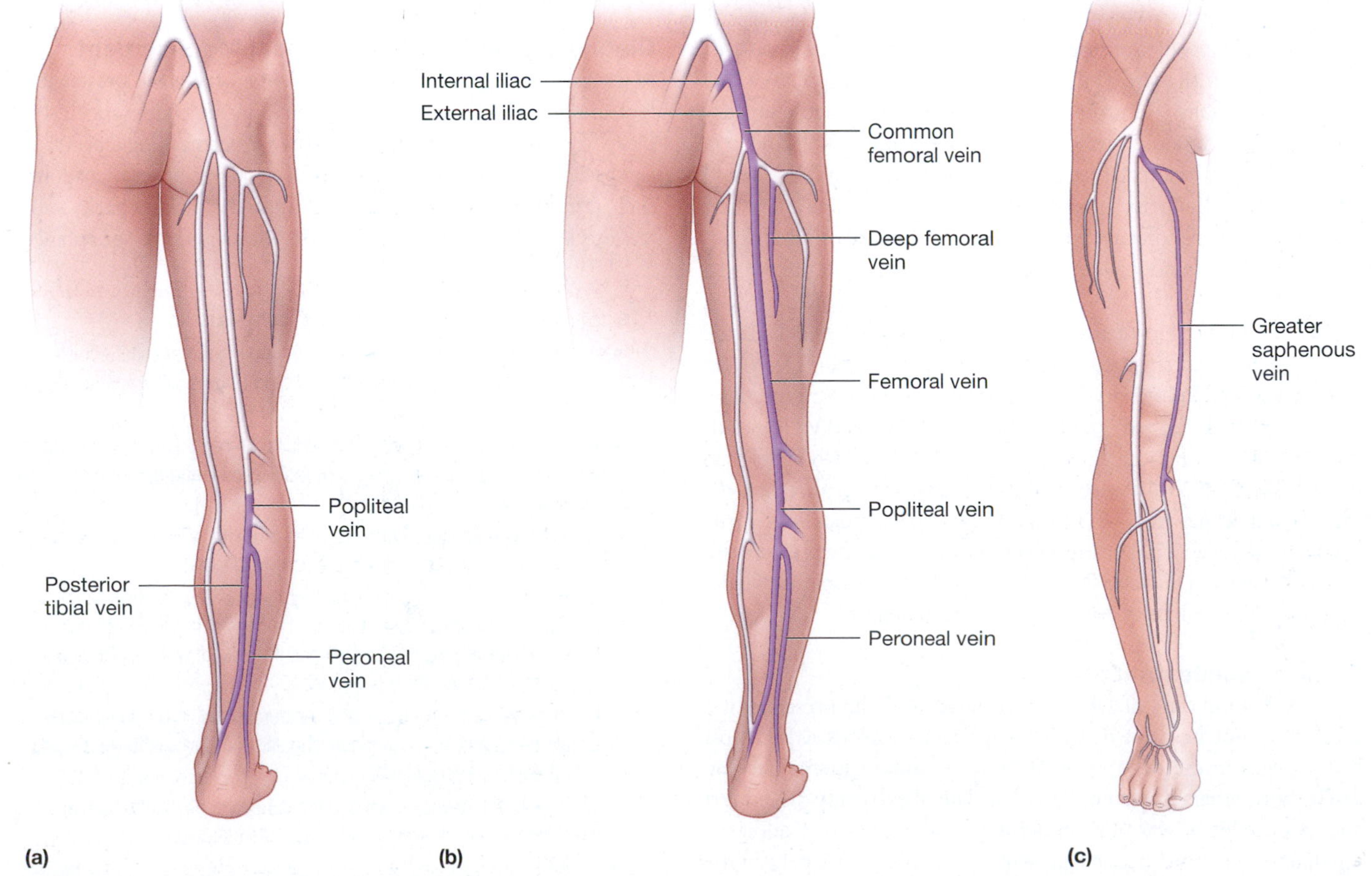

FIGURE 35–14 ◆ Common locations of venous thrombosis.

Weblink: VTE Prophylaxis

EVIDENCE-BASED PRACTICE VTE Prophylaxis: Nonpharmacologic and Mechanical Strategies to Prevent VTE

Clinical Problem

Patients at higher risk of developing VTE include older adults; the obese; the immobile; those with previous VTE; and those with stroke, heart failure, severe respiratory disease, cancer, severe infections, or recent surgery.

Nonpharmacologic strategies to decrease VTE risk include ambulation, graduated compression stockings (GCS), and mechanical devices such as intermittent pneumatic compression devices (IPCs). These nonpharmacologic strategies may be used in conjunction with anticoagulation therapy in many patients.

Research Findings

Nonpharmacologic methods of VTE prophylaxis have been shown to reduce symptomatic DVT in one or more patient groups (Geerts, 2009). They do not increase the risk of bleeding as anticoagulation does.

GCS have been found to be effective in VTE prophylaxis in some patient populations (Geerts, 2009). Challenges with the use of GCS include improper usage, incorrect size, and poor compliance with use because of patient discomfort. GCS have been associated with skin breakdown or ulceration, especially in older adults or patients with compromised skin integrity. Knee-high GCS are preferred over thigh-high GCS because of better fit, ease in application, and increased patient comfort (Hilleren-Listerud, 2009; Winslow & Brosz, 2008) leading to improved compliance with their use.

Intermittent pneumatic compression devices have also been found to be effective in some patient populations (Geerts, 2009). They are commonly used in the hospital setting, especially with surgical patients. However, IPCs are effective only when worn by a patient, activated, and functioning properly. They may be a barrier to early ambulation, as they must be removed for walking. In addition, the size, fit, pressure settings, and timing and mode of compression of IPCs have not been standardized. Furthermore, IPCs cannot be used with a preexisting DVT in the same limb.

Contraindications to the use of GCS and IPCs include the presence of peripheral arterial disease, any leg deformity, massive edema, peripheral neuropathy, gangrenous limb or gross limb cellulitis or local dermatitis or recent skin graft, and an ABI < 0.8. Use of the only the IPC is indicated with preexisting DVT in same limb.

Implications for Nursing Practice

For mechanical prophylaxis to be effective, the nurse must do the following:

1. Measure the patient to ensure proper fit of GCS and IPCs. Follow the manufacturer's recommendations for sizing. Re-measure when edema is noted and change sizes when indicated.
2. Check to ensure proper use and that there is no restriction to perfusion regularly.
3. Remove GCS and IPCs and fully assess the skin for redness or breakdown at least daily. More frequent assessment may be needed for some patients.
4. Educate patients and their families about the rationale, use, and care of GCS or IPC.

Critical Thinking Questions with answers can be found in the Osborn Student Resources at nursing.pearsonhighered.com.

Sources: Adapted from Geerts, W. (2009). Prevention of venous thromboembolism: A key patient safety priority. *Journal of Thrombosis and Haemostasis, 7* (Suppl.1), 1–8; Hilleren-Listerud, A. E. (2009). Graduated compression stocking and intermittent compression device length selection. *Clinical Nurse Specialist, 23*(1), 21–24; Winslow, E. H., & Brosz, D. L. (2008). Graduated compression stockings in hospitalized postoperative patients: Correctness of usage and size. *American Journal of Nursing, 108*(9), 40–50.

formation. The postpartum state, oral contraceptives, certain cancers, and dehydration all increase the risk for the development of DVT due to hypercoagulablity. Recurrent DVTs lead to valve damage, ultimately causing chronic venous insufficiency (Porth & Matfin, 2009).

Most hospitalized patients are at risk of developing DVT due to immobility, making risk assessment and prophylaxis an extremely important nursing management issue. The Evidence-Based Practice box discusses nonpharmacologic and mechanical strategies to prevent VTE.

Because of the significance of the problem of DVT and VTE, the U.S. Surgeon General issued a "Call of Action to Prevent Deep Vein Thrombosis and Pulmonary Embolism" (Worel, 2009). Several guidelines have been developed to address the issue of DVT and VTE, including those of the American College of Chest Physicians, who published its Eighth ACCP Conference on Antithrombotic and Thrombolytic Therapy guidelines in 2008. Despite these detailed guidelines, many hospitalized patients are not receiving adequate treatment to prevent DVT (Stevens & Douketis, 2010; Worel, 2009). The National Guidelines for VTE Prophylaxis box outlines these guidelines.

Clinical Manifestations

Signs and symptoms of DVT are variable, and the presence of a DVT may not be known until the patient develops a PE. Most DVTs begin in the deep veins of the calf. Some patients have no discomfort; others may complain of unilateral extremity discomfort and pain, edema, warmth, tenderness, and redness. In addition, a palpable vein cord may be present. *Homans' sign,* or pain in the calf when the foot is dorsiflexed, is not a reliable indicator of DVT (McCaffrey & Blum, 2009).

Diagnosis, Medical, and Surgical Management

A number of diagnostic tests assist in identifying the presence and location of DVT. These tests are outlined in the Diagnostic Tests for Deep Venous Thrombosis box (p. 1086). Pharmacologic agents that can be added to the DVT prophylaxis regime include anticoagulants, such as intravenous or subcutaneous unfractionated heparin, subcutaneous low molecular weight heparin, intravenous or subcutaneous

NATIONAL GUIDELINES for VTE Prophylaxis

- All patients should be evaluated for VTE risk upon hospital admission, when there is a change in level of care or providers, and prior to discharge.
- All patients should receive proper education regarding VTE risk, signs and symptoms, early and frequent mobilization, and appropriate treatment and prophylaxis methods.
- All hospitalized patients who are at high risk for VTE should receive anticoagulation prophylaxis unless contraindicated.
- Aspirin alone is not recommended for routine VTE prophylaxis following hip or knee arthroplasty but may be considered in combination with mechanical prophylaxis methods in patients without additional risk factors. Further study is needed.
- For all patients receiving spinal or epidural anesthesia, precautions should be taken when using anticoagulant prophylaxis to reduce the risk of epidural perispinal hematoma.
- The risk of VTE development continues beyond hospitalization, and the need for post-discharge anticoagulation should be assessed.

Source: Adapted from Institute for Clinical Systems Improvement (ICSI). (2010). Venous thromboembolism prophlaxis for the medically ill patient. (6th ed.). Retrieved from http://www.icsi.org/.

direct thrombin inhibitors, and oral warfarin. Aspirin has not been demonstrated to be effective in preventing DVT and is not recommended (McCaffrey & Blum, 2009). According to the Eighth ACCP Conference on Antithrombotic and Thrombolytic Therapy guidelines (2008):

- Strict bed rest for confirmed DVT is not needed.
- Patients may ambulate as tolerated.

Additional interventions for confirmed DVT include:

- Extremity elevation 10 to 20 degrees above the level of the heart
- Local application of moist heat
- Avoidance of massaging the affected extremity to prevent clots from breaking loose
- GCS.

Anticoagulation with short-term intravenous or subcutaneous unfractionated heparin or subcutaneous low molecular weight heparin followed by long-term warfarin therapy for 3 to 6 months is initiated. The goal for the international normalized ratio (INR) is 2 to 3. Treatment regimes for DVT can be done in the outpatient setting as well as for the hospitalized patient. The Pharmacology feature (p. 1064) outlines the pharmacologic treatment of VTE/DVT.

Some patients may require surgical intervention to prevent PE from occurring. Procedures include venous thrombectomy and interruption of the vena cava. However, thrombectomy is not commonly performed. Vena cava interruption is done percutaneously by placement of an inferior vena cava filter device that captures thrombi yet allows blood to flow through it (Figure 35–15◆). This is indicated for patients who have a contraindication to anticoagulation for DVT prophylaxis and treatment, such as the trauma patient or patients who have failed therapy by developing a clot while on anticoagulation. Complications of filter placement are rare. Trapped clots can eventually lead to venous congestion and obstruction of the vena cava. Collateral vessels develop to maintain venous flow.

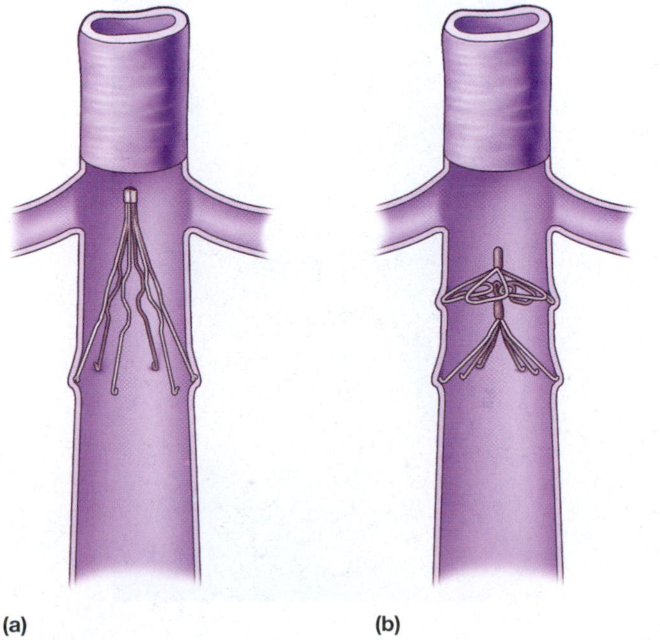

(a) (b)

FIGURE 35–15 ◆ Vena cava filters.

Nursing Management

Nurses play an active and important role in DVT prophylaxis and prevention. Nursing interventions include encouraging early ambulation whenever possible and assisting the patient in active and passive range of motion exercises, extremity elevation, and mechanical methods of prophylaxis such as graduated compression stockings, intermittent pneumatic devices, and venous foot pumps. The Evidence-Based Practice box discusses nonpharmacologic treatment of VTE. These mechanical devices increase venous outflow and/or reduce stasis in the leg veins (Worel, 2009). Accurate leg length and calf circumference measurements are required to size GCS correctly. Knee-high GCS are effective, less expensive, and easier to apply than are thigh-high GCS; therefore, using knee-high GCS may enhance patient compliance with wearing stockings. Intermittent and sequential compression devices decrease venous stasis and are often used in conjunction with GCS (Figure 35–16◆). However, patients with underlying peripheral arterial disease should use compression stockings carefully. It is important that these devices be correctly sized and applied and that they be removed for only short periods of time. Complications of compression devices are rare and may include skin blisters.

The Nursing Process: Patient Care Plan for Venous Thromboembolism box (p. 1087) outlines the nursing diagnoses and patient care

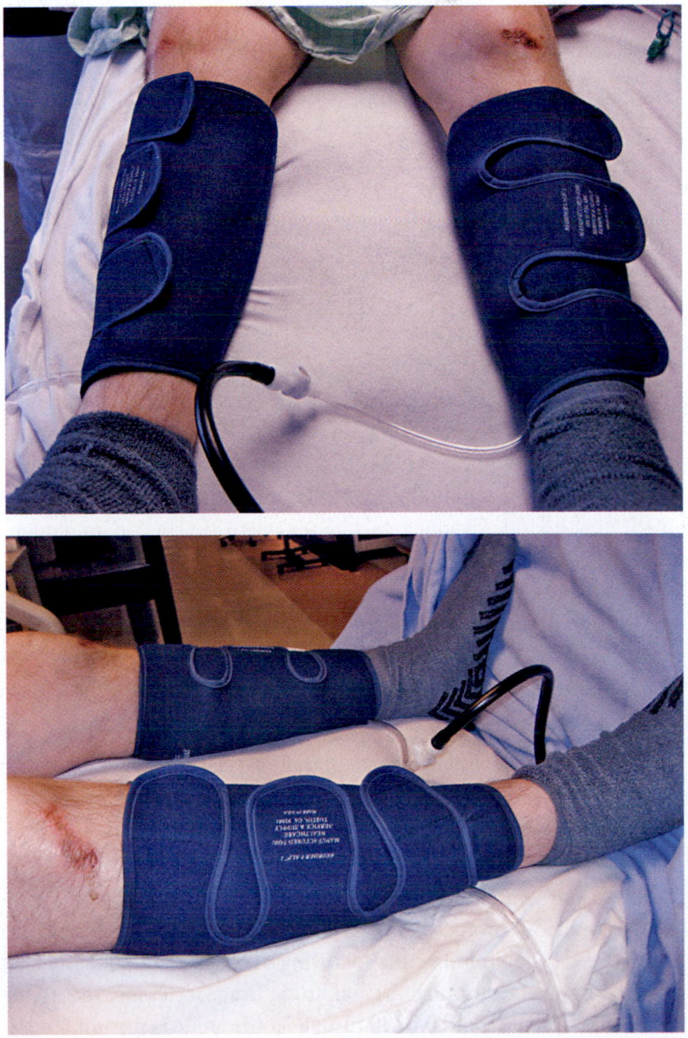

FIGURE 35–16 ◆ Intermittent and sequential compression devices.
Source: Cheryl Wraa.

DIAGNOSTIC TESTS for Deep Venous Thrombosis

Test with Normal Values	Expected Abnormality
Duplex Ultrasound	
Veins compressible; no visible clot.	Location and extent of clot or noncompressibility of the vein. Can identify floating or unstable clot. May be difficult to perform in an obese patient.
Venography (also called phlebography)	
Normal venography; no filling defects. No clot visualized.	Defines location and extent of the clot, which is seen as a filling defect. Identifies collateral circulation, if present.
CT Scan	
No clot visualized.	Useful to evaluate possible pelvic or abdominal thrombus. Useful for obese patients.
MRI	
No clot visualized.	Useful for suspected iliac vein or inferior vena caval thrombosis.
D-Dimer	
Less than 250 ng/mL.	Elevated in DVT/PE due to release of degradation products released into the circulation when fibrin undergoes fibrinolysis.
Venous Duplex Imaging	Provides anatomic extent of venous disease. Detects DVT or venous obstruction. Provides information about valve function.
Photoplethysmography	A venous refill time < 20 seconds is indicative of venous disease.
Ambulatory Venous Pressure	Pedal vein pressure is measured before and after exercise to assess the severity of venous disease.

needs that will provide a comprehensive plan of care for a patient experiencing a DVT.

Complications

One of the complications of DVT is PE, which is described in Chapter 27. Most thrombi come from the deep veins of the legs and can break loose spontaneously or be jarred loose by mechanical forces such as sudden standing, the Valsalva maneuver, or when the patient bears down to have a bowel movement. Pulmonary embolism may occur despite adequate anticoagulation. Clinical findings in PE may include dyspnea, tachypnea, pleuritic chest pain, cough, wheezing, syncope, hypotension, and cardiovascular collapse. The mortality associated with a large PE is 30% or more. A majority of patients with PE die within the first hour of symptom onset. Hypoxia occurs in these patients because of the imbalance or mismatch between blood flow and alveolar ventilation.

Safety Alert *Signs and symptoms of PE include dyspnea, tachypnea, anxiety, apprehension, tachycardia, chest pain, hemoptysis, hypoxia, collapse, shock, and cardiac arrest. Right ventricular failure is the cause of death in patients who die of PE. The nurse must monitor patients with DVT for these symptoms and notify the health care provider immediately if they occur.*

A second complication following acute DVT is postphlebitic syndrome, which is chronic venous insufficiency (CVI). As many as 50% of patients develop this disorder following a DVT (Stevens & Douketis, 2010). To prevent postphlebitic syndrome from occurring, the use of GCS with a pressure of 30 to 40 mmHg at the ankle is recommended for at least 2 years following the acute DVT episode. Chronic venous insufficiency occurs from vein pathology, such as venous valvular incompetence, causing venous stasis and increased venous pressure in the lower extremities. Symptoms of CVI include dependent swelling, pain, and skin changes such as hyperpigmentation (brownish discoloration of the skin), edema, dermatitis, ulcerations, or scarring from healed ulcerations (Figure 35–17◆). Patients may complain of cramping, heaviness, or aching of their legs.

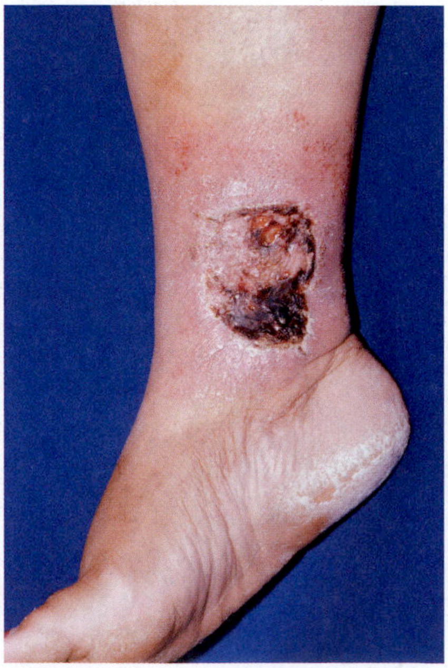

FIGURE 35–17 ◆ Chronic venous insufficiency.

Source: Ribotsky/Custom Medical Stock Photo, Inc.

NURSING PROCESS: Patient Care Plan for Venous Thromboembolism

Assessment of Cardiovascular Status Using Gordon's Functional Health Patterns:

- Nutrition Metabolic Pattern
- Activity Exercise Pattern
- Cognitive Perceptual Pattern

Subjective Data

Assessment of Peripheral Vascular Status

Do you have pain, tenderness, or swelling in your legs or arms?

When did this occur and how long have you had it?

What is your activity level?

Have you traveled long distances recently?

Are you feeling short of breath?

Do you have pain in your chest?

Assessment of Pain Related to Impaired Circulation

Where is your pain?

What brings it on?

What makes it go away?

How long have you had it, and is it getting worse or better?

Assessment of Bleeding Related to Anticoagulant Therapy

Do your gums bleed when you brush your teeth?

Do you notice any blood in your urine or stool?

Do you notice any increased or unusual bruising?

Assessment of Pulmonary Embolus Related to Embolization of Thrombus

Are you feeling short of breath?

Are you having chest pain?

Are you coughing up blood-tinged sputum?

When did these symptoms begin?

Assessment of Self-Care Activities

Has anyone explained your health problems to you?

How does this disease affect your daily life?

Objective Data

Assessment of Peripheral Vascular Status

Assess for contributing factors for deep vein thrombosis (DVT)/pulmonary embolism (PE) development: immobility, major surgery, trauma, paralysis, history of previous DVT/PE episodes.

Assess extremities for pain, tenderness, erythema, and swelling.

Assessment of Pain Related to Impaired Circulation

Use a pain scale (0–10) to quantify pain.

Assess the cultural and religious impact on the patient's responses.

Note increased pain to evaluate for disease progression or acute arterial obstruction.

Assessment of Bleeding Related to Anticoagulant Therapy

Assess aPTT or INR, and report subtherapeutic values and overtherapeutic ranges.

Stool guaiac negative.

Assess for bleeding in mouth, nose, and urine.

Assessment of Pulmonary Embolus Related to Embolization of Thrombus

Rate, depth, and ease of respiration.

Assess lung sounds for adventitious or diminished sounds.

Assess sputum for blood.

Assess oxygen saturation levels.

Assessment of Self-Care Activities

Assess knowledge of disease process and progression, risk factors, and need for compression stockings.

Assess knowledge of patient's understanding of treatment plan, including medications, if indicated.

Outcomes and Evaluation Parameters / Planning and Interventions with *Rationales*

1. NURSING DIAGNOSIS: Impaired Tissue Perfusion *related to DVT* (NANDA-I © 2012)

Outcomes and Evaluation Parameters

Outcomes: Patient has adequate blood flow to extremities. Patient does not develop pulmonary embolus clinical manifestations (Chapter 28).

Evaluation Parameters: Warm skin, absence of edema, and absence of pain. Normal respiratory patterns, normal heart rate, and absence of chest pain.

Planning and Interventions with *Rationales*

Apply properly fitting compression stockings *to promote venous return and decrease venous stasis.*

For Confirmed DVT

Measure the circumference of the affected extremity daily *to monitor progression and/or resolution of DVT.*

Maintain activity per order with affected limb elevated 10 to 20 degrees above the level of the heart *to reduce venous pooling and edema.*

Maintain hydration *to prevent increased blood viscosity.*

Explain the risk factors of venous thromboembolism (VTE), and the need for bed rest, limb elevation, compression stockings, and sequential compression; avoid rubbing/massaging calf *to prevent reoccurrences.*

Monitor results of laboratory testing and noninvasive studies *to assess treatment effectiveness.*

(*continued*)

NURSING PROCESS: Patient Care Plan for Venous Thromboembolism, *continued*

Outcomes and Evaluation Parameters	Planning and Interventions with *Rationales*
2. NURSING DIAGNOSIS: Readiness for Enhanced Comfort *related to impaired circulation* (NANDA-I © 2012)	
Outcome: Relief of pain. ***Evaluation Parameters:*** Patient states adequate relief of pain. Patient understands measures necessary to prevent pain.	Provide moist heat *to help relieve pain and inflammation.* Keep affected extremity elevated above the level of the heart *to promote venous return and decrease venous stasis.* Provide a supportive environment where patient is able to express pain level. Instruct the patient to inform the nurse if pain is not relieved *in order to revise the care plan.* Use pain control measures before the pain becomes severe *to enhance comfort.* Teach nonpharmacologic methods of pain control; that is, guided imagery and breathing exercises *to assist in relaxation and pain control.* Pain relief *to promote comfort.*
3. NURSING DIAGNOSIS: Fluid Volume Deficit, Potential for *related to bleeding* (NANDA-I © 2012)	
Outcomes: Therapeutic aPTT or INR maintained in therapeutic range. No bleeding. ***Evaluation Parameters:*** No signs of bleeding in mouth, nose, urine, or stool.	Initiate and continue anticoagulant therapy *to prevent further clot development.* Monitor aPTT and/or INR prior to adjusting heparin or administering Coumadin *to optimize anticoagulation.* Assess for signs of bleeding *to ensure prompt identification and treatment.* Teach dietary restrictions of vitamin K *to avoid interactions with Coumadin.*
4. NURSING DIAGNOSIS: Impaired Gas Exchange *related to VTE* (NANDA-I © 2012)	
Outcomes: No respiratory distress. Normal arterial blood gases. Normal oxygen saturation levels. ***Evaluation Parameters:*** No signs or symptoms of respiratory distress. No blood in sputum. No shortness of breath. No pain.	Instruct the patient of reportable conditions: signs and symptoms of pulmonary embolus. Auscultate breath sounds for *assessment of crackles, rhonchi, or diminished sounds.* Provide oxygen per order *to increase oxygen to the heart, lungs, and periphery.* Administer anticoagulants or thrombolytic therapy *to treat VTE.*
5. NURSING DIAGNOSIS: Deficient Knowledge of Self-Care Needs *related to disease* (NANDA-I © 2012)	
Outcome: Adequate knowledge level. ***Evaluation Parameters:*** Patient is able to discuss the disease process, risk factors, and current treatment plan. Verbalizes adherence to and compliance with treatment plan.	Provide factual information about the diagnosis, treatment, risk factor modification, medications, and treatment plan *to enhance compliance.* Explain all procedures and allow the patient to ask questions *to promote his understanding.*

Source: Adapted from Wilkinson, J. M., & Ahearn, N. R. (2009). *Prentice Hall nursing diagnosis handbook* (9th ed.). Upper Saddle River, NJ: Prentice Hall.

Another complication includes venous ulcerations, which are typically located near the medial malleolus or the lateral malleolus of the ankle but can occur anywhere below the knee. They are shallow, irregularly shaped, exudative wounds that are typically difficult to treat. Pain may be worse when the legs are in a dependent position. Walking or elevating the legs may improve the pain of venous ulcers. Venous ulcers, which often recur, affect the patient's quality of life by causing pain and discomfort, decreased mobility, increased visits to the health care provider, or hospitalizations, as well as the negative impact of managing issues related to a chronic condition: anxiety, fear, and depression.

Before venous ulcers are treated, concomitant PAD must be ruled out. Compression therapy is the primary therapy used to treat venous ulcers. Because compression therapy is contraindicated in PAD, an ankle–brachial index (ABI) should be performed prior to compression therapy. A finding of ≤ 0.9 indicates PAD.

Compression therapy is provided by using elastic or nonelastic dressings or wraps. An elastic dressing stretches with changes in leg size but will continue to compress, whereas a nonelastic dressing resists stretching. A rigid bandage, such as the **Unna's boot,** commonly used to treat venous ulcers, prevents edema while promoting healing and is worn for several days at a time.

The Unna's boot is being replaced in clinical practice by multilayer wrap compression, which is available in high and low compression pressures. An example of a multilayer wrap that provides graded compression is Profore.

Venous ulcers require treatment using absorbent compresses, compression dressings, topical steroids, topical zinc oxide, or in rare cases a broad-spectrum antifungal cream. The wound should be cleansed at each dressing change, and the patient should be instructed to avoid known skin irritants and allergens. The application of a mixture of local anesthetic cream may produce pain relief for sharp debridement, if needed. Adhesive hydrocolloid dressings have been found to be effective in healing venous ulcers. Topical antibiotics are generally not effective; a short course with a topical antimicrobial such as silver sulfadiazine may be beneficial. If signs of infection occur, such as pain, fever, and drainage from the ulcer, a culture should be obtained and the appropriate systemic antibiotic started. Infections most commonly include gram-positive organisms such as

Staphylococcus and *Streptococcus* and gram-negative organisms such as *Pseudomonas.*

An important component of wound assessment is ongoing documentation using photographs of the wound and measurements of the wound size. This can readily be achieved by using a digital camera and single-use rulers that are available from various manufacturers. Having this objective history of the wound appearance and size makes it easier to follow trends in therapy and healing. An in-depth discussion of wound healing is presented in Chapter 60.

Patients with venous leg ulcers need to maintain adequate nutritional status to promote healing. A dietary consultation may be indicated. If overweight, the patient should be counseled about weight loss. Sufficient amounts of protein, vitamins A and C, and zinc are important. In addition, decreased sodium intake is important to assist with managing edema. For patients with diabetes, tight glycemic control is essential to reduce infection and promote healing. An in-depth discussion of the nutritional aspects of wound healing is presented in Chapter 8. Surgical intervention for venous ulcers is rarely required because no definitive procedure has been found for treatment.

Collaborative Management

A multidisciplinary team approach including health care providers, nurses, pharmacists, physical therapists, and dietitians is needed in providing care for patients with VTE. In order to meet desired patient outcomes, it is essential that this interdisciplinary team communicate openly with one another in developing and evaluating care of the patient and family (IOM [Institute of Medicine], 2010). Patients may benefit greatly from a nurse- or pharmacist-directed anticoagulation program to assist them in taking and monitoring their warfarin, if prescribed. Physical therapy can educate the patient and family about an appropriate level of activity that will help prevent recurrence. The dietitian is essential for adjusting the patient's diet so that foods that interfere with anticoagulation medications, such as dark green vegetables, are avoided. Home health visits may be necessary for the patient undergoing outpatient treatment of DVT.

Health Promotion

To prevent DVT, patients should be taught the importance of regular walking, foot and ankle exercises, and foot elevation when hospitalized and during recovery from hospitalization. If patients are discharged home on a pharmacologic prophylaxis plan such as unfractionated heparin, warfarin or enoxaparin, or direct thrombin inhibitors, they need to be taught their medication regime, which may include learning how to do injections, follow-up monitoring, and reportable adverse effects. The Patient Teaching & Discharge Priorities for Use of Anticoagulant Medications box (p. 1090) presents suggestions for teaching the patient who is on anticoagulating medications. The most common complications of these medications include bleeding and heparin-induced thrombocytopenia. GCS should be worn to prevent venous pooling. The nurse needs to stress to patients that they should avoid prolonged sitting, standing, and crossing their legs. The Patient Teaching & Discharge Priorities for Deep Venous Thrombosis (p. 1091) outlines the discharge priorities that the nurse needs to include in the discharge teaching plan.

Lymphatic Disorders

The lymphatic system is composed of lymphatic vessels, lymph nodes, the spleen, and the thymus. This system filters bacteria and other particulate matter, thereby providing defense against disease.

Lymphangitis

Lymphangitis is an acute inflammation of the lymphatic channels most commonly caused by an infection in one of the extremities. In this condition, the associated lymph nodes become enlarged and tender. Recurrent episodes of lymphangitis can be associated with progressive lymphedema. Lymphedema is swelling caused by an accumulation of lymph fluid in the interstitial tissues.

Lymphangitis most commonly occurs following a streptococcal infection of the skin, at which time the associated lymph nodes become enlarged and tender. Additional symptoms of lymphangitis include throbbing pain, swelling, fever, chills, and reddened streaks from the area of the infection to the axilla or groin, depending on the site of the infection. Treatment includes antibiotics, analgesics, and anti-inflammatory agents.

Lymphedema

Etiology and Epidemiology

Lymphedema can be primary or secondary. Primary lymphedema is inherited as an autosomal dominant trait. Secondary lymphedema occurs as a result of an acquired disorder, such as a malignancy, radiation, surgical removal of a component of the lymphatic system, trauma, or infection. Malignancy is the most common cause of secondary lymphedema in the United States (Rockson, 2008). Figure 35–18◆ shows lower extremity severe lymphedema.

Pathophysiology

Lymphedema occurs when there is an obstruction causing excess lymph buildup within the system, which ultimately overloads the transport capacity of the lymphatic system. This can progress to fibrosis and irreversible tissue damage. Lymphedema is classified into three stages. In Stage I, the edema is pitting and is reversible with elevation of the affected limb. In Stage II, fibrosis has occurred and the edema is nonpitting and nonreversible. In Stage III, the affected limb is greatly enlarged and the skin is thickened.

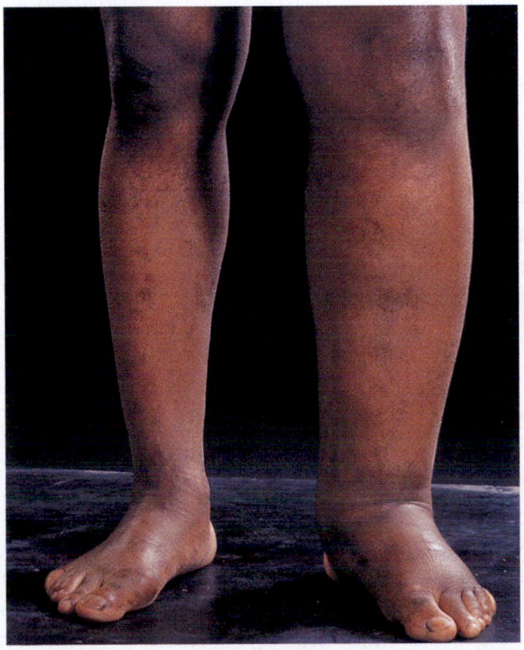

FIGURE 35–18 ◆ Severe lymphedema.
Source: MSNB/Custom Medical Stock Photo, Inc.

PATIENT TEACHING & DISCHARGE PRIORITIES for Use of Anticoagulant Medications

Medication Need	Teaching
All anticoagulant/antiplatelet agents	Take as directed by the health care provider. Do not skip doses. Consider an alert bracelet/necklace. Avoid activities that can cause injury or falling. Early warning signs of bleeding include bruising, nosebleeds, or bleeding gums. Serious bleeding can occur and includes: • Pink or brown urine • Red or black stool • Spitting up or coughing up bloody secretions or secretions that look like coffee grounds • Severe headache • Dizziness, fatigue, or weakness. Report any excessive bruising or bleeding to the health care provider.
Heparin and low molecular weight heparin	Patients need to be taught subcutaneous injection techniques. Frequent monitoring of laboratory work is generally not required for patients on low molecular weight heparin.
Warfarin/Coumadin	Patients need to take the exact dose as prescribed by their health care provider or pharmacist. They may need to take different doses of warfarin (Coumadin) on different days of the week. Many patients taking warfarin are monitored by an interdisciplinary anticoagulation clinic rather than their health care provider. Instruct patients to know who is monitoring their warfarin (Coumadin) and when they need to see them. If patients miss two or more doses in a row, they should call whoever is managing their medication for further instructions. Regular blood testing of the INR level is required. Instruct patients to know their optimal INR range. For many cardiovascular patients, it is between 2 and 3. Drug interactions can occur. Patients should use care when taking many over-the-counter drug preparations. The most likely drugs to affect the INR include aspirin, ibuprofen, cold remedies, antacids, and vitamin supplements. Herbal supplements can affect the INR, especially dan shen, garlic, *Ginkgo biloba,* ginseng, green tea, or kava. Food interactions can occur. Because the drug reduces the liver's ability to use vitamin K, any foods that change the amount of vitamin K in the body can affect the INR. These foods include Brussels sprouts, kale, green tea, asparagus, avocado, broccoli, cabbage, cauliflower, collard greens, liver, soybean oil, soybeans, certain beans, mustard greens, peas (black-eyed peas, split peas, chick peas), turnip greens, parsley, green onions, spinach, and lettuce. Patients may be advised to limit their alcohol intake. Warfarin (Coumadin) can cause birth defects; it should NOT be taken by patients planning to become pregnant.

Clinical Manifestations

Lymphedema is the interstitial accumulation of lymph fluid that occurs when the lymphatic system is impaired. The affected limb(s) become edematous with thickened skin. Patients may complain of heaviness or fullness of the affected extremity.

Diagnosis and Medical Management

Diagnosis of lymphedema is based on the patient's history and clinical presentation. The Diagnostic Tests for Lymphedema box outlines the typical tests that are done to assist in confirming the diagnosis of lymphedema. The patient should be asked about previous surgeries, radiation treatment, trauma, and infection. Medical treatment of lymphedema is directed toward controlling the fluid accumulation, maintaining skin integrity, and preventing infections. Bed rest, compression therapy, manual lymphatic drainage, short stretch compression wrapping, and limb elevation are the primary interventions for lymphedema.

Complications of Lymphedema

Complications of lymphedema include recurrent cellulitis and/or lymphangitis, DVT, severe functional impairment, cosmetic embarrassment, and (rarely) amputation. Complications following surgery are common and include partial wound separation, seroma, hematoma, skin necrosis, and exacerbation of foot or hand edema. Patients with chronic lymphedema have a risk of developing lymphangiosarcoma. Although rare, this cancerous tumor is highly aggressive, requires radical amputation of the involved extremity, and has a very poor prognosis.

Nursing Management

Patients with lymphedema require limb elevation; compression garments, which are custom fit garments that apply compression and prevent fluid from accumulating in the limb; and manual drainage or the use of a lymph pump to reduce edema. The affected extremity is placed into the sleeve of the lymph pump, which is then inflated to a preset

PATIENT TEACHING & DISCHARGE PRIORITIES for Deep Venous Thrombosis

Need	Teaching
Knowledge of disease process	Home care needs include verbal and written instructions for: Treatment plan, including anticoagulation Follow-up care Activity restrictions, if any.
Understanding of medications	Teach the purpose, dose, and possible adverse effects of all medications to increase compliance and to prevent over/underdosing. Anticoagulant teaching: reason and importance, how to perform injections (if low molecular weight heparin prescribed), taking medications at the same time each day, not skipping a dose, frequent follow-up and lab testing, avoiding anything that might cause trauma/bleeding such as vigorous tooth brushing, contact sports.
Disease prevention	Explain the risk factors for DVT/PE development to prevent reoccurrences. The Risk Factors box (p. 1083) presents a detailed list of risk factors for VTE. Avoid prolonged immobility, standing for long periods of time, car/airline flights > 6 hours; avoid constrictive clothing. Wear properly fitting and applied GCS. If these stockings are recommended long term, teach the patient to replace them every 3 months, because they lose their elasticity.
Reportable clinical manifestations	Instruct patient/family to report: Increase in pain, tenderness, or swelling of an affected extremity New onset pain, tenderness, or swelling in another extremity New onset shortness of breath, chest pain, anxiety, or restlessness New onset bleeding, headache, or mental status changes.
Family/support system	Assess availability of, knowledge of, and compliance with treatment plan. Assess discharge placement needs. Assess for need for professional home health needs. Assess need for follow-up appointments.

DIAGNOSTIC TESTS for Lymphedema

Test With Normal Values	Expected Abnormality
Lymphangiography	
No obstruction of lymphatic fluid flow.	Obstructions in lymphatic communication visualized.
Lymphoscintigraphy	
No obstruction of lymphatic fluid flow.	Obstructions in lymphatic communication visualized.

pressure to help drain the extremity. The lymph pump may be used daily to reduce edema. Surgical options include resection of skin and subcutaneous tissue, skin grafting, drainage procedures, removal of tissue containing abnormal lymphatics, and, less commonly, transplant of tissue from areas with normal lymphatic tissues to areas with abnormal lymphatic drainage. In rare cases, bypass of abnormal lymphatic tissue is attempted, in some cases using vein grafts. Such procedures, which are frequently unsuccessful, are usually performed only under experimental protocols. Surgery for lymphedema has met with limited success and requires significant experience and technical expertise. Complications of surgery include poor healing, infection, prolonged hospitalization, poor cosmetic results, and failure to reduce the edema (Rockson, 2008).

Health Promotion

The nurse should instruct the patient on the importance of excellent skin hygiene and infection prevention. Good skin care with mild soaps and moisturizing creams is needed. Because patients with lymphedema are at risk of infection, particularly fungal infections, they need to be taught to inspect regularly for signs and symptoms of infection and to report them promptly.

Gerontological Considerations

The prevalence of peripheral arterial disease, AAA, DVT, and CVI increases with age. Peripheral arterial disease, stroke, and myocardial infarction are the principal causes of death and disability in patients over age 50. Older patients with peripheral arterial disorders are at higher risk of coronary and cerebrovascular events, such as myocardial infarction and stroke. Older patients with acute and chronic venous disease are at higher risk of pulmonary embolus and death (Brotman & Jaffer, 2008; Moser & Riegel, 2009).

Peripheral vascular disease can cause functional limitations in older adults, greatly affecting their quality of life. Physical training, strength training, and exercise programs can improve functional status. Low-intensity exercise programs, such as walking, golf, and shuffleboard, can be of great benefit for older adults. Patients should be encouraged to continue to modify their risk factors for peripheral vascular disease

RESEARCH OPPORTUNITIES Related to Peripheral Vascular Disorders

Research	Clinical Impact
Effects of gene therapy on peripheral arterial disease	Decrease in tissue loss and enhanced healing
Herbal and complementary medicine to treat peripheral arterial disease	Lowers blood lipids and blood pressure
Wound care in arterial and venous ulcers	Rapid and enhanced healing
Pressure reduction surfaces and devices	Decrease in tissue loss
How do childhood obesity and hypertension affect the rate of development of end-organ damage?	Children's physiological response to obesity and hypertension is different than that of adults, especially older adults.
How does the meaning of living with a diagnosis of hypertension influence the patient's prognosis?	Knowing the meaning and significance of the diagnosis of hypertension to the patient will enhance teaching and learning opportunities.
What are the roles of heredity and environment in the prevention of hypertension?	Determine the role of genetics and the environment in the prevention and treatment of hypertension.

through smoking cessation and controlling their blood pressure and blood sugar levels.

Special nursing care considerations for older adults include a careful assessment of the cardiovascular and cerebrovascular systems. Myocardial ischemia and infarction can occur, leading to decompensation of the cardiovascular system. Stroke is a leading cause of death and disability in older adults. Therefore, teaching the patient and family members the signs and symptoms of transient ischemic attacks and impending stroke is essential.

Recovery from major vascular surgical procedures, such as AAA repair or femoropopliteal bypass, can be prolonged in older adults. Wound healing may be delayed in these patients; in addition, older adults may be more likely to develop surgical complications, such as atelectasis, pneumonia, and wound infection. Older patients are more likely to develop complications of immobility, so turning, repositioning, and ambulating the patient as early as possible to maintain pulmonary function and promote independence also are important aspects of care. Careful assessment of the patient's nutritional intake is essential, in that it affects wound healing and survival. Strict asepsis is critical because of the diminished immune response and increased susceptibility to infection.

Research

Peripheral vascular disorders affect millions of Americans, and the effects of these diseases can be limiting and potentially devastating. Research that further explores and defines nursing interventions and therapies for patients with peripheral vascular disorder is needed. Nursing research in the area of peripheral vascular disorders and the application of evidence-based practice is essential for the continued refinement of care for the patients with peripheral vascular disorders. The research topics related to peripheral vascular disorders are outlined in the Research Opportunities Related to Peripheral Vascular Disorders box.

CLINICAL PREPARATION READ DOCUMENT APPLY

READ: **History of Present Illnesses** >> Laboratory Study Results >> Critical Thinking Questions

As the on-coming nurse on the medical–surgical unit, you receive a report on Gregory Davis, a 68-year-old retired schoolteacher admitted 2 days ago with peripheral arterial disease, rest pain in the right forefoot, and a nonhealing ulcer on the distal aspect of the right great toe. He was admitted from the ED and gave a 2-week history of persistent and severe pain, which has kept him from sleeping at night. He also noted redness and drainage from what had previously been a stable callus over the distal great toe.

The night nurse tells you that Mr. Davis was stable throughout the night and was able to sleep at short intervals, although his pain level never decreased below 5/10 despite use of a morphine sulfate patient-controlled analgesia pump and bolus doses of 5 mg twice.

Medical–Surgical History

Mr. Davis's medical history includes intermittent claudication after walking two blocks, type 2 diabetes, hypertension, hypercholesterolemia, and coronary artery disease. He is allergic to penicillin. Currently, he is a nonsmoker for 1 year after smoking 1 pack per day for 50 years. He has an alcohol intake of one glass of red wine with dinner most nights. Past surgeries include three-vessel coronary artery bypass grafting 8 years prior and percutaneous transluminal angioplasty and stenting of the right external iliac artery 1 year ago.

Social History

Mr. Davis is married with two grown children and a 2-year-old granddaughter. He is active in his church group and plays golf three times per week, although he is unable to walk the course because of leg pain and now uses a cart.

READ: History of Present Illnesses >> **Physical Exam** >> Admitting Medical Records >> Laboratory Study Results

Current Medications

Atorvastatin (Lipitor) 40 mg po daily
Cilostazol (Pletal) 100 mg po bid
Aspirin 325 mg enteric-coated po daily
Metformin (Glucophage) 500 mg po bid
Benazepril (Lotensin) 20 mg po daily
Nitroglycerine 0.4 mg sublingual prn

Physical Exam

Physical exam findings reveal that Mr. Davis is alert, cooperative, and oriented to person, place, and time. He currently rates his pain as 5/10 in the right foot. Vital signs: BP 150/90 in the left arm, 160/100 in the right arm; HR 72; RR 18; temperature 37.5°C. His weight is 200 pounds. His height is 5′10″. He has a left carotid bruit. His neurological exam is normal. He has a well-healed midline sternal incision. Heart tones are regular with no murmur heard. Lungs are clear with diminished breath sounds at the bases bilaterally. His abdomen is soft and nontender with active bowel sounds. He has bilateral femoral bruits. His femoral pulses are faintly palpable bilaterally, and his popliteal, dorsalis pedis, and posterior pulses are absent bilaterally.

Dependent rubor is noted in the right foot, which blanches with elevation. Skin of the feet is dry and intact, except for the right great toe ulcer, which measures 1 cm. Capillary refill of the other toes is sluggish. Slight erythema is noted on the surrounding skin, and there is a small amount of serous drainage on the dressing. His toenails are thickened. 12-lead ECG: sinus rhythm with nonspecific ST segment changes.

Admitting Medical Orders

Vascular service
Admit to telemetry with continuous cardiac monitoring
Diagnosis: peripheral arterial disease with ulceration, right toe
Allergy: penicillin
Vital signs q4h
Bilateral lower extremity pulse checks q4h
Bed rest with bathroom privileges
1,800-calorie ADA diet
Accuchecks ac and hs
Call house officer: pulse < 60–130/minute; BP < 90–160 systolic; temperature > 38.5; urine output < 30 mL/hr x 2 hrs, respiratory rate 40/minute; glucose > 150
IV saline lock: flush with NS q8h
NS wet-to-dry dressing changes to right great toe q8h

Scheduled Medications

Atorvastatin (Lipitor) 40 mg po daily
Aspirin 325 mg enteric-coated po daily
Metformin (Glucophage) 500 mg po bid
Benazepril (Lotensin) 20 mg po daily
Nitroglycerine 0.4 mg sublingual prn chest discomfort/angina
Mylanta 30 mL q4h prn dyspepsia
Zolpidem (Ambien) 5 mg po qhs prn for sleep
Ativan 1 mg IV q6h prn anxiety
Milk of Magnesia 30 mL daily prn constipation
Tylenol 650 mg po/pr q4h prn for pain
Morphine sulfate PCA: 1 mg incremental dose q10min; if pain not well controlled, give morphine sulfate bolus 1–5 mg IV × 1

Ordered Laboratory Studies

CBC, basic metabolic panel, daily
Culture drainage right toe

Ordered Diagnostic Studies

12-lead ECG
PA and lateral chest x-ray
Carotid duplex today; also have vascular lab perform bilateral ABI
NPO at midnight for aortic angiography with runoff

READ: History of Present Illnesses >> **Laboratory Study Results** >> Critical Thinking Questions

Test	Admit	Day 2	Day 3
WBC	13.4/mm^3	14.0/mm^3	17.1/mm^3
RBC	3.66/mm^3	3.93/mm^3	3.67/mm^3
Hemoglobin	11.4 g/dL	12.1 g/dL	11.6 g/dL
Hematocrit	33.6%	35.8%	33.3%
Platelet count	172/mm^3	192/mm^3	221/mm^3
Sodium	137 mEq/L	134 mEq/L	135 mEq/L

Test	Admit	Day 2	Day 3
Potassium	3.7 mEq/L	3.8 mEq/L	3.8 mEq/L
Chloride	101 mEq/L	96 mEq/L	97 mEq/L
Calcium	7.9 mg/dL	8.6 mg/dL	8.2 mg/dL
Blood sugar	306 mg/dL	255 mg/dL	203 mg/dL
BUN	34 mg/dL	36 mg/dL	34 mg/dL
Creatinine	1.7 mg/dL	1.8 mg/dL	1.7 mg/dL

Pearson Nursing Student Resources

Log on to **nursing.pearsonhighered.com** *to download forms*

DOCUMENT:

>> Summary of Hospitalization
>> Pathophysiology Form
>> Laboratory Values
>> Laboratory Results Explanation

APPLY:

>> List of Potential Nursing Diagnosis
>> Concept Map
>> Critical Thinking Questions and Concept Map

CLINICAL PREPARATION, *continued*

APPLY: History of Present Illnesses >> Laboratory Study Results >> **Critical Thinking Questions**

1. What are the priorities of care for Mr. Davis?
2. What additional objective data would be helpful in assessing Mr. Davis?
3. What is the significance of the smoking history?
4. After morning rounds, Mr. Davis's health care provider orders an angiogram of the aorta and lower extremities. What is the rationale for these tests?
5. How will you prioritize Mr. Davis's nursing management following his angiogram?

Answers to Critical Thinking Questions can be found in Appendix D in the Osborn Student Resources at nursing.pearsonhighered.com.

NCLEX® PRACTICE

1. A nurse is suspicious that the patient has "white coat" hypertension. Which nursing intervention is indicated?

1. Retake the patient's blood pressure in the opposite arm.
2. Have the patient rest for 5 minutes and recheck the blood pressure.
3. Ask the patient to measure the blood pressure at home for several days.
4. Measure the blood pressure in both the sitting and standing positions.

2. A patient with peripheral arterial disease has intermittent claudication. Which intervention should the nurse include in this patient's plan of care?

1. Use moist heat.
2. Keep legs elevated above the level of the heart.
3. Teach the importance of regular and structured ambulation.
4. Remind that the legs will feel cool to the touch.

3. The nurse is instructing a patient with Raynaud's disease on self-management. Which topic should be included in this instruction?

1. Smoking cessation is the only treatment for this disease.
2. Dress warmly in cold weather.
3. Avoid physical exercise.
4. Prescribed medications have no effect on the disease.

4. A patient is postoperative after having an endovascular stent graft to repair an aortic abdominal aneurysm. Which nursing assessments are necessary to detect possible complications in caring for this patient? (select all that apply)

1. Urine output measurement hourly
2. Continous cardiac monitoring
3. Pedal pulse assessment daily
4. Temperature measurement every 12 hours
5. Breath and bowel sound assessment every 4 hours

5. A patient recovering from orthopedic surgery has developed a confirmed deep vein thrombosis in the left calf. Which intervention should the nurse include in this patient's care plan?

1. Massage the affected leg three times each day.
2. Apply cold packs to the affected leg for 15 minutes three times each day.
3. Complete bed rest with the left leg elevated.
4. Monitor status of compression stockings twice per shift.

6. A patient diagnosed with a deep vein thrombosis is started on low molecular weight heparin. What should the nurse instruct the patient about this medication?

1. Avoid increasing the amount of green leafy vegetables in your diet.
2. Watch for bleeding from your gums and easy bruising.
3. Make monthly appointments to have INR levels drawn.
4. Do not take antacids when taking this medication.

Answers to NCLEX Practice questions can be found in Appendix D in the Osborn Student Resources at nursing.pearsonhighered.com. Practice additional NCLEX questions online at the Student Resources site.

Pearson Nursing Student Resources Find additional review materials at: **nursing.pearsonhighered.com**

REFERENCES

ACCP Guidelines (8th ed.). (2008). Antithrombotic and thrombolytic therapy. *Chest, 133*(6 suppl).

Adams, M. P., & Koch, R. W. (2010). *Pharmacology: Connections to nursing practice.* Upper Saddle River, NJ: Pearson.

American Diabetes Association. (2011). High blood pressure (hypertension). Retrieved from http://www.diabetes.org/living-with-diabetes/complications/high-blood-pressure-hypertension.html

American Heart Association. (2008). Atherosclerosis. Retrieved from http://www.americanheart.org/presenter.jhtml?identifier=4440

American Heart Association. (2010). National Cholesterol Education Program. Retrieved from http://www.americanheart.org/presenter.jhtml?identifier=4638

American Heart Association. (2011). High blood pressure. Retrieved from http://www.americanheart.org/presenter.jhtml?identifier=4623

Brotman, D. J., & Jaffer, A. K. (2008). Prevention of venous thromboembolism in the geriatric patient. *Cardiology Clinics, 26*(2), 221–234.

Centers for Disease Control. (2010). Adult Obesity Facts: Obesity is common, serious and costly. Retrieved from http://www.cdc.gov/obesity/data/adult.html

Chang, A. K. (2008). Thoracic outlet syndrome. Retrieved from http://www.emedicine.com/emerg/TOPIC578.HTM/

Christman, S. K. (2009). Care of patients with peripheral vascular disease. In D. K. Moser & B. Riegel (Eds.), *Cardiac nursing: A companion to Braunwald's heart disease.* St. Louis: Saunders Elsevier.

Gardner, A. W., & Afaq, A. (2008). Management of lower extremity peripheral arterial disease. *Journal of Cardiopulmonary Rehabilitation and Prevention, 28*(6), 349–357.

Geerts, W. (2009). Prevention of venous thromboembolism: A key patient safety priority. *Journal of Thrombosis and Haemostasis, 7*(Suppl.1), 1–8.

Heidenreich, P. A., Trogdon, J. G., Khavjou, O. A., Butler, J., Dracup, K., Ezekowitz, M. D., et al. (2011). Forecasting the future of cardiovascular disease in the United States: A policy statement from the American Heart Association. *Circulation,123.*

Hilleren-Listerud, A. E. (2009). Graduated compression stocking and intermittent compression device length selection. *Clinical Nurse Specialist, 23*(1), 21–24.

Institute for Clinical Systems Improvement (ICSI). (2010). Venous thromboembolism prophlaxis for the medically ill patient. (6th ed.). Retrieved from http://www.icsi.org/

IOM (Institute of Medicine). (2010). *The future of nursing: Leading change, advancing health.* Washington, DC: The Academic Press.

Kee, J. L. (2010). *Laboratory and diagnostic tests* (8th ed.). Upper Saddle River, NJ: Pearson.

Leopardi, D., Hoggan, B. L., Fitridge, R. A., Woodruff, P. W. H., & Maddern, G. J. (2009). Systematic review of treatments for varicose veins. *Annals of Vascular Surgery, 23*(2), 264–276.

McCaffrey, R., & Blum, C. (2009). Venothrombotic events: Evidence-based risk assessment, prophylaxis, diagnosis, and treatment. *Journal for Nurse Practitioners, 5*(5), 325–333.

McCulloch, B. J. (2010). Renal artery interventions. In *Invasive cardiology: A manual for cath lab personnel.* Sudbury, MA: Jones & Bartlett Learning.

McDermott, M. M., Ades, P., Guralnik, J. M., Dyer, A., Ferrucci, L., Liu, K., et al. (2009). Treadmill exercise and resistance training in patients with peripheral arterial disease with and without intermittent claudication: A randomized controlled trial. *Journal of the American Medical Association, 301*(2): 165–174.

Moser, D. K., & Riegel, B. (2008). *Cardiac nursing: A companion to Braunwald's heart disease.* St. Louis: Saunders Elsevier.

Muir, R. L. (2009). Peripheral arterial disease: Pathophysiology, risk factors, diagnosis, treatment, and prevention. *Journal of Vascular Nursing, 27*(2), 26–30.

National Heart Lung and Blood Institute (NHLBI). (2011). The Seventh Report of the Joint National Committee on Prevention, Detection, Evaluation, and Treatment of High Blood Pressure (JNC 7). Retrieved from http://www.nhlbi.nih.gov/guidelines/hypertension/index.htm

Ogedegbe, G., Tobin, J. N., Fernandez, S., Gerwin, W., Diaz-Gloster, M., Cassells, A. N., et al. (2009). Counseling African Americans to Control Hypertension (CAATCH) trial: A multi-level intervention to improve blood pressure control in hypertensive Blacks. *Circulation: Cardiovascular Quality and Outcomes, 2,* 249–256.

Porth, C. M., & Matfin, G. (Eds.). (2009). *Pathophysiology: Concepts of altered health states* (8th ed.). Philadelphia: Wolters Kluwer/Lippincott Williams & Wilkins.

Rockson, S. G. (2008). Diagnosis and management of lympathic vascular disease. *Journal of the American College of Cardiology, 52,* 799–806.

Rooke, T. W., Hirsch, A. T., Misra, S., Sidawy, A. N., Beckman, J. A., Findeiss, L. K., et al. (2011). ACCF/AHA focused update of the guideline for the management of patients with peripheral artery disease (updating the 2005 guideline): A report of the American College of Cardiology Foundation/American Heart Association Task Force on Practice Guidelines. *Journal of the American College of Cardiology, 58*(19), 2020–2045.

Saigal, R., Kansal, A., Mittal, M., Singh, Y., & Ram, H. (2010). Raynaud's phenomenon. *Journal of the Association of Physicians of India, 58,* 309–313.

Sakamoto, S., Yokoyama, N., Tamori, Y., Akutsu, K., Hashimoto, H., & Takeshita, S. (2009). Patients With Peripheral Artery Disease Who Complete 12-Week Supervised Exercise Training Program Show Reduced Cardiovascular Mortality and Morbidity. *Circulation Journal; 73,* 167–173.

Stevens, S. M., & Douketis, J. D. (2010). Deep vein thrombosis prophylaxis in hospitalized medical patients: Current recommendations, general rates of implementation, and initiatives for improvement. *Clinics in Chest Medicine, 31*(4), 675–689.

Wilkinson, J. M., & Ahearn, N. R. (2009). *Prentice Hall nursing diagnosis handbook* (9th ed.). Upper Saddle River, NJ: Prentice Hall.

Winslow, E. H., & Brosz, D. L. (2008). Graduated compression stockings in hospitalized postoperative patients: Correctness of usage and size. *American Journal of Nursing,108*(9) 40–50.

Worel, J. N. (2009). Venous thromboembolism: What is preventing achievement of performance measures and consensus guidelines? *Journal of Cardiovascular Nursing, 24*(6), S14–S19.

Yung, L. M., Laher, I., Yao, X., Chen, Z. Y., Huang, Y., & Leung, F. P. (2009). Exercise, vascular wall and cardiovascular diseases: an update (part 2). *Sports Medicine: 39*(1), 45–63.

UNIT 8

Nursing Management of Patients with Gastrointestinal, Renal, and Urinary Disorders

Content in Unit 8 that addresses the **Institute of Medicine (IOM)** competencies, **Nursing Core Competencies (NCC)**, the **Quality and Safety Education for Nurses (QSEN)** competencies, and **Concepts** for concept-based learning is listed below.

Competencies	Feature or Text	Location
IOM, QSEN, NCC Providing patient-centered care	Cultural Considerations: Using Ginger for Nausea, page 1101	Chapter 36
	Nursing Process: Patient Care Plan for GI Disorders, pages 1116, 1124, 1132, 1147, 1156	Chapter 37
	Cultural Considerations Related to Colon Cancer, page 1153	Chapter 37
	Nursing Process: Patient Care Plan for Hepatic Disorders, pages 1171, 1181, 1188, 1193	Chapter 38
	Cultural Considerations in Patients with Cholelithiasis, page 1183	Chapter 38
	Nursing Process: Patient Care Plan for Chronic Renal Failure/Chronic Kidney Disease, page 1230	Chapter 39
IOM, QSEN, NCC Working in teams	Collaborative Management, pages 1116, 1123, 1129, 1136, 1155	Chapter 37
	Collaborative Management, pages 1169, 1179, 1186, 1192	Chapter 38
	Collaborative Management, page 1234	Chapter 39
IOM, QSEN, NCC Employing evidence-based practice	Evidence-Based Practice: Colon Cancer: Keys to Survival, page 1153	Chapter 37
	Evidence-Based Practice: Medications Used in Palliative Care of Patients with Liver Failure, page 1183	Chapter 38
	Evidence-Based Practice: Hemodialysis, page 1233	Chapter 39
IOM NCC Applying quality and safety improvement	Safety Alerts, pages 1102, 1104, 1107, 1108	Chapter 36
	Safety Alerts, pages 1113, 1128	Chapter 37
	Safety Alerts, pages 1164, 1165, 1178	Chapter 38
	Safety Alerts, pages 1227, 1229, 1232, 1235	Chapter 39
NCC Educating patients	Patient Teaching & Discharge Priorities for GERD, page 1122	Chapter 37
	Patient Teaching & Discharge Priorities for Cirrhosis, page 1182	Chapter 38
	Patient Teaching & Discharge Priorities, pages 1202, 1207, 1212, 1214, 1215, 1217	Chapter 39
Concepts covered in Unit 8 include:	Fluid and electrolyte balance Oxygenation Ingestion Elimination Infection	Inflammation Metabolism

Nursing Assessment of the Patient with Gastrointestinal, Renal, and Urinary Disorders

36 CHAPTER

Pamela Stetina
Cheryl Wraa

Outcome-Based Learning Objectives

After studying this chapter, the learner will be able to:

1. Illustrate anatomy and physiology of the gastrointestinal and urinary systems as related to patient assessment.
2. Compare and contrast the significant subjective and objective data that pertain to the gastrointestinal and urinary systems.
3. Apply the four components of the physical exam to a patient with gastrointestinal or urinary system issues.
4. Differentiate abnormal findings from normal findings of the physical assessment of the gastrointestinal and urinary systems.
5. Relate diagnostic and laboratory testing to the gastrointestinal and urinary systems.

KEY TERMS

anal canal p.1099
barium enema p.1103
colon p.1099
colonoscopy p.1103
endoscopic retrograde cholangiopancreatography (ERCP) p.1103
esophagus p.1097
flexible sigmoidoscopy p.1103
gastroparesis p.1103
iliopsoas p.1107
immunoglobulin A p.1098
intussusception p.1101
peristalsis p.1098
pyloric stenosis p.1101
rectum p.1099
renal calculi p.1105
tympany p.1106
ventral hernia p.1105

ABDOMINAL PAIN is a frequently presenting medical complaint. The symptoms may represent something very benign or something extremely serious and even life threatening. For example, abdominal pain can be caused by gastroenteritis or by an aortic aneurysm. The two diagnoses can be differentiated by a thorough history and physical examination. To perform a proper history and physical examination, the nurse must have a thorough understanding of the anatomy and physiology of the gastrointestinal (Figure 36–1◆) and urinary systems. The nurse will then be able to determine what is occurring with the patient.

Anatomy and Physiology

To perform a thorough assessment of the gastrointestinal and urinary system, the nurse must understand the anatomy and physiology of each system. This knowledge will assist the nurse in thinking critically and assimilating all data gathered during the assessment.

Gastrointestinal System

The primary functions of the gastrointestinal (GI) system are to transport and deliver nutrition and water and to support the function of cells throughout the body. The oral cavity or mouth is at the beginning of the GI tract. This is where food is taken in and the process of digestion starts. The act of chewing (mastication) and mixing with saliva starts the breakdown of the food and makes it a size acceptable for passage through the **esophagus,** a muscular tube that carries swallowed foods and liquids from the pharynx to the stomach.

There are three pairs of major salivary glands: the parotid, sublingual, and submandibular glands. These glands have several roles in the process of digestion. First, they secrete amylase, which begins the process of carbohydrate digestion. Next, they add an aqueous component to the food bolus, making it easier to swallow. Finally, they lubricate the mouth, facilitating the movement of the lips and tongue during swallowing. This aqueous environment assists in the distribution of the

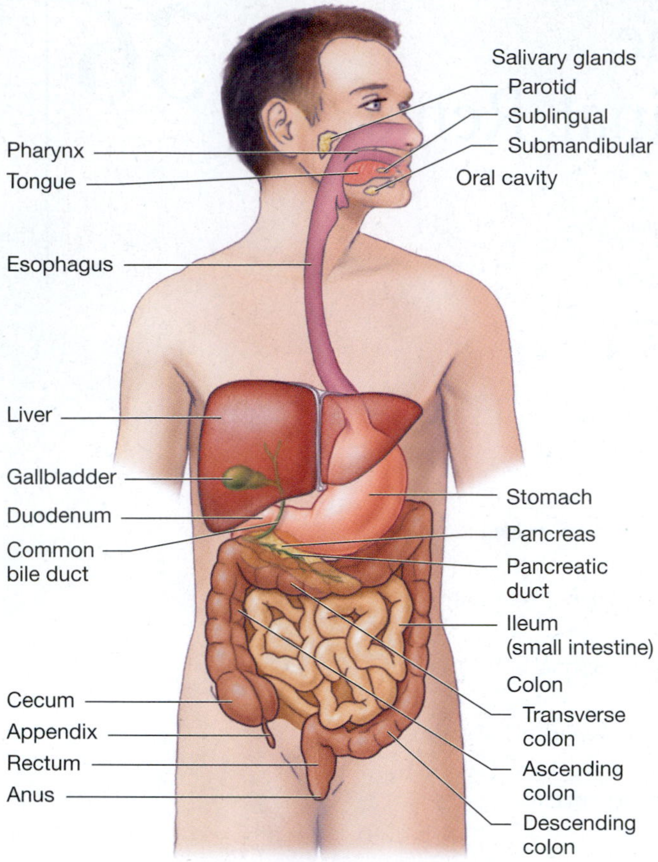

FIGURE 36–1 ◆ Organs of the gastrointestinal (GI) system.

food across the taste buds that are dispersed across the tongue, making the food palatable and therefore more pleasing to eat. Without these taste buds, food would have no taste and would be difficult to eat. An additional property of saliva is the reduction of bacteria in the oral cavity. Saliva contains large amounts of ions, such as chloride, bicarbonate, potassium, thiocyanate, hydrogen, and **immunoglobulin A,** an antibody that is necessary for destroying oral bacteria (Urden, Stacy, & Lough, 2010).

The act of swallowing is a complex process that includes both voluntary and involuntary processes. Voluntary processes involve using the teeth to masticate the food and using the tongue to move the food bolus backward toward the pharynx. Simultaneously, involuntary processes cause the soft palate to lift and cover the nasal passage while the epiglottis closes the opening to the larynx, preventing aspiration of food. A change in any of these intricate movements can cause problems with the first step of digestion.

The food bolus then moves through the esophagus, passing through the diaphragmatic hiatus into the abdominal cavity. There are two esophageal sphincters: the upper esophageal (pharyngoesophageal) sphincter, which is created by the cricopharyngeus muscle, and the lower esophageal (cardioesophageal) sphincter. The upper esophageal sphincter inhibits air from entering the esophagus during respiration, and the lower esophageal sphincter is an area at the distal end of the esophagus that controls the food entering the stomach and prevents reflux of gastric contents. After swallowing, the esophageal sphincter in the upper portion closes, which increases the normal pressure within the esophagus. This phenomenon, along with peristalsis, moves the food bolus down to the stomach. **Peristalsis** is a progressive wavelike movement that occurs involuntarily in hollow tubes of the body. It is caused by the coordinated contraction of the circular and longitudinal muscle fibers making up the musculature of the esophagus. The pressure changes in the esophagus prevent reflux of the food bolus into the pharynx as well as gastric contents from entering the lower portion of the esophagus. Gastroesophageal reflux disease (GERD) is a common condition in which acid from the stomach flows back into the esophagus, causing discomfort and, in some cases, damage to the esophageal lining. Commonly called "heartburn," it is a frequent patient complaint. Once the bolus has passed through the esophagus, the pressures return to normal. Gastroesophageal reflux disease is discussed in detail in Chapter 37.

The vagus nerve provides the parasympathetic innervation of the pharynx and the esophagus. Pharyngeal branches of the vagus nerve innervate the constrictor muscles of the pharynx with a small contribution by cranial nerves IX and XI. The upper esophageal sphincter and the upper portion of the esophagus are innervated by branches of the recurrent laryngeal nerves, which originate from the vagus nerve. Patients with injury to these nerves will have functional problems with their vocal cords as well as problems with the upper esophageal sphincter and motility of the esophagus, one of the causes of dysphasia (speech impairment resulting from a brain lesion or neurodevelopmental disorder). Problems with the upper esophageal sphincter can also cause an increased risk of aspiration and resulting respiratory complications.

The food bolus passes from the esophagus into the stomach. The stomach is a muscular container where food is released into the intestine at a controlled rate. The stomach starts with the lower esophageal sphincter and ends with the pylorus. In between these two structures, the stomach can be divided into four portions: the cardia, the fundus, the body, and the antrum (Figure 36–2◆). The cardia, the upper orifice of the stomach, connects with the esophagus. The fundus and body are the next portions of the stomach and lead to the antrum, which is a nearly closed cavity or chamber.

The stomach muscle wall has four layers: the serous outermost layer, a muscular layer, a submucosal layer, and an inner mucosal layer. The innermost layer contains multiple folds called rugae, which allow the stomach to increase as it fills. The stomach is innervated by the vagus nerve.

Several secretions occur within the stomach. For example, mucus is secreted to protect the surface of the stomach from the very acidic gastric juices. Parietal cells secrete hydrochloric acid (HCl) and intrinsic

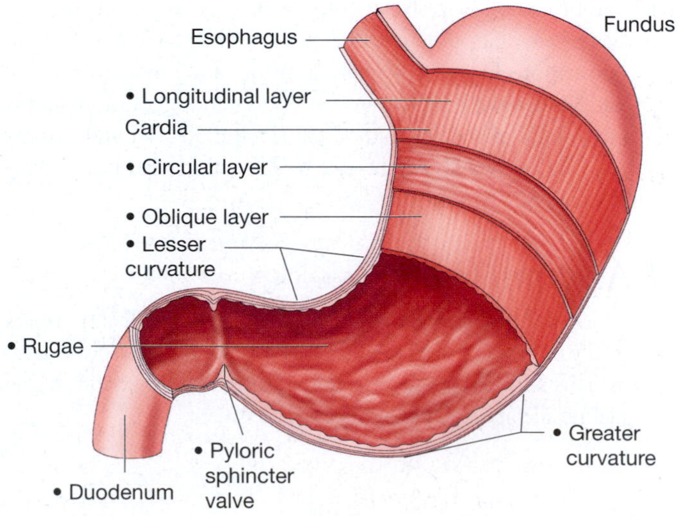

FIGURE 36–2 ◆ The stomach.

factor, chief cells secrete pepsinogen, and G cells secrete gastrin. Hydrochloric acid is very acidic, which helps with protein digestion as well as to decrease bacterial growth in the stomach. Intrinsic factor facilitates vitamin B_{12} absorption. Pepsinogen is an enzyme that converts to pepsin, a secretion that helps to digest proteins. Gastrin stimulates the secretion of HCl from the parietal cells. Finally, the gastric juices include fluids and electrolytes, including sodium and potassium.

The muscular function of the stomach mixes food with gastric juices into chyme. Chyme is secreted through the pylorus into the small intestine, where digestion and absorption occur.

The small intestine is approximately 22 to 23 feet (6.7 to 7 meters) long, but only about 1.3 to 1.5 inches (3.5 to 4 cm) in diameter. The surface of the small intestine is covered with small finger-like projections called villi. These, in turn, are covered with more projections called microvilli. By creating a larger surface area and a greater ability for absorption of nutrients before passing into the large intestine, the villi and microvilli enhance the digestion and absorption of nutrients, vitamins, electrolytes, and water. The small intestine is divided into three main sections: the duodenum, the jejunum, and the ileum.

The first section, called the duodenum, is about 12 inches (30 cm) long and is found almost entirely in the retroperitoneal space, the area behind the peritoneum and outside the kidney. The primary purpose of this portion of the gastrointestinal tract is to regulate digestion and the absorption of the luminal contents. The initial part of the duodenum receives the acidic chyme from the stomach, making this portion at risk for duodenal ulcers although the duodenum does secrete mucus to protect the duodenum. To assist digestion, the pancreas secretes approximately 500 milliliters of fluid per day (Fisher, Andersen, Bell, Saluja, & Bruinicardi, 2010). The pancreatic juice is secreted from acinic and duct cells. The acinic cells secrete amylase, proteases (such as trypsin), and lipases, which are responsible for the breakdown of carbohydrates, fats, and proteins. The duct cells secrete the water and electrolytes in the pancreatic juice. These cells keep a constant balance between the amount of bicarbonate/chloride and sodium/potassium that is secreted. The secretion of the pancreatic juice is the exocrine function of the pancreas. The endocrine function, although vital, is not discussed in this chapter; it is discussed in Chapter 45.

The pancreatic duct carries the pancreatic juice, joins with the bile duct, and enters the duodenum, where the contents assist the digestive process. The bile duct originates from the gallbladder, a muscular sac lying beneath and adjacent to the liver (Figure 36–3◆). A simplistic way of thinking of the gallbladder is as a conduit and storage receptacle for bile produced by the liver. The bile enters from the liver via the cystic duct and exits via the common bile duct, which then empties into the duodenum. Bile makes the fat molecules water soluble so the body may better utilize them.

The second and third portions of the small bowel are called the jejunum and the ileum. These portions of the small bowel lie in the peritoneum but are tethered to the retroperitoneum. The jejunum is 7 to 9 feet (2 to 3 meters) long; the ileum is about 10 to 12 feet (2.3 to 6 meters) long. The ileum is usually narrower than the duodenum or jejunum. Digestion and absorption are completed in the jejunum and ileum.

The large intestine starts at the ileocecal valve and ends at the anus; it is about 4 to 5 feet (1.2 to 1.5 meters) long and 2 inches (5 cm) in diameter. There are three anatomic and functional sections: the **colon** (the large intestine from the end of the ileum to the anal canal that surrounds the anus), the **rectum** (the lower part of the large intestine between the sigmoid colon and the anal canal), and the **anal canal** (the last part of the large intestine situated between the rectum and the anus). The colon

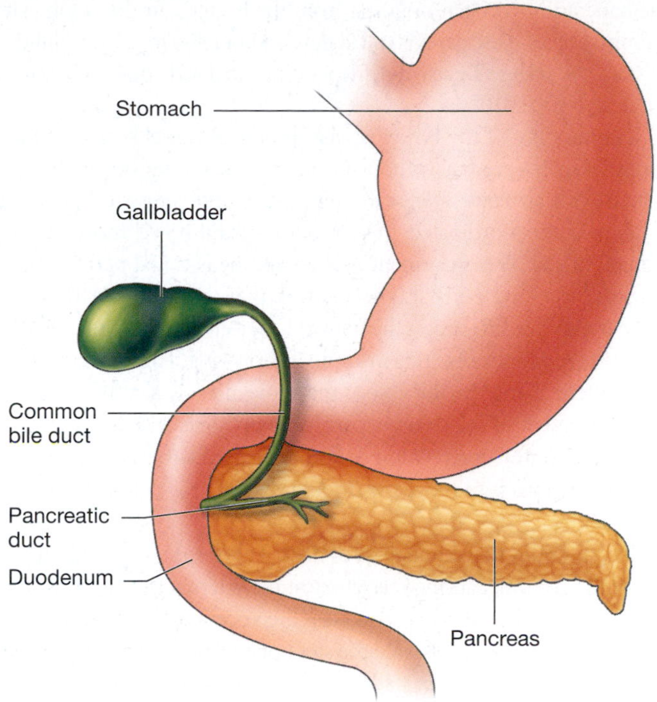

FIGURE 36–3 ◆ The pancreas and gallbladder.

and rectum have five layers: the mucosa, submucosa, inner circular muscle, outer longitudinal muscle, and serosa (Dunn & Rothenberger, 2010). The distal rectum also has inner smooth muscles, which join together to form the internal anal sphincter. The colon is also divided into sections, including the ascending, transverse, descending, and sigmoid colon. The ascending colon, on the right side of the abdomen, is fixed to the retroperitoneum. The cecum (part of the ascending colon at the connection with the small intestine) has the widest diameter and the thinnest muscle wall (Dunn & Rothenberger, 2010). The appendix is a projection off of the cecum. The transverse colon is freer but is attached by the omentum. The descending colon is the portion on the left of the abdomen. The sigmoid colon is the narrowest and most mobile portion of the colon (Dunn & Rothenberger, 2010). The rectum is about 8 inches (20.3 cm) long and ends at the anal canal. The anal canal is about 1 to 2 inches (2.5 to 5 cm) in length and ends at the internal and external sphincter.

The functions of the colon are primarily water absorption and electrolyte balance. This is why patients with diarrhea can have such imbalances in electrolytes; when diarrhea is present, the stool passes quickly through the colon, so there isn't time for the normal functions to take place. Normally, a large amount of water can be absorbed through the colon, up to 5,000 milliliters per day (Dunn & Rothenberger, 2010). Sodium, potassium, and chloride are transported along with this water. Ammonia is produced when there is bacterial degradation of protein and urea (Dunn & Rothenberger, 2010). This ammonia is absorbed and transported to the liver, where it is metabolized.

Stool is composed of approximately 30% bacteria, the most prominent being *Escherichia coli*, which is known to cause grave illness when it contaminates food sources (Dunn & Rothenberger, 2010). Intestinal gas is primarily from swallowed air, but also is produced by intraluminal production and diffusion of blood. Nitrogen and oxygen are derived from the swallowing of air, carbon dioxide comes from the breakdown of triglycerides and from the bicarbonate and hydrogen ions, and methane and hydrogen originate from the bacteria in the colon. The culmination of these gases is called flatus. About 400 to 1,200 milliliters of flatus is released each day, depending on food intake (Dunn & Rothenberger, 2010).

The motility of the bowel is what produces bowel sounds. Bowel sounds can be present without having a functioning bowel. For instance, with an ileus, there can be bowel sounds present, but as the motility is not coordinated, there is not resultant bowel movement or passing of gas. The movement of the intestine is called *peristalsis*. In the small intestine, peristalsis occurs with the contraction of the longitudinal muscles; this causes the bowel to shorten and the inner circular muscles to contract, resulting in luminal narrowing. This process moves the content along. In the colon, the movement is slightly different. The movement of the colon occurs more in bursts with low and high amplitude contractions (Dunn & Rothenberger, 2010). The purpose of the contractions is to move the stool mass along the colon to eventual elimination.

Defecation is the elimination of stool. This occurs with the stretching of the rectum, causing relaxation of the internal sphincter as stool enters the rectal canal. Defecation can then occur as the rectum shortens and peristaltic waves force the stool out of the rectum. A problem with any of these steps can lead to constipation or incontinence.

Other organs that are involved in the process of digestion are the liver, pancreas, and gallbladder. Both the liver and the pancreas are multifunctional. The liver is one of the largest organs and the largest gland. The liver has numerous functions; however, only key functions will be discussed here. One important function is the liver's role in metabolism of carbohydrates, fats, and proteins as well as storage and synthesis of vitamins. The production of bile also aids in digestion of fat. In addition, the liver has a role in the detoxification of drugs, hormones, and other damaging substances. The liver metabolizes bilirubin, which is a by-product of the breakdown of hemoglobin. Finally, the liver synthesizes clotting factors and plasma proteins (Urden et al., 2010). The gallbladder was discussed earlier as a storage sac for bile. The pancreas has both endocrine and exocrine functions. The exocrine functions were discussed earlier. Although it is not within the scope of this chapter to discuss all the endocrine functions of the pancreas, an understanding of them is important. They will be discussed in Chapter 45.

Related Structures

When the nurse examines the patient's abdomen, it is important to have knowledge of all structures within the abdomen, even those that are not related to the gastrointestinal system. The abdomen is the only major cavity of the body not encased in bony structures. Although the lower ribs lend some support to the posterior cavity, the anterior cavity receives its structure from the muscle wall. The abdominal wall muscles consist of the rectus abdominis, the internal and external obliques, and the transverse abdominis (Figure 36–4◆). These muscles support the abdomen, allow for movement, and, when contracted, increase the intra-abdominal pressure.

The major artery to be aware of and examine in doing an abdominal assessment is the aorta. This is the major artery descending from the heart through the diaphragm, through the abdominal cavity, and bifurcating at the lower abdomen into the right and left iliac arteries. The aorta is discussed more thoroughly in Chapter 35.

The spleen is found in the left upper quadrant of the abdomen and is protected by the lower left ribs. It is directly inferior to the diaphragm. The primary purpose of the spleen is to filter blood, destroy aged red blood cells, and return their by-products to the liver. Because of its vascular nature, when the spleen suffers trauma, the injury can be life threatening.

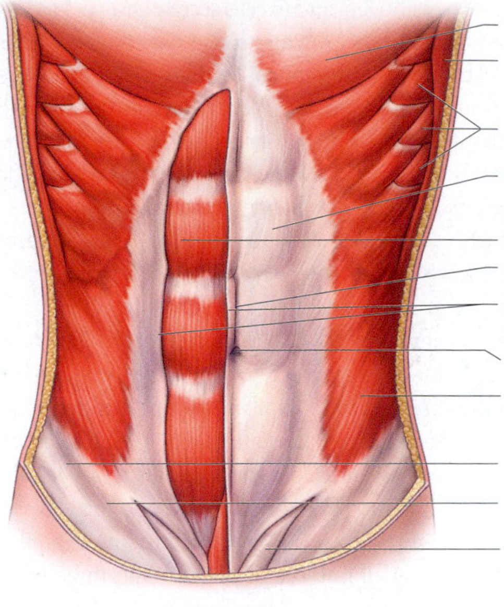

FIGURE 36–4 ◆ Abdominal muscles.

Urinary System

The organs of the urinary system lie within the abdomen. The kidneys and bladder lie within the space called the retroperitoneum. This is a space defined by the posterior peritoneum and the posterior body wall. Chart 36–1 lists the organs found in the peritoneal/retroperitoneal spaces.

The kidney is a complex organ, and its function is discussed in detail in Chapter 39. A pair of kidneys is located in the retroperitoneum, one on each side of the vertebral column. The right kidney is slightly lower than the left, owing to the location of the liver. The kidneys are protected by the rib cage. They are also protected by a tough fibrous capsule, cushioned by perirenal fat, and supported by the renal fascia. The kidney is divided into an inner medulla, containing renal pyramids, and

CHART 36–1 Organs in the Peritoneal and Retroperitoneal Spaces

Peritoneal Cavity	Anterior Retroperitoneal Space	Posterior Retroperitoneal Space
Omentum	Pancreas	Kidneys
Liver	Duodenum	Ureters
Stomach	Ascending colon	Adrenal glands
Gallbladder	Descending colon	
Spleen		
Jejunum		
Ileum		
Transverse and sigmoid colon		
Cecum		
Appendix		

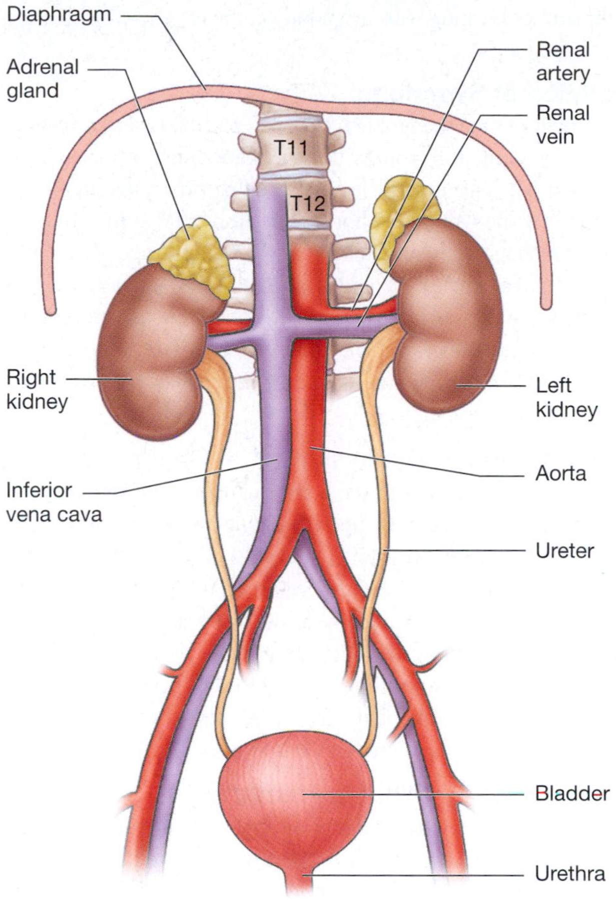

FIGURE 36–5 ◆ The renal system.

an outer cortex, containing glomeruli and collecting ducts (Urden et al., 2010). The kidney's functional unit is the nephron. The kidneys' primary roles are to maintain fluid and electrolyte balance, help to achieve acid–base balance, and remove metabolic wastes. The renal system also has an important role in control of blood pressure, bone metabolism, and red blood cell synthesis (Figure 36–5◆). Understanding these roles is crucial to assessing kidney function in patients.

The urinary system also includes a drainage system: the ureters, bladder, and urethra. As urine is formed in the kidneys, it flows through the ureters (small tubes) by peristalsis into the bladder. The peristaltic action helps prevent reflux of the urine back into the kidneys. The bladder, which is also muscular, holds the urine and has a capacity of 280 to 500 milliliters (Urden et al., 2010). When the bladder is stretched, the parasympathetic nervous system signals the smooth muscle of the bladder to contract and expel the urine through the urethra. When urine is expelled, the voluntarily controlled external sphincter and the autonomically controlled internal sphincter must open. The length of the urethra is 3 to 5 centimeters in women and approximately 20 centimeters in men.

The reproductive organs are also found in the abdomen, specifically the pelvic region, in both sexes. This system will be examined in Chapter 40.

History

A thorough history will help the nurse identify gastrointestinal and urinary symptoms as well as current or potential problems that may affect system function. Information learned from a thorough history and physical exam could help to prevent undesirable responses to current therapies and treatment plans. The essential assessment data included in the gastrointestinal and urinary history are outlined next.

Weblink: Ginger

Biographic and Demographic Data

Biographic and demographic data can provide a myriad of information to assist the nurse in narrowing the questions, thinking of potential causes of the problem, and formulating how to pose questions and educational plans to meet the patient's needs.

Biographical data should include age, gender, culture, and educational background. Age and gender are important in narrowing the potential causes of the patient's initial complaint. For instance, **intussusception,** the slipping of one part of an intestine into another part just below it, is a common cause of intestinal obstruction in children 2 years of age and younger but is not seen in adults (Hackam, Grikscheit, Wang, Newman, & Ford, 2010). The same is true of **pyloric stenosis,** narrowing of the pyloric orifice, which is a cause of regurgitation and poor feeding in infants, generally within the first month, but would not be the cause of similar complaints in adults. If pyloric stenosis does occur in adults, it frequently results from peptic ulcer disease, malignant compression of the gastric outlet, or pneumatosis intestinalis (gas in the bowel wall). Alternatively, if an infant were having left lower quadrant abdominal pain, the nurse would not be thinking about diverticulitis, which would be a common cause in adults, especially in people older than age 50, but not in children or adolescents (Dunn & Rothenberger, 2010).

The nurse may also glean important information from demographic data. If a patient lives in an agricultural area or has well water as a source of drinking water, *Giardia* and *Cryptosporidium* infections need to be considered in the case of ongoing diarrhea and abdominal cramping. However, this might not be the common differential diagnosis for a person who lives in a high-rise apartment in a city.

Cultural Considerations

Cultural background is important in understanding many aspects of communication and care because it may greatly influence the patient's perception of the complaint, whom to speak with in the family, and what interventions the patient may have sought on her own. Certain diseases may be more prevalent in some cultures. For example, in comparison to other ethnic groups, Japanese people have a higher rate of colitis but a lower rate of ulcers in North America (Andrews, 2008). Additionally, if the patient has recently traveled to her country of origin, this may provide a clue as to other causes not commonly seen. For example, certain types of parasites may be more prevalent in other countries than in the United States. The Cultural Considerations box highlights the issues that may arise with one culture's use of ginger for nausea.

CULTURAL CONSIDERATIONS Using Ginger for Nausea

It is important to consider the patient's cultural background and be sensitive to other therapies the patient might have relied on to decrease symptoms. Some Chinese patients may use ginger for nausea or morning sickness (Andrews, 2008). However, ginger may have gastrointestinal side effects such as heartburn and diarrhea, as well as increase bleeding times (U.S. National Library of Medicine, 2010). This could be catastrophic if the cause of the patient's initial complaint was an ulcer and the patient is at greater risk for internal bleeding.

Chief Complaint

It is important to allow the patient to express his concerns and explain the problem in his own words. Interruptions should be kept to a minimum, but the nurse should ask clarifying questions as needed. In addition, the nurse should keep an open mind, because sometimes information that is initially thought of as trivial can be the answer to the problem. For example, a patient with chest pain had a thorough cardiac work-up without any indication of the source of the chest pain. The condition remained troublesome, and at a later visit the patient mentioned an intake of a half gallon of ice cream on a daily basis. Although the symptoms are not common to lactose intolerance, the chest pain symptoms were resolved after a trial of stopping the ice cream for 2 weeks. This would not have been recognized if the interviewer had not listened to what the patient was saying and kept an open mind.

Safety Alert *Patient complaints of chest pain should be taken seriously and followed up. A thorough history and physical will help to determine whether the pain is cardiac or gastrointestinal in nature.*

Taking a history is a very important patient encounter. This process is a time when the nurse establishes a relationship with the patient. Therefore, it is vital for the nurse to develop good interpersonal skills and information-gathering skills early in nursing practice. Because there are core questions in taking a history, it is best to develop a systematic approach that fits one's personal style and comfort level. As a beginner, the nurse should try different methods she has observed others using. As the nurse becomes an expert, her individual style will emerge, allowing her to gather all important information and establish a relationship with the patient. Characteristics, duration, exacerbation or diminishment of symptoms, and what is wrong or feared by the patient define the chief complaint.

Present Symptoms

Asking the question "Tell me how your symptoms started" is an appropriate way for a nurse to start an interview. This open-ended question allows the patient to tell the nurse the history of the complaint. The nurse should allow the patient time to answer such questions while the nurse gives nonverbal feedback such as nodding. This can be followed by more clarifying questions, such as the following:

Are there any events that appear to make the symptoms return?

What has changed since the onset of your symptoms?

Does the pain get worse after you eat?

Has the character or intensity of the pain changed over time?

Can you do something that makes the diarrhea (or nausea or vomiting) start or go away?

These types of clarifying questions help the nurse hone in on the problem and further clarify the complaint. If pain is present, the nurse should ask the patient to describe it.

When interviewing adults, the nurse should have a number of adjectives in his repertoire to assist the patient. *Stabbing, crushing, dull, sharp, radiating, knifelike,* and *burning* are a few of the adjectives that can assist the patient in giving a better description of the symptoms. The nurse should listen carefully to the words the patient uses in characterizing the symptoms, which can lead to further clues. For example, a complaint of burning or gnawing pain can be associated with ulcers emanating from the duodenum or the stomach. However, these ulcers can be differentiated by the timing and the cause of the symptoms. For example, duodenal ulcers are generally postprandial and awaken the subject at night, whereas the pain of the gastric ulcer is precipitated by food. A complaint of burning with urination can be associated with a urinary tract infection.

Duration of Symptoms

The length of time the problem has been present is very revealing. Has the person waited 4 months to have something evaluated? Possibly there was a change in the characteristic that prompted the sudden attention. Are the symptoms short in duration but continue to return? Is something happening simultaneously with the return of the symptoms? For example, a female patient may have had mild symptoms of stress incontinence, such as urine leaking when coughing or sneezing, for some time but would just wear a panty liner. Now she is experiencing incontinence when she has the urge to void, so the problem has worsened and she is now seeking care.

Exacerbation or Diminishment of Symptoms

Many times a patient will try home remedies before presenting for evaluation of a problem. Be open to asking about alternative therapies such as acupuncture or herbal remedies. Did anything the patient tried make the symptoms better or worse? Why did the patient think a certain action would work? The answer to this question can lead into what the patient thinks is wrong. For instance, if the patient thinks that his obstructive symptoms were caused by constipation alone, the use of laxatives not only could be ineffective but also could make the symptoms worse by causing increased peristalsis.

What Is Wrong? What Is Feared?

This leads to a very important and sometimes missed area of exploration. What does the patient think is wrong with him? Many times, the patient will have a very good idea of what might be the cause of the problem without really knowing it. Other times, the possibility of exploring the patient's fears of what might be the cause allows the nurse the opportunity to allay the patient's anxieties. Does the patient's culture lead the patient to believe certain things? For example, if a patient of a certain culture believes that there are psychosocial or folk illnesses that have caused or contributed to an illness (Andrews, 2008), it might be difficult for the patient of this culture to believe that the illness (e.g., diarrhea) has a purely physical cause (such as poorly prepared foods).

Is any weight loss due to a fear of eating? Is the person eating frequently in order to make the symptoms subside? Weight loss can be associated with gastric ulcers because the patient is trying to avoid the pain by not eating. On the other hand, patients suffering from duodenal ulcers might gain weight as they are eating more frequently to avoid the symptoms. Does the patient notice a change in skin color or the color of the urine? This could be very important, as hepatitis A can lead to dark-colored urine.

By the end of this part of the interview, the nurse needs to have information regarding the following characteristics: location of symptoms, quality of the discomfort or pain, severity of the symptoms, onset and duration of the complaint, any changes to the symptoms, and what makes symptoms better or worse. If any of these questions are not answered, the nurse needs to use more focused questions. Some sample questions are listed in Chart 36–2.

Past Medical History

A patient's past medical history should always include certain elements; for example, childhood diseases, immunizations, major illnesses, hospitalizations, diagnostic procedures, surgeries, sexual history, medications, and allergies are all considered imperative in gathering data. If the

Weblink: Colonoscopy

CHART 36–2 Examples of History Questions

Location	Where does it hurt the most?
Severity	At the time it is the most painful, how would you rate the pain on a scale of 1 to 10, with 10 being the worst?
	Does the pain change as it becomes more severe?
Duration	How long does the pain last?
Quality	What does the pain feel like?
Onset	When did the pain start?
	What were the circumstances of the pain starting?
Aggravating Factors	What makes the pain worse?
Alleviating Factors	What do you do to make the pain better?
Changes	Have your symptoms changed over a period of time?
	Does your pain change from one episode to another?

patient is vague regarding the information or does not remember the name of a procedure, the nurse should assist the patient by giving the best description. For instance, a childhood illness may have required hospitalization or surgery, but the patient might not know whether she had pyloric stenosis or a bowel obstruction. A surgery for a repair of pyloric stenosis is more common in the first 6 months of life, whereas a bowel obstruction from intussusception can be seen in patients up to 2 years of age. Having knowledge regarding surgical procedures and age-related diseases can assist the nurse in helping the patient clarify her possible childhood history.

It is also important to consider where the patient was raised. Practices and availability of medical care and hospitalization will differ between industrialized nations and developing countries, and even sometimes in various places or cultures within the United States. In some circumstances, the availability of medical history might be difficult if not impossible to obtain.

Childhood Illnesses and Immunizations

A history of childhood illnesses should include any significant illnesses. For example, patients with a history of celiac disease and cystic fibrosis commonly will have experienced stooling problems and obstruction due to the bulking of the stool. A history of streptococcal infection, hypoplastic kidneys, or obstructive uropathy can lead to urinary tract or renal dysfunction as an adult.

The nurse should specifically ask about immunizations commonly given for hepatitis, hepatitis B, and hepatitis A. There is also a hepatitis D vaccine, although it is less common. A patient reporting a cholera vaccine may be less common unless there has been recent travel or the patient has been residing in another country.

Previous Illnesses and Hospitalizations

A history of major illnesses is important and may affect the chief complaint. For instance, a person whose diabetes is poorly controlled who presents with symptoms of a partial bowel obstruction may be having **gastroparesis,** a delayed emptying of food from the stomach into the small bowel. A patient with hypertension and diabetes may develop renal failure due to the vascular changes with decreased circulation to the kidneys. A history of Crohn's disease not only can be related to multiple surgeries but also signals the nurse to be aware of the potential for anal fissures and fistulas.

The nurse should ask the patient about medical problems for which the patient is currently being treated. The nurse should ask whether the patient has been given any diagnosis in the past. For example, a patient may be treated for recurrent hemorrhoids due to intermittent bright-red blood from the rectum. Chart 36–3 lists common major illnesses.

Diagnostic Procedures and Surgeries

A history of procedures is important in compiling the history of gastrointestinal and urinary diseases. Common endoscopic evaluations include **endoscopic retrograde cholangiopancreatography (ERCP),** which uses an endoscope that visualizes the pancreatic and biliary ducts with radiography following injection of a radiopaque material into the papilla of Vater; **flexible sigmoidoscopy,** in which a sigmoidoscope uses fiber optics to inspect the sigmoid colon; and **colonoscopy,** visualization of the lower gastrointestinal tract through a flexible endoscope inserted through the anus. Patients might not remember the name of the test but would probably recall what symptoms led to the test. For example, a person would not get an ERCP, which looks for gallbladder and pancreatic causes, if the chief complaint were blood in the stool.

In addition to invasive testing, radiologic testing might be utilized in a work-up of GI symptomatology. Upper GI studies as well as a **barium enema** are common radiologic tests. The upper GI series looks at the upper part of the GI tract (esophagus, stomach, and duodenum). X-rays are taken after the patient ingests barium. An upper GI study might be the test of choice in a patient complaining of reflux. The barium enema is used to obtain an x-ray of the large intestines. Radiographs are taken after the patient receives barium sulphate through an enema tube. A barium enema will assist in the evaluation of diverticular disease or possibly a tumor. For the renal system, a kidney–ureter–bladder (KUB) radiograph (a plain film that helps determine the position, size, and structure of the kidneys and urinary tract), intravenous pyelogram (IVP), renal ultrasound, computed tomography (CT), magnetic resonance imaging, and renal angiography may help with a diagnosis.

In obtaining a medical history from a patient with gastrointestinal symptoms, past surgeries play a major role. It is also important to correlate this information with the physical exam. At times, patients will forget a surgery, especially if it was many years ago. Therefore, correlating the history with scars on their abdomen is a helpful tool. When doing the abdominal examination, the nurse should confirm what operation relates to which scar. This can also trigger more information from the patient. The nurse should pay particular attention to the area around

CHART 36–3 Major Illnesses with GI Related Complaints

Celiac sprue	Diabetes	Hirschsprung's disease	Crohn's disease	HIV
Alcoholism	Hyperlipidemia	Cystic fibrosis	Cancer	Hepatitis (A, B, C)
Inflammatory bowel disease	Thyroid problems	Hypertension	Hypercholesteremia	Depressive disorders

CHART 36–4 Common Gastrointestinal Surgeries

Appendectomy	Removal of the appendix
Cholecystectomy	Removal of the gallbladder
Choledochojejunostomy	Opening between the common bile duct and the jejunum
Colostomy	Opening of the colon through the abdominal wall
Gastrectomy	Removal of part or all of the stomach
Ileostomy	Opening of the ileum through the abdominal wall
Pyloroplasty	Repair of the pylorus or to increase the opening
Vagotomy	Resection of the branch of the vagus nerve

the umbilicus, as laparoscopic scars are small and can be very faint. Chart 36–4 lists common gastrointestinal surgeries.

Sexual History

A person's sexual practices can have an effect on certain gastrointestinal and urinary complaints. Therefore, it is important for the nurse to become comfortable with asking patients not only about their sexual activity but also about their individual practices. The more self-conscious and uncomfortable the nurse is in asking these questions, the more reluctant the patient will be to self-disclose.

Anal intercourse can be related to disease of the anus and the rectum. Rectal cancer from human papillomavirus is important to identify and treat early. It is also possible to get other sexually transmitted infections, such as gonorrhea, in the rectum. If the question is never asked, the problem will be overlooked, with potential detrimental results for the patient. If a woman has frequent cystitis, it is important for the nurse to ask and teach her that urinating shortly after intercourse is important to flush any bacteria that might have entered the urethra.

Medications

The medication history should include what is prescribed, what is taken over the counter, and what is given to the patient by friends or family. Over-the-counter antacid is a commonly overused medication. What type and how often the medication is taken may also be important. The nurse should remember to include questions about laxatives and enemas, inquiring how frequently patients are using them. A frequent use of either laxatives or enemas can cause a decrease in bowel tone, thus causing an increase in constipation which leads to continued use of these treatments.

A history of frequent use of aspirin or nonsteroidal anti-inflammatory drugs (NSAIDs) is also significant. The nurse should make sure to ask about both. Some patients may be taking either of these frequently and then following it with an antacid to make the stomach pains subside so they can treat the discomfort from arthritis. NSAIDs, antihypertensive drugs that block angiotensin, and aminoglycoside antibiotics can cause an acute or chronic decline in kidney function.

Safety Alert *Acetaminophen may be used for pain and can be toxic to the liver if not used as directed.*

The nurse should remember to ask about the use of herbal remedies or supplements. Some of the medications can be toxic to the liver or have other adverse effects not known to the patient. If the medication is a combination of medicines, it is sometimes difficult to verify exactly what the patient is taking, especially if the supplement is a combination of different types of herbs. At times, further research is warranted to find all the different ingredients in a powder or tincture.

Allergies

A history of allergies should include not only the offending agent but also the allergic symptom it produces. Many patients mistake nausea for an allergic reaction when it is only a side effect. Any food or environmental allergies should also be explored. Food allergies are especially important when examining a patient for gastrointestinal symptoms. The nurse should ask whether there is a certain food that is avoided due to undesirable effects and what those undesirable effects are.

Family History

A thorough family history is important and should include a relevant health history of the patient's siblings, parents, and grandparents. However, some patients will include a medical history of a relative who is not related by blood. In other words, a patient may provide a medical history of an uncle, and the nurse may find out the uncle is married to the mother's sister. The nurse must make sure to clarify that only direct relatives should be included in the history. Some diseases of the gastrointestinal system that have hereditary components are Crohn's, familial polyposis, colon cancer, and malabsorption of nutrients such as fructose and folate. Adult onset diseases of the renal system with hereditary components include polycystic disease of the kidney, renal amyloidosis, and some renal cancers. Risk factors for chronic kidney disease are outlined in the Risk Factors box.

Social History

Social history includes any alcohol, tobacco, or recreational drug usage, including how often and how much of the substance is used or taken. For example, if a patient has a positive history of smoking, the nurse should ask how many cigarettes the patient smokes per day. The same is true for alcohol use to determine whether the patient is at risk for hepatic disease due to years of alcohol consumption. However, some patients may be reluctant to discuss these habits. The nurse should ask these questions in a matter of fact way so the patient does not feel stigmatized or judged. Patients also need to know that this information is confidential and used only to assist in their care.

Habits

Changes in a patient's normal routine can provide clues about the symptomatology of the complaint. This information will also help to guide the nurse's line of questioning. For example, the nurse should ask the patient about his diet and any fluctuations in weight. What is the patient's usual diet? Have there been any changes related to the patient's current complaint? Has the patient's appetite changed? A recent change in diet can affect gastrointestinal illnesses. An example is the patient who completes a liquid fast and then starts eating again. This sudden stimulation may cause a first attack of cholecystitis, an inflammation of the gallbladder.

RISK FACTORS for Chronic Kidney Disease

At-risk Groups: African American, first-degree family history of renal disease, history of polycystic kidney disease.

At-risk Disease Processes: Diabetes, hypertension, chronic glomerular disease, chronic infection, untreated urinary tract obstruction (i.e., enlarged prostate).

Stool patterns also should be included in this part of the history. What is the patient's normal stool pattern? For some patients, having bowel movements 1 to 2 times per week is very normal, whereas others need to have daily movement. Are there changes in consistency or color? Pencil-thin stools can be a concern for colon cancer but also can indicate large hemorrhoids. Is the act of defecation painful? Rectal fissures can be excruciating and may lead to constipation due to the fear of defecation.

The nurse should also ask about urinary habits. How often does the patient void? Does the patient get up at night to void (nocturia)? How much does the patient void? What does the urine look like? Have there been changes in the urinary pattern? Patients who are developing renal failure may experience a metallic taste in their mouth from the uremia, which may cause a decrease in appetite. Also, rapid weight gain accompanied by orthopnea may be a sign of fluid overload from renal failure.

Recent Travel

Any recent history of travel is significant information for the nurse to obtain. Certain gastrointestinal illnesses such as diarrhea are commonly linked to travel. Many travelers, both abroad and locally, experience traveler's diarrhea. This is a name commonly used for diarrhea experienced either while traveling or afterward, but it can be caused by many different agents, including viral, bacterial, and parasitic organisms, and is generally contracted through contaminated food or water. It can be self-limiting or cause problems for an extended period of time. Certain organisms such as *Vibrio cholerae* may be common only in certain areas, but *Giardia* can be found in most countries, including the United States. Therefore, it is important to get a complete history of travel, both recent and as far back as several years, if necessary.

Physical Examination

When performing the physical examination of the patient with abdominal complaints, the nurse must take a systematic approach to the examination. If it is done out of order, important findings may be obscured due to pain and the patient's subsequent inability to cooperate with the examination. The order is different from that used in assessing other systems. Inspection should come first, followed by auscultation, percussion, and finally palpation to avoid eliciting or increasing pain. It is important for the nurse to assess the patient's general state of health. Examining a patient who is experiencing pain from appendicitis is very different from examining a patient with complaints of mild diarrhea. However, positioning the patient for the optimal examination does not always mean that it is optimal for the examiner. For instance, a patient might not be able to lie flat in a supine position. A more comfortable position may be to have the knees bent. The nurse should work with the patient in establishing a comfortable position; this will make the examination more productive for both of them.

Inspection

The first element of the nurse's physical examination of the patient's abdomen is inspection. This is done initially by just watching the patient. Is the patient able to walk with a normal posture, or is the person walking hunched over, protecting her abdomen? When the patient is sitting, is the posture normal? Is the patient able to sit, or is the patient curled into a fetal position on the examination table or bed? Is the patient able to be still, or must the patient move about because of the colicky pain of **renal calculi** (kidney stones)? These observations are the first part of the data collection and contribute to the ongoing collection of data.

Inspection should include the mouth. Inspect the mucosa for redness, any lesions, and moistness. Inspect the teeth for dental caries, loose teeth, and tooth loss. If the patient has dentures, do they fit properly? The tongue should be inspected for any redness, inflammation, fissure, ulcerations, or lesions. The pharynx is evaluated by using a tongue blade to hold the tongue out of the way. Having the patient tilt her head back slightly assists the nurse in visualization of the soft palate, uvula, and movement of this structure. The nurse should inspect the uvula, tonsils, soft palate, and anterior and posterior pillars. He should have the patient say "aah," at which point the soft palate and uvula should rise symmetrically.

Inspection continues after the patient is lying flat and the abdomen is exposed. This might be difficult if the patient is unable to lie flat due to pain. However, inspection can be done with the patient in different positions, although this may not be as optimal.

Before the nurse touches the patient he can collect important data. The nurse should look at the contour of the patient's abdomen both obliquely and straight on. Is the abdomen symmetrical? Sometimes masses, fluid waves, or a change in contour can be seen. For example, a **ventral hernia,** a hernia through the abdominal wall, is very distinct in an oblique view, particularly when the patient contracts the abdominal muscles. The umbilicus is normally midline and inverted, but will become everted with pregnancy, ascites, or an underlying mass. It also can become enlarged and everted with an umbilical hernia. The nurse should observe the skin for any changes such as scars, color changes, hair patterns, or presence of striae. Hair patterns will vary between male and female patients. There can also be differences between different races. Female patients with hirsutism (excessive growth of hair in unusual places) may have increased hair growth along the pubic mons extending to the umbilicus. Asian women will have finer and scarcer hair patterns than Caucasian or African American women. The nurse should also be cognizant of coloration changes between skin tones. For example, what appears red on a light skin tone will have a different appearance on a darker skin tone. Observe the skin for redness with localized inflammation, jaundice with hepatitis, rashes, striae, or cutaneous angiomas (spider nevi) that occur with portal hypertension (high blood pressure in the veins of the portal system caused by an obstruction in the liver) or liver disease.

The inspection is the time to ask about scars and the surgery related to them. Sometimes readdressing questions during this time will assist the patient in recalling further information. It also allows the nurse to ask a question in a slightly different manner, eliciting further recollection from the patient.

Auscultation

Auscultation is the second step in the physical examination process. Since this is an important step, the nurse should become comfortable with auscultation and the sound of the abdomen. However, contrary to previous teaching, bowel sounds may mean very little in the realm of an abdominal examination. For example, a person can have acute peritonitis but still have bowel sounds. A patient with a postoperative ileus may have very loud bowel sounds, but the patient is distended and the bowels are not functioning in a coordinated manner. Complete absence of bowel sounds would be significant, but keep in mind that the nurse would have to listen for a minimum of 5 minutes in all four quadrants to be sure that bowel sounds are absent. That being said, bowel sounds should be auscultated prior to palpation, as the deep palpation can affect the frequency of bowel sounds. The nurse should listen over all four

Weblink: Renal Calculi
Weblink: Assessment of the Oral Cavity

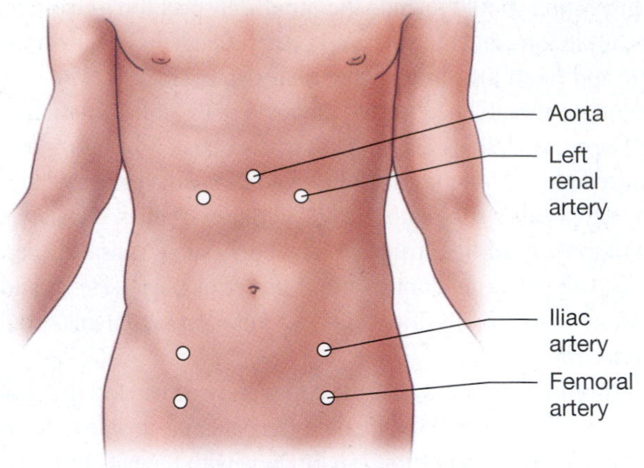

FIGURE 36–6 ◆ Sites for vascular sounds.

quadrants for a period of 2 to 5 minutes. He should note the frequency, pitch, and character of the bowel sounds. Are the bowel sounds hypoactive? Hyperactive? The nurse should ask the patient about passing flatus. Like all parts of the examination, auscultation should be correlated with the history.

The epigastrium and bilateral upper quadrants should be auscultated with both the diaphragm and the bell of the stethoscope. This is the area to listen for the aorta and renal arteries. The nurse is listening for a bruit or schussing sound, which is an indication of an abnormality. Both groins should also be auscultated for bruits of the iliac arteries. Figure 36–6◆ indicates sites to listen for vascular sounds.

A ticklish patient may not tolerate the touch of the stethoscope. Having the patient place the stethoscope where the nurse directs will enhance the examination of this type of patient. This technique not only distracts the patient, but also avoids tickling.

Percussion

Percussion, the third step in the physical examination process, is done by placing the nondominant hand flat on the surface of the patient's abdomen. The first joint of the index or third finger is then struck gently with the index or third finger of the dominant hand (Figure 36–7◆). The nurse should practice this on different types of surfaces and listen to the difference in the sound. A good example is on a melon or even a thigh. The nurse should be able to hear the difference. It is also important for the nurse to have his fingernails clipped short so as not to cause injury to himself or the patient.

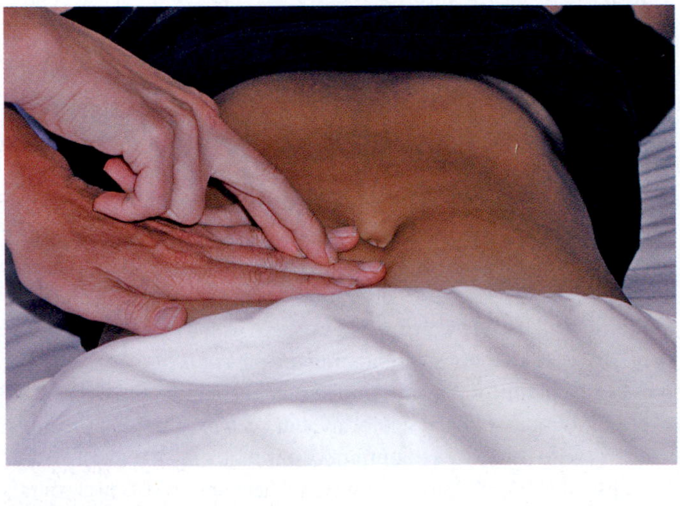

FIGURE 36–7 ◆ Percussion of abdomen.
Source: Cheryl Wraa.

Percussing the abdomen will elicit different sounds. There should be the hollow sound, similar to that of tapping on a watermelon, over the epigastric area and sometimes over the bowels. If this high-pitched, drum-like tone of medium duration is heard throughout the entire abdomen, it is called **tympany** and is produced by air in the intestine. This sound is indicative of an obstruction or distention of the abdomen.

The liver and a full bladder give off a dull sound, similar to that when percussing a piece of meat. The liver edges can be determined by percussing from the lower right abdomen to the edge of the rib. At the transition of the hollow sound to the dull sound, the nurse will find the liver edge. The nurse should measure this area by determining how many finger breadths it is from the costal margin.

The spleen can be measured in the same fashion. However, the edge of the spleen should not be below the costal margin. It is more likely found near the 10th left rib. If it is below the rib, this is an indication of an abnormal enlargement. Palpation of the area should be done with great care. Percussion can also elicit pain, particularly in patients with acute peritonitis (inflammation of the peritoneum).

The size of the bladder can be determined by percussion, especially if the patient has a full or distended bladder. For the nurse to percuss the kidney, the patient must be lying on one side or be in a sitting position. The nurse should make a fist and gently strike the patient with the ulnar surface of the fist in the costal vertebral angle. This should be jarring to the patient but should not elicit any pain. If this action causes pain, it is a sign of kidney infection or injury.

Palpation

Palpation, the final step in the physical examination process, should start with the patient's mouth and throat area. The nurse should palpate any lesions or abnormalities of the oral pharynx by using a gloved finger. Lesions of the cheek are better felt by placing one finger inside the mouth and one on the cheek. By isolating the lesion between the fingers, the nurse can better determine the lesion's size and shape.

Palpation of the abdomen should be done in a systematic pattern, starting with light palpation. This assists in the identification of muscle resistance and more superficial findings. In patients who are sensitive, even light palpation will cause muscle resistance. To relax the patient, the nurse may have the patient bend her legs, use a stethoscope to palpate, or have the patient place her own hand under the nurse's, using the patient's hand to press down. After the patient becomes relaxed, the nurse can slide his hand under the patient's hand. When using the stethoscope to palpate, the nurse should place the stethoscope on the abdomen and, while listening, press harder on the abdomen, eliciting any pain the patient might sense.

The next step is deeper palpation. The nurse should use the palmar surface of the hand and palpate in all four quadrants. If the patient has a complaint of abdominal pain, the nurse should palpate last the area the patient identified as painful.

The liver edge should be palpable. The nurse should recall where he first percussed the edges of the liver border and place his fingertips below this area. His hand should be placed lateral to the rectus muscle on the right hand side. The nurse then presses gently down and up toward the ribs (Figure 36–8◆). The nurse should have the patient take a deep breath. As the patient is inhaling, the liver edge will come down under

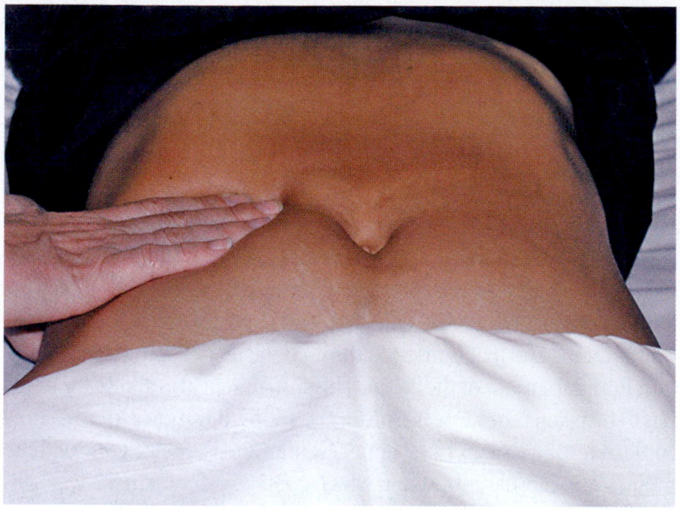

FIGURE 36–8 ◆ Palpation of abdomen.
Source: Cheryl Wraa.

the nurse's fingertips. A normal liver feels firm and has a clear edge. However, a cirrhotic liver will feel stiffer, and the edge will be irregular. The edge will also be palpable farther down on the abdomen.

To palpate the spleen, the nurse should be standing on the patient's right. The nurse reaches across with the left hand and places it on the lateral chest wall at the 10th rib. The nurse's hand should be placed below the costal margin. While supporting the rib with the left hand, the nurse gently palpates up toward and under the costal margin. As the patient takes a deep breath, the tip of the spleen might be palpated as it descends. The spleen is not always palpable, especially in adults. If it is easily palpated below the costal margin, the spleen is considered enlarged and the health care provider should be notified.

Both the kidneys should be palpated, but the right kidney is easily palpated and the left kidney is rarely felt. When palpating the right kidney, the nurse places his left hand on the right flank area with gentle pressure toward the abdomen and his right hand on the abdomen parallel to the costal margin. The nurse then presses his hands firmly together. The lower pole of the kidney should be felt as the patient takes a deep breath. At times, the patient will have a sharp sensation as the kidney pole passes through the nurse's hands. This is not considered a painful sensation.

The left kidney is rarely palpable. However, the nurse should examine this area for any abnormalities. The maneuver is the same. The nurse places his left hand along the flank area. In some patients, this can be accomplished from the right side of the table. However, if the patient is large or the left side cannot be reached in this fashion, this examination may be performed from the left side of the table (Figure 36–9◆). The kidneys should feel firm and smooth. It is considered abnormal if an irregular surface is palpated, the kidney extends significantly lower than the rib cage, or obvious trauma is noted.

The aorta is palpated in the area above the umbilicus and slightly to the left. The aorta may be difficult to palpate in the obese abdomen and can sometimes be seen as pulsating in the scaphoid abdomen. If the pulsation of the aorta is easily palpated, the nurse should attempt to gently isolate it between the thumb and finger.

Adjunctive Physical Examinations

Certain physical examinations are specific to conditions of the abdomen in particular. These adjunctive examinations will assist in narrowing or confirming the nurse's differential diagnosis.

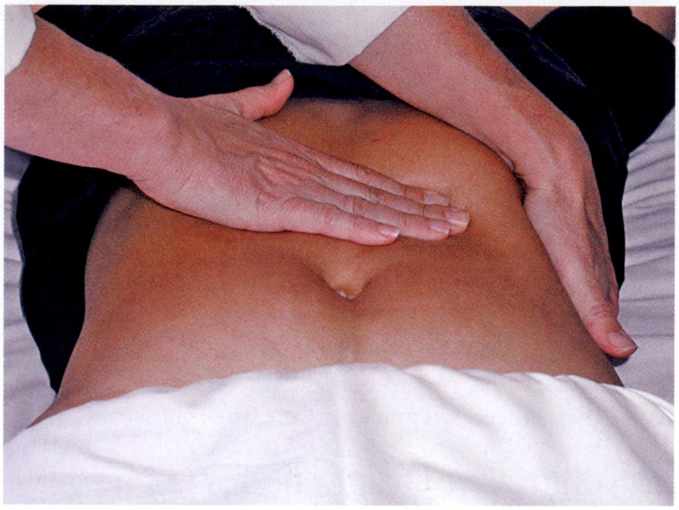

FIGURE 36–9 ◆ Palpation of kidneys.
Source: Cheryl Wraa.

Rebound Tenderness

Rebound tenderness describes tenderness that is greater when the pressure is released than when it is applied; it is a reliable sign of peritoneal inflammation. To perform this test, the nurse gently presses into the abdomen and then releases the pressure, starting light and then with greater firmness as the examination warrants. The nurse should start away from the area of pain and work toward the area identified by the patient as hurting the most. If the patient feels a great deal of discomfort away from the identified source, the nurse should stop. There is no further benefit in causing more pain to the patient.

Iliopsoas Sign

Iliopsoas refers to three muscles of the abdomen—psoas major, psoas minor, and iliacus—that pass from the abdomen through the pelvis and are partially responsible for hip flexion. When the iliopsoas sign test is positive, it indicates an inflammation of the psoas muscle, which lies lateral to the lumbar vertebrae and passes deep into the inguinal ligament to the lesser trochanter of the femur. The lumbar plexus of nerves is embedded in the psoas. The iliacus muscle lies along the lateral side of the psoas muscle and extends across the sacroiliac joint to attach to the iliac fossa. Clinically, the iliopsoas has relations to the kidneys, ureters, cecum, appendix, sigmoid colon, pancreas, lumbar lymph nodes, and nerves of the posterior abdominal wall. When there is intra-abdominal inflammation or disease of any of these structures, movement of the iliopsoas causes pain. To assess for the iliopsoas sign, the nurse asks the patient to lie flat and flex the leg closest to the nurse. With the nurse's hand flat against the lateral surface of the thigh, the patient pushes against the nurse's palm with some resistance applied. The test is positive if this causes the patient pain. The test is then repeated on the other side.

Safety Alert *The iliopsoas sign test should be performed cautiously in immobilized or older patients. It should not be performed in patients with hip replacement.*

Obturator Sign

The obturator sign test is positive in patients with inflammation along the obturator internus muscle. Positive tests can be related to appendicitis, diverticulitis, and pelvic inflammatory disease, to name a few

Weblink: Endoscopy Tutorial

conditions. The nurse should stand along the side of the bed while performing this test. The patient is asked to bend her knee and flex at the hip. While supporting the leg, the nurse then flexes the thigh to a right angle and externally and internally rotates the leg. This should be done on both sides. The test is positive if the patient experiences pain.

Murphy's Sign

The Murphy's sign test is positive when a person has inflammation of the gallbladder, as seen in cholecystitis. The nurse should stand on the right side of the bed and place his hand flat on the patient's abdomen with his fingertips just below the right costal margin. The patient then gently inhales. As the liver and gallbladder descend into the nurse's fingertips, the patient will feel pain when there is inflammation.

Noninvasive Diagnostic Testing

The use of noninvasive diagnostic testing is important in establishing the diagnosis of many abdominal complaints. Although it is not the goal of this chapter to provide education on all radiologic tests, a few will be listed.

Computed Tomography Scan of the Abdomen and Pelvis

The computed tomography (CT) scan is very versatile in the information it provides to the clinician caring for the patient. Abscesses, fluid collections, vascular disorders, obstructions, and trauma can be seen. For trauma, however, CT scans work better for injuries to solid organs, such as the liver and spleen, than to hollow organs, such as the bowel or bladder. This test can utilize intravenous, rectal, or oral contrast to enhance the images.

Safety Alert *Assess the patient for any allergies to iodine or contrast media and alert the health care provider if allergies exist prior to tests that use these substances.*

Ultrasound

Ultrasound is used for evaluation of the gallbladder, kidneys, and urinary tract, and at times the appendix. It can also be used for identification of free fluid in trauma patients with suspected intra-abdominal injury.

Kidney–Ureter–Bladder Versus Three-Way Abdominal Films

The abbreviation KUB stands for kidney, ureters, and bladder; it is also the term used for a plain film of the abdomen. This is obtained with the patient lying flat and the x-ray plate placed beneath. It helps to determine the position, size, and structure of the kidneys and urinary tract. It is useful in evaluating for the presence of calculi and masses. Also, this is an excellent test for obstruction, because it shows the air in the colon nicely. The three-way abdominal series not only incorporates the KUB view but also includes a picture of the abdomen with the patient on her side as well as one upright. This test helps to differentiate air fluid levels in the intestinal tract.

Invasive Diagnostic Procedures

Invasive procedures are uncomfortable and at times painful. For that reason, most of these procedures are done with conscious sedation.

Barium Enema

In this radiologic test, barium contrast is inserted in the rectum. The barium fills the colon and shows the contour of the intralumen. This test would enhance intraluminal processes such as colon cancer or diverticular disease.

Colonoscopy and Endoscopy

Colonoscopy and endoscopy allow the clinician to visualize the intraluminal space directly. The colonoscopy is a flexible tube with a small camera at the end that is inserted through the rectum and visualizes the intraluminal surface of the colon. This instrument also allows for biopsies to be taken. The same is true for the endoscopy; however, this similar flexible tube visualizes the upper GI tract and is inserted through the mouth. The capsule endoscopy, which contains a tiny camera, will help to diagnose problems in the small intestine.

Endoscopic Retrograde Cholangiopancreatography

Endoscopic retrograde cholangiopancreatography (ERCP) is a test similar to the endoscopy, but it includes a study of the pancreatic and bile ducts. This test is commonly used in evaluating for cholecystitis or pancreatitis. When the scope reaches the duodenum, the endoscopist locates the opening into the ducts or the ampulla. A small tube is placed in the ampulla, and contrast dye is injected that allows for visualization of the ducts. Removal of stones, biopsy, and sphincterotomy may be performed during this procedure.

Common Laboratory Studies

The significance of these laboratory tests will be discussed in more detail in Chapters 37 to 39. Chart 36–5 lists common studies used in the assessment of gastrointestinal, liver, pancreatic, renal, and urinary functions, as well as their clinical significance.

Gerontological Considerations

The older adult may have increased deposits of subcutaneous fat on the abdomen and hips as it redistributes away from the extremities. The musculature of the abdomen is thinner and has less tone. If the patient is thin, the nurse may be able to visualize peristalsis when the patient is lying supine. Also, the softer abdominal wall may make palpation of the organs easier. Because the lungs may be distended and the diaphragm depressed, the liver is palpated lower, appearing 1 to 2 centimeters below the costal margin with inhalation. Kidney function declines in the older adult but is adequate for functioning. The number of nephrons (filtering units) decrease, as does the overall amounts of kidney tissue. The kidney's blood vessels may become hardened with age and the kidneys will filter the blood more slowly. However, the older adult may have more difficulty compensating for sudden changes in the body. The slowness of the kidneys' response to changes can affect an elderly person's ability to concentrate urine and retain water. Dehydration occurs more readily as older adults tend to have less of a sense of thirst.

CHART 36-5 Common Laboratory Studies

Study	Clinical Significance
Studies of GI function	
• Stool culture	Detection of bacteria, ameba, or worms
	Large amounts of pus associated with ulcerative colitis, abscesses, and anorectal fistula
Studies of liver function	
• Alkaline phosphatase	↑ with biliary obstruction and hepatitis
• Aspartate aminotransferase (AST)	↑ with hepatocellular injury
• Alanine aminotransferase (ALT)	↑ with hepatocellular injury
• Lactate dehydrogenase (LDH)	↑ with hypoxic and primary liver injury
• Serum bilirubin	
• Indirect	↑ with hemolysis
• Direct	↑ with hepatocellular injury or obstruction
• Total	↑ with biliary obstruction
• Urine bilirubin	↑ with biliary obstruction
• Urine urobilinogen	↓ with obstructive liver disease
• Albumin	↓ with hepatocellular injury
• Globulin	↑ with hepatitis
• Prothrombin time	↑ with chronic liver disease or vitamin K deficiency
• Partial thromboplastin time	↑ with severe liver disease or heparin therapy
Studies of pancreatic function	
• Serum amylase	↑ with pancreatic inflammation
• Serum lipase	↑ with pancreatic inflammation
• Urine amylase	↑ with pancreatic inflammation
• Stool fat	Decreased pancreatic lipase increases stool fat
Studies of renal function	
• Blood urea nitrogen (BUN)	↑ with poor renal function
• Serum creatinine	↑ with damage to nephrons
• Urine osmolality	↑ fluid volume deficit
	↓ fluid volume excess
• Serum osmolality	↑ fluid volume deficit
	↓ fluid volume excess
• Urinalysis	See Chapter 39 for specific details

NCLEX® PRACTICE

1. An adult patient is experiencing left lower quadrant pain. The nurse realizes this patient might be demonstrating:
   1. acute appendicitis.
   2. intussusception.
   3. pyloric stenosis.
   4. diverticulitis.

2. The nurse is preparing to examine the abdomen of an adult patient. Which of the following should the nurse do first?
   1. Inspection
   2. Percussion
   3. Auscultation
   4. Palpation

3. When percussing a patient's bladder, the nurse hears a dull sound. Which of the following would this sound indicate?

1. An empty bladder
2. A bladder obstruction
3. Kidney stones
4. A full bladder

4. Which of the following is an abnormal assessment finding in an adult?

1. Positive bowel sounds in all four quadrants
2. Tympany percussed over the stomach
3. A negative obturator sign
4. A positive Murphy's sign

5. During the health history, a patient states that she has had no abdominal surgeries, but the nurse sees a large abdominal scar when performing the physical examination of her abdomen. What should the nurse do first?

1. Document what the patient stated.
2. Ask the patient what caused the abdominal scar.
3. Assume the patient doesn't want to talk about the scar and change the subject.
4. Palpate the scar.

6. The nurse explains to a patient with a possible kidney infection that the kidneys lie in the retroperitoneal area. Other structures that occupy this area are: (select all that apply)

1. the stomach.
2. the gallbladder.
3. the pancreas.
4. the duodenum.
5. the ureters.

Answers to NCLEX Practice questions can be found in Appendix D in the Osborn Student Resources at nursing.pearsonhighered.com. Practice additional NCLEX questions online at the Student Resources site.

Pearson Nursing Student Resources Find additional review materials at: **nursing.pearsonhighered.com**

REFERENCES

Andrews, M. M. (2008). Cultural competence in the health history and physical examination. In M. M. Andrews & J. S. Boyle, *Transcultural concepts in nursing care* (pp. 34–65). Philadelphia: Wolters Kluwer/Lippincott, Williams & Wilkins.

Dunn, K. M. B., & Rothenberger, D. A. (2010). Colon, rectum and anus. In F. C. Brunicardi (Ed.), *Schwartz's principles of surgery* (9th ed.). New York: The McGraw-Hill Companies, Inc. Retrieved from http://online.statref.com/document.aspx?fxid=18&docid=1101

Fisher, W. E., Andersen, D. K., Bell, R. H., Saluja, A. K., & Bruinicardi, F. C. (2010). Pancreas. In F. C. Brunicardi (Ed.), *Schwartz's principles of surgery* (9th ed.). New York: The McGraw-Hill Companies, Inc. Retrieved from http://online.statref.com/document.aspx?fxid=18&docid=1229

Hackam, D. J., Grikscheit, T. C., Wang, K. S., Newman, K. D., & Ford, H. R. (2010). Pediatric surgery. In F. C. Brunicardi (Ed.), *Schwartz's principles of surgery* (9th ed.). New York: The McGraw-Hill Companies, Inc. Retrieved from http://online.statref.com/document.aspx?fxid=18&docid=1500

Urden, L. D., Stacy, K. M., & Lough, M. E. (2010). *Critical care nursing: Diagnosis and management* (6th ed.). St. Louis: Mosby Elsevier.

U.S. National Library of Medicine. (2010). Ginger. Retrieved from http://www.nlm.nih.gov/medlineplus/druginfo/natural/961.html

Caring for the Patient with Gastrointestinal Disorders

CHAPTER 37

Pamela Stetina
Cheryl Wraa

Outcome-Based Learning Objectives

After studying this chapter, the learner will be able to:

1. Compare and contrast the different causes of stomatitis and describe the related nursing care.
2. Analyze the pathophysiology, clinical manifestations, and treatment with related nursing care of patients with peptic ulcer disease (PUD) and gastroesophageal reflux disease (GERD).
3. Generate a teaching plan for a patient with celiac disease.
4. Analyze the similarities and differences between different types of inflammatory bowel disease.
5. Delineate nursing care for a patient with colon cancer and intestinal obstruction.
6. Generate a nursing care plan for patients with an ileostomy, a colostomy, and a continent ileostomy.

KEY TERMS

THE GASTROINTESTINAL (GI) TRACT consists of a hollow tube extending from the mouth to the anus and includes the esophagus, stomach, small intestine, large intestine, and rectum, as well as the accessory organs involved in digestion such as the pancreas, liver, and gallbladder. Anatomy of the gastrointestinal tract is presented in Chapter 36, and disorders of the liver, gallbladder, and pancreas are discussed in Chapter 38. Because the major functions of the GI tract are to prepare ingested food for absorption, absorb nutrients, and eliminate wastes, disorders of this system can have devastating effects on a person's nutritional status, lifestyle, body image, and health in general. Most disorders of the GI tract can be classified as inflammatory, ulcerative, structural, or neural.

Disorders of the Mouth

Disorders of the mouth and esophagus have a variety of causes ranging from viral to nutritional. Diseases may be as common as gastroesophageal reflux disease or as serious as esophageal cancer.

Stomatitis

Stomatitis, the generalized inflammation of the oral mucosa, is classified according to the etiology. Similar to stomatitis is glossitis, or inflammation of the tongue, which is caused by many of the same factors that cause stomatitis; for this reason, they often coexist. These problems may be caused by a virus, bacteria, fungus, trauma, chemical agents, or nutritional deficiencies.

Pathophysiology

The oral mucosa consists of a thin, fragile layer of squamous epithelial cells with a rich blood supply. Cellular turnover is rapid, thus promoting quick healing but also providing an opportunity for cellular mutation and damage to these rapidly dividing cells. Because of the abundant blood supply and the fragility of the epithelial cells, the risks for infection, inflammation, and trauma are increased.

Etiology, Epidemiology, and Clinical Manifestations

Etiology of disorders of the mouth and esophagus include viral, bacterial, fungal, traumatic, and chemical causes, as well as nutritional deficiencies.

Viral Causes

Herpetic stomatitis is a very common inflammation of the oral cavity caused by a herpes simplex virus (HSV) infection, which is widespread in the United States. It is estimated that between 30% and 100% of the U.S. population has HSV-specific antibodies, which indicate a past or dormant infection, and that up to 20% of the adult population is shedding the virus at any given time. A previous infection of HSV (anywhere on the body) is the primary risk factor for all secondary manifestations of herpes simplex infection (Gerzevitz, Porter, & Dunphy, 2011).

Patients may note nonspecific symptoms followed by consistently sized vesicles that are most commonly found on the tongue, buccal and labial mucosa, gums, and occasionally the hard or soft palate. The vesicles rupture and progress to painful ulcerations (similar to aphthous ulcers, described later) and resolve in 10 to 14 days. Any condition that decreases the immune response, such as HIV infection, cancer, chemotherapy, immunosuppressive medications, or aging, can increase the likelihood of viral reactivation, causing recurrent stomatitis (Arduino & Porter, 2008; Gerzevitz et al., 2011).

Bacterial Causes

Aphthous stomatitis (contact stomatitis), commonly known as canker sores, is a common ulcerative condition limited to the oral cavity. An estimated 20% of the population is affected at some time, with a possible prevalence of up to 66%. Although the pathogenesis is unclear, an immunologic response is believed to be responsible for this type of stomatitis. Other possible causes and contributing factors are psychological stress, vitamin deficiencies, genetic predisposition, trauma, menstruation, allergies, and viruses. The prevalence is also higher in people with some gastrointestinal (GI) disorders, such as inflammatory bowel disease (Plewa, 2010), suggesting these disorders as a possible cause. Aphthous stomatitis initially begins with painful red macules or papules that then become painful ulcers covered by a grayish yellow membrane.

Vincent's stomatitis, also known as acute necrotizing stomatitis or "trench mouth," is an acute bacterial infection of the gingival oral mucous membranes most often caused by the bacteria *Borrelia vincentii*. It occurs in people with systemic conditions that decrease the tissue's resistance, as well as in patients with poor nutrition, extreme stress, and poor oral hygiene (Ubertalli, 2008). The clinical manifestations of Vincent's stomatitis include erythematous ulceration and necrosis of the gingival margins and oral mucosa. The interdental gingival papillae are red, are reduced in size, and appear raw and painful. There is a characteristic purulent gray exudate, and the person complains of pain, increased salivation, gums that bleed easily, and bad breath. There may also be systemic manifestations such as malaise, anorexia, and enlarged lymph nodes in the neck. Untreated, the tissue can become gangrenous (necrotic).

Fungal Causes

Oral candidiasis is extremely common and occurs largely as a result of a compromised immune system or a disruption of the normal oral flora; this type of stomatitis results from an overgrowth of the yeast-like fungus *Candida albicans*. The overgrowth can result from antibiotic therapy, which destroys the normal flora in the oral cavity, and from the chronic use of inhaled steroids. The overgrowth can also occur when the immune system is compromised by such things as cancer chemotherapy treatments, radiation treatments to the head, immunosuppressive medications (glucocorticoids, antirejection drugs), aging, diabetes, emotional stress, malnourishment, or HIV/AIDS. The manifestations of oral candidiasis include painful, white curdlike patches on the tongue, palate, and oral mucosa. Under the white patches, the surface of the tissue is red and sore, which may be all that is visible upon examination (Lustig & Schindler, 2010).

Traumatic Causes

Traumatic oral ulcers are very common and occur most often at the tongue margins and buccal mucosa. It is often difficult to differentiate traumatic ulcers from aphthous stomatitis other than by history and the report of pain; traumatic ulcers are usually not as painful as aphthous ulcers. Common traumatic causes include thermal injury (e.g., from hot food or beverage) and mechanical injury. Mechanical injury can result from ill-fitting dentures, malocclusion, broken teeth, and habitual cheek biting.

Chemical Causes

Chemical irritation can cause stomatitis. Common chemical irritants include foods that are spicy (hot pepper sauce), acidic (dill pickles), or salty (potato chips). Dental care products such as toothpaste as well as mouthwash that contains alcohol and peroxide can also act as chemical irritants. Cancer chemotherapy frequently causes stomatitis because, in addition to attacking cancer cells that are rapidly dividing, chemotherapy agents attack other rapidly dividing cells such as the mucous epithelial cells in the oral cavity. The chemical irritation from tobacco, whether smoking, dipping, or chewing, can result in nicotinic stomatitis (Gerzevitz, Porter, & Dunphy, 2011). Bulimia can be a risk factor for stomatitis because of the repeated exposure of the oral mucosa to stomach acid from vomiting.

Nutritional Deficiencies

Several vitamin deficiencies can cause stomatitis, particularly angular stomatitis (irritation and fissuring in the corners of the lips), glossitis, and cheilosis (scaling and fissures of the surface of the lips). Vitamin deficiencies, although rare in the United States, can be caused by malnutrition, malabsorption, alcoholism, restrictive dieting, and fad dieting. Stomatitis and glossitis are caused from deficiencies in many of the B vitamins: B_6 (pyridoxine), B_{12} (cobalamin), B_2 (riboflavin), niacin, folate, and iron (Gerzevitz, Porter, & Dunphy, 2011).

No Known Cause

Benign migratory glossitis, also known as geographic tongue, erythema migrans, and stomatitis areata migrans, is, as the name implies, a benign condition; it occurs in up to 3% of the population and is more frequently reported in people with psoriasis. It is characterized by the loss of papillae in some areas of the tongue. These areas are smooth and erythematous, giving the tongue a maplike appearance, hence the name *geographic tongue*. The areas can change in size, location, and appearance daily. Often, the person with this condition complains of soreness or burning of the tongue that is exacerbated by hot, spicy, or acidic foods (Kelsch, 2007).

Laboratory and Diagnostic Procedures

There are no specific diagnostic laboratory tests for diagnosing specific mouth sores, although a white blood cell count (WBC), nutritional indices (B_6, B_{12}, B_2, niacin, folate, and iron), anti-HSV antibodies, and Gram stain for fungus may be helpful to diagnose mouth disorders. Refer to the Laboratory and Diagnostic Tests box on page 1115.

Medical Management

Diagnosis of stomatitis is made by noting the history of current symptoms, including the presence of systemic illness or evidence of trauma (e.g., broken teeth, ill-fitting dentures), physical examination, culture, and/or biopsy. Medical management includes treatment of the causative factor, if known, and relief of symptoms.

Drug Therapy

The health care provider may order topical oral anesthetics such as 2% viscous lidocaine. The nurse should ensure that the patient rinses her mouth with the viscous lidocaine, then spits it out, because swallowing an anesthetic solution may impair the patient's ability to swallow. However, for a patient who has lesions in the upper esophagus, the solution may be swallowed to relieve the pain of these lesions. The nurse should inform the patient that the lidocaine may be used every 3 hours as needed. Using lidocaine before meals may help improve oral intake. Agents that coat the oral mucosa may also be helpful in relieving the discomfort of stomatitis. Agents such as magnesium hydroxide (Milk of Magnesia) and kaolin (Kaopectate) may relieve the pain, particularly of aphthous ulcers, while protecting the lesions from further irritation. Orders for a combination of equal parts of antihistamines such as diphenhydramine (Benadryl) and antacids such as aluminum-magnesium hydroxide (Maalox) may be added to an equal part of lidocaine to relieve a combination of symptoms and improve appetite/nutritional status, although the effectiveness of these rinses is not established through research (Gerzevitz, Porter, & Dunphy, 2011; Harris, Eilers, Harriman, Cashavelly, & Maxwell, 2008).

Safety Alert *Nurses should assess the patient's ability to swallow after administration of oral lidocaine to prevent any risk of aspiration or choking. Wilson, Shannon, and Shields (2011) suggest that the patient not ingest food for at least an hour after taking lidocaine.*

Anti-infective drugs (drugs that are used to treat infections and include antibiotics, antivirals, and antifungals) will be ordered for the patient with stomatitis caused by viruses, bacteria, or fungus and are dispensed in topical, oral, or intravenous (IV) formulations. Antibiotics such as oral penicillin V potassium (Pen-Vee K) are usually effective for Vincent's stomatitis, but IV antibiotics may be required for severe gangrenous cases (Gerzevitz, Porter, & Dunphy, 2011). Antifungal agents such as nystatin suspension are prescribed for Candida infection. The nurse instructs the patient to swish the suspension around in the mouth for about 2 minutes and then swallow it. The antifungal agent may also be taken as a lozenge, which is held in the mouth until it is dissolved, at which point the patient swallows the dissolved solution. The nurse should instruct the patient to abstain from eating or drinking for 30 minutes after taking the medication.

Antiviral agents are prescribed for herpes simplex stomatitis. Oral acyclovir (Zovirax) is used for patients with intact immune systems. Continued use decreases the frequency and severity of the acute episodes. IV acyclovir may be needed for patients with compromised immune systems, such as those with HIV/AIDS or those taking immunosuppressive medications. The Pharmacology feature box (p. 1114) outlines medications used to treat stomatitis.

Nursing Management

Nursing care of the patient with stomatitis focuses on assessing the condition of the oral mucosa and determining how these inflammatory conditions are affecting the patient's well-being, specifically the patient's nutritional status. The treatment of stomatitis and similar conditions is focused on treating the underlying cause, such as correcting vitamin deficiencies, removing the source of traumatic or chemical irritation, or medicating for the infecting organism.

For all causes of stomatitis, nursing care focuses on good oral hygiene. Frequent mouth care helps debride oral lesions and can decrease the patient's chance of developing a superinfection (a new infection occurring in a patient having a preexisting infection). Mouth care using a soft toothbrush, toothette oral swab, or water pick should be done frequently—at least twice daily. It is essential to teach patients to avoid harsh mouthwashes, particularly those that contain alcohol, because these can irritate the ulcerated mucosa. Bland rinses, such as normal saline, a sodium bicarbonate solution, or a mixture of the two may be used to promote oral care (Harris et al., 2008).

Another important nursing intervention for patients with stomatitis is nutritional assessment. It is often painful for patients to eat or drink when they have stomatitis, so the nurse should encourage a high-calorie, high-protein diet. Often, soft, bland foods are better tolerated, and cool or cold foods may be soothing. Acidic foods such as citrus juices and tomatoes should be avoided, as should spicy or hot foods. Weighing the patient daily can help establish the adequacy of the patient's caloric intake. Patients should also be taught to avoid tobacco (Harris et al., 2008).

Finally, nursing responsibilities include teaching the patient and the family that the medication does not cure the disease and that the virus remains latent in the body and may recur during times of physical or emotional stress.

Salivary Gland Disorders

The salivary glands create saliva, which is excreted into the mouth. Saliva moistens food and assists the patient with chewing, swallowing, and digestion of food. Saliva also contains antibodies to protect the mouth. These glands can become infected, occluded, or cancerous. Signs and symptoms of salivary gland infections include (1) dry mouth, (2) swelling of the face and neck, (3) foul taste, (4) pain of the face and neck, and (5) difficulty opening the mouth. Medical and nursing management of salivary gland infections are the same as that for stomatitis.

Oral Cancer

Epidemiology

Oral cancer, abnormal cells that arise from the flat cells in the oral cavity, can occur on any surface of the mouth, including the lips, tongue, and pharynx. The American Cancer Society (2010) estimates that approximately 36,540 people in the United States were newly diagnosed with oral cancer in 2010, with 7,880 expected deaths. Oral cancer is the eighth-leading cause of cancer in men. Of those diagnosed in 2010, about 61% will be alive in 5 years (American Cancer Society, 2010).

Etiology and Risk Factors

The most widely recognized risk factor for the development of oral cancer is tobacco use. Tobacco contains chemicals that are known carcinogens, causing mutations in cellular DNA. Smokeless tobacco is particularly hazardous because the chemicals are absorbed directly through the oral mucosa. The use of tobacco is associated with 80% of all cases of oral cancer. Other risk factors include drinking alcohol, combined drinking and smoking, betel quid chewing (an addictive chew common in Southeast Asia containing betel leaf, areca nut, and slaked lime), human papillomavirus (HPV), sunlight exposure, poor nutrition, and being male (American Cancer Society, 2011b). Most oral cancers are attributed to lifestyle choices.

PHARMACOLOGY Summary of Medications Used to Treat Stomatitis

Medication Category and Action	Application/Indication	Nursing Responsibility
Antibiotics		
Penicillin V potassium (Pen-Vee K) ***Action:*** Exerts bacteriocidal activity by destroying and inhibiting synthesis of the bacterial cell wall.	Vincent's infection; pneumococcal, streptococcal, and staphylococcal infections; endocarditis risk prophylaxis.	Monitor for adverse effects such as nausea, vomiting, and diarrhea. Monitor for hypersensitivity reaction: pruritus, urticaria, fever, edema, arthralgia, and anaphylaxis. Teach the patient not to take the drug if reactions occur. Give after a meal. Warn female patients that the antibiotic may render oral contraceptives ineffective. Teach the patient to take the medication as prescribed.
Metronidazole (Flagyl) ***Action:*** Enters pathogen and binds to DNA, RNA, and intracellular protein, resulting in absence of DNA repair and RNA synthesis, resulting in cell death.	Intestinal amebiasis, trichomoniasis, colorectal surgery prophylaxis, *H. pylori* eradication, Crohn's disease, pseudomembranous colitis, anaerobic bacterial infections.	Monitor for adverse effects: nausea, vomiting, anorexia, abdominal pain, dizziness, headache, peripheral neuropathy, seizures, and Candida overgrowth. Monitor liver function tests if hepatic dysfunction is present. Be aware of multiple drug interactions; monitor for drug toxicities (lithium, warfarin, disulfiram, and others). Instruct the patient not to consume alcohol while taking the drug and for at least 48 hours after the last dose.
Ciprofloxacin (Cipro) ***Action:*** Inhibits bacterial DNA gyrase and topoisomerase, affecting bacterial replication and DNA repair.	GI infection, infectious diarrhea, respiratory infections, urinary tract infections, skin infections, bone infections, and anthrax prophylaxis.	Monitor for adverse effects: nausea, vomiting, diarrhea, abdominal cramps, rash, headache, peripheral neuropathy, seizures, and signs of Candida overgrowth. Monitor for acute onset of joint pain: notify health care provider. Monitor kidney and liver function if renal or hepatic impairment is present. Monitor cardiac function. Be aware of multiple drug interactions; monitor for drug toxicities (theophylline, warfarin, antacids, and others). Give medication 4 hours before or after antacid or vitamin administration. Ensure adequate fluid intake (2 to 3 L/day). Warn the patient about possible photosensitivity and the need for sunblock. Be aware of extensive IV drug incompatibilities.
Antifungal		
Nystatin (Mycostatin, Nilstat) ***Action:*** Binds to sterols in the fungal cell membrane, weakening the cell membrane and allowing leakage of intracellular contents.	Local Candida infections (e.g., oropharyngeal, intestinal candidiasis).	Monitor for signs of contact dermatitis. Instruct the patient not to eat or drink for 30 minutes after treatment for oral candidiasis. Teach the patient to swish the oral suspension for at least 2 minutes.
Antiviral		
Acyclovir (Zovirax) ***Action:*** Decreases viral shedding, formation of new lesions, and healing time by interfering with viral DNA synthesis.	Mucosal and cutaneous herpes simplex virus.	Monitor for adverse effects: headache, nausea, vomiting, and diarrhea. Monitor renal function, especially with IV administration. Teach the patient to clean the area before topical administration and to avoid contact with eyes.

Sources: Adams, M. P., & Koch, R. W. (2010). *Pharmacology: Connections to nursing practice.* Upper Saddle River, NJ: Pearson; Wilson, B. A., Shannon, M. T., & Shields, K. M. (2011). *Pearson nurse's drug guide 2011.* New York: Pearson.

Laboratory and Diagnostic Procedures

To diagnose oral cancer, dyes, such as toluidine blue, and assessment using laser light will help detect abnormal areas (American Cancer Society, 2011b). Biopsy will detect the specific type of cancer. See the Laboratory and Diagnostic Tests box.

Pathophysiology

Most oral cancers are squamous cell carcinoma, arising from the flat cells that line the oral cavity. This form of cancer might not produce symptoms until the tumor is well advanced, usually after invasion of the adjacent tissues and metastasis to other areas have occurred. Symptoms may include sores, lumps, or thickening on the lips or mouth, pain, leukoplakia (white patch), erythroplakia (red patch), trouble chewing or swallowing, sore throat, and problems with teeth or dentures (National Cancer Institute, 2010).

Medical Management

Elimination of causative factors or sources of irritation, such as all forms of tobacco and alcohol, is the initial treatment for oral cancer. Biopsy of the lesion is needed to diagnose the type of cancer. Tumor staging usually requires additional studies such as magnetic resonance imaging (MRI) or computed tomography (CT). Treatment is based on the extent of the cancer and whether it has metastasized. Radiation therapy may be prescribed before surgery in order to shrink the tumor.

LABORATORY AND DIAGNOSTIC TESTS for Mouth Disorders

Test with Description, Rationale, and Normal Values	Expected Abnormality
WBC Normal: 4,500–10,000 µL (mm3) *Used to detect infection.*	WBC counts above 10,000 indicate the presence of infection and/or inflammation. May be present with stomatitis.
Pyridoxine (Vitamin B_6) Normal: 5–30 ng/mL *Used to detect vitamin B_6 deficiencies.*	Low levels indicate malnutrition, malabsorption, and anemia. May be present with stomatitis.
Vitamin B_{12} Normal: 200–900 pg/mL *Used to detect vitamin B_{12} deficiencies.*	Lower levels indicate pernicious anemia, malabsorption, or liver disease. May be present with stomatitis.
Riboflavin (Vitamin B_2) Normal: 3.5–20 ug/L *Used to detect vitamin B_2 deficiencies.*	Lower levels are associated with skin problems and anemia. May be present with stomatitis.
Niacin (Vitamin B_3) Normal: 1.2–2.9 ug/L *Used to detect vitamin B_3 deficiencies.*	Abnormalities are associated with fatigue, diarrhea, depression, and dermatitis. May be present with stomatitis.
Folate Normal: 3–16 ng/mL *Used to check for folic acid deficiencies.*	Decreased levels indicate anemia or malabsorption, and may be lowered in pregnancy. May be present with stomatitis.
Iron Normal: 50–150 mcg/dL *Used to identify iron excess or deficiency.*	Lowered iron indicates anemia, renal failure, or bleeding. May be present with stomatitis.
Anti HSV Antibodies Normal: < 1:10 *Used to detect the presence of HSV.*	Positive results indicate the presence of herpes simplex virus.
Gram Stain Normal: negative *Used to detect the presence of fungi.*	Positive smear indicates the presence of fungi.
Toluidine Blue Dye Normal: no abnormal tissue	Abnormal areas of tissue stain blue. Used to detect oral cancer.
Laser Light/Special Light (with acetic acid) Normal: no abnormal tissue	Abnormal areas of tissue are seen with a laser light or with a special light after the mouth has been rinsed with acetic acid.
Biopsy Normal: no abnormal tissue *Used to detect abnormal cells.*	Cells are abnormal and may indicate oral cancer.

Sources: American Cancer Society. (2011b). Oral cavity and oropharyngeal cancer. Retrieved from http://www.cancer.org/Cancer/OralCavityandOropharyngealCancer/DetailedGuide/index; Bio-Center Laboratory (2012). Vitamins. Retrieved from http://biocenterlab.org/tests/vitamins/vitaminb.shtml; Kee, J. L. (2010). *Laboratory and diagnostic tests with nursing implications* (8th ed.). Upper Saddle River, NJ: Prentice Hall.

Radiation and chemotherapy may be appropriate postoperatively or as a combined treatment modality, depending on the stage of the tumor and the patient's general health. Targeted therapies may also be used to treat oral cancer.

Excision of the tumor is usually the treatment of choice unless the tumor is very far advanced and considered unresectable. The goal of surgery is to remove the cancerous tissue, but the surrounding tissue and lymph nodes may also be removed to ensure that there is no local infiltration of cancerous cells. Surgery may include removal of all or part of the tongue (glossectomy), removal of the mandible or maxilla, or a radical neck dissection if the tumor is advanced (American Cancer Society, 2011b). Radical neck dissection is a disfiguring condition that involves the removal of lymph nodes and muscles in the neck. A tracheostomy will be performed during surgery to maintain adequate respiratory support and may become permanent depending on the extent of the neck dissection and subsequent respiratory function.

Nursing Management

Nursing management of the patient with oral cancer centers on the elimination of causative factors, the care of the oral mucosa, and maintenance of good nutritional status before and after surgery. The Nursing Process: Patient Care Plan box (p. 1116) outlines care for the patient with oral cancer.

NURSING PROCESS: Patient Care Plan for Oral Cancer

Assessment of Gastrointestinal Status Using Gordon's Functional Health Patterns:

- Nutrition Metabolic Pattern
- Cognitive Perceptual Pattern

Subjective Data	Objective Data
Assessment of Oral Mucosa How long have you had this mouth sore? Do you smoke or use smokeless tobacco? Do you drink alcohol? If so, how much?	**Assessment of Oral Mucosa** Visual inspection of the oral cavity including the tongue and under the tongue: • Lesions may appear as white patches or velvety red. • Inspect for poorly fitting dentures or teeth in disrepair.
Assessment of Nutritional Status Do you have difficulty swallowing? Are there any foods that cause discomfort? Are you having trouble eating? Is your appetite good? Have you recently lost weight without trying? If so, how much?	**Assessment of Nutritional Status** Body weight and appearance. Skin turgor. Skin and hair condition.
Assessment of Pain Do you have mouth pain? On a scale of 1–10, with 10 being the worst pain, how would you rate your pain? Do you take anything for the pain? What makes the pain better or worse? Do you have any cultural or religious ways to control your pain?	**Assessment of Pain** Grimacing when swallowing. Drooling (too painful to swallow secretions).

Outcomes and Evaluation Parameters	Planning and Interventions with *Rationales*
1. NURSING DIAGNOSIS: Tissue Integrity, Impaired *related to oral lesion* (NANDA-I © 2012)	
Outcome: Reduced oral cancer risk. ***Evaluation Parameters:*** No behaviors harmful to oral mucosa: • Tobacco cessation. • Limited alcohol consumption. • Dentures/dentition in good repair.	Assess for and educate about contributing factors for oral cancer. *To decrease future risk, cause less irritation of lesions present, and improve overall health.* Provide and teach about good oral hygiene.
2. NURSING DIAGNOSIS: Nutrition, Readiness for Enhanced *related to oral pain or anorexia* (NANDA-I © 2012)	
Outcome: Adequate nutrition. ***Evaluation Parameter:*** No weight loss.	Provide cool, soft foods or liquids that are high in calories. Cool or cold foods that are soft or liquid are soothing to the oral mucosa. Daily weight. Indicator of fluid and nutrition status. Assess need for dietary consult.
3. NURSING DIAGNOSIS: Pain, Acute *related to oral lesion* (NANDA-I © 2012)	
Outcome: Comfort level maintained. ***Evaluation Parameters:*** Reports adequate pain control. Consumes meals and snacks without pain.	Assess pain using the pain scale (1–10) *to increase consistency in quantifying pain.* Assess cultural and religious beliefs about pain and pain relief. Different cultures and religions may view pain as punishment or may have nontraditional ways of treating pain. Administer prescribed pain medications or oral anesthetics as ordered. *Adequate pain relief before meals will increase the ability to eat pain free.*

Source: Adapted from Wilkinson, J. M., & Ahearn, N. R. (2009). *Prentice Hall nursing diagnosis handbook* (9th ed.). Upper Saddle River, NJ: Prentice Hall.

Health Promotion

Eliminating tobacco use is the single most important factor in reducing the risk of oral cancer. Because use of smokeless tobacco is highest in males ages 15 to 22, the nurse should target this group for education. Smoking cessation, as well as limiting alcohol consumption, should be encouraged for everyone. Use of sunscreen on the face and lips can reduce the risk of carcinoma. Routine dental visits are also important in the early detection of oral cancers, as well as for keeping dentition in good repair.

Collaborative Management

The patient with disorders of the mouth faces many challenges and requires the collaboration of an interdisciplinary team. Patients with oral cavity issues may be under the care of nurses, social workers, oncologists, surgeons, infectious disease specialists, dentists, nutritionists, and primary care providers. In order to meet desired patient outcomes, it is essential that this interdisciplinary team communicate openly with one another in developing and evaluating care of the patient and family (IOM [Institute of Medicine], 2010).

It is critical to establish good nutrition, as these patients may have difficulty chewing and swallowing related to pain, ill-fitting dentures, or surgical procedures. Nutritionists can help assess foods that patients can tolerate, as well as evaluate their nutritional needs. Enteral nutrition may need to be instituted for patients receiving surgical procedures for oral cancer.

Primary health care providers and dentists will help evaluate the status of the oral cavity and address trauma, infection, or issues related to teeth and dentures. Patients with bacterial, viral, or fungal infection may need infectious disease specialists if traditional treatment is ineffective. Oncologists and surgeons are important additions in providing care to patients with oral cancer. Nurses will be critical in providing education, nursing care, and support to patients and families. Social services will also be instrumental in providing resources and support for patients with disorders of the mouth.

Disorders of the Esophagus

Hiatal Hernia

A **hiatal hernia** involves the herniation of the upper portion of the stomach into the thorax through the esophageal hiatus. There are two types of hiatal hernia. Ninety percent of hiatal hernias are **sliding (direct) hiatal hernias,** which occur when a portion of the fundus of the stomach moves upward through the esophageal hiatus into the thoracic cavity (Figure 37–1A◆) (Huether, 2010a). The second type is the **rolling (paraesophageal) hernia,** which is a protrusion of the greater curvature of the stomach through the esophageal hiatus (Figure 37–1B◆). Although hiatal hernias are believed to be very common, the majority of individuals who have a hiatal hernia have no symptoms.

Epidemiology, Etiology, and Pathophysiology

Hiatal hernias are more prevalent in Western countries than other areas, and their frequency increases with age. Up to 70% of patients who are 70 years of age will develop a hiatal hernia. It is thought that muscle weakening and a loss of elasticity are the primary factors that predispose older adults to have an increased risk of developing a hiatal hernia. Hiatal hernias are more common in women, and this may be due to the increased intra-abdominal pressures associated with pregnancy (Qureshi, 2009).

Several factors contribute to the development of a sliding hiatal hernia, including "a congenitally short esophagus, trauma, or weakening of the diaphragm at the gastroesophageal junction" (Huether, 2010b, p. 1459). The movement of the stomach upward occurs most often when the individual is lying down. Obesity and pregnancy exacerbate this type of hernia, as does anything that increases the intra-abdominal pressure, such as eating a large meal. When the individual assumes a standing position, the hernia slides back into the abdominal cavity. With this type of hernia, there is lower esophageal sphincter (LES) pressure resulting in gastroesophageal reflux (described later) and esophagitis. In a rolling hernia, the gastroesophageal junction remains in the normal position below the diaphragm, and reflux is unusual. However, there can be congestion of the mucosal blood flow in the portion of the stomach that is in the thorax, which can lead to gastritis and ulceration. In rare instances, there can be strangulation of the hernia, causing ischemia and hemorrhage; this requires surgical intervention (Huether, 2010a).

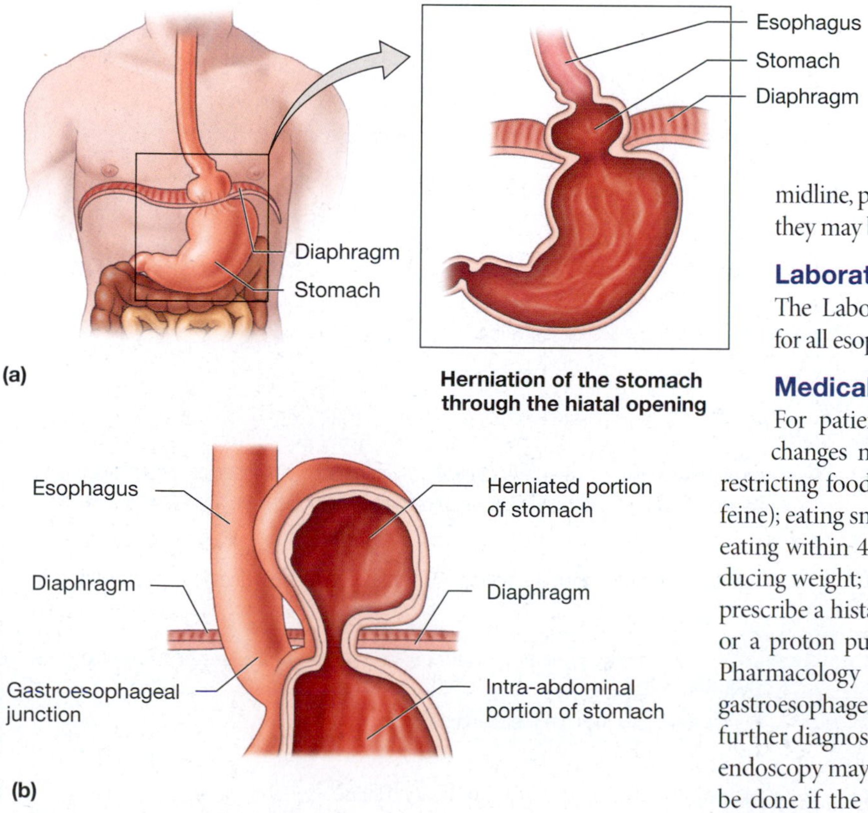

FIGURE 37–1 ◆ (A) Hiatal hernia and (B) Paraesophageal hernia.

Clinical Manifestations

Generally, both types of hiatal hernia are asymptomatic. If symptoms exist, the primary symptoms are reflux and heartburn. Patients often complain of feeling full, belching, and indigestion. Because the stomach herniates into the thoracic cavity near the midline, patients may complain of substernal chest pain and think they may be having a heart attack.

Laboratory and Diagnostic Procedures

The Laboratory and Diagnostic Tests box (p. 1118) lists tests for all esophageal disorders discussed in this chapter.

Medical Management

For patients with mild symptoms of hiatal hernia, lifestyle changes may provide symptom relief. These changes include restricting food that reduces LES pressure (such as alcohol and caffeine); eating small, frequent meals; not lying down after meals; avoid eating within 4 hours of bedtime; elevating the head of the bed; reducing weight; and smoking cessation. The health care provider may prescribe a histamine$_2$ (H_2)-receptor blocker (ranitidine, famotidine) or a proton pump inhibitor (PPI) (lansoprazole, omeprazole). The Pharmacology box (p. 1121) outlines medications used to reduce gastroesophageal reflux. If these medications fail to resolve symptoms, further diagnostic evaluation is indicated. A barium swallow or upper endoscopy may be performed to establish the diagnosis. Surgery may be done if the hernia becomes incarcerated or if severe symptoms persist even with medication. The most common surgical procedure for hiatal hernia is the Nissen fundoplication (Figure 37–2◆, p. 1119).

LABORATORY AND DIAGNOSTIC TESTS for Esophageal Disorders

Test with Description, Rationale, and Normal Values	Expected Abnormality
Upper Endoscopy Normal: no abnormalities *Used to visualize the esophagus directly for tissue abnormalities, including Barrett's epithelium.*	For GERD and tissue abnormalities, including Barrett's epithelium.
Ambulatory Esophageal pH Monitoring Normal: pH 5–6 *Used to evaluate GERD by use of a probe 5 cm above the LES to evaluate pH for 24 hours.*	pH less than 4, indicating acidity in the esophagus.
Barium Swallow Normal: no abnormalities *Used to detect ulcers, polyps, tumors, hiatal hernias, foreign bodies, varices, and strictures in the upper GI tract.*	Any abnormality, such as ulcers, polyps, tumors, hiatal hernias, foreign bodies, varices, and strictures. Esophageal dilatation may be present in achalasia. Narrowing of the esophageal lumen or abnormal mucosa may be seen with esophageal cancer.
Esophageal Manometry Normal: no abnormalities *Used to detect acid reflux and identify causes of heartburn or difficulty swallowing.*	Manometry will show incomplete relaxation of the lower esophageal sphincter (LES) with swallowing, increased resting LES pressure, and no esophageal peristalsis.
Computed Tomography (CT) Normal: no abnormalities *Used to detect lesions, tumors, and metastasis, vascular disease, infection, and bone destruction.*	Any lesions, tumors, or metastatic disease.
Magnetic Resonance Imaging (MRI) Normal: no abnormalities *Used to detect lesions, vascular problems, injury, edema, or tumors.*	Tumors, edema, or any other abnormality.
Red Blood Cell Count Normal: Male: 4.6–6 mcg/L Female: 4–5 mcg/L *Used to detect problems with RBCs, including anemia.*	Decreased levels indicate possible blood loss or anemia.
Hemoglobin Male: 13.5–18 g/dL Female: 12–15 mg/dL *Used to detect the oxygen-carrying capability of the RBCs.*	Lower levels indicate anemia and blood loss.
Hematocrit Male: 40–54% Female: 36–46% *Used to detect the volume of RBCs in the blood.*	Lower levels are associated with anemia and blood loss.
Serum Albumin Normal values: 3.5–5.0 g/dL; 52–68% of total protein *Used to detect albumin deficiency.*	Lower levels may be seen with malabsorption, certain malignancies, and malnutrition as well as in liver and renal disease, prolonged immobilization, and ulcerative colitis.
AST (Aspartate Aminotransferase) Normal: 8–38 units/L *Used to detect liver or cardiac damage.*	Ten times or more above the normal AST is released when there is cellular injury.
ALT (Alanine Aminotransferase) Normal 10–35 units/L *Used to detect liver disease.*	Over 300 units/L. Higher elevations indicate liver damage.
ALP (Alkaline Phosphatase) Normal is 42–136 units/L *Used to detect liver or bone disorders.*	Markedly elevated in severe liver or biliary disease.

Weblink: Achalasia

LABORATORY AND DIAGNOSTIC TESTS for Esophageal Disorders, *continued*

Test with Description, Rationale, and Normal Values	Expected Abnormality
Biopsy	
Normal: no abnormal tissue *Used to detect abnormal cells and tissue.*	Cells are abnormal, indicating the possibility of esophageal cancer, including Barrett's epithelium.

Sources: Fisichella, P. M., & Patti, M. G. (2009). Achalasia. Retrieved from http://emedicine.medscape.com/article/169974-overview; Huether, S. E. (2010a). Alterations of digestive function. In K. L. McCance, S. E. Huether, V. L. Brashers, & N. S. Rote (Eds.), *Pathophysiology: The biologic basis for disease in adults and children* (6th ed., pp. 1452–1515). St. Louis: Mosby; Kee, J. L. (2010). *Laboratory and diagnostic tests with nursing implications* (8th ed.). Upper Saddle River, NJ: Prentice Hall; Thomas, D. J. (2011). Abdominal problems. In L. M. Dunphy, J. E. Winland-Brown, B. O. Porter, & D. J. Thomas, *Primary care: The art and science of advanced practice nursing* (2nd ed., pp. 492–581). Philadelphia: F. A. Davis.

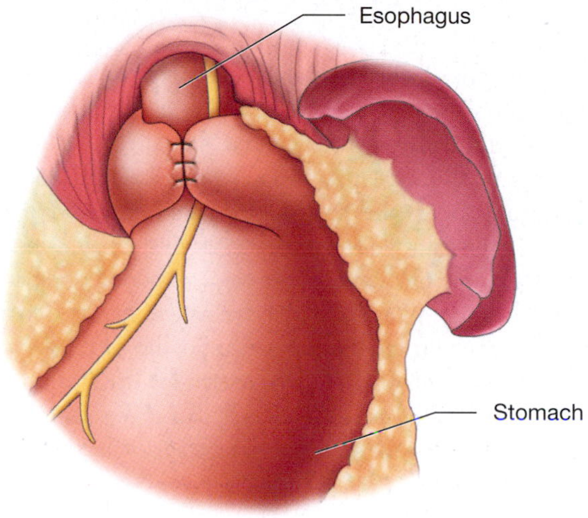

FIGURE 37–2 ◆ Nissen fundoplication.

This procedure strengthens the valve between the stomach and the esophagus by wrapping the upper curve of the stomach (fundus) around the esophagus and sewing it into place.

Gastroesophageal Reflux Disease

Epidemiology, Etiology, and Risk Factors

Gastroesophageal reflux is the backward flow of stomach contents (chyme) into the esophagus without associated vomiting. Gastroesophageal reflux is considered a disease when the symptoms are severe, mucosal damage has occurred, or symptoms occur frequently. Among the adult population in the United States, 10% complain of having heartburn daily; another 35% to 45% of these individuals have symptoms at least once a month. It is believed that the number of people experiencing reflux may actually be much higher, but because many H_2-receptor blockers are available without a prescription, a large number of cases go unreported. The incidence of gastroesophageal reflux disease (GERD) increases after age 50, but it can occur at any age, and its prevalence is equal across gender, ethnic, and cultural groups (Thomas, 2011).

Many factors increase the risk for developing GERD, such as obesity, pregnancy, and hiatal hernia. In addition, a number of foods and medications decrease the LES pressure and therefore increase the risk of GERD. These include alcohol, caffeine, chocolate, fatty foods, spicy foods, citrus fruit, onions, tomatoes, peppermint, beta-adrenergic blockers (e.g., Inderal), calcium-channel blockers (e.g., verapamil), estrogen, progesterone, diazepam (e.g., Valium), and theophylline. Nicotine also lowers LES, including the levels obtained via secondhand smoke (Thomas, 2011).

Pathophysiology

Gastroesophageal reflux disease is caused by relaxation of the LES. Normal LES pressure is 10 to 30 mmHg and is under muscular, hormonal, and neural control; in patients with GERD, the pressure is less than 10 mmHg. The decreased pressure allows for reflux of stomach contents into the esophagus, particularly during activity that increases intra-abdominal pressure, such as coughing, lifting, bending, straining, or lying supine (Thomas, 2011). Because the esophageal mucosa does not contain the same protective mechanism against the acidic stomach contents as does the stomach, mucosal damage and erosion result.

When the esophagus is exposed to gastric contents, an inflammatory response is initiated. Over time, with repeated exposure, this inflammation becomes chronic. The normal squamous epithelial cells are replaced with columnar epithelium, which is more resistant to damage by acidic stomach contents and supports healing of the erosions. However, this new epithelium, called **Barrett's epithelium,** is a premalignant tissue and increases the risk for esophageal cancer (Thomas, 2011). Another result of long-term exposure of the esophagus to stomach acid is the development of esophageal strictures.

Clinical Manifestations

The most common symptom of GERD is heartburn, which can be mild to severe. Additional symptoms that commonly occur are a sour taste in the morning on arising, regurgitation, dysphagia, coughing, belching, and chest pain. Atypical symptoms include asthma or a cough. There are usually no outward physical signs that the patient has GERD, although the stool may test positive for occult blood due to possible microhemorrhages in the irritated esophageal mucosa (Huether, 2010a; Thomas, 2011).

Laboratory and Diagnostic Procedures

The diagnosis of GERD is most often made by evaluating the patient's symptoms and predisposing risk factors. Unfortunately, the severity of the disease does not always correlate with the severity of the symptoms; in fact, severe disease may exist with few symptoms (Thomas, 2011). If symptoms persist after 4 weeks of conservative treatment and lifestyle changes, an upper endoscopy may be done along with other diagnostic procedures, such as ambulatory esophageal pH and barium studies (see the Laboratory and Diagnostic Tests box). Chart 37–1 details nursing care of the patient undergoing endoscopy.

Medical Management

The medical management of GERD involves educating the patient about causative factors and assisting the patient to make lifestyle changes. If the symptoms persist, additional tests will be done to try to identify an underlying cause.

Diet and Lifestyle Modifications

Lifestyle modifications including diet are key in the treatment of GERD. Many patients may have total symptom relief through these

CHART 37–1 Nursing Care of a Patient Undergoing Endoscopy

Pre-Procedure

- Ensure that there is a signed consent in the chart.
- Explain the procedure to the patient and answer any questions she may have.
- Ensure the patient has nothing to eat or drink (NPO) for 8 to 12 hours prior to test.
- Record the name of the person who will be driving the patient home after the test.
- Have the patient remove any jewelry, dentures, or eyeglasses.
- Ensure that the patient empties her bladder before the procedure.
- Take vital signs and start an IV for sedation.
- Explain that there may be a sensation of pressure as the endoscope is inserted and fullness in the stomach as air is injected to expand the stomach and allow for better visualization.

Postprocedure

- Assess vital signs.
- Check gag reflex, NPO until gag reflex returns.
- Monitor for signs of complications: pain, dyspnea, tachycardia, or subcutaneous emphysema in the neck.
- Tell the patient to expect flatus resulting from the instillation of air during the procedure.

efforts alone. Foods that lower LES pressure should be eliminated from the diet or eaten infrequently following use of medication to prevent symptoms. Because spicy foods may irritate the esophageal mucosa, they should be avoided as well. It is often helpful to eat small, frequent meals with the largest meal at midday. The patient should avoid eating anything within 4 hours of bedtime (Thomas, 2011), and the head of the bed should be elevated. Caffeine should be decreased or eliminated completely. Weight loss is important in patients who are overweight or obese. A regular exercise program such as daily walking can promote digestion as well as weight loss, thus diminishing symptoms. Tight garments or belts may increase symptoms by increasing intra-abdominal pressure and should be avoided. Smoking cessation should be considered a priority.

Medications

Medications for GERD can be purchased over the counter or prescribed. It is important to know whether the patient has been self-medicating, what the patient has used, and whether it has helped to relieve the symptoms. The most common medications include antacids, histamine$_2$-receptor blockers, and proton pump inhibitors, all of which are frequently used by individuals with GERD. These medications are very effective in treating GERD and have now been approved for long-term use. They may be needed for 6 months or longer. Proton pump inhibitors have been shown to heal the erosive lesions in addition to decreasing acid production.

Other medications such as metoclopramide (Reglan) promote gastric motility and speed gastric emptying but do not affect acid secretion. By enhancing gastric motility, the amount of time gastric contents have to potentially contact esophageal mucosa is reduced. Long-term use is not recommended, and use is associated with side effects such as fatigue, anxiety, ataxia, and even hallucinations. The Pharmacology box outlines medications used to treat gastroesophageal reflux.

Surgery

Although most patients respond favorably to lifestyle modification and drug treatment, some patients require surgery to resolve GERD. Surgery involves increasing the LES pressure to prevent reflux of gastric contents. Several laparoscopic procedures are used either to tighten the LES with sutures or to cause scar tissue to form in the muscles surrounding the sphincter. The most common antireflux surgical procedure is the Nissen fundoplication (see Figure 37–2).

Nursing Management

Nursing care for the patient with GERD focuses primarily on assessment, prevention of complications, and patient and family teaching.

Assessment

The nurse will ask whether the patient experiences a sour taste in the mouth upon waking or a burning sensation in the mouth or throat when bending or lying down. The nurse should conduct a thorough pain assessment, asking the patient about precipitating factors (such as tight clothing or foods), the quality of the pain (e.g., gnawing or burning), whether the pain radiates, the severity of the pain (using a 0 to 10 rating scale), and the timing of the pain (with food or on an empty stomach). The nurse should ask what the patient has tried to alleviate heartburn and/or pain and the effectiveness of these treatments. A diet history and assessment of knowledge related to GERD and treatment of GERD will focus on needed teaching. An abdominal assessment should be included; the nurse will be specifically evaluating for epigastric tenderness.

Nursing Diagnoses

Possible nursing diagnoses that apply to the patient with GERD include the following:

- *Pain* related to esophageal mucosal injury from contact with gastric secretions.
- *Knowledge, Ready for Enhanced* related to treatment and long-term consequences of GERD.

  NANDA-I © 2012

Planning

The goals for the patient with GERD are to eliminate pain and to have the patient express understanding of the disease process.

Outcomes and Evaluation

Outcomes and evaluation parameters include the following:

- The patient is free from heartburn per patient statement.
- The patient is free from pain.
- The patient verbalizes knowledge about GERD.
- The patient demonstrates management of GERD.

Interventions and Rationales

Nursing interventions and rationales for the patient with GERD include the following:

- Assess pain every 2 to 4 hours using the 0 to 10 pain rating scale. *Using the same scale at regular intervals increases consistency in quantifying pain.*
- Teach the importance of eating 4 to 6 small meals a day and of eliminating foods known to decrease LES pressure or cause irritation. *This decreases reflux.*
- Explain the conversion of squamous epithelial cells to columnar epithelial cells and the possibility of developing cancer if reflux goes

PHARMACOLOGY Summary of Medications Used to Treat Gastroesophageal Reflux

Medication Category and Action	Application/Indication	Nursing Responsibility
Histamine$_2$-Receptor Antagonists (H_2 Blockers)		
Ranitidine (Zantac) Famotidine (Pepcid) Cimetidine (Tagamet) Nizatidine (Axid) ***Action:*** Inhibits all phases of gastric acid secretion by blocking histamine receptors in gastric parietal cells; decreases volume and hydrogen ion concentration in gastric secretions.	GERD, duodenal ulcers, gastric ulcers, chronic hypersecretory conditions.	Monitor for adverse effects: rash, nausea, constipation, diarrhea, abdominal pain, dizziness, and headache. Monitor blood count. Monitor older patients and patients with hepatic or renal disease for CNS effects. Administer 2 hours before or after administration of antacids.
Proton Pump Inhibitors (PPIs)		
Lansoprazole (Prevacid) Omeprazole (Prilosec) Rabeprazole (Aciphex) Esomeprazole (Nexium) Pantoprazole (Protonix) ***Action:*** Decreases gastric acid by binding with H+, K+ ATPase in the gastric parietal cells.	Short-term treatment of GERD with erosive esophagitis (4 to 8 weeks), peptic ulcers, duodenal ulcers, or long-term treatment of chronic hypersecretory conditions. Treatment in combination with antibiotics for *Helicobacter pylori* (*H. pylori*).	Monitor for adverse effects: diarrhea, constipation, nausea, stomach pain, headache, and dizziness. Monitor for altered absorption of medications, vitamins, and minerals requiring an acid environment. Be aware of multiple drug interactions (e.g., warfarin, diazepam, phenytoin, digoxin, theophylline); monitor for signs of elevated serum levels. Instruct patient to take medication 30 minutes prior to meal. Do not crush or chew.
Antacids		
Aluminum hydroxide (Amphojel) Calcium carbonate (Tums) Calcium carbonate/magnesium hydroxide (Rolaids) Magnesium hydroxide (Milk of Magnesia) Magnesium hydroxide/aluminum hydroxide (Maalox, Mylanta) Magaldrate (Riopan) Sodium bicarbonate (Alka-Seltzer) ***Action:*** Neutralizes gastric acid by increasing gastric pH.	GERD, peptic ulcer disease, hyperacidity.	Monitor for constipation if taking calcium- or aluminum-based product, or for diarrhea if taking magnesium-based product. Monitor patients with renal or cardiac insufficiency for signs of accumulation of sodium, magnesium, or calcium from selected antacid. Monitor for hypophosphatemia if taking antacid containing aluminum. Be aware of multiple drug interactions; administer 2 hours before or after other oral medications if medication absorption may be affected.
Prokinetic Agent		
Metoclopramide (Reglan) ***Action:*** Increases gastric emptying and intestinal transit, apparently by working as a dopamine receptor antagonist; lowers esophageal sphincter tone; stimulation of medullary chemoreceptor trigger zone (CTZ) receptors for direct antiemetic effect.	Diabetic gastroparesis, GERD, as an antiemetic postoperatively, and in chemotherapy treatment.	Monitor for adverse effects: restlessness, fatigue, drowsiness, insomnia, headache, confusion, involuntary movements, and diarrhea. Monitor for drug interaction (levodopa, digoxin, narcotics, tetracycline, and others). Monitor electrolytes for hypernatremia and hypokalemia, especially in patients with cardiac insufficiency or hepatic disease. Administer oral dose 30 minutes prior to meals. Warn patient to avoid alcohol, sedatives, and other CNS depressants. Be aware of multiple IV drug incompatibilities and light sensitivity.

Sources: Adams, M. P., & Koch, R. W. (2010). *Pharmacology: Connections to nursing practice.* Upper Saddle River, NJ: Pearson; Wilson, B. A., Shannon, M. T., & Shields, K. M. (2011). *Pearson nurse's drug guide 2011.* New York: Pearson.

untreated over time. *This helps the patient understand the consequences of GERD.*

- Instruct the patient to avoid lying down after eating. *This minimizes reflux.*
- Educate the patient about the medication regimen and possible side effects. *This helps improve adherence to the medication regimen.*

Evaluation

The patient should have no heartburn or pain and should express and demonstrate knowledge of the disease process and management. Topics to be addressed with patients with GERD and/or their families are outlined in the Patient Teaching & Discharge Priorities box.

PATIENT TEACHING & DISCHARGE PRIORITIES for GERD

Need	Teaching
Knowledge of disease process and prognosis	Written and verbal instructions related to: Pathophysiology Risk factors Clinical manifestations Complications
Understanding of medications	Teach the purpose, dose, and possible side effects of all medications (see the Pharmacology Summary of Medications Used to Treat Gastroesophageal Reflux)
Modification of lifestyle	Written and verbal instructions related to diet, meal frequency, weight loss, exercise, and smoking cessation
Reportable clinical manifestations	Instruct patient to report: Chest pain Ongoing symptoms such as regurgitation and heartburn Dysphagia
Psychosocial concerns	Some symptoms, such as chest pain, may be frightening. Calm communication and education are crucial.

Health Promotion

The nurse should teach patients and community members that frequent heartburn may be a sign of GERD and that anyone who experiences this should seek treatment. The long-term consequences of untreated GERD can be serious and include esophageal strictures, Barrett's epithelium, and the possibility of esophageal cancer. See the Patient Teaching & Discharge Priorities for GERD box for some key teaching needs for patients with GERD.

Achalasia

Etiology, Epidemiology, and Clinical Manifestations

Achalasia is a motor disorder of the esophagus that is characterized by impaired peristalsis and failure of the LES to relax properly. This is caused by defective innervation of the smooth muscle of the esophagus and LES. Normally, the LES has tonic contractions with intermittent relaxation. Achalasia has a low prevalence of approximately 0.01%. The clinical manifestations include chronic and progressive dysphagia, regurgitation, and chest pain. The inability of food to pass forward can increase the risk for ulceration or aspiration pneumonia (Enestvedt, Williams, & Sonnenberg, 2011; Huether, 2010a; Kumar, Abbas, Fausto, & Mitchell, 2007).

Pathophysiology

In the patient with achalasia, the LES fails to relax in response to swallowing, and there is a loss of normal peristalsis. The etiology of this disorder is unknown, but it is believed to be a result of autoimmunity causing destruction of myenteric ganglion cells (Huether, 2010a). It results in a functional obstruction because the esophagus is unable to empty properly.

Laboratory and Diagnostic Tests

Upper endoscopy and barium swallow may be helpful in diagnosing achalasia (see the Laboratory and Diagnostic Tests box on page 1118). Fisichella and Patti (2009) also describe the use of esophageal manometry and esophageal pH monitoring (see the entry on ambulatory esophageal pH monitoring in the Laboratory and Diagnostic Tests box) as helpful in diagnosing achalasia and ruling out other diseases.

Medical Management

The traditional treatment of achalasia has been the use of esophageal dilation or myotomy. Esophageal dilation is done by using a balloon catheter (Figure 37–3◆). The pneumatic dilator (balloon) is placed across the LES, usually under fluoroscopy with local anesthesia. This causes small tears in the esophageal sphincter muscle fibers, thereby reducing the pressure. The health care provider performs a myotomy using a laparoscope to incise the circular muscle layer of the LES. A less invasive procedure is performed with the injection of botulinum toxin (botox) into the LES through an endoscopic procedure to relax the sphincter. The disadvantage of this procedure is that the effects of the treatment do not last longer than a year and the procedure may cause inflammatory complications such that a subsequent myotomy cannot be performed (Fisichella & Patti, 2009; Huether, 2010a).

Nursing Management

The nursing management for achalasia includes a detailed assessment of the patient's symptoms and nutrition. The focus then becomes teaching

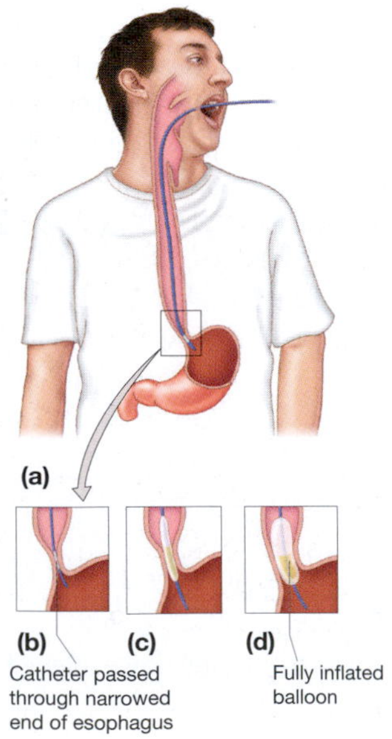

FIGURE 37–3 ◆ Esophageal dilation.

the patient about the disease process and helpful dietary changes. The nurse should determine the presence of primary symptoms, their duration, the factors that increase their frequency or intensity, and what measures the patient has taken to relieve them. A respiratory history is essential because of the potential for aspiration pneumonia. A complete nutritional assessment, including food tolerances and weight loss, will give the nurse an idea of the impact of the esophageal symptoms. The patient with achalasia may have halitosis (foul breath) because of food retained in the esophagus.

Nursing interventions for achalasia include advising the patient to try different foods because some may be better tolerated than others. Warm, soft foods or liquids are often better tolerated than a standard diet, and small, frequent meals may aid in esophageal emptying. Sleeping either with the head of the bed elevated or in a semi-sitting position can help prevent nocturnal reflux.

The nurse should educate the patient and family about what to expect regarding the procedure and symptoms that should be reported to the health care provider. The major nursing responsibility is to monitor the patient for respiratory distress and the return of swallowing after the procedure.

Esophageal Cancer

Epidemiology and Etiology

Esophageal cancer, which is caused by abnormal cell growth anywhere along the esophagus, is almost always fatal. The American Cancer Society (2012a) estimated approximately 17,460 people in the United States were newly diagnosed with esophageal cancer in 2011 with 15,070 expected deaths. Esophageal cancer is the seventh-leading cause of cancer death in men. The overall 5-year survival rate is less than 17% (American Cancer Society, 2010). The chances of survival increase if diagnosis occurs in the early stages. However, because the symptoms often go unrecognized or are associated with other, more benign conditions, esophageal cancer is usually not diagnosed until late in the course of the disease. The risk for esophageal cancer increases with age (over age 70) and is higher in men than women, particularly African American men (Edmondson & Schiech, 2008).

Pathophysiology and Risk Factors

Cancer can occur anywhere along the esophagus but is most common at the junction of the esophagus and stomach. There are two main types of esophageal cancers: squamous cell and adenocarcinoma. The most common type is squamous cell, which is linked to smoking, alcohol consumption, and chewing betel nuts. Adenocarcinoma is less common overall but is more common in Whites than other races. It is associated with the presence of Barrett's epithelium (columnar rather than squamous epithelium) resulting from chronic GERD (Huether, 2010a; Edmondson & Schiech, 2008).

Risk factors for esophageal cancer include age, gender, tobacco use, alcohol consumption, and GERD. Other risk factors include obesity and diets low in fruits and vegetables. Inadequate nutrition also plays a role in genetic mutation in the esophagus (Huether, 2010a).

Clinical Manifestations

The clinical manifestations of esophageal cancer are similar to those of GERD, hiatal hernia, and achalasia; they include dysphagia, heartburn, chest pain, and regurgitation. Dysphagia, as the most common and most diagnostic symptom, is usually progressive, beginning with difficulty swallowing solid food, especially meat, and then progressing to difficulty swallowing soft foods and liquids. The dysphagia usually progresses rapidly over the course of weeks or months.

Laboratory and Diagnostic Tests

Diagnosis of esophageal cancer is made with endoscopic visualization and biopsy. A barium swallow may be done initially. After diagnosis has been made, a CT scan or MRI is usually done to assess for metastasis to other organs. Other laboratory tests are done to assess for nutritional status and liver function and to detect liver metastasis. Refer to the Laboratory and Diagnostic Tests box on page 1118.

Medical Management

The goal of therapy for the patient with esophageal cancer is to control dysphagia and maintain or improve the patient's nutritional status. Surgery is the only definitive treatment and is preferred in patients who are otherwise healthy. Radiation, chemotherapy, and targeted therapies may offer additional treatment options alone or in addition to surgery.

Surgery for esophageal cancer involves removal of the affected area of the esophagus and possibly part of the stomach, as well as reanastomosis (reattachment) of the remaining esophagus to the stomach (Edmondson & Schiech, 2008). It may be done in conjunction with radiation and chemotherapy. Radiation and chemotherapy done preoperatively can shrink the size of the tumor, making removal easier. If the cancer is extensive, has invaded the local tissue, and has metastasized to distant organs, surgery is done for palliation to relieve pain and dysphagia. Laser treatment and stents may be done to keep the esophagus patent in patients who have had surgery, or they may be used as palliation. Tumors in the upper esophagus usually require a tracheostomy and possibly a radical neck dissection with laryngectomy. Chemotherapy drugs may enhance the effects of surgery. Targeted therapies that focus on the malignant cells are currently being studied (Edmondson & Schiech, 2008).

Nursing Management

Nursing care for the patient with esophageal cancer will focus on assessing the severity of the symptoms, providing support once diagnosis has been made, and educating the patient and family on lifestyle changes needed to facilitate palliative care. The Nursing Process: Patient Care Plan (p. 1124) presents the postoperative plan of care for patients with esophageal cancer. Nursing care also involves assessing the patient for side effects related to chemotherapy or radiation therapies, which is discussed in detail in Chapter 57.

Health Promotion

As was stated previously, many of the same risk factors exist for both hiatal hernia and GERD. Reducing obesity may reduce the incidence of these disease processes. Reduction of obesity will also reduce symptoms associated with hiatal hernia and GERD. The aforementioned changes in eating habits and smoking cessation may also help reduce symptoms. Changes in eating habits also help reduce symptoms associated with achalasia. Reducing symptoms of GERD, along with smoking cessation and limited alcohol consumption will help reduce the risk of esophageal cancer. Patients should be encouraged to seek treatment if they experience symptoms associated with GERD (i.e., heartburn) or hiatal hernia (i.e., belching) or have any difficulty in swallowing.

Collaborative Management

The patient with disorders of the esophagus may experience several challenges, which require the collaboration of an interdisciplinary team. The team may include nurses, social workers, oncologists, surgeons, gastroenterologists, nutritionists, and primary care providers. Communication is critical to ensure the best patient care. In order to

NURSING PROCESS: Patient Care Plan for Postoperative Esophageal Cancer

Assessment of Gastrointestinal Status Using Gordon's Functional Health Patterns:

- Nutrition Metabolic Pattern
- Activity Exercise Pattern
- Cognitive Perceptual Pattern

Subjective Data	Objective Data
Assessment of Airway and Gas Exchange	**Assessment of Airway and Gas Exchange**
Assessing level of consciousness (decreased mentation can be a sign of hypoxia): What is your name? What day is it? Do you know where you are? Do you remember why you are here?	Lung sounds. Oxygen saturation. Respiratory rate and character. Color of skin and nail beds.
Assessment of Pain	**Assessment of Pain**
What is your level of pain on a scale of 0 to 10, with 10 being the worst pain? Are you allergic to anything? Do you have any cultural or religious practices for dealing with pain?	Restlessness. Grimacing. Moaning or groaning. Shallow or increased respirations. Increased pulse or blood pressure.
Assessment of Nutrition	**Assessment of Nutrition**
How much weight have you lost? How long did you have difficulty swallowing? What have you been able to eat?	Body weight. Body mass index. Skin condition. Wound healing. Physical appearance. Serum albumin and CBC.

Outcomes and Evaluation Parameters	Planning and Interventions with *Rationales*
1. NURSING DIAGNOSIS: (a) Airway Clearance, Ineffective *related to proximity of surgery to the trachea and thoracic incision.* (b) Gas Exchange, Impaired *related to possibility of aspiration and general anesthesia* (NANDA-I © 2012)	
Outcome: Adequate oxygenation. ***Evaluation Parameters:*** Alert and oriented. Normal pulse oximetry and arterial blood gases. Clear lung sounds. Ability to cough to clear secretions. Unlabored respiration.	Assess level of consciousness. Indicates possible decrease in oxygenation and brain hypoxia. Monitor ABGs and oxygen saturation. *To evaluate gas exchange.* Assess mucous membranes and nail beds for signs of cyanosis. *Indicators of inadequate gas exchange.* Assess for diminished or adventitious breath sounds. Indicates possible aspiration or decreased inspiratory ability related to surgical pain. Encourage deep breathing and coughing and use of incentive spirometer at least every hour. *To promote lung expansion, mobilize secretions, and prevent atelectasis.* Assess the need for suctioning. *To maintain a patent airway.* Monitor respiratory rate and character. *To assess for respiratory distress.* Report respiratory distress to the health care provider. *Early intervention can prevent respiratory failure.*
2. NURSING DIAGNOSIS: Pain, Acute *related to surgery* (NANDA-I © 2012)	
Outcome: Comfort level maintained. ***Evaluation Parameters:*** Able to communicate level of pain and relief from medications. Able to take deep breaths without pain. Appears restful without restlessness or moaning.	Assess pain using pain scale (0 to 10) to quantify pain level. *To increase consistency in monitoring pain.* Assess level of pain 30 minutes and 1 hour after giving pain medication. *To assess effectiveness of medications.* Explore cultural and religious practices and beliefs about pain and illness. Different cultures and religions have varying beliefs about pain, suffering, and disease. Teach nonpharmacologic methods of pain control, such as guided imagery, music therapy, meditation, and breathing exercises. *This may augment pain relief.*

NURSING PROCESS: Patient Care Plan for Postoperative Esophageal Cancer, *continued*

3. NURSING DIAGNOSIS: Imbalanced Nutrition: Less Than Body Requirements *related to dysphagia and pain* (NANDA-I © 2012)

Outcome: Optimal nutrition. ***Evaluation Parameters:*** Maintains body weight or gains weight if underweight. Normal serum albumin. Skin is soft without evidence of dryness. Surgical incision healing. No evidence of skin breakdown.	Monitor body weight at the same time every day. Indicates a degree of adequate calorie intake and fluid balance. Assess skin condition and healing. Adequate dietary protein and calories are needed for wound healing and general skin condition. Monitor laboratory values, particularly serum albumin. Prepare and give parenteral or enteral nutrition as ordered. Assess for edema. The presence of edema is one indicator of low serum proteins. Check placement of feeding tube to prevent aspiration and help ensure adequate nutrition.

Source: Adapted from Wilkinson, J. M., & Ahearn, N. R. (2009). *Prentice Hall nursing diagnosis handbook* (9th ed.). Upper Saddle River, NJ: Prentice Hall.

meet desired patient outcomes, it is essential that this interdisciplinary team communicate openly with one another in developing and evaluating care of the patient and family (IOM [Institute of Medicine], 2010).

Gastroenterologists and primary care providers will help make the diagnosis of esophageal disease processes such as hiatal hernia, GERD, achalasia, and esophageal cancer; they will also provide medical management and follow-up care. A surgeon may be required if there are complications associated with hiatal hernia or if tightening of the LES is required for patients with GERD. A surgeon and oncologist may be needed to treat esophageal cancer.

Patients with diseases of the esophagus will need education about prevention, long-term management, and dietary changes. Nurses can facilitate educating patients about the disease process, lifestyle changes, medication regimen, and follow-up care. Pharmacists can also provide education about medication regimens and possible side effects. Nutritionists will help patients with dietary changes as well as provide education on reducing weight for patients with GERD, hiatal hernia, and achalasia. A collaborative effort is crucial in ensuring that patients with esophageal cancer have adequate nutrition both before and after surgery; this may need to be accomplished through enteral nutrition. Social services can help provide resources for these patients.

Disorders of the Stomach and Duodenum

The stomach is well suited for storing and mixing food with acid and enzymes. Alterations of the stomach lining or malignancies can cause painful and serious disease. The small intestine is the area for most of the digestion and absorption that occur in the digestive tract, with the large intestine absorbing the remaining water and concentrating feces. Diseases of the intestines may manifest themselves as diarrhea, constipation, changes in the character of the stool, or secondary diseases that arise as a result of poor nutrition.

Peptic Ulcer Disease

Peptic ulcer disease (PUD) is a generic term used for any ulceration in the digestive surfaces of the upper GI tract. This includes gastric and duodenal ulcers. The word *ulcer* itself denotes disruption in the protective mucosal lining, thereby exposing the submucosal tissue to gastric secretions and digestion of the submucosa (autodigestion).

Gastric Ulcers: Etiology, Epidemiology and Pathophysiology

Gastric ulcer, an erosion of the stomach lining that develops most often in the antrum, is most commonly seen in patients between the ages of 55 and 70, and occurs with equal frequency in men and women (Thomas, 2011). Gastric ulcers occur less frequently than duodenal ulcers but tend to heal more slowly.

Most gastric ulcers develop in the antrum, adjacent to the body of the stomach where acid is produced. Interestingly, gastric ulcers are associated not with increased acid secretion but rather with a defect in the mucosal barrier to hydrogen ions, allowing the ions to permeate the mucosa (Huether, 2010a). Chronic gastritis may precipitate gastric ulcers by preventing the mucosa's ability to produce a protective layer of mucus. ***Helicobacter pylori* (*H. pylori*),** a bacterium that infects the stomach and duodenum, is associated with peptic ulcers and gastritis and is thought to be responsible for 70% of gastric ulcers (Shrestha & Lau, 2009).

Another factor contributing to the formation of gastric ulcers is decreased prostaglandin secretion by the mucosa, thereby diminishing its protective ability. Medications such as nonsteroidal anti-inflammatory drugs (NSAIDs) inhibit prostaglandin formation. There is a strong association between the habitual use of these drugs and the development of gastric ulcers (Shrestha & Lau, 2009).

Duodenal reflux of bile is another contributing factor in the development of gastric ulcers. Bile salts decrease the electrical potential across the gastric mucosal membrane, allowing hydrogen ions to diffuse into the mucosa, where they disrupt permeability and cellular structure (Huether, 2010a). An inflammatory response is established and histamine is released, stimulating an increase in acid, pepsinogen, blood flow, and capillary permeability leading to edema and minute hemorrhages.

Duodenal Ulcers: Etiology and Epidemiology

Duodenal ulcers are erosions of the duodenal lining resulting from *H. pylori* infection and hypersecretion of acid and pepsin. They are the most common type of peptic ulcer in the United States and are found most often in younger people (ages 30 to 55) (Thomas, 2011). There is an association between people with type O blood and the development of duodenal ulcers, although the relationship is not yet clear (Huether, 2010a). As with gastric ulcers, duodenal ulcers occur equally in men and women.

Almost 75% of patients with duodenal ulcers are infected with *H. pylori* and have ulcers in the proximal duodenum (Thomas, 2011).

H. pylori thrives in the acid environment of the stomach, once thought to be inhospitable to any bacteria. *H. pylori* produces urease, the enzyme that catalyzes the hydrolysis of urea to ammonia (Thomson, Leung, Devlin, & Meddings, 2010). Ammonia is toxic to the gastric epithelial cells and causes an inflammatory response that induces cytokine production, leading to chronic gastritis.

Other factors that contribute to duodenal ulcer formation include hypersecretion of acid and pepsin related to a greater parietal cell mass or to breakdown of the mucosal defenses. There may also be an inadequate secretion of bicarbonate by the duodenal mucosa, which in turn would result in increased secretion of acid. Cigarette smoke stimulates acid production, and NSAIDs inhibit prostaglandins, contributing to increased acid and decreased mucosal defenses (Huether, 2010a; Thomas, 2011).

Clinical Manifestations

The common characteristic of both gastric and duodenal ulcers is pain that is located in the upper abdomen. The pain is intermittent and described as gnawing, burning, aching, or hunger-like (Le & Fantry, 2009). Traditionally, the pain of gastric ulcers was considered to be related to food consumption and relieved by antacids; the pain of duodenal ulcers, in contrast, was relieved by food and commonly occurred before a meal or at night. However, there is wide variability in individual experiences of ulcer pain, and the pattern of pain is not diagnostic. Both duodenal and gastric ulcers produce pain when the stomach is empty that is most often relieved by food or antacids.

Other manifestations, particularly in older adults, are not as easily associated with peptic ulcer disease (PUD). These patients may present with chest pain, dysphagia, or anemia. Anemia may be the presenting symptom in older adults, especially those taking NSAIDs. Typically, gastric ulcers tend to be chronic, whereas duodenal ulcers show periods of remission and exacerbation. Anorexia, weight loss, and vomiting are more common in patients with gastric ulcers, chiefly in those who are older adults (Huether, 2010a).

Complications

Complications of PUD include hemorrhage, perforation, and pyloric or gastric outlet obstruction. All of these complications can be life threatening, but they can be avoided with early diagnosis and treatment.

Bleeding is the most common complication of PUD, especially in older adults. It may occur from an erosion of a small vessel, producing a slow and insidious blood loss, or from an erosion of a larger vessel, leading to severe hemorrhage and shock. When erosion occurs in smaller vessels, anemia and occult blood in the stool may be the only clinical manifestations (positive guaiac). In the erosion of larger vessels, the patient may have bright-red emesis or emesis of partially digested blood, which has a "coffee-grounds" appearance. In addition, these patients usually have melena (dark, tarry stools).

Gastric outlet obstruction (also known as **pyloric obstruction**), which is the result of edema, inflammation, scarring of the pylorus, or a combination of these conditions, obstructs the flow of gastric contents from the stomach to the duodenum. As a slowly evolving process, it often begins with a feeling of epigastric fullness progressing to vomiting. If complete obstruction occurs, gastric acid, sodium, and potassium are lost in the vomitus, which can result in metabolic alkalosis and electrolyte imbalance.

The most serious complication of PUD is perforation. Perforation of the ulcer causes severe, sudden upper abdominal pain that radiates throughout the abdomen. Gastroduodenal contents containing acid, pepsin, bile, and pancreatic juice enter the abdominal cavity, causing peritoneal irritation and peritonitis, which triggers a massive inflammatory response. The classic manifestations of peritonitis—a rigid boardlike abdomen and absence of bowel sounds—happen almost immediately following the perforation. However, the older adult might not exhibit these classic signs; instead, she might have other nonspecific symptoms, thus delaying diagnosis and treatment.

Laboratory and Diagnostic Procedures

Definitive diagnosis is made by direct visualization of the mucosa in the esophagus, stomach, and duodenum using an endoscope. See Chart 37–1 (p. 1120) for the nursing care of a patient undergoing endoscopy. Tissue specimens can be taken during the endoscopic procedure to detect *H. pylori* and malignancy. Because the majority of peptic ulcers are caused by *H. pylori* infection, testing for the organism is often done. The Laboratory and Diagnostic Tests box outlines the different tests that can be used to detect *H. pylori*.

Medical Management

Treatment for PUD is aimed primarily at relieving symptoms, eradicating *H. pylori* infection, and preventing complications such as hemorrhage, obstruction, or perforation. The health care provider makes the diagnosis of PUD through patient history and physical examination. With a high suspicion of the disorder, an initial course of drug therapy will be ordered. If treatment does not provide relief or there is evidence of a complication, further diagnostic testing is done.

Medications

Most peptic ulcers can be successfully treated with medications. The goal of pharmacologic intervention is to eradicate *H. pylori*, and it has a success rate of 85% to 90%. The standard therapeutic regimen includes treatment with two antibiotics and a proton pump inhibitor for 7 to 14 days; it may also include the use of a bismuth preparation. Other medications that are used to treat PUD are antacids, prostaglandin analogs, H_2 blockers, and mucosal barrier fortifiers (Le & Fantry, 2009; Thomas, 2011). See the Pharmacology box (p. 1121) for *H. pylori* eradication.

Lifestyle Modifications

No food is considered ulcerogenic, so there are no specific dietary modifications that individuals with PUD should make. The individual can consume any food that does not cause discomfort, and foods that cause discomfort should be avoided. The patient should be advised not to take NSAIDs or aspirin (or products containing aspirin, such as Excedrin or Alka-Seltzer). Small amounts of alcohol do not cause harm, but large amounts should be avoided. Smoking should be discouraged because it slows the rate of healing; in addition, the recurrence rate of ulcers is increased in patients who smoke. Because *H. pylori* is found in saliva and feces, increasing the possibility of person-to-person transmission through oral-to-oral and fecal-to-oral routes, good hand hygiene should be encouraged. Higher rates of *H. pylori* infection have been found in people living in close contact and where sanitation is not good.

Surgery

Fortunately, with the discovery that *H. pylori* infection is the major cause of peptic ulcers and the development of medications to eradicate this organism, surgery is rarely necessary. However, surgery, such as gastrectomy, may be required to treat the complications of PUD if medical treatment fails. (For the nursing care of the patient having gastric surgery, see the Nursing Process: Patient Care Plan for Gastric Cancer and Gastric Resection, (p. 1132).)

LABORATORY AND DIAGNOSTIC TESTS for *Helicobacter pylori*

Test with Description, Rationale, and Normal Values	Expected Abnormality
Biopsy Urease Test A tissue specimen is obtained during endoscopy and placed in a gel-containing urea. *H. pylori* produces urease, which changes the color of the gel if the organism is present. Normal: No color change	Presence of *H. pylori.*
Biopsy Examination A tissue specimen is sent to the laboratory and examined under the microscope for evidence of *H. pylori.* Presence of *H. pylori* indicates infection. Normal: No evidence of *H. pylori.*	Presence of *H. pylori.*
Enzyme-Linked Immunosorbent Assay (ELISA) A blood sample is tested for antibodies (IgG) against *H. pylori.* The patient has been exposed to *H. pylori* either currently or in the past. Normal: No antibodies.	Current or past infection of *H. pylori.*
Urea Breath Test Radioactive carbon (C-13 or C-14) labeled urea is given in an oral preparation. *H. pylori* metabolizes urea and produces carbon that then travels to the lungs and is exhaled. The amount of radioactive carbon in the breath is measured.	*H. pylori* infection.

Source: Kee, J. L. (2010). *Laboratory and diagnostic tests with nursing implications* (8th ed.). Upper Saddle River, NJ: Prentice Hall.

PHARMACOLOGY Summary of Anti-Infective Medications

Medication Category and Action	Application/Indication	Nursing Responsibility
Anti-Infective Agents Amoxicillin (Amoxil) Clarithromycin (Biaxin) Metronidazole (Flagyl) Tetracycline Metronidazole, bismuth, and tetracycline combination (Helidac) ***Action:*** Treatment protocols: Triple therapy (2 antibiotics + 1 PPI) Quadruple therapy (2 antibiotics + 1 PPI + bismuth) Causes bacterial cell death by inhibition of DNA or bacterial protein synthesis.	Active or inactive peptic ulcer with positive *H. pylori* test.	Monitor for effectiveness: decrease in symptoms of pain, weight loss, and nausea/vomiting. Monitor for adverse effects: rash, diarrhea, and nausea. Instruct patient to complete course of medications as ordered; contact health care provider if patient has adverse reaction. Instruct patient not to crush extended-release forms of drug. Multiple drug interactions; monitor for signs of increased drug levels (theophylline, digoxin, warfarin, and others).

Sources: Adams, M. P., & Koch, R. W. (2010). *Pharmacology: Connections to nursing practice.* Upper Saddle River, NJ: Pearson; Wilson, B. A., Shannon, M. T., & Shields, K. M. (2011). *Pearson nurse's drug guide 2011.* New York: Pearson.

Nursing Management

Most patients with PUD are treated with medications at home unless complications occur; then, hospital admission is necessary. Nursing care focuses on assessing the patient's pain and educating the patient in managing the disease.

Assessment

Nursing assessment should include a general health history with a focused assessment on complaints of epigastric pain and heartburn, including the nature of the pain (burning, gnawing, aching, stabbing) and relationship to eating, the presence of any symptom associated with a complication (dysphagia, vomiting, and presence of blood in the vomitus), what relieves the pain, what makes the pain worse, and the pain rating on a 0-to-10 scale. The nurse should ask about what medications the patient uses, including NSAIDs or aspirin, and whether the patient smokes. The nurse should assess vital signs, conduct an abdominal assessment, and evaluate the patient's vomitus and stool for blood.

Nursing Diagnoses

The main nursing diagnoses to discuss for patients with peptic ulcer disease are as follows:

- *Pain, Acute* related to peptic ulceration and irritation of nerve endings.
- *Knowledge Deficit* related to disease process and management.

(NANDA-I © 2012)

Outcomes and Evaluation Parameters

Outcomes and evaluation parameters for the patient with PUD include the patient verbalizing an understanding of effective pain relief methods. In addition, the patient will verbalize the need for smoking cessation. Finally, the patient will verbalize how to manage the disease and prevent complications.

Interventions and Rationales

Interventions for the patient with PUD include assessing for pain using a 0 to 10 rating scale. Additionally, to establish a pattern to the pain and make a plan to control contributing factors, the nurse needs to determine the character and location of pain and its relationship to the patient's food intake, empty stomach, or other factors, in addition to what relieves the pain. The nurse needs to administer medications ordered to reduce acid secretion and monitor their effectiveness (see the earlier Pharmacology box for details, p. 1127). The nurse needs to stress the importance of following through with the prescribed medication regimen in order to increase the effectiveness of *H. pylori* eradication and decrease the risk of complications.

Patient and family education includes information about the symptoms of complications of PUD and the importance of calling the health care provider immediately if any should occur. The nurse should provide information about the importance of smoking cessation and methods to quit smoking.

Evaluation

The patient with PUD should express a decrease in pain, demonstrate no restlessness or facial grimacing, express knowledge regarding disease management and prevention of complications, and express the importance of smoking cessation.

Safety Alert *Approximately 30 million people in the United States take over-the-counter (OTC) and prescription NSAIDs daily for pain relief, headaches, and arthritis, but many people are unaware of their potential gastrointestinal complications (Cryer & Gerson, 2011). It is important for nurses to assess patient usage of NSAIDS, to ask patients about stomach problems, and to assess other personal risk factors such as a history of ulcers and alcohol use. Education related to NSAIDs and other risk factors may help prevent PUD.*

Health Promotion

The thrust of health promotion to prevent PUD is to advise people to avoid known risk factors. As with chronic gastritis and GERD, these risk factors include cigarette smoking, excessive and prolonged alcohol ingestion, the use of oral corticosteroids, and the excessive use of NSAIDs and aspirin. Chronic gastritis and GERD do contribute to ulcer formation, and patients should be encouraged to seek treatment for these disorders. Nurses should use every opportunity to refute the common misconception that ulcers are caused from eating spicy food; however, certain foods may precipitate symptoms in some individuals with PUD. The nurse should encourage patients to pay attention to their own reactions to foods they eat and tailor their diets accordingly.

Cancer of the Stomach

Epidemiology and Etiology

Gastric carcinoma (cancer in the stomach) is the second most common cancer in the world, though it is less common in the United States (Kumar et al., 2007). The American Cancer Society (2012b) estimated that approximately 21,320 people in the United States were newly diagnosed with stomach cancer in 2011, with 10,540 expected deaths. The overall 5-year survival rate is less than 26% (American Cancer Society, 2012b). It is more prevalent in men, with the highest incidences in Hispanics, African Americans, and Asian Americans; the disease is more prevalent in Japan (American Cancer Society, 2011c).

The majority of gastric cancer develops in the distal portions of the stomach and can be attributed to *H. pylori* infection. Family history, increased age, tobacco use, type A blood, gastric polyps, pernicious anemia, and dietary factors such as the use of nitrates (used to preserve meats) and smoked meats may also contribute to the development of gastric cancer (American Cancer Society, 2011c). Lack of hydrochloric acid in the stomach (**achlorhydria**), atrophic gastritis, and history of gastric resection are also known to be risk factors for gastric cancer.

Pathophysiology

The most common type of cancer that develops in the stomach is adenocarcinoma. Although stomach cancer can develop on any mucosal surface, it is most common in the antrum and distal portions of the stomach (Huether, 2010a). Early gastric cancer may involve the mucosa and submucosa and is usually asymptomatic. As the lesion progresses, it spreads to the gastric wall and regional lymph nodes. It may then advance to adjacent organs such as the liver, pancreas, and transverse colon. Because the stomach has a rich blood and lymphatic supply, the cancer spreads via the portal vein to the liver and through the systemic circulation to the lungs. Metastasis has also been found in bone, ovarian, and peritoneal tissue.

Clinical Manifestations

Regrettably, there are rarely any symptoms associated with gastric cancer. The patient may complain of anorexia, indigestion, heartburn, or early satiety, but these are vague, and often the patient does not consider them serious. The patient may self-diagnose and self-treat with over-the-counter medications such as antacids, H_2-receptor antagonists, or proton pump inhibitors. Weight loss occurs as the disease progresses, and the patient eventually becomes cachectic (physical wasting including loss of muscle mass and weight due to disease). When the patient's health fails, that is when the patient usually seeks medical attention and diagnosis is made. By this time, the disease is advanced and prognosis is poor.

Laboratory and Diagnostic Procedures

Definitive diagnosis of gastric cancer is done through upper endoscopy and biopsy. See Chart 37–1 (p. 1120) for the nursing care of a patient undergoing endoscopy. Other tests, such as an abdominal ultrasound and small bowel series, may be used to assess the extent of the cancer. See the Laboratory and Diagnostic Tests box.

Medical Management

The medical management of gastric cancer involves identification of the cancer, followed in most cases by surgical removal of the tumor.

Surgery

Surgical resection of the stomach is considered the treatment of choice if gastric cancer is diagnosed early, or it may be performed for palliation if the cancer is more advanced. A partial gastrectomy (removal of a portion of the stomach) can be done in several ways. The two most common partial gastrectomy procedures are the gastroduodenostomy (an operation known as Billroth I), whereby the lower portion of the stomach is removed and the remainder is anastomosed to the duodenum (Figure 37–4A ◆), and the gastrojejunostomy (known as Billroth II), which involves removal of a larger distal portion of the stomach and anastomosis of the remainder to the jejunum (Figure 37–4B ◆). In total gastrectomy,

LABORATORY AND DIAGNOSTIC TESTS for Stomach Disorders

Test with Description, Rationale, and Normal Values	Expected Abnormality
Abdominal Ultrasound Normal: no abnormalities *Used to examine the size and structure of organs.*	Will see abnormalities in tissue lining, size, and structure of organs.
Small Bowel Series Normal: no abnormalities *Used to detect ulcers, polyps, tumors, hiatal hernias, foreign bodies, varices, and strictures in the upper GI tract.*	Any abnormality, such as ulcers, polyps, tumors, hiatal hernias, foreign bodies, varices, and strictures.
Upper Endoscopy Normal: no abnormalities *Used to visualize the stomach for tissue abnormalities.*	Tissue abnormalities in the stomach will be seen.
Biopsy Normal: no abnormal tissue *Used to detect abnormal cells, such as cancer cells.*	Cells are abnormal, indicating possible stomach cancer.

Source: Kee, J. L. (2010). *Laboratory and diagnostic tests with nursing implications* (8th ed.). Upper Saddle River, NJ: Prentice Hall.

the removal of the entire stomach, the esophagus is anastomosed to either the duodenum or the jejunum (Figure 37–4C ◆).

Long-term complications of gastric surgery are not uncommon. The most common problem is dumping syndrome, whereby the pylorus is bypassed and a food bolus enters the duodenum or jejunum rapidly. Because chyme (partially digested food in the stomach containing gastric acid and digestive enzymes) is hyperosmolar, water is pulled into the intestinal lumen, causing a rapid decrease in blood volume. When the blood volume is decreased, a reflex sympathetic nervous system response is manifested by tachycardia, orthostatic hypotension, dizziness, flushing, and diaphoresis. Additional symptoms such as nausea, epigastric pain, cramping, diarrhea, and loud, hyperactive bowel sounds (borborygmi) can also occur. A later manifestation of dumping syndrome is a rapid rise in blood sugar with a resultant release of excessive amounts of insulin. The insulin causes a secondary hypoglycemia to occur about 1 to 3 hours after eating (Huether, 2010a). The symptoms can be managed by eating small, frequent meals. Carbohydrates should be reduced while the amounts of protein and fat are increased in order to help slow the transit time. Fluids at meal time should be restricted. The patient should be instructed to lie down for 30 to 60 minutes after eating to slow transit time further.

Removal of any portion of the stomach can affect vitamin and mineral absorption. For example, iron is primarily absorbed from the duodenum and proximal jejunum. With the extensive surgery coupled with the rapid gastric emptying, interference with iron absorption can manifest in anemia. Gastric resection may also decrease the amount of intrinsic factor produced by the parietal cells. Intrinsic factor is needed for the absorption of vitamin B_{12}, so the patient should be observed for pernicious anemia.

Radiation/Chemotherapy

Radiation or chemotherapy (Chapter 57) may be used to arrest metastatic or lymphatic spread of gastric carcinoma. It is considered palliative in patients with advanced disease to help shrink the tumor and provide some pain relief.

Targeted Therapy

Certain targeted therapies such as angiogenesis inhibitors or drugs that target epidermal growth factor receptors may be used to inhibit growth-promoting cells. Patients may have flulike symptoms related to this therapy.

Nutrition

Because of the location of the cancer, many patients will require a feeding tube, in the form of either a gastrostomy tube if the total stomach has been affected or, if there is a sufficient portion of the stomach remaining, a jejunostomy tube (Figure 37–5◆, p. 1131). Chart 37–2 indicates nursing care of the patient with a feeding tube.

Nursing Management

Nursing care of the patient with gastric cancer is mostly supportive. If there is no metastasis, surgical resection of the stomach is performed. For a detailed discussion on care of the patient with cancer, refer to Chapter 57. Application of the nursing process can facilitate a comprehensive approach to patient care. The Nursing Process box (p. 1132) covers the nursing management plan for patients with gastric cancer or having gastric resection.

Health Promotion

The nurse can educate the public about the contributing factors to the development of gastric cancer, such as avoiding or limiting foods containing nitrates, which include smoked meats, bacon, lunch meats, hot dogs, and any other meat product that does not require refrigeration. If a patient is known to have *H. pylori*, the nurse should encourage completion of the prescribed course of medications and return for follow-up to evaluate *H. pylori* eradication.

Collaborative Management

The patient with stomach problems may experience a myriad of changes that necessitate the collaboration and excellent communication of an interdisciplinary team. The team may include nurses, social workers, oncologists, surgeons, gastroenterologists, nutritionists, and primary care providers. In order to meet desired patient outcomes, it is essential that this interdisciplinary team communicate openly with one another in developing and evaluating care of the patient and family (IOM [Institute of Medicine], 2010).

As with disorders of the esophagus, primary care providers and gastroenterologists need to carefully assess and diagnose stomach problems. Patients with complications, such as bleeding, may need a critical care intervention.

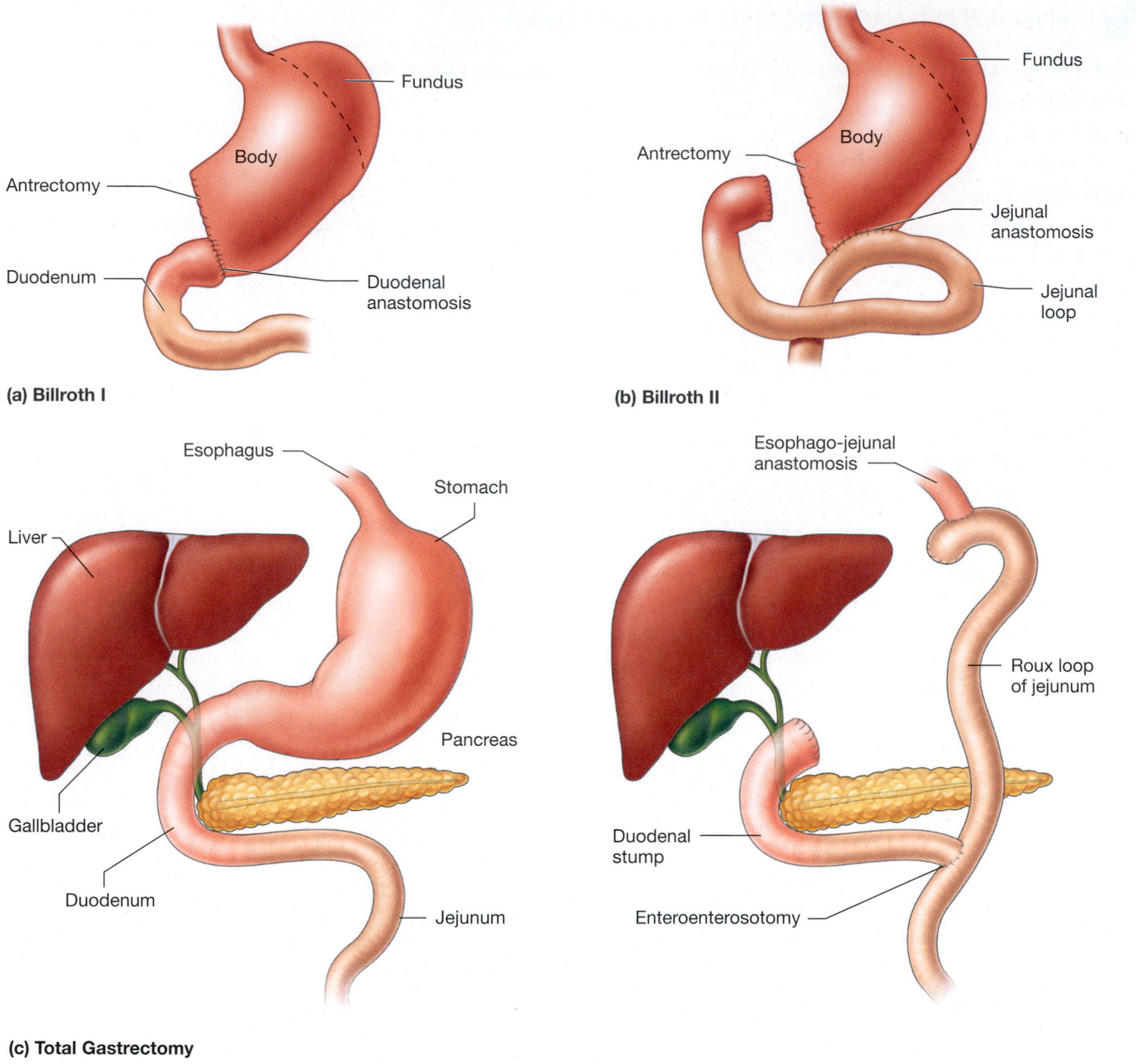

FIGURE 37–4 ◆ (A) Billroth I, (B) Billroth II, and (C) total gastrectomy.

Nurses will facilitate education regarding prevention, long-term management, needed lifestyle changes, and dietary changes. Pharmacists can provide education about medication regimens and possible side effects. Nutritionists will help patients with dietary changes and promote good nutrition before and after surgical procedures such as gastrectomy. Social services can help provide resources for these patients.

Malabsorption and Maldigestion Syndromes

Malabsorption is the failure of the small intestine to absorb nutrients from digested food, whereas **maldigestion** is the failure of chemical processes, such as inadequate pancreatic enzymes or bile salts, to break down food products. Maldigestive disorders result in the malabsorption of nutrients and thus are considered a form of malabsorption. In addition to absorptive failure, malabsorption can be caused by surgical resection of the stomach and intestines or by vascular disorders or intestinal diseases (Huether, 2010a).

Celiac Disease

Etiology and Epidemiology

Celiac disease, also known as gluten-sensitive enteropathy and celiac sprue, is an autoimmune disorder in the mucosal lining of the small intestine triggered when gluten (from wheat, rye, or barley) is ingested. Celiac disease can occur in individuals at any age and may affect as many as 1 in 133 people in the United States (Martin, 2008).

Pathophysiology

Development of celiac disease involves a genetic predisposition for the disease, gluten ingestion, and immune-mediated responses. When a genetically susceptible individual ingests a product that contains gluten, there is a T-cell mediated immune response, and chronic inflammation develops if ingestion is continued (Kumar et al., 2007). The microvilli

CHART 37–2 Nursing Care of the Patient with a Feeding Tube

The purpose of a gastrostomy tube or a jejunostomy tube is to provide complete nutrition through the alimentary system. It is safer and has fewer side effects than intravenous total parenteral nutrition (TPN), particularly when the patient is to have feedings at home.

Check Tube Placement

- Aspirate and check the pH of the aspirate.
- A pH of 5 or less indicates gastric placement.
- A pH of 7 or more usually indicates intestinal placement.

Irrigate Tube

- Gently instill 30 to 50 milliliters of water before and after each feeding or as ordered.

Cleanse Insertion Site

- Remove the old dressing (using clean gloves).
- Inspect the site for healing or signs of infection (drainage, redness, or swelling).
- Clean the site using saline or whatever solution is ordered, using sterile technique if the stoma is not yet healed or clean technique if the site is healed.
- Apply a fresh dressing using a drain sponge. (Do not cut gauze dressing; it will fray, and threads may enter the wound.)

Monitor for Intolerance to Feedings

- Assess the abdomen for distention.
- Auscultate bowel sounds.
- Palpate the abdomen to assess for tenderness.

Conduct Patient and Family Teaching

- Tube care (patient may clean site in the shower after stoma has healed).
- Feeding schedule.
- Monitoring for side effects of feeding.

and the brush border of the small intestine are destroyed by the release of cytokines. Continued ingestion of gluten will cause the eventual disappearance of the microvilli and the loss of brush border digestive enzymes, which results in malabsorption (Martin, 2008).

Clinical Manifestations

Although diarrhea is the most common symptom in patients with celiac disease, up to 38% of patients are asymptomatic because the small intestine can compensate if the degree of involvement is limited. In fact, most adults have signs and symptoms that are unrelated to the GI tract, such as symptoms of type 1 diabetes mellitus, chronic hepatitis, dental enamel hypoplasia (less quantity of enamel), iron deficiency anemia, neurological dysfunction, osteoporosis, and cardiomyopathy. Other gastrointestinal symptoms may include flatulence, weight loss, and borborygmus (stomach growling) (Martin, 2008; Presutti, Cangemi, Cassidy, & Hill, 2007).

Laboratory and Diagnostic Procedures

A biopsy of the small intestine is considered the gold standard for diagnosing celiac disease. Serologic tests for celiac disease are proving to be sensitive and specific. These include tests for immunoglobulin A endomysium antibodies (IgA EMA) and the IgA tissue transglutaminase (tTG) antibodies (Martin, 2008). See the Laboratory and Diagnostic Tests box on page 1133.

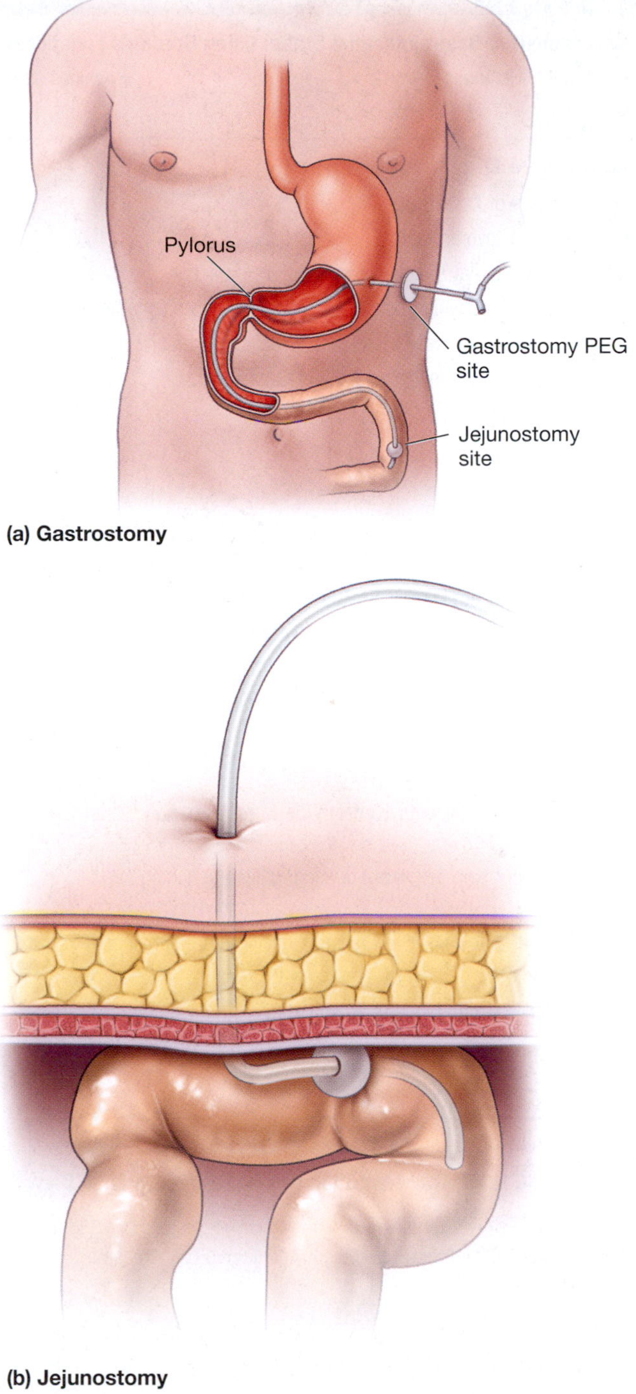

FIGURE 37–5 ◆ Gastrostomy and jejunostomy tube.

Medical Management

At the present time, the only treatment for celiac disease is a totally gluten-free diet. Gluten is found in wheat, barley, and rye grains (Chart 37–3). Some sources report that oats and corn products should also be avoided because they may be contaminated by being processed in machines that also process wheat, rye, and barley without interim cleanings and decontamination. Since additives, preservatives, and stabilizers may contain gluten, many foods, medicines, and other products (such as lipstick) may also cause symptoms (Martin, 2008; Presutti, Cangemi, Cassidy, & Hill, 2007).

NURSING PROCESS: Patient Care Plan for Gastric Cancer and Gastric Resection

Assessment of Gastrointestinal Status Using Gordon's Functional Health Patterns:

- Nutrition Metabolic Pattern
- Cognitive Perceptual Pattern
- Values and Belief Pattern

Subjective Data

Assessment of Nutrition

What are your favorite foods?

Describe a usual day's diet.

How much did you weigh before you found out about your cancer?

Had you noticed any weight loss before that? How much?

Do you feel full after eating a small amount?

Are you nauseated?

Assessment of Emotional Status

What have the doctors told you about your cancer?

Who do you count on for support?

Do you have any religious, cultural, or spiritual beliefs that help you deal with your cancer?

Assessment of Pain

On a scale of 0 to 10, with 10 being the worst pain, how would you rate your pain?

What does your pain feel like—burning, gnawing, aching, or stabbing?

Have you felt nauseated?

Did you vomit?

Did the vomit contain blood or brown fluid?

Objective Data

Assessment of Nutrition

Daily weights.

Intake and output (I&O).

General appearance.

Laboratory studies:

Serum albumin

H & H

Transferrin

Ferritin

TIBC

Electrolytes.

Assessment of Emotional Status

Family or friends visiting.

Clergy visiting.

Initiates conversations with the nursing staff.

Assessment of Pain

Vital signs.

Abdominal examination:

Distention?

Pain or tenderness on palpation?

Bowel sounds?

Soft or rigid?

Stool for occult blood.

Facial grimacing.

Restless, holding abdomen.

Outcomes and Evaluation Parameters / Planning and Interventions with *Rationales*

1. NURSING DIAGNOSIS: Nutrition Imbalanced: Less Than Body Requirements *related to removal of part of stomach* (NANDA-I © 2012)

Outcome: Adequate nutrition.

Evaluation Parameters: Body weight maintained or increased.

Healing incision.

Normal serum albumin.

Normal serum electrolytes.

Normal iron studies.

Normal hemoglobin and hematocrit.

See Chart 37–2 for nursing interventions for patients with feeding tubes.

Weigh daily at the same time and on the same scale to provide an accurate assessment of fluid balance and nutritional adequacy.

Measure and record accurate intake and output *to estimate fluid balance.*

Monitor laboratory indicators of nutritional status. These are better indicators of nutritional status than body weight alone.

Assess skin for breakdown. Can be an indicator of nutritional status, particularly protein.

Assess wound healing. Decreased protein and vitamin C can hinder wound healing.

Medicate for nausea and pain as needed before meals. Pain and nausea often produce anorexia and relief can increase the appetite.

Provide the patient with favorite foods or have family members bring home-prepared food when she is able to eat *to increase the patient's nutritional intake.*

Invite family or friends to visit at mealtime. *Gathering for meals is a social function for many families and may improve the patient's intake.*

NURSING PROCESS: Patient Care Plan for Gastric Cancer and Gastric Resection, *continued*

2. NURSING DIAGNOSIS: Grieving, Complicated *related to diagnosis of cancer with poor prognosis* (NANDA-I © 2012)

Outcome: Anxiety and fear controlled.

Evaluation Parameters: Verbalizes fears about cancer and death.

Communicates feelings with significant others.

Encourage family and significant others to spend as much time as possible with the patient, especially during difficult times such as visits from the health care provider and during chemotherapy and radiation treatments *to give purpose to the family and significant others and help them feel a part of the process.*

Allow the patient to express any feelings without negating any of these feelings. *Allowing the patient to have hope may aid in coping behavior.*

Inquire about the patient's cultural, religious, and spiritual beliefs about illness and death, and facilitate discussion with family and clergy where appropriate. *Spiritual and cultural beliefs can comfort the patient and family during this time.*

3. NURSING DIAGNOSIS: Pain, Acute *related to surgical incision and metastatic cancer* (NANDA-I © 2012)

Outcome: Pain relieved.

Evaluation Parameters: Able to communicate level of pain and therapies that relieve it.

Abdomen soft, nontender, and bowel sounds present.

No restlessness or facial grimacing.

Assess pain using a pain scale (0 to 10) to quantify pain *to increase consistency in pain measurement.*

Assess pain, character and location, and any related symptoms to give the nurse clues to the cause of the pain (i.e., incisional pain vs. infection, vs. peritonitis, vs. metastatic cancer).

Administer pain medications as ordered and assess pain level 30 minutes and 1 hour after administration *to evaluate the effectiveness of the pain medication.*

Source: Adapted from Wilkinson, J. M., & Ahearn, N. R. (2009). *Prentice Hall nursing diagnosis handbook* (9th ed.). Upper Saddle River, NJ: Prentice Hall.

LABORATORY AND DIAGNOSTIC TESTS for Malabsorption/Maldigestion Syndromes

Test with Description, Rationale, and Normal Values	Expected Abnormality
Biopsy Normal: no abnormal tissue	Cells in the mucosa are flattened with an absence of villi in celiac disease.
Celiac Disease (Serologic) Normal: negative *Used to detect celiac disease.*	Positive tests may indicate celiac disease.
Immunoglobulin A endomysium antibodies (IgA EMA) Normal: negative *Used to detect celiac disease.*	Positive tests may indicate celiac disease.
Immunoglobulin A transglutaminase (tTG) Normal: negative *Used to detect celiac disease.*	Positive tests may indicate celiac disease.
Lactose Breath Test Normal: negative *Used to detect lactase deficiency through the presence of hydrogen.*	The presence of hydrogen indicates a possible lactase deficiency.
Lipase Normal: 20–180 IU/L *Used to detect pancreatic problems.*	Elevated levels are seen in pancreatitis. Decreased levels may indicate pancreatic insufficiency.
Amylase Normal: 60–100 somogyi unit/dL *Used to detect pancreatic problems.*	Elevated levels may be seen in pancreatitis. Decreased levels may be seen in advanced chronic pancreatitis, chronic alcoholism, toxic hepatitis, or pancreatic insufficiency.
Urinary Amylase Normal: 6.5–48 units/hr *Used to detect pancreatic problems.*	Elevated levels indicate acute pancreatitis. Decreased levels indicate diminished renal function.
Fat in Stool Normal: 2–7 g/24 hours *Used to identify whether fat is in stool.*	Elevated levels indicate malabsorption or maldigestion. Increased levels may correspond to decreased lipase secretion.

Sources: Huether, S. E. (2010b). Structure and function of the digestive system. In K. L. McCance, S. E. Huether, V. L. Brashers, & N. S. Rote (Eds.), *Pathophysiology: The biologic basis for disease in adults and children* (6th ed., pp. 1420–1451). St. Louis: Mosby; Kee, J. L. (2010). *Laboratory and diagnostic tests with nursing implications* (8th ed.). Upper Saddle River, NJ: Prentice Hall; Martin, S. (2008). Against the grain: An overview of celiac disease. *Journal of the American Academy of Nurse Practitioners, 20*(5), 243–250. doi:10.1111/j.1745-7599.2008.00314.x; McQuaid, K. R. (2010). Gastrointestinal disorders. In S. J. McPhee & M. A. Papadakis (Eds.), *Current medical diagnosis and treatment* (49th ed., pp. 502–597). New York: McGraw Hill.

CHART 37–3 Common Sources of Gluten That Should Be Avoided by the Patient with Celiac Disease

Barley malt	Bleached flour	Bran
Beer	Brewer's yeast	Bulgur wheat
Bread flour	Couscous	Durum wheat
Coloring	Farina	Fillers
Edible starch	Gluten	Kamut
Food starch	Malt extract	Malt flavoring
Malt	Malt vinegar	Matzo
Malt syrup	Pasta	Pearl barley
Miso	Seitan	Semolina
Rye	Soba noodles	Spelt
Shoyu (soy sauce)	Wheat	Wheat germ
Vegetable starch	Wheat germ oil	Wheat grass
Wheat germ extract		
Seasoned French fries (coated with flour)		

Nursing Management

Support and education are the major nursing responsibilities in the care of individuals with celiac disease. Because the treatment is total elimination of gluten from the diet, the nurse needs to be well informed about foods that contain gluten in order to teach the patient diet modification. Potential hidden sources of gluten should be identified, such as canned or homemade cream soup, cream sauces, gravy, and some candies. Chart 37–3 lists the most common foods that contain gluten. Some items that contain gluten and are often overlooked include stamps, envelopes, and gummed labels, some toothpaste, some vitamins, and some laxatives. The nurse should be familiar with celiac-related resources, such as the numerous organizations and websites that provide support, information, and gluten-free products.

Lactose Intolerance

Etiology, Epidemiology, and Clinical Manifestations

Lactose intolerance is caused by a deficiency of lactase at the brush border of the small intestine, resulting in malabsorption. Lactase is an enzyme that aids in the breakdown of lactose, a disaccharide found in milk, into a monosaccharide, which can then be absorbed in the small intestine. The deficiency is usually the result of a congenital defect but also can be caused by several diseases of the intestine, including celiac disease. Lactase deficiency is very common. In fact, it may affect as many as 90% of Asians, 95% of Native Americans, 50% of Mexican Americans, and 70% of African Americans. Because of the lactase deficiency, there is undigested lactose in the intestines. This causes two issues. First, intestinal bacteria cause fermentation of the undigested lactose, which produces gas. Second, because lactose is a large molecule, it increases the osmotic gradient in the intestines. These two processes produce the symptoms of lactose intolerance, which include bloating, abdominal distention, flatulence, crampy pain, and diarrhea. However, many individuals may remain symptom free unless they ingest large amounts of milk and milk-containing foods at one time (Huether, 2010a; McQuaid, 2010).

Laboratory and Diagnostic Procedures

Lactase deficiency is diagnosed by using the lactose breath test. Refer to the Laboratory and Diagnostic Tests box on page 1133.

Medical Management

Elimination of lactose from the diet will relieve the symptoms of lactose intolerance. Therefore, individuals should avoid foods that cause symptoms. Some individuals may tolerate small amounts of lactose and may include in their diets foods that are lower in lactose, such as aged cheese and yogurt. There are lactase enzymes (Lactaid) available without a prescription to improve lactose tolerance; milk containing lactase is also available. Individuals who must avoid all dairy products, particularly women, may require calcium supplementation in order to get the minimum daily requirement of this mineral. The diet of most Americans contains more than adequate protein, so eliminating dairy products should not cause protein deficiency.

Nursing Management

Nursing care for the patient with a lactase deficiency centers on educating the patient and family about sources of lactose and appropriate nutritional alternatives. Lactose is most concentrated in milk, ice cream, and cottage cheese but is also found in other cheeses, milk chocolate, sherbet, custard, and cream soups. The nurse should teach the patient and family how to read labels in order to detect lactose in food.

Pancreatic Insufficiency

Etiology and Pathophysiology

Pancreatic insufficiency is a deficiency of pancreatic enzymes resulting in malabsorption of nutrients. Lipase, trypsin, chymotrypsin, and amylase are needed to digest fat, protein, and carbohydrates. If these pancreatic enzymes are insufficient, maldigestion occurs. A deficiency in pancreatic enzymes can be caused by pancreatitis, pancreatic cancer, cystic fibrosis, and pancreatic abscess (Huether, 2010a). However, there must be significant pancreatic damage before insufficiency results.

Clinical Manifestations

Pancreatic insufficiency results in maldigestion of all nutrients; however, because enzymes secreted by the intestinal brush border and salivary amylase help to digest carbohydrates and proteins, maldigestion of these nutrients is not profound. However, these enzymes do not aid in the digestion of fat, so there is a profound inability to digest fats, resulting in **steatorrhea** (fat in the stools) and weight loss (Huether, 2010a). There could also be problems with the absorption of fat-soluble vitamins.

Laboratory and Diagnostic Procedures

Pancreatic insufficiency can be determined by evaluating the function of the pancreas. Tests include lipase, amylase, urinary amylase, and evaluations for fat in the stool (Huether, 2010b). Refer to the Laboratory and Diagnostic Tests box on page 1133.

Medical and Nursing Management and Health Promotion

Pancreatic insufficiency is treated with supplemental pancreatic enzymes. The nurse should administer the enzymes (Viokase) before meals. The Pharmacology box outlines the use of supplemental enzymes. The nurse should teach the patient and family about the administration of the medication, to monitor for signs of vitamin deficiency, and to notify the health care provider if weight loss or steatorrhea occurs.

PHARMACOLOGY Summary of Medications Used to Treat Pancreatic Insufficiency

Medication Category and Action	Application/Indication	Nursing Responsibility
Digestive Enzymes		
Pancrelipase (Viokase) ***Action:*** Breaks down fats, proteins, and starches in the final stage of digestion for easier absorption.	Replacement related to malabsorption, cystic fibrosis, or other diseases causing insufficient pancreatic enzymes.	Monitor for adverse effects: nausea, anorexia, and diarrhea. Assess for improved nutritional status and decreased steatorrhea. Be aware of religious considerations; drug is pork based.

Short Bowel Syndrome

Etiology, Epidemiology, and Clinical Manifestations

Short bowel syndrome results when there is a reduction in the surface of the small intestine from surgical resection of the small bowel, typically because of tumors, Crohn's disease, infarction, trauma, and radiation enteritis (McQuaid, 2010). The degree of the resulting malabsorption depends on the location and extent of the resection. For example, if the duodenum, jejunum, or proximal ileum is removed, severe malabsorption usually occurs. The incidence of short bowel syndrome is rare; most estimates are based on patients requiring long-term home parenteral nutrition. It is estimated that there are approximately 10,000 to 20,000 patients in the United States who receive home parenteral nutrition for short bowel syndrome (Cagir, 2012).

The absorption of water, nutrients, vitamins, and minerals is hindered in the early postoperative period after small bowel resection. If a large portion of the small intestine is removed, the transit time is significantly reduced. With time, the bowel adapts by enlarging and lengthening the villi that remain, thereby increasing the surface area available for absorption. Some patients may achieve levels of digestion and absorption that are similar to what they experienced before the resection. However, a significant number of patients have considerable malabsorption that leads to diarrhea, weight loss, dehydration, and nutrient deficiencies (McQuaid, 2010).

Medical Management

Treatment for short bowel syndrome focuses on relief of symptoms and methods to maintain nutrition. To maintain nutrition, small, frequent feedings of high-calorie, high-protein foods are usually prescribed if the patient can tolerate oral feedings. If oral feedings are not tolerated, then enteral tube feedings or total parenteral nutrition (TPN) will be ordered. Supplementation with vitamins and minerals is frequently necessary.

If diarrhea is a continued problem, antidiarrheal medications, such as Lomotil, which slows intestinal motility, will be ordered. Proton pump inhibitors such as omeprazole (Prilosec) may be ordered for patients who have gastric reflux or hypersecretion of gastric acid postoperatively. See the Pharmacology box (p. 1121), which outlines the use of proton pump inhibitors, and the Pharmacology Summary of Medications Used to Treat Diarrhea box.

Nursing Management

Because the patient with short bowel syndrome is at risk for diarrhea, particularly in the early postoperative period, fluid and electrolyte imbalances are possible. The nurse should take vital signs frequently, monitor the condition of the patient's mucous membranes, weigh the patient daily, and keep an accurate record of intake and output including measuring the volume of diarrhea.

The patient is also at risk for nutritional deficits. The health care provider may order intravenous TPN to maintain the patient's nutritional status until the GI tract has recovered from surgical resection. The nurse monitors the patient's weight, laboratory values, central IV catheter, and insertion site. Once the patient's bowel sounds have returned, oral or enteral feedings may be started. It is important to monitor the patient's tolerance of the feeding once it is begun.

Educating the patient and family members is a major nursing responsibility. The patient will most likely have some problems with digestion and/or absorption for the rest of his life and will need guidance about the recommended diet and ways to maintain nutritional

PHARMACOLOGY Summary of Mediations Used to Treat Diarrhea

Medication Category and Action	Application/Indication	Nursing Responsibility
Antidiarrheal Agents		
Opioids: Codeine Camphorated opium tincture (Paregoric) Diphenoxylate/atropine (Lomotil) Loperamide (Imodium) **Other:** Bismuth subsalicylate (Pepto-Bismol) ***Action:*** Increases fluid and electrolyte absorption from the colon by slowing peristalsis. Reduces GI hypermotility by direct antibacterial effect and decreased prostaglandin synthesis.	Moderate to severe diarrhea. Traveler's diarrhea.	Monitor for signs and symptoms of dehydration and altered electrolyte levels. Observe for potential drowsiness. Instruct patient not to drive or perform other potentially hazardous activities until response to drug is known. Notify health care provider if no relief in 48 hours.

status. If the patient is able to tolerate oral feeding, small, frequent meals may be helpful. Resting in a reclining position after meals may help slow the GI transit time. The patient should be taught to monitor his body weight and to notify the health care provider if there is a consistent weight loss, which could signify either a fluid loss or inadequate calories.

Health Promotion

Patients with malabsorption and maldigestion syndromes face many challenges with nutrition. Patients should be encouraged to seek health care advice if they experience symptoms of food intolerance. Education regarding foods they can eat and how to read food labels is critical. In addition, education regarding replacement therapy, such as pancreatic enzymes, is crucial to the patient's well-being.

Collaborative Management

Diagnosing food intolerances and issues with malabsorption and maldigestion can prove challenging. Patients may need the collaborative interdisciplinary efforts of primary care providers, gastroenterologists, allergists, pharmacists, nutritionists, nurses, and social services. In order to meet desired patient outcomes, it is essential that this interdisciplinary team communicate openly with one another in developing and evaluating care of the patient and family (IOM [Institute of Medicine], 2010).

Allergists, primary care providers, and gastroenterologists may be needed to help diagnose the underlying disease. An allergist can help rule out food allergies; primary care providers and gastroenterologists can help narrow down the specific issue and conduct necessary laboratory and diagnostic studies.

Nurses and nutritionists will help patients learn to read food labels and create appropriate menus in order to avoid complications and issues associated with diseases such as celiac disease. Nurses and pharmacists will educate patients on any medication regimens. Finally, social services may be able to find resources such as support groups to help patients transition into dealing with lifelong changes.

Disorders of the Intestines

Appendicitis

Etiology and Epidemiology

The appendix is located near the ileocecal valve and is considered a true diverticulum of the cecum. The orifice opens into the cecum. Lymphoid cells in the mucosa of the appendix create a lymphoid pulp that aids immunologic function. The lymphoid tissue atrophies with age and can obstruct the appendix, leading to appendicitis.

Appendicitis commonly has the highest incidence in the 10- to 30-year-old age group. Men are twice as likely to have appendicitis in the 10 to 30 age range, but rates are equal for men and women over the life span (Thomas, 2011).

Pathophysiology

Obstruction is thought to be the primary cause of appendicitis (Thomas, 2011). Obstruction can be caused by hard feces (fecalith), calculi, lymphoid hyperplasia, an infectious process, or a benign or malignant tumor. Once the lumen of the appendix is obstructed, it becomes filled with mucus and distends, increasing intramural pressure. The increased pressure causes thrombosis and occlusion of the small vessels and stasis of the lymphatic flow. The wall then becomes ischemic and then necrotic, eventually leading to bacterial overgrowth and perforation (rupture).

Clinical Manifestations

Pain is the most common symptom of appendicitis. Classic signs and symptoms of appendicitis include right lower quadrant abdominal pain, anorexia, nausea, and vomiting. Rebound tenderness (pain that is worse after releasing pressure on the abdomen), rigidity (tightening of the abdomen), and guarding (not wanting to be touched in the area) may also be present. Patients may also flex the right knee with palpation to reduce pain (Thomas, 2011). A low grade fever may be present. A ruptured appendix is a serious complication of appendicitis and holds a high risk of peritonitis. When the appendix ruptures, there may be sudden cessation of pain followed by symptoms of peritonitis: abdominal pain, rigid boardlike abdomen, and absence of bowel sounds (Thomas, 2011).

Laboratory and Diagnostic Procedures

Clinical exam is the main diagnostic marker for appendicitis. Laboratory and diagnostic tests that may be supportive are a white blood count to identify leukocytosis, an abdominal x-ray, and a CT of the abdomen (Thomas, 2011). Refer to the Laboratory and Diagnostic Tests box.

Medical and Surgical Management

Medical management includes surgical removal of the appendix. The appendectomy is performed by laparoscopy or an open laparotomy. Approximately 58% of appendectomies in the United States are done laparoscopically (Smink & Soybel, 2011). The patient should be given prophylactic antibiotics prior to surgery to prevent wound infection and intra-abdominal abscess. For patients with a nonperforated appendix, a single preoperative dose is given. Because the flora in the appendix is that of the colon, a patient with a perforated (ruptured) appendix should receive broad spectrum antibiotics that cover gram-negative rods and anaerobic organisms. The antibiotics should be given prior to surgery and should be continued until no clinical evidence of infection exists.

Nursing Management

Nursing management of the patient with acute appendicitis includes management of fluid and electrolyte balance, pain, and infection. Prior to surgery, the patient requires adequate hydration with intravenous fluids and perioperative antibiotics. Preoperative nursing care and post-operative nursing care are discussed in Chapters 17 and 19, respectively. Nausea and vomiting are common after abdominal surgery. Antiemetics should be given if ordered. Early ambulation helps to restore peristalsis and prevent abdominal distention and gas pain after surgery. The patient should be monitored for signs and symptoms of peritonitis and wound infection.

Intestinal Obstruction

Etiology and Epidemiology

Intestinal obstruction is impairment of the forward movement of intestinal contents because of a mechanical cause (tumors [Figure 37–6C ◆]; adhesions [Figure 37–6A ◆]; Crohn's disease, which causes twisting or narrowing; diverticular disease, which causes narrowing; or foreign bodies) or a functional cause (surgery, anesthesia, medications) that can occur anywhere from the pylorus to the rectum and can be either partial or complete. Intestinal obstructions account for approximately 20% of hospital admissions for abdominal disorders (Schueler, Beckett, & Gettings, 2008). Functional bowel obstructions are also called paralytic ileus (a problem

LABORATORY AND DIAGNOSTIC TESTS for Disorders of the Intestines

Test with Description, Rationale, and Normal Values	Expected Abnormality
WBC Normal: 4,500–10,000 μL (mm³) *Used to detect infection.*	WBC counts above 10,000 indicate the presence of infection and/or inflammation.
Neutrophils (Segs) Normal: 50–65 *Used to detect the number of mature circulating neutrophils.*	Increased in acute infection and inflammatory processes.
Bands Normal: 0–5 *Used to detect the number of immature neutrophils.*	Increased in acute infection and inflammatory processes.
Monocytes Normal: 4–6 *Used to assess infection.*	Increased in viral disease, cancer, and monocytic leukemia.
Lymphocytes Normal: 25–35 *Used to assess infection.*	Increased in viral infection, leukemia, and chronic infection.
Red Blood Cell Count Normal: Male: 4.6–6 mcg/L Female: 4–5 mcg/L *Used to detect problems with RBCs, including anemia.*	Decreased levels indicate possible blood loss or anemia.
Hemoglobin Normal: Male: 13.5–18 g/dL Female: 12–15 g/dL *Used to detect the oxygen-carrying capability of the RBCs.*	Lower levels indicate anemia and blood loss.
Hematocrit Normal: Male: 40–54% Female: 36–46% *Used to detect the volume of RBCs in the blood.*	Lower levels are associated with anemia and blood loss.
Abdominal X-Ray Normal: no abnormalities *Used to examine structure of abdominal organs.*	In appendicitis, may see air-filled appendix, ileus, or a fecalith. In obstruction, may see distended loops of bowel; the entire large intestine will be distended to the level of the obstruction and gas and fluid will be seen in a small bowel obstruction. Will see free air in the presence of perforation.
Computed Tomography (CT) Normal: no abnormalities *Used to detect lesions, tumors, metastasis, perforation, vascular disease, infection, and bone destruction.*	Any abnormalities. May see perforation (free air in abdomen) and can visualize mechanical obstruction. Can see abscess and inflammation associated with diverticular disease. Can identify tumors or metastasis related to cancer.
Amylase Normal: 60–100 unit/dL *Used to detect pancreatic problems.*	Elevated levels may be seen in bowel obstruction as well as pancreatitis, making diagnosis challenging
Barium Enema Normal: no abnormalities *Used to detect problems in the large intestine.*	Any tumors, inflammatory disease, diverticula, fistulas, polyps, intussusception, or obstruction.

(*continued*)

LABORATORY AND DIAGNOSTIC TESTS for Disorders of the Intestines, *continued*

Test with Description, Rationale, and Normal Values	Expected Abnormality
Sodium Normal: 135–145 mEq/L *Used to evaluate sodium balance.*	Decreased levels may be associated with vomiting, diarrhea, or gastrointestinal suction. Increased levels may be associated with dehydration, severe vomiting, and diarrhea.
Potassium Normal: 3.5–5.3 mEq/L *Used to evaluate potassium balance.*	Decreased levels may be related to vomiting, diarrhea, dehydration, gastrointestinal suction, or malnutrition. Increased levels may be associated with renal failure or increased intake, acidosis, and burns.
Chloride Normal: 95–105 mEq/L *Used to evaluate chloride balance.*	Decreased levels are associated with vomiting, diarrhea, gastrointestinal suction, hypokalemia, hyponatremia, colitis, and alkalosis (metabolic). Increased levels are associated with dehydration, hypernatremia, and acidosis (metabolic).
Acid–Base Balance (Arterial Blood Gas) Normal: pH: 7.35–7.45 CO_2: 35–45 mmHg HCO_3: 24–28 mEq/L *Used to assess acid-base balance*	Decreased pH and increased CO_2 indicates respiratory acidosis. Increased pH and decreased CO_2 indicates respiratory alkalosis. Decreased pH and decreased HCO_3 indicates metabolic acidosis. Increased pH and increased HCO_3 indicates metabolic alkalosis.
Colonoscopy Normal: no pathology and normal mucosa *Used to detect polyps, the origin of lower intestinal bleeding, and for cancer screening of the colon.*	May see intestinal bleeding, diverticular disease, strictures, polyps, and tumors. Visualization of continuous inflammation (ulcerative colitis) or intermittent inflammation (Crohn's disease). Inflamed ileum (Crohn's disease). With biopsy, can diagnose colon cancer with 100% accuracy.
Sigmoidoscopy Normal: no abnormalities *Used "to examine the anus, rectum, and sigmoid colon [and] to detect blood, polyps, or tumor in the sigmoid colon" (Kee, 2010, p. 585).*	The presence of bleeding, polyps, tumors, or abnormal tissue.
Abdominal Ultrasound Normal: no abnormalities *Used to examine the size, structure, and position of organs; blood flow; and for cysts, tumors, or calculi.*	Will see abnormalities in the tissue lining or an abscess.
Stool for Occult Blood Normal: no blood *Used to detect blood in the stool.*	Positive results indicate bleeding, esophageal varices, peptic ulcer, gastrointestinal cancer, diverticulitis, or colitis.
Biopsy Normal: no abnormal tissue	Acute and chronic inflammation will be present in the tissue of patients with ulcerative colitis and Crohn's disease. A biopsy will see abnormal cells in patients with cancer; can diagnose colon cancer with 100% accuracy.
Barium Swallow with Small Bowel Follow Through Normal: no abnormalities *Used to detect ulcers, strictures, colonic distention, obstruction, and fistulas.*	Any abnormality, such as ulcers, polyps, tumors, hiatal hernias, foreign bodies, varices, and strictures. Esophageal dilatation may be present in achalasia. Narrowing of the esophageal lumen or abnormal mucosa may be seen with esophageal cancer.
Erythrocyte Sedimentation Rate (ESR) Normal: Male: 0–15 mm/hour ($<$ age 50); 0–20 mm/hour ($>$ age 50) Female: 0–20 mm/hr ($<$ age 50); 0–30 mm/hr ($>$ age 50) *Used to evaluate inflammation.*	Elevated in inflammatory processes (such as ulcerative colitis or Crohn's disease).

Weblink: Achalasia
Weblink: Inflammatory Bowel Disease

LABORATORY AND DIAGNOSTIC TESTS for Disorders of the Intestines, *continued*

Test with Description, Rationale, and Normal Values	Expected Abnormality
Glucose Normal: 70–110 mg/dL *Used to evaluate carbohydrate metabolism.*	Increased levels indicate diabetes mellitus, adrenal gland hyperfunction, stress, burns, infections, extensive surgery, or postgastrectomy (dumping) syndrome. Decreased levels are associated with hypoglycemia, adrenal gland hypofunction, malnutrition, or cirrhosis.
Serum Albumin Normal values: 3.5–5.0 g/dL; 52–68% of total protein *Used to detect albumin deficiency.*	Lower levels may be seen with malabsorption, certain malignancies, and malnutrition, as well as in liver and renal disease, prolonged immobilization, and ulcerative colitis.
BUN Normal: 5–25 mg/dL *Used to evaluate kidney function and dehydration.*	Increased levels indicate dehydration, gastrointestinal bleeding, renal disorders, or sepsis. Decreased levels indicate liver damage, overhydration, or malnutrition in negative nitrogen balance.
Creatinine Normal: 0.5–1.5 mg/dL *Used to detect kidney dysfunction.*	Increased levels are associated with acute and chronic kidney disease, shock, and intestinal cancer.
Pyridoxine (Vitamin B_6) Normal: 5–30 ng/mL *Used to detect Vitamin B_6 deficiencies.*	Low levels indicate malnutrition, malabsorption, anemia, and small bowel inflammatory disease.
Vitamin B_{12} Normal: 200–900 pg/mL *Used to detect vitamin B_{12} deficiencies.*	Lower levels indicate pernicious anemia, malabsorption, liver disease, pancreatic insufficiency, sprue, Crohn's disease, and gastrectomy.
Folate Normal: 3–16 ng/mL *Used to check for folic acid deficiencies.*	Decreased levels indicate folic acid anemia, vitamin B_6 deficiency anemia, malabsorption, malnutrition, malignancies, liver disease, celiac sprue, and may be lowered in pregnancy.
Iron Normal: 50–150 mcg/dL *Used to identify iron excess or deficiency.*	Lowered iron indicates anemia; cancer of the stomach, small or large intestines, rectum, and breast; bleeding peptic ulcer; renal failure; or chronic blood loss.
Anti-*Saccharomyces Cerevisiae* Antibodies (ASCA) Normal < 20 units (Quest Diagnostics, 2010) *Used to help diagnose inflammatory bowel disease in cases where it is difficult to distinguish the disease.*	Positive levels are associated with Crohn's disease.
Perinuclear Antineutrophil Cytoplasmic Antibodies (pANCA) Normal: negative *Used to help diagnose inflammatory bowel disease in cases where it is difficult to distinguish the disease.*	Positive levels are associated with ulcerative colitis.
C-Reactive Protein Normal: negative *Used to detect inflammation and the risk of coronary artery disease.*	Elevated with inflammation, such as that found in inflammatory bowel disease.
Carcinoembryonic Antigen (CEA) Normal: < 2.5 ng/mL (nonsmokers) < 5 ng/mL (smokers) *Used to evaluate treatment in gastrointestinal cancer, specifically colon and pancreatic cancers.*	Increased levels indicate a variety of cancers, emphysema, cirrhosis of the liver, pneumonia, heart disease, pancreatitis, inflammation, acute renal failure, and chronic smoking.

Sources: Fisichella, P. M., & Patti, M. G. (2009). Achalasia. Retrieved from http://emedicine.medscape.com/article/169974-overview; Kee, J. L. (2010). *Laboratory and diagnostic tests with nursing implications* (8th ed.). Upper Saddle River, NJ: Prentice Hall; Quest Diagnostics. (2010). Inflammatory bowel disease differentiation panel. Retrieved from http://www.questdiagnostics.com/hcp/intguide/jsp/showintguidepage.jsp?fn=HematOnc/Gastrointestinal/TS_IBD_Differention_Panel.htm; Thomas, D. J. (2011). Abdominal problems. In L. M. Dunphy, J. E. Winland-Brown, B. O. Porter, & D. J. Thomas, *Primary care: The art and science of advanced practice nursing* (2nd ed., pp. 492–581). Philadelphia: F. A. Davis.

of intestinal motility). Most bowel obstructions occur in the small intestines related to the smaller intestinal lumen (Huether, 2010a; Thomas, 2011).

Obstructions can be further classified by severity, extent, or location. Severity includes simple or strangulated effects (Trevino, 2010). Simple obstructions do not have any impairment of blood or nerves on the intestinal wall; strangulated obstructions include occlusion of the blood supply (Huether, 2010a). A strangulated bowel obstruction is extremely serious and requires immediate medical attention because impairment of arterial blood flow leads to ischemia, infarction progressing to gangrene, and perforation and death. This type of bowel obstruction is most often caused by hernias (Figure 37–6B◆), intussusception (telescoping of the bowel, Figure 37–6D◆), volvulus (twisting of the bowel, Figure 37–6E◆), or vascular occlusion. It can also result from surgical adhesions and tumor involvement.

The extent of an obstruction is either partial (incomplete obstruction) or complete. The location of the obstruction can be classified as distal or proximal. A final classification may involve whether the onset is acute or chronic (Huether, 2010a).

Pathophysiology

The pathophysiology of bowel obstruction is the same regardless of the cause. When the intestines are obstructed, fluid and gas accumulate near the obstruction. The fluid buildup is due to the inability to reabsorb water and electrolytes as well as increased secretions; the gas relates to bacteria and swallowed air. The continued accumulation of fluid leads to vomiting, dehydration, and possibly hypovolemic shock. The distention also presses against the diaphragm, increasing the risk for pneumonia and atelectasis. Finally, the patient is at risk for acid–base imbalances because of fluid shifts, electrolyte imbalances, and vomiting (Huether, 2010a; Thomas, 2011).

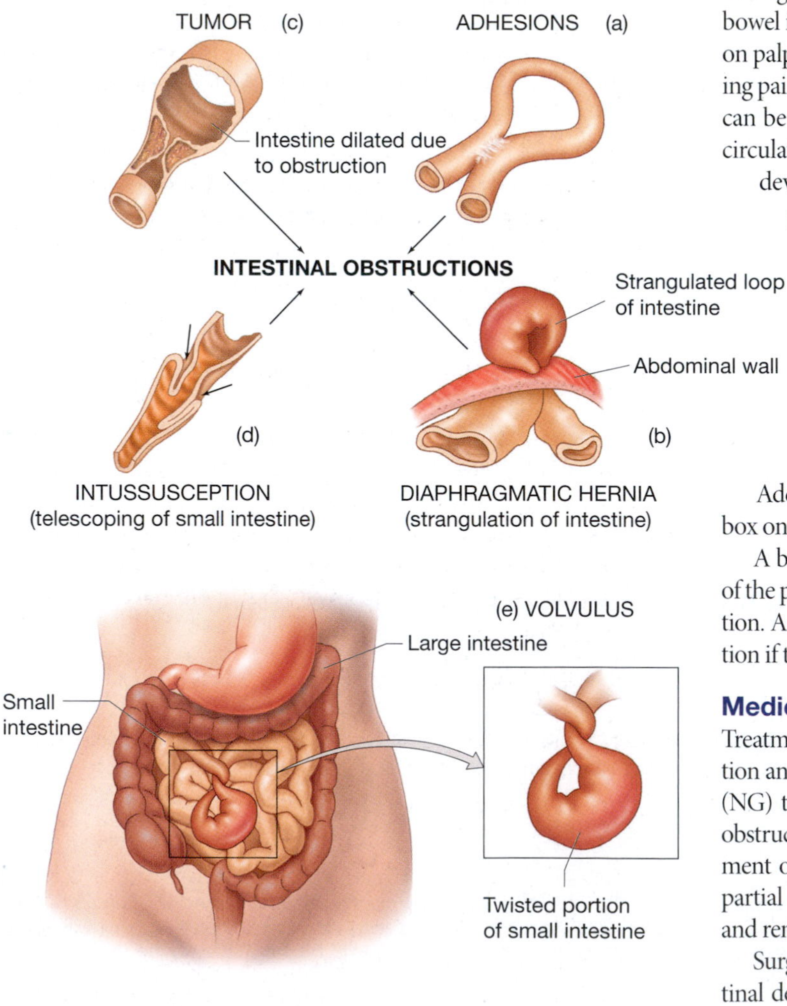

FIGURE 37–6 ◆ Causes of intestinal obstruction (A) Adhesions, (B) Hernias, (C) Tumors, (D) Intussusception, (E) Volvulus.

Clinical Manifestations

The manifestations of a bowel obstruction vary depending on the location, type of obstruction, and rapidity of development. The most common symptom is cramping or colicky pain that increases as the obstruction progresses. Initially, the cramping or pain may be intermittent, but it becomes constant with the progression of the obstruction or if the intestines become strangulated. If the obstruction is in the proximal small bowel, vomiting is common, and metabolic alkalosis can result from the loss of gastric acid. If the obstruction is in the distal small bowel, the pain is usually intense, and the patient may vomit fecal material (Huether, 2010a).

Abdominal assessment reveals distention resulting from the accumulation of gas, intestinal secretions, and distended and edematous loops of bowel. Early in the obstructive process, visible peristaltic waves may be seen on inspection. In addition, hyperactive, high-pitched tinkling bowel sounds may be heard on auscultation of the abdomen and may cease later in the course of the obstruction. However, with a paralytic ileus, there may be diminished or absent bowel sounds throughout the process. Severe and continuous pain may indicate bowel ischemia or perforation. Abdominal tenderness may be evident on palpation. If the obstruction is located in the large intestine, cramping pain and constipation are the most common manifestations. There can be massive dilation of the colon, causing pressure and impairing circulation, which leads to gangrene and perforation. If vomiting develops with a large bowel obstruction, it is usually late in the process or with an incompetent ileocecal valve (Thomas, 2011; Trevino, 2010).

Laboratory and Diagnostic Procedures

Bowel obstruction is determined by a careful history and physical exam. Confirmation of the diagnosis is made by x-rays and CT scan. A complete blood count with a differential white blood cell (WBC) count is done because a very elevated WBC count can indicate ischemia or impending strangulation. Additional tests are listed in the Laboratory and Diagnostic Tests box on page 1137.

A barium swallow is contraindicated in bowel obstruction because of the possibility of intestinal perforation or a worsening of the obstruction. A barium enema may be used to diagnose a large-bowel obstruction if there is no threat of perforation.

Medical Management

Treatment for bowel obstruction is centered on relieving the obstruction and resulting pressure in order to avoid perforation. A nasogastric (NG) tube is placed to decompress the bowel, possibly relieving the obstruction. Decompression of the bowel using an NG tube is the treatment of choice for small bowel obstructions and is very effective for partial obstructions. The tube is attached to low intermittent suction and removes the accumulated gas and fluid.

Surgery is needed if the obstruction does not respond to the intestinal decompression or if there is a complete mechanical obstruction or strangulation. Preoperatively, all patients will have an NG tube inserted to remove stomach contents and any fluid that accumulates in the stomach (unless there is a mechanical obstruction involving the stomach, in which case insertion of the NG tube is not possible). This will prevent vomiting and possible aspiration during surgery and the immediate postoperative period.

The health care provider will order intravenous fluids to hydrate and correct any electrolyte imbalances before surgery and concurrently with NG tube suction. Isotonic IV fluids (normal saline, lactated Ringer's) will be given at a rate that will correct fluid balance rapidly but without risk of causing cardiac problems. Because potassium is lost in nasogastric suctioning as well as through vomiting, potassium is usually added to the IV solution. Intravenous antibiotics will be given preoperatively and during surgery to prevent the possibility of infection and may also be given in the presence of strangulation (Thomas, 2011).

Surgery may involve several procedures including the lysing of adhesions, removal of infarcted or gangrenous bowel, removal of foreign bodies, or tumor resection. A bowel resection is done for most cases of obstruction, except when the cause of obstruction is adhesions. In that case, the adhesions are surgically released. A bowel resection involves removing the section of intestine that is involved, and usually an end-to-end anastomosis is performed to reattach the sections of bowel. If a large section of small bowel is removed, the patient may have malabsorption postoperatively.

Nursing Management

Nursing care for the patient with a bowel obstruction focuses on assessment of the patient's present condition, instituting fluid and electrolyte replacement, and performing bowel decompression through NG tube placement. If the bowel obstruction cannot be relieved, surgery will be necessary. The nurse prepares the patient for possible surgery, both physically and emotionally.

Assessment

Assessing for fluid and electrolyte balance and gastric perfusion is critical. The nurse will want to ask the patient about vomiting (how much and how long), urinary and bowel patterns, dizziness, and abdominal distention. A pain assessment, including what provokes or relieves the pain, the quality of the pain, whether the pain radiates, its severity (pain scale rating on 0 to 10 scale), and the timing of the pain, should also be included. The nurse will want to assess vital signs, including orthostatic vital signs; intake and output (IV fluids, urine output, NG tube output, and bowel elimination); and skin, as well as complete an abdominal assessment.

Nursing Diagnoses

Nursing diagnoses that apply to bowel obstruction include the following:

- *Fluid Volume, Deficient, Risk for* related to bowel obstruction and sequestration of fluid and nasogastric suction.
- *Tissue Perfusion, Ineffective Gastrointestinal* related to possible strangulation, volvulus, tumor, foreign body, or vascular congestion resulting from obstruction.

NANDA-I © 2012

Outcomes and Evaluation

Outcomes and evaluation parameters include the following:

- Normal fluid balance as evidenced by:
  - Normal vital signs with no orthostatic changes
  - Equal intake and output
  - Pink, warm skin with normal moisture
  - Normal bowel sounds and abdominal assessment.
- Adequate GI perfusion and return of peristalsis as evidenced by:
  - Normal bowel sounds
  - Normal bowel elimination
  - Normal abdominal assessment
  - No evidence of pain.

Interventions and Rationales

The nurse should assess the frequency and amount of vomiting prior to hospitalization to accurately assess fluid loss. The nurse should also assess urine frequency prior to hospitalization. A decrease in urination is a sign of fluid sequestering in the gut.

It is important to monitor orthostatic blood pressure and dizziness to assess hypotension and fluid volume deficit. The nurse should also monitor and record input and output from all sources every 2–4 hours. Urine output less than 30 milliliters per hour indicates inadequate glomerular filtration rate and is an indicator of inadequate fluid volume. Nasogastric tube drainage is figured into the fluid replacement needs.

The nurse administers IV fluids as ordered to replace lost fluids. Adequate fluid replacement is necessary to sustain tissue perfusion, particularly to the heart and kidneys. The patient's level of pain should be assessed every 1 to 2 hours using a scale of 0 to 10, with 10 being the worst pain. A change in the intensity or character of the pain can indicate ischemia, infarction, gangrene, or perforation of the bowel.

The nurse should monitor the patient's vital signs every 1 to 2 hours. Tachycardia can result from pain or a sympathetic response to tissue ischemia. Increased temperature may indicate impending sepsis from bowel perforation or gangrene. Falling blood pressure could signal shock; with a low blood pressure, it is difficult to perfuse the intestines, increasing the risk for infarction and possible perforation. The nurse should monitor bowel sounds, abdominal distention, and tenderness. Increasing abdominal girth and pain could signal perforation or sequestering of fluids in the intestines, causing congestion and impairing perfusion.

Diverticular Disease

Diverticular disease results from the occurrence of abnormal saclike outpouchings of the intestinal wall called diverticula. Diverticula can occur anywhere in the gastrointestinal tract except the rectum but usually occur in the distal large intestine. Diverticular disease includes **diverticulosis,** which is the presence of one or more diverticula, and **diverticulitis,** which is inflammation of the diverticula with possible rupture into the colonic lumen.

Pathophysiology, Etiology, and Epidemiology

There are inherent weak points in the intestinal wall where arteries penetrate the tunica muscularis of the large intestine (Huether, 2010a). It is at these points, particularly where pressures are normally high in order to push fecal material toward the rectum, that diverticula form. Diverticula themselves cause few problems; however, if undigested food or bacteria become trapped in the diverticula, they form a hard mass called a fecalith, and intraluminal pressure increases, resulting in compromise of the blood supply. This results in ischemia and inflammation of the diverticula and may lead to perforation (Thomas, 2011).

Diverticular disease is more common in developed countries such as the United States, England, Australia, and France than in undeveloped countries. The incidence of diverticular disease increases as people age and is quite common after age 60 but is rarely found in pediatric patients (Thomas, 2011).

Clinical Manifestations

Most people with diverticular disease are asymptomatic. When diverticulitis develops or the diverticulum hemorrhages, the clinical manifestations typically include left lower quadrant pain and fever with corresponding tachycardia and possible chills. The patient may also have nausea, vomiting, and bowel changes, causing either diarrhea or constipation. The pain is usually located in the left lower quadrant because most diverticula form in this portion of the colon. Abdominal distention and flatulence may also occur. On palpation, the abdomen may be tender over the left lower quadrant, and a mass may be palpated (Thomas, 2011). The complications of diverticular disease are relatively rare but can include hemorrhage, peritonitis, bowel obstruction, and fistula formation.

Laboratory and Diagnostic Procedures

Diverticular disease may be detected incidentally during diagnostic procedures for other problems or on routine colonoscopy. In the case of asymptomatic and uncomplicated diverticulosis, no other testing is usually indicated.

If symptoms develop, the health care provider will order a complete blood count (CBC) with a differential to assess for bleeding and infection. The stool may also be tested for occult blood. Refer to the Laboratory and Diagnostic Tests box on page 1137.

Neither a barium enema nor a sigmoidoscopy will usually be done during the acute phase of the process because of the risk of perforating an inflamed diverticulum. Ultrasonography is a noninvasive test that can detect an abscess or bowel thickening. A CT scan can be used not only to detect an abscess but also to assess inflammation. If a perforation is suspected, abdominal x-rays can show free abdominal air, which is characteristic of perforation.

Medical Management

The treatment for diverticular disease can range from dietary modifications to surgical resection of the colon. Dietary modifications for simple diverticulosis include teaching the patient to eat a high-fiber diet or to increase supplementary fiber. Patients with mild symptoms may be treated as outpatients; acutely ill patients will be admitted to the hospital (Thomas, 2011). Treatment for mild symptoms includes rest, drug therapy, and dietary modifications. Hospital admission is required for higher fevers, persistent (more than 3 days) abdominal pain, peritonitis, or dehydration (Nguyen, Chudasama, Dea, & Cooperman, 2009). Treatment for more severe diverticulitis includes IV fluids, IV antibiotics, possible nasogastric suction, and pain management. Surgery may be necessary if the patient develops peritonitis from a ruptured diverticulum, abscess, bowel obstruction, fistula, or uncontrolled bleeding.

Dietary Modifications

While the patient is in the acute phase of diverticulitis, a clear liquid diet is recommended. If hospitalized, the patient is usually kept NPO initially. The health care provider may insert a nasogastric tube as well. Once the acute phase has passed, dietary recommendations include eating a diet high in both soluble and insoluble fiber. The recommended fiber consumption for the general public of the United States is 25 to 30 grams, and this should be stressed for the person with diverticular disease. It was once thought that patients with diverticular disease should avoid foods containing small seeds, foods with skins (e.g., grapes), nuts, and corn because they may become lodged in a diverticulum and cause inflammation and an exacerbation of diverticulitis, but Nguyen et al. (2009) state this issue is not as significant as was previously thought. However, it is still wise to avoid these foods during active diverticulitis and eat them as tolerated otherwise (USCF Medical Center, 2011). For more information on the nutritional aspects of diverticular disease, see page 184 in Chapter 8, Nutrition.

Drug Therapy

Acute diverticulitis is treated with broad-spectrum antibiotics. For mild attacks of diverticulitis, oral metronidazole (Flagyl) and ciprofloxacin (Cipro) may be used; alternatively, metronidazole (Flagyl) and trimethoprim-sulfamethoxazole (Bactrim) may be used (Thomas, 2011). If the diverticulitis is severe and the patient is hospitalized, IV antibiotics effective against gram-negative bacteria and anaerobes will be used. Refer to the Pharmacology Summary of Anti-Infective Medications box in the section on peptic ulcer disease (p. 1127) for an outline of anti-infective agents.

Analgesics will be ordered for the patient with diverticulitis who is experiencing pain. If the pain is not severe, a mild analgesic is ordered. However, opioid analgesics such as meperidine hydrochloride (Demerol) or morphine may be necessary to relieve more severe pain.

Bulk-forming agents are usually prescribed and laxatives are avoided because they increase motility and intracolonic pressure, although stool softeners (e.g., Colace) may be used. See the Pharmacology box. Enemas are also contraindicated because they increase the intraluminal pressure of the colon and risk diverticular perforation.

Rest

Rest is advocated during acute diverticulitis. The patient should avoid any activity that increases the intra-abdominal pressure, thereby risking perforation; some of these activities are lifting, straining, coughing, sneezing, and bending.

Bowel rest may be necessary during the acute phase of the illness. Depending on the severity of the inflammation, the patient may be kept NPO. As feeding is resumed slowly, the health care provider may prescribe a low-roughage diet. This diet eliminates foods that are high in insoluble fiber, such as whole wheat foods, fruit, nuts, raw vegetables, and dried peas and beans. Fruit juices without pulp are usually permitted. On recovery, high-fiber foods are resumed.

Surgery

If the patient's condition does not improve within 3 days of treatment or deteriorates, surgical intervention may be needed. About 20% to 30% of patients with diverticulitis require surgical treatment (Thomas, 2011). Surgery usually consists of a bowel resection with anastomosis. If surgery is required during the acute phase, a temporary colostomy (in which the colon is brought to an opening on the abdomen) may be necessary until the inflammation has subsided. (See the Medical Management section for colon cancer for more information about colostomy.) The temporary colostomy is closed in 2 to 3 months. Refer to the Nursing Process: Patient Care Plan for the Patient With Colon Cancer Having Surgery (p. 1156) for more information on colostomy care.

Nursing Management

Because most patients with diverticular disease are symptom free, nursing care focuses on assessing the patient for clinical symptoms of diverticulitis and secondary complications, as well as assessing the diet for fiber content.

Assessment

Assessment of clinical symptoms includes asking the patient about bleeding from the GI tract (vomiting or bloody stool), nausea and

PHARMACOLOGY Summary for Diverticular Disease

Medication Category and Action	Application/Indication	Nursing Responsibility
Bulk-Forming Agents		
Psyllium seed (Metamucil) Methylcellulose ***Action:*** Improves bowel elimination by increasing stool bulk, which promotes peristalsis.	Constipation	Monitor for effectiveness—patient will have bowel movement. Monitor for adverse effects: nausea, abdominal cramps, or diarrhea. Be aware of drug interactions; monitor warfarin and digoxin levels. Instruct the patient to follow each dose with an additional glass of liquid.
Stool Softeners		
Docusate sodium (Colace) ***Action:***: Softens stool by drawing water into the colon.	Constipation, prevention of straining	Monitor for adverse effects: nausea, abdominal cramps, or diarrhea. Instruct the patient to increase fluid intake.
Pain Control		
Morphine sulfate ***Action:*** Binds with pain receptor sites.	Pain relief	Obtain baseline vital signs and hold if respirations are less than 12. Monitor vital signs. Monitor pain. Monitor safety. Teach the family to avoid other central nervous system depressants (e.g., alcohol).
Meperidine hydrochloride (Demerol) ***Action:*** Alters perception of pain	Pain relief	Obtain baseline vital signs and hold if respirations are less than 12. Monitor vital signs. Monitor pain. Monitor safety. Teach the family to avoid other central nervous system depressants (e.g., alcohol).

Source: Adams, M. P., & Koch, R. W. (2010). *Pharmacology: Connections to nursing practice.* Upper Saddle River, NJ: Pearson.

vomiting, and pain, as well as normal bowel and nutritional habits. The nurse should thoroughly assess the patient for severity of pain using a 0 to 10 pain rating scale and asking about the quality of the pain (dull, sharp, burning, aching, or stabbing), what provokes the pain, what relieves the pain, and the timing of the pain. Objective data include vital signs, a thorough abdominal assessment, and a stool assessment. The nurse can evaluate the patient for clinical signs of pain such as facial grimacing and restlessness.

Nursing Diagnoses

Nursing diagnoses that apply to diverticular disease include the following:

- *Tissue Integrity, Impaired* related to the acute inflammatory process of diverticulitis.
- *Pain, Acute* related to diverticulitis and a possible ruptured diverticulum.

  NANDA-I © 2012

Outcomes and Evaluation Parameters

Outcomes and evaluation parameters include the following:

- Normal intestinal tissue as evidenced by:
  - Normal vital signs
  - Normal bowel sounds in all quadrants
  - No abdominal distention
  - No abdominal tenderness or guarding
  - Formed, soft stool
  - Stool negative for blood.
- Patient will maintain comfort level as evidenced by statement of pain relief and display of no-pain behaviors (e.g., no facial grimacing).
- Patient will have a soft abdomen with no distention, pain, or tenderness

Interventions and Rationales

Nursing interventions and rationales for the patient with diverticular disease include the following:

- The nurse assesses vital signs every 4 hours for tachycardia and tachypnea, which may indicate increased inflammation resulting in increased vascular leak syndrome and a fluid shift. Increasing fever may indicate perforation and peritonitis as well as increasing inflammation.
- The nurse assesses the abdomen every 4 hours for bowel sounds. Decreasing bowel sounds may indicate peritonitis or bowel obstruction.
- The nurse measures the patient's abdominal girth and palpates the abdomen for tenderness and guarding. Increasing girth and/or tenderness and guarding can indicate a ruptured diverticulum, infection, peritonitis, or bleeding in the intra-abdominal cavity.
- The nurse examines stools for consistency and character and for evidence of blood, occult or visual. Diverticulitis can cause lower gastrointestinal bleeding.
- The nurse assesses pain using a 0-to-10 pain scale, with 10 being the worst pain, to increase consistency in quantifying pain.

- The nurse instructs the patient to inform her if the pain gets worse or is not relieved, which can indicate complications or the need for a change in pain medication.
- The nurse assesses for associated symptoms that could indicate a complication. Nausea and vomiting; a rigid, boardlike abdomen; and absent bowel sounds can indicate peritonitis.
- The nurse notifies the health care provider if pain increases or there are associated manifestations such as nausea, vomiting, or abdominal distention. This will promote early intervention.

Evaluation

The patient should have normal vital signs, normal bowel function, and a normal abdominal assessment. The patient should not present with any abdominal distention, tenderness, or guarding. The abdomen should be soft.

Health Promotion

Health promotion is the nurse's number-one responsibility. Primary prevention of diverticular disease can be accomplished the majority of the time through a high-fiber diet. Nurses can teach people in the community as well as patients in the hospital about the importance of a high-fiber diet. Nurses can work with local agencies to promote healthy eating, which includes a diet with 25 to 30 grams of fiber.

Inflammatory Bowel Disease

Inflammatory bowel disease (IBD) is an immunologic disease that results in idiopathic intestinal inflammation. It includes two distinct yet similar conditions: ulcerative colitis (UC), a disorder that involves chronic inflammation of the mucosal and submucosal layers of the colon and rectum, and Crohn's disease (regional enteritis), which involves all layers of the intestinal wall and can occur anywhere from the mouth to the anus but commonly affects the ileum. Ulcerative colitis and Crohn's disease have clinical manifestations in common as well as similar pathophysiology involving an inflammatory process. The cause of IBD remains under investigation, though it is now known that a constellation of factors contribute to the development of the disease. A combination of a genetic susceptibility and an abnormal immune response is linked with IBD (Huether, 2010a).

Ulcerative Colitis

Ulcerative colitis (UC) is a disorder that involves chronic inflammation of the mucosal and submucosal layers of the colon and the rectum. It usually begins in the rectum and advances proximally, involving only the large intestine and usually only the sigmoid colon and rectum (Huether, 2010a).

In UC, the inflammation begins at the base of the crypts of Lieberkühn with neutrophil infiltration and cytokine release (Thomas, 2011). This, in turn, causes congestion and edema leading to tissue friability and ulcer formation. The ulcers bleed easily, causing bloody stools, a characteristic manifestation of UC. Atrophy and narrowing of the colon result from chronic inflammation.

Crohn's Disease

Crohn's disease (CD) differs from UC in that it can occur in any portion of the gastrointestinal tract, from the mouth to the anus; however, it is usually limited to the ileum or ileocecal valve. Crohn's disease involves all layers (transmural) of the intestinal wall but usually begins in the submucosa, spreading to the mucosa and serosa while affecting some haustral segments and not others, producing what are called skip lesions (Huether, 2010a). The lesions are granulomatous with areas of inflamed tissue circumscribed by scar tissue, giving the intestinal lumen a cobblestone appearance. As the disease progresses, the chronic inflammation causes fibrosis and loss of intestinal flexibility, resulting in obstruction, abscess, and fistula formation (Thomas, 2011).

Malabsorption or malnutrition may develop in Crohn's disease for several reasons. First, Crohn's disease usually affects the jejunum and ileum, where many nutrients are absorbed, and the presence of inflamed tissues and ulcers impairs absorption. Second, surgical removal of part of the intestines may impair nutrient absorption (Day, 2008). Weight loss may occur because of malabsorption.

Epidemiology

Approximately 1.4 million people in the United States are believed to have IBD. The incidences of UC and Crohn's disease are similar. The age of onset is usually between ages 15 and 35, although it can occur at any time; men and women are affected by IBD equally. The incidence of IBD is higher in Caucasians but has been increasing in African Americans (Crohn's & Colitis Foundation, 2009a).

Etiology and Pathophysiology

The etiology of IBD is unknown, but there may be genetic and immunologic causes (Huether, 2010a). There also is a link to increased risk of Crohn's disease but decreased risk for ulcerative colitis in patients who smoke (Day, 2008).

Genetic Links

It is clear that some individuals are genetically predisposed to IBD even though fewer than 15% of cases are familial. The gene that encodes for a protein that possibly mediates epithelial cell-to-cell interactions is found on chromosomes 7 and 10 and has been linked to IBD; another gene on chromosome 16 is linked specifically to Crohn's disease (Thomas, 2011).

Immune Response

There may be impaired communication between an antigen in the gastric mucosa and the immune system. The impaired T-cell mediated response causes inflammation and disrupted epithelial lining in the gastrointestinal mucosa of the large intestine (Baumgart, 2008).

Clinical Manifestations

Ulcerative colitis and Crohn's disease have similar clinical manifestations that result from the inflammatory process in the intestines, and distinguishing between the two can be difficult. Symptoms may be nonspecific and persist for years before diagnosis is made. These include the following:

- Abdominal pain is usually present in both diseases and is characteristically a cramping type of sensation. The pain can be continuous or intermittent. It also can be localized to either the right or left lower quadrant or can be more diffuse, occurring over the entire lower abdomen.
- Diarrhea is usually present in both UC and Crohn's disease. People with these disorders may have as many as 10 bowel movements per day (Thomas, 2011). They can be loose and/or watery and may contain blood, although blood is more common in UC.
- Rectal urgency, incontinence, and tenesmus (a feeling that one constantly needs to pass stool) can be present in either UC or Crohn's disease (Thomas, 2011).
- Systemic manifestations include arthritis, mouth sores, uveitis (swelling and irritation of the middle layer of the eye), autoimmune hepatitis, and primary sclerosing cholangitis (swelling, scarring,

PHARMACOLOGY Summary of Medications for Irritable Bowel Disease

Medication Category and Action	Application/Indication	Nursing Responsibility
5-Aminosalicylic Acid Agents		
Sulfasalazine (Azulfidine) Mesalamine (Asacol, Pentasa) Olsalazine (Dipentum) ***Action:*** Reduces inflammation by inhibiting prostaglandin production in the gut.	Treatment of Crohn's disease, ulcerative colitis, and rheumatoid arthritis.	Monitor for adverse effects: headache, nausea, vomiting, diarrhea, and blood dyscrasias. Evaluate for aspirin hypersensitivity, which is contraindicated in these patients. Sulfasalazine is contraindicated in patients allergic to sulfa. Sulfasalazine is contraindicated in pregnancy. Monitor BUN and creatinine, especially in the presence of renal disease.
Corticosteroids		
Prednisone (Meticorten) Methylprednisolone (Medrol) Hydrocortisone (Cortef) ***Action:*** Decreases inflammation and immune response through inhibition of leukocytes and inflammatory mediators.	Inflammatory conditions, severe IBD.	Monitor for adverse effects: psychosis, insomnia, nausea, hypertension, impaired wound healing, and symptoms of gastric ulcer. Other possible long-term effects include osteoporosis, peptic ulcer disease, cataracts, and effects of hyperglycemia. Monitor electrolytes and blood sugar. Usually is started at the lowest dose possible. Warn the patient not to stop using the drug abruptly.
Immunomodulators		
Azathioprine (Imuran) Methotrexate (MTX) 6-mercaptopurine (6-MP) ***Action:*** Suppresses immune response by depressing T-cell function.	Severe IBD.	Understand that these drugs may be better tolerated than corticosteroids. Monitor for adverse effects: nausea, vomiting, and anorexia. Monitor CBC, kidney, and liver function. Observe for signs and symptoms of infection and thrombocytopenia, which may be dose limiting. Teach that drugs may take up to 2 months for effectiveness.
Biologic Response Modifier		
Infliximab (Remicade) Adalimumab (Humira) Certolizumab (Cimzia) ***Action:*** Monoclonal antibody that decreases inflammation by inhibiting TNF-α.	Moderate to severe IBD.	Monitor for adverse reactions: fever, chills, pruritus, urticaria, chest pain, hypotension, hypertension, dyspnea, nausea, abdominal pain, diarrhea, or decreased blood counts, specifically WBC and platelets. Stop the infusion and notify the health care provider if adverse reactions occur.

Sources: Adams, M. P., & Koch, R. W. (2010). *Pharmacology: Connections to nursing practice.* Upper Saddle River, NJ: Pearson; Day, M. W. (2008). Fight back against inflammatory bowel disease. *Nursing, 28*(11), 34–41. doi: 10.1097/01.NURSE.0000341078.53082.f8; Wilson, B. A., Shannon, M. T., & Shields, K. M. (2011). *Pearson nurse's drug guide 2011.* New York: Pearson.

and destruction of the bile ducts of the liver) (Huether, 2010a). It is believed that these extraintestinal manifestations are of an immunologic nature similar to the IBD.

Laboratory and Diagnostic Procedures

Diagnosis of IBD can be difficult, especially when symptoms are nonspecific. A key test for diagnosing IBD is colonoscopy. However, colonoscopy should be avoided in patients with severe inflammation (Thomas, 2011). Refer to the Laboratory and Diagnostic Tests box on page 1137 for additional tests.

Serologic tests are now available to help distinguish between UC and CD. They are not diagnostic in themselves but are used in conjunction with other tests. Two genetic markers have been developed for clinical use: anti-*Saccharomyces cerevisiae* antibodies (ASCA) and perinuclear antineutrophil cytoplasmic antibodies (pANCA) (Rowe, 2011).

Medical Management

The treatment goal for IBD is to eliminate the intestinal inflammation and control the intestinal inflammatory response in the future. Medical management with medications and dietary changes is the first course of treatment. Surgery is considered only if medical management fails.

Drug Therapy

Medications are used in the treatment of IBD to halt acute exacerbations and minimize or eliminate recurrences. The most common medications act locally to control inflammation and systemically to suppress the immune response. Drug classes include 5-aminosalicylic acid agents, corticosteroids, immunomodulators, and biologic response modifiers. See the Pharmacology box for medications used to treat IBD. Bulk-forming agents and stool softeners are discussed in the Pharmacology box on page 1143.

Diet Therapy

There is no specific diet to follow for patients with IBD, other than ensuring it is a well-balanced diet. Some patients with IBD report that certain foods exacerbate their condition. For example, milk and dairy products may increase abdominal pain and diarrhea in some patients and should therefore be avoided. Conversely, a diet high in fiber may lessen diarrhea and improve tenesmus and rectal urgency. If the patient is known to have strictures or severe acute symptoms, dietary fiber is contraindicated. Low residue diets are also recommended for CD when obstructive symptoms are present (Thomas, 2011). Studies are being conducted to assess whether probiotics, which are microorganisms that may be found in dietary supplements or food, help to treat IBD. (Refer to the Complementary & Alternative Therapies box on page 1150 for detailed information on probiotics.) A review by Cary and Boullata (2010) indicates that although studies show that probiotics have beneficial effects, there is a lack of randomized control studies to fully support their use.

During an acute exacerbation of IBD, particularly Crohn's disease, the patient is allowed no food at all. This "bowel rest" helps relieve symptoms, which supports the theory that some foods and bacteria may be antigenic, causing inflammation in the gut. Total parenteral nutrition (TPN) is usually prescribed during the period of bowel rest.

Surgery

Patients who do not respond to the maximum doses of medication and/or who have complications such as malnutrition, anemia, bowel obstruction, and severe weight loss are candidates for surgical intervention. The type of surgery will depend on the type of IBD and the location and extent of the lesions. As many as 75% of patients with CD and 25% of patients with UC will undergo surgery. Because surgery does not cure CD, up to 50% of patients will experience symptom reoccurrence, and 25% may need additional surgery (Day, 2008).

For patients with severe UC and some patients with Crohn's disease, the surgical option is usually a restorative proctocolectomy, also called an **ileal pouch anal anastomosis (IPAA),** in which the entire colon, including the rectum, is removed and a pouch is fashioned from the terminal ileum and then anastomosed to the anus (Figure 37–7◆). When healed, the pouch can hold enough fecal material to reduce bowel movements to 6 times a day (Crohn's & Colitis Foundation of America, 2009b). To allow time for the anastomosis to heal and the pouch to mature, a temporary loop ileostomy is done, which involves bringing a loop of the ileum to the abdominal surface and creating a stoma to allow for the drainage of stool into a collection device. After about 10 to 12 weeks, a second surgery is done to close the stoma and repair the bowel (Crohn's & Colitis Foundation of America, 2009b).

Another surgical procedure is proctocolectomy with ileostomy. In this surgery, an ileostomy is performed after removal of the entire colon, rectum, and anus. In a permanent ileostomy, fecal material is collected in an external collection bag. Fecal drainage is characteristically continuous and watery, because the large intestine is removed and this is where the majority of water is reabsorbed from feces.

Another option is a **continent ileostomy,** also known as **Kock ileostomy** or **Kock pouch** (Figure 37–8◆), in which the terminal ileum is folded back on itself during the ileostomy surgery and the inner wall is removed, thereby forming a reservoir and a nipple valve. The end is then brought through the abdominal wall to form a stoma. The nipple valve prevents leaking of fecal contents through the stoma, and the reservoir is emptied by a catheter inserted through the stoma. Generally, the continent ileostomy is not recommended as the first choice (Crohn's & Colitis Foundation of America, 2009b). Nursing care of the patient with an ileostomy is outlined in the Nursing Process: Patient Care Plan box for patients with IBD.

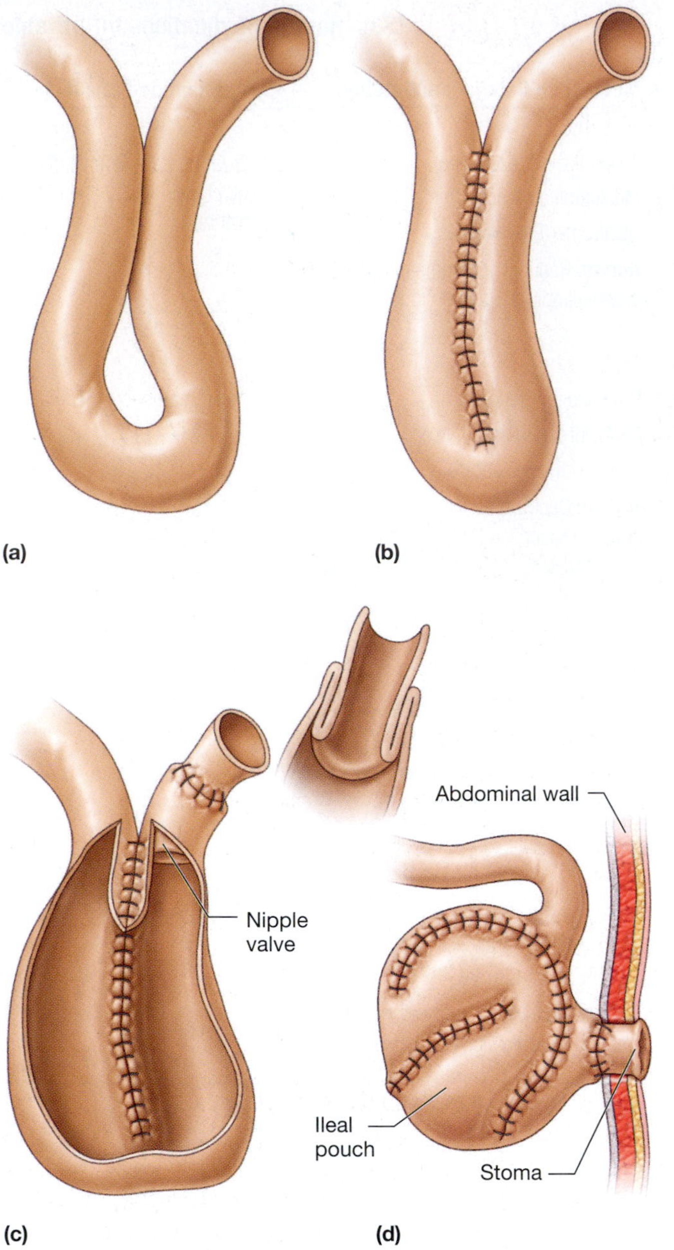

FIGURE 37–8 ◆ Kock ileostomy.

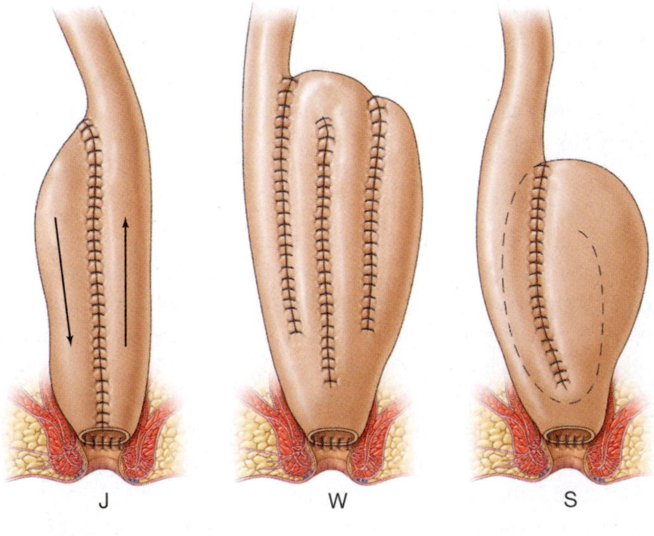

FIGURE 37–7 ◆ Ileal pouch anal anastomosis.

Nursing Management

Most patients with IBD are managed with medications, dietary changes, and stress reduction. Nursing care involves preparing the patient for diagnostic tests, managing the medication regimen, educating the patient about drug treatments and stress reduction, assessing the effectiveness

NURSING PROCESS: Patient Care Plan for Inflammatory Bowel Disease and Ileostomy

Assessment of Gastrointestinal Status Using Gordon's Functional Health Patterns:

- Nutrition Metabolic Pattern
- Elimination Pattern
- Cognitive Perceptual Pattern
- Self-Perception Self-Concept Pattern

Subjective Data

Assessment of Bowel Elimination

How many stools do you have a day?

What is the consistency and color?

Is there any blood?

Do you have any abdominal pain or cramping?

How long have you been having this problem?

When did it start?

Does stress in your life make it worse?

Does any food make the diarrhea worse?

Do you have any joint pain or fatigue?

Have you been treated before?

Do you take any home remedies, herbs, or over-the-counter medications?

Assessment of Body Image

How has this disease/surgery affected your life?

Are you able to continue working? Socializing with friends? Shopping?

Has this affected how you feel about your personal relationships? Sexual activity?

Assessment of Fecal Diversion (Ileostomy)

Are you having any cramping?

Are you passing any gas through the stoma?

How often are you emptying the bag?

Objective Data

Assessment of Bowel Elimination

Vital signs.

Examination of abdomen:

Bowel sounds

Palpation

Visual exam for contour, scars.

Visual inspection of stools.

Test stool for occult blood.

Assessment of Body Image

Facial expressions.

Body language.

Attitude toward stoma.

Assessment of Fecal Diversion (Ileostomy)

Vital signs.

Abdominal assessment:

- Stoma color
- Stoma drainage/bleeding
- Condition of skin surrounding stoma
- Condition of ostomy appliance.

Outcomes and Evaluation Parameters

Planning and Interventions with *Rationales*

1. NURSING DIAGNOSES: (a) Diarrhea *related to inflammatory bowel disease (IBD).* (b) Fluid Balance, Readiness for Enhanced *related to the diarrhea* (NANDA-I © 2012)

Outcome: Decreased diarrhea.

Evaluation Parameters: Number of stools decreased by at least half.

Consistency of stool: formed.

Absence of blood in the stool.

No abdominal cramping.

Take vital signs every 4 hours to assess for signs of dehydration such as tachycardia, tachypnea, or fever.

Weigh daily to assess for fluid losses.

Examine skin and mucous membranes for evidence of dehydration, such as poor turgor, dry mucous membranes, or dry, cracked tongue.

Maintain NPO if ordered to rest the bowel, which promotes healing and improves diarrhea.

Provide good perianal care with gentle cleansing agents, and apply protective cream or ointment to the area *to prevent skin breakdown.*

Administer ordered medications, assess their effectiveness, and monitor adverse effects:

5-ASA compounds (sulfasalazine, mesalamine, olsalazine) are anti-inflammatory drugs that reduce inflammation by inhibiting prostaglandin production in the gut.

Monitor for adverse effects, which include headache, abdominal pain, cramps, nausea, vomiting, diarrhea, skin rashes, blood dyscrasias, and decreased urine output (renal failure).

Teach the patient to take these medications after eating.

(*continued*)

NURSING PROCESS: Patient Care Plan for Inflammatory Bowel Disease and Ileostomy, *continued*

Outcomes and Evaluation Parameters	Planning and Interventions with *Rationales*
	Encourage increased fluid intake (2 L/day) to prevent kidney damage. Teach the patient to notify the health care provider if any of the adverse effects occur. Corticosteroids are adrenal hormones (prednisolone) that suppress the immune response and have anti-inflammatory properties. Monitor for side effects such as elevated blood glucose, fluid retention (edema, weight gain, hypertension, heart failure), gastric ulcers, hypokalemia (muscle weakness, nausea, dysrhythmias), and psychosis. These should be given only with meals to decrease the risk of ulcers and gastric distress. Teach the patient to increase foods high in potassium (citrus fruit, bananas, potatoes) and reduce intake of sodium (canned soup, bottled salad dressing, processed meats, cheese). Teach the patient NOT TO STOP THE MEDICATION ABRUPTLY (the dose must be tapered). Immunomodulators (azathioprine) suppress the immune system. Be sure to tell the patient that these drugs must be taken for 6 to 8 weeks before the full effect is seen. Monitor for adverse effects such as nausea, vomiting, and anorexia, as well as low WBC or platelet count. Infliximab, a monoclonal antibody that decreases inflammation by inhibiting TNF-α, is given every 2 to 3 months and must be given intravenously. 1. Monitor for adverse effects: fever, chills, pruritus, urticaria, chest pain, hypotension, hypertension, or dyspnea.
2. NURSING DIAGNOSIS: Disturbed Body Image *related to disease process and/or surgery* (NANDA-I © 2012)	
Outcome: Normal body image. ***Evaluation Parameter:*** Verbalizes acceptance of body image, demonstrates care for the stoma.	Assess the patient's current perception of self and demonstrate acceptance of where the patient is now. Acceptance of the patient's feelings can help establish a caring and trusting nurse–patient relationship. Provide an environment in which the patient feels comfortable talking about the disease and how it has impacted his life *to build caring nurse–patient relationship.* Encourage the patient to talk about ways this disease has affected personal, work, social, and sexual relationships *to provide understanding and demonstrate acceptance of the patient as a person.* Delineate possible treatment options, including graphic descriptions of surgery and postop possibilities *to give the patient a sense of control.* Provide names and phone numbers of IBS support groups. If possible, arrange for the patient to meet with someone who has the disease. *This shows the patient that she is not the only person facing this problem.*
3. NURSING DIAGNOSES: (a) Bowel Incontinence *related to fecal diversion.* (b) Skin Integrity, Impaired, Risk for *related to ostomy drainage.* (c) Knowledge, Deficient *related to fecal diversion* (NANDA-I © 2012)	
Outcome: Normal functioning ileostomy. ***Evaluation Parameters:*** Stoma color pink and moist. No bloody effluent. Effluent dark green and viscous initially, gradually turning yellow-brown. Skin around stoma free of irritation and inflammation. Ileoanal skin without irritation or inflammation. Able to communicate necessary stoma care, dietary modification, and stress reduction techniques.	Monitor stoma color. The stoma should be pink. It should also be moist with no obvious cyanosis or bleeding. In addition, the stoma should extend about 2 to 3 centimeters from the abdominal wall. Impaired circulation will cause the stoma to be dark, blue, or very pale. Assess stoma function. *Immediately postop there may be small amounts of blood.* Within 1 or 2 days the drainage will be dark green and viscous, gradually turning yellow-brown and developing an odor. Empty and measure the ileostomy drainage when the pouch is one-third to one-half full and explain the procedure to the patient each time. *Emptying the pouch when it is not too full eliminates the possibility of the seal in the pouch breaking and causing leaking. Explaining the procedure to the patient each time gets the patient more comfortable with self-care.*

NURSING PROCESS: Patient Care Plan for Inflammatory Bowel Disease and Ileostomy, *continued*

Assess the skin surrounding the stoma and around the perianal area. The skin should be pink and remain free of irritation, excoriation, or inflammation. *Ileostomy drainage is irritating to the skin because it contains bile salts and digestive enzymes that normally get reabsorbed in the large intestine.*

Apply a protecting skin barrier under the pouch *to prevent contact of drainage with skin.*

Report abnormal assessment findings such as poor stoma color, bulging or retracted stoma, or rash around the stoma. Poor stoma color indicates poor circulation to the section of bowel that forms the stoma; bulging can indicate herniation or prolapse.

Teach the patient and family members to assess the stoma and to treat it gently. Because there are no pain receptors in the stoma, it can become injured without feeling pain.

Teach the patient to notify the health care provider if there is a change in the stoma or if a rash develops in the skin surrounding the stoma.

Assess the patient's ability to manage the ileostomy including knowledge of ostomy care, what medications to avoid (laxatives, enteric coated, or capsules), and signs and symptoms to report.

Source: Adapted from Wilkinson, J. M., & Ahearn, N. R. (2009). *Prentice Hall nursing diagnosis handbook* (9th ed.). Upper Saddle River, NJ: Prentice Hall.

of the interventions, and caring for the patient during the surgical experience, should surgery be necessary. Support networks are vitally important for this very life-disrupting disease. A number of resource groups are available; the one recommended by most patients with IBD is the Crohn's & Colitis Foundation of America. See the Nursing Process: Patient Care Plan box (p. 1147) for the complete nursing care of the patient with IBD.

Irritable Bowel Syndrome

Irritable bowel syndrome (IBS) is a functional bowel problem of the large intestine that is accompanied by abdominal pain, discomfort, and altered bowel elimination.

Pathophysiology, Etiology, and Epidemiology

Population-based studies have estimated the prevalence of irritable bowel syndrome to be 10% to 20% and the incidence to be 1% to 2% per year (Lehrer, 2012). The cause and pathophysiology of IBS are not known. There is a theory that IBS is caused by an alteration in the colon's contractions or by a hypersensitivity to triggers, such as certain foods or stress (Thomas, 2011). Another theory is that increased serotonin concentrations related to decreased receptor sites influence the altered contractions as the body is signaling enterocytes to attempt to update the excessive serotonin (Grundmann & Yoon, 2010).

Clinical Manifestations

Abdominal pain and discomfort, as well as changes in stool patterns (may include constipation or diarrhea) with occasional gas and bloating, are common symptoms of IBS. The abdominal pain and discomfort may be relieved with defecation. Objective assessment reveals tenderness in the left lower quadrant or over the epigastric area (Thomas, 2011). Diagnosis is made based on the existence of the aforementioned symptoms for 6 months. In the presence of symptoms, further evaluation of IBS-specific symptoms are warranted, such as whether the symptoms abate following defecation; changes in stool frequency, consistency, and amount; bloating; passing mucus; or worsened symptoms with eating (Reed, 2010).

Medical Management

Treatment of IBS is based on eliminating potential triggers and controlling bowel patterns and motility (Grundmann & Yoon, 2010). This includes the use of lifestyle and dietary modifications and the possible use of pharmacologic measures. A complete diet and lifestyle history should be evaluated along with potential triggers. A slow increase in dietary fiber and hydration along with reducing caffeine and possible elimination of lactose may be helpful to patients with IBS (Thomas, 2011). Grundmann and Yoon (2010) suggest the use of psychological interventions such as stress management, biofeedback, cognitive behavioral therapy, and hypnotherapy to reduce stress triggers that may be related to IBS.

Drug therapy for IBS depends on the clinical manifestations. For patients with constipation, intermittent use of laxatives such as Milk of Magnesia may be appropriate, whereas patients with diarrhea will need antidiarrheals such as loperamide (Thomas, 2011). Antispasmodics may be helpful in reducing abdominal pain. Tricyclic antidepressants and selective serotonin reuptake inhibitors (SSRIs) reduce symptoms in IBS as a second-line treatment (Reed, 2010).

Nursing Management

Nursing care of the patient with IBS includes assessing the patient for symptoms of the disorder and asking the patient about possible triggers. Listening and good communication are essential in caring for patients with IBS (Reed, 2010). The other key nursing role is education regarding symptoms, avoidance of triggers, stress management, and drug therapy. Nurses can instruct patients in stress management techniques, such as deep breathing, imagery, and progressive muscle relaxation. Nurses can also encourage the use of support groups for IBS, such as the IBS support group online (http://www.ibsgroup.org/), and may refer the patient to counseling as needed.

COMPLEMENTARY & ALTERNATIVE THERAPIES Probiotics

Nancy Yilk

HISTORICALLY, THE HUMAN DIET has included a generous amount of fermented foods through the process of culturing or canning harvested crops. This provided sustainable food to families who did not have the modern conveniences of refrigeration or the ability to preserve foods by freezing them for future use. Still today, in many parts of the world, the preservation of food and use of vinegars to antiseptically clean foods and kill pathogens in drinking water is a way of life. The benefits of fermentation of vegetables and fruits are complementary to the gastrointestinal system by increasing the lactic acid balance with favorable fibers and healthy bacteria flora. The beneficial bacteria found in foods such as sauerkraut and yogurts have been used in one form or another for centuries with a good safety record. This historical integrity of gut balance has been influenced by the modernization of food production and our use of antibiotics.

Prebiotics are nondigestible fibers in foods that cause the gut flora to selectively stimulate one bacterium or a group of bacteria in the gastrointestinal environment with probiotics. Probiotics, meaning "for life," is a growing area of interest in the medical community and has increasing public awareness. Together, prebiotics and probiotics create a foundational symbiosis of flora integrity in the gut.

Probiotics have been shown to be effective in varied clinical conditions, including infantile diarrhea, necrotizing enterocolitis, antibiotic-associated diarrhea, relapsing *Clostridium difficile* colitis, *Helicobacter pylori* infections, inflammatory bowel disease, cancer, female urogenital infections, and surgical infections. Probiotic administration has been effective with antibiotic-associated diarrhea (AAD). One of the meta-analyses found that *S. boulardii*, *L. rhamnosus*, and multiple mixtures of two different probiotics were the most protective against AAD.

In a number of studies, probiotic cotreatment has not consistently been shown to prevent *Clostridium difficile* colitis (CDC). In the largest study to date, *S. boulardii*, in combination with vancomycin and metronidazole, was associated with a significant decrease in the risk of CDC recurrence.

A systematic review of trials suggests that infectious diarrhea, commonly called *traveler's diarrhea*, may be shortened in both adults and children by about 30 hours by the use of probiotics. In this Cochrane review of 23 studies including almost 2,000 participants (352 of which were adults), it was concluded that probiotics reduced the risk of persistent diarrhea compared with placebo or no probiotics at 3 days with a RR of 0.66 (95% CI 0.55–0.77) (Allen et al., 2010). The majority (18 out of 23 studies) of the probiotics tested were LABs (lactic acid bacteria), with two studies using *S. boulardii* (Verna, 2010).

The strongest evidence for the use of probiotics in IBD is in the prevention and treatment of pouchitis. After proctocolectomy with ileal pouch–anal anastomosis, pouchitis (acute and chronic inflammation of the ileal reservoir) is the most frequent long-term complication, occurring in up to 20% of patients at 1 year. Studies of the microflora in the pouch have revealed deficiency of Streptococcal species. These studies consistently show a decrease in incidence and relapse of inflammatory response. One uncontrolled trial in patients with mild active pouchitis who were treated with VSL#3 showed a remission rate of 69% (Gionchetti et al., 2007).

Researched clinical benefits are achieved with strain-specific microbial organisms, which are defined by their genus, species, and strain and delivered at adequate levels of probiotic microbes to confer health benefits. With the utilization of DNA testing, strains' names have changed in recent years, making it difficult to follow which strains contribute health benefits and their new identified names. Preparation of probiotic products with unknown strain composition cannot be credited as having the same health benefits. Unfortunately, study results often become commercialized by supplement manufacturers and their marketing teams, who assign health benefits to products that do not meet the rigors of strains of specific species or have sufficient colony forming unit (CFU) levels to deliver the same health benefits. Compounding this confusion for both health care providers and the public is that charting of probiotic strains in journals is often done using country of origin studies that do not correlate to the U.S. market, since some products are not available in the United States or have altered product names.

Probiotic Strains Available in the United States

Probiotic	Company/Food Product	Therapeutic Use/Benefits	Recommended Clinical Dose CFU (Colony Forming Units)
B. animalis DN 173 010	Activia yogurt	Prevention of antibiotic diarrhea in adults.	10^{10} cfu b.i.d.
		Alleviates symptoms of irritable bowel syndrome.	10^{10} cfu b.i.d.
		Increased gut transit time.	10^{10} cfu b.i.d.
B. infantis 35624	Algin	Alleviates symptoms of irritable bowel syndrome.	10^8 cfu o.d.
B. lactis HN019 (aka Howaru™)	Xymogen	Immune support.	10^8 cfu o.d.
	Metagenics	Increased gut transit time.	1.5 10^9 cfu o.d.
	Lifetime Kefir		
B. lactis HN019 performs with a high adherence to cultured intestinal epithelial cells and helps modulate immunity by positively influencing intestinal immune cell and cytokine balance. Additional HN019 proved to dose-dependently increase colon transit time and reduce frequency of digestive complaints. Antibiotic use occurred before and after (Chang et al., 2010).			
B. lactis BB12	YoPlus yogurt	Prevention of antibiotic diarrhea in children.	$10^7 + 10^6$ cfu/g of formula
S. thermophilus			
B. lactis Bl-01	Metagenics		
B. lactis Bl-07			
B. lactis Bl-01 and Bl-07 strains target support to small and large intestines. Symptom relief addresses bowel distress such as cramping or occasional urgent bowel movements. Supports normal gut transit time and positively influences intestinal immune cells and cytokine balance. Antibiotic use occurred before and after (EFSA Panel on Dietetic Products, Nutrition and Allergies, 2009).			
L. acidophilus La-14	Xymogen		
L. acidophilus La-14 targets the human mouth, intestinal tract, and vagina with excellent adhesion to human epithelial cell lines, competing with pathogens for adhesion and limiting the ability of enteric pathogens to colonize. This strain is vancomycin-sensitive. It does not contribute to antibiotic resistance (EFSA Panel on Dietetic Products, Nutrition and Allergies, 2009).			
L. acidophilus NCFM	Metagenics		

COMPLEMENTARY & ALTERNATIVE THERAPIES Probiotics, *continued*

Probiotic	Company/Food Product	Therapeutic Use/Benefits	Recommended Clinical Dose CFU (Colony Forming Units)
L. acidophilus NCFM targets the small intestine. It provides beneficial support to cramping with urgent bowel movements alternating with occasional constipation. Adjuvant therapy is available for urinary tract infection and vaginal candidiasis (Putaala et al., 2010).			
L. bulgaricus and/or *S. thermophilus*	All yogurts	Lactose intolerance.	
L. bulgaricus is a starter culture for commercial yogurts with live, active cultures listed on the labeling (Wolvers, Antoine, Myllyluoma, Schrezenmeir, Szajewska, & Rijkers, 2010).			
L. casei DN-114 001 Fermented milk with *L. delbrueckii ssp bulgaricus, S. thermophilus*	DanActive yogurt Actimel yogurt	Prevention of *C. difficile* diarrhea in adults. Prevention of antibiotic diarrhea in adults. Adjuvant therapy for *H. pylori* eradication.	10^{10} cfu b.i.d. 10^{10} cfu b.i.d. 10^{10} cfu b.i.d.
L. helveticus R0052 and *L. rhamnosus* R0011	Xymogen	Supports gut immune functions.	
L. helveticus R0052 and *L. rhamnosus* R0011 strains were clinically tested as a mixture due to their complementary synergy. This mixture has diverse health benefits with excellent adhesion to human epithelial cell lines, competing with pathogens for adhesion and limiting the ability of enteric pathogens to colonize. This strain is vancomycin-sensitive. It does not contribute to antibiotic resistance (EFSA Panel on Dietetic Products, Nutrition and Allergies, 2009).			
L. paracasei Shirota	Yakult	Prevention of nosocomial diarrhea in children.	10^{9} cfu b.i.d.
L. paracasei Shirota beneficially affects lowered immunity and can be used for support during and after antibiotic use (Wolvers et al., 2010).			
L. paracasei Lpc-37	Metagenics		
L. paracasei Lpc-37 encourages the growth of beneficial microflora, particularly in the small intestine, which beneficially supports diverse health concerns such as eczema and intestinal dysbiosis (microbial imbalance) (EFSA Panel on Dietetic Products, Nutrition and Allergies, 2009).			
L. plantarum 299v	Metagenics Good Belly yogurt		
L. plantarum 299v targets the small and large intestines. Preliminary research suggests that *L. plantarum* 299v may beneficially influence levels of IL-6 and IL-10, important cytokines that may affect intestinal function and comfort. Antibiotic use occurs before and after (EFSA Panel on Dietetic Products, Nutrition and Allergies, 2009).			
L. plantarum Lp-115	Metagenics Xymogen		
L. plantarum Lp-115 encourages the growth of beneficial microflora, particularly in the small intestine. This safe strain is frequently found in high numbers in lactic-acid-fermented foods such as olives and sauerkraut. Human studies indicated stimulation of specific immunity (IgG). The strain degrades oxalates by 40% (EFSA Panel on Dietetic Products, Nutrition and Allergies, 2009).			
L. reuteri ATCC 55730	BioGaia Stonyfield Yogurt	Treatment of acute infectious diarrhea in children. Prevention of nosocomial diarrhea in children. Colic in infants (*L. reuteri* drops BioGaia).	10^{10} –10^{11} cfu b.i.d. 10^{9} cfu b.i.d.
L. rhamnosus GG	Culturelle Danimals Yogurt Sauerkraut	Prevention of antibiotic diarrhea in children. Prevention of antibiotic diarrhea in adults.	10^{10} –10^{11} cfu b.i.d. 10^{10} –10^{11} cfu, b.i.d.
L. rhamnosus HN001	Metagenics	Treatment of acute infectious diarrhea in children. Prevention of antibiotic diarrhea in adults. Prevention of nosocomial diarrhea in children. Adjuvant therapy for *H. pylori* eradication. Alleviates symptoms of irritable bowel syndrome.	10^{10}–10^{11} cfu b.i.d. 10^{10}–10^{11} cfu b.i.d. 10^{10}–10^{11} cfu b.i.d. 6×10^{9} cfu b.i.d. 6×10^{9} cfu b.i.d.
L. rhamnosus HN001 is beneficial in the treatment of eczema and prevention of atopy (hereditary predisposition toward developing allergic hypersensitivity reactions); supportive in cases of erosive gastritis due to nonsteroidal anti-inflammatory drug use; supports intestinal hyperpermeability and intestinal dysbiosis (EFSA Panel on Dietetic Products, Nutrition and Allergies, 2009).			
L. rhamnosus R0011	Xymogen		
L. rhamnosus R0011 maintains the integrity of the intestinal barrier and increases the expression of mucins in the jejunum and ileum. It greatly modulates pro-inflammatory reactions. Studied in combination with species *L. helveticus* R0052 (EFSA Panel on Dietetic Products, Nutrition and Allergies, 2009).			
L. salivarius LS-33	Metagenics		

(*continued*)

Weblink: Probiotics—European Commission

Weblink: Probiotics and Prebiotics

COMPLEMENTARY & ALTERNATIVE THERAPIES Probiotics, *continued*

Probiotic	Company/Food Product	Therapeutic Use/Benefits	Recommended Clinical Dose CFU (Colony Forming Units)
L. salivarius LS-33 targets the small intestine, encouraging the growth of beneficial microflora (Putaala et al., 2010).			
Saccharomyces boulardii	Metagenics	Treatment of acute infectious diarrhea in children.	200 mg t.i.d.
	Xymogen	Prevention of antibiotic diarrhea in children.	250 mg b.i.d.
		Prevention of antibiotic diarrhea in adults.	1 g or 3×10^{10} cfu o.d.
		Prevention of *C. difficile* diarrhea in adults.	2×10^{10} cfu o.d.
		Adjuvant therapy for *H. pylori* eradication.	1 g or 5×10^{9} cfu o.d.
Saccharomyces boulardi is a beneficial, nonpathogenic yeast. Within the lumen of the intestine, it may degrade toxins of pathogens, interfere with pathogenic adherence, modulate normal microbiota, and preserve normal intestinal physiology. It may also indirectly restore normal short-chain fatty acid (SCFA) balance, increase secretory IgA (sIgA) levels, or act as an immune regulator by influencing cytokine levels (McFarland, 2010). It does not contribute to antibiotic resistance.			
Streptococcus thermophilus ST-21	Metagenics		
Streptococcus thermophilus ST-21 is normally blended with *Bifidobacterium* strains to support the large intestine's immunity and bowel functions (Wolvers et al., 2010).			
Tested as Mixture			
L. acidophilus CL 1265 & *L. casei* Lbc80r	BioK+	Prevention of antibiotic diarrhea in adults.	5×10^{10} cfu o.d.
Tested as Mixture			
L. rhamnosus GR-1 & *L. reuteri* RC-14	Fem Dophilus	Prevention and maintenance of remission for bacterial vaginosis.	
L. rhamnosus GR-1 and *L. reuteri* RC-14 have clinical success in passing through the intestine, ascending along the perineum into the vagina, and competing with pathogens for adhesion (EFSA Panel on Dietetic Products, Nutrition and Allergies, 2009).			
Tested as Mixture			
VSL3# *L. acidophilus* NCFB 1748	VSL#3	Alleviates symptoms of irritable bowel syndrome.	4.5×10^{11} cfu b.i.d.
L. acidophilus, L. plantarum, L. paracasei, Lactobacillus delbrueckii, Bifidobacteria (*B. breve, B. longum, B. infantis*), *Streptococcus thermophilus*		Prevention and maintenance of remission of pouchitis.	4.5×10^{11} cfu b.i.d.

Source: Guarner, F., Khan, A. G., Garisch, J., Eliakim, R., Gangl, A., Thomson, A., et al. (2008). Probiotics and probiotics. *World Gastroenterology Organisation Practice Guideline.*

Criteria for Table Each probiotic strain supports specific activities within the body. The scientific identification of strains with established health benefits ensures clinical reliability and predicted safety. Clinical reliability is ensured through the genetic identification of each strain; beneficial properties of each probiotic strain are verified by supportive scientific and clinical research; potency and high viability of each strain are verified through testing of acid and bile tolerance and cell adherence; potency and viability are guaranteed through date of expiration. The two predominant suppliers of well-researched strain-specific probiotics used in nutritional supplementation are Institut Rosell and Danisco; their strains are represented in the United States in the health care professional lines of Metagenics and Xymogen. Both companies have protocols to effectively communicate product recall information to health care providers.

Unless under medical observation, probiotics are contraindicated in the following circumstances: intravenous catheters; postsurgery for GI, oral, and allografts; patients with a history of myocarditis and endocarditis; patients with liver dysfunction, including diabetes; patients undergoing immunosuppressive therapy; and immune-deficient patients such as AIDS patients.

Sources: Allen, S.J., Martinez, E.G., Gregorio, G.V., & Dans, L.F. (2010). Probiotics for treating acute infectious diarrhea. *Cochrane Database of Systematic Review, Issue 11,* Art. No.: CD003048. Borchers, A. T., Selmi, C., Meyers, F. J., Keen, C. L., & Gershwin, M. E. (2009). Probiotics and immunity. *Journal of Gastroenterology, 44*(1), 26–46. Epub; Liu, C., Zhang, Z.Y., Dong, K., & Guo. X.K. (2010). Adhesion and immunomodulatory effects of *Bifidobacterium lactis* HN019 on intestinal epithelial cells INT-407. *World Journal of Gastroenterology, 16*(18), 2283–2290; EFSA Panel on Dietetic Products, Nutrition and Allergies (2009). Scientific opinion on the substantiation of health claims related to noncharacterized microorganisms pursuant to Article 13 of Regulation (EC) No 1924/2006 on request from the European Commission. *EFSA Journal, 7*(9), 1247. [64 pp.]. doi:10.2903/j.efsa.2009.1247. Retrieved from: www.efsa.europa.eu; Gionchetti, P., Rizzello, F., Morselli, C., Poggioli, G., Tambasco, R., Calabrese, C., et al. (2007). High-dose probiotics for the treatment of active pouchitis. *Diseases of the Colon and Rectum, 50*(12), 2075–2082; discussion 2082-4. Epub 2007 Oct 13; Guarner, F., Khan, A. G., Garisch, J., Eliakim, R., Gangl, A., Thomson, A., et al. (2011). Probiotics and prebiotics. *World Gastroenterology Organisation Practice Guideline,* Retrieved from: http://www.worldgastroenterology.org/assets/export/userfiles/Probiotics_FINAL_20110116.pdf?utm_source=wgofoundation&utm_medium=wdhd2012&utm_campaign=guidelines.; McFarland, L. V. (2010). Systematic review and meta-analysis of *Saccharomyces boulardii* in adult patients. *World Journal of Gastroenterology, 16*(18), 2202–2222; Putaala, H., Barrangou, R., Leyer, G. J., Ouwehand, A. C., Hansen, E. B., Romero, D. A., et al. (2010). Analysis of the human intestinal epithelial cell transcriptional response to *Lactobacillus acidophilus, Lactobacillus salivarius, Bifidobacterium lactis* and *Escherichia coli. Beneficial Microbes, 1*(3), 283–295; Sanders, M. E., Akkermans, L. M., Haller, D., Hammerman, C., Heimbach, J., Hörmannsperger, G., et al. (2010). Safety assessment of probiotics for human use. *Gut Microbes, 1*(3), 164–185. Epub 2010 Mar 4; Verna, E. C. (2010). Use of probiotics in gastrointestinal disorders: What to recommend? *Therapy of Advanced Gastroenterology, 3*(5), 307–319; Wolvers, D., Antoine, J. M., Myllyluoma, E., Schrezenmeir, J., Szajewska, H., & Rijkers, G. T. (2010). Guidance for substantiating the evidence for beneficial effects of probiotics: Prevention and management of infections by probiotics. *Journal of Nutrition, 140*(3), 698S–712S. Epub 2010 Jan 27.

Weblink: Cancer: Facts & Figures 2012

Colon Cancer

Epidemiology and Etiology

Colon cancer involves abnormal cells that grow in either the colon or the rectum. The American Cancer Society (2012c) estimates that approximately 103,170 people in the United States were newly diagnosed with colon cancer in 2011, and 40,290 with rectal cancer, with an expected 51,690 deaths for colorectal cancer. If the lesions are confined to the colon and rectum, the 5-year survival rate is as high as 91%. If there is spread to the adjacent tissues, the survival rate drops to 70%; and if there is involvement of distant sites, the survival rate is as low as 11% (American Cancer Society, 2010). Although early detection is vital, the American Cancer Society (2010) reports that only 39% of colorectal cancer is found early. The Cultural Considerations box outlines the disparity in the rates of cancer, including colon cancer, among different racial and ethnic groups. The Evidence-Based Practice box features research on the keys to survival of colon cancer.

There are numerous screening recommendations for colorectal cancer, including sigmoidoscopy every 5 years, colonoscopy every 10 years, double contrast barium enema every 5 years, or CT colonography every 5 years (American Cancer Society, 2010). Other tests may include a yearly fecal occult blood exam or a yearly fecal immunochemical test. Finally, a DNA stool test may be conducted. All of the tests are recommended to begin with patients at age 50, but it is generally thought that individuals with personal or family histories should begin screening earlier (American Cancer Society, 2010). Hopefully, the newer DNA stool test will promote early detection of colorectal cancer.

CULTURAL CONSIDERATIONS Related to Colon Cancer

According to the American Cancer Society (2011a), African Americans are more likely to develop and die from colon cancer than members of any other racial or ethnic population. Currently, the death rate from cancer among African American males is 32% higher than that among White males; for African American females, it is about 16% higher. Overall, racial and ethnic minorities face more obstacles in receiving health care services, including cancer prevention, early detection, and quality treatment. African American males have the highest incidence and mortality associated with colorectal cancers (Jemal, Siegel, Ward, Murray, Xu, & Thun, 2007).

Pathophysiology

As was previously mentioned, colorectal cancer is linked with increasing age. Other risk factors include IBD, a personal history of colorectal cancer or polyps, a family history of colorectal cancer, and several lifestyle factors (obesity, smoking, heavy alcohol consumption, inactivity, and dietary issues) (American Cancer Society, 2010). There is a strong association between the development of colon cancer and genetics. Researchers have linked an alteration in the p53 gene to 75% to 85% of colorectal cancers. Also, when there is an allelic deletion on chromosome 5, 17, or 18, the transformation from normal to malignant colon tissue is promoted (Huether, 2010a).

Adenomatous polyps, which result from a mutation on chromosome 5, are considered premalignant tissue, and most colorectal cancers develop from this type of polyp. The larger the polyp, the more likely it will transform into malignant tissue. Another hereditary type of cancer is hereditary nonpolyposis colon cancer (HNPCC), or Lynch Syndrome, which is more common on the right side of the colon and is associated with a DNA mutation (Huether, 2010a).

There appears to be a link between dietary factors and the development of colorectal cancer. Generally, diets that are high in fruits and vegetables are linked to lower incidence of colorectal cancer, whereas diets that are high in red and processed meats are linked to higher incidence of colorectal cancer (American Cancer Society, 2010). Other

EVIDENCE-BASED PRACTICE Colon Cancer: Keys to Survival

Clinical Problem

Colon cancer is the third highest of all cancers in both incidence and deaths for men and women, and the incidence generally increases after age 50. The survival rate can be as high as 91% when colon cancer is found early; however, only 39% of colorectal cancer is found early (American Cancer Society, 2010). The key to increasing survival is to identify risk factors in combination with early detection and screening. Risk factors associated with colon cancer include increasing age, inflammatory bowel disease, a personal history of colorectal cancer or polyps, a family history of colorectal cancer, genetics, and lifestyle factors such as obesity, smoking, heavy alcohol consumption, inactivity, and diet. There are numerous screening recommendations for colorectal cancer, as noted previously. Nurses must understand how to use evidence-based findings when caring for patients who are considered to be at risk for developing colon cancer as well as those who should begin screening.

Research Findings

Myers et al. (2007) reported targeted and tailored interventions increased colorectal cancer screening. The researchers felt that the underutilization of screening and the high rates of colon cancer incidence and mortality warranted the need for tailored interventions to improve screening use. The sample consisted of 1,546 adult participants divided into four research groups: a control group that received care without additional colon cancer information, a standard intervention group that received care plus colorectal screening information and intervention, a tailored intervention group that received the standard intervention plus two messages discussing barriers to flexible sigmoidoscopy and fecal occult blood screening, and a tailored intervention plus reminder phone call group that received the tailored intervention plus reminder phone calls. Results indicated that all intervention groups participated in colorectal screenings significantly more than the control group, but there were no significant differences between the intervention groups. However, the researchers stated that many of the participants did not receive phone calls because of incorrect and disconnected phone numbers and lack of availability, so it was difficult to truly assess the effectiveness of the intervention; the participants who did receive calls (72%) did show a significantly higher rate of screening use.

Implications for Nursing Practice

The study by Myers et al. (2007) indicates that any intervention providing more information for colorectal screening will improve utilization and screening. Education is clearly within the nurse's scope of practice. Nurses can take the initiative to educate about the various types of colorectal screening as well as discuss possible barriers to screening. Reminder phone calls may prove beneficial in increasing screening use. Nurses may also assess patient preferences for colorectal screening and encourage follow-up for the preferred method. Although not addressed in this study, education about screening should also include education about reducing risk factors.

Critical Thinking Questions with answers can be found in the Osborn Student Resources at nursing.pearsonhighered.com.

Sources: American Cancer Society. (2010). Cancer facts & figures 2010. Retrieved from http//www.cancer.org/acs/groups/content/@epidemiologysurveilance/documents/document/acspc026238.pdf; Myers, R. E., Sifri, R., Hyslop, T., Rosenthal, M., Verson, S. W., Cocroft, J., et al. (2007). A randomized controlled trial of the impact of targeted and tailored interventions on colorectal screening. *Cancer, 110*(9), 2083–2091.

nutrients that are associated with a lower risk for colon cancer are folic acid, vitamin D, and calcium. Obesity is linked to an increased risk despite the patient's physical activity level (American Cancer Society, 2008); however, physical activity will help decrease obesity, so inactivity is considered a risk factor (American Cancer Society, 2010). There is also an increased risk of colon cancer with alcohol consumption of 30 grams or more per day (Ferarri et al., 2007).

There is some research to indicate that the use of nonsteroidal anti-inflammatory drugs (NSAIDs), such as aspirin and ibuprofen, and hormone replacement therapy decreases colon cancer risk (American Cancer Society, 2007).

There is also evidence to indicate a link between C-reactive protein (CRP) and colon cancer. C-reactive protein is a protein released from the liver in response to local inflammation or tissue injury. (See Chapter 32 for a detailed explanation of CRP.) Inflammation is known to be a risk factor associated with colon cancer, and studies indicate that CRP is often elevated in patients with colorectal cancer. In fact, it may indicate a poorer prognosis than in those who do not have elevations (Kwon et al., 2010). The chronic inflammation of inflammatory bowel disease is also known to increase the risk for developing colon cancer.

Adenocarcinoma is the most common type of colon cancer, accounting for 95% of colon tumors. Adenocarcinomas grow irregularly and form hard, nodular areas (Thomas, 2011). Colon cancer is classified by the tissue type, lymph node involvement, and stage of metastasis (TNM). Chapter 57 (p. 1770) outlines two tumor classification systems. Colon cancer cells range from well differentiated to poorly differentiated. The cancer is spread first by local invasion and direct extension. Any tissue or organ in the neighboring area can be affected, such as the liver, duodenum, small intestine, pancreas, and abdominal wall. Because the lymph system is closely associated with the intestines, cancer is also easily spread to distant sites. It can also reach distant sites by way of the circulation. The most common sites for metastasis of colon cancer are the liver, lungs, brain, and bones.

Clinical Manifestations

Colon cancer is usually asymptomatic until it is advanced. Most types of colon cancer grow very slowly, taking up to 10 years before symptoms are present, and even those symptoms are vague and often misdiagnosed (Thomas, 2011). The symptoms will depend mostly on the location of the tumor and its stage of growth. The most common symptoms are a change in bowel habits, such as constipation or diarrhea, or a change in the caliber of the stools. The symptom that causes the most alarm and usually prompts the patient to see a health care provider is blood in the stool. As the disease progresses, there may be weight loss, fatigue, abdominal pain, and anorexia. Anemia may also be a manifestation that causes the patient to seek medical attention.

Tumors in the ascending colon are usually polypoid and extend along one wall of the ascending colon. Because they are bulky tumors, a palpable mass can usually be felt. They tend to develop necrotic areas and ulcerate, contributing to the slow blood loss and anemia (Huether, 2010a). Descending colon tumors are usually small, buttonlike, and tend to grow around the circumference of the colon. They also spread along the entire bowel wall rather than growing along one wall of the colon. Because of the circumferential nature of this type of colon cancer, obstruction is common. Constipation is the predominant symptom as the bowel lumen becomes smaller as the tumor grows (Huether, 2010a).

Laboratory and Diagnostic Procedures

The various screening methods for colorectal cancer were discussed earlier. However, because sigmoidoscopy will detect cancer in only the sigmoid colon and the rectum, most health care providers recommend colonoscopy along with a tissue biopsy (Thomas, 2011). A CT scan is done to detect possible metastasis in distant locations such as the liver or lungs. There are no laboratory tests that can establish the diagnosis of colon cancer; however, many tests, such as a CBC to detect anemia related to chronic blood loss, are used to detect manifestations of colon cancer (Thomas, 2011). Other tests include a C-reactive protein and carcinoembryonic antigen (CEA) to detect inflammation and to serve as a tumor marker, respectively.

Medical Management

Surgery is the treatment of choice for individuals with colon cancer because it offers the only known cure. Even when metastasis has occurred, surgical resection can improve the chance of survival. There are several different surgical procedures for the patient with colon cancer, depending on the stage, tumor size, and the patient's general health. Surgery can range from abdominoperineal resection with a colostomy to local excision. With advances in surgical technique and equipment, most patients do not require a colostomy, as was once the case.

The National Comprehensive Cancer Network (NCCN, 2011) identifies surgical procedures for both colon and rectal cancer. The main types of surgeries are polypectomy, colectomy, and resection. The type of surgery will depend on the cancer stage and location.

Polypectomy

Many polyps can be removed through local excision (polypectomy); pedunculated polyps are easier to remove than sessile polyps (NCCN, 2011). Local excision can be done by endoscopy or by laparoscopy. This surgical method is used if the tumor is small and well defined.

Colectomy

If more extensive surgery is needed, an open or laparoscopic colectomy may be performed; NCCN (2011) guidelines also recommend evaluating at least 12 lymph nodes. Laparoscopic colectomy generally can be performed if there is no advanced or metastatic disease and no cancer complications such as obstruction. Open colectomies may include right- or left-sided hemicolectomy. Right-sided hemicolectomy involves removing part of the right ileum, right ascending colon, and transverse colon; left-sided hemicolectomy removes part of the transverse colon up to part of the rectum (Wilkes, 2011).

Resection

Rectal cancer is often surgically treated with resection. Tumors of the rectum usually require removal of the rectum, sigmoid colon, and anus, necessitating a sigmoid colostomy for fecal elimination (NCCN, 2011).

Occasionally, an end-to-end anastomosis is not possible during colon resection or colectomy; in this situation, the patient requires a colostomy for the diversion of fecal material. The type and permanence of the colostomy depend on the tumor's location (Figure 37–9◆). If there is a large amount of inflammation or tissue trauma, a temporary colostomy is created to give the bowel time to heal; at a later date, the bowel is reanastomosed and the colostomy is closed. There are many types of colostomies, including transverse double-barrel, transverse loop, ascending, descending, and sigmoid. A transverse double-barrel colostomy is when there are two stomas on the abdominal surface. The distal colon is bypassed but not removed and may be reanastomosed. The distal stoma, also called a mucous fistula because it drains mucus from the distal colon, usually requires only a gauze dressing. The proximal stoma will have fecal discharge and will require the application of an ostomy appliance (bag) to collect feces (see Figure 37–10◆). A transverse loop colostomy brings a loop of bowel through the abdominal wall, at which point an ostomy is created (Phillips, 2007).

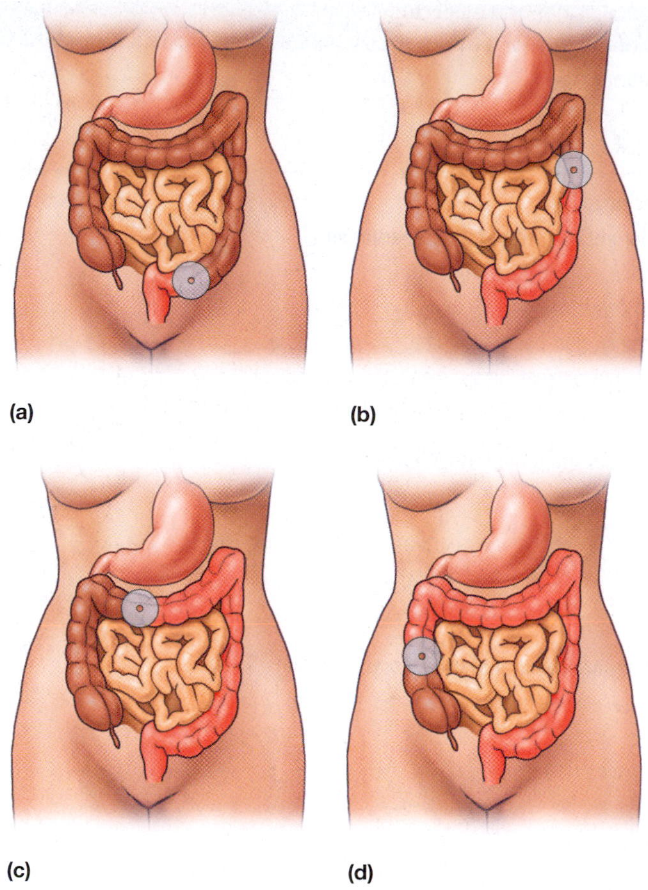

FIGURE 37–9 ◆ Colostomy sites.

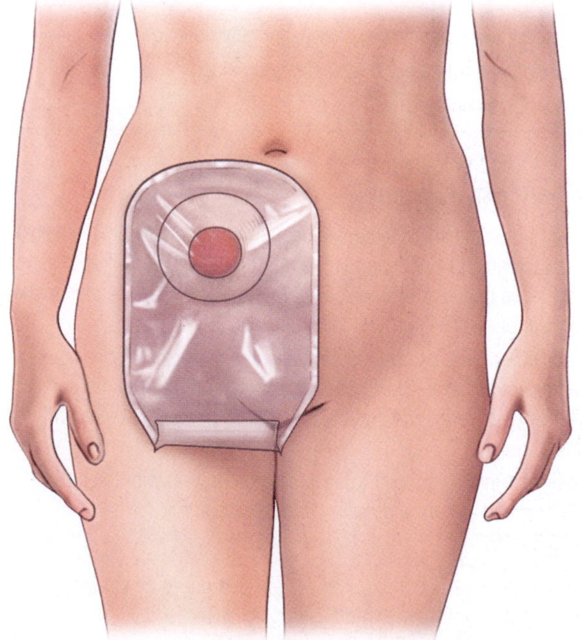

FIGURE 37–10 ◆ Patient wearing a colostomy bag.

Ascending colostomies, descending colostomies, and sigmoid colostomies are created on the basis of whether the tumor is on the right side, left side, or sigmoid part of the colon. Patients require the same care whether the colostomy is permanent or temporary. Nursing care of the patient with a colostomy is discussed in the Nursing Process box.

Chemotherapy and Radiation Therapy

Chemotherapeutic agents are used as an adjunctive therapy for colon cancer after colon resection. The patient is usually given a period of time to heal postoperatively before chemotherapy is started. Chemotherapy can be combined with radiation therapy to reduce the rate of recurrence. Radiation appears to prolong survival in patients with more advanced cancer, particularly rectal tumors. Radiation can also be used before surgery to shrink large tumors and make them easier to surgically resect (Wilkes, 2011).

Nursing Management

Early detection is key to improving the prognosis of patients with colon cancer. In addition to identifying patients with risk factors, tailored interventions may prove invaluable, as seen in the Evidence-Based Practice box (p. 1153). The health promotion section that follows discusses additional nursing management strategies.

Because the treatment of choice for patients with colon cancer is surgery, the focus of nursing care is on pre- and postoperative care and support in dealing with a possible colostomy, chemotherapy, or radiation treatment and possibly death. Emotional support throughout the course of the illness is paramount. See the Nursing Process: Patient Care Plan for Colon Cancer box. See Chapter 57 for more information about the care of the patient receiving radiation therapy or chemotherapy.

Health Promotion

Because there is a link between lifestyle choices and the development of colon cancer, nursing can encourage primary prevention of the disease by teaching and advising patients about lifestyle choices that may decrease the risk. Dietary modifications, including increasing the amount of dietary fiber and reducing the amount of fat, sugar, alcohol, and red and processed meat, can help reduce the risk of colon cancer. However, it is not enough simply to tell patients to modify their diet. The nurse must give specific information about what foods are high in fiber, such as fruits and vegetables, and those that are high in fat and sugar and should be eaten in limited quantities. It is important to consider cultural, economic, and religious factors in making the suggestions. Additionally, the nurse should talk to patients about exercise and reducing obesity in conjunction with dietary changes. Other important aspects of nursing care include teaching patients about the warning signs of colon cancer and when to seek treatment. The nurse should initiate a frank discussion with patients over age 40 about recommended screening and what each test involves.

Patients with abdominal pain, changes in bowel habits, or abdominal distention with rigidity should be encouraged to see a health care provider as these may be symptoms of more serious disease, such as obstruction or appendicitis.

Collaborative Management

Patients with intestinal disorders face many challenges, and will benefit from the assistance of an interdisciplinary team of health care providers. In order to meet desired patient outcomes, it is essential that this interdisciplinary team communicate openly with one another in developing and evaluating care of the patient and family (IOM [Institute of Medicine], 2010). The interdisciplinary team may consist of nurses, social workers, oncologists, surgeons, gastroenterologists, nutritionists, and primary care providers.

NURSING PROCESS: Patient Care Plan for Colon Cancer

Assessment of Gastrointestinal Status Using Gordon's Functional Health Patterns:

- Nutrition Metabolic Pattern
- Elimination Pattern
- Cognitive Perceptual Pattern
- Self-Perception Self-Concept Pattern

Subjective Data	Objective Data
Assessment of Perioperative Readiness	**Assessment of Perioperative Readiness**
What did the surgeon tell you about your surgery? Do you have any questions that you would like to ask?	Vital signs. Signed consent. Character of stool post bowel prep. Has the enterostomal therapy nurse seen the patient? Are all preop laboratory reports in the chart?
Assessment of Postoperative Pain	**Assessment of Postoperative Pain**
On a scale of 1 to 10, with 10 being the worst pain ever, how would you rate your pain? Are you allergic to any pain medications? Do you have any cultural or religious beliefs that might impact your pain control?	Vital signs. Restless and irritable. Facial grimacing when moving.
Assessment of Skin Integrity (Postoperative)	**Assessment of Skin Integrity (Postoperative)**
Ask the patient whether he has feeling around the stoma.	Assess the stoma and skin around the stoma for: Redness Color of stoma Swelling Drainage.
Assessment of Bowel Function	**Assessment of Bowel Function**
Are you passing any gas through the stoma? Do you feel any rumbling in your abdomen? Have you been nauseated?	Examination of abdomen: Bowel sounds Palpation Visual exam for contour, condition of stoma, and any drainage. Color, consistency, and frequency of colostomy drainage. Test stool for occult blood.

Outcomes and Evaluation Parameters	Planning and Interventions with *Rationales*
1. NURSING DIAGNOSIS: Fear *related to surgical procedure and diagnosis of cancer* (NANDA-I © 2012)	
Outcome: Ready for surgery. ***Evaluation Parameters:*** Signed consent. Lab reports in chart. Communicates fears and anxiety. Able to verbalize the nature and extent of the surgery.	Ask the patient to tell the nurse what will happen postoperatively. This helps the nurse assess the patient's understanding of the procedure and what to expect in the postoperative period. It also assesses whether the patient understands what she signed for on the informed consent. Administer the bowel prep as ordered and examine the stool to assess the effectiveness of the prep. Stool should be liquid and clear by the end of the prep. *The prep cleans the bowel and reduces the risk of infection postoperatively.* Contact the enterostomal therapist to arrange a preop visit with the patient *to help ease fear and anxiety about the possible colostomy.*
2. NURSING DIAGNOSIS: Pain, Acute *related to surgical incision* (NANDA-I © 2012)	
Outcome: Comfort level maintained. ***Evaluation Parameters:*** Communicates pain level and effectiveness of analgesia. Reports adequate pain control. No facial grimacing.	Use pain scale (1 to 10) to quantify level of pain in order to be consistent from nurse to nurse, and time to time, when assessing pain. Teach the patient to inform the nurse if the pain is not relieved. *Indicates the need to change the pain management plan.* Assess cultural and religious beliefs about pain and pain relief. Different cultures and religions may view pain as punishment or may have nontraditional ways of treating pain. Medicate the patient prior to ambulation. *Decreased pain increases exercise tolerance, and ambulation increases intestinal motility, preventing ileus, and enhances the respiratory effort, decreasing the chance of pneumonia.*

NURSING PROCESS: Patient Care Plan for Colon Cancer, *continued*

3. NURSING DIAGNOSIS: Skin Integrity, Impaired *related to colostomy and surgical incision* (NANDA-I © 2012)	
Outcome: Good skin and stomal integrity. ***Evaluation Parameters:*** Stoma pink and moist. Skin surrounding stoma pink, no excoriation.	Inspect the stoma and surrounding skin for color and edema. A healthy stoma is pink or beefy red and moist due to mucus production. The peristomal skin should be pink and show no signs of irritation, inflammation, excoriation, or rashes. *A bluish purple or dusky stoma indicates impaired blood flow to the stoma. Skin around the stoma can be irritated by the appliance, by a yeast infection, or from a leaking appliance.* Apply caulking agents (Stomahesive or Karaya paste) to maintain a leak-free secure ostomy appliance to prevent leakage onto skin. Ostomy drainage is very irritating to the skin and can cause skin breakdown. Assess the surgical incision for bleeding, redness, and draining at least every 4 hours. Change the dressing as ordered by the surgeon to keep the incision clean and dry, *which helps prevent an infected incision.*
4. NURSING DIAGNOSIS: Bowel Incontinence *related to surgery and fecal diversion* (NANDA-I © 2012)	
Outcome: Functioning colostomy. ***Evaluation Parameters:*** Stool from colostomy semiformed. Active bowel sounds.	Assess abdomen for bowel sounds, which indicate peristalsis has returned. *Bowel manipulation and anesthesia have the potential for causing an ileus.* Assess for nausea and vomiting, *which can also indicate an ileus.* Assess the characteristics of the colostomy drainage. Fecal-like drainage and flatulence from the stoma indicate the return of bowel function.

Source: Adapted from Wilkinson, J. M., & Ahearn, N. R. (2009). *Prentice Hall nursing diagnosis handbook* (9th ed.). Upper Saddle River, NJ: Prentice Hall.

Gastroenterologists and primary care providers will help make the diagnosis of intestinal diseases such as appendicitis, bowel obstruction, inflammatory bowel disease, irritable bowel disease, diverticular disease, and colon cancer. They will also provide medical management and follow-up care. They will also help promote education and screening for colorectal cancer. A surgeon may be required to treat any intestinal disease depending on the severity of the issue. An oncologist will be needed to consult with patients who have cancer.

Patients with diseases of the intestines will need education about prevention, long-term management, and dietary changes. Nurses can facilitate educating patients about the disease process, lifestyle changes, medication regimen, and follow-up care. A wound and ostomy nurse specialist will facilitate educating about stomas and stoma care as well as help with optimal placement of a stoma. A nutritionist will be instrumental in educating the patient regarding dietary changes, including preventive dietary changes for colon cancer. Social services can help provide resources, including support groups and ostomy supplies, for patients with intestinal disorders.

Disorders of the Rectum and Anus

Anorectal disorders include hemorrhoids, fissures, abscesses, and fistulas. These disorders are benign and fairly common.

Hemorrhoids

Hemorrhoids are swollen, inflamed veins in the anal canal. The cause is usually increased pressure exerted on the veins from straining when having a bowel movement or pregnancy. Hemorrhoids can be inside the anus or under the skin around the anus (external).

Clinical Manifestations

Symptoms may include (1) itching and burning, (2) swelling around the anus, (3) pain or discomfort, and (4) painless bleeding with bowel movement.

Medical Management

Most hemorrhoids are treated conservatively. Adding fiber to the diet is helpful for patients with bleeding from hemorrhoids as it softens the feces. The irritation and pruritus are treated with analgesic creams and warm sitz baths (sitting in warm water). For recurrent or very painful hemorrhoids, surgical removal may be necessary. Small hemorrhoids can be removed in an outpatient setting via rubber band ligation (a small rubber band is placed that strangles the hemorrhoid, which then dies and falls off); sclerotherapy, in which a chemical solution is injected into the hemorrhoid to shrink it; or coagulation therapy, in which a laser, infrared light, or heat is used to destroy the hemorrhoid. If the hemorrhoids are large, the patient may require surgical removal (hemorrhoidectomy).

Anal Fissure

An anal fissure is a tear in the lining of the anal canal. Most fissures are caused by local trauma to the canal (Breen & Bleday, 2011b).

Clinical Manifestations

After the tear occurs, the exposed internal sphincter muscle beneath spasms and causes severe pain. The spasm also pulls the edges apart and impairs healing of the fissure. Patients will complain of a tearing pain with bowel movements and may have a small amount of bright rectal bleeding. Anal fissures are diagnosed from the history and direct visualization of the rectum.

Medical Management

Medical management of anal fissures consists of three components:

1. Relaxation of the internal sphincter. Topical nitroglycerin may be used to increase local blood flow and reduce pressure in the internal anal sphincter. Injection of botulinum toxin into the anal sphincter can also be done to inhibit the release of acetylcholine from the nerve endings and stop the spasms.

2. Prevention of traumatic passage of stool by introducing fiber therapy to keep stools soft and formed. Also, the patient can take warm sitz baths after bowel movements to help relax the sphincter.
3. Pain control with topical anesthetic creams to soothe the inflamed tissue.

Surgical Management

If medical management of anal fissures fails, a lateral internal sphincterotomy may be performed to relax the internal anal sphincter. The fissure itself is not removed. The main complication from a sphincterotomy is the development of fecal incontinence.

Anal Abscesses and Fistulas

Anal abscesses are the acute manifestation of an infectious process, and the fistula is the chronic manifestation of the same perirectal process. Most abscesses and fistulas originate from an infected anal crypt gland (Breen & Bleday, 2011a). There are 8 to 10 anal crypt glands around the anal canal. An abscess develops when a gland becomes obstructed by debris that permits bacterial growth and abscess formation. The anal fistula is the connection between two epithelial structures and connects the abscess from the gland to the skin of the buttocks.

Clinical Manifestations

Patients with anal abscesses or fistulas usually complain of severe, constant pain in the anal region. They may also have a fever and general malaise. Purulent rectal drainage may be present if the abscess is draining spontaneously.

Medical Management

Anal abscesses are drained immediately. Approximately 50% of all patients with an anal abscess develop a fistula (Breen & Bleday, 2011a). Symptomatic fistulas may be removed surgically (fistulotomy), but the procedure is associated with a high rate of anorectal dysfunction and fecal incontinence.

Nursing Management

The nurse should have the patient describe the kind of pain and exact location and determine whether the patient has experienced rectal itching or pain with sitting, coughing, or bowel movement. The nurse also should ask whether the patient has had any signs of infection such as fever, malaise, or drainage from or around the anus. If the patient has required a surgical procedure, discharge instructions should include the following:

- Lie flat for 1 or 2 days after surgery to decrease swelling in the anal area; this position is also more comfortable than sitting.
- Increase fluids and fiber in the diet. Fiber supplements will produce bulky stool, which is easier to pass.
- Use pain medication as prescribed. A narcotic may cause constipation and a stool softener should be prescribed.
- Take sitz baths at least three times a day to keep the area clean.

Gerontological Considerations

During evaluation of the older patient with abdominal pain, the nurse must remember that medications such as glucocorticoids and beta-blockers, as well as comorbidities such as heart disease and diabetes, are more common and may mask signs and symptoms. According to Kendall and Moreira (2011), serious disorders that are common to consider in the older patient with abdominal pain are (1) mesenteric ischemia, (2) bowel obstruction/perforation, and (3) diverticular disease.

The incidence of digestive disorders increases with age. Johns Hopkins Medicine states that up to 40% of older adults experience

RESEARCH OPPORTUNITIES Related to Disorders of the Gastrointestinal Tract

Area	Clinical Impact
Physiological Research	
Use of complementary and alternative medicine in patients with gastrointestinal disorders.	Use of non-Western medicine for treatment of GI disorders may improve patient compliance because of fewer side effects and less cost, but more research is needed to validate its effectiveness.
Effectiveness of probiotics in inflammatory bowel disease.	Alternative therapies and probiotics may improve quality of life and decrease symptoms in patients with inflammatory bowel disease, but more research is needed.
Laparoscopic surgery for colon cancer.	Less invasive surgical techniques would decrease complications and patient length of stay.
Identifying symptoms for irritable bowel syndrome.	Better diagnosis of irritable bowel syndrome will lead to earlier treatment.
Effect of aspirin, vitamin D, and fish oil on preventing colon cancer, as well as the possible role of aspirin in treating colon cancer.	Additional preventive measures may decrease the risk for colon cancer, but more research is needed; nurses also need to be cautious regarding side effects of aspirin before recommending.
Emotional and Psychological Research	
Communicating about screening for colon cancer in culturally diverse groups.	Improved communication between health care providers and culturally diverse groups can increase screening in these groups and hopefully decrease mortality.
Quality of life after surgery for gastroesophageal cancer.	Understanding issues about quality of life can assist nurses to help patients cope better with life changes.
Effectiveness of hypnotherapy on patients with inflammatory bowel disease.	
Role of stress and coping factors on gastrointestinal disorders.	Improve psychological interventions to improve coping.

digestive symptoms such as abdominal pain, nausea, bloating, gas, fever, or rectal bleeding (McLaughlin, 2010). These symptoms can indicate diverticular disease, gallstones, or colon cancer. Loss of muscle strength due to aging may lead to diverticular disease. Older patients who eat a low-fiber or high-fat diet and are overweight and sedentary heighten the risk of diverticular disease.

Research

Research being done regarding gastrointestinal disorders is focused on less invasive approaches to surgical treatments; education regarding screening exams, particularly those with cultural barriers; and multiple alternative therapies. The Research Opportunities box describes current research opportunities for gastrointestinal disorders.

Summary

The gastrointestinal tract begins at the mouth and continues to the anus. Each part of the gastrointestinal tract plays an important role in breaking down food to a form that can be used to build and nourish cells and provide energy. It is essential that the nurse understands the function of the gastrointestinal tract to care for and educate the patient with GI disorders. The nurse is key in teaching lifestyle changes and necessary screening to promote a healthy GI tract.

CLINICAL PREPARATION READ DOCUMENT APPLY

READ: **History of Present Illness** >> Laboratory Study Results >> Critical Thinking Questions

As a nurse working on a GI floor in a large teaching hospital, you are receiving report about Angela Trent, a 55-year-old woman who was admitted 2 days ago with hematemesis and abdominal pain. She reported symptoms of increasing epigastric pain for approximately 3 weeks, and the use of Tums, which had been working most of the time. She also reported taking aspirin daily for prevention of heart disease. The bleeding has stopped now, and she has just returned from an EGD (esophagogastroduodenoscopy), which confirmed a gastric ulcer.

Medical–Surgical History

Ms. Trent's past medical history includes gastroesophageal reflux disease for which she was prescribed Prilosec, but she could not afford to purchase the medication, so she has been taking Tums instead.

Social History

Ms. Trent has a 10 pack-year history of smoking, having quit 3 months prior to this admission. She reports being a social drinker. She reports an intentional weight loss of 50 pounds during the last year.

Physical Exam

Ms. Trent's vital signs are temperature 37°C; heart rate 90 and regular; respirations 16 and unlabored; and blood pressure 100/60 sitting. Her skin is pale and dry. Her lungs are clear to auscultation, and her heart is regular with no murmurs or extra heart sounds noted at this time. Her bowel sounds are present in all four quadrants, and her abdomen is soft with tenderness noted in the epigastrium. She has a nasogastric tube set to low intermittent suction that is draining green fluid.

Ms. Trent's current nursing care, medication schedule, and laboratory study results follow.

READ: History of Present Illnesses >> **Physical Exam** >> Admitting Medical Records >> Laboratory Study Results

Admitting Medical Orders

Service: Medicine
Diagnosis: gastric ulcer
Allergies: none
Vital signs with oxygen saturation q15min × 4 then q1h × 2 then q4h
Activity: up to chair 4 times per day, may ambulate to bathroom
Diet: NPO, may have ice chips
Nasogastric tube to low intermittent wall suction; flush NG with 30 mL saline q8h
Call health care provider: temp > 38.5°C, HR >130 or < 60, RR > 30 or < 12, BP sys >160 or < 90, O_2 sat < 92%, urine output < 120 mL in 4 hours, change in neurological or abdominal exam, any Hct result that is 5 less than the baseline ED Hct
IV: D5NS IV at 125 mL/hr
I&O: q8h
Test each stool for occult blood
Test NG drainage for occult blood q8h

Medications

Omeprazole 40 mg per NG daily (note: clamp NG tube for 2 hours after administration)
Sucralfate 1 g susp daily (note: give through NG at least 3 hours after omeprazole and clamp for 1 hour after administration)

PRN Medications

Morphine 2–3 mg IVP every 3 hours

Ordered Laboratory Studies

Type and crossmatch for 2 units packed RBCs (PRBCs)
CBC, electrolytes, reticulocyte count daily

CLINICAL PREPARATION, *continued*

READ: History of Present Illnesses >> **Laboratory Study Results** >> Critical Thinking Questions

Test	Admission	Day 1	Day 2
CBC			
Hemoglobin (Hgb)	10.5 g/dL	9.5 g/dL	10 g/dL
Hematocrit (Hct)	31%	27%	30%
RBC	3.2 mm^3	2.7 mm^3	3 mm^3
Reticulocytes	2.0%	2.4%	2.4%
MCV	72 μm^3	68 μm^3	70 μm^3
MCH	27 pg	25 pg	26 pg
Platelets	150 mm^3	146 mm^3	148 mm^3
Electrolytes			
Sodium	135 mEq/L	135 mEq/L	140 mEq/L
Potassium	3.6 mEq/L	3.5 mEq/L	3.9 mEq/L
Calcium	9 mg/dL	9 mg/dL	9 mg/dL

Pearson Nursing Student Resources *Log on to* **nursing.pearsonhighered.com** *to download forms*

DOCUMENT:

>> Summary of Hospitalization
>> Pathophysiology Form
>> Laboratory Values
>> Laboratory Results Explanation

APPLY:

>> List of Potential Nursing Diagnoses
>> Concept Map
>> Critical Thinking Questions and Concept Map

APPLY: History of Present Illness >> Laboratory Study Results >> **Critical Thinking Questions**

1. What is the physiology mechanism behind the reason that aspirin causes peptic ulcers?
2. Why is omeprazole being given to Ms. Trent?
3. What is the impact of acute hemorrhage on the results of the CBC?

Answers to Critical Thinking Questions can be found in Appendix D in the Osborn Student Resources at nursing.pearsonhighered.com.

NCLEX® PRACTICE

1. The nurse suspects a patient has a fungal stomatitis when which clinical manifestation is assessed?
   1. Increased salivation and bad breath
   2. Painful red maculas with erythematous halos
   3. White curdlike patches on the tongue
   4. Oral ulcers covered with a grayish yellow membrane
2. The patient experiencing symptoms of gastroesophageal reflux disease (GERD) is diagnosed with Barrett's epithelium following endoscopic examination. How should the nurse explain the diagnosis to the patient?
   1. This is a precancerous tissue located in the esophagus. in the esophagus.
   2. This indicates the presence of esophageal strictures.
   3. This finding relates to fine tears in the distal esophagus common with GERD.
   4. This finding is reflective of ulcerated and inflamed esophageal tissue.
3. A patient is being evaluated for the presence of celiac disease. Which test would the nurse include as the most reliable when teaching the patient about diagnosis of this disease process?
   1. Gram staining of the stool
   2. Gastric pH analysis
   3. IgA tissue transglutaminase (tTG) antibodies
   4. Biopsy of the small intestine
4. A patient with a history of irritable bowel disease (IBD) has been recently diagnosed with Crohn's disease. Which manifestation specific to Crohn's disease, rather than IBD, disease does the nurse consider when planning care?
   1. Diarrhea can occur 10 to 20 times a day.
   2. Abdominal pain is cramping in nature.
   3. Malabsorption of nutrients often occurs.
   4. Incontinence of stool may be a problem.

5. A patient complains of having frequent episodes of belching and heartburn and is concerned that he may have gastroesophageal reflux disease (GERD). After completing the assessment, which of the following does the nurse determine could be a contributing factor to GERD? (select all that apply)
   1. Patient has a BMI of 21.
   2. Patient is lactose intolerant.
   3. Patient drinks citrus juice with meals.
   4. Patient eats a lot of high-fiber foods.
   5. Patient is a 1 pack per day cigarette smoker.

6. The nurse is planning care for a patient recently diagnosed with colon cancer. The patient is considering options for treatment. Which of the following should the nurse include in care? (Select all that apply.)
   1. Assess the patient's knowledge of surgical procedures.
   2. Assess the patient's ability to change the stoma device.
   3. Educate the patient about the importance of reporting constipation.
   4. Instruct the patient to limit red meat intake to 4 oz. per week.
   5. Encourage the patient to take a low dose aspirin every day.

Answers to NCLEX Practice questions can be found in Appendix D in the Osborn Student Resources at nursing.pearsonhighered.com. Practice additional NCLEX questions online at the Student Resources site.

Pearson Nursing Student Resources Find additional review materials at: **nursing.pearsonhighered.com**

REFERENCES

Adams, M. P., & Koch, R. W. (2010). *Pharmacology: Connections to nursing practice.* Upper Saddle River, NJ: Pearson.

Allen, S.J., Martinez, E.G., Gregorio, G.V., & Dans, L.F. (2010). Probiotics for treating acute infectious diarrhea. *Cochrane Database of Systematic Review, Issue 11,* Art. No.: CD003048.

American Cancer Society. (2008). Colorectal cancer facts and figures 2008–2010. Retrieved from http://www.cancer.org/acs/groups/content/@nho/documents/document/f861708finalforwebpdf.pdf

American Cancer Society. (2012a). Esophagus cancer. Retrieved from http://www.cancer.org/Cancer/EsophagusCancer/DetailedGuide/esophagus-key-statistics

American Cancer Society. (2012b). Stomach cancer. Retrieved from http://www.cancer.org/Cancer/StomachCancer/DetailedGuide/stomach-key-statistics

American Cancer Society. (2012c). Colorectal cancer. Retrieved from http://www.cancer.org/Cancer/ColonandRectumCancer/DetailedGuide/colorectal-cancer-key-statistics

American Cancer Society. (2010). Cancer facts & figures 2010. Retrieved from http://www.cancer.org/acs/groups/content/@epidemiologysurveillance/documents/document/acspc-026238.pdf

American Cancer Society. (2011a). Cancer facts & figures for African Americans 2011–2012. Retrieved from http://www.cancer.org/acs/groups/content/@epidemiologysurveillance/documents/document/acspc-027765.pdf

American Cancer Society. (2011b). Oral cavity and oropharyngeal cancer. Retrieved from http://www.cancer.org/Cancer/OralCavityandOropharyngealCancer/DetailedGuide/index

American Cancer Society. (2011c). Stomach cancer. Retrieved from http://www.cancer.org/Cancer/StomachCancer/DetailedGuide/index

Arduino, P. G., & Porter, S. R. (2008). Herpes simplex virus type 1 infection: Overview on relevant clinico-pathological features. *Journal of Oral Pathology & Medicine, 37,* 107–121.

Baumgart, D. C. (2008). What's new in inflammatory bowel disease in 2008? *World Journal of Gastroenterology, 14*(3), 329–330. doi: 10.3748/wjg.14.329

Bio-Center Laboratory. (2012). *Vitamins.* Retrieved from http://biocenterlab.org/tests/vitamins/vitaminb.shtml

Borchers, A. T., Selmi, C., Meyers, F. J., Keen, C. L., & Gershwin, M. E. (2009). Probiotics and immunity. *Journal of Gastroenterology, 44*(1), 26–46. Epub.

Breen, E., & Bleday, R. (2011a). Anal abscesses and fistulas. Retrieved from http://www.uptodate.com

Breen, E., & Bleday, R. (2011b). Anal fissures. Retrieved from http://www.uptodate.com

Brown-Guttovz, H. (2008). About irritable bowel syndrome. *Nursing, 38*(2), 28. doi: 10.1097/01.NURSE.0000309719.52056.fc

Cagir, B. (2012). Short-bowel syndrome. Retrieved from http://www.emedicine.medscape.com/article/193391-overview

Cary, V. A., & Boullata, J. (2010). What is the evidence for the use of probiotics in the treatment of inflammatory bowel disease? *Journal of Clinical Nursing, 19,* 904–916. doi:10.1111/j.1365-2702.2009.03123.x

Liu, C., Zhang, Z. Y., Dong, K., & Guo. X. K. (2010). Adhesion and immunomodulatory effects of Bifidobacterium lactis HN019 on intestinal epithelial cells INT-407. *World Journal of Gastroenterology, 16*(18), 2283–2290.

Crohn's & Colitis Foundation of America. (2009a). About the epidemiology of IBD. Retrieved from http://ccfa.org/about/press/epidemiologyfacts

Crohn's & Colitis Foundation of America. (2009b). Surgery for ulcerative colitis. Retrieved from http://www.ccfa.org/info/surgery/surgeryuc

Cryer, B. L., & Gerson, L. B. (2011). Nonsteroidal anti-inflammatory drugs. Retrieved from http://www.gastro.org/patient-center/diet-medications/nonsteriodal-anti-inflammatory-drugs-nsaids

Day, M. W. (2008). Fight back against inflammatory bowel disease. *Nursing, 28*(11), 34–41. doi: 10.1097/01.NURSE.0000341078.53082.f8

Edmondson, D., & Schiech, L. (2008). Esophageal cancer—A tough pill to swallow. *Nursing, 38*(4), 44–51.

EFSA Panel on Dietetic Products, Nutrition and Allergies (2009). Scientific opinion on the substantiation of health claims related to noncharacterized microorganisms pursuant to Article 13 of Regulation (EC) No 1924/2006 on request from the European Commission. *EFSA Journal, 7*(9), 1247. [64 pp.]. doi:10.2903/j.efsa.2009.1247. Retrieved from www.efsa.europa.eu

Enestvedt, B. K., Williams, J. L., & Sonnenberg, A. (2011). Epidemiology and practice patterns of achalasia in a large multicentre database. *Alimentary Pharmacology & Therapeutics, 33*(1), 1209–1214.

Ferrari, P., Jenab, M., Norat, T., Moskal, A., Slimani, N., Olsen, A., et al. (2007). Lifetime and baseline alcohol intake and risk of colon and rectal cancers in the European prospective investigation into cancer and nutrition (EPIC). *International Journal of Cancer, 121*(9), 2065–2072. doi:10.1002/ijc.22966

Fisichella, P. M., & Patti, M. G. (2009). Achalasia. Retrieved from http://emedicine.medscape.com/article/169974-overview.

Gerzevitz, D., Porter, B. O., & Dunphy, L. M. (2011). Eyes, ears, nose, and throat. In L. M. Dunphy, J. E. Winland-Brown, B. O. Porter, & D. J. Thomas (Eds.), *Primary care: The art and science of advanced practice nursing* (3rd ed., pp. 245–333). Philadelphia: F. A. Davis.

Gionchetti, P., Rizzello, F., Morselli, C., Poggioli, G., Tambasco, R., Calabrese, C., et al. (2007). High-dose probiotics for the treatment of active pouchitis. *Diseases of the Colon and Rectum, 50*(12), 2075–2082; discussion 2082-4. Epub 2007 Oct 13.

Grundmann, O., & Yoon, S. L. (2010). Irritable bowel syndrome: Epidemiology, diagnosis and treatment: An update for health-care practitioners. *Journal of Gastroenterology and Hepatology, 25,* 691–699. doi:10.111/j.1440-1746.2009.06120.x

Guarner, F., Khan, A. G., Garisch, J., Eliakim, R., Gangl, A., Thomson, A., et al. (2008). Probiotics and probiotics. *World Gastroenterology Organisation Practice Guideline.* Retrieved from http://www.worldgastroenterology.org/assets/export/userfiles/Probiotics_FINAL_20110116.pdf?utm_source=wgofoundation&utm_medium=wdhd2012&utm_campaign=guidelines

Harris, D. J., Eilers, J., Harriman, A., Cashavelly, B. J., & Maxwell, C. (2008). Putting evidence into practice®: Evidence-based interventions for the management of oral mucositis. *Clinical Journal of Oncology Nursing, 12*(1), 141–152. doi:10.1188/08.CJON.141-152

Huether, S. E. (2010a). Alterations of digestive function. In K. L. McCance, S. E. Huether, V. L. Brashers, & N. S. Rote (Eds.), *Pathophysiology: The biologic basis for disease in adults and children* (6th ed., pp. 1452–1515). St. Louis: Mosby.

Huether, S. E. (2010b). Structure and function of the digestive system. In K. L. McCance, S. E. Huether, V. L. Brashers, & N. S. Rote (Eds.), *Pathophysiology: The biologic basis for disease in adults and children* (6th ed., pp. 1420–1451). St. Louis: Mosby.

IOM (Institute of Medicine). (2010). *The future of nursing: Leading change, advancing health.* Washington, DC: The Academic Press.

Jemal, A., Siegel, R., Ward, E., Murray, T., Xu, J., & Thun, M. J. (2007). Cancer statistics, 2007. *CA: A Cancer Journal for Clinicians, 57*(1), 43–66.

Kee, J. L. (2010). *Laboratory and diagnostic tests with nursing implications* (8th ed.). Upper Saddle River, NJ: Prentice Hall.

Kelsch, R. (2007). Geographic tongue. Retrieved from http://www.emedicine.com/derm/topic664.htm

Kendall, J. L., & Moreira, M. E. (2011). Evaluation of the adult with abdominal pain in the emergency department. Retrieved from http://www.uptodate.com

Kumar, V., Abbas, A. K., Fausto, N., & Mitchell, R. N. (2007). *Robbins basic pathology* (8th ed.). Philadelphia: Saunders.

Kwon, K. A., Kim, S. A., Oh, S. Y., Lee, S., Han, J. Y., Kim, K. H., et al. (2010). Clinical significance of preoperative serum vascular endothelial growth factor, interleukin-6, and C-reactive protein level in colorectal cancer. *BMC Cancer, 10*, 203–210. doi:10.1186/1471-2407-10-203

Le, T. H., & Fantry, G. T. (2009). Peptic ulcer disease. Retrieved from http://emedicine.medscape.com/article/181753-overview

Lehrer, J. K. (2012). Irritable bowel syndrome. Retrieved from http://www.emedicine.medscape.com/article/180389-overview

Lustig, L. R., & Schindler, J. (2010). Ear, nose & throat disorders. In S. J. McPhee & M. A. Papadakis (Eds.), *Current medical diagnosis and treatment* (49th ed., pp. 179–214). New York: McGraw Hill.

Martin, S. (2008). Against the grain: An overview of celiac disease. *Journal of the American Academy of Nurse Practitioners, 20*(5), 243–250. doi:10.1111/j.1745-7599.2008.00314.x

McFarland, L. V. (2010). Systematic review and meta-analysis of *Saccharomyces boulardii* in adult patients. *World Journal of Gastroenterology, 16*(18), 2202–2222.

McLaughlin, A. (2010). Digestive disorders in the elderly. Retrieved from http://www.Livestrong.com/article/109339-digestive-disorders-elderly/.

McQuaid, K. R. (2010). Gastrointestinal disorders. In S. J. McPhee & M. A. Papadakis (Eds.), *Current medical diagnosis and treatment* (49th ed., pp. 502–597). New York: McGraw Hill.

Myers, R. E., Sifri, R., Hyslop, T., Rosenthal, M., Verson, S. W., Cocroft, J., et al. (2007). A randomized controlled trial of the impact of targeted and tailored interventions on colorectal screening. *Cancer, 110*(9), 2083–2091.

National Cancer Institute. (2010). General information about lip and oral cavity cancer. Retrieved from http://www.cancer.gov/cancertopics/pdq/treatment/lip-and-oral-cavity/Patient

National Comprehensive Cancer Network. (2011). Colon and rectal cancers. Retrieved from http://www.nccn.com/treatment-summaries/colon-rectal.html

Nguyen, M. C. T., Chudasama, Y. N., Dea, S. K., & Cooperman, A. (2009). Diverticulitis. Retrieved from http://emedicine.medscape.com/article/173388-overview

Phillips, N. (2007). *Berry & Kohn's operating room technique* (11th ed.). St. Louis: Mosby.

Plewa, M. C. (2012). Pediatric aphthous ulcers. Retrieved from http://emedicine.medscape.com/article/909213-overview

Presutti, R. J., Cangemi, J. R., Cassidy, H. D., & Hill, D. A. (2007). Celiac disease. *American Family Physician, 76*(12), 1795–1802.

Putaala, H., Barrangou, R., Leyer, G. J., Ouwehand, A. C., Hansen, E. B., Romero, D. A., et al. (2010). Analysis of the human intestinal epithelial cell transcriptional response to *Lactobacillus acidophilus, Lactobacillus salivarius, Bifidobacterium lactis* and *Escherichia coli. Beneficial Microbes, 1*(3), 283–295.

Quest Diagnostics. (2010). *Inflammatory bowel disease differentiation panel.* Retrieved from http://www.questdiagnostics.com/hcp/intguide/jsp/showintguidepage.jsp?fn=HematOnc/Gastrointestinal/TS_IBD_Differention_Panel.htm

Qureshi, W. A. (2009). Hiatal hernia. Retrieved from http://emedicine.medscape.com/article/178393-overview

Reed, L. (2010). Irritable bowel syndrome. *Practice Nurse, 40*(1), 15–20.

Rowe, W. A. (2011). Inflammatory bowel disease. Retrieved from http://emedicine.medscape.com/article/774566-overview

Sanders, M. E., Akkermans, L. M., Haller, D., Hammerman, C., Heimbach, J., Hörmannsperger, G., et al. (2010). Safety assessment of probiotics for human use. *Gut Microbes, 1*(3), 164–185. Epub 2010 Mar 4.

Schueler, S. J., Beckett, J. H., & Gettings, D. S. (2008). Intestinal obstruction. Retrieved from http://www.freemd.com/intestinal-obstruction/incidence.htm

Shrestha, S., & Lau, D. (2009). Gastric ulcers. Retrieved from http://emedicine.medscape.com/article/175765-overview

Smink, D., & Soybel, D. I. (2011). Acute appendicitis in adults: Management. Retrieved from http://www.uptodate.com

Thomas, D. J. (2011). Abdominal problems. In L. M. Dunphy, J. E. Winland-Brown, B. O. Porter, & D. J. Thomas (Eds.), *Primary care: The art and science of advanced practice nursing* (2nd ed., pp. 492–581). Philadelphia: F. A. Davis.

Thomson, A. B. R., Leung, Y. P. Y., Devlin, S. M., & Meddings, J. (2010). Duodenal ulcers. Retrieved from http://emedicine.medscape.com/article/173727-overview

Trevino, C. (2010). Small bowel obstruction: The art of management. *AACN Advanced Critical Care, 21*(2), 187–194. doi:10.1097/NCI.0b013e3181d99247

Ubertalli, J. T. (2008). Gingivitis. In R. S. Porter, & J. L. Kaplan (Eds.), *The Merck manual online.* Retrieved from http://www.merckmanuals.com/professional/sec08/ch095/ch095c.html?qt=vincent&alt=sh

UCSF Medical Center. (2011). Diverticular disease and diet. Retrieved from http://www.ucsfhealth.org/education/diverticular_disease_and_diet/

Verna, E. C. (2010). Use of probiotics in gastrointestinal disorders: What to recommend? *Therapy of Advanced Gastroenterology, 3*(5), 307–319.

Wilkes, G. M. (2011). Colon, rectal, and anal cancers. In C. H. Yarbro, D. Wujcik, & B. H. Gobel (Eds.), *Cancer nursing: Principles and practice* (7th ed., pp. 1205–1257). Boston: Jones and Bartlett Publishers.

Wilkinson, J. M., & Ahearn, N. R. (2009). *Prentice Hall nursing diagnosis handbook* (9th ed.). Upper Saddle River, NJ: Prentice Hall.

Wilson, B. A., Shannon, M. T., & Shields, K. M. (2011). *Pearson nurse's drug guide 2011.* New York: Pearson.

Wolvers, D., Antoine, J. M., Myllyluoma, E., Schrezenmeir, J., Szajewska, H., & Rijkers, G. T. (2010). Guidance for substantiating the evidence for beneficial effects of probiotics: Prevention and management of infections by probiotics. Journal of Nutrition, *140*(3), 698S–712S. Epub 2010 Jan 27.

Caring for the Patient with Hepatic and Biliary Disorders

CHAPTER 38

Pamela Stetina
Cheryl Wraa

Outcome-Based Learning Objectives

After studying this chapter, the learner will be able to:

1. Compare and contrast mode of transmission, pathophysiology, clinical manifestations, and treatment with related nursing care of patients with hepatitis.
2. Compare and contrast pathophysiology, clinical manifestations, and treatment with related nursing care of patients with cirrhosis.
3. Delineate nursing care for patients with cirrhotic complications.
4. Generate a nursing plan of care for a patient with liver cancer.
5. Generate a nursing plan of care for a patient with gallbladder disease.
6. Discuss care of the patient with a T-tube following cholecystectomy surgery.
7. Analyze the similarities and differences between acute and chronic pancreatitis, including nursing care.
8. Discuss the causes, clinical manifestations, and treatment for pancreatic cancer.
9. Develop a teaching plan for a patient with pancreatitis.

KEY TERMS

apudomas p.1195
asterixis p.1173
bile canaliculi p.1165
biliary dyskinesia p.1184
caput medusae p.1175
cholangiocarcinoma p.1179
cholecystectomy p.1186
cholecystitis p.1184
choledocholithiasis p.1182
cholelithiasis p.1182
cirrhosis p.1172
esophageal varices p.1173
exocrine pancreas p.1163
gluconeogenesis p.1173
hepatic encephalopathy p.1173
hepatitis A virus (HAV) p.1164
hepatitis B virus (HBV) p.1164
hepatitis C virus (HCV) p.1165
hepatitis D virus (HDV) p.1165
hepatitis E virus (HEV) p.1165
hepatitis G virus (HGV) p.1165
hepatocellular p.1164
hepatorenal syndrome p.1174
Kupffer cells p.1165
melena p.1173
pancreaticoduodenal (Whipple) resection p.1195
pancreatitis p.1189
paracentesis p.1177
portal hypertension p.1173
primary biliary cirrhosis p.1179
sclerosing cholangitis p.1179
sclerotherapy p.1178
steatorrhea p.1191
viral hepatitis p.1164

THE LIVER, GALLBLADDER, AND EXOCRINE PANCREAS (that part of the pancreas that acts as an exocrine gland producing pancreatic juice to secrete into the duodenum to aid in protein digestion) facilitate digestion by secreting hormones, enzymes, and other substances that are necessary for the breakdown of food (Figure 38–1◆, p. 1164). For example, the liver produces and secretes bile, a substance that contains salts, cholesterol, bilirubin, electrolytes, and water needed for the breakdown and absorption of fats. Bile is stored and concentrated by the gallbladder for release in response to cholecystokinin, which is a hormone secreted from the mucosa of the small intestines. Cholecystokinin, in turn, stimulates the gallbladder to contract and eject bile, as well as stimulating the pancreas to secrete alkaline fluid. In addition to alkaline secretions that help neutralize the acidity of the chyme, the pancreas secretes enzymes that hydrolyze proteins, carbohydrates, and fats. Trypsin, chymotrypsin, and carboxypeptidase are enzymes secreted in inactive form from the pancreas that digest proteins. Pancreatic amylase and lipase are enzymes in the pancreas that aid in the digestion of carbohydrates and fats, respectively. This chapter discusses disorders of the liver, gallbladder, and pancreas.

Disorders of the Liver

The liver is a complex organ with over 500 identified functions, including metabolic and regulatory functions. Because of its complexity, the clinical manifestations of liver problems can be varied and may include both physiological and psychological symptoms. Liver disorders can

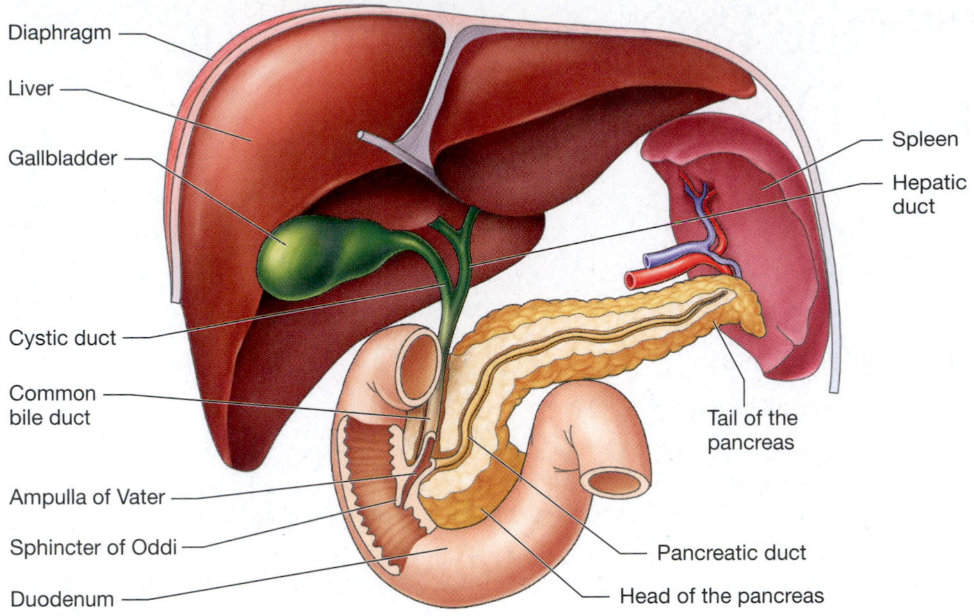

FIGURE 38–1 ◆ Liver and biliary system.

result from infectious organisms, toxic substances, and/or tumors that produce either localized or diffuse **hepatocellular** (pertaining to the cells of the liver) inflammation or destruction.

Hepatitis

Hepatitis, which is simply defined as inflammation of the liver, is a common problem throughout the world. It can be an acute or chronic infection that may be mild or life threatening, depending on the infectious agent and the rapidity of development. Inflammation of the liver may also be the result of lifestyle choices such as alcohol or drug abuse.

Etiology and Epidemiology

Some of the many causes of liver inflammation are viruses, bacteria, metabolic and vascular disorders, drugs, alcohol, and other toxic substances such as carbon tetrachloride (Thomas, 2011). Chart 38–1 lists the many causes of hepatic inflammation.

Safety Alert *Acetaminophen is well known as a nonopioid analgesic and antipyretic; it is also found in many other medications such as cold remedies and in combination with some opioid analgesics. However, acetaminophen can be toxic to the liver. It is imperative that nurses assess patients' use of acetaminophen and urge them to read labels for acetaminophen-containing products. The maximum safe dose of acetaminophen is 4 grams/day for adults, but preexisting liver disease, other drugs that may also affect the liver, and age should be taken into consideration in recommending doses. Patients with liver disease may not be able to take acetaminophen. To reduce toxicity to the liver, alcohol should not be taken concurrently with acetaminophen.*

Viral Causes

When most people hear the word *hepatitis,* they think of **viral hepatitis.** However, there are many types of viruses that are known to cause inflammation of the liver. Because of the diversity of liver function, the effects of hepatitis can be locally diffuse throughout the liver or can manifest as systemic disease.

Hepatitis A

Hepatitis A virus (HAV), a member of the picornavirus family, is a small RNA virus (Thomas, 2011). Many cases go undiagnosed because symptoms are often nonspecific, mild, and flulike. In the United States, there were an estimated 2,585 cases per 100,000 in 2008, which indicates a steady decline since 2000, when there were 13,397 cases per 100,000 reported (Centers for Disease Control and Prevention [CDC], 2010).

Transmission of HAV is usually through the fecal–oral route, meaning that the virus is contracted by drinking water contaminated with sewage, eating uncooked food washed in this water, eating shellfish harvested from contaminated water, or eating food contaminated by a person who is infected and did not wash his hands after using the toilet. Other methods of transmission include sexual transmission and the transfusion of infected blood. The incubation period (time between exposure and onset of symptoms) for HAV is anywhere from 4 to 6 weeks. The virus is typically found in the feces up to 2 weeks before symptoms occur and the week following the onset of symptoms, but it may remain as long as 3 months and is most contagious during this time (Huether, 2010). It takes about 4 weeks for the body to develop antibodies to HAV (anti-HAV antibodies). Serum immunoglobulin M (IgM) (an antibody produced by the body in response to an antigen) is seen in the acute phase of the illness and begins to decline about 3 months after exposure. Serum immunoglobulin G (IgG) (an antibody produced by the body that is an indicator of long-term immunity or resolving infection) levels are slower to peak but remain elevated years after exposure, conferring immunity against further infection by HAV. Hepatitis A usually causes no long-term damage, and a chronic state is unknown for HAV.

Hepatitis B

Hepatitis B virus (HBV) is a DNA virus that replicates in the liver. Hepatitis B occurs in most places in the world, but the rate of infection varies depending on location. HBV is a complex organism that has three basic components. The intact virus is sometimes called a Dane particle, which has a double-layered outer coat that carries the hepatitis B surface antigen (HBsAg), thereby allowing it to be detected by radioimmunoassay. Because of the protective coating, the core antigen (HBcAg) is not detectable in serum; however, a derivative of the core antigen, HBeAg, is detectable and serves as a marker of viral replication and infectivity (Huether, 2010).

CHART 38–1 Common Causes of Hepatic Inflammation

Viral
- Hepatitis A, B, C, D, E, G (HAV, HBV, HCV, HDV, HEV)
- Cytomegalovirus
- Epstein–Barr virus
- Herpes and varicella-zoster viruses
- Yellow fever virus

Nonviral
- Amebic infiltration
- Lyme disease
- Syphilis
- Bacteria

Toxins
- Ethanol (alcohol)
- Carbon tetrachloride
- Mushrooms *(Amanita phalloides)*
- Herbs (comfrey)

Metabolic Disorders
- Alpha$_1$-antitrypsin deficiency
- Wilson disease (copper metabolism)

Vascular Disorders
- Budd–Chiari syndrome
- Congestive heart failure
- Severe hypotension
- Shock

Drugs
- Acetaminophen
- Nonsteroidal anti-inflammatory drugs (NSAIDs)
- Amiodarone
- Anabolic steroids
- Birth control pills
- Chlorpromazine
- Erythromycin
- Halothane
- Methyldopa
- Isoniazid
- Methotrexate
- Statins
- Sulfa drugs
- Tetracyclines

Sources: Dugdale, D. C. (2010). Drug-induced hepatitis. Retrieved from http://www.nlm.nih.gov/medlineplus/ency/article/000226.htm; Lehne, R. A. (2010). *Pharmacology for nursing care* (7th ed.). St. Louis: Mosby; Thomas, D. J. (2007). Abdominal problems. In L. M. Dunphy, J. E. Winland-Brown, B. O. Porter, & D. J. Thomas (Eds.), *Primary care: The art and science of advanced practice nursing* (2nd ed., pp. 473–561). Philadelphia: F. A. Davis; Wilson, B. A. Shannon, M. T., & Shields, K. M. (2011). *Pearson nurse's drug guide 2011*. New York: Pearson; Wolf, D. C. (2010). Cirrhosis. Retrieved from http://emedicine.medscape.com/article/185856-overview.

Hepatitis B virus may be found in blood, semen, cervical secretions, saliva, and wound drainage, with the highest concentration occurring in blood and blood products. Viral transmission is through direct contact with blood and blood products, sexual contact, and contact with contaminated inanimate objects. High-risk groups include health care workers, particularly those working in a laboratory, blood bank, or hemodialysis setting where there is frequent contact with blood and blood products. IV drug users, homosexual men, and people with multiple sex partners are also at risk. Transmission can occur during pregnancy from mother to fetus if the mother is infected in the third trimester or at birth (Huether, 2010; Thomas, 2011).

The incubation period for HBV is longer than that for other hepatic viruses, lasting anywhere from 6 weeks to 6 months, during which time transmission is possible even when symptoms are absent (Thomas, 2011). Hepatitis B virus can exist in an asymptomatic carrier state, and/or it can create a chronic active state of infection, which can progress to cirrhosis and liver failure, thus requiring liver transplantation. Hepatitis B virus infection can lead to an increased risk for developing liver cancer as well.

Hepatitis C

Hepatitis C virus (HCV), once known as non-A, non-B virus, is a flavivirus with an incubation period of 35 to 72 days (Huether, 2010). It replicates at a very high rate, mutating readily, which causes the host immune system to have difficulty building a response (Mukherjee & Dhawan, 2010). This leads to a high rate of chronic infections. There are six different genotypes of HCV, three of them occurring most often in the United States. The most common genotype found in the United States is genotype 1; other genotypes occur in various areas of the world.

The rate of HCV infection has dropped drastically since 2000. The CDC reported that there were 3,197 new cases per 100,000 of HCV infection in 2000 but only 878 per 100,000 in 2008 (CDC, 2010). Hepatitis C virus is found predominantly in blood, blood products, and transplanted tissue. However, there is evidence that HCV can be transmitted sexually, particularly in people who have multiple sex partners. In fact, the risks of contracting hepatitis C appear to be similar for people who report drug use and those who report multiple sex partners (Daniels, Grytdal, & Wasley, 2009). The most common route of HCV transmission in the United States is injection drug use (CDC, 2010).

Safety Alert *In performing a patient assessment, it is important for the nurse to identify patients who have histories that put them at greater risk for contracting hepatitis C. Of the reported cases of acute hepatitis C in 2007 (Daniels et al., 2009), the most common risk factor identified was injection drug use (48%). Other risk factors included multiple sexual partners (42%), surgical procedures (20%), and occupational exposure to blood (2%).*

Weblink: Viral Hepatitis

Weblink: Drug-Induced Hepatitis

Weblink: Viral Hepatitis

Hepatitis D

Hepatitis D virus (HDV), also known as delta virus, is an RNA virus that is defective and must have HBsAg present for its replication; therefore, simultaneous infection with HBV is necessary for HDV (Huether, 2010). The incubation period lasts from 1 to 6 months, and transmission occurs in the same manner as transmission of HBV. IV drug users have a high rate of HDV infection, with a mortality rate of about 3% (Thomas, 2011).

Hepatitis E

Hepatitis E virus (HEV) is an RNA virus with an incubation period of 15 to 60 days (Huether, 2010). It is transmitted via the fecal–oral route and is similar to hepatitis A in clinical manifestations. Compared to HAV, however, the mortality rate for pregnant women who contract HEV is higher at 10% to 20% (Friedman, 2010). Hepatitis E virus is endemic in Southeast Asia, India, North Africa, and Mexico but is uncommon in the United States (Thomas, 2011).

Hepatitis G

Hepatitis G virus (HGV) is an RNA virus about which little is known. Transmission may occur percutaneously or through sexual contact. The virus has been detected in at least 50% of IV drug users, 30% of patients undergoing hemodialysis, and 15% of patients with chronic HBV or HCV (Friedman, 2010). Hepatitis G virus infection is associated with a chronic viremia (presence of a virus in the bloodstream). It should be noted that if patients with HIV are also infected with HGV, their survival rate is improved. It is thought that the HGV inhibits HIV reproduction (Friedman, 2010).

Pathophysiology

Once the liver is infected with any of the hepatitis viruses, an inflammatory response is initiated when the acini cells develop mononuclear inflammatory infiltrates. The inflammatory response causes edema within the liver and can obstruct the **bile canaliculi,** small channels adjacent to the hepatocytes that move bile toward the common bile duct. This intrahepatic obstruction of bile causes obstructive jaundice. There may also be liver cell necrosis, **Kupffer cell** (cells that line the liver sinusoids and are phagocytic cells) hyperplasia, and scarring. The cell-mediated immune response (cytokines, toxic T cells, natural killer cells) is responsible for the tissue injury that occurs. If the case of hepatitis is mild, there is little parenchymal damage. Hepatitis B and C usually cause the most severe liver inflammation and damage. Hepatitis C invades the liver cells, causing injury directly; therefore, the inflammation in the hepatocytes is directly related to the viral load (Thomas, 2011). Although rare, acute fulminating (sudden and severe) hepatitis may be caused by hepatitis B (also by coinfection with HDV), resulting in massive hepatocellular necrosis that leads to liver failure. One of the liver's most amazing features is its ability to regenerate itself so that some level of healing can occur. Even in severe cases of hepatitis, liver regeneration begins within 48 hours of the tissue injury (Huether, 2010).

For both HBV and HCV, asymptomatic carrier states may exist. Although these individuals may never develop an active disease process, they carry an increased risk for developing hepatocellular carcinoma (Thomas, 2011). Hepatitis B and C can produce chronic, active infections in which the immune system is unable to clear the virus completely. About 2% to 6% of individuals infected with HBV will go on to develop chronic infection, and about 75% to 85% of those infected with HCV will go on to develop chronic infection (Poole, 2009).

Other agents can also cause liver inflammation (hepatitis); 10% to 15% of chronic hepatitis is not directly related to any viruses (Poole, 2009). Bacteria and circulating bacterial endotoxins can invade the parenchyma during sepsis and cause liver injury. Some medications can also cause hepatitis. For example, toxic metabolites of acetaminophen can damage the liver's cellular structure, leading to inflammation (Thomas, 2011). The most common toxic substance that causes chemical hepatitis is alcohol. Liver inflammation can occur after drinking large quantities in a relatively short time or from chronic consumption (alcohol abuse).

Clinical Manifestations

Regardless of the cause, the clinical manifestations of hepatitis are frequently very similar. The severity of the symptoms can range from almost none to fulminating hepatitis, progressing to liver failure and death. The patient is usually asymptomatic during the incubation period of viral hepatitis. With HBV infection, there is evidence of HBeAg in the blood, indicating a high degree of infectivity. Later in the incubation period, HBsAg (hepatitis B surface antigen) appears. Following the incubation period, there are three phases in the clinical course of viral hepatitis: the prodromal phase, the icteric phase, and the convalescent phase (recovery).

Prodromal Phase

It is often difficult to determine the beginning of the prodromal phase. This phase of acute hepatitis occurs between exposure to the virus and the appearance of jaundice, a yellow color of the skin, mucous membranes, and eyes due to the increased bilirubin in the blood, because it starts about 2 weeks after exposure to the virus. Because the time of exposure is often unknown, the prodromal phase will vary depending on the incubation period. The prodromal phase can have either an insidious or a rapid onset. Symptoms may be vague, often flulike, with anorexia, nausea, vomiting, and malaise, as well as frequent occurrences of myalgia, arthralgia, and fatigue. Anorexia usually occurs early in this phase and is frequently accompanied by a distaste for smoking in patients who are smokers. Other manifestations may include mild but constant abdominal pain in the right upper quadrant (RUQ) or the epigastrium and a fever less than 103°F (39.4°C) (Thomas, 2011).

Icteric Phase

The icteric phase begins with the onset of jaundice, which usually occurs 5 to 10 days after the initial symptoms, although some patients never develop jaundice. The prodromal symptoms become worse with the onset of jaundice, but ongoing clinical improvement follows (Thomas, 2011). Owing to the increased levels of conjugated bilirubin, a product in the breakdown of hemoglobin that is conjugated by the hepatocytes and is excreted in bile, the urine may be dark during this phase (Huether, 2010).

The CDC (Daniels et al., 2009) reported that overall, 73% of persons infected with acute hepatitis A develop jaundice, 35% are hospitalized, and 0.8% die. Persons ages 5 to 14 and ages 15 to 39 were more likely to report the development of jaundice (84.8% and 80.1%, respectively), whereas persons younger than 5 years and persons age 60 or older were less likely (61.8% and 56.8%, respectively). The rate of hospitalization increased with age, with persons younger than 5 years less likely to be hospitalized (21%) than persons age 60 or older (53%).

Convalescent Phase

The convalescent, or recovery, phase is characterized by an increased sense of well-being, which usually begins after 2 to 3 weeks of acute illness. The phase is marked by additional signs of improvement such as increased appetite and energy level. In addition, the jaundice of the icteric phase and abdominal pain disappear. The time to complete clinical recovery varies depending on the type of hepatitis, but HAV is usually resolved in 9 to 10 weeks, while HBV recovery may take up to 16 weeks (Thomas, 2011).

Laboratory and Diagnostic Procedures

Tests that assess the degree of liver injury include alanine aminotransferase (ALT), aspartate aminotransferase (AST), alkaline phosphatase (ALP), gamma-glutamyltransferase (GGT), lactic dehydrogenase (LDH), serum bilirubin, and liver biopsy. (Refer to the Laboratory and Diagnostic Tests for Liver Disorders box on page 1167.) Specific serological tests for viral antigens, antibodies, or the virus itself are available (Chart 38–2).

Medical Management

The goals of medical treatment for hepatitis are to identify the cause of the inflammation, either infectious or chemical; provide symptomatic treatment; monitor the damage to the liver; and support the liver's ability to regenerate and heal itself. Laboratory and diagnostic tests give clues to the cause of hepatitis, assess the degree of liver injury, and indicate the degree of healing.

Vaccines are available for HAV and HBV. The vaccine for HBV became available in 1912 and the vaccine for HAV in 1995 (Daniels et al., 2009). Combination vaccines for HAV and HBV have existed since 2001.

Anyone in a high-risk group should be vaccinated against HAV and HBV. High-risk groups include health care workers, day care workers, employees at correctional facilities, injection drug users, male homosexuals, and anyone traveling to an area where HAV is endemic (Thomas, 2011). Patients on hemodialysis and household and sexual contacts of persons with HBV should be vaccinated as well. Vaccine for HAV is given in 2 intramuscular (IM) doses 6 to 12 months apart. The most common side effect is pain at the injection site. The HBV vaccine is given in a series of 3 IM doses, with the first dose followed in 1 month by the second one, and the third one given 5 months after the second dose. Side effects of HBV vaccine include pain at the injection site, fatigue, and headache.

Immune globulin (IG) is available for HAV and HBV postexposure prophylaxis. Postexposure prophylaxis is recommended for household and sexual contacts of people with HAV or HBV, health care workers after a needlestick injury, and others exposed to infected blood or body fluids. Postexposure prophylaxis for HAV is a single dose of IG, which

LABORATORY AND DIAGNOSTIC TESTS for Liver Disorders

Test with Description, Rationale, and Normal Values	Expected Abnormality
ALT (alanine aminotransferase)	
Normal 10–35 units/L	Over 300 units/L.
Used to detect liver disease by measuring an enzyme released from hepatocytes when the liver is injured.	Higher elevations indicate liver damage. ALT is more specific for the liver than other enzymes.
AST (aspartate aminotransferase)	
Normal 8–38 units/L	10 times or more above the normal.
Used to detect liver or cardiac damage by measuring an enzyme found in hepatocytes and cardiac cells, as well as skeletal muscle cells, kidneys, and the pancreas.	AST is released when there is cellular injury.
ALT/AST Ratio	
Normal: both ALT and AST are in the normal range	The ALT is more elevated than the AST in liver disease. Ratio changes reflect disease damage as well as alcohol consumption. In alcoholic cirrhosis, the AST is more elevated.
ALP (alkaline phosphatase)	
Normal is 42–136 units/L	Markedly elevated in severe liver or biliary disease.
Used to detect liver or bone disorders by measuring enzyme found in the liver and bone cells.	
Gamma-Glutamyltransferase (GGT)	
Normal: Male: 9–69 units/L Female: 4–33 units/L	Elevated levels indicate liver disease and alcoholism. Levels will elevate 12 to 24 hours after heavy alcohol consumption and may remain elevated for several weeks after cessation; some alcohol recovery programs use this to plan care for alcoholic patients.
Used to detect liver disease by measuring an enzyme found in the kidneys and liver.	
Lactic Dehydrogenase (LDH)	
Normal: 70–250 units/L	Elevated levels of LDH_5 indicate liver injury. Elevated levels of LDH indicate myocardial infarction, cerebrovascular accident, cancer, skeletal muscle disease, and acute hepatitis.
An enzyme used to detect cellular damage in cells with active metabolism, such as the heart, skeletal muscle, liver, brain, and red blood cells. LDH_5 is specific for liver injury.	
Bilirubin	
Normal: Indirect: 0.1–1.0 mg/dL Direct: 0.1–0.3 mg/dL Total: 0.1–1.2 mg/dL	Total and indirect bilirubin are elevated in obstructive jaundice (regardless of underlying cause), cirrhosis of the liver, and cancer of the liver. Indirect bilirubin is elevated with sickle cell, pernicious, and hemolytic anemias, cirrhosis, hepatitis, and transfusion reactions.
Used to detect unconjugated bilirubin and the presence of liver disease. Bilirubin is formed when hemoglobin is broken down; the liver conjugates the bilirubin and excretes in bile.	
Biopsy	
Normal: no abnormal tissue	Cells are abnormal, indicating hepatitis, cirrhosis, or liver cancer. In early cirrhosis, the histologic changes seen are micronodular. Histologically, there are hepatocellular necrosis and Mallory bodies (hyaline endoplasmic reticulum), which indicate the onset of fibrosis. Fatty infiltration and fibrosis are also seen.
A tissue sample is taken via a needle puncture of the liver. It is used to determine the type of liver disease or whether cancer exists.	
Serum Ammonia	
Normal: 15–45 mcg/dL	Compromised liver function causes ammonia levels to increase. Elevated in hepatic failure, hepatic encephalopathy, with a portacaval shunt (a surgical connection made between the portal vein and the inferior vena cava to decrease high blood pressure in the liver), and with a high-protein diet with liver failure.
Ammonia is nitrogenous waste from the breakdown of protein. Liver cells convert ammonia to urea for excretion by the kidneys.	
Prothrombin Time (PT)	
Normal: 10–13 seconds	Increased levels because compromised liver function will decrease clotting.
Prothrombin time measures clotting ability that is influenced by factors I (fibrinogen), II (prothrombin), V, VII, and X.	
Serum Albumin	
Normal: 3.5–5.0 g/dL; 52–68% of total protein	Diminished liver function will decrease albumin levels. Liver is unable to synthesize albumin and maintain oncotic pressure with low levels.
Albumin is synthesized by the liver and makes up more than half of the plasma proteins.	

(continued)

LABORATORY AND DIAGNOSTIC TESTS for Liver Disorders, *continued*

Test with Description, Rationale, and Normal Values	Expected Abnormality
Serum Glucose Normal values: 70–110 mg/dL *Stored in the liver as glycogen.*	Serum glucose may be decreased owing to inadequate glycogen storage related to decreased liver function.
Serum Cholesterol Normal values: <200 mg/dL *The liver synthesizes cholesterol.*	May be decreased in severe malabsorption. May be increased in biliary cirrhosis and cholangitis. Relates to increased fatty acids and triglycerides.
CBC Normal: Hemoglobin: Male: 13.5–18 g/dL Female: 12–15 mg/dL Hematocrit: Male: 40–54% Female: 36–46% RBCs: Male: 4.6–6 mcg/L Female: 4–5 mcg/L Platelets: 150,000–400,000 mcg/L *For patients with liver disease, the CBC is used to detect systemic problems related to the disease processes.*	These values may all be decreased due to bleeding, folate and B_{12} deficiency, and increased platelet and RBC destruction. Nutritional status may be compromised in patients with liver disease. Folic acid and B_{12} deficiencies are common in alcoholic cirrhosis. Esophageal varices cause bleeding. Splenomegaly, caused by portal hypertension, causes increased destruction of platelets.
Serum Electrolytes Normal: Sodium—135–145 mEq/L Potassium—3.5–5.3 mEq/L Magnesium—1.5–2.5 mEq/L Phosphorus—1.7–2.6 mEq/L Chloride—95–105 mEq/L Calcium—4.5–5.5 mEq/L *In patients with liver disease, used to evaluate the impact of disease on electrolytes.*	Decreased values indicate malnutrition, hemodilution, and altered renal excretion caused from cirrhosis. Serum electrolytes include sodium, potassium, magnesium, and phosphate; they are affected by malnutrition, fluid retention, and altered renal excretion, all due to cirrhosis.
Abdominal Ultrasound Normal: normal structures within the abdomen *Sound waves are reflected back from tissues and converted to electrical signs by a computer. It is used to determine the size of organs.*	The liver and spleen may be enlarged earlier in cirrhosis but are usually small and nodular in advanced disease. Enlargements occur related to intrahepatic obstruction and fibrotic changes in the liver.
Esophagogastroscopy Normal: normal structures *Endoscopic examination of the esophagus.*	Esophageal varices. Altered microcirculation and fragile collateral blood vessels.
Magnetic Resonance Imaging (MRI) Normal: no abnormalities *Used to detect lesions, vascular problems, injury, edema, or tumors (Kee, 2010).*	Tumors, edema, or any other abnormality (Kee, 2010).
Computed Tomography (CT) Normal: no abnormalities *Used to detect lesions, tumors, and metastasis; vascular disease; infection; and bone destruction (Kee, 2010).*	Any lesions, tumors, or metastatic disease (Kee, 2010).
Alpha-Fetoprotein (AFP) Normal: <15 ng/mL *Serves as a tumor marker for some cancers.*	Elevated levels may indicate cirrhosis or carcinoma of the liver, hepatitis, or testicular cancer.

Sources: Kee, J. L. (2010). *Laboratory and diagnostic tests with nursing implications* (8th ed.). Upper Saddle River, NJ: Prentice Hall; Thomas, D. J. (2011). Abdominal problems. In L. M. Dunphy, J. E. Winland-Brown, B. O. Porter, & D. J. Thomas (Eds.), *Primary care: The art and science of advanced practice nursing* (2nd ed., pp. 492–581). Philadelphia: F. A. Davis.

CHART 38–2 Specific Tests for Viral Hepatitis

Hepatitis A	**HAV-RNA** is viral RNA that is found in stool; RNA is detected in feces up to 2 weeks before symptoms begin.
	Anti-HAV IgM is found in serum during acute illness, peaking about 1–3 months after exposure and slowly decreasing. It is usually gone by 1 year after exposure.
	Anti-HAV IgG is found in serum during recovery and indicates immunity to the virus. It remains elevated for years.
Hepatitis B	**HBV-DNA** is viral DNA that is found in serum just before the second month and disappears by the fifth month.
	HBeAg is a marker for viral replication and appears about 2 months after exposure.
	HBsAg is the surface antigen on the virus and is usually detected 2 weeks after exposure and 1 week before HBeAg; it usually disappears by the fifth month. Persistent levels indicate either a chronic or a carrier state.
	Anti-HBc IgM is antibody to HBcAg and is found during acute illness and convalescence but may persist for years.
	Anti-HBs IgM indicates acute illness and infectivity.
	Anti-HBs IgG and **Anti-HBc IgG** both indicate recovery from acute illness.
Hepatitis C	**HCV-RNA** is viral RNA and indicates a replicating virus.
	Anti-HCV is antibody to the virus but does not indicate immunity.
Hepatitis D	**HDV-RNA** is viral RNA and indicates acute infection.
	HDAg is hepatitis D antigen and indicates acute infection.
Hepatitis E	**Anti-HEV** is antibody and indicates infection.

must be given within 2 weeks of exposure. For HBV, IG should be given as soon as possible, but it may be given up to 1 week after exposure, with a second dose given 1 month after exposure.

Although there is no vaccine for hepatitis C, treatment is initiated to prevent chronic HCV once the diagnosis is made. The goal of treatment is to get a sustained viral response, which means that HCV-RNA is undetectable 6 months after treatment is finished (Thomas, 2011). Standard treatment is with pegylated interferon alfa-2a or -2b subcutaneously and oral ribavirin for 48 weeks for genotype 1 and 24 weeks for genotype 2 or 3 (Holcomb, 2008). The side effects of this treatment regimen may include flulike symptoms, fatigue, muscle aches, headache, fever, nausea, depression, anxiety, and possible bone marrow suppression (Holcomb, 2008). Drinking a lot of water and getting adequate rest can minimize these effects. The National Guidelines box presents some practice guidelines for hepatitis C.

Complementary Therapies

Several herbal preparations have been shown to be beneficial to the liver. Milk thistle (Silybum marianum) is one of the oldest therapies for liver disease. Its active ingredient, silymarin, has demonstrated an ability to prevent liver destruction, reduce inflammation, and even promote new growth with minimal side effects (a slight laxative effect) (Ross, 2008). Another herbal preparation for hepatitis uses licorice root, which has anti-inflammatory properties. However, long-term use may cause hypertension and edema because of its chemical resemblance to aldosterone. Phytochemicals have been clinically evaluated as treatment for liver disease (see the Complementary & Alternative Therapies box on p. 1170).

Nursing Management

Nursing care for the patient with hepatitis involves supportive measures and education. Most patients with hepatitis are not hospitalized; their care is managed in their own homes. Patients who require hospitalization are those with fulminant hepatitis or with chronic hepatitis that has progressed to cirrhosis, liver cancer, or liver failure. The Nursing Process: Patient Care Plan box on page 1171 includes specific interventions and applications of the nursing process to a patient with hepatitis.

Collaborative Management

The patient with hepatitis may experience several challenges, which require the collaboration of an interdisciplinary team. The team may include the nurses, a social worker, a gastroenterologist, an infectious disease specialist, a nutritionist, and the primary care provider. In order to meet desired patient outcomes, it is essential that the interdisciplinary team communicate openly with one another in developing and evaluating care of the patient and family (IOM [Institute of Medicine], 2010). Gastroenterologists and primary care providers will help make the diagnosis of hepatitis; they will also provide medical management and follow-up care. An infectious disease specialist may be needed to help treat underlying infection.

Treatment for hepatitis is primarily supportive, regardless of the cause. The key aspects of therapy are rest, adequate nutrition, proper diet, and avoidance of alcohol. The diet recommended for patients with hepatitis is low in fat, cholesterol, and simple carbohydrates; a large portion of the calories should come from complex carbohydrates, such as whole grains, fruits, and vegetables (Holcomb, 2008). Depending on the level of functional liver impairment, increased protein intake may also be recommended. Working with a dietitian will help the patient to choose good sources of protein with lower fat concentrations such as egg whites, tofu, beans, and fat-free dairy products. Alcohol and other agents that are toxic to the liver must be avoided.

Patients with hepatitis will need education about prevention and long-term management. Patients who got hepatitis through IV drug use require counseling and additional resources to treat the addiction; social services may be able to help with these resources. Patients who contracted hepatitis through sexual activity may also need treatment and further assessment of additional sexually transmitted infection. Nurses can facilitate educating patients about the disease process, lifestyle changes, medication regimens, and follow-up care. Nutritionists will help patients with dietary changes.

Health Promotion

One of the primary nursing responsibilities with regard to viral hepatitis is a focus on prevention and reducing the spread of infection through

NATIONAL GUIDELINES for the Diagnosis and Treatment of Hepatitis C

Following are selected guidelines from Ghany, Strader, Thomas, and Steeff (2009) as presented on the website of the Agency for Healthcare Research and Quality.

Screening and Counseling

1. As part of a comprehensive health evaluation, all persons should be screened for behaviors that place them at high risk for hepatitis C (HCV) infection.
2. Persons who are at high risk should be tested for the presence of HCV infection.
3. Persons infected with HCV should be counseled on how to avoid transmitting HCV to others.

Diagnosis of Acute and Chronic HCV Infection and Interpretation of Assays

4. Patients suspected of having acute or chronic HCV infection should first be tested for anti-HCV.
5. HCV ribonucleic acid (RNA) testing should be performed in:
   a. Patients with a positive anti-HCV test
   b. Patients for whom antiviral treatment is being considered, using a sensitive quantitative assay
   c. Patients with unexplained liver disease whose anti-HCV test is negative and who are immune-compromised or suspected of having acute HCV infection.
6. HCV genotype should be determined in all HCV-infected persons prior to interferon-based treatment in order to plan for the dose and duration of therapy and to estimate the likelihood of response.

Utility of Liver Biopsy and Noninvasive Tests of Fibrosis

7. A liver biopsy should be considered in patients with chronic hepatitis C infection if the patient and health care provider wish information regarding the fibrosis stage for prognostic purposes or to make a decision regarding treatment.
8. Currently available noninvasive tests may be useful in defining the presence or absence of advanced fibrosis in persons with chronic hepatitis C infection but should not replace the liver biopsy in routine clinical practice.

Assessment Prior to Treatment and Monitoring during and after Therapy

9. Treatment decisions should be individualized based on the severity of liver disease, the potential for serious side effects, the likelihood of treatment response, the presence of comorbid conditions, and the patient's readiness for treatment.
10. For patients in whom liver histology is available, treatment is indicated in those with bridging fibrosis or compensated cirrhosis provided that they do not have contraindications to therapy.
11. The optimal therapy for chronic HCV infection is the combination of peginterferon alfa and ribavirin.
12. HCV RNA should be tested by a highly sensitive quantitative assay at the initiation of or shortly before treatment and at week 12 of therapy.

General Management Issues

13. All persons with chronic HCV infection who lack antibodies to hepatitis A and B should be offered vaccination against these two viral infections.
14. Persons with chronic HCV infection should be advised to abstain from alcohol consumption.
15. No recommendation can be made for the use of herbal supplements. There is no current evidence that herbal supplements have a role in the treatment of patients with acute or chronic HCV infection.

Source: Adapted from Ghany, M. G., Strader, D. B., Thomas, D. L., & Seeff, L. B. (2009). Diagnosis, management and treatment of hepatitis C: An update. *Hepatology, 49*(4), 1335–1374, doi:10.1002/hep.22759

COMPLEMENTARY & ALTERNATIVE THERAPIES Phytochemicals for Treatment of Liver Disease

Nancy Yilk

LIVER DISEASE IS A SERIOUS AILMENT and the scenario is worsened by the lack of precise therapeutic regimens. Currently available therapies for liver ailments are not suitable and systemic toxicity inhibits their long-term use. Medicinal plants have been traditionally used for treating liver diseases since centuries of use has shown that toxicity factors appear to be on the lower side.

Several phytochemicals have been identified that have significant hepatoprotective activity with minimal systemic adverse effects that could limit their long-term use. The scenario calls for extensive investigations that can lead to development of lead molecules of the hepatoprotective plants' properties and their future uses. These traditional herbal phytochemicals generally have strong antioxidative potential and cause induction of antioxidant enzymes like superoxide dismutase, reduced glutathione, and catalase. Additional mechanisms of hepatoprotection include stimulation of heme oxygenase-1 activity, inhibition of nitric oxide production, hepatocyte apoptosis, and nuclear factor-ℵB activation.

Out of the several leads obtained from plant sources as potential hepatoprotective agents, silymarin, andrographolide, neoandrographolide, curcumin, picroside, kutkoside, phyllanthin, hypophyllanthin, and glycyrrhizin have been established as potent hepatoprotective agents. The hepatoprotective potential of several herbal medicines has been clinically evaluated. Significant efficacy has been seen with silymarin, glycyrrhizin, and Liv-52 in treatment of hepatitis, alcoholic liver disease, and liver cirrhosis (Ghosh, Ghosh, Mandal, & Mandal, 2011).

Source: Ghosh, N., Ghosh, R., Mandal, V., & Mandal, S. C. (2011). Recent advances in herbal medicine for treatment of liver diseases. *Pharmaceutical Biology, 49*(9), 970–88. Epub 2011 May 19.

education. For all types of viral hepatitis, especially for HAV and HEV, good hand hygiene practices after using the bathroom and before handling food are crucial to prevent transmission. Because many types of hepatitis can be spread through sexual activity, education should include encouraging patients to use safer sexual practices, including barrier protection (condoms), abstinence, and monogamy. There is a high risk of transmitting viral hepatitis through shared needles and other equipment. Some communities therefore participate in a needle exchange program, in which used needles can be traded for sterile ones, thereby reducing the risk of viral hepatitis and HIV.

Nurses are influential in educating the public about vaccinations for HAV and HBV. The nurse should encourage all people in moderate- and high-risk groups to be vaccinated. Many public health departments offer these vaccines at a reduced cost or no cost for individuals at risk. Postexposure prophylaxis is available for people who have known or probable exposure to HAV or HBV.

NURSING PROCESS: Patient Care Plan for Hepatitis

Assessment of Hepatic and Biliary Status Using Gordon's Functional Health Patterns:

- Health Perception Health Management Pattern
- Nutrition Metabolic Pattern
- Activity Exercise Pattern

Subjective Data

Assessment of Fatigue

How long have you felt tired or fatigued?

Are you able to maintain your activities of daily living?

How much activity can you tolerate before you feel fatigued?

What makes you feel better?

Assessment of Nutritional Status

Are you having trouble eating?

Have you lost any weight?

How is your appetite?

Have you lost a taste for any foods?

Are there foods that you have a taste for?

Has your food consumption changed?

Do you drink alcohol? If so, how much/how often?

Assessment of Skin

Does your skin itch?

Have you been scratching your skin?

Have you noticed a change in the color of your skin?

Assessment of Infection Transmission

Have you ever had a blood transfusion?

Do you have any tattoos or body piercings?

Do you use injectable drugs?

Where have you traveled recently?

Have you eaten any raw fish or seafood?

Where do you work? Child care facility? Correctional facility? Hemodialysis unit?

Do you handle blood or body fluids for your job?

Has anyone you know been sick or had yellow skin?

Do you have multiple sex partners?

When did your symptoms begin?

Objective Data

Assessment of Fatigue

Musculoskeletal examination:

- Muscle strength
- Activity tolerance
- Vital signs
- Labs.

Assessment of Nutritional Status

Body weight and appearance

Skin turgor

Skin and hair condition.

Assessment of Skin

Examine skin for:

- Dryness
- Jaundice
- Bruises
- Lesions from scratching
- Petechiae.

Assessment of Infection Transmission:

Enlarged lymph nodes

Tender liver.

Outcomes and Evaluation Parameters	Planning and Interventions with *Rationales*
1. NURSING DIAGNOSES: (a) Fatigue. (b) Activity Intolerance *related to inadequate liver function* (NANDA-I © 2012)	
Outcome: Reduced fatigue. ***Evaluation Parameters:*** Ability to perform activities of daily living. Increased activity tolerance.	Encourage frequent rest periods during the day. *Energy conservation is necessary for tissue rebuilding and regaining well-being.* Facilitate the identification of essential activities and delegate tasks to others. *Energy conservation is necessary for tissue rebuilding and regaining well-being.* Encourage increased activity as fatigue improves. *A feeling of improvement can enhance well-being, self-concept, and a sense of control.*

(*continued*)

NURSING PROCESS: Patient Care Plan for Hepatitis, *continued*

Outcomes and Evaluation Parameters	Planning and Interventions with *Rationales*
2. NURSING DIAGNOSIS: Nutrition, Readiness for Enhanced *related to anorexia and reduced liver function* (NANDA-I © 2012)	
Outcome: Adequate nutrition. ***Evaluation Parameter:*** No weight loss.	Instruct the patient to eat foods that appeal to her, but stress the importance of high-calorie carbohydrates and proteins. *Carbohydrates are necessary for sufficient energy, and proteins are needed for healing.* Explain the importance of avoiding substances that can be toxic to the liver, such as alcohol and acetaminophen in order *to prevent further liver damage or inflammation.* Teach the patient to read food labels and choose foods that are low in fat and have adequate levels of vitamins and minerals, such as instant breakfast drink mix, *to improve nutritional status and promote healing.*
3. NURSING DIAGNOSIS: Skin Integrity, Risk for Impaired *related to jaundice and resultant pruritus* (NANDA-I © 2012)	
Outcome: Skin integrity maintained. ***Evaluation Parameters:*** Reports diminished itching. No bruising or petechiae. No lesions from scratching.	Instruct the patient to use cool, lightweight, nonrestrictive clothing and avoid woolens. *Clothing made from lightweight fabrics causes less itching.* Explain that a cool environmental temperature and cool water for bathing *may increase comfort related to pruritus.* Instruct the patient to keep her fingernails trimmed and well cared for *to decrease the likelihood of excoriating when scratching.* Instruct the patient to take antihistamine medication as ordered *to reduce pruritus.*
4. NURSING DIAGNOSIS: Infection, Risk for *related to the transmission of viral hepatitis* (NANDA-I © 2012)	
Outcome: No spread of the infection. ***Evaluation Parameter:*** Verbalizes modes of transmission and ways to prevent spread.	Use standard or universal precautions when handling blood or body fluids. *Viral hepatitis is transmitted by direct contact with infected feces, body fluids, and blood.* Explain that the time of highest infectivity is before symptoms appear, and that *good hand hygiene can prevent the spread of the disease.* Teach about safe and safer sex practices *to prevent the spread of the virus.* Encourage prophylactic treatment for close contacts and/or vaccination against HAV and HBV. *These measures decrease the risk of contracting the disease or decrease the severity of the illness.*

Source: Adapted from Wilkinson, J. M., & Ahearn, N. R. (2009). *Prentice Hall nursing diagnosis handbook* (9th ed.). Upper Saddle River, NJ: Prentice Hall.

Cirrhosis

Etiology and Epidemiology

Cirrhosis, the 12th-leading cause of death in the United States (Friedman, 2010), is an irreversible, progressive deterioration of the liver that results from chronic liver disease. Cirrhosis is the result of hepatocellular injury or inflammation that usually occurs over time. If the injury or inflammation is short lived, the liver is usually able to regenerate itself. However, severe acute injury, such as that seen in hepatitis, can result in cirrhosis. Cirrhosis may be brought about by a variety of causes including chronic hepatitis; alcoholism; prolonged, severe right heart failure; and long-term obstruction to biliary flow (Huether, 2010; Wolf, 2010). Refer to Chart 38–3 for the causes of cirrhosis.

Pathophysiology

Prolonged liver injury from toxins, inflammation, and metabolic derangements cause liver cell damage and cell death. The damaged or dead liver cells are repaired or replaced with tissue that is more fibrous than the original tissue. Fibrotic scarring is the result. Liver cells continue to regenerate but do so in an abnormal pattern. This abnormal liver regeneration creates nodules known as regenerative nodules. The fibrotic scarring and nodular development alter the normal lobular architecture, resulting in diffuse, disorganized fibrous bands and more regenerative nodules. The development of cirrhosis depends on several factors, including the length of time the liver is subjected to the injury, the severity of the injury, and the liver's reaction to the assault. As the liver repairs itself, there is distortion in the microcirculation. Collateral vessels develop in the newly regenerated nodule connecting the portal vein to the hepatic artery (Figure 38–2◆). This results in increased resistance to the flow of blood throughout the liver, causing portal venous hypertension because these vessels are inefficient (Thomas, 2011).

Cirrhosis can have a variety of causes, one of which is alcohol abuse. Alcohol ingestion decreases fatty acid utilization and increases fat deposits in the liver. The increase in fatty acids also leads to accumulation of triglycerides (Huether, 2010). This condition, called *fatty liver*, can sometimes be reversed if no further alcohol is consumed. Continued use of alcohol will cause continued liver damage, including fibrosis, regenerative nodules, and structural changes.

Prolonged obstruction to the flow of bile within the liver or biliary system can also cause cirrhosis. When the bile ducts within the liver are obstructed, the proximal hepatocytes are injured. There is an inflammatory response to the injury with inflammatory cells infiltrating the liver, leading to fibrosis and regenerative nodules. This is essentially the same pathway by which chronic hepatitis B and hepatitis C cause cirrhosis, that is, chronic inflammation leading to fibrosis and regenerative nodules.

CHART 38–3 Causes of Cirrhosis

Infectious and disease-related causes	Alpha$_1$-antitrypsin deficiency Autoimmune hepatitis Biliary cirrhosis Cholelithiasis Glycogen storage disease Hepatitis B and C Sclerosing cholangitis.
Hepatotoxins	Direct: • Alcohol • Carbon tetrachloride. Indirect: • Acetaminophen • Anabolic steroids • Mushroom toxin *(Amanita phalloides)* • Methotrexate • Tetracycline.
Genetic diseases	• Galactosemia • Hemochromatosis • Wilson disease.
Vascular disorders of the liver	• Budd-Chiari syndrome • Ischemic hepatitis • Right heart failure (chronic).

Sources: Adapted from Huether, S. E. (2010). Alterations of digestive function. In K. L. McCance, S. E. Huether, V. L. Brashers, & N. S. Rote (Eds.), *Pathophysiology: The biologic basis for disease in adults and children* (6th ed., pp. 1452–1515). St. Louis: Mosby; Wolf, D. C. (2010). Cirrhosis. Retrieved from http://emedicine.medscape.com/article/185856-overview.

Clinical Manifestations

Cirrhosis can be asymptomatic until liver function is severely affected; even then, the onset of symptoms is gradual. Cirrhosis may be found incidentally on the annual physical exam. The manifestations of cirrhosis can be nonspecific and are the result of the hepatocellular damage and portal hypertension. Initially, the patient might complain of fatigue, weakness, anorexia, and weight loss, which is caused by the decreased metabolic functions of the liver. Because the liver produces bile, which is needed for the digestion of fat and the formation of fat-soluble vitamins, impaired liver function may result in fat-soluble vitamin deficiency, particularly of vitamin K. Deficiency of vitamin K causes problems with blood clotting. Other metabolic functions of the liver include **gluconeogenesis** (the making of glucose from noncarbohydrate sources), glycogen storage, synthesis of albumin, clotting factors, and other blood proteins. When liver function is severely compromised and the liver is unable to make albumin, hypoalbuminemia (low albumin) leads to edema. Both ascites and peripheral edema develop in part because of the decrease in colloidal osmotic pressure. Because of the architectural changes in the cirrhotic liver structure, there is obstruction to the flow of bile out of the liver, causing jaundice of the skin and sclera. Chart 38–4 contains a list of clinical manifestations of cirrhosis and the physiological basis for each.

Complications

As cirrhosis progresses, severe systemic complications occur, the most significant of which are portal hypertension, hepatic encephalopathy, and hepatorenal syndrome. Each of these conditions has further clinical manifestations and complications, which are discussed next.

Portal Hypertension

As the internal architecture of the liver becomes distorted as a result of scarring, venous blood flow through the portal venous system is impeded. This increases the portal venous blood pressure from a normal of about 3 mmHg to at least 10 mmHg; this is known as **portal hypertension** (Huether, 2010). Because the portal veins carry blood from the GI tract, spleen, and pancreas to the liver, the obstruction of this blood flow from cirrhosis causes increased pressure in the vessels in the aforementioned organs. The increased pressure promotes the formation of collateral circulation, which normally has lower pressure. In turn, the increased blood flow to the collateral circulation causes varices (distended, tortuous, collateral veins) to develop, particularly in the esophagus and rectum.

Esophageal varices are thin-walled veins in the esophagus that are prone to rupture, causing massive, life-threatening hemorrhage. Rupture of esophageal varices can result from anything that increases the pressure in the vessel, such as coughing, or from trauma caused by something as simple as eating high-roughage food. However, bleeding from esophageal varices can be slow and chronic, leading to anemia and **melena,** the black or maroon, sticky, foul-smelling feces that result from the digestion of blood. When the varices rupture, there is hemorrhage and the patient vomits large volumes of dark-red blood. Contributing to the risk of hemorrhage is erosion by gastric acid, elevated venous pressure, and decreased clotting factors. Individuals who have recurrent esophageal bleeding from portal hypertension usually die within a year (Huether, 2010).

Another consequence of portal hypertension is splenomegaly (enlargement of the spleen). The splenic vein branches from the portal vein; therefore, when blood flow is obstructed through the portal vein, the subsequent increasing pressure in the splenic vein causes an enlarged spleen as well as the increased rate of blood cell destruction by the spleen. This contributes to the occurrence of thrombocytopenia anemia. More platelets are removed from circulation and sequestered in the spleen, leading to impaired clot formation, all of which contribute to esophageal bleeding.

Ascites is simply the accumulation of protein-rich fluid in the abdominal cavity. Portal hypertension is the primary cause of ascites, but hypoalbuminemia and accumulation of aldosterone aid in the fluid accumulation. The low serum albumin decreases the colloidal osmotic pressure in the blood vessels; this causes fluid to escape into the interstitial space, which decreases the circulating blood volume. In turn, this causes the kidneys to retain sodium and water to increase the blood volume, leading to an increase in hydrostatic pressure and accelerating portal hypertension and ascites formation (Huether, 2010).

Hepatic Encephalopathy

Hepatic encephalopathy, also known as portosystemic encephalopathy, is the result of an increased level of circulating neurotoxins. The most abundant neurotoxin is ammonia, which is an end product of protein digestion. Normally, the hepatocytes convert ammonia to urea, which is then excreted by the kidneys. However, when liver function is impaired, ammonia builds up in the blood and is shunted to the brain via the circulation (Huether, 2010). It is important to note that ammonia levels alone do not necessarily correlate with the severity of the problem. There are other neurotoxins that may cause or contribute to the problem, including gamma-aminobutyric acid (GABA), endogenous benzodiazepines, and false neurotransmitters (Kelso, 2008). Any of these toxins can cause additional symptoms of encephalopathy, including **asterixis,** a flapping tremor of the hands when the arms are outstretched, believed to be caused by the accumulation of substances

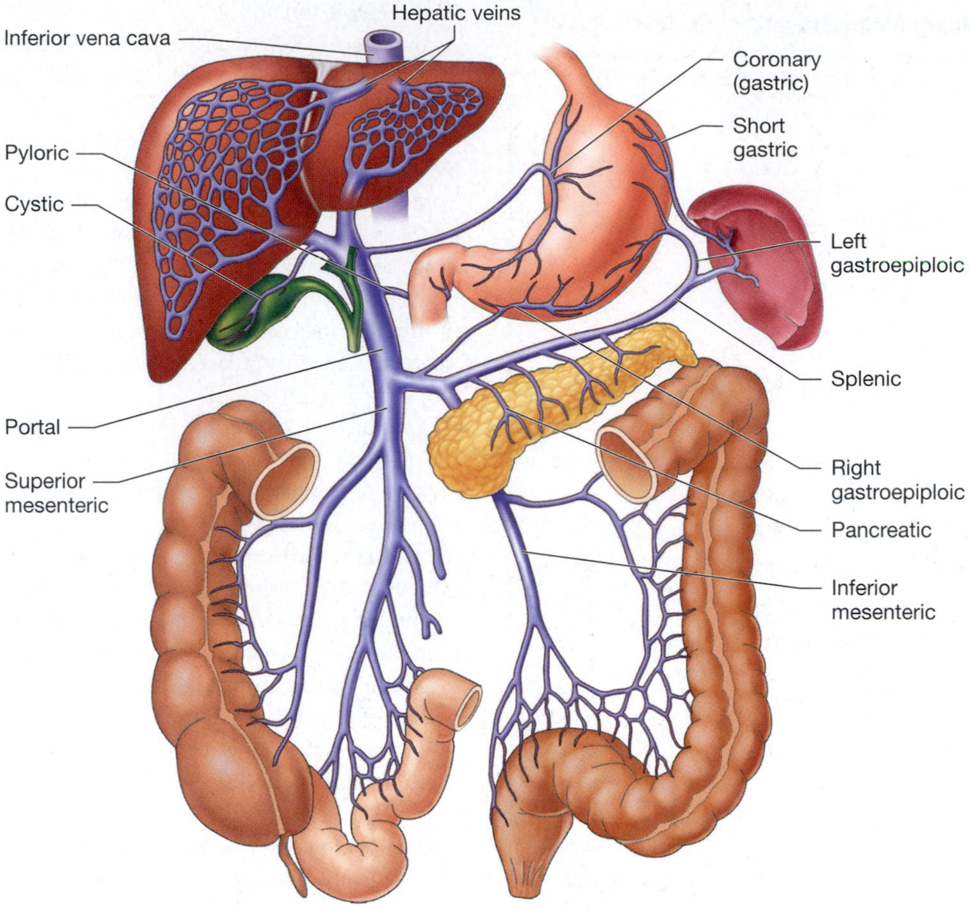

FIGURE 38–2 ◆ Portal circulation.

normally detoxified by the liver, agitation, restlessness, and changes in mentation (Huether, 2010).

Hepatorenal Syndrome

Hepatorenal syndrome is characterized by the occurrence of azotemia (elevation of blood urea nitrogen—BUN) in a patient with liver failure when other causes of renal failure have been excluded. The cause of this syndrome is unknown, but intense renal vasoconstriction and decreased renal blood flow are present while renal tissue is normal. Type I hepatorenal syndrome is acute and occurs rapidly; type II hepatorenal syndrome is chronic and progresses more slowly (Huether, 2010). The presence of oliguria (diminished urine output), sodium and water retention, hypotension, and peripheral vasodilation indicates a poor prognosis.

Laboratory and Diagnostic Procedures

Because cirrhosis has systemic consequences, nonspecific abnormalities may be found in many laboratory tests. For example, liver function tests—including ALT, AST, ALP, and GGT (which are indications of liver injury, not liver function)—not only are all usually elevated in patients with cirrhosis but also are elevated in patients with hepatitis, sclerosing cholangitis, or gallbladder disease, as well as because of some medications. Conversely, these lab results may be normal in the early stages of cirrhosis. Laboratory tests that help measure liver function include the serum albumin, prothrombin time, partial thromboplastin time, clotting time, bilirubin, and serum ammonia level. The definitive diagnosis of cirrhosis is made through liver biopsy. Other tests give indications of severity and associated complications. The Laboratory and Diagnostic Tests for Liver Disorders box (p. 1167) outlines the laboratory and diagnostic tests and anticipated results for patients with cirrhosis (Kee, 2010; Thomas, 2011).

Medical Management

The first priority in medical management for the patient with cirrhosis is to prevent or minimize complications such as portal hypertension, esophageal varices, hepatic encephalopathy, and hepatorenal syndrome. This is accomplished through holistic care that addresses the patient's physical, spiritual, and psychosocial needs.

Because alcoholism is a major cause of cirrhosis in the United States, it is important for nurses to encourage patients' efforts to abstain from alcohol. This requires the involvement of the family as well as other forms of support. Comprehensive treatment of cirrhosis includes medications, surgical intervention, diet, and counseling.

Treatment for Ascites

Most medications given to a patient with cirrhosis target the complications of cirrhosis. For example, most patients with cirrhosis have portal hypertension with or without ascites, low serum albumin, and increased renin-angiotensin-aldosterone secretion, complicated by the liver's inability to inactivate aldosterone; therefore, they require diuretic therapy. Spironolactone (Aldactone) is usually given because it inhibits aldosterone action and increases reabsorption of potassium, making it a potassium-sparing diuretic. The dose is usually 100 milligrams per day. Furosemide (Lasix), 40 to 160 milligrams per day, may also be given to augment diuresis (Friedman, 2010). The Pharmacology box (p. 1176) outlines the medications used to treat hepatic disorders.

CHART 38–4 Clinical Manifestations of Cirrhosis and Physiological Causes

Clinical Manifestation	Physiological Cause
Integumentary	
• Jaundice	Blocked outflow of bile from the liver due to structural change.
• Palmar erythema	Altered sex hormone metabolism (high estrogen).
• Spider angioma (abnormal blood vessels near the surface of the skin)	High capillary pressure; also may be related to high estrogen levels.
• Decreased body hair	Altered sex hormone metabolism.
• Pruritus	High levels of bile salts cause itching.
• Ecchymosis	↓ clotting factors, ↑ platelet destruction by spleen, ↓ vitamin K.
• **Caput medusae** (dilated and engorged paraumbilical veins seen on the abdomen)	Intrahepatic obstruction to portal blood flow.
• Edema.	Low serum albumin, high hydrostatic pressure, sodium and water retention.
Gastrointestinal	
• Esophageal varices	Intrahepatic obstruction to portal blood flow.
• Abdominal pain	Stretching of Glisson's capsule or ascites.
• Anorexia	Increased venous pressure in GI tract.
• Ascites	Intrahepatic obstruction to portal blood flow, hypoalbuminemia, ↑ renal absorption of sodium and water.
• Light-colored stools	Intrahepatic obstruction of bile flowing into the duodenum.
• GI bleeding	Esophageal varices rupture or bleed.
• Hemorrhoids.	Portal hypertension causes venous congestion.
Neurological	
• Hepatic encephalopathy	Hepatocytes are unable to convert ammonia to urea to be excreted by the kidney. May relate to GABA or other neurotoxins.
• Sensory disturbances	High serum ammonia levels are neurotoxic.
• Asterixis (flapping tremor of hands).	Caused by high serum ammonia levels.
Cardiovascular	
• Portal hypertension	Intrahepatic obstruction to portal blood flow.
• Bounding pulse	Increased fluid volume from sodium and water retention and ↑ aldosterone.
• Dysrhythmias.	Fluid and electrolyte imbalance.
Hematologic	
• Decreased clotting factors	Liver unable to synthesize clotting factors and vitamin K.
• Thrombocytopenia	Enlarged spleen causes ↑ destruction of platelets.
• Anemia.	↑ RBC destruction in spleen, bleeding.
Hepatic	
• Atrophic, nodular liver	Scarring.
• Splenomegaly.	Intrahepatic obstruction to portal blood flow causes engorgement of the spleen.
Respiratory	
• Dyspnea	Ascites cause pressure on the diaphragm.
Reproductive	
• Oligomenorrhea (infrequent menstruation—female)	Altered sex hormone metabolism.
• Testicular atrophy	Altered sex hormone metabolism (high estrogen).
• Gynecomastia (breast enlargement—male)	Altered sex hormone metabolism (high estrogen).
• Loss of libido.	Altered sex hormone metabolism.
Metabolic	
• Hypoalbuminemia	Liver unable to synthesize albumin.
• Hypokalemia	Altered renal excretion.
• Hypocalcemia	Related to low serum protein levels.
• Malnutrition	Impaired metabolism of nutrients.
• Muscle wasting.	Muscles are used as protein source.

PHARMACOLOGY Summary of Medications Used to Treat Hepatic Disorders

Medication Category and Action	Application/Indication	Nursing Responsibility
Antiviral Agents		
Interferons Peginterferon alfa-2b (PEG-Intron) Interferon alpha-2a (Pegasys) ***Action:*** Attach to uninfected cells and induce the production of protective antiviral proteins. When the virus attacks the cell, the pathogen will be inactivated. PG-Intron has a molecule of PEG attached which gives the drug an extended half-life.	Management of chronic hepatitis C.	Monitor for adverse effects: fatigue, muscle aches, headache, fever, and chills. Monitor complete blood count (CBC) with differential, platelets, and renal function. Monitor for severe reactions: suicidal ideation and hepatomegaly (enlarged liver). Be aware that the theophylline level may increase. Monitor drug level.
Noninterferons Adefovir (Hepsera) ***Action:*** Exerts antiviral effects by interfering with viral DNA.	Treatment of chronic hepatitis B.	Monitor for adverse effects: abdominal pain, diarrhea, dyspepsia, nausea, hematuria, and headache. Monitor electrolytes and renal and hepatic function, especially in the presence of liver or kidney dysfunction.
Lamivudine (Epivir) ***Action:*** Exerts antiviral effects by interfering with the viral RNA chain.	Treatment of chronic hepatitis B.	Monitor for adverse effects: neuropathy, insomnia, dizziness, fever, nausea, and diarrhea. Monitor liver and renal function, CBC with differential. Observe for lactic acidosis.
Oral ribavirin (Rebetol) ***Action:*** Antiviral effect thought to be due to interference with viral RNA synthesis.	Management of hepatitis C in combination with interferon alpha-2b.	Monitor for adverse effects: fatigue, elevated liver enzymes (transient), light-headedness, hypotension, risk for pneumonia, and jaundice. Monitor CBC with differential, platelet count, and liver function. Observe for development or worsening of cardiac or pulmonary dysfunction.
Diuretics		
Potassium sparing: Spironolactone (Aldactone) ***Action:*** Promotes diuresis through sodium and chloride excretion in distal tubule without loss of potassium.	Hepatic cirrhosis, ascites.	Monitor for adverse effects: hyperkalemia, menstrual irregularities, gynecomastia, and impotence. Monitor electrolytes and I&O. Be aware of multiple drug interactions (digoxin, heparin, warfarin, aspirin). Monitor for altered drug efficacy or toxicity. Monitor digoxin level if given concurrently.
Loop diuretic: Furosemide (Lasix) ***Action:*** Diuretic effect due to reduced reabsorption of sodium and chloride in loop of Henle, proximal tube, and distal tubule.	Edema associated with hepatic cirrhosis.	Monitor for adverse effects: hypotension, hypokalemia, hyponatremia, hypochloremia, and hypocalcemia. Be aware of multiple drug interactions (digoxin, insulin, NSAIDs, and others). Monitor for altered drug efficacy or toxicity. Be aware of ototoxicity. Monitor electrolytes and I&O. Be aware of multiple drug incompatibilities when given IV.
Hyperosmotic Laxative Lactulose ***Action:*** Increases ammonia excretion by acidifying colon contents and reducing diffusion of ammonia from colon to blood.	Prevention and treatment of hepatic encephalopathy.	Monitor for adverse effects: nausea, vomiting, diarrhea, and hypernatremia. Monitor electrolytes. Monitor fluid status.
Aminoglycoside Antibiotic Neomycin sulfate ***Action:*** Reduces blood ammonia by destroying ammonia-forming bacteria.	Cirrhosis, hepatic coma.	Monitor for adverse effects: diarrhea, nausea, and vomiting. Observe for severe adverse reactions: respiratory paralysis, ototoxicity, and nephrotoxicity. Monitor renal function and serum drug levels.

PHARMACOLOGY Summary of Medications Used to Treat Hepatic Disorders, *continued*

Medication Category and Action	Application/Indication	Nursing Responsibility
Synthetic Hormone Octreotide (Sandostatin) ***Action:*** Reduces portal blood flow by inhibiting release of vasodilatory hormone.	Variceal bleeding.	Monitor for adverse effects: nausea and diarrhea. Monitor electrolytes and blood glucose.
Sedative–Hypnotic Oxazepam (Serax) ***Action:*** Causes sedative effect by potentiating inhibitory neurotransmitter GABA.	Anxiety, acute withdrawal symptoms in chronic alcoholism, agitation.	Monitor for adverse effects: drowsiness, ataxia, paradoxical stimulant response, and sleep disturbances, especially in the elderly. Monitor for drug interactions (other CNS depressants, cimetidine, phenytoin, smoking, and others). Monitor for altered drug efficacy or toxicity. Be aware that prolonged use requires slow withdrawal of medication. Caution patient that the sedative effect is increased with alcohol.
Immunosuppressants Cyclosporine (Sandimmune, Neoral) Tacrolimus (Prograf, Protopic) ***Action:*** Inhibits the function of calcineurin. Diminishes the activity of T and B cells and suppresses the immune response. Mycophenolate (CellCept) ***Action:*** Inhibits DNA synthesis of B and T cells. Azathioprine (Azasan, Imuran) ***Action:*** Inhibits DNA synthesis, resulting in damage and chromosome breakage.	Adjunct therapy with corticosteroids to prevent transplant rejection, use for ulcerative colitis or rheumatoid arthritis. Prevent transplant rejection. Treatment of RA. Off-label use in autoimmune hepatitis and ulcerative colitis.	Monitor for adverse effects: hypertension, nausea, vomiting, infection, anemia, and thrombocytopenia. Observe for signs of toxicity: tremors, seizures, altered mental status, visual disturbances, nephrotoxicity, and neurotoxicity. Monitor CBC, liver, and renal function tests, electrolytes, and blood sugar. Be aware of multiple drug specific interactions (erythromycin, verapamil, cimetidine, ACE inhibitors, and others). Monitor for altered drug levels, nephrotoxicity, or leukopenia. Teach to avoid grapefruit juice which inhibits the metabolism of the drug. Monitor CBC weekly for first month. Report decreases in leukocyte or platelet counts that may represent bone marrow depression. Monitor for any signs of systemic infection. Monitor kidney and liver function. Use protective isolation when patient is hospitalized. Patient should not receive any vaccinations during therapy. Teach patient and family to take the drug in divided doses with meals to reduce gastric irritation. Tell the patient to avoid contact with crowds or persons with signs of infection.

Sources: Adams, M. P., & Koch, R. W. (2010). *Pharmacology: Connections to nursing practice.* Upper Saddle River, NJ: Pearson; Wilson, B. A., Shannon, M. T., & Shields, K. M. (2011). *Pearson nurse's drug guide 2011.* New York: Pearson.

Many medical therapies for patients with ascites involve a reduction in dietary sodium, which is usually accomplished by restrictions on the patient's fluid and sodium intake. Initially, the sodium restriction is quite severe, with sodium limits of no more than 400 to 800 milligrams per day. Once diuresis occurs, sodium intake may be increased slightly. Fluid restrictions are usually set to between 800 and 1,000 milliliters per day (Thomas, 2011).

Some patients with extensive ascites may have difficulty breathing because diuretic therapy was ineffective and the remaining fluid limits movement of the diaphragm. In these patients, a **paracentesis** (removal of fluid from the abdominal cavity) may be performed. After cleansing the lower abdomen, the health care provider will apply local anesthesia and insert a small bore needle into the peritoneal cavity. Vacuum tubing is connected to the needle, and fluid is drained into a collection bottle. Removal of 1 to 2 liters through paracentesis may be effective without increasing the risk of fluid and electrolyte imbalance. However, large-volume paracentesis, or the removal of 4 to 6 liters of fluid, may be needed and is usually effective in relieving the respiratory symptoms. This can be performed daily as well, but that increases the risk of fluid and electrolyte imbalance. Intravenous albumin may be given with a large-volume paracentesis to replace the proteins contained in ascitic fluid. If these are not replaced, a shift in oncotic pressure could cause a reduction in blood volume. Chart 38–5 covers nursing care of the patient undergoing paracentesis.

Although it is not a true surgical procedure, a transjugular intrahepatic portosystemic shunt (TIPS) may be used to relieve refractory ascites and portal hypertension. It involves insertion of a catheter into the jugular vein, through which an expandable stent is placed between the hepatic vein and the portal vein. The stent allows blood to flow from the portal vein into the hepatic vein, therefore bypassing the liver and effectively reducing portal pressure. The TIPS procedure has replaced a procedure that used peritoneovenous shunts (Friedman, 2010).

Treatment for Hepatic Encephalopathy

Hepatic encephalopathy is a complication of cirrhosis that mainly results from increased levels of ammonia causing a disturbance in mental

CHART 38–5 Nursing Care of the Patient Undergoing Paracentesis

Preprocedure

- Ensure there is a signed informed consent.
- Weigh the patient.
- Take vital signs and measure abdominal girth.
- Have the patient empty his bladder.
- Place the patient sitting in a high Fowler's position.
- Assemble the needed equipment.

During Procedure

- Monitor blood pressure, pulse, and respiratory rate and effort.
- Reassure the patient and family.

Postprocedure

- Monitor vital signs, especially blood pressure and respiratory effort.
- Monitor for bleeding or excessive drainage from the puncture site.
- Administer albumin if ordered.
- Send specimens to the laboratory for analysis if ordered.
- Change dressing as needed.
- Monitor for infection.

status. Lactulose, a nonabsorbable synthetic disaccharide that causes the contents of the colon to become more acidic, is the most commonly used medication to reduce ammonia levels in the blood. When the colon contents are more acidic, a nonabsorbable form of ammonia (NH_4+) is created that is excreted in feces. Lactulose also decreases the presence of bacteria in the colon that form ammonia when they digest protein in the stool (Thomas, 2011). The standard dose of this medication is 30 milliliters of liquid 3 to 4 times a day. The dose is titrated to a level that results in the patient having two or three loose stools per day. If the patient cannot take oral medication, then 300 milliliters of lactulose is mixed with about 700 milliliters of saline and given as a retention enema, with repetition every 4 to 6 hours (Friedman, 2010). Some patients may also receive neomycin sulfate, which destroys the ammonia-forming bacteria in the intestines, but this practice is used less now than it once was.

Patients with hepatic encephalopathy are often agitated and combative because of the increased level of ammonia and other toxic substances. Oxazepam (Serax), a benzodiazepine that is not metabolized by the liver, is used cautiously to treat marked agitation (Friedman, 2010). The standard dose is usually 10 to 30 milligrams by mouth or through a nasogastric tube. The Pharmacology box on page 1176 outlines the medications used to treat hepatic disorders.

Helicobacter pylori generates ammonia in the stomach. There is some evidence that eradicating the *H. pylori* can improve hepatic encephalopathy. The medication regimen for *H. pylori* eradication is discussed in Chapter 37.

Dietary protein is withheld from patients with hepatic encephalopathy during acute episodes. Once oral intake of food is resumed, protein is reintroduced slowly into the diet to a maximum of 60 to 80 grams per day. Vegetable protein is tolerated better than animal protein (Friedman, 2010).

Treatment for Esophageal Varices

Because many cirrhotic patients with esophageal varices are prone to developing bacterial infections, prophylactic antibiotic medication is often given. Quinolone antibiotics such as norfloxacin are preferred; the drug is given orally, via nasogastric tube, or intravenously twice a day for 5 to 7 days (McQuaid, 2010).

Medications used to reduce portal pressure may be given. The only such medication approved in the United States is octreotide (Sandostatin), which is given intravenously as a bolus followed by an infusion (McQuaid, 2010). It is unclear how the drug works, but it seems to reduce blood flow to the spleen and liver, thereby reducing portal pressure in patients with cirrhosis. Use of this drug in combination with endoscopic therapy has been shown to improve survival (Kelso, 2008).

Vitamin K is often given to patients with cirrhosis and esophageal varices because intrahepatic obstruction to bile flow (from the change in hepatic architecture) causes a vitamin K deficiency (because bile is needed to emulsify fats and vitamin K is fat soluble). The healthy liver produces clotting factors, many of which are vitamin K dependent, so the person with a cirrhotic liver demonstrates an abnormal prothrombin. The recommended dose of vitamin K is 10 milligrams given subcutaneously (McQuaid, 2010). In the case of severe bleeding from esophageal varices, a transfusion of red blood cells, fresh frozen plasma, or platelets may be given. The Pharmacology box on page 1176 outlines the medications used to treat hepatic disorders.

Bleeding from esophageal varices must be stopped as quickly as possible. The preferred method is banding. Banding, or variceal ligation, is done during endoscopy and involves the placement of tiny rubber bands on the varices to occlude blood flow. Another treatment done during endoscopy is **sclerotherapy.** This is done by injecting the varices with a chemical agent, most commonly ethanolamine or tetradecyl sulfate, that causes the vessel to become sclerotic. Banding has fewer complications than sclerotherapy, but the latter is preferred by some health care providers during active bleeding, which makes it difficult to visualize the varices for banding (McQuaid, 2010).

Balloon tamponade of bleeding varices may be used as a short-term measure when endoscopy or a TIPS procedure cannot be performed immediately (Kelso, 2008). A special three-lumen nasogastric tube (Sengstaken-Blakemore and Minnesota tubes) that has an esophageal balloon, a gastric balloon, and a lumen that opens into the stomach is inserted through the nose. Once in the stomach, the gastric balloon is inflated, applying pressure to the cardiac sphincter at the distal esophagus. Then the esophageal balloon is inflated, and tension is applied to the tube. This effectively applies direct pressure to any bleeding vessels. Complications of this treatment, such as aspiration, ulceration and perforation of the esophagus, and airway obstruction, are not uncommon, so this method is rarely used (Thomas, 2011).

Safety Alert *Ruptured esophageal varices are life threatening. Patients are at risk not only for major hemorrhage and hypovolemia, but also for respiratory complications such as aspiration. Nurses need to carefully monitor the patients with esophageal varices for bleeding and report any symptoms immediately to the health care provider.*

Treatment for Hepatorenal Syndrome

Liver transplantation is the treatment of choice for hepatorenal syndrome, but patients often do not survive waiting for an available liver. Drug therapy for hepatorenal syndrome is generally ineffective. An intravenous infusion of a long-acting vasoconstrictor (ornipressin) and albumin may improve the condition temporarily, but there are numerous ischemic side effects of this therapy (Friedman, 2010). Other combinations of albumin and vasopressors may also be used. The Pharmacology box earlier in the chapter (p. 1176) outlines the medications used to treat hepatic disorders.

Weblink: Liver Cancer

Weblink: Cancer Facts and Figures

Very few interventions are effective in treating hepatorenal syndrome. The molecular absorbent recirculating system (MARS), a type of modified dialysis, selectively removes substances that are bound to albumin and may prolong survival (Friedman, 2010). Patients with hepatorenal syndrome may also benefit from the TIPS procedure, as previously described.

Surgical Treatment for End-Stage Liver Disease

Liver transplantation is indicated for patients with end-stage liver disease resulting from cirrhosis, chronic hepatitis B and C, **sclerosing cholangitis** (an inflammatory disorder of the biliary tract that leads to fibrosis and strictures in the biliary system), **primary biliary cirrhosis** (an autoimmune disease in which inflammation and destruction of the intrahepatic biliary system results in fibrosis), small hepatocellular carcinoma, and some metabolic diseases in which the defect is in the liver. Absolute contraindications for liver transplant include active alcoholism or drug abuse, malignancy, and advanced cardiopulmonary disease (Friedman, 2010). Patients who have abstained from alcohol for less than 6 months and those infected with HIV are evaluated on an individual basis. Transplant is not usually considered until the patient demonstrates a deteriorating functional status, increasing bilirubin, decreasing serum albumin, refractory ascites, recurrent variceal bleeding, or worsening encephalopathy.

Survival rates for liver transplantation have steadily improved in the past 2 decades; the current 5-year survival is about 80%. The increased survival is due to advances in surgical technique and improved immunosuppression. Immunosuppression is accomplished with a combination of cyclosporine or tacrolimus, prednisone, azathioprine, and mycophenolate mofetil (Friedman, 2010). Side effects of the medications are numerous; they include infection, hypertension, hyperlipidemia, neuropsychiatric effects, and weight gain.

Nursing Management

Nursing management of the patient with cirrhosis involves a thorough assessment of risk factors (alcohol and substance abuse, sexual history, previous exposure to blood products during surgery, and employment history), education regarding lifestyle changes, and development of a plan of care to minimize complications. The Nursing Process: Patient Care Plan box (p. 1180) applies the nursing process to a patient with cirrhosis. The Patient Teaching & Discharge Priorities box (p. 1182) describes the discharge priorities for patients with cirrhosis.

Collaborative Management

Patients with cirrhosis face many challenges, and an interdisciplinary team approach is the most effective way to manage them. The team may include the nurse, a social worker, a gastroenterologist, a critical care specialist, a nutritionist, a pharmacist, and the primary care provider. In order to meet desired patient outcomes, it is essential that this interdisciplinary team communicate openly with one another in developing and evaluating care of the patient and family (IOM [Institute of Medicine], 2010).

The gastroenterologist and primary care provider will help make the diagnosis of cirrhosis and provide medical management and follow-up care. A critical care specialist may be needed in case of complications such as ruptured esophageal varices.

Nurses provide education about the prevention of cirrhosis and may make referrals to any needed social service resources, such as alcohol rehabilitation programs. Patients with cirrhosis will also need education about long-term management and medication regimens. Pharmacists should collaborate in teaching about medication regimens. Nutritionists can help patients with dietary changes.

The entire team will need to communicate well to assess for and treat any complications. Careful monitoring of the patient's status and laboratory and diagnostic results will facilitate identifying problems early. Ruptured varices can be life threatening, so prompt attention to bleeding and airway issues is a necessity.

Health Promotion

Because most cases of cirrhosis are preventable, educating the patient and community, especially children and young adults, about high-risk behaviors is essential. The most common cause of cirrhosis in the United States is alcohol abuse, so limiting alcohol intake, especially for women, is the number-one topic for health education. Hepatitis B and especially hepatitis C are risk factors for the development of cirrhosis. Prevention of bloodborne hepatitis is accomplished by sexual abstinence or safe sex practices and avoidance of injection drug use, as well as avoidance of unnecessary exposure to blood and bodily fluids. Patients should be educated about the availability of hepatitis A and hepatitis B vaccinations.

Liver Cancer

Etiology and Epidemiology

The American Cancer Society (2012) estimated that approximately 28,720 people in the United States would be newly diagnosed with liver cancer in 2012, with 20,550 expected deaths. Liver cancer is the fifth-leading cause of death in men and the eighth-leading cause in women in the United States (American Cancer Society, 2012a). It is the fifth-highest cancer in incidence and third-leading cause of death in the world. People with chronic hepatitis B or C are at high risk for developing primary liver cancer. In general, primary liver cancer is rare in the United States, though it is common in densely populated areas in southern Africa, Asia, and Greece (Huether, 2010). However, the liver is a common site of metastatic spread of cancer in other parts of the body.

Pathophysiology

Cancer of the liver develops from the liver's parenchymal cells (hepatocellular carcinoma) or from the cells in the bile ducts (**cholangiocarcinoma**). The most common type is hepatocellular carcinoma, which can be nodular, massive, or diffuse and is most closely related to cirrhosis or hepatitis B and C. Hepatocellular carcinoma metastasizes to the heart, lungs, brain, kidneys, and spleen. Cholangiocarcinoma is more common in southeast Asia, where liver fluke infestation is common, and has a metastatic profile similar to that of hepatocellular carcinoma (Huether, 2010).

Primary liver cancer arises when there is damage to the hepatocellular DNA. Both hepatitis B and C viruses can act as carcinogens, especially in the presence of cirrhosis. Exposure to mycotoxins, such as those produced by *Aspergillus flavus* (mold on corn, peanuts, and grain), causes the mutation of the p53 suppressor gene (Huether, 2010). Other risk factors for the development of liver cancer include smoking and heavy alcohol consumption.

Clinical Manifestations

The clinical manifestations of liver cancer are often general and nonspecific. Symptoms may include weakness, anorexia with weight loss, abdominal pain, fatigue, and fever (American Cancer Society, 2010). These usually occur early, but as the tumor enlarges or more of the liver becomes involved, manifestations include abdominal pain, ascites,

NURSING PROCESS: Patient Care Plan for Cirrhosis

Assessment of Hepatic and Biliary Status Using Gordon's Functional Health Patterns:

- Nutrition Metabolic Pattern
- Cognitive Perceptual Pattern

Subjective Data

Assessment of Fluid Volume

Have you noticed your ankles or feet swelling? For how long?

Have you noticed that your belly has gotten bigger? When did you notice this?

Have you vomited any blood?

Do you have hemorrhoids?

Assessment of Nutrition

Are you having trouble eating?

Have you lost any weight?

How is your appetite?

Do you drink alcohol? How much/how often?

Assessment of Skin

Does your skin itch?

Have you been scratching your skin?

Have you noticed a change in the color of your skin?

Assessment of Bleeding Potential

Have you vomited blood?

Have your stools been dark and tarry looking?

Have you noticed that you bruise easily?

Assessment of Mental Status

What is your name?

What is the date?

Do you know where you are?

Do you recall why you are here?

Objective Data

Assessment of Fluid Volume

Vital signs.

Abdominal assessment:

- Bowel sounds
- Contour
- Girth
- Liver size
- Tenderness
- Fluid wave.

Stool assessment.

Laboratory values:

- Serum albumin
- Serum electrolytes
- Hematocrit
- Creatinine
- BUN.

Peripheral edema.

Body weight.

Jugular venous distention.

Intake and output (I&O).

Urine specific gravity.

Assessment of Nutrition

Body weight and appearance.

Skin and hair condition.

Lab work: CBC, albumin, electrolytes.

Assessment of Skin

Examine skin for:

- Jaundice
- Lesions from scratching
- Dryness
- Bruises
- Petechiae.

Assessment of Bleeding Potential

Vital signs.

Test stool for occult blood.

Laboratory values:

- Coagulation studies
- Platelet count
- Hemoglobin and hematocrit.

Assessment of Mental Status

Assess cognitive function.

Reflexes.

Outcomes and Evaluation Parameters / Planning and Interventions with *Rationales*

1. NURSING DIAGNOSIS: Fluid Volume, Excess *related to portal hypertension and possible hepatorenal syndrome* (NANDA-I © 2012)

Outcome: Fluid status normal.

Evaluation Parameters: Decreasing abdominal girth.

No peripheral edema.

Normal laboratory results.

Weigh daily at the same time of day on the same scale, and monitor I&O. *This gives an accurate assessment of fluid status because a daily change in body weight can be attributed to water retention (or loss).*

Measure abdominal girth at the same location on the abdomen at least once a day, but preferably every 8 hours *to monitor progression of ascites.*

NURSING PROCESS: Patient Care Plan for Cirrhosis, *continued*

No evidence of active bleeding. No jugular venous distention. Urine specific gravity normal. Urine output at least 30 mL/hr.	Restrict dietary sodium to less than 2 grams per day and fluid as ordered; sodium may be restricted to as low as 400 mg/day. *Sodium promotes water retention, aggravating ascites and portal hypertension.* Monitor lab values and report abnormalities. *Low serum albumin can contribute to ascites and edema. Hyponatremia and hematocrit may indicate hemodilution. Rising BUN and creatinine can indicate impending hepatorenal syndrome.* Examine neck veins for distention and extremities for edema. *Distended jugular veins indicate fluid overload, and edema can result from excess fluid and low serum albumin.* Give prescribed diuretics *to reduce body water.*
2. NURSING DIAGNOSIS: Nutrition, Imbalanced: Less Than Body Requirements *related to anorexia, impaired protein metabolism, and reduced absorption of fat-soluble vitamins because of reduced liver function* (NANDA-I © 2012)	
Outcome: Adequate nutrition. ***Evaluation Parameter:*** No weight loss.	Provide a high-calorie, low-protein, low-sodium diet with 6 small meals per day as ordered. *Protein may be restricted if there is evidence of GI bleeding or encephalopathy in an effort to reduce nitrogenous waste products from protein metabolism.* Weekly weights after discharge. *Short-term fluctuations are usually associated with fluid balance, whereas long-term changes are a better indicator of nutritional status.* Explain the importance of avoiding substances that can be toxic to the liver, such as alcohol and acetaminophen, *in order to prevent further liver damage.* If there is no protein restriction, teach the patient to read food labels and choose foods that are high in protein and have adequate levels of vitamins and minerals, such as instant breakfast drink mix, *to improve nutritional status and prevent breakdown of skeletal muscle.*
3. NURSING DIAGNOSIS: Skin Integrity, Risk for Impaired *related to jaundice and resultant pruritus* (NANDA-I © 2012)	
Outcome: Skin integrity maintained. ***Evaluation Parameters:*** Reports diminished itching. No bruising or petechiae. No lesions from scratching.	Instruct the patient to use cool, lightweight, nonrestrictive clothing and avoid woolens. *Clothing made from lightweight fabrics causes less itching.* Explain that a cool environmental temperature and cool water for bathing *may increase comfort related to pruritus.* Hot water causes more pruritus. Instruct the patient to keep his fingernails trimmed and well cared for *to decrease the likelihood of excoriating when scratching.* Instruct the patient to take antihistamine medication as ordered to reduce pruritus. Use approved nondrying lotions *to reduce pruritus.*
4. NURSING DIAGNOSIS: Fluid Volume, Deficit: Risk for *related to the liver's ability to synthesize clotting factors, portal hypertension with resultant esophageal varices, and hemorrhoids* (NANDA-I © 2012)	
Outcome: No hemorrhage. ***Evaluation Parameters:*** Stool negative for occult blood. No vomiting blood. Coagulation studies normal. Hemoglobin and hematocrit normal. Vital signs normal.	Give vitamin K as ordered. *Vitamin K is synthesized in the liver and may be decreased in cirrhosis.* Teach the patient to use a soft toothbrush and avoid using dental floss *because decreased clotting factors make the patient more prone to bleeding.* Monitor for bleeding (stool, skin, urine, and mucous membranes) *because decreased clotting factors make the patient more prone to bleeding.* Instruct the patient to refrain from eating rough foods that can cause *trauma to the esophagus and cause varices to bleed.*
5. NURSING DIAGNOSIS: Confusion: Risk for *related to hepatic encephalopathy* (NANDA-I © 2012)	
Outcome: No disruption in mental status. ***Evaluation Parameters:*** Alert and oriented to person, place, and time. Able to perform simple computations. Behavior appropriate. Normal reflexes. Mini-Mental Status Exam (MMSE) score of 25 or better.	Administer Mini-Mental Status Exam (MMSE). *Hepatic encephalopathy can cause changes in mentation even in the prodromal phase.* Provide a low-protein diet as ordered *to reduce the nitrogen metabolites of protein digestion.* Administer medications to reduce ammonia level as ordered. *Lactulose, oral or enema, promotes diarrhea and the elimination of ammonia in the feces.* Monitor deep tendon reflexes. *As hepatic encephalopathy progresses, reflexes become exaggerated.*

Source: Adapted from Wilkinson, J. M., & Ahearn, N. R. (2009). *Prentice Hall nursing diagnosis handbook* (9th ed.). Upper Saddle River, NJ: Prentice Hall.

Weblink: Cancer Facts and Figures

PATIENT TEACHING & DISCHARGE PRIORITIES for a Patient with Cirrhosis of the Liver

Need	Teaching
Knowledge of disease process and prognosis	Home care needs include verbal and written instructions for: The treatment plan Follow-up care Nutritional and fluid needs.
Diet therapy	Many patients with cirrhosis have special dietary needs and restrictions, particularly related to protein, sodium, and fluid intake. Teaching should focus on each patient's specific dietary plan developed by the health care practitioner (Rolfes, Pinna & Whitney, 2012). Frequently, these patients develop abdominal ascites and fluid retention; the nurse should guide the patient in selecting low-sodium foods and in improving palatability of food (Rolfes et al., 2012). For the most part, patients with chronic liver disease are at risk for protein depletion (Rolfes et al., 2012). The nurse should reinforce the importance of consuming small, frequent meals that are high in food energy (Rolfes et al., 2012).
Drug therapy	The nurse should recognize that drug therapy is focused on the alleviation of symptoms and the prevention of complications, but it cannot reverse cirrhosis (Ryan, 2007). Current drug therapy is available to treat the complications of ascites, varices, spontaneous bacterial peritonitis, hepatic encephalopathy, and coagulation abnormalities (Ryan, 2007). Patients with liver disease may have several types of medications prescribed; commonly prescribed medications include beta-blockers, diuretics, and lactulose syrup. It is important for the nurse to provide teaching related to their expected effects and prescribed dosage, as well as any side effects in order to improve compliance and promote optimal patient outcomes. Emphasis should be placed on the importance of reporting side effects to the health care provider immediately for further evaluation.
Alcohol abstinence	Abstinence from alcohol is critical and should be reinforced during discharge teaching. The nurse should provide information regarding local support groups and counseling services to facilitate adherence to this critical component of the treatment plan.

Sources: Rolfes, S. R., Pinna, K., & Whitney, E. (2012). *Understanding normal and clinical nutrition* (9th ed.). Belmont, CA: Wadsworth Cengage; Ryan, L. (2007). Portal hypertension and cirrhosis. In M. A. Chisholm-Burns, B. G. Wells, T. L. Schwinghammer, P. M. Malone, J. M. Kolesar, J. C. Rotschafer, & J. T. Dipiro (Eds.), *Pharmacotherapy principles & practice* (pp. 323–336). New York: McGraw-Hill.

jaundice, and a palpable mass in the right upper quadrant. There may also be signs of liver failure such as portal hypertension.

Laboratory and Diagnostic Procedures

There are no specific tests for liver cancer, although most tumors can be identified by magnetic resonance imaging (MRI), ultrasound, and computed tomography (CT) scans. Once a suspicious area is found, a liver biopsy is done to determine the tumor type. The liver enzymes AST and ALT are measured and are usually elevated in people with liver cancer. Patients with advanced hepatocellular cancer will have an elevated alpha-fetoprotein (AFP) level. An elevated AFP level is strongly correlated with chronic hepatitis B infection, rapid tumor growth, and poorly differentiated tumors (Huether, 2010). Refer to the Laboratory and Diagnostic Procedures box on page 1167.

Medical Management

Surgical resection of the liver is possible only if the tumor is localized and is in a lobe of the liver that can be removed; for example, if the tumor is in the posterior section of the right lobe, it cannot be removed because the right hepatic vein is located in this area (Huether, 2010). Chemotherapy agents may be administered directly into the liver or systemically. Radiation and targeted therapies are also treatment options. Liver transplant is an option for small tumors without evidence of spread. Overall, the 5-year survival rate for patients with liver cancer is 14% (American Cancer Society, 2010).

Nursing Management

A goal of nursing care for patients with liver cancer is prevention whenever possible. Nurses can encourage alcohol abstinence and prevention of HBV and HCV. If a patient has a risk factor for liver cancer, such as chronic infection with HBV or HCV, the risk for developing liver cancer can be reduced if the patient abstains from alcohol. Most of the nursing interventions for a patient with liver cancer are similar to those for patients with cirrhosis and liver failure. Nursing care includes helping patients with liver cancer prepare for death, supporting the family, and providing comfort. Refer to Chapter 11 for nursing management at the end of life. See the Evidence-Based Practice box for specific medications for palliative care of patients with liver failure.

Disorders of the Gallbladder

The gallbladder is a saclike structure that concentrates and stores bile. Bile is produced by the liver and is necessary for the absorption of dietary fat and fat-soluble vitamins. Most gallbladder disorders result in obstructed bile flow from the liver to the gallbladder or from the gallbladder to the duodenum (Huether, 2010). The most common cause of obstructed flow is gallstones, or **cholelithiasis.** When a gallstone either forms in or migrates to the common bile duct, the resultant condition is called **choledocholithiasis.** Cirrhosis can obstruct the flow of bile from the liver to the gallbladder (Figure 38–3 ◆, p. 1184). Other causes of obstructed flow include tumors (rare) and abscesses.

Cholelithiasis

A combination of factors can cause gallstones to form, as described next. If the stone is large, it may obstruct flow from the gallbladder to the duodenum, causing pain.

EVIDENCE-BASED PRACTICE Medications Used in Palliative Care of Patients With Liver Failure

Clinical Problem

When a patient develops acute or chronic liver failure, the medications commonly used for palliation are metabolized abnormally, necessitating a careful and frequently changing dosing regimen. Decreased hepatic blood flow and the shunting of blood cause the medications to be metabolized more slowly and to have an increased bioavailability. For instance, benzodiazepines such as midazolam that are used for sedation may have an increased effect due to the presence of unmetabolized toxins, increased sensitivity to the drug, stimulation of the gamma-aminobutyric acid (GABA) receptors, and reduced cerebral blood flow (Rhee & Broadbent, 2007).

Research Findings

To facilitate care of the patient with liver failure, Rhee and Broadbent (2007) conducted an extensive literature search, as well as a review of major textbooks in pharmacology, palliative care, hepatology, and gastroenterology. From these data, they developed a table of functional groups of medications commonly used in palliative care, which lists the pharmacologic half-life with normal liver function and with cirrhosis. When data were available, the medications affected by cirrhosis were further broken down according to the Child–Pugh criteria of liver disease. This information may assist in the process of deciding which medications to use, reduce potential complications, and improve palliation of symptoms for patients with liver failure. As an example, here are the findings for opioid analgesics and nonopioid analgesics. Within the article, the complete table includes comments and recommendations for changes in dose and frequency with the references used for each drug.

Implications for Nursing Practice

It is important for the nurse to understand the degree of decreased function of the liver and to understand the effect it has on the metabolism of medications. Patients with end-stage liver disease require palliation. Knowing the expected increase in the half-life of analgesics will allow the nurse to administer medications safely.

Critical Thinking Questions with answers can be found in the Osborn Student Resources at nursing.pearsonhighered.com.

Source: Rhee, C., & Broadbent, A. M. (2007). Palliation and liver failure: Palliative medications dosages guidelines. *Journal of Palliative Medicine, 10*(3), 677–687.

Medication	Half-Life Normal Liver	Half-Life Cirrhosis	Half-Life Child–Pugh A	Half-Life Child–Pugh B	Half-Life Child–Pugh C
Opioid Analgesics					
Fentanyl	263 minutes	304 minutes			
Hydromorphone	2.5 hours	No data			
Methadone	18.8 hours	No data	11.3 hours	13 hours	35.5 hours
Morphine (IV)	1.7 hours	4.2 hours	3.4 hours	4.35 hours	4.47 hours
Morphine (oral)	3.3 hours	5.5 hours	6.4 hours	6.85 hours	4.4 hours
Morphine (SR)	4.01 hours	No data	7.36 hours		
Oxycodone	3.4 hours	13.9 hours			
Nonopioid Analgesics					
Aspirin	7.9 hours	7.3 hours			
Ibuprofen	2.2 hours	No data	1.9 hours		2.6 hours
Naproxen	14.14 hours	20.36 hours			

Etiology and Epidemiology

Gallstones result from a combination of factors including biliary stasis, inflammation of the gallbladder, and abnormal bile composition and reabsorption. There are two types of gallstones: those composed predominantly of cholesterol and pigmented gallstones (composed of several chemicals, including calcium bilirubinate and cholesterol). Cholesterol gallstones are the more commonly occurring, with about 80% of gallstones in the United States and Europe being this type. In Japan, 30% to 40% of gallstones are the pigmented type (Friedman, 2010).

Cholelithiasis is more common in women, but the incidence in both men and women increases with age. In fact, 20% of women and 10% of men have gallstones by the age of 65. Certain ethnic groups are at a higher risk for gallstones. For example, 75% of Native American Indian women over age 25 have gallstones (Friedman, 2010; Thomas, 2011). (See the Cultural Considerations box.) Other risk factors for the development of cholelithiasis are obesity, diabetes, hyperlipidemia, cirrhosis, and Crohn's disease. Rapid weight loss is also associated with gallstone formation, and there is an increased incidence after bariatric surgery. Many drugs can increase the risk for gallstone formation, such as clofibrate, ceftriaxone, and oral contraceptives.

CULTURAL CONSIDERATIONS in Patients with Cholelithiasis

Many factors influence the prevalence of cholelithiasis, including comorbidities, ethnicity, genetics, and gender. Cholelithiasis rates are higher in Western Caucasian, Hispanic, and Native American populations and lower in eastern European, African American, and Japanese populations (Afdhal, 2009).

Formation of gallstones is also reported to be more common in women. For example, in non-Hispanic White women, the prevalence was reported to be 16.6%, compared to 8.6% in non-Hispanic white men (Afdhal, 2009). Among Mexican American populations, the disparity is even greater, with 26.7% of Mexican American women developing symptomatic cholelithiasis, whereas only 8.9% of Mexican American men develop gallstones (Afdhal, 2009). This disparity is attributed to the fact that estrogens cause increased cholesterol secretion and progesterone promotes biliary stasis.

Pathophysiology

Cholesterol is a normal component of bile, but when the bile is supersaturated with cholesterol, the chances increase for cholesterol crystal formation. The cholesterol crystals aggregate to form larger stones. When these "macrostones" obstruct the cystic or common bile

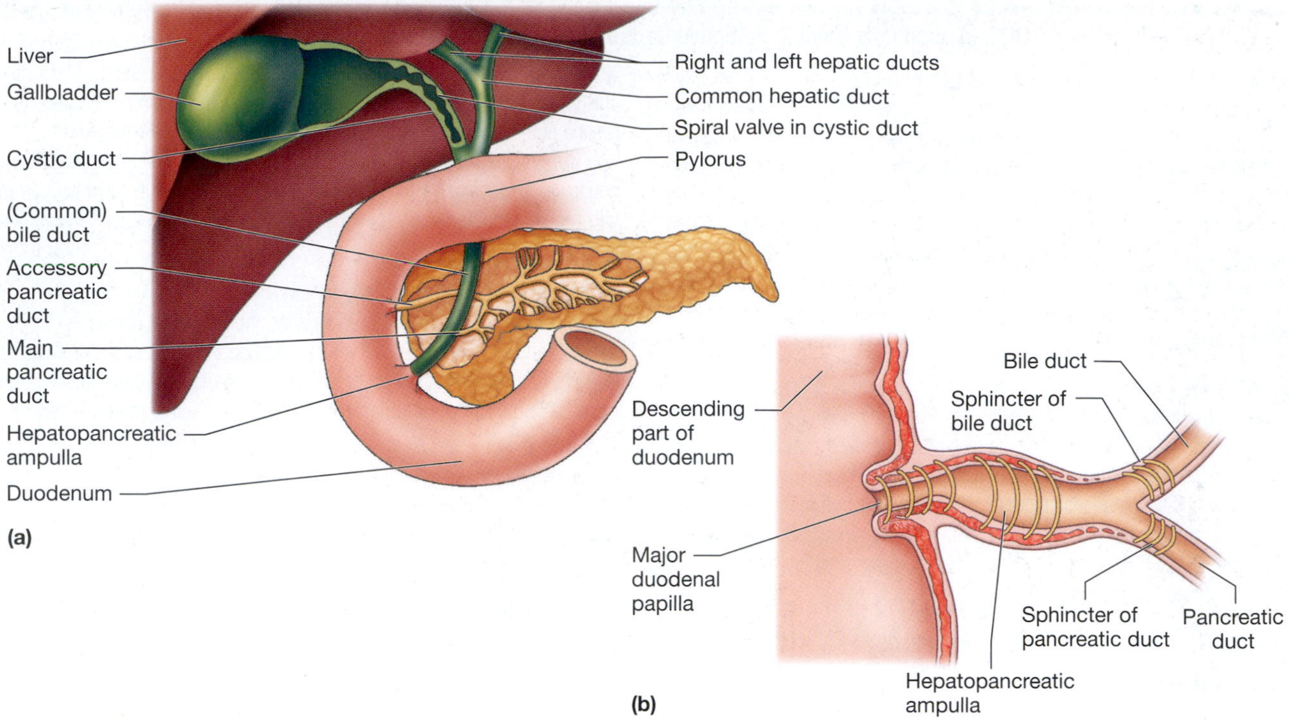

FIGURE 38–3 ◆ (a) Extrahepatic bile passages, gallbladder, and pancreatic ducts. (b) Entry of the pancreatic and bile ducts into the hepatopancreatic ampula, then into the duodenum.

duct, the gallbladder becomes inflamed and cholecystitis results (see the following text). It is unclear why the hepatocytes form bile with a high concentration of cholesterol, but the cause is most likely a combination of factors, including the presence of a defective enzyme that influences the liver cells' synthesis of cholesterol, decreased secretion of bile acids, and decreased reabsorption of bile salts from the ileum (Huether, 2010).

Clinical Manifestations

Although many patients with cholelithiasis are asymptomatic, the most common manifestation is epigastric and/or right upper quadrant pain. Often the pain associated with gallstones is steady and severe with radiation to the mid-upper back, right scapula, and shoulder. Most patients also complain of nausea and intolerance of fatty foods. Other symptoms include flatulence, bloating, abdominal distention, diarrhea, light-colored stool, and chest pain. If a stone becomes lodged in the common bile duct, the patient may develop jaundice as a result of hepatocyte damage from bile refluxing into the liver.

Cholecystitis

Cholecystitis is simply inflammation of the gallbladder and can be an acute or chronic problem. The most common cause of both acute and chronic cholecystitis is a gallstone lodged in the cystic duct. When the flow of bile out of the gallbladder is obstructed, the gallbladder becomes distended and an inflammatory response is initiated.

Pathophysiology, Etiology, and Epidemiology

In at least 90% of the patients with cholecystitis, cholelithiasis is the cause. If the gallstones are in the cystic duct, pressure in the gallbladder increases, causing ischemia of the mucosal wall and inflammation (Huether, 2010). Prolonged ischemia leads to necrosis; in severe cases, gangrene can result. In a severely inflamed gallbladder or in the case of gangrene, perforation with resultant peritonitis is possible. In patients who are immunosuppressed, infectious organisms such as cytomegalovirus and cryptosporidiosis can cause acute cholecystitis (Friedman, 2010). Chronic cholecystitis can result from persistent irritation of the gallbladder by either repeated bouts of acute cholecystitis or the constant presence of many small gallstones in the gallbladder.

Clinical Manifestations

The clinical manifestations of cholecystitis are similar to those of cholelithiasis. Pain is the predominant symptom and is usually severe and steady, lasting up to 12 to 18 hours (Friedman, 2010). As with gallstones, the pain is usually in the right upper quadrant and may radiate to the mid-upper back, right scapula, and shoulder. Unlike cholelithiasis, the patient with cholecystitis can have a fever and chills. The gallbladder may be palpable on abdominal exam if it is extremely inflamed, and there may be tenderness with possible guarding on palpation of the RUQ. Jaundice may be present as well.

Biliary Dyskinesia

Biliary dyskinesia, also called acalculous cholecystopathy, is a term applied to motility disorders of the gallbladder. Although they are uncommon disorders, the clinical manifestations are almost indistinguishable from those of other problems of the gallbladder. The most common clinical manifestation is episodic abdominal pain. The pain is usually epigastric or in the right upper quadrant and may radiate to the back and right scapula. As with the pain in cholelithiasis, the pain from biliary dyskinesia occurs following a fatty meal and may be accompanied by nausea and vomiting. The incidence of biliary dyskinesia in the United States is not known. It is known, however, that the condition occurs more frequently in females and in individuals 40 to 60 years of age (Thomson, 2011).

Laboratory and Diagnostic Procedures

The diagnostic test of choice for cholelithiasis is an *ultrasound of the gallbladder*. This test is noninvasive and can detect gallstones as well as the gallbladder's size and shape. It can also be used in conjunction with nuclear studies to assess the emptying of the gallbladder for patients who may have biliary dyskinesia (Kee, 2010). Other tests may be performed to identify possible complications or to rule out other possible causes of the symptoms. Refer to the Laboratory and Diagnostic Tests for Gallbladder Disorders box.

Medical Management

Patients with asymptomatic cholelithiasis are usually treated conservatively with dietary modifications and lifestyle changes. However, if the patient has frequent symptoms, very severe symptoms, or cholecystitis, surgery to remove the gallstone and the gallbladder is indicated.

Dietary and Lifestyle Management

For mild cases of cholelithiasis, diet (low fat) and lifestyle changes may be effective in managing the condition. For more severe cases, diet and lifestyle changes are only part of the treatment, which will include surgery. In either situation, dietary fat intake is limited. Patients with obstructed bile flow may require supplementation with the fat-soluble vitamins A, D, E, and K. For patients who are obese, a weight loss program that includes exercise is recommended. Other contributing factors such as hyperlipidemia and diabetes are treated to minimize the recurrence of gallstones.

LABORATORY AND DIAGNOSTIC TESTS for Gallbladder Disorders

Test with Description, Rationale, and Normal Values	Expected Abnormality
Ultrasound of the Gallbladder	
Normal: normal size and structures of the gallbladder	Enlarged structures, gallstones, and any obstruction.
Noninvasive test to assess the gallbladder's size and structure.	
Nuclear Scan of the Gallbladder	
Normal: no abnormalities	Obstruction, cholelithiasis, cholecystitis, or biliary dyskinesia. Highly sensitive for cholecystitis.
Uses a radioisotope to evaluate cholelithiasis, cholecystitis, and biliary dyskinesia.	
Bilirubin	
Normal: Indirect: 0.1–1.0 mg/dL Direct: 0.1–0.3 mg/dL Total: 0.1–1.2 mg/dL	Total and indirect bilirubin are elevated in obstructive jaundice (liver or biliary), cirrhosis of the liver, and cancer of the liver. Indirect bilirubin is elevated with sickle cell, pernicious, and hemolytic anemias; cirrhosis; hepatitis; and transfusion reactions; as well as hemolysis.
Bilirubin is formed when hemoglobin is broken down; the liver conjugates the bilirubin and excretes it in bile.	
Amylase	
Normal: 30–170 units/L	Elevated in the presence of pancreatitis, which may be related to a biliary obstruction.
Used to diagnose pancreatitis.	
Lipase	
Normal: 14–280 units/L	Is elevated in the presence of pancreatitis and acute cholecystitis.
Used to diagnose pancreatic disorders.	
ALT (alanine aminotransferase)	
Normal: 10–35 units/L	Over 300 units/L.
Used to detect liver disease by measuring an enzyme released from hepatocytes when the liver is injured.	Higher elevations indicate liver damage. ALT is more specific for the liver than other enzymes.
AST (aspartate aminotransferase)	
Normal: 8–38 units/L	10 times or more above the normal.
To detect liver or cardiac damage by measuring an enzyme found in hepatocytes and cardiac cells as well as skeletal muscle cells, kidneys, and the pancreas.	AST is released when there is cellular injury.
WBC	
Normal: 4,500–10,000 μL (mm^3)	WBC counts above 10,000 indicate the presence of infection and/or inflammation.
Used to detect infection.	
Cholecystogram	
Normal: no abnormalities in the gallbladder	Gallstones, tumors, or obstructions.
Used to detect problems in the gallbladder, including tumors, gallstones, or obstruction.	

Source: Kee, J. L. (2010). *Laboratory and diagnostic tests with nursing implications* (8th ed.). Upper Saddle River, NJ: Prentice Hall.

CHART 38–6 Nursing Care of the Patient With a T-Tube

- Attach the tube to sterile gravity drainage.
- Place the patient in Fowler's position to maximize gravity drainage.
- Monitor drainage and record the amount every 8 hours.
- The amount may be 500 milliliters on the first day, decreasing to about 200 milliliters by the third day.
- Drainage may be blood tinged at first but becomes green-brown.
- Drainage in excess of 500 milliliters by the third day is excessive, and the surgeon should be notified.
- Monitor the color of the stools.
- Pale stools indicate obstruction of flow of bile to the duodenum.
- Clamp the T-tube as ordered, and monitor the patient's response to the clamping.
- Keep the skin clean and free from bile drainage.
- Bile is irritating to the skin. Skin can be protected with zinc oxide, karaya (a gum from the Karaya tree that is used in lotions and acts as a protectant), or other barrier.
- Teach the patient how to care for the tube during activities of daily living.
- The patient may be discharged with the tube in place and should be informed of the signs of infection, such as fever, redness, swelling, or drainage from the site, as well as care for the tube, avoiding any direct pulling or traction on the tube.
- A daily shower is usually permitted, but a tub bath is not.

Surgical Management

Surgery is the treatment of choice for most patients with cholelithiasis, cholecystitis, and biliary dyskinesia. Removal of the gallbladder, or **cholecystectomy,** is done most often using the laparoscopic surgical method, which is minimally invasive, has fewer complications, and requires a much shorter length of hospital stay than the traditional open cholecystectomy. Patients with a very large or infected gallbladder may not be candidates for laparoscopic cholecystectomy and may require an open cholecystectomy. In addition, during the laparoscopic procedure, the surgeon may find it necessary to convert the procedure to an open cholecystectomy. If stones are located in the common bile duct, an exploration of this duct is done, and a T-tube is placed in the common bile duct to maintain patency, allowing bile to pass from the liver into the duodenum until the edema from surgery diminishes. Chart 38–6 outlines the nursing care of a patient with a T-tube.

Medications

Some patients with gallstones may not be good surgical candidates or may refuse surgery. In these cases, drugs are available to dissolve the gallstones by reducing the cholesterol content of the stone. Ursodiol (Actigall) or chenodiol (Chenix) may be used but are effective only if the gallstones contain a high concentration of cholesterol and are less than 1 centimeter in diameter. Treatment usually lasts at least 6 months, with success in fewer than 50% of patients (Chiang, Lee, & Santen, 2010). See the Pharmacology Summary of Medications Used to Treat Biliary Disorders.

Other drug treatment for cholelithiasis and cholecystitis includes antibiotics if an infection is suspected. Bile salts accumulate on the skin when the patient is jaundiced; this causes pruritus. Cholestyramine (Questran) binds these bile salts, which are then excreted in the stool. For acute cholecystitis, a narcotic analgesic may be needed to relieve the pain.

Ultrasound Therapy

Extracorporeal shock wave lithotripsy (ESWL) is a method to break up large gallstones by using ultrasound waves, usually in conjunction with oral dissolution therapy; however, ESWL is no longer widely used as fragments may not clear the bile duct. This puts the patient at risk for further problems such as pancreatitis (Friedman, 2010). After the procedure, the patient may have biliary colic pain when the gallbladder attempts to expel the stone fragments.

Nursing Management

Nursing care for patients with cholelithiasis or cholecystitis includes assessment, ensuring pain relief, preparing the patient for possible surgery, preventing infection, and educating the patient about future prevention, postoperative care, and dietary modifications. The nurse will complete a head-to-toe assessment preoperatively. See the Nursing Process: Patient Care Plan box for the patient with cholelithiasis and surgery.

Collaborative Management

The patient with gallbladder disorders may experience many challenges, especially related to nutrition, pain, and possible postoperative complications. These challenges require the collaboration of an interdisciplinary team. The team may include the nurse, a gastroenterologist, a surgeon, a nutritionist, a pharmacist, and the primary care

PHARMACOLOGY Summary of Medications Used to Treat Biliary Disorders

Medication Category and Action	Application/Indication	Nursing Responsibility
Gallstone-Solubilizing Agents		
Ursodiol (Actigall) Chenodiol (Chenix) ***Action:*** Dissolves gallstones by reducing the cholesterol content of the stone or blocking cholesterol production.	Prevention of gallstones, dissolution of noncalcified cholesterol gallstones, and primary biliary cirrhosis.	Monitor for adverse effects: nausea, vomiting, and dyspepsia. Be aware of drugs that reduce efficacy: bile acid sequestrants (medications used to bind certain components of bile in the gastrointestinal tract), aluminum antacids, estrogens, and some lipid-lowering agents.
Bile Acid Sequestrants		
Cholestyramine (Questran, LoCholest) Colestipol (Colestid) ***Action:*** Decreases pruritus by decreasing circulation bile acids and decreasing bile acid deposits in skin tissue.	Relief of pruritus secondary to partial biliary stasis.	Monitor for adverse effects: constipation, abdominal pain, nausea, vomiting, and indigestion. Be aware long-term use may require supplementation of fat soluble vitamins. Give 2 hours after or 4 hours before other drugs.

NURSING PROCESS: Patient Care Plan for Cholelithiasis and Surgery

Assessment of Hepatic and Biliary Status Using Gordon's Functional Health Patterns:

- Health Perception Health Management Pattern
- Nutrition Metabolic Pattern
- Activity Exercise Pattern
- Cognitive Perceptual Pattern

Subjective Data

Assessment of Pain—Preoperatively

What is your level of pain on a scale of 0 to 10, with 10 being the worst pain?

Are you allergic to anything?

Do you have any special cultural or religious practices for dealing with pain?

Do you have pain when you eat certain foods, particularly high-fat foods?

Have you ever had this type of pain before? If yes, how long did it last? What relieved the pain in the past?

Do you take oral contraceptives? Or hormone replacement therapy?

Could you possibly be pregnant?

Assessment of Nutrition

How is your appetite?

What have you eaten in the last 24 hours?

Are you nauseated?

Are there any foods that make you nauseated?

Have you lost a lot of weight lately?

Assessment of Postoperative Status

What is your level of pain on a scale of 0 to 10, with 10 being the worst pain?

Are you nauseated?

How active were you before surgery?

Are you having any trouble breathing?

Are you coughing and using your incentive spirometer?

Objective Data

Assessment of Pain—Preoperatively

Vital signs q4h:

- Temperature
- Blood pressure
- Pulse
- Respirations.

Abdominal examination:

- Bowel sounds
- Tenderness
- Guarding.

Restlessness.

Grimacing.

Moaning or groaning.

Shallow respirations.

Assessment of Nutrition

Height and weight measurements.

BMI.

Laboratory results:

- Bilirubin
- Serum albumin
- Glucose
- Cholesterol
- Urinalysis.

Assessment of Postoperative Status

Vital signs:

- Temperature
- Blood pressure
- Pulse
- Respirations.

Abdominal examination:

- Bowel sounds
- Tenderness
- Guarding
- Wound inspection.

Laboratory values:

- CBC
- Coagulation studies
- Bilirubin.

Respiratory assessment:

- Lung sounds
- Respiratory rate and rhythm.

Outcomes and Evaluation Parameters / Planning and Interventions with *Rationales*

1. NURSING DIAGNOSIS: Pain, Acute *related to cholelithiasis/cholecystitis* (NANDA-I © 2012)

Outcome: Comfort level maintained.

Evaluation Parameters: Able to communicate level of pain and relief with medications.

Able to take deep breaths without pain.

Appears restful without restlessness or moaning.

Assess pain using a pain scale (0 to 10) to quantify the pain level *to increase consistency in monitoring pain.*

Administer pain medication, usually meperidine or morphine, and assess the level of pain 30 minutes and 1 hour after giving medication *to assess the effectiveness of the medications.*

Explore cultural and religious practices and beliefs about pain and illness. *Different religions have varying beliefs about pain, suffering, and disease.*

Teach nonpharmacologic methods of pain control, such as guided imagery, meditation, and breathing exercises. *This may augment pain relief.*

Discuss foods that are high in fat and may cause nausea and GI distress even after surgery. *Foods high in fat stimulate contractions of the gallbladder and may cause pain if stones are present.*

(*continued*)

NURSING PROCESS: Patient Care Plan for Cholelithiasis and Surgery, *continued*

2. NURSING DIAGNOSIS: Nutrition: Readiness for Enhanced *related to anorexia, pain, and nausea from impaired bile flow* (NANDA-I © 2012)

Outcome: Adequate nutrition. ***Evaluation Parameters:*** No weight loss. Serum albumin normal. Fasting glucose normal. No reported nausea. No evidence of bleeding.	Obtain diet history, history of large rapid weight loss, and height and weight measurements *to help establish current nutritional status and possible imbalanced diet with fat-soluble vitamin deficiency.* Assess laboratory results and report any abnormal values to the patient's health care provider. *Bilirubin in the urine indicates an obstruction to bile flow and will be reflected in an elevated serum bilirubin. Patients with diabetes mellitus and high serum cholesterol are at risk for gallstones. Protein malnutrition is reflected in a low serum albumin.* Give supplemental vitamins as ordered. *Bile is necessary for the absorption of fat-soluble vitamins, so supplements may be necessary.* Educate the patient about avoiding foods that contain a large amount of fat. *Even after removal of the gallbladder, high-fat foods may cause nausea.* Refer to a dietitian for a low-fat diet plan that promotes slow weight loss. *Many patients with gallbladder disease are overweight or obese and will benefit from a sensible weight loss plan.*

3. NURSING DIAGNOSES: (a) Comfort: Readiness for Enhanced *related to surgical incision.* (b) Nutrition: Readiness for Enhanced *related to postoperative nausea.* (c) Airway Clearance, Ineffective *related to decreased lung expansion, immobility, and anesthesia.* (d) Infection: Risk for *related to surgical incision and ineffective airway clearance* (NANDA-I © 2012)

Outcome: Discharge 1 to 2 days postoperatively. ***Evaluation Parameters:*** Hemoglobin and hematocrit normal. Vital signs normal. No complaints of nausea. Bowel sounds and bowel movement. Eating soft foods without nausea. Lung sounds clear and patient eupneic.	Assess pain using a pain scale (0 to 10) to quantify the pain level, and administer pain medication as ordered or monitor the PCA (patient-controlled analgesia) if the patient has an IV pump *to increase consistency in monitoring pain.* Give antiemetics as ordered *to prevent vomiting that may result from anesthesia, pain, or pain medication.* Discuss the patient's previous activity level, and instruct her to resume normal activity slowly over 2 to 3 days after discharge. *An otherwise sedentary patient cannot be expected to be more active after surgery than before.* Give vitamin K as ordered. *Vitamin K is a fat-soluble vitamin and may be ordered postoperatively to prevent bleeding.* Position the patient in a semi-Fowler's position and ambulate as ordered when the patient is alert, as well as encourage the use of incentive spirometry. *Early mobility/ambulation promotes lung expansion and helps prevent postoperative pneumonia and deep vein thrombosis, as well as promotes intestinal motility. The upright position allows for enhanced lung expansion.* Monitor vital signs every 2 to 4 hours, then every 4–8 hours as ordered *to detect any complications. Tachycardia, increased respiratory rate, or elevated temperature can indicate pain, bleeding, or infection.* Examine the abdomen for the return of bowel sounds and signs of peritonitis, and assess the wound for drainage and infection. *Increasing abdominal tenderness, guarding, and rigid abdomen may be signs of an intra-abdominal leak of bile or blood.* Assess laboratory results for signs of over-/underhydration, bleeding, biliary obstruction, and infection, and notify the health care provider. *Early detection of complications of surgery, such as hemorrhage, infection, edema of the common bile duct, and fluid overload/dehydration, makes treatment more efficient.*

Source: Adapted from Wilkinson, J. M., & Ahearn, N. R. (2009). *Prentice Hall nursing diagnosis handbook* (9th ed.). Upper Saddle River, NJ: Prentice Hall.

provider. In order to meet desired patient outcomes, it is essential that this interdisciplinary team communicate openly with one another in developing and evaluating care of the patient and family (IOM [Institute of Medicine], 2010).

Communication is critical to ensure the best patient care. Primary care providers, gastroenterologists, and surgeons may need to diagnose and provide medical management for patients with gallbladder disorders. Nurses, pharmacists, and nutritionists collaborate to teach patients about dietary changes and medication regimens as well as about the disease process and prevention. Many patients with cholelithiasis and cholecystitis require removal of the gallbladder. Pre- and postoperative teaching and care are critical to prevent potential surgical complications, such as atelectasis or deep vein thrombosis.

Health Promotion

Several risk factors for cholelithiasis can be controlled, such as obesity, hyperlipidemia, and diabetes. Increasing exercise and maintaining a well-balanced, low-fat, low-calorie diet can modify obesity. However, rapid weight loss should be discouraged because it could contribute to gallstone formation. Hyperlipidemia can be controlled through medication; by a low-fat, low-cholesterol diet; and with at least 30 minutes per day of regular exercise. Good control of blood sugar in patients with diabetes may also decrease the recurrence of gallstones.

Disorders of the Exocrine Pancreas

Disorders of the pancreas that will be discussed are acute and chronic pancreatitis and cancer of the pancreas.

Acute Pancreatitis

Etiology

Pancreatitis, or inflammation of the pancreas, can be acute or chronic and is a potentially serious disease. Most cases of pancreatitis occur between ages 50 and 60, and the incidence is the same for men and women. Risk factors for the development of pancreatitis include alcoholism, biliary obstruction, peptic ulcers, trauma, extreme hyperlipidemia, hypertriglyceridemia, and the use of some medications (Huether, 2010). The mortality rate is higher in patients who develop complications such as shock, acute respiratory distress syndrome (ARDS), or renal complications.

Epidemiology

Many cases of acute pancreatitis are mild and self-limiting and do not require hospitalization. However, about 20% of patients develop severe pancreatitis, which can lead to necrosis of the pancreas. These patients must be hospitalized (Huether, 2010).

Pathophysiology

The precise cause of acute pancreatitis is unknown, but most cases are associated with either biliary tract obstruction or heavy alcohol use. It is believed that activated pancreatic enzymes, particularly trypsin, leak into the pancreatic tissue and begin the process of autodigestion (the pancreas begins to digest itself). If bile refluxes into the pancreas as a result of biliary obstruction, this activates the pancreatic enzymes and the process of autodigestion. Activated trypsin and lipase begin to break down the cell membranes, which results in edema, vascular leakage, hemorrhage, and necrosis. In response to this autodigestion, tissue necrosis factor-alpha (TNF-α), substance P, and many interleukins and kinins enter the systemic circulation, causing damage to tissue in the lungs, blood vessels, and kidneys, which results in increased mortality (Huether, 2010).

Clinical Manifestations

The most prominent manifestation of acute pancreatitis is sudden, severe, steady epigastric pain that may radiate to the right or left side of the back. The pain is worse when the patient is lying supine or with activity and is made better by sitting and leaning forward with the knees bent. The patient usually complains of nausea and vomiting. During a severe attack, the patient may appear anxious and sweaty (Thomas, 2011). The patient may also have abdominal distention, tenderness without rigidity, and decreased bowel sounds. Transient hyperglycemia may result from glucagon secretion from damaged cells in the pancreatic islets. Less common symptoms include Turner's sign (ecchymosis in the flanks) and Cullen's sign (bruising around the umbilicus), which may appear as a result of retroperitoneal bleeding (Andris, 2010).

More severe pancreatitis can lead to multiple organ system failure related to fluid shifting around the pancreas. These fluid shifts can lead to pleural effusions, ARDS, and shock (Andris, 2010). Manifestations of these complications include tachypnea, tachycardia, and hypoxia.

Laboratory and Diagnostic Procedures

The diagnosis of acute pancreatitis is based on a complete history and physical exam and elevated levels of serum amylase and lipase. Other tests, such as serum bilirubin and serum alkaline phosphatase, indicate obstruction of the common bile duct, which can result from stones or edema, resulting in acute pancreatitis. An elevated ALT level (three times above normal) in patients with symptoms of acute pancreatitis indicates a biliary pancreatitis (Thomas, 2011).

Imaging tests are ordered for the patient with acute pancreatitis, including an abdominal x-ray, computed tomography (CT) scan, and ultrasonography (see the Laboratory and Diagnostic Tests for Pancreatic Disorders box on page 1190).

Ranson's criterion is widely used to assess the severity of acute pancreatitis. Each diagnostic criterion is awarded a point. See Chart 38–7.

Medical Management

Treatment of acute pancreatitis involves resting the pancreas, which involves keeping the patient NPO (nothing by mouth). If the patient has persistent nausea and vomiting, a nasogastric tube may be inserted and connected to low intermittent suction. This keeps normal secretions from stimulating the pancreas to release digestive enzymes, therefore causing pain. Bed rest may be ordered until the acute phase has subsided. When the patient is free from pain, lab values are normal, and bowel sounds have returned, a diet of clear liquids is usually ordered. The diet is then advanced slowly to low fat. Fluid status is maintained to keep urine output at 30 mL/hr (Andris, 2010). Patients with severe pancreatitis may require large amounts of intravenous fluids to maintain the patient's fluid volume and may require the patient to be transferred to the intensive care unit (Thomas, 2011).

Medications

Pain relief is of primary importance and is usually achieved with narcotic analgesics. Meperidine originally was the drug of choice because it

CHART 38–7 Ranson's Criteria for Assessing Acute Pancreatitis Severity

At onset of symptoms:

- Age > 55
- White blood cells > 16,000/μL
- Blood glucose > 200 mg/dL
- Serum lactate dehydrogenase (LDH) > 350 units/L
- AST > 250 units/L

During the following 48 hours:

- Hematocrit drop of 10% or more
- Blood urea nitrogen (BUN) increase of 5 mg/dL or more
- Arterial PO_2 < 60 mmHg
- Serum calcium < 8 mg/dL
- Base deficit > 4 mEq/L
- Estimated fluid sequestration > 6 L

Number of Criteria	Mortality Rate (%)
0–2	1
3–4	16
5–6	40
7–8	100

Source: Ranson, J. H., Rifkind, K. M., Roses, D. F., Fink, S. D., Eng, K., & Spencer, F. C. (1974). Prognostic signs and the role of operative management in acute pancreatitis. *Surgical Gynecology and Obstetrics, 139*(1):69–81.

LABORATORY AND DIAGNOSTIC TESTS for Pancreatic Disorders

Test with Description, Rationale, and Normal Values	Expected Abnormality
Amylase Normal: 30–170 units/L *Used to diagnose pancreatitis.*	Amylase is elevated in the presence of pancreatitis, increasing hours after the onset of disease and increasing to two to three times normal. Levels return to normal within 2 to 4 days (Kee, 2010). May remain normal with chronic pancreatitis.
Lipase Normal: 14–280 units/L *Used to diagnose pancreatic disorders.*	Lipase is elevated in the presence of pancreatitis, increases rapidly, and remains elevated for up to 14 days (Kee, 2010). May remain normal with chronic pancreatitis.
Bilirubin Normal (Kee, 2010): Indirect: 0.1–1.0 mg/dL Direct: 0.1–0.3 mg/dL Total: 0.1–1.2 mg/dL *Bilirubin is formed when hemoglobin is broken down; the liver conjugates the bilirubin and excretes in bile.*	Total and indirect bilirubin are elevated in obstructive jaundice (liver or biliary), cirrhosis of the liver, and cancer of the liver (Kee, 2010). Indirect bilirubin is elevated with sickle cell, pernicious, and hemolytic anemias, cirrhosis, hepatitis, and transfusion reactions as well as hemolysis (Kee, 2010).
ALT (alanine aminotransferase) Normal: 10–35 units/L *Used to detect liver disease by measuring an enzyme released from hepatocytes when the liver is injured.*	An ALT three times above normal indicates biliary pancreatitis (Thomas, 2011).
ALP (alkaline phosphatase) Normal is 42–136 units/L *Used to detect liver or bone disorders by measuring enzymes found in the liver and bone cells.*	ALP is markedly elevated in severe liver or biliary disease. It may indicate pancreatitis caused by biliary obstruction.
WBC Normal: 4,500–10,000 μL (mm^3) *Used to detect infection.*	WBC counts above 10,000 indicate the presence of infection and/or inflammation.
C-Reactive Protein Normal: negative *Used to detect inflammation and the risk of coronary artery disease.*	C-reactive protein is elevated with inflammation, such as in pancreatitis; elevations after 48 hours may indicate pancreatic necrosis (Friedman, 2010).
Calcium Normal: Total: 9–11 mg/dL Ionized: 4.25–5.25 mg/dL *Used to evaluate calcium balance.*	Decreased levels may be associated with fat necrosis as calcium accumulates in the abdomen in patients with pancreatitis (Kumar, Abbas, Fausto, & Mitchell, 2007). Levels below 7 mg/dL are associated with a poorer prognosis (Friedman, 2010).
Serum Glucose Normal: 70–110 mg/dL *Stored in the liver as glycogen.*	Serum glucose may be elevated in patients with chronic pancreatitis who have developed diabetes (Friedman, 2010).
Urine Glucose Normal: negative *Used to assess for glycosuria.*	Glycosuria may indicate the patient with chronic pancreatitis has developed diabetes (Friedman, 2010).
Fat in Stool Normal: 2–7 g/24 hours *Used to identify whether fat is in stool.*	Increased fat related to pancreatic insufficiency.
Abdominal X-Ray Normal: no abnormalities *Used to examine structure of abdominal organs.*	Abdominal x-rays scan for masses, obstructions, and abscesses (Kee, 2010). They may show gallstones, a segment of small intestine in the left upper quadrant that is filled with air, or a gas-filled segment of transverse colon that ends in the area of pancreatic inflammation (Friedman, 2010).

LABORATORY AND DIAGNOSTIC TESTS for Pancreatic Disorders, *continued*

Test with Description, Rationale, and Normal Values	Expected Abnormality
Computed Tomography (CT) Normal: no abnormalities *Used to detect lesions, tumors, and metastasis; vascular disease; infection; and bone destruction.* *Used to detect necrotizing pancreatitis.*	Fluid collection in the pancreas is an ominous sign of necrotizing pancreatitis and is associated with higher mortality rates (Friedman, 2010). Presence of tumors or lesions.
Abdominal or Gallbladder Ultrasound Normal: normal structures within the abdomen and gallbladder *Used to determine the size and structure of organs.*	Ultrasounds are used to diagnose gallstones, an inflamed pancreas, and edematous common bile ducts (Andris, 2010). Evaluates abnormal structures.
Endoscopic Retrograde Cholangiopancreatography (ERCP) Normal: no problems in biliary and pancreatic ducts *Used to locate the cause of a biliary obstruction. It may be conducted in conjunction with CT, MRI, or endoscopic ultrasound.*	ERCP evaluates for dilated ducts, strictures, stones, pseudocysts. It detects bile duct stones and pancreatic duct obstruction (Friedman, 2010).
Magnetic Resonance Imaging (MRI) Normal: no abnormalities *Used to detect lesions, vascular problems, injury, edema, or tumors.*	MRI tests for tumors, edema, or any other abnormality.
Positive Emission Tomography (PET) Scan Normal: normal function and blood flow *Used to evaluate cell activity and blood flow; can detect benign and malignant tumors and lesions.*	Malignant lesions in pancreatic cancer.
Biopsy Normal: no abnormal tissue *Used to determine whether cancer exists.*	A biopsy determines if cells are abnormal, indicating pancreatic cancer.

Source: Kee, J. L. (2010). *Laboratory and diagnostic tests with nursing implications* (8th ed.). Upper Saddle River, NJ: Prentice Hall.

was thought that other opioids caused spasms in the sphincter of Oddi, but this is no longer considered to be the case (Andris, 2010; Thomas, 2011). In fact, meperidine is no longer the drug of choice for pancreatitis because of possible toxicities; morphine sulfate, hydromorphone, and fentanyl are currently used for pain control (Andris, 2010). Antibiotics such as Imipenem or cefuroxime may be prescribed if there is evidence of infection or, in the case of pancreatic necrosis, to prevent infection (Friedman, 2010). In the patient with severe pancreatitis who has been NPO for 7 to 10 days, total parenteral nutrition may be needed to maintain adequate nutritional status. Enteral nutrition may be given if the gut is functional. Patients who are hypocalcemic will be given calcium gluconate intravenously to prevent tetany. (See the Pharmacology box on p. 1185.)

Surgery

Surgery to debride the pancreas and surrounding tissue is indicated for patients who have infected necrotizing pancreatitis. This process may improve survival for patients with multiorgan failure if the pancreatitis does not respond to other treatment within 4 weeks. If pancreatic abscesses develop, then the patient may require a percutaneous or open surgical drainage. Occasionally, patients with acute pancreatitis develop pseudocysts, which require drainage if persistent pain develops or if there is ductal obstruction (Friedman, 2010).

Chronic Pancreatitis

Etiology and Epidemiology

Chronic pancreatitis is an irreversible process of gradual destruction of pancreatic tissue. Although 70% to 80% of the cases are attributed to chronic alcohol use, fewer than 10% of alcoholics develop chronic pancreatitis. Smoking may enhance alcohol's effect on the pancreas. Other causes of chronic pancreatitis include stones, cystic fibrosis, malnutrition, and heredity. Approximately 25% of cases of chronic pancreatitis have no identifiable cause (Friedman, 2010; Huether, 2010; Thomas, 2011).

Pathophysiology

There are several theories about the pathogenesis of chronic pancreatitis. One theory relates to pancreatic ductal obstructions caused by increased pancreatic proteins. Another theory, the toxic-metabolic theory, surmises that acinar cells in the pancreas are lost because of toxins. The oxidative stress theory proposes that free radicals damaged acinar cells due to inflammation. Finally, the necrosis–fibrosis theory describes the effects of chronic inflammation on the pancreas, including increased scarring in the pancreas (Kumar, Abbas, Fausto, & Mitchell, 2007).

Clinical Manifestations

The predominant manifestation of chronic pancreatitis is recurrent epigastric and left upper quadrant pain that may be referred to the left lumbar region and is less severe than the pain in acute pancreatitis. A physical exam may reveal abdominal tenderness. Other common symptoms may include anorexia, nausea, vomiting, weight loss, flatulence, and diarrhea. A late manifestation is **steatorrhea,** which is stools that are bulky, fatty, and foul from the lack of pancreatic enzymes (Thomas, 2011). Some patients may also exhibit signs of diabetes mellitus.

Weblink: Pancreatic Cancer

Laboratory and Diagnostic Procedures

Laboratory values for patients with chronic pancreatitis are usually similar to those of patients with acute pancreatitis; however, the amylase and lipase levels may be normal in chronic pancreatitis. Most patients with chronic pancreatitis (80%) will develop diabetes after having the disease for 25 years and have elevated blood sugar levels and glycosuria (Friedman, 2010). Stool samples are examined for fat.

The most sensitive test for chronic pancreatitis is the endoscopic retrograde cholangiopancreatography (ERCP). Newer tests that are less invasive and will show bile duct stones and pancreatic duct obstruction include magnetic resonance cholangiopancreatography (MRCP) and endoscopic ultrasonography with tissue sampling (Friedman, 2010). See the Laboratory and Diagnostic Tests box on page 1190.

Medical Management

Patients with chronic pancreatitis require lifelong changes in lifestyle. Abstinence from alcohol is mandatory because it often will precipitate an acute attack. A low-fat diet should be maintained because of the lack of the pancreatic enzyme lipase, which is responsible for fat synthesis. Smoking cessation should be part of the plan. During an acute exacerbation of chronic pancreatitis, the patient will be treated in much the same way as a patient with acute pancreatitis.

Medications

Although pain is a major manifestation of chronic pancreatitis, narcotic analgesia is avoided when possible because opioid addiction is common in these patients; alternative pain management with NSAIDs (nonsteroidal anti-inflammatory drugs) or acetaminophen may be utilized (Friedman, 2010). These patients will require nutritional supplementation with pancreatic enzymes (Chart 38–8). The supplements should be taken with meals. If the medication is not enteric coated, then an H_2-receptor antagonist such as ranitidine or a proton pump inhibitor such as omeprazole is given once or twice a day.

Surgery

Patients with chronic pancreatitis may need surgical intervention to eradicate biliary tract disease, to ensure that bile can freely flow into the duodenum, or to eliminate obstruction of the pancreatic duct. Pancreatic pseudocysts may need to be drained if they are over 6 centimeters in diameter (Friedman, 2010).

CHART 38–8 Pancreatic Enzyme Supplement Preparations

Pancreatic enzymes are purified from pig pancreases.	• Actions:
	  • Contains protease, lipase, and amylase
	  • Digests proteins, fats, and carbohydrates.
	• Contraindications:
	  • Allergy to pork protein
	  • Religious and cultural considerations related to kosher foods.
	  • Vegetarians

Conventional preparations	Viokase Ilozyme Cotazym
Enteric-coated preparations	Creon Pancrease Cotazym-S Ultrase

Nursing Management

The major focuses of nursing care for the patient with pancreatitis are pain control, nutrition, and health teaching about alcohol abstinence. The Nursing Process: Patient Care Plan box also outlines the nursing diagnoses and interventions for the patient with pancreatitis.

Collaborative Management

The patient with acute or chronic pancreatitis may experience many challenges, especially related to nutrition and pain. These challenges require the collaboration of an interdisciplinary team, which may include the nurse, social services, a gastroenterologist, a nutritionist, a pharmacist, and the primary care provider. In order to meet desired patient outcomes, it is essential that this interdisciplinary team communicate openly with one another in developing and evaluating care of the patient and family (IOM [Institute of Medicine], 2010). For example, endocrinologists may be needed for patients with chronic pancreatitis. Communication is critical to ensure the best patient care.

Primary care providers, gastroenterologists, and surgeons may need to diagnose and provide medical management for patients with pancreatitis. Patients with long-term pancreatitis who develop diabetes may need an assessment by an endocrinologist.

Patients with pancreatitis will need pain management collaboration by nurses, primary care providers, and pharmacists. Assessment and education about pain management is critical to providing patient care.

Nutritionists and nurses will need to educate patients about dietary needs. Patients with acute pancreatitis may be NPO and possibly have an NG tube placed. Nurses will need to provide care and education to these patients.

Since many patients have alcohol as a risk factor for pancreatitis, social services may be involved to provide resources for these patients. They may also provide information about support groups, such as Alcoholics Anonymous. Nurses also will want to educate about the role of alcohol in causing pancreatitis.

Health Promotion

Because most cases of pancreatitis are related to alcohol abuse, the focus of prevention is on abstinence from alcohol. After diagnosis, it is essential that patients with pancreatitis abstain from alcohol to prevent future painful episodes. The nurse should refer the patient to Alcoholics Anonymous or another support or treatment program.

Cancer of the Pancreas

Etiology and Epidemiology

The American Cancer Society (2012b) estimated that approximately 43,920 people in the United States would be newly diagnosed with pancreatic cancer in 2012, with 37,390 expected deaths. Pancreatic cancer is the 10th most common cancer and fourth-leading cause of death in men as well as in women in the United States. The overall 5-year survival rate for all stages is 6%. Risk factors include obesity, chronic pancreatitis, family history of pancreatic cancer, and cigarette smoking. Smoking (both personal and environmental exposure) is linked to 20% to 30% of pancreatic cancers. There is some evidence that exposure to other chemicals, high-fat diets, and diabetes mellitus increase the risk as well (Hodgin, 2011). The risk of developing pancreatic cancer increases with age.

NURSING PROCESS: Patient Care Plan for Pancreatitis

Assessment of Hepatic and Biliary Status Using Gordon's Functional Health Patterns:

- Nutrition Metabolic Pattern
- Cognitive Perceptual Pattern

Subjective Data

Assessment of Pain

What is your level of pain on a scale of 0 to 10, with 10 being the worst pain?

Are you allergic to anything?

Do you have any special cultural or religious practices for dealing with pain?

Describe the character of your pain: Burning? Steady? Does it radiate?

Is your pain worse when you are lying down?

Do you have pain when you eat?

Does vomiting relieve the pain?

Have you ever had this type of pain before? If yes, how long did it last? What relieved the pain in the past?

Do you have a history of gallbladder disease?

Do you drink alcohol? How much? How often?

Assessment of Nutrition

Are you nauseated?

Have you vomited?

Have you noticed any weight loss?

What is your usual diet?

Assessment of Fluid and Electrolyte Status

Do you feel dizzy or light-headed?

Objective Data

Assessment of Pain

General appearance:

- Looks distressed
- Sits with knees pulled toward chest
- Restlessness
- Grimacing
- Moaning or groaning
- Clenched fists.

Heart rate—tachycardia.

Shallow rapid respirations.

Abdominal tenderness or guarding.

Flank or periumbilical ecchymosis.

Diaphoresis.

Assessment of Nutrition

Height and weight measurements.

BMI.

Abdominal examination:

- Diminished or absent bowel sounds.

Laboratory results:

- Serum albumin
- Glucose
- Transferrin
- Hemoglobin and hematocrit (H&H)
- Amylase and lipase.

Assessment of Fluid and Electrolyte Status

Cardiac status:

- Rate and rhythm
- Pulmonary artery pressure
- Peripheral pulses
- Capillary refill.

Vital signs:

- Blood pressure
- Pulse
- Respirations.

Renal function:

- Hourly urine output
- Daily body weight.

Neurological function:

- Mental status
- Level of consciousness
- Behavior.

Laboratory values:

- Electrolytes
- Hematocrit
- BUN and creatinine.

Outcomes and Evaluation Parameters	Planning and Interventions with *Rationales*
1. NURSING DIAGNOSIS: Pain: Acute *related to pancreatitis* (NANDA-I © 2012)	
Outcome: Comfort level maintained. ***Evaluation Parameters:*** Able to communicate level of pain and relief from medications. Appears restful without restlessness or moaning.	Assess pain using a pain scale (0 to 10) to quantify the pain level *to increase consistency in monitoring pain.* Administer pain medication, usually morphine, hydromorphone, or fentanyl, and assess level of pain 30 minutes and 1 hour after giving medication. Notify the health care provider if pain is unrelieved *to assess the effectiveness of medications.* Explore cultural and religious practices and beliefs about pain and illness. *Different religions have varying beliefs about pain, suffering, and disease.*

(*continued*)

NURSING PROCESS: Patient Care Plan for Pancreatitis, *continued*

Outcomes and Evaluation Parameters	Planning and Interventions with *Rationales*
	Teach nonpharmacologic methods of pain control, such as guided imagery, music therapy, meditation, and breathing exercises. *This may augment pain relief.* Maintain a quiet, darkened, comfortable environment. *This can help decrease physical and mental stimulation, which can lead to decreased pancreatic secretions and less pain.* Maintain bed rest and position the patient in a sitting position *to decrease the pain caused by stretched abdominal muscles that are irritated by inflammation.* Close the patient's door during mealtime because *the smell of food can stimulate pancreatic secretions.* Place a nasogastric tube if ordered, and/or monitor drainage and relief of pain. *This helps to "rest" the pancreas and removes secretions that can stimulate the pancreas to produce enzymes.*
2. NURSING DIAGNOSIS: Nutrition, Imbalanced: Less Than Body Requirements *related to nausea, vomiting, pain, and possible lack of pancreatic enzymes for digestion* (NANDA-I © 2012)	
Outcome: Adequate nutrition. ***Evaluation Parameters:*** No weight loss. Serum albumin normal. Fasting glucose normal. Hemoglobin and hematocrit normal. No reported nausea.	Weigh daily on the same scale at the same time. *Fluctuations in weight from day to day are an indicator of fluid balance, but changes over a week reflect nutritional status.* Assess laboratory results and report any abnormal values to the patient's health care provider. *The pancreas produces enzymes that aid in the digestion of protein, fat, and carbohydrates. Protein malnutrition is reflected in a low serum albumin. Transferrin is a protein that transports iron, so this level may be low. The H&H may be decreased in cases of malnutrition. Serum glucose may be elevated if the pancreatitis affects the endocrine function of the gland.* Monitor the frequency, color, consistency, and odor of stools. *Lack of lipase from the pancreas results in poor fat digestion and steatorrhea results. The presence of steatorrhea indicates severe pancreatitis with impaired pancreatic function.* Provide oral hygiene at least every 2 hours while the nasogastric tube is in place *to decrease discomfort and maintain the integrity of the oral and nasal mucosa.* Offer small, frequent meals, beginning with clear liquids once bowel sounds return and pain is relieved. *Smaller meals reduce the secretion of pancreatic enzymes.* Monitor parenteral or enteral nutrition if ordered. Alternative nutrition may be ordered if the patient is NPO for longer than 7 to 10 days.
3. NURSING DIAGNOSIS: Fluid Volume Deficit *related to vascular leak syndrome resulting from inflammation and fluid accumulation in the abdominal cavity.* Potential for Electrolyte Imbalance *related to nasogastric suction* (NANDA-I © 2012)	
Outcome: Adequate fluid volume and electrolyte balance. ***Evaluation Parameters:*** Normal blood pressure with no orthostatic changes. Normal sinus rhythm on cardiac monitor. Stable daily weight with moist mucous membranes. Pulmonary artery pressure within normal (15–30 mmHg systolic, 8–12 mmHg diastolic). Cardiac output and cardiac index within normal (CO 3.5–7.5 L/min, CI 2.4–4.0 L/min/m^2). Brisk capillary refill. Good peripheral pulses. Urine output $\geq$ 30 mL/hr. Alert and oriented.	Evaluate cardiac status: heart rate and rhythm at least every 4 hours; orthostatic blood pressure, pulmonary artery pressure usually every 4 hours as indicated; peripheral pulses; capillary refill; skin color. *These assessments help establish fluid volume. The body compensates for diminished volume by increasing the heart rate to maintain cardiac output. Capillaries constrict to force more fluid into the general circulation and the signs are weak peripheral pulses and pale skin color. A decreased cardiac output means a decrease in the renal perfusion, decreased urine output, and possibly early prerenal renal failure.* Monitor renal function by measuring urine output every hour and notifying the health care provider if the level is less than 30 mL/hr. *Daily body weight is an indicator of fluid status.* Monitor neurological function by assessing the level of consciousness and behavior. *Cerebral perfusion may be diminished if there is a fluid volume deficit and the cardiac output is low. Electrolytes, particularly sodium, can cause confusion when the levels are low.* *Monitor laboratory values for electrolyte status and renal function. Electrolytes are lost in nasogastric suction or vomiting. The BUN and creatinine will rise if renal function is compromised.*

Source: Adapted from Wilkinson, J. M., & Ahearn, N. R. (2009). *Prentice Hall nursing diagnosis handbook* (9th ed.). Upper Saddle River, NJ: Prentice Hall.

Pathophysiology

Most pancreatic cancer is ductal adenocarcinoma, which develops from the exocrine cells in the ducts. Rarely, cancer develops in the endocrine cells; these types of tumors are called **apudomas.** Ductal adenocarcinoma begins in the ducts, slowly invades the glandular tissue, and then extends into the surrounding tissue (Huether, 2010). Roughly 60% to 70% of these cancers arise in the head or neck of the pancreas, although they can occur anywhere in the pancreas (Hodgin, 2011). When the tumor arises in the head of the pancreas, it usually causes obstruction of the common bile duct early in the course of the disease with resultant jaundice. Survival is longer in these patients, probably because they became symptomatic, and therefore sought treatment, earlier than those with cancer in the body or tail of the pancreas. Because of the vascular structure of the area, cancer cells infiltrate the portal vein, mesenteric artery, vena cava, and aorta, with metastasis to the liver (Huether, 2010).

Clinical Manifestations

Most cases of pancreatic cancer are asymptomatic until the tumor invades surrounding tissue or obstructs the common bile duct. Jaundice may be the first sign. Patients may also experience weight loss, which is often attributed to other gastrointestinal issues. Other signs may include anorexia, indigestion, weakness, early satiety, diarrhea, steatorrhea, pain, and many other GI symptoms. New onset diabetes may be present in 10% to 20% of patients with pancreatic cancer (Hodgin, 2011).

Laboratory and Diagnostic Procedures

Diagnosis of pancreatic cancer is done by history and physical examination. When there is a suspicion of pancreatic cancer, ultrasonography of the abdomen, a spiral CT, or an MRI is done to detect the tumor. Positive emission tomography (PET scan), ERCP, and MRCP may also be utilized to diagnose pancreatic cancer. See the Laboratory and Diagnostic Tests box on page 1190. A laparotomy with biopsy or a CT or ultrasound guided needle biopsy is performed to establish a definitive diagnosis and determine the extent of the disease (Hodgin, 2011). Tumor staging is based on the TNM system of classification, which is outlined in Chapter 57.

Medical and Surgical Management

Treatment of pancreatic cancer is varied, ranging from surgical intervention to palliation. If the tumor is limited to the head of the pancreas and there is no lymph node involvement or metastasis, then radical **pancreaticoduodenal (Whipple) resection** is done. The Whipple procedure involves removal of the head of the pancreas, the duodenum, a distal portion of the stomach, and the lower half of the common bile duct. Unfortunately, most pancreatic cancer is too advanced when first diagnosed for the Whipple procedure to be effective. Radiation and chemotherapy may be used after surgery to enhance recovery efforts or for palliation in patients with unresectable cancer.

Patients with pancreatic cancer require nursing care that focuses on palliation, comfort, and support. Chapter 57 presents the care of patients with cancer, and Chapter 37 discusses the care of patients with gastrointestinal surgery.

Gerontological Considerations

Enzyme secretions decrease in older adults along with other age-related changes such as fibrosis and atrophy. This can mean the patient may experience some difficulty digesting fat. The liver shrinks but retains

RESEARCH OPPORTUNITIES Related to Patients with Liver, Gallbladder, or Pancreatic Disorders

Research	Clinical Impact
Physiological Research	
Vaccine for hepatitis C	Development of a vaccine would decrease the number of people with chronic hepatitis C and possible liver failure.
Drugs to treat hepatitis C genotype most common in the United States	Effective drug treatment can help decrease the spread of hepatitis C and improve morbidity and mortality.
Drugs to reverse hepatic encephalopathy	Medications or other treatments would decrease the complications of cirrhosis, thereby improving the quality of life and longevity of patients with cirrhosis.
Effective treatments for hepatorenal syndrome	Patient comfort is enhanced with less dependence on narcotics.
Drugs to prevent esophageal varices	Medications for varices would decrease the complications of cirrhosis, thereby improving the quality of life and longevity of patients with cirrhosis and reduce the risk for rupture and hemorrhage.
Herbal preparations to boost liver function in patients with a compromised liver	Discovery of herbal preparations may improve liver function and reduce long-term complications associated with a compromised liver.
The management of pain in patients with pancreatitis	Pain management increases patient comfort and may promote healing.
Use of acupuncture as an adjunct to pain management in pancreatitis	Pain management increases patient comfort and may promote healing. The use of alternatives will reduce dependence on narcotics.
Clinical trials for the treatment of pancreatic cancer	Discovery of treatment for pancreatic cancer will help lower mortality.
Emotional and Psychological Research	**Clinical Impact**
Living with the Uncertainty of Chronic Hepatitis C	
Music therapy to reduce anxiety before, during, and after painful procedures such as paracentesis, ERCP, and surgical intervention	Nurses can help patients cope with an uncertain future and increase patient well-being.
Quality of life after liver transplant	The goal is to improve psychological interventions to help improve the patient's coping.
	Understanding the issues after liver transplant can help nurses plan interventions for patients to maximize their recovery.

normal function. However, blood flow to the liver is decreased, resulting in slower metabolism and an increased risk for drug toxicities. The aged also have more difficulty adjusting to disorders that may directly or indirectly affect the liver, such as infection. Although there are no age-related changes in the gallbladder or biliary ducts, the older adult is at higher risk for gallstones because the bile more readily forms stones (Stamm, Wiersema-Bryant, & Ward, 2011). Age also increases the risk of both pancreatitis and pancreatic cancer.

Research

Research is necessary for improvement in the care of patients with liver, gallbladder, and pancreatic disorders. The goal of research is to identify areas in practice in which innovations can positively affect the patient's health and well-being and then to develop and test interventions that address the identified problems. The Research Opportunities Related to Patients With Liver, Gallbladder, or Pancreatic Disorders box presents a list of research opportunities related to these disorders.

Summary

Liver and biliary function is complex. Dysfunction within this system affects many other body systems. The nurse must have an understanding of the anatomy and physiology of the system, diagnostic and treatment procedures, and excellent assessment skills to care for patients with disorders of the hepatic and biliary system.

CLINICAL PREPARATION READ DOCUMENT APPLY

READ: **History of Present Illness** >> Laboratory Study Results >> Critical Thinking Questions

As the nurse on a medical–surgical floor in a community hospital, you receive report about Stephen Meakin, a 60-year-old construction worker who was admitted 2 days ago with a diagnosis of cirrhosis of the liver.

Medical–Surgical History

According to his ex-wife, Mr. Meakin's past medical history includes hepatitis A infection as a young man. He has no history of any other diseases. He does not take any prescription medications but uses Tylenol occasionally for headache. He has had a "beer belly" for at least 20 years, but his ex-wife has noticed that it has been getting larger during the last week.

Social History

Mr. Meakin is a 60-year-old construction worker. He is divorced, lives alone in an apartment, and drinks 6 to 10 beers each night after work and more on the weekends. He has smoked three packs of cigarettes a day for the last 30 years.

Assessment

Mr. Meakin is confused and restless in bed. His vital signs are temperature of 37°C; pulse of 120 beats per minute; respirations 26 and labored; blood pressure of 140/76. He is slightly jaundiced and diaphoretic. His lungs are clear to auscultation, and gynecomastia is noted on the chest exam. His heart sounds indicate a regular rhythm, tachycardia, and no murmurs or gallops.

Mr. Meakin's abdomen is large and distended with hypoactive bowel sounds. It is tender to palpation with a positive fluid wave. His spleen is enlarged. His abdominal girth is 56 inches, and his stool tests positive for blood. He is confused and oriented to person only. He has asterixis and hyperactive reflexes.

READ: History of Present Illnesses >> **Physical Exam** >> Admitting Medical Records >> Laboratory Study Results

Admitting Medical Orders

Service: medicine
Diagnosis: cirrhosis of the liver
Allergies: none known
Vital signs q4h including oxygen saturation
Neurological checks q4h
Abdominal girth q shift
I&O q shift
Daily weight
Activity: bed rest
DVT prophylaxis: sequential compression device to lower extremities
Incentive spirometer: q1h while awake
Diet: sodium restriction: 2 g/day; fluid restriction: 1,500 mL/day; high-calorie, low-protein, 20 g/day diet
Call house officer: temp $>$ 38.5°C, HR $>$110 or $<$ 60, RR $>$30 or $<$ 12, BP sys $>$160 or $<$ 90, O_2 sat $<$ 92%, urine output $<$ 120 mL in 4 hours, change in neurological or abdominal exam, any Hct result that is 5 less than the baseline ED Hct
IV: D5NS IV at 10 mL/hr

Scheduled Medications

Multivitamin 1 po daily
Lactulose 30 mL po qid $\times$ 3 days then bid
Spironolactone (Aldactone) 100 mg po daily
Lasix 40 mg po daily
Oxazepam (Serax) 10 mg po tid

Ordered Laboratory Studies

Hgb and Hct
Electrolyte panel
Liver function tests
Serum ammonia qam
Chart and test stool for occult blood

READ: History of Present Illnesses >> **Laboratory Study Results** >> Critical Thinking Questions

Test	Admission	Day 1	Day 2
Hemoglobin (Hgb)	12.5 g/dL	12.0 g/dL	11.8 g/dL
Hematocrit (Hct)	38%	36%	34%
• Bilirubin—total	1.5 mg/dL	1.5 mg/dL	1.5 mg/dL
• Direct	0.6 mg/dL	0.6 mg/dL	0.6 mg/dL
Indirect	0.9 mg/dL	0.9 mg/dL	0.9 mg/dL
AST	400 unit/L	386 unit/L	352 unit/L
ALT	150 unit/L	149 unit/L	147 unit/L

Test	Admission	Day 1	Day 2
Alkaline phosphatase	150 unit/L	144 unit/L	144 unit/L
Electrolytes:			
• Sodium	138 mEq/L	140 mEq/L	141 mEq/L
• Potassium	3.5 mEq/L	3.4 mEq/L	3.5 mEq/L
• Calcium	8.6 mg/dL	8.8 mg/dL	8.8 mg/dL
Serum ammonia	50 μ/dL	58 μ/dL	46 μ/dL
Serum albumin	3.0 g/dL	3.2 g/dL	3.0 g/dL

Pearson Nursing Student Resources

Log on to **nursing.pearsonhighered.com** *to download forms*

DOCUMENT:

- >> Summary of Hospitalization
- >> Pathophysiology Form
- >> Laboratory Values
- >> Laboratory Results Explanation

APPLY:

- >> List of Potential Nursing Diagnoses
- >> Concept Map
- >> Critical Thinking Questions and Concept Map

APPLY: History of Present Illnesses >> Laboratory Study Results >> **Critical Thinking Questions**

1. What signs and symptoms of hepatic encephalopathy is Mr. Meakin manifesting?
2. Describe the pathophysiology of cirrhosis and how it relates to each of his clinical manifestations.
3. Why is Mr. Meakin on a low-protein diet?
4. Why is lactulose being given to Mr. Meakin?

Answers to Critical Thinking Questions can be found in Appendix D in the Osborn Student Resources at nursing.pearsonhighered.com.

NCLEX® PRACTICE

1. A patient is being evaluated for possible hepatitis C infection. Which question will best assist the nurse in identifying if a common method of exposure has occurred?

1. "Have you traveled outside the country recently?"
2. "Do you eat a lot of uncooked shellfish?"
3. "Have you ever had a tattoo?"
4. "Do you share eating utensils with anyone infected with hepatitis?"

2. Which of the following symptoms does the nurse expect to assess in the patient during the prodromal phase of hepatitis? (select all that apply)

1. Hypothermia
2. Increased appetite
3. Dark-colored urine
4. Constant epigastric pain
5. Muscle pain

3. A patient with cirrhosis of the liver has an albumin level of 2.5 gm/dL. The nurse should plan care for this patient to address the patient's risk for developing:

1. peripheral edema.
2. prolonged blood coagulation.
3. jaundice of the skin.
4. vitamin A malabsorption.

4. A patient with cirrhosis develops hepatic encephalopathy and is extremely confused and agitated. The nurse places priority on administering which ordered medication? (select all that apply)

1. Lactulose, Chronulac
2. Oxazepam, Serax
3. Propanolzole Protonix
4. Phytonadione, Vitamin K
5. Octreotide, Sandostatin

5. A patient diagnosed with liver cancer 3 months ago has elevated alpha-fetoprotein (AFP) levels. Which of the following interventions should the nurse incorporate into the plan of care?
   1. Provide supportive and comfort measures to the patient and family.
   2. Explain how the transhepatic portosystemic shunt (TIPS) will relieve symptoms.
   3. Prepare the patient and family for the likelihood of a liver transplant.
   4. Restrict dietary proteins and foods high in sodium.

6. Which of the following factors would the nurse identify as potentially leading to the development of stones in a patient diagnosed with cholelithiasis?
   1. The patient consumes a high-fiber diet.
   2. The patient recently was treated with aminoglycosides for a urinary tract infection.
   3. The patient has had rapid weight loss secondary to crash dieting.
   4. The patient is of northern European descent.

Answers to NCLEX Practice questions can be found in Appendix D in the Osborn Student Resources at nursing.pearsonhighered.com. Practice additional NCLEX questions online at the Student Resources site.

Pearson Nursing Student Resources Find additional review materials at: **nursing.pearsonhighered.com**

REFERENCES

Adams, M. P., & Koch, R. W. (2010). *Pharmacology: Connections to nursing practice.* Upper Saddle River, NJ: Pearson.

Afdhal, N. H. (2009). *Epidemiology of and risk factors for gallstones.* Retrieved from http://www.uptodate.com/contents/epidemiology-of-and-risk-factors-for-gallstones

American Cancer Society. (2012a). Liver Cancer. Retrieved from http://www.cancer.org/cancer/livercancer/detailedguide/liver-cancer-what-is-key-statistics

American Cancer Society (2010). *Cancer facts & figures 2010.* Retrieved from: http://www.cancer.org/acs/groups/content/@epidemiologysurveilance/documents/document/acspc-026238.pdf

American Cancer Society. (2012b). Pancreatic Cancer. Retrieved from http://www.cancer.org/cancer/pancreaticcancer/detailedguide/pancreatic-cancer-what-is-key-statistics

Andris, A. (2010). Pancreatitis: Understanding the disease and implications for care. *AACN Advanced Critical Care, 21*(2), 195–204. doi:10.1097/NCI.0b013e3181d94feb

Centers for Disease Control and Prevention (CDC). (2010). Viral hepatitis. Retrieved from http://www.cdc.gov/hepatitis/

Chiang, W. K., Lee, F. M., & Santen, S. (2010). Cholelithiasis. Retrieved from http://emedicine.medscape.com/article/774352-overview

Daniels, D., Grytdal, S., & Wasley, A. (2009). Surveillance for acute viral hepatitis—United States, 2007. *Morbidity and Mortality Weekly Report, 58*(S S03), 1–27. Retrieved from http://www.cdc.gov/mmwr/preview/mmwrhtml/ss5803a1.htm

Dugdale, D. C. (2010). Drug-induced hepatitis. Retrieved from http://www.nlm.nih.gov/medlineplus/ency/article/000226.htm

Friedman, L. S. (2010). Liver, biliary tract & pancreas. In S. J. McPhee & M. A. Papadakis (Eds.), *Current medical diagnosis and treatment* (49th ed.). Retrieved from http://online.statref.com/document.aspx?fxid=27&docid=314

Ghany, M. G., Strader, D. B., Thomas, D. L., & Seeff, L. B. (2009). Diagnosis, management, and treatment of hepatitis C: An update. *Hepatology, 49*(4), 1335–1374. doi:10.1002/hep.22759.

Ghosh, N., Ghosh, R., Mandal, V., & Mandal, S. C. (2011). Recent advances in herbal medicine for treatment of liver diseases. *Pharmaceutical Biology, 49*(9), 970–988. Epub 2011 May 19.

Hodgin, M. B. (2011). Pancreatic cancer. In C. H. Yarbro, D. Wujcik, & B. H. Gobel (Eds.), *Cancer nursing: Principles and practice* (7th ed.). (pp. 1580–1608). Boston: Jones and Bartlett Publishers.

Holcomb, S. S. (2008). Caring for a patient with chronic hepatitic C. *Nursing, 38*(12), 32–37. doi:10.1097/01.NURSE.0000342029.39505.aa

Huether, S. E. (2010). Alterations of digestive function. In K. L. McCance, S. E. Huether, V. L. Brashers, & N. S. Rote (Eds.), *Pathophysiology: The biologic basis for disease in adults and children* (6th ed., pp. 1452–1515). St. Louis: Mosby.

IOM (Institute of Medicine). (2010). *The future of nursing: Leading change, advancing health.* Washington, DC: The Academic Press.

Kee, J. L. (2010). *Laboratory and diagnostic tests with nursing implications* (8th ed.). Upper Saddle River, NJ: Prentice Hall.

Kelso, L. A. (2008). Cirrhosis: Caring for patients with end-stage liver failure. *The Nurse Practitioner, 33*(7), 24–30. doi:10.1097/01.NPR.0000325976.85753.dd

Kumar, V., Abbas, A. K., Fausto, N., & Mitchell, R. N. (2007). *Robbins basic pathology* (8th ed.). Philadelphia: Saunders.

Lehne, R. A. (2010). *Pharmacology for nursing care* (7th ed.). St. Louis: Mosby.

McQuaid, K. R. (2010). Gastrointestinal disorders. In S. J. McPhee & M. A. Papadakis (Eds.), *Current medical diagnosis and treatment* (49th ed.). Retrieved from http://online.statref.com/document.aspx?fxid=27&docid=298

Mukherjee, S., & Dhawan, V. K. (2010). Hepatitis C. Retrieved from http://emedicine.medscape.com/article/177792-overview

Poole, S. (2009). Update on the treatment and management of patients with hepatitis. *Journal of Infusion Nursing, 32*(5), 269–275. doi:10.1097/NAN.0b013e3181b42d30

Ranson, J. H., Rifkind, K. M., Roses, D. F., Fink, S. D., Eng, K., & Spencer, F. C. (1974) Prognostic signs and the role of operative management in acute pancreatitis. *Surgical Gynecology and Obstetrics, 139*(1):69–81.

Rhee, C., & Broadbent, A. M. (2007). Palliation and liver failure: Palliative medications dosages guidelines. *Journal of Palliative Medicine, 10*(3), 677–687.

Rolfes, S. R., Pinna, K., & Whitney, E. (2012). *Understanding normal and clinical nutrition* (9th ed.). Belmont, CA: Wadsworth Cengage Learning.

Ross, S. M. (2008). Milk thistle (*Silybum marianum*): An ancient botanical medicine for modern times. *Holistic Nursing Practice, 22*(5), 299–300. doi:10.1097/01.HNP.0000334924.77174.6d

Ryan, L. (2007). Portal hypertension and cirrhosis. In M. A. Chisholm-Burns, B. G. Wells, T. L. Schwinghammer, P. M. Malone, J. M. Kolesar, J. C. Rotschafer, & J. T. Dipiro (Eds.), *Pharmacotherapy principles & practice* (pp. 323–336). New York: McGraw-Hill.

Stamm, L. A., Wiersema-Bryant, L. A., & Ward, C. (2011). Gastrointestinal function. In S. E. Meiner (Ed.), *Gerontologic nursing* (4th ed, pp. 482–516). St. Louis: Mosby.

Thomas, D. J. (2011). Abdominal problems. In L. M. Dunphy, J. E. Winland-Brown, B. O. Porter, & D. J. Thomas (Eds.), *Primary care: The art and science of advanced practice nursing* (2nd ed., pp. 492–581). Philadelphia: F. A. Davis.

Thomson, A. B. R. (2011). Acalculous cholecystopathy. Retrieved from http://emedicine.medscape.com/article/172013-overview

Wilkinson, J. M., & Ahearn, N. R. (2009). *Prentice Hall nursing diagnosis handbook* (9th ed.). Upper Saddle River, NJ: Prentice Hall.

Wilson, B. A., Shannon, M. T., & Shields, K. M. (2011). *Pearson nurse's drug guide 2011.* New York: Pearson.

Wolf, D. C. (2010). Cirrhosis. Retrieved from http://emedicine.medscape.com/article/185856-overview

Caring for the Patient with Renal and Urinary Disorders

CHAPTER 39

Pamela Stetina
Cheryl Wraa

Outcome-Based Learning Objectives

After studying this chapter, the learner will be able to:

1. Describe the function of the kidney in relation to regulating fluid, electrolyte, and acid–base balance.
2. Analyze the various diagnostic tests used to determine kidney function and related diseases.
3. Compare and contrast the major diseases of the kidney.
4. Generate a nursing plan of care for patients with chronic renal failure.
5. Delineate complications seen in kidney, bladder, and urinary tract disorders.
6. Compare and contrast the underlying principles of hemodialysis and peritoneal dialysis.

KEY TERMS

anasarca p.1221
anuria p.1221
azotemia p.1208
end-stage renal disease (ESRD) p.1226
erythropoietin p.1199
hematuria p.1208
Kussmaul's respirations p.1221
oliguria p.1208
staghorn calculus p.1200

THE KIDNEYS PLAY AN IMPORTANT ROLE in maintaining constancy of the body's internal environment through multiple functions, including the following:

- Maintaining electrolyte balance, which is a major factor for normal nerve and muscle physiology.
- Helping to regulate the acid–base balance through the reabsorption and elimination or conservation of sodium, potassium, hydrogen, chloride, and bicarbonate ions.
- Producing **erythropoietin,** a hormone that stimulates the production of red blood cells in the bone marrow.
- Secreting *renin,* which converts angiotensinogen to angiotensin, which stimulates the release of aldosterone by the adrenal cortex. Aldosterone plays a part in the regulation of sodium and water reabsorption to help elevate blood pressure.
- Activating vitamin D and regulating calcium and phosphate conservation and elimination, which contribute to the metabolic functions of the skeletal system.
- Regulating the osmolality of the extracellular fluid through action of the antidiuretic hormone (ADH).
- Eliminating metabolic wastes: urea, uric acid, creatinine, and drugs and their metabolites.

Throughout the day, the two kidneys process approximately 180 liters of blood and combine the waste products to produce approximately 1 to 2 liters of urine. To put it another way, the kidneys filter a person's entire blood volume 60 to 70 times a day (Urden, Stacy, & Lough, 2010).

Physiology of the Renal System

To better understand the disease processes that affect the renal system, it is important to be familiar with the system's physiology. The *nephron* is the functional unit of the kidney, and each kidney contains approximately 1 million nephrons (Urden et al., 2010). Each nephron consists of a *glomerulus,* a compact tuft of capillaries where blood is filtered (Figure 39–1◆, p. 1200) (Porth & Matfin, 2009). The glomerulus is encased in a thin double-walled capsule called *Bowman's capsule.* The capillary walls of the glomerulus are very thin, and the blood pressure within them is higher than the pressure in Bowman's capsule; therefore, fluid from the plasma is filtered into the capsule. This fluid is called *filtrate.* In the healthy nephron, neither red blood cells nor protein should pass through the filter. Nutrients and water are then reabsorbed by the proximal convoluted tubule and taken back into the capillaries that surround the tubules. Sodium, chloride, and potassium are also reabsorbed, along with bicarbonate. The *loop of Henle* continues the reabsorption of sodium, chloride, and potassium. Water is also reabsorbed in the distal convoluted tubule (Porth & Matfin, 2009; Urden et al., 2010). The waste products of protein metabolism (urea and creatinine) along with substances that are present in excess in body fluids, such as hydrogen ions, are secreted into the tubules to be excreted. Finally, urine empties into the renal pelvis, moves down the ureters, is stored in the bladder, and then leaves the body through the urethra.

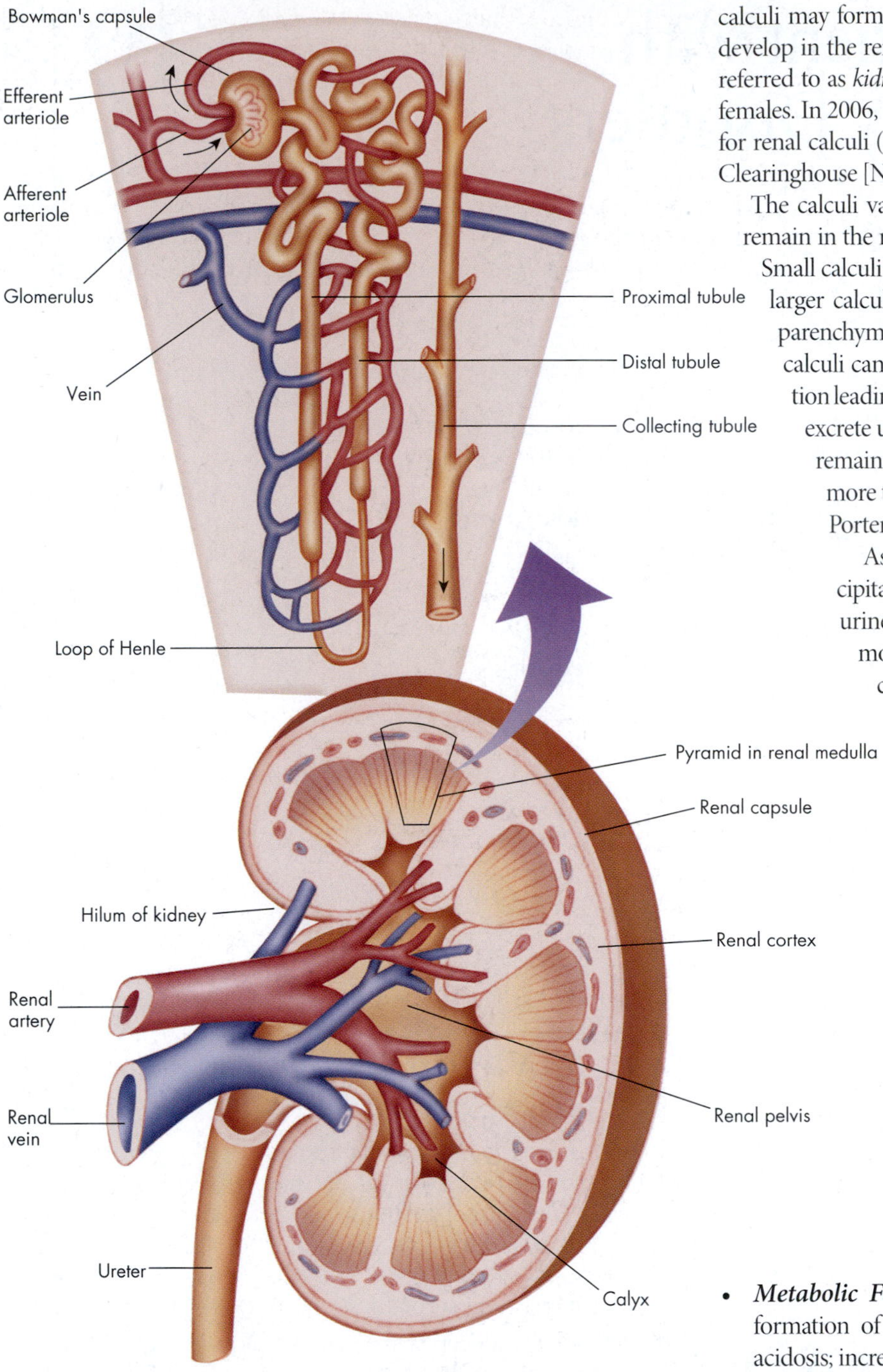

FIGURE 39–1 ◆ The kidney and nephron.

Disorders of the Bladder and Urinary Tract

The bladder stores urine and controls its elimination. Disorders that affect urine storage and elimination can result in incontinence or obstruction of urinary flow, which ultimately will affect renal function.

Nephrolithiasis

Etiology and Epidemiology

Renal and ureteral calculi are formed when substances supersaturate the urine and form a precipitate that aggregates and grows in size. The calculi may form anywhere in the urinary tract but most commonly develop in the renal pelvis or calyces of the kidneys and are generally referred to as *kidney stones*. They are more prevalent in males than in females. In 2006, 166,000 people in the United States were hospitalized for renal calculi (National Kidney and Urologic Diseases Information Clearinghouse [NKUDIC], 2010).

The calculi vary in size and may be single or multiple. They can remain in the renal pelvis or pass through the ureter to the bladder. Small calculi are often passed spontaneously in the urine, whereas larger calculi, when entering the ureter, may damage the renal parenchyma or become lodged and cause pressure necrosis. If the calculi cannot pass through the ureter, they will cause obstruction leading to hydronephrosis, as the kidney becomes unable to excrete urine. A **staghorn calculus** is a calculus or stone that remains in the renal pelvis and becomes so large that it fills more than one calyx, blocking the flow of urine (Thomas & Porter, 2007).

As was stated earlier, the calculi are formed from precipitation of substances that are normally dissolved in the urine. Eighty percent of patients form calcium stones, most commonly calcium oxalate and less commonly calcium phosphate (Curhan, Aronson, & Preminger, 2008). Other types include magnesium ammonium phosphate (struvite) and, occasionally, uric acid or cystine. The exact cause is unknown, but predisposing factors include the following:

- ***Infection:*** The pH changes that occur with infection provide a favorable medium for formation of calculi, especially magnesium ammonium phosphate (struvite). Infected tissue also provides a site for the development of calculi. Bacteria may serve as the nucleus in calculus formation; this commonly occurs in magnesium ammonium phosphate or staghorn calculi (*Professional Guide to Diseases*, 2009).
- ***Dehydration:*** The decrease in urine production causes calculus-forming substances to become concentrated and therefore able to form calculi more easily (*Professional Guide to Diseases*, 2009).
- ***Metabolic Factors:*** Conditions that predispose a person to the formation of calculi include hyperparathyroidism; renal tubular acidosis; increased excretion of oxalates, uric acid, and calcium; and an excess of vitamin D (Hall, 2009).
- ***Obstruction:*** Any condition that results in urinary stasis can increase the risk for calculi to form. Stasis also promotes infection, which increases the risk of stone formation.
- ***Heredity:*** There are several hereditary diseases by which the patient may develop renal calculi. Cystinuria and hyperoxaluria are two inherited metabolic disorders in which calculi tend to develop (Hall, 2009). Hypercalciuria is an inherited disease that causes calcium from food to be absorbed in excess and lost into the urine; this high level of calcium in the urine causes calcium oxalate or calcium phosphate crystals and the formation of calculi.

Clinical Manifestations

Pain is the primary symptom of renal calculi and is usually the result of obstruction. As the calculi attempt to pass, they may occlude the opening to the ureter, increasing the number and force of peristaltic contractions. Typically, the pain is severe and colicky and travels from the costovertebral angle to the flank to the perineal area and inner thigh (Thomas & Porter, 2007). If the calculi remain in the renal pelvis and calyces, the pain will usually be more constant and dull in nature. Because the pain is severe, nausea and vomiting usually occur. The patient may also have hematuria from damage caused by the calculi. Patients may also exhibit symptoms of urinary tract infection such as dysuria and urinary frequency.

Laboratory and Diagnostic Procedures

Tests that are helpful in the diagnosis of calculi are outlined in the Diagnostic Tests box.

Medical Management

Treatment of pain will be a priority for patients with renal calculi regardless of the size of the stone (Huether & Forshee, 2010; Thomas & Porter, 2007). Most renal calculi smaller than 4 millimeters in diameter can pass without invasive intervention. Treatment focuses on promoting the passage through vigorous hydration and pain control. Diuretics may be given to prevent urinary stasis and continuing calculus formation but should be used cautiously, as they may increase calcium excretion (National Institute of Diabetes and Digestive and Kidney Diseases [NIDDK], 2007a). The Pharmacology box on page 1206 presents medications used to treat bladder and urinary tract disorders.

If calculi are too large to pass, an endoscopic procedure, lithotripsy, or surgical intervention may be required. A cystoscope may be inserted through the urethra to retrieve calculi from the ureter, or a ureteroscope may be inserted through the ureter to remove calculi from the kidney. If the attempt to capture the stone is unsuccessful, electrohydraulic lithotripsy or laser lithotripsy may be used to break the stone into smaller particles that can pass naturally. Extracorporeal shock-wave lithotripsy is the use of acoustic shock waves that travel through soft tissues to shatter the calculi into fragments, which can then pass normally. When the procedure is performed with the patient immersed in a tank of water, it is called hydrolithotripsy. Surgical procedures involve an incision in the bladder, ureter, or kidney to directly remove the stone (Thomas & Porter, 2007).

Nursing Management

It is important to try to determine the composition of the calculi to prevent further formation. In managing the patient with renal or ureteral calculi, the nurse should have the patient strain all urine through a urine strainer; all solid material thus obtained is then sent to the lab for analysis. The nurse should encourage intake of fluids to facilitate passage and encourage the patient to walk to encourage movement of the stone. Renal calculi are very painful, and frequent monitoring of the pain level and administration of analgesics will assist with their passage. In the past, patients who tended to form calcium calculi were told to avoid foods high in calcium. However, recent studies have shown that foods high in calcium may help prevent calcium calculi, though taking calcium in pill form may increase the risk of developing calculi (NIDDK, 2007a).

DIAGNOSTIC TESTS for Renal Calculi

Test with Description, Rationale, and Normal Values	Expected Abnormality
Kidneys/Ureters/Bladder (KUB) Radiograph *Done to assess structure, size, and shape of tissues. Done before tests utilizing contrast, such as IVP.*	Will show if renal calculi are present.
Excretory Urography, Abdominal CT Scan Renal MRI scan *Done to detect any obstruction, abnormalities, tumors, and infection. Need to assess for allergies to CT contrast, or presence of metal items for MRI.* Normal results for all of these would be a negative result.	Any of these imaging tests will reveal the obstruction and help determine the size and location of the calculi.
Renal Ultrasonography *Used to identify the size of the kidneys and tissue abnormalities.*	May detect obstructive changes such as hydronephrosis.
Calculus Analysis *Done to determine the type of stone.*	Reveals the mineral content and assists in diagnosing the cause of calculi.
Urinalysis Normal: Specific gravity: 1.005–1.030 pH: 4.5–8.0 Blood: negative RBC: 1–2 Casts: occasional hyaline *Used to diagnose urinary system and kidney disease.*	Increased specific gravity and acid or alkaline pH. Hematuria. Crystals: calcium, urate, or cystine.
Blood Uric Acid Levels Normal: Male: 3.5–8.0 mg/dL Female: 2.8–6.8 mg/dL *Uric acid reflects purine metabolism.*	May be increased if uric acid is associated with calculi formation.

Patients may also need to avoid antacids that have a calcium base (NIDDK, 2007a).

Assessment

Assessment for the patient with renal or ureteral calculi includes the following:

- Any past history or family history of calculi, gout, or other renal problems
- Blood in the urine
- Painful, urgent, and frequent urination
- Decreasing urine output
- Severe pain in the back or pelvis, which can be dull, constant pain or intermittent, excruciating pain radiating anteriorly down to the vulva in women or the testes in men.

Nursing Diagnoses

Major nursing diagnoses for the patient with calculi include the following:

- *Pain, Acute* related to passing of calculi.
- *Urinary Elimination, Impaired* related to blockage of the ureter by the calculi.
- *Knowledge, Deficient* related to the disease process.

NANDA-I © 2012

Planning

Overall goals of treatment for calculi include pain control, passage and identification of the calculi, and understanding of potential causes of calculus formation and the possible need for dietary restrictions and increased fluid intake.

Outcomes and Evaluation Parameters

Outcomes and evaluation parameters for the patient with calculi include the following:

- Pain is decreased to a tolerable level as evidenced by the patient rating the pain as less than 3 on a 0 to 10 scale.
- The patient will not exhibit impaired urinary elimination as evidenced by voiding more than 2 liters of clear amber urine in 24 hours (NIDDK, 2007a).
- The patient will understand the disease process and plan of care as evidenced by her ability to articulate how calculi are formed and the need for dietary restrictions.

Interventions and Rationales

Nursing interventions and rationales for the patient with calculi include the following:

- The nurse will administer analgesics and antispasmodics as ordered. *Narcotic analgesia is warranted because of the severity of the pain. Antispasmodics relax tense muscles and reduce reflex spasms.*
- The nurse will monitor the volume and character of each void. The nurse will strain all urine for calculi and encourage intake of fluid (2 to 3 liters of fluid daily (NIDDK, 2007a). *Adequate urine output indicates proper kidney function. Increased fluid intake is necessary to flush the calculi through the kidney and ureters. The characteristics of the urine can indicate the presence of infection (odorous, cloudy) and hemorrhage.*
- The nurse will provide information to the patient and family about dietary limitations for specific calculi, the need for regular activity, adequate fluid intake, and signs and symptoms of recurrence, such as pain and hematuria. *The patient needs an understanding of preventive strategies in order to comply with the regimen.*

Evaluation

With successful treatment of calculi, the patient will have a tolerable level of pain as evidenced by a low pain rating on a 0 to 10 scale. The patient will void more than 2 liters of urine each day. The urine will be clear and without foul odor. The patient will be able to articulate an understanding of preventative measures and will agree to comply.

Topics that should be addressed with patients who have renal calculi and/or their families before discharge are presented in the Patient Teaching & Discharge Priorities box.

Cystitis and Urethritis

Epidemiology and Etiology

Acute cystitis accounts for more than ten million medical visits annually and has been reported to be the most common bacterial infection (Huether & Forshee, 2010). Cystitis is an inflammation of the urinary bladder and is more common in women than in men because the urethra is shorter in women and closer to the anus. The most common cause is the introduction of *Escherichia coli* from fecal material into the urethra. Other bacteria may include *Klebsiella*, *Pseudomonas*, and *Proteus* (Huether & Forshee, 2010). The bacteria then travel up to the bladder. Cystitis may also develop following sexual intercourse when

PATIENT TEACHING & DISCHARGE PRIORITIES for Renal Calculi

Need	Teaching
Prevention of further stones	Encourage patient intake of fluids to maintain a urine output of 2 to 3 liters a day. The patient's urine should be diluted and appear colorless.
Acidify urine	If the patient's urine is consistently alkaline, calcium phosphate or magnesium ammonium phosphate calculi may develop. Encourage the patient to drink fruit juices, especially cranberry juice.
Dietary restrictions with increased uric acid or increased oxalates	Uric acid calculi may develop with excessive ingestion of purine rich foods. Calcium oxalate stones may develop with diets high in oxalates. Instruct the patient/family who have or are at risk for uric acid stones to avoid alcohol and purine-rich foods such as anchovies, sardines, herring, mussels, liver, goose, kidneys, sweetbreads, yeast, and lentils. Patients prone to calcium oxalate calculi should limit their intake of beets, chocolate, nuts, rhubarb, spinach, strawberries, tea, and wheat bran.

organisms around the vaginal opening enter the urethra. Fungi and *Candida* may also cause cystitis (Thomas & Porter, 2007).

Urethritis is an inflammation of the urethra. As with cystitis, the most common causative microorganism is *Escherichia coli*. The term *urethritis* is more commonly used in reference to inflammation caused by sexually transmitted infections. Specific etiologies are further divided into gonococcal and nongonococcal causes (such as *Chlamydia*) (Terris & Sajadi, 2009). Chapter 43 includes a discussion of sexually transmitted diseases.

Clinical Manifestations

The signs and symptoms of cystitis include increased urinary frequency with a sense of urgency, burning with urination, and at times hematuria. Patients may also complain of suprapubic or low back pain and foul smelling urine.

Laboratory and Diagnostic Procedures

Urinalysis reveals bacteria, pus, and casts in the urine. Urine cultures will grow the specific type of bacteria that are the cause.

Nursing Management

Nursing management for the patient with cystitis and urethritis includes treatment of the source and education regarding ways to prevent recurrent infections. The nursing interventions and rationales include the following:

- The nurse should encourage the patient to increase fluids. Fluids assist in flushing bacteria out of the urethra.
- Treatment usually consists of an appropriate antibiotic. The patient should be instructed to take the entire prescription.
- Treatment may also include phenazopyridine, which produces an analgesic effect on the urinary mucosa, if urination is very painful (Wilson, Shannon, & Shields, 2011). The nurse should inform the patient that the phenazopyridine will turn urine a bright-orange color that may stain clothing.
- The nurse should discuss with the female patient the importance of cleansing the genital area from front to back to avoid contamination by fecal material.
- The nurse should encourage the female patient to void before and as soon as possible after having sexual intercourse. This will flush contaminates that may have entered the urethra.
- Women should also be encouraged to wear cotton underwear and to avoid tub baths (Thomas & Porter, 2007).
- The nurse should encourage male patients to have protected sex.

The Pharmacology box on page 1206 lists medications used to treat bladder and urinary tract disorders.

The Complementary & Alternative Therapies box discusses therapies for treating urinary tract infections.

Neurogenic Bladder

Epidemiology and Etiology

In the United States, incontinence affects 8.5% of women and 1.6% of men between the ages of 15 and 64. As the renal system creates urine, it is stored in the bladder to be released. For the system to function properly, muscles and nerves work together to hold urine in the bladder and then release it when desired. When the bladder becomes full, nerves carry messages to the brain to let it know. The nerves then carry messages from the brain to tell the muscles either to tighten (to block the release of urine) or to release (to allow the urine to flow out). Problems that affect the nerves' ability to relay these messages may cause difficulty with bladder control. This type of nerve dysfunction is known as neurogenic bladder. The incidence of neurogenic bladder varies depending on the cause (MDGuidelines, 2011). The most common causes of damage to nerves and nerve pathways are as follows:

- Diabetes: autonomic neuropathy
- Cerebral disorders: stroke, brain tumor, cerebral palsy
- Vaginal childbirth
- Infections of the brain or spinal cord
- Traumatic injury to the brain or spinal cord
- Multiple sclerosis, Parkinson's disease
- Heavy metal poisoning (National Institute of Diabetes and Digestive and Kidney Diseases [NIDDK], 2008; Pellatt, 2008).

COMPLEMENTARY & ALTERNATIVE THERAPIES Treating Urinary Tract Infections *Nancy Yilk*

URINARY TRACT INFECTION (UTI) affects predominantly women, infants, and older adults. In an effort to limit the repeated use of antibiotics in chronic reoccurring episodes of UTIs, compromised patients and their health care providers have reached out to supportive preventive care treatments.

Empirically, cranberries and especially cranberry juice have been used for decades as both a prevention and a treatment for UTIs. It was believed that the cranberries changed the alkaline–acid balance of the urinary tract. However, research has uncovered that the beneficial effects instead come from the anti-adherence benefits that enable uroepithelial cells to resist bacterial overgrowth. Cranberries contain phytochemicals of anthocyanidins, flavonols, flavan-3-ols, proanthocyanidins, and phenolic acid derivatives. The presence of these phytochemicals appears to be responsible for the health benefits of cranberries in the management of infections.

A stable and consistent delivery of a high concentration of these proanthocyanidins is crucial to success for the patient with chronic noncomplicated UTIs. Therefore, the use of supplementation is often easier and preferred to drinking high concentrations of juice. In a study comparing two commercial extracts that contain proanthocyanidins (PACs) at 4% and 20% for antimicrobial, antiproliferative, antiradical, and protective properties against oxidative stress on cell lines, both extracts showed antimicrobial activity, and both extracts showed a dose-dependent free-radical scavenging capacity. A protective effect on the cell damage was also revealed by reduction of intracellular active oxygen species release (Menghini et al., 2011).

For patients who do not respond to cranberries, the use of supplementation of D-mannose, a simple sugar, has shown to be beneficial in similar anti-adherence of *E. coli*. D-mannose is apparently the primary bladder cell receptor site for uropathogenic *E. coli*. In a study of urinary tract epithelial cells collected from voided urine from healthy women, a 2.5% concentration of D-mannose, D-mannitol, or alpha-methyl-D-mannoside completely inhibited *E. coli* adherence. The same concentration of D-lyxose, D-arabinose, D-fructose, and D-glyceraldehyde only partially inhibited adherence. Also, only partial inhibition was achieved by lower concentrations (0.1% to 1.0%) of mannose, mannitol, and mannoside, demonstrating D-mannose's beneficial benefits in UTIs (Head, 2008).

Probiotics have shown success in contributing to the resolution of UTIs. Refer to Chapter 37 for a discussion of strain-specific probiotics that have shown success in promoting urogenital health.

Bladder Control Problems

There are several different kinds of bladder control problems:

- ***Urinary Retention:*** When the body is unable to empty the bladder properly, this may be related to damaged nerves and pathways, infection, benign prostatic hyperplasia (BPH), kidney stones, surgical procedures, or strictures (National Institute of Diabetes and Digestive and Kidney Diseases (NIDDK), 2007b). The bladder then becomes too full, and urine may back up, resulting in hydronephrosis, stagnant urine leading to infection, and overflow incontinence.
- ***Poor Control of Sphincter Muscles:*** There are sphincter muscles that surround the urethra, keeping it closed to hold urine in the bladder. If the nerves or pathways to the sphincter muscles are damaged, the muscles will either become loose, allowing leakage, or remain tight, preventing the release of urine (NIDDK, 2008).
- ***Overactive Bladder:*** Involuntary contraction of the bladder muscles caused by damaged nerves and pathways may send inappropriate signals (Huether & Forshee, 2010; Porth & Matfin, 2009). Symptoms of an overactive bladder include urinary frequency, urinary urgency, and urge incontinence, the leaking of urine immediately following urgency (NIDDK, 2008).
- ***Incontinence:*** Incontinence is an involuntary loss of urine. There are several types, including the aforementioned overflow incontinence and urge incontinence. Other key types include (1) stress incontinence, which is the loss of urine with increased intraabdominal pressure, such as coughing, sneezing, or laughing, and (2) functional, which relates to cognitive or mobility impairment (Huether & Forshee, 2010).

Diagnostic Procedures

If the history and physical examination lead the patient's health care provider to suspect nerve damage, the tests outlined for neurogenic bladder in the Diagnostic Tests box are helpful in supporting the diagnosis.

Medical Management

The management of bladder control dysfunction depends on the type of dysfunction.

Urinary Retention

Urinary retention can occur when the bladder wall muscle is unable to contract or the sphincter muscle is unable to relax. The general treatment is to relieve the underlying cause or treat through intermittent catheterization. The amount of urine in the bladder can be measured with a bladder scanner or catheterization; however, catheterization may increase the risk for infection. Patients and/or their family members can be taught to perform intermittent catheterization at regular intervals to empty the bladder. If patients are unable to catheterize themselves and there is no other family member or caregiver to assist them, they may need to have an indwelling catheter that can be changed less often. There are several risks associated with indwelling catheters, including infection.

When the nerve signals sent to the sphincter muscles that squeeze the urethra shut and the bladder are not coordinated, the bladder and urethral sphincter may contract at the same time, making it difficult to pass urine easily. In these situations, medications may be used to reduce muscle spasms and help relax the sphincter. Baclofen (Lioresal) is used to prevent muscle spasms or cramping in patients with multiple sclerosis and spinal injuries. Bethanechol chloride (Urecholine) helps contract the detrusor muscle to aid with urination (Wilson et al., 2011). Alpha-adrenergic blockers such as terazosin (Hytrin) and doxazosin (Cardura) can be used to relax the sphincter and may also be used to treat BPH (see Chapter 42 for more information about BPH). Side effects can include low blood pressure, dizziness, and nasal congestion.

Urethral stents, which are small tubelike devices, can be inserted into the urethra and expanded to widen the opening for urine to flow out. This may be used to relieve strictures. Risks associated with stents include displacement of the stent and infection. Male patients may consider surgery to treat BPH.

If conservative treatment has failed and the patient is experiencing frequent urinary retention with damage to the kidney, urinary diversion may be needed. Urinary diversion is described in the next section, Cancer of the Bladder.

Overactive Bladder

The goal of treatment of overactive bladder is to protect the kidney and upper urinary tract, prevent infection, and prevent urinary incontinence by routinely evacuating the bladder. If the patient has an overactive bladder, bladder training may be the first course of treatment.

For bladder training, the patient keeps a diary that includes fluid intake, times the patient voids, and any episodes of urine leakage. The diary helps to identify any patterns and assists in planning to avoid incontinence. The patient plans to void at certain times of the day and, as she gains more control, may increase the interval of time between voiding (NIDDK, 2008). For women, Kegel exercises are also part of bladder training and are used to strengthen the muscles

DIAGNOSTIC TESTS for Neurogenic Bladder

Test with Description, Rationale	Expected Abnormality
Voiding Cystourethrography *Looks at voiding patterns using dye.*	Evaluates neurogenic bladder, incontinence obstruction.
Uroflow *Measures force of urinary stream.*	Diminished urine flow.
Cystometry *Looks at neuromuscular function of the bladder and urethral pressure profile.*	Evaluates stress incontinence, neurogenic bladder, and obstruction.
Sphincter Electromyography *Examines electrical activity of skeletal muscle. Distinguishes between muscle and nerve problems.*	Decreased sphincter and bladder tone. Poor nerve innervation.

Source: Kee, J. L. (2010). *Laboratory and diagnostic tests with nursing implications* (8th ed.). Upper Saddle River, NJ: Prentice Hall.

that hold urine in. The patient education for Kegel exercises includes the following:

- Have the patient identify the correct muscles by trying to stop the flow of urine (Thomas & Porter, 2007). Tightening the wrong muscles can put increased pressure on the muscles that control the bladder (NIDDK, 2008). Instruct the patient to squeeze the pelvic muscles and not to hold her breath.
- Hold these muscles for 2 to 3 seconds without tightening the stomach, buttocks, or thigh muscles. Then relax the muscles.
- Initially tell the patient to do a few sets and gradually work up to 3 sets of 10 repeats. If it is difficult to do the exercises in a sitting position, have the patient try the exercise lying down (NIDDK, 2008).
- Inform the patient that bladder control may not improve for 3 to 6 weeks. Some patients have noticed an improvement after the first few weeks (NIDDK, 2008).

Medications that help to relax the bladder muscles and prevent bladder spasms include anticholinergics such as oxybutynin chloride (Ditropan), hyoscyamine (Levsin), propantheline bromide (Pro-Banthine), and tolterodine tartrate (Detrol). The most common side effect is dry mouth, but larger doses can cause blurred vision, tachycardia, flushing, and constipation (Wilson et al., 2011). Administering time-release formulations helps to decrease the side effects. See the Pharmacology Summary of Drugs Used in Bladder and Urinary Tract Disorders box on page 1206.

Stress Incontinence

Like overactive bladder, stress incontinence may be treated by educating the patient about Kegel exercises, if the patient is female, or with electrical stimulation. Bladder control treatment may include electrical stimulation of the nerves that control the bladder and sphincter muscles. The stimulation may be delivered through the vagina, through patches placed on the skin or via a wire surgically placed near the coccyx and connected to a stimulator that can be placed under the skin. This device, marketed as the InterStim system, has been approved by the Food and Drug Administration (FDA) to treat urge incontinence, urgency-frequency syndrome, and urinary retention in patients for whom other treatments have failed (NIDDK, 2008).

If urinary incontinence is severe and other treatments have failed, a surgery known as augmentation cystoplasty may be considered. The surgery enlarges the bladder by replacing the diseased bladder with a section taken from the bowel. This improves the ability to store urine but may make it more difficult to empty, requiring regular catheterization (NIDDK, 2008).

Nursing Management

Nursing care for the patient with neurogenic bladder varies depending on the underlying cause and the method of treatment. It is very important for the nurse to explain and review the treatment plan with the patient frequently. Topics that should be addressed with patients who have neurogenic bladder and/or their families before discharge are outlined in the Patient Teaching & Discharge Priorities box.

Cancer of the Bladder

Etiology and Epidemiology

There are three main categories of tumors: supervision noninvasive, invasive into underlying muscles, and metastatic (Shelton, 2011). Approximately 90% of bladder tumors are transitional cell carcinomas that arise from the transitional epithelium of mucous membranes (Thomas & Porter, 2007). Tumors may develop on the surface of the bladder wall or within the wall. The American Cancer Society (2012a) estimated that approximately 73,510 people in the United States would be newly diagnosed with urinary bladder cancer in 2012, with 14,880 expected deaths. Cancer of the bladder is the fourth most common cancer in men and the ninth most common cause of death by cancer in men (American Cancer Society, 2012a). Bladder tumors are four times more common in men than in women, and the incidence is higher in Caucasian men than in African American men (American Cancer Society, 2012a). Bladder cancer also occurs more frequently in older adults (over age 65) (Shelton, 2011).

Smoking is an extremely important risk factor; approximately 50% of those diagnosed with bladder cancer are smokers. Occupational carcinogens are also linked to bladder cancer, including dyes, beta naphthylamine, and benzidine (Shelton, 2011; Thomas & Porter, 2007). Exposure to occupational carcinogens can occur in plants that manufacture dyes, paint, rubber, textiles, petroleum, and aluminum; it also includes exposure to diesel fumes. Other risk factors may include artificial sweeteners, nitrates, and exposure to certain chemotherapeutic agents (Shelton, 2011). There is a latent period between exposure and cancer development.

Clinical Manifestations

The first sign of bladder cancer is most commonly gross, painless, intermittent hematuria. Patients may also present with signs of urinary tract infections (such as urgency) or an actual infection (Shelton, 2011). Patients with invasive tumors may have pelvic pain (Thomas & Porter, 2007).

Laboratory and Diagnostic Procedures

There are no screening tools to detect bladder cancer early (American Cancer Society, 2012a). Bladder cancer is detected with cystoscopy and biopsy. IVP, CT, renal ultrasound, and MRI may also be conducted (Shelton, 2011). Tests that are helpful in the diagnosis of bladder cancer are listed in the Diagnostic Tests box (p. 1207).

Staging and Grading the Tumor

Bladder cancer is categorized according to stage (the tumor's anatomic progression or depth) and grade (the cell differentiation and aggressiveness). The TNM system is the most common staging system used. Refer to Chapter 57 for an explanation of the TNM staging system. Grading compares how abnormal the cancer cells appear in relation to normal tissue of the same type and how aggressive the cells seem to be. Well-differentiated cells resemble normal cells more closely, tend to be less aggressive, and grow slowly. Poorly differentiated cells do not resemble normal cells and are more aggressive.

Medical Management

Treatment will depend on the stage and grade of the cancer. If it has not invaded the muscle, the tumor can be removed by transurethral resection. Intravesicular chemotherapy, in which the bladder is directly washed with an antineoplastic, is also used to treat superficial cancer. Intravesical immunotherapy is similar to intravesicular chemotherapy except that the agent that is instilled to treat the cancer is Bacillus Calmette-Guérin (BCG), a form of inactivated tuberculosis bacterium. Bacillus Calmette-Guérin immunotherapy works by triggering the body's own immune system to destroy the cancer cells. This treatment is indicated for superficial tumors that have not invaded the muscle wall.

Tumors that are too large to be removed transurethrally, are located away from the bladder neck and ureteral orifice, or have not responded

PHARMACOLOGY Summary of Drugs Used in Bladder and Urinary Tract Disorders

Medication Category and Action	Application/Indication	Nursing Responsibility
Opioid Analgesics		
Morphine sulfate ***Action:*** Binds with and activates opioid receptors in the brain and spinal cord to produce analgesia and euphoria.	Treatment of pain.	Monitor vital signs, including pain level. Monitor for respiratory depression. Provide safe and timely reduction of pain and symptom levels. Barriers to effective pain management should be addressed, including inappropriate fears of risk of side effects, addiction, and respiratory depression. Patient teaching: Avoid other central nervous system depressants. Be careful with tasks requiring alertness.
Urinary Analgesic		
Phenazopyridine (Pyridium) ***Action:*** Azo dye that has local anesthetic action on urinary tract mucosa.	Symptomatic relief of pain, burning, frequency, and urgency caused by irritation of the urinary tract mucosa.	Instruct patient: The drug will turn urine a bright-orange color and can stain clothing. Stop use immediately, and contact the health care team if skin or sclera appears to have a yellowish color.
Anti-Infectives		
Cephalosporins Cefazolin (Ancef) (Kefzol) Cefuroxime (Zinacef) Ceftriaxone (Rocephin) Cefotaxime (Claforan) ***Action:*** Binds to one or more of the penicillin-binding proteins located on cell walls of susceptible organisms. This inhibits the final stage of bacterial wall synthesis, killing the bacteria.	Infections of genitourinary tracts.	Determine prior hypersensitivity to cephalosporins and penicillins. Perform culture and sensitivity tests prior to therapy. Monitor intake and output (I&O) pattern. Monitor patients for antibiotic-associated pseudomembranous enterocolitis. Avoid use of alcohol during and for 48 to 72 hours after taking drug. Have patients consume yogurt or buttermilk, which may help protect against intestinal superinfection by maintaining normal intestinal flora.
Sulfonamides sulfadiazine Sulfadoxine-pyrimethamine (Fansidar) Sulfisoxazole Trimethoprim-sulfamethoxazole ***Action:*** Believed to interfere with folic acid biosynthesis (required for bacterial growth) by inhibiting enzymes and prevents bacterial synthesis.	Acute, recurrent, and chronic urinary tract infections.	Obtain culture and sensitivity prior to administration. Monitor I&O. Fluid intake should be enough to create urinary output of at least 1,500 milliliters a day to prevent formation of crystals in the urine and stone formation. Monitor temperature. Assess for skin rashes. Observe patients with diabetes taking oral hypoglycemic medication for hypoglycemic reactions. Patient teaching: Sulfonamides may make hormonal contraceptives unreliable. Avoid exposure to ultraviolet light and excessive sunlight.
Quinolone antibiotics Ciprofloxacin (Cipro) Norfloxacin (Noroxin) ***Action:*** Inhibits DNA gyrase, an enzyme necessary for bacterial replication.	Urinary tract infections.	Obtain culture and sensitivity prior to administration. Assess for skin rash and GI symptoms. Patient teaching: Increase fluid intake while taking mediation. Do not take the following within 4 hours of antacids. Drug interactions include theophylline, sucralfate, iron, warfarin, and calcium, as well as antacids. Avoid exposure to excess sunlight or artificial UV light.
Aminopenicillin Ampicillin Amoxicillin ***Action:*** Binds to penicillin-binding proteins in bacterial cell wall causing bacterial lysis and death.	Urinary tract infections.	Obtain culture and sensitivity prior to administration. Determine previous hypersensitivity to penicillins and cephalosporins. Assess for urticarial rash: may be a sign of hypersensitivity. Assess for diarrhea to rule out pseudomembranous colitis. Patient teaching: Take medication as prescribed; do not miss a dose and continue until all medication is taken.

PHARMACOLOGY Summary of Drugs Used in Bladder and Urinary Tract Disorders, *continued*

Medication Category and Action	Application/Indication	Nursing Responsibility
Anticholinergic (parasympatholytic) Oxybutynin (Ditropan) ***Action:*** Exerts direct antispasmodic action and inhibits muscarinic effects of acetylcholine on smooth muscle.	Relieve symptoms associated with voiding in patients with neurogenic bladder.	Monitor patients for expected responses to therapy. Assess patients with colostomy or ileostomy for abdominal distention and onset of diarrhea—may be early signs of obstruction or toxic megacolon. Patient teaching: Patient should not drive or engage in potentially hazardous activities until the patient knows the effects of the medication. Patient should not overexert in hot environments; medication suppresses sweating and may cause heatstroke. Instruct patient that the drug may cause blurred vision and dry mouth.

PATIENT TEACHING & DISCHARGE PRIORITIES for Neurogenic Bladder

Need	Teaching
Prevention of calculi formation and infection from urinary stasis	Encourage the patient to increase fluid intake to prevent formation of calculi and infection.
Bladder evacuation	Teach the patient about bladder training as well as intermittent catheterization. To assist the female patient in learning self-catheterization, use a mirror.
Prevent infection	Teach the patient/family the importance of strict aseptic technique during catheterization. If the patient has an indwelling catheter, teach the need for cleaning the catheter insertion site with soap and water at least twice a day. Teach the patient/family to watch for signs of infection including fever and cloudy or foul-smelling urine.
Enterostomal care	If a urinary diversion procedure has been done, arrange for consultation with an enterostomal therapist.

DIAGNOSTIC TESTS for Bladder Cancer

Test with Description, Rationale, and Normal Values	Expected Abnormality
Urinalysis Normal: Blood: negative RBC: 1–2 *Used to diagnose urinary system and kidney disease.*	Red blood cells and hematuria.
Excretory Urography (IVP) Normal: normal size, structure, and function of kidneys, ureter, and bladder. *Done to evaluate the structure, size, and function of the kidneys, ureters, and bladder. Ask the patient about allergies to contrast or shellfish. Will generally need a bowel prep prior to the procedure.*	Damage to the bladder and surrounding structures by a tumor.
CT Scan *Used to detect tissue abnormalities in the kidney and urinary system.*	Displays renal lesions and the progression of the cancer.
Ultrasonography *Used to identify the size of the kidneys and tissue abnormalities.*	May detect metastasis outside of the bladder.

to intravesical therapy may be eligible for a partial cystectomy, although recurrence is common (Shelton, 2011). Tumors that have infiltrated the muscle require a radical cystectomy (removal of the entire bladder and lymph nodes). In men, this may also include removal of the prostate, part of the urethra, and the seminal vesicles; in women, the uterus, cervix, ovaries, fallopian tubes, and part of the vagina may be removed (Shelton, 2011). A urinary diversion referred to as an ileal conduit is created by using the intestinal tract (Figure 39–2◆). A segment of ileum is separated and formed into a tubular pouch, with the open end being brought to the skin's surface, forming a stoma. The ureters are then connected to the pouch. The patient will need to wear an external pouch to collect the urine.

Another urinary diversion option is the creation of a neobladder, or internal urine collection reservoir, formed from the small intestine and connected to the urethra. The patient learns to void normally through the urethra by tightening the abdominal muscles in a Valsalva-type

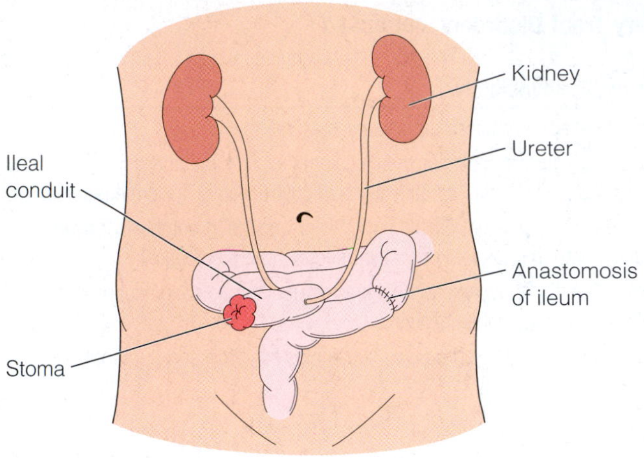

FIGURE 39–2 ◆ Ileal conduit.

maneuver and using the Credé maneuver (application of pressure to the lower abdomen). The advantage of the neobladder is that the patient can maintain a relatively normal lifestyle. However, the patient may experience short-term incontinence and may need to learn self-catheterization to completely empty the bladder (Shelton, 2011). Some patients may have an internal pouch made from sections of bowel with formation of a catheterizable stoma; the patient will pass a catheter through the stoma at scheduled intervals to empty the pouch.

Advanced bladder cancers will also require radiation therapy and chemotherapy. These modalities may be used before or after cystectomy. Radiation may be used as a primary treatment modality in patients who are not able to tolerate chemotherapy or have invading cancer without lymph node involvement (Shelton, 2011). Refer to Chapter 57 for nursing care of the patient undergoing radiation therapy and chemotherapy.

Nursing Management

For general nursing management of the postoperative patient, refer to Chapter 19. Following radical cystectomy, one of the most important postoperative nursing responsibilities is to monitor urine output. Urine output that drops below 30 mL/hr may indicate shock, hemorrhage, obstructed ureters, or renal dysfunction. Another intervention involves examining the appearance of the stoma, which should be beefy red in color. The nurse should encourage the patient to look at the stoma and involve the patient in its care as soon as possible. Nursing assessments for infection, tissue perfusion and cardiac output, gas exchange and airway clearance, bleeding, fluid volume status, skin integrity and oral mucous membranes, fatigue, nutrition, pain, body image disturbance, urinary elimination, and coping for the patient with cancer are covered in detail in Chapter 57. Prior to discharge, the nurse may make a referral for home health care or an enterostomal therapist to help coordinate the patient's care. Patients with an ostomy should be referred to resources such as the United Ostomy Association and the American Cancer Society.

Health Promotion

Several steps can be taken to maintain a healthy urinary system:

- Maintain good hygiene habits.
- Drink at least eight glasses of water a day to flush the bladder.
- Include dairy products in the diet (calcium).
- Urinate regularly.
- Control your blood pressure.
- Drink cranberry juice (fights bacteria).
- Avoid long-term use of medications such as aspirin and ibuprofen, which can damage the kidneys.
- Limit alcohol and drug intake.

Disorders of the Kidneys

There are numerous diseases of the kidneys, all of which cause loss of filtration capacity. Some are rapidly reversible; others cause permanent damage to the kidneys. Symptoms of renal failure often do not become evident until the level of renal function is less than 25% (Huether & Forshee, 2010). Treatment of most kidney disorders involves recognizing early signs and symptoms and correcting the underlying cause to protect kidney function (Kumar, Abbas, Fausto, & Mitchell, 2007).

Acute Glomerulonephritis

Epidemiology and Etiology

Glomerulonephritis occurs most often in patients who are ages 5 to 15 years. It has a male-to-female ratio of 2:1 and is the most common cause of chronic renal failure (also called kidney disease). Glomerulonephritis is a degenerative inflammation of the glomeruli and most commonly results from a previous streptococcal infection, usually of the respiratory tract. The streptococcal infection triggers antibody production against the streptococcal antigen. The antigen–antibody complexes become trapped in the glomeruli, causing an inflammatory response. Immune complexes in the glomerular basement membrane trigger an inflammatory response. This response triggers both chemical mediators and proliferation of macrophages and neutrophils. This furthers the inflammatory response and damages the epithelial and glomerular cells, subsequently increasing cellular permeability to red blood cells and protein (specifically albumin). Damage to the kidney may ultimately lead to renal failure (Huether & Forshee, 2010). Glomerular disease may be classified as primary (postinfectious, immunoglobulin A [IgA] nephropathy), secondary (lupus erythematosus, diabetes mellitus, Goodpasture's syndrome), or hereditary (Alport syndrome) (Kumar et al., 2007).

Clinical Manifestations

Acute glomerulonephritis may occur within 10 to 21 days after an untreated case of pharyngitis (Huether & Forshee, 2010). Symptoms include mild edema (usually around the eyes, feet, or ankles), **oliguria** (decreased urine output of less than 400 milliliters in a 24-hour period), proteinuria (the presence of protein in the urine), **azotemia** (an increase in the blood urea nitrogen caused when the kidneys are unable to excrete normally), and **hematuria** (the presence of blood in the urine) (Huether & Forshee, 2010).

Laboratory and Diagnostic Procedures

A detailed patient history and assessment of clinical symptoms are important for the diagnosis of acute glomerulonephritis. The Diagnostic Tests box lists tests that are helpful in determining the diagnosis of acute glomerulonephritis.

Goodpasture's Syndrome

A cause of acute or rapidly progressive glomerulonephritis is Goodpasture's syndrome, also known as antiglomerular basement membrane disease. In this disorder, circulating antibodies are directed

DIAGNOSTIC TESTS for Acute Glomerulonephritis

Test with Description, Rationale, and Normal Values	Expected Abnormality
Urinalysis	
Normal: Protein: 2–8 mg/dL; negative reagent strip Glucose: negative Red blood cells: 1–2 Casts: mixed hyaline *Used to diagnose urinary system and kidney disease.*	Presence of protein, red blood cells, and mixed cell casts related to increased permeability of the functioning glomeruli.
Serum Creatinine	
Normal: 0.5–1.5 mg/dL *Helps evaluate renal function.*	Elevated serum creatinine related to impaired glomerular filtration.
Urine Creatinine Clearance	
Normal: 85–135 mL/min *Used to estimate glomerular filtration rate (GFR)*	Decreased related to impaired glomerular filtration.
Serum Antistreptolysin-O Titer	
Normal: <100 international units/ml *Determines the effect of beta-hemolytic streptococcus in secreting antistreptolysin-O.*	Elevated related to recent streptococcal infection.
Throat Culture	
Normal: negative	May show group A beta-hemolytic streptococci related to recent streptococcal infection.

Source: Kee, J. L. (2010). *Laboratory and diagnostic tests with nursing implications* (8th ed.). Upper Saddle River, NJ: Prentice Hall.

against an antigen that is intrinsic to the glomerular basement membrane (GBM), resulting in acute glomerulonephritis. It is unknown what stimulus triggers the production of the circulating autoantibodies, although certain chemicals (hydrocarbons) and influenza are implicated in some patients. The disease is rare, accounting for an estimated 5% of all cases of rapidly progressive glomerulonephritis (Porth & Matfin, 2009). Between 60% to 80% of patients with Goodpasture's syndrome will have both renal and pulmonary symptoms (Stevenson, Sharma, & Verrelli, 2009).

Symptoms may include edema, hypertension, proteinuria, and hematuria (Huether & Forshee, 2010). Patients should also be evaluated for respiratory symptoms, such as cyanosis, crackles, tachypnea, and hemoptysis. Chest radiography will show consolidation (Stevenson et al., 2009). To diagnose the syndrome, there must be demonstration of anti-GBM antibodies in either the serum or the kidney. Normally, a renal biopsy is performed, as it provides information about the activity and chronicity of renal involvement.

The medical management of Goodpasture's syndrome includes plasmapheresis in conjunction with prednisone and cyclophosphamide. The plasmapheresis removes the circulating anti-GBM antibodies and other mediators of inflammation and inhibits antibody production (Kaplan, Appel, & Pusey, 2009; Porth & Matfin, 2009). Goodpasture's syndrome is typically associated with severe renal injury and, if untreated, progresses quickly to end-stage renal failure.

Alport Syndrome

Alport syndrome, or hereditary nephritis, is a progressive glomerular disease that is genetically heterogeneous with X-linked autosomal recessive and autosomal dominant variants. The disease is rare; its prevalence is approximately 0.2% in adults and 3% in children. The disorder occurs from mutations in genes encoding several members of the type IV collagen protein family, the predominant collagenous constituent of basement membranes. The secondary changes in glomerular basement membrane composition that occur because of the mutations predispose patients to the development of glomerulosclerosis (Saxena, 2008).

Patients with Alport syndrome will initially present with asymptomatic microhematuria and episodes of gross hematuria. Hypertension and proteinuria also occur. The disease is generally more severe in men than in women. Patients may also exhibit several extrarenal manifestations, including sensorineural hearing loss and eye changes such as slow deterioration of vision and dot and fleck retinopathy (abnormal pigment of the retina) (Saxena, 2008). Diagnosis is usually suspected with a family history of renal failure and deafness. Kidney biopsy and genetic testing may also be used to definitively diagnose Alport syndrome.

Medical Management

The goals of treatment for acute glomerulonephritis are relief of symptoms and prevention of complications as well as treating the underlying cause. Supportive care includes fluid restrictions, bed rest, dietary sodium restrictions, and correction of electrolyte imbalances. Medical treatment includes diuretics to reduce extracellular fluid and antihypertensives if needed. The Pharmacology box on page 1210 lists medications used to treat renal disorders.

Nursing Management

Although care for the patient with acute glomerulonephritis is primarily supportive, it is important for the nurse to monitor the patient and watch for signs of acute kidney injury (also known as acute renal failure). Critical assessments include strict monitoring of intake and output (I&O), daily weight, assessment of renal function through serum creatinine, blood urea nitrogen (BUN) levels, and

PHARMACOLOGY Summary of Drugs Used in Renal Disorders

Medication Category and Action	Application/Indication	Nursing Responsibility
Anti-Infectives		
Quinolone (Fluoroquinolones) antibiotics Ciprofloxacin (Cipro) Norfloxacin (Noroxin) ***Action:*** Inhibits DNA gyrase, an enzyme necessary for bacterial replication.	Urinary tract infections.	Obtain culture and sensitivity prior to administration. Assess for skin rash and GI symptoms. Patient teaching: Increase fluid intake while taking medication. Do not take within 4 hours of antacids. Drug interactions include theophylline, sucralfate, iron, warfarin, and calcium, as well as antacids. Avoid exposure to excess sunlight or artificial UV light.
Sorafenib (Nexavar) ***Action:*** Inhibits enzymes that promote uncontrolled tumor growth and angiogenesis.	Renal cell cancer.	Monitor for leukopenia, anemia, and thrombocytopenia. Monitor for hypertension, GI upset, joint pain, and fatigue. Monitor for skin reactions. Avoid drugs that decrease clotting (aspirin, warfarin). This has interactions with numerous other drugs, including phenytoin. Patient teaching: Report bleeding, pain, and rashes to health care provider.
Loop Diuretics		
Furosemide (Lasix) Bumetanide (Bumex) Torsemide (Demadex) ***Action:*** Decreases intravascular volume. Inhibits reabsorption of sodium.	Treatment of edema associated with kidney disease, including nephrotic syndrome.	Monitor for signs of hypokalemia: fatigue, depressed reflexes, muscle weakness, and rapid irregular pulse. Monitor blood pressure. Monitor serum and urine electrolytes. Monitor intake and output (I&O) ratio and pattern. Patient teaching: Consult health care team regarding allowable salt and fluid intake. Eat potassium-rich foods daily such as bananas and oranges. Report signs and symptoms of hypokalemia. Make position changes slowly to prevent dizziness or imbalance. Avoid prolonged exposure to direct sun.
Corticosteroids		
Dexamethasone Cortisone Betamethasone Budesonide Hydrocortisone Methylprednisolone Prednisolone Prednisone Triamcinolone ***Action:*** Anti-inflammatory and immunosuppression properties.	May be used in cancer therapy, in inflammatory conditions, and as an immunosuppressant.	Monitor blood pressure; report an ascending pattern. Monitor serum electrolytes and glucose. Monitor for signs of infection: Use of steroids may mask infection and delay healing. Long-term use: Monitor bone density. Patient teaching: Do not alter dosing regimen or stop medication suddenly. Appetite will improve and a slight weight gain is expected. Avoid alcohol, as it may contribute to steroid ulcer development. Report any symptoms of GI distress to the health care team.
Antihypertensives		
Refer to Chapter 35.	Refer to Chapter 35.	Refer to Chapter 35.

Source: Adams, M. R., & Koch, R. W. (2010). *Pharmacology connections to nursing practice.* Upper Saddle River, NJ: Pearson Education.

urine creatinine clearance. The nurse in a hospital setting will consult the dietary department to provide a high-caloric, low-protein, low-sodium, and low-potassium diet. Discharge priorities include instructing the patient that follow-up examinations are necessary to detect renal failure. The patient should have his blood pressure, urine protein, and renal function assessed for at least 1 year following the initial infection to detect recurrence. More detail will be given in the Nursing Management section for the patient with chronic glomerulonephritis.

Although the prognosis for acute glomerulonephritis is generally good, with normal kidney function returning after a period of time, repeated occurrences can lead to chronic glomerulonephritis.

Chronic Glomerulonephritis

Epidemiology and Etiology

Chronic glomerulonephritis is a slow, progressive disease caused by inflammation of the glomeruli that results in sclerosis and scarring. Approximately 30% to 50% of patients with end-stage renal disease have chronic glomerulonephritis. Chronic glomerulonephritis is twice as common in men as in women. Common causes of chronic glomerulonephritis include membranoproliferative glomerulonephritis, membranous nephropathy, focal segmental glomerulosclerosis, and rapidly progressive glomerulonephritis (Kumar et al., 2007). Systemic disorders include lupus erythematosus, Goodpasture's syndrome, and diabetes mellitus.

Clinical Manifestations and Diagnostic Tests

Chronic glomerulonephritis usually remains subclinical until the progressive phase begins, which may take years. At any time, the disease may become progressive, and the patient will exhibit hypertension, proteinuria, and hematuria. As the disease progresses, the patient may exhibit azotemia, nausea, vomiting, pruritus, dyspnea, and fatigue. During the late stages of the disease, mild to severe edema and anemia may develop. The ensuing severe hypertension may cause the heart to hypertrophy and may lead to heart failure, which will accelerate the development of renal failure, necessitating dialysis or kidney transplantation (discussed later in the chapter).

Tests that are helpful in the diagnosis of chronic glomerulonephritis include those outlined in the Diagnostic Tests box for acute glomerulonephritis on page 1209 with the addition of tests included in the Diagnostic Tests box for chronic glomerulonephritis below this.

Medical Management

The goals of treatment for chronic glomerulonephritis are control of hypertension with antihypertensives and a restricted-sodium diet, correction of electrolyte imbalances through dietary restrictions and supplements, and reduction of edema and prevention of heart failure with diuretics. For end-stage glomerulonephritis, treatment may include antibiotics for urinary tract infections, dialysis for renal failure, and possibly kidney transplantation. The Pharmacology box lists medications used to treat renal disorders.

Nursing Management

Because treatment for chronic glomerulonephritis is primarily supportive, the nurse's role includes close observation and monitoring of the patient's blood pressure, strict I&O, and daily weight to evaluate fluid retention and possible fluid overload. The nurse must monitor blood work for signs of electrolyte and acid–base imbalances. In the hospital setting, the nurse will consult the dietary department to plan a low-sodium, high-caloric diet with adequate protein.

Assessment

The nurse should inquire about the following items when taking the history of a patient with glomerulonephritis:

- Amount and frequency of urination
- Headaches, swelling of the lower extremities
- Recent high-risk episodes such as an infection, cardiovascular surgery, or significant trauma; ingestion of aspirin, antibiotics, or other drugs; and allergic response to food, drugs, or a blood transfusion
- Pain in the flank area
- Fatigue or longer than usual sleep periods
- Muscle cramps or difficulty breathing during exercise.

The nurse should assess the patient for the following physical findings:

- Oliguria (less than 400 mL/day of urine output)
- Abnormal urine color, clarity, or smell
- Lethargy
- Normal or high blood pressure
- Dyspnea
- Fine crackles with auscultation of the lung fields.

Nursing Diagnoses

Nursing diagnoses for the patient with glomerulonephritis include the following:

- *Fluid Volume, Excess* related to sodium and water retention.
- *Infection, Risk for* related to suppression of the normal cell metabolism and immune response.
- *Nutrition, Imbalanced: Less Than Body Requirements* related to anorexia, nausea, and restricted dietary intake.

NANDA-I © 2012

Planning

The overall goals for the patient with glomerulonephritis are to prevent further damage to the kidney and prevent renal failure.

DIAGNOSTIC TESTS for Chronic Glomerulonephritis

Test with Description, Rationale, and Normal Values	Expected Abnormality
Blood Urea Nitrogen (BUN) Normal: 5–25 mg/dL *Helps evaluate renal function or the presence of dehydration.*	Rising serum BUN related to renal insufficiency.
X-Ray or Ultrasonography Normal: normal structure of kidneys *Used to detect abnormalities.*	Shows smaller kidneys, possibly related to atrophy of the kidney.
Biopsy of the Kidney Normal: no abnormal cells *Used to assess kidney disease. Usually done by guided ultrasound or fluoroscopy.*	Abnormal tissue related to disease.

Outcomes and Evaluation Parameters

Outcomes and evaluation parameters for the patient with glomerulonephritis include the following:

- The patient will maintain serum electrolyte levels within acceptable limits.
- The patient will be normovolemic, as exhibited by vital signs and hemodynamic readings within acceptable parameters, clear lung sounds, minimal peripheral edema, normal skin turgor, and maintenance of weight gain and loss.
- The patient will not show signs of infection; this will be exhibited by a normal temperature; clean, dry access sites for lines and catheters; negative cultures; and completion of the antibiotic regime.
- The patient will be able to understand and agree to comply with dietary modifications and activity restrictions.

Interventions and Rationales

Nursing interventions and rationales for the patient with glomerulonephritis include the following:

- The nurse will continually assess for signs of infection and will document and report any signs to the health care team. *Uremic syndrome, the formation of thrombi in the capillaries and arterioles of the kidney (which may occur), suppresses normal cell metabolism and immune response, placing the patient at greater risk for infection.*
- The nurse will provide skin care and use preventive measures to protect against shearing or decubitus formation. Preventive measures include turning the patient every 2 hours, maintaining wrinkle-free linens, and using protective pads to cushion bony areas. The nurse will provide site care and dressing changes for intravenous lines according to hospital policy. *Skin integrity is compromised because of the edema and accumulation of waste products in the tissues caused by altered metabolism. Site care will assist in preventing the accumulation of moisture, which serves as a growth medium for infective organisms.*
- The nurse will collaborate with the other members of the health care team to implement a high-carbohydrate diet that provides small amounts of high-quality proteins; limits fluids, sodium, and potassium; and includes vitamin supplements. *A high-carbohydrate diet supplies calories for energy needs. Limiting proteins prevents protein catabolism, as the kidneys are unable to excrete the waste products at this time. Fluids and sodium are limited to prevent volume overload, while potassium is limited because the kidneys are unable to excrete it.*
- The nurse will administer diuretics as needed and ordered and document the results. *Diuretics may be given to reduce fluid overload and increase fluid volume through the kidneys in an attempt to prevent acute renal failure.*

Evaluation

With successful treatment of glomerulonephritis, the patient will remain free of infection, maintain fluid and electrolyte balance, and maintain her weight while following the diet regimen. Topics that should be addressed with patients who have glomerulonephritis and/or their families before discharge are described in the Patient Teaching & Discharge Priorities box below.

Pyelonephritis

Epidemiology and Etiology

In the United States, acute pyelonephritis accounts for approximately 200,000 hospitalizations annually, with uncomplicated infections occurring primarily in young women. Pyelonephritis is an inflammation related to an infection in the kidney; it affects the tissue, tubules, and renal pelvis. The infection is thought to ascend from the urethra through the ureters to the kidneys, even though some patients may not show symptoms of lower urinary tract infection (Porth & Matfin, 2009; Thomas & Porter, 2007). In severe infection, abscesses develop and can lead to necrosis, scarring, and renal failure. The most common causative bacteria are *Escherichia coli*, *Proteus*, and *Pseudomonas* (Huether & Forshee, 2010). Other causative bacteria include *Enterococcus*, *Staphylococcus aureus*, *Staphylococcus saprophyticus*, and *Klebsiella* (Thomas & Porter, 2007).

Women are at higher risk than men for urinary tract infections because of the shorter urethra in women and its proximity to the anus (Huether & Forshee, 2010). The bacteria can also be introduced by instrumentation such as catheterization, cystoscopy, or urologic surgery; obstruction; sexual intercourse; or by bacteria translocated by the blood. Risk factors for increased incidence of pyelonephritis are included in the Risk Factors box.

Clinical Manifestations and Diagnostic Tests

The signs and symptoms of pyelonephritis include urinary urgency, frequency, burning dysuria (painful urination), and hematuria. Because of the inflammatory response to the bacteria, the patient usually experiences fever, chills, flank pain, and fatigue. If the bacterial infection is not severe, the symptoms may subside within a few days, but a residual bacterial infection is common and, if untreated, may cause recurrence of symptoms. Tests that are helpful in the diagnosis of pyelonephritis are listed in the Diagnostic Tests box.

PATIENT TEACHING & DISCHARGE PRIORITIES for Glomerulonephritis

Need	Teaching
Nutrition	Have the patient and family work with a dietitian to plan a low-sodium, high-caloric diet with adequate protein.
Medications	Stress to the patient and family the importance of taking prescribed antihypertensives as scheduled, even if the patient is feeling better.
	Suggest that diuretics be taken in the morning to decrease disruption of sleep due to the need to void.
Skin care	Stress to the patient and family the importance of good skin care, as pruritus and edema may cause skin breakdown.
	Teach the patient and family how to assess ankle edema.
Avoidance of continued infections and scarring	Stress to the patient and family the importance of reporting signs of infection, particularly urinary tract infection, and of avoiding contact with people who have infections.
	Stress the importance of follow-up appointments to assess renal function.

RISK FACTORS for Pyelonephritis

Inability to empty the bladder. Examples include neurogenic bladder, urinary obstruction due to tumor, kidney stone, prostatic hyperplasia, or urinary stasis.

Being female. This is due to the proximity of the urinary meatus to the vagina and rectum.

Sexually active women. This is due to the increased risk of bacterial contamination from intercourse.

Pregnant women. Approximately 2.9% to 5% develop asymptomatic bacteriuria; if untreated, approximately 20% to 30% of these infections develop into pyelonephritis (Shoff, Green-McKenzie, Edwards, Behrman, & Shepherd, 2010).

Diabetes. This is due to the development of neurogenic bladder, which causes incomplete emptying and urinary stasis. Also, glucose in the urine may support bacterial growth.

Compromised renal function from other renal diseases increases the susceptibility.

Instrumentation.

Medical Management

Treatment for pyelonephritis consists of identification of the infecting organism and treatment with the appropriate antibiotics. Intravenous antibiotics may be used initially to control the growth of bacteria in more severe infection. Commonly used antibiotics include sulfa drugs, cephalosporins, amoxicillin, and fluoroquinolones (Thomas & Porter, 2007). If the patient is experiencing urinary urgency and frequency, urinary analgesics such as phenazopyridine are appropriate. See the Pharmacology Summary of Drugs Used in Renal Disorders on page 1210. If the infection was caused by an obstruction, surgery may be necessary to relieve the obstruction.

Nursing Management

Assessment

When taking a patient history, the nurse should consider the patient's age and sex; whether a female patient is sexually active; whether the patient has had a recent procedure such as catheterization, cystoscopy, or urologic surgery; and whether the patient has a history of neurogenic bladder (discussed earlier in the chapter). Physical assessment findings may include fever (usually 38.9°C or higher), burning with urination, general fatigue, hematuria, flank pain, and urinary frequency and urgency.

Nursing Diagnoses

Nursing diagnoses that apply to pyelonephritis include the following:

- *Infection, Risk for* related to insufficient knowledge to avoid exposure to pathogens, neurogenic bladder, or urinary obstruction.
- *Urinary Incontinence, Urge* due to infection.
- *Fatigue* due to inflammation and infection.

NANDA-I © 2012

Planning

The goals for the patient with pyelonephritis are to treat the infection and to prevent further infections.

Outcomes and Evaluation Parameters

Outcomes and evaluation parameters for the patient with pyelonephritis include the following:

- The patient is free from infection, as exhibited by follow-up urine culture that is free of growth.
- The patient does not experience urgency or urinary urge incontinence.
- The patient does not suffer fatigue, as exhibited by the ability to perform normal activities without tiring.

Interventions and Rationales

If the patient with pyelonephritis has a high fever, the nurse will administer antipyretics. When collecting urine for urinalysis and culture, the nurse should teach the patient the proper technique for obtaining

DIAGNOSTIC TESTS for Pyelonephritis

Test with Description, Rationale, and Normal Values	Expected Abnormality
Urinalysis Normal: Appearance: clear Odor: aromatic Specific gravity: 1.005–1.030 Protein: 2–8 mg/dL; negative reagent strip Glucose: negative Red blood cells: 1–2 White blood cells (leukocyte esterase): 3–4 Casts: mixed hyaline *Used to diagnose urinary system and kidney disease.*	Cloudy urine, foul smelling, lowered specific gravity, proteinuria, possible hematuria, positive WBC, casts.
Urine Culture Normal: negative *Done to detect microorganisms in urine.*	Bacteriuria: more than 100,000 organisms/mcL of urine.
X-Ray Films of the Kidneys, Ureters, and Bladder (KUB) *Done to assess the structure, size, and shape of tissues. Done before tests utilizing contrast, such as intravenous pyelogram (IVP).*	Any abnormal structure, size, or shape of tissue. May reveal any cause of obstruction: renal calculi, tumor, or cysts.

Source: Kee, J. L. (2010). *Laboratory and diagnostic tests with nursing implications* (8th ed.). Upper Saddle River, NJ: Prentice Hall.

a clean-catch urine specimen and should send the culture within 30 minutes of collection to prevent overgrowth of the bacteria. Additional nursing interventions and rationales for the patient with pyelonephritis include the following:

- The nurse should teach the patient the importance of completing the prescribed antibiotic therapy and of drinking 2,000 to 3,000 mL of fluid each day. *Stopping antibiotics early, even when symptoms have subsided, may allow the infectious agent to remain. Drinking plenty of fluid helps to empty the bladder of contaminated urine.*
- The nurse should teach the patient to plan activities in short increments to allow for rest time. *Planning for rest periods between activities will help prevent fatigue.*
- If the patient is having urinary urgency and burning with urination, the nurse should administer urinary analgesics. *Urinary analgesics relieve the pain of burning, frequency, and urgency arising from irritation of the urinary tract mucosa.*

Evaluation

With successful treatment of pyelonephritis, the patient should have a normal temperature, no burning or frequency with urination, and no growth on culture of the urine.

Health Promotion

Topics that should be addressed with patients who have pyelonephritis and/or their families before discharge are outlined in the Patient Teaching & Discharge Priorities box.

Hydronephrosis

Epidemiology and Etiology

Hydronephrosis (swelling of the kidney caused by retention of urine) is usually the result of another disease process, the most frequent cause being obstruction or blockage. If an obstruction occurs in the ureter, bladder, or urethra, the kidney can become extremely dilated with urine. The most common causes of obstruction are an enlarged prostate gland, urethral or ureteral strictures, and renal calculi. Other causes may include abdominal tumors, tumors of the ureter and bladder, blood clots, inflammatory disorders such as ureteritis or prostatitis, neurogenic bladder, and congenital abnormalities (Kumar et al., 2007). If the site of the obstruction is the urethra or bladder, then both kidneys are usually affected. If the obstruction occurs in one ureter, then the hydronephrosis will be unilateral. When the obstruction is in the urethra, distal to the bladder, the bladder dilates with urine first, acting as a buffer, which delays the hydronephrosis.

Hydronephrosis can be acute or chronic. Acute hydronephrosis is generally reversible; chronic hydronephrosis can lead to irreversible damage (Vourganti & Maniam, 2008). If the obstruction is severe and prolonged, fibrotic changes occur in the kidney, leading to a loss of function of the involved nephrons. The finding of hydronephrosis, which is often accidental, occurs when a radiograph or ultrasound of the abdomen is ordered for another reason.

Clinical Manifestations and Diagnostic Tests

Signs and symptoms of hydronephrosis vary depending on the cause of the obstruction and the extent of the blockage. Symptoms may be as mild as slight discomfort and slightly decreased urine flow. Other patients may experience severe, colicky renal pain or flank pain that radiates to the groin; this type of pain is generally found in acute hydronephrosis. Patients with chronic hydronephrosis generally complain of vague abdominal or back pain (Porth & Matfin, 2009). If the hydronephrosis is unilateral, affecting only one kidney, the pain is only on the affected side. If infection occurs because of stagnation of urine, the patient will develop fever, nausea, and pain on urination. Tests that are helpful in the diagnosis of hydronephrosis are presented in the Diagnostic Tests box.

Medical Management

Treatment of hydronephrosis consists of identifying and treating the cause of the obstruction in order to preserve renal function and prevent infection. Removal of the obstruction may include dilation for stricture of the urethra, prostatectomy for prostatic hypertrophy, or surgical removal of calculi or tumor. Inoperable obstructions may require drainage of the kidney using a nephrostomy tube.

Nephrostomy Tube

Nephrostomy tubes are placed percutaneously under fluoroscopy or surgically. The tube is placed through the flank area into the renal pelvis and secured to a closed drainage system to allow drainage via gravity flow. Before the procedure, several precautions are taken: The patient signs a consent form, and the health care provider corrects coagulopathy (bleeding disorder), gives a broad-spectrum antibiotic to prevent infection, and corrects uncontrolled hypertension. After the tube is placed, it is important for the nurse to assess it for kinks or clots that may impede drainage. The tube may need to be flushed with saline to maintain its patency. Careful monitoring of the patient for bleeding is essential after the procedure. The nurse should exercise caution to prevent dislodgement of the tube; although tubes can be replaced in mature tracts, new incisions may be required for newer tracts (Hautmann & Leveillee, 2008; Uppot, 2009).

Nursing Management

If the hydronephrosis has already affected the patient's renal function, a diet low in protein, sodium, and potassium is indicated to prevent progression of renal failure prior to surgery. (Refer to the earlier Nursing Management section for the patient with glomerulonephritis.) Prior to

PATIENT TEACHING & DISCHARGE PRIORITIES for Pyelonephritis

Need	Teaching
Prevention	Instruct female patients to wipe the perineum from front to back after defecation.
	Instruct female patients to void after sexual intercourse to flush the bladder and urethra.
Antibiotic therapy	Teach patients the signs and symptoms of infection: cloudy urine, burning with urination, urgency, frequency, and fever.
	Instruct the patient to complete the prescribed antibiotics even after symptoms subside.
Follow-up treatment	Stress the importance of completing the antibiotics.
	Stress that if symptoms return the patient needs to see the health care provider as soon as possible.
	Encourage follow-up care for high-risk patients as described previously under risk factors.

DIAGNOSTIC TESTS for Hydronephrosis

Test with Description, Rationale, and Normal Values	Expected Abnormality
Intravenous pyelogram (IVP) Normal: normal size, structure, and function of the kidneys, ureter, and bladder. *Done to evaluate the structure, size, and function of the kidneys, ureters, and bladder. Ask the patient about allergies to contrast or shellfish. Will generally need a bowel prep prior to the procedure.*	Identification of stricture or obstruction as well as kidney disease or tumors.
Renal Ultrasonography Normal: normal structure of kidneys *Used to detect abnormalities.*	Identification of fluid accumulation and areas of obstruction related to the inability of urine to drain, stricture, tumors, or calculi.
Renal Function Studies **Blood urea nitrogen (BUN)** Normal: 5–25 mg/dL *Helps evaluate renal function or the presence of dehydration.*	Increased related to decreased filtration.
Serum Creatinine Normal: 0.5–1.5 mg/dL *Helps evaluate renal function*	May rise related to nephron function loss.
Creatinine clearance Normal: 85–135 mL/min *Used to estimate glomerular filtration rate (GFR).*	Decreased related to decreased glomerular filtration.

the patient's diagnostic tests, the nurse should inquire about any allergies to dye or to foods that contain iodine such as shellfish. Hydronephrosis can be very painful; the nurse should administer pain medication as needed.

Nursing management of the patient who has had a nephrostomy tube placed includes the following:

- The nurse assesses for complications such as bleeding at the site, hematuria, and infection.
- The nurse assesses the patient's skin at the nephrostomy site for signs of inflammation, infection, bleeding, leakage of urine, and skin irritation.
- The nurse assesses tube patency. If the tube is obstructed, the patient will complain of pain and pressure.
- The nurse uses aseptic technique when replacing dressings.
- The nurse encourages oral intake of fluids to promote flushing of the kidney and nephrostomy tube.
- A nephrostomy tube should never be clamped.
- A nephrostomy tube should never be irrigated without specific orders.

Topics that should be addressed with patients who have hydronephrosis and their families before discharge are listed in the Patient Teaching & Discharge Priorities box.

Polycystic Kidney Disease

Etiology and Epidemiology

Polycystic kidney disease is a congenital anomaly that is characterized by multiple clusters of fluid-filled cysts that grossly enlarge the kidneys. The cysts are dilated kidney tubules. As the cysts enlarge and fuse, they may become infected or may collect blood after mild to severe trauma. The cysts compress and gradually replace the functioning renal tissue, leading to fatal uremia. The disease affects 300,000 to 600,000 people, with equal incidence in males and females (Grantham, 2008). Half of the children born to patients with polycystic kidney disease develop the disorder.

PATIENT TEACHING & DISCHARGE PRIORITIES for Hydronephrosis

Need	Teaching
Prevention	Teach older men, especially those with prostatic hypertrophy, to have routine prostate checkups. Also instruct them to recognize and report symptoms of hydronephrosis, such as colicky pain, blood in the urine, or urinary tract infections.
Nephrostomy tube care	Instruct the patient/family in the care of the nephrostomy tube. Teach the importance of checking for bleeding and patency. Stress the importance of immediately notifying the health care provider if the tube becomes dislodged.
Signs and symptoms of post-operative complications	Instruct the patient/family during hospitalization and at home after discharge about complications such as infection or bleeding. Instruct the patient/family to report any sign of impending hemorrhage and shock: tachycardia; cold, clammy skin; and a feeling of anxiousness or decreased level of consciousness.
Antibiotic therapy	If there was concurrent infection, instruct the patient to complete the prescribed antibiotics even after symptoms subside.

There are two main types of polycystic kidney disease: autosomal dominant (adult) and autosomal recessive (childhood). Childhood polycystic kidney disease, including perinatal and neonatal forms, results in a mutation in the PKHD1 gene and may cause stillbirth or early neonatal death. Adult polycystic kidney disease is inherited as an autosomal dominant trait that affects either PKD1 or PKD2. The disease usually becomes symptomatic around age 40 (Grantham, 2008; Kumar et al., 2007). In the adult form, renal deterioration is more gradual and progresses to fatal uremia. The patient will need treatment with dialysis, a kidney transplant, or both.

Clinical Manifestations

Adult polycystic kidney disease may go undiagnosed for some time because the symptoms—such as hypertension, polyuria, and urinary tract infections—are nonspecific. As the disease progresses, the patient will develop signs and symptoms related to the enlarging kidneys. These include flank pain and possible palpation of an abdominal mass, hematuria, retroperitoneal bleeding from a ruptured cyst, proteinuria, and abdominal pain.

Laboratory and Diagnostic Procedures

The diagnosis of polycystic kidney disease is made from both family history and examination revealing grossly enlarged and palpable kidneys. Tests that are helpful in the diagnosis of polycystic kidney disease are listed in the Diagnostic Tests box.

Medical Management

The goal of treatment for polycystic kidney disease is to preserve renal function and prevent infectious complications. Adequate control of hypertension is necessary to help prevent rapid deterioration in function. As the disease progresses, the patient will require dialysis. The Pharmacology box on page 1210 presents medications used to treat renal disorders.

Nursing Management

Young adult patients with polycystic kidney disease should be encouraged to seek genetic counseling. Approximately half of the children born to a patient with polycystic kidney disease will have the disease (Grantham, 2008). Because the disease is progressive, comprehensive patient teaching and emotional support are extremely important. For more detail, refer to the Nursing Management section for the patient with acute renal failure later in this chapter. Topics that should be addressed with patients who have polycystic kidney disease and/or their families before discharge are presented in the Patient Teaching & Discharge Priorities box.

Renal Infarction

Epidemiology and Etiology

Renal infarction is rare, and because patients present with complaints that mimic other conditions, such as pyelonephritis, the diagnosis is often missed. An occlusion of a renal blood vessel results in renal infarction and an area of necrosis in one or both kidneys. The location of the infarction depends on the site of the occlusion. In approximately 75% of infarctions, the vessel that becomes occluded is the renal artery (*Professional Guide to Diseases*, 2009). The embolic event is secondary to a predisposing cardiovascular disease such as mitral stenosis, atrial fibrillation, microthrombi in the left ventricle, rheumatic valvular disease, endocarditis, or a recent myocardial infarction.

DIAGNOSTIC TESTS for Polycystic Kidney Disease

Test with Description, Rationale, and Normal Values	Expected Abnormality
Ultrasonography, Tomography, and Radioisotope Scans Normal: normal structure of kidneys *Used to detect abnormalities.*	Enlargement of the kidneys and cysts caused by the fluid-filled cysts that displace the renal tissue.
Retrograde Ureteropyelography Normal: kidneys, ureters, and bladder *Done to evaluate the structure, size, and function of the kidneys, ureters, and bladder. Ask the patient about allergies to contrast or shellfish. Will generally need a bowel prep prior to the procedure.*	Enlarged kidneys with elongation of the renal pelvis, flattening of the calyces, and indentations. Enlargement is caused by the fluid-filled cysts that displace the renal tissue.
Urinalysis Normal: Protein: 2–8 mg/dL; negative reagent strip Red blood cells: 1–2 Casts: mixed hyaline *Used to diagnose urinary system and kidney disease.*	Presence of protein, red blood cells, and red blood cell casts related to impaired filtration.
Serum Creatinine Normal: 0.5–1.5 mg/dL *Helps evaluate renal function.*	Rising serum creatinine may indicate advanced renal insufficiency and decreased nephron function.
Blood Urea Nitrogen (BUN) Normal: 5–25 mg/dL *Helps evaluate renal function or the presence of dehydration.*	Rising serum BUN indicates advanced renal insufficiency.

PATIENT TEACHING & DISCHARGE PRIORITIES for Polycystic Kidney Disease

Need	Teaching
Asymptomatic stage	Monitor kidney function carefully: • Obtain a creatinine clearance test every 6 months. • Obtain a urine culture every 6 months and earlier if symptomatic.
Follow-up care	Patient/family at home: • Monitor filtration capacity and progression of the disease. • If infection is detected, patient should receive antibiotic treatment even if she is asymptomatic.

The degree of occlusion and rate of decreased blood flow to the kidney determine whether the event will be acute or become chronic as the narrowing progresses. Signs and symptoms include severe upper abdominal pain or constant flank pain with tenderness, fever, nausea, and vomiting; hematuria may also be present (Lopez & Glauser, 2010; *Professional Guide to Diseases*, 2009). Renovascular hypertension may occur several days after infarction due to the reduced blood flow, which stimulates the renin-angiotensin mechanism.

Renal infarction may also arise from renal vein thrombosis (RVT). A spontaneous renal vein thrombosis is rare in patients who are ambulatory but has been reported in patients with trauma, nephrotic syndrome, or lupus nephritis; those with inherited procoagulant defects; and women taking oral contraceptives (Laskowski & Schwing, 2009).

Clinical Manifestations

Pulmonary embolus may be the first clue that the patient has chronic RVT. Acute RVT typically presents with flank pain, microscopic or gross hematuria, a marked elevation in serum lactate dehydrogenase (LDH), and an increase in the size of the affected kidney on radiographic study. If the acute RVT is bilateral, the patient may present with acute renal failure.

Laboratory and Diagnostic Procedures

Any patient who is at risk for hypercoaguability should be further evaluated, especially patients with predisposing cardiovascular disease, flank trauma, or diseases that affect the kidneys. Renal venography will show the exact location and extent of obstruction, but it is a high-risk procedure because of the adverse effects of the dye load on renal function. Tests that are helpful in the diagnosis of renal infarction are listed in the Diagnostic Tests box.

Medical Management

Therapies designed to remove the occlusion in patients with renal infarction include administration of intra-arterial streptokinase, lysis of blood clots, catheter embolectomy, and anticoagulation therapy. If the infarcted area becomes infected or is very large, causing hypertension, surgical repair of the occlusion or removal of the kidney may be necessary. The patient may also receive pharmacologic therapy for hypertension.

Nursing Management

In caring for the patient with renal infarction, it is important for the nurse to monitor the patient's I&O, daily weight, and electrolyte levels to assess renal function. The nurse should encourage the patient to schedule follow-up appointments to monitor the return of renal function. More details can be found in the Nursing Management section for the patient with acute renal failure later in this chapter.

Nephrotic Syndrome

Etiology and Epidemiology

Nephrotic syndrome has a reported annual incidence of approximately 50 cases per 1 million adult population. The major cause of nephrotic syndrome is diabetes. Therefore, American Indians, Hispanics, and African Americans, who have high incidences of diabetes, also have an increased incidence of nephrotic syndrome. The syndrome is more common in males than in females (Cohen, 2011). It is the result of damage to the glomeruli blood vessels that filter wastes from the blood. The damaged glomeruli allow 3 grams or more of protein to leak into the urine during a 24-hour period. The protein loss creates a decrease in circulating protein, which allows fluid to accumulate in the body's tissue rather than in the vascular space. The cause of nephrotic syndrome may be unknown or can be the result of diseases such as diabetic nephropathy and amyloidosis.

Clinical Manifestations

Clinical manifestations of nephrotic syndrome include high levels of protein in the urine; low levels of protein in the blood; edema, especially around the eyes, feet, and hands; and high cholesterol.

Medical Management

Nephrotic syndrome is treated by addressing the underlying cause. The syndrome may go away once the underlying cause has been treated. However, if treatment does not maintain remission of the syndrome, the patient may develop chronic kidney disease that progresses to end-stage renal disease.

Renal Carcinoma

Epidemiology and Etiology

The American Cancer Society (2012b) estimated that approximately 64,770 people in the United States would be newly diagnosed with renal cancer in 2012, with 13,570 expected deaths. Renal cancer is the seventh most common cancer in men and eighth most common in women; it is the 10th-leading cause of death in men. Renal cell carcinoma of the kidney causes abnormal tissue growth and may lead to kidney disease. Approximately 85% of all primary renal cell carcinomas originate within the renal cortex. They are further divided by histology: clear (75% to 85%), chromophilic (15%), or chromophobic (5%); 5% to 8% of primary renal cell carcinomas are transitional cell carcinomas (Thomas & Porter, 2007). Renal carcinoma represents approximately 3% of all incidences of cancer (Wood, 2011). The Risk Factors box lists the risk factors that have been associated with renal carcinoma. The influence of genetic disorders on the risk of developing renal carcinoma is outlined in the Genetic Considerations box.

Weblink: Renal Artery Thrombosis Weblink: Renal Carcinoma Weblink: Renal Cell Carcinoma

DIAGNOSTIC TESTS for Renal Infarction

Test with Description, Rationale, and Normal Values	Expected Abnormality
Urinalysis Normal: Protein: 2–8 mg/dL; negative reagent strip Red blood cells: 1–2 Casts: mixed hyaline *Used to diagnose urinary system and kidney disease.*	Presence of protein, red blood cells, and red blood cell casts related to impaired filtration.
Serum Enzyme Levels Normal: LDH: 70–250 units/L ALP: 42–136 units/L AST: 8–38 units/L	Elevated lactate dehydrogenase (LDH), alkaline phosphatase, and aspartate aminotransferase results from tissue destruction.
Excretory Urography/Intravenous Pyelogram (IVP) Normal: normal size, structure, and function of kidneys, ureter, and bladder. *Done to evaluate the structure, size, and function of the kidneys, ureters, and bladder. Ask the patient about allergies to contrast or shellfish. Will generally need a bowel prep prior to the procedure.*	Reveals diminished or absent excretion of contrast, which indicates diminished or nonfunctioning kidney.
Isotopic Renal Scan Normal: no pathology *Uses nuclear radioisotope.*	Reveals absent or reduced blood flow to the kidneys, which indicates the area and extent of occlusion.
Angiography Normal structure of vasculature *Uses dye to visualize blood vessels.*	Highly diagnostic for renal infarction; reveals absent or reduced blood flow to the kidneys.
CT Scan Normal structures *May or not utilize contrast.*	Highly diagnostic for renal infarction; reveals abnormalities.

Sources: Kee, J. L. (2010). *Laboratory and diagnostic tests with nursing implications* (8th ed.). Upper Saddle River, NJ: Prentice Hall; Lopez, V. M., & Glauser, J. (2010). A case of renal artery thrombosis with renal infarction. *Journal of Emergencies, Trauma, & Shock, 3*(3), 302. Retrieved from http://www.onlinejets.org/text.asp?2010/3/3/302/66569.

RISK FACTORS for Renal Carcinoma

Cigarette Smoking: Smoking increases the risk of renal carcinoma.

Obesity: There appears to be a direct correlation between obesity and an increased risk of developing renal carcinoma.

Hypertension: Hypertension or antihypertensive drugs are associated with a higher risk of renal carcinoma.

Occupational Exposure to Toxic Compounds: Exposure to compounds such as cadmium, asbestos, and benzene has been suggested to increase the risk of renal carcinoma.

Source: American Cancer Society. (2012c). Kidney cancer (adult): Renal cell carcinoma. Retrieved from http://www.cancer.org/Cancer/KidneyCancer/DetailedGuide/kidney-cancer-adult-risk-factors.

GENETIC CONSIDERATIONS for Renal Carcinoma

Patients with certain inherited disorders show an increased risk of developing renal carcinoma (see Chapter 7). Some of these disorders are von Hippel-Lindau disease, hereditary papillary carcinoma, hereditary renal oncocytoma, and Birt-Hogg-Dube syndrome. About 40% of patients with von Hippel-Lindau disease develop renal carcinoma. The inherited papillary cancers are autosomal dominant, and patients develop multifocal tumors bilaterally. Patients with hereditary renal oncocytoma can also develop multifocal tumors bilaterally. Finally, Birt-Hogg-Dube syndrome is characterized by lesions that develop on the skin of the head and neck; patients with this syndrome have a predisposition to kidney neoplasms.

Source: Sachdeva, K., Jana, B. R. P., Javeed, M., Makhoul, I., & Curti, B. (2010). Renal cell carcinoma. Retrieved from http://emedicine.medscape.com/article/281340-overview.

Clinical Manifestations

Many patients are asymptomatic in the early stages of renal cancer. The most common presenting symptoms are hematuria, pain, and a flank mass. However, only 10% of patients present with these symptoms. Other symptoms may include abdominal mass, weight loss, and fatigue. Patients may also present with signs of metastatic renal cancer to the lungs, liver, bone, adrenal glands, or contralateral kidney. An increasing number of patients are being diagnosed with renal cancer as an incidental finding of a radiological procedure performed for another indication (Thomas & Porter, 2007; Wood, 2011).

Laboratory and Diagnostic Procedures

Laboratory and imaging procedures for diagnosing renal cancer include ruling out other kidney disease. An ultrasound, a CT, and an MRI may be conducted along with a detailed history (Wood, 2011). The imaging studies will help detect whether a mass exists. Angiography and intravenous pyelogram (IVP) studies may also be conducted (Huether & Forshee, 2010). Finally, a biopsy will help grade and stage the cancer.

Medical Management

Treatment of renal cancer consists of surgical removal. Radiation is often used for symptom management or palliation. However, chemotherapy has not been shown to be effective against renal cancer. Immunotherapy using natural killer cells, interferon-α, or recombinant interleukin-2 may be employed. Interleukin-2 is linked to several adverse reactions, such as capillary leak syndrome and cardiopulmonary toxicities. The newest treatment modalities involve targeted therapies (medications that block the growth and spread of cancer by interfering with specific molecules). Five drugs have currently been approved with more undergoing cinical trials; the approved drugs are sorafenib, sunitinib malate, temsirolimus, everolimus, and bevacizumab (Wood, 2011). Refer to Chapter 57 for the care of the patient with cancer.

Nursing Management

This nursing management section pertains to the immediate preoperative and postoperative care for the patient undergoing a nephrectomy (removal of a kidney).

Assessment

During the health history, the nurse should focus on the following:

- Any history of comorbidities such as diabetes, hypertension, or vascular disease
- Any concerns or fears the patient may have regarding normal kidney function after the surgery
- Concerns regarding activity and diet restrictions after the surgery
- Patient's level of weight loss, nausea or vomiting, and fatigue
- Patient's current and past history of smoking
- Any complaints of pain.

During the physical assessment, the nurse should focus on the following:

- Signs of fluid overload: peripheral edema and distended neck veins
- Hypertension
- Signs of hypovolemia: decreased blood pressure; pale, cool skin; agitation
- Adventitious breath sounds
- Dysuria, hematuria, oliguria, or polyuria
- Skin color, temperature, and turgor
- Any complaints of changes in weight, weakness, or fatigue.

Nursing Diagnoses

The primary nursing diagnoses for the patient undergoing nephrectomy are as follows:

- *Knowledge, Deficient* related to the procedure.
- *Pain, Acute* related to surgical manipulation.
- *Fluid Volume, Imbalanced, Risk for* related to the surgery and the function of the remaining kidney.
- *Gas Exchange, Impaired* related to anesthesia and pain.

NANDA-I © 2012

Planning

The overall goals for the patient undergoing nephrectomy include understanding of the procedure and the postoperative plan (cough and deep breathe, use of incentive spirometer, etc.), control of postoperative pain, and prevention of postoperative complications.

Outcomes and Evaluation Parameters

The major outcomes and evaluation parameters for the patient undergoing nephrectomy are as follows:

- The patient is able to verbalize understanding of the operative procedure.
- The patient is able to demonstrate the ability to cough and deep breathe, splint the incision site, use the incentive spirometer, and perform leg exercises.
- Postoperative pain is controlled as evidenced by the patient rating the pain at a tolerable level on a 0 to 10 scale. Patient maintains vital signs within normal limits.
- The patient's fluid and electrolytes will be balanced as exhibited by a urine output of at least 30 mL/hr. Electrolytes will be within normal limits.
- The patient will maintain adequate oxygenation as evidenced by unlabored respirations, clear breath sounds in all lobes, and arterial blood gases within normal limits.
- The patient will have normal bowel function as evidenced by normal, active bowel sounds; ability to eat a regular diet; and ability to have a regular bowel movement.

Interventions and Rationales

Nursing interventions and rationales for the patient undergoing nephrectomy include the following:

- The nurse should discuss with the patient where the incision will be made, whether the patient will have a chest tube or any drains, and the effects of positioning after surgery. *Knowledge of what to expect postoperatively will decrease the patient's fear and anxiety and increase the patient's ability to participate in postoperative care.*
- The nurse should teach the patient about postoperative pain management and let the patient know whether pain will be managed with patient-controlled analgesia or epidural infusion. This teaching includes discussing potential adverse effects and the importance of requesting pain medication before the pain becomes severe. *The patient will be able to better control pain with an understanding of the pain management plan.*
- The nurse will protect the remaining kidney by ensuring that the patient maintains adequate hydration. The nurse will monitor urine output and specific gravity and minimize the use of nephrotoxic medications. *Preservation of the remaining kidney is paramount. Appropriate hydration preserves renal function and the removal of waste products. Use of nephrotoxic drugs may damage the remaining kidney.*
- The nurse will assist the patient to perform incentive spirometry, encourage the patient to cough and deep breathe, splint the incision site, promote early ambulation, and check the patient's pulmonary status frequently. *Atelectasis (collapse of part of the lung) is an inherent risk of general anesthesia. Also, the patient with a flank incision is at risk because the intercostal muscles were spread and the 12th rib may have been removed. Pain involved with this incision limits deep breathing. If atelectasis develops and is not treated, it can lead to pneumonia.*
- The nurse should encourage early and frequent ambulation and encourage fluids and progression of diet as tolerated. The nurse assesses the abdomen for distention and bowel sounds and monitors nasogastric tube drainage if in place. *Manipulation of the bowel during surgery increases the risk of paralytic ileus.*

Evaluation

With successful treatment, the patient's pain will be controlled postoperatively, respiratory effort will be unlabored, and breath sounds will be clear in all lobes. The patient will be able to resume a normal diet and have return of normal bowel function. The patient will be able to take adequate food and fluid orally and will maintain normal fluid and electrolyte balance.

Acute Tubular Necrosis

Epidemiology and Etiology

The incidence of acute tubular necrosis is unreported, mainly owing to differences in definition of the disease. Acute tubular necrosis (ATN) results from damage to the renal tubular epithelium from a nephrotoxic or ischemic injury. Acute tubular necrosis is the most common form of intrinsic renal failure and accounts for the majority of acute kidney injuries in critically ill patients (Urden et al., 2010). The damage to the epithelium prevents normal concentration of urine, filtration of waste products, regulation of acid–base balance, electrolyte hemostasis, and fluid balance.

The common causes of ATN can be divided into two categories:

1. Toxic injury is the result of damage from nephrotoxins that cause uniform, widespread damage. Nephrotoxins are usually drugs, chemical agents, or bacterial endotoxins. Sources of nephrotoxins include rhabdomyolysis; nephrotoxic medications such as cephalosporins, some antineoplastic agents, aminoglycosides, and amphotericin B; contrast media; heavy metals such as arsenic, mercury, lead, or uranium; and street drugs such as phencyclidine (PCP) and heroin.
2. Ischemic injury occurs when perfusion to the kidneys is severely reduced. The damage to the tubular membrane is irregular and causes cast formation (protein cells that are held together by secreted mucoprotein in low flow, low pH or high salt concentrations which favor protein denaturation and precipitation) (Urden et al., 2010). Causes of ischemic injury include hemorrhage; severe dehydration; hypovolemic, septic, or cardiogenic shock; anaphylaxis; and transfusion reaction.

Clinical Manifestations

Acute tubular necrosis commonly occurs in patients who are debilitated or critically ill. It can be difficult to diagnose in the early stages because the effects of the primary disease or injury may mask the symptoms of ATN. There are four phases associated with acute tubular necrosis: the initiating, oliguric, diuretic, and recovery phases. The initiating phase involves a decreased glomerular filtration rate (GFR). The oliguric phase reflects further decreasing GFR with increased BUN and creatinine levels with changes in electrolytes. Oliguria is more common in ischemic damage and carries a higher mortality rate when present. In the diuretic phase, the GFR increases, and the patient may have polyuria (Urden et al., 2010). The recovery phase brings a slow return to normal laboratory levels and kidney function.

Laboratory and Diagnostic Procedures

Diagnosis of ATN includes an evaluation of kidney function, electrolyte abnormalities, and metabolic acidosis. Tests that are helpful in the diagnosis are outlined in the Diagnostic Tests box.

Medical Management

Treatment of ATN revolves around preserving kidney function and correcting the underlying cause. Treatment may include the use of diuretics as long as cardiac output is adequate; fluid replacement should be given as needed. Antibiotics will be given in the presence of infection; infection is linked to a higher mortality rate (60%) than is seen in cases with nephrotoxic causes (30%). Dialysis may also be used to treat ATN (Lerma, Agraharkar, & Kelly, 2011). The Pharmacology box on page 1210 presents medications used to treat renal disorders.

With appropriate treatment, renal function will slowly return; in fact, the glomerular filtration rate will be at 70% to 80% of normal within 1 to 2 years. Although most patients recover normal renal function, 33% will have residual renal insufficiency, and approximately 5% will require ongoing hemodialysis (Urden et al., 2010).

Nursing Management

Maintenance of fluid balance is important in the patient with ATN. Fluid overload is a common complication of therapy or may be related to acute kidney injury. Therefore, it is important for the nurse to accurately document the patient's daily weight; I&O, including loss from wound drainage; and dialysis balances. The nurse can ensure that the patient's electrolyte balance is maintained by monitoring laboratory results, enforcing restriction of foods containing sodium and potassium, and assessing for potassium content in prescribed medications such as penicillin.

The debilitated patient is vulnerable to infection. Because infection has a high mortality rate in patients with ATN, use of aseptic technique is paramount. The nurse should be certain to monitor for fever, chills, delayed wound healing, and flank pain. Encouraging the patient to cough and to breathe deeply will help to prevent pulmonary complications. For a more detailed review of additional interventions, refer to the Nursing Management section for the patient with acute renal failure later in this chapter.

Acute Renal Failure/Acute Kidney Injury

Epidemiology and Etiology

Acute renal failure has an annual incidence of approximately 100 cases per 1 million population. Only 1% of these patients present with acute renal failure at admission; hospital acquired renal failure has a higher incidence. This is believed to be related to the aging population with increased risks for failure, a high prevalence of nephrotoxic exposures possible in the hospital setting (medications, contrast, etc.), and the increased severity of illness in hospitalized patients (Peacock, 2011). Renal failure is the inability of the kidneys to clear the blood of urea and creatinine, the waste products of protein metabolism. Excretion of urea, which results from the breakdown of ammonia in the liver, is the primary method of ridding the body of nitrogen. If the body is unable to excrete the urea, it accumulates and toxicity develops. Creatinine is a by-product of muscle metabolism; an elevation indicates renal impairment (Kee, 2010).

Acute renal failure (ARF) is now also being referred to as acute kidney injury (AKI) (Dirkes, 2011). It develops suddenly and can often be reversed with treatment; however, if the condition that is causing the failure is not treated, the patient will progress to end-stage renal disease, uremic syndrome, and death. The causes of acute renal failure can be classified into three categories: prerenal, intrarenal, and postrenal. Chart 39–1 (p. 1222) lists causes in the three categories. The mortality rate remains high for acute renal failure, with rates ranging from 25% to

DIAGNOSTIC TESTS for Acute Tubular Necrosis

Test with Description, Rationale, and Normal Values	Expected Abnormality
Urinalysis	
Normal:	Presence of red blood cells and red blood cell casts related to impaired filtration.
Specific gravity: 1.005–1.030	Low specific gravity (1.010) related to decreased ability to concentrate urine.
Red blood cells: 1–2	Low osmolality.
Osmolality: 200–800 mOsm/kg (average)	
Used to diagnose urinary system and kidney disease.	
Serum Creatinine	
Normal: 0.5–1.5 mg/dL	Rising serum creatinine may indicate advanced renal insufficiency and decreased nephron function.
Helps evaluate renal function.	
Blood Urea Nitrogen (BUN)	
Normal: 5–25 mg/dL	Rising serum BUN indicates advanced renal insufficiency.
Helps evaluate renal function or the presence of dehydration.	
Arterial Blood Gases (ABG)	
Normal: pH 7.35–7.45	Metabolic acidosis related to impaired filtration:
Normal: HCO_3 24–28 mEq/L	pH < 7.35
Evaluates acid–base problems.	$HCO_3 < 24$ mEq/L
Electrolytes	
Sodium	Hypernatremia.
Normal: 134–145 mEq/L	
Potassium:	Hyperkalemia.
Normal: 3.5–5.3 mEq/L	
Phosphorus:	Hyperphosphatemia.
Normal: 1.7–2.6 mEq/L	
Calcium:	Hypocalcemia.
Normal: 4.5–5.5 mEq/L	
Done to evaluate electrolyte problems.	

90%, depending on the cause and the duration of renal failure prior to therapeutic intervention. Influencing factors include the increasing age of patients and the comorbid conditions that accompany aging, such as vascular disease and diabetes (Dirkes & Hodge, 2007).

Clinical Manifestations

Symptoms of acute kidney injury can be classified according to the phases associated with acute tubular necrosis (initiating, oliguric, diuretic, and recovery) (Goshorn, 2009; Huether & Forshee, 2010; Thomas & Porter, 2007). Generally, acute kidney injury is a sudden and critical event that will show evidence of the underlying cause followed by early signs of oliguria, azotemia, or **anuria** (a total loss of urine production). As the patient becomes more uremic, systemic signs and symptoms appear, including irritability, confusion, drowsiness, nausea, vomiting, pruritus, pallor, purpura, hypertension (although the patient may show hypotension at first depending on the underlying cause), **anasarca** (total body edema), and alterations in coagulation. Reduced tubular hydrogen excretion and decreased bicarbonate reabsorption result in metabolic acidosis (Goshorn, 2009). As a result of the acidosis, the patient's breath will have the odor of ammonia, and the patient may exhibit **Kussmaul's respirations,** which are deep, sighing respirations. The most immediately life-threatening electrolyte imbalance that occurs with acute renal failure is severe hyperkalemia (an excess of potassium in the blood). Elevated potassium levels can cause dysrhythmias and cardiac arrest. Sources of potassium should be identified and regulated if possible. Water and sodium imbalances are common, because the patient can neither conserve nor excrete sodium or water optimally. Hyponatremia and fluid overload are common. The kidney's ability to excrete phosphorus is impaired when the glomerular filtration rate drops. The resulting phosphorus retention leads to the formation of insoluble calcium phosphorus salts that can precipitate in soft tissue, forming diffuse tumorlike masses.

Laboratory and Diagnostic Procedures

Although not a diagnostic test, the RIFLE classification system helps identify acute kidney injury. See Chart 39–2 for the RIFLE classification system criteria.

The progress and severity of renal failure can be assessed by measurement of the glomerular filtration rate (GFR). The GFR is estimated through clearance tests of the waste product creatinine. When the GFR is impaired, the serum creatinine level rises, and the creatinine clearance rate falls. The formula is as follows (Kee, 2010):

$$\textit{Creatinine clearance} = \frac{\textit{Urine creatinine (mcg/dL)} \times \textit{Urine volume (dL)}}{\textit{Serum creatinine (mcg/dL)}}$$

The test involves a 12- or 24-hour urine collection and a blood sample. Normal levels are 85 to 135 mL/min. Values are slightly decreased in older adults because of reduced renal plasma flow with aging.

Weblink: Glomerular Filtration Rate: On-Line Calculator

CHART 39–1 Types of Acute Renal Failure

Category	Causes
Prerenal failure	Diminished blood flow to the kidneys causes prerenal failure. The decreased flow may result from: • Hypovolemia • Sepsis • Embolism, heart failure, severe vomiting, and diarrhea.
Intrarenal failure	Intrarenal (parenchymatous) failure results from damage directly to the kidney. The damage may be a result of: • Acute tubular necrosis • Acute poststreptococcal glomerulonephritis • Systemic lupus erythematosus • Malignant hypertension • Vasculitis • Sickle cell disease • Bilateral renal vein thrombosis • Nephrotoxins • Ischemia • Acute pyelonephritis.
Postrenal failure	Postrenal failure is the result of bilateral obstruction of urine outflow. Obstruction may be caused by: • Renal calculi • Clots • Tumors • Benign prostatic hyperplasia • Strictures • Blockage from catheterization.

A creatinine clearance rate of less than 40 mL/min suggests moderate to severe renal impairment (Kee, 2010). Glomerular filtration rate may also be estimated by using online calculators that utilize serum creatinine, age, gender, and race, such as the one found on the National Kidney Foundation website: www.kidney.org/professionals/kdoqi/gfr_calculator.cfm. Some estimations also include height and weight. Tests that are helpful in the diagnosis of acute renal failure are outlined in the Diagnostic Tests box.

Medical Management

The goal of treatment for acute renal failure is to identify and treat reversible causes. Supportive measures include the following:

- Maintain fluid balance. Depending on the underlying cause, the patient may initially be hypovolemic and should be treated for hypovolemia. However, patients should also be monitored for signs of fluid overload, such as edema. Free water may need to be restricted, and sodium should be monitored carefully.
- Maintain a protein intake of 0.8 g/kg per day (Goshorn, 2009). This may be adjusted based on the severity of the acute kidney injury.
- Provide nutrition to ensure a caloric intake of 25–35 kilocalories/kg of desirable body weight per day to reduce tissue catabolism (Goshorn, 2009).
- Monitor potassium. If hyperkalemia occurs, therapy can include hypertonic glucose and insulin infusions, administration of intravenous calcium gluconate, and oral or rectal administration of potassium exchange resin (e.g., sodium polystyrene sulfonate, or Kayexalate). If the patient continues to be hyperkalemic, dialysis may be necessary.
- Avoid exposure to or administration of nephrotoxic agents (see Chart 39–3).
- Adjust doses of all medications that are excreted by the kidneys.
- Avoid nonsteroidal anti-inflammatory drugs (NSAIDs), as well as angiotensin-converting enzyme inhibitors (ACE inhibitors), as they interfere with potassium regulation.
- Avoid magnesium-containing drugs (antacids).
- Control metabolic acidosis.
- Reduce the risk of hospital-acquired infection by using strict aseptic technique and removing indwelling urinary and vascular catheters when feasible.
- Use intermittent hemodialysis or continuous renal replacement therapy.

Continuous Renal Replacement Therapy

Continuous renal replacement therapy (CRRT), a mode of dialysis that may be used in the hospital to treat acute renal failure, is a way to remove solute and fluids slowly and continuously in a patient who may be hemodynamically unstable. Described simply, CRRT involves blood flowing from a vascular access point where the blood is removed and then purified by use of a hemofilter; the purified blood is returned

CHART 39–2 RIFLE Classification System for Acute Kidney Injury

Category	Criteria	
Severity Grade	**Glomerular Filtration Rate (GFR)**	**Urine Output Criteria**
Risk	Serum creatinine increased 1.5 times or GFR decreased > 25%	<0.5 mL/kg for 6 hours
Injury	Serum creatinine increased 2 times or GFR decreased > 50%	<0.5 mL/kg for 12 hours
Failure	Serum creatinine increased 3 times, GFR decreased > 75%, or serum creatinine ≥ 4 mg/dL	<0.5 mL/kg for 12 hours or anuria for 12 hours
Outcomes		
Loss	Complete loss of kidney function for > 4 wk	
End-Stage Kidney Disease	Need renal replacement for > 3 months	

Source: Dirkes, S. (2011). Acute kidney injury: Not just acute renal failure anymore? *Critical Care Nurse, 31*(1), 37–49.

DIAGNOSTIC TESTS for Acute Renal Failure

Test with Description, Rationale, and Normal Values	Expected Abnormality
Blood Urea Nitrogen (BUN)	
Normal: 5–25 mg/dL	Increased and may be an indicator of impaired glomerular filtration.
Helps evaluate renal function or the presence of dehydration.	*Not as reliable an indicator of renal damage as serum creatinine levels, because the BUN is easily changed by protein intake, blood in the gastrointestinal tract, and cell catabolism.*
Serum Creatinine	
Normal: 0.5–1.5 mg/dL *Helps evaluate renal function.*	Rising serum creatinine may indicate advanced renal insufficiency and decreased nephron function.
Serum Electrolyte Levels	
Potassium Normal: 3.5–5.3 mEq/L	Increased related to impaired filtration.
Sodium Normal: 135–145 mEq/L	Decreased, usually dilutional.
Phosphorus Normal: 1.7–2.6 mEq/L	Increased related to impaired filtration.
Calcium Normal: 4.5–5.5 mEq/L	Decreased related to inability to activate Vitamin D and in response to increased phosphorus.
Done to evaluate electrolyte problems.	
Urinalysis	
Normal: Red blood cells: 1–2	The kidneys have a decreased ability to concentrate urine and impaired kidney filtration.
Protein: 2–8 mg/dL; negative reagent strip	Presence of red blood cell casts and proteinuria.
Specific gravity: 1.005–1.030	Low specific gravity (1.010).
Osmolality: 200–800 mOsm/kg (average)	Low osmolality (less than 400 mOsm/kg).
Used to diagnose urinary system and kidney disease.	
Radiography	
Renal ultrasound	Changes may signify damage to the kidney.
Used to identify the size of the kidneys and tissue abnormalities.	May identify the cause of kidney dysfunction.
Computed tomography (CT) *should be done without contrast.*	
Used to detect tissue abnormalities in the kidney and urinary system.	
Retrograde Pyelography	
Looks at the size and structure of the kidneys, ureters, and bladder.	Will identify damage to the kidney as well as obstructions.
Isotopic Renal Scan	
Normal: no pathology *Uses nuclear radioisotope.*	Reveals absent or reduced blood flow to the kidneys, which indicates the area and extent of occlusion.

Source: Kee, J. L. (2010). *Laboratory and diagnostic tests with nursing implications* (8th ed.). Upper Saddle River, NJ: Prentice Hall.

via another vascular access point. The removed fluid, which is termed ultrafiltrate, is composed primarily of water, electrolytes, wastes, and some dialyzable medications. Indications for its use include hypervolemia, hyperkalemia, extremely elevated BUN or creatinine, metabolic acidosis, multiple organ dysfunction syndrome (MODS), and large fluid volume removal in hemodynamically unstable patients (Goshorn, 2009; Huether & Forshee, 2010; Urden et al., 2010). The following terms are commonly used with CRRT:

- ***Ultrafiltration:*** The process of removing excess water by creating a pressure differential between the blood and fluid compartments. Positive pressure in the blood path and negative pressure in the dialysate path cause the excess water to move from the patient to the dialysate. The negative pressure is a suctioning force applied to the membrane.
- ***Diffusion:*** Spontaneous movement of solutes from an area of higher concentration to an area of lower concentration.
- ***Convection:*** Movement of solutes through a membrane via an action called a solvent drag.
- ***Osmosis:*** Spontaneous movement of water from an area of lower concentration to an area of higher concentration.
- ***Hemofiltration:*** Movement of large amounts of fluid via ultrafiltration and some movement of solutes via convection.

CHART 39–3 Nephrotoxic Agents

Antibiotics	Heavy Metals	Solvents	Miscellaneous
Amphotericin B Gentamicin Kanamycin Neomycin Phenazopyridine Polymyxin B	Arsenic Lead Mercury	Carbon tetrachloride Ethylene glycol Methanol	Excessive use of acetaminophen Amphetamines Cyclosporine Phencyclidine (PCP) Heroin Silicon Nonsteroidal anti-inflammatory drugs Pesticides Poisonous mushrooms Iodinated radio-graphic contrast Some antineoplastic agents

- ***Replacement Fluid:*** Approximates normal plasma to meet the patient's needs. Fluids given may include lactated Ringer's solution, normal saline, albumin, bicarbonate, and electrolytes.
- ***Dialysate:*** Solution in dialysis that surrounds the patient's blood, separated by a filter, that allows solute to cross from one side to the other.

There are several forms of CRRT. The four most frequently used are as follows:

- ***Continuous Arteriovenous Hemofiltration (CAVH).*** The blood is circulated by the patient's own arterial pressure, so a pump is not necessary. There is no concentration gradient, so only filtration of fluid occurs. Electrolytes are eliminated only as they are pulled along with the fluid. Replacement fluid is infused into the venous port to approximate fluid removal or to maintain weight balance.
- ***Continuous Arteriovenous Hemodialysis (CAVHD).*** As with CAVH, the blood is circulated by the patient's own arterial pressure, so a pump is not necessary. Instead, CAVHD uses dialysate, which adds the filtering properties of dialysis, providing a better clearance of urea. The dialysate solution is infused along with the hemofiltered blood.
- ***Continuous Venovenous Hemodialysis (CVVHD).*** Diffusion and ultrafiltration are used to remove waste products. Dialysate is infused countercurrent to the blood flow in the outside compartment of the hemofilter to provide diffusion of wastes from the blood. CVVHD requires the use of a blood pump to control the flow at specific rates to optimize diffusion.
- ***Slow Continuous Ultrafiltration (SCUF).*** This form of CRRT is used primarily for fluid removal. No dialysate or replacement fluids are used as wastes; electrolyte balance and acid–base balance are not as critical an issue. SCUF is the hemofiltration therapy of choice when the only goal is fluid removal and the patient is not azotemic. SCUF may be used in patients who are refractory to diuretics.

The nurse's role in CRRT includes monitoring of fluid and electrolyte balance; hourly monitoring of vital signs, hemodynamic status, and I&O; and daily monitoring of weight. The amount of hourly ultrafiltrate that is removed depends on an hourly fluid-balance calculation and assessment of the patient's volume status. Excess fluid volume to be removed is ordered by the health care provider and is usually termed *net loss*; it may be ordered as 25 to 200 mL/hr more than hourly intake. This would be calculated as the patient's non-CRRT intake, such as intravenous infusions, medications, and feedings, plus fluid loss ordered by the health care provider minus non-CRRT system output, such as chest tube drainage, blood loss, and urine. Once the fluid volume has been calculated, the CRRT system is set to infuse and remove fluid; the system then monitors the amount of fluids infused and removed (Dirkes & Hodge, 2007). Assessment and care of the vascular access sites is very important, because the catheter's patency can affect the therapy's effectiveness.

Nursing Management

Fluid balance is critical for the patient with acute renal failure. The nurse should closely monitor and document the patient's I&O and daily weight. Intake of fluids should match the amount of urine output plus 500 to 750 milliliters a day for insensible losses; fluids will be restricted to 1 liter plus insensible loss (Urden et al., 2010). Strict measurement of output should include all body fluids, including wound drainage. Monitoring of intake includes the patient's nutritional status. A high-calorie, adequate-protein, low-sodium, low-potassium diet is key in preventing further progression of the disease; phosphorus may also be restricted (Rolfes, Pinna, & Whitney, 2009). Restrictions should be as follows:

- Sodium intake should only be what is needed to replenish losses, approximately 1,100 to 3,300 mg daily (Rolfes, Pinna, & Whitney, 2009).
- Protein intake should be 0.8 g/kg body weight per day to ensure adequate intake (Goshorn, 2009). Some patients may require further restrictions of 0.6 to 0.8 g/kg to minimize azotemia or nitrogen retention if not being dialyzed; if on dialysis, the patient may increase protein up to 2 g/kg daily (Rolfes, Pinna, & Whitney, 2009).
- Dietary potassium should be limited to 20 to 50 mEq/day to prevent hyperkalemia until urine volume increases during recovery (Goshorn, 2009).
- Erythropoietin may be needed to enhance erythropoiesis.
- Dietary phosphate may need to be restricted if hyperphosphatemia exists. Phosphate-binding antacids may be used to decrease the amount.

The patient with acute renal failure is susceptible to infectious complications. The nurse must rigorously use aseptic technique to prevent hospital-acquired infections. Complications of immobility can be prevented with frequent position changes, coughing and deep breathing, and passive range-of-motion exercises. The nurse should provide frequent mouth care to prevent stomatitis.

The patient who is uremic or has electrolyte imbalances or metabolic acidosis may be confused and unsteady. The nurse provides safety measures, such as having the bed in the low position with two to three side rails up to prevent falls and a sitter if necessary. In addition, the nurse should explain all procedures and keep lines of communication open.

Assessment

Focused nursing assessment during history taking should include the following:

- Amount and frequency of urination
- Change in urine color and smell
- History of headaches, dependent edema, or palpitations
- Pain around the flank or costal margin areas
- Nausea, loss of appetite, odd taste in mouth
- Weight gain or loss
- Weakness and fatigue
- Inability to concentrate or confusion
- Any job-related exposure to nephrotoxic agents
- Recent illness, surgery, or trauma
- Increased irritability.

A focused nursing assessment during physical exam should include the following:

- Abnormal urine color, clarity, or smell
- Oliguria (<400 mL/day), anuria (<100 mL/day), or nonoliguric (>400 mL/day)
- Lethargy, apathy
- Tremors
- Bounding, rapid pulse with normal or high blood pressure, distended neck veins
- Orthostatic hypotension
- Tachypnea, dyspnea, or adventitious breath sounds
- Kussmaul's respirations (found when patient is acidotic)
- Dependent edema (with hypervolemia), poor skin turgor (with hypovolemia)
- Arrhythmias (related to electrolyte imbalances).

Nursing Diagnoses

Key nursing diagnoses for the patient with acute renal failure include the following:

- *Fluid Volume, Excess* related to decreased glomerular filtration.
- *Infection, Risk for* related to anasarca and uremia.
- *Nutrition, Imbalanced: Less Than Body Requirements* related to nausea and poor taste in mouth.
- *Injury, Risk for* related to decreased sensorium and confusion.
- *Knowledge, Deficient* related to ARF and possible dialysis.

  NANDA-I © 2012

Planning

The overall goals for the patient with ARF are to identify and treat reversible causes, prevent further damage to the kidneys, and maintain fluid and electrolyte balance.

Outcomes and Evaluation Parameters

Patient outcomes and evaluation parameters for the patient with acute renal failure include the following:

- Serum electrolyte levels will be maintained as evidenced by results of laboratory findings within normal limits.
- Fluid volume will be maintained as evidenced by vital signs and hemodynamic readings within acceptable limits.
- The patient will maintain balanced nutrition as exhibited by limited weight loss without muscle wasting or edema.
- The patient will remain free of infection as exhibited by white blood count (WBC) being within the normal range, no increase in temperature, and no redness, edema, or drainage at the access sites for lines and catheters.
- The patient will be injury free as exhibited by no signs or symptoms of uremia, such as confusion and tremors.
- The patient will have a clear understanding of the disease process and the plan of care by expressing knowledge of, and commitment to comply with, treatments.

Interventions and Rationales

Nursing interventions and rationales for the patient with ARF include the following:

- The nurse will monitor and document electrolyte levels as ordered. *The kidneys have lost the ability to regulate electrolyte excretion and reabsorption. This is especially true of potassium, phosphate, calcium, and magnesium. The levels can change quickly, which may result in complications.*
- The nurse will monitor the ECG continuously, notify the health care team of any changes, and document the changes. *Electrolyte imbalances can cause dysrhythmias and cardiac arrest.*
- If hyperkalemia is detected, the nurse will notify the health care team and be prepared to administer the following, as ordered: *The kidneys' inability to excrete potassium released by normal cellular metabolism can cause very high potassium levels.*
  1. 50% glucose intravenously with IV insulin. *In an emergent situation, glucose and insulin may transport potassium into the cells, temporarily lowering the serum potassium level.*
  2. Calcium chloride or calcium gluconate intravenously. *To protect the heart from the effect of hyperkalemia on the cardiac rhythm, calcium competes with potassium for entry into cardiac cells.*
  3. Cation-exchange resins such as sodium polystyrene sulfonate (Kayexalate with sorbitol) orally or rectally as ordered. *Sodium polystyrene sulfonate removes potassium by exchanging it for sodium in the bowel. The sorbitol helps to remove the bound potassium from the bowel by acting as an osmotic diuretic.*
- The nurse will limit dietary and drug intake of potassium (penicillin VK or potassium-containing antacids) and magnesium-containing antacids. *The kidneys are unable to excrete the potassium or magnesium.*
- The nurse will assess for signs of fluid overload, such as weight gain, hypertension, tachypnea, adventitious breath sounds, peripheral edema, and low hematocrit. The nurse will also maintain a strict record of I&O. *During ARF, the kidneys are unable to maintain normal fluid balance, resulting in fluid overload during the oliguric stage and a potential for dehydration during the diuretic stage.*
- The nurse will restrict fluid intake to measure output plus 500 to 750 mL/day and compare intake and output records with daily weights. If fluid losses have increased or the patient is losing weight, the nurse will consult the health care team. *The kidneys are unable to eliminate excess fluids; therefore, intake must be restricted to replacement of lost fluids plus 500 to 750 mL/day to cover insensible losses (through lungs and skin).*

- The nurse will provide hard candies and frequent mouth care. *Restricting fluids may cause dry mouth and thirst. Hard candy will stimulate salivation, and mouth care will remove debris and add comfort.*
- The nurse will administer diuretics as ordered and document the results. The nurse will also administer vasodilators as ordered, such as low-dose dopamine. *Although there is controversy about their outcomes and effectiveness (Urden et al., 2010), diuretics may be administered during the prerenal phase in an attempt to prevent ARF by increasing fluid volume through the kidneys. However, if the kidneys are only marginally functioning, diuretics may cause ARF. Vasodilators expand the vascular bed, lessening the congestion and the risk of pulmonary edema. Low-dose dopamine increases renal perfusion by dopaminergic stimulation of the renal blood vessels.*
- The nurse will assess the patient for signs of infection (increased temperature, increased WBC, signs of infection at IV and catheter sites). The nurse will practice strict asepsis and provide site care and dressing changes according to policy. *The uremic syndrome that develops with ARF suppresses normal cell metabolism and immune response, placing the patient at increased risk for infection. Careful hand hygiene and the use of aseptic technique during procedures help to prevent infection. Site care prevents the accumulation of secretions that serve as growth media for infective organisms. Regular assessment of all site areas and general assessment of the skin will allow for early identification and treatment of infection.*
- The nurse will provide skin care and use preventive measures to protect against shearing or decubitus formation. Protective measures include turning the patient every 2 hours, maintaining wrinkle-free linens, and using protective pads to cushion bony areas. Provide site care and dressing changes for intravenous lines according to hospital policy. *Skin integrity is compromised because of the edema and accumulation of waste products in the tissues due to the altered metabolism. Site care will assist in preventing accumulation of moisture, which serves as a growth medium for infective organisms.*
- The nurse will collaborate with the other members of the health care team to implement a high-carbohydrate diet that provides small amounts of high-quality proteins; limits fluids, sodium, and potassium; and includes vitamin supplements. *A high-carbohydrate diet supplies calories for energy needs. Providing small but adequate amounts of high-quality proteins prevents protein catabolism, as the kidneys are unable to excrete the waste products at this time. Fluids and sodium are limited to prevent volume overload, while potassium is limited because the kidneys are unable to excrete it.*
- The nurse will monitor BUN, creatinine, uric acid, and pH levels as ordered. The nurse will also assess the patient for signs and symptoms of uremia (headache, confusion, change in mentation, pruritus, nausea and vomiting, weight loss with muscle wasting, Kussmaul's respirations, and seizures). *The accumulation of metabolic waste products and increasing acidosis reflect worsening kidney function. Uremia affects all systems in the body, but the changes may initially be subtle.*
- The nurse will assess the patient for signs and symptoms of hemorrhage. *Uremic syndrome places the patient at high risk for stress ulcers and coagulopathy.*
- The nurse will monitor the patient for anemia (hematocrit and hemoglobin levels) and administer erythropoietin, folic acid and iron supplements, or blood as ordered. *In ARF, the kidneys' ability to produce erythropoietin, a hormone that stimulates the production of red blood cells (RBCs), diminishes, resulting in anemia. Folic acid and iron supplements stimulate RBC production. Administration of packed red blood cells provides RBCs without causing fluid overload.*
- The nurse will provide information and teaching for the patient and family as needed regarding the process and stages of ARF, signs and symptoms that should be reported immediately, dietary modifications, activity restriction, and an explanation of any procedures, including dialysis. *Knowledge and understanding of the disease process and of the treatment plan help to decrease anxiety and may enhance recovery. If the patient is acutely ill, teaching may need to be done in small time frames.*

Evaluation

The patient with ARF should be able to verbalize his understanding of the disease process and the plan of care. With successful treatment, the patient will maintain serum electrolyte levels and vital signs within acceptable limits. The patient will not display signs of uremia. The patient will remain free of infection with clean, dry access sites for lines and catheters. The patient will have only limited weight loss and no signs of muscle wasting or edema.

Chronic Renal Failure/ Chronic Kidney Disease

Etiology and Epidemiology

Chronic renal failure, generally now referred to as chronic kidney disease (CKD), is generally not reversible and involves a progressive loss of kidney function. The symptoms of renal failure usually do not appear until renal capacity has decreased to 10% to 15% of normal. When a patient reaches this stage of failure, the patient is said to have **end-stage renal disease (ESRD)** (Huether & Forshee, 2010; Thomas & Porter, 2007). If the patient continues without treatment, uremic toxins accumulate and cause potentially fatal physiological changes in all of the major organ systems.

In the United States, over 500,000 patients have ESRD, and 350,000 of these patients are currently on dialysis (NKUDIC, 2010). The United States, Japan, Taiwan, and Mexico have the highest rates of ESRD in the world, with Taiwan's being the highest (U.S. Renal Data System, 2010).

Many patients who are developing kidney disease and early renal failure are unaware of their condition because of the lack of symptoms in the early stages. However, certain groups have been identified as being at risk for renal failure due to inherited susceptibilities or dangerous behaviors. Groups at risk for renal failure are listed in the Risk Factors box.

Diseases that lead to an increased risk of renal failure include the following:

- ***Diabetes:*** Almost 200,000 patients have ESRD attributed to diabetes mellitus (NKUDIC, 2010). The exact cause is unknown but may relate to hyperglycemia, hypertension, hyperperfusion, increased blood viscosity, and increased glomerular pressure that damage the nephrons (Jones, Brashers, & Huether, 2010).
- ***Hypertension:*** Hypertension is the second most common cause of ESRD, affecting approximately 128,000 patients (NKUDIC, 2010). Vascular changes in this disease cause a decrease in circulation to the kidneys, gradually damaging the nephrons. A term used to describe the renal changes occurring due to hypertension is *nephrosclerosis*.

RISK FACTORS for Renal Failure

Being African American: The members of this population are more likely to have ESRD; their rate is up to 3.9 times in general, and they are 6.7 times more likely to have ESRD related to hypertension (Thomas & Porter, 2007).

Gender: Men are at higher risk of having ESRD compared to women (about 1.4 times higher [Thomas & Porter, 2007]).

Age: Although ESRD can begin at any age, the risk increases after age 65 (Thomas & Porter, 2007).

Certain Hereditary Diseases: Polycystic kidney disease, an inherited condition, was discussed earlier in the chapter. About 25,000 patients have ESRD related to polycystic kidney disease (NKUDIC, 2010). Other hereditary diseases, such as Alport syndrome, have also been linked to ESRD (Thomas & Porter, 2007).

- ***Urinary Tract Obstruction:*** Diseases that obstruct the outflow of urine, such as an enlarged prostate in men, will cause back pressure and hydronephrosis. If not treated, the hydronephrosis will distort the kidney's shape and diminish its function.
- ***Chronic Glomerular Disease:*** Chronic glomerulonephritis is the third-leading cause of ESRD, affecting approximately 81,500 patients. Glomerulonephritis scars and eventually destroys the glomeruli's ability to function.
- ***Chronic Infection:*** Chronic infections such as pyelonephritis or tuberculosis will cause scarring and eventually destroy the kidney's ability to function.

Clinical Manifestations

The presence of any type of chronic kidney disease should be established as early as possible. The diagnosis may be based on the presence of kidney damage and level of renal function through measurement of the glomerular filtration rate (GFR). The National Kidney Foundation (2011) defines chronic kidney disease on the basis of two independent criteria: (1) kidney damage (structural or functional seen on laboratory, pathology, or imaging studies) for more than 3 months with or without a decreased GFR and/or (2) GFR less than 60 mL/min/1.73 m^2 for more than 3 months with or without kidney damage. The extent of the disease is classified according to the level of renal function. The National Kidney Foundation (2011) defines the stages as follows:

Stage 1: Kidney damage with normal or increased GFR, GFR $\geq$ 90 mL/min/1.73 m^2

Stage 2: Kidney damage with mild decrease in GFR, GFR is 60 to 89 mL/min/1.73 m^2

Stage 3: Moderate decrease in GFR, GFR is 30 to 59 mL/min/1.73 m^2

Stage 4: Severe decrease in GFR, GFR is 15 to 29 mL/min/1.73 m^2

Stage 5: Kidney failure, GFR $<$ 15 mL/min/1.73 m^2 or dialysis.

Diagnosis of chronic kidney disease is made through clinical assessment and a patient history of progressive debilitation with gradual deterioration of renal function. Early symptoms include complaints of fatigue (increasing with exertion), anorexia, and weakness. Patients may also complain of nausea, vomiting, a metallic taste in the mouth, irritability, insomnia, itching, and muscle cramps. Objective assessment may include pallor, dry skin, hypertension, bruising, and edema. These symptoms, along with other clinical manifestations, are often related to uremia and azotemia, as well as the kidney's failure to perform other functions, such as the production of erythropoietin and vitamin D and the kidney's tendency to overproduce renin (Murphy & Byrne, 2009; Thomas & Porter, 2007). Chronic kidney disease eventually produces changes throughout all body systems. Chart 39–4 lists the changes by body system.

Laboratory and Diagnostic Procedures

Tests that are helpful in the diagnosis of chronic kidney disease are the same as those listed for the diagnosis of acute renal failure (p. 1223) with the addition of those presented in the Diagnostic Tests for Chronic Renal Failure/Kidney Disease box.

Medical Management

Treatment of chronic renal failure is aimed at slowing the progression of the disease by treating any underlying condition that may be contributing to or causing the failure, treating specific symptoms, and minimizing complications. As the disease progresses, the health care provider must identify the patient's need for dialysis.

For patients with chronic renal failure, the administration of drugs or diagnostic contrast will adversely affect renal function. The use of drugs that lower the glomerular filtration rate (such as NSAIDs), aminoglycosides, antibiotics, and radiographic contrast should be avoided.

Medical Management to Slow Progression

To slow the progression of renal failure, health care providers employ protective mechanisms. This includes controlling hypertension. Antihypertensive therapy is given for both renal protection and cardiovascular protection because there is a marked increase in cardiovascular risk with chronic kidney disease. Patients are usually given angiotensin-converting enzyme (ACE) inhibitors or angiotensin II receptor blockers (ARBs). These drugs reduce glomerular pressure because systemic hypertension is reduced (Murphy & Byrne, 2009). The goal is a reduction in blood pressure to less than 130/80 mmHg. If the goal is not reached with the use of an ACE inhibitor or an ARB, then a diuretic is added and, if necessary, diltiazem, verapamil, or a beta-blocker (Thomas & Porter, 2007).

Safety Alert *ACE inhibitors and angiotensin II receptor blockers (ARBs) can cause a decrease in renal function and an increase in plasma potassium soon after the onset of therapy. Plasma creatinine and potassium should be checked within 1 to 2 weeks after initiating therapy (Murphy & Byrne, 2009).*

Patients with chronic kidney disease who are being treated conservatively (without dialysis) should be referred to a dietitian with planned follow-up. Deterioration of the patient's nutritional status often begins early in the course of the disease, and good nutrition plays a key role in slowing disease progression, preventing complications, and controlling waste products and electrolytes (Rolfes, Pinna, & Whitney, 2009). Patients who have protein malnutrition when starting dialysis have a poorer prognosis (Murphy & Byrne, 2009). For patients who are not undergoing dialysis, a low-protein diet consisting of 0.60 to 0.75 g/kg per day should be considered. When well monitored, a low-protein, high-energy diet maintains nutritional support while limiting the potentially toxic nitrogenous metabolites, development of uremic symptoms, and occurrence of other metabolic complications. Low-protein diets can decrease the effects of hyperphosphatemia, metabolic acidosis, and other electrolyte disorders. The patient who is on maintenance dialysis, either hemodialysis or peritoneal dialysis, should have a dietary protein intake of 1.2 g/kg per day with at least 50% of the protein being of high biologic value.

CHART 39–4 Body System Changes Due to Chronic Kidney Disease

Cardiovascular Changes	Respiratory Changes	Gastrointestinal Changes	Neurological Changes
Hypertension Cardiomyopathy Uremic pericarditis Hyperlipidemia Heart failure Peripheral edema Dysrhythmias	Increased susceptibility to infection Pulmonary edema Pleural effusions Uremic pleuritis Uremic pneumonitis Dyspnea due to heart failure Kussmaul's respirations due to acidosis	Inflammation and ulceration of gastrointestinal mucosa Gastritis Uremic colitis Uremic fetor: ammonia smell breath Anorexia Nausea and vomiting Constipation or diarrhea	Peripheral neuropathy Paresthesias Muscle weakness Shortened memory and attention span Drowsiness Irritability Altered mental status Coma Seizures
Endocrine and Reproductive Changes	**Hematopoietic Changes**	**Skeletal Changes**	**Integumentary Changes**
Infertility and decreased libido in both sexes Amenorrhea Impotence and decreased sperm production in men Increased aldosterone secretion due to increased renin production Increased blood glucose levels due to impaired carbohydrate metabolism and insulin resistance	Anemia Increase in bleeding and clotting disorders	Altered calcium and phosphorus metabolism, altered vitamin D production, and increased parathyroid hormone result in: Bone pain Pathologic fractures Calcifications in the soft tissue and vasculature	Yellowish bronze color Dry skin, hair, and nails Itching Purpura Ecchymosis Uremic frost (rare)

DIAGNOSTIC TESTS for Chronic Renal Failure/Kidney Disease

Test with Description, Rationale, and Normal Values	Expected Abnormality
Hemoglobin and Hematocrit	
Normal Hg: Male 13.5–18 g/dL; Female 12–15 g/dL *Examines oxygen-carrying capability of the RBCs.* Normal Hct: Male 40–54%; Female 36–46% *Examines concentration of RBCs in the blood.*	Decreased related to insufficient production of erythropoietin.
Arterial pH and Bicarbonate Levels	
Normal: pH 7.35–7.45 Normal: HCO_3 24–28 mEq/L *Evaluates acid–base balance.*	Decreased related to inability to secrete hydrogen and reabsorb bicarbonate.
Radiography	
Renal ultrasound *Used to identify the size of the kidneys and tissue abnormalities*	Reduced kidney size related to kidney damage.
Computed tomography *should be done without contrast to protect the kidneys.* *Used to detect tissue abnormalities in the kidney and urinary system.*	Characterization of the parenchyma and collecting systems.
Isotopic Renal Scan	
Normal: no pathology *Uses nuclear radioisotope*	Reveals decreased function and perfusion.
Kidney Biopsy	
Normal: no abnormal cells *Used to assess kidney disease. Usually done by guided ultrasound or fluoroscopy.*	Histologic identification of underlying pathology.

The energy expenditure and requirements of a nondialyzed patient with chronic renal failure are similar to those of healthy adults. A diet that provides approximately 35 kcal/kg per day has been shown to help minimize wasting; patients who are age 60 or older tend to be less physically active, so an intake of 30 to 35 kcal/kg per day may be sufficient (Rolfes, Pinna, & Whitney, 2009). Daily energy intake for the patient requiring dialysis is the same as that for the patient not having dialysis. It may be difficult for patients to achieve this level of energy intake, and nutritional supplements with high energy density may be necessary.

Medical Management of Complications of Renal Failure

Chronic kidney disease affects many body systems. Multiple complications may arise because of the loss of renal function. The patient should be monitored closely and have any complication treated.

Even though patients with mild to moderate kidney failure are able to maintain fluid balance, these patients are less able to respond to a rapid infusion of sodium and are prone to fluid overload. Most patients with renal failure who experience fluid overload respond to a combination of dietary sodium restriction and diuretic therapy with a loop diuretic given daily.

Hyperkalemia usually develops in the patient who is oliguric or has a GFR of 20 to 25 mL/min. Patients who continue to ingest a large amount of potassium in the diet, have illness or infection, or are taking medications that increase or spare potassium (ACE inhibitors, ARBs, potassium-sparing diuretics) are also at risk for hyperkalemia (Murphy & Byrne, 2009). Patients should be educated about foods that are high in potassium. For some patients, a low dose of Kayexalate (5 grams with each meal) can lower the serum potassium concentration (Thomas & Porter, 2007).

Patients with chronic kidney disease tend to retain hydrogen ions and progressively develop metabolic acidosis. Treatment of even mild acidemia is desirable, because the acidic state may lead to worsening bone breakdown. Also, uremic acidosis can diminish albumin synthesis, eventually causing loss of lean body mass and weakness (Murphy & Byrne, 2009). Treatment consists of administration of sodium bicarbonate 0.5 to 1 mEq/kg per day (Wilson, Shannon, & Shields, 2011). Sodium levels should be carefully monitored along with arterial blood gases. Phosphate retention starts early in renal disease owing to decreased filtration. The parathyroid gland hypersecretes parathyroid hormone (PTH) to correct both hyperphosphatemia and hypocalcemia, often resulting in secondary hyperparathyroidism (Murphy & Byrne, 2009). Dietary phosphate restriction may delay the development of secondary hyperparathyroidism, but this can be accomplished only by limiting protein intake, which may not be acceptable. In addition, some foods that contain phosphorus also contain calcium (e.g., milk), meaning that the patient needs to rely on calcium supplementation to improve calcium levels (Rolfes, Pinna, & Whitney, 2009). Vitamin D may be given to facilitate calcium absorption.

Phosphate binders are often given if dietary measures are unsuccessful or if the patient has persistent hyperphosphatemia. The most widely used phosphate binder is calcium carbonate. The dose ranges from 2.5 to 20 g/day and is increased gradually until the serum phosphate falls or hypercalcemia ensues (Thomas & Porter, 2007). Close monitoring of the serum calcium concentration is needed, as hypercalcemia is a common complication of this therapy.

Safety Alert *The nurse needs to teach patients who take phosphate binders that these medications are most effective when taken with meals to bind dietary phosphate.*

Another phosphate binder is sevelamer (Renagel). Sevelamer is a cationic polymer that binds with phosphate through ion exchange and does not contain calcium or aluminum (Wilson et al., 2011). It is used in patients who cannot tolerate calcium carbonate or who exhibit a persistent hyperphosphatemia. Other phosphate binders such as aluminum hydroxide, magnesium hydroxide, and calcium citrate should be avoided because of their side effects of aluminum toxicity, as well as hypermagnesemia with the magnesium hydroxide. All phosphate binders have limited binding capacity and should be used in conjunction with a carefully planned diet that restricts phosphorus when possible.

The anemia associated with chronic renal failure is due primarily to reduced production of erythropoietin. Although most patients with chronic kidney disease have anemia, the patient should be evaluated for other causes before a therapy to treat the anemia is instituted. In patients with end-stage renal disease, epoetin alfa (EPO) or darbepoetin alfa therapy helps to correct the anemia. The goal of treatment is for the hemoglobin to be 11 to 12 g/dL. Dosing is 80 to 120 units/kg subcutaneously or intravenously per week. The hemoglobin level should be tested weekly, and the dose or frequency should be adjusted as needed. Darbepoetin alfa, another erythropoietic agent, has a longer half-life and greater biologic activity than recombinant erythropoietin and can be scheduled weekly, every 2 weeks, or monthly. The recommended starting dose for patients with chronic renal failure is 0.45 mcg/kg per week subcutaneously or intravenously (Thomas & Porter, 2007). For an adequate response to erythropoietin or darbepoetin, the patient should have sufficient iron stores. Patients are most commonly given 325 milligrams of ferrous sulfate 3 times daily. Any vitamin B_{12} or folic acid deficiencies should be corrected prior to therapy (Wilson et al., 2011). Severe anemia may require the infusion of packed red blood cells. See Chapter 55 for a discussion of anemia.

Safety Alert *Nurses need to teach patients about the signs of thrombotic events, such as chest pain, difficulty breathing, shortness of breath, changes in mentation, and/or persistent headache (Wilson et al., 2011).*

A tendency to bleed is present in both acute and chronic kidney disease due to platelet dysfunction. If the patient is asymptomatic with regard to bleeding, no therapy is indicated. If the patient is actively bleeding or is scheduled for an invasive procedure, then therapy may consist of the administration of desmopressin acetate (DDAVP), which improves platelet function by increasing levels of factor VIII, administration of cryoprecipitate, and the initiation of dialysis (Thomas & Porter, 2007; Wilson et al., 2011). See Chapter 55 for a discussion of bleeding disorders.

Patients with advanced renal failure may present with uremic pericarditis. They will complain of fever, pleuritic chest pain, pericardial friction rub, and shortness of breath. This development is an indication to institute dialysis. With dialysis, most patients will have a resolution of chest pain and a decrease in the size of the effusion. See Chapter 33 for a discussion of pericarditis.

If end-stage renal disease goes untreated, the patient will develop uremic neuropathy with dysfunction of the central and peripheral nervous systems, including encephalopathy that may lead to seizures and coma. Signs of sensory dysfunction, such as restless leg or burning feet syndrome, are frequent presentations of uremic neuropathy. These signs and symptoms usually indicate the need to initiate dialysis. See Chapter 23 for a discussion of encephalopathy.

Nursing Management

With chronic kidney disease, management is aimed at slowing the progression of the disease to end-stage renal disease and avoiding complications. The nurse has a key role in educating the patient regarding control of underlying causes such as diabetes and hypertension. It is important for the nurse to explain why infection, volume depletion, and the taking of nephrotoxic medications must be avoided to prevent further deterioration of renal function. As the patient reaches end-stage renal disease, management moves to dialysis or renal transplantation. The Nursing Process: Patient Care Plan outlines nursing care for chronic renal failure (see p. 1230).

NURSING PROCESS: Patient Care Plan for Chronic Renal Failure/Chronic Kidney Disease

Assessment of Renal and Urinary Status Using Gordon's Functional Health Patterns:

- Health Perception Health Management Pattern
- Nutrition Metabolic Pattern
- Activity Exercise Pattern

Subjective Data

Assessment of Fluid Status

How much fluid have you been taking in?

Have you felt short of breath?

Have you gained weight? If so, how much?

Assessment of Nutritional Intake

Describe your usual intake pattern.

Is this intake sufficient?

Do you have religious dietary restrictions or practices?

Who prepares your meals?

How often do you exercise?

Do you feel you have enough energy?

Assessment of Activity Tolerance

Are you able to perform activities of daily living?

Do you experience pain or fatigue that interferes with activity?

Are there activities you feel you are unable to do?

Assessment of Knowledge of Disease Process

What causes renal failure?

What is the relationship of fluid and dietary restrictions to renal disease?

What is your understanding of renal failure?

What is your understanding of lifestyle changes to slow the progression of your disease?

Objective Data

Assessment of Fluid Status

Assess:

- Patient weight
- Skin turgor
- Presence of edema
- Blood pressure
- Respiratory effort and lung sounds.

Assessment of Nutritional Intake

Assess:

- General appearance
- Weight
- Hair, nails, and skin
- Muscle mass
- Edema.

Assessment of Activity Tolerance

Assess strength and balance.

Assess response to activity by taking vital signs at rest and then after performing an activity.

Assess coping strategies.

Assessment of Knowledge of Disease Process

Patient is able to articulate understanding of disease process.

Patient verbalizes understanding of and follows treatment regimen.

Outcomes and Evaluation Parameters	Planning and Interventions with *Rationales*
1. NURSING DIAGNOSIS: Fluid Volume, Excess ***related to compromised regulatory mechanisms secondary to renal failure*** **(NANDA-I © 2012)**	
Outcome: Neither fluid volume excess nor deficient volume will occur. ***Evaluation Parameters:*** Demonstrates no rapid weight changes. Absence of edema. Normal skin turgor. Reports no difficulty breathing.	Assess dietary intake and habits that may contribute to excess fluid volume *to identify potential sources of fluid such as foods high in sodium, medications that contain fluid, or the amount of fluid taken with medications.* Weigh daily at the same time on the same scale. *Daily weight will help identify fluid changes.* Teach the patient/family the rationale for restrictions. *Understanding promotes cooperation.* Teach and encourage the need for frequent oral hygiene *to minimize dry mouth associated with fluid restriction.*
2. NURSING DIAGNOSIS: Nutrition, Imbalanced: Less Than Body Requirements ***related to need for increased high biologic value protein*** **(NANDA-I © 2012)**	
Outcome: The patient will maintain adequate nutrition. ***Evaluation Parameter:*** Maintenance of weight without loss of muscle mass.	Facilitate education with a renal dietary consultant. *Consultation can ensure a diet that provides optimal caloric and nutrient intake. Nutrition plays a key role in slowing disease progression, preventing complications, and controlling waste products and electrolytes.* Promote the intake of protein foods with high biologic value: eggs, meats, and dairy products. *Complete proteins provide positive nitrogen balance needed for growth and healing. Protein requirements differ for patients not on dialysis versus those on dialysis.* Monitor laboratory data. *Assessing data will help identify early changes in nutritional status.* Encourage frequent oral hygiene. *Poor oral hygiene leads to bad breath and taste in the mouth, which decreases the appetite.* Provide the patient with printed material outlining the dietary needs and restrictions *to aid the patient in selecting the proper foods.*

NURSING PROCESS: Patient Care Plan for Chronic Renal Failure/Chronic Kidney Disease, *continued*

3. NURSING DIAGNOSIS: Activity Intolerance *related to fatigue, anemia, and altered metabolic state* (NANDA-I © 2012)

Outcome: Patient will have a balance of rest and activity and be able to perform self-care without fatigue. ***Evaluation Parameters:*** Alternates rest and activity. Reports a decrease in fatigue and an increased sense of well-being. Participates in self-care activities.	Promote independence in self-care as tolerated *to promote self-esteem.* Encourage rest between activities *to promote activity within patient's limits.* Assess factors that may be contributing to fatigue: fluid and electrolyte imbalances, anemia, and depression *to identify factors contributing to fatigue.*

4. NURSING DIAGNOSIS: Therapeutic Regimen Management, Ineffective *related to lack of knowledge of disease process and treatment* (NANDA-I © 2012)

Outcome: Understands cause of renal failure and need for treatment. ***Evaluation Parameters:*** Patient can explain fluid and dietary restrictions and their relationship to kidney failure. Patient expresses the importance of managing any underlying disease processes that increase the risk of renal failure such as diabetes and hypertension. Uses written information to clarify questions.	Assess understanding of the disease process and factors contributing to the disease process *to provide a baseline for teaching needs.* Assist the patient to identify ways to incorporate treatment into his lifestyle *to help build self-esteem and facilitate adherence to restrictions.* Assist the patient to obtain written information about renal disease *to give the patient information that can be reviewed at home.*

Source: Adapted from Wilkinson, J. M., & Ahearn, N. R. (2009). *Prentice Hall nursing diagnosis handbook* (9th ed.). Upper Saddle River, NJ: Prentice Hall.

Initiation of Maintenance Dialysis

For patients with chronic kidney disease, the decision to initiate maintenance dialysis or renal transplantation involves discussion between the patient and the health care provider with consideration of subjective and objective data. It is important to explore with the patient her perception of the current quality of life and the changes that will occur in participating in a therapy that is technologically complex, such as dialysis, or with the transplantation of an organ. With hemodialysis, the treatment regimen is based on two factors: the restriction of certain nutrients and the removal of waste metabolites from the blood by regular dialysis. The management is effective only if the patient adheres closely to the therapeutic regimen. Although hemodialysis can effectively contribute to long-term survival of patients with ESRD, the morbidity and mortality rates of patients on dialysis remain high, especially due to cardiovascular disease. Approximately 33% of patients on hemodialysis survive past 5 years of treatment, whereas 70% of recipients of kidney transplant are alive after 5 years (Denhaerynck et al., 2007).

Early recognition of chronic renal failure allows for reno-protective therapy such as rigorous blood pressure control and protective dietary changes as discussed earlier. Ismail (2010) identifies the following absolute clinical indications to initiate renal replacement therapy:

- Pericarditis
- Volume overload or pulmonary edema that is refractory to diuretics
- Increasing hypertension that is minimally responsive to antihypertensive medications
- Progressive uremic encephalopathy or neuropathy
- Persistent nausea and vomiting.

Additional indicators include plasma creatinine concentration above 12 mg/dL or blood urea nitrogen greater than 100 mg/dL and a GFR less than 10 mL/min (Thomas & Porter, 2007).

When the decision has been made to begin renal replacement therapy, discussion should commence with the patient regarding the advantages and disadvantages of hemodialysis, peritoneal dialysis (continuous or intermittent), and renal transplantation (living or deceased donor).

Hemodialysis

To perform hemodialysis, the patient must have vascular access. For acute access, a dual-lumen venous catheter may be used. The outflow openings are proximal to the inflow openings on the opposite side to avoid dialyzing the same blood that was just returned to the vessel. The subclavian, internal jugular, and femoral veins are usually used for this short-term access, and the catheters can be inserted at the bedside. Percutaneous catheters in the subclavian or jugular vein may be left in place for 1 to 3 weeks. Catheters placed in the femoral vein can remain for up to 1 week.

For patients who require long-term or maintenance dialysis, vascular access is imperative. There are various forms of access, including arteriovenous fistula and arteriovenous graft (Figure 39–3◆). All of these allow access to the arterial circulation and return to the venous circulation.

Arteriovenous (AV) graft is the most common form of access for treating chronic kidney disease. The graft consists of a GORE-TEX tube that is surgically implanted into the forearm. A surgical incision is made; an artery and vein are identified, a tunnel (either straight or U-shaped) is created, and the graft is anastomosed to the artery and vein. After the surgical site is closed, the graft creates a raised area that looks like a large peripheral vein. The graft takes 2 to 4 weeks to mature. During dialysis, two large-bore needles are placed for outflow from and inflow to the graft. When the needles are removed, pressure is required until the bleeding subsides.

An AV fistula is the preferred access because it is associated with fewer complications (McCann, Einarsdóttir, Van Waeleghem, Murphy & Sedgewick, 2008). It is formed by creating a surgical incision, identifying a peripheral artery and vein, and then anastomosing the two. The anastomosis may be side to side, end to end, or end to side. The high pressure from the arterial flow creates engorgement of the vein that, when healed, allows a large-bore needle to be inserted for dialysis (McCann et al., 2008). The fistula must mature and may require weeks to months before developing sufficient flow. AV fistulas also have the rare potential of creating arterial insufficiency due to the high arterial blood flow diverted for dialysis. The symptoms that occur are known as *vascular steal syndrome*. The extremity becomes pale, cool, and painful. The nurse may assess patency of the fistula by palpation or auscultation.

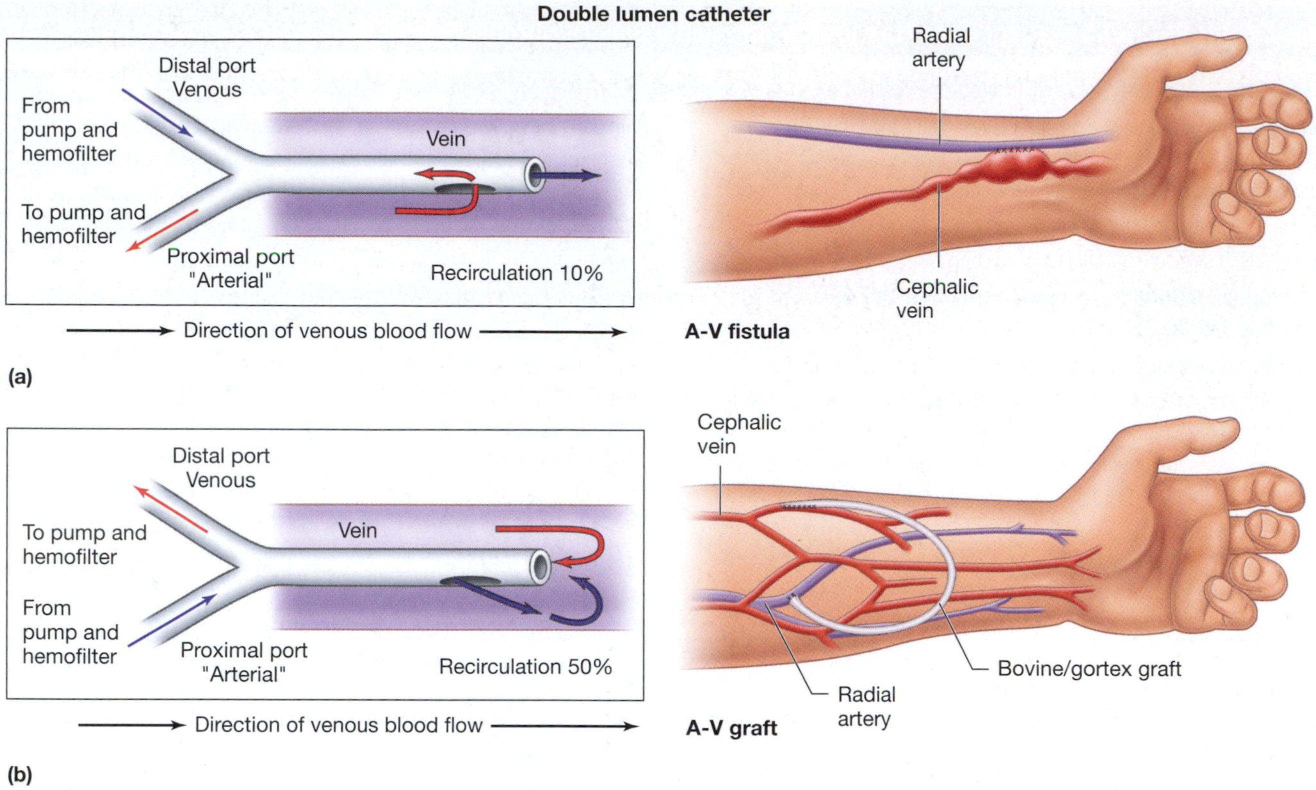

FIGURE 39–3 ◆ Types of vascular access.

A patent fistula has a thrill when palpated and a bruit when auscultated with a stethoscope. (See Chapter 29 for a description of a thrill and bruit.) The extremity should also be assessed and should be warm to the touch with good color.

The nursing responsibilities for vascular access devices are to protect the patency of the device and to prevent infection. Complications involving access devices are among the leading causes for hospitalization of patients on renal dialysis. Nursing management of complications of AV fistulas and grafts is described in Chart 39–5.

Safety Alert *The nurse should never do blood pressure measurements, blood draws, and intravenous lines on the arm that has the access device.*

Prior to dialysis, the nurse should evaluate the access site, labs, vital signs, and weight, as well as conduct a head-to-toe assessment (including lung sounds). Dialysis is initiated with the insertion of two large-bore needles, which are placed in the fistula or graft. Arterial blood is sent from the patient to the dialyzer with the assistance of a pump. Prior to dialysis, the machine is primed with saline so that no air is in the system. Heparin is added to the blood to prevent clotting. The blood then enters the dialyzer (a long plastic tube), which serves as a semipermeable membrane made of a synthetic material. Dialysis fluid, called dialysate, is pumped into the dialyzer. Through osmosis, diffusion, and ultrafiltration, exchanges of fluid, electrolytes, and toxins from the blood enter the dialysate. The dialysate and blood are pumped in opposite directions through the dialyzer to maintain a high osmotic and chemical gradient. After the blood leaves the dialyzer, it is returned to the patient via the venous line through the second needle. At the end of the procedure, the dialysis machine is filled with saline to return all of the patient's blood. Each dialysis treatment takes between 3 and 4 hours, and most patients require treatment 3 times a week. Although dialysis is very efficient, it does not remove all metabolites. After each dialysis treatment, electrolytes, toxins, and fluids increase. Contraindications to hemodialysis include hemodynamic instability, lack of access, and inability to anticoagulate. Chart 39–6 lists the complications of hemodialysis. The research topics related to chronic kidney

CHART 39–5 Nursing Management of Complications of AV Fistulas and Grafts

Complication	Nursing Management
Grafts and Fistulas	
Infection	Use aseptic technique when cannulating access.
Bleeding	Place gentle pressure on site. Monitor heparinization.
Thrombosis	Teach patients not to wear anything constrictive on the accessed arm. Teach patients that there should be no lab draws, IV starts, or blood pressures on the accessed arm.
Pseudoaneurysm	Avoid multiple cannulations in the same area. Pseudoaneurysms may need surgical resection.
Pain from vascular steal syndrome	Apply warm compresses and administer analgesia. Access may need revascularization.
Fistulas	
Inadequate blood flow	Teach patients to develop blood flow through daily exercises such as squeezing a ball while applying slight impedance to the flow distal to the access point.

CHART 39–6 Complications of Hemodialysis

Complication	Cause
Hypotension	Rapid removal of fluid
	Decreased cardiac output
Bleeding	Bleeding from access site after removal of needles
	Accidental disconnection of tubing
	Anemia and thrombocytopenia
	Heparinization
Muscle cramps	Unclear, possibly related to rapid removal of sodium and water
Hepatitis	Blood transfusions
	Poor infection control measures
Sepsis	Infection of the vascular access site
	Introduction of bacteria during dialysis due to poor technique or interruption of tubing
Disequilibrium syndrome (development of cerebral edema)	Rapid changes in the composition of the extracellular fluid due to removal of solutes (i.e., urea) from the blood more rapidly than from the brain

disease are outlined in the Research Opportunities box at the end of the chapter. The Evidence-Based Practice box below discusses the success of hemodialysis.

Peritoneal Dialysis

Peritoneal dialysis is the infusion of sterile dialyzing fluid through an implanted catheter in the abdominal cavity. The dialysate fluid bathes the peritoneal membrane that covers the abdominal organs and overlies the capillary beds. As occurs with hemodialysis, excess fluid and solutes travel via osmosis, diffusion, and active transport from the peritoneal capillary fluid through the capillary walls, through the peritoneal membrane, and into the dialyzing fluid (Urden et al., 2010). After a prescribed amount of time, the fluid is drained from the abdomen by gravity.

Peritoneal dialysis may be performed continuously or intermittently. Continuous ambulatory peritoneal dialysis (CAPD) requires multiple exchanges during the day and a continuous dwell overnight. The nighttime dwell can be accomplished by using an exchange device, which would perform two exchanges overnight. Continuous cyclic peritoneal dialysis (CCPD) has a continuous daytime dwell with an exchange device exchanging several cycles overnight. Intermittent peritoneal dialysis (IPD) has periods during which dialysate is in the abdomen (dwell time) and periods during which the peritoneal cavity has been drained (drain time).

Nursing Management

The amount of, concentration of, and dwell time for the dialysate are determined by the health care provider. In performing IPD, it is important to obtain baseline vital signs and weight for comparison at the end of the drainage. Measurement of abdominal girth and respiratory status is helpful as an indication of fluid retention. The nurse should assess for the presence of edema and obtain laboratory work for electrolytes, hematology, and blood glucose levels. In connecting or disconnecting the solution to the catheter, it is imperative to use aseptic technique to prevent entry of bacteria into the peritoneal cavity. Dialysate fluid should be at least body temperature to provide comfort and enhance exchange. When the fluid is removed, the nurse should assess its appearance. The outflow fluid should be straw colored and not be cloudy or blood tinged, which may indicate peritonitis. The nurse should compare the amount of dialysate infused to the outflow amount to determine whether less fluid drained out and the patient is fluid balance positive or whether there was more outflow volume than was infused and the patient is fluid balance negative. Notify the health care team if there is a significant difference either way.

EVIDENCE-BASED PRACTICE Hemodialysis

Clinical Problem

Registries within the United States and Europe show an increase in the prevalence and incidence of end-stage renal disease. Only 32% to 33% of patients on hemodialysis survive beyond their fifth year of treatment. In comparison, 70% of patients who have kidney transplants survive beyond their fifth year post transplant (Denhaerynck et al., 2007). The success of hemodialysis depends on following a regimen of fluid restriction, dietary guidelines, medication prescriptions, and attendance at hemodialysis sessions.

Research Findings

Denhaerynck et al. (2007) reviewed the literature, looking at the four aspects of success with hemodialysis. Results of adherence versus nonadherence to fluid restriction, dietary guidelines, medication prescriptions, and attendance at hemodialysis sessions varied greatly depending on how the study was conducted and which country the subjects were from. Most of the studies concentrated on adherence to fluid restriction; however, adherence to the entire prescribed medical regimen is crucial for achieving good therapeutic results and reducing morbidity and mortality. Fluid nonadherence can result in fluid overload and provoke shortness of breath, dizziness, anxiety, panic, lung edema, and hypertension. Nonadherence to medication and dietary regimens can result in elevated serum levels of phosphate, which plays a role in the development of secondary hyperparathyroidism and renal osteodystrophy. Elevated levels of phosphate also contribute to coronary artery disease, which significantly increases the risk for mortality. Skipping or shortening dialysis is associated with increased mortality. Denhaerynck and colleagues found in their review of the literature that "In studies in which the delivered dialysis dose was determined by assessing appointment nonadherence, the relationship between the dose and higher mortality or higher blood pressure was significant. Skipping at least one dialysis session per month has been associated with a 25% to 30% higher risk of death" (p. 230).

Implications for Nursing Practice

After reviewing the literature, Denhaerynck et al. (2007) believed that "The prevalence of nonadherence with the different aspects of the dialysis regimen seems considerable. However, assessment of nonadherence has 2 major obstacles: inconsistencies in definitions and invalid measurement methods" (p. 231). Despite these issues, the evidence suggests that the health care teams should stress the behavioral dimension of hemodialysis to guarantee the patient's adherence to the treatment regimen and adequate treatment results. Nurses are in an excellent position to affect the behavioral dimension by assessing adherence and by implementing adherence-enhancing interventions and patient teaching that have the ultimate goal of improving clinical outcomes.

Critical Thinking Questions with answers can be found in the Osborn Student Resources at nursing.pearsonhighered.com.

Source: Adapted from Denhaerynck, K., Manhaeve, D., Dobbels, F., Garzoni, D., Nolte, C., & De Geest, S. (2007). Prevalence and consequences of nonadherence to hemodialysis regimens. *American Journal of Critical Care, 16*(3), 222–235.

Weblink: Chronic Kidney Disease

Weblink: Healthy People 2020 Objectives for Kidney Disease

If it is anticipated that the patient will be doing CAPD or CCPD, the nursing focus is on teaching the patient and family how to perform the dialysis. Use of aseptic technique and recognition of signs and symptoms of infection (either infection at the catheter exit site or peritonitis) are particularly important aspects to be taught.

Kidney Transplantation

Kidney transplantation is the treatment of choice for end-stage renal disease because it improves the quality of life and reduces the mortality risk for most patients (Berns, 2009). Restoring kidney function reverses many of the pathophysiological changes that occur with renal failure. Transplantation eliminates the dependence on and restrictions associated with dialysis. Maintenance of a successful kidney transplant costs much less than the continued need for dialysis.

A kidney for transplantation may be from a living donor, such as a relative with compatible tissue type, or a human cadaver. The success of the transplant depends on careful tissue typing before the transplant and immunosuppression after the transplant. Rejection is the major complication related to transplant surgery. Rejection is potentially reversible and is treated with increased immunosuppression. Signs of rejection are oliguria, sudden weight gain, fever, a rise in BUN and serum creatinine, hypertension, and pain over the graft site. The long-term complications, which occur secondary to the use of immunosuppressive drugs, include infection, hypertension, chronic liver disease, bone demineralization, cardiovascular disease, cancer, cataracts, and gastrointestinal hemorrhage.

Nursing Management

The greatest risk to patients who have undergone transplantation is infection. Risk for infection occurs from invasive procedures, immunosuppression, and exposure to infected individuals. In caring for transplant patients, use of aseptic technique is paramount. It is important for the nurse to teach the patient and family that because of the immunosuppressive medications, the patient's response to infection will be muted. The nurse should teach them the importance of being sensitive to low-grade temperature elevation, any fever, and unexplained tachycardia. The nurse should also stress the importance of avoiding exposure to individuals who are known to have infections. See Chapter 19 for care of the postoperative patient. The National Guidelines box provides a listing of recommendations and resources for patients with chronic kidney disease.

Collaborative Management

To provide the best care for patients with chronic kidney disease, an interdisciplinary team is often needed. In order to meet desired patient outcomes, it is essential that this interdisciplinary team communicate openly with one another in developing and evaluating care of the patient and family (IOM [Institute of Medicine], 2010). Working with a renal dietitian is very beneficial. To slow progression of the disease, protein and phosphorus are restricted. Carbohydrates are increased to ensure that the patient has adequate caloric intake to prevent tissue catabolism. As the disease progresses, sodium intake is limited and fluids may be restricted. The kidneys' ability to excrete potassium is decreased; therefore, potassium intake is also limited. Providing a fact sheet listing foods that are to be restricted or limited is helpful. Sample menus help the patient plan daily menus that incorporate the restrictions. Patients may also benefit from psychological counseling to help them cope with a chronic illness and the uncertain future it entails.

Health Promotion

Chronic kidney disease is a significant public health problem and a source of poor quality of life for those afflicted. Although genetics has a large influence on the development and progression of chronic kidney disease, environmental influences and personal behaviors may also be involved. *Healthy People 2020* (www.HealthyPeople.gov) presents 14 objectives, with the goal of reducing new cases of chronic kidney disease and its complications, disability, death, and economic costs:

1. Reduce the proportion of the U.S. population with chronic kidney disease.
2. Increase the proportion of persons with chronic kidney disease who know they have impaired renal function.
3. Increase the proportion of hospital patients who incurred acute kidney injury who have follow-up renal evaluation in 6 months post discharge.
4. Increase the proportion of persons with diabetes and chronic kidney disease who receive recommended medical evaluation.

NATIONAL GUIDELINES for Chronic Kidney Disease

Topic	Recommendation
Screening and diagnosis	Assess markers of kidney damage in patients at high risk for chronic kidney disease (CKD): blood pressure twice a year (more frequently as needed), serum creatinine, estimated GFR every 1 to 2 years (more frequently as needed), albumin–creatinine ratio, urinalysis, lipid panel, electrolytes, and BUN.
Risk factor management and patient education	In patients at risk for CKD, evaluate and manage comorbidities (such as diabetes and hypertension) with each routine health exam and educate about lifestyle changes (such as smoking cessation and weight reduction) with each routine health exam.
Core principles of treatment	In patients with CKD: review medications, ensure that vaccinations are up to date, reduce sodium, incorporate self-management behaviors, and develop clinical action plans based on the stage of kidney disease at each routine health exam. Stage 1 treatment: Monitor GFR yearly. Educate about lifestyle changes. Treat hypertension. Stage 2 treatment: Refer to nephrologist. Continue education and treatment for hypertension. Stage 3 treatment: Refer to nephrologist to examine for abnormalities in parathyroid, vitamin D, calcium, and phosphorus. Avoid nephrotoxic drugs. Stage 4 treatment: Refer to nephrologist, provide CKD education. Avoid nephrotoxic drugs. Stage 5 treatment: Renal replacement (dialysis).

Source: Michigan Quality Improvement Consortium. (2008). Diagnosis and management of adults with chronic kidney disease. Retrieved from http://www.guideline.gov/content.aspx?id=24799.

5. Increase the proportion of persons with diabetes and chronic kidney disease who receive recommended medical treatment with angiotensin-converting enzyme inhibitors or angiotensin II receptor blockers.
6. Improve cardiovascular care in persons with chronic kidney disease.
7. Reduce the death rate among persons with chronic kidney disease.
8. Reduce the rate of new cases of end-stage renal disease.
9. Reduce kidney failure due to diabetes.
10. Increase the proportion of chronic kidney disease patients receiving care from a nephrologist at least 12 months before the start of renal replacement therapy.
11. Improve vascular access for hemodialysis patients.
12. Increase the proportion of dialysis patients wait-listed and/or receiving a deceased donor kidney transplant within 1 year of end-stage renal disease start (patients <70 years old).
13. Increase the proportion of patients with treated chronic kidney disease who receive a transplant.
14. Reduce deaths in persons with end-stage renal disease.

Gerontologic Considerations

The normal physiologic changes associated with aging have a significant effect on the renal system, making the older population at greater risk for renal and urinary disorders. In the United States, the highest incidence rate of end-stage renal disease occurs in patients older than 65 years of age. Age is an independent predictor of chronic kidney disease because the process of aging causes various structural and functional changes in the kidney. The kidneys become smaller, and there is a notable decrease (up to 30% to 50%) in glomerular number by age 70. A person's glomerular filtration rate peaks during the thirties at approximately 120 mL/min/1.73 m^2, and shows an annual mean decline of approximately 1 mL/min/y/1.73 m^2 to reach a mean value of 70 mL/min/1.73 m^2 at the age of 70. This rate of decline is also affected by race, gender, genetic variance, and other risk factors such as diabetes and hypertension (Arora & Batuman, 2011).

Safety Alert *Medications that are excreted primarily by the kidneys require modification of dosage and/or frequency. Older patients with chronic kidney disease who are taking digitalis must have careful dosage titration, as 80% to 90% of the drug is excreted by the kidneys (Wilson et al., 2011).*

Incontinence is a commonly reported problem in older adults (Friedman, 2011). Some of the age-related changes that may increase the risk of incontinence include decreased bladder capacity, increased frequency of urination, decreased muscle tone in women, and an enlarged prostate in men (Friedman, 2011). Other contributors to incontinence are chronic disease (such as diabetes), decreased mobility, cognitive impairment, and medications (Friedman, 2011). Health care providers should assess patients for incontinence.

The incidence of bladder cancer increases with age. The average age at diagnosis is 68 or 69 years. Men are 3 times as likely as women to develop bladder cancer. The risk factors are chronic bladder irritation and cigarette smoking, which contributes to over half of bladder tumors (Mauk, 2010).

As women experience the decline of hormones after menopause, the loss of estrogen affects the muscle tone of the genitals and causes thinning of the vaginal mucosa, which disrupts healthy vaginal flora. A randomized double blind controlled trial of intravaginal cream ovestin (estriol) was conducted in 102 postmenopausal females with chronic cystitis. The patients were divided into two groups. Group 1 ($n = 52$) received standard therapy; group 2 ($n = 50$) received standard therapy plus ovestin (daily intravaginal administration for 2 weeks, then twice a week). Final results were evaluated 1 year after therapy. Before the treatment, 94% of patients had subnormal levels of blood estradiol. One year after the treatment, positive results were achieved in 91.3% of patients in group 2 and 65.8% of patients in group 1 ($p < 0.001$). In group 2 patients, ovestin significantly reduced pollakiuria, nocturia, episodes of urgent urinary incontinence, and painful voiding. The percentage of patients with leukocyturia diminished from 100% to 8%, the percentage with bacteriuria decreased from 74% to 4%, the percentage with vaginal lactobacilli increased from 0% to 56%, and enterobacterial contamination of the vagina fell from 66% to 12%. Vaginal pH decreased from 6.0 to 3.6. The addition of ovestin to standard therapy reduced the number of cystitis recurrences 11-fold and the days of antibacterial therapy 12.4-fold. Side effects of ovestin (vaginal pruritus) were seen in 4% of the patients (Head, 2008).

Research

Research related to chronic kidney disease in which the nurse can participate focuses on improving the quality of life for the patient with chronic disease.

Weblink: National Kidney Foundation

RESEARCH OPPORTUNITIES Related to Chronic Kidney Disease

Research	Clinical Impact
Is it possible to regenerate kidney tissue (Imai, Tarundeep, Rosenberg, & Gupta, 2009)?	Discovering whether kidneys can regenerate will improve understanding of physiology as well as improve possible treatment options and patient outcomes.
When is the best time to start dialysis (Cooper et al., 2010)?	Starting dialysis at the optimal time may help improve patient outcomes.
What is the best screening to determine whether there are bone density issues in chronic kidney disease patients (National Kidney Foundation, n.d.)?	Early detection of bone density loss can promote early treatment and perhaps prevention of fractures.
What is the best indicator of adequate nutrition in chronic kidney disease patients (National Kidney Foundation, n.d.)?	Ongoing assessment of protein needs will help improve patient outcomes.
What screening indicators are most effective in patients with diabetes and chronic kidney disease (National Kidney Foundation, n.d.)?	Screening tools, such as albumin, may help improve outcomes and slow the progression of kidney disease.

READ: **History of Present Illness** >> Laboratory Study Results >> Critical Thinking Questions

Dale Johnson, a 72-year-old male, came to the emergency department (ED) complaining of right lower abdominal/groin pain. He stated that the pain was 8 on a 1-to-10 scale and had started suddenly after he returned from the airport, where he had lifted heavy luggage. He was found to have an incarcerated right inguinal hernia with bowel necrosis. He was taken to the operating room for bowel resection and repair of his hernia. He received 100 mL of normal saline IV and 300 mL of blood product in the ED. His output was 110 mL of urine via Foley catheter and 200 mL gastric content via nasogastric tube.

After surgical repair, Mr. Johnson was admitted to the medical–surgical unit. On postoperative day 1, his total urine output for the day was 230 mL. Despite receiving multiple fluid boluses, his urine output remained low, and he had a rise in his serum creatinine and BUN. On the morning of postoperative day 2, he was transferred to the ICU for fluid management and strict monitoring of his intake and output.

Medical–Surgical History

Mr. Johnson has no significant medical history and takes aspirin, multivitamins, fish oil, folic acid, and calcium daily. His family history is significant for adult-onset diabetes.

Social History

Mr. Johnson has never smoked. He occasionally drinks alcohol. He is married and lives with his wife.

Physical Exam

Mr. Johnson is in bed with the head of the bed up 30 degrees. He opens his eyes to voice and follows commands. He complains of lethargy and a mild headache. Breath sounds are clear bilaterally. His abdomen is soft and slightly tender at the surgical site. The surgical site is clean, dry, and intact. His bowel sounds are decreased. The extremities are warm with 3+ pulses to all. You note 2+ dependent edema to the lower extremities.

READ: History of Present Illnesses >> **Physical Exam** >> Admitting Medical Records >> Laboratory Study Results

Admitting Medical Orders

- Service: surgical ICU service
- Diagnosis: incarcerated right inguinal hernia, acute kidney injury
- Allergies: penicillin
- Diet: NPO
- Vital signs with oxygen saturation every 1–2 hours and prn
- Accu-Cheks: before meals and at bedtime
- Activity: bed rest; up to chair bid
- Call house officer if temp > 38.5°C; SBP >180 or < 90; pulse >110 or < 50 or resp rate > 30 or < 8; O_2 sat < 92%, urinary output < 30 mL/hr × 2 hours; blood sugar < 50 or > 150
- IVs: D5.45NS; titrate fluids to equal output plus 500 mL/day
- Foley to gravity drainage
- Strict I&O
- Weigh daily
- Respiratory care: incentive spirometer every hour when awake
- DVT prophylaxis: sequential compression device to lower extremities

Scheduled Medications

- Famotidine 20 mg IV bid
- Regular insulin SC sliding scale
- Hydromorphone 0.2 mg/mL concentration IV per PCA, incremental 0.2 mg, lock-out 6 min

PRN Medications

- Diphenhydramine 12.5 mg IV q6h prn itching

Ordered Laboratory Studies

- Electrolyte panel every am
- Complete blood count every am

READ: History of Present Illnesses >> **Laboratory Study Results** >> Critical Thinking Questions

Test	Day 1	Day 2	Day 3
WBC	17.8/mm^3	21.7/mm^3	12.3/mm^3
RBC	5.97/mm^3	5.80/mm^3	5.25/mm^3
Hgb	17.1 g/dL	16.8 g/dL	15.4 g/dL
Hct	51.1%	49.6%	46.2%
Platelets	867/mm^3	815/mm^3	658/mm^3
Na	138 mEq/L	139 mEq/L	140 mEq/L

Test	Day 1	Day 2	Day 3
K	4.0 mEq/L	4.2 mEq/L	4.9 mEq/L
Cl	104 mEq/L	106 mEq/L	109 mEq/L
Total CO_2	26 mEq/L	25 mEq/L	26 mEq/L
BUN	14 mg/dL	25 mg/dL	33 mg/dL
Creatinine	1.0 mg/dL	1.9 mg/dL	2.1 mg/dL
Glucose	175 mg/dL	151 mg/dL	173 mg/dL

DOCUMENT:

- >> Summary of Hospitalization
- >> Pathophysiology Form
- >> Laboratory Values
- >> Laboratory Results Explanation

APPLY:

- >> List of Potential Nursing Diagnoses
- >> Concept Map
- >> Critical Thinking Questions and Concept Map

APPLY: History of Present Illness >> Laboratory Study Results >> **Critical Thinking Questions**

1. What contributed to Mr. Johnson's acute renal failure?
2. What serum electrolyte changes would you expect to see?

Answers to Critical Thinking Questions can be found in Appendix D in the Osborn Student Resources at nursing.pearsonhighered.com.

NCLEX® PRACTICE

1. The urine output of a patient in cardiogenic shock has been 200 mL for the last 24 hours and the serum creatinine level is 1.5 mg/dL. Which of the following lab values indicates to the nurse that the patient may be in acute kidney failure?

1. BUN is 16 mg/dL.
2. Calcium is 8.7 mg/dL.
3. Sodium level is 152 mg/dL.
4. Potassium is 4.8 mEq/L.

2. A patient with suspected pyelonephritis has urine sent for analysis and culture. The nurse checks for which result to substantiate the diagnosis?

1. High specific gravity
2. Low leukocyte count
3. Casts in the urine
4. Negative for protein

3. A patient has been diagnosed with the onset of acute kidney injury. Which of the following does the nurse recognize as a prerenal precipitating cause in the patient?

1. Urinary calculi
2. Recent intravenous pyelogram with contrast dye
3. Congestive heart failure
4. Crushing injury

4. What should the nurse include in the plan of care for a patient in order to prevent the cardiovascular complications associated with chronic renal failure?

1. Apply a nondrying lotion to the skin.
2. Maintain a low-fat, low-carbohydrate diet.
3. Evaluate ankles for edema daily.
4. Restrict fluid and salt intake.

5. A patient has a neobladder created following a radical cystectomy due to bladder cancer. The nurse plans to teach the patient which technique to incorporate into the home management routine?

1. Bladder irrigation
2. Kegel exercises
3. Self-catheterization
4. Stoma wafer change

6. A patient receiving hemodialysis tells the nurse that the worst part of the treatment is the severe leg cramps that he gets a few hours after the procedure. Which of the following should the nurse offer to this patient as an explanation of this problem?

1. "The leg cramps are because of the blood transfusions that you receive."
2. "The leg cramps are because of an infection that will need to be treated."
3. "The leg cramps are because of the extra water and salt that is being removed."
4. "The leg cramps are because you aren't eating enough protein."

Answers to NCLEX Practice questions can be found in Appendix D in the Osborn Student Resources at nursing.pearsonhighered.com. Practice additional NCLEX questions online at the Student Resources site.

Pearson Nursing Student Resources Find additional review materials at: **nursing.pearsonhighered.com**

REFERENCES

Adams, M. R., & Koch, R. W. (2010). *Pharmacology connections to nursing practice.* Upper Saddle River, NJ: Pearson Education.

American Cancer Society. (2012a). Bladder cancer. Retrieved from http://www.cancer.org/cancer/bladdercancer/detailedguide/bladder-cancer-key-statistics

American Cancer Society. (2012b). Kidney cancer (adult): Renal cell carcinoma. Retrieved from http://www.cancer.org/Cancer/KidneyCancer/DetailedGuide/kidney-cancer-key-statistics

American Cancer Society. (2012c). Kidney cancer (adult): Renal cell carcinoma. Retrieved from http://www.cancer.org/Cancer/KidneyCancer/DetailedGuide/kidney-cancer-adult-risk-factors

Arora, P., & Batuman, V. (2011). Chronic kidney disease. Retrieved from http://emedicine.medscape.com/article/238798-overview#aw2aab6b2b5

Berns, J. S. (2009). Patient information: Dialysis or kidney transplantation—which is right for me? Retrieved from http://www.uptodate.com/contents/patient-information-dialysis-or-kidney-transplantation-which-is-right-for-me

Cohen, E. P. (2011). Nephrotic syndrome. Retrieved from http://emedicine.medscape.com/article/244631-overview#a0156

Cooper, B. A., Branley, P., Bulfone, L., Collins, J. F., Craig, J. C., Fraenkel, J. B. . . ., et al. (2010). A randomized, control trial of early versus late initiation of dialysis. *New England Journal of Medicine, 363*(7), 609–619.

Curhan, G., Aronson, M., & Preminger, G. (2008). Diagnosis and acute management of suspected nephrolithiasis in adults. Retrieved from http://www.uptodate.com/patients/content/topic.do?topicKey=~PEEs8wkDGf.awB&selectedTitle=1~150&source=search_result

Denhaerynck, K., Manhaeve, D., Dobbels, F., Garzoni, D., Nolte, C., & De Geest, S. (2007). Prevalence and consequences of nonadherence to hemodialysis regimens. *American Journal of Critical Care, 16*(3), 222–235.

Dirkes, S. (2011). Acute kidney injury: Not just acute renal failure anymore? *Critical Care Nurse, 31*(1), 37–49. doi: 10.4037/ccn2011946

Dirkes, S., & Hodge, K. (2007). Continuous renal replacement therapy in the adult intensive care unit. *Critical Care Nurse, 27*(2), 61–81.

Friedman, S. (2011). Urinary function. In S. E. Meiner (Ed.), *Gerontologic nursing* (4th ed., pp. 545–563). St. Louis: Mosby.

Goshorn, J. (2009). Acute renal failure. In M. L. Sole, D. G. Klein, & M. J. Moseley (Eds.), *Introduction to critical care nursing* (5th ed., pp. 475–508). St. Louis: Mosby.

Grantham, J. J. (2008). Autosomal dominant polycystic kidney disease. *New England Journal of Medicine, 358*, 1477–1485.

Hall, P. M. (2009). Nephrolithiasis: Treatment, causes and prevention. *Cleveland Clinic Journal of Medicine, 76*(10), 583–591. doi:10.3949/ccjm.76a.09043

Hautmann, S. F., & Leveillee, R. J. (2008). Nephrostomy. Retrieved from http://emedicine.medscape.com/article/445893-overview_

Head, K. A. (2008). Natural approaches to prevention and treatment of infections of the lower urinary tract. *Alternative Medicine Review, 13*(3), 227–244.

Huether, S. E., & Forshee, B. A. (2010). Alterations of renal and urinary tract function. In K. L. McCance, S. E. Huether, V. L. Brashers, & N. S. Rote (Eds.), *Pathophysiology: The biologic basis for disease in adults and children* (6th ed., pp. 1365–1401). St. Louis: Mosby.

Imai, N., Tarundeep, K., Rosenberg, M. E., & Gupta, S. (2009). Cellular therapy of kidney diseases. *Seminars in Dialysis, 22*(6), 629–635. doi:10.1111/j.1525-139X.2009.00654.x

IOM (Institute of Medicine). (2010). *The future of nursing: Leading change, advancing health.* Washington, DC: The Academic Press.

Ismail, N. (2010). Indications for initiation of dialysis in chronic renal failure. Retrieved from http://www.uptodate.com/contents/indications-for-initiation-of-dialysis-in-chronic-kidney-disease?source=search_result&selectedTitle=23%7E150

Jones, R. E., Brashers, V. L., & Huether, S. E. (2010). Alterations of hormonal regulation. In K. L. McCance, S. E. Huether, V. L. Brashers, & N. S. Rote (Eds.), *Pathophysiology: The biologic basis for disease in adults and children* (6th ed., pp. 727–780). St. Louis: Mosby.

Kaplan, A., Appel, G., & Pusey, C. (2009). Treatment of anti-GBM antibody (Goodpasture's) disease. Retrieved from http://www.uptodate.com/patients/content/topic.do?topicKey=~OaJEblyepxfF.0&selectedTitle=1~150&source=search_result

Kee, J. L. (2010). *Laboratory and diagnostic tests with nursing implications* (8th ed.). Upper Saddle River, NJ: Prentice Hall.

Kumar, V., Abbas, A. K., Fausto, N., & Mitchell, R. N. (2007). *Robbins basic pathology* (8th ed.). Philadelphia: Saunders.

Laskowski, I. A., & Schwing, L. (2009). Renal vein thrombosis. Retrieved from http://emedicine.medscape.com/article/460752-overview

Lerma, E. V., Agraharkar, M., & Kelly, B. (2011). Acute tubular necrosis. Retrieved from http://emedicine.medscape.com/article/238064-overview

Lopez, V. M., & Glauser, J. (2010). A case of renal artery thrombosis with renal infarction. *Journal of Emergencies, Trauma, & Shock, 3*(3), 302. Retrieved from http://www.onlinejets.org/text.asp?2010/3/3/302/66569

Mauk, K. L. (2010). *Gerontological nursing: Competencies for care* (2nd ed.). Sudbury, MA: Jones and Bartlett Publishers.

McCann, M., Einarsdóttir, H., Van Waeleghem, J. P., Murphy, F., & Sedgewick, J. (2008). Vascular access management 1: An overview. *Journal of Renal Care, 34*(2), 77–84.

MDGuidelines. (2011). Neurogenic bladder. Retrieved from http://www.mdguidelines.com/neurogenic-bladder

Menghini, L., Leporini, L., Scanu, N., Pintore, G., La Rovere, R., Di Filippo, E. S., et al. (2011). Effect of phytochemical concentrations on biological activities of cranberry extracts. *Journal of Biological Regulators & Homeostatic Agents, 25*(1), 27–35.

Michigan Quality Improvement Consortium. (2008). Diagnosis and management of adults with chronic kidney disease. Retrieved from http://www.guideline.gov/content.aspx?id=24799

Murphy, F., & Byrne, G. (2009). Chronic kidney disease stages 4–5: Patient management. *British Journal of Cardiac Nursing, 4*(2), 59–66.

National Institute of Diabetes and Digestive and Kidney Diseases (NIDDK). (2007a). Kidney stones in adults. Retrieved from http://kidney.niddk.nih.gov/kudiseases/pubs/stonesadults/

National Institute of Diabetes and Digestive and Kidney Diseases (NIDDK). (2007b). Urinary retention. Retrieved from http://kidney.niddk.nih.gov/kudiseases/pubs/UrinaryRetention/

National Institute of Diabetes and Digestive and Kidney Diseases (NIDDK). (2008). Nerve disease and bladder control. Retrieved from http://kidney.niddk.nih.gov/kudiseases/pubs/nervedisease/

National Kidney Foundation. (n.d.). KDOQI clinical practice guidelines research recommendations. Retrieved from http://www.kidney.org/professionals/kdoqi/pdf/KDOQIGuidelinesResearchUPDATE.pdf

National Kidney Foundation. (2011). About chronic kidney disease. Retrieved from http://www.kidney.org/professionals/KLS/aboutCKD.cfm

National Kidney and Urologic Diseases Information Clearinghouse (NKUDIC). (2010). Kidney and urologic diseases statistics for the United States. Retrieved from http://kidney.niddk.nih.gov/kudiseases/pubs/kustats/

Pellatt, G. C. (2008). Neurogenic continence. Part 1: Pathophysiology and quality of life. *British Journal of Nursing, 17*(13), 836–841.

Peacock, P. R. (2011). Management of acute complications of acute renal failure. Retrieved from http://emedicine.medscape.com/article/777845-overview#aw2aab6b3

Porth, C. M., & Matfin, G. (2009). *Essentials of pathophysiology: Concepts of altered health states* (2nd ed.). Philadelphia: Lippincott Williams & Wilkins.

Professional guide to diseases (9th ed.). (2009). Philadelphia: Lippincott, Williams, & Wilkins.

Rolfes, S. R., Pinna, K., & Whitney, E. (2009). *Understanding normal and clinical nutrition* (8th ed.). Belmont, CA: Wadsworth Cengage.

Sachdeva, K., Jana, B. R. P., Javeed, M., Makhoul, I., & Curti, B. (2010). Renal cell carcinoma. Retrieved from http://emedicine.medscape.com/article/281340-overview

Saxena, R. (2008). Alport syndrome. Retrieved from http://emedicine.medscape.com/article/238260-overview

Shelton, G. (2011). Bladder cancer. In C. H. Yarbro, D. Wujcik, & B. H. Gobel (Eds.), *Cancer nursing: Principles and practice* (7th ed., pp. 1080–1090). Boston: Jones and Bartlett Publishers.

Shoff, W. H., Green-McKenzie, J., Edwards, C., Behrman, A. J., & Shepherd, S. M. (2010). Pyelonephritis, acute. Retrieved from http://emedicine.medscape.com/article/245559-overview

Stevenson, F. T., Sharma, S., & Verrelli, M. (2009). Goodpasture syndrome. Retrieved from http://emedicine.medscape.com/article/240556-overview

Terris, M. K., & Sajadi, K. P. (2009). Urethritis. Retrieved from http://emedicine.medscape.com/article/438091-overview

Thomas, D. J., & Porter, B. O. (2007). Renal problems. In L. M. Dunphy, J. E. Winland-Brown, B. O. Porter, & D. J. Thomas, *Primary care: The Art and science of advanced practice nursing* (2nd ed., pp. 562–606). Philadelphia: F. A. Davis.

Uppot, R. N. (2009). Emergency nephrostomy tube placement for acute urinary obstruction. *Techniques in Vascular and Interventional Radiology, 12*, 154–161. doi:10.1053/j.tvir.2009.08.010

Urden, L. D., Stacy, K. M., & Lough, M. E. (Eds.). (2010). *Critical care nursing: Diagnosis and management* (6th ed.). St. Louis: Mosby.

U.S. Renal Data System. (2010). *USRDS 2010 annual data report: Atlas of chronic kidney disease and end-stage renal disease in the United States.* Bethesda, MD: National Institutes of Health, National Institute of Diabetes and Digestive and Kidney Diseases. Retrieved from http://www.usrds.org/atlas.htm

Vourganti, S., & Maniam, P. (2008). Hydronephrosis and hydroureter. Retrieved from http://emedicine.medscape.com/article/436259-overview

Wilson, B. A., Shannon, M. T., & Shields, K. M. (2011). *Pearson nurse's drug guide 2011.* New York: Pearson.

Wood, L. S. (2011). Renal cancer. In C. H. Yarbro, D. Wujcik, & B. H. Gobel (Eds.), *Cancer nursing: Principles and practice* (7th ed., pp. 1634–1649). Boston: Jones and Bartlett Publishers.

Nursing Management of Patients with Reproductive Disorders

9 UNIT

Content in Unit 9 that addresses the **Institute of Medicine (IOM)** competencies, **Nursing Core Competencies (NCC)**, the **Quality and Safety Education for Nurses (QSEN)** competencies, and **Concepts** for concept-based learning is listed below.

Competencies	Feature or Text	Location
IOM, QSEN, NCC Providing patient-centered care	Genetic Considerations: Sex Chromosome Disorders, page 1244	Chapter 40
	Genetic Considerations for Female Reproductive Disorders, page 1259	Chapter 41
	Nursing Process: Patient Care Plan for Prostate Cancer, page 1301	Chapter 42
	Nursing Process: Patient Care Plan for STIs, page 1326	Chapter 43
	Nursing Process: Patient Care Plan for Breast Cancer Post-Modified Mastectomy, page 1347	Chapter 44
IOM, QSEN, NCC Working in teams	Collaborative Management, page 1266	Chapter 41
	Collaborative Management, pages 1300, 1306	Chapter 42
	Collaborative Management, pages 1327	Chapter 43
	Collaborative Management, page 1346	Chapter 44
IOM, QSEN, NCC Employing evidence-based practice	Evidence-Based Practice: Using CAM, page 1281	Chapter 41
	Evidence-Based Practice for Prostate Cancer, page 1299	Chapter 42
	Evidence-Based Practice: Screening for Chlamydia, page 1315	Chapter 43
	Evidence-Based Practice: Lymphadema, page 1345	Chapter 44
IOM, NCC Applying quality and safety improvement	Safety Alerts, pages 1244, 1245 1248, 1250	Chapter 40
	Safety Alerts, pages 1256, 1267, 1272, 1274	Chapter 41
	Safety Alerts, pages 1289, 1296, 1305	Chapter 42
	Safety Alerts, page 1321	Chapter 43
NCC Applying ethical and legal responsibilities	Ethical Issues of Fertility Programs, page 1274	Chapter 41
	Ethical Issues for Brachytherapy, page 1298	Chapter 42
	Ethical Issues: Young Woman with an STI, page 1325	Chapter 43
	Ethical Issues in Cancer Genetic Testing, page 1339	Chapter 44
	Ethical Issues: Women and Research on Breast Disorders, page 1351	Chapter 44
NCC Educating patients	Patient Teaching & Discharge Priorities for Hysterectomy, page 1279	Chapter 41
	Patient Teaching & Discharge Priorities for Male Reproductive Disorders, pages 1292, 1294, 1296, 1304	Chapter 42
	Patient Teaching & Discharge Priorities for Post-Mastectomy Breast Cancer, page 1349	Chapter 44
Concepts covered in Unit 9 include:	Infection Cell division Elimination	Reproduction Sexuality Violence

CHAPTER 40

Nursing Assessment of the Patient with Reproductive Disorders

Patricia Caudle
Kathleen Osborn

Outcome-Based Learning Objectives

After studying this chapter, the learner will be able to:

1. Describe the structures and function of the male and female reproductive systems.
2. Identify pertinent subjective and objective data related to the reproductive systems and information about sexual function that should be obtained in an assessment.
3. Identify risk factors for reproductive system disorders.
4. Differentiate normal from abnormal findings obtained from the physical assessment for males and females.
5. Describe age-related changes in the male and female reproductive systems.
6. Discuss the implications for health promotion related to the reproductive systems of females and males.

KEY TERMS

andropause p.1251
cervicitis p.1248
colostrum p.1249
cremasteric reflex p.1250
cryptorchidism p.1250
endometriosis p.1245
endometrium p.1242
estrogen p.1241
friable p.1248
galactogenesis p.1241
hot flashes p.1251
hydrocele p.1250
hypogonadism p.1251
hypospadias p.1245
lactation p.1241
lithotomy p.1247
menarche p.1245
menopause p.1251
menses p.1242
moliminal p.1245
neutraceutical p.1251
orchidectomy p.1245
ovum p.1242
oxytocin p.1241
perianal p.1244
perimenopause p.1249
progesterone p.1241
prolactin p.1241
retroverted p.1249
varicocele p.1250
vasectomy p.1245

ASSESSMENT OF THE FEMALE AND MALE reproductive systems requires an understanding of the anatomy, an ability to communicate, a nonjudgmental attitude, gentleness, and a high degree of empathy and compassion. Most women and men consider the genital area very private, and many may be reluctant to talk about their concerns or allow examination by the nurse. The nurse should not be offended if the patient asks for a nurse examiner of the same gender. Privacy and confidentiality are very important and should be maintained at all times.

The female and male reproductive systems include sexual organs, the lower urinary system, and the anorectal area. This means that assessment of the reproductive system is complex and must include history and physical examination involving all three systems. This chapter outlines the important components of the female and male reproductive system assessment. Concepts discussed here introduce the learner to assessment skills needed to care for patients with disorders of the female and male reproductive systems that are discussed in Chapters 41 to 44.

Anatomy and Physiology of the Reproductive Systems

The Female Reproductive System

The female reproductive system includes the breasts and the external and internal genitalia. This section will describe the anatomy of the breasts and the genitalia as well as menstrual cycle physiology.

Breast

The female breast tissue extends from the second to the sixth rib on either side of the sternum and covers the pectoralis major muscle (Figure 40–1◆). The skin over the breasts is the same color as other skin and may have striae (stretch marks). On the anterior surface of each breast is the nipple, surrounded by the areola (pigmented skin around the nipple). The areola has sebaceous glands (skin glands that secrete sebum that lubricates the skin) that may be raised and more active during pregnancy (Montgomery's tubercles). Sebaceous glands

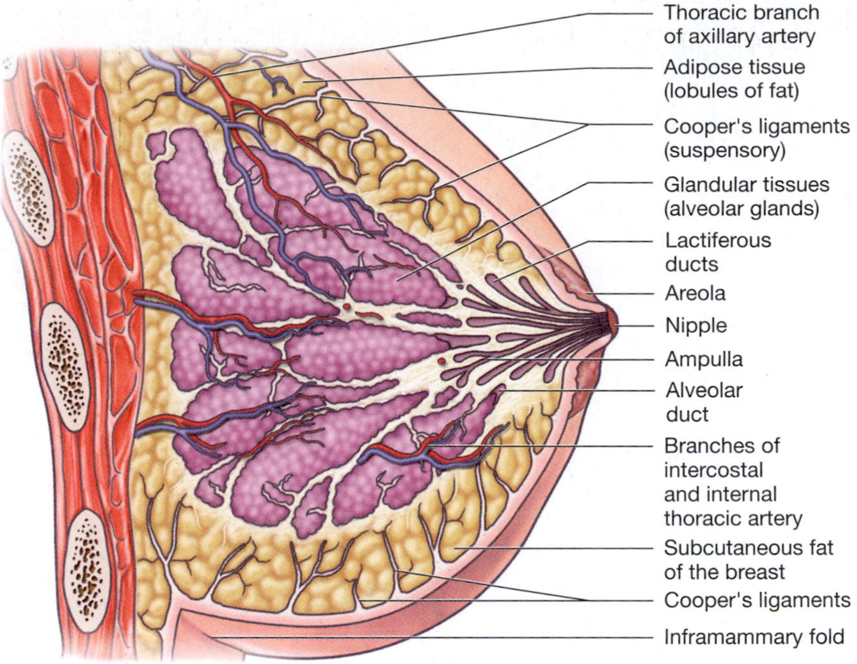

FIGURE 40–1 ◆ The female breast.

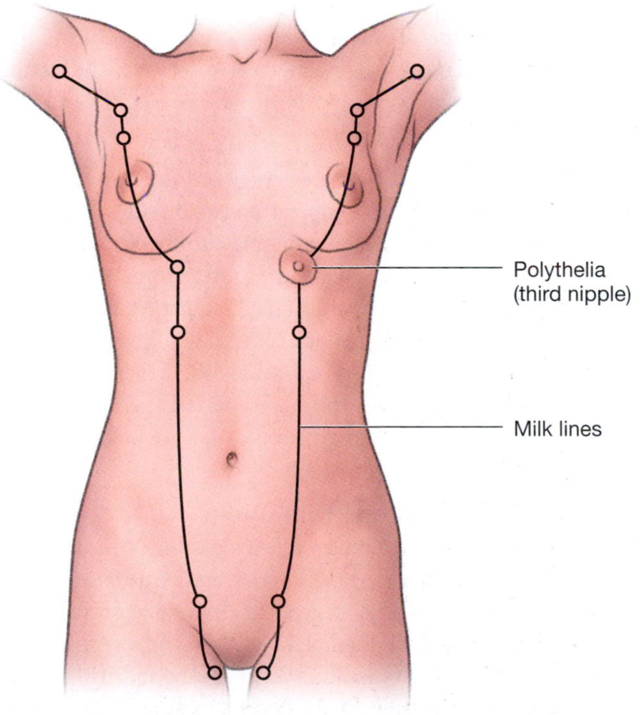

FIGURE 40–2 ◆ Supernumerary nipples.

help to moisturize the nipple to make it more pliable ("Montgomery's tubercles," 2011). Occasionally, additional nipples known as supernumerary nipples are seen along a line (the "milk line") from the axilla to the upper thigh on either side (Figure 40–2◆). These small nipples may be mistaken for moles. However, they are considered normal variants and are benign (Metzker, 2010).

Each breast is made up of glandular, connective, and adipose (fatty) tissue. The glandular tissue includes 15 to 20 lobes suspended from ducts that drain into sinuses. The sinuses are near the nipple and are drained by smaller ducts on the nipple surface. The lobes are further divided into lobules where the milk is produced during lactation. The connective tissue provides support via ligaments within the breast (also called Cooper's ligaments). Adipose tissue completes the structure of the breasts and determines their size (see Figure 40–1) (Gabriel & Maxwell, 2009).

Physiologically, breast tissue responds to **estrogen** (steroid female hormone produced by the ovary and placenta), **progesterone** (steroid female hormone produced by the ovary and placenta), **prolactin** (hormone produced in the anterior pituitary), and **oxytocin** (hormone produced in the hypothalamus and released by the posterior pituitary) in the processes of **galactogenesis** (the manufacture of milk from available nutrients) and **lactation** (breast-feeding) (Schauler & Potak, 2009). The cyclic changes in estrogen and progesterone levels each month cause changes in the breasts as they prepare for lactation, even though a pregnancy does not always occur. This cyclic exposure to hormonal change is thought to be a factor in the development of breast cancer (American Cancer Society [ACS], 2010b).

Lymph nodes drain the breasts to the axilla, clavicular area, and mediastinum; to the opposite breast; and into glands in the liver (Lymph nodes, 2012). The lymph nodes of the axilla and clavicular area are accessible to physical examination.

Female External Genitalia

The female external genitalia depicted in Figure 40–3◆ (p. 1242) have several components that are important to recognize during examination. These include the mons, the vulva (labia majora and labia minora), the clitoris (erectile tissue at the apex of the labia minora), the urinary meatus (urinary opening above the vaginal opening), and the introitus (opening to the vagina). The introitus is surrounded by an elastic line of connective tissue called the hymenal ring (Rosenblatt, 2010b). At the posterior aspect of the urinary meatus, a pair of Skene's glands can be found at 5 and 7 o'clock to the opening. Bartholin glands are found at 5 and 7 o'clock to the opening of the vagina.

Weblink: Breast Anatomy
Weblink: Lymph Nodes
Weblink: Supernumeray Nipple

Weblink: The Menstrual Cycle Fact Sheet

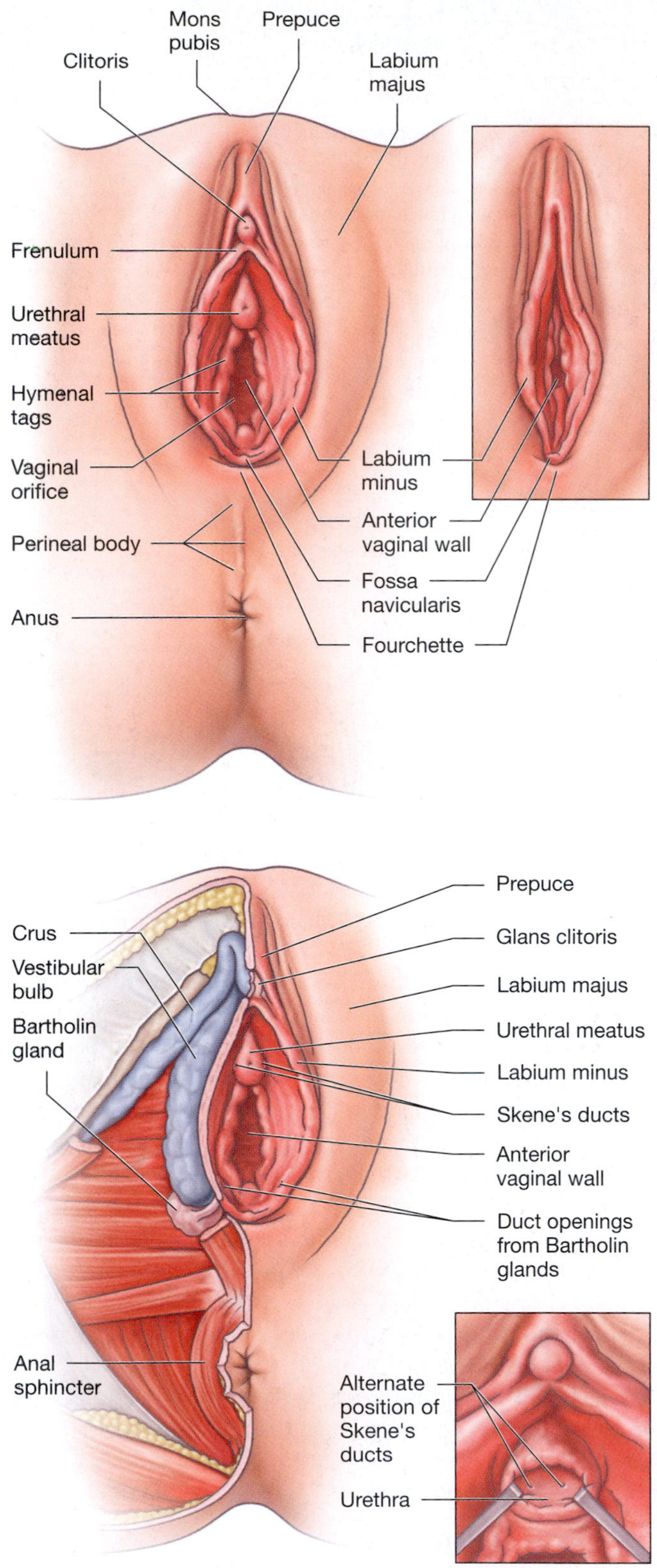

FIGURE 40–3 ◆ Female vulva including anus.

Female Internal Reproductive Organs

Internally, the female reproductive organs include the uterus (muscular, hollow organ where the embryo matures before birth), the fallopian tubes (hollow tubes from the uterus to the ovaries, where fertilization occurs), and the ovaries (female gonads). The opening to the uterus is the cervix, located at the internal end of the vagina (Rosenblatt, 2010c).

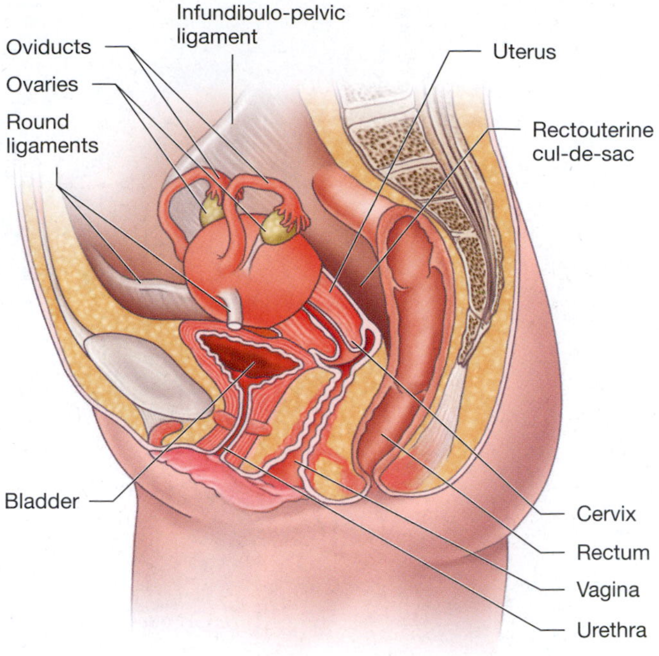

FIGURE 40–4 ◆ Female internal genitalia.

The vagina, a stretchable tube that extends from the cervix to the external opening and is covered by a mucous membrane. The uterus and vagina sit between the rectum and the bladder (Figure 40–4◆).

Lymph Nodes

The lymph nodes of the female external and internal reproductive organs that are accessible to examination are the superficial inguinal nodes, including the horizontal grouping and the vertical grouping. These nodes are found on each side of the groin. The horizontal grouping is below the inguinal ligament, and the vertical grouping lines up along the great saphenous vein (the long vein of the lower extremities). The horizontal group drains the lower abdomen, the superficial external genitalia, the anal canal, the perineum, and the lower vagina. The vertical group drains the upper leg (Bickley & Szilagyi, 2007).

Physiology of the Menstrual Cycle

The menstrual cycle is a complex physiological process that involves the hypothalamus, pituitary gland, ovaries, and **endometrium** (uterine lining). It is a physiologic process that normally occurs regularly for all women between the ages of 12 and 50. The menstrual cycle is usually 28 days long but varies from 25 to 45 days in length. The cycle begins with the first day of menses. **Menses**, or cyclic vaginal bleeding, is the result of the thickened uterine lining that was constructed during the previous cycle that is being sloughed or shed. As this occurs, the hypothalamus recognizes a need to secrete gonadotropin-releasing hormone (GnRH). This hormone stimulates the anterior pituitary to release follicle-stimulating hormone (FSH), which in turn stimulates a few of the follicles that exist on the ovary. From the follicles that first respond to the FSH, one follicle becomes dominant. This growing follicle produces and secretes estrogen. When estrogen peaks, it signals the anterior pituitary to release luteinizing hormone (LH). When LH peaks, ovulation occurs. That is, the dominant follicle extrudes the **ovum** (an egg or female germ cell). The ovum travels to the fallopian tube and into the uterus (Hall, 2012).

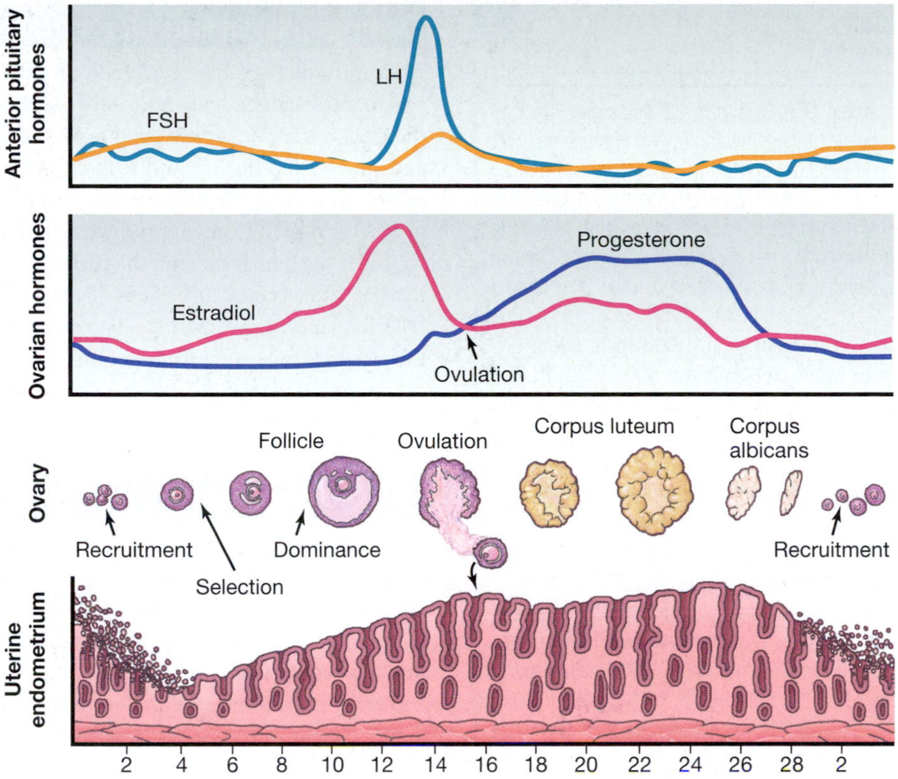

FIGURE 40–5 ◆ The menstrual cycle.

Under the influence of estrogen, the uterine lining, known as the endometrium, has been thickening before ovulation. After ovulation, the lining begins to proliferate; that is, it gets even thicker. It now has more nutrients available in the event that the ovum is fertilized and implantation into the uterine lining occurs (Hall, 2012).

After ovulation, the follicle remnants become the corpus luteum (yellow body), which secretes progesterone. Progesterone causes the "fluffing" of the uterine lining. If a fertilized ovum does not implant, then at the end of 12 to 14 days the corpus luteum regresses and progesterone decreases. When this happens, the uterine lining sloughs and menses begins (Hall, 2012). Figure 40–5◆ is a graph that shows when in the cycle each event occurs.

The Male Reproductive System

The male reproductive system includes the breast and external and internal genitalia. The male breast features a small nipple and an areola. There is a small amount of undeveloped breast tissue that may enlarge (gynecomastia) in response to certain medications. The male external genitalia are pictured in Figure 40–6◆. They include the penis and scrotum (skin pouch that contains the testes). The penis is made up of erectile tissue and contains the urethra (tube that drains urine from the bladder to the outside). At the end of the penis is the glans which has an expanded base called the corona. The glans is covered by the foreskin, a loose hood of skin. At the tip of the penis is the urinary meatus (opening of the urethra to the outside). Within the scrotum are the testis (organ that produces sperm), the epididymis (anatomic structure on the posterior of the testicle), and the spermatic duct. The spermatic duct is surrounded by blood vessels, and together they form the spermatic cord (Degeneres & Huether, 2010). As the spermatic cord ascends into the abdomen via the inguinal canal, it becomes the vas deferens (duct that carries sperm and semen to the seminal vesicles and prostate).

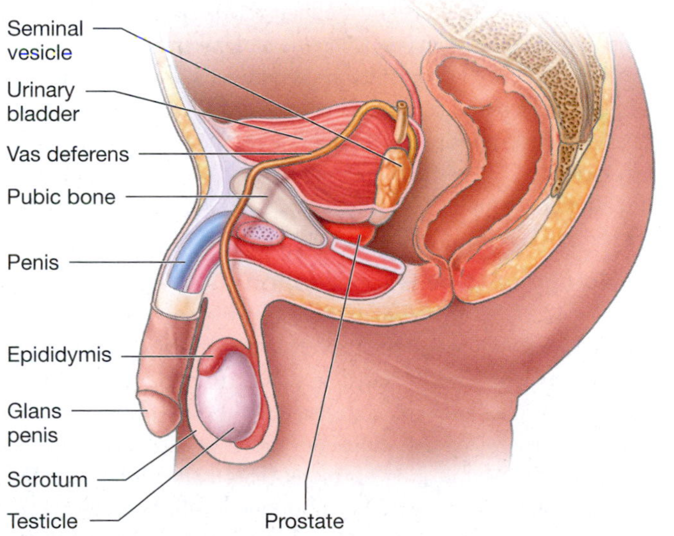

FIGURE 40–6 ◆ Male genitalia.

Sperm pass through the vas deferens to the seminal vesicles (fingerlike structures behind the prostate), which produce the majority of semen, and into the prostate (a gland at the bladder neck that the urethra passes through) to be mixed with prostate fluid before ejaculation during intercourse. The prostate is about 2.5 centimeters long with a median sulcus (groove) between two lateral lobes (Seidel, Ball, Dains, Flynn, Solomon, & Stewart, 2011). A third, anterior lobe is not palpable. The prostate is fibrous and firm to the touch.

The inguinal canal (tunnel for vas deferens) is medial to the inguinal ligament and has two openings: the external and internal inguinal rings. The external inguinal ring is accessible to examination. Inguinal

GENETIC CONSIDERATIONS
Sex Chromosome Disorders

Normal sperm occur in two types. One type has 22 autosomes and an X chromosome, and the other has 22 autosomes and a Y chromosome. Only one type of ovum is ready for fertilization, and it has 22 autosomes and an X chromosome. Therefore, it is the sperm's contribution to the coupling that will determine the sex of the child. In assessment of females and males, the nurse may examine individuals who have a sex chromosome disorder. The two most common examples are Klinefelter's syndrome and Turner's syndrome (Jorde, 2010).

Klinefelter's syndrome occurs in about 1 in 1,000 male births and usually involves an extra one or two X chromosomes (XXY or XXXY). This disorder is generally not identified until puberty when the male secondary sexual characteristics do not appear. Individuals with Klinefelter's syndrome have decreased testosterone, testicular atrophy, long legs and arms, feminine hair distribution, gynecomastia, a feminine voice, infertility, and mental retardation (Jorde, 2010).

Turner's syndrome is a monosomy disorder in which the sex chromosome has only one X chromosome and no corresponding X or Y. The phenotype (how the person will look or will display the abnormality) is female, but the ovaries do not develop, and female secondary sex characteristics such as breast development and pubic hair do not appear. This abnormality is rare, occurring in about 1 in 3,000 live births (Jorde, 2010). Other physical characteristics include short stature, webbing of the neck, amenorrhea (no menses), a wide chest, and heart defects.

Source: Jorde, L. (2010). Genes and genetic disease. In K. McCance & S. Huether, *Pathophysiology: The biologic basis for disease in adults and children* (6th ed., pp. 126–162). St. Louis: Mosby/Elsevier.

lymph nodes are located below the inguinal ligament in a horizontal configuration at the groin and along the femoral and great saphenous veins vertically on the upper thigh. The horizontal group drains the lower abdomen, buttock, external genitalia, anal canal, and **perianal** (situated or occurring around the anus) area. The vertical group drains the upper thigh. The testicles drain into lymph nodes in the abdomen. The abdominal lymph nodes are not accessible to palpation (Bickley & Szilagyi, 2007).

Physiology of Male Reproduction

Male reproductive physiology involves the hypothalamus, the pituitary gland, and the testis. The hypothalamus secretes gonadotropin-releasing hormone (GnRH) based on signals from the central nervous system and blood levels of testosterone. The GnRH travels to the anterior pituitary gland and causes the release of luteinizing hormone (LH) and follicle-stimulating hormone (FSH). Luteinizing hormone stimulates testosterone and other hormone synthesis in the Leydig cells of the testicle. The role of FSH in the male is not fully understood, although it appears to be necessary for sperm production. Leydig cells of the testis produce testosterone. Sertoli cells of the testis support and provide nutrients for spermatids (immature sperm) as they grow to become spermatozoa (mature sperm) (Degeneres & Huether, 2010). Information about sex chromosome disorders is presented in the Genetic Considerations box.

History

History, or what patients can tell about themselves and their health concerns, is the most important component of assessment. Much of what nurses do is based on what the patients are able to convey about how they feel and the symptoms they are having. This section discusses the health history related to the reproductive system.

Biographical and Demographic Data

After introductions have been completed, the patient is asked about age, marital status, occupation, address, and other data that will make the history specific to this patient. It is important to record the date and time of the history and to note the perceived reliability of the person providing the information. From this interview, clues begin to emerge related to any reproductive system problems. For instance, the older the female patient, the higher the risks are for breast, endometrial, and uterine cancer. See Chapters 41 and 44 for more about risks for cancer in women. The older the male patient, the higher the risks are for sexual dysfunction, prostate problems, and bladder cancer. See Chapters 42 and 44 for more about risk factors for cancer in men.

Chief Complaint

This section begins with the patient's reason for seeking medical care. The nurse should be aware from the beginning of the interview that emergent conditions must be reported as soon as the patient arrives, without waiting to complete the history. For example, a male complaining of severe scrotal pain of sudden onset may have testicular torsion and will lose the testicle without immediate attention by a surgeon. The female patient with very heavy vaginal bleeding who is weak might be experiencing a hemorrhage, and this needs to be reported right away. More information about testicular torsion is found in Chapter 42. More information about menstrual disorders and miscarriage is found in Chapter 41.

Safety Alert *Emergent conditions should be recognized and reported immediately. The nurse should not delay treatment with history taking when emergency medical treatment is needed.*

When the nurse has determined that there is no emergent condition, the patient is asked to describe the reproductive concern that has brought her or him into the health care system. The chief complaint is recorded in the patient's own words (Seidel et al., 2011). Once the chief complaint has been established, a description of the health concern follows. It is important to ask about the onset, location, duration, associated symptoms, any treatments tried, aggravating factors, and factors (other than treatments) that may alleviate the problem. For example, a male may complain of urinary frequency, urgency, difficulty beginning the urinary stream, and nocturia (frequency of urination at night) with gradual onset when he is describing symptoms of benign prostatic hyperplasia (BPH). See Chapter 42 for a complete description of BPH.

Current Medications

This section of the history should include a list of prescribed medications, illicit drugs, herbal remedies, over-the-counter drugs, home remedies, or vitamins that the patient is taking. It is important to record the name of the drug or herb, the dosage, and how often the patient is taking it. Some women who are taking birth control pills may forget to mention this, so it is a good habit for the nurse to ask women of childbearing age about birth control pills. The nurse should ask men with prostate problems whether they are taking saw palmetto. Men who are taking Viagra or similar medications may be hesitant to discuss this with the nurse. However, medications for erectile dysfunction have the potential for interacting with other drugs, such as cardiac medications, and causing harm; therefore, it is important to inquire about them.

Allergies

All patients should be asked about allergies to drugs, latex, foods, animals, insects, and environmental substances. If a patient has allergies, the medical record should be clearly marked so that the health care team is alerted.

Safety Alert *When a patient has a latex allergy, examination of that patient using latex gloves increases the risk for an adverse reaction, including anaphylactic shock. The nurse must be sure to ask about possible allergies before the examination begins.*

Past Medical History

This section of the history includes childhood and adult illnesses, immunizations, comorbid conditions, hospitalizations, diagnostic procedures and surgeries, and menstrual and obstetric histories. Here the discussion is about some parts of the patient's past history that may affect reproductive health.

Childhood Illnesses and Immunizations

Childhood diseases that affect the female patient's health or fertility or the health of her children need to be documented. For instance, any communicable disease that affected her health severely could affect her ability to have children. This could mean that she would need to prevent pregnancy or to have special care if she were to become pregnant. If a woman of childbearing age has not had rubella or been immunized for it, contracting rubella while she is pregnant could cause birth defects in her child.

The childhood disease of concern for men is mumps. This viral illness has the potential to affect the testicles, causing sterility. See Chapter 42 for further discussion of mumps orchitis.

Comorbid Illnesses and Hospitalizations

Medical comorbidities that may affect the reproductive system include diabetes, hypertension, hepatitis, and HIV. The male with diabetes or hypertension treated with certain antihypertensive drugs may experience impotence. Hepatitis and human immunodeficiency virus (HIV) are sexually transmitted infections (STIs) that may be life threatening. Females or males who have hepatitis or HIV may pass these diseases to their sexual partners. The nurse should determine whether the patient has been diagnosed and treated for a sexually transmitted infection such as chlamydia, gonorrhea, syphilis, or herpes. For women, it is also important for the nurse to ask whether they have ever had pelvic inflammatory disease (Kruszka & Kruszka, 2010). The nurse should ask about hospitalizations for any reproductive health concerns or chronic health problems and find out when the hospitalization occurred, what the problem was, and how it was treated.

Diagnostic Procedures and Surgeries

Past surgeries that may affect the woman who has a reproductive system problem may include breast surgeries, hysterectomy, bilateral tubal ligation, cervical laser surgery or cryosurgery, or any surgery for **endometriosis** (presence of uterine lining in sites other than within the uterus). See Chapter 41 for further discussion of surgeries of the reproductive system.

For women, procedures of particular interest in this section of the history include screenings or tests for breast cancer and cervical cancer. Mammograms, lump biopsies, or any other procedures for breasts would need to be dated and recorded in the history. It is also important to note the date of the last cervical cancer screening and the results of the Papanicolaou (Pap) test. If the patient has ever been diagnosed with cervical dysplasia or treated for an abnormal Pap test, it should be documented. Pap tests are discussed further in Chapter 43.

Men who have had prostate surgery may have increased incontinence or impotence. Other surgeries that may affect the male reproductive system or lower urinary system include **orchidectomy** (surgical removal of the testicles), **vasectomy** (surgical removal of a part or all of the vas deferens), or penile reconstruction due to epispadias (the urinary meatus is at the top or dorsal surface of the penis, between the penis and the bladder) or **hypospadias** (the urinary opening is on the ventral or bottom of the penis, between the scrotum and the distal end of the penis). See Chapter 42 for further discussion of surgeries of the reproductive system.

Menstrual History

For women, the menstrual and obstetric history should be included in the health history. The menstrual history should include age at **menarche** (first menstruation), length of time from first day of menstrual flow to first day of next menstrual flow (one cycle), number of days and characteristics of menses, regularity of cycles, **moliminal** symptoms (symptoms accompanying menstruation such as cramps, headache, breast tenderness, etc.), and the first day of the woman's last menstrual period. Older women need to be asked about menopause, including age at onset and symptoms such as hot flashes, vaginal dryness, night sweats, and insomnia (Danakas & Alvero, 2009).

Obstetric History

A woman's obstetric history includes the number of pregnancies, the number and date of premature and term births, and the number and date of spontaneous and therapeutic abortions. It is also important to determine whether the deliveries were spontaneous vaginal births or cesarean sections and whether there were any complications with either births or abortions (Barad, 2010).

Sexual History and Risks for Sexually Transmitted Infection

Healthy People 2020 has set 42 high-priority public health topic areas for this decade. Reducing the incidence of sexually transmitted disease is among the most important of the goals set to help improve the health of everyone in the United States (U.S. Department of Health and Human Services [DHHS], 2010). The steps toward achieving this goal include identifying people who are engaging in risky sexual behavior and helping them to choose safer practices. In working toward this goal, the nurse examiner can ask the patient about the last time the patient had intimate physical contact or sex with someone; whether the patient is content with his sex life; whether the patient has sex with men, women, or both; and whether the patient has any concerns about sexual health. Being in a mutually monogamous relationship decreases the risks for contracting or spreading sexually transmitted infection (Centers for Disease Control and Prevention [CDC], 2010a).

In settings where the patients may be at risk for sexually transmitted infection or HIV, more in-depth exploration of sexual practices may be indicated. The CDC has published a list of five areas to be explored along with counseling about the prevention of sexually transmitted infection and HIV. Chart 40–1 (p. 1246) lists specific questions that the CDC suggests using to elicit this history.

Family History

Explore the family history of women for mother, sister, maternal grandmother, or aunts with breast cancer. The occurrence of breast cancer in any of these relatives increases the risks for the patient (Latendrasse,

CHART 40–1 CDC Questions for Sexually Transmitted Infections

Exploring the Five Areas of Concern in the Prevention of Sexually Transmitted Infection (STI)

Partners

"Do you have sex with men, women, or both?"

"In the past 12 months, how many partners have you had sex with?"

Prevention of Pregnancy

"Are you or your partner trying to get pregnant?" If "no":

"What are you doing to prevent pregnancy?"

Protection from STIs

"What do you do to protect yourself from STIs?"

Practices

"To understand your risks for STIs, I need to understand the kind of sex you have had recently."

"Have you had vaginal sex, meaning 'penis in vagina sex'"? If "yes":

"Do you use condoms: never, sometimes, or always?"

"Have you had anal sex, meaning 'penis in anus sex'"? If "yes":

"Do you use condoms: never, sometimes, or always?"

"Have you had oral sex, meaning 'mouth on penis/vagina sex'"?

For Condom Answers

If "never": "Why do you not use condoms?"

If "sometimes": "In what situations, or with whom, do you not use condoms?"

Past History of STIs

"Have you ever had an STI?"

"Have any of your partners had an STI?"

Additional Questions to Identify Human Immunodeficiency Virus (HIV) and Hepatitis Risk

"Have you or any of your partners ever injected drugs?"

"Have any of your partners exchanged money or drugs for sex?"

"Is there anything else about your sexual practices that I need to know about?"

Source: Workowski, K., & Berman, S. (2010). Sexually transmitted disease treatment guidelines 2010. *Morbidity and Mortality Weekly Report, 59*(RR-12), 2–3.

McCance, & Morgan, 2010). This is also true of about 10% of cases of ovarian cancer.

There may be women whose mothers took diethylstilbestrol (DES) to prevent a miscarriage while pregnant with them. These daughters are at 40 times the risk of developing cancer of the vagina and cervix (CDC, 2010b). Therefore, it is important to ask women born between 1938 and 1971 whether they were exposed to DES while *in utero*.

Men should be asked whether their father or brother has prostate cancer. Early onset prostate cancer seems to occur in some families. African American men are particularly susceptible. See Chapter 42 for further discussion of inheritance of susceptibility to prostate cancer.

Social History

In this section of the history, the nurse examiner asks about the patient's work, hobbies, home situation, life experiences, leisure activities, support systems, and lifestyle. Work settings or hobbies may expose a person to hazardous materials that can increase the risk for infertility (female and male) and some forms of cancer. The nurse examiner should ask patients whether they work around hazardous conditions or materials such as excessive heat, radiation, heavy metals, or organic solvents and how they protect themselves (Seidel et al., 2011).

Another aspect of the social history involves the patient's relationships with others in the family or community. Patients facing diagnoses such as cancer of the reproductive organs will need support. Exploring the availability of support persons and discussing the patient's home situation will be important to the plan of care.

Cigarette Smoking and Substance Abuse

The nurse should explore patient habits such as cigarette smoking, alcohol use, or illicit drug use. There is evidence from cohort and case-control research that cigarette smoking and secondhand smoke increase the risks for cervical cancer (National Cancer Institute [NCI], 2010). Alcohol use and illicit drug use have been shown to increase the incidence of sexually transmitted infection and HIV (Abatangelo et al., 2010). Alcohol use as a contributor to the risk of breast cancer is discussed in Chapter 44.

It is best to ask directly, "Tell me about your use of alcohol" or "When was your last drink of alcohol?" If the patient answers in such a way that the nurse examiner is suspicious of problem drinking, then screening questions such as the CAGE questionnaire can be used to help identify alcohol abuse. CAGE stands for "cutting down, annoyance if criticized, guilty feelings, eye-openers" (Seidel et al., 2011).

The same direct approach should be used in questioning about illicit drug use. Direct questions, such as "Have you ever used any drugs other than those required for medical reasons?" and "Have you ever injected a drug?" work best to elicit this information from the patient (Bickley & Szilagyi, 2007).

Intimate Partner Violence

Violence affects people of all ages, both genders, and all religions, races, and socioeconomic groups. Intimate partner violence, whereby intimate partners inflict physical, sexual, or emotional injury, is very common (Torpy, Cassio, & Glass, 2010). In fact, *Healthy People 2020* lists injury and violence as top priority health issues in the United States (U.S. DHHS, 2010). People who suffer intimate partner violence are more likely to abuse alcohol and drugs and to have HIV or a sexually transmitted infection (Dunaif, 2012).

Intimate partner violence is difficult to discuss, but questions about abuse should be asked of all patients, both women and men. The only way to begin to change behavior is to uncover the abuse. Make it a habit to ask patients questions, such as "Are there times in your relationship that you feel unsafe or afraid?" or "Within the last year, have you been hit, kicked, punched, or otherwise hurt by someone you know?" (Seidel et al., 2011). Try to conduct the interview in private, away from family members or the patient's partner.

Physical Examination

After the history has been completed, the nurse examiner should ask the patient to disrobe and put on a gown for the physical examination. The gown should open in front for better access to the breasts and genitals of both the female and male patient. Assemble the equipment needed for the pelvic examination. The nurse examiner should step out of the room while the patient changes. The nurse examiner's hand hygiene and donning of gloves need to occur in the room, in front of the patient.

CHART 40–2 Equipment Needed for the Female Genital Examination

1. Examination gloves (latex or nonlatex, depending on whether the patient has a latex allergy)
2. A light source (gooseneck lamp or light that attaches to the speculum)
3. Speculum (choose size most appropriate for the patient)
4. Water-soluble lubricant
5. Pap smear equipment
6. Culture tubes for STIs or other bacterial infection

Female Examination

Chart 40–2 lists the equipment needed for the female examination. The nurse examiner should be accompanied by an assistant because of the intimate nature of this examination. This is true regardless of the gender of the nurse. During the physical assessment, the nurse should teach the patient about her body and about healthy lifestyles and choices.

Breasts

The breast examination is best done with the woman sitting at the end of the examination table. For inspection of the breast, she should be asked to open the gown so that her breasts are fully visible to the nurse examiner. The nurse examiner should inspect the breasts for size, shape, contour, dimpling, and inverted nipples; areas of increased vascularity; and erosion or inflammation of the nipple or areola. The inspection should be carried out while the patient's arms are at her side, then again when she raises her arms above her head or presses her hands to her hips to contract the pectoralis muscle. The woman should then be asked to lean forward, so that her breasts can move freely away from the chest wall. These maneuvers will move the breast and pull the suspensory ligaments in such a way that a tumor would cause dimpling or a bulge (Seidel et al., 2011).

The next portion of the breast examination is palpation. The nurse examiner asks the patient to lie down and raise one arm over her head. The nurse examiner places a small pillow or folded towel beneath the patient's shoulder on the side of the breast to be examined and palpates all the breast tissue. The palpation is done with the pads of the fingers in a circular pattern, in smaller circles as the nurse examiner nears the center of the breast. An alternative is the strip pattern, where the breast is palpated in linear strips that slightly overlap. All four quadrants of the breast are included, including the upper outer quadrant and the tail of Spence (a section of breast tissue that extends toward the axilla). End the palpation by gently squeezing the nipple between the thumb and forefinger to determine whether there is discharge from the nipple. The procedure is repeated for the other breast. The nurse examiner palpates for masses or tenderness. If there is nipple drainage, the nurse examiner collects a specimen on a slide and sends it to the laboratory for cytology (Seidel et al., 2011). To inspect the axilla for lesions, masses, or inflammation, the nurse examiner holds the patient's arm in a relaxed position and palpates for the axillary nodes by grasping the axillary fold and feeling for pectoral nodes along the pectoral muscle. Reaching high in the axilla with the fingers flat against the chest wall, the nurse examiner feels for the central nodes. Then the nurse examiner turns the examining hand and feels along the humerus for the lateral lymph nodes. Changing hands so that the arm is supported, the nurse examiner then uses the opposite hand to examine for subscapular nodes by feeling inside the posterior axillary fold and examines along the top and below the clavicle for supraclavicular and infraclavicular nodes. The entire procedure is then repeated for the opposite axilla (Seidel et al., 2011). If the woman has large, pendulous breasts, a bimanual (using both the nurse examiner's hands) examination of the breasts as she leans forward will help to palpate any masses.

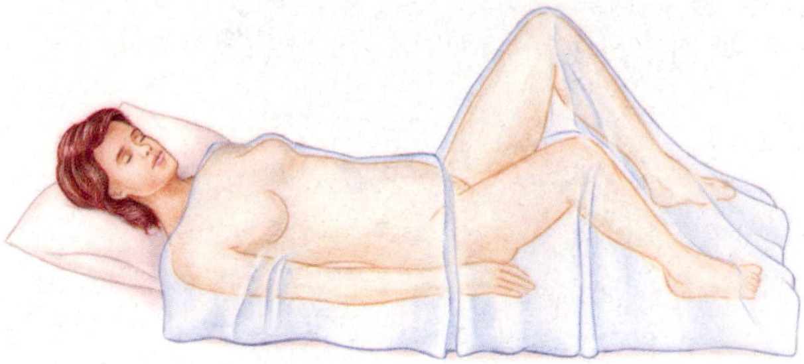

FIGURE 40–7 ◆ Female lithotomy position.

If the examination reveals a breast mass, nipple or areolar lesion, nipple discharge, abscess, or enlarged axillary nodes, these findings should be reported for immediate medical attention. While they are not emergent, it is very important that the problem be properly diagnosed and treated as soon as possible to prevent complications.

External Genitalia

While the patient is still lying down, the nurse examiner palpates the groin for swollen inguinal lymph nodes. When this is completed on both sides, the nurse examiner should help the patient to move down on the table and to put her feet into the stirrups for the external genitalia and internal genitalia examinations. Her buttocks should be right at the edge of the end of the examination table with her knees flexed and legs spread so that the external genitalia are accessible to examination. This is the **lithotomy** position (Figure 40–7◆). The nurse examiner should raise the head of the examination table to help the patient be more comfortable and drape her lower body and legs.

The nurse examiner should sit on a stool for the examination and lower the drape so that the nurse can see the patient's face during the examination. When ready to inspect the external genitalia, the nurse should tell the patient when she is going to touch her before the nurse moves a gloved hand to the vulva to spread the tissues for inspection of the entire vulva and perineum. The nurse inspects for lesions, warts, vesicles, changes in pigmentation, signs of abuse such as bruises or lacerations, swollen Bartholin glands, or vaginal discharge or blood at the introitus. Figure 40–8◆ (p. 1248) illustrates the technique for examining the Bartholin glands. The nurse asks the patient to bear down, as if to move her bowels, and observes for any bulges of cystocele (relaxation of the anterior vagina wall under the urinary bladder) or rectocele (relaxation of the posterior vaginal wall over the rectum) or prolapsed uterus at the introitus. Cystocele and rectocele are discussed in Chapter 41. If there are any bulges, the nurse palpates to differentiate the cystocele from the rectocele. The nurse also palpates the Bartholin glands at 7 and 5 o'clock to the introitus and palpates with one finger for the location of the cervix within the vagina to determine the location of the cervix (Seidel et al., 2011).

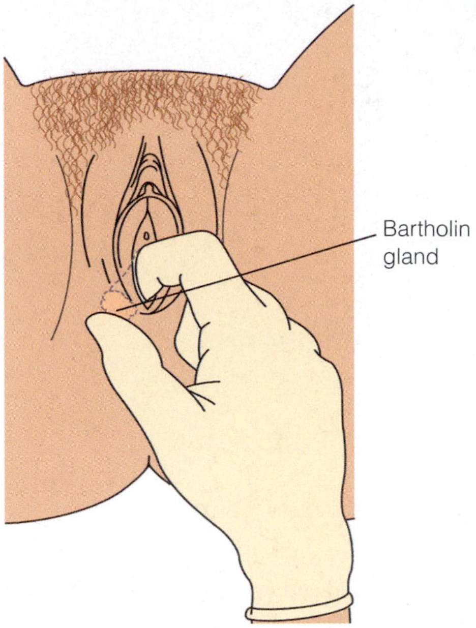

FIGURE 40–8 ◆ Palpation of the Bartholin glands.

Safety Alert *If very painful swelling of the Bartholin gland is discovered, the patient should be referred immediately to a gynecologist for treatment.*

Vagina and Cervix

The nurse places a small amount of water-soluble lubricant on the speculum and tells the patient that she is about to insert the speculum to visualize the cervix. A small amount of water-soluble lubricant will not interfere with the Pap smear or any tests for infection (Harmanli & Jones, 2010). The nurse grasps the speculum in the dominant hand, spreads the labia with the opposite hand, and inserts the speculum, pointing it down and back toward the cervix (Figure 40–9◆). The nurse opens the speculum to visualize the cervix and inspects for any lesions, warts, or increased vascularization on the cervix or the vaginal walls. The nurse inspects the cervical os (opening) for drainage and obtains specimens for Pap smear or STI cultures as appropriate (Figure 40–10◆). The nurse notes whether the cervix bleeds slightly on contact with the specimen collector. If blood is present, this means that the cervix is **friable** (easily damaged) and the nurse examiner should proceed gently. The nurse rotates the speculum to visualize the remainder of the vagina before removing it. Discard the speculum appropriately (Seidel et al., 2011).

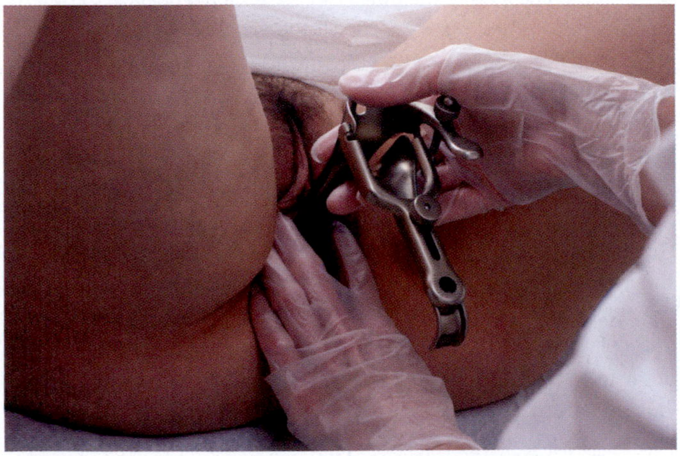

FIGURE 40–9 ◆ Speculum insertion.

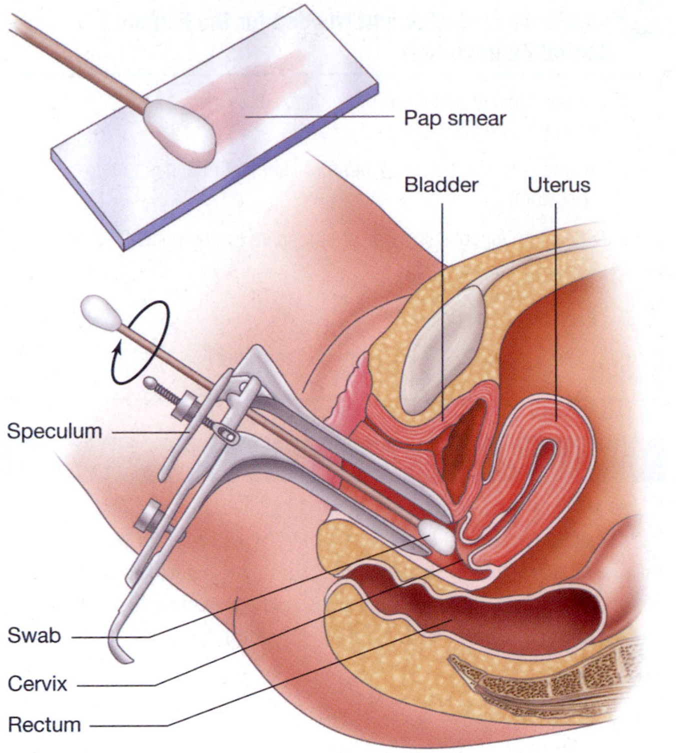

FIGURE 40–10 ◆ Obtaining Pap smear.

A friable cervix, discharge from the os, or cervical motion tenderness may indicate **cervicitis** (inflammation of the cervix) or pelvic inflammatory disease and should be reported to the medical provider for treatment.

Uterus and Adnexa

Next, the nurse lubricates the forefinger and long finger of the dominant hand for the bimanual examination. After explaining to the patient that the examination of the uterus and ovaries is next, the nurse inserts the lubricated fingers into the vagina and palpates the cervix for motion tenderness by moving it side to side. A bimanual examination is performed with one hand on the lower abdomen just above the symphysis (pubic bone) and the nurse's fingers in the vagina, pressing the cervix and uterus upward toward the abdominal hand to determine uterine tenderness, position, size, and shape. Figure 40–11◆ shows the bimanual exam of the female. The nurse moves the hands to the right adnexa, examines it bimanually for masses or tenderness, and then moves the hands to the left adnexa and repeats the examination for masses or tenderness (Seidel et al., 2011).

Safety Alert *Adnexal tenderness could be an indication of an ectopic pregnancy. Be very careful not to apply too much pressure, as the fallopian tube may rupture and hemorrhage. Report this finding immediately.*

Rectum

If the woman's history or examination indicates a reason, then a rectal examination should be done. The nurse puts on clean examination gloves and inspects the anal area for hemorrhoids, fissures, lesions, or warts. The nurse then lubricates the index and long fingers of the

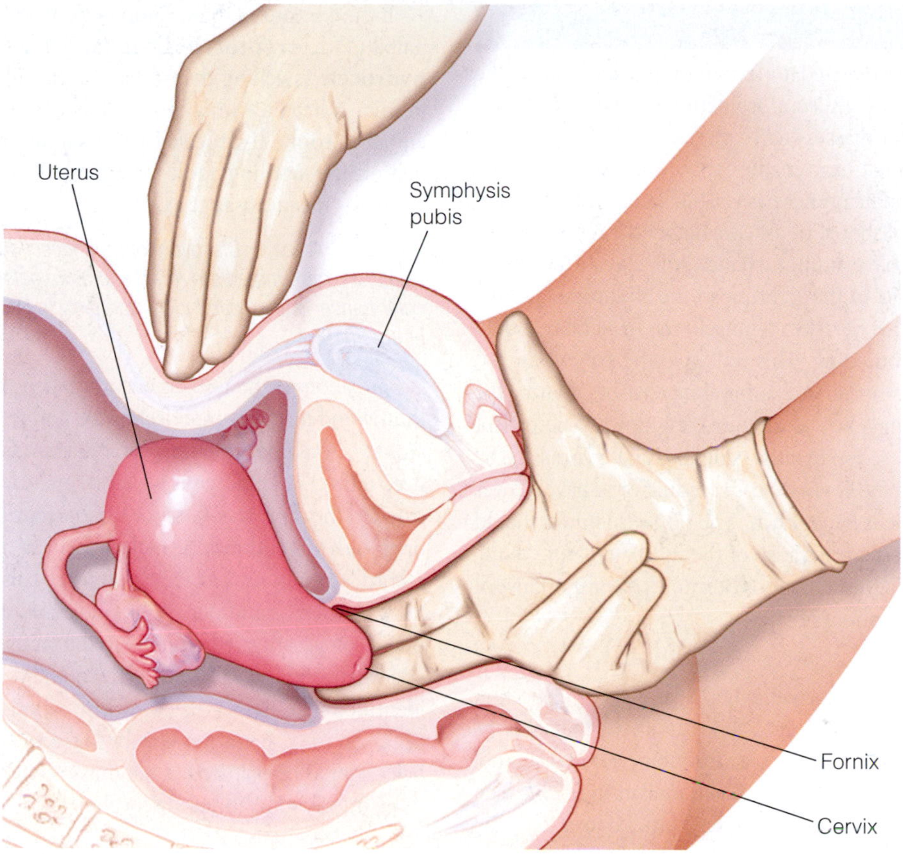

FIGURE 40–11 ◆ Bimanual exam female.

dominant hand and places the long finger over the anus and asks the patient to bear down as if for a bowel movement. As the anus opens, the nurse inserts the long finger. Placing the forefinger into the vagina, the nurse palpates for lesions, a **retroverted** (turned backward) uterus, or a fistula between the vagina and rectum. The nurse then removes the forefinger from the vagina and palpates the entire rectal wall with the long finger for rectal lesions. After removing the long finger from the anus, the nurse places any stool obtained on a hemoculture card to test for occult blood (Seidel et al., 2011).

The nurse helps the patient to move back on the table before sitting up, so that she is supported by the examination table. The nurse then helps her down from the examination table, gives her some tissue to remove the excess lubricant from the genitalia, and leaves the room to give her privacy to dress.

Laboratory and Imaging Results

Laboratory tests that are used to help diagnose female reproductive disorders may include, but are not limited to, blood tests for syphilis, herpes, and HIV; follicle stimulating hormone (FSH) serum levels; luteinizing hormone (LH) serum levels; and blood and urine testing for human chorionic gonadotropin (hCG). Use of these tests in the diagnosis of specific female disorders is discussed more fully in Chapters 41 and 44.

Imaging studies that are used in determining female reproductive disorders may include, but are not limited to, ultrasound; x-ray, colposcope, and laparoscope; and hysteroscope. These imaging studies are discussed according to how they are used in diagnosing various female reproductive disorders in Chapter 41.

Health Assessment for Adult Life Span

This discussion so far has been about the older teen and young adult female. In this section, physical changes related to pregnancy, **perimenopause** (years prior to menopause when changes in the menstrual cycle begin), and menopause will be discussed.

The breasts will enlarge during pregnancy, and a visible venous pattern may be seen by the end of the second month. **Colostrum** (first breast milk) may leak from the nipple around 3 months into the pregnancy. The sebaceous glands in the areola (Montgomery's tubercles) become more prominent. The nipple and areola become more darkly pigmented, and stretch marks may appear as the breasts grow (Blackburn, 2007).

In normal pregnancy, the introitus will be relaxed and the labia and clitoris will be slightly enlarged. There may be scars on the perineum if this is a second or later pregnancy. The cervical changes in pregnancy include softening and a bluish purple coloration by about 8 weeks' gestation. A woman who has previously given birth vaginally will have evidence of healed changes at the cervical os. The uterus grows as the fetus grows and will fill the abdomen to the xiphoid process by 38 to 40 weeks' gestation (Blackburn, 2007).

As a woman enters middle age, the glandular tissue of the breasts begins to atrophy. This causes the breasts to sag and become flaccid. The ducts around the nipples will become more palpable. Axillary hair will become sparse. The pubic hair becomes more sparse and gray. The labia become smaller and flaccid. The vagina narrows, and the mucosa will be pale and dryer due to a decrease in estrogen. The uterus and ovaries become smaller. During the menopausal years, if an ovary is palpable, it should be considered enlarged and should be reported (Bickley & Szilagyi, 2007).

Male Examination

The male breast should be inspected for lesions or gynecomastia. If the history or examination has revealed a problem with the male breast, the nurse should palpate for masses and tenderness.

The male external genital examination should occur in a warm, private room after the nurse examiner has washed and warmed the examining hands. The patient should be asked whether the room is warm enough. A cold room or cold examining hands will activate the **cremasteric reflex** (testicles rise in the scrotum to the abdominal cavity). The nurse should introduce herself or himself and, if female, should ask permission before proceeding. This will give the patient an opportunity to ask for a same-sex nurse examiner if he wishes. During the examination, the patient may be standing or lying down. The patient should be draped and gowned so that the genitalia can be visualized by having the patient hold up the gown if he is standing or to have a cover over his chest and legs if he is lying down. The nurse examiner should be accompanied by an assistant because of the intimate nature of the examination. The Cultural Considerations box notes the importance of respecting cultural attitudes about privacy.

External Genitalia

The examination of the male external genitalia consists of inspection followed by palpation. Chart 40–3 lists the equipment that may be needed. With the patient standing, the nurse examiner can sit on a stool in front of him and inspect the genitalia for lesions in the pubic hair, on the penis, or on the front or back of the scrotum. Lesions that may be seen include chancres (ulcers of syphilis), abnormal contour of the scrotum, cancer, warts, herpetic vesicles, or infestation by lice or other insects in the pubic hair. The dorsal vein of the penile shaft may be normally prominent. If the patient is not circumcised, the nurse should ask him to retract the foreskin so that the glans can be inspected. Smegma (white, cheesy material) is a normal finding under the foreskin. Inflammation of the glans is called balanitis. Inspection for the location of the urinary opening follows. Normally, it will be at the end of the penis and free of discharge. If the patient has reported discharge but it is not visible, he should be asked to strip the penis (compress or milk the penis) to bring discharge to the meatus for culture (Seidel et al., 2011).

Palpation of the penis is reserved for any abnormalities such as tenderness or plaque formation. The nurse should be aware that the male patient may develop an erection during the examination. This is often beyond his control, and the nurse should assure him that this is a normal occurrence (Seidel et al., 2011).

CHART 40–3 Equipment Needed for the Male Genitalia Examination

1. Examination gloves (latex or nonlatex, depending on patient allergy)
2. Water-soluble lubricant
3. Flashlight or other light source for transillumination

CULTURAL CONSIDERATIONS
Male Genital Examinations

Before proceeding with a male genital examination with the partner present, ask the partner whether he or she would prefer to leave. In certain cultures, the wife's presence during a genital examination of her husband would be considered taboo or against cultural mores.

If the contour of the scrotum appears suspicious, the nurse should palpate for **cryptorchidism** (an undescended testicle), scrotal **hydrocele** (swelling due to fluid accumulation in the scrotum), or hernia. A hernia with a loop of bowel in the scrotum can be differentiated from a hydrocele by transillumination (with a light source behind the swelling, look for a glow of clear fluid or no light penetrance) (Latendrasse et al., 2010).

Safety Alert *Discovery of an undescended testicle in a teenager would warrant immediate referral to a urologist. The incidence of testicular cancer is increased when the testicle is undescended (Latendrasse et al., 2010).*

Palpation of the testis is accomplished by grasping it between the thumb and forefinger and feeling for nodules or masses. The nurse examiner should be aware that too much pressure on the testis can cause deep pain. The epididymis is found on the posterior surface and is palpated in the same way. Cysts or tumors may be identified on the testicle or epididymis and may be malignant or benign. From the epididymis, a cord ascends toward the abdomen. This spermatic cord contains the vas deferens and nerves, blood vessels, and lymphatic vessels. The nurse palpates this structure up to the inguinal ring where it enters the abdomen. **Varicocele** (varicosities of the veins of the scrotum) may be identified here. These "bag of worms" abnormalities are more likely to occur on the patient's left side. Both sides of the scrotum and both testicles should be palpated (Latendrasse et al., 2010). See Chapter 42 for more information about varicoceles.

Hernia and Inguinal Lymph Nodes

Femoral and inguinal hernias may be detected by inspecting the inguinal and femoral areas for bulges. These bulges can be intensified by asking the patient to strain down or cough. To palpate for an inguinal hernia that has not presented as a loop of bowel in the scrotum, the nurse examiner should use the right forefinger to examine the patient's left external inguinal ring and the left forefinger to examine the patient's right external inguinal ring. This maneuver should start low enough in the scrotum to ensure that the nurse examiner's fingertip will reach the inguinal ring. While the examining finger is held against the ring, the patient should cough or strain down.

The superficial inguinal lymph nodes are palpated; if the nodes in the horizontal or vertical group are swollen or tender, this may indicate inflammation or malignancy of the scrotum or penis. Cancer or inflammation of the testicles would affect intra-abdominal lymph nodes that cannot be palpated (Bickley & Szilagyi, 2007).

Prostate

To palpate the prostate, a rectal examination is required. The patient will need to lean over the examining table or lie on his left side with his right knee drawn up (Figure 40–12◆). The anal area is inspected by spreading the buttocks. The nurse examiner should inspect for lesions, external hemorrhoids, or warts in this area. The nurse examiner should lubricate the forefinger of the dominant hand generously. To decrease discomfort, the nurse should tell the patient what is about to be done, have the patient bear down as if moving his bowels, and move the examining finger into the anal canal as it opens. The posterior surface of two lobes of the prostate is palpated through the anterior rectal wall. The nurse examiner should identify the median sulcus and note the size and firmness of the prostate and the presence of any masses or tenderness. When the examination is complete, the nurse examiner removes the finger from the anus and wipes the excess lubricant from the area (Seidel et al., 2011).

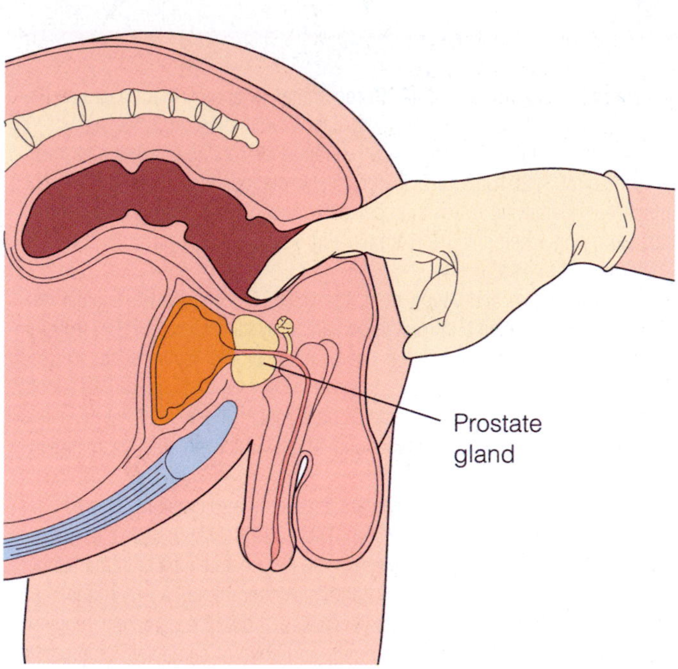

FIGURE 40–12 ◆ Digital rectal exam prostate.

Laboratory and Imaging Results

Laboratory tests that are specific for male reproductive disorders include, but are not limited to, blood tests for syphilis, herpes, or HIV; serum testosterone levels; prostate specific antigen; and sperm analysis. These diagnostic laboratory tests are discussed more fully with the specific disorders for which they are used in Chapters 42 and 43.

Imaging studies that are used in diagnosing disorders of the male reproductive system include ultrasound, CT scan, and direct visualization via laparoscope at the time of laparoscopic surgery. These diagnostic tools are discussed more fully in relation to specific male reproductive disorders in Chapter 42.

Health Assessment for Adult Life Span

This discussion so far has been about the older teen and young adult male. In older adult males, the penis decreases in size, the scrotum sags, and the testicles are lower in the scrotum and may be smaller. Pubic hair will become sparse and gray. Most men will develop an enlarged prostate (Bickley & Szilagyi, 2007).

Gerontological Considerations

As with all systems of the body, the reproductive system undergoes changes with aging. Psychologically, older adults experience reduced libido and decreased sexual satisfaction. However, this does not mean that men and women over age 65 are not sexual or that they do not enjoy sexual activity. It just means that sex is not as intense or frequent. In fact, Huang et al. (2009), in their study of 1,977 ethnically diverse women, discovered that more than 25% of participants over age 65 indicated that they were interested in sex, and 33% of those with interest reported having sexual intercourse within the last 3 months. The primary reasons given for decline in libido and sexual feelings among healthy older women were loss of or lack of interest from a significant other. Other research has shown that a healthy sex life contributes to psychological and physical well-being and may continue well into the eighth decade (Sexual Health Network, 2010a).

Typically, women experience **menopause** (normal cessation of menstruation) and the loss of estrogen in the early part of the fifth decade. The decrease in estrogen may cause symptoms such as **hot flashes** (intense heat sensation followed by sweating), which usually come and go during the first 5 years of menopause, and drying of the vaginal mucosa. Drying of the vaginal mucosa will make sexual intercourse and vaginal examinations uncomfortable. Less frequently, the woman may experience sleep disturbances, decreased ability to concentrate, and depression. Over time, decreased estrogen will contribute to loss of muscle mass and bone and increased fat in the abdomen (Nappi & Lachowsky, 2009; Rosenblatt, 2010a; Semmens, 2009).

Changes in the joints brought on by aging may necessitate a change in positioning for vaginal examinations. For women who cannot open their legs at the hips for the lithotomy position, a side-lying positioning with the top leg drawn up will allow for small speculum examination of the vagina and cervix. Another option is to have two assistants support the patient's legs during the examination (Bickley & Szilagyi, 2007).

Men experience **andropause** (decrease in testosterone) beginning gradually in about the third decade. Testosterone levels decrease enough to cause symptoms between ages 40 and 55. These symptoms may include weight gain, sleep disturbances, memory loss, diminished libido, hot flashes, erectile dysfunction, depression, loss of muscle and bone mass, fatigue, and night sweats. In many men, this **hypogonadism** (decreased production of hormones by the gonads) may also cause decreased frequency of morning erection and sexual thoughts (Wu et al., 2010). Corona and his colleagues (2010) studied 3,369 European men ages 40 to 79 and determined that 30% of the participants had erectile dysfunction (ED). The age group in which erectile dysfunction peaked for this group was 50 to 59 years. Although loss of testosterone is a natural result of aging, many men will seek methods to slow or stop the process. Methods used include pharmaceutical drugs, hormone replacement therapy, and **nutraceuticals** (foods used as medicine) such as saw palmetto, stinging nettle, and others. Drugs and testosterone replacement therapy carry risks such as breast enlargement, sleep apnea, stroke, and prostate cancer (Duncan, 2009). Chapter 42 discusses nutraceutical alternatives for prostate health in more detail.

Loss of mobility or inability to stand for long periods may necessitate that the older male lie down for the prostate examination. Lying on the left side, bent at the hips, and with the right leg drawn up so that the anal area is accessible to the nurse examiner is the recommended position (Bickley & Szilagyi, 2007).

Health Promotion

Health promotion means following a lifestyle that is conducive to health. The World Health Organization (WHO) (2011) defines sexual health as "the state of physical, emotional, mental and social well-being related to sexuality; it is not merely the absence of disease, dysfunction and infertility." Sexual health requires a healthy mind and body, open communications with the partner, and the capacity to enjoy and control sexual impulses according to social norms (Sexual Health Network, 2010b). To be sexually healthy is to have a positive body image and comfort with one's sexual identity. Sexual health is promoted by mutually monogamous relationships, free of coercion and violence, with uninfected partners. Nurses must recognize that sexual health is a right of all people and that those rights should be respected and protected (Sexual Health Network, 2010c). The National Guidelines box details other benchmarks used for sexual health.

NATIONAL GUIDELINES for Disease Screening and Self-Examination

Early detection of disease through screening examinations is a tactic for health promotion. For women, cervical and breast cancer screenings are recommended. The U.S. Preventive Services Task Force (USPSTF) recommends that sexually active women who have a cervix have screening Pap tests until age 65. At this point, the benefit of screening seems to diminish (USPSTF, 2003). The American Cancer Society (ACS) (2010a) recommends that screening Pap smears begin about 3 years after the initiation of sexual intercourse but no later than 21 years of age. If a liquid-based test is used, screening for women between the ages of 15 and 30 may be done every 2 years. After age 30, women who have had normal Pap tests 3 times in a row may be screened every 3 years regardless of the screening test type. Unlike the USPSTF, ACS recommends that Pap tests continue until age 70. The USPSTF and ACS agree, however, that there is no need for Pap tests in women who have had a total hysterectomy unless the surgery was done for cancer treatment or due to precancerous lesions.

For breast screening, the USPSTF recommends a screening mammogram every 2 years for women ages 50 to 74. Starting regular mammography screening before that age is a decision based on individual risk factors and the patient's perceptions of risk versus benefits. The USPSTF recommends that self-breast examination should not be taught based on evidence that teaching self-breast examination is of no benefit (Recommendation D) (USPSTF, 2010). The American Cancer Society (ACS) recommends annual mammograms beginning at age 40 along with clinical breast examination (ACS, 2010a).

Neither the USPSTF nor the ACS recommends routine screening for ovarian cancer (ACS, 2010a; USPSTF, 2004a). No diagnostic test has proven to be effective in identifying ovarian cancer early enough to warrant mass screening. More about screening for female reproductive cancers is discussed in Chapters 41and 44.

For adolescents and young men, the USPSTF recommends against testicular self-examination and routine screening by clinicians (USPSTF, 2004b). Studies demonstrate that routine examination of the testicles has caused more harm than benefit. The ACS, however, suggests that young men should be taught to self-examine the testicles on a regular basis and that clinicians should include testicular examinations in all cancer-related examinations (ACS, 2010e).

The USPSTF has found no evidence to recommend prostate screening for men age 75 and older (USPSTF, 2008). The ACS (2010a) suggests that more evidence is needed to support the screening for prostate cancer in men under 50 years of age who have no risk factors. African American men and men whose father or brother has prostate cancer should be screened regularly starting at age 45. More about the pros and cons of screening for prostate cancer is presented in Chapter 42.

NCLEX® PRACTICE

1. The nurse is instructing a patient about the menstrual cycle and hormone regulation. Which of the following should the nurse include in this instruction?

1. The next menstrual cycle begins on the last day of the current menses.
2. The uterine lining becomes thicker because of estrogen.
3. Ovulation is a result of estrogen release from the uterine lining.
4. After ovulation, the lining of the uterus becomes thinner.

2. A male patient seeks medical care for a new onset of impotence. Which of the following should the nurse assess in this patient?

1. Any chronic illnesses such as diabetes
2. Past medical history including mumps
3. History of sexually transmitted infections
4. Date of first sexual experience

3. A 35-year-old female is having difficulty conceiving. Which of the following can the nurse assess in this patient to aid in determining the cause of the infertility?

1. Smoking history
2. Occupations and hobbies
3. Amount of daily exercise
4. Amount of daily sleep and rest

4. While assessing the penis of an uncircumcised male, the nurse notes a white cheesy substance under the foreskin. The nurse realizes this finding is consistent with:

1. smegma.
2. syphilis.
3. inflammation.
4. hypospadius.

5. A 50-year-old female patient believes something is "drastically wrong" because she is "losing hair down there." Which of the following should the nurse respond to this patient?

1. "There could be something wrong."
2. "Hair loss over the mons and vulva is a normal part of the aging process."
3. "I suggest you schedule a complete physical immediately."
4. "Hair doesn't really serve a purpose there anyway."

6. A 70-year-old male patient tells the nurse that he "hates his annual physical" because every year he worries what his PSA level is going to be. Which response by the nurse is best?

1. "Do you want to be referred to a new health care provider?"
2. "What makes you worry about this test?"
3. "Do you think you have cancer?"
4. "Is there information about your health that your doctor should know?"

Answers to NCLEX Practice Questions can be found in Appendix D in the Osborn Student Resources at nursing.pearsonhighered.com. Practice additional NCLEX questions online at the Student Resources site.

REFERENCES

Abatangelo, L., Okereke, L., Parham-Foster, C., Parrish, C., Saglione, L., Zotte, D., et al. (2010). If pelvic inflammatory disease is suspected empiric treatment should be initiated. *Journal of the American Academy of Nurse Practitioners, 22* (2010), 117–122. doi:10.1111/j.1745-7599.2009.00478.x

American Cancer Society (ACS). (2010a). American Cancer Society guidelines for early detection of cancer. *Stay Healthy.* Retrieved from http://www.cancer.org/Healthy/FindCancerEarly/CancerScreeningGuidelines/american-cancer-society-guidelines-for-the-early-detection-of-cancer

American Cancer Society (ACS). (2010b). Breast cancer: Causes, risk factors, and prevention topics. *Learn About Cancer.* Retrieved from http://www.cancer.org/Cancer/BreastCancer/DetailedGuide/breast-cancer-risk-factors#top

American Cancer Society. (2010c). Breast cancer in men. *Learn About Cancer.* Retrieved from http://www.cancer.org/Cancer/BreastCancerinMen/DetailedGuide/breast-cancer-in-men-key-statistics

American Cancer Society. (2010e). Testicular cancer. *Learn About Cancer.* Retrieved from http://www.cancer.org/Cancer/TesticularCancer/DetailedGuide/testicular-cancer-detection

Barad, D. (2010). General gynecologic evaluation. *Merck Manuals.* Retrieved from http://www.merckmedicus.com/pp/us/hcp/framemm.jsp?pg=www.merck.com/mmpe/sec18/ch242/ch242b.html

Bickley, L., & Szilagyi, P. (2007). *Bate's guide to physical examination and history taking* (9th ed.). Philadelphia: Lippincott Williams & Wilkins.

Blackburn, S. (2007). *Maternal, fetal, & neonatal physiology: A clinical perspective* (3rd ed.). St. Louis: Saunders/Elsevier.

Centers for Disease Control and Prevention (CDC). (2010a). Clinical prevention guidance. *Sexually Transmitted Disease Treatment Guidelines 2010.* Retrieved from http://www.cdc.gov/mmwr/preview/mmwrhtml/rr5912a1.htm?s_cid=rr5912a1_w

Centers for Disease Control and Prevention (CDC). (2010b). DES update: Consumers. *About DES.* Retrieved from http://www.cdc.gov/des/consumers/about/index.html

Corona, G., Lee, D., Forti, G., O'Connor, D., Maggi, M., O'Neill, T., et al. (2010). Age-related changes in general and sexual health in middle-aged and older men: Results from the European Male Aging Study (EMAS). *The Journal of Sexual Medicine, 7*(4 Pt 1), 1362–1380.

Danakas, G., & Alvero, R. (2009). Menopause. *Ferri's Clinical Advisor.* Retrieved from http://www.merckmedicus.com/pp/us/hcp/thcp_ferri_content.jsp?pg=/ppdocs/us/hcp/content/ferri/B9780323056090000228/ferri-611A.htm

Degeneres A., & Huether, S. (2010). Structure and function of the reproductive systems. In K. McCance & S. Huether (Eds.), *Pathophysiology: The biologic basis for disease in adults and children* (6th ed., pp. 781–813). St. Louis: Mosby/Elsevier.

Dunaif, A. (2012). Chapter 6. Women's health. Retrieved from http://www.merckmedicus.com/pp/us/hcp/frame_textbooks.jsp?pg=http://www.accessmedicine.com/content.aspx?aid=2860110

Duncan, N. (2009). Male menopause? *Natural Solutions,* May/June, p. 54.

Gabriel, A., & Maxwell, P. (2009). Breast anatomy. eMedicine. Retrieved from http://emedicine.medscape.com/article/1273133-overview

Hall, J. (2012). Chapter 347. The female reproductive system: Infertility and contraception. Access Medicine/Harrison's Online. Retrieved from http://www.merckmedicus.com/pp/us/hcp/frame_textbooks.jsp?pg=http://www.accessmedicine.com/content.aspx?aid=2902937

Harmanli, O., & Jones, K. (2010). Using lubricant for speculum insertion. *Obstetrics & Gynecology, 116*(2, Part 1), 415–417. doi:10.1097/AOG.0b013e3181e750f1

Huang, A., Subak, L., Thom, D., Van Den Eeden, S., Ragins, A., Kuppermann, M., et al. (2009). Sexual function and aging in racially and ethnically diverse women. *Journal of American Geriatric Society, 57(80),* 1362–1368. doi:10.1111/j.1532-5415.2009.02353.x

Jorde, L. (2010). Genes and genetic disease. In K. McCance & S. Huether, *Pathophysiology: The biologic basis for disease in adults and children* (6th ed., pp. 126–162). St. Louis: Mosby/Elsevier.

Kruszka, P., & Kruszka, S. (2010). Evaluation of acute pelvic pain in women. *American Family Physician, 82*(2), 141–147.

Latendresse, G., McCance, K., & Morgan, K. (2010). Alterations of the reproductive systems. In K. McCance & S. Huether, *Pathophysiology: The biologic basis for disease in adults and children* (6th ed., pp. 816–922). St. Louis: Mosby/Elsevier.

Lymph nodes. (2012). Imaginis. Retrieved from http://www.imaginis.com/breast-health/lymph-nodes-2

Metzker, A. (2010). Supernumerary nipple. eMedicine. Retrieved from http://emedicine.medscape.com/article/1117825-overview

Montgomery's tubercles. (2011). The Free Dictionary by Farlex. Retrieved from http://encyclopedia2.thefreedictionary.com/Montgomery's+tubercles

Nappi, R., & Lachowsky, M. (2009). Menopause and sexuality: Prevalence of symptoms and impact on quality of life. *Maturitas, 63*(2009), 138–141. doi:10.1016/j.maturitas.2009.03.021

National Cancer Institute (NCI). (2010). Cervical cancer prevention (PDQ). Retrieved from http://www.cancer.gov/cancertopics/pdq/prevention/cervical/healthprofessional#top

Rosenblatt, P. (2010a). Effects of aging. *Merck Manuals.* Retrieved from http://www.merckmedicus.com/pp/us/hcp/framemm.jsp?pg=www.merck.com/mmhe/sec22/ch241/ch241f.html

Rosenblatt, P. (2010b). External genital organs. *Merck Manuals.* Retrieved from http://www.merck.com/mmhe/sec22/ch241/ch241b.html

Rosenblatt, P. (2010c). Internal genital organs. *Merck Manuals.* Retrieved from http://www.merck.com/mmhe/sec22/ch241/ch241c.html

Schauler, R., & Potak, D. (2009). Physiology of lactation. *UpToDate.* Retrieved from http://www.uptodate.com/patients/content/topic.do?topicKey=~S2USSLK5B.V5nVo

Seidel, H., Ball, J., Dains, J., Flynn, J., Solomon, B., & Stewart, R. (2011). *Mosby's physical examination handbook* (7th ed.). St. Louis: Mosby/Elsevier.

Semmens, J. (2009). Sexual problems and aging. *Clinical Advisors—Patient Handouts/Merck Medicus.* Retrieved from http://www.merckmedicus.com/pp/us/hcp/hcp_patient_resource_allhandouts_content_search.jsp?pg=/ppdocs/us/common/crs/aha/aha_intro_bha.htm

Sexual Health Network. (2010a). Love and relationships: Age-related changes. SexualHealth.com. Retrieved from http://www.sexualhealth.com/channel/view_sub/love-relationships/age-related-changes/

Sexual Health Network. (2010b). Men's sexual health. SexualHealth.com. Retrieved from http://www.sexualhealth.com/channel/view/men-sexual-health/

Sexual Health Network. (2010c). Women's sexual health. SexualHealth.com. Retrieved from http://www.sexualhealth.com/channel/view/women-sexual-health/

Torpy, J., Cassio, L., & Glass, R. (2010). Intimate partner violence. *Journal of the American Médical Association, 304*(5), 596. doi:10.1001/jama.304.5.596

U.S. Department of Health and Human Services (DHHS). (2010). Sexually transmitted disease: 2020 topics and objectives. HealthPeople.gov. Retrieved from http://www.healthypeople.gov/2020/topicsobjectives2020/overview.aspx?topicid=37

U.S. Preventive Services Task Force (USPSTF). (2003). Screening for cervical cancer. Retrieved from http://www.uspreventiveservicestaskforce.org/uspstf/uspscerv.htm

U.S. Preventive Services Task Force (USPSTF). (2004a). Screening for ovarian cancer. Retrieved from http://www.uspreventiveservicestaskforce.org/uspstf/uspsovar.htm

U.S. Preventive Services Task Force (USPSTF). (2004b). Screening for testicular cancer. Retrieved from http://www.uspreventiveservicestaskforce.org/uspstf/uspsprca.htm

U.S. Preventive Services Task Force (USPSTF). (2008). Screening for prostate cancer. Retrieved from http://www.uspreventiveservicestaskforce.org/uspstf/uspsprca.htm

U.S. Preventive Services Task Force (USPSTF). (2010). Screening for breast cancer. Retrieved from http://www.uspreventiveservicestaskforce.org/uspstf/uspsbrca.htm

Workowski, K., & Berman, S. (2010). Sexually transmitted disease treatment guidelines 2010. *Morbidity and Mortality Weekly Report, 59*(RR-12), 2–3.

World Health Organization (WHO). (2011). Sexual health. Retrieved from http://www.who.int/topics/sexual_health/en/

Wu, F., Tajar, A., Beynon, J., Pye, S., Silman, A., Finn, J., O'Neill, T. W., Bartfai, G., Casanueva, F. F., Forti, G., Giwercman, A., Han, T. S., Kula, K., Lean, M. E., Pendleton, N., Punab, M., Boonen, S., Vanderschueren, D., Labrie, F., Huhtaniemi, I. T.; EMAS Group. (2010).Identification of late-onset hypogonadism in middle-aged and elderly men. *The New England Journal of Medicine, 363(2),* 123–135. DOI: 10.1056/NEJMoa0911101

CHAPTER

41 Caring for the Patient with Female Reproductive Disorders

Patricia Caudle
Kathleen Osborn

Outcome-Based Learning Objectives

After studying this chapter, the learner will be able to:

1. Differentiate the epidemiology, etiology, pathophysiology, and clinical manifestations of the most common female reproductive disorders.
2. Generate nursing management goals when caring for women with reproductive disorders.
3. Generate nursing diagnoses relevant to women with reproductive disorders.
4. Apply the nursing process to the care of women with reproductive disorders.
5. Plan interventions that will enhance health education, health promotion, and disease prevention specific for female health.
6. Describe key components of the interview of a patient who has been victimized by intimate partner violence.

KEY TERMS

abortion p.1274
acanthosis nigricans p.1266
amenorrhea p.1264
anorgasmia p.1263
anovulation p.1265
Bartholinitis p.1255
bladder suspension p.1275
cervical polyps p.1267
colposcopy p.1275
cystocele p.1255
dysmenorrhea p.1259
dyspareunia p.1263
ectopic p.1259
embolization p.1258
endometrioma p.1259
endometriosis p.1258
fibroid tumor p.1257
fistula p.1257
galactorrhea p.1265
hysterectomy p.1278
Kegel exercises p.1256
leiomyoma p.1257
lichen sclerosis p.1255
metrorrhagia p.1258
mittelschmerz p.1258
myoma p.1257
oligomenorrhea p.1265
oophorectomy p.1278
ovarian torsion p.1260
perimenopause p.1272
pessary p.1256
polycystic ovary syndrome (PCOS) p.1265
premenstrual dysphoric disorder (PMDD) p.1268
premenstrual syndrome (PMS) p.1268
prolapse p.1257
rectocele p.1256
rectovaginal fistula p.1257
salpingectomy p.1278
salpingo-oophorectomy p.1278
tinea cruris p.1255
tinea pubis p.1255
vaginismus p.1263
vesicovaginal fistula (VVF) p.1257
vulvodynia p.1255
vulvovaginal candidiasis (VCC) p.1254

REPRODUCTIVE SYSTEM DISORDERS ARE VARIED and do not have age barriers. This chapter discusses the more common disorders, their clinical manifestations, and their treatment modalities, along with some prevention methods where applicable. Further information on general reproductive assessment can be found in Chapter 40.

Vulvovaginal Disorders

Inflammation of the vulva and vagina may or may not be due to sexually transmitted infection. In this section, the focus will be on those disorders of the vulva and vagina that are not always considered sexually transmitted, such as fungal vaginitis, vulvodynia, Bartholinitis, cystocele, rectocele, and uterine prolapse. Sexually transmitted infections will be covered in Chapter 43.

Vulvovaginal Candidiasis (VCC)

Description and Etiology

Vulvovaginal candidiasis (VCC) is a fungal infection, more commonly referred to as a yeast infection of the vagina and vulva. Other fungal organisms may cause yeast vaginitis, but *Candida albicans* is the most common. Approximately 75% of women will have an episode of yeast infection and about 45% of women will have two or more infections in their lifetime (Workowski & Berman, 2010). *Candida* organisms are typically found in the genital tract, the gastrointestinal tract, and the mouth. Symptoms develop when there is an overgrowth of *Candida* caused by multiple factors such as pregnancy, diabetes mellitus, and the use of antibiotics and/or corticosteroids that disturbs the pH, eradicates the normal bacterial flora, or causes a hormone imbalance in the vagina (Centers for Disease Control and Prevention [CDC], 2010). Other causes can include tight-fitting undergarments that maintain a moist environment for fungal growth and frequent douching that may alter the normal flora and pH balance that is needed to prevent it. The usual *Candida* flora is rarely passed from person to person (CDC, 2010), but can be transmitted through oral or genital sexual contact, when a disturbance in pH or hormone balance occurs.

Clinical Manifestations

Symptoms include a white, cheesy discharge, often with intense itching, a burning sensation, and painful urination. Vulvovaginal candidiasis is diagnosed by taking a specimen from the infected vagina and examining it under the microscope. The pseudohyphae and buds of yeast are easily detected (McCloskey, 2010).

Medical Management

The treatment of VCC is a 1-, 3-, or 7-day course of antifungal drugs taken orally, topically, or vaginally (CDC, 2010). Self-treatment is becoming common as more over-the-counter drugs become available. The CDC (2010) indicates that as many as two-thirds of women who self-treat do not have the disease, leading to an increasing number of resistant infections. Women who have recurrences of what they believe to be candidiasis should seek medical diagnosis to rule out another cause of their symptoms, such as a resistant fungal organism, HIV, or diabetes. Untreated infections may lead to persistent symptoms and an increased chance of passing the infection between partners. Wearing cotton undergarments that allow for better absorption of moisture and avoiding douching will decrease the incidence of *Candida* growth in prone individuals.

Health Promotion

Patient education is essential to the prevention and spread of VCC. The following facts are necessary components of the teaching plan:

- Observe for changes in color, odor, and amount of vaginal discharge, as well as itching or burning of the vulva and vagina.
- Wear light cotton underwear.
- If a presumed yeast infection does not improve with over-the-counter (OTC) treatment, seek medical care.
- Changes in the environment of the vagina may occur with changes in diet, medications, and a new sex partner who has ***tinea pubis*** (fungal infection of the pubic area).
- Recurrent vaginitis or vaginitis that is nonresponsive to treatment requires further consultation with a health care provider.
- Avoid douching.

Vulvodynia

Description and Etiology

Vulvodynia (also called vulvar vestibulitis or vulvitis) is either (1) chronic vulval pain that occurs without painful stimuli or (2) chronic burning, soreness, rawness, stinging, and irritation of the vulva (Ventolini, Barhan, & Duke, 2009). It is the most frequent cause of dyspareunia in women ages 14 to 50 (MacKay, 2011). It is underreported because women are reluctant to talk about it and there are very few outward signs of the disorder. Several experts believe that there is a genetic predisposition that makes the vulva react abnormally to inflammation. Others believe that some cases of vulvodynia are due to trauma to the nerves or muscle spasms (MedicineNet.com, 2011).

Clinical Manifestations

Women affected with this disorder will describe discomfort upon opening the labia minora, pain on beginning intercourse, pain on sitting, and pain that includes all glands and mucosal areas around the opening to the vagina (Ventolini, Barhan, & Duke, 2009).

Vulvodynia is difficult to diagnose because generally there is no physical evidence of the condition. Some women may suffer for years before the condition can be diagnosed and properly treated. Conditions that have been identified as contributing to vulvodynia include yeast vaginitis, sexually transmitted infections, seborrhea, psoriasis, **lichen sclerosis** (whitening and thinning of vulvar skin), **tinea cruris** (fungal infection of the trunk), and inflammation of the sweat glands (Latendresse, McCance, & Morgan, 2010).

Medical Management

Medical management depends on identifying a cause for the pain and then treating that cause. Treatment may include hydrocortisone creams, water barrier creams, water-soluble amitriptyline cream, estrogen cream, overnight lidocaine cream, or oral antidepressants and anticonvulsants. Health care providers have also performed nerve blocks and vestibulectomy, where the vestibule is removed along with the superficial muscles (MacKay, 2011; MedicineNet.com, 2010).

Health Promotion

Women need more information about this disorder and how to self-treat. Nurses may be instrumental in providing education and resources for women who are affected. The National Vulvodynia Association www.nva.org/ is an excellent resource for nurses and women interested in learning more about this disorder.

Weblink: National Vulvodynia Association

Bartholinitis

Description, Etiology, and Clinial Manifestations

Bartholinitis or Bartholin cyst is an inflammation of one or both of the Bartholin glands at the opening of the vagina. The usual cause is blockage of the gland duct by infection with such organisms as streptococci, staphylococci, and sexually transmitted pathogens (Latendresse, McCance, & Morgan, 2010). The blockage will lead to cyst formation, possible abscess, and severe pain. Once the infection is resolved, the cyst will persist and may become re-infected (MacKay, 2011).

Medical Management

Medical treatment begins with diagnosis of the condition and culture of any pus or drainage from the cyst. Appropriate antibiotics are given based on the culture and sensitivity tests if tenderness and cellulitis is evident. If an abscess forms, incision and drainage is needed. If the cyst is not abscessed but large and uncomfortable, a Word catheter may be surgically placed in the gland to facilitate drainage. Warm, moist compresses or warm sitz baths are soothing and help healing. Asymptomatic small cysts do not need to be treated (MacKay, 2011).

Cystocele

Description and Etiology

A **cystocele** occurs when the wall between the bladder and the anterior vagina weakens and the bladder protrudes into the vaginal vault (Figure 41–1◆). The most frequent cause is multiple vaginal deliveries

Weblink: Pelvic Organ Prolapse

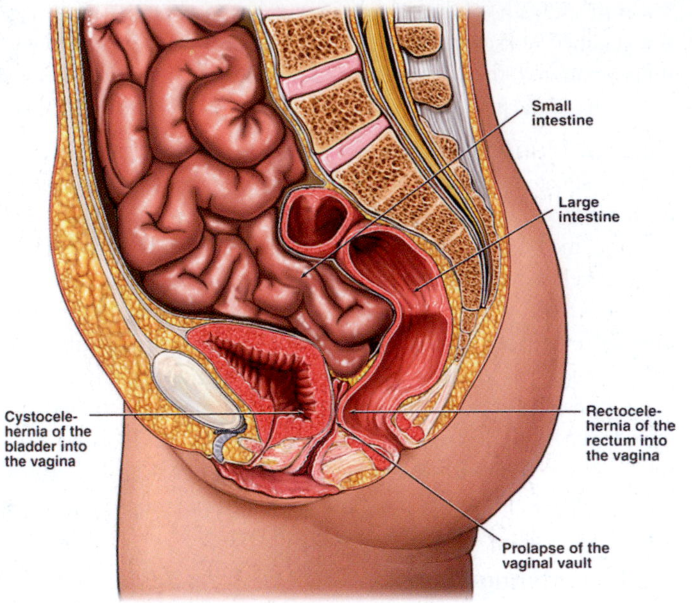

FIGURE 41–1 ◆ Cystocele with uterine prolapse.
Source: Nucleus Medical Art, Inc./Alamy

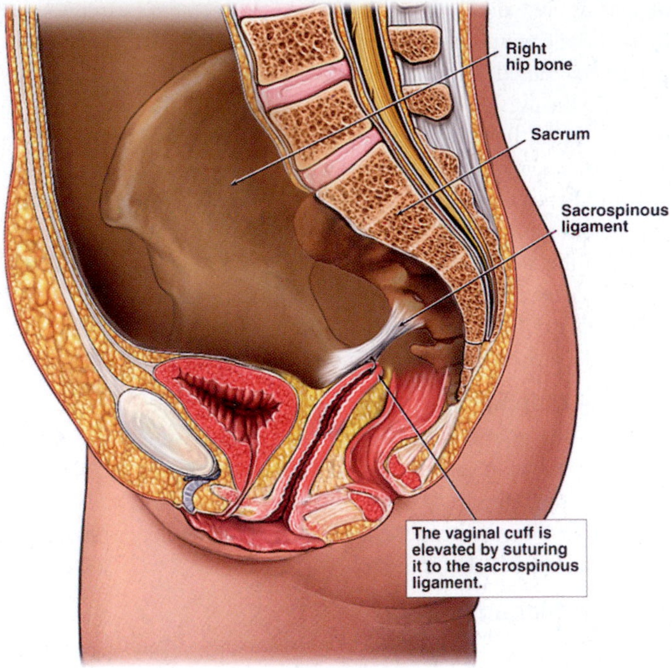

FIGURE 41–2 ◆ Rectocele.
Source: Nucleus Medical Art, Inc./Alamy

where the fascia, muscles, and perineal body are stretched and torn. Other related risk factors are pregnancy without vaginal birth, obesity, changes related to chronic disease such as diabetes, and genetic predisposition (Davis, 2010; Lazarou & Grigorescu, 2010; Norton, 2010). Refer to the Risk Factors for Pelvic Organ Prolapse feature for a list of causes. Like endometriosis, there is emerging evidence that a genetic component exists. The Genetics Considerations feature outlines this link (p. 1259).

Clinical Manifestations

Symptoms of cystoceles include urine leakage when the woman sneezes, coughs, or laughs, or incomplete emptying of the bladder. The woman will often describe a feeling of pelvic pressure. When cystoceles are large, the bladder may not empty completely, and the patient will be susceptible to urinary tract infections. A grading system has been developed to classify cystoceles. Chart 41–1 lists the stages of cystocele prolapse.

A **rectocele** occurs when the posterior vaginal wall is weakened and the rectum bulges into the vagina (Figure 41–2◆). The most frequent symptom is difficulty initiating a bowel movement, with resultant constipation, in addition to rectal pressure. This can occur in women who have had conditions that involve repetitive bearing down, such as chronic constipation, chronic coughing, or repetitive heavy lifting. Simple **Kegel exercises** (intermittent tightening of the perineal and vaginal muscles) will help to prevent the development of problems related to both rectocele and cystocele.

CHART 41–1 Classification of Cystocele Prolapse

Stage 0—no prolapsed cystocele

Stage I—lower portion of prolapsed cystocele is 1 cm above the hymen

Stage II—prolapsed cystocele is between 1 cm above and 1 cm below the hymen

Stage III—prolapsed cystocele more than 1 cm below hymen

Stage IV—total or complete anterior vaginal wall prolapse

Source: Adapted from ICS classification (POP-Q) system. Listed in Lazarou, G., & Grigorescu, B. (2010). Pelvic organ prolapsed. eMedicine. Retrieved from http://emedicine.medscape.com/article/276259-overview.

For women with mild to moderate symptoms, a pessary may be an option. A **pessary** is a device that, when inserted into the vagina, will help support the vaginal walls, reducing the bulging into the vagina; therefore, it is used for management of pelvic support defects such as cystocele, rectocele, and uterine prolapse. The pessary is also used before and after pelvic surgery such as hysterectomy to support the pelvic floor muscles. For those patients who are not good candidates for extensive surgery to repair defects of the pelvic floor, the pessary is an effective management option (Angelo, 2010). Pessaries should not be used if there is evidence of active pelvic infection such as vaginitis or pelvic inflammatory disease. Also, the pessary should be removed daily to prevent ulcers. Complications of pessaries include vaginal irritation, infection, discharge, pressure sores, or allergy to the components of the pessary.

Safety Alert *Patients must understand that although the pessary can be worn during sexual intercourse, it does not provide any method of birth control or protection against sexually transmitted infections. In addition, the patient must be taught effective placement and removal of the pessary and how to care for and clean it.*

Medical Management

Surgery can correct the issues of cystocele and rectocele when the symptoms are moderate to severe. Cystoceles and rectoceles are repaired using a procedure called a colporrhaphy, also referred to as an anterior/posterior (A&P) repair, depending on whether one or both procedures are done. The anterior wall repair, done for a cystocele, involves repair and resultant strengthening of the weakened area by either shortening the pelvic muscles providing greater support for the bladder or suspending the urinary bladder in the proper position. The posterior repair is used for the rectocele and tightens the pelvic floor muscles to provide greater support for the rectum. Risks are minimal but can include bleeding and infection.

Nursing Management

Postoperative nursing assessment includes monitoring vital signs, observing vaginal bleeding greater than simple spotting, noting signs of infection, and maintaining adequate hydration. The woman will have a Foley catheter for 1 or 2 days, and intake and output should be monitored accordingly. Stool softeners may be needed to avoid straining with bowel movements, and encouraging a well-balanced, high-fiber diet will assist in maintaining normal bowel function. Discharge instruction should include avoiding activities that might stress the incision, including intercourse or placing anything in the vagina, until released by the surgeon. Avoiding long periods of standing, coughing, and sneezing will also decrease strain on the surgical site. Adequate fluids and continuing a well-balanced, high-fiber, high-protein diet will aid in healing and regaining normal bowel function.

Uterine Prolapse

Uterine **prolapse** is another common structural disorder that occurs as a result of weakening of the pelvic floor musculature. The structures supporting the uterus are sometimes weakened during pregnancy and childbirth. There is an increased risk for uterine prolapse with obesity, chronic coughing, and straining during bowel movements. In addition, multiple pregnancies, congenital weakness, and loss of elasticity and muscle tone due to the aging process can contribute to the problem. As a result, the uterus is displaced downwardly into the vaginal canal. The uterus can prolapse enough to be seen outside the vagina. The prolapse pulls on surrounding structures and puts pressure on the bladder and rectum. This pressure can cause symptoms of incontinence or retention, and may be aggravated by coughing or lifting heavy objects. Generally, the treatment of choice is surgery to suture the uterus into place and tighten the musculature supporting it. Occasionally, a hysterectomy is done, although a pessary can be inserted into the vagina to support the uterus.

Fistula

Description, Etiology, and Clinical Manifestations

A **fistula** is an abnormal opening or tract between two structures caused by cancer, infection, injury, or surgery. Fistulas that affect the female reproductive system may occur between the vagina and the bladder or rectum, between the uterus and the peritoneal cavity, or between the bladder and the cervix or uterus (Mayo Clinic Staff, 2011; Spurlock, 2011; Vorvick, 2011a).

Vesicovaginal fistula (VVF) (fistula between the bladder and vagina) is caused by bladder injury during pelvic surgery, prolonged labor and difficult birth, or radiation (Chapter 57) and surgery for gynecologic cancers. This is the most prevalent form of female urogenital fistula (Spurlock, 2011). The primary symptom is urine passing from the bladder into the vagina continuously. Treatment if the problem occurs in the first few days following surgery or birth is suprapubic catheter or foley catheter, depending on where the fistula is, to divert urine drainage away from the fistula. Many VVFs will heal spontaneously if found early and treated this way. If the fistula occurs later or is allowed to become chronic, then surgical repair is needed.

Nursing management for patients with VVF includes patient education about fistulas, skin care, and catheter use. The patient will need assistance with sitz baths and the use of barrier ointments to protect the skin of the perineum. See Chapter 36 for care of patients with urinary problems and catheters.

Rectovaginal fistula (fistula between the vagina and rectum) may result from injuries in childbirth, as a complication of Crohn's disease, after pelvic surgery, or as a complication of radiation treatment to the pelvic area (Mayo Clinic Staff, 2011). Rarely, this type of fistula will occur as the result of severe infection in the rectum or vagina. Symptoms include stool and gas in the vagina; foul smelling vaginal discharge; recurrent urinary tract or vaginal infection; pain in the vagina, vulva, and perineum; and dyspareunia.

Medical Management

Medical treatment is surgery; however, before surgery is performed the skin and tissue around the fistula must be healthy. If infection is present, it must be treated with antibiotics and cured before surgery. A waiting period of up to 3 months before surgery may be required to assure that the tissues are healthy (Mayo Clinic Staff, 2011). In severe cases, a colostomy may be needed to divert stool away from the surgical area so that it can heal.

Nursing Management

Nursing management includes education about the condition, the planned surgery, and the importance of keeping the perineum clean. Washing the vaginal area and perineum with water only or using a premoistened, alcohol-free wipe rather than using harsh soaps or dry toilet paper will facilitate healing. Moisture barrier creams will help protect the skin (Mayo Clinic Staff, 2011). In addition, cool compresses and loose clothing will help the patient be more comfortable. Chapter 36 contains more information about the care of patients with colostomy.

Uterine and Ovarian Disorders

Uterine disorders such as fibroid tumors, endometriosis, and ectopic pregnancy, which are among the most common of the female reproductive disorders, are discussed in this section.

Uterine Fibroid Tumors

Description and Etiology

Fibroid tumors of the uterus, also known as **leiomyomas** and **myomas**, are the most common benign tumor of the womb (Figure 41–3◆) (Stoppler, 2010). In fact, they occur in about 50% of women and are the leading reason for hysterectomy in the United States. African American women are most often affected, with an occurrence rate 5 times that of White women (Latendresse, McCance, & Morgan, 2010). The tumors consist of smooth muscle tissue and may occur in the uterine cavity, in the uterine muscle, on the surface of the uterus, or attached to the uterus in clusters or as single tumors. Chart 41–2 lists the fibroid types by location.

The exact cause of fibroids is unknown. However, there is a family tendency and the growths respond to estrogen. The tumors usually grow slowly and begin to develop during the early twenties in

RISK FACTORS for Pelvic Organ Prolapse

Obesity	Pregnancy without vaginal birth
Menopause (loss of estrogen and atrophy)	Diabetic neuropathy
Pelvic tumors	Genetic factors

Multiple vaginal births (stretching and tearing of endopelvic fascia, levator muscles, and perineal body)

Source: Adapted from Davis, K. (2010). Pelvic floor dysfunction: Causes and assessment. *Practice Nursing, 21*(7), 340–346; Lazarou, G., & Grigorescu, B. (2010). Pelvic organ prolapsed. eMedicine. Retrieved from http://emedicine.medscape.com/article/276259-verview;___

Weblink: Uterine Fibroids

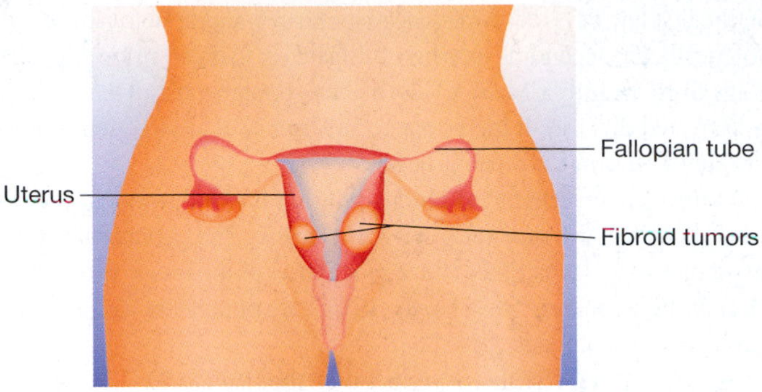

FIGURE 41–3 ◆ Uterine fibroid tumor.
Source: VEM/Photo Researchers, Inc.

CHART 41–2 Uterine Fibroid Types by Location

Submucosal—in the uterine cavity
Intramural—in the uterine muscle
Subserous—just under the surface lining of the uterus
Pedunculated—attached to the uterus via a stalk

Source: Mayo Clinic Staff. (2009). Uterine fibroids. Retrieved from http://www.mayoclinic.com/health/uterine-fibroids/DS00078.

susceptible women. Fibroids grow very rapidly during pregnancy due to the increase in estrogen. They recede after menopause when natural estrogen decreases (Latendresse et al., 2010; Stoppler, 2010). Many fibroids are small and asymptomatic, although some can grow to be very large. See the Risk Factors for Uterine Fibroid Tumors feature for a list of the most common causes.

Clinical Manifestations

Since fibroids often cause no symptoms, many remain undiscovered unless the patient has abnormal uterine bleeding, pelvic pain, and infertility or pregnancy loss. Uterine tumors can add pressure to surrounding organs, causing pain, constipation, and urinary problems. Abnormal uterine bleeding may present as **menorrhagia** (heavy bleeding) and **metrorrhagia** (irregular bleeding). Larger fibroids are more painful because of blood vessel compression and decreased blood flow and oxygen to the tumor (Latendresse et al., 2010).

Medical Management

Diagnosis is suspected when bimanual examination reveals an enlarged uterus. See Chapter 40 for more about the bimanual examination. Diagnosis is confirmed based on abdominal, transvaginal, or pelvic ultrasonography or hysteroscopy (passing a small fiber-optic device into the uterine cavity to view the lining) to help visualize the tumor and determine its exact location and size. The surgeon can then determine the best approach for treatment. The options for treatment of uterine fibroid tumors are many and depend on the size of the tumor, the age of the patient, and the severity of symptoms. Choice of options also depends on whether fertility needs to be preserved. Observational management is increasingly recognized as a reasonable course for women with asymptomatic or mildly symptomatic tumors. Conservative treatment involves drug therapy such as nonsteroidal anti-inflammatory drugs (NSAIDs) to control pain, birth control pills to decrease menstrual flow, and hormone therapy such as gonadotropin-releasing hormone agonists or androgenic drugs to decrease the size of the fibroids and the associated discomfort. Hormone therapy is often used to control growth before surgery or as a temporary measure when a woman is close to menopause (Stoppler, 2010). Refer to the Pharmacology feature for more about drug therapy (p. 1277).

Uterine fibroid **embolization** (clotting of the arterial blood supply to the fibroid) is a nonsurgical treatment done under intravenous sedation that shrinks the fibroid. This radiologic procedure entails placement of a line into the femoral artery, using x-ray video to trace the uterine blood supply, and then clotting the artery feeding the tumor with particles the size of sand grains (Stoppler, 2010). Patients usually experience pelvic pain immediately after the procedure. In women whose symptoms are severe, or the fibroid is very large, treatment can range from simple fibroid removal (myomectomy) to hysterectomy. Laser surgery is often used for myomectomy. The hysterectomy is used the most often for fibroid tumors. Justification for this recommendation includes the risk that large tumors could potentially mask other adnexal pathology and increase operative complication rates. This procedure will not preserve fertility.

RISK FACTORS for Uterine Fibroid Tumors

Obesity	Nulliparity
Onset of menarche before age 10	African American descent
Polycystic ovary syndrome	Diabetes mellitus
Hypertension	

Source: Latendresse, G., McCance, K., & Morgan, K. (2010). Alterations of the reproductive systems. In K. McCance & S. Huether (Eds.), *Pathophysiology: The biologic basis for disease in adults and children* (6th ed., pp. 781–815). St. Louis: Mosby/Elsevier; Stoppler, M. (2010). Uterine fibroids. eMedicinehealth. Retrieved from http://www.emedicinehealth.com/uterine_fibroids/article_em.htm.

Nursing Management

Nurses are responsible for monitoring sedated patients and should be prepared to manage sedation and the analgesia required immediately after the procedure. Nursing interventions include monitoring:

- Vital signs until the effects of anesthesia have worn off
- Vaginal bleeding including how often the pad is changed
- Pain and anxiety.

Pelvic Pain

Pelvic pain is discomfort in the lower abdomen that may be caused by problems in the female reproductive organs. Other causes may arise from the gastrointestinal system, the urinary system, or the musculoskeletal system; the pain also may be psychogenic. If the pain is gynecological, it may be cyclic (recurring at the same time during each cycle) or it may be separate and unrelated to the menstrual cycle. The most common gynecologic cyclic causes are dysmenorrhea, **mittelschmerz** (pain felt at ovulation due to peritoneal irritation from fluids from a ruptured follicle), and endometriosis (Barad, 2011). Causes that are not cyclic may include pelvic inflammatory disease, ruptured ovarian cyst, ectopic pregnancy, cancer, adhesions, miscarriage, and ovarian torsion.

Endometriosis

Description and Etiology

Endometriosis affects approximately 5.5 million women between the ages of 15 and 64 in the United States and Canada (McLeod & Retzloff, 2010). The exact incidence is difficult to determine because many women who are affected do not have symptoms or have not been diagnosed. Many women will have either infertility or pain for 6 to 12 years before a definitive diagnosis is made (Mao & Anastasi, 2010). Endometriosis is the third-leading cause for hospitalization related to the female reproductive system. The highest prevalence rates are among infertile couples where, depending on the study, rates vary from 5% to 50% (McLeod & Retzloff, 2010). Although it affects women from all ethnic groups and socioeconomic backgrounds, the incidence is higher among White women 25 to 34 years of age.

Endometriosis is a condition where endometrial-like cells that are normally found only in the uterus have grown in areas outside of the uterus. These **ectopic** (outside the usual site) growths respond to hormones of the menstrual cycle by growing and sloughing just as they do inside the uterus. These responses to hormones depend on the presence of a blood supply, glandular, and stromal cells within the ectopic implant. The bleeding that occurs each month from the implants will cause inflammation and the release of inflammatory products that cause pain, as well as eventual scarring and fibrosis. As the misplaced tissue grows, it can cover and grow into the ovaries and block the fallopian tubes, causing infertility (Latendresse et al., 2010; Mao & Anastasi, 2010).

The cause of endometriosis is unknown. However, there are several theories:

- Retrograde menstruation (where menstrual products move backward through the fallopian tubes and out into the pelvic cavity). This is not a complete explanation because it occurs in many women who do not develop endometriosis.
- Impaired cellular and humoral immunity occurs.
- Autoimmune response develops.
- Endometrial cells are spread via the lymph or vascular system (this explains lung and brain implants).
- Genetic predisposition exists (a mother or sister with endometriosis increases the risks to 4 to 8 times those of the general population) (Latendresse et al., 2010; Mao & Anastasi, 2010).

Endometrial implants may occur anywhere in the body, but are most frequently found in the pelvic and abdominal cavities attached to the ovaries, peritoneum, colon, small intestine, rectum, bladder, uterus, vulva, vagina, and cervix. Less frequently, the implants may be found in the pleural cavity, lungs, brain, and surgical scars (especially those made during gynecological surgical procedures) (Latendresse et al., 2010).

Larger nodules of endometriosis are called **endometriomas** and may attach deeply into uterosacral ligaments, the bladder, the bowel, and ureters. An ovarian endometrioma will appear as a cyst filled with thick, tarlike brownish fluid; a so-called "chocolate cyst" (Nelson & Baldwin, 2009).

Risk factors for endometriosis include a family history, menstrual flow of greater than 6 days, and menstrual cycle of less than 28 days. Women at risk for endometriosis experienced menarche at an early age and have very heavy menses; they also have periods that last more than 7 days.

Other risk factors that have been proposed include tall stature, low body mass index, no pregnancies, immune disorders, dioxin and PCB exposure, low birth weight, being one of a set of twins, and genetic predisposition (McLeod & Retzloff, 2010). Risk factors for endometriosis are presented in the Risk Factors feature. Refer to the Genetic Considerations feature for more about the heritable component of this disorder.

RISK FACTORS for Endometriosis

Early menarche	Shorter menstrual cycle
Nulliparity	Low birth weight
Woman is one of twins or triplets	Endometriosis in first-degree relative
Tall	Low body mass index
Dioxin/PCB exposure	Immune disorders

Source: Adapted from McLeod, B., & Retzloff, M. (2010). Epidemiology of endometriosis: An assessment of risk factors. *Clinical Obstetrics and Gynecology, 53*(2), 389–396.

GENETIC CONSIDERATIONS for Female Reproductive Disorders

Endometriosis
Incidence and severity of endometriosis is highest among women with female relatives who have endometriosis. Some genetic polymorphisms have been identified (Latendresse et al., 2010). There is a strong familial tendency and genetic component for cystocele and rectocele. Hispanic women have the highest risk for this disorder (Latendresse et al., 2010).

Ovarian Cancer
DNA mutations that turn on oncogenes and turn off tumor suppressor genes can cause this cancer. A mutation in the BRCA1 or BRCA2 genes is responsible for most inherited ovarian cancers. In fact, the lifetime ovarian cancer risk for women with a BRCA1 mutation is 35% to 70%, or as high as 70 women in every 100 who has this gene mutation. Ashkenazi Jewish women are 10 times as likely to have a mutation in these genes (ACS, 2010).

Polycystic Ovary Syndrome
Polycystic ovary syndrome is familial and transmitted as a modified autosomal dominant trait (Fitzgerald, 2011).

Clinical Manifestations

Endometriosis can produce mild symptoms of discomfort or severe pain. While the symptoms vary in severity, about 50% of women who will eventually be diagnosed with endometriosis will come to the health care provider with severe **dysmenorrhea** (painful menses) that becomes worse each month. The patient may also report deep dyspareunia, painful defecation and urination, lower abdominal and back pain, fatigue, malaise, and difficulty with sleep. Endometriosis is difficult to diagnose because it mimics other conditions and the degree of pain does not always correlate with the extent of the endometriosis (Nelson & Baldwin, 2009). Abnormal uterine bleeding may also occur. Endometriosis is associated with infertility because of adhesions that distort the pelvic anatomy and cause impaired ovum release and implantation. Many women who present for infertility will have endometriosis with mild symptoms (Mao & Anastasi, 2010). On examination, women with endometriosis usually have normal gynecologic findings. However, some may have an asymptomatic pelvic mass; or tender, irregular, mobile masses; or a fixed, retroverted uterus (Latendresse et al., 2010).

The most common abnormal objective finding is tenderness of the posterior vagina (Mao & Anastasi, 2010).

Medical Management

Endometriosis is diagnosed by direct visualization via laparoscopy and biopsy. Using pelvic ultrasound is helpful in identifying endometriomas and disease involving the bladder and bowel. However, ultrasound does not help with the diagnosis of peritoneal endometriosis (Nelson & Baldwin, 2009). Treatment ranges from palliative over-the-counter pain medications to prescription medications and surgery. Choices are made based on the severity of symptoms and the patient's desire for a pregnancy. The most commonly prescribed medication is oral contraceptives. Oral contraceptives and nonsteroidal anti-inflammatory drugs (NSAIDs) control dysmenorrhea and decrease menstrual bleeding. Continuous combined oral contraceptives will lead to amenorrhea and cessation of symptoms until the pills are discontinued. Other medications prescribed include high-dose progesterone, gonadotropin-releasing hormone (GnRH) agonists, and Danazol. These medications alter the production of hormones, causing the symptoms associated with endometriosis, or shrink the sites of adhesions that will reduce symptoms (Mao & Anastasi, 2010). See the Pharmacology feature (p. 1277). Laparoscopic surgery to examine reproductive organs and remove or obliterate endometrial implants is an alternative treatment. A hysterectomy may be indicated in extreme cases.

Nursing Management

Assessment

Nursing management for the patient with endometriosis is primarily about patient education. The patient needs to understand the disease process and the accompanying signs and symptoms. In addition, the patient needs to understand the treatment options and the use of medications that are prescribed to treat endometriosis. For example, NSAIDs and heat are often helpful for dysmenorrhea. Hormone medications such as Danazol and GnRH agonists may stop periods but can cause side effects similar to menopause (hot flashes and vaginal dryness). Sometimes these side effects will subside if patients take estrogen every day. Patients should not get pregnant while taking medications for endometriosis. Women who want to get pregnant may need surgery to treat their endometriosis before they can conceive. Even with surgery, women with endometriosis may still need fertility treatments. In addition, endometriosis can recur. Endometriosis pain will probably go away with the onset of menopause.

Nursing Diagnoses

Nursing diagnoses associated with endometriosis include:

- *Potential for Tissue Perfusion, Ineffective* related to prolonged and heavy periods.
- *Fatigue* related to anemia and chronic pain.
- *Chronic* and *Acute Pain* related to pelvic lesions.
- *Deficient Knowledge* related to management of symptoms and treatment options.
- *Ineffective Sexuality Pattern* related to dyspareunia.
- *Anxiety* and *Grieving* related to decreased fertility.

  NANDA-I © 2012

Outcomes

Expected outcomes associated with endometriosis is the occurrence of a normal menstrual pattern, regular menstrual cycles extending to 28 days, and menstrual bleeding that does not require more than 1 pad in 2 hours. Outcomes also include menstrual discomfort that is controlled and does not interfere with the patient's normal activities and the patient verbalizes understanding of management of the symptoms and treatment options. Finally, the patient seeks infertility counseling.

Planning and Interventions

Nursing interventions associated with endometriosis include:

- Monitoring of complete blood count (CBC) to determine changes in hemoglobin and hematocrit. Report a drop of 1 gram or more in the hemoglobin or a drop of 3% or more in the hematocrit.
- Encourage the patient to pace activities to avoid fatigue.
- Instruct the patient in pain management techniques, including use of NSAIDs and heat, along with relaxation techniques and diversion.
- Provide resources for information about endometriosis such as the Endometriosis Association (www.endometriosisassn.org/) and www.endometriosis.org/ for global news.
- Provide a nonjudgmental environment in which to discuss problems with dyspareunia and sexual dysfunction.
- Provide resources for further counseling, including infertility as indicated.

Ovarian Cysts

Benign ovarian cysts may occur at any time in a woman's reproductive years but most often occur during puberty or perimenopause when hormones are fluctuating. About one-third of hospital admissions for gynecological reasons are related to benign ovarian cysts (Latendresse et al., 2010). Follicular cysts occur when the dominant follicle does not rupture or when one or more of the other follicles do not recede after ovulation. Signs and symptoms of follicular cyst include bloating, tender breasts, and irregular menses with more bleeding than normal. These cysts usually regress over time and do not need treatment; however, they do recur. Some may be as big as 8 to 10 centimeters (Latendresse et al., 2010). Oral contraceptives at regular dosages will decrease the occurrence of follicular cysts (Nelson, 2009).

Corpus luteum cysts develop because of low luteinizing hormone levels that cause a lack of maturation of the corpus luteum after ovulation (Latendresse et al., 2009). Corpus luteum cysts are less common, but more painful, than follicular cysts. Hemorrhagic corpus luteum cysts may rupture and cause hemorrhage that requires emergency surgery (Nelson, 2009). Signs and symptoms are more likely to occur during the latter half of the menstrual cycle and include pelvic pain, as well as amenorrhea or delayed menses followed by heavier than usual bleeding. Corpus luteum cysts usually diminish without treatment, unless they rupture and bleed. Treatment to prevent recurrence is oral contractive pills (Latendresse et al., 2010).

Dermoid cysts (teratomas) are benign ovarian cysts that are made up of elements of all three germ layers of the embryonic period. Elements of these layers include skin, hair, sebaceous and sweat glands, muscle, cartilage and bone (Latendresse et al., 2010). Dermoid cysts are most likely to be found during pelvic examination because they do not always cause symptoms. These cysts are likely to become malignant, so surgical removal is recommended.

Ovarian cysts may cause **ovarian torsion** or the twisting of the ovary and fallopian tube. This causes a loss of blood flow to these organs (Schraga & Blanda, 2011). The ischemia from loss of blood flow will cause severe pelvic pain. Ovarian torsion is the fifth most common gynecologic surgical emergency in the United States (Schraga & Blanda, 2011).

Ectopic Pregnancy

Description and Etiology

An ectopic pregnancy is implantation of the products of conception outside the uterine endometrium (Figure 41–4◆). Approximately 2% of all pregnancies are ectopic (Dulay, 2010). The most common location for an ectopic pregnancy is the fallopian tube. Ectopics may also occur in such places as the cornua of the uterus, cervix, ovary, or abdominal organs.

Weblink: Ectopic Pregnancy

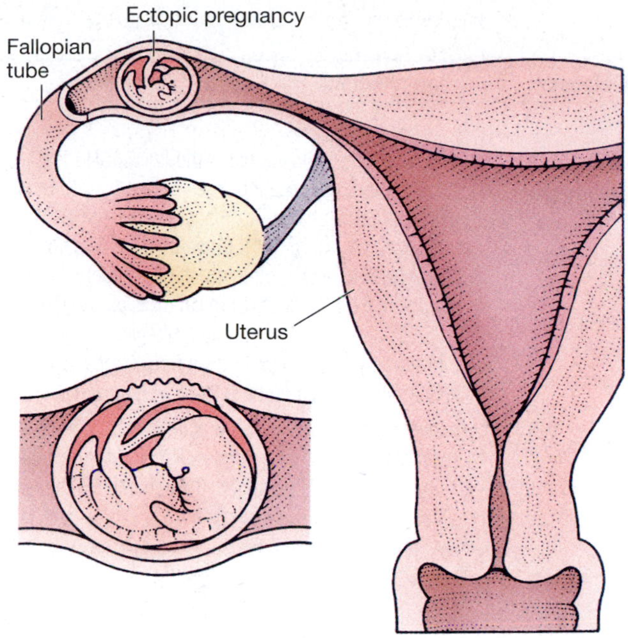

FIGURE 41–4 ◆ Ectopic pregnancy.
Source: © Dorling Kindersley.

RISK FACTORS for Ectopic Pregnancy

Prior ectopic pregnancy	History of pelvic inflammatory disease
History of tubal surgery	Intrauterine device use
Increasing age	History of infertility
Multiple sex partners	Cigarette smoking
Abnormally shaped uterus	Prior induced abortion
Use of fertility drugs or assisted reproductive technology	

Sources: Dulay, A. (2010). Ectopic pregnancy. Merck Medicus Online Medical Library. Retrieved from http://www.merckmedicus.com/pp/us/hcp/framemm.jsp?pg=www.merck.com/mmpe/index.html; Sepilian, V., & Wood, E. (2010). Ectopic pregnancy. eMedicine. Retrieved from http://emedicine.medscape.com/article/258768-overview.

Epidemiology

Causes of ectopic pregnancy are varied but often include problems that may leave scar tissue or prevent appropriate movement of the fertilized ovum down the fallopian tube and into the uterine cavity. These problems include pelvic inflammatory disease (PID), previous ectopic pregnancy, endometriosis, tubal surgery, and use of an intrauterine device (IUD) for birth control. Also contributing to the risk of ectopic pregnancy are procedures used in infertility treatments, including *in vitro* fertilization and embryo transfer. See the Risk Factors for Ectopic Pregnancy feature. Approximately 30% of women treated for ectopic pregnancy later have difficulty conceiving. Rates of recurrent ectopic pregnancy are between 5% and 20% (Sepilian & Wood, 2010).

Pathophysiology and Clinical Manifestations

Any condition that leaves residual scar tissue can cause partial or complete blockage of the fallopian tubes. The scar tissue impedes the passing of the fertilized egg into the uterus. As the cells divide, the gestational sac expands against the tubal wall. If allowed to continue, the tube expands until it ruptures, causing acute lower abdominal pain and internal bleeding.

Often, the patient will present with typical symptoms of pregnancy, including an elevated quantitative human chorionic gonadotropin (HCG), amenorrhea, and nausea, but with pelvic pain and in some cases light vaginal bleeding. The prime time for the manifestations of ectopic pregnancy is at approximately 7 weeks after a missed period, although rupture has occurred as early as 6 weeks' gestation (Dulay, 2010). These findings are very nonspecific and are certainly common to patients who may be having a spontaneous abortion, acute appendicitis, ovarian cyst or torsion, pelvic inflammatory disease, urinary tract infection, or renal calculi (Sepilian & Wood, 2010). Therefore, the positive HCG is very important to making the diagnosis of ectopic pregnancy. Because the implantation is not inside the uterus where space for the growth of the embryo is adequate, the growth puts pressure on the surrounding tissues and structures, causing discomfort and pain. If the fallopian tube ruptures, the patient experiences intense, sharp, unilateral pain, with pain referred to the shoulder as a result of irritation of the diaphragm by blood in the abdominal cavity. When this happens, there is a risk of hemorrhage and hypovolemic shock. This is treated as a medical emergency. Ruptured ectopic pregnancy is the cause of about 9% of pregnancy-related maternal deaths in the United States (Dulay, 2010).

Medical Management, Laboratory and Diagnostic Testing

Due to the life-threatening potential of ectopic pregnancy, all women of childbearing age who present with lower abdominal or pelvic pain should be tested for pregnancy. If the test is positive, then the patient will need a high-resolution transvaginal ultrasound to examine the ovaries, uterus, and fallopian tubes (Kirsch & Scoutt, 2010). Quantitative HCG is a serum test used to determine the duration of the pregnancy. Under normal circumstances, this value doubles every 48 hours in early pregnancy. If the HCG level fails to double, the pregnancy is not viable, and an ectopic pregnancy is assumed until proven otherwise. The transvaginal ultrasound will be accurate in determining the presence of an intrauterine pregnancy when the quantitative HCG has reached 1,500 to 2,000 mLU/m (Kirsch & Scoutt, 2010).

Medical treatment of ectopic pregnancy is preferred over surgical treatment. Methotrexate, a drug often used in cancer treatment, is the current drug of choice and will act on the ectopic cells as it does in cancer treatment: to destroy the cells. It is given if the ectopic is unruptured and no bigger than 3.5 centimeters by ultrasound, the patient is in stable condition, and no contraindications exist for the use of methotrexate (Sepilian & Wood, 2010). It is given intramuscularly and often as an outpatient procedure. Successful treatment may require more than one dose of methotrexate.

Failure of beta HCG levels to decrease by at least 25% from day 4 to day 7 after methotrexate administration indicates the need for an additional dose of methotrexate or surgery (Dulay, 2010). If surgery is indicated with a ruptured ectopic pregnancy, a laparoscopic approach is preferred. Surgery consists of repair of the tube if future pregnancies are desired. Removal of the tube may be necessary if repair is not possible or may be desired if future pregnancies are not planned.

Reproductive System Cancers

Reproductive system cancers include cervical, vulvar, endometrial, ovarian, and vaginal cancers. See Chart 41–3 for a comparison of these cancers. The Genetic Considerations feature contains information about the genetics for ovarian cancer (p. 1259). Chapter 57 has an in-depth discussion of the pathophysiology of cancer, treatment options, and prognosis.

CHART 41–3 Comparison of Female Reproductive Cancers

Etiology, Epidemiology, & Risk Factors	Assessment & Clinical Manifestations	Interventions
Cervical Cancer		
Incidence continues to decrease in U.S., thanks to Pap test. 90% Squamous cell. 10% Adenocarcinoma. Average age 30–50. Increased risk with human papillomavirus (HPV), smoking, immunosuppression, multiple partners, Chlamydia infection, taking oral contraceptives longer than 5 years, young age at first term pregnancy, genetic predisposition, and poverty. Occurs most often in Hispanic women (2 times more than White women). African American women have an incidence rate 50% higher than White women.	Preinvasion is often asymptomatic. Invasive shows postcoital bleeding and abnormal bleeding. Late symptoms include rectal bleeding, hematuria, back and leg pain, and anemia. Pap test is the single most reliable diagnostic test (it will show 90% of early cervical cancers). See Chapter 43 (p. 1323) for more about Pap tests. Other diagnostic tests include colposcopy, biopsy, and conization.	Regular Pap tests with or without HPV DNA testing to detect cervical changes before cancer. Best prevention is abstinence. Vaccine against HPV types 6, 11, 16, and 18 prevents cervical cancer. Preinvasive lesions often entail cryosurgery, laser surgery, or loop electrosurgical excision procedure (LEEP: an electrically charged thin wire is used to remove a thin layer of cells from the cervix). Typically done as an outpatient procedure. Invasive treatment is hysterectomy with internal (brachytherapy) or external radiation. May include chemotherapy if advanced. See Chapter 57 for discussion of these therapies.
Fallopian Tube Cancer		
Very rare. Accounts for 1–2% of gynecological cancers. About 300 to 400 women are diagnosed each year in the United States. Most of the time result of metastasis from other organs. Affects Caucasian women ages 50 to 60 most often, but may occur at any age. More common on women with no children. BRCA1 gene may be involved in the cause.	Symptoms mimic other gynecologic problems and include abnormal vaginal bleeding (especially after menopause), lower abdominal pain and pressure, and pelvic mass. Diagnosis is difficult. May be discovered as adnexal mass on pelvic exam or pelvic ultrasound. CA125 blood test is a tumor marker for this cancer and ovarian cancer.	Surgery—usually total abdominal hysterectomy. Chemotherapy is recommended after surgery.
Vulvar Cancer		
Accounts for 4% of female reproductive cancers and 0.6% of all cancers in women. Average age of those affected is 50 to 70. Those under 50 are linked to high risk type HPV. 90% squamous cell carcinoma. Other risks: smoking, HIV, lichen sclerosis, other genital cancers, and melanoma.	Lesion usually asymptomatic until 1–2 centimeters. Symptoms include vulvar pruritus, burning pain, tumor growth, raw surface, or white rough area in vagina. Diagnosed by biopsy with histologic evaluation using toluidine blue applied to detect dysplastic areas on the vulva.	Depends on the stage of cancer. Local, wide excision, or vulvectomy. External radiation.
Endometrial Cancer		
Most common gynecologic malignancy. Most common type: endometriod adenocarcinoma. Average age 50 to 69. More common in White women, but Black women are more likely to die from it. Risk factors include obesity, early menarche, late menopause, nullipara, infertility, diabetes mellitus, hypertension, family history, Tamoxifen therapy, and hormone imbalance, which is the most significant risk factor.	Symptoms include abnormal uterine bleeding or non-bloody vaginal discharge. Lower back pain, lower pelvic pain, uterine enlargement, and weight loss are later signs. Diagnosis by fractional curettage or endometrial biopsy.	Total abdominal hysterectomy with bilateral salpingectomy and oophorectomy. Radiation (brachytherapy or external beam) before or after surgery. Chemotherapy with advanced stage or recurrent.
Ovarian Cancer		
Ninth most common cancer among women; ranks fifth in cancer deaths. More common in White women. Risks include age, obesity, personal history of breast cancer, nullipara, infertility, and family history. About 50% of cases are diagnosed after age 60.	No definitive tests. Often diagnosed in late stage. Symptoms include abdominal swelling, pelvic pressure, abdominal pain, digestive and urinary complaints. Increased pain, weakness, and malnutrition are late signs.	Treatment varies from removal of the ovary to total hysterectomy. Chemotherapy. Hormone therapy to turn off estrogen production. Antineoplastic drugs. Radiation is controversial.

CHART 41–3 Comparison of Female Reproductive Cancers, *continued*

Etiology, Epidemiology, & Risk Factors	Assessment & Clinical Manifestations	Interventions
Vaginal Cancer		
Rare. Two types: squamous cell 70% (increased in ages 60 to 80) and adenocarcinoma 15%. Risks include young women of mothers who received diethylstilbestrol (DES) in 1945–1970 as a treatment for miscarriage. Also, HPV types 16 and 18, personal history of cervical cancer, smoking, and HIV.	Bleeding or discharge not related to menstruation, mass in the vagina, and pain during intercourse (dyspareunia). Pelvic pain is a late sign.	Treatment depends on the stage of the cancer and may include: • Surgery (to remove the cancer) • Radiation (to kill cancer cells and/or shrink tumors) • Chemotherapy (to kill the cancer cells).

Sources: American Cancer Society (ACS). (2010). Detailed guides for cervical, vulva, endometrial, ovarian, and vaginal cancer. *Learn about cancer.* Retrieved from http://www.cancer.org/Cancer/CervicalCancer/DetailedGuide/index; http://www.cancer.org/Cancer/VulvarCancer/DetailedGuide/index; http://www.cancer.org/Cancer/EndometrialCancer/DetailedGuide/index; http://www.cancer.org/Cancer/OvarianCancer/DetailedGuide/index; http://www.cancer.org/Cancer/VaginalCancer/DetailedGuide/index; University of California at San Francisco (UCSF) Medical Center Staff. (2011). Fallopian tube cancer. UCSF Medical Center. Retrieved from http://www.ucsfhealth.org/conditions/fallopian_tube_cancer/.

Sexual Disorders

Orgasmic Dysfunction

Description, Etiology, Epidemiology, and Clinical Manifestations

One phase of the sexual response cycle is the orgasmic phase. When there is difficulty reaching orgasm, it is called orgasmic dysfunction, or **anorgasmia**. Anorgasmia is considered to be one of the most common sexual problems among women; however, less than 20% of cases are related to physiological issues. Anorgasmia is frequently found to be psychological in nature and results from unresolved conflicts about sexual activity or marital conflict (Bridges, 2010). Primary dysfunction is when the woman has never had an orgasm following any means of sexual stimulation. Secondary dysfunction occurs when the woman has had orgasms in the past, but is unable to achieve them now.

Pathophysiology

Causes of anorgasmia can be disease that results in general debility such as multiple sclerosis, diabetes, spinal cord injuries, and hormonal conditions that affect sexual response. Drugs such as antidepressants, alcohol, and other central nervous system (CNS) depressants can also inhibit sexual response. Chart 41–4 outlines medications that interfere with sexual function.

CHART 41–4 Medications That Interfere with Sexual Function

Psychoactive Medications	
Antipsychotics	Barbiturates
Benzodiazepines	Selective serotonin reuptake inhibitors
Lithium	Tricyclic antidepressants
Cardiovascular and Antihypertensive Medications	
Antilipid medications	Beta-blockers
Clonidine	Digoxin
Spironolactone	Central nervous system agents
Anticholinergics	Antihistamines
H_2 blockers	Methyldopa
Amphetamines	Anorexic drugs
Narcotics	Phenytoin

Menopause and oophorectomy (surgical removal of the ovaries) create a hypoestrogenic state, which may increase the likelihood of orgasmic dysfunction. Testosterone decreases with menopause and oophorectomy, and, like in males, is considered an essential female hormone for sexual desire. Testosterone appears to have a direct role in sexual desire. However, studies are limited at this point, so no guidelines exist for testosterone replacement therapy for women with disorders of desire (Bridges, 2010).

Medical Management

Orgasmic disorders can be treated with Kegel exercises and masturbation. The purpose is to maximize stimulation and minimize inhibition.

Treatment of both physical and psychological circumstances may benefit from counseling therapy. When medical conditions prevent the patient's ability to reach orgasm, therapy may be directed at alternative ways of satisfaction, such as simply holding each other close, touching, or exploring individual ways that make each other feel satisfied. When secondary dysfunction is the cause, counseling is directed at the couple and the root of their discord.

Dyspareunia

Etiology, Epidemiology, and Clinical Manifestations

Dyspareunia, painful intercourse, can be a result of several physiological and psychological factors. Endometriosis is an example of a physiological cause, which is due to displaced endometrial tissue in the peritoneal cavity. Menopause is another physiological cause, resulting from a decrease in hormone production, which in turn decreases the normal lubricating mechanism of the vagina. In addition, the vagina may become somewhat smaller during menopause, causing a more difficult penetration. Other physiological causes may include an imperforate hymen or vaginal scarring.

Psychological causes may be related to early traumatic events such as sexual abuse or rape, triggering an involuntary reflex known as vaginismus. **Vaginismus** is a condition in which the vaginal muscles at the introitus contract very tightly, making vaginal penetration painful.

Medical Management

Hormonal treatment of endometriosis, often with danazol (Danocrine), an androgenic steroid, has been successful in regression of the displaced endometrial tissue. Hormone replacement therapy and lubricating gel can assist in the treatment of dyspareunia related to menopause. Psychological causes require counseling.

Nursing Management

Assessment

Use of the nursing process provides an effective framework to guide the nursing management for patients experiencing the various reproductive system disorders. During the nursing assessment, it is important to obtain a history from the woman about the type of reproductive disorder that is occurring. The nurse should be careful not to ask questions in a manner that alludes to bias toward heterosexuality or homosexuality. However, establishment of the patient's sexual orientation is necessary for appropriate evaluation and management. Nonjudgmental, direct questions best achieve this goal (Bickley, 2007). The interviewer must be careful to ensure privacy and confidentiality. During the interview, the nurse gains a complete history of the patient's symptoms include timing, situation, and duration. Questioning the patient about her insight into the cause also may be very helpful. It is important to collect history regarding the patient's chronic illnesses and injuries, and to gather a psychiatric history. Prescription and over-the-counter medications, as well as the use of recreational drugs and alcohol, must be listed accurately. Surgical interventions and malignancies such as breast cancer can alter self-image and cause decreased sexuality. The nurse should ask questions regarding the patient's relationships to determine the level of partner support and previous problematic or violent relationships.

A complete physical with a pelvic exam needs to be done to determine the existence of vaginismus, vulvar dystrophy, dermatitis, vaginal atrophy, infectious disease, scar tissue, postoperative changes, fibroids, masses, endometriosis, tenderness, or structural defects. The goal of the examination is detection of disease; however, the examination also provides an opportunity to educate the patient about normal anatomy and sexual function, and to reproduce and localize pain encountered during sexual activity (Bickley, 2007).

Nursing Diagnoses

Nursing diagnoses associated with female reproductive dysfunction include:

- *Disturbed Body Image* related to reproductive system disorder.
- *Ineffective Sexuality Pattern* related to reproductive system disorder.
- *Risk for Situational Low Self-Esteem* related to sexual difficulties.
- *Chronic Pain* related to reproductive system disorder.
- *Compromised Family Coping* related to reproductive system disorder.
- *Decisional Conflict* related to treatment options.
- *Deficient Knowledge* related to disease process.
- *Disturbed Thought Process* related to sense of inadequacy.
- *Fear.*

NANDA-I © 2012

Outcomes

Expected outcomes of care for patients experiencing reproductive dysfunction include:

- Enhanced knowledge related to sexual functioning
- Decreased anxiety and fear
- Acceptance of body image
- Adequate decision making regarding treatment options
- Improved family coping
- Adequate health seeking behaviors
- Adequate sexual functioning and identity
- Enhanced self-esteem related to sexual difficulties
- Adequate pain relief and ability to cope with pain.

Planning and Interventions

Care of the patient with sexual dysfunction requires education, support, and therapeutic interventions. Information regarding normal anatomy, sexual function, and the normal changes of aging, pregnancy, and menopause are important. Encourage discussion of sexual issues in the context of a medical condition or a new medication agent prescribed. Depression is frequently associated with reproductive disorders; therefore, psychological counseling may be necessary. Women with longstanding dysfunction, multiple dysfunctions, or history of sexual abuse need to be referred to a gynecologist and/or psychological counseling.

Health Promotion

Patients frequently have difficulty discussing sexual problems with their health care provider. However, up to 70% of couples have a problem with sex at some time during their relationship. Promoting good sexual health is dependent on providing an accepting environment in which patients can discuss their problems with sexual response. Encouraging patients to explain their problems openly and honestly with their health care provider can result in possible treatments. It is also important for couples to communicate regarding concerns. A mutually satisfying relationship that includes respectful and caring behaviors on the part of both partners provides the best hope for a gratifying sex life.

Menstrual Disorders

Menstrual disorders involve not only physical symptoms but emotional symptoms as well. Because the menstrual cycle is related to the woman's reproductive ability, any problems may be a cause of great concern. Almost all women will experience some form of menstrual disorder in their lifetime, such as missing a period, having heavy periods, or enduring painful periods. The most common disorders are discussed next.

Amenorrhea

Description, Etiology, Epidemiology, and Pathophysiology

Amenorrhea is defined as the absence of menstruation. It is considered primary when the girl/woman has not started her menstrual cycles by the age of 16 (Fitzgerald, 2011). It is secondary when menstruation has been present but ceases for more than 3 months and is not related to pregnancy. Secondary amenorrhea is more common than primary amenorrhea. Causes of amenorrhea are varied and may be related to stress, athleticism, weight changes, and disease/hormonal processes. Chart 41–5 outlines the various causes of amenorrhea.

Primary amenorrhea can be caused by a congenital absence of a part of the reproductive tract such as the ovaries, uterus, or vagina. Another cause could be the presence of the imperforate hymen. Imperforate hymen is a congenital defect in which the opening to the vagina does not form, and as a result there is no exit from the vagina. Imperforate hymen occurs in 1 in 1,000 women. A procedure using local anesthetic can correct the defect.

In adolescence, stress, eating disorders, exercise, and ovulation abnormalities can cause irregular periods. This is especially pertinent for the patient in whom fat comprises less than 10% of the body.

CHART 41–5 Causes of Amenorrhea

Hormone Alteration	
Thyroid disease: hypothyroidism	Pituitary dysfunction
Menopause	Pregnancy
Cushing's syndrome	Polycystic ovary syndrome
Chronic Disease	
• Liver failure	Renal failure
• Cancer (bronchogenic, renal cell CA)	Autoimmune diseases
• Chemotherapy	Pelvic radiation
• Central nervous system tumor	Diabetes
• Immunodeficiency	Inflammatory bowel disease
• Thyroid disease	Severe chronic depression
Structural Defects	
Imperforate hymen	Cervical stenosis
Transverse vaginal septum	
Congenital defect causing absence of ovaries, fallopian tubes, or uterus	
Medications	
Oral contraceptives	Antipsychotics
Antidepressants	Antihypertensives
Histamine H_2-receptor blockers	Opiates, cocaine
Exercise and Nutrition	
Anorexia or bulimia nervosa	Excessive exercise
Excessive weight loss	Malnutrition
Alterations in Growth and Development	
Constitutional delay of growth and puberty	Acromegaly
Congenital adrenal hyperplasia	Mumps
Genetic defects	

Bulimia, anorexia, obesity, and malnutrition may alter the hormone balance in the body, as some are produced by fat cells. This change in hormone production or utilization may cause amenorrhea. Excessive exercise, usually more than 20 hours a week for a prolonged number of weeks, triggers a reduction in reproductive hormones, particularly leptin. Decreased leptin can interfere with the production of luteinizing hormone, which is necessary for ovulation.

Clinical Manifestations

There is a triad of symptoms that has been identified in the female athlete that reflects the health issues of females who exercise more than 20 hours per week. The components are amenorrhea or oligomenorrhea, eating disorder (anorexia or bulimia), and decreased bone mineral density (Quinn, 2010). Alternatively, women who are obese also have a higher incidence of amenorrhea due to **anovulation** (absence of ovulation).

Medical Management

Elevated prolactin levels may inhibit ovulation and consequently cause amenorrhea. The elevated levels may be related to pituitary tumors and can cause breast milk production not related to pregnancy (**galactorrhea**) (Latendresse et al., 2010). Elevated prolactin levels need to be evaluated by an endocrinologist. Treatment of amenorrhea depends on the cause. Frequently, correcting pituitary disorders or thyroid disorders, or inducing appropriate nutrition and exercise levels, can result in normal menstruation.

Oligomenorrhea

Infrequent menstruation or menstrual cycles longer than 6 to 7 weeks is termed **oligomenorrhea** (Paradise, 2011). It is the pattern seen when the menstrual cycle is longer than 35 days but not long enough to be considered amenorrhea (Nelson & Baldwin, 2009). Oligomenorrhea usually indicates endocrine control changes in the menstrual cycle such as those seen during the first year after menarche and the last few years before menopause. Oligomenorrhea may also occur among women who are obese and women who have polycystic ovary syndrome (discussed later in this chapter) (Fitzgerald, 2011). Other medical problems that may cause oligomenorrhea include hypothyroidism, hyperprolactinemia, and liver disorders.

It is important to determine the underlying cause of oligomenorrhea and then treat that cause. In the cases where oligomenorrhea occurs as a result of excessive weight gain or polycystic ovary syndrome, unopposed estrogen is the cause. Without intervention, these women are at risk for endometrial hyperplasia and cancer. Exercise, weight loss, and the use of oral contraceptives or other endometrial suppressant drugs will help decrease the risk (Nelson & Balwin, 2009). This is further discussed in the section concerning polycystic ovary syndrome.

Polycystic Ovary Syndrome

Description, Etiology, and Epidemiology

Polycystic ovary syndrome (PCO or PCOS) is one of the most common endocrine disorders that affect women and one of the leading causes of infertility (Latendresse et al., 2010). Approximately 5 million women of childbearing age have PCOS (Eisenberg, 2011). In order to receive a diagnosis of PCOS, a woman must either have anovulation (no ovulation), elevated levels of androgen, or clinical signs of hyperandrogenism and polycystic ovaries. Polycystic ovaries do not have to be present for the syndrome to be diagnosed (Fitzgerald, 2011; Latendresse et al., 2010). The causes of PCOS are unknown at this time, but scientists are studying genetic mutations that may be at the root.

Pathophysiology

Genes involved in androgen biosynthesis and the insulin receptors in the ovaries have been identified as possible culprits (refer to the Genetic Considerations feature (p. 1259). High levels of androgen are the main feature of this disorder; however, insulin resistance, hyperinsulinemia, and glucose intolerance are also features (Fitzgerald, 2011). Higher levels of insulin cause an increase in androgen; androgen affects ovarian follicle growth and insulin causes more follicles to survive. Androgen excess and higher levels of insulin will suppress follicle-stimulating hormone (FSH) and cause an elevation in luteinizing hormone (LH). Increased LH leads to further increases in androgen production from the adrenals and ovaries. There is also an increase in free estradiol related to the higher levels of androgen. The higher estradiol will cause a further increase in LH and does not fully suppress FSH, so the follicles continue to grow but do not mature or produce an ovum. This causes a "string of pearls" phenomenon on ultrasound of the ovary because there are many fluid-filled follicles (Latendresse et al., 2010). The follicles of PCOS do not form ovum or eggs, so there is no ovulation and subsequent change in the follicle that will cause it to produce progesterone. Without progesterone, a woman's menstrual cycle is irregular or absent and the endometrium does not slough as it would normally.

Clinical Manifestations

The associated low or absent progesterone production, increased estrogen levels, and increased androgen production may produce the

Weblink: Polycystic Ovarian Syndrome Fact Sheet

following manifestations: hirsutism (excessive hair growth) and acne, **oligomenorrhea** (few periods), infertility due to anovulation, pelvic pain due to ovarian cyst formation, anxiety or depression due to appearance and infertility, obesity, and elevated lipids and blood glucose. The obesity, if present, is in the abdomen, causing increased waist circumference. **Acanthosis nigricans** (a velvety, brown-thickened skin of the neck, axilla, groin, and dorsum of the hand) is an indication of hyperinsulinemia and is often seen among obese women with PCOS. These women are prone to type 2 diabetes mellitus, dyslipidemia, hypertension, heart disease, stroke, and endometrial cancer (due to stimulation of the endometrium) (Bartoszek, 2009). On rare occasions, PCOS may produce the male characteristics of deepening voice.

Medical Management

Medical management of PCOS depends on the signs and symptoms. Many women with this syndrome do not know they have it until they discover they are infertile. The infertility work-up will reveal the problem and the patient may be given clomiphene to stimulate ovulation. If she does not ovulate, metformin is given to increase the chance for ovulation. Metformin, an oral hypoglycemic drug, will reduce hyperinsulinemia and high levels of androgen. If ovulation still does not occur, laparoscopic surgery to open the white membrane around the ovary and follicles has been successful for some women (MacKay, 2011).

For those obese women with PCOS, weight reduction and exercise are imperative for controlling the metabolic effects of this disorder. Metformin will help decrease the body mass index and improve cholesterol levels. In addition, low dose birth control pills are given to control hirsutism, acne, and other androgenic effects in women who do not desire pregnancy. Birth control pills also prevent endometrial hyperplasia and cancer by causing regular shedding of the endometrium (Bartoszek, 2009; MacKay, 2011). See the Pharmacology feature (p. 1277).

Nursing Management

Nursing interventions are directed toward education about the disorder and the treatment options. Women who adopt a healthy lifestyle by maintaining normal weight and getting regular exercise can help manage PCOS. Even 5% to 7% loss in body weight can restore a normal period and make a woman's cycle more regular (Bartoszek, 2009). Weight reduction will also decrease hirsutism, acanthosis nigricans, and high insulin levels. Diets that reduce the glycemic load seem to be the most beneficial. Regular exercise 30 to 60 minutes daily will enhance weight reduction and cardiovascular health. Group therapy where women can join with others with PCOS and combine exercise class, information sessions, and dietary advice are very helpful.

Resources for women looking for more information about PCOS include the Polycystic Ovarian Syndrome Association, Inc. (www.pco-support.org/) and the National Women's Health Information Center (www.womenshealth.gov/faq/polycystic-ovary-syndrome.cfm).

Collaborative Management

Polycystic ovary syndrome is a complex disorder that requires a team approach for optimum care. The syndrome may be treated by a gynecologist, a fertility specialist, or an endocrinologist, depending on the symptoms the patient is experiencing. The health care provider's care is supplemented by nurses, nutritionists, counselors, and community resources. If surgery is required, then anesthesiologists will direct general anesthesia. Open communication between specialists will enhance the potential for the woman with PCOS to maintain optimum health and avoid the severe complications that can occur. In order to meet desired patient outcomes, it is essential that this interdisciplinary team communicate openly with one another in developing and evaluating care of the patient and family (IOM [Institute of Medicine], 2010).

The gynecologist is usually the team leader and may direct infertility studies and perform surgery, if it is needed. Nurses assist in the many roles discussed earlier. In addition, nurses are responsible for managing sedation and analgesics if surgery is needed. The endocrinologist may be consulted if diabetes or adrenal problems complicate the disorder. Nutritionists help the patient understand and choose correct foods so that body weight can be controlled. Counselors help the woman with PCOS cope with body image issues. Community resources may include support groups, exercise centers, and organizations such as Weight Watchers.

Dysmenorrhea

Description, Etiology, Epidemiology, and Clinical Manifestations

Dysmenorrhea is defined as painful menstruation. It is generally described as cramping-type pelvic pain that begins shortly before or at the onset of the monthly menses. Most women experience the discomfort for approximately 3 days. Adolescents report the highest incidence of dysmenorrhea. Approximately 50% to 75% of women experience dysmenorrhea at some time in their lives and some (5% to 6%) have severe pain (MacKay, 2011). Dysmenorrhea is classified as primary, which is associated with increased uterine contractility, or secondary, which is caused by some form of pelvic pathology, such as endometriosis or fibroid tumors. Risk factors for dysmenorrhea include adolescent age, nulliparity, heavy menstrual flow, attempts to lose weight, depression and anxiety, family history, and smoking (Pinkerton, 2010).

Secondary dysmenorrhea is pain associated with a specific condition, such as endometriosis, pelvic inflammatory disease, cervical stenosis with obstruction, adenomyosis, or uterine fibroids. In contrast to primary dysmenorrhea, this discomfort is often characterized by dull, lower abdominal aching that radiates to the back and thighs, bloating, and pelvic fullness. The pain from secondary dysmenorrhea grows progressively worse each month (MacKay, 2011).

Pathophysiology

With primary dysmenorrhea, there is an increase in uterine muscle contractions due to an increase in the prostaglandin level in the second half of the menstrual cycle. Systemic response to increased prostaglandin levels is manifested in pain in the lower back and lower abdomen, nausea, diarrhea, headache, and weakness. It is seen only with ovulatory cycles because both estrogen and progesterone are necessary for it to occur. It is seen primarily in adolescents and women in their early 20s, with the incidence and severity often declining with age.

Laboratory and Diagnostic Testing

Evaluation of the patient with dysmenorrhea should include a history of symptoms and menstrual cycles, including age of menarche and level of flow. An abdominal exam alone is performed on the adolescent who is not yet sexually active unless an imperforate hymen is suspected. In contrast, a pelvic examination should be performed in females who have been sexually active to screen for sexually transmitted infections. A transvaginal ultrasound can be used to rule out anatomic abnormalities such as masses, ovarian cysts, and endometriosis. Laparoscopic surgery may be needed to further identify and define causes of dysmenorrhea (MacKay, 2011; Pinkerton, 2010).

CHART 41–6 Nonpharmacologic Therapies for Dysmenorrhea

Therapy	Rationale
Adequate rest and sleep	
Heating pad/hot bath and fetal position	Increases vasodilation
	Relaxes uterine muscle
	Decreases uterine ischemia
Lower back massage	Relaxes paravertebral muscles
	Increases pelvic blood supply
Effleurage (rhythmic rubbing)	Distraction and focal point
Exercise (especially walking and yoga)	Increases vasodilation
	Decreases ischemia
	Releases natural endorphins
	Decreases prostaglandins
	Decreases stress
Dietary changes:	
Decreased salt	Reduces fluid retention
Increased water intake	Natural diuretic

Source: Adapted from Stoppler, M., & Shiel, W. (2010). Menstrual cramps (dysmenorrheal). MedicineNet.com. Retrieved from http://www.medicinenet.com/menstrual_cramps/article.htm.

Medical Management

Management varies depending on the severity of the symptoms. Chart 41–6 shows the nonpharmacologic therapies most often prescribed. The pharmacologic therapies are listed in the Pharmacology feature (p. 1277). Being cognizant of the increased incidence of bleeding that occurs with certain pain relievers is essential.

Safety Alert *Do not use nonsteroidal anti-inflammatory drugs (NSAIDs) for patients with hemophilia, those with bleeding ulcers, those allergic to aspirin or other NSAIDs, or those taking anticoagulant medications. Be sure to take NSAIDs with milk or food to help prevent gastric irritation and possible bleeding.*

Management is directed at removing the underlying cause, often necessitating surgery to excise the displaced tissue or remove the fibroids. Pharmacologic pain-relief measures are the same as with primary dysmenorrhea.

Nursing Management

Nursing care is directed at educating the woman regarding the cause or treatment modalities. Patients should be advised to maintain a healthy diet and exercise level, take in plenty of fluids, and use heat and NSAIDs in moderation to help with symptoms. Patients need instructions to seek medical care if simple measures do not relieve the symptoms in order to determine the possibility of secondary causes. Also, patients should seek care for dysmenorrhea that occurs later in life, pain that occurs at other times besides the first couple of days of a period, any vaginal discharge, or abnormal bleeding between periods.

Menorrhagia

Description, Etiology, Epidemiology, and Clinical Manifestations

Menorrhagia is defined as excessive or prolonged menstruation that occurs at regular intervals (MacKay, 2011). The menses of young women may vary from month to month, and a single heavy period is not necessarily cause for concern. However, high-volume periods that last more than 7 days are cause for concern. The best measure to determine the volume of blood loss is to ask the woman to explain how her periods have changed compared to periods she considered normal (Nelson & Baldwin, 2009). Menorrhagia can be caused by endometriosis, pelvic inflammatory disease, intrauterine devices for birth control, uterine fibroids, pregnancy and pregnancy-related complications, polyps, endometrial hyperplasia, or functional ovarian cysts. Also, women with hypothyroid conditions can have very heavy periods. Health care providers will also check for clotting disorders (Latendresse et al., 2010).

Weblink: Menstrual Cramps†(Dysmenorrhea)

Medical Management

Treatment is dependent on the cause. For example, if a particular method of contraception is the cause, alternative contraceptive methods may be utilized as treatment. Fibroids may be surgically removed or medically shrunk. Infections may indicate the need for antibiotic drug therapy. Hemoglobin analysis can be used to determine the extent of blood loss. Other pertinent laboratory values include cervical tests for infection; *von Willebrand factor* (a genetic bleeding disorder), platelet count, and other coagulation studies; a thyroid-stimulating hormone to determine the presence of a hypothyroid condition; and serum or urine HCG to test for pregnancy (MacKay, 2011).

Cervical Polyps

Description, Etiology, Epidemiology, and Pathophysiology

Cervical polyps are benign growths attached to the endocervical canal. The cause of these polyps is unknown; however, chronic inflammation, clogged blood vessels, and abnormal response to estrogen do seem to have a role in their appearance (Vorvick & Storck, 2011a). Cervical polyps are fairly common among parous women over age 20. However, they are rare in the pre-menarche years. Cervical polyps occur as single lesions visible at the os. It is rare to see two or three at the same time.

Clinical Manifestations

Symptoms include yellowish vaginal discharge and abnormal vaginal bleeding. The bleeding is most likely to occur after douching or intercourse and between periods. Regular menses will be heavier than usual. Polyps also may cause postmenopausal bleeding. They appear as smooth, red growths at the os with an attachment. Cervical polyps must be differentiated from polyps or myomas that extend from the endometrium as these lesions are likely to be cancerous and to cause more bleeding when removed (MacKay, 2011).

Medical Management

Treatment involves removal of the polyp, usually in the outpatient setting. The polyp is grasped with a vaginal forcep and twisted until it comes off. Larger polyps may require electrocautery. All tissue removed is sent for pathologic evaluation even though only a very few will be precancerous or cancerous (Vorvick & Storck, 2011a). Polyps rarely grow back.

Metrorrhagia

Description, Etiology, Epidemiology, and Clinical Manifestations

Irregular, frequent menstrual periods of variable amounts of bleeding is called metrorrhagia (Nelson & Baldwin, 2009). A small amount of spotting may be seen around the time of ovulation and is considered normal. Use of low-dose oral contraceptives reduces the amount of

Video: Premenstrual Syndrome Weblink: Premenstrual Syndrome (PMS) Fact Sheet

hormones available in the body; this is associated with breakthrough bleeding or spotting. Pathologic causes of metrorrhagia include endometritis, STIs, pregnancy-related problems, ovarian cysts, or uterine fibroid tumors. Postmenopausal bleeding may be caused by uterine polyps, inappropriately prescribed hormone therapy, or uterine cancer. Early evaluation of this concern is extremely important.

Pathophysiology

If a pathologic cause is not identified, then dysfunctional uterine bleeding is considered the cause. This is usually due to anovulation and subsequent estrogen excess and progesterone deficiency. This results in hyperplasia of the endometrial lining of the uterus. Without adequate progesterone, sloughing of the lining does not occur; thus, the endometrial lining thickens under the influence of estrogen, and eventually begins to shed irregularly. This results in vaginal bleeding that is not in accordance with the woman's monthly cycle. Hormone imbalances can be caused by anovulation related to PCOS or perimenopause, stress, and emotional upheavals. However, of utmost concern is that abnormal bleeding from the vagina, whether menorrhagia or metrorrhagia, can be an indicator of neoplasm and should be evaluated urgently.

Medical Management

Treatment is directed at the cause, such as drug therapy for endometritis and STIs; removal or shrinkage of cysts and fibroids; dilatation and curettage for hyperplasia; and surgery, drug, or chemotherapy/radiation for cancers (MacKay, 2011). Pregnancy-related problems must be dealt with on an individual basis. Nursing care involves education regarding the causes of and treatments for metrorrhagia and addressing the fatigue associated with anemia and the relative dehydration.

Premenstrual Syndrome

Description and Epidemiology

Premenstrual syndrome (PMS) is a common, but complex, often misunderstood condition involving physical, psychological, and behavioral symptoms that occur regularly 7 to 14 days before the onset of menses. Premenstrual syndrome affects approximately 40% of women between ages 25 and 40. It may be severe in up to 8% of women affected (MacKay, 2011).

Etiology and Pathophysiology

The etiology and pathophysiology of PMS is poorly understood. There seems to be a biologic trigger that is exacerbated by psychosocial factors. Serotonin neurotransmitter is also considered to be a factor. It does appear there is a genetic or familial tendency associated with PMS. Additionally, estrogen and progesterone imbalances may play a role, as well as nutritional deficiencies such as folic acid, calcium, vitamin E, vitamin B_6, and magnesium (Barclift, 2010). Risk factors for PMS include age, family history, or personal history of depression, as noted in the Risk Factors feature.

RISK FACTORS for Premenstrual Syndrome

- Age between late 20s and early 40s
- Have at least one child
- Have a family history of PMS or depression
- Have a past medical history of either postpartum depression or a mood disorder.

Source: Barclift, S. (Reviewer). (2010). Premenstrual syndrome. Womenshealth.gov. Retrieved from http://www.womenshealth.gov/faq/premenstrual-syndrome.cfm.

CHART 41–7 Symptoms Commonly Associated with Premenstrual Syndrome

Abdominal bloating	Lower extremity edema
Breast tenderness	Weight gain
Depression	Irritability
Loss of concentration	Food cravings/binges
Headache	Fatigue
Backache	Mood swings

Source: Adapted from Barclift, S. (Reviewer). (2010). Premenstrual syndrome. Womenshealth .gov. Retrieved from http://www.womenshealth.gov/faq/premenstrual-syndrome.cfm.

Clinical Manifestations

The symptoms of PMS vary widely among women, so much so that it is difficult to define the condition. When present, the symptoms occur in the luteal phase, the time from ovulation until the start of the menstrual period of the cycle. Chart 41–7 shows the more common symptoms related to PMS, although symptoms can number up to 100 (Barclift, 2010). The diagnosis of PMS should meet specific criteria: symptoms occur in the luteal phase and resolve with menses, no symptoms occur during the follicular phase, and symptoms recur with repeated cycles (MacKay, 2011).

Medical Management

Management of PMS symptoms is difficult because of the diversity of symptoms in different women. Diet and exercise provide some relief for some women, along with the reduction of salt, sugar, and caffeinated beverages. The diet needs to be high in complex carbohydrates such as whole grains, limited in simple sugar, and limited in alcohol use to minimize hypoglycemia. Caffeine intake should be limited to decrease irritability. Women who exercise regularly appear to have fewer symptoms of anxiety and depression due to the increase in endorphin levels.

Health Promotion

Education is by far the most important part of management. The nurse can assist the woman in symptom evaluation, in cyclic relationships, and in counseling and support. Alternative and complementary therapies have been found to help manage symptoms for some women. For example, the use of black cohosh root helps relieve anxiety and depression by suppressing estrogen. Other alternative therapies include chasteberry, evening primrose oil, wild yam root, and dong quai (Barclift, 2010; Nihira, 2010). Medications may be used when other treatments fail to improve the PMS symptoms. Diuretics; prostaglandin inhibitors, which are the nonsteroidal anti-inflammatory drugs (NSAIDs); progesterone; and oral contraceptives have been shown to relieve symptoms. Serotonin reuptake inhibitors such as fluoxetine (Prozac or Sarafem) and paroxetine (Paxil) are used with success when mood disorders such as irritability, tension, anxiety, and depression are the dominant symptoms (MacKay, 2011). See the Pharmacology feature on page 1277.

Premenstrual Dysphoric Disorder

Description, Etiology, and Epidemiology

Premenstrual dysphoric disorder (PMDD) is recognized as a separate syndrome with similar, but more severe, symptoms than PMS that often overwhelm the woman (Nelson & Baldwin, 2009). Premenstrual dysphoric disorder is a severe form of PMS that, in order to be diagnosed, requires at least 5 of 11 criterion symptoms to occur 1 or 2 weeks before menses. It is estimated that 3% to 8% of women of reproductive age are affected with PMDD worldwide (Htay & Aung, 2011). No one race of women is affected more than others. The etiology of PMDD is a combination of biologic, psychological, environmental, genetic, and social factors (Htay & Aung, 2011). A predisposition for PMDD occurs in families; however, it is not clear whether this is related to genetics or environment (Latendresse et al., 2010).

Pathophysiology

It is reasonable to believe that PMDD has a hormonal basis because PMDD occurs when there is an abnormal tissue response to cyclic hormones of the normal menstrual cycle. In addition, serotonin, gamma aminobutyric acid (GABA), and norepinephrine seem to be involved in the mood symptoms of PMDD (Htay & Aung, 2011).

Clinical Manifestations

Symptoms include those of atypical severe depressive disorders (depressed mood, thoughts of suicide, panic attacks, interpersonal rejection, hypersensitivity, carbohydrate craving, and hypersomnia). Women have depressed mood with feelings of hopelessness, lack of interest, anxiety, tension, and feelings of being "on edge." Many women describe marked anger or irritability and increased interpersonal conflicts. Friends and family notice decreased interest in usual activities and hypersomnia. Patients also complain of lethargy, easy fatigability, and marked lack of energy with changes in appetite and food cravings. Women with PMDD state they feel overwhelmed and out of control. Physical symptoms include breast tenderness and swelling, headaches, joint and muscle pain, and bloating. Symptoms will begin to remit within a few days of onset of menses or after onset of the follicular phase of the next menstrual cycle (Barclift, 2010). There is a significant correlation between depression and PMDD; however, not all patients have depressive symptoms, so PMDD is not considered just a variant of depression.

Medical Management

Treatment of PMDD must incorporate lifestyle changes, nutritional supplements, stress management, and pharmacologic interventions. Lifestyle changes include aerobic exercise and dietary changes such as eating small frequent balanced meals rich in complex carbohydrates, decreasing caffeine and sodium, restricting alcohol, and eliminating smoking. Nutritional supplements that are recommended include folic acid, vitamin B_6, calcium citrate with vitamin D, magnesium, and vitamin E (Barclift, 2010). Nonpharmacologic treatments are also pertinent recommendations and include stress management, anger management, individual and couple's therapy, and patient education regarding the cause of, diagnosis of, and treatment for PMS and PMDD. Psychologists also recommend light therapy with 10,000 lux cool-white fluorescent light (Htay & Aung, 2011). Pharmacologic treatments include antidepressant and anxiolytic medications. Selective serotonin reuptake inhibitor (SSRI) antidepressants are considered first line. Fluoxetine 20 milligrams per day may be used during the luteal phase or throughout the full menstrual cycle (Htay & Aung, 2011). Alprazolam or another anxiolytic has also been shown to be effective in patients with PMS and PMDD. There is an issue with dependency on benzodiazepine-type medications, however, so this should only be used for a short-term treatment and only as a second-line therapy if SSRIs fail. Hormonal therapies that are used are the gonadotropin-releasing hormone agonists; these suppress ovulation and cause amenorrhea, thereby providing significant relief of symptoms in those who do not also have significant depressive symptoms. These medications can cause symptoms of menopause such as hot flashes, vaginal dryness, fatigue, and irritability, so use is limited. Danazol is a weak androgen that is sometimes prescribed for women with endometriosis and fibrocystic breast disease. It is also sometimes used to treat PMDD. Danazol can reduce symptoms, but has side effects of anovulation and masculinization. Gonadotropin-releasing hormone agonists and danazol have limited use due to the side effects and cost. See the Pharmacology feature (p. 1277).

Nursing Management

Ideally, all women should be screened for PMS and PMDD on a routine basis. Incorporate screening questions into a self-assessment that is routinely collected during intake. Much of the basic subjective data can be collected via a structured questionnaire. The following screening questions are effective:

- Do you ever have pelvic pain or cramps during or around the time of your period?
- Are you able to treat this pain so it does not bother you?
- Do you ever have other physical or mood discomforts during or around the time of your period?
- Are you able to treat these discomforts so they do not bother you?

Assessment of PMS and PMDD

Conduct a focused nursing assessment for women with PMS and PMDD for whom current treatments or self-care therapies are ineffective. An interview by a nurse can confirm self-report data as well as collect additional data. Start with a focused health history whenever possible to identify the individual woman's pattern of PMS or PMDD. The menstrual cycle may be divided into three phases: premenstrual, early menstrual (days 1 to 3 or days of heavy flow), and late menstrual (day 4 and onward or days of lighter flow).

The following areas should be assessed:

- Pattern of severity of PMS or PMDD across premenstrual and early menstrual phases
- Rating of overall distress caused by PMS or PMDD
- Pattern of severity of other cyclic discomforts across premenstrual and early menstrual phases
- Rating of overall distress caused by cyclic discomforts
- Influences on the cyclic pain symptoms; for example, work stress, diet, or exercise.

Identify the individual woman's pattern of symptom management by gathering the following information:

- Interventions, including self-care strategies
- Pattern of use across premenstrual and early menstrual phases
- Rating of relief obtained from intervention
- Rating of satisfaction with pain and symptom control
- Rating of adherence (i.e., consistent use of treatment).

Conduct a focused history and physical assessment using data from the history as a basis. The assessment data need to be organized into symptom patterns. Chart 41–8 provides a template for this organization.

Planning Expected Outcomes

Review assessment data together with the woman, and identify the outcomes important to the woman and amenable to nursing intervention.

CHART 41–8 Organization of Assessment Data for Premenstrual Syndrome and Premenstrual Dysphoric Disorder

Pelvic Pain	Abdominal cramps
	Nausea, vomiting
	Backache
	Change in bowel frequency
Perimenstrual Physical Discomforts	Fatigue
	Headaches
	Fluid retention
	Joint aches and pain
	Breast tenderness
	Leg and thigh discomfort
	Change in energy and appetite
Perimenstrual Mood Discomforts	Depression, irritability
	Tension, impatience
	Anxiety, anger
	Mood swings, hostility
	Guilt, tearfulness
	Feeling out of control
	Change in sexual desire

Expected outcomes for PMS and PMDD management may include the following:

- Improvements in PMS and PMDD symptoms' frequency, severity, distress, and pattern
- Increased comfort level (physical and psychosocial well-being)
- Successful use of treatments to manage symptoms
- Relief of pain and discomfort
- Enhanced role performance (work, family, friends, school, leisure)
- Patient understanding of the cost of various forms of treatment.

Review symptom patterns and establish expected outcomes through mutual goal setting with the woman. Use the assessment as an opportunity to educate the woman about managing pain and discomfort. Develop an individualized treatment plan, incorporating the multimodal treatment strategies and participant involvement through personal choice whenever possible.

Interventions for PMS and PMDD

Because PMS and PMDD are a complex mixture of physiological and psychological clinical manifestations, it is essential to implement a comprehensive plan that focuses on symptom management interventions. This plan will provide the patient with the knowledge and interventions to manage the disorder. The nurse, along with the patient, must identify goals of care and explore ways to best achieve the goals. To enhance coping, the nurse must provide an atmosphere of acceptance and give factual information concerning diagnosis, treatment, and prognosis. Mutual goal setting is essential for the plan to be successful.

Keeping a log of when incidents occur and what stressors increase the clinical manifestations will assist the nurse in identifying appropriate interventions. The patient needs to be instructed to self-monitor stressors and habits that impact the disorders and then identify effective interventions. Chart 41–9 outlines the pharmacologic and nonpharmacologic interventions for PMS and PMDD.

Evaluation

Following the interventions outlined in Chart 41–9, the nurse needs to assess the plan's effectiveness. Ideally, the same assessment tools should be used for both the initial assessment and the follow-up evaluation. The evaluation assesses the achievement of expected outcomes initially identified by the woman in collaboration with her health care provider. When a woman is referred to another health care provider for additional evaluation or treatment, the nurse should follow up on the woman's progress whenever possible and indicated.

Toxic Shock Syndrome

Description, Etiology, Epidemiology, and Pathophysiology

Toxic shock syndrome (TSS) is a potentially deadly condition caused by toxins produced by *Staphylococcus aureus* and *group A streptococcus* infection. The condition received a lot of attention when it was linked to tampon use in 1980 (Balentine, 2011). The incidence of this infection when it is associated with tampon use is about 1/100,000 women of reproductive age. Risk factors for this form of toxic shock include leaving a tampon in place for a long time, leaving diaphragms or contraceptive sponges in place too long or not cleaning these devices as directed, and use of postsurgery wound packing.

Clinical Manifestations

Symptoms of TSS include sudden onset of fever, chills, vomiting, diarrhea, low blood pressure, and a diffuse sunburnlike red rash. The symptoms, if not treated, will progress to worsening low blood pressure, confusion, headache, and seizures. Kidney, liver, and heart failure may develop. The death rate is about 5% to 15% of those affected (Balentine, 2011; Schwartz, 2011). About 1 to 2 weeks after the onset of the rash, skin peeling, especially of the palms and soles, will occur. Chart 41–10 outlines the signs and symptoms associated with TSS.

Medical Management

Hospitalization is imperative if there is a rapid progression of severe symptoms requiring intravenous fluids and antibiotics. The mortality rate will vary, depending on the organism involved. Although *S. aureus* is the primary organism involved, TSS has been associated with *Streptococcus pyogenes exotoxin*. The mortality rate with *S. aureus* is less than 3%, but with *S. pyogenes exotoxin* it is as high as 60% (Bush, Chaparro-Rojas, & Perez, 2009). Primary prevention techniques include avoiding the super plus tampons and/or changing them every 2 to 4 hours, as well as using the smallest size tampon that will absorb the menstrual flow without leakage for 2 to 4 hours. Once toxic shock has been diagnosed or suspected, the woman should avoid tampons altogether and use sanitary pads exclusively.

Diagnosis of TSS is based on fever, low blood pressure, rash that peels after 1 to 2 weeks, and at least three organs with signs of dysfunction. In some cases, blood cultures may be done for growth of *S. aureus* (Balentine, 2011). Treatment includes intravenous fluids, removal of any suspected source of infection, vasopressors to control hypotension, antibiotics, and dialysis as needed for acute renal failure.

CHART 41–9 Interventions for Premenstrual Syndrome and Premenstrual Dysphoric Disorder

Self-Monitoring Interventions

Tracking symptoms

Tracking stressors, function, and health status.

Pharmacologic Symptom Management

Over-the-counter (OTC) pain medication:

- Use nonsteroidal anti-inflammatory drugs (NSAIDs).
- Timing and strength of the medication are critical to pain relief.
- Take an adequate dose of medication at the first sign of pain or before bleeding occurs.
- Manufacturers' recommendations for OTC medications should not be exceeded.
- Read labels of other OTC medications taken concomitantly, particularly cold and sleep remedies that contain the NSAID.
- Be advised regarding appropriate duration of use because of the potential for gastrointestinal distress or other side effects.

Hormones:

- Combination estrogen–progestin oral contraceptives
- Progesterone intrauterine device.

Nutritional supplements:

- Folic acid—400 mcg/day
- Calcium with vitamin D: 1,200 mg/day (do not exceed 2,500 mg/day)
- Magnesium: 400 mg/day (do not exceed 500 mg/day)
- Essential fatty acids (Omega 3 and 6)
- Vitamin E 400 IU
- Vitamin B complex: B_6 50–200 mg/day, B_1 100 mg/day.

Antidepressant medication:

- Refer to a mental health professional as indicated for symptoms of anxiety, panic attack, or depression.

Topical/cutaneous symptom management:

- Heat application: heating pad, hot baths, and disposable heat wraps
- Therapeutic massage
- Acupressure and acupuncture
- Transcutaneous electrical nerve stimulation (TENS).

Behavioral/Cognitive Symptom Management

Behavioral relaxation:

- Breathing exercises
- Progressive muscle relaxation
- Stretching exercises
- Autogenic training.

Cognitive relaxation:

- Thought-stopping strategies
- Guided imagery
- Thought substitution
- Prayer
- Decreased negative self-talk
- Affirmations
- Meditation
- Biofeedback
- Mindfulness meditation
- Distraction.

Lifestyle Modifications as Indicated

General dietary modification:

- Decrease intake of caffeine, simple sugars, and salt.
- Eat frequent, small meals.
- Increase water and fluid intake to 6–8 glasses per day.
- Reduce alcohol intake.
- Increase intake of foods that can decrease symptoms such as:
  Those rich in essential fatty acids
  Those rich in B complex vitamins
  Those rich in calcium and magnesium.
- Use a daily multivitamin and mineral supplement.
- Use a premenstrual syndrome formula vitamin and mineral supplement during premenses.
- Quit smoking.
- Exercise. Encourage one or more of the following types of exercise as indicated and as can be tolerated:
  Regular aerobic exercise
  Nonaerobic exercise (e.g., yoga, t'ai chi, stretching/relaxation)
  Exercise modification across the menstrual cycle.

Environmental modification interventions:

- Environmental stress management
- Time management
- Social support.

CHART 41–10 Signs and Symptoms of Toxic Shock Syndrome

Sudden high fever

Low blood pressure

Vomiting and/or diarrhea

A macular rash similar to sunburn

Peeling of the skin on the hands and feet 1 to 2 weeks after the onset of the rash

Confusion/delirium

Muscle aches

Redness of eyes, mouth, and throat

Seizures

Headache

Sepsis, organ failure, and, in extreme cases, death.

Health Promotion

Patient education regarding toxic shock syndrome should include information regarding signs and symptoms of the disorder and when the patient should seek care. Women should be advised that superabsorbent tampons that are left in place for too long become a breeding ground for bacteria and put young women at risk for TSS. Women should also be advised that using a diaphragm or contraceptive sponge can cause TSS. A woman can reduce her chances of developing TSS by changing her tampon every 4 to 8 hours and using the lower absorbency tampon. It can also help to alternate using tampons and sanitary napkins whenever possible or using sanitary napkins exclusively.

Menopause

Description, Etiology, Epidemiology, and Pathophysiology

Menopause is the normal aging process by which the ovaries cease to function. The process can take 10 to 15 years as the regression of follicles within each ovary starts to accelerate after age 35. Symptoms begin as early as age 42 and end by age 58 with the average age being 51. More than 90% of women have ceased having periods by their early 50s. This process is accelerated by smoking. Once a woman has experienced 1 year of amenorrhea, she is considered menopausal. A hysterectomy is referred to as surgical menopause. **Perimenopause** is the time during which periods may increase, decrease, and become irregular as the function of the ovaries waxes and wanes. As the ovaries become nonfunctional, the follicles cease to respond by producing estrogen.

Clinical Manifestations

As the estrogen levels are depleted, a number of signs and symptoms appear. Irregular vaginal bleeding is common, and vasomotor symptoms manifest as hot flashes. Patients may experience vaginal drying and thinning of the mucosa; this causes atrophic vaginitis, which leads to dyspareunia. The same mucosal changes occur in the bladder as well, causing a decrease in bladder capacity and loss of tone. These changes can cause dysuria and frequency even when no infection is present. This is often a somewhat difficult time for many women psychologically, as they experience emotional lability and changes in sleep patterns.

Health problems can become an issue at this time of life because the cardiovascular, musculoskeletal, and endocrine systems are affected. Cholesterol levels may begin to change, increasing the cardiovascular risks. The high density lipoproteins (good cholesterol) decrease and the low density lipoproteins (bad cholesterol) increase. The loss of estrogen, which begins a steady decline in bone density, puts the woman at risk for osteopenia, osteoporosis, and the potential for fractures.

The symptoms that the perimenopausal or menopausal woman may present should be considered carefully before making a determination of menopause. For example, thyroid dysfunction, anemia, and depression can present with many of the same symptoms. Laboratory tests may be used to identify thyroid dysfunction or anemia. Tests to verify perimenopause or menopause include a serum estrogen level and serum FSH level. The FSH is elevated and the estrogen level is decreased with menopause.

Medical Management

The most significant concern for the woman presenting with menopausal symptoms is how to manage her symptoms. Women have received volumes of conflicting information regarding hormone therapy during menopause. Most women know that hormone therapy provides relief from symptoms, but they also know that there are increased risks of breast cancer, stroke, heart disease, deep venous thrombosis, and pulmonary emboli. Thus, women are very conflicted about using hormone therapy to help with symptoms. If women want to consider taking hormone therapy for short-term treatment of their menopausal symptoms, the risks and benefits should be explained fully. All options should be considered. Estrogen alone may be prescribed for the woman who has had her uterus removed. However, estrogen and progesterone must be prescribed for the woman who still has a uterus. Unopposed estrogen causes hyperplasia of the endometrial lining and places the patient at risk for endometrial cancer if the uterus is intact. Progesterone has side effects that are problematic including increased appetite, weight gain, irritability, depression, headache, and breast tenderness. There are numerous preparations of hormone therapy, combination preparations with estrogen and progesterone, and separate preparations and topical creams, gels, rings, and dermal patches. Vaginal creams are usually specific for atrophic vaginitis; however, they do not provide relief from vasomotor symptoms.

Safety Alert *One very important aspect of patient teaching for the woman considering hormone therapy is the high risk of fatal pulmonary emboli in the women who smoke and take hormone therapy.*

Other therapies are available; for example, antidepressants can be used to help with situational depression that can accompany menopause. Fluoxetine, paroxetine, and venlafaxine are sometimes effective alternatives to hormone therapy in managing symptoms. Vasomotor symptoms can be relieved even if the patient is not depressed. Selective estrogen receptor modulators (SERMs) such as raloxifene can be used to prevent bone loss in patients at risk for osteoporosis. See the Pharmacology feature (p. 1277).

Nonpharmacologic therapies can often be a better alternative for the woman with a family history of endometrial, ovarian, or breast cancer. Managing the environment and reducing caffeine and alcohol can reduce the effects of vasomotor symptoms. Vitamin E (800 international units) may also help reduce vasomotor symptoms. Kegel exercises and lubricants can aid in vaginal dryness and associated dyspareunia. Well-balanced nutrition, exercise, and good sleep habits can decrease anxiety and depression and maintain a sense of well-being. Weight-bearing exercise also reduces the loss of bone density and prevents weight gain. Aerobic exercise helps the patient manage her weight and improves cardiovascular health. The patient who takes calcium supplements and maintains a diet high in complex carbohydrates and vitamin B complex will maintain optimal weight and minimize symptoms. The American Cancer Society recommends yearly exams after age 40 to detect cancers. Health teaching should address alcohol and tobacco abuse, diet, and exercise. Recent research that improves practice related to women experiencing menopause is discussed in the Evidence-Based Practice feature (p. 1281). The Complementary & Alternative Therapies feature outlines alternative therapies for controlling the symptoms of menopause.

Reproduction Disorders

Infertility

Description, Etiology, Epidemiology, and Pathophysiology

Infertility is generally considered a viable diagnosis when a couple has been unable to achieve a pregnancy after 12 months of unprotected intercourse. This condition affects about 15% of the reproductive population (Latendresse et al., 2010). Primary infertility refers to a couple who has never been pregnant, whereas secondary infertility refers to a couple who has been pregnant in the past but has been unable to achieve another pregnancy. There are many significant religious and cultural considerations when discussing infertility with couples. For instance, the Roman Catholic Church deems technical procedures such as *in vitro* fertilization, donor insemination, and the freezing of embryos as unacceptable. In contrast, Protestant and Muslim groups support *in vitro* fertilization with the husband's sperm but are against the use of donor sperm (Greil, McQuillan, Benjamins, Johnson, Johnson, & Heinz, 2010).

Both male and female factors are involved with infertility. About one-third of cases are male related, one-third are female related, and one-third are a combination or unexplained (Eisenberg & Brumbaugh, 2011). In male infertility, the cause is most commonly related to a decreased sperm count, but could be related to retrograde ejaculation, impotence, hormone deficiency, a varicocele (distended testicular veins),

COMPLEMENTARY & ALTERNATIVE THERAPIES Phytotherapy

Nancy Yilk

PHYTOESTROGENS are a group of nonsteroidal compounds that originate as functional and structural aspects of plants that are similar with estradiol. There is a growing interest in the usefulness of phytotherapy in the treatment of symptoms and menopause-related diseases. Phytotherapy offers an option to women who want to improve their quality of life through relief of hot flashes and anxiety that occurs with menopause (Molla, Hidalgo-Mora, & Soteras, 2011).

A special extract of Siberian Rhubarb root, called ERr 731, has been in widespread use in Germany since 1993 by health practitioners to provide relief for the symptoms of menopause. In a German study to assess its efficacy and tolerability in everyday use, 363 menopausal women were enrolled at 70 German gynecological practices. By assessing results on the Menopause Rating Scale (MRS) after 6 months, researchers found the women's quality of life improved markedly. In 252 women, there was a significant decrease of the MRS total score from 14.5 points at baseline to 6.5 points (Kaszkin-Bettag, Beck, Richardson, Heger, & Beer, 2008).

A randomized, double-blind, placebo-controlled clinical trial (RTC) demonstrated that ERr 731 is highly effective in reducing anxiety in perimenopausal women. In this trial, 109 perimenopausal women with hot flash complaints and anxiety received either ERr 731 or placebo daily for 12 weeks. The Hamilton Anxiety Scale (HAS), the Menopause Rating Scale II, the Women's Health Questionnaire, and the Psychological General Well-Being Index were used to measure the women's anxiety, health state, and subjective psychological well-being. After 12 weeks, the HSA total score decreased significantly for somatic and psychic anxiety. After 12 weeks, a reduction in the severity of anxiety from "moderate" or "severe" to "slight" was observed in 33 of 39 ERr 731 women completing the double-blind phase, which correlated well with the reduction in the number and severity of hot flashes. This was reflected by a high rate of ERr 731 women reporting a marked improvement in their health state and general well-being (Kaszkin-Bettag, Ventskovskiy, et al., 2007).

Investigating long-term efficacy and safety of ERr 731 with a multicenter, prospective, 48-week observational study (OS I) followed by a 48-week OS II in perimenopausal women with menopausal symptoms taking ERr 731 demonstrated positive results. Of 109 women participating in a previous RCT, 39 women received ERr 731 and 41 women received placebo. Fifty-one women continued to take ERr 731 in OS II (23 women from the ERr 731 group and 28 women from the placebo group). The primary outcome criterion for long-term efficacy of ERr 731 was the change in the Menopause Rating Scale II score after 48 and 96 weeks. Women in the ERr 731 group in the RCT experienced a further decrease in their symptoms during OS I. Women who received placebo during the RCT and started taking ERr 731 in OS I reported a significant decrease in menopausal symptoms. After 18 weeks in OS I, their symptom scores were comparable to those of women who had taken ERr 731 for 12 weeks during the RCT. The symptom scores further decreased slightly in all women during OS II. At the end of OS II, all women had on average less than 1.4 slight hot flashes per day. ERr 731 is effective and safe in the long-term treatment of menopausal symptoms in perimenopausal women (Hasper, Ventskovskiy, Rettenberger, Heger, Riley, & Kaszkin-Bettag, 2009).

Sources: Hasper, I., Ventskovskiy, B. M., Rettenberger, R., Heger, P. W., Riley, D. S., & Kaszkin-Bettag, M. (2009). Long-term efficacy and safety of the special extract ERr 731 of Rheum rhaponticum in perimenopausal women with menopausal symptoms. *Menopause, 16*(1), 117–131; Kaszkin-Bettag, M., Beck, S., Richardson, A., Heger, P. W., & Beer, A. M. (2008). Efficacy of the special extract ERr 731 from rhapontic rhubarb for menopausal complaints: A 6-month open observational study. *Alternative Therapies in Health and Medicine, 14*(6), 32–38; Kaszkin-Bettag, M., Ventskovskiy, B. M., Kravchenko, A., Rettenberger, R., Richardson, A., Heger, P. W., et al. (2007). The special extract ERr 731 of the roots of Rheum rhaponticum decreases anxiety and improves health state and general well-being in perimenopausal women. *Menopause, 14*(2), 270–283; Molla, M. D., Hidalgo-Mora, J. J., & Soteras, M. G. (2011). Phytotherapy as alternative to hormone replacement therapy. *Frontiers in Bioscience* (School Edition), *3*, 191–204.

Note: Err731 is marketed in the United States as Estrovera™.

RISK FACTORS for Male Infertility

Heavy alcohol use	Drugs
Smoking cigarettes	Age

Environmental toxins, including pesticides and lead

Health problems, such as mumps, kidney disease, hormone problems

Radiation or chemotherapy for cancer

Source: Adapted from Eisenberg, E., & Brumbaugh, K. (Reviewers). (2011). Infertility: Frequently asked questions. Womenshealth.gov. Retrieved from http://www.womenshealth.gov/faq/infertility.cfm#top.

RISK FACTORS for Female Infertility

Age	Smoking
Excess alcohol use	Stress
Poor diet	Athletic training
Being overweight or underweight	Sexually transmitted infections

Health problems that cause hormonal changes such as PCOS and ovarian insufficiency

Source: Adapted from Eisenberg, E., & Brumbaugh, K. (Reviewers). (2011). Infertility: Frequently asked questions. Womenshealth.gov. Retrieved from http://www.womenshealth.gov/faq/infertility.dfm#top.

or scarring from a sexually transmitted infection. A man's risks for infertility is increased if he uses alcohol, drugs, or tobacco; has health problems or takes certain medications; or has been treated for cancer. The Risk Factors feature outlines risks for male infertility.

Female-related causes are most commonly related to ovulatory dysfunction. Other causes may include hormone imbalance, blocked fallopian tubes, uterine fibroids, ovarian cysts, or pelvic infections. Age has also been associated with fertility difficulties. In addition to age-related factors, the risks for female infertility include alcohol use, smoking, poor diet, and other factors listed in the Risk Factors feature. Couples at risk for infertility are those with multiple sexual partners, those with a sexually transmitted infection, those with endometriosis, men with a history of orchitis or a history of undescended testicles, past history of diethylstilbestrol (DES) exposure for both men and women, and those with chronic diseases such as diabetes or thyroid disorders.

Medical Management

Diagnosis is determined through a complete history and physical examination of both partners, in addition to the reported inability of a couple to conceive after 1 year of unprotected intercourse. The year time frame is often decreased in older couples due to the premium time frame for conception. The Diagnostic Tests feature presents the typical diagnostic tests for reproductive disorders.

Treatment for infertility must be directed at the cause. Sometimes all that is necessary is counseling regarding the timing of intercourse. Assisted reproductive therapies (ARTs)—for example, *in vitro* fertilization—have brought hope and success to many infertile couples. These procedures are expensive and have a modest success rate. Chart 41–11 (p. 1274) outlines the assisted reproductive therapies available to infertile couples. The Ethical Considerations feature discusses issues related to parenthood and infertility.

Weblink: Infertility Fact Sheet
Weblink: Assisted Reproductive Statistics
Weblink: Miscarriage

CHART 41–11 Assisted Reproductive Therapies

Reproductive Therapy	Indications	Procedure
In vitro fertilization (IVF) *In vitro* fertilization and embryo transfer (IVF-ET)	Blocked fallopian tubes; severe male infertility/sterility; cervix has an unfavorable environment due to acidic secretions. Shortens life span of sperm.	Ova retrieved from female and sperm from male; fertilization takes place in laboratory; fertilized eggs transferred a few days later to uterus in hopes of implantation (41% result in live births in women under 35. Only 12% are successful in women over 40) (SART, 2011).
Intrauterine insemination (IUI)	Mild to severe male infertility/sterility; cervical hostile environment. Unexplained infertility.	Husband or donor sperm are passed through a syringe or catheter into the uterus at the time of ovulation.
Intracytoplasmic sperm injection (ICSI)	Severe male infertility or failure to inseminate via IVF.	Harvest a single sperm and inject into ova and then inseminate via IVF.
Gamete intrafallopian transfer (GIFT)	Same as IVF but must have at least one tube patent.	Ova retrieved from ovary and fertilized in catheter with washed motile sperm; immediate transfer to fimbriated ends of fallopian tube.
Zygote intrafallopian transfer (ZIFT)	Same as GIFT.	Same as IVF but fertilized ova are transferred to fallopian tube during zygote stage.

Sources: Adapted from Eisenberg, E., & Brumbaugh, K. (2011). Infertility: Frequently asked questions. Womenshealth.gov. Retrieved from http://www.womenshealth.gov/faq/infertility.cfm#top; Society for Assisted Reproductive Technology (SART). (2011). All SART Member Clinics: Clinic summary report. SARTcors Online. Retrieved from https://www.sartcorsonline.com/rptCSR_PublicMultYear.aspx?ClinicPKID=0.

ETHICAL ISSUES of Fertility Programs

Do fertility programs have an ethical obligation to withhold services from persons who may not be good parents? Should fertility programs treat the individual as if they were adopting a child? This is the topic of the American Society of Reproductive Medicine (ASRM) Ethics Committee Report of 2009.

When a couple presents for fertility services, the focus is usually on the medical and physical aspects of infertility. Rarely do fertility clinics pay close attention to the home situation or child-rearing capabilities of the couple who has requested fertility assistance. The ASRM Ethics Committee (2009) recommends that fertility programs develop written policies related to the evaluation of potential parents. These policies should specify conditions such as uncontrolled psychiatric disease, drug abuse, or ongoing physical or emotional abuse that would indicate that an individual would not make a good parent. Such evidence would support the decision not to provide medical treatment for infertility. At the same time, fertility programs should guard against discriminating based on a disability that would not affect parenting skill. This type of evaluation necessitates home studies and psychological or social work consultation, much like the scrutiny required before adoption.

CHART 41–12 Classification of Spontaneous Abortions

Incomplete: Not all products of conception are expelled.

Complete: All productions of conception are expelled.

Threatened: Signs/symptoms of abortion are present and indicate the loss could happen.

Inevitable: Signs/symptoms of abortion cannot be stopped and the loss will eventually happen.

Missed abortion: Pregnancy is lost and products of conception have not been expelled.

Symptoms of all types of abortion include vaginal bleeding with or without abdominal cramping.

Source: Adapted from Vorvick, L., & Storck, S. (Reviewers). (2011b). Miscarriage. MedlinePlus. Retrieved from http://www.nlm.nih.gov/medlineplus/ency/article/001488.htm.

Abortion

Description, Etiology, and Epidemiology

An **abortion** or miscarriage may be spontaneous or induced. Spontaneous abortion is a naturally occurring loss of a pregnancy before 20 weeks' gestation, whereas an elective or induced abortion is the intentional termination of a pregnancy (Vorvick & Storck, 2011b). A miscarriage is considered a "lay term" for spontaneous abortion. The rate of spontaneous abortion is 15% to 20% for known pregnancies (Vorvick & Storck, 2011b). The risk for miscarriage is higher in women over age 35 or women who have had a miscarriage before.

Safety Alert *Because of the negative connotation associated with the term abortion, when asking the patient about her pregnancy history, it might be beneficial to ask whether she has ever had a spontaneous loss or an elective loss of a pregnancy, rather than use the single term abortion or miscarriage. A patient may say yes to a miscarriage, but may not include the fact that she has also had an elective abortion, because the lay public often confuses the terms.*

Pathophysiology

Spontaneous abortion has five classifications: incomplete, complete, threatened, inevitable, and missed (Chart 41-12). A threatened abortion is a condition such as vaginal bleeding that suggests that an abortion is about to happen (Vorvick & Storck, 2011b). Vaginal bleeding during pregnancy, with or without cramping, does not always end in spontaneous abortion; however, it is a significant warning sign. When spontaneous abortion does occur, it is usually because the fetus has chromosomal problems unrelated to the mother or father's genes (Vorvick & Storck, 2011b). Other causes of spontaneous abortion include maternal endocrine disease, such as thyroid disorders or diabetes; infection; maternal reproductive anomalies; or maternal immune response abnormalities. It is thought that up to 50% of pregnancies may be spontaneously lost before the woman knows she is pregnant.

Clinical Manifestations

Symptoms of all types of spontaneous abortion include cramping and vaginal bleeding associated with a pregnancy. Low back or abdominal pain, described as dull, sharp, or cramping, may be constant or intermittent. If tissue is passed, the abortion is usually considered inevitable.

On examination, the cervix is often thin and dilated, and there may be evidence of rupture of the amniotic membranes. Human chorionic gonadotropin (HCG) levels will begin to drop after a fetal death. Other laboratory tests that may be beneficial with a pregnancy loss include a complete blood count (CBC) to determine blood loss and a white blood count (WBC) to identify any infection. An ultrasound, transvaginal or abdominal, will assist with the diagnosis of fetal death and/or the presence of placental fragments that may have been retained in the uterus after a pregnancy loss. Nothing can be done to treat an abortion that is inevitable, although there are palliative interventions that may help maintain the integrity of a pregnancy by providing a quiet uterine environment. These interventions include bed rest and abstaining from intercourse.

Medical Management

When an abortion occurs, it must be determined that all placental fragments and products of conception were fully expelled. If not, a procedure called a dilation and curettage (D&C) may be performed to scrape the uterine lining clean of fragments. The amount of postprocedure uterine bleeding must be monitored. It is expected after a complete abortion or a D&C that the amount of bleeding is about the same as a normal menstrual period. Bleeding that continues longer, is heavier, or contains tissue fragments or any signs of infection, such as fever or foul-smelling vaginal discharge, should be reported to the health care provider. It is recommended that the couple wait at least one normal menstrual period before attempting to become pregnant again (Vorvick & Storck, 2011b).

The second type of abortion is elective or induced. This may be done if the woman does not desire a child or if medical tests determine that there is a potential for Down syndrome or a congenital illness such as cystic fibrosis. The woman herself may have an illness that would put the fetus or herself at risk for harm, such as a serious heart condition, cancer, or advanced diabetes. When done for medical necessity, the term *therapeutic abortion* is often used. *Roe v. Wade* is the hallmark case in 1973 that legalized abortion in the United States for any reason before the 24th week of gestation. Third-trimester abortions may be performed only when the life or health of the mother is endangered by the pregnancy.

Induced abortions may be completed through the use of drugs or surgery. Two surgical abortion methods are manual vacuum aspiration (MVA) and dilation and evacuation (D&E) (FamilyDoctor.org Editorial Staff, 2011). With MVA, a small cannula is inserted through the cervix. The products of conception are suctioned out of the uterus using a syringe. This procedure is best done during the 4th through 12th week of gestation. A D&E is normally used from the 4th through the 13th week of gestation. The cervix is dilated and a cannula is inserted into the uterus. This cannula is attached to a vacuum device that will remove the products of conception. The MVA and D&E procedures are done in an office setting.

A dilation and curettage (D&C) can be performed between the 6th and 16th weeks of gestation. The procedure involves dilating the cervix and scraping the lining of the uterus with a curette to remove the contents. The D&C for induced abortion is done under general anesthesia.

Medical abortion can be done with pharmaceuticals during the first 9 weeks of gestation. The most common medication used is mifepristone (blocks progesterone) followed in about 48 hours with misoprostol (causes contractions and emptying of the uterus). Vaginal bleeding after these medications is expected to last as long as 13 days, although some women will experience spotting and discharge for several weeks (FamilyDoctor.org Editorial Staff, 2011).

Complications of any abortion procedure include bleeding, infection, cervical or uterine tear, retained products of conception, or even missed abortion whereby the pregnancy continues. Along with these physical complications, the woman may experience emotional upset surrounding the circumstances, which may require counseling to come to terms with the decision or necessity of the abortion. Nursing care involves education on complications, referral as needed, and emotional support.

Diagnostic Tests and Pharmacologic Management

Diagnostic tests for reproductive disorders are listed in the Diagnostic Tests feature box on page 1276. A summary of medications used to treat female reproductive disorders is presented on page 1277.

Diagnostic and Surgical Procedures

Several surgical procedures are specific to women's health. These include exploratory laparoscopy, colposcopy, bladder suspension, salpingo-oophorectomy, and hysterectomy. An exploratory laparoscopy is a minimally invasive procedure that involves a small incision through which a laparoscope is inserted that allows visualization of the internal organs and structures to assess for disease processes. Carbon dioxide is instilled into the abdomen to elevate the abdominal wall and create a larger work area. After the procedure, the incision is sutured to secure the edges for healing. The patient may experience shoulder pain as the carbon dioxide dissipates from the abdomen. Instruct the patient to sit up and walk to promote gas diffusion and reduce pain. The nurse should be careful to assess the following:

- Incisions and any drainage
- Vital signs, bowel sounds
- Nutrition.

A **colposcopy** is a test to evaluate the cells of the cervix. A colposcope is a binocular magnifying tool used by the health care provider after a speculum has been placed in the vagina to allow for direct visualization of the cervix. Abnormal areas identified on the cervix may be biopsied and sent to the laboratory. This procedure can be done in an office setting. The patient is encouraged to take ibuprofen or extra strength Tylenol shortly before the procedure to help control the pain of the biopsy. It is important to remind the patient not to insert anything into the vagina, including not having intercourse, for 24 to 48 hours before the procedure, since spermicides, tampons, and semen can interfere with test results. Risks and complications are rare but can include slight spotting to heavy bleeding after the biopsy. The patient should be taught signs and symptoms of infection and that she should report any pelvic or abdominal pain.

A **bladder suspension**, or Burch procedure, is done to suspend the bladder and correct urinary incontinence. During childbirth, the bladder ligaments are sometimes weakened and cause the bladder to sink in the pelvic cavity, causing leakage of urine, or incontinence.

DIAGNOSTIC TESTS for Reproductive Disorders

Test	Expected Abnormality
Transvaginal Ultrasound	
Pelvic ultrasound	Positive for uterine mass, ectopic pregnancy, or ovarian cyst.
Determines the size and location of masses and helps with the decision for or against surgery.	Positive for fetal demise.
Determines presence of ectopic pregnancy.	
Urine Human Chorionic Gonadotropin (HCG)	
Serum HCG	Positive: indicative of pregnancy.
Quantitative HCG	A quantitative HCG that doubles in 48 hours is indicative of pregnancy that is continuing.
Serum HCG is most accurate. Quantitative HCG is helpful in determining the length of pregnancy, and serial quantitative HCG tests are performed to determine the possibility of spontaneous abortion or ectopic pregnancy.	A quantitative HCG that fails to double in 48 hours is indicative of fetal demise or ectopic pregnancy. Increased in hydatidiform mole.
Blood Culture	
Possible toxic shock syndrome.	Positive for *S. aureus* or *group A streptococcus.*
Follicle-Stimulating Hormone (FSH) (urine)	
Indicative for menopause.	Greater than 40 milliunits per liter.
Luteinizing Hormone (LH)	
Increased in polycystic ovary syndrome.	Greater than 150 milli-international units/mL.
Used in ovulation testing.	
Semen Analysis	
Determines the adequacy of volume, viscosity, sperm count, and motility.	Lower than normal sperm count or motility.
Antisperm Antibody Test	
Possible cause of infertility.	Presence of antisperm antibodies in serum.
Basal Body Temperature	
Determines ovulation if temperature rises of 0.5–1 degree is noted during the cycle.	Daily temperature of the woman before rising will slightly increase at ovulation.
Cervical Mucus	
Notes cyclic changes in mucus to determine whether sperm can pass. Ideally needs thin, stretchy mucus for optimal sperm movement.	Slippery, stretchy, and clear at ovulation.
Serum Progesterone	
Determines corpus luteum production of progesterone necessary for maintenance of a pregnancy. Used in evaluation of infertility. Aids in diagnosis of ovarian tumor.	Increased during the luteal phase.
Postcoital Test	
Evaluates sperm motility in cervical mucus.	Part of infertility work-up.
Commercial Urine Test for Ovulation	
Determines luteinizing hormone, which is necessary for ovulation.	Helps pinpoint ovulation for optimum fertilization.
Hysterosalpingogram	
Assesses patency of uterine cavity and fallopian tubes. Identifies fibroids, abnormal structure of uterus, or tumors.	Fluoroscopic and x-ray evidence of blocked fallopian tubes or abnormal uterus.
Hysteroscopy	
Hyperplasia, endometrial cancer, or polyps can be identified, or biopsy or removal of polyps can be done.	Allows visualization of entire endometrium. Biopsy or removal of polyps may be done via hysteroscopy.
Laparoscopy	
Direct visualization of the abdominal and pelvic cavity.	Insertion of a scope through the abdominal opening to view abdominal and pelvic organs. Diagnostic or curative.

Sources: Adapted from Jennings, V., & Arevalo, M. (2009). Fertility awareness-based methods. In R. Hatcher, J. Trussell, A. Nelson, W. Cates, F. Stewart, & D. Kowal (Eds.), *Contraceptive technology.* New York: Ardent Media; Kee, J. (2010). *Laboratory and diagnostic tests with nursing implication.* (8th ed.). Upper Saddle River, NJ: Pearson.

PHARMACOLOGY Summary of Medications Used to Treat Female Reproductive Disorders

Medication Category and Action	Application/Indication	Nursing Responsibility
Antibiotics		
Clindamycin (for streptococcal infection) ***Action:*** Acts on the bacterial ribosomal subunit. Bacteriostatic. Nafcillin (for penicillinase resistant staphylococcal infection) ***Action:*** Inhibits bacterial wall synthesis. Bacteriocidal.	Toxic shock syndrome	Risk of resistant bacteria. Risk for pseudomembranous colitis. Advise patient to report diarrhea. Pregnancy category B. Monitor for hypersensitivity reaction. Monitor renal, hepatic, and hematologic function during therapy.
Nonsteroidal anti-inflammatory drug (NSAID)		
Ibuprofen (Motrin) ***Action:*** Cyclooxygenase-1 (COX-1) inhibitor with anti-inflammatory, analgesic, and antipyretic effects.	Dysmenorrhea, premenstrual syndrome (PMS), premenstrual dysphoric disorder (PMDD), and fibrocystic breast disease.	Caution patient to take with food to avoid stomach irritation.
Antiestrogen Agents		
Aromatase inhibitors Anastrozole (Arimidex) Letrozole (Femara) ***Action:*** Inhibitor of the enzyme system that converts androgens to estrogens.	Blocks estrogen production by other tissues in women who are postmenopausal. May be used for leiomyomata. Often used in treatment of breast cancer in postmenopausal women.	Menopausal symptoms may increase. Monitor serum calcium.
Antineoplastic Antimetabolite		
Methotrexate (Rheumatrex) ***Action:*** Antimetabolic and folic acid antagonist, thereby interfering with mitotic processes.	Nonsurgical treatment of ectopic pregnancy.	Generally one or two doses given. Most adverse effects are seen in long-term use such as with rheumatoid arthritis. Methotrexate will be excreted in breast milk.
Abortifacients		
Mifepristone ***Action:*** Blocks progesterone receptors of uterus. Misoprostol ***Action:*** Prostaglandin that causes uterine contractions.	Abortifacient. Used with Mifepristone to help remove uterine contents.	Instruct on expected cramping and vaginal bleeding that may last for several weeks. ER care needed if hemorrhaging. Instruct on expected cramping.
Antiestrogen with Weak Androgen Effects		
Danazol (Danocrine) ***Action:*** Mild androgenic effects that suppress follicle-stimulating hormone (FSH) and luteinizing hormone (LH). Causes anovulation and amenorrhea.	Treatment of endometriosis and fibrocystic breast disease.	Monitor for masculinity effects, virilization, menstrual irregularities, hot flashes, vaginal dryness, and gastrointestinal (GI) distress. Pregnancy category X.
Infertility Agent		
Clomiphene citrate (Clomid) ***Action:*** Ovarian stimulant.	Drug of choice for female infertility caused by ovulatory dysfunction.	Monitor for increased levels of FSH and LH, as well as pregnancy. Monitor for rapid weight gain, nausea, vomiting, dyspnea, chest pain and report to health care provider immediately.
Female Hormones		
Estrogen ***Action:*** Steroid hormone secreted by the ovarian follicle. Available in natural and synthetic forms.	Treatment of menopausal symptoms from natural occurrence or surgical occurrence. Low doses can be used to control metrorrhagia and menorrhagia.	Monitor for irregular vaginal bleeding and breast tenderness. Increased potential for deep venous thrombosis, especially if patient is a smoker.
Progesterone ***Action:*** Steroid hormone secreted by the corpus luteum.	Prevents endometrial hyperplasia. Treatment for dysfunctional uterine bleeding.	Monitor for fluid imbalance. Monitor liver function, blood glucose, sodium, and chloride serum levels.

(*continued*)

PHARMACOLOGY Summary of Medications Used to Treat Female Reproductive Disorders, *continued*

Medication Category and Action	Application/Indication	Nursing Responsibility
Antidiabetic Agent		
Metformin (Glucophage, Fortamet) ***Action:*** Reduces insulin resistance and serum insulin levels. Reduces androgen serum levels.	Lowers testosterone production in the patient with polycystic ovary syndrome.	Monitor for hypoglycemia and GI distress. Pregnancy category B.
Antidepressants		
Fluoxetine (Prozac) pregnancy category C Paroxetine (Paxil) pregnancy category D ***Action:*** Selective serotonin reuptake inhibitor (SSRI). Venlafaxine (Effexor) pregnancy category C ***Action:*** Serotonin-norepinephrine re-uptake inhibitor (SNRI)	Approved for PMS and PMDD.	Avoid abrupt withdrawal of the medication. Monitor for suicidal ideation. Avoid alcohol. Take in the morning to avoid insomnia. Same as SSRIs.
Hormonal Agents		
Raloxifene (Evista) ***Action:*** Selective estrogen receptor modulator (SERM)	Primary use—prevention or treatment of postmenopausal osteoporosis. Increases bone mass density; reduces vertebral fractures.	Monitor for signs of thromboembolism. Educate patient to report gastric disturbances, headache, chest pain, or gynecologic abnormalities.

Sources: Adapted from Adams, M., & Koch, R. (2010). *Pharmacology: Connections to nursing practice.* Upper Saddle River, NJ: Pearson; Vernkataraman, R., & Sharma, S. (2011). Toxic shock syndrome: Treatment and medication. eMedicine. Retrieved from http://emedicine.medscape.com/article/169177-treatment.

This is a common complaint of women typically over 40 years of age that have given birth to one or more children. The bladder suspension can be done using an abdominal incision, or it can be done utilizing a laparoscope. Laparoscopic surgery causes less trauma and will require a shorter hospital stay. As with any surgery, bleeding is a complication that needs assessing. In addition, the patient is instructed that normal bladder function often does not return for up to 2 months.

Salpingo-oophorectomy is the procedure whereby the fallopian tubes and ovaries are removed. Removal of just the fallopian tube is a **salpingectomy**. **Oophorectomy** is the removal of just the ovary. These can be unilateral or bilateral depending on the pathology that requires the procedure. These surgeries are done for ectopic pregnancy, ovarian cysts, or cancers of the ovary. In the case of cancer of the endometrium or ovaries that is spreading, the salpingo-oophorectomy may be done in conjunction with a total abdominal hysterectomy and the procedure may be abbreviated as TAH-BSO (total abdominal hysterectomy and bilateral salpingo-oophorectomy). A procedure such as this creates surgical menopause. However, the symptoms can be more intense than the gradual menopause that occurs naturally. The patient may be treated for these symptoms with a variety of estrogen replacements if the surgery is not done for cancer. Remember that estrogen is generally not given to women with reproductive cancer because many of these types of cancer are estrogen dependent. The care of these patients is very similar to that of the patient with a hysterectomy.

Hysterectomy

Hysterectomy, a surgical procedure to remove the uterus, is the second most frequently occurring major surgery in women of reproductive age. An estimated 600,000 hysterectomies are performed each year in the United States (CDC, 2009). The surgery can be done as a total abdominal hysterectomy removing the uterus, ovaries, and fallopian tubes, or as a vaginal hysterectomy in which the uterus is removed through the vagina. Hysterectomies are performed primarily for uterine fibroids (leiomyoma, myoma), endometriosis, and uterine prolapse. Other reasons necessitating a hysterectomy include severe, chronic pelvic pain; long-term, chronic vaginal bleeding; or cancers involving the cervix, ovaries, or uterus.

A hysterectomy involves removal of the uterus, which can be done in one of three ways: through an abdominal incision, through the vagina, or through laparoscopic incisions in the abdomen. The reason for the removal will determine which procedure to use and whether other organs besides the uterus are to be removed. A partial hysterectomy is the removal of the upper portion of the uterus, leaving the cervix intact. A total hysterectomy involves removal of the entire uterus and the cervix. A radical hysterectomy is the removal of the uterus, the cervix, and the upper part of the vagina. The procedure chosen will depend on the extent of the pathology necessitating the surgery. For example, uterine fibroids may require only a partial hysterectomy, whereas extensive cancer could require a total or radical hysterectomy.

Nursing Management

Nursing care for the woman having a hysterectomy includes addressing the following nursing diagnoses:

- *Anxiety* related to fear of surgery and related diagnoses.
- *Risk for Infection* related to the surgical procedure.
- *Readiness for Enhanced Fluid Balance From Electrolyte Imbalance* related to urinary retention.
- *Potential for Altered Tissue Perfusion* related to hemorrhage.
- *Potential for Altered Tissue Perfusion* related to deep venous thrombosis.
- *Deficient Knowledge* related to surgical procedure and risks and benefits.
- *Acute Pain* related to incision.

PATIENT TEACHING & DISCHARGE PRIORITIES for Hysterectomy

Need	Teaching
Analgesics	Take analgesics as prescribed.
Patient	Encourage the patient to take analgesics as prescribed.
Family/support system	Advise the patient to report to the health care provider if analgesics are inadequate.
Activity	
Patient	Avoid lifting, straining, driving, or other strenuous activity for 2 to 4 weeks.
Family/support system	Assist the patient as needed to allow adequate rest and avoidance of strenuous activity.
Diet	Resume a regular, well-balanced diet as soon as desired.
Patient	Avoid spicy foods, caffeine, and alcohol, as they may irritate the bladder during healing.
Family/support system	Encourage a healthy diet.
Bladder care	
Patient	Increase oral fluids to 3 quarts per day and urinate regularly.
Family/support system	Assist the patient as needed.
Sexual Intercourse	
Patient	May resume sexual relations 6 weeks after surgery.

Source: Adapted from Trimble, E. (Reviewer). (2011). Hysterectomy. WomensHealth.gov. Retrieved from http://www.womenshealth.gov/faq/hysterectomy.cfm#f.

- *Fatigue* related to blood loss.
- *Disturbed Body Image* related to perceived loss of femininity.

NANDA-I © 2012

Risks associated with hysterectomy are the same as those related to any major abdominal surgical procedure, including reactions to medications, bleeding, infection, and bladder and bowel injury. Recovery is fastest with the vaginal or laparoscopic procedure; the patient also may experience less pain. The patient usually has a urinary catheter for 1 to 2 days while hospitalized; in addition, some health care providers order injectable heparin for those at higher risk for blood clots. Ambulation is essential as soon as feasible, and a regular diet is encouraged after bowel function returns. Discharge instructions should include no heavy lifting, regular diet, rest, and nothing in the vagina, including intercourse, until released by the health care provider in 6 to 8 weeks. Menopause is immediate for women who also have their ovaries removed during the hysterectomy, and estrogen replacement therapy should be discussed with the patient. Specific discharge instructions for a hysterectomy that the nurse should carefully review with the patient are outlined in the Patient Teaching & Discharge Priorities box.

Intimate Partner Violence

Sexual assault is an act of violence. It is defined as the forcible perpetration of a sexual act on a person without his or her consent. According to the CDC (2011), 1 in 6 women will be the victim of rape or attempted rape. In addition to the initial trauma, many women who have been raped experience long-term physical health problems, emotional distress, and are at risk for drug or alcohol abuse, as well as adopting risky sexual behaviors (Vivolo, Holland, Teten, Holt, and the Sexual Violence Review Team, 2010).

The immediate reactions to rape include shock, fear, confusion, and disbelief. Some who have been raped may deny the incident occurred or withdraw from rescuers. Those who have been raped may sustain physical injuries as well, which include bruising and lacerations to the genital area, head and neck injuries, and abdominal trauma.

Initial care of the woman who has been sexually assaulted centers on the person's safety. Treatment of the urgent and emergent injuries and emotional responses requires specifically trained professionals who have experience in dealing with those who have been sexually assaulted and can provide not only the crisis intervention that makes a difference at the time of the incident but also the continuing care over the course of her recovery. Readily available rape advocates, specially trained law enforcement personnel, and sexual assault nurse examiners (SANEs) should be involved with the patient from the very beginning of the patient's presentation. The importance of careful and meticulous evidence collection is the second priority after assuring the patient's safety and treatment of injuries. Sexual assault nurse examiners are specially trained to collect this evidence according to the protocol of the local jurisdiction. Sexual assault exams are for the express purpose of collecting evidence and have no bearing on the patient's medical care. The victim of a sexual assault must consent to the collection of evidence in total or in part. The collection process is laborious and time consuming, and many who have been victimized become exhausted and frustrated with the process without the appropriate support from the rape advocate and the sexual assault examiner. The evidence that should be collected and usually included in local protocols includes a history of the assault, collection of seminal fluid and possible sperm, combing pubic hair for foreign hair and matter, taking fingernail scrapings, collecting the patient's blood for typing and DNA screening, collecting torn or stained clothing, taking photographs of the injuries, and creating an accurate body map of the injuries. The handling of evidence is critical; therefore, the sexual assault nurse examiner carefully labels all evidence and seals it for transfer to law enforcement. This is referred to as "creating a chain of evidence," which is critical to maintaining the evidence's integrity. No unnecessary personnel should be involved in handling evidence.

Assessment findings of the victim of rape may be unpredictable. Emotionally, some victims of rape may be extraordinarily calm and controlled. Others may be hysterical and difficult to calm. Many cry uncontrollably and express anger and fear; others may be silent and withdrawn. Physical findings include oral, vaginal, and rectal injuries, bruises to the neck and arms, head injuries, and multiple scrapes and

Weblink: Sexual Assault Response Teams† Weblink: Violence Against Women

cuts. One of the most important findings in a woman who has been raped is a slight tear to the posterior fourchette of the vaginal opening. This small physical indication is frequently a sign of forced penetration. Many victims of rape show very few, if any, injuries because they cooperate with their attacker out of fear for their lives. All these women should be monitored carefully during evidence collection for delayed response to the assault. Decreasing level of consciousness or changes in vital signs will require evidence collection to be halted and the patient to be assessed for occult injuries. Most evidence collection protocols include toxicology and blood alcohol levels to determine whether the person who was raped was under the influence of drugs or alcohol, which may have impacted her ability to fight off her attacker. Screening for sexually transmitted infections is also part of the exam, and prophylactic treatment with antibiotics is offered to the patient. Additionally, the patient is offered emergency contraception. Victims of sexual assault should never be allowed to leave the hospital alone after treatment. Rape advocates should be available to ensure the patient's safety once released from the hospital. A safe house, family member's home, or women's shelter may be possible options for the patient.

Nurses can help prevent sexual assaults by educating young women about self-defense and avoiding risky situations. Encouragement of patients to participate in self-defense classes can improve their situational awareness and confidence. Female patients should also be encouraged to practice safe habits in lighting entrances to their home, locking doors, and avoiding opening doors to strangers. Women patients should protect their identification as a single occupant in phone books, in mailbox listings, and on answering machines. Remind patients of the dangers of walking in deserted areas, especially after dark. Encourage patients to pay attention to suspicious behaviors and avoid being alone in offices or elevators with unknown persons. In social situations, patients should avoid becoming intoxicated or accepting mixed drinks from casual acquaintances. All women should proceed very cautiously with online correspondence. Providing resources to female patients for obtaining whistles or pepper spray and encouraging them to keep it accessible will add to the general safety of women.

Many communities have rape crisis centers or phone lines that are staffed 24 hours a day. The programs provide counseling and advocacy and ensure appropriate treatment during medical and legal procedures. Victim financial assistance can be arranged to offset lost time from work and added expenses for medical care, psychological counseling, transportation, and housing. The National Sexual Violence Resource Center (NSVRC) (2009) lists several state and county guidelines for the treatment of adult victims of sexual assault. The CDC also has included guidelines for treatment in the 2010 Treatment Guidelines for Sexually Transmitted Disease (Workowski & Berman, 2010). These are summarized and outlined in the National Guidelines box. More

NATIONAL GUIDELINES for the Management of Adult Victims of Sexual Assault

Ensure local law enforcement is aware of the patient.

Forensic exam is useful up to 7 days post-assault.

The orifices used in the assault, the timing of the assault, prior and subsequent consenting sexual intercourse, use of condoms by the assailant, and whether or not ejaculation had occurred should be documented.

Signed consent is essential if any information is subsequently disclosed to the police. This should be with the understanding that the court may order disclosure of all information divulged during the legal proceedings.

Injuries requiring immediate attention will take precedence over any other examination.

If the assault is recent, accurately document injuries found on the genital inspection. Petechial hemorrhages on the palate should be sought with a history of forced oral penetration. Anal examination including proctoscopy should be performed if there is a recent history of forced anal penetration, noting any trauma.

A full screening for sexually transmitted infections at presentation is recommended.

Exam should include cultures for *Neisseria gonorrhoeae* and tests for *Chlamydia trachomatis* from any sites of penetration or attempted penetration.

Vaginal slides should be prepared for microscopy and yeasts, bacterial vaginosis, and *Trichomonas vaginalis*.

Blood should be drawn for syphilis serology.

Hepatitis B, HIV, and hepatitis C testing should be offered.

Sexually transmitted infection (STI) prophylaxis (Workowski & Berman, 2010):

- Ceftriaxone 250 milligrams IM plus Metronidazole 2 grams p.o. and Azithromycin 1 gram immediately. Or Cefixime 400 milligrams p.o. plus Metronidazole 2 grams p.o. and Azithromycin 1 gram immediately.
- Hepatitis B vaccination should be offered if the patient has not received it previously.
- A discussion about HIV infection should be part of the interview with the patient, as well as follow-up testing and counseling. The patient can be offered postexposure prophylaxis in line with the postexposure prophylaxis guidelines for occupational exposure. This should be started within 72 hours after a high-risk exposure.

Pregnancy prevention:

- Postcoital oral contraception can be issued if within 72 hours of the assault and no risk of preexisting pregnancy exists.
- Levonorgestrel 0.75 milligram for 2 doses 12 hours apart.

Counseling:

- Post-traumatic stress disorder is common following sexual assault; however, there is no evidence that brief psychological debriefing reduces this.
- Links with local victim support organizations, rape crisis groups, and local psychologists should be present to facilitate referral if needed.
- As psychological sequelae may develop months or years later, communication should be encouraged with the general health care provider to ensure continuity of care.

Sources: Adapted from National Sexual Violence Resource Center (NSVRC). (2009). Protocols and guidelines for sexual assault response teams (SART). Retrieved from http://www.nsvrc.org/projects/sart/protocols-and-guidelines-sexual-assault-response-teams-sart; Workowski, K., & Berman, S. (2010). Sexually transmitted disease treatment guidelines, 2010. *Morbidity and Mortality Weekly Report, 59*(RR12), 1–110.

EVIDENCE-BASED PRACTICE Using CAM During Perimenopausal and Menopausal Years

Clinical Problem

Many women, both in the United States and Canada, use complementary and alternative medicines (CAM) during their perimenopausal and menopausal years.

Research Findings

Lunny and Fraser (2010) conducted an "open" web survey via the Internet where 423 women between 40 and 60 years of age answered a self-administered questionnaire with 12 closed-ended questions about their use of CAM therapies. Of the women who participated, 385 (91%) reported use of CAM, with vitamins and minerals, relaxation, yoga/meditation, soy products, and prayer being the most frequently reported therapies. When compared by postmenopausal to early and late perimenopausal, it was discovered that postmenopausal women reported using St. John's Wort, support groups, and prayer more than the younger groups. Lunny and Fraser also determined that older women with more education and more somatic menopausal symptoms reported higher use of CAM therapies. These women may be reluctant to discuss the use of CAM with their health care provider, either because they think that it is unimportant or because they think their provider will criticize them.

Implications for Nursing Practice

This study emphasizes the importance of communication between women and health care providers about the use of CAM therapies. Improved communication has the potential of promoting shared decision making and decreasing the incidence of adverse drug–herb interactions.

Nurses can provide evidence-based information handouts, brochures, and reputable websites such as CAMline for women in waiting areas for clinics and in hospitals. It is very important that women have full information about these products and the potential for drug–herb interactions.

Critical Thinking Questions with answers can be found in the Osborn Student Resources at nursing.pearsonhighered.com.

Source: Lunny, C., & Fraser, S. (2010). The use of complementary and alternative medicines among a sample of Canadian menopausal-aged women. *Journal of Midwifery and Women's Health, 55*(4), 335–343. doi:10:1016/j.jmwh.2009.10.015

RESEARCH OPPORTUNITIES Related to Female Reproductive Disoders

Research Area	Clinical Impact
Clinical Trials	
Medications for PMS and PMDD	May help to relieve physiologic and mood problems associated with PMS and PMDD.
Education, technologies, drugs, and alternative therapies	Prevention, diagnostics, and therapeutics for girls and women.
Physiologic Research	
Research on why some fibroids grow to become problems and others do not	May help develop strategies to prevent fibroids and to develop new strategies to decrease the need for hysterectomy.
Ovarian cancer	Cause, treatment, prevention, and survival.
Menopause	Treatment options for prevention of symptoms.
Pregnancy	Prenatal care and prevention of complications and fetal abnormalities and death.
Infertility	Ability to have children.
Health Disparities and Diversity	
Cultural diversity, environmental exposures, effects of poverty, rural and inner city residence, physical and mental disabilities	Women are disproportionately affected by disease related to gender, culture, socioeconomic status, residence, and environmental exposures.

Source: Adapted from Office of Research on Women's Health. (2011). Annual NIH research priorities for women's health. Retrieved from http://orwh.od.nih.gov/research/priorities.html.

information for women victims of sexual violence is available from the National Women's Health Information Center (www.womenshealth.gov/violence/types/sexual.cfm).

Gerontological Considerations

As women age, they are more prone to some conditions and less prone to others. In general, the geriatric population is rapidly growing, and health issues need to be addressed by the health care providers. Information on the effects of aging on the female population is widely available. For example, much information exists on menopause and the effects it has on sexual desire and sexual response. There is a plethora of information on breast cancer and the need for screening mammography, even in the aging population. The National Institute on Aging provides information on many topics, including women's health issues.

Research

Research on women's health issues has been in the forefront for many years. Both the Office of Research on Women's Health and the National Institute on Aging are involved in research on menopause, fibroids, and cancer, to name only a few topics. The Research Opportunities box outlines potential research topics related to female reproductive disorders and trends in the care of women.

READ: **History of Present Illnesses** >> Laboratory Study Results >> Critical Thinking Questions

Helen Goldman is a 54-year-old woman admitted early yesterday morning for a scheduled total abdominal hysterectomy and bilateral salpingo-oophorectomy. Mrs. Goldman has had heavy menstrual periods all her life, but for the last 2 years she has felt confined to the house due to the amount of bleeding she experienced. Her health care provider has put her on various medications in an attempt to control the heavy bleeding without success. Mrs. Goldman also has several uterine fibroid tumors that cause severe discomfort. She and her health care provider decided a total abdominal hysterectomy with bilateral salpingo-oophorectomy was warranted.

During morning report, the nurse reports that the occlusive dressing on Mrs. Goldman's abdominal incision has been marked for a moderate amount of bleeding, but that it appears to have stopped as the drainage marks have gotten no bigger in the last 6 hours. Mrs. Goldman is scheduled for a hemoglobin and hematocrit this morning. She is currently receiving patient-controlled analgesia with morphine. You enter Mrs. Goldman's room at 0745 and begins the initial assessment: Temp: 99.4°F, P: 96, RR: 22, BP: 108/62. IV D5½ NS with 20 KCL infusing at 125 mL/hr, without signs of redness or swelling at the IV site. Lung sounds: clear to auscultation.

Mrs. Goldman is lying quietly in bed, her eyes closing as if she is very tired. She reports her pain is increasing and classifies it a 7 on a 1 to 10 scale. When her covers are pulled back to examine the dressing, you note bright-red blood oozing from the edges of the dressing. Further assessment reveals approximately 20 milliliters of bright-red blood staining the top sheet that was covering Mrs. Goldman. You push the patient call light and ask the secretary to please page the attending surgeon. The surgeon arrives and requests a suture kit and local anesthetic to put in retention sutures in an attempt to control the bleeding. The equipment arrives, and the surgeon removes the occlusive dressing to reveal an oozing incision, without redness, edema, slight ecchymosis, and edges that remain approximated with staples. The surgeon asks for the most recent laboratory work that was drawn earlier in the morning. After placing 6 retention sutures and observing that the oozing has stopped, the surgeon leaves the floor after writing orders for antibiotics every 6 hours.

Medical–Surgical History

Mrs. Goldman had three vaginal deliveries of live children. She had an appendectomy at age 15.

Social History

Mrs. Goldman lives with her husband and has three grown children who all live in the local area. She has never smoked or used illicit drugs. She has a glass of wine in the evening with her dinner. Mrs. Goldman runs an average of 20 miles per week.

READ: History of Present Illnesses >> **Physical Exam** >> Admitting Medical Records >> Laboratory Study Results

Physical Exam

Temp: 97.4°F P: 82 RR: 16 BP: 108/62
Oxygen sat 98% on RA
HEENT: normal
Heart: regular rate and rhythm, normal S_1, S_2
Lungs: clear to auscultation in all fields
Abdomen: soft, nontender, bowel sounds present
Normal neuro exam
No rash
Chest x-ray: clear
ECG: WNL
Weight: 130 lb
Height: 5.4 ft

Admitting Medical Orders

Surgical service
Admit to surgical floor
Admitting diagnosis was menorrhagia and uterine fibroid tumors
Status post total abdominal hysterectomy with salpingo-oophorectomy
No known allergies
Call house officer: pulse < 60–130/minute; BP < 90–160 systolic; temperature > 38.5; urine output < 30 mL/hour for 2 hours; > 30/minute
Ambulate qid beginning postoperative day 1
IV D5½ NS with 20 KCL at 125 mL/hr
Vital signs q4hours
Indwelling catheter to be inserted morning before surgery
Sequential compression device (SCD) to lower extremities until ambulating without assistance
Incentive spirometer q2h while awake
I&O q8hours
Progressive postoperative diet as tolerated post-nausea

Scheduled Medications

PCA: morphine sulfate 1 mg/mL, incremental dose 1 mg, lock out 6 minutes
Unasyn 2 grams IV q6h

PRN Medications

Phenergan 25 mg q6h prn nausea IM
Ativan 0.5–2 mg IV q6–8h prn anxiety (not to exceed 10 mg/24 hours)
Tylenol 650 mg PO/PR q4h for pain
Benadryl 25–50 mg IV q6hours PRN insomnia or itching

Ordered Laboratory Studies

CBC morning after surgery

READ: History of Present Illnesses >> **Laboratory Study Results** >> Critical Thinking Questions

Test	1 Day Prior to Surgery	4 Hours After Surgery	0500 Today
HGB	14.3 g/dL	11.9 g/dL	9.5 g/dL
HCT	43%	38%	32%
Platelets	230,000/mm^3	165,000/mm^3	90,000/mm^3

Test	1 Day Prior to Surgery	4 Hours After Surgery	0500 Today
WBC	8,000/mm^3	12,000/mm^3	14,000/mm^3
RBC	4.9/mm^3	4.1/mm^3	3.92/mm^3

Pearson Nursing Student Resources *Log on to* **nursing.pearsonhighered.com** *to download forms*

DOCUMENT:

>> Summary of Hospitalization
>> Pathophysiology Form
>> Laboratory Values
>> Laboratory Results Explanation

APPLY:

>> List of Potential Nursing Diagnoses
>> Concept Map
>> Critical Thinking Questions and Concept Map

APPLY: History of Present Illnesses >> Laboratory Study Results >> **Critical Thinking Questions**

1. What action would be your top priority?
2. What should you do next?
3. Based on this situation and the 3 days of lab values, which of the interventions outlined below should receive the highest nursing priority?
   - Assess incision q30min × 2, then q1h × 2, then q2h × 2, then prn for signs of bleeding or infection. Call surgeon if bleeding recurs.
   - IV at 200 milliliters q1h for 4 hours, then decrease to 150 milliliters per hour.
   - Administer analgesic as prescribed.
   - Unasyn 2 grams IV q6h.
   - Vital signs and oxygen saturation q4h.
   - CBC stat.
   - Call laboratory results to the health care provider.
   - Educate patient on safety measures for low hemoglobin and platelets.
   - Change patient linens to provide comfortable environment.
   - Encourage oral fluids and increased protein and iron in diet.

Answers to Critical Thinking Questions can be found in Appendix D in the Osborn Student Resources at nursing.pearsonhighered.com.

NCLEX® PRACTICE

1. A woman who has polycystic ovary syndrome wants to become pregnant. Which one of the following drugs would the nurse anticipate being included in the plan of care for this patient and thus require the development of a teaching plan?

1. Metformin
2. Birth control pills
3. Danazol
4. Lupron

2. The nurse is admitting a patient with a diagnosis of probable endometriosis. When planning care the nurse should anticipate the patient will most likely need preparation for which of the following procedures?

1. Urine hCG
2. Abdominal ultrasound
3. Laparoscopic surgery
4. Transvaginal ultrasound

3. A patient with uterine fibroids was told that the size of the fibroids has decreased. The nurse realizes that the decrease in size could be due to:

1. constant uterine bleeding.
2. decreased estrogen production.
3. pregnancy.
4. dietary changes.

4. A patient is diagnosed with an unruptured ectopic pregnancy. The nurse gathers educational material for this patient for which treatment that will most likely be selected?

1. surgical removal of the fallopian tube.
2. methotrexate.
3. a pessary.
4. low dose birth control pills.

5. The nurse is assessing a 24-year-old female's reproductive status. Which of the following factors revealed in an assessment interview should the nurse address in a teaching plan regarding this patient's risk of infertility?
   1. Type 1 diabetes mellitus
   2. Diagnosis of scoliosis
   3. Menses began at the age of 13
   4. Parents had 4 children, all live births

6. A patient is recovering from an exploratory laparoscopy. Which of the following nursing diagnoses is the priority for this patient?
   1. Nutrition, Imbalanced: Less than Body Requirements.
   2. Pain, acute.
   3. Impaired Mobility.
   4. Impaired Skin Integrity.

Answers to NCLEX Practice Questions can be found in Appendix D in the Osborn Student Resources at nursing.pearsonhighered.com. Practice additional NCLEX questions online at the Student Resources site.

Pearson Nursing Student Resources Find additional review materials at: **nursing.pearsonhighered.com**

REFERENCES

Adams, M., & Koch, R. (2010). *Pharmacology: Connections to nursing practice.* Upper Saddle River, NJ: Pearson.

American Cancer Society (ACS). (2010). Detailed guides for cervical, vulva, endometrial, ovarian, and vaginal cancer. *Learn About Cancer.* Retrieved from http://www.cancer.org/Cancer/CervicalCancer/DetailedGuide/index; http://www.cancer.org/Cancer/VulvarCancer/DetailedGuide/index; http://www.cancer.org/Cancer/EndometrialCancer/DetailedGuide/index; http://www.cancer.org/Cancer/OvarianCancer/DetailedGuide/index; http://www.cancer.org/Cancer/VaginalCancer/DetailedGuide/index

Angelo, T. (2010). Clinical advisors—Patient handouts: Vaginal pessary. *Merck Medicus.* Retrieved from http://www.merckmedicus.com/pp/us/hcp/hcp_patient_resource_allhandouts_content_search.jsp?pg=/ppdocs/us/common/crs/wha/wha_vagipess_wha.htm

Balentine, J. (2011). Toxic shock syndrome (TSS). MedicineNet.com. Retrieved from http://www.medicinenet.com/toxic_shock_syndrome/article.htm

Barad, D. (2011). Pelvic pain. MerckManuals Online Medical Library. Retrieved from http://www.merckmedicus.com/pp/us/hcp/framemm.jsp?pg=www.merck.com/mmpe/index.html

Barclift, S. (Reviewer). (2010). Premenstrual syndrome. Womenshealth.gov. Retrieved from http://www.womenshealth.gov/faq/premenstrual-syndrome.cfm

Bartoszek, M. (2009). Recognizing polycystic ovary syndrome in the primary care setting. *The Nurse Practitioner, 34*(7), 23–29.

Bickley, L. (2007). *Bates guide to physical examination and history taking* (9th ed.). Philadelphia: Lippincott Williams & Wilkins.

Bridges, D. (Reviewer). (2010). Female sexual problems. WebMD. Retrieved from http://www.webmd.com/sex-relationships/guide/womens-sexual-problems

Bush, L., Chaparro-Rojas, F., & Perez, M. (2009). Toxic shock syndrome (TSS). Merck Manuals Online Medical Library. Retrieved from http://www.merckmedicus.com/pp/us/hcp/framemm.jsp?pg=www.merck.com/mmpe/index.html

Centers for Disease Control (CDC). (2009). Women's reproductive health: Hysterectomy fact sheet. Retrieved from http://www.cdc.gov/reproductivehealth/WomensRH/00-04-FS_Hysterectomy.htm

Centers for Disease Control (CDC). (2010). Candidiasis. National Center for Zoonotic, Vector-Borne, and Enteric Diseases. Retrieved from http://www.cdc.gov/nczved/divisions/dfbmd/diseases/candidiasis/

Centers for Disease Control (CDC). (2011). Understanding sexual violence: Fact sheet. Retrieved from http://www.cdc.gov/violenceprevention/pub/SV_factsheet.html

Davis, K. (2010). Pelvic floor dysfunction: Causes and assessment. *Practice Nursing, 21*(7), 340–346.

Dulay, A. (2010). Ectopic pregnancy. Merck Medicus Online Medical Library. Retrieved from http://www.merckmedicus.com/pp/us/hcp/framemm.jsp?pg=www.merck.com/mmpe/index.html

Eisenberg, E. (Reviewer). (2011). Polycystic ovary syndrome (PCOS). Womenshealth.gov. Retrieved from http://www.womenshealth.gov/faq/polycystic-ovary-syndrome.cfm#b

Eisenberg, E., & Brumbaugh, K. (Reviewers). (2011). Infertility: Frequently asked questions. Womenshealth.gov. Retrieved from. http://www.womenshealth.gov/faq/infertility.cfm#top

Ethics Committee of the American Society for Reproductive Medicine. (2009). American Society for Reproductive Medicine: Defining embryo donation. *Fertility and Sterility, 92*(6):1818–1819. doi:10.1016/j.fertnstert.2009.10.026

Ethics Committee of the American Society for Reproductive Medicine. (2009). Child-rearing ability and the provisions of fertility services. *Fertility and Sterility, 92*(3), 864–867. doi:10.1016/j.fertnstert.2009.07.978

Familydoctor.org Editorial Staff. (2011). Ending a pregnancy. FamilyDoctor.org. Retrieved from http://familydoctor.org/online/famdocen/home/articles/846.html

Fitzgerald, P. (2011). Endocrine disorders. In S. McPhee & M. Papadakis (Eds.), *2011 Current medical diagnosis and treatment* (50th ed., pp. 1050–1139). New York: McGraw Hill/Lange.

Greil, A., McQuillan, J., Benjamins, M., Johnson, D., Johnson, K., & Heinz, C. (2010). Specifying the effects of religion on medical help-seeking: The case of infertility. *Social Science & Medicine, 71*(2010), 734–742. doi:10.1016/j.socscimed.2010.04.033

Hasper, I., Ventskovskiy, B. M., Rettenberger, R., Heger, P. W., Riley, D. S., & Kaszkin-Bettag, M. (2009). Long-term efficacy and safety of the special extract ERr 731 of Rheum rhaponticum in perimenopausal women with menopausal symptoms. *Menopause, 16*(1), 117–131.

Htay, T., & Aung, K. (2011). Premenstrual dysphoric disorder. eMedicine. Retrieved from http://emedicine.medscape.com/article/293257-overview

IOM (Institute of Medicine). (2010). *The future of nursing: Leading change, advancing health.* Washington, DC: The Academic Press.

Jennings, V., & Arevalo, M. (2009). Fertility awareness-based methods. In R. Hatcher, J. Trussell, A. Nelson, W. Cates, F. Stewart, & D. Kowal (Eds.), *Contraceptive technology.* New York: Ardent Media.

Kaszkin-Bettag, M., Beck, S., Richardson, A., Heger, P. W., & Beer, A. M. (2008). Efficacy of the special extract ERr 731 from rhapontic rhubarb for menopausal complaints: A 6-month open observational study. *Alternative Therapies in Health and Medicine, 14*(6), 32–38.

Kaszkin-Bettag, M., Ventskovskiy, B. M., Kravchenko, A., Rettenberger, R., Richardson, A., Heger, P. W., et al. (2007). The special extract ERr 731 of the roots of Rheum rhaponticum decreases anxiety and improves health state and general well-being in perimenopausal women. *Menopause, 14*(2), 270–283.

Kee, J. (2010). *Laboratory and diagnostic tests with nursing implications* (8th ed.). Upper Saddle River, NJ: Pearson.

Kirsch, J., & Scoutt, J. (2010). Imaging of ectopic pregnancy. *Applied Radiology, 39*(3), 10-2, 14-7, 21-2.

Latendresse, G., McCance, K., & Morgan, K. (2010). Alterations of the reproductive systems. In K. McCance & S. Huether, *Pathophysiology: The biologic basis for disease in adults and children* (6th ed., pp. 781–815). St. Louis: Mosby/Elsevier.

Lazarou, G., & Grigorescu, B. (2010). Pelvic organ prolapse. eMedicine. Retrieved from http://emedicine.medscape.com/article/276259-overview

Lunny, C., & Fraser, S. (2010). The use of complementary and alternative medicines among a sample of Canadian menopausal-aged women. *Journal of Midwifery and Women's Health, 55*(4), 335–343. doi:10:1016/j.jmwh.2009.10.015

MacKay, H. (2011). Gynecologic disorders. In S. McPhee & M. Papadakis (Eds.), *2011 Current medical diagnosis and treatment* (50th ed., pp. 721–753). New York: McGraw Hill/Lange.

Mao, A., & Anastasi, J. (2010). Diagnosis and management of endometriosis: The role of the advanced practice nurse in primary care. *Journal of the American Academy of Nurse Practitioners, 22*(2010), 109–116. doi:10.1111/j.1745-7599.2009.00475.x

Mayo Clinic Staff. (2009). Uterine fibroids. MayoClinic.com. Retrieved from http://www.mayoclinic.com/health/uterine-fibroids/DS00078

Mayo Clinic Staff. (2011). Rectovaginal fistula. MayoClinic.com. Retrieved from http://www.mayoclinic.com/health/rectovaginal-fistula/DS01065

McCloskey, C. (2010). Updated office testing skills for vaginal infections. *The Nurse Practitioner, 35*(2), 46–52.

McLeod, B., & Retzloff, M. (2010). Epidemiology of endometriosis: An assessment of risk factors. *Clinical Obstetrics and Gynecology, 53*(2), 389–396.

MedicineNet.com. (2011). Vulvodynia: Causes, symptoms, and treatments. Women's Health Center. Retrieved from http://www.medicinenet.com/vaginal_pain_vulvodynia/article.htm

Molla, M. D., Hidalgo-Mora, J. J., & Soteras, M. G. (2011). Phytotherapy as alternative to hormone replacement therapy. *Frontiers in Bioscience* (School Edition), *3*, 191–204.

National Sexual Violence Resource Center (NSVRC). (2009). Protocols and guidelines for sexual assault response teams (SART). Retrieved from http://www.nsvrc.org/projects/sart/protocols-and-guidelines-sexual-assault-response-teams-sart

National Women's Health Information Center (NWHIC). (2011). Violence against women: Sexual assault and abuse. Retrieved from http://www.womenshealth.gov/violence/types/sexual.cfm

Nelson, A. (2009). Combined oral contraceptives. In R. Hatcher, J. Trussell, A. Nelson, W. Cates, F. Stewart, & D. Kowal (Eds.),

Contraceptive technology (19th ed., pp. 193–270). New York: Ardent.

Nelson, A., & Baldwin, S. (2009). Menstrual disorders and related concerns. In R. Hatcher, J. Trussell, A. Nelson, W. Cates, F. Stewart, & D. Kowal (Eds.), *Contraceptive technology*. New York: Ardent Media.

Nihira, M. (Reviewer). (2010). Your guide to premenstrual syndrome, or PMS. WebMD/Women's Health. Retrieved from http://women.webmd.com/guide/premenstrual-syndrome

Norton, P. (2010). Genetics and the lower urinary tract. *Neurology and Urodynamics, 29*(4), 609–611.

Office of Research on Women's Health. (2011). Annual NIH research priorities for women's health. Retrieved from http://orwh.od.nih.gov/research/priorities.html

Paradise, J. (2011). Evaluation of oligomenorrhea in adolescence. *UpToDate*. Retrieved from http://www.uptodate.com/contents/evaluation-of-oligomenorrhea-in-adolescence

Pinkerton, J. (2010). Dysmenorrhea. Merck Manuals Online Medical Library. Retrieved from http://www.merckmedicus.com/pp/us/hcp/framemm.jsp?pg=www.merck.com/mmpe/index.html

Quinn, E. (2010). Amenorrhea in female athletes. About.com/Sports Medicine. Retrieved from http://sportsmedicine.about.com/od/women/a/Amenorrhea.htm

Schraga, E., & Blanda, M. (2011). Ovarian torsion in emergency medicine. eMedicine. Retrieved from http://emedicine.medscape.com/article/795994-overview

Schwartz, B. (2011). Bacterial and chlamydial infections. In S. McPhee & M. Papadakis (Eds.), *2011 Current medical diagnosis and treatment* (50th ed., pp. 1357–1400). New York: McGraw Hill Medical.

Sepilian, V., & Wood, E. (2010). Ectopic pregnancy. eMedicine. Retrieved from http://emedicine.medscape.com/article/258768-overview

Society for Assisted Reproductive Technology (SART). (2011). All SART member clinics: Clinic summary report. SARTcors Online. Retrieved from https://www.sartcorsonline.com/rptCSR_PublicMultYear.aspx?ClinicPKID=0

Spurlock, J. (2011). Vesicovaginal fistula. eMedicine. Retreived from http://emedicine.medscape.com/article/267943-overview

Stoppler, M. (2010). Uterine fibroids. eMedicinehealth. Retrieved from http://www.emedicinehealth.com/uterine_fibroids/article_em.htm

Stoppler, M., & Shiel, W. (2010). Menstrual cramps (dysmenorrheal). MedicineNet.com. Retrieved from http://www.medicinenet.com/menstrual_cramps/article.htm

Trimble, E. (Reviewer). (2011). Hysterectomy. WomensHealth.gov. Retrieved from http://www.womenshealth.gov/faq/hysterectomy.cfm#f

University of California at San Francisco (UCSF) Medical Center Staff. (2011). Fallopian tube cancer. UCSF Medical Center. Retrieved from http://www.ucsfhealth.org/conditions/fallopian_tube_cancer/

Vernkataraman, R., & Sharma, S. (2011). Toxic shock syndrome: Treatment and medication. eMedicine. Retrieved from http://emedicine.medscape.com/article/169177-treatment

Ventolini, G., Barhan, S., & Duke, J. (2009). Vulvodynia, a step-wise therapeutic prospective cohort study. *Journal of Obstetrics and Gynaecology, 29*(7), 648–650. doi:10.1080/01443610903095882

Vivolo, A., Holland, K., Teten, A., Holt, M., and the Sexual Violence Review Team. (2010). Developing sexual violence prevention strategies by bridging spheres of public health. *Journal of Women's Health, 19*(10), 1811–1814. doi:10.1089/jwh.2010.2311

Vorvick, L. (Reviewer). (2011a). Fistula. MedlinePlus. Retrieved from http://www.nlm.nih.gov/medlineplus/ency/article/002365.htm

Vorvick, L. (Reviewer). (2011b). Miscarriage—threatened. MedlinePlus. Retrieved from http://www.nlm.nih.gov/medlineplus/ency/article/000907.htm

Vorvick, L., & Storck, S. (Reviewers). (2011a). Cervical polyps. Medline Plus. Retrieved from http://www.nlm.nih.gov/medlineplus/ency/article/001494.htm

Vorvick, L., & Storck, S. (Reviewers). (2011b). Miscarriage. MedlinePlus. Retrieved from http://www.nlm.nih.gov/medlineplus/ency/article/001488.htm

Workowski, K., & Berman, S. (2010). Sexually transmitted disease treatment guidelines, 2010. *Morbidity and Mortality Weekly Report, 59*(RR12), 1–110.

CHAPTER 42

Caring for the Patient with Male Reproductive Disorders

Patricia Caudle
Kathleen Osborn

Outcome-Based Learning Objectives

After studying this chapter, the learner will be able to:

1. Differentiate the most common male reproductive disorders.
2. Discuss the etiology, pathophysiology, clinical manifestations, and treatments of testicular, prostatic, and penile disorders.
3. Interpret diagnostic test results for male reproductive disorders.
4. Generate nursing management goals when caring for males with reproductive disorders.
5. Generate nursing diagnoses and apply the nursing process to the care of patients with testicular cancer and prostate cancer.
6. Plan interventions that will enhance health education, health promotion, and disease prevention specific for male health.

KEY TERMS

benign prostatic hyperplasia (BPH) p.1293
bioavailable testosterone p.1307
bladder diverticula p.1294
buccal p.1307
dysuria p.1287
epididymitis p.1286
erectile dysfunction (ED) p.1305
germ cell p.1291
gynecomastia p.1291
hydrocele p.1290
hydronephrosis p.1294
impotence p.1291
orchiectomy p.1289
orchiopexy p.1289
orchitis p.1287
paraphimosis p.1303
penectomy p.1305
Peyronie's disease p.1303
phimosis p.1300
priapism p.1305
prostatectomy p.1298
prostatitis p.1292
prostatodynia p.1293
retrograde ejaculation p.1295
spermatocele p.1290
spermatogenesis p.1305
stromal cell p.1291
suprapubic catheter p.1299
testicular torsion p.1289
thermoablation p.1295
ureaplasmal p.1286
vasectomy p.1307

MALE REPRODUCTIVE DISORDERS are often complex, as they involve both sexual functioning and the urinary system. Figure 42–1◆ portrays the normal anatomy of the male genitourinary system. Disorders of the reproductive system may also be a source of embarrassment for the male. Nursing care should include both the physical and emotional aspects associated with these disorders. This chapter will differentiate some of the major male reproductive disorders and will discuss both medical and nursing management.

Testicular Disorders

Testicular disorders may arise from inflammation, infection, trauma, or cancer. The most common disorders are discussed here, along with appropriate treatment modalities and nursing care. Health education and prevention are important aspects of nursing care covered in this section.

Epididymitis

Epididymitis is an infection or inflammation of the ductus epididymidis, a crescent-shaped structure found on the posterior aspect of each testicle (Latendresse, McCance, & Morgan, 2010). The epididymis functions in the transport of sperm from the testicle to the vas deferens (Deneris & Huether, 2010).

Etiology and Epidemiology

An infection of the epididymis may originate at the prostate, the urethra, or the urinary bladder and migrate via the urinary system to the vas deferens and the epididymis (see Figure 42–1). Epididymitis is most likely to occur among men ages 20 to 39 (Davis & Nettleman, 2011). Infection of the epididymis in men younger than age 35 is likely to be the result of gonococcal, chlamydial, or **ureaplasmal** (bacteria that is part of the genital flora) organisms. In older men, infection is more likely to

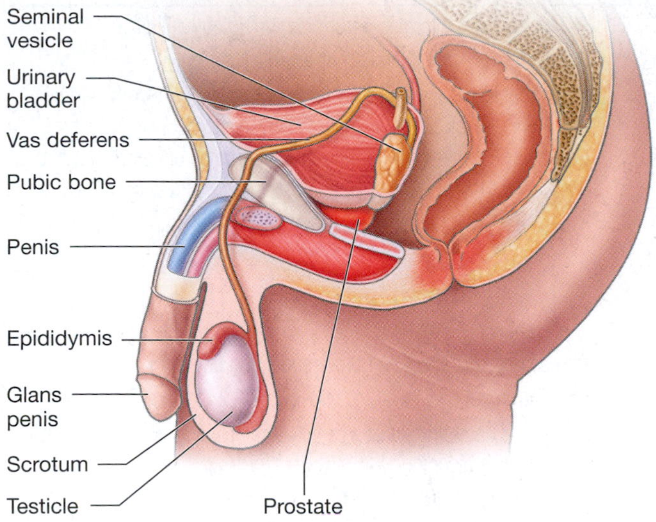

FIGURE 42–1 ◆ Normal anatomy of the male genitourinary system.

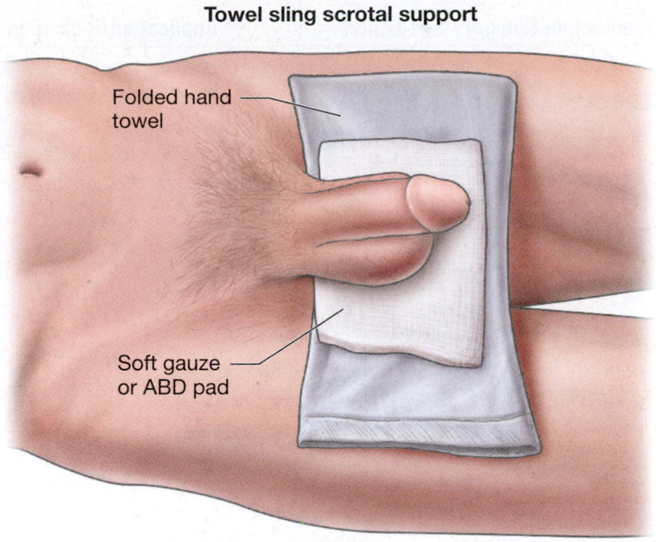

FIGURE 42–2 ◆ Scrotal supports.

be the result of prostatitis, instrumentation of the urinary system, or a structural lesion such as carcinoma of the testicle. In these cases, the coliform bacteria, especially *Escherichia coli*, are most frequently identified as causative (Trojian, Lishnak, & Heiman, 2009).

Clinical Manifestations

Symptoms of epididymitis include gradual onset of pain and swelling of the epididymis that may spread to the testicle, causing a large, tender scrotal mass (Trojian et al., 2009). When a sexually transmitted organism is the cause, **dysuria** (painful urination), penile discharge, fever, and pus in the urine or semen may be seen. Inguinal lymph nodes may be enlarged, especially on the side where the infection is located. The tests outlined in the Diagnostic Tests box can be used to determine a diagnosis of epididymitis.

Medical Management

Medical management of epididymitis includes antibiotics specific to the causative organism identified, analgesics, scrotal elevation, and cold packs (Trojian et al., 2009). See Chapter 12 for a discussion of pain assessment and management. The Pharmacology box presents medications used to treat male reproductive disorders.

Nursing Management

Nursing management for epididymitis includes encouraging the patient to maintain bed rest and elevating the scrotum with a towel sling. Elevation and the application of cold to the scrotum will help decrease swelling and pain. Figure 42–2◆ depicts one form of towel sling. Ambulation requires a soft scrotal support that keeps the scrotum close to the body. Patients need education about epididymitis, including possible complications such as sepsis, abscess, and infertility (Trojian et al., 2009). They also need to know about the medications prescribed, potential side effects, and how to avoid recurrence of the infection.

Orchitis

Etiology, Epidemiology, and Pathophysiology

Orchitis is an inflammation or infection of one or both testes. Infection may be caused by bacterial or viral agents. As with epididymitis, the usual causative bacteria include gonorrhea, chlamydia, and *Escherichia coli*. One form of orchitis with a viral cause is mumps orchitis, which may be seen 7 to 10 days after mumps parotitis in 25% to 40% of men who are affected with mumps (Shandera & Corrales-Medina, 2008). Mumps orchitis usually is unilateral (i.e., affecting only one testis) and

DIAGNOSTIC TESTS for Epididymitis

Test and Normal Values	Expected Abnormality
Urinalysis (first void)	
Normally will not have any white blood cells or bacteria	Elevated white count due to inflammatory/infectious process.
Cultures of Any Discharge	
Normally will be negative for bacteria *Sexually transmitted infections and coliforms may cause epididymitis.*	May be positive for chlamydia, gonorrhea, *Escherichia coli*, and so on.
White Blood Cells (WBC)	
Normal = 4,500–10,000/mm^3	Elevated white count. Shifts indicating acute infection and/or inflammation.

Sources: Adapted from Trojian, T., Lishnak, T., & Heiman, D. (2009). Epididymitis and orchitis: An overview. *American Family Physician, 79*(7), 583–587; Kee, J. (2010). *Laboratory and diagnostic tests* (8th ed.). Upper Saddle River, NJ: Pearson.

PHARMACOLOGY Summary of Medications Used to Treat Male Reproductive Disorders

Medication Category and Action	Application/Indication	Nursing Responsibility
Antibiotics Macrolides (Biaxin) Penicillin (Pen-Vee K) Fluoroquinolones (Cipro) Trimethoprim-sulfamethoxazole (Bactrim) Doxycycline (Doryx) ***Action:*** Varies with antibiotic; may be bactericidal or bacteriostatic. Specific type used depends on the causative agent and the drug's sensitivity to it.	Used for infections of susceptible organisms including sexually transmitted infections, epididymitis, orchitis, prostatitis, coliforms, and any postoperative infections.	Assess for drug allergies before beginning any antibiotic. Assess for any manifestation of allergic reaction. Assess for improvement of symptoms, especially decreased fever and pain. Educate the patient concerning the importance of completing the full course of antibiotics.
Nonsteroidal anti-inflammatory drugs (NSAIDs) Ibuprofen (Advil) Naproxen sodium (Aleve) ***Action:*** Prostaglandin synthetase inhibition.	Used for fever reduction, for pain relief, and for decreasing inflammation.	Assess for drug allergies before beginning any drug. Give with food. Assess for gastrointestinal side effects, including ulcer and gastrointestinal (GI) bleeding. Assess for relief of symptoms.
Chemotherapy Cisplatin (Platinol-AQ) Bleomycin (Blenoxane) Etoposide (VePesid) Docetaxel (Taxotere) ***Action:*** Alkylates DNA, RNA; inhibits enzymes that allow synthesis of amino acids in proteins; activity is not cell cycle phase specific. Miotic inhibitor.	Used for testicular cancer tumor eradication.	Assess for drug allergies. Prepare for anaphylactic reaction with first dose. Monitor renal and liver function tests for abnormalities related to chemotherapy side effects. Side effects of cisplatin include nausea, vomiting, alopecia, fatigue, azoospermia, peripheral neuropathy, ototoxicity, and nephrotoxicity. Bleomycin may cause pulmonary fibrosis, pneumonitis, and lung toxicity. Etoposide may cause hepatotoxicity and bone marrow toxicity. Taxotere may cause bone marrow suppression and neutropenia, severe fluid retention, and neurologic toxicity.
Antiemetics and Antidiarrheals (especially for side effects of chemotherapy): Ondansetron (Zofran) ***Action:*** Ondansetron blocks serotonic 5-HT3 receptor, decreasing nausea. Antidiarrheals work directly at intestinal muscle to decrease peristalsis or increase bulk.	Side effects of chemotherapy include vomiting and diarrhea. Ondansetron (Zofran) has been especially efficacious for this type of nausea.	Assess for drug allergies. Assess for untoward effects such as headache and dizziness. Assess for relief of symptoms.
Benign Prostatic Hyperplasia		
Alpha blockers: Doxazosin (Cardura) Terazosin (Hytrin) Tamsulosin (Flomax) Alfuzosin (Uroxatral) ***Action:*** Alpha blockers work by relaxing the bladder neck and prostatic smooth muscle tone.	Improves urinary flow; relieves hesitancy, urgency, and frequency.	Assess for drug allergies. Monitor blood pressure and heart rate. Assess for side effects such as dizziness, headache, and nausea. Observe for improvement of symptoms. Warn patients to limit Viagra and other ED medications to 25 milligrams at least 4 hours before or after using alpha blockers.
5-Alpha reductase inhibitors: Finasteride (Proscar) Dutasteride (Avodart) ***Action:*** Blocks the conversion of testosterone to androgen, thereby decreasing the size of the prostate.	Blocks conversion of testosterone to potent androgen, thereby reducing the size and growth of the prostate. It is more efficacious for men with larger prostates.	Assess for allergies before administering. Monitor for side effects such as decreased libido, ejaculatory problems, and lower prostate-specific antigen (PSA) levels.
Antimuscarinics Tolterodine (Detrol LA) Oxybutynin (Ditropan) ***Action:*** Relaxes smooth muscle in urinary tract. Exerts analgesic, anesthetic action on the urinary mucosa.	Radiation cystitis: helps relieve frequency and urgency. Relieves discomfort of bladder irritation.	Assess for allergies to any drugs. Monitor for side effects. Assess for relief of symptoms. Encourage diet low in irritants such as coffee, spicy foods, and alcohol. Encourage diet high in fluid intake and roughage to keep stool soft and movements regular.

PHARMACOLOGY Summary of Medications Used to Treat Male Reproductive Disorders, *continued*

Medication Category and Action	Application/Indication	Nursing Responsibility
Phenazopyridine (Baridium) Trypsin, castor oil, and balsam of Peru (Xenaderm) ***Action:*** Antispasmodic. Skin protectant.	For relief of proctitis (inflammation of the anus and rectum). Skin irritation due to radiation. Soothes and promotes healing.	
Hormone Replacement Therapy Testosterone (formulations: IM, Male sex hormone pellets, transdermal patches or gel, buccal tablets) Diethylstilbesterol (DES) Leuprolide (Lupron) (Lupron®) (Lupron Depot®)? ***Action:*** Antiandrogen. Luteinizing hormone-releasing hormone agonist.	Reduces side effects of testosterone deficiency. Slows or stops prostate cancer growth by lowering androgen levels to those of castration.	Potential for interaction with other drugs or herbals. Review with patient what he is taking. May increase fluid retention. Pregnancy Risk Factor X: use barrier contraceptive (see Chapter 41 for Pregnancy Risk Factor Categories). Monitor for side effects: feminization and loss of libido. Erectile dysfunction. Explain side effects. Help the patient find ways to cope. Monitor for side effects such as hot flashes, erectile dysfunction, and loss of libido.

Sources: Adapted from Adams, M., & Koch, R. (2010). *Pharmacology: Connections to nursing practice.* Upper Saddle River, NJ: Pearson; Lexi-Comp. (2010). Testosterone. *Merck Manuals Online Library.* Retrieved from http://www.merck.com/mmpe/lexicomp/testosterone.html#N1B826F.

may cause infertility. Men who have never had mumps and are exposed to the mumps virus require treatment.

Safety Alert *Men exposed to the mumps virus who have never had mumps should receive gamma globulin immediately to aid in decreasing the severity of the disease and preserving fertility.*

Clinical Manifestations

Symptoms and diagnostic testing for orchitis are the same as those for epididymitis. It is important to be aware that the symptoms of orchitis closely resemble those of testicular torsion, a surgical emergency described in the next section of this chapter.

Medical Management

Medical treatment for orchitis includes the use of antibiotics when appropriate, analgesics, and nonsteroidal anti-inflammatory drugs (NSAIDs) (see the Pharmacology box). Viral causes are treated with rest, fluids, and NSAIDs.

Nursing Management

Nursing management includes minimizing activity, elevation of the scrotum using a towel sling or soft support (see Figure 42–2, p. 1287), and cold compresses to decrease edema and pain. The goal of treatment is to prevent testicular atrophy, infertility, abscess, and impotence. Emotional support is important because of the reproductive and sexual activity concerns. In cases in which antibiotics are needed, teaching should stress the importance of completing the full course of medication prescribed.

Testicular Torsion

Epidemiology, Etiology, and Pathophysiology

Testicular torsion occurs when a mobile testicle causes a twisting of the spermatic cord, essentially closing off the blood supply to the testicle. Loss of blood supply to the testicle will cause ischemia, necrosis, and loss of the testicle if it is not relieved within 6 to 12 hours (Polt, 2009; Schmitz & Safranek, 2009).

Safety Alert *Sudden onset of scrotal/testicular pain without injury in an adolescent should be considered testicular torsion until proven otherwise. Surgical intervention to preserve the testicle should occur within 6 to 12 hours of occurrence.*

Annually, 1 in 4,000 males under the age of 25 experience testicular torsion (Wampler & Llanes, 2010). The process for the development of this problem begins with the congenital absence of attachment of the testicle to the tunica vaginalis. Without this attachment, the testicle hangs freely and can easily twist on the cord. The left testicle is more at risk because of the longer spermatic cord.

Clinical Manifestations

Clinical manifestations of testicular torsion include sudden, severe pain in one testicle, nausea, vomiting, and light-headedness. On examination, the testicle will be high in the scrotum due to the shortening of the spermatic cord. Figure 42–3 ◆ depicts the twisting and shortening of the spermatic cord. The affected testicle may also feel larger than normal, and the cremasteric reflex (the testicle rises in the scrotum when the thigh near the scrotum is stroked) will be absent (Schmitz & Safranek, 2009). Diagnosis is confirmed with Doppler ultrasound.

Medical Management

Medical treatment for testicular torsion is immediate surgery. The testicle and cord are untwisted; if the testicle is viable, it is anchored to the scrotum (**orchiopexy**) to prevent recurrence. If the testicle is nonviable, then it is removed (**orchiectomy**) (Polt, 2009). The patient will require analgesia before and after surgery. See Chapter 12 for a discussion of pain assessment and management.

Nursing Management

Nursing care of boys and men experiencing testicular torsion usually begins in the postoperative period and includes providing bed rest, observing for bleeding or drainage on the dressing, monitoring vital signs, administering analgesics, and providing scrotal support. The towel sling (see Figure 42–2) can be used while the patient is in bed. Ambulation will require a soft scrotal support that keeps the scrotum close to the

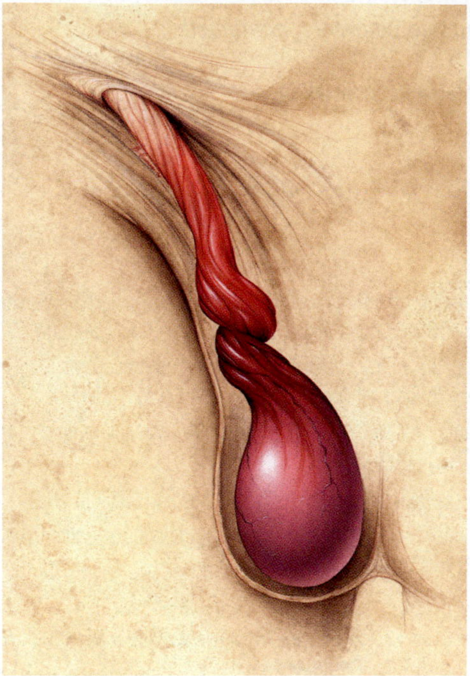

FIGURE 42–3 ◆ Testicular torsion.
Source: Brian Evans/Photo Researchers, Inc.

body. Education of the patient and his parents would include information about the analgesic action and side effects and the importance of follow-up visits with the urologist or surgeon. When orchiectomy is performed in a boy, a testicular prosthesis can be implanted, if desired, when he reaches ages 14 to 16 (Polt, 2009). This would also be an option for older men who have lost a testicle.

Hydrocele

Epidemiology, Etiology, and Pathophysiology

The space between the layers of the tunica vaginalis of the scrotum may fill with fluid, causing a **hydrocele** (Ferri & Wachtel, 2010). A hydrocele may fill with fluid from the peritoneum (communicating) or may be local (noncommunicating). In newborn males, a hydrocele develops when fluid that surrounds the testicles does not absorb after the closure of the tunica vaginalis *in utero*. In older males, hydrocele may develop after infection in the scrotum, injury, radiation, or testicular cancer. There are also incidences of idiopathic hydrocele among elderly males (Latendresse et al., 2010).

Clinical Manifestations

Clinical manifestations include scrotal swelling that transluminates (light source behind the swollen scrotum will cause a glow as the light penetrates the fluid). The swelling is not painful unless there is so much fluid that it causes increased pressure on the testes (Wampler & Llanes, 2010).

Medical Management

Medical management is usually conservative, as the fluid will be reabsorbed in time. Should the swelling increase to painful levels, the fluid can be aspirated or surgically drained to prevent damage to the testes. Surgical removal of the hydrocele may be followed by injection of a sclerosing agent to prevent recurrence (Latendresse et al., 2010).

Nursing Management

Nursing care depends on the extent of the hydrocele. For newborns with hydrocele, the care is the same as that for all newborns. For adults, elevation of the scrotum may help. If surgery is required, postoperative care is similar to the postoperative care for testicular torsion.

Spermatocele

Etiology, Epidemiology, and Pathophysiology

Spermatoceles are painless, sperm-containing cysts that occur on the upper portion of the testis near the epididymis. These cysts are thought to be caused by an occlusion of the efferent (outflow) spermatic ducts of the testis. Usually only one testis is affected, and the cyst is typically 1 centimeter or less in diameter (Wampler & Llanes, 2010).

Clinical Manifestations

While most spermatoceles go unnoticed, some become large enough to annoy the male. Others may be found coincidentally. On physical examination, the cyst is palpable and transluminates. Translumination helps differentiate this fluid-filled cyst from a solid nodule that is more likely to be testicular cancer. Diagnosis is verified by ultrasound (Wampler & Llanes, 2010).

Medical Management

Medical management for those rare spermatoceles that grow large enough to disfigure or cause pain is inguinoscrotal surgery to remove the mass. Wampler and Llanes (2010) explain that patients should be warned that there is a potential for infertility or chronic pain related to this surgery.

Varicocele

Epidemiology, Etiology, and Pathophysiology

A varicocele is an enlargement of the veins of the pampiniform plexus within the scrotum. It develops because of incompetent venous valves, just like varicose veins in the legs. (See Chapter 35 for more information about varicose veins.) Varicoceles are most likely to occur on the left because the left spermatic vein empties into the renal vein at a 90 degree angle, causing increased hydrostatic back pressure within the vein when the patient stands. Approximately 10% to 15% of males who have varicoceles also have fertility problems (Nowak & Patacsil-Trull, 2010). The cause is unknown, and there are no specific risk factors.

Clinical Manifestations

Signs and symptoms of varicocele include a "bag of worms" appearance to the scrotum that decreases in size when the patient is recumbent. The varicocele is usually not painful, but some men will notice a dull ache and fullness or pulling to the affected side of the scrotum after prolonged standing (Nowak & Patacsil-Trull, 2010).

Medical Management

Medical management is not necessary unless there are symptoms or infertility. Surgical treatment may be used to seal the affected vein and redirect blood flow to a normal vein if the varicocele is painful or the testicle is beginning to atrophy. Surgery to correct varicocele has improved semen quality and fertility. In fact, 40% to 60% of men who undergo varicocelectomy will have increased conception rates (White & Kim, 2011). In addition, the affected testicle will grow to match the size of the unaffected testicle once blood flow is improved (Nowak & Patacsil-Trull, 2010).

Testicular Cancer

Etiology and Epidemiology

Cancer that forms in the tissue of the testis usually occurs in men between the ages of 20 and 39. In fact, it is the most common form of cancer in Caucasian men between the ages of 15 and 34 (National Cancer Institute [NCI], 2010a). It was estimated that testicular cancer would occur in 8,480 men in the United States in 2010. Of these, approximately 350 will die of the disease (NCI, 2010d). Overall, the rate of occurrence has doubled in the last 40 years. Men of Scandinavian descent are at greatest risk, but other risk factors include familial history (especially siblings), prior personal history, cryptorchidism, smoking, Klinefelter's syndrome, natural exposure to gestational estrogen, and exposure to insecticides (NCI, 2010a; Wampler & Llanes, 2010).

There is currently no evidence that screening asymptomatic men can lead to early detection of testicular cancer (Ilic, Misso, & Wilt, 2009). Since this form of cancer affects very few men and there is a high cure rate, resources are best used to diagnose men suspected of having the disease.

Pathophysiology

Testicular cancer may arise from a **germ cell** (cell that produces sperm) of the testicle or from a **stromal cell** (cells of supportive or hormone-producing tissues). Germinal tumors account for 95% of testicular tumors and are generally divided into two groups: seminomas, which are slow growing, and nonseminomas, which are more aggressive. Nonseminomas have four subtypes: embryonal, yolk sac, choriocarcinoma, and teratoma (Latendresse et al., 2010). Teratoma subtypes are the least likely to metastasize, whereas choriocarcinomas are the most likely to metastasize (NCI, 2010c).

Clinical Manifestations

Most men who have testicular cancer will present with testicular swelling; scrotal heaviness; testicular pain; or a solid, painless, nontransluminating lump on the testicle. Some will have symptoms similar to those of epididymitis or orchitis. In fact, many testicular cancers are first diagnosed as epididymitis or orchitis and treated with antibiotics. When the lump does not resolve, further studies reveal the malignancy. Testicular tumors have also been found coincident to sports injuries to the groin or genitals. A small number of men may first seek medical advice because of **gynecomastia** (enlargement of the male breast) caused by testicular tumors that secrete beta human chorionic gonadotropin (HCG) (Wampler & Llanes, 2010). A few testicular cancers are not discovered until metastatic disease has occurred. Symptoms of metastatic disease secondary to testicular cancer may include back pain, chest pain, hemoptysis (vomiting blood), and weight loss. Chapter 57 has an in-depth discussion of the diagnosis and treatment of cancer.

Diagnostic Testing and Staging

The first line of diagnostic testing for testicular cancer after a lump is found is ultrasonography of the scrotum. Ultrasound is excellent for differentiating cancer from epididymitis, spermatocele, or hydrocele (Winter, 2009). Once the tumor is identified, a unilateral radical orchiectomy is performed after serum markers have been obtained. Serum markers such as human chorionic gonadotropin (hCG), alpha-fetoprotein (AFP), and lactate dehydrogenase are obtained in order to stage the cancer. When the pathology report confirms cancer, a careful search for any metastasis is done using a computed tomographic (CT) scan of the chest, abdomen, and pelvis (Wampler & Llanes, 2010). Fine needle biopsy or open biopsy is never done because of the danger of seeding the scrotum with the cancer cells and causing a more rapid dissemination of the cancer to the abdomen and lungs (NCI, 2010d).

Medical Management

Medical management decisions for testicular cancer depend on the type of tumor, the stage of the disease, and tumor markers. Seminomatous testicular tumors, Stages I and II, are treated by orchiectomy via an inguinal route and retroperitoneal node irradiation (NCI, 2010d). This combination will result in 100% cure rates. Side effects of radiation therapy include fatigue, skin changes, loss of appetite, nausea, diarrhea, and reduced sperm production. Sperm production from the remaining testicle does recover, but recovery will take 1 to 2 years after radiation. Seminomatous tumors at Stage III may be treated pre- and postorchiectomy with cisplatin-based chemotherapy that results in high cure rates (Harrison's, 2010). See the Pharmacology box (p. 1288).

Nonseminomatous testicular tumors in Stage I require inguinal orchiectomy of the affected testicle. If the cancer is limited to the testicle, then surveillance using periodic chest x-ray, physical examination, CT of the abdomen, and tumor marker studies is done. The cure rate for surgery under these conditions is about 95% (Harrison's Practice, 2010). Stage II of the nonseminomatous tumors requires chemotherapy. Cisplatin-based multiple-agent chemotherapy is highly effective, even in patients with metastatic disease. This newest chemotherapy for testicular cancers has decreased the need for wide lymphadenectomy (removal of lymph nodes), and cure is possible in 98% of patients (Harrison's, 2010). For Stage III, chemotherapy and postchemotherapy surgery are used to remove residual metastases. Cure rate depends on the extent of the metastases (Harrison's, 2010).

Follow-up medical surveillance is very important. For the first year, the patient is seen monthly. He is evaluated every other month in years 2 and 3, every 3 months in the third year, and every 6 months in the fourth and fifth years. The majority of recurrences will occur within the first 2 years, but relapse can occur even beyond that time. Examinations should include physical examination, tumor marker studies, chest x-ray, and CT scans of the abdomen and pelvis (NCI, 2010d).

Prognosis is generally favorable. About 95% of men with Stage I testicular cancer are cured. Stage II has a 5-year survival rate of 91% to 96%. Stage III has a 10-year survival rate of 66% to 94%, depending on the extent of the disease (Harrison's, 2010).

Nursing Management

Nursing care for men newly diagnosed with testicular cancer requires a high degree of emotional support. The men experiencing this cancer face altered sexuality, body image, role function, and fertility. They often fear loss of masculinity and must come face to face with their own mortality. Reassurance that orchiectomy does not cause **impotence** (problems associated with ejaculation or orgasm, in addition to erectile dysfunction) or infertility and that masculinity will remain intact is important. Open discussion of sexuality and the genitalia will allow the patient to express his worries without embarrassment. Review of the surgical procedure, the treatment planned, and the cure rates of these treatments will also help to alleviate fear. The nurse should keep communications with the patient clear, concrete, and open.

Preoperative teaching and preparation of the patient with testicular cancer is similar to preparation of all patients who undergo abdominal surgery. See Chapter 17 for a review of preoperative teaching and preparation. This is a very stressful time, so education will need to be repeated and reinforced.

Postoperatively, emotional support is needed. Anxiety and fear may require that the nurse continue to repeat information. If the surgery includes extensive retroperitoneal lymph node removal, the patient may be in the hospital for about a week. During the recovery time, routine care includes controlling pain, maintaining fluids, monitoring the incision for bleeding or infection, pulmonary toileting, and monitoring vital signs for elevated temperature or shortness of breath. (See Chapter 19 for postoperative care and Chapter 12 for pain assessment and management.) All postoperative patients are at increased risk for deep venous thrombosis and should begin to ambulate on the first day. Pain management before ambulation will ease the discomfort and help the patient to be more willing to move.

Patients who have seminomas will begin radiation therapy before discharge. Radiation therapy will involve the retroperitoneal area and will require education for the patient about what to expect. Side effects of irradiation include nausea, vomiting, diarrhea, fatigue, skin changes, and loss of appetite. An antidiarrheal and an antiemetic will be needed. Cisplatin-based multiagent chemotherapy will begin for patients with nonseminomas or cancers that have spread outside the testicle. Chemotherapy offers systemic therapy, reaching cancer cells anywhere in the body. Common side effects are nausea, hair loss, fatigue, diarrhea, vomiting, fever, chills, cough, mouth sores, and skin rash. Other, less common side effects include numbness, loss of reflexes, impaired hearing, and decreased to absent sperm production (Adams & Koch, 2010; NCI, 2010d). Nursing care will include emotional support, assistance with oral hygiene, antidiarrheal and antiemetic medications such as Zofran (ondansetron), and skin care. See the Pharmacology box (p. 1288).

Discharge priorities for the patient with testicular cancer are delineated in the Patient Teaching & Discharge Priorities box.

Prostate Disorders

The prostate gland is located under the urinary bladder at the bladder neck and in front of the rectum in men (see Figure 42–1, p. 1287). It is made up primarily of smooth muscle and collagen enclosed in a fibrous capsule. The urethra passes through the prostate. When semen moves through the prostatic portion of the urethra, the prostate secretes prostatic fluid that increases the pH of semen to help sperm survive in the more acidic female reproductive system (Deneris & Huether, 2010). Disorders of the prostate include inflammation, infection, hyperplasia, and cancer. This section discusses each of these disorders.

Prostatitis

Etiology and Epidemiology

Inflammation of the prostate gland (**prostatitis**) may be acute, chronic, infectious, or noninfectious. Chronic nonbacterial prostatitis is the most common of the prostatitis syndromes (Meng, Stoller, & Walsh, 2010). Prostatitis is one of the most common ailments seen in urology clinics; almost 2 million men are treated for it each year (Hedayati & Stehman, 2011). The National Institutes of Health has developed a consensus classification system for prostatitis, which is outlined in the National Guidelines box.

Pathophysiology

Acute prostatitis may arise from ascending urinary infection, rectal infection, or bloodborne pathogens. Gram-negative coliforms are the usual causative bacteria, especially *Escherichia coli, pseudomonas.* Less commonly, gram-positive organisms such asenterococci may be cultured from prostatic fluid (Meng et al., 2010).

Men who have chronic bacterial prostatitis may or may not have had an acute infection of the prostate before the onset of symptoms.

PATIENT TEACHING & DISCHARGE PRIORITIES for Testicular Cancer

Need	Teaching
Knowledge of disease process and prognosis	Home care needs include verbal and written instructions for: 1. The treatment plan, including continued radiation therapy or chemotherapy appointments 2. Follow-up care and appointments with the health care provider 3. Activity restriction.
Understanding of medications	If chemotherapy is to continue, patient/family is taught how to care for the infusion site using aseptic technique. Teach the purpose, dose, timing, and possible side effects of all medications.
Reportable clinical manifestations	Instruct the patient/family to report: 1. Bleeding or drainage at the incision site 2. Fever 101°F 3. Signs of deep venous thrombosis 4. Signs of pulmonary embolism or other lung problems.
Patient/family support system	Assess the availability of, knowledge of, and compliance with the treatment regimen. Assess the home environment for need for assistive devices. Assess for the need for professional home health services. Offer cancer support resources.
Emotional adjustment of the patient/family due to diagnosis of cancer	Answer questions honestly. Encourage verbalization of frustration and anger. Discuss adjustments that will need to be made at home.

NATIONAL GUIDELINES for the Classification of Prostatitis

I. Acute bacterial prostatitis
II. Chronic bacterial prostatitis
III. Chronic prostatitis/chronic pelvic pain syndrome
  A. Inflammatory
  B. Noninflammatory
IV. Asymptomatic inflammatory prostatitis (discovered incidentally)

Source: Adapted from NIH Consensus Classification System for Prostatitis in Sharp, V., Takacs, E., & Powell, C. (2010). Prostatitis: Diagnosis and treatment. *American Family Physician, 82*(4), 397–406.

Occasionally, the syndrome will be preceded by symptoms of a urinary tract infection. The organisms associated with chronic prostatitis, when they are found, are the same as those for acute prostatitis (Meng et al., 2010). Several other causes have been theorized, including increased levels of purine, uric acid, or pyrimidine that may have entered the prostatic ducts, causing inflammation. Some researchers believe it may be an autoimmune disorder (Meng et al., 2010; Ramakrishnan & Salinas, 2010).

Clinical Manifestations

The clinical presentation of prostatitis differs depending on the type the patient has contracted. Chart 42–1 summarizes the symptoms according to prostatitis type.

Laboratory and Diagnostic Procedures

Patients with acute prostatitis are very ill and can usually be diagnosed based on history and physical examination, including a gentle digital rectal examination (DRE) of the prostate. Chapter 40 describes the rectal examination more fully. The DRE, if too vigorous, has the potential for disseminating bacteria and causing sepsis. Urinalysis, urine culture, and complete blood cell count (CBC) are obtained to verify the diagnosis and guide the choice of antibiotic treatment (Sharp, Takacs, & Powell, 2010).

For chronic prostatitis, the diagnosis is based on a more involved urinalysis, such as the 2-glass (pre- and postprostatic massage urines) or the Meares and Stamey 4-glass. The 4-glass test is used to localize infection and includes collection and culture of the first voided urine, midstream urine, urine after prostate massage, and expressed prostatic fluids (Ramakrishnan & Salinas, 2010). Semen cultures may also be done. Blood tests will include CBC, C-reactive protein, and erythrocyte sedimentation rate. For older men, urine cytology is also recommended (Sharp et al., 2010).

Diagnosis of chronic prostatitis/chronic pelvic pain syndrome is usually done by excluding other possible causes of the patient's symptoms such as benign prostatic hyperplasia or bladder cancer. This can be done with urine cytology, post-void residual urine tests, transrectal ultrasound guided biopsy, cystoscopy (examination of the urethra and bladder via a fiber-optic scope), and semen analysis and culture (Ramakrishnan & Salinas, 2010; Sharp et al., 2010).

CHART 42–1 Clinical Manifestations of Acute and Chronic Prostatitis

Acute Prostatitis	Chronic Prostatitis
Flulike symptoms: fever, chills, myalgia, malaise; possible signs of sepsis	Recurrent episodes of infection
Pain in genitalia, pelvis, or low back	Symptoms same but milder
Dysuria, nocturia, urgency, frequency	Nonbacterial **prostatodynia** (chronic painful inflammation of the prostate)
Hematuria	Pain in pelvis
Painful ejaculation	Painful ejaculation
Tender, boggy, enlarged prostate	Tender, boggy, enlarged prostate

Source: Ramakrishnan, K., & Salinas, R. (2010). Prostatitis: Acute and chronic. *Primary Care Clinical Office Practice, 37*(3), 547–563. doi:10.1016/j.pop.2010.04.007

Medical Management

Medical management decisions depend on the type of prostatitis the patient has and the infective agent identified. Bacterial prostatitis is treated with appropriate antibiotics. The Pharmacology box (p. 1288) provides more details about antibiotic treatment and other drugs used in prostatitis. Antibiotics for patients with acute prostatitis are given orally for a period of 4 to 6 weeks in an attempt to cure the infection and prevent chronic prostatitis. If the patient becomes septic or develops a prostatic abscess, he may be admitted for care and be given intravenous (IV) antibiotic therapy until he is afebrile for 24 to 48 hours (Ramakrishnan & Salinas, 2010; Sharp et al., 2010). When the patient is discharged, oral therapy will continue for 4 to 6 weeks.

Some health care providers will prescribe other drugs such as alpha blockers (doxazosin, tamsulosin, terazosin) to relieve bladder spasm and improve cure rates when combined with antibiotics or NSAIDs and muscle relaxants to relieve pain and pelvic muscle spasms until the antibiotic can eradicate the infection (Ramakrishnan & Salinas, 2010). Symptomatic treatments may include sitz baths, prostate massage, acupuncture pelvic floor exercises, and microwave therapy. Microwave therapy is a transurethral heat treatment used often in benign prostatic hyperplasia, which is discussed later in this chapter.

Nursing Management

Nursing care for patients with prostatitis includes education about the disease, the medications used, and the treatments to help decrease pain and swelling of the prostate. If the patient is admitted for sepsis related to prostatitis, IV antibiotic therapy will be given. This will require education of the patient regarding the medication and its side effects and close monitoring of the patient for signs of worsening condition. The nurse will also help with sitz baths and other comfort measures. When the patient is discharged, he and his family will need education about the disease, the medications, the need to continue the antibiotic for 4 to 6 weeks as prescribed and why, and the importance of follow-up visits with the health care provider. The Patient Teaching & Discharge Priorities box lists some teaching points important for the patient with prostatitis.

Benign Prostatic Hyperplasia

Benign prostatic hyperplasia (BPH) is nonmalignant, nodular growth of prostatic tissue that eventually compresses the urethra, causing lower urinary tract symptoms (LUTS) (see Chart 42–2 for these symptoms) (Nash, 2010; Paolone, 2010). Benign prostatic hyperplasia is a common disorder of aging men, occurring in as many as 90% of men ages 85 and older (Latendresse et al., 2010; Paolone, 2010).

Etiology and Epidemiology

The exact cause of BPH is not known. One theory is that a growth factor imbalance occurs that causes an increase in epithelial cell growth and a decrease in cell death that leads to both epithelial cell and stromal

Weblink: Prosate Enlargement

PATIENT TEACHING & DISCHARGE PRIORITIES for Prostatitis

Need	Teaching
Patient/family/support system	Continue antibiotics as prescribed.
Patient/family/support system	Report continuation or worsening of symptoms to health care provider.
Patient	Regular voiding and complete emptying of bladder.
Patient	Increase fluids, such as water, to 64 to 128 ounces per day to flush the bladder.
Patient	Avoid beverages and foods that are irritating to the bladder: • Alcohol • Caffeine • Citrus juices • Hot/spicy foods.

hyperplasia (Nash, 2010). This imbalance is thought to be due to aging and changes in circulating androgens (Latendresse et al., 2010).

Pathophysiology

Nodules form at the transition zone, or innermost aspect of the prostate gland, along the urethra in response to the change in hormones (Nash, 2010). Because the prostate is expandable and elastic, urethral constriction may not occur until the prostate is significantly enlarged. Also, neuronal control over prostatic smooth muscle differs among men, making LUTS unpredictable (Paolone, 2010).

As the urinary urethra constricts, it causes increased pressure to urinate, thereby causing bladder distention, eventual hypertrophy of the detrusor muscle, **bladder diverticula** (outpouching areas of bladder wall due to increased urinary pressure), urinary stasis, infection, and bladder stone formation. If the obstruction is prolonged, **hydronephrosis** (backflow of urine into the renal pelvis) will occur and cause damage to the kidneys (Latendresse et al., 2010).

Clinical Manifestations

Clinical manifestations of BPH are varied. Some men who have BPH do not develop LUTS or acute urinary retention (O'Leary, 2009). Others will present with obstructive or irritative symptoms that significantly affect their quality of life. Chart 42–2 lists the signs and symptoms of BPH. The American Urological Association (AUA) has developed a symptom index tool that can be used to quantify the symptoms of BPH. Used both in diagnosing and for monitoring therapeutic response, the AUA Symptom Score is a seven-question exploration of symptoms that the patient can answer while waiting to be seen. The score allows the health care provider to match treatment options with the severity of the symptoms for each patient (Neal & Keister, 2009; Paolone, 2010).

Laboratory and Diagnostic Procedures

Diagnostic testing for BPH begins with the AUA Symptom Index. The next step is the history and physical examination, including evaluation for other medical conditions that may cause the symptoms and a digital rectal exam (DRE) of the prostate gland. Other tests that may be used include urinalysis, serum blood urea nitrogen and creatinine, postvoid residual urine measurement, and uroflow rate studies that assess voiding patterns. If hematuria, urinary tract infection, or signs of renal failure are discovered, then renal imaging, urine cytology studies, and cystoscopy need to be done. The prostate-specific antigen (PSA) is sometimes used to differentiate BPH from prostate cancer (Paolone, 2010). The PSA is described more fully in the section on cancer of the prostate, which appears later in this chapter.

CHART 42–2 Clinical Manifestations of Benign Prostate Hypertrophy

- Urinary hesitancy and intermittency
- Weak urine stream
- Nocturia, frequency, and urgency
- Sensation of incomplete bladder emptying
- Terminal dribbling of urine
- Overflow incontinence
- Complete urinary retention
- Hematuria if straining at urination is severe
- Enlarged, rubbery prostate that has lost the median furrow
- Full urinary bladder palpable on abdominal examination
- Urinary tract infection
- Bladder stones and diverticuli
- Renal damage, insufficiency, and failure after prolonged urinary retention.

Sources: Adapted from Ferri, F. (2009). Prostatic hyperplasia, benign. In F. Ferri, *Ferri's clinical advisor: Instant diagnosis and treatment. MerckMedicus.* Retrieved from http://www.merckmedicus.com/pp/us/hcp/thcp_ferri_content.jsp?pg=/ppdocs/us/hcp/content/ferri/B9780323056090000253/ferri-815F.htm; Neal, R., & Keister, D. (2009). What's best for your patient with BPH? *The Journal of Family Practice, 58*(5), 241–248; Paolone, D. (2010). Benign prostatic hyperplasia. *Clinical Geriatric Medicine, 26*(2), 223–239. doi: 10.1016/j.cger.2010.02.010

Medical Management

Patients with BPH who have developed LUTS seek medical advice because of the discomfort. Treatment will depend on the condition's impact on the patient's quality of life, the presence of comorbidities such as diabetes or heart disease, and the severity of the urinary problem (Nash, 2010). Treatment modalities vary from watchful waiting to radical surgery.

Medication and Treatments

Patients with mild symptoms who are willing to make some lifestyle changes can usually postpone medical or surgical intervention for a time. Lifestyle changes would include such things as decreasing fluid intake at bedtime to decrease nocturia, decreasing caffeine and alcohol intake because of the irritation to the urinary system, and limiting the use of prescription and over-the-counter drugs that may affect urination (DynaMed Editorial Team, 2010; Ferri, 2009). Chart 42–3 lists medications that may affect urination. Patients who choose watchful waiting are evaluated annually or when worsening symptoms occur.

CHART 42–3 Medications That Affect Urination

- Diuretics cause urinary frequency.
- Sympathomimetic agents such as ephedrine cause increased urethral sphincter contractility.
- Anticholinergic drugs such as atropine, spiriva, and vesicare cause decreased detrusor contractility.
- Antihistamines and antidepressants may cause lower urinary tract symptoms (LUTS) in older men.
- Over-the-counter drugs, especially cold remedies, cause LUTS by various mechanisms.
- Opiates (hydromorphone, oxymorphone, meperidine) may cause urinary retention and urinary tract spasms.
- Skeletal muscle relaxants (methocarbamol) may cause renal impairment.

Sources: Adams, M., & Koch, R. (2010). *Pharmacology: Connections to nursing practice.* Upper Saddle River, NJ: Pearson; Neal, R., & Keister, D. (2009). What's best for your patient with BPH? *The Journal of Family Practice, 58*(5), 241–248.

Medication therapy has replaced surgery as the most common treatment of BPH (Paolone, 2010). Two primary drug types are used to reduce LUTS: alpha-adrenergic antagonists and 5-alpha reductase inhibitors. Alpha-adrenergic antagonists work by relaxing the bladder neck and prostatic muscle tone, thereby relieving obstruction. Newer alpha-adrenergic antagonists selectively reduce the prostatic smooth muscle tone and do not affect the blood pressure (Adams & Koch, 2010).

The second class of medication for BPH is the 5-alpha reductase inhibitors that work by reducing the conversion of testosterone. This slows prostate growth; however, it takes 3 to 6 months of drug therapy to see the full effect (Neal & Keister, 2009). More about the different drugs used for BPH can be found in the Pharmacology box (p. 1288).

Many men wanting to prevent or decrease symptoms of BPH choose herbal remedies such as *Pygeum africanum* (African star grass), African plum tree bark, and Cernilton (Neal & Keister, 2009). The Complementary & Alternative Therapies box presents some of the alternative therapies that are available.

Surgery

Although many men with BPH respond to medication therapy, there are those who do not want to take the medication for life, who are unable to tolerate the medications, or whose prostate continues to enlarge. These men are candidates for more invasive therapy. The mainstay of surgeries for BPH is transurethral resection of the prostate (TURP), wherein a resectoscope is passed through the urethra, a cystoscope is passed through the resectoscope to visualize the bladder and urethra, and a removable loop of resectoscope cuts prostate tissue and coagulates bleeding vessels. Continuous irrigation is needed to prevent blood clotting. Postoperative side effects may include erectile dysfunction, **retrograde ejaculation** (backflow of semen into the bladder at ejaculation), and, in about 1% of cases, incontinence (Burke et al., 2010; Paolone, 2010).

Transurethral microwave heat treatment (TUMT) and transurethral needle ablation (TUNA) are forms of **thermoablation** (use of heat to destroy tissue) of the prostate. These are alternative operative therapies wherein microwave heat (up to 45°C) is used to coagulate prostate tissue. A microwave antenna is placed in the urethra, and radiofrequency is passed into the prostate via needles. The device is surrounded by a cooling jacket to protect the urethra. These outpatient procedures are cheaper than TURP, and there is less bleeding, but thermoablation does not remove as much tissue, and it usually has to be repeated in 1 to 2 years (Burke et al., 2011; Paolone, 2010).

Other treatments include transurethral vaporization of the prostate (TUVP) and transurethral incision of the prostate (TUIP). In TUVP, the urologist uses laser or electrical vaporization to destroy or remove prostate tissue. TUIP involves making surgical incisions in the prostate to enlarge the urethral opening. TUIP is less destructive than TURP and TUVP, making it a better choice for younger men. It is also less likely to cause retrograde ejaculation or erectile dysfunction (Burke et al., 2011; Paolone, 2010).

Acute urinary retention of BPH can rapidly become an emergent condition, requiring catheterization. If a standard catheter cannot be passed through the urethra, a stiffer catheter may be used. If the blockage still cannot be penetrated, the patient must undergo cystoscopy and the use of dilators to open the urethra and drain the bladder. Eventually,

COMPLEMENTARY & ALTERNATIVE THERAPIES Saw Palmetto Extract and Pollen Extract

Nancy Yilk

SAW PALMETTO EXTRACT (SPE) has been widely used for the treatment of lower urinary tract symptoms secondary to benign prostatic hyperplasia (BPH). Clinical studies of SPE have been equivocal, with some showing significant results and others not. These inconsistent results may be due, in part, to varying bioactivities of the SPE used in the studies.

A saw palmetto extract, SPET-085, effectively inhibits the enzyme that has been linked to BPH, and the amount of extract required for activity is very low compared to data reported for other extracts. SPET-085 exhibited the highest levels of bioactivity and is more effective than other SPEs tested. This study confirmed that SPET-085 has prostate health-promoting bioactivity that also corresponds favorably to that reported for the established prescription drug standard of therapy, finasteride (Pais, 2010).

A pollen extract of Cernilton was investigated in a multicenter, prospective, randomized, double-blind, placebo-controlled phase 3 study of the National Institutes of Health (NIH) comparing the standardized and monogrammed pollen extract (Cernilton) to placebo in men with prostatitis/chronic pelvic pain syndrome (CP/CPPS) attending urologic centers. The study assessed improvements in the pain domain of the NIH Chronic Prostatitis Symptom Index (NIH-CPSI). Participants were evaluated using the NIH-CPSI individual domains and total score, the number of leukocytes in post-prostatic massage urine, the International Prostate Symptom Score, and the sexuality domain of a life satisfaction questionnaire at baseline and after 6 and 12 weeks. Of 139 men, 70 were randomly allocated to the pollen extract and 69 to receive a placebo. Pain and quality of life (QoL), as well as the total NIH-CPSI score, were significantly improved after 12 weeks of treatment with Cernilton as compared to placebo. Decrease of the NIH-CPSI total score by at least 25%, or at least 6 points, was seen in the pollen extract versus placebo group in 70.6% and 50.0% of men, respectively. Compared to placebo, Cernilton significantly improved total symptoms, pain, and QoL in patients with inflammatory CP/CPPS without severe side effects.

Note: Cernilton is marketed in the United States as Cernitin 63™.

Sources: Adapted from Wagenlehner, F. M., Schneider, H., Ludwig, M., Schnitker, J., Brähler, E., & Weidner, W. (2009). A pollen extract (Cernilton) in patients with inflammatory chronic prostatitis-chronic pelvic pain syndrome: A multicentre, randomized, prospective, double-blind, placebo-controlled phase 3 study. *European Urology, 56*(3), 544–551. Epub 2009 Jun 3; Pais, P. (2010). Potency of a novel saw palmetto ethanol extract, SPET-085, for inhibition of 5alpha-reductase II. *Advances in Therapy, 27*(8), 555–563. Epub 2010 Jul 10 an overfull bladder will cause hydroureter, hydronephrosis, and renal failure (Andriole, 2010).

Nursing Management

When a patient with BPH comes to the hospital because of LUTS, bladder infection, urinary retention, or hydronephrosis, he is seeking relief and is anxious about any procedures that may have been planned with his health care provider. The nurse will need to do a careful assessment of the patient's condition, elimination patterns, and medications, as well as the patient's knowledge of his condition and any planned procedure. He and his partner or family will need to receive education about the procedure, medications that will be used, and what to expect from the procedure. Preoperative preparation is similar to that of other surgeries, which is discussed in Chapter 17.

If the patient is admitted with acute urinary retention, catheterization is needed. It is very important to maintain a closed, sterile system while the catheter is in place. As for any patient with a renal or urinary problem, intake and output records should be maintained. Chapter 39 describes care of the patient with urinary impairment.

Postsurgical care following a TURP will include maintenance of continuous bladder irrigation to decrease clot formation and bleeding. A three-way catheter is placed after surgery and a steady flow of saline is used to flush the bladder. The nurse should be sure that the catheter is secured to the patient's thigh to prevent injury to the urethra and bladder neck. The irrigation and drainage tubing should be checked often for kinks that would block flow. Clot formation will cause obstruction and fluid retention. If a clot should occlude the catheter, the system can be opened and direct irrigation with saline can be done, but this should be a sterile procedure and avoided unless absolutely necessary.

Monitoring for bleeding is very important. If the output becomes redder, the irrigation should be increased. Bright-red heavy bleeding indicates an arterial bleed, requiring the surgeon's assistance.

Safety Alert *The potential for hemorrhage is high for patients who have undergone TURP. The nurse needs to observe the urine output over time for a gradual change in the color of the output from red to normal urine color. If the output does not change, the surgeon needs to be notified.*

TURP is painful surgery, and bladder spasms frequently occur because the catheter irritates the bladder mucosa. The patient should be encouraged not to strain against the catheter or try to urinate around the catheter, as this will increase the spasm. Also, straining at stool will be very uncomfortable for the patient. Therefore, analgesia and stool softeners are indicated. Review Chapter 12 on pain assessment and treatment for more information about care of patients with postoperative pain.

Safety Alert *Use of continuous bladder irrigation adds to the risk for the patient absorbing too much fluid and developing dilutional hyponatremia (Paolone, 2010). Nurses should watch for symptoms such as lethargy, headache, confusion, seizures, and coma (Huether, 2010).*

Infection may be prevented by keeping the irrigation system closed and cleaning the urinary meatus with soap and water at least twice a day. The nurse should monitor the vital signs and the patient for any indication of infection. The patient should be encouraged to increase fluid intake to keep urine output at about 50 milliliters above the irrigation fluid being used. As with all patients who have had surgery, the nurse should encourage ambulation and pulmonary toilet (Chapter 27).

In 24 to 48 hours, the irrigation will stop if the bleeding has stopped. The catheter may be removed in 1 to 5 days (Andriole, 2010). The patient should be monitored for urinary retention and assisted as needed when he attempts to void. Some men prefer to stand to void. Some may be able to void if sitting in a warm bath.

Discharge planning and education should begin early so that the patient and his family have time to consider the information and ask questions. The Patient Teaching & Discharge Priorities box lists the discharge teaching needed for the patient with BPH who has experienced TURP.

PATIENT TEACHING & DISCHARGE PRIORITIES for TURP

Need	Teaching
Knowledge of disease process and prognosis	Home care needs including verbal and written instructions for:
	Urinary incontinence, lower urinary tract symptoms (LUTS), and sexual function, which will improve.
	Rest; avoid lifting heavy objects or sitting for long periods.
	Practice performing pelvic exercises, stopping urinary stream, and contracting and relaxing pelvic muscles.
	Follow up with the health care provider in 1 week.
Understanding of medication	Use of analgesic for bladder pain; how much and how often. Review dosage and possible side effects.
	Purpose, dose, and possible side effects of alpha-adrenergic blocker if ordered for improvement of voiding.
Safety	Pain medication and alpha-adrenergic blocker may cause hypotension, especially if used together.
	Rise slowly and move carefully to avoid falls.
Danger signs	Inability to void, shortness of breath, and bleeding from the urinary tract are signs of emergent conditions for which patient needs to come to the emergency department.
Family/support system	Assess availability of, knowledge of, and compliance with the treatment plan.
	Assess home environment for need of assistive devices.
	Assess for need for professional home health care.
Emotional adjustment	Answer questions honestly.
	Encourage verbalization of frustrations with LUTS.
	Encourage positive reinforcement from the family.

GENETIC CONSIDERATIONS for Prostate Cancer

There is a strong familial predisposition for 5% to 10% of all prostate cancers. Individuals whose father or brother has had the disease have twice the risk. Having two first degree relatives who have had prostate cancer increases the risk to 5 times those of men without affected family members.

Men with the BRCA2 gene (breast cancer) have a 20-fold increase in risk for prostate cancer.

Prostate cancer susceptibility genes may account for about half of early-onset disease (age 55 years or younger).

Source: National Cancer Institute (NCI). (2010a). Genetics of prostate cancer (PDQ). Retrieved from http://www.cancer.gov/cancertopics/pdq/genetics/prostate/healthprofessional.

Cancer of the Prostate

Etiology and Epidemiology

A man's lifetime risk for prostate cancer is 1 in 6, making this disease the most common cancer in men in the United States and the second leading cause of death after lung cancer (ACS, 2010h; NCI, 2010c). An estimated 218,890 new cases and 27,050 deaths occurred in 2010 in the United States due to prostate cancer (NCI, 2010c, 2010g). The incidence is increasing as the population ages. In fact, aging is the most powerful risk factor for prostate cancer. African American men have a 60% higher incidence rate of prostate cancer than do Caucasian men (NCI, 2010a). The Genetic Considerations box outlines the influence of mutated genes on developing prostate cancer. Other risk factors for this cancer are presented in the Risk Factors box.

Pathophysiology

The prostate has three zones—the central zone, peripheral zone, and transitional zone—surrounded by a fibromuscular casing. The peripheral zone is where prostate cancer usually originates, although the cause of prostate cancer is still unknown (Latendresse et al., 2010). Prostate cancer occurs in two forms: latent or slow growing and aggressive or fast growing. The aggressive form is more likely to occur in African American and younger men (ACS, 2010c).

Clinical Manifestations

Prostate cancer may be asymptomatic. Some men have the slow-growing type of prostate cancer for many years and die of other causes. Often signs and symptoms of prostate cancer are not noticed until after metastasis has occurred. Chart 42–4 lists the more common signs and symptoms of prostate cancer.

RISK FACTORS for Prostate Cancer

Age: most cases occur in men over age 65; 80% prevalence rate by age 80.

Ethnicity: African American men are at greatest risk.

Family history: especially first degree relative, including mother or sister with breast cancer.

Diet: high fat and red meat consumption.

Obesity

Smoking.

Sources: Adapted from National Cancer Institute (NCI). (2010c). Prostate cancer. Retrieved from http://www.cancer.gov/cancertopics/types/prostate; Wallace, M., Bailey, D., & Brion, J. (2009). Shedding light on prostate cancer. *The Nurse Practitioner, 34*(10), 25–33.

CHART 42–4 Common Signs and Symptoms of Prostate Cancer

- Frequent urination
- Trouble starting or holding back urine
- Dysuria
- Painful ejaculation
- Pain in the lower back, hips, or upper thigh if cancer has metastasized.
- Urinary retention
- Weak or interrupted urine stream
- Hematuria (rare)
- Nocturia

Source: Adapted from National Cancer Institute (NCI). (2010c). Prostate cancer. Retrieved from http://www.cancer.gov/cancertopics/types/prostate.

Diagnostic Testing and Staging

With the advent of prostate-specific antigen (PSA) as a screening tool, asymptomatic, early prostate cancer has been identified in many men. Prostate-specific antigen is a serum kinase that originates from the prostate epithelial cells. It is considered a tumor marker because it is produced in cancer cells (Virshup, 2010). However, it is not specific enough to diagnose prostate cancer as a single test because several non-malignant conditions can cause an increase in the PSA. A DRE is also used as a screening tool for finding prostate cancer, but it covers only a small portion of the prostate gland (Wallace et al., 2009). Used together, PSA and DRE increase the likelihood of identifying prostate cancer.

Controversy has arisen surrounding the use of PSA to diagnose prostate cancer. While a large number of prostate cancers have been identified with this tumor marker, many of these cancers are of the slow growing type and do not need to be treated aggressively. Overtreatment tends to occur, causing more harm than the slow growing cancer would have. In addition, there is evidence that some men with normal PSA levels do have cancer of the prostate. On the other hand, there has been a decrease in prostate cancer-specific death rates in the United States since PSA has been used as a screening tool (ACS, 2010f).

To make the PSA more reliable, several measures of progression are being used. PSA density measures the ration of serum PSA to prostate volume. PSA velocity measures how serum PSA levels change over time. PSA age-specific reference ranges have been established. In addition, total PSA, the combination of free and bound PSA, is being used. All of these approaches offer more specific tests for the detection of prostate cancer and for determining the response to cancer treatment (Djavan, Eckersberger, Finkelstein, Sadri, Taneja, & Lepor, 2010; Latendresse et al., 2010).

Once a possibility of prostate cancer has been established by PSA, DRE, or both, then transrectal ultrasound (TRUS)-guided biopsy is used to identify, stage, and grade the disease. There is one system for staging and one system for grading: the tumor, node, metastasis (TNM) staging system and the Gleason histologic grading system (Wallace et al., 2009). The TNM system is discussed in depth in Chapter 57.

The Gleason grading system is based on histologic patterns in the cellular structure of the prostate. The pathologist looks at the two most common patterns within the sample and gives a grade to the first and second most frequently occurring patterns. This gives a score such as 4 + 3 or 3 + 4, the 4 + 3 being the sample with the poorest prognosis. Gleason scores of less than 7 indicate a lower risk of metastasis, and scores higher than 7 indicate a higher risk (Wallace et al., 2009).

The PSA and the Gleason score are used in planning further medical diagnostic testing and intervention. If the PSA is less than 2.5 ng/mL and the man has few risks, then it is recommended that

Weblink: Genetics of Prostate Cancer

NATIONAL GUIDELINES for Treatment and Support of Patients With Prostate Cancer

Principles of Active Surveillance

Active surveillance means active monitoring of the course of the disease with the expectation of intervention if the cancer progresses.

Localized cancer monitoring includes:

- Prostate-specific antigen (PSA) assessment every 3 months, or at least every 6 months.
- DRE as often as every 6 months or at least annually.
- Needle biopsy of prostate repeated within 6 months of diagnosis if initial biopsy was < 10 cores or
- Needle biopsy of the prostate repeated within 18 months of diagnosis if initial biopsy was > 10 cores.

Cancer progression may have occurred if:

- Primary Gleason grade 4 or 5 is found with repeat prostate biopsy.
- PSA doubling time <3 years.

A repeat prostate biopsy is indicated for signs of disease progression by exam or PSA.

Source: Adapted from National Comprehensive Cancer Network (NCCN). (2010). Practice guidelines in oncology-v.3.2010 Prostate cancer. Retrieved from http://www.nccn.org/professionals/physician_gls/PDF/prostate.pdf.

he be retested every other year. If the PSA is between 2.5 and 4 ng/mL, a risk assessment is done looking at race, family history, previous biopsy results, and DRE. About 25% of these men will have prostate cancer. If the PSA is 4 ng/mL or higher, further evaluation is indicated (ACS, 2010f; Gaines, 2010). If the PSA is greater than 20 ng/mL, then bone metastasis is probable and a bone scan is recommended. CT scans are used only for men whose Gleason scores are between 8 and 10 (Swanson, 2010).

Medical Management

Once the diagnosis of prostate cancer has been established and the tests for staging and grading have been completed, the next step is medical intervention. Compounding factors include the patient's age and any comorbidities. If the tumor is slow growing and the patient's life expectancy is affected by other health issues, he may decline treatment and enter a period of watchful waiting in which no further testing is done. Men who probably have low risk cancers may choose a program of active surveillance (Gaines, 2010). In this case, regular serum PSA (free/total, velocity, and density), DRE, and TRUS-guided biopsy is done. The patient also is monitored for LUTS and signs that the cancer may have metastasized. TRUS-guided biopsy may be done every 3 years; however, these examinations are painful, and the patient may choose not to have them done. During this time, lifestyle interventions to improve diet, exercise, and stress management can be instituted. Group support also may be helpful. The National Guidelines box details the protocol for active surveillance.

Radiation therapy is used for localized tumors and can be delivered by external beam radiation or implant therapy (brachytherapy). Brachytherapy has fewer side effects than radical surgery or external beam radiation, including less frequent occurrence of erectile dysfunction and urinary incontinence. This therapy will cause swelling of the prostate that will alter urination patterns and can last up to 12 months (Wallace et al., 2009). External beam radiation occurs over about 6 weeks, and there are several side effects including cystitis (bladder inflammation), proctitis, and dermatitis (inflammation of the skin) that occur near the end of the treatment period and may last for as much as 6 weeks after the treatments have stopped. Long-term side effects may include erectile dysfunction (Wallace et al., 2009). External beam radiation is discussed in Chapter 57. Patients who choose either of the radiation treatments may need medication to help them to void and reduce the risk of urinary retention. Conversely, these patients may need medication to alleviate frequency and urgency. The Ethical Issues box discusses lack of informed consent for brachytherapy.

ETHICAL ISSUES for Brachytherapy

Guido and Watson (2010) explain that patient comprehension is required for valid consent for a procedure. There is a legal duty to make every effort to ensure that the patient fully understands the pros and cons of brachytherapy before signing the consent. The fact that a patient does not understand everything about brachytherapy before he signs the consent does not cancel or invalidate his signed consent. However, it does pose a potential malpractice liability if the patient decides to sue. If the nurse discovers that a patient does not understand everything about brachytherapy, it is the nurse's responsibility to contact her supervisor and the health care provider so that they are made aware of the patient's lack of understanding at the time the consent was signed. Once the procedure has been done, the lack of understanding at the time of consent cannot be rectified. However, this incident should generate in-service programs within the hospital where the incident occurred to educate and remind nurses of their responsibility to educate patients fully before obtaining their signature on the consent form. Informed consent means that the patient knows all the benefits and risks of the procedure before he signs the consent.

If the tumor is the more aggressive type and the patient is younger, he may choose radical **prostatectomy** or removal of the prostate, seminal vesicles, and adjacent tissues. This can be done as open surgery or by laparoscopic or robot-assisted open surgery. Robot-assisted laparoscopic radical prostatectomy offers smaller incisions, less blood loss, and shorter hospital stays but requires a high degree of skill for the surgeon and is more expensive (Wallace et al., 2009).

Hormone therapy (androgen suppression) or orchiectomy is used to decrease the level of testosterone, thereby slowing disease progression (Wallace et al., 2009). This therapy is being used in both localized disease and for advanced, symptomatic metastatic disease. Often, it helps to relieve the pain and other symptoms of advanced disease. However, there are dramatic and lasting side effects such as erectile dysfunction, loss of libido, weight gain, loss of body hair, lethargy, hot flashes, and genital shrinkage (Brown, 2010). Medications used to decrease testosterone include estrogen and the GnRH agonist.

Chemotherapy is a last resort in prostate cancer. It is used if the prostate cancer does not respond to androgen suppression. The drug used for chemotherapy is docetaxel (Taxotere) (Wallace et al., 2009).

New developments in the treatment of localized prostate cancer include thermal ablation that can target specific areas within the prostate or destroy the entire gland. This approach is focal and nerve-sparing, according to its proponents (Ward & Jones, 2010).

The United States Food and Drug Administration (FDA) has approved a vaccine called Provenge for use in treating advanced prostate cancer. This vaccine, the first designed to treat existing cancer, is made of the patient's own white blood cells (WBCs) that are activated by exposing them to a protein found in prostate cancer cells. Once activated, the WBCs are returned to the patient intravenously. This stimulates the immune system and causes it to attack the cancer. This vaccine will not cure the cancer, but it does offer a treatment option for men who have metastatic disease (ACS, 2010a).

EVIDENCE-BASED PRACTICE for Prostate Cancer

Clinical Problem

Early diagnosis and treatment of prostate cancer have increased the period of time during which the patient and his family must cope with treatment regimens for the cancer. The cancer introduces a threat to life, and the treatments cause severe side effects such as fatigue, incontinence, sexual dysfunction, threatened body image, emotional distress, and loss of masculinity. These insults to quality of life have a profound effect on the patient and his family. Sometimes the health care team does not recognize the toll this illness takes on the patient's partner, nor do they include the partner in the patient's care plan. This can have a devastating effect on the partner and the patient. Nurses are in an ideal position to recognize the need for emotional and psychological support for both the patient and his partner and to offer this support.

Research Findings

Evertsen and Wolkenstein (2010) conducted a descriptive study using two focus groups of women whose partners had undergone surgery for prostate cancer within the previous 1 to 18 months. The purpose of the study was to "explore the interaction of the female partner with the patient's physicians and her support needs associated with treatment of and recovery from prostate cancer" (p. 2). The participants shared that the health care providers did not seem "worried about me [emotionally]" (p. 3). The women expressed how they had to talk for their partner when "he shut down" (p. 4). One woman became ill with shingles and high blood pressure due to the stress of the ordeal caused by her husband's illness. Other themes from the group sessions included the need for support groups for patients' partners; the need for mandatory or prescribed support groups for male patients because they are less likely to ask for help; that patients' partners need more information about the disease, its treatment, and what to expect; that partners need more information about being a caregiver instead of a companion; partners' desire for more practical information about how difficult and long recovery may be; and partners' strong need for emotional support from family, friends, and others who have experienced the same diagnosis.

Implications for Nursing Practice

Partners of men with prostate cancer need support and guidance. Nurses should recognize that the problems partners face when their significant others are ill are not solely from the patient's diagnosis and treatment regimen. Partners should be given the opportunity to discuss problems with balancing their lives and maintaining emotional wellness. If there are problems within the relationship, such as lack of communication, these could undermine the couple's ability to cope with treatment-related issues, as well as take away energy needed for the patient to heal. Partners need more information about the disease and its treatment, and they need support groups in their community. Nurses can begin a discussion with the partner, explore what she or he finds stressful, and offer problem-solving guidelines. The patients and their partners need to know whether what they are going through is normal.

Anticipating problems when a treatment regimen is planned and initiating discussions with the patient and his partner will help them both to cope and problem solve.

Critical Thinking Questions with answers can be found in the Osborn Student Resources at nursing.pearsonhighered.com.

Source: Adapted from Evertsen, J., & Wolkenstein, A. (2010). Female partners of patients after surgical prostate cancer treatment: Interactions with physicians and support needs. *BMC Family Practice, 11*(19), 1–6. doi:10.1186./1471-2296-11-19

Nursing Management

The nurse's role in the diagnostic stage of prostate cancer may include assisting with the diagnostic examinations, educating the patient and his partner about the diagnostic tests and what to expect, performing physical care postbiopsy, and providing emotional support. If the patient and his partner choose active surveillance, the nurse may educate them concerning the timing of follow-up visits with the health care provider for DRE, PSA, and TRUS-guided biopsy. The nurse may also guide the patient in improving his diet, exercise regimen, and stress management. Referrals to groups in the local community for support of patients with newly diagnosed prostate cancer would also be appropriate. The patient's partner may have need of support as well. The Evidence-Based Practice box outlines women's experiences as the result of their partner's prostate cancer diagnosis and delineates holistic approaches to recognizing partners' needs.

Patients with prostate cancer may be seen in the emergency department for urinary retention. The nurse's role here is to offer emotional support, to educate about the catheter being used to relieve the retention, and to understand the need for slowed release of urine from a distended bladder. The patient and his partner will need emotional support and education about the catheter and the use of any incontinence pads or devices.

Since there are many treatment options, the patient and his partner will need to be educated about all of them, including the benefits and adverse effects of each approach. When the medical plan is for radiation therapy in the form of external beam radiation or brachytherapy, the nurse's role will be teaching about the procedure and the side effects. Chapter 57 discusses the various types of radiation therapy. The patient and his partner should be alert to signs of urinary retention secondary to prostate swelling and should seek care immediately if it occurs. The patient will need education about proctitis, cystitis, and dermatitis and demonstrations on how to use the skin protectant and the medications ordered (see the Pharmacology box, p. 1288).

Radical prostatectomy may be chosen. In this event, the preoperative preparation is much the same as that for other surgeries. Refer to Chapter 17 for preoperative preparation. The patient will need to know about the use of the **suprapubic catheter** (catheter inserted into the bladder via a surgical opening made above the pubic bone) and the pain management plan for him. He will need emotional support as he faces some of the complications such as urinary incontinence, erectile dysfunction (depending on the operative approach), possible rectal injury, and anal damage. Urinary incontinence is most likely right after surgery and will improve over the next 6 months to 2 years (Wallace et al., 2009).

Reinforcement of education and repeated information is needed for the anxious patient and his partner. The diagnosis is a difficult one and will change their lives substantially. The patient's body image is changing, and he will have many life adjustments to make. Cultural background and beliefs are important considerations in the approach to these men. The Cultural Considerations box list some aspects of the African American male culture.

Hormone therapy or orchiectomy may be done if the cancer has spread beyond the prostate. If orchiectomy is chosen, the surgery is quick, and normal recovery is uncomplicated. The loss of the testicles, however, may have a profound emotional effect on the patient. In addition, the loss of masculinity can mean depression due to altered body image and function. Hormone therapy in the form of diethylstilbestrol or luteinizing hormone-releasing hormone agonists will lower the testosterone level, but the side effects may be further debilitating to the patient. The nurse can help find ways of decreasing the side effects

CULTURAL CONSIDERATIONS
African American Male Culture and Health Care

African American males:

1. Are taught as young boys to act strong, autonomous, and aggressive. They are expected to control expressions of emotion and consider emotional displays as a sign of weakness and vulnerability.
2. Have difficulty expressing their feelings, thereby increasing inner stress and anxiety.
3. Are skeptical about health care treatments and distrust most health care providers.
4. Are less likely to seek health care until symptoms are severe.
5. View mental illness as a character weakness, not as a disease.
6. Have wives, mothers, grandmothers, or daughters who serve as gatekeepers to foster and monitor health for the man.

Consult this website for cultural competence training: http://www.hrsa.gov/culturalcompetence.

Sources: DeCuir, D., Wicks, M., & Rice, M. (2009). The health of African-American men. *The American Journal for Nurse Practitioners, 13*(11/12), 34–39; Halbert, C., et al. (2010). Racial differences in quality of life following prostate cancer diagnosis. *Urology, 76*(3), 559–564; Hamilton, J., Stewart, B., Crandell, J., & Lynn, M. (2009). Development of the ways of helping questionnaire: A measure of preferred coping strategies for older African-American cancer survivors. *Research in Nursing & Health, 32*(3), 243–259. doi:10.1002/nur.20321; Holt, C., Wynn, T., Litaker, M., Southward, P., Jeames, S., & Schulz, E. (2009). A comparison of a spiritually based and non-spiritually based education intervention for informed decision making for prostate cancer screening among church-attending African-American men. *Urologic Nursing, 29*(4), 249–258.

and offer support to the patient and his partner as they cope with the changes. Chemotherapy may be needed if the patient's disease has spread to other organs. Nursing care for cancer patients is discussed in Chapter 57.

The Nursing Process: Patient Care Plan box provides further information about treating a patient who has undergone radical prostatectomy. Refer to the Patient Teaching & Discharge Priorities box for information on discharge planning after radical prostatectomy (p. 1304).

Collaborative Management

Prostate cancer is a complex disease and requires a team approach for optimal care. The urologist is assisted by nurses, the oncologist, anesthesiologists, nutritionists, counselors, and community resources. In order to meet desired patient outcomes, it is essential that this interdisciplinary team communicate openly with one another in developing and evaluating care of the patient and family (IOM [Institute of Medicine], 2010). The health care team should include the patient's partner and family in all aspects of the plan of care.

The urologist is a specialist in the care of patients with renal and urinary disorders. The urologist is the team leader and responsible for surgery. Nurses assist in the many roles discussed earlier. The oncologist, a specialist in chemotherapy and /or the radiation oncologist for radiation treatment for cancer, will be called if the tumor has grown outside the prostate and metastasized to other organs. Anesthesiologists direct the general anesthesia or epidurals needed during surgery or as a palliative measure for severe pain. Nutritionists help the patient and his partner to choose nutritious foods that will help in healing and restoration of the body. Counselors help the couple to cope with this stressful life event. The counselor may help with problem-solving methods, stress relief, or biofeedback and relaxation techniques. Community resources include the different institutions that offer information, as well as support groups, such as the American Cancer Society and the National Cancer Institute. Other community resources may be home health care, physical therapy, massage therapists, and local support groups for the spouse or the couple.

Penile Disorders

There are a number of penile disorders, many of which may cause an alteration in sexual functioning. Treatment for the various disorders may range from simple medication to radical surgery. Psychological counseling is an integral part of the treatment and follow-up phases of care for patients with these conditions. The most common penile disorders are discussed in this section.

Phimosis and Paraphimosis

Phimosis (tight foreskin) occurs when the foreskin cannot be retracted over the penile glans (Figure 42–4◆). Phimosis is a natural occurrence at birth. As the baby grows and the penis develops, the foreskin loosens from the glans and becomes completely retractable by age 3 to 5 years. By age 17, very few boys will have persistent physiologic phimosis (Wan & Rew, 2010). Phimosis may occur at any age as the result of inflammation or infection secondary to poor hygiene. Treatment

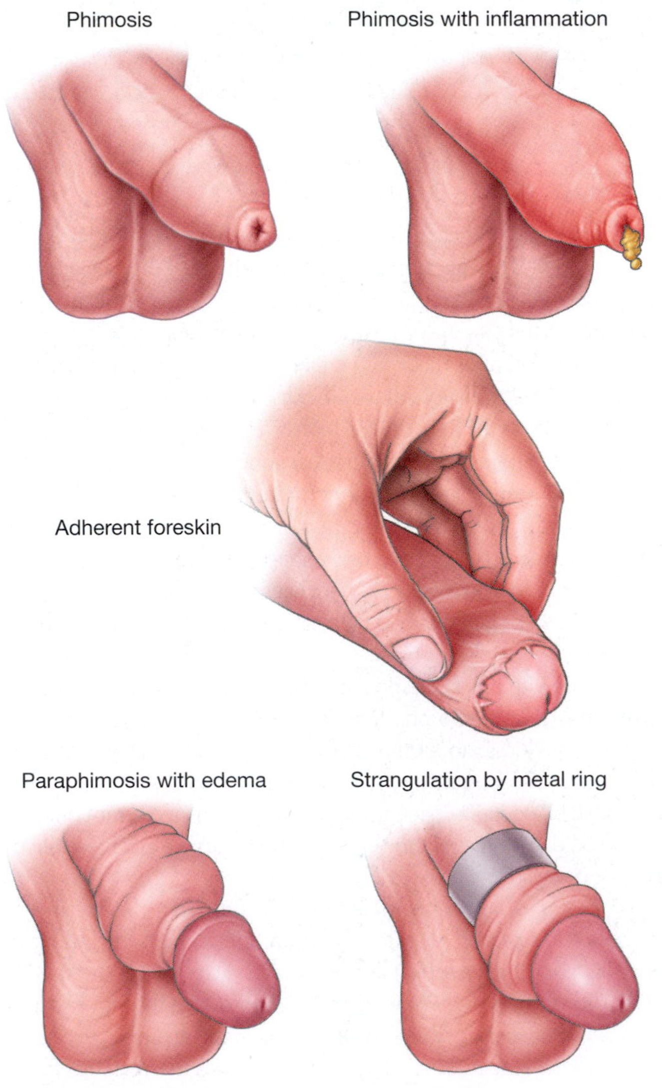

FIGURE 42–4 ◆ Phimosis and paraphimosis.

NURSING PROCESS: Patient Care Plan for Prostate Cancer After Radical Prostatectomy

Assessment of the Male Reproductive Status Using Gordon's Functional Health Patterns:

- Sexuality–Reproductive
- Coping Stress Tolerance
- Cognitive–Perceptual
- Elimination
- Self-Perception/Self-Concept

Subjective Data

Assessment of Anxiety and Fear

Tell me about your concerns.

Are you concerned that treatments may affect your quality of life?

Do you understand your diagnosis?

Do you understand your health care provider's plan for you?

Who are your support people?

Have you ever had cancer before?

How have you coped with stress in the past?

Are you aware that there will be a loss of sexual function that may or may not be permanent?

Assessment of Pain

Do you have pain?

Where is the pain?

Is it getting worse?

On a pain scale of 1 to 10, with 10 being the worst, how would you rate your pain?

Assess gender, cultural, and religious impact on patient response to pain.

Assessment of Knowledge

Tell me what you understand about your disease and the surgery planned.

Have you had surgery before?

Do you know what to expect after surgery?

What is your understanding about the catheter used after surgery?

Do you know how to use an incentive spirometer?

Do you know how to use support hose?

Assessment of Urinary Elimination

Preoperative:

What is your usual pattern of urination?

When was the last time you voided?

Does your bladder feel full?

Are you dribbling urine?

Postoperative:

Is the catheter uncomfortable?

Assessment of Bowel Elimination

When was your last bowel movement?

Are you using a stool softener or laxatives?

Assessment of Skin and Fluid Volume

Have you had problems with urine leaking from your catheter?

Are you able to keep your skin dry?

Are you thirsty?

Does your urine appear concentrated?

Have you had a fever or chills?

Does your urine appear cloudy or clear?

Objective Data

Assessment of Anxiety and Fear

Body language: look of concern or anguish.

Assessment of Pain

Body language, facial grimace, confusion, and anxiety may be signs of pain.

Assessment of Knowledge

Whether or not patient is able to answer questions correctly.

Whether patient asks questions that indicate lack of knowledge.

Assessment of Urinary Elimination

Preoperative:

Bladder distention, dribbling urine, or incontinence.

Postoperative:

Yellow, pink-tinged urine

Catheter and tubing intact and free of kinks

Catheter secured to inner thigh.

Assessment of Bowel Elimination

Frequency and consistency of bowel movements.

Type and amount of stool softeners and/or laxatives

Assessment of Skin and Fluid Volume

Inspect skin exposed to urine or tape.

Inspect incision and catheter site.

Check vital signs.

(*continued*)

NURSING PROCESS: Patient Care Plan for Prostate Cancer After Radical Prostatectomy, *continued*

Outcomes and Evaluation Parameters	Planning and Interventions with *Rationales*
1. NURSING DIAGNOSIS: Anxiety *related to diagnosis, treatment plan, and prognosis;* Ineffective Sexuality Pattern *related to prostate cancer and treatments;* Disturbed Body Image *related to diagnosis, orchiectomy, and side effects of other treatments* (NANDA-I © 2012)	
Outcome: Reduced stress and improved ability to cope. ***Evaluation Parameters:*** Appears more relaxed. States that he feels less anxious. Reiterates information about diagnosis, treatment, and prognosis in a calm manner.	Clarify information and help patient to cope by helping him to understand the disease, treatment, and prognosis. *Often, anxious patients are not able to understand as well.* Be there for him. *Quiet presence helps alleviate fear.* Offer support and open communication with him and his partner. *An atmosphere of acceptance and openness will help him to be more willing to talk.* Answer questions honestly and reiterate information often and in concrete terms. *Anxiety reduces cognition.* Encourage him to verbalize his concerns about sex and changes in his physical appearance. *Verbalizing fear is the first step in alleviating fear.*
2. NURSING DIAGNOSIS: Readiness for Enhanced Comfort *related to postoperative prostatectomy pain* (NANDA-I © 2012)	
Outcome: Comfort level maintained. ***Evaluation Parameters:*** Patient will be able to communicate pain level and therapies that help alleviate it. Pain is reduced and/or absent as evidenced by patient report and no pain behaviors. Nonpharmacologic method of pain control is effective, as evidenced by patient report and no pain behaviors. Patient reports satisfaction with pain management.	Instruct the patient not to strain against the catheter in an attempt to void. *Straining will cause bladder spasms and increased pain.* Instruct the patient to inform the nurse if the pain is not relieved. *This indicates the need to change the pain management plan.* Obtain a clear description of the location of the pain *to assist in developing a pain management plan.* Provide a supportive atmosphere so that the patient is comfortable asking for assistance with pain. *Open communications facilitate pain management.* Ask the patient about pain and encourage him to use the pain medication prescribed. *Men are more stoic and less likely to request medication for pain.* Use pain control measures before pain becomes severe *to increase comfort, decrease anxiety, and decrease the need for pain medication.* Record the patient response to pain medication. *Record of relief or lack of relief helps the health care team plan for better pain relief.*
3. NURSING DIAGNOSIS: Deficient Knowledge *related to the treatment plan and care needs* (NANDA-I © 2012)	
Outcome: Patient will be more cooperative and willing to participate in his care. ***Evaluation Parameters:*** Patient verbalizes understanding of the surgical procedure planned. Patient verbalizes understanding of the need for pulmonary toilet, support hose, and early ambulation, as well as the need for a catheter and the pain management plan. Patient demonstrates use of incentive spirometer. Patient verbalizes understanding of how, and why, to use support hose.	Provide education in simple terms. *Simplicity enhances the anxious patient's ability to learn.* Explain what to expect with surgery and the recovery period. *Knowledge assists the patient to be less fearful.* Explain that the urinary catheter is also a splint to help maintain the surgical reconnection of the urethra. *Knowing the reason for the catheter increases tolerance of the discomfort.* Explain what will be experienced. *Knowing a little about how it will feel will reduce fear.* Allow the patient to ask questions. *Open communication enhances learning.* Allow the patient to become familiar with the spirometer. *Handling equipment makes it familiar and easier to use after surgery.* Demonstrate how support hose are used. *Support hose are used to help prevent thrombosis and pulmonary embolism.*
4. NURSING DIAGNOSIS: Urinary Retention *due to urethral obstruction secondary to prostate enlargement* (NANDA-I © 2012)	
Outcome: Normal urinary output. ***Evaluation Parameters:*** Preoperative: Urinary retention relieved. Patient is dry and comfortable.	Preoperative: Usual pattern gives baseline. *Return to usual pattern is goal to work toward.* Relieve urinary retention. *Urinary retention will cause damage to the bladder and, if severe and prolonged, hydroureter, hydronephrosis, and renal failure.*

NURSING PROCESS: Patient Care Plan for Prostate Cancer After Radical Prostatectomy, *continued*

Postoperative: Output at 50 milliliters or more per hour. Balance intake and output. No retention related to kinks in catheter tubing. Patient does not strain against catheter. Catheter is secured to inner thigh at all times.	Postoperative: Maintain strict intake and output records. *High output is needed to clear blood from the bladder to prevent clots and obstruction. Output less than intake indicates retention.* Monitor color and amount of output. *Increased bleeding must be identified early and corrected.* Keep the catheter secured to the thigh and prevent dislodging. *Dislodging the catheter can cause damage to the urethra anastomosis or bladder neck.* Keep tubing coiled on the bed and free of kinks *to facilitate urine flow and prevent obstruction.* Use incontinence pads to keep the patient dry. *Urine is irritating and can cause skin breakdown.*
5. NURSING DIAGNOSIS: Potential for Pain, Acute *related to constipation and straining at stool* (NANDA-I © 2012)	
Outcome: Regular bowel movement (BM) without straining. ***Evaluation Parameter:*** Patient reports regular BM that is soft and passed without straining.	Administer stool softener and encourage increased fluids. *Straining at stool can cause bleeding and increased pain.*
6. NURSING DIAGNOSIS: Risk for Impaired Skin Integrity *related to urinary incontinence;* Risk for Infection *related to surgery and urinary retention;* Risk for Deficient Fluid Volume *related to blood loss* (NANDA-I © 2012)	
Outcomes: No skin breakdown. No infection at the incision. ***Evaluation Parameters:*** Skin is intact. Patient has no complaints of skin itching or burning. Vital signs are normal for the patient.	Inspect the skin and keep it clean and dry. *Clean, dry skin does not break down.* Monitor surgical wound and drain sites for infection or signs of healing. *Early identification of infection decreases morbidity.* Monitor vital signs for elevated temperature. *This is an indication of infection.* Monitor pulse and blood pressure for signs of blood loss. *High pulse and lower blood pressure indicate blood loss.* Assist in early ambulation. *Ambulation improves circulation and enhances healing.*

Source: Adapted from Wilkinson, J. M., & Ahearn, N. R. (2009). *Prentice Hall nursing diagnosis handbook* (9th ed.). Upper Saddle River, NJ: Prentice Hall.

in these cases includes antibiotics for infection and circumcision if the phimosis interferes with urination (Latendresse et al., 2010).

Paraphimosis occurs when a retracted foreskin becomes trapped over the glans (Figure 42–4, p. 1300). The retracted foreskin causes a tourniquet effect, decreasing circulation to the glans. Swelling develops swiftly, further tightening the foreskin band. Compressing the glans and moving the foreskin forward should be attempted as soon as possible. If the foreskin cannot be manually reduced, circumcision is needed and may have to be done as an emergency procedure to prevent ischemia and necrosis of the glans (Latendresse et al., 2010).

Nursing care includes educating the patient about hygiene, providing emotional support, monitoring vital signs for evidence of a worsening condition, and administering analgesics. Circumcision is usually an outpatient surgery and does not require hospitalization.

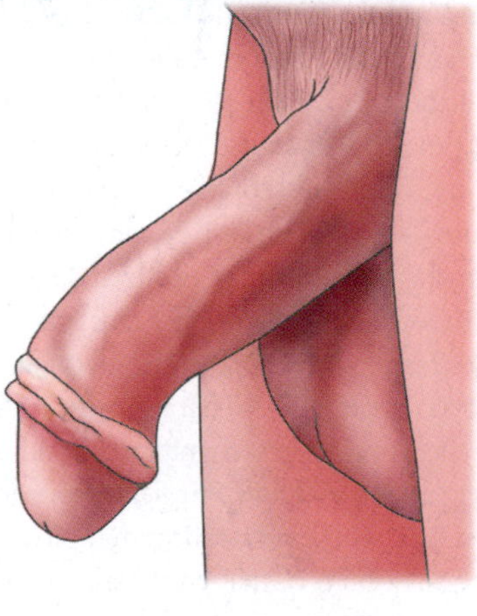

FIGURE 42–5 ◆ Peyronie's disease.

Peyronie's Disease

Peyronie's disease is a penile condition in which palpable, fibrous plaque forms on the corpora cavernosa. The plaque will cause abnormal curvature of the penis and painful, incomplete erections. Peyronie's disease affects middle-aged and older men (Wan & Rew, 2010) (Figure 42–5◆). The cause of this disorder is unknown.

There are no completely effective treatments for Peyronie's disease. Treatment with potassium paraaminobenzoate acid (Potaba) has had limited success. Surgery, which involves removing the plaque and repairing the corpora cavernosa with a graft, is a last resort that has offered relief of pain. However, erectile dysfunction may result from the surgery (Wan & Rew, 2010).

Nursing management would include emotional support, education about the condition and medications used, preoperative care, and postoperative care for those who have surgery. If the surgery is extensive, a suprapubic catheter may be placed so that the penis can heal more quickly.

PATIENT TEACHING & DISCHARGE PRIORITIES for Prostate Cancer After Radical Prostatectomy

Need	Teaching
Knowledge of self-care and need for follow-up visit with health care provider	Home care needs including verbal and written instructions for the following: May go home with the catheter in place. The patient and his partner need education about home care including maintaining patency of the tubing and cleansing the urinary meatus. Urinary incontinence may follow removal of the catheter but will improve. Rest; avoid lifting heavy objects, sitting for long periods, or straining at stool. Maintain increased oral intake at about 2 to 3 quarts a day, unless medically contraindicated. Practice pelvic exercises, which include stopping urinary stream and contracting and relaxing pelvic muscles. Follow up with the health care provider in 1 to 3 weeks.
Understanding of medication	Use of analgesic and antimuscarinic for bladder pain; how much, how often, and what the side effects may be. Purpose, dose, and possible side effects of alpha-adrenergic blocker if ordered for improvement of voiding.
Safety	Pain medication and alpha-adrenergic blocker may cause hypotension. Rise slowly and move carefully to avoid falls.
Danger signs	If the catheter comes out before it is supposed to; if the patient is unable to void after the catheter is removed; or if the patient experiences any shortness of breath, bleeding from the urinary tract, or high fever, he should be sent to his health care provider or emergency department.
Family/support system	Assess the availability of, knowledge of, and compliance with the treatment plan. Assess the home environment for need of assistive devices. Assess for the need for professional home health care. Seek support groups for the patient's spouse or partner to help with coping. Respite care may be needed.
Emotional adjustment	Answer questions honestly. Encourage verbalization of frustrations and fears. Encourage positive reinforcement from the family.
Institutional and community resources and support groups	Suggest National Cancer Institute and the American Cancer Society as resources. Offer community-based programs and support group addresses and phone numbers.

Urethral Stricture

The urethra, the most distal portion of the urinary tract (Figure 42–1, p. 1287), allows urine and semen to pass out of the body. Stricture within the urethra may occur as the result of trauma, an enlarged or nodular prostate, use of a cystoscope or other surgical instrument, or infection that causes scarring. Strictures will block the flow of urine and ejaculate. Urinary retention may occur and, if the stricture is severe enough, hydronephrosis may result. Signs and symptoms include decreased urinary stream, spraying of urine, urethral discharge, bladder infection secondary to retrograde urination, and urinary retention. Diagnosis is made by cystoscopy or urethrography (Latendresse et al., 2010).

Medical management includes surgical procedures to dilate or reconstruct the urethra. These procedures may be done under general or epidural anesthesia on an outpatient basis. Chapter 39 includes a discussion of the treatment for urinary disorders and treatments.

Nursing care depends on the extent of the stricture and surgical procedures to correct the stricture. Most patients will need pre- and postoperative teaching, analgesia, careful monitoring of vital signs, and observation for bleeding or drainage. See Chapter 12 for information about pain assessment and management. Many of these patients need emotional support if the stricture has become severe enough to warrant surgery.

Penile and Scrotal Injuries

Men are more likely than women to experience genital trauma. Scrotal injuries may be the result of infections, burns, or gunshot wounds. Testicular injuries are more likely to be blunt trauma that may cause hematoma or even rupture of the testicle. Penile injuries may occur from pant zippers, amputations, animal bites, gunshot wounds, battlefield injuries, or ruptures of the corpus cavernosum caused by severe bending of the penis during an erection (Armenakas, 2010).

Medical care includes identification of the extent of the injury and surgical repair as needed. In addition, antibiotic therapy and analgesia will be needed. Nursing care depends on the extent of the injury. Preoperative and postoperative education and emotional support are imperative.

Cancer of the Penis

Epidemiology and Etiology

Penile cancer is very rare in North America and Europe, accounting for fewer than 2% of cancers in men in the United States. Penile cancer is more common in some parts of Africa and South America, where it accounts for up to 10% of cancers in men (ACS, 2010b). More than 95% of penile carcinomas are squamous cell carcinomas (ACS, 2010b).

Causes of the various types of penile cancer are not known. Research has shown that human papillomavirus, especially types 16 and 18, can interfere with tumor suppressor genes, thereby allowing cancer to grow (ACS, 2010c). Human papillomavirus (HPV) has many different types. Some types will cause warts on the genitals; others are more virulent. The HPV types most associated with malignancies in both males and

RISK FACTORS for Penile Cancer

Poor local hygiene	Phimosis
UV light treatment for psoriasis	Smoking
Age (most cases occur in men over age 55)	AIDS
Not being circumcised	Human papillomavirus infection

Source: Adapted from American Cancer Society (ACS). (2010d). Penile cancer: What are the penile cancer risk factors? *Learn About Cancer.* Retrieved from http://www.cancer.org/Cancer/PenileCancer/DetailedGuide/penile-cancer-risk-factors.

females are types 16 and 18. Risk factors for penile cancer are listed in the Risk Factors box.

Medical and Nursing Management

Medical care for penile cancer is usually surgery. This may be circumcision or laser ablation for smaller lesions or partial or total **penectomy** (removal of part of or the entire penis) for larger lesions. When diagnosed early, a cure is probable. If the cancer has reached stage III or IV, however, a cure is less likely (NCI, 2010b). Radiation therapy is used if the cancer has not spread beyond the local lymph nodes. Chemotherapy, though rarely successful, is used when the cancer has spread widely. Chemotherapy is usually a combination of vincristine, bleomycin, and methotrexate.

Nursing care depends on the extent of the cancer. Preoperative and postoperative education and emotional support are imperative. Care of the patient undergoing cancer treatment is discussed in detail in Chapter 57.

Priapism

Etiology and Epidemiology

Priapism is a persistent penile erection unrelated to sexual stimulation. It is usually painful and may lead to permanent erectile dysfunction and penile necrosis if left untreated. Priapism is frequently idiopathic in etiology but is associated with neural or vascular abnormalities and pharmacologic agents. More common causes include thromboembolic events such as sickle cell disease (due to the collection of erythrocytes in the corporal bodies) and thalassemia. It can also occur with leukemia (due to an increased number of white blood cells) and multiple myeloma, trauma (pelvic, genital, or perineal), tumor (may be primary or metastatic), neurologic causes (spinal cord injury and anesthesia), cauda equina compression syndrome, and, finally, black widow spider bites. Medications that can cause priapism include sildenafil, as well as psychotropic drugs such as chlorpromazine, trazodone, haloperidol, quetiapine, and thioridazine. Cocaine, marijuana, ethanol abuse, and ecstasy can also cause priaprism.

The overall incidence of priapism is 1.5 cases per 100,000 person-years, which increases to 2.9 cases per 100,000 person-years for men older than 40 years (Dougherty, Richard, & Carey, 2009a). In one study, 38% to 42% of adult patients with sickle cell disease reported at least one episode of priapism (Cherian et al., 2006).

Pathophysiology

Priapism is the result of persistent engorgement of the corpora cavernosa of the penis, originating from a disturbance in the mechanisms that control normal penile detumescence. Typically, the ventral corpora spongiosum and glans penis remain flaccid in priapism. The most common pathophysiologic cause is full and unremitting corporeal veno-occlusion, in which venous stasis and deoxygenated blood pools within the cavernous tissue. This veno-occlusive priapism, if prolonged, results in fibrosis of the penis and a loss of the ability to achieve an erection. Fibrosis at the cellular level can occur within 24 hours.

Safety Alert *Priapism is considered a true urologic emergency due to the potential for compromised circulation to the penis. Any patient who has an erection for longer than 4 hours, especially if he has a predisposing illness (e.g., sickle cell disease), should seek treatment.*

Medical Management

The focus of medical management of priapism is to facilitate venous drainage from the corpora cavernosa. During the initial assessment, the presence of priapism is confirmed by the finding of an erect or semierect penis, with the ventral glans and corpus spongiosum rarely rigid. The presence of trauma and evidence of an underlying condition that may predispose the patient to priapism are evaluated. Initial treatment may include ice packs and prostatic massage, pain medication, and a urinary catheter if the patient is unable to void. Pharmacologic agents used to treat the priapism include phenylephrine and terbutaline. If these initial treatments are not effective, needle aspiration of the corpora cavernosa is indicated. Surgical intervention is the final mode of treatment if all else fails. Refractory priapism may require the placement of a corpus cavernosum-spongiosum shunt (Dougherty, Richard, & Carey, 2009b).

Male Sexual Functioning

To impregnate a female, a male must have normal **spermatogenesis** (manufacture of normal sperm in high numbers), and he must have the ability to transmit the sperm into a woman's vagina. This means that he needs to be able to have and sustain an erection and to have a normal ejaculation. If a male does not want to produce children but wishes to continue sexual relations, he can use condoms or undergo a sterilizing surgery called vasectomy (Nelson & Marshall, 2009). This section will explore selected topics related to male sexual function, including erectile dysfunction, male infertility, andropause, and vasectomy.

Erectile Dysfunction

Erectile dysfunction (ED) is the inability to achieve or sustain an erection firm enough for intercourse. It is estimated, based on imprecise data, that 10 to 20 million men over age 18 in the United States have had at least a few instances of ED. The prevalence increases to 50% of men ages 40 to 70 (Anawalt, 2010). Erectile dysfunction is also a common side effect of treatments for prostate cancer (Albaugh, 2010).

Epidemiology and Etiology

Erectile dysfunction may be primary (a man has never achieved erection) or secondary (a man has had erections but is no longer able). It is estimated that about 80% of ED events are physiological and the remaining events have a psychological cause, including but not limited to guilt, depression, performance anxiety, and fear of intimacy (Anawalt, 2010).

The major organic causes of ED include diabetes, stroke, atherosclerosis, spinal cord injuries, and complications of prostate surgery. Hormones, significant smoking, drugs, and structural problems may also contribute to ED. Chart 42–5 lists some drugs that may cause ED.

Laboratory and Diagnostic Procedures

Diagnostic tests for ED will include a complete history to reveal disease, congenital defects, medication use, and any associated psychological concerns. The physical examination focuses on secondary sexual

Weblink: Penile Cancer

Video: Erectile Dysfunction Etiology & Physiology

CHART 42–5 Drugs That May Cause Erectile Dysfunction

Clonidine	Spironolactone
Beta-blockers	Tricyclics
Selective serotonin reuptake inhibitors (SSRIs)	Alcohol
Cocaine	Opioids
Anticholinergics	

Source: Adapted from Anawalt, B. (2010). Male reproductive endocrinology: Introduction. *Merck Manuals Online Medical Library.* Retrieved from http://www.merckmedicus.com/pp/us/hcp/framemm.jsp?pg=www.merck.com/mmpe/index.html.

characteristics, any evidence of circulatory problems, anatomic abnormalities of the penis, and neurological deficits. Laboratory tests may include testosterone serum levels, prolactin levels, tests for diabetes, a lipid profile, and thyroid function tests, depending on the findings of the history and physical examination (Anawalt, 2010; Kamel, 2010). Chapter 40 on reproductive assessment details the male reproductive history and physical examination.

Medical Management

Medical management of ED depends on the underlying cause. Contributory drugs can be changed or discontinued, depression can be treated, and patients and their partners can be educated about ED, sexual intimacy alternatives to intercourse, and the need for continued open communication with each other (Morgan, 2009).

Devices are available to help achieve and sustain an erection. If mechanical devices are not acceptable to the patient and his partner, drug therapy may be used. The most popular of these drugs is sildenafil (Viagra), which enhances nitric oxide release needed for an erection. Sildenafil will cause coronary vasodilation and hypotension and should not be used with other nitrates such as nitroglycerine. In addition, it should be used in lower dosage and with extreme caution if the patient is taking an alpha blocker for BPH (Albaugh, 2010; O'Leary, 2009).

Other drugs may be injected into the urethra or into the penis to produce an erection. These medications have a higher incidence of injury to the penis and are more likely to cause priapism (an erection that lasts more than 4 hours). There are also penile prostheses that may be surgically implanted (Albaugh, 2010).

Collaborative Management

Collaborative management is indicated for men with ED. In order to meet desired patient outcomes, it is essential that the interdisciplinary team communicate openly with one another in developing and evaluating care of the patient and family (IOM [Institute of Medicine], 2010). The first member of the team is his sexual partner. A loving, accepting partner with whom the man with ED can maintain excellent communications is essential. Education, counseling, and emotional support may be provided by health care providers and nurses. Psychologists or counselors can help with mental and emotional issues that may affect the patient's ability to have an erection or result as a consequence of ED. Pharmacists may be involved in educating the patient about the medications ordered by the health care provider. This education includes how the medication works, the potential side effects, and how quickly the man may experience results. In addition, community support groups may have a role in providing holistic care for the couple on a long-term basis.

CHART 42–6 Causes of Male Infertility

Reversible Causes	Irreversible Causes
Varicocele	Klinefelter's syndrome
Heavy smoking	Congenital bilateral absence of vas deferens
Hypercholesterolemia	Spinal cord injuries
Some forms of erectile dysfunction	Antisperm antibodies
Hypogonadism	Some forms of erectile dysfunction
Obesity	Impaired spermatogenesis
Recreational drug use	
Alcohol intake	

Source: Stroller, M., Kane, C., & Meng, M. (2008). Urologic disorders. In S. McPhee & M. Papadakis, *2009 Current medical diagnosis and treatment* (48th edition, pp. 827–847). New York: McGraw-Hill/Lange.

Male Infertility

General information about infertility may be found in Chapter 41. Achieving a pregnancy requires both male and female contributions. When a couple cannot achieve a pregnancy after 1 year of unprotected intercourse, the male factor alone is the cause in about 20% of cases and will contribute in 30% to 40% of all couples who seek medical help for infertility (Nelson & Marshall, 2009). There are reversible and irreversible causes of male infertility, many of which are listed in Chart 42–6.

The most common test for evaluating male infertility is semen analysis. This test gives information about male hormone cycle integrity, spermatogenesis, and the patency of the genital tract (Kamel, 2010). Semen specimens are best collected after 3 days of sexual abstinence (Kee, 2010). Refer to Chart 42–7 for the parameters for semen analysis.

Medical care for infertility depends on the underlying cause and is highly specialized. Most of the medical interventions are completed on an outpatient basis from infertility clinics.

Andropause

Epidemiology and Etiology

Unlike women, men begin to decrease production of sex hormones at about age 30. The decrease is gradual, and the rate of decline varies greatly among individual men. On average, men in their seventh decade will have testosterone levels that are about 1/2 to 2/3 less than those of men in their twenties (Anawalt, 2010). Whether or not this age-dependent reduction in testosterone levels requires hormone replacement is under debate.

CHART 42–7 Semen Analysis Parameters

Volume	1.5 to 5 Milliliters
Sperm count	60 to 150 million/mL (conception has occurred as low as 10 million/mL)
Motility	at 3 hours > 60% are mobile
Morphology	70%
Viscosity	Liquid after 30 minutes
Antisperm antibody test	Negative to 1:32

Source: Adpated from Kee, J. (2010). *Laboratory and diagnostic tests* (8th ed.). Upper Saddle River, NJ: Pearson.

Physiologically, men ages 40 to 70 experience a decrease in total, free, and **bioavailable testosterone** (both free testosterone and testosterone that is loosely bound to albumin) and an increase in sex hormone-binding globulin (SHBG). The decrease in testosterone is associated with an increase in follicle-stimulating hormone (FSH) and a modest increase in luteinizing hormone (LH). These changes suggest an age-related change in the secretion of hypothalamic gonadotropin-releasing hormone (Anawalt, 2010). Unlike women in menopause who stop ovulating, men with lower levels of testosterone remain fertile.

Clinical Manifestations

Androgen decline in aging males (ADAM), or andropause, may cause mood changes, decreased libido, fatigue, decreased muscle mass, muscle weakness, increased abdominal fat, thinning of bones, decreased energy, slowed mathematical thinking, depression, decreased sense of well-being, sleep disturbances, and lower red blood counts (Laborde & Brannigan, 2010; Male hypogonadism, 2010). Androgen deficiency has also been shown to increase the risk for type 2 diabetes and metabolic syndrome (Laborde & Brannigan, 2010).

Diagnostic and Laboratory Procedures

After a thorough history and physical examination, laboratory measurement of bioavailable testosterone may be used to diagnose andropause in men over age 65. Serum levels of testosterone are highest soon after awakening, so test results should be evaluated based on the timing of the sample (Kee, 2010).

Medical Management

Testosterone replacement therapy will improve libido, muscle strength, sense of well-being, and mood (Adams & Koch, 2010). Testosterone may be administered via intramuscular injections, pellet implants, transdermal patch or gel, or **buccal** (mucosal lining of the mouth) tablets. It is important that candidates for testosterone replacement be carefully screened for prostate cancer. Testosterone replacement will not cause cancer, but an existing tumor will grow under its influence.

Contraindications to testosterone replacement therapy include history of cancer, hematocrit > 55%, untreated sleep apnea, obstructive urinary symptoms of BPH, and congestive heart failure (Laborde & Brannigan, 2010).

Potential side effects of testosterone replacement include acne, worsening BPH, elevated PSA levels, increased RBC count and hematocrit, lipid abnormalities, liver function test abnormalities, and sleep apnea (Adams & Koch, 2010).

Men experiencing andropause seem to benefit from counseling, decreasing stress, losing excess weight, increasing zinc intake, maintaining adequate nutrition, and weight training to build muscle mass.

Nursing Management

Nursing care of older men with andropause symptoms includes education about what andropause is and the lifestyle changes that can improve symptoms. If the patient elects to take testosterone replacement therapy, he should understand the potential side effects and how to use pellets, transdermal applications, or buccal tablets. See the Pharmacology box.

Vasectomy

Vasectomy is male sterilization surgery whereby the vas deferens on each side is identified and cut, and the cut ends are ligated or cauterized closed. Vasectomy is highly effective in preventing pregnancy if at least two semen-free ejaculates have been analyzed and documented. This is needed to ensure that the vas deferens was cut and closed and that all sperm have been cleared from the system. The procedure can be done in the health care provider's office under local anesthesia in about 20 minutes (Pollack, Thomas, & Barone, 2009).

Gerontological Considerations

Many nurses and other health care providers assume that because a man is older, he no longer has sexual needs. While it is true that growing older may be accompanied by illness or treatments that may diminish the sexual response, many men enter the senior years healthy. Today, people live longer, stay healthier, and are better informed about health concerns than ever before. Nurses are in an ideal position to have open discussions with older men about healthy sexual feelings and the normal male sexual response that changes with age.

RESEARCH OPPORTUNITIES Related to Male Reproductive Disorders

Research Area	Clinical Impact
Examination of why prostate cancer risks are higher for African American men.	African American men are much more likely to develop and die from prostate cancer.
Determination of whether selenium and vitamin E may help prevent prostate cancer.	Research is currently underway.
	Prevention of prostate cancer is much preferred to treating it.
Use of complementary and alternative therapies among patients with cancer.	Nurses should know more about complementary and alternative therapies so that they can give information about safety and efficacy to patients.
Prostate cancer outcomes study (PCOS) is examining the impact of treatments for prostate cancer on quality of life.	It is important for the patient to know all about his options and potential outcomes before choosing a treatment.
Identifying problems faced by partners of men with prostate cancer.	Nurses are recognized support persons, and patients' partners will turn to them when they need help dealing with decreased affection from or depression in their partner. Support of the partner helps in support of the patient.
Predicting the use of complementary and alternative therapies among patients with cancer.	Nurses need to ask patients about the complementary and alternative therapies they may be using such as herbs, vitamins, and homeopathic medications that may affect their medical care.

The sexual response for the older male has been described by Peate (2009) as less frequent and less orgasm driven. Older men experience a reduction in morning erections and spontaneous erections, diminished pre-ejaculatory sensation, rapid reduction in the erection, a decrease in the volume of ejaculation fluids, and less desire to ejaculate. The sexual response for men becomes more associated with affection, intimacy, bonding, and acceptance.

If the reduction in the sexual response is of concern to the male and his partner, then the nurse can explain that there are safe medical interventions that can assist the older man in continuing sexual relations. For instance, lower levels of testosterone can be replaced, drugs to enhance the erection and libido can be taken if there are no medical contraindications, or penile prosthesis can be implanted.

Research

To improve the care of males experiencing reproductive system abnormalities, it is imperative that nurses be knowledgeable and that research continue to refine this knowledge. The Research Opportunities box outlines potential research topics related to male reproductive disorders.

CLINICAL PREPARATION

READ DOCUMENT APPLY

READ: **History of Present Illnesses** >> Laboratory Study Results >> Critical Thinking Questions

You are receiving report on Allen Hyatt, a 60-year-old male patient who is 3 days postoperative from a suprapubic prostatectomy. Mr. Hyatt was first seen 2 weeks ago in his health care provider's office with complaints of increasing difficulty voiding during the past 4 months. The physical exam and elevated PSA strongly suggested prostate cancer, and a transrectal ultrasound guided biopsy was done. The results showed a T2, Gleason 2 + 2 tumor. The patient was given the option of radiation therapy or surgery. Mr. Hyatt opted for an immediate prostatectomy. He was admitted early yesterday morning for surgery.

You begin your shift rounds and greet Mr. Hyatt as you enter the room. You note an IV in the right forearm, without redness or edema, infusing at 100 mL/hr. A suprapubic catheter is in place and draining well. The outflow bag contains red-tinged fluid. Mr. Hyatt is in a semi-Fowler's position with the overbed table in front of him. The tray on the table contains unopened containers of apple juice, chicken broth, and coffee. When questioned about his untouched food, Mr. Hyatt states that he is just not hungry. You continue the assessment and examine the occlusive suprapubic dressing, which appears moist under the tape. Mr. Hyatt states that his pain on a 1 to 10 point scale, with 10 being the worst, is 6, mostly around the suprapubic catheter. You give him an analgesic and help him to a more comfortable position.

You change the suprapubic dressing around the catheter and note a thick yellow odorous discharge on the dressing with a streak of red on the gauze. You apply a sterile dressing to the site, which appears inflamed, with slight edema, minimal bruising, and pale yellow drainage at the catheter insertion site. A visible suture is holding the catheter in place. When you return to the nurses' station, you discover that the laboratory results for the patient have returned. You then notify the health care provider of the CBC values.

Medical–Surgical History

Mr. Hyatt's past medical history is on the chart and is remarkable for hypertension and insulin-dependent diabetes. Mr. Hyatt had all the "usual" childhood illnesses, including measles, mumps, and rubella. He had a broken arm requiring casting at age 15 as a result of a baseball injury. There were no major illnesses or medical events until he was in his 40s. At age 42, he was diagnosed with hypertension requiring 150 milligrams of irbesartan (Avapro) once daily. At age 48, he was diagnosed with diabetes, which was controlled with diet therapy until 3 years ago when he started taking a sliding-scale insulin lispro (Humalog) with meals. His blood sugars average in the 120s most days.

READ: History of Present Illnesses >> **Physical Exam** >> Admitting Medical Records >> Laboratory Study Results

Social History

He lives with his wife independently.
He has three adult children, all of whom live out of state.
He smoked for 30 years and quit about 10 years ago.
He drinks alcohol socially.

Physical Exam

Vital signs: temp 100°F, P 88, R 18, and BP 134/90
Cardiovascular: JVP not elevated; normal S_1 and S_2; regular rate and rhythm, no significant murmur, rub, or gallop; carotids 2+ without bruits
Lung sounds: clear
Bowel sounds: hypoactive in all four quadrants; abdomen is tense
HEENT: scleras anicteric, oropharynx clear
Neck: supple, no lymphadenopathy
Lungs: clear to auscultation bilaterally
Extremities: no edema
Neurological: normal, alert, and oriented × 3
CXR: normal
ECG: normal sinus rhythm with bundle branch block

Admitting Medical Orders

Diagnosis: cancer of the prostate; prostatectomy
Surgery/urology service
Admit to surgical floor
No known allergies
Vital signs and oxygen saturation q4h
Call house officer: pulse < 60–>130/minute; BP < 90–> 160 systolic; temperature > 38.5; urine output < 30 mL/hour × 2 hours, respiratory rate > 30/minute; oxygen saturation < 92%, blood sugar > 120
IV: D5W/2NS at 100 mL/hr
Clear liquids post nausea; advance to regular diet as tolerated
Ambulate qid beginning postoperative day 1
Sterile dressing change daily and prn beginning postoperative day 1
Three way indwelling catheter with continuous sterile NS bladder irrigation to maintain pink urine

Fingerstick glucose ac and at bedtime beginning on postoperative day 1
I&O q8h
Incentive spirometer q2h during the day and q4h at night
Sequential compression devices (SCDs) to lower extremities

Scheduled Medications

Humalog S_Q sliding scale per patient home routine
Unasyn (ampicillin sodium) 1.5 g IV daily
Avapro 150 mg po daily beginning postoperative day 1

PRN Medications

Demerol 100 mg IM q4h prn pain
Lortab 7.5 mg po q4h prn pain
Phenergan 25 mg IV or IM q4h prn nausea
Tylenol 325–650 mg q4h prn fever and pain, not to exceed 3000 mg per day

Ordered Laboratory Studies

CBC and glucose daily

READ: History of Present Illnesses >> **Laboratory Study Results** >> Critical Thinking Questions

Test	Postoperative Day 1	Postoperative Day 2	Postoperative Day 3
White blood cell count (WBC)	12,000/mm^3	15,000/mm^3	18,000/mm^3
Platelets	410,000/mm^3	380,000/mm^3	378,000/mm^3
Hemoglobin (HGB)	14 g/dL	12 g/dL	10 g/dL
Hematocrit (HCT)	48%	42%	39%

Test	Postoperative Day 1	Postoperative Day 2	Postoperative Day 3
Red blood cells (RBC)	4.92/mm^3	4.2/mm^3	3.5/mm^3
Platelets	298,000 mm^3	308,000 mm^3	310,000 mm^3
Hemoglobin A1c	7.2%	—	—
Serum glucose	114 mg/dL	105 mg/dL	114 mg/dL

Pearson Nursing Student Resources

Log on to **nursing.pearsonhighered.com** *to download forms*

DOCUMENT:

>> Summary of Hospitalization
>> Pathophysiology Form
>> Laboratory Values
>> Laboratory Results Explanation

APPLY:

>> List of Potential Nursing Diagnoses
>> Concept Map
>> Critical Thinking Questions and Concept Map

APPLY: History of Present Illness >> Laboratory Study Results >> **Critical Thinking Questions**

1. Which nursing assessment should take priority for this patient?
   a. Temperature 100°F
   b. Pain
   c. Weakness
   d. Pallor
2. Why should the nurse assess the suprapubic catheter when assessing the patient's pain?
   a. A foreign object in the bladder will cause pain for most men.
   b. If the catheter becomes dislodged, it can cause pain.
   c. Occlusion will trap urine and distend the bladder, causing increased pain.
3. What significance is there to the thick yellow drainage at the suprapubic insertion site?
   a. This is an infection that needs to be reported and treated.
   b. There is no significance to the drainage, but the skin should be protected from the wet dressing.
   c. The drainage is a sign that the catheter is dislodged; notify the health care provider.
4. What impact does the hemoglobin have on the patient's recovery?
   a. No effect
   b. Lower hemoglobin means decreased oxygen to tissues and poor healing
   c. Lower hemoglobin is an indication for increased oral fluids
5. What impact does diabetes have on the patient's recovery?
   a. Diabetes will slow the healing process.
   b. Diabetes will decrease the patient's susceptibility to infection.
   c. Diabetes will have no effect.
6. What significance does the temperature have at this point in the patient's postoperative course?
   a. Temperature of 100°F is always an indication of infection.
   b. This patient's temperature is due to dehydration.
   c. Low-grade fever within 24 hours of surgery is due to trauma and expected.

Answers to Critical Thinking Questions can be found in Appendix D in the Osborn Student Resources at nursing.pearsonhighered.com.

NCLEX® PRACTICE

1. The nurse is caring for a young male patient with an infection of the epididymis. The nurse realizes this infection is most likely the result of:
   1. inflammation from a sports-related injury.
   2. exposure to the mumps.
   3. sexually transmitted infections.
   4. *Escherichia coli* spread from the gastrointestinal tract.
2. A 30-year-old male patient is admitted with complaints of an enlarged scrotum which has become painful in the last 24 hours. Which of the following would the nurse expect to accompany these symptoms?
   1. Urinalysis that is negative for bacteria.
   2. A white blood cell count of 13,000/mm^3.
   3. Negative cultures of penile discharge.
   4. The patient reports that he is afebrile.
3. The nurse working in a urology clinic asks a male patient to complete an American Urological Association (AUA) Symptom Index Tool for the purpose of:
   1. assisting to diagnose sexual dysfunction disorders.
   2. determining risk factors for urinary tract malignancy.
   3. assessing the symptoms associated with incontinence.
   4. quantifying the symptoms of benign prostatic hypertrophy.
4. The nurse is providing care to a male patient with continuous bladder irrigation after a transurethral resection of the prostate (TURP). The care priority for this patient that addresses the goal of decreased bleeding and clot formation would be:
   1. running in 1 liter per hour of irrigation fluid.
   2. securing the catheter to the bedrail to promote drainage.
   3. manually irrigating the catheter several times per shift.
   4. checking the drainage tubing for kinks on a regular basis.
5. The nurse is providing care to a patient recovering from an orchiectomy for testicular cancer. Which of the following nursing diagnoses should the nurse include when planning this patient's care?
   1. *Risk for Infection*
   2. *Altered Mobility*
   3. *Disturbed Body Image*
   4. *Impaired Urinary Elimination*

   NANDA-I © 2012
6. The nurse is discussing the value of screening for prostate cancer with a male patient and his partner. The nurse should include which of the following in this discussion? (select all that apply)
   1. Elevation of PSA levels is the best method of determining the presence of a prostate cancer.
   2. Presence of a normal PSA value indicates that there is no prostate cancer.
   3. Combining PSA with DRE increases the chance that prostate cancer will be identified.
   4. U.S. prostate cancer deaths have decreased since PSA has been used as a screening tool
   5. A patient with an elevated PSA will require surgical intervention for prostate cancer.

Answers to NCLEX Practice Questions can be found in Appendix D in the Osborn Student Resources at nursing.pearsonhighered.com. Practice additional NCLEX questions online at the Student Resources site.

Pearson Nursing Student Resources Find additional review materials at: **nursing.pearsonhighered.com**

REFERENCES

Adams, M., & Koch, R. (2010). *Pharmacology: Connections to nursing practice.* Upper Saddle River, NJ: Pearson.

Albaugh, J. (2010). Addressing and managing erectile dysfunction after prostatectomy for prostate cancer. *Urologic Nursing, 30*(3), 167–178.

American Cancer Society (ACS). (2010a). FDA approves prostate cancer vaccine. *Learn About Cancer.* Retrieved from http://www.cancer.org/Cancer/news/News/fda-approves-prostate-cancer-vaccine

American Cancer Society (ACS). (2010b). Penile cancer. *Learn About Cancer.* Retrieved from http://www.cancer.org/Cancer/PenileCancer/DetailedGuide/index

American Cancer Society (ACS). (2010c). Penile cancer: What are the causes? *Learn About Cancer.* Retrieved from http://www.cancer.org/Cancer/PenileCancer/DetailedGuide/penile-cancer-what-causes

American Cancer Society (ACS). (2010d). Penile cancer: What are the penile cancer risk factors? *Learn About Cancer.* Retrieved from http://www.cancer.org/Cancer/PenileCancer/DetailedGuide/penile-cancer-risk-factors

American Cancer Society (ACS). (2010e). Prostate cancer. *Learn About Cancer.* Retrieved from http://www.cancer.org/Cancer/ProstateCancer/DetailedGuide/prostate-cancer-key-statistics

American Cancer Society (ACS). (2010f). Prostate cancer: Can prostate cancer be found early? *Learn About Cancer.* Retrieved from http://www.cancer.org/Cancer/ProstateCancer/DetailedGuide/prostate-cancer-detection

Anawalt, B. (2010). Male reproductive endocrinology: Introduction. *Merck Manuals Online Medical Library.* Retrieved from http://www.merckmedicus.com/pp/us/hcp/framemm.jsp?pg=www.merck.com/mmpe/index.html

Andriole, G. (2010). Benign prostatic hyperplasia. *Merck Manuals Online Medical Library.* Retrieved from http://www.merckmedicus.com/pp/us/hcp/framemm.jsp?pg=www.merck.com/mmpe/index.html

Armenakas, N. (2010). Genital trauma. *Merck Manuals Online Medical Library.* Retrieved from http://www.merck.com/mmpe/sec21/ch314/ch314c.html

Brown, M. (2010). Prostate cancer: How assessment of QOL can improve delivery of care. *British Journal of Nursing, 19*(17), 1080–1084.

Burke, N., Whelan, P., Goeree, L., Hopkins, R., Campbell, K., Goeree, R., & Tarride, J. (2011). Systematic review and meta-analysis of transurethral resection of the prostate versus minimally invasive procedures for the treatment of benign prostatic obstruction. *Urology, 185*(3), 1019–1027.

Cherian, J., Rao, A., Thwaini, F., Shergill, I., and Samman, R. (2006). Medical and surgical management of priapism. *Postgraduate Medical Journal, 82*(964), 89–94.

Davis, C., & Nettleman, M. (2011). Epididymitis. eMedicinehealth. Retrieved from http://www.emedicinehealth.com/testicle_infection_epididymitis/article_em.htm

DeCuir, D., Wicks, M., & Rice, M. (2009). The health of African-American men. *The American Journal for Nurse Practitioners, 13*(11/12), 34–39.

Deneris, A., & Huether, S. (2010). Structure and function of the reproductive systems. In K. McCance & S. Huether (Eds.), *Pathophysiology: The biologic basis for disease in adults and children* (6th ed., pp. 781–815). St. Louis: Mosby/Elsevier.

Djavan, B., Eckersberger, E., Finkelstein, J., Sadri, H., Taneja, S., & Lepor, H. (2010). Prostate-specific antigen testing and prostate cancer screening. *Primary Care Clinical Office Practice, 37*(3), 441–459. doi:10.1016/j.pop.2010.05.001

Dougherty, C. M., Richard, A. J., & Carey, M. J. (2009a). Priapism. eMedicine from WebMD. Retrieved from http://emedicine.medscape.com/article/777603-overview

Dougherty, C. M., Richard, A. J., & Carey, M. J. (2009b). Priapism: Treatment & medication. eMedicine from WebMD. Retrieved from http://emedicine.medscape.com/article/777603-treatment

DynaMed Editorial Team. (2010). Benign prostatic hyperplasia. Retrieved from http://dynaweb.ebscohost.com.ezproxy.midwives.org/Detail?id=AN+116944&sid=6320bb2f-84c5-4112-86ab-b48193bef747@sessionmgr12

Evertsen, J., & Wolkenstin, A. (2010). Female partners of patients after surgical prostate cancer treatment: Interactions with physicians and support needs. *BMC Family Practice, 11*(19), 1–6. doi:10.1186./1471-2296-11-19

Ferri, F. (2009). Prostatic hyperplasia, benign. In F. Ferri, *Ferri's clinical advisor: Instant diagnosis and treatment. MerckMedicus.* Retrieved from http://www.merckmedicus.com/pp/us/hcp/thcp_ferri_content.jsp?pg=/ppdocs/us/hcp/content/ferri/B9780323056090000253/ferri-815F.htm

Ferri, F., & Wachtel, T. (2010). Hydrocele. In F. Ferri, *Ferri's clinical advisor: Instant diagnosis and treatment.* St. Louis: Mosby/Elsevier.

Gaines, K. (2010). Controversies in prostate cancer screening and treatment. *Urologic Nursing, 30*(3), 165–166.

Guido, G., & Watson, A. (2010). Ethical and legal guidelines for nursing practice. In K. Osborn, C. Wraa, & A. Watson (Eds.), *Medical-surgical nursing: Preparation for practice.* Boston: Pearson.

Halbert, C., Coyne, J., Weathers, B., Mahler, B., Delmoor, E., Vaughn, D. (2010). Racial differences in quality of life following prostate cancer diagnosis. *Urology, 76*(3), 559–564. doi: 10.1016/j.urology.2009.09.090

Hamilton, J., Stewart, B., Crandell, J., & Lynn, M. (2009). Development of the ways of helping questionnaire: A measure of preferred coping strategies for older African-American cancer survivors. *Research in Nursing & Health, 32*(3), 243–259. doi:10.1002/nur.20321

Harrison's Practice: Answers on demand. (2010). Testicular cancer. Merck Medicus. Retrieved from http://www.unboundmedicine.com/hpmerck/ub/view/Harrisons_Practice/Testicular_Cancer/141203/1

Hedayati, T., & Stehman, C. (2011). Prostatitis. eMedicine. Retrieved from http://emedicine.medscape.com/article/785418-overview

Holt, C., Wynn, T., Litaker, M., Southward, P., Jeames, S., & Schulz, E. (2009). A comparison of a spiritually based and non-spiritually based education intervention for informed decision making for prostate cancer screening among church-attending African-American men. *Urologic Nursing, 29*(4), 249–258.

Huether, S. (2010b). The cellular environment: Fluids and electrolytes, acids and bases. In K. McCance & S. Huether (Eds.), *Pathophysiology: The biologic basis for disease in adults and children* (6th ed., pp. 96–125). St. Louis: Mosby/Elsevier.

Ilic, D., Misso, M., & Wilt, T. (2009). Screening for testicular cancer. *Cochrane Database of Systemic Reviews, 3*(CD007853). doi: 10.1002/14651858.CD007853

IOM (Institute of Medicine). (2010). *The future of nursing: Leading change, advancing health.* Washington, DC: The Academic Press.

Kamel, R. (2010). Management of the infertile couple: An evidence-based protocol. *Reproductive Biology and Endocrinology, 8*(21), 1–7. Retrieved from http://www.rbej.com/content/8/1/21

Kee, J. (2010). *Laboratory and diagnostic tests* (8th ed.). Upper Saddle River, NJ: Pearson.

Laborde, E., & Brannigan, R. (2010). Androgen deficiency in the aging male: The tip of the iceberg? *Urology Times, 38*(5), 44–46.

Latendresse, G., McCance, K., & Morgan, K. (2010). Alterations of the reproductive systems. In K. McCance & S. Huether (Eds.), *Pathophysiology: The biologic basis for disease in adults and children* (6th ed., pp. 781–815). St. Louis: Mosby/Elsevier.

Lexi-Comp. (2010). Testosterone. *Merck Manuals Online Library.* Retrieved from http://www.merck.com/mmpe/lexicomp/testosterone.html#N1B826F

Male hypogonadism. (2010). Sexual dysfunction in men. In *The Merck manual of geriatrics* (chapter 115). Retrieved from http://www.merck.com/mkgr/mmg/sec14/ch115/ch115c.jsp

Meng, M., Stoller, M., & Walsh, T. (2010). Urologic disorders. In S. McPhee & M. Papadakis (Eds.), *Lange current medical diagnosis and treatment* (4th ed., pp. 850–871). New York: McGraw-Hill.

Morgan, M. (2009). Considering the patient-partner relationship in cancer care: Coping strategies for couples. *Clinical Journal of Oncology Nursing, 13*(1), 65–73.

Nash, J. (2010). Benign prostatic hyperplasia: Risk factors and management. *Midlife and Beyond, 40*(7), 364–368.

National Cancer Institute (NCI). (2010a). Genetics of prostate cancer (PDQ). Retrieved from http://www.cancer.gov/cancertopics/pdq/genetics/prostate/healthprofessional

National Cancer Institute (NCI). (2010b). Penile cancer treatment (PDQ). Retrieved from http://www.cancer.gov/cancertopics/pdq/treatment/penile/healthprofessional

National Cancer Institute (NCI). (2010c). Prostate cancer. Retrieved from http://www.cancer.gov/cancertopics/types/prostate

National Cancer Institute (NCI). (2010d). Testicular cancer. Retrieved from http://www.cancer.gov/cancertopics/types/testicular/

National Comprehensive Cancer Network (NCCN). (2010). Practice guidelines in oncology–v.3.2010 Prostate cancer. Retrieved from http://www.nccn.org/professionals/physician_gls/PDF/prostate.pdf

Neal, R., & Keister, D. (2009). What's best for your patient with BPH? *The Journal of Family Practice, 58*(5), 241–248.

Nelson, A., & Marshall, J. (2009). Impaired fertility. In R. Hatcher et al. (Eds.), *Contraceptive technology.* New York: Ardent Media, Inc.

Nowak, B., & Patacsil-Trull, T. (2010). Varicocele. In F. Ferri, *Ferri's clinical advisor: Instant diagnosis and treatment* (p. 1065). St. Louis: Mosby/Elsevier.

O'Leary, M. (2009, June). By the way, Doctor: Will Levitra overcome the problems caused by finateride? *Harvard Health Letter,* p. 8.

Pais, P. (2010). Potency of a novel saw palmetto ethanol extract, SPET-085, for inhibition of 5alpha-reductase II. *Advances in Therapy, 27*(8), 555–563. Epub 2010 Jul 10.

Paolone, D. (2010). Benign prostatic hyperplasia. *Clinical Geriatric Medicine, 26*(2), 223–239. doi: 10.1016/j.cger.2010.02.010

Peate, I. (2009). Understanding the impact of ageing on male sexuality. *Nursing & Residential Care, 11*(10), 512–516.

Pollack, A., Thomas, L., & Barone, M. (2009). Female and male sterilization. In R. Hatcher et al. (Eds.), *Contraceptive technology* (19th ed., pp. 361–401). New York: Ardent Media, Inc.

Polt, C. (2009). Critical care: Getting to the root of testicular pain. *Nursing, 39*(6), 56cc7–11.

Ramakrishnan, K., & Salinas, R. (2010). Prostatitis: Acute and chronic. *Primary Care Clinical Office Practice, 37*(3), 547–563. doi:10.1016/j.pop.2010.04.007

Schmitz, D., & Safranek, S. (2009). How useful is a physical examination in diagnosing testicular torsion? *The Journal of Family Practice, 58*(8), 433–434.

Shandera, W., & Corrales-Medina, V. (2008). Viral and rickettsial infections. In S. McPhee & M. Papadakis (Eds.), *Lange 2009 Current medical diagnosis and treatment* (48th ed., New York pp. 1205–1255).

Sharp, V., Takacs, E., & Powell, C. (2010). Prostatitis: Diagnosis and treatment. *American Family Physician, 82*(4), 397–406.

Stroller, M., Kane, C., & Meng, M. (2008). Urologic disorders. In S. McPhee & M. Papadakis (Eds.), *2009 Current medical diagnosis and treatment* (48th ed., pp. 827–847). New York: McGraw-Hill/Lange.

Swanson, D. (2010). Prostate cancer. *Merck Manuals Online Medical Library.* Retrieved from http://www.merckmedicus.com/pp/us/hcp/framemm.jsp?pg=www.merck.com/mmpe/index.html

Trojian, T., Lishnak, T., & Heiman, D. (2009). Epididymitis and orchitis: An overview. *American Family Physician, 79*(7), 583–587.

Virshup, D. (2010). Biology, clinical manifestations, and treatment of cancer. In K. McCance & S. Huether (Eds.), *Pathophysiology: The biologic basis for disease in adults and children* (6th ed., pp. 360–395). St. Louis: Mosby/Elsevier.

Wagenlehner, F. M., Schneider, H., Ludwig, M., Schnitker, J., Brähler, E., & Weidner, W. (2009). A pollen extract (Cernilton) in patients with inflammatory chronic prostatitis-chronic pelvic pain syndrome: A multicentre, randomised, prospective, double-blind, placebo-controlled phase 3 study. *European Urology, 56*(3), 544–551. Epub 2009 Jun 3.

Wallace, M., Bailey, D., & Brion, J. (2009). Shedding light on prostate cancer. *The Nurse Practitioner, 34*(10), 25–33.

Wampler, S., & Llanes, M. (2010). Common scrotal and testicular problems. *Primary Care Clinical Office Practice, 37*(3), 613–626. doi:10.1016/j.pop.2010.04.009

Wan, J., & Rew, K. (2010). Common penile problems. *Primary Care: Clinics in Office Practice, 37*(3):627–642. doi: 10.1016/j.pop.2010.04.010.

Ward, J., & Jones, S. (2010). Classification system: Organ preserving treatment for prostate cancer. *Urology, 75*(6), 1258–1260. doi:10.1016/j.urology.2009.10.044

White, W., & Kim, E. (2011). Varicocele: Follow-up. eMedicine. Retrieved from http://emedicine.medscape.com/article/438591-followup

Wilkinson, J. M., & Ahearn, N. R. (2009). *Prentice Hall nursing diagnosis handbook* (9th ed.). Upper Saddle River, NJ: Prentice Hall.

Winter, T. (2009). There is a mass in the scrotum—what does it mean? *Ultrasound Quarterly, 25*(4), 195–205.

CHAPTER

43 Caring for the Patient with Sexually Transmitted Infections

Patricia Caudle
Kathleen Osborn

Outcome-Based Learning Objectives

After studying this chapter, the learner will be able to:

1. Differentiate the cause, mode of transmission, prevention, and treatment of sexually transmitted infections.
2. Generate nursing diagnoses specific to individual patients who present with sexually transmitted infections.
3. Design nursing care plans specific to individual patients with sexually transmitted infections.
4. Plan interventions that will enhance health education, health promotion, and prevention of sexually transmitted infections.
5. Determine outcome goals for nursing care and medical treatment for sexually transmitted infections.

KEY TERMS

bacterial vaginosis (BV) p.1319
buboes p.1319
chancre p.1317
chancroid p.1319
chlamydia p.1313
chorioamnionitis p.1319
condylomata acuminata p.1323
condylomata lata p.1318
diplococcus p.1315
endometritis p.1319
genital warts p.1323
gonorrhea p.1315
gummas p.1318
herpes simplex p.1312
human papillomavirus (HPV) p.1312
incubation period p.1315
juvenile-onset recurrent respiratory papillomatosis (JORRP) p.1323
lymphogranuloma venereum (LGV) p.1314
ophthalmia neonatorum p.1316
pelvic inflammatory disease (PID) p.1316
receptive sex p.1313
salpingitis p.1316
syphilis p.1317
trichomoniasis p.1325
vesicle p.1322

Weblink: List of STIs

SEXUALLY TRANSMITTED INFECTIONS (STIs) are transmitted via intimate body contact with another person and may be present without causing any obvious symptoms. An older term, *sexually transmitted diseases (STDs)*, is used to denote STIs that produce medical problems or that may be incurable (American Social Health Association [ASHA], 2010). Many resources will discuss STI/STD concurrently. However, the World Health Organization (WHO) refers to STIs only. The WHO has determined that there are more than 30 infections that may be passed during heterosexual or homosexual relations or close physical contact. In addition, several STIs may be passed from mother to child during pregnancy and birth (WHO, 2010b). Chart 43–1 lists diseases that are considered STIs by the Centers for Disease Control and Prevention (CDC).

CHART 43–1 List of Sexually Transmitted Infections and Related Conditions

Bacterial vaginosis	Chlamydia
Gonorrhea	Hepatitis
Herpes, genital	HIV/AIDS
Human papillomavirus (HPV)	Pelvic inflammatory disease (PID)
Syphilis	Trichomoniasis
Chancroid	Lymphogranuloma venereum (LGV)
Pubic lice infestation	Scabies

Source: Adapted from Centers for Disease Control and Prevention. (2010c). Sexually transmitted disease. Retrieved from http://www.cdc.gov/std/.

Public Health Concerns

STIs are a major public health problem, yet their occurrence is considered underreported. Currently, the CDC only requires that health care providers report incidences of chlamydia, gonorrhea, and syphilis. However, these three infections make up but a small part of the health burden of STIs. For instance, viruses such as **herpes simplex** and **human papillomavirus (HPV),** which need not be reported, have very high incidence rates. The CDC estimates that there are about 19 million new STI cases each year. The estimated cost of these infections is $16.4 million annually, not counting the costs of any complications or

Weblink: STI Prevention Weblink: Trends in STIs

CULTURAL CONSIDERATIONS for Sexually Transmitted Infections

- Racial groups with the highest burden of sexually transmitted disease are Blacks and Hispanics.
- Contributing factors are poverty, lack of access to good health care, high prevalence of STIs in communities, fewer attempts to seek medical care, stigma, and homophobia.
- Sexually active Black adolescent and young adult women are more likely to be infected than other populations.

Sources: Adapted from Centers for Disease Control and Prevention. (2010r). 2009 Sexually transmitted diseases surveillance/Trends in sexually transmitted disease in the United States: 2009 National data for gonorrhea, chlamydia, & syphilis. Retrieved from http://www.cdc.gov/std/stats09/trends.htm; U.S. Department of Health and Human Services. (2010). Sexually transmitted disease. HealthyPeople.gov. Retrieved from http://www.healthypeople.gov/2020/topicsobjectives2020/overview.aspx?topicid=37.

long-term sequelae of these diseases (CDC, 2010r). In addition, STIs increase the patient's risks for HIV infection and transmission, discussed later in this chapter.

As of 2009, there was evidence that some progress was being made in decreasing the spread of STIs. For example, gonorrhea infection rates were the lowest ever recorded. Likewise, syphilis cases among women and congenital syphilis (infection of an unborn child or newborn) had not increased for the last 4 years (CDC, 2010r). Despite this positive news, CDC surveillance data continued to show that Blacks and Hispanics had a much higher incidence of STIs than was found in Whites. The Cultural Considerations box discusses the STI burden among racial groups. Risk factors for STIs are listed in the Risk Factors box.

Women are disproportionately affected by STIs because of **receptive sex** (receiving semen orally, vaginally, or via the rectum), increased risk for infertility, and pregnancy. Each year about 24,000 women become infertile due to an STI (CDC, 2010r). Young women ages 14 to 25 are particularly vulnerable because the transformational zone and columnar cells of the cervical os are vulnerable to any organisms that may enter the vagina. (See Chapter 41 for the anatomy of the cervix.) From the cervix, infectious organisms can ascend into the upper genital tract and cause scarring of the fallopian tubes, leading to infertility. Many STIs can be passed from mother to fetus via the placenta or through direct contact with infected vaginal fluids during the birth process (WHO, 2010b).

Diagnosis is difficult with many STIs because the patient may be asymptomatic or the infection may mimic so many other diseases. In addition, treatment, even if it is correct, will not prevent re-infection.

RISK FACTORS for Sexually Transmitted Infections

- New sexual partner and/or multiple sexual partners
- Sex with a person who has sex with other persons
- Use of prostitutes or sex workers
- Exchange of sex for money or drugs
- Poverty or low socioeconomic status
- Participating in vaginal, anal, or oral sex
- Douching
- Young female under the age of 25
- Alcohol or drug use that leads to risky sexual behavior.

Source: Adapted from the CDC STD fact sheets. Retrieved from http://www.cdc.gov/std/.

All sexual partners and their partners must be examined and treated to prevent further spread of the condition. The sensitive nature of STIs also leads to situations charged with anger, anxiety, fear, shame, and guilt.

One of the 41 focus areas in *Healthy People 2020* is reducing or preventing sexually transmitted infections. Specifically, the goals of this focus area are promoting responsible sexual behavior, strengthening community capacity, and increasing access to high-quality services in an attempt to prevent STIs and their complications. The government recognizes that social, cultural, and behavioral factors play a role in the spread of these infections and that access to health care is critical to preventing the spread of disease. Interventions that have been suggested to meet the objectives include clinical recommendations such as:

- Increased screening of populations at risk
- Community intervention in the form of education and risk reduction programs
- The provision of consumer information.

Further information about the goals and objectives for STI prevention from the U.S. Department of Health and Human Services can be obtained at this website: www.healthypeople.gov/2020/topicsobjectives2020/overview.aspx?topicid=37.

Sexually Transmitted Infection Caused by Bacteria

The STIs caused by bacteria that we discuss in this chapter include chlamydia, gonorrhea, pelvic inflammatory disease (PID), syphilis, bacterial vaginosis, and chancroid. Chlamydia, gonorrhea, and syphilis are the most prevalent STIs in the United States, affecting thousands of individuals. Many people who are infected are asymptomatic. All three infections are highly contagious but, at the same time, are easily cured with antibiotics (Workowski & Berman, 2010).

Chlamydia

Description and Epidemiology

According to the CDC, chlamydia is the most frequently reported communicable disease (2010e; 2010k). In 2009, there were 1,244,180 reported cases of chlamydia, or 409 cases per 100,000 persons in the United States (CDC, 2010p). Chlamydia is one of the leading causes of preventable infertility and ectopic pregnancy (pregnancy that occurs outside the uterus) (Voelker, 2010). In a study conducted by Tu, Batteiger, Wiehe, and colleagues (2009), approximately 50% of teenage girls living in urban areas contracted chlamydia within 2 years of becoming sexually active. In fact, by age 15, about 25% of women have been diagnosed with an STI, most commonly chlamydia (STD Quarterly, 2010). Black people accounted for 48% of all reported chlamydia cases in 2009. This represents a rate that is 8 times higher than that in Whites and 3 times higher than that in Hispanics (CDC, 2010r). See Figure 43–1◆.

Etiology

Chlamydia is a sexually transmitted infection caused by *Chlamydia trachomatis*, a highly contagious bacterium that causes urethritis, nongonococcal urethritis, mucopurulent cervicitis, PID, and chronic pelvic pain (Jenkins & Kruse, 2010). It is transmitted via secretions contacted during vaginal, anal, and oral sex (CDC, 2010e).

Pathophysiology

C. trachomatis is an intracellular bacterium that uses the host cell to replicate (Kaloczi, Latendresse, & Morgan, 2010). It prefers the epithelial

Video: Gonorrhea

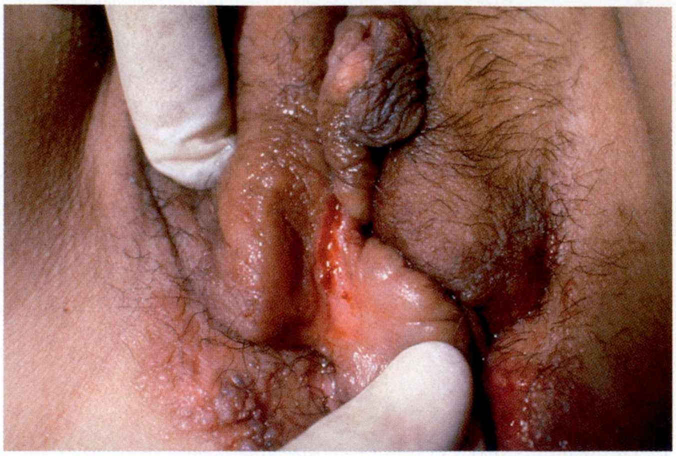

FIGURE 43–1 ◆ Chlamydia graphic from CDC.

Source: Courtesy, Director-General and Programme Manager Prevention of Blindness, World Health Organization.

cells of the mucosa of the urethra, cervix, epididymis, fallopian tubes, and hepatic capsule and, in the case of the newborn, the eyes, nasopharynx, lungs, rectum, and vagina. Infection with this organism will result in an inflammatory reaction that will cause permanent scarring. The untreated acute phase may progress to an asymptomatic chronic infection that may last for years (Kaloczi et al., 2010).

There are several forms of *C. trachomatis* including a strain that causes **lymphogranuloma venereum (LVG),** an STI that is more prevalent in Asian and African countries (Kaloczi et al., 2010). This strain of the chlamydia bacteria causes a skin lesion and spreads to lymphatic tissue, where it may cause inflammation and, eventually, abscesses of the inguinal lymph nodes.

Another strain of this organism will cause ocular trachoma. Ocular trachoma is an infectious disease of the upper eyelid and cornea that, if left untreated, will cause blindness due to corneal scarring and clouding (WHO, 2010a). This form of *C. trachomatis* occurs in developing countries and is rare in the United States.

Clinical Manifestations

Chlamydia is often asymptomatic in both women and men. When it is symptomatic, symptoms show up in 1 to 3 weeks after exposure (CDC, 2010e). The symptoms of an acute infection include dysuria, clear urethral discharge in men, and discharge that stains underwear and bedding. In men, the epididymis may become infected, causing scrotal pain, swelling, and fever. Infections of the rectum will cause rectal bleeding, mucous discharge from the anus, and occasionally diarrhea. In women, cervical edema, beefy red cervix, cervical motion tenderness, *friability* (damaged and bleeds easily), and profuse yellow discharge are evident. Figure 43–2◆ depicts the erythematous, friable cervix with yellow discharge. *C. trachomatis* may infect the Bartholin glands, causing purulent drainage and painful cyst formation. *C. trachomatis* also may be transmitted to the fallopian tube via sperm or uterine contractions. The scarring that develops as a result may cause PID, tubal infertility, or ectopic pregnancy (Kaloczi et al., 2010).

Reiter syndrome, a reactive arthritis, is a complication of untreated chlamydia infection that occurs most often in men. Signs and symptoms include urethritis, conjunctivitis, arthritis, and mucocutaneous lesions (Kaloczi et al., 2010).

Babies born to mothers who are infected with chlamydia may develop conjunctivitis and pneumonia. Chlamydial conjunctivitis will manifest as watery eyes at about 5 to 14 days after birth. Without treatment, this infection will progress to purulent discharge and red, swollen eyes. This form of conjunctivitis will not cause blindness (CDC, 2010a). Chlamydia pneumonia may be mild or severe and develops in 3 to 11 weeks after birth. Symptoms may include staccato cough, nasal congestion, dyspnea, and mild fever for mild cases. For severe cases, tachypnea, wheezing, bronchospasm, and periodic apnea are seen (Kaloczi et al., 2010).

Laboratory Tests

Several diagnostic tests are available to identify *C. trachomatis* in body fluid or urine. The most sensitive test for this organism is the nucleic acid amplification test (NAAT) (Healthwise Staff, 2009a). An example of a NAAT is the polymerase chain reaction test (PCR). Another important test is the nucleic acid hybridization test or DNA probe test. See the Diagnostic Tests box. The Evidence-Based Practice box discusses controversy related to testing for chlamydia.

Gonorrhea

Description and Epidemiology

Gonorrhea is the second most frequently reported STI in the United States (CDC, 2010l). Like chlamydia, gonorrhea can cause PID with complications such as tubal infertility, ectopic pregnancy, and chronic pelvic pain. A pregnant woman infected with gonorrhea may pass it to her baby during pregnancy, or it can be transmitted via scalp electrodes or during the birth process (Kaloczi et al., 2010).

In 2009, 301,174 cases of gonorrhea were reported, or 99.1 cases per 100,000 persons (CDC, 2010p). This was a decrease in reported cases compared to 2008. The Southern states, especially large cities in the South, continue to have the highest rate of reported cases of gonorrhea. Unlike chlamydia, gonorrhea affects more men than women. Gonorrhea rates are highest among the Black populaton (CDC, 2010l). In fact,

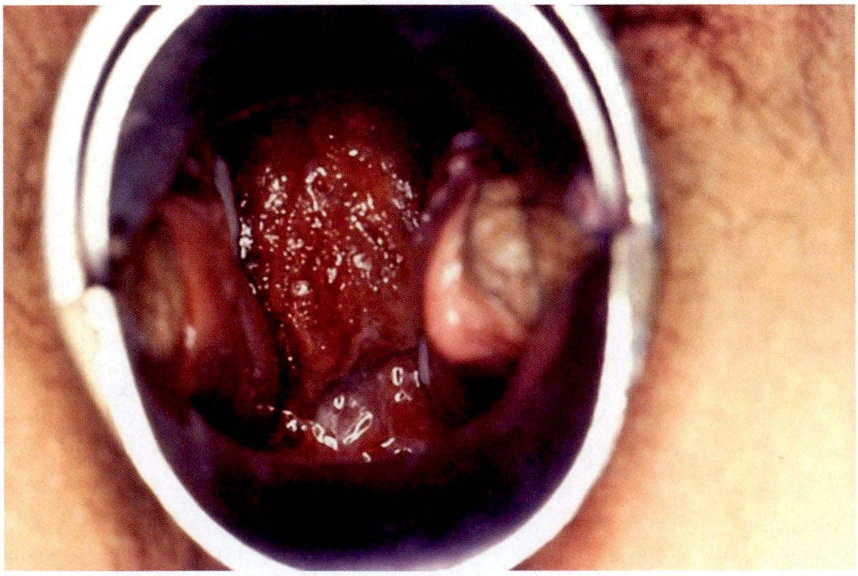

FIGURE 43–2 ◆ Chlamydia infection of the cervix.

Source: CDC/ Dr. Lourdes Fraw, Jim Pledger.

DIAGNOSTIC TESTS for Sexually Transmitted Infections

Test with Normal Values	Expected Abnormality
Tests for Chlamydia and Gonorrhea	
Nucleic acid amplification test (e.g., polymerase chain reaction [PCR] test). Should be negative.	Detection of genetic material of *Chlamydia trachomatis* or *Neisseria gonorrhoeae* bacteria in cervical cells, urethral cells, or urine.
Nucleic acid hybridization test (DNA probe). Negative.	Detection of genetic material (DNA) of *Chlamydia trachomatis* or *Neisseria gonorrhoeae* bacteria in urethral or cervical cells.
Tests for Syphilis	
Dark field microscopic exam of exudates from chancre.	Identification of *Treponema pallidum* spirochete—definitive diagnosis of syphilis.
Nontreponemal tests	Not definitive—need confirmation test for syphilis.
RPR	Confirms syphilis diagnosis.
VDRL	
Treponemal tests	
FTA-ABS	
MHA-TP	
Tests for Herpes and HPV	
Polymerase chain reaction (PCR) test for herpes. Should be negative.	Detection of herpes DNA from the lesion. Infection by herpes simplex type 1 or type 2.
Serologic type-specific herpes testing. Should be negative.	Detection of type 1 and type 2 herpes simplex. Very specific.
HCII HPV test, HCII Low-risk HPV test, Cervista HPV 16/18 test—should be negative.	Human papillomavirus infection—low-risk types and high-risk types 16 and 18. No one test will identify all types that cause cancer.
Papanicolaou test (Pap test). Should be negative.	Tests for cervical changes consistent with HPV infection, hyperplasia, and cancer of the cervix.

Sources: Adapted from Healthwise Staff. (2009a). Chlamydia tests. Quest Diagnostics. Retrieved from http://www.questdiagnostics.com/kbase/topic/medtest/hw4046/descrip.htm; Healthwise Staff. (2009b). Gonorrhea tests. Quest Diagnostics. Retrieved from http://www.questdiagnostics.com/kbase/topic/medtest/hw4905/descrip.htm; Kee, J. (2010). *Laboratory and diagnostic tests* (8th ed.). Upper Saddle River, NJ: Pearson; Workowski, K. & Berman, S. (2010). Sexually transmitted disease treatment guidelines, 2010. *Morbidity and Mortality Weekly Report, 59*(RR12), 1–110.

EVIDENCE-BASED PRACTICE Screening for Chlamydia

Clinical Problem

Chlamydia infections are the most common sexually transmitted disease in the United States. The highest risk is for sexually active individuals (PubMed, 2010).

Research Findings

The CDC currently recommends that all young women be screened for chlamydia annually because untreated chlamydia can lead to PID, tubal infertility, or ectopic pregnancy. A recent study, however, demonstrated that as many as 50% of adolescent girls who were treated for chlamydia had another chlamydia infection within a year. The study also determined, using genotyping, that 84% of these repeated infections were caused by the same organism (Batteiger et al., 2010).

Voelker (2010) and Batteiger et al. (2010) suggest that these findings indicate a need to screen young men. However, the U.S. Preventive Services Task Force (USPSTF) has concluded that current evidence does not support screening adolescent and young adult men (USPSTF, 2007). Both the CDC and USPSTF do recommend that all persons who are infected with chlamydia return to their health care provider in 3 months to be tested for re-infection.

Implications for Nursing Practice

Nurses are in a pivotal position to educate and encourage high-risk individuals to get tested and treated for chlamydia infections.

Critical Thinking Questions with answers can be found in the Osborn Student Resources at nursing.pearsonhighered.com.

Sources: Adapted from Batteiger, B., Tu, W., Ofner, S., Van Der Pol, B., Stothard, D., Orr, D., et al. (2010). Repeated *Chlamydia trachomatis* genital infections in adolescent women. *The Journal of Infectious Diseases, 201*(1), 42–51; U.S. Preventive Services Task Force (USPSTF). (2007). Screening for chlamydia infection. Retrieved from http://www.uspreventiveservicestaskforce.org/uspstf/uspschlm.htm; Voelker, R. (2010). Experts reconsider wisdom of limiting chlamydia screening only to women. *Journal of American Medical Association, 303*(9), 823–824.

Black people accounted for 71% of all gonorrhea cases in 2009, even though they comprise only 14% of the U.S. population. This rate is 20 times higher in Blacks than in Caucasians and 10 times higher than in Hispanics (CDC, 2010r). Figure 43–3◆ provides a graphic representation of cases in the United States.

Pathophysiology

Gonorrhea is a sexually transmitted infection caused by *Neisseria gonorrhoeae*, an anaerobic gonococcus. *N. gonorrhoeae* is a gram-negative, round bacteria that occurs in pairs. The **diplococcus** (paired bacteria) attaches to epithelial cells, then invades and destroys the cells. Humans are the only natural hosts (Kaloczi et al., 2010). The **incubation period** (time from exposure to symptoms) in men ranges from 12 hours to 3 months. Women who develop symptoms do so in about 10 days or within 1 to 2 days of menses (Kaloczi et al., 2010). However, about 50% of infected women will be asymptomatic.

Clinical Manifestations

Uncomplicated local gonorrhea in men may be asymptomatic or manifest as urethritis with dysuria and profuse mucopurulent discharge during the acute phase (CDC, 2010g). If left untreated, symptomatic gonorrhea will become asymptomatic after about 3 months (Kaloczi et al., 2010). Figure 43–4◆ shows how profuse the discharge may be from the urethra.

Women may be asymptomatic or may experience dysuria, increased vaginal discharge, abnormal periods, or painful intercourse (CDC, 2010g). The infection may mimic a bladder or vaginal infection. Examination of the cervix will reveal erythema, friability, cervical motion tenderness, and purulent cervical discharge. The Skene and

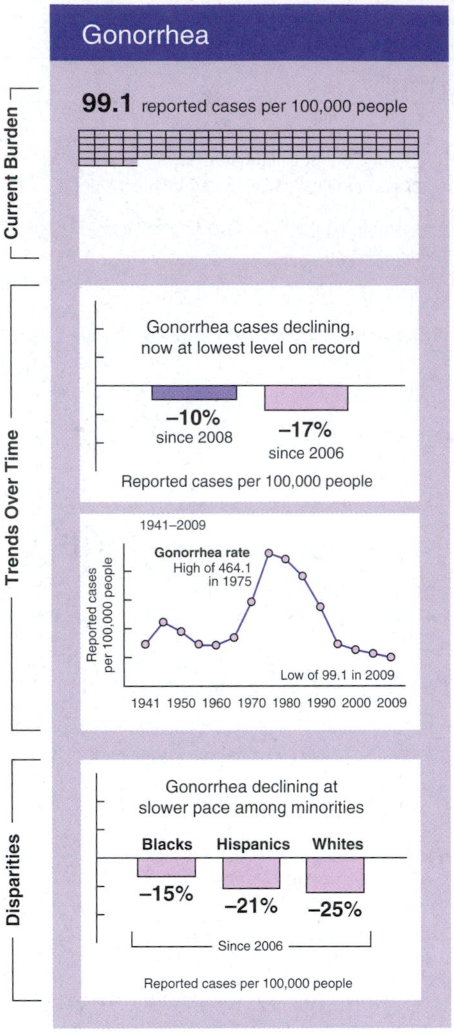

FIGURE 43–3 ◆ Gonorrhea graphic from CDC.

Source: Sexually Transmitted Disease Surveillance 2009. Available at www.cdc.gov/std/stats/.

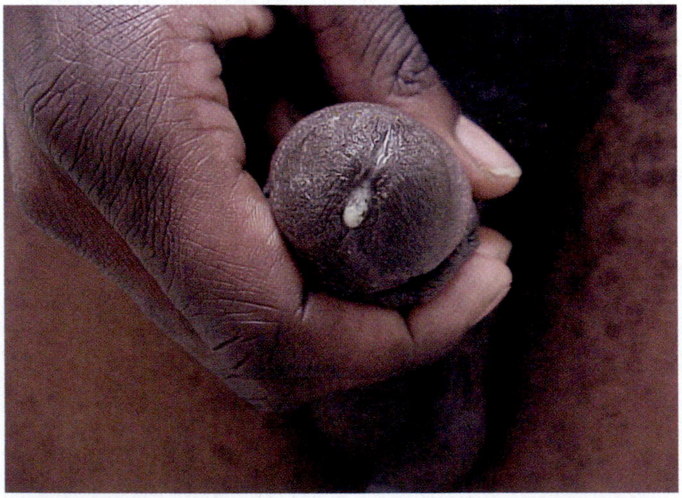

FIGURE 43–4 ◆ Penile discharge, gonorrhea.

Source: Cincinnati STD/HIV Prevention Training Center/CDC.

Bartholin gland ducts may also drain pus (Kaloczi et al., 2010). Refer to Chapter 40 for a review of the anatomy and pelvic examination.

N. gonorrhoeae may infect the anal and rectal areas of women who have a cervical infection with or without anal intercourse. However, it is more likely to occur in homosexual men after receptive anal intercourse (Kaloczi et al., 2010). The anorectal infection may cause itching, mucopurulent rectal discharge, rectal bleeding, soreness, and pain with defecation; it may also be asymptomatic (CDC, 2010g).

The throat may be infected with gonorrhea after oral–genital sex. Symptoms, if present, will mimic strep throat and include fever, cervical lymph node swelling, and tonsillitis (CDC, 2010g).

Complications of gonorrhea include prostatitis, epididymitis, urethral stricture, **salpingitis** (infection of the fallopian tubes), PID, and bartholinitis. Approximately 10% of women with untreated gonorrhea will develop PID (Kaloczi et al., 2010).

A rare but very serious complication of *N. gonorrhoeae* infection is disseminated gonococcal infection (NGI). This occurs when gonorrhea enters the bloodstream, and it affects men more often than women (Kaloczi et al., 2010). Signs and symptoms of NGI include fever, rash, joint swelling, and pain (Schwartz & Kapila, 2010).

Newborns of mothers with gonorrhea are at risk for bacterial **ophthalmia neonatorum** (eye infection). Gonococcal eye infection occurs less often than it used to because prophylactic eye ointment is now administered at birth; however, the rate continues to be 1 to 2 per 10,000 births (Caserta, 2009). Symptoms become evident in 2 to 5 days and include eyelid swelling and purulent discharge; if left untreated, ulceration and blindness can occur. These newborns are also at risk for anorectal infection or an abscess if fetal monitoring electrodes have been placed.

Laboratory Tests

Diagnosis of gonorrhea requires more than clinical signs and symptoms because the infection is often asymptomatic. Current testing methods use body fluids or urine. The most sensitive test is the nucleic acid amplification test (NAAT). Also available is the nucleic acid hybridization test (DNA probe), which uses cells collected from the urethra or cervix where the infection has occurred (Healthwise Staff, 2009b) (See the Diagnostic Tests box , p. 1315, for more about these tests.)

Pelvic Inflammatory Disease

Description and Epidemiology

Pelvic inflammatory disease (PID) is a multi-microbial disorder of the uterus, fallopian tubes, and ovaries that may involve any one or all of these organs. It is a common and serious complication of both chlamydia and gonorrhea infections. In fact, 85% of cases of PID are triggered by these STIs, and about 15% follow medical procedures such as hysteroscopy, dilatation and curettage, or intrauterine device placement (Strickland & Gibson, 2009). Many cases of PID go unrecognized and undiagnosed (Workowski & Berman, 2010). In recent years, hospitalizations and health care provider office visits for PID have decreased (CDC, 2010n). This decline has been attributed to the screening and treatment of young women for chlamydia (Workowski & Berman, 2010). However, in 2009, 100,000 PID cases were reported as the diagnosis for initial health care provider office visits (CDC, 2010q). Racial disparities are very evident in this population. For example, Black women have PID rates that are 2 to 3 times higher than those seen among White women (CDC, 2010n). Complications of PID include dyspareunia (painful intercourse), ectopic pregnancy, tubal infertility, chronic pelvic pain, pelvic adhesions, perihepatitis, and tubo-ovarian abscess (CDC, 2010h; Strickland & Gibson, 2009). PID can progress

RISK FACTORS for the Development of Pelvic Inflammatory Disease

Age (adolescent and young women)	Nonwhite women
Multiple sex partners	Sex with a male who has had many partners
History of sexually transmitted infection	Intercourse with a partner who has an untreated STI
Recent intrauterine device insertion	Nulliparity

to pelvic peritonitis, septicemia, and death (Workowski & Berman, 2010). Ectopic pregnancy caused by PID may also result in death if the fallopian tube ruptures. See Chapter 41 for more about ectopic pregnancy.

Etiology and Pathophysiology

Chlamydia and gonorrhea infection often trigger PID; however, vaginal bacterial flora including anaerobes such as *Gardnerella vaginalis, Haemophilus influenzae*, enteric gram-negative rods, and *Streptococcus agalactiae* contribute to the disease (Workowski & Berman, 2010). Also, cytomegalovirus (CMV), *Mycoplasma hominis, Ureaplasma urealyticum*, and *M. genitalium* have been identified in some cases. The enteric gram-negative rods, such as *Escherichia coli*, are more likely to occur in older women (Latendresse, McCance, & Morgan, 2010). These organisms ascend into the upper genital tract after gonorrhea, chlamydia, or both have caused damage to the columnar cells of the cervix. Other potential avenues of spreading infection include lymphatic drainage to the uterus and sperm that carry bacteria into the uterus and fallopian tubes. Women with bacterial vaginosis are much more likely to develop PID. *M. genitalium* has been identified as the cause of some cases of PID that have not been triggered by chlamydia or gonorrhea. The complications, including tubo-ovarian abscess and tubal infertility of PID, occur in 15% to 25% of women who have experienced only one episode of PID (Latendresse et al., 2010). Risk factors for the development of PID are outlined in the Risk Factors box.

Clinical Manifestations

Symptoms of PID vary from none to severe and may include lower abdominal pain, fever, foul-smelling vaginal discharge, painful intercourse, painful urination, and irregular menstrual bleeding. Women with symptomatic PID will describe pain in the lower abdomen that worsens with movement such as walking. Objective findings include fever (38.3°C); abnormal cervical or vaginal discharge; elevated white blood count (WBC), C-reactive protein (CRP), and erythrocyte sedimentation rate (ESR); and pain with palpation of the cervix, uterus, and adnexal areas. Symptoms worsen during or after menses (CDC, 2010h). Figure 43–5 ◆ demonstrates a swollen fallopian tube and ovarian adhesions resulting from PID.

Diagnostic Tests

PID is subtle in many cases and difficult to diagnose, since there are no precise tests for PID. Clinical signs and symptoms guide the health care provider in choosing what tests should be done. Usually, if there is clinical evidence of PID, the health care provider will perform tests for pregnancy, gonorrhea, and chlamydia. A pelvic ultrasound may be ordered to determine whether the fallopian tubes are enlarged or to identify an abscess. Occasionally, laparoscopy is needed to obtain cultures to confirm the diagnosis (CDC, 2010h). Refer to the Diagnostic Tests box (p. 1315) for more information about testing.

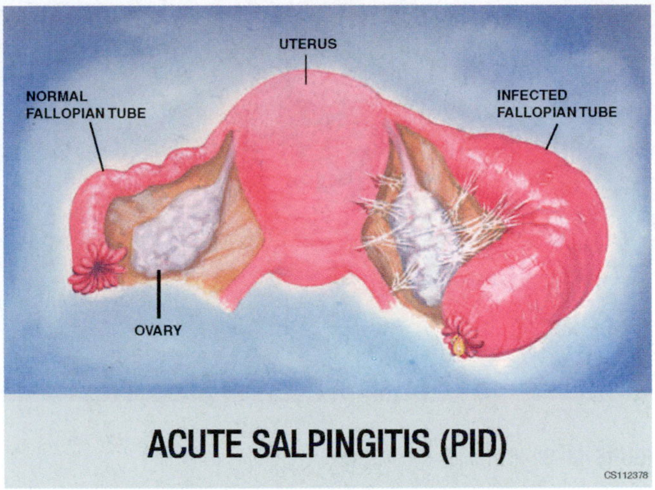

FIGURE 43–5 ◆ Pelvic inflammatory disease: Acute salpingitis.
Source: CDC.

Syphilis

Description and Epidemiology

Syphilis is an ulcerative bacterial disease that causes significant systemic health problems if untreated; furthermore, it facilitates the transmission of human immunodeficiency virus (HIV). Before penicillin became available in the 1940s, syphilis was a major global public health problem (Douglas, 2009). With the advent of penicillin, rates of syphilis in the United States decreased 90% by 1975. Since 1975, incidence of syphilis has increased periodically as societal mores have changed, but rates have been relatively low. According to the CDC (2010p), 44,828 cases of all stages of syphilis were reported in 2009, or 14.7 cases per 100,000 persons in the United States. In the 44 states and the District of Columbia where the gender of the sex partner is recorded, 62% of syphilis cases occurred among men who have sex with men (CDC, 2010o). People in Southern states, those in large cities, and Blacks have the highest incidence rates. Black populations had a syphilis rate increase from 17.2 to 19.2 per 100,000 in 2009 (CDC, 2010o). Between 2005 and 2009, primary and secondary syphilis cases among Black men ages 15 to 24 tripled. This rate increase contributed to the disproportionately high rates of HIV among these young men (CDC, 2010r). The rate of congenital syphilis has decreased from 10.4 to 10 per 100,000 live births. In 2009, 427 cases were reported (CDC, 2010o). Worldwide, syphilis continues to be a major problem.

Etiology and Pathophysiology

Syphilis is caused by *Treponema pallidum*, an anaerobic bacterium that looks like a corkscrew (Kaloczi et al., 2010). This organism is capable of infecting any organ or tissue in the body. It enters via microscopic abrasions and becomes systemic after an incubation period of 12 days to 12 weeks (average 3 weeks). Transmission from mother to fetus may occur as early as 9 weeks' gestation. Untreated primary and secondary syphilis in the mother will cause fetal death in 40% of cases (CDC, 2010o).

The course of untreated syphilis has four stages: primary, secondary, latent, and tertiary. Primary syphilis begins when *T. pallidum* enters and multiplies in epithelial cells. A **chancre** (painless, firm ulcer) occurs where the bacterium enters. From here, the bacterium migrates to the lymph system, and the body's immune system is stimulated (Kaloczi et al., 2010).

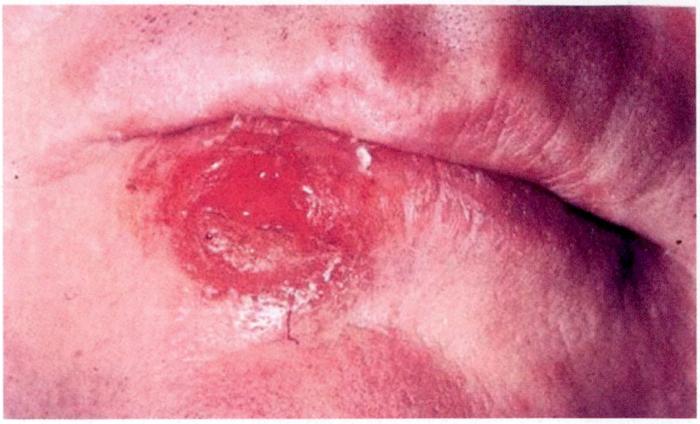

FIGURE 43–6 ◆ Primary syphilis: Chancre of the lower lip.
Source: Public Health Agency of Canada/CDC.

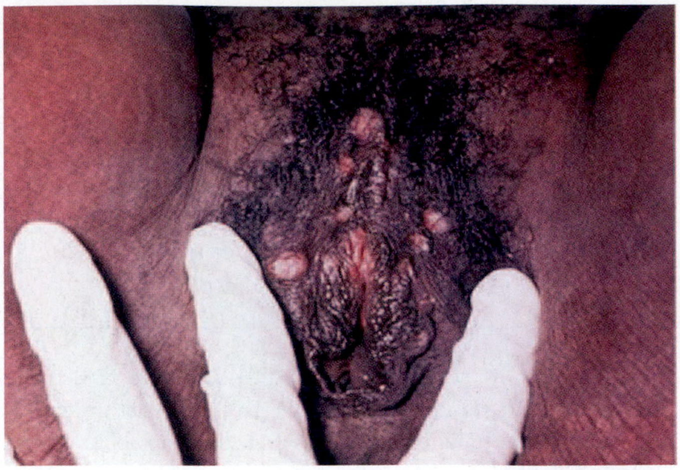

FIGURE 43–7 ◆ Secondary syphilis: Condylomata lata of the labia.
Source: Connie Celum, Walter Stamm, Seattle STD/HIV Prevention Training Center/CDC.

Secondary syphilis is systemic. The bacteria have spread to all major organ systems. The signs and symptoms of secondary syphilis are described in the following text. Eventually, during the secondary stage, the host's immune system is able to suppress the infection, and all signs disappear, even without treatment. This period is referred to as the latent period, and it may last for years (CDC, 2010i). The disease, which is detectable via blood tests, may be transmitted during this phase.

Tertiary syphilis is the most serious stage. Cardiovascular and neurological manifestations are severe and eventually cause death (CDC, 2010i).

A baby infected with syphilis may be born without symptoms; however, without treatment, severe mental and physical problems will develop in a few weeks. Congenital syphilis is more likely to occur if the mother has primary or secondary syphilis; however, the bacterium can be transmitted to the fetus even during the tertiary stage (Kaloczi et al., 2010).

Clinical Manifestations

Primary syphilis begins with the appearance of one or more chancres, typically on the penis, vulva, vagina, or anus (Keefe, 2010). Occasionally, *T. pallidum* enters via the skin of the hands or face, leaving a chancre that is dry, scaly, and papular (Kaloczi et al., 2010). Figure 43–6◆ depicts a chancre of the lower lip.

Secondary syphilis symptoms appear about 6 weeks after the chancre. Usually, this stage begins with low-grade fever, malaise, sore throat, hoarseness, anorexia, headache, joint pain, and papular rash over the trunk, palms, and soles of feet. **Condylomata lata,** a contagious lesion that looks like a flat wart, may develop over the vulva, perineum, groin, inner thigh, or anal area and occurs in both men and women (Figure 43–7◆). Other signs of secondary syphilis may include mucous patches in the mouth, lymph node swelling, itching, and alopecia (scalp hair loss). These manifestations heal in 2 to 10 weeks but recur periodically if the patient is not treated (McCutchan, 2008).

Latent syphilis is an asymptomatic stage that may last for many years. Tertiary syphilis, the last stage, may present with **gummas** (destructive skin, bone, or soft-tissue necrotic mass). These masses can damage the brain, nerves, eyes, heart, blood vessels, liver, bones, and joints. The untreated patient will die of neurological and cardiovascular complications (CDC, 2010i). The manifestations of tertiary syphilis are rare in the United States because antibiotic use will have cured the disease before it reaches this terminal stage.

Congenital syphilis may manifest as early (within the first 2 years of life) or late (after 2 years of life). Early manifestations include oral mucous patches, skin rash, "snuffles" or syphilitic rhinitis, growth restriction, and symptoms similar to those of secondary syphilis. Late manifestations include developmental delay, neurological problems, enlarged liver and spleen, bone marrow depression, bone and teeth involvement, skin lesions, hearing loss, and retinal inflammation. Late onset congenital syphilis is not contagious (Waseem & Aslam, 2009). Figure 43–8◆ demonstrates mucous patches and skin lesions of congenital syphilis.

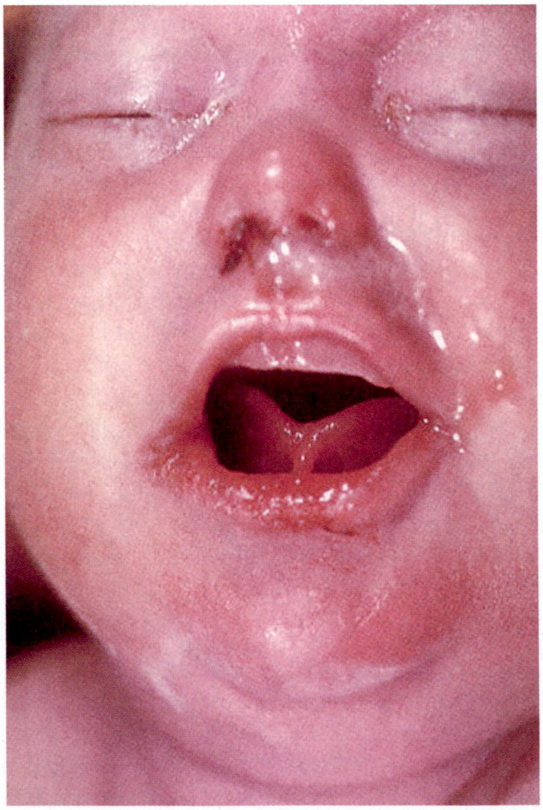

FIGURE 43–8 ◆ Congenital syphilis: Intraoral mucous patches and facial skin lesions.
Source: CDC.

Laboratory Tests

To diagnose syphilis, laboratory tests must be done. The only definitive laboratory test is dark field microscopic examination of drainage or tissue from a chancre for *T. pallidum*. However, presumptive diagnosis can be made with either nontreponemal tests or treponemal tests. Nontreponemal tests include the Venereal Disease Research Laboratory (VDRL) and Rapid Plasma Reagin (RPR) tests. False positive results occur frequently, so a positive nontreponemal test must be followed by a treponemal test to confirm the diagnosis. Refer to the Diagnostic Tests box for more information about these tests (p. 1315).

Bacterial Vaginosis

Description and Epidemiology

Bacterial vaginosis (BV) occurs when the normal flora (protective bacteria) is replaced by an overgrowth of opportunistic, harmful bacteria. Bacterial vaginosis is the most common vaginal infection in women between the ages of 13 and 50, including many pregnant women (CDC, 2010d).

Etiology and Pathophysiology

The cause of BV is unclear. The condition is associated with sexual activity but is not necessarily sexually transmitted. Activities or behaviors that may predispose women to BV include anything that would upset the normal flora (CDC, 2010d; McCloskey, 2010). Events that can lead to BV include:

- Having a new sexual partner
- Having multiple sexual partners
- Douching
- Wearing thong underwear (drags colon bacteria into the vagina).

Normal vaginal flora is predominantly lactobacilli. Bacteria that have been identified in women who have BV include *Haemophilus vaginalis, G. vaginalis*, genital mycoplasma, *Bacteroides*, and *Mobiluncus* species. These bacteria adhere to the vaginal walls and proliferate without causing inflammation (Kaloczi et al., 2010).

Bacterial vaginosis has been implicated in increased susceptibility to STIs such as HIV, herpes, chlamydia, gonorrhea, and PID. Having BV increases a woman's risk for infection after hysterectomy, abortion, or any instrumentation of the cervix. Having BV while pregnant increases the woman's risks for **chorioamnionitis** (infection of the layers of membrane around the fetus in the womb), preterm labor, low-birthweight newborns, and postpartum **endometritis** (inflammation of the uterine lining) (Kaloczi et al., 2010).

Clinical Manifestations

Clinical manifestations of BV include vaginal discharge that is smooth, thin, and grayish and has a "fishy" odor (McCloskey, 2010). Some women with BV will have dysuria or itching around the opening to the vagina (CDC, 2010d). However, many women with BV have no symptoms.

Bacterial vaginosis is diagnosed by examination of the vaginal discharge through evaluation of the pH, microscopic detection of clue cells, and an amine ("whiff") test (McCloskey, 2010). Health care providers treat BV with antibiotics. Male partners do not need to be treated. Bacterial vaginosis often recurs after even the best treatment (CDC, 2010d). See the Pharmacology box for specific antibiotics used for treating BV (p. 1320). Some women will use probiotic therapy to treat or prevent BV even though there is no evidence that this approach is effective. See the Complementary & Alternative Therapies box for more about probiotic use.

Chancroid

Description and Epidemiology

Chancroid is an ulcer-forming STI caused by the gram-negative bacillus *Haemophilus ducreyi* (Kaloczi et al., 2010). This STI does not occur often in the United States, although outbreaks have occurred in larger cities in populations where there is poverty, prostitution, and illicit drug use. In 2009, only 28 cases were reported in the United States (CDC, 2010m).

Etiology and Pathophysiology

H. ducreyi is transmitted via sexual intercourse and *autoinoculation* (person spreads infection to self via dirty hands). It is not spread from mother to fetus during pregnancy, during birth, or after birth. The incubation period is 3 to 10 days (Kaloczi et al., 2010).

Clinical Manifestations

The ulcers caused by *H. ducreyi* are found under the foreskin of the penis in men and in the labial folds of women. The infection begins as a papule that enlarges, then opens into a soft ulcer with a spreading border. The lymph nodes that drain the area will become inflamed and very tender. Men who are infected are most likely to develop inguinal **buboes** (abscesses of inguinal lymph nodes) in 7 to 10 days after the soft ulcer has appeared. Buboes rupture and drain. The drainage is highly infectious, and autoinoculation is probable (Kaloczi et al., 2010). Figure 43–9 ◆ shows chancroid with swollen inguinal lymph nodes.

Laboratory Tests

Special media are needed to grow *H. ducreyi* with 80% sensitivity. Since the media are not always available and the sensitivity is poor, health care providers will treat for chancroid based on clinical presentation and a negative test for both syphilis and herpes (Workowski & Berman, 2010). These patients should also be tested for HIV, because the ulcers caused by *H. ducreyi* place the patient at risk for contracting HIV/AIDS due to loss of skin integrity.

Medical Management for STIs Caused by Bacteria

All STIs caused by bacteria are curable with antibiotics. However, it is very important that the STI be identified so that the most efficacious

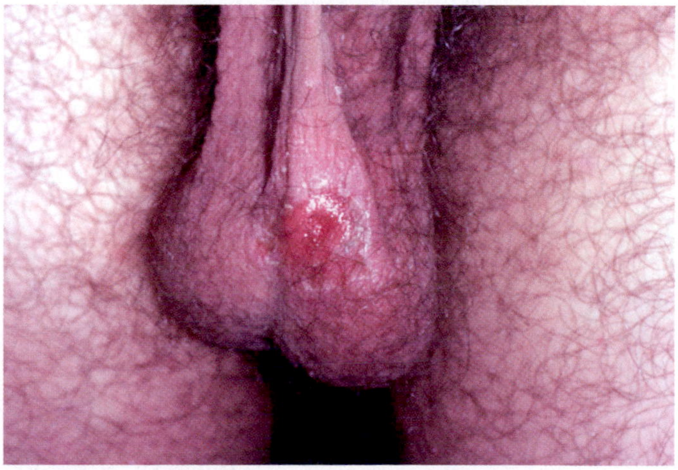

FIGURE 43–9 ◆ Chancroid.
Source: © Custom Medical Stock Photo/Alamy.

PHARMACOLOGY Summary of Medications Used to Treat Sexually Transmitted Infections

Medication Category and Action	Application/Indication	Nursing Responsibility
Antibiotics		
Azithromycin or erythromycin (Zithromax or ERY-C) ***Action:*** Disrupts cell wall synthesis of susceptible bacteria.	Chlamydia infection. Chancroid.	Large single dose given. Assess for drug allergies. Consider prevention for nausea. Take with food.
Doxycycline (Doryx) ***Action:*** Disrupts cell wall synthesis of susceptible bacteria.	Chlamydia infection.	Take with large glass of water. Not for patients under 18 years of age.
Ceftriaxone ***Action:*** Bactericidal. Inhibits cell wall synthesis.	Gonorrhea infection.	Increased risk for secondary infection such as yeast vaginitis.
Penicillin G ***Action:*** Disrupts cell wall synthesis of susceptible bacteria.	Syphilis.	Assess for allergy to penicillin. Intramuscular (IM) injection.
Metronidazole (Flagyl) ***Action:*** Anti-protozoan and anti-bacterial—especially anaerobes. Enters cell and binds with DNA, causing cell death.	Trichomoniasis. Bacterial vaginosis.	Caution patient not to drink alcohol while taking. Patient should refrain from sex during therapy. May be given orally or as vaginal gel or ovules.
Clindamycin (Cleocin) ***Action:*** Acts on the 50S bacterial ribosomal subunit. Bacteristatic.	Bacterial vaginosis.	Can be given orally or as vaginal gel or ovules.
Cefotetan Plus Doxycycline ***Action:*** Bacteriostatic; inhibits cell wall synthesis.	Pelvic inflammatory disease. Inpatient and outpatient RX same as chlamydia and gonorrhea.	Assess for any known reaction to penicillin or cephalosporin. Monitor closely for drug reaction in first 30 minutes of IV use.
Cefotetan + Clindamycin or Metronidazole ***Action:*** Same as above	Tubo-ovarian abscess.	IV medications. Monitor for drug reaction. Monitor for improvement in condition.
Antivirals		
Acyclovir Famciclovir Valacyclovir ***Action:*** Nucleoside analog that inhibits viral replication.	Herpes simplex types 1 and 2.	Should be started as soon as possible after onset of symptoms. Monitor for adverse effects.
Imiquimod (Aldara) ***Action:*** Induces cytokines including interferon. Podofilox ***Action:*** Antimitotic drug that destroys warts.	Genital warts.	Teach that this is a pregnancy category C drug and that the medication, applied as a cream, may weaken condoms. Teach the patient how to self-treat and that this is a pregnancy category C drug.
Gardasil and cervarix ***Action:*** Vaccines.	Prevention of human papillomavirus.	Teach that Gardasil is effective against HPV types 16, 18, 6, and 11. Cervarix is effective against HPV types 16 and 18. Both are given in a series of 3 IM injections. Tell the patient to expect mild pain, swelling, and redness at the injection site.

Sources: Adapted from Adams, M., & Koch, R. (2010). *Pharmacology: Connections to nursing practice.* Upper Saddle River, NJ: Pearson; Workowski, K., & Berman, S. (2010). Sexually transmitted diseases treatment guidelines, 2010. *MMWR, 59*(RR12), 1–110.

antibiotic can be used. Health care providers must also recognize that STIs do not always occur as a single infection. In fact, the CDC recommends that any individual identified as having a bacterial STI should be tested for STIs that may co-exist, particularly HIV. The CDC STI Treatment Guidelines 2010 (Workowski & Berman, 2010) also direct providers to treat both gonorrhea and chlamydia every time a patient is identified who has one of these infections.

The CDC recommends that women under the age of 26 should be screened annually for chlamydia and that all women who are treated for chlamydia be retested for infection in 3 months after treatment (Workowski & Berman, 2010). It is also recommended that expedited partner therapy (EPT) be implemented in states where it is permitted. For instance, a female infected with chlamydia may bring medication and health advice to her heterosexual partner so that both are treated at the same time (Saperstein & Firnhaber, 2010). Expedited partner therapy is not recommended for treatment of trichomoniasis because none of the cohort studies that compared traditional referral and EPT supported the use of EPT for

COMPLEMENTARY & ALTERNATIVE THERAPIES Probiotics for Treatment of Bacterial Vaginosis *Nancy Yilk*

BACTERIAL VAGINOSIS (BV) is the most common cause of vaginal discharge in women, and is responsible for 40% to 50% of clinical cases. Estimates of the prevalence of BV among women between the ages of 14 and 49 years in the United States has been found to be 29% (Allsworth & Peipert, 2007). Bacterial vaginosis is a common condition believed to be associated with susceptibility to STI. Bacterial vaginosis has been associated with herpes simplex virus' types 1 and 2 (HSV-1 and HSV-2) among women in the general U.S. population (Allsworth, Lewis, & Peipert, 2008).

The shift of vaginal flora was investigated in a double-blind, randomized, placebo-controlled study for effectiveness by using vaginal probiotic capsules for recurrent BV prevention. A pool of 120 healthy Chinese women with a history of recurrent BV were assigned randomly into two groups, with 58 women using daily vaginal prophylaxis capsules which contained 8 billion units of *Lactobacillus rhamnosus*, *L. acidophilus*, and *Streptococcus thermophilus*, and 62 women taking a placebo capsule.

Probiotic treatment resulted in lower recurrence rates for BV (15.8% vs. 45.0%) and *G. vaginalis* incidence through 2 months (3.5% vs. 18.3%). In both 2- and 11-month follow-up periods, women who received probiotics reported a lower incidence of both BV and *G. vaginalis* (Ya, Reifer, & Miller, 2010).

In a Brazilian study assessing depletion of the indigenous lactobacilli in BV, in which antimicrobial therapy is often ineffective, oral administration of probiotic *Lactobacillus rhamnosus* and *L. reuteri* was provided as an adjunct to antimicrobial treatment to improve cure rates. Sixty-four Brazilian women diagnosed with BV were randomly assigned to receive a single dose of tinidazole (2 g) supplemented with either 2 placebo capsules or 2 capsules containing probiotics every morning for the following 4 weeks. At day 28, end of treatment, the probiotic group had a significantly higher cure rate of BV (87.5%) than the placebo group (50.0%). In addition, according to the Gram-stain Nugent score, more women were assessed with "normal" vaginal microbiota in the probiotic group (75.0% vs. 34.4% in the placebo group). This study shows that probiotic lactobacilli can provide benefits to women being treated with antibiotics for an infectious condition (Martinez et al., 2009).

Sources: Allsworth, J. E., Lewis, V. A., & Peipert, J. F. (2008). Viral sexually transmitted infections and bacterial vaginosis: 2001–2004 National Health and Nutrition Examination Survey data. *Sexually Transmitted Diseases, 35*(9), 791–796; Allsworth, J. E., & Peipert, J. F. (2007). Prevalence of bacterial vaginosis: 2001–2004 National Health and Nutrition Examination Survey data. *Obstetrics & Gynecology, 109*(1), 114–120; Martinez, R. C., Franceschini, S.A., Patta, M.C., Quintana, S.M., Gomes, B.C., De Martinis, E. C., Reid, G. (2009). Improved cure of bacterial vaginosis with single dose of tinidazole (2 g), Lactobacillus rhamnosus GR-1, and Lactobacillus reuteri RC-14: a randomized, double-blind, placebo-controlled trial. *Canadian Journal of Microbiology, 55*(2), 133–138; Ya, W., Reifer, C., & Miller, L. E. (2010). Efficacy of vaginal probiotic capsules for recurrent bacterial vaginosis: A double-blind, randomized, placebo-controlled study. *American Journal of Obstetrics and Gynecology, 203*(2), 120.e1–6.

this infection. In addition, EPT is not appropriate for men having sex with men because of the danger of undiagnosed HIV and other comorbidities when these men are not seen by a health care provider. Syphilis treatment by EPT is not done because it requires an injection of penicillin. EPT is prohibited in nine states.

Since the rectum and throat are the sites where asymptomatic infection with bacterial STIs may occur in men having sex with men, the CDC recommends annual screening tests of these sites in men who have participated in receptive oral or anal sex (Klausner et al., 2009). Antibiotics used for the treatment of bacterial STIs are listed in the Pharmacology box.

Pelvic inflammatory disease presents a much more serious medical problem. The condition is curable, but it is often difficult to determine the causative agent. For this reason, at least two broad spectrum antibiotics are used. Some women with PID will need to be hospitalized and treated with intravenous antibiotics and analgesics. The Pharmacology box includes the antibiotics that may be used.

Nursing Management

Nurses are active in education programs for individuals and groups at risk for bacterial STIs. They also identify and refer persons with signs and symptoms of these diseases to local health care providers or the Health Department, depending on the state's reporting requirements.

When a woman is admitted to the hospital for treatment of PID, nurses administer antibiotics, analgesics, and sedatives as prescribed. Nurses teach and encourage these patients to maintain bed rest in the high Fowler's position to help control the spread of infection to the upper abdomen. Universal precautions must be strictly enforced if the patient has purulent vaginal drainage. Nurses should provide emotional support, education about the disease, drug therapy, and methods to prevent recurrence. The patient recovering from PID will begin oral antibiotics once the fever and pain have subsided. The patient is discharged on oral antibiotics when she has been afebrile for at least 24 hours. Nurses should stress the importance of follow-up care and evaluation with the health care provider within 2 days of discharge. More about nursing management appears in the following Nursing Process feature.

Safety Alert *The nurse should always ask the patient about allergies before administering any antibiotic. In addition, the nurse should always be prepared for an allergic reaction to any antibiotic administered.*

Health Promotion

Patient and partner education are essential to the prevention and spread of bacterial STIs. The following facts are necessary components of the teaching plan:

- STIs are most often transmitted during vaginal, anal, or oral sex.
- Ejaculation does not have to occur for infection to occur.
- Many of these infections can be passed from an infected mother to her baby during pregnancy and birth.
- The greater number of sex partners, the greater the risk of infection.
- Teenagers and young women are most at risk for STIs if sexually active.
- Sex partners must be treated in order to prevent recurrence and spread.
- Complications from STIs may include PID, ectopic pregnancy, and infertility.
- Routine screening for STIs should occur during yearly exams.
- A single dose of the appropriate antibiotic can cure some bacterial STIs.
- Prevention of STIs is accomplished by being in a long-term, mutually monogamous relationship with a partner who has been tested and is known to be uninfected.
- When used consistently and correctly, latex condoms can reduce the risk of transmission of bacterial STIs.

Video: Herpes

Sexually Transmitted Infections Caused by Viruses

Viral infections, unlike bacterial infections, cannot be cured with antibiotics. Viruses may be transmitted even when the infected individual has no signs or symptoms of infection. The severity of a sexually transmitted viral infection varies widely, from simple warts caused by human papillomavirus to immunodeficiency caused by human immunodeficiency virus. This section includes discussions of the most prevalent of the sexually transmitted viral infections in the United States, including genital herpes, human papillomavirus, hepatitis, and acquired immunodeficiency syndrome.

Genital Herpes

Description and Epidemiology

Genital herpes (herpes simplex virus [HSV]) is the most common ulcer-causing viral infection in the United States. In fact, about one in six people ages 14 to 49 have genital herpes (CDC, 2010f). This viral infection is more common in women because transmission from a male to a female is more likely than transmission from a female to a male due to the vagina's receptive nature during intercourse. The viral infection is often asymptomatic; in fact, persons without symptoms transmit most infections (Kaloczi et al., 2010).

Congenital HSV (infection in utero) infection is very rare. Neonatal HSV (infection in a newborn within the first 28 days of life) is more likely to occur. If untreated, neonatal HSV has only a 40% survival rate (Corey & Wald, 2009). Even with early recognition and intervention, those infants who survive have severe disabilities. The incidence of neonatal HSV varies from 1 case per 12,500 live births to 1 per 1,700 live births depending on the patient population studied (Corey & Wald, 2009).

Etiology and Pathophysiology

Herpes simplex virus (HSV) is a double-stranded DNA virus (Pinninti & Tolan, 2010). There are two types of HSV that cause genital infection. Type 1 HSV has historically been the source of cold sores or fever blisters on the mouth and lips. In contrast, type 2 HSV usually refers to herpes infection of the genitals. However, it is no longer uncommon to find HSV types 1 and 2 in both areas of the body, even though HSV-2 is most often recovered from genital herpes lesions. The incubation period for HSV is 3 to 7 days with a range of 1 day to 3 weeks (Salvaggio & Lutwick, 2010). The virus enters via abrasions of the skin or mucous membrane. Local cell destruction by the replication of the virus will lead to the skin manifestations (Salvaggio & Lutwick, 2010). The virus then spreads to sensory nerves and is transported to the dorsal root, where it stays. Herpes simplex virus is not destructive to the dorsal root even though it will reside there for life (Kaloczi et al., 2010). Reactivation of the virus causes similar, but not as severe, lesions on the skin innervated by the nerve affected. Reactivation is not predictable but seems to occur after exposure to ultraviolet light, stress, hormonal changes, immunosuppression, and other infections (Pinninti & Tolan, 2010). Some women may have reactivations as often as every menstrual period during the first 1 to 2 years. The incidence of reactivation decreases over time. HSV-2 is more virulent and will cause more reactivations than HSV-1.

Neonatal infections usually occur during the birth process when the fetus is exposed to cervical lesions. The risk of transmission is highest when the mother acquires HSV-2 infection during the latter part of the pregnancy (Corey & Wald, 2009). However, neonatal herpes occurs in fewer than 1% of infants delivered vaginally to women with HSV-2 shedding during labor and birth.

Disseminated infection is usually the cause of death in neonates who acquire HSV. This systemic spread of the virus may also affect immunocompromised persons. It is believed that HSV has the ability to further suppress the host's innate immunity (Pinninti & Tolan, 2010).

Clinical Manifestations

The first symptoms of HSV infection, if present, are fever, headache, malaise, and myalgia. Local cell destruction by the replication of the virus will cause pain, itching, dysuria, vaginal and urethral discharge, tender enlarged lymph nodes, and **vesicle** (blister) formation (Salvaggio & Lutwick, 2010). The vesicles rupture, leaving painful ulcers that will last 10 to 20 days. Although the vesicles and ulcers are very infectious, they do not cause scarring (Kaloczi et al., 2010). The lesions of genital herpes appear on the penis, scrotum, vulva, cervix, buttocks, or thighs. In people who participate in anal sex, the perineum, anus, and rectum may be sites of eruptions. Figure 43–10 ◆ shows a painful outbreak of HSV.

Reactivation of HSV infection does not cause systemic symptoms such as fever, and fewer vesicles and less pain occur. The patient will experience *prodromal* (early indication of impending disease) sensations in the form of tingling or itching before the lesions erupt. The recurrence is usually unilateral and will crust in 4 to 5 days. Complete healing will occur in about 10 days (Kaloczi et al., 2010).

Psychologically, genital herpes has a measurable impact. Mark, Gilbert, and Nanda (2009) assessed the psychological well-being and quality of life of women with new HSV diagnoses and found that anxiety and depression were common among their study's participants. These women also experienced feelings of isolation, difficulty in showing affection, and fear of spreading the disease to intimate partners.

The newborn infected with HSV may manifest symptoms in one of three patterns. About 45% will have lesions that are confined to the skin, eye, and mucosa (Corey & Wald, 2009). These children do not have central nervous system (CNS) symptoms but will have recurrent outbreaks of skin lesions during their early years. The second pattern, CNS associated infection, occurs in about 30% of cases studied and is manifested as poor feeding, lethargy, seizures, HSV DNA in cerebrospinal fluid, developmental delay, epilepsy, blindness, and cognitive disability.

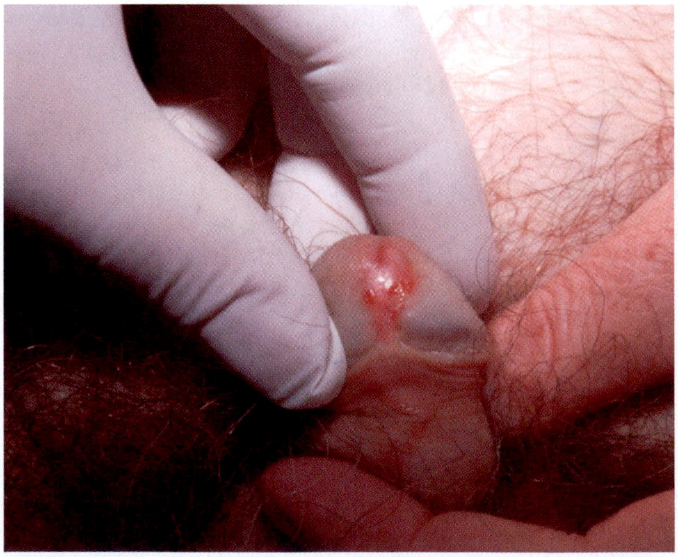

FIGURE 43–10 ◆ Herpes simplex of the penis.
Source: Phanie/SuperStock.

The third pattern, disseminated infection, has the highest mortality rate and occurs in about 25% of the cases studied. Disseminated infection of HSV will manifest just like bacterial sepsis, affecting many organs including the liver, lungs and brain.

Laboratory Tests

Identification of the vesicles and ulcers as genital herpes needs to be substantiated with laboratory testing. According to Workowski and Berman (2010), the tests of choice include the polymerase chain reaction (PCR) assay for HSV DNA and a serology test for type-specific glycoprotein G. Since the PCR assay will detect HSV only when the virus is shedding, false negatives are frequent. Serologic type testing, the most reliable, differentiates the two types of herpes simplex. The Papanicolaou test (Pap test) may reveal tissue changes consistent with HSV, but these findings are not diagnostic. See the Diagnostic Tests feature (p. 1315).

Human Papillomavirus

Description and Epidemiology

Human papillomavirus (HPV) infection is the most common STI in the United States. It is estimated that 50% of sexually active individuals will have genital HPV at some point in their lifetime (CDC, 2010b). This clearly indicates an epidemic. According to the CDC (2010b), the cancers attributed to HPV affect many people annually:

- 12,000 women are diagnosed with cervical cancer.
- 3,700 women are diagnosed with vulvar cancer.
- 1,000 men are diagnosed with penile cancer.
- 2,700 women and 1,700 men are diagnosed with anal cancer.

The populations at highest risk for HPV infection are gay and bisexual men and people with weak immune systems. In fact, men having sex with men are about 17 times more likely to develop anal cancer than men who only have sex with women (CDC, 2010b).

Etiology and Pathophysiology

Human papillomavirus is a circular, double-stranded DNA virus. About 120 different types of HPV have been identified, but only 40 of these types infect the genitals, mouth, and throat (CDC, 2010b; Kaloczi et al., 2010). The virus is passed via genital contact, especially during vaginal, anal, and oral sex. The incubation period is 2 to 3 months. In rare situations, HPV is passed to a newborn during the birth process, causing **juvenile-onset recurrent respiratory papillomatosis (JORRP).**

The HPV types can be divided into low-risk and high-risk types. Low-risk types are associated with benign warts called **condylomata acuminata.** High-risk types are found in cervical dysplasia and cancer of the cervix, vulva, vagina, penis, and anus. The virus enters the body via abrasions or other trauma to the epithelium. Epithelial cells infected with HPV are transformed as the virus changes the nucleus of the cell and the way the cell grows (Kaloczi et al., 2010).

Clinical Manifestations

Condylomata acuminata, or **genital warts,** affect about 1% of sexually active adults at any one time (CDC, 2010b). These painless growths may be flat, raised, or cauliflower-like and may appear on the penis, scrotum, groin, thighs, anus, perineum, mouth, vulva, vagina, or cervix. The warts may be itchy and, if large, may cause dyspareunia (painful intecourse) (Kaloczi et al., 2010). Figure 43–11◆ shows genital warts.

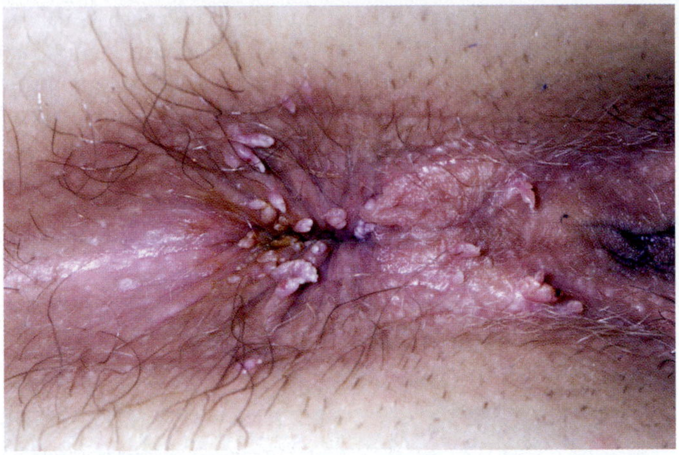

FIGURE 43–11 ◆ Human papillomavirus: Genital warts.
Source: Dr. P. Marazzi / Science Source/Photo Researchers

Cervical dysplasia and cervical cancer may be asymptomatic. In later stages, a vaginal discharge will develop, and the cancer will metastasize to the lymph nodes and other areas of the body. Cancer is discussed in Chapter 57, and penile cancer is discussed in Chapter 42.

Babies and children with JORRP will have multiple benign growths in the respiratory tract. These growths will occur on the larynx and cause hoarseness. In more severe cases, the airway will be blocked by growths. The lesions can be removed surgically but often recur or may disappear completely (Web MD, 2010).

Laboratory Tests

Currently, there are no tests to diagnose HPV in men (CDC, 2010b). For women, there is an HPV test that is used to find high-risk HPV infection. This test uses cervical cells collected during the Pap test to check for HPV DNA. The test is able to identify high-risk HPV types 16, 18, 31, and 45 (Healthwise Staff, 2010c).

The most important test to consider for HPV-related complications is the Pap test. As explained in Chapter 41, the Pap test is the best and most widely used test for the detection of cell changes on the cervix caused by HPV. Regular Pap tests are recommended for all women of childbearing age with a cervix.

Hepatitis

Hepatitis A, hepatitis B, and hepatitis C are viral diseases of the liver that are considered STIs by the CDC (CDC, 2010c; Workowski & Berman, 2010). The hepatitis virus can be transmitted via sexual contact. Hepatitis A may also be transmitted via the oral–fecal route or by eating or drinking contaminated food or water. Hepatitis B is transmitted in the same ways that HIV is transmitted, including any exchange of body fluids and contaminated needle use. Chapter 38 includes an in-depth discussion of hepatitis and other liver diseases.

Acquired Immunodeficiency Syndrome

Acquired immunodeficiency syndrome (AIDS) is a result of an infection with the human immunodeficiency virus (HIV). HIV/AIDS is transmitted primarily by sexual contact, but it also can be acquired through a transfusion with infected blood, by an infant through the childbirth process, via contaminated hypodermic needles, or through breast-feeding from an infected mother. The HIV virus attacks the immune system, placing the individual at high risk for opportunistic infections. Often unable to fight infections because of the compromised immune system, these individuals eventually succumb to one of them. Although certain medications have been successful at slowing the disease process, as of yet, there is no cure (Workowski & Berman, 2010).

The CDC (2010g) estimates there are 40,000 new cases of HIV/AIDS in the United States each year. The fastest growing affected population is heterosexual men and women under the age of 25. HIV/AIDS is a deadly combination; to decrease the incidence, a concerted effort must be made on the part of all people. Chapter 53 includes an in-depth discussion of HIV/AIDS.

Medical Management for STIs Caused by Viruses

Unlike STIs caused by bacteria, STIs caused by viruses cannot be cured with antibiotics. Although there are vaccines to protect against certain types of HPV, no vaccine exists for herpes simplex. Antiviral medications for herpes are palliative and may reduce the number of episodes of recurrence. In this section, the focus for medical management will be the diagnosis and treatment of herpes simplex virus (HSV) and the diagnosis, prevention, and treatment of human papillomavirus (HPV).

Herpes Simplex Virus (HSV): Diagnosis and Treatment

Diagnosis of HSV can often be made by visual exam; however, confirmation must be made using viral culture or serologic tests. Serologic tests will also determine whether the infection is type 1 or type 2 HSV. Viral cultures are not as reliable and do not type the virus (Workowski & Berman, 2010).

Although genital herpes causes recurrent outbreaks that are painful and worrisome, the condition is not life threatening unless the patient is immunosuppressed. Potentially lethal HSV infections can occur in patients with HIV/AIDS. Furthermore, HSV infections can make people more susceptible to HIV/AIDS if the open lesions come into contact with the HIV virus. HSV-2 can also make HIV-infected individuals more infectious because of the increased virulence and number of recurrences. Pregnant women with HSV-2 risk transmission of HSV to their infants during delivery; therefore, women with lesions caused by HSV-2 at term frequently deliver by cesarean. However, cesarean birth does not guarantee that the baby will be spared (Workowski & Berman, 2010).

Treatment of HSV-2 can be accomplished with antiviral medications (acyclovir or valacyclovir). These medications cannot cure HSV-2, but they can shorten and prevent outbreaks. Daily suppressive therapy is used for some patients who continue to have repeated outbreaks and to reduce transmission to uninfected partners. Treatment recommendations also include cleaning of lesions daily to prevent secondary infections, taking sitz baths to increase comfort, wearing loose cotton underwear, and taking analgesics for discomfort. Abstinence from sexual intercourse starting with the first sign of recurrence through complete healing of the lesions is recommended, along with use of condoms between episodes.

Human Papillomavirus (HPV): Diagnosis and Treatment

Most women are diagnosed with HPV based on the appearance of warts on the genital area or an abnormal Pap test. A Pap test, the primary method of screening for cervical cancer, detects precancerous changes in the cervix that may occur as a result of HPV infection. Genital warts caused by low-risk HPV can be treated with topical medications that are either self-administered or applied by health care providers, such as Podofilox solution or Imiquimod cream. Genital warts can also be removed with minor surgery, known as cryotherapy (destruction of abnormal tissue by freezing); with liquid nitrogen; or with a shave excision (slicing off thin layers from surface). Many genital warts resolve spontaneously (Workowski & Berman, 2010).

Currently, two vaccines have been approved for use in the prevention of specific types of HPV. Both Gardasil and Cervarix are given in three separate injections over a 6-month interval. Both are most effective if given before first sexual contact, and both are appropriate for girls ages 9 to 26. Gardasil adds an extra protection against most genital warts because it protects against HPV types 6 and 11 (low-risk types) and 16 and 18 (high-risk types). Gardasil may also be given to males ages 9 to 26 to prevent genital warts (CDC, 2010b). Gardasil has also been approved to prevent anal cancer (Snowden, 2010). The advent of the HPV vaccine does not change any of the recommendations for cervical cancer screening outlined in Chapter 41.

Nursing Management

Nurses can assist patients with viral STIs through education about the disease and drug therapy. Nurses should encourage compliance with drug therapy and safe-sex practices so that patients with viral STIs, including HIV, do not spread the disease to their partners. More about nursing management appears in the Nursing Process section later in this chapter.

Health Promotion

Patient and partner education are essential to the prevention and spread of diseases caused by viruses. The following facts are necessary components of the teaching plan:

- Any unusual discharge, sore, or rash, particularly in the groin area, should be a signal to refrain from having sex and to seek the care of a health care provider.
- Prevention of STIs is best accomplished by abstaining from sexual contact or by being in a long-term, mutually monogamous relationship with a partner who has been tested and is known to be uninfected.
- Condoms are not fully effective in preventing the spread of genital viral diseases. Therefore, persons with HSV and HPV should abstain from sexual activity with uninfected partners when lesions or other symptoms are present.
- An HPV- or HSV-infected person who does not have any symptoms can still infect sex partners by shedding virus between outbreaks.
- HPV infection can lead to cervical, vulvar, penile, and anal cancer.
- Avoidance of alcohol and drug use may also help prevent transmission of STIs, as these activities may lead to risky sexual behavior.
- It is important that sex partners talk to each other about their HIV status and history of other STIs so that preventive action can be taken if needed.
- Transmission of an STI cannot be prevented by washing the genitals, urinating, and/or douching after sex.
- Viral STIs that cause sores, ulcers, or breaks in the skin or mucous membranes disrupt barriers that provide protection against infections such as HIV.

As is the case with bacterial STIs, abstinence is the only sure way to prevent viral STIs. A mutually monogamous relationship with a partner who is free of viral infection is also protective.

Other Sexually Transmitted Infections

The CDC recognizes pubic lice, scabies, and trichomoniasis as STIs (2010c; Workowski & Berman, 2010). Pubic lice (pediculosis) and scabies are discussed in Chapter 59. In this section, trichomoniasis will be the focus.

Trichomoniasis

Description, Epidemiology, Etiology, and Pathophysiology

Approximately 7.4 million new cases of trichomoniasis occur each year in women and men, including 124,000 pregnant women (CDC, 2010j). **Trichomoniasis** is caused by a single-celled protozoan parasite, *Trichomonas vaginalis*. This parasite may infest the vagina and urethra and is transmitted during sexual contact.

Clinical Manifestations

Symptoms will appear within 5 to 28 days of exposure to the parasite (Kaloczi et al., 2010). Men may be asymptomatic, or they may experience urethral irritation, mild discharge, or slight burning on urination or after ejaculation. Women may be asymptomatic or may experience yellow-green vaginal discharge with a strong odor. Women may also have discomfort during intercourse, or they may have irritation and itching of the genital area (Figure 43–12◆) after urination. On inspection of the cervix, the health care provider may see small red ulcers on the vaginal wall and cervix. These ulcers are a potential entry point for HIV and other STIs.

Laboratory Tests and Medical Management

Trichomoniasis is diagnosed by clinical signs and identification of the one-celled parasite by microscopic examination of a saline wet preparation of the vaginal discharge (McCloskey, 2010).

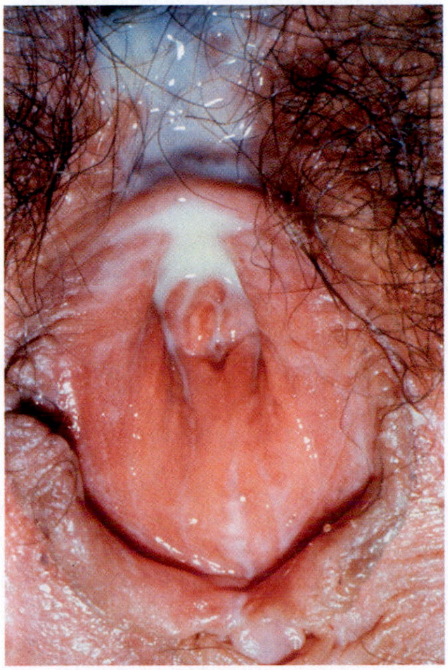

FIGURE 43–12 ◆ Trichomoniasis.

Source: National Medical Slide Bank/Custom Medical Stock Photo, Inc.

Medical treatment is intended to eradicate the parasite with metronidazole, clindamycin, or tinidazole oral medication or vaginal gels. Both partners must be treated at the same time to prevent re-infection. See the Pharmacology box (p. 1320) for more information about these medications.

Nursing Management

Care of patients with STIs is primarily aimed at promoting health education that prevents infections. Patients must receive the results of their testing as soon as possible and be encouraged to follow up for treatment. Nurses who are responsible for revealing test results for STIs to patients must be extremely careful to protect the patients' confidentiality. For example, leaving messages on phones or with domestic partners or other family members is strictly prohibited. The Nursing Process: Patient Care Plan box outlines nursing care specific to sexually transmitted infections.

Health Promotion

Health promotion for sexually transmitted infections should be directed at prevention. Once the disorder occurs, the care is directed toward symptom management, decreasing progression when possible, prevention of recurrence, and prevention of infection of other people. The care and education need to be individualized both to the type of STI and to the patient's needs. Specific information for patient and partner teaching about each type of STI, if available, is included in the relevant section in this chapter.

The CDC (Workowski & Berman, 2010) maintains that the primary preventive measure of sexually transmitted infections is to abstain from sexual intercourse and contact (including vaginal, anal, and oral sex) or to be in a long-term, monogamous relationship with an uninfected partner. Because neither of these measures is always followed, safer sex practices are the most common preventive measure.

ETHICAL ISSUES
A Case Study of a Young Woman with an STI

An ethical dilemma is a situation in which a patient's perspective may differ from that of a health care provider regarding the best medical decision to be made.

J. J. Vantoch, age 19, has just learned that she is infected with chlamydia. After taking her medication, she is being interviewed by a public health worker who must question her about her sexual contacts. The worker's goal is to identify, educate, and treat all persons in the community with the infection.

Ms. Vantoch is reluctant to reveal her contact. Her boyfriend is very dear to her, and she does not want to lose him. She is also concerned that her friends will reject her if she tells the worker about her boyfriend. In her mind, "No one likes an informer."

Critical Thinking Questions

Which of the following approaches will be most helpful in convincing Ms. Vantoch to divulge her boyfriend's identity?

1. Talk with her about how "bad" her boyfriend is to have given her this infection.
2. Educate her about how chlamydia may cause a more serious illness in her boyfriend, such as epididymitis or Reiter's syndrome.
3. Talk with her about expedited partner therapy and about advising her male partner to seek more education.
4. Respect her decision not to tell, and educate her about the high re-infection rate and the potential for PID and tubal infertility for her.

NURSING PROCESS: Patient Care Plan for Sexually Transmitted Infections

Assessment of Reproductive System Status Using Gordon's Functional Health Patterns:

- Sexuality–Reproductive
- Cognitive–Perceptual
- Role Relationship
- Coping/Stress Tolerance

Subjective Data

Assessment of Impaired Tissue Integrity

When did your symptoms begin?

Have you ever had this before?

Describe your symptoms.

Tell about the sexual habits of your sex partner or partners.

Assessment of Anxiety

Describe for me how you feel about this diagnosis.

What is your greatest concern?

Assessment of Knowledge

What do you know about the prevention/transmission of STIs?

Are you or have you ever been sexually active?

Do you have sex with men, women, or both?

Do you have more than one partner?

Do you want to get pregnant?

Do you use birth control? If so, what kind?

Do you use any protection from diseases such as condoms?

Assessment of High-Risk Behaviors

Are you aware of the dangers of unprotected sexual contact?

Are you concerned about either contracting or transmitting an STI?

Objective Data

Assessment of Impaired Tissue Integrity

Skin appearance (color, texture, temperature, discharge).

Describe lesions (type, location, distribution, size).

Assess for edema and pain.

Assessment of Anxiety

Verbal statements that indicate concern and anxiety.

Nonverbal clues such as facial expressions showing concern or worry, wringing of hands, or nervousness.

Is the patient withdrawn/quiet/apathetic?

Assessment of Knowledge

Patient's level of knowledge related to STIs.

Patient's willingness to learn more about the importance of and the types of protection.

Assessment of High-Risk Behaviors

Evidence of STI based on culture or serology results and/or clinical examination.

Outcomes and Evaluation Parameters	Planning and Interventions with *Rationales*
1. NURSING DIAGNOSIS: Impaired Tissue Integrity *related to effects of disease process of STIs* (NANDA-I © 2012)	
Outcome: Tissue integrity will be restored. ***Evaluation Parameters:*** Skin tissue will be without breaks or lesions. Skin tissue will be pink without redness, excoriation, pain, or damage.	Assess damaged skin. *Gives baseline data to determine the healing process.* Instruct the patient on healthy hygiene. *Keeping clean and dry will decrease organism growth.* Instruct the patient on the use of sitz bath or warm soaks *to cleanse the area, increase circulation, and increase healing.* Administer and do teaching on prescribed medications *to decrease organism growth and increase healing.*
2. NURSING DIAGNOSIS: Anxiety *related to diagnosis of sexually transmitted infection (STI)* (NANDA-I © 2012)	
Outcome: Patient's anxiety level will be reduced. ***Evaluation Parameters:*** Patient will verbalize feeling less anxious. Patient's affect will appear less stressed.	Assess patient concerns. *Gives baseline for intervention needs.* Provide open atmosphere and nonjudgmental attitude for communication/discussion *to maintain relaxed atmosphere and nonjudgmental attitude to encourage patient verbalization.* Identify support systems for patient *to identify whom patient can rely on for encouragement.* Answer questions honestly and openly *to provide a therapeutic environment.*
3. NURSING DIAGNOSIS: Deficient Knowledge *related to disease prevention/transmission* (NANDA-I © 2012)	
Outcome: Disease transmission will be reduced or prevented. ***Evaluation Parameters:*** Patient will verbalize understanding of ways to prevent/reduce transmission. Patient will verbalize understanding of need for partner treatment to reduce re-infection. Patient will verbalize increased knowledge of safer sex practices.	Assess knowledge level. *Must have baseline for teaching.* Teach ways to prevent/reduce disease transmission such as abstinence or condoms. *Both ways will decrease direct contact.* Encourage questions. *Giving information increases the chances of compliance.* Provide information regarding treatment of partners to reduce re-infection. *Important to reduce transmission.*

NURSING PROCESS: Patient Care Plan for Sexually Transmitted Infections, *continued*

4. NURSING DIAGNOSIS: Self-Neglect *related to ineffective health maintenance due to sexual behaviors* (NANDA-I © 2012)

Outcome: Patient will verbalize understanding of safer sex practices. ***Evaluation Parameters:*** Patient will verbalize understanding of the use of condoms. Patient will advise partner of need for treatment. Patient will avoid further exposure to sexually transmitted infection.	Assess understanding of how STIs are transmitted. *Must have baseline for teaching.* Assess understanding of the use of condoms. *Must have baseline for teaching.* Supply condoms as needed *to supply condoms for use with subsequent sexual contacts.* Encourage questions and frank discussion of risks of unprotected sexual contact. *Information provided in a nonjudgmental manner will increase potential for compliance.* Provide resources for pregnancy planning *to encourage the patient to prevent unplanned pregnancy.* Provide resources for the treatment of sexual partners *to emphasize the importance of partner treatment to prevent re-infection.*

Source: Adapted from Wilkinson, J. M., & Ahearn, N. R. (2009). *Prentice Hall nursing diagnosis handbook* (9th ed.). Upper Saddle River, NJ: Prentice Hall.

Once the infection is present, early treatment can help decrease its progression. Some STIs are curable, such as gonorrhea, syphilis, and trichomoniasis; others are only treatable. To prevent transferring infection to another partner, as well as enduring recurrence, safer sex practices are encouraged. Legal and ethical issues arise when treating patients for STIs. It is essential for the nurse to manage each situation with sound clinical judgment and sensitivity. This is the best approach to patient management. The Ethical Issues box demonstrates one approach that is both sensitive and ethical.

Collaborative Management

Sexually transmitted infections are a sensitive topic for many patients. Patients are reluctant to seek treatment for these issues and instead hope that they will resolve on their own. Nurses and health care providers must work together to help patients feel comfortable discussing their possible STIs and the source of these infections. Patients should be encouraged to disclose their infection to sexual partners; for some infections (i.e., HIV/AIDS, syphilis, gonorrhea, and chlamydia), the disease also may be reported to the public health department. On occasion, patients will realize that an STI is the result of an unfaithful partner. At that time, it may be reasonable to offer psychological counseling to the patient. In order to meet desired patient outcomes, it is essential that this interdisciplinary team communicate openly with one another in developing and evaluating care of the patient and family (IOM [Institute of Medicine], 2010).

Gerontological Considerations

Being older does not protect a person from sexually transmitted infections. Regardless of age, sex with someone who is infected will increase the risks of infection. Unfortunately, many health care providers overlook the possibility of an STI in an older adult because they believe that older people do not participate in risky sexual behavior. Therefore, many older adults who have STIs may be misdiagnosed. While it is true that sexual function does decrease with age, sexual interest continues. Older adults need encouragement and reminders to choose lifelong, healthy sexual behaviors.

Research

A goal of *Healthy People 2020* is to reduce the number of persons affected by sexually transmitted disease through health promotion education and improved access to quality health care (U.S. Department of Health and Human Resources [DHHS], 2010). Research is needed to help determine the best approaches to reach this goal. The Research Opportunities box lists some potential research topics.

RESEARCH OPPORTUNITIES Related to Sexually Transmitted Infections

Research	Clinical Impact
Sexually transmitted disease among people over age 50	Raise awareness, improve treatment
Expedited partner treatment	To raise provider awareness of pros and cons of this method of treating partners who are probably infected
Improving community resources for people at risk for STIs	To decrease the number of cases of STI in specific age, racial, and socio-economic groups
Effectiveness of abstinence only in the prevention of STIs among teenagers	To identify methods for prevention of STI among teenagers
Internet-based education program effectiveness	Education readily available to help prevent STIs

READ: **History of Present Illnesses** >> Laboratory Study Results >> Critical Thinking Questions

Kimberly Giroux is a 20-year-old female college student who was seen by her primary health care provider for lower abdominal pain. The health care provider suspects a tubo-ovarian abscess secondary to pelvic inflammatory disease and has sent Ms. Giroux to the hospital for diagnostic studies and care. On admission, Ms. Giroux tells the nurse that she has severe lower abdominal pain described as dull and continuous. She further describes the pain as 8 on a scale of 1 to 10, with 10 being the most intense pain. Ms. Giroux has been nauseated and has vomited twice today. She tells the nurse that she is wearing a perineal pad because "there is so much discharge" from her vagina. Ms. Giroux's last menstrual period was 2 weeks ago, but her periods are irregular. She denies any allergies to drugs.

Medical–Surgical History

Ms. Giroux is generally healthy and has never been in the hospital before. She denies use of any medication except Tylenol for fever or headache.

Social History

Ms. Giroux entered college last fall. She tells the nurse that she has been "burning the candle at both ends," partying 2 to 3 nights a week and studying to maintain her grade average. Ms. Giroux has a new boyfriend who is very popular in her circle of friends. She is very distressed to find out that sex with him, her first sexual partner, has resulted in this pelvic infection. Ms. Giroux admits drinking alcohol during the parties and when she is with her boyfriend. She denies use of tobacco or illicit drugs.

READ: History of Present Illnesses >> **Physical Exam** >> Admitting Medical Records >> Laboratory Study Results

Physical Examination

Temperature: 103°F (39.4°C) orally
Pulse: 126 beats per minute
Respiratory rate: 22 BP 110/70
O_2 Sat: 98% on room air
Weight: 125 pounds
Height: 5 feet 4 inches
HEENT: within normal limits
Heart: S_1S_2, tachycardia, regular rate and rhythm, no murmurs
Lungs: clear to auscultation in all fields
Abdomen: positive bowel sounds in all quadrants; flat, soft, tender with guarding in suprapubic area
Neuro exam: within normal limits
Skin: vulva and perineum erythematous and excoriated
Mental status: anxious, depressed, ashamed
Chest x-ray: normal
Pelvic ultrasound: thickened, fluid-filled fallopian tubes and right tubo-ovarian abscess
Cervical cultures (DNA probes) for *N. gonorrhoeae* and *C. trachomatis* are both positive.
Pregnancy test: negative

Admitting Medical Orders

Admit to Gynecologic Service
Admitting diagnosis: pelvic inflammatory disease
No known allergies
Call house officer: pulse < 60 & > 130 per minute; temperature > 38.5°C; urine output < 30 mL/hour for 2 hours; respiratory rate > 30 per minute
Ambulate PRN
Vital signs every 4 hours
Intake and output every 8 hours
IV D51/2 NS at 125 mL/hour

PRN Medications

Demerol 75 mg IV or IM every 6 hours prn abdominal pain
Phenergan 25 mg IV or IM every 6 hours prn nausea and/or vomiting

Scheduled Medications

Clindamycin 900 mg IV every 8 hours
Gentamycin loading dose (2 mg/kg) followed by maintenance dosing (1.5 mg/kg) every 8 hours

Ordered Laboratory Tests

CBC with differential; erythrocyte sedimentation rate; C-reactive protein

READ: History of Present Illnesses >> **Laboratory Study Results** >> Critical Thinking Questions

Test	On Admission	24 Hours After Antibiotics Started	48 Hours After Antibiotics Started
RBCs	4.3	4.32	
Hemoglobin	13 g/dL	12.8 g/dL	
Hematocrit	39%	38%	
RDW	12	12	
WBC	20,000/mm^3	20,500/mm^3	15,000/mm^3
Bands	20%	19%	12%
PMNs	80%	82%	78%
ESR	48 mm/h		25 mm/h

Test	On Admission	24 Hours After Antibiotics Started	48 Hours After Antibiotics Started
Serum creatinine and BUN	0.8 mg/dL and 10 mg/dL		0.9 mg/dL and 10 mg/dL
Cultures for gonorrhea and chlamydia	Both positive		
Pregnancy test	Negative		
C-Reactive Protein	28 mg/dL	24 mg/dL	19 mg/dL

DOCUMENT:

- >> Summary of Hospitalization
- >> Pathophysiology Form
- >> Laboratory Values
- >> Laboratory Results Explanation

APPLY:

- >> List of Potential Nursing Diagnoses
- >> Concept Map
- >> Critical Thinking Questions and Concept Map

APPLY: History of Present Illnesses >> Laboratory Study Results >> **Critical Thinking Questions**

1. Should this patient be in a private room? If so, why?
2. What is the top priority for this patient?
3. What are the potential side effects of the IV antibiotics ordered?
4. This patient needs emotional support. How should the nurse approach this aspect of her care?

Answers to Critical Thinking Questions can be found in Appendix D in the Osborn Student Resources at nursing.pearsonhighered.com.

NCLEX® PRACTICE

1. A female patient is diagnosed with a chlamydia infection. The nurse anticipates that this patient will most likely be treated with:
   1. Penicillin G.
   2. Flagyl (metronidazole).
   3. Zithromax (azithromycin).
   4. Cleocin (clindamycin).
2. A male patient comes into the clinic with a complaint of dysuria and a purulent urethral discharge. His vital signs are within normal limits. He had unprotected sex 2 weeks ago and his symptoms began 3 days ago. The most likely cause of his symptoms is:
   1. genital herpes.
   2. gonorrhea.
   3. syphilis.
   4. trichomoniasis.
3. A female patient is seen in the clinic for a recurrence of painful vesicles on her labia consistent with genital herpes.. The priority nursing diagnosis for this patient is:
   1. Potential for Social Isolation.
   2. Risk for Infection.
   3. Knowledge Deficit.
   4. Risk for Nutritional Deficit.
4. A patient is concerned that she may have contracted syphilis. The nurse would include in the plan of care to explain to the patient that she will likely need this test which is definitive for syphilis, before a diagnosis is made.
   1. RPR.
   2. VDRL.
   3. dark field microscopic examination.
   4. MHA-TP.
5. When discussing sexually transmitted infections (STIs) with a community group, a participant asks if STIs can be treated. The nurse can discuss which of the following that can be successfully treated with antimicrobial therapy? (select all that apply)
   1. Hepatitis
   2. Head lice
   3. HIV
   4. Chlamydia
   5. yphilis
6. A female student comes to the women's health center and expresses to the nurse that she is concerned that she may be at risk for contracting sexually transmitted infections. When planning education for this client, the nurse should consider which of the following data that increase risk for STI revealed by the patient during the health assessment interview? (select all that apply)
   1. is 21 years old.
   2. is from an affluent family.
   3. has had one sex partner.
   4. broke up with her last boyfriend because he was having sex with someone else.
   5. reveals a history of binge drinking.

Answers to NCLEX Practice Questions can be found in Appendix D in the Osborn Student Resources at nursing.pearsonhighered.com. Practice additional NCLEX questions online at the Student Resources site.

REFERENCES

Adams, M., & Koch, R. (2010). *Pharmacology: Connections to nursing practice.* Upper Saddle River, NJ: Pearson.

Allsworth, J. E., Lewis, V. A., & Peipert, J. F. (2008). Viral sexually transmitted infections and bacterial vaginosis: 2001–2004 National Health and Nutrition Examination Survey data. *Sexually Transmitted Diseases, 35*(9), 791–796.

Allsworth, J. E., & Peipert, J. F. (2007). Prevalence of bacterial vaginosis: 2001–2004 National Health and Nutrition Examination Survey data. *Obstetrics & Gynecology, 109*(1), 114–120.

American Social Health Association. (2010). Learn about STIs/STDs. Retrieved from http://www.ashastd.org/learn/learn_overview.cfm

Batteiger, B., Tu, W., Ofner, S., Van Der Pol, B., Stothard, D., Orr, D., et al. (2010). Repeated *Chlamydia trachomatis* genital infections in adolescent women. *The Journal of Infectious Diseases, 201*(1), 42–51.

Caserta, M. (2009). Neonatal conjunctivitis. *Merck Manuals Online Medical Library.* Retrieved from http://www.merckmedicus.com/pp/us/hcp/framemm.jsp?pg=www.merck.com/mmpe/index.html

Centers for Disease Control and Prevention (CDC). (2010a). Conjunctivitis (pink eye) in newborns. Retrieved from http://www.cdc.gov/conjunctivitis/newborns.html

Centers for Disease Control and Prevention (CDC). (2010b). Human papillomavirus (HPV). Retrieved from http://www.cdc.gov/hpv/

Centers for Disease Control and Prevention (CDC). (2010c). Sexually transmitted disease. Retrieved from http://www.cdc.gov/std/

Centers for Disease Control and Prevention (CDC). (2010d). Sexually transmitted diseases/Bacterial vaginosis CDC fact sheet. Retrieved from http://www.cdc.gov/std/bv/STDFact-Bacterial-Vaginosis.htm

Centers for Disease Control and Prevention (CDC). (2010e). Sexually transmitted diseases/Chlamydia fact sheet. Retrieved from http://www.cdc.gov/std/chlamydia/STDFact-Chlamydia.htm

Centers for Disease Control and Prevention (CDC). (2010f). Sexually transmitted diseases/Genital herpes CDC fact sheet. Retrieved from http://www.cdc.gov/std/Herpes/STDFact-Herpes.htm

Centers for Disease Control and Prevention (CDC). (2010g). Sexually transmitted diseases/Gonorrhea CDC fact sheet. Retrieved from http://www.cdc.gov/std/gonorrhea/STDFact-gonorrhea.htm

Centers for Disease Control and Prevention (CDC). (2010h). Sexually transmitted diseases/Pelvic inflammatory disease CDC fact sheet. Retrieved from http://www.cdc.gov/std/pid/STDFact-PID.htm

Centers for Disease Control and Prevention (CDC). (2010i). Sexually transmitted diseases/Syphilis CDC fact sheet. Retrieved from http://www.cdc.gov/std/syphilis/STDFact-Syphilis.htm

Centers for Disease Control and Prevention (CDC). (2010j). Sexually transmitted diseases/Trichomoniasis CDC fact sheet. Retrieved from http://www.cdc.gov/std/trichomonas/STDFact-Trichomoniasis.htm

Centers for Disease Control and Prevention (CDC). (2010k). 2009 Sexually transmitted diseases surveillance/Chlamydia. Retrieved from http://www.cdc.gov/std/stats09/chlamydia.htm

Centers for Disease Control and Prevention (CDC). (2010l). 2009 Sexually transmitted diseases surveillance/Gonorrhea. Retrieved from http://www.cdc.gov/std/stats09/gonorrhea.htm

Centers for Disease Control and Prevention (CDC). (2010m). 2009 Sexually transmitted diseases surveillance/Other sexually transmitted diseases. Retrieved from http://www.cdc.gov/std/stats09/other.htm

Centers for Disease Control and Prevention (CDC). (2010n). 2009 Sexually transmitted diseases surveillance/STDs in women and infants. Retrieved from http://www.cdc.gov/std/stats09/womenandinf.htm

Centers for Disease Control and Prevention (CDC). (2010o). 2009 Sexually transmitted diseases surveillance/Syphilis. Retrieved from http://www.cdc.gov/std/stats09/Syphilis.htm

Centers for Disease Control and Prevention (CDC). (2010p). 2009 Sexually transmitted diseases surveillance/Table 1. Cases of sexually transmitted disease reported by state health departments and rates per 100,000 population, United States, 1941–2009. Retrieved from http://www.cdc.gov/std/stats09/tables/1.htm

Centers for Disease Control and Prevention (CDC). (2010q). 2009 Sexually transmitted diseases surveillance/Table 43. Selected STDs and complications—initial visits to physicians' offices, National Disease and Therapeutic Index, United States, 1966–2009. Retrieved from http://www.cdc.gov/std/stats09/tables/43.htm

Centers for Disease Control and Prevention (CDC). (2010r). 2009 Sexually transmitted diseases surveillance/Trends in sexually transmitted disease in the United States: 2009 National data for gonorrhea, chlamydia, & syphilis. Retrieved from http://www.cdc.gov/std/stats09/trends.htm

Corey, L., & Wald, A. (2009). Maternal and neonatal herpes simplex virus infections: Current concepts. *The New England Journal of Medicine, 361*(14), 1376–1384. doi: 10.1056/NEJMra0807633

Douglas, J. (2009). Penicillin treatment of syphilis: Clearing away the shadow of the land. *Journal of the American Medical Association, 301*(7), 769–771.

Healthwise Staff. (2009a). Chlamydia tests. Quest Diagnostics. Retrieved from http://www.questdiagnostics.com/kbase/topic/medtest/hw4046/descrip.htm

Healthwise Staff. (2009b). Gonorrhea tests. Quest Diagnostics. Retrieved from http://www.questdiagnostics.com/kbase/topic/medtest/hw4905/descrip.htm

Healthwise Staff. (2009c). Human papillomavirus test. Quest Diagnostics. Retrieved from http://www.questdiagnostics.com/kbase/topic/medtest/tu6451/descrip.htm

IOM (Institute of Medicine). (2010). *The future of nursing: Leading change, advancing health.* Washington, DC: The Academic Press.

Jenkins, W., & Kruse, J. (2010). Chlamydia screening: How we can better serve patients. *The Journal of Family Practice, 59*(2), E10–E12.

Kaloczi, L., Latendresse, G., & Morgan, K. (2010). Sexually transmitted infections. In K. McCance & S. Huether, (Eds.), *Pathophysiology: The biologic basis for disease in adults and children* (6th ed., pp. 923–951). St. Louis: Mosby/Elsevier.

Kee, J. (2010). *Laboratory and diagnostic tests* (8th ed.). Upper Saddle River, NJ: Pearson.

Keefe, A. (2010). Syphilis: A public health issue. *Nurse Prescribing, 8*(3), 111–114.

Klausner, J. D., Bernstein, K. T., Pandori, M., San Francisco Dept of Public Health, Hall, C., Gibson, S., et al. (2009). Clinic-based testing for rectal and pharyngeal *Neisseria gonorrhoeae* and *Chlamydia trachomatis* infections by community-based organizations—five cities, United States. *Morbidity and Mortality Weekly Report, 58*(26), 716–719.

Latendresse, G., McCance, K., & Morgan, K. (2010). Alterations of the reproductive system. In K. McCance & S. Huether (Eds.), *Pathophysiology: The biologic basis for disease in adults and children* (6th ed., pp. 816–920). St. Louis: Mosby/Elsevier.

Mark, H., Gilbert, L., & Nanda, J. (2009). Psychological well-being and quality of life among women newly diagnosed with genital herpes. *Journal of Obstetrics, Gynecology, Neonatal Nursing, 38,*(3) 320–326. doi: 10.1111/j.1552-6909.01026.x

Martinez, R. C., Franceschini, S. A., Patta, M. C., Quintana, S. M., Gomes, B. C., De Martinis, E. C., Reid, G. (2009). Improved cure of bacterial vaginosis with single dose of tinidazole (2 g), Lactobacillus rhamnosus GR-1, and Lactobacillus reuteri RC-14: a randomized, double-blind, placebo-controlled trial. *Canadian Journal of Microbiology, 55*(2), 133–138.

McCloskey, C. (2010). Updated office testing skills for vaginal infections. *The Nurse Practitioner, 35*(2), 46–52.

McCutchan, A. (2008). Syphilis. *Merck Manuals Online Medical Library.* Retrieved from http://www.merckmedicus.com/pp/us/hcp/framemm.jsp?pg=www.merck.com/mmpe/index.html

Pinninti, S., & Tolan, R. (2010). Herpes simplex virus infection. eMedicine. Retrieved from http://emedicine.medscape.com/article/964866-overview

Salvaggio, M., & Lutwick, L. (2010). Herpes simplex. eMedicine. Retrieved from http://emedicine.medscape.com/article/218580-overview

PubMed. (2010). Chlamydia. Retrieved from http://www.ncbi.nlm.nih.gov/pubmedhealth/PMH0002321/

Saperstein, A., & Firnhaber, G. (2010). Should you test or treat partners of patients with gonorrhea, chlamydia, or trichomoniasis? Clinical inquiries. *The Journal of Family Practice, 59*(1), 46–48.

Schardt, D. (2010, April). Probiotics: "Good" bacteria to the rescue? *Nutrition Action HealthLetter*, 9–11.

Schwartz, R., & Kapila, R. (2010). Gonococcemia. eMedicine. Retrieved from http://emedicine.medscape.com/article/1055007-overview

Senok, A., Verstraelen, H., Temmerman, M., & Botta, G. (2009). Probiotics for the treatment of bacterial vaginosis. *Cochrane Database of Systematic Reviews, Issue 4.* doi: 10.1002/14651858.CD006289.pub2

Snowden, R. (2010). Gardasil approved to prevent anal cancer. *Learn About Cancer/News.* Retrieved from http://www.cancer.org/Cancer/news/News/gardasil-approved-to-prevent-anal-cancer

STD Quarterly. (2010). STD alert: 50% of urban teen girls acquire STDs within 2 years of first sexual activity. *STD Quarterly,* April 2010 Supplement of *Contraceptive Technology Update*, 1–3.

Strickland, J., & Gibson, E. (2009). Teach the teacher: Pelvic inflammatory disease. *Journal of Pediatric and Adolescent Gynecology, 22*, 387–389. doi:10.1016/j.jpag.2009.03.002

Tu, W., Batteiger, B., Wiehe, S., Ofner, S., Van Der Pol, B., Katz, B. et al. (2009). Time from first intercourse to first sexually transmitted disease among adolescent women. *Archives of Pediatrics and Adolescent Medicine, 163*(12), 1106–1111.

U.S. Department of Health and Human Services (DHHS). (2010). Sexually transmitted disease. HealthyPeople.gov. Retrieved from http://www.healthypeople.gov/2020/topicsobjectives2020/overview.aspx?topicid=37

U.S. Preventive Services Task Force (USPSTF). (2007). Screening for chlamydia infection. Retrieved from http://www.uspreventiveservicestaskforce.org/uspstf/uspschlm.htm

Voelker, R. (2010). Experts reconsider wisdom of limiting chlamydia screening only to women. *Journal of American Medical Association, 303*(9), 823–824.

Waseem, M., & Aslam, M. (2009). Syphilis. eMedicine. Retrieved from http://emedicine.medscape.com/article/969023-overview

Web MD. (2010). Recurrent respiratory papillomatosis. Lung Disease and Respiratory Center/WebMD. Retrieved from http://www.webmd.com/lung/recurrent-respiratory-papillomatosis

Wilkinson, J. M., & Ahearn, N. R. (2009). *Prentice Hall nursing diagnosis handbook* (9th ed.). Upper Saddle River, NJ: Prentice Hall.

Williams, N. (2010). Probiotics: Clinical review. *American Journal of Health-System Pharmacists, 67*, 449–458. doi:10.2146/ajhp090168

Workowski, K., & Berman, S. (2010). Sexually transmitted disease treatment guidelines, 2010. *Morbidity and Mortality Weekly Report, 59*(RR12), 1–110.

World Health Organization. (2010a). Initiative for vaccine research. Sexually transmitted infection/*Chlamydia trachomatis.* Retrieved from http://www.who.int/vaccine_research/diseases/soa_std/en/index1.html

World Health Organization. (2010b). Sexually transmitted infection. Retrieved from http://www.who.int/topics/sexually_transmitted_infections/en/

Ya, W., Reifer, C., & Miller, L. E. (2010). Efficacy of vaginal probiotic capsules for recurrent bacterial vaginosis: A double-blind, randomized, placebo-controlled study. *American Journal of Obstetrics and Gynecology, 203*(2), 120.e1–6.

Caring for the Patient with Breast Disorders

CHAPTER 44

Patricia Caudle
Kathleen Osborn
John M. Osborn, MD

Outcome-Based Learning Objectives

After studying this chapter, the learner will be able to:

1. Differentiate the most common benign and malignant breast disorders of women and men.
2. Discuss the etiology, pathophysiology, clinical manifestations, diagnostic studies, and treatment of breast disorders.
3. Generate nursing management goals when caring for patients with breast disorders.
4. Generate nursing diagnoses and apply the nursing process to the care of patients with breast disorders.
5. Plan interventions that will enhance health education, health promotion, and disease prevention among patients at risk for breast disorders.
6. Determine outcome goals for nursing care of patients with breast disorders.

KEY TERMS

ablate p.1343
atypia p.1332
cysts p.1332
duct ectasia p.1332
fat necrosis p.1332
fibroadenomas p.1332
fibrocystic breast changes p.1331
galactorrhea p.1332
gynecomastia p.1332
hyperprolactinemia p.1334
hypothyroidism p.1334
induration p.1341
inflammatory breast cancer (IBC) p.1341
lumpectomy p.1342
macromastia p.1332
mammography p.1342
mastalgia p.1332
mastectomy p.1344
mastitis p.1332
Mondor disease p.1332
neoadjuvant therapy p.1345
Paget's disease p.1339
papilloma p.1334
peau d'orange p.1341
phyllodes tumor p.1332
superficial thrombophlebitis p.1336
targeted therapy p.1345

BREAST DISORDERS occur in both women and men and may be benign or malignant. Breast disorders are typically manifested as masses, pain, inflammation, enlargement, or nipple discharge. Breast signs and symptoms may signal malignant or benign lesions; therefore, all must be carefully evaluated.

It is estimated that as many as 80% of women experience some form of benign breast complaint during their lifetime (Latendresse, McCance, & Morgan, 2010). Breast malignancies are the most commonly occurring cancer in women and the second leading cause of death after lung cancer in women in the United States (American Cancer Society [ACS], 2011a). The topic of this first section is common benign breast disorders.

Benign Breast Disease

Benign breast disease (BBD) is a term used to identify several benign alterations that may occur in the breast as a result of changes in hormones during the menstrual cycle. These benign changes may cause irregular lumpiness, cysts, sensitive nipples, itching, pain, or nipple discharge. These signs and symptoms can be very distressing to the woman because of the specter of breast cancer. All breast complaints must be evaluated closely because of the potential for breast cancer.

Many forms of histologic change in breast tissue may cause symptoms. Those that are nonproliferative such as fibrocystic changes, cysts, and benign tumors such as fibroadenomas are very common. In fact, it has been estimated that 50% to 80% of women experience these conditions (Giuliano & Hurvitz, 2011; Latendresse et al., 2010; Lee, 2009). Nonproliferative changes are caused by repeated hormonal fluctuations of the menstrual cycle that cause milk glands and ducts to enlarge and then decrease in size each month. Breast growth due to these cellular changes peaks during the luteal phase. In many women, the breasts may enlarge as much as 15% during the luteal phase (Lee, 2009).

Fibrocystic breast changes are characterized by an increase in glandular and fibrous tissues in the breast (Figure 44–1◆). This increase in fibrous tissue is palpable on examination and also may be seen on mammography. Fibrocystic changes are thought to be caused

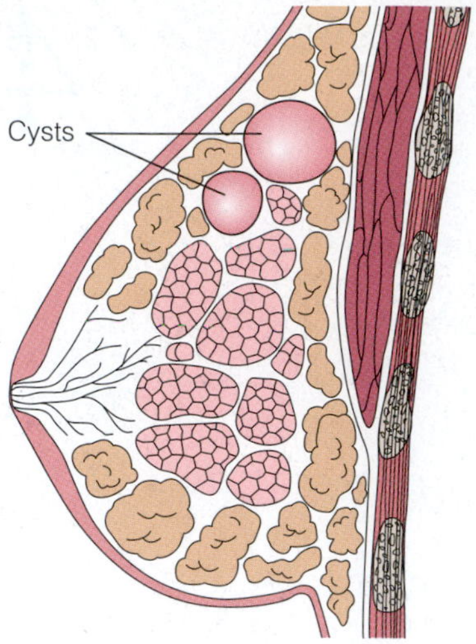

FIGURE 44–1 ◆ Fibrocystic breast changes.

by estrogen dominance, which is why the changes wax and wane with menses and usually disappear after menopause; however, the exact cause is unknown. When the fibrous tissue blocks milk ducts, fluid-filled cysts form. During the luteal phase of the menstrual cycle, fibrocystic changes may cause pain in the breasts. Typically, this condition affects women between the ages of 30 and 50.

Cysts (fluid-filled sacs) caused by blocked milk ducts are most likely to be noticed by the woman during the luteal phase of her menstrual cycle, when the cysts tend to enlarge. A cyst may or may not be tender or painful. If the cyst is near the surface of the breast, it is easier to determine whether it is fluid filled or solid. If the cyst is deeper, it may feel hard. Ultrasound and fine needle aspiration are needed to distinguish between fluid filled and solid masses.

Fibroadenomas are benign solid tumors that occur more often in Black women than other races during their 30s (Giuliano & Hurvitz, 2011). They rarely occur after menopause. Fibroadenomas are made of epithelial and connective tissue that grows under the influence of estrogen. They are round or oval, and they have clear boundaries and a rubbery texture.

Proliferative breast lesions without **atypia** (abnormality in a cell that may or may not be precancerous) may occur as a result of the proliferation of epithelial cells of the ducts and stroma (supporting tissue) without signs of malignancy. The cells in these lesions are without precancerous abnormalities (ACS, 2011a; Latendresse et al., 2010; Lee, 2009). When these changes occur, the risk for breast cancer increases about 1.5 to 2 times normal (ACS, 2011a). Chart 44–1 lists the types of proliferative lesions without and with atypia.

Proliferative breast lesions with atypia comprise a third group of BBD. These lesions are benign, but women who have these cellular changes in the breasts have an increased risk for breast cancer that is 4 to 5 times normal (ACS, 2011a). See Chart 44–1 for a list of proliferative breast lesions with atypia.

Several benign breast conditions do not fall into these categories. For example, congenital nipple inversion, **macromastia** (large breasts), **mastitis** (inflammatory breast disorder), **Mondor disease** (superficial thrombophlebitis of the breast), **phyllodes tumor** (tumor of large size that consists of both epithelial and stromal cells), mammary **duct ectasia** (chronic ductal inflammation and fibrosis), and **fat necrosis** (mass from trauma or surgery) (Latendresse et al., 2010). These conditions may be confused with or mask breast cancer. In the case of phyllodes tumor, about 10% to 25% will actually become malignant (Giuliano & Hurvitz, 2011; Latendresse et al., 2010).

CHART 44–1 Proliferative Breast Lesions with and without Atypia

Without Atypia	With Atypia
• Epithelial hyperplasia	• Atypical hyperplasia
• Sclerosing adenosis	• Ductal hyperplasia
• Complex sclerosing lesions	• Lobular hyperplasia.
• Single papillomas.	

Source: Adapted from Latendresse, G., McCance, K., & Morgan, K. (2010). Alterations of the reproductive systems. In K. McCance & S. Huether (Eds.), *Pathophysiology: The biologic basis for disease in adults and children* (6th ed., pp. 781–815). St. Louis: Mosby/Elsevier.

Mondor disease is a rare condition in which subcutaneous veins of the chest and breasts become inflamed and tender (Figure 44–2◆). Most cases are associated with breast surgery, and only 400 cases of Mondor disease have been reported worldwide (Schwartz, 2011). This is a self-limited disorder caused by pressure on a vein or direct trauma to the vein. However, Mondor disease has also been associated with breast cancer.

Phyllodes tumors are fibroepithelial, may be surrounded by a proliferation of connective tissue stroma, and grow to a large size (Latendresse et al., 2010). Some of these slow growing tumors may become malignant.

Duct ectasia is most likely to occur after menopause or during pregnancy and breast-feeding (Latendresse et al., 2010). In duct ectasia, the milk duct becomes dilated and filled with cellular debris. This will cause inflammation along the duct; in rare cases, the duct will rupture. These lesions are a frequent cause of nipple discharge that is sticky, thick, and sometimes bloody.

Health care providers agree that all clinical manifestations of the breast must be evaluated carefully to differentiate cancerous lesions from benign ones. The manifestations that warrant careful scrutiny include masses, **mastalgia** (breast pain), **galactorrhea** (nipple discharge), mastitis, and **gynecomastia** (enlargement of the male breast).

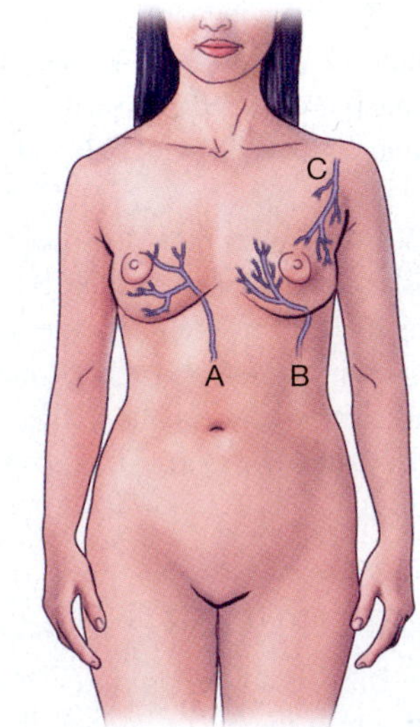

FIGURE 44–2 ◆ Mondor disease (superficial thrombophlebitis of the breast).
Source: http://emedicine.medscape.com/article/1087099-overview.

Breast Masses

A mass in the breast is the most frightening of the breast manifestations and the one sign most frequently associated with breast cancer. However, a mass may be caused by a multitude of benign disorders, including cysts, fibroadenoma, phyllodes tumor, fibrocystic changes, normal nodularity of the breast during the luteal phase, fat lobules, fat necrosis, inframammary lymph nodes, or infection (Giuliano & Hurvitz, 2011; Rodden, 2009). Benign tumors may be solid or fluid filled, smooth, soft or firm, and mobile; they also may have distinct borders. These masses change in size at different phases of the menstrual cycle and will disappear after menopause. However, lumps that are diagnosed as malignant may mimic the benign mass. Many malignant masses present as hard and fixed with irregular borders (Latendresse et al., 2010; Rodden, 2009). Chart 44–2 is a list of signs of benign and malignant breast masses.

Diagnostic Tests and Procedures

A thorough history, including individual risk factors for cancer, physical examination, imaging by ultrasound or mammography, and either surgical or nonsurgical biopsy, are considered necessary for all women who have a palpable breast mass (Lee, 2009). The Diagnostic Tests feature delineates all the modalities used to diagnose breast conditions.

CHART 44–2 Differentiation of Breast Masses by Clinical Exam

Benign Mass	Malignant Mass
No skin changes are noted. Breasts are symmetrical.	The mass is fixed to surrounding skin and soft tissue, causing skin dimpling and asymmetry of the breasts.
When palpated, the lump is smooth.	The mass is irregularly shaped.
The consistency of the lump is soft to firm.	The consistency is hard.
The lump is mobile beneath the skin.	The mass is immobile beneath the skin.
The margins are well defined and easily delineated.	The margins are poorly defined and irregular.
The mass is tender to palpation.	The mass is usually nontender.
Masses regress after menopause.	More common after age 50.

Source: Adapted from: Bickley, L. (2007). *Guide to physical examination and history taking* (9th ed.). Philadelphia: Lippincott Williams & Wilkins.

DIAGNOSTIC TESTS For Breast Disorders

Test with Description, Rationale, and Normal Values	Expected Abnormality
Mammogram (breast x-ray) *Used to detect suspicious changes in breast tissue.* No suspicious changes detected.	Calcifications, masses, thickening, abnormal ducts, or glandular tissue are possible signs of malignancy. Can detect breast lesion 2 years before it is palpable. Can detect about 90% of breast malignancies. Requires biopsy for confirmation.
Ultrasound *Used to detect abnormalities of the breast and to differentiate fluid from solid masses.* Normal sound wave pattern image of the breasts.	Masses, cysts, edema, and thickening of the breasts may be detected. Better than mammogram for women under 40 with dense breasts or with silicone implants.
Core Needle Biopsy Ultrasound-guided Stereotactic-guided Freehand *Allows for extraction of tissue for pathologic evaluation.* Normal or normal variations in tissue are normal.	Ultrasound and stereotactic-guided core needle biopsy 97% to 99% accurate in finding breast cancer. Freehand finds only 86% of breast cancers.
Surgical Biopsy *Surgical excision to remove suspicious tissue for pathologic evaluation.*	Find 98% to 99% of breast cancers.
BRCA1 and BRCA2 Genetics Testing *Blood sample.* Negative findings of genetic mutation of these genes.	Positive findings identify women and men at risk for breast cancer and other cancers.
HER2/Neu Oncogene *May be identified in a biopsy sample or the blood.* Negative for HER2 gives a better prognosis.	Positive HER2/neu findings associated with poor prognosis. Targeted therapy with trastuzumab (Herceptin) for this oncogene may control the cancer.
Estrogen or Progesterone Receptor Negative tumor tissue estrogen or progesterone receptors.	Tumors positive for estrogen or progesterone receptors respond to anti-estrogen therapy (e.g., tamoxifen).

Sources: Adapted from Agency for Healthcare Research and Quality (AHRQ). (2010a). Core-needle biopsy for breast abnormalities: Clinician's guide. Effective Health Care Program. Retrieved from http://effectivehealthcare.ahrq.gov/index.cfm/search-for-guides-reviews-and-reports/?pageaction=displayproduct&productID=406&mode=P; Agency for Healthcare Research and Quality (AHRQ). (2010b). Having a breast biopsy: A guide for women and their families. Effective Health Care Program. Retrieved from http://effectivehealthcare.ahrq.gov/index.cfm/search-for-guides-reviews-and-reports/?pageaction=displayproduct&productID=407; Kee, J. L. (2010). *Laboratory and diagnostic tests with nursing implications* (8th ed.). Upper Saddle River, NJ: Prentice Hall.

Medical Management

Once imaging and biopsy have determined that a mass is benign, the health care provider can offer either ultrasound or mammogram follow-up every 6 months for 2 years and then annually or full excision of the mass (Lee, 2009). Many women become very anxious when there is a breast mass and want it removed as soon as possible.

Mastalgia

Breast pain may wax and wane during the menstrual cycle or remain constant. Cyclic breast pain is more common among women ages 30 to 49 and is worse during the luteal phase (Rodden, 2009). This type of pain is usually described as soreness or as aching discomfort that is related to fibrocystic changes. Fibrocystic changes are due to estrogen and progesterone effects that cause swelling, lumpiness, and tenderness during the menstrual cycle (Mills, 2011). When perimenopause occurs and the hormones are off balance, the breasts can become more tender. Constant breast pain that is not associated with the menstrual cycle is more likely to be sharp, burning, and unilateral. Women in their perimenopausal and menopausal years are more apt to have this type of mastalgia. The cause is unknown (Rodden, 2009). Several drugs may cause mastalgia including some antipsychotic drugs, some antibiotics, drugs that contain hormones such as birth control pills, and clomiphene. Mastalgia without a mass is rarely a sign of breast cancer (Rodden, 2009).

Diagnostic Tests and Procedures

Even though mastalgia without a mass is probably benign, a careful history and physical examination are warranted. Family history of a close relative with breast cancer is an indication for ultrasound in women younger than age 40 to look for any evidence of malignancy. For older women with constant breast pain and risk factors for breast cancer, a mammogram is recommended (Rodden, 2009).

Medical Management

The patient should be reassured that mastalgia is usually self-limited. Bras that fit properly, cessation of smoking, and reduction in caffeine are usually suggested, along with decreasing fat and sodium intake. Massage with heat or ice also may help. If a medication may be causing the problem, it should be changed if possible. Evening primrose oil, which contains gamma-linolenic acid (omega 6 essential fatty acid), may be ordered, as some unclear scientific evidence exists that it is effective in reducing mastalgia (National Standard, 2011). Medications that have been somewhat effective, include danazol, bromocriptine, and tamoxifen. Topical afimoxifene gel and oral and topical nonsteroidal anti-inflammatory drugs (NSAIDs) are also effective (Rodden, 2009). Read more about these drugs in the Pharmacology feature.

Galactorrhea

Nipple drainage from a nonlactating breast may be benign or a sign of malignancy. Manipulation of the breast and nipple by the woman or her sexual partner, medications such as some antihypertensives and antipsychotics, or a loose fitting bra may cause benign nipple discharge that will continue as long as the stimulation occurs. Other causes of nipple discharge include duct ectasia, intraductal papilloma, carcinoma, pregnancy, and systemic disorders such as **hyperprolactinemia** (endocrine disorder caused by pituitary tumor) and **hypothyroidism** (endocrine disorder caused by low production of thyroid hormone). Like mastalgia, galactorrhea may also be a side effect of antipsychotic drugs, antihypertensive drugs, birth control pills, or hormone replacement therapy (Giuliano & Hurvitz, 2011).

Nipple discharge may be unilateral or bilateral, from one duct in the nipple, or from all the ducts in both nipples. Nipple discharge from a single duct in one breast that is serous or bloody may be a sign of cancer or a sign of a single, benign **papilloma** (epithelial soft, yellow or red growth attached to the duct wall) (Latendresse et al., 2010). Nipple discharge may be green, gray, yellow, brown, black, or white. It may be milky, clear, purulent, or sticky (Giuliano & Hurvitz, 2011; Rodden, 2009). Green or brownish discharge during the luteal phase of the menstrual cycle is most often due to fibrocystic changes. Milky discharge from multiple ducts may indicate pregnancy or hyperprolactinemia. Purulent discharge may occur when an abscess has formed secondary to mastitis (Giuliano & Hurvitz, 2011). Dirty white, greenish, or black discharge may indicate ductal ectasia (Mayo Clinic Staff, 2011b).

Diagnostic Tests and Procedures

Cytology of the nipple discharge is often done in an attempt to determine whether there is a malignancy in the breast. A negative cytology report, however, does not eliminate cancer as a possible cause (Giuliano & Hurvitz, 2011). Even if the cytology report is positive, further testing is needed to identify the type of cancer involved. Other laboratory tests that are done when there is galactorrhea may include a pregnancy test, thyroid function tests, and serum prolactin levels (Rodden, 2009). Diagnostic mammogram or ultrasound should be done for all women older than age 30 with unexplained galactorrhea.

Medical Management

The first recommendation is to stop any nipple stimulation. Any squeezing of fluid from the nipple will prolong the problem. Bras that fit well and changes in any possibly offending medications such as angiotensin-converting enzyme inhibitors and thorazine that a patient may be taking are important steps in stopping benign galactorrhea. If the condition persists, if there is any evidence of a possible malignancy, or if the patient is anxious about the discharge, a referral should be made to a breast surgeon for duct excision biopsy (Giuliano & Hurvitz, 2011; Rodden, 2009).

Mastitis

Mastitis, or inflammation of the breast tissue, occurs most often in lactating women. It has been estimated that about 33% of women who are breast-feeding develop mastitis (Balkam, 2010). Breast inflammation in lactating women may be noninfectious or infectious. Both types of mastitis are most likely to occur during the first 3 months after delivery among first-time mothers. Noninfectious redness and heat occur when the milk duct is not draining. The woman may or may not have fever. Infectious mastitis occurs when microorganisms invade the breast through a portal of entry such as a crack or a fissure in the nipple or through a milk duct. The usual causative agent in infectious mastitis is *Staphylococcus aureus* (Rogers & Cox, 2011).

Symptoms of infectious mastitis include breast tenderness, redness and heat (typically at the site of inflammation), and edema. The woman may also experience fatigue, malaise, fever, or chills. Mastitis due to bacterial infection can progress to abscess formation (Rogers & Cox, 2011). It is estimated that about 3% of women with infectious mastitis will develop an abscess (Balkam, 2010). The most serious form of infectious mastitis and abscess is caused by

PHARMACOLOGY Summary of Medications Used to Treat Breast Disorders

Medication and Action	Application/Indication	Nursing Responsibility
Antiestrogen Medications Tamoxifen (Nolvadex, Soltamox) Anastrozole (Arimidex) Letrozole (Femara) ***Action:*** Binds to estrogen receptors, produces agonist effects in bone and antagonist effects in breasts. Binding in breast tissue inhibits DNA replication.	Risk reduction of 86% for invasive breast cancer in men and women with estrogen receptor positive tumors. Reduces gynecomastia. Used to treat male gynecomastia.	Watch for side effects: deep vein thrombosis (DVT) and pulmonary embolism. Monitor baseline and changes in CBC. Administer analgesics for pain when discomfort occurs as the tumor responds to the medication.
Medications for Mastalgia Evening primrose oil (contains gamma-linolenic acid) ***Action:*** Essential fatty acid.	Improves cyclic mastalgia with minimal side effects.	Advise patient it may take months for full relief of symptoms.
Danazol ***Action:*** Exerts anti-estrogen effects. After 6 weeks of therapy, causes anovulation and amenorrhea.	Most effective medication for mastalgia. Also used in fibrocystic breast changes.	Pregnancy category X, obtain pregnancy test before administering.
Bromocriptine ***Action:*** Dopamine agonist; activates dopaminergic receptors in the hypothalamus. Ergot alkaloid.	Off-label use in mastalgia.	High side effect profile. Not tolerated well in most women.
Afimoxifene gel ***Action:*** Estrogen receptor blocker: topical form.	Effective in some cases of mastalgia.	Applied to breast; minimum side effects.
Nonsteroidal anti-inflammatory drugs (NSAIDs)—oral and topical gel ***Action:*** Analgesic, antipyretic. Inhibits COX-1 and COX-2, thereby blocking prostaglandin synthesis.	Used in mastalgia and other painful conditions.	Assess for history of stomach ulcers or gastrointestinal bleeding before giving; assess for effectiveness, fluid retention, and kidney and liver function.
Medications for Mastitis Dicloxacillin ***Action:*** Penicillinase-resistant penicillin—primarily used for staphylococcal infection; inhibits bacterial wall synthesis.	Antibiotic for infectious mastitis.	Check for allergy to penicillin before giving; obtain culture and sensitivity (C&S) before beginning this antibiotic; monitor for adverse reactions.
Cephalexin ***Action:*** Antibacterial; cell wall inhibitor.	Treatment of infectious mastitis.	Check for allergies before giving; obtain C&S prior to beginning treatment; monitor for allergies and suprainfection, especially diarrheal infection.
Clindamycin ***Action:*** Acts on the bacterial ribosomal subunit; bacteriostatic.	Antibiotic that may be used in mastitis.	Check for allergies before giving; obtain C&S prior to beginning treatment; monitor for allergies and diarrhea. Risk for development of pseudomembranous colitis exists that can be fatal.
Medications for Breast Cancer Treatment Trastuzumab (Herceptin) ***Action:*** Monoclonal antibody—binds to the CD3 protein, preventing the T cell from initiating an immune response.	Used in targeted therapy in HER2/neu breast cancer.	Obtain baseline labs; assess for toxicity—look for leukopenia and thrombocytopenia. Increases patient's susceptibility for infections.
Doxorubicin (Adriamycin) ***Action:*** Binds to DNA, causing strand splitting and inhibition of DNA synthesis. Cell cycle nonspecific.	Antibiotic antineoplastic.	Prevent patient from exposure to infections during periods of leukopenia. Monitor cardiac function. Monitor liver function tests, renal function tests, and CBC. Report signs of hepatic or renal dysfunction or bloody diarrhea.
Docetaxel (Taxotere) ***Action:*** Binds to tubulin; mitotic inhibitor.	Antineoplastic.	Prevent patient from exposure to infections during periods of leukopenia. Monitor I&O, blood pressure, and temperature daily. Monitor weight weekly. Monitor electrolytes and CBC. Assess for hand weakness and diminished DTRs. Walking may be impaired.

Sources: Adapted from Adams, M., & Koch, R. (2010). *Pharmacology: Connections to nursing practice.* Upper Saddle River, NJ: Pearson; Johnson, R., & Murad, M. (2009). Gynecomastia: Pathophysiology, evaluation, and management. *Mayo Clinic Proceedings, 84*(11), 1010–1015; Lee, E. (2009). Evidence-based management of benign breast disease. *The American Journal for Nurse Practitioners, 13*(7/8), 22–31; Rodden, A. (2009). Common breast concerns. *Primary Care Clinic Office Practice, 36*(1), 103–113. doi:10.1016/j.pop.2008.10.006; Rogers, V., & Cox, S. (2011). Obstetrics and obstetric disorders. In S. McPhee & M. Papadakis (Eds.), *2011 Current medical diagnosis and treatment* (50th ed., pp. 754–778). New York: McGraw-Hill Medical.

RISK FACTORS for Lactational Mastitis

Sore, cracked nipples	Wearing plastic-backed breast pads
Milk stasis	Blocked milk ducts
Infant mouth abnormalities	First baby, during first 3 months postpartum.

Sources: Adapted from Rogers, V., & Cox, S. (2011). Obstetrics and obstetric disorders. In S. McPhee & M. Papadakis (Eds.), *2011 Current medical diagnosis and treatment* (50th ed., pp. 754–778). New York: McGraw-Hill Medical; Spencer, J. (2008). Management of mastitis in breastfeeding women. *American Family Physician, 78*(6), 727–731, 732.

methicillin-resistant *S. aureus* (MRSA). The box above contains a list of risk factors for lactational mastitis.

In nonlactating women, mastitis is rare but may occur in those women with ductal ectasia when the ducts involved become plugged with fatty material (Kamal, Hamed, & Salem, 2009; Mayo Clinic Staff, 2011b). Mastitis of this type may become infected and progress to abscess (Giuliani & Hurvitz, 2011). Another form of mastitis is **superficial thrombophlebitis** (Mondor disease). This condition was described earlier. Figure 44–2 shows the venous channels affected by Mondor disease.

Mastitis in lactating and nonlactating women is not a risk factor for breast cancer. However, symptoms of inflammatory breast cancer closely resemble those of mastitis. This may cause delay in the diagnosis and treatment of this very aggressive form of breast cancer (ACS, 2011c; Kamal et al., 2009; Spencer, 2008). More about inflammatory breast cancer is presented later in this chapter.

Diagnostic Tests and Procedures

Laboratory tests or other diagnostic procedures are not usually indicated for mastitis in lactating women. However, if a lump appears before treatment or persists after treatment for infectious mastitis, then ultrasound will help identify the abscess and can be used to monitor treatment effectiveness (Balkam, 2010). If infectious mastitis is suspected, a culture and sensitivity (C&S) and a white blood cell (WBC) count from the milk should be obtained.

Medical Management

Mothers with milk stasis or mastitis should continue breast-feeding (Balkam, 2010; Rogers & Cox, 2011; Spencer, 2008). If breast-feeding is not emptying the breast, then removal with breast massage and expression of milk or using a breast pump after breast-feeding is advised. In some cases, a small white lesion will occur on the nipple. This is occlusive to the duct and should be removed with a sterile needle to help drain the duct (Spencer, 2008).

If an infection occurs, the antibiotics chosen should cover penicillin-resistant organisms and MRSA. The Academy of Breastfeeding Medicine (ABM) protocol recommends dicloxacillin or floxacillin (see Pharmacology feature, p. 1335). If the patient is allergic to penicillin, then cephalexin or clindamycin may be used. If the patient does not respond, then C&S should guide drug choice (Balkam, 2010). Abscesses should be surgically drained if necessary. Breast-feeding may continue as long as the baby does not come into contact with purulent discharge. It has been shown that breast milk from the breast with mastitis offers anti-inflammatory components that will protect the infant from infection (Spencer, 2008).

Mondor disease is treated with hot, moist compresses and NSAIDs for pain relief as needed. Patients should be reassured that the condition will not last long (Schwartz, 2011).

CHART 44–3 Substances and Drugs That Cause Gynecomastia

Estrogen therapy	Digitalis	Cimetidine
Spironolactone	Reserpine	Thiazide
Isoniazid	Tricyclic antidepressants	Amphetamines
Vincristine	Busulfan	Minocycline
Metronidazole	Haloperidol	Alcohol
Marijuana	Heroin	Methadone

Sources: Johnson, R., & Murad, M. (2009). Gynecomastia: Pathophysiology, evaluation, and management. *Mayo Clinic Proceedings, 84*(11), 1010–1015; Latendresse, G., McCance, K., & Morgan, K. (2010). Alterations of the reproductive systems. In K. McCance & S. Huether (Eds.), *Pathophysiology: The biologic basis for disease in adults and children* (6th ed., pp. 781–815). St. Louis: Mosby/Elsevier.

Gynecomastia

Gynecomastia is a benign enlargement of male breast tissue that may be caused by decreased testosterone activity, increased estrogen, or the use of one of many medications or substances. Chart 44–3 is a list of drugs and substances that have been linked to gynecomastia. It is estimated that 32% to 40% of all males experience gynecomastia at some time in their lifetime (Latendresse et al., 2010). During the male life span, gynecomastia may occur physiologically during the newborn period, adolescence, and the elderly years. Pathphysiologically, an imbalance between androgen and estrogen action in male breast tissue will cause the male breast to enlarge. Men who are obese will have a greater rate of conversion of androgen to estrogen, owing to aromatase that is present in adipose tissue (Johnson & Murad, 2009). This conversion is also seen in patients with estrogen-secreting tumors, gonadal failure, hyperthyroidism, or chronic liver disease. All unilateral gynecomastia should be considered a malignancy and evaluated carefully (Latendresse et al., 2010). Male breast cancer will be discussed more fully later in this chapter.

Diagnostic Tests and Procedures

Usually, gynecomastia is benign and self-limited (Johnson & Murad, 2009). Gynecomastia related to the newborn period resolves within the first month of life. When it occurs during adolescence, gynecomastia will resolve within 1 year.

Mammography may be used to distinguish benign from malignant lesions in the male breast. If the cause of benign gynecomastia is not clear, then laboratory tests are used to determine the presence of thyroid, gonadal, or liver problems.

Medical Management

Management depends on the cause of gynecomastia. If it is physiologic, it will simply resolve over time. Offending medications or substances may be changed or stopped as indicated. If gynecomastia persists or causes distress, then estrogen receptor modifiers such as tamoxifen will decrease the size of the breast. Other drugs that have been used include danazol and clomiphene, but the evidence that these drugs work is low, and the side effects are substantial (Johnson & Murad, 2009). Surgical removal of the breast tissue or liposuction has been used, but only as a last resort in men who are very anxious about their appearance.

Nursing Management

Nursing management of women and men with benign breast disorders depends on the disorder, the patient's emotional response, and the patient's general state of health. All the benign disorders have similar nursing management requirements.

Assessment

Nursing care begins with gathering a relevant history that includes characteristics of the breast disorder, when it began, how it has changed over time, and whether or not the problem changes during the menstrual cycle. It is also important to complete a risk assessment for breast cancer. This includes asking about family history, hormonal risk factors such as early menarche or late menopause, the timing and number of pregnancies, whether or not the woman is breast-feeding or has breast-fed in the past, and whether or not she has any history of malignancies. In addition, use of alcohol, use of tobacco products, and a complete drug history, including use of recreational drugs, would be pertinent. The nurse should identify any drugs or substances that would contribute to mastalgia, galactorrhea, or gynecomastia.

The patient's emotional status may be very fragile when there is a breast problem. Therefore, it is important for the nurse to assess for anxiety, worry, and fear. The nurse also should allow the patient to express concerns and ask questions regarding the breast condition. The nurse should be careful to ensure privacy and confidentiality during the interview so that the patient feels comfortable confiding in him.

Breast disorders in women and men affect self-image and may affect intimate relationships. Questions regarding relationships will help the nurse to determine the level of partner support available to the patient. As the interview progresses, the nurse can assess the patient's level of distress related to the breast disorder.

The physical examination of the breast should include inspection and palpation of the breasts and axilla so that the breast disorder is fully described in the chart. Clinical breast examination is described in Chapter 40.

Nursing Diagnoses

Nursing diagnosis associated with benign breast disorders include:

- *Disturbed Body Image* related to breast disorder.
- *Risk for Situational Low Self-Esteem* related to change in body image.
- *Acute Pain* related to mastalgia, tests, or procedures.
- *Decisional Conflicts* related to treatment options.
- *Deficient Knowledge* related to the disease process.
- *Disturbed Thought Process* related to sense of loss of body image.
- *Fear.*

NANDA-I © 2012

Outcomes

Expected outcomes of care for patients experiencing benign breast disorders include:

- Enhanced knowledge related to benign versus malignant breast disorders, medications, and tests and procedures
- Relief of symptoms or total cure of the disorder
- Decreased anxiety and fear
- Acceptance of body image
- Adequate decision making regarding treatment options
- Improved coping
- Adequate health-seeking behaviors
- Enhanced self-esteem related to change in body image
- Adequate pain relief and ability to cope with pain

Planning and Intervention

Nursing management requires education, support, and therapeutic interventions. The nurse must ensure that patients understand the terms *benign* and *malignant* and the types of diagnostic evaluations that will be used to make a definitive diagnosis. Patients will need to be prepared physically and emotionally for diagnostic procedures such as stereotactic biopsy (image- or mammographic-guided biopsy) or operative biopsy. Patients will be less anxious if they understand the test and how it is done. It is important for the nurse to give reassurance *without giving false reassurance* as patients with breast masses are waiting for these procedures and then waiting for the results. Nurses administer sedation and analgesics before and after these procedures.

Nursing management when the patient has mastalgia or galactorrhea may include suggesting a well-fitting bra; decreasing salt, fat, and caffeine in the diet; and using warm, moist compresses or cold packs to help relieve mastalgia. The patient will need education about the uses and potential side effects of any medications prescribed such as ibuprofen, evening primrose oil, danazol, or tamoxifen (see the Pharmacology feature on p. 1335).

Lactating women who have developed mastitis need help to continue breast-feeding, including positioning the infant for optimum drainage of the area of the breast involved. If the breast-feeding is not draining the breast well enough, the woman will need instructions on the use of breast pumps. Breast milk, expressed and spread on the nipple, or water-soluble lanolin will relieve dry, cracked nipples and prevent fissures and cracks that will allow bacteria into the breast. Pharmacologic treatment, such as antibiotics or analgesics, also may be used; if so, the patient will need education about their use and side effects. Lactating women should be reassured that the antibiotics they take will not harm their baby. Women with mastitis who develop an abscess may require operative incision and drainage. These patients will need sedation and analgesia before and after surgery. Postoperative care of patients with draining wounds of the breast may be needed. See Chapter 19 and Chapter 60 for a review of postoperative care of infected wounds and use of drains.

Breast Cancer

Breast cancer is defined as the formation of a malignant tumor as a result of an uncontrolled growth of abnormal cells in the breast tissue. Cancer invades surrounding breast tissue and may spread to other areas of the body (metastasize). Breast cancer occurs in both women and men, although at a much lower rate among men.

Epidemiology

Other than skin cancer, breast cancer is the most common cancer in women (ACS, 2011a). Breast cancer is the leading cause of cancer death for women ages 40 to 44 and the second-leading cancer cause after lung cancer for women (ACS, 2011a; Latendresse et al., 2011). It was estimated that 39,840 women would die from breast cancer in 2010 (ACS, 2011a). The odds for a woman to die of breast cancer are 1 in 35, or about 3% (ACS, 2011a).

There has been a decrease in the incidence of breast cancer since 2002, particularly among women over age 50. The decrease correlates with the decrease in use of hormone replacement therapy that occurred following the Women's Health Initiative research in 2002. This landmark study demonstrated that hormone replacement therapy increased risks for breast disease and heart disease (National Cancer Institute [NCI], 2011d). For women under age 50, deaths due to breast cancer

Weblink: Breast Cancer Statistics Weblink: Breast Cancer

have been decreasing since 1990 because of increased awareness, better screening modalities, and improved treatments (ACS, 2011a).

About 1,970 new cases of invasive breast cancer were expected to occur among men in the United States in 2010, and approximately 390 men were expected to die from this disease (ACS, 2011b). The lifetime risk for developing breast cancer in men is about 1 in 1,000 (ACS, 2011b). Looking at these statistics, it becomes very clear why one of the goals of *Healthy People 2020* is to "reduce the numbers of new cancers as well as the illness, disability, and death caused by cancer" (U.S. Department of Health and Human Services [USDHHS], 2011).

Risk Factors

A risk factor is anything that affects an individual's chance for developing a disease. Having a risk factor does not mean that the disease in inevitable; however, it is a good reason for taking preventive measures such as healthy diet, exercise, and screening tests. Several nonmodifiable risk factors are associated with increased risk of breast cancer including age, race, family history, age at first pregnancy, age of menarche, and age of menopause. Modifiable risk factors include obesity, hormone replacement therapy, alcohol consumption, and sedentary lifestyle.

Besides being female, age is the most important risk factor for breast cancer. According to the National Cancer Institute (NCI) (2011f), 1.9% of cases occur in women ages 20 to 34 and 22.6% of cases occur in women ages 45 to 54. Approximately 5.6% of all women in the United States will develop breast cancer between ages 50 and 70 years (NCI, 2011f). This means that a woman living in the United States has a 1 in 8 lifetime risk of developing breast cancer. This has gradually increased over the past three decades, in part due to longer life expectancy and more complete diagnosis through the use of mammography screening (ACS, 2011a).

Caucasian women are more likely than women of other races to develop breast cancer. However, Black women are more likely to have breast cancer at a younger age and to die from the disease (Latendresse et al., 2010). Asian, American Indian, and Hispanic women have lower incidences of breast cancer; however, breast cancer is the number one killer of Hispanic women (Centers for Disease Control and Prevention [CDC], 2011b). The Cultural Considerations feature lists the cultural groups affected by breast cancer.

Family history and genetics represent significant etiologic factors. Women with a family history of breast cancer, especially in a first-degree relative (mother, sister, or daughter), have an increased risk of developing breast cancer (Latendresse et al., 2010). In fact, it is believed that 5% to 10% of breast cancer cases are hereditary (ACS, 2011a).

Families with extensive history of breast (in women or men) and ovarian cancers are often screened for mutation of the BRCA1 and BRCA2 genes. These two genes are the most common causes of hereditary breast cancer and have been linked to the development of other organ cancers, as well (ACS, 2011a). The BRCA1 and BRCA2 are tumor suppression genes when they function normally. However, these genes can undergo mutation or alteration that causes increased susceptibility of the patient to breast, ovarian, and other cancers. Women with BRCA1 and BRCA2 gene mutations have a 40% to 80% lifetime risk of developing breast cancer. BRCA1 and BRCA2 gene mutations are also associated with early onset of breast cancer (Latendresse et al., 2010).

Other gene mutations that may contribute to hereditary breast cancer are listed in the Genetics Considerations feature (ACS, 2011a; Latendresse et al., 2010). Some cancers found in both women and men have too much HER2/neu, a gene that promotes tumor growth (ACS, 2011b).

Genetic testing can be used to identify individuals at risk for cancer. This can lead to ethical issues such as breach of confidentiality and insurance discrimination. The Ethical Issues feature offers information about how disclosure of a patient's genetic information may be handled.

Reproductive hormones, specifically estrogen and progestin, influence breast cancer risk. How this occurs is not fully understood. However, situations that expose a woman to higher levels of these hormones over long periods of time, such as early menarche, late menopause, no pregnancies, or delaying pregnancy until after age 30,

CULTURAL CONSIDERATIONS
Incidence of Breast Cancer

Cultural groups with the highest incidence of breast cancer include:

- Caucasians—126.5 per 100,000 women
- Blacks—118.3 per 100,000 women
- Asian/Pacific Islander—90 per 100,000 women
- Hispanic—86 per 100,000 women
- American Indian—76.4 per 100,000 women.

Mortality rates among cultural groups include:

- Caucasian—23.4 per 100,000 women
- Black—32.4 per 100,000 women
- Asian/Pacific Islander—12.2 per 100,000 women
- Hispanic—15.3 per 100,000 women
- Jewish women of Ashkenazi origin are more likely to have BRCA mutation.

Sources: Adapted from American Cancer Society (ACS). (2011a). Detailed guide: Breast cancer. *Learn About Cancer*. Retrieved from http://www.cancer.org/Cancer/BreastCancer/DetailedGuide/index; http://www.cancer.org/Cancer/BreastCancer/DetailedGuide/breast-cancer-risk-factors; http://www.cancer.org/Cancer/BreastCancer/DetailedGuide/breast-cancer-prevention; http://www.cancer.org/Cancer/BreastCancer/DetailedGuide/breast-cancer-diagnosis; http://www.cancer.org/Cancer/BreastCancer/DetailedGuide/breast-cancer-treating-general-info; http://www.cancer.org/Cancer/BreastCancer/DetailedGuide/breast-cancer-survival-by-stage; National Cancer Institute (NCI). (2011f). SEER Stat fact sheet: Breast. Surveillance epidemiology and end results: Cancer statistics. Based on 2009 SEER data submission posted 2010. Retrieved from http://seer.cancer.gov/statfacts/html/breast.html.

GENETIC CONSIDERATIONS for Breast Cancer

Several gene mutations have been associated with the development of breast cancer. Gene mutations may occur in these genes:

- BRCA1 and BRCA2 (tumor suppressor genes)
- ATM (normally helps repair damaged DNA)
- P53 (tumor suppressor gene)
- CHEK2
- PTEN (helps regulate cell growth)
- CDH1
- HER2 (oncogene)
- Bcl-2 and c-myc (proto-oncogenes).

Sources: Adapted from American Cancer Society (ACS). (2011a). Detailed guide: Breast cancer. *Learn About Cancer*. Retrieved from http://www.cancer.org/Cancer/BreastCancer/DetailedGuide/index; http://www.cancer.org/Cancer/BreastCancer/DetailedGuide/breast-cancer-risk-factors; http://www.cancer.org/Cancer/BreastCancer/DetailedGuide/breast-cancer-prevention; http://www.cancer.org/Cancer/BreastCancer/DetailedGuide/breast-cancer-diagnosis; http://www.cancer.org/Cancer/BreastCancer/DetailedGuide/breast-cancer-treating-general-info; http://www.cancer.org/Cancer/BreastCancer/DetailedGuide/breast-cancer-survival-by-stage; Latendresse, G., McCance, K., & Morgan, K. (2010). Alterations of the reproductive systems. In K. McCance & S. Huether (Eds.), *Pathophysiology: The biologic basis for disease in adults and children* (6th ed., pp. 781–815). St. Louis: Mosby/Elsevier.

Weblink: Genetics Risk Assessment and Counseling

Video: Breast Cancer Etiology and Pathophysiology

ETHICAL ISSUES in Cancer Genetic Testing

The International Society of Nurses in Genetics and other groups interested in the ethics of cancer genetic testing believe that relatives should be given information about genetics testing results if the patient who has had the tests gives her consent. However, there are instances when patient confidentiality can be overruled. The United States Bioethics Commission and other groups have set forth guidelines to help health care providers determine when it may be more ethical to disclose genetic information to a relative without the patient's consent. The main tenets of these guidelines include potential harm to the relative if not warned; whether the technology available can prevent, treat, or manage the cancer; cases in which only information needed to prevent harm is released; and if there is no other way to prevent harm.

Source: National Cancer Institute (NCI). (2011a). Cancer genetics risk assessment and counseling (PDQ). Retrieved from http://www.cancer.gov/cancertopics/pdq/genetics/risk-assessment-and-counseling/HealthProfessional/page6.

do increase risks (NCI, 2011e). The prolonged use of combination hormone replacement (estrogen and progestin) has also been shown to increase the risk of breast cancer (NCI, 2011d). In addition, a study sponsored by the NCI concluded that women who use oral contraceptives may increase the risk of breast cancer slightly; however, once the woman stops using oral contraceptives for 10 years or more, she has the same risk as the woman who never used oral contraceptives (NCI, 2011e).

Modifiable risk factors can be considered in the prevention of breast cancer. There is, of course, no guaranteed way to prevent breast cancer, but decreasing risk factors is an effective strategy. Obesity increases the risk of postmenopausal, but not premenopausal, breast cancer (ACS, 2011a). In postmenopausal women, circulating estrogen is primarily produced in fat tissue; therefore, having more adipose tissue increases estrogen levels and supports potential tumor formation. Extra weight in the waist area seems to hold higher risks for breast cancer than does extra weight in the hips and thighs. Researchers believe there are differences in the fat cells in these locations that would explain the difference in the risks (ACS, 2011a). Physical activity such as walking appears to have a protective effect on women with regard to breast cancer. This protective effect seems to come from alterations in free radical formation, oxidative damage, DNA repair capability, increased peristalsis, weight loss, and changes in estrogen and progesterone levels that occur with a daily 1-hour walk (Latendresse et al., 2010).

Alcohol consumption is consistently associated with increased breast cancer risk (Li et al., 2010). Li and colleagues (2010) assessed the relationship between alcohol consumption and postmenopausal breast cancer risk and found that alcohol consumption of any amount increased the likelihood of developing breast cancer, especially lobular hormone receptor-positive invasive breast cancer, which is discussed later in this chapter.

The risk factors for male breast cancer include aging, genetics, family history, alcohol consumption, and obesity. Men with breast cancer are more likely to be around 68 years old at diagnosis. If a male has a blood relative (male or female) with breast cancer, his risks are increased. Men may inherit the BRCA2 gene, which causes 1 in 10 cases of male breast cancer (ACS, 2011b). Men born with Klinefelter syndrome have lower levels of androgen and higher levels of estrogen, making them more prone to developing gynecomastia and breast cancer. Alcohol consumption and liver disease affect the liver's ability to regulate estrogen levels, thereby increasing risks for gynecomastia and breast cancer in men (ACS, 2011b). Obesity is a risk factor in men and women primarily because fat cells convert androgens to estrogen, thereby increasing estrogen levels (ACS, 2011b). The Risk Factors feature summarizes the risk factors for breast cancer for women and men.

Etiology and Pathophysiology

Breast tissue is made up of glands for milk production, called lobules, and ducts that connect the lobules to the nipple. Cancer arises from the epithelial cells that line the ducts and the lobules. These structures are present in both men and women but do not develop in men after puberty because of lower levels of estrogen and progesterone. However, many men have palpable breast tissue under the nipple (Deneris & Huether, 2010).

There are many forms of breast cancer:

- Carcinoma of the mammary ducts (papillary or intraductal)
- Infiltrating carcinoma (ductal [most prevalent of all breast cancer], mucinous, medullary, tubular, adenoid cystic, metaplastic, or squamous cell)
- Carcinoma of mammary lobules (lobular carcinoma *in situ*, infiltrating lobular, Paget disease, or inflammatory carcinoma
- Sarcoma of the breast (cytosarcoma phyllodes or fibrosarcoma).

In general, about 90% of breast tumors in both men and women arise from the ductal epithelium and about 10% are from within the lobular alveolar epithelium (Latendresse et al., 2010). The wide diversity of breast cancer types presents a challenge to scientists trying to explain how it begins and evolves.

Cancer *in Situ*

Breast cancers can be *in situ*, which is the term that describes a cancer confined to the ducts or lobules. Ductal carcinoma *in situ* (DCIS) is limited to ducts and lobules but may extend to the skin. DCIS cells have mutations in their chromosomes similar to those seen in invasive breast cancer, which suggests that both may arise from precancer stem cells. These cells seem pre-programmed to progress to invasion and metastasis (Latendresse et al., 2010).

Many oncologists do not consider lobular cancer *in situ* (LCIS) a true cancer; they consider it more of an indicator of increased risk of invasive cancer. LCIS begins in the terminal duct–lobular unit and appears as "noncohesive" clusters within the lobules (Latendresse et al., 2010). Unlike DCIS, LCIS will not cause calcifications or stromal invasion that would cause a mass to form. LCIS is less common than DCIS but more likely to occur in both breasts and in younger women. LCIS will progress to invasive cancer in 25% to 35% of women who have LCIS (Latendresse et al., 2010). Nearly all cancers at the *in situ* stage can be cured (ACS, 2011a).

Paget's Disease

Paget's disease is a rare form of breast cancer that is characterized by a chronic, crusting rash of the nipple that develops as a result of intraductal carcinoma. The cancer cells grow from the cancer mass into the duct and extend into the epidermis of the nipple and areola. This type of cancer accounts for 1% to 4% of breast cancer cases (Kao, 2011). Paget's disease has occurred in supernumerary nipples. Most Paget cells express HER2/neu. This is an oncogene that is present in 25% to 30% of breast cancers (Latendresse et al., 2010). Treatment targeting HER2/neu genes has been successful. Prognosis is good for Paget's disease when the cancer is localized in the nipple.

RISK FACTORS for Developing Breast Cancer

Nonmodifiable Risk Factors

Gender

100 times more common in women.

Age

About 1 out of 8 invasive breast cancer diagnoses are younger than age 45.

About 2 out of 3 women are age 55 or older.

Men with breast cancer are older, usually around 68 years of age.

Genetics

Women with mutated breast cancer genes BRCA1 and BRCA2 have an 80% chance of developing breast cancer during their lifetime.

The BRCA2 mutated gene causes 1 in 10 cases of male breast cancer.

Testicular disorders and Klinefelter syndrome increase the risks for male breast cancer

Ethnicity

Caucasian women are slightly more likely to develop breast cancer than are African American women.

However, African American women are more likely to die from this cancer.

Asian, Hispanic, and Native American women have a lower risk of developing and dying from breast cancer.

BRCA Mutations Most often Found in

Jewish women of Ashkenazi (Eastern European) population

African American women

Hispanic women

Family History of Breast Cancer

Having one first-degree relative (mother, sister, or daughter) with breast cancer approximately doubles a woman's risk.

Having two first-degree relatives increases her risk about fivefold.

A family history of breast cancer in a father or brother increases a woman's risk.

20% to 30% of women with breast cancer have a family member with this disease.

70% to 80% of women who get breast cancer do not have a family history.

One out of five men with breast cancer have a close male or female relative with the disease.

History of Breast Cancer

Someone who has had cancer in one breast has a three- to fourfold increased risk of developing a new primary cancer in the other breast or in another part of the same breast. This is different from a *recurrence* of the first cancer.

Modifiable Risk Factors

Childbirth

Having children later than age 30.

Not having any children.

Oral Contraceptive Use

Women now using oral contraceptives have a slightly greater risk.

Risk seems to decline once their use is stopped.

Hormone Replacement Therapy (HRT)

Combined HRT increases the risk of developing and may also increase the chances of dying from breast cancer.

Breast-Feeding

Some studies suggest that breast-feeding may slightly lower risk, especially if continued for 1.5 to 2 years.

Alcohol

One alcoholic drink a day creates a very small increase in risk.

Having 2 to 5 drinks daily creates about 1 1/2 times the risk.

Alcohol consumption is also a risk factor for male breast cancer

Overweight or Obese

Increased breast cancer risk exists, especially for women after menopause. Once the ovaries stop making estrogen, most of a woman's estrogen comes from fat tissue. Having more fat tissue after menopause can increase estrogen levels and thereby increase the risk.

Obesity is also a risk factor for male breast cancer because fat cells convert androgen to estrogen.

Physical Activity

Evidence is growing that physical activity in the form of exercise reduces breast cancer risk. The only question is how much exercise is needed. The Women's Health Initiative (WHI) found that as little as 1.25 to 2.5 hours per week of brisk walking reduced a woman's risk by 18%.

Walking 10 hours a week reduced the risk a little more.

Uncertain, Controversial, or Unproven Risk Factors

High-Fat Diets

Most studies found that breast cancer is less common in countries where the typical diet is low in total fat, low in polyunsaturated fat, and low in saturated fat.

Many studies of women in the United States have not found breast cancer risk to be related to dietary fat intake.

Night Work

Several studies have suggested that women who work at night may have an increased risk. This is a fairly recent finding, and more studies are in progress to look at this issue. According to some researchers, the effect may be due to disruption in melatonin, a hormone that is affected by light, but other hormones are also being studied.

RISK FACTORS for Developing Breast Cancer, *continued*

Nonmodifiable Risk Factors	Modifiable Risk Factors	Uncertain, Controversial, or Unproven Risk Factors
Abnormal Breast Biopsy Results The *proliferative lesions with atypia* (those with excessive growth of cells in the ducts or lobules of the breast tissue, and in which the cells no longer appear normal) increase risk 4 to 5 times. They include: Atypical ductal hyperplasia (ADH) Atypical lobular hyperplasia (ALH). **Menstrual Periods** Menstruating at an early age (before age 12). Menopause after age 55 has a slightly higher risk. **Previous Chest Radiation** Radiation therapy to the chest area as treatment for another cancer (such as Hodgkin's disease or non-Hodgkin's lymphoma) significantly increases risk for both women and men. Diethylstilbestrol (DES) exposure: Slightly increased risk.		

Sources: Adapted from American Cancer Society (ACS). (2011a). Detailed guide: Breast cancer. *Learn About Cancer.* Retrieved from http://www.cancer.org/Cancer/BreastCancer/DetailedGuide/index; http://www.cancer.org/Cancer/BreastCancer/DetailedGuide/breast-cancer-risk-factors; http://www.cancer.org/Cancer/BreastCancer/DetailedGuide/breast-cancer-prevention; http://www.cancer.org/Cancer/BreastCancer/DetailedGuide/breast-cancer-diagnosis; http://www.cancer.org/Cancer/BreastCancer/DetailedGuide/breast-cancer-treating-general-info; http://www.cancer.org/Cancer/BreastCancer/DetailedGuide/breast-cancer-survival-by-stage; American Cancer Society (ACS). (2011b). Detailed guide: Breast cancer in men. *Learn About Cancer.* Retrieved from http://www.cancer.org/Cancer/BreastCancerinMen/DetailedGuide/index; http://www.cancer.org/Cancer/BreastCancerinMen/DetailedGuide/breast-cancer-in-men-risk-factors; http://www.cancer.org/Cancer/BreastCancerinMen/DetailedGuide/breast-cancer-in-men-treating-by-stage; http://www.cancer.org/Cancer/BreastCancerinMen/DetailedGuide/breast-cancer-in-men-survival-rates.

Inflammatory Breast Cancer

Inflammatory breast cancer (IBC) is an entirely different form of breast cancer. It presents as an inflammation involving the skin of the breast. The inflamed breast looks like it is suffering from mastitis because it is red, it is warm, and it swells. However, the changes are caused by cancer cells blocking the lymph vessels in the skin (ACS, 2011b). The swelling rapidly causes **induration** (hardening of the skin surface) and a ***peau d'orange*** (orange peel) appearance of the breast surface. There is rarely an associated mass or lump, and IBC shows only as skin thickening or increased breast density on mammogram (Molckovsky, Fitzgerald, Freedman, Heisey, & Clemons, 2009). Inflammatory breast cancer is a rare form of cancer, seen as the cause for about 1% of all breast cancers. It is more likely to occur in Black women between the ages of 50 and 58 than in White women (ACS, 2011c; Molckovsky et al., 2009). Inflammatory breast cancer is very aggressive and is usually already at stage IIIB (locally advanced) or IV (metastatic) when it is diagnosed.

Invasive or Infiltrative Cancer of the Breast

Invasive or infiltrative cancer starts in the lobules or ducts but breaks through the walls to invade the surrounding fatty tissue of the breast. It can arise from anywhere within breast tissue but is most common in the upper outer quadrant. In contrast to colon cancer, which follows a step by step process, breast cancer is much more complex. Current research suggests that most invasive cancer (ductal type) may originate from pre-cancer stem cells (Latendresse et al., 2010). This model of cancer causation shows promise as a method for predicting which cells will become DCIS and eventually invasive cancer.

Once cancer is identified as invasive, it is staged. Staging has been developed and maintained through the cooperation of the American Joint Committee on Cancer (AJCC) and the International Union Against Cancer (UICC) (AJCC, 2010). The TNM staging system is most commonly used by doctors to guide treatment. It is based on the tumor (T), the spread to lymph nodes (N), and the presence of metastasis (M) (AJCC, 2010). The National Guidelines for the Staging of Breast Cancer feature outlines the TNM stages for breast cancer.

Clinical Manifestations

Early stage breast cancer (*in situ* cancer) typically produces no symptoms when the tumor is small and most treatable. Invasive breast cancer is usually a painless, hard, irregularly shaped, fixed mass. The lump is most often in the upper outer quadrant of the breast where the majority of glandular tissue is found. The mass may feel like a thickening in the breast tissue found during self-breast exam, while showering, or during a clinical breast examination. More advanced breast cancer will block the lymphatic ducts and cause *peau d'orange* skin changes. A cancer lesion may attach to and pull on Cooper ligaments, causing a dimpling on the breast surface. If the mass or lesion is in the center of the breast, the nipple may be retracted or inverted (Bickley, 2007; Latendresse et al., 2010). Enlarged axillary, supraclavicular, or infraclavicular lymph nodes may indicate cancer of the breast that has spread to the lymph nodes.

Inflammatory breast cancer may be seen as *erythema* (redness) over most of an enlarged, indurated breast with no palpable lump (Molckovsky et al., 2009). A persistent skin rash near the nipple area can signal Paget's disease, along with flaking or eruption near the nipple. Nipple abnormalities such as thickening, loss of elasticity, spontaneous discharge, erosion, inversion, or tenderness can occur less commonly (ACS, 2011a).

Breast cancer in men may present as a painless lump, discharge from the nipple, redness or scaling of the nipple or skin, nipple retraction,

Weblink: Breast Cancer Staging

NATIONAL GUIDELINES for the Staging of Breast Cancer

Stage	Tumor Size	Lymph Node	Metastasis
0	Tis (*in situ*)	No involvement	None
IA	T1 ≤2 centimeters	No involvement	None
IB	T0 or T1 ≤2 cm	Micrometastasis to 1 to 3 nodes	None
IIA	T0 or T1 ≤2 cm or not found	0 to 3 Axillary or internal mammary nodes	None
	Or—T2 > 2 cm but < 5 cm	No involvement	None
IIB	T2 2 to 5 centimeters	1 to 3 Axillary or internal mammary nodes	None
	Or—T3 > 5 cm but not in chest wall or skin	No involvement	None
IIIA	T0 to T2 5 cm or cannot be found	4 to 9 axillary or internal mammary nodes	None
	Or—T3 > 5 cm but no growth into chest wall or skin	1 to 9 axillary or internal mammary nodes	None
IIIB	T4 Any size with extension to chest wall or skin	No lymph involvement or 1 to 3 axillary Or tiny amount in internal mammary nodes Or 4 to 9 axillary nodes or enlarged internal mammary nodes	None
IIIC	Any T (size) or cannot be found	10 axillary, or spread to infraclavicular or supraclavicular nodes; or involves axillary and internal mammary nodes; or has spread to 4 axillary and small amounts in internal mammary nodes	None
IV	Any T (size)	Any type of nodal involvement	Yes (most common = bone, liver, brain, or lung)

Source: Adapted from American Joint Committee on Cancers (AJCC). (2011). *AJCC cancer staging manual* (7th ed.). Retrieved from http://www.cancerstaging.org/products/ajccproducts.html.

or skin dimpling (ACS, 2011b). Because male breast cancer is rare, the general public has given it little attention. Consequently, many men do not recognize the signs and may wait until lymph nodes are involved (Thomas, 2010).

Diagnosis of Breast Cancer

The key to survival from breast cancer is early detection and intervention, with a 5-year survival rate of 97% for women diagnosed in Stage I (ACS, 2011a). Early detection may be accomplished by self-breast examination (SBE), clinical breast examination (CBE), or regular screening mammograms. Neither SBE nor CBE has been shown to decrease risks for dying from breast cancer (CDC, 2011a). However, a woman who is familiar with how her breasts look and feel is much more likely to notice changes early and seek medical attention. Breast awareness can be increased through regular SBE. If a woman chooses SBE, the ACS (2011a) suggests the step-by-step approach presented in Chart 44–4. Not all women choose to do SBE, or they do it infrequently.

Clinical breast examination should be part of a regular physical examination. The ACS (2011a) recommends that women ages 20 to 39 have a physical examination and CBE every 3 years. After age 40, these examinations should occur annually.

Mammography

The CDC (2011a) maintains that mammography is the most effective way to detect breast cancer when it is at a treatable stage. **Mammography** is a low-dose x-ray procedure that allows visualization of the breast's internal structure. Mammography can identify cancer several years before physical symptoms develop. Modern screen-film units used today result in higher quality images with a considerably lower x-ray dose than the general-purpose x-ray equipment used in the past. Mammography can detect cancer before it can be felt by the woman or her health care provider. It can also detect microcalcifications that may indicate a cancerous lesion.

The NCI (2011c) and the CDC (2011a) recommend that all women over age 40 have a mammogram every 1 to 2 years. The National Cancer Institute cites studies showing that deaths from breast cancer can be reduced through regular mammogram screening, especially among women 50 years and older.

Terms associated with mammography include *screening* versus *diagnostic* and *film* versus *digital*. A screening mammogram simply indicates that the breast is being evaluated for any lumps or signs of potential cancer. A diagnostic mammogram is utilized when the screening mammogram or a clinical breast exam finds a suspicious area of the breast requiring closer evaluation. The diagnostic mammogram is often specific to the area in question and may utilize an enhancement mechanism to better view this area. Film mammography uses a film to both capture and display the breast tissue being evaluated. However, film mammography is limited with dense breast tissue, seen in women who may be at higher risk for breast cancer (Stephan, 2011). Digital mammography stores the electronic image in a way that allows for it to be enhanced, magnified, or manipulated to evaluate areas in question more fully.

Breast Ultrasound

Breast ultrasound is not as effective a screening tool as is mammography. Nonetheless, ultrasound is used more often in the office setting for further characterization and guided biopsy of breast masses and suspicious axillary nodes. Ultrasound is very useful in differentiating solid masses and cystic lesions. Sound waves bounced off of the cystic lesion reveal lobulated and non-echogenic lesions with well-defined borders. The surgeon can use ultrasound to aid in locating and excising nonpalpable breast lesions and achieving clean **lumpectomy** (surgical removal of a tumor and small amount of surrounding tissue) margins. In addition, the future may find

CHART 44–4 Self-Breast Exam

Beginning in their 20s, women should be told about the benefits and limitations of breast self-exam (BSE). Women with breast implants also can do BSE. It may be helpful, however, to have the surgeon help identify the edges of the implant so that the woman knows what she is feeling. Women who are pregnant or breast-feeding can also choose to examine their breasts regularly.

Establish a Regular Schedule

- Perform on day 4 to 7 of the menstrual cycle.
- If no periods, choose a regular day (i.e., the first of each month).
- Know how breasts normally look and feel and report any new breast changes to a health professional as soon as they are found.
- The best time to examine the breasts is when the breasts are not tender or swollen.
  - Look at the breasts in the mirror. Press the hands on the hips and see if this causes a change in the shape of the breast. Also look for any retraction of the nipple or skin changes.
- Lie down and place your right arm behind your head. The exam is done while lying down, not standing up, because when lying down the breast tissue spreads evenly over the chest wall and is as thin as possible, making it much easier to feel all the breast tissue.
- Use the finger pads of the three middle fingers on the left hand to feel for lumps in the right breast.
- Use overlapping dime-sized circular motions of the finger pads to feel the breast tissue.
- Use three different levels of pressure to feel all the breast tissue. Use each pressure level to feel the breast tissue before moving on to the next spot.
  - Light pressure is needed to feel the tissue closest to the skin.
  - Medium pressure is used to feel a little deeper.
  - Firm pressure is used to feel the tissue closest to the chest and ribs. A firm ridge in the lower curve of each breast is normal.
- Examine each underarm while lying with the arm slightly pulled away from the body. Raising the arm too high will tighten the tissue and make it harder to examine.

Important Points to Remember

- Many lumps are benign.
- Early detection through breast self-exam and mammography increases the survival rate.

Source: "How to Perform a Breast Self-Exam." Adapted and reprinted by the permission of the American Cancer Society, Inc. from http://www.cancer.org.

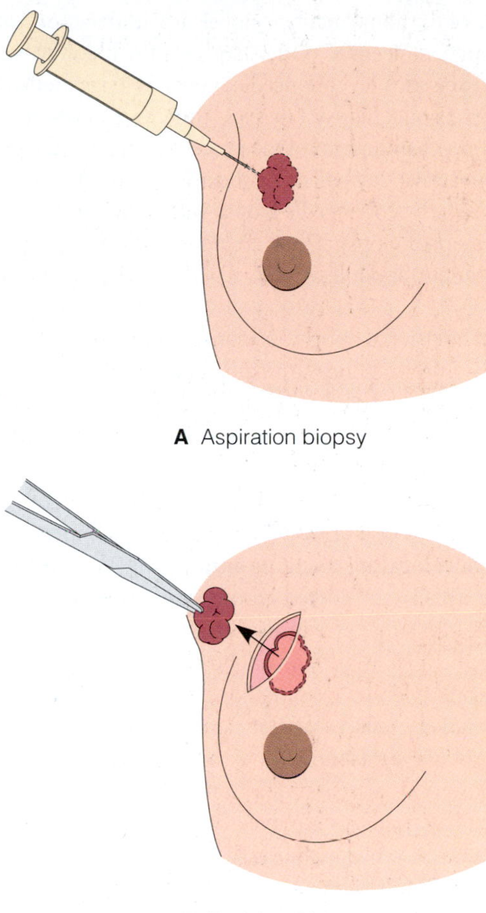

FIGURE 44–3 ◆ Types of breast biopsy. (A) In an aspiration biopsy, the needle is used to aspirate fluid or tissue from the breast. (B) In an excisional biopsy, tissue from the breast lesion is removed surgically.

ultrasound being used to **ablate** (minimally invasive removal of abnormal tissue) tumors.

Breast Biopsy

A breast biopsy is performed to evaluate a lump or cyst that is found to be of a suspicious nature on mammography (Figure 44–3◆). There are four primary types of biopsies: fine needle aspiration biopsy, *incisional biopsy* (surgical biopsy where a portion of the lesion is removed), *excisional biopsy* (surgical biopsy where the entire tumor is removed), and *stereotactic needle biopsy* (image-guided core needle biopsy). Each is unique and used for specific reasons. The different forms of biopsy are included in the Diagnostic Tests feature (p. 1333).

A fine needle aspiration (FNA) biopsy uses a fine gauge (typically 22- or 25-gauge) needle to pierce the skin and remove fluid from a cyst or remove cells from a solid mass. The tissue is removed by inserting the needle in the mass and aspirating fluid or cells, which are then sent to a pathology lab for analysis. The procedure is done under mammography or ultrasound guidance to pinpoint the exact location of the mass. This is usually an outpatient procedure, requiring no stitches, and many patients resume normal activities that same day. Prior to discharge from the outpatient facility, assessment of the puncture site, vital signs, and pain evaluation are done. Discharge instructions include signs and symptoms of infection, pain-relief measures, and health care provider follow-up appointment. Fine needle aspiration is considered the least invasive form of breast biopsy, with rapid results (ACS, 2011a). It is limited in that it samples only a small portion of tissue or cells.

Breast masses are often evaluated using an image-guided core needle biopsy (stereotactic biopsy) (Agency for Healthcare Research and Quality [AHRQ], 2010a). A stereotactic needle biopsy refers to the method in which the needle is guided into the abnormality. Stereotactic mammography is a three-dimensional mammography whereby the woman lies on her stomach on a mammography table with her breast protruding through a hole in the table. The breast is compressed as with a mammogram, at which point an image is taken. A tissue sample is extracted under a local anesthetic using a fine gauge needle. This procedure does not require surgery and is only mildly uncomfortable but will produce a biopsy sample similar to that of the surgical route (Singhal & Teh, 2011). The disadvantage is that the size of the abnormality is not clearly understood with this method. The patient needs to understand that the lesion will only be sampled, not excised. The core needle biopsy is less expensive than incisional or excisional biopsy, takes less time, and leaves only a tiny scar (ACS, 2011a). Limitations of the procedure include the possibility of a sampling error that will cause the examiner to miss the lesion. Missing the lesion by core needle biopsy will require follow-up such as surgical incisional biopsy. There are no special discharge instructions for the patient, and follow-up is scheduled with the health care provider.

A surgical incisional biopsy is considered the gold standard against which other methods are compared (ACS, 2011a). An incisional biopsy is performed when the lesion is large enough that removal through the small incision is not possible. A part of the lesion is removed in this case and sent for pathology evaluation, with follow-up surgery or treatment based on the pathology report. Surgical incisional biopsies involve a less than 2-inch incision in the breast done under local anesthetic or intravenous (IV) sedation, and, like FNA, are usually considered an outpatient procedure. Prior to the procedure, the surgeon will use mammography to locate and mark the specific area. Marking is done by several methods. If the abnormality can be felt by examination, the surgeon will mark the area using a marker or skin dye. If it cannot be felt by examination, the surgeon will use ultrasound to insert a small hollow needle into the mass, followed by insertion of a thin wire into the hollow bore of the needle. The needle is removed once the wire is placed. The patient is then taken to the operating room for removal of part of the abnormality (AHRQ, 2010b).

An excisional biopsy is done when complete removal of the abnormality and some surrounding tissue is planned. In this case, the pathologist will evaluate whether the margins of the lesion are free of abnormal cells, indicating that the entire lesion was removed. The nurse evaluates pain control, vital signs, incisional assessment, and the patient's emotional needs. In addition, a follow-up appointment is made with the health care provider.

Women or men who have close family members who have had breast cancer may elect to have a blood sample drawn to check for BRCA1 and BRCA2 mutations. The lifetime risk for women who have this harmful gene mutation to get breast cancer is 60%, or 600 out of 1,000 (NCI, 2011b). For men, the presence of this gene mutation increases the risks for breast cancer, testicular cancer, and early-onset prostate cancer. Genetic counseling is recommended before and after the test is done.

Medical and Surgical Management

Breast cancer treatment is usually multileveled. Most women will require some form of surgery, and this may be followed by radiation, chemotherapy, hormone therapy, or monoclonal antibody therapy.

A lumpectomy, removal of the cancerous growth and a small amount of surrounding normal tissue, is the least invasive form of surgery and is usually followed by 6 to 7 weeks of radiation (Figure 44–4A ◆). This is coupled with axillary node dissection and radiation therapy to improve long-term survival. Many women who choose lumpectomy and radiation therapy have experienced the same expected long-term survival rates as women who choose a more invasive surgery such as mastectomy (ACS, 2011a).

Other surgical techniques include a simple (also called a total) **mastectomy,** which is removal of the entire breast, or a modified radical mastectomy (see Figure 44–4B), which is removal of the entire breast along with the surrounding lymph nodes. This surgery does not include removal of the chest wall muscles, as is done in radical mastectomy. Radical mastectomy is very rarely used today because of the disfiguring nature of the surgery. Furthermore, radical mastectomy is not any more effective than lumpectomy with axillary dissection followed by radiation therapy (Giuliano & Hurvitz, 2011). A complication of axillary node dissection is the problem of lymphedema, a serious swelling of the arm caused by retention of lymph fluid (Armer, Shook, Schneider, Brooks, Peterson, & Stewart, 2009). The Evidence-Based Practice feature examines the problem of lymphedema in breast cancer survivors.

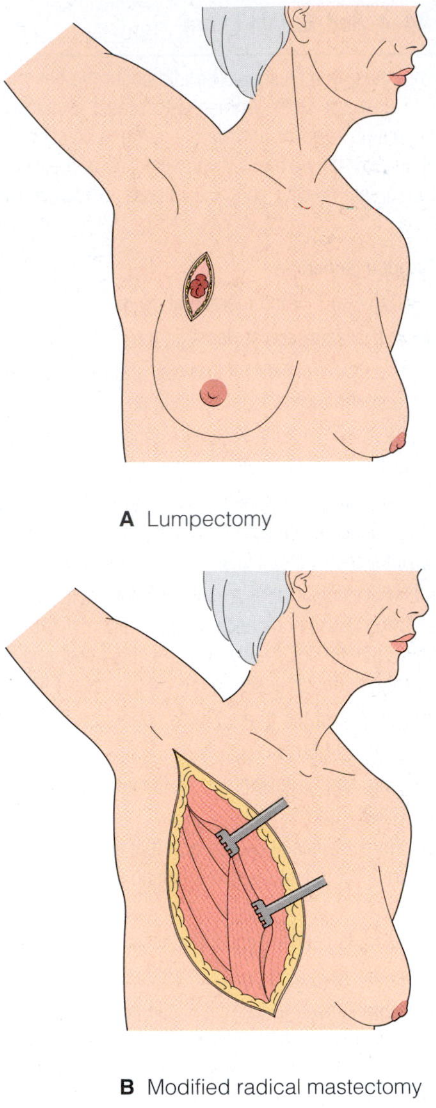

FIGURE 44–4 ◆ Types of mastectomy. (A) In a lumpectomy, only the tumor and a small margin of surrounding tissue are removed. (B) In a modified radical mastectomy, all breast tissue and the underarm lymph nodes are removed, but the underlying muscles remain.

Radiation is used to destroy cancer cells remaining in the breast tissue, chest wall, or underarm lymph nodes. Currently, technology increases the ability to target radiation therapy accurately and decrease the side effects from radiation therapy. Radiation therapy can be used in conjunction with surgery and chemotherapy to improve long-term survival in women with lymph node positive disease (ACS, 2011a). Use of radiation and chemotherapy after surgery is called adjuvant therapy

EVIDENCE-BASED PRACTICE Lymphedema in Breast Cancer Survivors

Clinical Problem

Lymphedema is caused by increased lymph fluid in the interstitial spaces of the limb adjacent to the area where lymph vessels and nodes have been removed or damaged. Without an intact lymph system, lymph cannot move into the bloodstream as it normally does. When a woman or man has breast cancer, the lymph vessels and nodes that drain the affected breast can be damaged by radiation or removed by surgery. It is estimated that half of breast cancer survivors develop lymphedema (Armer et al., 2009). Nurses can be instrumental in applying evidence-based education and self-care support to help many breast cancer survivors prevent or lessen lymphedema.

Research Findings

Armer and colleagues (2009) conducted a study that used self-care agency (the power to engage in self-care) to improve patient education that would decrease postsurgical lymphedema among breast cancer survivors. They describe the development of an educational program for nurses designed to improve supportive–educative nursing when working with patients at risk for lymphedema. Their premise was that patients can participate in self-care activities, such as avoiding weight gain and obesity, avoiding infections to the affected arm, and reducing hand use, that will help prevent lymphedema. Self-care agency depends not only on the education the nurse gives, but also on nursing support during the recovery phase.

Implications for Nursing Practice

Should lymphedema begin to develop, nurses can educate the patient about self-care methods that will improve lymph function, such as "deep breathing, abdominal massage, axillary clearance, and gentle lymphatic manipulation of the arm" (Armer et al., 2009 p. 7). These patients also benefit from learning about how to use compression sleeves, how to do skin care and avoid injury, lifestyle changes to control weight, and how to avoid any constriction to the arm or axilla.

Their study demonstrated how motivational interviewing that focuses on giving the patient the responsibility for daily self-care duties rather than being the nurse "expert in charge" is much more helpful to the patient. Self-care agency means that the patients are able to accept that the methods will help reduce lymphedema and that they believe that they are capable of doing the things necessary to prevent lymphedema.

Critical Thinking Questions with answers can be found in the Osborn Student Resources at nursing.pearsonhighered.com.

Source: Adapted from Armer, J., Shook, R., Schneider, M., Brooks, C., Peterson, J., & Stewart, B. (2009). Enhancing supportive–educative nursing systems to reduce risk of post-breast cancer lymphedema. *Self-Care, Dependent-Care & Nursing, 17*(1), 6–15.

(additional treatment done after the main treatment to decrease risk of recurrence). Radiation is discussed in detail in Chapter 57.

Chemotherapy is a systemic method of destroying cancer cells that may have migrated to other parts of the body. Chemotherapy also is used to reduce the size of a tumor to allow a more conservative, rather than radical, approach to surgery. Used in this way, chemotherapy is **neoadjuvant therapy** (therapeutic medicine such as hormone therapy given before the primary treatment such as radiation). Neoadjuvant therapy is used in the treatment of inflammatory breast cancer (Molckovsky et al., 2009). Chemotherapy is discussed more fully in Chapter 57.

Hormone therapy is used to block the effects of estrogen on the growth of breast cancer cells. It may be used as adjuvant or neoadjuvant therapy or when a cancer has reoccurred (ACS, 2011a). However, hormone therapy is effective only in those breast cancers that are estrogen receptor positive. Estrogen receptors' presence or absence is determined by pathology reports after biopsy. Tamoxifen, the most common medication used in breast cancer, blocks the estrogen receptor positive tumor's ability to utilize estrogen in both pre- and postmenopausal women and men. Another group of antiestrogen agents known as aromatase inhibitors (anastrozole, letrozole) has been successfully used to block estrogen production by tissues other than the ovaries in postmenopausal women (ACS, 2011a).

Targeted therapy occurs when medication is given that targets a specific gene found in some breast cancers. One gene that can be targeted is the HER2/neu oncogene. Tissue from biopsy is analyzed for HER2 positive or negative status (Markman, 2011). Trastuzumab (Herceptin), a monoclonal antibody, targets HER2/neu. Trastuzumab has been shown to improve survival for women and men with metastatic disease as well as late stage and recurrent disease (ACS, 2011a; Markman, 2011). See the Pharmacology feature (p. 1335). A complete discussion of monoclonal antibodies is found in Chapter 52. Additional information on aspects of the diagnosis and treatment of breast cancer may be found in Chapter 57.

Reconstructive breast surgery occurs after mastectomy for breast cancer. Advances in techniques have made breast reconstruction a more desirable procedure for women requiring mastectomy. Reconstructive surgery can be done at the time of the mastectomy or it can be delayed, based on the woman's preference. Immediate breast reconstructive surgery does not delay administration of chemotherapy or radiation, nor does it prevent detection of recurrent disease. It is beneficial to perform the breast reconstruction immediately after the mastectomy. An immediate breast reconstruction is more cost-effective, allows for a quicker recovery, and makes for reduced inconvenience, as well as greater satisfaction, for the patient (Imaginis, 2011).

Predicting Breast Cancer Survival

Breast cancer survival is dependent on multiple factors. Overall, 88% of women survive 5 years after diagnosis; for White women, the 5-year survival rate is 90.2%, and for Black women, it is 77.5% (NCI, 2011f). The 5-year survival rate is slightly lower among women who were diagnosed with breast cancer before age 40. This may be because tumors in this age group are more aggressive and less responsive to hormonal therapy (ACS, 2011a).

The stage of cancer at diagnosis also determines the patient's survival rate. Naturally, the survival rate is lower among women with a more advanced state of disease. Chart 44–5 lists the 5-year survival rate by stage of cancer at diagnosis for women and men.

The presence of additional illnesses, lower socioeconomic status, unequal access to medical care, and disparities in treatment may contribute to the observed differences in survival between lower and higher income breast cancer patients (ACS, 2011a). Chapter 57 provides an in-depth discussion of cancer staging and treatment.

Nursing Management

The patient with breast cancer requires a comprehensive interdisciplinary care plan to address the complex nature of the disease. The Nursing Process: Patient Care Plan feature (p. 1347) provides a complete

Weblink: Breast Cancer in Men Weblink: Breast Cancer

CHART 44–5 Five-Year Survival Rate by Stage of Cancer at Diagnosis for Women and Men

Women		Men	
Stage 0	93%	Stage 0	100%
Stage I	88%	Stage I	96%
Stage IIA	81%	Stage II	84%
Stage IIB	74%	Stage III	52%
Stage IIIA	67%	Stage IV	24%
Stage IIIB	41%		
Stage IIIC	49%		
Stage IV	15%		

Sources: Adapted from American Cancer Society (ACS). (2011a). Detailed guide: Breast cancer. *Learn About Cancer.* Retrieved from http://www.cancer.org/Cancer/BreastCancer/DetailedGuide/index; http://www.cancer.org/Cancer/BreastCancer/DetailedGuide/breast-cancer-risk-factors; http://www.cancer.org/Cancer/BreastCancer/DetailedGuide/breast-cancer-prevention; http://www.cancer.org/Cancer/BreastCancer/DetailedGuide/breast-cancer-diagnosis; http://www.cancer.org/Cancer/BreastCancer/DetailedGuide/breast-cancer-treating-general-info; http://www.cancer.org/Cancer/BreastCancer/DetailedGuide/breast-cancer-survival-by-stage; American Cancer Society (ACS). (2011b). Detailed guide: Breast cancer in men. *Learn About Cancer.* Retrieved from http://www.cancer.org/Cancer/BreastCancerinMen/DetailedGuide/index; http://www.cancer.org/Cancer/BreastCancerinMen/DetailedGuide/breast-cancer-in-men-risk-factors; http://www.cancer.org/Cancer/BreastCancerinMen/DetailedGuide/breast-cancer-in-men-treating-by-stage; http://www.cancer.org/Cancer/BreastCancerinMen/DetailedGuide/breast-cancer-in-men-survival-rates

care plan for the patient with breast cancer. The Patient Teaching & Discharge Priorities box (p. 1349) outlines the discharge teaching for the patient with breast cancer.

Further nursing care planning involved in postoperative care is found in Chapter 19.

Health Promotion

Patient and family education is essential for the prevention of breast cancer. The following facts are important components of the teaching plan:

- Clinical breast exam and self-breast exam
- Weight management
- Avoidance of excessive alcohol use
- Mammograms every 2 years after age 40
- Caution with use of hormone replacement therapy during menopause.

The United States (U.S.) Preventive Services Task Force recommends screening mammography, with or without clinical breast examination, every 2 years for women ages 50 to 74. This task force found evidence that mammography screening every 12 to 33 months significantly reduces mortality from breast cancer. Evidence is strongest for women ages 50 to 69, the age group generally included in screening trials. For women ages 40 to 49, the evidence is weaker that screening mammography reduces mortality from breast cancer. The decision to start regular mammography screening before age 50 should be made based on each individual woman's risks and potential benefits (U.S. Preventive Services Task Force, 2010).

Collaborative Management

Breast cancer is a complex disorder that requires a team approach for optimum care. In order to meet desired patient outcomes, it is essential that this interdisciplinary team communicate openly with one another in developing and evaluating care of the patient and family (IOM [Institute of Medicine], 2010). Breast cancer requires the expertise of gynecologists or other primary care providers to recognize the problem and to refer the patient to an oncologist, breast surgeon, and radiologist. The health care provider's care is supplemented by nurses, nutritionists or dietitians, counselors, and community resources such as social services. If surgery is required, then anesthesiologists will direct general anesthesia. Open communication among specialists will enhance the potential for the woman or man with breast cancer to maintain optimum health and avoid some of the severe complications that can occur. The surgeon is the team leader at the time of surgery and immediate recovery.

The oncologist becomes team leader for adjuvant care such as chemotherapy, targeted therapy, and hormone therapy as needed. The radiation oncologist will direct any localized radiation treatments, if these are needed.

Nurses assist in many roles, as discussed earlier. In addition, nurses are responsible for managing sedation and analgesics should surgery be needed. Pain management is a major responsibility for nurses in the care of patients with breast cancer. Nutritionists and dietitians help the patient understand and choose correct foods so that appropriate nutrition can be maintained.

Counselors may be engaged to help the survivors of breast cancer deal with body image issues. Community resources may include social services, support groups, exercise centers, and organizations such as the American Cancer Society. Support groups are especially helpful to families of patients with breast cancer as they learn to cope with the many changes that are occurring with their loved one. Care for the caregivers should be a major focus for nurses in the community and home setting.

Additional Surgical Procedures

Lumpectomy and mastectomy have been discussed in the Medical and Surgical Management section for breast cancer on pages 1344–1345. Additional common surgical breast procedures include cosmetic and reconstructive surgery. These procedures are performed to increase or decrease breast size, to lift the breast tissue, or for replacement after mastectomy. Augmentation or enlargement of the breast is generally done for cosmetic purposes. In contrast, breast reduction is often done for functional reasons because large breasts can cause back and shoulder pain and contribute to poor posture; in such cases, this surgery might be covered financially by insurance. A mastopexy is a surgical procedure performed to improve drooping (ptotic) breasts. Breast reconstruction following mastectomy also is possible.

Breast Augmentation

Mammoplasty (augmentation of the breast) involves the implantation of a manufactured silicone shell implant filled with silicone gel, saline, or, in some cases, a double lumen implant consisting of each of these substances. The implants are placed in a surgically created pocket that is either subglandular (beneath the breast tissue but in front of the muscle fascia) or submuscular (under the pectoralis muscle and sometimes the serratus anterior and upper part of the rectus abdominus muscles). The surgery is typically done on an outpatient basis either under local anesthesia and conscious sedation or under general anesthesia. Surgical incisions are made in one of four areas: around the periareolar margin, in or just above the inframammary fold, in the axilla, or in and around the

NURSING PROCESS: Patient Care Plan for Breast Cancer Post-Modified Mastectomy

Assessment of Reproductive System Status Using Gordon's Functional Health Patterns:

- Self-Perception/Self-Concept
- Cognitive–Perceptual
- Coping Stress Tolerance
- Sexuality–Reproductive
- Role–Relationship

Subjective Data

Assessment of Patient's Knowledge of the Disease

What do you know about breast cancer and the surgery planned?

Do you plan to have reconstructive surgery at the same time the modified mastectomy is done?

Do you understand what is involved in reconstruction after mastectomy?

Do you have questions about mastectomy and reconstruction?

Do you have questions about your treatment plan?

How would you manage the side effects of surgery and treatment?

Assessment of Pain

Are you experiencing pain?

Tell me your level of pain on a scale of 0 to 10, with 10 being the worst pain you have ever had.

Describe the location, intensity, and quality of your pain.

Assessment of Body Image Disturbance

What feelings do you have about the change in your appearance after modified mastectomy?

Will reconstructive surgery begin immediately after the mastectomy?

Do you feel less anxious with more or less information?

Tell me what you are feeling regarding your illness.

Who are your support systems?

Have you been socializing?

Assessment of Infection

Do you have any increased pain, redness, or drainage from surgical site?

Assessment of Coping

Do you feel saddened, angry, and vulnerable?

Have you been avoiding others or withdrawing from your usual routines?

Are you able to sleep?

Do you have family support that comforts you?

Objective Data

Assessment of Patient's Knowledge of the Disease

Is the patient withdrawn or quiet?

Is the patient reluctant to participate in conversation?

Is fear present?

Assessment of Pain

Are the pulse and blood pressure increased?

Does the patient seem unwilling to participate in care?

Is there any facial grimacing, guarding painful area, or restlessness?

Assessment of Body Image Disturbance

Does the patient seem to have reduced communicative efforts?

Does the patient seem to have withdrawn from social support?

Does the patient complain of insomnia? Does the patient seem to sleep?

Is the patient crying occasionally or often?

Is the patient unwilling to touch the affected breast?

Assessment of Infection

Does the patient have fever and chills?

Are there changes in the patient's white blood count (WBC)?

Is there drainage from the wound?

Are there positive wound cultures? What organisms are identified?

Is there evidence of decreased or delayed healing?

Assessment of Coping

Does the patient seem unwilling to participate in care?

Does the patient seem unwilling to interact with social support persons?

Is the patient able to sleep? Is the patient crying, lashing out, or angry?

Outcomes and Evaluation Parameters	Planning and Interventions with *Rationales*
1. NURSING DIAGNOSIS: Deficient Knowledge ***related to the disease process, medications, treatment options, and complications;*** **Fear** ***related to diagnosis, surgery, treatment, and prognosis*** **(NANDA-I © 2012)**	
Outcome: Increased understanding of diagnosis, disease process, and treatment. Decreased anxiety and fear. ***Evaluation Parameter:*** Patient asks pertinent questions related to the disease process, treatment, and symptoms.	Provide information to the patient regarding the disease process including the type of cancer. Provide information about medications that may be used such as analgesics, antiemetics, and intravenous fluids. Provide information about mastectomy and immediate reconstruction of the breast or, depending on the need for chemotherapy or radiation therapy, delayed reconstruction of the breast. Provide information about treatment modalities such as radiation and chemotherapy. Explain equipment and the environment. Encourage the patient to ask questions regarding the disease process, medications, and treatment options.

(continued)

NURSING PROCESS: Patient Care Plan for Breast Cancer Post-Modified Mastectomy, *continued*

Outcomes and Evaluation Parameters	Planning and Interventions with *Rationales*
	Explain all findings to the patient and encourage her to relate the changes in signs and symptoms. *To increase knowledge about the disease. To decrease anxiety and provide for less distress related to lack of knowledge of the treatment, thereby encouraging continuation of treatment. To reduce fear through helping the patient understand more about the surgery and the treatment plan.*
2. NURSING DIAGNOSIS: Acute Pain *related to breast cancer and surgical intervention* (NANDA-I © 2012)	
Outcomes: Comprehensive pain management. Patient reports intervention has alleviated pain. No facial grimacing or restlessness. Patient uses analgesic and nonanalgesic measures appropriately. ***Evaluation Parameters:*** Reduction in pain to patient acceptance. Patient reports pain is under control.	Perform a comprehensive pain assessment regularly. Provide for a quiet and restful environment. Reposition for comfort as needed. Provide for diversion with music, television, or relaxation techniques. Provide patient teaching regarding use of analgesics or PCA as appropriate. Advocate for patient when needed to change or increase pain medications. Encourage patient to use pain control measures before pain becomes severe and out of control. Encourage use of relaxation techniques or cutaneous stimulation. *Promotes comfort, reduces anxiety, promotes relaxation. Provides consistent pain control.*
3. NURSING DIAGNOSIS: Disturbed Body Image *and* Risk of Low Self-Esteem *related to anticipated physical effects of surgery and treatment modalities* (NANDA-I © 2012)	
Outcomes: Acceptance of body image changes. Development of attitude of realistic hope. ***Evaluation Parameters:*** Patient verbalizes feelings and fears about body image changes. Patient accepts social support. Patient reports decrease in worry and fear. Patient reports increase in psychological well-being.	Encourage verbalization of feelings about body image and level of self-esteem, perceptions, and fears *to reduce stress and anxiety.* Validate concerns. Encourage the patient to seek social support in the form of outreach groups *to feel less alone.* Encourage interaction with other women with breast cancer *to feel less alone.* Encourage patient to verbalize feelings of helplessness, and provide information regarding progress with treatments *to decrease stress level.* Assist in cosmetic enhancements to improve appearance *to promote positive body image.* Encourage the patient to touch the affected breast *to enhance acceptance of loss of breast.* Encourage family members to verbalize concerns regarding the diagnosis, treatment, and potential complications *to decrease stress level.*
4. NURSING DIAGNOSIS: Risk for Infection *related to surgery and neutropenia secondary to radiation therapy and chemotherapy* (NANDA-I © 2012)	
Outcome: Avoidance of infection. ***Evaluation Parameters:*** Healed wound. No fever. Diminishing or absent pain.	Instruct the patient and family members in hand hygiene *to prevent wound contamination.* Monitor the surgical site for signs of infection, such as redness, odor, drainage, and lack of healing, *that would indicate an infection.* Provide patient education about infection signs and symptoms and what to report to the surgeon *to institute medical intervention as soon as possible.*
5. NURSING DIAGNOSIS: Ineffective Coping *related to life changes brought about by diagnosis, surgery, and treatments* (NANDA-I © 2012)	
Outcomes: Development of effective coping behaviors. Development of attitude of realistic hope. ***Evaluation Parameters:*** Patient verbalizes feelings and fears about illness. Patient demonstrates effective coping strategies for living with cancer. Patient shows acceptance of social support. There is an interaction with individuals with similar change in body image. Patient discusses changes in body image. Patient demonstrates willingness to use strategies to enhance appearance. Patient actively participates in recovery.	Encourage the patient to verbalize feelings *as an effective coping strategy.* Consult a psychiatrist, psychologist, or spiritual counselor *for expertise in evaluating and enhancing coping strategies.* Encourage the patient to interact with Reach to Recovery volunteer *to develop hope for the future.* Encourage the patient to attend a breast cancer support group where she can draw on experiences of other women with breast cancer. Provide information on support groups available to the patient. Facilitate contact with individuals with similar change in their lives.

Source: Adapted from Wilkinson, J. M., & Ahearn, N. R. (2009). *Prentice Hall nursing diagnosis handbook* (9th ed.). Upper Saddle River, NJ: Prentice Hall.

PATIENT TEACHING & DISCHARGE PRIORITIES for Post-Mastectomy Breast Cancer

Need	Teaching and Follow-Up Treatment Plan
Knowledge of disease process and prognosis	Home care needs include verbal and written instructions for: Follow-up treatment plan: Physical therapy, chemotherapy, and hormone therapy. Follow-up care visits with surgeon and oncologist. Activity restrictions—avoid heavy lifting or strenous work using arm on the operative side for 4 to 6 weeks. Home care needs, follow-up treatment plan, and visits with oncologist instructions will help encourage the patient to participate in follow-up care.
Understanding of medications	The patient and family are taught about use of analgesics and oral tamoxifen (if tumor is estrogen receptor positive). This includes purpose, dose, and possible side effects of these drugs to prevent over- or underdosing.
Care of chest wound and reconstruction	The patient should learn the importance of keeping the wound(s) clean. Wounds should be kept dry for the first 48 hours; then they may be washed gently according to the surgeon's directions. Explain the use of any topical medications prescribed. Encourage the patient to look at the surgical wound daily for redness, drainage, or swelling. Check the patient's temperature daily. Report any evidence of infection, including increased pain or temperature of 100.4°F (38°C), to the health care provider immediately.
Disease prevention	Encourage the patient to avoid anyone with upper respiratory infections to prevent increased risk of infection, particularly while on chemotherapy.
Lymphedema prevention or control	Educate the patient about avoiding obesity, avoiding injury or infection to the affected arm, and reducing hand use to lower the risk for lymphedema. If edema begins, teach the patient use of deep breathing, abdominal massage, axillary clearance, gentle manipulation of the arm, use of the compression sleeve, proper skin care, and avoidance of constriction of the arm or axilla.

Source: Adapted from Armer, J., Shook, R., Schneider, M., Brooks, C., Peterson, J., & Stewart, B. (2009). Enhancing supportive–educative nursing systems to reduce risk of post-breast cancer lymphedema. *Self-Care, Dependent-Care & Nursing, 17*(1), 6–15.

umbilicus. Figure 44–5◆ (p. 1350) shows a patient both before and after an augmentation mammoplasty.

Complications are rare; they include hypertrophic scars, hematoma formation, infection, deflation or rupture of the implant, asymmetry of the breasts, temporary or permanent loss of sensation, and contracture of scar tissue. Formation of scar tissue around the implant is normal to "wall it off" as a foreign body. However, the scar tissue can sometimes thicken and contract, making a smaller pocket, which can then lead to breast firmness referred to as *capsule contracture*. The cause of this condition is usually unknown, but the incidence is thought to be increased by hematoma and seroma formation or subclinical infections. Treatment is usually surgical, incising the scar to allow the surrounding tissues to expand and create a larger pocket, thus allowing the implants to feel softer and drape more naturally. Recently, the Erchonia laser has been used to soften the capsules, resulting in a more natural feel and appearance of the breasts. The long-term effects of laser use are yet to be determined, and the results are variable among patients. Women with breast augmentation have the same incidence of developing a malignancy as those without implants and therefore should continue to do regular breast self-examination and mammograms (ACS, 2011a).

Breast Reduction

Breast reduction is usually done for complaints of pain and discomfort related to large breasts but can be done for cosmetic reasons as well. Breast reduction relieves pain in the back, neck, and shoulders; may improve the patient's feelings of self-worth; and potentially decreases anxiety and depression (Mayo Clinic Staff, 2011a). Breast reduction is a surgical procedure in which breast tissue and skin are removed from the center and lower parts of the breast. Usually the nipple and areolar complex are relocated superiorly, keeping the complex attached to the subcuticular breast tissues to retain circulation and sensation. In women with very large breasts, it may be necessary to remove the nipple and areolar complex completely during the procedure and relocate the complex as a full-thickness skin graft after the breast tissue and skin have been removed; the remaining breast tissue and skin are then sculpted to give a natural-looking breast appearance.

Breast reduction also can be performed using liposuction if much of the breast is made up of fat cells. Liposuction may or may not use ultrasonic energy to emulsify fat cells. This technique removes a significant volume of breast fat; in younger patients with good elasticity, it lifts the breast while leaving minimal scarring. However, liposuction for breast reduction is not indicated for older women or for women with very large breasts.

Breast reduction is usually done under general anesthesia and, depending on the patient's age and condition, can be done on either an outpatient or an inpatient basis. Complications include blood loss, infection, hematoma, asymmetry of breasts, loss of sensation, and hypertrophic scarring. In women of childbearing age, this surgical procedure may result in the inability to breast-feed. The scar from this procedure extends around the areola and straight down from the center of the inferior portion of the areola to the inframammary fold. Sometimes there is also a scar across the inframammary fold. Women tend to be extremely satisfied with the results of this procedure because of the increased comfort and appearance.

Mastopexy

Mastopexy is a surgical procedure performed in women who have nursed, have lost weight, or have breasts that have settled due to the

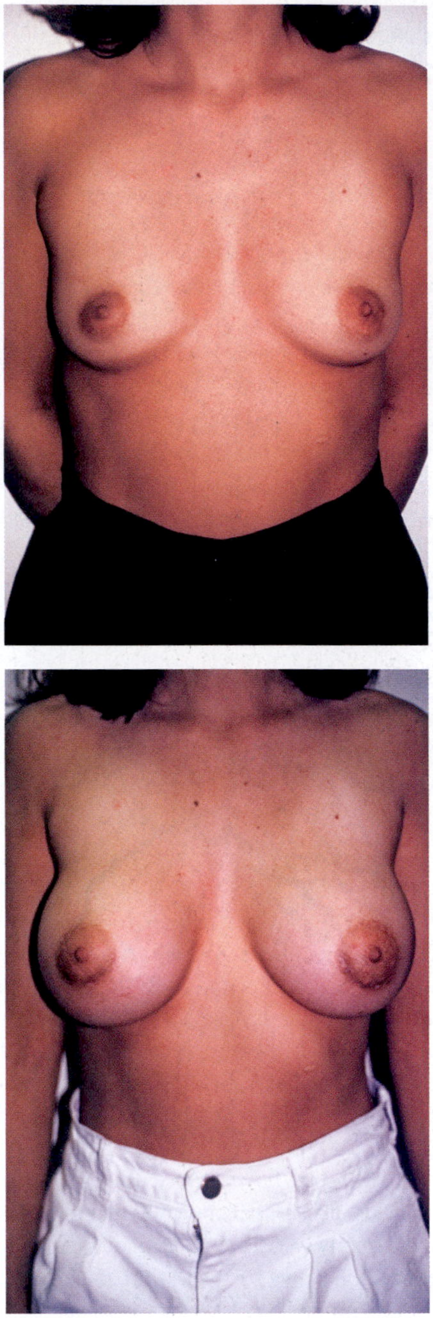

(a)

(b)

FIGURE 44–5 ◆ Breast augment (A) before and (B) after.
Source: JPD/Custom Medical Stock Photo.

aging process. This procedure lifts the nipple and areolar complex superiorly, excises excess skin, and reshapes the remaining skin without removing breast tissue. An implant may be inserted during a mastopexy to improve breast fullness and give a more natural shape. However, this procedure does have some degree of visible scarring.

Breast Reconstruction

Several approaches exist for reconstructing the breast following a mastectomy. The goal of breast reconstruction is to create a mound that gives a normal appearance in a bra or a bathing suit and improves the woman's self-image. It also is possible to re-create a pigmented circle with a small mound in the center that looks like a normal nipple and areola in thin clothing. However, it is not possible to restore the normal breast functions of lactation, nipple sensation, or nipple erectility. The process of reconstructing the breast can begin immediately when the mastectomy is being performed, or it can be delayed and begun in a separate surgery later. The timing is based on patient and surgeon preference, along with the possible need for chemotherapy and/or radiation.

Symmetry of the breasts is usually easier to achieve when doing bilateral reconstruction. No matter which technique is used, it is sometimes difficult to match a normal side that is too large, is ptotic, or has had other changes associated with the aging process. Sometimes a mastopexy, augmentation, or reduction is done on the normal side for symmetry. In some states, the law mandates that both breasts' procedures be covered by the patient's insurance carrier.

Tissue Expanders and Implant Reconstruction

Breast reconstruction using an implant is usually a multistep process. It begins after the mastectomy with the placement of a tissue expander under the skin and pectoral, serratus anterior, and rectus abdominus muscles in order to stretch the muscle and skin and create a pocket for subsequent placement of an implant. The tissue expander is minimally inflated on insertion and gradually filled with weekly injections of saline inserted into a self-sealing valve in the expander. This facilitates a gradual expansion of skin and muscle tissue until the desired breast size is reached (Figure 44–6◆). Once the size is reached, the expander is surgically removed and a permanent implant is inserted. Although not commonly used, some expanders are designed to be the permanent implant, thereby eliminating the need for a second surgery to remove the expander.

Tissue Transfer Reconstruction

It is possible to use the patient's own tissue to reconstruct the breast by using tissue transferred from other areas of the body. The three types of tissue used in transfers are the latissimus dorsi muscle of the back, the transverse rectus abdominus muscle (TRAM) of the lower abdomen, and the microvascular free flaps from the lower abdomen or buttocks. The placement of this tissue will replace skin and breast tissue removed during the mastectomy.

A latissimus dorsi flap consists of a skin island attached to the latissimus dorsi muscle, which gets its blood supply from axillary vessels to which it is attached. Usually an implant is inserted beneath muscle to augment the volume when a latissimus dorsi flap is used.

A TRAM flap consists of skin from the lower abdomen that is left attached to the rectus abdominus muscle for its blood supply. It is then tunneled up under the remaining abdominal skin and carefully inserted and sculpted into the deficient breast area to create a mound that resembles a breast. If there is sufficient abdominal tissue, this technique can be used to reconstruct both breasts at the same time, splitting the skin in the center and leaving each half attached to its respective rectus muscle. The main trade-off for this procedure is that it weakens the abdominal musculature. Implants may or may not be used with a TRAM flap, depending on the amount of fatty tissue available, the patient's preference for size, and the amount of volume required for symmetry.

Some patients may be better candidates for a microvascular free flap reconstruction, in which skin and fat are taken from either the abdomen or the buttock, along with their vascular supply. These are then sutured, using microvascular techniques, to the surrounding recipient vessels for circulation. Patients who smoke, patients with diabetes, and patients with some previous abdominal scars may not be good candidates for this procedure, because of the already compromised vascular supply to the skin and muscle.

Nipple–Areolar Reconstruction

Once the breast mound is reconstructed, several methods are available for reconstructing the nipple and areolar complex. The techniques used involve various combinations of local flaps, skin grafts, and sometimes tissue from the nipple on the normal side, if it is of adequate size. After the nipple and areola have been reconstructed, the final step is to use micropigmentation (tattooing) to darken the area to match the contralateral breast for unilateral reconstruction. This completes the reconstruction and helps to make women feel "whole" again.

Complications of breast reconstruction include wound infection, hematoma, dehiscence, asymmetry, rupture of the expander or implant, and capsule contracture. Wound infection may occur, especially if the woman is immunosuppressed due to the cancer itself and/or is under treatment with chemotherapy. Capsule contracture was discussed earlier in this chapter. Previous radiation may result in various degrees of fibrosis of the skin and muscle and may make expansion more difficult.

ETHICAL ISSUES
Women and Research on Breast Disorders

Nurses who conduct or assist with research among women concerning their breasts should be aware of the ethical issues involved. For instance, a group of women were approached to participate in research to determine whether light waves could be used as a noninvasive method for diagnosing breast disease (Armstrong & Morris, 2010). Research of this type must first be approved by an ethics committee within the institution where the research is being conducted. The ethics committee is responsible for ensuring that research conducted does not endanger the participants. Once the research has been approved, each potential participant must be fully informed of the risks and benefits of participating in the study. This information should fully disclose any anticipated painful procedures, expected touching of the breasts by research personnel, and any physical safety issues. Some women may object to male researchers handling their breasts, so the gender of the person who is conducting the experiment should be disclosed. The patient should be informed that she may withdraw from the study at any time and that leaving the study will not affect any health services she may receive. The participant must complete a signed consent form, proving that she understands everything about the procedure. Full disclosure prior to the research allows the woman to understand her rights and to determine for herself what is or is not acceptable as far as exposure of her breasts and the research being done.

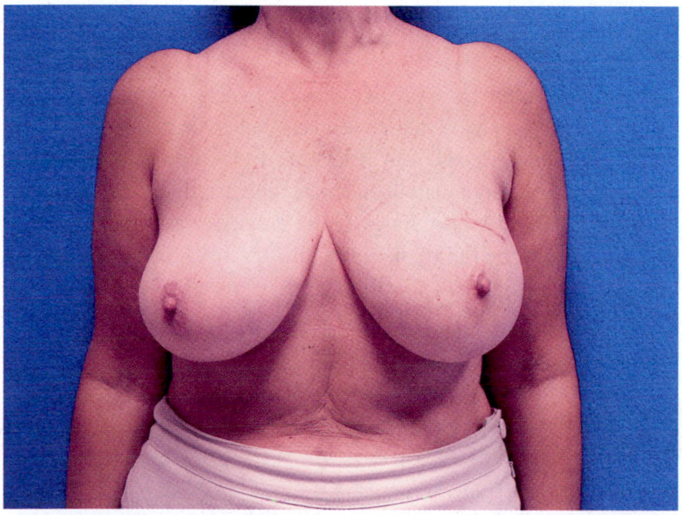
(a)

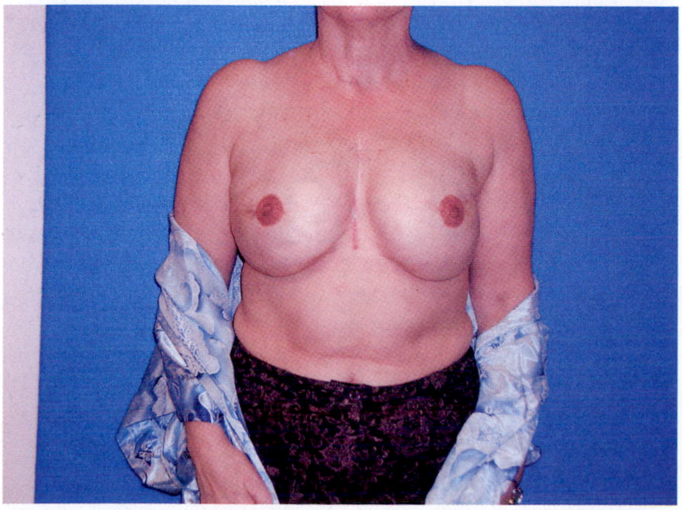
(b)

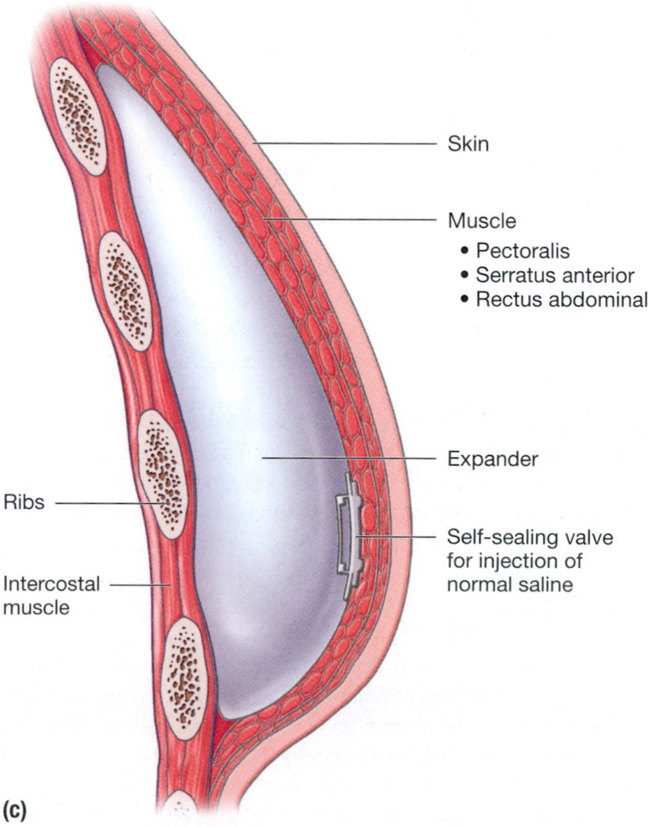

(c)

FIGURE 44–6 ◆ Tissue expander (C) and breast reconstruction photos (A) before, (B) after.
Source: (A) and (B): John M. Osborn MD.

RESEARCH OPPORTUNITIES for Breast Disorders

Research	Clinical Impact
Effect of continued trastuzumab use when metastatic disease has progressed	To determine whether or not continued use improves overall survival and quality of life.
Men's awareness of male breast cancer	To identify the level of male awareness of male breast cancer and to explore ways to increase awareness.
Increased public awareness of the hereditary causes of breast cancer	To identify level of awareness of genetic causation of some breast cancers.
Ethics of responsibility in decision making about treatment in breast cancer	Should surgeons make the decisions for patients? Do patients always want to make their own decisions?
Effect of complementary or alternative therapies for mastalgia	To determine which of the complementary therapies work best for women who suffer from mastalgia.
Effects of mastectomy on the shoulder	A side effect of mastectomy is shoulder changes, including scapular rotation. Interventions to restore normal scapulohumeral articulation are needed.
Coping with changes in body image	To improve supportive care for breast cancer survivors with body image changes.
Use of light waves for diagnosis of breast cancer	To improve early detection of breast cancer without radiation exposure.

Geronotological Considerations

Breast tissue responds to cyclic estrogen and progesterone. During the perimenopause years and menopause, cycle decreases in the production of these hormones cause the glandular tissue of the breasts to decline. At the same time, there is an increase in fat and connective tissue (Deneris & Huether, 2010). This makes the breast less firm, and it hangs lower on the chest.

Research has shown that the aging breast is more vulnerable to breast cancer than those of younger women. This is probably due to the cumulative effect of years of breast exposure to cyclic estrogen and other risk factors. Fortunately, the decrease in breast density related to aging makes mammography an excellent tool for early detection of cancerous lesions among older women.

Research

Women who suffer from breast disorders benefit from research that helps improve quality of life or validates better diagnostic tools and treatments. Research also can help identify the best approaches for public education about male breast cancer and hereditary causes of cancer. The Research Opportunities feature provides a list of a few related research topics. The Ethical Issues feature describes the importance of ethical considerations when working with women.

CLINICAL PREPARATION

READ DOCUMENT APPLY

READ: History of Present Illnesses >> Laboratory Study Results >> Critical Thinking Questions

John Kirklin is a 68-year-old retired pilot who has been admitted to the surgical oncology ward for right breast surgery to treat breast cancer. He has had four chemotherapy sessions to shrink the lesion, and the surgeon plans modified mastectomy to remove all diseased tissue.

The situation has been a huge shock to Mr. Kirklin, not only because he has been told he has cancer, but also because he is a man and "men don't get breast cancer." He tells you that his friends can't believe his diagnosis either. He expresses his feelings that all that is happening is "out of his control." He feels vulnerable for the first time in his life, and he is angry.

Medical–Surgical History

Mr. Kirklin was in good health until the discovery of his breast cancer. "I had to take care of myself while I was working as a pilot," he says. "It was not until I retired 4 years ago that I began to gain weight." He is not currently taking any medications.

Social History

Mr. Kirklin has been married to his wife, Joanne, for 38 years. They have a very good relationship, and Mrs. Kirklin is very supportive. Their two sons are also supportive.

Mr. Kirklin does not use tobacco, alcohol, or drugs of any kind.

Physical Examination

Vital signs: T 98.4°F orally, P 88, R 18, BP 130/80, BMI 29

Mr. Kirklin is overweight but appears in good health. His right nipple is retracted and scaly with a blood-tinged clear discharge. There is a 2 × 2 centimeter hard, fixed nodule under the nipple and areola. There is no axillary swelling.

His lungs are clear to auscultation, and his heart sounds are normal with regular rate and rhythm.

His abdomen is protuberant, bowel sounds are present, and there is no tenderness or masses.

READ: History of Present Illnesses >> **Physical Exam** >> Admitting Medical Records >> Laboratory Study Results

Admitting Medical Orders

Surgical Oncology Service
Admit to surgical ward
Diagnosis: Invasive ductal carcinoma, right breast
Estrogen receptor positive
No known allergies
Vital signs every 4 hours
NPO at midnight
Ambien 10 mg p.o. H.S.
Before surgery in a.m.: begin IV D5 1/2NS at 125 mL/hour
Atropine 0.6 mg IM and Demerol 75 mg IM 1 hour before surgery.

The next morning, Mr. Kirklin is prepared for surgery. You talk with him about the surgery and anesthesia, including the risks and benefits, then ask him whether he has any questions. Mr. Kirklin explains that his mother had breast cancer and died soon after the surgery. You listen as Mr. Kirklin tells about how he learned to cope with her illness and death. He acknowledges that he understands the risks and benefits and signs the consent form.

After surgery, Mr. Kirklin returns to the ward. He has had the mastectomy, and the good news is that the axillary sentinel node was negative for any cancer. His cancer is Stage I. Since the tumor was larger than 1 centimeter, the health care provider recommends continued chemotherapy for 4 more months and the addition of hormone therapy with tamoxifen for the next 3 years.

Mr. Kirklin receives standard postoperative care and goes home 2 days later.

READ: History of Present Illnesses >> **Laboratory Study Results** >> Critical Thinking Questions

Test	On Admission	Postoperative Day 1	Postoperative Day 2
White blood cell count (WBC)	5,000/mm^3	9,000/mm^3	8,500/mm^3
Platelets	410,000/mm^3	399,000/mm^3	401,000/mm^3
Hemoglobin (HGB)	14 g/dL	12.5 g/dL	12.6 g/dL

Test	On Admission	Postoperative Day 1	Postoperative Day 2
Hematocrit (HCT)	42%	37%	37.5%
Red blood cells (RBC)	4.92/mm^3	4.4/mm^3	4.3/mm^3
Tumor biopsy	Estrogen receptor positive		

Pearson Nursing Student Resources *Log on to* ***nursing.pearsonhighered.com*** *to download forms*

DOCUMENT:

>> Summary of Hospitalization
>> Pathophysiology Form
>> Laboratory Values
>> Laboratory Results Explanation

APPLY:

>> List of Potential Nursing Diagnoses
>> Concept Map
>> Critical Thinking Questions and Concept Map

APPLY: History of Present Illnesses >> Laboratory Study Results >> **Critical Thinking Questions**

1. What are Mr. Kirklin's risk factors for breast cancer? (choose 2)
   1. Use of alcohol and tobacco
   2. First-degree relative with breast cancer
   3. Being overweight
   4. Being a pilot
2. How can you best help Mr. Kirklin deal with his "feeling out of control"?
   1. Allow him to talk about his feelings in a nonjudgmental setting.
   2. Discourage discussion and tell him he needs to talk with his health care provider.
   3. Encourage him to participate in activities and decision making related to his care.
   4. Recommend that he call his minister.
3. How can you best help Mr. Kirklin deal with his anger?
   1. Help him identify the cause of the anger and verbalize his angry feelings.
   2. Discount his concerns about his diagnosis.
   3. Never validate the patient's anger.
   4. Encourage the patient to follow the doctor's orders without question.
   5. Leave the patient alone until he is ready to go home.
4. What is the goal of hormone adjuvant therapy for Mr. Kirklin?
   1. To help him feel better and stronger
   2. To prevent recurrence of the cancer in the other breast
   3. To kill undetected cancer cells
   4. To boost his immune system

Answers to Critical Thinking Questions can be found in Appendix D in the Osborn Student Resources at nursing.pearsonhighered.com.

NCLEX® PRACTICE

1. A Caucasian female, age 35, presents with tender, firm masses in both breasts that enlarge during the menstrual cycle. This patient probably has:
   1. breast cancer.
   2. fibrocystic changes.
   3. fibroadenoma.
   4. mastitis.
2. A 56-year-old woman presents with an erythematous, swollen right breast. She has no fever. The nurse suspects:
   1. infectious mastitis.
   2. ductal ectasia.
   3. ductal cancer *in situ.*
   4. inflammatory breast cancer.
3. Nursing care of the woman who has benign galactorrhea should include directions such as: (select all that apply)
   1. press the nipple to remove the discharge daily.
   2. stop taking nonsteroidal anti-inflammatory drugs.
   3. refrain from expressing the discharge from the nipple.
   4. decrease caffeine, high-fat foods, and sodium.
   5. stop wearing a bra until the symptoms resolve.
4. A female patient wants to reduce her risk of developing breast cancer. Which of the following should the nurse instruct this patient?
   1. "Do not have any children."
   2. "It is best to use oral contraceptives throughout the child-bearing years."
   3. "Limit dietary fat intake."
   4. "Have children before the age of 30."
5. The nurse is reviewing the technique for self-breast examination with a postmenopausal female. Which of the following should be included in this instruction?
   1. Do the exam at least one time each week.
   2. In postmenopausal women, the breast exam is only done if an abnormality is found.
   3. Always examine the breasts while lying down.
   4. If you feel a lump, prepare yourself emotionally for the diagnosis of breast cancer.
6. The nurse has determined that her patient who is scheduled for a mastectomy is worried about the physical effects of the surgery. Which of the following would help the patient to cope?
   1. Encourage verbalization of feelings, perceptions, and fears.
   2. Distract the patient and encourage watching television.
   3. Provide more education about the surgical procedure and what will be removed.
   4. Administer a sedative medication to calm the patient.

Answers to NCLEX Practice Questions can be found in Appendix D in the Osborn Student Resources at nursing.pearsonhighered.com. Practice additional NCLEX questions online at the Student Resources site.

Pearson Nursing Student Resources Find additional review materials at: **nursing.pearsonhighered.com**

REFERENCES

Adams, M., & Koch, R. (2010). *Pharmacology: Connections to nursing practice.* Upper Saddle River, NJ: Pearson.

Agency for Healthcare Research and Quality (AHRQ). (2010a). Core-needle biopsy for breast abnormalities: Clinician's guide. Effective Health Care Program. Retrieved from http://effectivehealthcare.ahrq.gov/index.cfm/search-for-guides-reviews-and-reports/?pageaction=displayproduct&productID=406&mode=P

Agency for Healthcare Research and Quality (AHRQ). (2010b). Having a breast biopsy: A guide for women and their families. Effective Health Care Program. Retrieved from http://effectivehealthcare.ahrq.gov/index.cfm/search-for-guides-reviews-and-reports/?pageaction=displayproduct&productID=407

American Cancer Society (ACS). (2011a). Detailed guide: Breast cancer. *Learn About Cancer.* Retrieved from http://www.cancer.org/Cancer/BreastCancer/DetailedGuide/index; http://www.cancer.org/Cancer/BreastCancer/DetailedGuide/breast-cancer-risk-factors; http://www.cancer.org/Cancer/BreastCancer/DetailedGuide/breast-cancer-prevention; http://www.cancer.org/Cancer/BreastCancer/DetailedGuide/breast-cancer-diagnosis; http://www.cancer.org/Cancer/BreastCancer/DetailedGuide/breast-cancer-treating-general-info; http://www.cancer.org/Cancer/BreastCancer/DetailedGuide/breast-cancer-survival-by-stage

American Cancer Society (ACS). (2011b). Detailed guide: Breast cancer in men. *Learn About Cancer.* Retrieved from http://www.cancer.org/Cancer/BreastCancerinMen/DetailedGuide/index; http://www.cancer.org/Cancer/BreastCancerinMen/DetailedGuide/breast-cancer-in-men-risk-factors; http://www.cancer.org/Cancer/BreastCancerinMen/DetailedGuide/breast-cancer-in-men-treating-by-stage; http://www.cancer.org/Cancer/BreastCancerinMen/DetailedGuide/breast-cancer-in-men-survival-rates

American Cancer Society (ACS). (2011c). Inflammatory breast cancer. Retrieved from http://www.cancer.org/Cancer/BreastCancer/MoreInformation/InflammatoryBreastCancer/index

American Joint Committee on Cancers (AJCC). (2010). *AJCC cancer staging manual* (7th ed.). Retrieved from http://www.cancerstaging.org/products/ajccproducts.html

American Joint Committee on Cancer (AJCC). (2012). TNM system quoted in American Cancer Society. (2012). Breast cancer. *Learn About Cancer.* Retrieved from http://www.cancer.org/Cancer/BreastCancer/DetailedGuide/breast-cancer-staging

Armer, J., Shook, R., Schneider, M., Brooks, C., Peterson, J., & Stewart, B. (2009). Enhancing supportive–educative nursing systems to reduce risk of post-breast cancer lymphedema. *Self-Care, Dependent-Care & Nursing, 17*(1), 6–15.

Armstrong, V., & Morris, N. (2010). Boundary setting in breast cancer research: A study of the experience of women volunteer research subjects. *Sociology of Health & Illness, 32*(1), 74–88. doi: 10.1111/j.1467-9566.2009.01182.x

Balkam, J. (2010). Painful breast lumps in nursing mothers. *American Journal of Nursing, 110*(12), 65–67.

Bickley, L. (2007). *Guide to physical examination and history taking* (9th ed.). Philadelphia: Lippincott Williams & Wilkins.

Centers for Disease Control and Prevention (CDC). (2011a). Breast cancer: Screening. Retrieved from http://www.cdc.gov/cancer/breast/basic_info/screening.htm

Centers for Disease Control and Prevention (CDC). (2011b). Cancer among women. Cancer prevention and control. Retrieved from http://www.cdc.gov/cancer/dcpc/data/women.htm

Deneris, A., & Huether, S. (2010). Structure and function of the reproductive systems. In K. McCance & S. Huether (Eds.), *Pathophysiology: The biologic basis for disease in adults and children* (6th ed., pp. 781–815). St. Louis: Mosby/Elsevier.

Giuliano, A., & Hurvitz, S. (2011). Breast disorders. In S. McPhee & M. Papadakis (Eds.), *2011 Current medical diagnosis and treatment* (50th ed., pp. 693–720). New York: McGraw-Hill Medical.

Imaginis. (2011). Breast reconstruction. Retrieved from http://www.imaginis.com/breast-health/breast-reconstruction#advantages-and-disadvantages-to-immediate-breast-reconstruction

IOM (Institute of Medicine). (2010). *The future of nursing: Leading change, advancing health.* Washington, DC: The Academic Press.

Johnson, R., & Murad, M. (2009). Gynecomastia: Pathophysiology, evaluation, and management. *Mayo Clinic Proceedings, 84*(11), 1010–1015.

Kamal, R., Hamed, S., & Salem, D. (2009). Classification of inflammatory breast disorders and step by step diagnosis. *The Breast Journal, 15*(4), 367–380. doi:10.1111/j.1524-4741.2009.00740.x

Kao, G. (2011). Mammary Paget disease. eMedicine. Retrieved from http://emedicine.medscape.com/article/1101235-overview

Kee, J. (2010). *Laboratory and diagnostic tests* (8th ed.). Upper Saddle River, NJ: Pearson.

Latendresse, G., McCance, K., & Morgan, K. (2010). Alterations of the reproductive systems. In K. McCance & S. Huether (Eds.), *Pathophysiology: The biologic basis for disease in adults and children* (6th ed., pp. 781–815). St. Louis: Mosby/Elsevier.

Lee, E. (2009). Evidence-based management of benign breast disease. *The American Journal for Nurse Practitioners, 13*(7/8), 22–31.

Li, C., Chlebowski, R., Freiberg, M., Johnson, K., Kuller, L., Lane, D., et al. (2010). Alcohol consumption and risk of postmenopausal breast cancer by subtype: The women's health initiative observational study. *Journal of the National Cancer Institute, 102*(18), 1422–1431. doi:10.1093/jnci/djq316

Markman, M. (2011). Breast cancer and HER2. eMedicine: Genomic medicine. Retrieved from http://emedicine.medscape.com/article/1689966-overview

Mayo Clinic Staff. (2011a). Breast reduction surgery. Mayo Clinic.com. Retrieved from http://www.mayoclinic.com/health/breast-reduction-surgery/MY00778

Mayo Clinic Staff. (2011b). Mammary duct ectasia. MayoClinic.com. Retrieved from http://www.mayoclinic.com/health/mammary-duct-ectasia/DS00751

Mills, D. (2011). Breast health: The mystery of breast pain—and how to solve it. Women to Women. Retrieved from http://www.womentowomen.com/breasthealth/breastpain.aspx

Molckovsky, A., Fitzgerald, B., Freedman, O., Heisey, R., & Clemons, M. (2009). *Approach to inflammatory breast cancer, 55*(1) 25–31.

National Cancer Institute (NCI). (2011a). Cancer genetics risk assessment and counseling (PDQ). Retrieved from http://www.cancer.gov/cancertopics/pdq/genetics/risk-assessment-and-counseling/HealthProfessional/page6

National Cancer Institute (NCI). (2011b). Fact sheet: BRCA1 and BRCA2: Cancer risk and genetic testing. Retrieved from *Canadian Family Physician* http://www.cancer.gov/cancertopics/factsheet/Risk/BRCA

National Cancer Institute (NCI). (2011c). Fact sheet: Mammograms. Retrieved from http://www.cancer.gov/cancertopics/factsheet/detection/mammograms

National Cancer Institute (NCI). (2011d). Fact sheet: Menopausal hormone replacement therapy use and cancer. Retrieved from http://www.cancer.gov/cancertopics/factsheet/Risk/menopausal-hormones

National Cancer Institute (NCI). (2011e). Fact sheet: Oral contraceptives and cancer risk: Questions and answers. Retrieved from http://www.cancer.gov/cancertopics/factsheet/Risk/oral-contraceptives

National Cancer Institute (NCI). (2011f). SEER stat fact sheet: Breast. In *Surveillance epidemiology and end results: Cancer statistics*. Based on 2009 SEER data submission posted 2010. Retrieved from http://seer.cancer.gov/statfacts/html/breast.html

National Comprehensive Cancer Network (NCCN). (2010). NCCN guidelines for patients: Breast cancer. Ductal carcinoma in situ (DCIS) (pp. 10–11). Retrieved from http://www.nccn.com/images/patient-guidelines/pdf/breast.pdf

National Standard. (2011). Evening primrose oil. Retrieved from http://naturalstandard.com.ezproxy.midwives.org/databases/herbssupplements/primrose.asp

Rodden, A. (2009). Common breast concerns. *Primary Care Clinic Office Practice, 36*(91), 103–113. doi:10.1016/j.pop.2008.10.006

Rogers, V., & Cox, S. (2011). Obstetrics and obstetric disorders. In S. McPhee & M. Papadakis (Eds.), *2011 Current medical diagnosis and treatment* (50th ed., pp. 754–778). New York: McGraw-Hill Medical.

Schwartz, R. (2011). Mondor disease. Medscape Reference. Retrieved from http://emedicine.medscape.com/article/1087099-overview

Singhal, H., & Teh, W. (2011). Breast stereotactic core biopsy/fine needle aspiration. eMedicine. Retrieved from http://emedicine.medscape.com/article/1845123-overview

Spencer, J. (2008). Management of mastitis in breastfeeding women. *American Family Physician, 78*(6), 727–731, 732.

Stephan, P. (2011). Digital mammography compares well with film mammography. Breast cancer. About.com. Retrieved from http://breastcancer.about.com/od/mammograms/a/digital_mammo.htm

Thomas, E. (2010). Men's awareness and knowledge of male breast cancer. *American Journal of Nursing, 110*(10), 32–40.

U.S. Department of Health and Human Services (USDHHS). (2011). Cancer. HealthyPeople.gov. Retrieved from http://www.healthypeople.gov/2020/topicsobjectives2020/overview.aspx?topicid=5

U.S. Preventive Services Task Force (USPSTF). (2010). Screening for breast cancer. Current as of 2009. Retrieved from http://www.uspreventiveservicestaskforce.org/uspstf/uspsbrca.htm

Wilkinson, J. M., & Ahearn, N. R. (2009). *Prentice Hall nursing diagnosis handbook* (9th ed.). Upper Saddle River, NJ: Prentice Hall.

UNIT

10 Nursing Management of Patients with Endocrine Disorders

Content in Unit 10 that addresses the **Institute of Medicine (IOM)** competencies, **Nursing Core Competencies (NCC),** the **Quality and Safety Education for Nurses (QSEN)** competencies, and **Concepts** for concept-based learning is listed below.

Competencies	Feature or Text	Location
IOM, QSEN, NCC Providing patient-centered care	Genetic Considerations Related to the Endocrine System, page 1362 Nursing Process: Patient Care Plan for Hypothyroidism, page 1374 Nursing Process: Patient Care Plan for Hyperthyroidism, page 1384 Nursing Process: Patient Care Plan for Acute Adrenal Insufficiency, page 1409 Nursing Process: Patient Care Plan for Diabetes, page 1454	Chapter 45 Chapter 46 Chapter 46 Chapter 46 Chapter 47
IOM, QSEN, NCC Working in teams	Collaborative Management, pages 1376, 1386, 1390, 1396, 1408, 1412 Collaborative Management, page 1453	Chapter 46 Chapter 47
IOM, QSEN, NCC Employing evidence-based practice	Evidence-Based Practice: Lifestyle Issues Experienced by Patients with Thyroid Diseases, page 1387 Evidence-Based Practice: Glycemic Control, page 1431	Chapter 46 Chapter 47
IOM, NCC Applying quality and safety improvement	Safety Alerts, pages 1363, 1364, 1365 Safety Alerts, pages 1372, 1383, 1385, 1388 Safety Alerts, pages 1429, 1432, 1438, 1441, 1449	Chapter 45 Chapter 46 Chapter 47
NCC Educating patients	Health Promotion related to endocrine disorders, page 1366 Patient Teaching & Discharge Priorities for Hypothyroidism, page 1376 Patient Teaching & Discharge Priorities for Hyperthyroidism, page 1392 Patient Teaching & Discharge Priorities for Growth Hormone Disorders, page 1396 Health Promotion related to prevention of Type 2 diabetes, page 1442 Patient Teaching & Discharge Priorities for Diabetes, page 1456	Chapter 45 Chapter 46 Chapter 46 Chapter 46 Chapter 47 Chapter 47
Concepts covered in Unit 5 include:	Metabolism Fluid balance	Thermoregulation

Nursing Assessment of the Patient with Endocrine Disorders

45 CHAPTER

Laurie Quinn
Annita Watson

Outcome-Based Learning Objectives

After studying this chapter, the learner will be able to:

1. Formulate a general description of the endocrine system and its function.
2. Explain the general structure and classification of hormones.
3. Differentiate between types of hormonal communication.
4. Evaluate subjective and objective data related to the general assessment of the endocrine system.
5. Explain the purpose, preparation, and nursing functions related to diagnostic testing of the endocrine system.

KEY TERMS

adrenocorticotropic hormone p.1358
androgens p.1360
antidiuretic hormone p.1357
autocrine communication p.1361
bloodborne communication p.1361
calcitonin p.1360
circadian rhythms p.1361
corticotrophin-releasing hormone p.1358
dopamine p.1358
endocrine glands p.1357
exophthalmos p.1363
gonadotropin-releasing hormone p.1358
glucocorticoids p.1360
growth hormone p.1358
growth hormone-releasing hormones p.1358
hormones p.1357
monoamines p.1360
negative feedback p.1361
neuroendocrine communication p.1361
oxytocin p.1358
paracrine communication p.1361
parathyroid hormone p.1360
peptide p.1360
positive feedback p.1361
prolactin p.1358
protein p.1360
receptors p.1357
somatostatin p.1358
thyroid-stimulating hormone p.1358
thyrotropin-releasing hormone p.1358
thyroxine p.1360
triiodothyronine p.1360
trophic p.1361

THE ENDOCRINE SYSTEM is a system of glands that regulate a living organism by means of biochemical messengers (**hormones**) synthesized within the organism. **Endocrine glands** are glandular structures that release hormones directly into circulating plasma (Gardner, Anderson, & Nissenson, 2011). The hormones communicate with target glands to elicit a specific biochemical response. This communication occurs in a variety of different ways by acting on the cellular **receptors** (molecules with binding sites for substances such as hormones) of distant target cells, neighboring target cells, and the cells that produce the hormone. The endocrine system controls and coordinates the body's metabolism, respiration, excretion, and reproduction, among other functions.

Anatomy and Physiology of the Endocrine System

The endocrine glands are distributed throughout the body (Figure 45–1◆). The primary organs (glands) involved in the endocrine system are as follows: hypothalamus, anterior pituitary, posterior pituitary, adrenal gland, thyroid gland, parathyroid glands, pancreas, ovaries, and testes. A summary of these organs, the hormones they produce, and their major functions is provided in Chart 45–1. Chart 45–2 lists some of the most common abbreviations used when discussing the endocrine system.

Hypothalamus and Pituitary

The hypothalamus and the pituitary form a unit that regulates the function of several endocrine glands, including the thyroid, adrenals, ovaries, and testes. The hypothalamus lies at the base of the brain in the diencephalon. The pituitary gland (hypophysis) is attached to the ventral side of the hypothalamus of the brain. The anterior pituitary (adenohypophysis) and the posterior pituitary (neurohypophysis) are embryologically and functionally distinct. The posterior pituitary is of neural origin, arising embryologically as an evagination (protrusion of some part or organ from its normal position) of the ventral hypothalamus and the third ventricle. The posterior pituitary is composed of nerve endings of neurons whose cell bodies originate in the supraoptic and paraventricular nuclei of the hypothalamus (Javorsky, Aron, Findling, & Tyrrell, 2011). The primary hormones of the posterior pituitary, **antidiuretic hormone** (ADH), which controls water

Video: Endocrine Glands

The endocrine glands secrete hormones which regulate various functions throughout the body

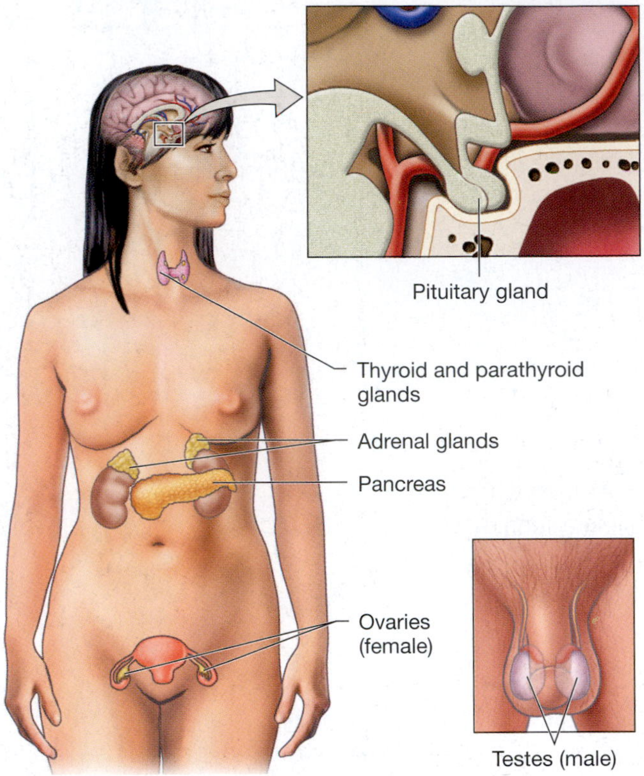

FIGURE 45–1 ◆ Location of the endocrine glands in the female and male bodies.

permeability in the kidneys, and **oxytocin,** which is involved in uterine contractions and milk let-down, are synthesized in the hypothalamus and are transported to the posterior pituitary via the hypothalamic-hypophyseal nerve tract, where they are stored in vesicles.

The anterior pituitary arises from Rathke's pouch, which is an ectodermal evagination of the oropharynx. The anterior pituitary is richly vascularized, receiving blood from a portal circulation connecting the median eminence of the hypothalamus and the anterior pituitary (Javorsky et al., 2011). The hypothalamus synthesizes a number of inhibiting and releasing hormones that regulate the secretion of anterior pituitary hormones. These hormones travel through the portal circulation, where they exert their effect on target cells in the anterior pituitary. These hypothalamic hormones include **corticotropin-releasing hormone** (CRH); **dopamine** (prolactin-inhibiting factor [PIF]); **growth hormone-releasing hormone** (GRH); **gonadotropin-releasing hormone** (GnRH); **somatostatin** (growth hormone inhibiting hormone [GH inhibiting hormone]); and **thyrotropin-releasing hormone** (TRH). The anterior pituitary hormones include **adrenocorticotropic hormone** (ACTH), **prolactin, growth hormone,** and **thyroid-stimulating hormone** (TSH).

These hormones act on specific cell types in the anterior pituitary to stimulate or inhibit the production of anterior pituitary hormones. CRH simulates the production of ACTH from the corticotrophs (cells of the anterior pituitary gland that secrete ACTH). Dopamine inhibits the production of prolactin from the somatotroph (cells of the anterior lobe of the pituitary gland that produce somatropins). GRH stimulates the production of growth hormone from the somatotrophs, whereas somatostatin inhibits the release of growth hormone from the somatotrophs. TRH stimulates the production of thyroid-stimulating hormone from the thyrotrophs (cells of the anterior lobe of the pituitary gland that produce thyrotropins).

CHART 45–1 Endocrine Gland Anatomy and Physiology

Site of Hormone Production	Hormones and Description
HYPOTHALAMUS	
Thyrotropin-releasing hormone (TRH)	Stimulates the anterior pituitary to produce and secrete thyroid-stimulating hormone (TSH).
Corticotropin-releasing hormone (CRH)	Stimulates the anterior pituitary to produce and secrete adrenocorticotropic hormone (ACTH).
Gonadotropin-releasing hormone (GnRH)	Stimulates the anterior pituitary to secrete follicle-stimulating hormone (FSH) and luteinizing hormone (LH).
Growth hormone-releasing hormone (GHRH)	Stimulates growth hormone (GH) release from the anterior pituitary.
Somatostatin	Inhibits GH and TSH release from the anterior pituitary.
Dopamine	Inhibits prolactin release from the anterior pituitary.
ANTERIOR PITUITARY	
Thyroid-stimulating hormone (TSH)	Stimulates production and release of T_3 and T_4.
Adrenocorticotropic hormone (ACTH)	Stimulates production and release of adrenocortical hormones (glucocorticoids, mineralocorticoids, androgens).
Luteinizing hormone (LH)	Stimulates ovulation, estrogen, and progesterone secretion in females and testosterone secretion in males.
Follicle-stimulating hormone (FSH)	Stimulates estrogen secretion and follicle maturation in females and spermatogenesis in males.
Prolactin (PRL)	Initiation and maintenance of lactation.
Growth hormone (GH)	Stimulates growth through IGF-1; also involved in intermediary metabolism.
POSTERIOR PITUITARY	
Antidiuretic hormone (ADH, vasopressin)	Increases water permeability of the distal nephron, thereby decreasing free water clearance; high concentrations cause an arteriolar vasoconstriction.
Oxytocin	Contraction of myoepithelial cells (contractile epithelial cells resembling smooth muscle cells that are present in glands and aid in secretion) of the mammary gland and uterine contractions.

CHART 45–1 Endocrine Gland Anatomy and Physiology, *continued*

Site of Hormone Production	Hormones and Description
Gland and Hormone	**Hormones and Description**
	ADRENAL GLAND (ADRENAL CORTEX)
Mineralcorticoids Aldosterone	Promotes sodium reabsorption along with potassium and hydrogen secretion in the kidney.
Glucocorticoids Cortisol	Involved in intermediary metabolism (the intermediate steps within the cells in which the nutrient molecules or foodstuffs are metabolized and converted into cellular components catalyzed by enzymes); promotes glycogenolysis, gluconeogenesis, proteolysis, lipolysis, and insulin resistance; inhibits bone formation and stimulates bone resorption; needed for vascular response to catecholamines; anti-inflammatory; suppresses immune function; necessary for integrity and function of the gastrointestinal tract; stimulates red blood cell production; alters mood and behavior.
Androgens	DHEA, androstenedione, small amounts of testosterone, and estrogen are released.
	ADRENAL GLAND (ADRENAL MEDULLA)
Epinephrine (80%)	Beta adrenergic effects: Epinephrine effects > norepinephrine effects Glycogenolysis Lipolysis Calorigenesis Increases insulin secretion Skeletal muscle vasodilation Bronchodilation
Norepinephrine (20%)	Alpha adrenergic effects: Epinephrine effects ~ norepinephrine effects Gluconeogenesis Decreased insulin secretion Increased mean arterial blood pressure Dilation of pupils Sweating Sphincter contraction
	THYROID GLAND
Thyroxine (T_4) Triiodothyronine (T_3)	Regulation of energy metabolism, growth, and development; maturation of tissues; essential for sympathetic nervous system function, cardiovascular function, and reproduction.
Calcitonin	Lowers serum calcium and phosphate levels primarily by inhibiting bone resorption.
	PARATHYROID GLAND
Parathyroid hormone (PTH)	Directly increases bone resorption and calcium mobilization from bone; increases reabsorption of calcium from the kidney; activates 1 alpha hydroxylase (necessary for the formation of active vitamin D).
Gland and Hormone	**Hormones and Description**
	PANCREAS
Insulin	Promotes the storage of glucose as glycogen in the liver and muscle. Promotes the formation of fat in the liver and adipose tissue. Promotes the formation of protein in the muscle and the liver from amino acid precursors. Promotes glycolysis. Enhances glucose transport into insulin-sensitive tissues, skeletal muscle and adipose tissues which allow glucose to enter via receptors on the surface of the tissue.
Glucagon	Increases hepatic glycogenolysis and gluconeogenesis. Stimulates ketogenesis.

CHART 45–2 Common Abbreviations Used in the Assessment and Treatment of Endocrine Disorders

ACE: angiotensin-converting-enzyme
ADH: antidiuretic hormone
CaSR: calcium-sensing receptor gene
CRH: corticotropin-releasing hormone
CSF: cerebrospinal fluid
CT: computerized tomography
DDAVP: 1-deamino-8-D-arginine vasopressin
DHEA: dehydroepiandrosterone
DI: diabetes insipidus
FTI: Free Thyroxine Index
GHD: growth hormone deficiency
GHRH: growth hormone-releasing hormone
IGF-1: insulin-like growth factor-1
IgGs: immunogammaglobulins
IPSS: inferior petrosal sinus sampling
MEN: multiple endocrine neoplasia syndromes
MRI: magnetic resonance imaging
OTC: over the counter
PTH: parathyroid hormone
PTU: propylthiouracil
RAAS: renin-angiotensin-aldosterone system
RAIU: radioactive iodine uptake
SIADH: syndrome of inappropriate antidiuretic hormone
SOMOSTATIN: hormone that inhibits the release of somatotropin (growth hormone)
SSKI: saturated solution of potassium iodide
T_3: triiodothyronine
T_4: thyroxine
TBG: thyroid-binding globulin
TgAb: antithyroglobulin antibodies
THBR: thyroid-binding ratio
TPO: thyroid peroxidase
TPOAb: antithyroid peroxidase antibodies
TRH: thyroid-releasing hormone
TSH: thyroid-stimulating hormone
USPSTF: U.S. Preventive Services Task Force

Thyroid Gland

The thyroid gland consists of two lobes connected by a thin isthmus that extends across the ventral surface of the trachea below the larynx (Porterfield & White, 2007). The thyroid produces two hormones, **triiodothyronine** (T_3) and **thyroxine** (T_4). The thyroid hormones influence a variety of physiological processes such as fetal and childhood growth, central nervous system development, energy expenditure, heat generation, myocardial contraction and relaxation, gastrointestinal motility, and lipid metabolism (Cooper & Ladenson, 2011). The thyroid also secretes **calcitonin,** a hormone whose primary function is to inhibit bone resorption (breakdown).

Parathyroid Glands

There are four parathyroid glands embedded in the thyroid gland. The parathyroid glands produce **parathyroid hormone** (PTH) that functions primarily to maintain normal calcium and phosphate balance by combined effects on the bones, kidneys, and intestinal tract.

Pancreas

The pancreas, which is located in the posterior portion of the upper abdomen, consists of two functionally distinct organs: the exocrine and endocrine pancreases. The exocrine pancreas is a major digestive organ, producing enzymes needed for the absorption of nutrients. The endocrine pancreas produces several hormones, including insulin, glucagon, somatostatin, and pancreatic polypeptide. These hormones have diverse functions; they are essential in carbohydrate, fat, and protein metabolism. These hormones and their functions are detailed in Chapter 46.

Adrenal Glands

The adrenal glands are located on the superior pole of each kidney. These structures are divided into two distinct organs: the adrenal medulla and the adrenal cortex, which compose the inner and outer layers, respectively. The medulla secretes catecholamines, and the cortex produces **glucocorticoids** (which play a major role in intermediary metabolism), mineralocorticoids, and **androgens** (male sex steroid hormones). Overall, the adrenal hormones are important regulators of metabolism and adaptation to stress (Porterfield & White, 2007).

Ovaries

The ovaries, together with the uterus and fallopian tubes, are located in the pelvis. These are the internal reproductive organs of the female. The primary hormones produced by the ovaries are estrogen and progesterone. These hormones and their functions are detailed in Chapter 40.

Testes

The testes, located in the scrotum, are the major reproductive organs of the male. The primary hormone produced by the testes is testosterone. These hormones and their functions are detailed in Chapter 40.

Principles of Endocrine Physiology

The primary secretory products of endocrine glands are hormones, which are chemical substances that exert a regulatory action on target cells. Hormones act as chemical messengers to stimulate, inhibit, and augment a number of biochemical and physiological processes. Some basic principles of endocrine physiology are detailed in the following paragraphs.

Hormone Classification and Release

The chemical composition of hormones varies widely. For example, hormones may be composed of **proteins** (large complex molecules made up of polypeptides, such as adrenocorticotropin [ACTH] and insulin), **peptides** (building blocks of protein, under 40 amino acids, such as vasopressin), **monoamines** (one amino group, such as epinephrine or norepinephrine), single amino acid derivatives (e.g., triiodothyronine [T_3]), steroids (e.g., cortisol), or lipids (e.g., prostaglandins) (Gardner et al., 2011). Generally, hormones synthesized from proteins, peptides, monoamines, and single amino acids are stored within the endocrine cells and are available when needed. However, steroid hormones are not stored in the endocrine cell; rather, they are synthesized when needed.

Hormone Receptors

The release of hormones from endocrine glands allows these hormones to exert their effect on target cells. These target cells have receptors specific for the hormone and are able to distinguish a specific hormone from others through binding to the receptor. The biologic activity of hormones is dependent on specific high-affinity receptors that are located on the surface, cytoplasm, or nuclei of target cells (Gardner et al., 2011). Protein, peptide, and monoamine hormones usually have cell surface receptors, while steroids and thyroid hormones have receptors in the cell nucleus. This binding of the hormone with specific receptors elicits cellular signaling mechanisms, culminating in the desired cellular response.

Hormone Communication

Hormones communicate with target cells in a number of different ways. For example, hormones may travel through the circulation and act on the cellular receptors of distant target cells. This is generally described as **bloodborne communication.** Hormones also may diffuse through interstitial fluids and act on cellular receptors in neighboring cells; this is termed **paracrine communication.** Thirdly, hormones may communicate with receptors on cells that produced the hormone; this is called **autocrine communication.**

Hormonal communication may be integrated with the nervous system; this is termed **neuroendocrine communication.** The nervous system and the endocrine system have much in common, such as the use of ligands or receptors to establish communication between cells (Gardner et al., 2011). There are, however, important differences between the two systems. The nervous system is a highly compartmentalized closed system that relies primarily on axons or cables (the nerves) to communicate between distant points, while the endocrine system relies on circulating plasma to communicate between distant points (Gardner et al., 2011). However, these two systems work synergistically to regulate overall physiological functioning by regulating responses to the internal and external environment. Growth and development, maintenance of homeostasis, adaptability to changes in the external environment, and reproduction occur through the combined efforts of these systems.

Hormone Transport

Hormones in the plasma circulate in either *free* or *bound* forms, which are uncomplexed or complexed to other molecules, respectively. The free or uncomplexed form of the protein is the biologically active form of the protein in the plasma. Homeostatic regulatory mechanisms work to maintain normal levels of the free hormone (Gardner et al., 2011). For example, it is the concentration of free thyroid hormone that stimulates or inhibits thyroid-stimulating hormone (TSH). The binding of hormones in the plasma allows for a reservoir where hormones can be released or bound to maintain normal levels, e.g., thyroid hormone may be released from protein-binding sites during hypothyroidism and bound to protein-binding sites during hyperthyroidism; thus precipitating an increase or decrease, in serum thyroid hormones.

Hormonal Rhythms

Hormones often are secreted in specific patterns or rhythms, which are important for normal endocrine function. Many of the rhythms have a 24-hour cycle; these are referred to as **circadian rhythms.** Rhythms that last more than 24 hours are referred to as infradian rhythms. Pulsatile rhythms (usually over 1/2 to 2 hours) are often imposed on circadian rhythms. Changes in, or the loss of, hormonal rhythms can be associated with disease states. Cortisol is an excellent example of a hormone that has a circadian rhythm, with plasma levels that are lowest in late evening and highest in the morning. The circadian rhythm of cortisol can be changed by a variety of factors, including changes in sleep patterns, physiological and psychological stress, and disorders such as Cushing syndrome.

Hormonal Feedback

A feedback system is a regulatory system that keeps certain body functions within a prescribed range to maintain homeostasis (Figure 45–2◆). Feedback loops describe the relationship between the plasma concentrations of hormones and their respective **trophic** hormones (e.g., hormones that exert their stimulatory or inhibitory effects on a target gland hormone).

Negative feedback refers to a reciprocal relationship between a target gland hormone and its respective trophic hormone. Negative feedback decreases the deviation from an ideal normal value, and is important in maintaining homeostasis. An example of negative feedback is the regulation of the body's blood calcium level. The parathyroid glands secrete parathyroid hormone, which regulates the blood calcium amount. If calcium decreases, the parathyroid glands sense the decrease and secrete more parathyroid hormone. The parathyroid hormone stimulates calcium release from the bones and increases the calcium uptake into the bloodstream from the collecting tubules in the kidneys. Conversely, if blood calcium increases too much, the parathyroid glands reduce parathyroid hormone production. Both responses are examples of negative feedback because in both cases the effects are negative (opposite) to the stimulus (The Hormone Foundation, 2011).

Positive feedback refers to a positive or linear relationship between a target gland hormone and its respective trophic hormone; in other words, an increase in a target gland hormone results in an increase in the respective trophic hormone. In positive feedback mechanisms,

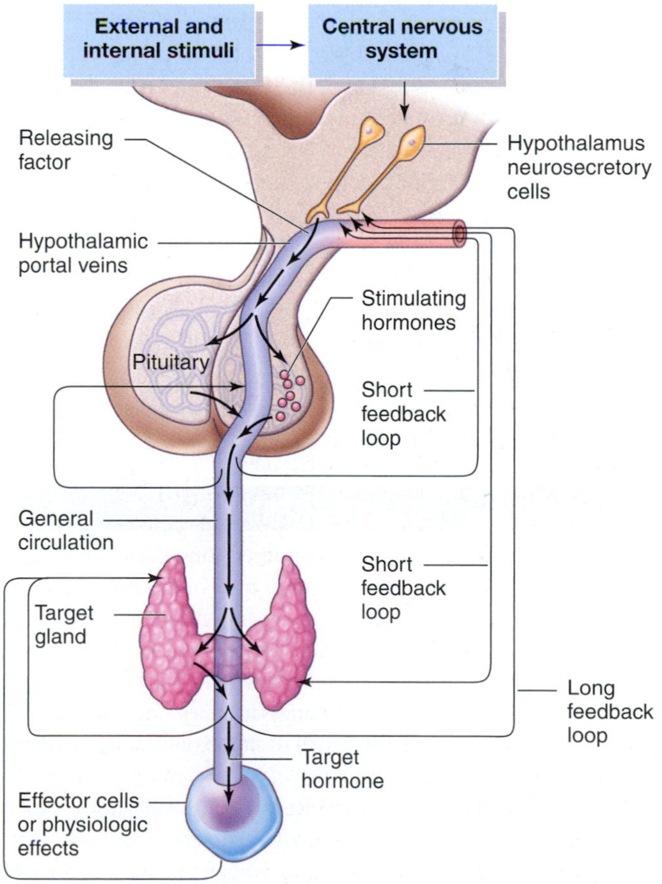

FIGURE 45–2 ◆ General feedback loops.

Weblink: Genetic Susceptibility

the original stimulus is promoted rather than negated. Positive feedback increases the deviation from an ideal normal value. Unlike negative feedback that maintains hormone levels within narrow ranges, positive feedback is rarely used to maintain homeostatic functions. An example of positive feedback occurs during the menstrual cycle. There is an increase in LH during the middle of the menstrual cycle, caused by a progressive increase in circulating concentrations of 17-β estradiol.

Feedback loops also can be *long-acting* or *short-acting* loops. The hypothalamus-anterior pituitary-target gland axis contains examples of each of these feedback loops. For example, corticotropin-releasing hormone (CRH) is secreted by the hypothalamus and acts on the anterior pituitary to produce adrenocorticotropic hormone (ACTH), which stimulates the secretion of glucocorticoids from the adrenal cortex. The relationship between the plasma concentration of glucocorticoids and CRH from hypothalamus is considered a long feedback loop, and the relationship between the concentrations of glucocorticoids and ACTH from the anterior pituitary is considered a short feedback loop.

Assessment of Endocrine Function

The endocrine system is a highly complex network composed of several glands, each producing one or more hormones with specific biochemical effects. Hormones have a variety of functions and influence almost all body systems. These functions include (but are not limited to) energy production, central nervous system development, growth and development, sexual maturation, and fluid and electrolyte imbalance. Since endocrinology covers numerous physiologic symptoms, there is no standard endocrine history and physical examination (Jameson, 2011). Because most endocrine glands are relatively inaccessible, the physical exam focuses on signs and symptoms of hormonal excess and deficiency along with direct examination of palpable glands (e.g., thyroid and gonads) (Jameson, 2011). Signs and symptoms of endocrine dysfunction lie on a continuum from vague, nonspecific complaints to life-threatening medical emergencies. Astute clinical skills are needed to identify the subtle signs and symptoms that may be associated with endocrine disorders (Jameson, 2011). Some of these subtle signs and symptoms (e.g., fatigue) may be common to several disorders. Therefore, knowledge of the prevalence and the pathophysiological determinants of disease is helpful in formulating a differential diagnosis (Jameson, 2011). Assessing for normal and abnormal hormonal variations entails a thorough assessment of the patient's history, along with a systematic, complete physical examination. Assessment should include examination of the patient's past medical history, family history, and current complaints; a general and functional health evaluation; and diagnostic testing.

History

The patient's health history is essential in eliciting information about the etiology of a patient's signs and symptoms. For example, a previous diagnosis of an endocrine disorder helps to determine whether current signs and symptoms are related to an exacerbation of an existing condition. The nurse asks the patient about previous hospitalizations, illnesses, surgeries and treatments, changes in appearance, sleep and rest patterns, elimination problems, sexual dysfunction, changes in diet or appetite, and medication usage.

Many endocrine systems are involved in energy metabolism; therefore, changes in appetite, weight, and activity tolerance are core symptoms of several endocrine disorders. A thorough nursing assessment of a patient's energy level is important in developing the ongoing plan of care. The patient is asked about her energy levels and ability to carry out activities of daily living (ADLs) independently. The patient may report not being able to "do what I used to" or may complain of generalized weakness and fatigue. Patients are more likely to report a gradual decline than an abrupt change in activity tolerance. Thyroid and adrenal dysfunction are common reasons for altered energy levels.

Along with a review of the entire medical history, the nurse evaluates the patient's family, occupational, and social histories. Disorders of the endocrine system may occur in a familial pattern. For example, there is a strong genetic basis for diabetes and thyroid disorders. Information regarding the genetic relationship to diabetes and thyroid disorders is shown in the Genetic Considerations box. Knowing this information should assist the nurse in conducting a more focused assessment. The patient's exposure to chemicals, use of drugs and alcohol, smoking, coping with stress, and behavioral patterns are all areas to be investigated.

Exposure to environmental toxins was discussed in the Genetic Considerations box as a potential source for the autoimmune endocrine disease type 1 diabetes mellitus and autoimmune thyroid disease. This phenomenon often is referred to as *endocrine disruption* and is defined by the U.S. Environmental Protection Agency (EPA) as "an exogenous agent that interferes with synthesis, secretion transport, metabolism, binding action, or elimination of natural blood-borne hormones that are present in the body and are responsible for homeostasis, reproduction, and developmental process (Diamante-Kandarakis, Bourguignon, Giudice, et al., 2009, p. 294). Endocrine disruption is receiving national and international attention in response to emerging concerns that substances in the environment may alter the function of endocrine systems and result in adverse effects to human health. The overall intent of the Endocrine-Disrupting Chemicals Exposure Elimination Act of 2011, introduced in the U.S. Congress in 2011, is to strengthen the regulation of chemicals that are found to be endocrine disruptors and increase the focus on research on these chemicals at the National Institute of Environmental Health Sciences (NIEHS) (Advocacy, 2011). This legislation was endorsed by the National Endocrine Society, who found it consistent with their 2009 position statement on endocrine-disrupting chemicals. The specific goals of this legislation are described in the National Guidelines box.

GENETIC CONSIDERATIONS
Related to the Endocrine System

"Epidemiological evidence suggests a common genetic background for both thyroid disease and diabetes mellitus" (Duntas, Orgiazzi, & Brabant, 2011, p. 4). However, at this time, identification of common genes is restricted almost exclusively to autoimmune causes, resulting in thyroid disease and diabetes mellitus (Huber, Menconi, Corathers, et al., 2008). With these genetic disorders, dysregulation of the immune system results in immune attacks on the endocrine glands, resulting in deficiency in the hormones secreted by them (Tomer, 2011). The most common autoimmune disorders are type 1 (T1) (juvenile) diabetes mellitus and autoimmune thyroid disease (AITH). These disorders frequently cluster within the same family, and may occur within the same person. It is likely that autoimmunity results from the impact of particular environmental factors on genetically susceptible individuals, resulting in loss of self-tolerance and thereby triggering disease (Yeung, 2011).

Health Assessment of Endocrine Function Across the Life Span

A number of endocrine disorders have their onset in childhood and adolescence, such as short stature caused by growth hormone (GH) deficiency. Other endocrine disorders, such as type 1 diabetes, are more

NATIONAL GUIDELINES Specific Goals of the Endocrine-Disrupting Chemicals Exposure Elimination Act of 2011

There are four specific goals of the Endocrine-Disrupting Chemicals Exposure Elimination Act of 2011. They are:

- Establish a research program through the National Toxicology Program (NTP) that is designed to strengthen the scientific information used by federal agencies to understand the effects of, and reduce human exposure to, EDCs.
- Establish an Endocrine Disruption Expert Panel under the NTP that will (A) consider, and report to the director on issues related to identification, classification, or evaluation of not more than 10 endocrine-disrupting chemicals or groups of endocrine-disrupting chemicals; (B) evaluate existing research aimed at understanding the biologic pathways in humans by which endocrine-disrupting chemicals operate and identify future research priorities as appropriate; and (C) maintain a list that identifies chemicals of concern for endocrine disruption effects.
- Establish the Endocrine Disruption Research Program at the National Institutes of Environmental Health Sciences to improve the understanding of how chemicals can disrupt the human endocrine system.
- Establish the framework for how federal agencies with jurisdiction over chemicals identified as endocrine disruptors by the NTP must respond.

likely to have their onset in childhood or adolescence. Younger patients with chronic endocrine disorders present special challenges when transitioning into adulthood. This underscores the need for a thorough health assessment as these patients begin treatment from adult health care providers.

The majority of common endocrine disorders, such as thyroid disease, occur in adulthood. Since there are a variety of physiological changes that occur with aging, the clinical presentation of endocrine disorders may be different in younger and older adults. For example, the initial clinical presentation of Graves' disease (a common form of hyperthyroidism) in older adults is far more likely to include new-onset atrial fibrillation than in younger adults. In contrast, older adults with hypothyroidism are more likely than younger adults to present with cardiovascular symptoms (e.g., heart failure) and neurological findings (e.g., confusion, impaired cognition, depression). Knowledge of age-related physiological changes and the impact of these changes on endocrine function are very helpful in assessing, diagnosing, and managing older patients.

Physical Examination

The physical exam begins with the measurement of vital signs (blood pressure, pulse, respiratory rate, and temperature), height, weight, and calculation of body mass index [weight (kg)/height (m^2)]. Abnormalities in body weight (e.g., obese or underweight) or height (e.g., short stature) are determined. The patient's behavior and communication skills are noted. If indicated, a brief assessment of cognitive function is performed.

Safety Alert *If cognitive impairment of the patient is suspected or indicated, the nurse should consider the patient's possible emotional and behavioral responses to the examination. The patient may be afraid of strangers, those conducting the examination, and the actual examination procedures used, thus projecting mistrusting and self-protective behaviors. Therefore, the nurse should use soothing and reassuring communication techniques when touching the patient and when speaking to her, as well as when conducting the examination. The nurse should complete the examination in a calm and quiet environment, away from other people, and do so as efficiently as possible. To avoid confusion, instructions and explanations of procedures should be kept short with the use of commonly understood words. Enlisting the aid of a family member when explaining what is happening during the examination may help keep the patient calm and cooperative.*

Skin, Hair, and Nails

The skin, hair, and nails are routinely assessed for changes that may be consistent with endocrine dysfunction. For example, disorders of the thyroid in particular are associated with changes in skin, hair, and nails. The temperature, color, hydration, pigmentation, and texture of the skin are inspected, at which time the nurse notes edema, lesions, masses, and hair texture and distribution. The nails are assessed for abnormalities such as brittleness, thickness, thickening, transverse grooving, onycholysis (separation from the nail bed), spooning, and clubbing.

Head and Neck

The head and neck examination is one of the most important assessments in determining endocrine dysfunction. This is because of the location of the hypothalamus, pituitary, and thyroid gland. The examination begins with the careful inspection of the face and neck for contours, symmetry, and masses. Changes in facial features in adults may be associated with growth hormone excess (acromegaly). The nurse assesses the patient's visual acuity and visual fields. For example, abnormalities in vision and loss of peripheral vision may be indicative of a pituitary tumor. The presence of **exophthalmos** (protrusion of the eyeball[s]) is consistent with a diagnosis of Graves' disease. The nurse then assesses symmetry and movement of the tongue, uvula, pharynx, and soft palate and notes the position of the trachea. The thyroid gland is palpated to determine the size and shape of the thyroid and to assess for tenderness, nodules, and masses (Figure 45–3◆).

Breasts

Endocrine disorders may be associated with changes in breast tissue, such as gynecomastia (enlargement of the male breasts). The nurse inspects the shape and symmetry of the breasts and examines them for masses, tenderness, thickening, or discharge.

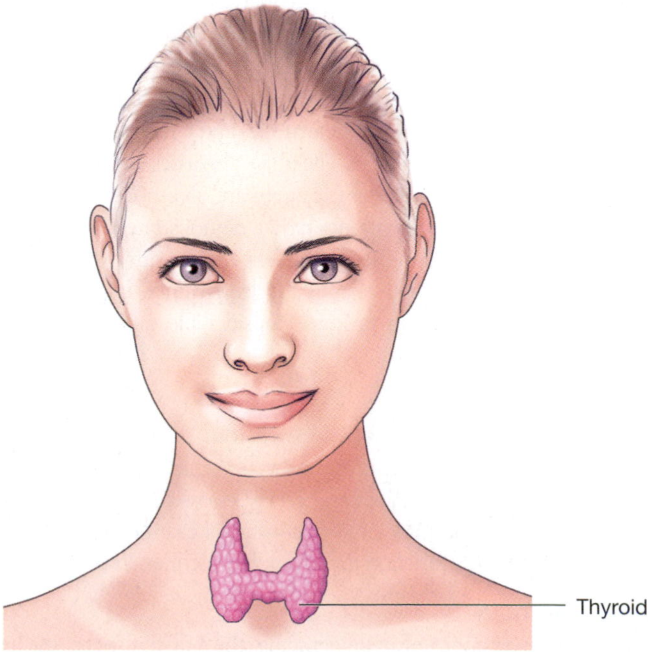

FIGURE 45–3 ◆ The thyroid gland.

Lungs

A thorough pulmonary examination is necessary in the assessment of endocrine function. Endocrine disorders may be associated with changes in the rate and quality of respirations. For example, a patient with diabetic ketoacidosis may have Kussmaul breathing (deep, rapid respirations). The nurse performs a visual inspection of the chest, noting symmetry of movement with respiration, the presence of retractions, and the use of accessory muscles. Lung sounds are auscultated for adventitious (abnormal) breath sounds.

Cardiac Examination

A thorough cardiac examination is necessary in the assessment of endocrine dysfunction. Disorders of the thyroid, in particular, are associated with changes in cardiac function. The nurse auscultates the heart for the presence of murmurs, clicks, snaps, and S_3 or S_4, and palpates for abnormal findings, such as pulsations, thrills, heaves, or lifts. Depending on the findings, a more extensive examination may be performed.

Safety Alert *Severe hyperthyroidism (thyrotoxicosis or Graves' disease) can cause tachycardia in excess of 150 beats per minute and is considered a medical emergency; beta-blockers are given to decrease the heart rate until ablation of the thyroid gland is accomplished.*

Abdomen

An examination of the abdomen can provide information on a number of abnormalities associated with endocrine dysfunction, such as adrenocortical disease. The nurse inspects the skin on the abdomen, noting its color, pigmentation, striae, abnormal hair distribution, distention, pulsations, and dilated veins. Changes in pigmentation and the presence of striae may be related to adrenocortical dysfunction. The nurse auscultates bowel sounds, noting frequency and character, and palpates the abdomen for the presence of masses, tenderness, or pain.

Musculoskeletal/Extremities/Neurological

A number of musculoskeletal changes are associated with endocrine dysfunction. For example, osteoporosis may be associated with a change in posture and a decrease in height from vertebral compression fractures. Therefore, the nurse notes the patient's posture and spinal alignment and palpates the spine for tenderness. The upper and lower extremities are inspected for general appearance, pigmentation pattern, skin texture, and hair distribution. For example, thyroid disorders may be associated with joint pain and stiffness, tremors, and myopathies. The nurse palpates the joints for deformities and tenderness and evaluates the patient's range of motion. The nurse also assesses the symmetry of muscle mass. Nervous system changes are common in endocrine dysfunction, since many hormones have a demonstrated influence on the central nervous system. For example, patients with hyperthyroidism may exhibit tremors of the hands. Electrolyte imbalances produced by endocrine disorders can produce considerable muscle weakness, spasms, and seizures.

Female Genitalia

Many endocrine disorders are associated with changes in reproductive function. In general, the nurse inspects the external genitalia and perineum, examines the vagina and cervix, assesses the size and position of the uterus, and performs a rectovaginal examination. In some settings, this may be a function for advanced practitioners only.

Male Genitalia

During the assessment of male genitalia, the nurse inspects the appearance of external genitalia; palpates the penis, testes epididymides, and vasa deferentia; and determines the presence of hernia or scrotal swelling. In some settings, this may be a function for advanced practitioners only.

Laboratory and Diagnostic Procedures

Disorders of endocrine function are generally caused by hyposecretion (decreased secretion of hormones), hypersecretion (increased secretion of hormones), or resistance of the target cells to the hormone (hormone resistance). Laboratory tests for endocrine function involve measurement of serum and urinary hormone levels and suppression and stimulation of hormones.

The measurement of serum or urinary hormones at any given time may be influenced by a variety of factors, including the half-life of the hormone, circadian rhythm, and clinical factors that influence the metabolism and clearance of hormones (e.g., renal and kidney disease). Radioimmunoassays are an important diagnostic tool in endocrinology, as they allow sensitive, specific, and quantitative measurement of hormones under both steady-state and dynamic conditions (Jameson, 2011). Hormonal measurements need to be interpreted in view of many factors. Although measurement of hormone levels may contribute to the diagnosis of an endocrine disorder, the results may not confirm a diagnosis.

The endocrine disorders, particularly those along the hypothalamic-anterior pituitary-target axis (e.g., adrenal, thyroid, ovarian, testes), are often referred to as primary (target gland), secondary (anterior pituitary), or tertiary (hypothalamus). For example, hypothyroidism can be caused by inadequate production of T_3 and T_4 from the thyroid gland (primary hypothyroidism), inadequate production of TSH from the anterior pituitary (secondary hypothyroidism), and inadequate production of TRH from the hypothalamus (tertiary hypothyroidism). Testing of thyroid function may involve an evaluation of the hypothalamic-anterior pituitary-thyroid gland axis, including measurement of circulating concentrations of TRH, TSH, T_3, and T_4.

If hormone *deficiency* is suspected, a stimulation test may be appropriate. During a stimulation test, the serum concentration of a hormone is measured before and after a stimulus (e.g., a drug) is administered. For example, an ACTH stimulation test may be performed to diagnose adrenal cortical insufficiency. During this test, a baseline measurement of serum cortisol is obtained, a dose of synthetic ACTH is administered, a serum cortisol level is obtained at a specified time, and the change in cortisol from baseline levels is calculated. A failure of the cortisol level to rise appropriately in response to ACTH may indicate primary adrenocortical insufficiency (i.e., the adrenocortical insufficiency is due to dysfunction of the adrenal cortex).

If hormone *excess* is suspected, a suppression test may be appropriate. In suppression testing, a hormone that is known to inhibit a hormone is administered. For example, a glucose suppression test may be performed to aid in the diagnosis of growth hormone excess (e.g., acromegaly or gigantism). During this test, a baseline measurement of serum growth hormone is obtained, 75 to 100 grams of oral glucose are administered, and growth hormone is drawn at specified times following the glucose challenge. Since growth hormone secretion is normally suppressed by hyperglycemia, the failure of the level of growth hormone to decrease during a glucose suppression test aids in the diagnosis of growth hormone excess.

The collection of urine over a longer period of time (e.g., 24 hours) may assist in the diagnosis of endocrine disorders. For example, a 24-hour urine collection for measurement of urinary catecholamines may be useful in the diagnosis of pheochromocytoma, a rare tumor of the adrenal gland. The release of catecholamines in pheochromocytoma may be episodic; therefore, the 24-hour urine collection for catecholamines may provide more information than a random urine or serum measurement.

Radiological Testing

The evaluation of endocrine function may include nuclear medicine studies (e.g., radioiodine [^{123}I] or technetium [99mTc]), computed tomography (CT) scans, magnetic resonance imaging (MRI) scans, and simple x-rays to visualize endocrine glands to assess them for size, atrophy, hypertrophy, or neoplasm.

Nursing Responsibilities During Endocrine Laboratory and Diagnostic Testing

Providing patient education, allaying patients' fears regarding the testing process and ensuring that testing is done appropriately are parts of the nurse's role in diagnostic assessment and evaluation of the endocrine system. Proper preparation for diagnostic testing is essential for ensuring accurate evaluation of endocrine system function. Testing may require special diets, fasting, or use of drugs to assess endocrine functioning. It is the nurse's role to assist the patient in preparing for these tests. The nurse should provide explanations on the purpose and procedures for all diagnostic tests and instruct the patient on the preparation for the test. This may include instructions on medications that should be withheld, foods that should be avoided during testing, and any special laboratory materials needed for specimen collection (e.g., containers for 24-hour urine collections). Special handling of the specimens also may be necessary (e.g., adding acid to the specimen or keeping the specimen on ice). These instructions are provided to the patient/family, and the nurse provides care in handling the specimens.

In relation to the detection of cross-sensitivity between iodinated radiographic contrast material and other iodine-rich substances, the nurse should assess the patient for allergies to iodine, shellfish, or contrast media prior to examination by CT (University of California, San Francisco, 2012). Additionally, pregnancy should be ruled out for female patients before any type of x-ray examination.

Safety Alert *If a patient is receiving a thyroid scan, he will be asked to take a drink or swallow a pill containing iodine. The test is then conducted in approximately 4 hours. It is imperative to let the imaging department know before the patient swallows the iodine if an allergy to iodine is present in order to prevent an adverse reaction to the medication used. If the patient is allergic to iodine, an alternative substance such as technetium may be used (Mathur, 2011).*

If the patient is to have an MRI, the nurse should inquire about claustrophobia, previous surgeries, implantable devices, and any previous injuries involving metals such as gunshot wounds or pellet injuries.

Safety Alert *It is important that the nurse notify the patient who is about to have an MRI of potential hazards if the patient is wearing something made of metal or has an implantation made of metal. A dangerous reaction may occur. The patient should be apprised that the MRI system has a very strong magnetic field that may be hazardous to individuals entering the MRI environment or MRI system room. The powerful magnetic field of the scanner can attract certain metallic objects known as 'ferromagnetic' objects, causing them to move suddenly and with great force toward the center of the MRI system. In order to reduce safety risks to the patient, she is asked to remove anything metallic, electronic, or magnetic that she is wearing. If she has mechanical implants of the same nature, she is asked to notify the individual taking the MRI. This often is done through a screening in which the health care provider asks about anything that might create a health risk or interfere with the imaging. Examples of those items or things that may create a health hazard include a pacemaker; implantable cardioverter defibrillator; neurostimulator; aneurysm clip; metal implant; implanted drug infusion device; foreign metal objects, especially if in or near the eye; shrapnel or bullet wounds; permanent cosmetics or tattoos; dentures/teeth with magnetic keepers; other implants that involve magnets; and medication patches (i.e., transdermal patches) that contain metal, or if they have certain metallic, electronic, magnetic, or mechanical implants, devices, or objects. Therefore, all individuals are required to fill out this form BEFORE entering the MRI environment or MRI system room. All individuals are advised that the MRI system magnet is ALWAYS on (MRIsafety.com, 2012). Steel oxygen tanks should not be allowed in the MRI room as they may be pulled into the machine (MRI Precautions, 2009).*

Safety precautions also need to be taken if the patient is having an MRI with contrast. The contrast material most often used is currently gadolinium contrast medium. This medium generally is very safe; however, it is necessary to question the patient as to whether he had any previous reactions during an MRI scan or if he has other allergies that may make him more reactive to an allergy to the contrast medium. Side effects or reactions are uncommon but may occur. The most common adverse reactions are brief headache, nausea (feeling sick), and dizziness for a brief time following the injection. This occurs in 1% to 5% of contrast injections. Infrequently, a feeling of coldness may occur at the injection site.

Severe (or anaphylactic) reactions are extremely rare. These severe reactions, which may involve difficulty breathing and swelling of the lips and mouth, occur in about 1 in every 10,000 people who have gadolinium (MRIsafety.com, 2012). These severe reactions generally respond very well to emergency drug treatment. This treatment is given while in the MRI department of the hospital or private radiology practice.

In patients with normal kidney function, most of the gadolinium contrast medium injected is almost entirely passed out in the urine within 24 hours. Patients with reduced kidney function or kidney failure (chronic or acute), or reduced function of the liver and kidneys, should not be exposed to this contrast medium. Nephrogenic systemic fibrosis (NSF), a debilitating disease resulting in skin contractures (or localized skin thickening and tightening) and internal organ damage, has occurred with some gadolinium-based contrast agents in a minority of patients who had preexisting severe kidney function abnormalities (MRIsafety.com, 2012).

Gerontological Considerations

The aging process affects nearly every gland in the endocrine system, causing age-related endocrine changes that include alterations in the secretion, circulating levels, metabolism, and biologic activity of hormones. There also is a loss of circadian (a 24-hour period) control of hormone secretion. For example, the hypothalamus is responsible for releasing hormones that stimulate the pituitary gland. During aging, there is either impaired secretion of some hypothalamic hormones or impaired pituitary response. These changes appear to influence the endocrine system's ability to respond to the body's internal environment. As a result, the body cannot respond as well either to internal or external stresses. Production of growth hormone may decrease. This may lead to a hormone imbalance that causes problems such as decreased lean muscle, decreased heart function, and osteoporosis. Aging is known to affect the pituitary gland and a woman's ovaries. These organs exhibit the most common endocrine change related to aging. In menopause, the ovaries stop responding to follicle-stimulating hormone and luteinizing hormone from the anterior pituitary. Ovarian hormone production of

Weblink: Thyroid Blood Tests

Weblink: MRI Information for Patients

Weblink: MRI Safety Information

Weblink: Endocrinology Tests Weblink: Endocrine Disorders Weblink: Endocrine Function

estrogen and progesterone slows down and then stops. Eventually, a woman stops having her periods altogether.

Although most glands decrease their levels of secretion, normal aging usually does not lead to a deficiency state. For example, while the adrenal cortex decreases its secretion of cortisol, negative feedback mechanisms maintain normal plasma levels (The Hormone Foundation, 2011). As the thyroid gland changes, there will be a decrease in the secretion of the thyroid hormones, which will lead to a decrease in the metabolic rate. One of the results from this is an unawareness of temperature. There will be an intolerance to cold, and hot days will not be noticed, thereby increasing the risk of heat stroke. A decrease in the secretion of the growth hormone causes a decrease in the muscle mass and an increase in the storage of fat. Blood and tissue concentrations of many other hormones remain unchanged (TSH, thyroid hormones, ADH, PTH, prolactin, and glucocorticoids).

Despite unchanging hormone levels, some endocrine tissues become less responsive to stimulation. For example, there is less GH (growth hormone) and insulin secreted after a carbohydrate-rich meal or during a glucose tolerance test. Peripheral tissues become less responsive to some hormones, particularly glucocorticoids and ADH. The failure to produce enough glucocorticoids can affect metabolism and produce an inability to deal with stress. In addition, a decline in production will also reduce the anti-inflammatory and immunosuppressive qualities that they give. This means that the elderly are more prone to pain and infections (The Hormone Foundation, 2011).

Increasing age is thought to be related to the development of type 2 diabetes. With aging, the target cell response time becomes slower, especially in people who might be at risk for this disorder. The pituitary gland function peaks in middle age, then gradually shrinks, thereby affecting the production of the hormones which control energy, metabolism, reproduction, and stress response. The pancreas secretes insulin which is critical to the metabolism of glucose. While insulin continues to be produced in sufficient quantities in most older adults, their muscle cells may become less sensitive to the effects of insulin. After age 50, the normal fasting glucose level rises 5 to 14 milligrams per deciliter every 10 years. Adult diabetes, type 2 occurs when the body develops resistance to insulin. It is usually managed through diet, exercise, and oral hypo-glycemic medications. Insulin injections become necessary if people stop producing insulin.

Critical Thinking Related to Assessment Data

Since endocrinology interfaces with multiple physiological systems, there is no standard endocrine history or physical examination (Jameson, 2011). Therefore, it is critical to begin with a thorough history of the patient's chief complaints. Since most glands are relatively inaccessible (with the exception of the thyroid and gonads), the examination needs to focus on the clinical signs and symptoms associated with hormonal excess or deficiency. The patients need to be evaluated in the context of presenting symptoms, review of systems, social and family history, and medication history (Jameson, 2011).

Examples of Data Collection

Data are acquired through the history and physical exam and enhanced with laboratory testing. With endocrine disorders, the history is the most essential piece of data collection. Many times, patients will have a constellation of symptoms that do not clearly fit into one hormone imbalance. The nurse is in a unique position to analyze the data to determine each symptom's relevance to the underlying disorder. Abnormal findings need to be reported to the primary care provider, and then the nurse needs to initiate patient education. With proper education, patients can be empowered to manage and improve their personal health.

Conducting the health history, physical examination, and preparation for and interpretation of laboratory tests and procedures takes experience and practice. It is not enough simply to ask the right questions and perform the physical exam. The nurse must critically analyze all of the data obtained, synthesize the data into a relevant problem focus, and then identify a plan of care for the patient based on this synthesis. Examples of plans of care based on assessment data are found in Chapters 46 and 47.

Health Promotion

Endocrine disorders comprise a number of diverse and distinct health problems. Health promotion in general is based on knowing and identifying the risk factors and overt symptoms of hormonal imbalances. Health promotion activities focus primarily on education regarding potential health risks, diagnostic testing, reproductive health, gender-related health, and the presence of endocrine disruptors,

Potential Health Risks

Patients should be apprised of potential health risks related to hormonal imbalance. These include type 2 diabetes, hypo- and hyperthyroidism, pregnancy issues, menopause, and cardiovascular issues.

Symptoms of Hormonal Imbalances

Symptoms of hormonal imbalances should be made known to the patient and the public. Common symptoms may consist of headache, reactions to temperature changes, dry cracked skin, excess perspiration, changes in mood, confusion or loss of consciousness for even a brief moment, hypotension, bradycardia, dehydration, depression or anxiety, eye problems, fatigue, weakness, and sleep.

Diagnostic Testing

The nurse should explain to the patient the types of tests that may be used to detect endocrine abnormalities, how they work, and what happens during the testing procedure. Diagnostic tests are used to measure the levels of various hormones in a patient's body; to learn if the endocrine glands are working properly; to determine the cause of an endocrinological problem; and to confirm an earlier diagnosis. Typical diagnostic tests and procedures include (BecomeHealthyNow.com. 2010; Dartmouth–Hitchcock, 2012; *Merck Manual*, 2009):

- 24-hour urine collection test
- ACTH stimulation test
- Bone density test
- CTH stimulation test
- Dexamethasone suppression test
- Fine needle aspiration biopsy
- Five-day glucose sensor test (for diabetes)
- HbA1c test (to determine average amount of sugar in blood over the last 2 to 3 months)
- Serum analysis

- Thyroid scan
- TSH blood test
- Comprehensive thyroid assessment
- Menopause Profile
- Adrenal stress index
- Radiological tests, such as nuclear medicine studies, computerized tomography scans, magnetic resonance imaging scans, and simple x-rays.

In addition to educational activities related to endocrine system changes, the patient/family should be advised of the need to complete an annual physical examination. This may alert patients to potential problems. Patients also should be counseled as to when to report aberrant symptoms to the health care provider. A discussion of what an aberrant symptom is needs to take place with the patient and family.

Summary

The endocrine system affects every part and function of the body. Therefore, endocrine disorders can cause changes in almost every bodily system. To discern the system or systems involved, the nurse must carefully assess each system for alterations in function and appearance. Some physical, mental, and emotional changes can be caused by more than one endocrine imbalance. Careful examination and laboratory testing are essential to accurate diagnosis and treatment.

NCLEX® PRACTICE

1. Results of imaging reveal that a 24-year-old female patient has a mass in the posterior pituitary gland. The nurse caring for this patient would monitor for disorders resulting from alterations in which hormones? (select all that apply)

1. Antidiuretic hormone
2. Calcitonin
3. Glucagon
4. Oxytocin
5. Corticotropin-releasing hormone

2. A young athlete states, "I don't know why everyone gets so upset about athletes taking steroids. They occur in our body naturally anyway." Which nursing response is accurate?

1. "Steroids are produced and released as the body needs them."
2. "Taking oral steroids is wasteful as they are eliminated from the gastrointestinal tract before being absorbed by the body."
3. "Introducing additional steroids into the body results in a lack of storage capacity for natural steroids in the endocrine cells."
4. "The only steroids that affect the body cells are those produced by the body."

3. The nurse manager believes that the nursing staff is healthier and provides better care to patients when there is minimal disturbance to the staff's circadian rhythms. Which action, made by the nurse manager, best supports this belief?

1. The manager assigns the same nurse to the same team as much as possible.
2. The manager does not ask staff members to switch shifts.
3. The manager insists staff members take two short breaks and one meal break each shift.
4. The manager does not ask staff members to come in on days off.

4. A nurse is taking a complete history from a patient new to the endocrinology clinic. The patient states, "I just can't do all of the things I used to do. I don't have the energy." The nurse should be aware of other indicators of disorder in which endocrine glands? (select all that apply)

1. Thyroid
2. Pancreas
3. Adrenal
4. Posterior pituitary
5. Parathyroid

5. During initial assessment, the nurse notes that the patient's eyeballs seem large and protuberant. How should the nurse document this finding?

1. As hypophthalmos
2. As Skene's disorder
3. As exophthalmos
4. As torsade

6. A nurse is conducting assessment of a patient in the endocrinology clinic. The skin of the patient's abdomen is blotchy and has multiple silvery, ribbon-like streaks present. The nurse is aware that these findings are most closely associated with which endocrine dysfunction?

1. Thyroid
2. Adrenocorticoid
3. Pancreatic
4. Parathyroid

Answers to NCLEX Practice Questions can be found in Appendix D in the Osborn Student Resources at nursing.pearsonhighered.com. Practice additional NCLEX questions online at the Student Resources site.

REFERENCES

Advocacy. (2011). Society leadership discusses common goals with NIEHS Director Birnbaum. *The Endocrine Society.* Retrieved from http://www.endo-society.org/advocacy/insider/2011/SocietyLeadershipDiscussesCommonGoals.cfm

BecomeHealthyNow.com. (2010). Endocrinology tests. Retrieved from http://www.becomehealthynow.com/category/productslabendo/

Cooper, D. S., & Ladenson, P. W. (2011). The thyroid gland. In D. G. Gardner (Ed.), *Greenspan's basic and clinical endocrinology* (9th ed., pp. 163–226). New York: McGraw-Hill.

Dartmouth-Hitchcock. (2012). Our care. Retrieved from http://patients.darmouth-hitchcock.org/endo/diagnostic_tests_and_procedures.html

Diamanti-Kandarakis, E., J. P., Bourguignon, L.C., Giudice, R., Hauser, G. S., Prins, A. M. Soto, R.T, et al., (2009). Endocrine disrupting chemicals: An Endocrine Society scientific statement, *Endocrine Reviews, 30*(4), 293–342.

Duntas, L. H., Orgiazzi, J., & Brabant, G. (2011). The interface between thyroid and diabetes mellitus. *Clinical Endocrinology.* Blackwell Publishing. Retrieved from www.ncbi.nlm.nih.gov/pubmed/21521298

Gardner, D. G., Anderson, M., & Nissenson, R. A. (2011). Hormones and hormone action. In D. G. Gardner & D. Shoback (Eds.), *Greenspan's basic and clinical endocrinology* (9th ed.). New York: McGraw-Hill.

Huber, A., Menconi, G., Corathers, S., Jacobson, E. M., & Tomer, Y. (2008). Joint genetic susceptibility to type 1 diabetes and autoimmune thyroiditis. *Hormone Research in Pediatrics, 29*(6), 697–725.

Jameson, J. L. (2011). Principles of endocrinology. In J. L. Jameson (Ed.), *Harrison's endocrinology* (pp. 1–14). New York: McGraw-Hill Medical.

Javorsky, B. R., Aron, D. C., Findling, J. W., & Tyrrell, J. B. (2011). Hypothalamus and pituitary gland. In D. G. Gardner & D. Shoback (Eds.), *Greenspan's basic and clinical endocrinology* (9th ed.). New York: McGraw-Hill.

Mathur, T. (2012). Thyroid blood tests. *MedicineNet.com.* Retrieved from http://www.medicinenet.com/thyroid_blood_tests/article.htm

Merck Manual. (2009). Endocrine disorders. Retrieved from http://www.merckmanuals.com/professional/endocrine_and_metabolic_disorders/principl

MRI Precautions. (2009). Gray Television, Inc. Retrieved from http://www.wowt.com/news/features/2/1851351.html

MRIsafety.com. (2012). MRI information for patients. Retrieved from http://www.mrisafety.co/safety_article.asp?subject=170

MRIsafety.com. (2012). MRI contrast agents and adverse reactions. Shellock, R D Services, Inc. Retrieved from http://www.mrisafety.com/safety_article.asp?subject5=172

Porterfield, S. P., & White, B. A. (2007). *Endocrine physiology* (3rd ed.). Philadelphia, PA: Mosby/Elsevier.

The Hormone Foundation. (2011). Endo 101: Factors that affect endocrine function. Retrieved from http://www.hormone.org/Endo101/page5.cfm

Tomer, Y. (2011). Genetic susceptibility to autoimmune endocrine disorders. American Autoimmune. Retrieved from http://www.aardaa.org/infocus_article.php?ID=27

University of California, San Francisco. (2012). Iodine allergy and contrast administration. *Department of Radiology & Biomedical Imaging.* Retrieved from http://www.radiology.ucsf.edu/patient-care/patient-safety/contrast/iodine-allergy

Yeung, S. C. J. (2011). Graves disease. Medscape Reference. Retrieved from http://emedicine.medscape.com/article/120619-overview

Caring for the Patient with Glandular and Hormonal Disorders

46 CHAPTER

Laurie Quinn
Annita Watson

Outcome-Based Learning Objectives

After studying this chapter, the learner will be able to:

1. Distinguish the common pathophysiological syndromes caused by underproduction and overproduction of hormones in the thyroid, parathyroid, pituitary, and adrenal glands and hypothalamus.
2. Analyze clinical manifestations, treatment, and nursing interventions for endocrine disorders.
3. Generate a plan of care for patients with each of the common endocrine gland disorders, including patient teaching and discharge needs.
4. Evaluate gerontological implications for the major endocrine disorders.
5. Determine implications for nursing research when caring for patients with glandular disorders.

KEY TERMS

acromegaly p.1392
acropathy p.1378
adrenal crisis p.1407
amiodarone-induced thyrotoxicosis p.1377
apathetic thyrotoxicosis p.1412
congenital hypothyroidism p.1371
cretinism p.1371
Cushing syndrome p.1410
dermopathy p.1378
diabetes insipidus (DI) p.1397
euthyroid p.1371
gigantism p.1392
goiter p.1371
goitrogens p.1370
Graves' disease p.1377
Hashimoto thyroiditis p.1371
hyperthyroidism p.1377
hypoparathyroidism p.1388
hypopituitarism p.1370
hypothyroidism p.1370
multinodular goiters p.1377
myxedema p.1370
myxedema coma/crisis p.1372
nephrogenic diabetes insipidus p.1397
ophthalmopathy p.1378
parathyroid hormone (PTH) p.1387
parathyroid hyperplasia p.1389
pheochromocytomas p.1402
pretibial myxedema p.1377
primary adrenal insufficiency p.1407
primary hyperaldosteronism (PH) p.1411
secondary adrenal insufficiency p.1407
secondary hyperaldosteronism (SH) p.1411
silent thyroiditis p.1377
subacute thyroiditis p.1377
syndrome of inappropriate ADH secretion (SIADH) p.1399
tetany p.1388
thyroid storm p.1378
thyrotoxicosis p.1377
thyrotoxicosis factitia p.1377
thyroxine (T_4) p.1370
triiodothyronine (T_3) p.1370

THE HUMAN BODY IS A COMPLEX ORGANISM that functions normally in part as a result of exquisite control by the endocrine system. All major organ systems and physiological processes such as growth, homeostasis, regulation of energy, and reproduction are regulated by the endocrine system and its interaction with other body systems (e.g., the nervous system). The general principles of the endocrine system are discussed in Chapter 45. This chapter focuses on disorders of the major endocrine glands: the anterior and posterior pituitary, thyroid, parathyroid, and adrenal glands.

Disorders of Thyroid Function

Disorders of the thyroid gland are among the most common diseases of the endocrine system (The Hormone Foundation, 2012). The majority of these disorders are related to hyperfunctioning or hypofunctioning of the thyroid gland. They can be broadly divided into hypothyroidism and hyperthyroidism. Thyroid disorders are subdivided into primary, secondary, and tertiary disorders. *Primary thyroid disease* is dysfunction occurring in the thyroid gland (excess or deficient thyroid hormone production, resulting in hypothyroidism or hyperthyroidism, respectively). *Secondary thyroid disease* is dysfunction occurring in the anterior pituitary (excess or deficient TSH production, resulting in hyperthyroidism or hypothyroidism, respectively). *Tertiary thyroid disease* is dysfunction occurring in the hypothalamus (excess or deficient TRH production, resulting in hypothyroidism or hyperthyroidism, respectively).

Anatomy and Physiology of the Thyroid Gland

The thyroid gland, which consists of a right and a left lobe connected by an isthmus, is located anterolateral to the trachea (refer back to

Figure 45–3, p. 1363). The normal thyroid gland is approximately 12 to 20 grams in size, soft in consistency, and highly vascularized. The functional unit of the thyroid gland is the thyroid follicle. This follicle contains colloid, which is composed of thyroglobulin, a protein essential for the synthesis of thyroid hormones. The thyroid gland produces two primary hormones: **triiodothyronine (T_3)** and **thyroxine (T_4).** A number of parafollicular cells are scattered throughout the thyroid gland; these are called C cells and secrete a hormone called calcitonin.

Thyroid function is regulated by the hypothalamic–anterior pituitary–thyroid gland axis. Thyroid-releasing hormone (TRH) is released from the hypothalamus; thyroid-stimulating hormone (TSH) is released from the anterior pituitary; and T_3 and T_4 are released from the thyroid gland. Thyroid-releasing hormone stimulates secretion of TSH, which stimulates secretion of T_3 and T_4 (see Figure 46–1◆). The secretion of hormones along the hypothalamic–anterior pituitary–thyroid axis is regulated by negative feedback. *Negative feedback*, as discussed in Chapter 45, is a control mechanism to stop the secretion of TRH and TSH when the body has enough thyroid hormone in the blood (The Hormone Foundation, 2012).

Thyroid hormones have multiple and diverse effects. These hormones are needed for maturation and differentiation; fetal and neonatal brain development; and neurologic function, growth, and metabolism. In addition, thyroid hormone has effects on sympathetic nervous system function, skeletal muscle, cardiovascular function, and reproduction (Porterfield & White, 2007).

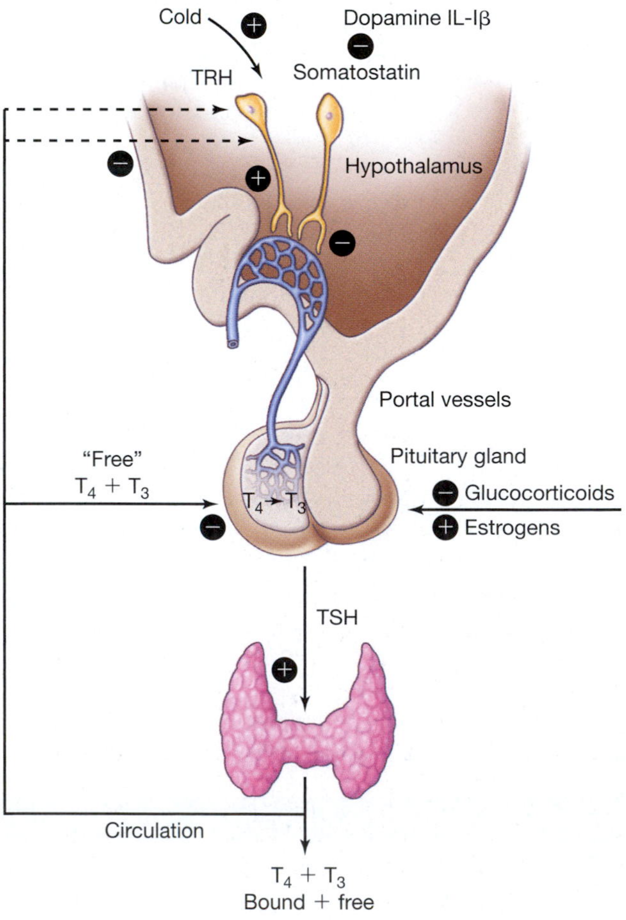

FIGURE 46–1 ◆ Diagram of the hypothalamic–pituitary–thyroid system.

Hypothyroidism

Hypothyroidism, also referred to as **myxedema,** is the condition in which the thyroid gland does not make enough thyroid hormone. As previously defined, this condition can be identified as primary, secondary, or tertiary (Jameson & Weetman, 2010).

Epidemiology and Etiology

The prevalence of hypothyroidism varies depending on the geographic location and environmental factors (iodine and **goitrogens** [foods and drugs that cause suppression of thyroid hormone productions] intake), as well as the genetics and age distribution, of the population (Cooper & Ladenson, 2011). Hypothyroidism is more frequent in older adults. The frequency of overt hypothyroidism has been reported to be approximately 6% in individuals over 65 years of age, with an increased prevalence among women (Bensenor, Goulart, Lotufo, Menezes, & Scazufca, 2011).

The most common cause of hypothyroidism in adults is autoimmune thyroiditis (Hashimoto thyroiditis), in which the immune system attacks the thyroid gland. Globally, the primary cause of hypothyroidism is iodine deficiency and iatrogenic issues (treatment of hyperthyroidism) (Jameson & Weetman, 2010). Other causes of hypothyroidism include pituitary and hypothalamic disease. Hypothyroidism originating from pituitary and hypothalamic disease is often diagnosed in the context of other disorders. Iatrogenic hypothyroidism can be drug-induced (e.g., antithyroid medications) or can occur following treatment (e.g., after iodine treatment) (Jameson & Weetman, 2010). Precipitating causative factors classified as primary, secondary, and tertiary hypothyroidism are listed in Chart 46–1.

Risk factors for hypothyroidism are listed in the Risk Factors box. In addition to those factors listed, excessive iodine intake, especially in someone with autoimmune thyroid disease, may result in hypothyroidism (Cooper & Ladenson, 2011). Genetic considerations for thyroid diseases are discussed in the Genetic Considerations box.

Pathophysiology

Thyroid function is dependent on the presence of two main thyroid hormones, thyroxine and triiodothyronine, which in turn are

CHART 46–1 Causes of Primary, Secondary, and Tertiary Hypothyroidism

Primary	Secondary
Autoimmune hypothyroidism (Hashimoto thyroiditis)	**Hypopituitarism** (e.g., tumors, pituitary surgery, irradiation)
Congenital hypothyroidism	Isolated TSH deficiency
Iatrogenic (e.g., ^{131}iodine treatment for hyperthyroidism, subtotal, or total thyroidectomy; external radiation to neck for cancer treatment)	
Medications (e.g., antithyroid drugs, lithium, amiodarone)	
Iodine deficiency	
Infiltrative disorders (e.g., amyloidosis, sarcoidosis)	

Source: Adapted from Jameson, J. L., & Weetman, A. P. (2010). Disorders of the thyroid gland. In J. L. Jameson (Ed.), *Harrison's endocrinology* (2nd ed., pp. 62–98). New York: McGraw-Hill Medical.

RISK FACTORS for Hypothyroidism

- Familial history of thyroid disease
- History of autoimmune disease
- Aging
- An inadequate supply of dietary iodine
- Previous treatment for hyperthyroidism (e.g., radioactive thyroid hormone, antithyroid drugs and surgeries).

GENETIC CONSIDERATIONS for Thyroid Disease

Patients should be advised of any familial predisposition to thyroid disease based on a family history of thyroid and autoimmune disorders so that other family members can be advised of this particular health risk. There is a genetic contribution to Hashimoto thyroiditis that must be considered when several members of a family have thyroid disease (Jameson & Weetman, 2010).

dependent on iodine to function appropriately. When iodine deficiency occurs, the thyroid is unable to secrete sufficient thyroid hormone. Thus, with an underactive thyroid gland, typically the blood level of T_4 (the main thyroid hormone) will be low, while the TSH level will be high. This means that the thyroid is not making enough hormone; the pituitary then recognizes it and responds appropriately as a compensatory mechanism by making more TSH in an attempt to force more hormone production out of the thyroid (Endocrineweb, 2011).

Thyroid-stimulating hormone is elevated in primary hypothyroidism as the pituitary responds to the relative lack of circulating T_3 and T_4; TSH is abnormal in all clinical and subclinical cases of primary hypothyroidism. As the disease progresses toward clinical or overt hypothyroidism, T_4 and T_3 become measurably decreased. In secondary and tertiary hypothyroidism, TSH, T_4, and T_3 levels are variably abnormal depending on the duration, cause, and severity of the disease. Since TSH is a trophic hormone (a hormone that controls the release of other hormones), a **goiter** (an enlargement of the thyroid gland) occurs. This is termed an endemic goiter, since it is caused by iodine deficiency (Cleveland Clinic, 2011; MedlinePlus, 2010a).

In the more rare case of hypothyroidism due to pituitary failure, the thyroid hormone T_4 will be low, but the TSH level will also be low. The thyroid is behaving "appropriately" under these conditions because it can only make hormone in response to TSH signals from the pituitary. Since the pituitary is not making enough TSH, the thyroid will never make enough T_4. In areas of severe iodine deficiency, there is increased hypothyroidism and **cretinism,** a severe form of hypothyroidism in children characterized by mental and growth retardation (Jameson & Weetman, 2010).

Congenital hypothyroidism, a condition of thyroid hormone deficiency present at birth, can result from a variety of pathophysiological processes. Defects in the anatomic location and structure of the thyroid, such as an ectopic thyroid gland (a gland located somewhere other than the normal position anterior to the laryngeal cartilages), thyroid aplasia (difficulty with language, affecting the ability to speak, read, or write), thyroid agenesis (a rare disorder where the thyroid fails to develop, resulting in hypothyroidism from birth), and thyroid hypoplasia (a rare disease in which the thyroid gland is incomplete, or is totally or partially underdeveloped), are causes of congenital hypothyroidism (Rastogi & LaFranchi, 2010). Inborn errors of metabolism can alter thyroid hormone synthesis, causing hypothyroidism. For example, thyrotropin receptor defects can alter thyroid hormone function, causing hypothyroidism. Additionally, transient hypothyroidism may be caused by maternal thyrotropin-blocking antibodies, maternal antithyroid medications, and iodine deficiency.

Hashimoto thyroiditis is a genetic immunological disease characterized by the development of autoantibodies, particularly directed toward thyroglobulin, resulting in lymphocytic infiltration and fibrosis of the thyroidal tissue. This leads to diminished production of thyroid hormones T_3 and T_4 and the development of hypothyroidism. The genetic relationship of Hashimoto thyroidism is discussed in the Genetic Considerations box.

Clinical Manifestations

The clinical signs and symptoms common to all forms of hypothyroidism are presented in Chart 46–2. The clinical signs and symptoms related to specific disorders are detailed in the following paragraphs. Figure 46–2◆ depicts a patient with hypothyroidism (myxedema).

In addition to the clinical signs and symptoms noted in Chart 46–2, Hashimoto thyroiditis usually presents with a goiter. Initially, the patient may be **euthyroid** (having normal thyroid function) or have mild hypothyroidism. As the hypothyroidism progresses, the patient may exhibit signs and symptoms of hypothyroidism. Hashimoto thyroiditis may be part of a syndrome of autoimmune endocrine diseases

CHART 46–2 Clinical Signs and Symptoms of Hypothyroidism

Signs	Symptoms
Dry skin	Tiredness
Bruising and delayed wound healing	Menstrual abnormalities
Cold extremities	Weakness
Hair loss	Cold intolerance
Bradycardia	Difficulty concentrating
Peripheral edema	Weight gain with poor appetite
Delayed relaxation phase of deep tendon reflexes	Constipation
	Hoarse voice
Carpal tunnel syndrome	

Source: Jameson, J. L., & Weetman, A. P. (2010). Disorders of the thyroid gland. In J. L. Jameson (Ed.), *Harrison's endocrinology* (2nd ed., pp. 62–98). New York: McGraw-Hill Medical.

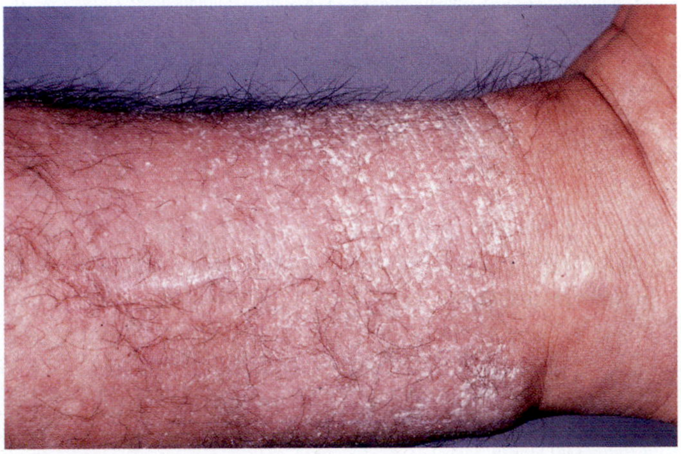

FIGURE 46–2 ◆ Patient with myxedema.
Source: Biophoto Associates/Photo Researchers, Inc.

(e.g., type 1 diabetes, adrenocortical insufficiency, vitiligo, and pernicious anemia) and have coexisting symptoms of these disorders (Jameson & Weetman, 2010).

Myxedema coma/crisis is a manifestation of severe hypothyroidism (Citkowitz, 2011). It is a medical emergency resulting from untreated or inadequately treated hypothyroidism. Patients with myxedema coma/crisis may present with or without coma (the term *myxedema coma* is a misnomer) and the usual clinical signs and symptoms of hypothyroidism, including hyperthermia, but these will be exacerbated (Gardner, 2011). This condition often is precipitated by some event such as infection, trauma, surgery, or neurological disorder in a patient with hypothyroidism.

Safety Alert *Immediately report to the health care provider signs of myxedema, a severe, life-threatening illness with symptoms including facial edema, thick tongue (macroglossia), mental confusion, irritability, severe mood swings, significant hypothermia (91°F to 95°F), severely slowed pulse and respirations, decreased blood pressure, profound neuromuscular weakness, anemia, and signs of psychosis.*

Laboratory and Diagnostic Procedures

Hypothyroidism typically can be diagnosed by measuring the serum-free T_4 and TSH concentrations. The patient with hypothyroidism is likely to have an elevated TSH level and a reduced free thyroxine level (FT_4). Testing for thyroid autoantibodies and measuring serum T_4 and TSH concentrations are usually sufficient to confirm the diagnosis of Hashimoto thyroiditis. Initially, the patient may present with a mildly elevated TSH and normal FT_4. When the disease progresses to overt hypothyroidism, the patient will present with decreased FT_4 and elevated TSH. The most important marker for Hashimoto thyroiditis is the presence of specific autoantibodies in serum, including antithyroid peroxidase antibodies (TPOAb) and antithyroglobulin antibodies (TgAb). Additional tests used to measure thyroid function include nuclear scans, CT scan, MRI, thyroid ultrasound, and needle biopsy with fine needle aspiration. These tests and procedures are discussed more fully in the Laboratory and Diagnostic Tests feature.

Medical Management

The treatment for hypothyroidism involves the replacement of thyroid hormone as indicated by the physiological functioning of the gland. In hypothyroidism, therapeutic actions are directed at stimulating the production of or replacing thyroid hormone. Most patients are treated on an outpatient basis. The synthetic thyroid hormone levothyroxine (T_4) typically is the drug of choice. The daily replacement dose usually is 1.6 µg/kg body weight (1.7 mcg/kg/day) (or approximately 100 to 150 µg or 100 to 125 mcg/day/70 kg). Adults under 60 years of age without cardiac disease may be started on doses of 50 to 100 µg (25 to 50 mcg/day). Initial and maintenance levels may be lower for older adults. The primary goal of treatment is restoration of a normal TSH concentration. Doses of levothyroxine are adjusted on the basis of TSH measurements.

Patients should consult with their pharmacist before combining any prescribed or over-the-counter (OTC) medication with levothyroxine. Other medications (e.g., estrogen, carbamazepine) may increase thyroid hormone requirements and should be considered if there is difficulty in normalizing serum TSH concentrations. Although administration

LABORATORY AND DIAGNOSTIC TESTS for Thyroid Function

Test, Description, Rationale, and Normal Values	Expected Abnormality
Thyroid Antibodies	
Thyroperoxidase antibodies (TPOAb) Antithyroglobulin antibodies (TgAb) *These blood tests are used to diagnose autoimmune hypothyroidism (Hashimoto thyroiditis) and autoimmune hyperthyroidism (Graves' disease). These can be present in both conditions.* Normal adult: Negative to 1:20; *antimicrosomal: Negative to 100.*	Increased (positive) titer indicates the presence of Hashimoto thyroiditis, carcinoma of the thyroid gland, and thyrotoxicosis (Graves' disease).
Thyroxine (T_4)	
A blood test used to assist in the diagnosis of hypothyroidism and hyperthyroidism. Measures both bound and unbound thyroid hormone; therefore, it can be altered by changes in carrier proteins such as thyroid-binding globulin (TBG) (e.g., estrogen-increased TBG during pregnancy) T_4 by column: 4.5–11.5 mcg/dL. T_4: (RIA): 5–12 mcg/dL Free T_4: 1.0–2.3 ng/dL Reported as thyroxine iodine: $T_{4\ by}$ column: 3.2–7.2 mcg/dL. Free thyroxin (FT_4) is more reflective of metabolic status.	Decreased level indicates hypothyroidism (cretinism, myxedema, and anterior pituitary hypofunction). Increased level indicates hyperthyroidism or acute thyroiditis. Elevated in Graves' disease.
Triiodothyronine (T_3)	
A blood test used to assist in the diagnosis of hypothyroidism and hyperthyroidism. It measures both bound and unbound thyroid hormone; therefore, it can be altered by changes in carrier proteins such as thyroid-binding globulin (TBG) (e.g., estrogen-increased TBG during pregnancy) and is more reflective of metabolic status. Normal adult value: 80–200 ng/dL	Decreased level indicates malnutrition, severe acute illness, and trauma. Increased level indicates T_3 thyrotoxicosis, Hashimoto thyroiditis, or toxic adenoma. Elevated in Graves' disease. Decreased level indicates hypothyroidism and thyroiditis. Increased level indicates hyperthyroidism.

LABORATORY AND DIAGNOSTIC TESTS for Thyroid Function, *continued*

Test, Description, Rationale, and Normal Values	Expected Abnormality
Free triiodothyronine (FT_3), also referred to as triiodothyronine resin uptake, is a blood test used to differentiate between hypo- or hyperthyroidism and to compare test results with T_3 to determine thyroid disorder. Normal adult: 25–35 relative percentage uptake.	
Thyroid-Stimulating Hormone (TSH) *A blood test used to suggest secondary hypothyroidism due to pituitary involvement.* Normal adult: 0.35–5.5 microinternational unit/mL.	Decreased level indicates secondary hypothyroidism with pituitary gland involvement, as well as anterior pituitary hypofunction. Increased level indicates primary hypothyroidism (thyroid gland involvement with a decreased T_4) thyroiditis (Hashimoto disease). Suppressed in Graves' disease.
Free Thyroxine Index (FTI) *This is a mathematical approximation of free T_4 using serum T_4 and thyroid-binding ratio (THBR). Results may be changed by drugs or physical conditions that alter the patient's thyroxine-binding globulin levels, or drugs that compete with endogenous T_4 and triiodothyronine (T_3) for protein-binding sites.* Normal: Free thyroxine index: 4–11.	Increased levels of FTI indicate hyperthyroidism. Decreased levels of FTI in hypothyroidism.
Radioactive Iodine Uptake (RAIU) *Measures concentration of radioactive iodine in the thyroid following oral ingestion of radioactive iodine. A scintillation counter is used to measure the uptake level of the RAIU.* This reflects the activity of the thyroid gland. Normal: Adult: 2 hours: 1–13% (thyroid gland); 6 hours: 2–25% (thyroid gland); 24 hours: 15–45% (thyroid gland).	Differentiates types of thyroidism. Decreased level indicates hypothyroidism (myxedema). Increased level indicates hyperthyroidism (Graves' disease) and thyroiditis. Can be helpful in diagnosing thyroid adenomas.
Scanning Devices Nuclear Scan/Radioactive Iodine Update (RAE-U) (radionuclide scan). *This scan is used to detect Graves' disease or an overactive thyroid gland.* The patient is given a small dose of radioactive iodine 124 in pill form. Several hours later, the amount of iodine in the bloodstream is measured. Normal: Thyroid gland of normal size, shape, and position.	In Graves' disease, the RAIU is elevated, and the entire gland becomes hot. In Hashimoto thyroiditis, the uptake is usually low, with patchy hot spots in the gland.
Computerized Tomography Scan (CT) *Used to evaluate the thyroid by detecting a goiter or larger thyroid nodules. It does not detect smaller nodules.* Normal: No evidence of goiter or large thyroid nodules.	Presence of goiter or large thyroid nodules.
Magnetic Resonance Imaging (MRI) *Used to detect size and shape of thyroid. It detects enlargement.* Normal: No enlargement of thyroid gland noted.	Abnormal size and shape of thyroid gland.
Ultrasound *Ultrasound of the thyroid is done to evaluate nodules, lumps, and enlargement of the gland. It is also used to detect whether a nodule is a fluid-filled cyst, or a mass of solid tissue.* Normal: No evidence of cysts, lumps, or gland enlargement.	Presence of cysts, masses, or enlarged gland.
Fine Needle Aspiration Biopsy *A fine needle aspiration biopsy is a procedure to remove thyroid cells to diagnose thyroid disease or thyroid cancer from palpable masses.* Normal: Thyroid tissue is normal in structure and the cells appear noncancerous under a microscope.	Abnormalities may represent diffuse thyroid disease such as a goiter or thyroiditis, noncancerous tumors, or thyroid cancer.

Sources: Anvita Health Wiki. (2012). Free thyroxine index (fT_4I). Retrieved from http://www.anvita.info/wiki/Free_Thyroxine_Index; Jameson, J. L., & Weetman, A. P. (2010). Disorders of the thyroid gland. In J. L. Jameson (Ed.), *Harrison's endocrinology* (2nd ed., pp. 62–98). New York: McGraw-Hill Medical; Kee, J. L. (2010). *Laboratory and diagnostic tests with nursing implications.* Upper Saddle River, NJ: Prentice Hall. Mayo Clinic, Mayo Medical Laboratories. (2012). Interpretive handbook. Retrieved from http://www.mayomedicallaboratories.com/interpretive-guide/index.html?alpha=F&unit_co...; MedlinePlus. (2010b). Growth hormone suppression test. Retrieved from http://www.nlm.nih.gov/medlineplus/ency/article/003376.htm; MedlinePlus. (2010c). T_3 test. Retrieved from http://www.nlm.nih.gov/medlineplus/ency/article/003687.htm.

of levothyroxine will bring thyroid hormone levels within normal limits, it may suppress TSH, which increases the risk of osteoporosis, a side effect that can be avoided by the ingestion of calcium carbonate. However, if the two preparations are taken together, the calcium can interfere with the absorption of thyroid hormone. Thus, patients should be advised to take any OTC vitamins, minerals, and antacids at least 4 hours earlier or later than thyroid hormone. Patients also need to be advised that they will be taking thyroid replacement hormone for life.

Treatment for myxedema coma/crisis includes supportive care (e.g., therapeutic warming), administration of intravenous fluids, administration of intravenous thyroid hormone, and recognition of signs and symptoms of further medical decompensation (e.g., cardiopulmonary failure). Many of these patients require intubation and mechanical ventilation (discussed in Chapter 28).

Nursing Management

Nursing care for patients with hypothyroidism is guided by the severity of the disease process and related symptoms. The nurse records the patient's signs and symptoms both during diagnosis and following treatment. Nursing care is directed at symptom management and improvement of the patient's physiological status using hormone replacement therapy. In the event of a myxedema crisis, the nurse, in consultation with the health care provider, needs to ensure respiratory support with administration of oxygen and ventilation, if needed. Additionally, intravenous fluids must be administered with caution, observing for plural effusion and congestive heart failure. The nurse needs to be prepared to administer fast-acting intravenous thyroid hormone to restore the body's thyroxine level. In addition, the patient must be slowly rewarmed to avoid causing refractory hypotension and increased oxygen demand. The patient also must be monitored for infection. See the Nursing Process: Patient Care Plan for Hypothyroidism, which details the nursing process used in caring for patients with hypothyroidism.

Discharge Priorities

Discharge priorities for the patient with hypothyroidism include ensuring that the patient understands the need for lifelong hormone replacement therapy and annual monitoring of hormone levels once a stable, therapeutic level of hormone has been reached. Some authorities advise patients to be wary of changing brands or suppliers of hormone replacement drugs because of the variability in bioavailability of the drug in different products (American Thyroid Association, 2010). If the brand name drug or generic drug is changed, the patient should be retested about 6 weeks after starting on the new medication (American Thyroid Association, 2010). Consultation with an endocrine specialist is advised, particularly if the patient is diabetic or pregnant. Specific teaching and discharge priorities are shown in the Patient Teaching & Discharge Priorities box.

NURSING PROCESS: Patient Care Plan for Hypothyroidism

Assessment of Endocrine Status Using Gordon's Functional Health Patterns:

- Nutrition Metabolic Pattern
- Elimination Pattern
- Activity Exercise Pattern
- Cognitive Perceptual Pattern

Subjective Data

Assessment of Current Body Characteristics

Is your pulse slower than normal?

Has your weight changed (increased or decreased) in recent months?

Do you feel energetic or fatigued much of the time? Are you sleeping a great deal but still feeling tired?

Has there been any change in your activity tolerance?

How would you describe your mental alertness and memory?

Describe your menstrual pattern. Has there been any change in the frequency or flow during your menstrual periods?

Assessment of Skin and Nail Characteristics and Wound Healing

Have you noticed any change in your skin, hair, or nails lately?

Are your nails brittle, thick, and often breaking or splitting?

Is your skin cold, dry, or itchy? Do you bruise easily? Do wounds heal slowly?

Assessment of Gastrointestinal Function and Disturbances

Have you observed any changes in your bowel habits?

Have you experienced frequent constipation or abdominal pain?

Is your cholesterol high?

Objective Data

Assessment of Current Body Characteristics

Weight gain

Edema around eyes and facial puffiness

Thick tongue

Bradycardia and dyspnea

Low body temperature

Enlargement of the thyroid gland (goiter)

TSH level high

FT_4 low

Unable to process thoughts rapidly

Assessment of Skin and Nail Characteristics and Wound Healing

Skin cool and dry

Evidence of itching skin

Brittle nails

Hair dry, sparse, coarse, and brittle

Generalized interstitial edema

Assessment of Gastrointestinal Function and Disturbances

Abdomen distended

Bowel sounds decreased

Weight gain

Increased TSH level

Decreased T_4

Presence of thyroid antibodies

NURSING PROCESS: Patient Care Plan for Hypothyroidism, *continued*

Assessment for Hypothermia	**Assessment for Hypothermia**
Are you feeling too cold or too hot? Do you feel anxious or restless?	Wearing multiple layers of clothing Cool and dry skin Hypothermia (in severe myxedema) with low body temperature
Assessment of Cognition Level and Memory Impairment	**Assessment of Cognition Level and Memory Impairment**
Do you feel mentally alert? Are your thought processes slowed? Is your short- or long-term memory impaired? Are you irritable or confused?	Responds appropriately to questions Able to follow directions Recalls objects when asked to Recognizes individuals by name and/or position

Outcomes and Evaluation Parameters	Planning and Interventions with *Rationales*
1. NURSING DIAGNOSIS: Fatigue and Activity Intolerance *related to hypometabolic state with decreased cardiac output* (NANDA-I © 2012)	
Outcome: Patient is able to manage self-care and explain rationale for therapeutic plan, including medication regime and instructions. ***Evaluation Parameters:*** Patient is able to repeat instructions for taking medications and can describe symptoms of both hypo- and hyperthyroidism. TSH and FT_4 levels return to normal range. **Outcome:** Patient does not use sedatives or opiates during the acute phase of the illness. ***Evaluation Parameter:*** Patient and health care team express awareness of the risks associated with the use of sedatives, opiates, or alcohol.	Instruct the patient on administration of hormone replacement medication, signs and symptoms of hypo- and hyperthyroidism, and self-care practices. *To ensure patient takes hormone replacement medication on an empty stomach for optimal absorption. To inform patient to be alert for signs of hypo- or hyperthyroidism.* Patient and health care providers are warned to avoid use of sedatives, opioids, analgesic medications, or alcohol products, which would further depress metabolic functions and increase risk of myxedema crisis. *To prevent further suppression of the patient's metabolic state and possible serious complications such as coma, particularly in the elderly.*
2. NURSING DIAGNOSIS: Risk for Impaired Skin Integrity *related to thyroid hormone deficiency* (NANDA-I © 2012)	
Outcome: Verbalizes satisfaction with improved condition of skin, hair, and nails, with less itching and breaking. ***Evaluation Parameters:*** Skin intact, soft, and moist with no evidence of patient itching or scratching. Patient's hair is soft and thick.	Avoid use of soaps, astringents, or other agents such as alcohol. Liberally apply emollient skin lotion. Consider using an alternating air mattress if needed. *To counteract drying of skin, hair, and nails due to hormone loss and to protect skin from injury.*
3. NURSING DIAGNOSIS: Constipation *related to lethargy, activity intolerance, and hypometabolic state* (NANDA-I © 2012)	
Outcome: Observed bowel function is normal with no reports of constipation or abdominal pain. ***Evaluation Parameters:*** Abdomen soft, not distended. Active bowel sounds. Patient's normal bowel pattern is resumed.	Administer stool softeners as prescribed. Gradually increase fluid intake and fiber in diet. Increase activity level with short, frequent walks and mild exercise. *To maintain or regain normal bowel function and to prevent bowel obstruction or megacolon.*
4. NURSING DIAGNOSIS: Hypothermia *related to metabolic dysfunction* (NANDA-I © 2012)	
Outcome: Patient is able to tolerate typical ambient temperatures without distress. ***Evaluation Parameters:*** Body temperature is within normal range. Patient appears comfortable with no reports of distress related to ambient temperature.	Monitor the environment to provide a warm room for patient comfort. *To minimize patient discomfort while the patient's body is adapting to the stabilization of hormone levels.*
5. NURSING DIAGNOSIS: Confusion, Acute *related to hypothyroidism* (NANDA-I © 2012)	
Outcomes: Patient oriented to time, place, and circumstances. Able to recall instructions regarding medications and activity prescriptions. Mood is stable. ***Evaluation Parameters:*** Alert and oriented. Evidence of effective short- and long-term memory. Family reports stable affect and mood.	Reduce stimuli and mental demands while hormone deficiency is replaced. Instruct family about potential mood swings, depression, and irritability. Provide instructions to the patient and family in writing as well as orally. *To minimize distress and disorientation while the patient's body is adapting to stabilization of hormone levels.*

Source: Adapted from Wilkinson, J. M., & Ahearn, N. R. (2009). *Prentice Hall nursing diagnosis handbook* (9th ed.). Upper Saddle River, NJ: Prentice Hall.

PATIENT TEACHING & DISCHARGE PRIORITIES for Hypothyroidism

Need	Teaching
Knowledge of disease process	Follow-up care, and ways of adjusting lifestyle patterns to conserve energy, are provided, with the understanding that hypothyroidism usually is a lifelong process.
Patient and family understanding of medication	The patient and family are taught to administer medications according to the established time schedule. Teach the purpose, dose, and possible side effects of all medications to increase compliance. Caution the patient to take medication on an empty stomach first thing in the morning, usually 30 minutes to 1 hour before breakfast, to avoid a reaction with another medication or food as they may affect the medication's absorption. Advise of foods that should be avoided if the patient is taking levothyroxine, fiber, and common daily supplements such as calcium. Advise the patient to notify the health care provider if there are changes in her health or diet, if she is taking new medications for other conditions, or if she is switching brands, as these changes can cause changes in thyroid hormone levels that require different medication doses. If patients change dose levels or thyroxine brands, they should be checked again at least 6 weeks later. Advise the patient to notify the health care provider if there is no symptom improvement when normal thyroid levels are reached; or when overdosing occurs. When overdosed, hyperthyroidism occurs and the patient is at a higher risk for abnormal heart rhythms, rapid heartbeat, and heart failure.
Disease prevention	Explain the need for follow-up checks with the health care provider to ensure that the medication dosage is correct, for a minimum of 6 to 12 months.
Patient and family	Instruct the patient and family on possible complications due to low production of thyroid hormones: goiter and enlarged heart (which may include shortness of breath, chest pain, general fatigue, an irregular heartbeat, and edema), as well as depression (Mayo Clinic Staff, 2011). Advise the patient and family of symptoms of myxedema crisis which may be triggered by stress or illness: extreme sensitivity to cold, unusual drowsiness, loss of consciousness, and decreased heart rate, blood pressure, and breathing. Instruct the patient and family to seek emergency care if any of these symptoms occur.
Cognition	Evaluate the patient's cognitive ability; if the patient is having difficulty problem solving or pursuing normal activities, based on knowing how to do them, instruct her to notify the health care provider.
Comfort and fatigue	Instruct the patient on ways to achieve physical comfort and prevent fatigue from occurring: maintain temperature of the environment, wear comfortable clothing suited to the immediate environment, and space and limit activities to prevent becoming overtired.
Emotional support of patient and family due to chronicity of disease	Answer questions regarding the disease condition. Reinforce lifelong commitment to taking medication. Explore the patient's feelings and concerns about this. Recommend community and Internet support groups or counseling as appropriate.

Health Promotion

Health promotion for patients with hypothyroidism most often revolves around instruction regarding medications for hormone replacement therapy since therapy will be required for the remainder of the patient's lifetime. Some patients find the notion of lifetime drug therapy difficult to accept. For this reason, the nurse should assess the patient's understanding of the disorder and the need for hormone replacement therapy. Other considerations include the patient's diet and activity. The thyroid gland requires iodine to manufacture thyroid hormone. Therefore, patients should be encouraged to eat a healthy diet, to purchase salt enhanced with iodine, and to ensure that iodine is ingested regularly. Relative to activity, patients should be advised that when thyroid medication is fully adjusted they should be able to resume a normal life and have a normal life expectancy; however, they should be cautioned that this may take some time after the initial doses. Most people need to build up the medication gradually until they reach a maintenance dose, increasing the dose in 3- to 4-week periods until thyroid hormone levels are normal.

Patients also should be advised of potential complications that may develop from taking too little or too much medication, as enumerated on the Patient Teaching & Discharge Priorities table. One complication that requires immediate attention is myxedema coma/crisis. They also should be advised of all of the other patient concerns and teaching areas reflected on the Patient Teaching & Discharge Priorities table.

Collaborative Management

Depending on the severity of the hypothyroidism, the patient with thyroid disease will benefit from the support of several members of the health care team. In order to meet desired patient outcomes, it is essential that this interdisciplinary team communicate openly with one another in developing and evaluating care of the patient and family (IOM [Institute of Medicine], 2010). Following diagnosis, the patient with hypothyroidism may benefit from instruction by the pharmacist regarding medication for replacement of thyroid hormone and medications to treat other symptoms such as anemia. The nutritionist or dietitian can provide helpful consultation on a healthy diet to address the hypometabolic needs of the patient's body during therapy until the patient becomes euthyroid. Patients should remain in continuous contact with their health care providers for assessment of medication dosage and response to the medication. The nurse remains focused on providing nursing care based on educational needs and the provision of emotional support when needed.

Hyperthyroidism and Thyrotoxicosis

Hyperthyroidism, a condition in which there is excess production of thyroid hormone, is caused by an increase in thyroid function for any reason. This condition may lead to **thyrotoxicosis,** a clinical syndrome that results when tissues are exposed to high levels of circulating thyroid hormone (Cooper & Ladenson, 2011).

Epidemiology and Etiology

The overall incidence of hyperthyroidism is estimated between 0.05% and 1.3%, with the majority consisting of subclinical disease. White and Hispanic populations in the United States have a slightly higher prevalence of hyperthyroidism in comparisons with Black populations. There also is a slight predominance of hyperthyroidism in females (Schraga, 2010).

The term *thyrotoxicosis* describes an excessive amount of circulating thyroid hormone; it is not synonymous with hyperthyroidism. Increased levels of hormone can occur despite normal thyroid function, such as in instances of inappropriate exogenous thyroid hormone or extreme release of stored hormone from an inflamed thyroid gland (Schraga, 2010).

A variety of conditions can cause thyrotoxicosis, including Graves' disease, toxic adenoma, toxic multinodular goiter, subacute thyroiditis, silent thyroiditis, drug-induced thyrotoxicosis, and thyrotoxicosis factitia (Cooper & Ladenson, 2011). Graves' disease accounts for approximately 60% to 70% of all cases of thyrotoxicosis, with the prevalence varying by population (Jameson & Weetman, 2010). The disease can occur at any age; however, the peak incidence is in the 20- to 40-year age group (Cooper & Ladenson, 2011). There is a strong genetic predisposition for Graves' disease; in fact, approximately 15% of patients with Graves' disease have a close relative with the disorder (Cooper & Ladenson, 2011).

Thyroid storm, a rare and potentially fatal complication of hyperthyroidism, typically occurs in patients with untreated or partially treated thyrotoxicosis who experience a precipitating event such as surgery, infection, or trauma. This phenomenon may occur at any age, but is most common in those in their third through sixth decades of life, and it predominantly affects those ages 20 to 40 years (Schraga, 2010).

Risk factors in the development of hyperthyroidism and thyrotoxicosis are listed in the Risk Factors box. The role of these factors in the development of hyperthyroidism is discussed in the following text.

Pathophysiology

Hyperthyroidism is a condition in which excessive levels of thyroid hormone stimulate the body's metabolic processes. In hyperthyroidism, serum T_3 usually increases more than does T_4, probably because of increased secretion of T_3 as well as conversion of T_4 to T_3 in peripheral tissues. In some patients, only T_3 is elevated (T_3 toxicosis). T_3 toxicosis may occur in any of the usual disorders that cause hyperthyroidism, including Graves' disease, multinodular goiter, and the autonomously functioning solitary thyroid nodule. If T_3 toxicosis is untreated, the patient usually also develops laboratory abnormalities typical of hyperthyroidism (i.e., elevated T_4 and ^{123}I uptake). The various forms of thyroiditis commonly have a hyperthyroid phase followed by a hypothyroid phase.

Thyrotoxicosis is an inclusive term that describes severe hypermetabolic conditions caused by the thyroid hormones. The pathophysiology of thyrotoxicosis varies dependent on the causative factor/s of the condition. **Graves' disease,** the most common cause of thyrotoxicosis, is an autoimmune disease of unknown cause. The T lymphocytes become sensitized to antigens in the thyroid gland during the development of Graves' disease and stimulate B lymphocytes to produce antibodies (IgGs) to these antigens (Porterfield & White, 2007). Additionally, antibodies are produced to the TSH receptor; these antibodies mimic the actions of TSH on TSH receptors, promoting growth and vascularity of the gland (Porterfield & White, 2007).

In toxic adenomas, there is autonomous hypersecretion of T_3 and T_4 from a functioning adenoma (i.e., a benign tumor of glandular origin). The pathologic process begins as a small functioning nodule that increases in size to produce excessive amounts of T_3 and T_4. The endogenous secretion of TSH is suppressed (Bauer & McPhee, 2010). As a result, there is reduced function of the contralateral thyroid lobe. Physical examination reveals a nodule on one lobe, with decreased thyroid tissue on the other side (Bauer & McPhee, 2010).

Multinodular goiters (multiple growths leading to enlargement of the total thyroid gland) may result in thyrotoxicosis if one of the nodules becomes autonomous from TSH regulation and excretes excessive amounts of T_3 and T_4 (Bauer & McPhee, 2010). This usually occurs in patients with long-standing multinodular goiter. Physical examination reveals a multinodular goiter of varying sizes. A condition called Jod-Basedow phenomenon, which is an iodine-induced thyrotoxicosis, can be seen in patients with multinodular goiter when they are given an iodine load (such as following a diagnostic test using radioiodine contrast media) (Jameson & Weetman, 2010).

Subacute thyroiditis and *silent thyroiditis* involve inflammation of the thyroid gland. Subacute thyroiditis (de Quervain thyroiditis) or silent thyroiditis may present with symptoms of mild to severe thyrotoxicosis following an acute release of T_3 and T_4. **Subacute thyroiditis** may follow an upper respiratory infection; the thyroid is tender, painful, and minimally enlarged. **Silent thyroiditis** is associated with an infiltrative process in the thyroid gland; the thyroid may be normal or slightly enlarged without tenderness or pain.

Amiodarone-induced thyrotoxicosis results from treatment with amiodarone, an antiarrhythmic drug that contains approximately 37% iodine by weight (Bauer & McPhee, 2010). In some patients, the thyrotoxicosis results from excessive iodine; in others, the thyrotoxicosis results from thyroiditis, which causes a release of T_3 and T_4.

Thyrotoxicosis factitia is a psychoneurotic disorder in which the patient induces thyroiditis by taking large quantities of T_4 hormone replacement (e.g., levothyroxine), usually for the purposes of losing weight. The patient is often female and a member of the health care field who can obtain thyroid medications easily (Bauer & McPhee, 2010).

RISK FACTORS for the Development of Hyperthyroidism and Thyrotoxicosis

- Personal or family history of thyroid or other autoimmune disease
- Recent pregnancy
- Exposure to excess iodine
- Medications (e.g., amiodarone).

Clinical Manifestations

The clinical signs and symptoms associated with hyperthyroidism, regardless of the cause, are listed in Chart 46–3. A number of clinical signs and symptoms are more specific to Graves' disease. Graves' disease is associated with one or more of the following features: goiter (often 2 to 3 times the normal size), exophthalmos (an abnormal protrusion of the eyeball), and **pretibial myxedema** (thickening of the skin commonly

CHART 46–3 Clinical Signs and Symptoms of Hyperthyroidism

Signs	Symptoms
Tachycardia	Hyperactivity
Atrial fibrillation	Irritability
Tremors	Dysphoria
Goiter	Heat intolerance
Warm, moist skin	Dyspnea on exertion
Proximal muscle weakness	Muscle cramps in back and lower extremities
Hyperreflexia	Weakness and fatigue
Eye changes: lid lag or retraction; stare, exophthalmos	Weight loss with increased appetite
Cornea erosion	Sight loss
Preorbital edema	Diplopia
Hair loss	Diarrhea
Thyroid **dermopathy** (skin disorder, also referred to as pretibial myxedema), inflamed indurated plaque with deep pink or purple color, and orange skin appearance.	
Acropathy – clubbing of hands and toes	

Sources: Adapted from Cooper, D. S., & Ladenson, P. W. (2011). The thyroid gland. In D. G. Gardner (Ed.), *Greenspan's basic and clinical endocrinology* (9th ed., pp. 163–226). New York: McGraw-Hill; Jameson, J. L., & Weetman, A. P. (2010). Disorders of the thyroid gland. In J. L. Jameson (Ed.), *Harrison's endocrinology* (2nd ed., pp. 62–98). New York: McGraw-Hill Medical.

over the anterior and lateral aspects of the lower legs) (Figure 46–2). In addition, a thrill (palpable increased blood flow in the thyroid) or a bruit (sound of increased blood flow in the thyroid) may be present on the thyroid gland, reflecting increased vascularity of the gland. **Ophthalmopathy** is often present in patients with Graves' disease and is characterized by eye changes that may include lid lag and retraction, periorbital edema, exophthalmos, diplopia (double vision), corneal involvement, and sight loss. A patient with Graves' disease is depicted in Figure 46–3◆.

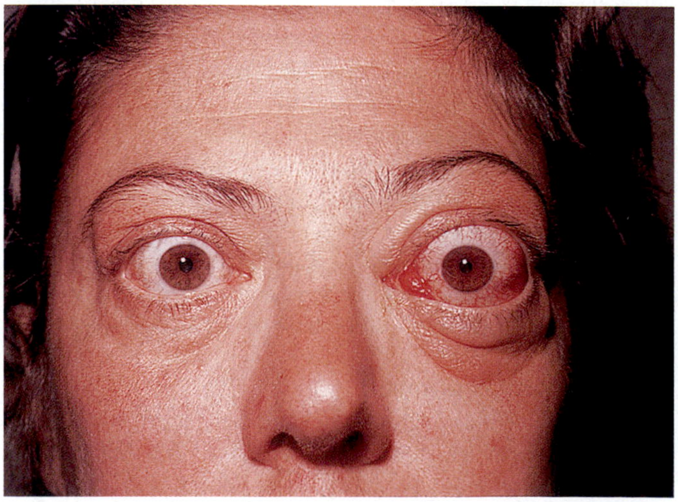

FIGURE 46–3 ◆ Patient with Graves' disease.
Source: Custom Medical Stock Photo, Inc.

Laboratory and Diagnostic Procedures

A combination of a suppressed TSH with an elevated FT_4 confirms the diagnosis of hyperthyroidism. The laboratory diagnosis of Graves' disease includes an elevated FT_4 and a suppressed TSH; however, the presence of thyroid peroxidase (TPO) antibodies helps to confirm the diagnosis. Approximately 5% of patients have a normal FT_4 but an elevated FT_3 in combination with a suppressed TSH. This condition is referred to as T_3 thyrotoxicosis.

The radioactive iodine uptake (RAIU) test may be used to help differentiate the etiology of hyperthyroidism. All tests are described in the Laboratory and Diagnostic Tests for Thyroid Function box (p. 1372).

Medical Management

Once the patient is diagnosed with Graves' disease, he must choose among the following three effective and safe initial treatment options: antithyroid drugs (ATDs), thyroidectomy, and ^{131}I (radioactive iodine) therapy.

Other factors influence the initial choice of therapy for the patient with Graves' disease. For example, radioactive ^{131}I therapy may be indicated for women planning a pregnancy in the future (Bahn et al., 2011). This is because treating hyperthyroidism during pregnancy without affecting the baby can be risky; it is usually best for women who plan to have children in the near future to have their thyroid condition permanently cured. Radioactive iodine is the most widely recommended permanent treatment (Endocrineweb, 2011). Treatment with radioactive iodine also is recommended for individuals with comorbidities that increase surgical risk, as well as those with previous surgery or radiation to the neck. Antithyroid drugs (ATDs) may be indicated for patients with a high likelihood of remission, older adults, or others with comorbidities that increase surgical risk or provide limited life expectancy. Surgery may be indicated for patients with symptomatic compression or large goiters (> 80 g) or when thyroid malignancy is documented or suspected (Bahn et al., 2011). (See the Pharmacology Summary of Medications Used to Treat Endocrine Disorders.)

Certain radiation procedures are necessary for the first few days following treatment with radioactive iodine. However, the exact guidelines vary among health care institutions. In general, patients are asked to avoid close and prolonged contact with children and pregnant women for several days following the procedure (Jameson & Weetman, 2010). This helps to prevent any transmission of residual isotope and radiation exposure from the thyroid gland in these two vulnerable populations (Jameson & Weetman, 2010).

If surgery is chosen as the initial therapy, a total or near-total thyroidectomy is the treatment of choice (Bahn et al., 2011). Complications of surgery can include bleeding, laryngeal edema, hypoparathyroidism, and injury to the laryngeal nerves; however, the more highly skilled and experienced is the team performing the surgery, the lower the rate of complications (Jameson & Weetman, 2010). Patients with significant comorbidities (e.g., severe cardiopulmonary disease, end-stage cancer) may not be appropriate candidates for surgery as they tend to have a poorer prognosis with higher morbidity and mortality (Bahn et al., 2011).

Complications

Thyroid storm is a life-threatening condition characterized by an exacerbation of all of the signs and symptoms of hyperthyroidism. Thyroid storm may occur in a patient with a history of Graves' disease who has discontinued the antithyroid medication or in a patient who has undiagnosed hyperthyroidism. The patient may present with a fever (a temperature $>$ 104°F), diaphoresis (profuse sweating), tachycardia,

PHARMACOLOGY Summary of Medications Used to Treat Endocrine Disorders

Medication Category and Action	Application/Indication	Nursing Responsibility
LEVOTHYROXINE		
Action: Converts to T_3 with actions identical to endogenous thyroid hormone. Increases the metabolic rate, thereby increasing oxygen consumption, respiration, and heart rate; increases the rate of fat, protein, and carbohydrate metabolism; and promotes growth and maturation.	Used to treat primary, secondary, and congenital hypothyroidism. Also used to treat a hypothyroid state resulting from the surgical removal of the thyroid gland, radiation, or antithyroid drugs.	Obtain a baseline weight, assess for allergies, and evaluate possible drug interactions. Monitor electrocardiogram and laboratory studies including serum T_4, T_3, and TSH levels. Monitor patient's pulse rate before each oral dose during dose adjustment periods; if the heart rate is faster than 100 beats per minute, hold the medication and contact the health care provider. Assess periodically for symptoms of hyperthyroidism and hypothyroidism. Monitor older adults during dose adjustments for angina, dysrhythmias, heart failure, and other cardiac adverse effects. Monitor patients who are taking anticoagulants for bleeding, and obtain regular laboratory results. Monitor blood glucose levels if the patient is diabetic because adjustment of antidiabetic drugs' doses may be required.
ESTROGEN		
(Hormone replacement therapy) ***Action:*** Conjugated estrogens bind to intracellular estrogen receptors that stimulate deoxyribonucleic acid (DNA) and ribonucleic acid (RNA) to synthesize proteins responsible for the biologic effects of estrogens.	May increase thyroid hormone requirements and should be considered for use if there is difficulty in normalizing serum TSH concentrations.	Obtain a drug history to determine possible drug interactions and allergies. Determine if the patient is pregnant or lactating prior to drug administration. Evaluate the patient's response to treatment; notify the prescriber of adverse symptoms such as breakthrough bleeding, excessive fluid retention, leg cramps, vomiting, diarrhea, or bloating.
CARBAMAZEPINE		
An antiepileptic drug ***Action:*** Affects the sodium channels in cortical neurons, slowing the propagation and spread of repetitive action potentials, which is characteristic of epilepsy.	Used to treat seizures and nerve pain such as trigeminal neuralgia and diabetic neuropathy. It also is used to treat bipolar disorder. Off label, it is used to treat central partial diabetes insipidus.	Evaluate the patient for response to medication and any adverse effects: drowsiness, dizziness, ataxia, nausea, and vomiting. Assess for gastric distress. Assess intake and output and vital signs. Withhold the medication if signs and symptoms of myelosuppression are noted: red blood cells less than 4 million/mm^3; hematocrit less than 32%; hemoglobin less than 11; and platelet count less than 100,000/mm^3.
CALCIUM CARBONATE		
Action: Works as a dietary supplement by supplying the body with calcium.	Used to treat and prevent calcium deficiencies and to avoid the development of osteoporosis. This side effect of decreased TSH is caused by the use of the antithyroid medication levothyroxine.	Monitor for side effects such as constipation and aggravation of kidney stones. Advise the patient to take antacids at least 4 hours earlier or later than thyroid hormone as they may interfere with thyroid hormone absorption. Do not administer with milk or any items with vitamin D as this may cause mild-alkali syndrome to occur. Early symptoms include headache, urinary frequency, anorexia, nausea, and fatigue. If the drug is continued in high doses, it may result in permanent renal damage.
PROPYLTHIOURACIL (PTU)		
Action: Inhibits the first step in the synthesis of thyroid hormone, and suppresses the peripheral conversion of T_4 to T_3.	Decreases thyroid hormone levels in hyperthyroid states caused by the overproduction of thyroid hormone. Also used to establish normal thyroid state prior to surgery or radioactive iodine treatment and for palliative control of toxic nodular goiter.	Monitor the patient for reduced signs and symptoms of hyperthyroidism. Instruct the patient to have regular follow-up visits to the health care provider since hyperthyroid activity may reoccur. Monitor white blood cell count. Monitor liver function.
METHIMAZOLE		
Action: Inhibits synthesis of thyroid hormone.	See the entry for propylthiouracil.	Monitor the patient for reduced signs and symptoms of hyperthyroidism. Instruct the patient to have regular follow-up visits to the health care provider since hyperthyroid activity may reoccur. Monitor white blood cell count and liver function. Instruct the patient to take at the same time daily at regular intervals.

(continued)

Medication Category and Action	Application/Indication	Nursing Responsibility
IODINE		
Saturated solution of potassium iodide ***Action:*** Inhibits release of thyroid hormone	Given to patients with hyperthyroidism prior to thyroidectomy or during a thyrotoxic crisis.	Advise the patient to drink all of the solution, to use a straw to avoid discoloration of the teeth, and not to withdraw the drug abruptly. Discourage use of OTC drugs without health care provider consultation.
RADIOACTIVE IODINE		
Sodium iodide [^{131}I], isotope ***Action:*** Radioactive iodine destroys thyroid tissue with the maximum benefit apparent in 3 to 6 months.	Used to treat hyperthyroidism by destroying thyroid tissue when patients wish to avoid surgery or for those who do not tolerate antithyroid drugs. Also used for thyroid cancer.	Instruct the patient to have thyroid hormone levels monitored regularly. Follow radiation precautions as directed. Advise the patient that therapeutic effects develop slowly over 2 to 3 months.
CALCITRIOL		
Active form of vitamin D_3 (Rocaltrol) ***Action:*** Promotes calcium absorption in the intestines and retention at the kidneys, thus increasing serum calcium levels. The rising calcium levels provide negative feedback to the parathyroid glands, reducing the secretion of PTH. Calcitriol provides negative feedback to the parathyroid glands.	Used to treat calcium deficiency with hypoparathyroidism.	Hepatic impairment and an accumulation of fat-soluble vitamins will increase the risk of toxicity from vitamin D supplementation. Monitor for adverse effects of vitamin D therapy: hypercalcemia, headache, weakness, dry mouth, thirst, increased urination, and muscular or bone pain. Monitor for signs of hypercalcemia such as deep bone and flank pain, anorexia, nausea, vomiting, thirst, constipation, lethargy, and psychosis.
BISPHOSPHONATE		
Fosamax, Didronel, Boniva, Aredia, Actonel, Skelid, Reclast ***Action:*** Bisphosphonates bind to hydroxyapatite in bone and suppress osteoclast activity, thus increasing bone mass.	Used to prevent and treat osteoporosis, as well as to increase bone density in hyperparathyroidism.	Administer medicine with a full glass of water to reduce the potential for esophageal irritation. Assess for calcium and vitamin deficiencies.
OCHREOTIDE		
Somatostatin analogue Sandostatin LAR analog (Injectable suspension) ***Action:*** Mimics the action of the growth hormone, HGH. Produces the same effects as the natural hormone somatostatin to suppress secretion of GH. It also suppresses secretion of serotonin, pancreatic peptides, gastin, vasoactive intestinal peptides, secretin, motilin, insulin, and glucagon.	Used to treat acromegaly.	Assess the patient's baseline height and weight and monitor regularly to determine drug effectiveness. Assess baseline and periodic vitamin B_{12} levels because the drug can reduce the absorption of B_{12}. Administer subcutaneously, as this is the preferred route. Allow the solution to reach room temperature before administering. Monitor serum glucose levels frequently because this drug can cause hypoglycemia. Monitor the patient's cardiac status, thyroid functionality, and electrolyte balance.
PEGVISOMANT		
Somavert ***Action:*** Acts as a GH receptor antagonist; suppresses secretion of the hormone.	Used to treat acromegaly.	Monitor the patient for side effects: nausea, vomiting, elevated liver enzymes, angina, chest pain, myocardial infarction, HTN, and flulike syndrome. Patients with diabetes should be monitored regularly to avoid hypoglycemia.
BROMOCRIPTINE		
Parlodel ***Action:*** As a dopamine D_2 and D_3-agonist, it works by activating postsynaptic dopamine receptors in the tuberoinfundibular and nigrostriatal pathways. It also inhibits the secretion of prolactin from the anterior pituitary.	Used for treatment of acromegaly and pituitary adenoma.	Assess the patient's baseline vital signs, especially blood pressure. Monitor for the presence of orthostatic hypotension, headache, nausea, vomiting, anorexia, or rash on the face and arms. Monitor for side effects: extreme drowsiness, falling asleep suddenly (even after feeling alert), confusion, agitation, hallucinations, paranoid delusions, or nightmares.
CABERGOLINE		
Action: As a dopamine receptor antagonist, it acts by blocking the release of prolactin from the pituitary gland.	Used to treat pituitary tumors and prolactinomas.	Monitor for side effects: nausea, vomiting, stomach upset, constipation, dizziness, light-headedness, tiredness, mental/mood changes, vision changes, painful menses, or breast pain. Monitor for serious allergic reaction: rash, itching/swelling (especially of the face/tongue/throat), severe dizziness, or trouble breathing. Notify the health care provider if these adverse reactions are present.

PHARMACOLOGY Summary of Medications Used to Treat Endocrine Disorders, *continued*

Medication Category and Action	Application/Indication	Nursing Responsibility
DESMOPRESSIN		
An ADH synthetic analogue ***Action:*** Increases the permeability of renal collecting tubules to water, thereby increasing the reabsorption of water.	Used to treat neurogenic diabetes insipidus by controlling acute symptoms of polyuria and polydipsia.	Obtain baseline data including blood pressure, weight, and intake and output. Continue to monitor blood pressure and weight during the dose regulation period. Monitor for early signs of water intoxication: nausea, slurred speech, headache, bloating, hallucinations, disorientation, muscle cramps, seizures, coma, and respiratory arrest. Advise the patient to decrease her fluid intake once treatment begins for diabetes insipidus. Monitor electrolytes, especially sodium levels. Weigh the patient daily and assess for edema. Monitor for treatment effectiveness by measuring the serum and urine osmolality; an increased urine osmolality and a decreased serum osmolality indicate effectiveness. Assess the nasal mucosa for irritation or ulceration during long-term therapy with nasal spray formulations.
CHLORPROPAMIDE		
Diabinese ***Action:*** Lowers the blood glucose acutely by stimulating the release of insulin from the pancreas, an effect dependent upon functioning beta cells in the pancreatic islets.	Used to treat type 2 diabetes. Off-label used to treat neurogenic diabetes insipidus.	Monitor for side effects: hypoglycemia, nausea, vomiting, and blood dyscrasias. Elderly patients may have an increased risk of hypoglycemia and drug interactions because of the long half-life.
CLOFIBRATE		
Atromid-S ***Action:*** Increases lipoprotein lipase activity to promote the conversion of very low density lipoprotein (VLDL) to low density lipoprotein (LDL), thereby reducing the VLDL.	Used to control the high cholesterol and triglyceride level in the blood. Used to stimulate residual ADH production in patients with partial central diabetes insipidus.	Monitor the patient and notify the health care provider for a serious allergic reaction (difficulty breathing; closing of throat; swelling of the lips, tongue, or face; or hives); chest pain or an irregular heartbeat; severe stomach pain with nausea and vomiting; fever and chills, a flulike feeling; blood in the urine or a decrease in urination; swelling of the ankles or legs; muscle cramps, muscle weakness, or muscle aches; joint pain; or sudden weight gain.
THIAZIDE DIURETICS		
Hydrodiuril ***Action:*** Acts by blocking Na+ reabsorption and increasing K+ and water excretion. When used in conjunction with clofibrate, the delivery of filtrate to the diluting segments of the nephron is reduced, which allows more sodium and water absorption in the proximal tubule.	Used to treat mild to moderate HTN and edema due to mild to moderate heart, liver, and renal failure. Used to treat partial central diabetes insipidus in conjunction with thiazide and potassium-sparing diuretics.	Monitor for therapeutic effectiveness; antihypertensive effects may be noted in 2 to 3 days. Monitor blood pressure before initiation of therapy and at regular intervals. Monitor the intake and output ratio and check for edema. Monitor serum potassium values and assess for symptoms of hypokalemia. Establish safety precautions if CNS effects or orthostatic hypotension occurs.
AMILORIDE-POTASSIUM SAVING DIURETICS		
Aldactone, Spironolactone Inspra ***Action:*** Acts by inhibiting the actions of aldosterone in the distal tubule and collecting ducts of the nephron. When these actions are blocked, sodium, chloride, and water excretion are increased and the body retains potassium.	Used for short-term preoperative treatment of primary hyperaldosteronism.	Obtain baseline and periodic determinations of serum electrolytes, CBCs, BUN, blood glucose, uric acid, and CO_2. Check the patient's blood pressure before the initiation of therapy and at regular intervals. Assess for signs of fluid and electrolyte imbalance, especially potassium levels. Monitor daily intake and output and check for edema. Report lack of diuretic response or development of edema. Weigh the patient under standard conditions before therapy begins and daily throughout therapy. Observe for and immediately report the onset of mental changes, lethargy, or stupor in patients with liver disease.

(*continued*)

Medication Category and Action	Application/Indication	Nursing Responsibility
HYPERTONIC 3% SODIUM CHLORIDE SOLUTION		
Action: Moves water from the cells into the vessels. Raises serum osmolality.	Used in the treatment of SIADH in the presence of severe symptomatic hyponatremia. This fluid restriction can be supplemented by intravenous hypertonic (3%) fluids.	Monitor the patient for neurological changes. If the hypertonic sodium is given too rapidly in a patient who has had hyponatremia for more than 24 to 48 hours, profound neurological changes can occur (Robertson, 2010). Therefore, protocols that guide the infusion rate, timing of biochemical measurements, and clinical (particularly neurological) monitoring procedures should be followed.
DEMECLOCYCLINE		
Declomycin ***Action:*** Causes diuresis through the inhibiton of ADH-induced water reaborption in the tubules and collecting ducts of the kidneys.	Used off label to treat SIADH due to its ability to causes diuresis.	Monitor for early signs of water intoxication. Monitor electrolytes, particularly sodium levels. Weigh patient daily and assess for edema, auscultate for lung sounds, and monitor blood pressure and heart rate.
LITHIUM		
Action: Precise action is unknown. It is hypothesized that it acts by changing neurotransmitter balance in specific brain regions. It also increases the synthesis of serotonin.	Used off label for the treatment of hyperthyroidism and SIADH.	Obtain baseline thyroid, kidney, and cardiac function, as well as electrolyte levels. Monitor for adverse effects: muscle weakness, lethargy, nausea, vomiting, polyuria, nocturia, headache, dizziness, drowsiness, tremors, and confusion. Assess daily for weight changes, presence of edema, changes in skin turgor, and sodium intake. Assess neurologic status, level of consciousness, gait, hand tremors, and motor reflexes.
ALPHA-ADRENERGIC ANTAGONIST		
Phenoxybenzamine (Dibenzyline) ***Action:*** Blocks the effects of alpha-adrenergic receptors, resulting in dilation of the blood vessels, causing blood pressure to decrease.	Used to treat high blood pressure and sweating caused by a tumor of the adrenal glands and pheochromocytoma.	Assess for full therapeutic effect, which should occur within 4 to 6 weeks of therapy. Administer the initial dose of medication at bedtime to minimize adverse effects such as postural hypotension and syncope. Monitor for drug-related adverse effects which include dizziness, fatigue, weakness, palpitations, orthostatic hypotension, and headache. Give medication with food to decrease the occurrence of possible faintness and dizziness; food may delay the absorption rate, but it does not affect the extent of absorption.
BETA-BLOCKERS		
Metoprolol (Lopressor, Toprol, Inderal) ***Action:*** Depresses myocardium. A selective beta-1 adrenergic antagonist that competes with endogenous catecholamines at adrenergic receptors in cardiac muscle. At high doses, it may affect beta-2 receptors in bronchial smooth muscle.	Used for symptomatic control of hyperthyroidism.	Assess vital signs, especially the apical pulse and blood pressure, before administering the drug. Report significant changes in rate, rhythm, or quality of pulse or blood pressure. Monitor blood pressure, heart rate, and ECG carefully during IV drug administration to determine the effects on the heart. Monitor hypertensive patients with congestive heart failure for symptoms of impending heart failure such as dyspnea on exertion, night cough edema, orthopnea, and distended neck veins. Do not withdraw the drug abruptly as this could precipitate thyroid storm. The drug masks hyperthyroidism in patients with thyrotoxicosis.
HYDROCORTISONE		
Action: Restores deficient levels of glucocorticoids and, to a lesser extent, mineralocorticoids.	Used to treat adrenocortical insufficiency (Addison's disease). Once proper dosing is achieved, its therapeutic effects should mimic those of endogenous corticosteroids.	Monitor for persistent backache or chest pain as compression and spontaneous fractures of long bones and vertebrae are potential adverse effects. Monitor for changes in mood and behavior, emotional instability, or psychomotor activity as this is an adverse effect. Do not discontinue the drug abruptly; gradual withdrawal of corticosteroids allows adrenal glands to resume normal function. Sudden withdrawal leads to acute adrenal insufficiency, hypotension, lethargy, renal failure, asthenia, nausea, and vomiting.
FLUDROCORTISONE		
Florinef ***Action:*** Acts on the distal tubules to promote sodium and water reabsorption, as well as increased urinary potassium excretion.	Used to treat adrenocortical insufficiency (e.g., Addison's disease).	Obtain weight and output ratio to monitor for the possible onset of fluid accumulation. Instruct the patient to report weight gain of 3 kg per week. Monitor and report blood pressure daily and report drug-induced HTN to the health care provider. Monitor for hypokalemia.

PHARMACOLOGY Summary of Medications Used to Treat Endocrine Disorders, *continued*

Medication Category and Action	Application/Indication	Nursing Responsibility
DEHYDROEPIANDROSTERONE (DHEA)		
Synthetic form of a hormone produced by the adrenal glands ***Action:*** DHEA is known as a "parent hormone" produced by the adrenal glands. It serves as a precursor to male and female sex hormones (androgens and estrogens) (MedlinePlus, 2012a).	Used in the treatment of adrenal insufficiency.	Because the body uses DHEA to make estrogen and testosterone, people with hormone-related cancers, such as breast, prostate, ovarian, adrenal, and testicular cancer, or a family history of these cancers should not take DHEA. DHEA may make other hormone-related conditions worse. High doses of DHEA may stop the body from making the hormone itself, and may be toxic to liver cells. People with diabetes should not take DHEA as it may increase insulin resistance.
VASOPRESSORS		
(e.g., Epinephrine) ***Action:*** A vasopressor is a nonselective adrenergic-agonist that stimulates both alpha- and beta-adrenergic receptors through the body, causing vasoconstriction and increasing blood pressure. Actions typical of the fight-or-flight response are induced.	Used to treat SIADH.	Establish baseline vital signs, including heart rate, respiratory rate, and blood pressure. Monitor blood pressure closely during the first 5 minutes of IV administration and continue to take measurements every 3 to 5 minutes until stable. When epinephrine is administered to patients with diabetes, monitor for hypoglycemia. Measure intake and output and inform the health care provider of any marked changes.
MITOTANE		
Action: Poisons cancer cells by forming links to proteins.	Used to treat advanced, inoperable, adrenocortical cancer.	Prevent exposure to people with infections or colds during periods of leucopenia. Monitor I&O ratio, blood pressure, and temperature daily. Weigh weekly to detect the presence of edema or ascites. Assess for hand muscular weakness and for signs of tetany. Check the patient's ability to ambulate, and supply support if necessary. Caution should be used in the event that a patient experiences trauma, infection, or other physiologically stressful events while taking mitotane, since this drug may seriously impair the patient's ability to increase hormone production in response to the stress.

Sources: Adams, M. P., & Koch, R. W. (2010). *Pharmacology: Connections to nursing practice.* Upper Saddle River, NJ: Pearson; Cleveland Clinic. (2011). Goiter. Disease & conditions. Retrieved from http://mmy.clevelandclinic.org/disorders/goiter/hic_goiter.aspx; Drugs.com. (2011a). Cabergoline. TEVA Pharmaceuticals USA Inc. Retrieved from http://www.drugs.com/pro/cabergoline.html; Drugs.com. (2011b). Spironolactone. Cemer Multum, Inc. Retrieved from http:///www.drugs.com/spironolactone.html; Drugs.com. (2012). Methimazole. Cemer Multum, Inc. Retrieved from http://www.drugs.com/mtm/methimazole.html; Mayo Clinic Staff. (2011). Hyperparathyroidism. Retrieved from http://www.mayoclinic.com/health/hyperparathyroidism/DS00385/METHOD=print; Medical News Today. (2012). What is diabetes insipidus? What causes diabetes insipidus? Retrieved from http://www.medicalnewstoday.com/articles/183251.php; MedlinePlus. (2012a). Calcitrol. Retrieved from http://www.nlm.nih.gov/medlineplus/druginfo/meds/a6823335.html; MedlinePlus. (2012b). Carbamazepine. Retrieved from http://www.nlm.gov/medlineplus/druinfo/meds/a682237.html; Monson, K., & Schoenstadt, A. (2009). Lithium uses. Retrieved from http://bipolar-disorder.emedtv.com/lithium;/lithium=uses-p2.html; University of Maryland Medical Center. (2011b). DHEA. Retrieved from http://www.umm.edu/altmed/articles/dehydroepianidrolesterone-000299,htm.

Weblink: Carbamazepine

Weblink: Dehydroepiandrosterone

atrial fibrillation, nausea, vomiting, diarrhea, tremors, agitation, and delirium. Thyroid storm occurs in severe hyperthyroidism and may be triggered by surgery, trauma, infection, postpartum status, or withdrawal of antithyroid drugs, resulting in severe tachycardia, heart failure, hyperthermia, and shock. Treatment of thyroid storm includes supportive measures (e.g., adequate oxygen and ventilation, administration of intravenous fluids, monitoring glucose and electrolyte levels, and control of dysrhythmias), administration of ATDs (i.e., PTU and methimazole) to inhibit the biosynthesis of thyroid, administration of hormones to block the release of thyroid hormone (i.e., SSKI), and control of adrenergic symptoms (e.g., propranolol) (Jameson & Weetman, 2010).

Safety Alert *Nurses should rely on the use of assessment skills to recognize the hypermetabolic state of thyroid storm so that treatment is not delayed. The cardinal signs of thyroid storm include high fever, marked tachycardia, atrial fibrillation, heart failure, neurological symptoms such as agitation and restlessness, and gastrointestinal symptoms such as nausea, vomiting, and diarrhea (Bray, 2012). Early recognition of these signs can improve outcomes and decrease mortality with thyroid storm.*

Nursing Management

The goal in nursing management of the patient with hyperthyroidism is to help the patient return to a euthyroid state. Instructing the patient on the actions, benefits, and side effects of ATDs is a key role for the nurse. The patient must understand that therapy should not be abruptly halted unless there are signs of serious side effects. Therefore, the patient should immediately contact the health care provider if ATDs are discontinued. The patient also must be advised to observe for worsening signs of hyperthyroidism and report such signs to the health care provider. If the patient is hospitalized, the nurse must note signs of significant change in the patient's condition, such as tachycardia, greatly increased body temperature, chest pain, shortness of breath, anxiety and

NURSING PROCESS: Patient Care Plan for Hyperthyroidism

Assessment of Endocrine Status Using Gordon's Functional Health Patterns:

- Health Perception Health Management Pattern
- Nutrition Metabolic Pattern
- Activity Exercise Pattern
- Self-Perception, Self-Concept Pattern

Subjective Data

Assessment of Cognition Level

What medications have you been taking?
Does your family have a history of any particular disease(s)?
Has your weight changed during the past year?
Is there unexplained change in body weight?
Do you feel anxious, nervous, or restless?
Have you noticed any insensitivity to changes in room temperature?
Are you "wound up" or "feeling like you are in overdrive"?
How much exercise are you getting?
Are you experiencing any muscle weakness?
Is there anything affecting your ability to be active?

Assessment of Understanding of Disorder

Have you lost or gained weight during the past year?
Did you take any specific steps to cause this change in your weight?
Describe your appetite for me.
How do you feel most of the time: anxious? calm?

Assessment of Ocular Characteristics and Function

Have you noticed any facial changes, swelling, redness, or protrusion of the eyes?

Assessment of Cardiac Function

Have you noticed any change in your pulse or heart rate?
Have you experienced any chest pain recently?
Have you observed any swelling in your feet?
What is your energy level?

Objective Data

Assessment of Cognition Level

Skin warm and diaphoretic
Hair loss
Agitation, hand tremors
Enlarged thyroid, exophthalmos of the eyes
Hyperthermia
Tachycardia (heart rate $>$100 beats/min)
Hyperreflexia
Elevated serum T_3, T_4

Assessment of Understanding of Disorder

Patient underweight for height
Clothing too large for size/frame

Assessment of Ocular Characteristics and Function

Eyes appear dry and reddened
Eyes protrude (exophthalmos)
Patient unable to close eyelids completely
Visible sclera

Assessment of Cardiac Function

Tachycardia with heart rate $>$ 100 beats/min
Atrial fibrillation
Edema
Cardiac enlargement
Chest pain

Outcomes and Evaluation Parameters	Planning and Interventions with *Rationales*
1. NURSING DIAGNOSIS: Anxiety and Restlessness, Fine Hand Tremors, and Insomnia *related to hypermetabolism* (NANDA-I © 2012)	
Outcome: Patient expresses relief from symptoms of excess thyroid hormone. ***Evaluation Parameters:*** Patient reports less anxiety and restful sleep through the night. Patient's tremors and blood levels of free T_3 and free T_4 decrease and stabilize. Patient is comfortable in an environment with a normal range in ambient temperature. Patient's vital signs are within normal range.	Decrease environmental stimuli and promote a restful environment. Eliminate chemical stimulants such as caffeine from diet. Administer antithyroid drugs as prescribed. *To eliminate stimulants that will exacerbate sleep deprivation and anxiety.*
2. NURSING DIAGNOSIS: Imbalanced Nutrition *related to anxiety, restlessness, and hypermetabolic state* (NANDA-I © 2012)	
Outcomes: Patient regains normal weight and reports resumption of appetite. Patient can describe symptoms of hypo- and hyperthyroidism. ***Evaluation Parameters:*** Patient's weight is maintained or returned to normal. Nutritional deficiencies are eliminated. Patient reports appetite and intake are satisfactory. Patient is able to describe symptoms of hypo- and hyperthyroidism.	Monitor weight daily. Offer the patient a well-balanced diet with nutritional supplements and nutritional consultation as needed. Teach the patient about the effects of hypo- and hyperthyroidism on weight. *To ensure patient regains health and lost weight if desirable and to enable patient to report early signs of change in metabolic state that might indicate a need for further medical intervention.*

NURSING PROCESS: Patient Care Plan for Hyperthyroidism, *continued*

3. NURSING DIAGNOSIS: Risk for Injury to Eyes *related to exophthalmos and inability to close eyelids completely* (NANDA-I © 2012)

Outcome: Eyes are moist and patient reports no eye pain or discomfort. ***Evaluation Parameter:*** No evidence of eye damage or corneal ulceration or abrasion.	Encourage the patient to flush the eyes with warm water at intervals while awake, to use artificial tears to keep the eyes moist, and to cover the eyes while sleeping and as needed if the patient is unable to close her eyes completely. *To keep eyes moist and to prevent corneal ulceration or abrasion.*

4. NURSING DIAGNOSIS: Decreased Cardiac Output *related to hypermetabolic state* (NANDA-I © 2012)

Outcome: Cardiac function within normal limits. Patient free from symptoms of pulmonary edema and heart failure. ***Evaluation Parameters:*** Assessment reveals that heart rate has decreased and stroke volume has increased. No dyspnea is present. No coughing and wheezing is present. Tissues are free from edema. Patient verbalizes feeling less tired and free of anxiety. Patient expresses having an appetite. Patient oriented to time, place, and person. No evidence exists of pink frothy sputum.	Evaluate vital signs frequently. Administer antithyroid and cardiac medications as prescribed. Maintain a restful, calm, supportive environment. Assess toleration of physical activity and work with patient to gradually increase activity as tolerated. *To reduce risk of congestive heart failure in patients with a hypermetabolic state.*

Source: Adapted from Wilkinson, J. M., & Ahearn, N. R. (2009). *Prentice Hall nursing diagnosis handbook* (9th ed.). Upper Saddle River, NJ: Prentice Hall.

irritability, disorientation, increased sweating, and weakness. The health care provider should be alerted so that immediate action can be taken to prevent thyroid storm.

Patients who choose radioactive iodine therapy as their treatment option need both instruction and reassurance about the benefits of this therapy, as well as any information about radiation precautions that must be taken during the first few days after therapy is initiated. The patient will need to know the signs and symptoms of hypothyroidism because radioactive iodine treatment is likely to result in hypothyroidism over a period of several weeks to months. The nurse should give written instructions regarding the signs of hypothyroidism and the need for regular evaluation of thyroid function to the patient at discharge.

If surgical intervention is planned for hyperthyroidism, the nurse prepares the patient for surgery and provides immediate postoperative care. Postoperatively, the nurse should pay particular attention to the patient's airway, because hemorrhage and swelling may compromise his respiratory status. The critical response team should be alerted as early as possible if there is any indication that the patient will need rapid intervention. The patient care plan for patients with hyperthyroidism is shown in the Nursing Process: Patient Care Plan for Hyperthyroidism feature.

Safety Alert *Following a thyroidectomy, it is essential that the patient be observed closely during the immediate postoperative period for signs of hemorrhage or swelling of the operative site, as well as damage to the vocal cords or parathyroid glands. The nurse should check behind the neck for signs of pooling blood.*

Discharge Priorities

Discharge priorities for the patient with hyperthyroidism include patient education about thyroid functioning, particularly symptoms of both hypothyroid disease and hyperthyroid disease because treatments for either condition may result in the opposite condition. The patient needs to understand the importance of having regular follow-up laboratory work to assess thyroid function because treatments for hyperthyroidism, including antithyroid drugs, radioactive iodine, and surgery, may result in a significant decrease or cessation in thyroid hormone production over time. On the other hand, administration of levothyroxine in dosages that are too high may lead to symptoms of hyperthyroidism. The patient also needs careful instruction about the need for follow-up after treatment for thyroid disorders until there is evidence that hormone levels are normal and have stabilized. Certain vulnerable patients with hyperthyroidism or hypothyroidism should be instructed to avoid additional stress or infections until their disease is under control.

Postsurgical patients should receive instruction about wound care and the need to report signs and symptoms of infection immediately to the health care provider. Hyperthyroidism in the older population is addressed in the Gerontological Considerations section later in the chapter (p. 1412). Complementary and alternative approaches to treatment for hyperthyroidism also may be considered by the patient. For example, meditation, massage therapy, and acupuncture may be beneficial in improving their sense of well-being. However, herbal therapies should be used with extreme caution at this time and only after consultation with the patient's primary health care provider, given the potential for drug interactions. Overall, complementary and alternative therapy should not be seen as a replacement for traditional medical therapy in thyroid disease. For more about the use of dietary supplements, see the Complementary & Alternative Therapies box.

Health Promotion

Although access to iodine is not an issue in developed countries such as the United States, optimal health requires a healthy diet, including a reliable source of iodine for the production of thyroid hormone. Patients may be encouraged to plan a healthy diet that includes fish and foods supplemented with iodine such as iodized salt. Health promotion for patients with thyroid disorders requires careful attention to prescribed medications such as hormone replacement therapy or ATDs. Patients may be advised to avoid additional stress when

COMPLEMENTARY & ALTERNATIVE THERAPIES Dietary Supplements

Nancy Yilk

THE DIETARY SUPPLEMENT HEALTH AND EDUCATION ACT OF 1994 (DSHEA) amended the Food, Drug, and Cosmetic Act to create the regulatory category called dietary supplements. This includes food products with fortified vitamins, minerals, amino acids, and botanical herbs, as well as manufactured products of these ingredients in stand-alone products. The DSHEA also gave the FDA authority to write current Good Manufacturing Practices (cGMP) that require manufacturers to evaluate the identity, purity, and composition of their ingredients and finished products (Phillips et al., 2011). Products are analyzed for toxic elements, and concentrations are measured accurately relative to reference values and concordance among the participants. Performance reports and certificates of completion are provided to participating manufacturers.

The measurement of water-soluble vitamins such as B and C groups, along with minerals, are more straightforward with less potential of miscalculations since most of these nutrients are relatively stable and are fortified at high levels in foods and dietary supplement products. Fat-soluble vitamins such as A, D, E, and K present more issues in testing measurements of their nutrients. The instability of fat-soluble vitamins makes their determination challenging for even the most experienced analyst. Analysis can be further complicated when vitamins are encapsulated or if the food or supplement has a high fat content or is not fortified. In addition, the weak chromophores of vitamins D and K make their determination even more difficult at the low levels found in many foods and supplements. Similar issues present themselves in measuring fatty acids and phytosterols calling for the further development of labs (Phillips et al., 2011).

The analysis of botanical dietary supplements brings greater challenges due to the complex nature of plants since they contain hundreds of chemical compounds. Variation of even a single constituent can vary greatly depending on which part of the plant is used in the product or the timing of harvest. Great attention to specifications of adventitious agents (pesticide, metals, weeds) and assessment of natural chemicals is desirable not just once but throughout the supplement's manufacturing process. Manufacturers with the highest quality control will test their products not just at the finish of the product but also throughout the product's shelf life for both the safety and stability of plant properties. Because dietary supplements often are complex mixtures, they pose analytic challenges; therefore, method validation may be difficult (Betz, Fisher, & Saldanha, 2007).

When the public hears of the health benefits of an herbal product, they may be unaware that one plant may have varying benefits depending on the part of the plant used: the leaf, root, or fruit. In addition, the benefits of plant properties can vary widely from nonexistent to beneficial depending on the time of harvest. The healing properties of plants grow with the plants' maturity. The plants' survival against the forces of nature, wind, lack of rain, too much rain, and harsh growing terrain devolves the healing properties in the secondary metabolites of the plants' growth. It is strengthened, however, by the stresses and challenges of survival. This is why wild harvested plant products are seen as having greater potential value. Harvesting a plant too soon can even result in plant properties that circumvent the plant from having any healing properties. As a simple comparative example of this, eating an unripe apple can make you feel sick, unlike eating a ripe apple that delivers nutrient benefits and nourishes the body. The ripe fruit has gone through its second stage of metabolization and reached maturity. This same process translates to herbs, leaves, roots, and berries that are used in herbology. Research results are reported on herbal products that are tested with a high supplication for a particular part of the plant. This part is fingerprinted to show the greatest benefits and then stabilized to maintain a consistent deliverable amount in each tablet or capsule throughout the product's shelf life.

Production of dietary products is a global event, with many of the advanced researched herbal products entering from Europe, China, and India—countries that have moved forward in the research of herbal medicines. The three countries best representing the world market are China, because it is the largest developing country and has a long tradition of herbal medicines; Germany, because it represents the biggest and most advanced herbal industry in developed countries; and the United States, because it is the largest developed country but has paid less attention to the herbal medicine industry than other developed countries.

References

Betz, J. M., Fisher, K. D., & Saldanha, L. G. (2007). The NIH analytical methods and reference materials program for dietary supplements. *Analytical and Bioanalytical Chemistry, 389*(1), 19–25. Epub May 31;

Phillips, M. M., Rimmer, C. A., Wood, L. J., Lippa, K. A., Sharpless, K. E., Duewer, D. L., et al. (2011). Dietary supplement laboratory quality assurance program: The first five exercises. *Journal of AOAC International, 94*(3), 803–814.

experiencing acute thyroid disease until such time as their condition stabilizes. In helping the patient develop insight and understanding of her health condition and developing a plan of disease improvement and healthy maintenance, the nurse will need to consider the cultural norms and values of individual patients. See the Cultural Considerations for Hyperthyroidism box.

CULTURAL CONSIDERATIONS for Hyperthyroidism

Patients with thyroid disorders may have to take long-term drug therapy or lifelong hormone replacement therapy. Chronic illness is not well accepted in some cultures; in addition, poor understanding of the outcomes of rejecting medical therapy may lead to life-threatening consequences. The nurse will need to assess the patient's and family's acceptance and understanding of the disease in order to tailor patient instruction and support appropriately. If patients are to be tested or treated with radioactive iodine, the nurse must be aware of the fear that this may trigger in some. For example, patients with Graves' disease may be treated with radioactive iodine; this may increase concerns of patients in caring for themselves and being around others, family, and the community.

Collaborative Management

Like patients with hypothyroidism, patients with hyperthyroidism will need the support of several members of the health care team. In order to meet desired patient outcomes, it is essential that this interdisciplinary team communicate openly with one another in developing and evaluating care of the patient and family (IOM [Institute of Medicine], 2010).

The pharmacist has a role in instructing hyperthyroid patients about their medications. A radiologist specializing in radiation therapy may administer radioactive iodine, which is the preferred treatment for hyperthyroidism. In some cases, the patient with hyperthyroidism may be referred to a surgeon for surgical removal of the thyroid gland if the patient is not a candidate for radioactive iodine therapy or if surgery is needed to remove a large goiter or malignant nodule. The nutritionist can provide helpful consultation on diet to address the hypermetabolic needs of the patient's body while therapy corrects and stabilizes thyroid hormones.

All members of the team play a significant role in helping the patient cope with and adapt to daily issues that may impede recovery of the patient with thyroid disorders. The Evidence-Based Practice feature addresses this need for identifying and recognizing the lifestyle issues experienced by patients with thyroid disease.

EVIDENCE-BASED PRACTICE Lifestyle Issues Experienced by Patients With Thyroid Diseases

Clinical Problem

Thyroid diseases affect people throughout their life. They include both metabolic changes and gland enlargement (goiter). There has been much discussion in the literature of recent improvements in the treatment of people afflicted with this disease; however, the literature on patient responses to treatment is limited. In discussing patient outcomes, the major focus has been on clinical patient outcomes resulting from the various forms of treatment: medication, radioactive iodine, and surgery (Endocrineweb, 2011a). There is a deficit of literature on the patients' adaptation or response to the treatments from a psychological and emotional response or quality-of-life perspective (Watt et al., 2006; Watt, et al., 2007; Watt, et al., 2008). However, this issue is gaining attention, as is the need to develop an assessment tool that addresses the quality-of-life issues experienced by patients.

Research Findings

At the present time, patient evaluation of health-related quality of living (HRQL) is being conducted by self-completed questionnaires that usually attempt to quantify various aspects of health. Professionals and patients have not found existing questionnaires helpful in eliciting the information needed to assess quality of life related to actual quality-of-life issues (Watt et al., 2006, 2007). Thus, in 2008, Watt et al. conducted a study in which they designed a questionnaire to evaluate HRQL in thyroid patients. This study was based on data gained from a 2006 review of questionnaires used to assess HRQL in patients in general. The study identified six HRQL questionnaires for thyroid patients. After data from these questionnaires was extracted, it revealed that the quality of life of thyroid patients was substantially impaired over a wide range of quality-of-life issues. These findings were validated in a subsequent study (2007) in which Watt et al. pursued the topic of identifying how thyroid diseases impact the patients' lives and to select the most relevant quality-of-life issues for a thyroid-specific questionnaire. Watt et al. (2007) found that 148 disease-related issues were rated as relevant during interviews with clinicians and patients. Patients rated issues about psychosocial problems and impact on daily life as more relevant, whereas clinicians focused on thyroid-characteristic issues. Fatigue and emotional susceptibility were found to be particularly relevant to patients.

In 2008, Watt et al. completed development of a scale structure of a patient-report outcome measuring thyroid-specific quality of life. The 98-item ThyPRO questionnaire was administered to patients with benign thyroid disease at two university hospitals. In total, 904 patients responded. A reliable scale structure displaying complete convergent and almost complete discriminate validity was established in general analyses and in distinct clinical subgroups of patients with benign thyroid disease. The validity and reliability of the ThyPRO scale questionnaire was affirmed in 2010 with a group of thyroid patients. Clinical validity was evaluated by whether the ThyPRO scales could detect expected differences in a cross-sectional study of 907 thyroid patients. Test–retest reliability was evaluated by intra-class correlations of two responses to the ThyPRO 2 weeks apart in a subsample of 87 stable patients. Results were found to be substantial and significant for both validity and reliability. This questionnaire is available for use in multiple settings, and has been cited by other researchers who are also interested in developing a questionnaire for use in measuring quality-of-life issues in patients with thyroid conditions (Giusti et al., 2011).

Implications for Nursing Practice

It is clear from the literature and the nursing research cited previously that patients with thyroid disorders experience problems or difficulties in adjusting to daily quality-of-life issues. When providing care to these patients, nurses must assess and identify how the patients are coping with a return to daily living expectations. Are they able to adjust? What do they worry about? What supportive measures can the nurse provide? Nurses must share the realization that there is more than a physical adjustment of caring for these patients with the entire health care team. It is important for the team to work together to identify and evaluate patients' total concerns regarding recovery from thyroid treatment and adaptation to a healthy lifestyle post-treatment.

Critical Thinking Questions with answers can be found in the Osborn Student Resources at nursing.pearsonhighered.com.

Sources: Giusti, M., Melle, G., Fenocchio, M., Mortara, L., Cecoli, F., Caorsim V., et al., (2011). Five-year longitudinal evaluation of quality of life in a cohort of patients with differentiated thyroid carcinoma. *Journal Zhejiang Universal Science12*(3), 163–173. doi: 10.1631/jzus.B1000382 PMCID: PMC3048930; Watt, T., et al. (2006). Quality of life in patients with benign thyroid disorders. A review. *European Journal of Endocrinology, 154*(4), 501–510; Watt, T., et al. (2007). Which domains of thyroid-related quality of life are most relevant? Patients and clinicians provide complementary perspectives. *Thyroid, 17*(7), 647–664) Watt, T., et al. (2008). Improving a newly developed patient-reported outcome for thyroid patients, using cognitive interviewing. *Quality of Life Review.* doi: 10.1007s11136-008-9364-z; Watt, T., et al. (2010). Validity and reliability of the novel thyroid-specific quality of life questionnaire, ThyPRO. *European Journal of Endocrinology, 162*, 161–167. doi: 10.1530/EJE-09-0521

Disorders of the Parathyroid Glands

The general functions of the parathyroid glands were discussed briefly in Chapter 45. The following paragraphs discuss disorders related to hypoparathyroidism and hyperparathyroidism.

Anatomy and Physiology of Parathyroid Glands

The parathyroid glands are four small, highly vascular glands located behind the thyroid gland. Anatomic variation in the number and location of parathyroid glands occurs with some frequency (Figure 46–4◆). Approximately the size of a grain of rice, the parathyroid glands secrete the **parathyroid hormone (PTH),** which is the most important mediator in a complex feedback loop that regulates calcium and phosphate physiology. The hormones involved in this feedback loop include PTH and calcitonin. Active vitamin D metabolite also is involved in the feedback loop. The target areas of the body include the intestinal mucosa, kidneys, and bone. The primary effect of PTH is to maintain the normal serum calcium concentration. The effect of PTH on the intestinal mucosa is indirect; PTH stimulates the production of the vitamin D metabolite, which increases the intestinal absorption of calcium.

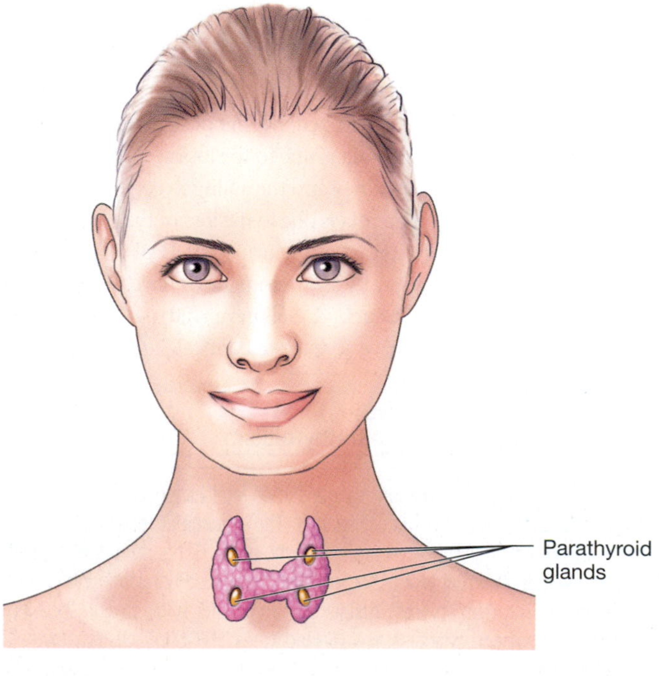

FIGURE 46–4 ◆ The parathyroid glands.

Parathyroid hormone has direct effects on the kidneys and bone. For example, PTH promotes calcium reabsorption in the distal tubule and the medullary thick ascending limb of Henle's loop. In addition, PTH stimulates the release of calcium from a rapidly exchangeable pool of calcium in bone (Shoback & Sellmeyer, 2010). These processes act in concert to maintain normal serum calcium concentrations.

Hypoparathyroidism

Hypoparathyroidism, the combination of symptoms that results from inadequate parathyroid hormone production, is a very rare condition. Most commonly, it occurs because of damage to or removal of parathyroid glands at the time of parathyroid or thyroid surgery. The decreased secretion or activity of parathyroid hormone (PTH) causes decreased levels of calcium (hypocalcemia) and increased levels of phosphorus (hyperphosphatemia) in the blood (Endocrineweb, 2011a).

Epidemiology and Risk Factors

Hypoparathyroidism affects both genders equally and generally is seen in children under age 16 and adults over age 40 (Parathyroid.com, 2012). Symptoms of hypocalcemia in older individuals should be explored fully because these are more likely due to nutritional deficiencies, renal failure, intestinal disorders, or neck surgery than to primary hypoparathyroidism. Risk factors for hypoparathyroidism include family history and heredity, neck surgery, and the presence of other disease. (See the Genetic Considerations box.) The disease may occur alone or concomitantly with other endocrine disorders.

Etiology and Pathophysiology

The primary causes of hypoparathyroidism are surgical, autoimmune, familial, or idiopathic. Of these, the most common cause is surgery on the neck (e.g., thyroidectomy, parathyroidectomy, cancer surgery) that results in destruction or removal of the parathyroid glands (Shoback et al., 2011). Idiopathic or acquired hypoparathyroidism is sometimes found in the setting of polyglandular endocrinopathies (sequential or simultaneous deficiencies in the function of several endocrine glands that have a common cause) (Shoback et al., 2011). There also are forms of pseudohypoparathyroidism that occur when there is resistance of the target organs to PTH (Shoback et al., 2011). In this chapter, discussion is focused on the more common forms of hypoparathyroidism.

Clinical Manifestations

Hypoparathyroidism is characterized by hypocalcemia and hyperphosphatemia. The hypocalcemia is due to the loss of PTH-stimulated calcium reabsorption at the kidney and the ability to generate active vitamin D. The hyperphosphatemia is due to the loss of the phosphaturic (excess excretion of phosphorous in the urine) effect of PTH. Patients with hypoparathyroidism may be asymptomatic or have latent or overt signs of hypocalcemia (Shoback & Sellmeyer, 2010). Patients with chronic hypocalcemia may have adapted to their calcium level and have few symptoms. When the hypocalcemia occurs rapidly, the symptoms can be profound. Hypocalcemia is characterized by increased neuromuscular excitability with widespread effects. Patients may complain of numbness and tingling sensations in the perioral area or in the fingers and toes. Muscle cramps are common in the back and lower extremities. Acute hypocalcemia may be associated with seizures and cardiac arrhythmias (Gardner, 2011).

Tetany, a constellation of symptoms caused by hypocalcemia, is characterized by painful carpal spasms and laryngeal stridor (Shoback & Sellmeyer, 2010). The presence of latent tetany may be demonstrated through the use of Chvostek's sign and Trousseau's sign (Shoback & Sellmeyer, 2010). Chvostek's sign can be elicited by tapping on the facial nerve anterior to the ear; twitching in the ipsilateral facial muscle is considered a positive test. Trousseau's sign can be demonstrated by inflating the blood pressure cuff above the systolic blood pressure and holding for 3 minutes. In individuals who have hypocalcemia, this results in painful carpal muscle contractions and spasms (Shoback & Sellmeyer, 2010).

GENETIC CONSIDERATIONS
for Development of Hypoparathyroidism

Hypoparathyroidism may present as genetic or familiar forms transmitted as an autosomal dominant or recessive trait. The autosomal recessive form of hypoparathyroidism is present in families who have PTH gene mutations that interfere with the normal processing of PTH. The autosomal dominant form of hypoparathyroidism, in contrast, results from mutations in the calcium-sensing receptor (CaSR) gene, which essentially inactivates PTH (Shoback, Sellmeyer, & Bikle, 2011).

Laboratory and Diagnostic Procedures

In hypoparathyroidism, serum calcium levels are decreased and serum phosphate levels are increased. Serum PTH may be inappropriately low, normal, or undetectable; however, the normal levels are inappropriately low in relation to the level of calcium (Shoback et al., 2011). Tests for these are in the Laboratory and Diagnostic Tests box (p. 1391).

Medical Management

Treatment of hypoparathyroidism is managed with supplementation of calcium, calcitriol (an active form of an artificial vitamin D), and high doses of oral vitamin D daily. Two or three grams of calcium are given daily to patients with primary hypoparathyroidism.

The health care provider must recognize that there may be normal atrophied tissue associated with hypoparathyroidism if the patient has undergone neck surgery for treatment of malignancy or for resection of parathyroid adenomas or hyperplasia of the PTH glandular tissue (Gardner, 2011). Following resection of the adenoma, it may take 1 to 2 days for the calcium and the PTH to return to normal.

Nursing Management

Nursing care for the patient with hypoparathyroidism is directed at hormone replacement: symptom management (e.g., joint pain, nausea and vomiting, constipation, and fatigue); management of potential complications and risk for injury (e.g., osteoporosis); and support of patient self-care. Patients need to be monitored carefully to avoid falls and potential fractures. Because primary disease lasts a lifetime, the patient requires thorough explanations about the condition and long-term treatment. Therefore, instruction on calcium and vitamin D supplements and their role in disease management should begin soon after diagnosis. The patient also may find support from networks established by other people who have the same disease; therefore, a nursing referral to community groups is suggested.

Safety Alert *Because acute hypoparathyroidism may result following surgery, the nurse must be aware of the potential for this complication and be vigilant regarding assessment of possible hypocalcemia.*

Discharge Priorities

Discharge priorities for the patient with parathyroid disease are focused on compliance with the prescribed medication regime and safety related to falls and fracture prevention. Follow-up home visits are warranted to assess how the patient has modified the environment for safety and to determine whether the patient needs further support in compliance with prescribed calcium and vitamin D supplementation.

Health Promotion

Vitamin D and calcium are essential nutrients in the human diet. Vitamin D is actually a hormone involved with the metabolism of bone and other tissues. Sources of vitamin D include both diet and exposure to sunlight, because vitamin D is synthesized by the skin. Patients living in northern climates are susceptible to vitamin D deficiency for several months of the year during which daylight hours are short. Thus, supplementation of the diet with vitamin D may be advisable, particularly for those with lower than desirable levels of calcium and those considered to be vulnerable to bone fractures. Brief daily periods of exposure to sunlight should be encouraged when this is feasible. Educational approaches to the immediate living environment and safety also should be considered. The home or immediate living environment should be free from clutter and obstacles that may cause the patient to fall. An inside and outside safety check should be completed to assist the patient in preventing falls. Modes of transportation also should be considered for patient safety.

Hyperparathyroidism

Hyperparathyroidism is an excess of parathyroid hormone in the bloodstream due to over-activity of one or more of the body's four parathyroid glands. The parathyroid glands produce parathyroid hormone, which helps maintain an appropriate balance of calcium in the bloodstream and in tissues that depend on calcium for proper functioning (Mayo Clinic Staff, 2011). There are two types of hyperparathyroidism: primary and secondary. In *primary hyperparathyroidism*, an enlargement of one or more of the parathyroid glands causes overproduction of the hormone, resulting in high levels of calcium in the blood (hypercalcemia). *Secondary hyperparathyroidism* is a result of another disease that causes low levels of calcium in the body. When calcium levels are too low, the body responds by increasing production of parathyroid hormone. This increase in parathyroid hormone causes more calcium to be taken from the bone and more calcium to be reabsorbed by the intestines and kidney. Medical conditions that cause low blood calcium levels or interfere with the body's ability to break down and remove phosphate can lead to secondary hyperparathyroidism. Too much phosphate causes changes in calcium levels. Kidney failure is a common cause of secondary hyperparathyroidism, as it can interfere with the body's ability to remove phosphate. Other causes of secondary hyperparathyroidism include calcium deficiency, cancer, malnutrition, and malabsorption.

Epidemiology

The prevalence of primary hyperparathyroidism is 1:1000 in the United States (Shoback & Sellmeyer, 2010). The incidence increases with age, and it frequently affects postmenopausal women (Shoback & Sellmeyer, 2010). The disease has a peak incidence in the third through fifth decades but also can occur in the young and in older adults (Potts, 2010).

Etiology

Primary hyperparathyroidism occurs because of some problem with one or more of the four parathyroid glands. The main causes of primary hyperparathyroidism include adenomas (benign tumors), hyperplasia (enlargement), and carcinomas (cancer) (Shoback & Sellmeyer, 2010). Of these, chief cell adenomas are the most common cause, accounting for 85% of cases (Shoback & Sellmeyer, 2010). Hyperplasia of two or more parathyroid glands accounts for most other cases. A cancerous tumor is a rare cause of primary hyperparathyroidism (Mayo Clinic Staff, 2011). Secondary hyperparathyroidism results from another condition that lowers calcium levels, causing the parathyroid glands to overwork to compensate for loss of calcium. These conditions include severe calcium deficiency, severe vitamin D deficiency, and chronic kidney failure. Chronic kidney failure is the most common cause of secondary hyperparathyroidism (Parathyroid.com, 2012).

Risk factors for primary hyperparathyroidism are shown in the Risk Factors for Primary Hyperparathyroidism feature. One risk factor for hyperplasia is genetically related, and is discussed in the Genetic Considerations for Hyperparathyroidism box.

RISK FACTORS for Primary Hyperparathyroidism

A woman who has gone through menopause
Prolonged, severe calcium or vitamin D deficiency
A rare, inherited disorder such as multiple endocrine neoplasia*
Have had radiation treatment for cancer that has exposed the neck to radiation
Have taken lithium, a drug used most often to treat bipolar disorder.

*Discussed in the Genetic Considerations box below.

GENETIC CONSIDERATIONS for Hyperparathyroidism

Parathyroid hyperplasia (enlargement or abnormality of all four glands) may be part of the autosomal dominant multiple endocrine neoplasia (MEN) syndromes. This is especially true for MEN1, which is caused by a mutation in the MEN1 gene that encodes for the protein menin (Shoback & Sellmeyer, 2010).

Pathophysiology

Primary hyperparathyroidism is a generalized disorder of calcium, phosphate, and bone metabolism resulting from increased secretion of PTH. In primary hyperparathyroidism, the parathyroid hormone production by extracellular calcium seems to be lost, resulting in a change in the set point. The set point is the serum calcium level that provides the negative feedback to control PTH secretion. An altered set point results in the need for a higher-than-normal serum calcium value to suppress PTH secretion and to retard cell proliferation. However, this is not the case in primary hyperparathyroidism from parathyroid hyperplasia. An increase in the cell numbers is probably the cause (Kim, 2011). "Low serum calcium levels stimulate PTH secretion. Excessive PTH leads to over-stimulation of osteoclast receptors resulting in overt bone resorption, with cortical bone affected more than cancellous bone" (Best Practice, 2011, p. 1). PTH also stimulates the kidneys to reabsorb calcium and to convert 25-hydroxyvitamin D_3 to its more active form of 1,25 dihydroxyvitamin D_3. This active vitamin D is responsible for the GI absorption of calcium. The chronic excessive resorption of calcium from bone caused by excessive parathyroid hormone can result in osteopenia (a condition where bone mineral density is lower than normal) (Kim, 2011).

Secondary hyperparathyroidism is a diffuse hyperplasia of the parathyroid glands due to a cause external to the parathyroid glands. Its pathophysiology is mainly due to hyperphosphatemia and vitamin D deficiency and resistance (Saliba & El-Haddad, 2009). Secondary hyperparathyroidism develops as a consequence of mineral metabolism disturbances and is characterized by elevated serum parathyroid hormone (PTH) and parathyroid hyperplasia. For example, several factors in chronic renal disease contribute to the development of secondary hyperparathyroidism, including decreased production of the active vitamin D metabolite which is essential for the intestinal absorption of calcium. This results in increased secretion of PTH and hyperplasia of the parathyroid glands. Individuals who are deficient in active vitamin D, regardless of the cause, can develop secondary hyperparathyroidism.

Clinical Manifestations

Patients with hyperparathyroidism may present in a variety of ways. For example, these patients may be asymptomatic; an abnormality on their routine laboratory tests (e.g., elevated serum calcium) and subsequent diagnostic work-up may indicate primary hyperparathyroidism. Patients may present with skeletal abnormalities (e.g., pathologic fractures) or kidney stones. Other symptoms may include systemic manifestations (e.g., weakness, fatigue, weight loss), neuropsychiatric and neuromuscular symptoms (e.g., depression, poor concentration, memory defects, peripheral sensory neuropathy, motor neuropathy, proximal and generalized muscle weakness), cardiac signs (e.g., hypertension, shortened QT interval on ECG), renal symptoms (e.g., stones, polyuria, metabolic acidosis), skeletal symptoms (e.g., pathologic fractures, osteopenia, joint pain), and gastrointestinal (e.g., peptic ulcer disease, nausea and vomiting, constipation) signs and symptoms.

Laboratory and Diagnostic Procedures

The measurement of serum PTH with a simultaneous measurement of serum calcium helps to establish the diagnosis of primary hyperparathyroidism (See the Laboratory and Diagnostic Tests box, p. 1391) (Gardner & Shoback, 2011). In patients with normal kidney function, an elevated serum PTH and elevated serum calcium are usually diagnostic of primary hyperparathyroidism. Additionally, studies may be performed to assess possible target organ damage from primary hyperparathyroidism, such as radiological studies (e.g., spine films); skeletal abnormalities such as osteopenia and osteoporosis may support the diagnosis of primary hyperparathyroidism. Patients with secondary hyperparathyroidism may have normal or decreased serum calcium levels. Serum phosphate may be reduced, urinary calcium may be low, and 1,25-dihydroxyvitamin D may be deficient. These patients often will have an underlying disorder that may contribute to the secondary hyperparathyroidism.

Medical Management

The definitive treatment for primary hyperparathyroidism is a parathyroidectomy (Potts, 2010). This type of surgery varies from minimally invasive to full neck exploration. If the patient has severe hypercalcemia (15 to 18 mg/dL), surgery is essential as soon as the PTH level is confirmed. Many patients with hyperparathyroidism are asymptomatic with mild hypercalcemia. These patients do not require emergent medical or surgical treatment (Potts, 2010); however, some women may choose to use estrogens, oral bisphosphonates, or selected estrogen response modulators to improve bone density (Shoback et al., 2011).

Nursing Management

Nursing management for the patient with hyperparathyroidism is focused on patient teaching about the disease; preparation and follow-up for surgical intervention, if appropriate; instruction about medications and ways to manage the disease without surgery; and the need for laboratory studies for regular follow-up. Nursing interventions include counseling about nutrition, ensuring that the patient receives sufficient fluid, taking safety precautions to minimize the risk for injury from falls, scheduling care to allow the patient with muscle weakness to receive as much rest as possible, and providing comfort measures to alleviate pain. Observe the patient's signs of pain and monitor him for effectiveness of analgesics and comfort measures. It also is necessary to auscultate the lungs regularly to check for signs of pulmonary edema if the patient is receiving large amounts of normal saline solution.

If the patient is having surgery, which usually is the treatment of choice, it is necessary to prepare the patient for surgery and provide postoperative care. Because the surgery is considered to be minimally invasive, it may be done in an inpatient or an outpatient setting. If performed in an inpatient setting, the patient is generally hospitalized for 1 to 2 days postoperatively. If surgery is performed in an outpatient setting, patients go home the same day. Postoperative care includes careful monitoring of the patient for complications of hemorrhage, infection, hypoparathyroidism, hypocalcemia, and damage to the laryngeal nerve. When the patient returns from surgery, the operative site is assessed carefully. The side and back of the neck, as well as the anterior dressing, should be observed for any bleeding; vital signs are monitored closely, and the patient is observed for any signs of respiratory distress. Accumulations of subcutaneous fluids must be watched carefully as they can contribute to infection and tissue necrosis. Typically, unless otherwise indicated, the patient is placed in a semi-Fowler's position postoperatively. This makes breathing easier, promotes drainage from the operative site, and decreases pressure on the skin and suture line. Postoperative neurological assessments may be completed according to agency protocol. More specifically, the patient's voice should be checked for hoarseness, as it might signify laryngeal nerve damage. In addition, the sensory and motor function may be temporarily or permanently impaired due to surgical manipulation.

Nursing focuses on preparing the patient for discharge and recovery from the onset of care. Specific discharge planning and postoperative instructions are included under Discharge Priorities.

Discharge Priorities

Discharge priorities for the patient with hyperparathyroidism include patient instruction on postsurgical care, including observation of the operative site and dressing changes as indicated by the health care provider. The importance of follow-up with laboratory studies to monitor serum calcium levels should be stressed, in concert with the importance of follow-up visits with the surgeon and endocrinologist. Surgical removal of the affected gland provides relief of major symptoms and problems related to hypercalcemia. Close follow-up is warranted to ensure that serum levels of calcium are maintained within recommended ranges. See the Patient Teaching & Discharge Priorities for Hyperparathyroidism box.

Health Promotion

Following surgery, the patient should feel a significant improvement in health status. With a return to normal or near-normal parathyroid functioning, the patient should maintain a healthy diet with good sources of calcium and vitamin D, which are essential for a healthy musculoskeletal system. Optimal synthesis of vitamin D in the body includes at least brief exposure to sunlight daily. Outdoor activities, such as walking, are beneficial to patients, as they address their need for vitamin D synthesis and provide cardiovascular benefits.

Collaborative Management

Patients with parathyroid disorders can benefit from care provided by a wide array of health care providers, including the pharmacist, the nutritionist, the endocrinologist, and the genetic counselor, as well as

LABORATORY AND DIAGNOSTIC TESTS for Parathyroid Gland Disorders

Test, Description, Rationale, and Normal Values	Expected Abnormality
Parathyroid Hormone	
Normal: Intact PTH 11–54 pg/mL PTH-C-Terminal PTH 50–330 pg/mL PTH-N-Terminal PTH 8–24 pg/mL *A blood test used to identify hypo- or hyperparathyroidism and to monitor the patient's response to PTH therapy.*	Decreased PTH serum indicates hypoparathyroidism, nonparathyroid hypercalcemia, Graves' disease, and sarcoidosis. Elevated PTH serum indicates primary and secondary hyperparathyroidism, hypercalcemia, chronic renal failure, or pseudohyperparathyroidism (a defect in tubular response). Decreased levels of PTH-C indicate hypoparathyroidism or nonparathyroid hypercalcemia. Increased levels of PTH-C indicate secondary hyperparathyroidism, tumors, hypercalcemia, and pseudohypoparathyroidism. Decreased levels of PTH-N indicate hypoparathyroidism, nonparathyroid hypercalcemia, certain tumors, and pseudohyperparathyroidism. Increased levels of PTH-N indicate primary and secondary hyperparathyroidism or pseudohypoparathyroidism.
Total Serum Calcium	
Normal: 4.5–5.5 mEq/L *A blood test used to check for serum calcium excess or deficit, to monitor calcium levels, and to detect calcium imbalance.*	A decreased level indicates hypoparathyroidism and chronic renal failure caused by phosphorous retention. It may also reflect diarrhea, malabsorption of calcium from the intestinal tract, extensive infections, or lack of calcium and vitamin D intake. An increased level indicates hyperparathyroidism; malignant neoplasm of the bone, lung, breast, bladder, or kidney; renal calculi; exercise; and prolonged immobilization. It may be influenced by vitamin D.
Ionized Serum Calcium	
Normal: Adult: 4.25–5.25 mg/dL *Usage same as above.*	A decrease is found in hypoparathyroidism; it also might lead to tetany symptoms related to lack of calcium and vitamin D intake. An increased level is found in hyperparathyroidism.
Serum Phosphorus	
Normal: 1.7–2.6 mEq/L *A blood test used to check phosphorous level, to monitor phosphorus levels during renal insufficiency or failure, and to compare phosphorus levels with those of other electrolytes (i.e., potassium, calcium).*	Decreased levels reflect hyperparathyroidism, hypercalcemia, and vitamin D deficiency. Increased levels indicate hypoparathyroidism or hypocalcemia (tetany). Decreased urinary output of less than 600 mL/day can increase the serum phosphorus level.
Skeletal Films	
Normal: Normal bony structure *X-ray of skeletal bones to detect abnormal size, structure, and shape of bone.*	Abnormal bone structure may be reflected in the white structure of the bones and may be indicative of hyperparathyroidism.
Bone Densitometry	
Normal: Is determined according to the patient's age, sex, and height: 1 standard deviation below peak bone mass level *Used to detect early and progressive osteoporosis by determining the density of bone mineral content.*	Loss of bone mineral content, early and progressive osteoporosis, indicated by greater than 2.5 standard deviations below peak bone mass level. Indicative of hyperparathyroidism.

Sources: Freitas, B. (2011). Imaging in primary hyperparathyroidism. Medscape Reference. Retrieved from http://emedicine.medscape.com/article/390728-overview; Kee, J. L. (2010). *Laboratory and diagnostic tests with nursing implications.* Upper Saddle River, New Jersey.

the registered nurse. In order to meet desired patient outcomes, it is essential that this interdisciplinary team communicate openly with one another in developing and evaluating care of the patient and family (IOM [Institute of Medicine], 2010).

Parathyroid problems are rare and typically should be dealt with by an endocrinologist and highly trained surgeons who have experience working with the parathyroid glands. The pharmacist will provide essential information on drug therapies and vitamin and mineral supplementation, not only to the patient but also to members of the health care team. All members of the team need to work together to assist the patient in coping with and adapting to daily issues which may impede recovery of the patient with parathyroid disorders.

Growth Hormone Disorders

Growth hormone is synthesized and secreted by the somatotrophs of the anterior pituitary. The release of growth hormone is mediated primarily by two hypothalamic hormones: growth hormone-releasing hormone (GHRH) and somatostatin (GH-inhibiting hormone), which stimulate the anterior pituitary to release and inhibit growth hormone, respectively. The primary function of growth hormone is to promote linear growth. The majority of the growth-promoting effects of growth hormone are mediated by insulinlike growth factor-1 (IGF-1), which is produced in the liver. Growth hormone has effects on carbohydrates, fats, and protein, such as increasing insulin resistance, raising blood

PATIENT TEACHING & DISCHARGE PRIORITIES for Hyperparathyroidism

Need	Teaching
Knowledge of disease process and prognosis (patient and family)	Home care needs include verbal and written instructions for: The treatment plan and follow-up care. Teach the patient and family about the disease process and the signs and symptoms of calcium imbalance, which include twitching or muscle spasms, irregular heartbeat, increased blood pressure, periods of sluggishness, loss of appetite, nausea, constantly thirsty, and periods of confusion or depression. Stress that the symptoms require immediate medical attention.
Understanding of medications	Teach the patient and family the action, dosage, route, and side effects of all medications.
Postoperative care	Teach the patient and family postoperative care. Describe incisional care and arrange for a follow-up visit with the surgeon. Instruct the patient on the appropriate activity level; encourage the patient not to lift heavy objects or engage in activities that stress the neck. Inform the patient that recalcification of bones will take some time.
Mobilization	Encourage the patient to maintain mobility as this will assist recalcification. Suggest that the patient avoid bed rest, which will not assist recalcification and may cause skin breakdown or pressure ulcers.
Activity level and rest	Encourage the patient to space activity throughout the day and use the energy levels as a guide to activity. Remind the patient to avoid contact sports or other activities that place him at risk for falls or fractures.
Dietary considerations	Describe any dietary considerations, including a diet low in calcium with limitation and avoidance of milk products. If on a potassium-depleting diuretic, advise that a diet high in potassium-rich foods is necessary (apricots, fresh vegetables, citrus fruits) if no potassium supplements are prescribed. Advise that a diet with adequate fiber and fluid will aid normal bowel function.

glucose levels, increasing lipolysis (the decomposition of fat), and enhancing protein synthesis. In this section, we review the main disorders of growth hormone that affect adults: hypersecretion and acromegaly. Growth hormone deficiency also is a disorder, but it affects children; therefore, it is not discussed in this section because of its pediatric focus.

Hypersecretion of Growth Hormone

The two primary disorders of growth hormone excess are acromegaly and gigantism. Since gigantism occurs in children, the majority of the discussion will focus on acromegaly. **Gigantism** refers to the development of disease prior to epiphyseal closure (prior to or during puberty); **acromegaly** refers to the onset of disease following epiphyseal fusion (after puberty). These disorders are almost always secondary to pituitary adenomas (Mayo Clinic Staff, 2010).

Epidemiology and Etiology

Gigantism is extremely rare, with approximately 100 reported cases to date in the United States (Ferry et al., 2011). Acromegaly is more common than gigantism, with an incidence of 3 to 4 cases per million people per year and a prevalence of 40 to 70 cases per million population (Ferry et al., 2011). However, sometimes the terms are used interchangeably and are differentiated by the time frame in which the disorder is diagnosed—childhood, adolescence, or young adult. For example, gigantism is usually diagnosed before puberty. In children, acromegaly results in an excessively tall stature and is called gigantism (Rightdiagnosis.com, 2011a). Primary gigantism typically is a rare disorder. However, it may concur with the context of a coexisting disorder or arise according to a pattern of familial inheritance. Acromegaly is a rare hormonal syndrome caused in at least 90% of cases by a benign GH-secreting pituitary adenoma (Eugster, 2012).

Due to the slow rate of tumor growth, acromegalic patients are often older than 50 years of age; however, when GH-hypersecretion occurs in teenagers it may cause gigantism. At diagnosis, tumors present as macroadenomas in more than 70% of cases, and in about 25% of cases they co-secrete prolactin (Mulinda, 2011). The majority of these tumors are sporadic and the relationship to predisposing genes is ongoing (Mayo Clinic Staff, 2012.). See the Genetic Considerations box for growth hormone disorders.

Pathophysiology

Gigantism and acromegaly are characterized by sustained hypersecretion of growth hormone (GH). Growth hormone secreted from the anterior pituitary somatotrophs is normally controlled by two hypothalamic factors. The growth hormone receptor hormone (GHRH) stimulates GH secretion and synthesis, is synthesized in the hypothalamus, and is transported via the hypothalamic pituitary portal system to the somatotrophs of the anterior pituitary. Several tissues, including the endocrine pancreas, produce somatostatin in response to the GH. Somatostatin inhibits GHRH secretion in a negative feedback pathway. Once released into circulation, GH stimulates the production of

GENETIC CONSIDERATIONS for Growth Hormone Disorders

Multiple groups have been identified in whom isolated GH excess is transmitted in an autosomal dominant fashion, resulting in an entity known as isolated familial somatotropinomas (Eugster, 2012). Thus, it behooves the health care professional to explore a genetic predisposition to pituitary disorders. Since the main causes of growth hormone excess are pituitary adenomas (benign tumors), the presence of several family members with pituitary tumors should prompt the health care professional to explore a genetic predisposition to pituitary adenomas or tumors, including multiple endocrine neoplasia type 1 (MEN 1), familial acromegaly, or familial isolated pituitary adenomas (Katznelson et al., 2011).

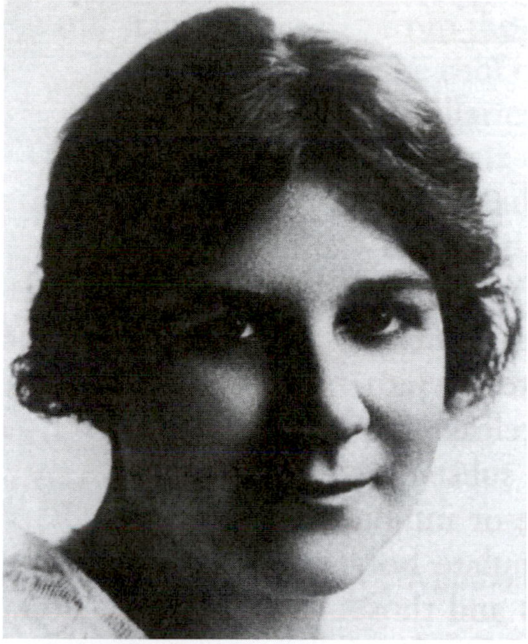

(A)

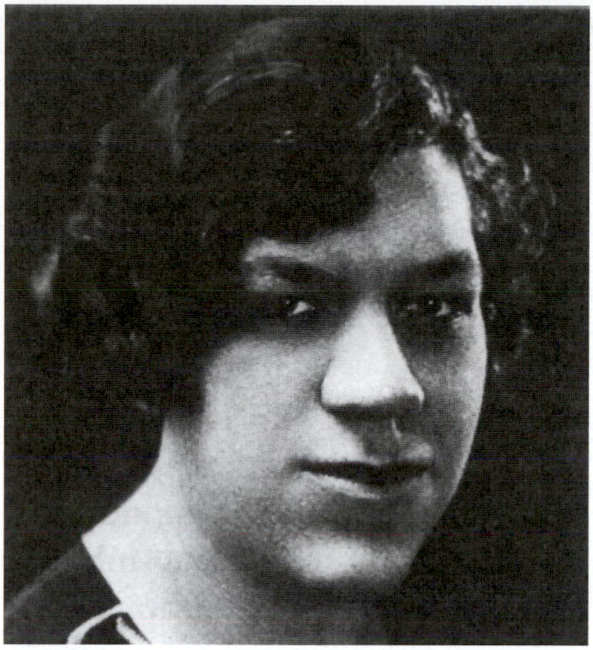

(B)

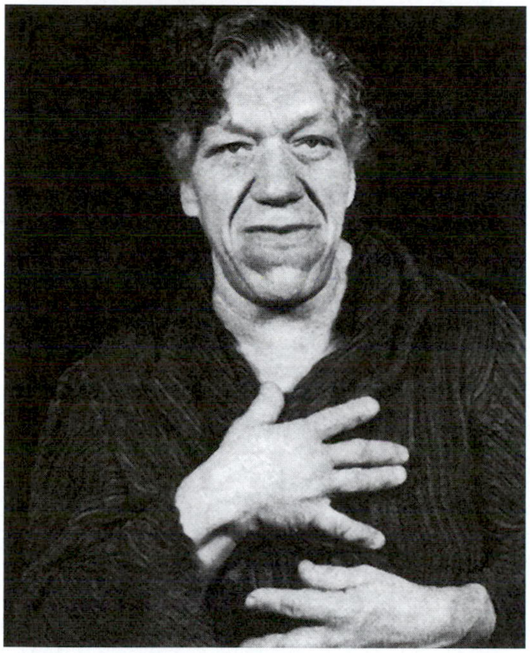

(C)

FIGURE 46–5 ◆ Patient with development stages of acromegaly.

Source: Published in American Journal of Medicine, Vol. 20, page 133, 1956, Dr. William H. Daughaday. Copyright Elsevier. With permission of Excerpta Media Inc.

insulinlike growth factor-I (IGF-I), also known as somatomedin C (SM-C). The main source of circulating IGF-I is the liver, though it is produced in many other tissues. IGF-I is the primary mediator of the growth-promoting effects of GH. More than 95% of acromegaly cases are caused by a pituitary adenoma that secretes excess amounts of GH (Khandwala, 2011, p. 1). Of these tumors, up to 40% have a mutation involving the alpha subunit of the stimulatory guanosine triphosphate (GTP)-binding protein. In the presence of a mutation, persistent elevation of cyclic adenosine monophosphate (cAMP) in the somatotrophs results in excessive GH secretion. The pathologic effects of GH excess include enlargement of the jaw; enlargement of the facial bone structure; enlarged hands and feet; large tongue; enlarged heart muscle, thyroid, liver, and kidney; insulin antagonism; nitrogen retention; and increased risk of colon polyps/tumors.

Clinical Manifestations

In adults, growth hormone excess (acromegaly) is characterized by local overgrowth of bone, especially in the skull and mandible (Figure 46–5◆). These patients have coarse features and large hands and feet with thick fingers and toes. There is no linear growth because the epiphyses of the long bones have fused after puberty. In children and adolescents, growth hormone excess (gigantism) is characterized by tall stature. These patients often have features similar to those of acromegaly, especially if the growth hormone excess persists beyond puberty into adulthood. Additional clinical manifestations of growth hormone excess may include excessive sweating, carpal tunnel syndrome, fatigue, lethargy, headaches, weight gain, paresthesias, joint pain, hypertension, diabetes, and cardiomegaly (enlargement of the heart). Growth hormone excess can be a chronic debilitating disorder with varying responses to different treatment modalities.

Laboratory and Diagnostic Procedures

The diagnosis of acromegaly or gigantism is made on the basis of clinical signs and symptoms and laboratory and diagnostic tests. A single measurement of serum growth hormone generally is not sufficient for the diagnosis of growth hormone excess, owing to the pulsatile or episodic release of growth hormone. Therefore, a glucose suppression test may be performed to aid in the diagnosis of growth hormone excess. See Laboratory and Diagnostic Tests for Growth Hormone Disorders on page 1394.

Patients with growth hormone excess may be hyperglycemic because of increased insulin resistance. Age- and gender-matched serum IGF-1 levels are elevated in the majority of patients with acromegaly. A computerized tomography (CT) or magnetic resonance imaging (MRI) scan may show pituitary tumors. In addition, radiographs may show enlargement of the sella turcica (the bony cavity in the skull that houses the pituitary) consistent with a pituitary tumor. Enlargement of the sinuses, hands, and feet may also be noted on radiograph scans (Gardner & Shoback, 2011; Lab Tests Online, 2012a).

LABORATORY AND DIAGNOSTIC TESTS for Growth Hormone Disorders

Description, Rationale, and Normal Values	Expected Abnormality
Growth Hormone (GH)	
Normal: Adult male: Less than 5 ng/mL Adult female: Less than 10 ng/mL Children: Less than 10 ng/mL. *A blood test used to determine the presence of human growth hormone deficit or excess.* *It aids in the diagnosis of gigantism or acromegaly.*	Decreased level indicates congenital acquired GH dwarfism in children and hypopituitarism. Increased level indicates acromegaly in adults and gigantism in children.
IGF-1 Concentrations (insulinlike growth factor-1, also known as somatomedin C)	
Normal: Normal IGF-1 levels depend on age and gender, and the reference numbers may vary slightly depending on which laboratory provides the results. Generally, they run between 100 and 300 ng/mL. *A blood test used to help diagnose the cause of growth abnormalities, monitor function, and monitor treatment of GH deficiencies and excesses. It is also used to detect a GH-producing pituitary tumor.*	If the IGF-1 concentration is decreased, it is likely that there is a GH deficiency or insensitivity to GH. Increased levels of IGF-1 usually indicate an increased production of GH. It is consistently elevated in acromegaly.
Glucose Suppression Test	
Normal: GH level of less than 1 ng/mL *A blood test used for the diagnosis of acromegaly and to determine remission after surgery. The test determines whether growth hormone production is suppressed by high blood sugar.*	The failure of growth hormone to decrease during a glucose suppression test aids in the diagnosis of growth hormone excess. Levels are nearly always elevated with acromegaly.
Computerized Tomography Scan (CT)	
Normal: No evidence of tumor *A specialized type of x-ray, brain imagery, that may be used to determine the presence of a pituitary tumor.*	Evidence of pituitary tumor.
Magnetic Resonance Imaging (MRI)	
Normal: No evidence of tumor *A scanning device used to detect the size and location of a pituitary tumor.*	Evidence of pituitary tumor.
Radiograph	
X-ray of skull to determine anomalies X-ray of hands	Reveals thickening of the skull and bones under the fingertips, and enlargement of nasal passages, with acromegaly.

Sources: Kee, J. L. (2010). *Laboratory and diagnostic tests with nursing implications.* Upper Saddle River, NJ: Prentice Hall; Lab Tests Online. (2012a). IGF-1. The test. American Association for Clinical Chemistry. Retrieved from http://labtestonline.org/understanding/analytes/igf1/ttab/test; MedlinePlus. (2011). Cortisol—urine. Retrieved from http://www.nlm.nih.gov/medlineplus/ency/article/003703.htm.

Medical Management

In 2011, the American Association of Clinical Endocrinologists published medical guidelines for clinical practice for the diagnosis and treatment of acromegaly (Katznelson, et al., 2011). These guidelines updated the 2004 guidelines by expanding recommendations based on current research studies. Altogether, 119 recommendations were made. Of particular note for future treatment care is Recommendation 119, which focuses on quality-of-life issues for patients with active acromegaly and those in remission. This recommendation has the potential to seriously impact the ways in which care is provided by the entire health care team. Refer to the National Guidelines at https://www.aace.com/files/acromegaly-guidelines.pdf for more information. Because the main causes of growth hormone excess are pituitary tumors, surgical intervention to remove these tumors is considered the initial treatment for most patients. This surgery is most successful with patients who have a small, localized mass. Somatostatin analogues (drugs that are a synthetic version of the hormone somatostatin) can be used as adjuvant treatment for preoperative shrinkage of larger tumors prior to surgery. Radiation therapy and pharmacologic intervention following surgery depend on the patient's response to the initial surgery. Transsphenoidal microsurgery (the surgical approach through the nose, along the front of the nasal septum, or under the lip and through the upper gum into the sphenoid sinus cavity) is the most common approach for removal of pituitary adenomas. This surgical procedure usually eliminates the need for a craniotomy and permits much shorter hospital stays.

Radiation may be selected as a treatment modality if the patient is not a good candidate for surgery. Radiation therapy also is used when surgical intervention is unable to remove all of the adenoma. With this method, however, reduction in growth hormone levels takes much longer, often a period of years (Melmed & Jameson, 2010). Unfortunately, since radiation therapy is associated with a high rate of late hypopituitarism and a slow rate of biochemical response, it is usually not a primary treatment (Melmed & Jameson, 2010). A number of promising targeted radiosurgery approaches are now available, including gamma knife and proton beam therapies; however, the long-term effects of these therapies are not known, and side effects have not been clearly identified (Melmed & Jameson, 2010). In these approaches, an MRI scan is used to create an image of the brain and the exact location of the tumor. The MRI is used to map locations for application of high-dose radiation beams, which are used to destroy tumor tissue while avoiding surrounding healthy tissue.

Octreotide is a somatostatin analogue medication that has proven effective in the treatment of growth hormone excess through suppression of growth hormone secretion. This medication can provide quick relief of the debilitating symptoms (Pituitary Network Association [PNA], 2012). Octreotide can provide long-acting suppression of GH in about 70% of patients; it also causes tumor shrinkage in 30% to 50% of patients. There are longer-acting somatostatin analogues (Sandostatin LAR and Lanreotide) that are preferred in the treatment of patients with acromegaly (Melmed & Jameson, 2010).

Bromocriptine and cabergoline are dopamine agonist medications (PNA). These medications lower GH secretion in about 15% of patients with acromegaly (PNA); however, GH lowering and tumor shrinkage are seen in only 10% to 15% of patients with acromegaly (PNA). Pegvisomant is a GH receptor antagonist that blocks the binding of GH to its receptor. The medication is administered by subcutaneous injections and normalizes IGF-1 in the majority of patients (Melmed & Jameson, 2010). See the Pharmacology feature on page 1379 for a complete description of these medications.

Nursing Management

Nursing management of patients with acromegaly is dependent on implementing the nursing process, the first phase of which is assessment. The patient should be assessed for both subjective and objective symptoms of acromegaly. These include verbalizations by the patient related to distress over physical appearance, anxiety over what is happening, and how it can be stopped and prevented from progressing. Objectively, the nurse should assess for progressive changes in facial features and in hat, glove, ring, or shoe size, all of which can be determined by asking the patient. The nurse should also ask the patient if he has had headaches or visual disturbances, which in acromegaly are caused by the growth of the adenoma, which exerts pressure on brain tissue and cranial nerves III, IV, and VI. The patient's history of altered sexual function should be determined, as should the presence of pain in the hands, feet, and spine. The nurse should ask the patient about any problems with chewing, swallowing, or talking, which may be caused by tongue, jaw, and teeth enlargement. She also should note the presence of a deepening of the voice, recurrent bronchitis, excessive sweating, heat intolerance, fatigue, and muscle weakness, as well as check for a family history of pituitary tumors. The nurse also should observe the patient's facial appearance, noting an enlarged supraorbital ridge, thickened ears and nose, or jutting of the jaw. If the patient has an enlarged tongue, the nurse should note any respiratory alterations. She should examine the patient's finger for skin thickening, and inspect the patient's torso, noting a barrel chest or kyphosis. In addition, the nurse should note any signs of bowed legs, assess the patient's skin for signs of oiliness or excessive sweating, assess the patient's hand strength, and test his vision for bitemporal hemianopia (defective vision or blindness in half of the visual field of one or both eyes) and loss of visual acuity. It is also important for the nurse to note if the patient has a deep, hollow-sounding voice. Because the patient undergoes some dramatic physical changes that can lead to permanent dysfunction, his self-concept and ability to perform expected roles may change. Therefore, he should be assessed for irritability, hostility, or depression. From this assessment data, diagnoses are made.

Nursing Diagnoses

Diagnoses based on assessment data include:

- *Disturbed Body Image* related to enlargement of body parts as manifested by enlarged hands, feet, and jaw.
- *Disturbed Sensory Perception* related to an enlarged pituitary gland as manifested by protrusion of the eyeballs.
- *Fluid Volume Deficit* related to polyuria as manifested by excessive thirst of the patient.
- *Anxiety* related to change in appearance and treatment as manifested by verbalization of the patient about body appearance, and the possibility of surgical treatment.
- *Ineffective Coping* related to change in appearance as manifested by verbalization of negative feeling about the change in appearance.
- *Knowledge Deficit* regarding development of disease and treatment as manifested by repeated questions by the patient regarding disease and treatment.

NANDA-I © 2012

Outcomes

Outcomes reflect the patient's desired response to nursing interventions, indicating resolution of nursing problems. In this situation with the acromegalic patient, they include the following: recognition and acceptance of body image as verbalized by the patient; improved sensory perception as indicted by reports of improved vision and improved comfort related to vision and position of eyeballs; ability to concentrate, remain oriented, and be free of sensory distortions; fluid and electrolyte status within normal range; increased skin turgor, reduced thirst; verbalizes feeling less anxious; and has increased understanding of the disease process and what is happening to his body. He acknowledges the possibility of surgery and appears receptive to learning about pre- and postoperative care. The patient verbalizes his coping deficits and expresses willingness to try new coping strategies.

Interventions and Rationales

Interventions are focused on helping the patient achieve desired outcomes and resolution of perceived problems (nursing diagnoses). They include assessing the patient's body changes and offering psychological support; assessing the patient's sensory perception status and administering medication, if ordered; and assessing the patient's fluid and electrolyte status and providing more fluids to the patient. Relative to the patient's anxiety level, the nurse might explain to the patient about progressive features of the disorder, allow the patient to talk about his concerns, and actively listen to the patient. The coping strategies engaged by the patient also should be discussed. The nurse needs to provide emotional support with explanation of and preparation for diagnostic tests and other components of the treatment plan. It is important to assess the patient's knowledge level regarding the disease's progression and treatment of the disorder. The nurse should clarify the patient's doubts and questions regarding hyperpituitary disorders.

Because most patients with acromegaly will undergo surgery, the nurse should prepare the patient for surgery and postoperative recovery from tumor resection. Preoperative nursing care includes instillation of antibiotic nose drops and discussion about mouth breathing, oral hygiene, early ambulation and activity, pain management, and medications. If the tumor is small and localized, it can be removed with transsphenoidal microsurgery. Nasal padding may be required for a brief period after surgery. Postoperative complications include increased intracranial pressure, meningitis, and transient diabetes insipidus. If and when symptoms of the complications develop, the nurse must notify the health care provider immediately.

Postoperative nursing care includes neurological assessment due to the risk of increased intracranial pressure and observations of temperature, pupils, vital signs, and fluid balance. The head of the patient's bed should always be elevated at a 30-degree angle to reduce headaches and pressure on the entry point in the sella turcica. To prevent leakage of cerebrospinal fluid, the patient should be cautioned to avoid coughing, sneezing, straining at stool, or other activities that would initiate the Valsalva maneuver. Leaking of CSF, which is signaled by complaints of persistent generalized or supraorbital headache, increases the risk of meningitis and warrants prophylactic antibiotics, bed rest, and continued elevation of the head of the patient's bed. Nasal drainage, if present, should be tested for glucose, which also indicates leakage of CSF.

Oral hygiene should be provided with caution to avoid trauma to the surgical site. The nurse should provide oral hygiene at 4-hour intervals and advise the patient not to use a toothbrush for up to 10 days. In addition, the nurse should take seizure precautions, such as keeping the bed lowered and side rails padded, and provide mild analgesia for pain. Because transient diabetes insipidus may occur following surgery due to loss of ADH stored in the pituitary, urine output and serum and urine osmolality should be monitored (see the section later on diabetes insipidus). The nurse should advise the patient to avoid exercise and unusual activities at home until cleared to do otherwise by the health care provider.

Discharge Priorities

Continued follow-up is required after initial treatment for acromegaly to ensure that the patient's hormone levels return to normal and that efforts are made to address any symptoms and complaints. Priorities for discharge also depend on the severity of the patient's condition prior to surgery, the patient's age, and other comorbidities. The Patient Teaching & Discharge Priorities box details components of the discharge plan for patients with growth hormone disorders.

Health Promotion

Patients with pituitary adenoma can have an improved quality of life with appropriate follow-up and case management. Patients should be instructed on signs of hypopituitarism, including severe chronic fatigue, central obesity, and reduced muscle mass, because they may experience this syndrome following treatment of the pituitary adenoma. Management of related endocrine disorders also is important. Referrals to support groups and organizations devoted to the needs of patients with pituitary problems may be another health promotion strategy to be considered.

Collaborative Management

A collaborative group of health care professionals is needed to thoroughly address the post-discharge and follow-up needs of the patient with acromegaly. This group may include (at minimum) the nurse, health care provider, and pharmacist. In order to meet desired patient outcomes, it is essential that this interdisciplinary team communicate openly with one another in developing and evaluating care of the patient and family (IOM [Institute of Medicine], 2010). For example, the patient may need to learn how to give subcutaneous injections. This may necessitate a meeting with the patient, family member(s), nurse, and pharmacist to learn this technique. Additionally, this disorder requires close follow-up to determine response to treatment. The patient and family may meet with the nurse to discuss follow-up appointments, along with clinical signs and symptoms that may prompt immediate consultation with health care providers.

Disorders of the Hypothalamus and Posterior Pituitary

Antidiuretic hormone (ADH) (vasopressin) is synthesized by the supraopticus and paraventricular nuclei of the hypothalamus and released by the posterior pituitary. The primary action of ADH is to increase the permeability of the distal convoluted tubule and collecting ducts of the kidney to water, thereby promoting the concentration of urine. The osmoreceptors that control thirst and osmotic regulation of ADH are located in the hypothalamus and are sensitive to small changes in serum osmolality. An increase in serum osmolality increases the release of ADH; in contrast, a decrease in serum osmolality decreases the release of ADH. There also are volume receptors in the atria and pulmonary

PATIENT TEACHING & DISCHARGE PRIORITIES for Growth Hormone Disorders

Need	Teaching
Knowledge of disease process and prognosis	Home care needs include verbal and written instructions for the treatment plan, the disease process, and the follow-up care and prognosis. These instructions will reinforce the need to follow the treatment plan and comply with therapy.
Understanding of medications	The patient and family are taught action, dosage, route, and side effects and how to administer medications. Instruct on administering an injectable medication, if appropriate.
Body image disturbance	Encourage the patient and family to express feelings about body image and how it is impacting their lives. Address anxiety concerns regarding changes in the thickness of skin and enlargment of the face, hands, and feet. Assist the patient to find support groups with similar disabilities if appropriate.
Ambulation and activities of daily living (ADL)	Encourage the patient to ambulate and complete ADLs. Discuss using assistive equipment in performing ADLs if necessary. Refer the patient with arthritic conditions to a physical therapist. Instruct the patient to avoid activities that increase intracranial pressure for up to 2 months after surgery.
Emotional and social support	Encourage the patient and family to express their feelings about the disease process. Help the patient identify socially intereractive activities he would like to be engaged in. Recommend counseling if appropriate.

venous system and baroreceptors in the carotid sinus and aortic arch. Decreased pressure and volume are associated with increased ADH, whereas increased pressure and volume decrease ADH. The two primary disorders of ADH secretion are diabetes insipidus and syndrome of inappropriate antidiuretic hormone.

Diabetes Insipidus

The primary defect in **diabetes insipidus (DI)** is defined as an inability of the kidneys to concentrate urine, resulting from an absolute or relative lack of circulating ADH. Diabetes insipidus is characterized by the passing of large amounts of dilute urine. If there is a partial or complete absence of ADH, the disorder is called *central diabetes insipidus*. If there is resistance of the renal tubules to the actions of ADH, this disorder is termed *nephrogenic diabetes insipidus*.

Epidemiology

The prevalence of congenital DI is 4 cases per 100,000 persons, and the incidence of this disorder is similar in men and women. The prevalence of the X-linked form of nephrogenic DI is 0.4 cases per 100,000 ("Diabetes Insipidus," 2011).

Etiology and Risk Factors

Diabetes insipidus is caused by a deficiency of antidiuretic hormone, also known as vasopressin, due to the destruction of the posterior portion of the pituitary gland where vasopressin is normally released, or by an insensitivity of the kidneys to that hormone. It can also be induced iatrogenically by various drugs. Diabetes insipidus can be genetic or acquired. The genetic form of central DI is inherited as an autosomal dominant or X-linked trait. The hereditary forms of central DI account for only 1% to 2% of all cases (Mayo Clinic Staff, 2010). The primary form of central DI is acquired, resulting from injury to the neurohypophysis, such as head trauma, neoplasms, and infections. Congenital nephrogenic DI is inherited as an X-linked disorder; however, nephrogenic DI also can be an autosomal recessive disorder ("Diabetes Insipidus," 2011). Nephrogenic DI primarily results from metabolic abnormalities (e.g., hypokalemia (low potassium) and hypercalcemia) or pharmacologic preparations that interfere with the actions of ADH (e.g., lithium or demeclocycline). The risk factors for nephrogenic DI include renal disease (e.g., chronic renal failure, chronic renal medullary disease, and pyelonephritis), electrolyte disturbances (e.g., chronic hypokalemia), drugs (e.g., demeclocycline, lithium), medical disorders (e.g., sickle cell disease), pregnancy, and genetic predisposition (Medical News Today, 2012). The risk factors for central DI include injury to the central nervous system, neoplastic or autoimmune disease, hypothalamic disease, pituitary surgery or ischemia, brain irradiation, infection (e.g., meningitis), cerebral edema, and intracranial hemorrhage and genetic predisposition.

Pathophysiology

Central DI can be permanent or transient depending on the underlying disorder. Only 15% of the ADH-secreting cells of the hypothalamus need to be present to maintain fluid balance under normal conditions (Else & Hammer, 2010). Destruction of the posterior pituitary alone does not result in permanent DI; destruction of the hypothalamus or part of the supraoptic hypophyseal tract must also occur (Else & Hammer, 2010). More commonly, central DI results transiently from an acute injury marked by neuronal shock and edema leading to inability to produce ADH (Else & Hammer, 2010). However, as the underlying abnormality (e.g., edema) improves, ADH secretion resumes.

The genetic form of **nephrogenic diabetes insipidus** results from a generalized defect in the V_2 class of the ADH (vasopressin) receptor, the aquaporin-2 water channel, or the renal tubules (Else & Hammer, 2010). Drug-induced DI can result from decreased sensitivity of the receptors to ADH and is usually reversible after the drug is withdrawn.

Clinical Manifestations

Diabetes insipidus is characterized by the excretion of a large volume of dilute and hypotonic urine. The clinical signs and symptoms of DI result from polyuria and polydipsia. Polyuria associated with DI is defined as urine volume of more than 3 liters in 24 hours (Medical News Today, 2012).

Damage to the hypothalamus-posterior pituitary region due to head trauma, surgery, or primary or metastatic tumor may result in decreased production of ADH, resulting in DI. Patients with the previous conditions or procedures should be monitored closely for the clinical signs and symptoms of DI, especially polyuria, to prevent hypovolemic shock.

Mortality is rare in adults as long as water is available. However, severe dehydration, hypernatremia, fever, cardiovascular collapse, and death can ensue in children, elderly people, or in those with complicating illnesses.

Laboratory and Diagnostic Studies

The diagnosis of DI is largely a diagnosis of exclusion since a variety of disorders can cause polyuria and polydipsia (e.g., diabetes mellitus, renal disease). See the Laboratory and Diagnostic Tests for Diabetes Insipidus and Syndrome for Inappropriate Diuretic Hormone (SIADH) box on page 1398.

The diagnosis of DI can be made without a water deprivation test; however, the water deprivation test can help to distinguish between central DI and nephrogenic DI (Medical News Today, 2012). The water deprivation test evaluates the release of ADH in response to volume depletion. In normal physiology, the release of ADH stimulates volume depletion, resulting in fluid volume expansion and urinary concentration. Patients with DI often are able to maintain fluid volume by drinking large quantities of fluid. When deprived of water, these patients have decreased fluid volume, hypernatremia (increased sodium), and dilute urine.

Medical Management

Diabetes insipidus treatment depends on the type and severity of patient illness. With central origin diabetes insipidus, the primary treatment involves replacement with ADH analogues. Desmopressin (1-deamino-8-D-arginine vasopressin, DDAVP) is the current drug of choice for long-term therapy of central DI and can be given intravenously, subcutaneously, orally, or intranasally. The secondary treatment of central DI includes chlorpropamide, carbamazepine, clofibrate, and thiazide diuretics (see the Pharmacology feature, p. 1379). In addition, with central type diabetes insipidus, replacing lost fluids is essential. This may be possible through oral intake; if not, intravenous solutions are used to maintain fluid balance.

The treatment of nephrogenic DI, which is the result of kidney disease and does not respond adequately to ADH, is challenging. Desmopressin is not a treatment option; instead, a diet low in salt to help reduce the amount of urine the kidney produces is recommended. In addition, the patient must drink enough water to avoid dehydration. Medications that improve ADH sensitivity and relieve symptoms (e.g., chlorpropamide and carbamazepine) may be used. Also, discontinuation of any offending drug or underlying pathology may reverse the condition.

LABORATORY AND DIAGNOSTIC TESTS for Diabetes Insipidus and Syndrome for Inappropriate Diuretic Hormone (SIADH)

Test with Description, Rationale, and Normal Value	Expected Abnormality
Urinary Osmolality	
Normal: Adult: 50–1,200 mOsm/kg; the average being 200–800 mOsm/kg *Test used to assess the kidney's ability to concentrate and dilute urine.*	Measurement of urinary osmolality can help to diagnose DI and differentiate between different causes of polyuria (e.g., hyperglycemia). If the urine osmolality is less than 200 mOsm/kg in the presence of polyuria, then diabetes insipidus is present. Increased value indicates SIADH.
Plasma Osmolality	
Normal: Adult 280–300 mOsm/kg Panic values = Less than 240 mOsm/kg and greater than 320 mOsm/kg *A blood test used to identify serum concentration by measuring the number of dissolved particles (electrolytes, urea, sugar) in the serum; thus, it monitors body fluid balance and determines the occurrence of fluid overload or dehydration.*	Decreased levels indicate excessive fluid intake, adrenal cortical hypofunction, and syndrome of inappropriate diuretic hormone (SIADH). Increased levels indicate diabetes insipidus and dehydration.
Antidiuretic Hormone (ADH)	
Normal: Adult: 1–5 pg/mL or 1–5 ng/L *A blood test used to detect a deficit or excess in ADH secretion, as well as identify the presence of body fluid deficit or excess.*	Decreased level indicates central diabetes insipidus. Increased level indicates SIADH.
Urinary Sodium	
Normal: Adult: 40–220 Eq/L/24 hours *A urine test used to monitor sodium level, detect sodium imbalance (hypo- or hypernatremia), and compare the sodium level with that of other electrolytes (i.e., calcium, potassium, chloride).*	Decreased level indicates Cushing syndrome or low sodium intake. Increased level indicates pituitary hypofunction, Addison's disease, dehydration, or high sodium intake.
Water Deprivation Test (also called water loading ADH suppression test)	
Normal value: Urine osmolality: 285–295 mOsm *A diagnostic test to determine the presence of excess secretion of antidiuretic hormone (ADH), also called SIADH. This test is designed to suppress the secretion of ADH from the posterior pituitary gland through water loading.* Urine osmolality is measured for 30 and 60 minutes following administration, and plasma osmolality is measured periodically. *Normally, as fluid intake increases, urine output increases and urine osmolality decreases.*	With SIADH, as water intake increases the urine output does not increase. As a result, the urine osmolality could be higher than serum osmolality. In central diabetes insipidus, urine osmolality remains less than plasma osmolality after dehydration; after administration of synthetic ADH, urine osmolality increases by more than 50% (Medical News Today, 2012). In nephrogenic diabetes insipidus, urine osmolality remains less than plasma osmolality; after the administration of synthetic ADH, urine osmolality increases by less than 50% (Medical News Today, 2012).

If the diabetes insipidus is caused by a tumor or abnormal growth on the hypothalamus or pituitary gland, surgery is recommended to remove the growth. The patient, then, is treated as a surgical patient with pre- and postoperative care as well as treatment for the diabetes insipidus. Treatment should be individualized, and patients should be monitored for the development of polyuria or hypo-osmolality. Fluid intake and output should be carefully recorded, and patients questioned about their thirst. Antidiuretic hormone therapy should be initiated. Desmopressin may be administered on an as-needed basis. Fluid balance is maintained by allowing the patient to drink according to her thirst; in addition, supplemental administration of hypotonic intravenous fluids may be used. The patient should be closely observed for hyponatremia. The patient also may be presumed to have anterior pituitary insufficiency and should receive corticosteroid replacement therapy (Cooperman, 2011; "Diabetes Insipidus," 2011; Loh & Verbalis, 2011; Mayo Clinic Staff, 2010).

Nursing Management

The primary goal in nursing care for hospitalized patients with central or nephrogenic DI is to prevent dehydration and shock, two potential complications of DI resulting from fluid loss (Cloe, 2012). This involves the administration of medications, intravenous and oral fluids, and electrolyte replacement. Additionally, if the patient has had surgery to remove a pituitary tumor, or is scheduled for surgery, pre- and postoperative care also is a primary focus. Preoperative care acknowledges the patient's anxiety related to body changes, fear of the unknown, brain involvement, and chronic, lifelong care implications of hypopituitary conditions following the procedure.

Postoperative care and teaching focus on pain control, ambulation, hormone replacement, activity, monitoring incision for drainage and bleedings, and neurological assessment and lung assessment. Patients are encouraged to avoid bending and straining for 2 months post-surgery, to use stool softeners, to avoid coughing, to use saline mouth rinses, and not to use toothbrushes for 7 to 10 days. The nurse should check for cerebral spinal fluid leak by assessing nasal drainage for the presence of glucose where the sella turcica was entered. If present, the nurse should notify the health care provider.

Potential nursing diagnoses to consider include *Deficient Fluid Volume*, *Risk for Impaired Skin Integrity*, and *Deficient Knowledge*. In light of these potential diagnoses, ongoing assessment includes monitoring intake and output, monitoring for increased thirst, monitoring daily weight, determining urine specific gravity, monitoring serum and urine osmolality, monitoring urine and serum sodium levels and serum potassium, and monitoring for signs of hypovolemic shock (e.g., tachycardia, tachypnea, hypotension). Ongoing assessment also includes assessing the patient for skin integrity, continence or incontinence, and other factors that may affect the patient's skin integrity, such as immobility, nutritional status, and altered mental status. In addition, the nurse must assess the patient's level of knowledge of DI cause and treatment, as well as the patient's readiness to learn. Nursing interventions are designed to alleviate the problems suggested by this assessment data and promote positive patient outcomes. The nurse should provide easy access to the bathroom, urinal, or bedpan; use skin barriers as needed; and keep the bed linen clean, dry, and wrinkle free. Consistent with the potential lack of knowledge, the nurse should provide written information concerning the diagnosis and treatment, meaning of the diagnostic tests, and instructions regarding the necessity of closely monitoring fluid balance, including daily weights, fluid intake and output, and maintenance of urine specific gravity.

Desired outcomes are skin integrity; knowledge of the disease process, medications, and specified interventions; and knowledge of how to prepare for home care. If the patient is recovering from surgery (e.g., removal of a pituitary tumor), instructions also should be provided on how to care for the wound and symptoms of surgical complications (e.g., increased drainage from wound, redness of wound, swelling around incision). Patients should continue to monitor their fluid status, take and record vital signs, and be aware of the symptoms of impending shock caused by dehydration: rapid and weak heartbeat, low blood pressure, high fever, feeling weak, and fainting (Cloe, 2012).

Patients with chronic DI have a lifetime commitment to managing this condition through medication and fluid regimens. The primary nursing care goal in the home setting, post-hospitalization, is to help patients manage these regimens effectively. An individualized discharge program needs to be developed based on the patient's knowledge of the disease and the patient's readiness to learn about the disease, treatment, and prognosis. Postoperative teaching focuses on pain control, ambulation, hormone replacement, and activity. Incorporated within the plan is the need for the patient to understand how fluid volume overload, fluid volume deficit, alteration in nutrients, and alteration in tissue perfusion affect his recovery and health status.

Discharge Priorities and Health Promotion

Discharge priorities for the patient with DI focus on patient instruction regarding the nature of the disease, as well as the importance of hydration and strategies to ensure the availability of fluid at all times. Postoperative instructions include ambulation, use of medications (e.g., hormone replacement), pain control, surgical wound management, and activity. Patients are cautioned to avoid straining, coughing, and sneezing to avoid incisional disruption. To assist with this, patients may take stool softeners and use saline mouth rinses, since they should not use a toothbrush for 7 to 10 days. Patients also are advised to seek medical care if the drainage from the nose increases; if severe headaches develop; if they have chills, a cough, or feel week and achy; if they have nausea; if a bandage becomes soaked with blood; if the skin is itchy, swollen, or has a rash; if patients have chest pain or trouble breathing; or if they have questions or concerns about the surgery, current condition, or care (University of Wisconsin Health, 2010).

If patients are taking antipituitary drugs to counteract excess hormone production, instructions should include signs and symptoms of the drugs' side effects. In addition, the route and timing of medications should be discussed and written down.

It is not uncommon for further treatment to be required if the tumor is not completely removed and continues to grow over time. Patients should be advised to continue follow-up evaluations with the endocrinologist so that additional treatment such as radiation therapy or medications can be used to reduce symptoms and to improve quality of life. Predictions regarding the course of care can be difficult, and therapies are initiated as needed: physical therapy for muscle strengthening, gait, balance, and mobility; occupational therapy for activities of daily living and safety recommendations; and speech therapy for language, speech articulation, and swallowing.

Patients should be instructed to always carry water with them, so they are never without it. The nurse should discuss ways in which this may change their social and professional habits and provide alternative solutions.

Patients and their families may need emotional support and strengthened methods of coping due to their unfamiliarity with, and the life-altering nature of, this disease. Referral to support groups and community resources, such as Family Village Library, also may be appropriate. Many resources are provided by the Diabetes Insipidus Foundation, Inc. via the Internet (www.familyvillage.wisc.edu/lib_di.htm). Social services also may be used to help connect patients and families with community resources.

The patient should always wear medical alert jewelry and carry a medical identification card so that, in an emergency situation, the patient's condition is known and the treatment can be appropriate and efficient.

Weblink: Diabetes Insipidus Online Resources

Syndrome of Inappropriate Antidiuretic Hormone (ADH) Secretion

Syndrome of inappropriate ADH secretion (SIADH) is a disorder of sodium and water balance characterized by hyponatremia, serum hypo-osmolarity, and impaired urinary dilution in the absence of renal disease or any identifiable nonosmotic stimulus known to release ADH (Esposito, Piotti, Bianzina, Malul, & Dal Canton, 2011). This results in a reduction in urinary output and fluid volume expansion.

Risk Factors and Etiology

SIADH occurs in patients who have central nervous system disorders; patients who have experienced shock, trauma, stress, or surgery; and patients with malignancies or pulmonary infections such as tuberculosis, bacterial pneumonia, or a lung abscess. Selected drugs, including narcotics, tranquilizers, barbiturates, general anesthetics, thiazide diuretics, hypoglycemic agents, antidepressants, and some chemotherapeutic agents, also are associated with rare cases of SIADH. A high percentage of patients with SIADH have a malignancy; this will often be a small cell or oat cell carcinoma lung cancer (Hannon & Thompson, 2010), but other forms of cancer also have been found to cause this disorder. Malignant cells can secrete ADH or ADH-like chemicals, which serve as an ectopic source of ADH. Seriously ill ventilated patients also may experience an increase in the release of ADH.

Pathophysiology

The hallmark of SIADH is excess ADH secretion despite plasma hypotonicity (lower osmotic pressure). The excess ADH in SIADH comes from the hypothalamus or an ectopic source (e.g., malignant tumors).

Irrespective of the source of ADH, the result is the same. There is decreased free water clearance due to increased free water reabsorption by the distal and collecting tubules; the subsequent dilution leads to hypotonicity and hyponatremia. Despite the hyponatremia, there is also a natriuresis (excessive loss of sodium in the urine) (Thomas, 2012). Diagnosis of SIADH is dependent on fulfillment of five cardinal features: (1) hypotonic hyponatremia, (2) natriuresis, (3) urine osmolality in excess of plasma osmolality, (4) absence of edema and volume depletion, and (5) normal renal and adrenal function (Porth & Matfin, 2009).

Clinical Manifestations

The clinical signs and symptoms of SIADH are related to hyponatremia, which may begin with fatigue, headache, nausea, and anorexia and proceed to altered mental status, seizures, coma, and death. Since hyponatremia may have many causes, the diagnosis of SIADH also is largely a diagnosis of exclusion. It cannot be made unless the patient is euvolemic (sufficient blood in the body) with normal renal, adrenal, and thyroid function.

Hyponatremia is a common and potentially life-threatening problem that occurs frequently in hospitalized patients. Patients with mild to moderate hyponatremia are often asymptomatic, especially if the hyponatremia develops slowly. However, patients with acute rapid-onset hyponatremia ($<$120 mEq/dL) occurring over 24 hours or less are often symptomatic. Patients with acute hyponatremia may present with nausea, vomiting, lethargy, restlessness, hyporeflexia, seizures, and altered sensorium. These findings are thought to result from cerebral edema as the hypotonic extracellular fluid volume shifts water into the cerebral cortical cells (Gardner, 2011).

Laboratory and Diagnostic Tests

The essential features of SIADH include decreased effective plasmatic osmolality ($<$275 mOsm/kg); increased urinary osmolality ($U_{osm} >$ 100 mOsm/kg during serum hypo-osmolality); increased urinary sodium (>40 mmol/L with normal dietary salt and water intake); and clinical euvolemia (the proper amount of blood in the body), as defined by the absence of signs of hypovolemia (e.g., orthostasis, tachycardia, decreased skin turgor, dry mucous membranes) or hypervolemia (e.g., ascites) (Esposito et al., 2011; Gardner & Shoback, 2011; Thomas, 2012). (See the Laboratory and Diagnosis Tests for Diabetes Insipidus and SIADH feature on page 1398.)

Medical Management

A thorough history is necessary to discriminate among various causes of hyponatremia. The treatment of SIADH depends on several factors, including the degree of hyponatremia along with the severity and duration of the symptoms. In patients with SIADH who have few symptoms, the objective is to gradually reduce body water and correct the hyponatremia through fluid restriction (Robertson, 2010). The fluid restriction is based on insensible (imperceptible loss through perspiration and breathing) and urinary fluid losses. Since insensible fluid losses are primarily replaced by the water content of food (300 to 700 mL/day), the typical fluid restriction usually is approximately 500 mL less than urinary output (Robertson, 2010). This fluid restriction can result in an increase in serum sodium of approximately 1% to 2% per day (Robertson, 2010). In the presence of severe symptomatic hyponatremia, this fluid restriction can be supplemented by intravenous hypertonic (3%) fluids. If the hypertonic sodium is given too rapidly in a patient who has had hyponatremia for more than 24 to 48 hours, profound neurological changes can occur (Robertson, 2010). Therefore, protocols that guide the infusion rate, timing of biochemical measurements, and clinical (particularly neurological assessment) monitoring procedures should be followed. In chronic SIADH, the hyponatremia can be treated with fluid restriction and medications (e.g., demeclocycline and lithium) that induce a reversible form of nephrogenic DI. Currently, vasopressin receptor antagonist medications are under development which may prove helpful in the treatment of SIADH (Esposito et al., 2011; Golay, 2011).

Nursing Management

The nursing management of the patient with SIADH primarily revolves around the recognition and treatment of hyponatremia. Symptoms and clinical manifestations are considered during the assessment phase of the nursing process, as are patient outcomes and nursing interventions.

Assessment

Assessment of the patient is critical in determining the multiple signs and symptoms representative of SIADH and this disorder's effect on body systems (e.g., neurologic, cardiovascular, pulmonary, gastrointestinal, and musculoskeletal). Vital signs reflect the body's response to excess fluids; thus, they need to be assessed regularly. For example the blood pressure may be increased or may be normal; the patient may be tachycardic. Neurological assessment determines the patient's response to fluid overload and potential electrolyte imbalances, which might include evidence of seizures and confusion. In addition, it is essential to know if the patient is experiencing any of the following signs and symptoms, which are all evident in a systemic reaction to SIADH: bounding pulse, pulmonary crackles, cramps, vomiting, decreased bowel sounds, muscle weakness, cramps, and absence of deep tension reflexes. Subjective assessment also includes questions of the patient regarding how he feels physically, such as if he has noticed any muscle weakness, lethargy or weakness in general, and/or restlessness. Emotional assessment is essential. Assessment of hydration, including skin turgor, mucous membranes, intake and output, daily weight, and monitoring for fluid overload, is essential. Based on the subjective and objective assessment data, nursing diagnoses are formulated.

Nursing Diagnoses

- *Excess Fluid Volume* related to excessive amount of antidiuretic hormone (ADH) secretion and compromised regulatory mechanism.
- *Risk for Injury* related to altered level of consciousness, confusion, with possibility of seizures.
- *Imbalanced Nutrition, Less Than Body Requirements* related to an inability to ingest or digest foods or absorb nutrients because of biologic factors (e.g., nausea and vomiting, anorexia).
- *Disturbed Thought Processes* related to physiological changes in the CNS, the brain's response to changes in osmolality.
- *Possible Ineffective Tissue Perfusion* related to cardiovascular disturbances caused by fluid and electrolyte imbalance.
- *Risk for Decreased Cardiac Output* related to cardiac dysrhythmias caused by electrolyte imbalance.
- *Ineffective Breathing Pattern* related to pulmonary congestion from fluid overload.
- *Potential Excess Fluid Volume* related to retention of free water, fluid replacement therapy.
- *Risk for Impaired Skin Integrity* related to immobility and edema.

- *Airway Compromise* related to low sodium serum level and/or seizure activity.
- *Knowledge Deficit* related to unfamiliarity with disease and treatment plan.
- *Ineffective Coping and Compromised Family Coping* related to the threat of disease and loss of control.

NANDA-I © 2012

Outcomes With Evaluation Parameters

The overriding outcome is that the patient will regain fluid and electrolyte balance and normal body fluid concentration. The patient's clinical status will reflect a decrease in excess fluid volume as measured by serum sodium levels: as they increase, the fluid volume decreases. The patient remains free from injury, maintains consciousness, and demonstrates orientation to time, place, and person. Balanced nutrition is achieved as evidenced by the patient's ability and willingness to eat foods without gastric upset and as recommended by the dietitian. Relative to disturbed thought processes, the patient will be able to think clearly as observed through his verbalization and problem-solving approaches. He is no longer confused; he recognizes people and knows where he is. Effective tissue perfusion is recognized through measurement of peripheral issues (e.g., lack of edema, strong peripheral pulses, dry skin [not clammy], and no numbness). Other indications of effective tissue perfusion include the patient's response to situations; he is alert and oriented, as well as appearing calm and restful. Bowel sounds are present; there is no evidence of nausea and vomiting. The heart rate and blood pressure are normal and the patient also demonstrates easy breathing without shortness of breath. If the patient has experienced an excess fluid level as a complication, the expectation is that this level will decrease and can be measured by serum sodium test and serum and urine osmolality.

The patient's skin should be intact, clear, and free from ulcers. The patient will understand the disease process and the treatment plan, with the evaluation parameter being verbalization of such and asking appropriate questions related to the disease and treatments, including self-care and the administration of medications. The patient and the family will identify coping strategies and discuss ways in which the illness is affecting them. They also will verbalize ways in which they can adjust and seek counseling, if needed.

Interventions and Rationales

Many interventions are designed to assist the patient and family in meeting desired outcomes, and they sometimes overlap, with one intervention meeting several objectives. Strict monitoring of intake and output is mandatory to determine fluid overload. The nurse should determine fluid balance every 8 hours, compare daily serial weights, and note rapid changes in weight; changes in weight of 0.5 to 1 kg/day suggest fluid imbalance. In addition, the nurse should evaluate hydration status every 4 hours, noting skin turgor and development of edema or crackles. He also should engage the patient in a plan to restrict fluids. Fluids generally are restricted to 1,000 mL/24 hours, or, if the condition is severe, it may be limited to 600 mL/24 hours. The nurse needs to enforce these restrictions and explore ways to maintain these restrictions with the patient. If thirst and a dry mouth are causing discomfort, alternatives such as hard candy, chewing gum, or a mouthwash could be offered. The nurse should work with the pharmacy to concentrate all medications in the lowest volume that is safe for the patient. In addition, he should arrange for a consultation with the dietitian to help plan for amounts of fluid throughout the day, as well as to find foods that sound appealing to the patient and have nutritional value to help the patient regain nutritional balance. The nurse needs to review serum sodium, serum osmolality, and urine osmolality to evaluate the patient's response to therapy. He should also monitor vital signs frequently and maintain a safe environment for the patient to prevent injury. This can be achieved by keeping the bed in the low position, with side rails up and padded, for seizure precautions. If a patient seizes, the nurse should remain with the patient until fully conscious, place the patient in a side-lying position, loosen restrictive clothing to promote breathing and prevent low oxygen levels, protect the patient's head from injury, note the duration and type of seizure, be sure not to restrain the patient, and move furniture away from the patient. If the patient is weak and has poor muscle strength, place her on the agency's fall prevention program.

The nurse must monitor the ECG for dysrhythmias resulting from electrolyte imbalance. He also must monitor the patient's neurological signs on a regular basis to determine CNS status. The nurse should encourage the patient to verbalize thoughts and make decisions in order to determine thought processes. He must monitor the status of tissue perfusion by checking peripheral pulses, peripheral edema, clammy skin, pain or numbness, and cardiovascular effects such as hypotension or angina, as well as cerebral issues such as lethargy, confusion, and restlessness. The nurse should also check the patient for gastrointestinal problems such as nausea, abdominal pain, or decreased or absent bowel sounds. The nurse should monitor the patient's breathing pattern and evaluate any difficulties present; in addition, he should assist the patient with breathing, if necessary, by inserting an oral or nasal airway or preparing the patient for endotracheal intubation, if it is needed. If the patient is able to maintain her airway and breathing, the nurse should position the patient so that the head of the bed is either flat or elevated no more than 10 degrees. This position enhances venous return and increases left atria filling pressure; in turn, this reduces the release of ADH. The nurse continues to monitor the patient's skin condition on a regular basis, assessing for pressure ulcer development secondary to edema and immobility. To help prevent skin breakdown, he should place patient on a decubitus prevention program approved by the agency, encourage mobility, and reposition every 2 hours to limit the complications of immobility. In addition, the nurse needs to prepare the patient for discharge. Specifics of preparation for discharge are detailed in the Discharge Priorities section.

Discharge Priorities and Collaboration

The discharge priorities for patients with SIADH include teaching the patient and family about medication administration and the importance of adherence. The nurse will need to make sure that the patient or significant others understand the medication regimen, including the dosage, route, action, adverse effects, and need for follow-up laboratory tests. He should instruct the patient to report changes in voiding patterns, level of consciousness, presence of edema, symptoms of hyponatremia, reduced neurological functioning, nausea and vomiting, and muscle cramping. If the patient is going home on fluid restriction, the nurse must discuss methods of limiting fluid intake and encourage the patient to weigh herself to monitor for fluid retention. The nurse should provide instructions on fluid restriction to the patient and/or family to prevent excess fluid retention. In addition, he should assess their ability to understand the instructions. The patient may also have any of a number of serious illnesses that may entail the collaborative resources of a home health team including (at minimum) a health care provider who is responsible for developing the treatment plan, a pharmacist who can assist the patient in understanding medications and how to take them, and a home health nurse. The nurse evaluates the patient's physical, mental, and emotional responses to the treatment program, collaborates with the patient in detecting complications of SIADH or other comorbidity issues, and indicates when to notify the health care provider if unusual symptoms occur. For example, with SIADH symptoms, the patient should be advised to report symptoms such as rapid weight gain, loss of consciousness, rapid heartbeat, and extreme weakness (IOM [Institute of Medicine], 2010).

Disorders of the Adrenal Glands

The adrenal glands are bilateral structures located on the superior poles of each kidney. The adrenal glands consist of two major divisions: the adrenal medulla and the adrenal cortex, which are located in the inner and outer portions, respectively. The adrenal cortex is divided into three layers. The inner layer of the adrenal cortex is the zona reticularis; the middle layer is the adrenal zona fasciculata; and the outer layer is the zona glomerulosa (Figure 46–6◆).

The adrenal medulla is part of the sympathetic nervous system. The major secretory products of the adrenal medulla are the catecholamines epinephrine and norepinephrine. In humans, approximately 90% of circulating epinephrine is produced in the adrenal medulla. In addition, approximately 7% of norepinephrine is produced in the adrenal medulla; the remainder originates from nonadrenal sympathetic nerve cells and synapses. These catecholamines bind with alpha- and beta-adrenergic receptors to exert their effects. In general, the release of catecholamines increases heart rate, cardiac output, and vasoconstriction, resulting in increased blood pressure. In addition, catecholamines have effects on extravascular smooth muscle in a variety of tissues. These include contraction and relaxation of the uterine myometrium; relaxation of the intestinal and bladder smooth muscle; contraction of smooth muscle in the bladder and intestinal sphincters; relaxation of tracheal smooth muscle; and papillary dilation. Catecholamines also have effects on metabolism, stimulating gluconeogenesis, glycogenolysis, and lipolysis. The primary disorders of the adrenal medulla are adrenomedullary hyperfunction or hypofunction. Each of the three layers of the adrenal cortex secretes a predominant type of hormone. The zona glomerulosa, for example, produces the mineralocorticoid aldosterone. The primary function of aldosterone is in the distal nephron: to promote Na^+ and water reabsorption and K^+ and H^+ excretion.

The zona fasciculata produces the glucocorticoid cortisol. This hormone has diverse effects on a variety of tissues. For example, cortisol increases gluconeogenesis and lipolysis, decreases protein synthesis, inhibits bone formation, stimulates bone resorption, suppresses the immune system, and is a potent anti-inflammatory. In addition, it stimulates red blood cell production and alters mood and behavior. Cortisol is necessary for the integrity of the gastrointestinal tract; it also is necessary for the vascular response to catecholamines.

The zona reticularis produces the androgen precursors dehydroepiandrosterone (DHEA), DHEA-sulfate, and androstenedione. These are converted peripherally into active androgens, providing approximately 50% of circulating androgens in women. The adrenal androgens have little effect on men; however, they promote pubic and axillary hair growth in women.

The adrenocortical feedback loop is illustrated in Figure 46–7◆. CRH secreted by the hypothalamus causes the secretion of ACTH from the anterior pituitary. ACTH, a trophic hormone, is responsible for the development of the adrenal cortex. Additionally, ACTH stimulates the release of glucocorticoids, mineralocorticoids, and androgens from the adrenal cortex. This hypothalamic–anterior pituitary–adrenocortical axis is maintained through negative feedback. The zona glomerulosa is controlled by the renin–angiotensin–aldosterone system (RAAS).

Pheochromocytoma

Pheochromocytomas are tumors arising from cells derived from the sympathetic preganglia of the adrenal medulla (Neumann, 2010). In general, pheochromocytomas are catecholamine-producing tumors located in adrenal or extra-adrenal sites (e.g., retroperitoneal, pelvis, and thorax) (Neumann, 2010).

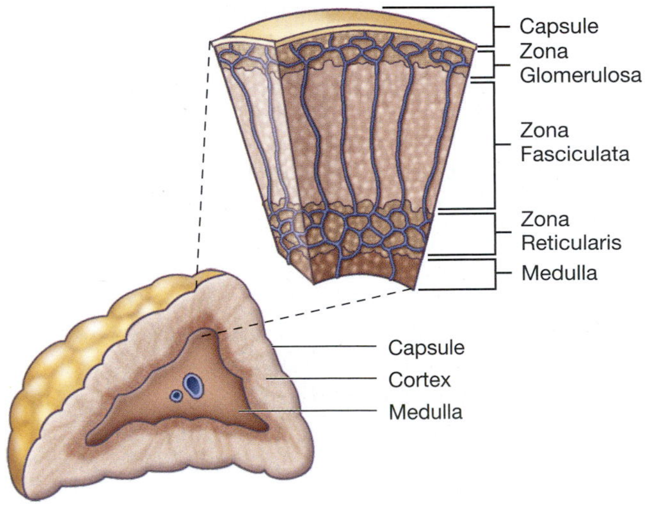

FIGURE 46–6 ◆ The adrenal gland.

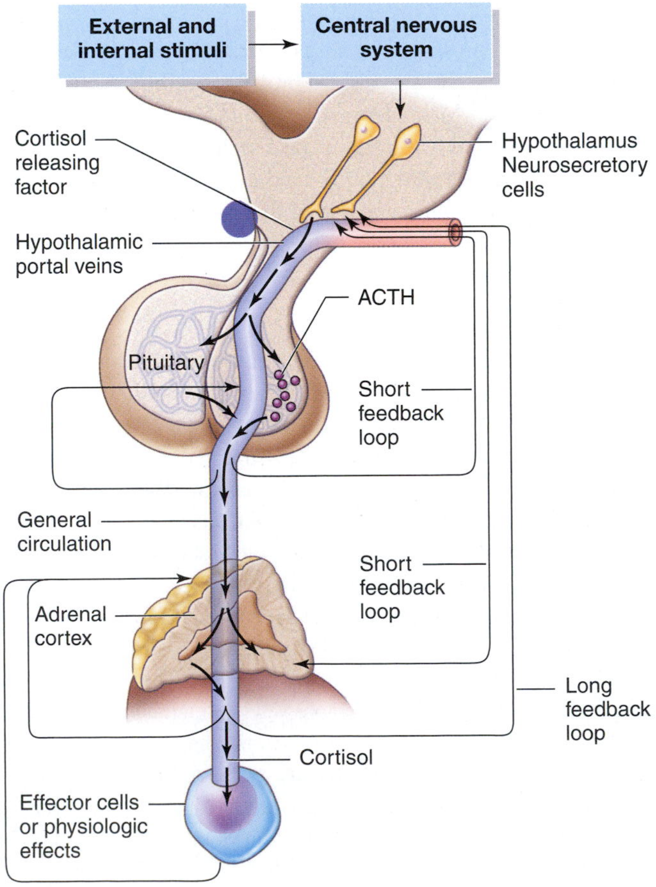

FIGURE 46–7 ◆ Adrenocortical feedback loop.

Epidemiology and Etiology

Pheochromocytomas occur in approximately 2 to 8 out of every 1 million persons per year (Neumann, 2010). Approximately 0.1% of hypertensive patients have a pheochromocytoma. The mean age at diagnosis is approximately 40 years, although they can occur at any age (Neumann, 2010).

Although the majority of these tumors have no defined cause, there is increasing evidence that approximately 25% of patients with pheochromocytomas carry a gene mutation consistent with a familial or genetic syndrome (Fitzgerald, 2011).

Clinical Manifestations

The clinical signs and symptoms of pheochromocytoma are variable and related to the hypersecretion of catecholamines (Neumann, 2010). The clinical features include headaches, excessive sweating, palpitations, tachycardia, sustained and paroxysmal hypertension, anxiety, and panic attacks. The most predominant symptom is hypertension, which may be episodic or sustained. A catecholamine crisis may lead to heart failure, pulmonary edema, dysrhythmias, and intracranial hemorrhage (Neumann, 2010). The duration of the episodic hormone release is variable, generally lasting for less than an hour, and is characterized by palpitations and tachycardia. These episodes may be precipitated by a number of factors, such as surgery, pregnancy, and medications (e.g., tricyclic antidepressants) (Neumann, 2010).

Laboratory and Diagnostic Testing

The diagnosis of pheochromocytoma is based on evidence of catecholamine excess through biochemical testing and localization of the tumor by imaging (Neumann, 2010). These include measurement of plasma and urinary catecholamines and their methylated metabolites: metanephrines (Neumann, 2010). A variety of methods have been used to localize the tumors, including CT (with contrast) and MRI scanning. Other scanning tests may include radioactive tracers (Neumann, 2010). See the Laboratory and Diagnostic Tests for Adrenal Function feature below.

Medical Management

Complete removal of the tumor is the primary goal of treatment for pheochromocytoma. The patient must be adequately prepared for surgery to avoid the effects of excess catecholamines during surgery (e.g., hypertensive crisis). This includes administering alpha-adrenergic blockers (phenoxybenzamine) for approximately 10 to 15 days prior to surgery (Neumann, 2010). Since patients with pheochromocytoma are vasoconstricted, they are instructed to increase salt intake and water intake to avoid orthostasis (hypotension when standing or moving after standing still for a long period of time) (Neumann, 2010). The blood pressure should be maintained below 160/90, and only moderate orthostasis should be present (Neumann, 2010). Beta-blockers may be added after alpha blockade for control of hypertension. Finally surgery is more successful in reducing blood pressure if symptoms have been of short duration.

Nursing Management

Nursing management for patients with pheochromocytomas includes pre- and postoperative care. On assessment of the patient, the nurse should validate presenting symptoms or those recently experienced by the patient in order to develop a plan of care. Assessment findings typically include hypertension, pounding headaches, hyperglycemia and glucosuria, tachycardia, apprehension, and palpitations; profuse sweating with cold extremities; nausea and vomiting; and dilated pupils. The nurse should monitor the patient's blood sugar and blood pressure, with the expectations that the patient will be hyperglycemic and hypertensive before sugery. Additional assessment variables include vital signs, hemodynamic parameters, and fluid and electrolyte status. The patient will undergo exams and tests which require instructions on preparation by the nurse, such as a 24-hour urine sample and a magnetic resonance imaging scan (MRI). Since these patients may undergo scans for localization of the pheochromocytoma, they should be clinically screened (e.g., for pregnancy and allergies to dyes) and informed about the diagnostic test, including a description of the procedure. Pharmacologic therapy will be instituted prior to surgery to decrease blood pressure and blood sugar. These medications need to be explained to the patient.

Following surgery, assessment includes blood sugar values (hypoglycemia expected) and blood pressure checks (hypotension expected). The nurse should be aware that the two major postoperative complications are severe hypotension and hypoglycemia. The blood pressure

LABORATORY AND DIAGNOSTIC TESTS for Adrenal Function

Test, Description, Rationale, and Normal Value	Expected Abnormality
Plasma ACTH	
Normal, contingent on time of day: 7 a.m. to 10 a.m.: 8–80 pg/mL 4 p.m.: 5–30 pg/mL 10 p.m. to Midnight: Less than 10 pg/mL *A blood test used to determine if a decreased plasma cortisol level is due to adrenal cortex hypofunction or pituitary hypofunction.*	A decreased level may signify adrenocortical hyperplasia, cancer of the adrenal gland, or hypopituitarism. An increased level may signify adrenalcorticol hypofunction (Addison's disease). Plasma ACTH is suppressed in ACTH-independent Cushing syndrome, while plasma ACTH is elevated in ACTH-dependent Cushing syndrome. Additionally, mean basal ACTH levels are generally higher in those with ACTH-independent Cushing syndrome of ectopic origin compared to pituitary origin.
Serum Cortisol	
Normal: Adult: 8 a.m.–10 a.m.: 5–23 mcg/dL 4 p.m.–6 p.m.: 3–13 mcg/dL *A blood test used to determine the presence of an elevated or decreased plasma cortisol level and altered adrenocortical function.*	A decreased level may signify adrenal cortical hypofunction (Addison's disease). An increased level may signify excess adrenal cortical hormone (Cushing syndrome), cancer of adrenal gland, or a benign tumor on the adrenal cortex.

(*continued*)

Weblink: Test for Cortisol in the Urine

LABORATORY AND DIAGNOSTIC TESTS for Adrenal Function, *continued*

Test, Description, Rationale, and Normal Value	Expected Abnormality
Urinary Free Cortisol Normal: 24–108 mcg/24 hours *A urine test used to assist in the diagnosis of adrenocortical hyperfunction.*	If elevated, it is indicative of: Too much adrenocortical hormone. Cushing syndrome. Adrenal or pituitary tumor. Decreased level may indicate Addison's disease, hypopituitarism, and/or congenital adrenal hyperplasia.
Plasma Catecholamines Normal: Epinephrine: Supine: Less than 50 pg/mL; Sitting: Less than 60 pg/mL; Standing: Less than 90 pg/mL. Norepinephrine: Supine: 110–410 pg/mL; Sitting: 120–680 pg/mL; Standing: 125–700 pg/mL. Dopamine: Supine and Standing: Less than 87 pg/mL. *A test used to detect the abnormality among the three main catecholamines (epinephrine, norepinephrine, and dopamine) in the blood.*	Increased level: Epinephrine and norepinephrine: Continuous elevation of epinephrine with pheochromocytomas. Pheochromocytoma: Total catecholamines: Greater than 1,000 pg/mL.
Urine Catecholamines Normal values: Free catecholamines: Less than 100 micrograms (mcg) or less than 590 nanomoles (nmol) Epinephrine: Less than 20 mcg or less than 109 nmol Norepinephrine: 15–80 mcg or 89–473 nmol Dopamine: 65–400 mcg or 420–2,612 nmol Normetanephrine: 105–354 mcg or 573–1,933 nmol Metanephrine: 74–297 mcg or 375–1,506 nmol Vanillylmandelic acid (VMA): Less than 9 milligrams (mg) or less than 45 micromoles (mcmol) *A 24-hour urine test used to assist in the diagnosis of health problems related to the abnormal amount of catecholamines in the urine.* *Fractional analysis of catecholamine levels (epinephrine, norepinephrine, and dopamine) is helpful for identifying certain adrenal medullary tumors and pheochromocytomas.*	Increased levels are indicative of pheochromocytoma.
Urine Metanephrines (Also measured in 24-hour urine catecholamines) Normal: Normotensive: 18 years and older; Male 44–261 mcg/24 hours; Female: 30–180 mcg/24 hours Hypotensive: All ages: Male < 400 mcg/24 hours; Female: < 400 mcg/24 hours *A test used to help detect and rule out pheochromocytomas in symptomatic patients.*	Elevated level is indicative of pheochromocytomas
Serum Metanephrines Normal: Free: 0.50 nmol/L Normetanephrine: Free: < 0.90 nmol/L *A blood test used to help detect and rule out pheochromocytomas in symptomatic patients.*	Elevated level is indicative of pheochromocytomas.
17-Ketosteroids (17KS) Normal Adult: Male: 5–25 mg/24 hours Female: 5–15 mg/24 hours Elderly: 4–8 mg/24 hours. *A urine test used to assist in the diagnosis of adrenocortical dysfunction.*	A decreased level may signify adrenal cortical hypofunction (Addison's disease) and hypopituitarism. An increased level may signify adrenocortical hyperfunction, Cushing syndrome, and adrenocortical carcinoma.

LABORATORY AND DIAGNOSTIC TESTS for Adrenal Function, *continued*

Test, Description, Rationale, and Normal Value	Expected Abnormality
Scanning Devices	
Computed Tomography	
Normal: No abnormalities *Used to visualize adrenal glands and identify abnormalities.*	Adenoma on adrenal gland.
Magnetic Resonance Imaging (MRI)	
Normal: No abnormalities found *Used to detect abnormalities on adrenal gland* *MRI with gadolinium enhancement; it may be performed to localize ACTH-secreting adenoma.*	Adenoma on adrenal gland with gadolinium enhancement and localization of the adenoma.
Inferior Petrosal Sinus Sampling (IPSS) with Corticotropin-Releasing Hormone (CRH) Stimulation	
Normal: Following CHR administration, a basal ratio of less than 3.0 is normal. Cortisol value of less than 50 mnol/L or 1.4 mcg/dL is normal.	Used to distinguish pituitary and ectopic ACTH-dependent Cushing syndrome.
Radioactive Tracer	
Normal: Absence of a tumor *A radioactive substance called a tracer is injected into a vein. Two different tracers may be used: ^{131}Iodine or ^{123}Metaiodobenzylguanidine (MIBG). A special scanner is used to find or confirm the presence of a tumor.*	A tumor on the adrenal gland.
Dexamethasone Suppression Test (DST)	
Normal: $<$ 5 mcg/dL Also called an ACTH suppression test or cortisol suppression test. *This blood and urine test is used to measure the response of the adrenal glands to ACTH. With the standard low-dose method, urine is collected over 3 days (stored in 24-hour collection containers) to measure cortisol. On day 2, the patient is given a low dose (0.5 mg) of dexamethasone by mouth every 6 hours for 48 hours. The urine is then tested on day 3 for cortisol with a normal value of $<$10 mcg/day.* *With the rapid or overnight screening test: Plasma cortisol: 8 a.m. is less than 10 mcg/dL; 4:00 p.m. is less than 5 mcg/dL. Urine 17-OHCS (5-hour specimen; less than 4 mg/5 hours)*	This test is considered a proactive stimulus test. If there is not a normal response on the low-dose test, abnormal secretions of cortisol is likely. This indicates Cushing syndrome. It also could be the result of a cortisol-overproducing tumor or a pituitary tumor.
Metyrapone Test	
Normal: Normal values are indication specific, patient specific, and technique specific. Some references report the normal as blood: 11-deocycortisol increased to greater than 7 mcg/dL; cortisol less than 10 mcg/dL; 24-hour urine: 17-hydroxycorticosteroid (OCHS) levels will be greater than two times the baseline level (Adler, 2012; Alina Hospitals & Clinics, 2012). *A blood and/or urine test used in the diagnosis of certain problems of the adrenal glands. Metyrapone is taken by mouth in one or more doses the day before the test is done. The next day, blood and/or urine samples are taken. The amount of hormones in the blood or urine is measured and studied.*	Abnormal values are indicative of adrenocortical hypofunction or insufficiency (Addison's disease).
Insulin-Induced Hypoglycemia	
Normal: In healthy people, blood glucose levels fall and cortisol concentrations increase. *This stress test is used to evaluate the response to stress, particularly when an ACTH deficiency is suspected as the cause.* *Glucose and cortisol levels are measured at predetermined intervals after an injection of insulin is used to stress the pituitary gland.*	With adrenal insufficiency, cortisol levels will remain low and glucose levels will fall, then recover slowly.

(*continued*)

Weblink: Cushing Syndrome Workup

Weblink: Cushing's Disease

LABORATORY AND DIAGNOSTIC TESTS for Adrenal Function, *continued*

Test, Description, Rationale, and Normal Value	Expected Abnormality
Blood Chemistry	
Determines electrolytes in intracellular fluids.	
Potassium: Adult: Normal: 3.5–5.3 mEq/L	Decreased levels indicate hyperaldosteronism and metabolic alkalosis. Increased levels indicate Addison's disease and acidosis.
Sodium: Adult: Normal: 135–145 mEq/L	Decreased levels indicate SIADH. Increased levels indicate dehydration, Cushing disease.
Chloride: Adult: Normal: 95–105 mEq/L	Decreased levels indicate hypokalemia, hyponatremia, adrenal gland insufficiency (Addison's disease), or metabolic acidosis. Increased level indicates dehydration, hypernatremia, hyperparathyroidism, adrenal gland hyperactivity, or metabolic acidosis.
Bicarbonate or CO_2: Adult: Normal: 22–30 mEq/L	Decreased levels indicate metabolic acidosis, dehydration, shock, and diabetic ketoacidosis. Increased levels indicate metabolic alkalosis, hypothyroidism, and potassium deficit.
Arterial Blood Gases *Usually ordered to assess disturbances of acid–base balance.* The basic components with normal values are: pH: 7.35–7.45 $PaCO_2$: 35–45 mm Hg PaO_2: 75–100 mm Hg SaO_2: greater than 95% SvO_2: greater than 70% HCO_3: 24–28 mEq/L BE base excesses: +2 to −2 mEq/L	A pH less than 7.35 indicates acidosis; a pH greater than 7.45 indicates alkalosis. When pH is elevated and $PaCO_2$ is reduced, respiratory alkalosis results; when pH is decreased and $PaCO_2$ is increased, respiratory acidosis results. When pH is decreased and HCO_3 and BE are decreased, it represents metabolic acidosis. When PH is elevated and HCO_3 and BE are elevated, it represents metabolic alkalosis. The combination of oxygen saturation, partial pressure of oxygen, and hemoglobin indicates tissue oxygenation. When there is an oxygen deficit, acidosis occurs. If a bicarbonate excess is present, metabolic alkalosis results. Decreased levels of HCO_3 indicate adrenal insufficiency or Addison's disease. Respiratory alkalosis is present in hyperthyroidism. Metabolic alkalosis is present with potassium loss, as in diuretic therapy.
Aldosterone Serum (fasting) Normal Adult: Less than 16 ng/dL (fasting) 4–30 ng/dL (sitting position) *Used to detect a deficit or excess of aldosterone and to compare with other tests for determining adrenal hypo- or hyperfunction.*	Decreased levels indicate adrenal cortical hypofunction and severe hypernatremia. Increased levels indicate adrenal cortical hyperfunction or primary hyperaldosteronism. Cancer of the adrenal gland.
Urinary Aldosterone Normal Adults: 6–25mcg/24 hours *Urine test that assists in the diagnosis of primary and secondary hyperaldosteronism.*	Decreased value may indicate primary adrenocortical insufficiency. An increased value may indicate primary hyperaldosteronism.
Renin (plasma) Normal adult with sodium diet: Supine: 0.2–2.3 ng/mL Upright/Sitting: 1.6–4.3 ng/mL On restricted sodium diet: Upright: 4.1–10.8 ng/mL Plasma renin levels are usually higher from 8:00 a.m. to noon and lower from noon to 6:00 p.m. *A blood (plasma) test that is used to identify primary and secondary hyperaldosteronism.*	Increased level indicates hyperaldosteronism.

Sources: Adler, G. K. (2012). Cushing syndrome workup. Medscape Reference. WebMD. Retrieved from http://emedicine.medscape.com/article/117365-workup; Allina Hospitals & Clinics. (2012). Metyrapone test. UpToDate, Inc. Retrieved from http://www.allina.com/CCS/doc/Consumer_Lab/49/150401.htm; Canterbury Health. (2012). Petrosal sinus sampling (Pss). Retrieved from http://www.cushings-help.com/petrossal.htm; Final Diagnosis. (2008). Cushing's disease: Hypercortisolism and pituitary adenoma. Retrieved from http://path.upmc.edu/cases/case556/dx.html; Golay, V. (2011). SIADH syndrome of inappropriate secretion of antidiuretic hormone. SlideShare, Inc. Retrieved from http://www.slideshare.net/VishalGolay/siadh-8611907; Kee, J. L. (2010). *Laboratory and diagnostic tests with nursing implications.* Upper Saddle River, NJ: Prentice Hall; Meditec. (2012). Normal lab values. Retrieved from http://www.meditec.com/resourcestools/medical-reference-links/normal-lab-values/; MedlinePlus. (2011). Cortisol—urine. Retrieved from http://www.nlm.nih.gov/medlineplus/ency/article/003703.htm; Science Clarified. (2012). Radioactive tracers. Advameg.Inc. Retrieved from http://www.scienceclarified.com/Qu-Ro/Radioactive-Tracers.html; Thomas, C. P. (2012). Symptom of inappropriate antidiuretic hormone secretion. Medscape Reference. Retrieved from http:/medicine.medscape.com/aticl246overview; WebMD. (2010). Catecholamines in urine. Retrieved from http://www.webmd.com/heart-disease/catecholamines-14697?page=2.

falls because of the sudden fall in circulating catecholamines once the tumor is removed. If hypotension occurs, fluids need to be administered. Glucose levels may fall as insulin is released following tumor removal (Tsegay, Ayango, Van Sell, & Miller-Anderson, 2008).

Along with blood sugar and blood pressure, the nurse monitors other vital signs, hemodynamic parameters, and fluid and electrolyte status. The nurse assesses the patient's postoperative site and checks for bleeding and infection. Pain assessment also is critical as pain and anxiety can trigger a hypertensive crisis. Therefore, the nurse must administer medication for pain and anxiety as ordered.

Postoperative teaching includes informing the patient that she may engage in light activity while at home after surgery and that she can remove any dressings and shower the day after the operation. Normal routine activities, such as driving, may be resumed within a week. When preparing for discharge, the nurse should explain that pheochromocytomas can recur, and that the prognosis is more favorable when tumors are detected early. Also, the nurse must explain that the patient will need to follow up with her health care provider at least twice a year for the next few years, and then annually until instructed otherwise.

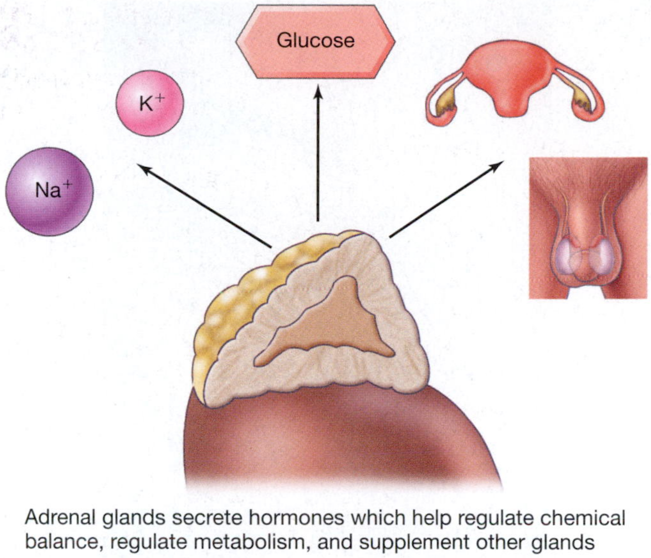

FIGURE 46–8 ◆ Adrenal gland hormone secretion.

Adrenocortical Hypofunction

Primary adrenal insufficiency is caused by dysfunction of the adrenal cortex, resulting in deficiency of adrenocortical hormones (e.g., mineralocorticoids, androgens, and glucocorticoids). **Secondary adrenal insufficiency** is caused by dysfunction of the anterior pituitary, leading to loss of ACTH production and resulting in deficiency of adrenocortical hormones.

Epidemiology and Etiology

The prevalence of primary adrenocortical deficiency is 110 to 144 cases per million people in developed countries (Betterle & Morlin, 2011). The disease is slightly more common in women and usually presents in the third to fifth decade (Else, Hammer, & McPhee, 2010).

Primary adrenocortical insufficiency is associated with progressive destruction of the adrenal cortex (Williams, 2010). Primary adrenocortical insufficiency has several causes, including autoimmune destruction of the adrenal cortex (Else et al., 2010), surgical removal of the adrenal gland, infections (e.g., tuberculosis, fungal, viral), hemorrhage, invasive disease (e.g., tumor metastasis), enzyme inhibitors (e.g., metyrapone, ketoconazole, aminoglutethimide), and disorders associated with defective adrenocortical hormone production (e.g., congenital adrenal hyperplasia) (Williams, 2010). Autoimmune adrenalitis, also known as Addison's disease, is the primary cause of primary adrenocortical insufficiency, accounting for 80% of cases (Williams, 2010). Secondary adrenocortical insufficiency may be caused by hypothalamic–pituitary disease or suppression of the hypothalamic pituitary axis. One of the most common causes of this suppression is the use of exogenous corticosteroids (e.g., prednisone).

Pathophysiology

In primary adrenocortical insufficiency, gradual destruction of the adrenal cortex may occur as a result of autoimmune, tuberculosis, or other infiltrative processes, resulting in decreased secretion of adrenocortical hormones. The basal glucocorticoid level may be normal but cannot increase in response to physiological stresses, such as trauma, surgery, or infection. With further destruction of the adrenal cortex, there is progressive loss of glucocorticoids, mineralocorticoids, and androgens; the clinical signs and symptoms of primary adrenal insufficiency then become apparent. The decreased cortisol leads to increased release of ACTH from the anterior pituitary. A rapid destruction of adrenal cortex may occur in some patients, as approximately 25% of patients present with adrenal crisis or impending crisis at diagnosis (Carroll, Aron, Findling, & Tyrrell, 2011).

Secondary adrenocortical insufficiency can occur following surgery or damage to the pituitary (e.g., removal of the pituitary, pituitary infarction). However, a major cause of secondary adrenocortical insufficiency is chronic exogenous glucocorticoid therapy. Many patients are treated with exogenous glucocorticoids (e.g., prednisone) for a number of chronic disorders. These medications increase the serum concentration of cortisol and suppress ACTH secretion from the anterior pituitary via negative feedback principles (see Figure 46–8◆).

Clinical Manifestations

The signs and symptoms of primary adrenocortical insufficiency are related to decreased production of glucocorticoids (i.e., cortisol), mineralocorticoids (i.e., aldosterone), and androgens. These may include fatigue, weakness, weight loss, anorexia, nausea, vomiting, abdominal pain, diarrhea, constipation, hypotension, dehydration, hypoglycemia, hyponatremia, hyperkalemia, and acidosis. Primary adrenocortical insufficiency is characterized by pigmentation changes such as freckling; diffuse darkening of skin; and creases of the hands, knuckles, and areola; bluish-black patches also may be noted on mucous membranes (Williams, 2010).

The clinical signs and symptoms of primary and secondary adrenal insufficiency are similar; however, there are a few exceptions. In secondary adrenocortical insufficiency, the pigmentation changes are not present because ACTH is not increased. Since the zona glomerulosa is regulated by the RAAS, mineralocorticoids are still produced; therefore, hypokalemia is not present, and hypotension is less prominent. Figure 46–9◆ depicts a patient with Addison's disease.

Acute adrenocortical insufficiency (**adrenal crisis**) is a life-threatening complication characterized by dehydration, fever, hyponatremia, hyperkalemia, vascular collapse, and death if not recognized and treated effectively. This crisis occurs in patients with chronic adrenocortical insufficiency and is often precipitated by physiologic stressors, such as trauma or infection.

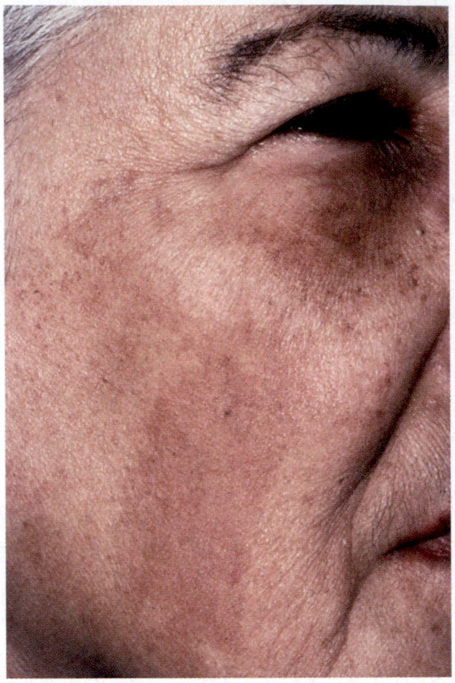

FIGURE 46–9 ◆ Patient with Addison's disease.
Source: BSIP/Science Source/Photo Researchers.

Laboratory and Diagnostic Studies

The laboratory abnormalities associated with adrenocortical insufficiency are related to the type (i.e., primary or secondary) and nature (acute versus chronic) of the adrenocortical insufficiency. The general laboratory approach to the diagnosis of adrenal insufficiency can be complex. Since urinary and basal plasma levels of adrenocortical hormones may be normal in partial adrenocortical insufficiency, provocative tests (those that establish the diagnosis before symptoms caused by disease damage are manifested) of adrenocortical function are necessary to establish the diagnosis of adrenocortical insufficiency and differentiate between primary and secondary dysfunction (Williams, 2010).

The rapid ACTH stimulation test assesses adrenocortical function and is the initial test in the evaluation of adrenocortical deficiency (Gardner & Shoback, 2011). Refer to the Laboratory and Diagnostic Tests box (p. 1403) for additional tests used to measure adrenal function.

Medical Management

Patients with adrenocortical insufficiency are treated with specific hormone replacement regimens to correct the glucocorticoid and mineralocorticoid deficiencies. The primary medication of choice is hydrocortisone (cortisol). Patients usually require mineralocorticoid replacement, which can be accomplished through the administration of fludrocortisone (0.05–1 mg/day) (Williams, 2010). Additionally, patients are advised to maintain adequate intake of sodium (3 to 4 grams/day) (Williams, 2010). In female patients, androgens produced in the adrenocortex are also decreased. Some health care providers will elect to replace the androgen deficiency with dehydroepiandrosterone (DHEA) 25 to 50 mg orally (Williams, 2010).

In adrenal crisis, the primary treatment is directed toward replacing glucocorticoids, as well as sodium and water deficits. This involves intravenous infusions of hydrocortisone, normal saline, and vasopressor medications (e.g., dopamine), if necessary. The high doses of hydrocortisone needed during treatment of adrenal crisis usually provide sufficient mineralocorticoid replacement. Electrolytes should be measured to assist in determining adjustments to drug dosages.

Complications of glucocorticoid therapy in the doses recommended for adrenocortical insufficiency result in few side effects; however, glucocorticoid replacement may cause gastritis. Patients are instructed to take the glucocorticoid replacement with meals. A number of OTC and prescription medications are designed to reduce gastric acidity. Patients should consult with their providers on the most appropriate medications. Mineralocorticoid replacement can be associated with side effects such as hypokalemia or hypertension. Periodic assessment of serum potassium, body weight, and blood pressure are useful to monitor the side effects of these medications.

Nursing Management

The diagnosis of adrenocortical hypofunction can be complex; this disorder can be chronic, evolving over a period of time, or can present as an acute crisis. The nurse may instruct the patient on testing procedures in an outpatient setting or collecting the specimens in a hospital setting. Careful attention to testing procedures is essential in performing the provocative stimuli test. If metyrapone or insulin-induced hypoglycemia is used to test the hypothalamic–anterior pituitary adrenocortical axis, careful monitoring of clinical status and established parameters (e.g., blood glucose) is essential.

The Nursing Process box explains the nursing process to be used in caring for patients with this disorder.

Discharge Priorities

Preparation of the patient with adrenocortical insufficiency for discharge must include instructions regarding the need to take hormone replacement therapy for life. Of particular importance is that the patient understands that stress or illness is likely to increase the need for hydrocortisone. In such situations, the patient should increase the dosage of hormone as advised by the health care provider. Persistence of vomiting or diarrhea indicates a need for urgent care, which may include intravenous saline and intravenous/intramuscular hydrocortisone. Flulike symptoms should never be ignored because they may be the initial indicators of adrenal crisis. The nurse should coordinate care with a home care or community health agency to ensure that the patients are receiving the proper care at home, particularly in terms of taking the medications as instructed and recognizing symptoms of complications which necessitate immediate notification of health care provider.

Health Promotion

The patient with a history of adrenocortical insufficiency should wear a medical identification bracelet or necklace and keep an identification card with medical instructions in the wallet or purse. A medical alert in the form of medical identification may enable health care personnel to respond to a patient's need for immediate hormone and fluid replacement, which could be life-saving. Knowledge about the disease is essential for self-management, particularly during illness or added stress. Therefore, the patient and a reliable family member should have appropriate follow-up with home care to ensure that they have adequate information and skill to manage the demands of the chronic form of the disease.

Collaborative Management

The pharmacist, rehabilitation professional, and home health nurse must be involved in providing follow-up care to the patient diagnosed with adrenocortical insufficiency. In order to meet desired

NURSING PROCESS: Patient Care Plan for Acute Adrenal Insufficiency

Assessment of Endocrine Status Using Gordon's Functional Health Patterns:

- Health Perception Health Management Pattern
- Nutrition Metabolic Pattern

Subjective Data

Assessment of Cognitive Level, Muscle Strength, and Ability to Perform ADLs Independently

Have you been taking any steroid medications, such as prednisone, cortisone, or any other steroid drugs?

What other medications, herbs, or dietary supplements have you been taking?

Have you been able to maintain your usual activities of daily living?

What has your appetite been like?

Have you noticed any food cravings lately?

How much salt or sodium do you get in your diet?

Have you experienced any nausea or vomiting?

Do you feel mentally alert?

Are you sleeping well?

Have you experienced any stress, trauma, or illness recently?

Assessment of Emergency Preparedness in the Event of Adrenal Insufficiency Crisis

Do you carry a medical identification card with a list of your medications on it?

Do you wear a medical ID bracelet or other jewelry?

Have you informed family members or caregivers of your history with corticosteroid drugs?

Tell me what your understanding is about how corticosteroid drugs affect your body.

Are you experiencing any pain?

Please describe the location and intensity.

Objective Data

Assessment of Cognitive Level, Muscle Strength, and Ability to Perform ADLs Independently

Low blood pressure

Orthostatic hypotension

Poor skin turgor

Tender abdomen

Face appears round, edematous

Muscle weakness noted

Low serum sodium, high potassium noted

Assessment of Emergency Preparedness in the Event of Adrenal Insufficiency Crisis

Blood pressure: 84/40

Temperature: 101°F

Heart rate: 124

Diaphoretic

Appears confused, disoriented as to time and place

Vomited during interview

No medic alert noted on patient on admission to ICU

Family members report patient has been taking corticosteroids for rheumatoid arthritis

Medications found in patient's purse

Outcomes and Evaluation Parameters	Planning and Interventions with *Rationales*
1. NURSING DIAGNOSIS: Deficient Fluid Volume and Hyponatremia *related to adrenal insufficiency* (NANDA-I © 2012)	
Outcome: Free of symptoms of adrenal insufficiency. ***Evaluation Parameters:*** Vital signs within normal limits. Patient is able to stand at the bedside without vertigo. Abdomen is soft, bowel sounds normal. Patient reports appetite has returned with no food cravings. Patient verbalizes feeling less fatigued. Skin turgor appears elastic. Serum sodium and sodium serum levels within normal range. No evidence of nausea, vomiting, or diarrhea.	Administer IV therapy, which may include 0.09% saline solution or 5% dextrose in saline, to improve fluid and electrolyte balance *to raise blood pressure and improve perfusion of oxygen to tissues.* Administer IV hydrocortisone for the first 48 to 72 hours, followed by oral administration for essential hormone replacement to be taken with meals *to provide hormones needed due to suppression of HPA axis due to long-term corticosteroid therapy and to prevent GI distress.*
2. NURSING DIAGNOSIS: Risk of Ineffective Therapeutic Regimen Management *related to knowledge deficit* (NANDA-I © 2012)	
Outcome: Prepared to care for self and to prevent insufficiency crisis. ***Evaluation Parameters:*** Patient wears a medical alert bracelet on next clinic visit and shows nurse her medical ID in purse. Patient reports notifying other health care providers (podiatrist, ophthalmologist, and dentist) of medication regimen. Patient is able to describe the rationale for safety precautions related to long-term use of corticosteroid drugs and the need for gradual tapering off of drugs when they are discontinued.	Develop a teaching plan with the patient and family to ensure adequate understanding of benefits and risks of corticosteroid therapy and measures to be taken for patient safety, including use of medical alert jewelry and ID card, notification of other health care providers, and need for gradual tapering off of corticosteroid medications when these are discontinued *to enable patient to manage self-care with better understanding of medications and side effects, to enhance safety of patient when undergoing medical procedures with other health care providers, and to alert health care providers to patient's history of corticosteroid use in the event of an emergency.*

Source: Adapted from Wilkinson, J. M., & Ahearn, N. R. (2009). *Prentice Hall nursing diagnosis handbook* (9th ed.). Upper Saddle River, NJ: Prentice Hall.

patient outcomes, it is essential that this interdisciplinary team communicate openly with one another in developing and evaluating care of the patient and family (IOM [Institute of Medicine], 2010). The patient must be advised about permanent hormone injections and the method of self-administration of intramuscular injections. The pharmacist also should be involved in providing instructions on how to take medications, which is particularly important during periods of stress and illness.

Adrenal Hyperfunction

Adrenocortical hyperfunction, also known as **Cushing syndrome,** is the clinical syndrome that results from chronic exposure to excessive circulating levels of cortisol. In addition to hypercortisolism, patients with adrenocortical hyperfunction have varying degrees of hyperaldosteronism and adrenal androgens.

Epidemiology

Cushing syndrome may occur spontaneously (e.g., ACTH-secreting pituitary adenomas) or from iatrogenic causes (e.g., chronic treatment with glucocorticoids such as prednisone). The general incidence of spontaneous Cushing syndrome is two to four cases per million people, and it is nine times more common in women than men (Else et al., 2010).

Etiology and Pathophysiology

Cushing syndrome is broadly divided into ACTH-dependent and ACTH-independent causes. *ACTH-dependent* causes are those associated with excess production of ACTH from pituitary (e.g., adenoma) or ectopic (e.g., ACTH produced by tumor) origin, resulting in excess production of glucocorticoids. *ACTH-independent* causes are from adrenocortical (e.g., tumor of adrenal cortex) or iatrogenic (e.g., medications, such as prednisone) origin, resulting in excess production of glucocorticoids.

Clinical Manifestations

The signs and symptoms of Cushing syndrome may include obesity, truncal obesity, thin arms and legs, moon face, buffalo hump, acne, hirsutism, striae, plethora, hypertension, severe fatigue and muscle weakness, hyperglycemia, easy bruising, gastrointestinal bleeding, emotional lability, depression, psychosis, osteoporosis, menstrual disorders, decreased libido, impotence, and kidney stones (Carroll et al., 2011). Figure 46–10◆ depicts a patient with Cushing syndrome.

Laboratory and Diagnostic Studies

Initial biochemical measurements are used to screen for the diagnosis of Cushing syndrome (Gardner & Shoback, 2011). Additional tests are used to confirm the diagnosis and to differentiate between the causes. A 24-hour urinary free cortisol collection and a low-dose dexamethasone suppression test provide a precise screening test. If the screening tests are consistent with the diagnosis of Cushing syndrome, a plasma ACTH may be performed to assist in distinguishing between the types of Cushing syndrome. If a diagnosis of ACTH-dependent Cushing syndrome is supported by the biochemical tests indicated previously, a pituitary MRI with gadolinium enhancement may be performed to localize the ACTH-secreting adenoma (Carroll et al., 2011). The most definitive means of distinguishing pituitary and ectopic ACTH-dependent Cushing syndrome is through the use of inferior petrosal sinus sampling (IPSS) with CRH stimulation (Carroll et al., 2011). In ACTH-independent Cushing syndrome of adrenocortical origin, localizing procedures such as MRI and CT are used. See the Laboratory and Diagnostic Tests for Adrenal Disorders feature on page 1403.

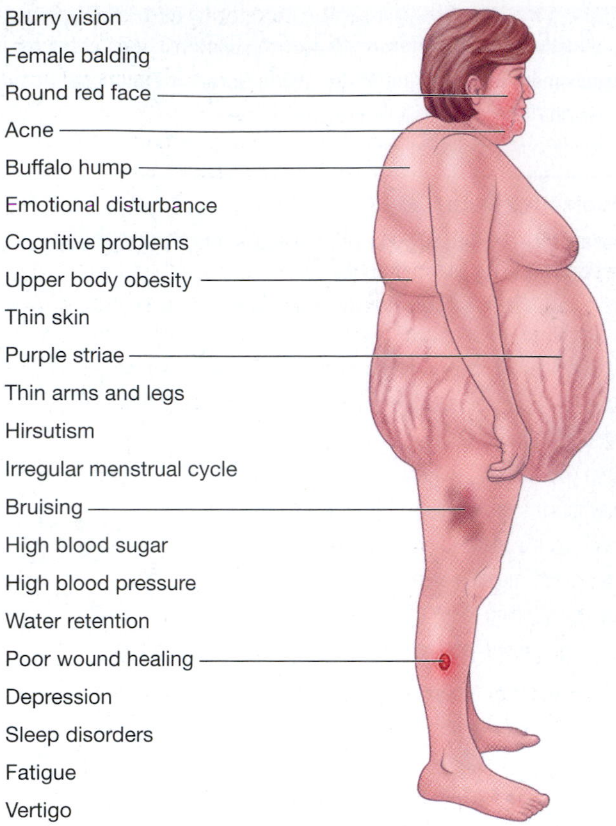

FIGURE 46–10 ◆ Patient with Cushing syndrome.

Medical Management

Medical management of Cushing syndrome is directed at the etiology of the disease. Since Cushing syndrome frequently has an iatrogenic cause, a thorough history of the patient's medication use is necessary as a first step in the diagnosis. Surgery is the primary intervention for tumors of the adrenal or pituitary glands or ACTH-secreting tumors. Transsphenoidal microsurgery is used to remove pituitary tumors that are stimulating excessive ACTH production. Radiation therapy also may be used for tumors in the pituitary or other locations. In some cases, surgery may be an option, and drugs may be used to counter the effect of excess production of adrenal hormones. One such drug is mitotane, an adrenal cytotoxic that destroys cell preparation, which suppresses cortisol production (Williams, 2010). Mitotane decreases the size of adrenal tumors and reduces symptoms caused by excess hormone secretion.

In patients for whom Cushing syndrome is caused by long-term administration of corticosteroid drugs, a plan for gradual withdrawal or reduction of medication is indicated. Corticosteroids cannot be withdrawn abruptly because this may trigger an adrenal crisis.

Nursing Management

The nursing care of patients being treated for Cushing syndrome depends on the treatment modality employed. Nursing care for patients with transsphenoidal surgery, indicated for those patients whose Cushing syndrome is caused by ACTH stimulation from the pituitary gland, has been described previously (p. 1394). Routine postoperative care is followed for patients undergoing removal of ACTH- or CRH-secreting tumors. This care encompasses the monitoring and recording of vital signs, including temperature, pulse, respirations, skin color/oxygen saturation, level of consciousness, wound sites and drains, urinary output, intravenous therapy rate/site, and pain source. Pain management is essential in postoperative care, as is prevention of postoperative nausea and vomiting and thromboembolic prophylaxis. The nurse assists the patient in positioning, as well as performing deep-breathing and coughing exercises to help maintain clear lungs and prevent pneumonia and atelectasis. Leg exercises, as well as moving and ambulation, are encouraged to prevent thrombus development. The patient should ambulate as soon as possible after surgery in accordance with the surgeon's orders.

Patients using medications to inhibit adrenocortical biosynthesis need to be monitored closely for tolerability of these medications so that appropriate adjustment can be made. For example, adverse reactions to the medication suggest intolerability. These include mood swings, weight gain, acne, facial flushing, nausea, insomnia, sodium and fluid retention, impaired wound healing, and menstrual abnormalities. Peptic ulcer, hypocalcemia, osteoporosis with possible bone fractures, loss of muscle mass, and possible masking of infections also are indications of the patient's intolerability of the medication (Adams & Koch, 2010). Adrenocortical insufficiency is a possible risk when using these medications, so close contact with the health care team is essential.

Discharge Priorities

The discharge priorities for the patient with Cushing syndrome are related to the type of treatment selected. For patients undergoing surgical procedures, the priority is optimal recovery from surgery along with education regarding postoperative instructions. Patients undergoing a total adrenalectomy will need lifelong treatment with glucocorticoid and mineralocorticoid replacement and need to follow the plan developed for preventing adrenocortical insufficiency. Patients using medications to block cortisol biosynthesis need careful monitoring of tolerability and side effects from these medications. It must be recognized that many patients are treated with oral medications because they have underlying illnesses (e.g., metastatic carcinoma). Older patients may be poor surgical risks; thus, medical management of Cushing syndrome may be the only treatment option. These vulnerable patients also may have other underlying issues that complicate their discharge priorities.

Hyperaldosteronism

Mineralocorticoids are produced in the zona glomerulosa of the adrenal cortex. Their synthesis and release are primarily regulated by the renin–angiotensin–aldosterone system (RAAS). Renin is an enzyme produced by the juxtaglomerular cells of the kidney. These cells are sensitive to changes in both blood volume and plasma sodium concentration. In the presence of hypovolemia or hyponatremia, the juxtaglomerular cells secrete renin, which acts on a substrate angiotensinogen to form angiotensin I. Angiotensin I is converted to angiotensin II by angiotensin-converting enzyme (ACE). Angiotensin II stimulates the release of aldosterone from the zona glomerulosa. In addition to the RAAS, the zona glomerulosa is controlled to a lesser degree by potassium and ACTH. The primary mineralocorticoid produced by the zona glomerulosa is aldosterone.

Epidemiology, Etiology, and Risk Factors

There are two major disorders of excess production of aldosterone: **primary hyperaldosteronism (PH)** and **secondary hyperaldosteronism (SH).** In primary hyperaldosteronism, the cause of excess aldosterone production resides within the adrenal cortex. In secondary hyperaldosteronism, the cause resides outside of the adrenal cortex. For example, secondary hyperaldosteronism occurs when aldosterone production is stimulated by excess secretion of renin by the juxtaglomerular apparatus of the kidney. This section focuses on primary aldosteronism.

The exact prevalence of PH is unclear. However, it appears to contribute more significantly than was previously thought to the prevalence of essential hypertension (HTN). Estimates suggest that the cause of essential HTN in 5 out of 105 people is due to PH (Uwaifo, 2012). In addition, the prevalence of PH may be higher in patients who have a low serum potassium level, the elderly, and in patients who have HTN that is resistant to single medication use (Uwaifo, 2012). Primary hyperaldosteronism occurs worldwide. Several reports suggest a higher prevalence in African Americans, persons of African origin, and possibly other Blacks (Uwaifo, 2012). Primary hyperaldosteronism caused by aldosterone-producing adenomas (APAs) is more common in women than in men; however, PH caused by idiopathic adrenal hyperplasia (IAH) is more common in men than women. The typical patient with APA is a woman ages 30 to 50 years. Idiopathic adrenal hyperplasia peaks in men in the sixth decade of life (Uwaifo, 2012).

The complete list of entities known to cause PH includes aldosterone-producing adenomas (APAs), aldosterone-producing renin-responsive adenomas (AP-RAs), bilateral adrenal hyperplasia or IAH, primary adrenal hyperplasia (PAH), and familal forms of PH (Uwaifo, 2012). As indicated in the demographic data, aldosteronomas are the most common causes of PH; however, recent data suggest that bilateral idiopathic adrenal hyperplasia also is becoming a major cause of PH (Uwaifo, 2012). The Hormone Foundation (2012) has identified several risks for primary aldosteronism (see the Risk Factors box).

Pathophysiology

Primary hyperaldosteronism primarily results from an aldosterone-producing adenoma (Conn syndrome) or bilateral adrenocortical hyperplasia (Williams, 2010). This chronic excess of aldosterone results in expansion of extracellular and plasma fluid volume. This increased volume is sensed by the juxtaglomerular apparatus, leading to suppression of renin production and low plasma renin activity.

Clinical Manifestations

Patients with primary hyperaldosteronism generally present with hypertension, muscle weakness, polydipsia, polyuria, headaches, and fatigue. The hypertension is often long-standing and refractory to multiple medications (Lal & Clark, 2010). Therefore, a detailed assessment of the medical history is indicated in the diagnostic work-up of a patient with suspected primary hyperaldosteronism.

Laboratory and Diagnostic Assessment

The diagnosis of primary hyperaldosteronism is suspected in any patient with unexplained hypokalemia (<3.2 mmol/L) or with hypokalemia while on diuretic therapy despite potassium supplementation (Lal & Clark, 2010). Other biochemical abnormalities may include hypernatremia, alkalosis, and hypochloremia. Elevated plasma and

RISK FACTORS for Primary Aldosteronism

- High blood pressure that requires more than three medications to manage
- High blood pressure that started at a young age (less than 30 years of age)
- A family history of stroke at a young age
- A low potassium level (called hypokalemia).

urine aldosterone levels with suppressed plasma renin activity assist in confirming the diagnosis. Failure to suppress plasma aldosterone with oral or intravenous salt loading also supports the diagnosis of primary hyperaldosteronism. Following the biochemical diagnosis, the location of the adenoma or bilateral hyperplasia can be confirmed through imaging studies such as adrenal MRI or CT.

Medical Management

Primary aldosteronism caused by an adenoma is usually treated by surgical removal of the adenoma. The laparoscopic approach is the preferred choice of surgery. If the underlying cause is bilateral hyperplasia, surgery is indicated only if the hypokalemia cannot be controlled with medical treatment, which usually involves the administration of an aldosterone antagonist (e.g., spironolactone) (Williams, 2010). The hypertension and hypokalemia associated with primary aldosteronism are typically controlled with spironolactone. Eplerenone is a less potent but more specific aldosterone antagonist that has minimal anti-androgen effects (Williams, 2010).

Nursing Management

The nurse caring for the patient with primary aldosteronism should perform routine postoperative management following laparoscopy. Postoperative care encompasses monitoring and recording vital signs, skin color/oxygen saturation, level of consciousness, wound sites and drains, urinary output, intravenous therapy rate/site, and pain source. Urinary output and fluid balance/hydration should be assessed and monitored, including the management of intravenous therapy as ordered, and an accurate record of intake and output documented. Pain management is essential. Initially, most patients receive intravenous analgesics but progress to oral medications rapidly due to limited pain (Hope, 2011). It is important for the nurse to document the administration of pain medications and the patient's response to the medications. The nurse also should monitor the patient for nausea and vomiting, which may result from anesthesia. Thromboembolic prophylaxis includes encouraging the patient to ambulate and the use of leg exercises. The nurse will assist the patient in positioning, as well as deep-breathing and coughing exercises to help maintain clear lungs and prevent pneumonia and atelectasis.

Patients usually are discharged 24 to 48 hours postsurgery; thus, it is important that discharge planning begins early in the recovery process. The patient should be instructed on the use and side effects of medication if a drug is prescribed. The nurse needs to review dietary restrictions with the patient if there are any, such as low sodium restriction. Typically, no activity restrictions are made other than to advise the patient to rest frequently the first week after surgery. The patient also may be advised on how to achieve a healthy status by maintaining an ideal weight, avoiding alcohol, and participating in regular aerobic exercise. These measures also will assist the patient in decreasing hypertension if it is still present. The nurse may recommend stress reduction strategies including meditation, biofeedback, yoga, and massage therapy.

Collaborative Management

Collaborative care for the patient with primary aldosteronism will involve the primary care provider, endocrinologist, surgeon, pharmacist, and nutritionist, as well as the nurse. The primary care provider, the endocrinologist, or the surgeon will assume coordination of care of all members of the health care team. The endocrinologist typically assumes responsibility for managing the medications related to the hormonal disturbances, and the surgeon follows the postoperative care of the patient that is related to the actual surgery. The pharmacist provides information regarding medications and assists the patient in developing an administration plan. The nurse continually assesses and evaluates the patient's physical, mental, and emotional status and response to the inpatient and outpatient care regimen. In order to meet desired patient outcomes, it is essential that this interdisciplinary team communicate openly with one another in developing and evaluating care of the patient and family (IOM [Institute of Medicine], 2010).

Patient support and instruction on these complex medical problems will help to allay anxiety and decrease stress. Instruction and involvement of family members is essential given that the patient may have to rely on family members for assistance in the event of a medical crisis.

Gerontological Considerations

There are many considerations in caring for older patients with endocrine disorders. Endocrine disorders in older adults tend to present with atypical, nonspecific manifestations and often are not recognized early. With many conditions, the symptoms may be blurred with other coexisting conditions, making it hard to diagnose the specific problem. Frailty and vulnerability to new medical conditions may affect their response to treatments and precipitate complications. Cognitive decline must also be considered as a factor affecting care of the elderly, especially when confronted with new conditions.

In considering the treatment of older patients with hypothyroidism, health care providers must be aware that this disorder may go unrecognized for a variety of reasons. These include mistaking the nonspecific signs and symptoms of this disorder as a part of the "normal aging process" or other medical conditions that may exist in older adults (Mitrou, Raptis, & Dimitriadis, 2011). Symptoms common to both the aging process and to hypothyroidism include anorexia, cognitive decline, cold intolerance, constipation, dry skin, fatigue, hearing loss, hoarseness, paresthesias, slowed reflexes, and weakness. The incidence of Graves' disease decreases with age, while other causes of hyperthyroidism (e.g., toxic multinodular goiter and toxic adenomas) increase. The clinical signs and symptoms of hyperthyroidism in older adults are often manifested in the cardiovascular system (e.g., atrial fibrillation, heart failure) and the central nervous system (e.g., depression, apathy, confusion). Older hyperthyroid patients may present with only symptoms of fatigue and weight loss; this condition is called **apathetic thyrotoxicosis.** This hypermetabolic rate also is associated with profound myopathy (muscle weakness), especially in the quadriceps, increasing the risk of falls (Greenspan, 2011).

Because older patients are particularly vulnerable to falls and bone fractures, the condition of hypoparathyroidism must be carefully managed during aging. Careful attention to nutrition, with a high intake of calcium and vitamin D, is important. Compliance with the medical regime is also important. The nurse will want to initiate a fall prevention program to decrease the risk of fractures. Patients should be encouraged to do a careful analysis of their home environment and remove throw rugs or other items that might put them at risk for a fall.

Older patients with acromegaly need considerations regarding their ability to care for themselves in the home environment. It is necessary to determine whether they can care for themselves or if they need assistance. Are they mobile; can they perform their own ADL; are they receiving any social stimulation? In the event of surgery, older patients and their families may need the resources of home health nurses. However, many older patients will not be candidates for surgical treatment

RESEARCH OPPORTUNITIES Related to Endocrine Disorders

Research Area	Clinical Impact
Improvement in clinical management of patients with endocrine disorders.	Improvement in quality of life of patients post-treatment for hormone disorder.
Develop and evaluate strategies aimed at improving adherence to chronic treatment regimes.	Provide patients with choices/alternatives to living with a chronic disease. Help them find ways to establish helpful coping mechanisms, and to enjoy a healthy and fulfilling life.
Study the impact of the genetic etiology of an endocrine disease.	Advance the knowledge base in order to guide patients in diagnostic and treatment choices.

and may be treated with medications and/or radiation. The family needs to become involved to ensure that the patient is receiving appropriate follow-up care. If necessary, family members may be taught how to administer medications and assess for side effects.

Older patients are more vulnerable to serious problems with adrenal insufficiency and may therefore require more frequent monitoring and observation. The nurse will want to instruct not only the patient, but also a spouse or other caregiver about signs and symptoms of impending crisis so that assistance can be obtained if the patient is unable to seek medical assistance in a timely way; for example, when there is infection or nausea and vomiting.

In summary, the older patients need special consideration when being treated for hormone disorders. Of primary importance is the need for emotional support; a safe environment in which to recover; assistance, if appropriate, in taking medications and resuming activities of daily living; and specific and clear directions as to their recovery protocol as they return to their optimal level of health.

Research

Significant advances have been made in the diagnoses and treatment of endocrine disorders in recent years since the development of new diagnostic imaging technologies, more sensitive hormonal assays, genetic analysis, and new synthetic hormone analogues and hormone agonists. The development of minimally invasive surgeries for pituitary, parathyroid, and adrenal tumors has been beneficial in the treatment of endocrine disorders. There have also been significant advances in the understanding of genetic factors underlying many endocrine disorders. The field of genetics, genetic counseling, and gene therapy all hold significant promise in endocrinology in the future. The advances that have been made have opened the doors to new research opportunities that will enhance the treatment and care of patients with endocrine disorders. The Research Opportunities feature outlines topics for future research.

CLINICAL PREPARATION READ DOCUMENT APPLY

READ: **History of Present Illness** >> Laboratory Study Results >> Critical Thinking Questions

Heather Birkin is a 49-year-old female who has been seen in your clinic for her primary health care needs for several years. On a recent visit, you note that she has gained approximately 20 pounds during the past year. She complains of constant fatigue, cold intolerance, and difficulty concentrating. She indicates that her performance at work has declined, that she does not feel as mentally alert as usual, and that she is slower to complete tasks than she was previously.

Medical–Surgical History

Ms. Birkin has had an unremarkable medical history, with the exception of a short episode of rheumatoid arthritis in her early 30s. The disease responded well to treatment, and she has been in remission since that time. Until now, she has maintained good physical health. She takes no medications except a daily multivitamin and an occasional aspirin. She has had no surgeries. Regular Pap smears and mammograms have been negative for disease.

Social History

Ms. Birkin does not smoke, and she drinks alcohol only rarely. She works as an administrative assistant in a local engineering firm. She is divorced and a single parent with two healthy adult children. She has engaged in regular exercise through walking and bicycling, but over the past several months has felt too tired to pursue these activities.

Ms. Birkin states that she has been feeling “a bit down,” which is unusual for her, and she has been increasingly irritable with her colleagues, her social acquaintances, and her family.

Physical Examination

Ms. Birkin’s physical examination reveals dry skin and hair that is dry and thinning in spots. Her thyroid gland appears enlarged upon palpation. The lungs are clear. The abdomen is slightly distended. Abdominal sounds are diminished; upon questioning, Ms. Birkin reports recent bouts of constipation. Vital signs are within normal limits.

Laboratory Studies

Based on a review of these symptons, the health care provider orders the following laboratory tests: thyroid-stimulating hormone (TSH) and thyroxin (free T_4). The TSH level is high, and the free T_4 level is low, indicating an underfunctioning thyroid.

CLINICAL PREPARATION, *continued*

Nursing Care

Ms. Birkin is given a prescription for thyroid hormone replacement therapy and instructed about its use. She is to take levothyroxine each day early in the morning on an empty stomach. Follow-up appointments are scheduled for 4-week intervals, progressing to 6-week during the next 6 months for continued evaluation of hormone levels to determine whether the dosage is adequate, symptoms abate, and the thyroid gland changes in size. Ms. Birkin is encouraged to increase her fluid and dietary fiber intake and to exercise to reduce constipation and aid in weight loss.

READ: History of Present Illnesses >> **Laboratory Study Results** >> Critical Thinking Questions

Test	Initial Screening	4-Week Follow-Up	8-Week Follow-Up
TSH	7.0 ng/mL	6.5 ng/mL	6.0 ng/mL
Free T_4 (Serum thyroxine)	0.5 mcg/dL	0.6 mcg/dL	0.7 mcg/dL

Pearson Nursing Student Resources *Log on to* **nursing.pearsonhighered.com** *to download forms*

DOCUMENT:

>> Summary of Hospitalization
>> Pathophysiology Form
>> Laboratory Values
>> Laboratory Results Explanation

APPLY:

>> List of Potential Nursing Diagnoses
>> Concept Map
>> Critical Thinking Questions and Concept Map

APPLY: History of Present Illness >> Laboratory Study Results >> **Critical Thinking Questions**

1. Identify Ms. Birkin's prevailing symptoms, with underlying rationale, that led to assessing her for hypothyroidism.
2. Explain the relevance of a low T_4 level and high TSH level in arriving at a diagnosis of hypothyroidism.
3. In developing an outpatient plan of care for the home setting, what key elements, with rationale, would you consider discussing with Ms. Birkin?

Answers to Critical Thinking Questions can be found in Appendix D in the Osborn Student Resources at nursing.pearsonhighered.com.

NCLEX® PRACTICE

1. A patient is admitted to the emergency department in adrenal crisis. The nurse should prepare to administer which treatment?
   1. A bolus of intravenous D_5W
   2. Intravenous hydrocortisone
   3. Intravenous diuretic such as furosemide (Lasix)
   4. Intravenous levothyroxine
2. A 13-year-old patient is diagnosed with an overproduction of a hormone produced by the anterior pituitary gland. The nurse should assess this patient for findings associated with which disorder?
   1. Gigantism
   2. Acromegaly
   3. Diabetes insipidus
   4. Infertility
3. A patient with hypothyroidism is prescribed levothyroxine. Which instruction should the nurse include when educating this patient?
   1. Take with a calcium-containing antacid.
   2. Take the medication first thing in the morning on an empty stomach.
   3. Expect the symptoms to subside immediately.
   4. Take this medication temporarily until the symptoms subside.

4. A patient who was recently treated with amiodarone is admitted with palpitations, hand tremors, muscle weakness, and muscle cramps. Which endocrine disorder should be considered as the cause of this patient's symptoms?
   1. Pheochromocytoma
   2. Hyperthyroidism
   3. Hypothyroidism
   4. Diabetes insipidus
5. The nurse is planning discharge teaching for a patient with diabetes insipidus. What is the priority instruction to this patient?
   1. The need for frequent rest periods
   2. Strategies to have access to fluids at all times
   3. Availability of high sodium foods
   4. Progressive ambulation activities
6. A nurse is concerned that a patient recovering from back surgery may be developing myxedema. Which assessment findings would support this concern? (select all that apply)
   1. Body temperature 94.6°F
   2. Slurring of speech
   3. Heart rate 126 bpm
   4. Respiratory rate of 24 breaths/min
   5. Severe irritability

Answers to NCLEX Practice Questions can be found in Appendix D in the Osborn Student Resources at nursing.pearsonhighered.com. Practice additional NCLEX questions online at the Student Resources site.

Pearson Nursing Student Resources Find additional review materials at: **nursing.pearsonhighered.com**

REFERENCES

Adams, M. P., & Koch, R. W. (2010). Pharmacology: Connections to nursing practice. Upper Saddle River, NJ: Pearson.

Adler, G. K. (2012). Cushing syndrome workup. Medscape Reference. WebMD. Retrieved from http://emedicine.medscape.com/article/117365-workup

Allina Hospitals & Clinics. (2012). Metyrapone test. UpToDate, Inc. Retrieved from http://www.allina.com/CCS/doc/Consumer_Lab/49/150401.htm

American Association of Clinical Endocrinologists (AACE). (2011). Acromegaly guidelines. *Endocrine Practice. AACE, 17* (suppl. 4), 1–44.

American Thyroid Association. (2010). Thyroid hormone treatment. Retrieved from http://www.thyroid.org/patients/patient_brochures/hormonetreatment.html

Anvita Health Wiki. (2012). Free thyroxine index (fT_4I). Retrieved from http://www.anvita.info/wiki/Free_Thyroxine_Index

Bahn, R. S., Burch, H. B., Cooper, D. S., Garber, J. R., Greenlee, M. C., Klein, I., et al. (2011). Hyperthyroidism and other causes of thyrotoxicosis: Management guidelines of the American Thyroid Association and American Association of Clinical Endocrinologists. *Endocrine Practice, 17*(3), 456–520. doi: Q707415233782R31 [pii]

Bauer, D. C., & McPhee, S. J. (2010). Thyroid disease. In S. J. McPhee & G. D. Hammer (Eds.), *Pathophysiology of disease: An introduction to clinical medicine* (pp. 549–569). New York: McGraw-Hill Medical.

Bensenor, I. M., Goulart, A. C., Lotufo, P. A., Menezes, P. R., & Scazufca, M. (2011). Prevalence of thyroid disorders among older people: Results from the Sao Paulo Ageing & Health Study. *Cadernos de Saude Publica, 27*(1), 155–161. doi: S0102-311X2011000100016 [pii]

Best Practice. (2011). Primary hyperparathyroidism. *BMJ Publishing Group Limited*. Retrieved from http://bestpracticebmj.com/best-practice/monograph/133/basispathophysiology.htm

Betterle, C., & Morlin, L. (2011). Autoimmune Addison's disease. *Endocrine Development, 20*, 161-c. doi: 000321239 [pii] 10.1159/000321239

Betz, J. M., Fisher, K. D., & Saldanha, L.G. (2007). The NIH analytical methods and reference materials program for dietary supplements. *Analytical and Bioanalytical Chemistry, 389*(1), 19–25. Epub May 31.

Bray, D. L. (2012). Thyroid storm and the AACN synergy model. *RN Journal*. Retrieved from http://www.rnjournal.com/journal_of_nursing/thyroid_storm_and_the_aacn_synergy_model

Canterbury Health. (2012). Petrossal sinus sampling (Pss). Retrieved from http://www.cushings-help.com/petrossal.htm

Carroll, T. B., Aron, D. C., Findling, J. W., & Tyrrell, J. B. (2011). Glucocorticoids and adrenal androgens. In D. G. Gardner & D. Shoback (Eds.), *Greenspan's basic and clinical endocrinology* (pp. 285–327.). New York: McGraw-Hill.

Citkowitz, E. (2011). Myxedema coma or crisis. Medscape Reference. Retrieved from http://emedicine.medscape.com/article/123577-overview

Cleveland Clinic. (2011). Goiter. Disease & conditions. Retrieved from http://mmy.clevelandclinic.org/disorders/goiter/hic_goiter.aspx

Cloe, A. (2012). Complications from neurogenic diabetes insipidus. Livestrong.com. Retrieved from http://www.livestrong.com/article/186668-complications-from-neurogenic-diabetes-insipidus/

Cooper, D. S., & Ladenson, P. W. (2011). The thyroid gland. In D. G. Gardner (Ed.), *Greenspan's basic and clinical endocrinology* (9th ed., pp. 163–226). New York: McGraw-Hill.

Cooperman, M. (2011). Diabetes insipidus. Medscape Reference. Retrieved from http://emedicine.medscaape.comm/article/117548-overview

Diabetes Insipidus. (2011). Harrison's practice. Retrieved from http://www.harrisonspractice.com/practice/ub/view/Harrisons%20Practice/141316/0/Diabetes_Insipidus

Drugs.com. (2011a). Cabergoline. TEVA Pharmaceuticals USA Inc. Retrieved from http://www.drugs.com/pro/cabergoline.html

Drugs.com. (2011b). Spironolactone. Cemer Multum, Inc. Retrieved from http:///www.drugs.com/spironolactone.html

Drugs.com. (2011c). Transsphenoidal surgery for pituitary tumors. Retrieved from http://www.drugs.com/e\cg/transsphenoidal-surgery-for-pituitary-tumors-aftercare-instruction

Drugs.com. (2012). Methimazole. Cemer Multum, Inc. Retrieved from http://www.drugs.com/mtm/methimazole.html

Else, T., & Hammer, G. D. (2010). Disorders of the hypothalamus and pituitary gland. In S. J. McPhee & G. D. Hammer (Eds.), *Pathophysiology of disease* (6th ed., pp. 523–547). New York: McGraw-Hill.

Else, T., Hammer, G. D., & McPhee, S. J. (2010). Disorders of the adrenal cortex. In S. J. McPhee & G. D. Hammer (Eds.), *Pathophysiology of disease* (6th ed., pp. 571–601). New York: McGraw-Hill.

Endocrineweb. (2011a). Hypothyroidism: Too little thyroid hormone. Retrieved from http://www.endocrineweb.com/conditons/thyroid/hypothyroidism0too-little-thyroid-hormo

Endocrineweb. (2011b). Thyroid problems and pregnancy. Retrieved from http://www.endocrineweb.com/conditions/thyroid/thyroid-problems-pregnancy

Esposito, P., Piotti, G., Bianzina, S., Malul, Y., & Dal Canton, A. (2011). The syndrome of inappropriate antidiuresis: Pathophysiology, clinical management and new therapeutic options. *Nephron Clinical Practice, 119*(1), c62–c73. doi: 000324653 [pii] 10.1159/000324653

Eugster, E. (2012). Pituitary gigantism. Retrieved from http://www.uptoPdate.com/contents/pituitary-gigantism

Ferry, Jr., R. J., Shim, M., Speiser, P. W., Windle, M. L., Bercu, B. B., & Kemp, S. (2011). Gigantism and acromegaly. Retrieved from http://emedicine.medscape.com/article/925446-overview#showall

Final Diagnosis. (2008). Cushing's disease: Hypercortisolism and pituitary adenoma. Retrieved from http://path.upmc.edu/cases/case556/dx.html

Fitzgerald, P. A. (2011). Adrenal medulla and paraganglia. In D. G. Gardner & D. Shoback (Eds.), *Greenspan's basic and clinical endocrinology* (9th ed., pp. 345–393). New York: McGraw-Hill Medical.

Freitas, B. (2011). Imaging in primary hyperparathyroidism. Medscape Reference. Retrieved from http://emedicine.medscape.com/article/390728-overview

Gardner, D. G. (2011). Endocrine emergencies. In D. G. Gardner (Ed.), *Greenspan's basic and clinical endocrinology* (9th ed., pp. 763–786). New York: McGraw-Hill.

Gardner, D. G., & Shoback, D. (Eds.). (2011). *Greenspan's basic and clinical endocrinology*. New York: McGraw-Hill.

Giusti, M., Melle, G., Fenocchio, M., Mortara, L., Cecoli, F., Caorsim, V., et al. (2011). Five-year longitudinal evaluation of quality of life in a cohort of patients with differentiated thyroid carcinoma. *Journals of Zhejiang University-Science, 12*(3): 163–173. doi: 10.1631/jzus.B1000382 PMCID: PMC3048930

Golay, V. (2011). SIADH syndrome of inappropriate secretion of antidiuretic hormone. SlideShare, Inc. Retrieved from http://www.slideshare.net/VishalGolay/siadh-8611907

Greenspan, A. (2011). *Orthopedic imaging: A practical approach* (5th ed.). Philadelphia: Lippincott Williams & Wilkins.

Hannon, M. J., & Thompson, C. J. (2010). The syndrome of inappropriate antidiuretic hormone: Prevalence, causes and consequences. *European Journal of Endocrinology, 162*(Suppl 1), S5–12. doi: EJE-09-1063 [pii] 10.1530/EJE-09-1063

Hope, W. W. (2011). Laparoscopic right adrenalectomy. Medscape Reference. Retrieved from http://emedicine.medscape.com/article/1894961-overview

IOM (Institute of Medicine). (2010). *The future of nursing: Leading change, advancing health.* Washington, DC: The National Academies Press.

Jameson, J. L., & Weetman, A. P. (2010). Disorders of the thyroid gland. In J. L. Jameson (Ed.), *Harrison's endocrinology* (2nd ed., pp. 62–98). New York: McGraw-Hill Medical.

Kaplow, R., & Hardin, S. (2007). *Critical care nursing: Synergy for optimal outcomes.* Sudbury, MA: Jones and Bartlett Publishers.

Katznelson, L., Atkinson, J. L., Cook, D. M., Ezzat, S. Z., Hamrahian, A. H., & Miller, K. K. (2011). American Association of Clinical Endocrinologists medical guidelines for clinical practice for the diagnosis and treatment of acromegaly—2011 update: Executive summary. *Endocrine Practice, 17*(4), 636–646. doi: 320L02N511745OG4 [pii]

Kee, J. L. (2010). *Laboratory and diagnostic tests with nursing implications.* Upper Saddle River, NJ: Prentice Hall.

Khandwala, H. M. (2011). Acromegaly. Medscape Reference. Retrieved from http://emedicine.medscape.com/article/116366-overview

Kim, H. J., Jung, T. S., Hahm, J. R., Hwang, S.J., Lee, S. M., Jung, J. H., Kim, S. K., & Chung, S. I. (2011). Thyrotoxicosis-induced acute myocardial infarction due to painless thyroiditis. *Thyroid, 21*(10), 1149–1151.

Lab Tests Online. (2012a). IGF-1. The test. American Association for Clinical Chemistry. Retrieved from http://labtestonline.org/understanding/analyses/igf1/ttab/test

Lab Tests Online. (2012b). T_3. American Association for Clinical Chemistry. Retrieved from http://labtestsonline.org/understanding/analyses/t3/tab/test

Lal, G., & Clark, O. H. (2010). Endocrine surgery. In J. L. Jameson (Ed.), *Harrison's endocrinology* (2nd ed., pp. 803–823). New York: McGraw-Hill Medical.

Loh, J. S., & Verbalis. J. A. (2011). Diabetes insipidus as a complication after pituitary surgery. Retrieved from http://www.medscape.com/viewarticle/558561

MayoClinic.com. (2012). Clofibrate (oral route). Retrieved from http://www.mayoclinic.com/health/drug-information/DR600441

Mayo Clinic, Mayo Medical Laboratories. (2012). Interpretive handbook. Retrieved from http://www.mayomedicallaboratories.com/interpretive-guide/index.html?alpha=F&unit_co

Mayo Clinic Staff. (2010). Hypothyroidism (underactive thyroid). Retrieved from http://www.mayoclinic.com/health/hypothyroidism/DSD993593/METHOD=print&DSECT

Mayo Clinic Staff. (2011). Hyperparathyroidism. Retrieved from http://www.mayoclinic.com/health/hyperparathyroidism/DS00385/METHOD=print

Mayo Clinic Staff (2012) Acromegaly. Mayo Foundation for Medical Education and Research. Retrieved from http://www.mayoclinic.com/health/acromegaly/DS00478/DSECTION=tests-and-diagnosis

Medical News Today. (2012). What is diabetes insipidus? What causes diabetes insipidus? Retrieved from http://www.medicalnewstoday.com/articles/183251.php

Meditec. (2012). Normal lab values. Retrieved from http://www.meditec.com/resourcesstools/medical-reference-links/normal-lab-values/

MedlinePlus. (2011). Cortisol—urine. Retrieved from http://www.nlm.nih.gov/medlineplus/ency/article/003703.htm

MedlinePlus. (2012a). Calcitrol. Retrieved from http://www.nlm.nih.gov/medlineplus/druginfo/meds/a6823335.html

MedlinePlus. (2012b). Carbamazepine. Retrieved from http://www.nlm.gov/medlineplus/druginfo/meds/a682237.html

MedlinePlus. (2010a). Goiter—simple. Retrieved from http://www.nlm.nih.gov/medlineplus/ency/article/001178.htm

MedlinePlus. (2010b). Growth hormone suppression test. Retrieved from http://www.nlm.nih.gov/medlineplus/ency/article/003376.htm

MedlinePlus. (2010c). T_3 test. Retrieved from http://www.nlm.nih.gov/medlineplus/ency/article/003687.htm

Melmed, S., & Jameson, J. L. (2010). Disorders of the anterior pituitary and hypothalamus. In J. L. Jameson (Ed.), *Harrison's endocrinology* (2nd ed., pp. 16–49). New York: McGraw-Hill Medical.

Mitrou, P., Raptis, S. A., & Dimitriadis, G. (2011). Thyroid disease in older people. *Maturitas, 70*(1), 5–9. doi: 10.1016/j.maturitas.2011.05.016

Monson, K., & Schoenstadt, A. (2009). Lithium uses. Retrieved from http://bipolar-disorder.emedtv.com/lithium/lithium=uses-p2.html

Mulinda, J.R. (2011). Pituitary Macroadenomas. *Medscape Reference.* Retrieved from http:/emedicine.medscape.com/article/123223-overview

Neumann, H. P. H. (2010). Pheochromocytoma. In J. L. Jameson (Ed.), *Harrison's endocrinology* (pp. 133–141). New York: McGraw-Hill Medical.

Parathyroid.com. (2012). Who gets parathyroid disease (hyperparathyroidism)? Retrieved from http://parathyroid.com/age.htm

Phillips, M. M., Rimmer, C. A., Wood, L. J., Lippa, K. A., Sharpless, K. E., Duewer, D. L., et al. (2011). Dietary supplement laboratory quality assurance program: The first five exercises. *Journal of AOAC International, 94*(3), 803–814.

Pituitary Network Association. (2012). Pituitary disorders. Retrieved from http://www.pituitary.org/disorders/acromegaly.aspx

Porterfield, S. P., & White, B. A. (2007). *Endocrine physiology* (3rd ed.). Philadelphia, PA: Mosby/Elsevier.

Porth, C. M., & Matfin, G. (2009). *Essentials of pathophysiology: Concepts of altered health states.* Philadelphia: Lippincott Williams & Wilkins.

Potts, J. T., Jr. (2010). Disease of the parathyroid gland. In J. L. Jameson (Ed.), *Harrison's endocrinology* (2nd ed., pp. 411–442). New York: McGraw-Hill Medical.

Rastoge, M. V., & La Franchi, S. H. (2010). Congenital hypothyroidism. *Orphanet Journal of Rare Diseases, 5*(17). Retrieved from http:www.ojrd.com/content/5/1/07

RightDiagnosis.com. (2011a). Symptoms of acromegaly. Retrieved from http://www.rightdiagnosis.co/a/acromegaly/symptoms.htm

RightDiagnosis.com. (2011b). Thyroid hypoplasia. Retrieved from http://www.rightdiagnosis.com/medical/thyroid_hypoplasia.htm

Robertson, G. L. (2010). Disorders of the neurohypophysis. In J. L. Jameson (Ed.), *Harrison's endocrinology* (2nd ed., pp. 50–61). New York: McGraw-Hill Medical.

Saliba, W., & El-Haddad, B. (2009). Secondary hyperparathyroidism: Pathophysiology and treatment. *Journal of the American Board of Family Medicine, 22*(5), 574–581.

Schraga, E. D. (2010). Hyperthyroidism, thyroid storm, and Graves disease. Medscape Reference. Retrieved from http://emedicine.medscape.com/article/767130-overview

Science Clarified. (2012). Radioactive tracers. Advameg. Inc. Retrieved from http://www.scienceclarified.com/Qu-Ro/Radioactive-Tracers.html

Shoback, D. M., & Sellmeyer, D. E. (2010). Disorders of parathyroid and calcium and phosphorus metabolism. In S. J. McPhee & G. D. Hammer (Eds.), *Pathophysiology of disease* (pp. 465–496). New York: McGraw-Hill Medical.

Shoback, D. M., Sellmeyer, D., & Bikle, D. D. (2011). Metabolic bone disease. In D. G. Gardner & D. Shoback (Eds.), *Greenspan's basic and clinical endocrinology* (pp. 227–284). New York: McGraw-Hill Medical.

The Hormone Foundation. (2012). Endo 101: Control of the endocrine system by negative feedback. Retrieved from http://www.hormone.org/Endo101/page3.cfm

Thomas, C. P. (2012). Symptom of inappropriate antidiuretic hormone secretion. Medscape Reference. Retrieved from http:/medicine.medscape.com/aticl246overview

Tsegay, E., Anyango, G., Van Sell, S. L., & Miller-Anderson, M. (2008). Pheochromocytoma: A rare tumor in adults and children. Retrieved from http://www.modernmedicine.com/modernmedicine/CE+Library/CNE-Pheochromocytoma-A-rare-tumor-in-adults-and-ch/ArticleStandard/Article/detail/523381?contextCategoryId=5796&ref=25

University of Maryland Medical Center. (2011a). Complementary medicine. Retrieved from http://www.umm.edu/altmed/articles/hyperparathyroidism-000086.htm

University of Maryland Medical Center. (2011b). DHEA. Retrieved from http://www.umm.edu/altmed/articles/dehydroepianidrolesterone-000299,htm

Uwaifo, G. I. (2012). Primary hyperaldosteronism treatment & management. Medscape Reference. Retrieved from http://emedicine.medscape.com/article/127080-treatment

Watt, T., et al. (2006). Quality of life in patients with benign thyroid disorders. A review. *European Journal of Endocrinology, 154*(4), 501–510.

Watt, T., Hegedus, L., Rasmussen, A. K., Groenvold, M., Bonnema, S. J., & Bjorner, J. B. (2007). Which domains of thyroid-related quality of life are most relevant? Patients and clinicians provide complementary perspectives. *Thyroid, 17*(7), 647–654.

Watt, T., et al. (2008). Improving a newly developed patient-reported outcome for thyroid patients, using cognitive interviewing. *Quality of Life Review.* doi: 10.1007s11136-008-9364-z

WebMD. (2010). Catecholamines in urine. Retrieved from http://www.webmd.com/heart-disease/catecholamines-14697?page=2

Wilkinson, J. M., & Ahearn, N. R. (2009). *Prentice Hall nursing diagnosis handbook* (9th ed.). Upper Saddle River, NJ: Prentice Hall.

Williams, G. H. (2010). Disorders of the adrenal cortex. In J. L. Jameson (Ed.), *Harrison's endocrinology* (pp. 99–141). New York: McGraw-Hill Medical.

Caring for the Patient with Diabetes

47 CHAPTER

Laurie Quinn
Annita Watson
With contributions by Cynthia Fritschi

Outcome-Based Learning Objectives

After studying this chapter, the learner will be able to:

1. Classify the risk factors for developing type 1 diabetes and type 2 diabetes.
2. Differentiate between the pathophysiology, clinical manifestations, and treatment of type 1 and type 2 diabetes.
3. Analyze the differences in the pharmacologic management of type 1 and type 2 diabetes.
4. Develop a plan for the nutritional management of type 1 and type 2 diabetes.
5. Generate a nursing plan of care for the patient with diabetes.
6. Explain the differences in the clinical signs and symptoms, diagnosis, treatment, nursing assessment, and management of diabetic ketoacidosis, hyperosmolar hyperglycemic syndrome, and hypoglycemia.

KEY TERMS

continuous subcutaneous insulin infusion (CSII) p.1433
dawn phenomenon p.1434
diabetes mellitus (DM) p.1418
diabetic ketoacidosis (DKA) p.1445
diabetic peripheral neuropathy (DPN) p.1450
gestational diabetes mellitus (GDM) p.1421
hemoglobin A_1c (A_1c) test p.1429
hyperosmolar hyperglycemic syndrome (HHS) p.1445
hypoglycemia unawareness p.1445
incretin mimetics p.1433
Kussmaul respirations p.1446
latent autoimmune diabetes in adults (LADA) p.1421
maturity-onset diabetes of the young (MODY) p.1421
neonatal diabetes mellitus (NDM) p.1421
prediabetes p.1423
secondary diabetes p.1422
Somogyi effect p.1434
type 1 diabetes mellitus p.1418
type 2 diabetes mellitus p.1419

DIABETES MELLITUS (DM) is a group of metabolic disorders characterized by abnormal fuel metabolism, all of which have hyperglycemia (high blood glucose) in common. These disorders result from defects in insulin secretion, insulin action, or both (American Diabetes Association [ADA], 2010a). Insulin, a hormone produced by pancreatic beta cells, has a critical role in carbohydrate, fat, and protein metabolism and is essential in maintaining normal blood glucose levels. Diabetes also is associated with the development of a number of debilitating complications including eye disease (retinopathy), kidney disease (nephropathy), nerve disease (neuropathy), stroke, cardiovascular disease (CVD), and peripheral vascular disease (PVD), all of which are discussed later in this chapter.

Approximately 25.8 million people, or 8.3% of the U.S. population, have diabetes, including 18.8 million who have been diagnosed and an estimated 7.0 million who are undiagnosed (Centers for Disease Control and Prevention [CDC], 2011). The prevalence of diabetes (diagnosed and undiagnosed cases) is projected to increase from 14% to 21% of all U.S. adults between 2010 and 2050. However, if the incidence of diabetes continues to rise and the rate of diabetes mortality remains relatively low, the prevalence will increase to 33% by 2050 (Boyle, Thompson, Gregg, Barker, & Williamson, 2010). The International Diabetes Federation (2009) predicted that there would be 285 million people worldwide with diabetes in 2010, increasing to 438 million in 2030 (International Diabetes Federation, 2009). The prevalence of diabetes differs by factors such as type of diabetes, race, ethnicity, and geographic location. These factors are discussed as they relate to each type of diabetes. The risk of developing diabetes is shown in Figure 47–1◆.

The most recent criteria for the diagnosis and classification of diabetes were published by the American Diabetes Association (ADA) in 1997, with periodic updates since then (ADA, 2010a). These criteria are based on the etiology of diabetes. In the past, classification was related to either age of onset (e.g., juvenile, adult) or pharmacologic treatment regimens (e.g., insulin, oral medications). These newer classification criteria allow for the diagnosis and classification of prediabetes and three major types of diabetes: type 1 diabetes, type 2 diabetes, gestational diabetes mellitus, as well asnd other types of diabetes. Type 1 diabetes and type 2 diabetes, the most common forms of diabetes, are the primary focus of this chapter.

Video: Diabetes Weblink: Overview of Diabetes Mellitus

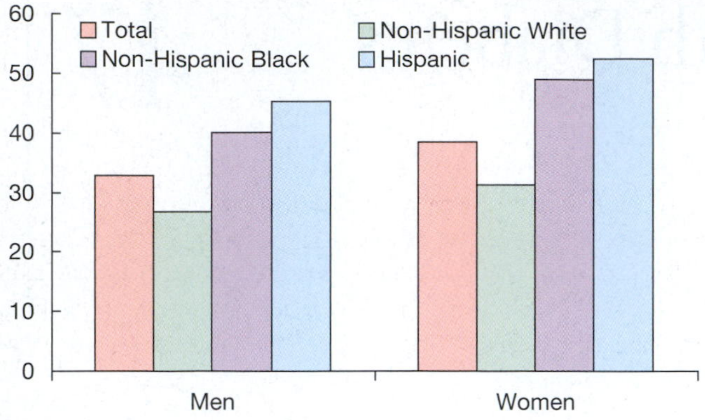

FIGURE 47–1 ◆ Estimated lifetime risk of developing diabetes for individuals born in the United States in 2000.

Source: CDC, 2011. http://apps.nccd.cdc.gov/DDTSTRS/FactSheet.aspx.

Types of Diabetes

The three major types of diabetes and prediabetes can be described as follows:

1. Type 1 diabetes is a chronic autoimmune disorder in which there is a complete lack of insulin production.
2. Type 2 diabetes is the most common form of diabetes, in which the body does not produce enough insulin or the cells ignore the insulin the body needs so that it can use glucose, the body's main fuel, for energy.
3. Gestational diabetes develops during pregnancy. It affects how cells use glucose.

Prediabetes (also referred to as "impaired glucose tolerance") is a health condition with no symptoms. In this condition, the individual's blood glucose levels are higher than normal but not high enough to be type 2 diabetes.

Type 1 Diabetes Mellitus

The distinguishing feature of **type 1 diabetes mellitus (DM)** is the complete lack of insulin production, which is caused by autoimmune destruction of the insulin-producing pancreatic beta cells. Therefore, people with type 1 diabetes need exogenous insulin to metabolize glucose and sustain life. Previous classifications of type 1 diabetes included juvenile diabetes mellitus, insulin-dependent diabetes mellitus, and type I diabetes (note the Roman numeral); these terms have become obsolete since the American Diabetes Association (ADA) adopted a new classification system in 1997 (ADA, 2008a).

Epidemiology and Etiology

Although type 1 diabetes can occur at any age, it is frequently diagnosed before 30 years of age. However, there is an adult form of autoimmune type 1 diabetes termed *latent autoimmune diabetes in adults* (LADA) (Appel, Wadas, Rosenthal, & Ovalle, 2009), which is discussed later in the chapter (p. 1421). Type 1 diabetes accounts for approximately 5% to 10% of all diagnosed diabetes in the United States (CDC, 2011). Approximately 1 in every 400 children and adolescents has type 1 diabetes, making it one of the most common severe chronic disorders of childhood (ADA, 2011b). Globally, there are large geographic and temporal variations in the incidence of type 1 diabetes, suggesting that there is an environmental contribution to the disorder. Individuals with type 1 diabetes are usually thin or of normal weight at diagnosis and have an abrupt onset of symptoms. Type 1 diabetes appears to result from an interaction among genetics, environment, and autoimmunity. Risk factors for type 1 diabetes are listed in the Risk Factors box, and a discussion of major causative theories follows.

RISK FACTORS for Type 1 Diabetes

Genetics. A familial predisposition exists.

Environmental. A variety of environmental triggers may initiate development (e.g., viral infections, dietary factors, and toxins).

Autoimmunity: Presence of circulating autoantibodies to pancreatic beta-cell components

Genetics

A familial predisposition to the development of type 1 diabetes does exist; however, the exact mode of genetic inheritance remains unclear. A sibling of a person with type 1 diabetes has a 6% risk of developing the disorder. In addition, the offspring of a father with type 1 diabetes has a greater chance of developing the disorder (6%) than the offspring of a mother (3%). Most significantly, however, there is a higher incidence for type 1 diabetes among monozygotic twins (25% to 50%) than among dizygotic twins (6%). If the development of type 1 diabetes were determined completely by genetic inheritance, the concordance rate would be 100%. The fact that the concordance rate among identical twins is 25% to 50% supports the theory that an environmental trigger initiates the transition from genetic predisposition to type 1 diabetes. The Genetic Considerations box discusses the genes involved in the development of type 1 diabetes.

Environmental

According to this theory, a triggering event in someone who is at risk for developing type 1 diabetes initiates a series of autoimmune events ending in the destruction of pancreatic beta cells. A variety of environmental triggers have been proposed as initiating events, including viral infections, dietary factors, and toxins; however, no single factor has been consistently associated with the risk of type 1 diabetes.

Congenital rubella syndrome is associated strongly with the development of type 1 diabetes, but this syndrome represents only a small number of cases (Gale, 2008). The observation that children frequently develop type l diabetes following a viral illness has provided anecdotal evidence that a virus may be the initiating event in type 1 diabetes. In particular, it has been postulated that enteroviruses may initiate the

GENETIC CONSIDERATIONS for Type 1 Diabetes

Approximately 40% to 50% of the genetic predisposition to the development of type 1 diabetes is conferred by genes on the short arm of chromosome 6, either within or in proximity to the Class II human leukocyte antigen (HLA) region of the major histocompatibility complex (MHC) (Kaufman & ADA, 2008). The inheritance of particular HLA alleles can account for more than half of the genetic risk of developing type 1 diabetes. HLA-DR and HLA-DQ are most strongly linked with type 1 diabetes. In type 1 diabetes, at least one allele of DR3 or DR4 is found in 95% of Caucasians, and individuals with both DR3 and DR4 are particularly susceptible to type 1 diabetes. Conversely, the DR2 allele is protective against type 1 diabetes (Kaufman & ADA, 2008).

Source: Kaufman, F. R., & American Diabetes Association. (2008). *Medical management of type 1 diabetes* (5th ed.). Alexandria, VA: American Diabetes Association.

development of type 1 diabetes in those who are genetically at risk for the disorder (Yeung, Rawlinson, & Craig, 2011).

Of the possible dietary etiologic factors, cow's milk proteins have received the main attention. Studies indicate an association between early exposure to dietary cow's milk proteins and an increased risk of type 1 diabetes, but the data remain controversial (Luopajarvi et al., 2008). Toxins that have gained attention as possible environmental triggers for type 1 diabetes are the N-nitroso compounds. Nitrate is found in vegetables, and nitrate and nitrite are found in meat products. In the intestines, nitrate is reduced to nitrite. Nitrite is transformed in the intestines by reaction with amines and amides to nitrosamines. Evidence such as this suggests that there is a relationship between nitrates and nitrites in type 1 diabetes; this relationship is under investigation.

Autoimmunity

A number of circulating autoantibodies that target specific pancreatic beta-cell components have been identified in individuals with type 1 diabetes. These include cytoplasmic islet cell antibodies (ICAs), insulin autoantibodies (IAAs), antibodies directed against the enzyme glutamic acid decarboxylase (GAD), and antibodies against islet tyrosine phosphatase (i.e., IA-2 and IA-2beta) (Kaufman & ADA, 2008). The presence of two or more antibodies, together with alterations in insulin secretion, is highly predictive of the development of type 1 diabetes within 5 years (Kaufman & ADA, 2008). Unaffected relatives are at risk for the development of type 1 diabetes.

Type 2 Diabetes Mellitus

Type 2 diabetes mellitus results from decreased insulin production by the pancreas and increased insulin resistance, which is characterized by an inability to use insulin effectively (ADA, 2011b; Mayo Clinic Staff, 2012c). Previous classifications of type 2 diabetes included terms such as *adult-onset diabetes, non–insulin-dependent diabetes mellitus* (NIDDM), or *type II diabetes*. These terms are no longer used.

Epidemiology and Etiology

Type 2 diabetes typically is diagnosed after the age of 30 years but is starting to occur more frequently in patients at younger ages. Type 2 diabetes accounts for approximately 90% to 95% of all diabetes, both nationally and globally (CDC, 2011). There has been a dramatic increase in the incidence of type 2 diabetes, especially in newly Westernized countries. However, only India and China exceed the United States in the number of individuals diagnosed with diabetes (International Diabetes Federation [IDF], 2009). People with type 2 diabetes often are overweight or obese at the time of diagnosis and have a strong family history of the disorder.

Insulin therapy and/or oral medications may be needed to control hyperglycemia (Mayo Clinic Staff, 2012b). Individuals with type 2 diabetes usually are not dependent on exogenous insulin to sustain life; however, some type 2 diabetics who have had diabetes for longer and produce less endogenous insulin may be dependent on insulin to sustain life.

There are numerous risk factors for type 2 diabetes (CDC, 2011; Diabetes Health Center, 2010; Mathur & Stöppler, 2012; Mayo Clinic Staff, 2012c; Type 2 Diabetes Risk Factors, 2012); these are outlined in the Risk Factors box. A brief discussion of the four risk factors that are most strongly associated with type 2 diabetes (marked with an asterisk in the box) by the American Diabetes Association (2012c) follows. Genetic origins for type 2 diabetes are described in the Genetic Considerations box (p. 1421).

Sedentary Lifestyle and Poor Dietary Patterns

A number of epidemiologic studies during the last two decades have demonstrated that high levels of physical activity protect against the development of type 2 diabetes. Two intervention studies have confirmed the value of lifestyle changes in the prevention of type 2 diabetes (ADA, 2010b). The classic Finnish Diabetes Prevention Study examined whether type 2 diabetes could be prevented through lifestyle modification in subjects with impaired glucose tolerance (IGT). In this study, subjects were assigned to either an intervention group or a control group. Subjects in the intervention group received individualized counseling aimed at weight reduction, dietary fat reduction, saturated fat reduction, increased dietary fiber, and increased physical activity. The risk of diabetes was reduced by 58% in the intervention group.

In the U.S. Diabetes Prevention Program (DPP), approximately 3,234 adults with elevated fasting and postload (time after glucose load) plasma glucose concentrations (i.e., those with prediabetes) were randomized into three groups: placebo, metformin (an oral hypoglycemic medication), or lifestyle modification program (Adams, 2011; CDC, 2011). The lifestyle modification program reduced the incidence of diabetes by 58%, and metformin reduced the incidence by 31% when compared with placebo. The study concluded that to prevent one case of diabetes during a 3-year period, 6.9 persons would have to participate in the lifestyle intervention program, and 13.9 would have to receive metformin. Therefore, the lifestyle intervention program was more effective than the metformin.

Poor dietary habits also play a major role in the development of type 2 diabetes. The American Diabetes Association (2012c) noted that during times of reduced caloric intake, such as in food shortages during wars, there was a decline in morbidity and mortality from type 2 diabetes (ADA, 2012c). The conclusion was that there appeared to be an association between the amount of caloric intake and development of type 2 diabetes. However, the independent effects of caloric restriction on prevention of type 2 diabetes are difficult to discern from the effects of reducing or maintaining normal body weight. The exact composition of diet in the prevention of type 2 diabetes also is not clear. High-carbohydrate and low-fat diets appear to cause insulin sensitivity to deteriorate, thus increasing the risk of type 2 diabetes, but high-fat and low-carbohydrate diets may decrease satiety and lead to higher energy intake. A study published in the journal *Diabetes Care* reported that having a high intake of certain foods can put an individual at risk for diabetes. For example, the people in the study ate a lot of red meat, low-fiber breads and cereals, eggs, and cheese, among other types of food (Type 2 Diabetes Risk Factors, 2012). A high-fat diet combined with high alcohol intake also may contribute to the development of diabetes.

Ethnicity

Approximately 15.7 million (10.2%) of all non-Hispanic (CDC, 2011) Whites ages 20 years or older have diabetes, while 4.9 million (18.7%) of all non-Hispanic Blacks ages 20 years or older are affected (CDC, 2011). After adjusting for population age differences, 7.1% of non-Hispanic Whites, 8.4% of Asian Americans, 11.8% of Hispanics, and 12.6% of non-Hispanic Blacks had diagnosed diabetes. There is insufficient data to calculate prevalence rates among all minority populations (e.g., American Indians, Alaska Natives) (CDC, 2011); however, adjusting for population age differences, 16.1% of the total adult population served by the Indian Health Service had diagnosed diabetes. These rates varied by region from 5.5% among Alaska Native adults to 33.5% among

RISK FACTORS for Type 2 Diabetes

Age: As a person ages, the risk of type 2 diabetes increases, especially after age 45. This is possibly because people exercise less, lose muscle mass, and gain weight as they age.

**Sedentary Lifestyle and Poor Dietary Habits:* Lack of physical activity and a high-calorie, high-fat, high-carbohydrate diet can lead to type 2 diabetes. The less active an individual is, the greater the risk. Physical activity helps to keep weight under control, uses up glucose as energy, and makes cells more sensitive to insulin.

**Obesity.* Weight greater than 130% of desirable body weight; a body mass index (BMI) greater than 25; and unequal weight distribution, especially in the upper body and abdomen, increase the risk of developing type 2 diabetes.

Intrauterine Development (also referred to as birth weight): There is a relationship between birth weight and developing diabetes: The lower the birth weight, the higher the risk of type 2 diabetes later in life (Stöppler, 2012). It is hypothesized that suboptimal early nutrition or poor growth in utero predisposes the fetus to type 2 diabetes later in life (Martin-Gronert & Ozanne, 2010).

Familial History (genetics): The risk increases if parents or siblings have type 2 diabetes. The general American population has a 1 in 9 lifetime risk of developing type 2 diabetes (Type 2 Diabetes Risk Factors, 2012). If your brother, sister, mother, or father develops type 2, your risk is doubled to a 1 in 4 chance of developing the condition (Type 2 Diabetes Risk Factors, 2012).

**Ethnicity:* African American, Alaska Native, American Indian, Asian American, Hispanic/Latino Americans, and Pacific Islanders have a higher tendency to develop type 2 diabetes than members of other races (CDC, 2011). Many people in these groups have a lower risk of developing type 2 diabetes when they do not live in a Westernized culture (Type 2 Diabetes Risk Factors, 2012).

**Metabolic Syndrome:* This cluster of conditions—increased blood pressure, a high blood sugar level, excess body fat around the waist, abnormal cholesterol levels—occurs together. If all or any of these components are present, the risk of developing type 2 diabetes increases.

Gestational Diabetes: Giving birth to a baby weighing more than 9 pounds increases a woman's risk of developing type 2 diabetes.

Prediabetes: When the blood glucose level is higher than normal but not high enough to meet the criteria for diabetes, the patient is said to have prediabetes. Left untreated, prediabetes often progresses to type 2 diabetes.

High Blood Pressure: An individual with 140/90 mmHg or above or being treated for high blood pressure is at risk.

Abnormal Cholesterol and Triglyceride Levels: HDL cholesterol level below 35 mg/dL or a triglyceride level above 250 mg/dL are risk factors.

Polycystic Ovary Syndrome (PCOS): This condition affects about 6% of women and results in the ovarian production of high amounts of androgens, particularly testosterone. Women with PCOS are at higher risk for insulin resistance (Gambineri, Patton, Altieri, et al., 2012). Other medical conditions associated with insulin resistance also are at risk.

History of Previously Impaired Glucose Tolerance (IGT) or Impaired Fasting Glucose (IFG): This is a situation in which the individual has had previous episodes of IGT and/or IFG.

Presence of Acanthosis Nigricans: This skin disorder is characterized by a dark, velvety rash or markings around the neck, armpits, and groin and under the breasts. It is often associated with a condition that increases the insulin level, such as being overweight, an endocrine disorder, or type 2 diabetes. If a patient's insulin level is too high, the extra insulin may trigger activity in skin cells, causing the characteristic skin changes. It is most common among people of African descent (WebMD, 2010).

History of Cardiovascular Disease: Diabetes has many of the same risk factors as cardiovascular disease: elevated triglycerides, lowered low density cholesterol levels, hypertension, and impaired fasting blood glucose (National Diabetes Information Clearinghouse [NDIC], 2007). Reciprocally, diabetes is a risk factor for cardiovascular disease.

Drug-Induced Diabetes: Pentamidine, nicotinic acid, glucocorticoids, and thiazides may induce type 2 diabetes (ThirdAge Media, 2012; Tufts University, 2012).

Endocrine Disorders: For example, Cushing syndrome, hyperthyroidism, pheochromocytoma, acromegaly, and glucagonoma may lead to diabetes (Type 2 Diabetes Risk Factors, 2012).

Genetic Diseases: Individuals with disorders such as Down syndrome, porphyria, hemochromatosis, Turner syndrome, and Klinefelter syndrome have a higher risk of developing type 2 diabetes (ADA, 2008a).

Urbanization: When certain populations migrate from rural to urban settings, they have an increased prevalence of type 2 diabetes when compared to relatives who remain in the original setting. Because urbanization is associated with changes in diet, physical activity, socioeconomic activity, and obesity, the risk of type 2 diabetes increases. For example, the Pima Indians of the Southwestern United States have a greater than 50% chance of developing type 2 diabetes in their lifetime, but their relatives in Mexico (who have a traditional lifestyle) have a very low risk of diabetes (Adams, 2011).

Socioeconomic Status (SES) and Education: Individuals in the lowest SES brackets have the highest risk of type 2 diabetes (Krishnan, Cozier, Rosenberg, & Palmer, 2010). Lower levels of education also are inversely related to diabetes risk (Dinca-Panaitescu et al., 2011).

American Indian adults in southern Arizona (CDC, 2011). There is wide variability in the risk of type 2 diabetes among different racial and ethnic groups.

Obesity

Obesity is strongly associated with the development of type 2 diabetes. There has been an increased emphasis on the role of central or visceral obesity (weight centered in the abdomen) in the development of type 2 diabetes. Central body obesity appears to be a prognostic marker for glucose intolerance, hyperinsulinemia (excess levels of circulating insulin), and hypertriglyceridemia (excess levels of circulating triglycerides). Type 2 diabetes and prediabetes are manifestations of an underlying disorder termed *metabolic syndrome* (Burant & ADA, 2008).

Metabolic Syndrome

Metabolic syndrome refers to a group of metabolic abnormalities that predispose individuals to cardiovascular disease and type 2 diabetes. The primary abnormalities that are in this syndrome are insulin resistance, glucose intolerance, hyperinsulinemia, hypertriglyceridemia and decreased HDL cholesterol, central obesity, and hypertension. The most common criteria used to define metabolic syndrome were developed by the Adult Treatment Panel III (ATP III) National Cholesterol Education Program Expert Panel on Detection, Evaluation, and Treatment of High Blood Cholesterol in Adults (Report of the Expert Committee on the Diagnosis and Classification of Diabetes Mellitus, 2003). Three or more of the following abnormalities must be present:

- High blood pressure (≥130/85 mmHg)
- Hypertriglyceridemia (≥150 mg/dL)
- Low high-density lipoprotein cholesterol (≤40 mg/dL in men; ≤50 mg/dL in women)
- Abdominal obesity (waist circumference ≥102 cm in men; ≥88 cm in women)
- Elevated fasting glucose (≥100 mg/dL).

Metabolic syndrome is also known as insulin resistance syndrome. Insulin resistance and hyperinsulinemia caused by these metabolic abnormalities lead to hyperglycemia, which is now known to occur at short intervals long before the diagnosis of diabetes. The effect of hyperglycemia from impaired glucose tolerance and insulin resistance sets off an inflammatory process in the vascular endothelial lining. Pro-inflammatory cytokines are released in the presence of hyperglycemia and start a cascade that further increases insulin resistance, increases hyperglycemia, and causes inflammatory damage to the endothelium.

Many people with metabolic syndrome will go on to develop type 2 diabetes within 5 to 10 years. However, the onset of type 2 diabetes can be delayed or in some cases prevented through a combination of weight loss, healthy diet, and exercise. Metabolic syndrome is identified as an independent risk factor for cardiovascular disease (Boudi, 2012).

Gestational Diabetes Mellitus

Gestational diabetes mellitus (GDM) is a condition in which the onset of diabetes occurs during pregnancy. The prevalence of GDM ranges from 2% to 10% for all pregnancies (CDC, 2011) but may reach 10% to 20% in high-risk populations (Galtier, 2010). Risk factors for GDM include previous GDM, advanced maternal age, obesity, family history of diabetes, and racial/ethnic origin (African Americans, Hispanic/Latino Americans, and American Indians are at higher risk). Women who are diagnosed with GDM need dietary treatment and possibly oral medications or insulin therapy to control hyperglycemia (Cheng et al., 2009). Uncontrolled hyperglycemia during pregnancy can result in fetal and maternal complications. Gestational diabetes resolves after childbirth; however, women with GDM have a 35% to 60% chance of developing diabetes in the 10 to 20 years following the pregnancy (CDC, 2011).

Other Specific Types of Diabetes

Other types of diabetes can result from certain specific genetic conditions, as occurs in monogenic forms of diabetes; surgery (e.g., pancreatectomy); drugs (e.g., corticosteroids); and infections

GENETIC CONSIDERATIONS
for Type 2 Diabetes Mellitus

A small number of cases of type 2 diabetes are caused by a single-gene defect, such as in mature onset diabetes of the young (MODY), which is described later in this chapter. The genetic component of the more common form of type 2 diabetes appears to be complex, involving the interactions of several genes and environmental factors (Groop & Lyssenko, 2009).

(e.g., congenital rubella), as well as other illnesses. The initial diagnosis and clinical presentation of the diabetes in this group vary with the underlying disorder.

Monogenic Diabetes

Epidemiology, Etiology, and Risk Factors

Monogenic diabetes accounts for 1% to 5% of all cases of childhood diabetes (NDIC, 2007). The monogenic forms of diabetes result from a single-gene mutation, whereas type 1 and 2 diabetes result from polygenic (multiple gene) defects. The two main forms of monogenic diabetes are **neonatal diabetes mellitus (NDM),** which occurs in newborns and young infants, and **maturity-onset diabetes of the young (MODY),** which usually first occurs during adolescence or early adulthood.

Clinical Manifestations and Pathophysiology

Although MODY, sometimes referred to as type 1.5 diabetes, is usually diagnosed in adolescence or early adulthood, it may remain undiagnosed until later in life (Ruhl, 2012). This inherited form of diabetes affects about 2% of people with diabetes (Porter, 202). It is caused primarily by defects in beta-cell function and secretion. There are eight different autosomal-dominant genetic mutations associated with MODY (Molven, Ringdal, Nordbø, et al., 2008). The gene mutations limit the pancreas's ability to produce insulin. This process leads to the high blood glucose levels that are characteristic of diabetes and, in time, may damage body tissues (What Is Maturity-Onset Diabetes of the Young [MODY], 2012).

Patients with MODY present clinically with a strong family history of diabetes, often through several generations. They may have only mild symptoms or no symptoms of diabetes, and their hyperglycemia may be discovered only during routine blood tests. MODY may be confused with type 1 or type 2 diabetes. However, people with MODY generally are not overweight and do not have other risk factors for type 2 diabetes, such as high blood pressure or abnormal levels of cholesterol or triglycerides.

Medical Management

Unlike people with type 1 diabetes, who always require insulin, people with MODY can often be treated with oral diabetes medications. Treatment varies depending on the genetic mutation that caused the MODY (Ruhl, 2012).

Latent Autoimmune Diabetes in Adults

Epidemiology, Etiology, and Risk Factors

Latent autoimmune diabetes in adults (LADA) is a genetically linked, hereditary autoimmune disease that is sometimes referred to as type 1.5 diabetes (Kapustin, 2012; Lightsey, 2011). With LADA, the body mistakes the pancreas as foreign and responds by attaching and destroying the insulin-producing beta islet cells of the pancreas (Latent Autoimmune Diabetes in Adults, 2012). This disease is seen commonly after age 30 in patients who usually have a normal body mass index without overt signs of metabolic syndrome (Kapustin, 2012). Latent autoimmune diabetes in adults accounts for 2% to 12% of all cases of diabetes (Nambam, Aggarwal, & Jain, 2010). Adults with LADA have positive circulating antibodies which attack islet cells, causing glutamic acid decarboxylase (GAD), reflecting the autoimmune nature of beta-cell destruction (Kapustin, 2012). Because these patients are older when first symptomatic, they often are diagnosed with type 2 diabetes.

Risk factors for LADA include age of onset (<59 [typically <35]), acute symptoms of diabetes, BI < 35 kg/m, personal history of autoimmune diseases such as autoimmune thyroid disease, and family history of autoimmune disease (Johnson, 2007; Kapustin, 2012).

Clinical Manifestations and Pathophysiology

Symptoms of LADA include age (patients usually are between 30 and 50 years old); have a lean build or normal to low body mass index; have not had a significant unexplained weight loss; do not present with ketoacidosis; have no known relatives with type 2 diabetes; and have a low C-peptide level.

Latent autoimmune diabetes in adults is thought to represent a slowly progressive beta-cell destruction process due to the presence of circulating islet autoimmunity. Patients with LADA demonstrate less aggressive beta-cell destruction than type 1 diabetes when initially diagnosed; however, most patients with LADA will require insulin within 3 years at the point of diagnosis. Latent autoimmune diabetes in adults is distinguished from type 2 diabetes by the presence of islet autoantibodies that are common to type 1 diabetes. Patients with type 1 diabetes commonly have one or more of four islet autoantibodies—islet cell antigens (ICAs), glutamic acid decarboxylase autoantibodies (GADAs), insulin antibodies, or tyrosine phosphatase protein; whereas patients with LADA typically only have one autoantibody. Latent autoimmune diabetes in adult patients have far less incidence of IA-2 and ICA autoantibodies than patients with type 1 diabetes (Lightsey, 2011).

Medical Management

"Diagnosis of LADA begins with a high level of suspicion" (Kapustin, 2012, p. 4). Clinical indicators of LADA should guide the health care provider to identify high-risk patients: those recently diagnosed with diabetes who are under the age of 50, who have acute diabetic symptoms (e.g., increased urinary output, thirst, hunger, and fatigue), have BMI less than 25 kg/m, or have a personal or family history of other autoimmune diseases. These indicators should trigger further screening. Performing a glutamic acid decarboxylase (GAD) antibody test is the most common method of diagnosing LADA, but not all patients have these antibodies; therefore, this one test alone is not sufficient to rule out LADA. The other test used in diagnosing LADA is C-peptides; a low level of C-peptides is associated with a higher degree of beta-cell destruction.

There is no single optimal treatment for LADA, nor are definitive treatment guidelines available as of this writing (Lightsey, 2011). It is, however, important to distinguish LADA from patients with type 2 diabetes to ensure that patients are not prescribed drugs that stimulate beta-cell insulin production, such as the sulfonylureas (e.g., glimepiride, glipizide, and tolazamide). The focus for management of patients with LADA is on controlling hyperglycemia and preventing complications. Strict glycemic control is used to prevent LADA from progressing to insulin-dependent diabetes. Dietary guidelines for patients with LADA are similar to those for patients with type 1. Patients with LADA should be advised to follow a healthy reduced-calorie diet and increase their physical activity according to an individualized program tailored to meet their individual needs. Patients also may be treated with oral antidiabetic medications which do not destroy beta-cell insulin production: biguanides, thiazolidinediones, meglitinides, and alpha-glucosidase inhibitor. Some health care providers do use insulin early in treatment in hopes of delaying beta-cell destruction (Latent Autoimmune Diabetes in Adults, 2012; Lightsey, 2011). Clinicians also should treat LADA patients for cardiovascular risk factors, as those patients have a similar risk for coronary heart disease and cerebrovascular disease as patients with type 2 diabetes (Lightsey, 2011; Myhill et al., 2008).

Secondary Diabetes

Secondary diabetes is the same as type 1 and type 2 diabetes in the regard that it is caused by the pancreas's inability to produce sufficient amounts of insulin. However, unlike other forms of diabetes, which are the result of genetic and environmental factors, secondary diabetes occurs as a reaction to other internal diseases or conditions (Health.com, 2011).

Epidemiology, Etiology, and Pathophysiology

This is a rare conditon; the Diabetes and Digestive and Kidney Diseases (NIDDK) estimates the incidence of secondary diabetes at 1% to 2% of total diabetes cases and the National Diabetes Education Program puts the figure at 1% to 5% of total diabetic cases (Ingenix Staff, 2008). Secondary diabetes can be caused by a wide range of health problems that damage, injure, interfere with, or destroy the pancreas. For example, secondary diabetes may develop from inflammation of the pancreas or cystic fibrosis. Some conditions increase the body's need for insulin, such as the overproduction of growth hormone or cortisol. Other outside factors that cause secondary diabetes include hyperthyroidism, Cushing syndrome, cystic fibrosis, hemochromatosis or any other damage done to the pancreas, hepatitis C, fatty liver disease, celiac disease, alcoholism, and cancer of the pancreas, liver, lungs, intestines, or stomach (Adamec, 2010).

Other diseases are not the only cause of secondary diabetes. Drugs taken to help alleviate diseases can also cause secondary diabetes, such as ones taken for high blood pressure, beta-blockers, diuretics, immune system suppressants, any hormone replacements such as steroids and estrogen, birth control pills, antipsychotics, antidepressants, and antiseizure, HIV, and chemotherapy drugs. Any of these drugs could affect the body's ability to produce insulin properly and lead to secondary diabetes (Adamec, 2010).

Secondary diabetes can also be caused by the body's reaction to certain surgeries. For example, any surgery involving the pancreas runs a high risk of causing secondary diabetes, as does the removal of the testes. Radiation therapy to treat cancer also can cause secondary diabetes (Health.com, 2011).

Clinical Manifestations, Laboratory Tests, and Medical Management

Patients with secondary diabetes manifest the same symptoms as those with primary diabetes. The standard diagnostic criteria for other forms of diabetes apply to secondary forms of diabetes. The signs and symptoms of the underlying condition usually are present; when present, they should increase the suspicion for diabetes and alert the patient to the need for blood glucose monitoring (Lingvay, 2010). The health care provider also may order blood tests for pancreatic enzymes to rule out pancreatitis, thyroid test to identify hyperthyroidism, or C-peptide tests to assess levels of insulin in the blood.

Treatment for secondary diabetes most often involves treatment of the underlying condition. In some cases, the diabetes is reversible if the underlying condition is found and treated expeditiously. Many causes of secondary diabetes are treated like type 2 cases, because their presentation is similar to the insulin resistance found in type 2 patients. In other patients, which may involve destruction of the insulin-making beta cells (such as those found in total pancreatectomy patients), the treatment may resemble that for many type 1 patients, and insulin injections may be required (Ingenix Staff, 2008; Lingvay & Raskin, 2010).

Prediabetes

Prediabetes is a term used to identify people with glucose intolerance who are at increased risk for developing diabetes. An estimated 79 million U.S. adults have prediabetes (CDC, 2011). The two types of abnormal glucose intolerance included in the classification of prediabetes are impaired fasting glucose (IFG) and impaired glucose tolerance (IGT). Impaired fasting glucose is a condition in which the fasting blood glucose level or hemoglobin (A_{IC}) level is higher than normal but not diagnostic of diabetes. Impaired glucose tolerance is a condition in which the blood glucose level 2 hours following an oral glucose load (during an oral glucose tolerance test) is higher than normal but not diagnostic of diabetes. People with prediabetes have an increased risk of diabetes (primarily type 2 diabetes), cardiovascular disease, and stroke; however, the abnormal blood glucose levels associated with prediabetes can be normalized with dietary modification, weight loss, and physical activity (ADA, 2011b). The Diabetes Prevention Program showed that about 11% of people with prediabetes developed type 2 diabetes within an average of 3 years of follow-up (ADA, 2011b). "Other studies show that many people with prediabetes develop type 2 diabetes in 10 years" (ADA, 2011b, p. 2).

Physiology of Fuel Metabolism

The pancreas, which is located in the posterior portion of the upper abdomen, is divided into the exocrine pancreas and the endocrine pancreas. The exocrine pancreas produces hormones primarily involved in digestion, whereas the endocrine pancreas produces hormones associated with endocrine function. Chapter 45 provides more information on the pancreas and the assessment of endocrine disorders.

The exocrine pancreas is composed primarily of small glands called acini; the endocrine pancreas is made up of small cells called islets of Langerhans. These islet cells are distributed throughout the exocrine pancreas and are divided into the alpha cells, beta cells, delta cells, and F cells. Alpha cells secrete the hormone glucagon, beta cells secrete the hormone insulin, delta cells secrete the hormone somatostatin, and F cells (or pancreatic polypeptide cells) secrete the hormone pancreatic polypeptide. Somatostatin (also produced in the gastrointestinal tract and hypothalamus) inhibits the release of insulin from the beta cells and glucagon from the alpha cells. Pancreatic polypeptide is a complex peptide hormone whose role is not entirely understood. In relation to diabetes, the most important of these hormones are insulin and glucagon, which are discussed in greater detail throughout the chapter. Figure 47–2 ◆ shows a diagram of the regulation of blood glucose levels by insulin and glucagon.

Interrelationships among insulin, glucagon, cortisol, growth hormone, and the catecholamines epinephrine and norepinephrine control fuel metabolism. The effects of insulin are most prominent in liver, adipose tissue, and muscle. The primary functions of insulin in these tissues include the synthesis of glycogen (the storage form of glucose) in liver and muscle, the synthesis of protein (a large complex molecule made up of one or more chains of amino acids) in liver and muscle, and the synthesis of triglycerides (molecules consisting of a glycerol backbone with three fatty acids) in adipose tissue and (to a smaller extent) in muscle.

Insulin is necessary for glycolysis, the biochemical pathway that results in the generation of high-energy compounds such as adenosine triphosphate (ATP) and nicotinamide adenine dinucleotide (NAD), and for glucose transport, the movement of glucose into

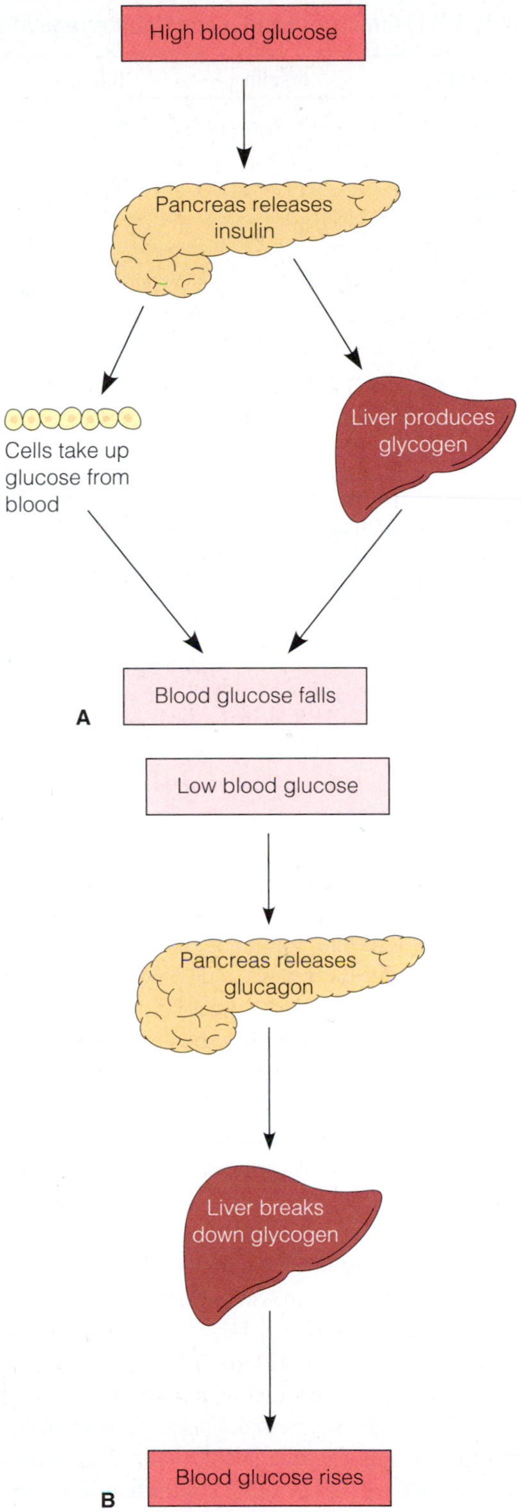

FIGURE 47–2 ◆ Regulation (hemostasis) of blood glucose levels by insulin and glucagon. (A) High blood glucose is lowered by insulin release. (B) Low blood glucose is raised by glucagon release.

insulin-sensitive tissues (most notably, skeletal muscle). Most important, insulin suppresses gluconeogenesis (formation of glucose from noncarbohydrate substrates), glycogenolysis (breakdown of glycogen to glucose), and lipolysis (breakdown of triglycerides to free fatty acids and glycerol). Insulin promotes glucose uptake and utilization in tissues. Skeletal muscle is the major site of insulin-mediated glucose disposal

CHART 47–1 Effects of Insulin and Counterregulatory Hormones on Intermediary Metabolism

Insulin Resistance	Insulin	Glucagon	Cortisol	Growth Hormone	Epinephrine/Norepinephrine
Glycogen synthesis	↑	↓			↓
Glycogenolysis	↓				↑
Gluconeogenesis	↓	↑	↑	↑	↑
Lipolysis	↓		↑	↑	↑
Ketogenesis	↓	↑			
Protein synthesis	↑		↓	↑	
Proteolysis	↓		↑		

Note: ↓ = inhibits or decreases; ↑ = stimulates or increases.

during the fed state (period following meals) and is critical for preventing hyperglycemia and maintaining glucose homeostasis.

Collectively, glucagon, cortisol, growth hormone, epinephrine, and norepinephrine are referred to as counterregulatory hormones because their actions oppose the effects of insulin. The functions of each of these hormones in intermediary metabolism are presented in Chart 47–1. The primary functions of glucagon include hepatic gluconeogenesis, glycogenolysis, lipolysis, and ketogenesis (formation of ketones [energy substrates] from free fatty acids). Cortisol, a hormone secreted by the adrenal cortex, causes protein catabolism and lipolysis, thereby providing precursors for gluconeogenesis and ketogenesis. Growth hormone, secreted by the anterior pituitary, causes lipolysis and provides precursors (glycerol and free fatty acids) for gluconeogenesis and ketogenesis. Of the catecholamines, epinephrine has the greatest role in fuel metabolism. This hormone is secreted by the adrenal medulla and is associated with glycogenolysis, gluconeogenesis, and lipolysis.

The primary metabolic goal after a meal is maintenance of normal blood glucose levels. Following the ingestion of carbohydrates, insulin levels rise, stimulating glucose uptake. Glucagon levels decrease, so there is a higher ratio of insulin to glucagon. Glucose is the primary oxidative fuel for all tissues during the absorptive state. Glucose that is in excess of the oxidative needs of the major tissues is stored as glycogen or lipids.

The primary goal of fuel metabolism during the fasted state is to provide glucose for the brain and nervous tissue. The fasted state generally is considered to be 10 to 12 hours without eating. The ratio of glucagon to insulin is higher during this time. Hepatic glycogenolysis and gluconeogenesis increase plasma glucose levels. Free fatty acids, released from adipose tissue lipolysis, are oxidized by muscle for energy. As fasting continues, insulin remains suppressed, glucagon levels remain elevated, and the principal source of hepatic glucose production is gluconeogenesis. In addition, ketones can be oxidized by the brain for energy.

In summary, normal fuel metabolism is regulated by a series of complex relationships among insulin, glucagon, and other counterregulatory hormones. Normal plasma glucose levels are tightly regulated by hepatic glucose production; glucose uptake and utilization by peripheral tissues (primarily skeletal muscle); and the actions of insulin and counterregulatory hormones, primarily glucagon. Insulin and glucagon have opposing effects on glucose metabolism. Higher glucagon levels and lower insulin levels facilitate hepatic gluconeogenesis and glycogenolysis during fasted states, thereby preventing hypoglycemia. Fasting plasma glucose levels are determined primarily by hepatic glucose production. Plasma insulin levels increase and glucagon levels decrease as blood glucose levels rise during the fasted state.

The hormonal-fuel relationships described previously are abnormal in all types of diabetes. In type 1 diabetes, there is a nearly complete loss of insulin production, whereas type 2 diabetes involves decreased insulin production and insulin resistance. Insulin resistance is generally described as the inability of either endogenous or exogenous insulin to achieve its normal biologic response in its target tissues. The abnormalities of fuel metabolism associated with diabetes result from a deficiency in insulin and an increase in glucagon and other counterregulatory hormones. These hormonal abnormalities most profoundly affect the muscle, liver, and adipose tissue. Hyperglycemia results from a decreased amount of effective circulating insulin to insulin-sensitive tissues, hepatic gluconeogenesis, and hepatic and muscle glycogenolysis (Hemphill, 2011). In type 1 diabetes, the increased mobilization of free fatty acids from adipose tissue leads to increased hepatic synthesis of ketone bodies, which can result in the acute complication of diabetic ketoacidosis, which is discussed later in the chapter. In type 2 diabetes, the amount of free fatty acids converted to ketone bodies usually is insufficient for development of diabetic ketoacidosis.

Pathophysiology of Type 1 Diabetes

The pathophysiology of type 1 diabetes is described in stages of development, as detailed in Figure 47–3◆. Environmental factors trigger an immune response with the development of ICAs, IAAs, and other islet cell antigens, such as GAD (Kaufman & ADA, 2008). These antibodies are markers of a progressive loss of pancreatic beta-cell mass, which can be helpful in the diagnosis of type 1 diabetes. As can be seen

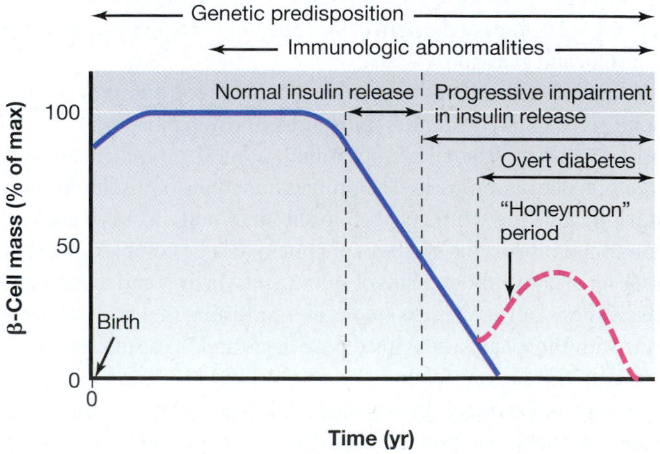

FIGURE 47–3 ◆ Proposed scheme of natural history of the beta-cell defect.

in Figure 47–3, when the beta-cell mass is reduced by 80% to 90%, marked impairments in insulin release and overt type 1 diabetes develop. This is followed by a period of endogenous insulin production called the honeymoon period. This "honeymoon period" represents the period of time during which exogenous insulin requirements are reduced. The clinical presentation of the honeymoon period varies from moderate reductions in insulin requirements to normalization of glucose tolerance (Aly & Gottlieb, 2009). This period is relatively short-lived, usually a few weeks to several months (Aly & Gottlieb, 2009), and is followed by loss of insulin production and dependence on exogenous insulin secretion.

How the environmental trigger actually initiates the cascade of events leading to pancreatic beta-cell dysfunction is still unknown. Two theories have been proposed to explain how an environmental trigger can initiate the autoimmune process. The first theory is that an environmental trigger, such as a virus, directly induces tissue damage and inflammation. This leads to the release of beta-cell antigens and the recruitment and activation of lymphocytes and additional inflammatory leukocytes to the tissue. The second theory, known as molecular mimicry, postulates that an environmental trigger, such as a virus, produces an immune response against autoantigens. This theory suggests that a susceptible host encounters an environmental trigger that has antigens that are immunologically similar to the host antigens; however, these antigens differ sufficiently to induce an immune response when presented to T cells. As a result, the tolerance to autoantigens breaks down, and the immune response cross-reacts with host structures to cause tissue damage and disease (Christen, 2010).

Pathophysiology of Type 2 Diabetes

Type 2 diabetes is a heterogeneous group of disorders characterized by decreased liver, muscle, and adipose tissue sensitivity to insulin and a defect in insulin secretion from the pancreatic beta cells. Often, both insulin resistance and a reduction in insulin secretion are present at diagnosis of type 2 diabetes, and the development of type 2 diabetes follows a typically evolving course, which can be divided into three distinct stages.

In the first stage, genetic factors probably influence both insulin sensitivity and insulin secretion. There is an initial period of hyperinsulinemia in which the pancreatic beta cells are able to overcome insulin resistance; although there is an underlying defect in insulin secretion, the pancreatic beta cells are able to produce high levels of insulin and maintain normal glucose tolerance (Figure 47–4◆). In the second stage, insulin resistance continues to increase, and this compensatory hyperinsulinemia becomes insufficient to maintain normal glucose homeostasis. Under conditions of insulin resistance, visceral adipose tissue is very sensitive to the effects

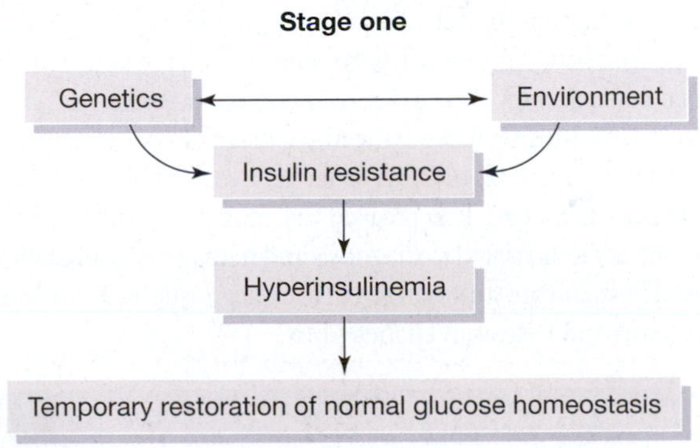

FIGURE 47–4 ◆ Stage 1 development of type 2 diabetes mellitus.

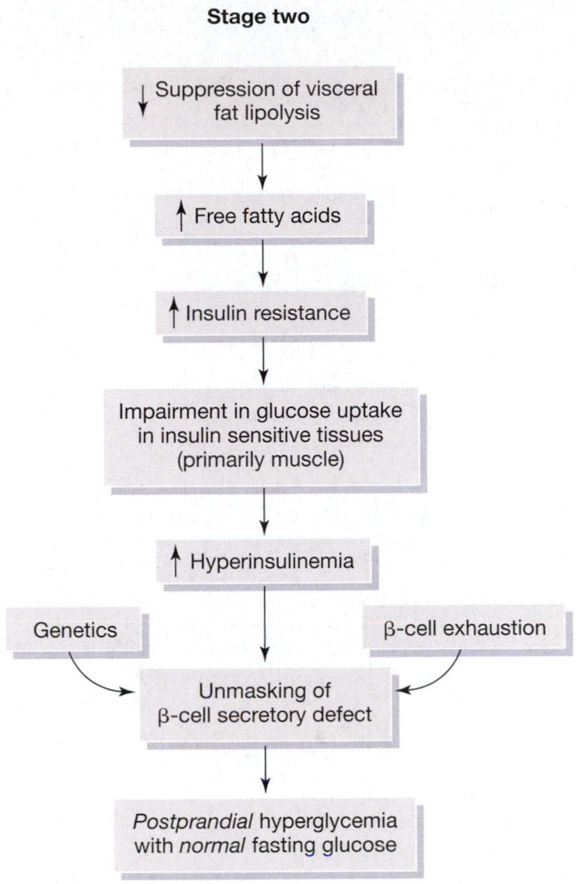

FIGURE 47–5 ◆ Stage 2 development of type 2 diabetes mellitus.

of catecholamines, and insulin resistance is associated with enhanced lipolysis. This leads to increased free fatty acid production and mobilization, exacerbating insulin resistance in liver and muscle tissue. In addition, impairments in insulin-mediated glucose uptake, particularly in muscle tissue, become evident. Insulin-mediated glucose transport into skeletal muscle, the major target for glucose disposal, becomes impaired. Fasting plasma glucose levels remain normal, but postprandial (after a meal) plasma glucose levels rise (Figure 47–5◆). Also in this stage, physiologic stress states that increase the production of hormones such as catecholamines, cortisol, growth hormone, and glucagon will cause hyperglycemia.

In the third stage, there is a further increase in insulin resistance. The restraining effects of insulin on hepatic glucose production become impaired, and plasma glucose levels increase. In addition, the worsening hyperglycemia has toxic effects on the pancreatic beta cells, and insulin secretion subsequently declines slowly over many years. With increasing insulin resistance, there is an even greater increase in free fatty acid production and mobilization, which causes a further increase in insulin resistance. Fasting and postprandial hyperglycemia result from increased insulin resistance, unrestrained hepatic glucose production, and glucose toxicity (Figure 47–6◆).

Clinical Manifestations of Type 1 and Type 2 Diabetes

In general, the clinical signs and symptoms of type 1 diabetes originate from hyperglycemia and ketosis (increased levels of ketone bodies), whereas the clinical signs and symptoms of type 2 diabetes originate from hyperglycemia. The following are signs and symptoms of diabetes without metabolic complications such as diabetic ketoacidosis (DKA)

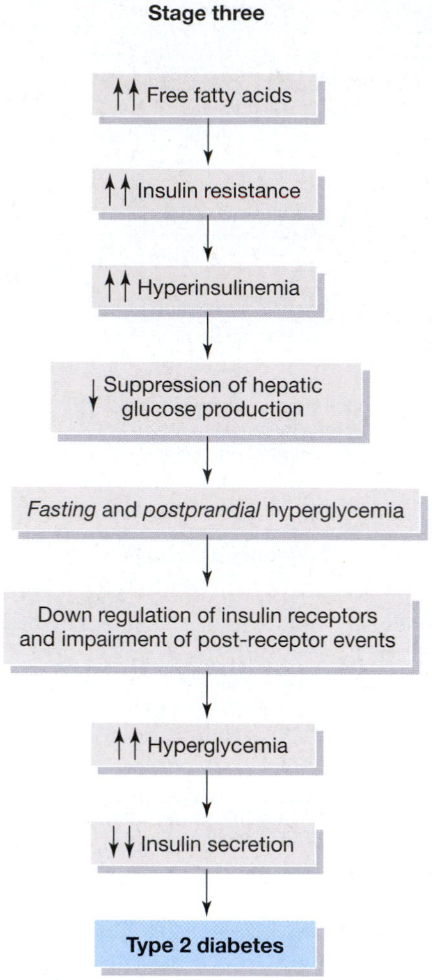

FIGURE 47–6 ◆ Stage 3 development of type 2 diabetes mellitus.

CHART 47–2 Common Complications of Diabetes

Clinical Complication	Site of Discussion
Eye: Retinopathy and glaucoma	Page 1449 and Chapter 64
Foot: Loss of sensation in the foot, skin dryness, cracking, and calluses	Page 1451–1452
Skin: Infections, itching, dermopathy, blisters	Chapter 59
Poor wound healing	Page 1443 and Chapter 60
Hearing loss	Chapter 63
Oral: Problems with teeth and gums	Page 1451
Heart disease	Page 1449 and Unit VII
Peripheral artery disease	Page 1450 and Chapter 35
Hypertension	Page 1430 and Chapter 29
Stroke	Page 1431, 1449, and Chapter 22
Gastroparesis	Page 1451 and Chapter 37
Neurogenic bladder	Page 1450 and Chapter 39
Diabetic diarrhea	Page 1450
Kidney disease	Page 1449 and Chapter 39
Ketoacidosis	Page 1445
Hyperosmolar hyperglycemic state (HHNS)	Page 1445
Neuropathy	Page 1450
Charcot deformity	Page 1451
Lower extremity ulceration	Page 1460
Sexual dysfunction	Page 1450 and Chapter 42

and hyperosmolar hyperglycemia state (HHS), which will be discussed later in the chapter:

- Glucosuria (glucose in urine) is associated with an osmotic diuresis, an increase in urine volume caused by an osmotic substance (glucose) in the renal tubules.
- Osmotic diuresis is associated with dehydration and volume depletion.
- Polyuria (increased urination) is the primary clinical manifestation of the osmotic diuresis.
- Nocturia is frequent urination at night associated with polyuria.
- Hypotension (low blood pressure) occurs as a result of dehydration and volume depletion.
- Tachycardia (increased heart rate) also occurs as a result of dehydration and volume depletion.
- Polydipsia (increased thirst) is a compensatory response to the dehydration and volume depletion.
- Polyphagia (increased appetite) results from the significant loss of calories that occurs through the loss of calories in the urine. For example, the amount of glucose in the urine can exceed 300 kcal.
- Weight loss occurs through dehydration, volume depletion, and the loss of calories in the urine.
- Fatigue is most likely related to alterations in carbohydrate, protein, and lipid metabolism, especially protein catabolism.

Complications of Diabetes

There are numerous common complications of diabetes. Many of these complications are discussed later in this chapter and others are fully discussed in other chapters throughout the book. Chart 47–2 shows a list of common complications with reference as to where they are discussed.

Laboratory Tests and Diagnostic Procedures

Diabetes is a chronic disease requiring frequent monitoring of blood glucose levels so that appropriate diagnoses are made and therapeutic goals can be accomplished through adjustments in diet, physical activity, and pharmacologic therapy. These determinations are performed in a clinical laboratory setting. Following the initial diagnosis of diabetes, patients are taught to measure blood glucose levels several times each day using portable glucose meters. This is called self-monitoring of blood glucose. The laboratory tests related to diagnosis and management of diabetes are discussed next and are summarized in the Diagnostic Tests for Monitoring Glycemia and Ketosis in Diabetes box.

Blood Glucose Levels

The fasting blood glucose level is measured following an overnight fast (no food or drink with the exception of water for 10 to 12 hours).

DIAGNOSTIC TESTS for Monitoring Glycemia and Ketosis in Diabetes

Test, Rationale, and Normal Values	Expected Abnormality
Blood Glucose Levels (fasting) Normal: Serum and plasma: 70–110 mg/dL Prediabetes: 100–125 mg/dL Older adult: 70–120 mg/dL *Used to confirm a diagnosis of prediabetic state or diabetic mellitus. Also used to monitor blood glucose levels for diabetic patients taking antidibetic agents.*	Decreased levels of serum glucose indicate a hypoglycemic reaction (too much insulin). Panic value: Less than 40 mg/dL. Increased levels of serum glucose indicate diabetes mellitus or diabetic acidosis. Panic value is greater than 700 mg/dL.
Oral Glucose Tolerance Test (OGTT), Serum or Intravenous Glucose Tolerance Test (IV-GTT) Normal values: Adult fasting: 70–110 mg/dL 0.5 hour: Less than 160 mg/dL 1 hour: Less than 170 mg/dL 2 hours: Less than 125 mg/dL 3 hours: Fasting level of 70–110 mg/dL. *Done to diagnose diabetes mellitus in individuals having high-normal or slightly elevated blood sugar values. The test may be indicated when there is a familial history of diabetes, in women having babies weighing 10 lbs or more, in individuals havaing extensive surgery or injury, and in individuals with obesity problems.*	In the standard OGTT, blood glucose levels are drawn before and 1/2, 1, 2, and 3 hours after ingestion of 75 grams of glucose (a glucose preparation dissolved in water). Decreased levels indicate hyperinsulinism. Increased levels indicate diabetes mellitus or latent diabetes. The diagnosis of prediabetes or diabetes is made on the basis of the 2-hour value (140 to $<$ 200 mg/dL and 200 mg/dL, respectively). The intermediate glucose levels (1/2, 1, and 3 or more hours) are used primarily for research purposes.
Hemoglobin A_1c ($HgbA_1c$ or HbA_1c) Normal: Range for an adult is 2% to 5% for a nondiabetic, 2.5% to 6% for diabetic control, and 6.1% to 7.5% for a high average. *A blood test used to determine an average blood glucose level during a 1- to 3-month period. Used to monitor the effectiveness of diabetic therapy and provide information regarding the presence of diabetes mellitus.*	An elevated HbA_1c indicates uncontrolled diabetes mellitus, hyperglycemia, and recently diagnosed diabetes mellitus.
Glycosylated Serum Proteins (GSPs) Normal: 212.5 μmol = 5.0 HbA_1c and 90 mg/dL glucose. *Fructosamine measures short-term control of blood sugar for the past 1 to 3 weeks. Each 75 μmol change equals a change of approximately 60 mg/dL blood sugar or 2% HbA_1c. It is used to measure glucose control.*	Higher levels reflect worsening glucose control.
Urine Glucose Normal: Negative *Used to evaluate the amount of glucose in the urine.*	Glucose is present in the urine when the blood levels are elevated.
Ketone Bodies, Acetone (urine) Normal: Adult: Negative *A random urine specimen is used to detect the presence of an acidotic state. Ketone bodies in the urine occur as a result of ketosis.*	Often reported as "trace," "small," "moderate," or "high," with higher levels reflecting a greater degree of ketosis. Positive results indicate diabetic acidosis (ketoacidosis).
Serum Ketones Normal: Acetone: Negative (less than 1 mg/dL) Ketones: 0.5–4 mg/dL *Ketones are composed of three compounds—acetone, acetoacetic acid, and beta-hydroxybutyric acid—which are products of fat metabolism. Ketone bodies result from uncontrolled diabetes mellitus. The test is used to detect the presence of ketone bodies and to identify the occurrence of diabetic ketoacidosis.*	In diabetic ketoacidosis, the serum acetone is greater than 50 mg/dL.
C-Peptide Normal value: Adult, fasting: 0.8–1.8 ng/mL *A serum test used to identify excess insulin administered and to assist in the diagnosis of insulin antibodies, insulinoma (tumor of the pancreas that secretes insulin), and the cause of hypoglycemia.*	Decreased level is indicative of type 1 diabetes mellitus. Increased level is indicative of insulinoma, type 2 diabetes mellitus, and latent autoimmune disease in adults.

(*continued*)

DIAGNOSTIC TESTS for Monitoring Glycemia and Ketosis in Diabetes, *continued*

Test, Rationale, and Normal Values	Expected Abnormality
Blood Urea Nitrogen (BUN)	
Normal value: 10:1 to 20:1	Decreased level indicates severe liver damage and overhydration.
A serum test that is used to detect a renal disorder or dehydration associated with increased BUN levels.	Increased level indicates dehydration or prerenal failure caused by diabetes mellitus.

Sources: Associated Regional and University Pathologists, Inc. (ARUP) Laboratories, 2012. Retrieved from http://www.aruplab.com/guides; Kee, J. L. (2010). *Laboratory and diagnostic tests with nursing implications* (8th ed.). Upper Saddle River, NJ: Prentice Hall.

Fasting blood glucose levels can be used in the diagnosis of prediabetes and diabetes. Additionally, the fasting blood glucose level is an important measurement in the daily monitoring of glycemic control.

Oral Glucose Tolerance Tests

Oral glucose tolerance tests (OGTTs) can be useful in confirming the diagnosis of diabetes in atypical clinical presentations of diabetes. Patients are asked to fast for approximately 10 hours prior to the OGTT and to make certain that their intake of carbohydrates is 150 g/day for the 3 days prior to the test (Pacini & Mari, 2007). In addition, they are asked to refrain from smoking during the test (i.e., during the periods of time between blood draws) and to participate in their usual activity on the day prior to the test (Pacini & Mari, 2007).

Self-Monitoring of Blood Glucose

The process of self-monitoring of blood glucose (SMBG) allows patients to measure blood glucose levels at any time. The information can be used to make immediate decisions (e.g., insulin dose prior to meals) or to make decisions on therapeutic changes based on blood glucose trends over time. Patients are instructed to perform preprandial blood glucose measurements (i.e., immediately prior to meals and snacks), postprandial blood glucose measurements (i.e., approximately 2 hours after a meal or snack), or when they experience clinical symptoms (e.g., hypoglycemia). Patients and health care providers can review the results of SMBG measurements together and discuss overall changes in management.

The process of SMBG involves measurement of capillary blood glucose levels using a variety of portable blood glucose meters (Figure 47–7◆). In this process, patients puncture their fingertip with a small lancet device, obtaining a drop of blood. (Some meters allow for testing on a less sensitive part of the body, such as the forearm; however, the results may not be as accurate as fingertip testing.) This drop of blood is placed on a strip that has been inserted in a small monitoring device. The blood reacts with an enzyme on the reagent strip; the meter shines a light on the strip and provides a digital readout of the blood glucose level (Garg & Hirsch, 2010). The normal range of blood glucose levels (non-fasting) is approximately 70 to 110 mg/dL (Kee, 2010).

Whether blood glucose levels are measured in a home, hospital, or clinic setting, the meters need to have the highest degree of accuracy. In hospitals and clinics, strict quality control procedures are needed to maintain the accuracy of these devices, which are used by multiple operators on several patients. Each hospital or clinic has detailed quality control procedures to ensure that the meters are measuring blood glucose levels accurately and the operators are performing the test correctly. At a minimum, the procedures will include checking the meters

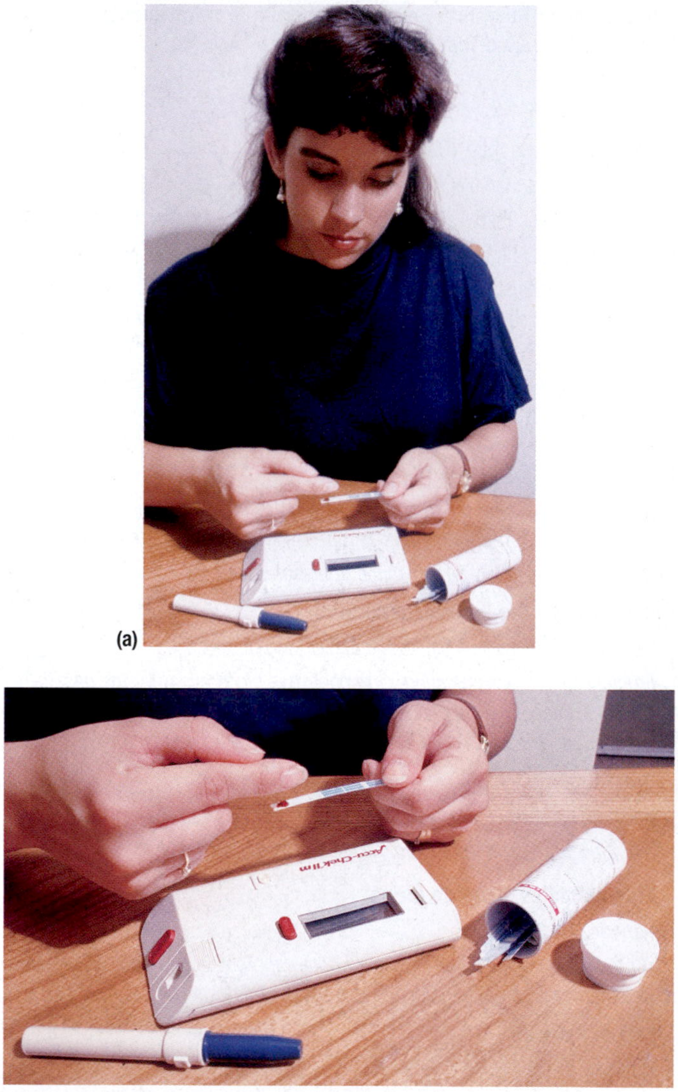

(a)

(b)

FIGURE 47–7 ◆ Blood glucose monitor.
Source: Tony Freeman/PhotoEdit Inc.

against high, normal, and low standard solutions and periodically assessing operator technique. In addition to strict quality control procedures, the following steps are important in obtaining accurate blood glucose levels (Garg & Naik, 2009):

- Strips must be current and properly stored at appropriate temperatures.
- The meter must be calibrated to the correct lot number of strips.
- The meter must be clean. This is particularly true of reflectance meters.

- An adequate amount of blood must be placed on the strip.
- The fingertip must be clean and dry prior to the puncture.

The timing of blood glucose measurements should correlate with the patient's meal status, clinical condition, and insulin regimen.

Safety Alert *A hospitalized patient eating four times per day (three meals and a bedtime snack) should perform a blood glucose measurement before each meal or snack. For example, calculation of the prebreakfast dose of rapid-acting insulin should be based on a glucose determination made shortly before breakfast, not several hours prior. Patients who are not eating also should have their glucose levels checked four times per day, but it may be more appropriate to check their blood glucose levels every 6 hours, depending on their insulin regimen. Patients who are more unstable may need determinations more frequently until they are stabilized.*

Continuous Blood Glucose Monitoring

During the past few years, blood glucose sensing devices have been developed that provide continuous intermittent measurement of the glucose level in interstitial fluid. For example, one continuous blood glucose monitoring system (Medtronic, Inc.) measures glucose levels in interstitial fluid every 10 seconds and provides an average blood glucose level every 5 minutes (Figure 47–8◆). The sensor is a small device with tubing and a small cannula; the cannula is inserted into the subcutaneous tissue, usually in the abdomen. Depending on the version of the sensor, the results may be transmitted to an insulin pump and read in real time or stored in the sensor to be downloaded later. Together, the patient and the health care provider discuss trends in the blood glucose patterns shown by the data and make mutually acceptable treatment decisions.

Hemoglobin A_1c Test

The primary laboratory test used for monitoring longer term glucose control is the **hemoglobin A_1c (Hgb A_1c)** test. A_1c is formed when glucose in the blood binds irreversibly to hemoglobin to form a stable glycated hemoglobin complex. Protein glycation is the nonenzymatic reaction of sugars with proteins. Because the normal life span of red blood cells is 90 to 120 days, the A_1c reflects the average blood glucose values of the previous 2 to 3 months and is directly proportional to the concentration of plasma glucose in the blood over the life span of the red blood cells. This test is the most widely used measure for assessment of glucose control (True, 2009).

Urinary Glucose

Self-monitoring of blood glucose has replaced the measurement of urinary glucose as the measure of glycemic control. The urinary measurement of glucose involves the semiquantitative measurement of glucose, usually in a single urine specimen. Urinary glucose is no longer used to routinely monitor glucose control; however, it is part of a routine urinalysis. Ordinarily, glucose should not be detectable in the urine. If glucose is present, further evaluation is warranted.

Urinary and Blood Ketones

Urinary ketone testing is an essential part of diabetes self-management for patients with type 1 diabetes, pregnancy with preexisting diabetes, and gestational diabetes (True, 2009). Patients use chemical reagents to provide an estimate of urinary ketones, usually ranging from "trace" to "large" amounts. Normally, ketones are not detectable in the urine.

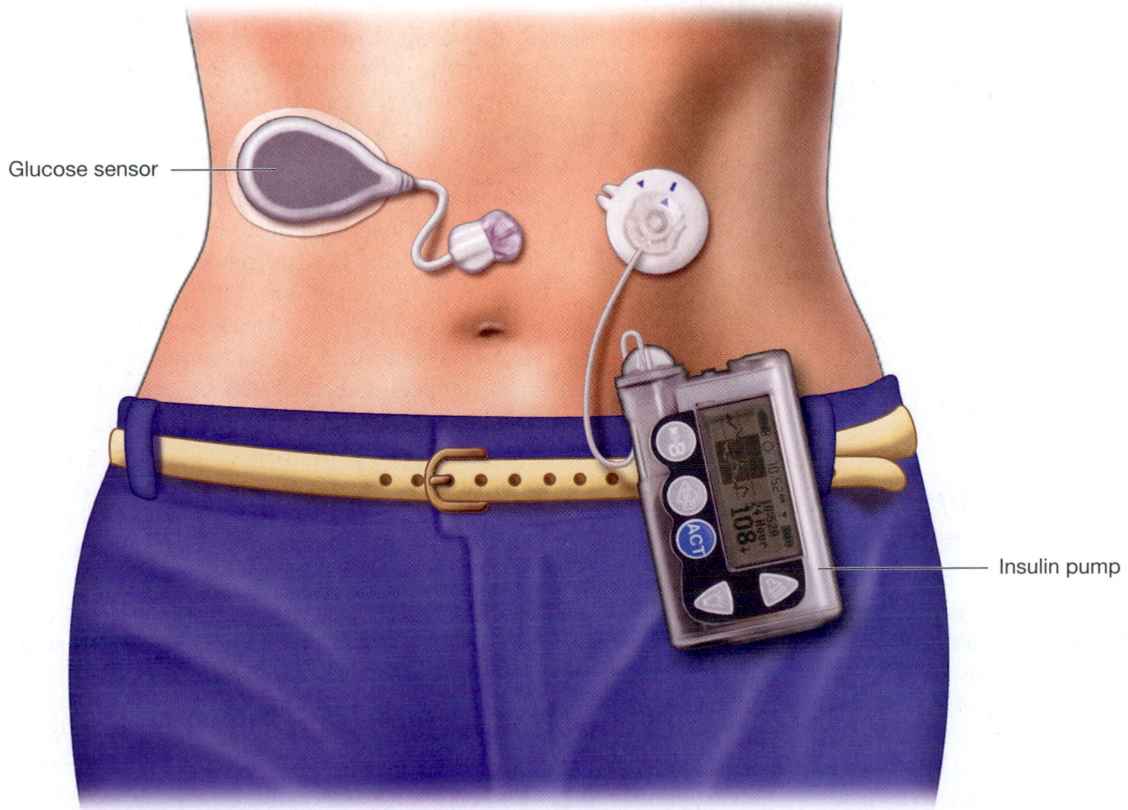

FIGURE 47–8 ◆ Continuous blood glucose monitoring system.

Weblink: Diabetes Medication

Urinary ketones may be present in nondiabetic individuals following fasting and in the first morning urine of pregnant women.

The presence of detectable amounts of urinary ketones in the urine of patients with diabetes reflects impending large amounts of serum ketones, which are associated with the development of diabetic ketoacidosis (DKA). It is recommended that patients with type 1 diabetes test their urine for ketones during times of stress or infection, when blood glucose levels are consistently elevated (>300 mg/dL), and when classic symptoms of DKA (e.g., abdominal pain, nausea, and vomiting) are present (Garg & Naik, 2009). In addition to urinary ketone assessment, bedside and self-testing kits can be used to quantify blood ketone (e.g., beta hydroxybutyrate) levels (Garg & Naik, 2009). See the Diagnostic Tests for Monitoring Glycemia and Ketosis in Diabetes box (p. 1427).

Diabetes Diagnosis

Through the laboratory tests just described, diabetes and other forms of glucose intolerance can be diagnosed using the criteria established by the ADA, which serve as a national guideline for diabetes diagnoses (ADA, 2010a). Typically, any one of the four criteria described in the National Guidelines for Establishing a Diagnosis of Diabetes may be used.

The following criteria are helpful in the diagnosis of diabetes:

- Glycosylated hemoglobin (Hemoglobin A_1c) 6.5% or higher. The test should be performed in a laboratory using a method that is National Glycohemoglobin Standardization Program (NGSP)-certified and standardized to the glycohemoglobin assay used in the DCCT (DCCT, 2003).
- C-peptide negative, meaning no insulin is produced.
- Urine tests positive for glucose and/or ketones (ADA, 2011a).

In the absence of unequivocal hyperglycemia, these criteria should be confirmed by repeat testing on a different day.

Prediabetes Diagnosis

Impaired glucose tolerance, also known as prediabetes, often occurs together with metabolic syndrome. Random blood glucose readings are sometimes normal, though a glucose tolerance test will show impaired glucose tolerance. Some people have impaired glucose tolerance but do not have metabolic syndrome, though many individuals have both metabolic syndrome and impaired glucose tolerance. Impaired fasting glucose is present when the fasting plasma glucose (FPG) is 110 to 125 mg/dL on two occasions. Impaired glucose tolerance is defined by a 2-hour plasma blood glucose level of $<$ 140 and $<$ 200 mg/dL following 75 grams of oral glucose (meaning that the tests are completed in 2-hour intervals) (ADA, 2010a; MedlinePlus, 2012).

Laboratory tests for the monitoring of short- and long-term glycemic control are detailed in the Diagnostic Tests for Monitoring Glycemia and Ketosis in Diabetes box (p. 1427).

NATIONAL GUIDELINES for Establishing a Diagnosis of Diabetes

According to the American Diabetes Association (2011a) guidelines, the following three tests are necessary in the diagnosis of diabetes:

- Fasting blood sugar over 126 mg/dL on more than one occasion with or without symptoms of hyperglycemia.
- Casual serum blood glucose over 200 mg/dL along with symptoms of hyperglycemia: for example, polydipsia (excessive thirst) or polyuria (excessive urination).
- Two-hour oral glucose tolerance test result of over 200 mg/dL (at 2 hours following consumption of 75 grams of glucose during an oral glucose tolerance test [OGTT]).

Medical Management

Medical management of diabetes typically involves insulin replacement therapy for patients with type 1 diabetes and insulin, oral medications, or a combination of both for patients with type 2 diabetes. Other medications may include antihypertensive and lipid-lowering drugs. Exercise, good nutrition, and lifestyle changes (e.g., smoking cessation) are other important aspects of treatment for diabetes. This combination of pharmacologic therapy and nonmedical therapy is directed toward normalization of blood glucose, blood pressure, and blood lipid levels.

Goals of Diabetes Management

The overall goal of diabetes management is the prevention of chronic long-term complications (which will be covered later in this chapter); however, there are distinctions between short-term and long-term goals. The short-term goals of diabetes management include prevention of severe hypoglycemia, hyperglycemia, and acute complications such as diabetic ketoacidosis (DKA) and hyperosmolar hyperglycemic state (HHS). Long-term glycemic goals include normalizing blood glucose levels and preventing systemic complications.

The current philosophy of diabetes management is based primarily on the results of two major classical studies: the Diabetes Control and Complications Trial (DCCT) (DCCT Trial Research Group, 1993) and the United Kingdom Prospective Diabetes Study (UKPDS) (United Kingdom Prospective Diabetes Study Group [UKPDS], 1998b). The DCCT and the UKPDS demonstrated in type 1 and type 2 diabetes, respectively, that any level of hyperglycemia is associated with the development of diabetes-related complications. In both of these studies, improvements in glycemic control were associated with reductions in microvascular complications (i.e., neuropathy, nephropathy, and retinopathy). Therefore, health care providers today emphasize tight glycemic control in managing diabetes. The Evidence-Based Practice box (p. 1431) discusses glycemic control and its relationship to diabetes-related complications in more detail.

In the UKPDS, hypertension was associated positively with the development of microvascular complications, and improved blood pressure control was associated with reductions in microvascular disease (UKPDS, 1998a). Although the DCCT (1993) and the UKPDS (1998b) demonstrated that improved glycemic control resulted in reductions in cardiovascular disease (CVD), these reductions did not reach statistical significance. This suggests that the development of diabetes-related CVD is caused by a variety of factors, including glycemic control, dyslipidemias (abnormally high level of lipids [cholesterol and other fat] in the blood), hypertension, and prothrombotic factors. The target glycemic and metabolic goals for patients with diabetes are as follows (McCarren & ADA, 2007):

- Glycemic goals:
  - A_1c: $<$ 7.0% (These goals are individualized; some patients may establish more stringent glycemic goals, such as a normal A_1c of $<$ 6%.)
  - Preprandial blood glucose: 90 to 130 mg/dL

EVIDENCE-BASED PRACTICE Glycemic Control

Clinical Problem

Patients with diabetes often develop severe diabetes-related complications (neuropathy, nephropathy, retinopathy, and an accelerated development of peripheral vascular disease, cardiovascular disease, and stroke). Nurses and other health care providers must apply evidence-based findings to reduce the development of these complications.

Research Findings

Two major studies have examined the relationship between glycemic control and the development of diabetes complications: the Diabetes Control and Complications Trial (DCCT Trial Research Group, 1993) and the United Kingdom Prospective Diabetes Study (UKPDS, 1998a, 1998b). The results of these studies changed diabetes management and are the primary foundation for current recommendations for glycemic control in diabetes.

The DCCT and UKPDS were prospective, randomized, controlled trials of intensive versus standard glycemic control of patients with type 1 and 2 diabetes, respectively. The DCCT demonstrated definitively that improved glycemic control is associated with sustained, decreased rates of microvascular complications (retinopathy, nephropathy, and neuropathy) in type 1 diabetes. The UKPDS demonstrated that, in patients with newly diagnosed type 2 diabetes, intensive use of medications (metformin, sulfonylureas, and insulin) and lifestyle interventions reduced the development of microvascular disease. In the UKPDS, there was a trend toward reduction in cardiovascular disease, as noted by a statistically nonsignificant reduction ($p = 0.052$) in the risk for combined fatal and nonfatal myocardial infarction and sudden death.

In both of these studies, the mean A_1c of the intensive group was approximately 7%. Therefore, the American Diabetes Association recommends a target A_1c of 7% or lower in patients with diabetes. Epidemiologic data have demonstrated an incremental benefit (although small in absolute terms) to lowering A_1c into the normal range (ADA, 2010b; Head to Head Comparator, 2011); however, this reduction must be balanced against the risk of hypoglycemia and other comorbidities. The recommendations of the ADA regarding glycemic control are as follows (ADA, 2010a):

- Lowering A_1c to an average of ~7% has clearly been shown to reduce microvascular complications of diabetes and possibly macrovascular disease. Therefore, the A_1c goal for nonpregnant adults in general is $< 7\%$.
- Epidemiologic studies have suggested an incremental benefit to lowering A_1c from 7% into the normal range. Therefore, the A_1c goal for selected individual patients is as close to normal ($< 6\%$) as possible without significant hypoglycemia.
- Less-stringent A_1c goals may be appropriate for patients with a history of severe hypoglycemia, patients with limited life expectancies, children, individuals with comorbid conditions, and those with long-standing diabetes with microvascular complications.

Implications for Nursing Practice

Attaining tight glycemic control in patients with diabetes requires maintaining a balance of diet, physical activity, and medications. This is not an easy task. Nurses are in a unique position to help patients self-manage their diabetes. Nurses need to develop strong assessment skills that examine the patient from clinical, cultural, behavioral, and psychosocial perspectives. Appropriate plans of care can be structured from this assessment.

Critical Thinking Questions with answers can be found in the Osborn Student Resources at nursing.pearsonhighered.com.

  - Postprandial blood glucose: < 180 mg/dL (The postprandial measurements are generally made 1 to 2 hours following the meal.)
- Blood pressure goals: < 130/80 mmHg
- Lipid goals:
  - Low-density lipoprotein (LDL) cholesterol: < 100 mg/dL
  - Triglycerides: < 150 mg/dL
  - High-density lipoprotein (HDL) cholesterol: > 40 mg/dL

Lifestyle changes such as increased exercising, smoking cessation, and dietary changes can contribute to lowering the levels of blood glucose and lipids. Most people with diabetes also require medication to lower their blood glucose level. The role of glucose-lowering drugs in type 1 and type 2 diabetes is discussed next.

Management of Type 1 Diabetes

The primary treatment for type 1 diabetes is insulin replacement therapy. To provide the insulin that the beta cells of the pancreas no longer make, the person takes insulin via injection or through an insulin pump.

Insulin Preparations

Until the mid-1980s, the insulin used in treatment of diabetes was produced from beef (bovine) and pork (porcine) sources. However, current insulin products are produced synthetically, and beef and pork insulin preparations are no longer manufactured or marketed in the United States. Synthetic human insulin is produced by recombinant DNA technology; the structure of recombinant human insulin matches the amino acid sequence of endogenous human insulin. Through amino acid rearrangement, substitution, and addition, insulin analogs have been developed that mimic the absorption and biologic activity of endogenous insulin secretion more precisely than traditional insulin preparations were able to do.

Insulin preparations are characterized by onset, peaks, and duration of action. Normal physiological insulin secretion involves both basal and meal-stimulated insulin release. Under normal physiological conditions, serum glucose and insulin responses are closely matched: When glucose levels rise, there is a corresponding rise in insulin levels. Under basal conditions (i.e., overnight, between meals, and during fasting), plasma glucose is maintained within a narrow range with a comparable response in insulin secretion. Following a meal, plasma glucose levels rise, and there is a rapid increase in insulin secretion. Therefore, insulin secretion often is referred to as basal or meal-stimulated. The goal of pharmacologic insulin therapy is to mimic this normal pattern of insulin secretion. Therefore, pharmacologic insulin preparations are often characterized by their ability to mimic basal or meal-stimulated properties. In clinical practice, the amount of insulin that is given to match the meal-stimulated insulin response is provided as an insulin bolus.

Commercial insulin preparations are divided into rapid-, short-, intermediate-, and long-acting preparations based on onset, peak (highest concentration of insulin), and duration of action. The comparative actions of each preparation are detailed in Chart 47–3.

The concentration of commercial insulin in the United States is 100 units/mL (U-100); however, regular insulin is also available as 500 units/mL (U-500). This concentration is typically used only in patients who are extremely insulin resistant.

CHART 47–3 Comparative Effects of Common Insulin Preparations

Type/Generic Name	Brand Name(s)	Onset (hours)	Peak (hours)	Duration (hours)
Rapid-Acting				
Insulin lispro (analog)	Humalog	<0.25	1–1.5	3–4
Insulin aspart	NovoLog			
Insulin glulisine	Apidra			
Short-Acting				
Regular	Humulin R Novolin R Humulin R (U-500)	0.5–1.0	1–5	6–10
Intermediate-Acting				
NPH (isophane)	Humulin N Novolin N	1–2	6–14	16–24
Long-Acting				
Insulin glargine	Lantus	1,1	Peakless	~ 24
Insulin detemir	Levemir	Gradual	6–8	~ 24
Combinations				
50% lispro protamine/50% insulin lispro	Humalog Mix 50/50	0.5–1	Dual** (NPA & lispro)	~18–24
70% NPH/30% regular	Humulin 70/30 Novolin 70/30	0.5–1	Dual** (NPH & R)	~18–24
50% NPH/50% regular	Humulin 50/50	0.5–1	Dual** (NPH & R)	~18–24
70% aspart protamine/30% aspart	NovoLog Mix 70/30	<0.25	Dual** (NPA & aspart)	~18–24
75% lispro protamine/25% lispro	Humalog Mix 75/25	<0.25	Dual** (NPA & lispro)	~18–24

Times are approximate, assume subcutaneous administration, and may vary with injection technique and factors influencing absorption (Merck Manual, 2011).
**Dual means combined insulins.

Five insulin analogs are currently available: lispro, aspart, glulisine, detemir, and glargine. Insulins lispro, aspart, and glulisine have rapid absorption profiles, whereas insulins detemir and glargine have delayed insulin absorption. The actions of insulins lispro, aspart, and glulisine most closely resemble basal insulin secretion.

Rapid-Acting Insulin

Rapid-acting insulins have an onset of action of approximately 15 minutes after injection and reach peak biologic action within approximately 1 to 2 hours. They are most effective in reducing postprandial hyperglycemia. Rapid-acting insulin preparations are routinely administered before a meal or snack; however, in certain situations these agents may be administered after a meal. For example, it is often difficult to predict the caloric intake of patients who are acutely or chronically ill because of changes in taste or appetite. In these situations, the actual amount of food consumed (particularly the carbohydrate content) can be determined, and then a postprandial dose of rapid-acting insulin can be administered. This method helps to reduce the potential for hypoglycemia, since the food intake and amount of insulin are more accurately matched.

Safety Alert *Because the onset of action of rapid-acting insulin preparations is so quick, they should be injected as close to the meal or snack as possible to avoid hypoglycemia. A critical role of the nurse is to be alert for signs and symptoms of hypoglycemia and educate patients and family about how to prevent and treat hypoglycemic reactions.*

Short-Acting Insulin

The only available short-acting insulin preparation is regular insulin, which is injected before meals. To match the peak action of insulin with the postprandial rise in glucose, regular insulin should be injected approximately 30 to 45 minutes before a meal. Regular insulin has been largely replaced by rapid-acting insulin analogs. Because the rapid-acting preparations have a more rapid onset of action and a greater peak effect, they resemble meal-stimulated endogenous insulin secretion more closely than regular insulin does.

Intermediate-Acting Insulin

The only intermediate-acting insulin preparation currently available is neutral protamine Hagedorn (NPH) insulin. With a slow onset of action, a prolonged peak effect, and a lengthened duration of action, NPH insulin traditionally has been used to provide basal insulin coverage (usually with two injections per day). However, the use of NPH as basal insulin is somewhat limited because of the high plasma insulin concentrations during peak action, which increase the risk of hypoglycemia.

Long-Acting Insulin

Long-acting insulin was produced to provide basal insulin coverage with relatively small peak biologic action. Glargine is a long-acting insulin analog that has no peak action, mirroring basal insulin secretion more precisely. Detemir, a long-acting insulin analog that has a relatively flat peak, also is used as basal insulin. Slight differences are seen in the onset, peaks, and duration of these preparations. These differences are detailed in Chart 47–3.

Premixed Insulins

Premixed insulins are combinations of rapid- or short-acting insulin preparations mixed with intermediate-acting insulin in specific proportions. The most common premixed insulin contains 70% NPH and 30% regular insulin (70/30). Other forms of premixed combinations are listed in Chart 47–3. These premixed insulins are helpful in patients who have difficulty mixing insulin doses; however, they do not permit easy adjustment of premeal and basal insulin. For example, if a patient using 70/30 insulin needed an increase in premeal regular insulin, it would be impossible to make this adjustment without also increasing the dose of NPH.

Incretin Mimetics

Exenatide injection (Byetta®) (Amylin Pharmaceuticals, Inc., 2011b) and Liraglutide (Victoza®) (Novo Nordisk Pharmaceuticals, 2011) are injectable medications that are used as adjunctive mealtime therapy to improve glycemic control in patients with type 2 diabetes mellitus. This medication belongs to a class of medications called **incretin mimetics.** An incretin mimetic enhances glucose-dependent insulin secretion from the pancreatic beta cells. Therefore, the greatest effect of incretin mimetics is a reduction in postprandial glucose levels. In addition, the incretins suppress elevated glucagon levels, promoting satiety, decreasing food intake, and slowing gastric emptying.

Exenatide and Liraglutide can be used in combination with metformin, sulfonylureas, and thiazolidinediones. The primary side effect of incretin mimetics is nausea, which may be minimized by increasing the medication dosage slowly. Exenatide should be administered subcutaneously 60 minutes prior to the morning or evening meals or the patient's two main meals that are separated by approximately 6 hours. Liraglutide is administered once daily at any time of day. The use of incretin mimetics decreases the rate at which orally administered drugs are absorbed. Therefore, oral medications that require rapid absorption and depend on threshold concentrations for effective action (e.g., antibiotics and oral contraceptives) should be administered 1 hour before the injection of mimetics.

Amylin Analog

Pramlintide acetate injection (Symlin) (Amylin Pharmaceuticals, Inc., 2011a) is a synthetic analog of human amylin, a hormone secreted by the pancreatic beta cells. Pramlintide can reduce postprandial blood glucose control by slowing gastric emptying, suppressing glucagon secretion, and promoting satiety. Pramlintide is injected subcutaneously immediately before meals (Gutierrez, 2008) and is indicated for improving glycemic control in type 2 diabetes. It also can be used as adjuvant mealtime therapy for the treatment of type 1 diabetes. Pramlintide may decrease the rate at which drugs affecting gastrointestinal motility and alpha-glucosidase inhibitors are absorbed. Such medications should be administered 1 hour before or 2 hours after administration of pramlintide.

Insulin Delivery Devices

The traditional method of delivering insulin is a disposable insulin syringe and needle. Recently, however, a variety of pens and insulin cartridges have been developed to add flexibility in insulin dosing and administration.

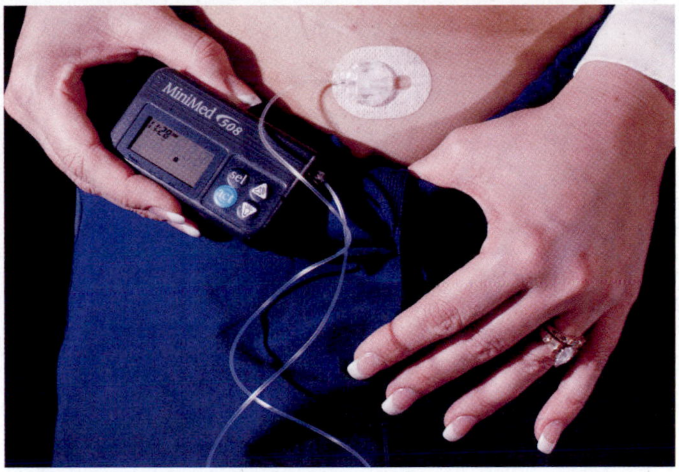

FIGURE 47–9 ◆ Insulin pump.
Source: Spencer Grant/Photo Researchers, Inc.

Continuous subcutaneous insulin infusion (CSII) is a method of intensive insulin therapy via pump that is used in the management of diabetes. An insulin pump is made up of a pump reservoir (syringe) filled with insulin, a small battery-operated pump, and a computer chip that allows the patient to program and deliver a specific amount of insulin on a regular basis (see Figure 47–9◆). The reservoir is connected to tubing with a needle or flexible cannula at the end, through which the insulin is delivered. The cannula is inserted subcutaneously, usually in the abdomen. The entire infusion set is changed routinely every 2 to 3 days.

The pump delivers insulin 24 hours a day at a programmed rate that is specific to the patient. Insulin pumps are designed to mimic the basal and meal-stimulated patterns of endogenous insulin secretion. During insulin pump therapy, a small amount of short- or rapid-acting insulin is infused continuously. This rate helps to maintain blood glucose levels within a normal range between meals and during the night.

The pump can be programmed to infuse differing basal rates throughout the 24-hour period. For example, a patient who exercises every day at a particular time may elect to decrease the basal rate during the exercise period. Before meals and snacks, the patient injects a specific calculated dose (bolus) of insulin through the pump. This dose of insulin is calculated on the basis of the premeal/snack blood glucose levels and the carbohydrate content of the meal/snack and reflects meal-stimulated insulin secretion.

The ADA publishes a product directory every January in its *Diabetes Forecast* magazine, thereby providing a resource for exploring the ever-changing spectrum of diabetes products (e.g., insulin pumps, sensors, pens, cartridges, and meters).

Insulin Regimens

The goal of insulin therapy in type 1 diabetes is the normalization of blood glucose levels. This is best achieved by using combinations of insulin in a manner that most closely resembles basal and meal-stimulated insulin release. Some of the options for insulin regimens in type 1 diabetes are presented next.

Twice-Daily Insulin Injection Regimen

In the twice-daily insulin injection regimen, regular or rapid-acting insulin (lispro) is combined with an intermediate-acting insulin (NPH)

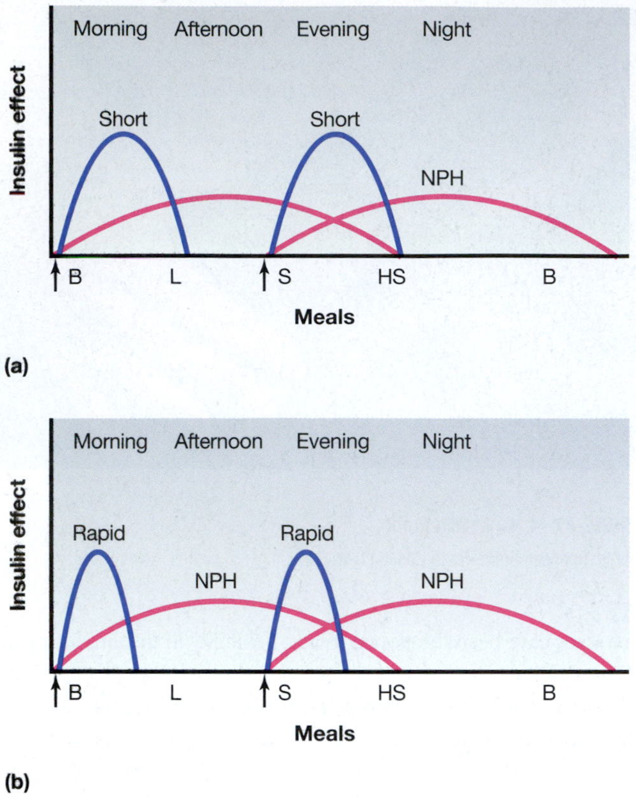

FIGURE 47–10 ◆ Twice-daily split and mixed insulin regimen.

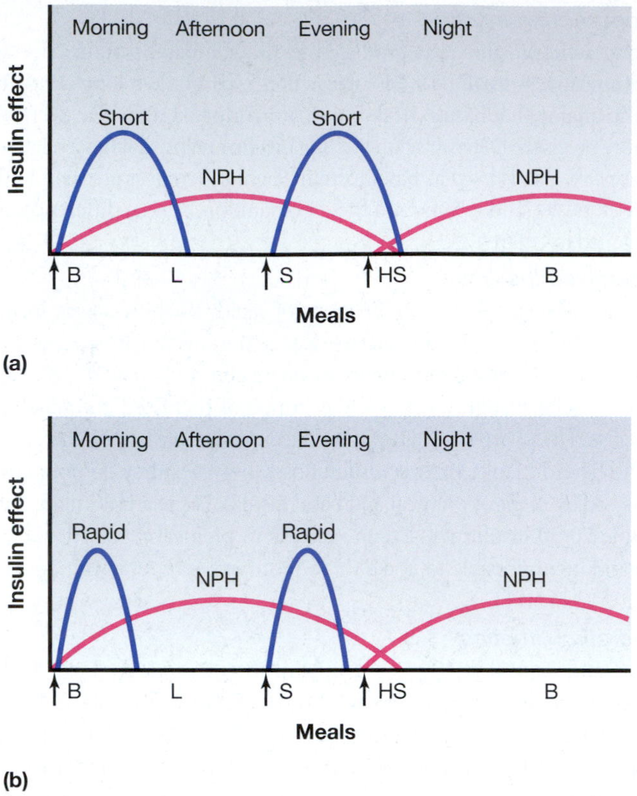

FIGURE 47–11 ◆ Three-times-daily insulin injection regimen.

prior to breakfast and prior to supper (Figure 47–10◆). Lispro peaks when the blood glucose level rises after breakfast and dinner, and the NPH insulin provides basal insulin coverage. Regular insulin peaks later, and the peaks are not as high. Because no rapid-acting insulin is provided at lunch, the peak of the NPH insulin helps to reduce blood glucose levels following lunch. Using this regimen, patients with type 1 diabetes can attain adequate glucose control. However, this regimen provides the patient little flexibility in changing mealtimes, and the peak effect of NPH predisposes patients to hypoglycemia if they skip meals.

Three-Times-Daily Insulin Injection Regimen

The three-times-daily insulin injection regimen (Figure 47–11◆) combines regular or rapid-acting insulin with NPH prior to breakfast, regular or rapid-acting insulin prior to dinner, and NPH prior to bedtime. The major difference between this method and the twice-daily method described previously is that the NPH is injected before bedtime. The movement of the NPH injection to bedtime means that the NPH will peak in the middle of the night, when the glucose is rising in response to the normal increase in endogenous growth hormone secretion. This method has value for individuals who have high fasting glucose levels on awakening.

Aside from chronically elevated blood glucose levels, fasting hyperglycemia has two major causes: the dawn phenomenon and the Somogyi effect. The **dawn phenomenon** is defined as fasting hyperglycemia without prior nocturnal hypoglycemia (Bilous, Donnelly, & Williams, 2010). The **Somogyi effect** is defined as fasting hyperglycemia with prior hypoglycemia (Garnero, 2012). The dawn phenomenon occurs when growth hormone, a counterregulatory hormone, is secreted during the night. Patients awake with elevated fasting blood glucose levels, precipitated in part by growth hormone. With pregnant women, the dawn phenomenon is even more exaggerated due to additional hormones released in the night (Garnero, 2011). When the NPH insulin is injected at bedtime, it will peak as the level of growth hormone rises.

Prior to initiating this regimen, it probably is best to assess whether the patient has dawn phenomenon or the Somogyi effect. In the Somogyi effect, also known as rebound hyperglycemia, there is a pattern of undetected hypoglycemia followed by hyperglycemia. Typically this happens in the middle of the night, but also can occur when too much insulin is circulating in the system. "The cause of the Somogyi effect is said to be man-made—that is, a result of insulin or diabetes pills working too strongly at the wrong time" (Garnero, 2011, p. 1).

When the hypoglycemia occurs, there is a release of glucose from the liver, which is associated with a rise in glucose and an elevated fasting blood glucose level. As a result, patients awake with an elevated fasting blood glucose level. The best way to assess for whether this is the Somogyi effect or the dawn phenomenon is to test the blood glucose levels in the middle of the night. If hypoglycemia is present in the middle of the night, it is likely that the elevated morning blood glucose level is rebound hyperglycemia or the Somogyi effect. If hypoglycemia is not present during this time, it is more likely that the elevated morning blood glucose level is a result of the dawn phenomenon.

Four-Times-Daily Insulin Injection Regimen

The insulin injection regimen described here requires four injections of insulin per day (Figure 47–12◆): a combination of NPH and rapid- or short-acting insulin at breakfast time, rapid- or short-acting insulin before lunch and dinner, and just NPH at bedtime. The premeal insulin helps to reduce the postprandial hypoglycemia. The NPH provides "basal" insulin.

Other Insulin Regimens

"Peakless" insulins, such as glargine, provide better basal insulin coverage. The multiple-dose regimen using glargine is widely used by patients

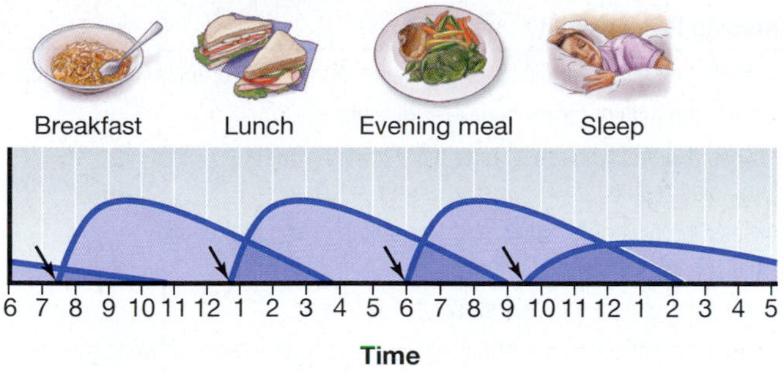

FIGURE 47–12 ◆ Four-times-daily insulin injection regimen.

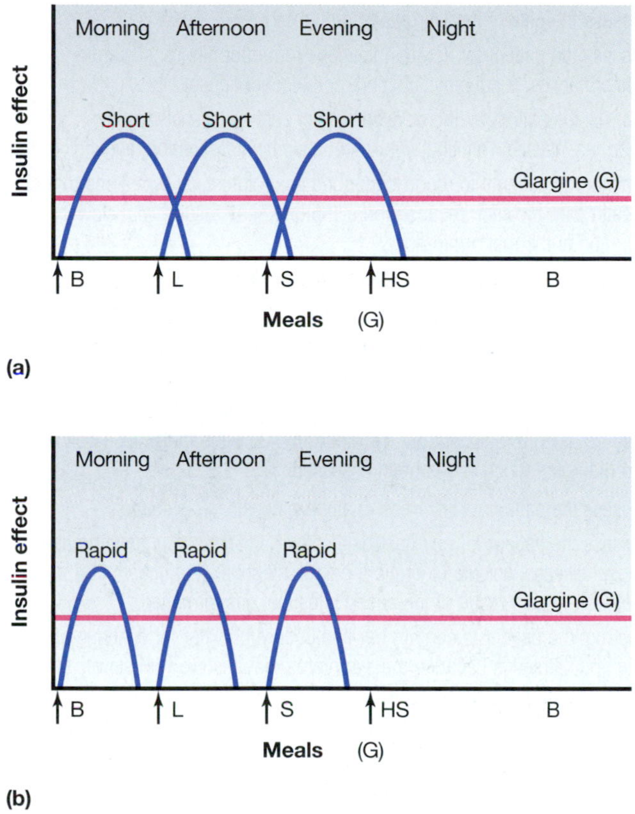

FIGURE 47–13 ◆ Multiple dose daily regimen.

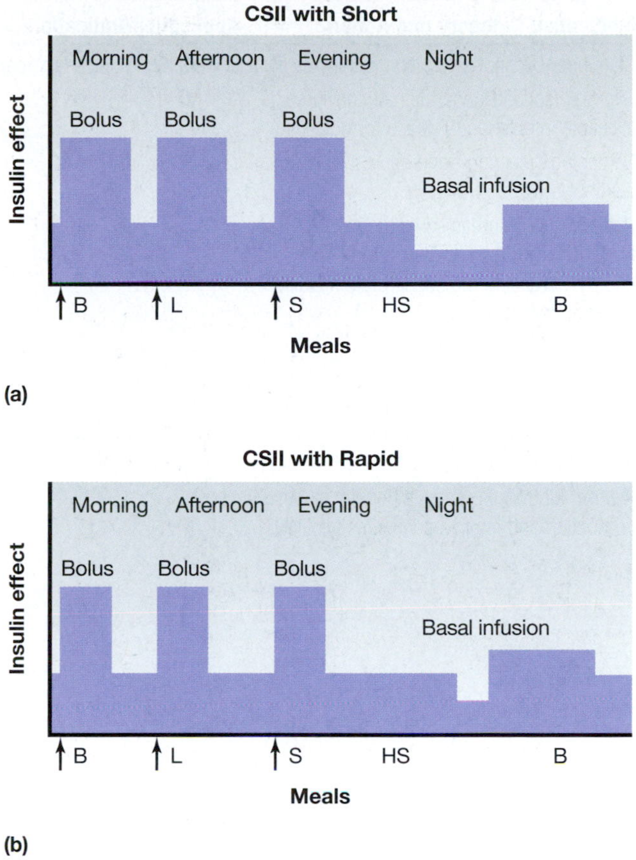

FIGURE 47–14 ◆ Continuous subcutaneous insulin infusion.

with diabetes and is illustrated in Figure 47–13◆. In this regimen, long-acting insulin (i.e., glargine) is used in combination with a rapid-acting insulin (lispro) prior to each meal. The glargine insulin has no peak; therefore, it resembles endogenous insulin more precisely.

One of the most effective ways to mimic normal insulin secretion is through the use of an insulin pump, which can provide continuous subcutaneous insulin infusion. The insulin pump, described earlier, is programmed to infuse rapid doses of short-acting insulin continuously at a basal rate, with patients determining bolus insulin injections prior to meals and snacks. The actions of the insulin pump are shown in Figure 47–14◆.

Nursing Management

The nursing management of insulin therapy involves (1) instructing patients in their prescribed insulin delivery technique (e.g., pen, syringe, insulin pump), (2) reviewing insulin delivery techniques with patients who have been on insulin therapy before their initial visit with the nurse, (3) instructing patients on their specific insulin regimens and assessing their understanding of the regimen, (4) instructing patients on the relationship between glucose monitoring and insulin regimens, (5) helping patients understand how prescribed adjustments in insulin therapy may affect glycemic control, and (6) understanding the signs and symptoms of hypoglycemia and hyperglycemia. The instructions specific to different medications are listed in the Pharmacology box on page 1436.

Management of Type 2 Diabetes

During the past decade, advances in the understanding of diabetes have caused reevaluation of the former standard of using diet and exercise as a first-line therapy in the treatment of type 2 diabetes and introducing pharmacologic therapy only when patients cannot meet their glycemic goals with diet and exercise alone. Some practitioners believe that early intervention with medication may improve glycemic control over time. Therefore, health care providers are increasingly recommending oral medications for patients with type 2 diabetes.

Oral Diabetes Medications

Six classes of oral medications are currently approved for the treatment of type 2 diabetes in the United States: sulfonylureas, meglitinides, alpha-glucosidase inhibitors, biguanides, thiazolidinediones, and dipeptidyl peptidase-4 (DPP-4) inhibitors. Broadly, these medications are grouped into those that enhance insulin secretion (sulfonylureas and rapid-acting secretagogues), those that reduce hepatic glucose production (biguanides), those that delay digestion and absorption of intestinal carbohydrate (alpha-glucosidase inhibitors), those that improve insulin

PHARMACOLOGY **Summary of Medications Used to Treat Type 2 Diabetes**

Medication Category and Action	Application/Indication	Nursing Responsibility
Glyburide (second-generation sulfonylurea) Glipizide (second-generation sulfonylurea; available in extended-release formulations) Glimepiride (second-generation sulfonylurea) ***Action:*** Sulfonylureas stimulate insulin secretion from the pancreatic beta cells and by increasing the sensitivity of insulin receptor cells.	Lowers blood glucose in patients with type 2 diabetes.	Assess the patient for allergies to other sulfonylureas or sulfa medications. Assess the patient for renal or liver disease. Assess patients who are at high risk for injury from hypoglycemia (e.g., older adults). Assess the patient for signs and symptoms of hyponatremia (chlorpropamide specific effect). Assess the patient for weight gain. Instruct the patient on the signs, symptoms, and treatment of hypoglycemia. Instruct the patient to avoid ingesting alcohol with medication to prevent a disulfiram reaction. Instruct the patient to take glipizide 30 minutes before meals.
Metformin (Biguanide) (available in extended-release formulations) ***Action:*** Metformin reduces hepatic glucose production and improves insulin sensitivity.	Lowers blood glucose in patients with type 2 diabetes.	Assess the patient for allergies to metformin. Assess the patient for contraindications to metformin (renal, cardiorespiratory, or hepatic dysfunction, and alcohol abuse). Assess the patient for the development of gastrointestinal symptoms, such as diarrhea, nausea, vomiting, flatulence, abdominal discomfort, and indigestion. Encourage patients to report continued gastrointestinal symptoms to their health care provider because the symptoms may resolve with slower titration of the metformin dose. Discuss with the patient the risk of lactic acidosis. Instruct the patient on the signs and symptoms of hypoglycemia. In general, metformin as monotherapy does not cause hypoglycemia. However, hypoglycemia may occur when metformin is combined with other medications. Discuss with patients the need to discontinue metformin prior to any procedure using a radiocontrast dye and to resume the medication only when normal renal function has been assessed.
Acarbose (alpha-glucosidase inhibitor) Miglitol (alpha-glucosidase inhibitor) ***Action:*** Alpha-glucosidase inhibitors reduce postprandial hyperglycemia by interfering with carbohydrate absorption from the GI tract. It acts locally in the GI tract by inhibiting the enzyme responsible for carbohydrate breakdown.	Lowers postprandial hyperglycemia in patients with type 2 diabetes.	Assess the patient for allergies to alpha-glucosidase inhibitors. Assess the patient for any gastrointestinal conditions (e.g., inflammatory bowel disease, colonic ulceration, partial intestinal obstruction) that may deteriorate as a result of increased intestinal gas formation. Instruct the patient to contact her health care provider for continued bloating and flatulence because the symptoms may resolve with slower titration of the alpha-glucosidase dose. Instruct the patient to take the medication with the first bite of each meal. Instruct the patient to recognize the signs and symptoms of hypoglycemia. In general, alpha-glucosidase inhibitors do not cause hypoglycemia when used as monotherapy. Hypoglycemia can occur when used in combination with other hypoglycemic medications. Instruct the patient on the treatment of hypoglycemia. Patients using alpha-glucosidase inhibitors need to treat their reactions with pure glucose, such as glucose gels, glucose tablets, or fruit juice, because the absorption of other carbohydrates may be delayed.
Repaglinide (Meglitinide) Nateglinide (Meglitinide) ***Action:*** Meglitinides cause a rapid increase in insulin secretion.	Lowers postprandial hyperglycemia in patients with type 2 diabetes.	Assess the patient for any allergies to meglitinide. Instruct the patient to take the medication at the start of the meal and to withhold the dose if no meal is eaten. Instruct the patient on the signs, symptoms, and treatment of hypoglycemia.
Sitagliptin (Dipeptidyl peptidase-4 [DPP-4] inhibitor) Saxagliptin DPP-4 inhibitors ***Action:*** Inhibits the enzyme responsible for breaking down incretins (DPP-IV). Inhibition of DPP-IV reduces the destruction of incretins. Levels of incretin hormones increase, thus decreasing blood glucose levels (Neumiller & Campbell, 2010).	Lowers postprandial hyperglycemia in patients with type 2 diabetes.	Assess the patient for allergies to DPP-4 inhibitors. Instruct the patient to notify the health care provider if a skin rash or other signs of allergic reactions develop.

PHARMACOLOGY Summary of Medications Used to Treat Type 2 Diabetes, *continued*

Medication Category and Action	Application/Indication	Nursing Responsibility
Pioglitazone (Thiazolidinedione) Rosiglitazone (Thiazolidinedione) ***Action:*** Thiazolidinediones lower blood glucose levels by increasing cellular sensitivity to insulin, thereby reducing insulin resistance.	Lowers postprandial hyperglycemia in patients with type 2 diabetes.	Assess the patient for the presence of liver disease. Monitor the patient for weight gain and fluid retention. Instruct the patient to contact the health care provider if the patient experiences shortness of breath with exertion or when lying down; fatigue and weakness; swelling of ankles, legs, and feet; rapid or irregular heartbeat; reduced ability to exercise; persistent cough or wheezing; swelling of abdomen; sudden weight gain; lack of appetite and nausea; or decreased alertness. These may be signs of heart failure. Instruct the patient to contact the health care provider if signs and symptoms develop of liver disease: nausea, vomiting, fatigue, jaundice, and dark urine. Instruct anovulatory premenopausal women (e.g., polycystic ovarian syndrome) that these medications may cause ovulation to resume and pregnancy to occur.
Exenatide (incretin mimetic) Liraglutide (incretin mimetic) ***Action:*** Exenatide reduces postprandial hyperglycemia.	Lowers postprandial hyperglycemia in patients with type 2 diabetes.	Assess the patient for any allergies to incretin mimetics. Instruct the patient on proper injection techniques. Instruct the patient to check the injection site for swelling and irritation. Instruct the patient to inject the medication prior to meals. Instruct the patient on the signs and symptoms of hypoglycemia. Instruct the patient on the treatment of hypoglycemia. Instruct the patient to contact the health care provider if gastrointestinal symptoms continue because slower titration of the dose may alleviate this problem.
Pramlintide (amylin analog) ***Action:*** Pramlintide reduces postprandial hyperglycemia.	Pramlintide is used in patients with type 1 diabetes and insulin-treated type 2 diabetes. Patients with type 1 diabetes are amylin-deficient. Patients with type 2 diabetes have a poor amylin response to a meal. Treatment with pramlintide can address each of these problems.	Assess the patient for any allergies to pramlintide. Assess the patient for gastroparesis (described later in the chapter) and hypoglycemic unawareness because these conditions may predispose the patient to severe hypoglycemia. Instruct the patient on proper injection techniques. Instruct the patient to check the injection site for swelling and irritation. Instruct the patient to inject medication prior to meals. Instruct the patient on the signs and symptoms of hypoglycemia. Instruct the patient on the treatment of hypoglycemia.

Sources: Adams, M. P., & Koch, R. W. (2010). *Pharmacology: Connections to nursing practice.* Upper Saddle River, NJ: Pearson; Amylin Pharmaceuticals Inc. (2011a). Amylin product information. Retrieved from http://www.amylin.com; Amylin Pharmaceuticals Inc. (2011b). Product information. Retrieved from http://www.byetta.com; Bailey, C. J. (2009). Metformin. In H. E. Lebovitz (Ed.), *Therapy for diabetes and related disorders* (5th ed., pp. 235–253). Alexandria, VA: American Diabetes Association; Bristol-Myers Squibb, Inc. (2011). Onglyza product information. Retrieved from http://www.onglyza.com/; Burant, C. F., & American Diabetes Association. (2008). *Medical management of type 2 diabetes* (6th ed.). Alexandria, VA: American Diabetes Association; Gutierrez, K. (2008). *Pharmacotherapeutics: Clinical reasoning in primary care* (2nd ed.). St. Louis, MO: Saunders Elsevier; Kaufman, F. R., & American Diabetes Association. (2008). Medical management of type 1 diabetes (5th ed.). Alexandria, VA: American Diabetes Association; Krentz, A. J., Patel, M. B., & Bailey, C. J. (2008). New drugs for type 2 diabetes mellitus: What is their place in therapy? *Drugs, 68*(15), 2131–2162. doi: 68155 [pii]; Merck Manual. (2011). Diabetes mellitus and disorders of carbohydrate metabolism. Retrieved from http://www.merckmanuals.com/professional/endocrine_and_metabolic_disorders/diabetes_mellitus_and_disorders_of_carbohydrate_metabolism/diabetes_mellitus_dm.html; Novo Nordisk Pharmaceuticals. (2011). Victoza product information. Retrieved from http://www.victoza.com.

sensitivity (thiazolidinediones and biguanides), and those that increase postprandial insulin secretion (DPP-4 inhibitors).

The general characteristics of medications within these classes are detailed in the Pharmacology box. More detailed information regarding drugs within each of these classes is provided in the following paragraphs.

Sulfonylureas

Sulfonylureas are indicated for the treatment of type 2 diabetes. Their primary mechanism is by stimulating insulin secretion from pancreatic beta cells. Second-generation compounds have largely replaced first-generation products, which are associated with more adverse events and interactions (Lebovitz, 2009a). The most common side effect of oral sulfonylureas is hypoglycemia, but it is important to note two specific issues. First, there is some cross-sensitivity with sulfa medications, suggesting that some patients who are allergic to sulfa will also be allergic to sulfonylureas. Second, the combination of chlorpropamide and alcohol can result in a disulfiram (medication used in the treatment of alcoholism) reaction characterized by warmth, flushing, headache, nausea, vomiting, sweating, and thirst (Lebovitz, 2009a).

Meglitinides

Meglitinides (see the Pharmacology box) are indicated as an adjunct to nutrition and exercise in patients with type 2 diabetes to reduce hyperglycemia. Meglitinides are a new class of insulin secretagogues that are structurally and pharmacologically distinct from sulfonylureas (Lebovitz, 2009a). Meglitinides cause rapid secretion of insulin from the pancreatic beta cells. Their rapid absorption pattern makes them ideal agents to be administered prior to each meal to reduce postprandial hyperglycemia. Because the meglitinides induce a rapid insulin response, hypoglycemia is a potential risk. Patients need to be counseled to eat within 20 minutes after oral administration to prevent hypoglycemia.

Alpha-Glucosidase Inhibitors

There is increasing emphasis on the contribution of postprandial hyperglycemia to the development of diabetes-related complications. Alpha-glucosidase inhibitors (see the Pharmacology box on page 1436) can reduce the postprandial rise in blood glucose levels and improve glucose control.

Alpha-glucosidase inhibitors are named for their ability to reversibly bind to alpha-glucosidase enzymes (i.e., sucrase, maltase, isomaltase, and glucoamylase) in the brush border of the small intestine. The alpha-glucosidase enzymes break down disaccharides and oligosaccharides into glucose and other monosaccharides that can be absorbed in the small intestine. The competitive reversible binding by the alpha-glucosidase inhibitors to these enzymes delays the absorption of carbohydrates from the gastrointestinal tract, which leads to a more even absorption of sugars throughout the gut. As a result, there is a blunting of the normally sharp rise in postprandial blood glucose levels that follows a meal.

The gastrointestinal side effects, such as softer stools, diarrhea, flatulence, and bloating, are self-limiting and can be reduced by starting with a low initial dose and titrating the dose slowly upward. Hypoglycemia can occur with alpha-glucosidase inhibitors; hence, patients need to be counseled to use pure glucose, such as fruit juices, glucose tablets, and glucose gels, to treat their reactions because the absorption of other carbohydrates may be delayed.

Biguanides

Biguanides (see the Pharmacology box on page 1436) such as metformin enhance the sensitivity of peripheral and hepatic tissues to insulin. This compound has multiple effects on the liver, reducing both hepatic glycogenolysis and gluconeogenesis and increasing glycogen synthesis. This reduction in hepatic glycogenolysis and gluconeogenesis results in decreased hepatic glucose production and lower blood glucose concentrations. The primary side effects of metformin are gastrointestinal disturbances, such as nausea, vomiting, and diarrhea. These side effects can largely be prevented through slow titration of the dosage. A rare but possibly life-threatening adverse reaction associated with metformin is lactic acidosis. In the presence of renal insufficiency, metformin is not excreted normally through the kidney and accumulates, raising the risk of lactic acidosis. Careful screening of patients who are at greatest risk for developing lactic acidosis is the best prevention.

Safety Alert *Radiological studies often are associated with nephrotoxic contrast dyes. The diabetic kidney is particularly vulnerable to these dyes. In patients treated with metformin, deterioration in renal function can result in the accumulation of lactic acid and development of lactic acidosis. Metformin should be withheld for at least 48 hours after procedures in which iodinated radio contrast dyes are used and restarted when serum creatinine levels are normal. In addition, metformin should be discontinued temporarily for any surgical procedure and should be reinstituted only after establishing that postprocedure renal function is normal.*

A number of medical conditions, such as heart failure, acute myocardial infarction, and septic shock, are associated with hypoxia, decreased tissue perfusion, and lactic acidosis. Metformin is contraindicated during these situations. Because patients who consume excess alcohol have a greater propensity for lactic acidosis, metformin should be used cautiously in chronic alcohol abusers. Impaired hepatic function also is associated with lactic acidosis; therefore, metformin should be used cautiously in such patients.

Thiazolidinediones

The thiazolidinediones (see the Pharmacology box on page 1436) are a unique class of antihyperglycemic medications that improve insulin sensitivity through multiple actions on gene regulation. These drugs, often termed *insulin sensitizers*, require the presence of circulating insulin to be effective. The action mechanisms of thiazolidinediones are not completely understood. Their effects are mediated through a family of nuclear receptors called the peroxisome proliferator-activated (PPAR) receptors. The PPAR receptors are responsible for the modulation of lipid homeostasis, adipocyte differentiation, and insulin action. In particular, thiazolidinediones bind and activate the PPAR isoform, improving blood glucose control through enhancement of hepatic and peripheral insulin sensitivity.

In 2010, the FDA restricted the use of rosiglitazone-containing medicines to patients with type 2 diabetes who cannot control their blood glucose on other medicines. These restrictions were placed in response to data suggesting an elevated risk of myocardial infarction in patients treated with rosiglitazone (U.S. Department of Health and Human Resources, 2010). Additionally, rosiglitazone is associated with an increased fracture risk (Lebovitz, 2009b).

Dipeptidyl Peptidase-4 Inhibitors

The newest class of oral diabetes medications is the dipeptidyl peptidase-4 (DPP-4) inhibitors (see the Pharmacology box on page 1436). These medications are a part of incretin-related therapies, which exert their effects by increasing meal-related insulin secretion and reducing postprandial blood glucose levels. Incretin hormones, including glucagonlike peptide-1 (GLP-1) and glucose-dependent insulinotropic polypeptide (GIP), are released by the intestine throughout the day, and levels are increased in response to a meal. These hormones are rapidly inactivated by the enzyme DPP-4. When blood glucose concentrations are normal or elevated, GLP-1 and GIP increase insulin synthesis and release from pancreatic beta cells. GLP-1 also lowers glucagon secretion from pancreatic cells, leading to reduced hepatic glucose production.

Two DPP inhibitors are available in the United States: sitagliptin (Januvia®) and saxagliptin (Onglyza®). One rare complication of sitagliptin is Stevens-Johnson syndrome (Chapter 59), a life-threatening hypersensitivity reaction affecting the skin (Burant & ADA, 2008).

Combinations of Oral Medications

Because medications used to control blood glucose have different mechanisms of action (e.g., augmenting insulin supply, decreasing insulin resistance, decreasing glucose absorption), these medications can be used in combination to maintain normal glycemic levels. Some of these combinations are sulfonylureas and metformin, sulfonylureas and alpha-glucosidase inhibitors, sulfonylureas and thiazolidinediones, and metformin and meglitinides. Additionally, a number of newer medications combine different medications into one pill. Examples of these medications include metformin and Glyburide (Glucovance), metformin and rosiglitazone (Avandamet), metformin and Glipizide (Metaglip), metformin and pioglitazone (ACTOplus Met), metformin and sitagliptin (Janumet), pioglitazone and glimepiride (Duetact), and rosiglitazone and glimepiride (Avandaryl). The specific properties of each of the classes (e.g., thiazolidinediones, sulfonylureas) are detailed in the Pharmacology box (p. 1436) earlier in this chapter.

Some general principles apply in combining oral medications (Riddle, 2009). First, when a patient fails oral monotherapy, combining drugs of different classes is usually more effective than stopping one and substituting another. Second, when a patient requires near-maximum doses of one medication, adding another drug is usually better than increasing the dosage of the original medication. Third, secondary failure of the two-drug combination in patients with type 2 diabetes is expected eventually. In these patients, a three-drug combination is potentially useful, but the addition of insulin to the existing regimen or insulin alone should be considered as an alternative.

Insulin Therapy for Type 2 Diabetes

The purpose of insulin therapy in patients with type 2 diabetes is to provide adequate insulin to supplement the reduction in insulin secretion and to overcome insulin resistance. Type 2 diabetes is a progressive disease in which patients respond to oral medications early in their disease but possibly require insulin treatment for adequate glucose control over time. Insulin therapy remains a viable and often necessary option for achieving optimal glucose control. When patients with type 2 diabetes require insulin therapy, any of the previously described regimens are useful.

Insulin also may be provided in combination with selected oral medications. The goal of this regimen is to suppress hepatic glucose production during the night. Theoretically, the patient awakens with a lower fasting blood glucose level, and the sulfonylureas are more effective during the day. In addition, insulin can be added to regimens consisting of metformin and thiazolidinediones. However, edema is a side effect of thiazolidinediones, particularly when combined with insulin. Both patients and health care providers should be cognizant of the risk of heart failure when thiazolidinediones are used in patients with type 2 diabetes.

Nursing Management

The nursing management of oral hypoglycemic therapy involves (1) instructing patients in their prescribed oral hypoglycemic medications; (2) reviewing oral hypoglycemic therapy with patients who have been on diabetes medications prior to the initial visit with the nurse; (3) instructing patients on the relationship between glucose monitoring and oral hypoglycemic medications; (4) helping patients understand how prescribed adjustments in oral medications may affect glycemic control; and (5) understanding the signs and symptoms of hypoglycemia and hyperglycemia.

Nutrition and Diabetes

Nutrition and physical activity are important in the management of diabetes. Historically, the American Diabetes Association attempted to identify the "ideal diabetes diet" based on estimated caloric needs and percentages of micronutrients (vitamins or minerals that are needed in small quantities) and macronutrients (protein, carbohydrates, and fat). Currently, medical nutrition therapy (MNT) in diabetes consists of meal planning approaches that are determined by clinical evidence; cultural, social, and ethnic preferences; and patient motivation. There is greater flexibility in allowable proportions of macronutrient content, particularly in the amount of carbohydrates, as long as both glycemic and lipid goals are met. See Chapter 8 for more information on nutrition.

The American Diabetes Association has extensively reviewed and revised its dietary guidelines (ADA, 2007), which include recommendations for the role of nutrition in the prevention of diabetes (primary prevention), the prevention of complications (secondary prevention), and the treatment of complications (tertiary prevention). These goals are outlined in the National Guidelines: MNT in Individuals at Risk for Diabetes or Prediabetes box.

NATIONAL GUIDELINES MNT in Individuals at Risk for Diabetes or Prediabetes

The goals for MNT for individuals at risk for diabetes or prediabetes are as follows:

- To decrease the risk of diabetes and cardiovascular disease (CVD) by promoting healthy food choices and physical activity, leading to moderate weight loss.
- To decrease the risk of diabetes and CVD through maintenance of this weight loss.

The goals of MNT for individuals with diabetes are as follows:

- Achieve and maintain blood glucose levels in the normal range or as close to normal as is safely possible.
- Achieve and maintain a lipid and lipoprotein profile that decreases the risk for the development of CVD.
- Achieve and maintain normal blood pressure levels in the normal range or as close to normal as is safely possible.
- Prevent or decrease the rate of the development of chronic diabetes complications by modifying nutrient intake and adapting healthy lifestyle changes.
- Address nutritional needs, taking into account each individual's personal and cultural references and willingness to change.
- Maintain the pleasure of eating by only limiting food choices where there is scientific evidence in support of excluding these choices from the diet.

The goals of MNT that apply to specific situations are as follows:

- Provide adequate calories to ensure normal growth and development in youth with type 1 diabetes, youth with type 2 diabetes, and pregnant and lactating women.
- Provide self-management training for safe conduct of exercise, including the prevention and treatment of hypoglycemia in individuals treated with medications that cause hypoglycemia.
- Provide self-management training for diabetes treatment during acute illness.

Source: American Diabetes Association. (2007). Nutrition recommendations and interventions for diabetes: A position statement of the American Diabetes Association. *Diabetes Care, 30*(Suppl 1), S48–65. doi: 30/suppl_1/S48 [pii] 10.2337/dc07-S048

Micronutrients and Macronutrients in the Diet

The ADA recommendations for treatment of prediabetes, diabetes, and diabetes complications are fairly extensive and beyond the scope of this chapter. However, the recommended micronutrients and macronutrients are summarized in Chart 47–4 (p. 1440). It is extremely important to note that the macronutrient content (i.e., carbohydrates, fats, and protein) is highly individualized and may need to be modified in response to the patient's lipid and blood pressure goals.

Medical Nutrition Therapy

There is no longer a single "diabetes diet"; patients work as partners with their diabetes care team to attain and maintain healthy eating habits that foster the goals of MNT. Primary considerations that need to be addressed in developing meal plans include glycemic and lipid goals, type of diabetes, and the pharmacologic treatment regimen being used. For patients with type 1 diabetes using intensive insulin therapy, such as CSII and multiple daily injections (MDIs), meals and physical activity can be coordinated with insulin doses. Meal planning for these

CHART 47–4 Diabetes-Specific Macronutrient and Micronutrient Recommendations

Carbohydrates (CHO)

- Dietary patterns including CHO from fruits, vegetables, whole grains, legumes, and low-fat milk are encouraged.
- Low-CHO diets, restricting total carbohydrate to < 130 g/day, are not recommended in the management of diabetes.
- Monitoring CHO (e.g., CHO counting, exchanges, experience) is an important strategy in the nutritional treatment of diabetes.
- The use of the glycemic index (i.e., a ranking system that evaluates the effect of CHO on blood glucose levels; higher glycemic index foods are associated with a higher postprandial rise in blood glucose) and load (i.e., a ranking system that takes into consideration the glycemic index and portion size) may provide a modest additional benefit over that observed when total CHO is considered alone.
- Sucrose-containing foods can be substituted for other CHO in the meal plan. If these foods are an addition to the meal plan, they can be covered with insulin or other glucose-lowering medications.
- Many more choices are available today than in the past for including the CHO intake into the diet of individuals with diabetes; however, care should be taken to avoid increased caloric intake.
- Sugar alcohols and nonnutritive sweeteners are considered safe as long as they are consumed within the daily intake levels established by the FDA.

Fat and Cholesterol

- Limit saturated fat to < 7% of total calories.
- Intake of trans fat should be minimized.
- Dietary cholesterol should be limited to < 200 mg/day.

Protein

- In diabetic patients with normal renal function, there is little evidence to suggest that the usual protein intake (15%–20% of caloric intake) should be modified.
- Ingested protein can increase the plasma insulin response without increasing blood glucose levels; therefore, protein should not be used to treat acute hypoglycemia or to prevent nocturnal hypoglycemia in patients with type 2 diabetes.
- High-protein diets are not recommended as a method for weight loss at this time.

Alcohol

- If adult patients with diabetes consume alcohol, their daily intake should be limited to a moderate amount (women: 1 drink per day; men: 2 drinks per day).
- Alcohol should be consumed with food to reduce the risk of nocturnal hypoglycemia in individuals using insulin or oral medications that enhance insulin secretion.
- Moderate alcohol consumption (ingested alone) has no acute effect on blood glucose and insulin concentrations; when CHO is combined with alcohol (i.e., in a mixed drink), the blood glucose level may rise.

Micronutrients

- Vitamin or mineral supplementation in patients with diabetes (compared with the general population) does not provide any additional medical benefits.
- Supplementation with antioxidants, such as vitamins E and C and carotene, is not advised; the benefits have not been established, and there are concerns about safety.
- Chromium supplementation is not recommended because the benefits have not been established.

Sources: American Diabetes Association. (2007). Nutrition recommendations and interventions for diabetes: A position statement of the American Diabetes Association. *Diabetes Care, 30* (Suppl 1), S48–65. doi: 30/suppl_1/S48 [pii] 10.2337/dc07-S048; Dietary Therapy of Diabetes Mellitus. (2011). Macronutrients and micronutrients in diabetes dietary therapy. Diabetes Treatment 1 Diabetes Mellitus Treatments. Retrieved from http://diabetesmellitustreatments.com/macronutrients-and-micronutrients-in-diabetes-dietary-therapy/?wpmp_switcher=mobile

patients can be relatively flexible. By contrast, meal planning for patients with more traditional insulin regimens (e.g., split-mixed insulin) needs to be consistent. Patients using split-mixed insulin dosing (NPH and short-acting insulin prior to breakfast and prior to dinner) cannot easily change the time of the insulin dose to accommodate meals.

Meal planning for patients with type 2 diabetes also depends on the treatment regimen. Diet, weight loss, and pharmacologic therapy need to be finely coordinated; otherwise, the amount of caloric intake needed to prevent and treat hypoglycemia may interfere with weight loss.

For patients with either type of diabetes, frequent blood glucose testing is necessary to determine the effectiveness of pharmacologic treatment combined with MNT.

Many patients who have been diagnosed with diabetes are taught a system of meal planning using the ADA's Exchange Lists, in which all foods are categorized into groups (e.g., bread/starches, meats, fruits, vegetables, fats) and are assigned portion sizes representing "1 exchange" or "1 serving." Each exchange has a specific amount of carbohydrates, proteins, and fats. Patients are prescribed a daily meal plan based on a total amount of daily calories (e.g., 1,200 calories per day) equaling a predetermined number of servings from each exchange group.

Although some health care providers continue to rely on the ADA Exchange Lists, they are no longer considered the best method of dietary planning. However, the principles of the exchange system may be used for easily determining CHO (carbohydrate) servings. Because one serving of CHO is 15 grams, patients may be given a meal plan with a specified number of CHO servings at each meal or snack. Books are available that list portion sizes of commonly eaten CHO-containing foods (McCarren & ADA, 2007). Individuals using insulin therapy may learn how to adjust their premeal rapid-acting insulin on the basis of the amount of CHO in the meal. Patients use the ratio of CHO quantity to an insulin dosage to calculate the dose of insulin they must take with meals or snacks. Most adults with type 1 diabetes require 1 unit of rapid-acting insulin (such as insulin lispro or aspart) for every 10 to 15 grams of CHO. The ratio may differ with each meal and may change with varying levels of physical activity. The following example shows how a patient with type 1 diabetes can calculate the correct insulin dose:

Prelunch blood glucose level: 104 mg/dL

Insulin-to-CHO ratio: 1:12

Prelunch insulin dose: 4 units

Food	CHO Amount (grams)
1 cup black bean chili	32
1 1/2 cups green salad with tomatoes	10
2 tbsp vinaigrette dressing	6
Total CHO grams:	48

Nutrition Facts

Serving Size 1 container (170 grams)

Amount Per Serving	
Calories 170	
	% Daily Values*
Total Fat 1.5g	**2%**
Saturated Fat 1g	**5%**
Cholesterol 10mg	**3%**
Sodium 130mg	**5%**
Potassium 300mg	**9%**
Total Carbohydrate 33g	**11%**
Fiber 0g	**0%**
Sugars 30g	
Protein 6g	**12%**
Calcium	**20%**
Vitamin B_{12}	**10%**
Riboflavin	**15%**
Phosphorus	**15%**

FIGURE 47–15 ◆ Example of food nutrition label.

As can be seen from the calculations, the total amount of CHO from a variety of food sources is 48 grams. Because the insulin-to-CHO ratio (grams) in the preceding example is 1:12, the premeal dose of rapid-acting insulin is 4 units.

Patients are instructed to read food labels (Figure 47–15◆) to determine the total amount of CHO in a food item. Serving size must also be monitored because food choices may contain several servings in one item (e.g., 2 servings of CHO in a 12-ounce soft drink). This method, which requires calculations before each meal, is an essential skill for patients who are using insulin pump therapy or intensive MDI therapy. The insulin:CHO ratio is determined through monitoring blood glucose levels before and after meals, frequent communication between all members of the health care team, and trial and error (Butler, 2011).

Nutritional Needs of Hospitalized Patients

As in any catabolic illness, the nutritional status of diabetic patients is compromised. In patients with diabetes, there is an added dilemma of providing adequate calories to maintain nutritional status and promote healing while maintaining glycemic control. The caloric needs of most hospitalized patients can be met through provision of 25 to 35 kcal/kg body weight (Alpers, 2008). Protein requirements are variable and depend on the degree of physiological stress. Mildly stressed patients with normal hepatic and renal function require 1.0 g/kg body weight, whereas moderately to severely stressed patients with normal hepatic and renal function may need 1.5 g/kg body weight (Williams, 2007).

The preferred route of feeding is the oral route; however, if adequate intake is not possible, then enteral or parenteral feedings are needed. CHO counting is integrated into the diet of the hospital patient in various ways. For example, in some hospital protocols, a specific amount of CHO is provided with each meal and an estimated insulin:CHO ratio is determined. Therefore, the nursing staff can administer the insulin dose immediately prior to the meal. In other hospital protocols, the estimated insulin:CHO ratio is determined and administered on the basis of the variable amount of CHO in the meal. In general, such protocols provide provisions for patients who have a poor appetite, nausea, vomiting, and other gastrointestinal disorders. In these cases, the nurse may administer the rapid-acting insulin dose at the end of the meal, when the nurse can observe the amount of CHO the patient has eaten.

Exercise and Physical Activity

Regular exercise and a physically active lifestyle provide numerous benefits for people with type 1 and type 2 diabetes as well as those at risk for developing diabetes. Results of a recent research trial clearly demonstrated that lifestyle interventions including regular exercise and dietary changes are essential to preventing the onset of diabetes in high-risk individuals (Roumen et al., 2011). Benefits for those who have already been diagnosed with type 1 or type 2 diabetes include lower blood glucose levels, improved insulin sensitivity, improvements in cardiovascular risks such as high blood lipid and blood pressure levels, improved cardiac conditioning, increased strength and flexibility, and improved personal well-being. Exercise also may help in weight loss when used in conjunction with a calorie-restricted diet (Horton, 2009).

Although the benefits of exercise outweigh the risks of exercise in most instances, many factors must be taken into account before initiating an exercise program. In nondiabetic individuals, metabolism of substrates is tightly balanced by neuroendocrine mechanisms to maintain normoglycemia. However, individuals with diabetes may have impaired neuroendocrine responses to exercise. Fuel mobilization from muscle and liver stores during exercise may be 20-fold higher than that during sedentary activity to maintain normal blood glucose levels. During exercise, glucose transport into working muscles is enhanced while cellular resistance to insulin is decreased. Plasma insulin levels decrease while levels of circulating counterregulatory hormones such as glucagon, cortisol, epinephrine, and norepinephrine increase to maintain glucose homeostasis and avoid hypoglycemia or hyperglycemia.

Safety Alert *In general, patients with diabetes using pharmacologic therapy are at greater risk for hypoglycemia during and following exercise. In fact, the hypoglycemic effect of exercise can persist for several hours; therefore, patient education about preventing and treating exercise-related hypoglycemia is essential.*

Individuals with type 1 diabetes can participate in all levels of physical activity, including leisure time activities and professional sports, if their metabolic control is good and they have no complications (Horton, 2009). For these individuals, the metabolic response to exercise may vary dramatically in relation to plasma glucose levels at the time of exercise, timing of the last food eaten, type of exercise, and level of insulin usage. The use of exogenous insulin plays a key role, potentiating hypoglycemia in individuals who are overinsulinized and hyperglycemia with possible ketosis in those who are underinsulinized. Individuals who have poor metabolic control are at risk for worsening of hyperglycemia and ketosis (ADA, 2011c). Guidelines for exercise in this population include the following (Exercise and Type 2 Diabetes: The American College of Sports Medicine and the American Diabetes Association: Joint Position Statement, 2010).

- Avoid exercise if blood glucose is > 250 mg/dL and ketones are present; use caution if blood glucose levels are > 300 mg/dL without ketosis.
- Ingest CHO-containing foods if blood glucose levels are < 100 mg/dL prior to exercise.
- Monitor blood glucose levels before, after, and more frequently during the postexercise period because the blood glucose-lowering effects of exercise may last many hours after exercise.
- Self-monitor blood glucose responses to different activity levels to determine appropriate changes to diet and insulin.
- Maintain a supply of CHO-containing foods that are readily available during and after exercise.

The use of intensive insulin therapies, such as MDI therapy or CSII, allows for greater flexibility in making appropriate adjustments to insulin and food, thus decreasing the risk of exercise-induced hypoglycemia or hyperglycemia. The importance of blood glucose monitoring and record keeping cannot be overemphasized because these are the primary means of monitoring glycemic responses to exercise and determining the necessary insulin and dietary changes required to avoid hypoglycemia or hyperglycemia.

For individuals with type 2 diabetes, regular exercise plays a key role in improving long-term metabolic control, owing to its positive impact on insulin resistance. Exercise, like insulin, decreases blood glucose levels by enhancing glucose uptake into skeletal muscles. Although exercise-induced hypoglycemia is less problematic in individuals with type 2 diabetes, those who are being treated with insulin or insulin secretagogues need the same precautions for prevention of hypoglycemia as individuals with type 1 diabetes.

Exercise and Diabetes Complications

The long-term complications associated with diabetes pose special concerns and require extra consideration when planning an exercise program. The ADA recommends that all individuals with diabetes undergo a detailed medical evaluation with appropriate diagnostic studies prior to beginning an exercise program (ADA, 2011c). Recommendations include use of a graded exercise test in high-risk individuals. A pre-exercise assessment for all individuals with diabetes should include an evaluation for peripheral vascular disease (PVD), retinal examination, evaluation of renal function, and assessment of autonomic and peripheral neuropathy. The presence of complications does not preclude participation in exercise but does require attention by members of the health care team.

Exercise Prescriptions

Exercise prescriptions should be individualized to each person, with an emphasis on enjoyment of the activity. Generally, an exercise program should include 5 to 10 minutes of warm-up, such as low-intensity walking or cycling; 5 to 10 minutes of gentle stretching; a period of aerobic activity, such as swimming, walking, or dancing; and 5 to 10 minutes of cool down. Moderate to vigorous aerobic activity should be based on individual preferences, current level of fitness, and risk factors. Individuals with type 2 diabetes should participate in a minimum of 150 minutes per week of exercise undertaken at moderate intensity or greater. Aerobic activities should be performed in 10-minute intervals and be spread throughout the week (Colberg, 2010). If weight loss is a goal, the frequency should be increased (Colberg, 2010).

Health Promotion

The nurse's role is essential in the primary prevention of type 2 diabetes and the secondary prevention of complications from type 1 and type 2 diabetes. Nurses are in a unique position to identify patients and their families who are at risk for diabetes, such as those adults and children who are obese and overweight. From this assessment, nurses can develop individualized programs to reduce the risk of type 2 diabetes. In addition, the nurse is in a pivotal position to help patients with both type 1 and type 2 diabetes integrate lifestyle and physical activity modifications to reduce the risk of complications.

Complementary and alternative medicine (CAM) is the term commonly used for certain health care products that are not considered to be part of conventional medicine. Approximately 2 to 3.6 million people in the United States use CAM for treatment of diabetes (Dham, Shah, Hirsch, & Banerji, 2006). Complementary and alternative medicine practices may include prayer, acupuncture, massage, biofeedback, yoga, and various plant remedies. Randomized clinical trials are needed to assess the efficacy of CAM practices, nonpharmacologic medications, and supplements (Dham et al., 2006). Most important, the nurse needs sound clinical judgment when patients report the use of CAM practices and supplements in treating diabetes. In particular, nurses and other health care professionals must understand that nonpharmacologic medications are supplemental therapy; some supplements claim to enhance insulin secretion, but they do not take the place of exogenous insulin. Because patients with type 1 diabetes lack the ability to produce insulin, claims that a supplement will increase insulin secretion in type 1 diabetes are misleading and can be dangerous. However, as knowledge is refined, there may come to be a place for these supplements in diabetes treatment. The Complementary & Alternative Therapies box provides guidelines for assessing the quality of supplements.

Management of Hospitalized Patients with Diabetes

For several decades, the management of diabetes in the hospitalized patient has focused on the treatment of the acute complications of diabetes: diabetic ketoacidosis (DKA) and hyperosmolar hyperglycemic state (HHS). Infection and the stress of illness or surgery, however, worsen glycemic control in patients with diabetes and often precipitates hyperglycemia. Hospitalized patients without diabetes who become hyperglycemic during an infectious process or the stress of illness or surgery should be evaluated for metabolic syndrome or prediabetes (McCulloch & Munshi, 2012). The following paragraphs focus on the treatment of hyperglycemia in patients who are acutely ill, along with general treatment strategies for DKA, HHS, and hypoglycemia.

Hyperglycemia in Acute Illness

Physiological stress that occurs with acute illness or surgery causes an increase in the counterregulatory hormones glucagon, cortisol, growth hormone, and catecholamines. These hormones increase insulin

COMPLEMENTARY & ALTERNATIVE THERAPIES Dietary Supplement Quality and Safety Criteria

Nancy Yilk

NEITHER HEALTH PROFESSIONALS NOR THE GENERAL PUBLIC have much understanding of what criteria should be used when selecting supplements on the basis of the manufacturing practices of the companies offering the products. Discerning whether the supplement manufacturers' products are represented with integrity to the purchaser can be put in a simple context: Are they simply in the industry for the money, or are they delivering products that truly support the research? To assess the quality of manufacturers, it is reasonable for purchasers to have a working knowledge of guidelines that are followed by professional health care manufacturers. Educating the public on high-quality manufacturing will move the industry forward because companies that truly support the integrative health care model will be rewarded economically by purchases of their products and other companies will not.

Following are reasonable guidelines, followed by a glossary of terms used in them, that can be used to assess a company's manufacturing policy. Answers to questions about which audits a company has formalized into policy should be stated in the company's manufacturing procedures or supplied by its representatives.

Production Process With Audits? FDA cGMP Food cGMP USP NSF NPA TGA

Date Last Verified? More than 1 year More than 3 years More than 5 years

Third Party Audit Site? Annual audit Biannual audit 3-year audit set as minimum

Raw Material Qualification and Testing? Testing of each batch
If not, at what frequency with written rationale?

______________ In-house, qualified laboratory or validated supplier certificate of analysis for identity and potency.

______________ Testing for microbiologic and heavy metal contaminants (NSF, USP, or AHPA limits), pesticides/herbicides (for applicable botanicals), aflatoxins (when applicable), melamine (when applicable), and potency (when applicable).

______________ All methodologies will be compendial methods and/or scientifically valid methods.

______________ Finished product testing for microbiologic contamination.

Potency Testing?

______________ Testing for finished products in place and in verified use.

______________ Evident industry knowledge of industry common adulterants.

______________ Evident industry knowledge of industry contaminates.

______________ Sufficient testing to guarantee the absence of adulterants and suppliers of adulterants.

Finished Product Verification and Testing? In addition to supplier certificate of analysis, identity is tested on each batch of raw materials or finished product and all other analytic tests (microbiology, heavy metals, pesticides/herbicides (nonorganic), solvents (concentrates)) are completed on at least every fifth batch/lot—or, if less than 5 lots, at least once annually.

Ongoing Testing? Product has a real-time stability program to ensure that all finished products meet label claims throughout the shelf life of the product.

Are They Voluntarily Involved With Third-Party Assessment Programs? If so, with which industry programs? Do they have their entire line of supplements listed or only a selected few? Some companies have entered into programs under pressure of meeting manufacturing criteria but will include only a small part of their line to be tested, excluding the products for whose quality they do not want to be held accountable. It is fair if their entire line is included in the testing protocols and they state how much of their line has actually been examined by testing.

Fish Oils? ______________ Use purity-certified essential fatty acids with country of origin?

Probiotics? ______________ Use third-party identity-certified strains to ensure targeted health benefits?

Taste & Tolerance Tests? ______________ Are products manufactured so that the pill or capsule is swallowable?

______________ Do liquids or gels taste good? (If the product is not tolerable, then compliance with dosage is greatly diminished.)

Therapeutic Doses? Does the product contain research-based doses of nutrients, or does the manufacturer engage in "label copy," which serves as a window dressing to increase marketing potential to the public? For example, research has indicated that CoEnzyme Q10 is successful at 100 mg to 200 mg, so having 5 mg of it in a formula is a biologic drop in the bucket to the body. The inclusion of this substance is simply window dressing used for marketing. Often, the practice is used to increase the base price without justification to the buyer. In herbal products, the formula may have a researched herbal in it, but the manufacturers will include the ingredient as part of a "proprietary blend" so that they do not have to be accountable to the dosage in testing. It is acceptable to suspect the intentions of manufacturers who use such practices.

Recall Protocol? Product has a reliable recall protocol that is communicated immediately via e-mail and mail to purchasing and dispensing health care providers and industry trade magazines. If the manufacturer sells directly to the public, does it have an established communication policy via U.S. mail or e-mail to purchasing clients and does it publish recall information in popular media sources, not just industry trade sources?

Glossary

- *Chemical Solvent Residue:* The solvents are classified as class 1 (solvents that are known to cause unacceptable toxicities, which should be avoided in the production), class 2 (solvents associated with less severe toxicity, which should be limited), and class 3 (less toxic solvents, which should be used where practical).
- *CoA:* A Certificate of Analysis (CoA), the formal report of the product's testing results, should contain the product name, brand, lot/batch number, brand/expiry/retest date, test, specifications for each test, and the actual test results. A signature of the quality unit certifies the validity of the certificate. The CoA typically includes tests for identity, impurities, and potency.

(*continued*)

COMPLEMENTARY & ALTERNATIVE THERAPIES Dietary Supplement Quality and Safety Criteria, *continued*

- *Dietary Supplement cGMP:* The requirements include provisions related to the design and construction of physical plants, cleaning, proper manufacturing operations, quality control procedures, testing the final product or incoming materials and in-process materials, handling consumer complaints, and maintaining records.
- *Economic Adulteration:* Product is adulterated if it omits a valuable constituent or substitutes another substance, in whole or in part, for a valuable constituent (for instance, tea tree oil diluted with olive oil or pomegranate spiked with Ellagic acid).
- *FDA:* The U.S. Food and Drug Administration (FDA) published the final rules for current Good Manufacturing Practices (cGMP) of Dietary Supplements in May 2007. These are published in Title 21 of the Code of Federal Regulations, Part 111 (21 CFR 111). The FDA has the authority to audit dietary supplement companies and take actions against any unsafe dietary supplement products.
- *Food cGMP:* Current food Good Manufacturing Practices (GMP) are published in Title 21 of the Code of Federal Regulations, Part 110 (21 CFR 110). GMPs describe the methods, equipment, facilities, and controls for producing processed food (buildings and facilities, equipment, production and process control, defect action level).
- *Heavy Metals:* Typically includes lead, arsenic, cadmium, and mercury.
- *Herbicides/Pesticides:* Herbicides and pesticides are defined as any substances or mixture of substances intended to prevent, destroy, or control any unwanted species of plants or animals causing harm during, or otherwise interfering with, the production, processing, storage, transport, or marketing of pure articles. The designation includes growth regulators, defoliants, desiccants, and any substances applied to crops before or after harvest to protect the product from deterioration.
- *Identity Testing:* Test the authenticity of the ingredients. USP provides monograph chapters for some ingredients that include appropriate identity testing methods. Other identity methods are developed by brands, and these methods must be verified.
- *In House or Qualified Quality Control Lab:* According to cGMP, a qualified lab is located in the finished product owner's facility, finished product manufacturing facility, and/or independent testing laboratory that is in cGMP compliance and provides testing service for brands.
- *Microbiologic:* Major sources of microbial contamination are associated with human or animal feces used as plant manure, contaminated irrigation water and/or process water, and poor worker hygiene and sanitation practices during harvesting, sorting, processing, packaging, and transportation. Good Manufacturing Practices (GMPs) are employed and adequate microbiologic specifications are established for nonsterile dietary supplements.
- *NPA:* The Natural Products Association (NPA) was the first organization to offer a third-party GMP certification program specific to the manufacturing of dietary supplements and dietary ingredients. The NPA GMP standard includes all of the current FDA GMP requirements and certain requirements from the NPA GMP standard.
- *NSF:* NSF International, The Public Health and Safety Company™, is a not-for-profit, nongovernmental organization. The NSF Good Manufacturing Practices (GMP) registration for brands of dietary supplement enables the company to become certified as complying with current FDA GMP requirements.
- *Pharmaceutical cGMP:* FDA cGMP regulations are enforced on prescription and OTC drug manufacturing processes.
- *TGA:* The Australian Government, Department of Health and Ageing, Therapeutic Goods Administration (TGA) regulates medical devices, complementary medicines, OTC medicines, prescription medicines, blood and tissues, IVDs, and other therapeutic goods. The TGA carries out a range of assessment and monitoring activities to ensure that therapeutic goods available in Australia are of an acceptable standard.
- *USP:* United States Pharmacopeia (USP), an official public standards-setting authority, sets standards for food ingredients and dietary supplements and also conducts voluntary verification programs for brand of dietary ingredients and dietary supplements. The onsite audit by USP ascertains information about the participating company's quality systems and critical manufacturing information.

resistance and hepatic glucose production and decrease glucose transport, resulting in hyperglycemia. Investigations into the relationship between hyperglycemia and poor recovery from both acute and chronic illness have gained momentum during the past few years. For example, hyperglycemia is known to interfere with recovery from infections and wound healing (Brealey & Singer, 2009).

Alterations in the immune response contribute to the severity of complications, such as lower extremity ulcers, along with the development of more severe infections (Bilous et al., 2010). Early in the last decade, a number of studies demonstrated that hyperglycemia was clearly associated with deleterious effects on recovery from critical illness, myocardial infarction, stroke, and cardiac surgery (Fowler, 2008). These studies provided momentum to design clinical protocols to normalize glucose levels in acutely ill hospitalized patients. The initial results of these clinical interventions suggested that normoglycemia was associated with decreased morbidity and mortality in critical illness. The long-term results of these interventions have been inconclusive, suggesting that the interventions may be of limited value in decreasing mortality rates (Brunkhorst et al., 2008; Wiener, Wiener, & Larson, 2008). Additionally, targeting normal glucose levels increases the risk of hypoglycemia (Finfer et al., 2009). As a result, a consensus conference on inpatient management of diabetes was convened to develop newer guidelines for glucose management, which is discussed in the following paragraphs (Moghissi et al., 2009).

Target Glucose Levels for Hospitalized Patients

The glucose goals for hospitalized patients are broadly divided into those for critically ill and those for non-critically ill hospital inpatients (Moghissi et al., 2009). In critically ill patients, insulin therapy should be initiated for treatment of continuing hyperglycemia beginning at a threshold of no greater than 180 mg/dL. Once this insulin therapy is initiated, a glucose range of 140 to 180 mg/dL is recommended for the majority of critically ill patients. There may be more stringent glucose goals, such as 110 to 140 mg/dL, in selected patients as long as these goals can be achieved without hypoglycemia. Critically ill patients need an intravenous insulin protocol that can achieve the desired glucose outcomes and does not cause significant hypoglycemia.

In non-critically ill inpatients, there is no clear evidence for specific blood glucose goals. If patients are treated with insulin, the premeal blood glucose should generally be 140 to 180 mg/dL. The preferred method to achieve desired glucose goals in non-critically ill inpatients is through scheduled subcutaneous insulin injections with basal, nutritional, and supplemental insulin correction doses.

Insulin Protocols Designed to Meet Treatment Goals in Hospitalized Patients

Evidence supports the use of intravenous insulin infusions in the intensive care unit (ICU) for hyperglycemic critically ill patients (e.g., during myocardial infarction, following surgeries) (Kansagara, Fu, & Freeman et al., 2011; Quaseem, Humphrey, Chou et al., 2011; Wiener et al., 2008). Various protocols are used to maintain target glucose levels during hospitalization. There is no single standard protocol because each individual's response to insulin depends on a variety of factors. In general, the protocols include infusion of glucose to help prevent hypoglycemia and wide fluctuations in blood glucose levels. Insulin infusion protocols have been found to be effective with patients who are NPO (nothing by mouth), those who are receiving parenteral nutrition, and those who are receiving enteral tube feedings. The use of an IV insulin infusion allows for greater flexibility in changing the insulin dosage and preventing hypoglycemia.

In addition, protocols are currently available for the use of subcutaneous insulin to meet target glucose levels, to transition from IV insulin infusions to subcutaneous insulin (especially when transferring from the ICU to noncritical care units), or to use subcutaneous insulin as a starting point to meet target glycemic control. Standardized insulin protocols have three major components: a premeal insulin dose (e.g., 3 units lispro), a basal insulin dose (e.g., 20 units Glargine qhs), and a correction factor (e.g., 5 units lispro). The correction factor is an additional amount of insulin that is provided with each meal based on the premeal blood glucose. For example, if a patient routinely uses 3 units of lispro before lunch but her pre-lunch blood glucose is 250 mg/dL, an additional 5 units of lispro may be administered. In the hospital setting, determination of the correction factor is based largely on predetermined protocols (Krikorian, Ismail-Beigi, & Moghissi, 2010).

Diabetic Ketoacidosis

Diabetic ketoacidosis (DKA) is a life-threatening complication precipitated by an acute or relative deficiency in insulin secretion (that changes in relationship to development of insulin resistance and level of blood glucose) and characterized by profound disturbances in metabolism of CHO, fat, and protein (ADA, 2010b; Kitabchi & Gosmanov, 2009). Typically, DKA is treated in the ICU. Patient care is aimed at correcting the following problems, which can be life threatening: severe dehydration, insulin deficiency, metabolic acidosis from ketosis and lactic acidosis, and depletion of electrolytes from osmotic diuresis. Additionally, the precipitating event needs to be identified and corrected.

Hyperosmolar Hyperglycemic Syndrome

Hyperosmolar hyperglycemic syndrome (HHS), also referred to as hyperosmolar hyperglycemic nonketotic syndrome (HHNS), is a life-threatening complication characterized by serum hyperosmolarity, dehydration, and hyperglycemia; it is usually restricted to patients who cannot recognize their thirst or express their need for water. Such patients may include the infirm; people who are neglected, very young, very old, or institutionalized; and those who have mental deficiencies. In addition, this syndrome is seen in patients with excessive unreplaced fluid losses, secondary to massive glycosuric diuresis, and following gastrointestinal fluid losses and limited fluid intake.

DKA and HHS have been considered complications of type 1 and type 2 diabetes, respectively. Although this is generally true, DKA and HHS can occur in both types of diabetes (Kitabchi & Gosmanov, 2009). The overlap is becoming more apparent as type 2 diabetes occurs with increasing frequency at younger ages.

Hypoglycemia

Hypoglycemia results from an imbalance between glucose production and glucose utilization that occurs when glucose use exceeds glucose production. Hypoglycemia results in a low blood glucose level ($<$60 mg/dL) and is associated with a variety of adrenergic and neuroglycopenic symptoms.

Hypoglycemia Unawareness

Hypoglycemia unawareness is defined as the loss of autonomic nervous system responses to low blood glucose. Symptoms such as tachycardia, sweating, or palpitations normally prompt patients to eat in order to prevent progression to severe hypoglycemia. Hypoglycemia unawareness results from altered counterregulation, particularly deficient glucagon and epinephrine responses to hypoglycemia. Subjects with hypoglycemic unawareness are clearly at risk for severe hypoglycemia and injury. The probability of hypoglycemic unawareness and its associated risks should be considered in patients with an increased emphasis on normalization of blood glucose control using intensive insulin regimens and oral hypoglycemic combination therapy.

Etiology and Precipitating Factors of DKA, HHS, and Hypoglycemia

A number of precipitating factors are associated with the development of DKA, HHS, and hypoglycemia. These are detailed in Chart 47–5.

Pathophysiology of Diabetic Ketoacidosis

The development of DKA is related to the effects of insulin deficiency on CHO, fat, and lipid metabolism. Although these derangements occur simultaneously, it is helpful to consider them individually in order to correlate the pathophysiology, clinical symptoms, and treatments.

Insulin Deficiency and Carbohydrate Metabolism

A relative or absolute insulin deficiency results in decreased glucose use by the peripheral tissues, particularly adipose tissue and muscle. Blood glucose levels increase as a result of decreased glucose transport, hepatic and muscle glycogenolysis, and hepatic gluconeogenesis. Glycosuria and osmotic diuresis occur when blood glucose levels exceed the renal threshold. The osmotic diuresis occurs because there is increased urine flow due to an abnormally high concentration of glucose that is reabsorbed incompletely by the proximal tubule. As water reabsorption occurs in the proximal tubule, secondary to sodium (Na^+) reabsorption, the concentration of glucose builds up, and its osmotic presence impedes the reabsorption of water. In addition, the failure of water to follow Na^+ causes the Na^+ concentration in the proximal tubular lumen to fall below that of the interstitial fluid. The concentration difference between the proximal tubular lumen and the interstitial fluid impedes some Na^+ reabsorption. Thus, both Na^+ and water reabsorption are impeded in an osmotic diuresis. This osmotic diuresis results in volume depletion and a reduced glomerular filtration rate (GFR). Reductions in GFR cause decreased renal excretion of glucose, further increasing the hyperglycemia.

Weblink: Hyperosmolar Hyperglycemia State

CHART 47–5 Common Precipitating Factors of Diabetic Ketoacidosis, Hyperosmolar Hyperglycemia Syndrome, and Hypoglycemia

Diabetic Ketoacidosis	Hyperosmolar Hyperglycemia Syndrome	Hypoglycemia
Infection	Undiagnosed diabetes	Excessive insulin
Cessation of insulin	Acute infection	Wrong type of insulin (e.g., administering rapid-acting instead of long-acting insulin)
Undiagnosed diabetes	Cerebrovascular accident	Missing meals or snacks
Myocardial infarction	Myocardial infarction	
Pancreatitis	Acute pancreatitis	
Trauma/shock	Acute pulmonary embolus	
Stroke	Hemodialysis	
	Peritoneal dialysis	
	Renal failure	
	Total parenteral nutrition	
	Medications (e.g., cimetidine, phenytoin, thiazide diuretics)	

Source: Gonzalez-Campoy, J. M. (2011). Hyperosmolar coma clinical presentation. Medscape Reference. Retrieved from http://emedicine.medscape.com/article/121693-clinical.

Adults with an intact thirst mechanism and normal renal function initially may become only mildly hyperglycemic during DKA, since their kidneys are able to excrete some of the filtered glucose load. Adults without intact thirst mechanisms (e.g., following a stroke) may not be able to compensate for their fluid loss and may become severely hyperglycemic. This loss of water and electrolytes leads to dehydration and hemoconcentration (increase in the concentration of red blood cells). There is a marked reduction in circulating blood volume, leading to peripheral circulatory failure progressing to shock, hypotension, and anuria. In addition, there is generalized tissue anoxia, with a shift to anaerobic metabolism, resulting in increasing concentrations of lactic acid in the blood. Coma and death result after the development of peripheral circulatory failure.

Insulin Deficiency and Fat Metabolism

Insulin deficiency results in mobilization of fat in the blood. The liver is flooded with free fatty acids, which are converted to ketone bodies (acetoacetate and beta-hydroxybutyrate). These ketone bodies are weak acids that are buffered after release from the liver, decreasing the body's buffering capacity. The developing ketonemia leads to progressive metabolic acidosis, which in turn initiates the characteristic deep and rapid respirations accompanied by an acetone odor to the breath (**Kussmaul respirations**). These Kussmaul respirations are a compensatory response to metabolic acidosis, designed to reduce the carbon dioxide level. As ketonemia exceeds the renal threshold for ketone body reabsorption, ketones appear in the urine. The ketones are excreted with sodium, which contributes to the net sodium loss. A severe metabolic acidosis results in depression of the respiratory vasomotor center, compromised cardiovascular output, and reduced vascular tone. This may result in cardiovascular collapse, with the generation of lactic acid, which adds to the existing acidosis.

Insulin Deficiency and Protein Metabolism

Insulin deficiency results in decreased protein synthesis and promotes net protein catabolism, particularly in muscle. This results in a net loss of nitrogen from the body and increased blood urea nitrogen (BUN) levels. This is accompanied by a net loss of potassium (K^+), particularly from muscle protein breakdown. Progressive dehydration results in protein catabolism, and additional K^+ is subsequently lost in the urine. The final result is a net body loss of K^+.

Counterregulatory Hormones

DKA causes increased plasma glucagon levels, resulting in accelerated rates of hepatic glucose production and ketogenesis. Catecholamines stimulate both hepatic and muscle glycogenolysis and adipose tissue lipolysis. The free fatty acids and glycerol resulting from the lipolysis are converted subsequently to ketones and contribute to glucose production in the liver through ketogenesis and gluconeogenesis, respectively. Cortisol increases proteolysis, providing amino acid precursors for gluconeogenesis. Growth hormone causes an increase in lipolysis, contributing to ketogenesis and glucose production. Catecholamines, cortisol, and growth hormone all cause insulin resistance and decreased peripheral glucose uptake.

Pathophysiology of Hyperosmolar Hyperglycemic Syndrome

The pathogenesis of HHS is similar to that of DKA, but there are specific differences. The pathogenesis of HHS includes hyperglycemia and severe dehydration, but does not include metabolic acidosis. Individuals with HHS have a significant reduction in glomerular filtration rate (GFR) related to dehydration and volume depletion. The reduction in GFR results in an inability to dispose of some of the excess glucose through the kidneys and potentiates hyperglycemia.

The metabolic acidosis does not develop, presumably because the underlying plasma insulin levels are sufficient to inhibit unrestrained lipolysis but not sufficient to normalize plasma glucose levels. Theoretically, the amount of free fatty acids that reach the liver is less than that in DKA, and the production of ketones is restrained. The emergent symptoms associated with metabolic acidosis are not present to prompt early medical intervention. HHS may evolve over a period of days to weeks, leading to more profound hyperglycemia, dehydration, and hyperosmolality than are seen in DKA.

Pathophysiology of Hypoglycemia

Glucose is the obligate fuel for the brain and central nervous system. The brain cannot synthesize or store glucose; therefore, it must rely on circulating blood glucose levels for survival. Normal blood glucose levels are maintained through the complex interplay among insulin, glucagon, and other counterregulatory hormones. In patients who do not have diabetes, plasma insulin levels decline as blood glucose levels decline, and serum insulin levels increase as plasma glucose levels increase. However, in patients using exogenous insulin and insulin secretagogues, plasma insulin levels are not appropriately suppressed. Therefore, blood glucose levels may decrease, but the insulin levels remain elevated.

Clinical Manifestations of DKA, HHS, and Hypoglycemia

DKA, HHS, and hypoglycemia have a variety of clinical signs and symptoms. In general, these result predominantly from hyperglycemia, dehydration, hyperosmolality, metabolic acidosis, and electrolyte disturbances. There is overlap between the signs and symptoms of DKA and HHS, with some exceptions. In addition, the degree of hyperglycemia, dehydration, and hyperosmolality is much more severe in HHS than in DKA. The general causes of these clinical signs and symptoms are listed in Chart 47–6.

Primary Laboratory and Diagnostic Procedures

Hyperglycemia in both DKA and HHS is due to a relative or absolute deficiency of circulating insulin. The hyperglycemia associated with HHS generally is greater than that in DKA (Chart 47–7, p. 1448). Because HHS is not associated with emergent symptoms of metabolic acidosis and many of the affected patients are unable to articulate their needs, the course of the disease may evolve over a longer period of time. The reduction in GFR during the severe dehydration of HHS decreases urinary loss of glucose, further increasing the blood glucose level.

Medical and Nursing Management of DKA, HHS, and Hypoglycemia

The overall treatment of DKA and HHS revolves around insulin treatment, fluid replacement, and the monitoring of electrolytes. The management of DKA and HHS includes the following:

- Identification of patients who require hemodynamic monitoring
- Protection of the airway in stuporous or comatose patients
- Insertion of a nasogastric tube in patients with a vulnerable airway
- Hourly measurement of serum glucose
- Frequent (every 1 to 4 hours) measurement of arterial blood gases (ABGs), serum ketones, and electrolytes

CHART 47–6 Signs and Symptoms of Diabetic Ketoacidosis, Hyperosmolar Hyperglycemic Syndrome, and Hypoglycemia

Diabetes Ketoacidosis

- Polyuria is caused by an osmotic diuresis induced by hyperglycemia.
- Polyphagia is caused by an inability to use energy substrates (CHO, protein, and fats) appropriately.
- As the metabolic acidosis progresses, polyphagia is generally replaced by anorexia, due to the effects of ketones.
- Polydipsia is a compensatory response to dehydration and volume depletion.
- Weight loss results from dehydration and altered utilization of CHO, protein, and fats.
- Fatigue occurs in response to altered CHO, protein, and lipid metabolism, especially protein catabolism, but other factors (e.g., dehydration) likely also contribute to fatigue.
- Blurred vision occurs in response to hyperglycemia. Fluid accumulates in the lens of the eye, causing refractory changes.
- Hypotension, tachycardia, and poor skin turgor result from dehydration and volume depletion.
- As the metabolic acidosis, dehydration, and volume depletion progress, orthostatic hypotension develops.
- Cardiac dysrhythmias result primarily from electrolyte disturbances, such as abnormal K^+.
- Nausea and vomiting are thought to result from the accumulation of serum ketones. The cause of abdominal pain is not certain but may be related to potassium depletion. Nausea and vomiting also may be related to the precipitating cause of DKA or HHS.
- Kussmaul respirations (deep, rapid respirations) are a compensatory mechanism to decrease partial pressure of carbon dioxide ($PaCO_2$).
- The red, flushed face seen along with Kussmaul respirations is due to the increased levels of $PaCO_2$, which have a vasodilating effect.
- Decreased mental status and coma are primarily due to dehydration and serum hyperosmolality.
- Hypothermia results from a variety of causes, the most common being peripheral vasodilation, severe dehydration, and, in DKA, metabolic acidosis. In addition, hypothermia may be a manifestation of the precipitating event (e.g., sepsis).

Hyperosmolar Hyperglycemic Syndrome

- Polyuria (as stated previously).
- Polyphagia (as stated previously).
- Polydipsia (as stated previously).
- Weight loss and dehydration (as stated previously).
- Fatigue (as stated previously).
- Blurred vision (as stated previously).
- Hypotension, tachycardia, and poor skin turgor (as stated previously).
- Cardiac arrhythmias (as stated previously).
- Decreased mental status and coma (as stated previously).
- Hyperglycemia, dehydration, and serum hyperosmolality are usually much more severe than in DKA. This results in cerebral dehydration, which is associated with neurological symptoms such as hemiparesis, seizures, and coma.
- Hypothermia results from a variety of causes, the most common being peripheral vasodilation and severe dehydration. In addition, hypothermia may be a manifestation of the precipitating event (e.g., sepsis).
- Vascular thrombosis results from severe dehydration. Patients with HHS are at greater risk because of the severity of dehydration and hyperosmolality.

Hypoglycemia

- The clinical symptoms of hypoglycemia are generally divided into autonomic and neuroglycopenic categories.
- The autonomic symptoms are subdivided into adrenergic (e.g., tremors, palpitations, nervousness, anxiety) and cholinergic (e.g., sweating and hunger) categories.
- The neuroglycopenic symptoms (irritability, confusion, drowsiness, weakness, difficulty speaking, unresponsiveness, unconsciousness, seizures, and coma) result from glucose deprivation in the central nervous system.

Weblink: Hyperglycemic Crises in Diabetes

CHART 47–7 Primary Laboratory Values in Diabetic Ketoacidosis, Hyperosmolar Hyperglycemic Syndrome, and Hypoglycemia

Diabetic Ketoacidosis	Hyperosmolar Hyperglycemic Syndrome	Hypoglycemia
Random plasma glucose (>250 mg/dL)	Random plasma glucose (usually > 600 mg/dL)	Random plasma glucose (usually < 60 mg/dL)
Arterial pH < 7.3	Arterial pH: >7.3	
7.25–7.30: associated with mild DKA	Serum bicarbonate: >15 mEq/L	
7.00–7.24: associated with moderate DKA	Anion gap: <12	
<7.00: associated with severe DKA	Serum ketones: negative or small	
Serum bicarbonate < 15 mEq/L (decreases with moderate to severe DKA)	Urine ketones: negative or small	
Anion gap: >10 (increases with moderate to severe DKA)	Serum osmolality: >340 mOsm/kg	
Serum ketones: positive		
Urinary ketones: positive		
Serum osmolality: variable		

Source: American Diabetes Association. (2012a). Hyperglycemic crises in diabetes. Diabetes Care. Retrieved from http://care.diabetesjournals.org/content/27/suppl_1/s94.long. doi:10.2337/diacare,27.2997./S94

- ECG monitoring for dysrhythmias (e.g., hypokalemia and hyperkalemia)
- Hourly assessment of urinary output, vital signs, and neurological status
- Chest x-ray and imaging studies as indicated
- Use of a flow sheet to monitor vital signs, urine output, glucose, ABGs, serum ketones, blood chemistries, electrolytes, and IV fluids
- Hourly assessment and documentation of clinical status as treatment progresses.

Insulin Treatment

The preferred method of insulin delivery in DKA and HHS involves regular insulin as a low-dose IV infusion. The continuous insulin infusion helps to prevent rapid changes in serum glucose along with hypokalemia and hypoglycemia. In addition, the insulin infusion allows for flexible adjustment of the infusion rate in response to changes in plasma glucose. An IV bolus injection of regular insulin is usually administered prior to beginning the insulin infusion. This bolus should be followed by a continuous infusion until the plasma glucose concentration is 250 to 300 mg/dL and the arterial pH is 7.3 or HCO_3^- is 18 mEq/L. Important points of this insulin therapy are as follows:

- Blood glucose levels need to be monitored hourly during the insulin infusion with a goal of reducing the plasma glucose gradually.
- The insulin infusion should be decreased to 2 to 3 units/hour until the blood glucose is 250 to 300 mg/dL and the bicarbonate (HCO_3 is > 18 mEq/L). The plasma glucose is likely to be corrected prior to the correction of acidosis.
- The insulin infusion should be continued in the presence of metabolic acidosis even if the glucose level is continuing to decline toward normal levels. Glucose should be administered at 5 to 10 g/hour intravenously to prevent hypoglycemia.
- Subcutaneous insulin should be given approximately 30 minutes prior to stopping the infusion to make certain that there is no delay that could cause relapse of DKA.

Fluid Therapy

The first goal of fluid therapy in DKA or HHS is the restoration of intravascular fluid volume, thereby maintaining adequate blood pressure, treating or preventing shock, and reestablishing renal perfusion. The use of isotonic normal saline (0.9 NS) is necessary as a first-line treatment in DKA and HHS. As hyperglycemia is corrected, water is shifted back into the intracellular space. This could potentially lead to circulatory collapse, if 0.9 NS, which remains in the intravascular space, is not administered concurrently with insulin.

After correction of the intravascular fluid losses, the second goal of fluid therapy is to restore the free water deficit by infusing hypotonic solutions such as 0.45 NS. As dehydration is corrected in HHS, normal renal perfusion is established and glucose is lost through urinary glucose disposal. Therefore, patients with HHS may have significant reductions in serum glucose during the process of rehydration alone, requiring less insulin to correct hyperglycemia.

In adult patients with no underlying comorbidities such as cardiac, renal, and liver disease, 1 to 2 liters of 0.9 NS should be infused for prompt correction of hypotension and hypoperfusion. After the initial fluid resuscitation, the infusion rate should be adjusted depending on the patient's intake, urinary output, and hydration status. The composition of the fluid is dependent on serum sodium and plasma osmolality measurements. In addition, the rate of fluid replacement depends on each patient's overall cardiopulmonary status and the presence of comorbidities.

Electrolyte Management

Phosphate replacement is not recommended routinely in either DKA or HHS, although other electrolytes such as magnesium and calcium may be supplemented as needed. The results of the admission serum K^+ level should be obtained prior to initiating K^+ replacement therapy. If the patient is anuric, the K^+ supplementation should be held and close ECG monitoring must be done along with frequent serum potassium assessment. Bicarbonate therapy is recommended only in the presence of life-threatening hyperkalemia, severe lactic acidosis, and severe acidosis (pH < 6.9).

Hypoglycemia Management

If the blood glucose level in DKA normalizes faster than resolution of the metabolic acidosis, the infusion of IV glucose ($D_{10}W$ or D_5W) is necessary for prevention of hypoglycemia. In HHS, the glucose level may decline fairly quickly; as renal function improves, urinary glucose disposal increases. Patients in this situation need close monitoring to avoid rapid shifts in blood glucose, serum osmolality, and hypoglycemia. This involves slowing the insulin infusion rate as the blood glucose levels decline and providing IV glucose as indicated. When patients with DKA and HHS treated with IV insulin infusions develop hypoglycemia, the lower blood glucose level can be treated with intravenous glucose ($D_{50}W$) if the patient is unable to eat and drink appropriately.

Occasionally, glucagon may be administered in the hospital setting. Since the major adverse effects of glucagon are nausea and vomiting, patients need to be positioned on their side following administration to prevent aspiration of stomach contents into the lungs. Adult patients with mild or documented asymptomatic hypoglycemia can be treated with 10 to 20 grams of glucose in the form of juice, soda, liquid glucose, or glucose tablets. If these patients are using alpha-glucosidase inhibitors, they need to be treated with 10 to 20 grams of pure glucose, such as glucose gels and glucose tablets; this is because there will be delayed absorption of other forms of CHO. Following treatment, the patient's blood glucose level should be checked, and treatment should be repeated every 15 minutes until the blood glucose level returns to normal (Goldstein, 2009).

Safety Alert *In hospital settings, insulin drips have long been used for DKA and HHS. Currently, insulin drips are also being used in non-DKA or non-HHS patients to maintain normal blood glucose levels. Nurses must assess patients on insulin drips frequently for signs and symptoms of hypoglycemia and assess blood glucose levels on a planned basis and anytime hypoglycemia is suspected. More intense insulin regimens require more frequent monitoring.*

Management of Complications of DKA and HHS

A number of complications can occur in patients with DKA and HHS. The most common complications include electrolyte imbalances such as hypokalemia, hypoglycemia, and hypercalcemia. The most emergent and dreaded complication of DKA is cerebral edema (Orlowski, Cramer, & Fiallos, 2008). Cerebral edema typically develops approximately 6 to 12 hours after therapy has begun, when the severe acidosis has been partially corrected, the blood glucose has been reduced, blood pressure is restored, and the patient appears to be recovering. This complication most commonly occurs in children (Orlowski et al., 2008).

Safety Alert *The development of cerebral edema is marked by abrupt changes in mental status, abnormal neurological signs, progression to coma, and brain herniation and death.*

A number of causes of cerebral edema have been proposed. These include a rapid fall in glucose with movement of water from the extracellular to intracellular space, causing brain swelling; a rapid decrease in plasma oncotic pressure resulting from the use of protein-free solutions; and altered cerebral pH with paradoxical cerebrospinal cord acidosis resulting from bicarbonate administration. The failure of serum sodium to rise despite correction of hyperglycemia is associated with an increased risk for cerebral edema. Whether this is a response to therapy or a physiological response to cerebral injury is unclear (Kitabchi & Gosmanov, 2009).

Although no one particular cause of cerebral edema in DKA has been identified, it appears prudent to avoid a rapid fall in plasma osmolality by using 0.9 NS as the initial hydrating solution, as in the protocol described previously. In addition, it appears prudent to allow the plasma glucose levels to fall slowly as described previously. If cerebral edema occurs, therapeutic measures include the use of mannitol and dexamethasone.

Chronic Complications of Diabetes and Associated Medical Treatment

Numerous chronic complications may develop as a result of having diabetes. These are discussed in the following text.

Diseases of the Heart and Blood Vessels

Coronary heart disease (Chapter 32), peripheral disease (PVD) (Chapter 35), and stroke (Chapter 22) are more common in people with diabetes, occur earlier, and are more severe. The rate of death from heart disease in adults with diabetes is about 2 to 4 times higher than that in adults without diabetes (CDC, 2011). Among adults ages 65 years or older, the risk for stroke is 2 to 4 times higher among people with diabetes than among those without diabetes, and approximately 68% of deaths among people are due to heart disease. About 67% of adults with diabetes have blood pressure readings ≥140/90 mmHg or use prescription medications for hypertension (CDC, 2011).

Kidney Disease

Diabetes is the leading cause of chronic kidney disease in the United States, accounting for 44% of new cases annually (CDC, 2011). In 2008, 48,374 people with diabetes began treatment for end-stage renal disease (ESRD) (CDC, 2011). In the same year, a total of 202,290 people with ESRD from diabetes were living on chronic dialysis or with a transplanted kidney. The risk of developing diabetic nephropathy is similar in type 1 and type 2 diabetes. The development of diabetic nephropathy is often asymptomatic and is usually detected through routine laboratory screening tests. The natural history of diabetic nephropathy is a progression from a period of hyperfiltration, characterized by an increased glomerular filtration rate (GFR), to ESRD, characterized by nephrotic range proteinuria (the primary indicator of nephrotic syndrome, in which an excessive amount of protein is excreted in the urine over a 24-hour period), decreasing GFR, and increasing creatinine. The development of diabetic nephropathy depends largely on the duration of the disease and the level of glycemic control. The first sign of developing nephropathy is the presence of microalbuminuria, the excretion of small amounts (>30 and < 300 mg/day) of the protein albumin into the urine (Burant & ADA, 2008). An estimated 20% to 30% of patients with type 1 diabetes have microalbuminuria approximately 15 years after diagnosis of the diabetes (Davis, Duka, & Bakris, 2009). Chapter 39 discusses the management of kidney disease. The ADA guidelines, as listed in the National Guidelines for Diabetic Nephropathy box, highlight the information that is considered to be the most important in the treatment of nephropathy (Burant & ADA, 2008).

Blindness and Other Visual Disorders

Diabetes remains the leading cause of new cases of blindness among adults 20 to 74 years old (CDC, 2011). Between the years 2005 and 2008, there were 4.2 million (28.5%) people in the United States with diabetes ages 40 years or older who had diabetic retinopathy. Of this group, 655,000 (4.4%) had retinopathy severe enough to cause severe visual impairment and blindness (CDC, 2011). The number of people with diabetic retinopathy is expected to increase threefold by 2050 (CDC, 2011). Other causes of severe visual impairment and blindness among patients with diabetes are cataracts, macular degeneration, and glaucoma. Visual disorders are discussed in more detail in Chapter 64.

NATIONAL GUIDELINES for Diabetic Nephropathy

- Optimizing glycemic control can prevent or delay the progression of diabetic nephropathy.
- Annual tests for microalbuminuria can detect early diabetic nephropathy.
- Regular blood pressure checks can identify hypertension; hypertension can damage the kidney, precipitate the onset of nephropathy, and accelerate the progression.
- Treatment of hypertension with medication, weight loss, and sodium restriction can prevent the development of diabetic nephropathy and decrease its progression.
- The increased risk of infections in patients with chronic hyperglycemia can result in infections, such as pyelonephritis, with decline in renal function. Patients need to report signs and symptoms of infection to their health care provider.
- Patients who have progressive diabetic nephropathy need to explore options such as dialysis and transplantation with their health care provider.

Source: Burant, C. F., & American Diabetes Association. (2008). *Medical management of type 2 diabetes* (6th ed.). Alexandria, VA: American Diabetes Association.

The national guidelines proposed by the ADA recommend that health care providers work closely with patients and families to identify possible visual complications of diabetes (Burant & ADA, 2008).

Neuropathy

About 60% to 70% of people with diabetes have mild to severe forms of nervous system damage (CDC, 2011). The results of such damage include, but are not limited to, peripheral neuropathy (e.g., impaired sensation or pain in the hands, legs, and feet) and autonomic neuropathy (e.g., delayed gastric emptying, bladder dysfunction, impotence, orthostatic hypotension, and cardiac abnormalities). Diabetic neuropathy can affect any area of the body and is referred to as diabetic polyneuropathy, autonomic neuropathy, or combinations of both. Autonomic neuropathy is associated with the development of gastroparesis, neurogenic bladder, diabetic diarrhea, impaired cardiovascular reflexes (e.g., orthostatic hypotension and tachycardia), and sexual dysfunction (e.g., impotence). Diabetic autonomic neuropathy also is associated with genitourinary tract disturbances. These may include bladder and/or sexual dysfunction. Neurogenic bladder is characterized by a pattern of frequent, small voiding and incontinence leading to urinary retention. An evaluation of bladder dysfunction should be performed in patients with diabetes who have recurrent urinary tract infections, pyelonephritis, urinary incontinence, or a palpable bladder (ADA, 2010b). In males, diabetic neuropathy may result in the loss of penile erection and/or cause retrograde ejaculation (ADA, 2010b). Therapy with selective phosphodiesterase-5 inhibitors (e.g., sildenafil, vardenafil) is now the first line of therapy for male erectile dysfunction (Mayo Clinic Staff, 2012; Snow, 2009). Erectile dysfunction is discussed in Chapter 42.

NATIONAL GUIDELINES for Diabetic Retinopathy

- Instruct patients to report visual symptoms promptly.
- Instruct patients about the relationship between hyperglycemia, hypertension, and diabetic retinopathy, focusing on risk factor control to preserve eyesight.
- Inform patients about the importance of an annual dilated examination.
- Inform patients that isometric exercise can raise intraocular pressure; as such, these exercises can worsen proliferative retinopathy.
- Inform patients about support programs and community services for patients with visual impairments and visual loss.

Source: Burant, C. F., & American Diabetes Association. (2008). *Medical management of type 2 diabetes* (6th ed.). Alexandria, VA: American Diabetes Association.

Cardiovascular autonomic neuropathy is associated with a variety of clinical manifestations, particularly resting tachycardia (>100 beats per minute) and orthostasis (a decrease in systolic blood pressure of >20 to 30 mmHg on standing) (ADA, 2010b). Patients with severe orthostasis (hypotension when standing or moving after standing still for a long time) may need fludrocortisone and/or compression stockings.

Polyneuropathy is most commonly seen in the legs, feet, and hands. This is called **diabetic peripheral neuropathy (DPN)** and is clearly a significant factor in the pathway leading to lower extremity ulceration, a potentially very serious complication of diabetes (Burant & ADA, 2008). Although DPN is predominantly associated with sensory loss, motor and autonomic nerve fibers also can be affected. Distal symmetric sensorimotor polyneuropathy is the most common form of DPN. As the name implies, it usually appears first in the distal portions of the extremities, moving proximally in a "stocking-glove" distribution (i.e., in the areas that would be covered by a stocking or glove), and encompasses both sensory and motor nerve damage. It affects both limbs.

Clinical symptoms associated with sensory nerve damage may include numbness, pain, burning, tingling, and eventual partial or total loss of sensation. The pain associated with DPN is first felt distally, in the lower legs, and usually worsens at night. The pain can be persistent or intermittent, occurring over periods of weeks or months. This pain is usually described as aching or burning. Improvement of pain without medication is usually accompanied by the loss of protective sensation and an increase in the risk of foot and lower limb injuries, including ulceration.

The primary treatment for neuropathy is pain management. Neuropathic pain is often refractory to traditional analgesic therapy and provides a challenge in pain management. Treatment of neuropathic pain is discussed in Chapter 12 (Casellini & Vinik, 2007; Zilliox & Russell, 2011).

Vascular and Neuropathic Complications Leading to Lower Extremity Amputations

Lower extremity amputations in patients with diabetes result from a combination of pathologic events working in tandem. Most diabetic lower extremity amputations originate from diabetic foot ulcers, peripheral arterial disease (PAD), PVD, peripheral neuropathy, minor trauma, deformity, increased plantar pressures, and infection contributing to the development and progression of these ulcers. In the United States, more than 60% of nontraumatic amputations are in patients with diabetes and usually result from the combination of PVD and neuropathy (CDC, 2011). In 2006, about 65,700 nontraumatic lower limb amputations were performed on people with diabetes (CDC, 2011).

Testing for sensory changes in the feet of diabetic patients is done with a Semmes-Weinstein monofilament (Feng, Schlosser, & Sumpio, 2011). The monofilament is a single nylon fiber attached to a handle that buckles under a specified amount of force. The patient is asked to

CHART 47–8 Diabetic Foot Screening Using the Semmes-Weinstein Monofilament

Plantar Sensory Testing

Fill in the following blanks with an "R," "L," or "B" to indicate positive findings on the right, left, or both feet, respectively:

Has there been a change in the foot since the last evaluation?	Yes___	No___
Is there a foot ulcer now, or history of foot ulcer?	Yes___	No___
Does the foot have an abnormal shape?	Yes___	No___
Are the nails thick, too long, or ingrown?	Yes___	No___
Does the patient currently perform daily foot care?	Yes___	No___

Risk Category		Action
0	No loss of protective sensation	0 and 1: Teach foot care guidelines.
1	Loss of protection sensation (no deformity, callus, preulcer, or history of ulceration)	
2	Loss of protective sensation with deformity, preulcer, callus, or corn	2 and 3: Refer immediately to primary care provider/foot care specialist.
3	History of plantar ulceration	

close her eyes, and the monofilament then is applied bilaterally to various points on the plantar surface of the toes and metatarsal heads, where discriminatory ability is best appreciated. The patient is then asked to give a verbal cue when the monofilament is felt. The inability to perceive the monofilament in any area is considered loss of protective sensation. A screening form can be used to document and track where there is loss of sensation (Chart 47–8).

Loss of protective sensation also can be established by testing the vibratory perception threshold (VPT), a technique that is used to measure sensory neuropathy. The simplest method uses a 128-Hz tuning fork that is rapped against the clinician's hand and then held to a bony prominence on the patient's foot or the hallux (big toe). The patient is asked to indicate when he stops feeling the vibration. A patient who is unable to feel vibration is considered at risk for ulceration.

Most diabetic foot problems can be prevented by instituting a regular, organized plan of foot care, but the first step is assessment of risk. Factors that have been associated with increased risk for lower extremity ulcers and amputations include: patients who have been diagnosed with diabetes for over 10 years; male gender; patients with poor glucose control; and patients with cardiovascular, retinal, or renal complications (Burant & ADA, 2008).

Conditions related to the feet that are associated with higher risk for amputations include:

- Peripheral neuropathy with loss of protective sensation
- Altered biomechanics in the presence of neuropathy
- Evidence of increased pressures (erythema, hemorrhage under a callous)
- Bony deformity
- Peripheral vascular disease
- A history of ulcers or amputation
- Severe nail pathology.

Charcot Deformity

Together, distal symmetric polyneuropathy (diabetic neuropathy that involves multiple nerves diffusely and symmetrically) and peripheral autonomic neuropathy can lead to neuropathic osteoarthropathy, or Charcot deformity (Khan, 2011; Lin, 2011). Neuropathic osteoarthropathy refers to bone and joint changes that occur secondary to loss of sensation. The underlying assumption is that autonomic neuropathy damages the sympathetic nerves innervating the small blood vessels of the lower extremities. This causes a loss of constrictive tone, resulting in vasodilation, increased peripheral perfusion, and expedited bone resorption and osteopenia. The salient features and therapy for Charcot deformity are detailed in Chart 47–9 (p. 1452).

Gastrointestinal Disturbances

Gastrointestinal disturbances are common in people with diabetes and may include esophageal disturbances, gastroparesis, diarrhea, and fecal incontinence (ADA, 2010b). Gastroparesis is a syndrome characterized by the impaired transit of food from the stomach to the duodenum in the absence of a mechanical obstruction. This condition is characterized by early satiety, nausea, vomiting, and abdominal discomfort. These symptoms are often accompanied by fluctuations in blood glucose levels due to delayed gastric emptying or retention of food products. These fluctuations are most pronounced in individuals who are being treated with insulin therapy. The action of the insulin may peak during periods of delayed gastric emptying, causing hypoglycemia; the absorption of food while the actions of insulin are waning may cause hyperglycemia.

Treatment of gastroparesis largely relies on diet and medications; nutritional support may be needed in the most severe cases. Improved glycemic control may improve gastric emptying. Frequent (six to eight per day) low-fat, low-fiber meals, especially liquids, may be indicated in gastroparesis (CDC, 2012). Metoclopramide, a dopamine agonist, improves gastric emptying time and has a central antiemetic action. Erythromycin is a motilin agonist that stimulates gastric motor activity and can provide some symptomatic relief in the treatment of gastroparesis (Vinik, Nakave, & Chuecos, 2009).

Diabetic Diarrhea

Diabetic diarrhea is characterized by the frequent passage of loose stools, occurring primarily after meals and during the night. Some patients have alternating periods of diarrhea and constipation. The cause of the diarrhea is unknown, and diagnosis is made after other causes of diarrhea (e.g., infection) are excluded. The treatment for diabetic diarrhea is largely empirical, involving the use of antidiarrheal agents such as loperamide (Vinik et al., 2009).

Oral/Dental Problems

The mouth and teeth are subject to problems exacerbated by diabetes. Infections and other problems such as receding gums and gum disease, or periodontal disease, are common afflictions among diabetics for many reasons. For example, diabetics often are plagued by diminished saliva production, which can hamper the proper cleansing of cavity-causing debris and bacteria from the mouth. Additionally, elevated blood sugar levels could lead to problems that promote cavities and gum disease. Good oral hygiene, including regular brushing, flossing, and rinsing, as well as the proper diabetes management, will help in preventing needless problems (Dental Problems & Treatments, 2012).

CHART 47–9 Stages, Clinical Findings, and Therapy for Charcot Deformity

Charcot Stage	Features	Clinical Findings	Therapy
1. Acute	Weakened ligaments are allowed to stretch beyond their normal range of motion, causing spontaneous dislocation of the foot. • Joint effusions and bone resorption also occur. • Easily confused with osteomyelitis.	**Physical Exam** Visible reddening of foot Warmth Edema Easily palpable pulses May require advanced imaging technologies because microfractures and joint effusions may be missed by x-ray.	Immediate elimination of weight-bearing on the affected limb. If compliance is questioned, hospitalization may be necessary. Continue until redness, edema, and foot temperatures return to normal.
2. Progressive	• Dislocation and fragmentation of bone • Further fracture • Osseous tissue and muscle have been weakened from nonuse and will need progressive return to full weight-bearing rather than an abrupt return.	Radiography usually shows fractures at the metatarsal joints.	Total non–weight-bearing. Crutches and walkers are not recommended, because they may overstress the contralateral limb. Use of a wheelchair is a better option. Total contact or walking casts ensure immobilization of the joint but can be walked on, thus undermining non–weight-bearing.
3. Advanced	• Collapse of the plantar arch from multiple fractures and joint collapse.	"Rocker-bottom" foot.	Prevention of foot ulcer and amputation. Referral for custom orthotic footwear. Surgical intervention may be warranted to reduce or excise bony prominences and/or ulcers, if present. Fusion of unstable joints or severely deformed feet may provide a safer base for accepting weight-bearing stress and reducing the risk for further ulceration and collapse.

Complications of Pregnancy

Elevated glucose levels prior to conception and during the first trimester of pregnancy in women with type 1 diabetes can cause major birth defects in 5% to 10% of pregnancies and spontaneous abortions in 15% to 20% of pregnancies (CDC, 2011). In addition, chronic hyperglycemia diabetes during the second and third trimesters of pregnancy can result in macrosomia (excessively large babies), resulting in neonatal and obstetrical risks (CDC, 2011).

Pregnant women who have been diagnosed with gestational diabetes mellitus require dietary treatment and possibly insulin therapy to control hyperglycemia. Uncontrolled hyperglycemia during pregnancy can result in fetal and maternal complications. Women who develop gestational diabetes mellitus have an increased risk for the development of type 2 diabetes.

Foot Problems

As described earlier in the chapter, people with diabetes have a high incidence of problems with, and amputations of, the feet.

Health Promotion

The ADA recommends that all patients with diabetes receive a thorough foot examination annually. The findings from this risk assessment should guide the plan for prevention and care of foot problems. The health care provider should assist the patient in changing any modifiable risk factors such as smoking, home foot care practices, activity levels, and glycemic control. A variety of home foot care practices have been devised that help to decrease the development of foot ulcers and the need for amputation in patients with diabetes and neuropathy. It is important to note practices that place the patient at higher risk for injury. These include walking without shoes, walking with ill-fitting shoes, decreased attention to daily inspections, and cutting toenails when vision is too poor to visualize the extremity. Activities such as jogging on concrete sidewalks may be contraindicated for patients with diabetes and neuropathy because they may result in trauma to the extremities. Poor glycemic control is associated with poor wound healing and infection. Care for the high-risk foot should not be delayed. Patient education for foot care is outlined in Chart 47–10.

Nursing Management

The nursing process provides a framework for caring for the patient with diabetes. There are differences in priorities in the outpatient and inpatient settings.

Outpatient Management of Diabetes

The primary role of the nurse in the outpatient setting is to assess the initial and ongoing needs of patients with respect to insulin regimens, medication, nutrition, physical activity, adherence to recommended guidelines of care for diabetes, and changes in health status. The patient needs to have testing of A_1c 2 to 4 times per year, ongoing MNT therapy evaluation and education, annual eye examination, foot examination 1 to 2 times per year by the health care provider and daily by the patient, annual nephropathy screening, regular blood pressure assessment, annual lipid profile and serum creatinine, and influenza and pneumococcal immunizations. Following the assessment, the nurse will diagnose the patient's needs and develop a plan that includes education or referral.

CHART 47–10 Patient Education for Foot Care

Inspection	The feet and interdigital areas should be checked daily for blisters, sores, cuts, and calluses. A magnifying glass or handheld mirror may be helpful in viewing the tops, sides, and bottoms of the feet. If patients have cognitive or visual impairments, a family member should be instructed in assisting or performing the foot examination. The shoes and socks also should be inspected for foreign objects, holes, or raised seams that could cause skin breakdown.
Daily Care	Feet should be washed with warm, soapy water and dried thoroughly; soaking of the feet in water is not advisable. The water temperature should be checked to avoid burns. Minor calluses may be gently removed with a pumice stone. Thick calluses should be inspected and reduced by a foot care specialist. Nails should be trimmed straight across and the edges filed. If a patient has any visual difficulty, he should not attempt to trim nails. Lotion should be applied daily or more often if skin is dry, avoiding the area between the toes.
Footwear	To prevent injury to their feet, patients should be taught never to go barefoot. The decreased sensation associated with neuropathy may cause an injury to go unnoticed. Shoes and slippers should be inspected before use to make certain that no objects (e.g., coins) have accidentally dropped into them. In addition, when purchasing shoes, patients should ensure that the size is correct. Patients should be advised to break their shoes in slowly, always wear socks or hose, and replace socks rather than attempting to darn them. Garters restrict blood flow and should be avoided.
Special Care	Patients should be taught not to use over-the-counter chemical agents to remove corns and warts. The irritation caused by such chemicals may result in irritation and subsequent ulceration. In addition, sharp instruments or razor blades should never be used to self-treat foot problems such as ingrown toenails. The health care provider should be notified if any problem arises (e.g., cuts, blisters, nonhealing wounds, signs of infection, redness, swelling).

For example, the nurse may need to provide education about insulin injection but refer the patient for MNT. The nurse implements the plan, evaluates its effectiveness, and modifies it as necessary.

Inpatient Nursing Management of Diabetes

The nursing care of hospitalized patients with type 1 or type 2 diabetes, regardless of their admitting diagnoses, involves ongoing attention to subjective and objective changes in diabetes status. The nurse often will be the first to assess improvement or deterioration in the patient's blood glucose control, which can hasten or delay recovery. The assessment data, which include sample questions specific to diabetes, are found in the Nursing Process: Patient Care Plan for Diabetes (p. 1454).

The nurse should also be aware of the discharge needs of patients who have diabetes. Some examples are listed in the Patient Teaching & Discharge Priorities box.

Collaborative Management

Optimal care of patients with diabetes requires a multidisciplinary team approach. Health care workers, nurses, and dietitians work as an interdisciplinary team to monitor blood glucose levels, make changes in medication or nutrition therapies, and assess the response to those changes. In order to meet desired patient outcomes, it is essential that this interdisciplinary team communicate openly with one another in developing and evaluating care of the patient and family (IOM [Institute of Medicine], 2010). Careful assessment and monitoring by the nurse is crucial in alerting other members of the health care team to changes in diabetes status. The health care provider may alter medications and treatment regimen in response to changes in the patient's status. The dietitian plays a key role in adjusting diets and nutrients. The physical therapist and occupational therapist also may be involved when there are mobility and self-care issues.

Health Promotion, Diabetes Education, and Cultural Implications

Diabetes care requires a complex balance between the patient and health care providers. The majority of diabetes management decisions are made by the patient, without the supervision of health care providers. Therefore, patients must be provided with the tools necessary to manage their disease.

Strategies of diabetes self-management education include providing the patient and significant other with the knowledge necessary for the successful management of diabetes. This information may include but is not limited to the following (Funnell et al., 2011):

- Describing the pathophysiology of diabetes and treatment options
- Incorporating nutritional management and physical activity into lifestyle
- Using diabetes medication(s) safely to achieve maximum therapeutic effectiveness
- Monitoring blood glucose and other parameters and interpreting and using the results to make self-management decisions
- Preventing, detecting, and treating acute and chronic complications
- Developing personal strategies to address psychosocial issues and concerns to promote health and behavior changes.

The behavioral context in which the patient learns diabetes self-management skills is based on the complex interplay between culture and perceptions of health and illness. The patient's culture and religious background provide the context in which the patient develops certain values, beliefs, behaviors, attitudes, self-care habits, and relationships with health care providers.

When engaged in teaching diabetes self-management, the nurse should assess the patient's beliefs about the causes of diabetes and diabetes complications, perceptions of the effect of diabetes and diabetes treatment on one's life, the role of family members in health care decisions and responsibilities, and the importance of customs and observances influencing the treatment plan. An understanding of such issues can form the basis of culturally sensitive self-management education. For information about how the diet of patients with diabetes is affected by the patient's culture, see the Cultural Considerations box.

The ADA website provides a number of useful materials about dietary instruction. The materials, which can be downloaded and printed, are available in a variety of languages and provide information

NURSING PROCESS: Patient Care Plan for Diabetes

Assessment of Endocrine Status Using Gordon's Functional Health Patterns:

- Nutrition Metabolic Pattern
- Activity Exercise Pattern
- Cognitive Perceptual Pattern

Subjective Data

Assessment of Blood Glucose Level

"I feel shaky."

"I am so thirsty, and I am urinating every few hours."

"I always feel hungry."

"I can't get any sleep because I am urinating all night long."

Assessment of Fluid Volume Alterations

"I feel weak and light-headed."

"My mouth is very dry, and I am always thirsty."

Assessment of Acid–Base Imbalances

"I'm breathing fast."

Complaints of headache, altered sleeping pattern, and occasional chest pain.

Assessment of Electrolyte Imbalances

Experience of muscle spasms.

Describes feelings of weakness, twitching, or confusion.

Objective Data

Assessment of Blood Glucose Level

Elevated blood glucose
Polyuria
Polyphagia
Weight loss
Fatigue
Diaphoresis
Tremors
Palpitations
Mood changes
Irritability
Unresponsiveness
Unconsciousness
Convulsions
Coma

Assessment of Fluid Volume Alterations

Hypotension
Orthostatic hypotension
Tachycardia
Poor skin turgor
Decreased urine output

Assessment of Acid–Base Imbalances

Decreased arterial pH
Increased anion gap
Decreased serum bicarbonate
Positive serum ketones
Positive urinary ketones
Kussmaul respirations
Acetone odor to breath
Red, flushed face
Decreased mental status

Assessment of Electrolyte Imbalances

Decreased serum potassium level (hypokalemia).

Outcomes and Evaluation Parameters / Planning and Interventions with *Rationales*

1. NURSING DIAGNOSIS: Risk for Unstable Blood Glucose *related to diabetic process* (NANDA-I © 2012)

Outcome: Patient will have an acute reduction in hyperglycemia. Patient will have resolution of hypoglycemia.

Evaluation Parameters: Evidence of a decrease in blood glucose levels. Common target blood glucose levels are:

Critically ill patients: 110–180 mg/dL

Non–critically ill patients: 90–130 mg/dL premeal; < 180 mg/dL at 2 hours postmeal.

Evidence of normalization of blood glucose levels.

In the event of hyperglycemia, administer medications to reduce blood glucose as ordered. These may include insulin, incretin mimetics, or oral diabetes medications alone or in combination.

In critically ill patients, insulin may be administered intravenously (see text).

All of the medications listed previously have a glucose-lowering effect.

In the event of hypoglycemia, administer medications or food to raise the blood glucose levels.

Examples of foods that raise blood glucose levels include:

3–4 glucose tablets

1/2 cup of fruit juice

5–6 pieces of hard candy.

Medications used to raise blood glucose levels include:

Dextrose 50% H_2O

Glucagon

All of the medications listed previously will increase blood glucose levels.

Check the blood glucose level prior to administering glucose-lowering medications.

Consult with the medical team if a change in dose may be indicated due to abnormally low (hypoglycemic) or high (hyperglycemic) values.

Because blood glucose levels are affected by factors such as medications (in general), diabetes medications, diet, exercise, and physiological stress, fluctuations in blood glucose levels are common in hospitalized patients.

NURSING PROCESS: Patient Care Plan for Diabetes, *continued*

	Sustained hyperglycemia in response to treatment may reflect a poor response to therapy, necessitating a change in treatment plan. As the illness resolves, blood glucose levels decline; this may result in hypoglycemia, necessitating a change in the treatment plan. Check blood glucose as ordered. The frequency and the timing of the blood glucose monitoring will differ depending on the therapy (see text). Monitor for signs and symptoms of hypoglycemia or worsening hyperglycemia; if either is suspected, test blood glucose levels immediately. Bedside blood glucose monitoring allows the nurse to verify whether the patient has hypoglycemia or hyperglycemia and treat accordingly.
2. NURSING DIAGNOSIS: Deficient Fluid Volume with Potential for Hypoglycemic Shock ***related to failure of regulatory mechanisms*** **(NANDA-I © 2012)**	
Outcome: The patient will have restoration of fluid volume. ***Evaluation Parameters:*** Resolution of hypotension. Resolution of orthostatic hypotension. Resolution of tachycardia. Improved skin turgor.	General measures include: Encourage fluid intake (in awake and alert patients). Rehydrate with 0.9 NS for intravascular fluid loss. Rehydrate with 0.45 NS for intracellular fluid loss (if indicated). 0.9 NS will reestablish extracellular fluid volume losses; 0.45 NS will restore intracellular volume losses. Monitor oral fluid intake. Monitor vital signs. Monitor urine output. To assess hydration status or adequacy of fluid replacement.
3. NURSING DIAGNOSIS: Risk for Acute Confusion ***related to alteration in acid–base balance*** **(NANDA-I © 2012)**	
Outcome: Patient will have resolution of acid–base imbalance. ***Evaluation Parameters:*** Normal arterial pH. Normal anion gap. Normal serum bicarbonate. Negative urinary ketones. Negative serum ketones. Improvements in mental status. Resolution of Kussmaul respirations, facial flushing, and acid odor to breath.	Administer intravenous insulin as ordered. Insulin will correct the metabolic acidosis. Obtain the following laboratory tests as ordered and monitor the results closely: ABGs, anion gap, serum ketones, urinary ketones, and serum bicarbonate. The timing of the laboratory tests will change based on the patient's acuity and response to treatment. The monitoring of these values will help to monitor the patient's response to treatment. Monitor for resolution of the following signs and symptoms: Kussmaul respirations; fruity odor to breath; red, flushed face; and mental status changes. Monitoring for resolution in signs and symptoms will help to assess the response to therapy.
4. NURSING DIAGNOSIS: Decreased Cardiac Output ***related to alteration in serum potassium levels (lower than normal), increased serum potassium levels, or higher than normal (hyperkalemia), decreased serum sodium levels (hypokalemia)*** **(NANDA-I © 2012)**	
Outcome: Normalization of serum potassium level. ***Evaluation Parameter:*** Serum potassium level is within normal limits.	Administer IV potassium (as ordered), usually in the form of potassium chloride or potassium phosphate. Total body potassium stores are often decreased in DKA or HHS. Patients often present with normal or increased potassium levels. Regardless, when exogenous insulin is administered, the serum potassium levels will decrease (see text). Administration of IV potassium is usually indicated to maintain normal potassium levels. Monitor patients for signs and symptoms of hypokalemia such as: Muscle weakness Anxiety Lethargy Depression Confusion Fatigue Muscle cramps Constipation Abnormal cardiac rhythms such as T-wave flattening, inverted T waves, prominent U wave, ST segment depression, ventricular arrhythmias (e.g., premature ventricular contractions), and atrial arrhythmias.

(*continued*)

NURSING PROCESS: Patient Care Plan for Diabetes, *continued*

Monitor patients for signs and symptoms of hyperkalemia such as:

Muscle twitching

Paralysis

Gastrointestinal hypermotility

Abdominal cramping

Diarrhea

Muscle cramps

Irritability

Anxiety

Abnormal cardiac rhythms such as tall peaked T waves, widened QRS, and ventricular fibrillation.

Monitoring for signs and symptoms of hypokalemia and hyperkalemia will help assess patient response to treatment.

Note: This list is not meant to be all inclusive but reflects common issues in the hospitalized patient with diabetes.

Source: Adapted from Wilkinson, J. M., & Ahearn, N. R. (2009). *Prentice Hall nursing diagnosis handbook* (9th ed.). Upper Saddle River, NJ: Prentice Hall.

PATIENT TEACHING & DISCHARGE PRIORITIES for Diabetes

Need	Teaching
Physiological teaching needs	In preparing the patient and family for discharge to home, the nurse's teaching should be individualized to each patient but at minimum should address the skills necessary for the patient to be able to self-manage diabetes in the outpatient setting. The patient should be able to do the following: • Demonstrate appropriate technique for monitoring blood glucose levels at home, and verbalize when testing should be done. • Describe the medication name, dosage, timing, side effects, and refill information. • Demonstrate appropriate technique for the preparation and administration of insulin injection (if patient requires insulin). • Verbalize target blood glucose goals and prepare a list as to when to call the health care provider. • Describe the signs, symptoms, and treatment for hypoglycemia. • Describe the signs, symptoms, and action to take for hyperglycemia. • Describe how to manage diabetes during illnesses such as the flu. • Verbalize basic understanding of healthy-eating concepts and timing of meals if the patient will be on insulin therapy. • Verbalize when to call a health care provider. If patients have been newly diagnosed with diabetes or prediabetes during this admission, have never received formal diabetes self-management education, or have had changes in their health or therapy, they should be referred for further outpatient diabetes education and follow-up.
Psychosocial teaching needs	Patients with diabetes must learn to cope with the daily stress of caring for a chronic disease. The incidence of depression and other psychological disturbances is much higher in people with diabetes than the general population. It is important for the nurse to assess psychosocial needs, family support, and coping skills to foster the patient's ability to self-manage diabetes while maintaining optimal quality of life. Discharge planning for patients who need further psychosocial support may include the following: • Referral for social work services • Information about local diabetes support groups • Referral for psychological evaluation.

on various ethnic and regional dietary habits. These are very important because a patient's adherence to dietary recommendations may increase when traditional foods, practices, and cultural and dietary customs are included in educational instruction.

Gerontological Considerations

Caring for older adults with diabetes requires special consideration of their needs and approaches to health maintenance. This heterogeneous population includes persons residing independently in their own homes, with family members, in assisted care facilities, and in nursing homes. Older adults with diabetes can be fit and healthy or frail with many comorbidities and functional disabilities. The overall goals of diabetes management in older adults are similar to those in younger adults and include management of both hyperglycemia and risk factors. However, in frail older patients with diabetes, avoidance of hypoglycemia, hypotension, and drug interactions due to polypharmacy are of even greater concern than in younger patients with diabetes.

In establishing a plan of care for older patients that has the immediate goal of achieving a normal life expectancy where possible, special

CULTURAL CONSIDERATIONS Related to Diet for Patients With Diabetes

Diabetes is a disease with noticeable racial and ethnic disparities (Vorderstrasse, 2012). For example, nearly 15% of Black U.S. residents have been diagnosed with diabetes, and Black people are twice as likely as non-Hispanic White people to develop the disease (CDC, 2011). Since diet is one of the cornerstones of diabetes management, it is imperative that the nurse help patients from unique cultural backgrounds integrate the disease and its treatment into their lifestyle and vice versa. Inherent in this caveat is the need to help patients adapt to a dietary plan tailored to assist in controlling diabetic symptoms (Anderson, Kendall, Perryman, & Prior, 2011; Vorderstrasse, 2012). In helping patients formulate a dietary plan that fits their own metabolism, nutrition, and lifestyle requirements, each individual's ethnic practices must be considered. Types of food eaten and methods of food preparation, as well as habits of eating, are common or unique to specific ethnicities. The cultural norms, beliefs, and practices that provide guidelines for the interpretation of food and eating must also be considered. Even motivated patients can struggle with diabetes self-management. Certain racial and ethnic groups face unique challenges due to strong cultural influences on diet. The influence of culture on dietary compliance is illustrated briefly with the following three ethnic groups: African Americans, Asian Americans, and Hispanics.

African Americans

The African American diet is based in part on certain health beliefs that have been passed down through generations and are still observed today. Some studies show that Black patients practice fewer dietary self-management behaviors than White patients, making this a salient issue for providers to address in this population (Melkus, Whittemore, & Mitchell, 2009). The traditional African American food—sometimes referred to as "soul food"—is diverse and flavorful with origins in Africa, the West Indies, and American southern states; however, it contains high-fat and high-sodium foods that are deleterious to diabetes. For some African Americans, soul food refers to meals made with fried chicken, pork chops, chitterlings, grits, cornbread, macaroni and cheese, gumbos, fried pogies, and hushpuppies. The use of okra in many of their foods, especially gumbo, is very important to African Americans, as it is believed to have spiritual and healthful properties. Thus, it should not be denied when developing a dietary plan for the African American with diabetes. Though many African Americans eat foods such as greens, beans, and rice, which are rich in nutrients, economic issues and deep-rooted dietary habits create challenges for changing behaviors and lowering disease risk in this population. For many, decreasing the cholesterol, fat, and sodium content of the diet and focusing on weight management are significant goals to reduce the risk of diabetes complications. Helping them modify recipes for foods they typically eat is valuable in achieving and maintaining adherence to recommended dietary changes (Dimensions of Culture, 2010; Vorderstrasse, 2012).

Asian Americans

Asian Americans are a diverse population, made up of individuals who are Chinese, Filipino, Asian Indian, Vietnamese, Korean, Japanese, and other Asian ancestry. Thus, it is important to remember that their beliefs, traditions, and practices vary among Asian cultures. It is important to assess each Asian patient as an individual possessing individual health needs and concerns. The adherence to traditional Asian practices varies depending upon the length of time the patient has lived in the United States. For example, the food choices of some Asians have changed due to their immigration to the United States. With each generation of Asian Americans living in the United States, there appears to be more adoption of U.S. lifestyle practices than adherence to native Asian practices. For example, the food choices of some have changed due to their immigration to the United States. Instead of their traditional plant- and fish-based diets, they are choosing foods with more animal protein, animal fats, and processed carbohydrates. They also are less physically active. With these two major lifestyle changes, their chance of developing and/or managing diabetes has increased. When discussing dietary changes with Asian Americans, it is important to note that their health care practices involve spiritual or supernatural traditions. It is very important to be knowledgeable of these traditions, one of which is to include the use of steamed herbs that may be mixed with wine; wine then must be considered in the dietary plan (Dimensions of Culture, 2010).

Hispanics

Food is a big part of Hispanic life; unfortunately, so is a high incidence of type 2 diabetes (Mitchell, 2012). Prevention and treatment programs for diabetes targeting this population must include foods commonly found in the traditional diet. The contemporary diet of Hispanics is heavily influenced by the traditional dietary patterns of their countries of origin. As such, there are many regional differences between Hispanic subgroups, both in terms of the composition of the diet and the way in which food is prepared. However, many still retain core elements of the traditional Hispanic diet, including a reliance on grains and beans and the incorporation of fresh fruits and vegetables in the diet. Family life traditionally has occupied a central place in Hispanic culture, and this has influenced current dietary behaviors. Meals tend to be prepared at home with families eating together. These habits influence the type and manner in which foods are prepared, signifying the need for family education as well as patient education. At this point, survey data indicate that Hispanics tend to eat more rice, but less pasta and ready-to-eat cereals, than their non-Hispanic White counterparts. However, as they have become enculturated into the mainstream U.S. population, their diet has changed to become higher in fat and cholesterol than what was included in traditional Hispanic diets (Mitchell, 2012). With enculturation, the changing nature of their diet, and their increasingly sedentary lifestyle, the prevalence of type 2 diabetes has increased (Mitchell, 2012). Nutritional education programs aimed at improving the quality of the Hispanic diet should be based on a combination of preserving some elements of the traditional Hispanic diet—including a reliance on beans, rice, and tortillas—and a change in others—such as reduced consumption of high-fat dairy products and less use of fat in cooking (Mitchell, 2012).

In order to assist patients of unique populations in developing diabetic dietary plans, it is essential to consider the cultural norms of each population. Understanding a patient's practice of cultural norms can allow providers to more easily build rapport and ensure effective patient–provider communication. However, it is important to remember that not all patients from diverse populations conform to commonly known culture-specific behaviors, beliefs, and actions. Generalizations may not apply; thus, patients must be assessed as unique individuals, with cultural norms providing a framework for assessment.

consideration must be given to the possibility that the older patient (McCulloch & Munshi, 2012):

- Comes from a poorer socioeconomic situation
- Experiences greater social isolation and loneliness
- Has a higher frequency of depressive illness or cognitive impairment
- Is a nursing home resident
- Relies heavily on informal or formal caregivers
- Experiences polypharmacy
- Is frail and has a limited life expectancy
- Has significant comorbidities that limit the ability to self-medicate and recognize or deal with hypoglycemia.

To individualize care and maintain glycemic targets in the context of these possibilities, the following factors are addressed next: nutrition and diet management, exercise, medication and testing, functional impairment, cognitive impairment, emotional distress, and education.

Nutrition and Diet Management

Nutrition and diet control are critical factors in managing diabetes. Many older adults are undernourished for a variety of physiological, psychological, social, and economic reasons. These may include, but are not limited to, changes in the senses of smell and taste and in the sensation of thirst; side effects of medications; inability to shop for food or prepare meals; cognitive impairment; depression, isolation, and loneliness; and inadequate resources to purchase food. For these patients, it may be necessary to modify their diet by changing the nutrient composition or density, modifying the food consistency, or using supplements (Halter, 2009).

Environmental factors also may need to be changed. The social environment in which food is prepared and eaten must be considered as well as the willingness of the person preparing the food to comply with dietary restrictions. Consultation with a dietitian may be helpful for the patient and family (Kalra, Kalra, & Saluja, 2012).

Exercise

Exercise is beneficial to help maintain physical function, reduce cardiac risk, and improve insulin sensitivity in patients with diabetes (McCulloch & Munshi, 2012). In older adults, exercise also improves body composition and arthritic pain, reduces falls and depression, increases strength and balance, enhances the quality of life, and improves survival. Patients with deconditioning (diminished muscle strength and balance) who are at risk for falls should be referred to an exercise physiologist and/or a physical therapist for muscle strengthening and balance training in a safe environment.

Medications and Testing

The older adult may receive oral hypoglycemia agents or insulin for treatment of diabetes. Pharmacologic therapy must be individualized on the basis of the patient's abilities and comorbidities. The goal of therapy is to maintain targeted glycemic controls. However, it may be necessary for the patient to take more than one medication to achieve this goal. It is vitally important that the patient and caregiver know what the medication is and its dose, route, and side effects. If the medication is insulin, it is important to evaluate whether or not the patient is physically and cognitively capable of using an insulin pen or drawing it up into a syringe. It is possible that a pharmacist, family member, or caregiver may prepare a week's supply of insulin in syringes and leave them in the refrigerator. Such a plan may allow an older patient to remain living independently at home.

Monitoring of blood glucose is an important component of diabetic self-management. This is accomplished through laboratory testing of A_1c at prescribed intervals and/or by home monitoring by the patient and/or caregiver. Some older patients may be able to conduct self-monitoring of blood glucose (SMBG), depending upon medications and the patient's functional and cognitive abilities (Standards of Medical Care in Diabetes, 2012).

Functional Impairment

Diabetes is associated with functional impairment and disability. The patient may suffer from vascular complications, acute metabolic decompensation, adverse effects of medication, and the effects of nutritional conditions and lifestyle behavior. These changes may have adverse rebound effects on the patient's vulnerability to other comorbidities, independence, and quality of life. Certainly, they will affect the patient's ability to care for self and manage the diabetes. Disabilities or functional impairments also contribute to emotional disturbances such as depression. Participation in activities should be encouraged, and the patient should be referred to an appropriate rehabilitation program if available.

Cognitive Impairment

Impaired cognitive function has been demonstrated in older patients with type 2 diabetes (McCulloch & Munshi, 2012). Older patients with diabetes and cognitive dysfunction may have difficulty performing self-management and following complicated treatment regimens. Cognitive function should be assessed in older diabetic patients when there is nonadherence with therapy, frequent episodes of hypoglycemia, and deterioration of glycemic control without obvious explanation.

Emotional Distress (Depression)

Emotional distress in the older patient with diabetes is frequently shown as depression. Depression has been associated with poor glycemic control and with accelerated rates of coronary heart disease in diabetic patients. Early identification of depression with a short screening tool and treatment may help achieve better glycemic control.

Education

Education for the older patient, the family, and the caregiver is critical to achieving the goals of self-management and achievement of a normal life expectancy when possible. Components of education include explanation of the disease process and treatment plan, medications (type, route, administration, side effects), the importance of physical activity and exercise, the implications of changes in behavior and mood, and knowledge of potential complications and actions to be taken.

To summarize, there are three key points to be addressed in caring for the older diabetic patient:

- Determine the glycemic goal and evaluate conformity and progress toward such.
- Prevent hypoglycemia, which may lead to impaired cognition and function.
- Provide individualized counseling regarding lifestyle modification, including a medical nutrition evaluation tailored to meet medical, lifestyle, and personal factors.

Research

Adult clinical care of diabetic patients has changed significantly over the last decade (ADA, 2012b). Research has given us new therapeutic agents and approaches to management. Research continues to focus on prevention and cure of diabetes. With knowledge of alternatives to current medical care, health care providers will be able to choose new therapies and introduce their patients to the possibilities of prevention in their family members (AllConferences.com, 2012).

Current research studies are exploring the possibility of transplantation of the cells responsible for insulin production and using stem cells to regenerate a patient's ability to produce insulin (Bluestone & Hebrok, 2012). The Diabetes Center of the University of California, San Francisco, reports the conduct of clinical trials of a vaccine that potentially could prevent type 1 diabetes (Bardi, 2012). The Center also is exploring research opportunities that focus on how undifferentiated epithelial cells develop into functional insulin-producing beta cells. This creates the possibility of recreating an insulin-producing cell in a Petri dish that could be given to people and correct the disease.

RESEARCH OPPORTUNITIES Related to Diabetes

Research Topic	Clinical Impact
Self-care management by older adults.	Improvement and increase in self-care management; assists patients in maintaining independence.
Depression related to onset and course of disease.	Identification and treatment of depression earlier in the disease process.
Identification of quality-of-life indicators for those with diabetes.	Once known, it is used to assist patients in self-care management and lifestyle changes.
Relationship of exercise to the prevention and control of type 2 diabetes.	Assists in the development of exercise programs and to prevent or reduce the impact of type 2 diabetes.
Preventable complications of diabetes.	Increased knowledge and distribution of education plans would assist in preventing complications.

The increasing incidence of diabetes in our society supports the need for prospective research on the prevention and cure of diabetes. Future research opportunities are presented in the Research Opportunities box.

Summary

Diabetes is a chronic disease; however, the occurrence and progression of diabetes-related complications can be decreased through intensive glucose, hypertension, and lipid control. In addition, there is mounting evidence that the number of people who develop diabetes can be decreased through lifestyle modification, including increased physical activity and weight maintenance or weight loss (if indicated). Acute complications of diabetes can be avoided through careful monitoring and attention to precipitating factors. When these acute complications occur, intensive medical management can decrease mortality and morbidity from these complications. Because the incidence of diabetes is increasing worldwide, health care professionals need to stay current with new treatment measures to address the personal, social, and economic problems associated with diabetes.

CLINICAL PREPARATION READ DOCUMENT APPLY

READ: History of Present Illnesses >> Laboratory Study Results >> Critical Thinking Questions

John McKenna is a 20-year-old college student who presented to the local emergency department (ED). He reported that he and several other students had a gastrointestinal virus over the past few weeks. The primary symptoms were nausea, vomiting, and diarrhea, which usually resolved within 24 to 48 hours. Mr. McKenna reported that he never completely recovered from his illness and that he had continued to feel tired and listless during the previous week. During the past 2 to 3 days, he noted increased thirst and increased urination along with fatigue. Mr. McKenna has been nauseated and vomiting during the last 2 hours and has vomited twice in the ED.

Mr. McKenna's laboratory values on admission to the ED are consistent with a diagnosis of DKA. The following medications were administered in the ED: an initial bolus of regular intravenous insulin (10 units) followed by an intravenous regular insulin drip of 6 units/hour. In addition, a potassium chloride (KCL) rider (20 mEq/hour) was initiated after it was established that the patient had adequate urinary output (>30 mL/hr).

Nursing care while Mr. McKenna was in the ED focused on assessing and providing interventions for any emergency needs (i.e., vascular fluid replacement) and obtaining the diagnostic laboratory values: arterial blood gases (ABGs), serum ketones, complete blood count (CBC), serum blood chemistries, serum electrolytes, and urinalysis (UA). The current nursing care plan for this patient calls for initiating fluid replacement therapy (0.9 normal saline [NS], 1 liter bolus); obtaining a capillary glucose reading; performing an electrocardiogram (ECG); and sending a stool specimen to the laboratory for culture and sensitivity. Mr. McKenna was transferred to the medical intensive care unit (MICU), where you are assigned to care for him.

Medical–Surgical History

Mr. McKenna's general medical history is noncontributory. There is no history of major medical illnesses, surgeries, or traumas. He does not use any medications but does report using an over-the-counter drug to stop diarrhea during the previous episode of the "flu." His mother (age 45) has rheumatoid arthritis; his father (age 50) has hypertension. He has three siblings: his brother (age 16) has no major illnesses, his sister (age 14) has no major illnesses, and his other brother (age 10) has type 1 diabetes.

Social History

Mr. McKenna reports social drinking (4 to 6 beers on weekends). He has never smoked cigarettes but smokes approximately 1 to 2 cigars every 2 to 3 months. He indicates that he has never used recreational drugs.

Physical Exam

Mr. McKenna is a thin, acutely ill male; 6′0″ and 155 lbs. The following clinical signs are noted: poor skin turgor, dry mucous membranes, facial flushing, and deep rapid breathing with fruity odor to the breath. His chest is clear to auscultation; his heart examination reveals tachycardia and is otherwise normal; the abdominal examination reveals a diffusely tender abdomen; the neurological examination reveals increasing lethargy; otherwise, his neurological status is normal. His vital signs are as follows: temperature is 37.2C. In a supine position, his blood pressure is 100/70, pulse 100 beats per minute, and respirations 32. In a standing position, his blood pressure is 90/60, pulse 115 beats per minute, and respirations are 32.

READ: History of Present Illnesses >> Physical Exam >> **Admitting Medical Records** >> Laboratory Study Results

Admitting Medical Orders

Admit to Medical ICU
Admitting diagnosis: newly diagnosed type 1 diabetes; diabetic ketoacidosis
Allergies: none noted
Vital signs q1h
Neuro checks q1h
Activity: bed rest with bathroom privileges
Intake and Output: q8h
Sequential compression stockings (SCDs) to lower extremities
Diet: NPO except ice chips until blood sugar below 250 mg/dL, then advance diet to 1800 calorie ADA as tolerated
Call house officer: HR < 60 or >120, systolic BP < 90 or >160, temperature $> 38.5^{\circ}C$, RR < 10 or > 30, urinary output < 240 mL in 8 hours, O_2 saturation $< 92\%$, glucose level < 70 or >130 mg/dL, serum sodium level < 135 or > 145, serum potassium level < 3.8 or > 4.5, increased lethargy per neuro checks
IVs: normal saline 0.45 at 100 mL/hr

Scheduled Medications

100 units of regular insulin/100 mL of 0.9 normal saline
Normal saline 0.45 with 20 mEq KCL at 100 mL/hr

PRN Medications

Phenergan for nausea 25 mg IV q4–6h prn
$D_{50}W$ 25 g IV prn if glucometer reading is less than 70 mg/dL

Ordered Laboratory Studies

Serum Na, Cl, HCO_3 q2h
Serum K every hour until acidosis is corrected
ABGs, CBC, chemistry panel, and serum acetone q4h
Glucometer readings q1h
Stool culture q24h x 3 days

Ordered Diagnostic Studies

ECG on admission and q4h

Clinical Course

Mr. McKenna has a relatively uneventful course during hospitalization with one exception. After approximately 8 hours of treatment, he is noted to be increasingly lethargic and confused. The two primary differential diagnoses for this condition are hypoglycemia and cerebral edema. A capillary blood glucose level taken at that time reveals a blood glucose level of 60 mg/dL, which confirms the hypoglycemia. Mr. McKenna is given 25 g of dextrose 50% in water ($D_{50}W$). After administration of the $D_{50}W$, he is alert and oriented, and the subsequent blood glucose reading is 100 mg/dL. The results of other pertinent tests at this time are shown in the following table.

Because Mr. McKenna's diabetic ketoacidosis has resolved and he is able to take fluids and food, the insulin drip is discontinued. Before discontinuation of the drip, Mr. McKenna is started on an insulin protocol with an initial starting dose of glargine 20 units subcutaneously. The premeal lispro dose will be titrated depending on the meal and his overall appetite. In general, an insulin:carbohydrate (CHO) ratio of 1:20 (1 unit of lispro insulin for each 20 mg of CHO) will be used.

The nursing care at this time is centered on (1) monitoring response to therapy and (2) patient education. In particular, patient education revolves around teaching survival skills (insulin injection, basic nutrition teaching, blood glucose monitoring, recognition and treatment of hypoglycemia) and helping to transition Mr. McKenna to an outpatient education program.

READ: History of Present Illnesses >> **Laboratory Study Results** >> Critical Thinking Questions

Test	Result on Admission	4 Hours Post-Admission	8 Hours Post-Admission
Serum glucose	450 mg/dL	250 mg/dL	60 mg/dL
Arterial $pH/PO_2/PCO_2$	7.1/105/22	7.2/100/35	7.4/100/38
Serum bicarbonate (HCO_3)	9 mEq/L	13 mEq/L	20 mEq/L
Serum Na^+	135 mEq/L	138 mEq/L	142 mEq/L
Serum K^+	5.3 mEq/L	5.0 mEq/L	4.8 mEq/L
Serum Cl^-	98 mEq/L	100 mEq/L	100 mEq/L
Serum acetone	1.16 dilutions	1.8 dilutions	Negative
Serum creatinine	1.4 mg/dL	1.2 mg/dL	—

Test	Result on Admission	4 Hours Post-Admission	8 Hours Post-Admission
Serum blood urea nitrogen (BUN)	25 mg/dL	20 mg/dL	—
Hemoglobin	17 g/dL	15 g/dL	14 g/dL
Hematocrit	47%	44%	42%
White blood count	15,000 cells/mm^3	10,000 cells/mm^3	5,000 cells/mm^3
Urine ketones	Large	Moderate	Negative
ECG	Normal sinus tachycardia	Normal sinus rhythm	Normal sinus rhythm
Stool (culture)	Negative		

Pearson Nursing Student Resources *Log on to* **nursing.pearsonhighered.com** *to download forms*

DOCUMENT:

- >> Summary of Hospitalization
- >> Pathophysiology Form
- >> Laboratory Values
- >> Laboratory Results Explanation

APPLY:

- >> List of Potential Nursing Diagnosis
- >> Concept Map
- >> Critical Thinking Questions and Concept Map

APPLY: History of Present Illness >> Laboratory Study Results >> **Critical Thinking Questions**

1. Mr. McKenna is suspected of having diabetic ketoacidosis (DKA). What are the four major biochemical derangements in DKA that you should assess for?
2. What are the clinical signs and symptoms (as noted in this scenario) that are derived from these biochemical derangements?
3. How do nursing interventions for DKA develop from identification of each of these derangements?
4. Mr. McKenna has mild to moderate DKA. How might clinical signs, symptoms, laboratory tests, and treatments differ if he had severe DKA?
5. Given the previous situation, what discharge plans would you anticipate for Mr. McKenna?

Answers to Critical Thinking Questions can be found in Appendix D in the Osborn Student Resources at nursing.pearsonhighered.com.

NCLEX® PRACTICE

1. A patient who was recently diagnosed with type 2 diabetes asks, "What does the type 2 mean? Is there more than one kind of diabetes?" Which nursing response is indicated?

1. "Type 2 diabetes is generally diagnosed in childhood, and type 1 is usually diagnosed in adults."
2. "The person with type 2 diabetes usually is born with it. Type 1 is a lifestyle disease."
3. "There are several types of diabetes. Type 1 is the most common."
4. "The person with type 1 diabetes doesn't make insulin. The person with type 2 diabetes makes insulin but doesn't use it well."

2. A nurse determines that a patient meets the criteria for prediabetes when which facts are identified on assessment?

1. The patient is 20 years old and requires therapy with oral hypoglycemic agents.
2. The patient was diagnosed with gestational diabetes during her last pregnancy.
3. Fasting blood sugar levels have been 118 mg/dL and 124 mg/dL on two tests.
4. Glycosated hemoglobin (Hemoglobin A_1c) is 6.9%.

3. The nurse identifies which patient to be most at risk to develop type 1 diabetes?

1. The adolescent who had chronic bacterial ear infections as a child
2. A school-age child whose mother has type 1 diabetes
3. A toddler with a monozygotic twin who has type 1 diabetes
4. A preschool-age child with a dizygotic twin who has type 1 diabetes

4. The nurse recognizes which assessment findings in a patient with type 2 diabetes are also associated with metabolic syndrome? (select all that apply)

1. Blood pressure averaging 132/86 mmHg over 6 months
2. Triglycerides of 180 mg/dL
3. High-density lipoprotein (HDL) cholesterol of 36 mg/dL
4. Fasting blood glucose of 90 mg/dL
5. Waist circumference of 118 cm

5. The nurse should incorporate which intervention in the plan of care for a patient receiving a meglitinide oral hypoglycemic agent?

1. Administer the medication at the same time every night, just before bed.
2. Check for signs and symptoms of hyperglycemia 1 hour after the meal.
3. Check for allergies to sulfa.
4. Instruct the patient to eat within 20 minutes of taking the medication.

6. The nurse should provide which education to a patient with type 2 diabetes who takes oral hypoglycemic agents and is planning to begin an exercise program?

1. "You will be at increased risk for hyperglycemia up to 2 hours after exercising."
2. "Avoid eating anything before you start exercising."
3. "Exercise may lower your blood sugar for several hours after completing the activity."
4. "Eat only simple carbohydrates if you become hypoglycemic after exercising."

Answers to NCLEX Practice Questions can be found in Appendix D in the Osborn Student Resources at nursing.pearsonhighered.com. Practice additional NCLEX questions online at the Student Resources site.

REFERENCES

Adamec, C. (2010). Medication causes of diabetes. Livestrong .com. Retrieved from www.livestrong.com/article/135530-media

Adams, M. P., & Koch, R. W. (2010). *Pharmacology: Connections to nursing practice.* Upper Saddle River, NJ: Pearson.

AllConferences.com. (2012). 2009 Advances in diabetes research. Retrieved from http://www.allconferences .com/conferences/20090220152711/

Alpers, D. H. (2008). *Manual of nutritional therapeutics* (5th ed.). Philadelphia: Lippincott Williams & Wilkins.

Aly, H., & Gottlieb, P. (2009). The honeymoon phase: Intersection of metabolism and immunology. *Current Opinion in Endocrinology, Diabetes, and Obesity, 16*(4), 286–292. doi: 10.1097/MED.0b013e32832e0693

American Diabetes Association. (2007). Nutrition recommendations and interventions for diabetes: A position statement of the American Diabetes Association. *Diabetes Care, 30* (Suppl 1), S48–S65. doi: 30/suppl_1/S48 [pii] 10.2337/dc07-S048

American Diabetes Association. (2008a). Diagnosis and classification of diabetes mellitus. *Diabetes Care, 31* (suppl. 1), S53–S60. doi: 10.2337/dco8-So55

American Diabetes Association. (2008b). Economic costs of diabetes in the U.S. in 2007. *Diabetes Care, 31*(3), 596–615. doi: 31/3/596 [pii] 10.2337/dc08-9017

American Diabetes Association. (2010a). Diagnosis and classification of diabetes mellitus. *Diabetes Care, 33* (suppl. 1), S62–S69. doi: 33/Supplement_1/S62 [pii] 10.2337/dc10-S062

American Diabetes Association. (2010b). Standards of medical care in diabetes—2010. *Diabetes Care, 33*(suppl. 1), S11–S61. doi: 33/Supplement_1/S11 [pii] 10.2337/dc10-S011

American Diabetes Association. (2011a). Executive summary: Standards of medical care in diabetes—2011. *Diabetes Care, 34* (suppl. 1), S4–S10. doi: 34/Supplement_1/S4 [pii] 10.2337/dc11-S004

American Diabetes Association. (2011b). Genetics of diabetes. Retrieved from http://www.diabetes.org/diabetes-basics/genetics-of-diabetes.html

American Diabetes Association. (2011c). Tight diabetes control. Retrieved from http://www.diabetes.org/living-with-diabetes/treatment-and-care/blood-glucose-control/tight-diabetes-control.html

American Diabetes Association. (2012a). Hyperglycemic crises in diabetes. Diabetes Care. Retrieved from http://care .diabetesjournals.org/content/27/suppl_1/s94.long. doi:10.2337/diacare,27.2997./S94

American Diabetes Association. (2012b). Recent advances. Retrieved from http://www.diabetes.org/news-research/research/recent/recent-advances/

American Diabetes Association. (2012c). Your risk. Retrieved from http://www.diaabetes-basics/prevention/risk-factors/

Amylin Pharmaceuticals, Inc. (2011a). Amylin product information. Retrieved from http://www.amylin.com

Amylin Pharmaceuticals, Inc. (2011b). Product information. Retrieved from http://www.byetta.com

Anderson, J., Kendall, P., Perryman, S., & Prior, S. (2011). Diet and diabetes. Retrieved from http://www.ext.colostate .edu/pubs/foodnut/09334.html

Appel, S. J., Wadas, T. M., Rosenthal, R. S., & Ovalle, F. (2009). Latent autoimmune diabetes of adulthood (LADA): An often misdiagnosed type of diabetes mellitus. *Journal of the American Academy of Nurse Practitioners, 21*(3), 156–159. doi: JAAN399 [pii] 10.1111/j.1745-7599.2009.00399.x

Associated Regional and University Pathologists, Inc. (ARUP) Laboratories. 2012. Retrieved from http://www.aruplab .com/guides

Bailey, C. J. (2009). Metformin. In H. E. Lebovitz (Ed.), *Therapy for diabetes and related disorders* (5th ed., pp. 235–253). Alexandria, VA: American Diabetes Association.

Bardi, J. (2012). A molecule central to diabetes is uncovered. *The Diabetes Center.* The Regents of the University of California, San Francisco. Retrieved from http://www.ucsf .edu/news/2012/08/12506/molecule-central-diabetes-uncovered

Bilous, R. W., Donnelly, R., & Williams, G. (2010). *Handbook of diabetes* (4th ed.). Hoboken, NJ: Wiley-Blackwell.

Bluestone, J., & Hebrok, M. (2012). UCSF diabetes symposium marks decade of research advances. Diabetes Center. Diabetes Health. Retrieved from http://www.ucsf.edu/news/2010/09/4458/ucsf-diabetes-symposium-marks-decade-research-advances

Boudi, F. B. (2012). Risk factors for coronary artery disease. Medscape Reference. Retrieved from http://medicine .medscape.com/article/164163-overview

Boyle, J., Thompson, T., Gregg, E., Barker, L., & Williamson, D. (2010). Projection of the year 2050 burden of diabetes in the US adult population: Dynamic modeling of incidence, mortality, and prediabetes prevalence. *Population Health Metrics, 8*(1), 29.

Brealey, D., & Singer, M. (2009). Hyperglycemia in critical illness: A review. *Journal of Diabetes Science and Technology, 3*(6), 1250–1260.

Bristol-Myers Squibb, Inc. (2011). Onglyza product information. Retrieved from http://www.onglyza.com/

Brunkhorst, F. M., Engel, C., Bloos, F., Meier-Hellmann, A., Ragaller, M., Weiler, N., et al. (2008). Intensive insulin therapy and pentastarch resuscitation in severe sepsis. *New England Journal of Medicine, 358*(2), 125–139. doi: 358/2/125 [pii] 10.1056/NEJMoa070716

Burant, C. F., & American Diabetes Association. (2008). *Medical management of type 2 diabetes* (6th ed.). Alexandria, VA: American Diabetes Association.

Butler, S. (2011). Introduction to carbohydrate counting. *NASN National Association of School Nurses, 26*(4), 257–259.

Casellini, C. M., & Vinik, A. I. (2007). Clinical manifestations and current treatment options for diabetic neuropathies. *Endocrine Practice, 13*(5), 550–566. doi: P53M48300742H475 [pii]

Centers for Disease Control and Prevention. (2011). *National diabetes fact sheet: National estimates and general information on diabetes and prediabetes in the United States, 2011.* Atlanta, GA: Author.

Centers for Disease Control and Prevention. (2012). Diabetes public health resource. Retrieved from www.cdc.gov/diabetes/consumer/proble

Cheng, Y. J., Gregg, E. W., Geiss, L. S., Imperatore, G., Williams, D. E., Zhang, X., et al. (2009). Association of A_1c and fasting plasma glucose levels with diabetic retinopathy prevalence in the U.S. population: Implications for diabetes diagnostic thresholds. *Diabetes Care, 32*(11), 2027–2032. doi: dc09-0440 [pii] 10.2337/dc09-0440

Christen, U. (2010). Enterovirus infection of human beta-cells activates dendritic cells and triggers innate antiviral responses: Are enteroviruses convicted now? *Diabetes, 59*(5), 1126–1128. doi: 59/5/1126 [pii] 10.2337/db10-0057

Colberg, S. R. (2010). Exercise and type 2 diabetes: American College of Sports Medicine and the American Diabetes Association: Joint position statement. Exercise and type 2 diabetes. *Medicine & Science in Sports & Exercise, 42*(12), 2282–2303. doi: 10.1249/MSS .0b013e3181eeb61c00005768-201012000-00018 [pii]

Davis, A., Duka, I., & Bakris, G. (2009). Diabetic nephropathy. In H. E. Lebovitz (Ed.), *Therapy for diabetes mellitus and related disorders* (5th ed., pp. 474–500). Alexandria, Virginia: American Diabetes Association.

DCCT Trial Research Group. (1993). The effect of intensive treatment of diabetes on the development and progression of long-term complications in insulin-dependent diabetes mellitus. The Diabetes Control and Complications Trial Research Group. *New England Journal of Medicine, 329*(14), 977–986. doi: 10.1056/NEJM199309303291401

Dental Problems & Treatments. (2012). A healthy smile is a beautiful smile! AtlanticDentists.com. Retrieved from http://www.atlanticdentists.com/dental-problems-and-treatments .php

Dham, S., Shah, V., Hirsch, S., & Banerje, M. A. (2006). The role of complementary medicine in diabetes. *Current Diabetes Reports 6*(3), 251–258. Retrieved from http://www.ncbi .nlm.nih.gov/pubmed/16898580

Diabetes Health Center. (2010). Type 2 diabetes risk factors. WebMD. Retrieved from http://diabetes.webmd.com/guide/risk-diabetes

Dietary Therapy of Diabetes Mellitus. (2011). Macronutrients and micronutrients in diabetes dietary therapy. Diabetes Treatment 1 Diabetes Mellitus Treatments. Retrieved from http://diabetesmellitustreatments.com/macronutrients-and-micronutrients-in-diabetes-dietary

Dimensions of Culture. (2010). Cultural group guides. Stratis Health. Retrieved from http://www.dimensionsofculture .com/culture-fact-sheets/

Dinca-Panaitescu, S., Dinca-Panaitescu, M., Bryant, T., Daiski, I., Pilkington, B., & Raphael, D. (2011). Diabetes prevalence and income: Results of the Canadian Community Health Survey. *Health Policy, 99*(2), 116–123. doi: S0168-8510(10)00224-1 [pii] 10.1016/j.healthpol .2010.07.018

Exercise and Type 2 Diabetes: The American College of Sports Medicine and the American Diabetes Association: JointPosition Statement. (2010). *Diabetes Care 33*: e147-e167; doi:2337/dc10-9990

Feng, Y., Schlosser, F. J., & Sumpio, B. E. (2011). The Semmes Weinstein monofilament examination is a significant predictor of the risk of foot ulceration and amputation in patients with diabetes mellitus. *Journal of Vascular Surgery, 53*(1), 220–226, e221–225. doi: S0741-5214(10)01495-3 [pii] 10.1016/j.jvs.2010.06.100

Finfer, S., Chittock, D. R., Su, S. Y., Blair, D., Foster, D., Dhingra, V., et al. (2009). Intensive versus conventional glucose control in critically ill patients. *New England Journal of Medicine, 360*(13), 1283–1297. doi: NEJMoa0810625 [pii] 10.1056/NEJMoa0810625

Fowler, J. M. (2008). Microvascular and macrovascular complications of diabetes. *Clinical Diabetes, 28*(2), 77–82.

Funnell, M. M., Brown, T. L., Childs, B. P., Haas, L. B., Hosey, G. M., Jensen, B., et al. (2011). National standards for diabetes self-management education. *Diabetes Care, 34*(Suppl 1), S89–S96. doi: 34/Supplement_1/S89 [pii] 10.2337/dc11-S089

Gale, E. A. (2008). Congenital rubella: Citation virus or viral cause of type 1 diabetes? *Diabetologia, 51*(9), 1559–1566. doi: 10.1007/s00125-008-1099-4

Galtier, F. (2010). Definition, epidemiology, risk factors. *Diabetes & Metabolism, 36*(6, Part 2), 628–651.

Garnero, T. (2011). Somogyi effect vs. dawn phenomenon. d.life.com. Retrieved from http://www.dlife.com/diabetes/blood_sugar_management/garnero_0106

Garg, S., & Hirsch, I. B. (2010). Self-monitoring of blood glucose. *International Journal of Clinical Practice, Suppl.*(166), 1–10. doi: IJCP2271 [pii] 10.1111/j.1742-1241.2009.02271.x

Garg, S. K., & Naik, R. G. (2009). Monitoring in diabetes. In H. E. Lebovitz (Ed.), *Therapy for diabetes mellitus and related disorders* (5th ed., pp. 144–160). Alexandria, VA: American Diabetes Association.

Goldstein, P. C. (2009). Assessment and treatment of hypoglycemia in elders: Cautions and recommendations. *Medsurg Nursing, 18*(4), 215–223, 241; quiz 224.

Gonzalez-Campoy, J. M. (2011). Hyperosmolar coma clinical presentation. *Medscape Reference.* Retrieved from http://emedicine.medscape.com/article/121693-clinical

Groop, L., & Lyssenko, V. (2009). Genetics of type 2 diabetes. An overview. *Endocrinology Nutrition, 56*(Suppl 4), 34–37.

Gutierrez, K. (2008). *Pharmacotherapeutics: Clinical reasoning in primary care* (2nd ed.). St. Louis, MO: Saunders Elsevier.

Halter, J. B. (2009). Diabetes in older adults. In H. E. Lebovitz (Ed.), *Therapy for diabetes mellitus and related disorders* (pp. 362–368). Alexandria, VA: American Diabetes Association.

Head to Head Comparator. (2011). Kombiglyze[TMXR] saxagliptin and metformin HCL extended. Retrieved from http://www.kombiglyzexr-hcp.com/head-to-head-study.aspx

Health.com. (2011). Secondary diabetes mellitus. Retrieved from http://www.health.com/health/library/mdp/0,,sts 14506,00.html

Hemphill, R. R. (2011). Hyperosmolar hyperglycemic state. Medscape Reference. Retrieved from http:/emedicine.medscape.com/article1914705-overview

Horton, E. S. (2009). Exercise. In H. E. Lebovitz (Ed.), *Therapy for diabetes mellitus and related disorders* (5th ed., pp. 192–200). Alexandria, VA: American Diabetes Association.

Hsu, W. C., Yoon, H. H., Gavin, J. R., Wright, E. E., Caballero, A. E., & Tenzer, P. (2007). Building cultural competency for improved diabetes care. *Primary Care Consortium Supplement to the Journal of Family Practice, 56*(9), S10–S40.

Ingenix Staff. (2008). Coding secondary diabetes mellitus. Advance for Health Information Professionals. Retrieved from http://health-information.advanceweb.com/article/coding-secondary-diabetes-mellitus.aspx

International Diabetes Federation. (2009). *IDF diabetes atlas* (4th ed.). Brussels, Belgium: International Diabetes Federation.

IOM (Institute of Medicine). (2010). *The future of nursing: Leading change, advancing health.* Washington, DC: The Academic Press.

Kalra, S., Kalra, B., & Saluja, S. (2012). Dietary management in geriatric patients of diabetes mellitus: Special considerations. *The Internet Journal of Geriatrics and Gerontology,* ISSN: 1937-8211. Retrieved from http://www.ispub.com/journal/the-internet-journal-of-geriatrics-and-gerontology/volume-5-number-1/dietary-management-in-geriatric-patients-of-diabetes-mellitus-special-considerations.html#sthash.GX0o5z5t.dpbs

Kapustin, J. (2012). Latent autoimmune diabetes in adults. *The Journal for Nurse Practitioners, 4*(9), 681–687.

Kansagara, D., Fu, R., Freeman, M., Wolf, F., & Helfand, M. (2011). Intensive insulin therapy in hospitalized patients: A systematic review. *Annals of Internal Medicine,154,* 268–282.

Kaufman, F. R., & American Diabetes Association. (2008). *Medical management of type 1 diabetes* (5th ed.). Alexandria, VA: American Diabetes Association.

Kee, J. L. (2010). *Laboratory and diagnostic tests with nursing implications* (8th ed.). Upper Saddle River, NJ: Prentice Hall.

Khan, A. N. (2011). Imaging neuropathic arthropathy (Charcot joint). Medscape Reference. Retrieved from http://emedicine.medscape.com/article/391989-overview

Kitabchi, A. E., & Gosmanov, A. R. (2009). Diabetic ketoacidosis and hyperosmolar hyperglycemic syndrome in adults. In H. E. Lebovitz (Ed.), *Therapy for diabetes mellitus and related disorders* (5th ed., pp. 124–136). Alexandria, VA: American Diabetes Association.

Krentz, A. J., Patel, M. B., & Bailey, C. J. (2008). New drugs for type 2 diabetes mellitus: What is their place in therapy? *Drugs, 68*(15), 2131–2162. doi: 68155 [pii]

Krikorian, A., Ismail-Beigi, F., & Moghissi, E. S. (2010). Comparisons of different insulin infusion protocols: A review of recent literature. *Current Opinion in Clinical Nutrition and Metabolic Care, 13*(2), 198–204. doi: 10.1097/MCO.0b013e32833571db

Krishnan, S., Cozier, Y. C., Rosenberg, L., & Palmer, J. R. (2010). Socioeconomic status and incidence of type 2 diabetes: Results from the Black Women's Health Study. *American Journal of Epidemiology, 171*(5), 564–570. doi: kwp443 [pii] 10.1093/aje/kwp443

Latent Autoimmune Diabetes in Adults. (2012). Health Grades Inc. Retrieved from http://www.rightdiagnosis.com/l/ltent_autoimmune_diabetes-in-adults/intro.htm

Lebovitz, H. E. (2009a). Insulin secretagogues, sulfonylureas, repaglinide, and nateglinide. In H. E. Lebovitz (Ed.), *Therapy for diabetes mellitus and related disorders* (5th ed., pp. 222–234). Alexandria, VA: American Diabetes Association.

Lebovitz, H. E. (2009b). Thiazolidinediones. In H. E. Lebovitz (Ed.), *Therapy for diabetes mellitus and related disorders* (5th ed., pp. 260–272). Alexandria, VA: American Diabetes Association.

Lightsey, R. F. (2011). Diagnosis and treatment of latent autoimmune diabetes in adults still evolving. Retrieved from http://www.clinicaladvisor.com/diagnosis-and-treatment-of-latent-autoimmune-diabetes-in-adults-still-evolving/article/203578/

Lin, H. C. (2011). Classification of diabetic neuropathy. Medscape Reference. Retrieved from http://emedicine.medscape.com/article/1170337-clinical

Lingvay, I. (2010). Secondary forms of diabetes mellitus. DOE *10.2310/7900.1160*

Luopajarvi, K., Savilahti, E., Virtanen, S. M., Ilonen, J., Knip, M., Akerblom, H. K., et al. (2008). Enhanced levels of cow's milk antibodies in infancy in children who develop type 1 diabetes later in childhood. *Pediatric Diabetes, 9*(5), 434–441. doi: PDI413 [pii] 10.1111/j.1399-5448.2008.00413.x

Martin-Gronert, M. S., & Ozanne, S. E. (2010). Mechanisms linking suboptimal early nutrition and increased risk of type 2 diabetes and obesity. *Journal of Nutrition, 140*(3), 662–666. Epub.

Mathur, R. (2012a). Diabetes mellitus. MedicineNet. Retrieved from http://www.medicinenet.com/diabetes_mellitus/page2.htm

Mathur, R. (2012b). Diabetes prevention. Retrieved from http://www.medicinenet.com/dibetes_prevention/page2.htm

Mathur, R. (2012c). Metabolic syndrome. MedicineNet. Retrieved from http://www.medicinenet.com/metabolic_syndrome/page3.htm

Mathur, R., & Stöppler, M.C. (2012). What is insulin resistance? MedicineNet.com. Retrieved from http://www.medicinenet.com/insulin_resistance/article.htm

Mayo Clinic Staff. (2012a.) Erectile dysfunction and diabetes: Take control today. Retrieved from www.mayoclinic.com/erectiledys

Mayo Clinic Staff. (2012b). Hypoglycemia. Mayo Clinic Foundation. Retrieved from http://www.mayoclinic.com/health/hypoglycemia/DS00198/DSECTION=symptoms

Mayo Clinic Staff. (2012c). Type 2 diabetes. Retrieved from http://www.mayoclinic.com/health/type-2-diabetes/DS00585/DSECTION=risk-factors

McCarren, M., & American Diabetes Association. (2007). *American Diabetes Association guide to insulin & type 2 diabetes.* Alexandria, VA: American Diabetes Association.

McCulloch, D. K., & Munshi, M. (2012). Treatment of type 2 diabetes mellitus in the elderly patient. UpToDate. Retrieved from http://www.uptodate.com.contents/treatment-of-type-2-diabetes-in-the-elderly-patient

MedlinePlus. (2012). Type 2 diabetes—risk factors. Retrieved from http://www.nlm.nih.gov/medlineplus/ency/article/002072.htm

G. D., Whittemore, R., & Mitchell, J. (2009). Type 2 diabetes in urban black and rural white women. *Diabetes Education, 35*(2):293–301.

Merck Manual. (2011). Diabetes mellitus and disorders of carbohydrate metabolism. Retrieved from http://www.merckmanuals.com/home/childrens_health_issues/hereditary_metabolic_disorders/disorders_of_carbohydrate_metabolism.html

Mitchell, B. D. (2012). Diet of Hispanics and Latinos. Advanog, Inc. Retrieved from http://www.faqs.org/nutrition/Hea-Irr/Hispanics-and-Latinos-Diet-of.html

Moghissi, E. S., Korytkowski, M. T., DiNardo, M., Einhorn, D., Hellman, R., Hirsch, I. B., et al. (2009). American Association of Clinical Endocrinologists and American Diabetes Association consensus statement on inpatient glycemic control. *Diabetes Care, 32*(6), 1119–1131. doi: dc09-9029 [pii] 10.2337/dc09-9029

Molven, A., Ringdal, M., Nordbø, A. M., Raeder, H., Støy, J., Lipkind, G. M. et al. (2008). Mutations in the insulin gene can cause MODY and autoantibody and -negative type 1 diabetes. *Diabetes, 57*(4), 1131–1135. Doe: 10. 2337/dbo7-1467.

Myhill, P., Davis, W. A., Bruce, D. G., Mackay, D. G., Zimmet, P., Davis, T.M.E., et al. (2008). Chronic complications and mortality in community-based patients with latent autoimmune diabetes in adults: The Fremantle diabetes study. doi: 10.1111/j.1464-5491.2008.02562.x

Nambam, B., Aggarwal, S., & Jain, A. (2010). Latent autoimmune diabetes in adults: A distinct but heterogeneous clinical entity. *World Journal of Diabetes, 1*(4), 111–115.

National Diabetes Information Clearinghouse. (2007). Monogenic forms of diabetes: Neonatal diabetes mellitus and maturity-onset diabetes of the young. Retrieved from http://diabetes.niddk.nih.gov/dm/pubs/mody/

Neumiller, J. J., & Campbell, R.K. (2010). Saxagliptin: A dipeptidyl peptidase-4 inhibitor for the treatment of type 2 diabetes mellitus. *American Journal of Health-System Pharmacy, 67*(18), 1515–1525. Retrieved from http://www.ajhp.org/content/67/17/1515 doi: 10.2146/ajhp090555

Novo Nordisk Pharmaceuticals. (2011). Victoza product information. Retrieved from http://www.victoza.com

Orlowski, J. P., Cramer, C. L., & Fiallos, M. R. (2008). Diabetic ketoacidosis in the pediatric ICU. *Pediatric Clinics of North America, 55*(3), 577–587, x. doi: S0031-3955(08)00088-6 [pii] 10.1016/j.pcl.2008.02.015

Pacini, G., & Mari, A. (2007). Assessment of insulin sensitivity from steady-state and dynamic tests. In M. Roden (Ed.), *Clinical diabetes research: Methods and techniques* (pp. 27–41). West Sussex, England: John Wiley & Sons.

Qaseem, A., Chou, R., Humphrey, L. L., Starkey, M., Shekelle, P, (2011). Venous thromboembolism prophylaxis in hospitalized patients: A clinical practice guideline from the American College of Physicians. *Annals of Internal Medicine, 155*(9),625–632.

Porter, J. (2012). Maturity onset diabetes of the young. Retrieved from http://www.diabetesmonitor.com/mody.htm

Report of the Expert Committee on the Diagnosis and Classification of Diabetes Mellitus. (2003). *Diabetes Care 24* (suppl. 1): 2003. Retrieved from http://care.diabetesjournals.org/content/26/suppl_1/s5.full.pdf

Riddle, M. C. (2009). Combination therapies with oral agents or oral agents and insulin. In H. E. Lebovitz (Ed.), *Therapy for diabetes mellitus and related disorders* (5th ed., pp. 332–342). Alexandria, VA: American Diabetes Association.

Roumen, C., et al. (2011). Predictors of lifestyle intervention outcome and dropout: The SLIM study. *European Journal of Clinical Nutrition, 65,* 1141–1147. Retrieved from http://www.nature.com/ejen/journal/v65/n10/full/ejen201175a.html

Ruhl, J. (2012). A rare form of "type 1.5" that is often misdiagnosed. Retrieved from http://www.phlaunt.com/diabaetes/14047009/php

Snow, K. J. (2009). Erectile dysfunction. In H. E. Lebovitz (Ed.), *Therapy for diabetes mellitus and related disorders* (pp. 563–571). Alexandria, VA: American Diabetes Association.

Standards of Medical Care. (2012). *Diabetes Care.* 35 Supp 11, 1–53.

Stöppler, M. C. (2012). Diabetes prevention (type 2 diabetes). MedicineNet.com.Retrieved from http://www.medicinenet.com/diabetesprevention

True, M. W. (2009). Circulating biomarkers of glycemia in diabetes management and implications for personalized medicine. *Journal of Diabetes Science and Technology, 3*(4), 743–747.

Tufts University. (2012). Diabetes mellitus: Diagnosis and pathophysiology. Tufts Open Courseware. Retrieved from http://oew.fufts.edu/Content/14/lecturenotes/265878

Type 2 diabetes risk factors. (2012). ThirdAge.Com. Retrieved from http://www.thirdage.com/hc/c/type-2-diabetes-risk-factors

United Kingdom Prospective Diabetes Study Group. (1998a). Effect of intensive blood-glucose control with metformin on complications in overweight patients with type 2 diabetes (UKPDS 34). UK Prospective Diabetes Study (UKPDS) Group. *Lancet*, *352*(9131), 854–865. doi: S0140673698070378 [pii]

United Kingdom Prospective Diabetes Study Group. (1998b). Intensive blood-glucose control with sulphonylureas or insulin compared with conventional treatment and risk of complications in patients with type 2 diabetes (UKPDS 33). UK Prospective Diabetes Study (UKPDS) Group. *Lancet*, *352*(9131), 837–853. doi: S0140673698070196 [pii]

U.S. Department of Health and Human Resources, U.S. FDA. (2010). FDA news release: FDA significantly restricts access to the diabetes drug Avandia. Retrieved from http://www.fda.gov/newsevents/newsroom/pressannouncements/UCM226975.htm

Vinik, A. I., Nakave, A., & Chuecos, M. (2009). Gastrointestinal disturbances. In H. E. Lebovitz (Ed.), *Therapy for diabetes mellitus and related disorders* (5th ed., pp. 532–557). Alexandria, VA: American Diabetes Association.

Vorderstrasse, A. A. (2012). Advance for NPs & PAs. Cultural issues in diabetes. Dietary counseling for black patients. Retrieved from http://nurse-practitioners-and-physician-assistants.advanceweb.com/Continuing-Education/CE-Articles/Cultural-Issues-in-Diabetes.aspx

What is maturity-onset diabetes of the young (MODY). (2012). Special edition—Uncommon diabetes diagnoses. Retrieved from http://www.diabetesincontrol.com/articles/54-feature/9986-what-is-maturity-onset-diabetes-of-the-young-mody

Wiener, R. S., Wiener, D. C., & Larson, R. J. (2008). Benefits and risks of tight glucose control in critically ill adults: A meta-analysis. *Journal of the American Medical Association*, *300*(8), 933–944. doi: 300/8/933 [pii] 10.1001/jama.300.8.933

Wilkinson, J. M., & Ahearn, N. R. (2009). *Prentice Hall nursing diagnosis handbook* (9th ed.). Upper Saddle River, NJ: Prentice Hall.

Williams, M. (2007). *Comprehensive hospital medicine: An evidence based approach*. Philadelphia: Saunders Elsevier.

Yeung, W. C., Rawlinson, W. D., & Craig, M. E. (2011). Enterovirus infection and type 1 diabetes mellitus: Systematic review and meta-analysis of observational molecular studies. *British Medical Journal*, *342*, d35. doi: 10.1136/bmj.d35 bmj.d35

Zilliox, L., & Russell, J. W. (2011). Treatment of diabetic sensory polyneuropathy. *Current Treatment Options in Neurology*, *13*(2), 143–159. doi: 10.1007/s11940-011-0113-1

Nursing Management of Patients with Musculoskeletal Disorders

UNIT 11

Content in Unit 11 that addresses the **Institute of Medicine (IOM)** competencies, **Nursing Core Competencies (NCC)**, the **Quality and Safety Education for Nurses (QSEN)** competencies, and **Concepts** for concept-based learning is listed below.

Competencies	Feature or Text	Location
IOM, QSEN, NCC Providing patient-centered care	Nursing Process: Patient Care Plan for patients with musculoskeletal disorders, pages 1489, 1494, 1503, 1509, 1515	Chapter 49
	Nursing Process: Patient Care Plan for the Orthopedic Surgical Patient, page 1551	Chapter 50
	Nursing Process: Patient Care Plan for Arthritis, page 1572	Chapter 51
IOM, QSEN, NCC Working in teams	Collaborative Management, pages 1497, 1502, 1508, 1514	Chapter 49
	Collaborative Management, pages 1523, 1525, 1540, 1543, 1546, 1555	Chapter 50
	Collaborative Management, pages 1581, 1588	Chapter 51
IOM, QSEN, NCC Employing evidence-based practice	Evidence-Based Practice: Prevention of Falls in the Acute Care Setting, page 1491	Chapter 49
	Evidence-Based Practice: Pin Site Care, page 1529	Chapter 50
	Evidence-Based Practice: Stump and Phantom Limb Pain, page 1550	Chapter 50
	Evidence-Based Practice: Treatment of Gouty Arthritis, page 1578	Chapter 51
IOM, NCC Applying quality and safety improvement	Safety Alerts, pages 1470, 1472, 1473, 1478, 1479	Chapter 48
	Fall Prevention, page 1489	Chapter 49
	Safety Alerts, pages 1525, 1528, 1532, 1534, 1546, 1550,	Chapter 50
	Safety Alert, page 1582	Chapter 51
NCC Educating patients	Patient Teaching & Discharge Priorities, pages 1511, 1513	Chapter 49
	Health Promotion, pages 1523, 1540, 1543, 1546, 1555	Chapter 50
	Patient Teaching & Discharge Priorities, pages 1575, 1579, 1584, 1587	Chapter 51
Concepts covered in Unit 11 include:	Mobility Stability Skin integrity Body image Grief Immunity	Metabolism Inflammation

CHAPTER

48 Nursing Assessment of the Patient with Musculoskeletal Disorders

Kara L. Gasiorowski
Cheryl Wraa

Outcome-Based Learning Objectives

After studying this chapter, the learner will be able to:

1. Describe the basic anatomy and physiology of the musculoskeletal system.
2. Organize the process of obtaining a history of the musculoskeletal system.
3. Analyze the normal and abnormal findings associated with a musculoskeletal assessment.
4. Critique normal and abnormal gaits.
5. Identify the musculoskeletal changes that occur throughout the life span.

KEY TERMS

abduction p.1471
adduction p.1471
ankylosing spondylitis p.1475
anteriorly p.1471
asymmetry p.1471
Bouchard's nodes p.1474
boutonnière deformity p.1474
bursae p.1468
crepitus p.1472
degenerative joint disease p.1477
dislocation p.1467
Dupuytren's contracture p.1475
fasciculations p.1470
gait p.1476
goniometer p.1470
gouty joint p.1470
Heberden's nodes p.1474
interphalangeal joint p.1474
metacarpophalangeal joint p.1474
muscle atrophy p.1470
nodules p.1470
pathologic fractures p.1481
posteriorly p.1471
range of motion (ROM) p.1467
strain p.1467
tenosynovitis p.1475
tremors p.1470

THE MUSCULOSKELETAL SYSTEM is composed of bones, joints, ligaments, tendons, and cartilage. Each of these parts plays a key role in maintaining a healthy, functioning system. The musculoskeletal system is definitively involved in determining a person's quality of life because it not only allows movement but also protects the inner organs, produces red blood cells, and supports the body.

At some time in their lives, people in every age group may be afflicted with either temporary or permanent disabilities related to musculoskeletal problems. Injuries can occur in all stages of life; however, children are particularly prone to accidents, and older adults are prone to falls and subsequent fractures.

Anatomy and Physiology of the Musculoskeletal System

Because of the importance of the musculoskeletal system and the number of patients with primary or secondary orthopedic problems, it is imperative for the nurse to understand how to conduct a musculoskeletal assessment. Each component of the musculoskeletal system must undergo a thorough and systematic evaluation to identify abnormalities so that they can be treated or further problems can be prevented.

Bones

Bones have many functions in the body. They provide the body's framework and support; protect internal organs from injury; store calcium, phosphorus, and other minerals; enable movement in conjunction with muscles; and, in long bones, produce red and white blood cells (Porth & Matfin, 2009).

Bones are composed of collagen fibers, which are made up of calcium and phosphate. The skeletal system develops from the middle layer of embryonic tissue. Development begins at approximately the fourth week in the embryo and continues to grow during the first two decades of life.

Bones have the ability to repair themselves after injury through a process of resorption and regeneration. The process involves formation of a hematoma that provides the basis for blood vessel and fibroblast infiltration, proliferation of osteoblasts, callus formation, ossification of the callus, and remodeling of the fracture site. The bone is made up of osteoblasts, which are cells that form the bone itself, and osteoclasts, which are cells that reabsorb bone during repair (for instance, repair of a fracture) (Porth & Matfin, 2009). As a person ages, bones become weaker and osteoblast activity starts to decrease.

CHART 48–1 Shape Types of Bones

Long Bones	Flat Bones	Short/Irregular Bones
Femur	Ribs	Vertebral column
Tibia	Scapula	Carpal
Fibula	Sternum	Tarsal
Humerus	Ilium	
Radius		
Ulna		
Clavicle		
Metacarpals		
Metatarsals		
Phalanges		

Bones in the human body can be classified into three shapes: (1) long bones, which have a tubular shaft and articular surfaces, or surfaces that form a joint, at each end; (2) flat bones, which are thin with broad surfaces; and (3) short or irregular bones that vary in size and shape (Bickley, 2009). Chart 48–1 provides examples of the three shapes of bones.

There are two types of bone: *cortical* and *cancellous* or trabecular bone. Cortical bone is the compact bone that forms the shaft of long bones and the hard outer layer of all bones. Cortical bone has a poor blood supply. Cancellous bone is the porous spongy bone that is typically found at the ends of long bones and has a rich blood supply.

Muscles

Muscles are contractile tissues that are attached by tendons to bone and other body parts. They are found in three types throughout the body. *Smooth muscle* is stimulated by the autonomic nervous system, meaning that it is not under voluntary or conscious control. Smooth muscle is found in the skin, internal organs, reproductive system, major blood vessels, and the excretory system. These muscles contract when necessary to perform the function of the particular organ system, such as peristalsis.

Skeletal muscles are connected to bones via tendons. The skeletal muscles, together with the bones to which they attach, allow the body to move, such as in walking or picking objects up with the fingers. Skeletal, or striated, muscles are called voluntary muscles because they are under conscious control and are supplied with nerves from the central nervous system.

Cardiac muscle, which comprises most of the heart, is under autonomic system control, not voluntary control. Like skeletal muscle, cardiac muscle is striated and contains actin and myosin filaments. The filaments are smaller and more compact than those in skeletal muscle cells and contain many large mitochondria, owing to the heart's continuous energy needs. The contractions of the cardiac muscle provide the heartbeat and the pumping of blood through the heart (Porth & Matfin, 2009).

Cartilage

Cartilage is an elastic, flexible connective tissue. The main function of cartilage is to act as a "cushioner." It covers the surfaces of joints, protecting them when they slide or move over one another, thus preventing damage and friction to the joints. For instance, costal cartilages join the ribs to the sternum and vertebrae. The articular cartilages, such as those in the shoulder or hip joint, protect the bone ends and allow easy movement of the joint. Once damaged, cartilage cannot be repaired (Weber & Kelley, 2007).

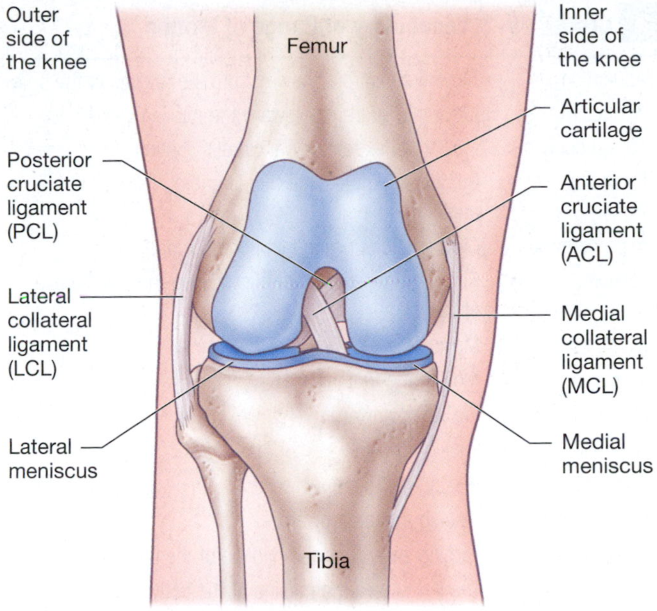

FIGURE 48–1 ◆ Ligaments of the knee joint.

Ligaments

Ligaments are a fibrous tissue that connects bones to other bones. They play a crucial role in the function of the skeletal joints by preventing **dislocations** (displacement of a bone from its normal position). An example is the knee joint connecting the femur with the patella, tibia, and fibula (Bickley, 2009) (Figure 48–1◆).

Tendons

Tendons connect muscle to bone. The dense tissue is composed largely of intercellular bundles of collagen fibers arranged in the same direction, which provides great tensile strength. Tendons can withstand tremendous pull in the direction of fiber alignment. If the musculotendinous unit is stretched to injury, this is called a **strain.** The most common sites for strains are the lower back and the cervical area of the spine (Porth & Matfin, 2009).

Joints

A joint is the structure where two or more bones come together. Joints are responsible for a person's **range of motion (ROM),** the extent and type of movement the person can make. In assessing joints, it is important for the nurse to understand and differentiate three different mechanical configurations of joints: spheroidal joints, hinge joints, and condylar joints. *Spheroidal joints* are located in the shoulders and hip. They have a ball-and-socket contour, which allows for a broad range of motion—not just in a back-and-forth direction, but also swiveling actions. *Hinge joints* are flat and slightly curved. The hinge joint allows movement in only one axis (namely, flexion and extension), as in the elbow. In *condylar joints,* such as the knee, the articulating ends of the

Weblink: Musculoskeletal System Structure and Function

CHART 48–2 Vocabulary of Range of Motion

Abduction	Moving an extremity away from the midline of the body
Adduction	Moving an extremity toward the midline of the body
Circumduction	Moving an extremity in a circular motion
Extension	Straightening the extremity of a joint; increasing the angle of the joint
Hyperextension	Moving a joint beyond its normal range
Flexion	Bending an extremity at a joint; decreases the angle of the joint
Eversion	Moving the foot outward
Inversion	Moving the foot inward
Pronation	Facing downward
Supination	Facing upward
Plantar flexion	Placing the foot downward
Dorsal flexion	Placing the foot upward
External rotation	Turning away from the midline of the body
Internal rotation	Turning toward the midline of the body

Sources: Adapted from Kozier, B., Erb, C., Berman, A., & Snyder, S. (2008). *Fundamentals of nursing. Concepts, process and practice* (8th ed.). Upper Saddle River, NJ: Pearson Prentice Hall; Magee, D. (2008). *Orthopedic physical assessment* (5th ed.). St. Louis, MO: Elsevier; Weber, J., & Kelley, J. (2007). *Health assessment in nursing* (3rd ed.). Philadelphia: Lippincott Williams & Wilkins.

bones are not connected directly but are linked by a strong fibrous capsule that surrounds the joint and is continuous with the periosteum. Additional support is provided by ligaments that extend between the bones of the joint (Bickley, 2009; Weber & Kelley, 2007). Figure 48–2◆ illustrates the three types of joints. Chart 48–2 defines the vocabulary that is used in describing the type of movement being evaluated.

Joints also can be classified according to material composition. *Fibrous joints* occur where bones are joined together with connective tissue, such as the sutures of the skull. There is no movement associated with a fibrous joint. *Synovial joints* are the most common type and most relevant in terms of injury and loss of range of motion. The synovial joints are the joints between bones that do not come into contact with one another but slide over one another, such as the knee. The bone surfaces of these joints are covered with cartilage, which allows the two bones to slide over one another and be freely movable. The bones of the joint are separated by a synovial capsule, which surrounds the joint and secretes synovial fluid, a lubricant that promotes the sliding movement of the bones.

Further aid to movement in the synovial joints is provided by the **bursae** (sacs containing viscous lubricating fluid; singular, *bursa*), which lie between the skin and the surface of the bone or joint, contain synovial fluid, and are located in areas where tendons, muscles, and bones have the tendency to rub against one another, such as the acromion process in the shoulder and in the wrists, knees, hips, and ankles. *Cartilaginous joints* are only slightly movable and are located between the vertebrae and the symphysis pubis. They are separated by a fibrous disk and joined by interosseous ligaments (Bickley, 2009; Weber & Kelley, 2007).

History

The nursing assessment of a patient presenting with a musculoskeletal complaint should start with a thorough history and physical assessment of the musculoskeletal system. A detailed history of the

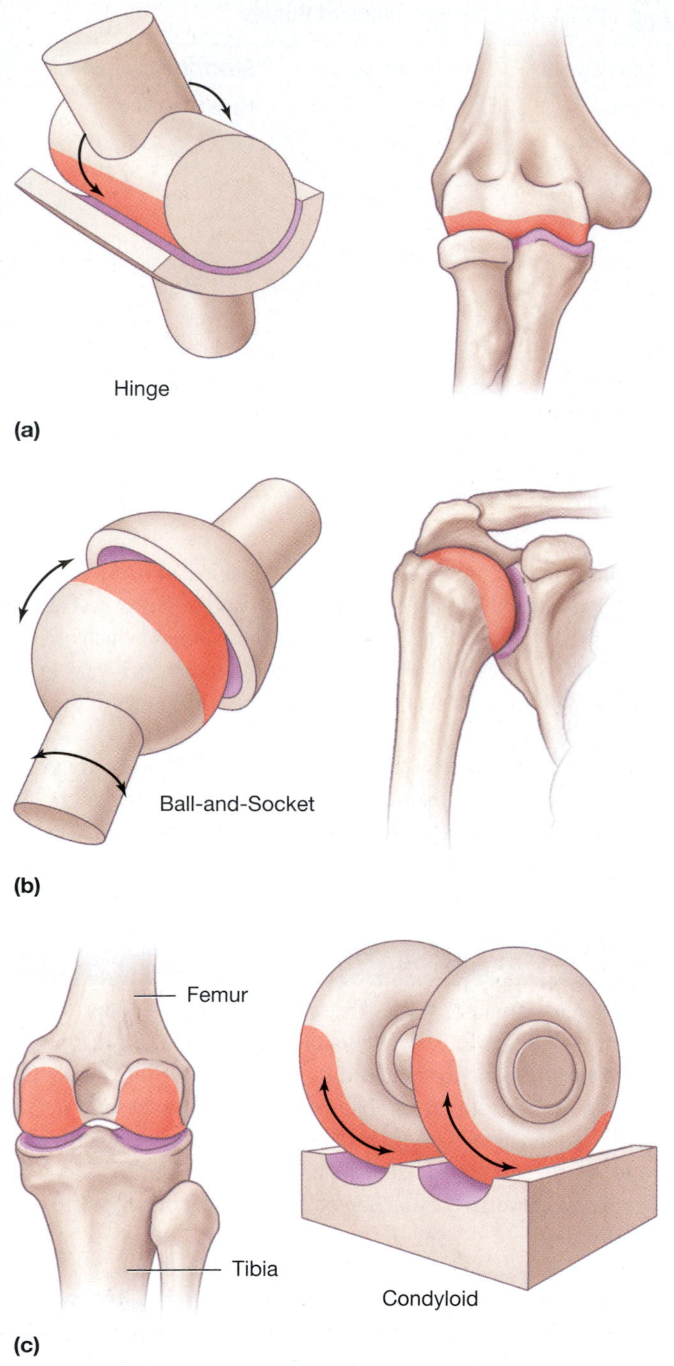

FIGURE 48–2 ◆ Types of joints: (A) hinge; (B) ball-and-socket; (C) condyloid.

system is vital in determining a patient's ability to function and perform activities of daily living (ADLs). This determination plays an important role in developing an effective plan of care, because disabilities related to musculoskeletal disorders can affect every aspect of a patient's life.

In gathering subjective data, the nurse should ask the patient a series of open-ended questions regarding past and present musculoskeletal illnesses, injuries, related diagnostic procedures, surgeries, and treatments. The questioning should start with the *chief complaint*, which is the symptom or condition that has compelled the patient to seek medical care. These questions should be formulated to allow the patient to describe her own impressions of the condition. Next, the patient's past medical history is important because previous injuries or disorders can have lingering effects on the musculoskeletal system, leading to new conditions. Chronic health conditions can also have a profound effect on the musculoskeletal system, and questions that reveal these disorders will help in the diagnosis of the presenting symptoms. Social history and psychosocial history add to the fullness of the patient's medical history by revealing lifestyle habits, such as smoking or level of exercise, and coping mechanisms that can be important in both the diagnosis and treatment of the condition.

History taking is an important part of assessment. During this time, the nurse establishes a caring relationship with the patient. It is important to let the patient describe her issues in her own words. The nurse should keep an open mind and listen carefully, as this information will direct clarifying questions.

Biographical and Demographic History

Biographical data should include the patient's age, gender, culture, and educational background. This information will assist the nurse in narrowing the questions, thinking of potential causes of the problem, and formulating how to pose questions and educational plans to meet the patient's needs. Demographic data may be helpful in determining causes of injury. For instance, a patient who has a job in which he is sitting and typing on a computer all day might complain of back and neck pain from sitting in a chair that does not support his back, or pain in the joints of the hand, wrist, or arm from the repetitive motion during typing, or pain from the improper height of the desk placing strain on the joints. Additional demographic questions are given in the section on past medical history.

Chief Complaint

The chief complaint may be defined by the characteristics, length of duration, and exacerbation or diminishment of symptoms and by what is wrong or feared by the patient. The nurse should ask open-ended questions, allowing the patient time to answer fully and giving encouragement with nonverbal cues such as nodding. Clarifying questions that may be useful include the following:

- What brings you to the facility/office/hospital today?
- How long have you had this symptom?
- How did it happen?
- Is there a mechanism of the injury? What was the force? What was the direction of the force?
- Has the symptom gotten worse since it first started? In what way has it gotten worse? When did it get worse? Did anything precipitate it getting worse? If so, what?
- Is pain associated with the symptom?
- Where is the pain, does it radiate anywhere, and how long does it last?
- What makes the pain better or worse?
- Have you taken any medication for the pain? What have you taken? How much? How often? Does the medication alleviate the pain? Does it reduce the intensity of the pain?
- How does the pain affect your daily lifestyle?
- What other treatments besides pain medication have you used?
- Do you have any other symptoms?
- Do you have any swelling or weakness?

Past Medical History

When obtaining a past medical history, the nurse may ask the following questions:

- Have you had any past surgeries? Where? When? For what reason?
- Do you have any permanent problems associated with past injuries or surgeries?
- Do you have any other health problems that could affect medication therapy or, due to respiratory problems or fatigue, inhibit ambulation or performance of ADLs?
- Do you have any chronic diseases such as diabetes, sickle cell anemia, or systemic lupus erythematosus (SLE)? These are important questions because diabetes can cause neuropathies that can affect ambulation, and sickle cell anemia and SLE can lead to osteoporosis and osteomyelitis (Weber & Kelley, 2007).
- Does anyone in your family have rheumatoid arthritis or osteoporosis? These diseases tend to be hereditary and may predispose a patient to these conditions (Weber & Kelley, 2007).
- Have you had a tetanus or polio vaccine recently? Recent tetanus and polio vaccines may cause joint stiffness. If the patient has never had a polio vaccination, ask whether the patient has traveled to a developing country recently; if so, the patient may have contracted the disease at that time.
- What medications do you take regularly? Include all over-the-counter (OTC) medications.
- Do you have any allergies? If so, to what? (Be specific: medications, environmental, latex.)
- *If the patient is female:* Have you started menopause? Are you on hormone replacement therapy? The lack of estrogen in a menopausal woman can lead to osteoporosis.

A social history provides additional information about the patient's lifestyle that may affect the potential disorder or complaint. The nurse should consider the following questions:

- Do you smoke? If so, how much and how often? Smoking raises the risk of osteoporosis.
- Do you drink alcohol? If so, how much? Excessive alcohol intake raises the risk of osteoporosis.
- Do you have a regular exercise regime? Can you describe it? Do you engage in exercise outside of a routine? How often? What type of exercise?
- Describe your occupation. Does it involve heavy lifting, pushing, or pulling, or do you sit at a desk all day? Heavy strenuous activities may precipitate back problems, while sitting may lead to posture anomalies, which can lead to other problems such as respiratory disorders.
- Do you use an assistive device such as a cane, walker, or brace? If so, which do you use? Why?
- Does your musculoskeletal problem affect your lifestyle or activities of daily living? If so, how?

The nurse should ask the patient how he copes with the injury or illness that constitutes the chief complaint and whether the illness or injury affects family and personal relationships. It is important to observe the patient's nonverbal cues and note whether the patient appears depressed, angry, or anxious when the history is taken.

Weblink: Muscle Testing Weblink: ROM Demonstrations

Physical Examination

In the physical examination, the nurse uses inspection and palpation to collect objective data. These data are recorded and made available to the health care team. An in-depth musculoskeletal exam is time consuming, but it is essential.

General Guidelines for Musculoskeletal Assessment

General guidelines for conducting a musculoskeletal assessment are as follows:

- Inspect for deformities.
- Inspect and palpate any swelling.
- Feel the area for increased temperature and observe for redness.
- Palpate for tenderness around a joint.
- Assess for range of motion.

Safety Alert *Do not force a body part past its normal range. Discontinue ROM when the patient complains of pain or discomfort.*

Inspection

The abnormal appearance of a joint may be due to a musculoskeletal or neuromuscular disease, dislocation, tumor, mass, degenerative change, contracture, or atrophy of the muscle. The nurse should compare corresponding paired joints for symmetry, contour, and size. The nurse observes for skin color, scars, shape of the site, deformities, **muscle atrophy** (shortening of a muscle), masses, or swelling. The nurse also inspects for **fasciculations** (abnormal contraction or shortening of a bundle of muscle fibers) and **tremors** (involuntary movement of a body part), which can be related to neuromuscular disorders.

Swelling may be caused by inflammation (reaction of tissue to irritation, injury, or infection), a hematoma (bleeding into the tissue from injury), intra-articular swelling or effusion (escape of fluid into the tissue), a swollen bursa, synovial membrane thickening, or a bony overgrowth. If there is swelling, the nurse should note the size and shape of the edematous area, the site, and the signs of inflammation such as redness. When inspecting a joint or bony structure, it is important to observe for alignment.

Palpation

The nurse needs to feel the patient's skin with the back of her fingers to assess the skin temperature. The nurse should note whether the skin is hot, warm, cool, or cold to the touch. Heat and redness over a joint may indicate inflammation or a septic joint (infection of a joint). Cold or cool temperatures of the skin on an extremity may suggest a circulation problem (Weber & Kelley, 2007). Next, the nurse assesses the skin texture and whether the skin is notably dry or moist. Excessive dryness may indicate an acute, **gouty joint** (inflammation of a big toe, heels, elbows, ankles, dorsum); moisture is often associated with a septic joint (Magee, 2008).

The nurse palpates the muscles surrounding the joint and bony articulations, noting any pain, tenderness, swelling, or masses. Normal bones, muscles, tendons, and joints are not tender to palpation. Tenderness around a joint may be due to arthritis, a septic joint, inflammation, bursitis, or osteomyelitis (Weber & Kelley, 2007). Tenderness over bony structures or muscles may result from strain, fracture, or infection. A "boggy" feeling over an edematous area may indicate an edematous synovial membrane, which can be indicative of a soft-tissue injury (Magee, 2008).

The nurse palpates for **nodules** (small raised areas) that may not be visible along the muscles that extend bony structures, such as the arm and elbow, and at pressure points, such as the feet and knees. Nodules are most commonly associated with arthritis. While palpating, the nurse inquires about any numbness, tingling, or weakness in a given area.

Range of Motion

The nurse assesses ROM of all joints by asking the patient to actively move the joints one at a time. The nurse compares each joint for flexibility and mobility and assesses the patient's ability to move the joint through its normal full range of motion. The nurse should familiarize himself with the normal ROM for each type of joint so as to be able to recognize any limitation. Range of motion may be decreased owing to pain, muscle spasms, weakness, and atrophy. Decreased ROM occurs in joints where there is inflammation, arthritis, lack of use, dislocation, masses, or pain.

Safety Alert *When assessing joints, muscles, and movements, always assess on both sides of the body for purposes of comparison.*

System Monitoring

A **goniometer,** which measures the angle of the joint in degrees, can assist in the assessment of ROM of a joint (Figure 48–3◆). To measure the joint angle, the nurse places the fulcrum of the goniometer exactly at the fulcrum of the joint and places the stationary arm of the goniometer to align with the part of the limb that will not be moved. The movable arm of the goniometer is placed along the part of the limb that will be moved. The nurse then holds the arms of the goniometer and asks the patient to move the limb while the nurse notes the measurement on the goniometer. The nurse will document, for example, "The right knee flexes from 20 to 60 degrees." This is important in describing the degree of decreased ROM from normal and provides a baseline for future measurement (Magee, 2008).

Testing Muscle Strength

The nurse measures muscle strength by placing a hand firmly against the patient's body part in question and asking the patient to push

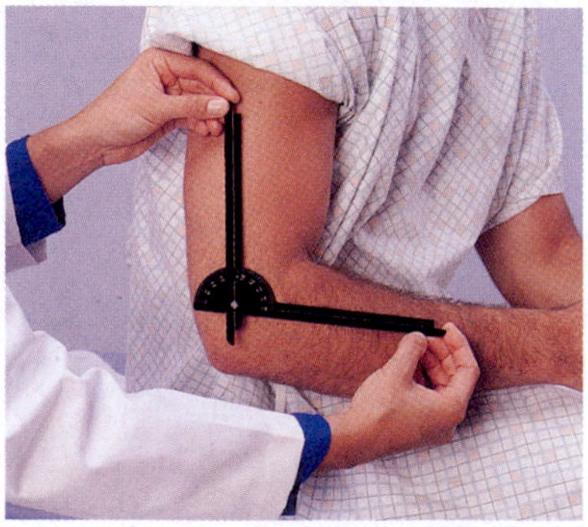

FIGURE 48–3 ◆ Goniometer.

CHART 48–3 Muscle Strength Grading

Functional Level	Grade
No evidence of contractibility (inability to contract muscles)—paralysis	0
Slight contractibility—severe weakness	1
ROM without gravity—passive ROM performed by examiner	2
Active ROM with gravity—moderate weakness	3
Complete active ROM against gravity with some resistance—minimal weakness	4
Complete ROM against gravity with resistance—normal	5

Sources: Adapted from Bickley, L. (2009). *Bates' guide to physical assessment and history taking* (10th ed.). Philadelphia: Lippincott; Kozier, B., Erb, C., Berman, A., & Snyder, S. (2008). *Fundamentals of nursing. Concepts, process and practice* (7th ed.). Upper Saddle River, NJ: Pearson Prentice Hall.

hard against the hand. The nurse performs the test on both sides and compares the findings, keeping in mind that the dominant side of the body will be stronger. The nurse then documents the patient's ability to push by describing the strength as *normal, slightly weak, weak,* or *severely weak,* or by recording that the patient was unable to push at all. Chart 48–3 describes a grading system for the documentation of muscle strength.

Head-to-toe Musculoskeletal Assessment

It is important to be methodical in assessing the musculoskeletal system so as not to miss any abnormalities. There is not one "right way" to conduct an assessment. The important thing is for the nurse to develop a method that is comfortable and thorough and to use it consistently.

Temporomandibular Joint

The temporomandibular joint (TMJ) is the hinge of the jaw. It is located anterior to the external ear and is constantly opening and closing when the person talks, eats, chews, and yawns (Bickley, 2009). Examination of the TMJ includes inspection and palpation. The patient should be in a sitting position for the exam. The nurse observes the mandible at rest and in motion. To assess the TMJ, the nurse places her index and middle fingers anterior to the patient's external ear, just in front of the tragus. The patient is asked to open his mouth as wide as possible. At this time, the nurse's fingers should slide into the "groove," or joint space. The nurse moves the patient's jaw back and forth, palpating for masses or nodules, while inspecting the area for redness and swelling, indicating inflammation.

The nurse then asks the patient to open and close the mouth. While the patient does this, the nurse notes the range of motion and questions the patient as to any tenderness. The nurse also listens for any "clicking" sounds. Soft clicking sounds without any complaints of discomfort or ROM difficulty may not be indicative of any problems; however, clicking sounds that are hard or grating, are accompanied by pain or discomfort, and are affecting range of motion can be indicative of arthritic changes or a possible dislocation (Magee, 2008).

Normal Findings

- The patient is able to open and close the mouth without difficulty about 2.5 to 5 cm (1 to 2 in.).
- Jaw moves laterally without pain or tenderness.
- Some clicking may be heard and felt during movement.

Source: Weber, J., & Kelley, J. (2007). *Health assessment in nursing* (3rd ed.). Philadelphia: Lippincott Williams & Wilkins.

Abnormal Findings (refer to Chapters 50 and 51)

- The patient is unable to open the mouth 2.5 to 5 cm (1 to 2 in.).
- A grating, clicking, or popping sound is noted with a TMJ problem, possibly a dislocation.
- The patient complains of pain, as well as tenderness with opening and closing of the mouth, which may indicate arthritis.
- Masses and/or nodules are felt during palpation.
- The patient has an inability to hold the mouth open.
- Decreased muscle strength is present.

Shoulders

The shoulder is a ball-and-socket joint formed by the junction of the humerus and the scapula. It is cushioned by cartilage and stabilized by a ring of fibrous cartilage. The shoulder is able to move in many directions because of the shoulder girdle, composed of the clavicle, humerus, and scapula as well as the surrounding musculature. Ligaments connect the bones and tendons join them to the surrounding muscles.

The patient should remain sitting in a chair for the shoulder assessment. The nurse will need to inspect the shoulders **anteriorly** (the front plane of the body) and **posteriorly** (the back plane of the body). The nurse observes for any swelling, change in skin color, deformity, atrophy, fasciculations, and **asymmetry** (unequal in size and proportion). Patients with scoliosis may have one shoulder higher than the other, causing asymmetry. The nurse inspects for swelling or redness over the joint capsule anteriorly or a bulge under the deltoid, which may be indicative of a problem in the bursa (Bickley, 2009).

The nurse assesses range of motion, including **abduction** (away from the midline of the body—in this case, raising the arm away from the body), **adduction** (moving toward the midline of the body—in this case, moving the arm across the front of the body), flexion, extension, hyperextension, internal rotation, and external rotation. The nurse explains that, to test the range of motion of the shoulders, the patient will be asked to perform seven movements (Figure 48–4◆, p. 1472):

1. The patient stands straight with arms at the sides. The nurse observes the area for symmetry.
2. To test for abduction, the nurse asks the patient to raise the arms to shoulder level.
3. To test for adduction, the nurse asks the patient to raise the arms above the head with the palms facing each other.
4. To test for flexion and extension, the nurse asks the patient to bend and straighten out the elbows.
5. To test for external rotation, the nurse asks the patient to place both hands behind the neck with elbows out to the side.
6. To test for internal rotation, the nurse asks the patient to place the hands behind the lower back.
7. As a final test, the nurse asks the patient to clasp the hands and bring them around the lower back as far as she can.

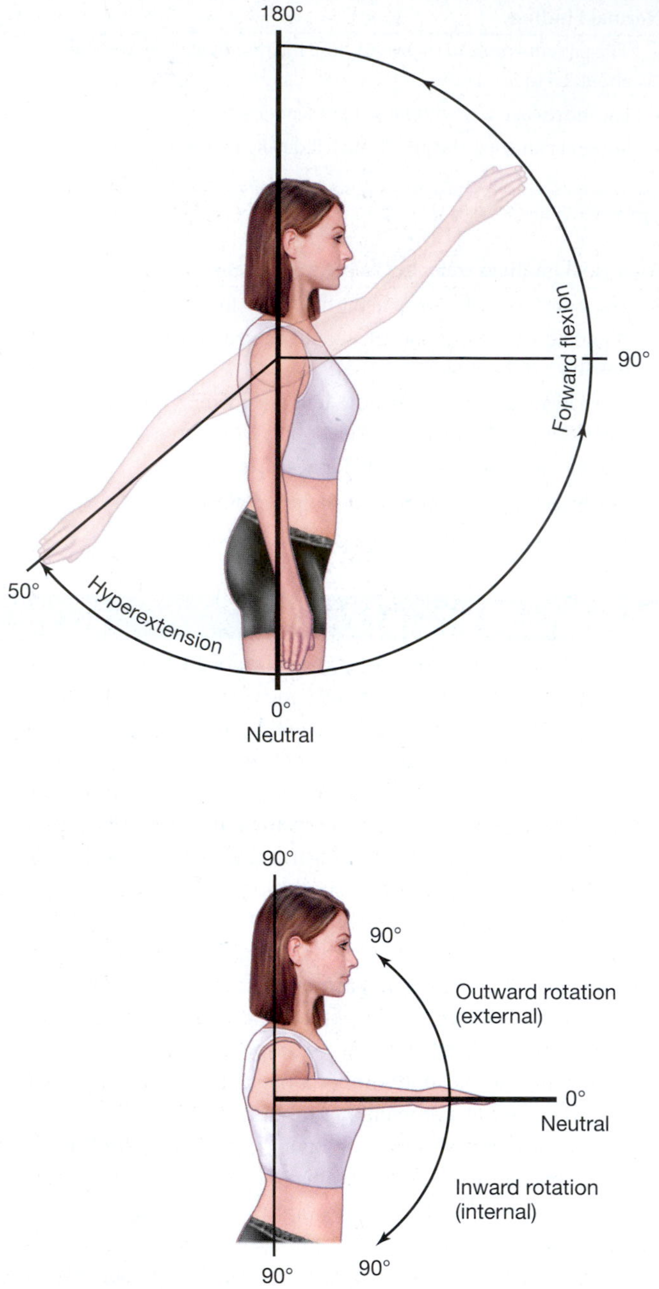

FIGURE 48–4 ◆ Shoulder ROM.

Normal Findings

The patient should be able to do the following:

- Raise the arms 90 degrees to the shoulder level.
- Flex the arms to 180 degrees and fully extend the arms.
- Hyperextend the arms behind the back 50 degrees.
- Place the hands behind the neck and lower back at 90 degrees without **crepitus** (grating produced by bone rubbing against bone), pain, or decreased ROM.
- Shrug the shoulders against resistance.

Source: Weber, J., & Kelley, J. (2007). *Health assessment in nursing* (3rd ed.). Philadelphia: Lippincott Williams & Wilkins.

Abnormal Findings (refer to Chapter 50)

- Pain and decreased ROM are associated with rotator cuff tears, tendonitis, sprains, and bursitis.
- Decreased ability to shrug shoulders or inability to shrug shoulders against resistance may indicate a lesion of cranial nerve XI.
- Weakness in performance of ROM exercises indicates joint disease or muscle disuse.
- Shoulder musculature that is flat or asymmetrical may be dislocated.
- Any redness, heat, or swelling may be associated with sprains, strains, degenerative joint disease, or arthritis.
- Atrophy is associated with nerve damage or disuse.

Sources: Bickley, L. (2009). *Bates' guide to physical assessment and history taking* (10th ed.). Philadelphia: Wolters Kluwer Health/Lippincott Williams & Wilkins; Magee, D. (2008). *Orthopedic physical assessment* (5th ed.). St. Louis, MO: Elsevier; Weber, J., & Kelley, J. (2007). *Health assessment in nursing* (3rd ed.). Philadelphia: Lippincott Williams & Wilkins.

While the patient is performing these tasks, the nurse palpates the joints for crepitus and questions the patient regarding any associated pain (Jarvis, 2008; Magee, 2008; Weber & Kelley, 2007).

To test the muscle strength of the shoulders, the nurse asks the patient to perform a number of movements and exercises. To assess the deltoid muscle, the patient holds the arms upward while the nurse pushes them down. To assess the biceps, the patient flexes the arm while the nurse tries to extend it. To assess the triceps, the patient extends the arm while the nurse tries to flex it. Finally, to assess the trapezius muscle, the patient shrugs the shoulders while the nurse tries to hold the shoulders down (Bickley, 2009; Weber & Kelley, 2007).

Normal Findings with Muscle Grading

- Muscle strength of 3 or greater (can move through the full range against gravity and hold the body part in the test position).
- Muscle strength greater in dominant side.
- Coordinated and painless movements.

Abnormal Findings (refer to Chapters 50 and 51)

- Muscle strength is less than 3.
- The patient is unable to push against resistance.
- Assistance is required to perform the exam.

Safety Alert *Some patients who complain of shoulder pain may be experiencing angina related to coronary artery disease or a myocardial infarction. It is essential to determine whether this is the origin of the shoulder pain and report it immediately to the health care provider as this may necessitate emergency assessment and management. It is also possible that the patient has already had a cardiac event. Further assessment is required.*

Elbows

The elbow is a complex joint where the humerus, radius, and ulna come together and are enclosed in a synovial capsule. The elbow can move in extension and flexion, using the joint of the humerus and ulna (humeroulnar joint), and in pronation (palm downward) and supination (palm upward), using the radius. The ulnar nerve passes through the elbow, around the medial epicondyle of the humerus (Bickley, 2009).

During inspection, it is best to support the patient's arm with the nurse's nondominant hand and flex the patient's elbow to approximately 70 degrees. This action prevents the patient's muscles from tightening during the examination. The nurse inspects the elbow for shape, deformities, size, redness, swelling, nodules, and bulging. With the tips of his middle fingers and thumb, the nurse palpates the patient's olecranon process and epicondyles and the grooves on either side of the olecranon process, assessing for heat, swelling, tenderness, and nodules (Weber & Kelley, 2007).

To test for range of motion, the nurse asks the patient to flex the elbow and bring the hand to the forehead, then extend or straighten the elbow (Figure 48–5◆). The nurse notes any deviations in the angle or deformities. The nurse asks the patient to hold the arm out and *supinate* (turn the palms up) and *pronate* (turn the palms down). The nurse then has the patient flex and extend the arm with resistance. The patient repeats flexion and extension, supinating and pronating the palms. The nurse assesses for deformities, tenderness, swelling, and nodules (Bickley, 2009; Magee, 2008).

Safety Alert *Never force a patient to perform ROM tests if the patient is unable or unwilling.*

Normal Findings

- Elbows are symmetrical without nodules, deformities, swelling, or redness.
- The patient is able to perform flexion, extension, supination, and pronation without evidence of swelling, tenderness, or any visible nodules.

Abnormal Findings

- Redness, swelling, or deformity over the olecranon process may indicate injury, arthritis, or bursitis (refer to Chapters 50 and 51).
- Inability to perform range of motion without pain, swelling, deformity, or nodules needs further investigation. Nodules noted during ROM exercises may indicate rheumatoid arthritis (an autoimmune disease that causes inflammation to the joints) or rheumatic fever (refer to Chapter 51). Pain and tenderness on movement may indicate tennis elbow, which is from overuse and inflammation of the forearm muscles where they attach to the elbow (refer to Chapter 50).
- Deformity or displacement of the joint during palpation or range of motion may indicate a fracture (broken bone) or dislocation of the elbow (refer to Chapter 50).

Wrists

The wrist joint contains the articulation of the distal radius, ulna, and double row of carpal bones intertwined to form a malleable hinge. Its movements include flexion, extension, abduction, adduction, and circumduction (Figure 48–6◆). The joint is surrounded by a capsule and strengthened by multiple ligaments.

The examination should start with the nurse inspecting and palpating the wrist. The nurse inspects the wrist for symmetry, size, shape, deformities, nodules, and swelling. The nurse palpates the wrist for nodules, movement, and tenderness by holding the patient's wrist between two hands and palpating the lateral and medial surfaces, as well as palpating the groove of each wrist joint with the nurse's thumbs.

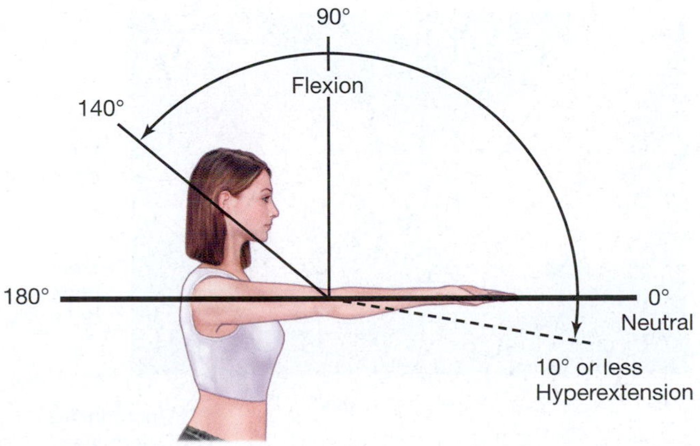

FIGURE 48–5 ◆ Elbow ROM.

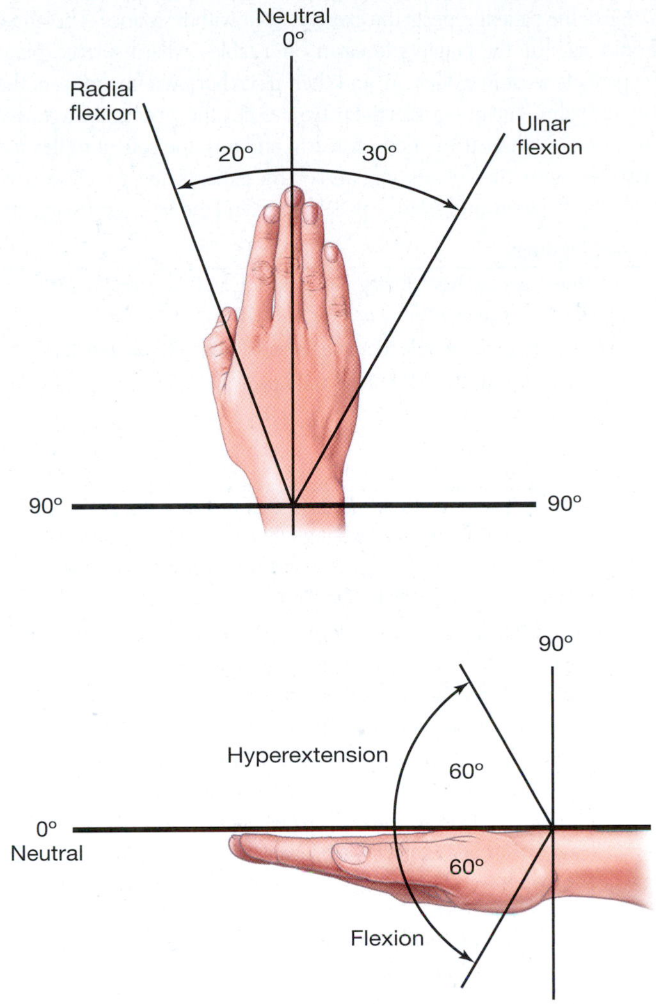

FIGURE 48–6 ◆ Wrist ROM.

Normal Finding

- The wrist is symmetrical, without any deformities, swelling, or nodules.

Abnormal Findings

- Swelling, tenderness, and nodules may indicate rheumatoid arthritis (refer to Chapter 51).
- Pain, tenderness, and a deformity may indicate an injury or trauma to the wrist (refer to Chapter 50).
- A round, painless, swollen, fluid-filled area may indicate a ganglion cyst.

Sources: Jarvis, C. (2008). *Pocket companion for physical examination and health assessment* (5th ed.). St. Louis: W. B. Saunders; Weber, J., & Kelley, J. (2007). *Health assessment in nursing* (3rd ed.). Philadelphia: Lippincott Williams & Wilkins.

Next, the nurse should test the patient's range of motion in the wrist. To test for flexion and extension, the nurse asks the patient to bend the wrist back and forth. To test for ulnar or radial deviations, the nurse asks the patient to hold the wrist straight out in front of the body, with the palm downward, and move the hand inward toward and outward from the body. Finally, the nurse should palpate the anatomic snuffbox, the hollow indentation seen on the radial aspect of the back of the hand when the thumb is fully extended.

Next, the patient repeats the exercises, but with resistance. The nurse should stabilize the patient's forearm on a table or hard surface, place the patient's wrist in extension, and then place her own fingertips in the patient's palm. The nurse asks the patient to flex the wrist against gravity. The nurse stabilizes the patient's forearm and asks the patient to flex the wrist. The nurse then places her hand on the patient's dorsal metacarpals, just below the wrist, and asks the patient to extend the wrist against gravity.

Normal Findings

- The patient should have 90 degrees of flexion and the ability to hyperextend to 70 degrees without pain or swelling.
- The patient should be able to move the wrists laterally and medially.
- The patient should be able to have full range of motion against resistance (Magee, 2008).

Abnormal Findings

- Inability to perform full ROM needs further investigation. An example of a common abnormal condition of the wrist is carpal tunnel syndrome (refer to Chapter 50). To assess for carpal tunnel syndrome, the patient is asked to perform three tests:
  1. *Thumb Abduction:* The nurse asks the patient to raise the thumb perpendicular to the palm. The nurse applies pressure to the distal phalanx. If the patient has difficulty performing this maneuver, the median nerve may be compressed.
  2. *Tinel's Sign:* With a finger, the nurse percusses lightly over the course of the median nerve, located in the medial, inner aspect of the wrist.
  3. *Phalen's Test:* The nurse asks the patient to place the back of each hand against one another while flexing the wrists 90 degrees for 60 seconds (Bickley, 2009; Magee, 2008; Weber & Kelley, 2007).

Abnormal findings include numbness, tingling, or pain at the wrist or fingers (refer to Chapter 50).

Hands and Fingers

The joints of the hands include the **metacarpophalangeal joint** (the joint between the metacarpal bones of the hand and the phalangeal bones of the fingers), the proximal interphalangeal joint, and the distal **interphalangeal joint** (the joints between the phalanx bones of the fingers). Because the bones in the fingers and hands have very little protection, they are susceptible to trauma and disability. Inspection and palpation are the techniques used in examination of the hands and fingers (Bickley, 2009).

The nurse inspects the palmar and dorsal surfaces of the hands and fingers for size, shape, deformity, color, swelling, nodules, and tenderness. The nurse then assesses the fingers at rest and while in motion. He should palpate the metacarpophalangeal joints at the distal fingers. Then the nurse palpates the proximal, middle, and distal interphalangeal joints using his thumb and index finger.

Normal Findings

- The fingers are in a straight line and symmetrical, without deformity, swelling, or nodules.
- Swelling, nodules, and complaints of tenderness are not noted on palpation.

Abnormal Findings (refer to Chapter 51)

- Swelling of the phalanges, in addition to stiff tender fingers, may indicate acute rheumatoid arthritis.
- Hard, painless nodules at the joints of the fingers may indicate osteoarthritis (progressive loss of cartilage at a joint). **Bouchard's nodes** are found over the proximal interphalangeal joints. **Heberden's nodes** are seen over the distal interphalangeal joints (Figure 48–7 ◆).

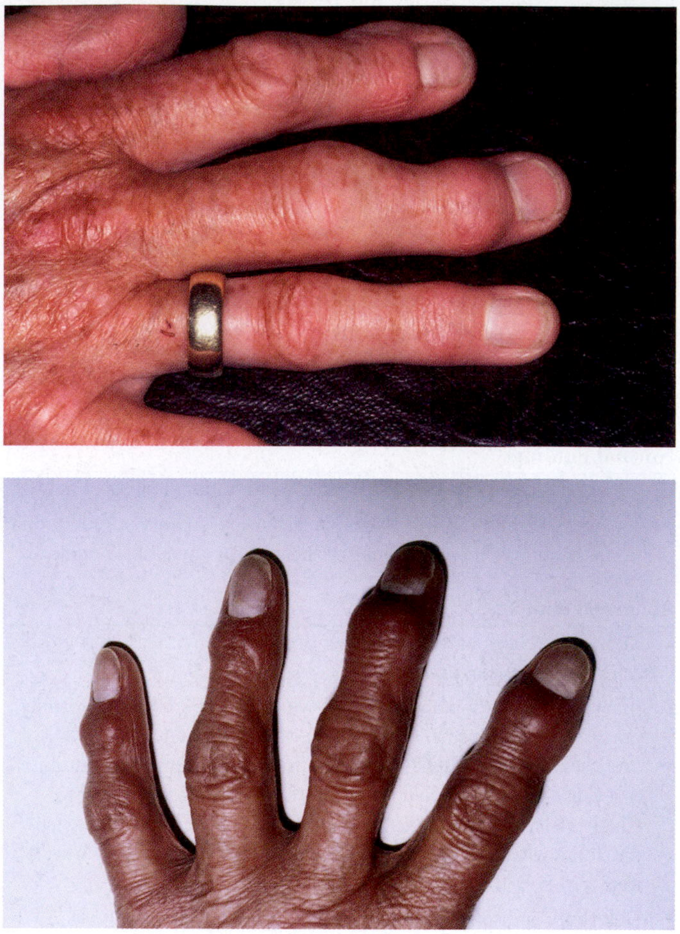

FIGURE 48–7 ◆ Bouchard's nodes and Heberden's nodes.

Source: (top) Hercules Robinson / Alamy; (bottom) Biophoto Associates / Science Source/Photo Researchers.

- "Swan neck" deformity is characterized by a hyperextension of the proximal interphalangeal joint with a fixed flexion of the distal joint.
- Swelling and thickening of the metacarpophalangeal joint exists.
- **Boutonnière deformity** is flexion of the proximal interphalangeal joint (Figure 48–8 ◆).

Sources: Bickley, L. (2009). *Bates' guide to physical assessment and history taking* (10th ed.). Philadelphia: Wolters Kluwer Health/Lippincott Williams & Wilkins; Weber, J., & Kelley, J. (2007). *Health assessment in nursing* (3rd ed.). Philadelphia: Lippincott Williams & Wilkins.

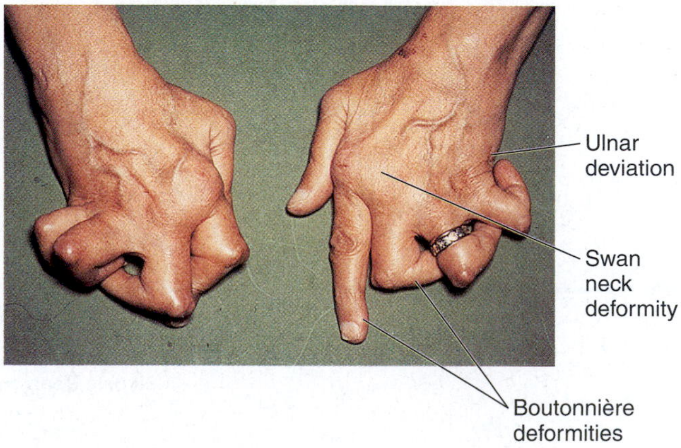

FIGURE 48–8 ◆ Deformities of the hand.

Source: Biophoto Associates / Science Source/Photo Researchers.

The nurse tests range of motion of the fingers and hands. To test for abduction, the nurse asks the patient to extend and spread the fingers apart. To test for adduction, the nurse asks the patient to make a fist. To text for flexion and hyperextension, the nurse asks the patient to bend the fingers down and then hold them up.

To test for flexion of the thumb, the nurse asks the patient to move the thumb across the palm and touch the fifth finger. To test for extension of the thumb, the nurse asks the patient to move the thumb across the palm away from the rest of the fingers. To test for abduction and adduction of the thumb, the nurse asks the patient to move the thumb anteriorly away from the palm, then back. To test for opposition, or movement of the thumb across the palm, the nurse asks the patient to touch each of the fingertips with the thumb.

Normal Findings

- The patient is able to perform all ROM exercises without pain or swelling.
- The thumb should move toward and away from the other fingers without difficulty.
- All fingers should abduct and adduct without pain and swelling.
- Hyperextension should occur without any difficulty at about 30 degrees.

Abnormal Findings (refer to Chapters 50 and 51)

- Inability to perform any of the ROM tests without discomfort, swelling, and deformity needs further investigation.
- Difficulty in extending the ring or fifth finger or inability to do so is a sign of **Dupuytren's contracture,** a slow thickening of the connective tissue in the palm of the hand.
- Slight flexion of a finger, pain on extension, swelling, and tenderness may be indicative of acute **tenosynovitis,** an infection of the flexor tendon sheaths.

Sources: Bickley, L. (2009). *Bates' guide to physical assessment and history taking* (10th ed.). Philadelphia: Wolters Kluwer Health/Lippincott Williams & Wilkins; Weber, J., & Kelley, J. (2007). *Health assessment in nursing* (3rd ed.). Philadelphia: Lippincott Williams & Wilkins.

Neck and Spine

The spine or vertebral column is composed of alternating vertebrae and fibrocartilaginous disks that are connected by ligaments and supported by muscles that extend from the skull to the pelvis. This provides axial support to the body. Each of the bony vertebrae is composed of an anterior body and a posterior arch made up of two pedicles and two laminae that are united to form the spinous process. On either side of the arch is a transverse process and superior and inferior articular processes. The articular processes articulate with the adjacent vertebrae to form synovial joints. The articular processes account for the degree of flexion, extension, or rotation possible in each segment of the vertebral column. The transverse and spinous processes act as levers for the muscles attached to them.

As the spinal column progresses from the head, the vertebral body size increases. The intervertebral disks connecting the vertebral bodies act as shock absorbers for stresses applied to the vertebral column. There are four distinct curvatures to the vertebral column: (1) the cervical curve, which is concave; (2) the thoracic curve, which is convex; (3) the lumbar curve, which is concave; and (4) the sacral curve, which is convex (Bickley, 2009).

Examination of the spine includes inspection and palpation. The patient stands straight with her arms at the sides. The nurse begins by examining the curvature of the cervical, thoracic, and lumbar areas from the right and left sides of the patient as well as behind the patient, observing for differences in the height of the shoulders and iliac crests.

Using a thumb, the nurse palpates the spinous processes of each vertebra and the paravertebral muscles on both sides of the spine and over the sacroiliac joint on the posterior superior iliac spines. If the patient complains of pain moving from the lower back down one or both legs, the straight leg test should be performed: With the patient in a relaxed, supine position, the nurse asks the patient to raise the affected leg until pain is felt, then lower the leg until the pain is relieved; at this point, the foot is dorsiflexed to reproduce the pain. Pain that shoots down one or both legs during dorsiflexion may indicate sciatic nerve involvement, a condition that may be caused by a herniated disk or pressure on the spinal cord (Magee, 2008; Weber & Kelley, 2007).

Normal Findings

- The cervical and lumbar curves should be concave; the thoracic and sacral curves should be convex when observed on either side of the patient.
- The spine is straight when observed from behind the patient.
- The shoulders, iliac crests, and gluteal folds should be aligned.

Source: Weber, J., & Kelley, J. (2007). *Health assessment in nursing* (3rd ed.). Philadelphia: Lippincott Williams & Wilkins.

Abnormal Findings (refer to Chapter 49)

- *Scoliosis:* Lateral deviation or curvature of the thoracic spine, with a downward slant of the thoracic cage on the affected side. The pelvis tilts upward on the opposite side, usually at the chest level. Noticed first in adolescence (Figure 48–9B◆).
- *Kyphosis:* An extreme thoracic curve (hunchback or humpback) that often occurs with aging (Figure 48–9D◆).
- *Lordosis:* Excessive inward curve of the spine. Patient appears to be swaybacked.
- Flattening of the lumbar spine may be indicative of a herniated disk at the lumbar area or **ankylosing spondylitis** (inflammation of the spine and the sacroiliac joints).
- Pain between the spinous processes may indicate arthritis, fracture or other trauma, infection, or herniated disks.
- Tenderness on palpation of the posterior superior iliac spine (the dimple just above the buttocks) may indicate ankylosing spondylitis.
- Pain on palpation of the paravertebral muscles may indicate degenerative changes or inflammation to the muscles.
- Pain radiating down one or both legs may indicate sciatic nerve involvement.

Sources: Bickley, L. (2009). *Bates' guide to physical assessment and history taking* (10th ed.). Philadelphia: Wolters Kluwer Health/Lippincott Williams & Wilkins; Magee, D. (2008). *Orthopedic physical assessment* (5th ed.). St. Louis, MO: Elsevier; Weber, J., & Kelley, J. (2007). *Health assessment in nursing* (3rd ed.). Philadelphia: Lippincott Williams & Wilkins.

Range of Motion of the Neck

To test the range of motion of the cervical spine, the nurse asks the patient to touch the chin to the chest (flexion) and then look up at the ceiling (extension). To test rotation of the neck, the nurse asks the patient to turn his head from side to side, looking over the shoulder. To test lateral bending of the neck, the nurse asks the patient to tilt his head and touch his ear to the corresponding shoulder.

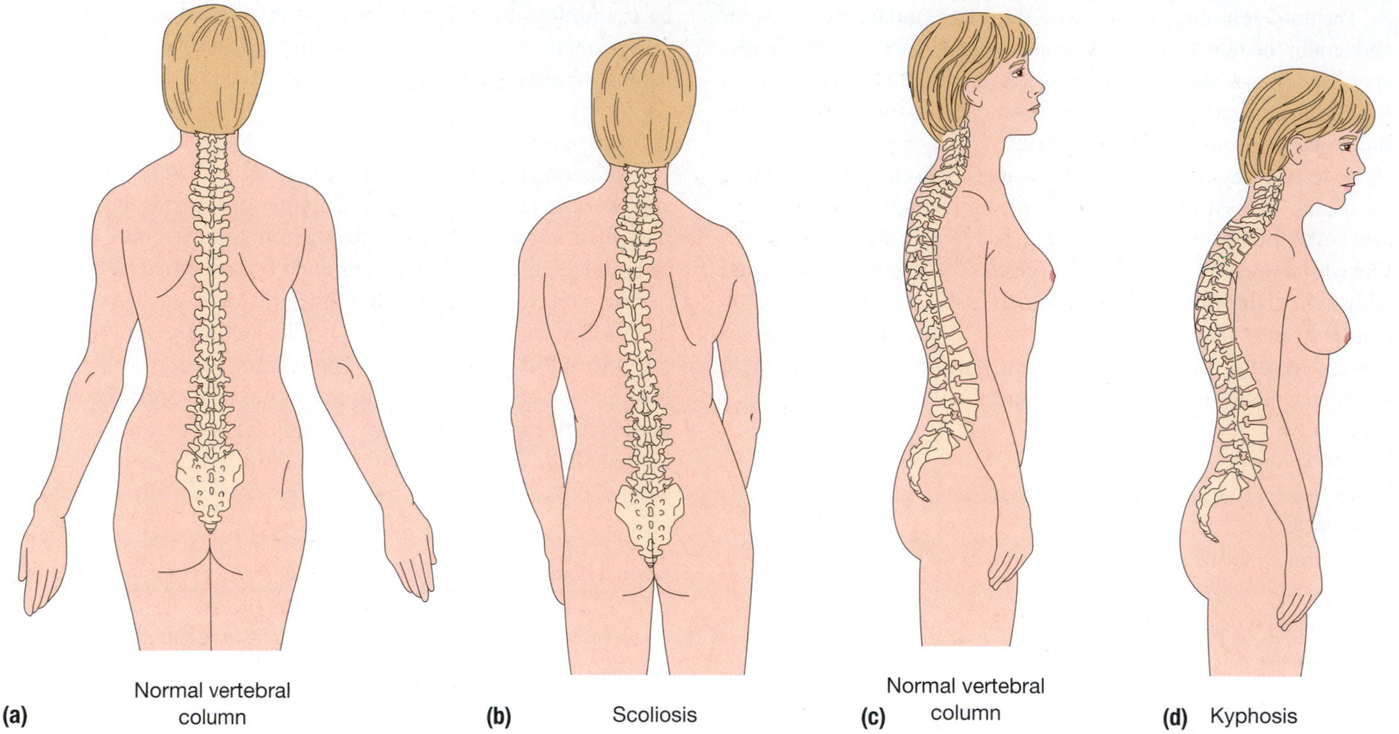

FIGURE 48–9 ◆ Normal spine and its deformities: (A) normal vertebral column, posterior view; (B) scoliosis; (C) normal vertebral column, lateral view; (D) kyphosis.

Normal Finding

- Full range of motion without pain.

Abnormal Findings (refer to Chapters 49 and 51)

- Decreased range of motion can result from arthritis, muscle spasms, or cervical strain.
- Pain in the neck, shoulders, and arms can be indicative of spinal cord compression.
- Numbness may indicate spinal cord compression.
- Neck pain with decreased ROM accompanied by fever and chills may be due to an infection, such as strep throat or meningitis.

Sources: Bickley, L. (2009). *Bates' guide to physical assessment and history taking* (10th ed.). Philadelphia: Wolters Kluwer Health/Lippincott Williams & Wilkins; Magee, D. (2008). *Orthopedic physical assessment* (5th ed.). St. Louis, MO: Elsevier.

Range of Motion of the Spine

To test for flexion, the nurse asks the patient to bend forward and touch the toes. To test for hyperextension, the nurse stabilizes the patient's hips from behind the patient and asks the patient to bend backward. To test for lateral bending of the spine, the nurse asks the patient to bend sideways. To test for rotation, the nurse asks the patient to twist the shoulders to the right and then to the left and vice versa.

Normal Findings

- The patient is able to perform full ROM exercises without pain or deformity.
- When the patient bends down to touch the toes, the back flattens.
- No exaggerated curvatures of the spine are noted.
- Muscles display symmetry.

Abnormal Findings (refer to Chapters 49 and 50)

- Pain on movement in the thoracic and lumbar areas can be due to muscle or soft-tissue injury, osteoarthritis, ankylosing spondylitis, and any congenital (describes a condition that was present at birth) conditions.
- Deformity of the thorax on bending indicates scoliosis.
- Lumbar lordosis indicates ankylosing spondylitis.
- Asymmetrical muscle movements, fasciculations, and decreased or exaggerated angles need further investigation.
- Pain radiating from the lower back to one or both legs may indicate nerve involvement.

Sources: Bickley, L. (2009). *Bates' guide to physical assessment and history taking* (10th ed.). Philadelphia: Wolters Kluwer Health/Lippincott Williams & Wilkins; Magee, D. (2008). *Orthopedic physical assessment* (5th ed.). St. Louis, MO: Elsevier; Weber, J., & Kelley, J. (2007). *Health assessment in nursing* (3rd ed.). Philadelphia: Lippincott Williams & Wilkins.

Hip

The hip is located inside the pelvis. The bones that make up the pelvis include the sacrum, pubis, ileum, and ischium. The hip joint is a ball-and-socket joint formed by the articulation of the rounded head of the femur and the cuplike acetabulum of the pelvis. It forms the primary connection between the bones of the trunk and pelvis and those of the lower extremity. Both joint surfaces are covered with a strong but lubricated articular hyaline cartilage. The hip is important because it bears the weight of the upper body and it contains the hip joint, which allows the leg to move freely.

To examine the hip, the nurse inspects the patient's anterior and posterior pelvis for bruising, asymmetry in height, and muscle atrophy and inspects the buttocks for symmetry. To observe the patient's **gait,** or way of walking, the nurse asks the patient to remove all clothing except underwear and observes the patient walking toward and away from the nurse while barefooted. If one of the patient's legs is longer than the other, the legs require measuring by having the patient lie down with the legs extended. The nurse measures each leg from the anterior superior iliac spine across the leg medially to the medial malleolus (Weber & Kelley, 2007).

The nurse observes for hip motion, knee flexion, and a heel-to-heel distance of 5 to 10 cm (2 to 4 in.) and inspects the spine for any abnormal curvatures. The nurse questions the patient regarding pain, specifically asking in which gait phase any pain occurs. With the patient standing, the nurse palpates the hips and pelvis for tenderness, crepitus, and nodules (Bickley, 2009; Weber & Kelley, 2007).

Normal Findings

- The pelvis, on anterior and posterior inspection, is symmetrical in height and shape.
- The buttocks are equal in size.
- The patient is able to bear weight on both legs without pain.
- The gait is rhythmic, nonstaggering, and without a limp.
- The feet are lifted off the ground and are then replanted firmly on the ground.
- The patient does not note crepitus during walking.
- The arm swing is in conjunction with the walking gait.
- During walking, the patient's hips are equal and move rhythmically with the gait.
- The patient is able to walk on the toes and on the heels without difficulty or pain.
- The legs are the same length.
- The knee is flexed while walking, except when the heel touches the ground.
- With the feet forward in a normal standing position, the heel-to-heel distance is 5 to 10 cm (2 to 4 in.).

Abnormal Findings (refer to Chapters 49 and 50)

- An asymmetric pelvis is indicative of hip dislocation, fractured hip, arthritis, **degenerative joint disease** (osteoarthritis), muscle weakness, or atrophy.
- Difficulty in ambulation with an irregular gait may indicate a dislocation or fracture of the hip, degenerative joint disease, or muscle weakness.
- Abnormal curvature of the spine during ambulation may indicate scoliosis or lordosis.
- Leg shortening could mean muscle deformities or hip fracture.
- Unequal leg length may indicate scoliosis.
- Wide heel-to-heel base may indicate a foot or cerebellar problem.

Source: Weber, J., & Kelley, J. (2007). *Health assessment in nursing* (3rd ed.). Philadelphia: Lippincott Williams & Wilkins.

Range of Motion of the Hip

To test ROM of the hip, the patient lies in the supine position (Figure 48–10◆). The nurse raises one of the patient's legs above the body while keeping the knee extended and then brings one knee to the chest while keeping the other leg extended. The exercise is repeated with the other leg. To assess for abduction and adduction, the nurse asks the patient to swing one leg laterally away from the body as far as possible while keeping the knee straight and then bring the leg back toward the midline of the body. This is repeated with the other leg.

To assess internal rotation, the nurse asks the patient to bend one knee and rotate the knee so that the knee moves inward toward the opposite leg and then to repeat this with the other knee. To assess external rotation, the nurse asks the patient to bend one knee and rotate the knee outward and then to repeat this with the other knee. To further test ROM, the nurse asks the patient to assume a prone position and swing one leg in the air and then to repeat this on the other side. The nurse then asks the patient to stand and swing one leg behind the body and then to repeat on the other side.

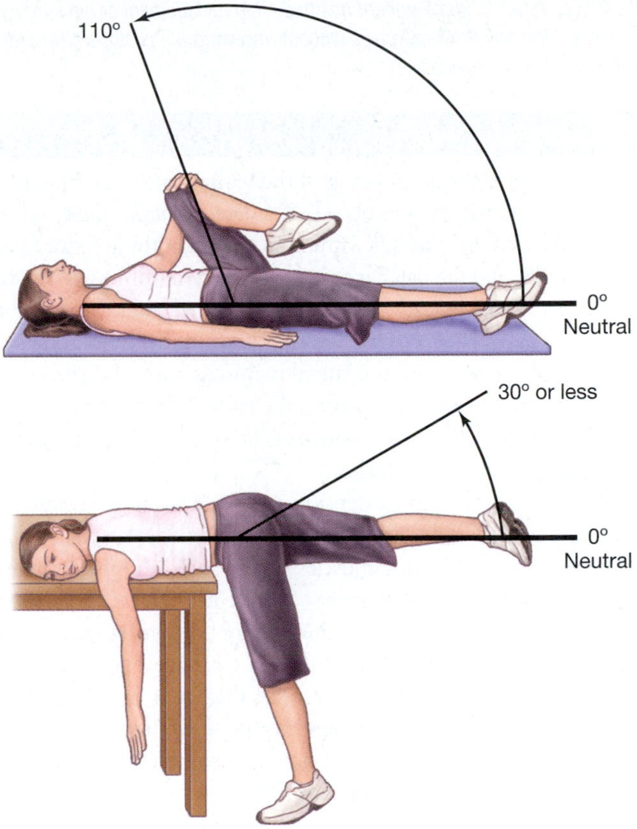

FIGURE 48–10 ◆ Hip ROM.

To assess muscle strength, the nurse places the patient in a supine position and asks the patient to raise an extended leg while the nurse tries to hold it down. The nurse then asks the patient to push both legs against the nurse's hands while the hands are placed on the outer side of the patient's knees (Bickley, 2009; Magee, 2008; Weber & Kelley, 2007).

Normal Findings

- The patient should be able to raise the legs to at least 90 degrees of flexion with the knee straight and to 120 degrees of flexion with the knee flexed.
- The patient should be able to adduct the leg 20 to 30 degrees and abduct it 45 to 50 degrees.
- The patient should be able to internally rotate to 40 degrees and externally rotate to 45 degrees.
- The patient should be able to hyperextend the leg at least 15 degrees.
- The patient should be able to move the extremities against resistance.

Sources: Magee, D. (2008). *Orthopedic physical assessment* (5th ed.). St. Louis, MO: Elsevier; Weber, J., & Kelley, J. (2007). *Health assessment in nursing* (3rd ed.). Philadelphia: Lippincott Williams & Wilkins.

Abnormal Findings (refer to Chapters 50 and 51)

- Deformity of one or both hips during flexion may indicate a hip deformity.
- Inability to flex knees may indicate a hip deformity.
- Inability to abduct hip is indicative of hip disease, such as arthritis.
- Inability to internally rotate the hip may be indicative of hip disease, such as arthritis.

Sources: Bickley, L. (2009). *Bates' guide to physical assessment and history taking* (10th ed.). Philadelphia: Wolters Kluwer Health/Lippincott Williams & Wilkins; Weber, J., & Kelley, J. (2007). *Health assessment in nursing* (3rd ed.). Philadelphia: Lippincott Williams & Wilkins.

Safety Alert *If the patient has had a hip replacement or hip surgery, do not perform any ROM exercises without reviewing the postoperative orders of the health care provider.*

Knees

The knee joint is the articulation of the femur, patella, and the tibia. The knee is actually two joints. (1) The *femoropatellar joint* consists of the patella, a bone that sits within the tendon of the anterior quadriceps muscle, and the patellar groove on the femur through which it slides, and (2) the *femorotibial joint* articulates the femur with the tibia. The joint is bathed in synovial fluid contained inside the joint capsule. The medial meniscus and the lateral meniscus are two cartilaginous menisci within the joint that protect the ends of the bones from rubbing against each other, act as shock absorbers, and deepen the tibial sockets where the femur attaches.

The knee allows flexion, extension, and slight rotation. The muscles that help move the joint are the quadriceps muscles on the front of the knee and the hamstring muscles on the back. Multiple ligaments help to stabilize the joint (Figure 48–11◆). The two cruciate ligaments located in the center of the knee, the anterior cruciate ligament (ACL) and the posterior cruciate ligament (PCL), are the major stabilizing ligaments of the joint. The PCL prevents the femur from sliding forward on the tibia, and the ACL prevents the femur from sliding backward on the tibia. Both of these ligaments also stabilize the knee in a rotational fashion; if they are damaged, the knee may become unstable when the person plants the foot and pivots, causing the knee to buckle and give way.

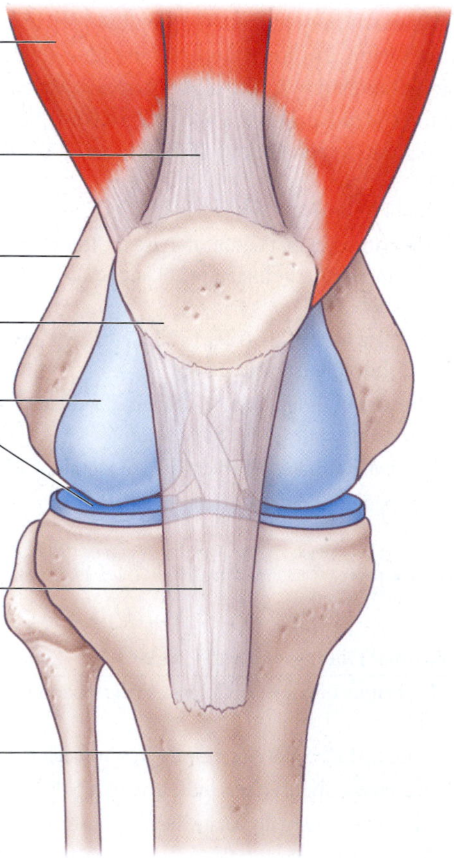

FIGURE 48–11 ◆ Knee joint.

Examination of the knee includes inspection and palpation. The nurse assesses the patient during ambulation for a rhythmic, smooth flow. The knee should be extended when the foot is striking the ground and flexed during the other phases of gait. The nurse asks the patient to first assume a supine position and then a sitting position. The nurse assesses the patient for symmetry of the knees, swelling, redness, size, shape, deformities, and alignment and for atrophy of the quadriceps muscles and the hollows on either side of the knee (Bickley, 2009; Weber & Kelley, 2007).

While the patient is sitting on the edge of the table with the legs dangling, the nurse palpates the knee for tenderness, heat, swelling, crepitus, and nodules. Beginning by palpating 10 cm (about 4 in.) above the patella, the nurse uses her fingers and thumb to move downward toward the knee (Bickley, 2009). If swelling is encountered, the following tests are performed with the patient in the supine position:

1. The *bulge sign* is used to detect fluid in the knee. The nurse places the hand on the medial aspect of the patient's knee and pushes upward two to four times to displace any fluid. Then the nurse places the hand on the lateral side of the patient's knee and looks for a bulge of fluid in the hollow area medial to the patella.
2. The *balloon sign* is performed by placing the thumb and index finger of one hand on each side of the patella while the other hand compresses the suprapatellar pouch against the femur. This allows the nurse to feel the fluid entering the spaces next to the patella.
3. The *ballottement test* is used to assess large amounts of fluid, particularly in the suprapatellar pouch. The nurse then presses against the sides of the patient's patella with the thumb and index finger of one hand while pushing the patella against the femur with the opposite hand. While the nurse presses on the sides of the patella, fluid is displaced in the suprapatellar pouch. While the patella is pushed against the femur, the fluid returns to the pouch and the nurse is able to feel a "wave" as the fluid returns to the pouch (Weber & Kelley, 2007).

Normal Findings

- The knees are symmetrical and the legs are the same length.
- The hollows are present on both sides of the patella.
- There is no redness, swelling, or tenderness.
- No deformities or nodules are noted.
- The muscles are firm and taut.
- No crepitus is felt or heard.

Abnormal Findings (refer to Chapters 50 and 51)

- Knees turn outward, called bowlegs or genu varum.
- Knees turn inward, called knock-knees or genu valgum.
- Irregular bony ridges may be indicative of osteoarthritis.
- Pain and tenderness may be indicative of bursitis.
- Heat may be indicative of osteoarthritis.
- Pain and crepitus may indicate a rough surface between the femur and the back of the patella.
- Pain on movement by means of quadriceps contraction may indicate a degenerative patella.

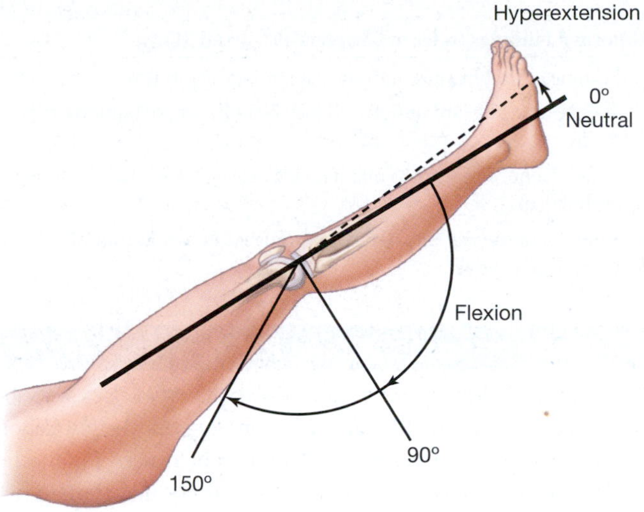

FIGURE 48–12 ◆ Knee ROM.

- Pain over a tendon or an inability to extend the leg may indicate a tear of a tendon or ligament.
- Thickness, warmth, and bogginess on the sides of the patella may indicate synovitis or osteoarthritis.
- Swelling or bulges of the lateral or medial aspects of the knee or above the knee may indicate an effusion (leaking of fluid into the knee) of the knee or synovial thickening.
- Inability to walk without stumbling or pushing the knee into extension may indicate a weakening of the quadriceps.

Range of Motion of the Knee

To test for ROM of the knee, the patient should be in a sitting position. To test for flexion, the nurse asks the patient to bend the knee. To test for extension and hyperextension, the nurse asks the patient to straighten the knee. To test for internal and external rotation, the nurse asks the patient to rotate the foot medially and laterally (Figure 48–12◆).

To test muscle strength, the nurse asks the patient to extend the leg as the nurse tries to bend it. This tests quadriceps muscle strength. Then the nurse asks the patient to flex the knee while the nurse tries to straighten it. This tests hamstring muscle strength.

Normal Findings

- The patient should be able to flex the knee to 120 to 130 degrees (Weber & Kelley, 2007).
- The patient should be able to extend the knee without difficulty and hyperextend the knee to 15 degrees.
- The patient should have full ROM against resistance.

Abnormal Findings (refer to Chapters 50 and 51)

- Difficulty with ROM may indicate osteoarthritis or a muscle or joint problem.
- Crepitus is noted in osteoarthritis.

The nurse should be aware that pain and abnormal or decreased ROM may also indicate a ligament injury or meniscus tear to the anterior or posterior cruciate ligaments and the medial and lateral collateral ligaments. Pain on the lateral sides of the knee, "popping" or "clicking" sounds with movement, patient complaints of the knee "locking," or difficulty in fully extending the knee may indicate damage to the meniscus. To assess for a torn meniscus, the nurse performs the McMurray test. With the patient in a supine position, the nurse asks the patient to flex one knee and hip. The nurse then cups one hand over the knee and places his index finger and thumb on opposite sides of the knee. With the other hand, the nurse grasps the patient's heel and rotates the lower leg and foot laterally and medially. The nurse gently and slowly extends the knee and notes any abnormal sounds (Weber & Kelley, 2007).

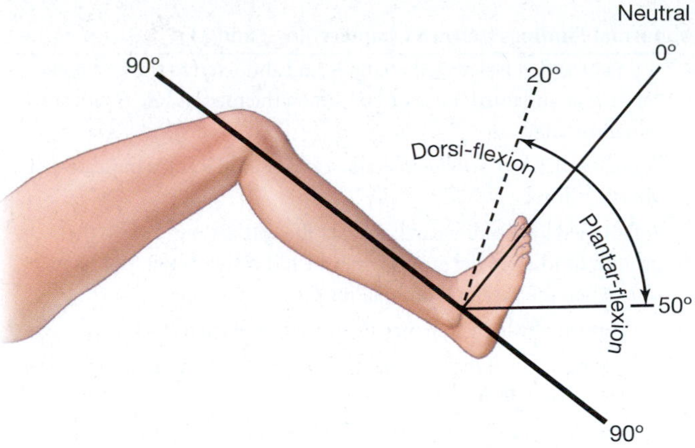

FIGURE 48–13 ◆ Ankle ROM.

Safety Alert *If the patient is complaining of severe pain, stop the assessment and notify the health care provider that the patient needs to have a McMurray test.*

Ankles and Feet

The ankle is the joint between the lower tibia, the fibula, and the talus. The feet are made up of many small bones. Both the ankle and foot have many ligaments and thick padding to cushion the foot against the body's weight during ambulation (Bickley, 2009).

After asking the patient to stand, walk, and sit, the nurse observes the patient's ankles and feet for shape, deformities, nodules, corns, calluses, bunions, and swelling and notes the position of the toes. The nurse asks the patient to walk barefoot and notes whether the patient can walk normally on the heels and on the toes. The nurse asks the patient to walk by placing one foot in front of the other, and then to walk backwards. The patient then sits with the feet dangling at the sides of the table, while the nurse observes the position of the patient's feet and toes and inspects for roundness and smoothness of the medial malleolus.

The nurse assesses ROM by asking the patient to point the toes toward the floor (plantar flexion), point the toes toward the patient's nose (dorsiflexion), turn the soles of the feet out and then in (eversion, inversion), and then flex and straighten the toes (Figure 48–13◆).

Normal Findings

- The toes should point straight ahead and be in alignment with the feet, though some may point slightly inward or slightly outward.
- No nodules, calluses, corns, or bunions are noted.
- The medial malleolus should be round and smooth.
- No pain is elicited on palpation.
- The Achilles tendon is without nodules or tenderness.

Abnormal Findings (refer to Chapters 50 and 51)

- A great toe that is deviated medially and abducted to the first metatarsal with an inflamed bursa or bunion on the medial side is indicative of hallux valgus.
- A hot, tender, red, swollen metatarsophalangeal joint is indicative of gouty arthritis.
- A flattened longitudinal arch, so that the sole is very close to the ground or touches the ground, may be indicative of flat foot (evident only when the patient is ambulating).
- An abnormally high arch may be indicative of cavus foot.
- Hyperextension of the metatarsophalangeal joint of the second toe is referred to as hammer toe.
- Painful thickening of the skin over a bony prominence is a corn.
- An area of thickened skin over a region of pressure points is a callus.
- A wart located over the thick skin of the sole of the foot is referred to as a plantar wart, or verruca vulgaris.
- Painful inflammation over the great toe may be indicative of gout.
- Tenderness between the ankle joints is indicative of arthritis, infection, or injury to the ankle.
- Painful movement may be indicative of arthritis.
- Pain or nodules around the Achilles tendon may be a result of rheumatoid arthritis, bursitis, or tendonitis.
- Pain at the calcaneus may be due to bone spurs.
- Pain and tenderness of the metatarsals and grooves may indicate arthritis or circulatory compromise.

Sources: Bickley, L. (2009). *Bates' guide to physical assessment and history taking* (10th ed.). Philadelphia: Wolters Kluwer Health/Lippincott Williams & Wilkins; Magee, D. (2008). *Orthopedic physical assessment* (5th ed.). St. Louis, MO: Elsevier; Weber, J., & Kelley, J. (2007). *Health assessment in nursing* (3rd ed.). Philadelphia: Lippincott Williams & Wilkins.

The nurse palpates with the thumbs at the anterior aspect of each ankle joint, the heel, and the posterior and anterior calcaneus. The nurse palpates the metatarsophalangeal joints, as well as in between them, for tenderness, and the Achilles tendon for tenderness, swelling, heat, and nodules (Bickley, 2009; Magee, 2008; Weber & Kelley, 2007).

Gait (Ambulation)

To assess gait, or ambulation, the nurse asks the patient to walk away from and toward the nurse using the heel-to-toe gait, swinging her arms. Then the nurse asks the patient to repeat the same procedure on tiptoes. The nurse observes the patient during the two phases of walking. The first is the stance phase of gait; this occurs when the foot is on the ground and the patient is weight bearing or walking on the foot. The second phase is the swing phase; this occurs when the patient moves the foot forward and is not bearing weight. The nurse observes for difficulty in weight bearing, gait anomalies, symmetry of legs, rate, rhythm, and arm motion.

The nurse inspects the patient during ambulation for the ability to walk heel to toe; the ability to swing the arms in conjunction with walking; base of support; posture; limping or leaning to one side; and inability to bear weight on one or both legs.

Normal Findings

- Smooth, rhythmic movement; arms swing in conjunction with walking.
- No leaning or limping noted; patient is able to keep balance.
- Toes point straight ahead.
- Patient is able to walk heel to toe.
- Back is straight with a wide base of support.

Abnormal Findings (refer to Chapters 49 and 51)

- Leaning or limping may indicate a neurological problem.
- Toes pointing inward or outward may be indicative of bunions or arthritis.
- Arms extended to sides to maintain balance may indicate a neurological problem.
- Shuffling or the inability to take coordinated steps may indicate Parkinson's disease.

Laboratory and Imaging Results

Most musculoskeletal disorders are assessed with radiological tests such as plain films, CT and MRI scans, and scans for bone density. Laboratory studies may include a complete blood count to assess for infection or blood loss and specific blood tests for arthritis and some genetic disorders. Refer to the specific laboratory and diagnostic test feature for the disorders covered in the following chapters.

Critical Thinking Related to Assessment Data

A person's quality of life can be significantly affected from injury or disorders of the musculoskeletal system. This system supports the body and is essential for a person's mobility and fine motor movement, as well as the person's ability to perform daily tasks and provide self-care. The muscles and bones also protect the internal organs; in addition, the bones produce red blood cells. During assessment, it is important for the nurse to recognize signs and symptoms of limb-threatening abnormalities. Any time an extremity feels cool to the touch or the nurse is unable to palpate pulses, it is considered a limb-threatening emergency; in this scenario, the nurse should notify the health care team immediately. Any disorder or injury to the musculoskeletal system interferes with the patient's mobility and ability to function normally. This disability may be temporary or permanent. Careful assessment of the musculoskeletal system will alert the nurse to changes and decrease potential permanent damage and disability.

Health Assessment for the Adult Life Span

Musculoskeletal disorders can result from individual behaviors as well as social and environmental factors. Regular physical exercise is a key factor to maintaining a healthy musculoskeletal system and should be included in the assessment. Many individuals do not participate in regular physical activities, such as jogging, bicycling, or walking. Physical activity is important for many reasons; as far as the musculoskeletal system is concerned, regularly scheduled physical activity increases muscle and bone mass. Weight-bearing activity can prevent thinning of bones as well as muscle atrophy. The increase in muscle mass coincides with a decrease in falling in older adults, which allows for independence and an ability to perform ADLs.

Obesity also affects the musculoskeletal system; people who are overweight, especially those who are obese, have a difficult time engaging in physical activity as they become short of breath and fatigued more easily. The extra weight also places a significant amount of strain on the musculoskeletal system. Cigarette smoking causes lung problems, which also can affect an individual's ability to participate in physical activity.

To maintain one's quality of life, it is important for everyone to engage in some degree of regular physical activity to help maintain a strong musculoskeletal system.

Gerontological Considerations

As "baby boomers" age, persons 50 years and older will soon make up the largest population group in the United States, so it is important to understand the numerous changes in the musculoskeletal system that occur with age. When assessing older patients with musculoskeletal ailments, the nurse needs to recognize several important aspects related to age:

1. Flexibility and strength tend to decrease as people age.
2. Because of changes to bone and muscle, older people may find it hard to maintain the various positions required for a proper assessment. Lying supine for a long period of time is difficult for patients with cardiopulmonary problems or with stiffness or pain in their joints.
3. Bones become weaker as calcium reabsorption lessens with age.
4. As the bones become weaker, fractures can become more prevalent.
5. Women who are menopausal or postmenopausal are subject to osteoporosis.
6. Articular hyaline cartilage becomes thinner at the joints, restricting ROM.
7. Osteoarthritic changes occur with age, particularly in postmenopausal women. Osteoarthritis causes smooth articular surfaces to become rough and painful.
8. Rheumatoid arthritis causes inflammation and decreased or limited movement of the fingers. The condition is painful and affects a person's ability to perform ADLs.
9. Older adults are prone to **pathologic fractures** (fractures that occur without trauma) due to thinning of the bones.
10. Skeletal muscle mass decreases with age, leading to cramping and severe pain.

Chart 48–4 describes differences in the older adult by system.

Weblink: ROM for the Elderly.

CHART 48–4 Assessing the Older Patient

System	Difference With the Older Adult
Shoulders	Inability to perform ROM without discomfort
Elbows	Inflammation, swelling, and decreased ROM due to arthritis
Wrist	Decreased ROM, swelling
Hands and fingers	Swelling and thickening of the metacarpophalangeal joint and the proximal interphalangeal joint, and decreased ROM, due to rheumatoid arthritis
	Heberden's nodules over the distal interphalangeal joint and Bouchard's nodes over the proximal interphalangeal joints due to osteoarthritis
Neck	May have difficulty performing ROM
Spine	Kyphosis
Hip	Decreased ROM, crepitus due to arthritis and degenerative joint disease
Knee	Bowleggedness due to loss of muscle control
Ankles	Decreased strength and ROM due to bone thinning and decreased muscle mass
Gait	Wider base of support; slower paced, nonrhythmic walking; use of assistive devices

Sources: Adapted from Magee, D. (2008). *Orthopedic physical assessment* (5th ed.). St. Louis, MO: Elsevier; Weber, J., & Kelley, J. (2007). *Health assessment in nursing* (3rd ed.). Philadelphia: Lippincott Williams & Wilkins.

NCLEX® PRACTICE

1. A patient's history reveals several "long bone" fractures. The nurse would assess for fractures in which body area? (select all that apply)
   1. Ankle
   2. Thigh
   3. Shoulder blade
   4. Back of the hand
   5. Middle of the chest

2. A nurse is assessing the social history of a 50-year-old female patient who presented with a musculoskeletal injury. Which question provides this information?
   1. "What were you doing when the accident happened?"
   2. "Do you use any assistive devices such as a cane or walker?"
   3. "Does anyone in your family have a history of rheumatoid arthritis or osteoporosis?"
   4. "Have you started menopause?"

3. The nurse is assessing the patient's right elbow range of motion when the patient winces. What action should the nurse take?
   1. Repeat the motion to see if the wincing recurs.
   2. Ask, "Does it hurt to move your elbow?"
   3. Stop the assessment and note the findings.
   4. Have the patient flex the wrist and repeat the elbow assessment.

4. The nurse documents a positive Phalen's test during the assessment of a patient's musculoskeletal system. Which teaching should the nurse provide?
   1. "Be careful not to stand in one position too long without moving around."
   2. "Take frequent breaks when performing tasks that require repetitive wrist movement."
   3. "Wear a compressive sleeve over your elbow when playing sports such as tennis."
   4. "A special brace that dorsiflexes your foot while you sleep is available to treat this condition."

5. The nurse is assessing a patient's feet. Which finding would the nurse document as normal?

1. Hallux valgus
2. Cavus foot
3. Verruca vulgaris
4. Rounded medial malleolus

6. The nurse has assessed the patient's hip range of motion. Which finding would the nurse document as normal?

1. Leg adduction 10 degrees
2. Leg abduction 25 degrees
3. External rotation 45 degrees
4. Internal rotation 20 degrees

Answers to NCLEX Practice Questions can be found in Appendix D in the Osborn Student Resources at nursing.pearsonhighered.com. Practice additional NCLEX questions online at the Student Resources site.

Pearson Nursing Student Resources Find additional review materials at: **nursing.pearsonhighered.com**

REFERENCES

Bickley, L. (2009). *Bates' guide to physical assessment and history taking* (10th ed.). Philadelphia: Wolters Kluwer Health/Lippincott Williams & Wilkins.

Jarvis, C. (2008). *Pocket companion for physical examination and health assessment* (5th ed.). St. Louis: W. B. Saunders.

Kozier, B., Erb, C., Berman, A., & Snyder, S. (2008). *Fundamentals of nursing. Concepts, process and practice* (8th ed.). Upper Saddle River, NJ: Pearson Prentice Hall.

Magee, D. (2008). *Orthopedic physical assessment* (5th ed.). St. Louis, MO: Elsevier.

Porth, C. M., & Matfin, G. (2009). *Essentials of pathophysiology: Concepts of altered health states* (2nd ed.). Philadelphia: Lippincott Williams & Wilkins.

Weber, J., & Kelley, J. (2007). *Health assessment in nursing* (3rd ed.). Philadelphia: Lippincott Williams & Wilkins.

Caring for the Patient with Musculoskeletal Disorders

CHAPTER 49

Kara L. Gasiorowski
Cheryl Wraa

Outcome-Based Learning Objectives

After studying this chapter, the learner will be able to:

1. Differentiate the etiology, pathophysiology, clinical manifestations, and medical and nursing management for bone diseases.
2. Evaluate the types of preventive measures necessary for patients with bone disease to avoid injury.
3. Differentiate the etiology, pathophysiology, clinical manifestations, and medical and nursing management for muscular diseases.
4. Compare and contrast the five types of myopathies, various treatment modalities, and nursing care of a patient diagnosed with a myopathy.
5. Analyze the causative factors, treatment modalities, and nursing care related to a patient diagnosed with fibromyalgia.
6. Organize the treatment and prevention needs of the gerontological population.

KEY TERMS

dermatomyositis p.1506
Gottron's sign p.1506
hypotonia p.1505
kyphosis p.1487
lordosis p.1487
osteoporosis p.1483
scoliosis p.1487
transcutaneous electrical nerve stimulation (TENS) p.1514

THE MUSCULOSKELETAL SYSTEM CONSISTS of the bones, muscles, ligaments, tendons, and other connective tissue. Organic materials (collagen fibers), inorganic materials (mineral salts), and water combine to form bone tissue, which provides protection for crucial internal organs, storage for calcium and other minerals, and sites for formation and development of the blood's cells (Copstead-Kirkhorn & Banasik, 2009).

Bone Disorders

Bone disorders can result from disuse, genetic or environmental influences, and traumatic injuries or accidents. Individuals with bone disease may experience loss of function and of independence. Therefore, the nurse must have a clear understanding of the effects of bone disease and how the particular disorder or disease will influence the individual.

Osteoporosis

Bone is composed primarily of a mineral-like matrix with varying degrees of density at various points within the structure. **Osteoporosis** is a skeletal disease that is characterized by low bone mass and deterioration of the bone tissue. Continuing deterioration results in bone fragility and susceptibility to fractures (MacLean et al., 2008).

Epidemiology

Osteoporosis is the most common of the metabolic bone diseases (Frazier & Drzymkowski, 2009). It is estimated that 44 million people in the United States are affected by low bone mass and osteoporosis independent of race or ethnic background. More than 50% of women 50 years of age or older will have an osteoporotic fracture during their lifetime. Statistically, approximately 4% of patients more than 50 years of age who have a hip fracture die while hospitalized, and 24% die within 1 year after the injury (MacLean et al., 2008).

In the past, osteoporosis was known primarily as a woman's disorder. However, research findings suggest that men are not immune to osteoporosis; in fact, 19% of men over 50 years of age have been diagnosed with osteoporosis, and 3.5 million men are at significant risk due to decreased bone mineral density. As with women, the changes in statistics are attributed to risk factors such as sedentary lifestyle, increased life expectancy, and history of fractures. In addition, advances in diagnostic screening in men have significantly improved. The most recent statistics state that osteoporosis affects at least 25% of women and 12% of men over 50 years of age (Majumdar et al., 2008).

Risk factors for osteoporosis can serve as a guide for early detection; however, caution is advised because some individuals with osteoporosis do not demonstrate known risk factors. After the age of 30, when peak

Weblink: Osteoporosis

CHART 49–1 Comparison by Gender of Risk Factors for Osteoporosis

Risk Factor	Women	Men
Age: increased age is at greater risk	X	X
Small, thin-boned body frame	X	X
Ethnicity: Caucasian and Asian	X	X
Family history of fractures and osteoporosis	X	X
History of maternal hip fracture		X
Low body weight and low body mass index		X
Absence of estrogen (i.e., menopause)	X	
Unusually fast decline in testosterone (e.g., prostate cancer)		X
Decreased libido and impotence		X
Sedentary lifestyle or prolonged immobility	X	X
Anorexia	X	
Diet low in calcium and vitamin D	X	X
Malabsorption conditions (e.g., inflammatory bowel disease or gastric surgery)	X	X
Cigarette smoking	X	X
Excessive use of alcohol	X	X
Fractures after the age of 50 years	X	X
Decreased bone mineral density	X	X
Use of certain medications, such as corticosteroids and anticonvulsants	X	X
Presence of certain chronic medical conditions such as chronic renal failure or diabetes	X	X

bone mass is reached, bone mass density begins to change. Loss of bone mass is a universal characteristic of humans; however, research suggests that racial, genetic, anthropometrical, sociocultural, economic, and nutritional differences all contribute toward the incidence and prevalence of osteoporosis (Pinheiro, Ciconelli, Martini, & Ferraz, 2009). See Chart 49–1 for a breakdown of risk factors for osteoporosis differentiated by gender.

Etiology and Pathophysiology

The disease process of osteoporosis is complex and insidious. It is a multifactor disorder that is 70% dependent upon genetic factors and 30% dependent upon environmental factors (Pinheiro et al., 2009). To understand the complicated etiology of osteoporosis, it is essential to review the remodeling–modeling process of bone tissue (refer to Chapter 50 for further explanation).

Genetic factors are linked to the maximal amount of bone mass a person has, which correlates with the amount of skin pigmentation. Caucasians have the least bone mass, and African Americans have the most (Porth & Matfin, 2009).

Over time, the processes that induce bone remodeling include damage to parts of bones in response to normal wear and tear, changes in body shape or weight, exercise, and local release of growth factors due to alterations in levels of hormones (Mayo Clinic, 2010). The age-related loss of bone occurs mainly in areas containing cancellous (trabecular) bone, such as the spine and neck of the femur, which are common sites for fractures in patients with osteoporosis.

Osteoporosis may be primary, or it may be secondary to an underlying disease. Primary osteoporosis is the major category and includes three types: (1) idiopathic, (2) Type I (postmenopausal), and (3) Type II (osteoporosis associated with the usual aging process). Idiopathic osteoporosis is uncommon and generally occurs in children and young adults with normal hormone levels. Type I osteoporosis, also known as postmenopausal osteoporosis, generally develops in women after menopause when the amount of estrogen in the body decreases. Type II osteoporosis, also known as senile osteoporosis, is associated with osteoporotic changes from the aging process; it affects the trabecular and cortical bone. In older women, Type I osteoporosis and Type II osteoporosis often occur together (Pinheiro et al., 2009).

In Type I (postmenopausal) osteoporosis, there is an increase in the activity of the *osteoclasts* and a decline in the activity of the *osteoblasts* (bone formation), leading to increased bone resorption. Menopause is associated with reduction of the estrogen that is needed for the bone formation process, causing a decline in bone mineral density and strength that results in thin, fragile bones.

Type II osteoporosis is a result of the normal aging process. As an individual ages, there is a decline in the number and activity of osteoblasts, which affects both cancellous (trabecular) and cortical bone. This type of osteoporosis is generally observed in adults who are 60 years of age or older. Both Type I and Type II osteoporosis can be observed in older women (McCance & Huether, 2009).

Research findings suggest that there is a degree of bone loss related to the amount and duration of glucocorticoid use in humans. It appears that there is an increased rate of bone reabsorption (increasing osteoclastogenesis and decreasing the level of osteoprotegerin) and a slower rate of bone remodeling (decreasing the osteoblast population). In addition, glucocorticoids decrease calcium absorption by the gastrointestinal tract. Long-term use of corticosteroid medications for treatment of rheumatoid arthritis, lupus, and asthma is damaging to bone (Mayo Clinic, 2010).

Diseases that may cause secondary osteoporosis include overactive thyroid, parathyroid, and adrenal glands, which accelerate bone remodeling and reduce bone density. Osteoporosis has also been found in individuals with chronic renal failure. In addition, eating disorders, which reduce the amount of calcium ingested, and weight-loss surgery due to loss of surface area available to absorb nutrients such as calcium may lead to secondary osteoporosis.

Regardless of the cause, osteoporotic changes occur in both cortical and cancellous bone. The hard, outer surface of the cortex (diaphysis and metaphysis) in cortical bone begins to thin, and increased intracortical porosity occurs within the bone. As the disease progresses, there is a loss of the trabeculae of the cancellous bone (spongy bone containing the red bone marrow located in the metaphysis of long bone). Further progress will result in thinning of the bone into the interior of the cancellous bone (spongy bone that contains both red and yellow marrow). Besides changes in the bone density, there is loss of trabecular connectivity. Any change in the process of bone turnover will result in changes in bone structure. As indicated, osteoporosis is a multifactorial and complex disease (Figure 49–1◆).

Clinical Manifestations

The clinical manifestations of osteoporosis may go undetected because individuals are often asymptomatic until the later stages. As the bone mass decreases in both cortical and cancellous bone, the bone becomes fragile and has a higher risk of fracturing. A fracture after minor trauma may be the first indication of having osteoporosis.

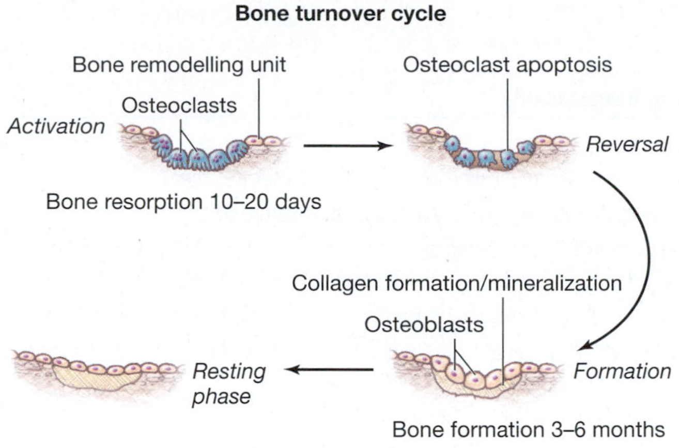

FIGURE 49–1 ◆ Bone turnover cycle.

Common sites for osteoporosis are the hand, wrist, spine, hip, knees, and feet. Fractures are common in the hip, vertebrae, and wrist. Signs and symptoms include fractures after a minor fall, exaggerated spine curvature, loss of height, pain aggravated by movement or jarring, pathologic fractures of the spine and femur, spontaneous wedge fractures, and vertebral collapse producing pain that radiates around the trunk.

Laboratory and Diagnostic Procedures

Assessment of bone mass is the primary measurement for osteoporosis. Because osteoporosis results from a decline in bone density, low bone mass is the most important measurement used to make a diagnosis and decide on the level of intervention. Therefore, bone mineral density tests are used to measure the bone density at various sites of the body. The DEXA is a dual-photon absorptiometry x-ray-based technique that allows measurement of any skeletal site, as well as the entire skeleton, because the technology corrects for soft tissue. Bone mineral content is measured and then compared to bone density values obtained in a reference population of the same race, gender, and age. Refer to the Laboratory and Diagnostic Tests for Bone Disorders box on page 1493 for additional tests.

Screening for osteoporosis is relatively inexpensive. In addition, in 1998, the Bone Mass Measurement Act required Medicare to reimburse for bone mineral density tests. Anyone who has risk factors for osteoporosis is strongly encouraged to have a bone mineral density test. Testing for osteoporosis, especially in females, should start at age 50, and is highly recommended for men ages 70 and older. In the presence of fracture or history of fracture after the age of 45, both men and women are recommended to have a bone mineral density test. It is recommended that men and women who have disorders or conditions that predispose them to low bone mineral density or who are on medications associated with bone loss (e.g., steroid therapy) have their bone mineral density assessed on a regular basis. In general, bone mineral density tests should be done every 2 years, but the frequency depends on the individual.

Biochemical markers are now available that evaluate the process of bone modeling and remodeling, which is useful in diagnosing osteoporosis. Biomarker response to therapy is useful for asymptomatic patients.

Medical Management

Management of osteoporosis is basically preventive in nature and begins in childhood. It is important to maintain an adequate supply of calcium and vitamin D throughout life to help maintain peak bone mass. Exercise stimulates bone formation as a result of the mechanical load exercise places on bones. Preventing osteoporosis requires a multidisciplinary approach; members of the team include a health care provider, a nurse, an exercise physiologist, a physical therapist, an occupational therapist, and a nutritionist.

The goal of treatment is to prevent further bone loss and maintain the individual's independence and functional ability. A holistic approach for medical management would involve screening, identification of underlying etiology, education, and pharmacologic and nonpharmacologic approaches (including exercise and complementary alternative strategies) (National Institutes of Health [NIH], 2010). See Chart 49–2 for nonpharmacologic patient management.

CHART 49–2 Nonpharmacologic Patient Management

Diet: Total daily intake of 1,200 to 1,500 mg/day of calcium

Exercise

- *Aerobic:* Walking and jogging to improve muscle mass and balance.
- *Anaerobic:* High impact exercises to stimulate bone growth.
- *Stretching:* Maintain muscle strength and balance.
- *Yoga:* Promote balance and coordination.

Kyphoplasty: A procedure in which a small balloon is inflated in the vertebral body to raise the height and is then stabilized with bone cement.

Vertebroplasty: A procedure in which bone cement is injected directly into a fractured vertebra.

Pharmaceutical strategies may include medications to manage the osteoporosis and pain associated with the disease. A health care provider may choose to treat the patient with a variety of medications: pain medication, anti-inflammatory medication (steroidal and nonsteroidal), bisphosphonates, calcitonin, calcium and vitamin D supplements, and parathyroid hormone. In addition, the medication regimen might be aimed at suppressing bone resorption and increasing bone formation (NIH, 2010).

Pharmacologic strategies include hormone replacement therapy for women who are postmenopausal and bisphosphonates to inhibit bone resorption. Calcium and vitamin D are important to bone mass. See the Pharmacology Summary for Bone Disorders box (p. 1486) for more information about medications to treat osteoporosis.

Nonpharmacologic strategies include diet and exercise. Protein, vitamins, and minerals are important to the production of the bone matrix. A diet that has less than the recommended dosage of protein, calcium, vitamins (C, D, and K), copper, manganese, and zinc will result in a lower bone mass density. (Refer to Chapter 8 for a discussion of nutrition.) Because bone responds to mechanical loading, strength training or exercises that include high impact forces is recommended.

Complementary and alternative strategies are palliative in nature. These strategies can provide the individual with the ability to deal with pain (acute and chronic) and stress. Strategies such as biofeedback, yoga, massage, and reflexology can aid the individual in relief of pain, as well as physical, emotional, and mental stress. These strategies can help increase the body's energy system to a state of well-being (NIH, 2010).

Nursing Management

Nursing care of the patient with osteoporosis is focused on the primary goals of maintaining independence and function, preserving bone mass, and preventing fractures. The majority of the strategies focus on education and behavioral changes.

PHARMACOLOGY Summary for Bone Disorders

Medication Category and Action	Application/Indication	Nursing Responsibility
Bone Resorption Inhibitor		
Bisphosphonates Alendronate (Fosamax) ***Action:*** Reduces the activity of cells that cause bone loss, slows rate of bone loss after menopause, and increases the amount of bone mass.	Prevention and treatment of osteoporosis.	Monitor serum calcium level before, during, and after treatment. Ensure adequate dietary intake of calcium and vitamin D. Teach the patient to take medication in the morning with a full glass of water. Orange juice, coffee, and mineral water reduce the drug's effects. To reduce esophageal irritation, teach the patient not to chew or suck on the pill. Teach the patient to wait at least 30 minutes after taking the medication before eating, drinking, or taking another medication. The patient should remain upright for 30 minutes after taking medication and until she has eaten the first food of the day as reflux will damage the esophagus.
Risedronate (Actonel) ***Action:*** Hinders excessive bone remodeling by binding to bone and reducing the rate at which osteoclasts are resorbed by bone.	Treatment of Paget's disease of bone when the serum alkaline phosphatase level is at least twice normal and the patient is symptomatic.	Administer supplemental calcium and vitamin D. Give calcium supplements and antacids at different times of day than risedronate to avoid impaired drug absorption. Teach the patient to take the medication at least 1 hour before the first food or drink of the day while in an upright position and with a full glass of water. Caution the patient to remain upright for at least 30 minutes after taking medication.
Osteoporosis Prophylactic		
Raloxifene (Evista) ***Action:*** Activates estrogen receptors, decreasing bone resorption while increasing bone mass and density.	Prevention of osteoporosis.	Assess distal extremities for impaired circulation and pain that may indicate thromboembolism. Discontinue drug at least 72 hours before and during periods of prolonged immobilization. Teach patient to avoid lengthy immobilization during travel because of the increased risk of thromboembolism.
Estrogen Replacement		
Cenestin Enjuvia Premarin ***Action:*** Binds to intracellular estrogen receptors to stimulate DNA and RNA to synthesize proteins responsible for biologic effects of estrogens.	Prevention of osteoporosis.	Estrogens should not be used in patients who have a history of breast cancer, cervical cancer, endometrial cancer, prostate cancer, or hepatic diseases. Increases risk of thromboembolism. Should be used with caution in patients with lipid disorders, as it may raise HDL cholesterol and triglycerides. Teach the patient to avoid lengthy immobilization during travel because of the increased risk of thromboembolism.
Calcium Supplements		
Calcium acetate (PhosLo) Calcium carbonate (Rolaids, Tums, etc.) Calcium chloride Calcium citrate Calcium gluconate ***Action:*** Restores normal serum levels that promote deposition of calcium in bone.	Helps restore bone strength and prevent fractures. Restores normal neuromuscular function and muscular contraction.	Assess for signs and symptoms of calcium imbalance. Hypercalcemia: drowsiness, weakness, headache, nausea, thirst and increased urination, decreased QT interval on ECG and inverted T waves. Hypocalcemia: facial twitching, muscle spasms, paresthesias, and seizures. Should not be given to patients with a history of renal calculi, digoxin toxicity, dysrhythmias, or hypercalcemia.
Vitamin D		
Calcitriol ***Action:*** Bone resorption inhibitor. Elevates serum calcium levels and decreases elevated blood levels of phosphate.	Decreases bone resorption and demineralization by promoting intestinal and renal reabsorption of calcium.	Should not be given to patients with hypercalcemia. Caution should be used in patients with renal failure who are at increased risk for vitamin D-induced hypercalcemia. Monitor for signs of hypercalcemia (listed previously). Monitor for signs of impaired liver function (yellowing of skin or sclera, pale bowel movements, and darkened urine). Hepatic impairment and an accumulation of fat-soluble vitamins will increase the risk of toxicity from vitamin D supplements.

PHARMACOLOGY Summary for Bone Disorders, *continued*

Medication Category and Action	Application/Indication	Nursing Responsibility
Antibiotics Broad Spectrum		
Cephalosporins Cefepime Carbapenems Imipenem-cilastatin ***Action:*** Inhibits bacterial cell wall synthesis.	Treatment for bone and soft-tissue infection.	Monitor laboratory results and infected sites for reduction in symptoms related to infection. Monitor the patient for symptoms of hypersensitivity reaction: wheezing; shortness of breath; swelling of face, tongue, or hands; and itching or rash. If symptoms are present, notify the health care team immediately. Instruct the patient to consume cultured dairy products with live active cultures to maintain normal intestinal flora. Instruct the patient to take the medication on schedule and to complete the entire prescription even if she is feeling better. Inform female patients on oral contraception that cephalosporins may reduce the effectiveness of oral contraceptives. Patients taking cephalosporins should not drink alcoholic beverages or alcohol-containing medicine; it may cause flushing, shortness of breath, nausea, chest pain, and blurred vision.

Source: Adams, M. P., & Koch, R. W. (2010). *Pharmacology: Connections to nursing practice.* Upper Saddle River, NJ: Pearson.

Assessment

The initial step in the nursing process is assessment. In a patient with osteoporosis, the focus of the assessment is on identification of risk factors and problems that may be associated with the disease. The nurse inquires about family history, previous fractures, dietary habits, exercise patterns, onset of menopause (if the patient is an older woman), and the use of alcohol, tobacco, corticosteroids, and caffeine. Assessment of the individual's general appearance and posture can provide useful information about the structure and motion of the skeletal system; therefore, the patient's height, weight, and body characteristics serve as objective data. In addition, assessing the spinal column for **lordosis** (accentuated curvature of the lumbar spine), **scoliosis** (a side-to-side curvature of the spine), **kyphosis** (exaggerated curvature of the thoracic spine), and spinal deformity (dowager's hump) may suggest osteoporotic changes.

The majority of patients with osteoporosis are older adults. The nurse is responsible for identifying limitations not associated with the aging process that need to be differentiated from those changes associated with osteoporosis. Older adults tend to have more than one medical condition; therefore, the nurse must expand the assessment to include other systems, such as cardiovascular and neurological. Chart 49–3 lists an assessment summary and cues for osteoporosis.

CHART 49–3 Nursing Assessment Cues for Assessing Osteoporosis

Assessment	Cues for Assessing
Cognitive ability	Impairments: what, when, how, and current management
Current activity level	Participation in activity: type, frequency, and duration Activities of daily living
Environment	Home environment
History of risk factors	Identify the risk factors for osteoporosis
History of fractures	When, how, and course of recovery
History of musculoskeletal disorders	What, when, course of treatment, and current management
Location of discomfort	When and how did it begin? Were there precipitating factors?
Range of motion	Ability and limitations
Neurological	Dementia? Delirium? Dizziness? Syncope? Orthostatic challenge
Impaired mobility	Assess gait, balance, posture, and center of gravity
Medical history	Past history of illnesses
Medications/recreational and prescribed	List of medications, dosage, and frequency
Pain	Verbalization of location, intensity, and description Precipitating factors and factors that relieve pain
Posture and general appearance	Observe for lordosis, scoliosis, and kyphosis Height and weight

Nursing Diagnoses

Nursing diagnoses for the patient with osteoporosis will be based on objective and subjective data collected during the assessment phase. Potential nursing diagnoses for osteoporosis include the following:

- *Pain* related to fracture and muscle spasm.
- *Injury, Risk for* related to additional fractures due to osteoporosis.
- *Constipation, Risk for* related to immobility and/or medications.
- *Knowledge Deficit, Risk for* related to disease process, treatment, and prevention.
- *Nutrition Imbalance, Risk for* related to increased calcium and vitamins needs.

NANDA-I © 2012

Outcomes and Evaluation Parameters

Outcomes for the patient with osteoporosis include relief from pain as verbalized by the patient. It is important for the patient to follow the treatment regimen to prevent further bone loss, increase strength and stability, and prevent additional fractures. The patient and family should institute preventive measures for safety in their environment. If sedentary, the patient may become constipated. However, the proper diet, mobility, and treatment regimen should improve bowel elimination with no signs of constipation or ileus.

Planning, Interventions, and Rationales

Educational interventions are focused on the (1) disease process, (2) risk factors, (3) medical management (pharmacologic interventions), (4) nonpharmacologic interventions, and (5) complementary and alternative strategies. It is very important for the patient to understand the disease process. Identification of risk factors is needed so that the patient can make an informed decision and modify any detrimental lifestyle behaviors. Depending on the clinical setting, monitoring the implemented strategies for changing behaviors may be achieved by asking the patient to keep a journal, followed by reinforcement of positive behavioral changes.

Teaching about the various prescribed medications is always essential to the educational component. Many of the medications prescribed for osteoporosis have a variety of side effects. It is important for the patient to be knowledgeable about side effects and strategies for prevention. Therefore, the nurse should review with the patient the medication's purpose, dosage, frequency, side effects, and special considerations. For example, some medications slow down gastrointestinal motility. As a result, individuals with osteoporosis have problems with constipation. It is prudent to educate the patient on monitoring the physiological response to new medications and combining medications. Because polypharmacy in the older adult is common, it is essential to assess the use of over-the-counter (OTC) drugs, vitamins, and minerals. Refer to the Pharmacology Summary for Bone Disorders box (p. 1486) for a summary of pharmacologic agents.

Educational interventions for nonpharmacologic strategies include exercise and diet. The patient with osteoporosis can benefit from learning about the positive effects of exercise on bone mass. If the patient with osteoporosis is active and wishes to remain active, an exercise physiologist can evaluate and prescribe an appropriate exercise program. However, if the patient has been sedentary for a significant period of time, consultation with a physical and occupational therapist may be the first step in intervening. Moderate exercise is best and can be achieved with walking, swimming, or riding a stationary bicycle.

Another lifestyle modification that may need to be implemented is dietary. After assessing the patient's diet, the nurse may determine that the patient could benefit from nutritional counseling and an adequate intake of calcium and vitamin D. Good dietary sources of calcium include low-fat dairy products, spinach, kale, beans and legumes, broccoli, tofu, fortified orange juice, salmon, and sardines. Natural sources of vitamin D include cod liver oil, fatty fish, and eggs (Hogan, DeLeon, Gingrich, & Willcutts, 2007). Calcium nutrition is important during the adolescent growth spurt and in postmenopausal women. For adults, the surgeon general recommends 1,000 to 1,200 milligrams of calcium per day depending on the age of the individual (NIH, 2010).

Immobility can be a result of osteoporosis. Slowing of gastrointestinal tract function can result from immobility and the effects of the medication. The nurse should educate the patient about strategies to prevent constipation (a high-fiber diet, exercise, and medication, if prescribed) and the potential risk of an ileus.

Other nursing interventions may include administration of prescribed pain medication, advocating, and encouraging. Through education and encouragement, the nurse can promote understanding about adequate pain relief so that the patient can focus on learning, participating, and maintaining functional ability and self-care (see Chapter 12 for a discussion of pain management).

The nurse can advocate for assistance in the home and self-care activities. For example, the nurse can encourage the wearing of splints or braces, if prescribed, to ensure proper musculoskeletal alignment. Education on protective pads worn on or around bony prominences can help to prevent fractures. The nurse promotes health by encouraging adherence to behavioral changes and lifestyle modifications to promote peak bone mass and functional ability.

Safety is an important consideration for patients with osteoporosis. Pain, weakness, and stiffness can place the individual at risk for falls, resulting in fractures. Reviewing a patient's home environment may reveal dangerous situations (e.g., rugs and furniture in the common travel paths), and even some simple alterations in that environment may prevent falls that can lead to costly and debilitating bone fractures.

Osteoporosis is associated with aging but is not part of the normal aging process. Risk factor reduction, adequate nutrition, and weight-bearing activities such as jogging, walking, jumping, and strength training can help preserve bone mass and strength. In addition, coordination and balance can be improved with endurance, strength, and flexibility training. If the goal is to maintain independence and the ability to perform daily activities, interventions aimed at improving muscle strength, coordination, and flexibility can lower the individual's risk for falling.

Fractures Associated With Osteoporosis

As an individual ages, muscle function declines, sarcopenia (decline in muscle mass) develops, and the rate of bone resorption and remodeling slows. These three factors in the aging process contribute to the process of bone loss and the loss of muscle strength and balance. For this reason, older adults are more likely than young people to fall and sustain fractures. For the older adult, common fracture sites include hips, vertebrae, and wrists (NIH, 2010).

Fractures are costly, debilitating, and have long-term implications. For example, a fracture of the spine and hip can leave the individual physiologically, psychosocially, and economically disabled during the recovery process. For a detailed discussion of the pathophysiology, clinical manifestations, diagnosis, and management of fractured bone, refer to Chapter 50.

Nursing Management

Nursing care of a fracture in the acute phase focuses on assessment, stabilization, and preparing the patient for surgery, if necessary. The majority of nursing management will focus on monitoring and preventing complications.

Sustaining a fracture may interfere with the patient's ability to provide self-care. During the hospitalization, the nurse may need to assist the patient with activities of daily living (ADLs). Family members may need to be educated on how to care for the patient, especially if the patient is discharged prior to rehabilitation.

The hip is a common site for fracture in older adults and patients with osteoporosis. The Nursing Process box provides a care plan for a patient with a fractured hip.

Fall Prevention

As stated earlier, screening for risk factors and falls assessment will identify the patients who are at risk for falls and fractures. The

NURSING PROCESS: Patient Care Plan for a Fractured Hip

Assessment of Musculoskeletal Status Using Gordon's Functional Health Patterns:

- Nutrition Metabolic Pattern
- Activity Exercise Pattern
- Cognitive Perceptual Pattern

Subjective Data	Objective Data
Assessment of Pain—Postoperative Vital signs Describe your pain: location, description, and pain scale score (0 to 10, with 10 being the worst) What is an acceptable pain scale score for you? Does anything make your pain worse? What helps with the pain (positioning, pain medication, nonpharmacologic interventions)?	**Assessment of Pain—Postoperative** Visual inspection of affected extremity: • Swelling and/or ecchymosis • Joint limitation • Skin temperature changes. Observable deformities? • Shortened? • Abducted/adducted? • Rotation? Vital signs (diaphoresis; blood pressure, pulse, and respiratory rate changes; pupillary dilation) Overt and covert expressions of pain (e.g., grimacing, restlessness)
Assessment of Impaired Physical Mobility Do you experience pain that interferes with your activities of daily living? Are there activities you feel you are unable to do?	**Assessment of Impaired Physical Mobility** Assess: • Strength and balance • Response to activity by taking vital signs at rest and then after they perform an activity • Coping strategies.
Assessment of Nutritional Intake Describe your usual intake pattern. Is this intake sufficient? Do you have religious dietary restrictions or practices? How often do you exercise? Who prepares your meals? Do you feel you have enough energy? Do you have any nausea with the pain medication?	**Assessment of Nutritional Intake** General appearance Weight Hair, nails, and skin Muscle mass Edema
Assessment of Skin Integrity Is the discomfort in the area of your surgical incision decreasing? Have you noticed any redness or drainage at the surgical site? Are you experiencing pain, itching, or discomfort to any area on the skin?	**Assessment of Skin Integrity** Assess the patient's skin and surgical site for redness, swelling, warmth, or drainage.

Outcomes and Evaluation Parameters	Planning and Interventions with *Rationales*
1. NURSING DIAGNOSIS: Pain *related to postoperative fracture repair* (NANDA-I © 2012)	
Outcome: Comfort level maintained. ***Evaluation Parameters:*** Reports adequate pain control. Participates in ADLs without pain.	Assess for pain using a pain scale from 0 to 10. Additionally, the description of the pain and location should be assessed *to maintain consistency in assessing the pain.*

(*continued*)

NURSING PROCESS: Patient Care Plan for a Fractured Hip, *continued*

	Assess cultural and religious beliefs about pain and pain relief. *In a dynamic system, there is an interaction and transaction between one's physiologic condition and one's cultural and religious beliefs. As a result, one's cultural and religious beliefs may impact how pain is perceived and treated. Treatment may involve strategies other than traditional Western medicine.*
2. NURSING DIAGNOSIS: Physical Mobility, Impaired *related to fractured hip* (NANDA-I © 2012)	
Outcomes: The patient will develop independence. The patient will be able to ambulate with minimal assistance. ***Evaluation Parameters:*** The patient will participate in physical therapy activities. The patient will be able to exercise without significant pain or activity intolerance.	While the patient is in bed, maintain neutral positioning of the hip with a trochanter roll and a pillow between the legs when turning. *Neutral positioning prevents stress on the fixation and minimizes external rotation. Supporting the legs with pillows during turning prevents adduction of the hip.* Teach the patient how to accomplish position changes by herself. *Teaching patients how to position themselves encourages their active participation in their care and prevents unwanted stress on the hip.* Teach the patient isometric exercises to maintain and increase strength of the quadriceps and gluteal muscles. *Strengthening of muscles assists with ambulation.*
3. NURSING DIAGNOSIS: Nutrition, Imbalanced: Less Than Body Requirements *related to increased need for calcium and vitamins* (NANDA-I © 2012)	
Outcome: The patient will maintain adequate nutrition to assist with healing. ***Evaluation Parameter:*** Maintenance of weight without loss of muscle mass.	Facilitate education with a dietary consultant. *Consultation can ensure a diet that provides optimal caloric and nutrient intake.* Encourage frequent oral hygiene. *Poor oral hygiene leads to bad breath and a bad taste in the mouth, which decreases the appetite.* Provide the patient with printed material outlining dietary needs and restrictions. *Aids the patient in selecting the proper foods.* Promote the intake of protein foods with high biologic value: eggs, meats, and dairy products. *Complete proteins provide the positive nitrogen balance needed for growth and healing.* If the patient has osteoporosis, encourage intake of foods rich in calcium: • Low-fat dairy products • Spinach • Kale • Beans and other legumes • Broccoli • Tofu • Salmon • Sardines. Also encourage foods rich in vitamin D: • Cod liver oil • Fatty fish • Eggs • Fortified foods such as milk and cereals. *Calcium adds strength and stiffness to bones. Vitamin D is essential for calcium absorption and normal bone mineralization.*
4. NURSING DIAGNOSIS: Skin Integrity, Impaired: Risk for *related to immobility and surgical incision* (NANDA-I © 2012)	
Outcome: Patient will achieve wound healing and not develop a pressure ulcer. ***Evaluation Parameters:*** The patient will relate minimal discomfort at the surgical site, and the incision will remain without signs of infection. The patient will show no signs of redness from pressure over bony prominences.	Monitor vital signs and lab results. *Temperature, pulse, and white blood cell count may increase in response to infection.* Maintain use of aseptic technique. *Use of aseptic technique avoids the introduction of infectious organisms.* Assess the surgical site for the appearance and character of drainage. *Redness, edema, and drainage at the surgical site indicate infection.* Reposition the patient at least every 2 hours and assess the skin for redness or change in sensation. Add padding to bony prominences. *Repositioning and adding padding relieves pressure on the bony prominences. Redness or a change in sensation on the skin may indicate the development of a pressure ulcer.*

Source: Adapted from Wilkinson, J. M., & Ahearn, N. R. (2009). *Prentice Hall nursing diagnosis handbook* (9th ed.). Upper Saddle River, NJ: Prentice Hall.

Evidence-Based Practice box includes recommendations for fall prevention strategies developed by the Institute for Clinical Systems Improvement.

Osteomyelitis

Osteomyelitis is an infection of the bone that requires aggressive early treatment to decrease the amount of bone or joint damage.

Epidemiology

In contrast to the silent onset of osteoporosis, osteomyelitis can have an acute, subacute (somewhat recent), or chronic onset. The acute and chronic forms can present the same clinical picture. The bones that are most commonly involved include the upper ends of the humerus and tibia and the lower end of the femur. Occasionally, the spinal vertebrae may be affected (Frazier & Drzymkowski, 2009).

Weblink: Preventing Falls in Acute Care Settings

Weblink: Prevention of Falls

EVIDENCE-BASED PRACTICE Prevention of Falls in the Acute Care Setting

Clinical Problem

Falls are a leading cause of hospital-acquired injury. The National Center for Injury Prevention and Control states that falls are the most common adverse event reported in hospitals (http://www.cdc.gov/ncipc/factsheets/adultfalls.htm).

The following guideline from the Institute for Clinical Systems Improvement provides an evidence-based summary of the clinical aspects of fall prevention and preventive strategies for those older people at high risk of falls.

Research Findings

Data on fall rates in acute care hospitals are incomplete. Reviews of available studies in acute care hospitals indicate that fall rates range from 1.3–8.9 falls/1,000 patient days and are higher in rehabilitation units, and units that care for elder adults or neurology patients (ICSI, 2012).

A cohort study of nine Midwestern hospitals stated that injury from falls was associated with older age, unassisted activities, bathroom falls, and falls in patient care areas outside of the patient's room (Krauss et al., 2007). A goal of the patient safety movement is the reduction and even elimination of falls that result in injury. Data have shown that best practice results have been achieved when there is organizational support for fall reduction across departments and disciplines.

Recommendations for Risk Assessment of Individuals at High Risk of Falls

The literature suggests that a patient's fall risk can be assessed with three questions:

1. Has the patient fallen in the last year?
2. Does the patient look as though he is going to fall? (Is there a detectable abnormality of gait or balance?)
3. Does the patient have an additional risk factor for an injurious fall such as visual impairment, impaired cognition, or multiple medications?

Screening

Several fall risk assessment tools have been developed and validated. There has been no consensus as to which of these tools is the best. Keep in mind that fall risk screening does not prevent falls but only helps to predict them.

Recommendations for Preventive Strategies

Identify patients who are at risk of falls by placing a visual identifier on the door to the patient's room and bathroom or a wristband on the patient. Members of the health care team from all departments, as well as visitors, should be educated in recognizing and understanding the identifiers.

Communication with and education of the patient and family is essential. The nurse should notify the patient and family of fall risk upon admission, if and when the risk changes, and upon discharge. The hospital's fall prevention program should be described to the patient and family. Expectations regarding the fall risk policy of the organization should be clarified, and ways in which the family can assist with fall prevention and how to contact staff when necessary should be discussed. These discussions should be documented in the patient's chart. Evidence shows that education is an integral piece to a fall prevention program. Multiple teaching methods including written, verbal, and DVD/video can help to deliver a consistent message and modify the patient's perceptions and knowledge (Hill et al., 2009).

Fall Prevention Measures

Patients who have been immobile, as well as older adults, have decreased muscle strength, impaired mobility, and impaired gait, which are some of the common risk factors that predict falls. These risk factors can be modified by physical therapy (Sherrington et al., 2008). Other interventions include the following:

- Wearing of shoes or nonskid footwear when ambulating
- Teaching the patient to rise slowly
- Performing early and regular ambulation of high-risk patients
- Repeating education of safety measures to family members
- Using assistive devices such as a walker or equipment recommended by physical therapy
- Using adequate lighting for ambulation
- Using elevated toilet seats and rails in the bathroom
- Using a gait belt or transfer belt during mobility.

Frequent rounding on high-risk patients, often referred to as the Four P's (position, plan assessment, personal needs, and placement), is a strategy that can decrease fall rates. Studies have shown that 45.2% of falls were toileting related (Tzeng, 2010). Components of safety and comfort rounds may include the following:

- Assessing pain
- Offering toileting assistance
- Repositioning
- Checking the position of the call light, telephone, television remote, urinal, and so on
- Offering fresh water
- Maintaining comfortable temperature and lighting of room
- Checking the area for environmental hazards
- Asking whether there is anything else the patient needs.

Implications for Nursing Practice

Nurses should screen older patients to evaluate their risk factors for falling and increased potential for fractures. Using the findings, the nurse will educate the patient and family regarding ways to decrease their risks and to increase mobility and safety within their environment.

Critical Thinking Questions with answers can be found in the Osborn Student Resources at nursing.pearsonhighered.com.

Sources: Institute for Clinical Systems Improvement. (2012). Prevention of falls (acute care) protocol (3rd ed.). Retrieved from http://www.icsi.org/falls_acute_care_prevention_of_protocol_24255.html; Krauss, M. J., Nguyen, S. L., Dunagan, W. C., Birge, S., Costanitnou, E., Caleca, B., & Fraser, V. J. (2007). Patient fall circumstances and injury across nine hospitals in a Midwestern healthcare system. *Infection Control Hospital Epidemiology 28*(5), 544–550; Hill, A., McPhail, S., Hoffmann, T., Hill, K., Oliver, D., Beer, C., Brauer, S., & Haines, T.P. (2009). A randomized trial comparing digital video disc with written delivery of falls prevention education for older patients in hospital. *Journal of the American Geriatrics Society, 57*(8): 1458–1463; Sherrington, C., Whitney, J. C., Lord, S. R., Herbert, R. D., Cumming, R. G., & Close, J. C. (2008). Effective exercise for the prevention of falls: a systematic review and meta-analysis. *Journal of the American Geriatrics Society, 58*(12): 2234–2243; Tzeng, H.M. (2010). Understanding the prevalence of inpatient falls associated with toileting in adult acute care settings. *Journal of Nursing Care Quality, 25*(1): 22–30.

Weblink: Osteomyelitis
Weblink: Muscular Dystrophy

The first line of defense for the bone is the skin; however, bones can become infected through the bloodstream, direct invasion (through trauma or surgery), and infections in adjacent bone or soft tissues. One in 5,000 children may experience acute osteomyelitis. In general, children tend to have a higher incidence of acute osteomyelitis, and adults tend to present with subacute and chronic osteomyelitis (King et al., 2010; Mayo Clinic, 2009). Individuals with diabetes have a 16% risk factor for acquiring osteomyelitis. The problem with osteomyelitis is that symptoms develop over time and may go unnoticed for several days to a week. Individuals who experience vertebral osteomyelitis have a 10% to 15% risk of developing neurological problems due to spinal cord compression from the inflammatory process (King et al., 2010).

Etiology and Pathophysiology

The cause of the inflammatory process results from pyogenic organisms such as *Staphylococcus aureus, S. epidermidis, Escherichia coli, Mycobacterium tuberculosis, Neisseria gonorrhoeae,* Pseudomonas, Salmonella, fungi, and mycobacteria. These organisms can affect anyone at any age. *S. aureus* is responsible for 90% of bone infections, followed by streptococcal bacteria. Individuals who are at risk for developing osteomyelitis include those who have a compromised immune system, diabetes, peripheral vascular disease, malignancies, or the presence of prosthetic hardware within the bone (Frazier & Drzymkowski, 2009).

Acute osteomyelitis falls into two categories: hematogenous and direct contact. Hematogenous osteomyelitis is an infection caused by bacterial infection from a distant site migrating by way of the bloodstream to the bone. It is most commonly seen in children. Two common bone sites provide a rich environment for organism growth: the vascular metaphysis of growing bones and the distal metaphysis. The pyogenic organism finds the rich blood supply of the growing bone's metaphysis an ideal environment for receiving needed nutrients for growth and proliferation. A sharp angle at the distal metaphysis structure slows the blood, causing stagnation and thrombosis formation. The thrombosis formation can result in ischemia, leading to necrosis and bacterial growth (King et al., 2010).

The other category of acute osteomyelitis, direct contact, results from direct trauma or surgery. Direct contact of bacteria or the implanting of bacteria from the outside environment can cause infection. For example, osteomyelitis can be diagnosed following a surgical procedure. In this case, the disease process is localized to a specific bone but can potentially spread to surrounding tissues. Osteomyelitis resulting from direct trauma, injury, or surgery involves many organisms, and the clinical manifestations tend to be more localized than those of hematogenous osteomyelitis (King et al., 2010).

Chronic osteomyelitis is typically associated with other disease processes that predispose the individual to bone infections. For example, individuals with diabetes have a higher incidence of osteomyelitis because of the poor circulation in the lower extremities and high level of blood sugar. Peripheral vascular disease, sickle cell anemia, and immune deficiency syndrome are just a few examples of other primary disease processes that predispose an individual to osteomyelitis (King et al., 2010).

In summary, osteomyelitis is a complex bone disorder with the potential for chronic and long-term effects. Therefore, the focus in the medical diagnosis must be on the accurate classification of the cause (direct or indirect) and the organism involved. In some cases, young, rapidly growing normal cells and cells that are subjected to inflammation and changes in their blood supply can exhibit characteristics that may indicate bone tumor.

Clinical Manifestations

Clinical manifestations of osteomyelitis include fever, edema at the involved site, warmth to touch, tenderness at the site, and movement or joint limitations (i.e., contractures) at the site. The patient may complain of fatigue and malaise. As the infection progresses, a subperiosteal abscess may develop. The purulent material causes pressure and eventual fracturing of small pieces of bone.

Laboratory and Diagnostic Procedures

Refer to the Laboratory and Diagnostic Tests for Bone Disorders box on page 1493.

Medical Management

Medical management of osteomyelitis in the acute phase focuses on treating the underlying cause for full recovery with minimal loss of function. Pharmacologic and surgical interventions are possible strategies. Management is geared toward preventing nonhealing of the wound, sepsis, immobility, and amputation.

Medical intervention may include immobilization of the affected bone and prescribing medications such as pain medicines and antibiotics. Pharmacologic interventions include the use of broad-spectrum antibiotics until organism sensitivity is obtained. Generally, antibiotics will be administered intravenously and may extend over a course of 4 to 6 weeks. Oral antibiotics may be prescribed following the completion of the intravenous (IV) antibiotics.

Surgery may be considered to incise the site and drain the abscess. In chronic osteomyelitis, surgery is recommended to remove the dead bone. The wound may require repeated debridement followed by frequent sterile dressing changes. It is suggested that patients be placed on drainage and secretion precautions.

Nursing Management

Nursing care of the patient with osteomyelitis focuses on rest, immobilization of the affected part, and administration of analgesics, antipyretics, and antibiotics. The affected extremity should be supported to facilitate adequate circulation, and proper alignment should be maintained to prevent contractures (Christensen & Kockrow, 2010). Preventive care includes monitoring the wound, performing prescribed wound care, preventing dehydration, reinforcing adherence to the antibiotic regimen, and performing regular follow-up. See the Nursing Process: Patient Care Plan for Osteomyelitis box on page 1494 for more details regarding pain, nutrition, mobility, and knowledge deficit.

Patient education focuses on information about the disease process, medications, signs of inflammation, and changes that might indicate worsening of the condition. If osteomyelitis is not treated properly, it can become chronic. In such cases, the individual may go home with an indwelling catheter or PICC line for antibiotics. The patient and family members will need education on how to care for the intravenous types of lines. The Patient Teaching & Discharge Priorities for Osteomyelitis box (p. 1495) lists other aspects of patient education.

Osteitis Deformans (Paget's Disease)

Osteitis deformans is a chronic disorder that causes irregular bone breakdown and formation, which in turn causes the bones to weaken. This results in pain, bone deformities, fractures, and arthritis.

LABORATORY AND DIAGNOSTIC TESTS for Bone Disorders

Test with Description, Rationale, and Normal Values	Expected Abnormality
Complete Blood Count	
Normal:	Increased WBC.
White blood cell: 4,500–10,000 µl	Decreased RBC, Hgb, and Hct with anemia in the presence of bone marrow suppression.
Hematocrit	
Male: 40–54% Female: 36–46%	
Hemoglobin	
Male: 13.5–18 g/dL Female: 12–15 g/dL	
Red Blood Cell	
Male: 4.6–6.0 µl Female: 4.0–5.0 µl	
Used to provide information on infection, malnutrition, and anemias.	
Serum Calcium and Phosphorous Levels	
Calcium 4.5–5.5 mEq/L	Decreased with malabsorption of calcium from the GI tract, as well as lack of calcium and vitamin D intake. Increased with malignant neoplasm of the bone, multiple myeloma, and multiple fractures.
Phosphorous 1.7–2.6 mEq/L	Decreased with malabsorption syndrome and hypercalcemia. Increased with hypocalcemia, bone tumors, and hypervitaminosis D.
Provide information on the level of calcium and phosphorus in relationship to malnutrition, osteomalacia, and abnormal levels in conjunction with hyper/hypo states.	
Urine Calcium	
Low-calcium diet: less than 150 mg/24 hours, less than 3.75 mmol/24 hours	Increased with osteoporosis and bone malignancies.
Average-calcium diet: 100–250 mg/24 hours, 2.50–6.25 mmol/24 hours	Decreased with vitamin D deficiency, malabsorption syndrome, and chronic renal failure.
High-calcium diet: 250–300 mg/24 hours, 6.25–7.50 mmol/24 hours	
Provides information on osteomalacia, malnutrition, and malabsorption as well as hyper/hypo states.	
Bone Aspirate Cultures	
Free of organisms.	Identification of causative organism.
Provides information on the infecting agent.	
MRI	
No bone or tissue abnormality.	Demonstrate swelling of overlying tissues.
Provides information regarding bone structure and soft tissue surrounding bone.	Demonstrate bone density loss or tumor.
	In osteomyelitis, this will differentiate soft tissue from bone marrow involvement.
CT Scan	
No bone or tissue abnormality.	Demonstrate bone loss, fracture, or tumor.
Provides information regarding bone structure and soft tissue surrounding bone.	Demonstrate soft tissue abscess or fluid collection.
Ultrasound	
No bone or tissue abnormality.	Demonstrate soft tissue abscess or fluid collection and periosteal elevation with infection.
Provide information regarding soft tissue surrounding bone.	
X-Ray	
No bone or tissue abnormality.	Demonstrate a swelling of overlying tissues.
Provides information regarding bone structure and soft tissue surrounding bone.	Demonstrate bone loss, fracture, or tumor.
Bone Scan	
No bone abnormality.	Detect the extent of the malignancy and help follow the planned therapy.
Provides information regarding bone structure.	

Epidemiology and Etiology

The cause of osteitis deformans is unknown. It can occur in just a portion of one bone, the entire bone, or many bones throughout the skeletal system. The most common sites are the pelvis and tibia. Other, less affected areas include the femur, clavicle, skull, and spine. The disease usually presents in patients older than 40 years of age and becomes more common with age (Frazier & Drzymkowski, 2009).

Pathophysiology

With osteitis deformans, the affected areas of bone produce new bone faster than old bone can be broken down. The disease usually occurs in

NURSING PROCESS: Patient Care Plan for Osteomyelitis

Assessment of Musculoskeletal Status Using Gordon's Functional Health Patterns:

- Nutrition Metabolic Pattern
- Cognitive Perceptual Pattern

Subjective Data

Assessment of Pain

On a scale of 1 to 10, with 1 being a little pain and 10 being the worst pain you have ever felt, at what level is your pain?

Do you routinely take pain medication at home? If yes, what is the name of the medication and why do you take it?

Are you allergic to any medications?

Assessment of Knowledge of Treatment Regimen

Do you understand which medications you are taking and when to take them?

Can you tell me what osteomyelitis is?

What is your weight-bearing status?

Assessment of Nutritional Intake

Describe your usual intake pattern.

Is this intake sufficient?

Do you have religious dietary restrictions or practices?

Who prepares your meals?

Do you feel you have enough energy?

How often do you exercise?

Objective Data

Assessment of Pain

Monitor the patient for:

- Facial grimacing
- Change in breathing pattern
- Change in blood pressure and/or pulse rate
- Diaphoresis
- Agitation

Assessment of Knowledge of Treatment Regimen

Patient takes medications as prescribed.

Patient demonstrates proper wound care.

Patient reports no elevation of temperature or recurrence of pain or other symptoms at the site.

Assessment of Nutritional Intake

General appearance

Weight

Hair, nails, and skin

Muscle mass

Edema

Outcomes and Evaluation Parameters	Planning and Interventions with *Rationales*
1. NURSING DIAGNOSIS: Pain, Acute *related to inflammation* (NANDA-I © 2012)	
Outcome: Pain level will be tolerable. ***Evaluation Parameter:*** Patient will not exhibit symptoms of pain and will verbalize pain control.	**Nonpharmacologic:** Reduce lighting and noise, and provide room for the patient's significant others. Cultural and spiritual factors such as prayer, ritual, and music can also increase the patient's comfort. *Promotes relaxation and comfort.* **Pharmacologic:** Medicate the patient with narcotics and nonsteroidal anti-inflammatory drugs as ordered. Assess for effectiveness. *Bone pain is usually severe.* Administer antipyretics and antibiotics as ordered. *Treatment of the underlying infection will lead to reduced pain.* Elevate and support the affected extremity. *Elevating the extremity reduces edema by enhancing venous return. Supportive positioning protects against muscle strain.* Teach the patient to report increasing or uncontrolled pain. *Increasing pain may indicate ineffective therapy or worsening infection.*
2. NURSING DIAGNOSIS: Knowledge, Deficient *related to treatment regimen* (NANDA-I © 2012)	
Outcome: The patient will comply with the therapeutic plan. ***Evaluation Parameters:*** The patient will take medications on time, demonstrate proper wound care, and report signs or symptoms of complications quickly.	Teach the patient and family the importance of adhering to the therapeutic regimen. *Knowledge regarding the reasons for the therapeutic plan and the consequences that may occur if not followed will motivate the patient to adhere.*
3. NURSING DIAGNOSIS: Nutrition, Imbalanced: Less Than Body Requirements *related to intake of optimal calories and protein to promote healing* (NANDA-I © 2012)	
Outcome: The patient will maintain adequate nutrition to assist with healing. ***Evaluation Parameter:*** Maintenance of weight without loss of muscle mass.	Facilitate education with a dietary consultant *to assess caloric and protein intake. Consultation can ensure a diet that provides optimal caloric and nutrient intake.* Provide the patient with printed material outlining the dietary needs and restrictions.

NURSING PROCESS: Patient Care Plan for Osteomyelitis, *continued*

Aids the patient in selecting the proper foods.

Promote the intake of protein foods with high biologic value: eggs, meats, and dairy products.

Complete proteins provide the positive nitrogen balance needed for growth and healing.

Promote the intake of foods high in protein and vitamins A, B, and C. Common food sources include meat, fish, poultry, fortified cereals, dairy products, dark green and yellow vegetables, citrus fruits/juices, potatoes, cauliflower, and tomatoes. *Promotes cell regeneration.*

Encourage frequent oral hygiene.

Poor oral hygiene leads to bad breath and a bad taste in the mouth, which decreases the appetite.

Source: Adapted from Wilkinson, J. M., & Ahearn, N. R. (2009). *Prentice Hall nursing diagnosis handbook* (9th ed.). Upper Saddle River, NJ: Prentice Hall.

PATIENT TEACHING & DISCHARGE PRIORITIES for Osteomyelitis

Need	Teaching
Nutrition:	Work with the dietitian to plan a high-protein diet rich in vitamins A, B, and C to promote cell regeneration.
Patient and family	
Medications:	Stress the importance of taking prescribed antibiotics as scheduled even if the patient is feeling better.
Patient and family	Teach the patient the signs and symptoms of any side effects that may occur.
Safety:	Stress the importance of a safe environment to prevent falls and possible fractures.
Patient and family	Teach the proper use of any assistive devices that may be required.
Avoidance of continued infections:	Stress the importance of reporting signs of infection.
Patient and family	Patients who need long-term antibiotics will require a special intravenous line such as a PICC. Educate the patient in maintenance of the catheter, emphasizing the importance of aseptic technique.
	Stress the importance of follow-up appointments to assess therapeutic effectiveness.

two stages: the vascular stage, in which bone tissue is broken down but the spaces are filled with blood vessels and fibrous tissue rather than new bone, and the sclerotic stage, in which the vascular fibrous tissue hardens and is similar to bone but is fragile, leading to pathologic fractures (Frazier & Drzymkowski, 2009).

Clinical Manifestations

Osteitis deformans symptoms include bone pain at the site. The pain can become disabling because it is unremitting and tends to be worse at night. Patients may experience edema or deformity at the affected site. If the ossicles of the ear are involved, hearing loss or deafness will occur. Complications of the disease include pathologic fractures, hypercalcemia, renal calculi, spinal cord injury, and occasionally development of bone sarcoma (Frazier & Drzymkowski, 2009).

Laboratory and Diagnostic Procedures

Radiographic imaging, bone scanning, and a bone marrow biopsy assist with diagnosis. Serum laboratory results will show an elevated alkaline phosphatase, and urinalysis will reveal an elevated hydroxyproline concentration. Both results indicate a high rate of bone production.

Medical Management

Treatment of osteitis deformans is symptom based. Treatment goals are the relief of pain and prevention of bone loss. Injections of the hormone calcitonin may be given to regulate the level of calcium in the blood and help prevent bone loss. A diet high in protein, calcium, and vitamin D also helps to prevent bone loss, especially if the use of bisphosphonate medications has been added to the treatment plan (Frazier & Drzymkowski, 2009).

Nursing Management

The goals of nursing management include education regarding the disease process and palliative treatment of symptoms. The nurse should teach the patient that exercise is an important part of the treatment plan to stimulate bone growth and maintain flexibility and strength. Maintaining a healthy weight is also important to avoid undue stress on affected bones.

Benign Bone Tumors

Bone tumor is an abnormal growth of the bone cells and can be benign or cancerous. The tumors can be from cartilage (chondrogenic), from bone (osteogenic), or from fibrous tissue (fibrogenic). Benign bone tumors do not spread to other tissues or organs.

Epidemiology

Generally, adults over the age of 40 years and children ages 10 years or younger are at the highest risk for developing bone tumors. Examples of benign bone tumors include aneurysmal bone cyst, osteochondroma, fibrous dysplasia, chondroblastoma, and osteoid osteoma.

Etiology and Pathophysiology

Bone tumors can be classified according to their origins or as benign or malignant. Benign bone tumors generally are not life threatening, present few symptoms, and do not result in death. A tumor in the bone causes the normal bone tissue to react by osteolytic response (bone destruction) or osteoblastic response (bone formation). Bone tissue cells are very active; new bone is constantly forming, and old bone is dissolving. Bone tumors result from an abnormal growth of cells that can originate from bone cells, cartilage, fibrous tissue, marrow, or vascular tissue.

Generally, benign tumors illustrate the geographical pattern by having a slow, symmetrical growth pattern. Slow erosion can cause bone destruction and may cause the adjacent normal bone to respond to the tumor by altering its normal pattern of remodeling. The bone's surface changes; in addition, the contours enlarge in the tumor areas. Because adjacent tendons and muscles provide structural support for the bone, the bone becomes weakened as the adjacent tissues are displaced, and fracture can result. Some examples of benign bone tumors include nonossifying fibroma, osteochondroma, osteoma, osteoblastoma, enchondroma (Ollier's disease), bone cyst, chondroblastoma, and giant cell tumor (McCance & Huether, 2009). Osteochondroma accounts for 35% to 50% of all benign tumors (Copstead-Kirkhorn & Banasik, 2009). Pathologic characteristics of bone tumors include bone destruction, bone attrition, expansion of the cortex, and periosteal response to changes in underlying bone (McCance & Huether, 2009).

Clinical Manifestations and Diagnostic Procedures

Benign bone tumors have two predominant clinical manifestations: Pressure around surrounding tissues may cause pain, and range of motion may be affected if the tumor becomes too large. Pain is usually the presenting symptom and is often worse at night or after exercise. At times, bone tumors produce no symptoms and are detected when the weakened bone fractures.

Radiographs, CT scan, radionuclide bone scan, and/or MRI can be used to diagnose the tumor.

Medical Management

The treatment for bone tumors, whether benign or malignant, is surgical excision. Surrounding muscle tissue and other tissue are often removed, and bone grafting may be needed. Amputation may be required depending on the tumor site and extent. Surgical removal alone is enough to treat benign bone tumors. Malignant tumors, however, require additional treatment, as described in the following section.

Bone Cancer and Bone Metastases

The most common types of primary bone cancer are osteosarcoma, chondrosarcoma, and Ewing's sarcoma (Frazier & Drzymkowski, 2009).

Epidemiology

In 2012, it was estimated that 2,890 new cases of bone and joint cancer would be diagnosed. Approximately 1,410 deaths are expected from these cancers. Chondrosarcoma and osteosarcoma are the most common forms of bone cancer, followed by chordoma, Ewing tumor, and malignant fibrous histiocytoma/fibrosarcoma (American Cancer Society [ACS], 2012a).

Osteosarcoma usually presents in young people between the ages of 10 and 30. However, a small percentage of cases (10%) develop in people who are older than 60 years of age (ACS, 2012b). Osteosarcoma has a greater incidence in males than in females and the tumor most often develops in the arm, leg, or pelvis.

Chondrosarcoma is a cancer of cartilage cells and is uncommon in people younger than 20 years of age. After the age of 20, the risk of developing the cancer continues to rise until the person reaches the age of 75. The incidence is equal for men and women (ACS, 2012a). Chondrosarcoma may present anywhere in the body where there is cartilage; the most common sites are the pelvis, leg, and arm bones. Chondrosarcoma also will occasionally present in the trachea, larynx, and chest wall.

Ewing's sarcoma is a primary malignant bone tumor that occurs in the pediatric and adolescent population. It usually occurs in the second decade of life, and approximately 80% of cases are in people younger than 20 years of age (Lahl, Fisher, & Laschinger, 2007). In contrast to osteosarcoma, in which there is no significant difference in incidence between the races, there is a significantly higher incidence of Ewing's sarcoma in Caucasian children when compared to children of the same age from the African American population (Lahl et al., 2007). Ewing tumors form in the cavity of the bone and most often present in the long bones of the leg and arm.

Etiology and Pathophysiology

Bone metastasis and primary bone cancer are two separate disease processes and are treated differently. Secondary tumors arise from cells that have broken off from the original tumor site, enter the lymph system or bloodstream, and travel to that specific area. Bone metastases are generally observed in patients who have had a relapse in their cancer. Approximately 75% of the bone metastases originate from carcinomas of the prostate, breast, kidney, and lung. To a lesser extent, cancers that spread to the bone can come from thyroid cancer, colon cancer, and melanoma. The bones most commonly affected are the pelvis, vertebrae, ribs, femur, and humerus (Frazier & Drzymkowski, 2009).

Malignant bone tumors that are primary tumors are rare and typically emerge from connective and supportive tissue cells. Primary malignant bone tumors account for greater than 85% of bone tumors in the pediatric population but are rarely seen after the age of 30 (Frazier & Drzymkowski, 2009).

The exact cause of bone cancer is unknown. Recent findings suggest that an individual's DNA can become defective or mutated. Oncogenes promote cell division, and tumor suppressor genes cause cells to die or slow down cell division. DNA mutations can activate oncogenes or inactivate tumor suppressor genes. Also, it has been determined that individuals with bone cancer can inherit mutations from their parents. As a result, cancerous cells form a tumor and invade and destroy adjacent bone tissue. The tumor's rate of growth and response to treatment depend on the type of cancer involved. Most bone cancers are not inherited but result from acquired mutations. For instance, radiation is used as a treatment for some cancers but can also cause cancer by damaging DNA. Bones that are exposed to radiation as a treatment are more likely to develop bone cancer later (ACS, 2012a).

Bone destruction from the tumor can result in one of three different types of patterns: (1) geographic, (2) moth-eaten, or (3) permeative. With the geographic pattern, the tumor edges have well-defined margins. In the moth-eaten pattern, the margins are less defined and are easily separated from the bone. When the margins are not clear and abnormal lytic bone merges with normal bone, this is suggestive of the permeative pattern (McCance & Huether, 2009). Bone tumors that are considered malignant include osteosarcoma, chondrosarcoma, chordoma, and Ewing tumor. Lymphoma and multiple myeloma also start in the bones but are not considered bone cancer because they develop in the lymph nodes and in the plasma cells, respectively.

Osteosarcoma, the most common primary bone cancer, usually presents between the ages of 10 and 15 years. It usually develops in the distal femur, followed by the proximal tibia and humerus. Most patients die within 2 years from metastasis to the lung. Risk factors include Paget's disease, parathyroid injections for osteoporosis, and radiation therapy for other forms of cancer (Frazier & Drzymkowski, 2009).

Ewing's sarcoma involves the pelvis and lower extremity. The tumor typically presents between the ages of 4 and 25 years of age. The tumor is invasive and extends into the soft tissue. Metastasis occurs early and usually involves the lungs and other bones (Frazier & Drzymkowski, 2009). Chondrosarcoma also involves the pelvis and lower extremity but usually presents in patients between the ages of 30 and 60 years old. The tumor grows slowly and is locally invasive (Frazier & Drzymkowski, 2009).

Clinical Manifestations

Because of the destruction and erosion of bone and the expansion of the tumor, pain is the primary symptom of bone cancer. The intensity of the pain can be mild to severe. If a fracture is sustained, the patient will have acute pain. As a result of swelling, the patient may experience range-of-motion (ROM) limitation and joint effusion. The area may be tender to palpation and warm to the touch with superficial blood vessels noticeable. Osteosarcoma begins with pain and swelling and a "sunburst" appearance on radiograph. Ewing's sarcoma presents with pain and swelling, fever, fatigue, anemia, and leukocytosis. On radiograph, the tumor has an "onion skin" appearance. Chondrosarcomas are slow growing, so the pain is intermittent and dull. The tumor presents a lobular pattern on radiograph.

Laboratory and Diagnostic Procedures

Radiographs are useful in demonstrating tumor activity and will show increases and decreases in bone density. Refer to the Laboratory and Diagnostic Tests for Bone Disorders box on page 1493 for additional tests.

Medical Management

The treatment of bone cancer is best achieved by a multidisciplinary team. The objective is to slow the growth of the tumor by destroying and removing the lesion. Depending on the specific type of bone tumor, treatment may involve chemotherapy, surgery, and/or radiation. Chapter 57 discusses chemotherapy and radiation. Chemotherapy may be administered before having surgery done and then again later to prevent metastases. A combination of therapies may be used to achieve the optimal response and minimize potential drug resistance. Immunotherapy and hormone therapy may also be used. Supportive care may be needed during the course of the disease and may involve case workers, social workers, and hospice.

Nursing Management

The care of the patient with bone cancer is challenging. Therapeutic management might include chemotherapy, radiologic therapy, surgery, and pharmacologic interventions. The primary focus of nursing care is relief of pain. Bone cancer pain tends to be worse at night and is localized. Refer to Chapter 12 for pain management. Surgery for bone cancer can range from removal of a small tumor to amputation or extensive resection such as a hemipelvectomy. Before surgery, the nurse should encourage the patient to eat foods high in protein and vitamins to promote wound healing. The patient and family should be taught exercises that, after surgery, will strengthen the affected limb and prevent contractures. Physical therapy will be instrumental in helping with this. Exercising should begin within 24 hours after surgery to maintain muscle tone and prevent edema and muscle atrophy. If a prosthesis is to be fitted after healing, the stump should be wrapped to promote proper shrinking and shaping. The change in the patient's body image can create emotional stress. The nurse should listen to the patient's concerns and provide referrals for counseling or a support group. Nursing care that focuses on preoperative and postoperative care may be implemented if a surgical procedure is indicated (refer to Chapter 50). For a detailed discussion of care for the patient with cancer, refer to Chapter 57.

Collaborative Management

The overall goal in the planning and implementation phase is to promote healing that results in restored function of the affected body part. This often requires the help of many in the health care system. In order to meet desired patient outcomes, it is essential that this interdisciplinary team communicate openly with one another in developing and evaluating care of the patient and family (IOM [Institute of Medicine], 2010). In the older population, fractures can result in prolonged recovery periods and increase the risk for morbidity. A goal is to promote physical mobility; therefore, rehabilitation is begun as soon as possible to restore function. Physical therapy provides the patient with the knowledge and skills required to prevent muscle atrophy and enhance mobility with the use of assistive devices such as a walker and crutches. Home health nurses evaluate the patient and home for additional fall risks and promote safety upon the patient's return to home. Because healing requires adequate nutrition, a nutritionist may be consulted to assess caloric and protein intake. Dietary planning is based on the patient's need for calories, protein, and vitamins to promote healing.

A social worker or case manager may be another key member of the multidisciplinary team, providing coordination of appropriate inpatient and outpatient care. When the patient is discharged, the home health nurse becomes important for following medical treatment in the home environment. With these disease processes, strict adherence to the medical regimen is imperative to prevent recurrence of disease. Therefore, it is essential for the home health nurse to reinforce education on medication and appropriate lifestyle changes.

Health Promotion

Health promotion strategies focus on education. For example, the community needs to be aware of safety measures that can be taken to prevent fractures at home, at work, and during leisure activities. An assessment of the home environment can reveal potential hazards for falling, especially for the older population. Pathways in the house should be cleared of furniture, throw rugs, and clutter. For the older adult, adequate lighting and proper footwear are essential steps in preventing unnecessary falls.

Muscular Dystrophies

Muscular dystrophies are a group of genetically based myopathies caused by a protein deficiency in muscle membranes. In other words, the person's DNA is not producing a particular protein, named dystrophin, which muscles and muscle membranes require to function properly. Therefore, a person with a muscular dystrophy has progressive muscle weakness leading to an inability to control any voluntary movement (Figure 49–2◆). The muscles eventually atrophy from nonuse. Skeletal muscles are not the only muscles affected by muscular

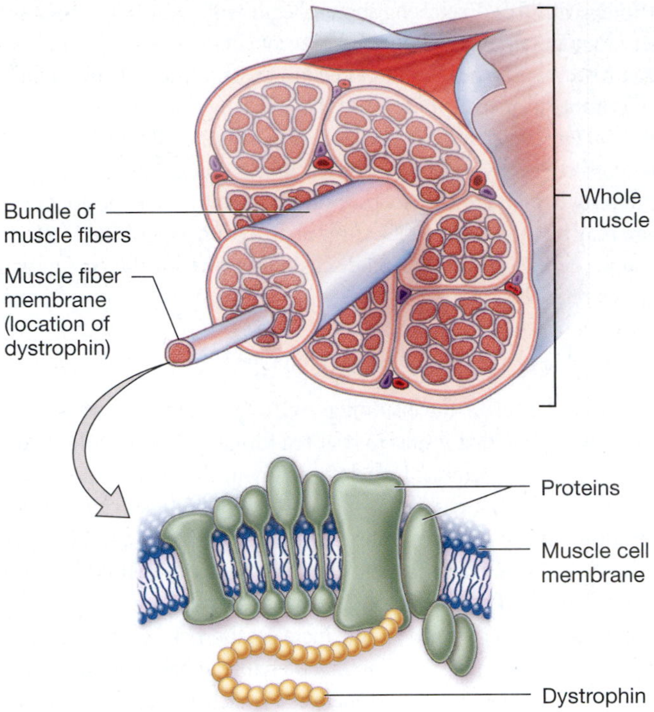

FIGURE 49–2 ◆ Muscle fiber membrane.

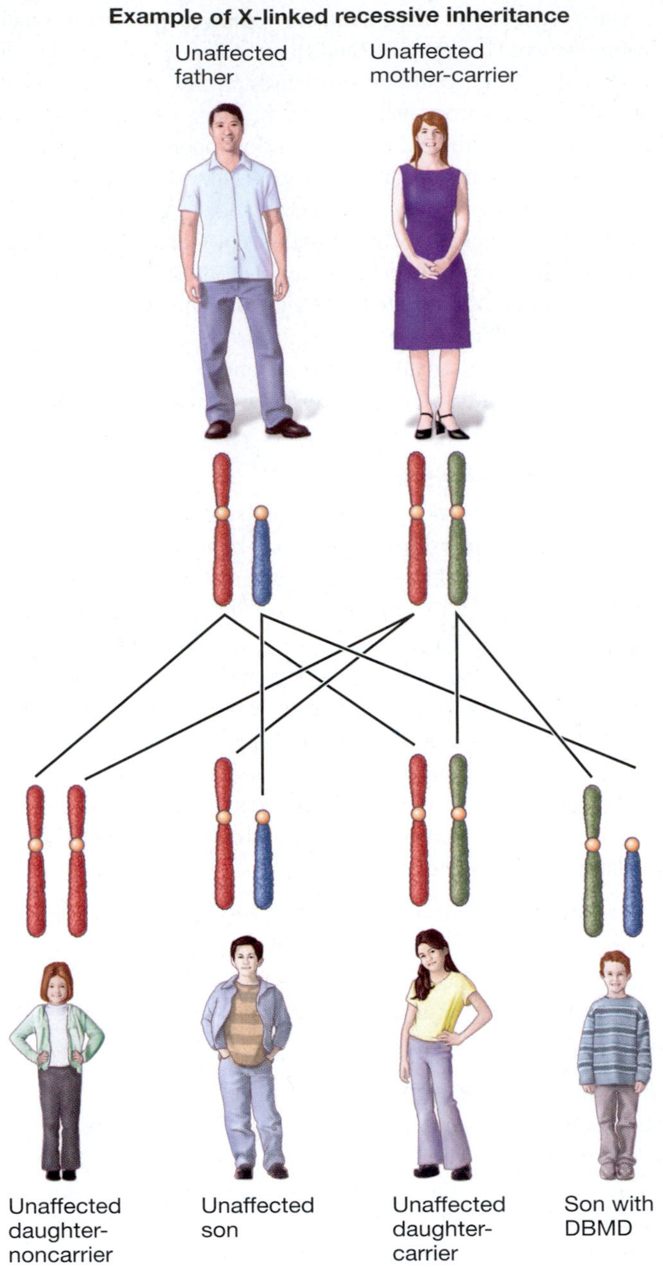

FIGURE 49–3 ◆ Muscular dystrophy inheritance pattern.

dystrophy; the cardiac muscle and diaphragm may be affected as well (Muscular Dystrophy Association [MDA], 2010a).

Genetics play the key role in whether a child develops muscular dystrophy (MD). Muscular dystrophy occurs when a gene on the X chromosome fails to make dystrophin. Most children afflicted with muscular dystrophy are males, because male children have only one X chromosome (from the mother). If that X chromosome is not producing dystrophin, then the child will develop MD. Female children receive X chromosomes from both parents, so even if one X chromosome is flawed, it is likely that the other X chromosome can provide the dystrophin, and these children will have few or no symptoms but will be carriers (Figure 49–3◆). Even though the incidence of MD is mostly in males, MD weakness develops in 2.5% to 20% of females. The incidence in male children is about 1 in 3,500 live male births (Centers for Disease Control and Prevention [CDC], 2010; MDA, 2010a).

Duchenne Muscular Dystrophy (DMD)

Etiology and Epidemiology

In children, especially male children, DMD is the most prevalent muscular dystrophy. In Duchenne muscular dystrophy, there is a complete absence of dystrophin. Muscle weakness and loss of muscle develop gradually. Signs usually first appear when the child is 2 through 6 years old, although symptoms generally are exhibited about age 3 (CDC, 2010). Weakness starts near the trunk, then progresses to the extremities about 3 to 5 years after the initial weakness is experienced. Most commonly, the lower extremities are affected before the upper extremities (Figure 49–4◆).

The weakness begins with the child having difficulty with simple tasks, such as maintaining balance, and leads to an inability to perform activities such as climbing stairs or getting up from a bed or chair. By school age, the child has an unsteady gait and falls quite often, perhaps appearing clumsy. The child uses the Gowers' maneuver to rise up from the floor (Figure 49–5◆). The Gowers' maneuver involves the child getting on his hands and knees, then raising his rear end, which allows the child to walk on his hands and knees, and then achieving a standing position (MDA, 2010a). Between the ages of 7 and 12, the child will lose the ability to walk and will use a wheelchair. Adolescents are usually unable to perform daily tasks, such as eating, with their arms, hands, or fingers. The course of the disease is progressive and usually fatal in the teens or early 20s. Death is usually due to respiratory or heart problems (CDC, 2010).

Becker Muscular Dystrophy (BMD)

Etiology and Epidemiology

Becker muscular dystrophy is a less common type of muscular dystrophy and is generally milder than DMD. In BMD, some dystrophin is produced, and the disease does not manifest itself until the teens or young adulthood when the person becomes weaker than usual when

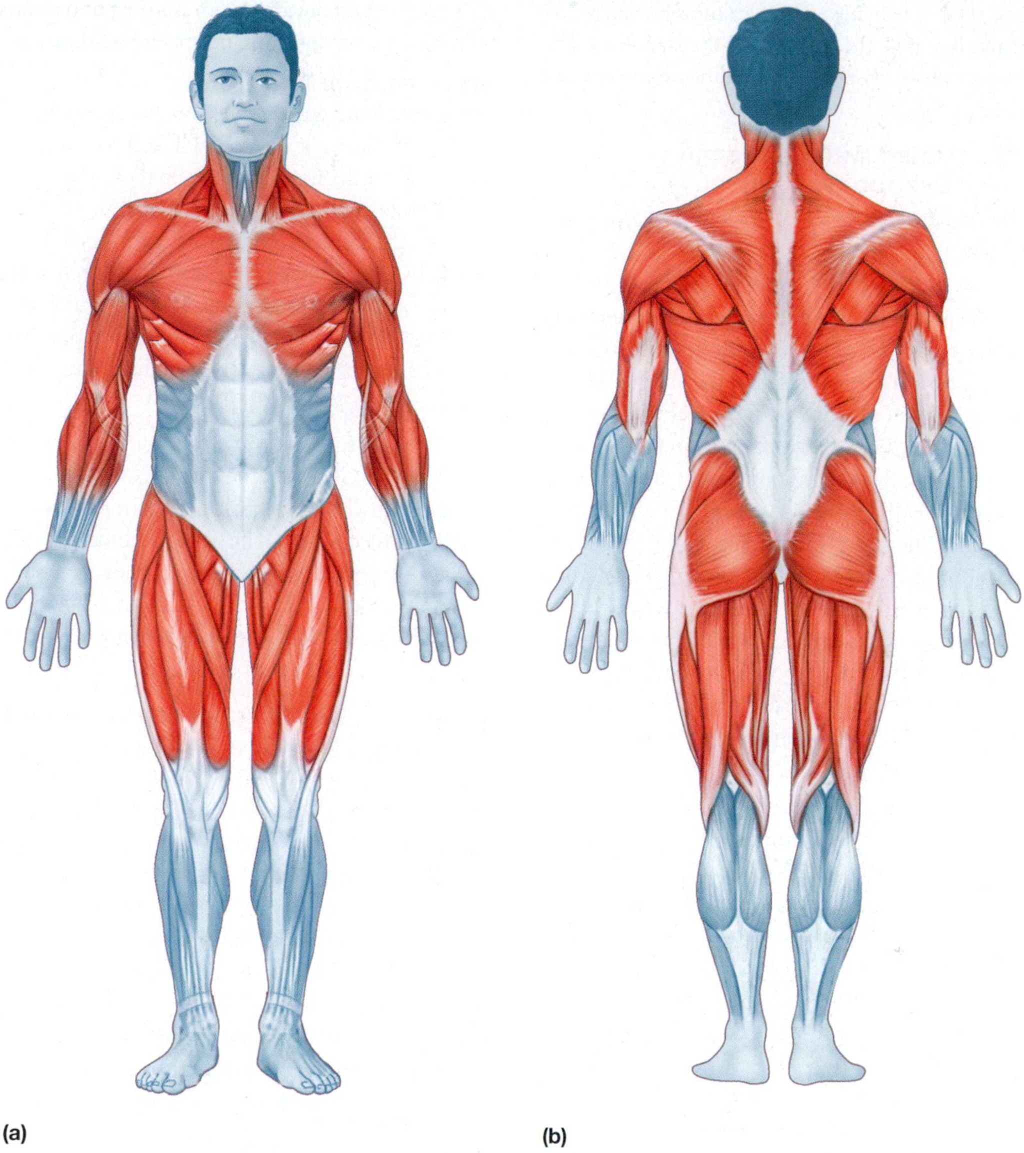

FIGURE 49–4 ◆ Muscles affected by muscular dystrophy.

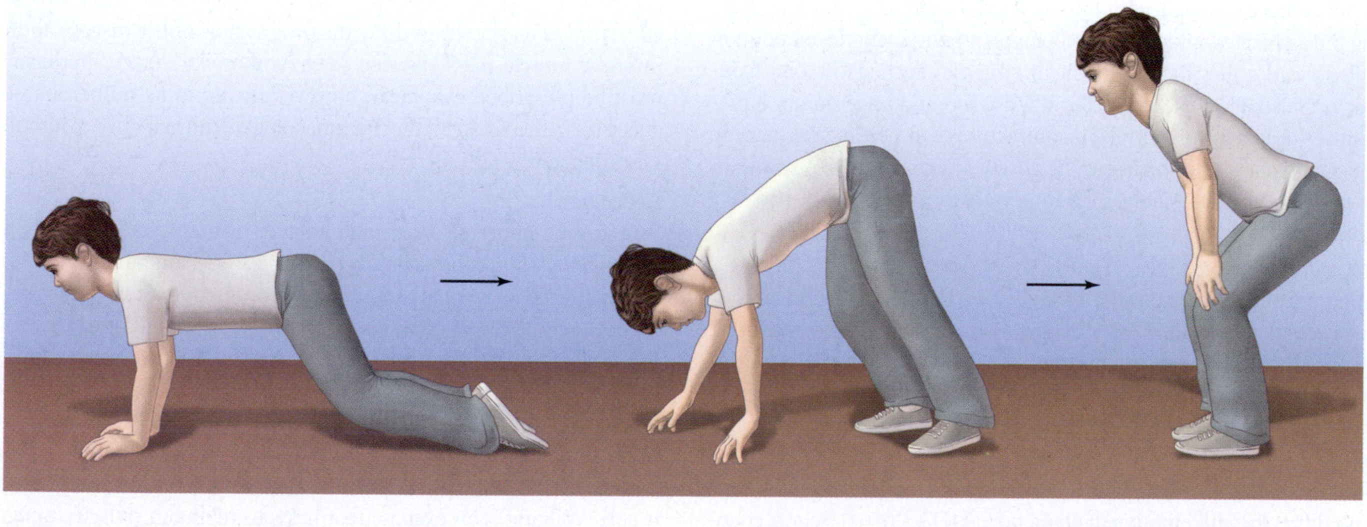

FIGURE 49–5 ◆ Gowers' maneuver.

engaging in physical exercise or activities. This weakness is usually first noticed in the pelvic and hip area, the thighs, and the shoulders. The severity and progression of the disease vary depending on the amount of dystrophin that is being produced.

Complications Associated with Duchenne or Becker Muscular Dystrophy

Both DMD and BMD may have several serious and sometimes life-threatening complications.

Cardiomyopathy

The most serious complications involve the cardiac and respiratory systems. As discussed in Chapter 33, cardiomyopathy is due to cardiac muscle weakening, which can be a direct result of the absence of dystrophin or an inadequate amount of dystrophin. Cardiomyopathy leads to heart failure, which is a major cause of death in patients with muscular dystrophy. Primary dilated cardiomyopathy and conduction abnormalities develop with DMD. Most MD patients do not become symptomatic until they are in their teens; the symptoms probably arise as a result of their lack of ability to exercise. Approximately 70% of people with BMD develop cardiomyopathy. As discussed in Chapter 33, patients with cardiomyopathy have shortness of breath, fluid in the lungs characterized by crackles or rhonchi, and lower extremity edema due to the heart muscle's inability to pump. Boys afflicted with muscular dystrophy often die from heart failure by the time they are in their 20s (CDC, 2010).

Respiratory Distress

Patients with muscular dystrophy have an increased risk for weakness of the diaphragm and other ancillary muscles that assist in ventilation (MDA, 2010a). If the diaphragm and other muscles are weak, the patient will have trouble expanding the chest to allow for effective inspiration and expiration. They will also have trouble coughing. Difficulty coughing coupled with weak, poor inspiratory/expiratory effort places MD patients at high risk for respiratory infections. Simply being in a room with someone who has a mild cold can predispose these patients to pneumonia. With progression of the disease, many of the patients will require long-term assisted mechanical ventilation or a tracheostomy. In addition, because patients with muscular dystrophy are prone to respiratory infections, it is extremely important for them to be current with their pneumococcal and flu vaccinations.

Muscle Atrophy and Contractures

When a muscle is weak and unused, it deteriorates and shortens, leaving the associated joint prone to being in a permanent flexed position called a *contracture*, the shortening of a muscle attached to a joint. Contractures can affect the knee, elbow, wrist, hip, and finger joints. If preventive measures are not taken, contractures can become permanent, causing total loss of mobility to the affected joint as well as discomfort. To prevent such contractures, it is important for all joints to be passively exercised.

Cognitive Effects

About one-third of the boys affected with Duchenne muscular dystrophy have some form of a progressive learning disability (MDA, 2010a). In addition, some children with DMD have some degree of mental retardation. Researchers believe that the lack of dystrophin in the brain affects the child's cognitive, behavioral, and intellectual abilities. Specific cognitive and intellectual skills that are affected are verbal skills, memory, attention, and focusing skills. In addition, some boys have difficulty with emotional interaction (MDA, 2010a). School counselors, psychologists, and neuropsychologists can educate the family in techniques that may assist with learning and interaction skills. People with BMD generally have a normal IQ for their age.

Spinal Abnormalities

Exaggerated curvature of the spine is prevalent in young adults with Duchenne muscular dystrophy. The three types of curvatures are lordosis (swayback), noticed mostly in those young men who are still able to ambulate; scoliosis, or a lateral curvature of the spine; and kyphosis (hunchback). Severe scoliosis can lead to respiratory problems, sleeping problems, and the inability to sit straight or remain seated for prolonged periods of time. Treatment for spinal curvatures consists of fusing vertebrae together to correct the curvature and may require attaching metal rods to the spine to help keep the spine in straight alignment.

Osteoporosis

Normally, muscles exert pressure on the bones they are attached to, which helps to maintain the strength of the bones. However, the weakening of muscles from muscular dystrophy can lead to weakening of bones, or osteoporosis. The bones become very thin and brittle, which can lead to pathologic fractures. In patients with muscular dystrophy, simple daily activities, such as lifting a heavy object or twisting, may cause a bone to break. Many patients in wheelchairs experience pathologic fractures due to their inability to bear weight.

Laboratory and Diagnostic Procedures

Diagnosis of muscular dystrophy is based on signs and symptoms noted specifically in toddlers in the prewalking or walking phase. Observance of the Gowers' maneuver is a telltale sign of muscular dystrophy. For other diagnostic tests, refer to the Laboratory and Diagnostic Tests for Muscular Disorders box.

Genetic testing may be done to look for a mutation in the dystrophin gene. The test first looks for large pieces of the gene that are missing or duplicated. If a deletion or duplication is found in the dystrophin gene, the diagnosis is confirmed. Between 65% to 70% of patients with DMD or BMD will have a deletion or duplication (CDC, 2010).

Pulmonary function tests and an electrocardiogram (ECG) may be done to evaluate the degree of respiratory or cardiac involvement.

Medical Management

At this time, there is no specific treatment for muscular dystrophy; however, modalities such as medications, exercise, and diet may enhance the patient's ability to move and function independently as long as possible.

Medications

A glucocorticoid such as prednisone, which has an anti-inflammatory effect, has been shown to delay the progression of the disease and to improve muscle mass (Frazier & Drzymkowski, 2009). Prednisone must be prescribed cautiously, however, owing to its numerous side effects, as discussed in the Pharmacology Summary for Muscular Disorders box.

Exercise

Exercise is important for people afflicted with muscular dystrophy. Ambulating should be encouraged because it maintains the motion of a joint and prevents the joint from contracting. Passive range-of-motion (PROM) exercises are helpful in preventing contractures of the joints if the patient cannot actively exercise. PROM exercises must be performed on each joint at least every 4 hours while the patient is awake to prevent the muscles and tendons associated with the joints from shortening or atrophying. A child who can walk should continue to walk, even if only short distances, for as many months or years as she is able. Walking is an exercise that helps to maintain muscle strength and mobility. If the child cannot or does not walk, the muscles will lose

LABORATORY AND DIAGNOSTIC TESTS for Muscular Disorders

Test With Description, Rationale and Normal Values	Expected Abnormality
Serum Creatinine Kinase (CK)	
Normal: male: 5–35 mcg/mL; female: 5–25 mcg/mL	Elevated.
Normally there are high levels of CK in muscle and low levels in serum. Increased levels in serum indicate muscle membrane breakdown with release of CK.	20 to 200 times higher with MD (CDC, 2010). >100 times normal with rhabdomyolosis.
Serum Potassium	
Normal: 3.5–5.3 mEq/L	Less than 3 mEq/L with hypokalemic myopathy.
To monitor electrolyte abnormalities.	
Urinalysis	
Normal:	Presence of myoglobin with rhabdomyolosis.
Protein: 2–8 mg/dL; negative reagent strip	
Glucose: negative	
Red blood cells: 1–2	
Casts: mixed hyaline	
Used to detect myoglobin in the urine when there is muscle breakdown.	
Muscle Biopsy	
Normal muscle tissue.	Absence of dystrophin.
Test for dystrophin.	
Electromyelogram (EMG)	
Normal electrical activity in muscles.	Decreased electrical conduction due to muscle damage.
Will differentiate between a myopathy and neuropathy.	

strength and atrophy more quickly. General aquatic therapy in warm water also maintains the muscle tone.

It is also important for patients with muscular dystrophy to maintain a reasonable body weight. Obesity can cause exacerbation or worsening of respiratory and cardiac dysfunction, whereas weight loss beyond a healthy weight can signify muscle wasting and decreasing energy stores and can further complicate an already weakened cardiac and respiratory system.

Myotonic Muscular Dystrophy (MMD)

Etiology and Epidemiology

Myotonic dystrophy, or Steinert's disease, is the most common adult form of muscular dystrophy. It affects at least 1 in 8,000 persons worldwide. Like Duchenne muscular dystrophy, it is caused by a defective gene that is transferred from one generation to another. The manifestations of myotonic dystrophy involve muscle wasting of the distal extremities, including the hands, forearms, and feet, and also the face and neck. The *myotonic* part of the term *myotonic dystrophy* refers to a delay in the relaxation phase after muscle contraction, as when a person is unable to release his hand after gripping something. Fifty percent of the cases of myotonic dystrophy are diagnosed by age 20; however, many cases are not diagnosed until 50 years of age (MDA, 2010a).

Clinical Manifestations

Myotonic dystrophy is a multisystem disease, affecting organs and tissues other than muscles. For example, myotonic dystrophy can affect the eyes, specifically in the manifestation of cataracts; the muscles involved in swallowing, resulting in dysphagia; the respiratory system, involving weakness of the diaphragm and an adverse reaction to anesthesia; the gastrointestinal system, including decreased peristalsis; and the endocrine system, resulting in alteration or inappropriate insulin secretion, increased carbohydrate metabolism, and excessive sleeping (MDA, 2010a). Unlike other dystrophies that can usually be diagnosed on the basis of muscle wasting symptoms alone, myotonic dystrophy is often diagnosed on the basis of the presentation of other symptoms. In some cases, the patient's initial complaint to the health care provider may be a change in vision or difficulty swallowing.

Laboratory and Diagnostic Procedures

Myotonic muscular dystrophy is diagnosed by a complaint of distal weakness and myotonia. Refer to the Laboratory and Diagnostic Tests for Muscular Disorders box on page 1501 for further tests. DNA testing will also delineate a diagnosis of myotonic dystrophy by finding an abnormality on chromosome 19. Some patients in the early stages of the disease have the "classic" look of myotonic dystrophy: muscle wasting of the face, jaw, neck, hands, feet, and forearms.

Medical Management

Treatment involves support of the wasting muscles. In addition, treatment will focus on avoiding complications such as constipation from decreased gastric peristalsis, aspiration from difficulty swallowing, and decreased visual acuity from resulting cataracts.

Medications used for myotonic dystrophy include phenytoin (Dilantin), mexiletine (Mexil), carbamazepine (Tegretol), quinine, and procainamide (Pronestyl). (Refer to the Pharmacology Summary for Muscular Disorders box on page 1507.) All of these medications may be useful in treating the delayed muscle relaxation that generally occurs in patients with myotonic dystrophy (Mayo Clinic, 2009).

Limb Girdle Muscular Dystrophy

Etiology and Epidemiology

Limb girdle muscular dystrophy, which primarily affects the pelvic and shoulder areas, is a genetic disease that causes protein defects in the biologic function of muscle. Limb girdle muscular dystrophy generally has a slow progression rate, but it may progress rapidly in some patients. Muscle weakness and wasting may begin at the upper extremities and progress to the lower extremities, or may have the opposite pattern of progression. The signs and symptoms are usually noted during childhood, but they can also begin during the teen years and into adulthood. The number of male and female cases is about equal, and frequency has been estimated to be 5 to 70 per 1 million population (Lopate, 2011).

Facioscapulohumeral Disease

Etiology and Epidemiology

Facioscapulohumeral disease (FSHD) is a rare type of muscular dystrophy that affects the face, shoulder girdle, and upper arms and is more common in females than males. It is the third-most common muscular dystrophy, with an estimated prevalence of 1 per 20,000 persons. Diagnosis is made on the basis of specific symptoms, which include weakness in the muscles that open and close the eyes; the muscles that allow a person to purse the lips, to smile, and to whistle; and the muscles that stabilize the scapula. Other affected muscles include the muscles of the hip girdle, foot, and abdomen. The diagnosis of FSHD is usually made by the time a person is in her 20s. The progression of this type of muscular dystrophy is insidious, with extended periods when the disease seems to be arrested (Sripathi, 2010).

Oculopharyngeal Muscular Dystrophy

Etiology and Epidemiology

Oculopharyngeal muscular dystrophy is a rare condition that generally strikes people who are in their 50s and 60s. The most prominent feature is bilateral ptosis, in which the eyelids droop to the level of, or below the level of, the pupil. The patient has a contraction of the occipitofrontal muscle (muscle at the forehead) that is evident on observation and tends to tip the forehead back to compensate for the ptosis, which can impair vision. The patient also has ocular muscle weakness, which prevents lateral eye movement, and weakness of the pharyngeal muscles (ineffective gag reflex), leading to dysphagia for solid foods.

Patients with oculopharyngeal muscular dystrophy also have weakness in their leg muscles and proximal hip girdle. The long-term problems associated with oculopharyngeal muscular dystrophy have less to do with the muscle weakness than with the dysphagia and the resulting possibility of aspiration pneumonia. With supplemental nutrition, modification to food consistency, and proper positioning, patients with this type of muscular dystrophy can have a good quality of life.

Nursing Management

Nursing care for patients with muscular dystrophy is aimed at supporting the patient's independence level, preventing complications, and preventing injury, as discussed in the Nursing Process: Patient Care Plan for Muscular Dystrophy box.

Muscular Dystrophy and Aging

As people with muscular dystrophy age, they experience many symptoms that adults without muscular dystrophy also experience. Eyesight often becomes poor. Cataracts are more prevalent in older adults, as is arcus senilis, a thin gray-white ring that surrounds the eye margin and may affect the vision. Peristalsis slows down, and appetite and nutritional caloric needs decrease with age. Because protein is so important for maintenance of healthy muscles, especially in a patient with MD, the nurse should take care to assist patients in meal planning or refer the patient to a dietitian. See the Patient Teaching & Discharge Priorities for Muscular Dystrophy box for more information.

Collaborative Management

Patients with muscular dystrophies require many types of care, involving a multidisciplinary team. The nurse, nutritionist, physical therapist, occupational therapist, and orthotics technician will assist the patient to maintain mobility for as long as possible. For the caregiver, assistance from a financial counselor, psychologist, and home health nurse, as well as access to respite care, will decrease the chance of severe caregiver role strain. In order to meet desired patient outcomes, it is essential that this interdisciplinary team communicate openly with one another in developing and evaluating care of the patient and family (IOM [Institute of Medicine], 2010).

Physical Therapy

Physical therapy is aimed at prolonging muscle strength and thus preventing contractures. Both active and passive ROM exercises are indicated, and walking is encouraged if possible to enhance strength and stamina. Physical therapy should also focus on gait training and transfer training. When the patient has lost the ability to ambulate, she needs to see a physical therapist for customization of a wheelchair, recommendations about devices that assist with ADLs, and help accomplishing tasks.

Occupational Therapy

Occupational therapy focuses on exercises that allow the patient with MD to perform ADLs such as eating, dressing, and brushing teeth. Whereas physical therapy focuses on gross motor movements, occupational therapy focuses more on the maintenance of fine motor movements.

Braces and Standing Walkers

Braces may be used to support the ankles and feet of an ambulatory child with MD. Braces are also utilized to prevent plantar flexion, a type of contracture. A standing walker can assist the patient to stand, thus promoting circulation and allowing the patient to bear weight on her joints.

Health Promotion

Because muscular dystrophy is a lifelong problem, health promotion involves exercise and good nutrition to keep as healthy as possible. A balanced diet supplemented with vitamins and amino acids can help the patient maintain a normal weight and manage the debilitating symptoms. The diet should include good sources of protein (fish, lean meats, and beans), foods that contain antioxidants (blueberries, cherries, tomatoes), and dark green vegetables. Maintaining adequate fluid balance is also important to maintain healthy cells, so six to eight glasses of water is recommended. Supplements that may be included are omega-3 fatty acids to enhance the immune system, calcium to support muscles and bones, coenzyme Q10 to support the immune and muscular system, probiotics to maintain the digestive tract, and glutamine as an energy source for the cells. The nurse should encourage the patient to have a dietitian perform ongoing assessment of his nutritional needs.

NURSING PROCESS: Patient Care Plan for Muscular Dystrophy

Assessment of Musculoskeletal Status Using Gordon's Functional Health Patterns:

- Health Perception Health Management Pattern
- Nutrition Metabolic Pattern
- Elimination Pattern
- Activity Exercise Pattern
- Role-Relationship Pattern

Subjective Data	Objective Data
Assessment of Muscle Strength Are you experiencing weakness in any muscle groups? Are you having difficulty walking or do you feel off balance?	**Assessment of Muscle Strength** Assess strength in the upper and lower extremities. Observe the patient as she ambulates.
Assessment of Nutritional Status Do you have difficulty swallowing? What types of food do you eat? Who prepares your meals?	**Assessment of Nutritional Status** Assess the patient's skin turgor and fragility. Assess for excessive loss of hair.
Assessment of Swallowing Ability Do you have difficulty swallowing? Do you ever choke on your food?	**Assessment of Swallowing Ability** Depressed cough and gag reflexes. Impaired swallowing.
Assessment of Breathing Do you have difficulty breathing? Do you feel short of breath?	**Assessment of Breathing** Ineffective chest excursion. Nasal flaring. Orthopnea. Use of accessory muscles to breathe.
Assessment of Elimination How often do you have a bowel movement? Is it difficult for you to have a bowel movement?	**Assessment of Elimination** Document frequency and quality of bowel movements.
Assessment of Self-Care Are you able to bathe yourself? Do you become fatigued with simple activities of daily living?	**Assessment of Self-Care** Observe the patient's ability to get in and out of the bath and wash her body or body parts.
Assessment of Cardiac Function Do you experience shortness of breath with physical activity?	**Assessment of Cardiac Function** Assess the patient's activity tolerance by noting the onset of shortness of breath or pain.
Assessment of Caregiver Role Are you having any difficulty with any of the caregiver tasks? How is your health? Are you having trouble sleeping? Do you have any concerns regarding your loved one's care?	**Assessment of Caregiver Role** Is the caregiver: • Experiencing headaches? • Losing or gaining weight? • Angry? • Feeling depressed?

Outcomes and Evaluation Parameters	Planning and Interventions with *Rationales*
1. NURSING DIAGNOSIS: (a) Activity Intolerance. (b) Impaired Physical Mobility ***related to muscle weakness*** **(NANDA-I © 2012)**	
Outcome: Ability to maintain enough muscle strength to ambulate as long as possible. ***Evaluation Parameter:*** Ability to stand with assistive devices.	Teach the family to perform PROM exercises. Have them do the exercises three times a day. *Maintains joint mobility and prevents contractures.* Administer prednisone if prescribed. *May improve muscle mass and prolong ambulation.* Teach the patient and family the need to maintain appropriate weight. *Obesity makes it difficult for the patient to move and support herself.* Teach the patient/family the importance of maintaining safety in the home by keeping it uncluttered *to prevent injury.*

(continued)

NURSING PROCESS: Patient Care Plan for Muscular Dystrophy, *continued*

Outcomes and Evaluation Parameters	Planning and Interventions with *Rationales*
2. NURSING DIAGNOSIS: Nutrition, Imbalanced: Less Than Body Requirements ***related to difficulty swallowing and muscle weakness*** **(NANDA-I © 2012)**	
Outcome: The patient/family will be able to understand the rationale for, and provide, well-balanced meals three times a day. ***Evaluation Parameters:*** The patient will not experience weight loss of 2.5 kg in a 24-hour period. The patient will drink at least one supplement per day.	Ensure a well-balanced meal high in protein, carbohydrate, fiber, vitamins, and minerals *to promote healthy bones, muscles, and tissues and to provide energy.* Weigh daily, using the same scale and the same type of clothing. *Weight loss may indicate muscle-mass wasting, as well as possible malnutrition.* Provide carbohydrate and/or protein supplements as needed. *Supplements assist in maintaining adequate nutrition, which is required to maintain a healthy musculoskeletal system.*
3. NURSING DIAGNOSIS: Aspiration, Risk for ***related to muscle weakness and difficulty swallowing*** **(NANDA-I © 2012)**	
Outcome: The patient will not aspirate. ***Evaluation Parameters:*** The patient will have an intact gag reflex. The patient will have clear lung sounds before and after eating and drinking.	Assess the patient's gag reflex prior to administering food or fluids. *A gag reflex that is not intact is a precursor to aspiration.* Assess lung sounds before and after meals/drinking. *A new onset of adventitious lung sounds may indicate aspiration.* Assess respiratory status before and after meals/drinking. *Shortness of breath, difficulty breathing, and increased respiratory rate may be indicative of aspiration.* Provide thickened liquids. *Thickened liquids are easier to swallow through the esophagus and into the stomach.* Teach the patient and family to eat small bites of food. *Patient is less likely to choke.*
4. NURSING DIAGNOSIS: Breathing, Ineffective ***related to muscle weakness*** **(NANDA-I © 2012)**	
Outcome: The patient will demonstrate effective breathing patterns. ***Evaluation Parameters:*** The patient will have eupneic respirations and normal color and will breathe without the use of accessory muscles. The patient will have an oxygen saturation level of between 90% and 100%.	Observe for dyspnea (difficulty breathing), pallor or cyanosis, rate and depth of respirations, and use of accessory muscles. *Tachypnea (rapid respiratory rate, usually greater than 24 per minute), bradypnea (slow respiratory rate, usually less than 10 per minute), and shallow respirations will indicate respiratory dysfunction.* Monitor oxygen saturation levels via pulse oximeter. *Levels below 90% may indicate hypoxia.* Encourage rest periods as needed *to allow for easier respirations.* Teach pursed-lip and deep breathing exercises *to expand lungs for maximum oxygen intake and expel carbon dioxide.*
5. NURSING DIAGNOSIS: Constipation, Risk for ***related to decreased peristalsis*** **(NANDA-I © 2012)**	
Outcome: The patient will not be constipated. ***Evaluation Parameter:*** The patient will not have difficulty having a bowel movement.	Provide a high-fiber diet. *Fiber adds bulk to the stool.* Encourage the patient to drink 2,500 mL of fluid per day (unless contraindicated by a medical condition). *Fluids help to maintain a soft stool.* Administer stool softener as ordered *to maintain a soft stool.* Reposition the patient every 2 to 4 hours *to facilitate peristalsis.*
6. NURSING DIAGNOSIS: Self-Care Deficit: Bathing/Hygiene ***related to muscle weakness*** **(NANDA-I © 2012)**	
Outcome: The patient will participate in all aspects of care and ADLs. ***Evaluation Parameter:*** The patient will be able to wash his body with minimal assistance.	Allow as much independence as possible, allowing the patient to assist in tasks that maintain or build self-esteem. *Maintenance of a positive attitude will allow for a better quality of life.*
7. NURSING DIAGNOSIS: Cardiac Output, Decreased ***related to muscle weakness*** **(NANDA-I © 2012)**	
Outcome: Patient will demonstrate increasing tolerance for physical activity. ***Evaluation Parameters:*** The patient will have audible S_1 and S_2 heart sounds. The patient will not have any cyanosis or pallor. The patient's capillary refill will be 3 seconds or less.	Monitor heart sounds. *Muffled heart sounds may be indicative of cardiomyopathy.* Assess color. *Pallor or cyanosis may be indicative of decreased cardiac output.* Assess capillary refill. *Capillary refill greater than 3 seconds may indicate decreased cardiac output.* Schedule rest periods between activities *to decrease the heart's workload.* Restrict fluids *to decrease the workload of the heart.*
8. NURSING DIAGNOSIS: Caregiver Role Strain, Risk for ***related to extent of care needed*** **(NANDA-I © 2012)**	
Outcome: The caregiver will demonstrate emotional health. ***Evaluation Parameters:*** Free of anger. Free of depression. Less frustrated. Verbalizes a sense of control and self-esteem.	Refer the patient/family to the Muscular Dystrophy Association and other local support groups. *Discussing concerns with others in the same situation provides a support network.* Allow the patient/family to verbalize fears/concerns. *This provides support.*

Source: Adapted from Wilkinson, J. M., & Ahearn, N. R. (2009). *Prentice Hall nursing diagnosis handbook* (9th ed.). Upper Saddle River, NJ: Prentice Hall.

PATIENT TEACHING & DISCHARGE PRIORITIES for Muscular Dystrophy

Need	Teaching
Safety: Setting (home)	Maintain a safe environment by having travel paths free of furniture and other items. Remove throw rugs, electrical wires, clutter, toys, and so on.
Proper nutrition: Patient	Eat a well-balanced diet including proteins, carbohydrates, minerals, and vitamins.
Self-care activities: Patient and family	Have the patient provide as much of her own care as possible to maintain independence, but rest when needed.
Maintain mobility: Patient and family	Move joints as much as possible.
Prevent constipation: Patient and family	Eat a diet high in fiber and drink at least 2,500 mL of fluid/day.

Myopathies

Myopathy refers to any disease of the muscle (National Institute of Neurological Disorders and Stroke [NINDS], 2010). There are various forms of myopathies, which can be inherited or can occur in later years (Chart 49–4). Myopathies can also be secondary complications due to endocrine disorders, metabolic disorders, muscle inflammation or infection, certain drugs, or gene mutations (NINDS, 2010).

The inflammatory myopathies are a group of acquired and treatable diseases of the skeletal muscle with moderate to severe muscle weakness. The three types of inflammatory myopathies are polymyositis, dermatomyositis, and inclusion body myositis.

Generalized Myopathy

Clinical Manifestations

The major clinical manifestation of generalized myopathy is weakness of the limbs. In some cases, exercise increases the weakness; in other cases, exercise improves the weakness or even causes it to disappear (NINDS, 2010). Affected muscle groups vary by patient.

Medical Management

Treatment varies according to the type of myopathy. Some patients may require symptomatic treatment only; others may require supportive care, such as braces or other orthotic devices, medications, or physical therapy (NINDS, 2010). The Pharmacology Summary for Muscular Disorders box (p. 1507) lists medications used to treat myopathies. The prognosis for myopathies again varies depending on the type. Some patients do not have a disrupted quality of life; for others, the myopathy may be disabling. Following are descriptions of specific myopathies, clinical presentations, and their specific medical management. Nursing management for the patient with myopathies is presented at the end of the section.

Congenital Myopathy

This type of myopathy is due to a chromosomal defect leading to **hypotonia,** an absence of muscle tone resulting in flaccid, weak muscles in infancy and weakness and delayed motor activity in later childhood years. Diagnosis of a congenital myopathy is made by muscle tissue sampling, which indicates changes in the structure and morphology of the muscle. Treatment is supportive.

Hypokalemic Myopathy

Acute periods of paralysis are referred to as hypokalemic and may be primary or secondary to excessive renal or GI losses. Attacks usually occur at night or in the early morning upon awakening. Hypokalemic myopathy can also be precipitated by a diet high in carbohydrates or from glucose or insulin given intravenously (Bethel, 2009). Hypokalemic paralysis can occur with diabetic ketoacidosis, chronic diarrhea, renal tubular acidosis, or other chronic conditions that cause hypokalemia, or after amphotericin B treatment.

CHART 49–4 Types of Myopathies

Type	Signs/Symptoms
Congenital	Chromosomal defect leading to hypotonia in infancy and weakness and delayed motor activity in later childhood years.
Hypokalemic	Common in older adults and due to an electrolyte imbalance caused by long-term diuretic use. Affects the proximal muscles of the legs, arms, trunk, and neck; may affect the thoracic muscles and diaphragm.
Mitochondrial	Affects the ocular muscles; may cause encephalomyopathies (a heterogeneous group of disorders that cause alterations of mitochondrial metabolism that result in muscle and nervous system dysfunction).
Steroidal	Chronic use of prednisone can lead to muscle weakness, as well as an increased risk for pathologic fractures.
Inflammatory:	Acquired diseases of the skeletal muscle.
• Polymyositis	Generalized muscle weakness.
• Dermatomyositis	Identified by a heliotrope (bluish-purplish in color) rash and muscle weakness.
• Inclusion body myositis	Progressive inflammation of the muscles, usually in men over 50 years of age.

Clinical Manifestations

Muscle weakness due to hypokalemic myopathy develops gradually and usually affects the proximal muscles of the legs, arms, trunk, and neck. Deep tendon reflexes are less active than normal or may be inactive (Bethel, 2009).

Medical Management

Potassium replacement therapy reverses hypokalemic myopathy within 1 month. Chronic hypokalemic myopathy may need to be treated with oral potassium supplements, and the nurse should encourage the patient to eat foods rich in potassium such as avocado, banana, cantaloupe, dates, figs, orange juice, potatoes, prunes, and some salt substitutes.

Mitochondrial Myopathy

Mitochondrial myopathy is named for the mitochondria, the cell part responsible for producing most of the energy that the cell needs to function. A mitochondrial disease can shut down some or all of the mitochondria, depleting the essential energy supply. Because muscle cells and nerve cells have especially high energy needs, muscular and neurological problems are common features of mitochondrial disease. Symptoms can include muscle weakness, exercise intolerance, hearing loss, trouble with balance and coordination, seizures, and learning deficits (MDA, 2010b).

Medical Management

Treatments aim at fixing or bypassing the defective mitochondria. These treatments are dietary supplements based on three natural substances involved in the production of the energy molecule ATP. One supplement is creatine, which normally acts as a reserve for ATP by forming a compound called *creatine phosphate*. When a cell's demand for ATP exceeds the amount its mitochondria can produce, creatine can release phosphate to rapidly enhance the ATP supply. Another substance is carnitine, which improves the efficiency of ATP production by helping import certain fuel molecules into mitochondria, and cleaning up some of the toxic by-products of ATP production. Carnitine is available as an over-the-counter supplement called L-carnitine. The third supplement is coenzyme Q10 (coQ10), which is a component of the electron transport chain that uses oxygen to manufacture ATP. Some mitochondrial diseases are caused by coQ10 deficiency, and there is evidence that coQ10 supplementation is beneficial in these cases (MDA, 2010b).

Steroid-Induced Myopathy

Long-term corticosteroid usage can lead to muscle weakness and increased risk for pathologic fractures. Steroid-induced myopathy is especially seen with prolonged high doses and/or in patients who take corticosteroids for more than 1 year (Bethel, 2009).

Medical Management

Unless contraindicated, the patient should be changed to a less frequent regime of corticosteroids as soon as possible. A daily exercise regimen is recommended to promote muscle tone.

Polymyositis

Polymyositis (PM) is a type of myopathy that occurs slowly over weeks and months. It is an autoimmune connective tissue disorder that causes damage to muscle fibers. Polymyositis usually affects proximal muscles and causes weakness to those muscles.

Polymyositis affects predominantly women and African Americans ages 45 to 65 years old. It is rare in patients younger than 20 years (Rosenkranz, 2010). The cause of PM is unknown, but it may be triggered by viral, bacterial, or parasitic agents, drugs, vaccinations, or even stress.

Clinical Manifestations

Symptoms that accompany polymyositis may be systemic as well as muscular. Generalized muscle weakness is the main complaint from patients. The weakness is most prevalent in the hips and thighs and begins as an "ache." The initial complaint that brings most patients to see the health care provider is weakness in the upper and lower extremities. Patients with PM also may experience fatigue, weight loss, and changes in nails or skin, including a rash or redness. Systemic involvement includes dysphagia, cardiac involvement, and respiratory involvement. Polymyositis may also occur with another connective tissue disorder; this is known as an overlap syndrome.

Laboratory and Diagnostic Procedures

Diagnosis of polymyositis is based on symptomology, the exclusion of other neuromuscular diseases, muscle biopsy findings, elevated serum CK levels (muscle enzymes), and an abnormal electromyography. The confirmatory diagnosis is made with five criteria: proximal muscle weakness, elevated CK, EMG changes, positive muscle biopsy, and a typical skin rash.

Medical Management

The treatment for polymyositis depends on the severity of the symptoms and the involvement of other systems. The goal of treatment is to improve the patient's quality of life, thus allowing the patient to carry out her normal ADLs. Various medications are used to treat polymyositis, including prednisone and immunosuppressive drugs, such as methotrexate and azathioprine (Imuran) (Rosenkranz, 2010). Refer to the Pharmacology Summary for Muscular Disorders box.

The prognosis is poor if the muscle weakness is progressive and severe. This may lead to aspiration pneumonia, dysphagia, malnutrition, and respiratory failure. The patient will benefit from physical therapy and a scheduled exercise routine. Frequent monitoring for progression of muscle weakness is warranted.

Dermatomyositis

Dermatomyositis, an autoimmune disease that affects the small blood vessels and capillaries in muscles, is identified by a heliotrope (bluish-purplish) rash and muscle weakness. Degeneration of the skin and muscle ultimately occur, leading to bilateral muscle weakness and some muscle atrophy, mostly of the proximal limb muscles. The heliotrope rash is noted on the eyelids, while an erythematous rash is noted on the chest, face, and neck. Gottron's rash, a reddish raised rash or papule, is noted on the metacarpophalangeal joints and the interphalangeal joints. The nail beds are thick and cracked. Dermatomyositis affects women more than men and is also observed in children, usually those ages 5 to 14 years (Rosenkranz, 2010).

Clinical Manifestations

The patient with dermatomyositis presents with one or more of the following signs: the heliotrope rash; Gottron's papules, which are violet-colored plaques at the finger joints; or **Gottron's sign,** a reddened smooth, scaly rash at the finger joints often accompanied by thickened fingernails and muscle weakness. However, the rash may be noted without muscle weakness. The weakness is a gradual process, usually

PHARMACOLOGY Summary for Muscular Disorders

Medication Category and Action	Application/Indication	Nursing Responsibility
Anticonvulsant		
Phenytoin (Dilantin) ***Action:*** Helps stabilize the neurons by regulating voltage-dependent sodium and calcium channels, inhibiting calcium movement across neuronal membranes, and enhancing sodium-potassium ATP activity in neurons and glial cells.	To treat delayed muscle relaxation with MMD (Mayo Clinic, 2009).	Preferred administration routes are oral and intravenous injection. If the patient has difficulty swallowing, open the rapid-release capsules and mix with food or fluid. To minimize gastric distress, give medication with or just after meals. If administering through a nasogastric tube, minimize drug absorption in tubing by diluting the suspension threefold with sodium chloride or sterile water. After administration, flush the tube with at least 20 mL of diluent. Long-term therapy may increase the patient's requirements for folic acid or vitamin D supplements.
Class IB Antiarrhythmic		
Mexiletine (Mexil) ***Action:*** Inhibits fast sodium channels in myocardial cell membranes.	To treat delayed muscle relaxation with MMD (Mayo Clinic, 2009).	Assess for signs of thrombocytopenia, which can occur within a few days of starting mexiletine therapy. Teach the patient to take the drug at evenly spaced intervals to avoid missing doses. To minimize gastric distress, give the medication with food.
Analgesic, Anticonvulsant		
Carbamazepine (Tegretol) ***Action:*** Slows nerve impulse transmission by blocking sodium channels, thus preventing sodium from entering the cell.	To treat delayed muscle relaxation with MMD.	Drug is metabolized by the liver, so use with caution in patients with impaired hepatic function. Monitor white blood cell and platelet counts. Decreased counts may indicate bone marrow depression. To minimize gastric distress, give medication with food. Teach the patient to wear sunscreen to prevent photosensitivity reactions. Teach the patient and family to notify the health care provider if the patient experiences unusual bleeding or bruising, fever, rash, or mouth ulcers.
Antiarrhythmic		
Procainamide (Pronestyl) ***Action:*** Inhibits sodium influx through cell membranes.	To treat delayed muscle relaxation with MMD (Mayo Clinic, 2009).	Teach the patient to swallow extended release tablets whole, without crushing or chewing them. If the patient has difficulty swallowing, have the patient crush regular-release tablets or open capsules and mix them with food or fluid. Teach the patient to take medication 1 to 2 hours after meals with a full glass of water. Teach the patient and family to notify the health care provider if the patient experiences unusual bleeding or bruising, fever, rash, or diarrhea.
Antipsoriatic, Antirheumatic		
Methotrexate ***Action:*** Inhibits dihydrofolate reductase, the enzyme that reduces folic acid to tetrahydrofolic acid. Inhibition of the acid interferes with DNA synthesis and cell reproduction.	Immunosuppressant to decrease inflammation in polymyositis (Rosenkranz, 2010).	Follow policy for preparing and handling drug. Avoid skin contact. Increase patient's fluid intake to reduce the risk of gastric distress. Assess the patient for signs of bleeding and infection.
Antimetabolite Immunosuppressant		
Azathioprine (Imuran) ***Action:*** May prevent proliferation and differentiation of activated B and T cells. Interferes with DNA and RNA synthesis.	Immunosuppressant to decrease inflammation in polymyositis (Rosenkranz, 2010).	Teach the patient to take oral drug with food or meals to minimize gastric distress. Therapy increases the risk of viral, fungal, bacterial, and protozoal infections. Monitor for signs of infection, especially in patients with cardiac insufficiency or hepatic disease. Administer oral dose 30 minutes prior to meals. Warn the patient to avoid alcohol, sedatives, and other CNS depressants. Be aware of multiple IV drug incompatibilities and light sensitivity.

(*continued*)

Weblink: Muscular Dystrophy
Weblink: Poliomyositis

PHARMACOLOGY Summary for Muscular Disorders, *continued*

Medication Category and Action	Application/Indication	Nursing Responsibility
Pregabalin		
Lyrica ***Action:*** Thought to act by increasing GABA levels by reducing the calcium channel function of neurons in the brain.	Used to manage neuropathic pain associated with peripheral neuropathy and postherpetic neuralgia. Used for pain associated with fibromyalgia (Arthritis Foundation, 2008).	Dose reduction with renal impairment is necessary to avoid toxicity. Administration with other CNS depressants can cause increased sedation. Monitor the patient for dizziness and drowsiness. Use with caution in patients with a history of abuse, as the drug can be physically and psychologically addictive.
Corticosteroid		
Prednisolone ***Action:*** Analog of hydrocortisone with 3 to 5 times greater potency. Effective as an anti-inflammatory agent.	Eaton-Lambert syndrome. Muscular dystrophy.	Evaluate the effectiveness in terms of decreased inflammation. Give at mealtime to decrease gastric irritation. Be alert to masked infection and delayed healing. Inspect the patient's oral cavity for Candida infection: white patches, black furry tongue, painful membranes and tongue. Patient teaching: Adhere to the prescribed dose; do not increase, decrease, or omit doses or change dose intervals. Report gastric distress or signs of ulcer. Do not breast-feed.

Sources: Adams, M. P., & Koch, R. W. (2010). *Pharmacology: Connections to nursing practice.* Upper Saddle River, NJ: Pearson; Arthritis Foundation. (2008). Fibromyalgia. Retrieved from http://www.arthritis.org/new-fibro-treatment.php; Mayo Clinic. (2009). Muscular dystrophy. Retrieved from http://www.mayoclinic.com/health/muscular-dystrophy/DS00200; Rosenkranz, H. (2010). Polymyositis in emergency medicine. Retrieved from http://emedicine.medscape.com/article/756355-overview.

developing over several months. The proximal limb muscles are affected and are weaker than the distal muscles. In addition, neck muscles are weak. Other muscles involved are those involved with swallowing, leading to possible dysphagia. Other complaints include myalgia and muscle tenderness. Other organs may also be involved, including the respiratory system, which may lead to interstitial lung disease; the cardiac system, which may lead to cardiomyopathy and conduction anomalies; and the gastrointestinal tract, leading to delayed emptying. Microvasculopathy (very small capillaries, veins, and arteries that do not allow for adequate perfusion) of the gastrointestinal tract occurs, leading to ulcerations and perforations of the intestine.

Laboratory and Diagnostic Procedures

Diagnosis of dermatomyositis is determined by signs and symptoms, elevated CK levels, an elevated eosinophil sedimentation rate, and an elevated antinuclear antibody titer. Muscle biopsy shows atrophy of muscle fibers, a decreased number of capillaries, and perivascular (around blood vessels) infiltrates.

Medical Management

Treatment of dermatomyositis is the same as that for polymyositis. The patient should be monitored for tumors, and should anticipate additional tests to rule out breast and lung cancer.

Inclusion Body Myositis

Inclusion body myositis (IBM), like the other myopathies, is an autoimmune disorder that is characterized by a progressive inflammation of the muscles. It occurs mostly in men over age 50 and is a common inflammatory myopathy in older adults (NINDS, 2011).

Clinical Manifestations

The patient complains of asymmetric muscle weakness, usually beginning in the wrists, finger flexors, and knee extensors. Muscle atrophy usually develops early compared to the other myopathies. In some cases, facial muscles are involved, as is dysphagia.

Medical Management

Elevated CK levels and muscle biopsies that show eosinophilic and cytoplasmic inclusion bodies are the main two diagnostic tools for IBM. As of this writing, there is no known treatment for IBM; however, prednisone and immune globulin have been shown to improve strength and improve function regionally. Sustained remission, however, has not been demonstrated. Prevention of foot drop and wrist drop is an important aspect in the maintenance of quality of life. This is achieved by bracing and physical therapy.

Nursing Management

The object of nursing care of patients with myopathies is to encourage as much independence as the patient can tolerate through teaching safety measures and the importance of adhering to the prescribed medication regime.

For further nursing management, refer to the Nursing Process: Patient Care Plan for Muscular Myopathies. For more information, see the Patient Teaching & Discharge Priorities for Muscular Myopathies box (p. 1510).

Collaborative Management

Collaborative management for patients with myopathies is the same as that for dystrophies. See the discussion of collaborative management for dystrophies on page 1502. Like collaborative management for dystrophies, it requires a multidisciplinary team. In order to meet desired patient outcomes, it is essential that this interdisciplinary team communicate openly with one another in developing and evaluating care of the patient and family (IOM [Institute of Medicine], 2010).

NURSING PROCESS: Patient Care Plan for Muscular Myopathies

Assessment of Musculoskeletal Status Using Gordon's Functional Health Patterns:

- Health Perception Health Management Pattern
- Nutrition Metabolic Pattern
- Activity Exercise Pattern
- Coping-Stress Tolerance Pattern

Subjective Data

Assessment of Muscle Strength

Have you experienced weakness in any extremity?

Have you had difficulty swallowing?

Assessment of Activity Tolerance

Do you become fatigued after performing simple tasks?

Assessment of Ability to Perform Self-Care

What activities are difficult for you to perform?

Do you require assistance with activities?

Assessment of Fall Risk

Do you have difficulty with balance?

Have you fallen recently?

Assessment of Swallowing

Do you ever choke on your food?

Do you have difficulty swallowing?

Assessment of Coping

Do you feel unusually fatigued?

Have you been able to communicate your concerns?

Objective Data

Assessment of Muscle Strength

Assess the patient's ability to perform ROM on all limbs.

Assess the patient's ability to perform resistance tests on all four limbs, flexion of the biceps, and extension of the triceps:

- Hand grip
- Flexion of the hip
- Adduction at the hip
- Abduction at the hip
- Extension at the hips
- Extension at the knee
- Flexion at the knee
- Dorsiflexion and plantar flexion.

Assessment of Activity Tolerance

Test the patient's muscle strength before and after performing simple tasks.

Assessment of Ability to Perform Self-Care

Observe the patient and evaluate his ability to perform ADLs.

Assessment of Fall Risk

Have the patient walk and observe for balance and muscle weakness.

Assessment of Swallowing

Have speech pathology do a swallow study.

Observe patient swallowing liquid and watch for coughing.

Assessment of Coping

Observe for:

- Decreased use of social support
- Destructive behavior toward self and others
- Inability to meet basic needs
- Inadequate problem solving
- Lack of goal-directed behavior
- Poor concentration.

Outcomes and Evaluation Parameters	Planning and Interventions with *Rationales*
1. NURSING DIAGNOSIS: Disuse Syndrome, Risk for *related to muscle weakness* (NANDA-I © 2012)	
Outcome: The patient is able to perform ROM on all extremities. ***Evaluation Parameter:*** The patient is able to perform resistance on all four limbs.	Provide a physical or occupational therapy referral as needed. *Physical therapists and occupational therapists are able to provide the patient with additional exercises for isotonic muscle movement.* Encourage the patient to eat a well-balanced diet (protein, carbohydrates, vitamins, and minerals) *to maintain a healthy musculoskeletal system.* Teach the patient and family the need to maintain appropriate weight. *Obesity makes it difficult for the patient to move and support himself.* Teach the patient/family the importance of maintaining safety in the home by keeping it uncluttered *to prevent injury.*
2. NURSING DIAGNOSIS: Activity Intolerance *related to muscle weakness* (NANDA-I © 2012)	
Outcome: The patient is able to perform ADLs without extreme fatigue. ***Evaluation Parameter:*** The patient and family have implemented an activity/rest period schedule.	Instruct the patient and family to pace activities per patient tolerance by assisting in devising an exercise plan that is tolerable and does not cause fatigue. *To decrease muscle fatigue and patient exhaustion.* Encourage the patient to eat a well-balanced diet (protein, carbohydrates, vitamins, and minerals) *to maintain a healthy musculoskeletal system.*

(continued)

NURSING PROCESS: Patient Care Plan for Muscular Myopathies, *continued*

Outcomes and Evaluation Parameters	Planning and Interventions with *Rationales*
3. NURSING DIAGNOSIS: If progressive, Self-Care Deficit: Bathing/Hygiene *and* Dressing/Grooming *related to muscle weakness* (NANDA-I © 2012)	
Outcome: The patient is able to perform ADLs without extreme fatigue. ***Evaluation Parameters:*** The patient has developed a schedule for performing ADLs. The patient will perform active ROM exercises on all joints three times a day.	Teach the patient/family to pace daily hygiene practices *to allow the patient to maintain independence.* Encourage active ROM exercises to all joints as prescribed *to maintain joint mobility.* Set up an exercise plan with the patient, keeping in mind the patient's limitations. *Exercise helps maintain a healthy musculoskeletal system.*
4. NURSING DIAGNOSIS: Falls, Risk for *related to muscle weakness* (NANDA-I © 2012)	
Outcome: The patient will not fall. ***Evaluation Parameters:*** The patient/family understands the importance of safety and will ensure safety measures are taken in the home. The patient demonstrates slower ambulation and verbalizes understanding about taking designated rest periods in between ambulation, if required.	Discuss with the patient/family safety issues in the home, such as throw rugs or other obstacles that may precipitate falls. *Such obstacles can lead to more serious injury.* Discuss with the patient/family the importance of taking time when ambulating. *May prevent serious injury and maintain level of independence.*
5. NURSING DIAGNOSIS: Swallowing, Impaired and/or Aspiration, Risk for *related to muscle weakness* (NANDA-I © 2012)	
Outcome: The patient will not aspirate. ***Evaluation Parameters:*** If required, the patient will see a speech pathologist. The patient and family demonstrate cutting foods into smaller pieces.	Refer to speech pathology. *Speech pathologists are able to detect various types of swallowing abnormalities.* Teach the patient and family to eat small bites of food. *Patient will be less likely to choke.* Provide thickened liquids to prevent aspiration. *Thickened liquids are easier to swallow directly into the esophagus and stomach.*
6. NURSING DIAGNOSIS: Coping, Ineffective *related to diagnosis* (NANDA-I © 2012)	
Outcome: The patient demonstrates effective coping. ***Evaluation Parameters:*** The patient: Takes actions to manage stressors. Shows self-restraint regarding compulsive or impulsive behaviors. Seeks information concerning illness and treatment. Reports decrease in negative feelings.	Allow the patient/family to verbalize fears and concerns. *Provides a support network.* Refer to local and national support systems. *Provide support of other people in similar situations.*

Source: Adapted from Wilkinson, J. M., & Ahearn, N. R. (2009). *Prentice Hall nursing diagnosis handbook* (9th ed.). Upper Saddle River, NJ: Prentice Hall.

PATIENT TEACHING & DISCHARGE PRIORITIES for Muscular Myopathies

Need	Teaching
Safety considerations	Pace exercise and performance of ADLs, including rest periods.
Importance of maintaining joint flexibility	Perform active ROM exercises on all joints three times a day.
Eat a well-balanced diet	Eat foods high in protein, vitamins, minerals, and carbohydrates.
Regular checkups	If symptoms worsen, see the health care provider immediately. Maintain follow-up appointments.

Health Promotion

Health promotion for patients with myopathies is the same as that for muscular dystrophies. See the section on collaborative management for muscular dystrophies on page 1502.

Other Musculoskeletal Disorders

Rhabdomyolysis

Etiology

Rhabdomyolysis is defined as a syndrome involving muscle necrosis or breakdown. The injured muscle fibers release myoglobin into the bloodstream. The myoglobin then alters the filtration in the kidneys, causing damage and kidney failure. The illness ranges in severity from elevations in muscle enzymes without any symptoms noted by the patient to severe life-threatening symptoms such as electrolyte imbalances and acute renal failure. Because rhabdomyolysis is thought of as a complication of a multitude of disease entities, there are no estimates of the incidence rate and prevalence. Some of the causes of rhabdomyolysis are trauma with muscle compression, surgical procedures in which there is a long period of muscle compression, immobilization due to a comatose or postictal state (usually occurring after seizure activity when the patient has been unconscious and unresponsive to stimuli) in which the patient is lying in one position for long periods of time, extreme physical exertion, snakebite, toxins, and viral, bacterial, or fungal infection (Bartelmo & Lockhart, 2008).

PATIENT TEACHING & DISCHARGE PRIORITIES for Rhabdomyolysis

Need	Teaching
Safety	Ensure that the home is free of obstacles. Take time with ADLs.
Monitor urine output	Inform the health care provider if urine output is low. If the patient is on a fluid restriction, explain the importance of maintaining the restriction so as not to overload the heart and lungs.
Follow-up care for kidney and electrolyte monitoring	Stress the importance of notifying the health care provider if the patient develops difficulty breathing, swelling, very dry skin, low urinary output, and discolored urine.

Clinical Manifestations and Diagnosis

The patient typically presents to the hospital with muscle pain (myalgia), fatigue, fever, nausea and vomiting, and dark-colored urine. The diagnosis of rhabdomyolysis is based on elevated serum CK levels (refer to the Laboratory and Diagnostic Tests for Muscular Disorders box on page 1501). Myoglobinuria (the presence of myoglobin in the urine) results when muscle tissue breaks down and the muscle substances enter the urine. It is an extremely abnormal condition. Myoglobin may be detected in the urine when the serum level is 1,500 to 3,000 ng/mL.

Complications

Numerous complications are associated with rhabdomyolysis:

- Acute renal failure due to tubular obstruction secondary to the myoglobulin pigments
- Electrolyte imbalance:
  - Hyperkalemia (elevated potassium levels in the blood) and hyperphosphatemia (elevated phosphate levels in the blood) can result due to the release of potassium and phosphate from the damaged muscles.
  - Hypocalcemia (low serum calcium level) due to deposited calcium salts in the muscle tissue. This electrolyte imbalance can be severe, and patients often show other symptoms associated with hypocalcemia, such as disturbances in cardiac conduction or blood coagulation.
  - Hyperuricemia (elevated uric acid level in the bloodstream) is a result of purine metabolism, resulting in an elevated serum uric acid concentration. Purines are present in nucleic acids, which are both obtained from endogenous and dietary sources.
  - Metabolic acidosis (electrolyte imbalance involving shift of the acid–base balance toward the acid side) can also occur.
  - Compartment syndrome (increased pressure in muscle compartment, which may lead to permanent disability of the associated joint) due to edema of a limb and muscle.

Medical Management

The treatment of rhabdomyolysis involves identifying and addressing the underlying cause. Prompt management and prevention of acute renal failure related to the muscle breakdown that causes the myoglobinuria is essential. Increased fluids are administered to hydrate the patient, thereby avoiding or preventing obstruction of the renal filtration process by the myoglobin, which could result in acute renal failure.

Nursing Management

Patients with acute or severe rhabdomyolysis are hospitalized and, owing to the severity of the kidney involvement, may be closely monitored in an intensive care unit (ICU). Nursing care will focus on hydration, strict fluid management, and close attention to the impact of possible abnormal electrolyte levels. Bicarbonate is given intravenously to prevent myoglobin from breaking down into toxic compounds in the kidney. Refer to Chapter 39 for nursing management of the patient in acute renal failure. See the Patient Teaching & Discharge Priorities for Rhabdomyolysis box for more information.

Eaton-Lambert Syndrome

Eaton-Lambert syndrome is an autoimmune disease that affects muscular activity and function. It is usually associated with small cell carcinoma of the lung and affects men more often than women. Eaton-Lambert syndrome is caused by a decrease in acetylcholine release. In addition, serum from patients with this syndrome contains circulating immunoglobulin antibodies that block calcium channels.

Clinical Manifestations

Patients with Eaton-Lambert syndrome complain of muscle fatigue primarily in the leg and trunk muscles. Other symptoms include occasional hyporeflexia, or weak tendon reflex; however, muscle contraction restores the tendon reflex. Autonomic symptoms are also present, such as dry mouth, impotence, decreased lacrimation and sweating, orthostatic hypotension, and decreased pupillary reaction to light accommodation.

Laboratory and Diagnostic Procedures

Diagnosis of Eaton-Lambert syndrome is made by electrophysiological responses to nerve stimulation. Affirmation of Eaton-Lambert syndrome is also determined by an elevated level of antibodies to the voltage-gated P/Q-type calcium channel. Elevations of these types occur in practically all cases that arise from lung cancer.

Medical Management

Patients with a diagnosis of lung carcinoma should be monitored frequently for muscle weakness. In some cases, the neuromuscular transmission improves after the tumor is removed. Drugs that increase acetylcholine release are also used, as well as drugs that control immune-mediated diseases. These drugs include prednisone and immune globulin. Refer to the Pharmacology Summary for Muscular Disorders box on page 1507.

Nursing Management

The object of nursing management of Eaton-Lambert syndrome is to teach the patient safety measures and adherence to their medication regime. If the cause of Eaton-Lambert syndrome is lung cancer, the nurse should provide symptomatic care and education.

Poliomyelitis

Poliomyelitis, also known as polio or infantile paralysis, is caused by a viral infection that spreads via infected oropharyngeal secretions or fecal matter. Outcomes for patients are often devastating, including effects such as difficulty breathing and flaccid paralysis of the legs.

Epidemiology and Etiology

Polio was epidemic around the world from the late 19th century to the 1950s, before development of effective vaccines. Although polio has been fairly well eradicated in the United States, many Third World countries are struggling to control the onset and outbreak of polio (CDC, 2011).

The polio virus infects the anterior horn cells of the gray matter of the spinal cord, which causes selective destruction of the motor neurons. The virus enters the body through the nasal and oral passages, crosses into the gastrointestinal tract, and enters the bloodstream, traveling to the central nervous system. The incubation period is 7 to 21 days. Polio is highly infectious, but up to 95% of patients who have the virus have no symptoms. Approximately 6% will have flu-like symptoms, and fewer than 1% will experience permanent paralysis. Of the patients who progress to paralysis, 5% to 10% die as a result of the virus affecting the respiratory muscles (CDC, 2010; Frazier & Drzymkowski, 2009).

Clinical Manifestations

The poliovirus damages the nerves that control muscles. Because of the nerve damage, patients with polio have extreme muscle weakness and at times paralysis of an extremity. The patient will present with a low-grade fever, discharge from the sinuses, and malaise. As the disease progresses, the patient will complain of muscle weakness, stiff neck, nausea and vomiting, and flaccid paralysis of the muscles involved. The muscles affected atrophy and decreased tendon reflexes and joint deterioration evolve. Many patients with polio require assistive devices, such as canes, walkers, and crutches. In some cases, the paralysis affects the respiratory muscles, causing death.

Medical Management

The best treatment for polio is prevention via immunization. Two forms of immunization are currently used against the polio virus: an injected polio vaccine (IPV) and a live, oral polio vaccine (OPV). Both vaccines are effective in preventing transmission of the disease from person to person, but in some cases the OPV can cause polio. For this reason, many health professionals recommend the IPV vaccine instead.

The vaccine schedule against polio varies for children and adults:

- ***Children.*** Children receive four doses of IPV at 2 months of age, 4 months of age, 6 to 18 months of age, and a booster at 4 to 6 years of age.
- ***Adults.*** For adults who have not previously received the vaccine, it is important to administer it if they (1) plan to travel to countries where polio is active, (2) work with the polio virus, or (3) care for patients with polio.

For the patient who actually has active polio, the treatment is supportive. Analgesics and moist heat application are administered for pain. In the acute phase, bed rest is indicated followed by physical therapy and evaluation for the use of assistive devices such as braces.

Post-Polio Syndrome

Patients who have had polio may later suffer from post-polio syndrome (PPS). In some patients who have had polio, some of the undamaged nerves grow branches that connect to muscles that have lost their nerve connection, allowing some movement to the muscle. However, it is now being found that the nerve connections are not as strong as was once thought and therefore start to break down again after a time. This breakdown causes renewed weakness of the muscle they control. The progressive weakness is not noted until 15 years or more after the initial disease and involves already affected muscles (Frazier & Drzymkowski, 2009; WebMD, 2009).

Clinical Manifestations

Manifestations of PPS include new muscle weakness, fatigue, and muscle and joint pain. Some patients may develop dysphagia, respiratory difficulty, and decreased ability to tolerate cold. Those at most risk for developing PPS are patients who had polio as a teenager or adult, still have muscle weakness, are female, and have had respiratory difficulty related to damage to the nerves that control breathing (WebMD, 2009).

Medical Management

Continuation of an active lifestyle is important for patients with PPS. The goals of treatment are to learn ways to stay active despite muscle weakness and to control muscle and joint pain with analgesics, heat and cold, and a balanced diet. However, the patient may require the use of assistive devices in order to maintain ADLs and the normal routine.

Nursing Management

Nursing care for polio and PPS is directed to supportive care, safety measures, and adherence to an exercise regimen.

Assessment

The nurse should listen to the patient's subjective complaints and ask about the following:

- The patient's medical–surgical history
- When the symptoms began
- Whether there are any accompanying symptoms
- Whether the symptoms have affected the patient's ability to maintain ADLs
- What type of exercise the patient engages in and how often the patient exercises
- Whether the patient has traveled to any Third World countries
- What type of medications the patient is taking, both prescription and OTC
- Whether the patient has had any respiratory difficulty, back pain, or dysphagia.

The nurse should objectively assess the patient by performing a physical examination. Important aspects of this examination are observation of the patient during ambulation, testing resistance of all four limbs, and auscultating lung sounds. The nurse should also have the patient bend forward and backward (if able) to test the strength of the back muscles.

Nursing Diagnoses

The primary diagnoses for the patient with poliomyelitis or PPS include the following:

- *Physical Mobility, Impaired.*
- *Fatigue.*

PATIENT TEACHING & DISCHARGE PRIORITIES for Post-Polio Syndrome

Need	Teaching
Need for exercise regime	Maintain and plan a daily exercise regime that promotes bone and muscle activity, but is not physically exhausting, such as walking or bike riding.
Eat a well-balanced diet	Plan a diet that includes vitamins, minerals, protein, calcium, and carbohydrates.
Maintain body mass index for height (ideal body weight)	Weigh weekly. If gaining weight, modify diet to decrease carbohydrates.
Rest periods	Rest if tired or in between activities and exercise programs.

- *Falls, Risk for.*
- *Airway Clearance, Ineffective.*
- *Disuse Syndrome, Risk for.*

NANDA-I © 2012

Outcomes and Evaluation Parameters

Outcomes for patients with polio or PPS include maintenance of a clear airway as exhibited by the patient's ability to swallow and cough, maintenance of current muscle use as exhibited by the patient's ability to perform scheduled exercises, and maintenance of functional alignment of all joints. The patient is at risk for falls because of muscle weakness. Outcome criteria would include no falls. Fatigue will be evaluated by the patient's ability to plan rest periods throughout the day to maintain strength.

Planning, Interventions, and Rationales

Patient education is key to the prevention of polio. Parents should be encouraged to have their children vaccinated, and any adult who has not been vaccinated for polio and is traveling to a Third World country is advised to receive the vaccine.

The patient with polio or PPS will be evaluated by the nurse for factors that increase the risk of muscle and joint complications, such as preexisting conditions like arthritis or surgery, that would reduce mobility. Muscle function depends on activity to maintain and increase muscle strength and maintain balance and muscle tone. Disuse will cause atrophy and lead to shortening of muscle fibers and reduced joint motion.

An active exercise program should be developed with the help of a physical therapist as the patient's condition permits, including complete ROM to all joints at least four times daily. Active exercise promotes maximum muscle contraction and helps to maintain muscle strength and endurance. Full ROM exercises to all joints stretch the surrounding muscle fibers and maintain the coordinated function of the joint structures.

It is important to plan rest periods between activities to prevent fatigue. Rest periods assist with endurance and the ability to participate in the plan of care.

The nurse administers analgesics and applies warm and cold compresses to areas of discomfort. Promoting comfort permits physical activity.

The nurse instructs the patient on the use of mobility aids (canes, braces, walkers). Educating the patient regarding the importance of mobility aids helps her adjust to using them. Mobility aids help to prevent injury and can offer the patient a sense of security.

Evaluation

Prognosis for the patient with poliomyelitis is fair depending on the muscles that are involved. The prognosis for PPS is good. Evaluation of the plan of care's effectiveness will include the patient's statement that pain is controlled and an assessment of muscle strength along with the patient's ability to participate in the exercise regimen. If the patient requires mobility aids, evaluation will include proper use of the device by the patient and a lack of falls or injury reported by the patient. For more information, see the Patient Teaching & Discharge Priorities for Post-Polio Syndrome box.

Muscle Cramps

Muscle cramps are sudden involuntary contractions in one or more muscles that last for a few seconds to minutes. Muscle cramps can be caused by a nerve that malfunctions, as in spinal cord injury, or from dehydration, lack of minerals in the body, overuse or straining of the muscle, and a decreased blood supply to the muscle (MedlinePlus, 2011).

The bundles of fibers that make up the muscle contract and expand to produce movement. It is important to keep the fibers stretched out so that they may respond vigorously during exercise. If the muscle is poorly conditioned, then it is more likely to become fatigued, which can change the spinal neural reflexes, causing cramping. Overexertion of the muscle depletes the oxygen supply to the muscle cells, leading to waste products that cause muscle spasm (American Association of Orthopaedic Surgeons [AAOS], 2010).

Exercise-induced muscle cramps are manifested by pain and involuntary muscle contractions that occur either during exercise or immediately after exercise. The pain is often spasmodic and episodic. Exercise-induced muscle cramps occur more frequently during hot weather as sweat drains the body of fluid, sodium, and other minerals such as potassium and calcium. The lack of these nutrients may cause the muscle to spasm. It is also thought that muscle cramps primarily occur over muscles that span two joints (AAOS, 2010).

Calcium plays an important role in the musculoskeletal system. One of its primary roles is in regulating muscle contraction and relaxation. A person who has hypocalcemia is at risk for muscle spasms of the face and extremities. Hypocalcemia also results in hyperactive deep tendon reflexes. Hypercalcemia, in turn, can cause generalized muscle weakness and flaccidity of the muscles.

Idiopathic muscle cramps are muscle cramps that occur with no particular etiology. The cramps are usually without accompanying weakness. Idiopathic muscle cramps generally affect healthy, middle-aged or older adults and generally occur during the nighttime or when the person is sleeping. The most common muscles affected are of the calf or foot muscles, causing plantar flexion to the afflicted foot.

Medical Management

Diagnosis of muscle cramps is made on the patient's subjective complaints and lack of any weakness or disability. The treatment is prophylactic, in that the patient is instructed to stretch before exercising and to maintain balanced nutrition and fluid intake. Patients who have night cramps should be encouraged to perform stretching exercises on the legs prior to falling asleep. When muscle cramps occur, the patient is instructed to stretch directly after the pain begins.

Nursing Management

The nursing plan of care for muscle cramps involves education regarding safety issues and measures to prevent the occurrence of cramps. Research into the efficacy of electrolyte-based drinks is addressed in the Research Opportunities Related to Muscular Disorders box.

The nurse should assess the patient's condition through a physical examination, observing the patient during ambulation and testing resistance on all four extremities. The nurse should monitor the patient's electrolyte levels and obtain a daily diary of the patient's intake and output. A history regarding the cramps can be elicited by asking whether the cramps occur only with exercise, whether they are relieved by stretching, and whether there is a family history of muscle cramps. Although most muscle cramps are benign, they can be signs of underlying disease such as spinal nerve irritation or compression, thyroid disease, or liver disease (AAOS, 2010). Older adults are prone to muscle cramps for reasons discussed in the Gerontological Considerations section later in this chapter.

Fibromyalgia

Fibromyalgia is a syndrome of chronic musculoskeletal pain. It is common in older adults and a major cause of disability. The exact cause is unknown. One theory suggests that stress is responsible for fibromyalgia. Other theories suggest that the patient has an abnormal amount of pain-related chemicals in the nervous system; that the patient has a conscious or subconscious tension, resulting in sleep disturbances; or that the patient has a lowered pain threshold.

Research has shown that patients with fibromyalgia have elevated levels of a nerve growth factor and a chemical signal called *substance P* in the spinal fluid. Also, the amount of serotonin, the chemical produced in the brain that has an effect on nerves, is low (Frazier & Drzymkowski, 2009). These patients become extremely sensitive to even minor pain. Fibromyalgia is not associated with any type of musculoskeletal disorder, nor does it predispose a patient to a musculoskeletal disorder, but it may coexist with certain rheumatologic diseases such as lupus or arthritis. The American College of Rheumatology (2010) uses criteria for classification of fibromyalgia. This criteria includes widespread pain for a minimum of 3 months and pain at 11 or 18 tender points on palpation. These points include the occipital, low cervical trapezius, supraspinatus, rib, epicondyle, and gluteal and knee areas.

Clinical Manifestations

The main signs and symptoms of fibromyalgia are pain in the back, neck, forearms, and knees. Patients with this condition not only complain of muscle and joint aches but also are extremely tender in the antecubital area, below the clavicles, in the posterior neck, in the posterior top of the buttocks, and in the lateral pelvis. Other symptoms are headaches, inability to sleep leading to daytime fatigue, dizziness, alternating constipation and diarrhea, generalized weakness, depression, numbness and tingling of the hands and feet, and memory loss. The onset of symptoms may be associated with psychological distress, trauma, or infection. The symptoms are aggravated by poor posture, strenuous exercise, and smoking (Frazier & Drzymkowski, 2009).

Laboratory and Diagnostic Procedures

The diagnosis of fibromyalgia is based on the patient's subjective symptoms, as well as a medical and surgical history. To date, there are no specific laboratory or diagnostic procedures to assist with the diagnosis.

Medical Management

The treatment of fibromyalgia is based on the patient's severity of pain, stress level, and overall health. Patients with fibromyalgia do not have any other associated musculoskeletal disorder; therefore, arthritis, inflammations, and bursitis should be ruled out. There is no cure for fibromyalgia, but treatment will help to alleviate symptoms and restore function. The plan of care will involve patient education, stress reduction, physical exercise, and medications to reduce pain and improve the quality of sleep.

The U.S. Food and Drug Administration has approved the use of pregabalin (Lyrica) for patients with fibromyalgia. Two double-blinded studies indicated that people using the medication showed rapid and sustained pain reduction and improved sleep patterns for 6 months (Arthritis Foundation, 2008).

A scheduled exercise plan is important for increasing the blood supply, oxygen, and nutrients to joints and muscles. Recommended exercises include walking, bike riding, swimming, and aerobic exercise. The patient with fibromyalgia may require assistance in eliminating or controlling the stress that is causing symptoms. Anxiety and depression must be controlled in order to control fibromyalgia. Sometimes an antidepressant may be ordered to assist the patient through the rough spots, which can promote the balance of pain-producing chemicals. A continuing medication regimen and an exercise plan are helpful in maintaining healthy muscles and joints.

Nursing Management

Nursing care for the patient with fibromyalgia should focus on assisting the patient to participate in a regimen that alleviates or minimizes discomfort, as well as suggesting methods to deal with the patient's current stressors. Education about the illness, the importance of sleep, use of pain management strategies, adaptation to the illness, and the importance of regular exercise should be the nurse's role in assisting patients with this illness. See the Nursing Process: Patient Care Plan for Fibromyalgia box and the section on fibromyalgia in the Gerontological Considerations section.

Alternative Treatments for Patients with Fibromyalgia

Massage therapy and relaxation techniques have been shown to help relieve the pain, stiffness, and sleep disturbances associated with fibromyalgia. Other alternative treatments used for patients with fibromyalgia include acupuncture, herbal products, reflexology, biofeedback, meditation and prayer, and **transcutaneous electrical nerve stimulation (TENS)** (pain relief via low-voltage electrical stimulation over a painful area). The Complementary & Alternative Therapies feature spotlights another popular pain relief method: acupuncture.

Collaborative Management

The care for patients with musculoskeletal disorders is complex and multifaceted. A nurse, nutritionist, physical therapist, occupational therapist, and orthotics technician will assist the patient to maintain mobility for as long as possible. In order to meet desired patient outcomes, it is essential that this interdisciplinary team communicate

NURSING PROCESS: Patient Care Plan for Fibromyalgia

Assessment of Musculoskeletal Status Using Gordon's Functional Health Patterns:

- Cognitive Perceptual Pattern
- Coping-Stress Tolerance Pattern

Subjective Data	Objective Data
Assessment of Pain On a scale of 1 to 10, with 1 being a little pain and 10 being the worst pain you have ever felt, at what level is your pain? Do you routinely take pain medication at home? If yes, what is the name of the medication and why do you take it? Are you allergic to any medications?	**Assessment of Pain** Pain is assessed during ROM to all joints. Pain is greater when bending and turning the neck. Monitor the patient for: • Facial grimacing • Change in breathing pattern • Change in blood pressure and/or pulse rate • Diaphoresis • Agitation.
Assessment of Coping Do you feel unusually fatigued? Have you experienced altered sleep patterns? Have you been able to communicate your concerns?	**Assessment of Coping** Observe for: • Decreased use of social support • Destructive behavior toward self and others • Inability to meet basic needs • Inadequate problem solving • Lack of goal-directed behavior • Poor concentration.

Outcomes and Evaluation Parameters	Planning and Interventions with *Rationales*
1. NURSING DIAGNOSIS: Pain, Acute or Chronic *related to muscle and joint pain* (NANDA-I © 2012)	
Outcome: Pain level will be tolerable. ***Evaluation Parameters:*** Diminished or absent level of pain through the patient's report. Absence of physiological indicators of pain.	Assess the patient's pain level on a scale of 1 to 10. Assess the pain level with bending the back, as well as ROM of all joints. *Determining a specific pain level in relation to certain movements is helpful in devising an exercise plan, as well as in prescribing a medication regime.* Assist the patient in developing an exercise plan that is not too strenuous. Teach the medication regime and the importance of adherence to the medication plan, as well as reporting of side effects related to NSAIDs: gastric upset, rectal or oral bleeding, bruising, or abdominal discomfort. If on Tylenol, monitor liver enzymes. *Long-term Tylenol use or high doses of Tylenol may cause liver damage.*
2. NURSING DIAGNOSIS: Coping, Ineffective *related to diagnosis* (NANDA-I © 2012)	
Outcome: The patient will demonstrate effective coping. ***Evaluation Parameters:*** The patient: Takes actions to manage stressors. Shows self-restraint regarding compulsive or impulsive behaviors. Seeks information concerning illness and treatment. Reports decrease in negative feelings.	Allow the patient/family to verbalize fears and concerns. *Provides a support network.* Assist the patient in finding ways to cope with stress: Refer to social services or a therapist to assist the patient in managing stressful situations. *Social services and/or therapy can assist the patient in dealing with stress via several techniques.* Refer to local and national support systems. *Provides support of other people in similar situations.* If the patient is placed on antidepressants, teach the patient the importance of maintaining the dose schedule and not to change or discontinue the medication without talking to her primary care provider. *Abruptly discontinuing antidepressants can exacerbate the symptoms of clinical depression.*

Source: Adapted from Wilkinson, J. M., & Ahearn, N. R. (2009). *Prentice Hall nursing diagnosis handbook* (9th ed.). Upper Saddle River, NJ: Prentice Hall.

openly with one another in developing and evaluating care of the patient and family (IOM [Institute of Medicine], 2010). Many of the musculoskeletal disorders are also very painful. It is important to work with a pain specialist to monitor and prescribe treatment for acute and chronic pain associated with muscular disease. For the caregiver, assistance from a financial counselor, psychologist, and home health nurse, in addition to access to respite care, will decrease the chance of severe caregiver role strain.

COMPLEMENTARY & ALTERNATIVE THERAPIES Acupuncture

Aeriel Ertel

ACUPUNCTURE IS THE PRACTICE of inserting fine needles into specific sites on the skin, called *acupuncture points*, for the purpose of producing a therapeutic response and relieving pain. Acupuncturists use several methods to stimulate acupuncture points (also known as acupoints, nodes, or sites). Sometimes they also stimulate larger areas of the skin using the following methods, either alone or in combination, during one session: needling, moxibustion (heat application), cupping (application of suction cups), acupressure massage techniques, and electrical stimulation. Historically, acupuncture has been used to treat most health problems, but it is best known in the West for its effectiveness in pain relief and musculoskeletal problems.

Needling, the most frequently used acupuncture method, can be combined with moxibustion or electrostimulation. Modern acupuncture needles are made from stainless steel, consisting of a shaft and a coiled handle to enable manipulation and prevent overpenetration. The needles are thin and flexible, with varying gauges and lengths.

When needling, the acupuncturist must locate the precise locations of the acupoints as well as the underlying anatomic structures. There are recommended needling depths and insertion angles for each point, but these must be adjusted for each patient, taking into account body shape and size, the patient's condition and current state, and the treatment goals. Patients sometimes experience momentary discomfort during insertion; however, once the needles are placed, there is no pain. Instead, a feeling of relaxation usually ensues.

Acupuncture originated in China over 5,000 years ago, and the first writings regarding it are close to 3,000 years old. As a medical practice, it developed alongside other methods such as massage and herbal medicine, which were used throughout Asia. Acupuncture spread from China throughout Asia, blending with local traditional medical practices in each country. Theories and schools of thought concerning the practice of acupuncture, based on the Chinese medical classics and the clinical experience of doctors, arose over the centuries among the countries of Asia. Practitioners in Japan and Korea developed innovations that contributed to the scope of practice. It may be more appropriate to say that while acupuncture has its roots in China, it forms an integral part of traditional Asian medicine.

While standardization of care is an ideal in modern cultures, the diversity in the practice of acupuncture is a strength of traditional Asian medicine. Centuries of clinical experience, often passed on in oral tradition, with core principles recorded in the medical texts enabled Asian doctors to adapt their medicine to meet the needs of whatever population they served.

Fundamental concepts in acupuncture include blood and Qi, which circulate along pathways (meridians) to nourish or regulate tissues, and acupuncture points (acupoints), which are located along the pathways. The acupoints can be stimulated to influence circulation and create a healing or analgesic response.

Diagnostic methods used to evaluate the problem involve observation, palpation, consideration of signs and symptoms, and the case history. Considering the details of a patient's history, symptoms, and metabolism reveal a pattern and give perspective on the chief complaint. These methods, as well as the acupoint selection and treatment strategy, can vary among practitioners depending on the emphasis in their training.

Acupuncture practice declined in China in the 19th century due to political and cultural changes. After 1949, however, Mao Zedong once again encouraged the use of acupuncture in China and it became widespread. Today in China, Korea, and Japan, the large hospitals have departments of traditional medicine, offering acupuncture and herbal medicines, alongside Western medicine departments. Many treatment plans integrate both acupuncture and Western medicine.

Acupuncture became well known in the United States after Nixon's trip to China in 1972 due to an emergency surgery. A *New York Times* reporter, James Reston, had an appendectomy in the Anti-Imperialist Hospital. Reston received acupuncture for postoperative pain with good results. He wrote of his experience in an article, "Now About My Operation in Peking." Today, there are a number of acupuncture colleges in the United States, and most states regulate and license acupuncture. The National Certification Commission for Acupuncture and Oriental Medicine (NCCAOM) provides national standards for examination and certification.

Although acupuncture has been used along with other traditional medical practices throughout Asia for millennia, there is no single physiological explanation for how it achieves therapeutic effects. Lacking a clear understanding of its mechanism, it is convenient to point to the placebo effect. However, the placebo effect is inadequate to explain acupuncture for several reasons. First, acupuncture is widely known to work on animals to relieve pain and bring about therapeutic effects. In fact, some American veterinarians currently offer acupuncture and Chinese herbal medicine in their small animal practices. However, there is no placebo response in animals. Nonetheless, physiological effects on animals have been repeatedly shown in laboratory studies where animal models are used in acupuncture research. Veterinary acupuncture has been used for at least a thousand years, as shown by ancient Chinese texts. Secondly, acupuncture analgesia has been used for many years in Chinese hospitals as a replacement for surgical anesthesia in appropriate cases; the patient in these cases is awake during the entire surgery. Acupuncture can also be used instead of novocaine in some dental procedures.

Basic research into acupuncture's mechanisms began in the Western world in 1986 with the postulation of the acupuncture endorphin hypothesis. Researchers in Europe and Canada provided a body of serious research over the next 20 years.

The advent of functional magnetic resonance imaging (fMRI) opened a new dimension of possibilities in the study of acupuncture. fMRI can show increases in blood oxygenation to discrete regions of the brain, indicating changes in activity. A stimulus such as shining a light in the eyes will cause changes in the visual cortex which are detected by the fMRI. Commonly used therapeutic indications for acupoints have been correlated with cerebrovascular reactions in corresponding regions of the brain when a specific point is needled while scanning with fMRI.

Sources: Hsu, P., & Peacher, T. (1977). *Chen's history of Chinese medical science.* Taiwan, Taipei: Modern Drug Publishers Co.; Kendall, D. (2002). *The dao of Chinese medicine.* London: Oxford University Press; Needham, J. (1982). *Science in traditional China.* Massachusetts: Harvard University Press; Pomeranz, G., & Gabriel, S. (Eds.). (1989). *Scientific bases of acupuncture.* Berlin: Bruce Springer-Verlag; Reston, J. (1971, July 26). Now about my operation in Peking. *New York Times*: p. 6. New York: New York Times Co.; Van Alphen, J., & Aris, A. (Eds.). (1997). *Shambhala.* Boston, MA: Oriental Medicine.

Health Promotion

All of the disorders discussed in this section have some type of permanent disability and/or an acute or chronic discomfort or weakness associated with them. Healthy living (i.e., not being overweight, eating a healthy diet, and following some type of exercise plan) is mandatory for preventing further complications in patients with these conditions. A scheduled exercise program is prescribed in order to maintain joint mobility, to increase circulation and oxygenation to the muscles and tissues, and to strengthen bone. Patients should maintain a weight that is appropriate for their height, because added weight causes stress to an already impaired musculoskeletal system. Maintenance of weight is predicated on a good exercise plan plus a diet low in fats.

The concept of the federal government's *Healthy People 2020* campaign is not just for healthy individuals but for everyone, even those with chronic or disabling conditions. It is a framework of national health objectives designed to identify preventable threats to health and establish goals to reduce these threats. The leading health indicators that correlate with this chapter are as follows: engage in an exercise program, abstain from tobacco use and substance abuse, maintain weight per body mass index (ideal weight), receive immunizations for polio if traveling to a Third World country, and maintain regular visits with a health care provider. Therefore, nursing responsibilities should include health teaching to include dietary management, weight control, abstinence from smoking, and a viable exercise program.

Gerontological Considerations

As patients age, there are many changes to the musculoskeletal system, as described in Chapter 48. Following are specific considerations for the muscular disorders that were discussed in this chapter.

Muscular Dystrophies

Some patients diagnosed with myotonic muscular dystrophy are over the age of 50, and patients diagnosed with oculopharyngeal muscular dystrophy are usually in their 50s or 60s. Nursing considerations for these patients include safety issues; this is because, as a person ages, muscle mass and muscle tone decrease. In addition to the weakness caused by the muscular dystrophy, the nurse must be aware of the normal aging process. Referrals to physical therapy or the use of assistive devices, such as canes or walkers, may be necessary.

Myopathy

It is common for myopathies to develop in people in their 50s and 60s. As with all patients with muscle diseases, safety concerns are a priority. The older a person becomes, the more brittle the bones become. Muscle mass and muscle tone decrease; combined with the effects of aging, the added muscle weakness associated with myopathy puts the patient at risk for falls and other injuries. In creating a plan of care for a patient diagnosed with a myopathy, safety must be a priority. For more information, see the Research Opportunities Related to Muscular Disorders box.

Many of these patients are diagnosed at an age when they might be contemplating retirement and future plans with their spouse. A medical diagnosis of a myopathy will alter their lifestyle, and many may become depressed. Nurses should anticipate patients reacting negatively to this new diagnosis and need to be aware of mood swings that are typical for a patient with a myopathy.

Muscle Cramps

In addition to the decreases in muscle mass and tone that are inherent to the aging process, many older adults do not drink enough fluids, owing to the fear and embarrassment of incontinence. Therefore, it is imperative that the nurse teach the older patient the importance of hydrating, exercising in moderate temperatures to prevent the onset of muscle cramps, and performing some mild stretching exercises. Before suggesting electrolyte-based drinks, the nurse should know the patient's laboratory values for sodium and potassium. Recommending use of these drinks on a daily basis may be detrimental to the health of patients with a history of hypernatremia or hyperkalemia. The older patient needs to eat a well-balanced diet with vitamins and minerals to maintain bone and muscle integrity. The nurse should encourage the patient to have regular checkups in which electrolyte levels are monitored.

Fibromyalgia

As people get older, sleep patterns change, and many older adults do not sleep soundly throughout the night. Inadequate sleep is exacerbated in patients diagnosed with fibromyalgia; therefore, besides the usual safety issues related to pain in the joints, they are particularly at risk for falls because of fatigue.

Older patients need to be aware that as the liver function decreases with age, medications are not filtered as quickly, leading to a faster rate of toxicity. This is particularly important when older adults take non-steroidal anti-inflammatory agents, which can lead to ulcerations of the stomach and intestinal wall. For example, Tylenol can cause altered liver function, which is especially dangerous to a patient who already has decreased liver function.

Last, chronic or acute pain, coupled with stress, may cause an older patient to feel hopeless, helpless, and alone, which can lead to depression.

Research

Current medical research into muscular and myotonic dystrophy is focusing on several areas, including "gene silencing," which attempts to "turn off" the cells that harbor the elongated stretch of DNA that is thought to cause a type of MD, and better DNA testing and mapping of the genetic defect (MDA, 2010a).

RESEARCH OPPORTUNITIES Related to Muscular Disorders

Research Area	Clinical Impact
Myopathies	
If the patient maintains his regular regime (at a slower pace), could the disease progression be delayed?	Maintenance of the patient's normal routine, to the extent possible, may promote a better quality of life.
How does a patient's support system affect the progression of the disease?	A positive family support system may prevent depression or poor self-esteem related to the disease.
Muscle Cramps	
In exercise-induced muscle cramps, will drinking one to two glasses of an electrolyte-based drink prior to exercising prevent muscle cramps?	A decreased incidence of muscle cramps due to dehydration, as well as longer endurance levels, may be a result.

CLINICAL PREPARATION READ DOCUMENT APPLY

READ: History of Present Illnesses >> Laboratory Study Results >> Critical Thinking Questions

As the nurse on a medical–surgical unit, you have been notified that you will be receiving a patient from the emergency department (ED). The ED nurse calls the unit and gives report on the patient being admitted. Helen Kwiatkowski, a 72-year-old female, was found by her daughter in her home on the floor of her bedroom approximately 12 hours after a fall. Mrs. Kwiatkowski states she does not clearly remember what led to the fall and is complaining of sharp, constant right hip discomfort.

Medical–Surgical History

Mrs. Kwiatkowski has a history of hypertension. She states that she has never had an operation.

Social History

Mrs. Kwiatkowski states that she has never smoked. She drinks alcohol occasionally. She walks for 20 minutes daily and takes a t'ai chi class on Tuesday afternoons.

Physical Exam

Mrs. Kwiatkowski is orientated to person, place, and time. Pupils are equal and react to light. Bilateral grasps are equal and strong. She rates her right hip pain at an 8 on a scale of 0 (no pain) to 10 (most pain ever). Vital signs: temp: 37.2C; BP: 180/90 mmHg; heart rate: 104 bpm; 22 respirations per minute, even and relaxed. Bilateral breath sounds are present and clear in all lobes; however, bilateral breath sounds are slightly diminished in the lower lobes. Right leg is adducted and internally rotated, but Mrs. Kwiatkowski denies numbness or tingling of her right foot. Right pedal pulses palpated less than left, but right pedal pulse is strong by Doppler. Mrs. Kwiatkowski states that she takes high blood pressure medication and on occasion an aspirin for joint discomfort.

READ: History of Present Illnesses >> **Physical Exam** >> Admitting Medical Records >> Laboratory Study Results

Admitting Medical Orders

- Service: orthopedic surgery
- Diagnosis: fracture right hip
- Allergies: no known allergies
- Vital signs: every 4 hours including oxygen saturation
- Call house officer: temp > 38.5°C, HR > 110 or < 60, RR < 12 or > 30, BP > 160 or < 90, O_2 sat < 92%, urine output < 120 mL in 4 hours, change in neurological exam, any Hct result that is 5 less than the baseline ED Hct
- Activity: bed rest
- Diet: nothing by mouth
- IVs: D5.45NS with 20 mEq of KCl at 100 mL/hr
- I&O: every shift
- Respiratory care: incentive spirometer every hour when awake
- DVT prophylaxis: sequential compression device to lower extremities bilaterally
- Treatments: skin traction to right lower extremity
- Consent to be signed for open reduction and internal fixation of right trochanter
- To the operating room tomorrow on call
- Insert Foley catheter
- Daily weight

Scheduled Medications

- Atenolol 50 mg po every day
- Preop medication per anesthesiologist

PRN Medications

- Phenergan 12.5–25 mg IV every 6 hours prn nausea
- Morphine 2–4 mg IV every 4 hours prn pain
- Ativan 0.5 mg IV every 6 hours prn anxiety
- Tylenol 650 mg PO every 4 hours for pain

Ordered Laboratory Studies

- Complete blood count and Chem panel every morning

READ: History of Present Illnesses >> **Laboratory Study Results** >> Critical Thinking Questions

Test	ED Initial	ED 2nd (4 hours)	On Admission to Floor
CBC			
Hemoglobin (Hgb)	10.5 g/dL	9.5 g/dL	9.5 g/dL
Hematocrit (Hct)	34%	33%	32%
RBC	3.2/mm^3	3/mm^3	3/mm^3
Reticulocytes	2.0%	2.4%	2.4%
MCV	72 μm^3	68 μm^3	68 μm^3
MCH	27 pg	25 pg	25 pg
Platelets	150/mm^3	146/mm^3	146/mm^3

Test	ED Initial	ED 2nd (4 hours)	On Admission to Floor
Electrolytes			
Sodium	135 mEq/L	135 mEq/L	140 mEq/L
Potassium	3.6 mEq/L	3.6 mEq/L	3.9 mEq/L
Calcium	9 mg/dL	9 mg/dL	9 mg/dL
BUN	14 mg/dL	14 mg/dL	16 mg/dL
Creatinine	0.8 mg/dL	1 mg/dL	1.2 mg/dL
Glucose	150 mg/dL	148 mg/dL	140 mg/dL

Pearson Nursing Student Resources *Log on to* **nursing.pearsonhighered.com** *to download forms*

DOCUMENT:

- >> Summary of Hospitalization
- >> Pathophysiology Form
- >> Laboratory Values
- >> Laboratory Results Explanation

APPLY:

- >> List of Potential Nursing Diagnoses
- >> Concept Map
- >> Critical Thinking Questions and Concept Map

APPLY: History of Present Illness >> Laboratory Study Results >> **Critical Thinking Questions**

1. What pertinent information can you assess as the medical–surgical nurse?
2. What are Mrs. Kwiatkowski's risk factors for sustaining a fracture?
3. What other lab tests might you, as the nurse, anticipate?
4. What are the goals of medical management for Mrs. Kwiatkowski?
5. What are two priority nursing diagnoses?
6. What are some postoperative instructions for Mrs. Kwiatkowski?

Answers to Critical Thinking Questions can be found in Appendix D in the Osborn Student Resources at nursing.pearsonhighered.com.

NCLEX® PRACTICE

1. A 60-year-old patient has been prescribed the bisphosphonate Fosamax to manage osteoporosis. What should the nurse teach the patient about taking this medication? (select all that apply)

1. "Take the medication just before bedtime with a full glass of water."
2. "Take the medication with an acidic drink like orange juice."
3. "Wait at least 30 minutes after taking the medication before eating."
4. "Chew up the pill very well and swallow with water."
5. "Take this medication at least 30 minutes before taking any other medications."

2. A nurse is providing a preventive health care seminar related to ways to decrease the effects of osteoporosis. Which of the following risk factors applies to both men and women?

1. Anorexia
2. Diet low in calcium and vitamin D
3. History of maternal hip fracture
4. Low body weight and low body mass index

3. A nurse has provided an overview of evidence-based care for prevention of institutional falls in older adults. Which statement made by a participant warrants further education?

1. "Most falls happen when patients are trying to get to the bathroom."
2. "Discussing fall risk with the patient and family may reduce the incidence of fall."
3. "None of our fall prevention strategies will work unless hospital administration supports our efforts."
4. "Falls are a leading source of injury to patients while they are hospitalized."

4. During the first prenatal appointment, a pregnant woman says, "My cousin has muscular dystrophy. How can I prevent my baby from having it, too?" What is the nurse's best response?

1. "Muscular dystrophy can be prevented by eating a healthy diet, avoiding cigarette smoke and alcohol, and taking vitamin B supplements during your pregnancy."
2. "As long as your baby is a girl, you won't have to worry about it."
3. "Muscular dystrophy is genetic and cannot be prevented."
4. "Prevention depends upon the type of muscular dystrophy."

5. During assessment of a 6-year-old boy, the clinic nurse observes Gowers' maneuver. Which assessment question should the nurse ask this child's parent?

1. "Has your son had any infections recently?"
2. "When was the last time your son had immunizations?"
3. "Have you noticed any balance problems?"
4. "How is your son's appetite?"

6. A patient is being admitted to the hospital from the emergency department with the diagnosis of rhabdomyolysis following a severe fungal infection. Which assessment findings would the nurse expect this patient to exhibit? (select all that apply)

1. Myalgia
2. Temperature of 38.4°C (101.2°F)
3. Fasting plasma glucose of 234
4. Dark-colored urine
5. Serum potassium of 4.0 mEq/L

Answers to NCLEX Practice Questions can be found in Appendix D in the Osborn Student Resources at nursing.pearsonhighered.com. Practice additional NCLEX questions online at the Student Resources site.

Pearson Nursing Student Resources Find additional review materials at: **nursing.pearsonhighered.com**

REFERENCES

Adams, M. P., & Koch, R. W. (2010). *Pharmacology: Connections to nursing practice.* Upper Saddle River, NJ: Pearson.

American Association of Orthopaedic Surgeons. (2010). Muscle cramp. Retrieved from http://orthoinfo.aaos.org/topic.cfm?topic=A00200

American Cancer Society. (2012a). Detailed guide: Bone cancer. Retrieved from http://www.cancer.org/Cancer/BoneCancer/DetailedGuide/bone-cancer-key-statistics

American Cancer Society. (2012b). Osteosarcoma. Retrieved from http://www.cancer.org/Cancer/Osteosarcoma/DetailedGuide/osteosarcoma-key-statistics

American College of Rheumatology. (2010). Fibromyalgia. Retrieved from http://www.rheumatology.org/practice/clinical/patients/diseases_and_conditions/fibromyalgia.asp

Arthritis Foundation. (2008). Fibromyalgia. Retrieved from http://www.arthritis.org/new-fibro-treatment.php

Bartelmo, J. M., & Lockhart, A. (Eds.). (2008). *Nursing: Understanding diseases.* Philadelphia: Lippincott Williams & Wilkins.

Bethel, C. (2009). Myopathies. Retrieved from http://emedicine.medscape.com/article/759487-overview

Centers for Disease Control and Prevention. (2010). Duchenne and Becker muscular dystrophy. Retrieved from http://www.cdc.gov/ncbddd/duchenne/

Centers for Disease Control and Prevention. (2011). Polio. Retrieved from http://www.cdc.gov/vaccines/vpd-vac/polio/in-short-both.htm

Christensen, B., & Kockrow, E. (2010). *Adult health nursing* (6th ed.). St. Louis: Mosby.

Copstead-Kirkhorn, L. E., & Banasik, J. L. (2009). *Pathophysiology* (4th ed.). St. Louis: Saunders.

Frazier, M. S., & Drzymkowski, J. W. (Eds.). (2009). *Essentials of human diseases and conditions* (4th ed.). St. Louis: Saunders.

Hill, A., McPhail, S., Hoffmann, T., Hill, K., Oliver, D., Beer, C., Brauer, S., & Haines, T. P. (2009). A randomized trial comparing digital video disc with written delivery of falls prevention education for older patients in hospital. *Journal of the American Geriatrics Society, 57*(8), 1458–1463.

Hogan, M. A., DeLeon, E., Gingrich, M. M., & Willcutts, K. (2007). *Nutrition and diet therapy* (2nd ed.), Upper Saddle River, NJ: Pearson Prentice Hall.

Hsu, P., & Peacher, T. (1977). *Chen's history of Chinese medical science.* Taiwan: Modern Drug Publishers Co.

Institute for Clinical Systems Improvement. (2012). Prevention of falls (acute care) protocol (3rd ed.). Retrieved from http://www.icsi.org/falls_acute_care_prevention_of_protocol_24255.html

IOM (Institute of Medicine). (2010). *The future of nursing: Leading change, advancing health.* Washington, DC: The Academic Press.

Kendall, D. (2002). *The dao of Chinese medicine.* London: Oxford University Press.

King, R. W., Johnson, D., Stearns, D. A., Talavera, F., Weiss, E. L., Halamka, J., et al. (2010). Osteomyelitis. Retrieved from http://www.emedicine.com/emerg/topic349/htm

Krauss, M. J., Nguyen, S. L., Dunagan, W. C., Birge, S., Costanitnou, E., Caleca, B., & Fraser, V. J. (2007). Patient fall circumstances and injury across nine hospitals in a Midwestern healthcare system. *Infection Control Hospital Epidemiology, 28*(5), 544–550.

Lahl, M., Fisher, V. L., & Laschinger, K. (2007). Ewing's sarcoma family of tumors: An overview from diagnosis to survivorship. *Clinical Journal of Oncology Nursing, 12*(1), 89–97.

Lopate, G. (2011). Lim-girdle muscular dystrophy. Retrieved from http://emedicine.medscape.com/article/1170911-overview#a0199

MacLean, C., Newberry, S., Maglione, M., McMahon, M., Ranganath, V., Suttorp, M., et al. (2008). Systematic review: Comparative effectiveness of treatments to prevent fractures in men and women with low bone density or osteoporosis. *Annals of Internal Medicine, 148*(11), 197–213.

Majumdar, S. R., Johnson, J. A., McAlister, F. A., Bellerose, D., Russell, A. S., Hanley, D. A., et al. (2008). Multifaceted intervention to improve diagnosis and treatment of osteoporosis in patients with recent wrist fracture: A randomized controlled trial. *Canadian Medical Association Journal, 178*(5), 569–575.

Mayo Clinic. (2009). Muscular dystrophy. Retrieved from http://www.mayoclinic.com/health/muscular-dystrophy/DS00200

Mayo Clinic. (2010). Osteoporosis. Retrieved from http://www.mayoclinic.com/health/osteoporosis/DS00128

McCance, K., & Huether, S. (2009). *Pathophysiology: The biologic basis for disease in adults and children* (6th ed.). St. Louis: Mosby.

MedlinePlus. (2011). Muscle cramps. Retrieved from http://www.nlm.nih.gov/medlineplus/musclecramps.html

Muscular Dystrophy Association. (2010a). Facts about Duchenne and Becker muscular dystrophies. Retrieved from http://www.mda.org/publications/fa-dmdbmd-what.html

Muscular Dystrophy Association (MDA). (2010b). Facts about mitochondrial myopathies. Retrieved from http://www.mda.org/Publications/mitochondrial_myopathies.html#whatare

National Institutes of Health. (2010). Osteoporosis. Retrieved from http://www.ncbi.nlm.nih.gov/pubmedhealth/PMH0001400/

National Institute of Neurological Disorders and Stroke. (2010). Myopathy. Retrieved from http://www.ninds.nih.gov/disorders/myopathy/myopathy.htm

National Institute of Neurological Disorders and Stroke. (2011). NINDS inclusion body myositis information page. Retrieved from http://www.ninds.nih.gov/disorders/inclusion_body_myositis/inclusion_body_myositis.htm

Needham, J. (1982). *Science in traditional China.* Massachusetts: Harvard University Press.

Pinheiro, M., Ciconelli, R., Martini, L., & Ferraz, M. (2009). Clinical risk factors for osteoporotic fractures in Brazilian women and men: The Brazilian Osteoporosis Study (BRAZOS). *Osteoporosis International, 20*(3), 399–408.

Pomeranz, G., & Gabriel, S. (Eds.). (1989). *Scientific bases of acupuncture.* Berlin: Bruce Springer-Verlag.

Porth, C. M., & Matfin, G. (2009). *Pathophysiology: Concepts of altered health states* (8th ed.). Philadelphia: Lippincott Williams & Wilkins.

Reston, J. (1971, July 26). Now about my operation in Peking. *New York Times.* Pg 6.

Rosenkranz, H. (2010). Polymyositis in emergency medicine. Retrieved from http://emedicine.medscape.com/article/756355-overview

Sherrington, C., Whitney, J. C., Lord, S. R., Herbert, R. D., Cumming, R. G., & Close, J. C. (2008). Effective exercise for the prevention of falls: A systematic review and meta-analysis. *Journal of the American Geriatrics Society, 58*(12), 2234–2243.

Sripathi, N. (2010). Facioscapulohumeral dystrophy. Retrieved from http://emedicine.medscape.com/article/1176126-overview#a0104

Tzeng, H. M. (2010). Understanding the prevalence of inpatient falls associated with toileting in adult acute care settings. *Journal of Nursing Care Quality, 25*(1): 22–30.

Van Alphen, J., & Aris, A. (Eds.). (1997). *Shambhala.* Boston, MA: Oriental Medicine.

WebMD. (2009). Post-polio syndrome. Retrieved from http://www.webmd.com/brain/tc/post-polio-syndrome-topic-overview

Wilkinson, J. M., & Ahearn, N. R. (2009). *Prentice Hall nursing diagnosis handbook* (9th ed.). Upper Saddle River, NJ: Prentice Hall.

Caring for the Patient with Musculoskeletal Trauma and Surgical Procedures

50 CHAPTER

Kara Gasiorowski
Cheryl Wraa

Outcome-Based Learning Objectives

After studying this chapter, the learner will be able to:

1. Analyze the incidence, prevalence, and prevention strategies for musculoskeletal trauma.
2. Discuss the components of the assessment appropriate for a patient who has had orthopedic surgery.
3. Examine the pathophysiological stages of bone healing, various types of fractures, and methods for fracture treatment.
4. Generate a nursing management plan and identify potential complications for musculoskeletal trauma and surgery patients.
5. Examine the types of precautions required to prevent hip dislocation in the postoperative hip replacement patient.
6. Compare and contrast the assistive devices utilized for orthopedic patients.
7. Critique the importance of optimal pain control in the postoperative orthopedic patient.

KEY TERMS

amputation p.1549
arthroplasty p.1536
avascular necrosis (AVN) p.1523
avulsion fracture p.1522
Buck's boots traction p.1528
burst fracture p.1528
chance fracture p.1528
compartment syndrome p.1556
continuous passive motion (CPM) devices p.1555
contusion p.1522
diaphysis p.1525
discectomy p.1544
dislocation p.1523
epiphysis p.1525
external fixation p.1529
fasciotomy p.1556
fat embolus p.1557
fracture p.1526
heterotopic ossification (HO) p.1558
intramedullary (I-M) rodding p.1530
laminectomy p.1544
metaphysis p.1525
open reduction internal fixation (ORIF) p.1530
osteolysis p.1541
osteonecrosis p.1559
PRICE p.1522
skeletal traction p.1529
skin traction p.1528
sprain p.1522
spinal fusion p.1545
strain p.1522
total joint replacement p.1536
traumatic amputation p.1549

MUSCULOSKELETAL TRAUMA INJURIES are a frequent occurrence in blunt trauma, such as motor vehicle crashes, falls, crush injuries, sports injuries, and auto versus pedestrian collisions. By employing prevention strategies, people decrease the effects of injuries to the muscles, tendons, ligaments, and bones. Many strategies have been designed to reduce or prevent injuries at home, in the workplace, at play, during sports, and on the road.

Musculoskeletal trauma results from injuries to the bones, joints, and soft tissues. Accidental trauma is caused by overuse, impact, sports injuries, and vehicle crashes. Motor vehicle crashes, bicycle and pedestrian injuries, and falls are the most common etiology for musculoskeletal trauma. Nonaccidental or inflicted trauma is seen as a result of domestic violence, child abuse, and altercations; it may take the form of blunt trauma, whereby impact is made between the body and an object or force, or penetrating trauma, which occurs when an object such as a knife or bullet enters the body. In the Major Trauma Outcomes Study, 48.6% of trauma patients had one or more musculoskeletal injuries (Browner & DeAngelis, 2008). The most common musculoskeletal injuries are strains, sprains, contusions, and fractures.

Types of Musculoskeletal Injuries

Understanding the mechanism and effect of an injury will assist the nurse in prioritizing the assessment and care of the patient with a

Weblink: Ankle Sprain.

musculoskeletal injury. Following are descriptions of common injuries found in musculoskeletal trauma.

Contusions

A **contusion** is an injury to soft tissue caused by trauma in which the skin is not broken. The trauma damages the small blood vessels, and a bruise results from blood leaking from the damaged vessels into the surrounding interstitial tissues, as well as from the body's inflammatory response to the injury causing edema at the site of the contusion. A contusion is characterized by pain, discoloration (bruising), and swelling.

Sprains and Strains

A **strain** is an injury to the muscle belly or its tendon attachment to bone, typically caused by excessive force or load on a joint or muscle. The associated pain may be described as dull or sharp pain that increases with movement of the muscle. It can take up to 24 hours for intramuscular bruising to become visible because the blood remains primarily within the muscle sheath, causing pain and local swelling (Anscomb, 2007).

Sprains are similar to strains but occur at the ligaments (strong fibrous bands of connective tissue) that attach bone to bone. Sprained ankles are among the most common musculoskeletal injuries in people of all ages, athlete and sedentary alike (Harvard Women's Health Watch, 2007). The most common type of ankle sprain occurs when the foot rolls inward, damaging the ligaments of the outer ankle (Figure 50–1◆). Medial ankle sprains, which affect the ligaments of the inner ankle, occur most often in contact sports and are most likely to cause chronic ankle instability with subsequent sprains. The severity of the sprain depends on the degree of damage to the ligaments and how unstable the joint becomes. Chart 50–1 describes the three grades for sprains. Often, a Grade 3 sprain is accompanied by an **avulsion fracture,** in which the

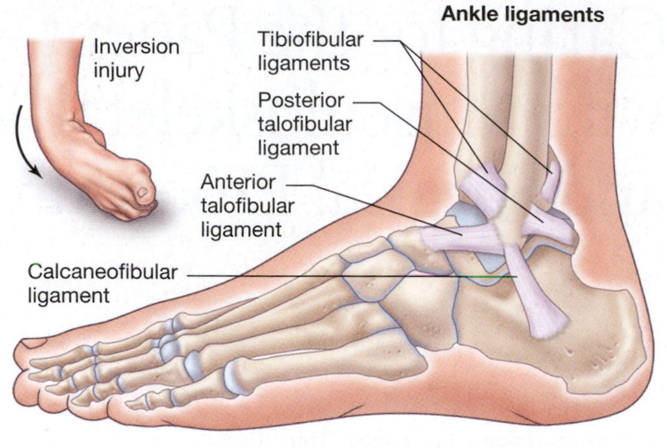

FIGURE 50–1 ◆ Ankle ligaments and inversion injury.

ligament breaks off a small piece of the bone at its attachment. The area may have an effusion (excess fluid in the joint) and ecchymosis; it also may be very tender to palpation. Although a Grade 3 sprain is a seemingly simple injury, relatively high numbers of individuals have persistent symptoms or recurrent problems despite treatment (Mabee & Mabee, 2009).

Medical Management

Strains and sprains are diagnosed by a physical exam and history. A radiograph of the affected extremity may be used to rule out an associated fracture. The initial treatment follows the acronym **PRICE:**

- ***Protection:*** Immobilize and prevent weight bearing. Grade 2 and 3 sprains are protected from further injury by splints, braces, or casts.
- ***Rest:*** Rest is important during the first 24 to 48 hours after the injury to prevent further damage.
- ***Ice:*** The use of ice has many benefits. Cold helps to relieve pain by reducing nerve conductivity, slowing metabolism of oxygen at the

CHART 50–1 Grades of Sprain Severity

Severity	Degree of Ligament Damage	Symptoms	Recovery Time	Treatment
Grade 1	Ligament stretched	Mild pain, swelling, and tenderness. Bruising uncommon. Joint stable with no difficulty bearing weight.	1–3 weeks	Mild injury PRICE (see Medical Management section)
Grade 2	Partial tear 20–75%	Moderate pain, swelling, and tenderness. Some bruising. Joint may have mild to moderate joint instability. Patient will have some decreased ROM and function. Patient will experience pain with weight bearing and walking.	3–6 weeks	PRICE Restrict weight bearing Splint Cast Brace
Grade 3	Complete tear or rupture	Severe pain, swelling, tenderness, and bruising. Unstable joint with loss of function and ROM. Patient will be unable to bear weight or walk.	Several months	PRICE Restrict weight bearing Splint Cast Brace May require surgical intervention

Source: Adapted from Harvard Women's Health Watch. (2007). *Recovering from an ankle sprain.* Retrieved from http://www.health.harvard.edu.

injury site, and reducing cell death and inflammation. An ice pack should be applied to the affected area with the limb elevated and should remain in place for 10 to 15 minutes. Ice packs should be used three to four times a day for the first 3 to 4 days postinjury. Contraindications to ice therapy are cold sensitivity (Raynaud's disease), skin lesions, and peripheral vascular disease.

- ***Compression:*** Compression aids in the control of edema at the injury site by applying direct pressure and increasing venous return. The pressure should be graduated. When patients begin to bear weight on the extremity, they should wear a compression bandage only when the foot is on the floor and not when it is elevated. Generally, patients only need a compression bandage for the first 4 to 5 days, after which the acute inflammatory phase should be over.
- ***Elevation:*** Elevation is effective only if the affected limb is raised above the level of the heart.

Medical attention should be sought immediately for any loss of function, loss of sensation, pallor, or pain that is disproportionate to the injury.

Nursing Management

The nursing management of strains and sprains initially focuses on protection of the limb and pain control. The most commonly used analgesic for sprains and strains is a nonsteroidal anti-inflammatory drug (NSAID). Patient teaching regarding exercises to help restore function and prevent injury are essential to the patient's recovery.

Assessment

The nurse should obtain a thorough history to help differentiate a soft-tissue injury from a fracture. The circumstances leading up to the injury and the mechanism of injury should be explored. Strains and muscle ruptures usually occur from a sudden stretch on a muscle that is actively contracting, such as during a sport or when lifting a heavy object. A sprain is usually the result of a sudden trauma such as tripping. A pop or snap felt at the time of injury could indicate ligament rupture or fracture. The nurse should inquire about previous injuries to determine whether the joint may have weakness. During the physical examination, the nurse compares both extremities to distinguish any deformity or asymmetry. Complete rupture of the muscle is identified by a break in the normal muscle outline, particularly with resisted movement. The nurse also evaluates the extremity for range of motion (ROM). It is normal to have decreased ROM and function as the swelling increases, so it is important for the nurse to determine a baseline, assessing the difference between active, passive, and resisted movement.

Nursing Diagnoses

The primary nursing diagnoses for sprains and strains are as follows:

- *Pain, Acute* related to tissue injury.
- *Physical Mobility, Impaired* related to injury.
- *Knowledge, Deficient* related to plan of care.

NANDA-I © 2012

Outcomes and Evaluation Parameters

The desired outcomes for the patient with a strain or sprain are relief of pain, protection of the joint, and return of strength and mobility. Following the PRICE regimen (described previously) will help to control pain and swelling. Rehabilitative ROM, stretching, and strengthening exercises, as described in Figures 50–2◆ and 50–3◆, will help to strengthen and protect the joint. Evaluation parameters include pain control as described by the patient, resolution of edema, and return of strength and range of motion.

Planning, Interventions, and Rationales

Administration of anti-inflammatory medication, elevation, application of an elastic bandage for compression, and application of an ice pack for 15- to 20-minute intervals four to five times a day will assist in decreasing the swelling and pain. Teaching the patient ROM, stretching, and strengthening exercises like those shown in Figures 50–2 and 50–3 will help the patient regain strength and mobility of the joint, hence restoring function and preventing further injury.

Collaborative Management

The treatment of sprains and strains often involves a multidisciplinary team. In order to meet desired patient outcomes, it is essential that this interdisciplinary team communicate openly with one another in developing and evaluating care of the patient and family (IOM [Institute of Medicine], 2010). Recovery from strains and sprains and prevention from further injury depend on rehabilitative training for strength, agility, and balance. Having the patient work with a physical therapist to teach the proper exercises for the injury is important. In addition, orthotic technicians are needed to properly fit braces and splints. If a patient is overweight, the excess weight can add stress to a musculoskeletal injury and make it difficult to participate in an exercise routine. In these cases, a dietitian can work with the patient to plan a safe and effective weight loss plan.

Health Promotion

Health teaching for patients with contusions, strains, and sprains centers on restoration of function and prevention of further injury. Balance training is found to reduce injury to the ankle and the knee. Some forms of balance training, such as t'ai chi, improve balancing ability and muscular contraction around the ankle joint, which is helpful in reducing injury in older adults who are balance impaired. Balance training in conjunction with strength and agility training has been used to enhance the neuromuscular responses to stabilize the knee joint in female athletes, thus reducing injury (Hrysomallis, 2007).

Dislocations

A **dislocation** is a displacement of a bone from its normal position in a joint. This causes injuries to the joint's ligaments and capsule. A compound dislocation occurs when soft tissue is torn and the joint is exposed to air, which can result in contamination and requires surgical intervention. The dislocation is very painful and requires reduction as soon as possible to reduce pain and avoid vascular and/or nerve damage. For example, a dislocated hip pulls against the soft tissue capsule that contains the vessels that feed the femoral head. This force can occlude the blood supply to the femoral head, which leads to severe complications such as **avascular necrosis (AVN),** in which the bone tissue dies owing to a temporary or permanent loss of blood supply to the bone. Dislocation may also cause significant neurological injury due to the nerve's proximity to the joint. For example, an anterior shoulder dislocation may cause axillary nerve injury. To avoid permanent injury, reduction of the bone to its normal position in the joint should be accomplished as soon as possible.

Range of motion, stretching, and strengthening: First 1–2 weeks

Ankle alphabet. With the heel on the floor, write all the capital letters of the alphabet with your big toe, making the letters as large as you can.

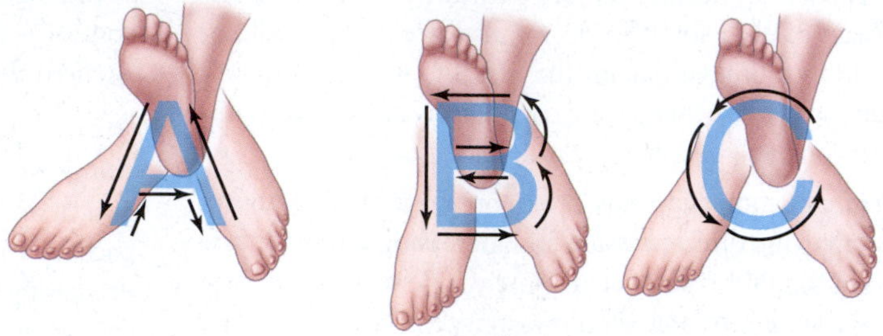

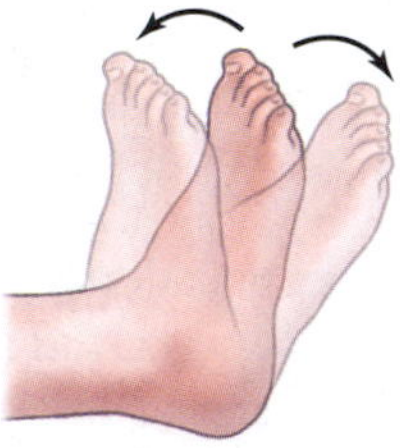

Flexes. Rest the heel of the injured foot on the floor. Pull your toes and foot toward your body as far as possible. Release. Then point them away from the body as far as possible. Release. Repeat as often as possible in the first week.

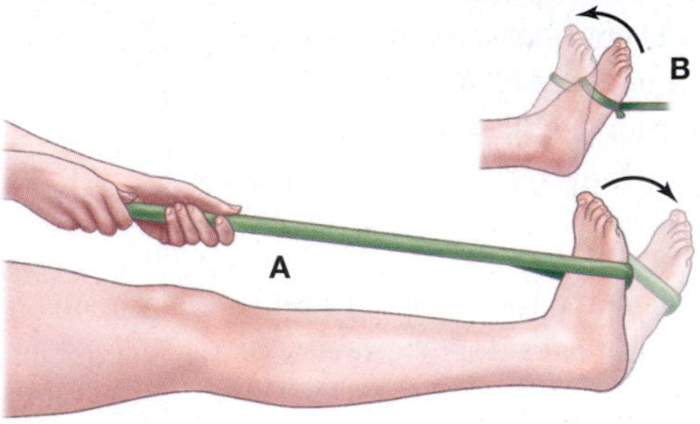

Press down, pull back. Loop an elasticized band or tubing around the foot, holding it gently taut (A). Press your toes away and down. Hold for a few seconds. Repeat 30 times. Tie one end of the band to a table or chair leg (B). Loop the other end around your foot. Slowly pull the foot toward you. Hold for a few seconds. Repeat 30 times.

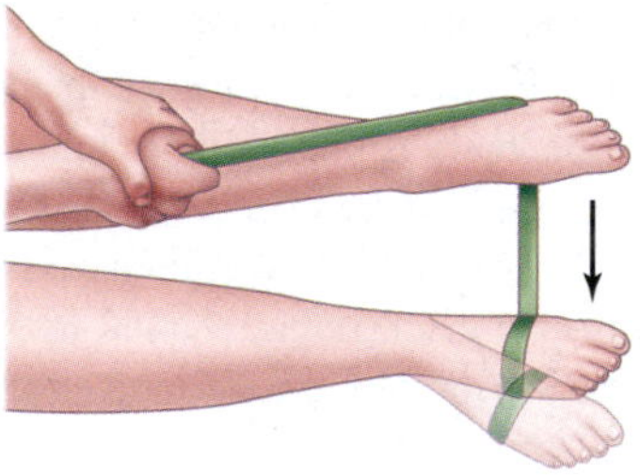

Ankle eversion. Seated on the floor, with an elasticized band or tubing tied around the injured foot and anchored around your uninjured foot, slowly turn the injured foot outward. Repeat 30 times.

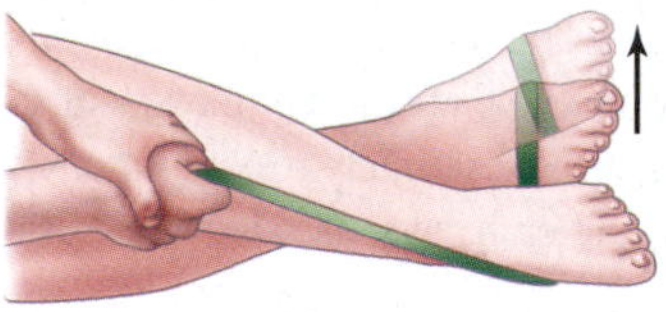

Ankle inversion. Seated on the floor, cross your legs with your injured foot underneath. With an elasticized band or tubing around the injured foot and anchored around your uninjured foot, slowly turn the injured foot inward. Repeat 30 times.

FIGURE 50–2 ◆ Range of motion, stretching, and strengthening of the ankle. Perform the first 1 to 2 weeks after injury.
Source: Harvard Women's Health Watch. (2007). Recovering from an ankle sprain. Retrieved from http://www.health.harvard.edu.

Stretching and strengthening: Weeks 3–4

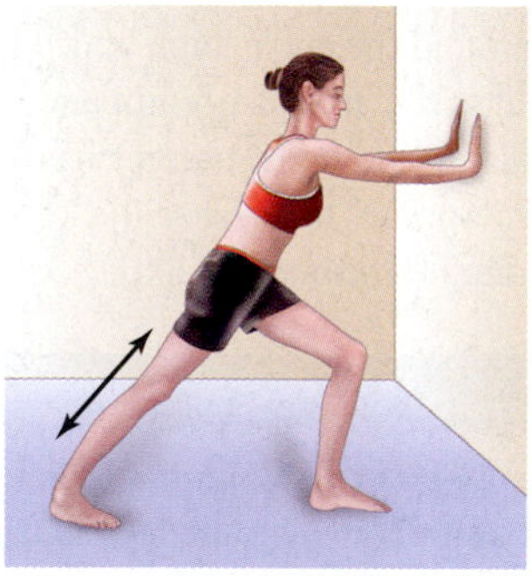

Standing stretch. Stand one arm's length from the wall. Place the injured foot behind the other foot, toes facing forward. Keep your heels down and the back knee straight. Slowly bend the front knee until you feel the calf stretch in the back leg. Hold for 15–20 seconds. Repeat 3–5 times.

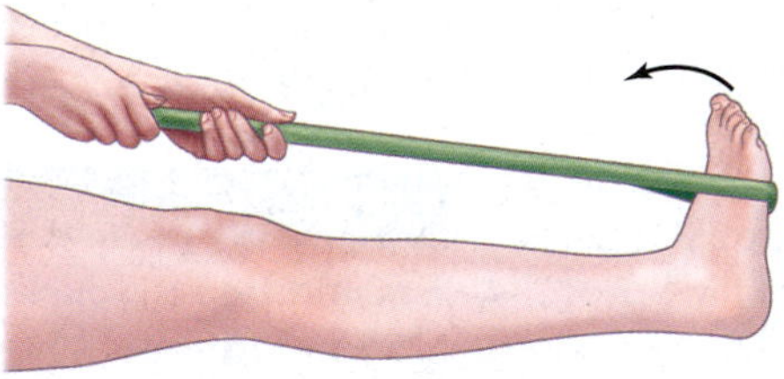

Seated stretch. Loop an elasticized band or tubing around the ball of the foot. Keeping the knee straight, slowly pull back on the band until you feel the upper calf stretch. Hold for 15 seconds. Repeat 15–20 times.

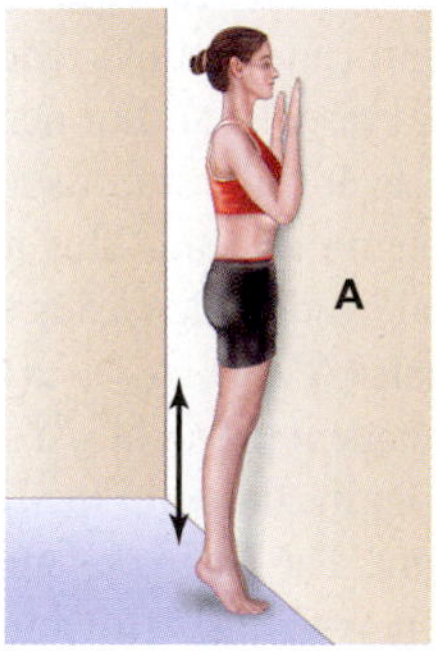

Rises. Stand facing a wall with your hands on the wall for balance (A). Rise up on your toes. Hold for 1 second, then lower yourself slowly to the starting position. Repeat 20–30 times. As you become stronger, do this exercise keeping your weight on just the injured side as you lower yourself down.

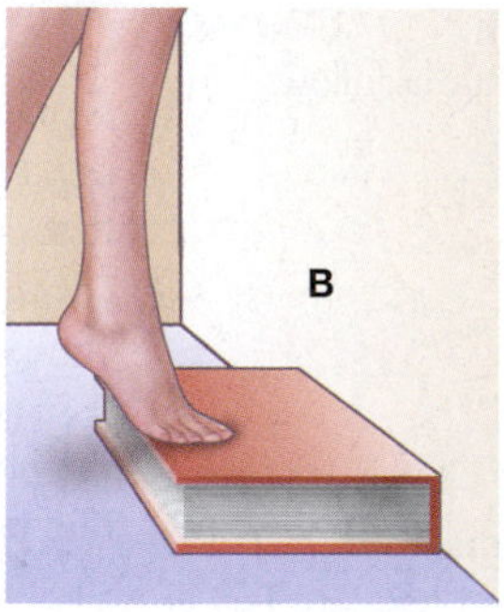

Stretches. Stand with your toes and the ball of the affected foot on a book or the edge of a stair (B). Your heel should be off the ground. Use a wall, chair, or rail for balance. Hold your other foot off the ground behind you, with knee slightly bent. Slowly lower the heel. Hold the position for 1 second. Return to the starting position. Repeat up to 15 times, several times a day. This exercise can place a lot of stress on the ankle, so get your clinician's go-ahead before trying it.

FIGURE 50–3 ◆ Stretching and strengthening exercises for the ankle. Perform 3 to 4 weeks after injury.
Source: Harvard Women's Health Watch. (2007). Recovering from an ankle sprain. Retrieved from http://www.health.harvard.edu.

Weblink: Joint Dislocation

Safety Alert *During the nursing assessment, if a dislocation is suspected, the nurse needs to notify the health care team immediately. A dislocation is considered an orthopedic emergency.*

Etiology, Epidemiology, and Clinical Manifestations

The cause of a dislocation is usually an injury that exerts force great enough to tear the joint ligaments such as a fall, motor vehicle crash, or sports-related impact. A fracture may also be associated with the dislocation. Although a dislocation can occur at any joint, shoulder dislocations are the most common with an estimated 11.2 cases per 100,000 person-years in the United States for traumatic shoulder dislocations (Wilson, 2011). Fracture dislocations of the hand account for 2% to 28% of all emergency department visits (BestPractice, 2010).

The patient will usually present with a deformity of the extremity. In addition, the patient will have severe pain and may have decreased sensation and/or circulation distal to the injury.

Diagnostic Procedures and Medical Management

A radiograph of the joint and surrounding bones may be done to rule out an accompanying fracture. Initial treatment consists of protection and reduction of the dislocation by a trained individual as soon as possible. Ideally, repositioning of the joint should occur within 15 to 30 minutes (Frazier & Drzymkowski, 2007). After that, the joint may be so edematous and painful that the reduction may be impossible without general anesthesia.

Nursing Management

Nursing management of a dislocation consists of assessment and protection of the extremity, pain control, and education to regain strength and mobility of the affected joint.

Assessment

The nurse completes a thorough examination of the involved extremity, including a peripheral nerve assessment to determine neurological impairment and frequent reassessment for any progression. Chart 50–2 describes common nerve involvement for specific dislocations. The nurse assesses capillary refill and pulses distal to the injury to determine vascular impairment.

Nursing Diagnoses

Primary nursing diagnoses for the patient with a dislocation include the following:

- *Acute Pain* related to tissue injury.
- *Risk for Injury* related to surrounding bone, vasculature, and nerves.
- *Impaired Physical Mobility* related to dislocation.

NANDA-I © 2012

Outcomes and Evaluation Parameters

The desired outcomes for the patient with a dislocation are relief of pain, prevention of damage to the nerves and vasculature, and restoration of strength and mobility of the affected joint. Evaluation parameters include control of pain as described by the patient, restoration of nerve and vascular function, and return of strength and mobility to the joint as exhibited by range of motion and strength assessment.

Planning, Interventions, and Rationales

As stated earlier, a dislocation is an orthopedic emergency. The nurse should quickly assess and immobilize the affected joint and extremity to prevent further damage and to recognize any vascular or nerve involvement. The patient will require intravenous pain medication because the pain is severe. The nurse should anticipate and prepare the patient for conscious sedation because this will most likely be needed for reduction. Postreduction, the patient will require a stabilization splint to prevent the joint from re-injury until the tissues have healed.

Collaborative Management

Collaborative management for the patient with a dislocation is the same as that for patients with sprains and strains.

Health Promotion

Teaching the patient ROM exercises to maintain mobility and strengthening exercises for the muscles that surround the joint is essential for optimal outcome. Repeated dislocation is potentially damaging to the joint. The nurse should review with the patient the proper use of splinting devices and the plan of care for timing or resumption of activities.

Fractures

A quick review of the basic anatomy of bones is helpful to understand terminology use in the description of fractures and injuries. Long bones are found in the upper and lower extremities and are classified as such because they have certain anatomic features in common, as shown in Figure 50–4◆ (p. 1526). The shaft of the long bone is mainly compact bone hollowed out to form a marrow-filled medullary canal. All long bones have an **epiphysis,** the bone end beyond the physis; growth plate; **metaphysis,** an area of widening between the diaphysis and physis; and **diaphysis,** the shaft between the metaphyses on each end. Bone ends typically form a joint with another bone end and are differentiated as proximal (closest to a person's head or core) and distal.

CHART 50–2 Peripheral Nerve Assessment

Injury	Nerve	Motor	Sensation
Wrist dislocation	Median distal	Thenar contraction with opposition	Index finger
Anterior shoulder dislocation	Musculocutaneous	Elbow flexion	Lateral forearm
Distal humeral shaft, anterior shoulder dislocation	Radial	Thumb, finger MCP extension	First dorsal web space
Anterior shoulder dislocation, proximal humerus fracture	Axillary	Deltoid	Lateral shoulder
Knee dislocation	Posterior tibial	Toe flexion	Sole of foot
Fibular neck fracture, knee dislocation	Superficial peroneal	Ankle eversion	Lateral dorsum of foot
Posterior hip dislocation	Sciatic nerve	Plantar dorsiflexion	Foot

Source: Adapted from American College of Surgeons. (2008). *Advanced trauma life support student course manual.* Chicago: American College of Surgeons.

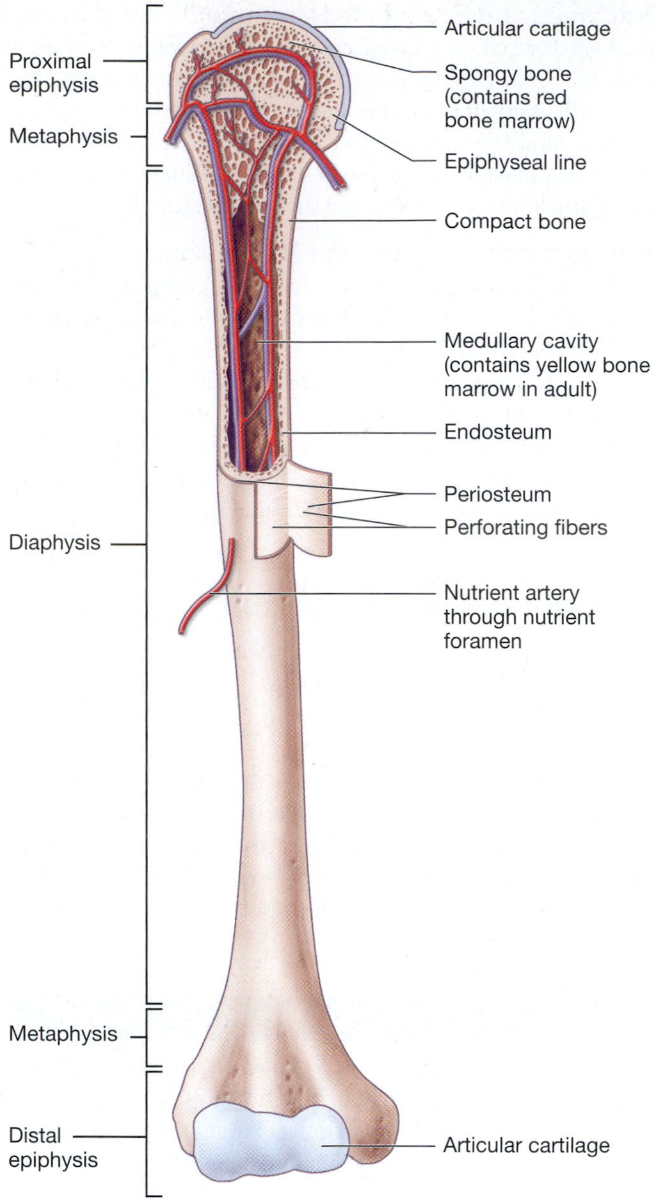

FIGURE 50–4 ◆ Long bone.

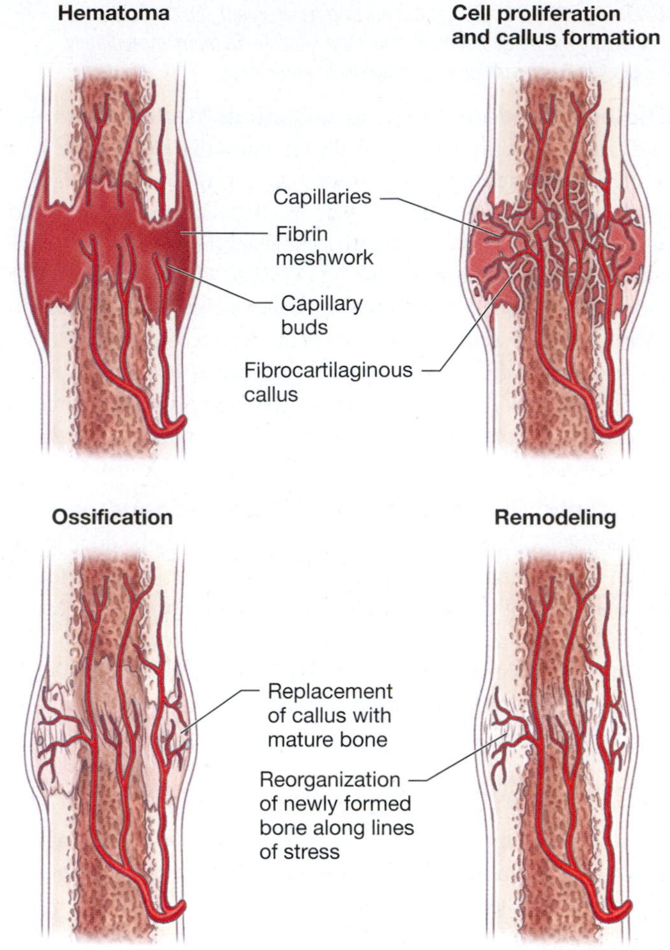

FIGURE 50–5 ◆ Bone healing.

Short bones are found in the wrist and ankle. They are irregularly shaped and, except for the compact bone on the surface, are spongy throughout. Flat bones are found where protection of underlying structures is needed, such as the skull and ribs, or to provide a large area for muscle attachment, such as the scapula. Flat bones consist of a layer of spongy bone between two layers of compact bone.

Healing of Fractures

A **fracture** is a discontinuity of the bone that may be complete or incomplete (Porth & Matfin, 2009). A fracture or break in the bone causes a healing cascade, beginning with the blood that leaks out at the fracture site. This hematoma is rich in osteoclasts, which make bone. Clotting factors that remain due to the hematoma initiate the formation of a fibrin meshwork that serves as a framework for the fibroblasts and new capillary buds. Granulation tissue is formed and gradually replaces the clot.

During cellular proliferation and callus formation, the osteoblasts, or bone-forming cells, multiply and differentiate into the fibrocartilaginous callus. This process begins distal to the fracture where there is greater blood supply. Within a few days, a cartilage "collar" is evident around the fracture site. The edges of the collar that are on either side of the fracture unite to form a bridge that connects the bone fragments. Initially, the callus is soft; however, within the third to fourth week of fracture healing, the bone calcifies as mineral salts are deposited. Ossification is the final laying down of bone after the fracture has been bridged and the fragments are united (Figure 50–5◆). Mature bone replaces the callus, and the fracture site feels firm and appears united on radiograph. At this point, a cast may be removed. The remodeling process involves resorption of the excess callus in the marrow space and the external aspect of the fracture. The process is directed by mechanical stress and weight bearing, thereby becoming stronger in relation to its function. Healing time depends on the site and type of the fracture and on the patient's underlying health. With fractures of the long bones, displaced fractures, and fractures with less surface area, strength and function usually return within 6 months after bone union is complete. Small nondisplaced fractures require less time to heal, and the patient will usually have full function within 2 to 4 weeks.

Classification of Fractures

Fractures are classified in various ways; the simplest is whether a fracture is open or closed. In a closed fracture, the soft tissue envelope, which may be damaged, does not communicate with the outside; in effect, there is no skin opening. An open fracture means there is a tear in the soft tissue, exposing the bone to the outside environment. All open fractures have the potential to be contaminated, which

CHART 50–3 Grading of Open Fractures

Grade	Description
Grade I	Wound less than 1 cm with minimal soft tissue injury. Wound bed is clean. Bone injury is simple with minimal comminution.
Grade II	Wound is greater than 1 cm with moderate soft tissue injury. Wound bed is moderately contaminated. Fracture contains moderate comminution.
Grade III	The following fractures automatically result in classification as Grade III: • Segmental fracture with displacement • Fracture with diaphyseal segmental loss • Fracture with associated vascular injury requiring repair • Farmyard injuries or highly contaminated wounds • High-velocity gunshot wound • Fracture caused by crushing force from fast-moving vehicle.
Grade IIIA	Wound less than 10 cm with crushed tissue and contamination. Soft tissue coverage of bone is usually possible.
Grade IIIB	Wound greater than 10 cm with crushed tissue and contamination. Soft tissue is inadequate and requires regional or free flap.
Grade IIIC	Fracture in which there is a major vascular injury requiring repair for limb salvage.

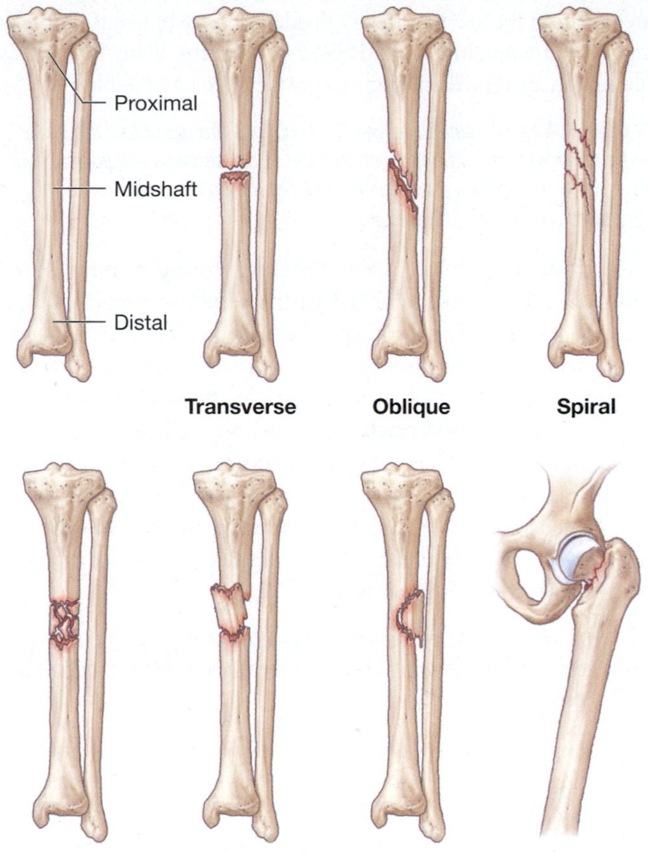

FIGURE 50–6 ◆ Classification of fractures by direction of fracture.

increases the morbidity (frequency of complications or poor outcome) and mortality (fatal outcome) of the injury. The time frames vary by institution, but many consider 6 to 8 hours the maximum time that a contaminated fracture can wait to be taken to the operating room and washed out, a process that is often referred to as an *inspection and debridement* (I&D) (Feliciano, Mattox, & Moore, 2008). During the I&D, the fracture and soft tissue are washed out with a pulsed lavage, typically with antibiotic solution. The soft tissue is inspected, debris is removed, and any damaged or necrotic tissue is debrided to try to reduce the possibility of infection. Chart 50–3 shows a grading classification for open fractures.

Grade I is typically an "inside-out" fracture, that is, one in which the end of the fractured bone pokes through the skin and returns. This is considered the cleanest fracture with limited risk for deep infection. A Grade II fracture occurs when a soft-tissue wound is greater than 1 cm with moderate contamination and soft tissue injury. A Grade III fracture has a greater than 10-cm wound opening, is severely contaminated, and involves comminution of the bone, soft tissue loss, and vascular injury (Wheeless, 2008).

There are other ways to classify fractures such as by appearance, apposition angulation, and mechanism of injury. Long bone fractures may be described by their appearance, which also gives some indication of the mechanism of injury. Descriptors such as *transverse, oblique, spiral, comminuted, segmental, butterfly,* and *impacted* are commonly used (Figure 50–6◆).

Transverse fractures are horizontal to the bone shaft and usually result from a direct blow. Healing of nondisplaced transverse fractures is usually uneventful because the muscle pulls and compresses the bone ends together, which is key in bone healing. Oblique fractures are diagonal and may allow shortening of the bone due to the muscle pulls. The diagonal configuration may allow the bone ends to slide down on each other. A spiral fracture is as described: spiral, and typically caused by rotatory torsion. Spiral fractures raise suspicions of inflicted injury in nonambulating children, because they typically occur as a result of limb twisting. Segmental fractures describe bone that is broken in more than one place. These fractures are difficult to manage without surgical intervention to stabilize the bone fragments. In butterfly fractures, large pieces of the bone are shaped like a butterfly with one side longer than the other. Impacted fractures occur when broken ends of bone are forced together. These fractures have a high rate of healing and limited pain because most pain of fractures comes from the innervated periosteum portion of the bone ends rubbing against each other. Impacted fractures do not readily move but need to be protected from displacing until healing occurs.

Fracture apposition describes the relation of the bone ends to each other; for example, if half of each bone end is touching the other, it is considered 50% opposed. If the bone ends are not in contact at all, the fracture may be referred to as 100% displaced or 0% apposition. Nondisplaced fractures keep anatomic alignment. Fracture angulation describes the angle at the fracture's apex in relation to the proximal fragment of bone. Some fracture descriptions are specific to the particular bone, such as spine and pelvis fractures.

Spinal fractures can occur in the 7 cervical vertebrae (frequently referred to as the C-spine), 12 thoracic vertebrae (T-spine), and 5 lumbar vertebrae (L-spine) and are classified as stable or unstable using a three-column theory. This theory divides the vertebrae into three columns: the anterior, middle, and posterior columns. If any two of these columns are disrupted, the spine is considered to be unstable.

Safety Alert *When two vertebral columns are disrupted, the spinal cord and nerve roots are no longer protected from serious neurological injury. Therefore, it is imperative that the nurse keep the patient in strict spinal immobilization per hospital protocol.*

An unstable spine is typically treated with complete bed rest with logrolling, a Roto Rest bed or Stryker frame bed, or surgical fixation. The special beds allow the patient to be turned without flexing the patient's spine. Changes in position are needed to avoid pressure areas and pooling of fluids. Some spine fractures are described by the mechanism of injury, such as a **burst fracture,** which occurs when an axial load is placed on the spine and a vertebra explodes out in all directions. This form of fracture may push bone fragments into the spinal canal and has the potential for neurological damage. Burst fractures are unstable, and patients with burst fractures need to be watched for any neurovascular changes in the lower extremities.

Safety Alert *During the nursing assessment, any changes in exam should be reported to the health care team immediately because deficits can become permanent.*

A **chance fracture** is one through bony and/or ligamentous portions of the spine caused by distraction of the vertebrae. This most often occurs in a person involved in a motor vehicle crash who was sitting in the back seat of a car with only a lap belt. The impact forces the person's upper body forward while the lap belt holds the person down, producing tearing through the spine. These injuries may not be visible on plain spine films, so any trauma patient with back pain should be assessed for injuries.

Some C-spine fractures or ligamentous injuries are unstable and require surgical treatment and/or treatment in cervical traction or a halo vest to prevent neurological compromise. Both the halo vest and cervical traction rely on two, four, or more pins to be placed in a ring around the patient's head and torqued to 6 to 8 pounds of pressure. This enables the pins to penetrate the skull's outer table, securing them in place. Care of the pin site includes watching for any drainage, erythema, or movement. Pin site care is discussed in more detail later in the chapter. For a detailed discussion of spine and spinal cord injuries, refer to Chapter 24.

Safety Alert *During the nursing assessment, clear drainage from a pin site or ear could be cerebrospinal fluid. The nurse must report the finding to the health care team immediately.*

A genetic disorder that predisposes patients to fractures is osteogenesis imperfecta. Refer to the Genetic Considerations box.

Medical Management

Initial management of an extremity fracture consists of immobilization that includes the joint above and the joint below the fracture. After the extremity has been splinted, the health care provider reassesses the patient's neurological and vascular status and accomplishes a plan for definitive care:

- Narcotics are generally needed for effective pain relief and should be given in small frequent doses. The patient will be further evaluated to determine the extent of the injury and whether it will require simple casting or surgical intervention for open reduction and internal fixation.

GENETIC CONSIDERATIONS Osteogenesis Imperfecta

Osteogenesis imperfecta (OI), commonly called brittle bone syndrome, is an extremely rare genetic disorder affecting type I collagen formation. There are several types of OI. Type I is the mildest form of the disease. Patients with type I OI are prone to fractures and have collagen deficiency; females with the disorder also have an increased risk of postmenopausal osteoporosis. Type II OI is nearly always fatal during the neonatal period due to birth injuries. Patients with type III (severe) OI have severe bone deformities, have sufficient but abnormal collagen, and are prone to bone fractures. Respiratory insufficiency related to rib fractures and thoracic cage deformity is a major complication in this group. The patient with type III OI may fracture a rib simply by coughing. Type IV, or "moderate OI with short stature," is similar to type III but has less skeletal deformity.

With this disease, the treatment of fractures is often complicated by delayed union.

- There are typically five treatment options for fractures: closed treatment with casting, traction, surgical treatment with external fixation, open reduction with internal fixation, and intramedullary rod. A combination of these options may also be used. There are risks, benefits, and indications for each, which are discussed next.

Casting, Bracing, and Splinting

The easiest and sometimes most cost-effective treatment for fractures is the cast. A cast is a rigid circumferential encasement device made of plaster or fiberglass. Casting material (plaster or fiberglass and Webril/cotton padding) is relatively inexpensive and readily available. However, casting does not completely keep bones from moving, and it may allow shortening or displacement of fractures. Patients may complain of hearing or feeling crepitus (crunching or grinding of their bone ends moving in the cast).

A cast must cover the joint above and the joint below a fractured long bone. This restricts joint motion for the length of time needed for fracture healing but renders those joints stiff when treatment is complete and frequently requires rehabilitation of atrophied muscles. This form of treatment is not optimal in the immediate postinjury period because it is rigid and does not allow for the swelling of tissues, which typically occurs for the first 3 days after a fracture. Fractures can be painful until the bone ends begin to granulate and get "sticky," which occurs around 10 to 14 days in the average, well-nourished, nonsmoking patient. Another problem with casting is there is no access to soft tissues to observe for pressure points or skin breakdown. Most cast material must stay dry, so it is difficult for the patient to bathe. Fiberglass casting tape used with a waterproof Gortex liner is now used for certain applications to allow casts in showers or chlorinated swimming pools.

A splint or brace is manufactured or made by the health care provider with casting material. It allows the fractured bone to rest within a firm surface to decrease motion but is not circumferential. The splint or brace is secured by straps or wrapped circumferentially with a bandage. This allows for adjustment if there is increased swelling and enables removal for visualization of the soft tissues.

Traction

Traction, a treatment option that is used in most underdeveloped countries, is not the treatment of choice in the United States because of the cost of long hospital stays and the complications associated with the immobilization involved with traction. The purpose of traction is to maintain alignment of the bone with an axial pull along the axis of the bone to counteract the pulls of the muscles. **Skin traction** or **Buck's boots traction** consists of straps or foam boots secured to lower extremities with a cord pulling no more than 6 pounds. Skin traction is frequently used for comfort in patients with a hip fracture. No more than 6 pounds should be placed on this kind of traction because pressure areas will develop. The nurse should examine the skin under the boot or bandage wrap every 4 to 6 hours for any reddened areas.

Skeletal traction entails placement of a skeletal pin that is drilled through the bone such as a distal femur or proximal tibia. The portions of the skeletal pin exiting the skin on either side of the limb are attached to a bail. A cord is secured to the bail and runs through pulleys to a weighted bag suspended at the end of the bed. The purpose of the weight is to pull along the axis of the bone to counteract the muscle forces (spasm) in an attempt to bring bones "out to length" and/or maintain anatomic alignment. A trapeze on the bed may help the patient move in the bed; however, a trapeze should not be used if the patient has a spine fracture.

Pin site care is an important nursing function. Skeletal traction pins are exposed to the environment where they protrude through the skin and can allow bacteria to travel down to the bone. Skeletal pins are generally not painful except when placed or removed or if the pin sites become infected. It is expected that the pin site will be red, tender, and have bloody or serosanguineous drainage for the first 24 to 72 hours. After that time, any tenderness or drainage should raise suspicions of infection. Pin sites should remain flat and not be allowed to tent on the pin. Pin releases are performed to keep the skin off the pin. The tent provides a warm, moist dark area where bacteria (always present at the pin–skin interface) can accumulate and grow. For more on pin site care, see the Evidence-Based Practice box.

Traction has high morbidity and mortality risks, especially in older adults. The problems with traction stem from the immobilization involved, which can produce complications such as skin breakdown, urinary tract infection, pneumonia, deep venous thrombosis (DVT), and pulmonary embolism (PE). The cost of hospitalization for traction in the United States far exceeds that of surgical treatment. Traction is labor intensive, involving setting up traction beds, repeating x-rays frequently, and changing the axis of the pull to change the angulation of the fracture.

External Fixation

External fixation refers to a form of treatment in which the bones or bone ends of a fracture are held in place by skeletal pins that are screwed into the bone and attached to a frame worn on the outside of the body. External fixation devices (EFDs) have become the treatment of choice for many fractures, especially when soft tissues are damaged and access is needed for wound care.

Unlike casting, external fixation allows for greater mobility and joint motion above or below the fracture. External fixation may be used for emergent stabilization of fractures or as definitive treatment. Scars are minimal compared to open reduction internal fixation or intramedullary rodding. For some patients, the pins may be removed in a clinic.

The most common complication of external fixation is pin site infection. Skeletal pins protrude through an opening in the skin, which creates a foreign body reaction. The body reacts by forming a bursal lining between the pin and skin. This protective membrane produces fluid to reduce the friction at the pin–skin interface. This fluid is easily contaminated by skin flora and needs to be allowed to drain out at the pin site to reduce the concentration of microorganisms (see the Evidence-Based Practice box).

Another complication of external fixation or skeletal traction is a plantar flexion contracture of the foot. Without support, the foot will rest in plantar flexion, and this can result in Achilles tendon shortening

EVIDENCE-BASED PRACTICE Pin Site Care

Clinical Problem

Infection of pin sites is one of the most common complications associated with the use of skeletal pins, wires, and external fixation (Walker, 2007). An infection at the pin site is painful and will delay mobilization of the patient. The infection may also lead to other severe complications, including osteomyelitis, nonunion of the bone at the fracture site, delayed fracture healing, loss of fracture alignment, or systemic infection. All of these complications can result in long-term pain and possible disability. Because of the significance of pin site care, it is important to base the care and technique on evidence.

Research Findings

Hydrogen peroxide was commonly used in the past to cleanse pin sites, especially to remove crusts from around the pin site. The use of hydrogen peroxide is now discouraged because it may cause damage to the healthy tissue surrounding the pin. It has also been associated with increased infection rates and the disruption of the skin's normal flora (Walker, 2007).

In 2005, the National Association of Orthopaedic Nurses (NAON) completed a systematic analysis of the research literature on skeletal pin site care and sought opinions of an expert panel to develop guidelines for skeletal pin site care (Holmes & Brown, 2005). These guidelines are still in use today. NAON found that there were two experimental studies regarding pin site care, but the studies explored different aspects: one explored cleansing solutions, and the other addressed frequency of site care. The panel also reviewed five case series studies; one of these, which reported comparison of two methods of site care, was judged to be of high quality. Using the methodology of expert consensus, the panel developed the following major recommendations:

- Pins located in areas with considerable soft tissue should be considered at greater risk for infection.
- After the first 48 to 72 hours, when drainage may be heavy, pin site care should be done daily or weekly for sites with mechanically stable bone–pin interfaces.
- Chlorhexidine 2 mg/mL solution may be the most effective cleansing solution for pin site care.
- Patients and their families should be taught pin site care before discharge from the hospital. They should be required to demonstrate whatever care needs to be done and should be provided with written instructions that include signs and symptoms of infection.

Implications for Nursing Practice

Guidelines reflect the state of current knowledge within the health care literature regarding the effectiveness of current practice. Clinical practice guidelines are developed by reviewing these findings and seeking the opinions of known experts in that field of practice. The expert consensus is vital in practice that has little or no research to review.

Although there was little research regarding care of the skin immediately surrounding the skeletal pin site, some of what had been done was judged to be of good quality and therefore useful. It is clear that (1) the solution used to cleanse pin sites should be chlorhexidine and (2) nurses should not use peroxide.

Critical Thinking Questions with answers can be found in the Osborn Student Resources at nursing.pearsonhighered.com.

Sources: Holmes, S. B., & Brown, S. J. (2005). Skeletal pin site care: National Association of Orthopaedic Nurses guidelines for orthopaedic nursing. *Orthopaedic Nursing, 24*(2), 99–107; Walker, J. A. (2007). Evidence for skeletal pin site care. *Nursing Standard, 21*(45), 70–76.

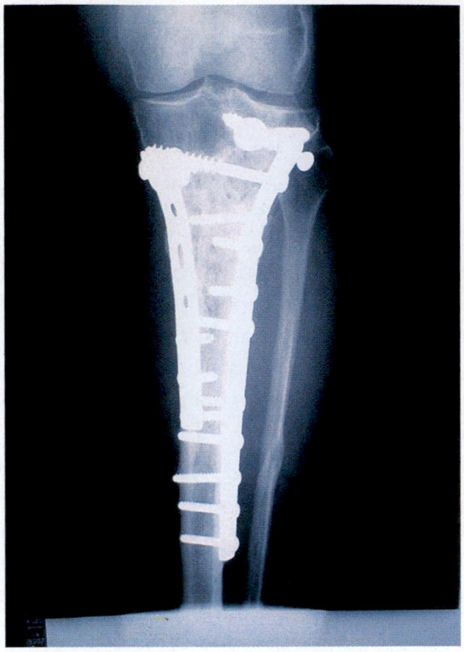

FIGURE 50–7 ◆ Open reduction internal fixation.
Source: Cheryl Wraa.

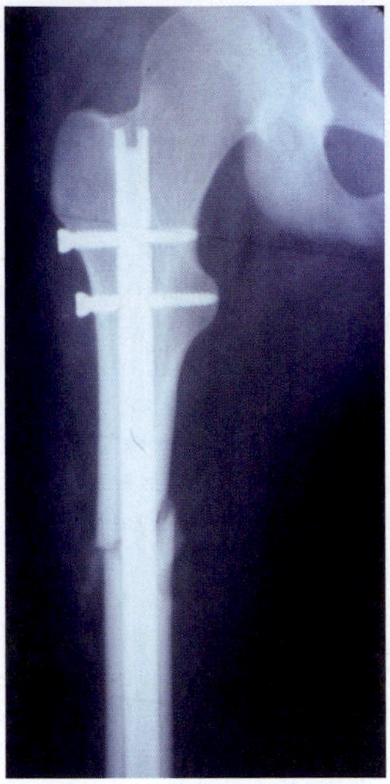

FIGURE 50–8 ◆ Intramedullary rodding.
Source: Cheryl Wraa.

or tightness. This deformity can be avoided with frequent stretching and the use of a foot plate.

Open Reduction Internal Fixation

A very common method of fracture fixation is **open reduction internal fixation (ORIF),** in which a fracture is exposed by an incision in the skin directly over the fracture. Implants such as plates (strips of metal), screws, and wires are placed directly on or in the bone to anatomically stabilize a fracture (Figure 50–7◆). This method of fracture fixation allows direct visualization of the fracture but can disrupt the circulation to the bone and leave large surgical scars.

Complications associated with ORIF are wound infection and hardware failure or breakage. Therefore, ORIF is not optimal for use with comminuted or osteoporotic bone or damaged or suboptimal soft tissues. Patients with conditions such as peripheral vascular disease, diabetes, and obesity frequently encounter healing problems. Screw heads may be prominent and irritate tissue, and hardware may need to be removed following healing.

Intramedullary Rod

Intramedullary (I-M) rodding refers to a method of fracture fixation that entails sliding a metal rod down the medullary canal of a long bone (Figure 50–8◆). This form of fixation allows for anatomic alignment and is helpful for segmental fractures. I-M rods allow for early weight bearing because they share the load and leave the joints free to move. They may need to be removed after healing is complete. The holes left by the screws are stress risers (a defect in the bone which concentrates stress in the area and increases the risk of failure of the bone at that site), and fractures may occur through them when an I-M rod is removed.

The benefits of this fixation method include smaller surgical scars in less obvious places than with other methods. For example, the rod in Figure 50–8 was placed through a 4-cm incision above the hip, and small stab incisions were made to place the screws. There is a slight increased risk of fat embolism with this method because of the pressure exerted in the canal by the reamer or from hammering the I-M rod down, which may force fat into the bloodstream.

Nursing Management

Nursing management of the patient with an extremity fracture involves relief of pain and frequent reassessment of the patient's neurovascular status. Patients with femur fractures require frequent monitoring of vascular status because femoral shaft fractures are associated with significant blood loss of up to 1,500 to 2,000 mL and the patient can develop hypovolemic shock (Feliciano et al., 2008).

Assessment

Initial assessment of an extremity fracture includes observation for deformities, breaks in the skin, and a thorough assessment of vascular and sensory status distal to the extremity. Frequent reassessment of neurovascular status is necessary to prevent complications.

Nursing Diagnoses

The primary nursing diagnoses for the patient with an extremity fracture include:

- *Pain, Acute* related to fracture.
- *Physical Mobility, Impaired* related to immobilization of fractured extremity.
- *Injury, Risk for* related to impaired mobility.
- *Fluid Volume, Risk for Deficient* related to blood loss from fracture.
- *Infection, Risk for* related to wounds, pin sites, and/or surgical sites.

NANDA-I © 2012

Outcomes, planning, intervention, and evaluation are discussed in the section on pelvic fractures.

Pelvic Fractures

Etiology

Pelvic fractures are frequently associated with other traumatic injuries from motor vehicle crashes. It is essential to know the mechanism of injury in pelvic fractures because this will assist the health care team

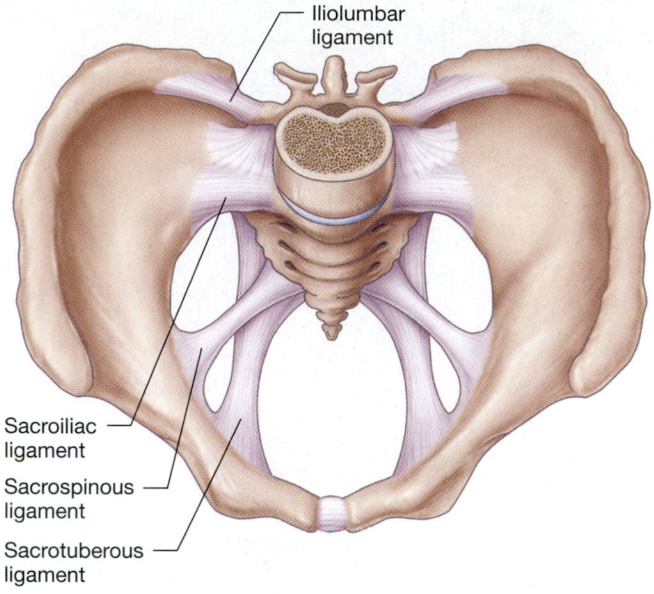

FIGURE 50–9 ◆ Ligaments of the pelvis.

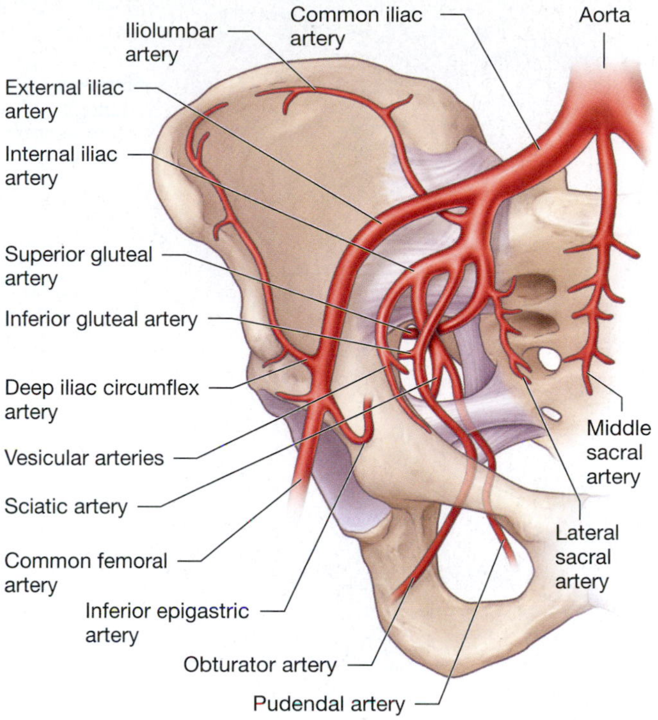

FIGURE 50–10 ◆ Vascular anatomy of the pelvis.

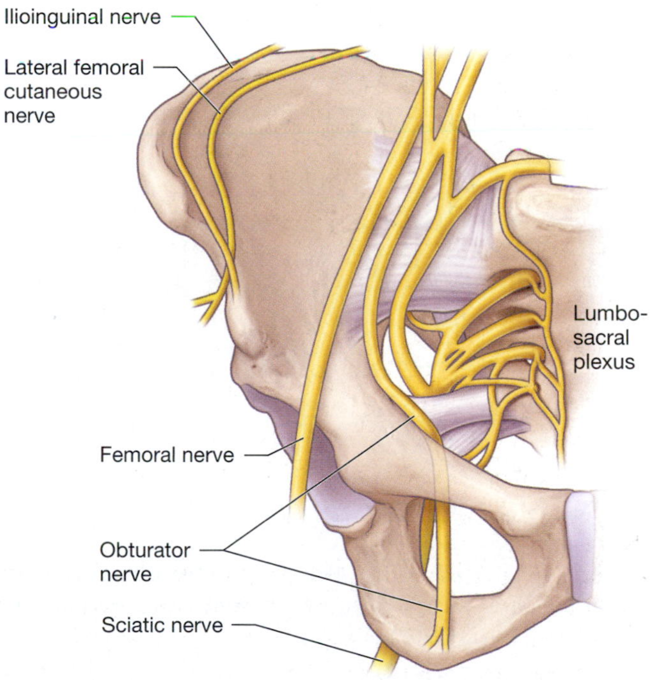

FIGURE 50–11 ◆ Neuroanatomy of the pelvis.

in anticipating additional injuries, especially when the patient was in a motor vehicle crash. Common additional injuries that are associated with pelvic fractures are femur fracture, bladder rupture, and risk for retroperitoneal bleeding. Simple fractures that are not displaced are considered to be stable fractures. Unstable fractures are fractures in which ligaments are torn, there are multiple fractures, or there is movement of the pelvic girdle with downward pressure when the patient is in a supine position. If the pelvic fracture is unstable, it may be treated with external fixation or internal fixation.

The pelvis consists of two innominate bones and the sacrum, which form a ring of bone. The bones are held in a structural unit primarily by the ligaments of the pelvis (Figure 50–9◆). The strongest ligamentous structures are in the posterior aspect of the pelvis at the sacroiliac (SI) joints. These ligaments have to hold up the weight-bearing forces from the lower extremities to the spine that are transferred to the SI joints. Major blood vessels are located on the inner wall of the pelvis (Figure 50–10◆). Whenever the pelvis is fractured, these arteries and associated veins can be damaged, and extensive bleeding will occur. The lumbar and sacral plexus of nerves run through the posterior pelvis and can be affected with pelvic trauma (Figure 50–11◆). Organs that can be injured during a trauma with pelvic fracture are the bladder and urethra, vagina, prostate, and gastrointestinal system.

A large amount of force is required to fracture the pelvis. Therefore, the nurse should simultaneously assess for other serious injuries. Three types of forces cause damage to the pelvis. The first and most common is lateral compression (Figure 50–12◆, p. 1532). Examples include a pedestrian hit on his side by a motor vehicle, a fall from a height in which the patient lands on his side, and a motor vehicle crash in which intrusion of the vehicle compresses the pelvis. The second most frequent force is from an anterior or posterior direction. This occurs from either direct contact with the iliac spine or force transmitted from the femur (Figure 50–13◆). An example of this mechanism occurs when a person's legs are spread apart in a motorcycle crash. The injury can involve ligament disruption only, and the injury usually manifests itself as a widened pubic symphysis and SI joints. The third type of force is vertical shear (see Figure 50–13). This type of injury is most commonly seen in patients who jumped from a height and landed on an extended lower extremity. The vertical shear injury disrupts the restraining ligaments of the hemipelvis, rendering it mechanically unstable.

One or more of these forces may have injured a patient at one time. It is important for the nurse to inquire as to the mechanism of injury to be able to anticipate the type of injury the patient may have sustained.

Epidemiology

In the United States, fractures of the pelvis comprise approximately 37 cases per 100,000 person-years with the highest incidence occurring

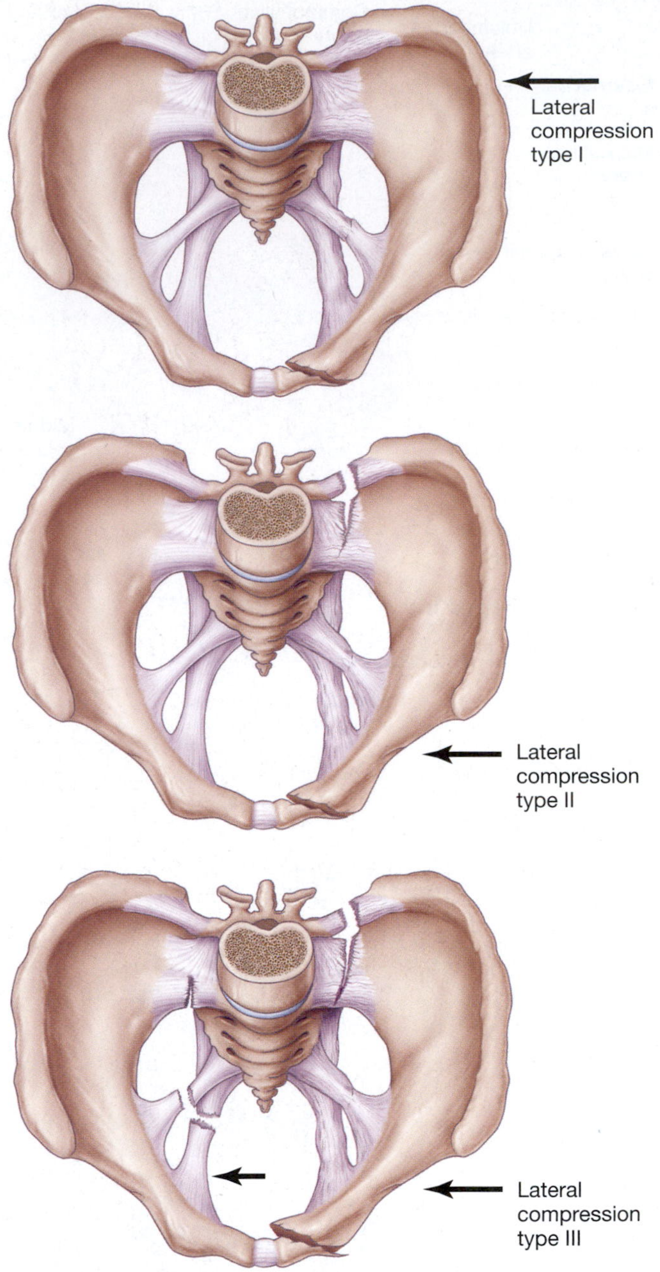

FIGURE 50–12 ◆ Lateral compression fractures.

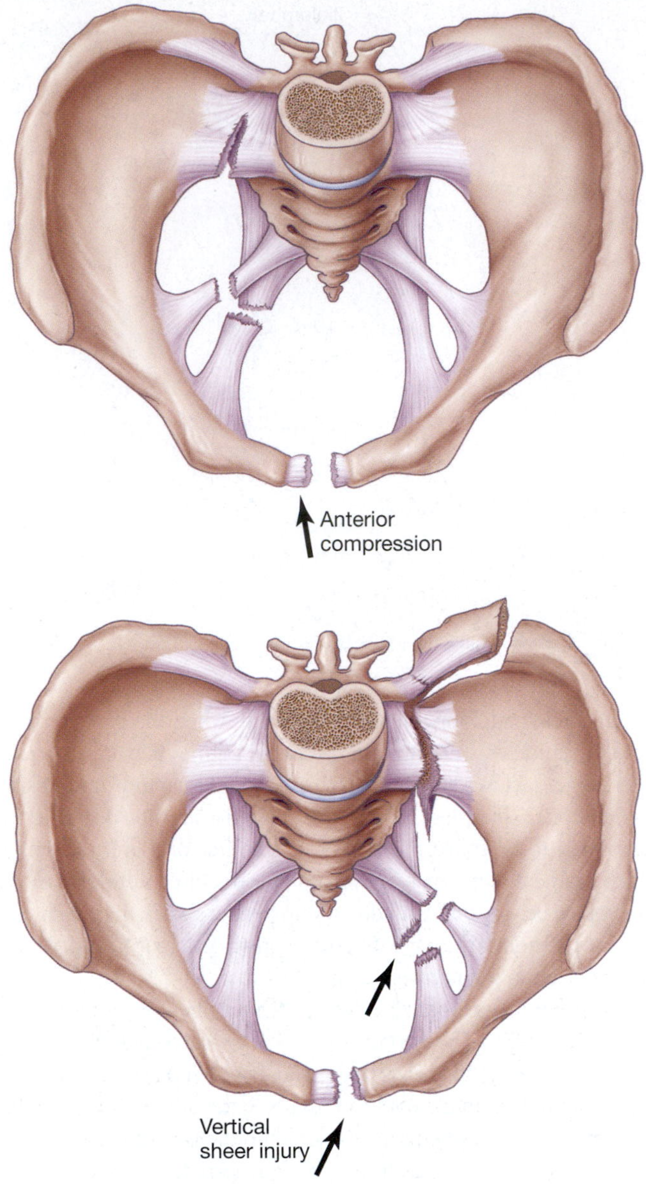

FIGURE 50–13 ◆ Anterior compression and vertical shear injuries.

in patients 15 to 28 years of age. Before age 35 years, hip fractures are more common in men; women sustain more pelvic fractures after 35 years of age (Russell, 2011).

Clinical Manifestations

During the physical examination, the nurse should inspect the pelvis to see whether there is a rotation of the iliac crest and/or any difference in leg length. When palpating, the nurse should exert gentle lateral compression and distraction of the iliac crests and inward compression of the symphysis pubis to determine pelvic stability.

Safety Alert *It is critically important for the nurse to be careful when moving the patient and maneuvering the pelvis so as not to cause damage to the vasculature or neural bundles.*

If the pelvis feels unstable, the nurse should alert the health care team so that others will not attempt to manipulate the pelvis and cause further damage or increased bleeding. The nurse should inspect the skin and skinfolds to identify any open fractures and observe the meatus to check for blood signifying a possible urethral injury.

Safety Alert *If there is blood at the meatus, do not attempt to insert a Foley catheter.*

The health care team will perform a digital rectal exam to evaluate for sensation, sphincter tone, presence of blood, and position of the prostate. Female patients will undergo a vaginal exam to look for tears in the vagina signifying an open fracture. The lower extremities should be evaluated for pulses, motor function, and sensation.

Diagnostic Tests

Initially, an anteroposterior (AP) radiograph of the pelvis will show most fractures and associated dislocations. However, this view does not allow the health care team to determine the degree of bone displacement, and small fractures may be missed. Additional views called inlet and outlet views may be obtained. The inlet view is taken at a 60-degree angle from the head toward the feet. This will show the posterior and cephalic displacement of fractures of the posterior arch, widening of the SI joint, and displacement of the anterior arch.

LABORATORY AND DIAGNOSTIC TESTS for Fractures

Test With Description, Rationale, and Normal Values	Expected Abnormality
Complete Blood Count	
Normal: White blood cell: 4,500–10,000 µl Hematocrit: Male: 40–54% Female: 36–46% Hemoglobin: Male: 13.5–18g/dL Female: 12–15g/dL Red blood cell: Male: 4.5–6.0 µl Female: 4.0–5.0 µl *To obtain a baseline and monitor for bleeding.*	Decreased RBC, Hgb, and Hct with bleeding
CT Scan	
No bone or tissue abnormality. *Provide information regarding bone structure and soft tissue surrounding bone.*	Demonstrate bone loss, fracture, or tumor. Demonstrate soft tissue injury or fluid collection. *Pelvic fractures*: assists with the diagnosis of crushing, shearing injuries; SI joint displacement; acetabular injuries; and posterior osseous ligamentous structure of the pelvis. The scan will also assist in diagnosing associated visceral injuries and bleeding.

The outlet view is a 45-degree angle taken from the foot of the bed directed toward the head. This helps in identifying a displacement or leg-length discrepancy, disruptions of the SI joints, and sacral factures. Other diagnostics are listed in the Laboratory and Diagnostics Tests for Fractures box.

Medical Management

The most important factors that direct management of pelvic injury are the patient's hemodynamic status and stability of the pelvic ring. In the patient who is both hemodynamically and mechanically unstable and in whom the bleeding is thought to be from the pelvic fracture, external stabilization of the pelvis is a priority. The main sources of bleeding are the presacral venous plexus and fractured bony surfaces. External stabilization with a pelvic binder decreases the hemorrhage by reducing the volume of the pelvic basin and bringing together the fracture ends. Pelvic binders are cloth and go around the pelvis circumferentially (Figure 50–14◆). They are simple to apply, are inexpensive, and can be placed in the prehospital setting. Potential complications of the binder include skin necrosis if the binder is left in place for a long period or applied too tightly. If a binder is applied too tightly in the care of lateral compression injuries with sacral fractures, it may cause visceral or neural injury.

The source of bleeding from pelvic fractures is usually venous; however, arterial injury can occur and account for hemodynamic instability in some patients. For the patients who remain hemodynamically unstable after external stabilization, pelvic angiography may be performed to identify and embolize (introduction of a substance into the vasculature to obstruct the vessel) the source of the bleeding. Patients who are hemodynamically stable but exhibit an arterial blush on CT scan, signifying bleeding at the site, may also undergo angiography for embolization.

Minimally displaced pelvic fractures that have ligamentous stability of the pelvic ring are treated with protected weight bearing on the affected side and pain medication. If displacement at the fracture site occurs when the patient begins to bear weight, further surgical treatment may be necessary. Fractures that have marked displacement of the anterior ring without complete posterior ring disruption are usually treated with reduction and surgical anterior ring stabilization. Patients who have complete disruption of the posterior ring will require surgical stabilization of both the anterior and posterior pelvic ring.

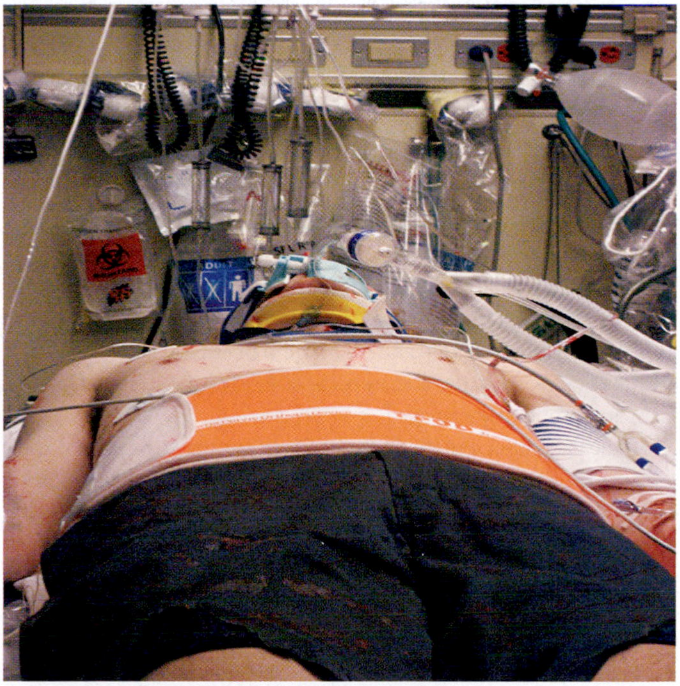

FIGURE 50–14 ◆ Pelvic binder.
Source: Cheryl Wraa.

Nursing Management

Initial nursing management of the patient with a pelvic fracture includes frequent reassessment for potential complications, pain control, and keeping the patient still if a binder has been applied. If the patient requires surgical stabilization, postfixation nursing management

Weblink: Glucosamine

includes pain control, as well as continued assessment for complications such as bleeding, infection at the incised site, DVT, PE, and pneumonia.

Assessment

Initial nursing management of the patient with a pelvic fracture includes continued assessment of the patient for concomitant injuries, as well as signs and symptoms of potential complications.

Nursing Diagnoses

The primary nursing diagnoses for the patient with a pelvic fracture include:

- *Pain, Acute* related to fracture.
- *Physical Mobility, Impaired* related to fracture.
- *Injury, Risk for* related to fracture and impaired mobility.
- *Fluid Volume, Deficient, Risk for* related to blood loss from fracture.
- *Infection, Risk for* related to wounds.

NANDA-I © 2012

Outcomes and Evaluation Parameters

The desired outcomes for the patient with a fracture of any type are relief of pain, prevention of damage to the nerves and vasculature, and restoration of strength and mobility. Evaluation parameters include control of pain as described by the patient, restoration of nerve and vascular function as demonstrated by exam, and return of strength and mobility as noted by assessment.

Planning, Interventions, and Rationales

With all fractures, the nurse should quickly assess and immobilize the affected extremity or pelvis to prevent further damage and to recognize any vascular or nerve involvement.

The patient will require intravenous pain medication because fracture pain is severe. In the postresuscitative phase, pain control is critical to assist with rehabilitation and resumption of normal activities of daily living. Patients are better able to participate in physical therapy if their pain is appropriately managed.

If the patient presents with an open fracture, the nurse should apply a sterile dressing immediately to help protect the wound from further contamination. Postoperatively, the nurse should monitor any wounds, dressings, or splints for signs of infection such as warmth and redness, drainage with a foul odor, purulent drainage, increased pain, and fever. If signs of infection are noted, the nurse should notify the health care team immediately.

For the patient who has an unstable pelvic fracture, the nurse should anticipate the need for a blood transfusion and ensure that the patient has been typed and crossmatched for blood products. If the patient is placed in a pelvic binder, the nurse should assess the position of the binder and ensure smooth, direct contact between the patient and the binder to avoid skin breakdown.

The nurse has a critical role in monitoring the patient for signs that indicate the onset of hypovolemic shock and the need for resuscitative measures. An orthopedic trauma patient who has experienced fractures of the pelvis or long bones is at risk for significant bleeding. The nurse should monitor the patient's hemodynamic status including vital signs and laboratory values. A patient may lose as much as 20% of her blood volume before exhibiting signs and symptoms of shock. The nurse should monitor the vital signs for an increase in heart rate, a decrease in blood pressure, an increase in respiratory rate, and a decrease in urine output. Laboratory results will show a decrease in the hemoglobin and hematocrit. Refer to Chapter 54 for a detailed discussion of shock.

Rehabilitation is an important aspect of the care of the patient with a fracture. The patient should be mobilized as soon as possible to prevent further complications. Physical therapy should begin early to prevent contractures and increase mobility and strength to the extremity.

Surgical Procedures

Patients undergoing musculoskeletal surgery generally fall into two categories: (1) those who have experienced increasing pain or disability over time, causing them to seek a surgical resolution to their complaints, and (2) those who have had a traumatic event. The patient who enters the hospital for an elective orthopedic procedure often has the benefit of preoperative teaching and preparation for the procedure. In contrast, the patient who has experienced a traumatic event may present unique challenges for the nurse, both preoperatively and postoperatively. The nurse is in a key position to recognize potential problems and prevent complications that have a direct impact on the patient's ability to improve or maintain functional status and return to a productive lifestyle. Orthopedic surgical patients face recovery from the sequelae of surgery and anesthesia as well as potential complications specific to the orthopedic problem encountered.

The orthopedic surgeon performs a physical assessment and diagnostic testing to determine whether the diseased or traumatized bone or joint requires surgical replacement or simple repair. Repair may include removal of bone and ligament particles, smoothing of joint surfaces, reconnection of torn ligaments, or replacement of ligaments with allograft (cadaver) or autograft (tissue from another area to replace damaged ligaments or bone). Replacement of the joint may include repair as well as the implantation of a new joint.

Traumatic injuries play a large part in the need for orthopedic surgery in patients of all ages. Congenital deformities are generally repaired in the pediatric population. Spinal surgery for scoliosis is usually performed in the early adolescent period, whereas spinal surgery for disk repair or laminectomy is performed in young and middle adulthood. Hip fractures are a common traumatic injury for older adults, as is joint replacement surgery. The life of an artificial joint and the surrounding bone tissue is shorter than that of a natural joint, with current artificial hips and knees lasting approximately 15 to 20 years, after which the artificial joint may need to be replaced (MedlinePlus, 2010). Knowledge of biographic and demographic data including cultural considerations is important in planning appropriate care for the patient (see the Cultural Considerations box). Older patients are at risk for postoperative delirium. Knowledge of the patient's prior experiences, abilities, and accomplishments can assist the nurse in providing patient-specific interventions to maintain orientation and prevent cognitive function alterations.

Safety Alert *A medication specific to patients with joint problems is glucosamine, which decreases joint discomfort and increases flexibility. In particular, many older adults take glucosamine. This drug may affect serum glucose levels and interact with insulin effects. The nurse should monitor serum glucose if the patient has been taking glucosamine (Mayoclinic.com, 2011).*

It is not within the scope of this chapter to review all types of orthopedic surgery. However, selected orthopedic surgical approaches that require hospitalization will be covered. See the Nursing Process: Patient Care Plan for the Orthopedic Surgical Patient on page 1551.

CULTURE CONSIDERATIONS
Concerning Surgical Procedures

The patient's cultural history should be included in the plan of care. If the patient has specific requirements regarding the gender of the nurses and caretakers assigned to his care, these should be accommodated whenever possible. Knowledge of a patient's pain expression also should be included in the plan of care. Cultural accommodations for activities of daily living (ADLs) and cultural dietary accommodations may be necessary and should be communicated. The patient should be offered spiritual affiliation if desired. Some cultures, such as the Jewish or Hmong cultures, may request that an amputated limb be made available to them for burial where the person will eventually be buried (Ehman, 2007).

Upper Extremity Surgery

Upper extremity surgeries include total shoulder or elbow joint replacement, rotator cuff repair, and open reduction or stabilization of fractures of the humerus, radius, or ulna. Most elective upper extremity surgeries below the elbow are performed on an outpatient basis. However, shoulder and elbow surgery may require one or more inpatient hospital days to ensure that nerve entrapment does not occur from postoperative edema. Reduction and stabilization of fractures are discussed in detail later in this chapter.

The shoulder is a ball-and-socket joint that is made up of three bones: the upper arm bone (humerus), shoulder blade (scapula), and collarbone (clavicle) (Figure 50–15◆). The top of the humerus fits into the small socket (glenoid) of the shoulder blade to form the shoulder joint (glenohumeral joint). The socket of the glenoid is surrounded by a soft tissue rim (labrum). The articular cartilage and a thin inner lining (synovium) of the joint allow the smooth motion of the shoulder joint. The upper part of the shoulder blade (acromion) projects over the shoulder joint. One end of the collarbone is joined with the acromioclavicular (AC) joint (joint with the shoulder blade), and the other end of the collarbone is joined with the sternum by the sternoclavicular joint. The joint capsule, which is a thin sheet of fibers that surrounds the shoulder joint, allows a wide range of motion yet provides stability. The rotator cuff is a group of four muscles—the supraspinatus, infraspinatus, teres minor, and subscapularis—that, along with the tendons, attaches the upper arm to the shoulder blade. A saclike membrane (bursa) between the rotator cuff and the shoulder blade cushions and helps lubricate the motion between these two structures. The rotator cuff stabilizes the humeral head in the glenoid fossa. The muscles attached to the rotator cuff enable arm motion that allows an individual to take part in activities such as throwing or swimming.

Rotator Cuff Repair

Etiology and Epidemiology

Rotator cuff tears can occur from a single traumatic injury (Figure 50–16◆, p. 1536). These patients often report recurrent shoulder pain for several months and can recall the specific injury that triggered the onset of the pain. A cuff tear may also happen at the same time as another injury to the shoulder, such as a fracture or dislocation. Most rotator cuff tears are the result of overuse of the muscles and tendons over a period of years. People who are especially at risk for overuse are those who engage in repetitive overhead motions such as baseball, tennis, weight lifting, and rowing. Rotator cuff tears are most common in people over the age of 40 (American Academy of Orthopaedic Surgeons [AAOS], 2007e). Partial-thickness or full-thickness tears may occur. Partial-thickness rotator cuff tears are associated with chronic inflammation and the development of spurs on the underside of the acromion or the acromioclavicular joint. Full-thickness tears are most often the result of impingement; partial-thickness rotator cuff tears result from heavy lifting or falls.

Clinical Manifestations

Clinical manifestations of rotator cuff tears include the following:

- When the tear occurs with an injury, there may be sudden acute pain, a snapping sensation, and an immediate weakness of the arm.
- Over time, atrophy or thinning of the muscles about the shoulder occurs.

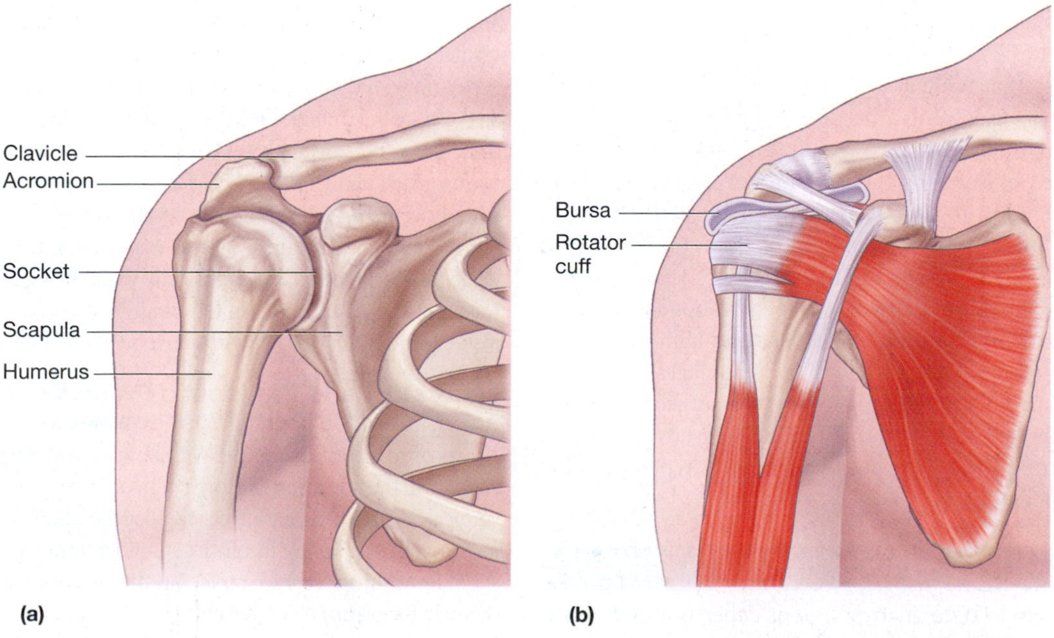

FIGURE 50–15 ◆ Shoulder anatomy.

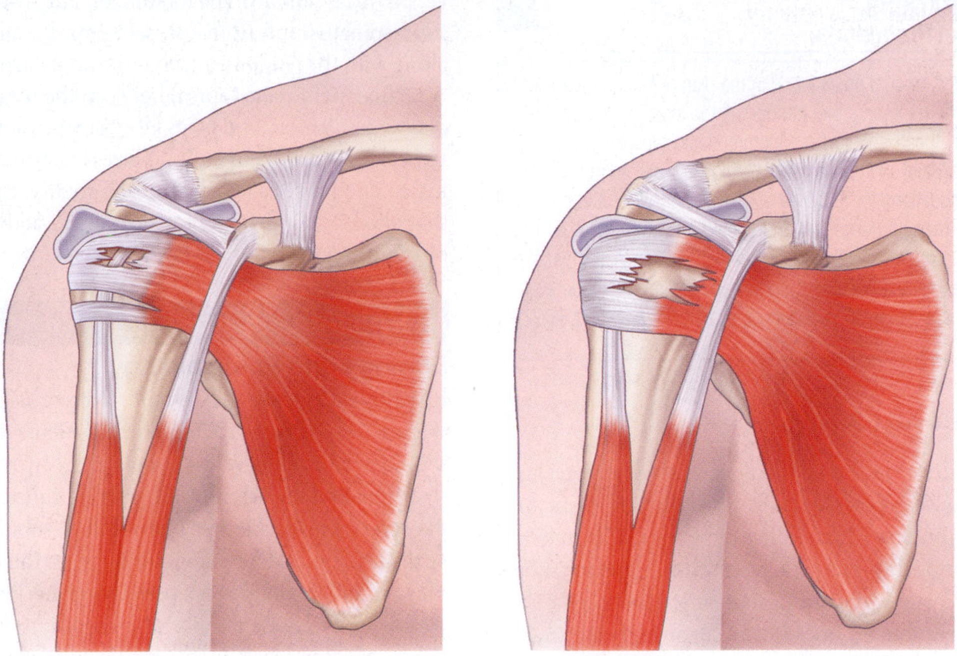

(a) (b)

FIGURE 50–16 ◆ Rotator cuff tears. (A) Impingement with partial tear. (B) Full-thickness tear.

- Pain in the front of the shoulder radiates down the arm when lifting the arm or when lowering the arm from a fully raised position.
- Weakness is felt when lifting or rotating the arm.
- Crepitus (crackling sensation) occurs when moving the shoulder into a certain position.

Symptoms may develop right away after a trauma, such as a lifting injury or a fall on the affected arm, or they may develop gradually with repetitive overhead activity or as the result of long-term wear.

Laboratory and Diagnostic Tests and Medical–Surgical Management

The type of surgical repair depends on the size, shape, and location of the tear. A CT or an MRI scan may be used to identify the extent of the tear. A partial tear (see Figure 50–16A) may require only a trimming or smoothing procedure, called a *débridement*. A complete tear (see Figure 50–16B) within the thickest part of the tendon is repaired by suturing the two sides of the tendon back together. If the tendon is torn away from where it inserts into the bone of the humerus, it is repaired directly to bone (AAOS, 2007e). There are two approaches to the surgical procedure: open and arthroscopic. With an arthroscopy, the orthopedic surgeon inserts a pencil-thin device with a small lens and lighting system into tiny incisions to look inside the joint. The images inside the joint are relayed to a TV monitor, allowing the surgeon to make a diagnosis. Other surgical instruments can be inserted to make repairs, based on findings. Many of these surgical repairs can be done on an outpatient basis.

Shoulder Arthroplasty

Arthroplasty refers to restoration of a joint either by **total joint replacement,** by replacement of a joint with a prosthesis, or by resurfacing bone and removing damaged bone and cartilage.

Etiology and Epidemiology

Total replacement of the shoulder and elbow is not as commonly performed as total replacement of the hip and knee. An indication for the surgery is severe pain resulting from rheumatoid arthritis, osteoarthritis, avascular necrosis, or post-traumatic arthritis. Osteoarthritis and rheumatoid arthritis can destroy the shoulder joint and surrounding tissue. Arthritis is discussed in detail in Chapter 51.

Clinical Manifestations

Clinical manifestations of joint degeneration include pain that progressively worsens and is aggravated by activity. When the glenohumeral shoulder joint is affected, the pain is centered in the back of the shoulder and frequently intensifies with changes in the weather. If the acromioclavicular joint is involved, the pain is focused in the front of the shoulder. A person with rheumatoid arthritis of both shoulders may have pain in all these areas. Limited motion is another problem. It may become more difficult for persons with this disorder to lift their arm to comb their hair or reach up to a shelf. A clicking or snapping sound may be heard with movement. As the joint degeneration progresses, any movement of the shoulder causes pain. Night pain is common, and sleeping may be difficult. The involved arm is typically weak owing to muscle atrophy, is tender to touch, and has limited range of motion. A grating sensation inside the joint may be felt with movement (AAOS, 2007b).

Laboratory and Diagnostic Procedures and Medical–Surgical Management

X-rays of an arthritic shoulder will show a narrowing of the joint space, changes in the bone, and the formation of bone spurs (osteophytes). The surgical approach used to treat the degeneration of the glenohumeral joint involves replacing the entire shoulder joint with a prosthesis (total shoulder arthroplasty) or replacing the head of the upper arm bone (hemiarthroplasty) (see Chart 50–4).

The goal of surgery is to restore the best possible function to the joint by removing scar tissue, balancing muscles, and replacing the

CHART 50–4 Shoulder Arthroplasty

- An incision of approximately 6 to 10 inches in length is made to expose the shoulder joint.
- The humeral head is dislocated from the socket.
- The head of the humerus is shaved/removed to shape the bone to fit the implant, and the bone canal is drilled to prepare for the prosthesis implant.
- The implant is inserted into the humerus.
- The glenoid socket is shaved to create a smooth articular surface. It may also be shaved and a concave disk implanted to replace the glenoid socket surface. Holes may be drilled into the glenoid surface to secure the implanted glenoid socket.
- Debris (torn ligaments, bone fragments, and clots) are removed, and ligaments are adjusted.
- The surgical site is sutured closed after the joint is tested for smooth motion.

joint surfaces. Figure 50–17◆ shows the artificial joint components including the humeral ball (which is made of metal) and the glenoid component (which is made of plastic).

The most common surgical procedure used to treat arthritis of the acromioclavicular joint is a resection arthroplasty. A small piece of bone from the end of the collarbone is removed, leaving a space that later fills with scar tissue. Surgical treatment of arthritis of the shoulder is generally very effective in reducing pain and restoring motion (AAOS, 2007b).

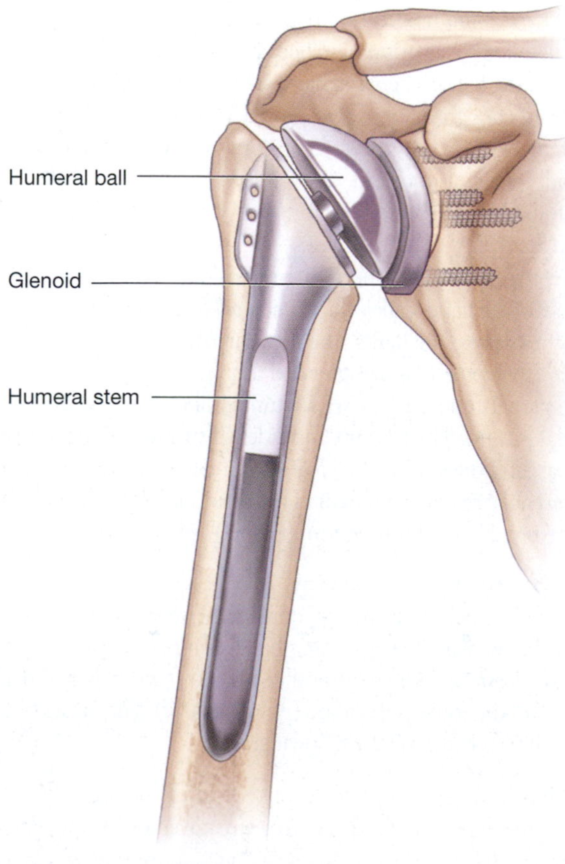

FIGURE 50–17 ◆ Shoulder arthroplasty.

Shoulder range of motion is started immediately after the procedure, and patients are usually discharged from the hospital 3 days after surgery if they are comfortable and have a good range of passive motion. The recovery of strength and function may continue to improve for up to 1 year after surgery (Matson & Warme, 2010).

Shoulder Subluxation and Dislocation Repair

The epidemiology, etiology, and nonsurgical treatment of joint dislocation are discussed on page 1523. This section discusses surgical repair of an unstable shoulder joint.

Clinical Manifestations

Shoulder instability including subluxation (the humerus slips slightly out of its socket then immediately goes back into place) and shoulder dislocation are potentially painful and disabling conditions. Subluxation and dislocation both represent problems that occur when the humeral head does not stay centered correctly in the socket (or *glenoid*). These problems may manifest themselves with pain from doing the normal activities of daily living or the inability to lift the arm without dislocating the joint.

Laboratory and Diagnostic Procedures and Medical–Surgical Management

Diagnosis of shoulder subluxation or dislocation is made on the basis of the patient history and physical examination. An x-ray of the affected joint may be done to rule out fractures. The treatments for these conditions vary widely depending on the severity of symptoms and signs. Many patients will improve with the appropriate bracing and physical therapy discussed earlier in the chapter. For patients who require surgery, arthroscopic surgery is used to diagnose the exact nature of the joint instability. The goal of surgery is to reestablish the stability of the humeral head in the shallow glenoid socket without compromising the shoulder motion. Using the scope, the surgeon can evaluate the entire shoulder joint and can usually treat the conditions leading to the instability. Infrequently, patients may require an open surgery, using an incision about 8 to 13 cm (3 to 5 inches) long to correct the problem. The procedure can usually be performed within a few hours under general (or nerve block) anesthesia.

Patients undergoing arthroscopic shoulder stabilization will usually require a sling for 2 to 3 weeks, and may perform simple range-of-motion exercises daily. In addition, outpatient physical therapy for reestablishing pain-free motion and strengthening the shoulder muscles will be needed for a few months. The patient can usually return to most forms of normal activity within 6 weeks, although return to some kinds of sports may take longer.

Elbow Repair

The elbow is a hinge and ball-and-socket joint made up of the humerus, ulna, and radius. The positioning and interaction of the bones in the joint allow for a small amount of rotation as well as hinge action. The primary stability of the elbow is provided by the ulnar collateral ligament on the medial (inner) side of the elbow. As muscles contract and relax, two unique motions occur:

- The hinge joint allows the elbow to bend and straighten (flexion and extension, respectively).
- Rotation through the ball-and-socket joint allows the hand to be rotated palm down and palm up (pronation and supination, respectively).

Etiology

Common causes of pain and injury to the elbow joint include sprains, strains, fractures, dislocations, bursitis, arthritis, and tumors. Injury, acute or from overuse, is the most common cause of elbow pain (WebMD, 2011). One of the most common injuries to the elbow occurs on the lateral, or outer, side of the elbow; this injury is referred to as lateral epicondylitis (tennis elbow) (AAOS, 2007d).

Clinical Manifestations

The most common clinical manifestations of elbow damage are pain and loss of range of motion. Patients also report a "grating" or "locking" sensation in the elbow. The grating is due to loss of the normal smooth joint surface because of cartilage damage or wear. The locking is caused by loose pieces of cartilage or bone that dislodge from the joint and become trapped between the moving joint surfaces, blocking motion. As the disease progresses, joint swelling may also occur. The swelling may cause numbness in the ring finger and small finger due to ulnar nerve pressure. Finally, if the elbow cannot be moved through its normal range of motion, it may stiffen into a position in which it is bent (flexion) (AAOS, 2007d).

Laboratory and Diagnostic Procedures and Medical–Surgical Management

An MRI is performed of the elbow to assess the extent of the damage. Arthroscopy, which removes loose bodies or inflammatory or degenerative tissue in the joint, provides symptom improvement at least in the short term. It also attempts to smooth irregular surfaces. Multiple small incisions are used to perform the surgery. This can be done as an outpatient procedure, and recovery is reasonably rapid.

If the joint surface has worn away completely, the most definitive treatment is joint replacement. For patients who are too young or too active to have prosthetic joint replacement, however, there are other surgical options. For example, if loss of motion is the primary symptom, the surgeon can release the contracture and smooth out the joint surface. At times, a new surface can be made from the patient's own body tissues. These procedures can provide years of symptom improvement (AAOS, 2007d).

Elbow Dislocation

Etiology and Epidemiology

Elbow dislocations are common injuries that typically occur when a person falls onto an out-stretched hand. It is the most common dislocation in children and the second-most common in adults (Halstead, 2011). On impact, the force is sent to the elbow, and there is usually a turning motion in this force that can rotate the elbow out of its socket. Because the elbow is stabilized with the combined effects of bone surfaces, ligaments, and muscles, any or all of these structures can be injured to different degrees when it dislocates. There are three basic types of elbow dislocation: simple, complex, and severe dislocation. A simple dislocation does not have any major bone injury. A complex dislocation can have severe bone and ligament injuries. With a severe dislocation, the blood vessels and nerves that travel across the elbow may be injured. If this happens, there is a risk that the arm will have to be amputated.

Clinical Manifestations

A complete elbow dislocation is extremely painful; after experiencing one, the arm will look deformed and may have an odd twist at the elbow. A partial elbow dislocation can be harder to detect; because the elbow is only partially dislocated, the bones can spontaneously relocate, and the joint may appear fairly normal. The elbow usually will move fairly normally, but it is painful. Bruising may exist on the inside and outside of the elbow where ligaments may have been stretched or torn. Partial dislocations can recur repeatedly if the ligaments never heal. If the artery is injured, the hand will be cool to the touch and may have a white or purple hue due to the diminished blood supply. The nurse must check the pulses on the injured side. If nerves were injured during the dislocation or from subsequent swelling, some or all of the hand may be numb and unable to move. Over time, following a dislocation, there is an increased risk for arthritis in the elbow joint if the alignment of the bones is not good, the elbow does not move and rotate normally, or the elbow continues to dislocate.

Laboratory and Diagnostic Tests and Medical–Surgical Management

Dislocation is diagnosed by physical exam. An x-ray of the affected joint may be done to check for fracture.

An elbow dislocation should be considered an emergency injury. The goal of immediate treatment is to return the elbow to its normal alignment, and the long-term goal is to restore function to the arm. With a complex elbow dislocation, surgery may be necessary to restore bone alignment and repair ligaments. Blood vessel or nerve injuries will also need surgical repair.

After surgery, the elbow may be protected with an external hinge. This device protects the elbow from dislocating again. Late reconstructive surgery can successfully restore motion to some stiff elbows. This surgery removes scar tissue and extra bone growth. It also removes obstacles to movement.

Carpal Tunnel Repair

The wrist is an extremely complex joint that provides the mobility to give the hand a full range of motion while at the same time providing the strength for heavy gripping. There are 15 bones from the end of the forearm to the hand. The wrist has 8 small bones, called carpal bones. These bones are grouped in two rows across the wrist. The proximal row begins with the thumb side of the wrist and is made up of the scaphoid, lunate, triquetrum, and pisiform bones. The distal row of carpal tunnel bones is made up of the trapezium, trapezoid, capitate, and hamate bones.

The proximal row connects the radius and the ulna (forearm) to the bones of the hand, called the *metacarpal bones*. These long bones *lie* within the palm of the hand. The metacarpals attach to the phalanges, which are the bones in the fingers and thumb.

The carpal tunnel is a narrow, tunnel-like structure in the wrist (Figure 50–18◆). The bottom and sides of this tunnel are formed by wrist (carpal) bones, and the top of the tunnel is covered by the transverse carpal ligament. The median nerve and tendons travel from the forearm into the hand through this tunnel.

Etiology and Epidemiology

With carpal tunnel syndrome, tendons in the wrist swell and put pressure on the median nerve, causing hand numbness and pain. Carpal tunnel syndrome is more common in women than in men and affects up to 10% of the entire population (AAOS, 2007c). The causes of carpal tunnel syndrome include the following:

- Heredity
- Repetitive motions of the hands or wrist over a very long period of time
- Hormonal changes related to pregnancy and menopause

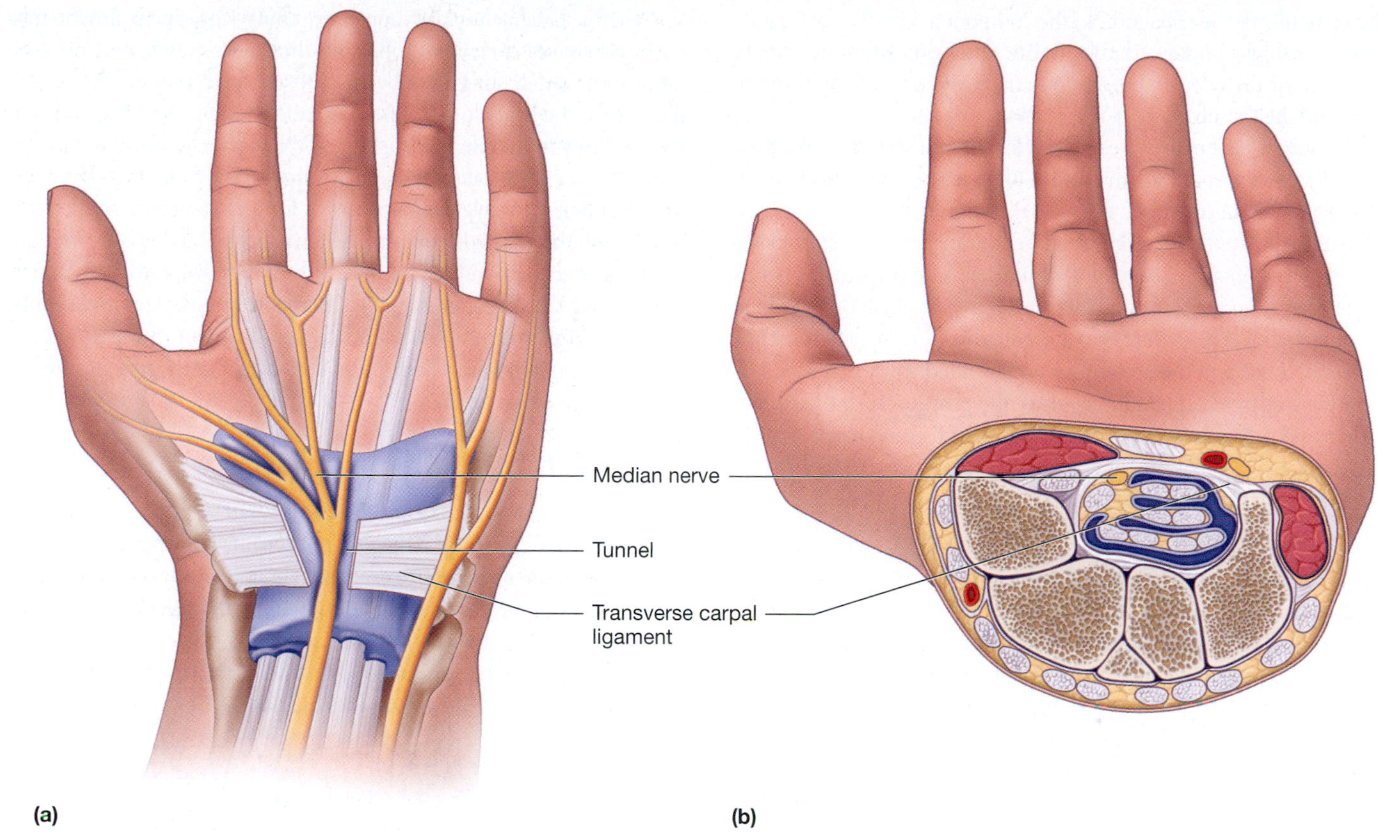

FIGURE 50–18 ◆ Carpal tunnel syndrome.

- Diabetes, rheumatoid arthritis, and thyroid gland imbalance
- In some cases, idiopathic measures.

Clinical Manifestations

The clinical manifestations are pain, numbness, and tingling in the hand. Patients describe an electric-shock-type pain in the fingers or hand. The thumb side of the hand is usually most involved. Movement of the hand and wrist, such as when holding an object (e.g., a phone) or when reading or driving, makes the pain occur. Shaking the hand often helps to decrease symptoms. Clinical manifestations are initially intermittent, but over time they may become constant. Fine motor coordination such as is needed to button a button can be difficult. When the condition is very severe, muscles in the palm may become visibly wasted.

Laboratory and Diagnostic Tests and Medical–Surgical Management

Carpal tunnel syndrome is diagnosed by physical exam. An x-ray of the wrist may be done to rule out other disease processes such as arthritis. Treatment begins with a brace or splint worn at night to keep the wrist in a natural position. Splints can also be worn during activities that aggravate symptoms. Anti-inflammatory medications such as nonsteroidal anti-inflammatory drugs (NSAIDs) help with pain relief. As the disease progresses and the individual becomes more disabled, surgery may become necessary. The decision whether to have surgery is based primarily on the severity of the symptoms. In more severe cases, surgery is considered sooner because other treatment options are less helpful. In very severe cases, surgery may be recommended to prevent irreversible damage. The surgeon uses an endoscope to access and open the top of the carpal tunnel, which increases the size of the tunnel and decreases pressure on the nerve. Typically the surgery is done on an outpatient basis under local anesthesia. Recovery is gradual; on average, grip and pinch strength generally return by about 2 months after surgery. Complete recovery may take up to 1 year, although it may be longer if the nerve is severely affected before treatment is attempted (AAOS, 2007c).

Wrist Arthroplasty

Etiology and Epidemiology

Both osteoarthritis and rheumatoid arthritis affect the strength of the fingers and hand, making it difficult to grip or pinch. In the United States, approximately 1 person in 7 develops wrist arthritis. Rheumatoid arthritis is the most common type of arthritis affecting the wrist (Lakshmanan, 2011). Refer to Chapter 51 for a detailed discussion of arthritis. The typical candidate for wrist replacement surgery has severe arthritis. However, the surgery is limited to individuals who do not need to use their wrist to meet heavy demands in daily use. The primary reasons for wrist replacement surgery are to relieve pain and to maintain function in the wrist and hand. It may also improve the patient's ability to perform daily living activities.

Surgical Management

Surgery for carpal tunnel syndrome consists of removal of the worn-out ends of the bones and their replacement by an artificial joint (prosthesis). During surgery, an incision is made on the back of the wrist. The damaged ends of the lower arm bones are removed, along with the first row of carpal bones. The radial component of the prosthesis is then inserted into the center of the radius bone on the outside of the lower arm. The carpal component is then inserted into the center hand bone (third metacarpal) or screwed into the remaining row of carpal bones.

Bone cement may be used to hold the components in place. Wrist arthroscopy surgery is often combined with other procedures to correct deformities or disorders in the tendons, nerves, and small joints of the fingers and the thumb.

After surgery, the patient wears a cast for the first several weeks, then wears a protective splint for the next 6 to 8 weeks. The patient needs to perform gradual exercises for several weeks to restore movement and, eventually, to increase power and endurance. Wrist arthroplasty can improve motion to about 50% of normal. The physical demands that are placed on the wrist prosthesis will have an effect on how long the implant lasts. The patient might need to avoid using a hammer or pneumatic tools, and the amount of weight lifted must be limited. A fall on the outstretched hand may break the prosthesis, so the patient should avoid activities such as roller sports, which could result in a fall. The average wrist replacement can be expected to last 10 to 15 years with careful use (AAOS, 2007f).

Nursing Management

Initial assessment during the initial postoperative period should focus on the potential problems of hypovolemia, bleeding complications, hypoxemia, and neurovascular compromise. Refer to the Nursing Process: Patient Care Plan for the Orthopedic Surgical Patient on page 1551. After upper extremity surgery, the nurse must perform a neurovascular assessment that includes all digits of the hand, specifically the thumb and fourth and fifth fingers, to test for ulnar nerve function (Figure 50–19◆). To check motor integrity related to the ulnar nerve, the nurse asks the patient to make an "OK" sign (a circle) with the thumb and index finger. The assessment of function of the operative extremity should be compared to that of a noninvolved site.

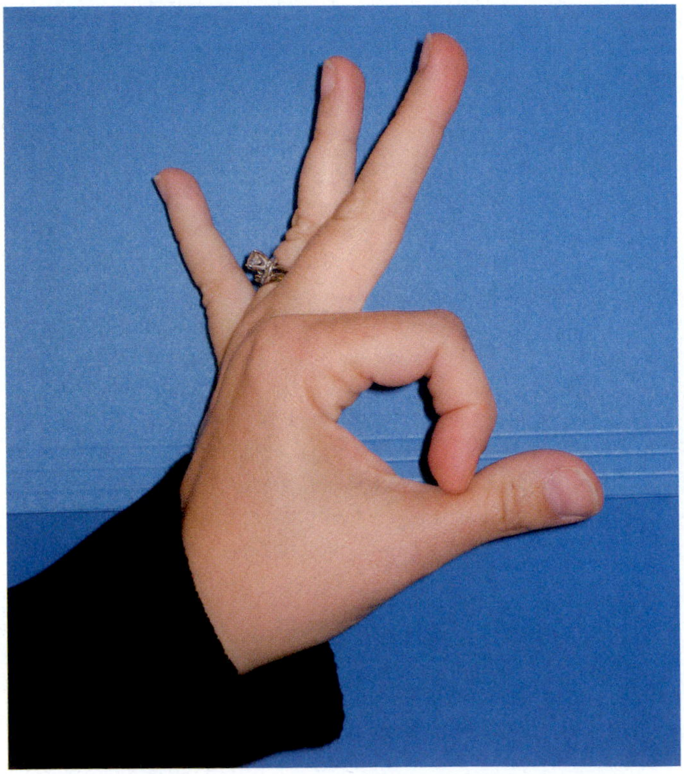

FIGURE 50–19 ◆ OK sign for ulnar integrity.
Source: Cheryl Wraa.

When a patient has had upper extremity surgery, treatment frequently involves slings, immobilizing dressings, splints, and binders postoperatively. A sling may be used to elevate the extremity above the level of the heart to decrease edema formation, as well as to keep the extremity immobile. An elastic and Velcro shoulder immobilizer is generally used with rotator cuff repair surgery. The patient may remove the immobilizer for hygiene purposes or for performing prescribed exercises with the affected arm until the formal physical therapy program begins. The patient with a shoulder arthroplasty will have a shoulder immobilizer or sling after surgery. External fixator devices and splints may be utilized to immobilize and retain alignment of the arm. The length of immobilization depends on the severity of the type of surgery and the surgeon's preference.

Collaborative Management

An exercise program will help the patient regain motion and strength in the involved extremity. This program begins with passive motion, advances to active and resistive exercises, and is typically coordinated by the surgeon and the physical therapist. In order to meet desired patient outcomes, it is essential that this interdisciplinary team communicate openly with one another in developing and evaluating care of the patient and family (IOM [Institute of Medicine], 2010).

Health Promotion

Complete recovery may take several months. A strong commitment to rehabilitation is important to achieve a good surgical outcome. The surgeon will examine the outcome to advise when it is safe to return to work and take part in sports activities that involve raising the arm over the head. Refer to the Discharge Planning for the Orthopedic Surgical Patient section on page 1555.

Lower Extremity Surgery

Total Hip Arthroplasty

The hip joint is formed where the top of the femur meets the acetabulum, or socket of the pelvic bone (Figure 50–20◆). The top of the femur is ball shaped and fits into the socket formed by the acetabulum. The bones are covered by a layer of smooth cartilage that cushions and protects the bones and allows easy motion. Also surrounding the joint is the synovial lining, which produces a moisturizing lubricant. Ligaments connect the bones of the joint and hold them in place. The ligaments also add strength and elasticity for movement. Large muscles attached by tendons keep the joint stable.

Etiology and Epidemiology

The most common cause of severe hip pain is arthritis, which is a result of joint injury causing inflammation and joint damage (Arthritis Foundation, 2011). It is estimated that 40 million people in the United States have some form of arthritis (Arthritis Foundation, 2011). The three most common types of arthritis that cause joint pain are osteoarthritis, rheumatoid arthritis, and trauma-related arthritis. Other conditions leading to total hip replacement include fracture, dysplasia, and malignancy.

Pathophysiology

Osteoarthritis causes the surfaces of the joint to become rough. This condition occurs when injury to a joint causes a breaking down of cartilage tissue. In turn, that breakdown causes pain, swelling, and deformity. The causes of osteoarthritis of the hip are not known,

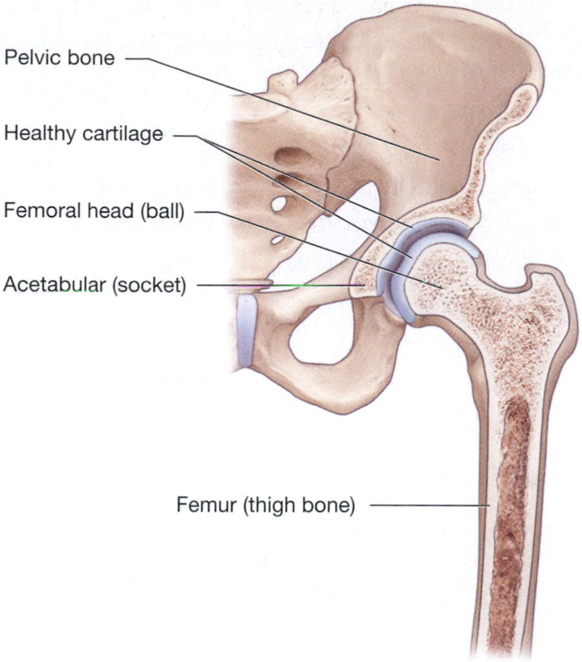

FIGURE 50–20 ◆ Hip joint.

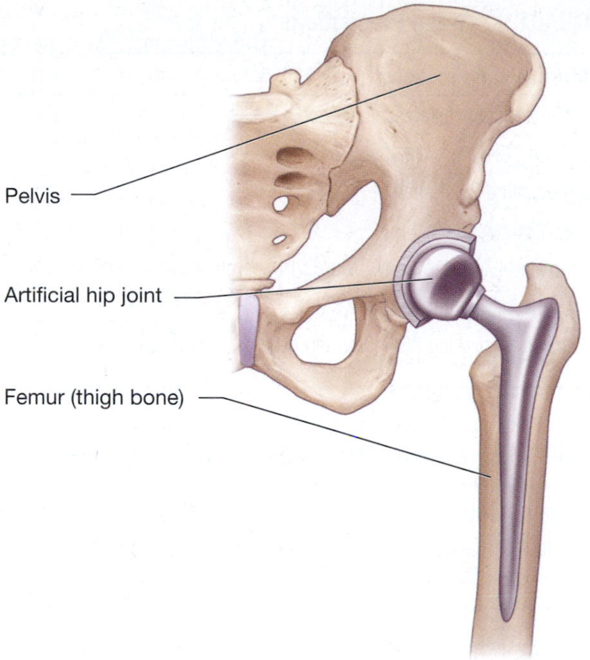

FIGURE 50–21 ◆ Artificial hip joint.

although increasing age and being overweight contribute to the joint injury.

Clinical Manifestations

Initially, arthritis or inflammation in the hip may cause discomfort to the groin, buttock, or thigh and stiffness to the joint when arising in the morning. The pain will increase when the person is active and decrease with rest. As the cartilage deteriorates and the bones of the joint rub directly against each other, the person will experience pain with movement and may lose the ability to rotate, flex, or extend the hip.

Laboratory and Diagnostic Tests and Medical–Surgical Management

An x-ray of both hips may be done to compare the joints and evaluate the extent of damage. When conservative treatment fails to provide adequate relief from pain, radiographs show destruction of the joint, and mobility is impaired, total hip replacement is considered. Hip replacement surgery involves removal of the femoral head, creation of a "posthole" in the femur for the implant or femoral stem, acetabular repair with implant of the cup and liner, and placement of the femoral head on the stem (Figure 50–21◆ and Chart 50–5). Hip replacement surgery may involve the use of cement, particularly if the bone quality is poor. Bone cement ingredients may include antibiotics but are primarily polymers that improve adhesion. This is particularly useful for patients who have high potential for delayed healing or infection. The use of cement may decrease the healing time after surgery, as bone growth and regeneration to secure the joint are not necessary. If the patient has the potential for repeated surgery, however, the use of cement will require a greater area of revision and removal of bone in the later surgeries, and this must be considered when determining whether cement should be used. Older patients who will not require further surgery for joint repair or replacement are more likely to receive surgery that includes the use of cement.

If the patient is active, the artificial hip joint may need to be replaced in 15 or 20 years. **Osteolysis** describes the state of previously repaired joints whose components have worn out or become damaged. If the patient requires a revision total hip surgery, or redo, it is a more complex procedure; in general, the surgery takes longer and there is more blood loss.

CHART 50–5 Hip Replacement Surgical Procedure

- The open surgical incision is 10 to 14 inches in size.
- Minimally invasive hip replacement incisions are made—one or two 1- to 2-inch incisions.
- The femoral head is dislocated from the acetabular socket.
- The acetabular socket is shaved to resurface and shape the bone to receive the shell implant (a domelike surface, which may include a liner).
- The femoral head is removed and shaved to shape the bone. The femoral canal is drilled to receive the implant stem.
- The stem of the implant is inserted into the femur.
- A surgical drain is implanted, and the surgical site closed with sutures.

Nursing Management

Initial assessment during the postoperative period should focus on the potential problems of hypovolemia, bleeding complications, hypoxemia, and neurovascular compromise. Refer to the Nursing Process: Patient Care Plan for the Orthopedic Surgical Patient on page 1551. In addition, after hip arthroplasty, the patient will be placed on hip precautions (Chart 50–6). The type of precautions required depends on the approach that was utilized. For instance, if a posterior approach was used, the patient will be placed on posterior hip precautions. The goal of the precautions is to prevent the hip from dislocating posteriorly. Anterior hip precautions involve avoiding activities that allow the hip to dislocate anteriorly. Chart 50–6 outlines the specific precautions for both posterior and anterior approaches.

Collaborative management and health promotion for the orthopedic surgical patient are discussed on page 1555.

CHART 50–6 Hip Precautions

Posterior Hip Precautions	Anterior Hip Precautions
Use a hip abductor pillow while in bed.	Use a hip abductor pillow while in bed.
Do not bend the hip more than 90 degrees.	Take mini-steps when walking.
Use an elevated toilet seat.	Do not assume a straddle position (as in mounting a horse).
Do not sit in low chairs.	Do not twist or turn the body away from the operative side.
Do not twist or turn the body toward the operative side.	Do not turn the leg and foot outward.
Do not turn the leg and foot inward.	Do not lift the operative leg up and out.
Keep the operative leg straight when getting up and use one's arms to push up.	

CHART 50–7 Home Modifications for Hip Surgery Patients

- Securely fastened safety bars or handrails for the bath and shower
- A stable armchair with a firm seat cushion allowing the knees to remain lower than the hips
- A raised toilet seat
- A shower bench or chair
- A sock aid and a long-handled shoe horn for putting on and taking off shoes and socks without excessive bending at the hip
- A reacher to access items without bending at the hip
- Removal of all loose carpets and electrical cords from walkways
- Moving of food and household items up to waist level to prevent bending.

Discharge Planning

The general considerations for discharge planning for the orthopedic surgical patient are discussed on page 1555. Home modifications specific for hip surgery are discussed in Chart 50–7.

Knee Injuries and Disorders

The knee is the largest joint in the body and one of the most easily injured. It is made up of four bones: the femur, the tibia, the fibula, and the patella (Figure 50–22◆). The knee contains four main ligaments: the inner medial collateral ligament (MCL), the outer lateral collateral ligament (LCL), the anterior cruciate ligament (ACL), and the posterior cruciate ligament (PCL). The function of the ligaments is to help control motion by connecting bones and by bracing the joint against abnormal types of motion. The knee muscles that go across the knee joint are the quadriceps (front of knee) and the hamstrings (back of knee). Another important structure, the meniscus, is a wedge of soft cartilage between the femur and the tibia that serves to cushion the knee and helps it absorb shock during motion.

Common sports injuries occur with the ligaments. For example, ligaments may be stretched, predisposing the joint to dislocation. Ligaments may also be torn if overextension or trauma occurs. Ligaments do not regenerate. If they are torn and disability or frequent dislocations occur, they must be repaired or replaced. The ACL and the MCL are frequently injured in sports. The PCL may also be injured.

Anterior Cruciate Ligament (ACL) Injury

Etiology, Epidemiology, and Clinical Manifestations

Changing direction rapidly, slowing down when running, and landing from a jump may cause tears in the ACL. Athletes who participate in skiing or basketball, as well as those who wear cleats, such as football players, are susceptible to ACL injuries. It is estimated that 200,000 ACL-related injuries occur in the United States annually, with approximately 95,000 ruptures and approximately 100,000 ACL reconstructions (Gammons, 2011). At the time of injury, the patient may hear an audible pop when changing directions or landing from a jump. The patient will experience pain, swelling, and instability of the knee joint.

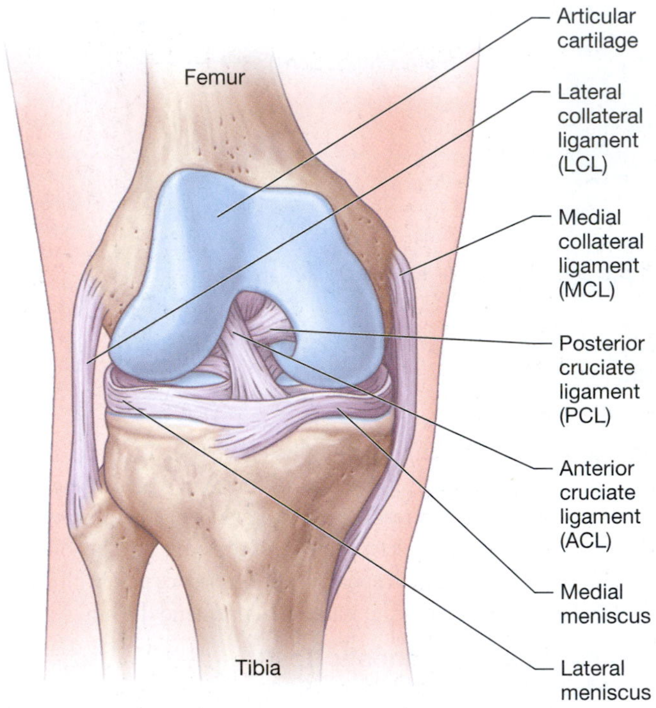

FIGURE 50–22 ◆ Knee anatomy.

Laboratory and Diagnostic Tests and Medical Management

Initially, an x-ray of the knee may be done to rule out a fracture. In addition, an MRI is done to evaluate the extent of injury. The ACL is not usually repaired because of failure over time with this approach. Instead, the ACL is generally replaced by a substitute graft made of tendon. The sources of tendon include patellar, hamstring, or quadriceps tendon autograft (from patient); or patellar tendon, Achilles tendon, semitendinosus, gracilis, or posterior tibialis tendon allograft (taken from a cadaver). There also are synthetic grafts available. The surgery procedure is described in Chart 50–8. The goal of ACL reconstruction surgery is to prevent instability and restore the function of the torn ligament, creating a stable knee. Patients treated with surgical

CHART 50–8 Anterior Cruciate Ligament Repair Surgery

- May be done as an open repair or endoscopic procedure.
- An open repair requires a 6-inch or greater incision.
- Endoscopic repair utilizes 1-inch incisions (two to three) as well as a surgical drill inserted into the incisions to prepare the bone to receive the graft.
- Debris is removed (torn ligaments, particles, clots, bone fragments).
- Meniscus and cartilage injuries are trimmed or repaired, and the torn anterior cruciate ligament (ACL) stump is then removed.
- Ligaments are typically replaced with allograft, autograft, or synthetic graft. If bone attachments are necessary, surgical drills may be utilized to prepare the bone for graft attachment.
- An ACL graft is placed in almost the same position as the torn ACL.
- The graft may be secured with sutures or screws.
- The open repair entrance site is sutured closed, and a drain may be inserted for blood collection.
- Before the surgery is complete, the surgeon will verify that the knee has full range of motion.
- Elastic support or immobilizer may be used postoperatively for simple repairs, to contain movement, and to prevent surgical site stress.
- Continuous passive motion (CPM) devices may be used postoperatively for extensive repairs or anterior cruciate ligament surgeries to prevent shortening of the ligament and prevent joint stiffening and loss of range of motion.
- ACL repairs are usually done on an outpatient basis.

reconstruction of the ACL have long-term success rates of 82% to 95%. Recurrent instability and graft failure are seen in approximately 8% of patients (AAOS, 2007a).

Meniscus Injury

The meniscus is a wedgelike rubbery cushion located where the femur and tibia meet at the knee joint (see Figure 50–22). The meniscus helps the knee joint carry weight, glide, and turn in many directions. It also keeps the femur and tibia from grinding against each other.

Etiology and Epidemiology

Meniscal tears can occur with twisting, pivoting, and decelerating motions of the knee. These injuries often occur in combination with other injuries such as a torn anterior cruciate ligament. As the cartilage weakens and wears thin over time, a degenerative tear can occur without any significant trauma. Injuries to the meniscus are among the most common knee injuries, with acute tears involved in 61 cases per 100,000 persons. The male-to-female ratio is approximately 2.5:1. In the older adult population, the rate of degenerative meniscal tears is 60% (Baker, 2011).

Clinical Manifestations

Clinical manifestations of meniscus injury typically include a "popping" sensation when the tear occurs, followed by inflammation, stiffness and swelling, pain, buckling, and fluid collection. Without treatment, a fragment of the meniscus may loosen and drift into the joint, causing it to slip, pop, or lock. The knee may lock at a 45-degree angle, until it is manually moved or otherwise manipulated.

Laboratory and Diagnostic Tests and Medical Management

The joint is evaluated with an MRI and/or arthroscopy. Initially, the treatment includes rest and pain medication. If the tear does not heal on its own and the knee becomes painful, stiff, or locked, a surgical repair may be necessary. The surgeon can examine the area arthroscopically and trim off damaged pieces of cartilage. A cast or brace is typically used to immobilize the knee after surgery. A course of rehabilitation exercises is then necessary before resuming previous activities.

Nursing Management

Assessment during the initial postoperative period should focus on the potential problems of hypovolemia, bleeding complications, hypoxemia, and neurovascular compromise. Refer to the Nursing Process: Patient Care Plan for the Orthopedic Surgical Patient on page 1551. In addition, after lower extremity surgery, the nurse must perform a neurovascular assessment that includes all toes on the affected side.

Patients who have had lower extremity surgery frequently are treated postoperatively with splints, slings, immobilizing dressings, and binders. The extremity needs to be kept immobile and should be elevated above the level of the heart to decrease edema formation. The patient may remove the immobilizer for hygiene purposes or for performing prescribed exercises with the affected joint until the formal physical therapy program begins. The length of immobilization depends on the severity of the type of surgery and the surgeon's preference.

Collaborative Management

An exercise program will help the patient to regain motion and strength in the involved extremity. This program begins with passive motion and advances to active and resistive exercises. It is typically coordinated by the surgeon and the physical therapist. In order to meet desired patient outcomes, it is essential that this interdisciplinary team communicate openly with one another in developing and evaluating care of the patient and family (IOM [Institute of Medicine], 2010).

Health Promotion

Complete recovery may take several months. To achieve a good surgical outcome, the patient must be strongly committed to rehabilitation. The surgeon will examine the outcome to advise when it is safe for the patient to return to work and sports. The general considerations for discharge planning for the orthopedic surgical patient are discussed on page 1555 later in this chapter.

Total Knee Replacement

Epidemiology, Etiology, and Clinical Manifestations

A total knee replacement is performed for patients whose joints have been damaged by progressive arthritis, trauma, or other rare diseases that are destructive to the joint, such as some autoimmune diseases. In the United States, the most common reason for replacement of the joint is severe osteoarthritis (Shiel, 2011). As the joint deteriorates, the patient will experience progressively increasing pain and stiffness of the joint.

Laboratory and Diagnostic Tests and Medical Management

An MRI of the affected knee is used to evaluate the extent of damage. As osteoarthritis wears away a knee joint's articular cartilage, arthroplasty (replacement) is a common and generally successful procedure that improves knee motion and allows a patient to resume relatively normal activities without pain (Figure 50–23◆). The surgeon resurfaces the knee joint, replacing damaged and worn weight-bearing surfaces with a prosthesis made of metal alloys, ceramic material, or high-density plastic parts that may be joined to bone by acrylic cement. Up to three bone surfaces may be replaced during the total replacement of the knee: the lower condyles of the femur, the top surface of the tibia, and the back surface of the kneecap. Chart 50–9 presents the surgical procedure.

Weblink: Knee Joint Replacement

Weblink: Lumbar Laminectomy

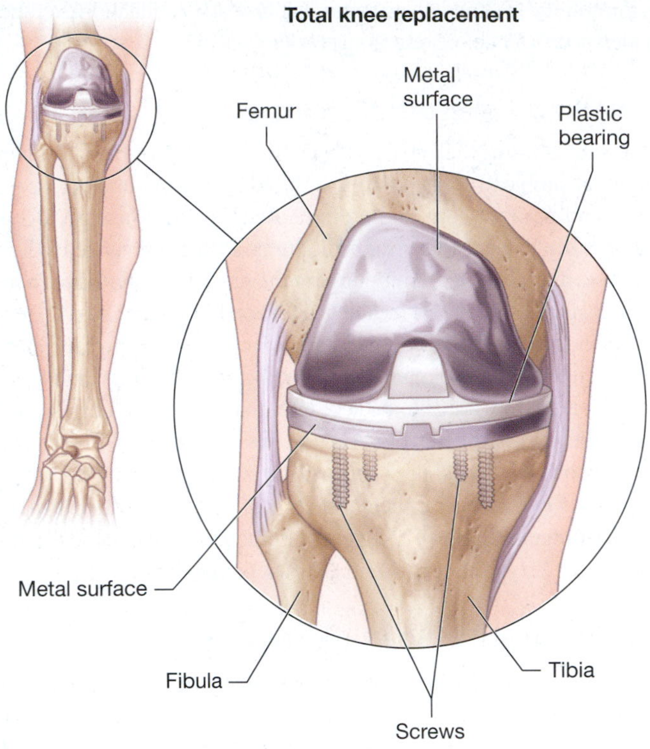

FIGURE 50–23 ◆ Knee arthroplasty.

CHART 50–9 Knee Arthroplasty

- A thigh tourniquet is applied to decrease bleeding during surgery.
- An incision approximately 10 inches in length is made in the anterior knee.
- The femoral head and tibia are surgically shaved to prepare for the prosthetic implant.
- The patella is shaved or replaced to allow free movement after the prosthesis is implanted.
- Debris in the surgical site is removed.
- A drain may be inserted to remove blood from the surgical area.
- The prosthesis is implanted.
- The surgical site is sutured closed.
- Continuous passive motion (CPM) may be utilized postoperatively using progressive angles of flexion and extension as prescribed by the health care provider.

Nursing Management

Refer to the Nursing Process: Patient Care Plan for the Orthopedic Surgical Patient on page 1551. For total knee replacement, early mobilization is important. Initially, there is a bulky dressing around the knee and a drain to remove any fluid buildup. The drain will be removed in a day or two. A CPM exercise machine that will slowly and smoothly straighten and bend the knee is typically used after surgery. Although pain after surgery is quite variable and not entirely predictable, it can be controlled with medication. The hospital stay may last from 3 to 7 days. The goal for discharge is to have the patient be able to get into and out of bed independently, bend the knee up to approximately 90 degrees, extend the knee fully, walk with crutches or a walker, and demonstrate knowledge of the prescribed home exercises.

Spinal Surgery

Epidemiology and Etiology

Back pain is the cause of more lost work hours than any other medical condition and is the second leading cause of work absences in the United States. The National Guidelines box on page 1546 outlines the recommendations for the diagnosis and treatment of low back pain. Most back pain occurs in people between the ages of 45 and 64, and it is more common among men than women (eMedicineHealth, 2011). The spine can be divided into three categories: the vertebral bony column, intervertebral disks, ligaments, and muscles; the spinal cord and nerves; and the spinal cord vasculature. The bony vertebral column consists of 33 vertebrae separated and cushioned by the intervertebral disks. The bony vertebrae and disks are joined together by ligaments. The disks allow a degree of flexibility to the spine. They temporarily flatten out and bulge when compressed, acting as shock absorbers. However, if the disk is under an extreme load, the central nucleus can rupture through the surrounding cartilaginous fibers, resulting in a herniated disk, which places pressure on the nerve root. Approximately 25% of people who have back pain have a herniated disk. The most common site of back pain is in the lower back with more than 95% of operations being performed on the fourth and fifth lumbar vertebrae (eMedicineHealth, 2011).

Spinal surgery is also done to stabilize or straighten the spinal column, as in kyphosis or scoliosis, and for fractures of the vertebrae. Of fractures that result in spinal cord injury, approximately half occur in the thoracic, lumbar, and sacral areas. The other half occur in the cervical vertebra (Reiter, 2011)

Clinical Manifestations

Pressure on the nerve roots from a herniated disk or displacement from a vertebral fracture will cause severe pain, possible paresthesia (decrease in sensation), and, if the spinal cord is affected, paralysis distal to the injury.

Diagnostic Tests and Medical–Surgical Management

Fractures and compression to nerve roots and the spinal cord are assessed through x-ray, CT scan, and MRI. **Discectomy** is surgery in which the diseased disk is removed. **Laminectomy,** in contrast, is surgery in which only part of the disk, usually only the herniated portion, is removed. It is called a laminectomy because the surgeon must cut through the lamina to access the herniated disk. During the procedure, the surgeon will make an incision over the vertebrae and down to the bony arches of the vertebrae. The ligament joining the vertebrae, along with all or part of the lamina, is removed so that the surgeon can see the involved nerve root. The surgeon will then pull the nerve root back toward the center of the spinal column and remove part of the disk or the entire disk. The incision will be closed, and the large back muscles will protect the spine and nerve roots. Traditional discectomy or laminectomy surgical procedures usually involve a 3- to 4-day hospital stay.

Minimally invasive surgery can be done through arthroscopic procedures and with the use of lasers. Procedures that are done arthroscopically include the following:

- ***Foraminotomy:*** This procedure is used to relieve pressure on nerves being compressed by the intervertebral foramen, the space where a nerve root exists in the spinal canal. The compression can be caused by bone, a bulging disk, or scar tissue. A small incision is made, and the scope is placed. With the use of small surgical instruments and/or a laser, the bone or tissue that is compressing the nerve is removed. The patient is ambulated within 2 hours of the procedure.

- ***Laminotomy:*** This procedure is used to relieve the pressure on the spinal canal for the exiting nerve roots and spinal cord by increasing the amount of space available. The pressure may be caused by bone spurs, spinal stenosis, arthritis, a bulging or herniated disk, or scar tissue. The procedure is done in the same manner as the foraminotomy. The patient is able to ambulate within 2 hours of the procedure.
- ***Percutaneous Arthroscopic Discectomy:*** This procedure involves the removal of a bulging or herniated disk that is pressing on a nerve root or the spinal cord. The procedure is done in the same manner as the foraminotomy. The patient is able to ambulate within 2 hours of the procedure.

Spinal fusion (fusing vertebrae together with bone graft or plates and screws so that an area of the spine cannot move) surgery may be performed after traumatic, unstable injuries to stabilize the spine and prevent further injury and loss of function (Figure 50–24◆). In some cases, spinal fusion may also be performed to treat vertebral fractures, kyphosis, or scoliosis. Bone grafts are used like cement to weld the vertebrae together, or the bones are held together by plates and screws so that they can no longer move. If an autologous bone graft is used, the piece of bone is generally taken from the iliac crest during the back surgery. Allograft bone donations are obtained from donor banks or stored in the operating room in a refrigerator or freezer. Allograft bones are obtained from cadavers and are sterilized and frozen or stored in sterile packaging. There are several types of spinal fusion surgery options:

- ***Posterolateral Gutter Fusion:*** The procedure is done through the back.
- ***Posterior Lumbar Interbody Fusion (PLIF):*** The procedure is done from the back and includes removing the disk between two vertebrae and inserting bone into the space created between the two vertebral bodies.

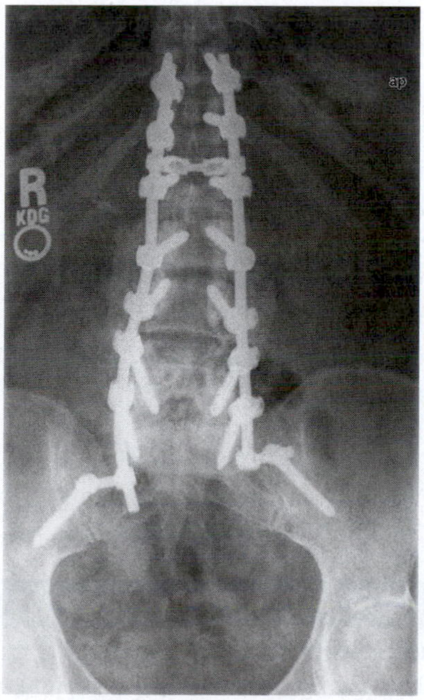

FIGURE 50–24 ◆ Spinal fusion with plates and screws x-ray.
Source: Karen Cooper, RN, MSN, CCRN, CNS.

- ***Anterior Lumbar Interbody Fusion (ALIF):*** The procedure is done from the front and includes removing the disk between two vertebrae and inserting bone into the space thus created.
- ***Anterior/Posterior Spinal Fusion:*** The procedure is done from the front and the back.

Nursing Management

Refer to the Nursing Process: Patient Care Plan for the Orthopedic Surgical Patient on page 1551. Additionally, for patients undergoing spinal surgery, until the bones fuse after surgery, the patient may need to wear a brace to maintain alignment of the spine. The operative site must remain in strict anatomic alignment. For example, if the patient who has had back surgery is to be turned, the patient's back must remain in a straight line during turning so that there is no torque or twisting of the operative site. The surgeon may order the patient to be flat in bed for a specified amount of time after surgery. Before getting the patient out of bed, the nurse must place a back brace on the patient while the patient is lying flat. This is done by logrolling the patient, applying the pieces of the brace, and securing the Velcro straps. A thoracolumbosacral orthosis (TLSO), the type of brace generally utilized (Figure 50–25◆), is

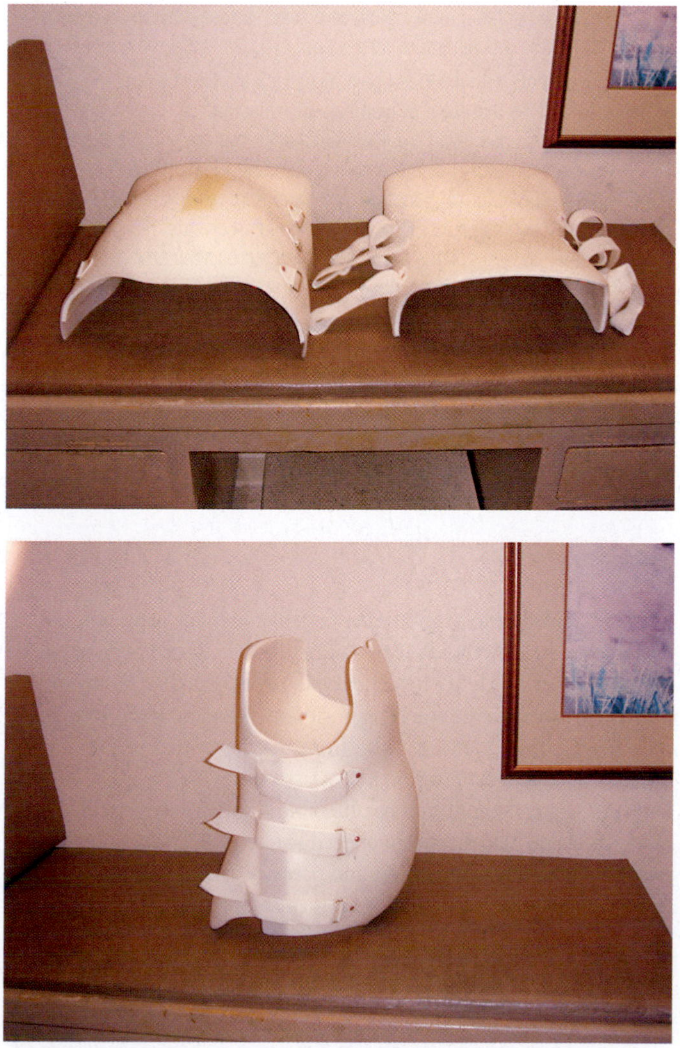

FIGURE 50–25 ◆ Thoracolumbosacral orthosis brace (TLSO).
Source: Karen Cooper, RN, MSN, CCRN, CNS.

NATIONAL GUIDELINES Diagnosis and Treatment of Low Back Pain

In 2007, the American College of Physicians (ACP) and the American Pain Society (APS) released clinical practice guidelines for the diagnosis and treatment of low back pain. The recommendations included the following:

1. Clinicians should conduct a focused history and physical examination to help place patients with low back pain into one of three broad categories: nonspecific low back pain, back pain potentially associated with radiculopathy or spinal stenosis, or back pain potentially associated with another specific spinal cause. The history should include assessment of psychosocial risk factors; these predict the risk of chronic disabling back pain.
2. Clinicians should not routinely obtain imaging or other diagnostic tests in patients with nonspecific low back pain.
3. Clinicians should perform diagnostic imaging and testing for patients with low back pain when severe or progressive neurologic deficits are present or when serious underlying conditions are suspected on the basis of history and physical examination.
4. Clinicians should evaluate patients with persistent low back pain and signs or symptoms of radiculopathy or spinal stenosis with MRI (preferred) or CT only if they are potential candidates for surgery or epidural steroid injection (for suspected radiculopathy).
5. Clinicians should provide patients with evidence-based information on the expected course of low back pain, advise patients to remain active, and provide information about effective self-care options.
6. For patients with low back pain, clinicians should consider the use of medications that have proven benefits in conjunction with back care information and self-care. Before initiating therapy, clinicians should assess the severity of the baseline pain and functional deficits, as well as the potential benefits, risks, and relative lack of long-term efficacy and safety data on the medication. For most patients, first-line medication options are acetaminophen or nonsteroidal anti-inflammatory drugs.
7. For patients who do not improve with self-care options, clinicians should consider the addition of nonpharmacologic therapy with proven benefits: for acute low back pain, spinal manipulation; for chronic or subacute low back pain, intensive interdisciplinary rehabilitation, exercise therapy, acupuncture, massage therapy, spinal manipulation, yoga, cognitive-behavioral therapy, or progressive relaxation (Shekelle, 2008).

specially created from a mold of the patient and made of durable plastic, using Velcro straps to hold the two sides together. The TLSO is also used as the postoperative brace for other types of back surgery. To ensure that the patient can achieve a standing position without bending, two people should assist the patient to move from the flat-in-bed position in the raised bed to the erect position.

Postoperative complications after spinal surgery may include transient bowel and bladder dysfunction due to edema of the spine causing compression of the sympathetic and parasympathetic nerve tracts. The nurse will monitor the patient for return of bowel sounds, and the patient should not receive a diet until bowel sounds return. A patient who has difficulty emptying the bladder after surgery may require intermittent urinary catheterization.

The nurse must monitor the spinal dressing for both bleeding and possible cerebrospinal fluid (CSF) leak. A CSF leak may occur if the dura is opened during the surgical procedure. During spinal surgery, the dura of the spinal cord is invaded, and there is potential for the surgical site to leak CSF. A CSF leak appears as a clear fluid that forms a halo around any serous drainage on the dressing. These leaks increase the potential for development of meningitis and often cause a postoperative headache that is worse when the patient is upright. The surgeon should be notified if a CSF leak is present or suspected. A blood patch may be used to treat the CSF leak from the surgical site. In this procedure, an anesthesiologist injects 5 to 20 milliliters of unclotted blood into the surgical site (into the epidural space). After the blood patch is performed, the patient should remain flat in bed for 2 hours to ensure that the blood does not migrate and is allowed to clot and prevent further CSF leakage.

Safety Alert *The nurse should report any cerebrospinal fluid leak in the spinal surgery patient immediately and institute precautions to prevent meningitis.*

If the patient has had back pain for many years, it may be difficult to manage the postoperative pain. Chronic pain follows different neural pathways than acute pain. Refer to Chapter 12 for an in-depth discussion of pain assessment and treatment. Alternative therapies such as low level laser treatment, described in the Complementary & Alternative Therapies box, are interventions that can help relieve the patient's pain.

Collaborative Management

Exercise to strengthen the core muscles helps ensure the health of the spinal column. Therefore, having the patient work with a physical therapist to design a safe and effective exercise regimen postoperatively is essential. Others may also be involved. In order to meet desired patient outcomes, it is essential that this interdisciplinary team communicate openly with one another in developing and evaluating care of the patient and family (IOM [Institute of Medicine], 2010).

Health Promotion

Obesity adds strain to the spinal column. If the patient is overweight, a dietitian can work with the patient to develop a safe weight loss plan. Discharge planning for the patient undergoing orthopedic surgery is discussed on page 1555. In addition, for patients who have had spinal surgery, the following instructions should be given:

- If the health care team instructed the patient to wear a back brace or cervical collar, the patient must wear it at all times when out of bed unless instructed otherwise. The brace does not need to be worn while the patient is showering; however, the patient must take care not to bend or twist when not wearing the brace.
- The nurse should encourage the patient to do as much walking as possible and instruct the patient to not sit for prolonged periods of time.
- The nurse should teach the patient to avoid activities that include bending, twisting, or lifting anything greater than 10 to 20 pounds.

Ankle and Foot Surgeries

Etiology and Epidemiology

The act of walking can put up to 1.5 times a person's body weight on her foot. The movement of the foot (which has 26 bones) and ankle is supported by the muscles and tendons. The ankle joint comprises the talus and the ends of the tibia and fibula. It is supported by three groups

COMPLEMENTARY & ALTERNATIVE THERAPIES Low Level Laser

Nancy Yilk

SOON AFTER THE DISCOVERY OF LASERS in the 1960s, it was realized that laser therapy had the potential to improve wound healing and reduce pain, inflammation, and swelling. The term *low level laser therapy* (LLLT) has become widely recognized and implies the existence of the biphasic dose response or the Arndt–Schulz curve (Chung, Dai, Sharma, Huang, Carroll, & Hamblin, 2011). In recent years, LLLT and Cold Lazer (CL), or photobiomodulation, have found their way into integrative therapies such as chiropractic, acupuncture, and physical therapy. First used mainly for wound healing and pain relief, the medical applications of LLLT have broadened to include diseases such as stroke, myocardial infarction, and degenerative or traumatic brain disorders. The biomechanisms of LLLT operate both on a cellular and a tissue level (Hashmi, Huang, Osmani, Sharma, Naeser, & Hamblin, 2010).

Injury of a major nerve trunk frequently results in considerable disability associated with loss of sensory and motor functions. Spontaneous recovery of long-term severe incomplete peripheral nerve injury is often unsatisfactory. The function of denervated muscles can be restored, not completely but to a very substantial degree, by laser treatment initiated at the earliest possible stage postinjury. Post-traumatic nerve repair and prevention of muscle atrophy represent a major challenge of restorative medicine. Considerable interest exists in the potential therapeutic value of laser phototherapy for restoring or temporarily preventing denervated muscle atrophy as well as enhancing regeneration of severely injured peripheral nerves. In peripheral nerve injury, laser phototherapy has an immediate protective effect. It maintains functional activity of the injured nerve for a long period, decreases scar tissue formation at the injury site, decreases degeneration in corresponding motor neurons of the spinal cord, and significantly increases axonal growth and myelinization.

The effectiveness of low-power laser irradiation (780 nm) in the treatment of patients suffering from incomplete peripheral nerve and brachial plexus injuries for 6 months up to several years was studied in a randomized, double-blind, placebo-controlled trial. The 18 subjects were randomly assigned to placebo (non-active light: diffused LED lamp) or low-power laser irradiation (wavelength, 780 nm; power, 250 mW) groups. In the study, 21 consecutive daily sessions of laser or placebo irradiation were applied transcutaneously for 3 hours to the injured peripheral nerve. Clinical and electrophysiological assessments were done at baseline, at the end of the 21 days of treatment, and 3 and 6 months thereafter. The analysis of motor function during the 6-month follow-up period compared to baseline showed statistically significant improvement ($p = 0.0001$) in the laser-treated group compared to the placebo group. No statistically significant difference was found in sensory function. Electrophysiological analysis also showed statistically significant improvement in recruitment of voluntary muscle activity in the laser-irradiated group ($p = 0.006$), compared to the placebo group. This pilot study suggests that in patients with long-term peripheral nerve injury, noninvasive 780-nm laser phototherapy can progressively improve nerve function, which leads to significant functional recovery (Rochkind, Drory, Alon, Nissan, & Ouaknine, 2007).

Low back pain (LBP) is a common musculoskeletal disorder that is highly prevalent in the general population. Management of this pathology includes numerous interventions depending on pain severity: analgesic, nonsteroidal anti-inflammatory drugs, or steroid injections. However, the duration of symptom relief is limited. To evaluate the short-term effectiveness of high-intensity laser therapy (HILT) versus ultrasound (US) therapy in the treatment of LBP, 30 patients with LBP were randomly assigned to a HILT group or a US therapy group. Study participants received 15 treatment sessions of HILT or US therapy over a period of 3 consecutive weeks (5 days/week). Findings obtained after 15 treatment sessions with the experimental protocol suggested greater effectiveness of HILT than of US therapy in the treatment of LBP, proposing HILT as a promising new therapeutic option for the rehabilitation of LBP (Fiore et al., 2011).

References

Chung, H., Dai, T., Sharma, S. K., Huang, Y. Y., Carroll, J. D., & Hamblin, M. R. (2011). The nuts and bolts of low-level laser (light) therapy. *Annals of Biomedical Engineering, 40*(2), 516–533.

Fiore, P., Panza, F., Cassatella, G., Russo, A., Frisardi, V., Solfrizzi, V., et al. (2011). Short-term effects of high-intensity laser therapy versus ultrasound therapy in the treatment of low back pain: A randomized controlled trial. *European Journal of Physical and Rehabilitation Medicine, 47*(3), 367–373. Epub 2011 Jun 8

Hashmi, J. T., Huang, Y. Y., Osmani, B. Z., Sharma, S. K., Naeser, M. A., & Hamblin, M. R. (2010). Role of low-level laser therapy in neurorehabilitation. *Physical Medicine and Rehabilitation, 2*(12 Suppl 2), S292–305.

Rochkind, S., Drory, V., Alon, M., Nissan, M., & Ouaknine, G. E. (2007). Laser phototherapy (780 nm), a new modality in treatment of long-term incomplete peripheral nerve injury: A randomized double-blind placebo-controlled study. *Photomedicine and Laser Surgery, 25*(5), 436–442.

of ligaments. Most injuries of the foot and ankle are caused by overuse, poor conditioning, and improperly fitting shoes.

Ankle pain is most commonly due to a sprain but also can be caused by arthritis, gout, bone fracture, tendonitis, infection, poor structural alignment of the leg or foot, or chronic ankle joint instability from a severe injury or multiple injuries. During a fall or jump, the foot is likely to turn inward (inversion), which might stretch or tear ligaments. The ankle joint is held together and protected from abnormal movement by the ligaments.

Tendon Injuries

Tendons connect muscle to bone. Two tendons run along the outer aspect of the ankle and foot to help stabilize the ankle joint. These tendons are called the peroneal tendons (Figure 50–26◆). Peroneal tendon injuries can be acute or chronic and occur most often in patients who participate in sports that involve repetitive ankle motion. The tendon may have an acute tear or fray from overuse. The tendons can also sublux out of their normal position.

The largest and strongest tendon of the lower leg is the Achilles tendon. The tendon connects muscles in the lower leg with the calcaneus bone. A complete or partial tear of the Achilles tendon is called a rupture (Figure 50–27◆, p. 1548). Jumping, pivoting, or sudden acceleration to a run can stretch the tendon beyond its capacity and cause a tear.

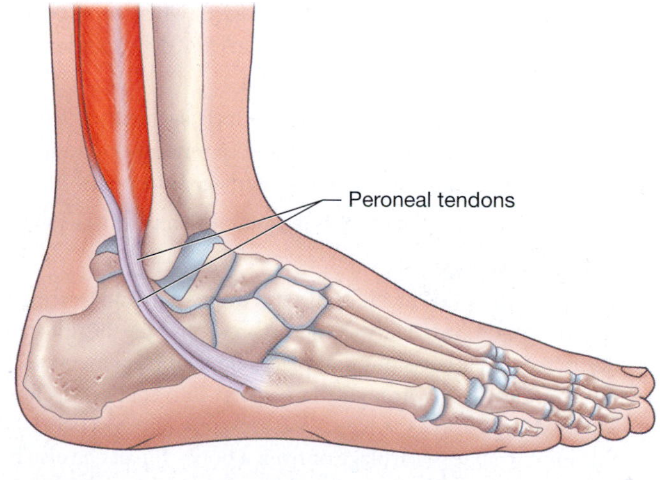

FIGURE 50–26 ◆ Peroneal tendons.

Clinical Manifestations

Injury to the tendons or ligaments of the ankle will cause severe pain, swelling, and difficulty with mobilization, because weight bearing will increase the pain. Without proper healing, the joint will become unstable, injury will reoccur, and the patient will develop chronic

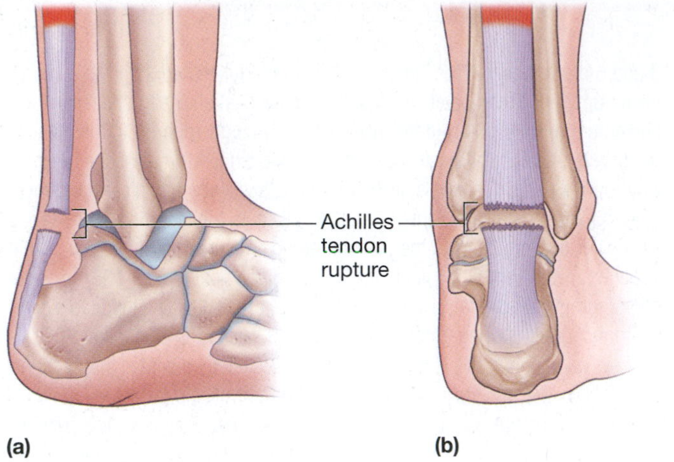

FIGURE 50–27 ◆ Achilles tendon rupture.

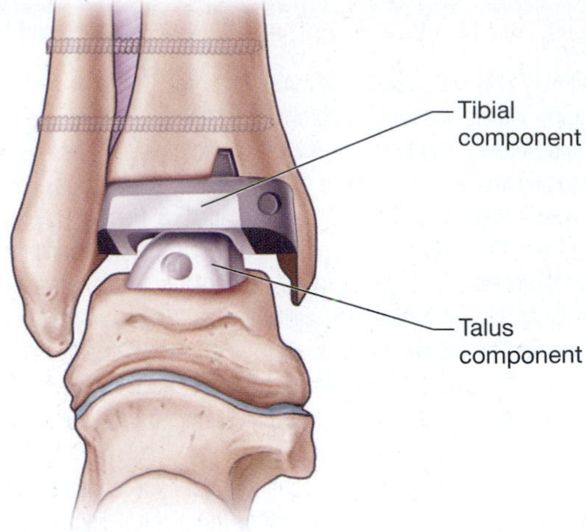

FIGURE 50–28 ◆ Ankle arthroplasty.

ankle pain. Other causes of chronic ankle pain include arthritis of the joint, synovitis (inflammation of the joint lining), an injury to the nerves that pass through the ankle, and development of scar tissue after a sprain, which takes up space in the joint and places pressure on the ligaments.

Symptoms of chronic ankle pain include pain on the lateral side of the ankle, swelling, stiffness, difficulty walking on uneven ground or in high heels, tenderness, and repeated ankle sprains.

Diagnostic Procedures and Medical–Surgical Management

Damage to the ankle or foot bones is identified with x-ray and CT scan. However, an MRI may be used to more accurately identify damage to the ligaments, tendons, and soft tissue. If conservative treatment does not bring relief, surgery may be required. Surgical treatment for ankle injuries is rare, but it is used for injuries that fail to respond to nonsurgical treatment and for persistent instability after months of rehabilitation and nonsurgical treatment.

Surgical options for ankle or foot injuries include the following:

- ***Arthroscopy:*** A surgeon examines the joint to see whether there are any loose fragments of bone or cartilage or whether part of the ligament is caught in the joint, then cleans any debris and makes repairs.
- ***Reconstruction:*** A surgeon repairs the torn ligament or tendon with sutures or uses other ligaments and/or tendons found in the foot and around the ankle to repair the damaged ligaments.
- ***Arthroplasty:*** A surgeon replaces the joint with an artificial joint.

Ankle Arthroscopy

Arthroscopy of the ankle includes surgical evaluation and treatment for multiple conditions. During the arthroscopy, the health care provider makes small incisions and places fiber-optic cameras with miniature surgical tools through the incision into the joint. These tools are used to perform the repair. Arthroscopy removes debris in the ankle joint from torn cartilage or from a bone chip. It can also be used to repair or reattach tendons and ligaments damaged during a severe sprain.

Ankle Reconstruction

Ankle reconstruction is the repair of the torn ligament or tendon with sutures, or the use of other ligaments and/or tendons found in the foot and around the ankle to repair the damaged ligaments. The procedure may be done through arthroscopic surgery or as an open procedure.

Ankle Arthroplasty

Ankle arthroplasty is the replacement of the joint with an artificial joint (Figure 50–28◆). Although ankle replacement is done much less frequently than knee or hip replacement, it can reduce the pain from arthritis. To fit the metal socket in place, the ends of the tibia and the fibula are shaped first. Following that, the top of the talus is shaped so the metal talus component can be inserted. After the bones have been prepared, all the different pieces of the artificial ankle joint are put into place. To make sure that the ankle socket or the tibial component fits tightly, two screws are placed through the fibula and the tibia just above the artificial ankle joint. To prevent any motion that could loosen the artificial joint, bone is grafted between the fibula and the tibia to fuse them. The graft material is taken from the bone that was removed earlier during the shaping procedure.

Surgeries of the Foot

Etiology and Epidemiology

The most common foot surgeries are for the treatment of bunions and hammer toes. A bunion, also called hallux valgus, is a turning outward of the big toe (Figure 50–29◆). The first metatarsal becomes prominent on the inner border of the foot. This bump is the bunion and is made up of bone and soft tissue. The larger the bunion becomes, the more pressure is exerted on the joint while walking and the more pain develops. The big toe may angle toward and even move under the second toe. The deformity may even progress to force the second toe out of alignment, at times overlapping the third toe, and the foot will appear deformed. As the bunion progresses, arthritis may develop in the joint.

A hammer toe is a deformity of the second, third, fourth, or fifth toe. The toe is bent at the middle joint and resembles a hammer (Figure 50–30◆). Initially, hammer toes are flexible and can be corrected with simple measures; if left untreated, however, they become fixed and require surgery. Hammer toe results from shoes that do not fit properly or a muscle imbalance. Muscles work in pairs to straighten and bend the toes. If the toe is bent and held in one position for a long period of time, muscles tighten and cannot stretch out.

Clinical Manifestations

Bunions are painful and can make it difficult to wear shoes and affect mobility. Bunions can be caused by polio or arthritis but most commonly are caused, as with hammer toe, by ill-fitting shoes that squeeze the toes into an unnatural position.

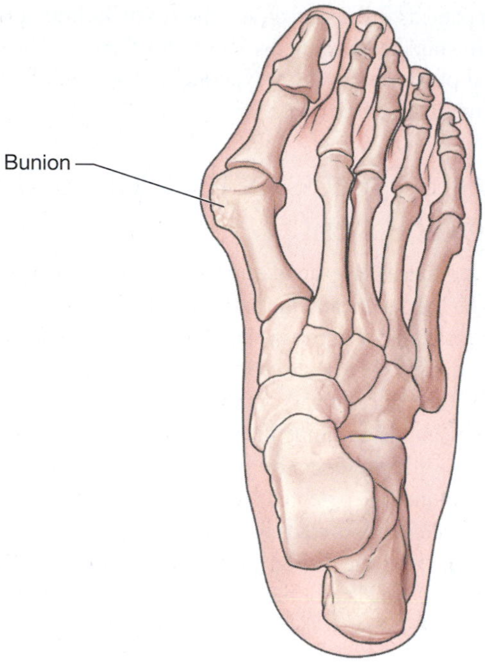

FIGURE 50–29 ◆ Bunion.

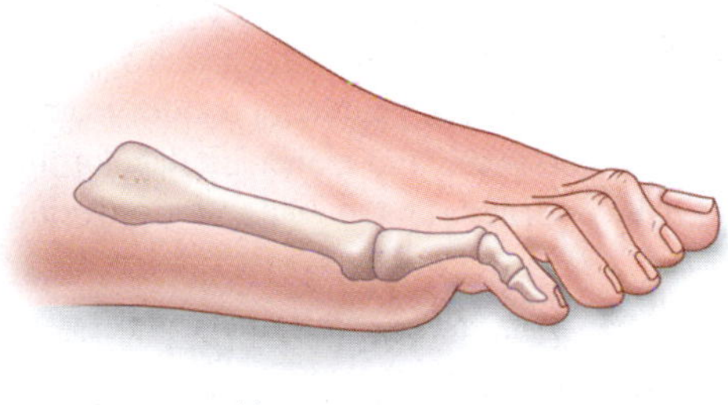

FIGURE 50–30 ◆ Hammer toe.

Diagnostic Tests and Medical Management

An x-ray of the affected foot may be done to rule out fracture. Multiple surgical procedures may be done alone or in combination, depending on the degree of deformity. The goal of surgery is to restore anatomic alignment, relieve pain, and correct the deformity. Maintenance of the correction relies on the underlying pathology and the establishment of good alignment and stability (Haas, 2009). The procedures include the following:

- ***Repair of the Tendons and Ligaments Around the Toe:*** With a bunion, the tissues may be too tight on one side and too loose on the other, creating an imbalance that causes the big toe to drift toward the others. This procedure shortens the loose tissues, lengthens the tight ones, and is usually combined with an osteotomy.
- ***Osteotomy:*** The surgical cutting of bone and realignment of the joint.
- ***Exostectomy:*** Removal of the excess bone on the toe joint; used only for an enlargement of the bone with no drifting of the big toe.
- ***Arthrodesis:*** Removal of the damaged joint surfaces, followed by the insertion of screws, wires, or plates to hold the surfaces together until it heals.
- ***Resection Arthroplasty:*** Removal of the damaged portion of the joint to create a flexible "scar" joint.

Nursing Management

Refer to the Nursing Process: Patient Care Plan for the Orthopedic Surgical Patient on p. 1551. Additionally, the patient's weight-bearing status, which will be determined by the surgeon, will depend on the extent of the repair. Some patients will be allowed to bear weight with crutches; others will be placed in an immobilizer for as long as 6 weeks. If the surgery was extensive, such as remodeling of the ankle, a cast may be applied to promote healing by preventing the patient from moving the joint too early. The ankle should be elevated and iced to minimize swelling and prevent increased pain.

Amputation

Etiology and Epidemiology

Amputation is the surgical removal or traumatic loss of a body part. The majority of new amputations occur due to complications of vascular disease, especially from diabetes. In the upper extremities, amputation is rare and often associated with trauma, meningococcemia, and osteosarcoma. Upper extremity amputation accounts for approximately 69% of traumatic amputations (National Limb Loss Information Center [NLLIC], 2008). Osteosarcoma necessitates the removal of the bone in which the cancer is present. Chapter 49 discusses osteosarcoma and other types of bone cancer. In the lower extremities, peripheral vascular disease, diabetes, and gangrene are the frequent causes for elective amputation. Below knee amputation (BKA) is preferred to above knee amputation (AKA) because balance and coordination are more stable with BKA, gait is more natural, and there is a better potential for revisions, if needed. Above knee amputation requires more energy to ambulate. The AKA patient must raise the hip and swing the prosthesis and leg forward for clearance because the leg plus prosthesis must remain straight. In the older adult, this may be a safety risk; if so, wheelchair mobility is a safer practice.

Traumatic amputation is a sudden loss of a body part and may require more extensive removal of tissue, bone, and muscle than amputation due to vascular insufficiency. Traumatic amputations are upsetting to patients as well as staff. Many emergency service members bring the amputated part to the hospital in hopes of possible reattachment. Traumatic amputation may be associated with increased potential for phantom limb pain, body image disturbance, and grief or loss disturbance than amputation resulting from a chronic disease process.

Surgical reattachment of a severed limb is done only under certain circumstances because the surgery is difficult. It is not attempted with a digit of the hand unless it is a thumb or index finger needed for function and the wound has clean borders. Reattachment of crush-type amputations are not attempted because of the poor outcome. Only cleanly separated traumatic amputations in patients without significant risk factors for impaired healing, such as smoking, are considered for reattachment. For adults, it is nearly impossible for nerves to regenerate in the lower extremity, and the reattached limb may be painful and dysfunctional (Feliciano et al., 2008). In addition, complete amputation and a prosthesis could allow a patient to return to normal activities in days to weeks, whereas reconstruction of mangled limbs can span years with a huge psychological strain and impact on function and occupation.

Surgical Management

Chart 50–10 describes the surgical procedure for amputation.

CHART 50–10 Surgical Amputation

- A tourniquet (pneumatic or other restrictive device) is applied above the area to be amputated.
- A skin flap is prepared by excising the skin from the muscle and folding it back (away from the area to be amputated).
- A guillotine device or saw is used to perform the amputation.
- The skin flap is utilized to close the surgical wound.

Nursing Management

Refer to the Nursing Process: Patient Care Plan for the Orthopedic Surgical Patient. Additionally, because many amputations are the result of peripheral vascular insufficiency, the patient must be monitored closely for skin integrity, with particular care given to prevent pressure ulcer development. If the amputation involved part of the lower extremity, the patient's remaining heel should be floated off of the mattress with pillows or a heel protection device. In the immediate postoperative period, stump care usually involves elevation of the stump and compression wrapping of the extremity to prevent edema. A figure-of-eight method beginning at the distal stump is utilized to wrap the stump.

Safety Alert *The nurse should elevate the stump for the first 24 hours to prevent postoperative edema. After 24 hours, the patient should keep the stump flat while in bed or extended while out of bed in a chair to prevent contracture of the nearest joint.*

For the patient with an amputation, there are as many physical and mobility issues to deal with as there are emotional issues. The patient may need to learn wound care of the stump and have trouble just looking at it. The patient may have bizarre sensations such as feeling as though the amputated foot is cold or itchy when it is not there. These are called phantom limb sensations. Patients may need to retrain their brains to distinguish where their body ends. The Evidence-Based Practice box provides information regarding stump and phantom limb pain. Most patients will need to grieve the loss of the limb, and counseling should be initiated prior to discharge. Prostheses will be made, and a great deal of physical and occupational therapy may be needed to adapt to a missing limb or digit.

Nursing Process for the Orthopedic Surgical Patient

The nurse formulates the plan of care for the orthopedic patient in conjunction with the patient and the health care team. The nursing process provides the framework to ensure that all aspects of patient management are being addressed. The nurse caring for the patient after surgery must consider the time since surgery (number of postoperative days) in setting priorities and determining the patient's progress toward discharge. Pain control in the postoperative period is a major area of focus, because pain can indicate potential problems or prevent the patient from completing exercises and reaching goals that are necessary to recover and rehabilitate. (See the section on assessment of pain in the Nursing Process: Patient Care Plan for the Orthopedic Surgical Patient). General postoperative assessment is discussed in Chapter 19.

Nursing Management

The nursing assessment of the patient is both holistic and focused. The nurse must rely on the patient's report to provide the necessary information to accurately determine the patient's current status. The Nursing Process: Patient Care Plan box provides examples of subjective and objective assessment and evaluation data for the patient with a musculoskeletal disorder as a foundation for providing care to this population.

Neurovascular Assessment

The neurovascular assessment is a requirement in the assessment of patients with musculoskeletal injury and surgery. The neurovascular assessment should be performed bilaterally so that the affected extremity can be compared to the unaffected extremity. If the patient undergoes

EVIDENCE-BASED PRACTICE Stump and Phantom Limb Pain

Clinical Problem

A significant problem following amputation is acute stump pain and phantom limb pain. Up to 90% of amputees report phantom limb pain during the first year following surgery (Borghi et al., 2010). Pain in the affected limb prior to surgery is correlated to the degree of stump and phantom limb pain postoperatively.

Research Findings

Phantom limb pain is a complex pain syndrome that is described as burning, aching, or electric shock type pain. If pain is inadequately controlled during the preoperative and postoperative period, the risk of phantom limb pain may increase (Hanley, Jensen, & Smith, 2007). Borghi and colleagues (2010) found that perineural infusion of a high concentration of local anesthetic solution placed before or during surgery and continued postoperatively for 4 to 83 days (median duration 30 days) decreased the incidence of severe phantom limb pain to only 3% at the end of a 12-month evaluation period.

Another therapy that has proven to help decrease phantom limb pain is mirror therapy (Chan et al., 2007; Diers, Christmann, Koeppe, & Flor, 2010). Phantom limb pain may be induced by a conflict between visual feedback and proprioceptive representation of the amputated limb. The patient attempts to perform movements with the amputated limb while viewing the reflected image of the movement of the intact limb. The decrease in pain is thought to be due to the activation of mirror neurons in the hemisphere of the brain that is contralateral to the amputated limb. Visual input of what appears to be movement of the amputated limb may reduce the activity of the systems that perceive pain.

Implications for Nursing Practice

Studies show a significant reduction in acute postoperative stump pain and the development of phantom limb pain with pre-, intra-, and postoperative analgesia via infusion. Patient education regarding the infusion and knowledge regarding the effects and side effects of the medication used is of great importance. Having the infusion started preoperatively and continue during the postoperative period appears to benefit the patient, especially with regard to phantom limb pain 12 months following surgery.

Critical Thinking Questions with answers can be found in the Osborn Student Resources at nursing.pearsonhighered.com.

Sources: Borghi, B., d'Addabbo, M., White, P. F., Gallerani, P.,Toccaceli, L., Raffeli, W., et al. (2010). The use of prolonged peripheral neural blockade after lower extremity amputation: the effect on symptoms associated with phantom limb syndrome. *Anesthesia Analgesia 111*(5): 1308–1315; Chan, B. L., Witt, R., Charrow, A. P., Magee, A., Howard, R., Pasquina, P. F. et al. (2007). Mirror therapy for phantom limb pain. *New England Journal of Medicine 357*(21): 2206–2207; Diers, M., Christmann, C., Koeppe, C., Ruf, M., & Flor, H. (2010). Mirrored, imagined and executed movements differentially activate sensorimotor cortex in amputees with and without phantom limb pain. *Pain 149*(2): 296–304; Hanley, M. A., Jensen, M. P., Smith, D. G., Ehde, D. M., Edwards, W. T., & Robinson, L. R. (2007). Preamputation pain and acute pain predict chronic pain after lower extremity amputation. *Journal of Pain 8*: 102–109.

NURSING PROCESS: Patient Care Plan for the Orthopedic Surgical Patient

Assessment of Orthopedic Status Using Gordon's Functional Health Patterns:

- Health Perception Health Management Pattern
- Nutrition Metabolic Pattern
- Activity Exercise Pattern
- Cognitive Perceptual Pattern

Subjective Data	Objective Data
Assessment of Airway and Gas Exchange	**Assessment of Airway and Gas Exchange**
Are you having difficulty breathing? Do you feel like you are getting enough air? Do you use an inhaler or have a history of lung problems? Can you take a deep breath and cough?	Lung sounds Adequate incentive spirometry and cough Presence of any sputum? Oxygen saturation, arterial blood gas analysis Respiratory rate, depth, effort Mental status
Assessment of Neurovascular Status	**Assessment of Neurovascular Status**
Can you move your (name part distal to surgery)? Where do you feel me touching you? Is this sharp or dull? Are you in pain? Can you describe your pain using a scale of 0 to 10? Do you have any numbness or tingling?	Strength of movement Sensation Pulses Color of skin Skin temperature Capillary refill time
Assessment of Fluid Volume Status	**Assessment of Fluid Volume Status**
Are you thirsty? Do you need to urinate? When was the last time you urinated? How much? What was the color (pale or dark)? Do you feel cold? How is your breathing? Do you feel anxious? Do you feel that your heart is beating faster than normal?	Urine output, color, specific gravity Blood loss from surgical drains/dressing Intake and output balance Heart rate (HR), blood pressure (BP), respiratory rate (RR) Blood urea nitrogen (BUN)/creatinine Hemoglobin (Hgb) and hematocrit (HCT) Skin turgor, capillary refill
Assessment of Pain	**Assessment of Pain**
Can you describe your pain for me using a 0 to 10 scale with 0 being no pain and 10 being the worst pain you have ever had? Using that 0 to 10 scale, what is your comfort level? What number on that 0 to 10 scale is your goal for your pain at this point in your recovery?	Patient pain score Patient pain score goal Type of pain-relief modality
Assessment of Wound Status and Potential for Infection	**Assessment of Wound Status and Potential for Infection**
Are you having more or less pain in your (name surgical site) today? Do you feel as though you have fever or chills? Are you having urinary frequency or urgency?	Temperature and vital signs Wound drainage appearance, odor Suture site redness, edema, warmth Urine appearance, odor Wound/urine culture results White blood count (WBC) results
Assessment of Functional Status	**Assessment of Functional Status**
How do you feel today? Are you able to bathe and perform your postoperative exercises unassisted, or do you need some help? How far did you walk today and yesterday?	Amount in feet that patient is able to ambulate Time in hours that patient is out of bed Amount of persons needed to get patient out of bed or to assist with ambulation Assistive devices needed for mobility
Assessment of Skin Integrity	**Assessment of Skin Integrity**
Are you able to turn and position yourself? Do you have any painful areas or sensations of pressure while you are in bed? Do you have any reddened areas that you are aware of?	Skin appearance Patient position Presence of pressure relief device

(continued)

NURSING PROCESS: Patient Care Plan for the Orthopedic Surgical Patient, *continued*

Subjective Data	Objective Data
Assessment of Patient's Understanding of Treatment Plan and Continuing Care Needs Do you have any questions about your plan of care? What are your goals for today? Do you have anyone at home to assist you? Tell me about your home so that I have a good understanding of it.	**Assessment of Patient's Understanding of Treatment Plan and Continuing Care Needs** Observation of activities Verbalization of continuing care plan

Outcomes and Evaluation Parameters	Planning and Interventions with *Rationales*
1. NURSING DIAGNOSIS: Gas Exchange, Impaired *related to anesthetic or narcotic effect, fluid overload, pulmonary or fat emboli, pneumonia, or preexisting pulmonary or cardiovascular disease exacerbation* (NANDA-I © 2012)	
Outcome: Airway open. Adequate gas exchange. ***Evaluation Parameters:*** Breath sounds clear, without evidence of snoring or stridor. Oxygen saturation > 94% or as ordered by health care provider. Arterial blood gas demonstrates PaO_2 > 80 mmHg and $PaCO_2$ 35–45 mmHg. Respiratory rate 12–20 per minute, unlabored with good chest expansion. Alert and oriented to person, place, time, and situation.	Initially, a jaw-thrust maneuver may be necessary to maintain an open airway if the patient has snoring breath sounds indicating airway obstruction from the tongue. If this maneuver is necessary, the patient may require additional reversal agents such as naloxone or flumazenil. The anesthesiologist or surgeon may need to be contacted for orders for these medications. Airway adjuncts may be indicated. *To maintain open airway.* Assess the patient for adequacy of respiratory rate and depth, auscultate breath sounds, and monitor oxygen saturation. Analyze arterial blood gas when results are available. *Indicates gas exchange is adequate.* Assess patient's level of consciousness and orientation to person, place, time, and situation. *Confusion, agitation, restlessness, or difficult arousal may indicate hypoxia.* Encourage the patient to perform incentive spirometry (ICS) every 1–2 hours for 10 breaths while awake. Have the patient cough and deep breathe after utilizing ICS. Assist the patient out of bed (OOB) to the chair and ambulating at least three times a day. *To promote adequate gas exchange, promote airway clearance, and prevent atelectasis.*
2. NURSING DIAGNOSIS: Neurovascular Dysfunction, Peripheral: Risk for *related to edema, vascular insufficiency, nerve damage, or surgical complication* (NANDA-I © 2012)	
Outcomes: Absence of neurovascular deficits. Skeletal structures in alignment. ***Evaluation Parameters:*** Full strength. Sensation intact. No numbness, tingling, or pain. Pulses 2–3+ palpated. Skin warm, pink, and dry. Capillary refill time < 3 seconds.	Perform neurovascular assessment every 2–4 hours. Assess bilateral extremities. *To give indication of normal findings for patient.* Elevate the limb above the level of the heart in a position of function. *To decrease edema formation and prevent contracture.* Evaluate sensation using a dermatome chart for patients with epidural anesthesia/catheters and patients with spinal surgery. *Dermatome chart describes level of anesthesia or deficit.* Evaluate strength and range of motion during planned postoperative activities. *Postoperative exercise improves circulation, improves healing, and prevents contractures and deconditioning.*
3. NURSING DIAGNOSIS: (a) Fluid Volume, Deficient *related to blood loss and inadequate fluid intake.* (b) Fluid Volume, Imbalanced: Risk for *due to impaired renal function and fluid intake in excess of output* (NANDA-I © 2012)	
Outcome: Adequate and balanced intake and output. ***Evaluation Parameters:*** Vital signs within normal limits. Intake and output balance. Lungs clear. Urine output adequate. BUN and creatinine normal. Hgb and HCT stable. Drainage from wound < 50 milliliters in 24 hours, or other parameter determined by surgeon.	Strict intake and output (I&O) to include all PO liquids, IV fluid intake, and urine, gastric, and wound drainage output. Maintain shift and ongoing totals. Assess wound drainage. Frankly bloody drainage may be present on the first postoperative day, but should change to serosanguinous after that. Notify the health care provider of excessive blood loss. *To give an accurate reflection of fluid balance.* Obtain vital signs as ordered. *Tachycardia and low blood pressure may indicate hypovolemia. Increased respiratory rate or adventitious breath sounds may indicate volume overload.* Monitor laboratory studies for signs of hypo-/hypervolemia. *The hemoglobin and hematocrit, BUN, and creatinine levels provide information on volume status.*

NURSING PROCESS: Patient Care Plan for the Orthopedic Surgical Patient, *continued*

4. NURSING DIAGNOSIS: Pain, Acute *related to surgical procedure, compartment syndrome, osteoarthritis, or cerebrospinal fluid (CSF) leak (in spinal surgery patient)* (NANDA-I © 2012)

Outcome: Patient will have pain controlled and will be able to participate in all aspects of rehabilitation program.

Evaluation Parameter: Pain scale score at or below the predetermined comfort level score.

Medicate the patient for pain score greater than pain goal level. Notify the health care provider if symptoms are unrelieved by ordered medication.

Patients have a right to pain control within their desired comfort level. Pain that is not relieved may indicate development of complications such as compartment syndrome.

Place the spinal patient in a supine position if he complains of headache. *CSF leak headache increases with drainage and an upright position.*

5. NURSING DIAGNOSIS: Infection, Risk for and Delayed Wound Healing *related to age, open surgery, compound fracture, and comorbid condition* (NANDA-I © 2012)

Outcomes: Wound/bone healing within expected time frame.

No evidence of infection.

Evaluation Parameters: Surgical incision is clean, dry, and wound edges are well approximated, without redness.

Urine clear, no odor.

Vital signs within normal limits (WNL).

WBC count $<$ 11,000/mcL.

Obtain vital signs as ordered or every 4 hours, including temperature.

To provide early indication of changes indicating infection.

Assess the surgical site and drainage each shift.

To provide early indication of changes indicating infection.

Monitor lab values, especially WBC count.

Elevations in WBC may indicate infection.

6. NURSING DIAGNOSIS: Self-Care, Readiness for Enhanced *related to surgery, pain, immobility, or decreased mental status* (NANDA-I © 2012)

Outcome: Patient able to care for self.

Evaluation Parameters: Able to perform postoperative exercises including transfers, ambulation, and pulmonary toilet at prescribed intervals.

Able to ambulate with walker 50 feet with steady gait; able to ambulate unassisted for 50 feet with steady gait.

Able to complete toilet and hygiene functions unassisted.

Patient should be assisted out of bed as soon as feasible. Follow the health care provider orders/clinical pathway instructions for mobility and activities. If the health care provider does not order progressive mobilization of the patient, notify the health care provider to obtain activity orders. *To prevent deconditioning and maintain or improve functional status.*

7. NURSING DIAGNOSIS: Skin Integrity, Risk for Impaired *related to decreased sensorium and immobility* (NANDA-I © 2012)

Outcome: Patient will have no evidence of skin breakdown.

Evaluation Parameters: Skin surface is clean, dry, pink, and intact.

Patient position change is performed or observed at least every 2 hours while in bed or every 15 minutes while seated.

Turn and position the patient at least every 2 hours while in bed (logroll, maintaining spinal alignment in patient with spinal surgery). Float heels off of the bed with pillows or a heel-lift device. Follow hospital protocol for use of pressure relief mattresses and overlays. *To prevent pressure ulcer development.*

Assess skin integrity and document each shift and with each change in position. Assess areas over bony prominences, where prostheses, casts, traction, or splints contact.

To provide early detection of potential for skin breakdown.

8. NURSING DIAGNOSIS: (a) Knowledge, Deficient of Self-Care Needs and Treatment Plan *related to postoperative delirium. (b)* Therapeutic Regimen Management, Ineffective *related to postoperative exercises, administration of deep venous thrombosis (DVT) prophylaxis, and self-care activities without assistance related to age, obesity, decreased functional capacity, and lack of home support* (NANDA-I © 2012)

Outcome: Patient is able to discuss a realistic plan for self-care after hospital discharge.

Evaluation Parameters: Patient verbalizes knowledge of plan of care and goals.

Patient demonstrates ability to perform postoperative exercises correctly in the appropriate frequency.

Patient verbalizes a plan for assistance with activities of daily living (ADLs) and ongoing therapeutic requirements, if needed.

Patient demonstrates ability to ambulate at least 100 feet and perform self-care activities.

Assess the patient's readiness to learn and provide patient education regarding patient procedures, activities, medications, and care needs. *Assessment of patient readiness enables the nurse to provide education at appropriate times.*

Begin discharge planning on admission. Encourage the significant other/family's participation in the plan. Evaluate care needs compared with patient abilities. Patient/significant other should be able to verbalize/demonstrate essential activities prior to discharge. *To ensure that sufficient time is allotted to provide education and training so that patient/family are able to perform activities after discharge.*

Prior to discharge, ensure that the patient understands the plan of care, is able to verbalize important aspects in her own words, and can verbalize a plan for obtaining medications, equipment, and assistance in the home environment. *To help ensure compliance with the treatment plan.*

Source: Adapted from Wilkinson, J. M., & Ahearn, N. R. (2009). *Prentice Hall nursing diagnosis handbook* (9th ed.). Upper Saddle River, NJ: Prentice Hall.

spinal surgery, the nurse performs the neurovascular assessment on the parts of the body distal to the surgical site. The neurovascular assessment includes assessment of the five Ps: pain, pulse, paresthesia, paralysis, and pallor. A complete assessment of circulation, motor, and sensory functions must be performed. In addition, the nurse should anticipate performing the neurovascular assessment in conjunction with vital signs. The nurse should report any neurovascular compromise or deterioration to the health care team immediately.

The neurovascular assessment should proceed systematically. Activities that may cause pain should be performed last. The nurse should first inspect the extremities for general appearance including color and presence of edema. Skin color should be described as pink or normal, pale, or cyanotic. Red or ruddy skin may indicate venous engorgement. Skin temperature and presence of moisture should be assessed. Normally the skin is warm and dry. Coolness of the skin may indicate decreased circulation. Excessive warmth or heat may be an early sign of infection or cellulitis. Moist skin is frequently found in the skinfolds of obese persons and may require interventions to prevent fungal infection or skin maceration. Moist skin may also indicate venous insufficiency, excessive effort, or fever.

The pulse strength provides information about blood supply to the affected extremity and surgical site. The nurse should palpate pulses most distal to the surgical site. If no pulse is present, the nurse should obtain Doppler pulses and systematically attempt to palpate the presence of a pulse in a proximal direction. For example, if no dorsalis pedis or posterior tibial pulse is present, the nurse should next palpate for a popliteal pulse. Pulses in the lower extremities include the dorsalis pedis, posterior tibial, and popliteal. Pulse points in the upper extremities include the radial and brachial. The pulse should be described as grade 0–4 or as a Doppler pulse (Chart 50–11).

Skin turgor indicates hydration status and also helps describe the fullness of tissue in the operative extremity. After surgery, the inflammatory process causes vasodilation of vessels supplying the site, which results in tissue swelling. Because the body part may be immobilized after surgery, venous return is decreased because of decreased muscle pump action. Skin turgor may be described as normal/brisk, slow, or tense. To test turgor, the nurse should compress the skin of the distal extremity between the nurse's thumb and index finger to form a tentlike projection and then release it. The skin should return to its normal state briskly. Slowed skin turgor indicates low volume status or dehydration. Tense skin cannot be tested. The nurse should assess edema in the surgical area regularly. Right after surgery, edema is a normal occurrence owing to tissue manipulation during surgery, but it gradually diminishes over time. If skin is tense or the extremity edematous, the patient should be instructed to elevate the part above heart level and perform appropriate exercises to increase muscle pump action and venous return. Patients who have had shoulder or arm surgery should perform finger exercises or hand squeezes with a rubber ball. Patients who have had lower extremity surgery should perform dorsiflexion and plantar flexion (foot pumps). The reoccurrence of edema may indicate infection.

Capillary refill testing is used to evaluate arterial filling in the small vessels supplying the skin. If the capillary refill is normal, the circulation in the larger vessels is assumed to be intact. Capillary refill is described in seconds. Either a nail bed or distal skin may be tested. The nurse depresses the nail bed or skin with one finger until the skin blanches. The nurse then releases it and observes the test site for the time it takes for skin color to return to normal. Normal capillary refill time is less than 3 seconds. Delayed capillary refill (greater than 3 seconds) indicates decreased tissue perfusion.

The sensory and motor assessments evaluate nerve function. Before testing sensation, the nurse should have the patient close her eyes, or the area to be tested should be obstructed from the patient's view with the bed sheets. This will prevent the patient from giving information based on what she sees instead of what she actually feels. If the patient underwent extremity surgery, testing of sensation distal to the surgical site is required. If the patient underwent spinal surgery or epidural anesthesia, a more comprehensive evaluation utilizing dermatomes should be performed. Nerve impulses may be delayed because of surgical complications or compression of nerves by postoperative edema. When assessing sensation, the nurse should apply light touch and ask the patient *where* she feels the touch instead of expressing it as a yes-or-no question. If repeatedly asked, "Do you feel this?" the patient may say yes just because she feels that is the expectation and therefore will give inaccurate responses.

The nurse assesses motor strength by asking the patient to perform specific activities. These activities involve testing the patient's ability to move the part, the strength of the part in moving against gravity, and the strength of the part against resistance. Motor strength should be graded on a scale of 0 to 5. If the patient is unable to move the part, the score is 0. If full strength is demonstrated and is equal to the unaffected part, the patient should receive a score of 5.

Weight-Bearing Status

Many musculoskeletal conditions will require a specific weight-bearing status. This is a directive on how much weight the clinician would—or would not—like the patient to put on an extremity (Chart 50–12).

CHART 50–11 Pulse Strength Chart

0	No palpable pulse
1+	Weak, barely palpable, or easily obliterated
2+	Palpable
3+	Strong, easily palpable
4+	Bounding

CHART 50–12 Weight-Bearing Status

NWB	Non weight bearing	Should not put any weight on the extremity (not even to push up in bed).
TDWB, TTWB	Touch down or toe touch	Allowed to let toe touch the ground for balance and allows leg to be rested on the ground but no weight should be placed on it.
PWB	Partial weight bearing	Usually a percentage of the person's weight, for example, 25% to 50%.
WBAT	Weight bearing as tolerated	The patient may begin to put weight on the extremity as pain recedes.
FWB	Full weight bearing	Allowed to walk normally on the extremity; does not require crutches.

Mobility

Patients with musculoskeletal trauma may have mobility issues. Even a sports injury may require crutches and a change in weight-bearing status. Many assistive devices, such as wheelchairs, walkers, crutches, canes, and reachers, are available. Wheelchairs need to be fit to the patient and can be equipped with elevating leg rests and reclining backs. Manual, one-side drive, and electric wheelchairs are available depending on the patients' abilities and how long they will be expected to use a wheelchair.

Walkers are frames with four posts and handgrips usually made of aluminum. They may be required by older patients, as well as those who are large or have difficulty with balance and need to have restricted weight bearing. Walkers may have wheels on the front legs for patients who cannot lift them.

Crutches are devices used in pairs to aid ambulation by transferring weight to the upper extremities. Crutches come in two types—axillary crutches and forearm (also referred to as Loftstrand or Canadian) crutches. The axillary crutches can be made of wood or aluminum. When patients are fitted for axillary crutches (allowing for four finger widths between the axilla and crutch top), they should be encouraged not to rest their armpits on the crutch. Most of the weight can be carried on the palms of the hands if there is no injury to the hand or arm. If such an injury exists, a platform crutch may be more appropriate. The patient's weight for these crutches is limited to 113 kg (250 pounds) for most manufacturers of wooden crutches. It is very important to teach the patient the proper use and to observe the patient using the crutches. The forearm crutch is made of a lightweight metal (aluminum or titanium) that has a flexible cuff that fits around the arm an inch below the elbow and above the handgrip, which is at the height of the bent wrist. The wrap around the arm and the handgrip enable the patient to rest his hands while giving support to the body. Forearm crutches act as a support and are made to take some, but not all, of the body's weight.

A cane is a wooden or metal stick with a curved graspable handle at the top. A cane should be used on the side opposite the injury to "unload" an extremity or aid with balance. In addition, it should be measured to fit to the palm of a nearly fully extended arm when laterally placed 8 to 12 inches from the foot.

A reacher is an assistive device made of metal with a handle control that can reach and grab an item so the patient does not have to stretch or bend to pick up or move the item.

Collaborative Management

A multidisciplinary team approach is necessary to optimize care for the orthopedic surgical patient. The surgeon determines the patient's activity prescription, and the nurse works collaboratively with the physical therapists to enable the patient to perform activities to the level of her capabilities. In order to meet desired patient outcomes, it is essential that this interdisciplinary team communicate openly with one another in developing and evaluating care of the patient and family (IOM [Institute of Medicine], 2010). It is important that any required restrictions on activity and precautions to prevent hip dislocation or spinal torque be determined and followed. Because many patients will have comorbid conditions, this collaboration ensures patient safety. Adequate nutrition is necessary for wound healing and to maintain patient strength. The clinical dietitian is a valuable team member to provide input regarding adequate caloric intake for patients with cardiovascular, endocrine, or renal disease, who may have to adhere to dietary restrictions. Because many patients who have had hip replacement surgery and amputation may require home care assistance and assistive devices or skilled care after discharge, the assistance of discharge planners and/or social workers is helpful. Individual patients may also require psychiatric consultation, depending on the patient's response to the surgery or the event that caused the surgery to be necessary. Spiritual support for patients during hospitalization may also help patients adapt successfully to their current situation and maintain a positive outlook necessary to participate fully in rehabilitation efforts.

Health Promotion

The greatest impact that nurses can have regarding musculoskeletal injuries and surgery relates to prevention. Patients who have musculoskeletal surgery generally receive explicit instructions on how to prevent the recurrence of their injury. It would be a great service to older adults to provide information on home safety before they become injured and need surgery. Safety devices to prevent injury, such as bathroom safety bars, should be made available to older adults by their health plans; alternatively, landlords should be required to install them.

Another way in which health care providers can improve care is by reviewing the patient's medications at each visit and in pharmacies. Over-the-counter medications should be included in the pharmacy medication lists so that better prevention of polypharmacy reactions can be achieved.

Health promotion includes regular exercise. Walking not only is an excellent cardiovascular exercise but also maintains bone mass. Obesity is increasing in the United States, and education on the effects of obesity on knee and hip joints may assist in promoting the maintenance of appropriate weight. Planned exercise is an important part of the recovery plan for the orthopedic surgical patient. Specific exercises, often called therapeutic exercises, will be prescribed to promote and maintain range of motion and function. The plan of care for the patient should include specific measurable goals. Because orthopedic surgery is generally performed to improve function or repair a defect, typical goals include range of motion, strengthening of the limb, and the ability to participate in the rehabilitation exercise program. Specificity and measurability are important so that it is clear whether the patient has attained the goal or not. For example, if the goal is that the patient will be able to ambulate independently 50 feet by day 2 after surgery and the patient ambulates with assistance for only 20 feet, there is an objective starting point for the analysis of why the goal was not accomplished. The patient should be encouraged to continue the exercises prescribed in the hospital after discharge. In addition, an overall general health exercise program should be encouraged to ensure cardiovascular and bone health.

Hormone replacement therapy to prevent osteoporosis remains controversial. Women who are postmenopausal should be encouraged to perform exercises and maintain their calcium levels; supplements or oral bisphosphonates may assist in preventing bone loss. Women should receive education by their health care providers on the options available.

Discharge Planning for the Orthopedic Surgical Patient

Many therapeutic modalities are commonly ordered for patients undergoing orthopedic surgery. **Continuous passive motion (CPM) devices** (machines into which the affected extremity or joint is placed to perform slow, continuous passive range of motion to avoid stiffness and prevent a decrease in range of motion) may be utilized to prevent loss of range of motion of the joint in patients who have knee surgery. Sequential compression devices or compression stockings may be utilized for patients who are at risk for DVT. Cryotherapy units or ice bags may be utilized to decrease pain and swelling in the joint after surgery.

Physical therapy as well as active and passive range of motion may be required to prevent loss of function and to maintain strength and range of motion in the orthopedic patient. Teaching the patient and family how and when to use these devices is critical to the patient's rehabilitation.

Knowledge of where the patient resides, including the residence's physical aspects such as number of stairs or size of bathrooms (whether the bathroom is large enough for the patient to turn around in with a walker, for example), is necessary to plan for the patient's safe discharge. The presence of children or significant others who are willing to assist the patient after hospitalization will influence the discharge plan. Older patients who have had joint replacement surgery frequently require skilled nursing care beyond hospitalization. If the hospitalized older adult is a primary caregiver for a spouse now left at home without assistance, the patient will need to make arrangements to provide care for the spouse during the current hospitalization. Anxiety related to home and financial concerns can impede the patient's recovery and rehabilitation.

Postoperative precautions and exercises may also be taught prior to surgery. These precautions and exercises depend on the surgical site (back, lower extremity, upper extremity, and pelvis). In some cases, the patient may be asked to perform general exercises such as walking to build endurance, specific exercises to improve circulation, or other exercises to increase strength and range of motion.

Environment

The nurse should discuss the physical environment of the patient's home. Specific accommodations may be necessary, and the patient should plan for these prior to discharge. For example, the patient may require a hospital bed after surgery; if so, the patient may need help from friends and/or family members to accomplish this. Throw rugs should be removed to prevent falls. Postoperative equipment such as cryotherapy, hospital bed, elevated toilet seat, or CPM devices should be ordered and confirmed to be in the patient's home prior to discharge. If the patient will have activity restrictions or precautions after surgery, the physical environment in the home may need simple alterations to accommodate them, such as moving articles used for activities of daily living to an accessible area. If the patient's residence prevents him from performing activities prescribed for recovery or affects his ability to obtain access to health care appointments or supplies, the nurse must help the patient develop an alternative plan for home care. If friends or family are unable to help provide the patient with an alternative living situation for the recovery period, a discharge planner or social worker may help place the patient in a rehabilitation, assisted living, or skilled nursing facility.

Complications of Musculoskeletal Trauma and Surgery

Compartment Syndrome

Compartment syndrome is a condition whereby increasing pressure within the muscle compartments compromises circulation and the function of soft tissues, nerves, and vessels in that compartment. This leads to anoxia of the tissue and necrosis, which in turn leads to more edema in the compartment and a subsequent increase in pressure. The swelling within an anatomic compartment restricts blood flow. Compartment syndrome can occur due to increasing internal pressure (for example, from bleeding into the compartment by fractured bone and torn muscle tissue or edema) or from the external pressure applied by the trauma itself, casts, dressings, burns, or even clothing. The most commonly affected compartments are those of the tibia (lower leg), forearm, upper arm, hand, foot, and thigh.

In an anatomic compartment, the fascia or an external device such as a cast prohibits expansion of the compartment as edema and engorgement increase. This causes compression of vascular and nervous system structures. As edema and engorgement increase, pain increases and is unrelieved by narcotic pain medication administration. The affected area will be swollen and tense. Pain significantly increases with extension or flexion of the affected part. There may be changes in the patient's neurovascular assessment, indicating that compartment syndrome is present. The patient may have pain, paresthesia, pulselessness, paralysis, and/or pallor of the part. If compartment syndrome in an extremity is suspected, the extremity should not be elevated but should be maintained at the level of the heart to improve perfusion. Normal tissue pressure is less than 15 mmHg. Numerous devices may be utilized to determine tissue or compartment pressure. If the tissue or compartment pressure is greater than 30 mmHg, compartment syndrome should be suspected.

Compartment syndrome is cyclical and builds until a surgical release of the fascial envelope is performed. If pressure is not reduced, irreversible muscle damage and nerve damage can occur within hours. Compartment syndrome can also lead to life-threatening complications such as rhabdomyolysis and renal failure (refer to Chapter 49).

The signs and symptoms of compartment syndrome include pain out of proportion to the injury (or pain with passive stretch of the muscle within that compartment), pallor, poor capillary refill, paresthesia, and pulselessness in the affected extremity. Pain that seems out of proportion to the injury or is not relieved by analgesia is the earliest of the symptoms.

Neurovascular assessment is the best way to note early symptoms because it is typically a clinical diagnosis; however, if there is doubt, intracompartmental pressure can be measured with a transducer. This pressure reading is then compared to the patient's diastolic pressure. A difference of 30 mmHg is essential for tissue perfusion. Normal compartment pressures are 0 to 8 mmHg, and a pressure of more than 30 to 45 mmHg will cause tissue necrosis if the patient's diastolic reading is low. There are also devices available that can be inserted through the skin to measure the actual compartment pressure.

When the nurse suspects compartment syndrome, all sources of pressure should be removed, and the health care team should be notified emergently to prevent permanent disability or loss of limb. Treatment of compartment syndrome requires release of the constriction to accommodate swelling. If a cast is causing the restriction, it should be bivalved (cut down both sides).

If the constriction is at the fascial level, the patient will require surgery. In this situation, the patient is taken to the operating room for an emergent **fasciotomy,** which is an incision along the length of the fascia to decompress the compartment. This procedure opens the fascial envelope along the entire length of the muscle. The muscle is allowed to expand, frequently protruding out through the open incision. It will be left open and covered with wet saline dressings for several days until the skin edges can be approximated again. Any necrotic tissue will be debrided. Skin grafts or amputations may be required for severe cases.

Rhabdomyolysis

Rhabdomyolysis occurs when the injured skeletal muscle fibers break down and leak inflammatory mediators, such as myoglobin and creatinine kinase, into the circulation. It is most commonly seen with crush injuries but can occur with any massive soft-tissue injury. Refer to Chapter 49 for an in-depth discussion of rhabdomyolysis.

Venous Thromboembolism

Venous thromboembolism (VTE) includes both deep venous thrombosis (DVT) and pulmonary embolism (PE). Deep venous thrombosis is a blood clot in the venous circulatory system, typically in the lower extremity. Pulmonary embolism is a blood clot that has broken free from a site, travels through venous circulation, and ends up through the right side of the heart to the lungs, where it lodges in one or both branches of the pulmonary artery to obstruct or partially obstruct circulation. While DVT may not present signs and symptoms, PE is the third most common cause of death in patients who survive the first 24 hours after trauma (Paffrath et al., 2009). The most common signs and symptoms are anxiety or a feeling of impending doom coupled with dyspnea. Refer to Chapter 27 for a detailed discussion of PE.

Risk factors for DVT in the orthopedic surgical population include immobility of a limb, long surgical times in a single position, hypercoagulability of blood due to activation of the clotting cascade from surgical stimulation and from being NPO, as well as endothelial disruption from the surgery or trauma itself. The three factors of venous stasis, hypercoagulability, and vessel injury make up Virchow's triad for VTE risk. Virchow's triad is discussed in Chapter 35.

Other risk factors have been identified that reflect the hypercoagulable state. Higher levels of homocysteine and plasminogen activator-1 levels correlate with DVT in a study of patients with spinal cord injury (Aito, Abbate, Marcucci, & Cominelli, 2007). Because patients undergoing total hip and total knee repair or replacement surgery are at high risk for DVT, current standards of practice include providing DVT prophylaxis in these patient populations. A recent analysis of 14,679 patients who developed DVT and PE revealed the following significant risk factors: male, blunt trauma, age greater than 40, number of operative procedures, and severity of injury (Paffrath et al., 2009).

Prevention strategies to decrease the incidence of DVT include the administration of heparin (unfractionated or low molecular weight), the use of antiembolism stockings, and the use of sequential compression devices.

In spite of appropriate therapy, the incidence of DVT in orthopedic patients is still high, and nurses must be diligent in assessing patients for signs and symptoms. The DVT symptoms may be nonspecific; for example, the patient may complain of pain in an extremity, which may become swollen, edematous, and tender at or distal to the clot. Although the legs are the most common site for DVT, immobile arms are also at risk to develop clots. Pain associated with DVT may increase with exercise of the part. A positive Homans' sign is associated with lower leg DVT. Homans' sign is considered positive when plantar and dorsiflexion on the affected side cause calf pain. Deep venous thrombosis is discussed in detail in Chapter 35.

Symptoms of VTE may range from dramatic to nonspecific. The patient with pulmonary embolism may have acute onset of chest pain, shortness of breath, decreased sensorium, and pink, frothy sputum. Typically, the patient with pulmonary embolism will demonstrate tachycardia and tachypnea. Arterial blood gases may be normal or demonstrate hypoxia. Oxygen saturation may be normal or decreased in pulmonary embolism. Pulmonary embolism is discussed in detail in Chapter 28.

CHART 50–13 Classic Triad for Signs and Symptoms of Fat Embolus

Early Findings	Later Findings	Last Component
Hypoxemia Dyspnea Tachypnea	Neurologic abnormalities: Confusion Altered LOC Focal deficits Possible seizures	Petechial rash found most often on the head, neck, anterior thorax, subconjunctiva, and axillae.

Source: Weinhouse, G. (2008). Fat embolism syndrome. Retrieved from http://www.utdol.com/online/content/topic.do?topicKey=cc_medi/13397&selectedTitle=1~27&source=search_result.

Fat Embolism Syndrome

Fat embolism syndrome (FES) occurs when fat globules released from long-bone fractures enter the circulatory system. Up to 90% of long-bone fractures have some release of fat emboli associated with the fracture, although only 3% to 4% progress to FES (Feliciano et al., 2008). In the most severe cases, the emboli can produce multiple-organ failure from both a direct embolic effect and from activation of the inflammatory cascade. The most commonly noted triad of symptoms is acute respiratory failure, neurological dysfunction, and a petechial rash (Chart 50–13). Acute respiratory failure may be the only symptom in many patients.

Pulmonary complications in the orthopedic surgical patient may be related to a variety of causative factors. **Fat embolus** is a complication specific to orthopedic injuries involving long bone fracture. In this condition, fat globules from the bone marrow travel into the venous system and to the pulmonary vessels. Fat then blocks the pulmonary vessels and inactivates surfactant, which promotes the development of acute respiratory distress syndrome (ARDS). The patient will develop respiratory distress: tachypnea, air hunger, and hypoxia. Other signs and symptoms associated with fat embolus are fever, tachycardia, restlessness, decreased mental status, and petechiae. Arterial blood gas findings demonstrate an initial decrease in $PaCO_2$ followed by increased $PaCO_2$ and low PaO_2. Other diagnostic tests such as chest x-ray and ventilation/perfusion scan are nonspecific for fat embolus. Patients with suspected fat embolus should be intubated and placed on mechanical ventilation with positive end-expiratory pressure (PEEP). Treatment is largely supportive until the condition resolves. A detailed discussion of the diagnosis and management of ARDS is found in Chapter 28.

Pulmonary embolus may also cause respiratory insufficiency and is usually associated with deep venous thrombosis. Signs and symptoms are similar to those of fat embolus; however, pulmonary embolus is not generally associated with the development of ARDS.

After arrival on the medical–surgical floor, the patient should be monitored closely for the first 4 to 12 hours to ensure that the vital signs remain stable and the respiratory rate and effort are appropriate. Routine vital signs and respiratory status are then observed for the remainder of the patient's hospitalization. Incentive spirometry is typically ordered for the postoperative period to promote lung expansion and prevent respiratory complications such as atelectasis and pneumonia. Typically, the patient is encouraged to perform incentive spirometry every 1 to 2 hours while awake. Coughing and deep breathing should follow use of the incentive spirometer to assist in the removal of secretions from smaller airways. Patients are now assisted out of bed as soon as they are able, depending on the type of surgery. Sitting in a chair enables the patient to expand the thorax to a greater degree than being in bed and also acts to promote respiratory function. Pneumonia is a serious complication, particularly for the older postoperative patient. The patient may be at risk for aspiration pneumonia related to decreased mental status, use of nasogastric (NG) tubes, or preexisting medical conditions such as stroke or dysphagia. Elevations in temperature should alert the nurse to the potential that the patient has atelectasis or pneumonia. Aggressive pulmonary toilet is needed to remove secretions and improve airway exchange.

Cast Syndrome

Cast syndrome or superior mesenteric artery syndrome (SMAS) can be fatal. This syndrome occurs when there is compression of the superior mesenteric artery at the duodenum. This compression occurs from anterior pressure such as a body cast or brace paired with pressure posteriorly resisted by the descending aorta and spine (Karrer & Jones, 2010). This compression impedes the blood flow to the bowel, causing ischemia and eventually necrosis of the gastrointestinal tract and vessel walls, which can result in hemorrhage and death. This condition is most often seen in children in body casts or hip spica casts; however, it also is seen in adults with casts or back braces, especially if they have had a spine injury or surgery in which there is any hyperextension of the lumbar spine or distraction injuries of the spine.

The first symptoms of SMAS are vague abdominal pain, pressure, distention, and irritability; this is followed by nausea, projectile vomiting, and bowel obstruction. The condition may occur postoperatively or days or weeks later, especially with very young children growing larger in hip spica casts. Early treatment is essential; the first step is cutting a bivalve (cutting both sides of the cast to relieve pressure), window (cutting a section of the cast away from a pressure point), or complete removal of the cast or brace. Decompression of the stomach is achieved with a nasogastric (NG) tube to provide continuous intermittent suction.

Complex Regional Pain Syndrome

Complex regional pain syndrome (CRPS), formerly known as reflex sympathetic dystrophy (RSD), is a diffuse persistent pain usually associated with vasomotor, trophic, and bony changes and limited mobility of an extremity following a local injury. Early referral to physical therapy for movement and pain clinic personnel who specialize in this disorder is crucial.

Pressure Ulcers

Maintaining skin integrity and prevention of pressure areas are key to orthopedic nursing. Providing adequate nutrition and hydration and keeping the skin clean and dry are measures aimed at promoting good skin turgor. Patients with orthopedic injuries are at particular risk for the development of preventable pressure ulcers. For example, patients who have had hip surgery are at particular risk for heel pressure ulcers. The heels should be floated off of the mattress utilizing pillows. If the pillows are insufficient to maintain the heels off the bed, assistive devices such as heel lift boots or specialty pressure relief beds or mattresses may be utilized. The best tool to prevent pressure ulcer development is repositioning the patient at least every 2 hours. Frequent assessment of the skin allows early detection of potential impairments in skin integrity that require more aggressive interventions. The orthopedic patient may also develop pressure ulcers in areas where prosthetic devices, casts, splints, or traction causes friction. If the nurse finds evidence of friction, extra padding may be needed, or adjustment of the splint, prosthesis, or cast may be necessary. Refer to Chapter 60 for a detailed discussion of pressure ulcers.

Osteomyelitis

Osteomyelitis is infection of the bone itself. The incidence of osteomyelitis is highest in patients who have had compound fractures, external fixator devices, and open orthopedic procedures. This infection may be related to invasion by bacteria, fungus, or virus. Tuberculosis infection may occur in the bone tissue as a result of exposure to tuberculosis. The patient may complain of deep bone pain. Failure of the surgical site or pressure ulcer to heal may be the first indication that osteomyelitis is present. Confirmation that osteomyelitis is present may be obtained from MRI, CT, x-ray, bone biopsy, or bone scan. Treatment for osteomyelitis requires long-term (generally 6 weeks of) antibiotic therapy. Refer to Chapter 49 for more details.

Hardware Infection

Late complications of orthopedic surgery include infection of the surgical hardware. The decision to remove the hardware depends on the impact on patient mobility, pain level, age, and potential complications such as neurovascular injury, deformity, and inability to replace the implant, which may have significant impact on the patient's mobility and ability to continue working in his current occupation. In cases of external fixator devices or screw implants, removal of hardware is less complicated and does not necessarily affect the patient's activities of daily living. If the bone has healed and the screws or plates are no longer necessary for joint or bone stability, the surgery has far less impact on patient mobility and ability to carry out activities of daily living, as well as occupational activities.

Joint Dislocation

Dislocation of the surgical joint may occur due to overextension. Complications of dislocation include pain, decreased range of motion, and neurovascular compromise. Strict adherence to joint precautions can prevent complications of dislocation. Signs and symptoms of joint dislocation include swelling, pain, immobility, and shortening (the extremity appears shorter than the unaffected extremity).

Heterotopic Ossification

Heterotopic ossification (HO) is the development of bone tissue in areas where bone tissue is not normally present. Myositis ossificans progressiva, which develops in childhood, is the progressive development of bone tissue (ossification) in soft tissues throughout the body. The life span of patients with myositis ossificans progressiva is severely shortened, and patients frequently die in the second or third decade from complications associated with compression of vital organs from lesions. Heterotopic ossification is a late complication that may be seen in musculoskeletal and spinal cord injury. The exact mechanism of this bone formation is not known, but it is thought to be an inflammatory reaction of intramuscular and connective tissue after injury or surgery. Sepsis or infection may predispose the patient to the development of HO. Symptoms associated with HO depend on the site and size of the lesion. In spinal cord injury, the site of the anomalous bone lesion is always lower than the level of injury. Frequent sites of post-traumatic HO are the soft tissues surrounding the hips, knees, shoulders, or elbows. Patients may be asymptomatic if the lesion is small; in contrast, they may experience pain, decreased range of motion, and signs of inflammation or infection if the lesion is large or interferes with joint motion. Signs and symptoms in an extremity with a heterotopic lesion may include pain, swelling, redness, and fever. Because these signs and symptoms are similar to those of venous thrombosis, the patient will have radiologic studies such as a bone scan and x-rays to determine whether the patient has heterotopic ossification, as well as testing for VTE through tests such as D-dimer and ultrasound flow studies of the extremity.

Treatment of heterotopic ossification includes administration of nonsteroidal anti-inflammatory medications and indomethacin for pain, in addition to focused radiation to the joint. These medications may decrease the development of heterotopic ossification as well. Etidronate disodium may be administered to patients prone to the development of heterotopic ossification to prevent lesion formation and is administered preoperatively and postoperatively when the HO lesions are surgically excised.

Osteonecrosis or Avascular Necrosis

Osteonecrosis (avascular necrosis), the death of bone tissue, may occur at any time after injury to bone because of impairment of circulation. Patients at high risk of osteonecrosis include those taking steroids, receiving radiation therapy, or living with alcohol dependence. Many medical conditions such as sickle cell anemia, HIV, gout, and osteoporosis may predispose the patient to osteonecrosis.

Psychological Issues

Orthopedic injuries are very painful. Broken bones hurt until they stop moving, which may take 14 days or longer. Pain management is paramount for injured patients for many reasons, including comfort level, adequate ventilation, rehabilitation, and sleep assistance. Most patients, including children, will require narcotics. Children have historically been undermedicated for pain, which can have long-term implications. Physiological predictors of post-traumatic stress disorder (PTSD) in children have shown that the strongest of the physiological correlations appears to be patients' perception of their pain. The worse the degree of early pain, the more likely that the patient will exhibit PTSD after the injury (Norman, Stein, Dimsdale, & Hoyt, 2008). Orthopedic patients frequently have physical therapy ordered and will need to get out of bed as soon as possible to prevent the complications of bed rest and immobilization. It is helpful to have patients premedicated 30 to 60 minutes prior to physical therapy.

The psychological impact and sequelae of musculoskeletal trauma are not well known. More factors are involved than just the trauma of the injury itself; there are medical treatments, loss of mobility, loss of school or work time, financial burdens, and even changes in self-concept. Post-traumatic stress disorder, depression, and other psychological sequelae in both adults and pediatric patients can be seen months after physical recovery.

A greater awareness of psychological repercussions from trauma, especially inflicted or disfiguring injuries, is needed. There are early identifiable risk factors for post-traumatic maladjustment: panic during or immediately after the trauma, re-experiencing symptoms, avoidance, sleep disturbance, injury from an assault, previous trauma and psychiatric history, and blaming someone else for the injury (Davydow, Katon, & Zatzick, 2009).

Gerontological Considerations

The nurse should be aware of specific gerontological considerations for patients with musculoskeletal trauma. Hip and wrist fractures are the most common types of fractures in older patients. Conditions such as osteoporosis or tumor may predispose the older adult to a pathologic or insufficiency fracture. In such a fracture, the bone is not strong enough for its function, and it breaks through the weakened framework with little trauma. Fractures in the older adult may occur prior to, or as a result of, a fall. A high mortality rate is associated with hip fracture in older adults; about 30% of people with a hip fracture will die in the following year or experience significant functional loss. However, a study in 2009 showed that the rates of hip fractures in older adults and subsequent mortality are declining in the United States (Brauer, Marcelo, Cutler, & Rosen, 2009). Although the rates of hip fracture are on a downward trend, it is still a public health concern because of the aging population and the risk of incidence increasing unless additional measures are taken.

Prevention of fractures is a key nursing initiative. Fall prevention, nutrition evaluation, and encouraging screening and osteoporosis treatment for older patients are essential for good quality-of-life outcomes.

Older patients have other considerations such as sensory and metabolic deficits and delays in medication absorption and healing. Constipation is a major concern for older adults who sustain musculoskeletal fracture and are immobilized, as well as among those who require narcotics or undergo surgery. There are also psychosocial issues for older adults such as fear of becoming infirm, being in pain, running out of money, having to be dependent on family, asking for help, changing appearance (such as concerns that assistive devices make them look old), sexuality, being alone, and that the road back to recovery may be too much. They may grieve over loss of function, friends, or lifestyle. Most will lose a functional level after a hip fracture; for example, if they were ambulatory within their community, they may be ambulatory only at home after the injury.

Research

Multiple physiological and psychosocial opportunities for research are available in the realm of musculoskeletal surgical complications and therapies. It is an exciting time in nursing research, and important practice changes are beginning to rely on new evidence. All of the areas listed in the Research Opportunities box lend themselves to study that may affect the future of orthopedic nursing care.

RESEARCH OPPORTUNITIES Related to Orthopedic Nursing and Musculoskeletal Surgical Procedures

Research Area	Clinical Impact
Physiological Research	
The management of pin sites placed for skeletal traction and external fixation.	Nurses do not have sufficient evidence on which to base best care of pin sites to prevent infection.
Use of alternative methods to manage pain on the orthopedic unit.	Nurses could use alternative methods of pain management such as acupuncture, acupressure, and massage to help manage pain.
Development of guidelines to manage pain treatment when patients are transferred to rehab/extended care facilities or home.	There are no guidelines and reports exist of poor pain control of patients after discharge from acute care.
Psychosocial, Ethical, and Legal Research	
Effectiveness of discharge teaching and plans of care and reality of resource availability in the home or community for postoperative patients or those with musculoskeletal injuries.	Many patients are discharged quickly without sufficient resources in place or without understanding plans of care. For example, what is ordered for home and what actually occurs may not be the same. Identify areas for improvement in teaching information and methods, as well as community resources for the postoperative or injured orthopedic patient, especially older adults and uninsured and underinsured individuals. Prevent the return of underinsured patients who use the emergency department for their health care. Decrease return visits and get patients into the appropriate health care systems, decreasing costs.
Musculoskeletal Surgical Procedures	
Prophylactic antibiotic therapy is commonplace for orthopedic surgical procedures. Studies could be performed comparing the infection rates in low-risk patients, as well as comparing the use of prophylactic antibiotics versus placebo.	Is the use of prophylactic antibiotic therapy necessary, or should it be reserved for patients who are at high risk of infection?
Which therapy is more effective in preventing deep venous thrombosis (DVT): sequential compression devices or elastic compression stockings? Many institutions utilize both. Is this overkill or an added expense, or is it truly useful? Research studies could compare the use of sequential compression devices alone versus the use of elastic compression stockings alone versus the use of both.	Possible cost savings exist for the institution and the patient.
Is there a difference in discharge date or ability to participate in postoperative activities in patients who receive regional/epidural anesthesia versus those who receive general anesthesia? Are there differences between the two groups in the perceived ability to participate in postoperative activities? Are there differences in the postoperative pain scores between the two groups? Is there a difference in the pain scores reported between patients receiving pain-controlled analgesia (PCA) versus those who received epidural anesthesia?	Possibility of decreased hospital stay exists for the patient.
Is there a difference in the range of motion or the distance ambulated between patients who receive preoperative exercise counseling prior to elective joint replacement and those who do not?	Possibility of decreased hospital stay exists for the patient. Decreased rehabilitation time is also a possibility.

CLINICAL PREPARATION

READ DOCUMENT APPLY

READ: History of Present Illness >> Laboratory Study Results >> Critical Thinking Questions

Kelly Lovett is a 17-year-old female who was involved in a high-speed, single-vehicle frontal crash and had a negative toxicology/drug screen. Multiple injuries include a concussion and a forehead laceration that has been sutured. Ms. Lovett has had her right open tibia fracture washed out with application of an external fixator. She has had an IM rod placed in her right femur fracture. Head CT was negative. Her admitting diagnoses include multiple trauma, right femur fracture, right open tibia/fibular fracture with soft tissue loss, chest contusion, loss of consciousness at the scene, and a forehead laceration.

Medical–Surgical History

Ms. Lovett takes no medications. Previous surgeries include an appendectomy at age 10.

Social History

Ms. Lovett is a junior in high school and lives with her parents. She denies smoking, drinking, or use of illicit drugs.

Physical Exam

Ms. Lovett opens her eyes to voice and is oriented. Pupils are equal, round, and reactive to light and accommodation. The suture line on her forehead is clean, dry, and intact. Breath sounds are equal bilaterally with equal chest rise. She complains of pain to the right chest wall with deep breath, no crepitus noted. Heart sounds are normal. Abdomen is soft and nontender with diminished bowel sounds in all quadrants. Right thigh is edematous. External fixator to right lower leg is intact; pin sites exhibit slight redness and small amount of serous drainage. Motor and sensory to extremities are intact. Peripheral pulses are slightly decreased in the right lower extremity. Ms. Lovett complains of pain in the right leg at a 6 on a 0-to-10 scale.

READ: History of Present Illnesses >> **Physical Exam** >> Admitting Medical Records >> Laboratory Study Results

Admitting Medical Orders

Service: trauma service with orthopedic consultation
Diagnosis: concussion, right femur fracture, right open tibia/fibular fracture with soft tissue loss, chest contusion, forehead laceration
Allergies: amoxicillin
Vital signs with oxygen saturations q4h × 24 hours
Call house officer: temp > 38.5°C, HR >130 or < 60, RR > 30 or < 12, BP sys >160 or < 90, O_2 sat < 92%, urine output < 120 mL in 4 hours, change in neurological or abdominal exam, any Hct result that is 5 less than the baseline ED Hct, any change in neurovascular exam of the right lower extremity
Activity: patient's weight-bearing status is touch down to right leg; up to chair with assistance
Diet: advance diet as tolerated
Intravenous fluids: D5/0.45 NS with 20 mEq of KCl at 100 mL/hr
Foley catheter to gravity drainage
I&O: every shift
Respiratory care: incentive spirometer every hour when awake
DVT prophylaxis: sequential compression device to left lower extremity
Wound care: pin site care tid, clean forehead laceration with half-strength H_2O_2 and apply bacitracin, elevate right lower extremity

Scheduled Medications

Hydromorphone PCA 0.2 mg/mL, incremental dose 0.4 mg, lock-out 10 minutes
Vancomycin 1 g IV q12h
Docusate capsule 100 mg by mouth twice daily
Enoxaparin 30 mg subcutaneously q12h

PRN Medications

Phenergan 12.5–25 mg IV q6h prn nausea
Ativan 0.5–1 mg IV q6h prn anxiety
Ondansetron 4 mg IV q12h if needed for nausea

Ordered Laboratory Studies

CBC every morning
Chem 7 panel every other day
Trough Vancomycin level prior to third dose of Vancomycin

READ: History of Present Illnesses >> **Laboratory Study Results** >> Critical Thinking Questions

Test	Preop	Postop, Immediate	Postop, 4 Hours
WBC	28.5/mm^3	19.3/mm^3	22.4/mm^3
RBC	4.40/mm^3	4.33/mm^3	4.65/mm^3
Hemoglobin	13.9 g/dL	12 g/dL	14.5 g/dL
Hematocrit	41%	40%	43%
Platelet count	412/mm^3	357/mm^3	399/mm^3
APTT	20.3 seconds		
INR	0.98		
Sodium	140 mEq/L		

Test	Preop	Postop, Immediate	Postop, 4 Hours
Potassium	3.6 mEq/L		
Chloride	109 mEq/L		
Carbon dioxide	23 mEq/L		
Urea nitrogen	11 mg/dL		
Creatinine blood	0.8 mg/dL		
Glucose	179 mg/dL		
Calcium	8.1 mg/dL		
Lipase	17 unit/dL		

Pearson Nursing Student Resources *Log on to* ***nursing.pearsonhighered.com*** *to download forms*

DOCUMENT:

>> Summary of Hospitalization
>> Pathophysiology Form
>> Laboratory Values
>> Laboratory Results Explanation

APPLY:

>> List of Potential Nursing Diagnosis
>> Concept Map
>> Critical Thinking Questions and Concept Map

APPLY: History of Present Illness >> Laboratory Study Results >> **Critical Thinking Questions**

1. On initial admission to the floor postoperatively, which complications should you assess for?
2. In what position should the right leg be placed?
3. How can you distinguish the difference between expected postoperative pain and the pain caused by compartment syndrome?
4. What areas of assessment must be performed immediately upon a patient's admission to the nursing unit after orthopedic surgery?
5. What types of precautions are necessary for a patient who has had a total hip replacement?
6. How are pulmonary complications prevented during the postoperative period?
7. What assessments and actions do you perform for a confused older postoperative patient?

Answers to Critical Thinking Questions can be found in Appendix D in the Osborn Student Resources at nursing.pearsonhighered.com.

NCLEX® PRACTICE

1. The nurse is planning a health promotion program for sports injuries. Which information is the most important for the nurse to emphasize in this program?

1. How to use new equipment
2. Prevention of injuries
3. Why sports need to be supervised
4. How injuries are related to the time of day

2. A patient has been advised that it will be 6 weeks before his cast can be removed. What information should the nurse provide when the patient asks why it takes so long to "get this cast off?"

1. "Just before the cast is removed, fibroblasts in your system will heal the fracture."
2. "While your bone is healing a callus will form."
3. "It is important to wait to remove the cast until the stage of calcification has been reached."
4. "Before your cast can be removed, ossification of the fracture must occur."

3. A victim of a motor vehicle crash has an open fracture of the left femur. What is the priority of care for this patient?

1. Provide pain relief.
2. Prevent damage to surrounding tissue.
3. Decrease the potential for contamination.
4. Cast the affected bone immediately.

4. The nurse is providing care to a patient who was just brought to the emergency department with a fractured pelvis and femur. What is the priority for this patient's care?

1. Monitoring hemodynamic status
2. Arranging for a traction set-up
3. Palpating the stability of the iliac crests
4. Administering oral narcotic analgesics

5. The patient who had a right above-the-knee amputation tells the nurse, "I keep wanting to scratch my right foot." How should the nurse respond to this statement?

1. "That feeling is a side effect of your pain medication."
2. "You are experiencing something called phantom limb sensations."
3. "Your leg was amputated, and it isn't there anymore."
4. "I can get a psychiatrist for you to talk to about this feeling."

6. A patient has undergone surgery for a fractured tibia. The nurse plans to complete a neurovascular assessment. Which aspects will be included? (select all that apply)

1. Pain level
2. Pulse quality
3. Sensation and movement
4. Color of extremity
5. Level of consciousness

Answers to NCLEX Practice Questions can be found in Appendix D in the Osborn Student Resources at nursing.pearsonhighered.com. Practice additional NCLEX questions online at the Student Resources site.

Pearson Nursing Student Resources Find additional review materials at: **nursing.pearsonhighered.com**

REFERENCES

Aito, S., Abbate, R., Marcucci, R., & Cominelli, E. (2007). Endogenous risk factors for deep-vein thrombosis in patients with acute spinal cord injuries. *Spinal Cord, 45*(9), 627–631.

American Academy of Orthopaedic Surgeons (AAOS). (2007a). ACL injury: Does it require surgery? Retrieved from http://orthoinfo.aaos.org/topic.cfm?topic=A00297

American Academy of Orthopaedic Surgeons (AAOS). (2007b). Arthritis of the shoulder. Retrieved from http://orthoinfo.aaos.org/topic.cfm?topic=A00222

American Academy of Orthopaedic Surgeons (AAOS). (2007c). Carpal tunnel syndrome. Retrieved from http://orthoinfo.aaos.org/topic.cfm?topic=A00005#Anatomy

American Academy of Orthopaedic Surgeons (AAOS). (2007d). Osteoarthritis of the elbow. Retrieved from http://orthoinfo.aaos.org/topic.cfm?topic=A00421

American Academy of Orthopaedic Surgeons (AAOS). (2007e). Rotator cuff tears. Retrieved from http://orthoinfo.aaos.org/topic.cfm?topic=A00064

American Academy of Orthopaedic Surgeons (AAOS). (2007f). Wrist joint replacement (wrist arthroplasty). Retrieved from http://orthoinfo.aaos.org/topic.cfm?topic=A00019

American College of Surgeons. (2008). *Advanced trauma life support course manual.* Chicago: American College of Surgeons.

Anscomb, S. (2007). Managing sprains and strains. *Practice Nurse, 33*(5), 44–49.

Arthritis Foundation. (2011). Arthritis and related diseases. Retrieved from http://www.arthritis.org/faq.php

Baker, B. S. (2011). Meniscus injuries. Retrieved from http://www.emedicine.medscape.com/article/90661_overview

BestPractice. (2010). Joint dislocation. Retrieved from http://www.bestpractice.bmj.com/best-practice/monograph/583/basics/edpidemiology.html

Borghi, B., d'Addabbo, M., White, P. F., Gallerani, P.,Toccaceli, L., Raffeli, W., et al. (2010). The use of prolonged peripheral neural blockade after lower extremity amputation: the effect on symptoms associated with phantom limb syndrome. *Anesthesia Analgesia 111*(5), 1308–1315.

Brauer, C., Marcelo, C., Cutler, D., & Rosen, A. (2009). Incidence and mortality of hip fractures in the United States. *Journal of the American Medical Association, 302*(14), 1573–1579.

Browner, B. D., & DeAngelis, J. P. (2008). Emergency care of musculoskeletal injuries. In C. M. Townsend, R. D. Beauchamp, B. M. Evers, & K. L. Mattox (Eds), *Sabisston text book of surgery.* St. Louis: Saunders.

Chan, B. L., Witt, R., Charrow, A. P., Magee, A., Howard, R., Pasquina, P. F., et al. (2007). Mirror therapy for phantom limb pain. *New England Journal of Medicine, 357*(21): 2206–2207.

Chung, H., Dai, T., Sharma, S. K., Huang, Y. Y., Carroll, J. D., & Hamblin, M. R. (2011). The nuts and bolts of low-level laser (light) therapy. *Annals of Biomedical Engineering, 40*(2), 516–533.

Davydow, D., Katon, W., & Zatzick, D. (2009). Psychiatric morbidity and functional impairments in survivors of burns, traumatic injuries, and ICU stats for other critical illnesses: A review of the literature. *International Review of Psychiatry, 21*(6), 531–538.

Diers, M., Christmann, C., Koeppe, C., Ruf, M., & Flor, H (2010). Mirrored, imagined and executed movements differentially activate sensorimotor cortex in amputees with and without phantom limb pain. *Pain 149*(2), 296–304.

Ehman, J. (2007). Religious diversity: Practical points for health care providers. Retrieved from http://www.uph.upenn.edu/pastoral/resed/diversity_points.html

eMedicineHealth. (2011). Lumbar laminectomy. Retrieved from http://www.emedicinehealth.com/lumbar_laminectomy/article_em.htm

Feliciano, D. V., Mattox, K. L., & Moore, E. E. (Eds.). (2008). *Trauma* (6th ed.). New York: McGraw-Hill.

Fiore, P., Panza, F., Cassatella, G., Russo, A., Frisardi, V., Solfrizzi, V., et al. (2011). Short-term effects of high-intensity laser therapy versus ultrasound therapy in the treatment of low back pain: A randomized controlled trial. *European Journal of Physical and Rehabilitation Medicine, 47*(3), 367–373. Epub 2011 Jun 8

Frazier, M. S., & Drzymkowski, J. W. (Eds.). (2007). *Essentials of human diseases and conditions* (4th ed.). St. Louis: W. B. Saunders.

Gammons, M. (2011). Anterior cruciate ligament injury. Retrieved from http://www.emedicine.medscape.com/article/89442-overview#a0199

Haas, Z. (2009). Optimizing outcomes in bunion surgery. *Clinics in Podiatric Medicine and Surgery, 26*(3), 443–457.

Halstead, M. E. (2011). Elbow dislocation. Retrieved from http://www.emedicine.medscape.com/article/96758-overview

Hanley, M. A., Jensen, M. P., Smith, D. G., Ehde, D. M., Edwards, W. T. & Robinson, L. R. (2007). Preamputation pain and acute pain predict chronic pain after lower extremity amputation. *Journal of Pain, 8*: 102–109.

Harvard Women's Health Watch. (2007). Recovering from an ankle sprain. Retrieved from http://www.health.harvard.edu

Hashmi, J. T., Huang, Y. Y., Osmani, B. Z., Sharma, S. K., Naeser, M. A., & Hamblin, M. R. (2010). Role of low-level laser therapy in neurorehabilitation. *Physical Medicine and Rehabilitation, 2*(12 Suppl 2), S292–305.

Holmes, S. B., & Brown, S. J. (2005). Skeletal pin site care: National Association of Orthopaedic Nurses guidelines for orthopaedic nursing. *Orthopaedic Nursing, 24*(2), 99–107.

Hrysomallis, C. (2007). Relationship between balance ability, training and sports injury risk. *Sports Medicine, 37*(6), 547–555.

IOM (Institute of Medicine). (2010). *The future of nursing: Leading change, advancing health.* Washington, DC: The Academic Press.

Karrer, F. M., & Jones, S. (2010). Superior mesenteric artery syndrome. Retrieved from http://www.emedicine.com/ped/topic2175.htm

Lakshmanan, P. (2011). Wrist arthritis. Retrieved from http://www.emedicine.medscape.com/article/1933090-overview#aw2aab6b2b6aa

Mabee, J., & Mabee, C. (2009). Acute lateral sprained ankle syndrome. *The Internet Journal of Family Practice, 7*(1).

Matson, F. A., III, & Warme, W. J. (2010). Total shoulder joint replacement for shoulder arthritis: Surgery with a dependable, time-tested conservative prosthesis and accelerated rehabilitation can lessen pain and improve function in shoulders with arthritis. Retrieved from http://www.orthop.washington.edu/uw/shoulderreplacement/tabID__3376/ItemID__62/Articles/Default.aspx

Mayoclinic.com. (2011). Glucosamine. Retrieved from http://www.mayoclinic.com/health/glucosamine

MedlinePlus. (2010). Knee joint replacement. Retrieved from http://www.nlm.nih.gov/medlineplus/kneereplacement.html

National Limb Loss Information Center (NLLIC). (2008). Amputation statistics by cause. Retrieved from http://www.amputee-coalition.org/fact_sheets/amp_stats_cause.html

Norman, S. B., Stein, M. B., Dimsdale, J. E., & Hoyt, D. B. (2008). Pain in the aftermath of trauma is a risk factor for post-traumatic stress disorder. *Psychology Medicine, 38*(4), 533–542.

Paffrath, T., Wafaisade, A., Lefering, R., Simanski, C., Bouillon, B., Spanholtz, T., et al. (2009). Venous thromboembolism after severe trauma: Incidence, risk factors, and outcome. *Injury, International Journal of Care of the Injured, 41*(1), 97–101.

Porth, C. M., & Matfin, G. (2009). *Essentials of pathophysiology: Concepts of altered health states* (2nd ed.). Philadelphia: Lippincott Williams & Wilkins.

Reiter, G. T. (2011). Vertebral fracture. Retrieved from http://www.emedicine.medscape.com/article/248236-overview

Rochkind, S., Drory, V., Alon, M., Nissan, M., & Ouaknine, G. E. (2007). Laser phototherapy (780 nm), a new modality in treatment of long-term incomplete peripheral nerve injury: A randomized double-blind placebo-controlled study. *Photomedicine and Laser Surgery, 25*(5), 436–442.

Russell, G. V. (2011). Pelvic fractures. Retrieved from http://www.emedicine.medscape.com/article/1247913-overview#a0103

Shekelle, P. (2008). Diagnosis and treatment of low back pain: A joint clinical practice guideline from the American College of Physicians and the American Pain Society. What's new? What's different? Retrieved from http://www.guideline.gov/expert-commentary.aspx?id=16452

Shiel, W. C. (2011). Total knee replacement. Retrieved from http://www.medicinenet.com/total_knee_replacement/article.htm

Walker, J. A. (2007). Evidence for skeletal pin site care. *Nursing Standard, 21*(45), 70–76.

WebMD. (2011). Elbow injuries. Retrieved from http://www.webmd.com/a-to-z-guides/elbow-injuries-topic-overiew

Weinhouse, G. (2008). Fat embolism syndrome. Retrieved from http://www.utdol.com/online/content/topic.do?topicKey=cc_medi/13397&selectedTitle=1~27&source=search_result

Wheeless, C. (2008). Gustillo classification of fracture. Retrieved from http://www.wheelessonline.com/oa2/60.htm

Wilkinson, J. M., & Ahearn, N. R. (2009). *Prentice Hall nursing diagnosis handbook* (9th ed.). Upper Saddle River, NJ: Prentice Hall.

Wilson, S. R. (2011). Shoulder dislocation in emergency medicine. Retrieved from http://www.emedicine.medscape.com/article/823843-overview#a0199

CHAPTER 51

Caring for the Patient with Arthritis and Connective Tissue Disorders

Kara Gasiorowski
Cheryl Wraa

Outcome-Based Learning Objectives

After studying this chapter, the learner will be able to:

1. Differentiate autoimmune disease from connective tissue disease.
2. Outline the etiology, pathophysiology, clinical manifestations, nursing management, and prevention of the various types of arthritis.
3. Explain the four highest priority nursing diagnoses for rheumatoid arthritis and osteoarthritis.
4. Generate a nursing management plan for patients experiencing arthritis.
5. Describe the clinical manifestations and nursing management for connective tissue disease.
6. Generate a nursing management plan for patients experiencing connective tissue disease.

KEY TERMS

ankylosing spondylitis (AS) p.1579
circinate balanitis p.1578
dactylitis p.1576
entheses p.1576
gouty arthritis p.1577
Lyme disease p.1586
osteoarthritis (OA) p.1564
psoriatic arthritis p.1574
reactive arthritis p.1578
rheumatoid arthritis (RA) p.1565
septic arthritis p.1580
Sjögren's syndrome (SS) p.1587
subcutaneous nodules p.1565
systemic lupus erythematosus (SLE) p.1582
tophi p.1577

Weblink: Osteoarthritis

ARTHRITIS AND OTHER RHEUMATIC DISEASES limit the activities of many adults and is the most common cause of disability in the United States (Centers for Disease Control and Prevention [CDC], 2011). People may believe that arthritis is a single disorder, but arthritis actually refers to a group of disorders that cause pain, stiffness, and swelling in the joints. The first part of this chapter discusses the various types of arthritis and the nursing management for patients experiencing arthritis.

Connective tissue consists of cells surrounded in an extracellular matrix of fibers, which serves to add strength and support, bind, and protect the various organs of the body. Three types of fibers make up the various connective tissues found in the body: collagen fibers, reticular fibers, and elastic fibers. Any inflammation of these tissues in joints can cause connective tissue disorders. Inflammation may be the result of an infection or injury, have a genetic component, or have no known cause. As with arthritis, connective tissue disorders can affect the joints and limit mobility.

Arthritis

Arthritis is a common descriptive term that applies to a group of rheumatic diseases that involve damage to the joints of the body. The most common forms of arthritis—osteoarthritis, rheumatoid arthritis, psoriatic arthritis, gouty arthritis, and reactive arthritis—are discussed in this chapter. It is estimated that by the year 2030, 67 million Americans 18 years of age and older will be diagnosed by a health care provider as having arthritis (CDC, 2010b).

Osteoarthritis

Epidemiology and Etiology

Osteoarthritis (OA), or degenerative joint disease, is the most common form of arthritis. It is a chronic condition that accompanies aging and most commonly affects weight-bearing joints. Osteoarthritis is a leading cause of joint pain and disability in older adults. In fact, 70% of people age 40 and older and 80% of those age 65 and older are afflicted with this chronic condition (FamilyPracticeNotebook.com, 2010). Osteoarthritis was previously thought to be a normal consequence of aging; however, it is now realized that OA results from a complex interplay of multiple factors, including joint integrity, genetic predisposition, local inflammation, mechanical forces, and cellular and biochemical processes. The disease can occur as a primary idiopathic disorder that is localized or generalized (i.e., involves more than three joints). Secondary OA is due to an underlying cause such as congenital defects of joint structure, single severe trauma or multiple traumas, inflammatory diseases, or metabolic disorders.

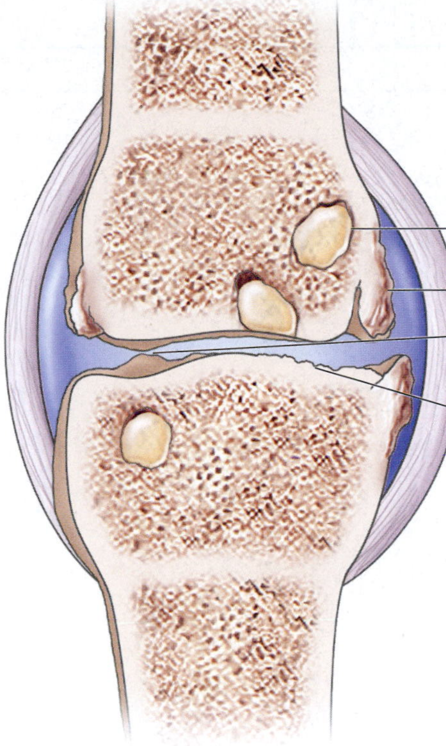

FIGURE 51–1 ◆ Joint degeneration with OA.

Pathophysiology

Joint degeneration in OA occurs on the articular surfaces of the cartilage with bony formations at the edges of weight-bearing joints, such as the knees and hips. Osteoarthritis may also involve the joints of the fingers at the proximal interphalangeal joints (Figure 51–1◆) and can affect the wrists, elbows, ankles, spinal vertebrae, and joints of the pelvis. Osteoarthritis results in significant changes in both the composition and the mechanical properties of cartilage. Early in the disease, the cartilage contains more water and fewer concentrations of proteoglycans, the large molecules that afford elasticity and stiffness and allow cartilage to resist compression. There is also a decrease in local synthesis of new collagen and an increase in the breakdown of existing collagen. It is thought that the changes are a result of the release of cytokines that stimulate production and the release of enzymes that are destructive to joint structures. This damage predisposes the cartilage tissue to more injury and impairs the cells' ability to repair the damage by producing new collagen and proteoglycans (Porth & Matfin, 2009).

Clinical Manifestations

Patients with OA will complain of a brief interval of morning stiffness, pain on motion of the affected joint, and joint bone deformity (FamilyPracticeNotebook.com, 2010). The joints that are most frequently affected are the lower back, knees, feet, and hips (Baumann, 2009). Other clinical manifestations of OA include fatigue, generalized weakness, anorexia, cold intolerance, and parasthesia. Over time, the patient may experience joint changes such as enlargement of the joint, limited movement, stiffness, swelling, redness, localized heat around the joint, shiny stretched skin over and around the joint, and **subcutaneous nodules** (firm nodules under the skin caused by inflammation). Other objective symptoms are weight loss, elevated temperature, crepitus (creaking or crackling) of joints, deformities or contractures, and cold and clammy extremities.

Laboratory and Diagnostic Procedures

Diagnosis of OA is typically made by an overall clinical impression, including the patient's age, history, findings on physical examination, and radiographic findings (Kalunian, 2011). Diagnosis of arthritis can be confirmed through plain radiographs of the affected joint, computed tomography (CT), and magnetic resonance imaging (MRI). See the Diagnostic Tests box for these diagnostic tests as well as the radiologic tests used to identify OA and the expected abnormalities that are found with these tests.

Medical and Surgical Management

Initially, the best treatment for OA in weight-bearing joints is rest. As the condition becomes more progressive, medications may be taken to alleviate discomfort of the affected joints. These medications include classifications such as nonsteroidal anti-inflammatory drugs (NSAIDs), cyclooxygenase-2 (COX-2) inhibitors, and antimalarials to relieve symptoms. The Pharmacology box on page 1567 outlines medications used to treat arthritis and other connective tissue disorders. A multidisciplinary approach may include a nutritionist to help with weight reduction and a physical therapist to develop an exercise program that includes range-of-motion exercises.

Once the patient has exhausted medical, nutrition, and exercise options, surgical intervention should be considered if the patient's quality of life is further compromised. There are three kinds of surgical procedures that can improve the health of patients suffering from osteoarthritis: synovectomy, arthrodesis, and reconstructive surgery. A synovectomy is the removal of the swollen synovial casing before damage to the bone and cartilage occurs. Arthrodesis is fusion of the joint. An arthrodesis is done when there is severe destruction of the joint's surfaces. Joint replacements, usually total knee or total hip replacements, are done when these weight-bearing joints have been completely damaged. The patient must be aware of her options in order to make an informed decision. For a detailed discussion of orthopedic surgery, refer to Chapter 50.

Nonpharmacologic interventions for arthritis include the use of heat to reduce muscle spasms and cold to reduce inflammation and pain. In addition, there are multiple alternative therapies to treat symptoms of arthritis, as described in the Complementary & Alternative Therapies box (p. 1570).

Nursing Management

The nursing process provides a framework to create a comprehensive plan of care for the patient with OA, utilizing the problem-solving approach. The nurse begins with general assessment and then concentrates on the clinical manifestations specifically related to OA. See the Nursing Process: Patient Care Plan for Arthritis box on page 1572.

Because OA is a chronic disease, discharge instructions are important to ensure compliance with the health care plan. For more details, see the Patient Teaching & Discharge Priorities box on page 1575.

Rheumatoid Arthritis

Epidemiology and Etiology

Rheumatoid arthritis (RA) is a chronic inflammatory process that mainly affects the synovial joints. It is a systemic disorder that affects many tissues, including peripheral joints and surrounding muscles, ligaments, tendons, and blood vessels. Rheumatoid arthritis is thought to be an autoimmune disorder that not only involves tissue hypersensitivity but also has a genetic component. Antiglobulin antibodies combine

DIAGNOSTIC TESTS for Osteoarthritis

Test, Normal Values, and Rationale	Expected Abnormality
Bone Density	
Normal density	Increased.
Confirmation of bone on bone contact.	Asymmetrical joint cartilage loss.
Erythrocyte Sedimentation Rate (ESR)	
Male:	Increased.
<50 years old: 0–15 mm/hour	
>50 years old: 0–20 mm/hour	
Female:	
<50 years old: 0–20 mm/hour	
>50 years old: 0–30 mm/hour	
Presence of inflammatory disease.	
Rheumatoid Factor	
Less than 1:20 titer; less than 1:40 chronic inflammatory disease; 1:20–1:80 positive for RA and other conditions; >1:80 positive for RA	Negative.
To detect antibodies found in rheumatoid arthritis	
Radiologic Test	
X-Ray	
Normal joint surfaces	Degenerative changes.
Articular surfaces are worn where bone rubs against bone.	Narrowing of bone space.
Computed Tomography (CT)	
Normal bone and soft tissue	Bone spurs.
Bone cyst and sclerosis are common with disease progression.	
Magnetic Resonance Imaging (MRI)	
Normal bone and soft tissue	Reactive bone edema.
Very sensitive test to bony and soft tissue changes.	Soft tissue swelling.
Able to identify early degenerative changes.	Bone fragments within the joint.

Source: Kee, J. L. (2010). *Laboratory and diagnostic tests with nursing implications* (8th ed.). Upper Saddle River, NJ: Prentice Hall.

with immunoglobulin in the synovial fluid and form complexes. Neutrophils are then attracted to the joint space and cause destruction.

Rheumatoid arthritis most commonly affects women between ages 20 and 40 and is present in 2% to 3% of the population. It is noted worldwide as affecting three times more women than men. Although it can occur at any age, the peak incidence is between ages 25 and 55 (Frazier & Drzymkowski, 2009).

Pathophysiology

Rheumatoid arthritis begins with an inflammatory process in the synovial membrane and joint capsule, with swelling causing the infiltration of lymphocytes, macrophages, and neutrophils that perpetuate the inflammatory response. The inflammation leads to destruction of cartilage and the joint surfaces, which leads to deformity. The inflammatory response has four signs: redness, heat, swelling, and pain. In some RA patients, pannus tissue forms in the joint, causing a loss of bone and cartilage. Pannus tissue is an abnormal layer of tissue with an extensive network of new blood vessels that develops in the synovial membrane (Figure 51–2◆).

Clinical Manifestations

Joint inflammation and deformity occur in the affected joints. With RA, patients experience remissions (during which the disease process is inactive) and exacerbations (flare-ups or times when the disease becomes active) of the disease. During exacerbations, patients may experience

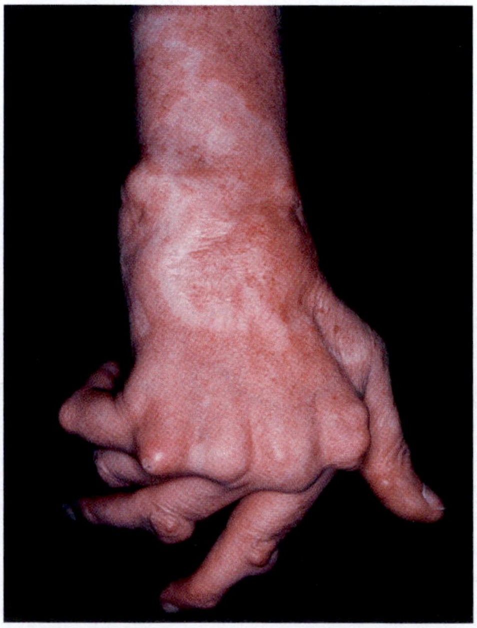

FIGURE 51–2 ◆ In some RA patients, pannus (development of an extensive network of new blood vessels in the synovial membrane that is destructive) is experienced.

Source: Princess Margaret Rose Orthopaedic Hospital/Photo Researchers, Inc.

PHARMACOLOGY Summary of Medications Used to Treat Arthritis and Connective Tissue Disorders

Medication Category and Action	Application/Indication	Nursing Responsibility
Nonsteroidal Anti-Inflammatory Drugs		
Ibuprofen (Motrin, Advil) Diclofenac (Voltaren) Naproxen (Naprosyn) Sulindac (Clinoril) ***Action:*** Exerts anti-inflammatory, analgesic action by inhibition of prostaglandin synthesis; inflammatory cell chemotaxis decreases release of superoxide radicals and increases the scavenging of these products at the inflammatory sites.	Rheumatoid arthritis, osteoarthritis, ankylosing spondylitis, and mild to moderate pain. Off-label use: psoriatic arthritis, systemic lupus.	Monitor for adverse effects: nausea, vomiting, diarrhea, constipation, gastric bleeding, blurred vision, and tinnitus. Warn the patient that alcohol and smoking increase the incidence of gastrointestinal (GI) bleeding. Monitor for exacerbation in patients with asthma or existing renal, liver, or hematopoietic dysfunction.
Cyclooxygenase-2 (COX-2) Inhibitor		
Celecoxib (Celebrex) ***Action:*** Inhibits COX-2 and prostaglandin synthesis to reduce inflammation. Relieves pain and inflammation in the joints and smooth muscle tissue.	Rheumatoid arthritis, osteoarthritis, and ankylosing spondylitis.	Monitor for adverse effects: dyspepsia, abdominal pain, nausea, headache, hepatotoxicity (nausea, vomiting, itching, abdominal pain), and GI bleeding (tarry stools, upper GI distress). Be aware of drug interactions with other anticoagulants (warfarin). Monitor hematocrit (HCT), hemoglobin (Hgb), electrolytes, and liver and renal function. Be aware of increased risk of myocardial infarction, stroke, and cardiovascular thrombosis, especially in the presence of existing cardiovascular disease. Give 2 hours before or after antacids.
Disease-Modifying Antirheumatic Drugs (DMARDs): Antineoplastic		
Methotrexate (MTX, Rheumatrex) ***Action:*** Blocks enzyme responsible for converting folic acid to reduced folate, which interferes with DNA synthesis, repair, and cellular replication in actively proliferating tissues.	Severe, disabling rheumatoid arthritis. Off-label use: psoriatic arthritis, systemic lupus.	Monitor for adverse effects: headache, rash, nausea, vomiting, diarrhea, stomatitis, and alopecia. Observe for signs of severe adverse effects: bone marrow suppression; liver, lung, kidney, or GI toxicities. Monitor the complete blood count (CBC), renal and hepatic function, metabolic profile, and chest x-ray at regularly scheduled intervals. Be aware of multiple drug interactions (acetylsalicylic acid (ASA), NSAIDs, digoxin, and phenytoin). Observe for altered drug efficacy or toxicity. Advise the patient of increased toxicity with alcohol and caffeine consumption. Contact the health care provider before using over-the-counter (OTC) drugs. Warn the patient of photosensitivity and to use sun block.
Immunosuppressants		
Cyclosporine (Sandimmune, Neoral) Mycophenolate (CellCept) Azathioprine (Imuran) ***Action:*** Suppresses immune response by inhibiting lymphocyte replication or disrupting helper T cells. Inhibits DNA synthesis, resulting in DNA damage.	Treatment of rheumatoid arthritis is unresponsive to conventional therapy, systemic lupus, and psoriatic arthritis. Severe RA and SLE.	Monitor for adverse effects: hirsutism, hypertension, nausea, vomiting, and infection. Observe for signs of toxicity: tremors, seizures, altered mental status, visual disturbances, nephrotoxicity, and neurotoxicity. Monitor CBC, magnesium, potassium, blood sugar, liver, and renal function tests. Be aware of multiple drug interactions (digoxin, NSAIDs, erythromycin, verapamil, cimetidine, and allopurinol).
Cyclophosphamide (Cytoxan) ***Action:*** Forms cross-links in DNA preventing cancer cell replication. Affects both B and T cells.	Off-label use: treatment of severe rheumatoid arthritis, SLE.	Monitor for adverse effects: dizziness, nausea, vomiting, alopecia, hyperkalemia, and hyponatremia. Monitor for severe adverse effects: leukopenia, pulmonary emboli, interstitial pulmonary fibrosis, nephrotoxicity, and hemorrhagic cystitis.

(*continued*)

PHARMACOLOGY **Summary of Medications Used to Treat Arthritis and Connective Tissue Disorders, *continued***

Medication Category and Action	Application/Indication	Nursing Responsibility
Rituximab (Rituxan, MabThera) ***Action:*** Binds to the CD3 protein, preventing the T cell from initiating an immune response.	Treatment of SLE.	Monitor leukocyte and platelet counts, HCT, electrolytes, and renal function including urinalysis. Assess frequently for adverse effects as this drug has a high potential for toxicity. Report to the health care provider dramatic or persistent decreases in leukocyte or platelet counts, which may represent irreversible bone marrow depression to the prescriber. Monitor for cytokine release syndrome: flulike symptoms, dyspnea, chest pain, pulmonary edema, dysrhythmias, and renal impairment. Report any signs immediately. Monitor kidney function, and assess fluid status. Monitor for abnormal bleeding signs such as easy bruising, bleeding gums, petechiae, melena, epistaxis, hematuria, hemoptysis, and hematemesis. Hospitalized patients should be placed in protective isolation to prevent infection.
Disease Modifying		
Sulfasalazine (Azulfidine) ***Action:*** Inhibits the mediators of inflammation in the colon—prostaglandins and leukotrienes.	First-line treatment for rheumatoid arthritis.	Monitor for adverse effects: rash, headache, nausea, vomiting, and bloody diarrhea. Observe for serious adverse effects (bone marrow suppression, hepatitis). Monitor CBC and renal and liver function tests.
Disease Modifying		
Etanercept (Enbrel) Infliximab (Remicade) ***Action:*** Exact mechanism for reducing symptoms of RA unknown. Reduces the migration of neutrophils and eosinophils and probably inhibits the synthesis of histamine and prostaglandins.	Rheumatoid arthritis management, psoriatic arthritis, and ankylosing spondylitis.	Monitor for adverse effects: infection, nausea, headache, injection/infusion site reactions, blood dyscrasia, demyelinating diseases, and sepsis (especially in poorly controlled diabetes and other predisposing diseases). Monitor CBC, chest x-ray, urinalysis, and C-reactive protein. Black box warning with adalimumab and TB with infliximab, sepsis, and invasive fungal infections, lupuslike syndrome, positive antinuclear antibodies, tumor lysis syndrome, heart failure exacerbations, or Stevens-Johnson syndrome. Be aware of drug interactions (methotrexate, azathioprine, and leflunomide).
Antimalarials		
Hydroxychloroquine (Plaquenil) Chloroquine (Aralen) Quinacrine ***Action:*** Exact mechanism in use with RA is not known. Reduces the migration of neutrophils and eosinophils and likely inhibits the synthesis of histamine and prostaglandins.	Treatment of rheumatoid arthritis and SLE.	Monitor for adverse effects: hypotension, nausea, diarrhea, pruritus, irritability, headaches, weakness, hair loss, or bleaching. Monitor electrocardiogram (ECG), CBC, and liver and kidney function. Observe for potential exacerbation of disease when given in the presence of blood, liver, GI, or neurological disorders. Monitor for irreversible retinal damage. Advise the patient of the importance of regular eye exams. Be aware of multiple drug interactions (antacids, cimetidine, and methotrexate). Give with food to decrease adverse GI effects.
Glucocorticoids		
Prednisone (Meticorten) Prednisolone (Delta-Cortef) ***Action:*** Dampens the immune response and inhibits the synthesis of inflammatory mediators. Decreases the number of circulating lymphocytes, eosinophils, monocytes, and basophils. Inhibits movement of macrophages and leukocytes to areas of inflammation. Decreases production of inflammatory cytokines. Decreases formation of prostaglandins.	Acute exacerbation of rheumatoid arthritis and pulse therapy. Inflammatory connective tissue disorders.	Monitor for adverse effects: mood swings, anxiety, insomnia, nausea, vomiting, weight gain, acne, and delayed wound healing. Observe for increased risk of GI bleeding and, in rheumatoid arthritis patients, pneumonia. Monitor blood count, glucose, and electrolytes. Be aware of drug interactions (theophylline and warfarin). Monitor for toxicity or decreased efficacy. Warn the patient of the potential need for dose adjustment if ill or if stress increases. Do not abruptly stop using the drug.

PHARMACOLOGY Summary of Medications Used to Treat Arthritis and Connective Tissue Disorders, *continued*

Medication Category and Action	Application/Indication	Nursing Responsibility
Antigout Agents		
Colchicine ***Action:*** Exerts anti-inflammatory effect; decreases pain and swelling by interrupting the inflammatory response. Reduces uric acid; has no direct anti-inflammatory or analgesic action.	Treatment of acute gout, prophylaxis, and recurrent gouty arthritis. Off-label use: scleroderma. Treatment of chronic gout.	Observe for early signs of toxicity (colchicine): weakness, anorexia, nausea, vomiting, diarrhea (especially in the presence of cardiac, renal, or hepatic disease), nausea, sore throat or mouth, fever, fatigue, unusual bleeding, or bruising (bone marrow depression). Monitor serum uric acid, CBC, electrolytes, urinalysis, and renal and hepatic function. Monitor the IV site to prevent extravasation when colchicine is given IV.
Allopurinol (Aloprim, Zyloprim) Probenecid (Benemid) ***Action:*** Reduces uric acid formation by inhibiting the action of xanthine oxidase responsible for the formation of uric acid.		Monitor for drug interactions (vitamin B_{12}, erythromycin, NSAIDs, and others with colchicine; theophylline, ampicillin, thiazide diuretics, and others with allopurinol; some antibiotics, vitamin C, and cranberry juice with probenecid). Advise the patient to increase fluid intake. Give after a meal to reduce gastric distress.
Calcium Channel Blocker		
Nifedipine (Adalat Procardia XL) Nicardipine (Cardene) ***Action:*** Selectively blocks calcium channels in vascular smooth muscle, causing a decrease in the amount of intracellular calcium available for muscle contraction.	Decrease Raynaud's symptoms.	Monitor blood pressure before administration and 30 minutes to 1 hour after. Patient may experience severe hypotension if taking other drugs known to lower blood pressure. Do not give the drug if the patient's systolic blood pressure is below 90.
Selective Serotonin Reuptake Inhibitor (SSRI)		
Fluoxetine (Prozac) ***Action:*** Blocks uptake of the neurotransmitter serotonin at the neuronal presynaptic membrane. This enhances the actions of serotonin.	Off-label use to decrease Raynaud's symptoms	Assess for signs and symptoms of adverse reactions such as nausea, vomiting, insomnia, or restlessness. Instruct the patient to take exactly as prescribed and do not discontinue without approval from the health care provider. Instruct the patient not to consume alcoholic beverages as it may cause sedation. Instruct the female patient to notify the health care provider immediately if she becomes pregnant.
Antibiotics		
Doxycycline (Vibramycin) ***Action:*** Protein synthesis inhibitor which inhibits bacterial protein synthesis.	Treatment of Lyme disease.	Obtain baseline and intermittent cultures to confirm susceptibility to the drug. Administer the drug with 8 ounces of water on an empty stomach at least 1 hour before or 2 hours after meals. Do not give immediately before sleep as esophagitis and esophageal ulceration are associated with bedtime administration. Monitor for diarrhea. Monitor for hypersensitivity reaction: rash, edema, difficulty breathing (anaphylaxis).
Amoxicillin (Amoxil, Trimox) ***Action:*** Inhibits bacterial wall synthesis by binding penicillin-binding proteins. The drug is bacteriocidal and inactivated by penicillinase.		Give medication with 8 ounces of water on an empty stomach at least 1 hour before or 2 hours after meals. Monitor for diarrhea. Same as doxycycline.

Sources: Adams, M. P., & Koch, R. W. (2010). *Pharmacology: Connections to nursing practice.* Upper Saddle River, NJ: Pearson; Gladman, D. (2011b). Pathogenesis of psoriatic arthritis. *UpToDate.* Retrieved from http://www.uptodate.com/patients/content/topic.do?topicKey=~nKkKMlvosxl56.&selectedTitle=1~78&source=search_result; MayoClinic.com. (2011). Lyme disease: Symptoms. Retrieved from http://www.mayoclinic.com/health/lyme-disease/DS00116/DSECTION-2; MedicineNet.com. (2011c). Systemic lupus erythematosus (SLE or lupus). Retrieved from http://www.medicinenet.com/systemic_lupus/article.htm.

fatigue, low-grade fever, anorexia, joint pain and swelling due to inflammation, and symmetrical joint deformity. The joints of the hands and feet are most often affected (Ferri, 2011).

Rheumatoid arthritis not only affects the joints but also may affect organs of the entire body. Glands may become swollen, and the patient's mouth may become dry. Other organs affected may include the lungs, blood, and spleen. Rheumatoid arthritis can cause rheumatoid nodules in the lungs, leading to pleuritis. There is a decrease of red blood cells, causing anemia, and a decrease of white blood cells due to spleen enlargement. Vasculitis may occur, which results in an impairment of

COMPLEMENTARY & ALTERNATIVE THERAPIES Using CAM to Reduce Inflammation

Nancy Yilk

BASED ON A 2011 STUDY, 40% to 60% of Americans use CAM therapies to support their health goals. This is not surprising, given the public's increasing awareness of CAM studies and the easy access to find CAM products. Relief from pain due to inflammation initially compels many people to use CAM therapies. Of the population of patients in the study, 33% cite pain as the primary reason, with patients in rheumatology tending to be higher than the general population, ranging from 28% to 90% who self-select to use alternative therapies such as nutritional supplementation. These patients often self-prescribe these products and often do not disclose their use to their health care professionals (Ernst, 2011). Even after seeking help from their health care providers and receiving prescribed medications, they often continue using these natural products, viewing them as adjunct therapy. They do not understand the possibility of drug interactions (Efthimiou, Kukar, & MacKenzie, 2009).

To understand the proper use of nutritional therapies in the treatment of inflammatory concerns, it is best to start with the dietary intake requirement of polyunsaturated fatty acids (PUFAs) and their relationship to inflammation and pain signaling. Like essential vitamins and minerals that must be supplied from dietary intake since the body lacks the ability to synthesize them, certain PUFAs are therefore referred as essential fatty acids (EFAs). The PUFAs are grouped into the following categories: n-3 (omega-3) series of fatty acids represented by a-linolenic acid (ALA), eicosapentaenoic acid (EPA), and docosahexaenoic acid (DHA); and n-6 fatty acids (omega-6) represented by linoleic acid (LA), g-linolenic acid (GLA) (omega-9), and arachidonic acid (AA). Omega-6 PUFAs, with the exception of performed conversion on GLA, are generally considered bad for the patient's health because prostaglandins, inflammatory eicosanoids, and inflammatory cytokines, such as interleukin-1 and -6, are derived from omega-6 PUFAs. The beneficial effects of n-3 PUFAs on various inflammatory diseases have been explained by the antagonistic action of n-3 PUFAs toward the arachidonic acid cascade. Both basic and clinical studies have shown that a dietary intake of PUFAs' n-3 series, which are abundant in fish oil, results in a reduction in the pain associated with rheumatoid arthritis, dysmenorrhea, inflammatory bowel disease, and neuropathy. In addition, levels of n-6 series polyunsaturated fatty acids are high in patients with chronic pain (Tokuyama & Nakamoto, 2011).

Historically, the human diet was low in calories, consisting of fish, plants, eggs, nuts, seeds, and game meat. This diet contained 20% to 25% fat with a ratio of PUFAs 1–2:1 of omega-6 to omega-3. The evolutionary development of the human physiology was greatly influenced by our historical diet, which contributed to the brain's development. Industrialization of food production and changing farming practices have created an increase in dietary omega-6 plant oils, dominated by soy and corn oil, in both animal feed and human-consumed processed foods. The real-time consequence of dietary PUFA ratios in Western diets has altered the equilibrium of this evolutionary ratio to current levels of 20–30:1. Influencing this ratio further is the fact that a large amount of fish consumption is from farmed fish that have a current imbalance of omega-3, resulting in higher levels of arachidonic acid (AA) (Gómez Candela, Bermejo López, & Loria Kohen, 2011).

Re-establishing the need for EFA ratios from both diet and supplementation affords the body the ability to effectively deal with pain and inflammation at a foundational level that is not achievable with many of the marketed products for arthritis and pain.

Supplementation	Clinical Benefits
EFA n-3 series (ALA) Flax oil	ALA from flax oil has not been found to be therapeutically beneficial in human studies related to inflammation or pain reduction.
EFA n-3 series (EPA/DHA) Source: Fish oil or algae	n-3 PUFAs suppress the production of inflammatory cytokines and eicosanoids. Such anti-inflammatory action by PUFAs is believed to result in pain suppression. The physiological and pharmacologic functions of DHA that support the proposal include (1) an anti-inflammatory effect viathe suppression of the arachidonic acid cascade, (2) inhibition of voltage-gated sodium channels, (3) agonistic action toward transient receptor potential vanilloid 1 (TRPV1) that is closely associated with the onset of inflammation, and (4) inhibition of calcium channels. Furthermore, the investigators have elucidated that one of the actions contributing to the antinociceptive mechanisms of DHA is not performed directly on the opioid receptor, but indirectly through the release of an endogenous opioid peptide beta-endorphin (Tokuyama et al., 2011).
EFA (GLA) Evening primrose oil	There has currently been limited success in using GLA for treatment of RA and the dry eyes of Sjorgen by affecting increased levels of PGE1. Note: Studies with success were performed with the brand name EPO marketed as Efamol. Borage oil and black currant oil have not shown desirable increased levels of PGE1.
Green-lipped mussel (GLM) *Perna canaliculus*	GLM has an anti-inflammatory activity associated with the omega-3 EFA contained within its lipid fraction of furan fatty acids (F-acids). These naturally but rarely detected fatty acids show potent radical-scavenging ability and are essential constituents of plants and algae. Based on these data, it has been proposed that F-acids could be potential antioxidants, which may explain the protective properties of fish and fish oil diets against chronic inflammatory diseases. Lyprinol, a stabilized GLM lipid extract, has shown properties that significantly improved antinociception (Brien, Prescott, Coghlan, Bashir, & Lewith, 2008).
Glucosamine HCL	The Glucosamine/chondroitin Arthritis Intervention Trial (GAIT), a 1,583-patient, 6-month trial sponsored by the National Institutes of Health (NIH) using Glucosamine HCL, failed to show significant improvement in the Western Ontario and McMasters Universities (WOMAC) Osteoarthritis Index in the overall patient population for glucosamine, chondroitin, or their combination (Chisholm, 2011).
Glucosamine sulphate	The Glucosamine Unum In Die (once-a-day) Efficacy (GUIDE) trial, a 318-patient, 6-month European trial sponsored by industry, showed a small improvement in the total WOMAC Index score over placebo for glucosamine sulfate (Chisholm, 2011).
Chondroitin sulphate	Chondroitin is used in combination with other ingredients, including manganese ascorbate, glucosamine sulfate, glucosamine hydrochloride, or N-acetyl glucosamine. Research from a couple of decades ago showed that chondroitin sulfate helped arthritis pain when taken with conventional medicines, such as aspirin, for pain and swelling. Later research showed chondroitin reduced arthritis pain slightly and performed best when used as a complementary ingredient in combination formulas.

COMPLEMENTARY & ALTERNATIVE THERAPIES Using CAM to Reduce Inflammation, *continued*

Supplementation	Clinical Benefits
Curcumin	Curcumin, the active compound in the East India herb turmeric, has a long history of use in Ayurvedic medicine as a treatment for inflammatory conditions. Extensive research within the past two decades has shown that curcumin mediates its anti-inflammatory effects through the downregulation of inflammatory transcription factors (such as nuclear factor kappaB), enzymes (such as cyclooxygenase 2 and 5 lipoxygenase), and cytokines (such as tumor necrosis factor, interleukin 1, and interleukin 6). Researched success was achieved with a proprietary complex of curcumin with soy phosphatidylcholine Meriva®. These results show that Meriva® is clinically effective in the management and treatment of osteoarthritis and suggest that the increased stability and better absorption of curcumin induced by complexation with phospholipids have clinical relevance, setting the stage for larger and more prolonged studies (Belcaro, Cesarone, Dugall, Pellegrini, Ledda, Grossi, et al., 2010).
Boswellia	5-Loxin® is a novel Boswellia serrata extract enriched with 30% 3-0-acetyl-11-keto-beta-boswellic acid (AKBA), which exhibits potential anti-inflammatory properties by inhibiting the 5-lipoxygenase enzyme. 5-Loxin® reduces pain and improves physical functioning significantly in OA patients; in addition, it is safe for human consumption. 5-Loxin® may exert its beneficial effects by controlling inflammatory responses through reducing proinflammatory modulators, and it may improve joint health by reducing the enzymatic degradation of cartilage in OA patients (Sengupta, Alluri, Satish, Mishra, Golakoti, Sarma, et al., 2008).
Devil's claw	Devil's claw (*Harpagophytum procumbens*), a traditional South African tribal herbal remedy, is used for rheumatic conditions. To date, 14 clinical trials have assessed its efficacy/effectiveness in OA. To assess the effectiveness, safety, and tolerability of Harpagophytum (Atrosan®) in the treatment of arthritis and rheumatic conditions, an open study of 8 weeks' duration (259 patients) was performed in the United Kingdom. There were statistically significant reductions in mean pain scores for hand, wrist, elbow, shoulder, hip, knee, and back pain. Quality-of-life measurements (SF-12) were significantly increased from baseline and 60% of patients either reduced or stopped concomitant pain medication. Harpagophytum is an effective and well-tolerated serious treatment option for mild to moderate degenerative rheumatic disorders that provides improved quality-of-life measures (Warnock, McBean, Suter, Tan, & Whittaker, 2007).

References

Belcaro, G., Cesarone, M. R., Dugall, M., Pellegrini, L., Ledda, A., Grossi, M. G., et al. (2010). Efficacy and safety of Meriva®, a curcumin-phosphatidylcholine complex, during extended administration in osteoarthritis patients. *Alternative Medicine Review, 15*(4), 337–344.

Brien, S., Prescott, P., Coghlan, B., Bashir, N., & Lewith, G. (2008). Systematic review of the nutritional supplement Perna Canaliculus (green-lipped mussel) in the treatment of osteoarthritis. *Quarterly Journal of Medicine, 101*(3), 167–179. Epub 2008 Jan 25.

Chisholm, T. (2011). Glucosamine for osteoarthritis. Select carefully for best results. *Advance for Nurse Practioners and Physician Assistants, 2*(4), 25–26.

Efthimiou, P., Kukar, M., & MacKenzie, C. R. (2010). Complementary and alternative medicine in rheumatoid arthritis: No longer the last resort! *Humanity and Social Sciences Journal, 6*(1), 108–111. doi: 10.1007/s11420-009-9133-8

Ernst, E. (2011). Herbal medicine in the treatment of rheumatic diseases. *Rheumatic Diseases Clinics of North America, 37*(1), 95–102. Epub 2010 Dec 3.

Gómez Candela, C., Bermejo López, L. M., & Loria Kohen, V. (2011). Importance of a balanced omega 6/omega 3 ratio for the maintenance of health. Nutritional recommendations. *Nutricion Hospitalaria, 26*(2), 323–329.

Sengupta, K., Alluri, K. V., Satish, A. R., Mishra, S., Golakoti, T., Sarma, K. V., et al. (2008). A double blind, randomized, placebo controlled study of the efficacy and safety of 5-Loxin for treatment of osteoarthritis of the knee. *Arthritis Research & Therapy, 10*(4), R85. Epub 2008 Jul 30.

Tokuyama, S., & Nakamoto, K. (2011). Lipid mediators and pain signaling—Unsaturated fatty acids and pain. *Biological & Pharmaceutical Bulletin, 34*(8), 1174–1178.

Warnock, M., McBean, D., Suter, A., Tan, J., & Whittaker, P. (2007). Effectiveness and safety of Devil's claw tablets in patients with general rheumatic disorders. *Phytotherapy Research, 21*(12), 1228–1233.

blood supply and potentially causes necrosis of tissues of the nail beds and dermal ulcers (Ferri, 2011).

Laboratory and Diagnostic Procedures

Diagnostic imaging is important for patients to undergo to determine the presence and severity of rheumatoid arthritis (Ferri, 2011). The Laboratory and Diagnostic Tests box on p. 1575 outlines the tests commonly used to diagnose rheumatoid arthritis.

Medical Management

Rheumatoid arthritis is a chronic condition without a cure. However, certain measures are used to control this disease and treat symptoms, such as pain control, maintaining joint function, reducing damage to joints, and reducing deformity (Ferri, 2011). Early intervention will improve outcomes, so patients should be treated as soon as possible to reduce complications. Treatment includes pharmacologic interventions, rest, exercises, safeguarding joints, and patient education. Sometimes it is more effective to use a blend of medications to treat the discomfort associated with RA, such as NSAIDs and corticosteroids. Other drugs also may be considered depending on the patient's severity of disease and the response to the disease. Common medications given include antineoplastics (methotrexate) or antimalarials (Plaquenil). Patient education regarding medication should include information about each medication's actions, adverse effects, and interactions with food or other medications. Some of these medications are long acting, and the patient needs to be compliant and take the medications as directed to maximize their effect. See the Pharmacology box on page 1567 for a summary of medications used to treat arthritis and connective tissue disorders.

Because many patients with RA are young, surgical intervention may be an appropriate option to include in discussions about treatment options for maintaining or improving the quality of life. Surgical treatment options for patients with RA include synovectomy, arthrodesis, and/or reconstructive surgery, which were discussed earlier in the chapter (p. 1565). Information is critical when all of the alternatives for treatment are being considered.

Nursing Management

The nursing process provides a framework to create a comprehensive plan of care for the patient with RA. During a subjective assessment, the patient may complain of joint stiffness, pain, and swelling. There also may be complaints of being tired and fatigued. Some patients experience weight loss due to anorexia. An objective assessment may include subcutaneous nodules over bony prominences and symmetrical, bilateral involvement of joints, which can cause crepitus in the affected joints. Over time, some patients experience contractures and muscle

NURSING PROCESS: Patient Care Plan for Arthritis

Assessment of Musculoskeletal Status Using Gordon's Functional Health Patterns:

- Health Perception Health Management Pattern
- Nutrition Metabolic Pattern
- Activity Exercise Pattern
- Cognitive Perceptual Pattern

Subjective Data	Objective Data
Assessment of Pain	**Assessment of Pain**
Do you have pain? Is it constant or intermittent? What brings it on and what makes it go away? What intensity is the pain (numeric, colors, or faces), including location, character?	Range-of-motion limitations Amount of joint swelling or deformity Blood uric acid levels (relates to gout)
Assessment of Mobility	**Assessment of Mobility**
Do you experience stiffness in your joints? Do you fall often? Are you able to care for yourself?	Observe balance when the patient is walking. Observe the patient performing activities of daily living.
Assessment of Ventilation for Patients With AS	**Assessment of Ventilation for Patients With AS**
Are you having difficulty taking a deep breath? Are you feeling short of breath?	Observe patient for: Altered chest excursion Shallow respirations Increased respiratory rate
Assessment of Fatigue	**Assessment of Fatigue**
How often do you feel fatigued? How far are you able to walk or how long are you able to exercise before you become fatigued?	Observe the patient during physical therapy to monitor fatigue levels.
Assessment of Powerlessness	**Assessment of Powerlessness**
Are you able to care for yourself? How often do you need help? Has your ability to care for yourself changed recently?	Observe patient's demeanor when discussing self-care. Observe if the patient tries to care for self or relinquishes care to others.
Assessment of Nutrition	**Assessment of Nutrition**
What kinds of foods do you eat on a daily basis? Have you gained or lost weight in the last year? Do you eat at home or in restaurants? Who prepares the meals? What is your knowledge of foods containing purines (relates to gout)?	Weights at specified interval Meal selections Verbalizing foods consumed that are high in purines (relates to gout)
Assessment of Infection	**Assessment of Infection**
Do you have increased pain? Do you have a fever? Are any of your joints reddened or inflamed?	Head-to-toe assessment with focus on the specific area of patient complaint.
Assessment of Therapeutic Regimen	**Assessment of Therapeutic Regimen**
Explain your dietary needs. Explain why and when you take your medications.	Patient is able to verbalize the appropriate foods for consumption. Patient verbalizes weight loss or maintenance. Patient verbalizes decrease in joint discomfort.
Assessment of Patient's Perception of Body Image	**Assessment of Patient's Perception of Body Image**
How are you feeling regarding the physical changes in your body? Are you embarrassed by the appearance of your joints?	Patient tries to hide the affected joints.

NURSING PROCESS: Patient Care Plan for Arthritis, *continued*

Outcomes and Evaluation Parameters	Planning and Interventions with *Rationales*
1. NURSING DIAGNOSIS: Comfort, Readiness for Enhanced Pain, Chronic *related to bone rubbing against bone, inflammation, or deformity (relates to osteoarthritis and rheumatoid arthritis);* Pain, Acute *related to uric acid crystal deposits in affected joints (gout)* (NANDA-I © 2012)	
Outcome: Comfort level maintained. ***Evaluation Parameters:*** Uric acid levels are within normal limits (relates to gout). Pain is controlled with or without nonpharmacologic therapies or with or without medication. Joint swelling decreased.	Assess pain on a scale (0 to 10), with 10 being the worst. Monitor uric acid levels (relates to gout, p. 1577). Alternative pain interventions: position, elevation, ice for inflammation and heat for stiffness, and distraction. Medicate as ordered by the health care provider. *With osteoarthritis, the patient will experience stiffness of the affected joints as well as swelling and pain.* *With gout, as there is an increase in blood uric acid levels, uric acid crystals form in joints causing discomfort, usually affecting one affected joint, which will be warm and swollen.*
2. NURSING DIAGNOSIS: Mobility and Weakness: Physical, Impaired *related to stiffness;* Falls, Risk for *related to malaise and weakness* (NANDA-I © 2012)	
Outcome: The desired outcomes for the patient with OA include control of pain and stiffness, maintenance of quality of life, and ability to perform self-care activities. ***Evaluation Parameter:*** These include the patient's expression that the pain and stiffness are controlled, the patient reports no falls, and the patient is able to perform daily self-care activities.	Medications are instituted to help with the relief of the symptoms. The nurse needs to teach the patient to read the adverse effects of the medication and take precautions, such as having food in the stomach before taking the drug *to prevent gastrointestinal upset.* Nonpharmacologic interventions include the use of heat *to reduce muscle spasms* and cold *to reduce inflammation and pain.* For the prevention of contractures, the patient should be active in exercise, sleep on a firm mattress, and use splints. *Splints and/or supportive devices may be useful in maintaining alignment and promoting function.* A physical activity program should range from passive and active range of motion to swimming. *Exercise is critical in minimizing the complications of immobility.* A fall protocol should be implemented with frequent observation of the patient, toileting often, offering nourishments, and responding quickly to the patient's call light. *This will assist in keeping the patient safe while hospitalized.* The family should also be made aware of the risk of falls and should be taught how to keep the patient safe while at home, such as by removing scatter rugs, removing clutter, and providing assistance when the patient is ambulatory. The installation of safety devices in the home, such as guardrails in the bathrooms and shower areas, will assist the patient in living independently, as well as in gaining confidence in her abilities. *This will assist in keeping the patient safe while at home.*
3. NURSING DIAGNOSIS: Breathing Pattern, Ineffective *related to changes in rib cage affecting lungs* (NANDA-I © 2012)	
Outcome: Patient will demonstrate effective breathing patterns. ***Evaluation Parameter:*** Uncompromised respiratory status as evidenced by depth of inspiration and ease of breathing.	Teach the patient the importance of exercise to maintain flexibility and lung capacity. *Lung capacity is enhanced by swimming or aerobic activities.*
4. NURSING DIAGNOSIS: Activity Intolerance *related to fatigue (relates to rheumatoid arthritis)* (NANDA-I © 2012)	
Outcome: Patient will not be fatigued. ***Evaluation Parameter:*** The patient will be able to do activities of daily living without becoming fatigued.	For rheumatoid arthritis, it is necessary to provide rest during times when the disease process flares up. Provide scheduled activities with planned rest periods *to prevent fatigue.*
5. NURSING DIAGNOSIS: Powerlessness *related to changes in disease process, loss of mobility, financial status, and role of the family* (NANDA-I © 2012)	
Outcome: The patient will not feel helpless. ***Evaluation Parameter:*** The patient will participate with care and be as independent as possible.	As a person loses function, powerlessness may follow. Empowerment is critical to the patient's well-being. Encourage the patient to verbalize any concerns, and listen actively. Utilize reflective communication. *Will assist the patient to discover how best to function.* Encourage the patient to be as independent as possible and to be proud of accomplishments made. *Assists the patient to have a sense of control.*

(*continued*)

NURSING PROCESS: Patient Care Plan for Arthritis, *continued*

Outcomes and Evaluation Parameters	Planning and Interventions with *Rationales*
6. NURSING DIAGNOSIS: Nutrition: Imbalanced, More Than Body Requirements ***related to increased intake of foods high in purine (relates to gout) and increased calories;*** **Less Than Body Requirements** ***related to fatigue and anorexia (relates to rheumatoid arthritis)*** **(NANDA-I © 2012)**	
Outcome: Patient maintains adherence to a low-purine diet. ***Evaluation Parameters:*** Patient will be able to verbalize appropriate meal planning with foods low in calories and purine. Weight loss at reasonable amount weekly based on baseline weight (about 1–2 pounds per week). RA: Patient will maintain a healthy weight.	Obtain a sample of the patient's meal choice selections in a week to determine baseline calorie and purine intake. For osteoarthritis, consulting a nutritionist will help provide a low-calorie, balanced, appealing diet plan to reduce weight. *It is important to realize that weight reduction is a slow process, and weight loss may take a long period of time depending on the amount the patient needs to lose.* For rheumatoid arthritis, consulting a nutritionist will help provide a balanced, appealing diet plan to maintain weight. *Knowledge regarding foods with high nutritional value is important to maintain a healthy weight.* For gout, create a low-purine weight loss meal plan to include foods of the patient's culture in order to decrease uric acid, such as grains, fruits, vegetables, and beans. Teach the patient to avoid the following foods high in purines: cheese, wine, organ meats, and shellfish. Encourage the patient to drink plenty of liquids, about 2,000–3,000 milliliters daily, *to reduce potential creation of kidney stones.* Encourage the patient to have an alkaline-ash diet *to increase the urine pH, to decrease the precipitation of uric acid, and to improve the action of gouty medications.*
7. NURSING DIAGNOSIS: Infection ***related to septic joint*** **(NANDA-I © 2012)**	
Outcome: Decrease of infectious signs and symptoms such as redness, warmth at the joint, and pain. ***Evaluation Parameter:*** Evaluation includes absence of infection exhibited by decreased pain and swelling, normal temperature, normal white blood cell count, and negative wound cultures.	The nurse must support and immobilize the affected joint in a splint. *Because the inflammatory process can cause scar tissue within the joint, it is important to splint the joint in a functional position.* Analgesics are prescribed *to control pain.* After the infection has responded to antibiotic therapy, anti-inflammatory medication such as NSAIDs may be used *to limit joint damage.*
8. NURSING DIAGNOSIS: Therapeutic Regimen Management, Effective. ***related to patient understanding and compliance*** **(NANDA-I © 2012)**	
Outcome: Patient will adhere to the therapeutic regimen. ***Evaluation Parameter:*** Patient verbalizes compliance to the prescribed therapeutic regimen.	Patient will verbalize compliance with the following: Foods low in purine (relates to gout) and calories Compliance to medication Comfort Management of weight loss or maintenance Exercise: passive and active range of motion. *Compliance to the above therapeutic regimen will empower the patient to take control of the disease by utilizing gained knowledge about therapeutic treatment.*
9. NURSING DIAGNOSIS: Body Image, Disturbed ***related to disfigurement of joints*** **(NANDA-I © 2012)**	
Outcome: Patient will be accepting of changes in body. ***Evaluation Parameter:*** Patient is able to openly discuss feelings surrounding joint disfigurement.	Provide an atmosphere in which a rapport can be built with the patient by listening actively. Time must be made for the patient to feel comfortable to verbalize feelings or concerns. *Allow the patient time to express feelings and build trust.* Assist the patient in making realistic short- and long-term goals; support the patient by providing referrals to local chapters of the American Arthritis Association and other organizations. *Speaking with others who have the same disease allows the patient to discuss feelings in a nonjudgmental environment.*

Source: Adapted from Wilkinson, J. M., & Ahearn, N. R. (2009). *Prentice Hall nursing diagnosis handbook* (9th ed.). Upper Saddle River, NJ: Prentice Hall.

atrophy. Refer to the Nursing Process: Patient Care Plan for Arthritis on page 1572.

Because RA is a chronic disease, discussing discharge priorities is essential. For more information, see the Patient Teaching & Discharge Priorities box for the patient with rheumatoid arthritis.

Psoriatic Arthritis

Epidemiology and Etiology

Psoriatic arthritis is an inflammatory process associated with psoriasis. For a detailed explanation of psoriasis, refer to Chapter 59. Initially, psoriatic arthritis was considered a variant of

PATIENT TEACHING & DISCHARGE PRIORITIES for Osteoarthritis

Need	Teaching
Because the joints affected are weight bearing, it is important not to contribute to stress of those joints by additional weight.	Encourage patients who are obese to reduce weight.
Increase mobility. Maintain range of motion.	Promote the patient to participate in an exercise program (stretching, passive and active range of motion, swimming, t'ai chi).
Do not exacerbate symptoms. Joint protection.	Modify work or home environment to accommodate limited weight bearing.
Reduce pain and avoid complications of drug therapy.	Teach about each drug classification, how to take the medication, drug interactions, adverse effects, and how to report any complications to the health care provider.

LABORATORY AND DIAGNOSTIC TESTS for Rheumatoid Arthritis

Test, Normal Values, and Rationale	Expected Abnormality
Laboratory Tests	
Rheumatoid Factor Normal: Less than 1:20 titer; less than 1:40 chronic inflammatory disease; 1:20–1:80 positive for RA and other conditions; >1:80 positive for RA *To detect antibodies found in rheumatoid arthritis.*	Positive
Anticitrulline Antibody Normal: Negative *Indicates presence of RA in the absence of rheumatoid factor. With RA, proteins may be changed to citrulline as part of the process that leads to inflammation of the joint (Stoppler, 2008).*	Positive
Antinuclear Antibodies Normal: Negative at 1:20 dilution *Indicates presence of RA.*	Positive
Erythrocyte Sedimentation Rate (ESR) Normal: Male: <50 years old: 0–15 mm/hour >50 years old: 0–20 mm/hour Female: <50 years old: 0–20 mm/hour >50 years old: 0–30 mm/hour *Presence of inflammatory disease.*	Increased
Radiologic Test	
X-Ray Normal: Normal joint surfaces *Articular surfaces are worn where bone rubs against bone.*	Degenerative changes Narrowing of bone space

Source: Kee, J. L. (2010). *Laboratory and diagnostic tests with nursing implications* (8th ed.). Upper Saddle River, NJ: Prentice Hall.

PATIENT TEACHING & DISCHARGE PRIORITIES for Rheumatoid Arthritis

Need	Teaching
Pain control	Teach the patient about medications that assist in managing pain.
Maintaining joint function	Active range of motion. Passive range of motion. Gentle exercise, such as swimming or moving joints in a Jacuzzi.
Rest	Alternate activities with periods of rest. Elevate affected joint to optimize circulation.

rheumatoid arthritis, but it is now recognized as a distinct clinical entity (Gladman, 2011b).

Psoriatic arthritis does not favor either gender. Among patients with psoriasis, estimates of prevalence vary from 4% to 6% up to 30%. Psoriatic arthritis carries an incidence of approximately 6 per 100,000 per year and a prevalence of approximately 1 to 2 per 1,000. The exact cause of psoriatic arthritis and of psoriasis itself is not known. It is thought that certain genetic, immunologic, and environmental factors contribute to the disease. Psoriasis is known to occur in families; approximately 40% of patients with psoriasis have a family history of the disease in first-degree relatives (Gladman, 2011b).

Psoriatic arthritis had not been considered an autoimmune disease, but a number of immune abnormalities have been identified in patients with psoriasis and psoriatic arthritis:

- Elevated serum levels of immunoglobulins and antinuclear antibodies.
- T-cell expression of HLA-DR molecules and receptors for interleukin-2 with a variety of adhesion molecules and the secretion of proinflammatory cytokines.
- Enhanced proliferative activity and platelet-derived growth factors in fibroblasts from the synovium (Gladman, 2011a).

Environmental factors that have been associated with the development of psoriasis and psoriatic arthritis include bacterial and viral infections and trauma (Gladman, 2011a). Patients who develop psoriatic arthritis frequently have a history of trauma to that joint prior to the onset of the disease. It is not clear how the trauma is related to psoriatic arthritis.

Pathophysiology

Psoriatic arthritis is an autoimmune disease with a known human leukocyte antigen (HLA)-associated risk factor. Psoriatic arthritis causes inflammation of insertion sites of tendons, ligaments, and joint capsules, as well as swelling of the digits. This disease occasionally develops even in the absence of detectable psoriasis. Psoriatic arthritis may occur at higher frequencies when skin involvement is more severe, especially when pustular psoriasis is present; however, recent studies suggest that this might not be the case (Hammadi, 2010).

Clinical Manifestations

Patients with psoriatic arthritis present with pain and stiffness in the affected joints. The stiffness worsens with prolonged immobility and is alleviated with physical activity. The affected joints will be tender, will be painful when the joint is stressed, and will present with effusions (abnormal fluid buildup). Most patients with psoriatic arthritis present with polyarthritis (i.e., involving five or more joints simultaneously); next most common is oligoarthritis (involving one to four joints simultaneously). Distal arthritis (affecting the distal joints of the fingers or toes) and arthritis mutilans (severe, deforming, and destructive) affect smaller percentages of patients (Gladman, 2011a). Other common features of psoriatic arthritis are soft-tissue inflammation at the site of tendon insertions into the bone and **dactylitis** (a uniform swelling of the soft tissues between the metacarpophalangeal and interphalangeal joints). With dactylitis, there is diffuse swelling of the entire digit, which is often referred to as "sausage digit." Dactylitis occurs in approximately one-half of patients with psoriatic arthritis and is associated with an increased risk of progressive joint damage (Gladman, 2011a). The patient may also have nail involvement characterized by pits in the nail plate and onycholysis (separation of the lateral edges of the nail plate from the nail bed).

Laboratory and Diagnostic Procedures

There is no specific diagnostic laboratory test for psoriatic arthritis. Approximately one-third of patients have an elevated sedimentation rate and leukocytosis showing an inflammatory response. Rheumatoid factor (RF) is found in only 2% to 10% of patients with psoriatic arthritis. The presence of joint damage is seen radiologically in two-thirds of patients at diagnosis. Radiologic findings show both erosive changes and new bone formation in the distal joints. Magnetic resonance imaging (MRI) reveals inflammation in the adjacent bone marrow and soft tissues with the appearance of inflammation of **entheses** (inflammation at the insertion site of ligaments, tendons, and fascia into bone) in joints that may not be clinically inflamed. These findings suggest that enthesitis is the primary lesion in psoriatic arthritis. Psoriatic arthritis is also associated with decreased bone mineral density, which may lead to osteoporosis and increased risk of fractures (Chapter 49).

Medical Management

The first line of treatment for psoriatic arthritis is typically the administration of nonsteroidal anti-inflammatory medications (NSAIDs). The use of both selective cyclooxygenase-2 (COX-2) inhibitors and nonselective NSAIDs is common, and the choice is usually according to health care provider or patient preference. This class of drug controls the mild inflammatory features of psoriatic arthritis. The combination of nonselective NSAIDs with an antiulcer drug may reduce the risk of gastroduodenal damage from the drug. Antiulcer drugs are discussed in Chapter 37.

If the arthritis does not respond to NSAIDs and the patient exhibits polyarticular involvement, the patient may benefit from early use of disease-modifying antirheumatic drugs (DMARDs). Also, patients whose psoriasis and arthritis are of equal severity may benefit from medications used for control of psoriasis. Although there is a lack of evidence of its efficacy, methotrexate has been the drug of choice for psoriatic arthritis (Gladman, 2011a). The most serious potential side effects of methotrexate are liver toxicity, bone marrow suppression, and interstitial lung disease. Because of the liver toxicity, patients must not consume alcohol when taking methotrexate. If the patient refuses to abstain from alcohol, sulfasalazine may be used as long as there is no known allergy to sulfa drugs. If the disease does not improve after 3 months of treatment with a DMARD, then an antitumor necrosis factor (anti-TNF) agent may be introduced. Etanercept and infliximab have received regulatory approval for the treatment of psoriatic arthritis. See the Pharmacology box on page 1567 for a summary of medications used to treat arthritis.

Any patient with psoriasis who has the complaint of joint discomfort should be evaluated for psoriatic arthritis. The patient's goals include relief of pain, treatment of the infection, rehabilitation of the joint after the infection subsides, and knowledge of the treatment regimen. Evaluation parameters include control of pain as expressed by the patient, absence of signs and symptoms of infection, and the patient's ability to articulate the plan of care. Patients may obtain complete relief of joint tenderness and swelling and, with continued use of medication, avoid a relapse. Patients who present with mild disease, less disability, and male gender have a greater likelihood of achieving remission (Gladman, 2011a). Assessment and protection of the affected joint are important to the success of treatment.

Nursing Management

Nursing management focuses on the same issues as with all types of arthritis: early recognition, pain relief, and protection of the joint from

Weblink: Gout

further damage. The nurse may support and immobilize the affected joint in a splint. Because the inflammatory process can cause scar tissue within the joint, it is important to splint the joint in a functional position. Analgesics are prescribed to control pain, and anti-inflammatory medications such as NSAIDs may be used to control joint inflammation. Refer to the Nursing Process: Patient Care Plan for Arthritis box on page 1572.

Gouty Arthritis

Epidemiology and Etiology

Gouty arthritis is a condition in which there is an imbalance in purine metabolism, which increases uric acid in the joints and leads to the formation of uric acid crystals (MedlinePlus Medical Encyclopedia, 2011). Gout can affect any joint but most commonly affects the joints of the feet, especially the hallus (great toe). According to the National Institutes of Health, approximately 275 people out of 100,000 are affected (MedlinePlus Medical Encyclopedia, 2011). Gouty arthritis accounts for 5% of cases of arthritis (National Institute of Arthritis and Musculoskeletal and Skin Diseases [NIAMS], 2009a). Primary gout, which occurs alone, is most commonly seen in men over age 30 and postmenopausal women. Secondary gout, which is associated with other medical conditions or medications such as diuretics, occurs in older adults (Frazier & Drzymkowski, 2009).

The cause of primary gout is unknown, but the disorder is thought to have a hereditary component with a defect in purine metabolism. Primary gout is more common in men than in women and is more common in individuals who are overweight. Onset of an acute attack of gout sometimes follows excessive eating or drinking (MedlinePlus Medical Encyclopedia, 2011). Risk factors include heredity, an enzyme defect, and exposure to lead (MedlinePlus Medical Encyclopedia, 2011).

Pathophysiology

With gouty arthritis, there is an imbalance in purine metabolism. Instead of the uric acid crystals being excreted through the kidneys, they accumulate in the joints. These crystals are needlelike, causing excruciating pain, usually in the joints of the elbows, wrist, fingers, knees, ankles, and toes; 75% of patients are affected in the great toe (Figure 51–3◆) (NIAMS, 2009a). Gout follows an intermittent course, and a patient can be free from symptoms for years between attacks.

Clinical Manifestations

Gout progression has four stages: asymptomatic hyperuricemia, acute gout episode, interval gout, and advanced chronic tophaceous gout (Mandell, 2008). During the asymptomatic stage, there is an elevation of uric acid in the blood but no symptoms. In the second stage, acute gout episode, an increasing number of uric acid crystals accumulate in the space of the joints. Uric acid crystals can also settle in cartilage in the earlobes, where they are referred to as **tophi.** During this stage, the patient experiences a sudden onset of severe pain, usually in the night. Other manifestations include increased swelling and inflammation, which cause the affected part to feel hot. Some patients will experience knifelike pain in the earlobe, elbow, or feet. This sudden attack can be triggered by stress, illness, or the consumption of alcohol or drugs. Without treatment, this phase can last from 3 to 10 days. Interval gout is the period of time during which the condition is in remission. The fourth stage, chronic tophaceous gout, occurs when uric acid crystals continue to accumulate and patients develop stiff and swollen joints. This stage is uncommon unless the illness is not treated, which results in disabling effects such as permanent damage to the joints and kidneys (Mandell, 2008).

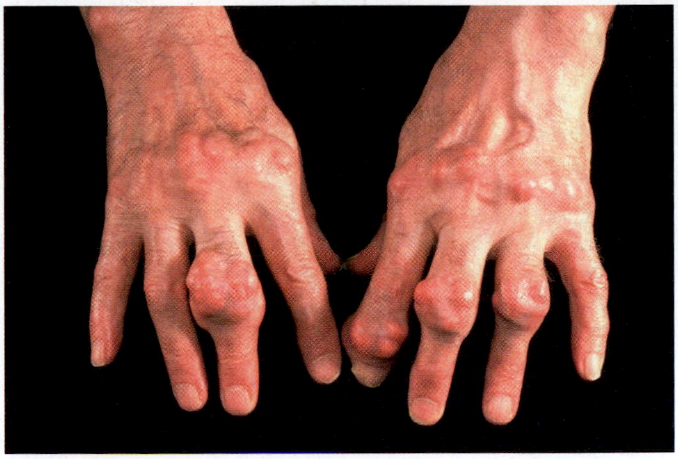

FIGURE 51–3 ◆ Instead of the uric acid crystals being excreted through the kidneys, they accumulate in the joints. These crystals are needlelike, causing excruciating pain, usually in the joints of the elbows, wrists, fingers, knees, ankles, and toes, with 75% of patients affected in the great toe.

Source: Medical-on-line/Alamy

Laboratory and Diagnostic Procedures

Elevated blood levels of uric acid occur in some individuals with gouty arthritis, but levels of uric acid are normal in approximately 10% of people during an acute attack of gouty arthritis. Moreover, they are elevated in 5% to 8% of the general population, so the presence of an elevated level does not necessarily mean that gout is the cause of an inflamed joint. X-ray examination of the joint is primarily used to assess underlying joint damage, especially in patients who have had multiple episodes of gouty arthritis. The most useful and accurate test is joint aspiration. A needle is inserted into the joint to withdraw a sample of fluid, which is examined to see whether gout crystals or bacterial infection is present. Sometimes other crystals can be found in the joint fluid, such as calcium pyrophosphate, which is caused by an entirely different condition called pseudogout ("like gout"). Joint aspiration is the ultimate method of being certain of a diagnosis of gouty arthritis, ruling out other causes such as an infection in the joint (eMedicineHealth, 2011).

Medical Management

Medical management of gouty arthritis focuses on mitigating the clinical manifestations. Medications that are used specifically for gout include colchicine and allopurinol. These drugs reduce uric acid production, thus reducing the inflammatory process. It is important to monitor uric acid levels while the patient is on medication (Frazier & Drzymkowski, 2009). See the Pharmacology box on page 1567 for a summary of medications used to treat gouty arthritis.

Patients with gout must adhere to a dietary regimen to reduce the consumption of purines. Foods that should be avoided are dried beans and peas, organ meats, wheat germ, rich foods such as gravies, anchovies, and other seafood. Patients should consume a moderate amount of protein. The recommendation is to eat only 200 grams of meat, poultry, or fish twice weekly and to eliminate organ meats. Alcohol consumption should be limited to 1 drink 3 times a week. Beer ingestion should be completely discontinued, as beer has a high purine count and increases gout risks regardless of amount (Hogan, 2007). A high-protein, low-carbohydrate diet is not recommended because this can worsen the

EVIDENCE-BASED PRACTICE Treatment of Gouty Arthritis

Clinical Problem

An acute attack of gouty arthritis is very painful. The drug colchicine has been used to decrease the symptoms related to gout but has gastrointestinal side effects that may increase the patient's distress.

Research Findings

A comparison was done with a sample size of 43 patients to determine whether colchicine was more effective than placebo (Schlesinger, Schumacher, Catton, & Maxwell, 2009). Patients who had taken colchicine experienced a reduction of the following symptoms: pain (34%) and tenderness on palpation, swelling, and redness (30%). However, all patients on colchicine (100%) developed vomiting and/or diarrhea.

Implications for Nursing Practice

The actual medication improved acute gout attacks but caused adverse gastrointestinal effects in all who took it. These effects were related to the dosage frequency necessary to reduce pain, swelling, and other symptoms causing the gout attack. Encouraging patients to maintain a low purine diet and avoid excessive use of alcohol in order to prevent an acute attack may be a better alternative for the patient.

Critical Thinking Questions with answers can be found in the Osborn Student Resources at nursing.pearsonhighered.com.

Source: Schlesinger, N., Schumacher, M. C., Catton, M., & Maxwell, L. (2009). Colchicine for acute gout. *Cochrane Database of Systematic Reviews*, 2006, Issue 4. Retrieved from http://mrw.interscience.wiley.com/cochrane/clsysrev/articles/CD006190/frame.html.

symptoms. Because fat intake should also be limited, patients should select low-fat meats and use nonsaturated oils. Increasing fluid intake is critical to dilute urinary uric acid crystals. Patients should consume between 2 and 3 liters of fluid daily (Hogan, 2007). See the Evidence-Based Practice box for a discussion of the research on the treatment of gouty arthritis. Long-term goals should be focused on patients becoming compliant to medication and dietary regimens.

Nursing Management

The Nursing Process: Patient Care Plan for Arthritis box (p. 1572) outlines the nursing management of the patient with gouty arthritis.

Health Promotion

Because gouty arthritis is caused by indulging in foods that are high in purines, it can be controlled by eating a well-balanced, low-calorie, low-purine diet and by reducing alcohol consumption. Foods to be avoided are alcohol, organ meats, dried beans and peas, wheat germ, seafood, and rich foods such as gravies and anchovies. These foods will increase uric acid in the blood and can lead to uric acid crystal buildup, which most often results in accumulation of uric acid crystals in the joint of the great toe. Pain medications are not the treatment of choice for gouty arthritis; rather, antigout medications and dietary therapy are used to reduce the uric acid level.

The main vulnerability factor for acquiring gouty arthritis is an increased uric acid level in the blood. Guidelines for reducing the incidence of gouty arthritis are featured in the National Guidelines box.

NATIONAL GUIDELINES for Reducing the Incidence of Gouty Arthritis

Healthy People 2020 is a set of government objectives that encourages a healthy lifestyle. Its main goal is to improve the quality of the nation's health by creating a framework for public health prevention priorities and actions (U.S. Department of Health and Human Services [DHHS], 2010). It is important, in caring for a patient with gouty arthritis, to provide the proper education that will enhance the patient's health. With gout, there is an increase of uric acids from purine metabolism, and diets that are high in purine can cause gout. Two of the health indicators identified by *Healthy People 2020* are overweight/obesity and substance abuse. People who are overweight are typically consuming foods that are high in purines; therefore, this population of people is more at risk for gouty arthritis. It is imperative for the patient to understand that behavioral changes will reduce, if not eliminate, this disease process and promote a healthy lifestyle. If the patient consumes an increased amount of alcohol, uric acid will be metabolized from the liver and passed in the bloodstream to be excreted in the kidneys.

Therefore, it is important to remember two factors in caring for a patient with gout: The increased consumption of foods high in purines results in high uric acid in the blood, and the decreased ability to excrete uric acids from the kidneys causes a buildup of uric acid crystals in the tissues. Healthy lifestyle choices can make the difference between one acute attack of gouty arthritis and a lifetime of gout attacks.

Source: U.S. Department of Health and Human Services (DHHS). (2010). *Healthy People 2020.* Retrieved from http://www.healthypeople.gov.

Reactive Arthritis

Epidemiology and Etiology

Reactive arthritis is a type of arthritis that develops soon after or during an infection somewhere else in the body (Yu, 2010). This disease is more common in men than in women. Men between ages 20 and 40 more frequently develop reactive arthritis. When the trigger is a sexually transmitted infection, men with this condition still outnumber women by 9%. Foodborne infections do not discriminate between genders in transmitting reactive arthritis; however, women experience a milder case with remissions and exacerbations (NIAMS, 2009b).

Reactive arthritis is a noncontagious disease. However, it can be triggered by a communicable infection (NIAMS, 2009b). Reactive arthritis usually begins between 1 and 3 weeks after the person becomes infected. Without treatment *Chlamydia trachomatis*, an organism that is spread through sexual contact, can cause reactive arthritis and a respiratory infection known as *Chlamydia pneumoniae*. Gastrointestinal infections such as *Salmonella*, *Shigella*, *Yersinia*, and *Campylobacter* also are responsible for causing reactive arthritis (NIAMS, 2009b).

Pathophysiology

Reactive arthritis develops approximately 2 to 6 weeks after a genitourinary or gastrointestinal infection. Approximately 10% of patients do not have a preceding infection (Lozada, 2010). The mechanism of how the inciting organism interacts with the host cells is not known. It is unclear whether the antigens cross-react with self-proteins, stimulating a Th2-cell-mediated autoimmune response.

Clinical Manifestations

Clinical manifestations of reactive arthritis include inflammation of joints, entheses, the axial skeleton, and mucous membranes; gastrointestinal tract upset; conjunctivitis; unilateral uveitis of the eye (inflammation of the uvea, the middle layer of the eye); and skin lesions called **circinate balanitis,** which are white plaques that grow centrifugally and eventually cover the entire surface of the glans penis in males.

PATIENT TEACHING & DISCHARGE PRIORITIES for Reactive Arthritis

Need	Teaching
Pain control	Teach the patient about medications that assist in managing the patient's pain.
Maintaining joint function	Active and passive range of motion.
	Gentle exercise, such as swimming or moving joints in a hot tub or whirlpool bath.
Rest	Alternate activities with periods of rest.
Adherence to therapeutic regimen	Elevate affected joint to optimize circulation.
	Of importance are adherence to the antibiotic regimen, support of the affected joint, and adherence to weight-bearing and activity restrictions during the inflammatory process to prevent permanent damage to the joint.
Aseptic technique	If joint fluid was surgically drained, the nurse teaches the patient aseptic techniques for dressing changes and wound care.

Asymmetrical joint swelling often occurs, especially in the lower extremities (knees and ankles) (Yu, 2010).

Laboratory and Diagnostic Procedures

There is no specific laboratory test that can be used to diagnose reactive arthritis. The diagnosis is based on recognition of the combination of arthritis with inflammation of the eyes and the genital, urinary, and/or gastrointestinal systems. The Laboratory and Diagnostic Tests box provides more information on tests for undifferentiated spondyloarthropathy, the family of related disorders that includes reactive arthritis and psoriatic arthritis. The spondyloarthropathies are linked by common genetics, the human leukocyte antigen (HLA) class I gene HLA-B27, and a common pathology (Brent, 2011).

Medical Management

Treatment of reactive arthritis involves symptom control and prevention. The medications that are most commonly used are (1) nonsteroidal anti-inflammatory drugs to reduce joint inflammation, (2) glucocorticoids to reduce severe joint inflammation, (3) topical glucocorticoids to reduce skin lesions and promote healing, (4) anti-infectives to treat infections, (5) immunosuppressants to suppress the immune system when previous medications have not been effective, and (6) tumor necrosis factor inhibitor drugs to reduce a protein involved with inflammation when other medication therapies are ineffective (NIAMS, 2009b). See the Pharmacology box on page 1567 for a summary of medications used to treat arthritis and connective tissue disorders.

Physical activity is needed to promote range of motion in the affected joints. Range-of-motion exercises reduce stiffness and promote flexibility. Using hydrotherapies can also assist the patient in maximizing movement of the joints of the body, especially the limbs and spine.

Nursing Management

The nursing management for the patient with reactive arthritis is the same as management for patients with other arthritis conditions. Refer to the Nursing Process: Patient Care Plan for Arthritis on page 1572. Discharge priorities for the patient with reactive arthritis are described in Patient Teaching & Discharge Priorities box above.

Ankylosing Spondylitis

Epidemiology and Etiology

Ankylosing spondylitis (AS) is a type of arthritis that affects the spine and the sacroiliac joints. This systemic inflammatory disease is usually progressive and affects primarily the spinal column (Figure 51–4◆). Like reactive arthritis, AS is classified as a spondyloarthropathy. The patient may also experience fatigue, weight loss, fever, and diarrhea as well as eye pain and photophobia due to uveitis (Frazier & Drzymkowski, 2009). In the United States, AS affects 129 out of 100,000 people, mainly adolescents and young adults. It is most common among Native Americans but also affects other ethnicities (American College of Rheumatology, 2008). It is more

LABORATORY AND DIAGNOSTIC TESTS for Undifferentiated Spondyloarthropathy

Test, Normal Values, and Rationale	Expected Abnormality
Erythrocyte Sedimentation Rate (ESR)	
Normal:	Elevated
Male: <50 years old: 0–15 mm/hour	
>50 years old: 0–20 mm/hour	
Female: <50 years old: 0–20 mm/hour	
>50 years old: 0–30 mm/hour	
Sedimentation rate increases with an acute inflammatory process, acute and chronic infections, and rheumatoid diseases.	
C-Reactive Protein (CRP)	
Normal: Not present or for N high sensitivity CRP, < 0.175 mg/L	Elevated
C-reactive protein is produced in the liver in response to tissue injury and inflammation. It appears in the blood 6 to 10 hours after an acute inflammatory process and tissue destruction.	

Source: Kee, J. L. (2010). *Laboratory and diagnostic tests with nursing implications* (8th ed.). Upper Saddle River, NJ: Prentice Hall.

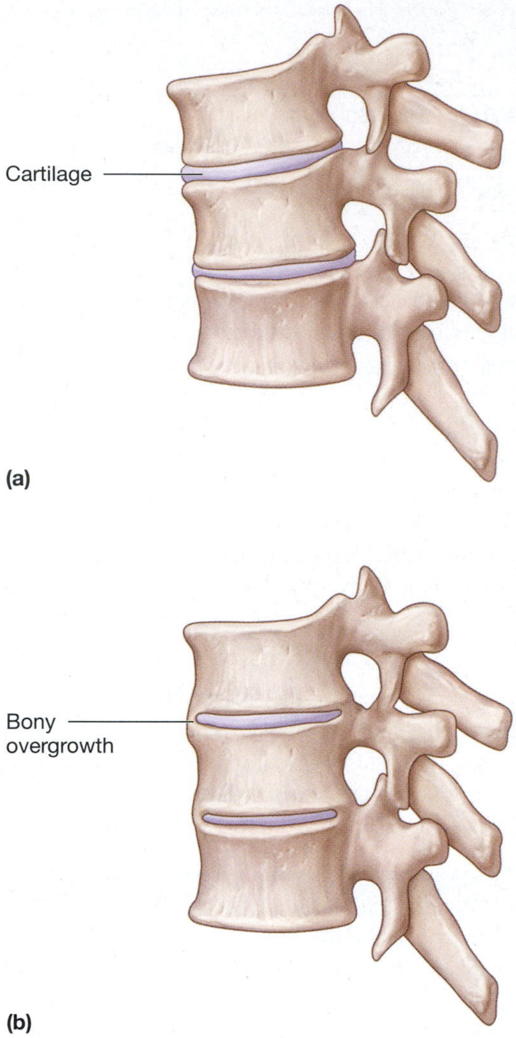

FIGURE 51–4 ◆ Bony overgrowth of ankylosing spondylitis. (A) Normal vertebrae. (B) Vertebrae with bony overgrowth typical of ankylosing spondylitis.

common in men than in women and typically begins in the sacroiliac area and adjacent soft tissues (Frazier & Drzymkowski, 2009).

It is not certain how a patient gets AS. However, there is a common genetic marker, called HLA-B27, in affected individuals. Some individuals become predisposed after bowel or urinary tract infections (American College of Rheumatology, 2008).

Pathophysiology

Ankylosing spondylitis is a chronic inflammatory disease that commonly involves the axial skeleton and sacroiliac joints. Peripheral joints and entheses with certain extra-articular organs, including the eyes, skin, and cardiovascular system, may also be involved to a lesser degree. The pathology is known as enthesitis (inflammation where tendons or ligaments insert into the bone); chronic inflammation leads to fibrosis and ossification at the sites of enthesitis (Brent, 2011).

Clinical Manifestations

Ankylosing spondylitis usually occurs first in the sacroiliac area. The patient may experience low back pain and stiffness in the morning that improves with activity. An early sign is a loss of flexibility in the lumbar spine. Arthritis can occur in attaching joints, tendons, and ligaments in the shoulder, hips, and feet. As the inflammation increases and healing occurs, new bone growth fuses the bones together such as in the ribs and vertebrae (American College of Rheumatology, 2008). With the resulting restriction of the ribs, lung capacity may be impaired as well as normal functioning in activities of daily living. As the condition advances, there can be eye inflammation, and the valves of the heart can be affected (American College of Rheumatology, 2008). The patient may also have a history of inflammatory bowel disease (Chapter 37) or a family history of arthritis (Frazier & Drzymkowski, 2009).

Laboratory and Diagnostic Procedures

Laboratory tests used in diagnosing AS include sedimentation rate, indicating inflammation (refer to the Laboratory and Diagnostic Tests for Undifferentiated Spondyloarthropathy box on page 1579), and HLA-B27 assay, indicating an increase to confirm the diagnosis of AS. Diagnostic tests that are helpful to confirm the diagnosis are x-rays and bone scans (American College of Rheumatology, 2008).

Medical Management

Early detection, diagnosis, and treatment of AS are the best plan in controlling it (American College of Rheumatology, 2008). Medications that are helpful in treating AS include nonsteroidal anti-inflammatory medications and methotrexate (an oncology chemotherapeutic agent). See the Pharmacology box on page 1567 for a summary of medications used to treat arthritis and connective tissue disorders.

Rest is just as important as physical activity, and the patient needs to plan rest periods during the day. The patient requires an ample amount of sleep during the night as well (American College of Rheumatology, 2008).

Nursing Management

Nursing assessment for AS includes evaluating the specific joint and back manifestations described earlier. The assessment also must include an in-depth assessment of other organs that may be affected. Refer to the Nursing Process: Patient Care Plan for Arthritis box on page 1572. Patient teaching and discharge priorities are the same as those for reactive arthritis (refer to the Patient Teaching & Discharge Priorities box on page 1579).

Septic Arthritis

Epidemiology and Etiology

Nongonococcal bacterial arthritis (**septic arthritis**) is the most destructive form of acute arthritis and can result from trauma, direct inoculation of bacteria during joint surgery, or hematogenous (via the blood) spread of infection from another part of the body. It also may occur when an infection from an adjacent bone extends through the cortex into the joint space (Goldenberg & Sexton, 2011).

The annual incidence of septic arthritis is estimated to be 2 to 5 per 100,000 persons. Predisposing factors include being over age 80; having rheumatoid arthritis, diabetes, or skin infection; having had recent joint surgery; having a prosthetic joint; and oral carriage of *Staphylococcus aureus* (Goldenberg & Sexton, 2011; Kherani & Shojania, 2007). Each of the predisposing factors has a modest impact on the risk; however, combinations of the factors lead to a substantially increased risk.

Pathophysiology

In the majority of cases, septic arthritis arises from hematogenous spread of bacteria to the joint. Common sources of the infection include intravenous drug use, indwelling catheters, and an underlying immunocompromised state such as HIV infection. Bacteria are more likely to localize in a joint with preexisting arthritis,

CHART 51–1 Causes of Septic Arthritis

Organism	Clinical Clues
S. aureus	Healthy adult with skin breakdown, previously damaged joint, or prosthetic joint
Streptococcus	Healthy adult, splenic dysfunction
Neisseria gonorrhoeae	Healthy sexually active adult, associated tenosynovitis, vesicular pustules, and negative synovial fluid culture and Gram stain
Aerobic or anaerobic gram-negative bacteria	Immune-compromised patients, gastrointestinal infection
Mycobacterium species	Immune-compromised patient with recent travel to or residence in an endemic area
Fungal	Immune-compromised patients
Spirochete	Exposure to ticks

Source: Adapted from Goldenberg, D., & Sexton, D. (2011). Bacterial (nongonococcal) arthritis in adults. *UpToDate.* Retrieved from http://www.uptodate.com/patients/content/topic.do?topicKey=~hcmhzYL2SL2ACJ&selectedTitle=7~147&source=search_result.

and patients with rheumatoid arthritis are especially susceptible (Goldenberg & Sexton, 2011). Any microbial pathogen can cause septic arthritis, but organisms such as *S. aureus* and *Streptococcus* more commonly cause joint infections than do gram-negative bacilli. Most joint infections are monomicrobial; rare polymicrobial infections occur in patients with penetrating trauma that involves the joint space. Initially, the bacteria deposit in the synovial membrane and produce an acute inflammatory response. The bacteria quickly enter the synovial fluid, creating purulent joint inflammation. Within 1 week, the synovial membrane develops hyperplasia (an increase in the number of normal cells), and the cytokines and proteases that were released cause cartilage degradation and inhibit cartilage synthesis. With large effusions, pressure necrosis can result in further cartilage and bone loss. Chart 51–1 outlines causes of infectious arthritis with clinical clues.

Clinical Manifestations

Patients with septic arthritis present with a single swollen and painful joint. Joints that are commonly affected are the knee (>50% of cases), wrist, ankles, and hips (Goldenberg & Sexton, 2011). Systemic chills, fever, and leukocytosis are usually present. There may also be evidence of an associated skin, urinary, or respiratory infection.

Laboratory and Diagnostic Procedures and Medical Management

The definitive diagnostic test for septic arthritis is the identification of bacteria via a culture of the synovial fluid obtained from joint aspiration. The infection is treated with broad-spectrum intravenous antibiotics initially and then with organism-specific antibiotics when the culture results are available. Intravenous antibiotics are continued until symptoms disappear. Therapy typically lasts 3 to 4 weeks, with approximately 2 weeks of intravenous antibiotics and the remainder with oral antibiotics. Progressive range-of-motion exercises will be needed once the infection has subsided. The patient also is treated with antipyretics and pain medication as necessary.

Nursing Management

Nursing management for septic arthritis focuses on early recognition, pain relief, and protection of the joint from further damage. The nursing process provides a framework for organizing and managing the care of patients with septic arthritis. Refer to the Nursing Process: Patient Care Plan for Arthritis on page 1572. Discharge priorities are the same as those for patients with reactive arthritis (page 1579).

Collaborative Management

To achieve optimal functioning, patients with arthritis need a multidisciplinary team approach, including health care providers, nurses, social workers, physical therapists, pharmacists, occupational therapists, psychologists or psychiatrists, and dietitians. In order to meet desired patient outcomes, it is essential that the interdisciplinary team communicate openly with one another in developing and evaluating care of the patient and family (IOM [Institute of Medicine], 2010).

Utilizing the multidisciplinary team to assist the patient in maintaining function is essential. Physical therapy and occupational therapy can assist the patient in remaining functional. Ongoing physical therapy will help to increase range of motion in the joints. The occupational therapist assists the patient with exercises that will enhance fine motor movements. The social worker and a psychologist/psychiatrist are used to help the patient adjust to a chronic illness. Respiratory therapy will assist the patient in maintaining lung function if the spine and ribs are involved. The patient can enhance lung capacity through swimming or aerobic activities. Finally, a comprehensive plan for nutrition is important for teaching the patient and family about dietary restrictions. The pharmacist helps the team coordinate the medication regimen.

Specialists must be incorporated in caring for a patient with reactive arthritis depending on symptoms. These specialists might include an ophthalmologist for eye disease, a gynecologist for female genital disease, a urologist to treat genitourinary disease in both males and females, a dermatologist for skin lesions, an orthopedist for surgical intervention with joint disease, a rheumatologist for arthritis, and a physical therapist for promoting joint function.

Health Promotion

The nurse should encourage patients who have arthritis to remain as independent as possible. Independence may be achieved by using assistive devices such as splints, walkers, or canes for performing activities of daily living and ambulation. It is important to encourage patients to pace activities with rest in order to prevent fatigue. The nurse can teach patients to use body mechanics for body posture to help patients achieve better balance and not add additional stress to the joints. Allowing patients to verbalize their frustrations may help them to adapt to their disabilities. The nurse should also encourage patient self-determination so that the patient with arthritis can achieve the highest possible level of function. Providing patients with knowledge is critical when patients need to make decisions about all types of treatment choices. See the Gerontologic Considerations section on page 1589 for more information.

Health teaching should include education regarding the adverse effects of NSAIDs because gastrointestinal upset and gastric bleeding are common. Black, tarry stools are a sign of gastric bleeding.

Safety Alert *Ringing in the ears (tinnitus) is a toxic side effect of aspirin use. The nurse should monitor these adverse effects with patients who are taking a high dosage of aspirin.*

Connective Tissue Disorders

Connective tissue disorders are not just one disease, but a collection of more than 100 unique conditions that can destroy the connective tissue of the joints and may have results ranging from daily pain to complete immobility. Common connective tissue disorders include lupus erythematosus, scleroderma, Lyme disease, and Sjögren's syndrome. It is projected that 37% of the population in the United States, or 1 million people, have a genetic connective tissue disorder (WrongDiagnosis.com, 2011). Making a definitive diagnosis of a connective tissue disorder can be very difficult because signs and symptoms are often vague.

Systemic Lupus Erythematosus

Epidemiology and Etiology

Systemic lupus erythematosus (SLE) is a chronic inflammatory autoimmune disease that attacks connective tissue or organs. The disease is characterized by remissions and exacerbations; the exacerbations, also known as flare-ups, are common during the spring and summer months. Systemic lupus erythematosus affects mostly women and first appears when they are of childbearing age (Frazier & Drzymkowski, 2009). The etiology is unknown, but SLE is thought to result from a defect in the body's immunologic mechanism, a genetic predisposition, or an environmental stimulus. Chapter 53 includes a complete discussion of the immune mechanisms related to SLE.

Pathophysiology

A significant feature of SLE is the body's ability to form antibodies against many different tissue components. For a patient who is genetically susceptible, multiple predisposing factors are associated with SLE. These include physical or mental stress, exposure to sunlight or ultraviolet light, viral or streptococcal infections, pregnancy, and abnormal estrogen metabolism. A lupuslike syndrome can also be aggravated or triggered by specific medications such as procainamide, anticonvulsants, hydralazine, and, less commonly, sulfa drugs, penicillins, and hormonal contraceptives. For unknown reasons, certain immune complexes get deposited in blood vessels, among collagen fibers, and on organs. This causes inflammation, necrosis, and permanent damage in the major organs, including the kidneys, brain, eyes, lymphatic system, gastrointestinal tract, lungs, and skin.

Clinical Manifestations

Subjective assessment of SLE includes weakness, sensitivity to light, and pain in the joints. Objective assessment may reveal elevated temperatures; butterfly rash on the face and the palms of the hands, a type of Raynaud's disease; weight loss; and dysfunction in one or any of the organs of the renal, gastrointestinal, cardiac, respiratory, or neurological system. Raynaud's disease is discussed in Chapter 35. With gastrointestinal involvement, patients often experience ulcers in the mouth and nasopharyngeal areas. In fact, 90% of patients with SLE experience joint pain similar to that of reactive arthritis. In addition, renal complications such as glomerulonephritis are common. Central nervous system changes occur, such as headaches, irritability, and depression.

Laboratory and Diagnostic Procedures

Two specific tests are used to confirm the diagnosis of SLE: lupus erythematosus preparation (LE prep) and antinuclear antibodies (ANAs). Other laboratory tests include anti-DNA, anti-Sm antibody, serum complement test, and complement proteins C3 and C4. For more details, see the Laboratory and Diagnostic Tests box.

Medical Management

There is no cure for SLE; therefore, the goal of treatment is to relieve symptoms and protect organs by decreasing inflammation and/or the level of autoimmune activity in the body. Many patients with mild symptoms may need no treatment or only intermittent courses of anti-inflammatory medications. Patients with more serious illness involving damage to internal organs may require high doses of corticosteroids in combination with other medications that suppress the body's immune system (MedicineNet.com, 2011c). See the Pharmacology box on page 1567 for a summary of medications used to treat arthritis and connective tissue disorders.

Patients with SLE need more rest during periods of active disease. It is important for the nurse to work with the patient and family to develop a plan that addresses sleep quality and the effects of underlying depression, lack of exercise, and self-care coping strategies on overall health. During these periods, carefully prescribed exercise is still important to maintain muscle tone and range of motion in the joints.

Nonsteroidal anti-inflammatory drugs (NSAIDs) such as aspirin, ibuprofen (Motrin), naproxen (Naprosyn), and sulindac (Clinoril) are effective in reducing inflammation and pain in muscles, joints, and other tissues. Corticosteroids are more potent than NSAIDs; therefore, they are used to restore function when the disease is active and are particularly helpful when internal organs are involved. Corticosteroids can be given by mouth, injected directly into the joints and other tissues, or administered intravenously. Unfortunately, corticosteroids have serious side effects when given in high doses over prolonged periods, and the health care provider must monitor the activity of the disease in order to use the lowest doses that are safe (MedicineNet.com, 2011c). Hydroxychloroquine (Plaquenil) is an antimalarial medication that has been found to be particularly effective for SLE patients with fatigue, skin disorders, and joint disease. Hydroxychloroquine has also been found to be significantly effective in reducing the frequency of abnormal blood clots in SLE patients. For resistant skin disease, other antimalarial drugs such as chloroquine (Aralen) or quinacrine are considered and can be used in combination with hydroxychloroquine (MedicineNet.com, 2011c).

Immunosuppressive medications are used for treating patients who have more severe manifestations of SLE such as damage to internal organs. Some immunosuppressive medications are methotrexate (Rheumatrex, Trexall), azathioprine (Imuran), cyclophosphamide (Cytoxan), chlorambucil (Leukeran), and cyclosporine (Sandimmune). All immunosuppressive medications can seriously depress blood cell counts and increase risks of infection and bleeding. Most recent research is indicating benefits of rituximab (Rituxan) in treating lupus. Rituximab is an intravenously infused antibody that suppresses a particular white blood cell, the B cell, by decreasing the number of these cells in the circulation. B cells have been found to play a central role in lupus

LABORATORY AND DIAGNOSTIC TESTS for Systemic Lupus Erythematosus

Test, Normal Values, and Rationale	Expected Abnormality
Lupus Erythematosus (LE) Prep	
Normal: negativa, no LE cells	Elevated
Presence of systemic lupus erythematosus (SLE).	
Antinuclear Antibody (ANA)	
Normal: negative at 1:20 dilution	Elevated
Presence of autoantibodies in blood.	
Anti-DNA	
Normal: negative at 1:20 dilution	Present
Conclude whether there are antibodies in the genetic materials in the cell.	
Anti-Sm Antibody	
Normal: negative	Present
Antibodies present on the ribonucleoprotein on the cell nucleus.	
Serum Complement Test	
Normal: 75–160 unit/mL	Decreased
Presence of total group proteins, which can be consumed in immune reactions.	
Complement Proteins C3 and C4	
Normal:	Increased with early SLE
C3: Male: 80–180 mg/dL	Decreased with SLE
Female: 76–120 mg/dL	Decreased
C4: 15–45 mg/dL	
Examine specific levels of proteins present.	
Urinalysis (UA)	
Normal:	Hematuria
Protein: 2–8 mg/dL; negative reagent strip	Proteinuria
Glucose: negative	
Red blood cells: 1–2	
Casts: mixed hyaline	
Evidence of kidney involvement.	

Source: Kee, J. L. (2010). *Laboratory and diagnostic tests with nursing implications* (8th ed.). Upper Saddle River, NJ: Prentice Hall.

activity; when they are suppressed, the disease tends toward remission (MedicineNet.com, 2011c).

Recently, mycophenolate mofetil (CellCept) has been used as an effective medication for lupus that is associated with kidney disease. Mycophenolate mofetil helps to reverse active lupus kidney disease (lupus renal disease) and helps to maintain remission after the disease is established. Additionally, it has fewer side effects than the traditional immunosuppressive medications (MedicineNet.com, 2011c). The Pharmacology box on page 1567 discusses these medications.

In SLE patients with serious brain or kidney disease, plasmapheresis is sometimes used to remove antibodies and other immune substances in order to suppress immunity. Some SLE patients develop seriously low platelet levels, thereby increasing the risk for spontaneous bleeding. Because the spleen is believed to be the major site of platelet destruction, surgical removal of the spleen is sometimes performed to improve platelet levels. Plasmapheresis has also been used to remove proteins (cryoglobulins) that can lead to vasculitis. End-stage kidney damage from SLE requires dialysis and/or a kidney transplant (MedicineNet.com, 2011c). Plasmapheresis is discussed in Chapter 16.

Nursing Management

The goals of nursing management for SLE are to limit complications from the disease, which vary for each patient. The nursing process provides the framework for the development of the plan of care.

Assessment

Nursing management of the patient with SLE includes ongoing assessments for signs of infection and any dysfunction of the renal, gastrointestinal, cardiac, respiratory, and neurological systems. It is essential to observe patients for signs or symptoms of organ complications. The nurse should watch for signs of cardiac involvement such as chest pain or murmurs. With respiratory involvement, a patient may experience increased respirations, dyspnea, tachypnea, or orthopnea. Diarrhea, abdominal pain, or distention may indicate gastrointestinal disturbances. Renal involvement may manifest itself as weight gain, scanty urine, and decreased specific gravity. Ataxia (lack of coordination) or ptosis (drooping of upper eyelids) may indicate neurological involvement. The nurse should notify the health care provider immediately about any hematologic signs such as malaise, weakness, chills, and/or epistaxis.

Nursing Diagnoses

Nursing diagnoses related to the patient with SLE are listed in priority order:

- *Injury, Risk for* related to weakness.
- *Comfort, Readiness for Enhanced* related to joint and/or nerve pain.
- *Activity Intolerance* related to weakness and anemia.
- *Skin Integrity, Impaired* related to photosensitivity.
- *Oral Mucous Membrane, Impaired* related to mouth and nasopharyngeal ulcers.
- *Nutrition: Imbalanced, Less Than Body Requirements* related to anorexia and weight loss.
- *Fluid Volume, Excess* related to kidney dysfunction and/or corticosteroid use.
- *Anxiety* related to fear of the disease process.
- *Therapeutic Regimen Management, Readiness for Enhanced* related to exacerbation of disease process.
- *Knowledge deficit* regarding disease process and therapeutic regimen.
- *Fatigue* related to inflammation and weakness.
- *Fall risk* related to muscle weakness and ataxia.
- *Mobility: Physical, Impaired* related to weakness and ataxia.

NANDA-I © 2012

Outcomes and Evaluation Parameters

Outcomes for the patient with SLE include adaptation to the physical and psychological changes brought about by the disease. The goal is to reduce or limit complications of SLE. The evaluation parameters include the patient's verbalizing an understanding of the changes that are occurring and identifying strategies to cope. The patient should also be able to explain the current therapeutic regimen and identify strategies to prevent complications and reduce side effects of medications.

Planning, Interventions, and Rationales

Planning for care of the patient with SLE includes developing a comprehensive health maintenance plan. Interventions include teaching the patient about ways to reduce injuries, controlling discomfort, balancing rest with activity, maintaining skin integrity, reducing oronasopharyngeal ulcers, improving diet, restoring fluid volume, reducing anxiety, and complying with the medication regimen.

In implementing care, one of the most important measures for the nurse to promote is rest. Patients should try to sleep between 8 and 10 hours a night. Therefore, the nurse should encourage the patient to pace activities and plan rest. The patient should avoid stress, and an unhurried environment is preferred. Teaching the patient and family the importance of rest and decreased stress is paramount.

It is important to provide passive or active range of motion to promote joint movement. The nurse should ensure that the patient has not sustained any injuries or falls, determine whether the patient experiences pain normally, and assess whether the patient remains physically active within his ability to do so. Additionally, the nurse needs to promote proper skin care, which includes good hygiene, use of mild soap, use of sunscreen when outdoors, and avoidance of exposure to sunlight. The nurse should observe the patient's skin and oropharyngeal cavities to determine whether they are intact and without lesions. It is important to encourage mouth care a couple times a day if the patient has mouth ulcers and to suggest that the patient change the consistency of her diet to reduce irritation and promote nutritious meals while the patient has stomatitis.

The diet should be well balanced, including all of the food groups, which will promote good nutritional status as well as counteract nutritional interactions with corticosteroids if the patient is taking them. A diet low in sodium is encouraged for patients who have edema, which could indicate renal involvement. The nurse should encourage the intake of vitamin C, as it is essential in the biosynthesis of collagen and increases total collagen synthesis. The patient's daily weight, intake, and output should be recorded to help determine fluid volume balance. The nurse should ascertain whether the patient maintains his weight, maintains fluid balance, and can tolerate the diet of choice. It is important to keep the patient calm and allow the patient to verbalize concerns about the disease process.

With the proper diet and precautions, the patient may remain in a state of remission while simultaneously keeping the organs intact and healthy. Refer to the Patient Teaching & Discharge Priorities for Systemic Lupus Erythematosus box.

PATIENT TEACHING & DISCHARGE PRIORITIES for Systemic Lupus Erythematosus

Need	Teaching
Safety	Stress the need to reduce injuries. Teach the patient and family ways to reduce risks in their environment to prevent falls.
Integrity of oral mucosa	Explain the importance of reducing irritation of the nose, mouth, and throat to reduce oronasopharyngeal ulcers. Avoid foods that irritate the mouth (acidic); avoid irritation from gum chewing; brush with a soft-bristled brush and floss daily; avoid picking the nares; keep nasal mucous membranes moist using a neti pot or Vaseline.
Rest	Encourage the patient to balance rest with activity.
Skin integrity	The patient should maintain skin integrity to prevent integumentary involvement. This includes good hygiene with mild soap, use of sunscreen when outdoors, and avoidance of exposure to sunlight.
Diet	Provide the patient with a plan for a balanced diet to maintain health.
Adequate fluid volume	Stress the importance of restoring fluid volume to prevent dehydration.
Low stress	Encourage the patient to reduce stress to prevent a flare-up of systemic lupus erythematosus (SLE). Encourage the patient to take advantage of resources such as support groups and meditation.
Medications	Teach the patient and family the importance of the patient's medications and the need to comply with the medication regimen to prevent further organ damage.

Scleroderma

Epidemiology and Etiology

Progressive systemic sclerosis (scleroderma) is a progressive disease that is characterized by inflammatory and then degenerative and fibrotic changes in the skin, blood vessels, synovial membranes, skeletal muscles, and internal organs. Scleroderma affects women four times more than men, with peak incidence between ages 35 and 50 (Frazier & Drzymkowski, 2009; Porth & Matfin, 2009). Scleroderma affects people of all ethnic backgrounds; however, those of European descent are afflicted more than African Americans (Porth & Matfin, 2009). The cause of scleroderma is unknown, but it is believed to be autoimmune.

Pathophysiology

With scleroderma, the immune system stimulates the production of an excess of fibroblasts, resulting in fibrotic changes in connective tissue throughout the body. Scleroderma can involve any of the following systems: integumentary, circulatory, joints, alimentary canal, cardiac, respiratory, renal, and/or gastrointestinal tract. As the disease becomes more involved, the acronym CREST identifies a group of symptoms affiliated with the disease's advancement with a poor recovery or chance of remission. C stands for calcium deposits in organs; R stands for Raynaud's type symptoms; E stands for esophageal dysfunction; S stands for sclerodactyly (thickening, induration, and tightening of the skin of the fingers); and T stands for telangiectasia, which is a vascular lesion formed by dilation.

Clinical Manifestations

Subjective clinical findings that point to scleroderma are verbalized by the patient who complains of joint pain and muscle weakness. Objective clinical findings are hard skin that fixes to underlying structures, causing general body movements to be rigid, and telangiectasias on the lips, fingers, face, and tongue. Some patients develop dysphagia and Raynaud's type symptoms, which include recurrent vasospasm of the fingers and toes, usually in response to stress or cold exposure. The vasospasm causes numbness and pain in the affected area.

In limited scleroderma, the hardening of the skin is limited to the hands and face. Diffuse scleroderma also involves the trunk and proximal extremities. The diffuse scleroderma is a severe and progressive disease with early onset of organ involvement, including the gastrointestinal tract, heart, lungs, and kidneys (Frazier & Drzymkowski, 2009; Porth & Matfin, 2009).

Laboratory and Diagnostic Procedures

Initially, the diagnosis of scleroderma is based on the clinical manifestations of the illness. Tests that help to evaluate the presence or extent of any internal disease include upper and lower gastrointestinal examinations; chest x-rays, lung function testing, and CAT scanning to examine the lungs; and ECG, echocardiograms, and sometimes heart catheterization to evaluate the pressure in the arteries of the heart and lungs.

Medical Management

Because scleroderma is a chronic disease, medical management focuses on symptom control and improving the patient's quality of life. Medications are utilized to assist the patient with symptoms of the disease. Corticosteroids help with the inflammation, and salicylates or narcotics are used for joint discomfort. For Raynaud's type symptoms, vasodilators are used to increase circulation. Most commonly, immunosuppressants are administered. Low-dose aspirin is frequently prescribed to prevent tiny blood clots in the fingers, especially in patients with a history of fingertip ulcerations. Medications that dilate the arteries, such as nifedipine (Procardia, Adalat) and nicardipine (Cardene), or topical nitroglycerin applied to the side of the affected digit is frequently used to treat moderate Raynaud's disease. In addition, gently applied finger splints can protect tender tissues. A class of medications that is typically used for depression, the selective serotonin reuptake inhibitors, such as fluoxetine (Prozac), can sometimes improve the circulation of the affected digit. Hand warming and protection from cold temperatures may be all that is necessary for mild Raynaud's disease. In cases of severe Raynaud's disease, surgical procedures, such as those used to interrupt the nerves of the finger that stimulate constriction of the blood vessels (digital sympathectomy), may be necessary. Ulcerations of the fingers can require topical or oral antibiotics (MedicineNet.com, 2011a).

Medications used to treat esophagus irritation and heartburn are omeprazole (Prilosec), esomeprazole (Nexium), and lansoprazole (Prevacid). Antacids can also be helpful. Elevating the head of the bed can reduce the backflow of acid into the esophagus that causes inflammation and heartburn. Avoiding caffeine and cigarette smoking also helps (refer to Chapter 37). Increased fluid intake and fiber intake are good general measures to help with constipation (MedicineNet.com, 2011a).

Medications that are used to suppress the overly active immune system include azathioprine and methotrexate. Serious inflammation of the lungs (alveolitis) can require immune suppression with cyclophosphamide (Cytoxan) along with prednisone. Approximately 10% of patients with the CREST variant of scleroderma have pulmonary hypertension (Chapter 28), which is often treated with calcium antagonist medications, such as nifedipine, and anticoagulation (MedicineNet.com, 2011a).

Irritated, itchy dry skin can be helped by emollients such as Lubriderm, Eucerin, or Bag Balm. Colchicine may be helpful in decreasing the inflammation and tenderness that periodically accompany the calcinosis nodules in the skin.

Telangiectasias, such as those on the face, can be treated with local laser therapy. Sun exposure should be minimized, as it can worsen telangiectasias (MedicineNet.com, 2011a). See the Pharmacology box on page 1567 for a summary of medications used to treat arthritis and connective tissue disorders.

Nursing Management

The nursing process provides the framework necessary to develop a comprehensive health care plan for the patient with scleroderma. The goals of nursing care involve control of pain and support of the patient and family.

Assessment

As with all of the joint diseases, nursing assessment focuses on the extent of joint range of motion and pain. With scleroderma, the nurse must also assess for organ involvement. The lungs, heart, skin, and gastrointestinal system must be assessed for involvement. Chapter 6 outlines the essential components of the nursing assessment for each of these organs.

Nursing Diagnoses

Nursing diagnoses for the patient with scleroderma include the following:

- *Pain, Chronic* related to joint pain.
- *Skin Integrity, Impaired* related to skin lesions.

- *Body Image, Disturbed* related to flat affect, skin lesions, and telangiectasias.
- *Falls, Risk for* related to limited motion and rigidity.
- *Therapeutic Regimen Management, Ineffective* related to noncompliance with medications.
- *Mobility: Physical, Impaired* related to rigidity and limited movement.
- *Anxiety* related to poor prognosis.

NANDA-I © 2012

Outcomes and Evaluation Parameters

Outcomes include adaptation to the physical and psychological changes brought about by scleroderma. The goal is to reduce complications. Evaluation parameters include the patient's ability to verbalize understanding of the changes that are occurring and identifying strategies to cope. The patient should also be able to verbalize understanding of the therapeutic regimen and strategies to reduce complications.

Planning, Interventions, and Rationales

When the nurse is planning the treatment for the patient with scleroderma, the goal is to support the patient and family and improve the quality of life, because there is no cure. When implementing the care, the nurse must be knowledgeable about which organs are involved and the associated clinical manifestations. The nurse must continually monitor the function of all vital organs, such as the heart, lungs, and kidneys, to determine the degree of organ dysfunction. It is important to explain the purpose of each medication, as well as the importance of compliance. It is also important to advise the patient about the adverse effects of all of the medications.

The nurse should inspect the patient's skin and oropharyngeal areas regularly to maintain skin integrity. Because skin manifestations are common in scleroderma, it is essential that the patient be taught to use mild soap and lotion on the skin. The use of emollient lotions is helpful, as is strict adherence to sunscreens. The nurse should stress that the patient should avoid exposure to the cold because it may cause vasoconstriction of vessels, thereby decreasing peripheral circulation. If there is lung involvement, the nurse should provide education on the importance of not smoking and should encourage deep breathing exercises to improve oxygenation.

Finally, the nurse should discuss with the patient the physical changes that scleroderma cause to help the patient be better able to cope with changes in body image as the disease progresses. The nurse should also explain which symptoms need to be reported to the health care provider and stress the importance of regular medical examinations.

Lyme Disease

Epidemiology and Etiology

Lyme disease is a bacterial infection that affects the organs and joints. Lyme disease is caused by *Borrelia burgdorferi*, bacteria that are found in infected black-legged ticks, which are also known as deer ticks. There are two species of black-legged ticks: *ixodes scapularis* located in the Northeast and north central United States, and *ixodes pacificus* in the western parts of the United States. These ticks are much smaller than the ticks that animals such as dogs and cattle typically carry. Ticks feed by placing their mouth on the host and sucking the host's blood. The bacteria that cause Lyme disease are transferred slowly over a couple of days of feeding (CDC, 2010a).

The disease got its name from the city of Lyme, Connecticut, where in 1975 a group of children and adults spontaneously developed a debilitating arthritis. The Centers for Disease Control and Prevention (CDC) was alerted to this phenomenon, and research into the progression of illness and disease vectors was instituted. The investigation concluded that deer ticks were transmitting a degenerative disease to humans (CDC, 2010a).

In 2006, 19,931 cases of Lyme disease were reported in the United States, a national average of 8.2 cases per 100,000 persons. In the United States, Lyme disease is heavily concentrated in the areas of the Northeast, Southeast, and West Coast. Individuals who live in rural areas near trees and overgrown shrubs may be at risk for Lyme disease. Outdoor activities, such as hiking, camping, gardening, working in forestry, and wildlife/parks management in specified areas, expose participants to a higher risk of being infected (CDC, 2010a).

Pathophysiology and Clinical Manifestations

An infected tick attaches to a human, sucks the person's blood, and transfers the disease from the bacteria in the tick's saliva. There are three stages of the disease, which can affect many systems of the body. Chart 51–2 describes pathophysiology and clinical manifestations of the three stages of the disease.

Laboratory and Diagnostic Procedures and Medical Management

A blood test is used to detect the presence of antibodies from the bacterium to corroborate the diagnosis of Lyme disease. For early-stage Lyme disease, oral antibiotics are the standard treatment. These usually include doxycycline for adults and children older than 8, or amoxicillin or cefuroxime axetil for older adults, younger children, and pregnant or breast-feeding women. These drugs often cure the infection and prevent complications. A 14- to 21-day course of antibiotics is usually recommended. If the disease has progressed to the early disseminated phase, intravenous antibiotic for 14 to 28 days is an effective treatment plan for eliminating infection, although it may take some time to recover symptomatically (MayoClinic.com, 2011).

The flulike symptoms are treated with supportive measures, depending on the presenting symptoms. For example, fever is treated with antipyretics and rest, and the joint pain is treated with NSAIDs and rest.

Nursing Management

The nursing process provides the framework for the management of patients with Lyme disease. Nursing management focuses on treatment of the infection and education of the patient and family on ways to avoid exposure to ticks and possible reinfection.

Assessment

Assessment of the early localized disease, the first stage, which occurs between days 7 and 10, includes evaluating for a growing rash called erythema chronicum migrans (ECM), which looks like a bull's eye on the affected part. In addition, the nurse will assess for flulike symptoms: headache, confusion, forgetfulness, stiff neck, irregular heartbeat, achy and swollen joints, and swollen lymph glands (Frazier & Drzymkowski, 2009).

During the second stage, which occurs a couple of weeks to months after the patient is infected, the nurse needs to focus the assessment on the neurological system. Assessment findings could include severe headaches, poor motor balance, and temporary facial paralysis. During the late stage of the disease, which can occur from months to years after being infected, the musculoskeletal system is attacked. Arthritis is a complication of this disease. Approximately 5% of the people infected will develop chronic arthritis (CDC, 2010a).

CHART 51–2 Three Stages of Lyme Disease

Early Localized Days to 1 Month After Bite	Early Disseminated Days to 10 Months After Bite	Late or Chronic Disease Months to Years After Bite
Erythema chronicum migrans (reddened area where the tick bite occurred, resembling a bull's eye) caused by the bacteria occurs in 70% to 80% of patients. As the inflammatory reaction begins, fatigue, malaise, lethargy, headache, stiff neck, myalgias, arthralgias, and regional or generalized lymphadenopathy occur.	Carditis caused by systemic spread of the bacteria occurs in approximately 5% of untreated patients. Manifestations include conduction defects, mild cardiomyopathy, or myopericarditis. Neurological disease occurs in approximately 15% of untreated patients. Manifestations include lymphocytic meningitis; encephalitis; cranial neuropathy (most often facial, can be bilateral), peripheral neuropathy, or radiculoneuropathy; or myelitis. Musculoskeletal involvement occurs in approximately 60% of untreated patients. Manifestations include migratory polyarthritis and/or polyarthralgias (pain in several joints). Skin involvement concerns multiple erythema chronicum migrans lesions. This rash appears 1 day to a month after the tick bite. It is caused by an infection from the Lyme bacteria. The patient may also develop erythema nodosum, an inflammation of the fat cells under the skin characterized by tender red nodules. Lymphadenopathy is regional and/or generalized in response to the bacteria. Eye involvement or inflammation of any part of the eye. Inflammation of the liver, liver function test abnormalities, and hepatitis. Inflammation of the kidneys. Microhematuria and asymptomatic proteinuria.	Musculoskeletal symptoms caused by systemic spread of the bacteria. Approximately 60% of untreated patients develop intermittent monoarticular (affecting one joint) or oligoarticular (affecting several joints) arthritis; approximately 10% of untreated patients develop persistent monoarthritis, usually affecting the knee. Neurological disease caused by the inflammatory process. Incidence is rare but may be exhibited by chronic, often subtle, encephalopathy, encephalomyelitis, and/or peripheral neuropathy.

Source: Adapted from Hu, L. (2011). Clinical manifestations of Lyme disease. *UpToDate.* Retrieved from http://www.uptodate.com/patients/content/topic.do?topicKey=~9197/aelfkcit3&selectedTitle=2~133&source=search_result.

Nursing Diagnoses

The following are the high-priority nursing diagnoses for the patient with Lyme disease:

- *Infection, Risk for* related to tick contamination.
- *Pain, Acute* related to neurological symptoms of the disease.
- *Knowledge, Deficient* related to unfamiliarity of Lyme disease.

NANDA-I © 2012

Interventions, Outcomes, and Evaluation Parameters

Nursing interventions for Lyme disease depend on the stage of the disease and the patient's clinical manifestations. For example, early in the disease process, the management would focus on treating the flu-like symptoms and the acute infection. The later stages of the disease are more complex, and the nursing care will depend on what systems are involved. For example, if there is neurological involvement and muscle weakness, the nurse must focus on protecting the airway and preventing patients from falling or injuring themselves. The outcome of care is to have the patient free of infection as exhibited by a decrease in symptoms. It is imperative that the patient and family understand ways to protect themselves from exposure and reinfection by using insect repellent. During this phase of the nursing process, the evaluation parameters involve the patient and family's ability to articulate understanding about the disease and its cause, signs, symptoms, treatment, and prevention. For discharge planning and teaching, see the Patient Teaching & Discharge Priorities box below.

Sjögren's Syndrome

Epidemiology and Etiology

Sjögren's syndrome (SS) is an autoimmune disease. In this disorder, SS immune cells attack and destroy the glands that produce tears and saliva (Frazier & Drzymkowski, 2009). In the United States, SS affects 1 million to 4 million people. The ratio of affected women to men is typically 9 to 1 (Borenstein, 2007). Sjögren's syndrome is found more commonly in patients with a family history of other autoimmune illnesses.

Pathophysiology

Sjögren's syndrome is caused by inflammation of the glands that produce tears (lacrimal glands), leading to decreased water production

PATIENT TEACHING & DISCHARGE PRIORITIES for Lyme Disease

Need	Teaching
Knowledge of disease process	Encourage understanding of the infectious process of Lyme disease. Early detection is critical for the early treatment and prevention of complications.
Prevention	Individuals who live in highly infected areas should be taking precautions to reduce the risk of getting infected. Teach the patient the importance of using insect repellant when out of doors in high risk areas.
Medications	Encourage compliance with the medication regimen. If the patient is infected, it is imperative to continue to take the entire prescription as ordered by the health care provider.
Complications	Teaching is needed about the progression of the disease.

for tears and eye dryness. Inflammation of the glands that produce the saliva in the mouth (salivary glands, including the parotid glands) leads to mouth dryness (MedicineNet.com, 2011b). Sjögren's syndrome is not considered a connective tissue disease when it involves the glands affecting the eyes and mouth only. However, when SS is associated with rheumatoid arthritis, it is considered a connective tissue disease (MedicineNet.com, 2011b).

Clinical Manifestations

The two symptoms that are the hallmark of Sjögren's syndrome are dry eyes and dry mouth (Sjögren's Syndrome Foundation, 2012). The disease can also cause dryness in other body organs. In the kidneys, renal calculi, tubular acidosis, nephrogenic diabetes insipidus, and hypokalemia can occur secondary to tubular damage caused by interstitial nephritis. In the gastrointestinal tract, dryness of the pharynx and esophagus may cause difficulty swallowing and esophagitis with reflux. In the pulmonary system, dryness of the tracheobronchial mucosa may cause a persistent dry cough. In the cardiac system, orthostatic symptoms may occur and are related to dysfunction of the autonomic control of blood pressure and heart rate that is associated with increased severity of SS. Many patients have debilitating joint pain and fatigue. The symptoms can wax and wane and even go into remission. Some patients may have only mild symptoms; others are severely affected and experience a poor quality of life.

Laboratory and Diagnostic Procedures

According to the Sjögren's Syndrome Foundation (2012), 70% of individuals with SS will have an elevated antibody (ANA), which measures antibodies that react against normal components of the cell nucleus. Sjögren's syndrome antigens (SSA and SSB) are also elevated; with 70% of the population having SSA and 40% having SSB, the rheumatoid factor is elevated, measuring positive. The erythrocyte sedimentation rate is also elevated, indicating an active inflammatory process. Immunoglobulins measure normal blood proteins and are also elevated with SS (Sjögren's Syndrome Foundation, 2012).

Other tests that may be used are the Schirmer's test, measuring tear production; Rose Bengal and Lissamine green, using dyes to observe abnormal cells on the surface of the eye; slit lamp exam, magnifying the volume of tears of the eye by viewing it in its resting state; parotid gland flow, measuring the amount of saliva produced over a certain period of time; salivary scintigraphy, measuring salivary gland function; sialography, an x-ray of the salivary duct system; and lip biopsy, used to confirm lymphocytic infiltration of the minor salivary glands (Sjögren's Syndrome Foundation, 2012).

Medical Management

There is no cure for SS at this time. However, symptoms can be treated. Patients can use moisture replacement therapies for symptoms of dryness. Increasing fluid intake, using oral sprays, and chewing sugarless gum may help with oral dryness. Wearing sunglasses to protect the eyes and using artificial tears also are recommended (Frazier & Drzymkowski, 2009). Many classifications of medications are helpful, such as nonsteroidal anti-inflammatory drugs for musculoskeletal symptoms and corticosteroids and immunosuppressive therapies for severe complications (National Institute of Neurological Disorders and Stroke, 2011).

Nursing Management

The nursing process, with its problem-solving approach, will lead the nurse to understand the disease process while prioritizing care for the patient with SS.

Assessment

In subjective assessments, patients will complain of feeling dryness in the mouth, mucous membranes, and skin. Objective assessments include irritation, a gritty feeling, or painful burning in the eyes; dry mouth; dysphagia; swelling of saliva glands; and dryness of nasal passage or throat, or vagina or skin (National Institute of Neurological Disorders and Stroke, 2011). There are periods of remissions and exacerbations. Exacerbations usually occur after an illness.

Patients also may experience blurred vision, recurrent mouth infections, swollen parotid glands, hoarseness, dysphasia, debilitating fatigue, and joint pain (National Institute of Neurological Disorders and Stroke, 2011).

Nursing Diagnoses

Nursing diagnoses for the patient with Sjögren's syndrome include the following:

- *Nutrition: Imbalanced, Less Than Body Requirements* as related by dysphasia.
- *Pain, Chronic* related to dried secretions in mucous membranes and joint pain.
- *Knowledge, Deficient* related to unfamiliarity of educational resources.
- *Communication: Verbal, Impaired* related to hoarseness.
- *Self-Care, Readiness for Enhanced* related to debilitating fatigue.
  NANDA-I © 2012

Interventions, Outcomes, and Evaluation Parameters

Interventions for the patient with Sjögren's syndrome include protecting the affected tissues, assisting in preventing complications, avoiding irritation to the tissues, monitoring for signs and symptoms of infection, and assessing for the development of complications. Outcomes for the patient with SS include relief of symptoms of dryness in the oral cavity and eyes. Evaluation parameters include adequate nutritional status, pain abatement, awareness of educational resources, ability to communicate effectively, and self-care.

Collaborative Management

To achieve optimal functioning, patients with connective tissue disorders need a multidisciplinary team approach, including health care providers, nurses, social workers, physical therapists, pharmacists, occupational therapists, psychologists/psychiatrists, and dietitians. In order to meet desired patient outcomes, it is essential that the interdisciplinary team communicate openly with one another in developing and evaluating care of the patient and family (IOM, 2010).

The multidisciplinary team approach is essential to assist the patient in maintaining function. Physical therapy and occupational therapy can assist the patient in remaining functional. Ongoing physical therapy will help to increase range of motion and maintain mobility. The occupational therapist assists the patient with exercises that will enhance fine motor movements. The social worker and a psychologist or psychiatrist can help the patient adjust to a chronic illness. A comprehensive plan for nutrition is important for teaching the patient and family about dietary needs to maintain weight and health. The pharmacist helps the team coordinate the medication regimen.

Health Promotion

For patients with connective tissue disorders, adequate health teaching is an important part of the plan of care. It is essential that the patient understands the medications, such as the different classifications, actions, adverse effects, and any interactions with food or other medications. In addition to understanding the medications, it is important that the patient understand the disease process, diagnosis, prognosis, and treatments available. The nurse should teach the patient ways to avoid sun, fatigue, infections, and changing medication doses. Female patients should avoid becoming pregnant without approval from the health care provider due to the effects of some medications used to treat connective tissue disorders and the close monitoring they will need as the risk of fetal loss is much higher than in the general population. The nurse should promote regular exercise to maintain the patient's mobility and prevention of fatigue by scheduling rest periods throughout the day. Patients with chronic diseases should wear medic alert bracelets.

It is important to teach individuals ways to prevent disease. For instance, many things can be done to promote protection from Lyme disease. During the summer months, people should avoid areas where ticks are likely to be found, especially wooded and grassy areas. Long sleeve shirts, long pants, and socks should be worn in areas of high tick concentration. In addition, tucking pants into socks and tucking shirts into pants will minimize exposure of the skin. Wearing light-colored clothing will make it easier to see ticks so that they can be removed before the person gets bitten. It is important to use tick repellents, such as DEET. However, individuals should be careful not to overuse these products and should follow the directions for use. If left on for long periods, repellents may cause skin irritation. Once individuals are finished being outdoors, they should remove their clothing and wash it. In addition, they should examine their body thoroughly and remove any attached ticks by very carefully using tweezers. Once the tick has been removed, the area of the skin where the tick was found should be cleaned with antiseptic. It is important to check pets to be certain that they do not have ticks. Tick collars can be put around the neck of the pets; in addition, some pet medications can help repel ticks.

Gerontological Considerations

In the United States, the number of people over the age of 65 years is expected to grow to 71.5 million by the year 2030, and the number of those who will be older than 85 years is expected to increase to 21 million by the year 2050 (Bruckenthal, 2010). Nurses will need to understand the normal physiologic changes that occur with aging and the increased risks of pain related to the disorders discussed in this chapter. Pain is a barrier to healthy aging, and nurses are in a unique position to assist older adults to remain active, manage pain, and promote well-being (Baumann, 2009). Teaching health promotion is critical to maintaining well-being, and diet and exercise should be the priorities of education. There have also been evidence-based studies to demonstrate that the integration of complementary therapies into the care of older patients enhances conventional pain management (Bruckenthal, 2010). For instance, glucosamine sulfate and chondroitin sulfate are popular supplements that many older adults use to treat arthritis, as described in the Complementary & Alternative Therapies feature earlier in the chapter.

Arthritis and connective tissue disorders are debilitating conditions that affect the whole person. The goal of nursing management is to treat the patient holistically and attempt to control the signs and symptoms of the disorder. For the older patient, safety is critical; in addition, assisting the patient with activities of daily living is important while maintaining the patient's dignity. Families may need to be involved in caregiving as a patient becomes incapacitated.

Research

Research opportunities for arthritis and other connective tissue disorders focus on early recognition and the ability to alter the inflammatory response. Refer to the Research Opportunities box.

Summary

Arthritis and connective tissue disorders are chronic and sometimes debilitating diseases. The nurse must have excellent assessment skills for evaluation of these patients. The nurse is also integral in helping the patient and family learn and plan for their long-term care so they will remain as functional as possible.

RESEARCH OPPORTUNITIES Related to Arthritis and Connective Tissue Disorders

Research Area	Clinical Impact
Research of osteoarthritis is focusing on joints that have sustained trauma. Investigators can study the pathogenic mechanisms as they begin in tissues that were healthy and can observe how the processes lead to cartilage breakdown, bone proliferation, and synovial inflammation. Investigators have access to the affected tissue, since many patients with joint trauma have surgical repair.	Understanding the pathogenic mechanisms of cartilage breakdown, bone proliferation, and synovial inflammation may lead to better medications and treatments to stop the progression of OA.
Research for rheumatoid arthritis is focused on the ability to detect RA prior to the onset of symptoms; identifying predictors to determine patient-specific medical interventions to slow or stop the RA process and permit the joint to heal; identifying the triggers that cause antibodies to produce inflammation in the joints; and developing methods to stop or reverse the immune system response.	Earlier identification and treatment could decrease the extent of damage to the joints. Development of medications that could stop the inflammatory response would prevent the damage to joints and progression of the disease.
Research for scleroderma is aimed at understanding how the immune system and vasculature malfunction and how fibrosis begins and progresses, as well as the interrelationships among these facets of the disease.	Research about disease mechanisms provides a basis for identifying new therapies and tests for earlier detection and treatment.
Research for lupus includes identifying the genes that increase susceptibility; biomarkers for diagnosing, monitoring, and treating lupus; and how lupus damages organs.	Knowing genetically what makes a patient susceptible to the disease would allow for earlier screening and treatment. Understanding the disease mechanisms provides a basis for identifying new therapies for treatment.

CLINICAL PREPARATION READ DOCUMENT APPLY

READ: **History of Present Illness** >> Laboratory Study Results >> Critical Thinking Questions

Eric Auliff is a 48-year-old Caucasian male who works as a bartender in San Francisco. He is divorced and has two children who are in high school. Mr. Auliff states that 1 week ago, he had a minor crash while he was riding his motorcycle. He suffered only minor injuries, including abrasions to his left leg and arm and a small laceration to the left knee. He did not seek medical attention after the crash. Approximately 1 week after the crash, he presented to his orthopedic surgeon complaining of increased pain and swelling of his left knee. The health care provider aspirated the joint, sent the fluid for cultures, and admitted Mr. Auliff to the orthopedic floor with a diagnosis of septic arthritis.

Medical–Surgical History

Mr. Auliff had a left anterior cruciate ligament repair 3 years ago after injuring his knee skiing. He states that he has developed arthritis in that joint.

Physical Exam

You receive Mr. Auliff on hospital day 3. He is awake, alert, and oriented. He states that the left knee pain is a 5 on a 1-to-10 scale. His vital signs are within normal limits. Breath sounds are equal bilaterally; his abdomen is soft and nontender with active bowel sounds. The left knee appears edematous and is warmer to touch than the right knee. Mr. Auliff has good motor and sensory abilities to all extremities, and his distal pulses are strong and equal. He has one peripheral IV in the left forearm.

READ: History of Present Illnesses >> **Physical Exam** >> Admitting Medical Records >> Laboratory Study Results

Admitting Medical Orders

Service: Orthopedic Surgery
Diagnosis: septic arthritis, left knee
Allergies: none known
Vital signs: every 6 hours including neurovascular checks to the left lower extremity
Call house officer: temp > 38.5°C, HR > 110 or < 60, RR > 30 or < 12, BP sys > 160 or < 90, urine output < 120 mL in 4 hours, and change in neurovascular exam to left lower extremity
Weight-bearing status: touch-down weight to left lower extremity
Activity: up to chair 4 times a day, may ambulate to bathroom using crutches. When in bed, left knee must be braced in a functional position.
Diet: regular
IV: saline lock
I&O: every shift
Respiratory care: use incentive spirometer hourly when awake
DVT prophylaxis: low-molecular-weight heparin, sequential compression devices to lower extremities when in bed

Scheduled Medications

Ceftriaxone 1 gm IV every 12 hours
Ibuprofen 400 mg PO every 8 hours
Enoxaparin 30 mg subcutaneously every 12 hours
Docusate sodium 100 mg po twice daily

PRN Medications

Oxycodone 5/500 mg PO every 6 hours as needed for pain

Ordered Laboratory Studies

CBC every morning

READ: History of Present Illness >> **Laboratory Study Results** >> Critical Thinking Questions

Test	Day 1	Day 2	Day 3
WBC	$12/mm^3$	$11/mm^3$	$10/mm^3$
RBC	$4.55/mm^3$	$4.50/mm^3$	$4.50/mm^3$
Hemoglobin	15 g/dL	15 g/dL	15 g/dL
Hematocrit	52%	52%	52%

Test	Day 1	Day 2	Day 3
Platelet count	250,000 µL	250,000 µL	250,000 µL
APTT	35 seconds		
INR	1.2		
Fluid aspirate culture			streptococcus

Pearson Nursing Student Resources *Log on to* **nursing.pearsonhighered.com** *to download forms*

DOCUMENT:

- >> Summary of Hospitalization
- >> Pathophysiology Form
- >> Laboratory Values
- >> Laboratory Results Explanation

APPLY:

- >> List of Potential Nursing Diagnoses
- >> Concept Map
- >> Critical Thinking Questions and Concept Map

APPLY: History of Present Illness >> Laboratory Study Results >> **Critical Thinking Questions**

1. What types of precautions are necessary for a patient with a septic joint?
2. Why is adherence to weight-bearing and activity restrictions important during the inflammatory process?
3. What key discharge teaching should be done to maintain optimal joint function?

Answers to Critical Thinking Questions can be found in Appendix D in the Osborn Student Resources at nursing.pearsonhighered.com.

NCLEX® PRACTICE

1. A patient has been diagnosed with systemic lupus erythematosus (SLE). What should the nurse include when teaching this patient about this diagnosis?

1. "Systemic lupus erythematosus is a complication of rheumatoid arthritis."
2. "The symptoms you experience are caused by chronic inflammation that affects the joints."
3. "This disease affects both connective tissues and organs."
4. "The major finding associated with SLE is psoriasis-like lesions on the skin."

2. A nurse is providing education to a patient who has just been started on Rheumatrex (methotrexate) for treatment of rheumatoid arthritis. What information should the nurse include in this education? (select all that apply)

1. "This medication may create a metallic taste in your mouth."
2. "Be certain to use sunblock when taking this medication."
3. "You should follow a low-fat, low-calorie diet while taking this medication"
4. "Do not drink caffeine-containing beverages with this medication."
5. "You may take aspirin for any breakthrough pain you might have while taking this medication."

3. A patient is admitted with circinate balanitis and uveitis. Which nursing assessment question is appropriate?

1. "Have you had a recent gastrointestinal infection?"
2. "Have you ever been told you had a positive rheumatoid factor?"
3. "Have you noticed any changes in your fingernails?"
4. "Have you had a recent tick bite?"

4. The nurse has completed the assessment of a patient with osteoarthritis. Which nursing diagnoses would likely be applicable to this patient? (select all that apply)

1. *Impaired Physical Mobility*
2. *Readiness for Enhanced Self-Care*
3. *Imbalanced Nutrition: Less Than Body Requirements*
4. *Fluid Volume Deficit*
5. *Chronic Pain*

5. A patient is diagnosed with gout. The nurse should instruct this patient to avoid which foods? (select all that apply)

1. Lettuce
2. Peas
3. Broccoli
4. Chicken
5. Wheat germ

6. Which nursing intervention would the nurse provide for a patient who has been diagnosed with systemic lupus erythematosus (SLE)?

1. Allow the patient to rest as much as possible during the day.
2. Order citrus juice and fruit on each dietary tray to increase vitamin C intake.
3. Control fluid intake by restricting fluids to those served with meals.
4. Ask the family to bring the patient chewing gum to help moisten the oral cavity.

Answers to NCLEX Practice Questions can be found in Appendix D in the Osborn Student Resources at nursing.pearsonhighered.com. Practice additional NCLEX questions online at the Student Resources site.

Pearson Nursing Student Resources Find additional review materials at: **nursing.pearsonhighered.com**

REFERENCES

Adams, M. P., & Koch, R. W. (2010). *Pharmacology: Connections to nursing practice.* Upper Saddle River, NJ: Pearson.

American College of Rheumatology. (2008). Ankylosing spondylitis. Retrieved from http://www.rheumatology.org/public/factsheets/as.asp

Baumann, S. (2009). A nursing approach to pain in older adults. *Medsurg Nursing, 18*(2), 77–82.

Belcaro, G., Cesarone, M. R., Dugall, M., Pellegrini, L., Ledda, A., Grossi, M. G., et al. (2010). Efficacy and safety of Meriva®, a curcumin-phosphatidylcholine complex, during extended administration in osteoarthritis patients. *Alternative Medicine Review, 15*(4), 337–344.

Borenstein, D. (2007). Epidemiology, diagnostics and management. Medscape Today. Retrieved from http://www.medscape.com/viewarticle/423760

Brent, L. H. (2011). Ankylosing spondylitis and undifferentiated spondyloarthropathy. Retrieved from http://www.emedicine.medscape.com/article/332945-overview

Brien, S., Prescott, P., Coghlan, B., Bashir, N., & Lewith, G. (2008). Systematic review of the nutritional supplement Perna Canaliculus (green-lipped mussel) in the treatment of osteoarthritis. *Quarterly Journal of Medicine, 101*(3), 167–179. Epub 2008 Jan 25

Bruckenthal, P. (2010). Integrating nonpharmacologic and alternative strategies into a comprehensive management approach for older adults with pain. *Pain Management Nursing, 11*(2 suppl): S23–31.

Centers for Disease Control and Prevention (CDC). (2010a). Lyme disease. Retrieved from http://www.cdc.gov/ncidod/dvbid/lyme/ld_statistics.htm

Centers for Disease Control and Prevention (CDC). (2010b). Prevalence of arthritis. Retrieved from http://www.cdc.gov/arthritis/data_statistics/arthritis_related_statistics.htm#1

Centers for Disease Control and Prevention (CDC). (2011). Arthritis. Retrieved from http://www.cdc.gov/arthritis

Chisholm, T. (2011). Glucosamine for osteoarthritis. Select carefully for best results. *Advance for Nurse Practioners and Physician Assistants, 2*(4), 25–26.

Efthimiou, P., Kukar, M., & MacKenzie, C. R. (2010). Complementary and alternative medicine in rheumatoid arthritis: No longer the last resort!. *Humanity & Social Sciences Journal, 6*(1), 108–111. doi: 10.1007/s11420-009-9133-8

eMedicineHealth. (2011). Gout. Retrieved from http://www.emedicinehealth.com/gout/article_em.htm

Ernst, E. (2011). Herbal medicine in the treatment of rheumatic diseases. *Rheumatic Diseases Clinics of North America, 37*(1), 95–102. Epub 2010 Dec 3

FamilyPracticeNotebook.com. (2010). Osteoarthritis. Retrieved from http://www.fpnotebook.com/Rheum/Osteoarthritis/Ostrthrts.htm

Ferri, F. F. (2011). *Ferri's clinical advisor 2011*. St. Louis: Elsevier.

Frazier, M. S., & Drzymkowski, J. W. (Eds.). (2009). *Essentials of human diseases and conditions* (4th ed.). St. Louis: Saunders Elsevier.

Gladman, D. (2011a). Clinical manifestations and diagnosis of psoriatic arthritis. *UpToDate.* Retrieved from http://www.uptodate.com/patients/content/topic.do?topicKey=~FFX.7DwCxZDGbF&selectedTitle=2~150&source=search_result

Gladman, D. (2011b). Pathogenesis of psoriatic arthritis. *UpToDate.* Retrieved from http://www.uptodate.com/patients/content/topic.do?topicKey=~nKkKMlvosxl56.&selectedTitle=1~78&source=search_result

Goldenberg, D., & Sexton, D. (2011). Bacterial (nongonococcal) arthritis in adults. *UpToDate.* Retrieved from http://www.uptodate.com/patients/content/topic.do?topicKey=~hcmhzYL2SL2ACJ&selectedTitle=7~147&source=search_result

Gómez Candela, C., Bermejo López, L. M., & Loria Kohen, V. (2011). Importance of a balanced omega 6/omega 3 ratio for the maintenance of health. Nutritional recommendations. *Nutricion Hospitalaria, 26*(2), 323–329.

Hammadi, A. A. (2010). Psoriatic arthritis. eMedicine.com. Retrieved from http://www.emedicine.com/MED/topic1954.htm

Hogan, M. A. (2007). *Nutrition & diet therapy* (2nd ed.). Upper Saddle River, NJ: Pearson.

Hu, L. (2011). Clinical manifestations of Lyme disease. *UpToDate.* Retrieved from http://www.uptodate.com/patients/content/topic.do?topicKey=~9197/aelfkcit3&selectedTitle=2~133&source=search_result

IOM (Institute of Medicine). (2010). *The future of nursing: Leading change, advancing health.* Washington, DC: The Academic Press.

Kalunian, K. C. (2011). Pathogenesis of OA: Diagnosis and classification of OA. Retrieved from http://www.utdol.com/online/content/topic.do?topicKey=osteoart/3785&selectedTitle=1~150&source=search_result

Kee, J. L. (2010). *Laboratory and diagnostic tests with nursing implications* (8th ed.). Upper Saddle River, NJ: Prentice Hall.

Kherani, R., & Shojania, K. (2007). Septic arthritis in patients with preexisting inflammatory arthritis. *Canadian Medical Association Journal, 176*(11), 1605–1608.

Lozada, C. J. (2010). Reactive arthritis. Retrieved from http://www.emedicine.medscape.com/article/331347-overview

Mandell, B. (2008). Clinical manifestations of hyperuricemia and gout. *Cleveland Clinic Journal of Medicine, 75*(5), S5–S8.

MayoClinic.com. (2011). Lyme disease: Symptoms. Retrieved from http://www.mayoclinic.com/health/lyme-disease/DS00116/DSECTION-2

MedicineNet.com. (2011a). Scleroderma. Retrieved from http://www.medicinenet.com/scleroderma/article.htm

MedicineNet.com. (2011b). Sjögren's syndrome. Retrieved from http://www.medicinenet.com/sjogrens_syndrome/article.htm

MedicineNet.com. (2011c). Systemic lupus erythematosus (SLE or lupus). Retrieved from http://www.medicinenet.com/systemic_lupus/article.htm

MedlinePlus Medical Encyclopedia. (2011). Acute gouty arthritis. Retrieved from http://www.nlm.nih.gov/medlineplus/ency/article/000422.htm

National Institute of Arthritis and Musculoskeletal and Skin Diseases (NIAMS). (2009a). Arthritis: Causes and risk factors—Gout. Retrieved from http://nihseniorhealth.gov/arthritis/causesandriskfactors/01.html

National Institute of Arthritis and Musculoskeletal and Skin Diseases (NIAMS). (2009b). Reactive arthritis. Retrieved from http://www.niams.nih.gov/hi/topics/reactive/reactive.htm

National Institute of Neurological Disorders and Stroke. (2011). Sjögren's syndrome information page. Retrieved from http://www.ninds.nih.gov/disorders/sjogrens/sjogrens.htm

Porth, C. M., & Matfin, G. (2009). *Essentials of pathophysiology: Concepts of altered health states* (2nd ed.). Philadelphia: Lippincott Williams & Wilkins.

Schlesinger, N., Schumacher, M. C., Catton, M., & Maxwell, L. (2009). Colchicine for acute gout. *Cochrane Database of Systematic Reviews*, 2006, Issue 4. Retrieved from http://mrw.interscience.wiley.com/cochrane/clsysrev/articles/CD006190/frame.html

Sengupta, K., Alluri, K. V., Satish, A. R., Mishra, S., Golakoti, T., Sarma, K. V., et al. (2008). A double blind, randomized, placebo controlled study of the efficacy and safety of 5-Loxin for treatment of osteoarthritis of the knee. *Arthritis Research & Therapy, 10*(4), R85. Epub 2008 Jul 30

Sjögren's Syndrome Foundation. (2012). About Sjogren's syndrome. Retrieved from http://www.sjogrens.org/home/about-sjogrens-syndrome/symptoms

Soppler, M. C. (2008). Citrulline antibody. Retrieved from http://www medicinenet.com/citrulline_antibody/article.htm

Tokuyama, S., & Nakamoto, K. (2011). Lipid mediators and pain signaling—Unsaturated fatty acids and pain. *Biological & Pharmaceutical Bulletin, 34*(8), 1174–1178.

U.S. Department of Health and Human Services (DHHS). (2010). *Healthy People 2020*. Retrieved from http://www.healthypeople.gov

Warnock, M., McBean, D., Suter, A., Tan, J., & Whittaker, P. (2007). Effectiveness and safety of Devil's claw tablets in patients with general rheumatic disorders. *Phytotherapy Research, 21*(12), 1228–1233.

Wilkinson, J. M., & Ahearn, N. R. (2009). *Prentice Hall nursing diagnosis handbook* (9th ed.). Upper Saddle River, NJ: Prentice Hall.

WrongDiagnosis.com (WD.com). (2011). Prevalence and incidence of connective tissue disorders. Retrieved from http://www.wrongdiagnosis.com/c/connective_tissue_disorders/prevalence.htm

Yu, D. (2010). Reactive arthritis. Retrieved from http://www.utdol.com/online/content/topic.do?topicKey=spondylo/7349&selectedTitle=1~86&source=search_result

Nursing Management of Patients with Immunologic, Inflammatory, and Hematologic Disorders

12 UNIT

Content in Unit 12 that addresses the **Institute of Medicine (IOM)** competencies, **Nursing Core Competencies (NCC)**, the **Quality and Safety Education for Nurses (QSEN)** competencies, and **Concepts** for concept-based learning is listed below.

Competencies	Feature or Text	Location
IOM, QSEN, NCC Providing patient-centered care	Nursing Process: Patient Care Plans for Immune Response Disorders, pages 1626, 1640	Chapter 53
	Nursing Process: Patient Care Plans for Shock and Sepsis, pages 1682, 1690	Chapter 54
	Nursing Process: Patient Care Plans for Blood Disorders, pages 1724, 1739, 1751	Chapter 56
	Nursing Process: Patient Care Plan for Cancer, page 1790	Chapter 57
IOM, QSEN, NCC Working in teams	Collaborative Management, pages 1630, 1636, 1639, 1663	Chapter 53
	Collaborative Management, pages 1680, 1689	Chapter 54
	Collaborative Management, pages 1723, 1731, 1734, 1738, 1750	Chapter 56
	Collaborative Management, page 1815	Chapter 57
IOM, QSEN, NCC Employing evidence-based practice	Evidence-Based Practice: Barriers and Facilitators to HIV Treatment, page 1665	Chapter 53
	Evidence-Based Practice: Management of Bleeding Following Trauma, page 1681	Chapter 54
	Evidence-Based Practice: Sickle Cell Crisis, page 1741	Chapter 56
	Evidence-Based Practice: Heparin-Induced Thrombocytopenia, page 1754	Chapter 56
	Evidence-Based Practice: Fatigue in Relation to Cancer, page 1819	Chapter 57
IOM, NCC Applying quality and safety improvement	Safety Alerts, pages 1596, 1598, 1608, 1610, 1611, 1615,	Chapter 52
	Safety Alerts, pages 1622, 1623, 1624, 1625, 1650, 1651	Chapter 53
	Safety Alerts, pages 1673, 1675, 1676, 1685	Chapter 54
	Safety Alert, page 1711	Chapter 55
	Safety Alerts, pages 1721, 1726, 1730, 1743, 1749	Chapter 56
	Safety Alerts, pages 1776, 1778, 1789, 1811	Chapter 57
IOM, QSEN, NCC Applying ethical and legal responsibilities	Ethical Issues Related to Patients in Shock, page 1681	Chapter 54
	Ethical Issues Related to Nutrition in Patients with Cancer, page 1819	Chapter 57
	Ethical Issues Related to Nursing Care of the Patient with Cancer, page 1820	Chapter 57
NCC Educating patients	Patient Teaching & Discharge Priorities, page 1663	Chapter 53
	Patient Teaching & Discharge Priorities, pages 1725, 1740, 1752	Chapter 56
	Patient Teaching & Discharge Priorities, page 1821	Chapter 57

Concepts covered in Unit 12 include:

Body image	Grief and loss	Inflammation
Cell development/abnormalities	Immunity	Metabolism
Cell proliferation	Infection	Thermoregulation
Cellular regulation		

CHAPTER

52 Nursing Assessment of the Patient with Immunologic and Inflammatory Disorders

Renée Holleran

Outcome-Based Learning Objectives

After studying this chapter, the learner will be able to:

1. Describe the function of the organs, tissues, and cellular components of the immune system.
2. Discuss the significance of self antigens versus non self antigens and immune tolerance.
3. Differentiate cell-mediated immunity and humoral immunity in relation to the type of lymphocytes involved, response to antigens, and role in immune protection.
4. Compare and contrast the actions of cytokines, lymphokines, interleukins, interferons, complement, and tumor necrosis factor on immune function.
5. Explain the action and significance of antigen presentation in B-cell activation, stimulation of immunoglobulin production, and secondary immune response.
6. Apply the assessment skills of inspection, palpation, percussion, and auscultation in evaluating body systems and determining the status of immune function.
7. Interpret and relate immune-related laboratory tests when assessing immune function.

KEY TERMS

acquired immunity p.1599
active acquired immunity p.1599
agglutination p.1604
anergy p.1615
antibodies p.1595
antigen p.1594
antigen–antibody complex p.1602
apoptosis p.1598
B cells p.1599
caspases p.1598
cell-mediated immune response p.1599
chemotaxis p.1601
chyle p.1596
complement p.1601
cytokines p.1601
fragment antigen binding (FAB) portion p.1602
fragment crystalline (FC) portion p.1602
human leukocyte antigens (HLAs) p.1598
humoral immune response p.1601
immune complex p.1601
immune tolerance p.1594
immunity p.1594
immunoglobulin p.1601
interferon p.1601
interleukin p.1601
lymphokines p.1601
monoclonal antibody p.1604
natural immunity p.1597
neutralization p.1602
nongranulocyte p.1595
non-self antigen p.1599
opsonization p.1601
Peyer's patches p.1596
phagocytosis p.1595
plasma cells p.1602
polyclonal response p.1604
precipitation p.1604
self antigen p.1599
T cells p.1599
T-helper cells p.1599
tissue factor (TF) p.1601
toll receptors p.1598
tumor necrosis factor (TNF) p.1601

AN INTACT AND FUNCTIONING IMMUNE SYSTEM is critical for the body's survival. The immune system protects the body from the invasion of microorganisms and foreign substances and eliminates damaged or mutant cells such as cancer cells. The protective process of response to a foreign substance is referred to as **immunity.** To function successfully, the immune system must be able to differentiate between "self" cells and an infinite number of "non-self" substances and foreign cells such as bacteria, viruses, or tumor proteins. Any substance that the immune system recognizes as foreign is referred to as an **antigen.** The ability to differentiate self from non-self is referred to as **immune tolerance.** Loss of immune tolerance is the basis for numerous immune disorders, which are discussed in Chapter 53.

The immune system includes central and peripheral lymphoid tissues and immune cells that defend the body against disease through natural and acquired immunity, as well as the inflammation process. Chart 52–1 provides an overview of the immune response (Rote, 2010; Rote & Huether, 2010).

CHART 52–1 Overview of Inflammation and Natural and Acquired Immunity

	Key Features
Inflammation	Initial response to injury of any kind. Includes cells, such as neutrophils and macrophages, and chemical mediators, such as histamine, complement, and clotting cascade. Inflammation produces the symptoms of redness, swelling, heat or fever, pain, and loss of function.
Natural Immunity	Natural immunity involves organs such as the skin and lymphatic system as well as the body's immune tolerance to self antigens. Mechanical processes such as coughing and sneezing can help remove debris from the body. Gastric pH helps protect the stomach from bacteria. Mucous membranes function as a lubricant, a physical barrier, and the body's first line of defense against toxins and infection.
Acquired Immunity	This system of cells, such as B and T cells, protect through immunoglobulins and cell-mediated immune response. Antibodies produced by B cells can attach to antigens and stimulate **phagocytosis.** T cells regulate the production of antibodies and release other lymphokines that direct immune cells to eliminate antigens or destroy mutant cells.

Natural immunity is provided by specific organs, cells, and chemicals that are present at birth or shortly afterward. However, the immune system in the prenatal and neonatal stages is immature and susceptible to environmental and chemical toxins (Rote & Huether, 2010). Acquired immunity includes antibodies, immunocompetent T cells and B cells, and cytokines that remove antigens that the body considers nonself (Rote & Huether, 2010). Immune cells also include a variety of white blood cells such as macrophages, neutrophils, and eosinophils. This chapter focuses on the anatomy and physiology of normal immune function and assessment of the immune system. A complete description of inflammation is available in Chapter 53.

Genetic factors play a key role in immune function. Abnormalities in gene development that affect the immune system will be discussed in Chapter 53 as they relate to the development of specific disease processes.

Anatomy of the Immune System

The major components of the immune system are the bone marrow, the lymphatic system (including lymph nodes and lymphatic circulation), and the spleen. These organs and tissues are located throughout the body and thus provide a systemic immune response.

Bone Marrow

The development of the immune system begins in the body's bone marrow. As illustrated in Figure 52–1◆ (p. 1596), bone marrow is rich in *stem cells,* which are able to differentiate into a variety of cell lines that are critical for immune function. Stem cells have the capacity to produce any type of cell that they are chemically directed to make. For example, stem cells differentiate into white blood cells such as granulocytes, lymphocytes, and monocytes. Granulocytes become neutrophils, eosinophils, and basophils. Lymphocyte precursors in bone marrow become B- and T-cell lines. Monocytes differentiate from white blood cell precursors to circulate in the blood and ultimately mature into macrophages. Bone marrow stem cells also differentiate into red blood cells (erythrocytes) and platelets (thrombocytes) (Rote & McCance, 2010).

Granulocytes

Granulocytes are the lineage of white blood cells that differentiate into neutrophils, basophils, and eosinophils. They are named granulocytes because their cell cytoplasm contains granules of chemicals such as histamine. These granules can be seen on Gram stain and are used to identify and count the cells microscopically.

Neutrophils

Neutrophils, also referred to as polymorphonuclear neutrophils (PMN), make up over 55% of the leukocyte count in the blood and are important phagocytic cells. Their function is to consume cellular debris, immune complexes, and bacterial and viral particles (Rote & McCance, 2010). Neutrophils are the first group of white blood cells to arrive at the site of injury or cell death. They have a short life span of approximately 72 hours or less. The various types of neutrophils and their percentage in the blood are described in the Diagnostic Tests to Assess Immune Function feature in this chapter.

Basophils

Basophils migrate from the bloodstream into tissue and mature into mast cells. When a body cell is injured, mast cells in the immediate vicinity release large quantities of histamine, stimulating the inflammatory response (Rote & McCance, 2010).

Eosinophils

Eosinophils comprise a very small portion of the total number of white blood cells. The presence of parasites stimulates them to increase their numbers. The number of eosinophils also increases in the presence of allergies. Eosinophils are responsible for increasing the immune and inflammatory response.

Nongranulocytes

Nongranulocytes are highly effective phagocytic white blood cells that can engulf large numbers of foreign antigens, such as bacteria. Their cell lineage includes monocytes and lymphocytes. These cells are identified microscopically by their large nucleus and the lack of granules in their cytoplasm.

Monocytes

The primary function of monocytes and macrophages is phagocytosis. These cells arrive at the site of cell injury hours to days after neutrophils. Macrophages have a longer life span, have a higher tolerance for an acidic environment, and are capable of consuming a large amount of debris for an extended period of time compared to other monocytes (Rote, 2010).

Lymphocytes

Lymphocytes differentiate into T cells and B cells. Microscopically, T and B cells appear similar, with a large nucleus and no granules in the cytoplasm. T cells are responsible for regulating and initiating the immune response. The primary function of B cells is the production of antibodies such as immunoglobulins (Ig): IgE, IgG, IgA, IgM, and IgD (Rote, 2010). **Antibodies,** proteins that bind to antigens and immobilize or destroy them, are discussed further later in the chapter.

Deficiencies in functional bone marrow and stem cells can lead to immune deficiency disorders. Primary immunodeficiencies of the B cells become apparent at 7 to 9 months after birth. The antibody titers received from the mother decrease, and the infant with immunodeficiencies is unable to produce mature and adequate levels of B cells (Newman & McGrath, 2010).

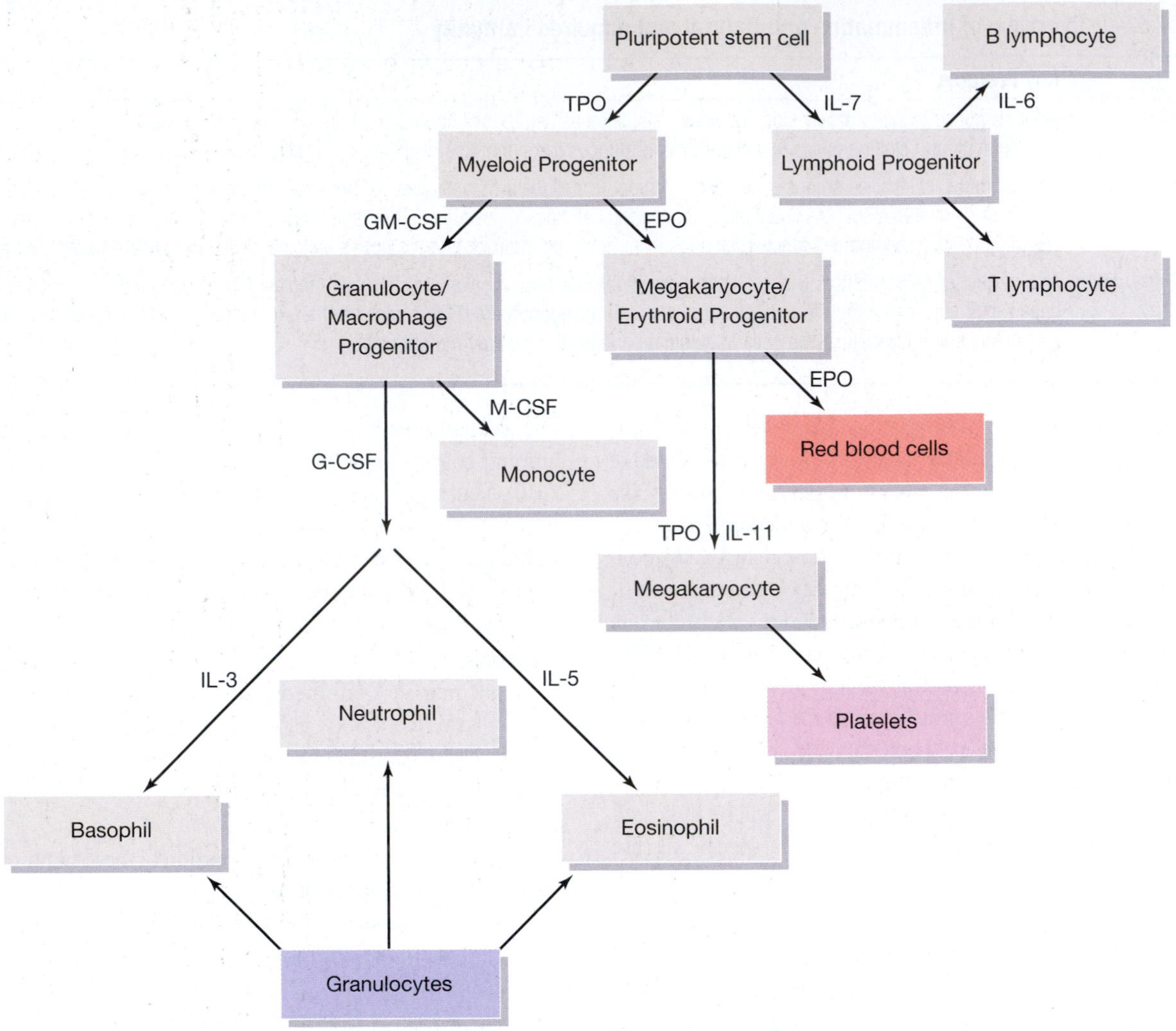

FIGURE 52–1 ◆ Cell line differentiation in bone marrow.

Lymphatic System

The lymphatic system is comprised of vessels, lymph nodes, and lymph tissue. This system of vessels drains lymph fluid through the entire body and returns it to venous circulation in the chest. The vessels drain this lymph fluid, referred to as **chyle** (a milky fluid composed of serous fluid, white cells, and fatty acids), into the thoracic and lymphatic ducts in the mediastinum. The lymph vessels follow the same route as veins and arteries and run parallel to veins. Chyle then drains from the mediastinum into the heart through the superior vena cava.

Lymph nodes and lymph tissue filter debris from the breakdown of cells, bacteria, viruses, and fungal antigens. Lymphocytes such as T and B cells are found in lymph nodes. Lymph nodes and tissue contain or house macrophages that ingest cells, bacteria, and debris. Two-thirds of fixed lymph tissue is located in the abdomen surrounding the intestinal tissue and is referred to as **Peyer's patches.** This is important because the vessels that deliver blood to the intestines facilitate the entry of large molecules of digested materials into the circulatory system. Vessels that are able to absorb large food particles may also allow the entry of viral and bacterial particles. Hence, immune protection by Peyer's patches is vital (Twite & Gaspard, 2007). A high concentration of lymph tissue also is located in the lungs. Alveolar macrophages function with lymph tissue to protect the lungs from bacteria, viruses, and debris from the outside environment (DeFranco, Locksley, & Robertson, 2007).

Lymph nodes are consolidated groups of lymph tissue that are found throughout the body. Lymph nodes located in the neck, axilla, and groin may be palpated. Like lymph tissue, they contain macrophages and lymphocytes and are able to filter and remove dead cells, bacteria, and other debris from the system, as well as assist in triggering the immune response (Figure 52–2◆).

During infection, inflammation, malignancy, or injury, lymph nodes in the area of injury will become swollen (lymphadenopathy). An example of lymphadenopathy is the swelling of lymph nodes in the axilla and neck during pneumonia (Rote & McCance, 2010).

Safety Alert *Patients with compromised immune function such as those with HIV/AIDS or cancer patients on chemotherapy need to have their lymph nodes examined even if no other complaint is present. Nodes swollen by cell debris of any kind warrant further investigation.*

Tonsils and Adenoids

Tonsils and adenoids are consolidated lymph tissue located in the throat. They remove and filter debris, bacteria, and viruses from the upper airways and mouth. Like all consolidated lymph tissue, they contain B and T cells as well as macrophages (DeFranco et al., 2007).

Video: Lymph Nodes

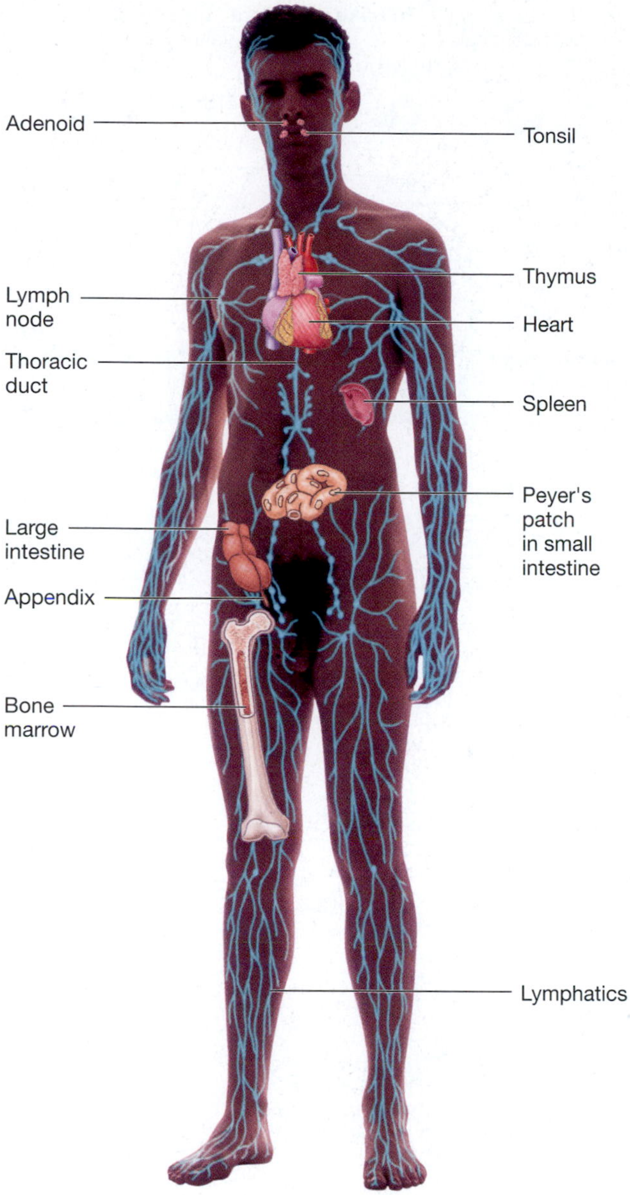

FIGURE 52–2 ◆ Lymphatic system with lymph nodes.

Spleen

The spleen plays a significant role in immune function as part of the lymphatic system. It is composed of white and red pulp. Red pulp is made up of multiple types of red blood cells such as platelets, granulocytes, and plasma. White pulp contains lymphocytes. The majority of the spleen is composed of red pulp. The spleen is involved in hematologic filtration, sequestering of red and white cells, and the immune response. The white pulp of the spleen is rich in lymphocytes that become active in the immune response. The red pulp is responsible for filtering out aged or damaged red blood cells. The spleen may also sequester red and white blood cells and platelets and thus decrease the cell levels circulating in the blood. The spleen may become enlarged in acute inflammatory or infectious disease processes because of the stimulation of the immune response. An enlarged spleen (splenomegaly) can be involved in a plethora of disease processes, such as trauma, cancer, infection, portal hypertension, thrombosis, cysts, and mononucleosis. This assessment finding warrants further investigation (Rote & McCance, 2010).

Physiology of the Immune System

The physiology of the immune system includes the function of the lymphatic tissues, cells, and chemicals that provide protection from infectious agents, antigens, and mutated cells and enable the body to differentiate self from non-self. The immune response includes both natural and acquired immunity.

Natural Immunity

Natural immunity, also referred to as innate immunity, is provided by a group of body organs, cells, and chemicals that are present at birth or shortly thereafter. **Natural immunity** is defined as the organs, cells, and secretions of the body that provide protection from foreign proteins, chemicals, and other non-self particles. Natural immunity includes the integumentary system, the lymphatic system, and secretions such as lysozymes, immunoglobulins, and subcellular receptors such as toll-like receptors. The white blood cells and chemicals of the inflammatory response are an important part of natural immunity. All of these components of natural immune function are present at birth (Figure 52–3◆).

Physical and Chemical Barriers

Physical and chemical barriers provide the first line of defense in immune protection. Physical barriers include the skin and the mucous membranes. Chemical barriers include lysozymes, acidic pH of the stomach, and toll receptors, all of which are discussed in the following text.

Skin

Natural immunity starts with the skin, the largest organ of the human body. It acts as a barrier to debris, bacteria, and other organisms. The skin also protects soft organs and tissue from changes in the

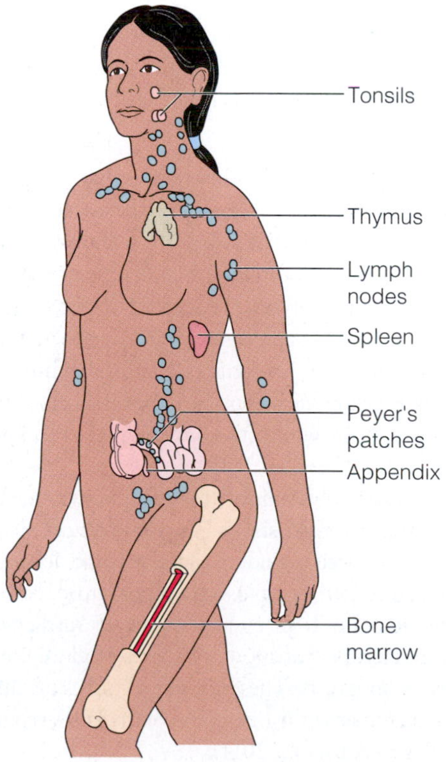

FIGURE 52–3 ◆ Immune system with organs.
Source: Michael Freeman/Phototake NYC.

environment. Bacteria are always present on the surface of the skin in varying quantities. However, the limited amount of moisture in the skin and its pH protect it from bacterial growth. Therefore, intact skin is critical to the organism's survival. Even small breaks in the skin's integrity can lead to large wounds or infections either locally or systemically because organisms are able to enter the body (Rote & Huether, 2010).

Safety Alert *Careful examination of the skin is an essential part of every physical assessment of patients. Patients may require education about maintaining skin integrity. When a rash or skin breakdown occurs, patients should be instructed to report to their health care provider the onset of the symptoms, location of the rash or breakdown, and any treatment modalities they have used to deal with it.*

Mucous Membranes

Mucous membranes also form part of the first line of defense in natural immunity. Mucous membranes assist in protecting the body from attack by removing dirt and debris from the body. Ciliated cells in the trachea remove bacteria and environmental toxins from the trachea using a wavelike motion of their cilia. Mucous membranes in the mouth secrete lysozymes and immunoglobulins that are mildly antibiotic and assist in protecting the mouth from bacterial infection (Sommer, 2007). Good oral hygiene is essential in preventing infections in the oral cavity.

Safety Alert *Patients who are receiving supplemental oxygen by mask or ventilator need frequent oral care. Although oxygen administration can be humidified, patients may not be able to keep the oral mucosa moist and clean. Gentle swabbing with soft swabs and water or mouthwash can help keep the mouth moist. Patients receiving oxygen by mask may require assistance with brushing their teeth, gums, and tongue. Patients on a ventilator are dependent on the nurse for oral care. The CDC issued guidelines in 2004 that remain relevant today promoting good oral care to assist in the prevention of ventilator-associated pneumonia (Tablan, Anderson, Besser, Bridges, & Hajjeh, 2004).*

Gastric pH

Immune protection is also provided in the stomach. The pH of the stomach ranges from approximately 1.0 to 3.0. This is so acidic that most bacteria, fungi, and viral particles are unable to survive.

Toll Receptors

Finally, **toll receptors** are a class of proteins that play a major role in natural immunity. Humans are born with these toll receptors, which provide an important form of innate protection for the body because they act as a gate or point of initiation of certain cell functions (Figure 52–4 ◆). Toll receptors are located on the surface of many types of immune and tissue cells and are able to initiate immune responses when pieces of bacterial cell walls attach to them. Some toll receptors are shaped to accept the lipopolysaccharide portion of the cell wall of bacteria, while others are shaped to accept the wall of a fungal cell (Rote & Huether, 2010).

Toll receptors not only stimulate the immune system, they also can signal a cell to start **apoptosis,** or programmed cell death. Infected cells can often be induced to undergo apoptosis and destroy themselves (McCance & Grey, 2010). Apoptosis is a programmed cascade event.

Caspases are a family of cysteine proteases further divided into initiator and executioner functions. Caspases produce the phenotypic changes seen in apoptosis. These include cytoskeletal disintegration, DNA fragmentation, and the disruption of the DNA repair molecular machinery (Nduka & Parrillo, 2011).

Additionally, cells stimulated by the attachment of a lipopolysaccharide piece of bacterial wall are able to stimulate the release of tumor necrosis factor, a key chemical in initiating immune and

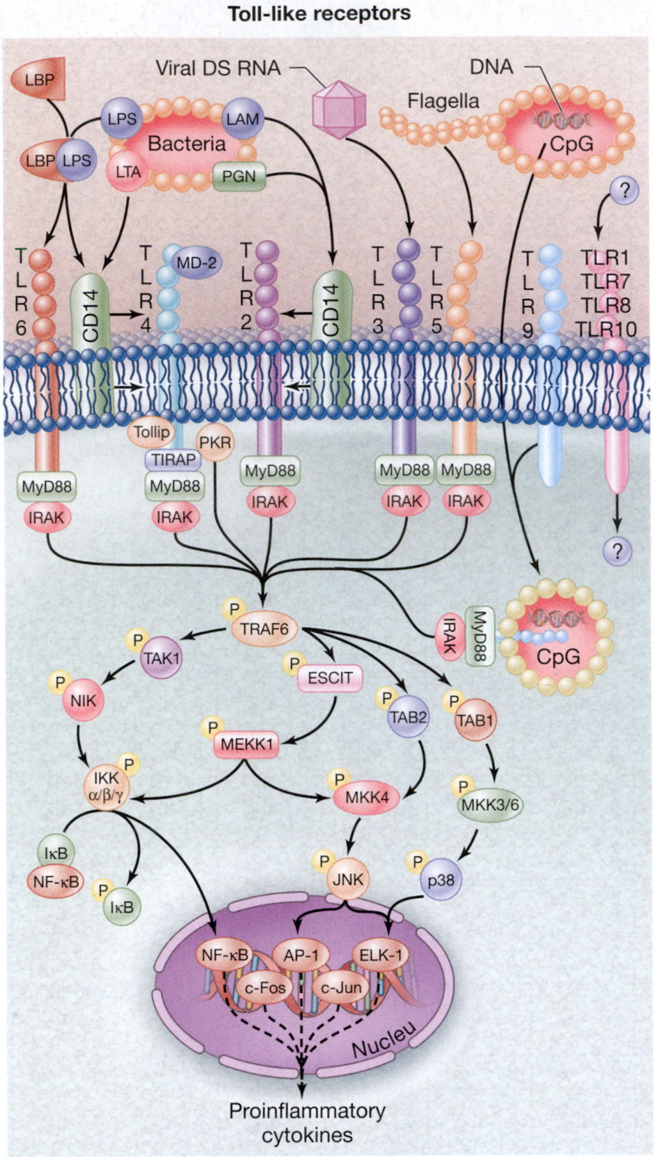

FIGURE 52–4 ◆ Toll receptors.

inflammatory responses. This response is critical in alerting the system to the presence of non self antigens such as bacteria (DeFranco et al., 2007; Rote, 2010).

Self Versus Non-Self

Self is defined as all cells of the body and the receptors on those cells that are recognized as unique to that individual. Major histocompatibility complex (MHC) receptors on cells are an example of a marker used by the immune system to determine whether a cell belongs to the organism or not. Additionally, **human leukocyte antigens (HLAs)** are protein markers on the cell wall of white blood cells that alert the immune system to the appropriateness of a cell belonging to the system. These markers are tested for matching in organ transplant because an exact HLA match will minimize the immune response and the risk of transplant rejection (Rote, 2010).

Non-self is any protein, antigen, or the stimulatory part of any foreign cell that the immune system does not recognize as self. Antigens are foreign substances that can signal the immune system to mount a response and eliminate the foreign cell, bacteria, virus, or fungus (DeFranco et al., 2007).

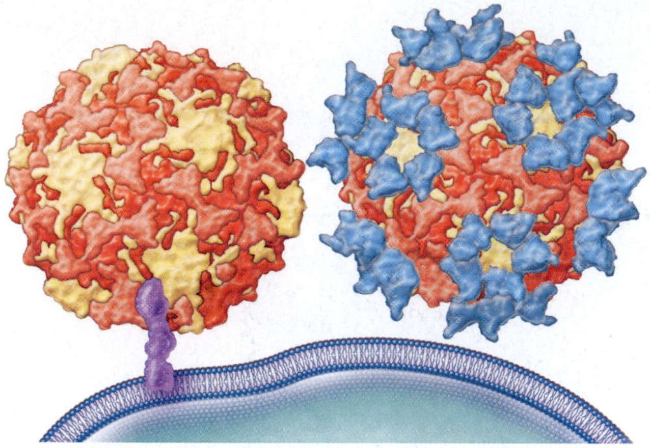

FIGURE 52–5 ◆ (A) Self versus (B) non-self.

Bacteria, viruses, fungi, and amoebic parasites are major threats to the survival of the human body. The immune system is constantly looking for cells and proteins that are not-self. Cancer cells frequently lack specific markers; thus, the immune system may or may not recognize the mutant cell as non-self (Figure 52–5◆). If the immune system does not identify the mutated malignant cells, a tumor may develop. Chapter 57 discusses the development of a cancerous tumor.

Immune Tolerance

Immune tolerance is defined as the immune system's ability to tolerate all *self antigens* while retaining the ability to mount an immune response to **non-self antigens** (foreign antigens). Immune tolerance begins during embryonic development of the immune system. Lymphocytes that react with self antigens are selectively eliminated as the immune system develops. This leaves the newborn with B-cell and T-cell lines that do not attack self antigens. **Self antigens** include HLAs and MHC, as well as several other antigenic particles that are often cell receptors. When the body reacts to self-receptors or other cell parts as an antigen, autoimmune disease may result (DeFranco et al., 2007). Chapter 53 discusses autoimmune diseases.

Inflammatory Response

The inflammatory response is an important part of the body's response to any injury and an integral part of the immune response. White blood cells such as neutrophils and macrophages travel to the site of injury in response to the chemicals of inflammation such as histamine, complement, and bradykinin. Inflammation presents with symptoms of redness, edema, pain, and heat from increased blood flow to the area of injury (Sommer, 2007).

The inflammatory response is seen in cell injury, allergy reactions, anaphylaxis, and many disease processes. Cells and chemicals of the inflammatory response also stimulate the activity of T cells and B cells to mount an immune response.

Acquired Immunity

Acquired immunity can be described as the ability of the immune cells to correctly produce antibodies, regulate the immune response, and respond only to non-self antigens (DeFranco et al., 2007). This immunity is considered acquired because the body develops the ability to regulate the immune system and produce antibodies after exposure to antigens in the environment. Active immunity is acquired by either contracting the disease or through a vaccination, such as childhood rubella vaccination or flu shots received by adults (Atkinson, Wolfe, & Hamborsky, 2011). **Active acquired immunity** involves the production of antibodies by the immune system in response to specific foreign antigens, such as bacteria. Acquired immunity involves lymphocyte cells and chemicals that remove antigens that are considered non-self and confer long-term permanent protection against the disease for which the antibodies have been produced.

Lymphocytes are white blood cells that include *T cells* and *B cells*. **T cells,** or T lymphocytes, are involved in the cellular immune response and are responsible for stimulating and regulating the immune response. The **B cells,** or B lymphocytes, are involved in the humoral immune response and are responsible for the creation and release of antibodies and development of long-term immune protection. Figure 52–6◆ (p. 1600) describes immune cell differentiation from precursor cells.

Cellular Immune Response

The cellular immune response is initiated by T cells (Figure 52–7◆, p. 1600). These cells are responsible for stimulating or decreasing the immune response through the production of chemicals called cytokines that can directly destroy cells, help macrophages find the antigen and consume it, and protect cells from viral attachment (Twite & Gaspard, 2007).

T Cells

T-cell precursors in the bone marrow differentiate into specific types of T cells. Immature T cells travel from the bone marrow via the bloodstream to the thymus gland and other lymphatic tissues. During childhood, T cells mature and differentiate primarily in the thymus. After puberty, the thymus gland shrinks, and T-cell differentiation and maturation occur predominantly in other lymphatic tissue such as the white pulp of the spleen and the lymph nodes.

T cells are the regulatory cells of the immune system whose function is to start and stop the immune processes. These processes include phagocytosis, cytokine secretion, and activation of B cells (Sommer, 2007). The functions of T cells are known as the **cell-mediated immune response.** There are an extensive number of T-cell types, which are named by their function or by the identifying markers on the cell membrane (DeFranco et al., 2007; Rote, 2010). The most significant T cells and their roles in immune function are discussed in the following text.

T-Helper Cells

T-helper cells are also known as CD4 cells because there are CD4 receptors on the surface of this group. T cells are further divided into T-helper 1 and T-helper 2 cell lines. T-helper 1 cells help upregulate immune activity and produce chemicals called cytokines that stimulate cytotoxic cells to destroy mutant and cancer cells. T-helper 1 cells produce cytokines that are chemotactic (i.e., they move toward the area of infection). CD4 receptors have been identified as the type of receptor that the human immunodeficiency virus (HIV) attaches to and uses to enter the T cell, thereby severely affecting immune function; this is discussed in detail in Chapter 53 (Rote, 2010; Sommer, 2007).

T-helper 2 cells stimulate B cells to make antibodies to specific antigens. This is accomplished through the release of chemicals such as interleukins and the antigen presentation process (DeFranco et al., 2007). Memory T cells retain a "chemical memory" of virus particles encountered by these cells. The next exposure to the "remembered" virus results in a quick immune response. For example, memory

Weblink: Immunity: Natural and Acquired

Weblink: Categories of Acquired Immunity

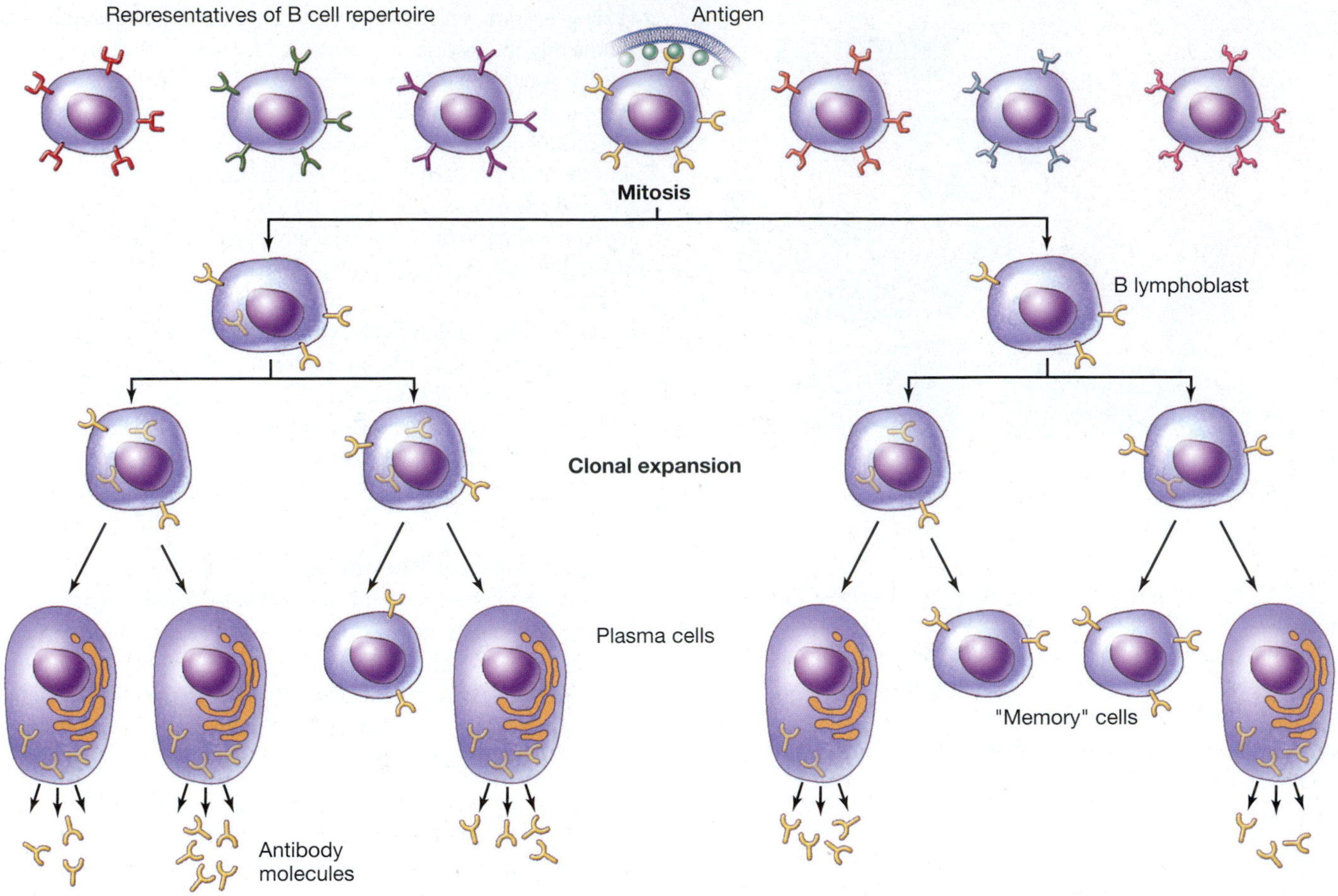

FIGURE 52–6 ◆ Immune cell differentiation from precursors.

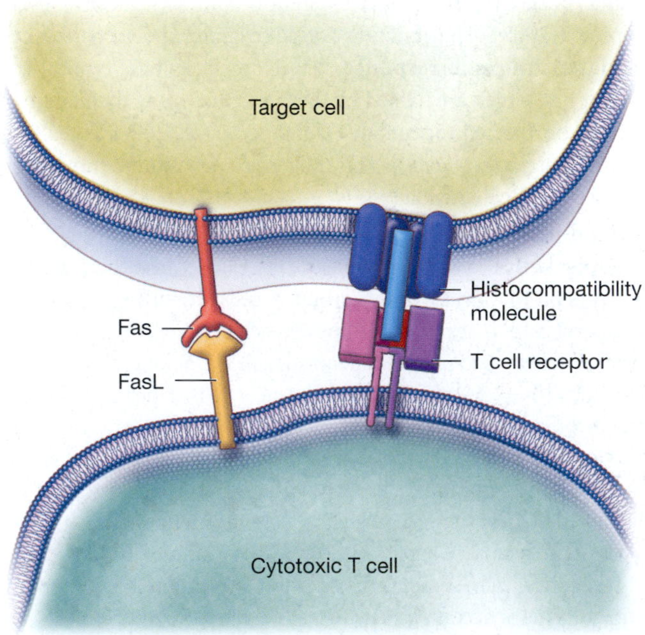

One method by which cytotoxic T cells induce their targets (e.g., virus-infected cells) to commit suicide (apoptosis)

FIGURE 52–7 ◆ T cell.

T cells are responsible for protection against rhinoviruses, one group of cold viruses. The first exposure to a rhinovirus usually results in cold symptoms such as sore throat, sneezing, and cough. The memory T cells retain a memory of that specific rhinovirus that lasts for a lifetime. On second exposure to that same virus, the memory T cells are able to stimulate a rapid immune response, thus minimizing or preventing signs and symptoms of infection. Frequent infections with rhinovirus occur because the virus mutates rapidly, creating a new virus antigen. Thus, the memory T cells must go through the process of developing a memory for each new rhinovirus. More than 200 rhinoviruses have been identified. Children have more colds than adults because children have not been exposed to as many virus antigens and therefore have not developed the same immune memory as adults (Sommer, 2007).

Suppressor T Cells

Suppressor T cells, also called CD8 cells, slow or stop the immune response. This *downregulation*, the primary role of suppressor T cells, is an important part of regulation of the immune system because it provides the ability to stop the production of antibodies and cell destruction once the threat of infection has been overcome (DeFranco et al., 2007).

Natural Killer Cells

Natural killer cells, also referred to as "null cells," are types of T cells that lack CD4 or CD8 external receptors but are able to directly kill cells or send cytokine messages to start the process of apoptosis. Natural killer cells are usually directed to initiate cell death by T-helper 1 cells (Rote, 2010).

Chart 52–2 describes lymphocyte function in greater detail.

CHART 52–2 Lymphocyte Functions

Lymphocyte	Functions
B cell	Antibody production.
Plasma cell	Antibody production, responsible for primary antibody response.
Memory cell	Antibody production, responsible for secondary antibody response.
T-cell lines	Regulation, stimulation, and downregulation of immune system through the use of chemical mediators. Null cells and natural killer cells may destroy infected cells directly.
T-helper cells (CD4) T-helper 1 T-helper 2 Memory T-helper cells	Stimulate and upregulate immune function. Assist in antigen presentation. Activate B cells to make antibodies (T-helper 2); stimulate natural killer cells (T-helper 1); nonspecific immune memory function (memory T-helper cells).
Suppressor T cells (CD8)	Can slow or downregulate immune function. Slow release of inflammatory cytokines.
Natural killer cells	T-cell line is able to chemically kill infected cells and tumor cells.

Sources: DeFranco, A. L., Locksley, R., & Robertson, M. (2007). *Immunity: The immune response in infectious and inflammatory disease.* Sunderland, MA: Sinauer Associates; McCance, K. L., & Grey, T. C. (2010). Altered cellular and tissue biology. In K. L. McCance & S. E. Huether (Eds.), *Pathophysiology: The biological basis for disease in adults & children* (6th ed., pp. 46–95). St. Louis: Mosby Elsevier.

Cytokines and Lymphokines

Cytokines are chemical messages produced by cells to communicate with other cells in the body. Cytokines have a plethora of functions such as chemotaxis and opsonization. **Chemotaxis** is the movement of additional white blood cells to an area of inflammation in response to the release of chemical mediators by neutrophils, monocytes, and injured tissue. **Opsonization** is the chemical coating of an antigen or cell that makes that cell more attractive to phagocytes. Cytokines that are made by lymphocytes are called **lymphokines** and include interleukins and interferons. Other examples of cytokines are tumor necrosis factor, tissue factor, and growth inhibitory factor (DeFranco et al., 2007). A variety of cytokines and their functions are described in Chart 52–3 (p. 1602) (Rote, 2010).

Interleukins

Interleukins are lymphokines that enable the cells of the immune system to communicate and coordinate the immune response. Interleukins are crucial to the immune response. Interleukin-1 and interleukin-6 are proinflammatory and stimulate the release of chemicals such as tumor necrosis factor and tissue factor that begin the inflammatory response. Interleukin-12 slows and helps stop the immune and inflammatory responses (Sommer, 2007).

Interferons

Interferons are proteins made and released by T cells when they are exposed to a virus. This group of lymphokines protects other cells from viral attack by inhibiting the production of the virus within infected cells, preventing the spread of the virus to other cells, and enhancing the activity of macrophages, natural killer cells, and cytotoxic T cells. In addition, interferons can inhibit the growth of certain tumor cells. Interferons made by recombinant technology are used to treat a variety of disease states. One example of this is alpha interferon, which is used to slow the growth of new blood vessels in some cancerous vascular tumors (Rote, 2010).

Tumor Necrosis Factor

Tumor necrosis factor (TNF) is a small peptide that is produced by a variety of cells, including granulocytes and lymphocytes. Tumor necrosis factor is critical in the stimulation of the initial inflammatory response, specifically the activity of macrophages and granulocytes. It also is important in telling cells to initiate apoptosis when mutations occur. This function is important in inhibiting tumor development and growth. Chronic inflammation has been implicated in the development of some types of cancerous tumors due to cell changes that occur with a long-term inflammatory response (DeFranco et al., 2007). Therefore, TNF is vital in inhibiting tumor development and growth.

Tissue Factor

Tissue factor (TF) is another cytokine that is important in immune function and inflammation. Tissue factor is a very significant cytokine that contributes to the body's protective inflammatory response (Sommer, 2007). Tissue factor can be released by a variety of injured tissue cells, macrophages, and platelets. Its function is to stimulate platelets to stick together and form the beginning of a clot. This is critical in stopping blood loss from injured blood vessels.

Complement Proteins and Function

Complement is a group of small proteins made in the liver and present in blood that can interact with cells and each other for a variety of functions. Complement proteins are important in the inflammatory and immune responses. Complement 3b is an opsonin (chemical that coats or attaches to an antigen or cell). After attachment, the cell or antigen becomes highly visible to neutrophils and macrophages. This stimulates the phagocytic cells to approach and consume the cell or antigen. Complement 3a and complement 5a are chemotactic and can chemically summon phagocytic cells such as neutrophils as well as T cells and B cells to the area of infection (DeFranco et al., 2007).

Complement can be activated by immune complexes attached to cell membranes or antibodies attached to cell membranes. When this occurs, complement fragments form a complex either around an attached antibody or directly to receptors on the cell membrane or wall. This complex of complement is capable of directly lysing (breaking down) a cell wall and killing the organism or cell (Rote, 2010). Figure 52–8◆ diagrams the classic complement pathway and the alternative pathway. Both pathways end in cell lysis.

Humoral Immune Response

The **humoral immune response** involves the antibodies produced in the B cell lineage. Antibodies are proteins that bind to antigens and immobilize or destroy them. The attachment of the antibody to the antigen is called an **immune complex.** The immune complex helps stimulate the immune response and can provide long-term protection from bacterial, viral, and fungal antigens.

B Cells

B cells are white blood cells that differentiate in bone marrow and enter the blood (Figure 52–9◆, p. 1605). B cells are responsible for the production of antibodies, which are also called **immunoglobulins.** B cells differentiate in the blood into either plasma B cells or memory B cells. B cells may be stimulated directly by some antigens or by T cells to make antibodies. Once stimulated, B cells make antibodies during

CHART 52–3 Cytokines and Their Functions

Cytokine	Functions
Tumor necrosis factor (TNF)	Stimulates immune and inflammatory responses. Participates in destroying cancer cells. Can activate macrophages and granulocytes. Contributes to the wasting syndrome seen in cancer. Can stimulate apoptosis.
Interleukin (IL)	
IL-1	Inflammatory mediator that activates T cells, induces fever, and assists in upregulating the immune system.
IL-2	Inflammatory mediator that promotes T-cell growth and replication and activates T cells and natural killer cells.
IL-3 (multiple colony-stimulating factor)	Stimulates the proliferation of hematopoietic precursor cells.
IL-4	Stimulates growth of T cells, B cells, mast cells, and eosinophils.
IL-5	Stimulates growth of B cells and eosinophils.
IL-6	Acts synergistically with IL-1 and TNF to increase inflammation. Stimulates growth of B cells and differentiation into plasma and memory cells. Can induce fever.
IL-7	Stimulates growth of T and B cells.
IL-8	Chemotactic factor for neutrophils and T cells.
IL-9	Mild stimulation of precursor cells of the T-cell line and red blood cell.
IL-10	Stimulates B cells and antibody production. Slows cytokine release by T cells and natural killer cells.
IL-12	Stimulates gamma-interferon production. Promotes cell-mediated immune response.
IL-16	Chemotactic factor for T cells, monocytes, and eosinophils.
IL-17	Stimulates release of IL-6, IL-8, and granulocyte colony-stimulating factor.
IL-18	Upregulates natural killer cell function. Stimulates the release of gamma interferon.
Interferons	
Alpha-interferon	Can slow and inhibit viral replication. Also activates natural killer cells.
Beta-interferon	Blocks viral replication.
Gamma-interferon	Blocks viral replication, activates macrophages, and enhances natural killer cell function and differentiation of B cells.
Colony-stimulating factors	Enhance differentiation and activation of white blood cell lines. Cells stimulated include macrophages and granulocytes. Erythropoietin stimulates differentiation and growth of red blood cells.

Sources: DeFranco, A. L., Locksley, R., & Robertson, M. (2007). *Immunity: The immune response in infectious and inflammatory disease.* Sunderland, MA: Sinauer Associates; McCance, K. L., & Grey, T. C. (2010). Altered cellular and tissue biology. In K. L. McCance & S. E. Huether (Eds.), *Pathophysiology: The biological basis for disease in adults & children* (6th ed., pp. 46–95). St. Louis: Mosby Elsevier; Porth, C. (2008). *Essentials of pathophysiology* (7th ed.). Philadelphia: Lippincott Williams & Wilkins.

their entire life span. Memory B cells can produce immunoglobulins more quickly and in greater numbers when an antigen surfaces the second time (Sommer, 2007).

Plasma Cells and Antibodies

Plasma cells are differentiated B cells that are found in the plasma and are responsible for production of specific antibodies. Plasma cells produce the antibodies in response to a primary or initial exposure to an antigen. The most common groups of antibodies are immunoglobulin G (IgG), immunoglobulin A (IgA), immunoglobulin M (IgM), immunoglobulin D (IgD), and immunoglobulin E (IgE).

Some B cells produce antibodies that are secreted into saliva, lung, and intestinal tissue. These antibodies, usually IgA, are referred to as secretory antibodies because they are found in secretions such as tears and saliva. Secretory antibodies provide immune defense at the pathogen's portal of entry (DeFranco et al., 2007). Antibodies have multiple shapes and functions, as described in Chart 52–4.

Antibodies have one or more binding sites for attachment to antigens. The antibody is composed of a **fragment antigen binding (FAB) portion,** which is capable of being shaped to receive a specific antigen. Deoxyribonucleic acid (DNA) within B cells is capable of creating many millions of combinations of FAB portions of antibodies to help protect the body from the invasion by pathogens (DeFranco et al., 2007).

The **fragment crystalline (FC) portion** of the antibody is capable of attaching to the membrane of infected cells, mutant cells, or foreign pathogens (bacteria or viruses) and assisting macrophages to eliminate them (Rote, 2010). Figure 52–10◆ (p. 1605) provides a visual representation of an immunoglobulin and the FAB and FC binding sites.

Antibody Functions

Antibodies function by attaching to an antigen at the FAB portion. This creates an **antigen–antibody complex** (also called an immune complex, as was mentioned earlier in the chapter) and is important in stimulating a strong immune response and destruction of the antigen. The antibody–antigen complex can attract other phagocytic cells such as neutrophils and macrophages to help eliminate the antigen. Each antibody is specifically shaped for only one type of antigen. When there is an exact fit between antigen and antibody, a strong antibody response results. If the fit is not exact, this type of antibody may not be able to bond as effectively with the antigen, resulting in a less profound immune response (Sommer, 2007).

Antibodies clustered around an antigen block its activity by neutralization, opsonization, agglutination, and precipitation. **Neutralization**

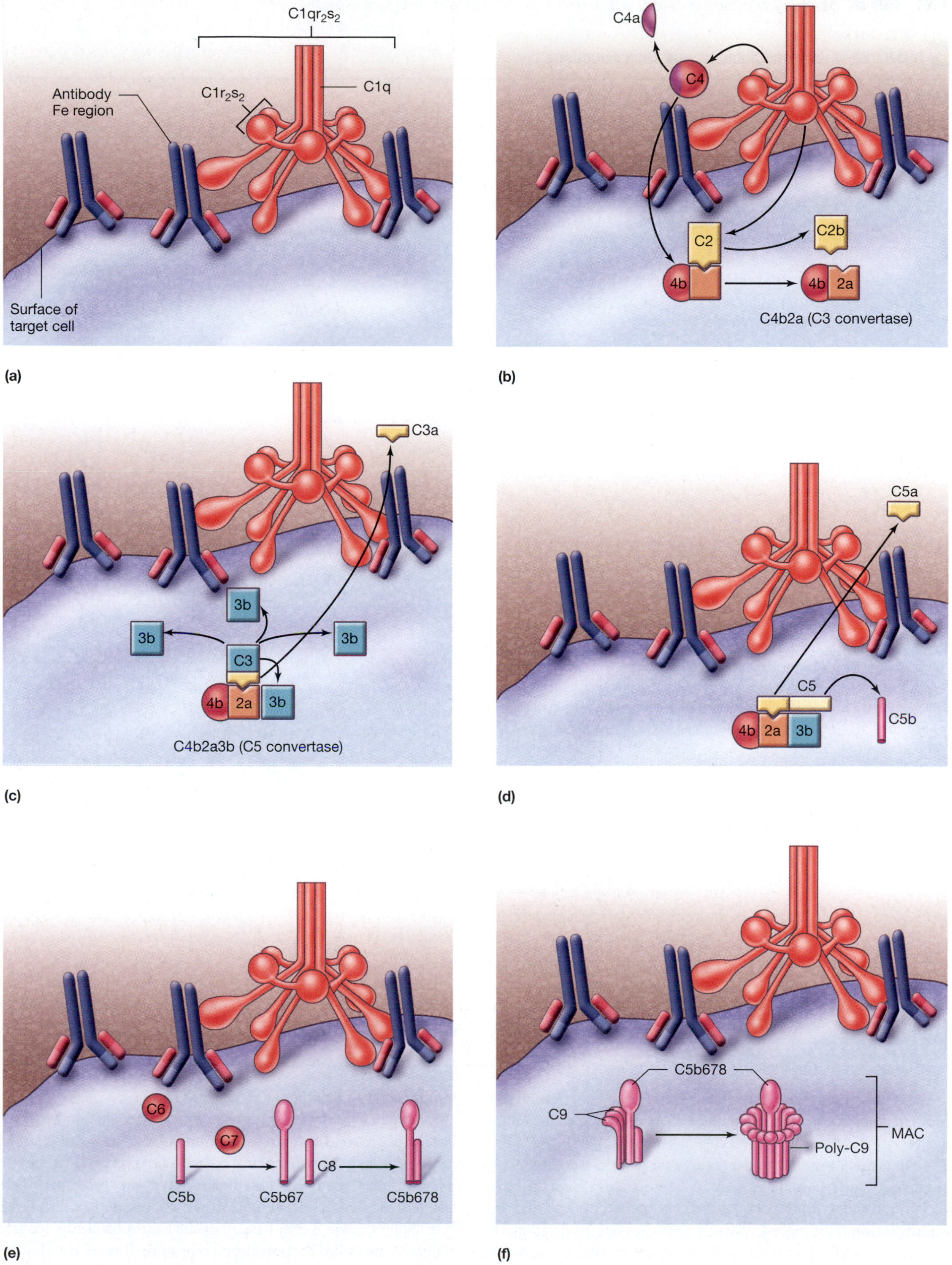

FIGURE 52–8 ◆ Complement cascade.

CHART 52–4 Immunoglobulins and Their Functions

Class of Immunoglobulin	Primary Function	Structure
IgG	The majority of circulating immunoglobulins are IgG. They are capable of most immune functions, such as agglutination, opsonization, neutralization, activation of complement, and precipitation. They can cross the placenta; major IgG is found in neonatal blood.	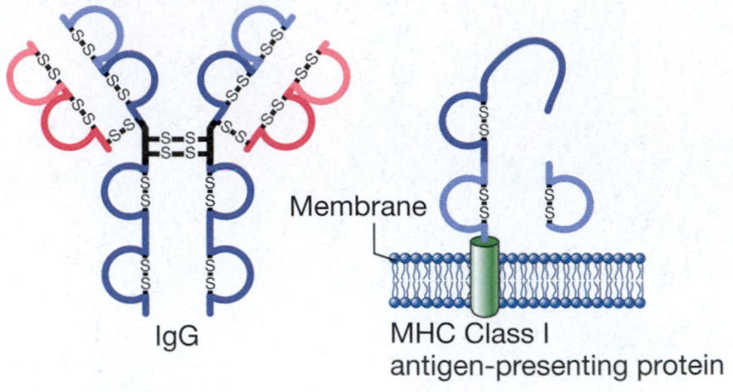
IgM	This is the first antibody produced in primary immune response. This antibody is first produced during embryonic development.	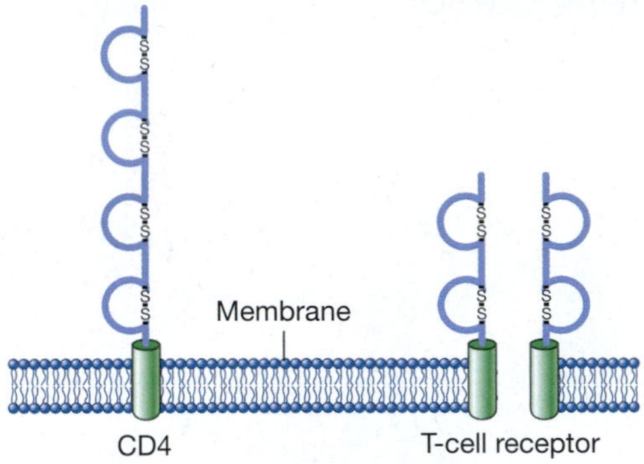
IgA	This immunoglobulin is most commonly found in secretions such as saliva. Its major function is to protect the eyes, mouth, nose, intestine, and lung from colonization and disease caused by viruses and bacteria. Secretory immunoglobulin, class IgA2, is most often found in lacrimal, saliva, intestine, lung, and nose secretions. It neutralizes bacterial and viral antigens.	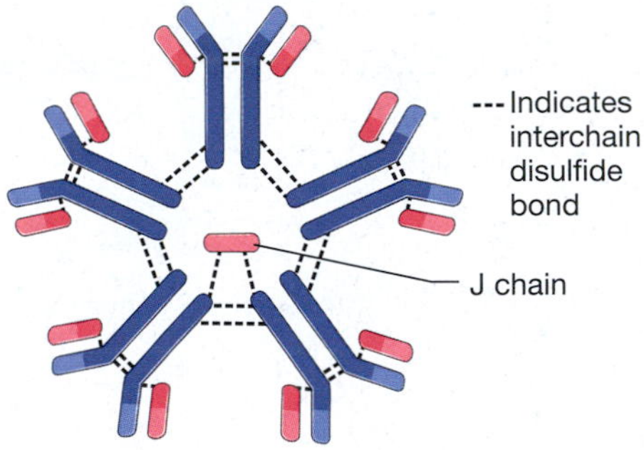
IgD	This is the least understood immunoglobulin. It attaches to B cells and acts as an antigen. IgD is present in small quantities in blood.	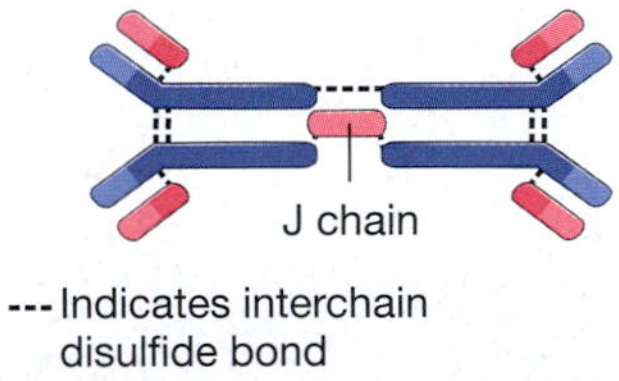
IgE	This is the primary antibody in allergic responses. The least concentration of IgE is found in serum.	

Sources: DeFranco, A. L., Locksley, R., & Robertson, M. (2007). *Immunity: The immune response in infectious and inflammatory disease.* Sunderland, MA: Sinauer Associates; McCance, K. L., & Grey, T. C. (2010). Altered cellular and tissue biology. In K. L. McCance & S. E. Huether (Eds.), *Pathophysiology: The biological basis for disease in adults & children* (6th ed., pp. 46–95). St. Louis: Mosby Elsevier; Porth, C. (2008). *Essentials of pathophysiology* (7th ed.). Philadelphia: Lippincott Williams & Wilkins.

is the process of changing the charge or shape of the antigen and blocking its ability to attach to another cell. As described earlier in the chapter, opsonization is the act of coating an antigen and making the cell or antigen more attractive to consume for phagocytic cells such as macrophages and neutrophils. Figure 52–11◆ demonstrates the formation of an immune complex that utilizes the process of opsonization. **Agglutination** is the process in which antibodies surround and attach to the antigen and clump together. Again, this stimulates the immune cells to locate the complex and consume or destroy it. **Precipitation** occurs when an immune complex precipitates out of circulation and thus becomes more easily found by neutrophils and monocytes for phagocytosis (DeFranco et al., 2007).

Monoclonal Antibodies

When antibody production begins in response to an antigen, B cells become plasma cells and start to make antibodies. The normal antibody response includes variations in the antibodies produced because the multiple antigenic properties on the antigen cause a spectrum of B cells to proliferate. This results in more than one clone of the initial B cells, even though all the B cells were stimulated to proliferate by the same antigen. This is called the **polyclonal response** (Rote, 2010). However, researchers Kohler and Milstein (1975) developed a B-cell clone that produced a single antibody capable of binding with only one antigen, called a **monoclonal antibody**. The monoclonal antibodies are antigen specific and can be produced in large quantities in a laboratory.

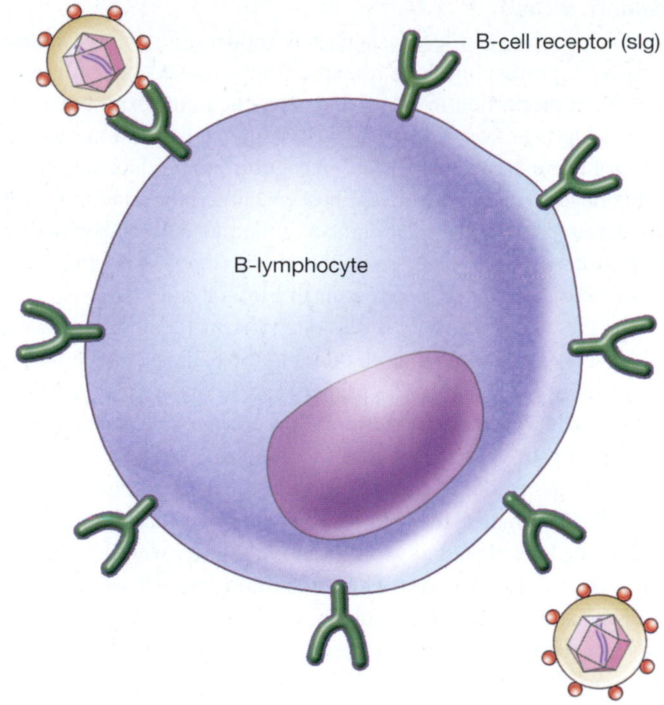

FIGURE 52–9 ◆ B cell.

Monoclonal antibodies are created by fusing rapidly growing plasma cells with antibody-producing B cells from the spleen of animals (usually mice) that have been injected with a specific antigen. One example of rapidly growing plasma cells is malignant myeloma cells. These are used because they proliferate rapidly and can live for a very long period of time in culture medium. This fusion process results in a hybridoma cell that produces a large quantity of monoclonal antibodies that target a single antigen involved in a disease process (Dunne, 2007).

Knowledge of how monoclonal antibodies develop has had a profound effect on disease research, diagnosis, and treatment modalities. In cancer research, for example, monoclonal antibodies are continually being developed to react against specific antigens on cancer cells and enhance the patient's immune response (Weiner, Dhodapkar, & Ferrone, 2009). They have been used extensively in cancer drug therapy to inhibit specific tumor growth factor (Tol & Punt, 2010). For example, Cetuximab is a monoclonal antibody used to treat metastatic colorectal cancer in combination with chemotherapy or when a patient is nonresponsive to chemotherapy treatment (Tol & Punt, 2010; Weiner et al., 2009).

Monoclonal antibodies are also a vital part of early detection of viral infections. Monoclonal antibodies can be labeled with a fluorescent dye or enzyme and targeted for a specific viral pathogen, which allows visualization and identification of the pathogen with fluorescent microscopy (Dunne, 2007). Thus, monoclonal antibody technology enables the clinician to diagnostically test for viral antigens, diagnose pathologic disease in its infancy, and, through evidence-based treatment, improve patient outcomes (Rote, 2010).

Antigen Presentation and Recognition

B cells must be activated, or told to make specific antibodies; this is accomplished through the mechanism of antigen presentation. When a foreign antigen enters a host, the macrophages found in tissue or monocytes found in blood ingest the bacterium or virus and then digest the antigen. The macrophage expresses a portion of the digested antigen

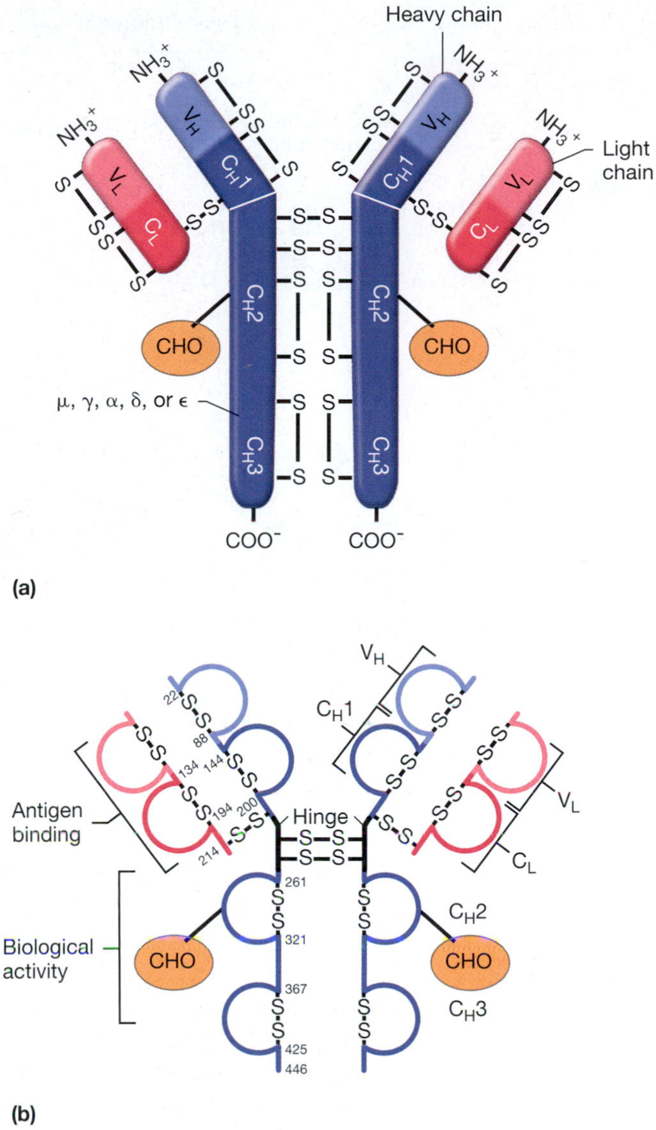

FIGURE 52–10 ◆ Immunoglobulin with FAB and FC binding sites.

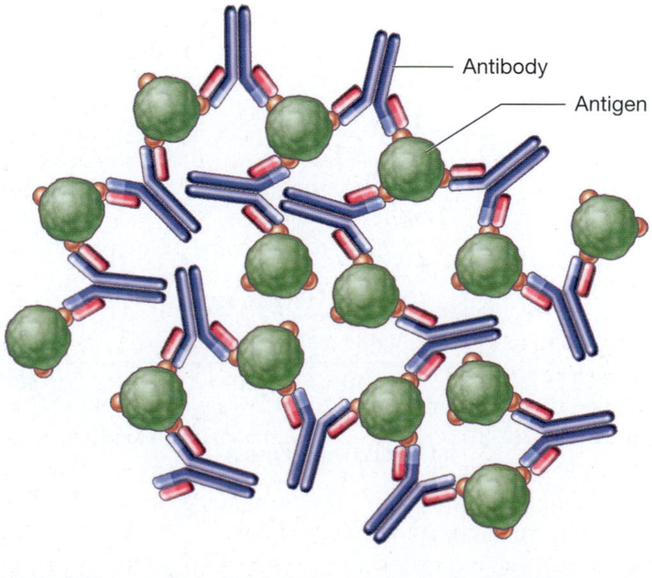

FIGURE 52–11 ◆ Immune complex and the process of opsonization.

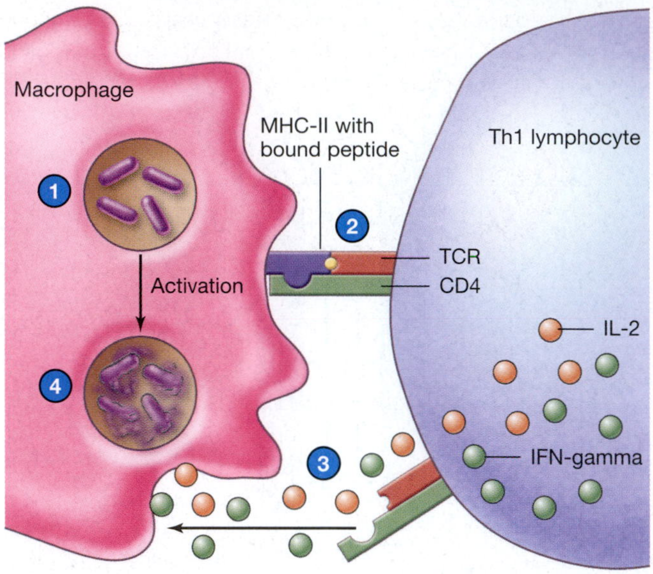

FIGURE 52–12 ◆ Antigen presentation (sequential graphic).

on its cell surface in the form of a small protein receptor with a part of the bacterial wall attached. T cells are often found near macrophages and can chemically bind to the receptor and accept the antigen onto their surface. T cells then present the antigen to the B cells that have a receptor to match the shape of the antigen. Linking of the T cell and B cell at the site of the antigen activates the B cell to make the appropriately shaped antibody to attach to the antigens (Rote, 2010). Figure 52–12◆ depicts the process of antigen presentation by a T cell to a B cell and the creation of antibodies.

Another mechanism of antigen recognition occurs when B cells are able to recognize antigens that may attach to surface receptors on the B cells and directly stimulate antibody production. This method of recognition often occurs during a secondary response. It is also possible for antigens to directly stimulate plasma B cells by attaching to receptors on the cell surface (Sommer, 2007).

Memory B Cells

The first exposure to a specific antigen is known as a *primary immune response*. A primary immune response results in evidence of immunoglobulin production in 4 to 8 days after the initial exposure to an antigen. During this period, some B cells differentiate into memory B cells that retain the ability to quickly recognize and produce antibodies to the antigen. The second time the host encounters the same antigen, it produces antibodies in greater numbers and more quickly than during the primary exposure. This stronger immune response, referred to as the *secondary immune response*, occurs in 1 to 3 days.

The presence of memory B cells often means the host will have a milder set of symptoms or no response to the pathogen. An example of a memory B-cell response is primary and secondary exposure to a rhinovirus. During the first exposure to the antigen, cold and flu symptoms are at their peak for the first 4 to 5 days. The primary immune response requires 7 to 10 days to produce sufficient lymphokines and antibodies to eliminate the virus and the symptoms that accompany it because the level of antibodies in the blood is lower with the primary response. The next exposure of the same rhinovirus activates memory B cells, and the production of antibodies specific to that antigen is quick and more robust in the secondary response. The person will have minimal or no cold symptoms (Figure 52–13◆) (Porth & Sweeney, 2007).

Effects of Age on the Immune System

The major protection of the newborn against antigens occurs through the transfer of maternal IgG antibodies across the placenta during fetal development, especially during the last weeks of pregnancy (Rote, 2010). Hence, infants born prematurely may be significantly immune deficient. Immunoglobulin G antibodies remain active in the newborn for the first several months while the infant's production of immunoglobulins, specifically IgM, rises rapidly and attains adult levels by approximately 1 year of age (Sommer, 2007). Infant serum IgA levels are first detected approximately 2 weeks after birth and attain adult levels by 7 years of age. Further immune protection can be attained through the transfer of maternal IgA in the colostrum during breast-feeding. Research has indicated that these antibodies provide

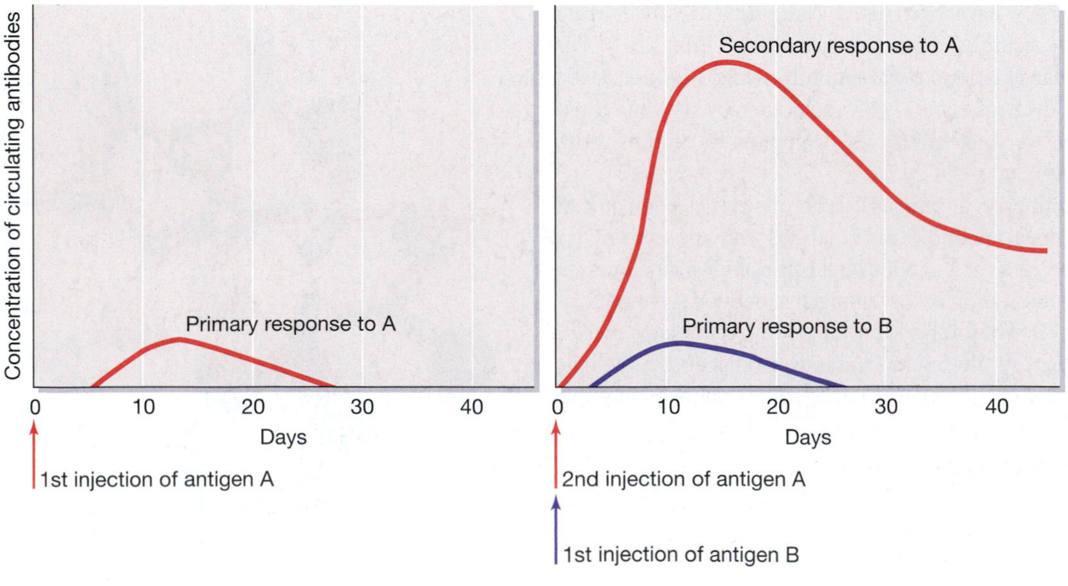

FIGURE 52–13 ◆ Primary and secondary immune response curves.

local immunity for the intestinal system and in underdeveloped countries decrease diarrheal infections (Sommer, 2007).

The thymus is also a major contributor to immune development because it generates mature immunocompetent T cells during infancy and childhood. By the time the patient reaches puberty, at which point the mature immune cells are sequestered in the peripheral lymphoid tissues, the thymus atrophies and is replaced by adipose tissue. Failure of the immune system to develop normally *in utero* will result in primary immune deficiencies that usually become evident in the first year of life. The effects of aging on the immune system for older individuals are discussed in the Gerontological Considerations section later in this chapter.

Genetic Implications

Nurses need to stay informed about the discoveries of genetic research to be able to identify and assess individuals at risk. Nurses also need an adequate understanding of the genetic research to be able to teach patients and families about the risk factors, tests, and treatment options associated with a familial or genetic disease. Patients who are at high risk for inherited diseases such as cancer or immune abnormalities will greatly benefit from this information.

Research has focused on discovering which genes are linked to the development of specific diseases such as immune disorders like asthma, systemic lupus erythematosus (SLE), and cancer. The major task ahead is to create the bridges from genomic discoveries to disease prevention and improved treatment (Hamilton, 2009).

Currently, genotyping is done at only a few research centers; however, it is not unrealistic to envision this becoming a common aspect of the clinical work-up for patients with immune alterations (Hamilton, 2009). DNA mutations and alterations in gene functioning have major ramifications for identifying and treating disease processes that affect the immune system and all other body systems. Genetics is discussed in Chapter 7.

History

Immune function assessment begins with a thorough health history and physical examination. Listening carefully to the patient's complaints about current and past medical problems provides valuable clues to the functioning of the patient's immune system. A thorough history guides the clinician to focus on specific physical findings and order appropriate diagnostic tests. Chart 52–5 outlines essential information about the immune system assessment.

The most common complaints related to the immune system and lymphatic tissues involve infection, allergy response, enlarged lymph nodes, and lymphedema (Bickley, 2009). Assessment should include recent exposure to any infectious diseases. Risk factors that affect immune function include a genetic familial history of immune-related diseases as well as lifestyle choices and habits that increase exposure to communicable diseases. Sexually transmitted infections are discussed in Chapter 43. Substance abuse behaviors that may alter immune function are discussed in Chapter 13.

Inflammation is often the first physical finding that is activated during an immune response. Indicators of inflammation should be assessed, including questions about fever, malaise, swelling, redness, cough with or without pain, and decreased function of a limb or part of the body. The nurse should inquire about the presence of rashes, skin cracks, or open wounds with serous drainage, bleeding, or pus that may indicate infection. The nurse should also ask whether the patient is experiencing night sweats or cough with or without sputum. If sputum is present, the patient should be asked to describe its color. Various colors of sputum indicate infection with different types of organisms. It also is important to gain information about the duration and frequency of infections. Incurable or recurrent infections are often the first indicator of significant impaired immune function. An example of this is frequent and recurrent oral or vaginal *Candida* infections, as is often seen in patients with HIV infection.

Chief Complaint

The integration of the immune system throughout the body's other systems means that alterations in immune function can present themselves in a variety of manifestations. Pain is one of the most common first complaints with immune abnormalities, owing to the presence of inflammation. For example, enlarged lymph nodes in the presence of viral or bacterial infection may be very tender and painful. Detailed assessment of pain is a vital aspect of the history and physical examination and should be quantified using a specific pain scale. Chapter 12 includes examples of pain assessment scales.

CHART 52–5 Key Criteria for Assessment of the Immune System

Assessment	Nursing Implications
Complete health history	Current complaint, prior diseases, immunizations, chronic disease, known immune disease, nutritional status, functional status.
Family health history	Familial genetic disorders or a family history of cancer, heart disease, asthma, and so on.
Social history	Abuse of alcohol or drugs, smoking, diet, sexual behaviors, and occupation can impact the immune function or increase exposure to sexual diseases.
Medications	Drug interactions or side effects can affect the immune system (e.g., corticosteroids suppress immune function).
Physical Assessment	
Inspection	Ensure skin and mucous membranes are intact, examine all rashes and wounds, and note any exudate.
Palpation	Palpate lymph nodes in the neck, groin, and axilla. Palpate the abdomen and kidneys.
Percussion	Percuss the thorax and abdomen.
Auscultation	Auscultate the lungs and heart. Abnormal breath sounds or murmurs can be associated with infections or allergic reactions.

Sources: Bickley, L. S. (2009). *Guide to physical examination and history taking* (10th ed). Philadelphia: Wolters Kluwer/Lippincott Williams & Wilkins; DeFranco, A. L., Locksley, R., & Robertson, M. (2007). *Immunity: The immune response in infectious and inflammatory disease.* Sunderland, MA: Sinauer Associates; Porth, C. (2008). *Essentials of pathophysiology* (7th ed.). Philadelphia: Lippincott Williams & Wilkins.

Past Medical History

The past medical history should include a history of childhood diseases and immunizations, prior hospitalizations, and diagnostic and surgical procedures. In addition, the nurse should obtain a medical history of chronic diseases such as hepatitis, diabetes, chronic obstructive pulmonary disease, or renal failure. This is significant because chronic diseases can impair immune function. The nurse should ask questions about diseases specifically related to immune disorders such as cancer or autoimmune diseases such as systemic lupus erythematosus or rheumatoid arthritis. All patients should be assessed for allergies to medications, food, and environmental antigens such as pollen or pet dander (Bickley, 2009).

It also is important to obtain a surgical history. The nurse should inquire about surgical procedures involving lymph node removal, trauma, or organ transplant. Loss of lymph nodes will alter lymphatic drainage and decrease immune function. Organ transplant requires lifelong immunosuppressive medications that result in immune suppression and an increased risk for infections. Finally, if the patient was involved in a previous trauma, it is crucial to determine whether blood products were administered. Blood products contain foreign antibodies that can alter normal immune response. Also, before 1985, blood transfusions were not screened for HIV. Blood infusion safety is discussed in detail in Chapter 16.

Knowledge of the patient's immunization status also is important in preventing illness and promoting optimal health. The nurse should inquire about childhood diseases such as chickenpox, measles, mumps, or whooping cough and about the patient's immunization history and currency. Additionally, the nurse should inquire about past or present exposure to tuberculosis and the dates and results of tuberculin tests such as a tine test or purified protein derived (PPD) test, as well as any diagnostic chest x-rays. It is important to elicit information on recent international travel or a history of living in another country, especially developing countries, because a traveler is at risk of being exposed to multiple strains of resistant organisms (Bickley, 2009).

Medication History

Medications can significantly affect the immune system. It is essential to obtain a complete list of all medications, including over-the-counter (OTC) medications and herbal supplements, that the patient is currently taking. Common OTC medications such as nonsteroidal anti-inflammatory drugs (e.g., ibuprofen, cyclooxygenase-2 inhibitors, and aspirin) that are taken in large quantities can cause significant decreases in leukocytes and neutrophils. Prescription medications the patient is taking to treat ongoing medical problems can result in profound immune suppression. Drugs such as corticosteroids or cytotoxic agents such as cyclophosphamide are immunosuppressive and significantly increase the patient's susceptibility to infection. Antibiotics given in large doses or administered over a prolonged period of time can also affect immune function and result in hemolytic anemia, leukopenia, and neutropenia, as well as agranulocytosis.

Interactions between various medications must be considered before patients are treated with additional medications for the current complaint. Ultimately, health care providers must consider the patient's current medications before adding any additional pharmacologic or nonpharmacologic interventions. Some medications, such as antibiotics, interfere with the action of others. Herbal supplements can also have significant drug interactions; therefore, patients should be questioned regarding herbal supplement use. The addition of new medications to the patient's treatment regime should prompt discussion with a consulting pharmacist to identify any potential medication interactions, along with laboratory values that may signal immune deficiency.

Family History

Many of the diseases that affect the immune system are associated with a specific gene alteration. These familial genetic diseases include malignancies such as breast and colon cancer, autoimmune diseases such as SLE, and allergic responses such as atopic dermatitis (Porth & Sweeney, 2007). The nurse should ask whether any members of the patient's family have been diagnosed with cancer or any other diseases involving the immune system, such as rheumatoid arthritis or allergic asthma. It is important to know whether members of the patient's immediate family (parents, grandparents, siblings) are deceased and the cause of death. Genetic predisposition plays a critical role in the development of many diseases in addition to those that affect the immune system, such as heart disease, emphysema, and diabetes. This information helps identify the patient's risk factors for disease development and can direct the physical examination and diagnostic work-up.

Social History

It is important to ask about the patient's occupation. Exposure to certain environmental substances can affect the action of the immune system. For example, asbestos and coal dust cause cell changes that can lead to cancerous tumors (Porth & Sweeney, 2007). In addition, occupational allergies can be directly related to the frequency and strength of exposure to certain products. One example is the increased incidence of latex allergies among health care workers who have daily exposure to latex products (National Institute for Occupational Safety and Health, 2007).

The nurse should inquire about lifestyle habits such as smoking, alcohol and drug use, and sexual practices, all of which can place the patient at an increased risk for developing diseases that affect immune function. Illicit use of injection drugs and having multiple sexual partners are examples of risky behavior that can lead to hepatitis and HIV, as discussed in Chapter 53.

Safety Alert *Questions about lifestyle habits such as alcohol and drug use and sexual practices are sensitive. These issues should be addressed in a private setting, away from family or friends. It is also best to ask sensitive questions toward the end of the patient history after the nurse has had an opportunity to establish rapport with the patient.*

It is important to obtain information related to the patient's social support system. Having family and friends who can provide psychological and physical care during illness and assist the patient in managing medications and follow-up treatment may improve patient compliance with the prescribed treatment regime. Diagnoses such as cancer or HIV infection are devastating and provoke high anxiety. Chronic diseases, such as SLE or rheumatoid arthritis, can dramatically alter the patient's lifestyle and occupational choices. Nurses are in an ideal position to identify issues related to lack of social support and to provide resources and referrals to address this issue, in an effort to decrease the risk of depression and isolation that can result.

Physical Examination

Lymphatic tissues and cells of the immune system are located throughout the body. The immune system affects every other body system. Often signs of immune abnormalities are subtle. Therefore, a thorough

CULTURAL CONSIDERATIONS
When Examining the Lymph Node System

Cultural factors can affect the patient's views about health, the medical exam experience, and treatment options. Some cultural groups make decisions based on leadership or authority. For example, the patient may prefer that the head of the family or clan be present when the patient's diagnosis, treatment, or prognosis is discussed. Knowledge about the patient's cultural attitudes can help the nurse facilitate taking the history and completing the physical examination. For example, concerns about modesty may be an issue during examination of lymph nodes in the breast and groin areas for women in Asian, Hispanic, American Indian, or Alaskan Native cultural groups, and may be sensitively addressed by assigning a same-gender health care provider and covering the perineum during the exam (Bickley, 2009).

physical examination involves inspection, palpation, percussion, and auscultation of various body systems to identify any abnormal function. Careful examination and palpation of immune tissue, especially the lymph nodes, are particularly important because enlarged and painful lymph nodes may indicate infection, inflammation, or malignancy. The Cultural Considerations box provides a reminder of the nurse's need to be sensitive to the patient's cultural values when conducting the examination. Figure 52–2 (p. 1597) describes the location of lymph nodes and the tissues that are drained by part of the lymph system.

Inspection

Inspection is always the first step in a physical examination. The nurse should begin by looking globally at the patient. Does the patient look fatigued, feverish, or pale? Is the patient well nourished, thin, or obese? Fever indicates an acute infection. Fatigue and weight loss may be associated with chronic disease processes. Inadequate nutrition affects the ability of the immune cells to function normally and causes immunosuppression. Rapid and significant weight loss that is unintentional is a serious concern because of its association with malignant diseases. An unintentional weight loss of 10 pounds or more in a month also indicates the need for a nutritional consult. Optimal nutrition is essential for immune function. Loss of protein reserves results in atrophy of lymphoid tissue and decreased antibody and T-cell response. Decreased vitamin and mineral intake affects the proliferation and maturation of immune cells and suppresses immune function. Malnutrition lowers the body's resistance to disease and increases morbidity and mortality from infection (Bickley, 2009). An extensive discussion on the importance of nutrition for body function can be found in Chapter 8. General inspection also includes careful examination of the skin and mucous membranes because they are the first line of defense in protecting the body from invasion by microorganisms.

Inspection should be directed to the area of complaint. For example, if the complaint is related to symptoms of a persistent cough and sore throat, the nurse should inspect the mucous membranes of the throat and the lymph nodes of the neck (see Figure 52–2, p. 1597). Superficial lymph nodes should not be visible; the presence of edema, erythema, and red streaks is indicative of inflammation and infection (Bickley, 2009). Additionally, the nurse should observe for edema at the extremities and at lymph node sites. Edema may be localized and related to a wound or infectious process that causes swelling in an extremity or related changes in normal circulatory flow. Areas of edema that are red and warm indicate inflammation. The nurse should note any signs of lymphedema, nonpitting edema at the site of lymph nodes that indicates inadequate drainage from lymphatic vessels and excessive accumulation of fluid in the interstitial spaces around the lymph vessels. This can occur for a variety of reasons including congenital abnormalities in the development of the lymphatic system (Milroy's disease), blocked lymphatic channels due to infection or malignancy, or surgical removal of lymph nodes related to trauma or prior malignancy. The presence of lymphedema should prompt questions related to the onset and duration of the swelling (Bickley, 2009).

Palpation

The nurse should palpate lymph nodes for size, tenderness, warmth, and mobility (see Figure 52–2, p. 1597), noting whether any are edematous, and ask the patient whether it is painful to have the nodes palpated. Superficial lymph nodes are normally pain free and nonpalpable. Enlarged lymph nodes from acute infection are tender, are slightly firm, and move freely. In contrast, malignancy is indicated when enlarged nodes are nontender, hard, asymmetrical, and nonmobile (attached to the underlying tissues) (Bickley, 2009). If the nodes are enlarged or tender, the nurse should focus the physical assessment on the structures surrounding the enlarged node. For example, if lymph nodes in the neck are bilaterally edematous, tender, firm, and freely movable, infection of the head and throat may be indicated. If the complaint is in the lower extremities, the groin lymph nodes should be palpated for edema and tenderness. Additionally, any edema in the extremities should be palpated to determine the extent and level of pitting. A thorough examination also involves palpation of the abdomen, which contains a large number of immune tissues, assessing for pain and/or a mass.

Percussion

Percussion is helpful in determining whether there is inappropriate fluid or a mass in an organ, indicating disease. For example, percussion over the lung is done to determine whether fluid is present that would change the normal resonant sound of the lung tissue to a dull sound, which may indicate infection. Kidneys are percussed to determine whether there is tenderness in the area, indicating possible infection or tumor (Bickley, 2009). Abnormalities in percussion sounds warrant further investigation and collaborative discussion with the health care provider for further diagnostic testing.

Auscultation

Lung sounds such as coarse and fine crackles indicate fluid from infection or edema. Heart sounds, including valve sounds and murmurs, give indications about the function of the organ. Cardiac valve dysfunction with murmurs is not uncommon in autoimmune diseases such as SLE or rheumatoid disease (Bickley, 2009). Abdominal auscultation is done to assess bowel sounds. For example, a loss of bowel sounds may indicate an ileus or infarcted bowel.

Integumentary Assessment

Skin should be assessed during every physical exam. Healthy skin is intact and free from areas of redness, swelling, rashes, purpura, or lesions that may indicate inflammation, an allergic reaction, or infectious processes. The nurse should examine the skin and identify any nodules, lumps, or wounds that are present. These abnormalities should be evaluated for symptoms of infection such as redness, inflammation, streaking lines, edema, or drainage. Signs of rash or petechiae, red or purple spots caused by damage to capillary blood vessels, indicate an allergic response or infection. A variety of autoimmune diseases, such as scleroderma, have signs or symptoms seen on the skin. Patients with scleroderma often have firm, hard skin and may have a somewhat immobile facial expression. Chapter 53 includes discussions of allergies and autoimmune diseases. Skin abnormalities are extensively discussed in Chapter 59.

While examining the skin, the nurse should give special attention to bony prominences where redness can indicate the first stage of skin breakdown, and to skin folds under the breast and in the groin, where small cracks in the skin may go undetected. The nurse should also inspect the mucous membranes, which should be pink, moist, and free of lesions.

Safety Alert *A patient who is obese may have difficulty cleansing skinfolds, especially on the back, on the thighs, and under a pendulous abdomen. Skinfolds that are not cleaned regularly place the patient at increased risk for development of candidiasis (yeast) infection or boils that can go undetected. The patient may also be embarrassed by lack of cleanliness and feel very uncomfortable with a skinfold examination. A caring and nonjudgmental attitude on the nurse's part is vital in helping the patient feel accepted and building a therapeutic relationship.*

Neurological Assessment

The brain is protected from injury and invasion by the bones of the cranium and by the blood–brain barrier, which is the mechanism of tight connections between endothelial cells in blood vessels that prevent many particles from diffusing into the brain. The brain does not have lymph tissue; however, protection is provided by lymph nodes in the neck (Rote, 2010). Therefore, examination of the immune system associated with the head and neck involves inspection and palpation of the lymph nodes located in front of and behind the ear, along the jaw and under the chin, the anterior and posterior neck, and the supraclavicular area. Palpation of the periauricular lymph nodes is done to assess lymph nodes that drain lymph fluid from the head (Figure 52–14◆). The technique for palpation of the lymph nodes of the neck can be seen in Figure 52–15◆. Swollen, tender, red nodes in these areas may reflect infection in the face, neck, or head.

Many autoimmune diseases have a neurological component. Physical examination of immune function in the neurological system includes assessment of the face's symmetry. The nurse should examine the face for the presence of facial droop or a facial expression that is frozen or not responsive to emotion. Disorders of the immune system that affect the neurological system include Guillain-Barré, myasthenia gravis, and cerebral vascular accident. Bell's palsy also can present with an asymmetrical facial expression. Patients presenting with fever and stiffness of the neck should be assessed for meningitis. Extremities should be assessed for numbness, tingling, or unilateral or bilateral paralysis. Unit V provides information on neurological abnormalities and a description of a full neurological assessment.

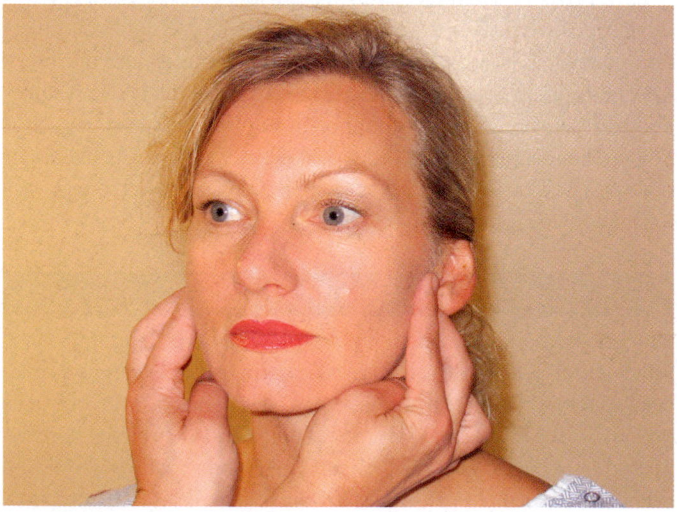

FIGURE 52–14 ◆ Palpation of the preauricular lymph nodes.

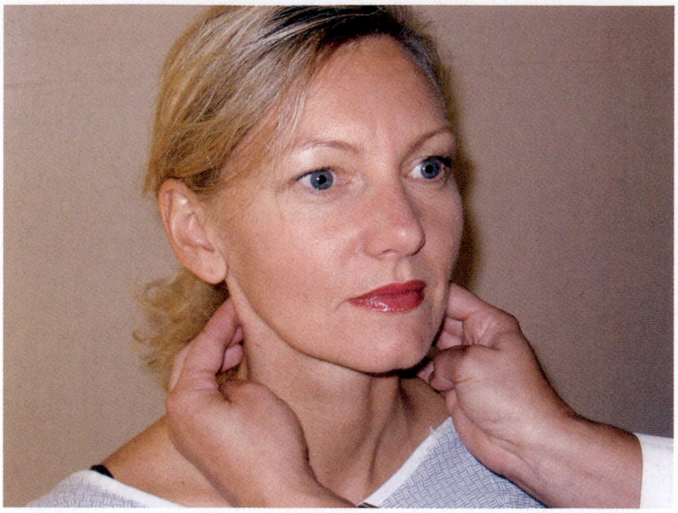

FIGURE 52–15 ◆ Palpation of the posterior superficial cervical chain lymph nodes.

Cardiovascular Assessment

The lymphatic vessels associated with the heart and vascular system are enmeshed; a lymphatic vessel is located next to each combination of artery and vein. Chyle drains into the right atrium from the lymphatic and thoracic ducts, then mixes with blood and is delivered from the heart into the body's circulation. Protection is also provided by the presence of immune cells, including B cells, T cells, macrophages, neutrophils, and basophils, along with circulating immunoglobulin. The vascular system allows rapid delivery of immune cells and chemicals to all areas of the body (Sommer, 2007). A functioning cardiovascular system is essential for proper immune function.

Assessment of immune function in the cardiovascular system itself primarily focuses on laboratory data and the patient's clinical presentation. Elevated white blood cell counts often occur with inflammation from an ischemic cardiac event such as acute myocardial infarction or an infectious process such as endocarditis. See Unit VII for a full discussion of cardiac abnormalities.

Respiratory and Chest Assessment

The respiratory system utilizes several natural mechanisms along with immune tissues to help protect the body. The upper airway contains the tonsils, which are made up primarily of lymphoid tissue that helps to trap and process antigens. The cough reflex helps to remove debris from the bronchial airways. Ciliated cells in the trachea and airways move cells, debris, and bacteria toward the mouth and away from the alveoli. Fixed macrophages are present in lung tissue to phagocytize bacterial cells and debris. The lungs are rich in vascular tissue; hence, the circulating immune cells provide protection against debris, viruses, and bacteria (Rote, 2010). Situations that damage the cilia and alter

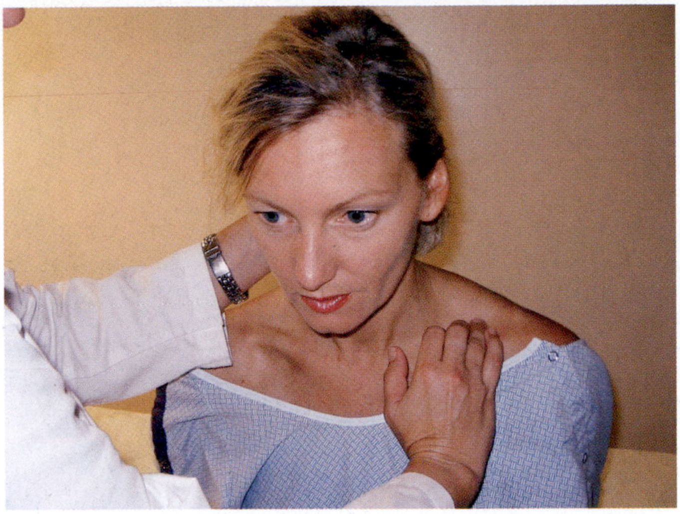

FIGURE 52–16 ◆ Palpation of the supraclavicular lymph nodes.

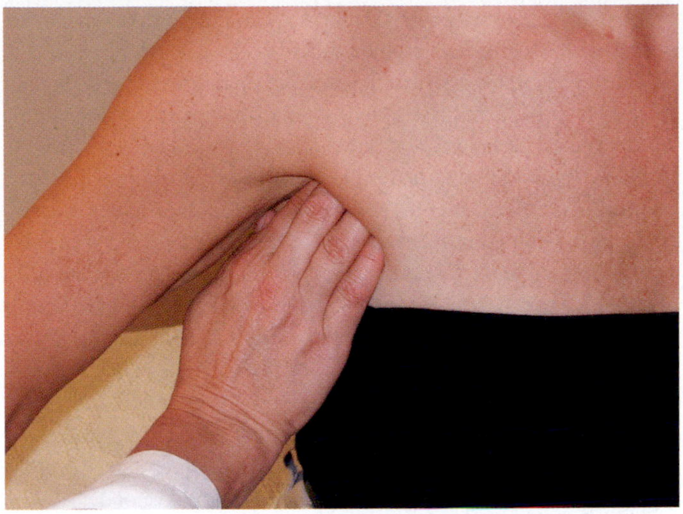

FIGURE 52–17 ◆ Palpation of axillary lymph nodes.

pulmonary tissue, such as smoking or inhalation burn injuries, place the patient at increased risk for infection. Medical treatment for acute respiratory failure that requires mechanical intubation bypasses all of the natural defense mechanisms; this is one of the primary reasons for extubation as soon as is feasible.

Competent immune function is critical in the respiratory system because of the variety and quantity of microorganisms to which the pulmonary tissues are exposed every day. Lung sounds should be auscultated. Patients with infectious processes may have coarse or fine crackles or a friction rub of the pleura. A friction rub indicates inflammation of the pleura, which may be associated with infection. Patients who present with a complaint of pain with cough or difficulty breathing should be evaluated for elevated white blood cell counts. Because the lungs' ability to clear debris and bacteria is so important, the quality and quantity of secretions must be assessed. Secretions that are green, yellow, or brown should be evaluated by laboratory culture to detect an infectious process.

Assessment of the respiratory system and structures of the chest involves inspection and palpation of the lymph nodes in the supraclavicular area, axilla, and breast. Figure 52–16◆ demonstrates the appropriate hand position for examining supraclavicular lymph nodes. Palpation and detection of enlarged supraclavicular nodes are of particular concern. Supraclavicular nodes are the last nodes of a chain of ducts, such as the thoracic duct, that drain the upper abdomen, lungs, breasts, and arms and are often the site of metastatic disease (Bickley, 2009).

The majority of lymphatic breast drainage flows into the axillary nodes. Palpation of axillary nodes is shown in Figure 52–17◆. The lymph nodes of the breast are located deep in the tissue and are rarely palpable. Axillary nodes that are enlarged, painful, and mobile indicate infection located in the breast or arm or systemic disease such as systemic syphilis. In contrast, axillary lymph nodes that are enlarged, painless, asymmetrical, and fixed to underlying tissue are indicative of malignant diseases such as breast cancer and Hodgkin's lymphoma (Bickley, 2009).

Gastrointestinal Assessment

Immune function is supported through a variety of natural protective mechanisms within the gastrointestinal (GI) system. The act of emesis can rid the stomach of toxins and bacteria. The stomach produces hydrochloric acid and maintains a pH of approximately 3.00. This acidic environment protects the body from most pathogens. However, *Helicobacter pylori*, one of the few organisms that can tolerate an acidic environment, is the cause of many gastric ulcers. *H. pylori* can withstand the acidic environment and starts to grow on the cell walls of the stomach. This growth is followed by an increase in bacteria that leads to destruction of the stomach's protective cell wall and ultimately causes formation of an ulcer (Rote, 2010). Gastric ulcers also may occur because of the secretion of additional acid as part of the stress response with illness. It is important to address stress as a potential patient problem.

Safety Alert *A critical assessment of the protection of the entire gastrointestinal system is essential for all patients hospitalized for more than a day or two. The stress of illness as well as immobility places the gastric mucosa at risk of degradation. The consequence of loss of protection can be GI bleeding and/or a stress ulcer. Proton pump inhibitors or H_2-receptor blockers are necessary for many patients.*

The highly vascular vessels of the small and large intestines are responsible for absorption of large molecules of digestion. Large numbers of bacteria are always present in the intestines. In fact, some bacteria are needed to assist in the breakdown of food molecules. The structure of the intestine protects the body's internal environment from pathologic bacteria. In addition, two-thirds of all fixed lymph tissue is located in the abdomen and is referred to as gut-associated lymphatic tissue (GALT) (Sommer, 2007). Gut-associated tissue (GALT) includes the tonsils, adenoids, Peyer's patches, and lymphoid aggregates such as the appendix. When the appendix is inflamed and infected, it produces pain in the right lower abdominal quadrant, and the inflammation can result in severe peritonitis if rupture occurs before the appendix can be surgically removed.

Accessory organs of the GI tract such as the liver and spleen also provide protection from antigens. Fixed macrophages in the liver filter out and consume bacteria and cellular debris. The liver also is responsible for the filtering of toxins. The spleen, located in the upper left abdominal quadrant, houses a large network of B and T cells and macrophages that filter antigens from the blood; the spleen is important in immune function for fighting systemic infection.

Assessing the immune function of the GI system should include inspection, auscultation, percussion, and palpation of all four abdominal quadrants. Inspection assesses symmetry of the abdomen and quality of the skin. Lack of symmetry or taut skin can indicate a mass or infection. Auscultation of the abdomen should be done before percussing or palpating the abdomen so that the presence or absence of bowel sounds or pain is not affected. Auscultation enables identification of bowel abnormalities, such as absent bowel sounds associated with paralytic ileus or mechanical obstruction. Percussion of the abdomen focuses on areas of tympany and dullness. Tympany usually indicates the presence of gas. Dullness is noted over tissue, tumor, or fecal material in the gastrointestinal tract. Chapter 6 demonstrates the appropriate hand position for percussion of the abdomen. Areas of dullness should then be palpated for a mass. Pain upon palpation should be further assessed for quality, degree, and duration. Pain can be related to infection or a disease process affecting the underlying tissue (Bickley, 2009).

To assess the spleen, the nurse places the patient on the right side and percusses down the midaxillary line from an area of resonance over the lung to dullness over the spleen. The spleen is normally not detected on palpation. If detected, the spleen should not be percussed more than 6 to 8 cm (about 2 to 3 in.) above the left costal margin. An enlarged spleen is diagnosed if there is a greater than 8-cm finding above the costal margin (Bickley, 2009). Additional information on GI assessment can be found in Chapter 36.

Genitourinary System

Organs of the genitourinary system provide natural immune protection for the body through several mechanisms. For example, the mechanical flow of urine can wash debris from the urethra. The kidneys filter out drug metabolites. In addition, vaginal secretions contain immunoglobulins and other immune cells that can provide some protection from bacteria, fungi, and viruses (Rote, 2010).

Immune assessment of the genitourinary system includes inspection, percussion, and palpation to identify the presence of infection or malignant tumors. External genitalia should be free from swelling and drainage. Skin should be intact and free from lesions and redness around the anus and upper inner thigh area. Percussion of the kidneys and bladder is not usually necessary unless the patient complains of specific flank pain, difficulty emptying the bladder, or an urge to urinate without voiding. Palpation of the bladder should be pain free, and the bladder should be soft. Kidneys may be palpated by pressing one hand on the anterior surface of the abdomen below the ribs and pushing gently with the other hand from the back in the same location below the ribs. Chapter 36 discusses kidney assessment, and Chapter 39 addresses abnormalities of the genitourinary system.

Lymph nodes in the groin should be inspected and palpated with either the genitourinary or musculoskeletal system exam. Figure 52–18◆ demonstrates appropriate patient draping of the groin area and hand position for palpation during the inguinal lymph nodes examination. Normally, inguinal nodes are small, mobile, and difficult to palpate. The superior and inferior inguinal lymph nodes receive drainage from the upper and lower leg, the vulva and lower third of the vagina in females, and the penis and scrotal surface in males. Enlarged, tender, firm, and freely movable nodes indicate an infection or inflammatory process in any of these tissues and warrant further investigation. Additionally, assessment for the presence of lymphedema should be included.

Musculoskeletal Assessment

Musculoskeletal assessment focusing on the immune system includes inspection and palpation of joints and limbs for evidence of swelling, inflammation, or infection. The nurse should assess for the presence of pain with range of motion and any limitation of joint motion. Autoimmune diseases such as rheumatoid arthritis and SLE include joint pain and swelling as a significant finding. An extensive discussion of musculoskeletal assessment can be found in Chapter 48.

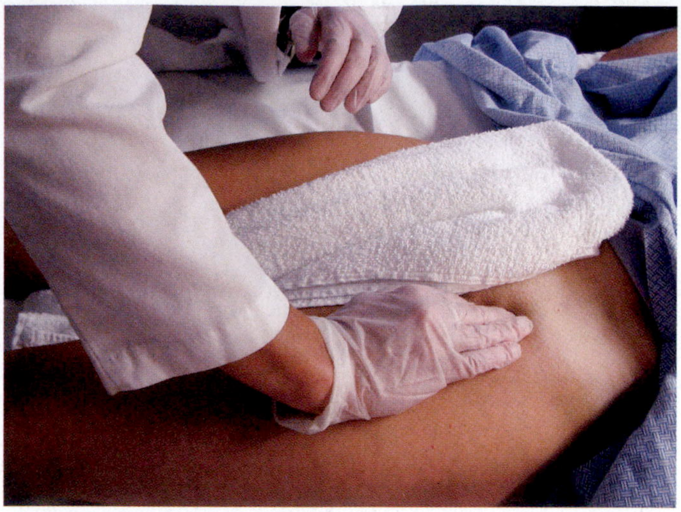

FIGURE 52–18 ◆ Palpation of inguinal lymph nodes with draping.

Common Laboratory and Diagnostic Tests

In addition to physical examination of immune tissues and various body systems, laboratory tests are required to evaluate the phagocytic, cellular, and antibody functions of the immune system. These tests are generally ordered when an abnormality such as an infection or a specific complaint related to an organ function is identified.

Laboratory Tests

An initial complete blood count (CBC) with manual differential is essential for identifying immune system abnormalities and providing a baseline to expand upon. An elevated total white blood count (total WBC) often indicates infection, inflammation, or, in some cases, blood disease such as leukemia. Low white blood cell counts indicate immunosuppression, as seen with various cancers or infections such as HIV, and warrant a complete work-up. For example, a patient with symptoms of an undiagnosed HIV infection may have a low total WBC and a very low total lymphocytes count on the CBC differential. This would prompt the health care provider to follow up with further tests to determine the level of CD4 cells and HIV antibody testing as described in Chapter 53.

White blood counts are differentiated into total lymphocytes, monocytes, neutrophils, bands (immature neutrophils), basophils, and eosinophils. All specific cell types are described as a percentage of total white cells. Neutrophils comprise approximately 70% of the total WBC and are the first cells to respond to a trauma, infection, or inflammation. Immature neutrophils are called bands. An increase in the number of bands in the serum circulation (>7%) indicates that the body is mounting a major inflammatory response; for example, fighting an infection, such as an abscess. Thus, an elevated band number occurs when the number of mature neutrophils is depleted and the immature neutrophils increase (Rote, 2010).

The CBC also includes information on platelets. Diseases such as systemic lupus erythematosus (SLE) may first present as thrombocytopenia on the CBC and prompt further testing. Another example is autoimmune thrombocytopenia, an autoimmune disease process in which the body identifies its own platelets as foreign and destroys them. Platelet abnormalities are of special concern because patients with platelet counts that are significantly decreased ($<$100,000 mm^3) have an increased risk of bleeding.

Decreased hemoglobin and hematocrit levels also occur in immune abnormalities. Anemia can result from autoimmune diseases. In addition, one of the first indications of a tumor can be decreased hemoglobin or hematocrit when there is no evidence of gross bleeding (Lefever-Kee, 2010). Abnormalities of lymphocyte counts on the CBC can be further evaluated by tests that examine specific T-cell and B-cell counts and immune function. This information is summarized in the Diagnostic Tests box (p. 1614).

Immune Function Tests

Specific serum tests examine the function of the immune system. Erythrocyte sedimentation rate (also known as a "sedimentation rate" or "sed rate"), C-reactive protein, antinuclear antibody tests, anti-IgG, IgG levels, IgM levels, enzyme-linked immunosorbent assay, and Western blot are all examples of serum tests designed to look at one specific chemical or antigen and the body's response to it.

The erythrocyte sedimentation rate (ESR) is a serum test that is used to diagnose acute and chronic inflammation and autoimmune diseases. The test does not diagnose a specific disease but is a sensitive and early indicator of a widespread inflammatory, autoimmune, or malignant disorder. An elevated level is the abnormal finding. In addition, the ESR is used to test autoimmune diseases such as rheumatoid arthritis. A protein called rheumatoid factor is often present in the serum of patients with rheumatoid disease in greater quantities than in individuals without autoimmune diseases (Lefever-Kee, 2010).

A test that is often ordered in conjunction with the ESR is the C-reactive protein (CRP) test. The CRP is a glycoprotein produced by the liver in response to acute inflammation. It is a more rapid and sensitive indicator of acute inflammation than the ESR. However, both CRP and ESR are unable to determine the cause of the inflammation. CRP levels decline rapidly from serum when inflammation has subsided (Lefever-Kee, 2010). Increased levels of CRP can be found in immune-related diseases such as SLE, rheumatoid arthritis, Crohn's disease, and inflammatory bowel disease, but are not always consistently elevated for reasons unknown. The test has proven most helpful in the diagnosis of acute flare-ups of inflammatory immune diseases and in monitoring response to medical therapy (Lefever-Kee, 2010). Elevated levels are also found in acute bacterial infection, in rheumatic fever, during the second half of pregnancy, and in acute myocardial infarction (Lefever-Kee, 2010). The major focus of recent research related to CRP has centered on its role in acute myocardial infarction (Chapter 32).

Immune function tests look for the presence of an antibody to a specific antigen. However, antigen testing can be inconclusive for the following reasons: (1) antigens are often destroyed by the time a test has been ordered, (2) antigens are present in only small quantities, or (3) antigens are hidden inside cells. Because of the difficulty in measuring antigens, the health care provider will test the serum for antibodies. Diagnosis for specific autoimmune diseases such as SLE, scleroderma, or rheumatoid arthritis involves testing for a variety of antibodies. Antinuclear antibodies (ANAs) are immunoglobulins (IgG, IgM, IgA) that react with the nuclear portion of leukocytes, forming auto-antibodies against the host's DNA and ribonucleic acid (RNA). The presence of these is indicative of SLE and warrants further testing for anti-DNA antibodies, which are further diagnostic of SLE. Total ANA levels can also be elevated in scleroderma, rheumatoid arthritis, cirrhosis, leukemia, and malignancy (Lefever-Kee, 2010; Porth & Sweeney, 2007).

Other antibody tests evaluate infection with a specific bacterium or virus such as hepatitis or HIV. An example of this is the enzyme-linked immunosorbent assay (ELISA) and the Western blot tests, which detect the presence of antibodies created in response to infection with the HIV antigen. Many of the tests currently used to assess immune function utilize monoclonal antibodies as the mechanism to bind the autoantibodies present in the patient's blood (Lefever-Kee, 2010). The Diagnostic Tests box describes the diagnostic laboratory tests used for assessment of the immune system and related nursing implications.

Computerized Axial Tomography

Immune system diseases can affect any body system. Therefore, computerized axial tomography (CT) scans are frequently used to diagnose immune system abnormalities. CT scans are most often used to identify areas of gross morphology and sites of possible tumors. These CT scans provide important information about organs and vascular function and enable identification of disease abnormalities.

Specific CT tests may require a contrast agent to enhance the films and help identify small tumors or abnormalities. The nurse must have an understanding of why the test is ordered and any patient preparation that is required to ensure optimal results. Patient teaching about the process is essential to alleviate fears about the unknown testing process.

Health Promotion

Health promotion related to the immune system is focused on risk factor identification and management of allergies and infections. Education needs to include information on lifestyle choices and habits that increase the risk for communicable disease transmission. For example, there are more than 19 million new cases of sexually transmitted infections each year that are preventable with education and compliance with risk factor prevention such as abstinence, condoms, or alternative sexual barriers (CDC, 2010). Finally, identification of genetic risk factors for allergies or environmental exposures such as food or insect vectors can prevent mild to life-threatening allergic reactions.

Gerontological Considerations

With aging, there is a decline in the ability of the immune cells to mount an immune response and a decrease in the production and response of these cells to chemical signals of inflammation. The most significant changes occur in relationship to T-cell function, which is primarily responsible for protection against infections and tumors (Rote, 2010). The number and percentage of T cells, both T-helper and suppressor T cells, decrease with age. Additionally, the ability of lymphocytes to produce interleukins diminishes as the body ages (Doerflinger, 2009). The decline in T-cell numbers and function results in greater susceptibility to infection. Influenza and pneumococcal pneumonia are two diseases from which most adults are relatively protected until they reach age 55 to 60. After that time, the slower response of T cells and B cells can result in severe infections.

Another effect of aging on the adult immune system is a delayed or decreased hypersensitivity reaction. When allergy testing is done in older adults, there may be a depressed ability to mount an inflammatory

DIAGNOSTIC TESTS to Assess Immune Function

Test, Normal Value, and Rationale	Expected Abnormality
Complete Blood Count with Differential WBC Count Red blood cells (RBC): Males: 4.6–6 µL Females: 4–5 µL Hemoglobin (HGB): Males: 13.5–18 g/dL Females: 12–15 g/dL Hematocrit (Hct): Males: 40–54% Females: 36–46%	RBC count and hemoglobin/hematocrit (Hgb/Hct) are important in determining the presence of anemia, blood loss, and hydration status, as well as the number of red blood cells and white blood cells, including neutrophils, basophils, and monocytes.
White blood count (WBC) 4,500–10,000 µL	The differential white blood count (WBC) total percentages will equal 100%. The percentages vary depending on the type of disease process. For example, with acute bacterial infection, the percentage of neutrophils will be elevated, whereas in acute allergy or parasite infection, basophils will have an increased percentage.
Neutrophils: 50–70% (total) Segments: 50–65% (mature neutrophils)	The largest group of granulocytes is first on the scene. High counts of >67% of total WBC indicate inflammation or infection. Low counts may indicate systemic infection or abscess. If neutrophils are low and bands are very high, abscess or systemic infection must be evaluated. Life span is <72 hours.
Bands: 0–5% (immature neutrophils)	Immature neutrophils may have banded rather than segmented nuclei. An elevation in this count (more than 10% of total WBC count) may indicate a large bacterial infection such as an abscess, pneumonia, or sepsis.
Basophils: 0.4–1.0%	Basophils are granulocytes that migrate out of circulation to become mast cells. Mast cells can release histamine in response to injury or cell death, a first step in inflammation.
Eosinophils: 1–3%	Eosinophils are granulocytes that become elevated in allergic and parasitic conditions.
Monocytes: 4–6%	Monocytes are nongranulocyte white blood cells that migrate out of circulation to become macrophages. Macrophages' primary role is to phagocytize cell debris, bacteria, viruses, and fungal cells.
Lymphocytes: 25–35%	Lymphocytes usually comprise about 25–33% of total WBC. If the lymphocyte level is severely elevated, consider infection or lymphoma.
Lymphocytes (T and B cells) (blood) 600–2,400/cells/µL 4–16%, 50–159 T cells 60–80% B cells 4–16% *T- and B-cell counts are used to monitor changes when treating immunosuppressive diseases.*	Low numbers (<500) may indicate acquired immunodeficiency syndrome (AIDS) or other immunodeficiencies. If the lymphocyte level is severely elevated, consider infection or lymphoma.
Antinuclear Antibodies (ANA): Negative Anticipate additional serum exams for immune function. *Few autoimmune diseases are diagnosed with one serum exam.*	Measures the number of antibodies made to parts of the patient's cells' nuclei. Indicates autoimmune disease.
Assays of IgG, IgA, IgM, IgD, IgE Adult: IgG: 650–1,700 mg/dL IgA: 70–400 mg/dL IgM: 40–350 mg/dL IgD: 0–8 mg/dL IgE: Less than 40	Serum assays of level of IgG in the blood can help identify patients with deficiencies. IgG is the major immunoglobulin, and IgG deficiency is relatively common.

DIAGNOSTIC TESTS to Assess Immune Function, *continued*

Test, Normal Value, and Rationale	Expected Abnormality
Erythrocyte Sedimentation Rate (ESR or sed rate), Westergren Method	
Males < 50 years: 0–15 mm/hr	An increased rate implies inflammation, a common finding in many immune diseases.
Females < 50 years: 0–20 mm/hr *Many immune diseases begin with multiple infections, fatigue, or vague symptoms.* *Immunoglobulin testing is an indication that immune function may be impaired. It is important to follow risk reduction behaviors.*	Sed rate may be elevated in inflammatory diseases such as rheumatoid arthritis, chronic infection, cancer, and other immune problems. Care should be taken to assess patients for increased risk of infection.
C-Reactive Protein (CRP)	
Titer: >1:2 *C-reactive protein may be elevated early in the acute inflammatory process and tissue destruction related to bacterial infection, tissue ischemia, tissue necrosis, and flare-ups in autoimmune diseases.*	Measures acute inflammation 6–10 hours postinjury and/or tissue destruction. CRP is an early nonspecific test for inflammation.

Sources: DeFranco, A. L., Locksley, R., & Robertson, M. (2007). *Immunity: The immune response in infectious and inflammatory disease.* Sunderland, MA: Sinauer Associates. Lefever-Kee, J. (2010). *Laboratory and diagnostic tests: Nursing implications* (8th ed.). Upper Saddle River, NJ: Pearson; McCance, K. L., & Grey, T. C. (2010). Altered cellular and tissue biology. In K. L. McCance & S. E. Huether (Eds.), *Pathophysiology: The biological basis for disease in adults & children* (6th ed., pp. 46–95). St. Louis: Mosby Elsevier; Porth, C. (2008). *Essentials of pathophysiology* (7th ed.). Philadelphia: Lippincott Williams & Wilkins.

response to the antigen that is injected. This is referred to as **anergy**; it results from the diminished ability of the T-cell line to produce chemical mediators of inflammation. Individuals who show evidence of anergy are at greater risk of developing cancer and have higher rates of mortality in general (Sommer, 2007).

Aging also results in a decreased ability on the part of immune cells to identify self antigens, while at the same time there is an increase in the number of autoantibodies produced. This results in higher incidences of autoimmune disease with aging (Rote, 2010). Research supports the hypothesis of an increased DNA mutation with aging, resulting in higher numbers of abnormal cells, and that the immune system fails to recognize and eliminate these mutant cells. This in part accounts for the greater incidence of tumors and cancers in older adults (Eggert, 2011; Sommer, 2007). Chart 52–6 summarizes the clinical effects of aging on the immune system.

Safety Alert *Older adults might not demonstrate the classic symptoms of infection and inflammation such as fever. As a result of decreased immune function, older adults may instead become hypothermic when they have a systemic infection. The white blood cell count is usually elevated, but the increase might not be as noticeable as in a younger person. Symptoms such as altered level of consciousness and confusion should be carefully assessed and evaluated in any older patients, especially those from settings such as skilled facilities, where the incidence of urinary tract infections may be high (Porth, 2008).*

CHART 52–6 Gerontological Considerations and the Effect on the Immune System

Clinical Signs	Effect
Decreased percentage of T cells	Increase risk of infection, tumor.
Decreased percentage of T-helper cells	Delayed initiation of the immune response.
Decreased percentage of suppressor T cells	Delayed downregulating of the immune response.
Decreased interleukin production	Slows inflammatory and immune responses to infection.
Decreased number of interleukin receptors on cells	Slows inflammatory and immune responses.
Delayed stimulation of T cells and B cells	Slows inflammatory response and may decrease ability to recognize cancer cells.
Decreased primary and secondary production of antibodies	Reduced response to infectious organisms. Increased severity of infections (i.e., pneumonia).
Delayed hypersensitivity response	Decreased allergic response, increased severity of infections.
Increased autoantibody production	Increased exacerbations of autoimmune disease.

Sources: Doerflinger, D. M. (2009). Older adult surgical patients: Presentation and challenges. *AORN Journal, 90,* 223–244; McCance, K. L., & Grey, T. C. (2010). Altered cellular and tissue biology. In K. L. McCance & S. E. Huether (Eds.), *Pathophysiology: The biological basis for disease in adults & children* (6th ed., pp. 46–95). St. Louis: Mosby Elsevier; Porth, C. (2008). *Essentials of pathophysiology* (7th ed.). Philadelphia: Lippincott Williams & Wilkins.

Critical Thinking Related to Immunologic and Inflammatory Disorders

Critical thinking is essential in order to prioritize the most significant clinical manifestations that need further investigation. Immunologic and inflammatory disorders can range from conditions as benign as the common cold to life-threatening reactions such as anaphylaxis. It is imperative that the nurse be able to distinguish normal from abnormal, benign from serious. The nurse must rely on critical thinking skills in interpreting the patient's symptoms and assessment findings to determine possible and potential patient diagnoses and to consider the appropriate actions to take. Analysis of these data allows the nurse to make a diagnosis and then follow up with an intervention. It is imperative that the nurse communicate and collaborate with other members of the health care team in developing and implementing a plan of care.

Because immunologic and inflammatory disorders can be simple or very complex, the nurse must be able to distinguish simple from severe symptoms. For example, when the patient reports symptoms of an infection such as a fever and swollen lymph glands, the nurse must possess knowledge of the difference between a minor and a major infection and assess the patient for each of them. Being able to identify additional risk factors, such as a compromised immune system, that would put the patient at greater risk for complications is an important component of critical thinking. Effective critical thinking skills include being curious and not making any assumptions. Regardless of the health problem, each symptom identified should be thoroughly described in order for the nurse to gain a full understanding. The nurse can say to the patient, "Tell me more about the problem," or "How did it start?" The patient usually proceeds with a discourse about the symptoms. The nurse then uses skillful interview techniques to explore and investigate each symptom further. Any symptom analysis is incomplete without a thorough description of its characteristics.

Summary

A fully competent immune system is essential to protect the human body from disease and disability. An alteration in the immune system's ability to eliminate pathogens, distinguish self from non-self, or identify and eliminate the proliferation of mutant cells results in immune-associated diseases. Immune tissues and cells are intricately associated with all body systems; therefore, a thorough assessment of immune function involves assessment of multiple body systems, as well as evaluation of cellular components of the immune system such as neutrophils and B and T cells and the development of specific antibodies. Abnormalities of the immune system can affect any system in the body, and often present through an inflammatory response.

NCLEX® PRACTICE

1. A patient is diagnosed with an immune deficiency disorder. The nurse explains to the patient that this problem is likely due to a malfunction of which of the following body structures?

1. Lymph nodes
2. Spleen
3. Bone marrow
4. Adenoids

2. The spouse of a patient diagnosed with an autoimmune disorder asks the nurse if the patient is allergic to something. The nurse bases the response to the patient's spouse on the fact that this disease process was caused by:

1. the body reacting to self receptors as an antigen.
2. the body's ability to tolerate all self antigens.
3. the body's ability to respond to non-self antigens.
4. adequate B and T cells that do not attack self antigens.

3. A patient is receiving a transfusion of plasma cells. The nurse is aware that these cells will contribute to which of the following?

1. Prodution of antibodies in response to exposure to an antigen
2. Stopping or slowing the immune process
3. Sending messages to start the process of programmed cell death
4. Stimulation of cells to destroy cancer cells

4. When planning care for a patient diagnosed with liver cirrhosis, the nurse should consider that this element of immunity will be altered:

1. Tumor necrosis factor
2. Interferons
3. Complement
4. Interleukins

5. The nurse is assessing a patient admitted due to the presence of an elevated temperature of unknown cause for several days. Which blood tests would the nurse anticipate being performed in the initial assessment of this patient? (select all that apply)

1. ESR
2. ANA
3. RBC
4. WBC
5. CRP

6. The nurse is caring for a patient with an infection. Which of the following explains how the patient's body will create specific antibodies to fight the infection?

1. T-cell activation
2. Antigen presentation
3. Linking of T cells
4. Linking of B cells

Answers to NCLEX Practice Questions can be found in Appendix D in the Osborn Student Resources at nursing.pearsonhighered.com. Practice additional NCLEX questions online at the Student Resources site.

Pearson Nursing Student Resources Find additional review materials at: **nursing.pearsonhighered.com**

REFERENCES

Atkinson, W., Wolfe, C., & Hamborsky, J. (Eds.). (2011). *Centers for Disease Control and Prevention: Epidemiology and prevention of vaccine preventable diseases.* Washington, DC: Public Health Foundation.

Bickley, L. S. (2009). *Guide to physical examination and history taking* (10th ed.). Philadelphia: Wolters Kluwer/Lippincott Williams & Wilkins.

Centers for Disease Control and Prevention (CDC). (2010). Trends in sexually transmitted disease in the United States: 2009 national data for gonorrhea, chlamydia and syphilis. Retrieved from http://www.cdc.gov/std/stats09/trends2009.pdf

DeFranco, A. L., Locksley, R., & Robertson, M. (2007). *Immunity: The immune response in infectious and inflammatory disease.* Sunderland, MA: Sinauer Associates.

Doerflinger, D. M. (2009). Older adult surgical patients: Presentation and challenges. *AORN Journal, 90*(2), 223–244.

Dunne, M. (2007). Infection, inflammation, and immunity. In C. M. Porth (Ed.), *Essentials of pathophysiology* (pp. 229–246). Philadelphia: Lippincott Williams & Wilkins.

Eggert, J. (2011). The biology of cancer: What do oncology nurses really need to know? *Seminars in Oncology Nursing, 27*(1), 3–12.

Hamilton, R. (2009). Nursing advocacy in a postgenomic age. *Nursing Clinics of North America, 44*(4), 435–446.

Kohler, G., & Milstein, C. (1975). Continuous cultures of fused cells secreting antibody of predefined specificity. *Nature, 256,* 495–497.

Lefever-Kee, J. (2010). *Laboratory and diagnostic tests: Nursing implications* (8th ed.). Upper Saddle River, NJ: Pearson.

McCance, K. L., & Grey, T. C. (2010). Altered cellular and tissue biology. In K. L. McCance & S. E. Huether (Eds.), *Pathophysiology: The biological basis for disease in adults & children* (6th ed., pp. 46–95). St. Louis: Mosby Elsevier.

National Institute for Occupational Safety and Health. (2007). Latex allergy: A prevention guide. Retrieved from http://www.cdc.gov/niosh/98-113.html

Nduka, O. O., & Parrillo, J. E. (2011). The pathophysiology of septic shock. *Critical Care Nursing Clinics of North America, 23*(1), 41–66.

Newman, K. M., & McGrath, J. M. (2010). Understanding the inflammatory response of the neonate: Clinical implications for caregivers in the neonatal intensive care unit. *Newborn Infant Nursing Review,10*(4), 165–176.

Porth, C. (2008). *Essentials of pathophysiology* (7th ed.). Philadelphia: Lippincott Williams & Wilkins.

Porth, C., & Sweeney, K. (2007). Alterations in immune response. In C. M. Porth (Ed.), *Essentials of pathophysiology* (pp. 293–319). Philadelphia: Lippincott Williams & Wilkins.

Rote, N. (2010). Adaptive immunity. In K. L. McCance & S. E. Huether (Eds.), *Pathophysiology: The biological basis for disease in adults & children* (6th ed., pp. 217–255). St. Louis: Mosby Elsevier.

Rote, N., & Huether, S. E. (2010). Innate immunity: Inflammation. In K. L. McCance & S. E. Huether (Eds.), *Pathophysiology: The biological basis for disease in adults & children* (6th ed., pp. 183–216). St. Louis: Mosby Elsevier.

Rote, N. S., & McCance, K. L. (2010). Structure and function of the hematologic system. In K. L. McCance & S. E. Huether (Eds.), *Pathophysiology: The biological basis for disease in adults & children* (6th ed., pp. 952–988). St. Louis: Mosby Elsevier.

Sommer, C. V. (2007). The immune response. In C. M. Porth (Ed.), *Essentials of pathophysiology* (pp. 134–149). Philadelphia: Lippincott Williams & Wilkins.

Tablan, O., Anderson, L., Besser, R., Bridges, C., & Hajjeh, R. (2004). Guidelines for preventing health-care–associated pneumonia, 2003. *Morbidity and Mortality Weekly Reports, 53*(RR03), 1–36. Retrieved from http://www.cdc.gov/mmwr/preview/mmwrhtml/rr5303a1.htm

Tol, J., & Punt, C. (2010). Monoclonal antibodies in the treatment of metastatic cancer: A review. *Clinical Therapeutics, 32*(3), 437–453.

Twite, K., & Gaspard, K. (2007). Disorders of the white blood cells and lymphoid tissues. In C. M. Porth (Ed.), *Essentials of pathophysiology* (pp. 247–266). Philadelphia: Lippincott Williams & Wilkins.

Weiner, L. M., Dhodapkar, M., & Ferrone, S. (2009). Monoclonal antibodies for cancer immunotherapy. *Lancet, 373*(9668), 1033–1040.

CHAPTER

53 Caring for the Patient with Immune Response Disorders

Renée Holleran

Outcome-Based Learning Objectives

After studying this chapter, the learner will be able to:

1. Differentiate the nursing management for patients wibth immune hypersensitivity responses and immune deficiencies.
2. Compare and contrast the immune hypersensitivity responses related to allergy, autoimmune, and alloimmune disorders.
3. Describe the pathophysiology, clinical manifestations, and laboratory data for the human immunodeficiency virus (HIV) and acquired immune deficiency syndrome (AIDS).
4. Generate a plan for the nursing management of the patient with HIV/AIDS to decrease the incidence of opportunistic infections.

KEY TERMS

acquired immunodeficiency syndrome (AIDS) p.1644
acute graft rejection p.1637
allergen p.1619
allergic response p.1618
allergy p.1619
alloimmune response p.1618
anaphylaxis p.1622
atopic p.1621
autoantibodies p.1632
autoantibody tests p.1632
autoimmune diseases p.1630
autoimmune response p.1618
CD4+ T cells p.1646
chronic graft rejection p.1637
flare p.1621
graft versus host disease (GVHD) p.1637
highly active antiretroviral drug therapy (HAART) p.1653
histamine p.1619
host versus graft disease (HVGD) p.1636
human immunodeficiency virus (HIV) p.1645
hyperacute rejection p.1637
IgE antibodies p.1619
immediate hypersensitivity reaction p.1619
immune deficiencies p.1618
immune hypersensitivity p.1618
immune hypersensitivity response p.1618
integrase p.1646
Kaposi's sarcoma p.1651
neoantigens p.1631
plasmapheresis p.1635
Pneumocystis jiroveci pneumonia p.1647
reverse transcriptase p.1646
sensitization p.1619
systemic lupus erythematosus (SLE) p.1632
tissue-specific antigens p.1619
type I (IgE-mediated) hypersensitivity p.1619
type II (tissue-specific) hypersensitivity p.1619
type III (immune complex–mediated) hypersensitivity p.1619
type IV (cell-mediated) hypersensitivity p.1620
type-specific hypersensitivity reactions p.1618
viral load p.1645
wasting syndrome p.1650
Western blot (WB) p.1651
wheal p.1621

IMMUNE DISORDERS result from a loss of regulation of some aspect of the immune system. They fall into two general categories: immune hypersensitivities and immune deficiencies. **Immune hypersensitivity** occurs when the immune system over-responds to an antigen from the environment, from the individual himself, or from another person. Hypersensitivity disorders fall into three broad categories based on the type of triggering antigen: allergic, autoimmune, and alloimmune reactions. An **allergic response** occurs when the antigen is from the external environment, in contrast to an **autoimmune response,** which is triggered by a self antigen. An **alloimmune response** occurs when the antigen is from another human. Within each of these categories are four specific mechanisms by which the immune system over-responds, referred to as **type-specific hypersensitivity reactions.**

Immune deficiencies occur when all or some part of the immune system fails to develop or is damaged through disease processes. The end result is an inability to mount an appropriate immune response. Immune deficiencies are discussed on pages 1643–1665.

Immune Hypersensitivities: Allergic, Autoimmune, and Alloimmune Responses

An **immune hypersensitivity response** occurs when the immune system does not maintain self-tolerance; in other words, when it overreacts to the presence of a foreign antigen. This process also initiates the mechanisms of inflammation that result in destruction of healthy tissue. Hypersensitivity reactions can be categorized according to the type of antigen (allergy, autoimmune, alloimmune), the time sequence of the reaction (immediate or delayed), and the mechanism of immunologic response. When an antigen is environmental or external in origin, it is referred to as an **allergy.** An example of this type of hypersensitivity reaction is allergies to common weeds and pollen, known as "hay fever." In autoimmune reactions, the body fails to recognize self antigens and begins to destroy its own proteins. Clinical disorders associated with autoimmune reactions include multiple sclerosis and systemic lupus erythematosus. An alloimmune response occurs when the immune system reacts against the antigens in or on the tissue from another individual, as may occur with grafted tissue and organ transplants.

A hypersensitivity response that occurs within seconds to hours is categorized as an **immediate hypersensitivity reaction.** An anaphylactic reaction, which is a severe, potentially life-threatening reaction to something the patient is allergic to, such as a bee sting, is a prime example of this type of response. A *delayed hypersensitivity reaction* can take several hours to days, as exemplified by a contact dermatitis (inflammation of the skin) reaction. The way in which the immune system responds to an antigen and the time sequence of the reaction are determined by the mechanism of immunologic response. These responses, which are categorized as types I through IV, are discussed next.

Mechanism of Hypersensitivity Immune Response

Four distinct mechanisms or types of immunologic reactions are involved in allergic, autoimmune, and alloimmune reactions: type I (IgE-mediated allergic reactions), type II (tissue-specific-mediated reactions), type III (immune complex–mediated reactions), and type IV (cell-mediated reactions). The type I, II, and III hypersensitivity responses involve antigen–antibody interactions and are known as *immediate hypersensitivity reactions.* The type IV response is an antigen–lymphocyte interaction and involves a delayed hypersensitivity reaction. All these responses can cause damage to body tissues.

Type I (IgE-Mediated) Hypersensitivity Reaction

Type I (IgE-mediated) hypersensitivity, also known as anaphylactic hypersensitivity, is the most common of the hypersensitivity disorders; it involves the production of antigen-specific IgE antibody after exposure to an **allergen** (a foreign antigen that causes a hypersensitivity reaction). Common allergens include plant pollen, pet dander, foods, and drugs. **IgE antibodies** are produced by the plasma cells in response to the foreign antigen (see Chapter 52 for more information on allergens). The process of creating antibodies that match the antigen is called **sensitization.** The IgE antibodies connect to receptors on mast cells in the connective tissue. The process of sensitization may take only one exposure or several exposures to the allergen depending on the level of IgE production. This explains why many allergic responses take time to develop.

When a hypersensitivity reaction occurs, the allergen binds to IgE antibodies on the mast cell and causes degranulation of mast cells and release of histamine. **Histamine** is a compound that causes smooth muscle contraction, vasodilation, and increased vascular permeability; it primarily affects the skin, mucous membranes, and lung. The histamines are responsible for the clinical symptoms associated with type I reactions such as redness, itching, mucus production, and bronchial constriction. The reactions can be localized in tissue or may be systemic, as with an anaphylactic response. The severity of the clinical symptoms depends on the sensitivity of the individual, the amount of allergen exposure and mediator release, and the entry route of the allergen. For example, an allergen injected via an insect sting elicits a very rapid hypersensitivity response (Porth & Sweeney, 2007; Rote, 2010).

Type II (Tissue-Specific) Hypersensitivity Reaction

Type II (tissue-specific) hypersensitivity reactions involve **tissue-specific antigens,** which are proteins located in the cell membrane of some tissues such as blood, nerves, lungs, and kidneys. Type II reactions are mediated by IgG or IgM antibodies and occur when the immune system fails to recognize a host's self antigen or antigens on donated red blood cells (RBCs). IgG or IgM antibodies interact with the tissue-specific antigen on a target cell's plasma membrane to form antibody–antigen complexes. Type II reactions can occur in several ways. This explains the variety of clinical signs and symptoms observed in this type of reaction.

The hallmark of type II hypersensitivity reactions is that they are limited to tissues or organs that have tissue-specific antigens. One example is Goodpasture's syndrome, in which antibodies are formed against the tissue-specific antigen found in the basement membrane of the glomeruli in the kidneys and the alveoli in the lungs. The result is destruction of these tissues and the associated clinical symptoms of renal failure and lung damage. Another example is myasthenia gravis, in which the immune system fails to recognize the tissue-specific antigen on nerve ending receptor sites and binds to acetylcholine receptors on the muscle, causing faulty muscle enervation. Type II hypersensitivity reactions are responsible for Rh-hemolytic disease of the newborn and antibody–antigen reactions involving RBC destruction such as incompatibility reactions in blood transfusions (Porth & Sweeney, 2007; Rote, 2010).

Blood Transfusion Reactions

Blood transfusion reactions are an example of a type II hypersensitivity antibody–antigen reaction that results in activation of the complement cascade and initiation of a systemic inflammatory response. Inflammatory cascades and the systemic inflammatory response result in the lysis of target cells and are discussed in great detail in Chapter 54. All RBCs except type O have type-specific antigens on their surface. The B lymphocytes produce antibodies specific to all other blood antigens. If the patient has type A blood, each blood cell is coated with antigen A and carries B antibodies. An individual with type B blood has B antigens on the surface of each RBC and carries A antibodies. If a patient with type A blood is erroneously given type B blood, the individual receives A antibodies that attach to the A antigen and form an immune complex (Figure 53–1◆). This immune complex stimulates the complement cascade that produces lysis of the cell, resulting in cell death.

The major clinical problems with blood transfusion reactions relate to the stimulation of an overwhelming systemic inflammatory response and shock state. Oxygen-carrying capacity is lost because the patient's own RBCs are destroyed, as are the RBCs in the transfused blood. Additionally, the cellular debris following cell lysis contains large proteins that may block the tubules of the glomeruli in the kidney and can produce acute tubular necrosis (Rote, 2010).

The ABO blood antigen is only one example of many antibodies and antigens for which blood is tested prior to blood transfusion. Another important factor is the Rhesus (Rh) factor. This factor is significant because of the severity of the clinical response such as anaphylactic reaction and refractory shock. An extensive discussion of blood products, testing, and key safety factors in blood administration can be found in Chapter 16.

Type III (Immune Complex–Mediated) Hypersensitivity Reaction

Type III (immune complex–mediated) hypersensitivity reactions also involve IgG and IgM antibody–antigen immune

Weblink: Allergic Reaction

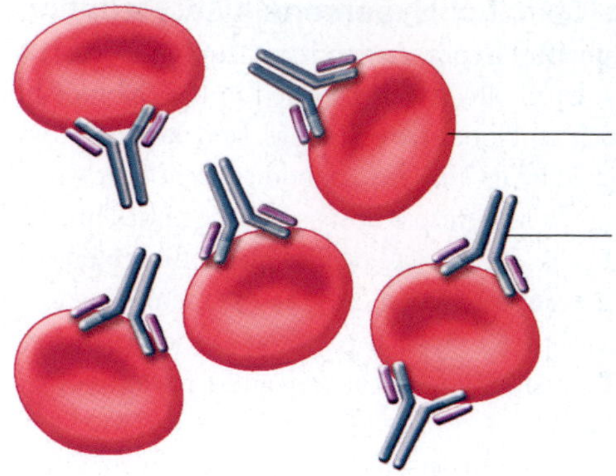

If a patient with type A blood is given type B blood, the anti-A antibodies in the type B blood attach to the A antigen.

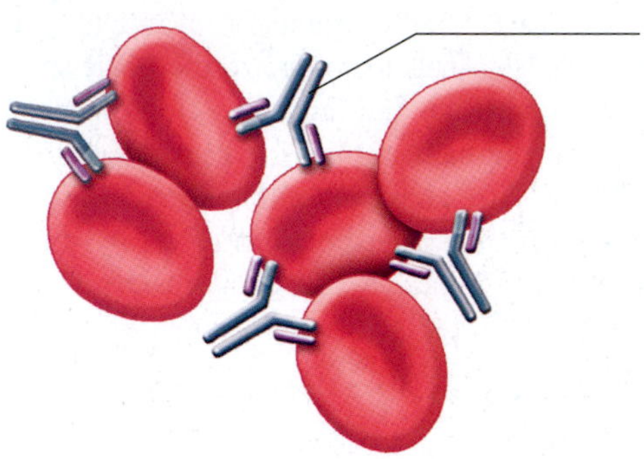

The anti-A antibodies cross-link the blood cells, resulting in agglutination and cell death.

FIGURE 53–1 ◆ Red blood cell immune complex.

complexes. However, they differ from type II reactions because the antigen in type III reactions is soluble and released into circulation instead of staying localized at a specific cell surface. The antigen can travel and be deposited in extravascular tissue, such as joints, and then an antibody–antigen reaction can occur. In other instances, the antibody–antigen reaction can happen in the circulation, which results in the immune complex being deposited in tissue, such as the glomeruli. In either case, damage to the tissues results because the immune complex stimulates the complement cascade and the mediators of inflammation. Neutrophils attempt to phagocytize large immune complexes; in the process, lysosomal enzymes are released at the tissue site, further stimulating the inflammation process and damaging the surrounding tissues.

As a result of the mobility of the type III antigen–antibody complex, systemic or local responses also can occur, although the reactions are not organ specific. Serum sickness is an example of a systemic response. Immune complexes are produced in the circulation in response to a foreign antigen and to some drugs such as sulfonamides and penicillin. The clinical symptoms of serum sickness include rash, fever, lymphadenopathy, arthralgias, and myalgias; they result from the immune complexes being deposited in the walls of small blood vessels, kidneys, and joints throughout the body (Porth & Sweeney, 2007; Rote, 2010).

Type IV (Cell-Mediated) Hypersensitivity Reactions

Type IV (cell-mediated) hypersensitivity reactions differ from the other three types of hypersensitivity reactions in that the response is delayed instead of immediate, onset being 24 to 48 hours after antigen exposure. Furthermore, these reactions are mediated by the T cells of the immune system instead of by antibodies. Type IV reactions occur as a result of an overreaction between normal cell-mediated mechanisms and an antigen that triggers the T cells to destroy the target cell directly or to release cells to produce lymphokines. The lymphokines activate phagocytic cells, especially macrophages at the inflammatory site. Examples of these types of reactions are seen with exposure to poison ivy, poison oak, and purified protein derivative (Rote, 2010).

Immune Hypersensitivity

The four mechanisms of immune response described previously can be seen in all three categories of antigen reaction: allergic, autoimmune, and alloimmune. These different categories and mechanisms of response account for the variety of clinical manifestations seen with hypersensitivity response.

Antigen Reaction: Allergic, Autoimmune, and Alloimmune

Allergy Reaction

Etiology and Epidemiology

The hallmark of allergy reactions is the IgE-mediated antibody–antigen response. An allergic reaction involves a type I hypersensitivity response in which an environmental antigen stimulates an overproduction of IgE antibodies that attach to mast cells. The interaction of these antibodies with an allergen, such as an environmental or foreign antigen, stimulates the release of histamine and proinflammatory mediators from mast cells. This release results in the irritating and uncomfortable symptoms associated with allergies including itching eyes, nose, and throat; cough; congestion; runny nose; watery eyes; and often bronchospasm. If the hypersensitivity reaction is severe, as with an anaphylactic reaction, the allergic response can be life threatening.

Allergic disease affects millions of people in the United States, and the incidence is increasing every year (Asthma and Allergy Foundation of America, 2011). Current research is focused on risk factors that may be responsible, including those listed in the Risk Factors for Respiratory Allergies box. See also the Genetic Considerations box. Studies to date have been disappointingly inconclusive (Centers for Disease Control and Prevention [CDC], 2011a). No clear evidence of a single causative factor has been identified, and it is most probable that

RISK FACTORS for Respiratory Allergies

Genetic predisposition
Frequency of viral infections
Increased use of antimicrobial cleansing products in the home
Early childhood exposure to allergens
Dietary factors
Air pollution and environmental factors
Dust mites
Pet exposure
Cockroaches.

GENETIC CONSIDERATIONS
for the Allergic Hypersensitivity Response

Research continues to demonstrate a link between individual genes and factors in the environment that trigger allergic reactions (Holloway, Yang, & Holgate, 2010; Seibert, 2010). Specific mutant genes linked to environmental triggers cause a hypersensitivity response, for example, the identification of an asthma susceptibility gene *ADAM33*. This gene, when exposed to environmental triggers such as secondhand smoke, can result in early onset asthma.

The identification of these genes and their triggers allows for the development of prevention strategies so that patients at risk can decrease their vulnerability. It is also important to remember the link between genes and the environment in hypersensitivity.

the occurrence of allergic diseases will be found to be a result of multiple factors (CDC, 2011a; Rote, 2010).

Pathophysiology

Normally, millions of IgE molecules of different specificities are attached to each mast cell. It is thought that individuals who are **atopic** (produce a hypersensitivity response) have a genetic predisposition to produce greater than normal levels of IgE (Dunne & Ledeboer, 2009). With each re-exposure to a triggering antigen, there is increased IgE production, increased mast cell degranulation, and increased release of histamine. The histamine causes vasodilation in local blood vessels. Additionally, endothelial cells pull apart, and localized swelling occurs. This process can allow the allergen to enter the bloodstream. If this occurs, a systemic allergic response can result because basophils in the bloodstream also are stimulated to release histamine. This is the basis for an anaphylactic reaction (p. 1622) (Rote, 2010).

Clinical Manifestations

Clinical manifestations of the allergic response occur in tissues such as skin, mucous membranes, the lungs, and the gastrointestinal (GI) tract because these tissues are highly vascular and have an abundance of mast cells as part of a fully competent immune system. A wide variety of allergic hypersensitivity reactions and clinical manifestations exist. Chart 53–1 describes some of the common allergens and their associated symptoms.

Skin Allergies

Allergic responses are commonly manifested on the skin. This is the basis for skin testing for allergies. A wheal and flare response is typical of a localized allergic response on the skin from exposure to an allergen, such as the resin of a star thistle plant, which binds with IgEs and causes immediate degranulation of the mast cells in the subcutaneous tissue. The clinical manifestation of the allergic response is a **wheal,** or small, round, raised blister filled with watery fluid, which is surrounded by a **flare** or round area of redness. This reaction occurs from the release of histamine, which causes local vasodilatation, redness, swelling, itching, and heat (Porth & Sweeney, 2007).

Other skin reactions, such as allergic contact dermatitis or a poison ivy reaction, are cell-mediated type IV delayed hypersensitivity reactions (Figure 53–2◆, p. 1622). On first exposure, the protein in poison ivy (which is the allergen) stimulates immune and memory T cells (sensitization). A second or later contact with the poison ivy resin stimulates sensitized T cells. The reaction reaches maximum intensity in 24 to

CHART 53–1 Common Allergens

Common Allergen	Characteristics	Symptoms
Pollen	Allergen is the dry pollen that is present in the air. Early spring: tree pollen (oak, elm, poplar). Early summer: rose pollen, grass pollen (Timothy, red-top). Early fall: weed pollen (ragweed).	Sneezing, runny nose, congestion, itching of the nose, eyes, ears, throat, and mouth
Animal dander	Allergen is the protein found in the saliva, dander, or urine of an animal with fur, not the "hair" of the animal.	Sneezing, itching, runny nose, swollen itchy eyes and throat
Dust mites	Allergen is the microscopic droppings of mites found in bedding, upholstery, and carpets. Most common trigger of year-round allergies and asthma.	Congested or runny nose, sneezing (especially in the morning), itchy watery eyes, coughing, wheezing
Mold	Allergen is the spores that are disseminated by the fungi. Molds thrive in humid areas such as bathrooms and basements.	Sneezing, runny nose, congestion, itching of the nose, eyes, ears, throat, and mouth
Insect stings	Allergen is the protein in the venom of the insect sting. Majority of sting reactions in the United States are caused by yellow jackets, honeybees, paper wasps, hornets, and fire ants.	Flushing, itching, hives, swelling at the site of the bite *Potential anaphylactic reaction:* light-headedness, feeling of impending doom, swelling in the throat, wheezing, severe bronchoconstriction, nausea, vomiting, drop in blood pressure, shock = medical emergency
Medications Common: antibiotics	Allergen is the protein in the medication or the substance with which the medication is made.	Rash, hives, general itching, tingling or itching of the mouth/palate, potential anaphylactic reaction as previously described
Food allergies Most common: nuts, fish, shellfish, milk, chicken eggs, kiwi, seeds	Allergen is the protein in the food particle. The majority of reactions develop within the first hour. Generally, the longer it takes for symptoms to develop, the less severe the reaction.	Oral itching or tingling in the mouth/palate, lip swelling, swelling of the face, generalized flushing, itching, nausea, vomiting, and potential anaphylactic reaction as previously described

Sources: American College of Allergy, Asthma and Immunology. (2011a). Be S.A.F.E.: Managing allergic emergencies. Retrieved from http://www.acaai.org/patients/resources/anaphylaxis/managing-allergic-emergencies/Documents/BeSAFEBrochure.pdf; American College of Allergy, Asthma & Immunology. (2011b). Latex allergy. Retrieved from http://www.acaai.org/allergist/allergies/Types/latex-allergy/Pages/default.aspx; World Allergy Organization. (2011). White book on allergy. Retrieved from http://www.worldallergy.org/UserFiles/file/WAO-White-Book-on-Allergy_FINAL.pdf.

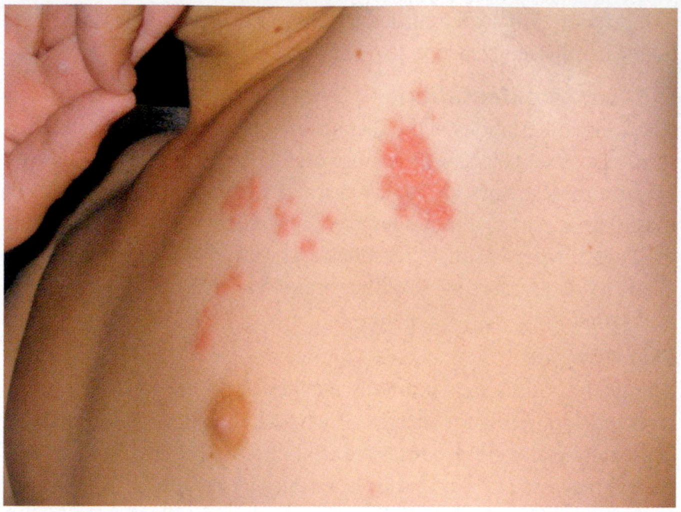

FIGURE 53–2 ◆ Skin allergy type IV response.
Source: Debra Brady

72 hours and results in clinical symptoms of blistering vesicles and red, scaled areas (Rote, 2010).

Latex Allergy

Latex allergies can occur as a type I allergic reaction or as a type IV (cell-mediated) reaction in response to contact with products containing natural latex. Type I reactions occur rapidly after exposure, usually within minutes. The release of IgE antibodies is responsible for the symptoms, which can include redness of the exposed skin, urticaria, asthma, itching, and conjunctivitis, which also may progress to anaphylactic shock (Rote, 2010). Exposure to the proteins that act as antigens in latex can occur through use of gloves on skin or IV catheters into the bloodstream. Type I reactions can be life threatening because of their bronchial constrictive effect on the airway and vasodilation of blood vessels, which decreases perfusion pressure (World Allergy Organization, 2011).

Safety Alert *A latex reaction can occur during a surgical procedure. Symptoms of reaction in the anesthetized patient include flushing, facial edema, wheezing, bronchospasm, laryngeal edema, tachycardia, hypotension, and, in extreme cases, cardiac arrest.*

A latex allergy also can manifest as a type IV delayed reaction, much like contact dermatitis, in which symptoms present between 4 and 48 hours after exposure. Symptoms of this type of latex allergy include dryness at the site of exposure, itching, and cracking of the skin. These symptoms are followed by redness, swelling, and scabbing of the fissures and cracks in the skin, usually within a day or two of the initial symptoms. This type of reaction is often seen in health care workers who handle latex equipment and use latex gloves. The increase in incidence of type IV latex reactions has coincided with the advent of standard precautions, which has increased the use of gloves. Estimates of the number of sensitized health care workers range from 8% to 17%. As with any antigen, the more often an individual is exposed to the antigen, the more likely that the individual will become sensitized to that antigen. Powder in gloves has been removed in hospital settings to reduce the risk of aerosolized exposure to latex. These exposures can be dangerous to the sensitized individual and result in a life-threatening anaphylactic response (National Institute for Occupational Safety and Health [NIOSH], 2011). All hospitals now provide latex-free gloves, and most institutions provide latex-free disposable products of all kinds, such as IV tubing, blood tubing, ventilator equipment, and aerosol tubing.

Identifying individuals who are at risk for latex allergy is essential to preventing the allergic response. Factors such as working in any industry that uses latex or rubber components (health care workers, housekeepers, hairdressers) increases the risk, as does a history of hay fever or asthma, and/or allergies to certain foods such as banana, avocado, kiwi, and strawberry. The proteins found in these foods have a structure similar to that of latex proteins and can trigger an allergic response. Patient populations with increased risk factors include those with neural tube defects such as myelomeningocele or spina bifida, those who require chronic bladder catheterization such as patients with spinal cord trauma or neurogenic bladders, and those who have had multiple surgeries. All of these situations involve multiple contacts with latex products, which enhance the risk of developing latex allergies. Any individual who is identified as part of these high-risk groups or who can describe a contact dermatitis type reaction after exposure to latex should be considered at risk for a latex allergy (NIOSH, 2011).

Safety Alert *Patients with neural tube deficits have a high risk of developing latex allergies. Latex-free products should always be used in caring for patients with neural tube deficits even when prior latex allergy has not been identified (American College of Allergy, Asthma and Immunology, 2011a).*

Latex-free products are to be used in all hospital settings with latex-sensitive individuals. These products are usually provided on special carts containing disposable equipment that is entirely latex free. The latex-sensitive patient's room should have a latex allergy alert sign posted. Health care workers with latex sensitivity must stringently adhere to the same precautions using powder-free and latex-free gloves and equipment. Special barrier creams are available to use on the hands for added protection. Symptoms of latex allergy need to be reported per agency protocol to the employee health center.

Food Allergies

Food allergy reactions most commonly involve mucous membranes and the GI tract but can quickly lead to an anaphylactic response. Food allergies can cause anaphylactic reactions, which may require treatment in the emergency department. Common food allergies seen in the United States include allergies to egg, milk, peanut, tree nuts (e.g., walnuts, pecans), wheat, crustacean shellfish, and soy (Marcason, 2011). Food allergies, in particular allergies to peanuts and tree nuts, can be fatal (Finkelman, 2010). The peanut protein antigen, for example, attaches to the IgE antibody, causing the mast cells to degranulate and release histamine. The sensitive individual experiences early symptoms of allergy such as tracheal and oral itching, swelling, redness, nausea, and vomiting. The response can be limited to itching on the interior of the mouth and the GI tract, or it can be as profound as a severe anaphylactic reaction.

Safety Alert *One of the most common early symptoms of an allergic reaction is itching in the mouth and palate. It is important to assess this in individuals complaining of allergy symptoms or who are receiving a new drug such as an antibiotic or vaccine.*

Anaphylactic Reaction

Anaphylaxis is a hypersensitivity response that can manifest as symptoms ranging from itching, erythema, vomiting, and breathing difficulties to severe laryngeal edema, respiratory distress, vascular collapse, shock, and death (Figure 53–3◆). Anaphylaxis can be a localized or systemic hypersensitivity response to an antigen that can quickly progress to a medical emergency if not recognized and treated appropriately.

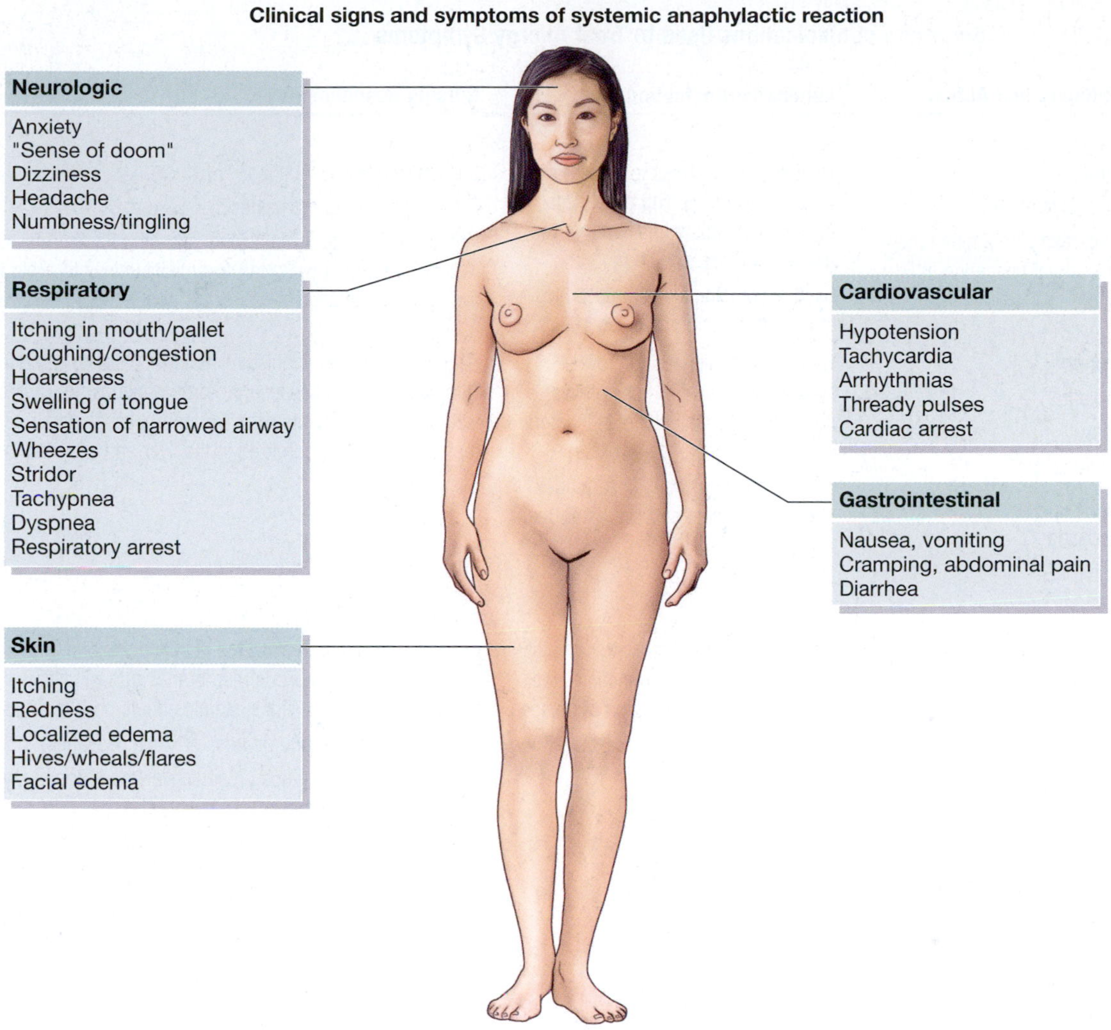

FIGURE 53–3 ◆ Anaphylaxis symptoms.

Combinations of presenting symptoms may vary in an individual experiencing an anaphylactic reaction depending on the number of IgE antibodies on the mast cells, the number of mast cells that degranulate and release histamine, and the release of other proinflammatory mediators such as bradykinin and serotonin. Symptoms of anaphylactic response are usually immediate (occurring within 30 minutes of exposure), although the oral route of allergen exposure can have a 2-hour delay. A secondary response, or biphasic reaction, is seen in approximately 20% of patients with anaphylaxis and can occur 4 to 8 hours after the initial remission of symptoms due to secondary mediators of inflammation such as bradykinin. In general, the anaphylactic reaction is more life threatening if the hypersensitivity response is immediate (Rote, 2010).

The result of a severe systemic anaphylactic reaction is a form of shock called *distributive shock* that results in massive vasodilation, loss of blood pressure, and inadequate distribution of blood supply and oxygen to all body tissues. Concurrent smooth muscle bronchoconstriction and laryngeal edema initially cause inspiratory and expiratory wheezing and difficulty breathing, which may progress to complete airway obstruction. Death can result from full circulatory collapse, severe bronchial constriction, or a combination of both. Nursing care focuses on early recognition of anaphylactic symptoms, airway management, and collaborative aggressive medication treatment to stem the continuum of anaphylactic response and prevent death.

Safety Alert *Patients can be in extreme danger when breath sounds diminish after wheezing because the airways are completely constricted and no air is being inspired or expired due to edema.*

Treatment of anaphylaxis focuses on immediate administration of intramuscular adrenaline. Adrenaline's alpha-receptor agonist activity reverses vasodilation and decreases edema. Its beta-receptor activity relaxes smooth muscle, thus dilating bronchioles; suppresses histamine release; and increases myocardial contractility. Administration of supplemental oxygen, establishment of intravenous (IV) access, and administration of IV fluid to support intravascular volume in patients with hypotension are also essential. Corticosteroids are a key aspect of ongoing drug therapy and work to control inflammatory mediators. Other medications that may be included in treatment are antihistamines and inotropic and antiarrhythmic agents.

Medical Management

Successful medical treatment for individuals with allergic hypersensitivity focuses on avoidance of triggering allergens, prevention of a hypersensitivity response, and relief of allergy symptoms. Therefore, identifying the causative allergens is primary to effective management of allergic disease. This involves obtaining a thorough patient history and diagnostic studies, followed by creation of a drug therapy and treatment regime for allergy symptom management. For severe allergy problems, this treatment plan may include allergy desensitization shots.

PHARMACOLOGY Summary of Medications Used to Treat Allergy Symptoms

Medication Category and Action	Application/Indication	Nursing Responsibility
Antihistamines		
First generation: Diphenhydramine (Benadryl) ***Action:*** First-generation histamine receptor blocks the effects of histamine at H_1 receptors.	Treatment of allergies to provide symptomatic relief of itching eyes, nose, throat; runny nose; and watery eyes; and to decrease swelling. Used in combination with decongestants and for cold and sinus treatment.	Causes significant sedation. Monitor patient for drowsiness. Instruct patients to avoid alcohol and other central nervous system (CNS) depressants when taking antihistamines to avoid the cumulative effects of sedation.
Second generation: Fexofenadine (Allegra) Cetirizine (Zyrtec) Desloratadine (Clarinex) Loratadine (Claritin) ***Action:*** Less sedating. Longer half-life.	Treatment of allergies to provide symptomatic relief of itching eyes, nose, throat; runny nose; and watery eyes; and to decrease swelling. Used in combination with decongestants and for cold and sinus treatment.	Second-generation antihistamines are contraindicated in patients with dysrhythmias because the drug prolongs the Q-T interval. Use with caution in patients with liver and/or renal impairment because these drugs are metabolized in the liver and excreted in the kidneys.
Intranasal Corticosteroids		
Fluticasone (Flonase) Beclomethasone (Beconase) ***Action:*** Applied directly to nasal mucosa. Does not have systemic side effects of steroids given orally or parenterally.	First-line treatment of allergic rhinitis to decrease local inflammation, swelling of tissues, and irritation of mucosa.	Instruct the patient to clear the nose, shake inhaler thoroughly, and assess for broken mucous membranes that will allow medication into the bloodstream, causing systemic effects prior to administration. May cause burning and dryness of nasal passages. Instruct the patient to use preservative-free saline spray or petroleum jelly to decrease dryness.
Decongestants and Sympathomimetics		
Pseudoephedrine (Sudafed, Actifed) PO Phenylephrine (Neo-Synephrine, Sinex) Intranasal ***Action:*** Stimulates alpha-adrenergic receptors in the sympathetic nervous system, causing nasal passages to constrict.	Treatment of congestion. Dries mucous membranes and decreases drainage.	Assess for nasal excoriation and bleeding. Monitor the patient for psychosocial/emotional changes; may cause agitation. Monitor vital signs; can increase heart rate and/or blood pressure. Oral sympathomimetics are contraindicated in patients with hypertension. Monitor blood glucose in patients who are diabetic because oral dose can increase glucose levels.

Source: Adams, M., & Koch, R. W. (2010). *Pharmacology connections for nursing practice.* Upper Saddle River, NJ: Pearson.

Safety Alert *A thorough history of any allergies the patient may have is essential before the nurse administers any medication. Individuals with a family history of hypersensitivity reaction are at greater risk for allergic response. Awareness of a patient's allergies is especially crucial with IV medications, such as antibiotics, because the antigen goes directly into the bloodstream, bypassing the local response delay, and can stimulate an immediate severe anaphylactic reaction.*

Laboratory and Diagnostic Procedures

Allergy symptoms are very disruptive and uncomfortable and can be expensive to treat. In the extreme, they can be life threatening. Therefore, it is important to identify the specific triggering allergen(s) to which the atopic individual may be sensitized so that contact with the allergen can be avoided and a plan can be developed to treat the symptoms most effectively. Allergy testing includes blood and sputum laboratory tests to determine total IgE and allergen-specific IgE, as well as skin tests with small amounts of allergens to evaluate sensitivity.

Blood Tests

Initial laboratory tests to detect lymphocyte, eosinophil, and immunoglobulin abnormalities commonly include a complete blood count (CBC) with white blood cell differential (WBC). This provides a total lymphocyte and eosinophil count. The eosinophil count is usually elevated with type I hypersensitivity reactions and is one of the indicators used to confirm a diagnosis of allergy. Nasal smears, sputum, and bronchial secretions may also be tested for the presence of eosinophils, which indicate probable allergy.

The allergen-specific IgE antibody is the most important serological marker for the diagnosis of allergic disease. It is also used to confirm exposure (World Allergy Organization, 2011). This test can measure IgE antibodies to numerous allergen specificities in one test. If a positive response occurs to a specific allergen, then a clinical history and more testing to specific antibodies can be used to confirm the diagnosis. This method has been found to be the most cost effective way to identify a specific allergen in vitro (World Allergy Organization, 2011).

Skin Tests

Skin testing involves introducing small amounts of various allergens into the skin through either intradermal injection or a scratch (prick test) on the individual's back. The prick test is the less sensitive of the two tests, but it also carries a lower risk of systemic reaction. It is performed by placing a small drop of allergen onto the skin, then pricking through it to introduce the allergen. If the individual is sensitive to a specific allergen, IgE antibodies activate mast cells to degranulate, histamine is released, and a localized reaction is produced, causing a wheal and flare of at least 3 mm. Allergy medications may suppress the skin reaction and result in a false-negative reading. Therefore, allergy medications including antihistamines and corticosteroids are generally stopped for 48 to 96 hours prior to allergy testing (World Allergy Organization, 2011).

The profound danger with skin testing is that even a small amount of skin test allergen can cause a systemic anaphylactic response in a severely allergic individual, which requires immediate and emergent attention. Therefore, skin testing should never be performed if the individual is experiencing respiratory abnormalities such as bronchospasm.

Safety Alert *Nursing care of the patient in the outpatient allergy testing clinic focuses on assessment for symptoms of anaphylactic response, respiratory assessment, airway management, and rapid treatment of anaphylactic emergency. Skin tests should never be undertaken if emergency equipment and medications to treat anaphylactic reaction are not available.*

Pharmacologic Management of Allergies

Drug therapy is the primary focus of allergy management. The vast majority of allergies are mediated by an IgE interaction between an allergen and receptors on the IgE antibody that stimulate the release of histamine. The goal of medications that relieve allergy symptoms is to decrease histamine release and its effects on the mucosa, skin, and tissues. A wide variety of allergy medications are available. Health care providers may suggest over-the-counter (OTC) products or write specific drug prescriptions. Frequently, the medication the patient uses is determined by insurance coverage. The Pharmacology Summary of Medications Used to Treat Allergy Symptoms box describes common allergy medications for symptom management. Major categories of drugs that provide symptomatic relief include antihistamines, sympathomimetic and decongestant drugs, corticosteroids, mast cell stabilizers, and antipyretic drugs.

The wide variety of allergy medications available often leads to confusion about which medication to take to alleviate symptoms or how to dose the medications correctly. Therefore, a primary role for members of the health care team is providing patient education on the appropriate dosing of allergy medications and the adverse effects that can occur if medication directions are not followed.

Desensitization Immunotherapy

Desensitization, or giving "allergy shots," involves introducing small doses of the triggering allergen to the sensitive individual in increasing amounts over a long period of time, with the goal of decreasing the severity of the allergic reaction. The exact mechanism by which desensitization occurs is not fully understood. It is thought that desensitization may work by inducing the production of blocking antibodies that bind with the allergen and neutralize it so that it cannot bind with IgE and degranulate mast cells. Desensitization injections also may stimulate the production of suppressor T lymphocytes, which suppress the production of IgE and inhibit hypersensitivity (Rote, 2010). However, this form of treatment does have a significant risk of systemic anaphylaxis.

Nursing Management

Nursing care of patients with allergies is focused on helping patients and families identify and avoid allergy triggers, providing education about medications for symptom relief, and offering instruction in strategies to prevent a severe allergy hypersensitivity response. Nursing care also involves early recognition and emergent treatment of anaphylactic reaction. Application of the nursing process will facilitate a comprehensive approach to the assessment and care of the patient with allergies. The Nursing Process: Patient Care Plan for Anaphylactic Response box (p. 1626) provides information and sample questions to be used in obtaining a thorough assessment and history of the allergies. Nursing diagnoses are developed from the assessment data. The care plan also provides detailed outcome goals and evaluation parameters, as well as the nursing interventions (with rationales) used to achieve these outcomes.

Weblink: Asthma and Allergy Foundation

Health Promotion

The health care team can further promote patient health and safety by encouraging patients with a history of anaphylactic reactions to wear a medical alert bracelet or other form of medical identification tag that identifies allergies to medications, foods, or other substances. This type of ID alerts health care providers to potential problems in the event of an emergency. Additionally, instructing patients with a history of anaphylactic reaction to carry a self-administered epinephrine kit to use in the event of an anaphylactic reaction is essential. Kits, such as the EpiPen (Figure 53–4◆), are easy to use and can save lives in an anaphylactic emergency (American College of Allergy, Asthma and Immunology, 2011a).

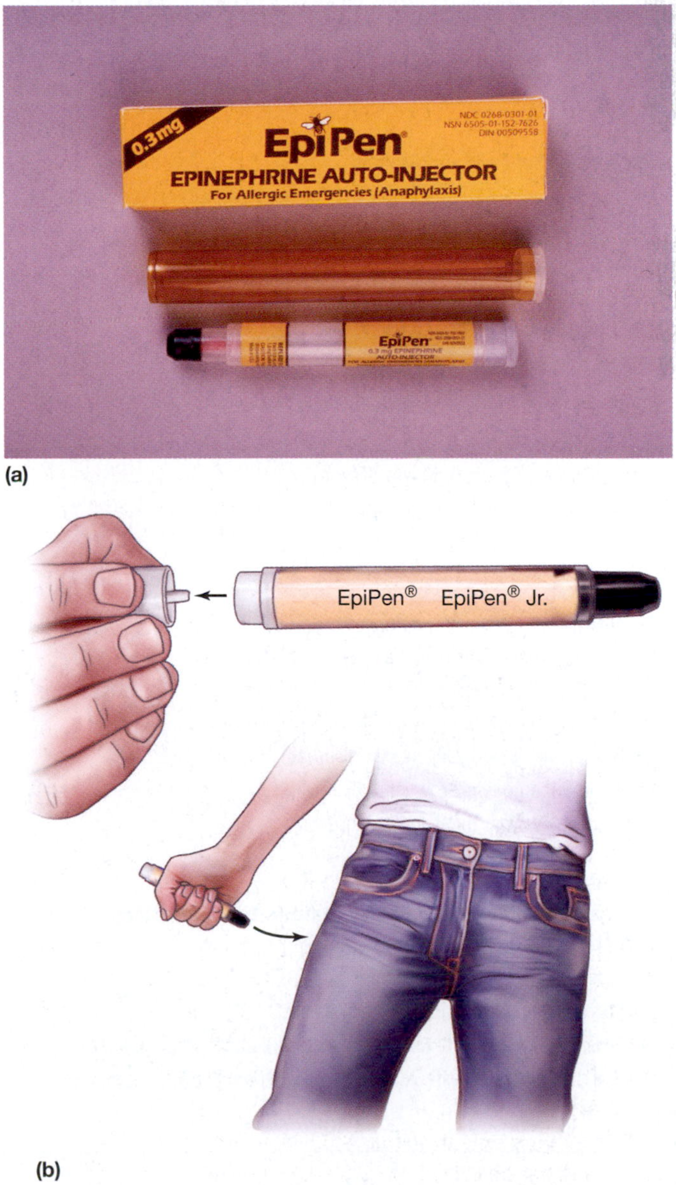

FIGURE 53–4 ◆ EpiPen.

NURSING PROCESS: Patient Care Plan for Anaphylactic Response

Assessment of Immune Status Using Gordon's Functional Health Patterns:

- Health Perception Health Management Pattern
- Nutrition Metabolic Pattern
- Activity Exercise Pattern
- Cognitive Perceptual Pattern
- Self-Perception Self-Concept Pattern

Subjective Data

Assessment of Airway and Gas Exchange

Are you allergic to any medications, food, or other substances?

Did you come in contact with something you are allergic to?

How much of the substance were you exposed to?

How long ago did you first notice itching, swelling, or breathing changes?

Has this ever happened to you before?

Did you take anything to treat your allergies?

Assessment of Cardiac Output

Do you feel dizzy or weak?

Have you fainted?

Assessment of Pain and Anxiety

What is your pain level on the 0-to-10 scale, where a 0 is no pain and 10 is the worst pain imaginable?

Are you feeling anxious?

Do you take pain or antianxiety medications routinely at home?

What helps when you have anxiety?

Do you have any medication allergies?

Do you have cultural or religious practices that impact your pain or anxiety?

Assessment of Fluid/Volume Status

Do you feel dizzy, tired, or thirsty?

Assessment of Potential Allergy Response

Do you have any allergies to medications, foods, plants, animals, or other materials (such as latex)?

Do you have any history of previous allergy reactions such as rash, itching, tingling, or swelling in your mouth, or breathing difficulties?

Have you undergone allergy testing?

Does anyone in your family have allergies?

Do you take any allergy medications?

Assessment of the Patient's and Family's Education Needs Regarding Allergy Response

What causes your allergy symptoms?

How do you avoid triggering your allergies?

What can you do to alert health care providers about your allergies?

What should you carry with you if you have experienced an anaphylactic reaction?

Objective Data

Assessment of Airway and Gas Exchange

Edema (e.g., face, eyes, tongue, extremities)

Work of breathing (e.g., increased rate, use of accessory muscles, gasping, loudness, grunt)

Lung sounds (e.g., stridor, wheezes [inspiratory, expiratory, or both], absent breath sounds)

Oxygen saturation (e.g., $< 94\%$ on room air)

Vital signs (HR > 100, RR > 22 or < 8, SBP < 90, or mean arterial pressure [MAP] < 60)

Skin (e.g., red, rash, wheal, and flare)

Assessment of Cardiac Output

Blood pressure (SBP < 90, MAP < 60)

Heart rate > 100

Are peripheral pulses present?

Is skin color pale, red, or mottled?

Assessment of Pain and Anxiety

Facial grimaces with movement

Taut or anxious facial expression

Restlessness and irritability

Vital signs (HR > 100, BP > 140)

Skin pale, cool, or moist

Assessment of Fluid/Volume Status

Blood pressure (SBP < 90, MAP < 60 mmHg)

Heart rate > 100

Urine output < 30 mL/hr

Assessment of Potential Allergy Response

Gather baseline data on:

Airway

Vital signs

Rash

Itching

Edema

Lung sounds

Assessment of the Patient's and Family's Education Needs Regarding Allergy Response

Verbalizes education needs

Identifies mode of receiving educational material

Actively participates in education discussion

NURSING PROCESS: Patient Care Plan for Anaphylactic Response, *continued*

Outcomes and Evaluation Parameters	Planning and Interventions with *Rationales*
1. NURSING DIAGNOSES: (a) Ineffective Airway Clearance *related to bronchial and/or laryngeal spasm and edema;* (b) Alteration in Gas Exchange *related to bronchial and/or laryngeal spasm and edema* (NANDA-I © 2012)	
Outcomes: Clear airway. Adequate gas exchange. ***Evaluation Parameters:*** Patent airway. Even, unlabored respirations. $<$ 22/minute. Clear breath sounds. O_2 saturation $>$ 94% on room air. IV access available. Emergency medications available and administered as prescribed. No alteration in level of consciousness. Alert and oriented to person, place, and time. Pulse oximetry and ABGs within normal limits. Intubation equipment available and functioning. Endotracheal tube appropriately placed. Equal chest wall expansion and breath sounds. Transfer to the appropriate level of care.	Assess for airway edema, stridor, wheezes, and decreased breath sounds. *Maintaining an open airway is the highest priority.* Position for comfort, typically high or semi-Fowler's. *Promotes lung expansion and respiratory effort.* Assess respiratory rate, pattern, work of breathing, and chest wall movement. *Rapid, shallow respiratory rate and increased work of breathing indicate hypoxemia from airway obstruction and the need for ventilatory support.* Auscultate lungs for wheezes, stridor, and decreasing or absent breath sounds. *Stridor indicates a narrowing airway. Decreased breath sounds are ominous and indicate airway obstruction. Absence of breath sounds indicates complete airway obstruction.* Report respiratory distress to the health care provider. *Medical intervention may be indicated to prevent respiratory failure.* Administer humidified oxygen (O_2) as prescribed. *Supplemental O_2 increases the alveolar gas concentration and diffusion of O_2 to the cells and tissues of the body.* Establish intravenous (IV) access with large-bore IV. *To enable administration of emergency medications and fluid.* Do not delay administration of emergency medications by non-IV route while establishing IV access. *Many emergency medications can be given SQ or IM if IV access is not available and are crucial for controlling airway edema and enabling gas exchange.* Administer medications as prescribed: subcutaneous epinephrine 1:1,000, 0.3–0.5 mL as ordered, repeat every 20–30 minutes as needed. *A potent bronchodilator and vasoconstrictor to counteract the effects of histamine.* Diphenhydramine (Benadryl) 50 mg IV. *Competes with histamine for H_1-receptor sites, blocking the bronchial constrictive effects of histamine released from mast cells.* Corticosteroid: Methylprednisone (Solu-Medrol) 125 mg IV. *Blocks the proliferation of inflammatory mediators that increase airway obstruction.* Ranitidine (Zantac) 50 mg IV. *Inhibits histamine at H_2 receptor sites on the parietal cells in the stomach, which decreases acid production. *Combined use of H_1 antagonists and H_2 blocker results in enhanced relief of symptoms and improved outcomes.* Assess for changes in level of consciousness (agitation, confusion, delirium, stupor, and coma). *Cerebral function is very sensitive to decreases in oxygenation; this indicates tissue hypoxemia.* Perform frequent respiratory assessment, continuous monitoring of pulse oximetry, and arterial blood gases (ABGs). *Status can deteriorate quickly. A secondary or delayed response can also result from secondary mediators of inflammation such as bradykinin several hours after the initial incident.* Prepare for possible endotracheal intubation, gather intubation supplies, and collaborate with respiratory therapy (RT) for ventilator setup. *Intubation requires a team approach; gathering and checking equipment early prevents delay in intubation.* If intubation is required, collaborate with the health care provider and RT to monitor the ventilator and maintain ventilator settings. *To maximize oxygenation and ventilation, support cellular oxygenation, and prevent tissue hypoxemia and ischemia.* Assess respiratory function. *To verify bilateral breath sounds postintubation.*

(*continued*)

NURSING PROCESS: Patient Care Plan for Anaphylactic Response, *continued*

Outcomes and Evaluation Parameters	Planning and Interventions with *Rationales*
	Obtain chest x-ray postintubation. *To verify appropriate placement of the endotracheal tube (ETT) in the trachea 2 to 4 cm above the carina.* Test arterial blood gases (ABGs). *To evaluate oxygenation.* Patients with severe anaphylactic response requiring intubation will be cared for in the intensive care unit (ICU) setting. The focus of care is controlling airway edema, normal ABGs, and extubation as soon as it is safe for the patient.
2. NURSING DIAGNOSIS: Risk for Decreased Cardiac Output *related to vasodilation with anaphylactic shock* (NANDA-I © 2012)	
Outcome: Tissue perfusion maintained. ***Evaluation Parameters:*** Blood pressure and heart rate within normal limits, MAP > 60 mmHg. (Chapter 31 explains MAP.) Capillary refill < 3 seconds; skin pink, warm, and dry; palpable peripheral pulses.	Assess blood pressure, MAP, and heart rate frequently. Evaluate for a drop in blood pressure and increased heart rate (HR). *Indicates shock. Histamine and inflammatory mediators cause peripheral vasodilation, and capillary membrane permeability results in decreased volume of blood to the heart, drop in blood pressure, and decreased tissue perfusion. HR increases to try and meet cellular oxygen needs and compensate for tissue hypoxia.* Assess peripheral perfusion for weak, thready pulses; pale or mottled skin color; decreased skin temperature; and slow capillary refill. *Indicates decreased blood flow in the capillaries, a sign of impaired tissue perfusion as shock progresses and cardiac output decreases.* Assess for circulatory failure. Report abnormal vital sign changes and assessment findings to the health care provider. *Medical intervention with IV fluids and medications may be immediately necessary to prevent circulatory failure.* Administer IV fluids. *To increase cardiac output and promote circulation and tissue perfusion.* Administer vasoactive IV medications as prescribed. *To vasoconstrict peripheral blood vessels, increase MAP > 60, and support perfusion of vital central organs.*
3. NURSING DIAGNOSIS: Pain and Anxiety *related to air hunger/hypoxia and emergency treatment procedures* (NANDA-I © 2012)	
Outcome: Comfort level maintained. Anxiety controlled. ***Evaluation Parameters:*** Patient reports pain level < 3 or at acceptable level. States what they are anxious about. Cooperative with emergency medical treatment. Premedicated for procedures as prescribed. Pain and anxiety assessed and treated while intubated.	Assess pain level using an objective scale. *Increases consistency in quantifying pain.* Remain with patient, provide calm reassurance, and explain all treatments. *Air hunger is extremely frightening to the patient; anxiety will increase respiratory rate and oxygen demand and hinder the patient's ability to cooperate with treatment.* Advocate for pain and sedation medications for the intubation procedure if blood pressure is stable. *Endotracheal intubation is uncomfortable; anxiety increases sympathetic nervous system stimulation and oxygen demands.* Assess pain and anxiety while intubated using objective scales and alternative communication techniques (pointing to scale, writing board, and hand signs). *An endotracheal tube can cause pain at the back of the throat. Breathing through a small ETT can induce anxiety. Pain and anxiety will increase oxygen demands. The ETT prevents the patient from communicating verbally, but the nurse must still be able to address the patient's needs.* Administer medication as prescribed. *To maintain comfort and decrease anxiety.*
4. NURSING DIAGNOSIS: Deficient Fluid Volume *related to anaphylactic shock* (NANDA-I © 2012)	
Outcome: Fluid volume and tissue perfusion are maintained. ***Evaluation Parameters:*** Blood pressure normal. MAP > 60 mmHg. Urine output = or > 30 mL/hr.	Assess and continuously monitor blood pressure, MAP, HR, and urine output. *Anaphylactic shock results in vasodilation of blood vessels and decreased intravascular fluid volume that is clinically evident as decreased blood pressure, MAP, and urine output. Heart rate increases to compensate for decreased volume status. Patients with severe anaphylactic response and fluid volume deficits will need ICU level care.* Place the urinary catheter and monitor hourly urine output and fluid intake. *Decrease in blood pressure and MAP < 60 will decrease the glomerular filtration rate and place the patient at risk for prerenal failure. The kidneys receive 25% of the cardiac output. A urine output of less than 30 mL/hr indicates decreased perfusion to the kidneys and fluid volume deficit. Trending hourly fluid volume intake and output is essential with fluid resuscitation therapy.*

NURSING PROCESS: Patient Care Plan for Anaphylactic Response, *continued*

	Administer IV fluids as prescribed. *To increase intravascular volume and tissue perfusion.* Report decreased blood pressure, MAP, and urine output to the health care provider. *Medical intervention may be indicated to correct fluid volume deficit.*
5. NURSING DIAGNOSIS: Risk for Injury *related to allergy hypersensitivity response* (NANDA-I © 2012)	
Outcome: Identification of allergy triggers and prevention of anaphylactic response. ***Evaluation Parameters:*** Allergies identified in patient's medical record. Allergy triggers are communicated to the health care team and avoided.	Obtain a thorough patient and family allergy history at the time of admission and prior to administering new medications to the patient. *To prevent administering a medication or treatment, or using equipment to which the patient has an allergy. Safe nursing practice requires allergy assessment prior to medication administration.* Document patient allergies and inform other members of the health care team (health care provider, pharmacy, nursing staff). *To facilitate communication and prevent the prescribing of medication or treatments or use of equipment to which the patient is allergic. Follow agency protocol for placing allergy alerts in the medical record, electronic patient database, the nursing Kardex (Rand), and on the patient's arm band. To alert members of the health care team to the patient's allergies.* Assess for symptoms of hypersensitivity reaction when administering any medications to the patient. *A history of allergy response increases the risk of future hypersensitivity responses.*
6. NURSING DIAGNOSIS: Deficient Knowledge Regarding Allergies and Prevention of Anaphylactic Response (NANDA-I © 2012)	
Outcome: Patient avoids allergy trigger and has no further anaphylactic reactions. ***Evaluation Parameters:*** Verbalizes understanding of allergy signs and symptoms, as well as anaphylactic allergen triggers. Consistently follows plan to avoid allergy triggers. Identifies symptoms of allergy response. Seeks appropriate medical attention for allergy symptoms. Informs health care providers of allergy status. Purchases and wears a medical alert tag. Carries an epinephrine self-medication emergency syringe. Keeps appointments and completes allergy testing if indicated.	Assess the patient's and family's learning needs, readiness to learn, and preferred method of education (verbal, written, audiovisual). *To present information at a time and in a manner the patient and family can understand. Hypersensitivity reactions have a genetic link; therefore, families must be informed about potential hypersensitivity reactions and how to prevent them.* Provide information on allergy management self-care as presented in Chart 53–2 (p. 1630), and assist the patient and family in developing a plan to eliminate exposure to the triggering allergen and decrease symptoms and progression of allergy sensitivity. *To promote self-care and help the patient and family eliminate allergy triggers.* Instruct the patient to monitor response to medications, foods, and insect stings by self-assessing for mouth/pallet itching, swelling, rash, and itching of skin or eyes. *To identify symptoms of allergy response.* Instruct the patient to seek immediate medical attention for airway swelling or shortness of breath with exposure to the triggering allergen. *Promotes seeking early medical treatment of potential life-threatening anaphylactic response.* Instruct the patient to inform future health care providers of the allergy and anaphylactic response. *Prevents future exposure to the allergen and anaphylactic response.* Instruct the patient to purchase and wear a medic alert bracelet that lists the triggering allergen and history of anaphylactic response. *Alerts health care providers to allergen and anaphylactic response, especially in an emergency situation when the patient may not be able to speak for herself.* If the anaphylactic triggering allergen is an insect, plant, or food, instruct the patient to carry emergency epinephrine at all times. *To self-administer epinephrine for an anaphylactic reaction.* Encourage follow-up appointments with the primary care health care provider to determine the need to see an allergist and undergo IgE allergen-specific diagnostic testing. *To determine triggering allergens so that exposure to them can be eliminated.*

Sources: Adapted from Adams, M., & Koch, R. W. (2010). *Pharmacology connections for nursing practice.* Upper Saddle River, NJ: Pearson. American College of Allergy, Asthma and Immunology. (2011a). Be S.A.F.E.: Managing allergic emergencies. Retrieved from http://www.acaai.org/patients/resources/anaphylaxis/managing-allergic-emergencies/Documents/BeSAFEBrochure.pdf; American College of Allergy, Asthma and Immunology. (2011b). Latex allergy. Retrieved from http://www.acaai.org/allergist/allergies/Types/latex-allergy/Pages/default.aspx; Simons, F., & Camargo, C. (2011). Anaphylaxis: Rapid recognition and treatment. *Up-to-Date.* Retrieved from http://www.uptodate.com; Wilkinson, J. M., & Ahearn, N. R. (2009). *Prentice Hall nursing diagnosis handbook* (9th ed.). Upper Saddle River, NJ: Prentice Hall; World Allergy Organization. (2011). White book on allergy. Retrieved from http://www.worldallergy.org/UserFiles/file/WAO-White-Book-on-Allergy_FINAL.pdf.

CHART 53–2 Self-Care Allergy Management

Allergens and Education Goal for Self-Care	Actions for Self-Care
Allergen: Pollen and mold	Remain inside on days when pollen counts are high.
Goal: Minimize exposure to pollens and molds.	Wear a mask during high-exposure times (windy days, when grass is being cut).
	Avoid contact with freshly cut grass, dry leaves, and weeds.
	Avoid damp, moist structures like basements.
	Clean showers and tubs several times a week.
	Avoid sprays and perfumes.
Allergen: Dust mites and animal dander	Replace cloth window coverings with pull shades.
Goals: Reduce dust in the home, school, and work environment.	Use a hypoallergenic mattress and pillow.
Eliminate animal dander from the home environment.	Replace carpet with wood, tile, or linoleum.
	Wash the floor, dust, and vacuum several times a week.
	Wear a mask when cleaning.
	Minimize upholstered furniture, throw pillows/rugs, and tufted bedspreads.
	Change the air filter frequently on the air conditioning/heating system.
	Choose a pet that does not have fur or feathers such as a fish or reptile.
Allergen: Insect stings	Quickly leave an area where bees, wasps, or yellow jackets are present.
Goal: Minimize exposure to insect venom.	Before sitting, carefully check grass areas to avoid ants or other insects.
	Carry a self-administered epinephrine kit when picnicking, hiking, or camping.
Allergen: Foods	Identify specific foods to avoid by keeping an allergy food journal, noting triggering foods and allergy symptoms.
Goal: Eliminate foods from diet that may cause allergy symptoms.	Develop a list of foods to avoid and share it with anyone who cooks in the household.
	Read labels when buying food and avoid allergy-triggering substances.
	Ask questions regarding ingredients in food when eating out to avoid allergy triggers.
Allergen: Medication	Make of list of medication allergies and inform any health care providers of allergies.
Goal: Avoid allergy-triggering medications.	Wear a medical alert tag for history of anaphylactic medication response.
	Review over-the-counter (OTC) medications with pharmacists to check for potential allergy.

Sources: American College of Allergy, Asthma and Immunology. (2011a). Be S.A.F.E.: Managing allergic emergencies. Retrieved from http://www.acaai.org/patients/resources/anaphylaxis/managing-allergic-emergencies/Documents/BeSAFEBrochure.pdf; American College of Allergy, Asthma and Immunology. (2011b). Latex allergy. Retrieved from http://www.acaai.org/allergist/allergies/Types/latex-allergy/Pages/default.aspx.

Collaborative Management

Optimal care of the patient with an allergic hypersensitivity response involves a collaborative approach among the health care provider, the nurse, and the pharmacist. Allergy diagnosis and development of an effective treatment plan are done by the health care provider. In order to meet desired patient outcomes, it is essential that this interdisciplinary team communicate openly with one another in developing and evaluating care of the patient and family (IOM [Institute of Medicine], 2010).

Nursing care involves extensive patient education on avoiding allergy triggers and teaching about allergy symptoms that require immediate medical attention. The nurse also educates the patient on medications, monitors the effectiveness of the treatment, and ensures that the patient's medical records reflect current allergy status. The pharmacist is an important member of the team who can advise patients about medication treatment options and provide extensive patient education on drug effects.

All members of the health care team have a role in identifying patients with allergies, providing appropriate education on allergy triggers and medications for symptom relief, and preventing anaphylactic response in multiple health care settings. Providing patient education to promote self-care regarding signs and symptoms of anaphylactic reaction is essential and is addressed in Chart 53–2.

Autoimmune Hypersensitivity Response

The ability to differentiate self antigens from foreign antigens is referred to as *immune tolerance*. Recognition of self antigens is vital for normal immune function because it prevents the immune system from destroying the host. When the immune system fails to recognize self antigens, an autoimmune response occurs. This is the basis for **autoimmune diseases,** which can affect any tissue in the body. The triggering mechanisms for a breakdown of tolerance are varied among autoimmune diseases. In most instances, the exact mechanism that stimulates an autoimmune response is unknown (Rote, 2010).

Epidemiology and Etiology

A genetic predisposition to autoimmune disease is supported by the association of various autoimmune abnormalities within family groups.

The peak time of development of autoimmune disease is ages 15 to 45. Sex hormones appear to have some relationship to the frequency and manifestation of the autoimmune disease systemic lupus erythematosus because it occurs 10 times more frequently in women than men (Porth & Sweeney, 2007).

Pathophysiology

Normally, immunologic tolerance is formed in humans during their embryonic development. During this developmental period, some lymphocytes can be created that are not able to differentiate between self antigens and non-self antigens; these are referred to as autoreactive lymphocytes. To attain immune tolerance, the immune system must suppress or eliminate these autoreactive lymphocytes.

The loss of immune tolerance is the basis for all autoimmune diseases. Multiple mechanisms may be involved in the loss of tolerance; in most instances, however, the exact process is unknown. Research has focused on the following theories: (1) exposure to a previously sequestered antigen, (2) development of a neoantigen, (3) complications of an infectious disease, (4) emergence of a forbidden clone, and (5) alteration of a suppressor T cell (DeFranco, Locksley, & Robertson, 2007). The theories behind these mechanisms are explained in the following text. Current research indicates that development of autoimmune disease is probably multifactorial and involves a combination of the mechanisms as well as the effect of an original insult, environmental influences, and genetic factors (Asthma and Allergy Foundation, 2011). Chapter 52 provides a discussion about immunity.

Sequestered Antigens

Sequestered antigens are normal self antigens found in cells that have not come into contact with the immunologic tissue during fetal development. Therefore, the immune system does not recognize them as self antigens. These sequestered antigens are tissues that are not drained by the lymphatic system and therefore do not usually come into contact with immunologic cells. Examples include receptors on the cornea of the eye and the testicles. These are referred to as *immunologic privileged sites*. Although these tissues lack lymphatic tissues, they are vascular. Therefore, if trauma occurs, immunologic cells will be delivered to the site. This can initiate an autoimmune response because the immune system has not recognized these antigens from previous exposure (Porth & Sweeney, 2007; Rote, 2010).

Neoantigens

Neoantigens are created by the developing fetal immune system while it is in the process of eliminating autoreactive lymphocytes. During the process of eliminating these autoreactive lymphocytes, some pieces of the lymph receptors may not be destroyed. These small bits of immune garbage are neoantigens, and they can hide in lymph tissues. They may attach at a later time to receptors on normal cells, triggering an autoimmune response (DeFranco et al., 2007; Rote, 2010).

Complications of Infectious Disease: Molecular Mimicry

When a foreign antigen invades the body and is destroyed by the immune system, small pieces of the cell wall of the bacterial or viral invader can remain in the circulation. If these foreign antigen proteins attach to a normal cell, the complex makes the host cell look like the cell of the foreign antigen, and this triggers the autoimmune response. Group A streptococcus bacteria are the most commonly studied bacteria that can initiate this response. An example of this is the streptococcal bacteria that attach to the cells of heart valves and stimulate the immune system to attack and destroy the heart valve tissue (Rote, 2010). Chapter 33 discusses the impact of this process on heart valve function.

Forbidden Clone

A clone is a second cell produced by replication of a cell. A *forbidden clone* is a mutant cell that is a type of autoreactive lymphocyte that should be eliminated. The theory about forbidden clones revolves around the concept that, during normal embryonic development, the original autoreactive lymphocyte is eliminated by the embryo's immune system but a copy (clone) remains hidden, usually in lymphoid tissue. These cells can emerge at a later date and attach to self antigens, thereby triggering an autoimmune response and destroying normal self cells. This is an important area of research because the exact triggering mechanisms of many autoimmune diseases, such as systemic lupus erythematosus (SLE) or rheumatoid arthritis, are unknown (DeFranco et al., 2007; Rote, 2010).

Suppressor Cell Dysfunction

A major function of suppressor T cells is to control inappropriate immune responses. There are many different lines of suppressor T cells. If a single group of these T cells is dysfunctional, a tissue-specific autoimmune response can occur. If several lines of suppressor T cells are dysfunctional, generalized autoimmune disease can occur. An example of this is SLE. It is thought that T-cell dysfunction is partly responsible for the large variety of autoantibodies seen in SLE because the T cells do not suppress the production of antibodies created by B cells against normal cells (DeFranco et al., 2007).

Specific genetic markers may also play a role in autoimmune disease, as discussed in the Genetic Considerations for Autoimmune Disease box.

Clinical Manifestations

Autoimmune disorders can affect any tissue in the body and are manifested in a variety of clinical symptoms depending on the system that is the target. The initiation of an autoimmune disorder is commonly associated with the onset of another illness or profound physical or psychological stressor, such as severe flu, pregnancy, or death of a significant other. It also is significant to note that once individuals have developed one autoimmune disorder, they are at increased risk for developing manifestations of other autoimmune diseases (Rote, 2010). Chart 53–3 lists the most common autoimmune disorders, target antigens, and symptoms.

Medical Management

Medical management of autoimmune disorders involves determining the diagnosis, medication treatment plan, and symptom management for disease complications. The difficulty in differentiating autoimmune diseases is that many of them have multiple self antigens and require a significant number of tests prior to making a diagnosis with confidence.

GENETIC CONSIDERATIONS for Autoimmune Disease

Insulin-dependent diabetes mellitus (IDDM) is caused by T cell-mediated autoimmune response that destroys the β-cells of the pancreas and stops the production of insulin. An inheritable human leukocyte antigen (HLA) accounts for about 50% of IDDM. Research continues on to identify other genetic, environmental, and cell factors that contribute to the development of this disease and may in the future lead to the disease's prevention before it occurs (Friday, Trucco, & Pietropaolo, 2010).

CHART 53–3 Autoimmune Disorders by Body System

Disease/System	Probable Antigen	Organ or Tissue	Symptoms
Blood			
Immune thrombocytopenic purpura	Platelet surface	Blood	Bruising, purpura, bleeding
Autoimmune hemolytic anemia	Erythrocytes	Blood	Fatigue, dizziness, anemia, dark urine
Respiratory System			
Goodpasture's syndrome	Septal membrane of alveoli (basement membrane)	Lungs, alveoli	Shortness of breath, respiratory failure, decreased gas exchange
Renal System			
Immune complex glomerulonephritis	Various immune complexes	Glomeruli, kidney	Acute renal failure, inflammation, fever, pain
Goodpasture's disease	Glomeruli basement membrane	Glomeruli, kidney	Decreased renal function, anuria, oliguria, pain
Connective Tissue/Systemic Diseases			
Systemic lupus erythematosus	Antigens from DNA, organelles, cytoplasm, and possible extracellular sites	Joints, muscle, skin, kidney, heart, lung	Rash, joint pain, arthralgias, fatigue, fever, impaired renal function, increased risk of infection, heart valve disease
Rheumatoid arthritis	Immunoglobulin G, collagen	Joints	Pain and swelling in joints
Scleroderma	Nuclear antigens, immunoglobulin G	Multiple organs, including skin, joints	Hard, shiny painful skin, immobile masklike face
Endocrine System			
Graves' disease (hyperthyroidism)	TSH receptors on membrane of thyroid cells	Thyroid, metabolic	Myxedema, exophthalmos, increased metabolic rate
Insulin-dependent diabetes	Islet cells, insulin, receptors on pancreatic cells	Pancreas, metabolic	Hyperglycemia, polyuria, thirst, weight loss, ketosis
Addison's disease	Surface antigen on steroid-producing cells in adrenal gland	Adrenal gland	Hypotension, fatigue
Primary myxedema	Microsomes	Thyroid	Orbital and facial edema, fatigue

Sources: DeFranco, A. L., Locksley, R., & Robertson, M. (2007). *Immunity: The immune response in infectious and inflammatory disease.* Sunderland, MA: Sinauer Associates; Rote, N. (2010). Alterations in immunity and inflammation. In K. L. McCance & S. E. Heuther (Eds.), *Pathophysiology: The biological basis for disease in adults and children* (6th ed., pp. 256–292). St. Louis: Mosby; Sommer, C. (2009). Innate and adaptive immunity. In C. M. Porth & G. Matfin (Eds.), *Pathophysiology: Concepts of altered health states* (8th ed., pp. 347–376). Philadelphia: Wolters Kluwer/Lippincott Williams & Wilkins.

Laboratory and Diagnostic Procedures

The focus of the diagnostic work-up for autoimmune disorders is serum tests. These tests include autoantibody testing, complement levels, and protein electrophoresis. **Autoantibody tests** evaluate the level of autoantibodies in the blood to specific self antigens. One of the primary tests is the antinuclear antibody (ANA). This is a monoclonal antibody (see Chapter 51) that attaches to **autoantibodies** that are made in response to self antigens from the nucleus. A positive ANA test indicates that autoantibodies to nuclear proteins are present and increases the likelihood of a diagnosis of autoimmune disease. For example, patients with SLE often have high levels of ANA and high levels of anti-DNA autoantibodies. A differential diagnosis of an autoimmune disease is usually based on cumulative evidence from several test results (see the Diagnostic Tests for Autoimmune Disease box) (Rote, 2010).

Drug Therapy

The wide variety of autoimmune disorders presents a challenge in treating with drug therapy. The goals of drug therapy are to suppress the immune system in general and to control symptoms related to specific self antigens if possible. These medications are discussed in the Pharmacology Summary of Medications Used to Treat Autoimmune Disorders and for Immunosuppressive Drug Therapy box (p. 1638). Other treatments to decrease autoantibody production include the use of monoclonal antibodies (Chapter 51) and *plasmapheresis,* which is discussed in Chart 53–4 (p. 1635).

Systemic Lupus Erythematosus

Systemic lupus erythematosus (SLE) is an example of a systemic type III hypersensitivity autoimmune disease; it is characterized by damage to joints and soft organs as a result of the effects of autoantibodies and antibody–antigen activity (immune complex responses). Patients with SLE have symptoms as varied as joint pain, fever, malaise, recurrent infections, renal failure, and endocarditis with valve dysfunction. Cardiac valve disease is discussed in Chapter 33. Renal failure is discussed in Chapter 39.

Epidemiology and Etiology

The cause of SLE is unknown, but research indicates that the development of autoantibodies most likely results from a combination of factors including genetics, hormonal influences, immune abnormalities, and environmental factors (Rote, 2010). A genetic predisposition is clearly involved in that certain families show a larger number of members with SLE than does the population at large, and there is evidence of SLE development in identical twins (National Institute of Arthritis and Musculoskeletal and Skin Diseases [NIAMSD], 2009). It is possible that as many as four genes are involved in SLE development (Faulhaber & Aberg, 2009). The disease is known to affect women more often than men, and researchers are exploring the role of hormones in expression of SLE (NIAMSD, 2009) because the greatest incidence of the disease occurs in women ages 15 to 45.

DIAGNOSTIC TESTS for Autoimmune Disease

Test, Normal Values, and Rationale for Abnormality	Expected Abnormality
IgG Levels	
Adult: 650–1,700 mg/dL *IgG is elevated in autoimmune diseases.*	IgG levels are elevated in autoimmune diseases such as rheumatoid arthritis (RA) and systemic lupus erythematosus (SLE). Individuals with autoimmune disease generally produce too many IgGs that can form antibody complexes with host cells and stimulate destruction of the host's cells. Nursing assessment includes monitoring lab trends to determine the presence of the disease process and effective treatment.
Antinuclear Antibody (ANA)	
Adult: Negative @ 1:20 dilution *Measures level of autoantibody to protein found in the cell nucleus.*	Elevated levels of ANA and specific patterns of staining indicate that the body is making antibodies to self proteins. SLE is the most frequent cause of ANA, but results of the test should be compared with those of other SLE tests and the patient's symptoms.
Anticardiolipin Antibodies (ACA)	
(serum), Antiphospholipid Antibodies, Cardiolipin Antibodies, Cardiolipin, IgM Cardiolipin Antibodies. Adult: Negative *Increased level of antiphospholipid antibodies indicates a risk of increased clotting.*	Increased level of autoantibodies to the patient's own DNA indicates a positive test. Patients with SLE, RA, and antiphospholipid syndrome have increased levels of the antiphospholipid antibody. The antibodies attach to phospholipids (one example is the IIB) on the platelet surface and stimulate clotting activity at the platelet level. Patients with SLE are at increased risk of clotting abnormalities such as thromboembolism.
Anti-DNA Antibody	
Adult: $<$ 1:10 titer	The patient produces increased autoantibodies to her own DNA because the T and B cells in patients with SLE are reacting to antigens that are normally viewed as self, in this case DNA.
Rheumatoid Factor	
Adult: Less than 1:20 titer *Measures an autoantibody to the FC portion of IgG. These antibodies bind to synovial tissue and with complement stimulate phagocytosis of joint and bone tissue. High levels are found in patients with RA and Sjögren's syndrome.*	Autoimmune diseases such as RA, sarcoidosis, syphilis, and SLE, as well as viral infections, liver disease, and other chronic inflammatory diseases, all stimulate a positive test.
IgE Antibodies	
Adult: Less than 40 mg/dL *A group of six respiratory and food allergies that promote immediate allergic responses.*	Patients with high IgE levels usually exhibit indications of allergic response. The individual capable of attaching IgE to test antigens will exhibit symptoms of allergy to triggers.
Erythrocyte Sedimentation Rate (ESR or sed rate)	
Male: Western Method: Less than 50 years: 0–15 mm/hr Greater than 50 years: 0–20 mm/hr Female: Less than 50 years: 0–20 mm/hr Greater than 50 years: 0–30 mm/hr *Measures the amount of settling of RBCs over 1 hour. Often first indicator of an acute inflammatory process or chronic inflammatory diseases.*	Autoimmune diseases such as RA, inflammatory diseases, infections, carcinomas, and SLE all have increased sed rates. Chronic inflammation occurs in autoimmune disease when the host's immune system consumes or attacks cells that it views as non-self.

(*continued*)

DIAGNOSTIC TESTS for Autoimmune Disease, *continued*

Test, Normal Values, and Rationale for Abnormality	Expected Abnormality
Complement 4 (C4) Level	
Adult: 15–45 mg/dL *Level of C4 is decreased in patients with SLE and inborn C4 deficiency. Complement is a necessary part of a healthy immune system.*	Inborn C4 deficiency, SLE. Patients with inborn C4 deficiency do not make enough C4. In SLE and RA, patients make C4, but it is consumed in the phagocytic process of the immune system attacking self antigens.
Platelet Count	
Adult: 100,000–400,000 µL	Decreased platelets, increased risk of bleeding and/or leukopenia. Decreased platelets occur because immunoglobulins can attach to the antigens on the surface of the platelet and stimulate phagocytosis and activation of complement. Platelets can decrease in patients with SLE to less than 100,000/mm^3, leading to development of bleeding abnormalities such as prolonged clotting time, purpura, petechiae, or oozing from invasive line insertion sites.
Blood Urea Nitrogen (BUN)	
Adult: 5–25 mg/dL *Can be slightly higher in the older adult.*	Increased creatinine indicating renal injury can occur in SLE because IgG attaches to renal cell surfaces, creating an immune complex that is then attacked by macrophages. This leads to decreased renal function at the tubular and cellular levels and is evidenced by increasing creatinine levels.
BUN: Creatinine Ratio	
Adult: 10:1 to 15:1	
Urinalysis	
Color: Clear *Appearance:* Clear *Glucose:* Negative *Ketones:* Negative *Blood:* Negative *Microscopic Examination* *RBC:* 1–2 per low power field *WBC:* 3–4 *Casts:* Occasional hyaline	Urinalysis can be useful in the diagnosis of renal disease. Specific gravity can be low in renal disease because of the inability to concentrate urine. Protein in the urine is a sensitive indicator of renal dysfunction. Damage to the kidneys occurs with SLE when IgG attaches to renal tubule cells. This immune complex stimulates macrophages to phagocytize the renal cells, leading to abnormal glomerular basement membrane function and the glomeruli's inability to appropriately reabsorb sodium and proteins. Decreased renal function can eventually lead to renal failure, a major complication of SLE.
Biopsy of Skin and/or Kidney	
	Changes in kidney function can be diagnosed with a renal biopsy. Antibodies adversely affect the tissue.

Sources: Lefever-Kee, J. (2010). *Laboratory and diagnostic tests: Nursing implications* (8th ed.). Upper Saddle River, NJ: Pearson; Rote, N. (2010). Alterations in immunity and inflammation. In K. L. McCance & S. E. Heuther (Eds.), *Pathophysiology: The biological basis for disease in adults and children* (6th ed., pp. 256–292). St. Louis: Mosby.

Racial factors may also play a role in SLE development because it occurs more frequently in African Americans, Hispanics, and Caucasians. Additionally, researchers have found that Hispanics and African Americans have a higher incidence of kidney damage and death rates when compared to Caucasians with SLE (NIAMSD, 2009).

Environmental factors that may act as triggers for autoantibody production include ultraviolet light from the sun as well as interior lights, thermal burns, drugs, and possibly some viral triggers (Rote, 2010). It has also been shown that drug-induced SLE syndrome can occur with exposure to certain medications such as procainamide, hydralazine, isoniazid, quinidine, methyldopa, and phenytoin (NIAMSD, 2009).

Pathophysiology

The development of SLE is characterized by the formation of autoantibodies or antigen–antibody complexes that can damage a variety of tissues by identifying them as foreign cells and attempting to destroy them. This results from hyperactivity of B cells that are polyclonal and produce different types of autoantibodies (Faulhaber & Aberg, 2009). Several autoantibodies have been identified in SLE including ANAs, such as anti-DNA, and antibodies against surface antigens on RBCs and platelets. Autoantibodies produced against these blood cells cause their destruction and lead to the clinical conditions of anemia and thrombocytopenia.

Clinical Manifestations

Systemic lupus erythematosus may present with a variety of symptoms that do not point to a specific, easily identified disease process. This is what makes diagnosis of SLE very time consuming and challenging. This difficulty in diagnosis is related to the potential number of autoantibodies and the wide range of organs that can be affected. Laboratory tests to diagnose SLE are described in the Diagnostic Tests for Autoimmune Disease box (p. 1633).

Symptoms that are often seen early in SLE include swollen joints, fatigue, unexplained fever, red rash (commonly a "butterfly" shape over the cheeks), arthritis, arthralgias, unexplained hair loss, photosensitivity, swollen lymph nodes, and edema in the legs or around the eyes. As the disease progresses, SLE can affect several organ systems. Although

CHART 53–4 Plasmapheresis: A Treatment for Autoimminue Disease

Plasmapheresis is the technique of removing only the plasma portion from the blood. Plasmapheresis is typically used in processing a voluntary blood product donation. The donor's blood is circulated through a machine that removes plasma and returns normal saline and RBCs back to the donor. Donated plasma contains clotting factors that can be used to help patients who have massive hemorrhage and are unable to clot their own blood effectively. Because the plasma also contains antibodies that are removed from the blood during the pheresis process, plasmapheresis can also be used as a treatment in a number of autoimmune diseases. By taking the immunoglobulins, immune complexes, and autoantibodies that are present in plasma out of the blood, plasmapheresis decreases the immune factors that are stimulating the autoimmune response.

Myasthenia gravis is an autoimmune disease that can be treated with plasmapheresis. The process of filtering out the plasma also filters out large numbers of autoantibodies that are believed to be stimulating the myasthenia crisis. Plasmapheresis is usually used only to treat myasthenia crisis. Drug therapy remains the mainstay of therapy for patients who are not in crisis. Plasmapheresis has also been indicated for patients with Guillain-Barré syndrome and rapidly progressing acute glomerulonephritis.

Nursing care of the patient receiving therapeutic plasma exchange or plasmapheresis includes patient education about the process of plasmapheresis itself and the rationale that is applicable for treatment of the patient's specific disease process. A needle or catheter is inserted into one of the patient's veins; the blood is then drawn from the vein and saline and red cells are returned through the same catheter. Potential complications include hematoma at the needle insertion site, dizziness following donation, nausea, and hypotension. Specially trained nurses at major blood centers operate the pheresis machines and complete the treatment as ordered by the health care provider.

Source: Hung, S. W. (2009). Disorders of motor function. In C. M. Porth & G. Matfin (Eds.), *Pathophysiology: Concepts of altered health states* (8th ed., pp. 1260–1298). Philadelphia: Wolters Kluwer/Lippincott Williams & Wilkins.

many patients have symptoms only in joints or skin, as many as 40% will have renal symptoms. Patients with SLE may develop nephritis or inflammation of the kidneys. The effect of this inflammation may temporarily or permanently reduce the kidney's ability to filter nitrogenous wastes such as blood urea nitrogen and creatinine. Some patients with SLE will require short- or long-term hemodialysis related to the damage to their kidneys (Rote, 2010). Chapter 39 discusses hemodialysis.

Other organ systems that can become involved include the blood, blood vessels, lungs, or the neurological system. Anemia, leukopenia, and thrombocytopenia have all been noted in patients with SLE. These blood disorders are discussed in Chapter 55. Vasculitis and inflammation of blood vessels also occur in SLE. Swelling in blood vessels may affect the blood's ability to circulate and place the patient at risk for developing blood clots. Development of endocarditis, myocarditis, or pericarditis is also a potential risk for SLE patients. Valves may be damaged or destroyed in the patient with endocarditis. Patients with valve damage may present with chest pain or shortness of breath (Chapter 33).

Neurological manifestations of SLE include headache, memory loss, visual changes, changes in behavior, and stroke. Evaluation of neurological symptoms may be complicated by some of the side effects of medications used to treat the disease. Furthermore, the stress of living with a complex disease such as SLE may add to some neurological symptoms (NIAMSD, 2009).

Medical Management

There is no cure for SLE; however, many patients have fewer flares (exacerbations of SLE) with adequate drug therapy. The goal of therapy is reducing inflammation and the immune response. Primary therapy for SLE is pharmacologic, the mainstay of therapy being corticosteroids. Drugs such as prednisone, dexamethasone, methylprednisolone, and hydrocortisone have all been used to treat SLE. However, the side effects often interfere with patient compliance. The short-term side effects of corticosteroids include weight gain, increased appetite, edema, and emotional instability.

Patients with only joint pain and arthritis pain may be treated successfully with nonsteroidal anti-inflammatory drugs (NSAIDs) such as ibuprofen, naproxen, indomethacin, sulindac, piroxicam, and oxaprozin. These drugs reduce the pain, swelling, and immobility of joint arthralgias by blocking various chemicals of inflammation. To treat neurological symptoms, immunosuppressive drugs may be used. Drugs such as cyclophosphamide (Cytoxan) or azathioprine (Imuran) have been used to decrease the action of some immune cells and block the growth of immune cells. See the Pharmacology Summary of Medications Used to Treat Autoimmune Disorders and for Immunosuppressive Drug Therapy box (p. 1638) for a complete description of these drugs.

Another class of drugs used to treat SLE is antimalarial drugs. Hydroxychloroquine (Plaquenil) and chloroquine (Aralen) are antimalarial drugs that have been effective in treating SLE. The exact mechanism of action for these drugs in SLE is unknown; research has centered on the effect of these drugs on suppressing immune function (DeFranco et al., 2007). When taken continuously, antimalarial drugs have been helpful in preventing flares. See the Pharmacology Summary of Medications Used to Treat Autoimmune Disorders and for Immunosuppressive Drug Therapy box (p. 1638) for a complete description of these drugs.

Nursing Management

Nursing care of the patient with autoimmune disease focuses on educating patients and families about the disease process and medications as well as providing interventions to promote symptom control and management. The goal of nursing care is to provide an individualized plan of care that promotes patient comfort and maximizes patient independence and self-care activities. The nursing process provides an excellent template for accomplishing this goal.

Assessment

Nursing assessment begins with listening carefully to the patient's concerns and developing a supportive therapeutic relationship. The nursing assessment includes a thorough history of symptoms with focus on patient reports of fatigue, rashes, pain including headaches, and swollen joints. The history will guide the nurse in performing an in-depth physical examination of all systems because of the varied organs and tissues that can be affected by SLE.

Nursing Diagnoses

Common nursing diagnoses associated with SLE include the following:

- *Pain.*
- *Fatigue.*
- *Impaired Mobility.*
- *Ineffective Tissue Perfusion.*
- *Urinary Elimination Impaired.*

- *Decreased Cardiac Output.*
- *Coping, Readiness for Enhanced Coping Ineffective.*

NANDA-I © 2012

Planning, Interventions, and Outcome and Evaluation Parameters

Planning nursing care of patients with SLE should focus on the specific problems the patient describes as well as assessment findings. Frequent reassessment to identify potential problems such as joint or renal impairment is done on an ongoing basis. Patient teaching regarding the importance of adhering to medication regimens, reporting side effects, and assisting the patient to identify flares of the disease early are vital nursing interventions. The remainder of nursing care centers on symptom control and psychosocial support. Outcome and evaluation parameters include control of symptoms, effective medication regime, and prevention of disease flares.

Health Promotion

The teaching plan includes helping individuals with SLE understand the importance of obtaining health care regularly, not just during disease flares. The patient needs to be taught to receive regular physical examinations, blood pressure checks, and laboratory work to enable the health care team to identify problems early and help prevent disease exacerbation. Annual gynecological and breast exams for women and prostate-specific antigen (PSA) tests for men are recommended, as are annual influenza vaccinations. An eye exam should be done yearly to screen for visual changes if the patient is taking corticosteroids or antimalarial medications.

Learning to recognize the early warning signs of an SLE crisis is also vital in preventing it or reducing the intensity. Warning signs include increased fatigue, pain, rash, fever, abdominal discomfort, headache, and dizziness (NIAMSD, 2009). Maintaining a healthy lifestyle by eating well-balanced and nutritious meals, exercising daily, and controlling stress is important in preventing SLE exacerbations. Developing an effective support system for emotional support, to improve coping skills, and to boost morale also is an essential part of this process.

Collaborative Management

Accurate diagnosis, early treatment, patient education on medications and disease management, and development of an individualized plan of care designed to empower the patient are critical for successful living with an autoimmune disease such as SLE. A team approach that involves health care providers or various specialties, nurses, and social workers is essential in creating an effective treatment plan that enables the patient to have a productive and rewarding life in spite of the devastating impact of an autoimmune disease. In order to meet desired patient outcomes, it is essential that this interdisciplinary team communicate openly with one another in developing and evaluating care of the patient and family (IOM [Institute of Medicine], 2010).

Health care providers specifically manage the multiple phases of the diagnosis and medical treatment plan. This involves medication management, laboratory testing, and monitoring and treatment of disease progression. Nursing care, described earlier, includes symptom management, education related to medications used for symptom control, and education on early signs and symptoms of disease exacerbation. The social worker assists with home management, respite care for caregivers, and financial concerns.

Alloimmune Hypersensitivity Response

The alloimmune response is a type of immune reaction in which the host's immune system responds to an antigen from another human or another species. This is the type of response that occurs when tissues or organs are transplanted. It is a normal immune response, because the immune system is reacting to foreign antigens. Therefore, matching the antigens between the donor and recipient of transplanted cells and suppressing the immune response are the key concepts in preventing organ and tissue transplant rejection.

Epidemiology and Etiology

The advancements in surgical technique and immunosuppressive medications have substantially improved the success of organ and tissue transplants. Organs that can currently be transplanted include the kidneys, liver, pancreas, heart, and lungs. Blood and numerous other body tissues including skin, bone, cartilage, corneas, veins, and bone marrow also can be transplanted. An *autograft* is a transplant of tissue or whole organ from one part of an animal (including humans) to the same animal. A transplant between identical twins is an *isograft*. A transplant that occurs from one animal to another or one human being to another is called an *allograft*. When the tissue or organ is transplanted from a nonhuman animal to a human, it is called a *xenograft*. An important goal with any graft is to minimize the risk of an alloimmune response that results in rejection of the transplanted tissue or organ (Rote, 2010).

Different mechanisms of hypersensitivity immune response are involved in alloimmune reactions. The type IV (cell-mediated) response is the type of alloimmune reaction involved in transplant rejection. The T cells are primarily responsible for this type of response. Antibody-mediated responses and complement also play a significant role in alloimmune reaction.

Physiology

The antigen system that is primarily responsible for alloimmune reaction is the HLA system. There are six different HLA markers: HLA-A, HLA-B, HLA-C, HLA-D, HLA-DR, and HLA-DQ. These create identifying protein markers that are on cell surfaces throughout the body and differentiate self from non-self. Each of these markers is capable of creating multiple different gene subtype combinations that are the basis for HLA inheritance in families. Identical twins will have the same HLA markers; family members will have similar HLA markers. HLA matching is critical in organ transplant and is the ideal marker for the genetic study of diseases (Rote, 2010).

To maximize the potential for graft acceptance, there must be a donor–recipient match between HLA subtypes. This match is vital because an organ that is transplanted (kidney, lung, or heart) is rich in donor vascular tissue, white blood cells, and lymphatic tissue, all of which carry HLA subtype antigens and thus are able to trigger an alloimmune response. Wherever possible, an exact or extremely close HLA match is essential to prevent the host's immune system from reacting against the donor's graft. Tissues such as corneas, cartilage, and veins have minimal concentrations of immune tissue with specialized HLA antigens; therefore, only blood typing and crossmatching are required in matching a donor and recipient.

Graft Rejection

Host versus graft disease (HVGD) occurs when the recipient's immune system reacts against the foreign antigens on the cells of the graft. This can occur in allograft tissues or organs such as the kidney, lung, and heart. HVGD is classified as hyperacute, acute, or chronic. Type II and type IV hypersensitivity reactions occur in most types of rejection. The

T cells involved in rejection are T-helper cells (CD4) and T-cytotoxic cells (CD8). Consequently, T-cell activity must be suppressed to prevent rejection. T-cell suppression is the primary target of immunosuppressive therapy for transplant recipients.

Hyperacute rejection occurs when the recipient has a preexisting antibody to the antigen in the graft tissue. The graft may turn white immediately or during the next several hours as vascular stasis occurs in the transplanted tissue. This is a result of the antigen–antibody complexes that stimulate the release of proinflammatory mediators and of complement. Complement, a primary mediator in the antigen–antibody reactions, attracts tissue-destroying neutrophils and macrophages and stimulates the coagulation cascade, which results in coagulation in the microvasculature of the graft tissue (Rote, 2010). Hyperacute rejection, which is rare, occurs because of previous exposure to an antigen, such as with prior blood transfusions, organ transplants, or multiple pregnancies (Rote, 2010).

Acute graft rejection is a type IV (cell-mediated) immune response that occurs approximately 2 weeks to a month after transplant. This type of delayed hypersensitivity response occurs when the recipient's T cells are activated against the unmatched HLA antigens on the transplanted donor tissue. The result is destruction of the transplant tissue by T cells and inflammatory mediators. Immunosuppressive drugs may delay the response.

The symptoms exhibited during acute rejection are consistent with an inflammatory response; they include fever, swelling, tenderness, and redness over the graft site. The result will be progressive organ failure evidenced in laboratory findings such as an elevation in creatinine with kidney transplant rejection or an increase in liver enzymes with liver transplant rejection. Acute rejection can be slowed or reversed with changes in immunotherapy treatment.

Chronic graft rejection, which may occur a few months to years after transplant, involves a slow progressive failure of the transplanted organ. Although improvements in immunotherapy have made significant strides in prevention or slowing of acute tissue rejection, chronic graft rejection continues to be a major problem. The exact mechanism of chronic graft rejection is not well understood. It is thought to involve T-cell-mediated cytotoxic cells and macrophages that damage the endothelial cell lining of blood vessels, causing thickening and fibrosis of the microvasculature (Rote, 2010). Over time, the organ slowly fails as evidenced by clinical symptoms and elevation of laboratory values that reflect organ function.

Graft Versus Host Disease

In **graft versus host disease (GVHD),** donor-grafted tissue contains functional immune cells that respond to the recipient's tissue antigens. As a result, the grafted tissue supersedes the immune function of the recipient and produces antibodies against the host tissue, initiates cytotoxic responses, and begins to attack tissue in the host. Patients who experience this type of immune reaction are usually severely immunocompromised.

Graft versus host disease is most often seen in bone marrow transplants (see Chapter 55 for a complete description of bone marrow transplant). It occurs because before the bone marrow transplant procedure, the host's immune system function is reduced or eliminated by radiation and/or chemotherapy. When the donor marrow is introduced, T lymphocytes in the donor marrow recognize that the recipient's HLA antigens are foreign and initiate an immune attack against cells rich in HLA antigens. Sites of initial GVHD symptoms include skin, liver, intestines, and, of course, the recipient's immune system cells. The response may be as mild as a rash on the skin or as severe as liver failure. Graft versus host disease can be prevented through the use of immunosuppressive therapy to eliminate or destroy T cells in the donated tissue (Porth, 2009).

Clinical Manifestations

The clinical manifestations of alloimmune hypersensitivity response can occur through two different mechanisms. The more common mechanism is HVGD, which involves the recipient's immune system reacting against the donor tissue. As discussed earlier, graft rejection is classified as hyperacute, acute, or chronic on the basis of various symptoms and the amount of time that has elapsed since transplant. The second mechanism of alloimmune hypersensitivity response, GVHD, occurs when the immune cells in the donor's tissue mount a reaction against the host.

Medical Management

Medical management of the patient with alloimmune response is targeted at preventing graft rejection and at early identification and suppression of immune activity that could lead to graft failure. As with other forms of autoimmune diseases, this involves depressing immune function. Immunosuppressive drug therapy is the focal point of alloimmune medical treatment.

Immunosuppressive Therapy

Immunosuppressive therapy will vary according to the type of organ or tissue being transplanted and institutional/health care provider protocols. For information on specific organ transplants, refer to the chapters related to the organ being transplanted—such as heart, lungs, liver, and kidney—that stimulate the inflammatory and immune response. Another focus of the treatment is to minimize the toxic effects of immunosuppressive drugs, which include nephrotoxicity, electrolyte abnormalities, hypertension, hepatotoxicity, hyperglycemia, and the hematologic effects of leukopenia, thrombocytopenia, and anemia (Adams & Koch, 2010). Therefore, patients must have frequent laboratory tests to evaluate blood chemistry, liver function, kidney function, and hematology cell production in order to monitor the effects of medication and allow for dose adjustments.

Initial immunotherapy begins prior to the transplantation procedure. High doses of immunosuppressive agents are used before surgery and for a short time after surgery. These doses are then tapered to maintenance levels. Common drugs used and the implications for nursing care are found in the Pharmacology Summary of Medications Used to Treat Autoimmune Disorders and for Immunosuppressive Drug Therapy box (p. 1638). If rejection develops, high-dose steroids and antilymphocyte therapy such as monoclonal antibodies are frequently used.

Nursing Management

The goal of nursing management for the patient with alloimmune response is prevention of transplant rejection and promotion of optimal quality of life and independence. Nursing care of the patient with tissue transplant must focus on educating patients and families about the importance of immunosuppressive therapy, including side effects and precautions, and the signs and symptoms of transplant rejection. The nursing process provides an excellent template to assess, treat, and evaluate patients with tissue transplant and subsequent alloimmune response. The Nursing Process: Patient Care Plan for Organ Transplant box (p. 1640) applies the nursing process to the most common nursing diagnosis associated with alloimmune response and graft rejection.

PHARMACOLOGY Summary of Medications Used to Treat Autoimmune Disorders and for Immunosuppressive Drug Therapy

Medication Category and Action	Application/Indication	Nursing Responsibility
Nonsteroidal Anti-Inflammatory Drugs (NSAIDs)		
Ibuprofen	Drug of choice for patients with autoimmune disease such as lupus with little or no organ involvement.	Assess pain level. Various NSAIDs affect people differently. After a time they may develop a tolerance, requiring a change to a new drug in the class.
Naproxen Indomethacin ***Action:*** Reduce the pain, swelling, and immobility of joint arthralgias by blocking the release of prostaglandins and leukotrienes responsible for inflammation and pain.	Patients with serious organ involvement or disease flares will require steroid anti-inflammatory drugs and immunosuppressive medications.	Monitor for bleeding, GI upset, and decreased renal function. Instruct the patient to take NSAIDs with food or milk to decrease GI symptoms.
Antimalarial Drugs		
Hydroxychloroquine sulfate (Plaquenil) Chloroquine (Aralen) ***Action:*** The exact mechanism of action for these drugs in SLE is unknown. They are effective in suppressing some immune function related to lupus and controlling mild inflammatory symptoms.	Low doses are used to manage mild symptoms of lupus including rheumatoid arthritis, skin rashes, mouth ulcers, fatigue, and fever. May enable the reduction of a total daily dose of corticosteroids.	Instruct the patient that medications may take several weeks to become effective in controlling symptoms. Monitor for vision changes; this can cause retinal damage.
Glucocorticosteroids		
Steroids: prednisone, dexamethasone, methylprednisolone, and hydrocortisone ***Action:*** Interfere with inflammatory response and antigen presentation. Block cytokine genes, thereby impairing synthesis of IL-1, -2, -3, and -6. Inhibit TNF.	Used to control exacerbations of autoimmune diseases. For transplant patients, used in combination with calcineurin inhibitors such as cyclosporine, and antimetabolites and cytotoxic agents such as azathioprine as triple-drug immunosuppressive therapy to prevent transplant rejection.	Monitor laboratory tests: serum glucose, lipid levels. Administer insulin as prescribed. Monitor wound healing. Promote skin integrity (change position frequently, avoid adhesive tape). Provide patient education on diet and body changes: low-fat, low-cholesterol diet with low calorie between-meal snacks. Monitor changes in strength; provide a physical therapy consult as needed. Administer medication with food; collaborate with health care provider for orders for hydrochloric acid (H_2) receptor blockers or antacids for gastric complaints. Monitor for signs and symptoms of infection. Instruct the patient on techniques to avoid infection (perform hand hygiene frequently, avoid crowds and ill individuals).
Calcineurin Inhibitor		
Cyclosporine (Sandimmune and Neoral)	The mainstay of immunosuppressive therapy; used as part of triple-drug immunosuppressive therapy to prevent transplant rejection.	Monitor and report abnormal laboratory tests: serum creatinine, BUN, potassium, serum transaminases, bilirubin, and glucose levels.
Reduce transcription of IL-2.	Now also commonly used to treat autoimmune diseases such as lupus.	Administer antiemetic and antidiarrhea agents as prescribed. Monitor and report serum cyclosporine trough levels and changes in neurological status for dose adjustments. Provide patient education on frequent oral care, such as dental cleaning every 6 months or more frequently if gingival hyperplasia occurs.
Impair cytokines that are required for T-cell activation (more potent than cyclosporine).		
Azathioprine (AZA, Imuran) ***Action:*** Inhibit aspects of lymphocyte replication, which decreases leukocytes.	Used in combination with cyclosporine and steroids as triple-drug immunosuppressive therapy to prevent transplant rejection.	Monitor and report symptoms of infection (hyperthermia or hypothermia, chills, malaise) and/or jaundice.

PHARMACOLOGY Summary of Medications Used to Treat Autoimmune Disorders and for Immunosuppressive Drug Therapy, *continued*

Medication Category and Action	Application/Indication	Nursing Responsibility
Cyclophosphamide (Cytoxan) ***Action:*** Inhibit proliferation of B- and T-cell lines.	Azathioprine is one of the most widely used immunosuppressive drugs for lupus.	Monitor and report abnormal labs: CBC, serum transaminases, and bilirubin.
Methotrexate (Rheumatrex) ***Action:*** Decrease leukocytes.	Cytoxan is reserved for treating lupus with kidney disease or other internal organ involvement.	Monitor fluid intake and urine output daily.
Sirolimus (Rapamune) ***Action:*** Selectively inhibit proliferation of B and T lymphocytes.	Rheumatrex is predominantly used for lupus arthritis.	Assess gastrointestinal disturbances and administer antiemetics and antidiarrheal agents as ordered.
Mycophenolate Mofetil (CellCept) ***Action:*** Selectively inhibit proliferation of B and T lymphocytes.	Sometimes used as an alternative to cyclophosphamide for lupus with kidney involvement.	Assess gastrointestinal disturbances and administer antiemetics and antidiarrheal agents as ordered.
Monoclonal and Polyclonal Antibodies		
Alemtuzumab (Campath) ***Action:*** Monoclonal antibody targeting CD3 receptor on T cells.	Organ and tissue transplant immune suppression.	Monitor and report fever, chills, nausea and vomiting, and headache.
Basiliximab (Simulect) ***Action:*** Downregulates T-cell activity.	Used in combination with cyclosporine and corticosteroid therapy to prevent transplant rejection.	Administer antiemetics and antipyretics as ordered.
Daclizumab (Zenapax) ***Action:*** A specific lymphocyte immunoglobulin that is a lymphocyte-selective immunosuppressant agent.	To prevent or delay onset or to reverse acute renal allograft rejection.	Monitor and report abnormalities in respiratory status (dyspnea, increased respiratory rate, decrease in pulse oximetry readings, abnormal breath sounds).
Infliximab (Remicade) ***Action:*** Composed of sterile, purified, concentrated immunoglobulin G (IgG) from serum of horses immunized with human thymus lymphocytes.	To decrease acute disease symptoms by placing the disease in remission.	Administer oxygen as ordered.
Muromonab-CD3 (Orthoclone OKT3) ***Action:*** The immune globulin lymphocytes bind with the patient's antigen reactive T lymphocytes and decrease or alter killer T-cell function.	To prevent or delay onset or to reverse acute renal allograft rejection.	Monitor pulse oxygen saturation and arterial blood gases (ABGs); report abnormalities. Monitor for signs/symptoms of infection.

Sources: Adams, M., & Koch, R. W. (2010). *Pharmacology connections for nursing practice.* Upper Saddle River, NJ: Pearson; National Institute of Arthritis and Musculoskeletal and Skin Diseases (NIAMSD). (2009). Handout on health: Systemic lupus erythematosus. Retrieved from http://www.niams.nih.gov/Health_Info/Lupus/default.asp.

Collaborative Management

The essence of collaborative care is exemplified in the care of transplant patients. A strong interdisciplinary team approach and a committed family support system are essential to help prepare the patient for transplant and monitor the patient's medications, treatments, and follow-up care after transplant. In order to meet desired patient outcomes, it is essential that this interdisciplinary team communicate openly with one another in developing and evaluating care of the patient and family (IOM [Institute of Medicine], 2010). Prior to transplant, the patient is interviewed by a health care provider from the transplant team to determine his appropriateness for transplant. An additional screening is done by a psychologist to determine whether the patient is mentally prepared to receive a transplant and understands the required treatment regime and can comply with it. A pretransplant nurse coordinator is responsible for scheduling all of the required preliminary tests and appointments.

At the time of transplant and immediately following, other members of the multidisciplinary team become involved. These include a team of transplant surgeons and other health care provider specialists, depending on any complicating factors. Transplant unit nurses care for the patient immediately after surgery and educate and prepare the patient and family for the responsibilities associated with discharge home. These include teaching about monitoring vital signs and preventing infection, medication administration and compliance, laboratory tests trending, and follow-up appointments.

The pharmacist has a crucial role in medication education and working with the health care provider to tailor the medication treatment plan. Additionally, a dietitian provides teaching on nutritional needs and dietary restrictions specific for the organ being transplanted. For example, patients with renal transplant receive teaching regarding a low-sodium diet. The social worker and discharge planner assist in helping the family with financial concerns, arranging any home care needs, and connecting with community resources.

NURSING PROCESS: Patient Care Plan for Organ Transplants

Assessment of Immune Status Using Gordon's Functional Health Patterns:

- Health Perception Health Management Pattern
- Nutrition Metabolic Pattern
- Activity Exercise Pattern
- Cognitive Perceptual Pattern
- Self-Perception Self-Concept Pattern
- Sexuality-Reproductive

Subjective Data

Assessment of Knowledge

Do you have a way in which you best learn information (e.g., reading, watching a video on the subject, or having 1:1 instruction)?

Who in your family is going to help you at home with your medications, vital sign monitoring, and follow-up appointments?

Is this a good time to do some of your teaching or are you too tired or in pain?

Assessment of Infection

Do you have any pain?

Do you have a temperature?

Are you having any "flulike" symptoms (body aches, fatigue, cough, sore throat, stiff neck)?

Do you have any rashes?

Do you have any burning with urination?

Do you have any redness or tenderness anywhere?

Do you have any sores anywhere?

Do you have any unusual or foul-smelling drainage (e.g., from vagina, penis, rectum, ears)?

How long have the symptoms been going on?

What have you done to treat the symptoms?

Have you taken any over-the-counter (OTC), prescription, or herbal medications for symptom relief?

Assessment of Skin and Oral Mucosa

Do you have any red, sore, or open areas on your skin?

Do you have any redness or drainage from your surgical incision?

Do you have any sores in your mouth?

Are you able to bathe and do oral care daily?

Do you have acne?

Do you use a sun block?

Assessment of Post-Transplant Self-Care

Are you taking your medications, and are you able to keep your clinic appointments?

Are you able to eat a balanced, nutritious diet?

Have you gained or lost weight?

Are you easily fatigued or can you participate in daily light, low-impact exercise, such as walking?

Are you experiencing any sexual difficulties you would like to discuss?

Are you seeing family and friends regularly?

Are you planning to travel anywhere out of the area?

Objective Data

Assessment of Knowledge

Patient is awake, alert, and oriented.

Patient does not show signs of pain or discomfort (e.g., pain level assessed at tolerable for patient, vital signs stable).

Appropriate person from family is present.

Patient and family verbalize readiness to learn.

Assessment of Infection

Head-to-toe assessment with focus on the specific area of the patient complaint; report any abnormal findings (e.g., abnormal vital signs, pain, "flulike" symptoms, rashes, redness, discharge, sores, drainage, bloody stools, and urinary discomfort).

Fever.

Heart rate > 100.

CBC with differential.

Assessment of Skin and Oral Mucosa

Redness on pressure points (coccyx, heels, elbows).

Skin tears: around wound site, IV sites, lab draw sites where tape has been applied.

Incision site: redness, drainage, foul odor, proximity of suture line, intact staples/sutures.

Skinfolds, especially with patients who are obese: redness, breakdown.

Oral membrane: open sores in mouth, white coating on tongue indicating possible candidiasis infection.

Assessment of Post-Transplant Self-Care

Keeps follow-up lab and medical appointments.

Weight (above or below goal weight).

Contacts transplant coordinator with travel plans.

Outcomes and Evaluation Parameters / Planning and Interventions with *Rationales*

1. NURSING DIAGNOSIS: Deficient Knowledge *related to therapeutic regimen and self-care, immunosuppressive medications, signs/symptoms of transplant rejection, and discharge follow up* (NANDA-I © 2012)

Outcomes: Successful recovery without graft rejection or complications.

Patient and family demonstrate self-care activities to prevent graft rejection.

Assess the patient's and family's level of understanding of information, participation in teaching sessions, initiation of self-care activities, and medication administration technique.

NURSING PROCESS: Patient Care Plan for Organ Transplants, *continued*

Evaluation Parameters: Participates in learning sessions and asks questions. Verbalizes education needs to reduce risk of graft rejection and maintain health. Develops plan to meet follow up care needs and initiates lifestyle changes. Verbalizes understanding to notify transplant coordinator immediately of any health problems. Verbalizes rationale for and doses of specific immunotherapy medications and follow up lab tests and appointments. Accurately self-doses all immunosuppressive therapy drugs prior to discharge. Demonstrates self-care by adhering to treatment regime including immunosuppressive drug therapy. Verbalizes signs and symptoms of transplant rejection. Reports any symptoms of transplant rejection early to transplant coordinator.	Assess knowledge level and lifestyle expectations of the patient and family. *To determine educational needs and clarify expectations.* Provide information via multiple modalities including written, video, presentations by transplant team, and demonstration/return demonstration. *Provides individualized learning plan, enhances learning experience, and provides resources postdischarge.* Instruct the patient and family about the importance of adhering to the medical treatment regime including follow up appointments and the frequent need for laboratory testing draws to assess the effectiveness of immunosuppressive drug therapy. *To prevent complications of graft rejection or medication side effects.* Review immunosuppressive medication doses, side effects, and administration schedule. *To provide information about why and how immunosuppressive drugs are administered.* Observe the patient self-administering medications appropriately. *To assess appropriate medication administration.* Instruct about signs and symptoms of rejection: fatigue/general malaise, "flulike" feeling, fever, sudden weight gain, delayed wound healing, pain in or around specific organ transplanted, or changes in normal function. *To identify early signs of rejection.* Instruct to notify the transplant coordinator immediately for any of the previous symptoms. *To initiate prompt medical treatment.*
2. NURSING DIAGNOSIS: Risk for Infection *related to immune suppression medications* (NANDA-I © 2012)	
Outcome: No infection. ***Evaluation Parameters:*** The patient and family verbalize understanding of signs/symptoms of infection and notify the transplant coordinator immediately of any health problems. Patient and family demonstrate understanding of self-care by following plan to minimize infection risk. Daily log completed and brought to follow up appointments. Patient performs vital sign monitoring accurately and records information in daily log appropriately.	Instruct the patient and family about signs and symptoms of infection: fever, chills, "flulike" feeling, cough with or without sputum, sore throat, shortness of breath, rashes, burning with urination, foul discharge from penis or vagina, loose or bloody stools, or any redness/tenderness or drainage from the incision; swollen lymph nodes; any new or unusual pain, stiff neck, or sores in the mouth or on the tongue. *To identify early signs/symptoms of infection, facilitate early medical treatment, and minimize risk of rejection.* Instruct the patient to notify the transplant coordinator immediately. *To initiate prompt medical treatment.* Instruct the patient and family on ways to minimize the risk of infection including performing hand hygiene frequently, avoiding crowded areas, and avoiding contact with people who are sick. *To minimize exposure to infectious organisms.* Perform weekly self-exam to assess for swelling of lymph nodes. *To detect symptoms of infection early.* Drink 6 to 8 glasses of water a day and empty your bladder frequently, avoid bubble baths, urinate after sex, and wear cotton crotch underwear. *To prevent urinary tract infections.* Wear a mask and gloves when working in the garden. *To avoid fungi and bacteria in the soil.* Do not handle pet waste or litter box. *Cat litter can transmit infectious organisms.* Swim only in pools with chlorine. *Lakes and ponds have multiple infectious organisms.* Cook all meats thoroughly before eating and wash fruits/vegetables well. *To decrease bacteria.* Instruct the patient in self-care practices to monitor for complications and how to document them in a daily log: temperature, weight before breakfast, blood pressure, pulse, changes in medications, and changes in health status. *To identify early signs of complications and provide trend information to the transplant team.* Observe the patient taking her own temperature, pulse, blood pressure, and weight and recording these prior to discharge. *To assess skill and ensure accuracy of readings and need for additional teaching.*

(continued)

NURSING PROCESS: Patient Care Plan for Organ Transplants, *continued*

3. NURSING DIAGNOSIS: High Risk for Impaired Skin Integrity *related to opportunistic infections of the mucous membranes* (NANDA-I © 2012)

Outcome: Intact mucous membranes.

Evaluation Parameters: Verbalizes importance of oral care.

Practices self-care by performing oral care according to plan.

Takes antibiotics prior to any dental work.

Inspect the patient's gums, mouth, and tongue daily and report abnormalities. *To facilitate appropriate medical treatment.*

Provide frequent oral care. *To keep mucous membranes moist and promote patient comfort.*

Instruct the patient about the importance of oral care; encourage frequent oral care during the day and regular dental checkups and inspection of gums, mouth, and tongue daily. *Immunosuppression increases the risk of opportunistic infections. Medication side effects can cause hypertrophy of the gums.*

Patient should inform dentist of immunosuppressed status. *To facilitate prescription of antibiotics prior to any dental work.*

Patient should always take antibiotics prior to dental work. *To minimize risk of blood infection from dental work.*

4. NURSING DIAGNOSES: (a) High Risk for Impaired Skin Integrity *related to post-transplant status and necessity for lifelong immunosuppressive medication.* (b) Imbalanced Nutrition: Less Than Body Requirements *related to decreased or inappropriate nutritional intake.* (c) Activity Intolerance *related to postoperative transplant status.* (d) Risk for Sexual Dysfunction *related to immunosuppressive medications and fatigue.* (e) Social Isolation *related to decreased social interaction during transplant process, feelings of being "different."* (f) Deficient Knowledge *related to travel planning* (NANDA-I © 2012)

Outcomes:

a. Intact skin and oral mucous membranes.
b. Maintains optimal weight.
c. Practices self-care by participating in appropriate daily exercise.
d. Verbalizes concerns and questions regarding sexual function.
e. Develops/maintains social support system.
f. Communicates travel plans, identifies transplant center closest to destination, and continues with scheduled medication regime.

Evaluation Parameters:

a. No evidence of pressure ulcers, skin tears, or sores on mucous membranes.

   Verbalizes instructions for postop wound care. Practices self-care by following postop care instructions.

   Verbalizes importance of skin care. Practices self-care by performing skin care daily.

b. Lifestyle adapted to prevent transplant rejection and maintain optimal quality of life.

   Verbalizes and demonstrates lifestyle changes to adhere to medication and treatment regime, prevent infection, and promote optimal physical and mental health.

Develops dietary plan and follows it at home.

c. Able to tolerate appropriate daily exercise.
d. Verbalizes ability to be intimate.
e. Verbalizes satisfaction with social support system.
f. Able to identify the transplant center closest to the destination and continues with scheduled medication regime during travel.

a. Assess for alteration in skin integrity and reposition frequently. *To promote skin integrity. Broken skin provides entry for bacteria.*

   Avoid the use of adhesive tape. *To minimize the risk of skin tears.*

   Instruct in postoperative home care, such as care of the wound site and monitoring for redness and drainage. These signs indicate infection. Gently clean the skin around the incision daily with soap and water. *To decrease bacteria and risk of infection.*

   Do not apply lotion over the wound. *Increases the risk of infection.*

   Avoid heavy lifting/strenuous exercise. Do not lift more than 20 pounds for 6 to 8 weeks. *To prevent damaging the suture/incision.*

   Get adequate rest and fluids. *To promote healing.*

   Discuss the importance of bathing daily, using a mild soap, and applying lotion to dry skin. *To decrease bacteria on skin and, hence, risk of infection and to maintain skin integrity.*

   Discuss care of acne that can develop as a side effect of medication: no picking at acne, use of acne soap, or use of over-the-counter (OTC) benzyl peroxide lotion in 5% or 10% if acne persists. *To maintain skin integrity and decrease risk of infection.*

   Instruct in the necessity of treating skin carefully, avoiding strong sunlight, and wearing sun block with an SPF of 15 or higher. *Steroid medications result in fragile skin that tears and burns easily. Broken skin provides entry for bacteria.*

   Assist as needed with oral care every 2–4 hours, keep mucous membranes moist, and brush teeth with a soft brush three times daily. *To maintain a moist oral mucosa and decrease risk of infection. Brushing teeth removes the bacteria much more effectively than oral swabs.*

   Assist as needed with lip care and application of lip balm. *To prevent drying and cracking and promote patient comfort.*

   Discuss and help problem solve difficulties with medication compliance and scheduling of appointments or laboratory tests.

   Provide referrals to collaborative services (dietary, social services, and transplant coordinator) as needed. *To promote compliance and optimal post-transplant care.*

NURSING PROCESS: Patient Care Plan for Organ Transplants, *continued*

b. Discuss the importance of selecting nutritious foods. Collaborate to create healthy menu options to make at home. *To promote healthy food choices and wound healing and maintain health.*

   Determine optimal weight and plan to attain weight goal. *Medications can result in weight loss or weight gain (especially prednisone, which stimulates appetite). Malnutrition impairs immune function; excessive weight places additional strain on all body organs.*

   Collaborate with a dietitian if the patient has special diet needs. *To promote optimal nutrition.*

c. Discuss the importance of gradually increasing daily exercise and allowing rest periods between activities. *To promote increasing mobility and avoid excessive fatigue.*

   Collaborate with the patient to develop a low-impact exercise plan that can be implemented when cleared by the health care provider. *To encourage activity, promote overall health, decrease sedentary lifestyle, and prevent osteoporosis.*

   Discuss the risks of contact sports and strenuous exercises for a patient with a new transplant. *To provide rationale for low-impact exercises and promote health.*

d. Offer information on possible sexual dysfunction related to immunosuppression medications and encourage discussion if the patient has questions. *Medications can cause erectile dysfunction, decreased libido, and impaired orgasmic ability.*

e. Encourage family/friends to visit, call, and send cards and pictures. Encourage the patient to phone and write notes to family/friends. *To decrease social isolation.*

f. Provide information on community resources including support groups/transplant clubs. *To provide support and guidance with problem solving.*

   Discuss the importance of notifying the transport team of travel plans. *To facilitate communication, plan for missed appointments, and coordinate with the transplant center at the point of destination for any care needs.* Instruct the patient to always hand-carry immunosuppressive medications if traveling by plane. *To avoid missing medication doses if luggage is lost.*

Sources: Adapted from Carpenito-Moyet, L. (2008). *Nursing care plans and documentation* (5th ed.). Philadelphia: Lippincott Williams & Wilkins; Porth, C. (2009). Disorders in immune response. In C. M. Porth & G. Matfin (Eds.), *Pathophysiology: Concepts of altered health states* (8th ed., pp. 400–426). Philadelphia: Wolters Kluwer/Lippincott Williams & Wilkins; Wilkinson, J. M., & Ahearn, N. R. (2009). *Prentice Hall nursing diagnosis handbook* (9th ed.). Upper Saddle River, NJ: Prentice Hall.

Post-transplant care involves the addition to the team of a post-transplant nurse coordinator. This nurse provides the patient and family with continual support and is the primary point of contact for them regarding questions, medications, any symptoms or complications, and follow up appointments. The post-transplant coordinator functions as a very specialized case manager to provide triage for any patient problems and determine what members of the transplant team the patient needs to see. Additionally, the patient continues to be followed on a regular basis by the transplant surgeon and several other members of the team to optimize a successful transplant.

Immunodeficiencies

Immune deficiencies occur when the immune system experiences abnormalities in function that result in a decreased or compromised ability to appropriately respond and protect the host from an antigenic attack. Primary immune deficiencies are the result of genetic abnormalities in the embryonic development of the immune system. Symptoms of primary deficiencies usually appear shortly after birth. Secondary immunodeficiency occurs when the immune system is damaged and unable to mount an appropriate immune response due to a variety of factors that range from normal aging to infections that eliminate immune cells and severely impair function, as in HIV. In this section, we will briefly review the abnormalities related to primary immune deficiency and related disorders.

Primary Immune Deficiencies

Primary immune deficiencies are categorized according to the type of immune cell that is genetically malformed or dysfunctional. These categories include phagocytic cell dysfunction, B-cell (humoral) deficiencies, T-cell (cell-mediated) deficiencies, and combined B-cell and T-cell deficiencies.

Phagocytic Dysfunction

Several primary immune deficiencies have been identified that relate to abnormal function of phagocytic cells, most commonly neutrophils. For genetic reasons, neutrophils may not develop in adequate numbers, or they may be dysfunctional. An individual who is unable to make an appropriate number of neutrophils cannot mount an adequate immune response. If the neutrophil DNA is dysfunctional, not enough neutrophils will be able to migrate to the site of injury or infection and appropriately protect the host from foreign antigens (Rote, 2010).

B-Cell (Humoral) Deficiencies

There are two different kinds of B-cell deficiencies. In the first group of disorders, B-cell precursors are unable to differentiate into plasma cells. This deficiency results in inadequate immunoglobulin levels (IgG, IgA, IgM, IgD, IgE) and recurrent infection. Immunoglobulins are discussed in Chapter 52. The second type of B-cell disorder is the more serious one. In this disease, also known as Bruton's disease, the B cells are unable to differentiate into mature B cells. As a result, no plasma cells can be found in circulation, and no immunoglobulins are produced, causing major immune deficits including lack of immunologic memory (Rote, 2010).

T-Cell (Cell-Mediated) Deficiencies

The function of T cells is to regulate the immune response. T-cell deficiencies most commonly result in opportunistic infections (OIs). Therefore, these abnormalities do not commonly manifest themselves immediately after birth. This type of deficiency is suspected when an infant has repeated OIs such as candidiasis of the oral, vaginal, or rectal mucosa. There are a wide variety of T-cell-mediated deficiencies, which are differentiated by the type of T cells affected. One extreme example of T-cell-mediated dysfunction is the rare disorder called DiGeorge syndrome. In this disease, because the thymus does not develop properly, T cells are unable to mature and appropriately stimulate an immune response to a foreign antigen. The result is susceptibility to OIs, symptoms of which begin to appear shortly after birth (Porth & Sweeney, 2007; Rote, 2010).

Combined B-Cell and T-Cell Deficiencies

Several variations of combined immunodeficiency syndrome have been identified; these involve a mutation in one or more of the many genes that involve lymphocyte development and response. This results in low or absent levels of B lymphocytes and T lymphocytes in serum, as well as low or absent levels of IgG and IgA. Subsequently, the diseases that result from these deficiencies range from moderate to fatal in severity. The most severe form of congenital B- and T-cell deficiencies is severe combined immunodeficiency (SCID). This deficiency results from multiple genetic abnormalities that cause all white blood cell lines to fail to develop normally from a stem cell, leading to the absence of all immune function. Infants with this genetic defect have failure to thrive, chronic diarrhea, and multiple OIs that usually result in death before 2 years of age. More recently, bone marrow transplant has been used successfully to treat infants identified with SCID at birth or within the first 3 months of life (Sommer, 2009). Bone marrow transplant is discussed in Chapter 57.

Secondary Immune Deficiencies

Multiple factors contribute to secondary immune deficiencies; the most significant of these are listed in Chart 53–5. Immunosuppressive

CHART 53–5 Common Causes of Secondary Immunodeficiency

Drug-Induced Immunodeficiency: chemotherapy drugs, corticosteroids
Age: infants and older adults
Malnutrition: dietary deficiency, cirrhosis, cachexia
Stress
Medical Treatments: surgery, anesthesia, radiation
Injury: trauma, burns
Diseases: AIDS, diabetes mellitus, chronic renal disease, malignancies, alcoholic cirrhosis, SLE

therapy for treatment of autoimmune diseases and prevention of organ transplant rejection, in addition to chemotherapy agents, are the most prevalent medications that contribute to secondary immune deficiencies. Suppression of the immune system places these patients at a high risk for OIs, which are infections from microorganisms that are not usually considered pathogens but cause disease if the immune system is impaired. Therefore, a primary focus of nursing care for patients who are immune suppressed is prevention of infection.

Other factors that can contribute to immune suppression are age and nutrition status. Aging results in decreased thymus and T-cell functioning, which contribute to increased levels of autoimmune disease and malignancies in the older adult. Infants have decreased function because the immune system is still in the process of maturing.

Nutrition also plays a key role in immune function. Prolonged malnutrition with low protein intake contributes to a decrease in lymphatic tissue, atrophy of the thymus gland, and altered cell-mediated immune response. Without appropriate nutritional intake, general cell function is impaired and increases the susceptibility to infection (Rote, 2010).

Major injuries such as trauma and burns destroy immune system tissues such as the skin and can result in shock states that damage cell function. Medical treatment requiring surgery that removes immune tissue and organs such as the lymph nodes, the spleen, or the thymus also impairs immune response. Additionally, radiation treatment suppresses immune function by destroying the lymph tissue directly or by causing atrophy of bone marrow function and depressing stem cell production of lymphocytes.

Numerous diseases significantly affect immune function by altering immune tissue or cells and leaving the individual susceptible to secondary infections. A primary example of the impact of disease on the immune system is evident in human immunodeficiency virus (HIV) infection, which is the subject of the remainder of this chapter.

Human Immunodeficiency Virus and Acquired Immunodeficiency Syndrome

Acquired immunodeficiency syndrome (AIDS) is the syndrome of opportunistic infections that occurs as the final stage of infection with the human immunodeficiency virus. AIDS was first recognized as a new disease entity in 1981, when previously healthy young homosexual males in Los Angeles and New York were diagnosed with *Pneumocystis carinii* (now known as *Pneumocystis jiroveci* when it occurs in humans, to distinguish it from nonhuman variants) and a rare cancer, Kaposi's sarcoma. The diagnoses were extremely disturbing because these disease entities had previously been seen only in individuals who were severely immunosuppressed, older, or debilitated. The presence of these entities in so many people who did not fit that profile indicated an unknown disease that was causing profound immune impairment (CDC, 1981a, 1981b).

During the course of the next few years, thousands of cases were diagnosed, primarily among homosexual males and users of illicit injection drugs. Research, initially stymied because of the social stigma associated with homosexuality and illicit drug use, began to accelerate rapidly as more members of other population groups were diagnosed with AIDS. These individuals included hemophiliacs and other blood transfusion recipients, women through heterosexual contact with infected individuals, and infants of infected mothers. An understanding of the epidemic proportions of AIDS was beginning to dawn as cases were reported in multiple countries and almost all continents by the mid-1980s (UNAIDS, 2011). At the end of 2010, over 34,000,000 people around the world were living with AIDS (UNAIDS, 2011).

Etiology

The **human immunodeficiency virus (HIV),** the virus that infects CD4 T cells and is the agent responsible for causing AIDS, was identified in 1984. It became apparent that AIDS was the most severe and final stage in a continuum of illnesses associated with HIV infection, which fatally impairs immune function. Subsequent research has identified two specific strains of HIV: HIV type 1 (HIV-1) and HIV type 2 (HIV-2). Virtually all of the cases in the United States are HIV-1. This strain is associated with acute and rapid progression from HIV infection to a diagnosis of AIDS. HIV-2 was identified in West Africa in 1986 and may have been present decades earlier. It is the dominant strain in Africa. HIV-2 involves a slower, milder progression to AIDS than HIV-1, with increased infectiousness at the end of the disease process. Both HIV-1 and HIV-2 have the same modes of transmission and are associated with the same opportunist infections (CDC, 2011b).

Epidemiology

Of the 34 million people living with HIV/AIDS worldwide, the majority are women and are under the age of 15. Resource-poor countries have been especially devastated by HIV/AIDS. Sub-Saharan Africa, which is home to 71% of the world's HIV/AIDS population, is the most affected region in the world (UNAIDS, 2011). The spread in these countries has been attributed primarily to heterosexual transmission, migration patterns, and limited use of condoms, as well as significant mother-to-infant transmission. These factors have been fueled by poverty, lack of health care resources to diagnose HIV infection, lack of HIV prevention education, and inadequate access to antiretroviral treatment (UNAIDS, 2011).

The rate of HIV/AIDS infection in the United States has remained relatively stable since 1999 (CDC, 2010a). The CDC estimates that about 1,000,000 people have an HIV infection, but one in five are unaware that they are infected. Groups at risk for HIV infection in the United States include gay males, bisexual males, and other men who have sex with men; heterosexuals, especially women; and injection drug users. African Americans and Hispanics/Latinos are disproportionally affected by HIV in the United States (CDC, 2010a).

The sad reality of HIV/AIDS infection in the 21st century is that in countries with meager economic resources, AIDS continues to be a devastating and rapidly fatal illness, predominantly affecting individuals 15 to 45 years of age in the prime of life and reproductive capacity. In economically stable countries, where there is access to antiretroviral treatment and public health resources, HIV/AIDS is transitioning to a chronic disease process that involves an increasing proportion of older, nonwhite, and female patients.

RISK FACTORS for HIV Infection

Unprotected sex (sex without a male or female condom) with an HIV-infected male or female

Sharing of injection equipment

Blood product recipient (especially prior to screening in 1985)

Infants born to mothers with HIV infection

Breast-feeding or rechewing food by an infected mother.

Source: Centers for Disease Control and Prevention (CDC). (2011c). How is HIV passed from one person to another? Retrieved from http://www.cdc.gov/hiv/resources/qa/transmission.htm.

Weblink: HIV Fact Sheet

Weblink: HIV Transmission

Transmission

HIV is transmitted by contact with infected body fluids that have lymphocytes that can harbor HIV. These fluids include blood, semen, vaginal secretions, and breast milk. For transmission to occur, there also must be a sufficient viral load and a susceptible host. **Viral load** is the number of copies of HIV antigens in a sample of blood. An infected individual with a high viral load (in the first months after initial infection or during an AIDS-related illness) has an increased ability to transmit HIV. Additionally, prolonged or repeated exposure to infected fluids will greatly increase the risk of transmission (Rote & Huether, 2010).

It is important to understand that HIV is not spread through casual contact such as working with someone, shaking hands, hugging, or dry kissing. Repeated studies have failed to demonstrate transmission of the virus through sweat, tears, saliva, urine, emesis, sputum, respiratory droplets, or feces. Studies on vector transmission by insects have also been found to be not valid.

Transmission to Health Care Workers

Health care workers, by virtue of the work they perform, have always been at risk for exposure to the HIV virus. However, since the beginning of the HIV/AIDS epidemic, only a small number of health care workers have been infected or have themselves infected patients (CDC, 2011f). The use of standard precautions in caring for patients as well as the implementation of safer work equipment such as blunt needles has contributed to the prevention of not only HIV but also other diseases. Prevention includes the following:

- Routinely using barriers such as goggles and gloves
- Immediately washing hands and any surfaces that may have been contaminated by fluids
- Carefully handling and disposing of sharp instruments before and after any invasive procedure (CDC, 2011f).

The areas in which nurses work, whether it is an inpatient or outpatient environment, should have a post exposure policy (PEP) to manage any significant exposure to potentially infectious body fluids. Guidelines are available at www.cdc.gov/mmwr/preview/mmwrhtml/rr5409a1.htm#tab1; these should be monitored closely, since they are routinely updated.

Pathophysiology

HIV belongs to a class of viruses made up of ribonucleic acid (RNA). Every virus is an obligate parasite (a parasite that cannot live independently) that requires a living cell as the host. RNA viruses also are called retroviruses because, to reproduce, they must be transcribed back into

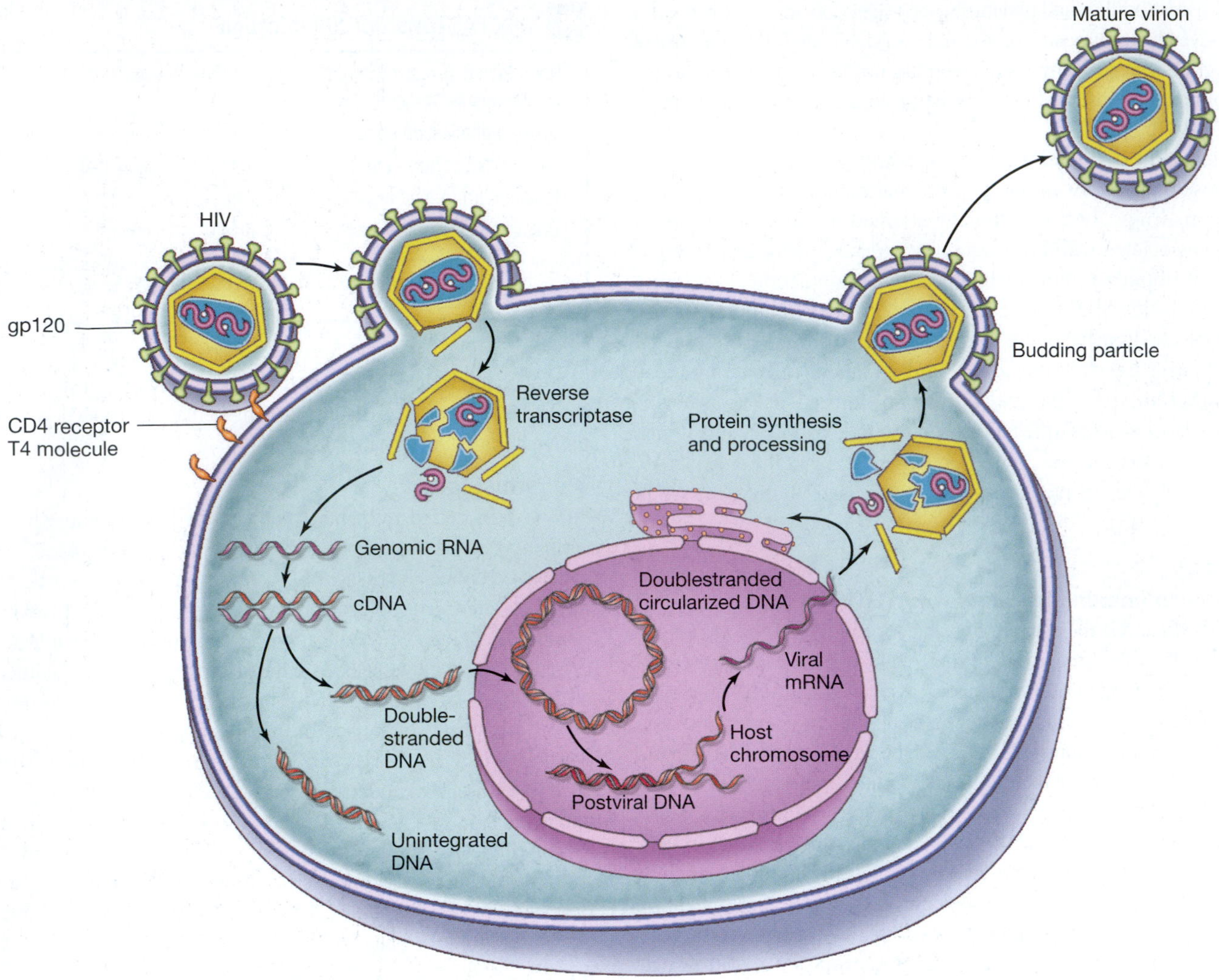

FIGURE 53–5 ◆ HIV infecting CD4+ T cell.

DNA through the action of an enzyme called **reverse transcriptase,** which uses RNA as a template to catalyze formation of DNA. This causes the conversion of RNA into double-stranded DNA. The new DNA is then inserted into an infected cell's genetic material using an **integrase,** which is a viral enzyme that catalyzes integration of DNA into chromosomes.

After the viral particle enters the cell, reverse transcriptase creates a DNA particle from the RNA. The DNA particle enters the nucleus and inserts itself into the host's DNA. HIV DNA can then direct proteins and enzymes to replicate the HIV portion and create more HIV particles. Figure 53–5◆ illustrates this process. It is important to understand the viral replication process because medications to control HIV infection are directed at different aspects of HIV replication. It is also important to realize that the viral material in the cell can remain dormant for years.

HIV is a highly infective virus for several reasons. It replicates easily and rapidly and mutates frequently. These mutations make it extremely difficult to create a consistently effective drug or a vaccine because the shape of the HIV molecules changes frequently (Rote & Huether, 2010).

HIV is devastating to the host's immune system, specifically the **CD4+ T cells,** which are T cells with CD4 receptors that react to antigens by stimulating B cells and killer T cells. CD4+ T cells exist to help regulate the immune system. If an individual is unable to initiate an immune response because of the loss of T cells, even the most benign infection can be deadly. Eventually, the immune system function and CD4+ T cells are overwhelmed by the virus and destroyed through several mechanisms. Every new HIV particle attaches to the cell membrane and buds outward as it breaks free of the host cell. When many HIV particles are released, holes develop in the plasma membrane. Cytoplasm and organelles can leak out, killing the cell. Lymphoid tissue also can house infected T cells and viral particles. Over time, the degradation of the lymph system by HIV sheds additional virus into the blood. This has been shown to be a factor in the progression of the disease. Also, macrophages and monocytes can be infected with HIV. Macrophages become a reservoir for HIV because the molecule can replicate within the cell. Trauma, inflammation, and infection at the site of the macrophage can cause rupture of the macrophage and the release of HIV into surrounding tissue (DeFranco et al., 2007; Rote & Huether, 2010). Additionally, as part of the normal immune response, antibodies to HIV attach to infected T-helper cells and stimulate the activation of the complement cascade. This results in the direct lysis of the cell membrane and death of the infected cell. Cell lysis also releases any completed viral particles into the host's system, further adding to the viral load.

Research is continuing to explore other mechanisms by which HIV destroys infected cells. Apoptosis (programmed cell death) of infected cells is one theory currently being researched. Additionally, increased

CHART 53–6 Stages of HIV Infection

HIV Stage 1	No AIDS-defining condition and either CD4+ T-lymphocyte count of > 500 cells/μL or CD4+ T-lymphocyte percentage of total lymphocytes of > 29.
HIV Stage 2	No AIDS-defining condition and either CD4+ T-lymphocyte count of 200–499 cells μL or CD4+ T-lymphocyte percentage of total lymphocytes of 14–28.
HIV Stage 3 (AIDS)	CD4+ T-lymphocyte count of < 200 cells/μL or CD4+ T-lymphocyte percentage of total lymphocyte of < 14 or documentation of a AIDS-defining condition.
HIV Stage UNKNOWN	No information available about CD4 + and T-lymphocyte count.

production of cytokines may be implicated in the destruction of infected T-helper cells. Finally, superantigen and autoimmune responses also are being studied as possible mechanisms of cell destruction in HIV infection (DeFranco et al., 2007).

Stages of HIV Infection

HIV infection has been divided into four stages (CDC, 2011c) as shown in Chart 53–6.

Clinical Manifestations

The clinical manifestations of HIV/AIDS vary and may affect almost any organ in the body. The specific clinical manifestations related to the OIs are outlined next.

The OIs occur in HIV-infected individuals as the virus destroys sufficient numbers of CD4+ T cells and the body is not able to protect itself. As CD4+ counts drop to < 200 cells/μL, the incidence of OI accelerates rapidly. Malignancies occur because of impairment in the immune system's ability to recognize and destroy abnormal cells that are regulated, in part, by T-cell function.

Diseases associated with HIV/AIDS result from impairment of the immune system that leaves the HIV-infected individuals susceptible to OIs and malignancies. Diseases also can be the direct result of the effects of HIV on specific tissue, as seen in AIDS-related GI and neurological dysfunction. Chart 53–7 describes the clinical manifestations of the most common opportunistic diseases associated with HIV/AIDS, as well as the diagnostic tests and medical treatment the nurse needs to anticipate coordinating as part of collaborative care. The last column lists critical assessment issues that need to be the focus of nursing assessment. This information provides more detail on specific AIDS-related diseases to enhance the nurse's understanding of these clinical manifestations.

Pneumocystis Jiroveci Pneumonia

***Pneumocystis jiroveci* pneumonia** is an opportunistic fungal respiratory infection that can develop in severely immunosuppressed individuals. It rarely moves outside of the pulmonary system. In the early years of the AIDS epidemic, 75% of HIV-infected patients developed this infection (which was known at the time as *Pneumocystis carinii*) at some point in their illness. Advances in understanding of the disease and treatment with prophylactic antibiotic therapy and corticosteroids have resulted in a decrease in the incidence of this infection. *P. jiroveci* is a fungal infection that proliferates in the alveoli, causing bronchial consolidation. Chest x-ray results will indicate bilateral patchy infiltrates. The symptoms of *P. jiroveci* are those of acute respiratory failure, with arterial oxygen levels decreasing to less than 70% and increased effort needed to breathe. If left untreated, *P. jiroveci* will result in respiratory arrest and death (Bennett, 2011; Kang & Crogan, 2009).

Mycobacterium Tuberculosis

Mycobacterium tuberculosis (TB) is another prevalent bacterial disease that is predominantly associated with pulmonary infection but also can be manifested in blood and cerebrospinal fluid (CSF). Unlike *P. jiroveci* respiratory infections, TB usually occurs early in the continuum of HIV infection, often preceding a diagnosis of HIV infection. Additionally, because the HIV infection impairs the immune system so severely, people infected with HIV and TB have a much greater risk of developing active TB and becoming infectious, compared to people not infected with HIV (CDC, 2011g).

In patients who have TB, purified protein derivative (PPD), the laboratory test for detecting TB, will test positive early in HIV infections. As the immune system fails with the progression of HIV disease, patients who have TB will usually have negative PPD tests because the appropriate immune response cannot be mounted to the PPD antigen. Conclusive diagnostic testing for TB is done by chest x-ray and acid-fast bacillus testing of sputum, blood, or CSF.

Hepatitis Virus B and C

Hepatitis virus B (HVB) and hepatitis virus C (HVC) are common opportunist infections in HIV-infected individuals because both are transmitted through shared body fluids such as blood, semen, and vaginal secretions. In addition, high-risk behaviors promote the spread of both infections. Hepatitis is more easily transmitted because fewer hepatitis viral particles are required to initiate an infection than is the case with HIV. Transmission by large or repeated exposures to contaminated blood by skin punctures is the most common mode of infection with HVB and HVC. Hence, the CDC estimates that 50% to 90% of HIV-positive injection drug users are also infected with HVC. Coinfection with HVC is present in approximately one-quarter of HIV-infected persons in the United States. There has also been an increase in HVC and HIV infection in men who have sex with men (CDC, 2010c).

The hepatitis virus affects liver function including metabolism of drugs, production of clotting factors, production of glucose and albumin, and filtering of waste, all of which contribute to the wasting syndrome in HIV. A combined HIV/HVB infection will increase morbidity and mortality due to the diminished function of both the immune system and the liver (CDC, 2010c).

Mycobacterium Avium Complex

Another leading OI is *Mycobacterium avium* complex (MAC), which includes a group of organisms (*M. avium, M. intracellulare*, and *M. scrofulaceum*). These organisms are usually found in food, water, and soil. They can cause respiratory infections but most often are found in the GI tract, bone marrow, and lymph nodes. *Mycobacterium avium* complex infections are a major cause of severe weight loss and chronic diarrhea. Severe weight loss in persons with AIDS and a MAC infection is associated with T-cell counts less than 100 and high mortality rates.

Other opportunistic pathogens such as cytomegalovirus (CMV) and candidiasis also affect the GI tract. Cytomegalovirus and MAC infections result in changes to the GI lining that cause anorexia, chronic diarrhea, GI malabsorption, and significant weight loss. These are all symptoms of wasting syndrome.

CHART 53–7 HIV/AIDS: Common Opportunistic Diseases

Clinical Manifestation by Body System	Possible Opportunistic Infection or Disease	Diagnostic Tests and Findings	Medical Treatment	Nursing Critical Assessments
Respiratory				
1. Increased respirations, nonproductive cough, dyspnea on exertion, adventitious breath sounds, increased hypoxemia	1. *Pneumocystis jiroveci* pneumonia	1. CD4 < 200 cells/μL, chest x-ray (bilateral patchy infiltrates), sputum culture or bronchoalveolar lavage (+ culture growth for *P. jiroveci*)	1. Antibiotic therapy (trimethoprim-sulfamethoxazole [TMP-SMZ]), bronchodilator therapy	1, 2, & 3 Respiratory rate, work of breathing, auscultate breath sounds, pulse oximetry saturation, sputum color/amount, monitor arterial blood gases (ABGs), to determine need for oxygen and ventilation support
2. Dyspnea, productive cough, blood-tinged sputum, 1 & 2 General body system: fever, night sweats, fatigue, weight loss are common to almost all respiratory opportunistic infections	2. *Mycobacterium tuberculosis* (TB)	2. TB skin test, chest x-ray, sputum for AFB stain and culture	2. Isoniazid (INH), ethambutol (Myambutol), rifampin (Rifadin), pyrazinamide	
3. Increasing shortness of breath, eventually progressing to respiratory failure	3. Kaposi's sarcoma	3. Chest x-ray, bronchoscopy examination and biopsy	3. Chemotherapy, radiation, alpha-interferon to decrease tumor size	
Gastrointestinal (GI)				
1. Inflamed oral mucosa, GI pain/cramping, bloody diarrhea, weight loss	1. Cytomegalovirus (CMV)	1. Stool specimen for examination and culture, endoscopy exam, biopsy, and culture	1. Medications: foscarnet (Foscavir), ganciclovir (Cytovene), cidofovir (Vistide)	1 & 2 Daily fluid intake and output, diarrhea, daily weight, oral intake (calorie count) Laboratory tests: complete blood count (CBC), electrolytes, blood urea nitrogen (BUN), serum albumin and transferrin levels
2. Anorexia, diarrhea, nausea, vomiting, weight loss, abdominal pain	2. *Mycobacterium avium* complex (MAC)	2. Stool specimen and culture, small bowel biopsy with AFB stain and culture	2. Antibiotic treatment when T cells < 100 cells/μL clarithromycin (Biaxin), azithromycin (Zithromax), ciprofloxacin (Cipro), rifampin (Rifadin)	
3. White patches in mouth, throat, or tongue that bleed if scraped, redness in oral cavity, → pain and difficulty swallowing, progressing to esophagus	3. Oral candidiasis	3. Microscope exam and culture of lesion scraping	3. Antifungals: Clotrimazole troches or Nystatin topical, po/IV fluconazole (Diflucan), clotrimazole (Lotrimin), itraconazole, amphotericin B (Fungizone)	3. Oral cavity, pain with swallowing, oral intake ability
4. Anorexia, weight loss >10%, chronic diarrhea, fever > 30 days unknown origin, chronic weakness, decreased muscle mass	4. HIV wasting (HIV causes changes to GI cells)	4. Rule out other causes: stool specimen and culture, endoscopy exam biopsy and culture	4. Symptom management • Diarrhea: octreotide acetate (Sandostatin) • Skin breakdown: barrier creams • Nutrition: appetite stimulant (Megestrol) • NV: antiemetic, Dronabinol • Oral nutritional supplement: Advera	4. Daily fluid I&O, diarrhea, daily weight, po intake (calorie count) Laboratory tests: CBC, electrolytes, BUN, serum albumin and transferrin levels

CHART 53–7 HIV/AIDS: Common Opportunistic Diseases, *continued*

Clinical Manifestation by Body System	Possible Opportunistic Infection or Disease	Diagnostic Tests and Findings	Medical Treatment	Nursing Critical Assessments
Neurological				
1. Forgetfulness, decreased attention and concentration, progressive impaired motor function	1. HIV encephalopathy (virus causes dysfunction of neural cells)	1. Rule out opportunistic infections or malignancy: cultures of blood, CSF; CT scan, MRI	1. Antiretroviral therapy, comfort measures, symptom management for any other clinical manifestations	1. Orientation, ability to remember medications, level of self-care with ADLs, gait, and risk of falling
2. Headaches, sensory and visual deficits, dizziness, aphasia, seizures, personality changes	2. Primary brain lymphoma	2. Tests listed in 1	2. Chemotherapy/radiation	2. Same as in 1
3. Headache, decreased level of consciousness, fever, stiff neck, visual changes, seizures	3. Cryptococcal meningitis	3. CT scan, CSF analysis, serum antigen test	3. Antifungal medications: amphotericin B (Fungizone), fluconazole (Diflucan), flucytosine (Ancobon), itraconazole (Sporanox)	3. Level of consciousness, neurological function, symptoms of infection (fever, stiff neck, WBC)
4. Pain, numbness in extremities, general weakness, decreased deep tendon reflexes, impotence	4. HIV peripheral neuropathy (caused by HIV demyelinating disorder)	4. Rule out other potential causes by the previous tests	4. Neurontin for pain	4. Neurological function, pain, changes in sexual patterns
Skin				
1. Nonblanching, flat or raised purple-brown lesions Progression of various shapes and sizes	1. Kaposi's sarcoma	1. Biopsy of lesion	1. Liquid nitrogen or cryotherapy to skin lesions, radiation of lesions, chemotherapy, or alpha-interferon to decrease tumor size	1. Inspect the skin for raised or flat purple-brown lesions of various sizes, pain or discomfort, and changes in any other body system such as GI or respiratory
2. Ulcer lesions of oral and nasal mucosa or ulcer lesions of the genital and perianal mucosa	2. Herpes simplex virus type 1 (HSV1) oral, herpes simplex virus type 2 (HSV2)	2. Viral culture	2. Antiviral medications: acyclovir (Zovirax), famciclovir (Famvir), valacyclovir (Valtrex), foscarnet (Foscavir)	2. Ask the patient about pain/discomfort of the mouth or perianal area; inspect the mucous membranes of the mouth, nose, and perianal area
Eyes				
Visual changes: "seeing spots," unilateral visual loss → bilateral loss → blindness	Cytomegalovirus (CMV)	Ophthalmoscope examination	T-cell counts < 50 cells/μL = antiviral (ganciclovir or foscarnet), not curable infection, medication must be taken for life; side effects of medications are significant and can interfere with highly active antiretroviral drug therapy (HAART)	Decreased vision ability, visual fields, presence of "spots," ability to read medication labels and identify drug and dose to take
Female Genitalia/ Sexual Health				
1. Genital itching, bleeding between menses, redness/swelling of external genitalia, white or yellow cheeselike discharge	1. Vaginal candidiasis	1. Microscopic examination and culture of lesion scraping	1. Antifungal medications: fluconazole (Diflucan), clotrimazole (Lotrimin), severe/incurable infection with previous medications = amphotericin B (Fungizone)	1. Sexual health risk factors include multiple sex partners, unprotected sex, changes in genitalia, or new discharge; color of genitalia and presence of redness, vaginal discharge

(*continued*)

CHART 53–7 HIV/AIDS: Common Opportunistic Diseases, *continued*

Clinical Manifestation by Body System	Possible Opportunistic Infection or Disease	Diagnostic Tests and Findings	Medical Treatment	Nursing Critical Assessments
2. Bleeding between menses or after intercourse; foul-smelling, blood-tinged vaginal discharge	2. Cervical intraepithelial neoplasia or cervical cancer	2. Cervical colposcopic examination and cone biopsy	2. Chemotherapy and radiation	2. Sexual health risk factors as previously noted; changes in menses bleeding or unusual vaginal discharge

Source: Carpenito-Moyet, L. (2008). *Nursing care plans and documentation* (5th ed.). Philadelphia: Lippincott Williams & Wilkins.

Wasting Syndrome

Wasting syndrome, one of the hallmark clinical manifestations of AIDS-related diseases, is defined as follows:

- A loss of lean body tissue from increased protein metabolism
- Changes in metabolic rates
- Anorexia and diarrhea.

Diagnostic criteria for wasting syndrome include chronic diarrhea for more than 30 days, weight loss of greater than 10% from baseline, and chronic weakness. Antiretroviral therapy and the production of lactic acid can be contributing causes (Faulhaber & Aberg, 2009). Wasting syndrome is associated with severe debilitation in the advanced stages of AIDS.

Candidiasis

Candidiasis is a fungal opportunist infection that affects virtually all patients with AIDS. Oral candidiasis creates white patches in the mouth that can extend into the esophagus and stomach. This can make swallowing difficult and painful and can significantly decrease oral intake because of discomfort. This places the patient at even greater risk for malnutrition and fluid and electrolyte imbalance. Also of concern is the fact that oral lesions can allow dissemination of the candidiasis into the bloodstream, causing a life-threatening fungal infection.

Safety Alert *Frequent and thorough oral assessment and care by the nurse is essential for the patient with oral candidiasis to maintain intact mucous membranes and prevent the spread of systemic infection by oral lesions.*

Candidiasis infection in skinfolds can lead to extensive skin breakdown. This is extremely uncomfortable for the patient and can lead to the development of a systemic fungal infection (see Figure 53–6◆). Vaginal candidiasis in HIV-infected women is a frequent and recurrent problem. Women with AIDS also have a higher incidence of pelvic inflammatory disease (PID). As a result of their immune-suppressed state, HIV-infected women with PID frequently require inpatient treatment with IV antibiotics.

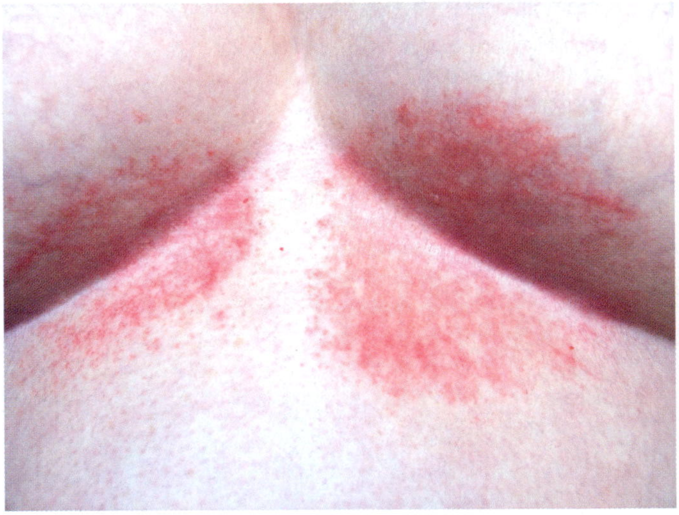

FIGURE 53–6 ◆ Candidiasis in skinfolds.
Source: ISM/Phototake NYC.

Herpes Zoster and Herpes Simplex

Herpes zoster and herpes simplex viral infections are common in patients with HIV or AIDS. Herpes infections recur in any individual who has been infected because the virus remains in human DNA neurons. Stress, infections, and surgery can all stimulate a recurrence of shingles (herpes zoster) and/or cold sores (herpes simplex). For HIV-positive individuals, the risk of repeated exacerbations of herpes is increased because of the decreased ability to mount an immune response.

Other Infectious Organisms and Disease Processes

Opportunistic infections also are responsible for many of the neurological changes associated with AIDS. The majority of individuals with AIDS have neurological alterations at some point during the disease process. Cryptococcus is a fungus that causes a meningitis infection, mental changes, and seizures. TB and CMV infections are also implicated in neurological alteration. Additionally, CMV causes retinitis, which is the leading cause of blindness in patients with AIDS.

AIDS dementia complex is a major factor in decreased neurological function. AIDS dementia is thought to be caused not by an opportunistic pathogen, but by actual changes to the neural cells due to the HIV infection. The brain cells infected by HIV are predominantly the monocyte-macrophage CD4 cells. It is believed that HIV causes the release of chemicals that result in destruction of the cell and interfere with the neurotransmission needed for normal cerebral function (Faulhaber & Aberg, 2009). The clinical manifestations of these changes are a progressive decline in cognitive, motor, and behavioral functions. Initially, memory deficits will occur, progressing to confusion, hallucinations, seizures, coma, and death.

Oncologic Manifestations

Patients with HIV/AIDS have an increased incidence of cancer. As cell-mediated immunity declines, malignant cells are not identified and destroyed internally, as they would be by an intact immune system. This leads to the development of the secondary cancers included in the CDC's classification of AIDS diseases: Kaposi's sarcoma, B-cell lymphoma (non-Hodgkin's), primary lymphoma of the brain, and invasive cervical carcinoma.

Kaposi's sarcoma, a malignancy involving the endothelial layer of the blood and lymphatic vessels, is the most common AIDS-related cancer. This is not surprising given that lymphatic tissues are an integral part of the immune system where HIV infection resides and replicates. Raised or flat cutaneous lesions can appear anywhere on the body and are deep purple to brown and/or pink in color. The lesions can progress rapidly and cause extensive disfigurement, disruption in skin integrity, venous stasis, lymphedema, and pain. Lesions also can develop in internal organs rich in lymphatic tissue, such as the lining of the GI tract, and the lungs. This can lead to extensive tissue damage, organ failure, and death.

Safety Alert *Kaposi's sarcoma often develops on the face, resulting in extensive disfigurement and increasing feelings of social isolation and depression in the patient with AIDS. Nursing interventions are focused on addressing issues of altered body image and social isolation to maximize self-acceptance and support and decrease the risk of depression.*

Lymphomas are malignancies of the lymphoid tissue that can be located anywhere in the body. The two lymphomas commonly associated with AIDS are non-Hodgkin's lymphoma and primary lymphoma of the brain. AIDS-related lymphomas differ from lymphomas found in the general population in that they are more aggressive tumors and tend to develop outside the lymph nodes, most commonly in the brain. Primary brain lymphoma is rapidly growing and is highly resistant to treatment. Common sites of non-Hodgkin's lymphomas are the bone marrow, liver, GI tract, mucous membranes, and the skin. Chemotherapy is frequently not successful in treating AIDS-associated non-Hodgkin's lymphoma because of the patient's immunosuppressive status and the complications that occur with OIs.

Laboratory and Diagnostic Procedures

Since as many as one in five HIV-infected people do not know that they are HIV positive, the CDC now recommends routine testing (CDC, 2010b). Tests that screen for HIV antibodies in the blood have a high degree of reliability and are used in diagnosing HIV infection. Testing for HIV antibodies also can be done on oral fluids and urine. The HIV antibody testing process described in the Diagnostic Tests box (p. 1652) produces highly accurate results that take 1 to 2 weeks to complete and involves pretest and post-test counseling.

The CDC recommends HIV screening in all health care settings for adults, adolescents, and pregnant women (CDC, 2011d). Increased screening fosters earlier detection of HIV infection, identifies and counsels persons with unrecognized HIV infection to enable treatment, and reduces transmission of HIV. Routine screening as a part of a diagnostic work-up for illness can facilitate earlier diagnosis and treatment with HAART (highly active antiretroviral therapy).

For pretest counseling, the nurse should do the following:

- Establish a therapeutic relationship with the patient.
- Inform the patient of the benefits of testing.
- Provide information about the test and testing procedures, including the fact that all positive tests are confirmed with a second test.
- Let the patient know that she may have to return for a second visit.
- Encourage annual screening for all patients with risk factors for HIV exposure.
- Provide education about HIV transmission and prevention.
- Inform the patient that if there is a diagnosis of HIV, there are specific tests that will be done on a routine basis to monitor disease progression and medication effectiveness.

Tests that determine the presence of a viral load (i.e., the number of copies of HIV antigens in a sample of blood) also have been developed. However, these tests are labor intensive, expensive, and not used for routine HIV screening. The exception to this is the presence of clinical symptoms consistent with acute retroviral syndrome during the window period when antibody testing will be negative (CDC, 2011d). Viral load levels are routinely monitored in patients with confirmed HIV infection to determine antiretroviral medication needs.

In 2002, the FDA approved the OraQuick Rapid HIV-1 Antibody test; it has subsequently approved three other rapid HIV tests that screen for HIV antibodies and return results in 15 to 60 minutes (CDC, 2011d). The benefit of these tests is that results are available very quickly and can be immediately discussed with the individual, who is also informed that all positive tests are sent for confirmation by further antibody testing. The rapid HIV tests have a high degree of specificity (99%) and can be used in routine screening in emergency departments and labor and delivery suites.

Rapid HIV tests also have been studied as an outreach screening tool for high-risk groups such as those in chemical dependency programs, homeless shelters, gay youth drop-in centers, or prostitute support programs. The benefit of this type of screening is that it provides immediate results and enables increased rates of post-test counseling, which can help to prevent HIV transmission and initiate appropriate early treatment. The major disadvantage of rapid HIV testing is that there is a slightly higher rate of false-positive tests. In addition, all positive tests must be confirmed with **Western blot (WB)** tests, which are tests with great sensitivity and specificity for HIV (CDC, 2011d; Faulhaber & Aberg, 2009).

HIV testing is confidential. Most states require written informed consent documentation prior to testing. However, in 2011 the CDC released revised recommendations for HIV testing of adults, adolescents, and pregnant women in health care settings; these recommendations represent a radical departure from existing testing practices, which focused on testing at-risk populations only. The revised CDC recommendations advocate HIV screening as a routine part of medical care for patients, similar to screening for other treatable conditions (CDC, 2011d; Stein, Grimes, Malow, Stratford, Spielberg, & Holtgrave, 2011). Individuals are notified that testing will be performed unless the patient declines, a process that is referred to as *opt-out screening*. Persons at high risk for HIV should be screened annually. The guidelines also recommend that general consent for medical treatment be considered sufficient for testing, so there's no need for a separate written HIV testing consent. Additionally, prevention counseling should not be required with diagnostic testing or HIV screening in health care settings. The ethical considerations surrounding HIV testing are discussed in the Ethical Issues box.

The rationale for the CDC recommendations is that undiagnosed HIV-infected individuals frequently visit health care settings such as hospitals or acute care clinics years before a diagnosis but are not tested for HIV in all health care settings. This results in a delay in effective antiretroviral treatment. Additionally, individuals who are aware of their positive HIV status significantly reduce sexual behavior that might transmit HIV, so early screening has the potential to substantially decrease the number of new HIV infections in the United States (CDC, 2011d). Routine prenatal HIV screening with streamlined counseling and consent procedures has substantially increased the number of pregnant women tested and has contributed to significant declines in perinatal HIV transmission rates (CDC, 2011d). This success has not been mirrored in the general population, where HIV screening is rarely

DIAGNOSTIC TESTS for HIV and Patient Counseling

Test, Normal Values, and Rationale for Abnormality	Expected Abnormality
Enzyme Immunoassay (EIA; previous test was the ELISA)	
Adults: Negative *Detects the presence of serum antibodies that bind to HIV antigens. Test requires two visits, testing, and then discussion of the results/counseling process. Results take 2 to 3 days.*	EIA results that are negative for antibodies are reported as negative tests. EIA tests that are positive are repeated. If the second EIA test is positive, a Western blot test is ordered.
Western Blot (WB) Test	
Adults: Negative *Antibody test with great sensitivity and specificity used to confirm the presence of HIV antibodies. Results take 1 to 3 days.*	Western blot test confirms the presence of HIV antibodies. A positive result is reported as HIV-antibody positive (seropositive) and confirms a diagnosis of HIV infection.
Rapid HIV Antibody Tests	
OraQuick (OraQuick Advance) Rapid 1. HIV-1/HIV-2 antibody test 2. Reveal G2 rapid HIV-1 antibody test 3. Uni-Gold Recombigen HIV test 4. Multispot HIV-1/HIV-2 rapid test *Immunoassay screening tests for HIV antibodies that provide results in 10 to 60 minutes*	All rapid HIV tests detect antibodies with sensitivities similar to those of EIAs, do not require instruments, and are interpreted visually. HIV antigens are fixed to the reagent strip; if HIV antibodies are present in the blood specimen, they affix to the antigen. The kit's colorimetric reagent binds to these antibody–antigen complexes to create a color change that is a visual indicator positive for antibodies. Results are available in approximately 20 minutes. A negative test requires no further confirmation test. A positive test is then confirmed by a Western blot test. The health care provider provides results in the same visit as the test to decrease the rate of patients failing to return for confirmatory HIV test results. This reduces barriers to early diagnosis of HIV and increases access to treatment and prevention services. • Initially used predominantly in community-based programs and sex-worker outreach clinics for rapid identification of HIV and in labor and delivery in acute care settings to minimize risk of perinatal transmission. Increased use in all health care settings encouraged as part of CDC recommendations to increase HIV screening (CDC, 2011d).
Ongoing Tests	
CD4+ T cells and viral load tests Adults: CD4 > or = to 500 cells/mm^3 *Rationale for CD4+ T-cell count test: HIV attaches to CD4+ T cells, infecting them, destroying them, and decreasing the number of CD4+ cells.*	Measures a person's immune status. CD4 low (<500 cells/μL) indicates decreased T-cell numbers and increased risk for opportunistic diseases. HIV attaches to CD4+ T cells, infecting them, destroying them, and decreasing the number of CD4+ cells, which impairs immune response; provides measurement of HIV progression to AIDS and effectiveness of highly active antiretroviral drug therapy (HAART) (p. 1653).
Viral Load Test	
Adults: Viral load levels of less than 10,000 copies/mL are considered "low" and copies greater than 100,000 are considered "high."	Done via polymerase chain reaction (PCR), HIV RNA, or bDNA tests to measure the actual amount of viral particles present in a blood sample. High levels indicate rapidly multiplying HIV, one marker of progression of HIV to AIDS; may also be done if the patient is on HAART (p. 1653) that is ineffective owing to drug resistance and/or lack of compliance with treatment regime.

Sources: Centers for Disease Control and Prevention (CDC). (2011d). Implementation of routine HIV testing in community health settings: Issues for community health centers. Retrieved from http://www.cdc.gov/hiv/topics/testing/resources/guidelines/pdf/routineHIVtesting.pdf; Stein, R., Grimes, T. S., Malow, R., Stratford, D., Spielberg, F., & Holtgrave, D.R. (2011). Introduction to special supplement. Monitoring and evaluation of HIV counseling, testing and referral (CTR) and HIV testing services. *AIDS Education and Prevention.* Jun;23(3 Suppl):1-6.

performed and the number of new HIV infections has remained stable in the United States (CDC, 2011d).

Tests that monitor the progression of HIV infection include CD4+ T-cell counts and viral load assay tests. CD4+ T-cell counts, as previously discussed, are essential in assessing for decreased immune function and the diagnosis of AIDS. Equally important are viral load tests such as the HIV RNA polymerase chain reaction (qPCR) test or the branched chain DNA (bDNA) test, which measure the viral activity and provide results that are reported as the number of "copies" per milliliter. Viral load testing is done at the time of HIV diagnosis as a baseline and then every few weeks to months depending on the initiation or type of drug treatment therapy. Viral load levels of less than 10,000 copies/mL are considered "low," and those greater than 100,000 copies/mL are considered "high" (Adams & Koch, 2010). HIV-infected individuals with HIV RNA levels of less than 20,000 copies/mL have a low risk of disease progression (Bartlett & Lane, 2007). As the HIV infection progresses, the CD4+ T-cell counts decline and the viral load increases, resulting in susceptibility to OIs and malignancies.

Testing for HIV resistance to antiretroviral drugs in patients being treated for HIV infection is currently possible. This is an important tool

ETHICAL ISSUES Related to HIV Infection

A significant ethical issue that the nurse in the acute care setting may encounter when caring for a patient with a newly diagnosed HIV-positive antibody status is the issue of sexual or needle-sharing partners at high risk for HIV infection. The HIV-infected patient may be very hesitant, embarrassed, or fearful about disclosing an HIV-positive test result to partners. This creates an ethical dilemma in that it places the partners at risk for undiagnosed HIV infection, limits their choices for testing and potential treatment if needed, and violates their rights to know their risk for infection.

The nurse must abide by the ethical principle of respect for autonomy and confidentiality while at the same time encouraging the patient to employ the ethical principle of veracity (truthfulness) in informing partners. The nurse may encourage the patient in making this ethical choice by developing a therapeutic relationship, asking about support systems and partners, listening to concerns, reviewing benefits of early screening for partners, and obtaining a social service referral to access resources for partner notification. State legislation requires health departments to offer anonymous partner notification services to newly reported HIV-infected persons. These services inform current partners (and former partners, if known) of HIV-infected individuals of their possible exposure and offer counseling, testing, and referral services (CDC, 2011d).

The importance of notifying sexual and needle-sharing partners of their exposure to HIV is also enforced by the federal Ryan White CARE Reauthorization Act of 1996, which requires health departments to show "good faith" in notifying marriage partners of HIV-infected persons. The nurse can provide emotional support and obtain referral resources to help newly diagnosed HIV-infected patients and spouses communicate and address this difficult situation.

in determining antiretroviral therapy. Genotyping and phenotyping assays are available. Genotyping assays detect drug resistance mutations that are present in reverse transcriptase and protease genes. Phenotyping assays measure the ability of the virus to grow in different antiretroviral drug concentrations. Information on drug resistance is important in identifying patients who are not responding to their antiretroviral medication regime and in guiding decisions about changes in therapy (Faulhaber & Aberg, 2009).

Medical Management

There is no cure for HIV infection. Development of an HIV vaccine to prevent HIV infection or control HIV progression to AIDS has not been successful thus far. However, advances in antiviral medication treatments have slowed the progression of HIV infection and provided new opportunities and challenges for medical treatment of the patient with HIV/AIDS. Initial medical treatment involves identification of patients at risk, followed by diagnostic testing and counseling. Individuals who are positive for HIV infection may be started on antiretroviral therapy. Medical management also involves identification and treatment of OIs and symptom control that optimizes comfort and quality of life for the patient with HIV/AIDS. Recent research has found that pre-exposure prophylaxis can reduce HIV risk among men who have sex with men. The results of this study and its implications to HIV management are discussed in the Research section later in the chapter.

Antiretroviral Drug Therapy for HIV Infection

Antiretroviral drugs are pivotal in delaying the progression of HIV to AIDS. The goal of drug therapy is to decrease the viral load (HIV RNA level < 55,000 copies/mL), increase or maintain CD4+ T-cell counts at greater than 200 cells/mL (greater than 500 cells/μL preferred), and delay the onset of HIV symptoms and OIs. A variety of antiretroviral agents are now available for use in treatment.

The complexity of the medications involved and concerns about appropriate treatment for patients who are asymptomatic with low HIV RNA levels and an adequate CD4+ T-cell count have created some confusion about when to initiate antiretroviral therapy. Antiretroviral drugs have serious adverse effects, and drug resistance can develop with prolonged use or nonadherence, requiring changes in therapy that may limit future treatment options. To address these concerns, the U.S. Department of Health and Human Services published guidelines for the use of antiretroviral agents in HIV-1-infected adults and adolescents in July 2003, with subsequent revisions in 2006 (Bartlett & Lane, 2007). Viral load and CD4+ T-cell levels are essential parameters in deciding to initiate or change antiretroviral therapies. In general, treatment should be offered to persons who have HIV RNA levels > 55,000 copies/mL or < 350 CD4+ T cells/μL.

The gold standard of treatment for HIV is referred to as **highly active antiretroviral drug therapy (HAART),** which involves combinations of various antiretroviral drugs that interfere with different aspects of the HIV replication cycle. Combination therapy has the greatest effect in controlling HIV proliferation and minimizing the development of drug resistance. Antiretroviral drugs are grouped according to the mechanism of action against HIV (see Figure 53–7◆, p. 1654).

Nucleoside reverse transcriptase inhibitors are a group of drugs that prevent viral replication by blocking the attachment of the nucleoside to the replicated DNA molecule. The nonnucleoside reverse transcriptase inhibitors make up another group of drugs that also prevent viral replication, but through a different mechanism. These drugs prevent the bond between a nucleotide and the growing DNA molecule of HIV. An additional group of drugs, the protease inhibitors, stop the replication of new RNA by inhibiting the action of protease enzymes, which are responsible for the synthesis of reverse transcriptase. A more recent class of medication, fusion inhibitors, is also available; these drugs work by preventing HIV from binding to CD4+ T cells and infecting healthy cells. Chart 53–8 (p. 1655) provides additional information on specific medications and adverse effects that can be used in patient teaching.

Central to the treatment of HIV/AIDS is adherence to the prescribed antiviral medication regime. If antiviral medications are not taken properly or consistently, CD4+ T-cell counts will decrease and viral loads of HIV will significantly increase, leading to greater risk of OI (Adams & Koch, 2010). Furthermore, resistance to these medications can develop if the treatment regime is not followed (Adams & Koch, 2010). Essential to creating strategies to improve adherence is a supportive therapeutic relationship between the patient and the provider and a negotiated treatment plan that the patient commits to that considers his daily routines and meal schedules as well as medication side effects (Bartlett & Lane, 2007).

Lack of adherence to medication treatment is a major concern in HIV treatment. The focal issues have been the complexity of dosing schedules, the volume of pills that the patient must manage, and the serious adverse effects of these medications, including fatigue, loss of appetite, diarrhea, and nausea and vomiting (Bartlett & Lane, 2007). Other issues that have been identified include socioeconomic factors such as homelessness, lack of insurance or finances, or lack of transportation to clinic appointments. Psychological factors also have been implicated including mental illness, poor coping skills, and failure to understand that self-care has a high priority.

Pharmaceutical companies have responded to these issues by developing combination antiviral medications to decrease the volume of pills patients must manage, therefore simplifying medication schedules. Research is ongoing in this area.

Weblink: Antiretroviral Therapy for HIV Infection

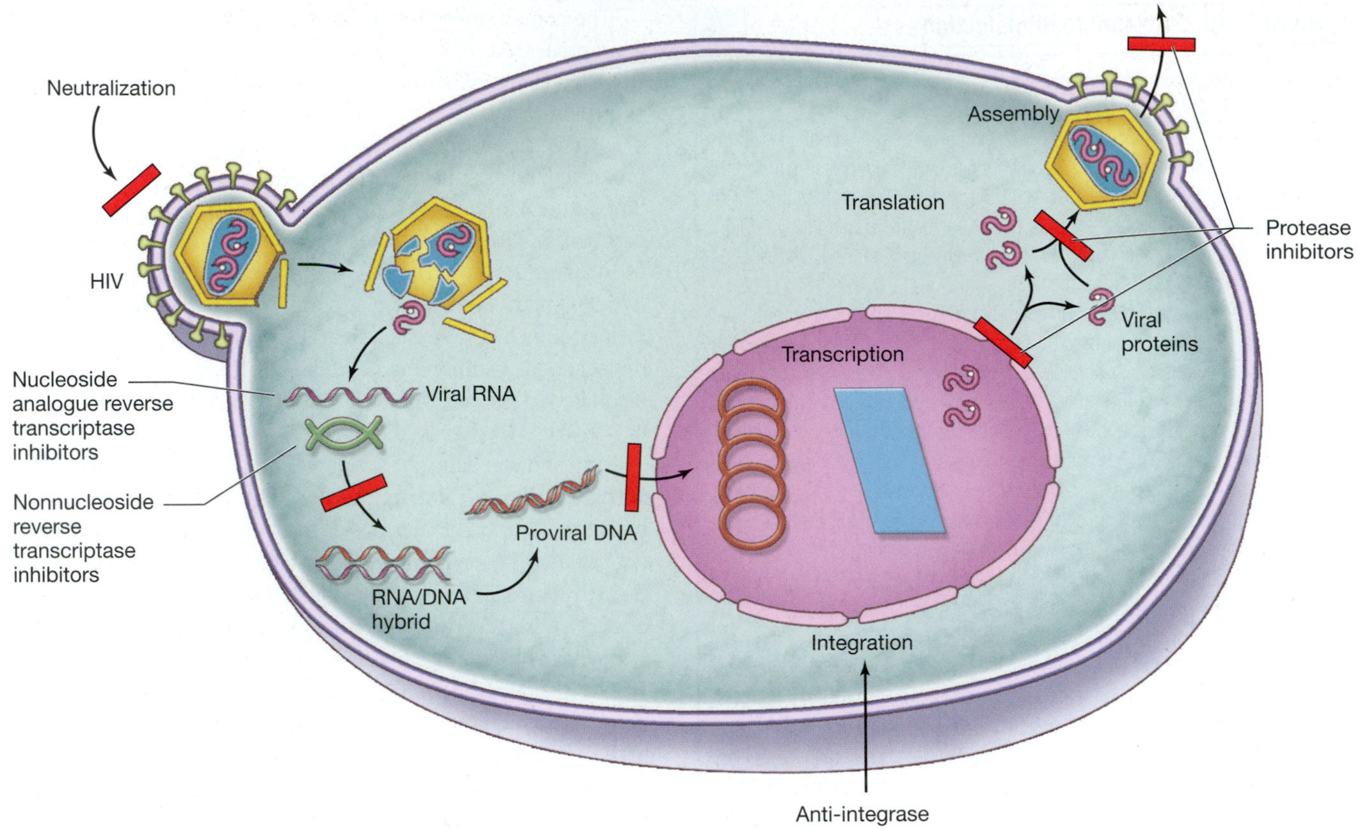

FIGURE 53–7 ◆ HIV replication and targets of antiretroviral therapy.

Nurses play a pivotal role in medication adherence through extensive patient and family education and follow up regarding medication side effects and concern. Additionally, nurses can facilitate the coordination and development of a patient-centered plan of care that addresses the socioeconomic, psychological, and physiological factors that affect treatment adherence.

Treatment of Opportunistic Infections and Symptom Management

The medical treatment for OIs and symptom management was summarized in Chart 53–7 (p. 1648). Drug therapy is the mainstay of treatment of OIs. The development of resistant organisms in an immunosuppressed individual is challenging and frequently involves treatment with new and innovative combinations of antibiotic therapy. Symptoms requiring treatment may be the result of antiretroviral drugs, treatment of OI, or proliferation of HIV, resulting in greater loss of immune function. In addition to infection, commonly treated symptoms include diarrhea, anorexia and weight loss, skin breakdown, pain, and depression. Nurses have an essential role in ongoing assessment of the patient's response to treatment and facilitating symptom management in order to promote optimal patient outcomes.

Nursing Management

Nurses need to understand the causes of HIV infection, signs and symptoms, diagnostic tests, and possible medical interventions in order to plan collaboratively for patient care. This will enable the nurse to provide appropriate nursing interventions and promote comfort measures that enhance the quality of life for patients with HIV/AIDS throughout the course of the disease. The nursing care of the patient with AIDS involves multiple physical as well as psychological and social support issues. Because the immune system is impaired, any part of the body can be the target of an OI or cancer, making nursing care especially challenging. Because there is currently no cure for HIV, a diagnosis of HIV/AIDS is psychologically devastating to patients, the vast majority of whom are 15 to 45 years of age and have not previously confronted issues of mortality. HIV/AIDS also carries a social stigma that may result in rejection by family and friends and social isolation at a time when the patient faces issues of grief and fear of dying and may also need assistance in complying with treatment or maintaining self-care. Nurses have a primary role in addressing these needs and providing skilled, compassionate care that is respectful to the individual's values, culture, and right to make individual choices (American Nurses Association, 2011).

The nursing process provides a template to assess, treat, and evaluate patients with HIV/AIDS. Use of the nursing process will facilitate creation of individualized care plans that optimize symptom management, patient comfort, and family support. Because of the complexity of HIV infection, multiple nursing diagnoses apply. Some of the most common nursing diagnoses that affect patients with HIV/AIDS, outcome goals, evaluation parameters, and appropriate nursing interventions are found in the Nursing Process: Patient Care Plan for HIV/AIDS . Research into Health Locus of Control (HLOC) gives insight into which life perspectives may lead a person to seek out the use of Integrative Healthcare (IH). Using the theory of Health Locus of Control to help patients with HIV/AIDS is addressed in the Complementary & Alternative Therapies box (p. 1661).

CHART 53–8 HIV/AIDS Infection Antiretroviral Agents

Drug Therapy	Drug Action	Application/Indication	Nursing Responsibilities
Protease Inhibitors			
Nelfinavir (Viracept) Ritonavir (Norvir) (keep refrigerated) Lopinavir and ritonavir (Kaletra) Indinavir (Crixivan) (Take 1 hour before or 2 hours after eating.)	Stop the replication of new RNA by inhibiting the action of protease enzymes, which are responsible for the synthesis of reverse transcriptase.	One of the three categories of drugs that are combined to interfere with different aspects of the HIV replication cycle, referred to as HAART (p. 1653).	Monitor the patient for anemia, anorexia/nausea, diarrhea, headache, fever, and malaise. Monitor labs: triglycerides, ALT, AST, alkaline phosphatase, creatine kinase and uric acid levels, and thrombocytopenia. Instruct the patient to take with food due to bitter taste and not to mix with juice, which increases the bitterness. Inform the patient of potential redistribution of body fat centrally (the "protease paunch"), facial atrophy, breast enlargement, and "buffalo hump" (a pad of fat on the back between the shoulders).
Non-Nucleoside Reverse Transcriptase Inhibitors			
Delavirdine (Rescriptor) Nevirapine (Viramune) Efavirenz (Sustiva) (Not to be used during pregnancy or breast-feeding. Women of childbearing years need a pregnancy test prior to taking this drug.)	Prevent viral replication, but through a different mechanism than protease inhibitors. These drugs prevent the bond between a nucleotide and the growing DNA molecule of HIV.	One of the three categories of drugs that are combined to interfere with different aspects of the HIV replication cycle, referred to as HAART (p. 1653).	Monitor the patient for fatigue, rash, headache, painful peripheral neuropathy (reversible with lower doses), insomnia, nightmares (usually resolve in 2 weeks), or retinal changes (eye exam recommended every 6 to 12 months). Monitor for increase in ALT, AST, alkaline phosphatase. Monitor creatinine levels of patient with renal insufficiency. Instruct patient to maintain adequate hydration and not to take with antacids.
Nucleoside Reverse Transcriptase Inhibitors			
Zidovudine (AZT, ZDT, Retrovir) (Take 1 hour before or 2 hours after meals.) Lamivudine (3TC, Epivir) Didanosine (ddl, Videx) (Take 1 hour before or 2 hours after meals. Two tablet doses, of which 1 is a buffer, must be chewed or dissolved to ensure an adequate buffer for absorption.) Stavudine (d4T, Zerit) Tenofovir Disoproxil Fumarate (DF, Viread) Abacavir (Ziagen) (Alcohol increases abacavir levels 41%.) Some reported fatal hypersensitivity reactions.)	Prevent viral replication by blocking the attachment of the nucleoside to the replicated DNA molecule.	One of the three categories of drugs that are combined to interfere with different aspects of the HIV replication cycle, referred to as HAART (p. 1653).	Monitor for bone marrow suppression: neutropenia, anemia, and granulocytopenia. Monitor ALT and AST. Monitor creatinine clearance in the patient with renal impairment. Monitor for malaise, insomnia, nightmares (subside in about 2 weeks), painful peripheral neuropathy (reversible with lower medication doses), visual changes (eye exam recommended every 6 to 12 months), GI intolerance, and nausea and vomiting.
Fusion Inhibitor			
Enfuvirtide (Fuzeon) (subcutaneous injection twice daily)	Interferes with entry of HIV-1 into host cells by inhibiting the fusion of the virus and cell membranes.	Treatment of advanced HIV disease with evidence of resistance to other therapies.	Monitor for irritation at injection site, nausea, insomnia, and peripheral neuropathy. Instruct the patient to keep medication refrigerated, reconstitute according to directions, and rotate injection sites.

Source: Adams, M., & Koch, R. W. (2010). *Pharmacology connections for nursing practice.* Upper Saddle River, NJ: Pearson.

NURSING PROCESS: Patient Care Plan for HIV/AIDS

Assessment of Immune Status Using Gordon's Functional Health Patterns:

- Health Perception Health Management Pattern
- Nutrition Metabolic Pattern
- Elimination Pattern
- Activity Exercise Pattern

Subjective Data

Assessment of Infection

Have you been running a temperature?

Have you had chills or periods of sweating?

Are you having any "flulike" symptoms (body aches, fatigue, cough, sore throat, stiff neck)?

Have you been coughing up any sputum? If so, what color is it?

Have you noticed any rashes?

Do you have pain anywhere?

Do you have any burning with urination?

Do you have any redness or tenderness anywhere?

Do you have any sores anywhere?

Do you have any unusual or foul-smelling drainage (e.g., from vagina, penis, rectum, ears)?

How long have you had these symptoms?

What have you done to treat the symptoms?

Have you taken any over-the-counter (OTC), prescription, or herbal medications for symptom relief?

Have you been taking your antiviral medications as prescribed?

Assessment of Airway and Gas Exchange

Are you having difficulty breathing?

Have you been coughing?

Are you coughing up any sputum?

If so, what color is it?

Assessment of Nutrition

Do you have an appetite?

What are you eating and how often do you eat?

Are you losing weight?

Are you experiencing nausea or vomiting?

Are you having any difficulty chewing or swallowing?

Assessment of Diarrhea

How many bowel movements are you having a day?

What is the consistency and color of the stool?

Are you taking any medications to stop diarrhea?

How many glasses of water/liquid are you drinking per day?

Are you experiencing abdominal pain or cramping?

Is the area around your rectum sore or bleeding?

What type of foods do you typically eat during the day?

Objective Data

Assessment of Infection

Abnormal vital signs (e.g., temp > 101 or < 97, HR > 100, BP < 90 or MAP < 60)

Skin: rashes, wounds, sores, redness, heat, or edema

Oral cavity: sores, white patches, poor dental hygiene

Drainage: color, amount, and foul smell from any wounds, incisions, or mucous membranes

Urine: amber, cloudy, amount of time indwelling urinary catheter is in place

Pain with palpation

Invasive lines/catheters: amount of time they have been in place, redness, drainage at insertion site

Laboratory tests: complete blood count with differential to evaluate white blood cell (WBC) count (neutrophils 12,000/mm^3; bands $> 10\%$);

CD4 T-cell count: < 500/cells/uL;

HIV viral load count: $> 25{,}000$ copies/mL;

Cultures: blood, sputum, stool, urine, wound (+ for bacterial or viral pathogens)

Assessment of Airway and Gas Exchange

Respiratory rate

Work of breathing: use of substernal and/or intercostal muscles with inspiration/expiration

Unequal chest wall movement

Oxygen saturation

Adventitious breath sounds: wheezes, fine or coarse crackles

Decreased level of consciousness (LOC) (lethargy, confusion, stupor)

Skin changes: mottled extremities, central cyanosis

Arterial blood gases (ABGs)

Assessment of Nutrition

Daily weight

Laboratory tests: serum protein, albumin, transferrin levels, hemoglobin/hematocrit (Hgb/Hct), electrolytes

Oral cavity: edema, white patches indicating Candida infection, open lesions, loose or decaying teeth

Assessment of Diarrhea

Vital signs (low BP, rapid HR may indicate dehydration)

Measurement of the number, volume, and consistency of bowel movements per day

Perianal area: red, excoriated

Skin turgor: tenting

Urine output: < 720 mL/day

Laboratory tests: abnormalities in electrolytes, phosphorus, magnesium, Hgb, red blood cells (RBCs)

Stool culture: pathogens

NURSING PROCESS: Patient Care Plan for HIV/AIDS, *continued*

Assessment of Oral Mucous Membranes

Are you having any difficulty or pain with chewing and swallowing?

Do you have any sores in your mouth?

Are you brushing your teeth at least twice a day?

Do you use a lip balm to protect your lips and keep them moist?

Assessment of Oral Mucous Membranes

Oral cavity: edema, white patches, open lesions, loose or decaying teeth, purple lesions

Outcomes and Evaluation Parameters

Planning and Interventions with *Rationales*

1. NURSING DIAGNOSIS: Risk for Infection *related to immunodeficiency from HIV infection* (NANDA-I © 2012)

Outcome: No infection.

Evaluation Parameters: Vital signs within normal parameters.

Alert and oriented.

Clear lungs.

Intact skin or mucous membrane without edema, pain, redness, or drainage.

Wounds/incisions healing.

No discomfort with urination.

Invasive line and catheter sites are not red or draining.

Symptoms of infection identified early and prompt treatment initiated.

WBC within normal limits.

Cultures negative for organisms.

Medications given on time.

Antibiotic therapy sensitive to infecting organism as evidenced by decreasing fever, WBC, and sputum production.

Patient continues HAART regime.

Health care providers and family perform hand hygiene frequently prior to and following patient contact.

Intake & output (I&O) balanced; patient maintaining or gaining weight.

No new skin or mucous membrane breakdown.

Invasive lines and catheters secured.

No invasive line or catheter-induced infections.

Catheters and invasive lines removed promptly when no longer of benefit in patient treatment.

Patient performs activities of daily living (ADLs).

Patient out of bed (OOB) and/or turned every 2 hours.

Lungs clear.

Patient and family can verbally identify signs and symptoms of infection.

Patient and family report early symptoms of infection to health care providers.

Patient environment is clean.

Has others handle pet cleanup.

Uses recommendations for food handling.

Assess for symptoms of infection: fever, chills, diaphoresis; tachycardia, tachypnea, hypotension; decline in neurological status; dyspnea, cough, adventitious breath sounds; white patches in oral cavity or painful swallowing; redness, swelling, or drainage from wounds or vaginal or perianal area; open lesions on face, lips, or perianal area; urinary frequency, urgency, or burning sensation; pain in any location.

Promotes early detection of infection.

Notify health care provider of symptoms of infection. *Early detection and treatment help prevent progression to refractory sepsis. Infections increase patient mortality.*

Monitor WBC count and differential. *Elevated or abnormally low WBC counts indicate possible infection.*

Obtain cultures of blood, sputum, urine, wound drainage, skin lesions, mouth, and stool as ordered prior to the start of the first dose of antibiotic. *Assists in identifying infecting organisms and targeting appropriate treatment. Obtaining culture prior to starting antibiotics increases the potential to capture the organism in the culture.*

Administer antimicrobial and HAART medications as prescribed. *Treats current infection or prevents additional opportunistic infections (OI). Decreases rate of HIV replication and increases CD4 counts.*

Prevent infection by washing hands before and after all patient contacts; instruct the patient/family to perform hand hygiene frequently, especially after toileting and prior to eating or handling medications. *Reduces risk of OI cross-contamination.*

Maintain fluid and nutritional intake, strict I&O, and calorie count. *Dehydration and malnutrition impair immune function and wound healing.*

Maintain skin and mucous membrane integrity with frequent turning and oral care every 2 hours. *Skin and mucous membranes are the first line of immune defense; lesions allow OI portal of entry.*

Maintain sterile technique during all invasive procedures (urinary catheterization, IV line placement). Perform meticulous care of any invasive lines or catheters; change out catheters according to agency policy.

Maintain a closed system for drains. Discontinue catheters/invasive lines as soon as possible. *Prevents hospital-acquired infections.*

Anchor catheters/tubes (IV lines, urinary catheters) securely. *Reduces trauma to tissue and decreases risk of introducing pathogens from in and out movement of catheter.*

Assist with mobility, out of bed three or more times a day unless contraindicated and/or turning every 2 hours. *Prevents skin breakdown, deep venous thrombosis, constipation, and pulmonary stasis, which may increase length of hospitalization and infection risk.*

Assist with inspirometer, coughing, and deep breathing every 1 to 2 hours when awake. *To prevent pulmonary stasis, which increases risk of OI.*

Instruct the patient and family about signs and symptoms of infection and infection prevention and the need to report possible infection. *Enables early detection and treatment.*

(*continued*)

NURSING PROCESS: Patient Care Plan for HIV/AIDS, *continued*

Outcomes and Evaluation Parameters	Planning and Interventions with *Rationales*
	Maintain cleanliness/personal hygiene. Clean household surfaces with disinfectant. *Decreases presence of potentially infective organisms.* Avoid handling animal waste or cleaning cages. *Infectious organisms such as CMV are in animal feces.* Clean and cook foods thoroughly (scrub skins of fruits and vegetables, cook meat and eggs). *To eliminate pathogens.* Avoid exposure to others' body fluids and do not share eating utensils. *Patient/family teaching to minimize exposure to OI is essential to preventing infection.*
2. NURSING DIAGNOSIS: (a) Ineffective Airway Clearance *related to (1) opportunistic pulmonary infection, increased bronchial secretions or (2) stasis of secretion from decreased ability to cough from general weakness.* (b) Risk for Impaired Gas Exchange *related to pulmonary secretions from opportunistic infections* (NANDA-I © 2012)	
Outcomes: Clear airway. Adequate gas exchange. ***Evaluation Parameters:*** Respiratory rate 12 to 20 breaths/min. Unlabored breathing without use of accessory muscles. Clear breath sounds. Alert and oriented. Skin is pink, warm. Normal ABG values. Pulse oximetry saturation > 94%. Appropriate medical treatment as needed. Patient cooperative with oxygen administration. Sputum culture obtained. Antibiotic therapy sensitive to infecting organism as evidenced by decreasing fever, WBC, and sputum production. Patient able to cough and clear secretions. Patient verbalizes understanding and performs pulmonary self-care. Patient reports decreased breathing problems. Patient has energy to cough and clear secretions. Secretions cleared. Airway and ventilation maintained.	Assess for rapid shallow respirations. *Indicates hypoxia and poor gas exchange.* Assess for use of accessory muscles. *Indicates increased work of breathing and progression to respiratory failure.* Assess for abnormal or absent breath sounds. *Indicates pulmonary infiltrates or consolidation that decreases gas exchange.* Assess for cough and sputum; note amount, color, and consistency of sputum. *A yellow, green, or tan color indicates presence of infecting organism.* Assess level of consciousness (restless, confused, somnolence). *Altered level of consciousness is an early indicator of hypoxia and decreased perfusion to the brain.* Assess dusky, cyanotic skin color. *Indicates tissue hypoxia.* Monitor ABGs and pulse oximetry oxygen saturation. *To assess adequacy of gas exchange.* Report respiratory distress to health care provider. *Enables prompt initiation of appropriate medical treatment.* Administer humidified oxygen as prescribed. *Supplemental oxygen increases the alveolar gas concentration and diffusion of oxygen to the cells and tissues of the body. Humidification helps loosen secretions and promote airway clearance.* Obtain sputum sample for culture. *To identify specific infecting organism so appropriate antibiotic is prescribed.* Administer antibiotic therapy as prescribed. *To treat infectious organism.* Maintain fluid intake of 3 L/day unless contraindicated. *To decrease viscosity of secretions.* Administer mucolytics and bronchodilators as prescribed. *To thin secretions and dilate airways, thus increasing gas exchange.* Maintain the head of the bed > 30 degrees at all times unless contraindicated. Instruct the patient to turn, cough, deep breathe, and use the inspirometer every 1 to 2 hours when awake. *Facilitates breathing, increases gas exchange, and prevents atelectasis and pulmonary secretion stasis.* Encourage adequate rest periods. *Prevents excessive fatigue, which impairs ability to breathe.* Perform tracheal suctioning as needed. *Removes secretions if patient is unable to do so, clears airway, and improves gas exchange.* Assist with endotracheal intubation; maintain ventilator settings as prescribed. *Maintains airway and gas exchange.*
3. NURSING DIAGNOSIS: Imbalanced Nutrition: Less Than Body Requirements *related to decreased oral intake associated with anorexia, nausea/vomiting, and impaired absorption and utilization of nutrients from effects of HIV infection* (NANDA-I © 2012)	
Outcome: Maintained or improved nutritional status. ***Evaluation Parameters:*** Gains weight. Adequate hydration. Normal electrolytes, albumin, hemoglobin/hematocrit, transferring levels.	Assess for significant weight loss or weight below normal for patient's height, weight, and age. *Indicates malnutrition.* Assess diet weight loss and diet history, as well as food likes, dislikes, and intolerances. *Identifies education needs and allows for an individual dietary plan.*

NURSING PROCESS: Patient Care Plan for HIV/AIDS, *continued*

Oral and esophageal opportunistic infections treated appropriately, as evidenced by no pain with swallowing and pink, nonedematous mucous membranes. Laboratory values improving and trending toward normal ranges. Intake of daily calories is nutritious and meets or exceeds body requirements. Patient and family use diet plan, report increased intake, and weight is increased. Nutritious food is available to the patient. Eats meals with others weekly. Decreased nausea and increased intake. Decrease in rate of weight loss.	Assess and report abnormalities of the oral cavity, mucous membranes, and swallowing. *To identify treatable OIs (oral candidiasis, esophagitis) that interfere with intake and facilitate medical treatment with oral candidiasis.* Monitor fluid and electrolytes, serum protein, albumin, transferrin levels, and hemoglobin/hematocrit energy level. *Low levels indicate inadequate intake/malnutrition, which places the patient at increased risk for infection.* Consult with the dietitian to determine the patient's nutritional needs. *To obtain information on calorie needs and facilitate meal planning.* Monitor daily intake with calorie count. *To provide data on total daily calorie intake.* Consult with health care provider and dietitian on high-calorie supplements. *To increase calorie intake when larger volumes of food cannot be tolerated.* Collaborate with patient/family to create a plan to increase intake: 1. Eat 6 to 7 small protein-rich foods. *To decrease nausea from feeling "over full" and to increase calorie intake.* 2. Select soft foods if patient has difficulty swallowing (eggs, ice cream, cooked vegetables, and pureed meats). *To decrease swallowing pain.* 3. Rest prior to meals. *To conserve energy for eating.* 4. Hold liquids 1 hour prior to eating. *To reduce satiety.* 5. Encourage the patient to eat meals with family/friends. *To increase social interaction and provide encouragement to eat.* Assess the need for community resources and consult a social worker or community liaison regarding financial assistance if the patient cannot afford food. *To provide resources on nutritious foods.* Administer prescribed medications: 1. Antiemetics. *To decrease nausea.* 2. Appetite stimulants (dronabinol, megestrol acetate). *To counteract anorexia effects of disease and medications.* 3. Cytokine inhibitors (thalidomide). *To improve appetite by suppressing TNF production (used only in cases of severe wasting syndrome).* Consult with health care provider and dietitian about enteral or parenteral nutrition if patient is unable to gain weight. *Provides additional nutritional support (used with severe wasting syndrome).*
4. NURSING DIAGNOSIS: Bowel Incontinence and Diarrhea ***related to HIV infection and/or opportunistic infections in the GI tract*** **(NANDA-I © 2012)**	
Outcome: Normal bowel habits. ***Evaluation Parameters:*** One to two soft-formed stools per day. Fluid and electrolyte status maintained. Factors contributing to acute episodes of diarrhea identified and avoided. Weight increasing. Opportunistic infection treated appropriately as exhibited by decreasing incidence of diarrhea, as well as normal stool cultures. Adequate fluid status maintained as evidenced by urine output > 720 mL/day, good skin turgor, and stable blood pressure. Normal electrolytes, Hgb, and RBCs. Decreased abdominal cramping and acute episodes of diarrhea. Perianal skin intact. Patient and family use diet plan, report decreased episodes of diarrhea, and weight is increased.	Assess for frequency and volume of loose stools and for abdominal cramping. *To determine the amount of diarrhea, fluid volume loss, and level of abdominal discomfort.* Identify factors that cause and alleviate diarrhea. *To help individualize care and create an effective plan.* Weigh daily and document amount. *To trend weights as part of an intervention assessment.* Obtain stool cultures. *Identifies opportunistic infections.* Administer antimicrobial therapy as prescribed. *To eliminate or control infecting organisms.* Instruct the patient to have fluid intake of >3 L/day unless contraindicated. *To prevent hypovolemia.* Monitor and report abnormal laboratory values (potassium, sodium, calcium, phosphorus, magnesium, Hgb, RBCs). *Chronic diarrhea and small intestinal inflammation may impair electrolyte absorption and absorption of vitamins necessary for Hgb and RBC formation.* Administer anticholinergics, antispasmodics, and opioids as prescribed. *To decrease intestinal motility and spasms.* Assess for perianal excoriation. *To determine the need for skin barrier creams or application of an external drainage bag to protect the skin.*

(*continued*)

NURSING PROCESS: Patient Care Plan for HIV/AIDS, *continued*

Outcomes and Evaluation Parameters	Planning and Interventions with *Rationales*
	Instruct the patient/family in diet measures to decrease bowel hyperactivity. *To help rest the bowel and possibly decrease diarrhea.* Eliminate bowel-irritating foods such as raw vegetables, nuts, and fried or fatty foods. *To reduce stimulation to the bowel.* Avoid coffee and nicotine. *These are bowel stimulants.* Encourage nonspicy, bland diet (BRAT diet = bananas, rice, apples/applesauce, toast). *Carbohydrates are easier to digest and cause less stimulation of the bowel. BRAT diet helps firm stool.*
5. NURSING DIAGNOSIS: Impaired Oral Mucous Membrane *related to immunologic deficit and presence of opportunistic infection/malignancy such as candidiasis, herpes, or Kaposi's sarcoma; malnutrition and/or dehydration; side effects of drugs and chemotherapy; or ineffective oral hygiene* (NANDA-I © 2012)	
Outcome: Integrity of mucous membranes maintained. ***Evaluation Parameters:*** Patient reports no oral discomfort. Mucous membranes are pink, moist, and intact. Oral and esophageal opportunistic infections are treated appropriately and effectively. Identified dental problems are treated appropriately. Medications are effective as evidenced by decreasing symptoms of infection or irritation. Lips and surrounding skin are intact. Tumors or growths in the oral cavity are treated appropriately as evidenced by the decreased size of lesion and increased patient comfort. Patient reports decreasing oral discomfort and participates in oral care. Patient practices oral hygiene self-care instructions. Family/friends support oral hygiene self-care practices. Patient has decreased oral pain. Moist pink mucous membranes.	Assess the patient for oral pain and difficulty with chewing or swallowing. *Indicates problem in oral cavity that affects patient comfort and impacts oral intake.* Assess oral cavity for ulcerations, redness, or white patches, especially on the side of the tongue. *Indicates probable oral candidiasis or progressing esophagitis.* Report symptoms of candidiasis. *To initiate medical treatment.* Obtain cultures or oral lesions as prescribed. *To identify opportunistic pathogens and target medical treatment.* Assess for swelling of gingiva, as well as loose or decaying teeth. *Indicates poor oral hygiene; increases risk of infection from dental source.* Refer to dental consultation if necessary. *To treat oral decay.* Administer medications as prescribed: antifungals, antibiotics. *To treat infections.* Assess for cracks or fissures at the corners of the mouth and on the lips. *Indicates sources of oral discomfort.* Assess for purple lesions or tumors. *Indicates possible Kaposi's sarcoma or lymphoma.* Assist with oral care every 2 hours. Rinse oral mucosa with saline and dilute hydrogen peroxide solution. *Decreases spread of lesions.* Use a soft toothbrush or sponge-tipped swab, nonabrasive toothpaste, and lip moisturizer. Brush teeth a minimum of twice a day. *Decreases acid formation from retained food, moistens mucous membranes, prevents infection, and promotes comfort.* Avoid lemon glycerin swabs and alcohol-based mouthwashes. *Acid irritates lesions and alcohol-based products dry mucous membranes.* Encourage use of commercial salivary product or hard candy or gum. *Neutralizes acids by increasing saliva flow and protects mucous membranes.* Instruct the patient and family in aspects of oral hygiene. *To promote comfort and self-care.* Collaborate with the patient/family to plan a menu that avoids salty, spicy, acidic, or abrasive foods. *To decrease aggravation of oral lesions.* Avoid extremely hot or cold foods. *Mucous membranes are sensitive to temperature extremes.* Instruct the patient to have fluid intake of $>$ 2,500 mL/day if not contraindicated. *To maintain hydration and keep mucous membranes moist.* Encourage the patient to avoid smoking. *To decrease drying and irritation to mucous membranes.*

Sources: Adapted from Carpenito-Moyet, L. (2008). *Nursing care plans and documentation* (5th ed.). Philadelphia: Lippincott Williams & Wilkins; Faulhaber, J., & Aberg, J. A. (2009). Acquired immunodeficiency syndrome. In C. M. Porth & G. Matfin (Eds.), *Pathophysiology: Concepts of altered health status* (8th ed., pp. 427–447). Philadelphia: Wolters Kluwer Health/Lippincott Williams & Wilkins; Wilkinson, J. M., & Ahearn, N. R. (2009). *Prentice Hall nursing diagnosis handbook* (9th ed.). Upper Saddle River, NJ: Prentice Hall.

COMPLEMENTARY & ALTERNATIVE THERAPIES Health Locus of Control

Nancy Yilk

COMPLEMENTARY AND ALTERNATIVE MEDICINE (CAM) involves a wide range of therapies including philosophical beliefs about health and illness. These perspectives are then supported with treatment therapies and lifestyle choices. Over the last decade, a greater acceptance has occurred in both the public and health care systems regarding the use of these therapies as an integrative model. This new acceptance, noted in public dialogue as integrative or functional medicine, is influencing an updated terminology to those who are practitioners and the public seeking its modulates. Research into Health Locus of Control (HLOC) gives insight into which life perspectives a person may follow to seek out the use of Integrative Healthcare (IH).

Health Locus of Control (HLOC) is a psychological concept concerning control beliefs in relationship to an individual's illness, injuries, and health. Developed as a social learning theory in 1954 by Rotter, this concept is based on the general approach of locus of control (LOC). The root word for authority, *author*, could be used to shed light on understanding the original terms used in considering a person's access of control during decision making. *Internal* LOC places authority within the people who believe they and their actions are the greatest influences in their life; *external* LOC places the authority with the influences of other people; and *chance* LOC places the authority to fate, which determines people's life blessings or challenges.

In an effort to add depth to the use of HLOC in understanding patient decision making, a German study further defined the external expression of HLOC. Previous analysis of HLOC was predominantly done in a health care setting in which patients received care, while nonclinical studies of general population sampling have been rare in regards to public health care. Among a sampling of 4,075 participants in northern Germany, individuals ages 18 to 64 were randomly selected from registration office files and completed the standardized German questionnaire which assesses HLOC. This model revealed a breakdown of external LOC to two additional latent variables, formal help and informal help. The following statements are examples of patient HLOC decision making used in seeking both formal and informal assistance (Otto, Bischof, Rumpf, Meyer, Hapke, & John, 2011).

HLOC	Statement of Belief/Perspective of an Individual's Decision Making Regarding Health
Internal	"My health is influenced by my actions even when I don't feel well."
	"When I know enough about myself I can help myself when I am sick."
	"It is up to me whether or not I get better when I am sick."
	"It's my responsibility to take the steps to remain healthy."
Formal Help	"When I have a medical concern, I usually go to the doctor."
	"Medical testing will help doctors know how to get me better when I'm sick."
	"Regarding my health, I only do what my doctor tells me to do."
Informal Help	"When I feel physically well, I owe this to all the advice and help of others."
	"When I don't feel well, I seek out the advice of others."
	"I can avoid getting sick when I take the advice of my friends and family."
	"When I don't feel well, others know better than me how I feel."
Chance	"No matter what I do, I'm just going to get sick again."
	"If I didn't have bad luck I wouldn't have any luck at all."
	"Being sick is my cross to bear, there isn't anything I can do, it's God's plan."
	"Being ill is payback for what I do in my life as my destiny."

In a study of 65 healthy graduate students, those with a greater internal HLOC measured by using the Multidimensional Health Locus of Control Scale (MHLC) were more likely to believe that their own actions directly relate to their health than those attributing health externally (to others or chance). Having greater control over personal health is a commonly reported reason for seeking CAM treatment, with previous studies finding a positive correlation between internal HLOC and CAM use.

Specifically, the study explored whether having a philosophical congruence with CAM, or being dissatisfied with conventional medicine, influences the choice to use CAM treatments. Philosophical congruence with CAM was measured with items such as "Most complementary therapies stimulate the body's natural therapeutic powers," and "I believe complementary medicine enables me to take a more active part in maintaining my health." Dissatisfaction with conventional medicine was measured with items such as "I don't trust medical doctors and hospitals, so I use them as little as possible," and "I have a lot of confidence in the medical doctor I see most often."

Three factors emerged during factor analysis rather than the anticipated two: (1) Philosophical congruence with CAM; (2) dissatisfaction with conventional; and (3) holistic balance that life is holistic in its nature.

The holistic balance factor represents the more holistic views associated with CAM and includes the following items: "Physical and mental health are maintained by an underlying energy or vital force," "Health and disease are a reflection of balance between positive life-enhancing forces and negative destructive forces," and "The body is essentially self-healing and the task of a health care provider is to assist in the healing process."

The holistic balance score was significantly correlated with philosophical orientation congruent with CAM, and dissatisfaction with conventional health care was mostly influenced by the increased belief in holistic balance which avails greater congruence with CAM (McFadden, Hernández, & Ito, 2010).

Integral to the use of Integrative Health is the coaching of patients in adopting lifestyle changes regarding exercise, diet, and continued healthy behavior that feel more natural to those individuals with internal HLOC who proactively seek out solutions to their health behavior. The success of this group's use of integrative CAM could be explained within the transtheoretical model of change, which organizes change in five stages:

1. *Precontemplation:* Individual has the problem (whether he recognizes it or not) and has no intention of changing.
2. *Contemplation:* Individual recognizes the problem and is seriously thinking about changing.
3. *Preparation for Action:* Individual recognizes the problem and intends to change the behavior within the next month. Some behavior change

(*continued*)

COMPLEMENTARY & ALTERNATIVE THERAPIES Health Locus of Control, *continued*

efforts may be reported, such as taking supplements when she remembers, eating better than she did before, and exercising on weekends. However, the defined behavior change criterion has not been reached (i.e., consistent healthy eating and exercise).

4. *Action:* Individual has enacted consistent behavior change (i.e., consistent healthy eating and active exercise) for less than 6 months.
5. *Maintenance:* Individual maintains new behavior for 6 months or more. Internal HLOC individuals are more inclined to be in the action phase when they first begin integration of complementary health practices into their daily lives. For external HLOC, family and friends serve as an influencing factor in use of Integrative Health.

A Japanese study explored the psychological and behavioral mechanisms of CAM use in Japanese cancer patients using two applied behavioral models: the transtheoretical model (TTM) and theory of planned behavior (TPB). Questionnaires were distributed to 1,100 patients at three cancer treatment facilities in Japan, and researchers used data on 521 cancer patients in the final analysis. The questionnaire included items based on TTM and TPB variables, as well as three psychological batteries. According to the TTM, 88 patients (17%) were in precontemplation, 226 (43%) in contemplation, 33 (6%) in preparation, 71 (14%) in action, and 103 (20%) in maintenance. The model, derived from structural equation modeling, revealed that the stage of CAM use was significantly affected by the pros, cons, expectations from family, norms of medical staff, use of chemotherapy, period from diagnosis, and place of treatment. The primary factor for the stage of CAM use was the expectation from family.

Positive Attitudes for CAM	**The Items Represented the High-Perceived Availability and Importance of CAM Use for the Patients**
	CAM is important to retain physical strength.
	Hospital care alone is not enough.
	Convenience is an important determinant of starting to use CAM.
	The cost of CAM is important.
Pros	**The Items Represented Patients' Perceived Positive Outcomes of CAM Use**
	The use of CAM leads to the cure of disease.
	The use of CAM halts the progression of disease.
	The use of CAM boosts physical and immune strength.
	CAM has fewer side effects compared with medical care.
Cons	**The Items Represented Patients' Perceived Negative Outcomes of CAM Use**
	The use of CAM has a bad influence on medical care.
	The use of CAM deteriorates disease.
	I am aware of the side effects of CAM.
	I am aware of the dependence liability of CAM.
Expectation from Family	**The Items Represented Patients' Perceived Expectations and Recommendations From Family**
	My family/friends believe that I should be actively engaged in the use of CAM.
	My use of CAM is influenced by the opinions of my family/friends.
Norms of Medical Staff	**The Items Represented Patients' Perceived Expectation, Recommendation From Patients' Medical Staff, or Their Norms**
	My doctors/nurses believe that I should be actively engaged in the use of CAM.
	My use of CAM is influenced by the opinions of my doctors/nurses.

The findings revealed the existence of a number of psychologically induced potential CAM users. Psychological variables including positive attitude for CAM use and perceived family expectation greatly influence CAM use in cancer patients (Hirai et al., 2008).

References

Hirai, K., Komura, K., Tokoro, A., Kuromaru, T., Ohshima, A., Ito, T., et al. (2008). Psychological and behavioral mechanisms influencing the use of complementary and alternative medicine (CAM) in cancer patients. *Annals of Oncology, 19*(1), 49–55. Epub 2007 Oct 26.

McFadden, K. L., Hernández, T. D., & Ito, T. A. (2010). Attitudes toward complementary and alternative medicine influence its use. *Explore (NY), 6*(6), 380–388.

Otto, C., Bischof, G., Rumpf, H. J., Meyer, C., Hapke, U., & John, U. (2011). Multiple dimensions of Health Locus of Control in a representative population sample: Ordinal factor analysis and cross-validation of an existing three and a new four factor model. *BMC Medical Research Methodology, 11*, 114.

Rotter, J. B. (1954). *Social learning theory and clinical psychology.* New York: Prentice Hall.

Discharge Priorities

Because of the chronic nature of HIV/AIDS, the process of discharging a patient from the hospital is complex. The nurse must address the medication schedule, physical care needs, and emotional issues surrounding the diagnosis. If followed carefully, current treatments can prolong and give quality to the person's life. Additionally, caregiver issues must be addressed. The Patient Teaching & Discharge Priorities box and Chart 53–9 outline the important information that is essential for patients with HIV/AIDS and their partners and caregivers that must be provided on discharge.

Health Promotion

Counseling regarding HIV encompasses two components: provision of information and prevention counseling. Counseling should be offered in an open, nonjudgmental manner and in the language that the individual is best capable of understanding. The counseling should include

PATIENT TEACHING & DISCHARGE PRIORITIES for the HIV-Infected Individual With AIDS

Need	Teaching
Knowledge of disease process	Provide verbal and written instructions on ways HIV can be transmitted (unprotected sex, sharing of needles, exposing others to blood or body fluids) to help the patient avoid infecting others.
Understanding of medications	Have the patient administer medications on schedule and verbalize the importance of compliance with HAART therapy to control disease progression and decrease the risk of developing drug resistance. Teach the purpose, dose, and possible side effects of all medications to increase compliance and prevent over- or underdosing. Explain the importance of a follow up laboratory appointment schedule to monitor medication effectiveness.
Prevention of opportunistic infections	Teach the signs and symptoms of infection and strategies to avoid exposure to opportunistic infections. Encourage avoidance of people with communicable diseases such as colds or flu.
Reportable clinical manifestations	Instruct the patient/family to report: • Symptoms of infection (fever, malaise, aching joints) • New or worsening rash or sores • Difficulty eating or swallowing • Nausea, vomiting, or diarrhea that lasts for more than 2 days • New or worsening pain • Weight loss.
Ongoing care	Explain the purpose of clinic and laboratory follow up appointments for ongoing monitoring of medication effectiveness and assessment of CD4+ T-cell and viral load counts. Provide schedule and contact information for appointments following discharge. Explain the value of regular health screenings including checkups with monitoring of weight and dental care.
Family/support system	Assess the availability of a support system to provide emotional support and to assist with medications and transportation to appointments. Collaborate with the discharge planner/case manager RN (if available) and assess needs for discharge to home or extended care. Assess the need for home assistive devices. Assess the need for a home health care provider.
Emotional adjustment of patient/family due to chronic nature of disease	Answer questions honestly. Encourage verbalization of feelings, fears. Discuss the possibility of depression and encourage discussion of this with the health care provider.

verbal as well as written information or audiovisual materials that the individual can take home and review. The CDC's revised recommendations for HIV testing released in 2006 change some of the previous recommendations for prevention counseling for individuals who take rapid HIV tests in a health care setting. The recommendations indicate that prevention counseling should not be required with HIV diagnostic testing or as part of an HIV screening program in health care settings such as emergency departments, urgent care clinics, inpatient services, substance abuse treatment clinics, public health and community clinics, correctional facilities, and primary care settings (CDC, 2011d). In 2011, these guidelines were again revised to strongly recommend that HIV screening become a routine part of patient care in community health care settings (CDC, 2011d). This is an effort to continue to remove barriers to HIV screening in busy health care settings. However, the CDC continues to support prevention counseling in all settings for persons at high risk for HIV and in nonmedical settings such as community-based organizations, outreach settings, or mobile vans (CDC, 2011d).

The CDC still recommends that patients in all settings receive information regarding HIV testing, HIV infection, and the meaning of results. Patients must be informed of the HIV screening in a face-to-face discussion or through written or audiovisual material. Information provided should include the testing process, the meaning of test results, ways HIV is transmitted and how to prevent it, and where to obtain further testing and services. Ongoing HIV counseling is vital for individuals who test positive for HIV. Overwhelming feelings of fear, anxiety, depression, and social isolation frequently occur with an HIV diagnosis. Nurses are in an optimal position to develop therapeutic relationships that support the HIV-positive patient, to review risk factors for transmitting HIV infection, and to encourage compliance with follow up testing and antiretroviral therapy. Nurses also can help facilitate referrals to social services for assistance with financial concerns and community and psychological support services.

It is important that HIV-infected patients and their families and friends understand the routes of transmission of HIV to prevent infection and alleviate fears of casual transmission. The information provided can address these issues and alleviate fears that may interfere with social support for the patient with HIV/AIDS.

Collaborative Management

A multidisciplinary collaborative approach to preventing HIV infection and transmission and providing treatment for patients with HIV/AIDS is essential. A variety of individuals using different educational approaches in varied settings can most effectively communicate the facts about HIV/AIDS. In order to meet desired patient outcomes, it is essential that the members of this interdisciplinary team communicate

CHART 53–9 Patient and Partner Teaching Guide on Preventing HIV Transmission

- Practice abstinence or mutual monogamy or limit the number of sexual partners.
- Do not have unprotected sex. Use latex condoms (animal skin condoms do not prevent HIV transmission). For latex allergies, use female condoms that are latex free.
- Do not lubricate the condom with spermicidal agent nonoxynol-9 or use spermicidal agent nonoxynol-9 because this may increase vaginal tissue damage and the risk of HIV infection.
- Do not use oil-based sex lubricants because this can damage the condom. Water-based lubricants are safe to use.
- Do not reuse male or female condoms.
- Always use a condom with other methods of birth control. Cervical caps or diaphragms will decrease the risk of pregnancy but not HIV transmission.
- Always use dental dams for oral female genital or anal stimulation.
- Avoid anal intercourse or manual anal intercourse "fisting" to prevent injury to tissues.
- Use safer sex practices, such as mutual masturbation, to decrease damage to mucous membranes.
- If entering a mutually exclusive monogamous relationship, both partners should undergo HIV testing. There is a window period of up to 6 months before HIV antibody testing is positive, so the previous guidelines should be followed during the window period when HIV status is unknown.
- If you are HIV antibody positive, inform previous, current, and prospective sex partners and drug-using partners of your HIV status. Follow the previous guidelines.
- If you are HIV antibody positive, inform health care providers of your HIV status. Laws protect the confidentiality of this information. This information helps direct your medical treatment.
- If you are HIV antibody positive, do not share items that may be contaminated with blood such as needles, syringes, drug preparation equipment ("works"), sex toys, razors, or toothbrushes.
- If you are HIV antibody positive, do not donate blood, plasma, sperm, or body organs.

Guidelines for Safer Use of Injection Equipment

If you use injection drugs, consider stopping and entering a treatment program. If you cannot make that choice, use the following guidelines to limit your risk of HIV and other disease transmission.

- Use sterile needles and syringes.
- Do not share your needles, syringes, or drug preparation equipment ("works").
- Access needle and syringe exchange programs, when available, to exchange used needles and syringes and obtain sterile ones.
- If injection equipment is shared, clean it thoroughly before use: Rinse the syringe and needle twice with tap water, fill the syringe with full-strength household bleach for 30 seconds, shake and squirt out, repeat the bleaching process a second time, then rinse again twice with tap water.
- Do not share your drug preparation equipment. If it is shared, clean it thoroughly with bleach and water.
- Do not share your bleach or rinse water.

Sources: Centers for Disease Control and Prevention (CDC). (2010a). HIV in the United States. Retrieved from http://www.cdc.gov/hiv/resources/factsheets/PDF/us.pdf; Centers for Disease Control and Prevention (CDC). (2010b). Sexually transmitted diseases treatment guidelines 2010. *Morbidity and Mortality Weekly Report, 59*(12), 1–109; Centers for Disease Control and Prevention (CDC). (2010c). Sexually transmitted diseases guidelines, 2010. Retrieved from http://www.cdc.gov/std/treatment/2010/hepC.htm.

openly with one another in developing and evaluating care of the patient and family (IOM [Institute of Medicine], 2010). Effective treatment of individuals with HIV infection and AIDS requires coordination between various members of the health care team such as health care providers, nurses, social workers, dietitians, and community workers at various levels of care from clinics to home care to acute care.

The health care provider is primarily responsible for diagnosis and development of the medical treatment plan. The nurse's role is centered on providing emotional support and monitoring and managing disease symptoms. Nurses also provide education on medications and the importance of complying with the medication regimen, having ongoing laboratory tests and appointments, and minimizing the risk of OIs. Social workers offer assistance in addressing financial concerns, managing personal care needs, and accessing community referrals and social networks in the community and acute care setting. Dietitians also have a significant role in monitoring nutritional needs and developing specialized nutritional plans that may include supplements in light of HIV complications and wasting syndrome (American Dietetic Association [ADA], 2010). For more on nutrition and how it affects patients with HIV/AIDS, see the Evidence-Based Practice box.

For patients who have been diagnosed with HIV/AIDS, collaborative care includes assessment of physical status as well as the knowledge level of the patient, partner, family, and friends in order to address their education needs. The promotion of self-care, independence, and adherence to the prescribed treatment plan is the primary goal in the care of the patient with AIDS. With antiretroviral therapy, HIV infection is transitioning into a chronic disease. Many HIV-infected individuals are able to maintain home and work functions for several years and are regularly followed by their health care provider or an AIDS outreach clinic. As the disease progresses, care needs increase and the patient becomes increasingly dependent on family and friends to provide support. Social workers, community support services, home health care nurses, community health nurses, and hospice nurses are often able to provide complex in-home nursing care that enables patients to remain comfortable at home.

Nurses are pivotal in providing ongoing patient and family education and making appropriate referrals to a variety of community-based organizations that can supply support such as meals, housekeeping, transportation, or shopping. Nurses also have additional information on national resources that the patient or family can access, such as the National Association of People with AIDS, CDC National AIDS Hotline, and the National Association on HIV Over Fifty. (For a discussion of AIDS in people over age 50, see the Gerontological Considerations section) At the point at which the patient's symptoms cannot be managed at home or a caregiver is not available, a transfer to skilled nursing care or an acute care facility is needed to ensure patient safety and comfort.

The primary mode of HIV/AIDS prevention is education and lifestyle modification for at-risk groups. Nurses, other health care providers, social workers, community health educators, and schools play a central role in providing education about HIV/AIDS and infection prevention. Instructing individuals and communities on safer sex practices

EVIDENCE-BASED PRACTICE Barriers and Facilitators to HIV Treatment

Clinical Problem

Today, many people live long lives with HIV. These people have become known as people living with HIV (PLWH). As discussed earlier, the CDC now strongly recommends routine screening for HIV not only to prevent transmission, but also to begin early HAART treatment and thus improve the quality of patients' lives. However, there still remain barriers to screening for HIV and, once HIV infection has been identified, barriers to treatment.

Williams, Amico, and Konkle-Parker (2011) used a qualitative design involving participants in group sessions discussing their experiences in order to identify some of the barriers and facilitators to HIV treatment. The study took place in a local public infectious disease clinic in Mississippi. There were a total of five focus group sessions that lasted about 1.5 hours each. Twenty-five HIV-positive people participated. Participants were asked specific questions related to how their HIV diagnosis affected their lives.

Research Findings

The recordings from the group sessions were analyzed to identify themes related to barriers and facilitators to HIV treatment. Five barriers to HIV treatment identified in the study were as follows:

- Competing demands (for example, those of employment and child care)
- System of care, how easy or hard it was to get needed care as well as those who were providing the care
- Stigma, concern about the implications of being diagnosed with HIV, and then being treated for it
- Experience of the negative effects of the disease (for example, possibility of being abandoned by friends and family)
- Beliefs about the need for care, especially if the patient was currently not symptomatic.

Facilitators to care identified in the study included the following:

- Support from friends, family, and clinical staff
- Activation around care (for example, acceptance of the diagnosis)
- Positive aspects of a health care visit
- Perceived vulnerability of not getting treatment.

Implications for Nursing Practice

Although it has been 30 years since HIV/AIDS became known to the world, there continue to be significant challenges in the care of PLWH. This study found some important barriers and facilitators to providing care to these people. The development of support systems and providing education about the potential consequences of not obtaining appropriate and timely care are only two examples of how nurses can make a difference in the lives of people living with HIV.

Critical Thinking Questions with answers can be found in the Osborn Student Resources at nursing.pearsonhighered.com.

Source: Williams, B., Amico, K. R., & Konkle-Parker, D. (2011). Qualitative assessment of barriers and facilitators to HIV treatment. *Journal of the Association of Nurses in AIDS Care, 22*, 307–312.

and ways to decrease disease transmission with injection drug use is essential. Chart 53–9 provides a teaching guide for individuals and partners regarding practices to decrease HIV transmission risk that can be used by a variety of HIV/AIDS prevention educators.

Collaborative care of HIV-infected patients also involves extensive education of patients, family, and friends regarding antiretroviral medications and prevention of OIs, as discussed earlier in Chart 53–7 (p. 1648). Collaborative care includes identifying potential risk factors for HIV infection in patients who have not been diagnosed with HIV and patient knowledge of how HIV is transmitted.

Gerontological Considerations

In the United States, 15% of all reported AIDS cases occur in adults over 50 years of age. Older adults are at increased risk for contracting HIV/AIDS because of declining immune system function with aging. However, AIDS is associated with youth, sexual activity, and IV drug use, factors that are generally not linked with the older population. Sexual contact is the most common form of HIV transmission, yet there is a prevalent misconception that older adults are not sexually active. Because older adults are beyond childbearing years, they often fail to use condoms when engaging in sexual activity. Additionally, older adults may have had a history of IV drug use that results in latent HIV infection. They also can be current IV drug users; however, given the more conservative nature of their social group and the socially unacceptable nature of this addiction, this issue may be hidden or denied. As a consequence, there is denial on the part of older adults and the health care community that older adults are at risk for HIV infection, and the potential for misdiagnosis and subsequent failure to treat with antiretroviral therapy is significant (Vance, 2011).

Nurses must be aware that the older adult is also at risk for HIV/AIDS and assess the risk factors by means of a thorough nursing history. It is essential to advocate for the patient by asking the medical team about possible HIV antibody testing when a diagnosis is unclear and the patient has risk factors and symptoms consistent with an AIDS-related illness.

Research

Research in the area of immune disease disorders is multifaceted. The fact that allergies affect such a large portion of the population makes identification of genetic and environmental factors that contribute to the development of allergies a major priority (see the Genetic Considerations box, p. 1621). A greater understanding of the association between allergies and the development of other pulmonary diseases also is a major priority.

Nurses are involved in many areas of study including coordinating clinical research sites, data collection, drug studies, and clinical outcomes research. The Research Opportunities box (p. 1666) provides information on some of the current areas of medical and nursing research under investigation as well as additional areas of current medical and nursing research related to allergies.

Summary

The HIV/AIDS epidemic means that nurses throughout the health care system will be called on to care for patients with HIV infection. Foundational to nursing is providing care in a compassionate, committed, and nonjudgmental manner. Care for the patient with AIDS involves a wide spectrum of activities from a gentle touch that communicates compassion to education on a complex medication regimen and multiple interventions to treat OIs and malignancies. Nurses also play a central role in providing emotional support to patients and families during the dying process and facilitating the discussions on end-of-life care. The complexity of HIV infection presents multiple care needs that nurses, using the nursing process, are well equipped to address. Nurses are an essential part of a collaborative care approach to optimizing treatment for the patient with AIDS.

RESEARCH OPPORTUNITIES Related to Immune Response Disorders

Research Area	Clinical Impact
Hypersensitivity	
Pursue development of new classes of allergy medication.	Decrease IgE stimulation and the inflammatory response; symptom control and improved functional ability.
Identify genetic factors associated with the development of allergies.	Development of new therapies that more specifically target the allergy trigger and overproduction of IgE.
Identify environmental factors associated with the development of allergies.	Development of new therapies that more specifically target the allergy trigger and overproduction of IgE.
Identify genetic and environmental links between allergies and the development of asthma.	Control of IgE stimulation to prevent development of asthma.
Determine pharmacologic action of herbal and complementary therapy in the treatment of allergy.	Identifying the effective or harmful action of herbal medications in the treatment of allergy response to promote new treatments and deter the use of unproven therapies.
Autoimmune Diseases	
Stem cell cloning to develop new methods for delivery of monoclonal antibodies.	Improved drug therapy by reducing side effects of monoclonal antibody therapy.
Identification of genetic factors that contribute to development of autoimmune diseases such as myasthenia gravis and Goodpasture's syndrome.	Enable gene alteration to prevent and treat autoimmune disease.
Identification of environmental triggers such as pesticides or radiation exposure that contribute to the development of autoimmune disease.	Control of exposure to environmental triggers to prevent altered immune function.
Development of medications, such as monoclonal antibodies for use in preventing transplant rejection.	Improved ability to transplant organs and reduce incidence of rejection.
Identification of additional antibodies and markers to better match tissue and organs for transplant.	Reduced transplant rejection through improved matching of host and recipient.
Examination of HLA markers and the importance of a maximal match versus optimal match to prevent transplant rejection.	To better predict which transplants have a higher risk of rejection and optimize antirejection drug therapy treatment.
HIV/AIDS	
Development of a vaccine to protect against infection after exposure with HIV.	Reduce active cases of HIV and AIDS through prevention with vaccine.
Epidemiologic studies that focus on areas of the world where the incidence of HIV is increasing and the risk factors noted in those areas.	Reduce cases of HIV through education of populations at greatest risk worldwide.
Development of new classes of antiretroviral medications.	Improve survival, slow progression of HIV infection, and maximize development of antiretroviral medications.
Development of a DNA bank of genes, HIV genes, and enzyme codes.	Promote research and development of better therapies and vaccines.
Clinical trials of high-dose combination therapy to extend life in advanced AIDS patients.	Improve quality and delay further progression of disease for advanced AIDS patients, and decrease development of resistance.
Comparative studies on HIV viral loads, initiation of antiretroviral therapy, and development of drug resistance.	Guide the appropriate initiation of antiretroviral therapy to help prevent development of drug resistance.
Study of adherence, quality of life, and satisfaction with combination drug therapy among patients with multiple years of HIV diagnosis.	Improve teaching of medication therapy and increase compliance for newly diagnosed HIV patients starting therapy. Prevent drug resistance.
Comparative studies on the effectiveness of complementary therapies for HIV disease progressive management.	Provide new drug treatments to control pain and improve the patient's quality of life.
Prevention of HIV/AIDS by taking antiviral medications.	Research has found that high-risk groups, particularly men who have sex with men, may be at less risk of getting HIV when taking prophylactic antiviral medications. Whether this will continue to be a significant intervention will continue to be monitored.

Sources: College of Allergy, Asthma and Immunology. (2011a). Be S.A.F.E.: Managing allergic emergencies. Retrieved from http://www.acaai.org/patients/resources/anaphylaxis/managing-allergic-emergencies/Documents/BeSAFEBrochure.pdf; American College of Allergy, Asthma and Immunology. (2011b). Latex allergy. Retrieved from http://www.acaai.org/allergist/allergies/Types/latex-allergy/Pages/default.aspx; Centers for Disease Control and Prevention. (2011a). Asthma. Retrieved from http://www.cdc.gov/asthma/faqs.htm; Centers for Disease Control and Prevention. (2011b). HIV-2 surveillance—United States, 1987–2009. *Morbidity and Mortality Weekly Report, 60*(29), 985–988. Retrieved from http://www.cdc.gov/hiv/resources/brochures/at-risk.htm; Centers for Disease Control and Prevention. (2011c). How is HIV passed from one person to another? Retrieved from http://www.cdc.gov/hiv/resources/qa/transmission.htm; Centers for Disease Control and Prevention. (2011d). Implementation of routine HIV testing in community health settings: Issues for community health centers. Retrieved from http://www.cdc.gov/hiv/topics/testing/resources/guidelines/pdf/routineHIVtesting.pdf; Centers for Disease Control and Prevention. (2011e). Interim guidance: Preexposure prophylaxis for the prevention of HIV infection in men who have sex with men. *Morbidity and Mortality Weekly Report, 60*(3), 65–68; Centers for Disease Control and Prevention. (2011f). Occupational HIV transmission and prevention among health care workers. Retrieved from http://www.cdc.gov/hiv/resources/qa/transmission.htm; Centers for Disease Control and Prevention. (2011g). TB and HIV coinfection. Retrieved from http://www.cdc.gov/tb/topic/TBHIVcoinfection/default.htm; DeFranco, A. L., Locksley, R., & Robertson, M. (2007). *Immunity: The immune response in infectious and inflammatory disease.* Sunderland, MA: Sinauer Associates.

READ: **History of Present Illness** >> Laboratory Study Results >> Critical Thinking Questions

Javier Bernal is a 42-year-old Spanish-speaking, thin, anxious-appearing male in moderate discomfort due to abdominal pain that he first noticed 2 weeks ago and described as dull. He does not have a regular doctor and has presented to the emergency department (ED) with abdominal pain. Mr. Bernal requests a Spanish-speaking interpreter. He states, via an interpreter, that he has had increased abdominal pain during the past 5 days, has lost more than 20 pounds during the last 3 months, does not have an appetite, and is having increasing difficulty swallowing because of "sores" in his mouth. He has been unable to take solid foods for the past 3 days owing to painful swallowing and has taken very little juice or water during the past 24 hours. He denies nausea or vomiting.

Mr. Bernal is being admitted by internal medicine to the medical–surgical unit. He states that he did not want to come to the doctor earlier because he does not have the money to pay the bill. He came to the ED today "because the pain was getting very bad, and I am afraid something is wrong with me." Upon admission to the floor, he is awake and alert. He states that he is continuing to have pain in his abdomen despite medication.

READ: History of Present Illnesses >> **Physical Exam** >> Admitting Medical Records >> Laboratory Study Results

Medical–Surgical History

- No known allergies
- Medications: none
- Denies history of cancer or family history of cancer
- Denies history of abdominal trauma or injuries, gastric reflux disease, hernia, or colitis
- Positive history of fatigue, intermittent fever, chills, and night sweats during the past 6 months
- Genital herpes onset age 19, intermittent recurrence, most recent occurrence 1 year prior
- Surgeries: appendectomy at age 22 in Mexico

Social History

- Immigrated to the United States 2 years previously, unmarried, lives with his brother and his brother's family; employed in lawn care and home maintenance business
- Drinks 1–2 beers daily
- Smokes 1/2 pack of cigarettes per day × 25 years
- Prior IV drug use; none in the past 7 years
- Intermittently sexually active with various partners

Physical Exam

- Vital signs: BP 101/45, HR 108, RR 22, temp 36.8°C, O_2 sat 95% on room air
- Pain: 6/10
- Neurological: alert and oriented × 3, worried expression on face, neurological exam normal, communicates with minimal English, primary language is Spanish
- HEENT: oral mucous membranes are red and inflamed, multiple white lesions present on oral mucosa and extending to the posterior oral pharynx; tonsils slightly enlarged, poor dental care, four teeth missing on anterior and left lateral upper jaw; submandibular lymph nodes bilaterally enlarged and tender to palpations; ears and eyes normal
- Neck: cervical lymph nodes enlarged bilaterally, right greater than left, tender to palpation; full range of neck motion present
- Respiratory: denies shortness of breath; unlabored respirations; equal chest wall expansion; no chest deformities evident or palpated; lungs clear
- Cardiovascular: tachycardia with occasional irregular beat, S_1, S_2, no murmur, pulses palpable in all extremities, capillary refill WNL
- GI/GU: abdomen slightly distended but soft, palpable mass lower quadrants, bowel sounds present in all quadrants, abdomen painful to light palpation in all quadrants, greatest area of pain in lower quadrants; denies painful urination, normal size genitals, uncircumcised, no drainage from penis, with no evidence of lesions
- Skin: intact, dry; poor skin turgor; no evidence of discoloration, rash, or bruising
- 12-lead ECG: showed sinus tachycardia, occasional PVCs, and no other abnormalities
- Abdominal CT: results indicate a pelvic mass in the retroperitoneal space above the bladder; size estimated at 20 cm by 15 cm

Admitting Medical Orders

- Medical Service
- Consults: Surgical, Social Services, Oncology
- Admit to medical–surgical floor with telemetry monitoring
- Admitting diagnosis: abdominal pain, pelvic mass, r/o abdominal malignancy, oral and esophageal candidiasis
- Allergies: none
- Full code status
- Strict I&O
- Vital signs and oxygen saturation q4h
- Daily weight
- Diet: clear liquids
- Ambulation ad-lib
- Incentive spirometer q1–2h
- Sequential compression devices (SCDs) to lower extremities when in bed
- Call house officer: BP $<$ 90 systolic or diastolic $>$ 90; HR $>$ 120 and $<$ 60, RR $>$ 30; temp $>$ 38.2°C: oxygen saturation $<$ 92%
- IV: 0.9% saline with 20 mEq of KCl via infusion pump at 500 mL/hr × 1 liter, then decrease rate to 125 mL/hr

Scheduled Medications

- Diflucan 200 mg po daily
- Protonix 40 mg po daily
- Nystatin 5 mL q6h, swish & swallow

PRN Medications

- Morphine sulfate 2–4 mg IV push q2h prn for severe pain
- Vicodin 1–2 tabs (5/500) po q6h prn for moderate pain
- Ativan, 0.5–1 mg po q4h prn anxiety
- Ondansetron 4 mg IV q6h prn nausea

Ordered Laboratory Studies

- CBC with differential on admission
- Blood count daily
- Complete metabolic panel (CMP), amylase, lipase, PO_4, PT/INR/PTT, UA, CD4 cell count
- HIV antibody test (health care provider has completed consent for testing with patient and this is documented on chart)

Ordered Diagnostic Studies

- 12-lead ECG
- Abdominal CT

READ: History of Present Illnesses >> **Laboratory Study Results** >> Critical Thinking Questions

Test	Day 1	Day 2	Day 3
Sodium	148 mEq/L	142 mEq/L	138 mEq/L
Potassium	2.9 mEq/L	3.9 mEq/L	4.2 mEq/L
Chloride	113 mEq/L	99 mEq/L	99 mEq/L
Venous carbon dioxide	22 mEq/L	25 mEq/L	25 mEq/L
Blood urea nitrogen (BUN)	42 mg/dL	22 mg/dL	19 mg/dL
Creatinine	1.1 mg/dL	0.9 mg/dL	0.7 mg/dL
Blood glucose	143 mg/dL	124 mg/dL	133 mg/dL
Calcium	7.9 mg/dL	7.8 mg/dL	7.9 mg/dL
Total protein	5.2 g/dL		
Amylase	72 units/L		
Lipase	27 units /L		
Magnesium	1.9 mEq/L	2.0 mEq/L	2.1 mEq/L
Phosphorus	3.1 mg/dL		
Albumin	2.9 g/dL	2.9 g/dL	2.9 g/dL
Alkaline phosphatase	225 units/L	197 units/L	192 units/L
Total bilirubin	1.2 mg/dL		
AST (SGOT)	64 units/L	99 units/L	104 units/L
ALT (SGPT)	52 units/L	80 units/L	92 units/L

Test	Day 1	Day 2	Day 3
WBC	1,700/mm^3	1,600/mm^3	1,600/mm^3
Hemoglobin	10.1 g/dL	9.8 g/dL	9.8 g/dL
Hematocrit	30.2%	29.8%	29.8%
RBCs	4.0/mm^3	3.9/mm^3	3.9/mm^3
Neutrophils	88%		
Lymphocytes	2%		
Monocytes	3%		
Platelets	227,000/mm^3	208,000/mm^3	87,000/mm^3
PTT	34 seconds		
PT	13.1 seconds		
INR	1.22 seconds		
CEA		> 11 ng/mL	
CD4 count	170 cells/uL		
HIV antibody	Positive		
ABGs			
PO_2	92 mmHg		
Oxygen saturation	95%	94%	
pH	7.34		
PCO_2	39 mmHg		

Pearson Nursing Student Resources *Log on to* ***nursing.pearsonhighered.com*** *to download forms*

DOCUMENT:

- >> Summary of Hospitalization
- >> Pathophysiology Form
- >> Laboratory Values
- >> Laboratory Results Explanation

APPLY:

- >> List of Potential Nursing Diagnoses
- >> Concept Map
- >> Critical Thinking Questions and Concept Map

APPLY: History of Present Illness >> Laboratory Study Results >> **Critical Thinking Questions**

1. What information was obtained that suggested the need for HIV testing?
2. Review the laboratory findings from the ED. Which ones are abnormal, what is the possible rationale for these abnormalities, and how are these abnormalities evidenced in physical assessment findings?
3. EIA and Western blot tests are ordered to confirm the diagnosis. The CD4 count results are 187 cells/μL. What is the rationale for ordering this test, and what is the significance of the result?
4. Mr. Bernal is HIV positive, but does he have AIDS, according to the CDC guidelines?
5. What additional treatment should you anticipate for Mr. Bernal on the basis of his HIV test results and CD4 results?

Answers to Critical Thinking Questions can be found in Appendix D in the Osborn Student Resources at nursing.pearsonhighered.com.

NCLEX® PRACTICE

1. The nurse suspects that the patient has developed an immune hypersensitivity response. The symptoms displayed by the patient would be based on which of the following?

1. When hypersensitivity occurs, the immune system loses self-tolerance and immune deficiencies result.
2. Hypersensitive reactions are determined by the type of antigen, the time sequence of the reaction, and the immunologic response.
3. The primary mechanism of a hypersensitive response is a genetic disorder that occurred during the embryonic development of the immune system.
4. Hypersensitive responses are usually the result of opportunistic infections which activate a primary response from the T and B cells.

2. A patient who has experienced a hypersensitivity response determined to be autoimmune asks the nurse for information about this response. The nurse should include which of the following to describe the processes that differentiate the immune hypersensitivity response resulting from an autoimmune mechanism from those resulting from an allergic or alloimmune mechanism?

1. "The primary trigger for a hypersensitive reaction is a genetic defect."
2. "The origin for an alloimmune reaction is from the host's DNA."
3. "The trigger for an autoimmune response is a self antigen."
4. "Once activated, the hypersensitive response is identical regardless of trigger."

3. A nurse is teaching a student group about the difference between acquired immune deficiency syndrome (AIDS) and human immunodeficiency virus (HIV). Which of the following should the nurse include when covering this material? (select all that apply)

1. "HIV is the end disease manifestation of AIDS."
2. "AIDS is a syndrome of opportunistic infections that occurs as a final stage in patients infected with HIV."
3. "HIV transmission is limited to contact with infected body fluids that have lymphocytes that can harbor HIV."
4. "AIDS precedes HIV and allows for the progression of the virus's entry into the host's lymphocytes."
5. "HIV and AIDS treatment has progressed so that these conditions are no longer a concern."

4. The nurse caring for a population of patients diagnosed with HIV/AIDS is aware that, to decrease the incidence of opportunistic infections, care may involve which of the following? (select all that apply)

1. Providing subjective assessment to promote the early detection of infection within any body region
2. Using prophylactic antibiotics to prevent the development of infection
3. Having health care providers and family members wash hands before and after patient contact to reduce the risk of opportunistic infection cross-contamination
4. Encouraging hydration and maintenance of weight to support the immune system
5. Offering a regular review of safe sex practices and ensuring that condom use is consistent and correct

5. The nurse explains to a student that if a patient has formed antibodies against pollen, this process is referred to as:

1. hypersensitivity.
2. sensitization.
3. autoimmunity.
4. anaphylaxis.

6. A patient asks the nurse for advice about treating seasonal allergies. What action should the nurse take?

1. Tell the patient that he should use only medications that require a prescription to treat allergy symptoms.
2. Tell the patient that he shouldn't drive while on allergy medications.
3. Inform the patient that insurance will not cover any medication for allergy symptom treatment.
4. Review the patient's chart for his medical history and current medication list.

Answers to NCLEX Practice Questions can be found in Appendix D in the Osborn Student Resources at nursing.pearsonhighered.com. Practice additional NCLEX questions online at the Student Resources site.

Pearson Nursing Student Resources Find additional review materials at: **nursing.pearsonhighered.com**

REFERENCES

Adams, M., & Koch, R. W. (2010). *Pharmacology connections for nursing practice.* Upper Saddle River, NJ: Pearson.

American College of Allergy, Asthma and Immunology. (2011a). Be S.A.F.E.: Managing allergic emergencies. Retrieved from http://www.acaai.org/patients/resources/anaphylaxis/managing-allergic-emergencies/Documents/BeSAFEBrochure.pdf

American College of Allergy, Asthma and Immunology. (2011b). Latex allergy. Retrieved from http://www.acaai.org/allergist/allergies/Types/latex-allergy/Pages/default.aspx

American Dietetic Association (ADA). (2010). Position of the American Dietetic Association: Nutrition intervention and human immunodeficiency virus infection. *Journal of the American Dietetic Association, 110*(7), 1105–1119.

American Nurses Association. (2011). Position statement: AIDS/HIV disease and socio-culturally diverse populations. Retrieved from http://nursingworld.org

Asthma and Allergy Foundation of America. (2011). Allergy facts and figures. Retrieved from http://www.aafa.org/display.cfm?id=9&sub=30#prev

Bartlett, J. G., & Lane, H. C. (2007). Guidelines for the use of antiretroviral agents in HIV-1-infected adults and adolescents. Developed by the DHHS Panel on Antiretroviral Guidelines for Adults and Adolescents—A working group of the Office of AIDS Research Advisory Council. Retrieved from http://aidsinfo.nih.gov/contentfiles/AdultandAdolescentGL.pdf

Bennett, N. J. (2011). *Pneumocystis* (*carinii*) *jiroveci* pneumonia. Medscape. Retrieved from http://emedicine.medscape.com/article/225976-overview

Carpenito-Moyet, L. (2008). *Nursing care plans and documentation* (5th ed.). Philadelphia: Lippincott Williams & Wilkins.

Centers for Disease Control and Prevention (CDC). (1981a). Opportunistic infections and Kaposi's sarcoma in homosexual men. *Morbidity and Mortality Weekly Report, 30.* Retrieved from http://aids-info.net/micha/hiv/aids/cdc81.htm

Centers for Disease Control and Prevention (CDC). (1981b). Pneumocystis pneumonia—Los Angeles. *Morbidity and Mortality Weekly Report, 30,* 250. Retrieved from http://aids-info.net/micha/hiv/aids/cdc81.htm

Centers for Disease Control and Prevention (CDC). (2010a). HIV in the United States. Retrieved from http://www.cdc.gov/hiv/resources/factsheets/PDF/us.pdf

Centers for Disease Control and Prevention (CDC). (2010b). Sexually transmitted diseases treatment guidelines 2010. *Morbidity and Mortality Weekly Report, 59,* 1–109.

Centers for Disease Control and Prevention (CDC). (2010c). Sexually transmitted diseases guidelines, 2010. Retrieved from http://www.cdc.gov/std/treatment/2010/hepC.htm

Centers for Disease Control and Prevention (CDC). (2011a). Asthma. Retrieved from http://www.cdc.gov/asthma/faqs.htm

Centers for Disease Control and Prevention (CDC). (2011b). HIV-2 surveillance—United States, 1987–2009. *Morbidity and Mortality Weekly Report, 60*(29), 985–988. Retrieved from http://www.cdc.gov/hiv/resources/brochures/at-risk.htm

Centers for Disease Control and Prevention (CDC). (2011c). How is HIV passed from one person to another? Retrieved from http://www.cdc.gov/hiv/resources/qa/transmission.htm

Centers for Disease Control and Prevention (CDC). (2011d). Implementation of routine HIV testing in community health settings: Issues for community health centers. Retrieved from http://www.cdc.gov/hiv/topics/testing/resources/guidelines/pdf/routineHIVtesting.pdf

Centers for Disease Control and Prevention (CDC). (2011e). Interim guidance: Preexposure prophylaxis for the prevention of HIV infection in men who have sex with men. *Morbidity and Mortality Weekly Report, 60*(3), 65–68.

Centers for Disease Control and Prevention (CDC). (2011f). Occupational HIV transmission and prevention among health care workers. Retrieved from http://www.cdc.gov/hiv/resources/qa/transmission.htm

Centers for Disease Control and Prevention (CDC). (2011g). TB and HIV coinfection. Retrieved from http://www.cdc.gov/tb/topic/TBHIVcoinfection/default.htm

DeFranco, A. L., Locksley, R., & Robertson, M. (2007). *Immunity: The immune response in infectious and inflammatory disease.* Sunderland, MA: Sinauer Associates.

Dunne, M., & Ledeboer, N. (2009). Mechanisms of infectious disease. In C. M. Porth & G. Matfin (Eds.), *Pathophysiology: Concepts of altered health status* (8th ed., pp. 324–346). Philadelphia: Wolters Kluwer Health/Lippincott Williams & Wilkins.

Faulhaber, J., & Aberg, J. A. (2009). Acquired immunodeficiency syndrome. In C. M. Porth & G. Matfin (Eds.), *Pathophysiology: Concepts of altered health status* (8th ed., pp. 427–447). Philadelphia: Wolters Kluwer Health/Lippincott Williams & Wilkins.

Finkelman, F. D. (2010). Peanut allergy and anaphylaxis. *Current Opinions in Immunology, 22*(6), 783–788.

Friday, R. P., Trucco, M., & Pietropaola, M. (2010). Genetics of type 1 diabetes mellitus. *Diabetes, Nutrition & Metabolism, 12,* 3–26.

Hirai, K., Komura, K., Tokoro, A., Kuromaru, T., Ohshima, A., Ito, T., et al. (2008). Psychological and behavioral mechanisms influencing the use of complementary and alternative medicine (CAM) in cancer patients. *Annals of Oncology, 19*(1), 49–55. Epub 2007 Oct 26.

Holloway, J. W., Yang, I. A., & Holgate, S. T. (2010). Genetics of allergic disease. *Journal of Allergy and Clinical Immunology, 125*(2), S81–S94.

Hung, S. W. (2009). Disorders of motor function. In C. M. Porth & G. Matfin (Eds.), *Pathophysiology: Concepts of altered health states* (8th ed., pp. 1260–1298). Philadelphia: Wolters Kluwer/Lippincott Williams & Wilkins.

Institute of Medicine (IOM). (2010). *The future of nursing: Leading change, advancing health.* Washington, DC: The Academic Press.

Kang, Y., & Crogan, N. L. (2009). An evidence-based review of infectious diseases. *Geriatric Nursing, 30,* 272–286.

Lefever-Kee, J. (2010). *Laboratory and diagnostic tests: Nursing implications* (8th ed.). Upper Saddle River, NJ: Pearson.

Marcason, W. (2011). What are the current guidelines for diagnosing food allergies? *Journal of the American Dietetic Association,* doi:10.1016/j.jada.2011.01.025.

McFadden, K. L., Hernández, T. D., & Ito, T. A. (2010). Attitudes toward complementary and alternative medicine influence its use. *Explore (NY), 6*(6), 380–388.

National Institute of Arthritis and Musculoskeletal and Skin Diseases (NIAMSD). (2009). Handout on health: Systemic lupus erythematosus. Retrieved from http://www.niams.nih.gov/Health_Info/Lupus/default.asp

National Institute for Occupational Safety and Health (NIOSH). (2011). *Latex allergy: A prevention guide* (NIOSH Publication No. 98-113). Retrieved from http://www.cdc.gov/niosh/topics/latex/

Otto, C., Bischof, G., Rumpf, H. J., Meyer, C., Hapke, U., & John, U. (2011). Multiple dimensions of Health Locus of Control in a representative population sample: Ordinal factor analysis and cross-validation of an existing three and a new four factor model. *BMC Medical Research Methodology, 11,* 114.

Porth, C (2009). Disorders in immune response. In C. M. Porth & G. Matfin (Eds.), *Pathophysiology: Concepts of altered health states* (8th ed., pp. 400–426). Philadelphia: Wolters Kluwer/Lippincott Williams & Wilkins.

Porth, C., & Sweeney, K. (2007). Alterations in immune response. In C. M. Porth (Ed.), *Essentials of pathophysiology* (pp. 293–319). Philadelphia: Lippincott Williams & Wilkins.

Rote, N. (2010). Alterations in immunity and inflammation. In K. L. McCance & S. E. Heuther (Eds.), *Pathophysiology: The biological basis for disease in adults and children* (6th ed., pp. 256–292). St. Louis: Mosby.

Rote, N., & Huether, S. E. (2010). Infection. In K. L. McCance & S. E. Heuther (Eds.), *Pathophysiology: The biological basis for disease in adults and children* (6th ed., pp. 293–335). St. Louis: Mosby.

Rotter, J. B. (1954). *Social learning theory and clinical psychology.* New York: Prentice Hall.

Rotter, J. B. (1982). *The development and application of social learning theory. Selected Papers.* New York: Praeger.

Seibert, D. C. (2010). Genetics and disease prevention: Complementary and contradictory? *Journal for Nurse Practitioners, 6,* 507–516.

Simons, F., & Camargo, C. (2011). Anaphylaxis: Rapid recognition and treatment. *Up-to-Date.* Retrieved from http://www.uptodate.com

Sommer, C. (2009). Innate and adaptive immunity. In C. M. Porth & G. Matfin (Eds.), *Pathophysiology: Concepts of altered health states* (8th ed., pp. 347–376). Philadelphia: Wolters Kluwer/Lippincott Williams & Wilkins.

Stein, R., Grimes, T. S., Malow, R., Stratford, D., Spielberg, F., Holtgrave, D.R. (2011). Introduction to special supplement. Monitoring and evaluation of HIV counseling, testing and referral (CTR) and HIV testing services. *AIDS Education and Prevention.* Jun;23(3 Suppl):1-6.

United Nations Program on HIV/AIDS (UNAIDS). (2011). Report on the global AIDS epidemic: Executive summary. Retrieved from http://www.unaids.org/globalreport/Global_report.htm

Vance, D. E. (2011). Aging with HIV: A cross-sectional study of comorbidity prevalence and clinical characteristics across decades of life. *Journal of the Association of Nurses AIDS Care, 22*(1), 17–25.

Wilkinson, J. M., & Ahearn, N. R. (2009). *Prentice Hall nursing diagnosis handbook* (9th ed.). Upper Saddle River, NJ: Prentice Hall.

Williams, B., Amico, K. R., & Konkle-Parker, D. (2011). Qualitative assessment of barriers and facilitators to HIV treatment. *Journal of the Association of Nurses in AIDS Care, 22*(2), 307–312.

World Allergy Organization. (2011). White book on allergy. Retrieved from http://www.worldallergy.org/UserFiles/file/WAO-White-Book-on-Allergy_FINAL.pdf

Caring for the Patient with Inflammatory Response, Shock, and Severe Sepsis

54 CHAPTER

Renée Holleran

Outcome-Based Learning Objectives

After studying this chapter, the learner will be able to:

1. Compare and contrast the etiologies of anaphylactic, cardiogenic, hypovolemic, neurogenic, and septic shock.
2. Describe the cellular alterations that occur in shock.
3. Identify the factors that place a patient at risk of developing shock.
4. Generate a plan for the emergency care of the patient in shock including identification of the underlying cause; management of the patient's airway, breathing, and circulation; and listing appropriate pharmacologic interventions.
5. Generate a plan for the acute care of the patient in shock, including oxygen management, circulatory management, nutritional management, skin care, and pain and sedation management.
6. Compare and contrast systemic inflammatory response syndrome (SIRS), sepsis, and severe sepsis based on the definitions used by the American College of Chest Physicians/Society of Critical Care Medicine.
7. Prioritize the treatment of the patient with SIRS and identify strategies to prevent the development of SIRS.
8. Differentiate the etiologies, epidemiology, and management of organ dysfunction as an end result of shock and severe sepsis; prioritize the treatment of the patient with organ dysfunction; and identify strategies to prevent its development.

KEY TERMS

afterload p.1674
end-organ perfusion p.1678
insulin resistance (IR) p.1673
ischemia-reperfusion injury p.1675
multiple organ dysfunction syndrome (MODS) p.1689
organ dysfunction p.1671
PIRO model p.1672
protein C p.1685
sepsis p.1672
septic shock p.1672
severe sepsis p.1681
shock p.1671
systemic inflammatory response syndrome (SIRS) p.1672
systemic vascular resistance (SVR) p.1673

Shock

SHOCK HAS BEEN DESCRIBED as the "rude unhinging" of the machinery of life. **Shock** in and of itself is not a disease but a clinical manifestation of the body's inability to perfuse tissues adequately (Cheek, Martin, & Morris, 2010; Holleran, 2010). Shock has multiple etiologies, including alterations in the circulating volume of blood or plasma in the body, alterations in the heart's capability to pump, and alterations in peripheral vascular resistance. Regardless of the cause of shock, the systemic response is harmful and often leads to multiple **organ dysfunction** (altered organ function in a critically ill patient) and death. It is important to have an understanding of the causes of shock so that it can be prevented or, if it occurs, can be rapidly recognized to prevent life-threatening complications.

Epidemiology

Defining shock and how to treat it did not really begin until the late 19th and early 20th centuries. During World War I, surgeons and physiologists thought that a toxin was released from traumatized tissues that caused shock. In 1964, shock was diagnosed when the patient had acute circulatory insufficiency and thus a cardiac output that was inadequate to provide perfusion to major organs. Nurses and health care providers waited for specific clinical manifestations such as a systolic

Video*: Shock

blood pressure less than 90 mmHg or an increase in heart rate before shock management began. Research was conducted to see how much volume must be lost before the patient was considered to be in "shock." Shock was looked at in pieces instead of as a systemic response to a particular insult to the body whether from an injury, disease, or infection (Grenvik, Ayres, Holbrook, & Shoemaker, 2000).

In recent years, the traditional definition and management of shock have been challenged. In 1992 and again in 2003, the American College of Chest Physicians and Society of Critical Care Medicine developed a consensus definition for **sepsis** (the body's response to infection) and multiple organ failure. One of these definitions described **systemic inflammatory response syndrome (SIRS),** a systemic response of the immune system that can be triggered by both infectious and noninfectious causes. Although SIRS was originally associated with sepsis, other researchers, particularly those who dealt with critically injured patients, recognized that SIRS is probably the first phase of shock (Vincent, Martinez, & Silva, 2011).

Despite the consensus on the definitions of SIRS and sepsis, confusion remains about when a patient may be septic and require care. What is important is to be able to recognize patients at greatest risk as quickly as possible so that the most appropriate care can be provided. The **PIRO model** has been developed to predict mortality in patients who are septic. The components of the PIRO model are as follows:

- P: predisposing factors
- I: infection
- R: response
- O: organ dysfunction.

Nearly 20% of all patients admitted to ICUs are diagnosed with severe sepsis, and sepsis remains the leading cause of death in noncardiac ICUs (Levy et al., 2010). Risk factors such as age, preexisting illness, and inappropriate antibiotic use can increase the risk of death from sepsis (Levy et al., 2010). These risk factors are explained in more detail on page 1676.

Etiology

The etiologies of shock have been classified in various ways. The most common classification is according to the cause of the shock syndrome; for example, sepsis from infection is referred to as **septic shock** (Cheek, Martin, & Morris, 2010). Another classification is related to the amount of circulating volume in the body and how it is affected by the shock syndrome, for example, low-volume shock, also known as absolute hypovolemia (Barkman & Pooler, 2009; Holleran, 2010). This classification system is outlined in Chart 54–1. The following subsections describe the etiology of shock based on the cause.

Anaphylactic Shock

Anaphylactic shock results from an antigen–antibody reaction. The body becomes hypersensitive to a specific agent such as a medication. When this happens, vasodilation of blood vessels occurs, causing pooling of blood. Because the blood has pooled in the periphery, perfusion to the tissues is markedly diminished or absent. In addition, other body systems will react to the toxin (for example, an antigen). In particular, the pulmonary system will respond with vasoconstriction, causing respiratory distress and the potential for respiratory arrest (Cheek et al., 2010). Chart 54–2 lists the causes of anaphylactic shock. Chapter 53 includes a more detailed discussion of anaphylaxis.

CHART 54–1 Shock Syndromes

Shock Syndrome	Etiology
Low-volume shock (absolute hypovolemia)	Major loss of blood or circulating body fluid such as plasma.
High-space shock (relative hypovolemia or distributive shock)	Injury or toxin affects the blood vessels, which results in the redistribution of blood and fluid. For example, in spinal shock, damage to the sympathetic nervous system causes vasodilation and alteration in blood distribution.
Mechanical (obstructive) shock	A condition that slows or obstructs blood flow into or out of the heart. Examples include cardiac tamponade, tension pneumothorax, and vena cava obstruction.

Cardiogenic Shock

When the heart is unable to pump effectively, cardiac output drops to such an extent that cardiogenic shock occurs. Myocardial infarction is one of the most common causes of damage to the heart; this damage may cripple the heart's ability to function and eventually cause cardiogenic shock. The incidence of cardiogenic shock is near 7% in ST-segment elevation myocardial infarction (STEMI) and has remained constant for the last 20 years (Vis, Piek, & Henriques 2011). Refer to Chapter 32 for a detailed description of STEMI. Despite advances in technological care, the mortality rate of cardiogenic shock remains high. Chart 54–2 lists causes of cardiogenic shock.

Hypovolemic Shock

Hypovolemic shock results from significant fluid loss that alters the amount of circulating volume in the body. Fluid loss can be loss of blood, plasma, or other body fluids. Hemorrhagic shock, which involves loss of blood, is the most common type of shock encountered when a person has suffered multiple system traumas. Hemorrhagic shock can also be the result of upper and lower gastrointestinal bleeding, ruptured aortic aneurysm, hemorrhagic pancreatitis, gunshot or stab wounds, and pelvic and long-bone fractures. Fluid loss that is not hemorrhagic can be caused by diarrhea, vomiting, and inadequate replacement of fluid lost because of heat stroke, burn wounds, and "third spacing," or leaking of plasma into the interstitial space, which can occur with intestinal obstruction, pancreatitis, and cirrhosis. Chapter 61 discusses "third spacing" of fluid.

The loss of intravascular volume causes a reduction in preload. *Preload* refers to the force that stretches the ventricles to an initial length. The resting force on the heart is determined by pressure in the ventricles at the end of diastole. Factors that affect preload are the volume of blood in the ventricle at the end of diastole, cardiac output, and venous vascular resistance (Holleran, 2010). If any of these factors are inadequate, it affects the amount of blood returning to the circulation. When blood is lost or is unavailable because of sequestration, the ability to carry oxygen to the cells is also lost because of the decrease in hemoglobin. Chapter 31 includes a discussion of preload. Chart 54–2 contains a summary of the most common causes of hypovolemic shock.

Neurogenic Shock

Neurogenic shock results from an imbalance between the sympathetic and parasympathetic stimulation of vascular smooth muscle, which results in vasodilation. The body's circulating blood volume generally remains unchanged. However, injury or medications that affect the spinal cord or medulla will cause an imbalance between the sympathetic

CHART 54–2 Causes of Specific Shock Syndromes

Shock Syndrome	Causes
Anaphylactic shock	Insect bites
	Medication allergies
	Food allergies
	Latex allergies
	Idiopathic reactions
Cardiogenic shock	Myocardial infarction
	Myocardial contusion
	Ruptured ventricles
	Ruptured papillary muscles
	Cardiomyopathy
Hypovolemic shock	Traumatic injury (abdominal trauma, chest trauma, orthopedic trauma)
	Gastrointestinal bleeding
	Vomiting and diarrhea
	Osmotic diuresis
	Diabetic ketoacidosis
	Thermal injuries
Neurogenic shock	Spinal cord or medulla trauma
	Anesthetic agents
	Severe emotional stress
	Severe pain
Septic shock	Bacterial infections
	Viral infections
	Immunosuppression
	Technology (indwelling urinary or intravenous catheters, feeding tubes)
	Antibiotic misuse

and parasympathetic nervous systems. Because of this imbalance, clinical symptoms usually associated with shock may not occur in neurogenic shock. For example, the patient may be hypotensive but not tachycardic. Chart 54–2 contains a list of the causes of neurogenic shock. Chapter 24 includes an in-depth discussion of spinal cord injuries and neurogenic shock.

Septic Shock

Sepsis is the body's response to infection. *Septic shock* is defined as severe sepsis refractory (does not respond to the usual medical management) hypotension or hypotension that does not respond to resuscitation and alterations in organ perfusion (Cheek et al., 2010; Guthrie-Chu, 2009). Impaired perfusion will cause lactic acidosis, oliguria, and alterations in mental status. Septic shock occurs when an infectious agent or infection-induced mediator causes systemic decompensation. Because of the body's response to the vasoactive mediators, there is decreased **systemic vascular resistance (SVR)** (arterial systolic pressure; normal SVR is 900 to 1,400 dyn•s/cm^5), as well as maldistribution of the blood into the microcirculation, causing compromised tissue perfusion and cellular dysfunction (Cheek et al., 2010; Guthrie-Chu, 2009). Chapter 31 includes a detailed discussion of SVR. Despite advances in antibiotic and antiviral therapies, the number of cases of septic shock, particularly in hospitals, continues to rise. The mortality rate from septic shock is about 50% and increases when the patient has comorbid risk factors such as immunosuppression, age, or preexisting diseases such as diabetes (Vincent et al., 2011). Chart 54–2 outlines the causes of septic shock.

In summary, multiple etiologies may place the patient at risk for developing shock. It is important for the nurse to be cognizant of any or all of these when a patient presents with symptoms that may indicate the initiation of the "rude unhinging of the machinery of life." Critical interventions must begin as early as possible to prevent irreversible shock leading to death.

Weblink: Septic Shock

Safety Alert *The primary treatment for all shock syndromes is early recognition of factors that may place the patient at risk for developing shock. Be aware of specific risk factors that can cause particular shock syndromes. For example, a patient with an indwelling urinary catheter is at risk for becoming septic; the sepsis can then predispose the patient to septic shock.*

Pathophysiology

Shock is a syndrome that results from inadequate tissue perfusion. As was previously discussed, shock has multiple causes that produce alterations in circulating volume, alterations in cardiac pump function, or alterations in peripheral vascular resistance, leading to impairment of cellular metabolism. This results in impaired oxygen use and impaired glucose use.

Oxygen consumption is an expression of the rate at which oxygen is used by tissues, usually given in microliters of oxygen consumed in 1 hour by 1 milligram dry weight of tissue.

Shock leads to an imbalance in electrolytes and water. As a response to the metabolic changes that are triggered, sodium moves intracellularly, causing water to follow and potassium to exit the cell, thereby altering nervous, cardiovascular, and muscular cell function. These systems then become impaired. Additionally, water is drawn from the vascular space to compensate for water drawn into the cells, further reducing circulating blood volume. Cells will shift from aerobic to anaerobic metabolism to compensate for oxygen loss. This causes metabolic acidosis, which affects enzyme activities and cellular functions such as repair and division. Cellular damage causes enzymes to be released, which will destroy noninjured cells.

Glucose metabolism is impaired in a manner similar to that of oxygen metabolism. The result is insulin resistance. This phenomenon has been observed in patients with sepsis and those who are critically ill or injured. The stress response that is initiated by an illness or injury triggers gluconeogenesis to supply glucose energy to assist in healing. The liver and kidneys produce more glucose in response to epinephrine, norepinephrine, glucagons, and cortisol, which are part of the body's stress response (Mizouk, 2009). **Insulin resistance (IR)** has been described as unresponsiveness of anabolic processes to the normal effects of insulin and possibly tissue insensitivity to insulin. The severity of IR is thought to be the result of an increased production of serum cytokines (Ball, de Beer, Gomm, Hickman, & Collins, 2007; Mizouk, 2009). Insulin resistance and glucose toxicity impair cellular growth and metabolic processes. In addition, IR has been associated with multiple organ failure, nosocomial infections, and renal injury (Ball et al., 2007; Mizouk, 2009).

Overall, the pathophysiology of shock has a profound effect on all of the body systems. This is well illustrated in Figure 54–1◆. Because of inadequate tissue perfusion, the body turns to anaerobic metabolism to produce energy. In addition, other pathophysiological pathways are initiated that affect all body systems because of the release of toxins as well as the body's inability to manage these toxins effectively. Ultimately,

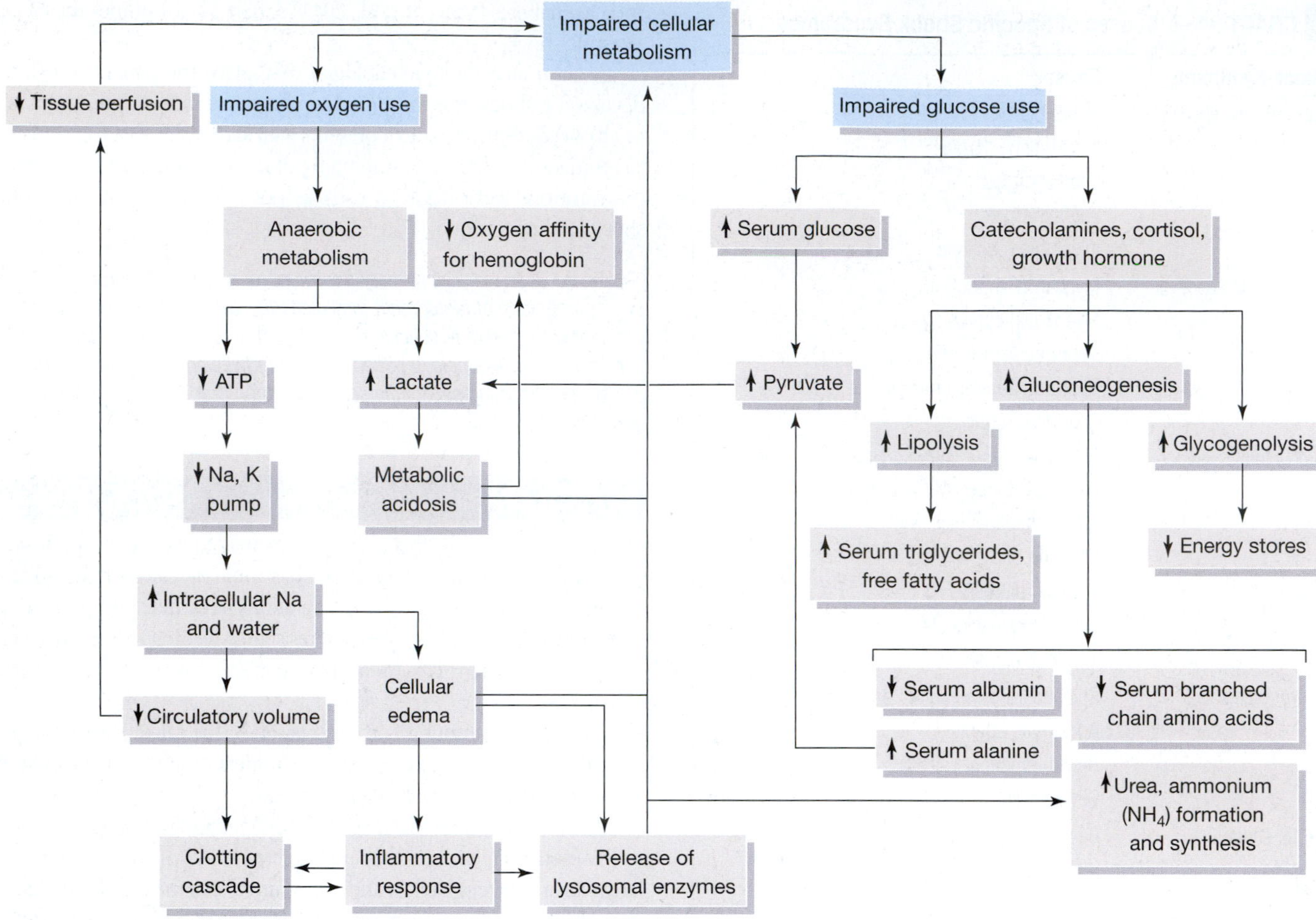

FIGURE 54–1 ◆ A network of cascading events in response to inflammation.

if the anaerobic state is not corrected, the toxins will cause multiple organ failure and death.

As previously discussed and as illustrated in Figure 54–1, inadequate perfusion and a reduction in available oxygen will trigger cellular and systemic responses. Alteration in cellular metabolism causes alteration in ATP production, failure of the sodium–potassium pump, redistribution of cellular ions, and interstitial fluid shifts. Blebs (small blisters) develop on cell walls and eventually rupture, releasing cellular enzymes and causing further damage to other cells.

Research continues to demonstrate that specific triggers such as infection, illness, and injury trigger a systemic inflammatory response syndrome (Barkman & Pooler, 2009; Levy et al., 2010). In response, the immune system activates a complement cascade system that causes macrophages to respond. When macrophages respond to an "insult," they cause the release of substances that contribute to platelet aggregation, causing clot formation, which "plugs" the vessel and at times causes vasodilation. Examples of these substances include cytokines, thromboxane, prostaglandins, and a slow-reacting substance of anaphylaxis. The end result is further tissue damage due to inadequate perfusion.

The brain is dependent on both oxygen and glucose. When either of these substrates is not available to the brain in sufficient amounts, an alteration in cerebral perfusion occurs. The patient will display an altered mental status, which may progress to coma and death.

Cardiac output declines because of an alteration in both preload and afterload. **Afterload** is the initial resistance that the ventricles must overcome to develop enough force to open the semilunar valves and propel the blood into the systemic and pulmonary systems. In addition, specific toxins such as myocardial depressant factor are released from damaged cardiac cells and a hypoperfused pancreas, causing further myocardial dysfunction and hypoxia. Ultimately, these factors can lead to cardiac dysrhythmia and acute lung injury.

Urinary output decreases because of the shift of sodium, which pulls water into the cells to conserve fluid. Decreased blood flow to the kidneys impairs their ability to detoxify the substances that result from anaerobic metabolism. Inadequate blood flow to the gastrointestinal (GI) tract causes the activation of circulating neutrophils that provoke multiple organ failure. The integumentary system responds by diverting blood from the skin. Pale, fragile skin affords little protection and places the patient at risk for hypothermia and further system disruptions.

A change in blood flow to the vital organs (brain, heart, and kidneys) triggers baroreceptors to release catecholamines, thus increasing the heart rate and cardiac output and causing further vasoconstriction and tissue injury. See Chapter 35 for an explanation of the normal regulation of blood pressure. Skeletal muscle, which is a major reservoir of amino acids, begins to break down and release acids, resulting in muscle weakness and wasting.

The "unhinging of the machinery of life" continues until it causes irreversible changes and eventual death. What is unfortunate is that many of the interventions used for the treatment of shock actually contribute to the development of further complications such as third spacing, ischemia-reperfusion injury, ventilator-associated pneumonia (VAP), multiple organ dysfunction syndrome (MODS), and in some cases death. VAP is the second most common hospital-acquired infection among patients who are mechanically ventilated (Cunha & Bronze, 2011).

Ischemia-reperfusion injury is a multifactorial process that occurs when anaerobic metabolism is initiated by hypoperfusion and hypoxia that leads to an oxygen deficit in endothelial, parenchymal, or immune competent cells (Krau, 2007). The energy deficit that results from prolonged ischemia can lead to irreversible tissue damage through apoptosis or necrosis of parenchymal cells. Reperfusion can also cause secondary tissue damage and organ dysfunction.

During the reperfusion phase, superoxide anions are generated from available oxygen. Superoxide anions are further reduced to hydrogen peroxide and hydroxyl ions, referred to as free oxygen radicals. These free oxygen radicals induce lipid peroxidation, membrane disintegration, and DNA damage, causing apoptosis and necrosis of endothelial, parenchymal, and immune cells (Mizouk, 2009). Ischemia-reperfusion injury is one of the major triggers of MODS (Krau, 2007).

Because of the serious and widespread effects of any shock syndrome, early recognition of symptoms and appropriate interventions are the primary management strategies for shock (Cheek et al., 2010; Holleran, 2010).

Medical Management

The assessment of the patient who may be in shock must include a high index of suspicion because the body's initial ability to compensate may mask the clinical signs of shock. Patient risk factors such as significant injuries, catastrophic illness, age, and allergies must be quickly acknowledged. It is interesting that the very young and the aged have similar risk factors for developing shock, including compromised immune systems due to age; fluid shifts; and an integumentary system that may not afford needed protection. Inadequate tissue perfusion and hypoxia will manifest itself in a variety of ways, as summarized in Chart 54–3.

Safety Alert *Even though some specific clinical manifestations, such as hypotension and tachycardia, are associated with shock, physical fitness, preexisting illness, certain injuries (e.g., spinal cord trauma), and medications (e.g., beta-blockers) can mask the anticipated symptoms.*

The Emergency Period of Shock Care

The emergency period of care for the patient in shock begins as soon as the risk for shock has been identified. The primary goal of shock management is to identify the cause and intervene to prevent the pathophysiology that results from ischemic and anoxic cell injury (Campbell, 2008; Holleran, 2010). The patient's care will be directed at identifying and correcting the cause of the shock, maintaining oxygen perfusion, controlling active bleeding, supporting the patient's circulatory status, maintaining the patient's body temperature, managing pain, and providing emotional support.

Prehospital Care and Transport

Patients who are in shock have been identified as being in "load and go situations," which means that they must be transported as quickly as possible to the nearest hospital (Campbell, 2008; National Association of Emergency Medical Technicians [NAEMT], 2011). The prehospital care provider needs to focus on the critical interventions that need to be performed to save the patient's life while preparing for and initiating rapid transport (Figure 54–2◆). A brief primary assessment includes evaluating the patient's ABCDE: A = airway with cervical spine protection if trauma is suspected, B = breathing, C = circulation, D = disability, and performing E = exposure and environmental management.

CHART 54–3 Clinical Manifestation of Inadequate Tissue Perfusion and Hypoxia

System	Clinical Manifestation
Neurological	Altered mental status
	Irritability
	Seizures from hypoxia
	Coma.
Pulmonary	Increased respirations
	Crackles from fluid shifts
	Decreased oxygen saturation despite an increase in oxygen administration.
Cardiovascular	Increased heart rate
	Decreased or absent peripheral pulses
	Cardiac dysrhythmia.
Gastrointestinal	Nausea and vomiting
	Absent bowel sounds.
Genitourinary	Decreased urinary output
	Increased specific gravity.
Integumentary	Cool clammy skin
	Mottling
	Cyanosis
	Development of decubitus ulcers.
Musculoskeletal	Generalized weakness
	Wasting
	Inability to wean from ventilator due to muscle wasting.

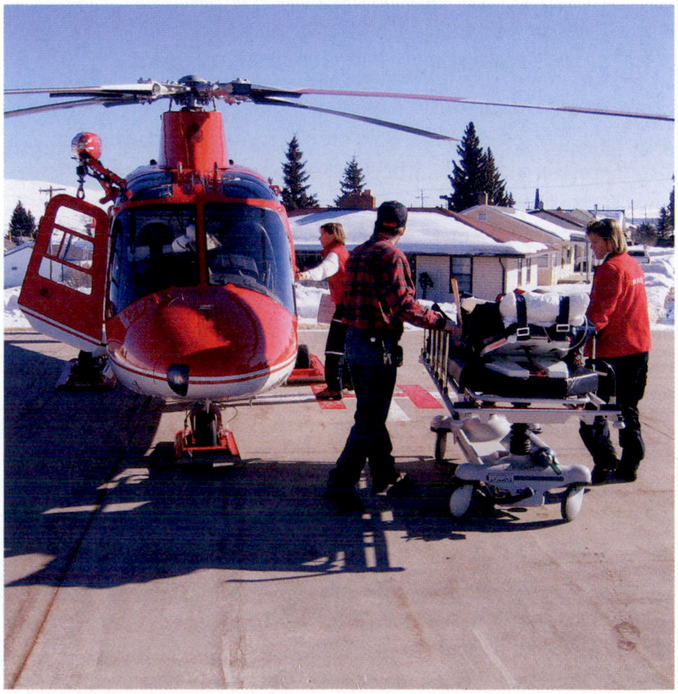

FIGURE 54–2 ◆ Rapid transport for a patient in shock.
Source: Renee Holleran

CHART 54–4 Indications and Contraindications for the Use of Pneumatic Antishock Garments with Shock

Indications	Contraindications
Suspected pelvic fractures with hypotension	Penetrating thoracic trauma
Profound hypotension (systolic blood pressure less than 60 mmHg)	Stabilization of an isolated lower extremity fracture
Suspected intraperitoneal hemorrhage	Evisceration of abdominal organs
Suspected retroperitoneal hemorrhage	Impaled objects in the abdomen
	Pregnant abdomen
	Traumatic arrest

Only critical interventions such as airway management should be executed before transport. Additional interventions such as obtaining intravenous (IV) access, immobilization measures (such as the application of a traction splint), warming the patient, and performing a secondary assessment should be accomplished during transport (Campbell, 2008; NAEMT, 2011). Chapter 67 discusses the rapid primary and secondary assessments for the patient at risk for shock.

If an active source of blood or fluid loss is identified, it should be managed as much as possible before and during transport. (Fluid resuscitation is discussed in the next section, p. 1678.) Pelvic and long-bone fractures may result in loss of large volumes of blood. Chart 54–4 contains a summary of the indications and contraindications for use of PASGs in the prehospital setting (Campbell, 2008; NAEMT, 2011).

In summary, the prehospital care of the patient in shock involves early recognition of the risk of shock and rapid transport of the patient to definitive care. The health care provider should perform a primary assessment and initiate critical interventions. There should be no additional delays in getting the patient to a center that can provide appropriate and lifesaving care.

Safety Alert *The patient in shock should be rapidly transported to a facility that can provide definitive care. For example, a trauma patient in shock should be transported to a trauma center when possible.*

Emergency Department Care

The care of the patient in shock in the emergency department demands a collaborative approach. It begins with performing a primary assessment and initiating critical interventions to support the patient's airway, breathing, and circulation (ABC). Interventions that were performed in the prehospital environment need to be reevaluated and considered in resuscitating the patient; for example, it is important to determine how much fluid the patient received during transport. A secondary assessment is then performed, including exposing the patient to identify any obvious signs of illness or injury that may be the source of the shock. An in-depth discussion of the primary and secondary assessments is contained in Chapter 67. The Risk Factors box contains a summary of the most common risk factors for the development of shock.

RISK FACTORS for the Development and Source of Shock

Indication	Source of Shock
Active bleeding anywhere on the body	Hemorrhage
Abdominal bruising	
Long-bone deformities	
Open fractures	
Amputations	
"Coffee-ground" emesis	
Penetrating trauma	
Purpura	Sepsis
Rashes	
Decubitus	
Gangrene	
Indwelling urinary catheters	
Indwelling IV ports	
Feeding tubes	
Burns	Hypovolemia
Dehydration	
Hypotension	Neurogenic
Bradycardia	
Spinal cord injury	

The source of the clinical insult needs to be identified immediately. When there is no obvious indication, other pieces of the patient history and risk factors must be considered, such as the patient's age or medications that the patient may have been prescribed. For example, certain medications may place a patient at risk of shock, particularly septic shock. These include medications that cause immunosuppression and antibiotic and antiviral therapies. The pathophysiological changes initiated by the body's response to shock cause the patient to become hypoxic. Therefore, the patient will require airway and ventilatory support. This may be as simple as administering oxygen by a 100% nonrebreather mask or as complex as advanced airway management. A chest radiograph can reveal a possible infection, a source of blood or other fluid loss, or even an obstructive reason for shock such as a cardiac tamponade. Chapter 25 discusses respiratory assessment and management.

The patient's circulatory status needs to be assessed. Peripheral and central pulses should be palpated to determine perfusion. The body will divert blood from the periphery to enhance oxygenation of the brain, heart, and kidneys. The patient's skin will be pale, cold, and clammy. Therefore, the patient will need to be kept warm by increasing the room temperature, covering the patient with warm blankets, or using a commercial device to deliver heat.

A 12-lead ECG should be obtained to rule out myocardial injury as the source of shock. Prolonged ischemia related to hypotension can also place the patient at risk of a myocardial infarction. Chapter 30 discusses the 12-lead ECG, and Chapter 32 discusses myocardial infarction. Blood studies are obtained to provide baseline assessment data, identify the physiological effects of the shock state, identify a source of infection, and evaluate the effects of specific treatments. Blood studies should include complete blood count (CBC) with a differential, serum electrolytes, whole blood glucose, blood urea nitrogen (BUN), serum creatinine, coagulation studies, liver function studies, and lactate levels. For the patient with suspected hemorrhagic shock, a type and screen or type and cross should be obtained.

When sepsis is suspected, specific laboratory tests should be performed to identify the source of the sepsis. Examples are blood cultures, urine cultures, cultures of any suspected wounds or appliances, and cerebrospinal fluid cultures. The Diagnostic Tests for Shock box contains a description of these tests. Additional radiography studies are required for diagnosis and may include computed tomography (CT) scans, magnetic resonance imaging (MRI), and angiography.

DIAGNOSTIC TESTS for Shock

Test with Description, Normal Values, and Rationale	Expected Abnormality
White Blood Cells Total (WBC)	
Adult: 4,500–10,000 µL (mm^3)	Increase in white blood cells.
An increased white blood cell count may indicate a stress response as well as an infection.	
White Blood Cell Differential	
Neutrophils: Adult: 50–70 Segments: Adult: 50–65 Bands: Adults: 0–5	Segments are mature neutrophils and bands are immature neutrophils. Bands increase quickly during an acute infection.
An increase in neutrophils will help differentiate an infection as the cause of the shock.	
Hemoglobin	
Adult: Male: 13.5–18 g/dL Female: 12–15 g/dL	Increased with fluid loss and shock compensation. Decreased with too much fluid or blood loss due to hemorrhage. Resuscitation can cause hemodilution, resulting in a low hemoglobin count.
Adequate hemoglobin is needed to ensure adequate oxygen delivery.	
Platelet Count	
Adult: 150,000–400,000 µL	Increase in number of platelets.
Platelets increase as a stress response.	
Serum Electrolyte Levels	
Sodium: Adult: 135–145 mEq/L Potassium: Adult: 3.5–5.3 mEq/L	Decreased sodium levels. Increased potassium levels.
Movement of sodium into the cell displaces potassium from the cell.	
Glucose (blood)	
Adult: 60–100 mg/dL	Increased blood glucose level.
Glucose metabolism is impaired.	
Blood Urea Nitrogen (BUN)	
Adult: 5–25 mg/dL Can be slightly higher in the older adult.	Increased BUN.
Urea is formed as an end product of protein metabolism and is excreted by the kidneys. An elevated BUN can indicate prerenal failure, renal failure, or dehydration.	
Arterial Blood Gases	
Adult: pH: 7.35–7.45 $PaCO_2$: 35–45 mmHg PaO_2: 75–100 mmHg SaO_2: > 95% SVO_2: > 70% HCO_3: 24–28 mEq/L Base Excess (BE): +2 to −2 mEq/L	Respiratory alkalosis. Metabolic acidosis. Hypoxia.
Increase respirations to blow off CO_2 to decrease metabolic acidosis. *Metabolic acidosis results from anaerobic metabolism.* *Hypoxia results from inadequate tissue perfusion.*	

(continued)

DIAGNOSTIC TESTS for Shock, *continued*

Test with Description, Normal Values, and Rationale	Expected Abnormality
Serum Lactate Levels	
Adult: 0.5–2.0 mmol/L	Elevated levels.
These reflect tissue perfusion. An increased level indicates inadequate tissue perfusion and anaerobic metabolism. A higher lactate level indicates a higher degree of shock and potential for death.	
Partial Thromboplastin (PTT)	
Adult: 60–70 seconds	Prolonged.
PTT occurs due to cellular dysfunction and abnormal clotting cascade. More profound if disseminated intravascular coagulation is present.	
Blood Cultures	
Adult: negative	Presence of bacteria.
Blood cultures should not be used without a good reason. Patients who are febrile, older adults, IV drug abusers, and patients with neutropenia, prosthetic heart valves, or indwelling devices are examples of patients who should have blood cultures drawn.	
Urinalysis	
Color: clear	Presence of bacteria.
Appearance: clear	Protein in the urine is a sensitive indicator of renal dysfunction.
Glucose: negative	
Ketones: negative	
Blood: negative	
Microscopic Examination:	
RBC: 1–2 per low power field	
WBC: 3–4	
Casts: occasional hyaline	
Chest Radiograph	
Adult: normal tissue; no pathologic findings	Presence of pneumonia.
Obtained to identify pneumonia, which may be a source of infection in septic shock. May also demonstrate acute lung injury, which is the result of inadequate perfusion to the lungs in shock.	Presence of ALI.
Computed Tomography (CT)	
Adult: normal tissue; no pathologic finding	Depends on the cause of the shock.
A CT would be performed to identify sources of blood or volume loss.	A CT scan could also identify pockets of pus as sources of potential infection contributing to sepsis and/or septic shock.

Resuscitation

Because shock involves alterations in circulating volume, cardiac function, or peripheral vascular resistance, the primary purposes of circulatory resuscitation are as follows:

- To restore oxygen transport and cellular uptake of oxygen
- To mitigate against oxygen debt accumulation and decrease the use of anaerobic metabolism to supply cellular energy
- To restore preresuscitation oxygen deficit
- To prevent the metabolic derangements that lead to SIRS, MODS, and eventually multiple organ system failure (MOSF). These complications are discussed later in the chapter.

It is important to remember that circulatory resuscitation may involve both volume resuscitation and the use of vasoactive medications to maintain adequate **end-organ perfusion,** the perfusion of the end organs such as the integumentary system.

Large-bore IV lines need to be inserted. Central IV access may be obtained with a catheter that will also allow the insertion of devices for hemodynamic monitoring. It is imperative to ensure that aseptic technique is used to prevent the possibility of introducing infection and increasing the risk of sepsis. Chapter 16 discusses the various types of intravenous catheters and their indications for use.

Fluid Resuscitation

Over the last 30 years, research has challenged the methods once commonly used for fluid resuscitation in shock. Researchers have discovered many pertinent issues that must be considered in resuscitating the patient in shock. First, hypotension may actually be a protective mechanism, especially in the patient who has sustained a penetrating injury or internal trauma. Increasing a patient's blood pressure multiplies the chances that clots that have been formed will dislodge; depending on the resuscitation fluid, increasing the blood pressure also dilutes circulating volume and in turn increases clotting time (Jacobs, 1994; Keel & Trentz, 2005; Kowalenko, Stern, Dronen, & Wang, 1992; Martin, Bicknell, Pepe, Burch, & Mattox, 1992; McSwain et al., 2011; Tisherman, 2010). Chart 54–5 contains a summary of some of the complications of massive fluid resuscitation (Ackerman, 1994; Alexander, 1996; Edelman,

CHART 54–5 Complications of Massive Fluid Resuscitation

Hypothermia
Dilution of clotting factors
- Hypercoagulopathy

Metabolic derangements
- Acidosis
- Hypocalcemia
- Hypomagnesia
- Hypophosphatemia
- Hypokalemia

Organ dysfunction and extravascular fluid shifts
Adult lung injury (ALI)
Sepsis
Acute renal failure
Pneumonia
Ventilator-assisted pneumonia (VAP)
Increased length of stay
Increased mortality.

White, Tyburski, & Wilson, 2007; Fernandes et al., 2007; McSwain et al., 2011; Rueden & Dunham, 1994; Tisherman, 2010).

Fluids that are used for resuscitation include lactated Ringer's solution, normal saline, hypertonic saline, blood, and blood products such as fresh frozen plasma. The type of fluid used will depend on the provider's preference, because the research has not clearly identified one more favorably over the others. The initial amount of fluid will range from 2 to 3 liters for an adult if the cause of the shock is unknown. If the patient has sustained blood loss, then administration of blood and blood products will be needed. Infusion therapy and blood administration are discussed in depth in Chapter 16. It is important to remember that patients who have lost more than 2 liters of blood should not receive excessive fluid resuscitation from either colloids or crystalloids until surgical management of bleeding has been initiated because such treatment dilutes the existing volume and further diminishes the oxygen-carrying capacity. In contrast, a patient who is septic and hypotensive may require early fluid boluses to maintain a systolic blood pressure greater than 90 mmHg (Tisherman, 2010).

Because of the complications of massive fluid resuscitation, as noted in Chart 54–5, the effects of fluid resuscitation must be closely monitored. The nurse should insert a urinary catheter to measure urinary output. Adequate hydration in an adult should yield a urinary output of 30 to 50 mL/hr or 0.4 to 1.0 mL/kg of body weight per hour. Adequate fluid resuscitation is also evaluated by a decrease in heart rate, presence and strength of the patient's central and peripheral pulses, patient's improving level of consciousness, and the return of bowel sounds.

Hemodynamic monitoring can be used to monitor the effectiveness of resuscitation. This may include measuring central venous pressure (CVP) or the insertion of a pulmonary artery catheter (PAC). However, any additional invasive procedures may leave the patient at risk of infection and sepsis (Casserly, Read, & Levy, 2011). An in-depth discussion of the use of hemodynamic monitoring is included in Chapter 31.

Pharmacologic Support

Shock resuscitation may require pharmacologic support. Different medications may be used for different shock states. The purpose of the medication may be to augment blood flow to the brain, heart, and kidneys or to fight the infection that caused the sepsis leading to shock. The medications that are typically used in selected shock states are listed in the Pharmacology box (p. 1688) (Adams & Koch, 2010).

Pain Management

Pain management is often neglected for the patient in shock. Analgesics and sedation agents can cause hypotension and respiratory depression, furthering complications. However, research has adequately demonstrated the consequences of poor pain management, which include increased peripheral vascular resistance, increased consumption of myocardial oxygen, increased metabolic rate, increased levels of circulating stress hormones, hypercoagulability, decreased gastric motility, and hopelessness (Tanabe, Semonin Holleran, & Reddin, 2010). Pain management should never be neglected in providing care for the patient in shock.

Appropriate use of analgesics and sedative agents can only serve to support patients. Chapter 12 provides an in-depth discussion of the assessment and management of pain.

Additional Interventions

Depending on the cause of the shock, other interventions may be indicated. For example, the patient who has suffered a spinal cord injury will need to be appropriately immobilized during transport and in the emergency department. Chart 54–6 contains a summary of additional

CHART 54–6 Additional Interventions for the Management of the Patient in Shock

Shock State	Additional Interventions
Hypovolemic	Direct pressure for active bleeding
	Surgery to control bleeding
	Immobilization of any long bones to decrease bleeding
	Ultrasound of chest and abdomen to discover bleeding
	For the patient with traumatic injury, may perform a FAST (focused abdominal ultrasound for trauma) exam to discover abdominal bleeding
	CT of abdomen or chest
	Endoscopy or colonoscopy to discover blood loss.
Cardiogenic	Obtain cardiac enzymes
	Fibrinolytic therapy
	Angioplasty
	Intra-aortic balloon pump (IABP) insertion.
Neurogenic	Spinal immobilization
	Spinal stabilization using halos or tong devices
	Warming measures to maintain body temperature.
Obstructive	Tension pneumothorax
	• Needle decompression
	• Chest tube insertion.
	Cardiac tamponade
	• Pericardiocentesis
	• Cardiac window.

interventions that may be indicated to manage shock depending on the source of the clinical insult.

Acute Care Period of the Patient in Shock

The unstable patient in shock will generally be admitted to the critical care unit. The care that was initiated will be continued, including support of the patient's oxygenation and circulatory status. Some type of shock monitoring should be established. This may include monitoring of the patient's CVP, pulmonary artery pressure monitoring with PACs, monitoring of oxygen transport and consumption, cardiovascular indices, and respiratory monitoring. Central venous pressure and PACs are discussed in Chapter 31.

The complications related to the body's response to shock pose additional problems in the acute period. Nutritional support is an important intervention during the acute care period for the management of the patient in shock from injury, illness, or infection. This is discussed later in the chapter (also see Chapter 8). Skin care, as well as promoting and maintaining mobility, are important in the acute period. Skin breakdown and immobility can lead to further risk of the development of sepsis. If this occurs, pain management and sedation will be required (see Chapter 12).

In addition, the psychosocial needs of patients and their families must be anticipated and dealt with. Depending on the cause of the shock state and the progression of clinical manifestations, both the patient and the family may have to face death or long-term disabilities. End-of-life issues are discussed in more depth in Chapter 11.

In conclusion, the medical management of the patient in shock is directed at early recognition of the risk factors that threaten the development of shock. Once the clinical manifestations of shock are evident, it is imperative that the source of the clinical insult be found and critical interventions be initiated to prevent the complications that come from impaired cellular and glucose metabolism. Prevention is the primary way to keep patients from suffering the potential irreversible consequences of shock.

Nursing Management

The nursing management of the patient in shock begins with an in-depth assessment of the patient, including identifying any current and past medical history that places the patient at risk for developing shock. Mechanisms of injury that may place the patient at risk for hemorrhagic or hypovolemic shock or an infection should be quickly identified so that the body's systematic compensatory response can be decreased or eliminated. Frequent monitoring and assessment of trend changes in vital signs and clinical manifestations of inadequate tissue perfusion and hypoxia, especially level of consciousness, skin color and temperature, and urinary output, can provide the most reliable information in the early identification of shock.

Once the source of shock or clinical insult has been identified, nursing care is focused on the specific cause. Fluid resuscitation and administration of blood and blood products will be required in the management of a patient in hemorrhagic or hypovolemic shock. This will require careful monitoring of organ perfusion including the presence of peripheral pulses, maintenance of a perfusing blood pressure, and correction of acid–base balance.

Many patients experiencing shock have suffered injuries that limit their mobility and place them at risk for skin breakdown and deep venous thrombosis (DVT). Range-of-motion (ROM) exercises, turning and positioning the patient at least every 2 hours, and meticulous skin care are needed to prevent sources of infection.

Vasopressor medications that may be used to maintain end-organ perfusion will also place the patient at risk for injury to the extremities because of the vasoconstrictive properties of these medications, which markedly diminish blood flow distally. Careful monitoring and early recognition of decreased blood flow can assist in early intervention and prevention.

Emotional and spiritual support of the patient and the family is essential for the patient in shock. If the patient has sustained severe enough injury, death may be imminent; in this situation, the family must be allowed time to be with the patient. End-of-life decisions may need to be made in a limited period of time (see Chapter 11).

Pain management can be very challenging in the shock patient. Hypotension is a common clinical manifestation of inadequate tissue perfusion, and it may impede adequate pain management because of fear that medications will make the patient's symptoms worse. The nurse must play an advocacy role to ensure that the patient's pain and anxiety is sufficiently managed. The Nursing Process: Patient Care Plan box (p. 1682) contains a summary of the nursing care provided for the patient in shock.

Evidence-based practice has suggested some specific guidelines for the resuscitation and management of the patient in shock. The Evidence-Based Practice box contains a summary reviewing some of this evidence.

Collaborative Management

To achieve optimal recovery and return to society, the patient in shock requires a multidisciplinary team that includes prehospital providers, health care providers, nurses, respiratory therapists, pharmacists, social service personnel, physical therapists, and nutritionists. In order to meet desired patient outcomes, it is essential that the members of this interdisciplinary team communicate openly with one another in developing and evaluating care of the patient and family (IOM [Institute of Medicine], 2010). To prevent the complications related to shock and its sequelae, nurses and health care providers must be alert to the risk factors that can contribute to the development of shock. Once the source of shock has been identified, care is directed at managing that source and assisting the body to maintain physiological functions such as cerebral and renal perfusion. This may be done through such interventions as fluid resuscitation or pharmacologic management. Because a patient in a shock state has compromised body systems, the pharmacist's assistance is necessary to ensure that the appropriate medications are correctly prescribed and administered.

The physical therapist helps to maintain a normal range of motion by providing passive and active exercises when the patient is able. Physical therapy is begun as soon as possible to decrease complications such as muscle wasting that can contribute to additional healing problems.

A comprehensive plan for nutrition is important in enhancing healing, regaining strength, and preventing additional complications such as infection. The nutritionist works with the health care team from the time of admission through discharge to ensure proper nutritional support. The primary focus of nutritional support is providing exogenous energy and protein to minimize gluconeogenesis, catabolism (protein oxidation), and the loss of lean tissue associated with injury. Patients in shock are in a hypermetabolic state. This requires nutritional support that prevents malnutrition and its consequences (Cheek et al., 2010). Before nutritional support can be initiated, a nutritional assessment must be completed. This assessment includes the patient's social, medical, and dietary history before the illness, injury, or infection. Additional

EVIDENCE-BASED PRACTICE Management of Bleeding Following Trauma

Clinical Problem

The management of bleeding following trauma to prevent hemorrhagic shock is a serious challenge. Recognition and management of potential sources of bleeding must begin early to prevent the sequelae of shock such as sepsis and organ dysfunction.

Research Findings

Neveleff and Kraiss (2010) developed an evidence-based paper that describes how to improve perioperative hemostasis in the surgical trauma setting. The paper is based on a review of the current evidence related to specific methods used to achieve hemostasis.

Options to achieve hemostasis include the following:

- Topical hemostasis, which falls into four categories:
  - Mechanical hemostats
  - Active hemostats
  - Fibrin sealants.
- Systemic management
  - Administration of vitamin K
  - Reversal of drugs that may increase bleeding such as heparin
  - Administration of fresh frozen plasma
  - Administration of platelets
  - Transfusion
  - Administration of Factor VII.
- Lowering of the patient's body temperature

Implications for Nursing Practice

The paper by Neveleff and Kraiss (2010) provides evidence-based information about local and systemic methods to improve hemostasis in the surgical and trauma settings. First, nurses need to quickly recognize a patient who is at risk of bleeding based on mechanism of injury or medical history, such as a patient who is taking an anticoagulant such as warfarin or aspirin. Ongoing nursing assessment needs to include identification of uncontrolled bleeding and clinical manifestations of hemorrhagic shock such as altered mental status, hypotension, tachycardia, and decreased urinary output. The nurse needs to be familiar with the interventions, both local and systemic, that can be used to achieve hemostasis. The nurse is also responsible for ensuring that these interventions are safely administered; for example, the nurse must check blood and blood products according to institutional policy to prevent any adverse events. The management of hemorrhagic shock requires a collaborative approach by both nursing and health care provider colleagues.

Critical Thinking Questions with answers can be found in the Osborn Student Resources at nursing.pearsonhighered.com.

Source: Neveleff, D., & Kraiss, L. (2010). Implementing methods to improve perioperative hemostasis in the surgical and trauma settings. *AORN Journal, 5*, S1–S15.

factors such as the patient's normal appetite, medications, food allergies, and the use of supplements or special diets must be included in the nutritional assessment. The patient's culture should also be considered. Currently, various prescribed regimes are available to provide nutrition to patients who are severely ill, injured, or septic (Bertolini, Luciani, & Bioli, 2007). Nutrition is discussed further in Chapter 8.

Finally, family dynamics are often affected by prolonged hospitalization and change in role function within the family structure. There are times when end-of-life decisions must be made, and social service personnel will play an important role in supporting the nursing and medical staff with implementing difficult decisions.

Ethical Considerations

Identification of end points in the resuscitation of patients in shock is difficult. Guidelines for futile resuscitation are limited, and the concept of palliative care in the resuscitation of trauma patients is now being proposed. The Ethical Issues box describes ethical issues in the care of the patient in shock.

ETHICAL ISSUES Related to Patients in Shock

Mosenthal and Murphy (2003) first pointed out the need for trauma surgeons to consider the integration of palliative care and trauma care. Two issues in particular make it important to consider incorporating palliative care. First, despite aggressive resuscitation, research continues to demonstrate that 10% to 15% of all trauma patients will die. Others may suffer disabling effects that may greatly diminish their quality of life. Second, a severe injury in the older adult involves a greater risk of death than does a similar injury in a young person. Life-prolonging technology and the availability of health care resources make it mandatory that resuscitation end points and guidelines be developed to ensure that compassionate care is given at the end of life for these patients. This issue continues to challenge all nurses and other health care providers who care for critically injured trauma patients (Toevs, 2011).

Systemic Inflammatory Response, Sepsis, and Severe Sepsis

The year 1991 was the first time the American College of Chest Physicians (ACCP) and the Society of Critical Care Medicine (SCCM) organized a conference to provide a conceptual and practical framework for defining the systemic inflammatory response to infection. The members of this conference developed and introduced definitions of sepsis, SIRS, and septic shock. These groups reconvened in 2001 and 2008 to include additional representation from European intensive care societies (Levy et al., 2010). The guidelines are currently being reviewed again.

Systemic inflammatory response syndrome is an organized immune response that can be triggered by infectious or noninfectious clinical insults including burns, pancreatitis, acute respiratory distress syndrome, surgery, and trauma (Cheek et al., 2010). *Sepsis* is a clinical syndrome defined as the presence of SIRS associated with a confirmed infectious process (Cheek et al., 2010; King, 2007). Septic shock is a state of acute circulatory failure characterized by persistent hypotension unexplained by other causes (for example, despite the fact that adequate fluids have been administered). It is important to remember the differences between a pediatric patient and an adult patient in describing septic shock. Septic shock in pediatric patients is manifested by tachycardia with signs of decreased perfusion including altered peripheral pulses, altered mental status, and capillary refill greater than 2 seconds. Chart 54–3 earlier in the chapter (p. 1675) outlines the clinical manifestations of shock in the adult patient.

Severe sepsis is defined as sepsis (the presence of a confirmed infection and a systemic inflammatory response) with single or multiple organ failure (Guthrie-Chu, 2009). Severe sepsis is associated with three integrated responses: activation of inflammation, activation of coagulation, and impairment of fibrinolysis. The patient is hypotensive, which causes hypoperfusion abnormalities such as arterial hypoxemia, acute oliguria, and coagulation abnormalities.

NURSING PROCESS: Patient Care Plan for Shock

Assessment of Shock Status Using Gordon's Functional Health Patterns:

- Nutrition Metabolic Pattern
- Activity Exercise Pattern
- Coping-Stress Tolerance Pattern

Subjective Data

Assessment of Circulation and Perfusion

How did you get injured?

When did your symptoms begin?

Do you feel dizzy, light-headed, anxious, or thirsty?

Do you have any other preexisting health problems such as heart, lung, or kidney disease?

Do you take any medications that may affect your blood pressure?

Do you take any medications that may affect your heart rate?

Do you take any medications that affect your immune system?

Do you take any medications that may make you bleed?

Assessment of Airway

Are you feeling short of breath?

Are you having difficulty breathing?

Do you feel like you are getting enough air?

Assessment of Nutrition

How is your appetite?

Has it changed recently?

Have you experienced any weight loss?

Assessment of Anticipatory Grieving

Do the patient and/or family realize the gravity of the illness or injury?

Do the patient and/or family have any support systems?

Do the patient and/or family have any spiritual beliefs that may assist them at this time?

Are there any cultural practices that are important to them at this time?

Objective Data

Assessment of Circulation and Perfusion

Oxygen saturation.

Work of breathing.

Peripheral and central pulses, presence, rate, and quality.

Blood pressure, mean arterial pressure, pulse pressure, respiratory rate, and temperature.

Skin color, moisture, and temperature.

Urinary output.

Assessment of Airway

Assess breath sounds.

Assess respiratory rate, rhythm, depth, and symmetry.

Monitor oxygen saturation.

Monitor arterial blood gas (ABG) values.

Assessment of Nutrition

24-hour caloric intake.

Daily weight.

Presence of bowel sounds.

Nausea and vomiting.

Flatus.

Assessment of Anticipatory Grieving

Observe family interaction with the patient.

Observe how the patient reacts to the illness or injury.

Observe how the staff is interacting with the patient and family.

Observe for anger, crying, physical threatening, or inability to cope with the situation.

Outcomes and Evaluation Parameters / Planning and Interventions with *Rationales*

1. NURSING DIAGNOSES: (a) Tissue Perfusion Ineffective *related to alterations in circulating volume.* (b) Fluid Volume Deficient *related to alterations in circulating volume.* (c) Cardiac Output, Decreased *related to alterations in circulating volume and cardiac pump function* (NANDA-I © 2012)

Outcome: Improved tissue perfusion.

Evaluation Parameters: Presence of peripheral pulses by palpation or Doppler.

Capillary refill < 3 seconds.

Maintenance of a perfusing blood pressure.

Improved mental status.

Glasgow Coma Scale (GCS) 15.

Follows commands.

No restlessness/fatigue.

Oxygen saturation is within normal limits.

Control of blood and fluid loss.

Adequate hydration.

Adequate urine output.

Corrected acid–base balance.

Improved core body temperature.

Adequate cardiac output and blood pressure.

Assess peripheral pulses and compare to central pulses. *Decrease in or loss of peripheral pulses indicates decreased tissue perfusion.*

Assess skin color and temperature. *Capillary refill indicates body's attempt to compensate for decreased perfusion by diverting blood flow from the periphery to the central circulation.*

Assess the patient's GCS and ability to follow commands.

Monitor restlessness and confusion *as an indication of decreased cerebral perfusion and worsening shock state.*

Assess for obvious signs of bleeding, *which will cause blood loss and alter circulating volume.*

Apply direct pressure and pressure dressings, assist with clamping of bleeding vessels, and prepare the patient for operative intervention *to prevent blood and volume loss.*

Apply pelvic binder to help manage large-volume loss from such injuries as an open book pelvic fracture *to stabilize the fracture and help prevent blood and volume loss.*

Initiate large-bore IV catheters.

NURSING PROCESS: Patient Care Plan for Shock, *continued*

	Assist with insertion of central venous access. Insert or assist with insertion of intraosseous needles *to replace volume and blood loss to maintain adequate circulation and improve perfusion.* Administer appropriate isotonic solution at 20 mL/kg and increase as indicated by patient's urinary output of 0.5 mL/kg/hr *to maintain adequate circulation and improve perfusion.* Prepare for administration of blood and blood products *to replace lost blood and increase oxygen to the tissues.* Administer O-negative blood if needed immediately (male patients and women beyond childbearing age may receive O-positive blood). Administer blood components such as fresh frozen plasma and platelets *to maintain adequate circulation and improve perfusion.* Place warm blankets on the patient. Use a commercial warming device. Use warm fluids and blood *to prevent hypothermia, maintain adequate circulation, and improve perfusion.* Obtain 12-lead *ECG to assess the status of the myocardium.* Increase cardiac contractility by administering a fluid bolus. Initiate medications to improve contractility: • Dopamine hydrochloride • Dobutamine hydrochloride • Amrinone lactate. Initiate medications to decrease afterload: • Nitroprusside sodium • Nitrates. Initiate medications to increase afterload: • Norepinephrine bitartrate • Epinephrine. *To improve cardiac output.* Prepare the patient for interventions that may increase reperfusion to an injured myocardium (e.g., percutaneous transluminal coronary angioplasty [PCTA] or insertion of an intra-aortic balloon pump [IABP]) *to improve cardiac output.*
2. NURSING DIAGNOSIS: Airway Clearance, Ineffective ***related to altered level of consciousness, obstruction by secretions, and aspiration of foreign matter*** **(NANDA-I © 2012)**	
Outcome: Patient will maintain a patent airway. ***Evaluation Parameters:*** Regular rate, depth, and pattern of breathing. Bilateral chest expansion. Effective cough and gag reflex.	Open and clear the airway. *Patient may have secretions in mouth.* Insert oro- or nasopharyngeal airway. *Patient may have adequate respiratory drive but needs support to keep airway open.* Prepare to assist with endotracheal intubation. *Level of consciousness is too low to protect and maintain the airway.*
3. NURSING DIAGNOSIS: Imbalanced Nutrition Risk for: Less Than Body Requirements ***related to decreased appetite secondary to treatments, fatigue, environment, and increased protein and vitamin requirements for healing*** **(NANDA-I © 2012)**	
Outcome: Patient will ingest daily nutritional requirements for activity level and metabolic needs. ***Evaluation Parameters:*** Patient maintains adequate weight. Patient maintains adequate caloric intake.	Communicate the need for adequate caloric intake of carbohydrates, fats, protein, vitamins, minerals, and fluids. *Adequate nutrition can reduce the risk of complications and promote healing.* Consult with the nutritionist to establish appropriate daily caloric requirements. *Consultation helps to ensure optimal intake.* Offer small frequent meals *to help prevent gastric distention.* Determine the patient's food preferences and arrange to have those foods provided. Encourage the family to bring allowed foods from home. Eliminate any offensive odors. Control pain and nausea. Provide a relaxed atmosphere during meals. *These interventions can improve appetite and lead to increased intake.*

(*continued*)

NURSING PROCESS: Patient Care Plan for Shock, *continued*

4. NURSING DIAGNOSIS: Coping, Readiness for Enhanced Grieving (NANDA-I © 2012)

Outcome: Patient and/or family are able to make decisions about care. ***Evaluation Parameters:*** Patient and family verbalize realistic perception of the patient's condition and chances of survival. Spiritual care is provided as identified by the patient and family. End-of-life decisions are made by the patient and/or family to ensure a painless and dignified death.	Provide the patient and the family with information about their illness or injury, especially related to outcomes *to assist the patient and family with grieving.* Allow the family to see the patient as soon as possible, especially if the patient is near death. Explain to the family what the patient looks like and how comfort has been provided for the patient *to assist the patient and family with grieving.* Provide requested spiritual care by contacting appropriate personnel. Respect cultural rituals related to the patient and family beliefs. Consult with personnel such as the ethics committee when problems arise with end-of-life decisions *to assist the patient and family with grieving.* Help the staff to recognize signs and symptoms of their own grief and provide them with resources *to assist them with the grieving process.*

Source: Adapted from Wilkinson, J. M., & Ahearn, N. R. (2009). *Prentice Hall nursing diagnosis handbook* (9th ed.). Upper Saddle River, NJ: Prentice Hall.

Epidemiology and Etiology

Sepsis kills millions of people worldwide, and studies have shown that the mortality rate due to sepsis is as high as one in four (Khan & Divatia, 2010). In the United States, sepsis is the 11th-leading cause of death overall and the leading cause of death in noncardiac care units (Kochanek, Xu, Murphy, Minino, & Kung, 2011). Since the time of Hippocrates, medicine has observed the consequence of sepsis and sought treatments to alleviate its deadly consequences (Porter, 1997).

Many factors have contributed to sepsis remaining a leading cause of death, including immunosuppression from medications such as chemotherapy and diseases such as human immunodeficiency virus (HIV). Chronic health problems (e.g., renal and liver disorders), traumatic injury, bone marrow suppression, surgical or invasive procedures, and sequential infections treated with multiple antibiotics are other significant risk factors for the development of SIRS and severe sepsis. Substance abuse and malnutrition may also contribute to SIRS and sepsis (King, 2007).

Pathophysiology

The innate immune system and the adaptive immune system both respond to a clinical insult. The innate immune system is the first line of defense and can be activated within minutes. The adaptive immune system is more specific in defending the body from microbes but takes longer to be initiated. When the immune system suffers a clinical insult, such as a devastating injury or exposure to a pathogen, a chain of events is initiated that is intended to activate receptors. These receptors, in turn, activate intracellular signaling pathways and transcription factors, resulting in expression of the gene immune response (Cheek et al., 2010). These defense mechanisms initiate an inflammatory response to the intruder. Research has determined that there are specific host immune responses to each pathogen that are mediated by various sets of pathogens associated with molecular patterns and pattern recognition receptors. In other words, there is no one particular medication or medical management strategy that can treat all patients with SIRS and sepsis (Cheek et al., 2010; Guthrie-Chu, 2009).

A comprehensive theory that helps explain the body's response to a critical illness or injury encompasses the hypothesis that the body starts out "fighting" an invader or responding to an insult such as an injury by having a hyperinflammatory response. A second response may occur due to infection or the degree of the injury that has occurred. If the event that initiated the response resolves quickly, the patient typically recovers. However, comorbid factors such as age, disease, extensive injury, and sometimes even the management of the infection or injury can cause a hypoinflammatory state. This state may be reversed, in a process that may take weeks or months, or it may progress to organ dysfunction (Cheek et al., 2010; Guthrie-Chu, 2009).

Three principal actions occur within the body in sepsis: inflammation, coagulation, and fibrinolysis. Inflammation is a complex systemic response to mechanical, ischemic, chemical, or microbial triggers that activate an immediate inflammatory and immune response. The purpose of the inflammatory response is to protect the body from further injury and promote rapid healing. When the infection occurs, endotoxins and exotoxins are produced that initiate a cellular response. This cellular response sparks a cascade of events that results in inflammation and cellular injury (Cheek et al., 2010; Guthrie-Chu, 2009; King, 2007). As a result of the release of histamine, prostaglandins, bradykinin, activated protein C, and other mediators, vasodilation occurs near the injured area with vasoconstriction of arterioles. This results in increased microvascular permeability, allowing exudate to form at the site. Neutrophil activation and adhesion are initiated, which promotes phagocytosis in order to clean the area and prepare for healing. Inflammation is further increased by the activation of the antigen–antibody response to the infectious agent, resulting in the release of cytokines including tumor necrosis factor (TNF) and interleukins 1L, 6L, and 8L (Cheek et al., 2010). Inflammation normally localizes an infection and kills the invading organism, but when inflammation is extreme, it results in vascular congestion, endothelial injury and dysfunction, and overstimulation of the coagulation system (Cheek et al., 2010).

The coagulation cascade is activated by the endothelial injury described previously, leading to clot formation. The cytokines activate TNF, and the endothelial injury activates Factor XII, resulting in the activation of clotting factors that cause thrombin generation. Normally, this cascade is helpful in the healing process because it helps repair damaged vessels. To prevent the proinflammatory mediators from damaging the normal tissues and organs, anti-inflammatory mediators are released to keep the infection at a local level. Normally, with infection the body suppresses fibrinolysis (clot breakdown) to allow time to destroy the antigen. In sepsis, coagulation produces thrombi that become emboli, which ultimately block microvasculature throughout the body, causing cellular death and organ dysfunction. Another reason for increased formation of thrombi in sepsis is the decrease in circulating activated protein C (APC). When thrombin binds with thrombomodulin, protein C becomes activated. **Protein C** is a normal component of the anticoagulant system, and in the presence of sepsis it attempts to achieve homeostasis by decreasing inflammation and coagulation and increasing fibrinolysis. A low serum level of APC is associated with sepsis, coagulopathy, multiple organ dysfunction, and increased mortality (Cheek et al., 2010). Figure 54–1 (p. 1674) provides an illustration of this process. Chapter 55 discusses the normal clotting cascade, the function of these factors, and their relationship to the normal immune function.

When sepsis occurs, the regulatory mechanisms have failed and uncontrolled inflammation overwhelms the body's normal protective responses. Excess coagulation, exaggerated inflammation, and abnormal fibrinolysis spread beyond the specific area of infection. This leads to systemic vasodilation, hypotension, and a generalized increase in vascular permeability, extravascular sequestration, and increased cellular aggregation with microvascular obstruction and greatly accelerated coagulation. The accelerated coagulation and suppressed fibrinolysis increase the disposition of fibrin clots, causing microvascular hypoperfusion and resulting in decreased blood flow to vital organs such as the lungs and kidneys. When blood flow to more than one organ system is compromised, severe sepsis develops. This may lead to multiple organ failure and death. In a healthy state, the body will break up these clots through fibrinolysis.

Cellular dysfunction that occurs in sepsis has multiple causes. The mechanisms that contribute to cellular dysfunction include cellular ischemia, disruption of cellular metabolism due to the effects of inflammatory mediators such as cytokines, and the toxic effects of free radicals. Unfortunately, in an effort to compensate for the shock state, cells undergo changes that reduce cellular energy, damage cell walls, and release other toxic substances; this can lead to irreversible shock even if the underlying cause of the clinical insult is eradicated (Cheek et al., 2010).

When the body suffers a clinical insult from such things as traumatic injury or infection, the immune system will respond. When there is an imbalance in this immune response, a devastating inflammatory response can occur that results in tissue injury, vascular collapse, multiple organ failure, and eventually, in some patients, death.

Infection causes a generalized inflammatory response system that initiates the continuum of SIRS to sepsis to severe sepsis (sepsis with organ dysfunction), leading to septic shock. Systemic mediators, which are bloodborne communicators, are activated in this hyperinflammatory response and lead to microcoagulation, consumption of platelets, and inhibition of clot lyses (fibrinolysis). A secondary problem includes uncontrolled alterations in vascular tone, vasodilation in large vessels (where pressure is measured), and both vasodilation and vasoconstriction in small vessels where oxygen delivery takes place. This alteration, along with microvascular clotting, limits oxygen delivery and may lead to ischemia in distant organs. This evolution may eventually lead to multiple organ dysfunction (MOD) syndrome, which is diagnosed when two or more organ systems fail (Barkman & Pooler, 2009; Cheek et al., 2010). Recent research has demonstrated that certain infectious agents interact with specific receptors (toll-like) in the body. Toll receptors are discussed in Chapter 52. In addition, severe gene polymorphisms have been associated with increased susceptibility to sepsis. Controlling both of these issues should assist in the management of sepsis and septic shock (Barkman & Pooler, 2009; Cheek et al., 2010; Guthrie-Chu, 2009).

Clinical Manifestations

The clinical manifestations of shock were discussed earlier in the chapter. However, because septic shock results from the body's response to an infectious agent, septic shock may initially manifest with different clinical manifestations from other forms of shock. For example, the patient may be febrile and chilling; the skin may be flushed and warm to the touch; and peripheral pulses may be bounding as the body attempts to fight the causative agent, although patients who are in advanced stages of sepsis, who are immunocompromised, or who have an immature or aged immune system may not be able to activate an adequate response to fight the infectious agent. Clinical manifestations are similar to those described in Chart 54–3 (p. 1675), although these patients quickly deteriorate.

Safety Alert *A patient suspected of being in septic shock who is hypothermic is in an advanced stage of sepsis, is at great risk of dying, and should be monitored very closely.*

Laboratory and Diagnostic Procedures

The Diagnostic Tests for SIRS and Septic Shock box contains a summary of the laboratory tests that can be used to diagnose SIRS and septic shock.

Medical Management

The Surviving Sepsis Campaign was launched in 2004 and updated in 2008 and 2010. The guidelines of the campaign incorporate best evidence-based practice into two therapies. The first therapy, titled the Sepsis Resuscitation Bundle, must be completed within 6 hours of the diagnosis. The second therapy, titled the Sepsis Management Bundle, must be completed within 24 hours (Khan & Divatia, 2010). Current elements of the sepsis resuscitation bundle include measurement of serum lactate; obtaining blood cultures; administration of broad-spectrum antibiotic within 3 hours of emergency department admission and within 1 hour of non-emergency department admission; treatment of hypotension and/or elevated lactate levels with 20 mL/kg of crystalloid or equivalent fluid; administration of a vasopressor for hypotension not responding to fluid resuscitation to maintain a mean arterial pressure (MAP) $>$ 65 mmHg; and achievement of a central venous pressure (CVP) $>$ 8 mmHg and achievement of a central oxygen saturation ($SCVO_2 > 70\%$) or mixed venous oxygen saturation ($SvO_2 > 65\%$).

The challenges associated with the medical management of the patient with SIRS, sepsis, or septic shock prompted an international conference. In 2003 and again in 2008, critical and infectious disease experts across the world developed management guidelines that could be used by all providers who come into contact with patients who may be at risk for sepsis (Dellinger et al., 2008). These guidelines are once again being reevaluated, beginning in 2010. The guidelines (see the National Guidelines box, p. 1687) contain evidence-based and consensus recommendations for the initial resuscitation, diagnosis, and management of sepsis and severe sepsis. It is important to continuously review these guidelines as they are updated.

In addition, the consensus group began an educational campaign that has been adopted worldwide to prevent sepsis, promote earlier recognition of risk factors, and provide a universal evidence-based approach to the management of sepsis (Dellinger et al., 2008). The Surviving Sepsis Campaign describes the management of a patient with suspected or confirmed sepsis, beginning with recognition by the

DIAGNOSTIC TESTS for SIRS and Septic Shock

Test, Normal Values, and Rationale	Expected Abnormality
White Blood Cell Count Adult: 4,500–10,000 μL *An increase in white blood cell count indicates the body's fight against the causative agent. This is also known as leukocytosis.* *A decrease in white blood cells, also known as leukopenia, can occur as part of the body's inflammatory response.*	White blood count will reflect an inflammatory process in order to fight the infectious agent. Thus, WBC can be either elevated or decreased depending on the response.
Blood Glucose Adult: 60–100 mg/dL *In infection, glucose production is increased to provide additional energy. This will continue to occur until the liver fails.*	There can be an increase in the blood glucose or hyperglycemia.
Blood Cultures Adult: negative *Blood cultures will identify the causative agent. Cultures require time for growth. Antibiotic therapy is typically withheld until appropriate cultures have been obtained.*	Positive if there is an infectious cause of the sepsis.
Arterial Blood Gases Adult: pH: 7.35–7.45 $PaCO_2$: 35–45 mmHg PaO_2: 75–100 mmHg SaO_2: > 95% SVO_2: > 70% HCO_3: 24–28 mEq/L Base Excess (BE): +2 to −2 mEq/L *Arterial blood gases are a measure of the patient's metabolic state. Respiratory alkalosis occurs with increased respirations to decrease CO_2, which is how the lungs compensate for metabolic acidosis, which results from anaerobic metabolism because of the lack of energy substrates to the cells.* *Metabolic acidosis results from the anaerobic metabolism from the hypoxia that results from inadequate tissue perfusion.*	Respiratory alkalosis. Metabolic acidosis. Hypoxia.
Serum Lactate Levels Adult: 0.5–2.0 mmol/L *Serum lactate level is elevated, which reflects tissue perfusion; increased level indicates inadequate tissue perfusion that results in lack of energy substrates and anaerobic metabolism.*	Elevated levels.
Coagulation Studies Platelet count: Adult: 150,000–400,000 μL Fibrin degradation products: Adult: 2–10 mcg/mL *These reflect activation of the clotting cascade and signal development of disseminated intravascular coagulation (DIC). Chapter 56 contains a complete discussion of DIC.*	Decrease in platelet numbers as shock progresses. Increased prothrombin time (PT), increased partial thromboplastin time (PTT), increased INR, and increased fibrin split products.

patient or the family and management in the emergency department and the critical care unit. Early, goal-directed therapy is the cornerstone of the initial management of the patient with sepsis (Surviving Sepsis Campaign, 2008).

The management of the patient in severe sepsis or septic shock should begin before the patient is admitted to the critical care unit. As with any patient in shock, the patient's airway, breathing, and circulation need to be assessed, and critical interventions are initiated. The major focus during resuscitation of these patients is to prevent the consequences of tissue hypoperfusion and hypoxia. In addition, the source of the infection must be quickly identified and appropriately treated to stop the cause of the sepsis.

Another important responsibility is the surveillance and application of guidelines for the use of antimicrobial agents that are used to manage sepsis and prevent development of antimicrobial resistance. Antibiotic use should be reevaluated every 48 to 72 hours to ensure that the correct medications are being administered and that no toxic side effects are occurring. (See the Pharmacology box on p. 1688.)

The Surviving Sepsis Campaign (2008) has provided important evidence-based guidelines that are being used all over the world to

NATIONAL GUIDELINES for the Initial Management of Sepsis

Initial Resuscitation	Guideline
Goal-directed during the first 6 hours	Maintain with fluids and vasopressors: • Central venous: 8–12 mmHg • MAP $>$ 65 mmHg • Urine output > 0.5 mL kg^{-1} hr^{-1} • Central venous (superior vena cava) or mixed venous oxygen saturation $>$ 70%
Diagnosis	Appropriate cultures of suspected sources of infection.
Antibiotic therapy	Antibiotic therapy should be initiated within 1 hour of recognition of severe sepsis, after appropriate cultures are obtained. The antibiotic regimen should be reassessed every 48–72 hours on the basis of microbiologic and clinical data, with the aim of using the appropriate antibiotic to prevent the development of resistance and toxicity.
Source control	Drainage of abscesses. Debridement of necrotic tissue. Removal of infected devices.
Fluid therapy	Fluid resuscitation may consist of colloids or crystalloids. No evidence is available to support one over the other. Fluid challenge over 30 minutes of 500–1,000 mL monitoring vital signs and urinary output. More fluid may be required depending on the patient's response.
Vasopressors	Maintain mean arterial pressure (MAP) $\geq$ 65 mmHg. When the appropriate fluid challenge fails and there is a need to restore end-organ perfusion, therapy with vasopressors may be started. Norepinephrine or dopamine is preferably given through a central catheter. Epinephrine should be used as the first alternative vasopressor when blood pressure does not respond to norepinephrine or dopamine. Do not use low-dose dopamine for renal protection. An arterial line should be placed for monitoring.
Inotropic therapy	In patients with low cardiac output despite adequate fluid resuscitation, dobutamine may be used to increase cardiac output. However, it is not recommended to increase cardiac index to predetermined supernormal levels.
Steroids	IV steroids are recommended for patients in septic shock when the patient's blood pressure does not respond to adequate fluid and vasopressor resuscitation. Hydrocortisone is recommended over dexamethasone.
Recombinant human activated protein C (rhAPC)	Recommended for adult patients who are at high risk of death and have no absolute contraindication related to bleeding risk, or have a relative contraindication that outweighs the risk of the treatment.
Mechanical ventilation of sepsis-induced acute lung injury (ALI) and acute respiratory distress syndrome (ARDS)	Low tidal volume 6 mL/kg predicted based on body weight. Avoid high plateau pressures and allow $PaCO_2$ to increase above normal to minimize plateau pressures and tidal volumes. Maintain mechanically ventilated patient in semi-recumbent position. For patients with ALI/ARDS, apply at least a minimal amount of positive end-expiratory pressure. Use a weaning protocol to get the patient safely off the ventilator. Noninvasive ventilation may be considered in patients who are hemodynamically stable, able to protect their airway, and expected to quickly recover. To decrease the days of mechanical ventilation and ICU length of stay, a conservative fluid strategy is used for patients with established ALI/ARDS who are not in shock. Do not routinely use a pulmonary arterial catheter for routine monitoring of ALI/ARDS.
Sedation, analgesia, neuromuscular blockade in sepsis	Protocols should be used to manage the patient and ensure adequate sedation and pain management while avoiding the consequences of immobility and too much medication. Intermittent bolus sedation or continuous sedation with predetermined end-points is recommended. Avoid neuromuscular blocking agents when possible to prevent problems with immobility.
Glucose control	Maintain blood glucose $<$ 150 mg/dL after initial stabilization. Use a validated protocol to manage glucose control.
Bicarbonate therapy	Not recommended for treatment of hypoperfusion-induced lactic acidemia with pH $>$ 7.15.
Renal replacement	Intermittent hemodialysis or continuous venohemofiltration is considered equivalent.
Deep venous thrombosis	Medical and mechanical treatment is based on the severity of the patient's condition. Use low-dose unfractionated heparin (UFH) or low-molecular weight heparin (LMWH) unless contraindicated.
Stress ulcer prophylaxis	Use H_2 blockers or proton-pump inhibitors. Patient must be monitored closely to prevent ventilator-associated pneumonia (VAP).
Consideration for limitation of support	Advance care planning and end-of-life issues must be considered and addressed.

Source: Surviving Sepsis Campaign. (2008). Guidelines for management of severe sepsis and septic shock. Retrieved from http://www.survivingsepsis.org/About_the_Campaign/Pages/AbouttheCampaign.aspx.

PHARMACOLOGY Summary of Medications Used to Treat Shock, Severe Sepsis, and MODS

Medication Category and Action	Application/Indication	Nursing Responsibility
Antibiotics		
Broad-spectrum antibiotics are used initially because the infectious agent is generally not known. Antibiotics should be chosen by using the following guidelines: • What community the patient lives in or has come from • Epidemiology of sepsis in the hospital or community • Suspected agents: Fungi Gram-positive bacteria Highly resistant gram-negative bacilli Methicillin-resistant *Staphylococcus aureus* Vancomycin-resistant enterococcus Penicillin-resistant pneumococcus ***Action:*** Will depend on the type of antibiotic that is prescribed by the clinician.	Choice of antibiotic should be based on the epidemiology of sepsis in the hospital and the community. Identification of the site of source or site of infection will direct the type of antibiotic approved. Only one antibiotic at a time, or monotherapy, is recommended.	Assess history of drug allergies. Assess clinical manifestations of allergic reaction. Assess relief of clinical manifestations to determine drug effectiveness 48–72 hours after initiation of the antibiotic therapy.
Corticosteroids		
Hydrocortisone Methylprednisone ***Action:*** Stimulates ACTH to increase cortisol. Stabilizes leukocyte lysosomal membrane. Inhibits phagocytosis and release of allergic substances. Reduces capillary dilation and permeability. Modifies immune response to various stimuli.	Treat adrenal insufficiency associated with septic shock. Treat inflammatory response related to spinal cord injury.	Assess relief of clinical manifestations. Carefully assess side effects: • Infection due to depressed immune response • Blood glucose • Gastric bleeding • Problems with wound healing.
Vasopressors		
Norepinephrine Dopamine Vasopressin ***Action:*** Reverse the vasodilation and reduced systemic vascular resistance. Promote alpha and beta sympathetic activity. Increase inotropy and chronotropy. Stimulate vasopressor receptors.	Vasopressors should not be used until appropriate fluid challenge fails to restore adequate blood pressure and organ perfusion. Vasopressin may be considered when fluid resuscitation and high-dose vasopressors have not worked.	Assess relief of clinical manifestations by monitoring MAP and urinary output. Assess the potential side effects of the medications such as peripheral vasoconstriction.
Insulin Therapy ***Action:*** Inducts euglycemia and anti-inflammatory effect. Protects endothelial and mitochondrial function.	Controls hyperglycemia, improves lipid levels, and has anti-inflammatory, anticoagulant, and anti-apoptotic actions.	Assess patient glucose to maintain glucose level <150 mg/dL (8.3 mmol/L).
Recombinant		
Activated coagulation factor VII (rFVIIa) ***Action:*** Promotes coagulation.	Facilitates cell membrane binding.	Assess for bleeding.

Source: Adams, M. P., & Koch, R. W. (2010). *Pharmacology: Connections to nursing practice.* Upper Saddle River, NJ: Pearson.

begin to reduce the morbidity and mortality related to sepsis and septic shock (Levy et al., 2010).

Nursing Management

Nurses play a key role in the prevention and early recognition of sepsis. It is important to be aware of potential sources of infection such as the presence of urinary catheters, central venous or arterial catheters, and continuous ventilator support. Meticulous hand hygiene and the use of strict aseptic technique when managing any break in skin integrity, such as wounds or invasive lines, can help prevent infection. Patients who take steroids or other immunosuppressive medications must be taught how to recognize signs and symptoms of infection such as spiking of a fever and chilling.

Nurses also should ensure the use of standard precautions, especially excellent hand hygiene, to prevent the transmission of microorganisms in the areas in which they work (Smith & McInnis, 2007).

Nursing care of the patient with sepsis is summarized in the Nursing Process: Patient Care Plan for Severe Sepsis box (p. 1690). It is based on the management of the patient's airway and breathing to improve oxygenation and circulation. Circulatory support may include fluids as well as vasopressors to maintain a perfusing blood pressure and prevent additional complications.

Collaborative Management

The care of the patient with sepsis requires a multidisciplinary approach to increase the patient's chances of survival. The nurse plays an important role in the early recognition of the risk of sepsis as well as recognizing its early signs of appearance. Health care providers who participate in the management of the patient with sepsis include specialty health care providers such as a critical care intensivist, surgeons, and infectious disease specialists; nurses; pharmacists; and respiratory and physical therapists. In order to meet desired patient outcomes, it is essential that the members of this interdisciplinary team communicate openly with one another in developing and evaluating care of the patient and family (IOM [Institute of Medicine], 2010).

The health care providers who care for the patient with sepsis are responsible for identifying the cause of the sepsis. This may involve performing surgery to drain an abscess or remove an injured organ. The intensivist is responsible for managing the patient's cardiovascular and pulmonary systems. Nurses are responsible for the continuous monitoring and administration of medications and fluids as well as the emotional and spiritual support of the patient and his family. Pharmacists participate in the evaluation of the appropriate antibiotics and vasoactive medications to fight the cause of the sepsis and maintain the patient's vital signs. Because many patients with sepsis require intubation and mechanical ventilation, the respiratory therapist will assist in the management of the patient's oxygenation. Finally, the physical therapist will be responsible for supporting the nursing staff in providing range-of-motion (ROM) exercises for sedated patients and moving patients out of bed when possible to prevent further complications from immobility.

Multiple Organ Dysfunction Syndrome

Multiple organ dysfunction syndrome is the result of severe sepsis. A critical injury or a disease process that initiates a massive systemic inflammatory response can also activate it. It does not need to be triggered by an infectious process. Despite recognition of this disease process since the mid-1970s, mortality from multiple organ dysfunction syndrome remains high, ranging from 60% to 100% (Rote, 2010).

Etiology

Multiple organ dysfunction syndrome (MODS) is a spectrum of organ dysfunction in a patient who has SIRS or septic complications. Two or more organ systems may be involved (Cheek et al., 2010; Guthrie-Chu, 2009). Triggers that can initiate MODS include multiple injuries, burns, hemorrhagic or hypovolemic shock, acute pancreatitis, acute respiratory distress syndrome (ARDS) or acute lung injury (ALI), and acute renal failure. Patients who are at risk for the development of MODS include patients with chronic diseases; those of advanced age; patients who have diabetes, cancer, pulmonary contusions, and widespread necrosis; and those with chronic infections who are being treated with immunosuppressant therapies. It remains a mystery why all patients with these risk factors do not develop MODS. Research is being directed at identifying biomarkers that place patients at greater risk of developing both sepsis and MODS (Cheek et al., 2010).

Clinical Manifestations and Diagnosis

The clinical manifestations of MODS depend on the area or areas of the body affected. Primary or early MODS is difficult to monitor. Examples of primary MODS in a trauma patient may include the primary cerebral edema seen in a head injury or ARDS that develops after a thoracic injury (Barkman & Pooler, 2009). Secondary or late MODS has a specific pattern of injury that can be observed and measured.

In summary, the clinical manifestations of MODS are the result of inflammatory mediator damage, tissue hypoxia, and hypermetabolism. The clinical manifestations of organ dysfunction are summarized in Chart 54–7 (p. 1692) (Cheek et al., 2010).

Laboratory and Diagnostic Procedures

The laboratory and diagnostic tests used to evaluate MODS are specific to the organ systems that are failing. For example, hyperbilirubinemia and increased serum aspartate transaminase, serum alanine aminotransferase, lactic dehydrogenase, alkaline phosphatase, and ammonia levels are indicative of liver failure. Patchy infiltrates on a chest radiograph are seen with ARDS. Decreased or absent urinary output reflects renal failure. The Diagnostic Tests for MODS box (p. 1693) contains information on laboratory tests that are monitored in the patient with MODS.

Medical Management

The primary focus for the management of MODS is prevention. Rapid recognition of the source of infection or management of the cause of shock or sepsis is one way to decrease the risk of the secondary insult. For example, nosocomial infections from invasive lines or catheters, or from poor hand hygiene, must be managed. After the initial injury or infection has been treated, care is directed at controlling infection, providing adequate tissue oxygenation, restoring and maintaining vascular volume, and supporting individual organ function. Antibiotics must be chosen carefully and closely monitored (Cheek et al., 2010). Because tissue hypoxia is a major problem, intubation and mechanical ventilation may be required. Oxygen saturation should be maintained between 88% and 92%. However, mechanical ventilation can lead to additional

NURSING PROCESS: Patient Care Plan for Severe Sepsis

Assessment of Shock Status Using Gordon's Functional Health Patterns:

- Health Perception Health Management Pattern
- Nutrition Metabolic Pattern
- Elimination Pattern
- Activity Exercise Pattern

Subjective Data

Assessment of Airway and Gas Exchange

Do you feel short of breath?
Are you getting enough air?
Do you breathe better sitting up?
Have you had a cough?
Are you coughing anything up and, if so, what color is it and how much?
Have you had a fever or chills?

Assessment of Fluid Volume Deficit

Are you thirsty?
How much fluid have you taken in?
What kind of fluids have you been drinking?
When was the last time you urinated?
Do you feel weak, dizzy, or light-headed?
Do you have any appetite?

Assessment of Infection

Have you had an infection in the last 2 weeks?
How often do you urinate? Do you feel you completely empty your bladder each time?
Do you have pain or burning on urination?
Have you been running a fever?
Do you have a cough?
Are you coughing up any sputum? If so, what color is it?
Do you have a history of infections? If so, what kind? How were they treated?
Are you taking any medications such as steroids or antibiotics?
Have you had an organ transplant?
Have you recently traveled outside of the country? If you have, where? Were you told of possible diseases such as avian flu where you traveled?

Assessment of Tissue Perfusion

Is it getting harder to breathe?
Are you more tired than before?
Does your chest hurt?
Are you having pain anywhere?

Objective Data

Assessment of Airway and Gas Exchange

Work of breathing
Increased rate, use of accessory muscles, and retractions
Lung sounds
Oxygen saturation and ABGs
Skin color, moisture, and temperature
Capillary refill < 3 seconds

Assessment of Fluid Volume Deficit

Decreased or absent peripheral pulses
Weak central pulses
Cool and clammy skin
Pale skin
Decreased or absent urinary output
Altered mental status
Alterations in vital signs
Tachycardia, decreased pulse pressure, decreased mean arterial pressure
Poor skin turgor
Dry mucous membranes

Assessment of Infection

Fever
Chills
Flushed skin
Presence of purpura or petechiae
Abscess
Burns
Presence of an indwelling urinary catheter
Feeding tube
Long-term intravenous access device
Pressure ulcer
Presence of wounds
White blood count

Assessment of Tissue Perfusion

Lung congestion
Oxygen saturation and ABGs
Work of breathing
Central and peripheral pulses
Cardiac rate and rhythm
Urinary output
Urine color
Level of consciousness
Abdominal distention and tenderness
Bowel sounds
Jaundice of eyes and skin
Enlarged liver
Muscle strength
Mobility

Outcomes and Evaluation Parameters	Planning and Interventions with *Rationales*
1. NURSING DIAGNOSES: (a) Gas Exchange, Impaired Risk for *related to inadequate tissue perfusion.* (b) Airway Clearance, Ineffective *related to altered mental status from inadequate tissue perfusion* (NANDA-I © 2012)	
Outcome: Adequate gas exchange. ***Evaluation Parameters:*** Normal arterial blood gases. Decreased respiratory rate because of a decreased need to compensate for metabolic acidosis; 12–20 breaths per minute.	Assess for symptoms of increased work of breathing, which indicate inadequate tissue perfusion: oxygen saturation, ABGs, length of capillary refill, skin temperature, and color *to assess tissue perfusion.* Monitor ABGs and oxygen saturation to assess adequacy of gas exchange and level of shock state. *When the body responds to shock, it will divert blood from the periphery and direct it to the brain, lungs, and kidneys.*

NURSING PROCESS: Patient Care Plan for Severe Sepsis, *continued*

Adequate perfusion for the patient to become alert and oriented. Clear breath sounds.	Monitor for changes in mental status such as restlessness and confusion. *Indicators of inadequate gas exchange with resultant cerebral hypoxia.* Observe for pallor and cyanosis, especially in the mucous membranes. *Indicators of inadequate gas exchange with resultant tissue hypoxia.* Administer 100% oxygen by nonrebreather mask. *To increase available oxygen and decrease tissue hypoxia.* Report respiratory distress and hypoxia to the health care provider. *Intubation and mechanical ventilation may be needed to deliver greater amounts of oxygen and maintain adequate tissue perfusion.*
2. NURSING DIAGNOSIS: Fluid Volume, Deficient ***related to alterations in circulating blood volume due to impaired vascular function from the effects of endotoxins on vasomotor tone*** **(NANDA-I © 2012)**	
Outcome: Adequate circulating fluid volume. ***Evaluation Parameters:*** Adequate peripheral perfusion. Normal capillary refill time. Normal urinary output (minimum of 30 mL/hr). Improvement in mentation. Heart rate 60–100 beats per minute with normal sinus rhythm. Blood pressure systolic greater than 100 mmHg.	Insertion of large-bore intravenous catheters *to provide fluid resuscitation.* Infuse intravenous fluids as directed, typically 20 mL/kg as an initial bolus that may be repeated several times *to optimize perfusion.* Insert central venous catheter and arterial catheter *to measure central venous pressure and monitor central arterial pressure.* Insert a urinary catheter *to measure hourly urinary output. These measures help with assessment of adequacy of fluid resuscitation.* Monitor the effectiveness of the use of prescribed vasopressors, *which are used to improve blood pressure and support circulation.* Monitor heart rate, blood pressure, and quality of central and peripheral pulses *to assess adequacy of fluid resuscitation.* Report signs of inadequate perfusion (e.g., hypotension, tachycardia, and low urinary output) to the health care provider *so that additional interventions such as administration of other vasopressor agents can be started to improve circulation.*
3. NURSING DIAGNOSIS: Infection ***related to a focus of infection*** **(NANDA-I © 2012)**	
Outcomes: Identification of focus of infection. Infection resolved. ***Evaluation Parameters:*** Decrease or absence of fever. Removal of the source of the infection, for example, draining of an abscess or removal of an invasive catheter. Normal white blood cell count and differential.	Measure and monitor the patient's body temperature using the most appropriate method; for example, rectal, esophageal, or bladder. *Effects of treatment can also be monitored.* Perform measures to decrease the patient's fever such as administration of an antipyretic or application of a cooling blanket. *To prevent side effects of fever such as dehydration and increased metabolic demand.* Note the presence of a source of an infection, for example, indwelling urinary catheter, draining wound, rigid abdomen, and colored sputum. *To determine cause and infection site.* Obtain blood cultures by drawing blood from two peripheral sites, preferably not from an existing intravenous catheter. *To diagnose the presence of bloodstream infection.* Obtain cultures from other sites such as urine, sputum, cerebrospinal fluid (CSF), or other body fluids to identify source and infectious agents. *To identify source of infection.* Use aseptic technique when changing dressings or drawing blood from invasive lines *to prevent introduction of further sources of infection.* Perform hand hygiene frequently and use infection control measures when indicated *to prevent introduction of further sources of infection.* Instruct the patient's family about hand hygiene *to prevent further introduction of infection.* Report to the health care provider changes in temperature as prescribed *so appropriate interventions and medications can be given to manage a fever.* Administer antibiotics per health care provider's orders *to flight infection.*

(*continued*)

NURSING PROCESS: Patient Care Plan for Severe Sepsis, *continued*

Outcomes and Evaluation Parameters	Planning and Interventions with *Rationales*
4. NURSING DIAGNOSIS: Tissue Perfusion, Ineffective *related to organ dysfunction* (NANDA-I © 2012)	
Outcome: Prevention of further organ failure and treatment instituted. ***Evaluation Parameter:*** Effective prevention of multiple organ dysfunction.	Initiate prescribed treatments including fluid resuscitation and vasopressor and antibiotic administration. *To hemodynamically stabilize the patient and treat the cause of infection.* Carefully monitor intake and output. *To evaluate for adequate fluid resuscitation.* Turn and position the patient frequently *to prevent skin breakdown and development of DVT.* Monitor for bleeding that may occur due to altered clotting mechanisms. *To prevent hemorrhage.* Prepare the patient and family for end-of-life decisions. *To prepare the family for possible death.*

Source: Adapted from Wilkinson, J. M., & Ahearn, N. R. (2009). *Prentice Hall nursing diagnosis handbook* (9th ed.). Upper Saddle River, NJ: Prentice Hall.

CHART 54–7 Clinical Manifestations of MODS

Pulmonary

Dyspnea, patchy infiltrates, refractory hypoxemia, respiratory acidosis, and abnormal O_2 indices

Pulmonary hypertension

Gastrointestinal

Abdominal distention and ascites

Intolerance of enteral feedings

Paralytic ileus

Gastrointestinal bleeding

Mucosal ulceration

Bacterial overgrowth in stool

Liver

Increased bilirubin level

Increased liver enzymes

Increased serum ammonia level

Jaundice

Hepatomegaly

Metabolic/Nutritional

Decreased lean body mass

Muscle wasting

Severe weight loss

Negative nitrogen balance

Hyperglycemia

Hypertriglyceridemia

Increased serum lactate levels

Decreased serum albumin

Renal

Increased serum creatinine level and BUN

Oliguria, anuria, or polyuria related to acute tubular necrosis

Cardiovascular

Hyperdynamic

Decreased:

Pulmonary capillary wedge pressure

Systemic vascular resistance

Right atrial pressure

Increased:

Oxygen consumption

Cardiac output

Cardiac index

Heart rate

Hypodynamic

Increased:

Systemic vascular resistance

Right atrial pressure

Left ventricular stroke work index

Decreased:

Oxygen delivery and consumption

Cardiac output

Cardiac index

Central Nervous System

Lethargy

Altered level of consciousness

Fever

Hepatic encephalopathy

Coagulation and Hematologic

Thrombocytopenia

Disseminated intravascular coagulation

Immune

Infection

Decreased lymphocyte count

Anergy

Source: Adapted from Rote & McCance (2010a, 2010b).

DIAGNOSTIC TESTS for MODS

Test, Normal Values, and Rationales	Expected Abnormality
Serum Lactate Level Adult: 0.5–2.0 mmol/L	Metabolic acidosis results from inadequate tissue perfusion and anaerobic metabolism.
D-dimer Adult: Greater than 250 ng/mL	Levels increase with MODS. Indication of coagulopathy that is present in MODS.
Liver Enzyme Tests Alkaline phosphatase (ALP): Adult: 42–136 unit/L Alanine aminotransferase (ALT or SGPT): Adult: 10–35 unit/L Lactic dehydrogenase (LD/IDH): Adult: 100–190 IU/L Gamma-glutamyl transferase/transpeptidase (GGT/GGTP): Adult: Male: 4–23 IU/L Female: 3–13 IU/L *Liver enzyme tests are a group of tests that measure the function of the liver.*	Liver is frequently one of the first organs to fail in MODS. Therefore, the liver function tests would be elevated.
Arterial Blood Gases Adult: pH: 7.35–7.45 $PaCO_2$: 35–45 mmHg PaO_2: 75–100 mmHg SaO_2: > 95% SVO_2: > 70% HCO_3: 24–28 mEq/L Base Excess (BE): + 2 to −2 mEq/L *Arterial blood gases are a measure of the patient's metabolic state. Respiratory alkalosis occurs with increased respirations to decrease CO_2, which is how the lungs compensate for metabolic acidosis, which results from anaerobic metabolism because of the lack of energy substrates to the cells.*	PO_2 decreased. Metabolic acidosis results from the anaerobic metabolism from the hypoxia, which results from inadequate tissue perfusion.

problems such as VAP, which may lead to the secondary assault that triggers the onset of MODS.

Adequate volume resuscitation and vascular support need to be ongoing. Volume resuscitation decreases the risks of complications from hemoconcentrated blood due to shifts in interstitial spaces. Replacing and maintaining volume also improves the supply and demand imbalance that occurs with hypermetabolism. Vasopressors such as epinephrine or norepinephrine may be used to increase systemic vascular resistance and improve cardiac output and oxygenation. Any problem that increases oxygen demand such as fever needs to be managed. Excessive body temperatures may require cooling measures such as hypothermia blankets, as well as medications such as acetaminophen. Patients may require analgesia and sedation to decrease pain and anxiety, thus decreasing oxygen demand. Nutrition through enteral feeding helps maintain the gut barrier and reduces the translocation of bacteria, thus reducing the incidence of infection and other complications. Glucose levels are tightly controlled because of the effect of high glucose levels on tissue and organ function. Individual organs will require support, which will be based on the organ or organ systems that have been affected.

Nursing Management

Nursing care for the patient with MODS includes early recognition of the risk factors for the development of MODS and close monitoring of interventions initiated to treat the patients, such as invasive lines and catheters. Meticulous skin care and aseptic technique must be used in inserting and changing any lines. The nurse should ensure that everyone who comes in contact with the patient uses meticulous hand hygiene and aseptic technique to prevent the risk of infection.

Frequent monitoring and assessment to observe trends in changes in vital signs and clinical manifestations will provide the most reliable information about early signs of MODS. Nursing care needs to be focused on decreasing oxygen demand, which includes pain and anxiety management as well as spacing activity to allow for long periods of rest. The nurse should assess for signs of pain and anxiety and medicate as needed. Tachycardia related to pain and anxiety increases oxygen consumption due to the stress imposed on the body by pain. Positioning of the patient is important to prevent the complications that occur with immobility such as skin breakdown, pulmonary congestion, and pooling of blood and secretions. Hypermetabolism causes loss of muscle, so it is important to prevent additional loss of movement. Patients should receive active and passive ROM exercises to retain strength and joint motion.

Emotional support for both the patient and the family is essential. Because of the high mortality rate associated with MODS, it is important for the nurse to help the family prepare for difficult decisions about end of life. As discussed in Chapter 11, the nurse needs to be aware of any religious or cultural needs the patient and family may have related to death and dying.

Administration of vasopressors will place the patient at risk of injury to fingers, hands, toes, and feet due to peripheral vasoconstriction. Frequent assessment of peripheral circulation is needed. Additionally, fluid resuscitation and shunting of blood and nutrients can lead to edema. Therefore, skin impairment can occur and is another source of infection. Positioning and use of special beds may decrease the risk of these complications.

Health Promotion

The primary emphasis in the treatment for shock is prevention. Early recognition of factors that place a patient at risk for the development of a shock syndrome may greatly reduce patient morbidity and mortality. See the Complementary & Alternative Therapies box for a discussion of the use of beta-glucans to strengthen the immune system. Traumatic injury contributes to the risk for all types of shock because of organ system injury. Adopting injury prevention strategies may help decrease the incidence of shock. Examples of injury prevention and control strategies can be found in the Emergency Nurses Association's Trauma Nursing Core Course (ENA, 2007). Examples include the following:

- Engineering and technologic interventions (e.g., high-mounted rear brake lights)
- Enforcement and legislative interventions (e.g., state seat belt and helmet laws)
- Placing children in properly fitted and located car seats
- Education and behavioral interventions (e.g., school- and hospital-based education programs).

Sepsis and septic shock have become a serious problem in the United States. Prevention strategies to reduce the incidence of septic shock include the following (Masur, 2003):

COMPLEMENTARY & ALTERNATIVE THERAPIES Beta-Glucans

Nancy Yilk

AMONG POLYSACCHARIDES that act as immunostimulants, beta-glucans were found to be the most effective against infectious diseases and cancer. Beta-1,3-D glucan is a complex carbohydrate, comprised of sugar molecules, that has been demonstrated to have powerful immune-boosting and anticancer effects. The role of beta-1,3-D glucans from yeast, fungi, mushrooms, and seaweed as biologic immunomodulators has been well documented in the past 40 years. Beta-glucan has been isolated from a variety of fungi such as shiitake (Lentinus edodes) and maitake (Grifola frondosa) mushrooms, from yeast cell walls including brewers' and bakers' yeasts (Saccharomyces cerevisiae), and from oat and barley bran. Traditionally, beta-glucans are considered to be a stimulator of cellular immunity (El Khoury, Cuda, Luhovyy, & Anderson, 2012).

In vitro studies demonstrated that beta-glucans can enhance the functional activity of macrophages and activate the antimicrobial activity of mononuclear cells and neutrophils. The differences between soluble and insoluble beta-glucans are significant in regards to application, mode of action, and overall biologic activity (Rondanelli, Opizzi, & Monteferrario, 2009).

In addition, beta-1,3-D glucans improve the body's immune system defense against foreign invaders by enhancing the ability of macrophages, neutrophils, and natural killer cells to respond to and fight a wide range of challenges such as bacteria, viruses, fungi, and parasites. *In vitro*, animal and human studies have shown that beta-1, 3-D glucans can enhance the responsiveness and function of immune cells, stimulating both humoral and cellular immunity. In addition, beta-glucans have been extensively used as protection against infection. Using several experimental models, beta-glucans have been shown to protect against both bacterial and protozoan infections and enhance antibiotic efficacy in infections with antibiotic-resistant bacteria. The protective effect of beta-glucans was shown in experimental infections with *Leishmania major* and *L. donovani*, *C. albicans*, *Toxoplasma gondii*, *Streptococcus suis*, *Plasmodium berghei*, *Staphylococcus aureus*, *Escherichia coli*, *Mesocestoides corti*, *Trypanosoma cruzi*, *Eimeria vermiformis*, and *Bacillus anthracis* (Rondanelli, 2009).

The identification of antigen-recognizing receptors in the innate immune system significantly helped the understanding of the initiation and regulation of the innate immune response. Dectin-1 was recently identified as the most important receptor for beta-glucan. Recognition of beta-glucan by dectin-1 triggers effective immune response, including phagocytosis and proinflammatory factor production, to eliminate infecting fungi, which especially benefits immunocompromised patients against opportunistic fungal infection. In addition, dectin-1 is involved in the adaptive immune response, as well as autoimmune diseases and immune tolerance (Sun & Zhao, 2011).

Few human studies have examined the immune function of beta-glucans in surgical patients. Three clinical studies demonstrated that pretreatment of high-risk surgical patients with intravenous yeast β-(1,3; 1,6)-D-glucan decreased the infection incidence, shortened the intensive care unit length of stay, and improved survival in comparison to a saline placebo injection. Postoperative infections that frequently complicate high-risk surgical procedures were studied in three multicenter, double-blind clinical trials; researchers evaluated the effects of beta-glucans on patients undergoing high-risk abdominal and thoracic surgery. Patients who received beta-glucans had significantly fewer postoperative infections compared to those treated with a placebo. The investigators concluded that beta-glucans could potentially decrease life-threatening postoperative infections (El Khoury et al., 2012).

To further understand the benefits of beta-glucans and the distinctions of β-glucans from source plant material, in vivo studies of a variety of beta-glucans were studied for their responses to pathogen infections in animals. This study was designed to compare the effect of pretreatment with N-acetylcysteine (NAC) and beta-glucans on inflammatory response in a rat model of sepsis. The results demonstrated that prophylactic administration of NAC or beta-glucans similarly ameliorated sepsis syndrome by reducing the proinflammatory cytokines and increasing the anti-inflammatory cytokine levels, as well as through accession of cellular antioxidants, which protect cells from oxidative stress, thereby recruiting inflammatory cells into tissue (Senoglu, Yuzbasioglu, Aral, Ezberci, Kurutas, Bulbuloglu, et al., 2008).

References

El Khoury, D., Cuda, C., Luhovyy, B. L., & Anderson, G. H. (2012). Beta- glucan: Health benefits in obesity and metabolic syndrome. *Journal of Nutrition and Metabolism.* Epub 2011 Dec 11. doi:10.1155/2012/851362

Rondanelli, M., Opizzi, A., & Monteferrario, F. (2009). The biological activity of beta-glucans. *Minerva Medical, 100*(3), 237–245.

Senoglu, N., Yuzbasioglu, M. F., Aral, M., Ezberci, M., Kurutas, E. B., Bulbuloglu, E., et al. (2008). Protective effects of N-acetylcysteine and beta-glucan pretreatment on oxidative stress in cecal ligation and puncture model of sepsis. *Journal of Investigative Surgery, 21*(5), 237–243.

Sun, L., & Zhao, Y. (2011). The biological role of dectin-1 in immune response. *Cellular Immunology, 270*(2), 183–187. Epub 2011 May 10.

CHART 54–8 Summary of Action Plan to Combat Antimicrobial Resistance

- Conduct a national public health education campaign to promote appropriate antimicrobial use as a national health priority.
- Develop and facilitate the implementation of educational and behavioral interventions that will assist clinicians in appropriate antimicrobial prescribing.
- Evaluate the effectiveness (including cost effectiveness) of current and novel infection control practices for health care and extended care settings and in the community.
- Promote adherence to practices proven to be effective.
- Support demonstration projects to evaluate comprehensive strategies that use multiple interventions to promote appropriate drug use and reduce infection rates, in order to assess how interventions found effective in research studies can be applied routinely and most cost effectively on a large scale.

- Age-appropriate vaccinations
- Reduction of the incidence of antibiotic-resistant pathogens in ICUs
- Aseptic management of invasive lines
- Aseptic management of indwelling catheters, feeding tubes, and central lines
- Frequent hand hygiene (hand hygiene has become a major quality indicator in hospitals, clinics, and any place patient care is given)
- Efforts to limit antibiotic resistance through policies to prescribe them and surveillance of their use.

Chart 54–8 contains a summary of an action plan that is being implemented to combat antimicrobial resistance.

Gerontological Considerations

The changes related to age can present additional challenges for the care of the older patient in shock as well as put them at greater risk for the development of shock. A decrease in cardiac output by almost half, as well as a decreased response to endogenous catecholamines, will impair an older patient's ability to respond to the redistribution of blood and fluids. Changes in blood pressure and heart rate in older adults are different from those seen in other age groups. Many of the medications prescribed to older adults, such as beta-blockers, will also affect physiological responses. Age causes diminished perfusion to all organs. This may manifest itself in altered mental status and an inability to concentrate urine. Both are important subtle signs of the early stages of shock. As age advances, the immune system becomes less able to provide protection from diseases (Kaplow & Hardin, 2007). In the older adult, sepsis can result from diseases such as pneumonia or urinary tract infections.

Shock resuscitation in the older adult must be closely monitored. These patients are prone to develop complications such as congestive heart failure and pulmonary edema. Also, nutrition and skin care are important areas of focus for the older patient in shock. Preexisting medical problems, appliances such as indwelling catheters, and feeding tubes are all things that can contribute to problems in the care of the older patient in shock, as listed in Chart 54–9.

CHART 54–9 Gerontological Considerations Related to Shock

Pulmonary
- Decreased blood flow to the lungs, so older adults already have a preexisting oxygen deficit.
- Decreased elasticity and strength for ventilation and less able to compensate for metabolic acidosis by increasing ventilations.

Cardiac
- Decrease in cardiac output related to age, which will decrease the body's ability to compensate for alterations in volume from shock.
- Baroreceptor sensitivity decreases, decreasing the body's ability to compensate for fluid volume changes.
- Diminished perfusion to all organ systems.
- Medications such as beta-blockers will alter the heart's response to shock.

Neurological
- Normal mental status may be altered owing to decreased blood flow to the brain.
- Previous disease such as a stroke will alter the patient's level of consciousness.

Renal
Age decreases blood flow to the kidneys, decreasing their ability to concentrate urine and detoxify.

Integumentary
- Skin is less elastic.
- Less fat and more easily injured.
- Less able to maintain normothermia and at greater risk of becoming hypothermic.

Medications
Numerous medications can alter the body's response to a clinical insult as well as leave the patient at greater risk of developing shock: beta-blockers, steroids, antibiotics, and antivirals.

Research

Research related to shock management is needed to identify areas in which practice could improve and to evaluate and test selected interventions. Resuscitation end-points and the identification of genetic markers that assist in the identification of patients at risk to develop sepsis are needed (Cheek et al., 2010). As was pointed out earlier in this chapter, research continues to challenge how shock has been managed. The death from sepsis that progresses to septic shock continues to increase each year. Research must be focused at multiple methods of prevention and management. Current research ideas and their clinical impact are listed in the Research Opportunities Related to Shock, SIRS, Sepsis, and Severe Sepsis box (p. 1696). Keeping up with the constant changes in the literature is important to ensure that the patient is receiving the best and most effective care.

RESEARCH OPPORTUNITIES Related to Shock, SIRS, Sepsis, and Severe Sepsis

Research Area	Clinical Impact
Physiological Research	
Identity of specific markers that indicate a systemic shock response.	Earlier diagnosis and identification of high-risk patients.
Identification of the most appropriate solution for initial and continued fluid resuscitation: hypertonic saline, lactated Ringer's solution, or normal saline.	Development of an algorithm for appropriate fluid resuscitation for the type of shock and nursing interventions to mediate the progression.
Determination of whether fluid resuscitation should be controlled based on the source of the clinical insult. The theory exists that hypotension may actually be a protective mechanism.	
Hypothermia and minimal fluid resuscitation.	Development of nursing guidelines for monitoring the patient's response to fluid resuscitation.
Medications effective against bacteria and viruses without causing additional systemic damage, for example, ketolides, which bind to two sites on bacteria preventing the development of resistance.	Antibiotic resistance is a growing problem, with an expanding number of resistant organisms occurring. Preventing resistance would help mitigate this issue.
Use of extracorporeal membrane oxygenation therapy (ECMO).	ECMO can potentially remove mediators that initiate destructive cascades in such shock states as sepsis.
Ethical Issues	
Identification of futile resuscitation parameters.	Development of guidelines for the end-points of resuscitation.
Staging of shock and sepsis to identify irreversible futile resuscitation parameters.	Development of nursing guidelines for withdrawal of support.
Genetic studies that identify a person's predisposition to developing sepsis.	Several gene polymorphisms have been associated with an increased susceptibility to sepsis.
Vaccinations.	Development of a vaccination that prevents SIRS when a patient has been exposed to an infectious agent.

CLINICAL PREPARATION READ DOCUMENT APPLY

READ: **History of Present Illness** >> Laboratory Study Results >> Critical Thinking Questions

As a nurse in a critical care unit, you have been notified that you will be receiving a new patient from the emergency department (ED). The ED nurse calls the following report: David Knudsen is a 19-year-old college student who was brought to the ED by his friends. His friends said that he has been vomiting for the past 24 hours. This morning he was confused. Mr. Knudsen states that he does not feel well and has been "hot and cold." According to his friends, there has been a recent outbreak of a viral infection on campus. They do not know what the name of the infection is, only that they had heard that it was occurring. Mr. Knudsen is awake and alert but complaining of a headache. The ED nurse states that he has a petechial rash on his lower extremities and he has received a dose of ceftriaxone 2 grams intravenously. His blood pressure is 100/70; heart rate 120; respiratory rate 28; and his temperature is currently 38.2°C orally.

Procedures Since Admission

Within a few hours of admission in the critical care unit, Mr. Knudsen's mental status begins to deteriorate. You notify the critical care resident of this change. Mr. Knudsen's level of consciousness continues to deteriorate; therefore, the resident decides to intubate using sedation and neuromuscular blocking agents. Mr. Knudsen is placed on a ventilator. A triple lumen line is inserted to administer 1 liter of normal saline since Mr. Knudsen's blood pressure is staying around 90 systolic and his pulse is in the 130s to 150s. The resident also inserts an arterial line.

READ: History of Present Illnesses >> **Physical Exam** >> Admitting Medical Records >> Laboratory Study Results

Medical–Surgical History

- No known allergies
- Taking no medications
- No prior medical history other than normal childhood illnesses

Social History

- Mr. Knudsen is a freshman at college; he is on the swimming team
- States that he drinks beer on the weekend with his friends
- Denies the use of illicit substances
- Denies cigarette smoking

Physical Exam

- Vital signs: BP 88/40; P 130; RR 36; T 104.0°F
- Oxygen saturation: 90% on room air initially and then dropped to 86% on room air
- HEENT: normal, braces on both upper and lower teeth
- Heart: rapid rate; normal S_1, S_2
- Lungs: bilateral basilar crackles
- Abdomen: flat, soft nontender

Neurological exam: Mr. Knudsen is lethargic but can be aroused with minimal stimulation. He is not able to answer simple questions but will raise his arms and legs when asked. His pupils are 4 mm, equal, round, and reactive. He complains of pain with neck movement.
Skin: flushed and hot to the touch
Chest radiograph: basilar infiltrates
ECG: sinus tachycardia
Weight: 180 lbs (80 kg)
Height: 6′
Extremities: petechial rash on both lower extremities that does not blanch
DP and PT pulses 2+

Admitting Medical Orders

Medical ICU Service
Floor: Medical Intensive Care Unit
Diagnosis: meningitis and septic shock
No known allergies
Foley
NG tube to low wall suction
Bed rest
Intake and output
Isolation: respiratory isolation
Ventilator settings:
TV 480
RR: 16
Oxygen: 60%
Mode: Assist/control
Peep: 5
Vital signs: every 15 minutes until stable, then every 1 hour
Neurological checks every 30 minutes
IV: 0.9 normal saline at 100 mL/hr. Maintain systolic blood pressure at 100 mmHg with normal saline fluid bolus of 500 mL × 1 bolus
NPO until further notice
Call house officer: pulse < 60 and > 100/minute; BP < 90 and > 160 systolic; temperature > 38.5; urine output < 30 mL/hour for 2 hours, RR > 30/minute; oxygen saturation < 92%
Sequential compression devices (SCDs) to lower extremities

Scheduled Medications

Ceftriaxone 2 grams IV once a day
Esomeprazole 40 mg IV daily
Norepinephrine drip (4 mg/250 mL of normal saline) at 2–12 micrograms per kilogram to maintain a systolic blood pressure at 100 mmHg

PRN Medications

Fentanyl 20–50 micrograms IV q2h for sedation and analgesia
Ativan 2–4 milligrams IV q4h for sedation
Acetaminophen 650 mg suppositories q4h for fever greater than 102°F

Ordered Laboratory Studies

STAT blood cultures were obtained in the emergency department
CSF studies: cell count, protein, glucose levels sent from the ED
Cultures: sputum, nasopharyngeal, cerebrospinal fluid (CSF)
Latex agglutination
Enzyme-linked immunosorbent assay (ELISA)
CBC, INR/PTT, Ca, Mg, phosphorous, electrolyte panel daily
UA

Ordered Diagnostic Studies

CT scan of head; repeat with changes
Lumbar puncture

READ: History of Present Illnesses >> **Laboratory Study Results** >> Critical Thinking Questions

Test	Day 1	Day 2	Day 3
Sodium	141 mEq/L	139 mEq/L	138 mEq/L
Potassium	4.0 mEq/L	3.5 mEq/L	3.8 mEq/L
Chloride	100 mEq/L	113 mEq/L	113 mEq/L
Venous carbon dioxide	17 mEq/L	18 mEq/L	22 mEq/L
Calcium	6.6 mg/dL	7.0 mg/dL	8.6 mg/dL
Blood urea nitrogen	30 mg/dL	25 mg/dL	18 mg/dL
Creatinine	2.0 mg/dL	1.5 mg/dL	1.0 mg/dL
Blood glucose	150 mg/dL	138 mg/dL	120 mg/dL
Total proteins	4.5 g/dL		
Magnesium	2.0 mg/dL	2.0 mg/dL	2.0 mg/dL
WBC	22,000/mm^3	10,000/mm^3	10,500/mm^3
Hemoglobin	14.0 gm/dL	13.4 gm/dL	14.7 gm/dL
Hematocrit	40.8%	38.7%	43.1%
RBC	4.69 m/mm^3	4.49 m/mm^3	4.97 m/mm^3
Platelets	128 K/mm^3	137 K/mm^3	269 K/mm^3
ABGs			
PO_2	78 mmHg	100 mmHg	150 mmHg
O_2 saturation	88%	94%	98%
pH	7.27	7.30	7.35
PCO_2	36.5 mmHg	30 mmHg	28 mmHg

Test	Day 1	Day 2	Day 3
HCO_3	24 mEq/L	22 mEq/L	24 mEq/L
CSF	Positive for group B streptococcus		
CT scan	Cerebral edema		
ELISA	Antiviral immunoglobulin		
INR	1.18	1.2	1.25
PTT	32 seconds	32.6 seconds	33 seconds
Sputum culture		Negative	
Nasopharyngeal culture		Positive for group B streptococcus	
CSF culture		Positive for group B streptococcus	
Latex agglutination	Certain antibodies in body fluids		
UA	Within normal limits		

Pearson Nursing Student Resources *Log on to* **nursing.pearsonhighered.com** *to download forms*

DOCUMENT:

- >> Summary of Hospitalization
- >> Pathophysiology Form
- >> Laboratory Values
- >> Laboratory Results Explanation

APPLY:

- >> List of Potential Nursing Diagnoses
- >> Concept Map
- >> Critical Thinking Questions and Concept Map

APPLY: History of Present Illness >> Laboratory Study Results >> **Critical Thinking Questions**

1. Upon his initial admission to the critical care unit, for what complications should you assess Mr. Knudsen?
2. How is meningitis transmitted and how can you protect yourself?
3. Why would a medication such as Levophed be started to maintain Mr. Knudsen's blood pressure?

Answers to Critical Thinking Questions can be found in Appendix D in the Osborn Student Resources at nursing.pearsonhighered.com.

NCLEX® PRACTICE

1. A patient is diagnosed as being in shock after starting a new medication. The nurse would report that this patient is most likely experiencing which of the following types of shock?
   1. Cardiogenic
   2. Anaphylactic
   3. Neurogenic
   4. Septic
2. A patient in shock is demonstrating signs of insulin resistance. The nurse explains to the patient's family that this is because of:
   1. the stress response.
   2. undiagnosed diabetes mellitus.
   3. excessive body weight.
   4. undiagnosed metabolic syndrome.
3. A patient in shock is demonstrating an alteration in level of consciousness. The nurse realizes that this is most likely due to:
   1. respiratory acidosis.
   2. low circulating blood volume or hypoglycemia.
   3. renal failure.
   4. hypertension.
4. The nurse is triaging victims of a multivehicular collision. Which of the following patients would be the most prone to developing shock?
   1. A 45-year-old male with a fractured femur
   2. An 86-year-old female with abdominal injuries
   3. A 55-year-old male with an injured arm and shoulder
   4. A 38-year-old male with cervical spine injuries
5. A patient in shock has lost more than 2 liters of circulating blood volume. Which of the following should be provided to this patient as initial treatment?
   1. Normal saline
   2. Packed red blood cells
   3. Fresh frozen plasma
   4. Dextrose 5% and water
6. The nurse is providing care to a patient in shock with an alteration in tissue perfusion and an increased afterload. Which of the following should be provided to this patient?
   1. Dopamine hydrochloride
   2. Nitroprusside sodium
   3. Epinephrine
   4. Norepinephrine bitartrate

Answers to NCLEX Practice Questions can be found in Appendix D in the Osborn Student Resources at nursing.pearsonhighered.com. Practice additional NCLEX questions online at the Student Resources site.

Pearson Nursing Student Resources Find additional review materials at: **nursing.pearsonhighered.com**

REFERENCES

Ackerman, M. (1994). The systemic inflammatory response, sepsis and multiple organ dysfunction. *Critical Care Nursing Clinics of North America, 6,* 243–250.

Adams. M. P., & Koch, R. W. (2010). *Pharmacology: Connections to nursing practice.* Upper Saddle River, NJ: Pearson.

Alexander, D. (1996). New concepts in shock management. *Air Medical Journal, 15*(2), 85–91.

Ball, C., de Beer, K., Gomm, A., Hickman, B., & Collins, P. (2007). Achieving tight glycaemic control. *Intensive and Critical Care Nursing, 23*(3), 137–144.

Barkman, A., & Pooler, C. (2009). Heart failure and circulatory shock. In C. Porth & G. Matfin (Eds.), *Pathophysiology: Concepts and altered health states* (8th ed., pp. 606–637). Baltimore: Lippincott Williams & Wilkins.

Bertolini, G., Luciani, D., & Bioli, G. (2007). Immunonutrition in septic patients: Philosophical view of the current situation. *Clinical Nutrition, 26,* 25–29.

Campbell, J. E. (2008). *International trauma life support for prehospital care providers* (6th ed.). Upper Saddle River, NJ: Pearson/Prentice Hall Health.

Casserly, B., Read, R., & Levy, M. (2011). Hemodynamic monitoring in sepsis. *Critical Care Nursing Clinics of North America, 23,* 149–169.

Cheek, D. J., Martin, L. L., & Morris, S. E. (2010). Shock, multiple organ dysfunction syndrome, and burns in adults. In K. L. McCance & S. E. Huether (Eds.), *Pathophysiology: The biologic basis for disease in adults and children* (6th ed., pp. 1969–1726). Maryland Heights, MO: Mosby Elsevier.

Cunha, B. A., & Bronze, M. S. (2011). Nosocomial pneumonia. *Medscape Reference: Drugs, Diseases, and Procedures.* Retrieved from http://emedicine.medscape.com/article/234753-overview

Dellinger, R. P., Levy, M. M., Carlet, J. M., Bion, J., Parker, M. M., Jaeschke, R., Reinhart, K., et al. (2008). Surviving Sepsis Campaign international guidelines for management of severe sepsis and septic shock. *Critical Care Medicine, 36*(1), 296–327.

Edelman, D., White, M., Tyburski, J., & Wilson, R. (2007). Post-traumatic hypotension: Should systolic blood pressure of 90–109 mmHg be included? *Shock, 27*(2), 134–138.

El Khoury, D., Cuda, C., Luhovyy, B. L., & Anderson, G. H. (2011). Beta-glucan: Health benefits in obesity and metabolic syndrome. *Journal of Nutrition and Metabolism,* Epub 2011 Dec 11. doi:10.1155/2012/851362

Emergency Nurses Association (ENA). (2007). *Trauma nursing core course.* Des Plaines, IL: Author. Retrieved from http://www.ena.org

Fernandes, T., Pontieri, V., Loretti, A., Teixeira, D., Abatepaulo, F., Soriano, F., et al. (2007). Hypertonic saline solution increases the expression of heat shock protein 70 and improves lung inflammation early after reperfusion in a rodent model of controlled hemorrhage. *Shock, 27,* 172–178.

Grenvik, A., Ayres, S., Holbrook, P., & Shoemaker, W. (Eds.). (2000). *Textbook of critical care* (4th ed.). Philadelphia: W. B. Saunders.

Guthrie-Chu, C. (2009). Sepsis and septic shock. Evidenced based monographs. Retrieved from http://www.nursingconsult.com/nursing/evidence-based-nursing/monograph?monograph_id=207869&filter=as&loe=&sortorder=title-a&pageno=1&parentpage=search&searchId=1196179791&searchTerm=Definition+of+Septic+Shock&page=&bestBetId=&search_type=allresults

Holleran, R. S. (2010). Shock emergencies. In P. Howard & R. Steimmann (Eds.), *Sheehy's emergency nursing: Principles and practice* (6th ed., pp. 445–456). St. Louis: Mosby Elsevier.

Institute of Medicine (IOM). (2010). *The future of nursing: Leading change, advancing health.* Washington, DC: The Academic Press.

Jacobs, L. (1994). Timing of fluid resuscitation in trauma. *New England Journal of Medicine, 331*(17), 1153–1154.

Kaplow, R., & Hardin, S. R. (2007). *Critical care nursing: Synergy for optimal outcomes.* Boston: Jones and Bartlett.

Keel, M., & Trentz, O. (2005). Pathophysiology of polytrauma. *Injury, 36*(6), 691–709.

Khan, P., & Divatia, J. V. (2010). Severe sepsis bundles. *Journal of Critical Care Medicine, 14*(1), 8–13.

King, J. (2007). Sepsis in critical care. *Critical Care Clinics of North America, 19,* 77–86.

Kochanek, K., Xu, J., Murphy, S., Minino, A., & Kung, H. C. (2011). Deaths: Preliminary data for 2009. *National Vital Statistics Reports.* Retrieved from http://www.cdc.gov/nchs/data/nvsr/nvsr59/nvsr59_04.pdf

Kowalenko, T., Stern, S., Dronen, S., & Wang, X. (1992). Improved outcome with hypotensive resuscitation of uncontrolled hemorrhagic shock in a swine model. *Journal of Trauma, 33*(3), 349–353.

Krau, S. D. (2007). Making sense of multiple organ dysfunction syndrome. *Critical Care Nursing Clinics of North America 19*(1), 87–97.

Levy, M. M., Delinger, R. P., Townsend, S. R., Townsend, S. F., Linde-Zwirble, W., Marshall, J., et al. (2010). The Surviving Sepsis Campaign: Results of an international guideline-based performance improvement program targeting severe sepsis. *Intensive Care Med, 36*(2), 222–231.

Martin, R., Bicknell, W., Pepe, P., Burch, J., & Mattox, K. (1992). Prospective evaluation of preoperative fluid resuscitation in hypotensive patients with penetrating truncal injury: A preliminary report. *Journal of Trauma, 33*(3), 354–362.

Masur, H. (2003). Strategies to reduce the incidence of antibiotic-resistant pathogens in the ICU. Retrieved from http://www.medscape.com

McSwain, N. E., Champion, H. R., Fabian, T. C., Hoyt, D. B., Wade, C. E., Eastridge, B. J., et al. (2011). State of the art of fluid resuscitation 2010: Prehospital and immediate transition to the hospital. *Journal of Trauma Injury, Infection and Critical Care, 70*(5), S2–S10.

Mizouk, B. A. (2009). The multiple organ dysfunction syndrome. *Disease-a-Month, 55,* 476–526.

Mosenthal, A. C., & Murphy, P. A. (2003). Trauma care and palliative care: Time to integrate the two? *Journal of the American College of Surgeons, 197*(3), 509–516.

National Association of Emergency Medical Technicians (NAEMT). (2011). *PHTLS. Prehospital trauma life support* (7th ed.). St. Louis: Mosby/JEMS.

Neveleff, D., & Kraiss, L. (2010). Implementing methods to improve perioperative hemostasis in the surgical and trauma settings. *AORN Journal, 5*(5), S1–S15.

Porter, R. (1997). *The greatest benefit to mankind.* New York: W. W. Norton.

Rondanelli, M., Opizzi, A., & Monteferrario, F. (2009). The biological activity of beta-glucans. *Minerva Medical, 100*(3), 237–245.

Rote, N. (2010). Alterations in immunity and inflammation. In K. L. McCance & S. E. Heuther (Eds.), *Pathophysiology: The biological basis for disease in adults and children* (6th ed., pp. 256–292). St. Louis: Mosby.

Rote, N., & McCance, K. (2010a). Alterations in erythrocyte function. In K. L. McCance & S. E. Heuther (Eds.), *Pathophysiology: The biological basis for disease in adults and children* (6th ed., pp. 989–1013). St. Louis: Mosby.

Rote, N., & McCance, K. (2010b). Alterations in leukocyte, lymphoid, and hemostatic function. K. L. McCance & S. E. Heuther (Eds.), *Pathophysiology: The biological basis for disease in adults and children* (6th ed., pp. 1014–1061). St. Louis: Mosby.

Rueden, K., & Dunham, C. M. (1994). Sequelae of massive fluid resuscitation in trauma patients. *Critical Care Nursing Clinics of North America, 6,* 463–472.

Senoglu, N., Yuzbasioglu, M. F., Aral, M., Ezberci, M., Kurutas, E. B., Bulbuloglu, E., et al. (2008). Protective effects of N-acetylcysteine and beta-glucan pretreatment on oxidative stress in cecal ligation and puncture model of sepsis. *Journal of Investigative Surgery, 21*(5), 237–243.

Smith, M. A., & McInnis, L. A. (2007). Antimicrobial resistance in critical care. *Critical Care Clinics of North America, 19*(1),53–60.

Sun, L., & Zhao, Y. (2011). The biological role of dectin-1 in immune response. *Cellular Immunology, 270*(2), 183–187. Epub 2011 May 10.

Surviving Sepsis Campaign. (2008). Guidelines for management of severe sepsis and septic shock. Retrieved from http://www.survivingsepsis.org/About_the_Campaign/Pages/AbouttheCampaign.aspx

Tanabe, P., Semonin Holleran, R., & Reddin, C. (2010). Pain. In P. Howard & R. Steimmann (Eds.), *Sheehy's emergency nursing: Principles and practice* (6th ed., pp. 127–147).

Tisherman, S. A. (2010). What is the best approach to fluid management, transfusion therapy, and the end points of resuscitation in trauma? In C. S. Deutschman & P. J. Neligan (Eds.), *Evidenced-based practice of critical care* (pp. 591–598). Philadelphia: Saunders Elsevier.

Toevs, C. C. (2011). Palliative medicine in the surgical intensive care unit and trauma. *Surgical Clinics of North America, 91*(2), 325–331.

Vincent, J., Martinez, E. O., & Silva, E. (2011). Evolving concepts in sepsis definitions. *Critical Care Nursing Clinics of North America, 23*(2), 29–39.

Vis, M. M., Piek, J. J., & Henriques, J. P. (2011). Cardiogenic shock: Role of revascularization. *Minerva Cardioangioliga, 59*(1), 75–87.

Wilkinson, J. M., & Ahearn, N. R. (2009). *Prentice Hall nursing diagnosis handbook* (9th ed.). Upper Saddle River, NJ: Prentice Hall.

CHAPTER

55 Nursing Assessment of the Patient with Hematologic Disorders

Dawn Lambie
Renée Holleran

Outcome-Based Learning Objectives

After studying this chapter, the learner will be able to:

1. Explain how the hematologic system functions in an adult.
2. Describe the types, characteristics, and functions of blood cells.
3. Describe appropriate nursing assessment responsibilities related to the hematologic system in the adult patient.
4. Analyze laboratory tests used to evaluate the hematologic system.
5. Distinguish between normal and abnormal test results for the hematologic system.
6. Discuss the meaning of "shift to the left."

KEY TERMS

absolute neutrophil count (ANC) p.1711
basophil p.1704
chyle p.1705
eosinophil p.1704
erythrocyte p.1703
granulocyte p.1703
hematocrit p.1710
hematology p.1700
hematopoiesis p.1701
hemoglobin p.1703
hemostasis p.1705
humoral immune response p.1704
leukocyte p.1703
lymphatic system p.1704
lymphocyte p.1703
mean corpuscular hemoglobin (MCH) p.1711
mean corpuscular hemoglobin concentration (MCHC) p.1711
mean corpuscular volume (MCV) p.1710
monocyte p.1704
myelosuppressive p.1709
neutropenic p.1710
neutrophil p.1704
plasma p.1702
platelet p.1704
red blood cell distribution width (RDW) p.1711
reticulocyte p.1703
reticuloendothelial system (RES) p.1704
stem cell p.1701
thrombocyte p.1704

THE HEMATOLOGIC SYSTEM is a very complex body system. Just as cardiology is the study of the heart, **hematology** is the study of blood. Just as the tissue of the heart makes up the cardiovascular system, blood is the tissue that makes up the hematologic system. The hematologic system can have problems inherent to itself, but it can also be a valuable source of information that reflects problems in other organ systems. Whether the gathering of hematologic data is for the purpose of evaluating the hematologic system itself or for the purpose of assessing other body systems, the nurse needs to understand the functions, structure, diagnostic tests, terminology, and nursing responsibilities that are relevant to the hematologic system. The nurse gathers this information through the assessment process, relying on both subjective and objective data.

Subjective assessment is accomplished by interviewing the patient or someone accompanying the patient (e.g., family member, friend) to obtain data regarding the patient's illness or reason for being seen by the health care provider. Objective assessment is an assessment obtained by means other than a patient interview, such as laboratory tests, x-rays, or vital signs. In an objective assessment, the data are retrievable without being dependent on the patient providing the information.

Anatomy and Physiology of the Hematologic System

The anatomy of the hematologic system can best be understood by describing its components. The most obvious is blood, comprising a wide variety of cells and supportive fluids. Additionally, there are other organ systems that contribute to the conceptual understanding as well as to the overall function of the hematologic system. These include the lymphatic system, the spleen (a lymphatic organ), the liver, and the reticuloendothelial/mononuclear phagocyte system (Porth & Matfin, 2009).

Blood is considered a type of connective tissue with two important responsibilities. First, blood and its associated vessels and organs provide a transport system that delivers nutrition, oxygen, and secretory products such as hormones throughout the body, as well as wastes to the kidneys and liver for disposal. Second, the immunologic products of the hematologic system are critical to the body's defense against infections and other foreign materials. In performing the two primary responsibilities related to being a transport system, blood also functions to maintain body temperature, control pH (to maintain a range of 7.35 to 7.45), remove toxins from the body, and regulate body fluid electrolytes (Kee, 2010). The contribution each component of the hematologic system makes to these functions is discussed in the following text.

Bone Marrow

Any discussion about the hematologic system should begin with the *bone marrow*. Bone marrow is the soft material found in the center of bones, and it is the origin of all blood cells. Bone marrow, one of the largest organs of the body, makes up about 4% to 5% of a person's total body weight. It consists of islands of cellular components (red marrow) separated by fat (yellow marrow). The **stem cell,** the precursor cell of all blood components (red blood cells, white blood cells, and platelets), resides in the bone marrow. When the proper stimulating signal is received, the stem cells undergo a series of cell division and differentiation resulting in the release of mature or nearly mature cells into the systemic circulation, as depicted in Figures 55–1◆, 55–2◆, and 55–3◆. This process is called **hematopoiesis.** See Chapter 56 for a thorough discussion of hematopoiesis.

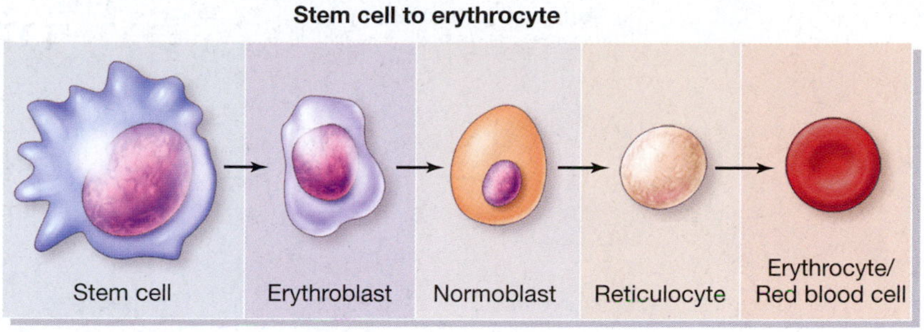

FIGURE 55–1 ◆ Stem cell to erythrocytes.

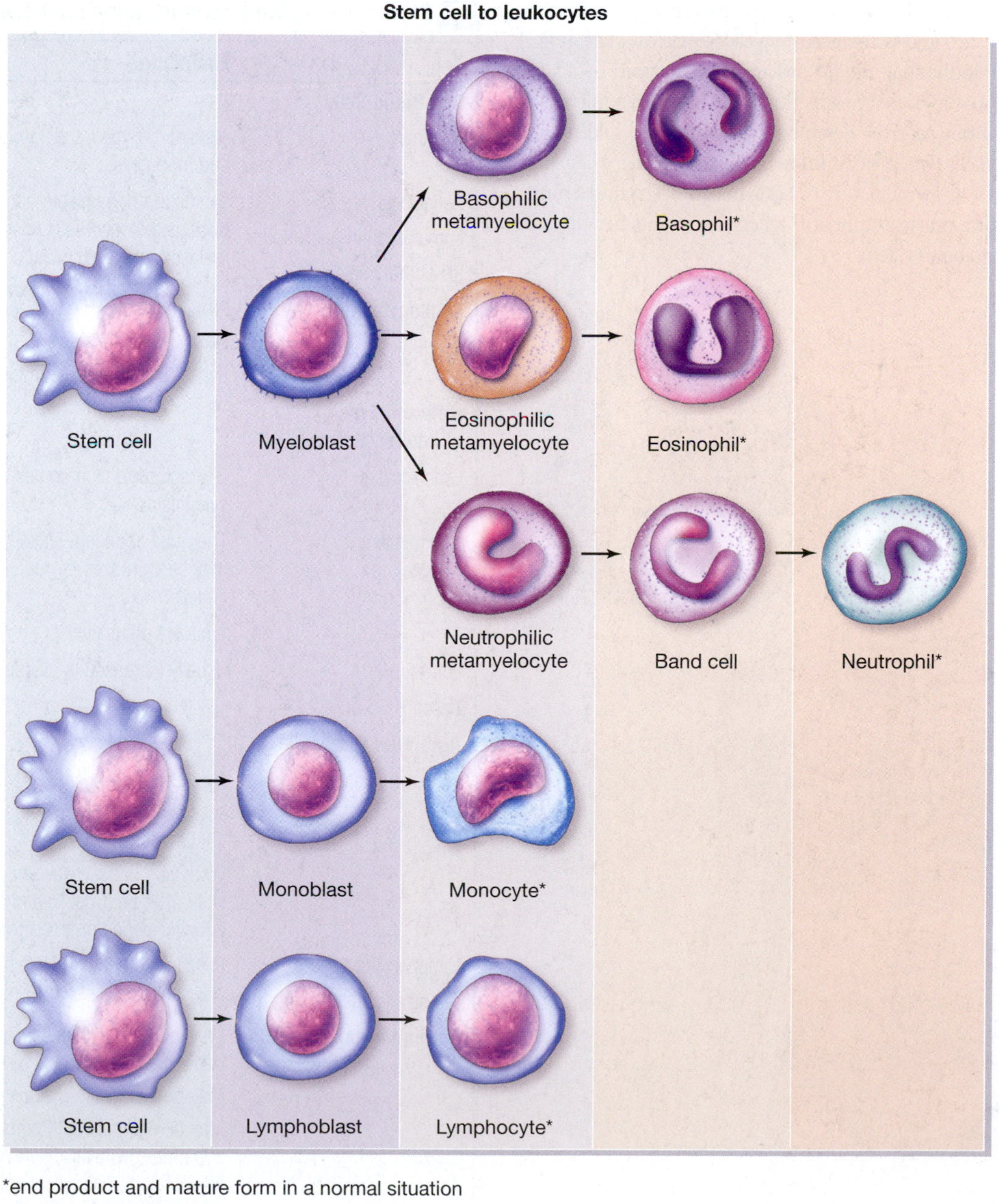

FIGURE 55–2 ◆ Stem cell to leukocytes.

Weblink: Image Bank of Blood Diseases

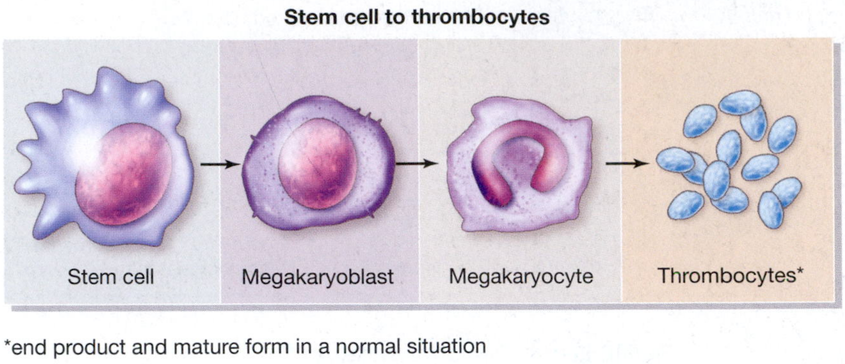

FIGURE 55–3 ◆ Stem cell to thrombocytes (end product and mature form in a normal situation).

In children, all skeletal bones are involved in the production of stem cells. With aging, marrow activity decreases and usually is limited to the pelvis, ribs, sternum, and vertebrae. As a person ages, the proportion of red marrow diminishes and is replaced by yellow marrow (fat); however, in the healthy individual, the fat can again be replaced by active (red) marrow if more blood cell production is required. In adults with diseases that cause bone marrow destruction, the liver and spleen also can produce blood cells by a process known as *extramedullary hematopoiesis.* Figure 55–4◆ shows a picture of bone marrow. The nurse must always consider bone marrow function when discussing any disease related to the hematologic system.

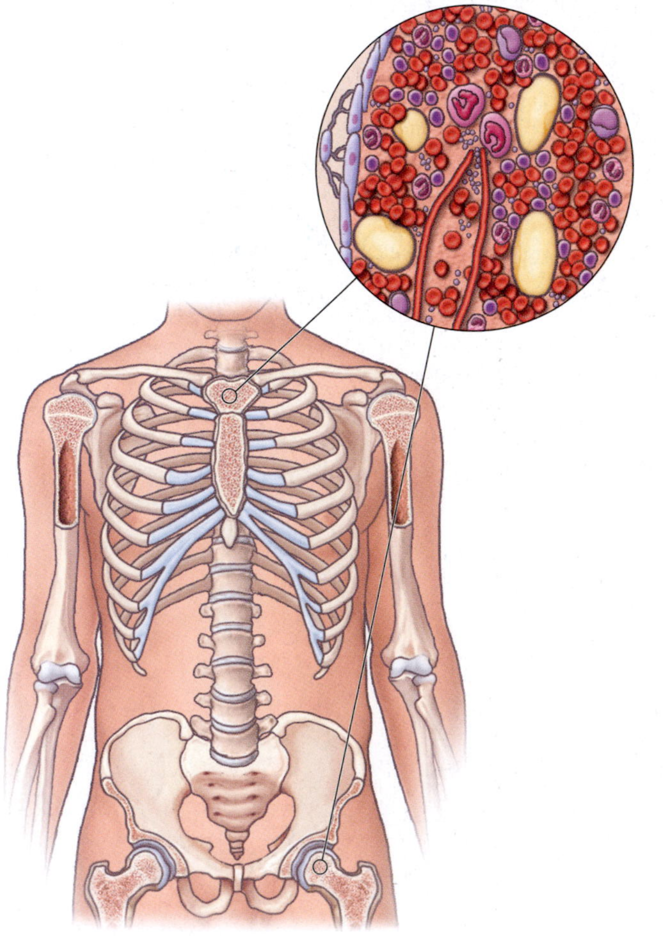

FIGURE 55–4 ◆ Bone marrow.

Types of Blood Cells

Blood is a fluid tissue that contributes about 7% to the total body weight of a person with a volume (in an average-sized adult) of about 4 to 6 liters. It is composed of 55% plasma and 45% blood cells (Porth & Matfin, 2009). **Plasma** is the straw-colored liquid in which the blood cells are suspended; it consists of approximately 90% water, with the remaining 10% being proteins, carbohydrates, electrolytes, and vitamins. A microscopic analysis of blood reveals a wide variety of blood cells that are broadly categorized into three major cell lines: erythrocytes, or red blood cells (RBCs); leukocytes, or white blood cells (WBCs); and thrombocytes, or platelets. Each cell line has its own characteristics and functions, as summarized in Chart 55–1.

CHART 55–1 Characteristics and Functions of Blood Cells

Cell	Function(s)
Red Blood Cells	
Erythrocytes	Transport oxygen and carbon dioxide to and from cells.
Reticulocytes: Immature, non-nucleated RBCs that contain RNA.	Synthesize hemoglobin after loss of the nucleus, so new RBCs continue to be released into the circulation.
Leukocytes (WBCs)	Protect the body against foreign matter. Leukocytosis: increase in the total number. Leukopenia: decrease in the total number.
Different Types of Leukocytes	
Granulocytes	Characterized by granules within their cytoplasm.
Neutrophils	The most abundant leukocyte; neutrophils may be increased or decreased in systemic infection. Work via phagocytosis.
Eosinophils	Usually increased in allergic diseases.
Basophils	
Agranulocytes	
Monocytes/macrophages	Monocytes give rise to macrophages. May be increased in infections and/or hematologic disorders. Work via phagocytosis; they do cleanup work after neutrophils and may circulate for a longer period of time than the neutrophils.
Lymphocytes T- and B-cell subsets	Function to fight viral infection; may be increased or decreased in infectious illness.
Thrombocytes/Platelets	Prevent blood loss by forming a platelet plug at the site of injury until a stable clot forms. May be increased in times of stress. May be decreased (thrombocytopenia) in bone marrow failure, autoimmune disease (idiopathic thrombocytopenia purpura), or disseminated intravascular clotting (DIC).

Note that reticulocytes are immature red blood cells, typically making up about 1% of the red blood cells in the human body. Also note that *leukocyte* is a broad term applied to the various cells of the immune system, including granulocytes (basophils, eosinophils, and neutrophils), monocytes, and lymphocytes (T cells, B cells, and natural killer cells).

Erythrocytes (Red Blood Cells)

Erythrocytes, or red blood cells, make up about 40% of the total blood volume. The RBC is produced in the bone marrow, and its function is to become filled with hemoglobin, maintain the chemical integrity of hemoglobin, and carry and distribute hemoglobin to the rest of the body's tissues. **Hemoglobin** is an iron-containing protein in RBCs that transports oxygen around the body. When oxygen combines with hemoglobin, the resulting oxyhemoglobin is bright red.

The normal shape of the red blood cell, a biconcave disk, is the optimal shape to perform this function. A biconcave disk can best be described as a donut or lifesaver shape. The cell has a diameter of approximately 8 μm and is very flexible; therefore, it is able to pass easily through capillaries that may be as small as 2.8 μm. Red blood cells also have a very thin membrane, which allows the oxygen and carbon dioxide to easily diffuse. A photograph of RBCs is shown in Figure 55–5 ◆. Their disk shape allows for optimal filling by the hemoglobin and ideal transport to body tissues through the circulatory system. The shape also provides a large surface that facilitates the absorption and release of oxygen molecules. With age, RBCs become increasingly fragile and are damaged by passing through narrow capillaries.

Red blood cells live about 120 days and then are ingested by phagocytic cells (those that engulf and ingest foreign particles, cell waste material, and bacteria) in the liver and spleen. The RBCs are eventually broken down by the spleen into the blood pigments bilirubin and iron. These components are then transported to the liver, where the iron is recycled for use by new erythrocytes. Approximately 3 million RBCs die and are scavenged by the liver each second.

There are approximately 4 to 6 million erythrocytes per microliter of healthy blood (although there are variations between males and females) (Kee, 2010). In the laboratory, RBCs are counted as the total number of RBCs in 1 mm^3 of blood. The typical red blood cell count is 4,600,000 to 6,000,000 cells per cubic millimeter for males and 4,000,000 to 5,000,000 cells per cubic millimeter for females. The number of RBCs is a measure of the blood's oxygen-carrying capacity. Hemoglobin accounts for approximately 95% of mature RBC composition.

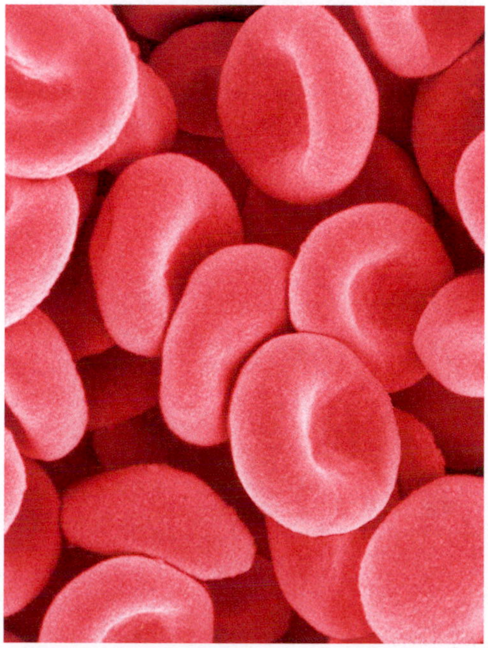

FIGURE 55–5 ◆ Red blood cells (erythrocytes).
Source: © Micro Discovery/CORBIS All Rights Reserved.

The bone marrow releases immature forms of RBCs into circulation that are referred to as **reticulocytes.** Reticulocytes are juvenile RBCs produced by erythropoiesis that spend about 24 hours in the marrow before entering the peripheral circulation. They contain some nuclear material, which consists of remnants of RNA. When measured in the laboratory, the percentage of reticulocytes provides an index of the rate of RBC production. Normally reticulocytes account for approximately 1% of the circulating red blood cells (Porth & Matfin, 2009). Reticulocytes persist for a few days in the circulation before forming the slightly smaller, mature red cell. The release of reticulocytes occurs as a normal response to an increased demand for RBCs, such as is the case with bleeding or possibly with disease.

In certain disorders such as sickle cell anemia, the RBC has a different shape and is more rigid than normal cells, causing difficulty transporting hemoglobin to the tissues. Two major consequences occur when red blood cells sickle: hemolysis (destruction) of the sickled cells and vessel occlusion. The rigidity of the cells causes obstruction of the microcirculation and ischemic injury to the tissues. This rigidity also makes the cells more prone to hemolysis or destruction while they are circulating through the spleen. The pain associated with sickle cell disease is due to vessel occlusion, resulting from ischemia. This can occur anywhere in the body (Porth & Matfin, 2009). (See Chapter 56 to learn more about sickle cell anemia).

Leukocytes (White Blood Cells)

The principal cells of the immune system are the **leukocytes,** or white blood cells. The WBCs generally are not present, except in a very small amount, in the bloodstream unless they are needed for defense against an infecting organism. They remain in the bone marrow, lungs, liver, spleen, and lymph nodes as developing and mature cells. The WBCs are separated into two major categories: **granulocytes** (or polymorphonuclear leukocytes [PMN]) and agranulocytes. Granulocytes are further divided into neutrophils, basophils, and eosinophils as determined by their staining properties in the laboratory. Agranulocytes are made up of monocytes and lymphocytes. Leukocytes have longevity of a few hours to a few days. There are approximately 4,500 to 10,000 leukocytes per microliter of blood.

Lymphocytes

Leukocytes are composed of approximately 25% to 35% **lymphocytes,** whose purpose is to recognize and respond to foreign antigens. Lymphocytes that produce antibodies include the T cells, B cells, and natural killer cells.

Approximately 60% to 80% of blood lymphocytes are T cells, and 10% to 20% are B cells. A common misconception is that the "B" in B cells refers to bone marrow, since these cells arise from bone marrow tissue. In actuality, the "B" stands for "bursa of Fabricius," a gland in birds where the cells mature and the first such tissue found in vertebrates. Immature B cells are produced by the bone marrow and released into the bloodstream. Upon interacting with an antigen, or protein, the B cells become activated into plasma cells, which are responsible for the production of antibodies, or immunoglobulins. All antibodies formed by the plasma cell are programmed to recognize only one unique protein structure: the antigen that stimulated the original B cell. (See Chapter 53 on immune response disorders for further discussion.) The process, referred to as the **humoral immune response,** is the mechanism in which organisms gain immunity to previously encountered substances.

T cells (lymphocytes) complete their maturation in the thymus gland and function in the peripheral tissues to produce cell-mediated immunity, as well as aiding in antibody production. Both T-cell and B-cell activation are triggered by the recognition of the antigen by unique surface receptors.

Both T cells and B cells destroy antigens (a foreign substance that is not naturally present and should not be in the body) and produce "memory cells" and antibodies. Memory cells attack disease-causing organisms if there is a subsequent invasion. This second response is much quicker than the first, thus preventing symptoms of the disease from occurring (Porth & Matfin, 2009).

A type of lymphocyte called natural killer cells (NK cells) are functionally distinct from T and B cells. Like cytotoxic T cells, they contain granules filled with potent chemicals; however, unlike cytotoxic T cells, they do not need to recognize a specific antigen before being activated. They are a major component of the innate immune system and play an important role in the rejection of tumors and cells infected by viruses.

Basophils

Basophils make up approximately 0.4% to 1.0% of the total white blood count (Kee, 2010). Along with the mast cells, basophils release heparin (anticoagulant), histamine (vasodilator), and other inflammatory mediators into the bloodstream. They participate in the destruction of bacteria with lysozyme and strong oxidants and play an exceedingly important role in allergic reactions (Porth & Matfin, 2009). An increased or higher percentage of basophils in the blood may indicate an inflammatory condition somewhere in the body.

Neutrophils

Neutrophils make up approximately 50% to 70% of leukocytes, and because their nuclei are divided into three to five lobes, they are typically referred to as polymorphonuclear leukocytes (Kee, 2010). Neutrophils are primarily responsible for maintaining a normal host defense against pathogens and are the first leukocytes to respond to organisms that invade the body. They act by carrying out the process of phagocytosis and also by releasing enzymes such as lysozyme that destroy certain bacteria. Neutrophils respond more quickly to infection than do monocytes. However, when monocytes reach the site of infection, they arrive in much larger numbers and, therefore, can phagocytize many more microbes than neutrophils are able to. Neutrophils also clear up cellular debris after an infection. Chapters 52 and 53 discuss the immune response.

Eosinophils

Eosinophils make up approximately 1% to 3% of the leukocytes. They liberate heparin, histamine, and serotonin in allergic reactions, intensifying an inflammatory response. The current belief is that they release enzymes or chemical mediators that detoxify agents associated with allergic reactions (Porth & Matfin, 2009). A higher than usual percentage of eosinophils in the blood may indicate a parasitic infection somewhere in the body. Eosinophils attach themselves to the parasite by special surface molecules and release hydrolytic enzymes and other substances that kill the parasite.

Monocytes and Tissue Macrophages

Monocytes and tissue macrophages arise from a common precursor in the bone marrow. **Monocytes** are the largest of the white blood cells and make up about 4% to 6% of the total leukocyte count. Monocytes and macrophages are a part of the **reticuloendothelial system (RES)** (also known as the mononuclear phagocytic system), whose function is to engulf and digest microbes and other foreign substances (Kee, 2010). The RES also removes senescent cells from circulation and provides phagocytic cells for both inflammatory and immune responses. Monocytes migrate from the blood to various tissues where they mature into macrophages. Macrophages, also known as scavengers, can either stay in one tissue or migrate from an organ via lymphoid tissues. Examples of tissue macrophages include Kupffer cells in the liver, alveolar macrophages in the lung, and microglial cells of the central nervous system. Macrophages are activated when their membrane comes into contact with an antigen. Once the microbe is ingested, the cell generates digestive enzymes and toxic oxygen and nitrogen products, thus killing the invading antigen.

The phagocytic white cells have a life span of about 2 to 4 months, which allows the macrophages to remain at the affected site for a relatively long time, sometimes until the antigen is destroyed. The macrophage response time works in concert with that of the first responders, neutrophils, which can rapidly surround and identify sources of infection but live for only about 12 hours (Rote & McCance, 2010b).

Thrombocytes (Platelets)

Thrombocytes, or **platelets,** are large cell fragments that are disk shaped and approximately 2 to 4 µm in diameter. They have many granules but no nucleus, and they live for 5 to 9 days. There are approximately 150,000 to 400,000 platelets per microliter of blood. The platelet membrane is covered with a glycocalyx, consisting of glycoproteins, glycosaminoglycans, and several coagulation factors absorbed from the plasma (Rote & McCance, 2010b). Glycoproteins act as a receptor in platelet function. Specifically, glycoprotein IIb/IIIa binds fibrinogen and forms bridges between adjacent platelets when activated, a process referred to as *aggregation*. Platelet activation and its role in hemostasis are discussed in the following text.

Figure 55–6◆ shows a Wright-stained smear of normal blood.

Lymphatic System

The **lymphatic system,** consisting of organs, ducts, and nodes, is responsible for removing excess fluid, proteins, and large particles from the interstitial (between cells) spaces back to the bloodstream (Porth & Matfin, 2009). The ducts (called lymph vessels) are thin tubes that run

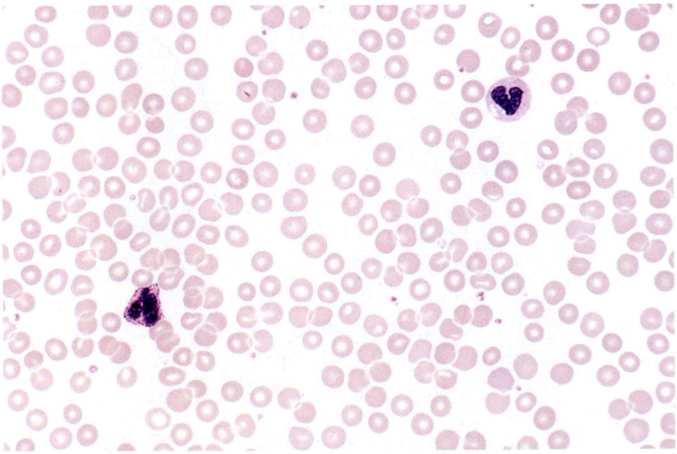

FIGURE 55–6 ◆ Wright-stained smear of normal blood.
Source: Corbis Images.

throughout the body in much the same way as blood vessels and with a similar structure to the capillary walls; however, instead of blood, they transport lymph fluid. Lymph fluid is formed from the natural diffusion of fluid across the semipermeable cell membranes of blood vessels and peripheral tissues into the interstitial space. The main functions of the lymphatic system are the following:

- Collect and return interstitial fluid, and thus help maintain fluid balance.
- Defend the body against disease by producing lymphocytes.
- Absorb lipids from the intestine and transport them to the blood.

Essentially, the lymphatic system is the body's highway and delivery system. Blood volume is maintained in every organ of the body as a result of the presence of lymph vessels. Lymph fluid is carried via the lymphatic system to every system in the body and then is returned to the circulatory system. Foreign objects such as bacteria and viruses also are carried through the body by the lymphatic system. When interstitial fluid volume rises, the increasing pressure drives the fluid into the lymphatic capillary walls. The walls of the capillaries are very permeable, allowing fluid to drain easily from the tissue into the lymphatic capillaries. The lymphatic capillaries, the entry point into the lymphatic vascular system, join to form the larger diameter lymphatic vessels, which ultimately drain into the subclavian veins of the neck. Once incorporated into the bloodstream, the lymphatic fluid can be appropriately processed by the liver, spleen, kidneys, and other organs.

Lymph nodes are small aggregates of lymphoid tissue located along the lymphatic vessels throughout the body. Each node processes lymph fluid from a discrete, adjacent anatomic site (Porth & Matfin, 2009). The human body has hundreds of clusters of lymph nodes placed strategically in the axillae, in the groin, and along the great vessels of the neck, thorax, and abdomen. The functions of the lymph nodes include removing foreign material from lymph before it enters the bloodstream and acting as the center for proliferation of immune cells. The lymph nodes are encapsulated structures where the lymph or chyle is juxtaposed (in proximity) to capillary blood vessels. The lymph nodes function as filters and reservoirs, acting as incubators for white blood cells. White blood cells, particularly B cells and T cells, mature and proliferate in the lymph nodes as they gain exposure to antigens absorbed from the interstitial fluid. During times of infection, these nodes can become swollen and tender as active lymphocytes, phagocytes, and invading bacteria and viruses initiate inflammation and the immune response; hence, the term *swollen glands*. Swollen glands can be palpated in the neck, axilla (armpit), or groin. However, there also are lymph nodes that cannot be palpated in the abdomen, pelvis, and chest. The lymph fluid distributes immune cells and other factors throughout the body (Rote, 2010).

The lymphatic system also contains certain hormones, protein, and gastrointestinal fat depending on the original location of the interstitial fluid. For instance, interstitial fluid, and consequently lymph fluid, surrounding the gastrointestinal tract is milky and turbid with a high percentage of fat. This lymphatic fluid is known as **chyle.** Microscopic evaluation of lymph fluid reveals a close resemblance to blood, but lymph fluid is much more dilute.

Spleen

The spleen is a large, ovoid secondary lymphoid organ located in the upper left corner of the abdominal cavity. It generally cannot be palpated because it is under the ribs. The spleen stores blood (20 to 40 mL of RBCs), removes old blood cells, and, as one of its primary roles, filters and destroys antigens before they can enter the systemic circulation (Rote & McCance, 2010b). The spleen is able to remove old or defective erythrocytes from circulation. Most notably, the spleen is able to catabolize the hemoglobin released from decaying erythrocytes and return the iron component (heme) back to the bone marrow. Patients suffering from hematologic disorders that result in high turnover of erythrocytes frequently present with an enlarged spleen (splenomegaly). Additionally, the spleen stores approximately one-third of the total volume of platelets.

Liver

The liver is the largest visceral organ of the body that performs multiple functions. (See Chapter 38 for further discussion of disorders of the liver.) For example, the liver produces bile; metabolizes hormones and drugs; synthesizes proteins, glucose, and blood-clotting factors; stores vitamins and minerals; changes ammonia produced by deamination of amino acids to urea; and converts fatty acids to ketones. As it relates to hematology, the liver stores blood and plays an important role in the clotting mechanism of blood (discussed in the following text). The liver produces the coagulation factors that are necessary for fibrin clot formation; in addition, the liver can produce anticoagulants so that there is not too much clotting.

Normal Clotting Mechanism: Hemostasis

Hemostasis is defined as the stopping of blood flow. Under normal conditions, hemostasis is regulated by a complex array of activators and inhibitors that maintain blood fluidity and prevent blood loss from the vascular space. The balance between the forces that cause blood to solidify or to remain fluid is very delicate and involves several interacting systems.

Intact blood vessels are central to moderating blood's tendency to clot. The endothelial cells of intact vessels prevent thrombus formation by secreting tissue plasminogen activator (t-PA) and by inactivating thrombin and adenosine diphosphate (ADP). Injury to vessels overwhelms these protective mechanisms, and hemostasis occurs. A blood vessel must incur an injury in order for hemostasis to be initiated. Hemostasis then proceeds in two phases: primary and secondary hemostasis. Figure 55–7 ◆ shows the normal sequencing of hemostasis, starting with the injury (called the *vascular phase*).

Primary Hemostasis

Primary hemostasis is characterized by vascular contraction, platelet adhesion, and formation of a soft aggregate plug. Primary hemostasis begins immediately after endothelial disruption. After the injury occurs, the initial, temporary response is vasoconstriction. This is the body's adaptive mechanism that tries to stop or at least minimize blood loss following injury to a vessel. Vasoconstriction slows blood flow, thereby enhancing platelet adhesion and activation. This promotes the ability of platelets to gather at the site of injury. First, the platelet is attracted to the exposed subendothelial layer of collagen and adheres to it. To accomplish this, the platelet undergoes a shape change. Second, the platelets release ADP, which stimulates other platelets to stick together at the wound site. Aggregation then occurs when the platelets adhere to each other to form a beginning plug. Finally, coagulation occurs and fibrin forms around the platelet aggregate to initiate repair (Porth & Matfin, 2009).

Weblink: Hemostasis Animation Video

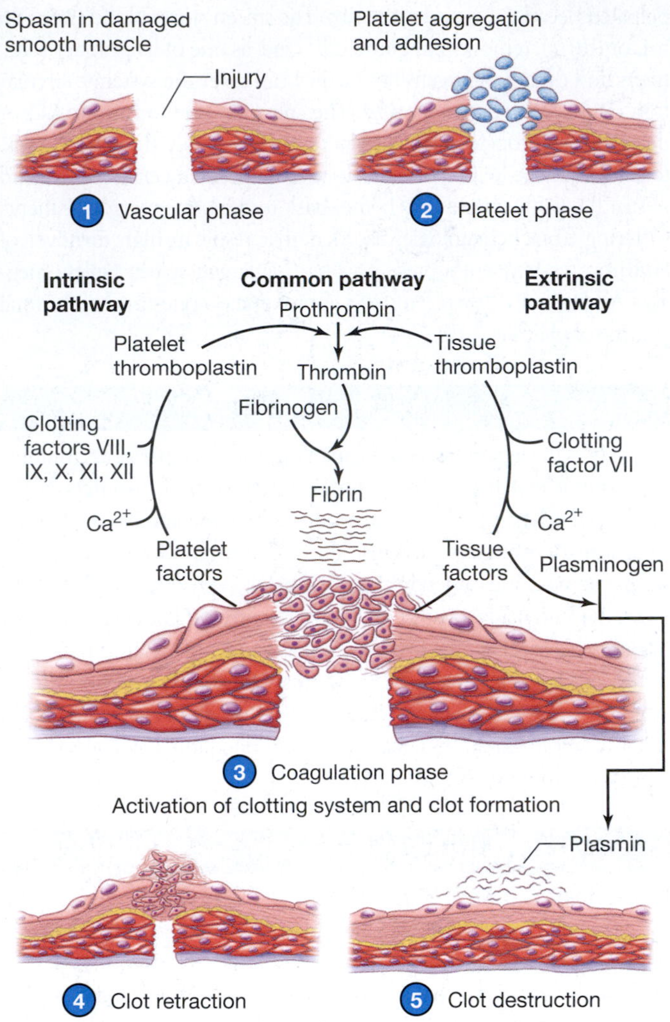

FIGURE 55–7 ◆ Hemostasis progression.

CHART 55–2 Sequential Steps of Hemostasis

A. Blood Vessel Spasm

1. Cutting a blood vessel causes a release of neural reflexes and humoral factors that result in muscle spasm.

B. Platelet Plug Formation

2. Platelets come into contact with the injured vessel wall, causing adhesion of the exposed edges of damaged blood vessels, forming a net with spiny processes protruding from their membranes.
3. Platelet aggregation occurs soon after adhesion, resulting in a platelet plug to stop the bleeding.
4. Platelet adhesion and aggregation stimulate the activation of the clotting cascade.

C. Blood Coagulation

5. Damaged tissues release tissue thromboplastin, which activates the first in a series of factors leading to the production of prothrombin activator.
6. Prothrombin activator converts prothrombin into thrombin, which, in turn, catalyzes a reaction that converts fibrinogen into fibrin. Fibrin forms a meshwork that cements the platelets and other blood components together. The amount of prothrombin activator formed is proportional to the amount of tissue damage.
7. Once a clot forms, it promotes still more clotting through a positive feedback system. Fibroblasts invade the area and produce fibers throughout the clots.
8. A clot that forms abnormally in a vessel is a thrombus; if it dislodges, it is an embolus.
9. Within 20–60 minutes after a clot has formed, clot retraction begins, causing the edges of the broken blood vessel to pull together, thus assisting with hemostasis.
10. Shortly after the formation of a clot, dissolution begins. Clots dissolve by fibrinolysis. The process involves the activation of plasmin by plasminogen, which then digests the fibrin strands of the clot. This allows blood flow to be reestablished and permanent tissue repair to take place.

Primary hemostasis is short lived. The immediate postinjury vascular constriction abates quickly. If flow is allowed to increase, the soft plug could be sheared from the injured surface, possibly creating emboli.

Secondary Hemostasis

Secondary hemostasis is responsible for stabilizing the soft clot and maintaining vasoconstriction. This phase is initiated when the cascade system of coagulation is activated by substances released at the time of injury. Depending on the type of stimulus or injury to the vessel, one of two clotting pathways is followed. These are referred to as intrinsic and extrinsic pathways, the end result from either pathway being the conversion of prothrombin to thrombin. Thrombin is necessary for fibrinogen to be converted into fibrin, the stabilizing protein that anchors the fragile platelet plug to the site of injury, thereby preventing further bleeding and allowing the injured vessel to heal. Primary and secondary hemostasis are summarized in Chart 55–2.

Coagulation Factors and the Cascade System

Coagulation factors circulate in the plasma as cofactors or as procoagulants; when activated, some of the components are needed for clot formation. The coagulation factors are generated in the liver cells, except for Factor VIII (or at least the von Willebrand's portion), which is produced in multiple organs, possibly the endothelial cells and megakaryocytes. The coagulation cascade system, as shown in Figure 55–8◆, is the model typically referred to in describing the mechanism of coagulation (Rote & Huether, 2010).

Damaged tissue releases Factor III which, with the aid of Ca^{2+}, will activate Factor VII, thus initiating the extrinsic mechanism. Factor XII from active platelets will activate Factor XI, thus initiating the intrinsic mechanism. Both active Factor VII and active Factor XI will promote cascade reactions, eventually activating Factor X. Active Factor X, along with Factor III, Factor V, Ca^{2+}, and platelet thromboplastic factor (PF_3), will activate prothrombin activator. Prothrombin activator converts prothrombin to thrombin, which converts fibrinogen to fibrin. Fibrin initially forms a loose mesh, but then Factor XIII causes the formation of covalent cross links, which convert fibrin to a dense aggregation of fibers. Platelets and RBCs become caught in this mesh of fibers, thus forming a blood clot.

As previously described, coagulation is actually a cascade of events. In the normal scenario, one enzyme activates the following proenzyme until the mesh fibrin network is developed, established, and functioning; a blood clot is formed; and the bleeding stops.

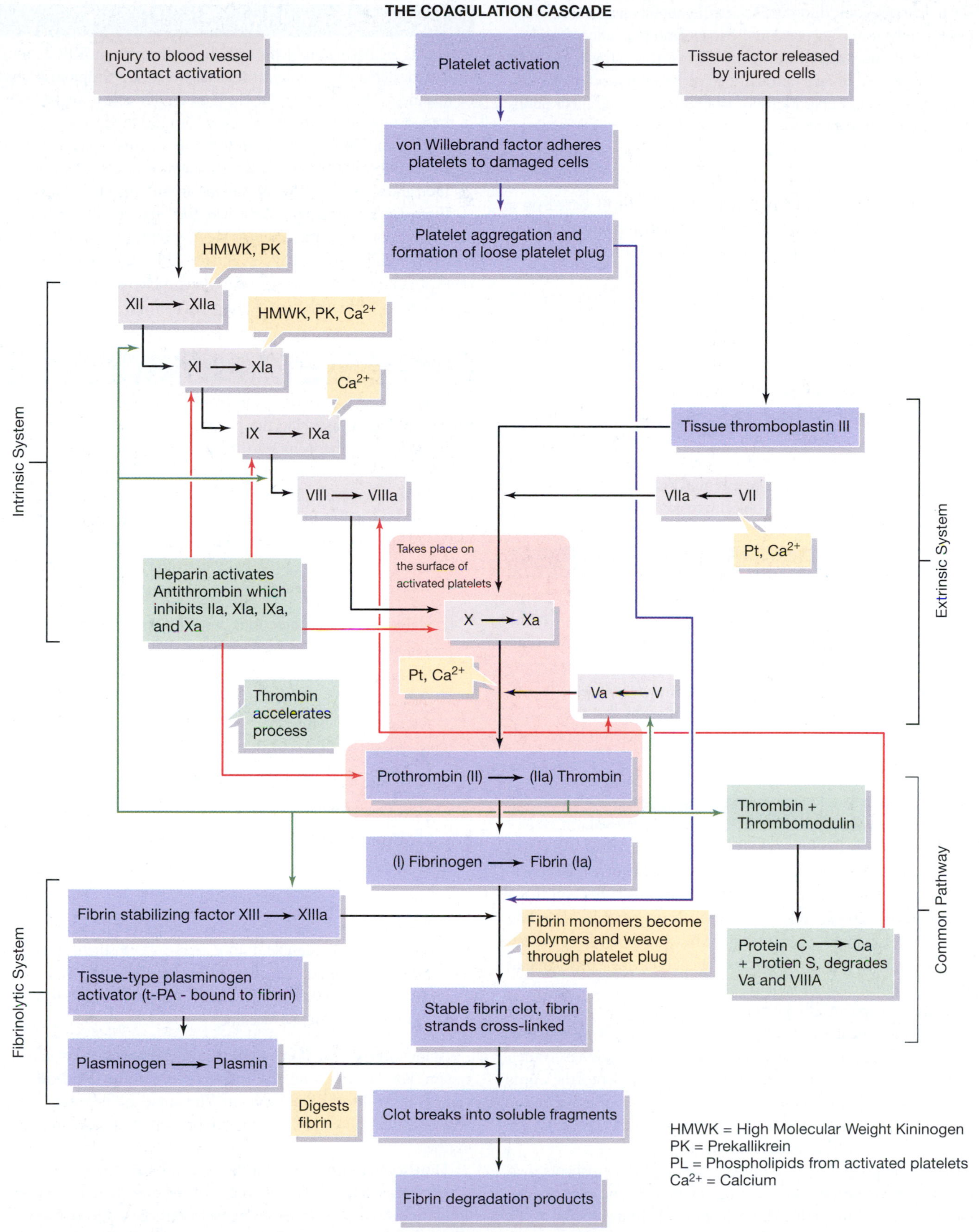

FIGURE 55–8 ◆ Coagulation cascade.

Weblink: Coagulation Cascade

Hereditary bleeding disorders, such as hemophilia, are caused by deficiencies in the factors involved in the coagulation cascade. Also, identification of the intrinsic pathway versus the extrinsic pathway and what factors are involved in each (as described earlier) is important because this information has implications for laboratory tests and medications that are ordered for patients.

History

Much of the evaluation of the hematologic system is based on a complete health history. In assessing a patient for hematopoietic system status, it is important to be thorough and to consider the presenting symptoms, chief complaint, and family history. Many hematologic conditions cause few symptoms; therefore, the use of extensive laboratory tests often is required to diagnose a hematologic disorder. Hematologic disorders are discussed in depth in Chapter 56.

A thorough history will help the nurse identify symptoms related to abnormalities with the hematologic system as well as current or potential problems. Information learned from a thorough history and physical exam could help prevent undesirable responses to current therapies and treatment plans. The essential assessment is contingent on obtaining both subjective and objective data.

Biographic and Demographic Data

Assessment of biographic and demographic data includes information regarding age, race, gender, and ethnicity, all of which can affect the susceptibility to some hematologic disorders. For example, African Americans have a higher incidence of sickle cell anemia than Caucasians, and a family history of coagulation disorders increases the risk for the individual. Particular patients may not know that they have a "hematologic" problem but may know that they have problems with prolonged bleeding.

Chief Complaint

The current issue is the focus of why the patient is being evaluated. Unless the patient already has some knowledge of her hematologic system from previous evaluations, the patient usually will not know that a hematologic problem exists. The patient will report generally not feeling well. From the questions asked during the history taking, the nurse can begin to determine whether or not the patient is having a problem that arises from the hematologic system.

The chief complaint tells the nurse, in the patient's own words, what problem(s) the patient is currently experiencing. In this way, it focuses the history-taking process and prioritizes treatment regimens. When the chief complaint is documented, the nurse actually writes the words that the patient has used to describe the complaint. For example, the patient may state, "I always feel tired, no matter how early I go to bed" or "It is all I can do to get through the day."

It also is important for the nurse to determine the patient's own perception of her health status in order to assist the patient with developing a plan for future health promotion. The nurse should assess risk factors such as smoking and alcohol intake, as well as the patient's dietary history. Other assessment factors include elimination pattern, activity–exercise pattern, sleep–rest pattern, and cognitive–perceptual pattern. Knowledge of these areas helps the nurse in determining the patient's current health status as well as helping to eliminate risk factors and promoting health restoration.

Presenting Symptoms

If patients are having problems with the erythrocyte, or RBC, component of the hematologic system, the usual presenting symptom is fatigue or weakness. The patient might say, "I used to be able to make my bed in the morning after I got up, but now I am too tired to even do that." Another common presenting symptom of a hematologic problem is shortness of breath. In this situation, patients may complain that they get tired and short of breath just walking around their own house.

If patients are having problems with the leukocytes, neutrophils, or WBC component of their hematologic system, they usually present with increasing episodes of illness and fevers. Finally, patients who present with unusual bleeding may be having problems with their platelets or thrombocytes or with their clotting mechanism.

Past Medical History

The history provides information from the patient's perspective and understanding. In assessing the patient, the nurse asks questions to determine what is happening to the patient, that is, what the patient is feeling and experiencing. In comparison to other systems (e.g., cardiovascular, nervous, reproductive), it is very unusual to ask questions about the hematologic system directly, since these questions are suggestive of changes in the composition and characteristics of the blood cells. Generally, questions are asked that would reflect the status of the hematologic system. Several such questions are as follows:

1. Have you ever had any prior problems with your blood, such as anemia, bleeding disorders, or blood diseases such as leukemia?
2. What medicines have you been taking, including prescription and over-the-counter (OTC) drugs and herbals, many of which can interfere with clotting?
3. Have you been feeling fatigued?
4. Have you been getting sick more often than usual?
5. Have you been having fevers?
6. Have you had any bloody or black stools?
7. Have you ever vomited brown or red liquid?
8. Have you had your spleen removed?
9. Have you had surgery or a major injury requiring medical intervention, for example, tumor removal, prosthetic heart valve placement, surgical excision of duodenum, and partial or total gastrectomy? Did any health care professional tell you that it took a long time to stop the bleeding?

Many surgical procedures affect the functioning of the hematologic system. For example, iron absorption occurs in the duodenum, and vitamin B_{12} is absorbed in the ileum. The nurse should discuss wound healing complications and bleeding in the context of past surgeries and injuries.

Diseases that involve any of the hematologic organs will result in hematologic disorders. For example, cancer suppresses bone marrow, and liver disease affects the clotting factors. Kidney disease also greatly affects the hematologic system because it results in poor production of erythropoietin. Erythropoietin is a hormone produced by the kidney that promotes the differentiation and production of red blood cells in bone marrow. It starts the production of hemoglobin, the molecule within red blood cells that transports oxygen. Gastrointestinal (GI) disorders such as Crohn's disease also affect blood cell production and function because the GI tract is the primary source of the nutrients needed for blood cell development and because GI diseases carry a high propensity for bleeding. Similarly, any surgical manipulation of the component hematologic organs can have deleterious consequences. Assessment findings of previous gastrectomy, colectomy, or splenectomy warrant a further diagnostic work-up.

Family History

Many hematologic disorders have familial patterns. Genetic information offers clues as to possible hematologic problems that are known to be common in specific populations. For example, sickle cell anemia is found in individuals with an African background. Thalassemia often can be found in patients with a Mediterranean background. Hemophilia is found more frequently in Caucasian males than in African American males. Tay-Sachs disease is found primarily in Jewish people of central and eastern European descent, and it is now also prevalent in non-Jewish populations, including people of French-Canadian/Cajun heritage (Boss & Huether, 2010).

Familial patterns also can be the result of similar environmental exposure or behavior modeling within the family. For example, patients with families who engage in smoking, eat poor diets, or are not very active are more prone to engage in similar behaviors. A nurse should never make an assumption about patients' genetic heritage, but should always ask patients about their background. The Cultural Considerations box discusses how culture can affect the function of the hematologic system.

Risk Factors

The traditional profile of poor health maintenance behaviors (smoking, excessive alcohol intake, poor dietary pattern, and a sedentary lifestyle) has an extremely negative impact on the hematologic system and is the basis for development of risk factors. Excessive alcohol use results in vitamin deficiencies and may cause GI damage that can suppress hematopoiesis. Poorly balanced diets also subject patients to insufficient quantities of iron, protein, vitamin B_{12}, and folate, all of which are critical in the production of blood cell lines.

Alterations in the hematologic system can come from a variety of sources including medications, diseases, behavior patterns, family history, and surgical interventions. Examples of risk factors associated with drugs and medications are discussed in the following text. The presence of any of these risk factors places the patient at risk of hematologic system derangement. Many risk factors have only a temporary effect, in which the derangement subsides once the risk factor is eliminated or resolved (e.g., temporary dietary deficiency); others can result in permanent damage (e.g., bone marrow disease). When a patient presents with hematologic system risk factors, the interdisciplinary health team should provide appropriate assessment of existing alterations and education to prevent further damage. The Risk Factors box highlights medications affecting the hematologic system.

CULTURAL CONSIDERATIONS Related to the Hematologic System

As the number of patients from other cultures entering the health care system increases, the nurse should be prepared to care for diverse groups of people by becoming aware of the influence of culture on patients' perception of their disease and how it affects their lives. This can be done through courses or through observation of other cultures. For example, a nurse may have the opportunity to visit other countries with a focus on health care practices. A great deal of variation is seen in the cultural habits of different demographic areas. Beliefs and values related to health, illness, and death, as well as daily habits, nutritional preferences, and health practices, may exist that are culturally important to patients and a part of their daily lives. For example, certain cultures only eat vegetarian foods, which can affect the amount of iron available to produce adequate RBCs.

RISK FACTORS of Drugs and Medications Affecting the Hematologic System

Many drugs have a deleterious effect on the hematologic system. Mechanisms of action include bone marrow suppression, which stunts the development of all three cell lines; suppression of the clotting cascade; and inflammatory process suppression, which affects WBC efficacy. Of particular concern are any drugs that are specifically termed **myelosuppressive,** or suppressive of the bone marrow function. Drugs in this category, most notably chemotherapy drugs, will result in *pancytopenia,* or suppression of all three blood cell lines. Examples of more common drugs affecting blood function, specifically platelets, are salicylic acid (aspirin), clopidogrel (Plavix), eptifibatide (Integrilin), and ibuprofen (Advil, Motrin).

Additionally, a patient can have an idiosyncratic reaction to any medication that may affect blood studies. For example, some individuals develop prolonged clotting times while taking antibiotics. Patients also may not understand the interactions when taking multiple medications or the impact of complementary drugs and/or diet; for example, when a patient is placed on warfarin, the amount of vitamin K taken needs to be minimized because it is an antidote for warfarin and will affect its ability to prolong clotting.

Social History

The nurse needs to obtain a social history in order to identify potentially harmful habits and activities. For instance, does the patient smoke and drink? If so, how much and how often? Is the patient exposed to potentially traumatic events through occupation and/or leisure activities? Does the patient live alone or with others? If with others, who are they? These details are important to determine, as they may identify risk factors that make the patient more prone to hematologic disorders or complications from other disease factors.

Physical Examination

A complete physical examination is required to thoroughly assess the effects of hematologic system dysfunction. Because blood cells affect every major organ and body system, only a comprehensive examination can ensure that all possible derangements are identified. Generally, early indicators of hematologic derangement such as fatigue or bleeding can be identified during inspection. Although these signs can also be indicative of temporary and benign situations, keen health care providers will often act on these early indicators to progress toward more definitive diagnostic work-ups. If further physical examination, such as auscultation or palpation, yields additional evidence of hematologic derangement, the health care provider should again move toward more definitive diagnostic tools such as laboratory and/or radiological assessments.

Inspection

Simple observation allows the health care provider to observe the patient's general appearance and exertional effort, both of which yield clues in an assessment of the hematologic system. Patients who are short of breath, are fatigued, or exhibit poor stamina and poor mental acuity may be at risk of anemia or infection. Fever is a very serious sign that

Weblink: Complete Blood Count

warrants prompt attention even in the absence of other clinical signs. For patients who are **neutropenic** (decreased neutrophil supply), fever is often the only observable indicator of infection.

Skin

Changes in skin color often indicate erythrocyte disorders such as anemia (pale, loss of pallor), liver failure (yellow, jaundice), polycythemia vera (pink, flushed), or rapid breakdown of erythrocytes (brown, dark). Platelet and/or clotting derangements often produce tiny capillary bleeds that manifest as petechiae, purpura, or ecchymosis. The appearance of these skin changes, especially in the absence of recent identifiable injury, should be reported immediately so that a laboratory analysis can be performed. In patients with known hematologic deficiencies, assessment of the skin must be included during all routine assessments and whenever laboratory values or assessments of other body systems suggest hematologic derangement.

Head and Neck

The structures of the head, particularly the eyes and mouth, provide useful evidence in the evaluation of the patient with known, potential, or suspected hematologic derangement. Using a penlight, gloved hand, and tongue depressor, the nurse should thoroughly assess the gums, lips, tongue, and teeth. Symptoms that warrant further collaboration and intervention include tenderness, increased or decreased saliva, inflammation, reddening, ulcerations, and bleeding. These symptoms are most worrisome in patients with neutropenia because they indicate signs of infection. Pernicious anemia and iron deficiency anemia also produce a characteristic symptom of smooth tongue texture and pale gums. The neck should be inspected for signs of lymph node enlargement or tenderness, especially in the submaxillary, tonsillar, or supraclavicular regions.

Eyes

The nurse should assess the sclera for color and swelling. The appearance of yellow, jaundiced sclera warrants immediate reporting to the health care provider because this indicates an accumulation of bile pigment due to rapid or excessive hemolysis. It also is a sign of liver disease.

Chest

Structures in the chest that yield clues to hematologic system health include the heart and the lymph nodes. The heart is a sensitive indicator of most abnormalities; for example, the heart rate will increase (tachycardia) in response to both infection and anemia. The lymph nodes in the mediastinum or the axilla will become enlarged and tender in the presence of infection, lymphoma, and other metastatic cancers.

Abdomen

Abdominal tenderness is a general complaint, the appearance of which warrants a more detailed work-up. The first task is to isolate (if appropriate) the source of the tenderness, so as to identify which organ is involved. An enlarged spleen (splenomegaly) or liver (hepatomegaly) is a general indicator of increased blood cell destruction, the cause of which must be identified. Additionally, liver tenderness may be associated with clotting system abnormalities. Further blood studies are warranted whenever a complaint of abdominal tenderness is found.

Laboratory and Diagnostic Procedures

A variety of laboratory tests provide a thorough analysis of blood component status. Health care providers should evaluate laboratory tests not only for the relative quantity of components, but also for the size and character of each cell type. Most commonly, health care providers of any specialty rely on automated blood counts of peripheral cells (i.e., the complete blood count); however, microscopic evaluation of either peripheral blood or bone marrow aspirate yields additional information about size, character, and quality of blood cells. Specific blood abnormalities are discussed through the book with each disorder.

Automated Blood Cell Analysis: Complete Blood Count

The automated blood count provides a highly accurate report of the number of blood cells (RBCs, WBCs, and platelets) in a given volume of peripheral blood. This section discusses each component of the complete blood count including normal/abnormal values and clinical implications.

Erythrocyte Evaluation

The CBC provides a total number of erythrocytes, morphologic analysis of blood cells, and hemoglobin analysis. The total RBC count is reported as RBC $\times 10^6/\mu L$ with normal values ranging from 4.0 to 6.0 depending on gender and ethnicity (Kee, 2010). Physiological increases in the RBC count occur with living in high altitude or after increased physical training, as a response to an increased need for oxygen. Pathologic reasons for an increase in the RBC count (polycythemia vera) are chronic obstructive lung disease and, in children with congenital heart disease who are cyanotic, as a response to chronic hypoxia. A decreased RBC count can be due to:

- Abnormal loss of erythrocytes (bleeding)
- Abnormal destruction of erythrocytes
- Lack of needed hormones and elements for the production of erythrocytes
- Bone marrow suppression.

However, quantity alone is not a reliable indicator of red blood cell adequacy and function. For that reason, the RBC count is almost always evaluated in conjunction with hemoglobin analysis and morphologic indices (Kee, 2010).

Recall that hemoglobin (Hgb or Hb), which is measured in grams, is the functional protein of the red blood cell that enables RBCs to carry out their primary function of oxygen transport. Hemoglobin is reduced in cases of nutritional deficiency, bleeding, anemia, or hemodilution. Volume depletion (dehydration) or polycythemia vera, in turn, causes hemoglobin increases. The **hematocrit** value represents the percentage of hemoglobin in a given volume of whole blood that is occupied by packed RBCs, or the concentration of hemoglobin. However, this value is highly susceptible to fluid status changes such as dehydration; therefore, when making determinations about anemia, most clinicians tend to rely on hemoglobin. If a hematocrit value is not reported, it can be estimated by multiplying the hemoglobin by 3.

Red blood cell indices reflect the volume, color, and character of individual red blood cells, thus providing valuable data about the quality of these cells. The indices include these measurements: mean corpuscular volume, mean corpuscular hemoglobin, mean corpuscular hemoglobin concentration, and red cell distribution width.

The **mean corpuscular volume (MCV)** is a measure of the size of the RBCs. If the MCV is less than 80 μm^3, the erythrocytes are *microcytic*, or smaller than normal. This occurs with iron deficiency anemia, lead poisoning, and thalassemia major and minor. An MCV of greater than 98 μm^3 indicates that the erythrocytes are larger than normal (*macrocytic*) (Kee, 2010). Macrocytic RBCs occur with liver disease, pernicious anemia, and folic acid deficiencies. The MCV can be used as a predictor of mortality in advanced cirrhosis. If the MCV is in the normal range, the term *normocytic* is used. Anemia due to acute blood loss results in normocytic anemia (Kee, 2010).

The **mean corpuscular hemoglobin (MCH)** measurement is the amount of Hgb present in one cell; the **mean corpuscular hemoglobin concentration (MCHC)** is the proportion of each cell that is occupied by hemoglobin, indicating efficacy of interaction of the hemoglobin molecule with the erythrocyte. These two indices are discussed together because both are tests to determine whether the erythrocytes have a normal amount of Hgb (are normal color or *normochromic*), less Hgb (decreased color or *hypochromic*), or more Hgb (increased color or *hyperchromic*). Iron deficiency anemia is the most common cause of hypochromic anemia.

The **red blood cell distribution width (RDW)** is a direct measurement of the homogeneity, or consistency, of red blood cell size. Immature cells are larger than mature cells and will result in RBC size variations. Additionally, the shape of red blood cells is highly influenced by the configuration of the hemoglobin molecule. Diseases such as sickle cell anemia and thalassemia, both diseases of hemoglobin, result in variations in the size of the molecule. An increased RDW indicates a relatively heterogeneous population of red blood cells, indicating the presence of either abnormal or immature cells. The RDW is used to differentiate the various types of anemias.

The MCV, MCH, and MCHC measurements are primarily used in the classification of anemia. As discussed in Chapter 56, *anemia* is a broad term applied to any situation resulting in a decrease in hemoglobin or erythrocytes. Anemia can be classified further (substantially) according to the underlying etiology (for example, whether it is blood loss, iron deficiency anemia, or sickle cell anemia). These RBC indices are most useful in delineating the likely cause.

Safety Alert *A drop in hemoglobin level below 10 or a serial decrease in hemoglobin on consecutive reports may indicate anemia and should be reported to the health care provider immediately.*

Leukocyte Evaluation

Leukocyte evaluation can be summarized by the white blood cell count value, which has a normal value of 4,500 to 10,000 cells per microliter. Normal values suggest that a patient has a sufficient number of cells to support host immune defense systems. However, the distribution of those WBCs is of significant clinical importance. White blood cells, or leukocytes, are a large heterogeneous group of cells, each with a unique role in host defenses, as described earlier. Of these, the neutrophils are the first responder cells responsible for the initial detection of foreign antigens and initiation of the immune response cascade. However, the total neutrophil count is a summary value that combines immature (blasts), juvenile (bands), and fully mature stages of the neutrophils.

Only the fully mature neutrophils, and to some degree the juvenile subpopulations, are useful in defense. The bone marrow may be stimulated to release a large number of relatively immature cells and juvenile cells as a compensatory mechanism to combat severe infection. During this situation, the total WBC count increases, but the rise is due to the proliferation of juvenile cells. This phenomenon is termed a shift to the left and should be reported to the health care provider. In an otherwise healthy individual, this shift to the left may be an early sign of an otherwise undetected infection. However, if the total WBC count remains within normal limits or even slightly below normal and a shift to the left occurs, the patient may be left with insufficient host defenses. This can occur with bone marrow disease, immune system insufficiencies, or immunosuppressive therapies such as chemotherapy.

The **absolute neutrophil count (ANC)** is a useful measurement revealing the proportion of white blood cells that can be utilized in first response immune interactions. To calculate the ANC, add the bands to the neutrophils and multiply by the total WBC count. Values greater than 1,500 indicate normal immune defense. Some laboratories provide this number directly; however, it can be easily calculated from the white blood cell differential.

The WBC differential is a determination of each of the five types of WBCs in 100 WBCs. This is a separate test from the CBC and generally must be specifically ordered by the health care provider. In contrast to the automated CBC, the CBC with manual differential must be performed by a laboratory scientist who conducts a microscopic analysis of a blood smear. Bands and neutrophils (also called polymorphonuclear cells or stabs, depending on the nomenclature used by the laboratory) are reported as a percentage of the total WBC count. See Chapters 52 and 57 on immunology and cancer, respectively, for further discussion.

Safety Alert *A decreased number of neutrophils indicates that the patient is at severe risk of infection and without sufficient defenses to prevent sepsis. The nurse should immediately assess the patient for signs of infection, initiate appropriate interventions, and report at once to the health care provider.*

Platelet Evaluation

The platelet count is a useful indicator of bleeding risk because platelets are responsible for initiation of the clotting cascade. Fortunately, the platelet count requires little further calculation because its final value reported on the CBC can be used as an immediate indicator of platelet activity. Normal values range from 150,000 to 400,000. Increased platelet counts (thrombocytosis) occur with malignant tumors, especially if they are metastatic lesions, as well as with polycythemia vera and splenectomy. Low platelet counts (thrombocytopenia) may be idiopathic, related to cancer, due to an autoimmune disease, or the result of a viral infection. Low platelet counts are also common with acquired immunodeficiency disease (AIDS) (Kee, 2010).

Safety Alert *Platelet levels below 30,000 indicate that the patient may be at imminent risk of internal bleeding, especially cranial bleeds. In this event, report to the health care provider immediately and implement bleeding precautions.*

Coagulation Studies

As discussed earlier in relation to the clotting cascade, numerous components interact in a complex sequence of steps in response to endothelial injury (refer to Figure 55–8, p. 1707). Insufficiencies in activity or supply in any of the components will result in abnormal bleeding. A variety of coagulation studies are utilized to identify individual insufficiencies. Generally, longer time values indicate insufficient clotting factors or overactivity of clot-inhibiting therapy (such as heparin, warfarin, or aspirin).

Bone Marrow Examination

Examination of the bone marrow may be required for several clinical scenarios, including the following:

- Evaluation of unexplained peripheral blood cytopenias (decreased blood cell counts)
- Evaluation of unexplained excessive peripheral blood cell counts
- Evaluation of suspicious cells in the peripheral blood

- Staging or further analysis of leukemia or lymphoma
- Evaluation of fever of unknown origin
- Evaluation of patient iron stores when other tests are ambiguous.

Bone marrow aspiration removes a small amount of bone marrow *fluid* through a needle inserted into a bone. In contrast, a bone marrow biopsy removes *bone* with the marrow inside and is obtained with a visual inspection of the marrow structure. A health care provider acquires bone marrow samples from the posterior superior iliac spine of the pelvis or the sternum, using local anesthesia.

Although there may be variations in technique among health care providers, if the biopsy is obtained from the iliac spine, the patient generally is placed into the lateral decubitus position with the top leg flexed and the lower leg straight. This position allows for optimal exposure of the iliac crest while providing stabilization with the lower leg. Oftentimes, the nurse can assist the patient and health care provider in maintaining this optimal position.

Once the site has been sterilized and anesthetized with local anesthetic, a small skin incision is made through which the bone marrow aspiration and biopsy needles are inserted. The bone marrow needle consists of an outer shell surrounding a stylet. Once the stylet has penetrated the marrow, it is removed; a syringe is then attached to the shell allowing for aspiration of 2 to 3 mL of bone marrow. The bone marrow biopsy is done in much the same fashion with a specialized needle that is able to extract small amounts of bone. After the procedure, the nurse applies a small gauze square with mild pressure to prevent bleeding, and assesses the patient for pain and bleeding. The presence of either should be reported to the health care provider.

Bone marrow examination specifically evaluates the specimen for adequacy of volume and appropriate production of bone marrow cells. Specific results include the following:

- Evaluation of the adequacy of marrow development of each hematopoietic cell line.
- Morphologic examinations of the cells to ensure that structures are consistent with normal cells.
- Infiltration of the bone marrow by inappropriate cells. Normally, only early precursors of blood cell lines should be observed in the

LABORATORY TESTS for Hematologic Conditions

Test	Normal Values
Red Blood Cell Indices	
Erythrocyte	Adult: Male: 4.6–6.0 Female: 4.0–5.0 Million/µL × 10^{12}/L{SI units}
Hemoglobin	Adult: Male: 13.5–18 g/dL Female: 12–15 g/dL
Hematocrit	Adult: Male: 40–54% Female: 36–46%
Mean corpuscular volume (MCV)	Adult: 80–98 µm^3
Mean corpuscular hemoglobin (MCH)	Adult: 27–31 pg
Mean corpuscular hemoglobin concentration (MCHC)	Adult: 32–36%
White Blood Cell Count Differential	
WBC count	Adult: 4,500–10,000 µL
Neutrophils	Adult: 50–70% Segments: 50–65% Bands: 0–5%
Lymphocytes (MCV)	Adult: 25–35
Monocytes	Adult: 4–6
Eosinophils	Adult: 1–3
Basophils	Adult: 0.4–1.0
Platelet	Adult: 150,000–400,000
Prothrombin time (PT)	Adult: 10–13 seconds
Activated partial thromboplastin time (aPTT)	Adult: 20 to 35 seconds
International normalized ratio (INR)	2.0–3.0
Fibrinogen	Adult: 200–400 mg/dL
Fibrin split products	Adult: 2–10 mcg/mL

Source: Kee, L. J. (2010). *Laboratory and diagnostic tests.* Upper Saddle River, NJ: Pearson.

marrow. The presence of other cells may indicate disease, most likely some type of malignancy.
- Fibrosis.

Gerontological Considerations

The effects of aging on the hematologic system currently are under study. It is thought, however, that the amount of red marrow and the number of stem cells decrease with aging but that the marrow is not completely depleted even in very old adults. The remaining stem cells retain their functional capacity to divide; however, as they decrease in number, they are gradually replaced by nonfunctional fat cells. This, in turn, potentially decreases the marrow's ability to respond to the body's need for blood cells in the advent of injury or disease (Rote & McCance, 2010a). The older adult is more vulnerable to possible problems with clotting, oxygen transport, and fighting infection, especially during periods of increased demand.

Laboratory parameters, as they relate to the hematologic system of aging patients, usually are not much different than those of a younger patient (Kee, 2010). Although it is recognized that hemoglobin levels tend to decrease after middle age, more so in men than women (Favero, 2010; Tussing-Humphreys & Braunschweig, 2011), aging changes do not usually occur with the WBC count or platelet count. It has been suggested that there may be some T-cell function loss and that this may account for the poor response to immunizations in the older population (Rote & McCance, 2010a).

If an older adult is anemic, this is often due to disease processes in other systems as opposed to the hematologic system, such as GI bleeding or malnutrition. The nurse needs to bring abnormal values in these areas to the health care provider's attention because further evaluation may be necessary. Thinking that changes in these parameters are due solely to aging may result in an incorrect interpretation of the laboratory test, which could then lead to incorrect management of the problem. It often is the duration of the disease process, not the person's age, that leads to illness, morbidity, and mortality.

Health Promotion

The hematologic system affects every organ in the body, without exception. Therefore, its maintenance must be incorporated into any health promotion strategy. A review of the risk factors of hematologic disorders should help the nurse determine what health promotion activities should be taken. Individuals can do a great deal to maintain and optimize the health of their hematologic system. For example, patients should be advised to examine their genetic history to determine whether there is any family history of bleeding disorders. Eating a well-balanced diet that is rich in iron, vitamin B_{12}, and proteins ensures that the bone marrow is supplied with the requisite building blocks for blood cells. Direct patient teaching by the nurse or referral to a registered dietitian can be of tremendous benefit to patients trying to navigate a plethora of food choices. The effect of nutrition on the hematologic system is discussed in detail in Chapter 56.

Exercise is critical for maintaining a healthy hematologic system, both because it encourages production of blood cells from the marrow (resulting in reduced fatigue and less shortness of breath) and because it reduces the risk of cardiovascular disease. With increased exercise, the patient is at decreased risk of coagulation disorders.

Excessive alcohol consumption damages the hematologic system on several fronts: (1) impaired nutrition, because beneficial calories are substituted with alcohol; (2) damage to the GI tract, resulting in bleeding and impaired absorption of vitamin B_{12}, iron, and folate; and (3) damage to the liver, resulting in decreased coagulation factors and erythrocyte processing. The nurse plays a critical role in identifying opportunities to promote lifestyles that ensure the health of the hematologic system. Patients should be advised that diet may be a contributing factor for anemia. Refer to Chapter 56 on blood disorders for additional information on health promotion.

Critical Thinking Related to the Hematologic System

It is imperative that the nurse becomes familiar with the components of the laboratory tests and other examinations that are used to evaluate the hematologic system. The nurse must be able to do the following:

- Explain the purpose of the tests to patients and/or their families.
- Explain to the patients and/or their families why the hematologic system is being evaluated for a patient in a particular situation.
- Identify normal and abnormal values of a complete blood count.
- Differentiate normal versus abnormal laboratory values according to the reference ranges for the laboratory performing the test. These reference points must be available; if they are not provided on the laboratory report, the nurse can call the laboratory and ask for the normal reference ranges for that particular test.
- Identify situations in which evaluation of the hematologic system would be appropriate or inappropriate.

Tracking laboratory values over a time period to determine trending in abnormalities is an essential nursing measure and requires critical thinking. An isolated abnormal finding may not be significant; however, if the value continues to trend toward abnormality, it becomes significant.

The nurse must rely on critical thinking skills when interpreting patients' symptoms and assessment findings to determine possible and potential patient diagnoses and to consider the appropriate action(s) to take. Analysis of these data allows the nurse to make a diagnosis and then follow up with any required interventions. It is imperative that the nurse communicate and collaborate with other members of the health care team in developing and implementing a plan of care for patients with any hematologic findings outside of the normal range.

Critical thinking is essential in order to prioritize the most significant clinical manifestations that need further investigation. Problems with the hematologic system can range from conditions like anemia, which can be easily managed, to life-threatening disorders that affect the blood's ability to clot. It is imperative that the nurse be able to distinguish normal from abnormal, benign from serious. The nurse must rely on critical thinking skills in interpreting the patient's symptoms and assessment findings to determine possible and potential patient diagnoses and to consider the appropriate actions to take. Analysis of these data allows the nurse to make a diagnosis and then follow up with an intervention. It is imperative that the nurse communicate and collaborate with other members of the health care team in developing and implementing a plan of care.

Because the hematologic system impacts all of the body's systems, assessing the patient for hematologic disorders requires that the nurse evaluate the whole patient. Identification of pertinent risk factors such as taking medications that impact clotting is an important component in using critical thinking skills when assessing the hematologic system.

Effective critical thinking skills include being curious and not making any assumptions. Regardless of the health problem, each symptom identified should be thoroughly described in order for the nurse to gain a full understanding. The nurse can say to the patient, "Tell me more about the problem," or "How did it start?" The patient usually proceeds with a discourse about the symptoms. The nurse uses skillful interview techniques to explore and investigate each symptom further. Any symptom analysis would be incomplete without a thorough description of its characteristics.

NCLEX® PRACTICE

1. The nurse is explaining stem cell transplants to a group of students. The nurse should include which statement about the function of stem cells?

1. The stem cell is a primitive cell located in the bone marrow that is the precursor of red blood cells, white blood cells, and platelets.
2. The liver and spleen can produce stem cells during intramedullary hematopoiesis when disease has caused bone marrow destruction.
3. The primary function of stem cells is to transport oxygen, hormones, and waste products.
4. The stem cells are no longer required for good health as the patient ages.

2. The nurse educator is teaching a class of new nurses about the functions of the hematologic system in the adult. Which of the following statements made by one of the participants indicates the need for further instruction?

1. "White blood cells usually remain in the bone marrow, lungs, liver, spleen, and lymph nodes, unless they are needed."
2. "Immature reticulocytes will persist for several days in the circulation before becoming a small, mature red blood cell."
3. "The cells of the reticuloendothelial system initiate the inflammatory and immune responses."
4. "Leukocytes are responsible for maintaining fluid balance in all body tissues."

3. The nurse is planning to care for a patient who is newly diagnosed with anemia. The nurse anticipates performing which of the following laboratory tests to better classify the anemia?

1. PT, aPTT, PLT
2. HGB, HCT, ANC
3. RBC, RDW, WBC
4. MCH, MCV, MCHC

4. Which of the following laboratory test results should the nurse immediately report to the health care provider?

1. HCT 28%
2. PLT 400,000/μL
3. WBC 10,000/μL
4. MCH 30 pg/dL

5. During shift report, the nurse is told that a patient's laboratory values indicate a shift to the left. The receiving nurse understands that this phenomenon indicates:

1. the measurement of the proportion of white blood cells that are available for use in a first-response immune reaction.
2. an increase in the total white blood cell count because of the proliferation of juvenile band and immature blast cells.
3. a quantitative method of indicating the efficacy of interaction between the hemoglobin molecule and the erythrocyte.
4. that there are insufficiencies in either activity or supply in one or more of the components of the clotting cascade.

6. When describing the hemostasis mechanism to a group of students, which statements does the nurse recognize as describing the correct sequence of events that would occur in a patient when the normal hemostasis mechanism is activated?

1. Soft aggregate plug formation, vasoconstriction, fibrin conversion into fibrinogen, initiation of the intrinsic coagulation mechanism
2. Vascular contraction, platelets release ADP, prothrombin conversion into thrombin, fibrinogen conversion into fibrin
3. Platelet adhesion, onset of primary hemostasis pathway, Factor XI activates Factor XII, initiation of the extrinsic coagulation mechanism
4. Start of intrinsic clotting pathway, Factor III and Factor V release, platelet thromboplastic factor release, Factor X activates Factor XI

Answers to NCLEX Practice Questions can be found in Appendix D in the Osborn Student Resources at nursing.pearsonhighered.com. Practice additional NCLEX questions online at the Student Resources site.

Pearson Nursing Student Resources Find additional review materials at: **nursing.pearsonhighered.com**

REFERENCES

Boss, J., & Huether, S. E. (2010). Alterations of neurologic function in children. In K. L. McCance & S. E. Heuther (Eds.), *Pathophysiology: The biological basis for disease in adults and children* (6th ed., pp. 665–695). St. Louis: Mosby.

Favero, H. (2010). Care of the adult chronic kidney disease patient in the perianesthesia setting. *Journal of Perianesthesia Nursing, 25*(3), 162–170.

Kee, L. J. (2010). *Laboratory and diagnostic tests*. Upper Saddle River, NJ: Pearson.

Porth, C., & Matfin, G. (2009). *Pathophysiology: Concepts of altered health states*. Philadelphia: Wolters Kluwer/Lippincott Williams & Wilkins.

Rote, N. (2010). Adaptive immunity. In K. L. McCance & S. E. Heuther (Eds.), *Pathophysiology: The biological basis for disease in adults and children* (6th ed., pp. 217–253). St. Louis: Mosby.

Rote, N., & Huether, S. E. (2010). Innate immunity: Inflammation. In K. L. McCance & S. E. Heuther (Eds.), *Pathophysiology: The biological basis for disease in adults and children* (6th ed., pp. 183–216). St. Louis: Mosby.

Rote, N., & McCance, K. L. (2010a). Alterations of leukocyte, lymphoid, and hemostatic function. In K. L. McCance & S. E. Heuther (Eds.), *Pathophysiology: The biological basis for disease in adults and children* (6th ed., pp. 1014–1061). St. Louis: Mosby.

Rote, N., & McCance, K. L. (2010b). Structure and function of the hematologic system. In K. L. McCance & S. E. Heuther (Eds.), *Pathophysiology: The biological basis for disease in adults and children* (6th ed., pp. 952–988). St. Louis: Mosby.

Tussing-Humphreys, L., & Braunschweig, C. (2011). Anemia in postmenopausal women: Dietary inadequacy or nondietary factors. *Journal of the American Dietetic Association, 111*(4), 528–531.

CHAPTER

56 Caring for the Patient with Blood Disorders

Renée Holleran
Dawn Lambie

Outcome-Based Learning Objectives

After studying this chapter, the learner will be able to:

1. Describe the physiology of hematopoiesis, thrombopoiesis, and hemostasis.
2. Explain the pathophysiological alterations in erythropoiesis, thrombopoiesis, and hemostasis that give rise to specific hematologic disorders.
3. Compare and contrast the causes, clinical presentation, and therapeutic management of the various types of anemias and hemostasis disorders.
4. Analyze laboratory values, correlate them with physical signs and symptoms, and thus distinguish between various hematologic disorders.
5. Generate a nursing care plan for management of the patient with thrombocytopenia.
6. Compare and contrast the hallmark clinical presentation of bleeding disorders and clotting disorders.

KEY TERMS

absolute iron deficiency p.1727
anemia p.1718
anemic hypoxia p.1719
aplastic anemia p.1759
autoimmune hemolytic anemia p.1743
deoxyhemoglobin p.1720
differentiation p.1717
disseminated intravascular coagulation (DIC) p.1756
elemental iron p.1730
erythropoiesis p.1718
erythropoietic stem cells (proerythroblast) p.1717
erythropoietin p.1718
ferritin p.1727
functional iron deficiency p.1727
glucose-6-phosphate dehydrogenase (G6PD) deficiency p.1742
hematopoiesis p.1717
hematopoietic stem cells (HSC) p.1717
heme iron p.1729
hemoglobin p.1719
hemoglobinopathy p.1734
hemolytic anemia p.1738
hemophilia p.1755
hemosiderin p.1727
hemostasis p.1743
heparin-induced thrombocytopenia (HIT) p.1753
hereditary spherocytosis (HS) p.1742
iron deficiency anemia (IDA) p.1727
megakaryocytic stem cells p.1717
megaloblast p.1732
megaloblastic anemia p.1732
myeloid progenitor cell p.1717
nonheme iron p.1729
pernicious anemia p.1733
progenitor cells p.1717
Schilling test p.1733
sickle cell anemia p.1736
thalassemia p.1734
thrombopoietin p.1748
von Willebrand's disease (vWD) p.1753

HEMATOLOGY IS THE STUDY OF BLOOD and blood disorders. Although blood contains both plasma and blood cells (see Chapter 55), hematology focuses on the cellular components of blood, specifically the erythrocytes (red blood cells), leukocytes (white blood cells), and thrombocytes (platelets). The normal function of these cellular components is described in Chapter 55. Hematologic disorders arise when normal functioning is disrupted by disease, genetics, or environmental factors. The study of blood and blood disorders is best approached by a systematic review of different blood components. This chapter focuses specifically on two cell lines: thrombocytes and erythrocytes. Refer to Chapters 52 and 53 for an in-depth review of the nursing care for patients with leukocyte disorders.

Some hematologic disorders are acute medical conditions that require immediate medical attention; others are chronic, resulting in the need for permanent lifestyle adjustments. Acute hematologic disorders include acute anemia, thrombocytopenia, and disseminated intravascular coagulation. These acute disorders usually are not independently occurring disease states; rather, they are serious side effects that result when another underlying disease process is present. Chronic hematologic diseases include sickle cell disease, thalassemia, and hemophilia.

Most nurses are likely to care for patients with acute blood disorders, because chronic diseases tend to be well managed in the outpatient setting. However, patients with chronic hematologic disorders may be hospitalized for other illnesses such as infection, trauma, or cardiac problems. Also, physiological stressors can severely exacerbate chronic diseases, potentially leading to acute attacks. However, such attacks can often be prevented by diligent initial assessment paired with continual observation for deviation from the baseline. If a patient does have an acute attack, the nurse must ensure that immediate intervention and coordination with the interdisciplinary health care team occur to prevent serious injury. For all of these reasons, it is critically important for the nurse to include any existing or potential hematologic disorder in a patient's care plan.

Hematopoiesis: Development of Blood Cells

Hematopoiesis (Rote & McCance, 2010c) is the process of blood cell development, beginning with the immature hematopoietic stem cell in the bone marrow and extending to complete cellular maturation in the peripheral bloodstream. Problems that can occur during hematopoiesis account for many of the hematologic disorders that are discussed in this chapter; therefore, a review of the normal physiological processes involved in hematopoiesis is a useful foundation for the study of hematologic disorders.

Blood contains many specialized cell lines, including erythrocytes (red blood cells), leukocytes (white blood cells), and platelets. Despite their variation in appearance and function, all of the cell types in the blood are generated from the **hematopoietic stem cells (HSCs).** The HSCs reside largely in the spongy bone marrow of the femurs, hips, ribs, sternum, and other long bones, although a small volume of HSCs circulates in the peripheral bloodstream. The HSCs may be thought of as the common ancestor cell of all blood cell lines. Although they eventually give rise to mature red blood cells (RBCs), platelets, and white blood cells (WBCs), the HSCs themselves do not possess the full capabilities of oxygen transportation, clotting, or immune response associated with their more mature progeny, the erythrocytes, platelets, and leukocytes. The *pluripotent* HSCs found in the bone marrow and the blood should not be confused with embryonic *totipotent* stem cells, which are found in developing embryos and can develop into any cell in the human body.

The goal of hematopoiesis is not only to produce large numbers of cells when needed, but also to produce well-differentiated cells. **Differentiation** is the process by which immature precursor cells (such as the hematopoietic stem cells) produce generations of increasingly specialized cells, ultimately resulting in a fully functioning mature cell (such as a mature erythrocyte or thrombocyte). Differentiation also is associated with increasing morphologic distinction, acquisition of a specialized cellular structure and membrane proteins, and narrowing of the variety of blood cells that can be produced by a given cell. The hematopoietic cascade shown in Figure 56–1◆ is a common and useful illustration of this process.

From the HSCs, the next level of specificity is the lymphoid or myeloid **progenitor cells,** which are blood line–specific stem cells. The common lymphoid progenitor cell eventually gives rise to the lymphoid cells of the immune system, specifically the natural killer cells, the T cells, and the B cells. Refer to Chapter 53 for a discussion of disorders related to these cell lines. The common **myeloid progenitor cell** further differentiates into the granulocyte–macrophage stem cell, the megakaryocytic stem cell, and the erythropoietic stem cell (proerythroblast). The granulocyte–macrophage stem cell will eventually give rise to the granulocytes (neutrophils, eosinophils, basophils) or the monocytes (monocytic cells of the immune system and macrophages).

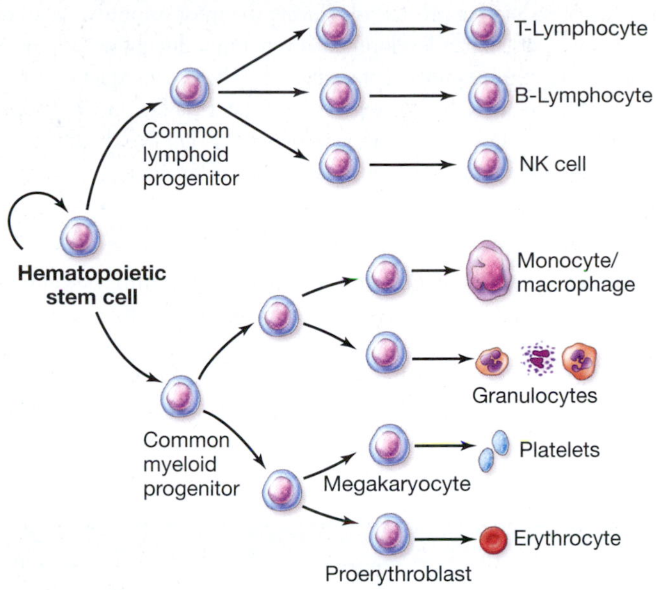

FIGURE 56–1 ◆ The hematopoietic cascade.

Immune system disorders related to these cell lines are discussed in Chapter 53. Of interest to this chapter are the **megakaryocytic stem cells,** which eventually will develop the platelets, and the **erythropoietic stem cells (proerythroblasts),** which will develop into mature erythrocytes or red blood cells.

The process of hematopoiesis is stimulated on an as-needed basis. Cellular and chemical signals, generated when the body requires increased production of blood cells, interact with cells undergoing hematopoiesis, beginning with the HSCs. An HSC receives a chemical signal to produce a particular cell line, to self-replicate to increase available HSCs, or even to undergo apoptosis (programmed cell death). Conversely, the absence of these chemical signals or the presence of inhibitory signals is associated with decreased levels of hematopoiesis. This elegant system of feedback regulation ensures that energy reserves are allocated efficiently and not wasted on production of already abundant cells. Common types of chemical signals that regulate hematopoiesis include soluble factors such as cytokines, direct cell-to-cell interaction, and contact with the extracellular matrix of the blood-forming organs. Specific signals include hormones such as erythropoietin in the case of RBC production and thrombopoietin and interleukins in the case of platelet cell production.

Research has expanded our understanding of the complexity, variety, and intricate interplay that exists among these cellular and chemical signals. A major field of research is directed at understanding these signals in an effort to expand the production of small numbers of highly pluripotent HSCs for clinical transplantation and for other scientific studies. Exogenous administration of hematopoiesis-stimulating chemicals is already a cornerstone of treatment for many diseases. Future treatment options will almost certainly evolve to incorporate medications derived from a growing understanding of these chemical signals. Specialized hematopoiesis of the RBC line (erythropoiesis) and platelet-forming cell lines (thrombopoiesis) are discussed later in the chapter as they relate to anemia and thrombocytopenia. As will be seen throughout this chapter, problems during hematopoiesis account for a large proportion of hematologic disorders. Successful hematopoiesis requires precise interaction and a delicate balance between numerous cells, chemical factors, and the physiological environment. Because

Weblink: Anemia

hematopoiesis plays a pivotal role during the most primitive stages of embryonic and cellular development, even minor disruptions can have far-reaching and amplified consequences. These consequences thus become the focus of hematology. This chapter builds on the pathophysiological foundation of hematopoiesis just outlined, highlighting alterations in the process that give rise to clinical disorders.

Anemia

Anemia is defined as a decrease in the total body erythrocyte volume, usually measured by a decrease in hemoglobin protein, a decreased hematocrit, and/or a decreased RBC count. The primary function of the erythrocytes is the transportation of oxygen on the hemoglobin molecules; thus, insufficiencies in the erythrocytes translate into an inability to maintain sufficient oxygen delivery to the tissues. Anemia is the most common blood disorder.

Generalized Anemia

Anemia is a condition in which there are not enough healthy red blood cells to carry oxygen to the body's tissues. Anemia can be temporary or chronic, and it can range from mild, with vague symptoms, to a severe and life-threatening condition.

Etiology and Epidemiology

Comprehensive mortality and morbidity rates for all causes of anemia are difficult to ascertain for two reasons. First, anemia is considered to be widely underdiagnosed; this is because patients often fail to seek diagnostic evaluation for symptoms of fatigue and shortness of breath, which are both symptoms of anemia. Second, anemia is not a disease in and of itself but rather is a clinical condition that results from some underlying pathologic disease process that often complicates a statistical tabulation. Anemia can be triggered by (1) loss of blood volume, (2) altered production of erythrocytes (hypoproliferative disorders), or (3) altered (increased) destruction of red blood cells. The various underlying etiologies have unique clinical presentations, which trigger a differential diagnostic work-up. After resolution of immediate life-threatening situations such as hypoxia or blood loss, treatment is tailored to address the primary hematologic disorder causing the anemia.

Normal Physiology of Red Blood Cell Development

A detailed overview of erythrocyte development, or erythropoiesis, is described next as a foundation for discussing various causes of anemia. Understanding the root causes of these diseases not only illuminates each cause, but also aids in patient education and the judicious application of treatment options.

Erythropoiesis

Erythropoiesis (Rote & McCance, 2010c), the process of hematopoiesis of erythrocytes (red blood cells), is stimulated primarily by the presence of erythropoietin, which acts on HSCs to produce the myeloid progenitor cell, thus starting the cascade toward RBC production. **Erythropoietin** is a hormone produced by the juxtaglomerular cells of the kidneys during periods of *hypoxia*, or decreased blood oxygen levels. Erythropoietin production also is modulated by other factors, including thyroid-stimulating hormone, adrenal cortical steroids, adrenocorticotropic hormone, and human growth hormone (HGH). All of these factors are produced during periods of increased growth, and their promotion of erythropoietin ensures that enough oxygen will be available to growing tissues.

As was discussed earlier, hematopoiesis results in cellular differentiation. During erythropoiesis, the pluripotent hematopoietic stem cell undergoes increasing differentiation, producing first the myeloid stem cell, then the pronormoblast, then the basophilic normoblast, the polychromatophilic normoblast, the orthochromatic normoblast, and the reticulocyte (Figure 56–2◆). The reticulocyte, or juvenile erythrocyte, is morphologically identifiable by its distinct reticulum in the cytoplasm. The reticulocyte circulates for approximately 3 days in the bone marrow before being released into the peripheral bloodstream, where, after approximately 24 hours of undergoing changes in its cytoplasm, the reticulocyte will mature into a fully developed erythrocyte. Note, however, that high levels of erythropoietin (which occur, for example, during hypoxic states or infection) may stimulate early release of reticulocytes from the bone marrow into the peripheral bloodstream. This is reflected on a complete blood count.

At the end of its designated life span (approximately 120 days), the aging erythrocyte (senescent erythrocyte) begins to display cell surface proteins, which trigger phagocytosis in the reticuloendothelial system. As described in Chapter 52, the reticuloendothelial system comprises phagocytic cells in the lymph nodes, spleen, and liver that clear the body of waste. Circulating macrophages consume the senescent erythrocyte and the hemoglobin, recycling the precious iron molecule by transporting it back to the body's iron stores.

Dietary elements play a key role in RBC production. In fact, RBC development is highly dependent on sufficient quantities of metals (iron, cobalt, and manganese), vitamins (B_{12}, B_6, C, E, folate, riboflavin, pantothenic acid, and thiamin), amino acids, and carbohydrates. Deficiencies in any of these dietary elements can negatively affect erythropoiesis. Although cellular growth requires all of the elements, vitamin B_{12}, folate, and iron play particularly pivotal roles in erythropoiesis. Folate and vitamin B_{12} are required for the extensive DNA synthesis that

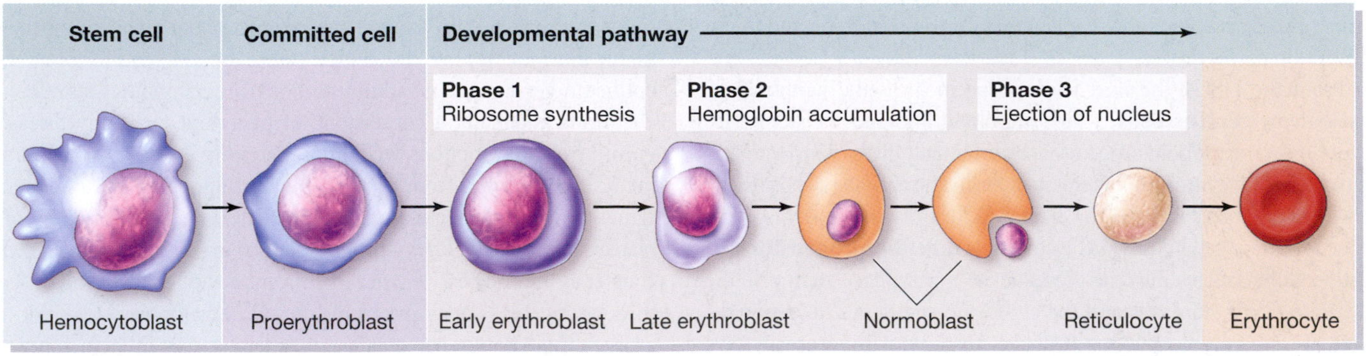

FIGURE 56–2 ◆ Erythropoiesis.

occurs with erythropoiesis. All proliferating cells require iron; however, the iron requirements of erythroid cells in the late basophilic erythroblast through reticulocyte stages, when hemoglobin is synthesized and accumulates, are much greater than the iron requirements of all other cell types (Gaspard, 2009). Diseases such as megaloblastic anemia and iron deficiency anemia result when supplies of iron are insufficient to support erythropoiesis.

Hemoglobin Development

Hemoglobin, the core functional protein of the red blood cell, shuttles oxygen between tissues, allowing blood to transport 100 times more oxygen than could be transported in plasma alone. In erythropoiesis, hemoglobin first becomes detectable in the myeloid progenitor cell, with each subsequent cell generation gaining more and more hemoglobin molecules. Ultimately, the mature erythrocyte contains approximately 250 million hemoglobin molecules. Hemoglobin fulfills its oxygen-carrying function by binding iron to the four heme regions of the molecule. Closer observation of hemoglobin reveals that hemoglobin protein actually is made up of four parts: two identical hemoglobin alpha chains and two identical hemoglobin beta chains. Iron binding is achieved when the hemoglobin alpha and beta chains form precise geometric configurations that allow iron to sit tightly in a lock-and-key style fit on the heme groups.

Healthy, functional hemoglobin conforms to one of two configurations. Which configuration the hemoglobin takes on depends on whether or not an O_2 molecule is bound to the heme, the pH of the environment, and the amount of a mediating chemical (2,3-diphosphoglycerate). The combination of these factors varies in hypoxic states versus well-oxygenated states. This interaction is the foundation of the oxygen-release or oxygen-carrying mechanism of hemoglobin. An alteration to the geometric shape of hemoglobin is the underlying cause of many hematologic disorders such as thalassemia and sickle cell disease, which are discussed in detail later in the chapter. The amount of hemoglobin in blood is a common clinical test used to diagnose disease. Although there are variations due to altitude, accepted values for hemoglobin for adult males are 13.8 to 18 g/dL, and those for adult females are 12 to 15 g/dL.

Decreased erythrocyte volume results in **anemic hypoxia,** or decreased oxygen availability to the tissues specifically because of a decreased concentration of functional hemoglobin or a reduced number of red blood cells. Anemic hypoxia should be distinguished from *hypoxic hypoxia*, in which oxygen deprivation occurs from defective oxygenation in the lungs, as caused by abnormal pulmonary function, airway obstruction, or a right-to-left shunt in the heart (Gaspard, 2009; Semonin Holleran, 2009). For the purposes of this chapter, anemic hypoxia will be referred to as hypoxia. The clinical presentation of the patient with anemia is primarily due to the effects of hypoxia.

Clinical Manifestations

The most common sign of anemia is generalized fatigue, as measured by the patient's report. The severity, pattern, and quality of fatigue are clinically significant findings that can contribute to the identification of an underlying etiology. In mild anemia, fatigue such as exertional dyspnea or lack of endurance may manifest upon only activity. With increasing severity of fatigue as hemoglobin levels drop, patients may report an inability to engage in activities of daily living (ADLs). Several fatigue severity scales that provide a rapid assessment of fatigue-related impairments have been validated in numerous research studies and are readily available for clinicians (Becherer & White, 2010; Bookbinder, 2010; Gaspard, 2009). One such fatigue scale, the Brief Fatigue Inventory, is shown in Figure 56–3◆.

CHART 56–1 Common Signs of Anemia

Abnormal paleness or lack of color of the skin
Increased heart rate (tachycardia) and respiratory rate (tachypnea)
Breathlessness, or difficulty catching a breath (dyspnea)
Lack of energy, or tiring easily (fatigue)
Dizziness, or vertigo, especially when standing
Headache, irritability
Decreased hemoglobin, decreased hematocrit, decreased RBCs

In addition to fatigue, physical manifestations of anemia can be grossly attributed to two major processes (Chart 56–1). The primary insult (hypoxia due to low erythrocyte volume) inflicts its own symptoms, whereas a secondary group of symptoms may arise from the body's attempt to compensate for the hypoxia. While every body system requires oxygen and thus is affected by anemia, the most notable evidence of hypoxia due to low erythrocyte volume can be observed in the cardiovascular system, the respiratory system, and, in severe cases, the neurological system (Gaspard, 2009; Rote & McCance, 2010a; Wilson, 2010).

1. ***Cardiovascular System Manifestations of Anemia:*** With mild anemia, patients may not report noticeable cardiovascular changes other than mildly increased fatigue. In moderate cases, the heart and vascular system will attempt to compensate for decreased oxygen density by increasing the pulse rate (tachycardia). Sustained hypoxia or severe anemia can overcome the cardiovascular system, resulting in angina or even acute myocardial infarction.
2. ***Respiratory System Manifestations of Anemia:*** Anemic patients may present with varying degrees of respiratory difficulty. With mild cases of anemia, patients may experience exertional dyspnea or orthopnea.
3. ***Neurological System Manifestations of Anemia:*** Mild anemia typically does not result in neurological compromise. However, as hemoglobin levels drop and hypoxia increases (as in severe hemoglobin deficiency), patients may report headache, difficulty concentrating, vertigo, irritability, and eventually confusion.

Compensatory Mechanisms

In addition to the clinical presentation that results from hypoxia directly, nurses must be aware of the manifestation of compensatory mechanisms. Biochemical detection of hypoxia in the bloodstream triggers a series of adaptive physiological compensatory mechanisms designed to slow organ damage. Despite the efficacy of these compensatory mechanisms, the reader should note that the oxygen requirements of tissues do not decrease over time. Hence, prolonged anemia and hypoxia can result in irreversible tissue damage if left unresolved. Immediately upon detection of hypoxia, the body adapts with the following four processes:

1. ***Decreased Hemoglobin Oxygen Affinity:*** Oxygen-starved, hypoxic peripheral tissues extract hemoglobin-bound oxygen from blood at high rates. Recall from the discussion earlier in

Brief Fatigue Inventory

STUDY ID# ____________ HOSPITAL # ____________

Date: ____/____/____ **Time:** ____________

Name: ______________ ______________ ______________
Last First Middle Initial

Throughout our lives, most of us have times when we feel very tired or fatigued. Have you felt unusually tired or fatigued in the past week? Yes ☐ No ☐

1. Please rate your fatigue (weariness, tiredness) by circling the one number that best describes your fatigue right now.

0 1 2 3 4 5 6 7 8 9 10
No Fatigue — As bad as you can imagine

2. Please rate your fatigue (weariness, tiredness) by circling the one number that best describes your usual level of fatigue during the past 24 hours.

0 1 2 3 4 5 6 7 8 9 10
No Fatigue — As bad as you can imagine

3. Please rate your fatigue (weariness, tiredness) by circling the one number that best describes your worst level of fatigue during past 24 hours.

0 1 2 3 4 5 6 7 8 9 10
No Fatigue — As bad as you can imagine

4. Circle the one number that describes how, during the past 24 hours, fatigue has interfered with your:

A. General activity
0 1 2 3 4 5 6 7 8 9 10
Does not interfere — Completely Interferes

B. Mood
0 1 2 3 4 5 6 7 8 9 10
Does not interfere — Completely Interferes

C. Walking ability
0 1 2 3 4 5 6 7 8 9 10
Does not interfere — Completely Interferes

D. Normal work (includes both work outside the home and daily chores at home)
0 1 2 3 4 5 6 7 8 9 10
Does not interfere — Completely Interferes

E. Relations with other people
0 1 2 3 4 5 6 7 8 9 10
Does not interfere — Completely Interferes

F. Enjoyment of life
0 1 2 3 4 5 6 7 8 9 10
Does not interfere — Completely Interferes

FIGURE 56–3 ◆ Brief Fatigue Inventory scale.

the chapter that the configuration of the hemoglobin chains determines oxygen-binding capacity. Furthermore, the geometric configuration is driven by a number of environmental factors. Hypoxia creates an environment that causes the hemoglobin to form into an arrangement referred to as the **deoxyhemoglobin** configuration (Figure 56–4◆).

The result of this configuration is twofold. First, the heme iron atoms have a low binding affinity for oxygen, meaning that an oxygen (O_2) molecule is less likely to remain bound to the hemoglobin of an RBC. Second, the deoxyhemoglobin configuration stimulates the production of 2, 3-diphosphoglycerate (2, 3-DPG), which ultimately works to sustain the deoxyhemoglobin

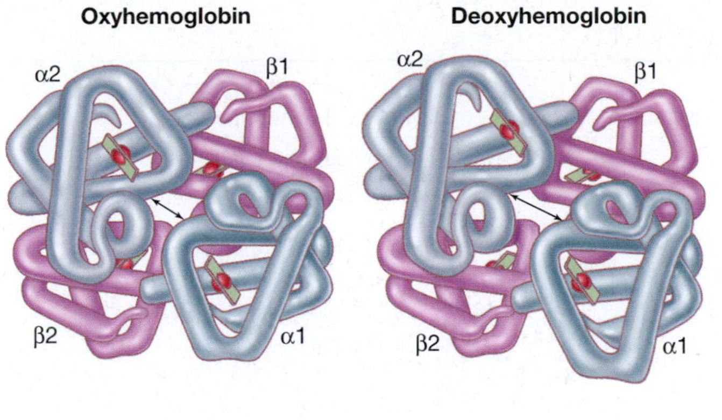

FIGURE 56–4 ◆ Hemoglobin and deoxyhemoglobin, the oxygen transporter.

configuration. Both processes result in increased oxygen release to surrounding tissues. This process results in a *shift to the right,* a phrase used to summarize a graphical illustration of hemoglobin oxygen saturation as a function of oxygen partial pressure (Figure 56–5◆). In cases of decreased hemoglobin oxygen affinity, any given partial pressure of oxygen is associated with less oxygen saturating the hemoglobin molecule. This translates to more unbound oxygen available to tissues, an effective short-term compensatory mechanism against hypoxia.

2. ***Cardiovascular Compensation:*** In cases of severe anemia (measured by hemoglobin < 7 g/dL), the resulting tissue hypoxia triggers cardiovascular compensation. First, the cardiac output increases in an effort to circulate more blood. This increased heart rate is matched by a decrease in peripheral vasculature resistance to first allow blood to flow more quickly and then to reduce the oxygen demands of the heart muscle.
3. ***Redistribution of Blood Flow:*** Another compensatory mechanism is redistribution of blood flow. In hypoxic anemic states, the body selectively vasoconstricts blood vessels to reroute oxygenated blood toward certain vital organs and away from less critical areas. Blood is shunted away from skin and toward the heart, brain, and other critical organs. While this shunting preserves critical organs as long as possible, oxygen deprivation in the "less critical" organs can result in intermittent claudication and pain.
4. ***Increased Erythropoietin to Stimulate RBC Production:*** Of note, during the redistribution of blood flow, selective vasoconstriction shunts blood away from the kidneys, which are hardly noncritical organs. However, detection of hypoxia by the kidneys results in increased production of erythropoietin. Recall from the earlier discussion that erythropoietin is the critical cytokine that triggers erythropoiesis, which ultimately increases RBC mass. Thus, the shunting of blood away from the kidneys is an adaptive attempt at long-term resolution of anemia.

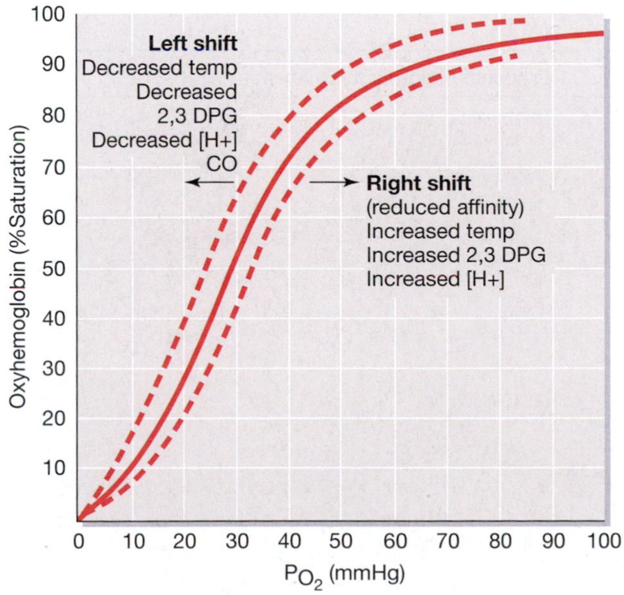

FIGURE 56–5 ◆ Deoxyhemoglobin curve.

Laboratory and Diagnostic Procedures

An assessment of the patient with anemia involves analysis of laboratory studies. Common laboratory tests used in the diagnosis of anemia are the complete blood count (CBC) to detect hematologic alterations and arterial blood gases (ABGs) to detect acid–base disturbances used in the evaluation of hypoxia.

Complete Blood Count

The complete blood count typically includes the following laboratory values pertinent to the study of red blood cells: hemoglobin (Hgb), hematocrit (Hct), red blood cells, reticulocyte mean corpuscle volume (MCV), and mean corpuscle hemoglobin (MCH). Normal values for these tests are summarized in Chart 56–2.

Hemoglobin values, as described in Chapter 55, reflect the amount of hemoglobin protein measured in a volume of blood. Hemoglobin is decreased in cases of anemia of any etiology, hemorrhage, and hemodilution. Hemodilution occurs when excessive fluid (i.e., water and plasma) significantly dilutes a volume of blood, which can occur in situations such as water toxicity and excessive intravenous (IV) infusion. A significant drop in hemoglobin values (>3 g/dL) over a short time period (<24 hours) may indicate active bleeding.

Safety Alert *It is essential that the nurse report any significant drop in hemoglobin values (>3 g/dL over less than 24 hours) to the health care provider. This may indicate active blood loss. This finding is of particular concern if blood loss is not readily visible (i.e., in vomiting or stool), suggesting internal bleeding. Patients should be immediately assessed for level of consciousness, lung sounds, and acute areas of pain.*

The hematocrit is the ratio of erythrocyte volume to volume of whole blood, or the concentration of red blood cells (see Chapter 55). Hematocrit values follow the same pattern established by hemoglobin values: They decrease with excessive hydration (hemodilution), anemia, and hemorrhage.

The total RBC count reflects the total volume of erythrocytes in a volume of blood. Total RBC values also tend to follow the directional patterns of hemoglobin and hematocrit. However, the total RBC value does not adequately indicate the quality or morphology of the erythrocytes. For these reasons, the morphologic RBC indices are often used in determination of anemia etiology, whereas the hemoglobin/hematocrit (H/H) ratio is more commonly used in the monitoring of anemia. Morphologic indices, as described in Chapter 55, including MCV, MCH, MCHC (mean corpuscular hemoglobin concentration), and average concentration of hemoglobin in each red blood cell, are useful tools in describing the blood cell structures characteristic of each type of anemia. The Diagnostic Tests box features tests for anemia.

The number of reticulocytes reflects the number of juvenile erythrocytes present in the peripheral bloodstream. The number of

CHART 56–2 Signs and Symptoms of Acute Blood Loss

% Blood Loss	Approximate Volume in Adult (5,000 mL [79 kg])	Signs and Symptoms	Physical Syndrome
<20	<1,000	BP may be normal. HR may be normal. Urine output may be normal. Possible restlessness.	Vasovagal reaction (peripheral vasoconstriction)
20–30	1,000–1,500	BP > 90 mmHg systolic. HR 100–120 bpm. RR > 24. Urine output 25–30 mL/hr. Anxiety and dyspnea on exertion.	Orthostatic hypotension, tachycardia on exertion
30–40	1,500–2,000	BP 70–90 systolic. HR > 120 beats/min. Cool, pale skin. RR increased. Urine output 5–15 mL/hr. Syncope on sitting and standing.	Orthostatic hypotension, tachycardia at rest
40	>2,000	BP < 90 systolic. HR > 140 beats/min. Cold, clammy skin. RR increased/hyperventilation. Urine output minimal. Confusion, shortness of breath.	Shock

Sources: Cheek, D., Martin, L., & Morris, S. (2010). Shock, multiple organ dysfunction syndrome and burns in adults. In K. L. McCance & S. Huether (Eds.), *Pathophysiology: The biologic basis for disease in adults and children* (pp. 1696–1726). St. Louis: Mosby Elsevier; Manji, R. A. (2009). The history and evolution of circulatory shock. *Critical Care Clinics, 25*(1), 1–29.

reticulocytes increases in most types of sustained anemia as erythropoiesis accelerates as a compensatory mechanism. Decreases in the number of reticulocytes are associated with bone marrow suppression or deficient production of erythrocytes. If a finding of decreased reticulocytes accompanies decreased total WBC count and decreased platelet count, a further examination including a bone marrow aspiration may be warranted in the work-up for leukemia, aplastic anemia, or some other life-threatening bone marrow failure.

Severity of Anemia

The severity of anemia symptoms is generally in direct proportion to the level of erythrocyte depletion as measured by the hemoglobin

DIAGNOSTIC TESTS for Anemia

Test and Normal Values and Rationale for Abnormality	Expected Abnormality in Anemia
Hemoglobin Women: 12–15 g/dL Men: 13.5–18 g/dL *Decreased hemoglobin production due to decreased erythrocyte production*	Decreased
Hematocrit Women: 36–46% Men: 40–54% *Decreased concentration of hemoglobin protein due to decreased erythrocyte production*	Decreased
Total RBC count Males: 4.6–6.0 million cells/μL Females: 4.0–5.0 million cells/μL *Reflects decreased total erythrocyte volume*	Decreased
Reticulocytes 0.5–1.5% of RBC count *Varies according to underlying etiology (acute or chronic, bone marrow involvement)*	Depends on etiology

volume and hematocrit in the CBC. Delineating between severity states of anemia is somewhat arbitrary; a review of the literature reveals little agreement as to the exact hemoglobin values that constitute mild, moderate, or severe anemia states. Additionally, the nurse should not rely solely on laboratory tests but must always incorporate physical and subjective findings when developing nursing interventions. Nonetheless, such delineation is a useful tool for discussion. Normal hemoglobin volume is defined as greater than 12 g/dL. Mild anemia is measured by a hemoglobin value of 10 to 12 g/dL, whereas moderate anemia is measured by a hemoglobin volume of 7 to 11 g/dL. Severe anemia is commonly defined by a hemoglobin volume of < 7 g/dL and a hematocrit of less than 25%. Body system changes typically become more pronounced with increasing severity of anemia (Rote & McCance, 2010a).

Medical Management

Care of the patient with anemia first requires resolution of hypoxia. If left unresolved, hypoxia can become a life-threatening medical emergency as critical organs are deprived of oxygen, instigating a cascade of cellular breakdown, tissue damage, organ failure, and possibly death. (See Chapter 28 for a review of care for acute hypoxia.) If the hypoxia is associated with active and significant blood loss, an additional emergent priority is often the replacement of blood volume to attain erythrocyte levels sufficient to sustain oxygen delivery, discussed later in the section on anemia from acute blood loss.

In otherwise healthy patients without underlying hematologic disorders, these emergency interventions resolve not only the hypoxia, but also the anemia. After the cardiovascular, respiratory, and neurological risks of emergent hypoxia and blood loss have been addressed, the focus shifts to determining the underlying cause of the anemia, usually via laboratory studies and a thorough history. Specific treatments and nursing interventions are then tailored to the underlying disease process. These specific treatments and nursing interventions are discussed later in the chapter as they relate to each classification of anemia. However, some signs and symptoms and their correlating nursing interventions are common to all forms of anemia. These are discussed in the Nursing Process: Patient Care Plan for Generalized Anemia (p. 1724). When older patients are involved, the nurse should be aware of additional considerations, as outlined in the Gerontological Considerations section (p. 1759).

Nursing Management

Nursing care for the patient presenting with anemia focuses on two goals: (1) prevention of complications secondary to decreased oxygen-carrying capacity and (2) thorough assessment to identify underlying etiologies. Decreased oxygen-carrying capacity carries the immediate risks associated with hypoxia: neurological and cardiac insults. Patients also frequently report activity intolerance and fatigue with sustained hypoxia, both of which must be addressed to prevent cardiovascular, respiratory, musculoskeletal, and digestive side effects.

Thorough assessments provide insight into the underlying etiology of anemia. Nurses are responsible for close monitoring of patient symptoms, alterations in laboratory values, and physical changes that may indicate the source of decreasing erythrocyte volume. Once these etiologies have been identified, the nurse, as part of the interdisciplinary health care team, is responsible for initiating interventions unique to that diagnosis. The Nursing Process: Patient Care Plan for Generalized Anemia (p. 1724) summarizes the interventions and rationales appropriate for patients presenting with initial signs and symptoms of anemia. This care plan is then enhanced with the nursing care indicated for specific underlying etiologies, which are discussed throughout the chapter.

Discharge Priorities

Management of anemia needs to continue after hospital discharge and may require long-term lifestyle and dietary change. It is essential that the patient and family be given the necessary information to make these changes. The Patient Teaching & Discharge Priorities box (p. 1725) outlines important information that should be conveyed to patients with generalized anemia.

Health Promotion

Treatment of anemia often involves alterations to the patient's diet and activity level. Part of the assessment of the patient with anemia must include an evaluation of nutrition intake, especially iron, folate, vitamin B_{12}, and proteins because these are all required for erythropoiesis. Nurses play a critical role in helping patients identify dietary sources of these vital nutrients. The sections of this chapter on iron deficiency anemia and megaloblastic anemias provide specific information about diets that will provide these nutrients.

Activity level also must be addressed as part of a complete patient care plan. Anemia frequently is associated with fatigue and dyspnea, which may decrease a patient's ability to participate in ADLs or to maintain prior physical activity levels. However, mobility and exercise should be maintained to prevent cardiovascular and musculoskeletal deconditioning. If either of these processes occurs, the patient may run the risk of further exacerbating the fatigue and dyspnea. Nurses play a pivotal role in assisting patients in identifying appropriate activity goals and incorporating activity into the daily patient care plan.

Collaborative Management

Comprehensive care of the patient with anemia requires the collaboration of an interdisciplinary team that may include dietitians, physical and occupational therapists, respiratory therapists, pharmacists, health care providers, and nurses. In order to meet desired patient outcomes, it is essential that the members of this interdisciplinary team communicate openly with one another in developing and evaluating care of the patient and family (IOM [Institute of Medicine], 2010). A dietitian can provide excellent resources to patients on how to identify and treat dietary deficiencies that exacerbate anemia and how to conserve energy when preparing meals. Additionally, the scientific grounding of the dietitian can help patients evaluate the numerous health benefits claimed in food advertising.

Respiratory therapists are experts in the diagnosis of hypoxia, especially in delineating anemic hypoxia from hypoxia of respiratory etiology. Their expertise is particularly valuable in evaluating the judicious use of oxygen therapy. Physical and occupational therapists play a key role in mobility preservation. Consultation with a physical and occupational therapist should be made early (within a few days of admission) so that exercise techniques can be incorporated early on before debilitating severe anemia takes hold. The pharmacist's knowledge of pharmacokinetics and drug–drug and drug–food interactions is of tremendous benefit in creating a patient care plan, and a pharmacist's guidance should be sought whenever medications are to be evaluated or prescribed.

NURSING PROCESS: Patient Care Plan for Generalized Anemia

Assessment of Hematologic Status Using Gordon's Functional Health Patterns:

- Health Perception Health Management Pattern
- Activity Exercise Pattern
- Cognitive Perceptual Pattern

Subjective Data

Assessment of Fatigue

Have you been short of breath? How long?

Do you have difficulty with energy throughout your day?

What makes it worse? What makes it better?

Do you have difficulty tolerating activity?

Do you have difficulty with everyday chores?

Do you feel weak, dizzy, or light-headed?

Assessment of Hypoxia

Do you feel short of breath?

Do you have chest pain?

Do other areas of your body ache? How often?

Do you feel dizzy or light-headed?

Objective Data

Assessment of Fatigue

General: pallor, malaise, fatigue

Neurological: level of alertness, mental acuity

Respiratory: dyspnea, ventilation depth, tachypnea, work of breathing

Cardiovascular: tachycardia

Laboratory values: alterations to CBC (decreased Hgb, Hct, RBCs)

Assessment of Hypoxia

Dyspnea	Tachypnea
Decreased O_2 saturation	Decreased hemoglobin and hematocrit
ABGs	Cyanosis
Tachycardia	Hepatomegaly/splenomegaly

Outcomes and Evaluation Parameters / Planning and Interventions with *Rationales*

1. NURSING DIAGNOSES: (a) Activity Intolerance *related to decreased oxygen delivery to neuromuscular and cardiovascular systems.* (b) Self-Care Deficit *related to fatigue and weakness impacting ability to participate in ADLs.* (c) Deficient Knowledge *related to dietary causes, underlying etiologies, and patient self-management techniques* (NANDA-I © 2012)

Outcomes: Free of shortness of breath. Able to perform ADLs.

Patient reports appropriate self-care techniques.

Patient demonstrates knowledge of appropriate dietary modifications if indicated, lifestyle changes, and self-management techniques.

Evaluation Parameters: Patient report of lack of dyspnea upon exertion. Patient report of subjective decrease in bothersome fatigue effects as measured by fatigue scale scores. Unlabored respirations < 24/min.

Patient/family verbalizes or demonstrates plan for accommodating self-care activities. Patient able to perform ADLs at a developmentally appropriate level. Patient demonstrates energy conservation techniques such as activity planning, appropriate exertion levels, and assistive devices as needed.

Patient reports knowledge of diet modification (increased iron, folate, vitamin B_{12}) if appropriate. Patient demonstrates plan to incorporate appropriate activity level into daily care. Patient verbalizes understanding of underlying causes of anemia and fatigue.

Assess a normal activity pattern throughout the day *in preparation for activity modification techniques (see below).*

Provide assistance with activities *to minimize shortness of breath.*

Modify activities to coincide with the patient's biologic energy cycles. *Patients should maintain a minimum level of activity to prevent cardiovascular and musculoskeletal decompensation. However, patients may be discouraged by fatigue. Planning activities at points in the day with normally higher energy levels maintains patient participation in the activity.*

Determine the patient's previous knowledge of or skills related to her diagnosis and the influence on willingness to learn. *New information is assimilated into previous assumptions and facts and may involve negotiating, transforming, or stalling.*

Provide developmentally appropriate patient education that addresses the underlying disease process, diet modification, medications, and activity modification. *Symptoms of anemia may require long-term management that is optimized by patient compliance.*

2. NURSING DIAGNOSES: (a) Impaired Gas Exchange *related to an insufficient hemoglobin oxygen delivery system, which can progress to cardiovascular, respiratory, neurological, and metabolic alterations.* (b) Risk of Injury: Falls *related to weakness, dizziness, and possible compromised mental acuity* (NANDA-I © 2012)

Outcomes: Blood morphology and chemistry return to patient baseline.

Patient remains free of injury from falls.

Evaluation Parameters: Lab tests normal

Hematocrit:

- Males: 40.7–50.3%
- Females: 36.1–44.3%.

Hemoglobin:

- Males: 13.8–17.2 g/dL
- Females: 12.1–15.1 g/dL.

Monitor oxygen saturation levels and ABGs *as indicators of hypoxemia.* Administer supplemental oxygen when indicated *to maximize hemoglobin delivery of oxygen. However, use only when indicated by lab values.* Hyperoxygenation suppresses erythropoiesis. Administer blood transfusions for severe cases of anemia when ordered *to correct emergency deficiencies in oxygen delivery capacity.* Monitor for signs such as a falling hematocrit level, pain, pulmonary edema, fever, hypotension, and hemolysis *as indicators of transfusion reactions (hemolysis and fluid overload).*

NURSING PROCESS: Patient Care Plan for Generalized Anemia, *continued*

RBC count:

- Males: 4.7–6.1 million cells/μL
- Females: 4.2–5.4 million cells/μL.

ABG PaO_2: <90 ± 10.

ABG pH: 7.35–7.45.

O_2 sat: >90% (depending on concurrent respiratory disease and age).

Patient experiences no injuries from falling. Environment is adjusted to minimize risk of falls. Patient verbalizes understanding of and demonstrates compliance with fall risk reduction plan.

Monitor for risk factors from falls such as unsteady gait, difficulty with transfers, and orthopnea to *identify physiological and behavioral indicators of fall risk.* Adjust the environment to minimize the risk of falls by placing necessary items within reach of the patient, positioning the bed in a low and locked position, and maintain frequent observation in an effort *to reduce additional risks of falls.* Reinforce patient instruction to call for assistance with ambulation if *indicated to avoid injury.* Assess vital signs (pulse, respirations, and blood pressure) prior to ambulation *to identify possible need to alter the mobility plan.*

Source: Adapted from Wilkinson, J. M., & Ahearn, N. R. (2009). *Prentice Hall nursing diagnosis handbook* (9th ed.). Upper Saddle River, NJ: Prentice Hall.

Anemia from Acute Blood Loss

Anemia from acute blood loss describes the loss of RBC volume that occurs when RBCs leave the circulating vascular space. Anemia from blood loss comprises a heterogeneous group of disorders ranging from "slow bleeds" to rapid trauma. Appropriate care of these patients focuses on determining the underlying cause, preventing immediate cardiovascular and hematologic emergencies, and, if appropriate, treating the underlying disease.

Pathophysiology and Etiology

In discussing the mechanisms responsible for anemia due to blood loss, three parameters should be included: underlying cause, rapidity of onset, and volume lost. Underlying causes include obvious bleeding such as trauma or menorrhagia (excessive menstrual bleeding) as well as less visible causes such as disorders of the gastrointestinal mucosa, slow cranial bleeding, and internal hemorrhage. Nurses should not rely solely on visible blood as an indication of bleeding; instead, they should be aware of the system's clinical presentation of blood loss, as discussed later in the chapter. Bleeding that results from chronic conditions including Crohn's disease, diverticulitis, and rheumatoid arthritis frequently is associated with inflammation; this causes a functional iron deficiency and thus anemia. This syndrome is discussed in the section on anemia of chronic disease.

The rapidity of the blood loss affects the body's ability to respond with compensatory mechanisms, which, in turn, relates to clinical presentation. With slow bleeds, which occur over the course of days to weeks, baroreceptors in the peripheral vascular system detect decreased

PATIENT TEACHING & DISCHARGE PRIORITIES for Generalized Anemia

Need	Teaching
Knowledge of dietary modifications	This is of particular importance in iron deficiency anemia and megaloblastic anemias. Consult with a dietitian to provide the patient and family with effective tools and resources regarding meal planning, appropriate foods, and guidance on food label reading. Teach patients to eat frequent small meals to prevent fatigue.
Fatigue management	Reinforce teaching regarding the daily fatigue scale. Teach patients to discuss the results and trends of the fatigue scale self-assessment with the health care provider. Reinforce teaching regarding activity modification to maintain and preserve energy levels. Reinforce teaching that energy levels may decrease as a physiological response to the disease process, and remind patients that asking for assistance and/or adjusting previous work/home activity schedules may be necessary. Suggest appropriate exercise activities for patient status including brief walks, chair exercises, and bed exercises. Reinforce education regarding mobility as an effective means of prevention of cardiovascular and musculoskeletal deconditioning.
Understanding of medications	For iron supplementation, teach patients the correct timing of administration and possible side effects (constipation). Reinforce key teaching points regarding hydration, constipation management, and iron absorption (see Chart 56–5, p. 1730). For hematopoietic growth factors, reinforce the administration schedule for subcutaneous injections, which may include appointments with the health care provider. Reinforce education regarding possible side effects of subcutaneous hematopoietic growth factors including bone pain and injection site soreness.
Disease prevention	Explain the need for maintenance of hemoglobin levels to ensure adequate oxygenation to tissues, thus decreasing risk of cardiac disease and infection.
Safety	Stress the importance of a medical alert bracelet to identify a problem with the blood to health care providers (for example, if the patient is on Coumadin or another type of blood thinner).
Reportable clinical manifestations	Instruct the patient/family to report any change in exercise and/or activity tolerance and any onset of new pain, especially chest pain, headaches, or abdominal pain.

pressure and respond by increasing plasma volume to preserve cardiovascular status. With this increase in volume, the heart and vascular system can generate enough blood pressure to maintain peripheral perfusion in the critical organs of the heart, lungs, brain, and kidneys. This process can result in a form of dilution anemia, in which the RBC mass is diluted by the increase in plasma volume. Hypoxia from this dilutional anemia is prevented by the compensatory mechanisms discussed earlier, including decreased hemoglobin oxygen affinity (shift to the right) and increased erythropoietin to stimulate RBC production. When the blood loss is rapid, occurring over the course of hours to days, total blood volume (including both RBCs and plasma) can decrease so severely as to cause hypovolemic shock. Hypovolemic shock is a medical emergency associated with high mortality and requires immediate emergency management interventions (see Chapter 54).

The third consideration is the total volume lost. With blood losses of up to 20% of total blood volume (Thomas, 2010), the compensatory mechanism of peripheral vasoconstriction initiates to shift blood flow to organs responsible for maintaining cardiovascular function and preventing hypoxia and hypovolemia. When blood loss becomes more pronounced, the body lacks sufficient circulating blood volume to support the vascular system or maintain adequate hydration and oxygenation of vital organs. The body's first attempt is to intensify cardiovascular compensatory mechanisms (tachycardia). However, with blood loss of 40% or more, all compensatory mechanisms rapidly become overwhelmed, and symptoms of shock are imminent.

Clinical Manifestations

Clinical presentation of the patient with blood loss is directly correlated to the *rapidity, location,* and *volume* of blood loss. Thorough assessment must include laboratory hematologic findings as well as cardiovascular measurements (pulse, blood pressure, and respiratory rate), integumentary signs (pallor, temperature, and diaphoresis), and renal and neurological changes. The action of multiple compensatory mechanisms may mask signs of anemia unless a multifaceted assessment is completed.

When acute blood loss is suspected, the patient should be carefully monitored for changes in cardiovascular, integumentary, renal, and neurological status. These changes are summarized in the Nursing Process: Patient Care Plan for Generalized Anemia (p. 1724) and include tachycardia, tachypnea, decreased level of alertness, pallor, decreased urinary output, and diaphoresis. These start to become apparent with acute, rapid blood loss or when slow blood loss exceeds 20% of baseline. Additionally, bleeds of relatively small volume (i.e., less than 20%) into closed spaces can cause swelling, tenderness, severe pain, sudden changes in neurological status, and eventually death. Bleeding into the cranial vault, the pericardium, the pleural space, or musculoskeletal compartments is a medical emergency that requires prompt attention by the medical team. Please refer to specific chapters addressing these systems for a full discussion.

Bleeding into the gastrointestinal (GI) tract is often first detected via an observation of fecal occult blood (hidden blood) in the stool. Fecal occult blood tests are cost-effective and rapid indicators of GI bleeding and therefore are widely used as screening tools. Melena (black tarry stools) appears when bacteria have had enough time to break blood down into component chemicals. In the case of lower GI bleeding, blood may not be in the colon long enough for bacterial breakdown; therefore, the presence of melena should not be the only indicator used to detect GI bleeding.

Laboratory and Diagnostic Procedures

For sudden blood loss, hematocrit values might not accurately indicate the severity of the problem because RBC mass is lost at the same rate as total blood volume; thus, the percentage of RBCs in the blood is unaffected. (Recall that hematocrit measures the percentage of RBCs in a volume of blood.) However, after 2 to 3 days when the body is able to initiate the compensatory mechanism of increasing plasma volume, RBCs become diluted, as reflected by decreasing erythrocyte, hemoglobin, and hematocrit values, as described in Chart 56–2.

Safety Alert *Any patient who reports sudden pain in the abdominal area, retroperitoneal area, or musculoskeletal fascial compartments or a change in level of consciousness should be immediately assessed for blood pressure, pulse, and respiratory rate changes. These may indicate bleeding into a closed space, which requires immediate medical intervention. Do not rely on changes in laboratory values because these may not accurately reflect blood loss.*

Medical Management

The immediate goal of treatment for acute blood loss is prevention of cardiovascular collapse and hypoxia. Most patients who present with slow bleeds have normal kidney function, normal bone marrow function, and an adequate supply of iron. For these patients, the increased erythropoietin production is sufficient to compensate for lost RBCs; thus, additional treatment with blood products is unwarranted. Attention then turns to identification of the underlying disease process and reducing or stopping the blood loss. A thorough history will assist the clinician in identifying possible causes such as GI bleeding from the intake of nonsteroidal anti-inflammatory drugs (NSAIDs). Transfusion of red blood cells may be indicated for some patients to prevent cardiovascular system collapse. These patients are identified by a sudden decrease in hematocrit by more than 3%, significant observable hemorrhage, a hematocrit of $< 25\%$, or severe impending hypovolemia.

Nursing Management

Nursing priorities in the care of patients who are suspected of having acute blood loss are multifaceted, evolving with the degree of blood loss and stage of treatment. The first goal is careful observation for early indicators of blood loss, especially in patients who present with high-risk diagnoses. Postoperative patients are at particular risk of bleeding from new incisions (both internal and external) and should be carefully monitored for changes in level of consciousness, cardiovascular changes from baseline, excessive blood loss from incision sites, and reports of pain.

Other high-risk populations include but are not limited to patients who present with abdominal pain of known or unknown etiology, patients with musculoskeletal trauma, and patients with deficient platelet function. Monitoring of these patients should involve comprehensive assessment of hematologic laboratory studies, trends in urine output, trends in cardiovascular indicators (blood pressure, pulse, and respirations), integumentary changes, pain descriptions, and musculoskeletal changes.

If transfusions are administered, nursing goals revolve around the safe administration of blood products and monitoring the patient for signs and symptoms of fluid overload or a transfusion reaction (see Chapter 15). Once the source of the blood loss has been identified, nursing interventions, including patient education, assessment, and treatment administration, become specific to the underlying disease process. Nursing interventions related to anemia are outlined in the Nursing Process: Patient Care Plan for Generalized Anemia (p. 1724). Generally, once the source of blood loss has been identified and resolved, no further treatment of anemia due to acute blood loss is warranted.

Iron Deficiency Anemia

Iron deficiency anemia (IDA) is the most common underlying cause of anemia worldwide. Although iron deficiency is more common in developing countries, a significant incidence was observed in the United States during the early 1990s among certain populations, such as toddlers and females of childbearing age (Becherer & White, 2010).

Recall from the discussion on hematopoiesis that iron is required for the heme portion of the hemoglobin protein. Thus, erythrocyte production is slowed when iron-dependent hemoglobin supplies are depleted or insufficient. The erythrocytes that are produced are morphologically distinct because of their small size (microcytic) and pale color (hypochromic). Signs and symptoms of anemia appear when iron supplies are depleted to the point at which the physiological needs of erythropoiesis cannot be met. Depletion of iron stores can be a result of a variety of underlying causes including dietary intake insufficiency, blood loss, or malabsorption disorders. The responsibilities of the health care provider are first to address any emergent symptoms of anemia, such as hypoxia, and then to determine and correct the underlying cause of the iron deficiency.

Iron Metabolism

Alterations in iron metabolism have consequences in many forms of anemia, including iron deficiency anemia, anemia of chronic disease, thalassemia, and hemolytic spherocytosis. Estimates of total iron body stores in healthy adults vary from 2.5–4.5 grams in women to 3.5–5.5 grams in men. International differences in body size and normal values account for the variation in commonly reported values.

Iron is distributed throughout the body in both active metabolic forms and storage forms. Hemoglobin typically houses 2,100 mg of iron, representing the most significant active metabolic form. Other active forms include myoglobin (200 mg); metabolic tissues of the liver, spleen, and bone marrow (150 mg); and the iron transportation system (3 mg). Iron also exists in two "storage forms" within cells: as **ferritin** (700 mg) and as **hemosiderin** (300 mg). These storage forms are metabolically inactive, meaning they do not directly contribute to erythropoiesis, oxygen transport, or immune or neurological function; rather, they act like iron reservoirs.

Approximately 1 mg of iron is lost on a daily basis from a variety of mechanisms, in particular via cell desquamation (the shedding of the outer epidermal layer). To maintain bodily functions, the body requires about 25 mg of iron daily, which is partially derived through dietary absorption (1 mg) via the intestines. However, the majority of the daily iron requirement is supplied from the storage forms (Gaspard, 2009; Rote & McCance, 2010a; Tussings-Humphrey, 2011). For this reason, serum ferritin is commonly included in the analysis of IDA.

As iron is consumed, it is absorbed via the intestinal cells of the duodenum and jejunum and immediately forms a complex with iron transport proteins known as transferrins, which deliver the iron molecule to the target cells (growing erythrocytes, placenta cells, liver cells, spleen, and bone marrow). The amount of transferrin-bound iron is commonly used for measurement of iron levels. Iron molecules that will not be immediately used for erythropoiesis are converted to the storage forms ferritin and hemosiderin. The key chemicals of iron metabolism are described in Chart 56–3.

The rate of intestinal cell absorption is regulated by physiological needs. Absorption *increases* with decreased iron stores, detection of a low peripheral erythrocyte count, increased erythropoietic activity in the bone marrow (i.e., pregnancy, growth spurts), or hypoxemia. Conversely, intestinal iron absorption *decreases* in the presence of inflammation, a process that contributes to the "anemia of inflammation" or "anemia of chronic diseases" (Gaspard, 2009). The body produces a variety of systemic signals (neurotransmitters, hormones, and cytokines) in response to these stimuli. Hepcidin, produced by the liver, has been identified as the key regulatory hormone of iron absorption, adjusting the rate of iron absorption in response to total iron body reservoirs. Although the exact molecular mechanism remains to be elucidated, an emerging body of research suggests that these systemic signals act on the intestinal cells of the duodenum and jejunum to alter iron absorption through regulation of the iron transport proteins (Rote & McCance, 2010a).

Pathophysiology

Iron deficiency anemia results from one or more processes: (1) excess iron loss, (2) iron absorption abnormalities, (3) reallocation of iron stores, and (4) insufficient dietary intake. Excess iron loss, iron absorption abnormalities, and insufficient dietary intake are classified as **absolute iron deficiencies** indicating insufficient amounts of total body iron. Reallocation of iron stores is referred to as a **functional iron deficiency.** In this condition, there is a failure to supply enough

CHART 56–3 Key Chemicals of Iron Metabolism

Chemical	Function	Physiological Consequences
Ferritin	Storage form	Used as measurement of iron status. A high ferritin level indicates adequate status.
Hemosiderin	Storage form	Measurement of iron status. A high hemosiderin level indicates adequate status, although this test is rarely performed because of the prevalence of ferritin.
Transferrin	Delivers iron to the target cell	High levels of iron-bound transferrin indicate adequate iron status.
Hepcidin	Hormone that regulates iron absorption	Inhibits iron absorption. Increases macrophage consumption of iron. Increases (stimulated by infection, inflammation, and malignancy) result in decreased iron available for erythropoiesis. Decreases cause iron overload.

Weblink: Iron Deficiency Anemia

iron to the bone marrow for erythropoiesis, despite adequate total body iron stores. Each of these etiologies is associated with some underlying behavioral or pathologic process:

1. ***Excess Iron Loss:*** Blood loss, which involves loss of the iron housed in the hemoglobin, is the leading cause of iron deficiency (Thomas, 2010). Chronic blood loss is most commonly attributed to gastrointestinal bleeding. Causes of GI bleeding include peptic ulcer disease, diverticulitis, hemorrhoids, esophageal varices, tumors, steroids, small tears along the rectum, and use of NSAIDs (see Chapter 37). Many of these processes can exist for long periods of time, evading detection by the patient and cumulatively allowing for a substantial loss of blood and iron. One milliliter of blood contains about 0.5 mg of iron. A steady blood loss of as little as 3 to 4 mL per day, which often goes undetected by the patient, results in 1.5 to 2 mg of lost iron daily. This loss places excess demand on daily iron needs, resulting in a negative iron balance. Menstrual bleeding, which typically results in 40 to 80 mL of daily blood loss, also is associated with IDA, in part explaining the prevalence among women.
2. ***Iron Absorption Abnormalities:*** Iron absorption abnormalities refer to any clinical situation that decreases the rate of intestinal absorption. As discussed earlier, absorption relies on the intricate interplay between intestinal cells, systemic cell signals, the iron transport system, and the storage forms of iron. Gastrointestinal tract abnormalities, such as surgical manipulation, Crohn's disease, and celiac disease, reduce the intestinal wall surface available for iron absorption. Liver disease also can result in IDA because transferrin is synthesized in the liver and the storage forms (ferritin and hemosiderin) partially reside in the hepatic cells of the liver. Additionally, several studies are beginning to examine IDA that stems from genetic alterations in the iron transport proteins and intestinal absorption systemic signals, specifically hepcidin (Gaspard, 2009; Rote & McCance, 2010a).
3. ***Reallocation of Iron Stores:*** Reallocation of iron stores refers to situations in which total body iron supplies are at normal levels but the iron molecule is unavailable for erythropoiesis. In chronic inflammatory conditions, available iron is preferentially allocated to increased macrophage production. Again, hepcidin has been identified as the key hormone regulating macrophage consumption of iron. In fetal development, iron is preferentially delivered to the developing fetus; however, maternal erythropoiesis may be affected.
4. ***Insufficient Dietary Intake:*** When any of the preceding situations occurs, demand for iron can exceed iron intake. Initially, the storage forms of iron act as buffers to adequately supply the body's active metabolic needs. The efficiency of the storage forms means that early iron deficiency often is asymptomatic and therefore goes unreported by the patient. Hemoglobin and erythrocyte values are decreased only mildly, if at all. However, serum ferritin values may decrease from normal. Eventually, depletion of the storage forms can quickly outpace dietary intake, and the serum ferritin concentration falls. Erythropoiesis is impaired, producing pale (hypochromic), small (microcytic) erythrocytes. The decreased oxygen delivery capacity of these impaired erythrocytes results in the signs and symptoms of anemia.

Clinical Manifestations

Iron deficiency anemia can have an insidious progression, often with no reportable symptoms despite falling iron stores. As iron depletion proceeds, IDA produces the signs common to all anemias and eventually manifests with morphologic, neurological, and integumentary symptoms that are unique to iron depletion. A laboratory analysis will reveal both qualitative and quantitative changes to RBC components. Often, IDA is first detected in the primary care setting during routine physicals or when patients seek evaluation for bothersome symptoms. The U.S. Preventive Services Task Force (2006) and the Centers for Disease Control and Prevention (CDC) (2007) have issued national guidelines to assist practitioners in the early identification and treatment of these patients in an effort to prevent severe negative outcomes related to iron deficiency (see the National Guidelines box). In the acute care setting, iron deficiency most often presents as a consequence of bleeding, decreased oral intake of iron, or chronic disease.

Because the body's highly efficient iron storage system provides a rich reservoir for active metabolic needs, early IDA often does not produce bothersome symptoms. As with all anemias, the severity of the symptoms correlates to the degree of hemoglobin deficiency; this, in turn, correlates to the volume of total iron body stores. As erythropoiesis becomes increasingly hampered, the patient may present with the general manifestations of anemia such as fatigue, pallor, shortness of breath, cold intolerance, headache, and activity intolerance. When iron stores fall critically low such that epithelial cell production is affected, the patient may present with symptoms that are uniquely indicative of IDA including pica (clay eating), glossitis (tongue inflammation), gastric atrophy, stomatitis, ice eating (pagophagia), and leg cramping (Rote & McCance, 2010a). Presentation of any of these symptoms along with mild activity intolerance warrants further evaluation of iron status.

Laboratory and Diagnostic Procedures

Laboratory tests in IDA reveal decreased erythrocytes common to all anemias. Hemoglobin and hematocrit levels also decrease in accordance with the severity of the anemia. Additionally, low levels of iron in the heme produce morphologically distinct erythrocytes. The MCV, MCHC, and MCH morphological indices are all decreased, indicating a microcytic (small), hypochromic (light) cell suggestive of IDA. These erythrocyte changes are shown in Figure 56–6◆.

Definitive diagnosis requires bone marrow aspiration, which reveals absent marrow stores of iron. However, other laboratory findings are

NATIONAL GUIDELINES for Screening for Iron Deficiency Anemia

Recommendation: Routine screening for iron deficiency anemia in asymptomatic pregnant women.

Recommendation: Routine iron supplementation for asymptomatic children ages 6 to 12 months who are at increased risk for iron deficiency anemia.

Recommendation: Periodic screening for anemia among high-risk populations of infants and preschool children, pregnant women, and nonpregnant women of childbearing age.

Recommendation: Universal iron supplementation to meet the iron requirements of pregnancy.

Sources: Centers for Disease Control and Prevention (CDC). (2007). Recommendations to prevent and control iron deficiency in the United States. Retrieved from http://www.cdc.gov/nchs/fastats/anemia.htm; U.S. Preventive Services Task Force. (2006). Screening for iron deficiency anemia, including iron supplementations for children and pregnant women: Recommendation statement. *American Family Physician.* Retrieved from http://www.aafp.org/afp/20060901/us.html.

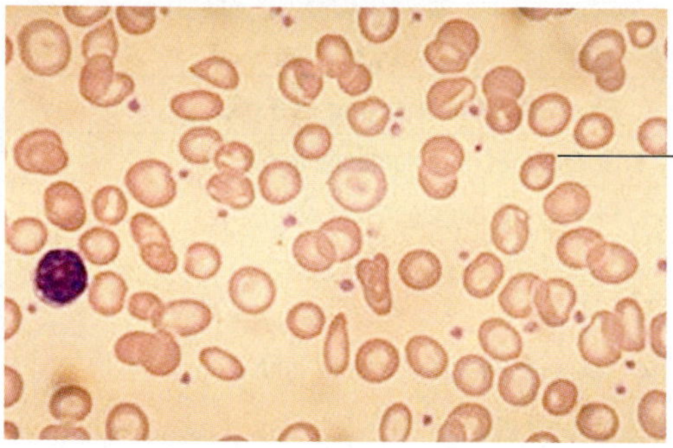

FIGURE 56–6 ◆ Peripheral smear showing microcytic erythrocytes of IDA.
Source: Annita B. Watson.

sufficient to begin treatment of IDA, most notably low serum iron, serum ferritin, and serum transferrin, as well as an elevated total iron binding capacity (TIBC). Serum iron levels fall as total body iron decreases; however, this value is highly sensitive to recent changes in diet. A decrease in serum ferritin is a more accurate indicator of iron stores. Serum transferrin (also referred to as TIBC) increases as a compensatory attempt to harvest more iron from the intestines; thus, its value *increases* in IDA. These laboratory findings are summarized in the Diagnostic Tests box .

Medical Management

Treatment of iron deficiency anemia addresses three goals: alleviation of immediate distress caused by anemia, identification of the underlying etiology, and replacement of iron if indicated. Immediate distress of anemia includes hypoxia and activity intolerance, as discussed in the earlier section on generalized anemia. A comprehensive patient assessment should include GI symptoms, menstrual patterns in female patients, or dietary changes because these will assist the practitioner in identifying the underlying etiology.

Because the majority of chronic blood loss is due to GI bleeding, a fecal occult stool is often ordered, especially in the absence of adolescent growth spurts, menses, and pregnancy. A fecal occult stool test is an important and cost-effective first step in early detection of GI bleeding, particularly since melena requires a relatively large blood loss of 50 to 75 mL from the intestinal tract. More invasive exploratory procedures may be indicated to first determine the source of the bleeding (e.g., cancerous tumors, polyps, ulcers), and also to stop hemorrhage if detected.

Weblink: Screening for IDA

Dietary Modifications

Replacement of iron stores is first attempted with dietary alterations (Chapter 8). Dietary iron is consumed in one of two forms: **heme iron,** which is available in red meats and fish, and **nonheme iron,** which is available in vegetables, cereals, and fortified foods. A significant chemical difference exists between the two forms that affects their utility in treating IDA with dietary modification. Heme iron is considered readily *bioavailable*, meaning that its molecular configuration is readily used in erythropoiesis. More important perhaps, heme iron is much better absorbed (15% absorption rate) in the intestinal tract than nonheme iron (<5% absorption rate). Furthermore, heme iron is rarely reduced by the presence of other substances in the intestinal tract. Nonheme iron absorption, by contrast, is reduced by tannins (found in tea), calcium, polyphenols, and phytates (found in legumes and whole grains). Ascorbic acid is the only common food element known to increase nonheme iron bioavailability.

Consideration of bioavailability and food–food interactions should be included in patient education about dietary modifications (American Dietetic Association, 2009; Wilson, 2010).

Oral Iron Supplementation

Iron supplementation may be indicated if dietary modification alone is insufficient to correct iron stores, especially in severe cases of iron deficiency anemia (serum ferritin level that falls > 10 from baseline).

DIAGNOSTIC TESTS for Iron Deficiency Anemia

Test, Normal Values, and Rationale for Abnormality	Expected Abnormality in IDA
Hemoglobin Women: 12–15 g/dL Men: 13.5–18 g/dL	Decreased. In the early stages of IDA, hemoglobin will not be affected. In severe cases, low iron stores decrease hemoglobin production.
Hematocrit Women: 36–46% Men: 40–54%	Decreased.
Serum Iron (Fe) 50–1,450 mcg/dL (11–25 μmol/L)	Decreased. Indicates decreased serum iron concentration. However, it may be artificially increased by recent dietary ingestion or hemolytic states.
Serum Ferritin Women: 25–235 ng/mL Men: 15–445 ng/mL *Highly sensitive measurement of total body iron stores.*	Decreased. The plasma ferritin value often falls to under 10% of its baseline level with significant iron deficiency.
Serum Transferrin (also referred to as total iron binding capacity [TIBC]) 200–430 mg/dL *Iron transport protein. Production is increased in response to low iron stores or increased iron needs.*	8.5 μg/mL.

Weblink: Treatment of IDA

CHART 56–4 Common Oral Iron Supplement Formulations

Generic Name	Tablet (mg) (Elemental Iron Content [mg])	Elixir Iron Content (mg in 5 mL)
Ferrous sulfate	325 mg (65 mg elemental iron)	300 mg (60 mg elemental iron)
	195 mg (39 mg elemental iron)	90 mg (18 mg elemental iron)
Extended-release ferrous sulfate	525 mg (105 mg elemental iron)	
Ferrous fumarate	325 mg (107 mg elemental iron)	
	195 mg (64 mg elemental iron)	100 mg (33 mg elemental iron)
Ferrous gluconate	325 mg (39 mg elemental iron)	300 mg (35 mg elemental iron)

Source: Adams, M. P., & Koch, R. W. (2010). *Pharmacology: Connections to nursing practice.* Upper Saddle River, NJ: Pearson.

Supplemental iron is available in two forms: ferrous and ferric. Ferrous iron salts (ferrous fumarate, ferrous sulfate, and ferrous gluconate) are the best absorbed forms of iron supplements (Rote & McCance, 2010a). For adults who are not pregnant, the CDC recommends taking 50 to 60 mg of oral elemental iron (the approximate amount of elemental iron in one 300-mg tablet of ferrous sulfate) twice daily for 3 months for the therapeutic treatment of IDA. **Elemental iron** is the amount of iron in a supplement that is available for absorption (Chart 56–4).

Iron supplements can have gastrointestinal side effects, including constipation and upper epigastric pain, which contribute to patient noncompliance. Patient education should include techniques that can avoid such complications and also enhance iron absorption (see Chart 56–5). Switching to a milder oral preparation such as ferrous gluconate tablets (325 mg with 39 mg of elemental iron) of carbonyl iron (Ircon) may be indicated if these techniques continue to prove unsuccessful.

The patient's response to oral iron supplementation may be measured by an increase in peripheral reticulocytes as soon as 4 days after initiation of therapy, and by a rise in hemoglobin, hematocrit, and serum ferritin within 2 to 3 weeks. Patients should be advised to continue therapy for 2 to 3 months to fully restore depleted iron storage reservoirs (National Institutes of Health, 2011).

Parenteral Iron Supplementation

Parenteral iron supplementation may be indicated for patients who require more rapid correction of depleted iron stores or patients with chronic kidney disease. However, significant side effect profiles of parenteral preparations have been reported including nausea, congestive heart failure, anaphylaxis, liver necrosis, and severe headache. A number of different intravenous (IV) preparations are currently available and each carries with it specific administration recommendations. Monitoring and test dose guidelines are listed in Chart 56–6.

CHART 56–5 Patient Education Regarding Oral Iron Supplements

Supplemental iron tablets should be taken 3 to 4 times daily per your health care provider's prescription.

Some patients experience heartburn, nausea, or constipation when taking iron supplements. To help avoid these side effects, take iron tablets with a snack or full meal and at least 8 ounces of fluids.

Do not lie down for at least 1 hour after taking iron pills.

Your health care provider may prescribe a stool softener for you to help with constipation.

Taking iron tablets with vitamin C (i.e., orange juice, strawberries) will help your body better absorb the iron.

Safety Alert *During any administration of IV iron supplementation, if the patient reports any signs and symptoms of hypersensitivity or allergic reaction, the nurse needs to stop the infusion, stay with the patient, monitor the airway, and call the health care provider immediately.*

Nursing Management

Nursing care of the patient with iron deficiency anemia focuses on management of symptomatic hypoxia consistent with all anemias. This includes providing patient education regarding prevention, detection, and management of iron deficiency and monitoring of possible complications from iron supplementation. Management of hypoxia related to anemia is a collaborative process and is addressed

CHART 56–6 Recommendation for Parenteral Infusion of Iron Supplementation

Name (Generic and Trade)	Comments	Test Dose	Infusion Guidelines
Iron dextran injection (INFeD, DexFerrum)	Appropriate for single-dose administration. Intramuscular route available.	25 mg slow IV push, then 1 hour monitoring required on first infusion	100 mg over 2–5 minutes IV push *OR* Dilute dose in 250–1,000 mL 0.9% NS over 1–6 hours
Sodium ferric gluconate in sucrose (Ferrlecit)	Recommendation by the National Kidney Foundation for 125 mg repeated in 8 doses. Suggested as an alternative for patients hypersensitive to iron dextran.	Not required; at health care provider's discretion 25 mg IV slow push or 25 mg in 50 mL of NS IV over 60 minutes	100 mg over 2–5 minutes IV push *OR* Dilute dose in 250–1,000 mL 0.9% NS over 1–6 hours
Iron sucrose injection (Venofer)		Not required; at health care provider's discretion 25 mg IV slow push	100 mg IV over 5 minutes *OR* Dilute dose in 100 mL 0.9% NS over 15 minutes

in the Nursing Process: Patient Care Plan for Generalized Anemia box (p. 1724). Once IDA has been identified, the nurse must provide patient education that can prevent recurrence. Because chronic GI blood loss is a major culprit, patients should be taught about the risk factors for GI bleed and early signs and symptoms (see Chapter 37).

Nursing care also must focus on promotion of safe and effective iron supplementation. As was discussed earlier, the efficacy of oral and IV iron supplementation depends on a variety of factors including timing of administration and management of bothersome side effects. To prevent noncompliance, patients should be advised about these risks before beginning iron supplementation and should be taught the management techniques listed in Chart 56–5. Particularly with regard to oral supplementation, nurses should perform thorough abdominal assessments for heartburn and constipation. Encouraging proper positioning (high Fowler's or sitting), mobilization, and fluid intake will help minimize the occurrence of digestive problems. Patient education should include dietary recommendations that will reinforce postdischarge behavior. Although a dietitian should be consulted whenever dietary recommendations are provided, nurses should also reinforce dietary teaching whenever possible.

Collaborative Management

The comprehensive care of the patient with IDA benefits from the collaboration of nurses, pharmacists, and dietitians. In order to meet desired patient outcomes, it is essential that the members of this interdisciplinary team communicate openly with one another in developing and evaluating care of the patient and family (IOM [Institute of Medicine], 2010). Pharmacists should be consulted to prevent drug–drug and drug–food interactions that may inhibit iron absorption. In the acute care setting, dietitians coordinate inpatient meal planning to ensure that sufficient quantities of iron are supplied. However, their planning efforts require nursing staff to accurately assess and document patient intake of meals and snacks. Often, dietary intake is negatively affected by the patient's financial and social limits, such as shopping and meal preparation challenges. Long-term comprehensive care must then involve social workers and discharge planners who can assist the family with financial concerns and identification of community resources.

Anemia of Chronic Disease

Anemia is a common consequence of chronic diseases. The most common chronic diseases associated with anemia are cancer, chronic kidney failure, autoimmune disorders, and infectious diseases such as acquired immunodeficiency syndrome (AIDS). The prevalence of anemia of chronic disease (ACD) varies significantly depending on the underlying chronic disease and tends to increase with the disease's severity and the patient's age. In rheumatoid arthritis, anemia is the most common nonmusculoskeletal side effect, reported in 30% to 60% of patients. In cancer, anemia is reported in 30% to 90% of patients (Swanson, 2011), and estimates in chronic kidney disease report a prevalence as high as 80% (Rote & McCance, 2010a).

Recognition of ACD contributes to difficulties in statistical analysis. Health care providers sometimes dismiss fatigue and general malaise indicative of anemia as psychosocial consequences of chronic disease. However, numerous studies report decreased side effects and improved quality of life and survival rates when hemoglobin levels are vigilantly monitored and maintained at therapeutic levels above 10 g/dL, the criteria recommended by both the National Kidney Foundation's Kidney Disease Outcomes Quality Initiative (KDOQI) (National Kidney Foundation [NKF], 2010) and the National Comprehensive Cancer Network's clinical practice guidelines (National Comprehensive Cancer Network, 2008).

Pathophysiology

As was mentioned earlier, anemia results from the inflammatory or infectious processes of chronic diseases including chronic kidney disease, cancer, rheumatoid arthritis, and chronic inflammatory bowel disease. Chemical signals produced by invading bacteria or a virus, a tumor, or the body itself attack erythropoietic cells and organs to negatively affect erythrocyte production and iron metabolism through a variety of mechanisms:

1. ***Decrease in Iron Absorption:*** Iron availability is diminished by a decrease in the rate of intestinal iron absorption. Chronic disease also can decrease appetite, further diminishing iron absorption. This process contributes to absolute iron deficiency.
2. ***Diversion to Macrophages:*** As the body attempts to fight infection, cytokines divert available iron to the production of macrophages characteristic of chronic disease, resulting in a functional iron deficiency.
3. ***Increased Hemolysis of Erythrocytes:*** An increase in RBC hemolysis is stimulated by cytokines produced during inflammation and infection. Circulating macrophages then scavenge the liberated iron, again contributing to a decrease in circulating erythrocytes and functional iron deficiency.
4. ***Decreased Erythropoietin Production and Response:*** Erythropoiesis also is affected by a blunting of erythropoietin in chronic kidney disease or secondary to malignancy or infection. These diseases result in decreased production of erythropoietin and in the desensitization of the myeloid progenitor cell to the stimulating effects of erythropoietin. As a result, erythropoiesis rates fail to increase to meet the increased physiological demands imposed by disease and infection.
5. ***Impaired Erythropoiesis in the Bone Marrow:*** Malignant tumors and infections first deplete iron and vitamin supplies and then crowd the bone marrow, leaving few resources for erythropoiesis. They also trigger apoptosis of the myeloid progenitor cells.

The simultaneous actions of these mechanisms ultimately result in measurable decreases in erythrocytes, hemoglobin, and hematocrit along with hypoxia, activity intolerance, and fatigue.

Clinical Manifestations

The physical signs and symptoms associated with ACD tend to be indistinguishable from those associated with generalized anemia because both result directly from decreased circulating erythrocytes. Anemia also can exacerbate symptoms that are specific to the underlying disease process. In both cancer and chronic kidney disease, hematocrit and hemoglobin levels maintained below 10 mg/dL for more than 6 weeks are associated with increased myelosuppression, infection, left ventricular hypertrophy, and congestive heart failure. Cognitive and emotional complications include headaches, loss of concentration, depression, and impaired memory (Adams & Koch, 2010).

Laboratory and Diagnostic Procedures

Anemia of chronic disease is distinguished by its etiology (association with an underlying chronic disease process) and its presentation in laboratory studies. In general, ACD presents as mild anemia with hemoglobin levels typically between 8 and 9.5 g/dL. The CBC will show decreased total erythrocytes and decreased reticulocytes, indicating diminished erythropoiesis. The morphology of erythrocytes and iron status laboratory values will vary between ACD with absolute iron deficiency and ACD with functional iron deficiency. Typically, erythrocytes in ACD present first as normochromic and normocytic and then, with increasing iron depletion, progress to being hypochromic and hypocytic, reflected by the MCHC, MCV, and MCH morphology indices. Ferritin levels in ACD with functional iron deficiency are increased, but they decrease from baseline with absolute iron deficiency. Transferrin levels are decreased in all iron deficiency stages of ACD.

Medical Management

The goal of therapy in ACD is maintenance of hemoglobin and hematocrit at sufficient levels to promote disease healing and prevent systemic complications. The target range for hemoglobin and hematocrit are Hgb 11 g/dL (Hct 33%) to Hgb 12 g/dL (Hct 36%) as prescribed by the National Anemia Action Council, National Comprehensive Cancer Network, and National Kidney Foundation practice guidelines. Maintenance of hemoglobin and hematocrit values at these ranges has been correlated with decreased rates of mortality and morbidity (National Anemia Action Council, 2011; National Comprehensive Cancer Network, 2008; NKF, 2010).

The ultimate resolution of anemia in chronic disease can be accomplished only with resolution of the underlying disease, such as cancer, chronic inflammation, or chronic kidney disease. Unfortunately, there is no definitive permanent cure for most of these diseases, so management of anemia may become a lifelong challenge. There are three primary options to maintain optimal hemoglobin and hematocrit values: blood transfusion, iron supplementation, and exogenous erythropoietin. These options, along with indications and monitoring guidelines, are discussed next.

The judicious use of blood transfusion is an option in correcting acute anemia associated with chronic disease. Blood transfusion is reserved for patients with severe anemia (Hgb < 8) or those with obvious signs of bleeding such as visible loss of blood or a significant drop in hemoglobin/hematocrit in a relatively short period of time. The risks of blood transfusion, especially repeated transfusions over the course of many months to years, may outweigh the benefits to the patient. Repeated blood transfusions place the patient at risk for fluid overload and iron overload. Patients also can become sensitized to the proteins found in donated blood, increasing their risk for transfusion-related allergic reactions. See Chapter 16 for a complete discussion of transfusion-related side effects.

Iron supplementation for ACD is reserved for patients with absolute iron deficiency. When ferritin levels indicate sufficient iron stores (greater than 100 ng/mL), as is the case in functional iron deficiency, iron supplementation exposes the patient to the possible effects of iron overload, including tissue damage and acute cardiovascular events. When ferritin and transferrin levels show iron depletion, iron supplementation has shown some benefit in maintaining normal hemoglobin levels. Iron supplementation may also be indicated for patients being treated with erythropoietic agents.

Erythropoietic agents are medications composed of the exogenous forms of erythropoietin, the primary stimulating hormone of erythropoiesis produced in the kidneys. The use of erythropoietic agents for the correction of ACD is reserved for patients with chronic kidney disease and patients undergoing chemotherapy or immunosuppressive therapy. These medications work in much the same way that natural erythropoietin does: by stimulating differentiation and proliferation of the hematopoietic cascade. In chronic disease, erythropoietic agents also have been found to preferentially stimulate iron absorption by the erythroid progenitor cell over macrophages. Guidelines for use vary among diseases; refer to the chapters on kidney failure (Chapter 39) and cancer (Chapter 57) for guidelines.

Nursing Management

Anemia complicates an already difficult diagnosis of chronic disease. Conversely, prevention, detection, and early treatment of anemia can improve the patient's quality of life and clinical outcomes. Nurses play a key role in recognizing early signs of anemia, especially in the acute hospitalized patient. Nursing priorities for the care of the patient with any chronic disease should include assessment of activity tolerance and assessment of integumentary signs such as pallor, respiratory difficulty, and cognition, as described in the Nursing Process: Patient Care Plan for Generalized Anemia presented earlier in the chapter (p. 1724). Detection of any such signs indicates the need for immediate implementation of nursing interventions to reduce the patient's risk of falls and hypoxia.

Frequent analyses of laboratory values also assist the nurse in detecting underlying bleeding and/or iron deficiency. Patient education and establishment of the therapeutic patient–nurse relationship are particularly important for these patients, who may be experiencing depression and exhaustion brought on by their underlying disease process. Patient education priorities include proper medication administration, increasing awareness of side effects of therapy, safety interventions, and signs and symptoms of worsening anemia.

Megaloblastic Anemias: Folate Deficiency, Vitamin B_{12} Deficiency, and Pernicious Anemias

Megaloblastic anemia results from impaired DNA synthesis of the erythrocyte RBC precursors. The impaired DNA synthesis results in production of large, immature red blood cells termed **megaloblasts.** Because of their immaturity and large size, these megaloblasts are often sequestered in the bone marrow rather than being released into the peripheral bloodstream. If released, megaloblasts are subject to an increased rate of hemolysis owing to structural defects in their membranes. Both processes—bone marrow sequestration and increased hemolysis—result in a decreased total RBC count, or anemia. Most commonly, megaloblastic anemia is caused by deficient dietary intake of folic acid or vitamin B_{12} (cobalamin) or by malabsorption of vitamin B_{12} (pernicious anemia). These processes account for the vast majority of megaloblastic anemias; however, other causes have been implicated, as summarized in Chart 56–7.

Etiology and Pathophysiology

The exact chemical roles of vitamin B_{12} and folate in erythropoiesis are still under investigation, although a great deal of research is being focused on the subject. What is known is that folate plays a critical role in the biochemical reactions involved in cell development, especially erythropoiesis. Folate is the natural form; folic acid is the synthetic form found in supplements and fortified food. Laboratory studies show that an absence of folate suppresses the proliferation of maturing erythrocytes. Furthermore, folate is absorbed as an inactive dietary form and must be converted to an active form before being used in DNA synthesis.

CHART 56–7 Common Causes of Megaloblastic Anemia

Major Causes

Insufficient dietary intake of folic acid

Insufficient dietary intake of vitamin B_{12} (cobalamin)

Deficiencies in gastric intrinsic factor leading to malabsorption of vitamin B_{12} (pernicious anemia)

Other Causes

Intestinal malabsorption due to chronic GI inflammatory processes or surgical shortening

General malnutrition

Liver disease

Chronic hemolytic anemias

Anticonvulsant medications such as phenytoin that interfere with folate absorption

Drugs that have antifolate activity including trimethoprim

Chemotherapies with DNA suppression activity

Alcohol abuse

Vitamin B_{12} (cobalamin), an essential nutrient found in animal proteins, is responsible for this conversion of inactive folate to active folate. This inextricable relationship is the reason vitamin B_{12} and folate deficiencies have similar clinical presentations and often occur simultaneously. Once absorbed, vitamin B_{12} and folate are either transported directly to the bone marrow for erythropoiesis or stored in the liver and, to a small degree, in the pancreas.

Vitamin B_{12} requires the action of gastric intrinsic factor (IF) before being absorbed into the intestinal mucosa and bloodstream. Intrinsic factor is a substance secreted by the gastric parietal mucosa. Megaloblastic anemias that result from deficiencies in IF are termed **pernicious anemias.**

Clinical Manifestations

Folate deficiency anemia, vitamin B_{12} deficiency anemia, and pernicious anemia typically progress slowly with symptoms manifesting gradually over years and months rather than days. In addition to the clinical signs common to all anemias, megaloblastic anemias present with characteristic signs and symptoms and laboratory test results.

The Nursing Process: Patient Care Plan for Generalized Anemia (p. 1724) delineates the most common signs of anemia, including fatigue, activity intolerance, exertional dyspnea, tachycardia, and hypoxia. Although this chapter focuses on the pivotal role of vitamin B_{12} and folate in erythropoiesis, both substances also are required for all DNA synthesis. In the absence of sufficient folate and vitamin B_{12} (either from dietary insufficiency or pernicious anemia), the patient can manifest gastrointestinal and integumentary signs and symptoms. These result from the absence of these vitamins in the production of epithelial cells. GI symptoms include a swollen and sore tongue (classically described as "smooth and beefy red"), anorexia, and nausea. Integumentary signs include hyperpigmentation over the hands and knuckles. Neurological symptoms that occur with vitamin B_{12} deficiencies include peripheral neuropathy, unsteadiness, lack of coordination, ataxia, confusion, and memory loss. Reflexes may also be diminished, and a positive Babinski's sign may be observed. (Refer to Chapter 20 for a discussion of neurological assessment.) These result from loss of myelination of nerve cells, in which vitamin B_{12} plays a critical role. Unfortunately, these symptoms often are permanent and irreversible.

Folate deficiency is clinically indistinguishable from vitamin B_{12} deficiency with the exception of neurological insults, which are not common in folate deficiency. Because nervous system findings are atypical, their appearance is clinically significant and warrants analysis for vitamin B_{12} deficiency or underlying neurological disease processes. The most common problem specifically associated with folate deficiency is neural tube defects, such as spina bifida, in newborns of mothers who had inadequate folate intake during pregnancy. Folate deficiency has also been linked to increased homocysteine (an amino acid found in the blood) levels, which in turn increases the risk of cardiovascular disease and thrombosis.

Laboratory and Diagnostic Procedures

Megaloblastic anemias result in changes to the CBC and RBC morphological studies. The hallmark diagnostic finding indicating megaloblastic anemia is macrocytosis or MCV (typically over 110 μm^3). Patients present with the decreased hemoglobin value typical of anemia as well as a decreased reticulocyte count. Increased hemolysis can result in decreased erythrocyte levels. To specifically diagnose megaloblastic anemia and its etiology, vitamin B_{12} and/or folate levels may need to be evaluated. An analysis of vitamin B_{12} and folate levels assists in establishing a definitive diagnosis. For example, a serum vitamin B_{12} level of < 100 pg/mL and a serum folate level of < 3 ng/mL are diagnostic of vitamin B_{12} deficiency and folate deficiency, respectively.

The next task is to determine the cause of the vitamin B_{12} deficiency and/or folate deficiency. A thorough nutritional history assists in isolating dietary causes; however, problems with absorption can be identified by using a **Schilling test,** in which the patient is given an oral dose of radioactively labeled vitamin B_{12}. A 24-hour urine collection is then measured for vitamin B_{12} excretion. Normally, urinary excretion is at least 8% to 40% of total radioactively labeled vitamin B_{12}, indicating that the substance was absorbed and metabolized. If urinary excretion is lower than 3%, this may indicate an inability to absorb vitamin B_{12}; in this case, a second stage of the test is performed. In this stage, the patient again is given an oral dose of radiolabeled vitamin B_{12} but now with a parenteral dose of intrinsic factor. A 24-hour urine collection is repeated, and results are compared with those of the first urine collection. An increase in urinary excretion of radiolabeled vitamin B_{12} with the addition of IF suggests pernicious anemia.

Analysis then turns to identifying the cause of pernicious anemia. Radiologic examinations, histories, endoscopies, and occasionally surgical exploration may reveal conditions such as celiac disease, tropical sprue, gastric shortening, Crohn's disease, blind loops, and diverticuli, all of which contribute to decreased intestinal production of intrinsic factor. Another diagnostic exam involves the insertion of a nasogastric tube to measure gastric acid secretion. Insufficiencies in gastric acids point to gastric parietal cell problems, which also contribute to insufficient IF and vitamin B_{12} malabsorption.

Medical Management

The first task of medical management is to remove or alter any factors that are contributing to folate and/or vitamin B_{12} deficiency, such as suppressive medication regimes. Dietary causes of both folate deficiency and vitamin B_{12} deficiency can be effectively treated with counseling, diet modifications, or vitamin supplementation. Recommended doses of folate supplements start with daily oral administration of 1 mg of folic acid for 4 months and maintenance with 0.4 mg in a multivitamin for patients with an underlying cause or inadequate diet. Folate deficiencies due to malabsorptive processes require treatment of the underlying cause. Intravenous folate should always be considered in

Weblink: Cooley's Anemia Foundation

the management of alcoholism to help minimize some of the painful side effects of recovery.

Vitamin B_{12} supplementation is usually achieved via dietary modifications rather than by administering the vitamin in pill form. The latest Recommended Dietary Allowance (RDA) for vitamin B_{12} is 2.4 mcg/day for persons ages 14 to 70 years; the average diet in the United States contains about 5 mcg daily. The prevalence of foods fortified with vitamin B_{12} means that increased intake can be readily achieved. However, the assistance of a dietitian is extremely valuable to ensure proper intake of recommended doses (see the Collaborative Management section that follows).

Vitamin B_{12} deficiency in the patient with absorption problems is usually managed with parenteral supplementation. The treatment schedule begins with parenteral 1,000 mcg vitamin B_{12}, followed by 1,000 mcg intramuscularly once a month for the rest of the patient's life. The efficacy of this approach is well documented. Patients report increased strength and stamina soon after institution of regular doses. Blood cell morphology begins to show normal red blood cells within hours of treatments with subsequent remission of the anemia during the next several weeks (Adams & Koch, 2010).

Oral vitamin B_{12} supplementation has been available since 1968; however, it is not widely used for two reasons: (1) fear of noncompliance and (2) lack of understanding of alternate biochemical pathways for vitamin B_{12} absorption. However, there is growing evidence that oral administration may be just as effective as parenteral administration if given in appropriate doses (Bryan, 2010).

Nursing Management

The nurse caring for the patient with megaloblastic anemias has the following priorities:

Continued Assessment for Signs and Symptoms of Hypoxic Distress in Severe Cases: The Nursing Process: Patient Care Plan for Generalized Anemia (p. 1724) provides assessment guidelines and nursing interventions appropriate for use in managing megaloblastic anemia.

Prevention of Mechanical Injury from Neurological Changes: In addition to the harm caused by hypoxia, these patients are at increased risk of falls and injury secondary to ataxia and lack of balance coordination. Patients with peripheral neuropathy secondary to vitamin B_{12} deficiency have diminished peripheral sensations, which increase their risk of injury. Nurses must include an assessment of progressive nerve damage and sensation; most importantly, they must ensure that the patient's environment is safe so as to limit injury.

Identification of High-Risk Populations: Because vitamin B_{12} is found primarily in meats, vegetarians, especially vegans, are at higher risk for vitamin B_{12} deficiency. The rate of folate deficiency is also a concern in women of childbearing age and in older adults. With this knowledge in hand, nurses may emphasize assessment of dietary histories and patient education to target these high-risk groups.

Patient Education and Reinforcement Regarding Dietary Modifications and/or Supplementation: Patient education regarding dietary modifications is discussed in the next section. For patients who require supplementation, nursing reinforcement and encouragement can be pivotal to ensuring compliance with a lifelong regime. Nurses should assess patients for compliance, efficacy, and safety of the intramuscular vitamin B_{12} injections and provide feedback as to its action. This can be accomplished by reviewing hematologic studies with the patient and indicating improvements when indicated. A major discharge priority for patients with megaloblastic anemia is verbalization of an understanding of dietary modifications and, if indicated, safe performance of medication self-administration techniques.

Collaborative Management

Collaboration with the health care team is important to ensure a comprehensive multifaceted approach to correction of underlying causes. In order to meet desired patient outcomes, it is essential that the members of this interdisciplinary team communicate openly with one another in developing and evaluating care of the patient and family (IOM [Institute of Medicine], 2010).

Dietitians play a critical role in providing accurate and appropriate patient education. Patients can become easily confused with food labels, such as "excellent" or "good," designed for advertising purposes. Handouts and food plans should be provided for clarification. Food sources for vitamin B_{12} and folate can be found in Chapter 8.

Collaboration with the pharmacist should not be overlooked. A number of drugs can interfere with vitamin B_{12} or folate absorption and metabolism. The pharmacist is able to monitor drug regimens to prevent such deleterious drug–food interactions. Additionally, the pharmacist can provide materials to help with the administration of parenteral supplements.

Hemoglobinopathies

Hemoglobinopathy is a term used to describe a class of red blood cell disorders characterized by abnormal hemoglobin, which can result in a variety of clinical problems including hypoxia, accelerated RBC destruction, and decreased RBC production. All of these diseases result from genetic mutations in the coding sequences that control the component hemoglobin chains. Classification of these diseases is often based on the type of genetic alteration (point mutation, base pair, or deletion). The disorders also are commonly classified on the basis of the molecular and chemical effect of the alteration. Alterations include decreased oxygen-binding capacity and structural defects that decrease the life span of the red blood cells.

As with most genetic disorders, the severity of clinical symptoms depends on the role of the gene involved and on the inheritance pattern. Homozygous patients frequently present with severe debilitating disease, whereas heterozygous patients can often live asymptomatically unless they are affected by acute illness or environmental stress.

More than 800 distinct diseases have been attributed to hemoglobinopathy, of which thalassemia and sickle cell disease are the most prominent. These diseases are discussed in the following sections.

Thalassemia

The term **thalassemia** refers to a group of hematologic disorders characterized by the genetic inheritance of a mutated hemoglobin-coding gene that appears most frequently in persons of Southeast Asian, African, and Mediterranean descent (PubMed, 2010a). The hallmark of thalassemia is a structural change in the hemoglobin molecule that subjects affected red blood cells to increased rates of hemolysis. The thalassemias are chronic disease states that are usually detected during infancy or adolescence. Cure of these anemias is not the goal for the acute care nurse; the focus is on prevention of disease complications and treatment of symptoms.

Pathophysiology

Recall from the earlier discussion of hemoglobin synthesis that oxygen binding occurs when alpha and beta chains form precise geometric configurations that allow iron to sit tightly in a lock-and-key style fit on the heme groups. Thalassemia arises when the alpha and beta chains are of unequal proportions, which ultimately reduces the rate of RBC maturation in the bone marrow. Cells that do survive bone marrow development and enter the bloodstream are recognized in the spleen as structurally abnormal and are subject to higher rates of hemolysis.

The thalassemias are broadly divided into two groups: alpha thalassemias or beta thalassemias, depending on the type of inherited gene mutation. Beta thalassemias result from reduced beta chains; the alpha thalassemias result from reduced alpha chains. The diseases are also characterized by their gene inheritance pattern: homozygous carriers, defining the inheritance of two defective genes, or heterozygous carriers, defining the inheritance of only one defective gene. Each combination of gene inheritance is associated with distinct clinical features (PubMed, 2010b).

Clinical Manifestations

Alpha thalassemias are generally milder than the beta thalassemias and often present without symptoms or with very mild symptoms that respond well to supportive care when indicated. The severity of symptoms in patients with beta thalassemias depends heavily on the inheritance pattern (see the Genetic Considerations box). The term *beta-thalassemia minor* describes the inheritance of only one defective gene and one normal gene (heterozygous); the term *beta-thalassemia major* is used for the inheritance of two defective genes (homozygous).

Patients with beta-thalassemia minor are able to produce small amounts of normal hemoglobin and therefore are frequently asymptomatic owing to long-term physiological adaptation. These patients are carriers of the genetic trait; therefore, genetic counseling may be offered for patients of reproductive age. Beta-thalassemia major (also called Cooley's anemia) results from complete lack of the beta protein in the hemoglobin chain manifesting as severe, life-threatening anemia. Symptoms that result from the increased rate of hemolysis include jaundice, hepatomegaly (enlarged liver), and splenomegaly (enlarged spleen). Pronounced pallor, tachycardia, and lethargy result from a critical lack of oxygen-binding capacity. The bone marrow is constantly in a state of increased erythropoiesis in an attempt to compensate for hemolysis and hypoxia, resulting in bone marrow expansion, recognized as thickening of facial bones and abnormal skeletal growth (Cunningham, 2010). The physiological demands imposed by beta-thalassemia major can be so serious that many children who acquire the disease do not survive into adulthood. *Beta-thalassemia intermedia* was a term coined by Sturgeon and colleagues in 1955 to describe a small group of patients who do not fit neatly into either the beta-thalassemia major or beta-thalassemia minor paradigm. These patients have symptoms that are hematologically too severe to be called "minor" and too mild to be called "major." These individuals are homozygous for thalassemia genes but maintain hemoglobin levels of 7 to 10 g/dL without regular transfusions.

GENETIC CONSIDERATIONS for Thalassemia

Individuals of Southeast Asian, Africa, or Mediterranean descent have a genetic predisposition to thalassemia. Patients with alpha-thalassemia and beta-thalassemia minor are often asymptomatic and not identified; however, patients with beta-thalassemia major usually require transfusions beginning early in life (Cunningham, 2010).

Alterations in laboratory values for thalassemia patients depend on the form of the inherited mutation and the inheritance pattern. In addition to alterations in hemoglobin and red blood cells, clinicians should monitor for alterations in bilirubin, which provide indications of hemolytic effects in the liver. Chart 56–8 summarizes the changes in laboratory values and clinical symptoms relative to the type of thalassemia (Gaspard, 2009).

In addition to clinical presentation directly related to thalassemia, the constant need for transfusion to maintain adequate RBCs often leads to transfusion-related complications and iron overload. Excessive iron comes from the patient's own hemolyzed red blood and the transfused blood, as well as increased iron absorption from food as a compensatory mechanism to combat anemia. The excess iron is stored in the spleen, liver, endocrine organs, and heart, causing splenomegaly, hepatomegaly, cirrhosis, hormone imbalances, and cardiomyopathy, all of which can become fatal.

Medical Management

Patients with alpha thalassemias and those with beta-thalassemia minor are usually asymptomatic and usually do not require medical intervention. Patients with thalassemia major, however, may require frequent transfusions of packed RBCs, often beginning early in life, to correct falling hematocrit and hemoglobin levels that result from rampant hemolysis. Transfusion doses are titrated to maintain therapeutic hemoglobin levels between 7 and 10 g/dL or to correct severe symptoms.

The leading cause of death among patients with thalassemia has shifted from hemoglobin-deficient anemia to iron overload associated with chronic blood transfusion therapy (Cunningham, 2010). Therefore, the patient's iron levels must be carefully monitored to prevent iron overload. Two common methods used to monitor iron are the

CHART 56–8 Laboratory Values and Clinical Presentation of the Thalassemias

	Alpha Thalassemia	Beta-Thalassemia Minor	Beta-Thalassemia Intermedia	Beta-Thalassemia Major
Hemoglobin	Normal	>10 g/dL (normal)	7–10 g/dL	<7 g/dL
Red blood cell appearance	Microcytic and Hypochromic			
Red blood cells		Usually normal	Usually normal or decreased	Severely decreased
Jaundice	Usually absent	Usually absent	Usually absent or mild	Severe
Splenomegaly	Usually absent	Usually absent	Usually absent or mild	Severe
Skeletal changes	Absent	Usually absent	Usually absent or mild	Severe

Weblink: Sickle Cell Disease Association of America
Video: Sickle Cell Anemia

serum ferritin test and liver biopsy. Iron chelation therapy with drugs such as desferrioxamine (Desferal) is administered intravenously or subcutaneously in an effort to bind and neutralize excessive iron from patients' bodies. Hydration and oxygenation complement transfusion and chelation therapy in an effort to rid the body of excess erythrocyte waste and maintain oxygen levels (Cunningham, 2010).

Nursing Management

Nursing assessment of patients with thalassemia focuses on the hemolytic and hypoxic effects manifested in the integumentary, gastrointestinal, lymphatic, and cardiovascular systems. Patients should be observed for jaundice in the skin and eyes due to RBC destruction and for pallor from hemoglobin-deficient anemia. Abdominal pain and liver and spleen tenderness are indicators of thalassemia and should be included in a comprehensive assessment. Cardiovascular signs and symptoms of activity intolerance and hypoxia should also be assessed as indicators of both hemoglobin deficiency and iron accumulation in the cardiac muscle.

Nursing interventions based on the preceding assessments should prioritize activity alterations, pain management, and collaboration with the multidisciplinary team. The Nursing Process: Patient Care Plan for Generalized Anemia (p. 1724) should be implemented in the care of these patients. If transfusion therapy is warranted, the nurse plays a critical role in managing the administration of blood products, including assessing for signs of a transfusion reaction such as fluid overload, fever, and anaphylaxis (Chapter 16).

Sickle Cell Anemia

Etiology and Epidemiology

Sickle cell anemia is the term given to a group of genetically based RBC diseases all characterized by misshapen "sickle-shaped" red blood cells. The source of the sickling is a malfunctioning hemoglobin molecule that twists the entire RBC from a soft, pliable, round doughnut shape into a long, hard, sticky elongated cell (Figure 56–7 ◆).

Sickle cell anemia is perhaps the best-known of the chronic erythrocyte disorders. It is estimated that more than 70,000 people in the United States suffer from sickle cell disease, with about 1,000 babies born annually with the disease. Sickle cell disease occurs most frequently in African Americans and Hispanic Americans. About 1 in every 500 African Americans has sickle cell disease. It also affects people of Arabian, Greek, Maltese, Italian, Sardinian, Turkish, and Indian ancestry (see the Genetic Considerations box) (Gaspard, 2009; PubMed, 2010a; Wilkie, 2010).

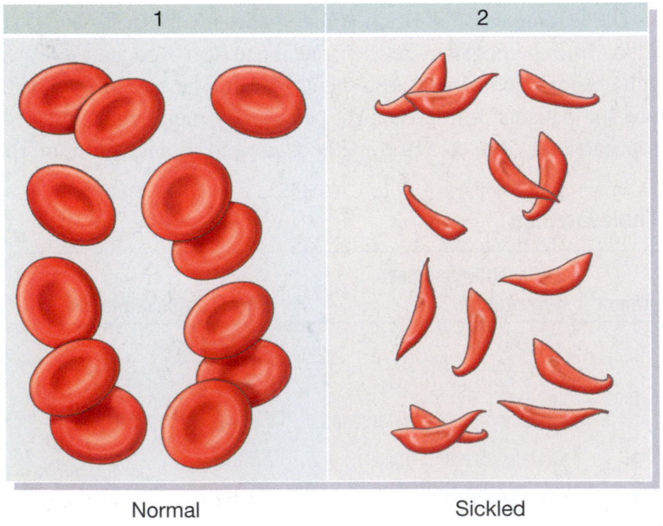

FIGURE 56–7 ◆ Red blood cells from sickle cell anemia.

Pathophysiology

Patients with sickle cell anemia acquire sickle hemoglobin (HbS), a mutated version of the normal form of hemoglobin A. Recall from the discussion on hemoglobin development and function earlier in the chapter that oxygen binding results in a geometric alteration of the hemoglobin molecule. In normal hemoglobin, the oxygenated state and the deoxygenated state coexist without deleterious side effects. However, HbS causes affected cells to take on a rigid, elongated sickle shape upon release of the oxygen molecule rather than the normal, flexible round configuration. Under normal circumstances, deoxygenated sickled cells make up only a small proportion of total blood volume, with minimal physical effects. However, any stress that results in oxygen deprivation increases the proportion of sickled cells. Figure 56–8 ◆ shows grouped RBCs shown in profile and normal RBCs compared to a sickle RBC.

Sickle cells possess "sticky membranes" and unusual shapes that occlude small blood vessels (a condition called *erythrostasis*), which serve to further potentiate oxygen deprivation. Sickled cells also are trapped by the spleen, further reducing circulating red blood cells and contributing to hypoxia. Initially, the hypoxia will stimulate increased erythropoiesis, thus reversing the cycle. However, if the hypoxia becomes extreme, widespread vessel occlusion leads to a syndrome termed *sickle cell crisis*. These crisis states are responsible for the severe pain of sickle cell disease. Pain, in turn, increases the demand for oxygen, hinders mobility and respiration, and taxes the cardiovascular system. Together, the sequence of events escalates into a cycle of deoxygenation and RBC sickling. Gone unchecked, the resultant thrombosis and acidosis progress to organ failure and eventually death.

Crisis Syndromes of Sickled Red Blood Cells

The critical situations that may be seen in patients with sickle cell anemia are termed vaso-occlusive crisis, sequestration crisis, aplastic crisis, and hyperhemolytic crisis. These are described next.

Vaso-Occlusive Crisis

Vaso-occlusive crisis is the occlusion of small vessels by long, hard chains of stacked sickled cells. This occlusion prevents oxygenation of surrounding tissues and tissue downstream of the occlusion. Oxygen deprivation in arterial vessels causes ischemic attacks and infarction. Oxygen deprivation to venous vessels leads to swollen, tender tissues as a result of the buildup of fluids and wastes. Both arterial and venous occlusions are marked by severe pain.

GENETIC CONSIDERATIONS for Sickle Cell Disease

Sickle cell disease is acquired through genetic inheritance in families of African, Hispanic, Arabian, Greek, Italian, Sardinian, Maltese, Turkish, and Indian ancestry. Patients who inherit the sickle cell gene from one parent (heterozygous HbS/HbA) usually do not exhibit symptoms and are termed sickle cell carriers. Patients who inherit the sickle cell gene from both parents (homozygous) are subject to severe sickle cell crises. Because both homozygous and heterozygous patients can pass their genes on to their children, sickle cell carriers typically are offered some type of genetic counseling prior to childbearing (Gaspard, 2009; Wilkie, 2010).

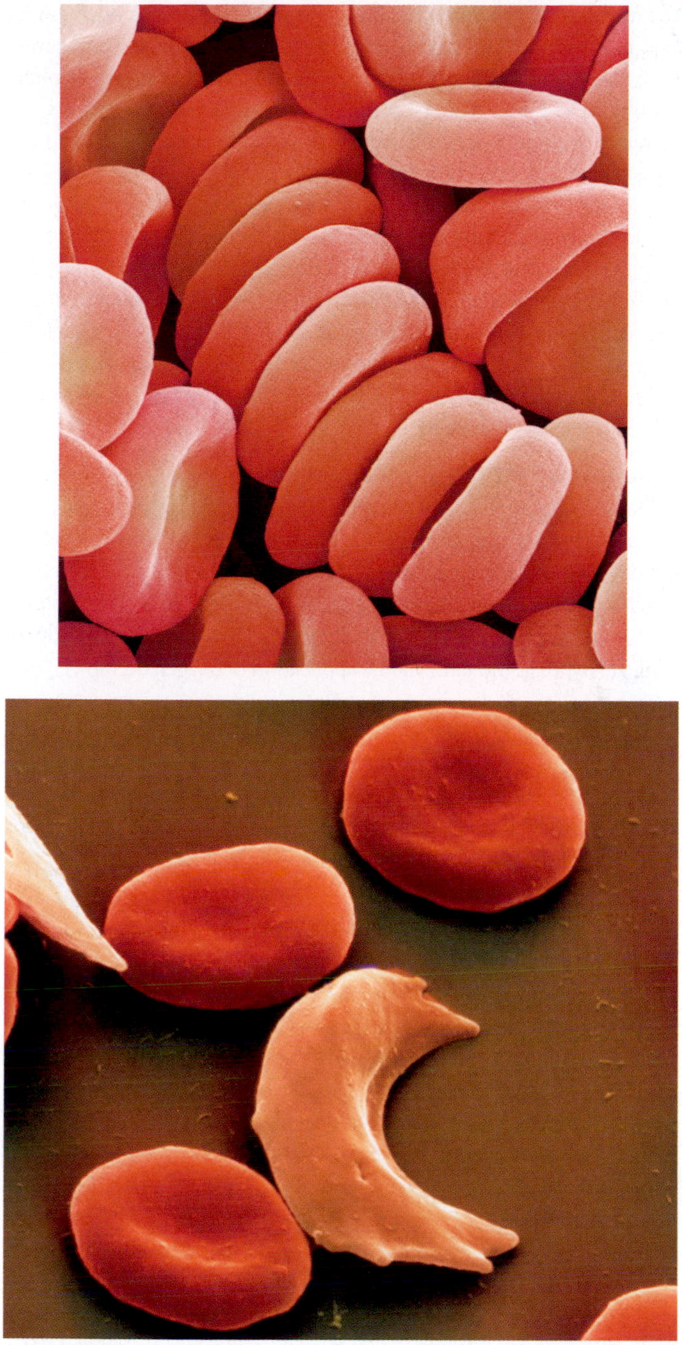

FIGURE 56–8 ◆ (top) RBCs in profile, forming rouleaux and (bottom) normal RBCs compared to a sickled RBC.

Source: (top) Andrew Syred/Photo Researchers, Inc.; (bottom) Oliver Meckes & Nicole Ottawa/Photo Researchers, Inc.

Sequestration Crisis

Sequestration crisis occurs when sickled RBCs overwhelm and clog the spleen. As a result, circulating blood volume decreases, manifesting as decreased blood pressure; this in turn stagnates blood flow and causes deoxygenation. Sequestration crisis manifests as a painful, tender, grossly enlarged spleen.

Aplastic Crisis

The destruction of large numbers of RBCs in the spleen by sickle cell anemia places an extraordinarily high demand on the amount of bone marrow available to replenish available circulating erythrocytes into the bloodstream. This extraordinary demand overwhelms the bone marrow regulatory feedback mechanism, resulting in complete bone marrow shutdown, akin to a system overload. This complete bone marrow shutdown is referred to as aplastic crisis. As a result of aplastic crisis, reticulocytes (juvenile RBCs) are not produced, causing a severe drop in hemoglobin, up to 1 g/dL per day, manifesting in severe lethargy, malaise, and deoxygenation.

Hyperhemolytic Crisis

Hyperhemolytic crisis is a rare complication. As the name implies, hyperhemolytic crisis involves a massive increase in RBC destruction. As in aplastic crisis, hemoglobin rates drop rapidly. However, if the bone marrow is still intact, reticulocyte production is increased.

Clinical Manifestations

The extent and severity of the disease depend on two criteria: the inheritance pattern (homozygous for HbS or heterozygous HbS/HbA) and the presence of deoxygenating triggering factors. Patients who are heterozygous HbS/HbA (termed sickle cell carriers) often live asymptomatic lives because the normal hemoglobin produced by HbA sufficiently prevents sickling crisis. Homozygous patients also usually live asymptomatic lives unless they are subjected to stressors such as infection, pain, blood loss, or high altitudes. Sickle cell crisis occurs when the patient is subjected to such stressors or prolonged hypoxia. Peripheral tissue and organ damage become more apparent, and oxygen deprivation and blood stagnation increase with prolonged sickle cell crisis. Although every body system eventually can become affected, certain signs and symptoms are most frequently observed:

- Persistent, usually painful, erection of the penis due to veno-occlusion causes both severe pain and embarrassment for male patients.
- Acute renal failure results primarily from arterial occlusion in the renal capillaries, which, in turn, leads to focal areas of hemorrhage or necrosis. Additionally, myoglobin and RBC waste products from extremely high RBC destruction can overload renal tubules, causing renal failure.
- Acute chest syndrome (ACS) results from a variety of causes. The causes directly pertaining to sickle cell crisis include pulmonary tissue infarction due to capillary occlusion and hypoventilation secondary to rib/sternal bone infarction. Treatment of sickle cell crisis can also exacerbate ACS. Examples include hypoventilation secondary to narcotic administration and pulmonary edema induced by narcotics or fluid overload. Regardless of the cause, the resultant hypoxia severely increases hemoglobin sickling, making the appearance of ACS an ominous sign in the patient with sickle cell anemia.
- Splenomegaly (enlarged spleen) results from splenic sequestration.
- Avascular necrosis (AVN), also known as ischemic necrosis, osteonecrosis, or aseptic necrosis of the large joints, results from interruption of the arterial supply of the femoral head. Patients with AVN have severe chronic joint pain, decreased weight-bearing ability, and joint malformation.
- Hemolytic anemia, or acute anemia caused by the accelerated breakdown of red blood cells, is characterized by splenomegaly, jaundice, and decreased urine output. Hemolytic anemia is discussed in greater detail later in this chapter.

As the microvasculature becomes increasingly occluded, major organs begin to suffer irreversible damage from hypoxia and thrombosis. Evidence of organ failure includes decreased level of consciousness (decreased cerebral tissue perfusion), decreased urine output and increased serum creatinine (decreased renal tissue perfusion), chest pain (decreased cardiopulmonary tissue perfusion), and abdominal pain (decreased liver, colon, and spleen perfusion).

Laboratory and Diagnostic Procedures

Laboratory studies analyzing RBC morphology are used to monitor for the prevalence of sickle cell hemoglobin. Hemoglobin electrophoresis analysis can reveal the presence of HbS in patients with sickle cell disease. Slide smears of peripheral blood samples can reveal partially or completely sickled cells, as the proportion of sickled cells to normal cells increases during crisis states. Hemoglobin values will be normal in patients with the sickle cell trait but below 7 g/dL during deoxygenation states or in homozygous patients. As sickling progresses, the patient also will display evidence of increasing RBC breakdown manifested by decreased numbers of RBCs and increased amounts of bilirubin.

Medical Management

The cornerstone of sickle cell disease management is prevention of sickle cell crisis by ensuring adequate oxygenation via avoidance of triggering events at all times. Because patients are usually diagnosed when they are children, prevention of sickle cell crisis states should always involve collaboration with parents. Any patient presenting to the acute care setting with a known history of sickle cell disease warrants particular attention to oxygenation and hydration status. In the unfortunate event that sickle cell crisis develops, supportive care must be implemented to prevent severe pain, organ failure, and death.

Treatments should include administration and monitoring of supplemental oxygen, analgesics for vaso-occlusive crisis, hydration, and, if indicated, blood cell transfusions to reverse hypoxia. Pharmacologic treatments to prevent sickle cell crisis are being researched. Avenues for investigation include drugs such as hydroxyurea, butyrate, and arginine that stimulate the body to make normal types of hemoglobin, drugs to increase oxygenation to small blood vessels (Poloxamer 188, Flocor), drugs that make sickled cell membranes less "sticky," and gene therapies (Gaspard, 2009; Wilkie, 2010).

Nursing Management

Prevention of sickle cell crisis is a primary goal for any patient admitted with sickle cell disease, regardless of the primary admitting diagnosis. Situations that are most likely to cause HbS chains to sickle and stack include dehydration, blood stagnation, decreased pH (acidosis), and decreased PaO_2. Disease management therefore focuses on maintenance of adequate hydration, maintenance of oxygenation to prevent acidosis and decreased PaO_2, and prevention of hypercoagulability.

Effective nursing management of patients with sickle cell disease involves first identifying high-risk factors and then implementing effective preventive nursing and medical interventions. If sickle cell crisis occurs, the medical team must quickly mobilize to treat pain and eliminate the triggering factors. Finally, all patients with sickle cell disease must be regularly assessed for evidence of organ and tissue dysfunction. In addition to the Nursing Process: Patient Care Plan for Generalized Anemia presented earlier (p. 1724), the Nursing Process: Patient Care Plan for Sickle Cell Anemia outlines specific nursing interventions aimed at preventing these sickling crisis states, addressing sickle cell crisis, and providing continued assessment of long-term sequelae.

Collaborative Management

Nursing collaboration with the multidisciplinary team is an effective means to address the complex needs of the patient with sickle cell disease. In order to meet desired patient outcomes, it is essential that the members of this interdisciplinary team communicate openly with one another in developing and evaluating care of the patient and family (IOM [Institute of Medicine], 2010). Interdisciplinary team members should include pharmacists, physical and occupational therapists, respiratory therapists, medical specialists such as hematologists, and the patient's primary health care provider.

Because pain is a major factor in sickle cell crisis, analgesia is certain to play a role in the acute hospitalization. Pharmacologic expertise can help to ensure that appropriate and effective options are readily available and implemented (Wright & Adeosun, 2009). Emerging trends in the management of sickle cell disease suggest that nonpharmacologic interventions (such as massage for pain management) and long-term physical exercise plans can help to prevent many of the complications related to sickle cell disease.

Discharge Planning

Physical, occupational, and rehabilitation therapists can provide assistance in the acute care setting but, more important, can provide patient education and referrals in preparation for discharge (see the Patient Teaching & Discharge Priorities box, p. 1740) (Wilkie, 2010). Respiratory therapy, particularly during acute chest syndrome, can help to mitigate hypoxia and pain via the application of oxygen therapy.

Health Promotion

The patient's primary health care provider may benefit from consultation with a hematologist who specializes in sickle cell disease. The Evidence-Based Practice box (p. 1741) discusses other interventions that can be used with patients who have sickle cell disease.

Hemolytic Anemias

Etiology

Hemolytic anemia is a term applied to a wide range of diseases characterized by increased RBC destruction (hemolysis). Hemolysis begins in the peripheral bloodstream with the recognition by phagocytes of dying or damaged red blood cells. The spleen, liver, and reticuloendothelial system then complete degradation. Normally, the rate of hemolysis is balanced by the rate of erythropoiesis; thus, a consistent volume of oxygen-carrying red blood cells is maintained in the peripheral circulation.

Infection, toxins, certain medications, injury, and other environmental stressors can all trigger minor increases in hemolysis, which result in a decrease in circulating red blood cells, triggering hypoxia. In healthy patients, this hypoxia stimulates increased erythropoietin production, accelerated erythropoiesis, and compensation of hypoxia. Clinically significant hypoxia, characterizing hemolytic anemia, results when the hemolysis persists or is so extensive that erythropoiesis cannot sufficiently compensate. Hemolytic anemia should be distinguished from anemia due to bone marrow disorders (Chart 56–9, p. 1741). In the latter, clinically significant hypoxia results from sluggish erythropoiesis; this cannot compensate for normal hemolysis.

Pathophysiology

Several pathophysiological processes can result in the anemia of hemolytic etiology just described. Commonly, causes of hemolytic anemia are grouped according to such processes. Certain causes are due to intrinsic defects in the erythrocyte, which decreases its ability to survive the normal RBC life span of 120 days. Deficiencies in metabolic, protective enzymes are the first intrinsic cause of hemolytic anemia. The most common defect of this type is glucose-6-phosphate dehydrogenase deficiency. A second intrinsic defect results from fragility and instability in

NURSING PROCESS: Patient Care Plan for Sickle Cell Anemia

Assessment of Hematologic Status Using Gordon's Functional Health Patterns:

- Activity Exercise Pattern
- Cognitive Perceptual Pattern

Subjective Data

Assessment of Tissue Perfusion

Have you been short of breath?

Are you dizzy?

Are you having chest pain?

Have you had any nausea or vomiting or abdominal pain?

Do your arms or legs hurt?

Assessment of Pain of Sickle Cell Disease

Are you feeling any pain? If so, where?

What makes it worse? What makes it better?

Can you describe it?

How have you treated sickle cell pain in the past?

Objective Data

Assessment of Tissue Perfusion

Integumentary: skin temperature cool, pale

Pulses: diminished, weak peripheral pulses

Renal: decreased urinary output, concentrated urine (high specific gravity)

Cerebral: restless, anxious, decreased level of alertness

Cardiopulmonary: tachypnea, tachycardia, angina, oxygen saturation decreased

Gastrointestinal: pain and tenderness with or without palpation

Laboratory values: hemoglobin <7, positive HbS, RBCs decreased, bilirubin elevated

Assessment of Pain of Sickle Cell Disease

General: pallor, malaise, fatigue

Fever: assess for possible sites of infection

Neurological: level of consciousness (ominous sign of intracranial bleeding)

Lung sounds: crackles, diminished lung sounds

Respiratory: cough, dyspnea, ventilation depth

Cardiovascular: poor capillary refill, tachycardia, hypotension

Pain: location, quality, onset, and alleviating factors

Abdominal: painful, swollen left upper quadrant

Genitourinary: priapism

Neuromuscular: painful swollen joints, especially hips

Renal: renal lab values, urinary output volume and character

Lab values: hemoglobin (presence of sickle cell disease) A2 and F hemoglobin

Full blood count (FBC) to detect anemia, and reticulocyte count

Outcomes and Evaluation Parameters / Planning and Interventions with *Rationales*

1. NURSING DIAGNOSIS: Risk for Ineffective Tissue Perfusion: Cerebral, Renal, Cardiopulmonary, and Abdominal Organ *related to vaso-occlusive crisis* (NANDA-I © 2012)

Outcomes and Evaluation Parameters

Outcome: Free of injury due to peripheral hypoxia.

Evaluation Parameters: Cerebral: Patient remains alert and oriented.

Cerebral: Pupil response remains unchanged from baseline. Gross reflex assessment remains unchanged from baseline.

Renal: Urinary output remains adequate for patient (at least 30 mL/hr for nondialysis patients). Electrolyte blood studies and urinalysis remain within normal limits. Patient remains free of edema.

Cardiopulmonary: Peripheral pulses remain intact compared to baseline. Patient remains free of chest pain. Lung and chest auscultation do not reveal adventitious or irregular sounds. Oxygenation status remains within normal limits as measured by SpO_2 saturation above 90% or within normal baseline parameters for patient and ABGs pH 7.3–7.5, $PaCO_2$ 35–45 mmHg.

Abdominal: Gastric motility remains intact. Patient remains free of nausea, vomiting, severe cramping, and diarrhea.

Planning and Interventions with *Rationales*

Frequently monitor neurological signs including level of consciousness, Glasgow Coma Scale, pupillary changes, and cranial nerves *to detect changes in level of consciousness and nerve damage.*

Assess for signs of edema and urine output (color, amount) *as indicators of renal function.*

Monitor blood studies (renal function tests, electrolytes) and urine tests (creatinine, protein) *as indicators of renal function.*

Encourage oral fluid intake and administer intravenous fluid (as ordered) *to maintain fluid balance, hydration, and renal cell perfusion.*

Administer hypotonic fluids such as dextrose 5% in water or in 0.45% normal saline. *Hypotonic fluids entering RBCs will reduce tendency of hemoglobin to crystallize into sickle shape and will promote dilution of already sickled cells and occluded vessels.*

Report changes and trends in renal output and renal lab studies immediately to the health care provider *to ensure timely interventions are implemented.*

Assess peripheral pulses *as indicators of peripheral tissue perfusion.*

Assess cardiac sounds *to detect irregular heart rhythms.*

Assess jugular vein distention and peripheral edema *as indicators of cardiac muscle status.*

Encourage the patient to avoid strenuous activity t*o decrease cardiac workload and oxygen demands.*

(*continued*)

NURSING PROCESS: Patient Care Plan for Sickle Cell Anemia, *continued*

Outcomes and Evaluation Parameters	Planning and Interventions with *Rationales*
	Assess for adventitious or diminished breath sounds. *Indicates decreased gas exchange and hypoxia.* Monitor respiratory rate and depth *to assess for respiratory distress.* Collaborate with respiratory therapist to administer high-flow oxygen therapy as ordered *to maximize oxygen availability in peripheral tissues.* Collaborate with health care provider to obtain ABGs when SpO_2 sat falls below 80% *as a more accurate analysis of acid–base balance.* Provide incentive spirometry every hour *to prevent atelectasis.* Collaborate with health care provider for administration of oxygen for SpO_2 states of less than 90% *to prevent acidosis. However, do not administer* O_2 *for patients who are not hypoxic, because this may suppress bone marrow production of RBCs.* Assess for abdominal pain and tenderness *as indicators of gastric perfusion.* Perform abdominal auscultation *as an indicator of gastric perfusion.* Monitor for nausea, appetite, vomiting, and diarrhea *as indicators of gastric function.* Offer small frequent meals *to minimize distention.*
2. NURSING DIAGNOSIS: Pain *related to vaso-occlusive crisis* (NANDA-I © 2012)	
Outcomes: Maintenance of adequate oxygenation and acid–base balance. Maintenance of comfort level. ***Evaluation Parameters:*** Able to communicate pain level and therapies that help alleviate it. Pain reduced and/or absent as evidenced by patient report and no pain behaviors: grimacing. Nonpharmacologic method of control is effective as evidenced by patient report and no pain behaviors. Reports satisfaction with pain management program.	Collaborate with the patient to determine preferred pain control modalities. *Patients with chronic sickle cell disease are most familiar with personalized effective treatment options. Collaboration also promotes trust and therapeutic relationships.* Assess pain including rating and character frequently and reassess after any pain intervention *to provide early detection of pain and to measure effectiveness of interventions.* Administer pain medication on a fixed schedule *to maintain consistent blood levels.* Administer RBCs per health care provider order in specific situations such as symptomatic anemia, a hematocrit reading 7 points below baseline, orthostasis, and a reticulocyte count of zero. *RBC transfusions provide nonsickled oxygen-carrying hemoglobin, increase oxygenation, and treat aplastic crisis.* Monitor for signs such as a falling hematocrit level, pain, pulmonary edema, fever, hypotension, and hemolysis *as indicators of transfusion reactions (hemolysis and fluid overload).*

Source: Adapted from Wilkinson, J. M., & Ahearn, N. R. (2009). *Prentice Hall nursing diagnosis handbook* (9th ed.). Upper Saddle River, NJ: Prentice Hall.

PATIENT TEACHING & DISCHARGE PRIORITIES for Sickle Cell Anemia

Need	Teaching
Disease process	Discuss cause of disease.
Patient/family	Discuss triggers and risks of sickle cell crisis.
Prevention/management of sickle cell crisis	Discuss activities or scenarios that can exacerbate a hypoxic state, emphasizing oxygenation and hydration.
Patient/family	Teach family to recognize key physical symptoms of sickle cell crisis.
	Discuss appropriate use of oxygenation.
	Discuss appropriate use of pain medication to control pain.
Pharmacologic management	Discuss appropriate use of pharmacologic treatments including side effects and recommended dosing schedule.
Patient/family	Consult with pharmacist for drug-specific teaching.
Nutrition	Discuss role of balanced nutrition, emphasizing need for key elements: vitamin B_{12}, folate, and iron.
Patient/family	Refer patient to a dietitian for assistance in meal planning.
Physical exercise	Discuss and explore appropriate physical exercise options that would maintain muscle/bone/cardiovascular strength but limit risks of hypoxia.
Patient/family	Refer the patient/family to physical, rehabilitation, and occupational therapy for outpatient consultation.

EVIDENCE-BASED PRACTICE Sickle Cell Crisis

Clinical Problem

Painful sickle cell crisis not only is a dreaded consequence of the disease but also presents a host of medical management problems to the health care team. Uncontrolled sickle cell crisis places the patient at risk of stroke, heart attack, and organ ischemia as well as unrelenting pain. Numerous interventions have traditionally been applied in an attempt to control pain and increase oxygenation, thus reversing erythrocyte sickling and decreasing blood viscosity. Nurses and health care providers should be aware of the barriers to the management of pain in sickle cell disease (SCD).

Research Findings

Wright and Adeosun (2009) conducted a review of the literature and found that there are three barriers to pain management in patients with SCD: the manifestations of vaso-occlusive pain, the sociocultural factors affecting pain assessment, and the concerns regarding addiction and pseudoaddiction (Wright & Adeosun, 2009). It was found that the pain of SCD manifested itself in many ways and is very individualized. The patient's ethnicity and other sociocultural factors can influence the patient's ability to receive adequate pain management. Members of ethnic minority groups and Black patients were found to have less access to care as well as trust issues related to the health care system in general. Finally, the perception that patients with SCD are narcotic dependent can provide a barrier to adequate pain management.

Implications for Nursing Practice

This study provides strong evidence supporting the idea that there are barriers to pain management in patients with SCD. It is important for nurses and the health care team to foster a trusting patient relationship with the patient with SCD. The pain from SCD is experienced differently by different individuals, and pain management should be individualized. Narcotics may play a role in pain management and should be used in adequate doses so that patients do not experience poor pain management.

Critical Thinking Questions with answers can be found in the Osborn Student Resources at nursing.pearsonhighered.com.

Source: Wright, K., & Adeosun, O. (2009). Barriers to effective pain management in sickle cell disease. *British Journal, 18*(3), 158–161.

CHART 56–9 Differences in Hemolysis in Hemolytic Anemia and Bone Marrow Disorders

Normal Hemolysis and Bone Marrow Function	Hemolytic Anemia	Anemia Due to Bone Marrow Disorders
Hemolysis matched by erythropoiesis	Increased hemolysis, normal erythropoiesis	Normal hemolysis, decreased erythropoiesis

the membrane structure, which is the hallmark of hereditary spherocytosis. A third type of intrinsic defect, which results in increased hemolysis, is the hemoglobinopathies, such as those that occur in sickle cell anemia and thalassemia. However, the primary clinical effects are more closely attributed to hemoglobin abnormalities rather than hemolysis; therefore, these disorders were discussed separately.

Extrinsic causes include situations in which the red blood cell is structurally and chemically normal but an unfavorable external environment leads to increased hemolysis. These causes include infections, certain medications, autoimmune processes, toxins, and malignancies. Hemolytic anemias from these extrinsic causes are classically grouped together as the acquired hemolytic anemias. The hemolytic anemias also are commonly classified as being intravascular or extravascular, referring to the primary site of hemolysis. In intravascular hemolysis, damaged RBCs are destroyed in the peripheral circulation and are associated most commonly with mechanical trauma and toxins. In extravascular hemolysis, the primary site of destruction is in the spleen and liver. Normally, a red blood cell has enough flexibility to maneuver through the spleen and liver several times in the course of its life span. However, membrane defects (including antibody binding) cause some red blood cells to get trapped and eventually become phagocytosed and destroyed.

Clinical Manifestations

In addition to unique signs and symptoms associated with individual disease processes, the hemolytic anemias share common physical findings. Consistent with hypoxia of anemias, the patient may complain of fatigue, activity intolerance, and shortness of breath. Severity of hypoxic symptoms correlates with severity of hemolysis. Patients with chronic disorders such as enzyme deficiencies may present with hypoxic symptoms only during periods of acute exacerbation. Jaundice, hemoglobinuria (red-brown urine), splenomegaly, and hepatomegaly (particularly in combination with poor liver function) are additional indicators of persistent hemolysis. Decreased, concentrated urine output is an indication of acute renal failure due to occlusion by lysed red blood cells and is an emergent sign requiring immediate intervention.

Laboratory and Diagnostic Procedures

Although the initial causes may vary, hemolytic anemias share some common trends in laboratory studies. Early stages of hemolytic anemia may reveal reticulocytosis (elevated reticulocyte count) in response to accelerated erythropoiesis. RBC counts will be decreased according to the severity of the hemolysis. Plasma haptoglobin levels also may be decreased (especially in intravascular hemolytic anemias) as liberated globin from lysed red blood cells binds all available haptoglobin. As haptoglobin molecules become overwhelmed, a large portion of the hemolyzed hemoglobin is excreted as unconjugated bilirubin. The level of unconjugated bilirubin in hemolysis is typically 70 to 85 μmol/L (4 to 5 mg/dL) and may be higher if liver function is impaired. If the marrow cannot compensate to replace the RBCs (as indicated by a decreased reticulocyte count), the anemia will worsen. Other indicators supporting a diagnosis of hemolytic anemia are increased lactate dehydrogenase (LDH) and serum AST (SGOT), both due to accelerated RBC destruction (Chart 56–10) (Gaspard, 2009; Rote & McCance, 2010a).

Medical Management

The first goal in the emergent management of the patient presenting with symptomatic hemolytic anemia is the stabilization of oxygenation status. Oxygen is administered to prevent critical organ hypoxia. However, administration of oxygen should be carefully titrated to prevent suppression of erythropoiesis. Intravenous infusions serve both to maintain fluid volume for cardiovascular status and to preserve renal function by flushing the body of excess waste and unconjugated bilirubin. Another goal is the amelioration of rampant hemolysis. If appropriate, triggering agents such as drugs or toxins should be immediately

CHART 56–10 Signs and Symptoms of Hemolytic Anemia

Physical Assessment	Laboratory Values
• Fatigue • Activity intolerance • Shortness of breath • Tachycardia • Tachypnea • Jaundice (severe cases) • Hemoglobinuria (severe cases) • Decreased urine output • Splenomegaly	• Reticulocytes: increased (reticulocytes decrease in severe hemolytic anemia or with failing bone marrow) • Red blood cells: decreased • Serum erythropoietin: increased • Serum haptoglobin: decreased • Unconjugated bilirubin: increased • Lactate dehydrogenase: increased • Hepatomegaly

removed. If the cause is extravascular and the patient presents with splenomegaly, a splenectomy (surgical removal of the spleen) may be indicated (Gaspard, 2009; Rote & McCance, 2010a). However, splenectomy usually is indicated only for certain forms of hemolytic anemia that have no identifiable triggering agents or in severe cases of acquired hemolytic anemia.

Once the patient is stabilized and the risk of imminent organ failure has subsided, attention turns to identification of the underlying pathophysiological process. A CBC and RBC morphology can help rule out or point to bone marrow involvement. Liver function tests can assist in distinguishing hemolytic anemia from nonhematologic causes such as liver failure. A thorough patient history that emphasizes family history and possible toxin and drug exposure also provides important diagnostic clues.

Nursing Management

Nursing care of the patient with hemolytic anemia has three main goals: avoidance of triggering factors in susceptible patients, prevention of complications, and treatment of complications should they occur. High-risk patients such as those with enzyme deficiencies, membrane deficiencies, or hemoglobinopathies, as well as patients with a history of autoimmune hemolytic anemia, may initially arrive in the acute care setting without symptoms of rampant hemolysis. To minimize the risk of hemolysis, the nurse should carefully review patient histories to identify high-risk individuals.

Once a patient has been identified as being at high risk of hemolytic anemia, the interdisciplinary team can collaborate to ensure that potential triggering agents are removed from the patient's environment, if appropriate. High-risk patients should be monitored closely for signs of generalized anemia, including increasing fatigue, activity intolerance, and hypoxia, as described earlier in the Nursing Process: Patient Care Plan for Generalized Anemia (p. 1724). Assessments that reveal decreased urinary output, hemoglobinuria, left flank pain (from splenomegaly), and fever suggest hemolytic anemia in particular. Analysis of laboratory values revealing reticulocytosis, decreased RBCs, increased bilirubin, and increased lactate dehydrogenase will further confirm hemolytic anemia.

Nursing interventions should then focus on minimizing the effects of blood cell hemolysis. The patient is at high risk for renal failure; therefore, the nurse should prioritize interventions to maintain renal blood flow. These interventions include encouraging oral intake of fluids and administration of IV fluid and blood component therapy as ordered. Frequent monitoring of urinary output, skin turgor, peripheral edema, and lung sounds will assist the nurse in determining fluid needs. Uncomfortable itching from excessive bilirubin, decreased oxygenation, and activity intolerance all increase the patient's risk for skin breakdown. Nurses should implement aggressive wound prevention protocols such as frequent turning, alleviation of pressure, and frequent skin lubrication to prevent skin breakdown. A third area of concern is pain related to splenomegaly and intravascular occlusion from lysed red blood cells. The nurse must perform frequent pain assessments and offer comfort measures, antipyretics, and analgesics (as ordered) to minimize pain.

Glucose-6-Phosphate Dehydrogenase Deficiency

Glucose-6-phosphate dehydrogenase (G6PD) deficiency is the most common enzyme deficiency contributing to hemolytic anemia. Inherited as an X-linked disorder, glucose-6-phosphatase dehydrogenase (G6PD) deficiency affects 400 million people worldwide. Deficiencies in the enzyme are genetically encoded and relatively common especially in individuals of African American and Mediterranean descent. Pyruvate kinase deficiency also results in hemolytic anemia, but this occurs less frequently. Enzymatic deficiencies in erythrocytes increase the red blood cells' sensitivity and susceptibility to oxidative stress. Normal metabolism is associated with oxidative stress and produces an accumulation of free radicals and other substances that can disrupt function and growth. Enzymes such as G6PD and pyruvate kinase neutralize such free radicals, thus protecting the RBCs. Free radical accumulation is accelerated by a variety of situations that cause oxidative problems, including exposure to certain drugs (malarial drugs, sulfonamides, nitrofurantoins, and chloramphenicol), dehydration, sepsis, and diabetic ketoacidosis. Therapeutic management involves removal of the triggering agent and supportive care until the hemolysis subsides. Because of the relatively high occurrence of G6PD deficiency in certain ethnic groups, susceptible patients should be screened for the deficiency before being given oxidant drugs. Once a patient has been diagnosed and triggering agents have been identified, most patients with G6PD deficiency can live asymptomatically (MedScape, 2012).

Hereditary Spherocytosis

Another cause of hemolytic anemia is defects in the red blood cell membrane. The RBC membrane is a specialized lattice structure of proteins arranged to produce strength, resilience, elasticity, and durability as the red blood cell navigates the peripheral bloodstream. The ability to survive the 120 days typical of the RBC's life span is highly enhanced by this strong exoskeleton. Genetic disorders, including hereditary spherocytosis, hereditary elliptocytosis, hereditary pyropoikilocytosis, and hereditary stomatocytosis, all encode proteins that weaken the lattice structure and produce malformed erythrocyte membranes. For example, in **hereditary spherocytosis (HS),** RBCs lack spectrin, a key membrane protein, which then forces the RBCs into an unstable spherical shape rather than the normal, more stable concave form. Hereditary spherocytosis is a genetic disorder that appears in individuals of northern European descent, affecting approximately 1 in 1,000 to 2,500 patients. The mutated spherical shape of HS cells increases their rate of splenic destruction, resulting in higher rates of hemolysis (Gaspard, 2009; Rote & McCance, 2010a).

Clinical Manifestations

Clinical presentation of HS varies with disease severity and inheritance pattern. Autosomal dominant forms and homozygous gene patterns produce persistent anemia, jaundice, and splenomegaly beginning early in life; patients with these forms are frequently diagnosed as children. Heterozygous gene patterns can produce carrier states, in which patients are able to develop sufficient compensatory mechanisms and remain asymptomatic. Pallor, activity intolerance, and hypoxia may appear only when erythropoiesis is unable to compensate for hemolysis, as occurs in severe infections, the presence of certain toxins, renal involvement, or bone marrow involvement. Rampant hemolysis of HS red blood cells will be indicated by splenomegaly and jaundice. These may be accompanied by biliary disease and cholecystitis.

Acquired Hemolytic Anemias

Acquired hemolytic anemias develop when an unfavorable external environment leads to increased hemolysis of structurally and chemically normal red blood cells. Such an environment can be mediated by three distinct pathophysiological processes: mechanical causes, infectious agents and toxins, and autoimmune reactions. Mechanical causes of hemolytic anemia describe any situation in which normal red blood cells are subjected to extreme or repeated shearing forces, heat, or osmotic attack. Such forces can be generated when red blood cells are exposed to foreign bodies such as prosthetic heart valves, hemodialysis filters, shunts, and cell savers (used during surgery). Mechanical trauma such as prolonged high-impact exercise or pressure also can result in RBC destruction, particularly in the extremities. Prolonged exposure to heat above 49°C can also cause RBC lysis, underscoring the potential dangers of blood-warming devices.

Certain toxins and infectious agents also can cause chemical reactions within the red blood cell or within the RBC membrane, causing premature lysis and hemolytic anemia. Drugs that are known to contribute to shortened RBC life spans include lead, copper, interferon-alpha, nitrites, dapsone, and arsenic. Infectious agents cause acquired hemolytic anemia through several different mechanisms, including direct invasion by parasites (malaria), release of bacterial toxins (*Clostridium perfringens* and *Haemophilus influenzae* type B), and promotion of splenic sequestration.

Immune-mediated hemolytic anemia is one of the most common causes of acquired hemolytic anemia; it is further divided into autoimmune hemolytic anemia and alloimmune hemolytic anemia. **Autoimmune hemolytic anemia** describes any situation in which the patient's own healthy immune system generates antibodies against proteins on his own red blood cells (autoantibodies). These autoantibodies are generally divided into two types: warm antibody hemolytic anemia and cold antibody hemolytic anemia. In the warm antibody type, the autoantibodies attach to and destroy red blood cells at temperatures equal to or in excess of normal body temperature. In the cold antibody type, the autoantibodies become most active and attach red blood cells only at temperatures well below normal body temperature. The warm antibody hemolytic anemia accounts for more than 80% of all disease cases. In either type of anemia, the mechanisms that trigger the generation of autoantibodies remain unclear. Possible causes include alteration to immune system development and stimulation by the microbial infections. Alloimmune hemolytic anemia occurs most commonly after prolonged exposure to donated RBC transfusion or after pregnancy. Other causes include malignancy, drugs, autoimmune disorders, systemic lupus erythematosus, and viral infection.

CHART 56–11 Major Factors Central to Hemostasis

Factor	Clotting Cascade Pathway*
I Fibrinogen	Both
II Prothrombin	Both
III Tissue factor	Tissue factor (extrinsic)
IV Calcium	Both
V Proaccelerin	Both
VI Accelerin	Both
VII Proconvertin, cothromboplastin	Tissue factor (extrinsic)
VIII Antihemophilic factor A	Contact activation (intrinsic)
IX Christmas factor	Contact activation (intrinsic)
X Stuart–Power factor	Both (common pathway)
XI Plasma thromboplastin	Contact activation (intrinsic)
XII Hegman factor	Contact activation (intrinsic)
XIII Fibrin stabilizing factor	Both

*Refer to discussion on clotting cascade in the text.

Sources: Gaspard, K. L. (2009). Disorders of red blood cells. In C. M. Porth & G. Matfin (Eds.), *Pathophysiology: Concepts of altered states* (pp. 278–300). Philadelphia: Wolters Kluwer Health/Lippincott Williams & Wilkins; Rote, N. S., & McCance, K. L. (2010c). Structure and function of the hematologic system. In K. L. McCance & S. Huether (Eds.), *Pathophysiology: The biologic basis for diseases in adults and children* (pp. 952–988). St. Louis: Mosby Elsevier.

Safety Alert *Correct crossmatching of blood involves ensuring that the RBC antibodies from donors will not stimulate autoimmune reactions in the recipient. Nurses must monitor blood cell transfusions very carefully, checking for correct crossmatch before infusion and watching extremely closely for signs and symptoms of hemolytic anemia.*

Treatment of acquired hemolytic anemias must first address identification and removal of triggering agents. If immune-mediated reactions are suspected, a Coombs' test will be ordered. The Coombs' test detects the presence of circulating antibodies against RBC surface proteins. The presence of any antibodies is an abnormal result indicative of immune-mediated hemolytic anemia. Any of the alterations to laboratory values listed in Chart 56–11 also will support a diagnosis of hemolytic anemia.

Supportive care of patients with acquired hemolytic anemias should focus on mitigating the immune response by the use of immunosuppressive agents and corticosteroids. If mechanical forces are suspected, peripheral blood smears will reveal ruptured blood cells. Treatment for these cases is tailored to the particular trauma involved. Nursing management is consistent with that presented earlier for hemolytic anemia and generalized anemia. Additionally, nurses should include an assessment for hemolytic anemia whenever a patient presents with a history of the risk factors outlined previously.

The Pharmacology box for anemia lists medications used to treat the various types of anemia along with their actions, applications, and nursing responsibilities.

Hemostasis: Regulation of Bleeding and Thrombosis

Hemostasis is the critical biologic process that mitigates blood loss due to injury to a blood vessel. Hemostasis is achieved via very complex and tightly controlled interactions among regulatory mechanisms, cellular components, vessel structures, hormones, plasma

PHARMACOLOGY Summary of Medications Used to Treat Anemia

Medicine Category and Action	Application/Indication	Nursing Responsibility
Erythropoietic agents *Action:* Provides exogenous source of erythropoietin, which stimulates differentiation and proliferation of the hematopoietic cascade. Also stimulates iron absorption by the erythroid progenitor cells.	Anemia of chronic disease, renal failure, or cancer. Indicated with hemoglobin less than 20.	Assessment of laboratory values to assess efficacy of treatment. Assessment of side effects such as bone pain related to therapy. Patient education regarding self-administration techniques, if appropriate.
Oral iron supplementation *Action:* Provides additional iron supply to increase amount of elemental iron available for hemoglobin synthesis.	Iron deficiency anemia when dietary modification is insufficient.	Assessment of drug allergy history prior to administration. Assessment of clinical manifestations of complications such as upper epigastric pain and constipation. Patient education regarding techniques to enhance iron supplement absorption and prevent or treat constipation.
Parenteral iron supplementation *Action:* Stimulates release of iron from plasma, which replenishes depleted iron stores in bone marrow.	Severe iron deficiency anemia requiring rapid correction or for patients with chronic kidney disease.	Assessment of drug allergy history. Patient education regarding infusion procedure and potential/expected reactions. Monitoring for signs and symptoms of hypersensitivity and anaphylaxis during and after infusion.
Vitamin supplementation: folates and vitamin B_{12} *Action:* Corrects deficiency in key elements required for hemoglobin synthesis.	Serum vitamin B_{12} level less than 100 pg/mL and serum folate level less than 5 ng/mL.	Patient education regarding necessity for vitamin supplementation. Referral to dietary consult to identify additional sources of bioavailable vitamins in foods. Assessment of vitamin therapy efficacy such as patient report of energy.

proteins, and other chemicals. Although it might appear that hemostasis is activated only occasionally (i.e., with visible injuries), in actuality the microvasculature is constantly subjected to "mini-traumas" from normal changes in blood pressure and seemingly insignificant physical contact with the environment. Failure of any of the hemostasis mechanisms leads to abnormal clotting, abnormal bleeding, or in some cases both. A review of the normal processes of hemostasis assists the nurse in understanding diseases that result from deviations in normal hemostasis.

Hemostasis Concepts

The process of hemostasis is a very tightly regulated and elaborate system of interacting proteins, cellular components, and chemical reactions. A discussion of some of the key concepts involved in hemostasis is a useful introduction to the chemical pathways that utilize them.

Cascades

The term *cascade* is an appropriate and important concept throughout hemostasis. In the absence of injury, the chemical components of hemostasis (factors, protein receptors) normally exist in an "inactivated" state in the bloodstream or on cell surfaces. However, injury sets off a chain of events that activates these chemical components. This activation process proceeds in a very specific sequence in which the activation of one chemical component triggers the activation of the next chemical component. For instance, tissue factor transforms Factor VII into Factor VIIa. When Factor VIIa reaches sufficient quantities, it triggers the activation of Factor X into Factor Xa. Each step in the cascade can proceed only if the prior step produced sufficient quantities of activated factors. This concept helps to explain the bleeding (or insufficient clotting) tendencies that accompany certain diseases, such as liver failure, hemophilia, and von Willebrand's disease, which result in insufficient production of factors.

Factors

Factors are proteins present in the bloodstream that, when activated, help facilitate the next step of the coagulation cascade. Most factors are synthesized in the liver in a chemically inactive form. When the chemically inactive form comes into contact with its very specific catalyst, chemical and structural changes occur that convert the inactive form to the active form. Classically, the suffix "*a*" has been used to differentiate the active form of the factor from the inactive form, and Roman numerals are used as a consistent label for all factors. Once in the active form, the factor can function as a very specific catalyst for the activation of the next step of the cascade. Deficiencies in any of the clotting factors from liver disease, vitamin K deficiency, or genetic causes manifests as a disorder of hemostasis. Chart 56–11 (p. 1743) lists the major factors central to hemostasis. The role of each factor is addressed in the discussion about the clotting cascades.

Hemostasis Pathways

Maintenance of normal blood flow requires hemostasis mechanisms to accomplish four critical goals: (1) recognition of the injury, (2) clot formation, (3) cessation of bleeding, and (4) clot lysis. Injuries to blood vessels are detected simultaneously by a number of body systems including the autonomic nervous system (which controls pain and vasoconstriction) and the hematologic system. Vasoconstriction in the target area reduces the chance of blood loss from the injured site. More important perhaps, the mechanical (squeezing) action also helps to release chemicals that initiate clot formation. The clot begins as a soft, pliable plug that typically is used to slow minor bleeding (primary hemostasis), but it then progresses to become a strong meshlike cover, encasing the injured vessel while it heals (secondary hemostasis). Once the injured vessel is healed, the clot must be removed to maintain a smooth surface on the blood vessel. The following section describes the hemostasis pathways,

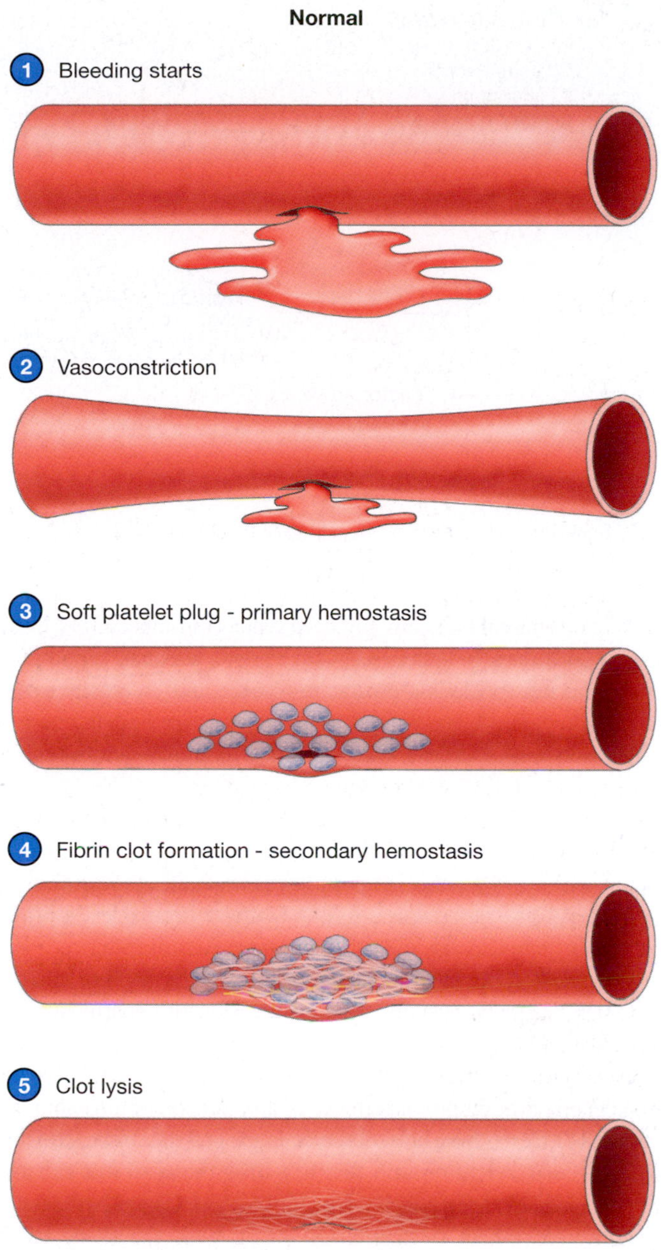

FIGURE 56–9 ◆ Stages of hemostasis.

beginning with formation of the soft plug (mediated by platelets) and continuing on to the formation of the meshlike cover (accomplished via the clotting cascade) and finally termination of the clot (a process termed *fibrinolysis*). Figure 56–9◆ provides a graphic illustration of the stages of hemostasis.

Platelet Plug Formation: Primary Hemostasis

Under normal circumstances, circulating platelets neither stick to each other nor adhere to vessel walls. When injury to a vessel occurs, injured blood vessels interact with circulating platelets, ultimately leading to the formation of a clump of platelets, called the soft platelet plug, in a process known as *primary hemostasis*. The catalyst for primary hemostasis is the release of substances from the exposed subendothelial layer that interact with protein receptors on platelets' surfaces, inducing chemical and configurational changes, a process termed *activation*.

Once activated, individual platelets undergo geometric and chemical changes that allow them to form a soft platelet plug. Formation of the platelet plug occurs rapidly via four distinct actions:

1. *Adhesion:* Adhesion refers to the sticking of platelets onto the injured vessel wall. Adhesion is initiated when von Willebrand's factor forms a bridge between exposed collagen from the subendothelial layer of the vessel wall and proteins (glycoprotein Ib) on the platelet surface. Patients afflicted with von Willebrand's disease lack sufficient quantities of the factor and can suffer uncontrolled bleeding.
2. *Aggregation:* On activated platelets, protein receptors (specifically IIb and IIa) seek out and bind to neighboring platelet membranes. Additionally, activated platelets adhere to fibrinogen, a chemical secreted into the bloodstream by the liver. Fibrinogen has the ability to form fibrous meshlike networks between platelets.
3. *Secretion:* The third function of activated platelets is the secretion of substances (a process called degranulation). Adenosine diphosphate (ADP) and serotonin recruit additional platelets to the site of injury and also stimulate more vasoconstriction. Other substances, including fibronectin, thromboxane A_2, thrombospondin, arachidonic acid, and platelet Factor V, stimulate the platelet membrane to form pseudopods (elongated shapes) and interact with fibrinogen, which help to stabilize the platelet plug. This soft platelet plug can form within seconds in the individual who does not lack any of the required chemical factors. Its primary goal is the immediate abatement of minor bleeding; however, the temporary plug can be easily sheared off unless stabilized. Intracellular calcium, which is required for factor activation in the clotting cascade, also is released from the platelets.
4. *Assembly:* Finally, activated platelet cell surfaces promote the assembly of enzymes necessary for the initiation of the clotting cascade. For example, von Willebrand's factor bound to the platelet can also bind coagulation factor VIII, a component of the clotting cascade (discussed next).

Clotting Cascade: Secondary Hemostasis

While vasoconstriction and platelets act rapidly to minimize blood loss, sustained turbulent blood flow at the site of injury can shear the platelet plug. The clotting cascade describes the sequential activation of factors that ultimately lead to the formation of a fibrin sheath, which stabilizes the platelet plug. Rather than being a single cascade of events, the term *clotting cascade* actually describes two distinct series of events: the contact activation (or intrinsic) pathway and the tissue factor (or extrinsic) pathway. If successful, each pathway results in the activation of Factor X to Factor Xa, which begins the final stage of clotting, the common pathway.

The molecular mechanisms underlying the clotting cascade have been the focus of intense research for several years, most likely because of the role of clotting and hemostasis in diseases such as cardiovascular disorders, thrombosis, and stroke. Scientific advancements have reshaped the classic understanding of and terminology used with the clotting cascade process. Traditionally, the two pathways were thought to act independently to form the fibrin net. Now, however, it is widely recognized that deficiencies in one pathway cannot be compensated for by the other pathway, suggesting some degree of interaction. Second, the terms *intrinsic pathway* and *extrinsic pathway* have been replaced by the terms *contact activation* and *tissue factor*, respectively, describing the discovery of the initiating events of each pathway.

Contact Activation

The Intrinsic Pathway The contact activation pathway describes the clotting cascade branch initiated by the contact between circulating plasma

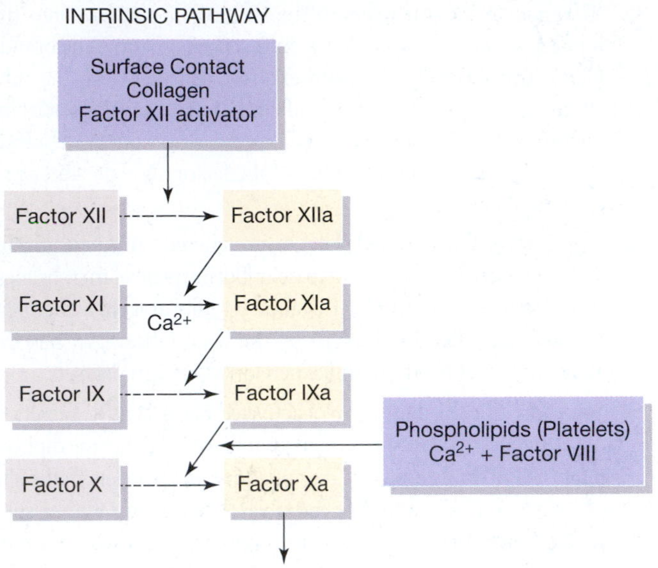

FIGURE 56–10 ◆ The contact activation (intrinsic) pathway.

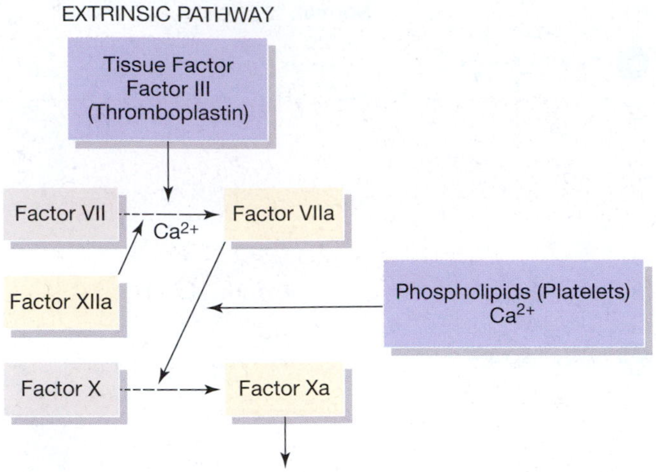

FIGURE 56–11 ◆ The tissue factor activation (extrinsic) pathway.

proteins and the negatively charged surface of the injured subendothelial layer. Figure 56–10◆ describes the activation steps. Hageman factor (Factor XII) sets off the cascade by contacting the subendothelial layer, which causes it to become Factor XIIa (activated factor), setting off the series of activations culminating with Factor VIIa, which then leads to the common pathway (Rote & McCance, 2010c).

Tissue Factor

The Extrinsic Pathway The extrinsic pathway describes the branch of the clotting cascade pathway initiated by tissue factor (TF), also called tissue thromboplastin, a substance released from injured cells of the subendothelial layers. In the presence of calcium and lipids released from platelets, tissue factor first activates Factor VII into Factor VIIa. Then tissue factor interacts with the newly activated Factor VIIa to activate Factor X into Factor Xa, the beginning step of the common pathway (Figure 56–11◆).

The Common Pathway

Both the contact activation and tissue factor pathways converge with the activation of Factor X into Factor Xa (Figure 56–12◆). In the presence of calcium and lipids from activated platelets, Factor Xa converts prothrombin (Factor II) to thrombin (Factor IIa). Thrombin is an extremely powerful component in coagulation, playing three main roles. First, thrombin interacts and amplifies the contact activation (intrinsic) and tissue factor (extrinsic) pathways to form a positive feedback loop, ensuring that coagulation continues. Second, thrombin interacts with fibrinogen to make fibrin strands (polymers). Last, thrombin activates fibrin stabilizing factor (Factor XIII). In the presence of calcium, again released from platelets, Factor XIIIa and the fibrin strands weave through the platelet plug, forming a strong mesh (termed the *fibrin mesh*), effectively sealing the site of injury and halting bleeding.

Termination of Clotting

The processes of platelet plug formation (primary hemostasis) and coagulation (secondary hemostasis) ultimately result in the formation of a fibrin mesh that effectively halts bleeding. However, if left unchecked, continued fibrin formation can lead to vessel occlusion by expanding clots, thrombosis, blood stasis, and embolism. These molecular processes are the underlying causes behind serious diseases such as embolic stroke, cardiovascular disease, and deep venous thrombosis (DVT). To prevent such damage and to maintain smooth, adequate blood flow, hemostasis must include a process to regulate and eventually terminate clotting when it is no longer required. This termination phase of coagulation hinges on the action of three inhibitors: antithrombin, tissue factor pathway inhibitor, and protein C.

Antithrombin is a naturally occurring protein circulating in the bloodstream that neutralizes the actions of thrombin and activated Factors Xa, Xia, XIIa, and IXa. As injuries heal and vasoconstriction begins to subside, blood flow begins to return to normal levels, bringing antithrombin to the site of coagulation. Antithrombin is a key target in the pharmacologic treatment of thrombosis, because its activity is significantly accelerated by the anticoagulant heparin (Rote & McCance, 2010c).

Tissue factor pathway inhibitor (TFPI) neutralizes Factor X, halting progression of the common pathway and production of thrombin. Increased TFPI levels have been observed in the presence of heparin and low-molecular-weight heparin, and new drug therapies that enhance the action of TFPI are being developed (Rote & McCance, 2010c).

Activated protein C neutralizes Factor V of the tissue factor (extrinsic) pathway and Factor VIII of the contact activation (intrinsic) pathway. The activation of protein C occurs with the binding of thrombin to the subendothelial layer of the vessel wall; thus, accelerated thrombin production results in accelerated protein C activation and an effective braking mechanism for coagulation.

Additional chemicals such as nitric oxide, prostacyclin, and thromboxane also limit excessive contributions to coagulation control by limiting platelet aggregation, activation, adhesion, and vasoconstriction. Activation of these components is the target of many anti-inflammatory drugs including nonsteroidal anti-inflammatory drugs (NSAIDs), aspirin, and COX-1 inhibitors.

Fibrinolysis: Clot Elimination

Once the endothelial layers of the blood vessel membrane have healed, the fibrin clot should be removed to optimize blood flow. The last phase of hemostasis is fibrinolysis, or the dissolution of the fibrin strands. Tissue plasminogen activator (t-PA), which is released by the endothelial cells during coagulation, and urokinase cause the activation of plasminogen to plasmin. Plasmin is a powerful enzyme that first digests fibrin strands into fibrin degradation products (FDPs), themselves

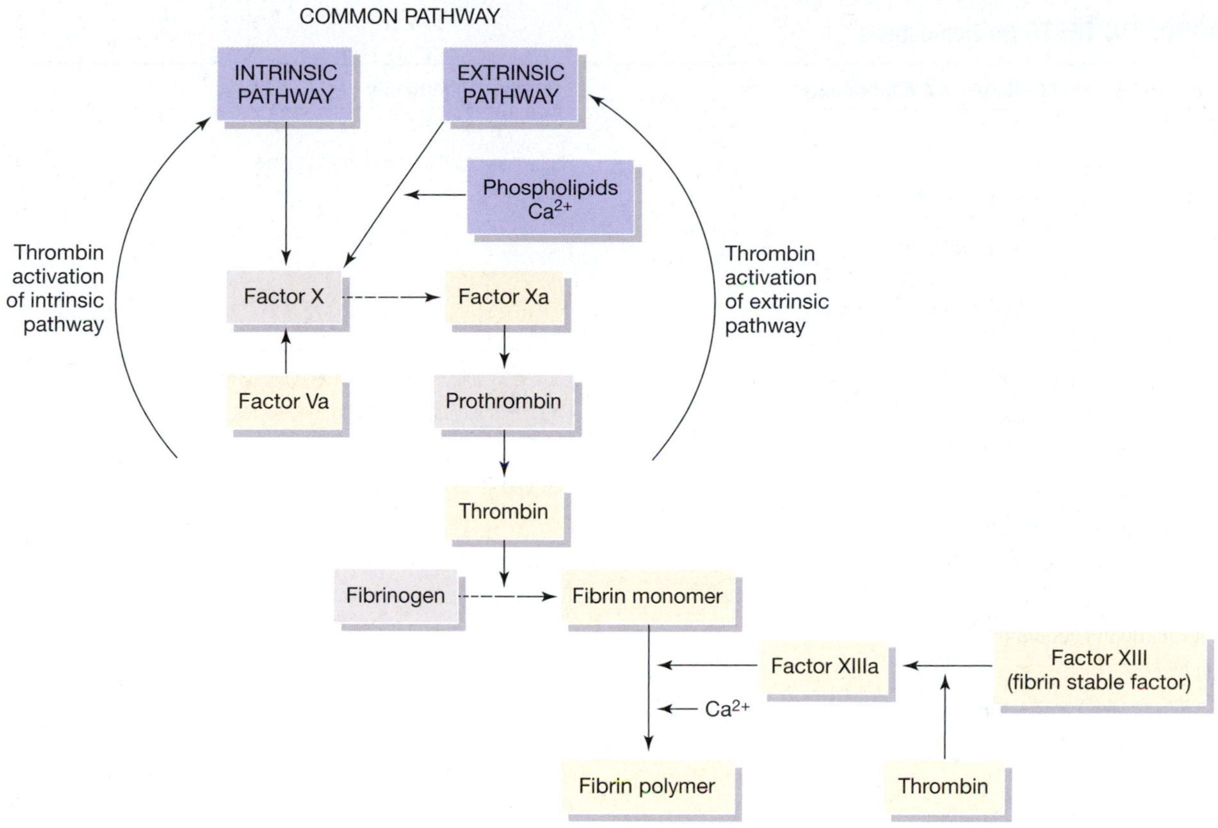

FIGURE 56–12 ◆ The common pathway.

extremely powerful promoters of fibrinolysis. These FDPs are able to inhibit thrombin activity, which slows clot formation, and to accelerate plasmin production. As with most of the chemical elements in the coagulation cascade, medical research has developed drug treatments that exploit the natural activity of t-PA and urokinase in the management of thrombosis.

Laboratory and Diagnostic Procedures

Several blood tests are available to measure the efficacy of platelet plug formation (primary hemostasis), coagulation (secondary hemostasis), and fibrinolysis. The platelet count, usually part of the CBC, describes the number of circulating platelets in a volume of blood. Normal values range from 150,000 to 400,000 per microliter of blood. Values less than 150,000 define thrombocytopenia and imply impaired clotting by platelets. However, spontaneous bleeding rarely occurs at levels above 50,000. Values greater than 400,000 are labeled thrombocytosis and imply excessive platelet clotting.

Bleeding time measures the efficacy of vasoconstriction and platelet response. In the bleeding time test, a blood pressure cuff is inflated around the arm to a specific pressure and then small incisions are made in the patient's arm. Normally, clot formation begins within 3 to 7 minutes.

Clotting time studies measure the amount of time required for a volume of blood to form a stable clot. Prothrombin time (PT) is measured in seconds and reflects the amount of time it takes to form a clot after the addition of tissue factor, thus measuring the tissue factor (extrinsic) pathway. Because of variations in tissue factor batches among laboratories, the International Normalized Ratio (INR) value was developed; it is now widely used as a standardized interpretation of the test. Many of the components measured by the prothrombin time require vitamin K for their synthesis; thus, diseases or dietary alterations that affect vitamin K also affect PT values. The activated partial thromboplastin time (aPTT), also expressed in seconds, measures the efficacy of the contact activation (intrinsic) pathway in clot formation. The normal values for these tests are in the Diagnostic Tests box on page 1748.

Fibrin degradation products (FDPs), especially D-dimer, measure the volume of these powerful fibrinolysis activators. Values are increased during sepsis, disseminated intravascular coagulation (or any coagulation event), and pregnancy.

Disorders of Hemostasis

When the tight regulation of hemostasis is disrupted by disease, drugs, or environmental factors, the affected patient can present with abnormal bleeding, abnormal clotting, or in some cases both. Like all blood disorders, disorders of hemostasis can be either acquired (as in response to sepsis or bone marrow suppression therapy) or chronic (as in genetic disorders of hemophilia and von Willebrand's disease). Disorders of hemostasis also can be categorized according to the deficient or errant component. Disorders of the platelet and vessel wall can be categorized as disorders of primary hemostasis and include thrombocytopenia, hemolytic uremic syndrome, and von Willebrand's disease. Disorders involving factor deficiencies affecting coagulation can be categorized as secondary hemostasis disorders and include liver disease, vitamin K deficiency, and hemophilia.

Disorders of Primary Hemostasis

Disorders of primary hemostasis include any problems that affect platelets or platelet interaction with the subendothelial vessel layer. All of these disorders result in prolonged bleeding times, resulting from

DIAGNOSTIC TESTS for Hemostasis

Test, Normal Values, and Rationale for Abnormality	Expected Abnormality
Platelets 150,000–400,000/mm^3 *Measures number of platelets in volume of blood.*	Reduction indicates thrombocytopenia.
Bleeding Time 3–7 minutes *Measures primary hemostasis efficacy*	
Prothrombin Time (PT) 10–13 seconds (significant variation in normal values between laboratories) *Measures efficacy of extrinsic pathway*	Increased values indicate thrombotic tendencies. Reduction indicates bleeding tendencies.
International Normalized Ratio (INR) 2.0–3.0 INR	Elevated in coumadin therapy.
Partial Thromboplastin Time (aPTT) Varies (compare with control); 20–35 seconds *Measures efficacy of intrinsic pathway.*	Increased values indicate thrombotic tendencies. Reduction indicates bleeding tendencies.
Fibrin Degradation Products (FDP) 2–10 mcg/mL *Measures efficacy of fibrinolytic system.*	
D-Dimer Greater than 250 ng/L *Measures efficacy of fibrinolytic system.*	Increased during sepsis, disseminated intravascular coagulation, and pregnancy.

slowed platelet plug formation. Qualitative problems or reduction of platelets from normal values are classified as the various thrombocytopenias and represent a significant portion of all disorders of hemostasis. Diseases resulting from abnormal interaction between the subendothelial layer of the vessel, although less common, also result in abnormal bleeding times and describe any disease process that affects platelet aggregation, adhesion, or secretion. Hemolytic uremic syndrome and von Willebrand's disease are discussed in the following text as exemplars of this class of primary hemostasis disorders.

Thrombocytopenia

Thrombocytopenia is defined as a decrease in the number of circulating platelets from the normal value of 150,000/μL. Although significant, spontaneous bleeding usually is not observed until levels fall below 50,000/μL. It is one of the most common hematologic problems experienced by patients and warrants a thorough understanding by nurses and other health care providers. The causes of thrombocytopenia are numerous, but like most hematologic disorders, it can be divided into two broad categories: thrombocytopenia due to impaired or suppressed production of platelets and thrombocytopenia due to accelerated destruction of platelets. The major patient care issue associated with thrombocytopenia is an increased tendency to bleed.

Normal Physiology of Platelets

An understanding of the normal physiology of platelet development provides an effective foundation for a discussion about platelet disorders. Platelets are not cells with independently functioning nuclei and cytoplasmic structures like white blood cells and red blood cells; rather, they are shed fragments of the megakaryocyte. Development of platelets proceeds in much the same fashion as that of red blood cells and white blood cells. Recall from the discussion of hematopoiesis at the beginning of the chapter that all cellular elements of the blood arise in the bone marrow from the hematopoeitic stem cell before undergoing differentiation, maturation, and release into the peripheral bloodstream (see Figure 56–1, p. 1717).

The complete pathway from HSC to fully mature platelet release into the peripheral bloodstream is called *thrombopoiesis*. The primary regulating substance in thrombopoiesis is thought to be the hormone **thrombopoietin,** produced by the liver and kidneys. Thrombopoietin directs the HSC to produce the megakaryocyte, the precursor to fully functioning platelets. Thrombopoietin additionally stimulates the megakaryocyte to undergo mitosis and reproduce itself (thus exponentially increasing the potential for platelet quantities) and, most important, triggers the fragmentation of the megakaryocyte into small particles. These particles are the platelets, which are then released into the peripheral bloodstream and generally survive an 8- to 12-day life span. Senescent (aging) platelets begin to express cell surface proteins, which trigger the platelets' destruction by macrophages in the spleen and reticuloendothelial system. Alterations to thrombopoiesis can have deleterious effects on hemostasis ranging from increased bleeding to increased thrombosis.

Pathophysiology

Thrombocytopenia has been attributed to several underlying causes, which can be broadly divided into suppressed production or accelerated destruction. The pathophysiology of each class and representative disease processes are discussed in the following text.

Impaired Production of Platelets

A number of disease processes as well as environmental factors impede thrombopoiesis and result in thrombocytopenia. Diseases such as leukemia, lymphoma, multiple myeloma, metastatic cancers, and aplastic anemia are associated with global suppression of hematopoiesis, which will thus include suppressed platelet production. Additionally, most of the treatment approaches (chemotherapy and radiation) that are used in cancer and other bone marrow diseases independently suppress thrombopoiesis. Exposures to viruses have resulted in selective suppression of the megakaryocyte, including exposure to human immunodeficiency virus (HIV) and Epstein–Barr, rubella, and mumps viruses. A third mechanism for impaired platelet production is liver disease resulting in insufficient quantities of thrombopoietin, vitamin B_{12}, and vitamin K (Rote & McCance, 2010b). Finally, exposure to certain drugs, especially large quantities of alcohol and thiazide diuretics, can suppress megakaryocyte production.

Accelerated Destruction of Platelets

Thrombocytopenia due to accelerated destruction can be subdivided into two categories: autoimmune causes and nonautoimmune causes. Autoimmune-accelerated destruction of platelets describes any situation in which the patient appropriately develops antibodies against invading pathogens, which then inappropriately attach to surface proteins of circulating platelets. When these antibody-bound platelets reach the spleen, they are prematurely removed, causing thrombocytopenia. This autoimmune response has been observed following exposure to systemic lupus erythematosus, rheumatoid arthritis, HIV, and excessive transfusions, as well as certain drugs including depakote and heparin (Rote & McCance, 2010b).

Nonautoimmune processes contributing to early platelet destruction include exposure to prosthetic heart valves, thrombotic thrombocytopenic purpura (TTP), sepsis, and hemolytic uremic syndrome. In these situations, the thrombocytopenia can be attributed to increased utilization of platelets by the underlying disease process. As the platelets (appropriately) respond to vessel damage caused by these processes, they are removed from circulation, manifesting as a decreased platelet count.

Clinical Manifestations

A diagnosis of thrombocytopenia often is made after observation of active bleeding, underscoring the need for vigilant assessment. Figure 56–13◆ provides a graphical representation of bleeding sites throughout the body. Increased bleeding and a decreased platelet count are the primary diagnostic indicators of thrombocytopenia.

Safety Alert *Patients who present with platelet counts less than 20,000 μL are at imminent risk of internal bleeding. A drop in the platelet count below this level should be immediately reported to the health care provider as part of a comprehensive assessment including neurological, respiratory, cardiovascular, and abdominal symptoms. The patient should be prepared for possible platelet transfusion.*

The primary physical manifestations of thrombocytopenia are the appearance of mucosal and cutaneous bleeding and prolonged bleeding after invasive procedures. The degree of symptom severity correlates with the platelet count. Below 100,000/mm^3, patients may experience prolonged bleeding after surgery or after any invasive procedure such as IV catheterization or dental treatments. Patients do not typically present

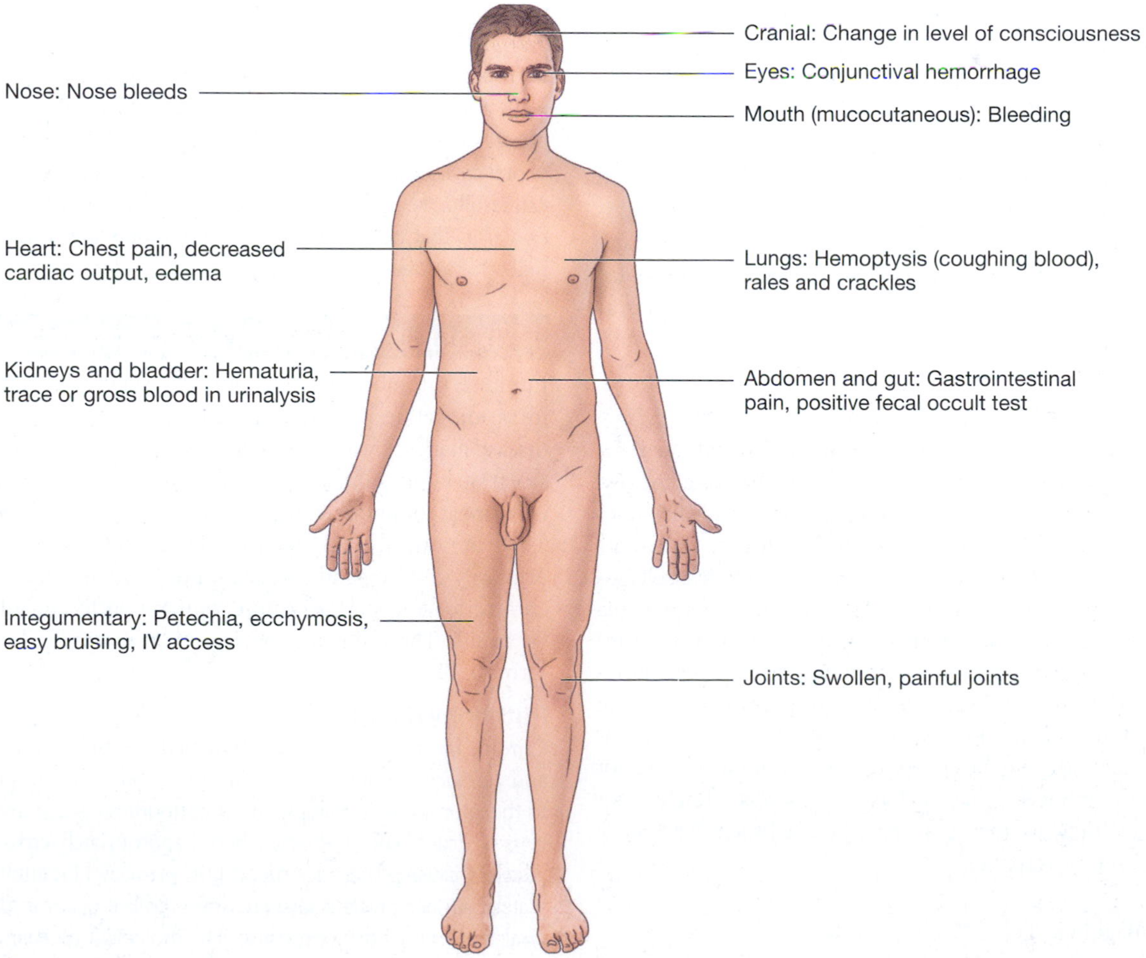

FIGURE 56–13 ◆ Assessment of bleeding sites.

with mucosal or cutaneous bleeding until platelet counts decrease to 50,000/mm^3 or lower. Mucosal bleeding can be observed in the gums, especially following aggressive brushing or flossing; in the urinary tract; or from the nares. Patients also may report blood-tinged sputum after coughing or blood in the stool. Cutaneous bleeding appears as discoloration of the skin and can often be mistaken for a rash. Cutaneous bleeding can be described as a continuum from small pinpoint lesions (petechiae), to larger group patches (purpura), to ecchymosis, or large (centimeters) patches of active bleeding into the skin.

At a platelet count of 20,000/mm^3, the patient is considered at risk for spontaneous bleeding. Although anemia due to acute blood loss should be addressed, a greater concern is bleeding into closed spaces such as the cranium, pleural space, pericardial space, or abdomen. At critically low platelet values, patients should be assessed frequently for changes in level of consciousness, respiratory status, cardiovascular status, or abdominal pain.

Laboratory and Diagnostic Procedures

Thrombocytopenia is a disease of primary hemostasis reflected in the platelet count and bleeding time. PT, aPTT, and INR are of little diagnostic value in the evaluation of thrombocytopenia because they focus on secondary hemostasis.

Medical Management

Management of thrombocytopenia must address any underlying etiology. If the thrombocytopenia results from impaired production due to bone marrow suppression, a watchful waiting approach and protective measures usually are the first line of management. Exogenous thrombopoietin to stimulate platelet production currently is in investigational stages. Platelet transfusion may be administered in these populations. If the thrombocytopenia is attributable to accelerated destruction of platelets, the causative factors must be identified and addressed. For example, drug-induced thrombocytopenia can be addressed by cessation of the offending drug. In immune-mediated accelerated destruction, immunosuppressive treatment may be initiated to reduce antibody production. Options may include corticosteroids, splenectomy, and IV immunoglobulin. Specific treatments for immune-mediated thrombocytopenia and heparin-induced thrombocytopenia are addressed later.

Nursing Management

Nurses in a variety of clinical settings must be familiar with the risks, early signs, and management of thrombocytopenia and bleeding disorders because they can occur as a side effect of a vast array of diseases and treatments. Often, thrombocytopenia is first detected by astute nursing observation and assessment, followed up by effective collaboration. Nursing interventions for the patient with thrombocytopenia focus on early detection, risk reduction, management of medical interventions, and patient education. Common bleeding precautions used to minimize risk of bleeding in high-risk patients are listed in Chart 56–12. The Nursing Process: Patient Care Plan for Thrombocytopenia and Bleeding Disorders outlines appropriate care for patients with thrombocytopenia and bleeding disorders. Teaching for patients with bleeding disorders is addressed in the Patient Teaching & Discharge Priorities box (p. 1752).

Collaborative Management

Patients who have thrombocytopenia require the coordinated efforts of a multidisciplinary team to prevent exacerbation of injury and to optimize recovery. In order to meet desired patient outcomes, it is essential that this interdisciplinary team communicate openly with one another in developing and evaluating care of the patient and family (IOM [Institute of Medicine], 2010). Pharmacists play a key role in the management of thrombocytopenia because of their expertise in drug side effect profiles and drug–drug interactions. The guidance of a pharmacist can assist the multidisciplinary team in identifying drugs that might exacerbate thrombocytopenia and finding alternative treatments that have the same efficacy but fewer deleterious side effects.

Especially in cases of bone marrow suppression, optimal nutrition plays a key role in patients' recovery from thrombocytopenia. Many patients with thrombocytopenia suffer from decreased appetite or fear of oral cavity injury (and bleeding) from chewing or swallowing, which can result in severe nutritional deficits. A dietitian can develop a nutrition plan that both maximizes key nutrients and minimizes further injury to the oral mucosa.

CHART 56–12 Bleeding Precautions

Although exact bleeding precautions vary among clinical sites, the following measures are widely implemented to minimize the risk of injury to patients:

- Avoid intramuscular and subcutaneous injections.
- Hold firm pressure to venipuncture sites for a minimum of 5 minutes.
- Minimize venipunctures and invasive procedures.
- Provide a soft toothbrush or tooth sponges for mouth care.
- Avoid rectal suppositories, thermometers, enemas, and other rectal/vaginal manipulation.
- Prevent constipation and straining with stools.
- Use an electric razor only.
- Maintain a safe environment to avoid injury.
- Assist with ADLs and ambulation as necessary to avoid injury.
- Avoid medications with antiplatelet activity (e.g., aspirin and aspirin-containing products, NSAIDs).

Immune Thrombocytopenia Purpura

Immune thrombocytopenic purpura (ITP) (previously referred to as idiopathic thrombocytopenic purpura) is an autoimmune disease marked by a decrease in the number of platelets due to destruction by antibodies produced against a patient's own platelets. It is the most common of the immune-mediated thrombocytopenias. There are two distinct forms of ITP: an acute form, which affects primarily children and neonates and is usually self-limiting, and a chronic form, which lasts more than 6 months and affects primarily adults. The following discussion primarily addresses chronic forms of ITP.

Pathophysiology

Chronic forms of ITP can be subdivided into two categories: *secondary* and *primary.* Secondary immune thrombocytopenic purpura refers to the appropriate development of antibodies against invading pathogens or drugs. The antibodies then inappropriately cross-react against platelets, causing their destruction. In primary ITP, antibodies against platelet surface proteins also are observed but occur in the absence of viral, bacterial, or drug exposure. The molecular mechanisms that give rise to either type of ITP are not clearly elucidated and are a focus of current research studies.

NURSING PROCESS: Patient Care Plan for Thrombocytopenia and Bleeding Disorders

Assessment of Hematologic Status Using Gordon's Functional Health Patterns:

- Health Perception Health Management Pattern
- Nutrition Metabolic Pattern
- Activity Exercise Pattern

Subjective Data

Assessment of Abnormal Bleeding

Do you have any history of disease?

Do you have recent history of exposure to viruses such as measles, mumps, varicella, or rubella?

Are you currently being treated with any medications? If so, which?

Do you take any over-the-counter (OTC) drugs, herbs, or street drugs?

How much alcohol do you drink on a daily basis?

Have you noticed any increased bleeding?

Assessment of Patient Self-Management

What do you understand about thrombocytopenia?

Do you have any particular fears about thrombocytopenia?

What signs and symptoms might you observe that cause you concern?

Objective Data

Assessment of Abnormal Bleeding

Skin: petechiae, ecchymosis

Mucosa: color, tenderness, increased bleeding

Conjunctivae: bleeding

Urine: color

Neurological: level of consciousness (ominous sign of intracranial bleeding)

Lung sounds: crackles, diminished lung sounds

Abdominal: painful, swollen

Laboratory values: platelets less than 100,000/μL; compare to previously recorded studies

Assessment of Patient Self-Management

Skin color and condition, absence of petechiae

Mucosa membrane color

Urine and stool color

Level of consciousness

Level of agitation and restlessness

Comprehension

Vital signs within normal values

Lab values: platelets less than 100,000/mm^3; compare to previously recorded studies

Verbalization of condition

Outcomes and Evaluation Parameters / Planning and Interventions with *Rationales*

1. NURSING DIAGNOSES: (a) Risk for Injury *related to increased intracranial pressure, abdominal bleeding, pericardial bleeding, and/or bleeding into pleural space.* (b) Impaired Skin Integrity *related to abnormal bleeding into cutaneous areas and mucosal surfaces* (NANDA-I © 2012)

Outcomes and Evaluation Parameters

Outcomes: Free of injury due to bleeding. Free of serious injury due to internal bleeding. Minimal or no bleeding observed.

Evaluation Parameters: Laboratory: Hemoglobin and hematocrit values remain within normal limits. Platelet, aPTT, PT, and INR values remain within normal limits.

Vital signs: Vital signs remain within baseline normal limits for patient.

Cerebral: Patient remains alert and well oriented. Pupils remain equal, round, and reactive to light. Gross reflex assessment remains unchanged from baseline.

Abdominal: Patient denies abdominal pain. Bowel sounds at baseline are present in all four quadrants. Urine color clear and free of hematuria.

Free of blood in stool.

Respiratory: Patient denies chest pain or shortness of breath. Clear breath sounds and absence of respiratory distress are present.

Integument: Free of petechiae and ecchymosis. Free of bleeding from gums, mucosa, and catheter sites.

Planning and Interventions with *Rationales*

Frequently monitor laboratory values for signs of precipitous decrease in hemoglobin *to detect changes in the level of circulating red blood cells.*

Frequently monitor laboratory values for signs of increased bleeding times *to detect tendencies to bleed.*

Assess vital signs, especially blood pressure, as indicators of vascular space volume. *In the event of bleeding, blood volume leaves vascular space.*

Report critical values immediately because *the health care provider may wish to initiate blood product transfusion.*

Frequently monitor neurological signs including level of Glasgow Coma Scale, pupillary changes, and cranial nerves *to detect changes in level of consciousness and nerve damage.*

Monitor restlessness and confusion as *indicators of increased intracranial pressure and/or decreased oxygenation due to bleeding.*

Frequently assess (inspection, auscultation, palpation, percussion) abdominal status and seek patient report of abdominal pain *to detect signs of bleeding into abdominal cavity and hypoxia in abdominal structures due to blood loss.*

Assess abdomen for pain, tenderness, or distention as *indicators of internal abdominal bleeding.*

Assess for adventitious or diminished breath sounds. *Indicates decreased gas exchange and hypoxia.*

Monitor respiratory rate and depth *to assess for respiratory distress.*

Frequently assess urine and stool color. *Possible early indicator of systemic internal bleeding. Detection of early signs allows for timely administration of platelet transfusion.*

(continued)

NURSING PROCESS: Patient Care Plan for Thrombocytopenia and Bleeding Disorders, *continued*

Outcomes and Evaluation Parameters	Planning and Interventions with *Rationales*
	Frequently assess skin and mucosa membrane for evidence of color change, tenderness, and bleeding. *For clinical manifestations of bleeding.* Frequently assess urine and stool color. *Possible early indicator of systemic internal bleeding. Detection of early signs allows for timely administration of platelet transfusion.* Assess vital signs, especially blood pressure, as *indicators of vascular space volume. In the event of bleeding, blood volume leaves the vascular space.*
2. NURSING DIAGNOSIS: Deficient Knowledge *related to management of thrombocytopenia* (NANDA-I © 2012)	
Outcome: Patient and family verbalize understanding of required skills and knowledge in the management of thrombocytopenia. ***Evaluation Parameters:*** Patient verbalizes understanding of bleeding precautions including avoidance of contact sports, use of razors, and oral care. Patient reports signs and symptoms that warrant immediate attention by the health care provider. Patient reports understanding of medications that should be avoided including aspirin and other drugs specific to the patient's history.	Frequently reinforce patient education regarding bleeding precautions *to minimize risk of injury.* Educate the patient and family about tests and procedures *to increase understanding of the disease process.* Educate the patient and family concerning the disease, treatment, and potential complications *to increase understanding of the disease process.* Collaborate with the multidisciplinary team to *reinforce pharmaceutical, nutritional, and rehabilitation/educational interventions.*

Source: Adapted from Wilkinson, J. M., & Ahearn, N. R. (2009). *Prentice Hall nursing diagnosis handbook* (9th ed.). Upper Saddle River, NJ: Prentice Hall.

PATIENT TEACHING & DISCHARGE PRIORITIES for Bleeding Disorders

Need	Teaching Objective
Disease process	Discuss cause of disease.
Patient/family	Assist the patient/family in recognition of cutaneous, GI, and genitourinary tract bleeding.
	Refer the patient/family to appropriate support groups.
Pharmacologic management	Practice and discuss self-administration of blood factors or supplementation as ordered.
Patient/family	Consult with a pharmacist for drug-specific teaching.
Nutrition	Discuss the role of balanced nutrition emphasizing the need for key elements: vitamin B_{12}, folate, vitamin K, and iron.
Patient/family	Discuss the need to reduce exposure to alcohol and thiazide medications.
	Refer the patient to a dietitian for assistance in meal planning.
Physical exercise	Discuss and explore appropriate physical exercise options that would maintain muscle/bone/cardiovascular strength but limit risks of trauma.
Patient/family	Refer the patient/family to physical, rehabilitation, and occupational therapy for outpatient consultation.
Safety	Discuss the need to avoid sharp objects or sports that would cause injury.
	Advise use of electric razors.
	Advise evaluation of the home setting to eliminate sharp corners or fall hazards.
Patient/family	Advise the patient/family to alert dentists and other medical professionals to bleeding risks.
	Discuss signs and symptoms that require emergency intervention.

Clinical Manifestations

The physical manifestations of ITP are similar to those presented earlier in the discussion about thrombocytopenia. Primary ITP can be distinguished from secondary ITP by the absence of recent infection or drug exposure. Additionally, splenomegaly usually is observed only in secondary forms. Laboratory values will reveal decreased platelet levels and perhaps anemia (due to bleeding).

Medical Management

Management of ITP has two primary goals: removal of the triggering event (if identifiable) and abatement of the immune response. In cases of secondary ITP, the underlying disease process must be treated and resolved so that the body is rid of the invading antigen that is responsible for antibody production. In the case of drug-induced ITP, immediate cessation of the drug is warranted.

Attention then turns to abatement of the immune response, which usually is attempted with immunosuppressive therapy. Steroids such as prednisone are the first choice in asymptomatic patients with decreased platelet counts of less than 50,000/mm^3. If steroids prove ineffective or major bleeding occurs, intravenous immunoglobulin (IVIG) is administered. Intravenous immunoglobulin has been associated with significant rates of hypersensitivity reactions; therefore, administration should be monitored closely. Splenectomy will be considered if patients continue to require significant doses of steroids or immunosuppressive therapy after several months (Kline, 2010). The Nursing Process: Patient Care Plan for Thrombocytopenia and Bleeding Disorders (p. 1751) is appropriate for use in the patient with ITP.

Heparin-Induced Thrombocytopenia

Heparin-induced thrombocytopenia (HIT) is an example of drug-induced, immune-mediated thrombocytopenia. Although the frequency of HIT is relatively rare, 3% of patients treated with unfractionated heparin form thromboses, and 0.5% of patients exposed to diluted heparin flushes for IV therapy management experience thrombocytopenia (Kannan, 2010; Szokol, 2010). Its incidence is steadily increasing, which is thought to be due to the ubiquitous use of heparin for DVT, pulmonary embolism, acute myocardial infarction, and IV catheter maintenance. Heparin-induced thrombocytopenia occurs frequently in patients undergoing cardiovascular or orthopedic surgeries, because heparin is widely utilized to prevent thrombosis in these high-risk populations.

Pathophysiology

Patients on heparin therapy (including intermittent IV catheter flushes) can develop antibodies to heparin that cross-react against their own platelets. Specifically, heparin can induce the production of the antiheparin platelet factor 4 (AHPF4) antibody. This antibody causes two reactions. First, as with the autoimmune-mediated thrombocytopenia, this antibody recognizes and binds to platelets, a process that causes their accelerated destruction in the spleen. Second and perhaps more significant, when the AHPF4 antibody binds to platelets, it can induce platelet activation, thus initiating the clotting cascade, coagulation, and possibly thrombosis (Kannan, 2010; Szokol, 2010).

Clinical Manifestations

A decrease in platelet count, particularly following heparin therapy, often is the only indication of HIT. The onset of thrombocytopenia or a drop from baseline values typically occurs within 5 to 14 days after starting heparin therapy. Platelet counts of 80,000 to 100,000/mm^3 or counts that drop by 30% or more suggest thrombocytopenia. Initially, the patient might not present with thrombotic complications such as DVT or thrombosis, despite the presence of HIT. However, thrombosis eventually does occur in approximately 35% to 75% of patients with HIT. HIT-related thrombosis leads to DVT, stroke, and cardiac events, which, in turn, carry amputation rates as high as 20% and mortality rates of 30% to 50% (Kannan, 2010; Szokol, 2010).

Medical Management

Heparin-induced thrombocytopenia can be extremely difficult to manage because (1) its presentation is insidious, (2) heparin is normally the drug of choice for the management of thrombosis, and (3) cessation of heparin therapy alone has proven to be an ineffective approach. Diligent observation and early intervention with appropriate drug therapies are the cornerstones of treatment for HIT. Baseline platelet levels should be measured and frequently monitored for all patients who have recently been exposed to any form of heparin, including low-molecular-weight heparin, unfractionated heparin, and heparin flushes. Patients who receive unfractionated heparin warrant even greater monitoring. Although abnormal bleeding can be observed in HIT, the absence of abnormal bleeding should not be ruled out with HIT. Clinical diagnosis of HIT is made on the basis of reduction of the platelet count, correlation with heparin administration, and when other causes (drugs, viruses, and bone marrow involvement) have been excluded (Kannan, 2010; Szokol, 2010). Laboratory tests also are available that can detect the presence of the antiheparin platelet factor 4 (AHPF4) antibody.

Once HIT is suspected, heparin therapy (including catheter flushes and low-molecular-weight heparin) should be stopped immediately. A nonheparin anticoagulant such as direct thrombin inhibitors (lepirudin, argatroban, or bivalirudin) often is recommended as a first-line defense followed by warfarin therapy if existing thrombosis is suspected. Direct thrombin inhibitors carry risks similar to those of bleeding, as do other anticoagulants, and should be monitored by using aPTT and INR.

Nursing Management

Nurses play a key role in the prevention and management of HIT. Nurses should carefully monitor the platelet counts of any patient who is receiving any form of heparin treatment. The rise of the incidence of HIT has made the prophylactic use of heparin flushes to maintain IV catheter patency a controversial issue, especially in light of the availability of alternatives. Alternative options to maintain catheter patency include positive pressure valves, valved vascular access devices, use of normal saline for flushing, and specially coated central lines. Further research is needed in this area to develop national guidelines.

If HIT is suspected, the nurse's responsibilities include the careful administration of antithrombotic therapy, monitoring of appropriate laboratory values, and assessment of bleeding risk. If bleeding also is suspected, the nurse should implement appropriate care plans to prevent anemia, hemorrhage, or injury. The Nursing Process: Patient Care Plan for Thrombocytopenia and Bleeding Disorders (p. 1751) provides details appropriate for use in this population. Other therapies for HIT are discussed in the Evidence-Based Practice box.

von Willebrand's Disease

von Willebrand's disease (vWD), the most common inherited bleeding disorder, affects 1% to 2% of the population worldwide. vWD results from mutations in the essential clotting factor, von Willebrand's factor, which plays key roles in both primary and secondary hemostasis. Clinical presentation of von Willebrand's disease depends on the extent and location of the genetic mutation and varies widely, but von Willebrand's disease is most commonly associated with mucosal and cutaneous bleeding and prolonged bleeding times. Emerging epidemiologic studies reveal that the prevalence of the disease is underestimated and that many cases, especially in women, go undiagnosed, with symptoms often being attributed to idiopathic menorrhagia (prolonged menstrual bleeding) (Kline, 2010).

Pathophysiology

The von Willebrand's factor protein plays two roles in clot formation. In primary hemostasis, von Willebrand's factor acts as a binding bridge between platelets and the damaged subendothelium at the site of vascular injury. In secondary hemostasis, von Willebrand's factor protects Factor VIII, which is important in the contact activation (intrinsic) pathway, from degradation and delivers it to the site of injury.

von Willebrand's disease is a heterogeneous group of disorders all involving disturbances in the von Willebrand's disease gene. The normal von Willebrand's disease gene is a very large, complex structure that usually produces a mature protein of more than 2,050 amino acids. Disturbances to this protein sequence can result in structurally

EVIDENCE-BASED PRACTICE Heparin-Induced Thrombocytopenia

Clinical Problem

Intravenous therapies are a crucial component of most hospitalized patient treatments, underscoring the importance of maintaining patent IV access. Nurses have traditionally maintained IV access with a combination of regular site assessment and manual instillation of a flush solution into the IV catheter site. Without proper nursing maintenance, IV access sites can easily become occluded because of the body's natural tendency to form fibrin sheaths over any foreign object. This normally beneficial mechanism has evolved to isolate harmful pathogens; however, formation of the fibrin sheath also blocks the indwelling end of the intravenous catheter. This blockage, in turn, prevents instillation of medications and blood withdrawal, thus requiring the instillation of a new IV access site, possible patient discomfort or injury related to installation, and delay in treatment.

For many years, heparinized saline flushes have been used to prevent fibrin clot formation. However, mounting evidence has revealed a growing incidence of heparin-induced thrombocytopenia (HIT). In HIT, exposure to heparin appropriately stimulates antibody formation against the heparin molecule. However, the same antibody that is formed against heparin has also shown efficacy activity against platelets. Heparin-induced thrombocytopenia is the depletion of platelets as a result of an autoimmune activity. Nursing practice must incorporate techniques that have shown efficacy in preserving IV access but that do not place the patient at additional risk of injury.

Research Findings

A number of studies are beginning to evaluate the efficacy of heparinized saline flushes compared to plain saline flushes in the maintenance of IV access. In a large study, 361 IV lock sites were assigned to either saline or heparin use exclusively. Sites were flushed every 12 hours with either 3 mL of normal saline or 3 mL of a diluted (10 units/mL) solution of heparin. At the conclusion of the study, there was no statistically significant difference in incidence of extravasation, phlebitis, clotting, or blood return between the groups.

A similar study at the Mayo Clinic was conducted in the obstetric population, who are particularly prone to clotting disorders because of hematologic changes during pregnancy. In this study of 73 patients, results indicated no statistically significant differences in IV lock patency or in phlebitis between heparin and normal saline flushes. Similar results appear in arterial line maintenance. In a New Zealand intensive care unit, 65 patients were randomly assigned to receive either normal saline (NS) or heparinized saline (HS) (3 mL/hr as a continuous flush) to maintain their arterial lines needed for monitoring and blood sampling. Each patient's nurse was asked to score the function of the line at the end of each nursing shift. At the conclusion of the study, nursing assessment of line function revealed no difference between flush solutions.

Implications for Nursing Practice

The studies discussed here provide evidence for limiting patient exposure to heparin in IV access flushes. The primary goal of routine flushes is to ensure patency and delivery of medications and therapies. Clearly, this goal can be achieved via the use of saline without the additional exposure to risk of potentially life-threatening heparin-induced thrombocytopenia. For patients who do not show evidence of IV line occlusion, nurses should collaborate with their interdisciplinary team to limit flush solutions to saline only.

Critical Thinking Questions with answers can be found in the Osborn Student Resources at nursing.pearsonhighered.com.

Sources: Fujita, T., Namiki, T., Suzuki, T., & Yamamoto, E. (2006). Normal saline flushing for maintenance of peripheral intravenous sites. *Journal of Clinical Nursing, 15*(1), 103–104; Whitta, R. K., Hall, K. F., Bennetts, T. M., Welman, L., & Rawlins, P. (2006). Comparison of normal or heparinised saline flushing on function of arterial lines. *Critical Care Resuscitation, 8*(3), 205–208.

abnormal von Willebrand's factor, too little von Willebrand's factor (most common), or too much von Willebrand's factor, accounting for more than 40 different variations of von Willebrand's disease. Insufficiencies in patients with von Willebrand's disease cause delayed platelet plug formation, prolonged bleeding times, and impaired fibrin clot formation. Alternatively, excess production of von Willebrand's factor can lead to thrombosis.

Clinical Manifestations

The severity of von Willebrand's disease varies widely depending on the extent and location of the genetic derangement. The exact genetic derangements have yet to be elucidated, but patients can present with a wide variation of bleeding tendencies. In an attempt to classify von Willebrand's disease according to disease severity, the International Society on Thrombosis and Hemostasis proposed a simplified classification of von Willebrand's disease (Kline, 2010; Sadler, 1994), which has since been adopted by both researchers and clinicians worldwide. The classification system is based on the amount and characteristics of detectable von Willebrand's factor in the bloodstream by laboratory tests and on clinical presentation. Chart 56–13 describes the variations in clinical presentation of each classification of von Willebrand's disease.

As suggested in Chart 56–13, some patients may appear generally asymptomatic with only mildly increased bleeding tendencies, whereas others with the most severe forms (type 3) experience joint bleeding and hemorrhage. Because type 3 von Willebrand's disease requires inheritance of two copies of the mutated von Willebrand's gene, it is the rarest form of the disease. Other indicators of von Willebrand's disease include prolonged bleeding after minor cuts, bleeding from the gums, and mucocutaneous bleeding (petechiae, ecchymosis).

von Willebrand's disease will manifest as prolonged bleeding times and a reduction of von Willebrand's factor in the blood. The von Willebrand's factor quantity is directly measured by using an ELISA test that can provide a quantitative measurement. Platelet count will appear normal. PT, aPTT, and INR should also be normal.

Medical Management

Treatment for von Willebrand's disease is based on the current presenting symptom. In the event of problematic uncontrolled bleeding or as prophylaxis before invasive procedures, the patient can be treated with replacement of the deficient vWF. Desmopressin is used as the first-line treatment of von Willebrand's disease. Desmopressin vasopressin analog (DDAVP), a synthetic hormone usually given by injection or nasal spray, induces production of vWF and leads to a subsequent increase in Factor VIII levels. DDAVP is administered at a dose of 0.3 μg/kg, with effects starting within 30 to 60 minutes and lasting for several hours. Because DDAVP is a synthetic hormone, hypersensitivity reactions including tachycardia, headache, and facial flushing are potential side effects of infusion.

Plasma-derived vWF-containing concentrates are used as a second-line treatment when the patient's desmopressin level is unknown to achieve a vWF:Rco $> 30\%$ in minor bleeding episodes and $> 50\%$ in major bleeding episodes (Singleton, Kruse-Jarres, & Leissinger, 2010). Cryoprecipitate can—and should—be used only when vWF-containing concentrates are not available (Singleton, Kruse-Jarres, & Leissinger, 2010).

CHART 56–13 Classifications of von Willebrand's Disease

Classification	Clinical Presentation
Type 1	Partial quantitative deficiency of von Willebrand's factor Mildly decreased clotting ability
Type 2A	Qualitative defect Mildly dysfunctional ability of von Willebrand's factor to bind platelets Primary hemostasis defect affecting platelet plug formation
Type 2B	Qualitative defect Moderately dysfunctional ability of von Willebrand's factor to bind platelets Primary hemostasis defect affecting platelet plug formation
Type 2M	Qualitative defect Severely dysfunctional or absent ability of von Willebrand's factor to bind to platelets Primary hemostasis defect affecting platelet plug formation
Type 2N	Qualitative defect Mildly dysfunctional ability of von Willebrand's factor to bind to Factor VIII Secondary hemostasis defect affects fibrin clot formation
Type 3	Severe or total deficiency of von Willebrand's factor affecting both platelet plug formation and fibrin sheath formation Patients can present with chronic mucosal and cutaneous bleeding, and/or joint bleeding Sometimes misdiagnosed as hemophilia

Source: Sadler, J. E. (1994). A revised classification of von Willebrand disease. For the Subcommittee on von Willebrand Factor of the Scientific and Standardization Committee of the International Society on Thrombosis and Haemostasis. *Thrombosis and Haemostasis, 71*(4), 520–525.

Nursing Management

As with other bleeding disorders, nursing responsibilities for patients with von Willebrand's disease include implementation of bleeding precautions, environmental risk reduction, and diligent assessment. Although platelet values tend to be normal in these patients, patients with severe disease can present with prolonged bleeding times (aPTT). The Nursing Process: Patient Care Plan for Thrombocytopenia and Bleeding Disorders (p. 1751) is appropriate for use in these patients because it outlines physiological assessments and nursing interventions that can be applied in vWF. Because von Willebrand's disease is a chronic lifelong condition, discharge priorities for these patients emphasize education, which reinforces prevention of injury.

Disorders of Secondary Hemostasis

Disorders of secondary hemostasis are processes that disrupt the formation of the fibrin sheath via errors in the tissue factor (extrinsic) pathway or the contact activation (intrinsic) pathway. The most common cause of these disorders is deficiencies in the quantity or quality of the clotting factors. Whereas disorders of primary hemostasis usually appear within minutes of injury and in superficial sites (mucosa, integumentary), bleeding associated with disorders of secondary hemostasis can occur days to weeks after injury and in the deep subcutaneous layers, the muscles, and the joints. Several disorders of secondary hemostasis have been identified; the most common are vitamin K deficiency and hemophilia, which is discussed next.

Hemophilia

Hemophilia is perhaps the best-known disease of hemostasis. It affected approximately 20,000 persons (primarily male) in the United States as of 2011 (CDC, 2012). **Hemophilia** is a chronic condition that arises from the inheritance of mutated genes controlling Factor VIII or Factor IX. Characteristic presenting symptoms include uncontrolled bleeding, particularly into large muscle groups and joints.

Weblink: National Hemophilia Foundation

Pathophysiology

Patients with hemophilia inherit mutated copies of the genes that control clotting Factor VIII or IX (PubMed, 1980). Recall from the previous discussion on normal hemostasis that both Factor VIII and Factor IX are required in the contact activation (intrinsic) pathway for the eventual activation of Factor X, leading to the common pathway and the conversion of fibrinogen to fibrin. Therefore, the lack of either of these factors may significantly alter formation of the fibrin sheath, clot formation, and, ultimately, clinical bleeding. Patients with hemophilia who inherit altered clotting Factor VIII are considered to have hemophilia A; inheritance of altered clotting Factor IX is referred to as hemophilia B. Both diseases are recessive X-linked genetic disorders with implications for gender-based inheritance.

Clinical Manifestations

The severity of hemophilia is related to the amount of clotting factor in the blood and is graded on a continuum from mild to severe. Mild hemophilia is characterized by insufficient clotting factor. The clinical presentations of hemophilia A and hemophilia B are identical; differentiation between the two disorders requires chemical assays of blood samples.

The clinical presentation of hemophilia is prolonged bleeding and an inability to form clots in response to injury, both of which can persist for days to weeks. For patients with severe disease who completely lack any Factor VIII or Factor IX, such bleeding can have serious, life-threatening consequences. In contrast to disorders of primary hemostasis, which cause increased bruising and superficial hemorrhages in the integumentary (petechiae), patients with hemophilia typically suffer from bleeding deep in the tissues. Typical bleeding sites include joints and organs. If left uncontrolled, the internal bleeding can cause severe pressure on closed compartments.

Serious consequences of internal bleeding into closed spaces include increased intracranial pressure, hemiarthrosis (bleeding into the joints)

GENETIC CONSIDERATIONS for Hemophilia

Hemophilia results from inheritance of defective genes controlling the clotting system. Because hemophilia is an X-linked recessive genetic disorder, the severity of the disease depends on whether the patient received one or two defective copies of the gene from his or her parents and whether the patient is male or female. Males bear only one X chromosome, passed from the mother. If this chromosome contains the mutated hemophilia gene, the male will be affected by the disease. Females, who bear two X chromosomes, one from each parent, may inherit either one or two copies of the defective gene. With only one defective copy and one normal copy of the gene, the female will not show clinical symptoms of the disease but will be a genetic carrier. Females need to inherit two mutated genes, one from each parent, to display the disease (PubMed, 1980).

leading to compartment syndrome, and oropharyngeal bleeding (into the esophagus). The eventual sequelae following each of these situations can cause lifetime disability. Increased intracranial pressure can cause ischemia and brain tissue damage. Bleeding into the joints predisposes the patient to arthritis, synovial tissue damage, and joint malformation. Oropharyngeal bleeding may occlude the airway so severely as to require intubation.

Laboratory and Diagnostic Procedures

Although the clinical presentations of hemophilia A and hemophilia B are identical, treatment options vary; therefore, laboratory analysis is critical in developing an effective care plan. Patients with hemophilia have usually been diagnosed as children, before admission to the acute care setting. For patients who are known to have hemophilia, diagnostic tests such as the CBC are used to determine the degree of blood loss. Bleeding and clotting studies, a platelet count, bleeding time, PT, aPTT, and INR are indicated for any patient who is suspected of having hemophilia. Because Factor VIII and Factor IX are disorders of the intrinsic pathway, the patient typically will have a prolonged aPTT with all other tests normal. Specific assays that detect blood levels of Factor VIII and Factor IX are used to distinguish between the two forms of hemophilia.

Medical Management

Medical management of hemophilia revolves around *factor replacement therapy*, that is, the administration of exogenous (donated or manufactured) Factor VIII and Factor IX. (See the Pharmacology Summary of Medications Used to Treat Clotting Disorders box, p. 1758.) Previously, factor replacement therapy was achieved via fresh frozen plasma (FFP); however, possible exposure to viruses and risk of volume overload combined with the availability of commercially prepared factors has decreased the use of FFP. For mild episodes or as prophylaxis before procedures, purified FVIII (clotting Factor VIII) concentrates, intermediate purity FVIII (contains some vWF or von Willebrand factor), and cryoprecipitate may be used. For hemophilia B, purified FIX (clotting Factor IX) concentrates may be used. In addition, fresh frozen plasma may be used when FIX concentrates are not available (Singleton, Kruse-Jarres, & Leissinger, 2010).

In the event of bleeding, antifibrinolytics are sometimes used. These medications slow the fibrinolytic system, thus extending the effect of already-formed fibrin sheaths and slowing the inhibitory effects of fibrin degradation products. However, these medications have shown significant clinical efficacy only in mucosal and oral bleeding. Another principle of hemophilia treatment is the prevention of deleterious sequelae and further injury. Toward that goal, aspirin and other platelet-interfering drugs are avoided.

Nursing Management

For the nurse caring for the hospitalized patient with hemophilia, cure is not the goal. Instead, disease management focuses on reduction of environmental factors that increase risk and on management of the administration of the replacement factors. Bleeding precautions as shown in Chart 56–12 (p. 1750) should be initiated with particular emphasis on maintaining a safe environment. Nursing interventions applicable to the care of the patient with hemophilia include assessing the patient's risk for injury (addressed with implementation of the Nursing Process: Patient Care Plan, p. 1751), managing pain due to hemiarthrosis, and patient education. Pain should be assessed regularly, including the level and quality of the pain. In addition, analgesics should be administered to manage pain.

Complex Disorders of the Blood

The following section discusses some of the complex disorders of the blood that may be encountered in clinical practice. The identification and management of these can be particularly challenging. However, rapid recognition of these disorders is imperative to prevent life-threatening complications and even death.

Disseminated Intravascular Coagulation

Disseminated intravascular coagulation (DIC) is triggered by an injury or event leading to persistent activation of the clotting cascade. It manifests as widespread clot formation and thrombosis. Situations that are known to trigger DIC include sepsis, trauma (including surgery), malignancy, toxin exposure, and obstetric complications. Under normal circumstances, the clotting pathways act only transiently until vessel damage is healed. However, the aforementioned situations can cause such widespread, persistent endothelial injury that the clotting pathways are required to respond with equal perseverance to seal off injured blood vessels. Eventually, this situation leads to two phenomena—the depletion of the clotting factors and the activation of the fibrinolytic system—that lead to uncontrolled bleeding. The complexity of the pathology and the simultaneous appearance of bleeding and massive thrombosis make DIC a very challenging clinical problem.

Pathophysiology

Disseminated intravascular coagulation is commonly associated with sepsis, trauma, cancer, or obstetric emergencies (Figure 56–14◆). Sepsis and trauma both appear to cause DIC by widespread release of coagulation-promoting cytokines or intracellular chemical signals. In sepsis, these cytokines are released by the body in response to systemic infections with gram-negative or gram-positive bacteria and, in some cases, viruses. In severe trauma, multiple mechanisms lead to DIC, including endothelial damage and widespread hemolysis, which cause cytokines to be released in much the same manner as in sepsis. In cancer, malignant tumors release tissue factor and other coagulation-promoting chemicals, ultimately leading to thrombosis. In obstetric emergencies, release of placental fluid or massive blood loss during childbirth is responsible for initiation of the clotting pathways (Rote & McCance, 2010b).

Emerging research reveals that, following initial injury by any of the mechanisms previously listed, DIC appears to follow a specific sequence of molecular events (Rote & McCance, 2010b). First, all of the previously noted mechanisms cause endothelial layer damage, which in turn causes massive release of tissue factor, initiating the tissue factor (extrinsic pathway) branch of the clotting cascade. The persistence of the injury results in prolonged activation of the clotting cascade. Second, thrombin production is greatly amplified. Recall that thrombin is an extremely powerful promoter of coagulation. Studies show that abnormal thrombin amplification is caused by defects in the regulators that normally inhibit thrombin (antithrombin, tissue factor pathway inhibitor, and protein C). The cause and nature of these defects are still under investigation (Rote & McCance, 2010b).

These derangements cause widespread coagulation fibrin deposits and thrombosis in the microvasculature. The thrombosis occludes small vessels leading to cyanosis, tissue hypoxia, and necrosis. Eventually, blood flow begins to affect the microvasculature of organs, especially the kidneys, lungs, and heart. As coagulation proceeds

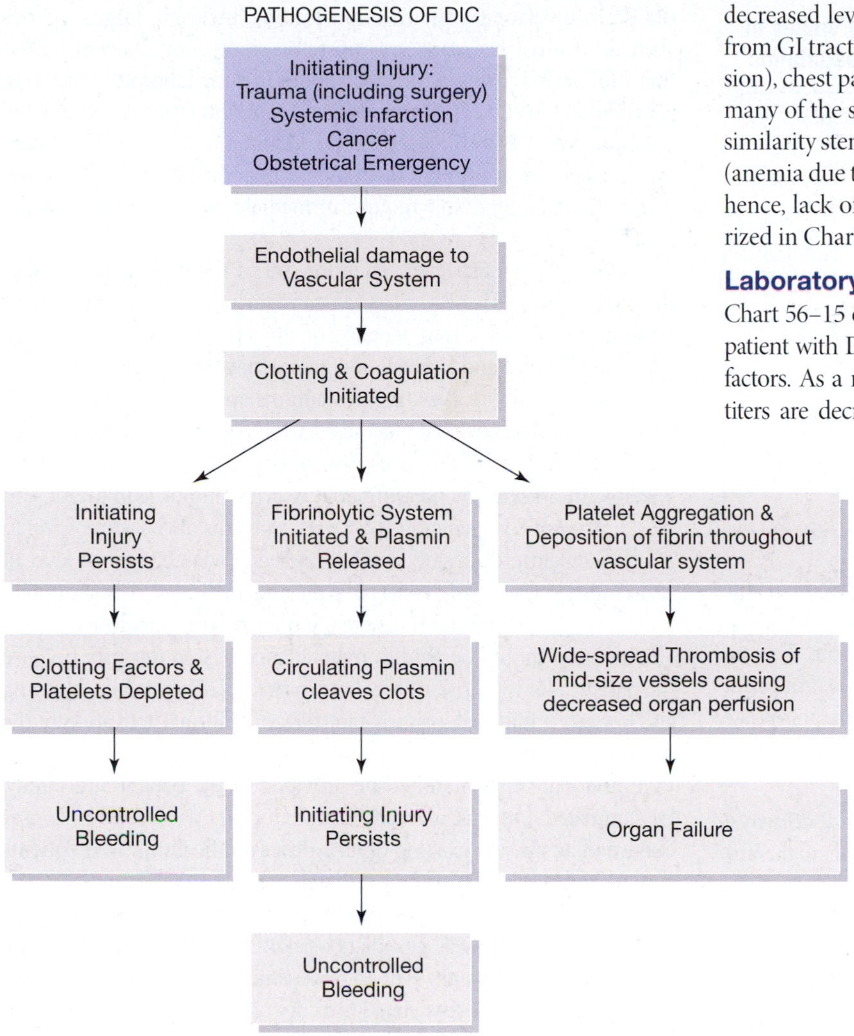

FIGURE 56–14 ◆ Pathogenesis of DIC.

unchecked, the body's supply of clotting components is exhausted and eventually depleted, resulting in a bleeding disorder.

Clinical Manifestations

As suggested by the pathophysiology just discussed, DIC presents with paradoxical widespread thrombosis and bleeding. Laboratory values reveal prolonged clotting times and consumption of coagulation factors.

Bleeding, although a later consequence of DIC, often is the first and most obvious sign detected. It frequently is manifested at mucocutaneous sites and as prolonged oozing from puncture sites. Refer to Figure 56–13 (p. 1749) to see common bleeding sites. As DIC progresses, bleeding in the gastrointestinal (GI) tract, central nervous system (CNS), heart, and genitourinary tract can occur. These are manifested as melena, a change in level of consciousness (hemorrhagic stroke), chest pain and shortness of breath, and hematuria, respectively. Extreme hypotension, tachycardia, a decreased level of consciousness, and critically low urine output (<30 mL/hr) all indicate hemodynamic shock due to blood loss (Rote & McCance, 2010b). Thrombosis can be more difficult to observe. Mild cyanosis, parasthesia (numbness), pain, and weakened pulses, especially in the extremities, are all indicators of microvasculature thrombosis. As the thrombi spread to affect the organs, patients can present with a decreased level of consciousness (ischemic stroke), abdominal pain from GI tract occlusion, decreased urinary output (poor renal perfusion), chest pain (cardiac), and respiratory difficulty (lung). Note that many of the signs of thrombosis also are indicators of bleeding. The similarity stems from the tissue hypoxia that can result from bleeding (anemia due to acute blood loss) and thrombosis (lack of circulation; hence, lack of oxygenation). Clinical indicators of DIC are summarized in Chart 56–14.

Laboratory and Diagnostic Procedures

Chart 56–15 outlines the expected changes in laboratory values in the patient with DIC, which primarily reflect the consumption of clotting factors. As a result, platelet counts and fibrinogen and clotting factor titers are decreased, leading to prolonged PT, aPTT, and INR. The D-dimer test indicates excessive fibrinolysis, the end point of excessive activation of the clotting pathways.

Medical Management

Complete removal of the underlying injury is required for the total resolution of DIC. All other treatments are used to mitigate the damage of thrombosis or bleeding until the sepsis, trauma, cancer, or obstetric emergency subsides. The cornerstone principle that guides treatment options is the cessation of rampant coagulation pathways. Common treatments include the following:

- ***Anticoagulant Therapy:*** Anticoagulants such as unfractionated or low-molecular-weight heparin can prevent the formation of new thrombi. Low doses are titrated carefully and monitored to prevent exacerbation of possible bleeding in DIC. New anticoagulants that specifically target thrombin (thrombin inhibitors) are being studied for their potential use in DIC.

CHART 56–14 Clinical Indicators of Disseminated Intravascular Coagulation

History
Sepsis
Trauma
Blood transfusion
Liver dysfunction
Malignancy
Recent pregnancy (retained placenta)

Signs
Bleeding from mucosa or catheter sites
Petechiae, ecchymosis, and purpura
Decreased sensation in extremities
Extremities cool to the touch
Altered level of consciousness
Hemoptysis

Symptoms
Pain described as swelling, sharp
Shortness of breath/tachypnea
Fatigue
Hypotension, tachycardia

CHART 56–15 Expected Changes in Laboratory Values in the Patient With Disseminated Intravascular Coagulation

Platelet Count	Decreased (<100,000 μL)
PT, aPTT	Prolonged
INR	Increased
Fibrinogen	Decreased
Clotting Factors: V, VIII, X, XIII	Decreased
Fibrin degradation products and D-dimer	Positive* (most sensitive)
Clotting inhibitors: antithrombin III and protein C	Decreased

*D-dimers and FDP can become elevated whenever the coagulation and fibrinolytic systems are activated. This occurs in a variety of conditions; therefore, the tests are not specific for any one diagnosis.

- ***Replacement Therapy:*** Patients who are at risk of hemodynamic collapse from excessive bleeding may be candidates for transfusion of platelets, FFP, or concentrations of coagulation factors. The use of these treatments is reserved for patients who are at imminent risk owing to depletion of clotting factors, because inappropriate use may exacerbate development of thrombosis (Rote & McCance, 2010b).
- ***Restoration of Anticoagulant (Antithrombin) Pathways:*** Administration of antithrombin agents is a relatively new therapy approach that shows significant promise.

Drugs used to treat DIC and other clotting disorders are shown in the Pharmacology box.

Nursing Management

Disseminated intravascular coagulation should be considered a medical emergency, the priorities being circulation and oxygenation, especially with respect to major organs such as the heart, lungs, CNS, and kidneys. The most effective nursing intervention is anticipation of DIC in any patient with infection, trauma (including large surgeries such as GI surgeries), cancer, or obstetric emergency. Diligent assessment for early indicators of DIC should include laboratory analysis, mucocutaneous bleeding, neurological function, and peripheral circulation. Normal findings should be documented as a baseline comparison against continual assessments. Abnormal findings should also be documented and require immediate collaboration with the health care provider.

Once DIC is suspected, attention turns to mitigating any life-threatening sequelae. Priorities of care include implementation of bleeding precautions, maintenance of fluid balance, maintenance of acid–base balance and oxygenation, maintenance of skin integrity, and psychosocial support. Bleeding precautions are listed in Chart 56–12 (p. 1750). Fluid balance derangements, which occur as a result of bleeding as well as thrombotic occlusion of the cardiovascular and renal systems, are assessed by measurement of urine output, skin turgor, and blood pressure. Oxygenation (hypoxia) problems also occur, owing to microvasculature occlusion, and are indicated via changes in level of consciousness, cyanosis, reports of pain, and analysis of ABGs. Supplemental oxygen often is administered to prevent severe acidosis.

Attention should be paid to maintenance of skin integrity because the patient is at high risk of breakdown due to ischemia and bleeding and because additional wounds can trigger additional activation of the clotting pathways.

Emotional support should be provided to the patient and family. Disseminated intravascular coagulation occurs as a serious consequence of an already existing disease process. The family and patient's coping strategies may already have been exhausted by the initial injury or infection, and the addition of DIC and its treatment can cause extreme stress, especially since a diagnosis of DIC often requires transfer to an intensive care unit. Nursing assessment should always include coping ability and patients' stated fears or concerns. Nurses should seek the collaboration of social workers, chaplains, and other professionals to assist both the patient and family.

Disseminated intravascular coagulation requires the application of multiple nursing skills, including the administration and monitoring of transfusion therapy, oxygen therapy, and anticoagulant

PHARMACOLOGY Summary of Medications Used to Treat Clotting Disorders

Medicine Category and Action	Application/Indication	Nursing Responsibility
Immune suppressive medications: Steroids Intravenous immunoglobulin ***Action:*** Suppression of immune response including autoimmune response.	Autoimmune thrombocytopenia (idiopathic) in asymptomatic patients with decreased platelet counts less than 50,000/mm^3. IVIG is indicated in patients for whom steroids have proven ineffective or who have significant bleeding due to lack of platelet activity.	Assessment of laboratory values to monitor efficacy. Assessment of and patient education regarding signs and symptoms of infection, since steroids will reduce immune system protection. Assessment of serum glucose levels secondary to steroid elevation. Assessment and patient education regarding mood shifts.
Clotting factor replacement therapy: Indirectly via hormone stimulation Desmopressin Direct factor replacement ***Action:*** Induces production of deficient clotting factors. (Desmopressin induces production of von Willebrand's factor.) Immediately replenishes deficient or depleted stores of clotting factors.	von Willebrand's disease, hemophilia, disease with uncontrolled bleeding or prophylaxis prior to invasive procedures. Direct factor replacement therapy is reserved for patients who cannot tolerate desmopressin.	Desmopressin has potent antidiuretic effects; therefore, fluid intake should be adjusted downward to decrease the potential occurrence of water intoxication and hyponatremia. Assessment of serum electrolytes, neurological status, cardiovascular status, urinary output, and edema are to be closely monitored. Assessment taken of immune-mediated hypersensitivity reaction (Singleton, Kruse-Jarres, & Leissinger, 2010).

therapy. Monitoring of transfusion therapy should include the basic skills outlined in Chapter 16. Oxygen therapy is used to prevent acid–base derangement and to correct hypoxia due to insufficient tissue perfusion. However, oxygen therapy must be closely monitored via oxygenation saturation and ABG levels. Additionally, oxygen therapy can dry delicate mucosal tissue, thus reinforcing the need for careful skin assessment. Anticoagulant therapy is usually addressed with heparin infusions, which require careful monitoring of laboratory values (aPTT, INR) and signs and symptoms of bleeding.

Aplastic Anemia

Aplastic anemia is a relatively rare disorder characterized by severe pancytopenia (low levels of or absence of red blood cells, white blood cells, and platelets) in both the peripheral bloodstream and bone marrow. Incidence rates are less than 2 persons per million in the United States; however, rates are higher in patients of Asian or European descent (Mayo Clinic, 2007). The severe depletion of defensive immune cells, oxygen-carrying red blood cells, and clotting platelets is a life-threatening condition, requiring the urgent implementation of protective interventions.

Pathophysiology

Aplastic anemia is thought to be caused by damage to the HSCs, resulting in their inability to reproduce and differentiate. In many cases, the cause of the damage is unknown (idiopathic); in other cases, aplastic anemia results from toxic exposure, infectious processes, or another disease process (Rote & McCance, 2010b). Toxins that are known to cause aplastic anemia include benzene, certain insecticides, kerosene, and heavy metals. Infections associated with aplastic anemia include Epstein–Barr virus, HIV, and cytomegaloviruses. Unfortunately, some therapeutic medications also may cause the pancytopenia of aplastic anemia. These drugs include chloramphenicol, certain antiepileptics, chemotherapeutic agents, and psychotropics (especially clozapine) (Bakhshi & Abella, 2008).

The diversity of causes implies that the underlying mechanisms may be equally diverse. Molecular research has shown that in most acquired diseases, the suppression of the hematopoietic stem cell is mediated by T cells that induce apoptosis (cell death) of the HSC (Rote & McCance, 2010b). However, the mechanism that causes these T cells to attack the HSC is unknown and under investigation. Drug-induced aplastic anemia has been associated with deficiency in a protein responsible for removing drug metabolites from cells; hence, affected cells may have abnormally high intracellular levels of drugs that interfere with cell function. Congenital aplastic anemia may result from chromosomal abnormalities causing early HSC death.

Clinical Manifestations

Regardless of the underlying cause, the hallmark of aplastic anemia is pancytopenia and the absence of HSCs from the bone marrow. Patients commonly will present with evidence of mucocutaneous bleeding, easy bruising, and oozing from puncture sites due to thrombocytopenia, as well as hypoxia due to severe anemia. Patients may report frequent infections due to WBC depletion. Laboratory analyses will reveal correlating laboratory values such as depressed platelet, WBC, and RBC counts. Peripheral blood smears will reveal lack of reticulocytes as well. Measures of increased iron stores and increased serum ferritin will reveal excess iron, since the vital element is not being used for RBC production. Aplastic anemia is definitively diagnosed with a bone marrow aspiration study that reveals a hypocellular marrow space that is often replaced with fatty deposits.

Medical Management

Stem cell transplant is the curative treatment for aplastic anemia. Transfusion with donated stem cells will presumably repopulate the hypocellular bone marrow with healthy hematopoietic stem cells, which will then produce fully functioning red blood cells, white blood cells, and platelets. Immunosuppressive therapy is another common approach to aplastic anemia, particularly in patients who are not candidates for stem cell transplantation. Patients who are severely ill may not benefit from the additional complications that preparation for a transplant could incur. Immunosuppressive agents such as antithymocyte globulin (ATG) and cyclosporine A (CsA) depress T-cell action on the HSCs. Blood transfusions with packed RBCs and platelets are administered to replace much needed blood elements. Prophylactic antibiotics and antifungals may be ordered to protect the severely neutropenic patient. Iron chelation therapy may be administered to reduce excess iron stores (Rote & McCance, 2010b).

Nursing Management

The patient with aplastic anemia benefits from nursing interventions designed for anemia, thrombocytopenia, and infection prevention. A common cause of death among these patients is infection; therefore, prevention of infection is a priority. Careful hand hygiene should be both stringently practiced and enforced and should be taught to the patient. All instruments and items that come in contact with the patient should be cleansed before and after each use.

The patient should be frequently assessed for signs of infection including general malaise, oozing or inflammation around puncture sites, cough, or pain. Bleeding due to thrombocytopenia and hypoxia due to anemia also are results of pancytopenia of aplastic anemia. The Nursing Process: Patient Care Plans for generalized anemia and thrombocytopenia (pp. 1724 and 1751) describe appropriate nursing interventions for use in this population. Homeopathic therapy also may be of benefit.

Gerontological Considerations

The frail older adult is at increased risk of anemia for several reasons, ranging from the physiological changes associated with aging and the prevalence of comorbidities to nutritional deficiencies and sometimes the psychosocial consequences of aging. Agreement surrounding the prevalence of anemia in the older adult varies greatly, perhaps due to inconsistencies in the reporting of anemia. The most comprehensive study to date has been the third *National Health and Nutrition Examination Survey (NHANES) 1988–1994* (National Center for Health Statistics, 2008), which evaluated anemia in the community-dwelling adult. In persons 65 years and older, anemia was present in 11.0% of men and 10.2% of women, with the prevalence rising to more than 20% in people 85 years and older.

Nutritional deficiencies account for a large portion of anemia seen in older adults due in part to decreased appetite and difficulty in chewing. However, social processes such as meal preparation and financial constraints also may negatively affect an older adult's ability to consistently consume a well-balanced diet. Comorbidities such as cardiovascular disease, lung disease, cancer, and kidney failure can also lead to anemia because of their effects on the organs of erythropoiesis, namely, the bone marrow and the erythropoietin-stimulating system of the kidneys. Perhaps most damaging to the effective treatment of anemia in

COMPLEMENTARY & ALTERNATIVE THERAPIES Homeopathic Therapy

Nancy Yilk

AS PART OF A LARGER STUDY, a descriptive cross-sectional survey assessing the use of complementary and alternative medicine (CAM) in patients with hematologic cancers involved data contributed from 68 patients with hematologic cancers from 12 European countries. Among the participants, 26.5% used some form of CAM after the cancer diagnosis. The most common therapy used was homeopathy (38.9%). The use of CAM in patients with hematologic malignancies is common; therefore, clinicians should assist patients who want to use CAM to make an appropriate decision and communicate with them about CAM use in an open and nonjudgmental manner (Molassiotis et al., 2005).

The term *homeopathy* comes from the Greek words *homeo*, meaning similar, and *pathos*, meaning suffering or disease. Homeopathy seeks to stimulate the body's ability to heal itself by giving very small doses of highly diluted substances. This therapeutic method was developed by German health care provider Samuel Christian Hahnemann at the end of the 18th century. Homeopathic medicines are used by patients with cancer, often alongside conventional treatment. Because cancer treatments can cause considerable morbidity, patients may use homeopathic medicines to help with adverse effects of these treatments. Researchers reviewed randomized controlled trials (RCTs) of homeopathic medicines in participants of all age groups and all stages of disease who had a clinical or histological diagnosis of cancer in which the intervention was aimed at preventing or treating symptoms associated with cancer treatments.

Eight controlled trials (seven placebo controlled and one trial against an active treatment) with a total of 664 participants met the inclusion criteria. Three studied adverse effects of radiotherapy, three studied adverse effects of chemotherapy, and two studied menopausal symptoms associated with breast cancer treatment. Two studies with low risk of bias demonstrated benefit: one with 254 participants demonstrated superiority of topical calendula over trolamine (a topical agent not containing corticosteroids) for prevention of radiotherapy-induced dermatitis, and another with 32 participants demonstrated superiority of Traumeel S (a proprietary complex homeopathic medicine) over placebo as a mouthwash for chemotherapy-induced stomatitis. No serious adverse effects or interactions were reported attributable to the homeopathic medicines used (Kassab, Cummings, Berkovitz, van Haselen, & Fisher, 2009).

In addition, CAM can be an effective treatment for musculoskeletal injuries. Management of these injuries usually employs the RICE (rest, ice, compression, and elevation) approach to limit excessive inflammation. NSAIDs are also commonly used to limit inflammation and to control pain which may not be desirable to patients with blood disorders. Traumeel S (Traumeel), a mixture of extracts from medicinal plants and minerals, is widely used in humans to relieve trauma, inflammation, and degenerative processes (Porozov, Cahalon, Weiser, Branski, Lider, & Oberbaum, 2004). Traumeel has been found to have a bioregulatory effect in treating the symptoms associated with acute musculoskeletal injuries, including pain and swelling. Traumeel is a fixed combination of biologic and mineral extracts, which aims to apply stimuli to multiple targets to restore normal functioning of regulatory mechanisms. Traumeel has shown comparable effectiveness to NSAIDs in terms of reducing symptoms of inflammation, accelerating recovery, and improving mobility, with a favorable safety profile. While continued research and development is ongoing to broaden the clinical evidence of Traumeel's use in acute musculoskeletal injury and to further establish its benefits, current information suggests that Traumeel may be considered an anti-inflammatory agent that is at least as effective and appears to be better tolerated than NSAIDs (Schneider, 2011).

To assess the use, effectiveness, and safety of a homeopathic preparation (Traumeel) compared with conventional therapies in the treatment of trauma and injuries, German health care providers who were using homeopathy in addition to conventional medicine included patients in a multicenter, prospective, comparative observational cohort study of patients with various musculoskeletal injuries. Patients treated with Traumeel were compared with patients managed conventionally. The primary outcome measure was the rate of resolution of the principal symptoms (i.e., pain and inflammatory symptoms) at the end of therapy.

In all, 69 Traumeel-treated and 64 conventionally treated patients met the selection criteria. The most common diagnoses were acute injuries (sprains, strains, contusions, etc.) of the ankles, knees, and hands. There were no significant differences between the demographic and anamnestic baseline characteristics of the two groups. Complete resolution of the principal symptom at the end of therapy occurred in 41 (59.4%) patients in the homeopathy group versus 37 (57.8%) patients in the conventional group. No adverse events were reported in the Traumeel group compared to six adverse events (6.3%) in the conventional group. Health care provider-assessed tolerability was significantly better in the Traumeel group ($P = 0.001$).

Traumeel is as effective as conventional medicines in the management of mild to moderate injuries in this population. Traumeel was safe in use and judged by health care providers to be better tolerated than conventional medicines. This study contributes to the case for a broad clinical effectiveness of Traumeel in the treatment of acute injuries and trauma (Schneider, Schneider, Hanisch, & van Haselen, 2008).

The anti-inflammatory effects of a homeopathic remedy, Traumeel S, have been observed in experimental and clinical studies; however, its antioxidant properties have not been elucidated. The aim of the present study is to evaluate the antioxidant effects of Traumeel S on peripheral blood neutrophils in patients with periodontitis.

The study was performed using venous blood of 22 individuals with chronic periodontitis and 21 healthy subjects. The antioxidant effects of Traumeel S on the production of reactive oxygen species by unstimulated neutrophils, as well as those stimulated with unopsonized *Escherichia coli,* were investigated using luminol- and lucigenin-dependent chemiluminescence (CL).

Polymorphonuclear leukocytes of periodontitis patients produced higher levels ($p<0.01$) of light output of lucigenin-dependent chemiluminescence and significantly reduced ($p<0.01$) light output of luminol-dependent chemiluminescence than analogous cells of healthy subjects. Traumeel S significantly (by approximately 50%) reduced superoxide-induced oxidation of lucigenin by unstimulated polymorphonuclear leukocytes of periodontitis patients, as well as those stimulated with unopsonized *E. coli,* and had a tendency to intensify luminol-dependent chemiluminescence. Preincubation of the unstimulated polymorphonuclear leukocytes of healthy subjects with Traumeel S, as well as those stimulated with unopsonized *E. coli,* exerts no inhibitory action on the luminol- and lucigenin-dependent chemiluminescence of the previously mentioned cells.

This study indicated that Traumeel S may significantly reduce production of superoxide anion by unstimulated and stimulated peripheral blood polymorphonuclear neutrophils of periodontitis patients (Žilinskas et al., 2011).

References

Kassab, S., Cummings, M., Berkovitz, S., van Haselen, R., & Fisher, P. (2009). Homeopathic medicines for adverse effects of cancer treatments. Cochrane Database of Systematic Reviews. Retrieved from http://summaries.cochrane.org/CD004845/homeopathic-medicines-for-adverse-effects-of-cancer-treatments

Molassiotis, A., Margulies, A., Fernandez-Ortega, P., Pud, D., Panteli, V., Bruyns, I., et al. (2005). Complementary and alternative medicine use in patients with haematological malignancies in Europe. *Complementary Therapies in Clinical Practice, 11*(2), 105–110.

Porozov, S., Cahalon, L., Weiser, M., Branski, D., Lider, O., & Oberbaum, M. (2004). Inhibition of IL-1beta and TNF-alpha secretion from resting and activated human immunocytes by the homeopathic medication Traumeel S. *Clinical and Developmental Immunology, 11*(2), 143–149.

Schneider, C. (2011). Traumeel—an emerging option to nonsteroidal anti-inflammatory drugs in the management of acute musculoskeletal injuries. *International Journal of General Medicine, 4*, 225–234.

Schneider, C., Schneider, B., Hanisch, J., & van Haselen, R. (2008). The role of a homeopathic preparation compared with conventional therapy in the treatment of injuries: An observational cohort study. *Complementary Therapies in Medicine, 16*(1), 22–27. Epub 2007 Jul 12.+

Žilinskas, J., Žekonis, J., Žekonis, G., Šadzevičienė, R., Sapragonienė, M., Navickaitė, J., et al. (2011). Inhibition of peripheral blood neutrophil oxidative burst in periodontitis patients with a homeopathic medication Traumeel S. *Medical Science Monitor, 17*(5), CR284–CE291.

RESEARCH OPPORTUNITIES Related to Bleeding Disorders

Research Area	Clinical Impact
Physiology	
Manipulation of cellular signaling pathways (biotherapy) to promote normal hematopoiesis or to suppress abnormal hematopoiesis	Establish effective methods of treatment and ultimately a cure for certain hematologic disorders that result from altered hematopoiesis. Results of molecular science are the first step in drug development for clinical trials.
Discovery and elucidation of the mechanisms that control clotting	Development of treatment protocols to prevent thrombotic disease.
Emerging Treatment Protocols (in Clinical Trials)	
Cord blood infusion for treatment of diseases of hematopoiesis	Cord blood banking is an emerging option for parents. These studies evaluate efficacy, cost, and quality of life to determine whether cord blood transfusion will become a recommended option for high-risk families.
Bone marrow transplant	Bone marrow transplant is currently the only definitive cure for most chronic hematologic disorders. However, risks are substantial. This research develops safe and effective protocols.
Novel applications of existing protocols	Drugs and treatment protocols in current clinical trials increase our understanding of both chronic and acute diseases and help establish effective treatments.
Manipulation of clotting factors to treat thrombotic diseases such as cardiovascular disorders, stroke, and DVT	The efficacy of oral vitamin B_{12} supplementation compared to parenteral is notable. Oral supplementation is cheaper and generates much less patient anxiety. Several trials are being conducted to quantitatively and qualitatively measure efficacy.
Quality-of-Life (QOL) Research	
Evaluation of QOL for adult patients with chronic hematologic disease compared to other diseases	Establish domains of QOL.
	Benchmark QOL in hematology against other diseases with well-understood QOL implications.
Evaluation of QOL across the life span for aging patients with hematologic disorders	As care advances, the average life span of patients with chronic hematologic disorders increases, which has physiological, social, and medical implications.
Complementary/Alternative Approach	
Guided imagery and other nonpharmaceutical techniques to manage sickle cell pain	Studies impact of complementary approaches on disease management and experience.

the older adult is the unfortunate practice of dismissing patient reports of decreasing activity intolerance as a "normal part of aging." Although some decline in endurance and cardiovascular capacity may occur with age, symptoms such as ataxia, worsening angina, severe dyspnea, and certainly abnormal laboratory studies warrant further evaluation.

The consequences of anemia in the older adult have been associated with significant morbidity, further highlighting the need for vigilance. Anemia late in life has been correlated with an increased rate of falls and decreased muscle strength (Tussings-Humphreys, 2011). Tachycardia due to the compensatory mechanisms in sustained anemia also has been correlated with increased mortality. In chronic kidney failure in the older adult, sustained decreased hematocrit levels have been associated with left ventricular hypertrophy, increased morbidity and mortality, and poor quality of life (Rote & McCance, 2010a, 2010b). The nurse plays a vital role in patient advocacy as part of providing adequate and unbiased care to the older adult.

Research

Research is essential to improve the care, quality of life, and survival of patients with hematologic disorders. The goal of research is to identify areas in which practice could improve and to evaluate and test methods for these improvements. The Research Opportunities box lists both medical and nursing research topics related to hematologic disorders that are still under investigation. Electronic databases are a source for finding specific studies related to these topics.

Summary

Hematologic disorders comprise a broad class of diseases affecting the cells and components of the blood. The functions performed by the cells of the bloodstream include oxygen transportation, hemodynamic stability, and response to injury, all of which are necessary for the adequate functioning of body systems.

Although some diseases of the hematologic system are chronic, acute illnesses (including infection) and surgery, as well as many common medications, can alter the functioning of the blood. Derangements in the hematologic system affect not only the blood, but every system in the body including vital organ functions. For these reasons, assessment of hematologic functioning is required for every patient regardless of the admitting diagnosis. Nurses should include signs and symptoms of hypoxia, oxygenation, and bleeding as part of every assessment and seek consultation as necessary.

CLINICAL PREPARATION READ DOCUMENT APPLY

READ: **History of Present Illness** >> Laboratory Study Results >> Critical Thinking Questions

Judith Sullivan is a 60-year-old female being treated on your unit. She was admitted from the emergency department (ED) with a diagnosis of gastrointestinal bleeding in the lower GI tract. Ms. Sullivan reports that she noticed changes in the color, odor, and consistency of her bowel movements two days before being seen in the emergency department. In the ED, a fecal occult stool test was positive for blood. She denies any change in her diet. She denies any travel. Ms. Sullivan has not had any major surgery or major procedures since her admission.

Medical–Surgical History

Ms. Sullivan's past medical history is unremarkable except for well-controlled non–insulin-dependent type 2 diabetes. She has no prior history of chronic GI inflammatory processes.

Social History

Ms. Sullivan is widowed and lives by herself. She has no close relatives in the area. Ms. Sullivan reports drinking alcohol only occasionally (defined as 1 to 2 glasses of wine per month) and a history of smoking 1 pack of cigarettes per day times 10 years, although she reports having quit more than 15 years ago.

READ: History of Present Illnesses >> **Physical Exam** >> Admitting Medical Records >> Laboratory Study Results

Physical Exam

When you assess Ms. Sullivan, she is alert and well oriented to person, place, time, and purpose. You perform a head-to-toe physical assessment, which results in the following findings:

Cranial nerves intact
Small conjunctival hemorrhage in the left eye; patient reports it appeared 1 week ago
Mild pallor noted in skin tone
Oral mucosa clear; however, gums appear slightly pink; patient reports that she noticed faint pink streaks when she brushes her teeth
Lung sounds clear, heart sounds clear
Vital signs: 38.2°C, BP 120/80, pulse 82 beats per minute, respirations 16
Abdomen: firm with hypoactive bowel sounds in all four quadrants; tense and tender to touch

You notice that Ms. Sullivan has shortness of breath when moving from lying to sitting and requires your assistance when moving from sitting to standing. She reports that her fatigue has been increasing during the past few weeks. She is reporting less energy throughout the day. As you continue, you notice that her peripheral pulses are intact, although you note that her extremities are cool and pale. She has small petechiae on her forearms, and you notice that her IV site is oozing small amounts of blood.

Admitting Medical Orders

Admit to general medical unit
Diagnosis: gastrointestinal bleeding in the lower GI tract; rule out anemia
Allergies: none noted
Vital signs and O_2 sat: q4h
Activity: ambulate with assistance
Diet: clear liquid
Call house officer: HR < 60 or > 120, systolic blood pressure < 90 or > 160, RR < 12 or > 30, temperature > 38.5°C
IVs: normal saline via IV infusion at 125 mL/hr
Intake and output q shift

Scheduled Medications

Potassium 10 mEq IV × 3 doses over 1 hour each; recheck serum potassium 1 hour following replacement
Metformin HCl tablet 500 mg 2 times daily with food
Polyethylene glycol/electrolytes 4 L starting at 1600; patient to drink 8 oz q 10 min until clear

PRN Medications

None noted

Ordered Laboratory Studies

CBC, Chem 7, and reticulocytes daily
Stools for occult blood daily

Ordered Diagnostic Studies

Accu-Cheks q ac and at bedtime
Colonoscopy in a.m.

READ: History of Present Illnesses >> **Laboratory Study Results** >> Critical Thinking Questions

Test	On Admission	Day 1	Day 2
Hematocrit	28 g/dL	29 g/dL	33.2 g/dL
Hemoglobin	7%	8%	10%
Reticulocytes	0.45%	0.45%	0.43%
Platelets	75,000 μL	75,000 μL	70,000 μL
Sodium	135 mEq/L	140 mEq/L	140 mEq/L

Test	On Admission	Day 1	Day 2
Potassium	3.0 mEq/L	3.5 mEq/L	3.5 mEq/L
Chloride	95 mEq/L	100 mEq/L	100 mEq/L
CO_2	22 mEq/L	24 mEq/L	25 mEq/L
Serum glucose	110 mg/dL	114 mg/dL	115 mg/dL
Occult stool test	Positive	Positive	Positive

Pearson Nursing Student Resources *Log on to* ***nursing.pearsonhighered.com*** *to download forms*

DOCUMENT:

- >> Summary of Hospitalization
- >> Pathophysiology Form
- >> Laboratory Values
- >> Laboratory Results Explanation

APPLY:

- >> List of Potential Nursing Diagnoses
- >> Concept Map
- >> Critical Thinking Questions and Concept Map

APPLY: History of Present Illness >> Laboratory Study Results >> **Critical Thinking Questions**

1. What syndromes do Ms. Sullivan's lab values reflect?
2. Is the bone marrow attempting to compensate? Which laboratory value reflects bone marrow?
3. Which signs or symptoms correlate with and can be accounted for by the platelet count?
4. Which signs or symptoms can be correlated to the hemoglobin and hematocrit?
5. Which protective mechanisms should the nurse employ? Why would the nurse implement them?

Answers to Critical Thinking Questions can be found in Appendix D in the Osborn Student Resources at nursing.pearsonhighered.com.

NCLEX® PRACTICE

1. A patient sustained multiple fractures to both femurs and several ribs. The nurse realizes the priority assessments are based on this patient's risk for developing:

1. infection.
2. low platelet count.
3. reduction in hematopoietic stem cells.
4. reduction in red blood cells.

2. A patient has missed receiving a vitamin B_{12} injection for 2 months. The nurse realizes this patient is at risk for developing:

1. reduced red blood cell production.
2. reduced white blood cell production.
3. reduced platelet production.
4. increased red blood cell destruction.

3. While conducting a physical examination, the nurse suspects a patient is experiencing iron deficiency anemia. Which of the following did the nurse assess in this patient?

1. Fatigue
2. Fever
3. Tachycardia
4. Pica

4. A patient with anemia due to acute blood loss has a normal hematocrit level. The nurse realizes this is due to:

1. a compensatory mechanism.
2. RBC mass being lost at the same rate as total blood volume.
3. an increase in plasma volume.
4. diluted RBC volume.

5. The nurse is caring for a patient with thrombocytopenia. Which of the following should be included in this patient's care?

1. Monitor volume of urine output.
2. Provide nutrition consult for high protein diet.
3. Encourage increased activity.
4. Perform frequent skin and oral mucosa assessment.

6. A patient with hemophilia is being evaluated in the emergency department after being in a motor vehicle crash. The nurse realizes that this patient's injuries will be:

1. immediate and transient.
2. minimal.
3. persistent and last for days or weeks.
4. superficial.

Answers to NCLEX Practice Questions can be found in Appendix D in the Osborn Student Resources at nursing.pearsonhighered.com. Practice additional NCLEX questions online at the Student Resources site.

Pearson Nursing Student Resources Find additional review materials at: **nursing.pearsonhighered.com**

REFERENCES

Adams, M. P., & Koch, R. W. (2010). *Pharmacology: Connections to nursing practice.* Upper Saddle River, NJ: Pearson.

American Dietetic Association. (2009). Position of the American Dietetic Association: Vegetarian diets. *Journal of the American Dietetic Association,109*(7), 1266–1282.

Bakhshi, S., & Abella, E. (2008). Aplastic anemia. *Emedicine.* Retrieved from http://www.emedicine.com/MED/topic162.htm

Becherer, S. A., & White, A. (2010). Iron deficiency anemia in the pediatric emergency department. *Journal of Emergency Nursing, 36*(2), 130–133.

Bookbinder, M. (2010). Symptom management in palliative care and end of life care. *Nursing Clinics of North America, 45*(3), 271–327.

Bryan, R. H. (2010). Are we missing vitamin B_{12} deficiency in the primary care setting? *Journal for Nurse Practitioners, 6,* 519–523.

Centers for Disease Control and Prevention (CDC). (2007). Recommendations to prevent and control iron deficiency in the United States. Retrieved from http://www.cdc.gov/nchs/fastats/anemia.htm

Centers for Disease Control and Prevention (CDC). (2012). Hemophilia homepage. Retrieved from http://www.cdc.gov/ncbddd/hemophilia/data.html

Cheek, D., Martin, L., & Morris, S. (2010). Shock, multiple organ dysfunction syndrome and burns in adults. In K. L. McCance & S. Huether (Eds.), *Pathophysiology: The biologic basis for disease in adults and children* (pp. 1696–1726). St. Louis: Mosby Elsevier.

Cunningam, M. J. (2010). Update on thalassemia: Clinical care and complications. *Hematology/Oncology Clinics of North America, 24*(1), 215–227.

Fujita, T., Namiki, T., Suzuki, T., & Yamamoto, E. (2006). Normal saline flushing for maintenance of peripheral intravenous sites. *Journal of Clinical Nursing, 15*(1), 103–104.

Gaspard, K. L. (2009). Disorders of red blood cells. In C. M. Porth & G. Matfin (Eds.), *Pathophysiology: Concepts of altered states* (pp. 278–300). Philadelphia: Wolters Kluwer Health/Lippincott Williams & Wilkins.

IOM (Institute of Medicine). (2010). *The future of nursing: Leading change, advancing health.* Washington, DC: The Academic Press.

Kannan, M. (2010). Diagnostic strategy in heparin induced thrombocytopenia. *Eastern Journal of Medicine,14,* 78–83.

Kassab, S., Cummings, M., Berkovitz, S., van Haselen, R., & Fisher, P. (2009). Homeopathic medicines for adverse effects of cancer treatments. Cochrane Database of Systematic Reviews. Retrieved from http://summaries.cochrane.org/CD004845/homeopathic-medicines-for-adverse-effects-of-cancer-treatments

Kline, N. E. (2010). Alterations in hematologic function in children. In K. L. McCance & S. Huether (Eds.), *Pathophysiology: The biologic basis for diseases in adults and children* (pp. 1062–1090). St. Louis: Mosby Elsevier.

Manji, R. A. (2009). The history and evolution of circulatory shock. *Critical Care Clinics, 25*(1), 1–29.

Mayo Clinic. (2007). Myelodysplastic syndromes. Retrieved from http://www.mayoclinic.com/health/myelodysplastic-syndromes/DS00596

MedScape. (2012). Glucose-6-phosphate dehydrogenase deficiency. Retrieved from http://emedicine.medscape.com/article/200390-overview

Molassiotis, A., Margulies, A., Fernandez-Ortega, P., Pud, D., Panteli, V., Bruyns, I., et al. (2005). Complementary and alternative medicine use in patients with haematological malignancies in Europe. *Complementary Therapies in Clinical Practice, 11*(2), 105–110.

National Anemia Action Council. (2011). Iron deficiency anemia. Retrieved from http://www.anemia.org/patients/information-handouts/iron-deficiency/

National Center for Health Statistics. (2011). National Health and Nutrition Examination Survey. Retrieved from http://www.cdc.gov/nchs/nhanes.htm

National Comprehensive Cancer Network. (2008). Cancer and chemotherapy-induced anemia, V.3.2009. Retrieved from http://www.nccn.org

National Institutes of Health, Office of Dietary Supplements. (2011). Iron deficiency anemia. Retrieved from http://www.nhlbi.nih.gov/health/health-topics/topics/ida/treatment.html

National Kidney Foundation (NKF). (2010). Anemia and chronic kidney disease. Retrieved from http://www.kidney.org/atoz/pdf/anemia.pdf

Porozov, S., Cahalon, L., Weiser, M., Branski, D., Lider, O., & Oberbaum, M. (2004). Inhibition of IL-1beta and TNF-alpha secretion from resting and activated human immunocytes by the homeopathic medication Traumeel S. *Clinical and Developmental Immunology, 11*(2), 143–149.

PubMed (1980). Hemophilia and von Willebrand's disease: Genetic considerations. Retrieved from http://www.ncbi.nlm.nih.gov/pubmed/6770741

PubMed. (2010a). Sickle cell disease: What increases your risk? Retrieved from http://www.webmd.com/a-to-z-guides/sickle-cell-disease-what-increases-your-risk

PubMed. (2010b). Thalassemia. Retrieved from http://www.ncbi.nlm.nih.gov/pubmedhealth/PMH0001613/

Rote, N. S., & McCance, K. L. (2010a). Alterations of erythrocyte function. In K. L. McCance & S. Huether (Eds.), *Pathophysiology: The biologic basis for diseases in adults and children* (pp. 989–1013). St. Louis: Mosby Elsevier.

Rote, N. S., & McCance, K. L. (2010b). Alterations of leukocyte, lymphoid, and hemostatic function. In K. L. McCance & S. Huether (Eds.), *Pathophysiology: The biologic basis for diseases in adults and children* (pp. 1014–1061). St. Louis: Mosby Elsevier.

Rote, N. S., & McCance, K. L. (2010c). Structure and function of the hematologic system. In K. L. McCance & S. Huether (Eds.), *Pathophysiology: The biologic basis for diseases in adults and children* (pp. 952–988). St. Louis: Mosby Elsevier.

Sadler, J. E. (1994). A revised classification of von Willebrand disease. For the Subcommittee on von Willebrand Factor of the Scientific and Standardization Committee of the International Society on Thrombosis and Haemostasis. *Thrombosis and Haemostasis, 71*(4), 520–525.

Schneider, C. (2011). Traumeel—an emerging option to nonsteroidal anti-inflammatory drugs in the management of acute musculoskeletal injuries. *International Journal of General Medicine, 4,* 225–234.

Schneider, C., Schneider, B., Hanisch, J., & van Haselen, R. (2008). The role of a homeopathic preparation compared with conventional therapy in the treatment of injuries: An observational cohort study. *Complementary Therapies in Medicine, 16*(1), 22–27. Epub 2007 Jul 12.+

Semonin Holleran, R. (2009). Air and surface patient transport. In P. K. Howard & R. Steimmann (Eds.), *Sheehy's emergency nursing: Principles and practice* (pp. 83–98). St. Louis: Mosby Elsevier.

Singleton, T., Kruse-Jarres, R., & Leissinger, C. (2010). Emergency department care for patients with hemophilia and von Willebrand disease. *Journal of Emergency Medicine, 39*(2), 158–165.

Sturgeon, P., Itano, H. A., & Bergren, W. R. (1955). Genetic and biochemical studies of intermediate types of Cooley's anemia. *British Journal of Haematology, 1*(3), 264.

Swanson, K. L. (2011). The nurse practitioner's role in the management of rheumatoid arthritis. *Journal for Nurse Practitioners, 7,* 858–862.

Szokol, J. W. (2010). Heparin-induced thrombocytopenia. *Seminars in Cardiothoracic and Vascular Anesthesia,14*(1), 73–74.

Thomas, J. (2010). Anemia and blood transfusion practices in the critically ill: A prospective cohort review. *Heart and Lung, 39*(3), 217–225.

Tussings-Humphreys, L. (2011). Anemia in postmenopausal women: Dietary inadequacy or non-dietary factors. *Journal of the American Dietetic Association, 111*(4), 528–531.

U.S. Preventive Services Task Force. (2006). Screening for iron deficiency anemia, including iron supplementations for children and pregnant women: Recommendation statement. American Family Physician. Retrieved from http://www.aafp.org/afp/20060901/us.html

Whitta, R. K., Hall, K. F., Bennetts, T. M., Welman L., & Rawlins, P. (2006). Comparison of normal or heparinised saline flushing on function of arterial lines. *Critical Care Resuscitation, 8*(3), 205–208.

Wilkie, D. J. (2010). Sickle cell disease: An opportunity for palliative care across the life span. *Nursing Clinics of North America, 45*(3), 375–387.

Wilkinson, J. M., & Ahearn, N. R. (2009). *Prentice Hall nursing diagnosis handbook* (9th ed.). Upper Saddle River, NJ: Prentice Hall.

Wilson, C. (2010). Iron deficiency in women and its potential impact on military fitness. *Nursing Clinics of North America, 23*(2), 645–659.

Wright, K., & Adeosun, O. (2009). Barriers to effective pain management in sickle cell disease. *British Journal, 18*(3), 158–161.

Žilinskas, J., Žekonis, J., Žekonis, G., Šadzevičienė, R., Sapragonienė, M., Navickaitė, J., et al. (2011). Inhibition of peripheral blood neutrophil oxidative burst in periodontitis patients with a homeopathic medication Traumeel S. Medical Science Monitor, *17*(5), CR284–CE291.

Caring for the Patient with Cancer

57 CHAPTER

Dawn Lambie
Renée Holleran

Outcome-Based Learning Objectives

After studying this chapter, the learner will be able to:

1. Identify the prevalence and incidence of cancer, list the common risk factors, and describe the correlation to development of malignancy.
2. Discuss the pathophysiology of cancer.
3. Compare and contrast the five common types of solid tumor cancer (prostate, breast, colorectal, lung, and brain) and cancers of the hematopoietic and lymphatic system.
4. Generate a detailed nursing plan of care for patients with cancer of the prostate, breast, colon or rectum, lung, brain, hematopoietic system, and lymphatic system.
5. Compare and contrast current approaches to treating fatigue, nutrition, and pain, and explain the importance of improving quality of life for patients with cancer.
6. Analyze the rationale for treatment modalities such as surgery, radiation therapy, chemotherapy, biotherapy, and transplantation.

KEY TERMS

absolute neutrophil count (ANC) p.1811
allogeneic bone marrow p.1813
anorexia p.1789
autologous BMT p.1813
benign p.1769
biopsy p.1780
biotherapy p.1812
bone marrow transplantation (BMT) p.1813
cachexia p.1815
carcinogen p.1767
carcinogenesis p.1767
carcinoma *in situ* p.1770
chemotherapy p.1801
cytokines p.1789
cytoreductive therapy p.1780
dysplasia p.1767
engraftment p.1814
hyperplasia p.1767
hypertrophy p.1767
malignant p.1769
metaplasia p.1767
metastasis p.1771
nadir p.1811
neoplasm p.1767
neutropenia p.1811
oncogene p.1768
palliative p.1780
peripheral blood stem cell (PBSC) transplantation p.1813
radiation p.1778
staging p.1770

FEW WORDS EVOKE AN EMOTIONAL RESPONSE as dramatic as the word *cancer* does. The impact is both physiological and psychological, since the disorder can cause considerable changes in the lifestyles of both patients and families. The diagnosis of cancer in a family member will often lead to changes in the emotional status, finances, division of responsibility, and social activities of the entire family (Rosen, 2009). Nurses need to be aware of their own feelings and attitudes toward cancer and cancer care in order to be supportive of patients and their families.

For the past two centuries, nurses have dedicated their lives to changing the experience of illness, with ensuing changes in nursing practice. Leaders in cancer nursing have directed their efforts toward prevention, detection, education, and the creation of a specialty within nursing that embraces the whole of the human being who has cancer. Sadly, many in our society continue to perceive malignancy as incurable and accompanied by dread and hopelessness. Of critical importance is the role of nurses in the continued development of cancer screening, detection, and prevention programs. These programs have already demonstrated improved survival rates and quality of life for patients undergoing cancer treatment.

Following the first National Cancer Nursing Research Conference in 1973, oncology nurses identified the need to form a national organization to support their profession. Cancer nursing was first recognized as a subspecialty in the nursing profession in 1975 with the incorporation of the Oncology Nursing Society (ONS). Since its inception, ONS has grown to a membership of more than 35,000 registered nurses and other health care providers. The organization is dedicated to maintaining excellence in patient care, education, research, and administration in oncology nursing (ONS, 2011). An effective oncology nurse must possess a broad base of knowledge about the pathophysiology and psychosocial aspects of the disease and its treatment. Patients rely on nurses for support and assistance throughout all phases of their illness, from diagnosis to end-of-life care.

Weblink: "2009 National Vital Statistics Report"

Epidemiology

The focus of therapeutic research on cancer is to discover a cure. In contrast, the focus of epidemiological research is to prevent cancer (McCance, 2010). Understanding basic epidemiologic terminology will help the nurse reach a sound interpretation of literature about cancer and its causes. In addition, this knowledge will assist the nurse in identifying target population groups for education, prevention, and screening programs.

Incidence is the number of newly diagnosed cases of cancer in a specific time period in a defined population. It will be expressed as a rate per 100,000 persons, allowing for comparison between different populations. For example, when evaluating the number of estimated cases of breast cancer in Minnesota for the year 2005 (3,240) and the number in California for that year (19,790), researchers must consider the states' respective populations or the numbers are meaningless (American Cancer Society [ACS], 2008a).

Prevalence is the measurement of all cancer cases at a designated point in time. The number is divided by the total population living at the time. The prevalence rate is very useful in planning the creation of health care facilities, determining necessary staffing, and designing and implementing screening programs (McCance, 2010).

Mortality is the number of deaths from cancer in a specific period of time and within an identified population. The total number of persons dying of cancer is divided by the total population living at that time. Since 1930, the United States has been collecting mortality data. The estimated number of cancer deaths in the United States in 2009 was 562,875 persons (Centers for Disease Control and Prevention [CDC], 2011). However, death certificates typically identify a single cause of death, leading to inaccuracy in the reporting of cancer deaths. For instance, although the identified cause of death might be pneumonia, the person might have been so debilitated by the progression of lung cancer that a pneumonia infection became fatal. Mortality figures are very useful in determining the impact of treatment, whereas incidence figures are more helpful in determining the cause of cancer.

Survival is the observation of persons with cancer over time and the likelihood of their dying over given time periods. This information, the link between incidence and mortality data, provides useful measures of the end result of treatment. In addition, survival information may provide evidence of improvement over time in the management of cancer.

Cancer Statistics

Based on data from cancer deaths between 2004 and 2008 and a 5-year overall survival rate, it is estimated that approximately 577,190 Americans will die from cancer in the year 2012 (Siegel, Naishadham, & Jemal, 2012). Overall, cancer death rates have declined by 1.8% per year in men and by 1.6% per year in women (Siegel et al., 2012). Refer to Chart 57–1 for details. Figure 57–1 ◆ represents the number of cancer cases and deaths according to gender. The most common sites of cancer for both sexes are the genital, digestive, respiratory, breast, and urinary areas. This information is important for nurses to understand in order to develop and implement patient education regarding cancer prevention.

CHART 57–1 Estimated Cancer Cases and Cancer Deaths, 2012

Estimated Cancer Cases			Estimated Cancer Deaths*		
Total	Female	Male	Total	Female	Male
1,638,910	790,740	848,170	577,190	275,370	301,820

Source: Siegel, R., Naishadham, D., & Jemal, A. (2012). Cancer statistics 2012. Retrieved from http://cacancerjournal.com.

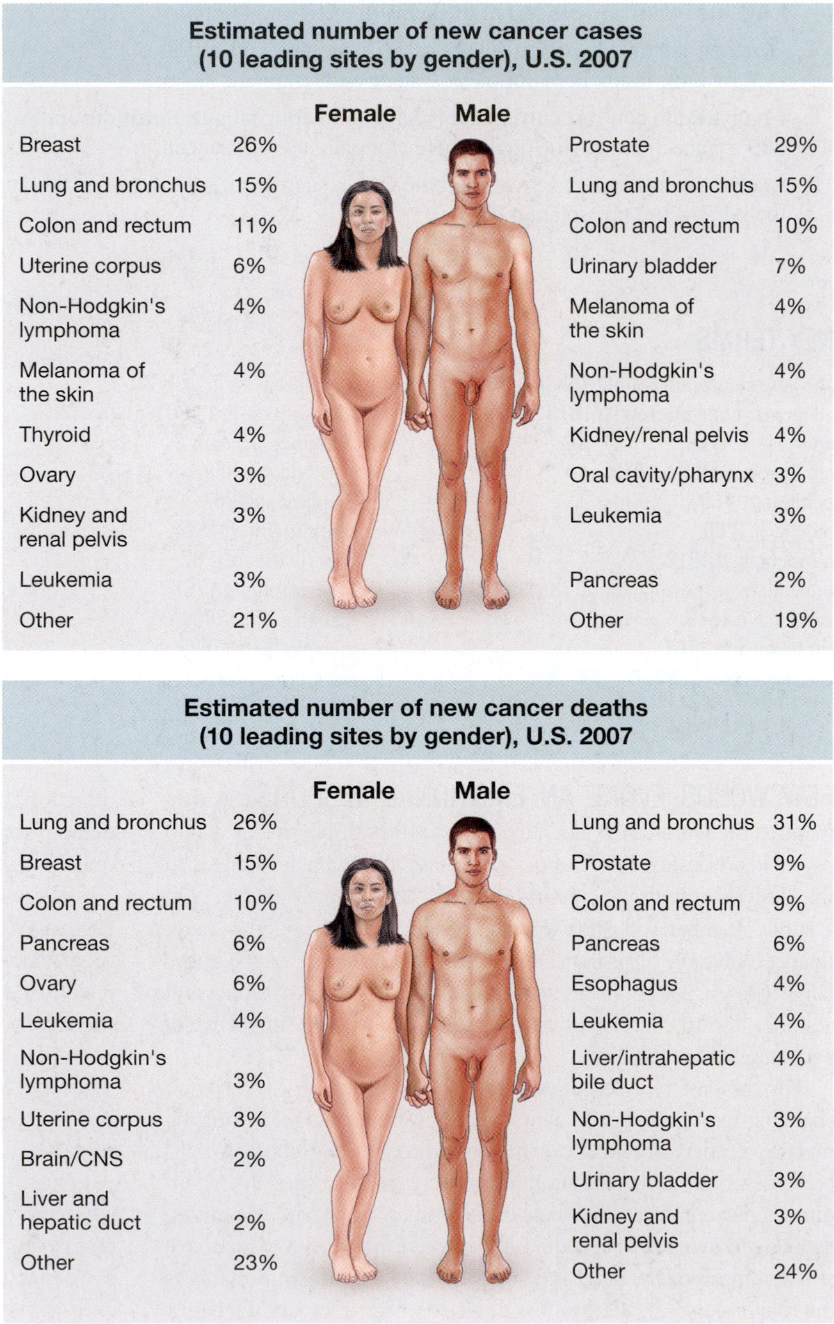

FIGURE 57–1 ◆ Epidemiology of cancer.

Etiology and Pathophysiology

Cancer is not an unruly growth of immature cells, as many people believe. Rather, it is a logical, coordinated process in which normal cells undergo changes and develop special functions. An understanding of the morphology and biochemistry of the normal cell is crucial in building an appreciation of the disease itself.

Proliferative Growth Patterns

Cancer cells do not have the usual limitations on cell proliferation placed by the host. In fact, *proliferation* and *cancer* are not always synonymous terms. Likewise, proliferation does not always imply the presence of cancer. Abnormal cellular growth may be *nonneoplastic* or *neoplastic*.

Nonneoplastic Growth Patterns

There are four common nonneoplastic growth patterns: hypertrophy, hyperplasia, metaplasia, and dysplasia. They are not neoplastic conditions but may precede the development of cancer. **Hypertrophy** refers to an increase in a cell's size. Situations that create hypertrophy include increased workload, stimulation by hormones, and compensation from loss of other tissue. **Hyperplasia** refers to an increase in tissue mass due to a reversible increase in the number of cells of a certain tissue type. This is a normal physiological response in times of rapid growth and development such as pregnancy and adolescence. Abnormality occurs when the volume of cells produced is larger than the physiological demand. **Metaplasia** occurs when one mature cell type is substituted for another type not typically found in the involved tissue. A stimulus such as inflammation, vitamin deficiencies, irritation, and chemical agents can induce metaplasia. If the stimulus is removed, the process is reversible. Otherwise, it will progress to **dysplasia,** which occurs when there are alterations in normal mature cells. These alterations can include variation from normal cell size, shape, or organization or replacement of one mature cell type with a less mature cell type. External stimuli are the usual impetus for creating dysplasia, but if removed the process may be reversible. These external stimuli can include radiation, inflammation, toxic chemicals, and chronic irritation.

An irreversible change in the structure of an adult cell that deteriorates to a more immature level is known as *anaplasia*. This type of cellular change is the classic finding of cancer. Anaplastic cells no longer have the ability to implement their unique functions and overall are chaotic in their nature.

Neoplastic Growth Patterns

The term **neoplasm** means "new growth." Inherent in this definition is the understanding that there is an abnormal tissue mass that goes beyond the normal cell boundaries and results in the cell's inability to perform its normal function. Neoplasms can be destructive to the host because they occupy space and they battle for nutrients crucial to maintain the host's life. There are two categories of neoplasm: benign and malignant. Papillomas and warts are examples of benign neoplasms. Malignant neoplasms, referred to as *cancer*, have the potential to destroy the host and include solid tumors and leukemias. Refer to Chart 57–2 for a comparison between benign and malignant tumors.

CHART 57–2 Differences Between Benign and Malignant Neoplasms

Benign	Malignant
Usually slow growing, expansive	May proliferate rapidly or grow slowly, infiltrative patterns
Localized or encapsulated	Spread (metastasize) throughout the body invading nearby tissue
Fibrous capsule	No enclosing capsule
Rarely recur after removal	May recur even after treatment
Usually regular in shape	Irregular shape with poorly defined border
Well differentiated	Poorly differentiated
Slight vascularity	Moderate to significant vascularity

Sources: McCance, K., & Grey, T. (2010). Altered cellular and tissue biology. In K. L. McCance & S. E. Huether (Eds.), *Pathophysiology: The biologic basis for disease in adults and children* (6th ed., pp. 46–92). St. Louis: Mosby Elsevier.

Characteristics of Cancer Cells

Metabolism for normal cells is achieved through aerobic glycolysis, in which oxygen is the crucial element in maintenance of cellular activity. Malignant cells utilize higher rates of aerobic glycolysis with a resulting decrease in oxygen needed for survival. This difference in metabolism may be due to differences in intracellular enzyme structure and quantity (Virshup, 2010).

Cancer cells differ according to the cell type from which they derive. It is incorrect to apply a standard definition to all cancer cells (Virshup, 2010). Some tumors may retain useful functions and closely resemble normal tissue, whereas others are chaotic enough that the tissue of origin cannot be determined. Certain cellular characteristics that are typical features of cancerous tissue include a local increase in the number of cells, loss of normal arrangement of cells, dissimilarity of cell shape and size, increase in nuclear size and total DNA seen by an increase in the density of staining, increase in mitotic activity, and abnormal mitoses and chromosomes.

Cancer cells are chaotic cells with significant cellular proliferation and assorted sizes and shapes. *Progression* is a term used to explain the dividing of cancer cells and the invasion and destruction of nearby tissue. It is important to understand that progression refers to an increase of abnormal biologic properties, not always a progression in tumor size. The increase in biologic activities is related to the tumor's malignant capabilities or its lack of differentiation. Therefore, cancer can be considered an aberrant cell mass.

Carcinogenesis

Carcinogenesis is defined as the process of tumor development (Virshup, 2010). Normal cells are altered, resulting in the development of cancerous cells. Carcinogenesis is a multistep process that is in constant unrest and is influenced by a variety of forces. A **carcinogen** (initiating agent) is a chemical, biologic, or physical agent that has the potential of changing the molecular structure of the genetic component (DNA) of a cell. The cell's transformation is due to direct contact with the carcinogen, and the result is permanent and irreversible. A co-carcinogen (promoting agent) changes the expression of the genetic information of the cell that assists in cellular transformation. Examples of co-carcinogens include hormones, drugs, and plant products. A complete carcinogen (e.g., radiation) is capable of performing functions of both an initiating agent and promoting agent. Anticarcinogens (reversing factors) are substances found in most diets, particularly in vitamins C, A, and E and in selenium. These substances may interfere with the effects of initiating agents and prevent cancerous growths.

Scientists have yet to definitively prove that the first event in carcinogenesis is a mutation; regardless of the cause, however, there is an irreversible alteration in the genetic code of cells (Virshup, 2010). A cause for most human cancers has yet to be determined (Virshup, 2010). A number of theories have been proposed to explain the development of cancer, but no single idea has been accepted. Many of the theories of carcinogenesis discuss three common stages: initiation, promotion, and progression. In 1947, the Berenblum theory attempted to explain the first two stages; over time, however, the third stage of progression was proposed to further explain the complex phenomenon of cancer development (Merkle, 2009). Figure 57–2 ◆ illustrates the stages of initiation, promotion, and progression. This theory suggests that the process of changing a normal cell into a cancer cell involves three stages in which all activity occurs in the cell's DNA.

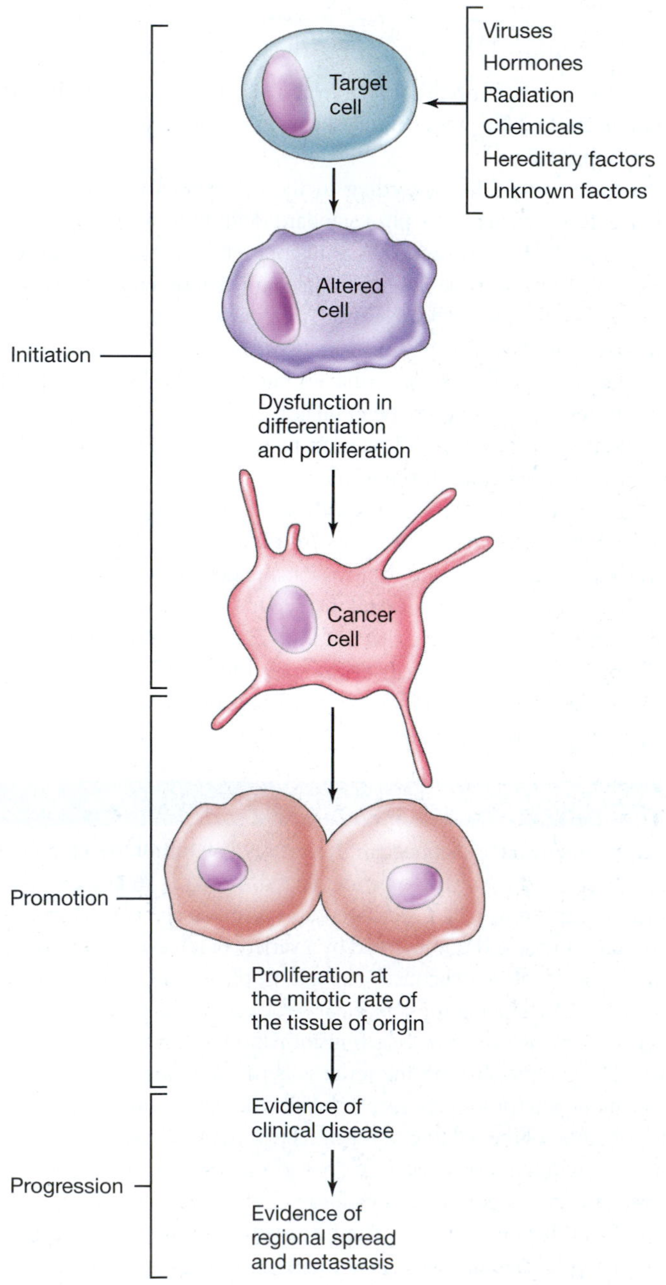

FIGURE 57–2 ◆ Cellular changes with cancer.

In the first stage, initiation, a carcinogen alters a particular gene, resulting in damaged DNA. The three possible outcomes of this transformation are:

- Repair of the gene with no cancer development
- The occurrence of permanent changes but no cancer development unless the cell is exposed to a co-carcinogen later
- Transformation into a cancer cell if the initiating agent is a complete carcinogen.

An **oncogene** is a slightly altered form of a normal gene that is responsible for cell growth and repair and has been associated with the development of cancer when activated (Virshup, 2010). Tumor suppressor genes hinder cellular growth, thus causing cellular death. An example of this is the p53 tumor suppressor gene on chromosome 17. This gene prohibits cells with DNA damage from multiplying. Mutations to the p53 gene have been identified in half of all human cancers (MacDonald, 2011).

In promotion, the second stage, co-carcinogens produce either reversible or irreversible destruction to the proliferative mechanism of the cell (Merkle, 2009). Cancerous cell formation occurs with irreversible cell damage. Progression, the final stage, involves morphologic changes within cells that begin to demonstrate malignancy and the evolution of metastatic potential. This last stage is irreversible.

In humans, the process of carcinogenesis is much more complex than in any laboratory model and frequently occupies many years of an individual's life (Merkle, 2009). Distinguishing among the three phases is difficult because of the presence of the latent period. Occurring between the initial exposure to a carcinogen and the evidence of detectable malignancy, this period is devoid of specific clinical or subjective findings. Adding to the difficulty in determining the beginning and end of the stages is the absence of tests to detect latent transformed cells. This explains why it is impossible to predict whether the risk of cancer exists in subsets of a population group.

Tumor Growth

Malignant tumors grow in an uninhibited way and do not adhere to the normal process of cell reproduction (Virshup, 2010). As the body loses cells or increases tissue function demands, there is a natural increase in the number of cells and cell replacement. Cell development approximates cell destruction (Virshup, 2010). Cancer cells do not reproduce faster than normal cells; in fact, many are slow growing in comparison to regular cells, such as those of the bone marrow and those located in the epithelial lining. All tumors contain cells that ignore the restraints typical of proliferation, but not all cancer cells proliferate indefinitely. This erratic behavior results in cell growth beyond normal margins and an increase in pressure on surrounding organs. In addition, cells may be noted to actually invade surrounding tissues and structures.

Tumor Nomenclature

Tumors receive their names according to the originating tissue type, as seen in Chart 57–3. The identification of the tissue is often difficult owing to the variety of possible cell types within one malignancy. Within a cluster of neoplastic cells, there may be benign cells as well, making identification even more difficult (Merkle, 2009). Tumors are classified according to cell type, originating tissue, whether they are malignant or benign, degree of differentiation, site, and function (Virshup, 2010).

CHART 57–3 Nomenclature and Classification of Neoplasms

Tissue of Origin	Malignant Tumor	Benign Tumor
Epithelial		
Squamous cells	Squamous cell carcinoma	Squamous cell papilloma
Basal cells	Basal cell carcinoma	No benign tumor for this type of cell
Liver cells	Hepatocellular carcinoma	Hepatocellular adenoma
Melanocytes	Malignant melanoma	Nevus
Renal epithelium	Renal cell carcinoma	Renal tubular adenoma
Glands	Adenocarcinoma	Adenoma
Endothelial/Related Tissue		
Lymphoid tissue	Lymphatic leukemia	No benign tumor for this type of cell
	Malignant lymphoma	No benign tumor for this type of cell
	Reticular cell sarcoma	No benign tumor for this type of cell
Bone marrow	Multiple myeloma	No benign tumor for this type of cell
	Leukemia	No benign tumor for this type of cell
	Ewing's sarcoma	No benign tumor for this type of cell
	Lymphosarcoma	No benign tumor for this type of cell
Lymph vessels	Lymphangiosarcoma	Lymphangioma
Mesothelium	Malignant mesothelioma	No benign tumor for this type of cell
Meninges	Malignant meningioma	Meningioma
Neural and Retinal Tissue		
Nerve fibers and sheaths	Neurofibrosarcoma	Neurilemoma, neurofibroma
	Neurogenic sarcoma	No benign tumor for this type of cell
Nerve cells	Neuroblastoma	Ganglioneuroma
	Spongioblastoma	Glioma
Muscle Tissue		
Smooth muscle	Leiomyosarcoma	Leiomyoma
Striated muscle	Rhabdomyosarcoma	Rhabdomyoma
Connective Tissue		
Fibrous tissue	Fibrosarcoma	Fibroma
Embryonic fibrous tissue	Myxosarcoma	Myxoma
Fat	Liposarcoma	Lipoma
Bone	Osteogenic sarcoma	Osteoma
Cartilage	Chondrosarcoma	Chondroma
Synovial membrane	Synovial sarcoma	Synovioma
Other		
Placenta	Chorion-epithelioma	Hydatidiform mole
	Embryonal carcinoma	Dermoid cyst
	Embryonal sarcoma	No benign tumor for this type of cell
	Teratocarcinoma	No benign tumor for this type of cell

Sources: Merkle, C. J. (2009). Neoplasia. In C. M. Porth & G. Matflin (Eds.), *Pathophysiology: Concepts of altered health status* (8th ed., pp. 156–196). Philadelphia: Wolters Kluwer/Lippincott Williams & Wilkins; Virshup, D. M. (2010). Biology, clinical manifestations, and treatment of cancer. In K. L. McCance & S. E. Huether (Eds.), *Pathophysiology: The biologic basis for disease in adults and children* (6th ed., pp. 396–435). St. Louis: Mosby Elsevier.

The degree of differentiation refers to the cell's maturity. Undifferentiated tumors are those that have completely lost identity with the tissue of origin. Well-differentiated and moderately differentiated tumors possess cells that continue to demonstrate characteristics of the tissue of origin.

Histogenetic Classification

The suffix *-oma*, Greek for "tumor," is used for both benign and malignant tumors. **Benign** tumors are those whose prefix designates specific tissue, whereas **malignant** tumors use the root *carcin* (epithelial tissue) and *sarc* (connective tissue). Other cancer types include lymphomas (lymphatic system), gliomas (glial cells of the central nervous system), and leukemias (blood-forming organs, usually bone marrow). Examples of benign tumors are fibromas and adenomas, which are located in fibrous and glandular tissue. The only exceptions to this are melanoma and hepatomas. Melanomas are malignancies of the melanocytes, and hepatomas are malignancies of the liver. Specific connective tissue sarcomas use several different prefixes that represent the anatomic location of the tumor (Merkle, 2009). These include the following:

- *Osteo-* (bone)
- *Chondro-* (cartilage)
- *Lipo-* (fat)
- *Rhabdo-* (skeletal muscle)
- *Leiomyo-* (smooth muscle).

Preinvasive epithelial tumors with glandular or squamous cell origins are called **carcinoma *in situ*.** They typically occur in the cervix, skin, oral cavity, bronchus, breast, and esophagus. Carcinoma *in situ* neoplasms have not invaded the basement membrane of the epithelial site; thus, the surrounding tissues are left untouched by malignant cells (Merkle, 2009).

Classifying Degree of Malignancy

Examination of tumor tissue under the microscope is the only way to classify, or grade, the degree of malignancy. Four grades are used as a standardized method of communicating the appearance of the cells and their potential for spread and growth. Using a standardized language allows practitioners to determine treatment options while providing prognostic information. A grade 1 tumor is small in size, more differentiated than other grades, and the least malignant. Grade 4 tumors are those with cells that appear more abnormal, are usually very aggressive in nature, and are considered to have a high degree of malignancy.

Staging is the portion of the classification system that describes the extent of the tumor and evidence of metastasis throughout the body. (Metastasis is discussed in the following text.) The TNM system is used to describe the presence and extent of local, regional, and distant disease. *T* refers to primary tumor size, *N* refers to the absence or presence of regional lymph nodes, and *M* refers to the absence or presence of distant metastases. Details of the TNM classification system are found in Chart 57–4. It is important to understand that not all malignancies will have similar degrees of grading and classification; ultimately, the labels will be determined by the pathologist upon examining the tissue specimens.

CHART 57–4 TNM System of Tumor Classification and Staging

Primary Tumor Size (T)	
T0	No evidence of a primary tumor or lesion
Tis	Carcinoma *in situ*
T1	Lesion contained in organ of origin
T2	Localized lesion with deep growth into adjacent structures
T3	Advanced lesion limited to a region of the original organ
T4	Advanced lesion spreading into adjacent organs
Regional Lymph Nodes (N)	
N0	No evidence of disease in lymph nodes
N1	Evidence of disease in regional lymph nodes but not likely metastatic
N2, 3, 4	Increasing involvement of regional lymph nodes
Anatomic Extent of Metastasis (M)	
M0	No evidence of metastasis
M1, 2, 3	Worsening degrees of metastatic involvement, including distant lymph nodes and functional impairment

Sources: Merkle, C. J. (2009). Neoplasia. In C. M. Porth & G. Matfin (Eds.), *Pathophysiology: Concepts of altered health status* (8th ed., pp. 156–196). Philadelphia: Wolters Kluwer/Lippincott Williams & Wilkins; Virshup, D. M. (2010). Biology, clinical manifestations, and treatment of cancer. In K. L. McCance & S. E. Huether (Eds.), *Pathophysiology: The biologic basis for disease in adults and children* (6th ed., pp. 396–435). St. Louis: Mosby Elsevier.

Route of Tumor Spread

Cells that are experiencing the transformation process have abnormal or decreased anchorage dependence. Anchorage dependence is necessary for cells to be able to divide or spread. Anchorage independence is the inability of the cell to maintain cellular or extracellular matrix attachments. Cancer cells do not require a surface on which to attach and multiply. Missing this cellular characteristic that inhibits proliferation will result in cancerous cell growth in new regions, known as metastases (Virshup, 2010).

Cancer may invade local tissues or spread to distant areas by hematogenous or lymphatic routes. As tumors grow locally, their cells extend to and invade lymph nodes found in the same anatomic region, resulting in distant metastases. Some tumors are known to metastasize to distant organs before or during involvement with local lymph nodes (Merkle, 2009).

Direct

Direct spread is the ability of a tumor to invade and eradicate adjoining tissue (Merkle, 2009). The following processes enhance this process:

- Tumor angiogenesis factor stimulates new capillary growth, which allows for continued tumor growth due to adequate nutrition and oxygen. Once a tumor reaches 2 mm^3 in size, it requires additional blood supply to grow. The new vascular growth provides not only the essential elements for growth but also a route for tumor cells to leave the primary site (Merkle, 2009).
- Mechanical pressure and increased rate of tumor growth occur when intratumor pressure causes fingerlike projections to be pushed into adjacent tissue. Uncontrolled tumor growth creates expanding masses that apply pressure on local tissues.
- Cell motility and loss of cellular adhesiveness promote tumor cell distribution because of the slippery nature of the cancer cell, which enhances movement.
- Tumor-secreted enzymes may be associated with the degree to which cells have the potential to invade surrounding tissues and destroy the normal tissue barriers. An example of this is plasminogen activator; this activates plasminogen to plasmin, which can break down the extracellular matrix.

Serosal seeding is another mechanism by which tumor cells demonstrate direct spreading (Merkle, 2009). Embolization of tumor cells occurs after malignant cells invade local tissues and infiltrate body cavities. These cells then attach to the serosal surface of organs within the involved cavity. The most common sites for serosal seeding to occur are the lung and ovary. Penetration of the parenchyma of the organ is unlikely to occur despite the presence of tumor cells within the surface of organs in the pleural and peritoneal cavities. Seeding of malignant cells may occur as needles are withdrawn during biopsies (defined later in the chapter); in addition, manipulation of a tumor during the

CHART 57–5 Common Sites of Metastases of the Four Most Frequently Occurring Cancers

Origin	Site of Metastasis
Breast	Bone, lung, liver, brain, lymph nodes
Prostate	Bone, lung, liver, bowel, kidney, lymph nodes
Lung	Bone, liver, kidney, brain, bone marrow, lymph nodes
Colorectal	Lung, liver, brain, lymph nodes

operative procedure may release cells into the vascular supply and into the circulation.

Metastatic

Metastasis is defined as the spread of cancerous cells from a primary site of origin to a distant site (Merkle, 2009). It is extremely important to recognize the effect of metastasis and that a benign tumor does not exhibit this type of behavior. The capability of malignant cells to travel to distant sites and invade adjacent tissues is very powerful and often deadly. Chart 57–5 lists the four most common cancers and their metastatic sites.

French health care provider Joseph Claude Recamier was the first to use the term *metastasis* in 1829 (Hawkins, 2001). Previously, researchers thought that tumors spread by direct extension and by invasion of lymph nodes. At that time, it was thought that distant metastasis was caused by new tumor growth unrelated to the primary tumor. Recamier was the first health care provider to prove that metastasis was caused by malignant cells separating from the primary tumor and traveling through the bloodstream and lymphatic system to distant anatomic locations (Liotta, 1992).

The metastatic process, although commonly evident clinically, is a unique, intricate series of events. A cancer cell released from a primary tumor has a long and difficult task in order to survive long enough to establish residency in a distant anatomic site. It is believed that only 1 in 10,000 tumor cells that separate from the primary tumor are able to endure long enough to begin the metastatic process (Merkle, 2009).

Understanding the mechanism of metastasis is important to increase our appreciation of metastatic patterns; however, metastasis is known to be unpredictable. Mechanisms of metastasis include (1) angiogenesis, (2) migration, (3) cell attachment, (4) cell invasion, and (5) growth factors.

Angiogenesis is the creation of new blood vessels due to migration and proliferation of endothelial cells from existing blood vessels. Although angiogenesis is a favorable occurrence in wound healing, ovulation, and embryogenesis, it is not so desirable when it promotes the development of malignancies. Vascular endothelial growth factor (VEGF) is an essential component for the growth and proliferation of cancer cells. New blood vessels provide nutrients, protein growth factors, and oxygen to the tumor mass. With the development of angiogenesis inhibitors (e.g., Avastin), this vital process for tumor growth can be slowed or stopped, affording patients better treatment options (Merkle, 2009).

Because vessels created by angiogenesis tend to have permeable walls, malignant cells enter easily, allowing access to the circulatory and lymphatic systems (migration). Tumor masses produce motility factors that enable cells to move with more ease throughout the circulatory and lymphatic systems. Once in the circulation, cancer cells cluster in the first vascular bed distal to the original site. After blood circulates through the heart, the pulmonary vascular bed is the first one encountered. Intestines drain their blood supply into the liver, thus exposing it to malignant cells. Understandably, the most common site of metastasis is the lung, followed by the liver.

Another common vehicle for the transportation of malignant cells is the lymphatic system. Tumor emboli, which form as a result of circulating tumor cells, may become trapped in lymph nodes. Not all lymph nodes will be hosts for these deadly cells. In fact, cancerous cells will bypass several lymph nodes before settling into a distant nodal site; this is known as "skip" metastasis (Merkle, 2009).

Normally, cells adhere to one another and to the extracellular matrix (ECM). The nurse must understand that tumor cells form temporary attachments to ECM components and to other cells that are not part of their origin. Cell-to-cell adhesion is altered, resulting in tumor cells attaching to cells of a different origin. For example, breast cancer metastasizing to the bone occurs when a breast tissue cell relocates to, and attaches to, the bone. This form of cell attachment is assisted by cell surface receptors such as CD44. The other type of cellular attachment is adhesion to the ECM, which promotes cellular growth and endurance. Anchorage dependence is necessary for cells to attach to surfaces that nurture their proliferation.

Cell invasion is essential for the metastatic process. Tumor cells may pass through vascular walls into a blood vessel (intravasation) or out of a blood vessel (extravasation). Thus, cancer cells are able to reach normal tissue, despite numerous mechanical barriers. Basement membrane invasion occurs when cancer cells leave the primary tumor, penetrate the blood or lymphatic vessels, and exit from the vasculature.

Growth factors contribute substantially to the metastatic process. Angiogenesis is potentiated or impeded by growth factors. In addition, tumor proliferation produces a decreased reliance on exogenous growth factors. The existence of growth factors at the metastatic site is imperative for continued growth of cancerous cells.

The phenomenon of metastasis is uniquely complex as it navigates through normal body controls and regulatory functions. The process often is associated with worsened prognosis and increased mortality. Understanding the metastatic process will assist researchers in discovering and developing new and more effective treatment options.

Commonly Occurring Cancers

Nurses who care for patients with cancer need to develop a knowledge base that is extensive and ever changing. Discoveries that change the diagnosis, treatment, and prognosis of this devastating disease are continuous. This fluidity demands that nurses continue the quest for more information to assist them in developing their nursing practice. Cancers are located in solid organs (e.g., lung, breast, prostate cancers) or in the hematopoietic and lymphatic systems (e.g., lymphoma and leukemia). Chart 57–6 (p. 1772) presents general information, clinical findings, diagnostic techniques, prognosis, and treatment modalities to assist the nurse in gaining a better understanding of the most commonly occurring cancers. A more in-depth discussion of the current diagnostic studies and treatment modalities is presented later in this chapter.

Prevention, Screening, and Detection

Surviving cancer is, in part, a result of improved therapies and earlier detection. The 5-year survival rate has improved from 2004 to 2008 (Siegel et al., 2012). Represented in these statistics are those people who are living 5 years after diagnosis, including those who are disease free, in remission, or in treatment with evidence of disease.

CHART 57–6 Commonly Occurring Cancers

Cancer		Clinical Findings	Diagnostic Technique	Prognosis	Treatment
Breast	Noninvasive (carcinoma *in situ*): confined to the ducts and/or lobules Invasive (infiltrating): cancerous cells penetrate tissue outside of ducts (80%) or lobules (10%) Inflammatory: swelling, erythema, and invasion of dermal lymphatics	Mass: hard, irregular, nontender Thick breast or axilla Nipple discharge Nipple retraction or inversion Dimpling or puckering of skin Changes in size, shape, and texture of breast	Mammogram Self-breast exam Biopsy, fine-needle or core needle Pathology testing: cytologic or histologic	Tumor size and presence of lymph node(s) have important roles in predicting survival. Presence of hormone receptors has a negative impact on survival. There remain percentages (20%) of those who develop recurrence.	Surgery: • Lumpectomy • Mastectomy • Breast reconstruction. Radiotherapy: external beam Chemotherapy: • Adjuvant • Hormonal. High-dose chemotherapy with transplantation (for advanced cancer)
Colon and rectum	Majority are adenocarcinomas Rectum: 40–50% Descending sigmoid colon: 20–35% Cecum and ascending colon: 16% Transverse colon: 8%	Changes in bowel habits Blood in stool Flatulence Indigestion Weight loss Fatigue	Barium enema Colonoscopy	Distant metastases negatively impact survival. Once treatment has been completed, follow-up treatment is advised (physical examination, colonoscopy, CEA levels).	Surgery: colon resection with temporary or permanent colostomy Chemotherapy Radiotherapy for involvement in the perineum or viscera
Prostate	Adenocarcinomas (95%) Endogenous hormones and environmental factors may be causative factors	*Early:* Painful urination Frequency Hematuria *Late:* Pain (bone, joint, back) Fatigue Weight loss	Prostate-specific antigen (PSA) Direct rectal examination (DRE) Transrectal ultrasound (TRUS) Biopsy	Transitional zone involvement is less aggressive. Metastatic disease negatively impacts survival.	Surgery: radical prostatectomy Radiotherapy: external beam or brachytherapy Cryotherapy Chemotherapy Expectant management ("watchful waiting")
Lung	Small cell anaplastic carcinoma Non–small cell: squamous cell carcinoma Adenocarcinomas Large cell anaplastic carcinoma Mixed cell types	Change in cough Chest pain Respiratory ailments not treated with antibiotics Dyspnea Wheezing Hemoptysis Weight loss Fatigue Dysphagia	History and physical examination Chest x-ray (anterior, posterior, lateral) CAT scan MRI CBC with differential Platelet count Chemistry panel Bronchoscopy	Prognosis for 5-year survival after surgical resection is best in patients who have carcinoma *in situ.* Prognosis for 5-year survival after surgical resection is worst for those patients who have cancer that has invaded the lymph nodes or other distant organs or structures.	Surgery Laser therapy (used for relief of complications associated with endobronchial lesions) Radiotherapy: external beam Brachytherapy Chemotherapy
Multiple myeloma	Most common in African Americans, males, age $\geq$ 70 Malignancy of B cell Immunodeficiency due to depressed antibody-mediated immunity	Findings are related to excess of Bence-Jones proteins Infections: Pneumonia Urinary tract infection (UTI) Systemic Skeletal: Pain worse with movement Hypercalcemia Pathologic fractures Vertebral collapse	Serum electrophoresis to determine Bence-Jones proteins Serum immunoglobulin electrophoresis Bone marrow biopsy: increase in abnormal, atypical, immature B cells Radiographic: osteolytic lesions in bones	Incurable, sometimes treatable. One-third of patients do not respond to therapy and die within weeks of diagnosis.	Chemotherapy Corticosteroids Immunotherapy Bone marrow transplant (autologous) Radiation therapy

Weblink: Video: Leukemia

CHART 57–6 Commonly Occurring Cancers, *continued*

Cancer		Clinical Findings	Diagnostic Technique	Prognosis	Treatment
		Renal failure: Proteinuria Obstructed distal and proximal tubules Hyperuricemia Blood/bone marrow dysfunction: Anemia Hyperviscosity Coagulation disorders Neurologic: Spinal cord compression Peripheral neuropathy			
Leukemias					
Acute lymphocytic leukemia (ALL)	Most common in children *Etiology:* Radiation Chemicals Drugs Viruses	*Anemia:* Malaise Fatigue *Neutropenia:* Fever Bone pain Thrombocytopenia: Bleeding Bruising CNS involvement (10%) due to meningeal infiltrates	Peripheral blood smear: • CBC with differential • Bone marrow biopsy	Complete remission: 80–90% Cure: 30–40% Children achieve cure at rate of 60–85%	Chemotherapy: Induction therapy to achieve remission CNS treatment if needed Postremission therapy Bone marrow or stem cell transplantation
Acute myeloid leukemia (AML)	*Etiology:* Radiation Chemicals Drugs Viruses Certain genetic disorders increase incidence of acquiring AML	*Anemia:* Malaise Fatigue *Neutropenia:* Fever Bone pain *Thrombocytopenia:* Bleeding Bruising Anemia is usually present when the health care provider sees the patient for the first time Recurrent infections are not resolved with antibiotics	Peripheral blood smear: • CBC with differential • Bone marrow biopsy	Patients over 70 years of age are intolerant of induction therapy. WBCs $>100,000/mm^3$ related to increased mortality during first week of therapy.	Chemotherapy: Induction therapy to achieve remission Postremission therapy Biotherapy: monoclonal antibodies Bone marrow or stem cell transplantation
Chronic lymphocytic leukemia (CLL)	B-cell lymphocytes undergo a malignant transformation Few cases are of the T-cell line	25% of patients are symptom free Evidence of disease found on routine examination and laboratory work Frequent respiratory and skin infections	Peripheral blood smear: • CBC with differential • Flow cytometry to evaluate immunophenotype of cells • Bone marrow biopsy (for prognostic information)	Survival is often determined by the severity of disease when diagnosed. No pattern of predictability of the disease course.	Often difficult to decide when to begin treatment. Treatment is aimed at alleviation of symptoms, not cure.

(*continued*)

CHART 57–6 Commonly Occurring Cancers, *continued*

Cancer		Clinical Findings	Diagnostic Technique	Prognosis	Treatment
					Treatment for complications: Antibiotics IV immunoglobulin Chemotherapy Splenectomy or radiotherapy (rarely done) Bone marrow or stem cell transplantation
Chronic myeloid leukemia (CML)	Myeloproliferative disorder Presence of Philadelphia chromosome Three stages: 1. Chronic 2. Accelerated 3. Blast crisis	*Chronic Phase:* Fatigue Pallor Dyspnea Anemia Night sweats Weight loss Sternum pain *Accelerated:* Chronic symptoms recur after treatment. *Blast Crisis:* Aggressive and terminal phase that includes above symptoms with increased severity.	Peripheral blood smear: CBC with differential Bone marrow biopsy	Chronic phase lasts 3–4 years. Once blast crisis occurs, median survival is $<$6 months. 85% of patients die during blast crisis from complications such as bleeding and infections.	Chemotherapy Biotherapy: interferon Bone marrow or stem cell transplantation
Lymphomas					
Non-Hodgkin's disease	Similar to Hodgkin's disease, but without the Reed-Sternberg cell *Etiology:* Infections Autoimmune disorders Environmental factors Typically female, Caucasian, and approximately 55 years of age	Painless lymphadenopathy (cervical or supraclavicular region) As disease worsens, swelling and obstructive symptoms occur	Lymph node biopsy Chest x-ray Bone marrow biopsy Serum blood analysis: • Hepatitis B and C • CBC with differential • Chemistries	Indolent disease has most favorable prognosis. Highly aggressive disease requires high-dose therapy that increases risk of life-threatening complications.	Chemotherapy Biotherapy: monoclonal antibodies Bone marrow or stem cell transplantation
Hodgkin's disease	Presence of Reed-Sternberg cells *Etiology:* Viral exposure Epstein–Barr virus most common Woodworking Most common in young adults, age 26–31 years Occasional peak in prevalence at age 60 years	Lymphadenopathy: Cervical Supraclavicular Mediastinal Fever Night sweats Weight loss	Lymph node biopsy Staging laparotomy if receiving radiation Chest x-ray Bone marrow biopsy Serum blood analysis: • CBC with differential • Chemistries	If early stage, 20-year survival is near 80%. If receiving salvage therapy after relapse, survival is 80–95%.	Radiotherapy Chemotherapy Bone marrow or stem cell transplantation

Sources: McCance, K. (2010). Cancer epidemiology. In K. L. McCance & S. E. Huether (Eds.), *Pathophysiology: The biologic basis for disease in adults and children* (6th ed., pp. 360–395). St. Louis: Mosby Elsevier; Merkle, C. J. (2009). Neoplasia. In C. M. Porth & G. Matfin (Eds.), *Pathophysiology: Concepts of altered health status* (8th ed., pp. 156–196). Philadelphia: Wolters Kluwer/Lippincott Williams & Wilkins; Virshup, D. M. (2010). Biology, clinical manifestations, and treatment of cancer. In K. L. McCance & S. E. Huether (Eds.), *Pathophysiology: The biologic basis for disease in adults and children* (6th ed., pp. 396–435). St. Louis: Mosby Elsevier.

NATIONAL GUIDELINES American Cancer Society (ACS) Goals and Objectives for 2015

Goals

Age-adjusted mortality rates reduced by 50%.

Age-adjusted incidence rates reduced by 25%.

Measurable improvement in the quality of life from the time of diagnosis through the balance of life.

Objectives

Proportion of adults who use tobacco products reduced to 12%.

Proportion of youth who use tobacco products reduced to 10%.

Proportion of persons who follow the ACS guidelines for consumption of fruits and vegetables increased to 75%.

Proportion of adults who follow the ACS guidelines for appropriate level of physical activity increased to 90%.

Proportion of youth who follow the ACS guidelines for appropriate level of physical activity increased to 60%.

Proportion of school districts that provide school health education increased to 50%.

Proportion of all persons who use at least two or more protective measures to reduce the risk of skin cancer increased to 75%.

Proportion of women (ages 40 or older) who have ACS recommended breast screening increased to 90%.

Proportion of persons (ages 50 or older) who have ACS recommended colorectal screening increased to 75%.

Proportion of men (ages 50 or older) who follow ACS recommended guidelines for prostate cancer increased to 90%.

Regular screening may result in earlier detection of cancers of the breast, colon, rectum, cervix, prostate, testes, oral cavity, and skin. Earlier detection allows for diagnosis at an early stage of tumor development, which may lead to a more positive outcome for the patient. In 1999, the American Cancer Society set goals that would significantly lower cancer incidence and mortality rates and improve the quality of life of cancer survivors by 2015 (see the National Guidelines box). One example of efforts aimed at accomplishing these goals is the American Cancer Society's collaborative work with the American Heart Association and the American Diabetes Association called "Everyday Choices for a Healthier Life" to focus attention on prevention and early detection of cancer. These three organizations are examining tobacco use, obesity, physical inactivity, and underutilization of effective screening tests.

The U.S. Department of Health and Human Services' *Healthy People 2020* objectives support monitoring trends in cancer incidence, mortality, and survival to better assess the progress being made in decreasing the burden of cancer in the United States. Cancer is identified as the third area of focus out of 28 in the objectives. The objectives of 2020 also emphasize the need for evidence-based screening for cervical, colorectal, and breast cancers. These screening tests are included in the U.S. Preventive Services Task Force Recommendations. The overall goal for cancer care is to reduce the number of cases along with the disability, illness, and death associated with the disease. Suggestions for reaching these reductions include (1) smoking cessation, (2) diet modification, (3) early detection via screening programs, and (4) current cancer treatment options. To affect the morbidity and mortality associated with cancer, early diagnosis and treatment are pivotal (U.S. Department of Health and Human Services, 2010).

Nurses play a crucial role in educating the public about cancer prevention, risk factors, and early detection. By teaching members of our society strategies to prevent cancer, how to reduce the risk of developing a malignancy, and the important tests used for detection early in the disease process, when it is easier to treat, nurses may help to reduce the fear associated with cancer. It is unknown whether individuals will consider adapting behaviors and practices with ongoing health education. Influencing factors include perceived susceptibility, the cost of behavior changes, and the actual health message delivered (Virshup, 2010).

Barriers exist that impede or prevent the success of cancer screening programs. Barriers that are associated with health care providers include the lack of time and expertise needed to integrate inclusive cancer screening programs. Barriers experienced by patients include lack of transportation, poor financial status, or no support to access the screening programs. Our health care system struggles with the lack of resources to support a comprehensive screening program. Diverse populations are experiencing additional barriers to cancer screening programs. Access to screening programs is less common for those who are poor or less educated, those for whom English is a second language, and members of certain minority groups. To create and implement cancer screening programs, the nurse must be open to a variety of issues that may affect the program's success.

Nurses are becoming more involved in cancer detection and screening programs. However, assisting individuals in selecting the appropriate cancer prevention and detection options can be done only when the nurse understands the principles of each type of cancer (Eggert, 2011).

Definitions

To develop sound cancer prevention and early detection programs, an understanding of the terminology used is essential. With this knowledge, nurses can assist individuals in making appropriate choices of cancer prevention and early detection strategies.

Cancer Screening

Cancer screening is the use of tests to look for evidence of cancer in someone who does not have signs or symptoms of the cancer (McCance, 2010). Examples are mammograms screening for breast cancer and fecal occult blood tests to screen for colon and rectal cancer. A positive cancer-screening test does not indicate a definitive diagnosis of cancer; rather, it indicates that more testing needs to be done. The term *early detection* is used interchangeably with *cancer screening*.

Cancer Prevention

Cancer prevention has three levels. *Primary prevention* refers to preventing diseases via immunizations and avoidance of known carcinogens. This form of prevention reduces the risk of developing cancer (e.g., educating youth regarding the effects of tobacco use) with the understanding that there is no guarantee that an individual will not show signs of malignancy in the future. *Secondary prevention* involves early detection and treatment of subclinical disease in individuals who have no signs or symptoms of a malignancy. Examples include Pap smears and colonoscopies. *Tertiary prevention* is the management of a disease with the goal of preventing progression, recurrence, or complications. Examples include monitoring for recurrence with the use of tumor markers and detecting further primary tumors early in individuals who are long-term survivors of cancer.

Screened Individuals

Individuals who are undergoing cancer screening tests are not considered patients. Only when an abnormal screening test is discovered is the

Weblink: Seven Steps to Reduce Your Cancer Risk

individual considered a patient. For example, women routinely undergo clinical breast exams and mammography. Women with negative results are not labeled as patients. Wellness is the main focus of all cancer prevention levels.

Target Population

The target population consists of individuals who have certain characteristics that make them suitable for screening. Oncology experts use the following characteristics to determine a target population: (1) gender, (2) family history, (3) presence of risk factors, (4) ethnicity, and (5) age (McCance, 2010).

It is important for the nurse to be aware of these characteristics so that the nurse can accurately educate the patient and family about the importance of recommended screening tests. Having an appreciation of the cultural beliefs and practices that influence a person's decision to be screened for cancer will give the nurse insight into how the individual approaches health and wellness. The Cultural Considerations box provides a few examples of how culture can affect health practices.

Risk Factors

The presence of interacting cellular, genetic, immunologic, and environmental forces that have the potential to create malignancy is frequently described in terms of *risk factors*. Assessing cancer risk is a common and crucial thread in all three levels of cancer prevention. Making appropriate screening recommendations is extremely difficult if there has not been an accurate and complete assessment of cancer risk. A screening program should incorporate an education portion that includes a discussion of the seven warning signs of cancer (Chart 57–7).

Safety Alert *Nurses are responsible for assessing patients for the seven warning signs of cancer and alerting the health care provider or encouraging the patient to seek medical evaluation. Ongoing education about the seven warning signs of cancer is essential for patients and their families so that they will understand the importance of recognizing unusual symptoms and seeking early medical attention.*

Risk factors are categorized according to whether they originate from outside the host (exogenous) or within the host (endogenous) (see the Risk Factors box). Both endogenous and exogenous risk factors cause cancer by damaging the genes that regulate normal cell growth or by perpetuating the growth of existing abnormal cells. Endogenous factors include age, genetic background (see the Genetic Considerations

CULTURAL CONSIDERATIONS
Related to Health Practices

Temporal orientation (perceived importance of detecting health problems early) and perceptions of internal control and physical space can affect the incidence of screening for mammograms. In comparison to Caucasian women, African American women have an increased sense of fatalism related to breast cancer. This belief about the inevitability of dying if they have the disease prevents many African American women from undergoing regular mammogram screening (Wilson, 2011).

The leading cause of death among Korean Americans is cancer, and breast cancer is the most common cancer in Korean American women. The mortality rate for females has increased by 280% since 1983. Because of these staggering numbers, mammogram screening is recommended beginning at the age of 30 for Korean American women, which is a decade earlier than for Caucasian women (Eun, 2009).

Greek women experience an increase in fatigue while undergoing adjuvant radiotherapy for breast cancer. Initially, the patient's fatigue is felt to be minimal, but it gradually increases to the point at which the patient has significant changes in health status. One known intervention to reduce the effect of fatigue is to participate in exercise activities. Because exercise is not a common behavior of many Greek women, nurses are asked to explore culturally appropriate alternatives (Zender, 2009).

Rates of breast and cervical cancer screening are low among Chinese, Japanese, and Vietnamese American women. Given that Asian Americans have a high rate of liver and stomach cancer combined with infrequent screening practices for breast and cervical cancer, nurses have an opportunity to assist with health promotion and education (Barton Burke, 2010).

Filipino American women typically demonstrate avoidance when dealing with a cancer diagnosis. However, several factors improve their willingness to participate in screening activities: supportive family members, suggestions from familiar health care providers, health insurance, and the personal attributes of physical symptoms, family history, past diagnosis, and health literacy (Barton Burke, 2010).

CHART 57–7 CAUTION: Seven Warning Signs of Cancer

Change in bowel or bladder habits
A sore that does not heal
Unusual bleeding or discharge from any body orifice
Thickening or a lump in the breast or elsewhere
Indigestion or difficulty swallowing
Obvious change in a wart or mole
Nagging cough or hoarseness

RISK FACTORS for Cancer

Exogenous	Endogenous
Drugs and chemicals: Environmental and occupational factors influence the carcinogenicity of a number of chemicals and drugs. For instance, tobacco smoke and asbestos exposure have synergistic effects, increasing the risk for smokers who are exposed to asbestos.	*Age:* Incidence increases with age.
Lifestyle behaviors: Tobacco is the most deadly carcinogen.	*Genetic predisposition:* Occasional genetic link.
Nutrition: Diets low in fiber and high in fat.	*Hormones:* Influence the process of carcinogenesis.
Sexual activity: Women who engage in sex with multiple partners and begin having sexual relations early in life have an increased risk of cancer.	*Immune dysfunction:* Immunocompetence is essential for identification of antigens (malignant cells).
Alcohol: Large consumptions of ethyl alcohol are linked to certain cancers of the head and neck, breast, and bladder.	
Radiation: Ionizing and ultraviolet radiation can cause cancer.	
Viruses: Several different cancers have been linked to viruses.	
Psychosocial: Stress and the relationship to neoplasms is still being investigated.	

Weblink: Cigarette Smoking

GENETIC CONSIDERATIONS Related to Cancer

Our understanding of the link between genetics and the development of cancer is partly attributable to the worldwide Human Genome Project, which began in 1990. The goal of the project was to locate, map, and sequence more than 100,000 genes that make up the human genome. There are three main categories of genetic cancer. First, inherited cancer syndromes typically are autosomal dominant and possess many different genes that regulate cell growth and gene repair. Diagnosis is usually done at an early age, and the syndromes frequently are associated with multiple primary tumors. An example is the breast/ovarian cancer syndrome in which chromosome 17 houses a mutated tumor suppressor gene (BRCA1). The risk of developing breast and ovarian cancer is significantly increased if a female carries BRCA1. Next, a group of genetic disorders that are typically nonmalignant have been known to predispose a person to developing malignancy. For example, the presence of ataxia-telangiectasia can be correlated to the development of breast cancer and leukemia. Finally, familial "clustering" occurs when there is an increased prevalence of cancer than would be expected statistically; however, the specific genetic factors have yet to be determined. Breast cancer is the most common example of a cancer that appears to cluster in families.

Sources: Adapted from American Cancer Society (ACS). (2008a). Cancer facts and figures 2008. Retrieved from http://www.cancer.org/downloads/STT/2008CAFFfinalsecured.pdf; American Cancer Society (ACS). (2008b). Seven steps to reduce your cancer risk. Retrieved from http://www.cancer.org/docroot/COM/content/div_NE/COM_1_1x_Seven_Steps_To_Take_To_Prevent_Cancer.asp?sitearea=COM; Eggert, J. (2011). The biology of cancer: What oncology nurses really need to know. *Seminars in Oncology, 27*(1), 3–12.

box and immune competence. Exogenous factors include tobacco, radiation, diet, chemicals, and infections.

Age

As we age, the likelihood of developing a malignancy increases. Up to age 39, the probability is between 1% and 2%; from ages 40 to 61, the chance increases to 8% to 9%. The lifetime incidence of cancer is higher for men (43.39%) than for women (38.25%). Because of breast cancer, a woman's chance of developing cancer before the age of 60 is slightly increased. Men have demonstrated a higher incidence of cancer (33%) between the ages of 60 and 79 compared to women (22%) (Eggert, 2011).

The concept of aging as it relates to cancer development can be incorporated into the discussion of other risk factors; however, to truly understand the impact of the aging process, it is important to examine the theories that attempt to explain the changes. First, over time, we are exposed to a cumulative increase in the number of carcinogens, which increases the chance of a malignancy emerging. Next, cells that have aged may be less tolerant of the genetic abnormalities that occur with cancer and become unable to initiate damage repair. Finally, as we age, our immune system does not function as efficiently, thus opening the door for abnormal cellular growth associated with cancer formation.

Hormones

Cancer of the brain, breast, endometrium, and prostate occur in target tissues, that is, those that are hormone responsive. Hormones have not been proven to have a direct carcinogenic effect. Rather, they support carcinogenesis by preparing target tissues so that they are ripe for the carcinogen insult, by permitting the carcinogenesis to continue, or by modifying the growth of an established tumor. The length of time during which tissue has been exposed to a hormone may influence carcinogenesis.

Immune Dysfunction

The immune system is an intricate network of surveillance that controls the proliferation of potential cancer cells. The immune system screens the human body for these cells and activates forces to eliminate them before a tumor can develop. Humoral factors are those that produce antibodies in the battle against cancer cells; cellular factors include sensitized lymphocytes and macrophages. Frequently, cancer cells contain antigens that are different from the person's own antigens; this results in destruction of the cancer cells by the immune system. The normal immune system can detect and destroy approximately 10 million cancer cells at one time. However, tumors that replicate faster than the rate at which the immune system can work will continue to grow unrestrained. Because of improvements in technology, today's diagnostic procedures can recognize a mass measuring only 1 cm in diameter. However, a tumor that is 1 cm in diameter contains at least 1 billion cells.

Most often, cancers occur in individuals whose immune systems are impaired because of malnutrition, chronic disease, advancing age, and/or stress. People with immunodeficiency are more susceptible to developing malignancy than are people whose immune system is intact. See Chapter 53 for a discussion of the immune system.

Drugs and Chemicals

Millions of chemicals have been registered with the Chemical Abstracts Service, and more than 50,000 are thought to be used regularly in business and industry. Although the importance of monitoring and regulating these substances has been generally acknowledged, fewer than 1,000 chemicals or exposures have been examined to determine their role in the development of cancer (Eggert, 2011). Great effort has been given to publishing and organizing data on cancer risk attributed to chemical carcinogens.

Chemical carcinogens are chemicals that contain compounds or elements that alter DNA. An awareness of the relationship between chemical exposures and disease began as early as the 1700s (Eggert, 2011). Men employed as chimney sweeps developed an increased incidence of scrotal cancer, and the cause was thought to be the continued exposure to soot from coal burned as fuel. Although it is easy to attribute chemical carcinogens to occupational exposure, the vastness of environmental exposures makes it difficult to connect a given case of cancer to a particular exposure. The Occupational Safety and Health Act of 1970 authorized the Occupational Safety and Health Administration (OSHA) to impose restrictions on the amount of exposure to known carcinogens. Threshold limit values (TLVs), or the maximum allowable exposure, are difficult to determine because identification of carcinogens in the environment and workplace is very time consuming (McCance, 2010). The U.S. Department of Health and Human Services publishes a list (*The Tenth Report*) of known human carcinogens biannually.

Agents that are used to combat cancer have been known to increase the risk of causing secondary malignancies. Years after receiving agents such as chlorambucil and cyclophosphamide, people have experienced a notably increased likelihood of developing leukemia. Individuals who require immunosuppressive agents to prevent transplant rejection are known to have a higher likelihood of developing secondary malignancies.

Tobacco

The carcinogenic effect of tobacco is demonstrated in several different compounds that promote the growth of malignant cells over time. There appears to be a direct relationship between the numbers of years a person has smoked, the number of cigarettes smoked per day, and the age when smoking began. Choosing to indulge in smokeless tobacco is not without risk. The use of chewing tobacco places a person at higher risk for developing head and neck cancer. By eliminating smoking as a lifestyle choice, a person can live longer and reduce the risk of lung cancer by approximately 50% (Eggert, 2011). Other health-related issues also are positively affected by smoking cessation, such as a reduction in the risk of cardiac disease and complications from pregnancy.

Approximately one in five Americans is addicted to tobacco products (ACS, 2011a). According to the ACS, there has been a dramatic increase in successful quit attempts in individuals who seek assistance with smoking cessation. However, with inadequate health insurance coverage and the cost of treatment programs, many individuals remain addicted to tobacco products. In 2007, the Centers for Disease Control and Prevention's *Morbidity and Mortality Weekly Report* concluded that there continues to be a need for states to assist with funding of smoking cessation and counseling programs (CDC, 2011). Thirty-four states provide some type of coverage to assist people who wish to quit using tobacco products; these programs cover over-the-counter (OTC) products, prescription drugs, or counseling services. Seventeen states, in contrast, offer no tobacco treatment coverage services.

The past several years have shown the effect of publicity associated with tobacco use. Smoking cessation campaigns across the country have become more common in the last few years. The ACS has identified school health education as critical to the effort to assist young people in developing and maintaining health practices that reduce cancer risk. Litigation by lung cancer victims or their families against tobacco companies has increased the attention paid to a behavior our society appears to be increasingly identifying as dangerous and life threatening. See Chapter 6 for a complete discussion of smoking and its risks.

Nutrition and Physical Activity

Approximately 20% of all cancer deaths are attributed to nutrition and physical activity factors (ACS, 2011b). The association between certain foods and eating habits and the incidence of some cancers is becoming better known and publicized. The link between high-fat foods and an increase in the development of colon, breast, and prostate cancers has been known for almost a decade. There is currently an alarming rate of obesity and overweight among adolescents 12 to 19 years of age (ACS, 2011b). In the past 20 years, the prevalence of obesity in African American girls has tripled. Overall, two-thirds of U.S. adults (20 years and older) are overweight or obese.

Diets that have a high fiber content appear to provide protection against colon cancer. The exact mechanism of protection remains unknown, but fiber is known to reduce the concentration of fecal bile acids, dilute colon contents, and decrease colon transit time, which helps in decreasing the time colonic contents are exposed to carcinogens (Palmquist, 2011). Rich sources of dietary fiber include fruits, vegetables, legumes, and whole-grain breads and cereals. Foods with vitamins C and D, beta-carotene, and selenium seem to repair cellular damage caused by free radicals, which are known to destroy the genetic makeup of cells; increasing the ingestion of these foods helps to create a cellular environment that resists malignancy development.

Regular physical activity reduces the risk of death due to coronary heart disease and the risk of stroke, colon cancer, breast cancer, diabetes, and hypertension (Erye, Kahn, Robertson, & Committee AAACW, 2004). By keeping physically fit, people tend to control their weight better, which reduces the risk of developing cancer related to excess weight. The ACS publishes guidelines for nutrition and physical activity for cancer prevention that can assist in identifying important healthy behaviors (ACS, 2011b).

Sexual Activity

Never before has the correlation between sexual practices and cancer risk been more obvious and concerning. The development of genital cancer is strongly related to sexual practices. In fact, studies have identified an association between sexual activity and AIDS and between sexual activity and cancers of the cervix, vagina, and vulva (Sanchez, 2011). Sexually transmitted infections (STIs), becoming sexually active at a young age, having had multiple sexual partners, and having had high-risk sexual partners all have been implicated in the development of cervical cancer. Viruses such as herpes simplex virus (HSV) and human papillomavirus (HPV) have also been known to increase the incidence of cervical cancer.

Penile cancer, although rare (occurring in 1 in 100,000 men), is more common in men who are uncircumcised, those who are infected with HPV, and those who use tobacco. It is speculated that males who are uncircumcised are prone to more incidence of smegma, which leads to irritation and inflammation of the penis (Sanchez, 2011). Exposure to HPV from multiple sexual partners, sexual intercourse at a young age, and unprotected sex will make a person more likely to develop malignancy. Smoking creates harmful chemicals that are absorbed into the bloodstream and disseminated throughout the body, resulting in damage to the DNA of cells. Cells of penile tissue are not immune to this destructive process. Chapter 42 presents a more detailed discussion of this rare but devastating cancer.

Safety Alert *It is important for the nurse to assess patients for risky lifestyle practices that increase their chances of developing cancer. Educating patients and their families about smoking cessation, about limiting the use of alcohol, and about safe sexual practices as they relate to the incidence of developing cancer (and other diseases) may contribute to changing or preventing undesirable lifestyle practices.*

Alcohol

Consumption of ethyl alcohol is known to cause cancers of the oral cavity, pharynx, larynx, esophagus, liver, and breast (ACS, 2008b). Men should refrain from consuming more than 2 drinks per day, and women should consume no more than 1 drink per day. When combined with tobacco use, alcohol is the leading etiologic factor in developing squamous cell carcinoma of the oral cavity, larynx, and esophagus. It is quite possible that alcohol behaves as a co-carcinogen or has a synergistic effect with tobacco (Merkle, 2009).

Radiation

Waves and particles of energy, or **radiation,** are known to cause cancer. Radiation has the potential to be a complete carcinogen, possessing both initiating and promoting properties. Ionizing radiation has electromagnetic waves that are powerful enough to remove electrons from molecules, thereby weakening the cell by altering its biochemical behavior. Radiation also causes mutation of the cell's DNA, which can weaken the cells' defense against a carcinogen or cause cell death. Although these changes take only seconds, the development of a malignancy may take years. The degree of damage to the cells is related to the dose of radiation received.

Historically, radiation exposure was first recognized after the invention of the x-ray in 1895. People working with x-ray generators were noted to have skin reactions resulting in a skin sore, which led to the first diagnosis of radiation-caused cancer in 1902 (ACS, 2008a). In 1911, leukemia was first reported among radiation workers.

Ionizing radiation includes x-rays, gamma rays, cosmic rays, and radioactive materials such as alpha particles, beta rays, and protons. Even though each form of radiation has a different energy level, all are capable of causing cellular destruction. The three types of ionizing radiation are natural background radiation, nonmedical synthetic radiation, and medical radiation. Natural background radiation is present in cosmic rays from the solar system and radioactive elements found in the soil. This form of radiation is the major contributor to worldwide radiation exposure. Nonmedical synthetic radiation was created by aboveground nuclear weapons testing, mostly done before 1962, and some commercial and occupational sources. Medical radiation is found in diagnostic x-rays and radiation therapy. Radiation therapy is used to treat certain forms of cancer and involves the use of doses that are thousands of times higher than those of x-rays (McCance, 2010). The amount of exposure during radiographic examinations depends on the machine that is used and the capability of the technician. Although the amount of exposure to the average hospital nurse who may assist a patient during an x-ray is slight, nurses need to step away from the area close to the x-ray machine (Merkle, 2009).

Exposure to high-dose ionizing radiation can cause a variety of problems including leukemia, bone cancer, leukopenia, and damage to the reproductive cells. The thyroid gland and the bone marrow are the most sensitive to radiation, whereas the kidney, ovaries, and bladder are the least sensitive. Health care workers whose job involves exposure to radiation must wear film badges, which absorb radiation on a photographic film and are developed each month to determine the amount of cumulative radiation exposure. Individuals who are pregnant are usually not assigned to departments that require exposure to radiation because of the fetus's susceptibility to the negative effects of radiation.

Ultraviolet radiation is composed of electromagnetic waves that are less powerful but still able to produce carcinogenic effects (Merkle, 2009). Ultraviolet radiation is present in the form of sunlight and industrial sources such as welding arcs and germicidal lights (McCance, 2010). Despite the vast amount of documentation linking sunlight to the development of skin cancer, many people still place the importance of tanned skin above the consequence of having cancer. Ultraviolet light is able to penetrate tissues, so the skin is potentially defenseless. The people who are at greatest risk for acquiring either basal or squamous cell cancer of the skin and melanoma are fair-skinned Caucasians and outdoor workers.

Detecting skin cancers early is pivotal to decreasing mortality rates and diminishing the extent of surgical interventions. The nose, cheeks, and ears are common sites for basal and squamous cell cancers to appear. These tumors appear as waxlike, pale nodules or scaly, reddened patches. Melanomas have the appearance of moles and erupt anywhere throughout the body. Melanomas also have the tendency to change color, shape, and size while forming localized ulcerations that may bleed. Pictures that assist the reader in better understanding how these tumors appear are found in Chapter 59. Chart 57–8 lists the warning signs of melanoma.

Radon, a colorless and odorless radioactive gas, is released when uranium decays. It is contained in soil and rocks and is located in underground mines and basements. The carcinogenic risk of radon is approximately the same as that associated with breathing secondhand smoke. According to the ACS, most radon-induced cancers are lung cancers and occur more commonly in people who smoke.

CHART 57–8 Warning Signs of Melanoma: The ABCD Rule

Asymmetry
Border irregularity
Change in color or pigmentation
Diameter greater than 6 mm

Viruses

Only recently has the relationship between viruses and cancer development in humans been established. Viruses are believed to infect the host DNA, which changes the portion that regulates normal cell proliferation and repair (proto-oncogene). In addition, cell mutation is initiated (Eggert, 2011). Cancer occurs only after a prolonged incubation or latency period (usually years), which makes it very difficult for researchers to connect a viral exposure with a specific cancer (McCance, 2010). Viral carcinogens can be either slow acting or fast acting, but all are tissue specific. Slow-acting viral carcinogens include adenoviruses and herpes viruses. Human T-cell leukemia/lymphoma virus (HTLV) is an example of a fast-acting carcinogen. People become particularly vulnerable to viral carcinogens as they advance in age or their immune system begins to function inadequately.

The relationship between certain viruses and the incidence of cancer has been demonstrated in the literature. The hepatitis B virus has been linked to malignancy of the liver, and the Epstein–Barr virus (EBV) has been known to increase the incidence of nasopharyngeal cancer. The human papillomavirus is associated with cancer of the genitalia, especially in women. It is strongly suspected that HPV is linked to cervical cancer. Kaposi's sarcoma is known to be caused by the presence of the cytomegaloviruses (CMVs), which are frequently seen in patients with the HIV virus.

Psychosocial Aspects

How a person's state of mind affects her immune and hormonal systems has not yet been fully determined, nor is it easily explained. It has been suggested that stressors such as death of a loved one, life changes, and personality variables may have significance in the development of cancer. However, most reports of the link between the mind and cancer are subjective, and more research needs to be done to explain how the relationship works (McCance, 2010).

Diagnosing Cancer

The most effective decisions about cancer treatment are based on the results of accurate diagnostic findings performed by a multidisciplinary team. A person with cancer typically undergoes a battery of tests to determine the location, extent, and tumor type of the malignancy. Diagnostic modalities need to be individualized to the patient and may include a thorough history and physical examination, appropriate imaging tests, invasive procedures such as biopsies, laboratory studies, and pathology examination of tissue or blood. New diagnostic techniques have provided the opportunity for the development of sophisticated plans of treatment that positively affect patient survival. Once a diagnosis of cancer has been confirmed, further diagnostic studies may be necessary to stage the cancer (see p. 1781); staging is important in determining an appropriate treatment plan.

The nurse needs to prepare the patient and family for each test and procedure. This includes explaining the rationale for the test or procedure and any preparation the patient needs to complete beforehand. The preparation depends on the procedure; examples include eliminating food and drink (NPO) for a certain number of hours before testing and administering bowel-cleansing agents such as enemas or oral preparations. During this time, patients and families are likely to be experiencing a tremendous amount of anxiety. Even though the term *cancer* might not have been mentioned, they may be experiencing fear about what the possibilities might be. During the diagnostic phase, it is critical for the nurse to offer ongoing support to patients and their families.

History and Physical Examination

Early detection of cancer can be done through screening; this is how some patients discover their diagnosis. Other patients end up in the health care provider's office after noticing unusual symptoms or after a wellness examination during which suspicious symptoms were detected. Nurses perform a comprehensive health history and systems assessment that can be combined with the history and physical exam done by the health care provider. The information obtained by both disciplines provides a holistic view of the patient's health condition and needs. Listening to patients report their health history gives the nurse a perfect opportunity to identify risk factors pertinent to the individual and may elevate the suspicion of malignancy. Further diagnostic evaluation will be determined on the basis of the assessment findings that identify potential diagnoses. The Diagnostic Tests box illustrates the tests done to evaluate for cancer, monitor treatment success and effects, and determine recurrence of disease. Chapter 52 discusses the use of monoclonal antibodies in the patient with an altered immune system, and Chapter 41 explains the Pap test in more detail.

Cancer Treatment Modalities

Multiple treatment modalities are available to patients who have been diagnosed with cancer. Each modality has certain risks, side effects, and chances for success. The nurse can assist the patient and family in obtaining information about treatment options so that they can make informed decisions about the plan of care.

Surgery

Surgical approaches to cancer have existed for centuries. In 1809, Ephraim McDowell demonstrated modern surgical approaches when he excised a 22-pound ovarian tumor from a woman who lived an additional 30 years. He performed 12 more ovarian resections, which became a hallmark in the advancement of elective surgery for cancer (Hill, 1979). Further surgical efforts built on the work of surgeons such as McDowell; however, in the 1950s, it was noted the mortality rates associated with radical procedures were not improving. The evidence was mounting that the benefit of surgery alone as treatment for all tumors needed to be evaluated.

Surgeries in patients with cancer may be performed to establish a diagnosis and to treat the disease. A histologic diagnosis is pivotal in establishing a definitive diagnosis of cancer along with a staging of the tumor, which determines the extent and type of the cancer. Understanding the diagnosis will allow the health care team to design a plan of care unique to each individual and his disease. Diagnosis is accomplished by obtaining tissue samples from an incisional biopsy, excisional biopsy, needle biopsy, or endoscopy. A **biopsy** is a procedure in which a portion of tissue is examined for the presence of abnormal cells. The technique that is used depends on the tumor's location, size, and growth characteristics.

Primary Treatment

Primary treatment for cancer involves removing the malignancy and a margin of surrounding normal tissue. Reducing the amount of total body tumor burden and improving the survival rate are the goals of this surgical approach. Wide excision (en bloc dissection) approaches are used to remove the primary tumor along with regional lymph nodes, intervening lymphatic channels, and involved adjacent structures. Examples of wide excisions are radical neck dissection, radical mastectomy, and abdominal-perineal resection. Local excision is used for skin cancers and consists of the simple excision of a tumor and a small amount of surrounding tissue.

It is important for the patient to be taught both the benefits and the burdens of undergoing surgery for cancer. The patient and family need to understand the potential complications, the expected length of recovery, and the degree of disfigurement, if any, associated with the procedure. In addition, the benefits of other treatment options such as chemotherapy, radiotherapy, and conservative surgical approaches need to be presented. Patients can then make informed decisions about the type of treatment they wish to receive.

Adjuvant Treatment

Adjuvant treatment is aimed at improving outcomes by providing additional cancer therapy. **Cytoreductive therapy** (debulking) is surgery used to remove a large tumor burden, which will reduce the quantity of cancer cells. Then other therapies are used on the remaining tumor burden. Occasionally, prophylactic surgery will be performed on diseased organs that are known to have a high incidence of developing a subsequent cancer.

Salvage Treatment

Salvage treatment is an extensive surgical approach that is used when there has been local recurrence since prior surgery. An example of this technique would be mastectomy after breast conservation done by lumpectomy and radiation therapy (Virshup, 2010).

Palliative Treatment

Palliative surgery is a useful therapy for patients with advanced cancer. The purposes of a palliative surgical procedure are to reduce or prevent disease- or treatment-related symptoms and to alleviate suffering when a cure is not possible or when the patient has decided to forgo other treatments. Before recommending palliative surgery, the surgeon will consider the rate of tumor growth, the person's projected life expectancy, and the expected treatment outcomes.

Combination Treatment

Combination treatment involves several different treatment modalities to minimize the change in the patient's appearance and functional ability. When chemotherapy, radiation therapy, or biotherapy is used during the preoperative, intraoperative, or postoperative periods, tumor resectability as well as the overall treatment outcomes may improve (Virshup, 2010).

Reconstructive Treatment

Patients who undergo surgical procedures that leave a deficit in function or appearance may be candidates for reconstructive surgery. The goal of this treatment option is to improve function or obtain a more acceptable cosmetic effect. Discussions about possible reconstructive surgery will occur before the primary surgery so that the patient can make a fully informed decision. Cancers of the breast, skin, and head and neck are the most common cancers for which reconstructive surgery is indicated (Virshup, 2010).

Preoperative Care

Planning care for the surgical oncology patient should be considered comparable to planning the nursing care for any surgical patient. However, an awareness of the problems and complications exclusive to patients who have been diagnosed with cancer is essential so that the nurse can provide compassionate holistic care. The health care team will assess the patient's emotional and physical status to predict how well the patient will tolerate surgery and the recovery period. The patient's functional status may be evaluated by using several validated

LABORATORY AND DIAGNOSTIC TESTS for Cancer

Test, Normal Values, and Rationale for Abnormality	Expected Abnormality
Sodium Adult:135–145 mEq/L **Potassium** Adult: 3.5–5.3 mEq/L	Elevated/lowered sodium, elevated potassium, elevated creatinine and blood urea nitrogen (BUN), elevated liver function tests. Assess for abnormality of liver, kidney, or bone related to malignancy or treatment.
BUN Adult: 5–25 mg/dL *Can be slightly higher in older adults.* **BUN: Creatinine Ratio** Adult: 10:1 to 20:1	Urea is formed as an end product of protein metabolism and is excreted by the kidneys. An elevated BUN can indicate pre-renal failure, renal failure, or dehydration.
LIVER ENZYME TESTS **Alkaline Phosphatase** Adult: 42–136 WI **Alkaline Aminotransferase** Adult: 10–35 UL **Lactate Dehydrogenase** Adult: 100–190 IU/L **Gamma-Glutamyl Transferase/**Transpeptidase Adult: Male: 4–23 IU/L Female: 3–13 IU/L	Elevation in liver of enzymes can indicate a liver tumor. It can also be an indication of damage from chemotherapy.
COMPLETE BLOOD COUNT (CBC) **White Blood Cells Total (WBC)** Adult: 4,500–10,000 μL (mm^3) **White blood cell differential:** **Neutrophils** Adult: 50–70 **Segments** Adult: 50–65 **Bands** Adults: 0–5 **Hemoglobin** Adult: Male: 13.5–18 g/dL Female: 12–15 g/dL **Platelet Count** Adult: 150,000–400,000	Lowered WBC, platelets, RBC, Hgb, and Hct. May have elevated WBC with leukemia.
Hemoccult Test Positive (blue color) result indicates the need for further diagnostic studies.	Assess for the presence of blood in stool for screening purposes.
Bone Marrow Biopsy (aspiration) Adult: WBC, RBC, Glucose	Assess for hematologic abnormalities. Abnormal numbers, size, and shape of WBCs, RBCs, and megakaryocytes.
Pap Smear Negative	Assess for premalignant changes and cervical cancer. Abnormal-appearing cervical cells, precancerous or malignant.

(*continued*)

LABORATORY AND DIAGNOSTIC TESTS for Cancer, *continued*

Test, Normal Values, and Rationale for Abnormality	Expected Abnormality
Urine Protein Immunoelectrophoresis	
Normal urine protein: 2–8 mg/dL	Assess urine protein and immunoglobulin levels seen in multiple myeloma. Increased levels of heavy-chain M proteins (Bence-Jones proteins).
Serum Protein Immunoelectrophoresis	
No monoclonal antibodies are detected. *Cells related to these types of cancer produce a type of protein called a monoclonal immunoglobulin, which can be detected with this test. However, some people have monoclonal immunoglobulins but do not have cancer. This is called monoclonal gammopathy of unknown significance (MGUS) (Dugdale, 2011b).*	Assess serum protein and immunoglobulin levels seen in multiple myeloma. Increased levels of heavy-chain M proteins. Abnormal results may be due to certain types of cancer such as multiple myeloma or chronic lymphocytic leukemia.
Urine Catecholamines	
All of the catecholamines are broken down into inactive substances that appear in the urine: Dopamine becomes homovanillic acid (HVA). Norepinephrine becomes normetanephrine and vanillylmandelic acid (VMA). Epinephrine becomes metanephrine and VMA. The following normal values are the amount of the substance found in the urine over a 24-hour period: Dopamine: 65–400 micrograms (mcg)/24 hours Epinephrine: 0.5–20 mcg/24 hours Metanephrine: 24–96 mcg/24 hours (some laboratories give the range as 140–785 mcg/24 hours) Norepinephrine: 15–80 mcg/24 hours Normetanephrine: 75–375 mcg/24 hours Total urine catecholamines: <100 mcg/24 hours VMA: 2–7 milligrams (mg)/24 hours (Dugdale, 2011a).	Assess for neuroblastoma and pheochromocytoma. Increased levels of epinephrine, norepinephrine, metanephrine, and vanillylmandelic acid.
CA125 (antigen, tumor marker)	
< 35 units/mL	Assess response to treatment in ovarian, pancreatic, breast, colon, lung, and liver cancer. Elevated in ovarian cancer and nonmalignant conditions that cause inflammation of the pleura (e.g., endometriosis, pelvic inflammatory disease [PID], pancreatitis).
CA19-9 (tumor marker)	
37 units/mL	Assess the response to treatment in pancreatic, colorectal, and gastric cancer. Elevated in colorectal, pancreatic, stomach, and bile duct cancer.
PSA (prostate-specific antigen, tumor marker)	
Less than 5.0 ng/mL	Assess the response to treatment of prostate cancer. Also used for screening at-risk persons. Elevated in prostate cancer and benign prostate enlargement.
CEA (carcinoembryonic antigen, tumor marker)	
Smokers: <4.0 ng/mL Nonsmokers: <2.5 ng/mL	Assess the response to treatment of breast, colorectal, and lung cancer. Elevated in breast, GI tract, liver pancreas, cervix, bladder, testes, kidney, and lung cancer.
HCG (human chorionic gonadotropin, tumor marker)	
Negative	Assess the response to treatment of testicular and certain uterine cancers. Elevated in germ cell cancers (ovarian and testicular) and pregnancy.
AFP (α-fetoprotein)	
<15 ng/mL	Assess the response to treatment of testicular, liver, and certain ovarian cancers. Elevated in liver and germ cell cancer, benign liver disease, and pregnancy.
Lactate Dehydrogenase (LDH)	
Adult: 100–190 international unit/L	Most helpful in monitoring treatment effect. Elevated in most cancers.

LABORATORY AND DIAGNOSTIC TESTS for Cancer, *continued*

Test, Normal Values, and Rationale for Abnormality	Expected Abnormality
Neuron-Specific Enolase (NSE)	
Range: 5.4–12.9 ng/mL	Most helpful in small-cell lung cancer (SCLC) and neuroblastoma to assess response to treatment. Elevated in lung, thyroid, kidney, testicle, and pancreatic cancer, neuroblastoma, Wilms' tumor, and melanoma.
IMAGING STUDIES	
Least invasive diagnostic studies performed first.	
Radiographic: X-Ray, CT Scan, Mammogram, Barium Swallow/Enema.	Detects abnormal masses in abdomen, chest, pelvis, and breast.
Performed during initial diagnostic workup and to monitor effectiveness of treatment.	
Ultrasonic Studies	
Echoes of high-frequency sound waves to visualize internal structures are helpful in distinguishing between benign cysts and malignancies. Some techniques involve inserting an ultrasound wand into a body cavity (e.g., rectum) to visualize surrounding organs (e.g., prostate).	Used to detect tumors in peritoneal space, pelvis, abdomen, prostate, and breast.
Magnetic Resonance Imaging (MRI)	
Use of a magnetic field and radio-frequency waves to align hydrogen nuclei in tissues.	Detects tumors in the brain, chest, and abdomen.
Nuclear Medicine Scans	
Radioactive isotopes are injected or ingested and then traced to the tissues where the isotope is attracted. Monoclonal antibodies are occasionally used to tag antigens known to be associated with malignancies. Organs with disease frequently show signs of increased or abnormal uptake of the material.	Common organs evaluated include the brain, thyroid, and liver.
Positron Emission Tomography (PET)	
Normal: negative for tumors	Tumors have more rapid rates of glycolysis compared to the tissue of origin. Gamma camera tomography maps structures and identifies malignancies. Studies glucose metabolism in body tissues and differentiates the rates of tissue metabolism. Images are obtained by detection of positron emissions from radionuclides.
INVASIVE DIAGNOSTIC STUDIES	
Pathology	
Cells are obtained via surgical incision, biopsy, or cytologic examination techniques.	These cells are examined for malignancy and, if positive, are graded, which assists the health care provider in prescribing an appropriate plan of care.
Biopsy	
See above.	Detects the presence of abnormal tissue cells obtained from the site of suspicious growth.
Endoscopy	Hollow metal tubes equipped with a light are used to visualize body cavities for diagnostic and therapeutic purposes. These tubes, known as scopes, are instruments named for the body area they visualize. Direct visualization provides the health care provider with the opportunity to examine the anatomic location and obtain samples of tissue or secretions that can be used to diagnose malignancy.

Sources: Kee, J. L. (2010). *Laboratory and diagnostic tests.* Upper Saddle River, NJ: Pearson; McCance, K. (2010). Cancer epidemiology. In K. L. McCance & S. E. Huether (Eds.), *Pathophysiology: The biologic basis for disease in adults and children* (6th ed., pp. 360–395). St. Louis: Mosby Elsevier; Merkle, C. J. (2009). Neoplasia. In C. M. Porth & G. Matfin (Eds.), *Pathophysiology: Concepts of altered health status* (8th ed., pp. 156–196). Philadelphia: Wolters Kluwer/Lippincott Williams & Wilkins.

scales, such as the Karnofsky Performance Scale, the Eastern Cooperative Oncology Group (ECOG) scale, and the World Health Organization scale. Chart 57–9 explains the scoring indicators in the Karnofsky Performance Scale, which is one of the hallmark tools used in cancer treatment. These scales reflect the patient's ability to care for self and carry out normal activities. This information will assist the health care team in developing a comprehensive plan that will maximize the patient's recovery capability (Grant, 2010).

The presence of other medical problems, such as heart disease or lung disease, may complicate postoperative recovery. In addition, physical debilitation due to advanced disease or type of symptoms present requires special attention. Improving the patient's physical well-being

CHART 57–9 Karnofsky Performance Scale

100	Normal; no complaints; no evidence of disease
90	Ability to carry on normal activity; minor signs or symptoms of disease
80	Normal activity with effort; some signs or symptoms of disease
70	Ability to care for self; inability to do normal activity or do active work
60	Occasional assistance necessary, but able to care for most needs
50	Considerable assistance and frequent medical care necessary
40	Disabled; special care and assistance necessary
30	Severely disabled; indication for hospitalization although death not imminent
20	Very sick; hospitalization necessary; active supportive treatment necessary
10	Moribund; fatal processes progressing rapidly
0	Death

includes treating symptoms such as pain, malnutrition, fatigue, insomnia, depression, and headaches. Managing a patient's symptoms in the preoperative period will affect the patient's response to surgery and recovery. The nurse needs to identify comorbidities and other symptoms before surgery and individualize the postoperative plan of care as needed.

During the preoperative period, the nurse focuses on assessment and intervention by becoming more familiar with the patient's knowledge of and adaptation to her situation. The nurse who knows the purpose of the surgical procedure can better understand the patient's behaviors. For instance, behaviors of patients who were recently diagnosed with cancer are different from behaviors of patients with metastatic disease who undergo palliative surgery for relief from spinal cord compression. The nurse must understand what kind of surgery will be performed in order to plan for appropriate preoperative preparation such as bowel preparation or nutritional support. Knowing which procedure will be performed will also alert the nurse to the location and size of the surgical incision and what type of indwelling device may be needed during the postoperative period. With this information, the nurse can engage each patient in education that is customized for that patient's particular situation.

The diagnosis of cancer can have a dramatic impact on patients and their loved ones. Many feel hopeless, powerless, and depressed. Often patients will be apprehensive about the upcoming surgery, demonstrating anger, anxiety, and perhaps panic (Grant, 2010). The nurse develops a therapeutic relationship with the patient and family or significant others by maintaining an open, honest, and caring approach to communication. A trusting relationship can assist the patient in maintaining a realistic sense of hope.

Age and physical status play an important role in accepting the diagnosis of cancer and postoperative recovery and rehabilitation (Grant, 2010). Patients in early adulthood to middle age typically have more physical endurance; however, they may have many emotional concerns. This is the most productive time in their lives for their careers, education, child rearing, and sexual activity. Some patients may fear a loss of job security, financial independence, and reproductive ability. They may also fear disfigurement and have worries about role adjustment. Older patients may fear burdening their family, both physically and financially, and are faced with recognizing their own mortality. It is important for nurses to use a caring approach when listening to the patient's concerns and to support the patient with appropriate information and resources.

Nursing Management

Postoperative nursing care of the oncology patient varies according to the type of cancer, type of surgery performed, previous therapies, and comorbidities. A comprehensive plan of care encompasses the patient's physical and psychological needs. Such plans of care can be found in Chapters 17 through 19, where care of the surgical patient is discussed. The oncology nurse knows that patients have unique medical and emotional needs that require an understanding of the overall management of the cancer patient.

Radiation Therapy

Radiation therapy is the use of ionizing rays or particles to treat cancer. More than 50% of all patients with cancer will be treated with radiation therapy during the course of their illness. The use of radiation in the treatment of disease, or radiotherapy, has been used since 1895 when radium, radioactivity, and x-rays were discovered. In 1898, the first successful radiation therapy treatment for cancer was used. Unfortunately, a host of complications occurred owing to the delivery of large doses in a single treatment. During the early and mid-1900s, scientists studied the effects of radiation on tissues. Results of these studies were responsible for the inception of fractionalization, or dividing of the total dose of radiation into several small doses. During the 1950s, several discoveries aided the advancement of radiotherapy, including the use of vacuum tubes, which allow for higher energy to be delivered to deeper tissues, and linear accelerators, which provided deeper penetration with less scatter to normal tissues (Iwamoto, 2001).

Radiation is a localized treatment that can be used alone or in combination with other treatments such as chemotherapy and surgery. Prescribing radiation therapy in the treatment of cancer serves several purposes: (1) to make a curative attempt to eradicate the disease; (2) to control metastatic activity, allowing the patient relief of symptoms; (3) to prevent microscopic disease associated with specific primary tumors; and (4) to improve a patient's quality of life by relieving or reducing symptoms seen with advanced cancer (Virshup, 2010). Chart 57–10 illustrates the symptoms of advancing disease targeted by radiation therapy.

Ionizing radiation destroys the ability of cancer cells to multiply and grow. This is accomplished by delivering energy that is potent enough to break the chemical bonds in molecules, leading to cellular damage or death. The nucleolus of a cell is penetrated by the ionizing rays or particles and interacts with its water content to form hydroxyl (free) radicals. The cells' DNA is then damaged, which results in the disruption of chromosomal strands. Cellular death depends on the ability of the chromosomal damage that can or cannot be repaired (Virshup, 2010).

Therapeutic radiation includes electromagnetic and particulate radiation. Electromagnetic sources are x-rays and gamma rays (energy rays without mass). Machines are the delivery mechanism for x-rays; radioactive materials are responsible for emitting gamma rays. Electromagnetic sources penetrate deep into tissue layers before releasing their energy and causing cellular damage. Particulate radiation contains mass, which prohibits it from penetrating into deep tissue, but delivers energy into the cells close to the surface (Virshup, 2010).

The health care provider will determine the radiosensitivity of the cancer cells, or target tissue, before prescribing the course of radiation therapy. *Radiosensitivity* is the measurement of potential susceptibility of

CHART 57–10 Symptoms Relieved by Radiation Therapy

Symptom	Etiology
Hemorrhage	Primary tumor
Fatigue	
Weakness	
Pallor	
Lowered blood pressure (BP)	
Elevated heart rate (HR)	
Pain	Bone metastasis
Vascular obstruction	Primary tumor
Alterations in pulses	
Cool, discolored skin	
Gastrointestinal obstruction	Primary tumor
Abdominal pain	
Nausea and vomiting	
Absent bowel sounds	
Kidney and ureter obstruction	Primary tumor
Flank pain	
Lower abdominal pain	
Difficulty urinating	
Tracheal obstruction	Primary tumor
Dyspnea	
Reduced oxygen saturation	
Spinal cord compression	Primary tumor
Numbness, tingling	
Difficulty moving	
Neurological symptoms	Brain metastasis
Headache	
Seizures	
Impaired speech	

cells to ionize radiation and how rapidly destruction will occur. Rapidly dividing cells (e.g., mucosal cells), either benign or malignant, are more sensitive. Cells that are slow to divide or nondividing (e.g., muscles or neurons) are radioresistant (Virshup, 2010). Because all body tissue has a degree of radiosensitivity, nurses caring for patients with cancer must understand how various tumor types will respond to radiation therapy.

A health care provider who is trained in radiation oncology (radiation oncologist) will determine the maximum radiation dose possible that will not harm normal tissues surrounding the target area. Various factors are considered in calculating the dose for any given patient: the patient's age, tumor size and stage, evidence of metastasis, and overall prognosis if radiation therapy is used as part of the treatment plan (Virshup, 2010). The total dose of radiation is divided into smaller doses (fractionalization) and delivered daily for several weeks. The rationale for the fractionalization is to maximize malignant cell kill, which occurs when cells enter mitosis, and to minimize damage to surrounding tissue and allow for repair to begin.

Administration of Radiation Therapy

Radiotherapy can be delivered in several ways. Teletherapy (external-beam) requires the use of a machine at a predetermined distance from the body. Brachytherapy (internal radiation) is performed using a sealed radioactive source placed in or near the malignancy. Occasionally, radioactive materials are delivered systemically via the oral or intravenous route. The most common cancer treated in this manner is that of the thyroid.

External Radiation Therapy

External radiation therapy can be used alone or with surgery to enhance the patient's chance of survival. Typically, when radiation is used alone, it is with the intent of achieving cure. Cancers that are known to respond to radiation alone include cancers of the prostate, uterus, cervix, pelvis, skin, and oral cavity, as well as early Hodgkin's disease. When cancers of the brain, spinal cord, muscle, and bone are treated with radiation therapy (high doses), there is typically minimal effect; however, these patients are likely to develop unwanted side effects (e.g., local skin burns, loss of function). When radiation is used in combination with surgery, the goal is either cure or palliation of distressing symptoms. Cancers that can be cured with both therapies include head and neck, breast, uterus, bladder, testes, and bone cancers.

For patients who undergo both surgery and radiation and are anticipating a curative outcome, administration of radiation may be done before or after surgery. Advantages of preoperative radiation include decreasing the tumor size, which increases the likelihood of successful removal of the entire mass; obliteration of cancerous cells beyond the surgical field; and elimination of lymph nodes where malignancy could form. Nurses who care for patients receiving preoperative radiation therapy will need to pay special attention to wound healing because a side effect of radiotherapy is delay in normal tissue repair.

The delivery of postoperative radiation therapy is intended to eliminate residual tumor and subclinical disease. Although higher doses may be delivered, treatment is delayed until postoperative wound healing is finished.

Before beginning any radiation therapy, the patient will need to undergo the treatment-planning phase. The purpose of this phase is to ensure the best way to deliver the treatments needed. After a radiation oncologist examines the patient, localization of the tumor will begin. A simulator machine is used to localize the tumor, and the anatomic area that will receive radiation (port) is marked with either ink or permanent tattoos. Figure 57–3◆ illustrates a simulator used in the treatment-planning phase and a linear accelerator, which delivers the radiotherapy. Precise identification of the area that will receive the radiation is critical to minimize tissue damage. Other examination procedures, such as computed tomography (CT) scans, magnetic resonance imaging (MRI), intravenous pyelogram (IVP), or barium enemas, may be used depending on the area being treated (Virshup, 2010).

Ports, or their position, may be changed on different days to ensure the delivery of safe and optimal radiation therapy. During treatment, the patient may have to be placed in difficult and uncomfortable positions; however, immobilization is important for accurate delivery of radiation. Devices to assist with immobilization or positioning may be necessary and are made specifically for the individual patient. Figure 57–4◆ shows immobilizers used to assist with positioning. Certain patient populations, such as children and older adults, may require special molds, casts, boards, or belts to help them maintain proper positioning. The nurse educates patients that the planning phase may take several hours and encourages patients to request pain medication as needed to promote comfort.

Patients receiving external radiation therapy should expect to have treatments daily (weekends excluded) for several weeks. For patients receiving palliative radiotherapy, fewer treatments will be given at higher doses. The actual treatment takes approximately 5 minutes; however,

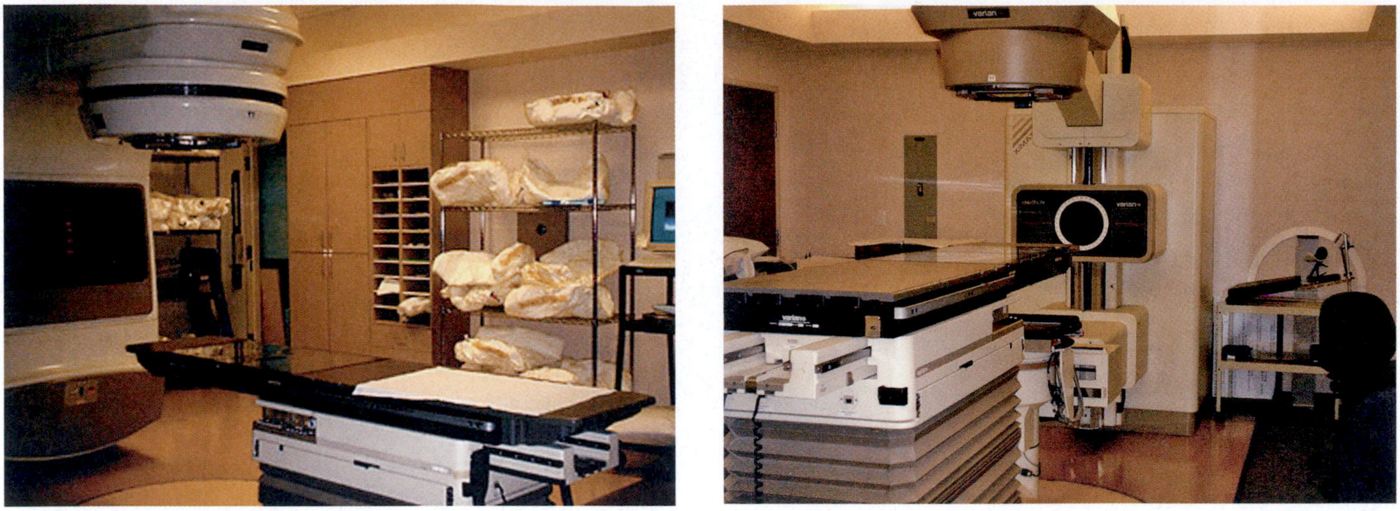

FIGURE 57–3 ◆ Accelerator and simulator for radiation therapy.
Source: Roseville Radiation Center.

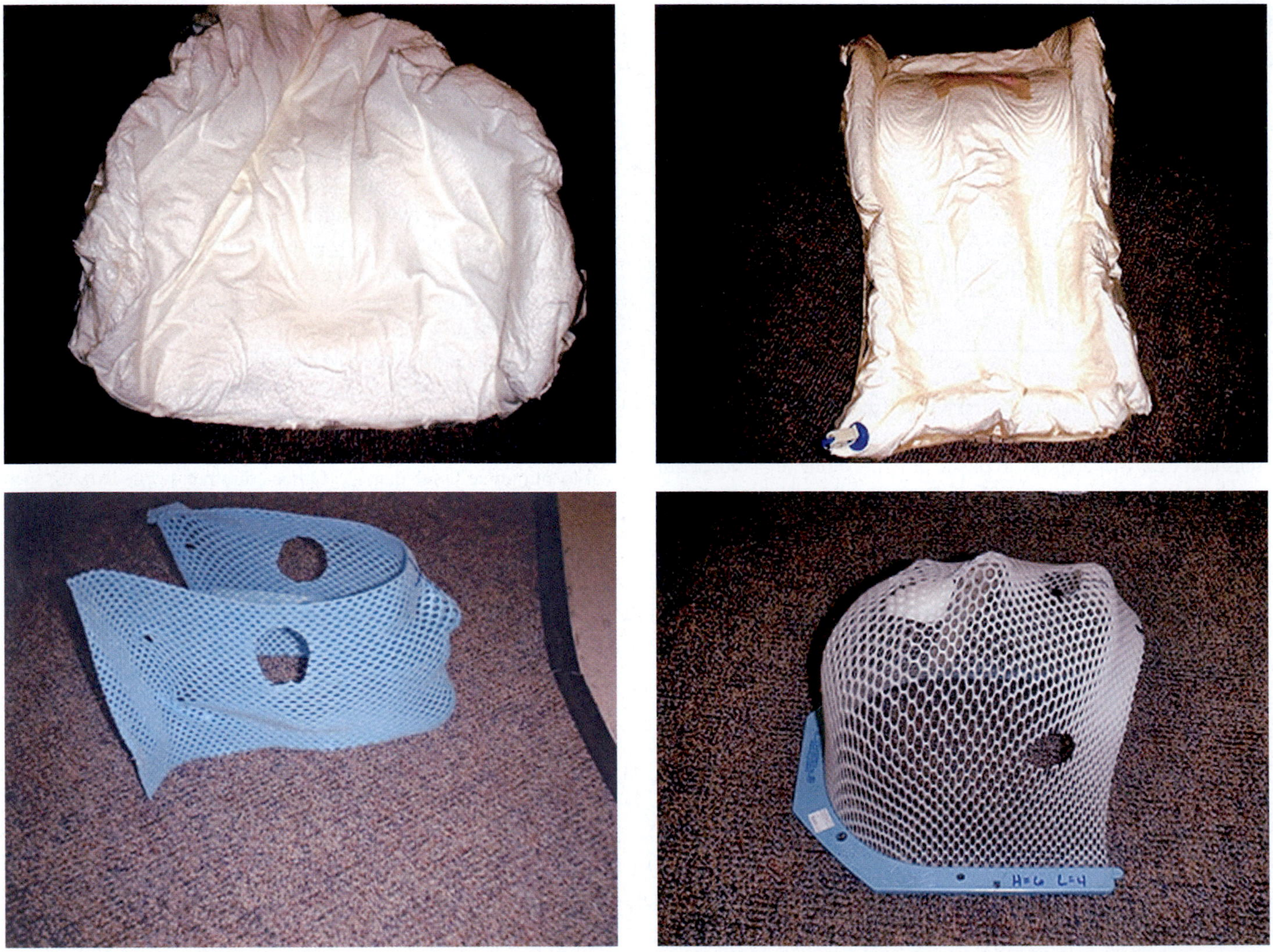

FIGURE 57–4 ◆ Immobilizers for radiation therapy.
Source: Roseville Radiation Center.

CHART 57–11 Unique Approaches in Radiation Therapy

Approach	Purpose
Intraoperative radiation therapy (IORT)	Control of local recurrence by directly visualizing and treating tumors.
Radiosensitizers	Medication used to enhance the effect of radiation.
Radiopharmaceuticals	Intravenous delivery of radioactive substances to treat pain from multiple osteoblastic bony metastases.
Stereotactic external-beam irradiation	Three-dimensional beam distribution, which provides high-dose treatment for small intracranial volumes. Treatment in other body areas is currently being done.

Source: Adapted from Virshup, D. M. (2010). Biology, clinical manifestations, and treatment of cancer. In K. L. McCance & S. E. Huether (Eds.), *Pathophysiology: The biologic basis for disease in adults and children* (6th ed., pp. 396–435). St. Louis: Mosby Elsevier.

more time is needed to properly position the patient. Total body irradiation is delivered to patients who have leukemia and are preparing for bone marrow transplantation, owing to the multiple areas that may be harboring leukemic cells.

Several unique approaches to external radiotherapy are being used for specific cancers. Chart 57–11 identifies the various approaches.

Photodynamic Therapy

An innovative approach to cancer treatment is photodynamic therapy (PDT) (Virshup, 2010). Photodynamic therapy uses light-sensitive molecules (photosensitizers) that form oxygen radicals after exposure to light. The radicals alter the DNA, cytoplasm, and cell membrane, resulting in cellular damage or death. Cancers of the skin, lung, esophagus, superficial bladder, and head and neck are currently the focus of this treatment. In addition, PDT has been used for purging bone marrow before autologous donor transplantation for leukemia and lymphoma (Virshup, 2010).

Porfimer sodium is the most commonly used photosensitizer. A laser treatment is given 48 hours after administration of the agent; tumor masses require 48 hours to acquire a sufficient quantity of the photosensitizer. Nurses caring for patients receiving PDT must be careful to educate patients and their families about the extreme photosensitivity caused by this agent and the precautions necessary to prevent skin damage from sources such as examination lights and sunlight.

Internal Radiation Therapy

Brachytherapy (internal radiation therapy) uses sealed radioactive sources (implants) that are placed into or on a tumor. The term *brachytherapy* means "near treatment." This approach allows for a high concentration of radiation to be delivered to a specific site in a short period of time. The major disadvantages are the need to access the tumor by invasive procedures and the skill required of the personnel who administer this particular therapy (Virshup, 2010). Brachytherapy may also be used in combination with external radiation therapy to enhance the overall effect on the tumor. Using this technique, a high dose of radiation can be delivered to a small malignant mass while very little is delivered to adjacent tissues. The therapy can be received over a period of several days using a low dose rate (LDR) or over a few minutes using a high dose rate (HDR) (Virshup, 2010). Cancers of the prostate, brain, tongue, lips, lung, breast, esophagus, vagina, cervix, endometrium, rectum, and bladder may be treated with brachytherapy.

Placement of implants into the body cavity or structure is done via special applicators. Radioactive material contained in applicators such as ribbons, wires, seeds, capsules, needles, or tubes is encapsulated to prevent body fluids from becoming contaminated. Placement occurs away from the nursing unit in the operating room, treatment room, or radiation department. After placement of the applicator, the patient returns to her hospital room, and the radioactive isotope is inserted. This approach, called afterloading, is used to minimize the unnecessary risk of exposing hospital employees to the radioactive material. The implant is left in place anywhere from a few hours to several days, during which the patient remains hospitalized and isolated.

The technique of HDR brachytherapy is another approach used to deliver radiotherapy. It involves positioning the applicator in the cavity of a tumor, then loading the applicator with pellets or tubes with a wire by remote control. The applicator is unloaded at the end of the treatment, which lasts minutes. Figure 57–5◆ illustrates the use of brachytherapy for prostate cancer. The HDR technique is done weekly for several weeks and does not necessitate hospitalization (Virshup, 2010).

Educating patients and their families about the implant, including the process, effects, and strategies to manage its effects, is an important role of the nurse. Before implantation, patients should be taught about symptom management, activity restrictions while the implant is in place, what causes current symptoms, and how the implant could change those symptoms. Once the implant is in place, patients need to be informed about when to notify the health care provider and potential side effects of the treatment, along with the customary management issues.

Radiation Precautions

Understanding the need to protect health care providers from the risk of injury is of extreme importance in caring for patients who receive radiation therapy. Adhering to radiation safety guidelines is necessary to minimize the risk of occupational radiation exposure. Placement of internal radiation sources should be done in specially designed rooms that prevent leakage of radioactivity. Individuals working in these areas must wear a personal monitor (e.g., a film badge) to measure their radiation dose. Badges contain photographic film and are worn on the topmost layer of clothing covering the front of the person's torso; they can be used to determine whether the person has received a cumulative amount of radiation that may put the person at risk. The exchange of badges among employees should never be done because such a practice prevents accurate determination of the amount of exposure. Each month badges are read for the amount of exposure, and a new one is provided to the employee (Mallick, 2009).

Planning is extremely important in caring for a patient who is exposed to radiation sources that emit gamma rays because these patients expose their caregivers over a varying period of time. Providers need to limit the time spent with these patients to prevent injury to themselves and others. Danger of exposure is reduced as the radioactive substance reaches its half-life (the point in time when radioactivity of a substance has decreased by half). Essential considerations in minimizing exposure to radiation are time, distance, and shielding. Chart 57–12 (p. 1788) explains these principles and related nursing responsibilities.

Nursing personnel have the opportunity to educate patients and their families about the precautions needed and to alleviate fears associated with radiation therapy. Nurses need to recognize their own fears or concerns before they can develop and implement an effective plan

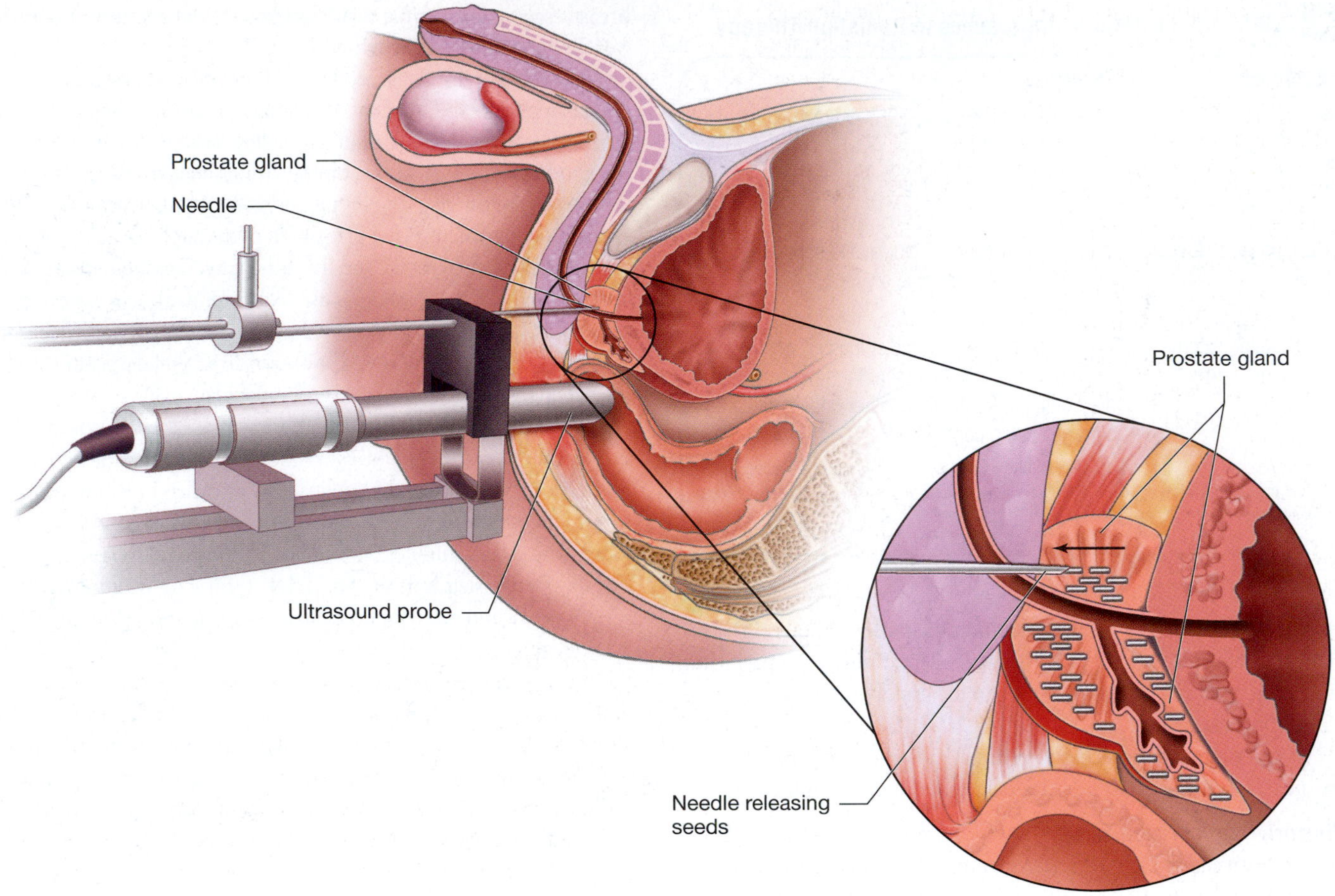

FIGURE 57–5 ◆ Brachytherapy applicator.

CHART 57–12 Principles for Minimizing Radiation Exposure

Principle	Nursing Responsibilities
Time:	Minimize time in proximity.
Exposure directly related to time spent within specific distance of source of radiation	Organize care activities; assemble supplies before entering room. Before leaving room, place patient care items within reach. Rotate staff assignments. Use 1/2 hour of patient contact per shift as a recommended guideline. Encourage patient self-care activities.
Distance:	Private room required.
Maximize distance from source	Perform duties as far away from source as possible.
Inverse square law: doubling the distance decreases exposure by one-fourth	Never touch a source; use long-handled forceps. Visit from the doorway if possible.
Shielding:	Place a shield at bedside if needed.
Type of shielding and its thickness depend on the type of source	Provide nursing care behind the shield. Do not use lead aprons used in x-ray departments.

Sources: King, C. A. (2011). Health care worker safety in surgery. *AORN Journal, 94*(5), 457–468; Klein, L. W. (2010). Occupational health hazards in the interventional laboratory. Time for a safe environment. *Journal of Radiology Nursing, 29*(2),75–82.

of care for their patients. Attending in-services or educational sessions about radiation safety practices combined with a skills laboratory for practicing appropriate patient care activities will help to clarify misconceptions and assist the nurse in providing comprehensive quality care. National and state regulations mandate the monitoring of radiation levels, which provides for a safe workplace (Sedhom & Yanni, 1985).

Radiation Side Effects

Nurses play an important role in assessing, planning, implementing, and evaluating outcomes used to prevent or minimize the side effects associated with radiotherapy. Collaborating with the radiation oncology team allows for an opportunity to provide continuity and quality patient care, which will maximize efforts aimed at relief of side effects.

Radiation therapy is a localized treatment that produces site-specific and general side effects that can be distressing to the patient and family.

Side effects experienced by most radiation therapy patients include skin changes, loss of appetite, fatigue, and bone marrow suppression. Radiation alters capillary blood flow, leading to detectable skin changes. Skin reactions may occur within 2 weeks of beginning treatment. Erythema may be noted, ranging from mild, light pink to deep and dusky red (Mallick, 2009; Virshup, 2010). Desquamation, first dry then moist, may occur in some patients. Moist desquamation is known to cause the epidermal layers of the skin to slough, leaving an area that is raw, painful, and draining serous exudate. Patients who have skinfolds, particularly in the axilla or groin, are more likely to develop skin reactions that progress to moist desquamation. These patients need education focused on maintaining good hygiene and understanding when to alert their health care provider for signs of skin infection.

Safety Alert *The nurse needs to assess the patient's skin during the course of radiotherapy for signs of reactions (redness, erythema, and desquamation). The nurse must report signs of skin breakdown to the health care provider so that possible treatment can be initiated. If skin reactions are minimized, the patient will experience less suffering and fewer (if any) complications and will be more likely to continue with the therapy.*

Anorexia (loss of appetite) can be due to the cancer or to the prescribed treatment. Although it is not completely clear what causes anorexia, contributing factors include inactivity, medications, and altered ingestion and digestion of food. Another explanation for anorexia may be found in the release of tumor necrosis factor (TNF) and interleukin-1 (IL-1). These **cytokines** (regulatory proteins that are released by cells as part of the immune response), which have an appetite-suppressing effect, are released from macrophages while they are attempting to defeat a cancer. Loss of appetite usually peaks 4 weeks into treatment and subsides shortly after treatment ends. If anorexia persists, weight loss may occur, resulting in the development of fatigue. The Nursing Process: Patient Care Plan for Cancer box (p. 1790) lists detailed nursing interventions and expected outcomes related to anorexia.

Many patients who receive radiotherapy experience fatigue. The exact causative mechanism is unknown, although it is thought to be the result of tumor breakdown, which releases by-products into the bloodstream (Mallick, 2009; Virshup, 2010). Another explanation for the development of fatigue is the increase in basal metabolic rate consuming the body's energy stores. Fatigue typically begins during the third or fourth week of treatment and gradually wanes once the treatment has been completed (Mallick, 2009; Virshup, 2010). Several other symptoms resulting from the alteration in energy production compound the effect of fatigue on cancer patients. These include pain, anorexia, infection, dyspnea, anemia, and depression.

The loss of energy and the feeling of tiredness tend to be cumulative and have a significant impact on patients' quality of life. Patient education regarding the side effects of radiation begins before treatment and continues during and after completion of treatment. Teaching patients that side effects should be expected may decrease their fear that treatment is ineffective. It is important to design nursing care with energy conservation in mind. Clustering patient care activities together will allow for prolonged periods of rest for patients who are experiencing fatigue. Teaching patients and their caregivers these principles will assist the patient in coping with the fatigue when he is discharged home.

Bone marrow suppression occurs because of the prevalence of bone marrow being affected in nearly every treatment port. The common areas of suppression include pelvis, sternum, ribs, spine, metaphysis of long bones, and the skull (Virshup, 2010). The nursing care required is complex and challenging. Complete blood counts (CBCs) should be monitored at regular intervals during therapy or more frequently if concerning symptoms occur such as infection, bleeding, and fatigue. Providing patient and family education about precautions for neutropenia, thrombocytopenia, and anemia is essential and frequently requires reinforcement throughout the radiotherapy course.

The nurse plays a valuable role in helping the patient cope with side effects produced by radiotherapy. It also is important to recognize how the side effects will affect the patient's quality of life and that socializing may be difficult if not impossible. Many side effects are specific to the area where radiation is delivered. Site-specific side effects are found in Chart 57–13.

Nursing Management

A comprehensive plan of care will encompass the patient's physical and psychological needs. The Nursing Process: Patient Care Plan for Cancer box identifies the appropriate nursing diagnosis and provides a detailed plan of care for the oncology patient. The nursing management sections for patients receiving chemotherapy and biotherapy provide details pertinent to patients who are receiving cancer-related treatments, including radiation therapy.

CHART 57–13 Site-Specific Side Effects of Radiation Therapy

Site	Side Effects
Head and neck	Stomatitis (irritation of the oral mucosa): • *Mild:* generalized erythema, few ulcerations, and small white patches • *Severe:* convergent ulcerations with bleeding and white patches covering > 25% of oral cavity
	Xerostomia (dryness of the mouth)
	Tooth decay and caries
	Osteoradionecrosis
	Hypopituitarism
	Taste changes
Chest	Esophagitis
	Cough
	Radiation pneumonitis
	Lung fibrosis
Abdomen	Gastritis
	Nausea and vomiting
Pelvis	Diarrhea
	Cystitis
	Erectile dysfunction
	Vaginal stenosis
	Ovarian failure
	Cessation of spermatogenesis
Brain	Cerebral edema
	Alopecia
	Changes in hair texture and color

NURSING PROCESS: Patient Care Plan for Cancer

Assessment of the Patient With Cancer Using Gordon's Functional Health Patterns:

- Health Perception Health Management Pattern
- Nutrition Metabolic Pattern
- Elimination Pattern
- Activity Exercise Pattern
- Cognitive Perceptual Pattern
- Self-Perception Self-Concept Pattern
- Sexuality-Reproductive
- Coping-Stress Tolerance Pattern

Subjective Data

Assessment of Infection

Have you had fevers, chills, or body aches?
Have you noticed drainage from your skin?
Have you noticed changes in your urine odor?
Have you experienced painful urination?

Assessment of Tissue Perfusion and Cardiac Output

Are you feeling breathless with minimal exertion?
Are you having chest discomfort?
Have you noticed weight gain or swelling?
Have you experienced feeling cold?

Assessment of Gas Exchange and Airway Clearance

Are you able to do your normal activities without breathlessness or fatigue?
Have you noticed a congested sounding cough? If so, describe your sputum.

Assessment of Bleeding

Have you noticed unusual bruising?
Have you noticed any blood in your urine or stools?
Have you noticed any bleeding from your mouth or gums?
Have you experienced dizziness or light-headedness?

Assessment of Fluid Volume Status

How frequent (if any) are your diarrhea episodes?
Are you able to drink fluids?
Do you feel dizzy or light-headed when you change positions?
Are there any remedies that have helped?
Have you noticed an increase in your weight?
Do you become breathless?

Assessment of Skin Integrity and Oral Mucous Membranes

Have you noticed pain in your mouth?
Have you noticed sores in your mouth?
Have you noticed areas of skin breakdown?
Have you noticed hair loss?
Do you have pain, drainage, or swelling in areas of skin breakdown?

Assessment of Fatigue

Do you feel unusually tired?
Do you perform your normal activities?
Do you have difficulty performing your normal activities?
How many hours per night do you sleep?
How is your appetite?
Do you have help at home?

Objective Data

Assessment of Infection

Signs of infection (e.g., dysuria, foul-smelling urine, elevated temperature, exudate from skin breakdown, elevated white blood cell [WBC] count)

Assessment of Tissue Perfusion and Cardiac Output

Poor-quality pulses
Weight gain and edema
Increased respiratory rate
Presence of crackles in lungs

Assessment of Gas Exchange and Airway Clearance

Abnormal arterial blood gases (ABGs) and oxygen saturation
Abnormal lung sounds, rate and depth of respirations
Changes in amount and characteristics of sputum
Changes in mental status

Assessment of Bleeding

Blood studies (platelets, hemoglobin, and hematocrit) results are lowered
Oozing from venipunctures
Unusual amount of bruising
Bleeding gums after oral hygiene
Hematuria and guaiac-positive stools
Change in mental status or behavior
Change in vital signs

Assessment of Fluid Volume Status

Poor skin turgor, dry mucous membranes
Elevated heart rate with position changes
Output exceeds intake
Multiple diarrhea episodes
Presence of edema and weight gain
Crackles in lungs

Assessment of Skin Integrity and Oral Mucous Membranes

Presence of mouth sores
Reports of pain in mouth while drinking citrus juices
Poor oral intake
Presence of skin breakdown and hair loss
Presence of skin redness
Signs of pain or infection

Assessment of Fatigue

Monitor hemoglobin, hematocrit, RBCs, and electrolytes
Monitor for adequate nutritional intake
Monitor for presence of pain or edema
Monitor energy expenditure

NURSING PROCESS: Patient Care Plan for Cancer, *continued*

Assessment of Nutrition How has your appetite been? Have you lost weight? Have you been able to perform your normal activities?	**Assessment of Nutrition** Weight loss Decreased albumin and prealbumin levels Poor dietary intake per calorie count and clinical nutrition consult
Assessment of Pain Are you experiencing pain? If so, describe where the pain is located, what it feels like, if it radiates anywhere else, and what makes it better or worse. Rate pain on scale of 0–10.	**Assessment of Pain** Unwilling to participate in care Facial grimacing Guarding or protecting of painful site Using increasing doses of pain medication
Assessment of Body Image Disturbance What feelings do you have about the change in your appearance? Have you been participating in your care and normal activities? Have you been socializing?	**Assessment of Body Image Disturbance** Isolating behaviors Avoidance Not involved with personal care
Assessment of Urinary Elimination Do you have difficulty urinating? What is the color of your urine? Do you have pain upon urination? What is your typical fluid intake throughout the day?	**Assessment of Urinary Elimination** Presence of hematuria Foul-smelling urine Presence of fever Complaints of pain with urination
Assessment for Impaired Swallowing Have you had difficulty swallowing? Do you have pain with swallowing?	**Assessment for Impaired Swallowing** Reports of pain with swallowing Inability to swallow bolus of food or fluids Refusing food or fluids
Assessment of Sexual Dysfunction Are you satisfied with your sexual functioning? Are you experiencing difficulty with sexual function?	**Assessment of Sexual Dysfunction** Minimal communication between patient and partner Lack of touching and closeness between patient and partner
Assessment of Growth and Development Parents report delayed progress in school. Appears to be of short stature.	**Assessment of Growth and Development** Height and weight lower than normal Motor abilities abnormal Cognitive testing abnormal
Assessment of Coping Do you feel saddened? Have you been withdrawing from your normal activities and routines? Have you been sleeping well? If not, why? Do you have a support system that comforts you?	**Assessment of Coping** Withdrawn behavior Unwilling to participate in care Insomnia Frequent episodes of crying, anger, aggressive behavior
Assessment of Knowledge What have you been told about your disease and treatment? How would you manage side effects of treatment? What symptoms would you contact your health care provider for?	**Assessment of Knowledge** Assess understanding of diagnosis and recommended treatments Assess understanding of potential side effects and related remedies

Outcomes and Evaluation Parameters	Planning and Interventions with *Rationales*
1. NURSING DIAGNOSIS: Risk for Infection ***related to skin reactions, skin breakdown, multiple invasive lines, and myelosuppression*** **(NANDA-I © 2012)**	
Outcome: No evidence of infection. ***Evaluation Parameters:*** Skin integrity is maintained. Urine appearance is clear, yellow, and possesses no foul odor. Invasive line sites are free from signs of infection. Patient demonstrates appropriate self-care behaviors.	Perform hand hygiene before and after working with patient. *Prevents spread of infection.* Monitor and record vital signs. *Elevated temperature and heart rate may indicate infection.* Assess for signs of infection and notify health care provider immediately: • Increased WBCs • Changes in temperature; > 101°F (38.3°C)

(*continued*)

NURSING PROCESS: Patient Care Plan for Cancer, *continued*

Outcomes and Evaluation Parameters	Planning and Interventions with *Rationales*
	• Presence of chills, diaphoresis • Presence of myalgias • Cough, with or without sputum • Purulent drainage from site of skin reactions, intravenous site, or invasive line sites • Pain with urination, frequency with urination, foul-smelling urine • Mental status changes • Diarrhea. *Identifies need for prompt treatment.* Obtain cultures and sensitivities before administering antibiotic therapy. *Identifies organism responsible for infection, which directs appropriate treatment.* Administer antibiotics, antifungals, and antivirals as prescribed. Note the presence of drug allergy. *Treatment of infection and prevention of drug reaction.* Initiate measures to reduce infection: • Ensure a private room if absolute neutrophil count (ANC) $< 1{,}000/mm^3$. • Avoid contact with those who have known or recent infection or recent vaccination. • Maintain strict hand hygiene. • Avoid rectal or vaginal procedures (temperatures, examinations, medications). • Administer stool softeners to prevent straining. • Maintain meticulous hygiene. • Avoid use of straight-edge razor. • Avoid raw meat and fish, fresh fruit and vegetables, fresh flowers and plants. • Provide clean liquids daily (e.g., denture cleaning solution, respiratory equipment fluid, drinking water). • Change solutions per protocol. • Avoid intramuscular injections. • Use strict aseptic technique when inserting medical devices (e.g., urinary catheters). *Infection control practice.* Instruct the patient and family about infection prevention measures. *Reduces the risk of infection and encourages good infection control practices.*
2. NURSING DIAGNOSIS: Ineffective Tissue Perfusion *and* Decreased Cardiac Output *related to chemotherapy-induced cardiac toxicity and capillary leak syndrome* (NANDA-I © 2012)	
Outcome: Normal tissue perfusion and cardiac output. ***Evaluation Parameters:*** Adequate peripheral perfusion as evidenced by: • Extremity pulses present by palpation and/or ultrasound • Capillary refill < 3 seconds in distal extremities • Color and temperature normal to extremities. Adequate urinary output evidenced by at least 30 mL/hr. Normal neurological function. No evidence of heart failure.	Evaluate baseline cardiac studies (e.g., echocardiogram, ECG, MUGA scan). *Provides baseline cardiac function to allow for future comparison.* Calculate and document cumulative dose of chemotherapeutic agents, if appropriate. *Provides ongoing information regarding maximum lifetime dosage.* Assess for signs of congestive heart failure and report to the health care provider: • Dyspnea • Tachycardia • Distended neck veins • Pedal edema • Crackles • Nonproductive cough • Extra heart tones (S_3) • Hepatomegaly. *Allows for prompt treatment.*

NURSING PROCESS: Patient Care Plan for Cancer, *continued*

Monitor vital signs for changes and report them to the health care provider, such as:

- Tachycardia
- Tachypnea
- Hypotension or hypertension.

Allows for prompt treatment.

Assess for syncope, dizziness, and weakness. *Indicates inadequate perfusion.*

Monitor serum electrolytes. *Provides additional sources for alteration in cardiac function.*

Administer medications to support cardiac function (e.g., diuretics, inotropic agents, vasodilators, oxygen). *Maximizes cardiac function.*

Position flat or with legs elevated. *Maximizes blood return to heart.*

Encourage the patient to adhere to dietary modifications (e.g., fluid restriction, sodium restriction, no alcohol, no tobacco). *Maximize cardiac function.*

Instruct the patient and family that cardiac effects may be irreversible. *Allows for time to consider lifestyle changes.*

Collaborate with the oncologist to achieve reduced dosing of chemotherapy if ejection fraction is < 55%. *Minimizes exposure to toxic effect of antineoplastic agents.*

Monitor peripheral perfusion by assessing:

- Capillary refill (<3 seconds)
- Pulses present and strong throughout
- Skin dry, color pink, and temperature warm.

Provides information about the quality of circulation.

Monitor urinary output for normal (>30 mL/hr). Report abnormal findings to the health care provider. *Indicates adequate renal perfusion and allows for prompt treatment if necessary.*

Monitor neurological status and report abnormalities to the health care provider. *Indicates possible perfusion abnormalities and need for prompt intervention.*

3. NURSING DIAGNOSIS: Risk for Impaired Gas Exchange *and* Ineffective Airway Clearance *related to chemotherapy, biotherapy, and transplant-induced pulmonary toxicity* (NANDA-I © 2012)

Outcome: Adequate gas exchange and airway clearance.

Evaluation Parameters: Normal ABGs.

No dyspnea: unlabored respirations < 24/minute.

Normal neurological status.

Normal breath sounds.

No signs of impaired tissue oxygenation.

Oxygen saturation is within normal limits.

Assess for adventitious or diminished breath sounds. *Indicates decreased gas exchange.*

Note depth, rate, rhythm, and effort of respiration. *Assesses for respiratory distress or increased work of breathing.*

Note the presence of cough, amount, color, and consistency of sputum. *Assesses for development of respiratory infections or pulmonary edema.*

Monitor ABGs and oxygen saturation via pulse oximetry. *Determines adequacy of gas exchange.*

Monitor restlessness and confusion. *Indicators of inadequate gas exchange with resultant brain hypoxia.*

Assess skin and mucous membranes for color (dusky, ashen, or cyanotic). *Indicators of tissue hypoxia and need for prompt intervention.*

Instruct patient to cough and deep breathe. *Increases gas exchange.*

Administer humidified oxygen therapy as prescribed. *Promotes airway clearance.*

Monitor for complaints of chest pain and report to the health care provider. *May indicate an acute pulmonary event such as pulmonary embolism, pleural effusion, or pneumothorax.*

Instruct the patient and family about symptoms of pulmonary toxicity and to report findings to the health care provider. *Allows for prompt intervention.*

Instruct the patient and family regarding the possibility of irreversible pulmonary effects. *Allows the patient to consider initiating lifestyle changes consistent with pulmonary function.*

(*continued*)

NURSING PROCESS: Patient Care Plan for Cancer, *continued*

Outcomes and Evaluation Parameters	Planning and Interventions with *Rationales*
4. NURSING DIAGNOSIS: Potential for Deficient Fluid Volume ***related to bone marrow suppression, hepatotoxicity, hepatic veno-occlusive disease (VOD), and hematologic laboratory abnormality induced by cancer treatments*** **(NANDA-I © 2012)**	
Outcome: No evidence of bleeding. ***Evaluation Parameters:*** Platelet count will be within normal limits. Hemoglobin and hematocrit will be within normal limits. Hemodynamic status will be maintained. Patient will demonstrate appropriate self-care behaviors.	Monitor platelet counts and report a count of $< 50{,}000/\text{mm}^3$ to the health care provider. *Identifies the need for prompt treatment.* Monitor liver function tests and coagulation studies. *Identifies the need for prompt treatment.* Assess for bleeding and report findings to the appropriate health care provider: • Decrease in hemoglobin and hematocrit • Prolonged bleeding or oozing from invasive procedures, venipunctures, cuts, or scratches • Presence of petechiae or ecchymosis • Presence of frank or occult blood in emesis, stool, or sputum • Presence of blood from any body orifice • Change in mental status • Change in vital signs (e.g., heart rate, BP) • Skin color pale, temperature cool. *Early detection aids in early treatment.* Perform venipunctures once daily for all laboratory tests. *Minimizes the risk of bleeding.* Avoid taking rectal temperatures; avoid use of suppositories or enemas. *Minimizes the risk of bleeding.* Apply direct pressure to injection and venipuncture sites for a minimum of 5 minutes. *Minimizes bleeding.* Instruct the patient regarding ways to minimize the risk of bleeding: • Perform oral hygiene with a soft toothbrush or toothettes. • Avoid use of commercial mouthwashes. • Avoid straight-edge razors. • File nails with an emery board. • Avoid foods that are difficult to chew. *Provides for appropriate self-care behaviors.*
5. NURSING DIAGNOSES: (a) Risk for Deficient Fluid Volume ***related to nausea, vomiting, diarrhea (due to pelvic radiation & cancer), hepatic VOD, and capillary leak syndrome.*** **(b) Risk for Excess Fluid Volume** ***related to hepatic VOD*** **(NANDA-I © 2012)**	
Outcomes: Adequate hydration. Absence of skin breakdown. Normal electrolytes. ***Evaluation Parameters:*** Normal serum electrolytes. Skin surrounding anus remains intact. Cessation of diarrhea episodes. No evidence of dehydration or fluid overload. Absence of skin breakdown. Normal electrolytes.	Assess bowel pattern. *Determines baseline.* Record frequency of diarrhea and vomiting episodes. *Indicates degree of fluid loss.* Establish and maintain IV access. *Allows for fluid volume replacement if needed.* Administer IV fluids per protocol. *Determines the need for fluid administration to prevent dehydration or the need to restrict fluids to prevent fluid overload.* Record accurate intake and output. *Determines adequacy of fluid volume replacement.* Monitor daily weights using the same scale and with the same clothing. *Indicates fluid retention or loss.* Monitor serum electrolyte values, hemoglobin and hematocrit, liver function tests, and coagulation studies and notify health care provider of critical abnormalities. *To monitor hematologic changes associated with fluid changes.* Monitor for presence of edema. *Indicates fluid retention.* Measure abdominal girth daily and apply landmark indicators to abdomen. *Indicates presence of accumulating ascites and allows for accuracy and consistency in measurements.* Restrict sodium and water intake. *Prevents fluid retention in extracellular spaces.*

NURSING PROCESS: Patient Care Plan for Cancer, *continued*

Monitor lung sounds. *Evaluates for fluid accumulation in lung, which may require prompt treatment.*

Place the patient in a semi-Fowler's position to avoid the patient lying flat. *Allows for optimal ventilation in the presence of ascites.*

Assess for excoriation of skin surrounding the anus. *Identifies the need for interventions.*

Instruct the patient to cleanse the area frequently. *Prevents skin breakdown.*

Instruct the patient to notify the health care provider if skin breakdown occurs. *Allows for prompt treatment.*

Administer antidiarrhea medication per protocol. *Reduces frequency of diarrhea episodes.*

Instruct the patient to use a low-residue diet and limit fat content. *Reduces the amount of diarrhea.*

6. NURSING DIAGNOSIS: Impaired Skin Integrity *related to alopecia, stomatitis, xerostomia, skin reactions due to radiation therapy, invasive procedures and lines, biotherapy-induced dry desquamation, rashes, pruritus, edema, cancer diagnosis, and treatment* (NANDA-I © 2012)

Outcomes: Maintain or restore skin integrity.

Cope with hair loss.

Mucous membranes are intact.

Evaluation Parameters: Minimal skin changes noted.

Appropriate self-care behaviors are demonstrated.

Skin infections are absent.

Social interaction is maintained.

Intact oral mucous membranes are maintained.

Nutritional status is maintained.

Patient is not suffering.

Skin integrity is maintained or restored.

Inspect the oral cavity daily. *Provides information needed to determine if the treatment is necessary.*

Instruct the patient regarding proper oral care:

- Brush and floss teeth as tolerated.
- Use moistening gauze or toothettes instead of a toothbrush if needed; for instance, if platelet count is low ($<40{,}000/mm^3$).
- Rinse with normal saline four times per day.
- Avoid commercial mouthwashes.
- Cleanse mouth before and after meals.

Prevents trauma and maintains oral hygiene.

Administer cytoprotectives as ordered (e.g., Ethyol). *Promotes comfort and reduces incidence of mucous membrane breakdown.*

Provide bland and soft diet. *Allows for ease of chewing and swallowing and reduces discomfort.*

Administer saliva substitutes and moisten food as needed. *Allows for ease of swallowing.*

Instruct the patient to report signs of stomatitis:

- Burning
- Pain
- Areas of redness
- Open lesions on the lips
- Pain with swallowing
- Intolerance to temperature extremes.

Identifies the beginning stages of mucous membrane breakdown and facilitates prompt treatment.

Assist in oral hygiene during mild stomatitis:

- Normal saline rinses every 2 hours, every 6 hours during sleep.
- Use soft toothbrush or toothette.
- Avoid use of dentures except for meals.
- Maintain proper fit of dentures.
- Moisten lips with lubricating ointment.
- Avoid eating foods that are spicy, those with temperature extremes, and those that are difficult to chew.

Promotes hygiene, minimizes trauma, and provides for comfort.

Assist in oral hygiene during severe stomatitis:

- Discontinue use of dentures.
- Rinse with prescribed agent or irrigate oral cavity with mixture of saline, anti-*Candida* agent (Mycostatin), and topical anesthetic agent.

(*continued*)

NURSING PROCESS: Patient Care Plan for Cancer, *continued*

Outcomes and Evaluation Parameters	Planning and Interventions with *Rationales*
	• Position the patient properly for irrigations. • Provide an oral suction device as needed for management of excessive secretions. • Use gauze or a toothette with irrigation solution for cleansing. • Lubricate lips. *Promotes hygiene and comfort.* Assess patient's ability to chew and swallow, and presence of gag reflex. *Identifies risk for aspiration.* Encourage use of pureed diet or liquid diet. *Promotes comfort and maintains nutrition.* Monitor for signs of infection and notify health care provider immediately. *Facilitates prompt treatment.* Obtain tissue cultures as needed. *Provides evidence of infection.* Administer analgesics, topical and systemic, as prescribed. *Promotes comfort.* Discuss patterns of hair loss and regrowth with patient and family. *Provides information so preparations for loss can begin and provides an understanding of the temporary nature of alopecia.* Encourage expression of concerns related to hair loss. *Facilitates coping.* Reduce or prevent hair loss: • Cut long hair before treatment. • Use mild shampoo and conditioner in small amounts. • Gently pat hair dry. • Avoid electric curlers, curling irons, dryers, clips, barrettes, hair sprays, hair dyes, or other hair chemicals. • Avoid excessive brushing or combing; use wide-tooth comb. • Use scalp tourniquets or hypothermia as appropriate. *Prevents hair loss as long as possible by decreasing the uptake of chemotherapy. Also maintains presence of hair as long as possible by reducing weight and manipulation.* Encourage the patient to avoid actions that traumatize the scalp: • Keep scalp lubricated to reduce itching (use vitamins A and D). • Use sunscreen or hat when exposed to ultraviolet rays. *Prevents breakdown of the skin.* Offer ways to cope with hair loss: • Obtain wigs or hairpieces before hair loss. • Take photograph of hair to wig shop to improve matching of hair color. • Contact the American Cancer Society for available resources. • Wear scarf, hat, or other head covering as needed. *Reduces changes in appearance.* Assess skin integrity. *Provides baseline information.* Instruct the patient regarding skin care of the area within the treatment field: • Cleanse with lukewarm water. • Avoid use of soap, powders, deodorants, and fragrances. • Avoid shaving. • Keep skinfolds dry and clean. • Use devices to protect the skin from sun, heat, and cold. • Avoid use of restrictive or tight-fitting clothing. • Avoid use of tape. • Avoid massaging, vigorous rubbing, or scratching. *Minimizes skin trauma and provides protection.*

NURSING PROCESS: Patient Care Plan for Cancer, *continued*

	Instruct the patient regarding skin care if dry desquamation occurs: • Cleanse with lukewarm water. • Avoid use of soap, powders, deodorants, cosmetics, ointments, and fragrances. • Avoid shaving. • Avoid rubbing or scratching. • Avoid hyperthermia or hypothermia treatments. • Avoid use of adhesive tapes. • Avoid exposure to sunlight or cold weather conditions. • Avoid use of restrictive clothing; use of cotton materials is preferred. • Apply hydrophilic moisturizing lotion or ointment two to three times per day (e.g., vitamins A and D ointment or Aquaphor). *Prevents further skin damage and drying and aids in healing.* Instruct the patient regarding skin care if moist desquamation occurs: • Notify the health care provider if blistering occurs. • Keep blisters intact. • Avoid frequent cleansing of the area. • Apply saline irrigations or cold compresses three to four times per day. • Apply dressings as prescribed (e.g., Vigilon). • Apply zinc oxide or silver sulfadiazine with nonstick dressing if radiation treatments are being held. • If area is draining, apply thin layer of gauze. *Provides for healing, decreases inflammation, and prevents infection.* Administer antihistamines per protocol. *Relieves itching associated with pruritus.* Apply cold towels to affected area. *Relieves itching associated with pruritus.* Instruct the patient to maintain room humidity between 30% and 40%. *Relieves itching associated with pruritus.*
7. NURSING DIAGNOSIS: Activity Intolerance *related to fatigue, bone marrow suppression, anorexia, and hepatotoxicity* (NANDA-I © 2012)	
Outcome: Able to perform activities of daily living (ADLs). ***Evaluation Parameters:*** Maintain ADLs and minimize fatigue. Serum laboratory studies within normal limits. Adequate energy levels are maintained. Patient shows no evidence of suffering or discomfort. Adequate diet with recommended calorie and protein intake is maintained.	Encourage frequent rest periods. *Energy is conserved and replenished.* Encourage more sleep hours at night. *Restores energy levels.* Encourage the patient to reorganize daily schedule of activities and seek assistance with shopping, cooking, housework, and so on. *To minimize energy expenditure.* Encourage a temporary decrease in work hours. *Decreases physical and psychological stress and provides for rest.* Assess nutritional intake for adequate protein and calorie intake. *Provides source of energy.* Administer blood products per protocol. *Provides adequate oxygen availability, which will decrease fatigue.* Monitor fluid and electrolyte balance. *Provides information regarding nerve transmission and muscle function.* Assess for sources of discomfort and suffering. *Minimizes energy expenditure.*
8. NURSING DIAGNOSIS: Imbalanced Nutrition: Less Than Body Requirements *related to chemotherapy and biotherapy-induced nausea, vomiting, hepatotoxicity, anorexia, and effects of pre- and post-transplant treatment* (NANDA-I © 2012)	
Outcome: Adequate nutritional status and maintenance of body weight. ***Evaluation Parameters:*** Patient experiences fewer episodes of nausea and vomiting. Adequate calorie intake maintained. Serum laboratory studies within normal limits. Adequate energy levels are maintained. Prescribed diet is tolerated.	Monitor accurate intake and output and record. *Indicates trends in intake pattern.* Perform nutritional assessment: • Calorie count • Ability to swallow

(*continued*)

NURSING PROCESS: Patient Care Plan for Cancer, *continued*

Outcomes and Evaluation Parameters	Planning and Interventions with *Rationales*
	• Food preferences • Patterns and behaviors related to eating • Ethnic and cultural preferences. *Indicates adequacy of nutrition.* Monitor serum albumin, prealbumin, glucose, magnesium, sodium, and iron. *Assesses adequacy of nutritional intake.* Assess for signs of malnutrition: • Muscle wasting • Edema • Changes in hair condition • Changes in skin. *Indicates adequacy of nutrition.* Consult nutritionist to determine appropriate needs for individual. *Assists in establishing or maintaining adequate nutrition.* Provide meticulous oral care. *Prevents infection and promotes appetite.* Administer antiemetics and appetite stimulants per orders. *Assists in improving appetite by reducing nausea and vomiting.* Encourage small frequent meals that are high in calories and protein. *Such meals are more suitable for digestion and better tolerated.* Encourage adequate fluid intake, while limiting fluids during mealtime. *Prevents the development of satiety.* Increase activity level as tolerated. *Activity stimulates the appetite.* Provide environment suitable for eating: • Pain free • Relaxed environment • Presentation of food tray. *To increase appetite.* Monitor tube feedings or IV total parenteral nutrition per protocol. *Determines tolerance of nutritional delivery system.* Administer cytoprotectives as ordered (e.g., Ethyol). *Promotes comfort and improved nutrition by preventing dry mouth.* Provide discharge teaching to patient and family regarding nutritional needs. *Maintains nutritional status at home.*
9. NURSING DIAGNOSIS: Pain *related to skin reactions, cough from chest radiation, chemotherapy-induced pancreatitis, chemotherapy- and biotherapy-induced peripheral neuropathy and bone pain, mucositis, invasive procedures, and disease process* (NANDA-I © 2012)	
Outcome: Pain is controlled. ***Evaluation Parameters:*** Patient verbalizes pain level and previous interventions that were successful in alleviating pain. Pain is reduced or absent as evidenced by patient denying presence or by nonverbal behaviors: no facial grimacing, restlessness, and so on. Patient reports complementary strategies of pain control are effective.	Assess pain using pain scale (0–10) to quantify pain level. *Provides consistency for evaluating pain.* Assess discomfort characteristics: • Location • Quality • Frequency • Duration • Alleviating therapies. *Provides baseline for assessing change.* Assess other factors contributing to pain: • Fear • Fatigue • Anger • Anxiety. *Provides data about factors that decrease the patient's tolerance to pain.*

NURSING PROCESS: Patient Care Plan for Cancer, *continued*

	Ensure adequate fluid intake. *Minimizes frequency and intensity of cough.* Instruct the patient to avoid irritants such as smoke. *Minimizes cough.* Instruct the patient regarding the use of humidification in the air. *Minimizes cough.* Administer analgesics according to protocol. *Provides pain relief.* Monitor for side effects of analgesics and treat accordingly. *Ensures tolerance of analgesics.* Encourage the use of a pureed diet or liquid diet. *Promotes comfort and maintains nutrition.* Monitor for signs of infection and notify the health care provider immediately. *Facilitates prompt treatment.* Administer analgesics before a procedure or treatment that may cause discomfort. *Controls increased pain level related to procedures and treatments.* Instruct the patient to notify the nurse when pain is not relieved or when pain begins to occur again. *Indicates the need for additional pain management therapies or the administration of analgesics earlier in the pain cycle.* Collaborate with the patient and the multidisciplinary team when changes in pain management are necessary. *Increases the patient's sense of control and allows for agreement and input from all team members.* Instruct the patient and family about complementary strategies to relieve pain and discomfort: • Guided imagery • Relaxation techniques • Distraction • Cutaneous stimulation. *Helps reduce anxiety and promotes relaxation.*
10. NURSING DIAGNOSIS: Disturbed Body Image ***related to skin reactions, alopecia, long-term venous access devices, decreased sexual function, role changes, and other cancer treatments*** **(NANDA-I © 2012)**	
Outcome: Social integration. Normal social interactions and acceptance of body image changes. ***Evaluation Parameters:*** Participates in self-care activities. Demonstrates interest in appearance. Resumes or continues interactions with others in established social network. Explores alternative ways of expressing concern and affection with partner.	Assess patient's feelings about body image and level of self-esteem. Validate concerns. *Provides baseline for evaluating changes and determining effectiveness of interventions.* Advocate for participation in activities and decision making. *Facilitates a sense of control.* Encourage patient to verbalize concerns. *Begins coping process.* Provide personalized care. *Prevents depersonalization.* Discuss patterns of hair loss and regrowth with patient and family. *Provides information so that preparations for loss can begin and provides an understanding of the temporary nature of alopecia.* Assist in self-care when fatigue, nausea, vomiting, or other distressing symptoms occur. *Improves self-esteem by ensuring physical well-being.* Help the patient in selecting cosmetic devices that increase the sense of attractiveness. *Promotes positive body image.* Offer ways to cope with hair loss: • Obtain wigs or hairpieces before hair loss. • Take photograph of hair to wig shop to improve matching of hair color. • Contact the American Cancer Society for available resources. • Wear scarf, hat, or other head covering as needed. *Reduces changes in appearance.* Encourage dialogue between the patient and partner regarding sexual function and alternatives. *Allows for affection and acceptance.*

(*continued*)

NURSING PROCESS: Patient Care Plan for Cancer, *continued*

Outcomes and Evaluation Parameters	Planning and Interventions with *Rationales*
11. NURSING DIAGNOSIS: Impaired Urinary Elimination *related to radiation therapy* (NANDA-I © 2012)	
Outcomes: Minimize cystitis. Able to urinate normally. ***Evaluation Parameters:*** Laboratory studies within normal limits. No evidence of discomfort or suffering. Adequate fluid intake maintained. Normal urinary patterns.	Assess for hematuria. *Indicates possible infection or cystitis.* Monitor fluid intake and encourage adequate intake. *Decreases incidence of cystitis.* Monitor for signs of urinary tract infection. *Promotes prompt treatment.* Obtain urine analysis and culture. *Evaluates for infection.* Assess for pain with urination. *Determines presence of symptoms needing further treatment.* Administer antibiotics, bladder analgesics, and antispasmodics as ordered. *To treat infection and pain.* Evaluate patient's understanding of cause of cystitis and measures to relieve symptoms. *Provides evidence of need for education.*
12. NURSING DIAGNOSIS: Risk for Impaired Swallowing *related to esophagitis or pharyngitis* (NANDA-I © 2012)	
Outcome: No difficulties with swallowing. ***Evaluation Parameters:*** Adequate nutritional status is maintained. Adequate pain management is maintained. Full course of radiation therapy is completed.	Instruct the patient to eat a soft, bland, or liquid diet that is high in protein and calories. *Facilitates swallowing and promotes adequate nutritional intake.* Administer anesthetic and coating mouth rinses before eating. *Relieves discomfort associated with swallowing.* Administer analgesics per protocol. *Relieves discomfort associated with swallowing and allows for patient to continue with therapy.*
13. NURSING DIAGNOSES: (a) Risk for Sexual Dysfunction *related to radiation therapy of the pelvis.* (b) Altered Sexuality Patterns *related to late effects of transplantation* (NANDA-I © 2012)	
Outcome: Maintains sexual functioning as desired. ***Evaluation Parameters:*** Patient and partner understand the rationale for treatment. Patient and partner maintain effective communication. Sexual functioning is improved.	Assess level of dysfunction via patient interview. *Determines baseline and need for interventions.* Encourage the patient to discuss concerns with partner. *Facilitates effective communication.* Facilitate consultation with urologist as needed, including patient education regarding rationale. *Provides treatment and education.* Monitor for symptoms that affect libido. *Allows for treatment and understanding of changes.* Assess for fear, anxiety, diminished self-image, and depression. *Indicates need for resources for coping.* Facilitate communication about sexual issues. *Promotes open communication between patient and partner.* Instruct the patient on hygiene and contraceptive measures. *Prevents infections and pregnancy.*
14. NURSING DIAGNOSIS: Delayed Growth and Development *related to late effects of transplantation in children* (NANDA-I © 2012)	
Outcome: Normalized growth and development. ***Evaluation Parameters:*** Growth patterns are normal according to standardized charts. Educational needs are being met. Identifies need to access support systems. Actively participates in recovery.	Monitor patient's growth according to standard charts. *Helps determine if growth patterns are impaired.* Evaluate normal growth and development behaviors consistent with patient's age. *Indicates need for possible treatment.* Monitor for learning disabilities. *Indicates need for special educational resources.* Administer growth hormone per protocol. *Assists in normalizing growth and development patterns.* Provide educational and emotional resources to the patient and family. *Improves coping and ability to function with deficits.*
15. NURSING DIAGNOSIS: Ineffective Coping *related to alopecia, fatigue, biotherapy-induced depression, anxiety, transplant process, role changes, lifestyle changes, diagnosis of cancer* (NANDA-I © 2012)	
Outcome: Patient will demonstrate effective coping skills. ***Evaluation Parameters:*** Demonstrates effective coping strategies for living with cancer. Identifies need to access support systems. Actively participates in recovery.	Assess the patient's and family's understanding of the diagnosis, recommended treatment, and prognosis. *Provides information about the need for further teaching if not consistent with actual diagnosis, treatment, or prognosis.* Encourage the patient to express feelings. *Effective coping strategy.*

NURSING PROCESS: Patient Care Plan for Cancer, *continued*

	Monitor aggressive behaviors. *May indicate ineffective coping.* Assess the patient's and family's support systems. *Indicates need for recommendations.* Consult psychiatrist, psychologist, or spiritual counselor. *Provides expertise that will evaluate for effective coping and make recommendations for assistance.* Encourage family to use memory prompts with patient for orientation in regard to time, date, and location. *Allows for reorientation and participation in care.*
16. NURSING DIAGNOSIS: Deficient Knowledge ***related to radiation therapy, chemotherapy, biotherapy side effects, and self-care needs*** **(NANDA-I © 2012)**	
Outcome: Understand the use of radiation therapy for cancer and the self-care behaviors necessary to manage side effects. ***Evaluation Parameters:*** Patient verbalizes an understanding of the purpose for therapy; side effects, and measures used to minimize side effects; and protective measures. Patient demonstrates appropriate self-care behaviors. Patient understands the use of biotherapy and chemotherapy for cancer and the self-care behaviors necessary to manage side effects. Patient understands the use of transplantation for cancer and the self-care behaviors necessary to manage side effects. Patient demonstrates appropriate self-care behaviors.	Assess the patient's expectations and concerns about therapy. *Determines baseline knowledge.* Instruct the patient and family about: • The purpose of using radiation therapy to treat cancer • Routines such as consultation, simulation, treatment schedules, routine appointments, and follow-up • Expected length of each visit • Appearance of equipment and environment. *Decreases anxiety associated with treatment.* Instruct the patient and family about the effects and side effects associated with radiation therapy. *Decreases anxiety associated with treatment.* Instruct the patient and family about measures used to minimize side effects. *Provides for less distress associated with treatment, which maximizes chance of patient continuing with therapy.* Instruct the patient and family about visiting restrictions and isolation requirements associated with internal radiation therapy. *Provides for an understanding of the need to protect others.* Instruct the patient and family about: • The purpose of using chemotherapy, biotherapy, and transplantation to treat cancer • Routines such as appointments and follow-up treatments • Expected length of each visit • Appearance of infusion equipment and vascular access devices. *Decreases anxiety associated with treatment.* Assess the patient's expectations and concerns about transplantation. *Determines baseline knowledge.* Instruct the patient and family about the effect and side effects associated with transplantation and associated conditioning. *Decreases anxiety associated with treatment.* Instruct the patient and family about measures used to minimize side effects. *Provides for less distress associated with treatment, which maximizes chance of patient continuing with therapy.*

Sources: Adapted from Bender, C., & Rosenzweig, M. (2004). Cancer. In S. Lewis, M. Heitkemper, & S. Dirksen (Eds.), *Medical–surgical nursing assessment and management of clinical problems* (6th ed.). St. Louis: Mosby; Iwamoto, R. (2001). Radiation therapy. In S. Otto (Ed.), *Oncology nursing* (4th ed.). St. Louis: Mosby; Keller, C. (2001). Bone marrow and stem cell transplantation. In S. Otto (Ed.), *Oncology nursing* (4th ed.). St. Louis: Mosby; Oncology Nursing Society. (2001). *Chemotherapy and biotherapy guidelines and recommendations for practice.* Pittsburgh: Author; Rokita, S. (2004). Oncology: Nursing management in cancer care. In S. Smeltzer & B. Bare (Eds.), *Brunner & Suddarth's textbook of medical–surgical nursing* (10th ed.). Philadelphia: Lippincott Williams & Wilkins; Wikle-Shapiro, T. (1998). Nursing implications of bone marrow and stem cell transplantation. In J. K. Itano & K. N. Taoka (Eds.), *Core curriculum for oncology nursing* (3rd ed.). Philadelphia: W. B. Saunders; Wilkinson, J. M., & Ahearn, N. R. (2009). *Prentice Hall nursing diagnosis handbook* (9th ed.). Upper Saddle River, NJ: Prentice Hall.

Chemotherapy

Chemotherapy is defined as the systemic administration of cytotoxic drugs to treat cancer. In one form or another, this systemic therapy has been present for centuries. Current practice can be linked to the early 1900s when studies were conducted using laboratory rodents to determine the effectiveness of potential chemotherapeutic agents in treating cancer (DeVita, 1997). During World War I and World War II, soldiers were exposed to mustard gas, which was discovered to cause bone marrow and lymphoid suppression. This discovery led to the use of mustard agents in the treatment of Hodgkin's and other lymphomas for the first time in 1940. The use of chemotherapy became a standard of practice in the treatment of cancer in the 1970s.

The American Cancer Society estimated that 1,437,180 new cases of cancer would be diagnosed in 2008 (ACS, 2008a) and that half of these would be treated with systemic chemotherapy. Given the prevalence of cancer, nurses need to understand the purpose of

Weblink: Chemotherapy Side Effects

CHART 57–14 Uses of Chemotherapeutic Agents in Treating Cancer

Type of Therapy	Use	Purpose
Adjuvant	Used in combination with other cancer treatment modalities	To treat micrometastasis
Neoadjuvant	Used before surgical resection of tumor	To shrink tumor in order to maximize surgical resection capabilities
Primary	Used for localized cancer when other treatment options are not as effective	To maximize chance of cure or disease control
Induction	Used for cancers for which other alternatives do not exist	To maximize chance of cure or disease control
Combination	Use of two or more chemotherapeutic agents	To allow each medication to enhance the effect of the other or to act synergistically with it

administering chemotherapy and how it is used. The primary reasons for prescribing chemotherapy are to prevent tumor cells from multiplying, spreading to adjacent tissues, or metastasizing (Virshup, 2010). Therapy aims to provide a cure, control spread of the disease, or relieve suffering. Chemotherapy may be used in several different ways, and oncologists prescribe treatment for patients with specific goals in mind. Chart 57–14 explains the five different ways of using chemotherapy and their purposes. Improvement in overall survival rate and increased periods of disease-free intervals can be attributed to the ongoing development of chemotherapy approaches to cancer treatment. The past five decades have been exciting for nurses who care for patients with cancer due to the dynamic state of chemotherapy research and the subsequent development of a host of new agents.

Principles of Chemotherapy

Every time a malignancy is exposed to a chemotherapeutic agent, a percentage of tumor cells are destroyed. The aim is destruction of as many cells as possible, up to 99% depending on the dose. Completely eradicating all tumor cells is virtually impossible, but the hope is to leave as few cells as possible so that the immune system can finish the job. Chemotherapy is thought to kill a fixed percentage of the total number of cancer cells. This cell-kill hypothesis, shown in Figure 57–6◆, suggests that if a drug has a 90% cell-kill rate and the tumor has 1,000 cells, there would be only 100 cancerous cells remaining at the end of the first treatment. The next treatment would leave the number of cells at 10; this is the rationale behind scheduling chemotherapy in multiple courses over a period of time.

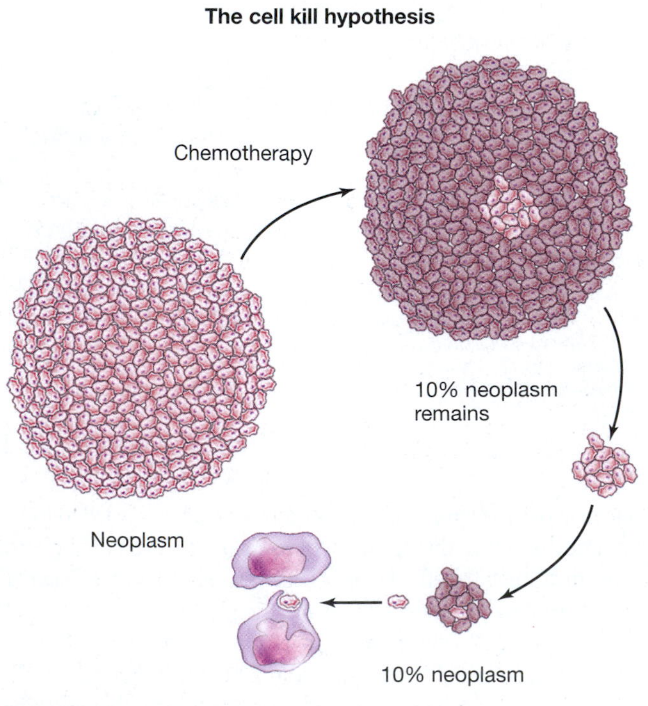

FIGURE 57–6 ◆ Cell-kill hypothesis.

Both cancerous cells and normal cells replicate via the various phases in the cell cycle. The cell cycle time is that time necessary for one tissue cell to divide and reproduce two identical daughter cells. The cycle for any cell has four phases, each with its own important role. These are the G_1 phase, in which RNA and protein synthesis occur; the S phase, in which DNA synthesis occurs; the G_2 phase, which is the premitotic phase in which DNA synthesis is completed and mitotic spindles form; and finally mitosis (M phase), the phase in which cell division occurs. Phase G_0, which is the resting or dormant phase, occurs after mitosis and before the next G_1 phase (Virshup, 2010). G_1 cells are particularly dangerous because they are not actively dividing but have the potential to replicate. Chemotherapeutic agents are meant to interrupt the cell replication at pivotal points within the cycle and are most effective when they target cells that are actively dividing.

Because the goal of chemotherapy is to reduce the number of malignant cells in both the primary tumor site and the metastatic tumor site, it is important to discuss the factors that determine the response of cancer cells to chemotherapy. First, the mitotic rate of the tumor affects the response of chemotherapy owing to the rapid proliferation of cancerous cells. The more rapid the mitotic rate, the greater the response to chemotherapy. Tumor size affects response because the smaller the number of cancer cells, the better the response to treatment. In addition, when the tumor cells are young, a larger percentage of proliferating cells are vulnerable to chemotherapy.

Certain anatomic sites offer protection from the effects of chemotherapy. Few agents, such as nitrosoureas and bleomycin, cross the blood–brain barrier, which lends the brain protection from the effects of chemotherapy. Furthermore, the presence of resistant tumor cells reduces the likelihood of chemotherapy producing a positive effect. This is accomplished when mutation of cancer cells results in variant cells that are resistant to chemotherapy and when certain cancer cells are unable to convert the drug to an active form (Virshup, 2010). The majority of chemotherapeutic agents are most effective when they can work against dividing cells, not against cells in a resting phase (as in G_0). As the tumor grows, more cells become inactive and convert to the resting phase. The presence of noncycling cells and drug resistance are the main difficulties encountered in the development of chemotherapeutic agents.

Classification

Chemotherapeutic drugs are classified or categorized according to their structure and mechanism of action. Agents that act during a specific cell phase are classified as cell-cycle phase-specific drugs and are known to destroy cells that are actively dividing. Certain agents act on the S phase affecting DNA and RNA synthesis; others act on the M phase, which terminates spindle formation. Chemotherapeutic agents that are active throughout the entire cell cycle are called cell-cycle phase-nonspecific drugs. These agents exert a longer acting effect on cells, leading to cell death or damage. Combining these two types of chemotherapeutic agents increases the number of susceptible tumor cells that are destroyed during a treatment period and reduces the adverse affects on normal cells, which may improve the patient's response to treatment (Virshup, 2010). The Pharmacology box (p. 1804) lists common antineoplastic (and biotherapy) agents used to treat cancer along with their common side effects and the related nursing interventions. This list is not meant to be comprehensive; rather, it gives an overview of information the nurse needs when planning care for a patient with cancer.

Administration and Safe Handling

Chemotherapeutic drugs are administered in a variety of locations and by a variety of routes. These agents can be given to patients who are in the hospital, in an outpatient infusion center, or in the home. Depending on the type of agent used, they may be given by the oral, intravenous, intramuscular, subcutaneous, arterial, intracavitary, or intrathecal routes. An oncology nurse knows, through experience and training, that the route is determined by the drug used, dose, type, location, and extent of tumor. Special education and training are essential in order to develop a safe practice for administering chemotherapy. The ONS, together with OSHA, has developed guidelines for the administration and handling of chemotherapy and biotherapy (Occupational Safety and Health Administration, Office of Occupational Medicine, 1995).

Safety Concerns

With the development of numerous chemotherapeutic agents in recent years has come heightened awareness of the hazards associated with those agents. Exposure to these agents can occur by inhalation, absorption, or digestion. Individuals who handle chemotherapeutic agents need to be given training regarding the hazards and how to implement safeguards that will protect themselves and others. Hospitals and regulatory agencies recognize the risk to health care professionals and have developed precautions for those involved in the preparation, administration, and disposal of chemotherapeutic agents (Adams & Koch, 2010; Virshup, 2010). Chart 57–15 (p. 1808) lists the common precautions that should be taken by anyone who cares for patients receiving chemotherapy, including suggestions that would apply in home care settings. Typically, nurses do not prepare chemotherapy agents; however, it is important to understand the safety precautions implemented by others to appreciate the seriousness of agents the nurse will be asked to administer. Education of all staff is an ongoing process that should include a discussion of unique patient care situations, introduction of new equipment, and reproductive issues such miscarriages and fetal deformities (Adams & Koch, 2010; Virshup, 2010).

Dose Calculations

Chemotherapeutic agents are dosed on the basis of the body surface area (BSA) in adults and children. Pharmacists who prepare chemotherapy agents use equations to determine the appropriate dose for a patient on the basis of the patient's height and weight. To maintain accurate dosing, it is crucial for the nurse to monitor weight changes throughout the course of chemotherapy and communicate this information to the pharmacist. A patient's weight changes frequently during treatment because of drug-induced side effects such as nausea, vomiting, anorexia, and fatigue. Other factors that are considered in determining the dose of chemotherapy agents include renal function and other comorbidities (e.g., chronic obstructive pulmonary disease, heart failure, and renal failure).

Administration

The oncologist prescribing chemotherapy selects a route of administration that will deliver the optimal amount of drug to the tumor. A variety of methods are used to meet this goal. Chart 57–16 (p. 1809) explains the routes of administration along with specific nursing concerns for each. The nurse should understand that the decision to use a specific delivery method and route is based on the pharmacokinetics of the drug to be used, as well as characteristics of the patient and the cancer (Adams & Koch, 2010; Virshup, 2010).

Oral and intravenous (IV) routes are the most commonly used. All delivery methods have associated inherent risks. Intravenously administered agents pose a particular concern associated with the risk of irritation to the vessel wall and extravasation (leaking of drug into the tissue surrounding the infusion site) causing local tissue damage. Chemotherapeutic drugs that cause severe local tissue breakdown and necrosis are called *vesicants* (Adams & Koch, 2010). Nurses need to be alert to symptoms that are common with extravasation such as pain, swelling, redness, and appearance of vesicles on the skin. Agency policy will identify nursing actions that are required once symptoms of extravasation have been recognized. Often, IV drugs are delivered via central vascular access devices. Refer to Chapter 16 for detailed information on these types of devices along with the nursing implications.

Chemotherapy Side Effects and Toxicities

Chemotherapy produces effects on both normal cells and cancer cells. Side effects or toxic effects are the result of the destruction of normal cells that produce specific signs and symptoms and are classified as acute, delayed, or chronic. Chart 57–17 (p. 1811) lists the effects found in each category (Adams & Koch, 2010). Cells with rapid growth rates are more susceptible to damage, resulting in noticeable signs and symptoms. Examples of cells that are affected by this process are epithelium, bone marrow, hair follicles, and sperm. The body will respond to the products of cellular destruction by demonstrating fatigue, anorexia, and taste alterations.

Gastrointestinal System Effects

Nausea and vomiting are the most common gastrointestinal (GI) side effects. Within 1 hour of beginning therapy, the patient may experience vomiting that may last up to 24 hours or more. Drugs that can reduce or eliminate nausea and vomiting are an essential part of the treatment plan for patients receiving chemotherapeutic agents and may also be given before therapy starts and for several days after it ends. Antiemetics include serotonin blockers, which block serotonin receptors located in the GI tract and chemoreceptor trigger zone (CTZ) in the medulla, dopaminergic blockers that block dopamine receptors of the CTZ, phenothiazines, sedatives, corticosteroids, and histamines.

Nurses are responsible for being aware of the types of drugs their patients are receiving so that they can anticipate what interventions may be needed to relieve suffering from nausea and vomiting. Some patients will require antiemetic therapy for several days after chemotherapy and will need to be encouraged to comply with their prescribed medication regime to lessen the emetic effects of the chemotherapy. Other interventions such as relaxation techniques, guided imagery, and altering the patient's diet may also assist in reducing nausea and vomiting. Monitoring for signs of fluid volume deficit and electrolyte imbalances should be ongoing nursing interventions, and abnormal findings need to be reported to the health care provider so that additional treatment

PHARMACOLOGY Summary of Medications Used for Cancer Treatment

Medication Category and Action	Application/Indication	Nursing Responsibility
Biologic Response Modifiers (Immunostimulants)		
INTEFERONS		
Interferon alfa-2b (Intron-A) Peginterferon alfa-2a (Pegasys, Sylatron) Interferon alfacon-1 Interferon alfa-2b ***Action:*** Antiviral and antitumor properties. Stimulate immune system or stop tumor growth. Enhance lymphocyte and antibody production. Assist with destruction of macrophages and natural killer cells. Inhibit cell replication by increasing phases of cell cycle.	α-Interferon approved for use in hairy-cell leukemia, Kaposi's sarcoma, chronic hepatitis B or C. PegINF alfa-2a also used to treat melanoma with nodal involvement.	Monitor for depression. Notify health care provider for possible consultation to social services and/or psychiatry. Monitor for flulike symptoms (e.g., fevers, chills, malaise, headache, anorexia). Monitor for evidence of dehydration (e.g., concentrated urine, poor skin turgor, and dry mucous membranes). Monitor electrolytes. Monitor for signs of infection (e.g., fever, increased sputum, dyspnea, urgency, and frequency). Implement neutropenic precautions as necessary. Implement safety precautions during activity. Administer antidiarrheals.
INTERLEUKIN-2		
Aldesleukin (Proleukin) ***Action:*** Activates cytotoxic T lymphocytes and promotes other actions of the immune response.	Metastatic renal cell carcinoma.	Monitor for severe flulike symptoms (e.g., fevers, chills, rigors, malaise, headache, anorexia). Monitor for capillary leak syndrome (e.g., generalized edema, decreased urine output, hypotension). Monitor for evidence of dehydration (e.g., concentrated urine, poor skin turgor, dry mucous membranes). Monitor electrolytes. Monitor for signs of infection (e.g., fever, increased sputum, dyspnea, urgency, and frequency). Implement neutropenic precautions as necessary. Implement safety precautions during activity. Administer antidiarrheals.
Monoclonal Antibodies and Targeted Therapies		
MONOCLONAL ANTIBODIES (MABs)		
Action: Cell-specific, MABs kill the cell or target it for action by other phases of the immune system. Also, some MABs are used to dampen overactive inflammatory cells. *Selected examples:* Rituximab (Rituxan) binds to CD20 Cetuximab (Erbitux) Trastuzumab (Herceptin)	Targets certain lymphomas and leukemias. Colorectal cancer, squamous cell cancer of head and neck (in combination with radiation). Breast cancer with over-expression of HER2 protein, HER2-positive breast cancer after surgery.	Monitor CBC and differential. Monitor for signs of bleeding (e.g., bruising, bloody stool/urine, hypotension, tachycardia). Monitor for signs of infection (e.g., fever, increased sputum, dyspnea, urgency, and frequency). Implement neutropenic precautions as necessary. Monitor for signs of hypersensitivity reaction (changes in BP, rash, edema, facial flushing, dyspnea). Monitor for evidence of dehydration (e.g., concentrated urine, poor skin turgor, dry mucous membranes). Monitor electrolytes. Administer antiemetics as needed. Administer antidiarrheals as needed. Monitor for signs of decreased cardiac output or inadequate tissue perfusion (e.g., diaphoresis, pale color, poor-quality pulses, chest pain, edema, crackles, and decreased urine output).
TARGETED THERAPIES		
Selected examples: Bevacizumab (Avastin) ***Action:*** An angiogenesis-inhibitor that restricts the ability of tumors to establish a new blood supply. Imatinib (Gleevec) ***Action:*** Inhibits tyrosine kinase, a key enzyme required for cell growth.	Metastatic colorectal, non-small-cell lung cancer, HER2 negative breast cancer, malignant glioblastoma. Gastrointestinal stromal tumors (GISTs), acute lymphoblastic leukemia.	Monitor renal function tests (e.g., creatinine, BUN, creatinine clearance). Encourage the use of oral saline rinses and avoid the use of mouthwashes. Provide a list of community resources for wigs, hats, caps, etc. Instruct the patient about reproductive issues and provide resources as needed.

PHARMACOLOGY Summary of Medications Used for Cancer Treatment, *continued*

Medication Category and Action	Application/Indication	Nursing Responsibility
Antineoplastic Agents		
Alkylating Agents		
NITROGEN MUSTARDS		
Bendamustine (Treanda) Chlorambucil (Leukeran) Cyclophosphamide (Cytoxan) Estramustine (Emcyt) Ifosfamide (Ifex) Mechlorethamine (Mustargen) Melphalan (Alkeran) ***Action:*** Disrupt DNA replication and RNA transcription by cross-linking DNA strands. Cell cycle nonspecific.	Ovarian, breast, lung, testicular, and head and neck cancer. Multiple myeloma, leukemias, lymphoma, sarcoma.	Monitor CBC and differential. Monitor for signs of bleeding (e.g., bruising, bloody stool/urine, hypotension, tachycardia). Monitor for signs of infection (e.g., fever, increased sputum, dyspnea, urgency, and frequency). Implement neutropenic precautions as necessary. Monitor for evidence of dehydration (e.g., concentrated urine, poor skin turgor, dry mucous membranes). Monitor electrolytes. Administer antiemetics as needed. Administer antidiarrheals as needed. Encourage the use of oral saline rinses and avoid the use of mouthwashes. Provide a list of community resources for wigs, hats, caps, etc. Monitor for signs of seizures and implement seizure precautions. Monitor renal function tests (e.g., creatinine, BUN, creatinine clearance). Instruct the patient to drink plenty of fluids prior to and during treatment. Administer bladder protectant as needed (Mesna). Instruct the patient about reproductive issues and provide resources as needed.
NITROSOUREAS		
Carmustine (Bicnu, Gliadel) Lomustine (CeeNu, CCNU) Streptozocin (Zanosar) ***Action:*** Block enzymes needed for synthesis of purine, resulting in immediate cell death. Similar actions to nitrogen mustards; cross blood–brain barrier. Cell cycle nonspecific.	Lymphomas, multiple myeloma, CNS tumors, malignant melanoma, pancreatic cancer.	Monitor CBC and differential. Monitor for signs of bleeding (e.g., bruising, bloody stool/urine, hypotension, tachycardia). Monitor for signs of infection (e.g., fever, increased sputum, dyspnea, urgency, and frequency). Implement neutropenic precautions as necessary. Monitor for evidence of dehydration (e.g., concentrated urine, poor skin turgor, dry mucous membranes). Monitor electrolytes. Administer antiemetics as needed. Instruct the patient to drink plenty of fluids prior to treatment. Administer bladder protectant as needed (Mesna). Monitor renal function tests (e.g., creatinine, BUN, creatinine clearance). Monitor serum osmolarity and electrolytes. Monitor dyspnea and cough.
MISCELLANEOUS ALKYLATING AGENTS		
Busulfan (Myleran) Carboplatin (Paraplatin) Cisplatin (Platinol) Dacarbazine (DTIC-Dome) Oxaliplatin (Eloxatin) Procarbazine (Matulane) Temozolomide (Temodar) Thiotepa ***Action:*** Causes damage to the DNA of the cancer cell by attaching an alkyl group to the DNA.	Various forms of cancer, leukemia, lymphoma.	Monitor CBC and differential. Monitor for signs of bleeding (e.g., bruising, bloody stool/urine, hypotension, tachycardia). Monitor for signs of infection (e.g., fever, increased sputum, dyspnea, urgency, and frequency). Implement neutropenic precautions as necessary. Monitor for evidence of dehydration (e.g., concentrated urine, poor skin turgor, dry mucous membranes). Monitor serum osmality and electrolytes. Monitor for peripheral neuropathy/visual disturbances and otoxicity.

(*continued*)

Medication Category and Action	Application/Indication	Nursing Responsibility
Antimetabolites		
Methotrexate (Rheumatrex, Trexall) Pemetrexed (Alimta) Pralatrexate (Folotyn) Capecitabine (Xeloda) Fluorouracil (5-FU, Adrucil, Carac, Efudex) Cytarabine (Cytosar, Depot-Cyt) Gemcitabine (Gemzar) ***Action:*** Hinder the synthesis of DNA by blocking the use of necessary enzymes. Cell cycle phase-specific (S phase).	Leukemias, lymphomas, myelodysplasia syndrome, breast and colon cancer.	Monitor CBC and differential. Monitor for signs of bleeding (e.g., bruising, bloody stool/urine, hypotension, and tachycardia). Monitor for signs of infection (e.g., fever, increased sputum, dyspnea, urgency, and frequency). Implement neutropenic precautions as necessary. Monitor for evidence of dehydration (e.g., concentrated urine, poor skin turgor, dry mucous membranes). Monitor break in skin integrity (e.g., rashes, blistering on palms and feet). Monitor liver and renal function and electrolytes. Administer antiemetics as needed. Instruct patient to drink plenty of fluids prior to treatment. Encourage the use of saline rinses and avoid the use of mouthwashes. Provide ice water during drug administration. Administer analgesics as needed. Provide a list of community resources for wigs, hats, caps, etc. Encourage the use of sunscreen year-round.
Antitumor Antibiotics		
Bleomycin (Blenoxane) Dactinomycin (Actinomycin-D, Cosmegen) Daunorubicin (Cerubidine) Daunorubicin liposomal (DaunoXome) Doxorubicin (Adriamycin) Doxorubicin liposomal (Doxil, Evacet) Epirubicin (Ellence) Idarubicin (Idamycin) Mitomycin (Mutamycin) Mitoxantrone (Novantrone) ***Action:*** Interfere with function and synthesis of nucleic acids, resulting in disruption of RNA and DNA replication. Cell cycle nonspecific.	Various solid tumors. Lymphomas and acute lymphocytic leukemia, soft-tissue sarcomas, multiple myeloma, Wilm's tumor.	For vesicants: IV push over 6–10 minutes, flushing with 75–100 mL solution. Premedicate with diphenhydramine, cimetidine, and dexamethasone. Monitor for signs of hypersensitivity reaction (changes in BP, rash, edema, facial flushing, dyspnea). Monitor neurological status (motor weakness, paresthesia). Provide a list of community resources for wigs, hats, caps, etc. Monitor CBC and differential. Monitor for signs of bleeding (e.g., bruising, bloody stool/urine, hypotension, and tachycardia). Monitor for signs of infection (e.g., fever, increased sputum, dyspnea, urgency, and frequency). Implement neutropenic precautions as necessary. Monitor electrolytes. Administer antiemetics as needed. Encourage the use of saline rinses and avoid the use of mouthwashes. Provide ice water during drug administration. Administer analgesics as needed. Administer appetite stimulants as needed. Monitor for signs of decreased cardiac output or inadequate tissue perfusion (e.g., diaphoresis, pale color, poor-quality pulses, chest pain, edema, crackles, decreased urine output). Monitor for cough and dyspnea. Instruct the patient about potential darkening of previously irradiated areas. Provide a list of community resources for wigs, hats, caps, etc.
Natural Products		
VINCA ALKALOIDS		
Vinorelbine (Navelbine) Vincristine (Oncovin) Vinblastine (Velban) ***Action:*** Inhibit mitosis, resulting in immediate cell death (cytocidal). Cell cycle phase-specific (M phase).	Breast, testicular, non-small-cell lung, ovarian, and head and neck cancers. Lymphomas, acute lymphocytic leukemia (ALL), chronic myelogenous leukemia (CML).	For vesicants: IV push over 6–10 minutes, flushing with 75–100 mL solution. Monitor for local skin changes. Monitor CBC and differential. Monitor for signs of bleeding (e.g., bruising, bloody stool/urine, hypotension, and tachycardia).

PHARMACOLOGY Summary of Medications Used for Cancer Treatment, *continued*

Medication Category and Action	Application/Indication	Nursing Responsibility
		Monitor for signs of infection (e.g., fever, increased sputum, dyspnea, urgency, and frequency). Implement neutropenic precautions as necessary. Monitor neurological status (motor weakness, paresthesia). Monitor liver function tests. Administer laxatives, stool softeners. Administer analgesics as needed. Provide a list of community resources for wigs, hats, caps, etc.
TOPOISOMERASE INHIBITORS Etoposide (Vepesid) Irinotecan (Camptosar) Topotecan (Hycamtin) Teniposide (Vumon) ***Action:*** Alters DNA replication by inhibiting topoisomerase I. Cell cycle phase-specific.	Colorectal, non-small-cell lung, and ovarian cancer. ALL.	Monitor CBC and differential. Monitor for signs of bleeding (e.g., bruising, bloody stool/urine, hypotension, and tachycardia). Monitor for signs of infection (e.g., fever, increased sputum, dyspnea, urgency, and frequency). Implement neutropenic precautions as necessary. Administer atropine as needed to reduce cholinergic-induced diarrhea. Monitor for signs of dehydration (e.g., concentrated urine, poor skin turgor, dry mucous membranes). Provide a list of community resources for wigs, hats, caps, etc.
Taxanes Cabazitaxel (Jevtana) Docetaxel (Taxotere) Paclitaxel (Taxol) Mitotic inhibitors	Ovarian, breast, and prostate cancer. Kaposi's sarcoma.	Monitor for hypersensitivity reactions. Monitor CBC and differential. Monitor for signs of bleeding (e.g., bruising, bloody stool/urine, hypotension, and tachycardia). Monitor for signs of infection (e.g., fever, increased sputum, dyspnea, urgency, and frequency). Implement neutropenic precautions as necessary. Monitor and report promptly severe or persistent diarrhea or vomiting. Monitor for signs of dehydration (e.g., concentrated urine, poor skin turgor, dry mucous membranes).
Hormones and Hormone Antagonists **HORMONES** Dexamethasone (e.g., Decadron) Diethylstilbestrol (DES, Stilbestrol) Ethinyl estradiol (e.g., Estinyl) Fluoxymesterone (Halotestin) Medroxyprogesterone (Provera, Depo-Provera) Megestrol (Megace) Prednisone (e.g., Deltasone) Testosterone enanthate (Delatest) ***Action:*** Interfere with proteins and hormone receptors throughout the cell cycle. Cell cycle nonspecific.	Prostate, breast, and endometrial cancers.	Monitor CBC and differential. Monitor for signs of infection (e.g., fever, increased sputum, dyspnea, urgency, and frequency). Implement neutropenic precautions as necessary. Monitor blood pressure. Instruct the patient to lower sodium intake. Instruct the patient to observe for swelling in the ankles, lower extremities, and hands. Instruct the patient to avoid discontinuing medication unless advised by the health care provider. Instruct the patient about signs of feminization and masculinization.
HORMONE ANTAGONISTS Abiraterone (Zytiga) Anastrozole (Arimidex) Bicalutamide (Casodex) Degarelix (Firmagon) Exemestane (Aromasin)		

(*continued*)

PHARMACOLOGY Summary of Medications Used for Cancer Treatment, *continued*

Medication Category and Action	Application/Indication	Nursing Responsibility
Flutamide (Eulexin) Fulvestrant (Faslodex) Goserelin (Zoladex) Histrelin (Supprelin LA, Vantas) Letrozole (Femara) Leuprolide (Eligard, Lupron, Viadur) Nilutamide (Nilandron) Raloxifene (Evista) Tamoxifen Toremifene (Fareston) Triptorelin (Trelstar) ***Action:*** Interfere with proteins and hormone receptors throughout the cell cycle. Cell cycle nonspecific.		

Sources: Adams, Holland, & Urban (2013); Wilson, Shannon, & Shields (2012).

CHART 57–15 Safe Handling of Chemotherapeutic Drugs

Drug Preparation

Prepare in a biologic safety cabinet (BSC):

- Vented system to outside environment
- Provides vertical laminar airflow to carry contaminated air away from the BSC operator
- Blower that operates continuously
- Located in low traffic area
- Used only with trained individuals.

Hand hygiene before donning personal protective equipment (PPE).

Wear appropriate PPE:

- Gloves that are powder free with long cuffs (change every 30 minutes)
- Gowns
- Face shields or goggles.

PPE should be replaced if torn, punctured, or soiled.

Use a plastic-backed sterile absorbent pad on the work surface.

Maintain sterile technique.

Use appropriate technique when opening ampules.

When reconstituting drugs in vials, use dispensing pins with venting devices to avoid aerosolization.

Use tubing and syringes with Luer-lock fittings.

Avoid overfilling of syringes.

Prime all tubing with normal saline or dextrose before adding cytotoxic drug.

Label each container "Cytotoxic Drug."

Place container in sealed bag before transport.

Dispose of all material that has come into contact with cytotoxic drug into appropriate receptacle.

Drug Administration

Explain to the patient that protective wear minimizes the exposure of health care providers to the harmful effects of chemotherapeutic drugs.

Wear appropriate PPE.

Implement High Alert Medication Safety practice.

Administer drugs in a safe and unhurried environment, working at eye level.

Use Luer-lock fittings on all intravenous tubing, needles, and syringes used for delivery of cytotoxic drugs.

Place a disposable, absorbent, plastic-backed pad under the work area to collect droplets of the drug.

Implement standard precautions when handling the blood, vomitus, or excreta of a patient who has received cytotoxic drugs within the last 48 hours.

Disposal of Supplies and Drugs

Do not recap needles or break syringes.

Place all used supplies in a leakproof, puncture proof, labeled container.

Keep containers in all areas where preparation and administration of cytotoxic drugs occur.

Environmental service personnel trained in safe handling procedures should remove containers.

Personnel should wear appropriate PPE.

Containers should be disposed of according to hazardous waste regulations.

In home situations:

Place containers in an area away from children and pets until retrieved by an appropriate agency.

Check county and state regulations.

Arrange with a medical supply company, health care provider's office, or private waste management company for proper disposal.

Sources: Occupational Safety and Health Administration, Office of Occupational Medicine. (1995). *Controlling occupational exposure to hazardous CPL2-2.20B CH-4.* Washington, DC: U.S. Department of Labor; Singleton, L., & Connor, T. (1999). An evaluation of the permeability of chemotherapy gloves to three cancer chemotherapy drugs. *Oncology Nursing Forum, 26*(4); The Joint Commision. (2008). *High alert medication: Strategies for improving safety.* Chicago, IL: Joint Commission Resources.

CHART 57–16 Routes of Administration

Route		Nursing Implications
Oral	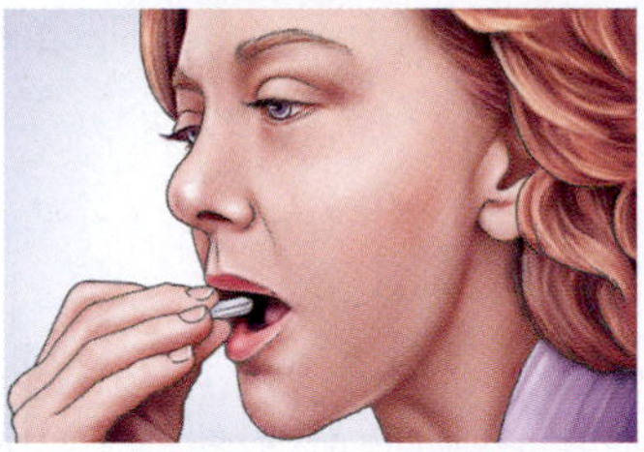	Educate the patient about the significance of complying with the prescribed schedule, optimal dosing, and patient safety. Devise educational strategies such as individualized medication sheets to reinforce information. Educate the patient about strategies to reduce the potential for side effects (e.g., taking drugs with emetic potential with meals, taking drugs that require adequate fluid intake early in the day). Coordinate educational sessions with an oncologist and pharmacist, since nurses may have minimal patient contact.
Subcutaneous	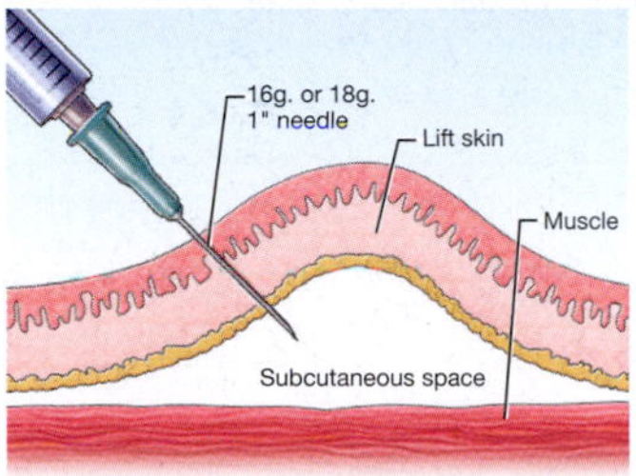	Educate the patient and/or caregiver to give injections and allow for return demonstration. Encourage the patient to rotate injection sites and keep a written log.
Intramuscular	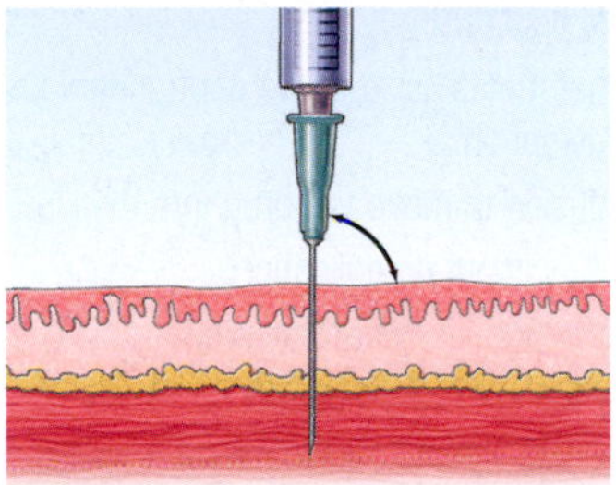	Same as subcutaneous.
Intravenous (may be given via central venous catheters or peripheral venous access) • Push • Piggyback • Side-arm • Infusion	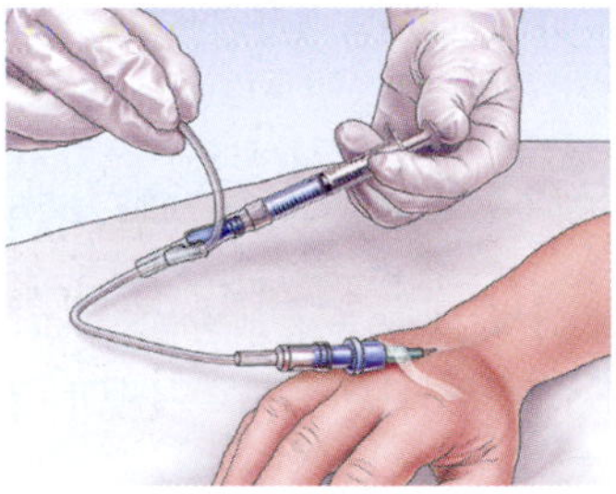	Administered directly into the vein via a syringe. Administered using a secondary bag and tubing while primary infusion is running concurrently. Administered into the side port of a running IV infusion. Drug is added to an appropriate size IV bag. All medications administered via the IV route should have the blood return of the vein evaluated at regular intervals during the infusion (as determined by agency policy).
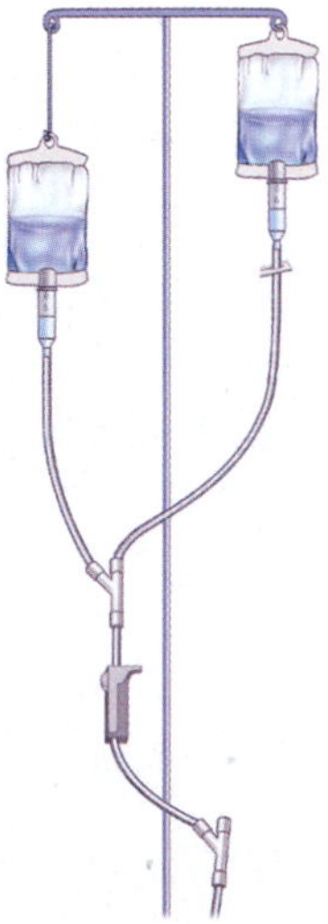	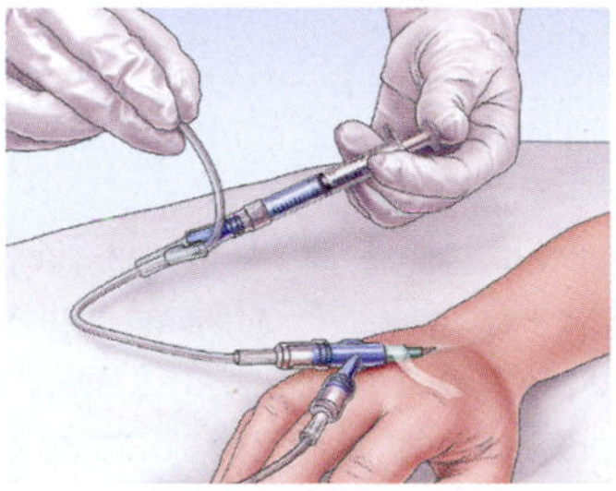	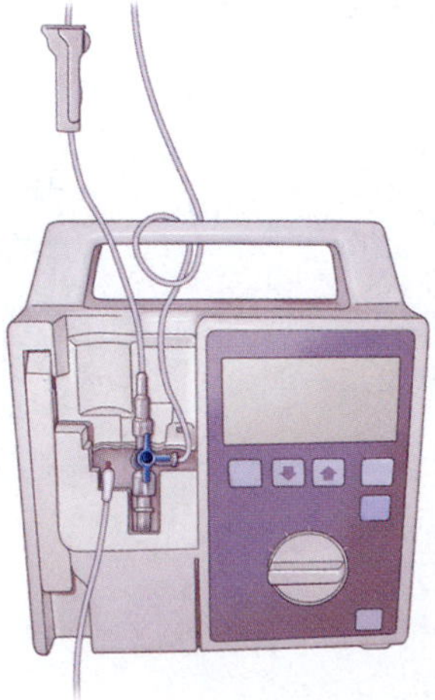

(continued)

CHART 57–16 Routes of Administration, *continued*

Route		Nursing Implications
Topical	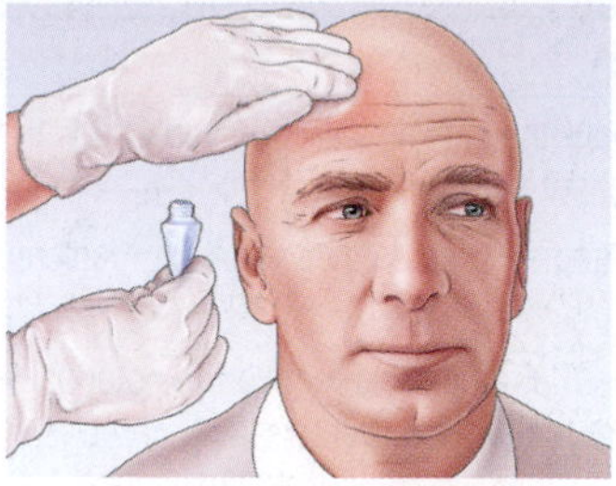	Educate the patient to cover the surface area with a thin layer of medication, then wear loose-fitting clothing. Wear gloves during the application and perform hand hygiene after the procedure. Educate the patient to avoid touching the medication.
Intracavitary	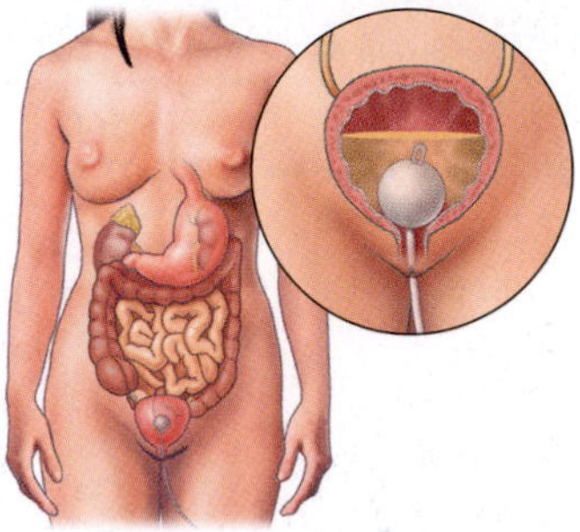	Instill medication into either the bladder (via a catheter) or the pleural cavity (via a chest tube). Administer premedication to reduce local irritation.
Intrathecal	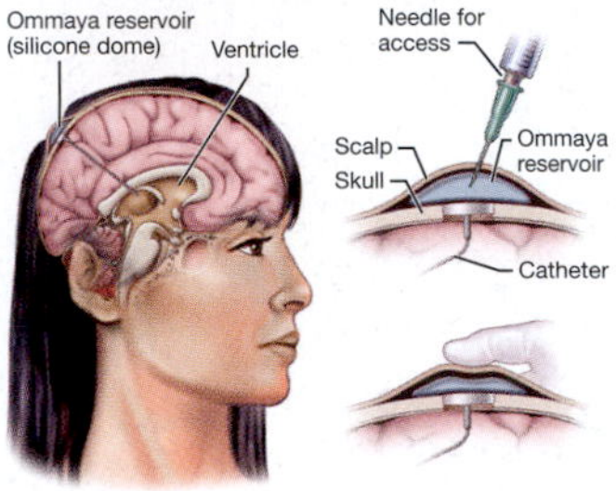	An Ommaya reservoir, which is implanted subcutaneously, is used to gain access to ventricular cerebrospinal fluid (CSF). Used to treat cancers that metastasize to the central nervous system (CNS) (breast, lung, GI, leukemia, and lymphoma). Does not depend on diffusion to move the drug into the CSF. May last months to years without complications. Sterile technique used throughout the procedure. Usually administered by a health care provider. Evaluate for neurotoxicities.
Intra-arterial	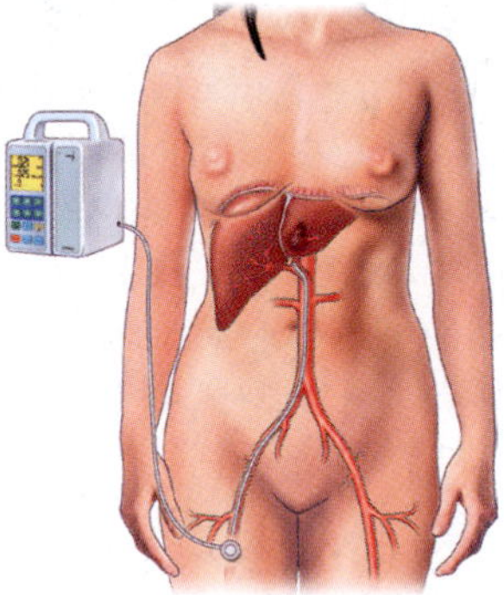	Catheter placement into artery near inoperable tumor (liver, bladder, brain, head and neck, cervix, and bone). Use infusion pump. Monitor vital signs, color and temperature of extremity, and signs of local bleeding throughout therapy. Monitor appropriate laboratory studies (e.g., liver function tests) for organ toxicity. Educate patient about the care of the catheter and pump if to be used at home.
Intraperitoneal	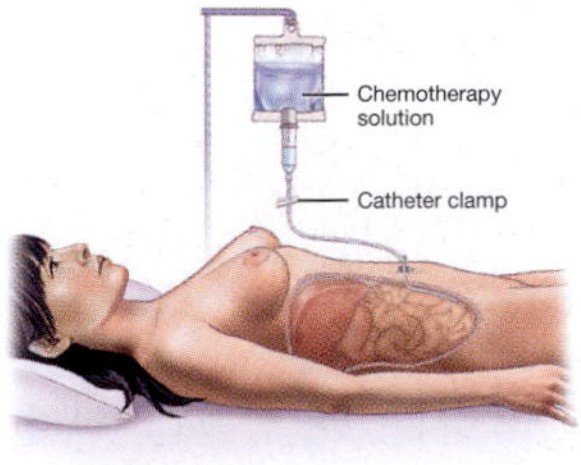 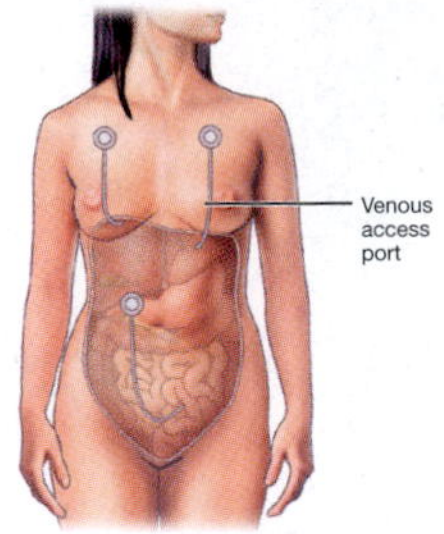	Administration of drug via implantable port or external suprapubic catheter into the abdominal cavity. Used typically for peritoneal metastases due to ovarian cancer. Heat infusate solution to body temperature before infusing. Infuse 1–2 liters of fluid and allow to "dwell" for 1–4 hours before draining. Monitor for abdominal pressure, pain, fever, and electrolyte imbalance after infusing. Measure abdominal girth.

Source: Adapted from Mellinger, (2010). Safe handling of chemotherapy in the perioperative setting. *AORN Journal*, *91*(4), 435–553.

CHART 57–17 Classification of Chemotherapy Toxicities

Classification	Toxicity
Acute	Vomiting, allergic reactions, cardiac dysrhythmias
Delayed	Mucositis: mouth sores, gastritis, diarrhea alopecia, bone marrow suppression
Chronic	Cardiac: reduced contractility
	Hepatic: elevated liver enzyme tests
	Renal: elevated creatinine and BUN

can be started in order to reduce the chance of significant weight loss and malnutrition.

Other GI toxicities are due to the rapid rate of proliferation of the cells that line the GI tract. These include stomatitis (inflammation of the oral cavity), anorexia, mucositis (inflammation of the mucosal lining), and diarrhea. Constipation can occur in some patients receiving chemotherapeutic agents that slow motility of the large intestine and may be due to reduced food intake secondary to persistent nausea and vomiting (Eilers, 2011).

Pancreatitis (inflammation of the pancreas) occurs with certain types of chemotherapeutic agents, radiotherapy to the left side of the abdomen, diabetes, tumor lysis syndrome (TLS), and the presence of intrahepatic catheters (Virshup, 2010). Common signs and symptoms include abdominal pain, fever, tachycardia, and nausea and vomiting. When a patient is suspected of having pancreatitis, the nurse should review laboratory data for elevated serum amylase, lipase, and hypoglycemia. If not successfully treated, pancreatitis can put the patient at risk for developing shock, leading to possible death. Nurses administering chemotherapy agents that are known to cause pancreatitis should be alert to potential signs and symptoms and collaborate with the oncologist to begin prompt treatment.

Although not common, hepatotoxicity occurs due to the direct toxic effect to the liver as a result of the metabolism of antineoplastic drugs. The likelihood of developing liver dysfunction related to chemotherapy is increased if the patient has a history of prior infections or damage (cirrhosis, hepatitis), cancer of the liver, radiotherapy to the right side of the abdomen, alcoholism, intrahepatic chemotherapy, and advancing age (Virshup, 2010). Clinical findings associated with hepatotoxicity are those consistent with liver dysfunction, including jaundice, ascites, fatigue, malaise, anorexia, nausea and vomiting, right upper quadrant pain, dark orange urine, and bleeding tendencies. In addition, results of laboratory tests used to determine hepatic function such as liver function tests and coagulation studies will be abnormal.

Genitourinary System Effects

A few chemotherapy agents damage kidneys because of the accumulation of end products after cell lysis and the direct effect during excretion. Chemotherapy can cause tumors to undergo rapid cell lysis, which causes an increase in uric acid production and urinary excretion resulting in kidney damage. In addition, the release of intracellular contents into the circulation causes increased levels of serum potassium and phosphates and decreased levels of serum calcium. Nurses need to be aware of the renal effect of the chemotherapy agent being administered and monitor serum blood urea nitrogen (BUN), creatinine, electrolytes, and creatinine clearance. Abnormal findings need to be reported to the health care provider so that adjustments in drug dosing can be considered. Prevention of uric acid crystals can be accomplished by ensuring adequate hydration, determining alkalinization of the urine, and administering drugs aimed at reducing serum uric acid.

Hemorrhagic cystitis is bladder mucosal damage that occurs as a result of inflammation and irritation from the metabolism of by-products of chemotherapeutic agents. The development of hemorrhagic cystitis is associated with administration of certain alkylating agents and prior radiotherapy to the pelvis or bladder. Nurses need to be alert to the few but important signs and symptoms that may produce suffering for most of these patients. These include dysuria, frequency, nocturia, oliguria, and hematuria.

Cardiopulmonary System Effects

Certain chemotherapeutic agents have toxic effects on the cardiopulmonary system that may produce permanent functional changes for the patient. Patients who are to receive antitumor antibiotics should have a cardiac evaluation before treatment to determine baseline cardiac function. During therapy, the nurse needs to monitor for heart failure and signs of decreased cardiac output. A decrease in pulmonary function is a lifelong effect associated with long-term chemotherapy. Nurses need to evaluate the patient for changes in pulmonary function, including pulmonary function tests (Virshup, 2010).

Hematopoietic System Effects

The majority of chemotherapy agents cause a disruption in the normal functioning of the immune system. *Myelosuppression* is the term used to define a depression of bone marrow function. WBCs, RBCs, and platelets are susceptible to bone marrow suppression from chemotherapy. Neutropenia (reduced neutrophils) and thrombocytopenia (reduced platelets) along with the presence of anemia (reduced hemoglobin and hematocrit) are the main factors that limit the doses of chemotherapy given to a patient (Virshup, 2010).

Neutropenia is defined as a reduction in the number of circulating neutrophils, whereas leukopenia is defined as a reduction in the number of circulating WBCs. The importance of monitoring the neutrophils in patients who are receiving chemotherapy lies in the ability of neutrophils to protect the host from bacterial invasion. Assessing the laboratory data includes monitoring the WBC count and calculating the **absolute neutrophil count (ANC).** Refer to Chapter 55 for additional information. An ANC of less than 500 is considered to put the patient at severe risk of infection (Virshup, 2010). It is important for the nurse to understand that neutropenia can occur when the total WBC is within normal range; therefore, knowing the ANC allows a correct assessment of the neutrophil status.

The term **nadir** refers to the point at which the lowest blood count is reached. When a patient receives chemotherapy, the nadir occurs approximately 7 to 10 days after treatment, at which point the patient is most susceptible to infection. Providing ongoing patient education regarding the signs of infection and when to report findings to the health care provider is critical. A detailed discussion of nursing management of patients who are experiencing side effects from chemotherapy is found in the Nursing Process: Patient Care Plan for Cancer box earlier in this chapter (p. 1790).

Safety Alert *When caring for patients receiving chemotherapy or biotherapy, the nurse should evaluate the laboratory data for the presence of anemia, thrombocytopenia, and neutropenia. Calculation of the ANC will provide the most accurate picture of the patient's risk for infection. The nurse should notify the health care provider immediately if the patient demonstrates signs of infection.*

Weblink: Biotherapy

The availability of drugs used to stimulate the bone marrow has allowed patients to continue with chemotherapy despite the associated side effects. Granulocyte colony-stimulating factor (G-CSF) and granulocyte-macrophage colony-stimulating factor (GM-CSF) stimulate the bone marrow to produce WBCs at a more rapid pace in order to reduce the duration of neutropenia. Erythropoietin (Epogen, Procrit) is used to increase the production of RBCs, thus playing a pivotal role in preventing the anemia-induced symptoms associated with chemotherapy. The benefit of administering these agents is a reduction of the incidence of infection, thus allowing for continuing the prescribed chemotherapeutic drug regime.

Reproductive System Effects

Both testicular and ovarian functions can be affected by antineoplastic drug therapy. Before receiving chemotherapy, the patient needs to be aware of the risks of sterility and early menopause. Men, who may experience an absence of spermatozoa that can be either permanent or temporary, should be given an option to bank sperm; likewise, women should be given the opportunity to preserve ova before the start of treatment if there is a risk of damage or sterility. Education for both patients and their partners about the potential risk to reproductive functions and appropriate protection behaviors (e.g., reliable birth control) should be provided as part of the treatment decision process (Virshup, 2010).

Neurological System Effects

Neurological effects are usually reversible and disappear after completion of chemotherapy treatments. Toxicities can arise as direct or indirect damage to the central nervous system (CNS), peripheral nervous system, cranial nerves, or a combination of the three. Peripheral neuropathies, loss of reflexes, hearing loss due to damage of the acoustic nerve, and paralytic ileus are some of the more commonly occurring effects. The nurse needs to educate the patient and family about the importance of patient safety, detection of signs and symptoms, when to notify the health care provider of evidence of toxicity, and how to get referrals for coping strategies.

General Effects

The incidence of fatigue has been identified in research frequently enough to be considered a major concern in cancer symptom management (Virshup, 2010). It is one of the many side effects seen during cancer therapy that can affect a person's ability to function. Several factors contribute to the degree of fatigue experienced by patients receiving chemotherapy. These include immobility, malnutrition, stress, lack of sleep, anemia, hypoxia, infection or febrile states, pain, and multiple cancer therapies (e.g., biotherapy, chemotherapy, radiation therapy, and surgery). The nurse needs to encourage patients to balance activity and rest, optimize nutritional intake, and consider physical therapy consultation if necessary.

Nursing Management

Managing patients with cancer undergoing chemotherapy is complex and challenging. Nurses must be able to perform assessments that include the patient's immune status, pain control, hemodynamic stability, and emotional coping. The ability to differentiate between toxic effects (e.g., heart failure), which can be irreversible, and expected side effects (e.g., nausea and vomiting), most of which can be managed successfully with other drugs, is one of the unique features of an oncology assessment.

The Nursing Process: Patient Care Plan for Cancer box earlier in this chapter (p. 1790) identifies the appropriate nursing diagnosis and provides a detailed plan of care for the oncology patient regardless of the type of treatment being given.

Biotherapy

Biotherapy (biologic therapy) consists of treatment with agents whose origin is from biologic sources (mostly mammal) and/or agents that affect biologic responses (Virshup, 2010). Historically, cancer treatment has included surgery, radiotherapy, and chemotherapy or a combination of two or more of these therapies. Biotherapy has emerged since the 1980s as another treatment option for cancer patients receiving high-dose chemotherapy and transplantation. Nurses caring for patients receiving biotherapy need to thoroughly understand the immune system before they can begin to comprehend the rationale behind this unique treatment modality and the primary agents that are currently being used. (Refer to Chapters 52 and 53 for a review of the immune system.) Although the mechanism of action varies with each type of biologic response modifier (BRM), the goal is the same: to destroy or halt the malignant growth of a tumor. A therapeutic effect is accomplished by altering the immunologic relationship between the tumor and the host (patient) (Eggert, 2011; Virshup, 2010). Direct antitumor effects; restoration, augmentation, or modulation of host immune system mechanisms; and disrupting tumor cells' ability to metastasize or differentiate may affect host and tumor response. In addition, these agents, specifically monoclonal antibodies (mAbs), are used in diagnosing cancer by using low-dose radioisotopes tagged to mAbs that can detect tumors using special scanning equipment (Adams & Koch, 2010).

The popularity of biotherapy research has led to the development of nonspecific immunomodulating agents and new agents that include monoclonal antibodies, hematopoietic growth factors, interferons (INF), and interleukins. The latter three agents are part of a group of agents called cytokines, which are protein products from cells that function as cell regulators to enhance the production and functioning of the immune system. For example, lymphokines are products of lymphocytes, and monokines are products of monocytes; interleukins are proteins that act as messengers between cells. Cytokines are described in Chapter 53. Nonspecific agents surfaced when early research identified Bacille-Calmette-Guerin (BCG) and *Corynebacterium parvum*. When injected into humans, these agents work as antigens that stimulate the immune response, which should destroy malignant cells. Very positive outcomes have been demonstrated with multiple trials on animal and human models. Bacille-Calmette-Guerin is known to be effective as a treatment for localized bladder cancer and appears to have promise in the treatment of malignant melanoma.

The Pharmacology chart presented earlier in the chapter (p. 1804) lists biotherapy agents along with specific clinical indicators, administration information, and side effects. Only agents that the Food and Drug Administration (FDA) has approved for use are discussed; however, it is important to realize that multiple agents are under investigation that may be determined to be beneficial for use in patients with cancer in the future.

Side effects discussed in this chapter are those generally common to all agents. When administering biotherapy agents, the nurse is responsible for knowing the specific agent being given and becoming familiar with side effects specific to that drug. If side effects are not treated successfully or become too burdensome to the patient, the therapy may be dose limited, i.e. increase in dose or level of treatment are prevented. Other concerns in administering biologic therapy include safe handling of the drugs (determined by agency policy), rate of administration, length of time the drug is stable once reconstituted according to the manufacturer's package insert, whether special infusion filters or equipment is needed, and compatibility with other medications.

Oncology nurses are becoming more familiar with administering BRMs as more agents become available for commercial use. Nurses caring for patients who are receiving biotherapy need to be familiar with the many unique details of this form of therapy and should be comfortable with and excited about a field of cancer treatment that is changing rapidly. Nurses must expand their knowledge and understanding of new treatment options for cancer patients because new discoveries are frequently being made. There is much satisfaction to be gained from being involved with developing new standards of care and mentoring new nurses in the field of cancer nursing.

Nursing Management

Biotherapy agents differ from chemotherapeutic agents in action and toxicity patterns but, at the same time, have many of the same side effects. Nurses can use their knowledge of chemotherapy-induced side effects to assist them in planning care for patients receiving biotherapy. A comprehensive plan of care encompasses the patient's physical and psychological needs. (Refer to the Nursing Process: Patient Care Plan for Cancer, p. 1790.)

Transplantation: Bone Marrow and Peripheral Blood Stem Cells

Survival rates for cancer patients have improved owing to treatments such as surgery, radiotherapy, and chemotherapy. Despite this promising outcome, many cancers that initially respond to therapy tend to reappear. **Bone marrow transplantation (BMT),** the transfer of hematopoietic cells from the bone marrow of one person into another person or from the recipient's own bone marrow, has been used to treat a variety of diseases. Bone marrow transplantation offers patients with cancer the ability to receive intensive chemotherapy or radiation therapy when resistance to or failure of standard treatment occurs (Virshup, 2010). Another option, **peripheral blood stem cell (PBSC) transplantation,** is becoming more widely used instead of the traditional bone marrow transplantation. Peripheral blood stem cell transplantation is accomplished by circulating the patient's blood cells through a machine that removes the stem cells from the blood and then returns the blood back to the patient. Both forms of treatment improve long-term survival, making transplantation one of the most promising cancer therapies.

Transplantation has been performed for more than a century, but only since the mid-1960s have the chances of survival really improved. In the 19th century, bone marrow was fed or injected into patients with grim results.

Indications for Transplantation

The majority of transplants are performed for malignant disorders, although success has been demonstrated for use in patients with nonmalignant diseases (Virshup, 2010). Several factors determine the type of transplant that will provide the best chances for survival. These include the type and stage of disease, the patient's age and performance status, and donor availability.

Types of Bone Marrow Transplantation

The types of BMT are based on where the donor cells originate. **Autologous BMT,** in which the transplanted bone marrow comes from the recipient, is used for disorders in which the patient's bone marrow has adequate stem cells that can produce functioning erythrocytes, leukocytes, and platelets. The patient's own bone marrow or stem cells are harvested and placed in frozen storage to be reinfused into the patient when the conditioning regime (chemotherapy or radiation with chemotherapy) is completed (Virshup, 2010). In the past decade, more autologous BMTs have been performed, typically for hematologic malignancies. **Allogeneic bone marrow** comes from a histocompatible donor. These include syngeneic (identical twins), related (blood relative), and unrelated donors. Allogeneic bone marrow is used for patients with hematologic malignancies, marrow failure, severe combined immunodeficiency syndrome (SCIDS), and certain inherited metabolic disorders. The majority of allogeneic transplants are done for acute myelogenous leukemia (AML), acute lymphocytic leukemia (ALL), and chronic myelogenous leukemia (CML).

Sources of Cells for Transplantation

In 1987 the National Marrow Donor Program (NMDP) was established to allow for easier access to unrelated donors. The registry contains information on more than 4 million individuals who have had tissue typing and expressed a desire to donate bone marrow. In 1999, the NMDP established a central registry of core blood banks so that transplant centers could search for these donors more easily. When a donor is chosen, she does not know who will be the recipient, nor does the recipient know who has made such a generous donation.

Peripheral Blood Stem Cells

Traditionally, stem cells have been harvested from within the bone marrow cavity. The use of stem cells in peripherally circulating blood was first performed in the late 1950s (Santos, 2000). It has become more common since effectiveness was demonstrated in 1986 (Voss, Armitage, & Kessinger, 1993). The use of PBSC transplantation for hematopoietic support following high-dose chemotherapy is now the standard of practice for several malignant and nonmalignant diseases.

Autologous PBSC collection involves two phases: mobilization and apheresis. Mobilization involves stimulating the production of PBSCs with the administration of G-CSF or GM-CSF, possibly with chemotherapy. Apheresis is the collection of PBSCs through a double-lumen central venous catheter that is placed into the patient's vein. Blood is run through a cell separator that is programmed to collect either lymphocytes or low-density leukocytes and return other blood components to the patient. Apheresis usually takes one to three sessions, each lasting 3 to 4 hours. When collection is completed, the stem cells are placed into a blood bag and cryopreserved, remaining frozen at −196°C until needed for transplantation.

Allogeneic PBSC collection involves the same phases as those of autologous transplantation. The donor receives G-CSF for approximately 4 to 5 days, which is adequate for mobilization of PBSCs. Side effects that the donor may experience include bone pain, headache, fatigue, nausea, and insomnia (Rice, 2009). Apheresis is usually done via a peripheral line inserted into the antecubital veins using the cell separator. Nurses need to instruct the donor about the importance of keeping follow-up doctor appointments, since the most significant side effect is a drop in platelet count of up to 50%, which places the donor at risk for bleeding.

Bone Marrow Harvesting

The process of obtaining bone marrow for transplantation is called *harvesting*. For an autologous donor, the procedure occurs in the operating room, likely under general anesthesia. Multiple punctures are made in the posterior or anterior iliac crest to obtain the necessary amount (500 to 700 mL) of marrow needed for transplant. Once the marrow has been obtained, it is mixed with heparin, filtered to remove bone fragments and fat, and placed into a blood bag. At this point, the bone marrow is purged, which is the process of removing any remaining malignant cells from the marrow. Once the purging step is completed, the marrow is placed into a blood bag and frozen just like PBSCs.

Allogeneic bone marrow harvesting involves the same process as autologous harvesting minus the purging. After the marrow is harvested from the donor, it is immediately transfused into the recipient. Nursing care of the donor includes routine postoperative care (Chapter 19). In addition, donors need to be informed that they may expect pain at the donor sites for approximately 1 week. This pain is usually remedied by nonnarcotic analgesics. The psychological and emotional needs of donors are as important as their physical needs. Nurses need to encourage donors to express their concerns related to the success or failure of the transplant and provide support as needed.

Umbilical Cord Blood

Collection and storage of umbilical cord blood (UCB), which is rich in stem cells, is being used in transplantation. Cord blood is obtained by withdrawing blood via the umbilical vein immediately after the umbilical cord has been clamped. The blood is then cryopreserved, as is done with PBSCs or bone marrow. Because the use of UCB is a new approach in transplantation, it is not clear how the long-term effect on the rate of relapse of the disease will be demonstrated. In addition, there are ethical issues specific to the use of UCB such as the timing of consent and identifying links between mother and baby, which may be the focus of clinical, ethical, and regulatory scrutiny.

The Transplantation Process

Selection of the appropriate donor and recipient is crucial so that graft rejection and other serious complications are avoided. Criteria for the selection of a marrow or stem cell donor are few but very important. First, histocompatibility as measured by HLA and mixed lymphocyte culture testing must be determined. The donor's health status is evaluated to minimize the risks associated with donating and to prevent infecting the recipient with diseases such as hepatitis and HIV. Next, the donor's psychosocial profile is evaluated in an attempt to predict his attitudes and feelings toward the procedure and unknown outcomes. Finally, the donor's age is taken into consideration because of the amount of marrow needed for transplantation. Younger donors tend to be smaller in size, which limits the amount of marrow available for harvest (Rice, 2009).

A multidisciplinary approach is needed to evaluate the patient before he receives either bone marrow or stem cells. The pretransplant management consists of a detailed evaluation, including laboratory tests, procedures, and consultations, that is performed to determine the recipient's physical and psychosocial status (Rice, 2009). It is important to remember the patient's family members and friends, who may be asked to provide assistance during the transplantation process and recovery.

Once the initial evaluation is complete, the patient will undergo conditioning, which is the process of preparing the patient to receive bone marrow or stem cells. Conditioning serves three vital purposes: to eliminate malignant disease, to kill the current immunologic state, and to develop space in the marrow cavity for the transplanted stem cells as they begin reproducing. The conditioning regime consists of high dose chemotherapy with or without radiotherapy and results in severe myelosuppression. With conditioning complete, the bone marrow or stem cells may be infused. An autologous transplant is done by rapid IV push using syringes or by hanging the bag of cells and infusing over 20 to 30 minutes. During the procedure, patients may experience mild dyspnea from the volume being infused and nausea and vomiting from the preservatives in the solution. Allogeneic marrow or stem cells are infused slowly over 1 to 5 hours. Patients may experience side effects similar to those seen in a blood transfusion, as discussed in Chapter 16 (Rice, 2009).

Establishment of new bone marrow is referred to as **engraftment** (Virshup, 2010). The time required for complete engraftment depends on the source of the stem cells. Typically, bone marrow engrafts within 3 weeks, whereas stem cells take 11 to 16 days and cord blood takes 26 to 42 days. Of utmost concern are the pancytopenia and immunosuppression that are experienced during the period immediately after the transplant. Nurses must be very diligent at monitoring post-transplant patients for signs of infection and bleeding.

Nursing care of the patient undergoing bone marrow transplantation has evolved with the development of transplantation approaches and therapies. The challenging needs of the acute care patient highlight the complexity of this field of nursing. Because the ages of BMT patients can range across the life span, the nurse must possess skills for managing infants as well as older adults (Rice, 2009).

Complications of Transplantation

Patients who become transplant recipients are at risk for life-threatening complications, primarily because of the effects of the conditioning regime. Complications associated with the conditioning regime are numerous and can include bleeding, infection, nausea and vomiting, diarrhea, mucositis, and graft-versus-host disease (GVHD) (Rice, 2009). Several months to several years after transplant, the patient may experience late effects such as chronic GVHD, avascular necrosis, osteoporosis, cataracts, gonadal dysfunction, growth failure, hypothyroidism, secondary malignancies, need for revaccinations, and changes in quality of life.

Nurses who care for patients undergoing transplantation need to be aware of the signs of graft failure and GVHD. Graft failure (rejection) occurs very rarely, but its significance requires nurses to be astute in their ability to assess patients for signs of infection and bleeding. Graft rejection is confirmed by serial bone marrow biopsies and will require the patient to undergo another transplant, or death will be the result. Graft-versus-host disease occurs after allogeneic transplants and is the result of an immune-mediated reaction of the new stem cells reacting to the recipient's body.

Nursing Management

Caring for patients receiving transplantation is complex and challenging, requiring a systematic approach to assessment along with the ability to remain flexible when implementing a plan of care. The patient's condition changes day to day and even hour to hour, requiring the nurse to adapt to these variations quickly and competently. Transplant centers have begun to develop unique care models as a result of competition among health care institutions, a desire to improve outcomes, and the need to decrease costs (Rice, 2010). Involving the patient and family members in all aspects of care has created an environment that is more personal and individualized while reducing costs and rehospitalizations. The nurse has the opportunity to assist the patient in becoming more confident and competent in self-care. A comprehensive plan of care will encompass the patient's physical and psychological needs (refer to the Nursing Process: Patient Care Plan for Cancer box earlier, p. 1790).

Collaborative Management

A collaborative care approach is optimal for management of patients with cancer. Cancer can be acute, with fairly rapid deterioration and death, or chronic, with recurring remissions and exacerbations, requiring lifelong management. A multidisciplinary team approach, including the skills of health care providers, nurses, radiologist, oncologists, physical and occupational therapists, psychologists/psychiatrists, and pharmacists, will facilitate the best possible quality of life for the patient and family. In order to meet desired patient outcomes, it is essential that the members of this interdisciplinary team communicate openly with one another in developing and evaluating care of the patient and family (IOM [Institute of Medicine], 2010). The patient may need psychosocial counseling to assist in lifestyle adjustments necessitated by a chronic disease. The occupational therapist helps to facilitate realistic occupational goals, while the physical therapist assists in the maintenance of optimum conditioning given the activity restrictions. Because much of the treatment for cancer varies depending on where the patient lives or is treated, medications may vary as well, so the pharmacist has an important role in educating the patient about how to manage the medications and their side effects. In addition to the nursing care described previously, the nurse plays a pivotal role in coordinating the efforts of the health care team. In the inpatient setting, the nurse facilitates communication between the members of the team and the patient and family.

Cancer Emergencies

Oncologic emergencies occur as a result of the disease process or side effects of treatment. On occasion, patients will present to the health care provider with a variety of distressing complaints, and evaluation determines that the patient has a malignancy. Regardless of the cause of the emergency, catastrophic results can occur if prompt and effective interventions are not initiated (Virshup, 2010). The two main categories of emergencies are structural and metabolic (Virshup, 2010). Chart 57–18 (p. 1816) presents the important emergencies along with a definition, clinical findings, and treatment options. Oncology nurses understand the importance of continuously monitoring their patients for both subtle and obvious changes that may indicate the development of these potential life-threatening emergencies.

Living with Cancer: Supportive Therapies and Symptom Management

The diagnosis of cancer does not have to be equated with miserable suffering and death. During the past 30 years, a person's chance of surviving cancer has improved owing to (1) a better understanding of the disease, (2) changes in dose-limiting treatment toxicities, (3) new targeted therapies, (4) improved screening and early detection programs, (5) evidence-based practice, (6) improved supportive interventions, and (7) changes in sociocultural factors (U.S. Department of Health and Human Services, 2010). Although these factors have given patients with cancer an improved chance of survival, patients also may have to live with a variety of symptoms or complications that have the potential to be distressing. Nurses caring for cancer patients need to be aware of the potential problems, perform accurate assessments, and determine appropriate nursing interventions to alleviate any suffering or distress.

It is not uncommon for patients to consider the use of complementary and alternative medicine (CAM) therapies throughout the course of cancer treatment. Such therapies range from patients taking herbal and vitamin supplements to health care providers prescribing hypnotherapy (see the Complementary & Alternative Therapies box, p. 1818). Often, patients choose not to reveal these therapies to their health care providers. Of particular importance is determining the use of herbal and vitamin supplements that may interact negatively with concurrent use of traditional treatment options. Nurses need to provide patients with education in the use of CAM while respecting the individual's right to make decisions.

Patients face multiple challenges throughout their cancer experience. One of the most difficult issues (for patients and nurses) is the ethics of cancer care. Nurses have opportunities to develop relationships with their patients who have cancer and their families as they go through diagnosis and treatment. This relationship provides the nurse with an understanding of the goals and values the patient possesses as they relate to the cancer experience. Collaborating with the multidisciplinary team is important to determine a plan of care that honors and respects these goals and values.

Nutrition

The nutritional status of cancer patients can be altered in a variety of ways. Emotional stress from impaired nutritional intake coupled with the metabolic demand of cancer and its treatment can have a profound effect on the patient. Nurses cannot ignore how eating can be a part of a patient's social presence and often is a source of enjoyment (Smith, 2009).

Weight loss in patients with cancer is likely to result in poor clinical and psychological outcomes (Smith, 2009). The nurse can recognize the syndrome of cancer **cachexia** by the presence of anorexia, weight loss, muscle and adipose tissue wasting, hyperlipidemia, and other metabolic derangements. It is present in 80% of those who die of cancer (Cunningham, 2004). Figure 57–7◆ (p. 1817) illustrates how profoundly cachexia affects the human body. Cachexia is the result of altered absorption and changes in metabolism, such as protein, fat, and carbohydrates (National Cancer Institute, 2011). It is important for the nurse to remember that cachexia can be present in patients who have adequate caloric and protein intake but are failing to absorb the necessary nutrients.

For those patients receiving chemotherapy, inadequate nutrition is of utmost concern. One of the most dreaded side effects of chemotherapy is nausea and vomiting. Uncontrolled nausea and vomiting can eventually result in cachexia preceded by anorexia and weight loss (Virshup, 2010). Oncology nurses are vital in ensuring that the nutritional needs of these patients are being met. Recognizing the early signs of cachexia and implementing effective interventions are key in slowing or reversing the progression of cachexia syndrome.

Nutritional screening is the process of evaluating patients for the risk of developing malnutrition. The goal of screening is to identify patients who are at risk, prevent or treat malnutrition early, and individualize the nutritional plan of care (Smith, 2009). Working together with a nutritionist, the nurse can perform an effective nutritional screening evaluation by determining food intake, noting the presence of symptoms,

CHART 57–18 Oncologic Emergencies

Emergency	Findings	Treatment
Metabolic		
Disseminated intravascular coagulation (DIC) (see Chapter 54)	Signs of bleeding and clotting	Elimination of triggering event Supportive measures (transfusion of blood products)
Hypercalcemia: serum calcium levels $>$ 9–11 mg/dL	Lethargy Altered mental status Nausea and vomiting Anorexia Polydipsia Constipation	Hydration Diuresis to enhance the excretion of calcium Pharmacology: bisphosphonates (inhibit the action of osteoclasts) Increased mobilization
Malignant pleural effusion; accumulation of fluid in the pleural cavity	Dyspnea at rest or activity Cough (nonproductive) Chest pain Malaise Weight loss Fear of suffocation, anxiety	Radiation or chemotherapy aimed at the primary tumor Insertion of chest tube with drainage capability Pleurodesis
Sepsis (see Chapter 54)	Fever Chills Decreased blood pressure Rapid respiratory rate Mental cloudiness	Recognition of impending shock is key Infection control practices Private rooms Hemodynamic monitoring while in the intensive care unit (ICU) Antibiotic therapy
Syndrome of inappropriate antidiuretic hormone (SIADH): endocrine paraneoplastic syndrome causing water imbalance (see Chapter 46)	Hyponatremia Decreased serum osmolality Water retention Increased urine osmolality Normal skin turgor Normal blood pressure	Treat underlying cause Fluid restriction Diuretic therapy
Hypersensitivity reaction (anaphylaxis): immunologic response to foreign substance or antigen; may be life threatening	Occurs within minutes of receiving certain chemotherapy agents Dyspnea Agitation Hypotension Laryngeal edema and spasm	Prevention is the key Careful monitoring of blood pressure, pulse, and oxygen saturation during infusion Emergency equipment needs to be available
Tumor lysis syndrome: rapid lysis of malignant cells resulting in renal (e.g., acidosis), electrolyte (e.g., hyperuricemia, hyperkalemia), cardiac, and neurologic complications	Nausea and vomiting Edema Flank pain Hematuria Changes in blood pressure Lethargy Muscle twitching and weakness	Prevention is the key Pretreatment hydration Pharmacologic therapy (diuretics, xanthine oxidase inhibitors, sodium bicarbonate) Supportive measures for potential organ failure
Structural		
Increased intracranial pressure: volume of the brain, CSF, and cerebral blood volume increase (see Chapter 20)	Signs and symptoms of increased intracranial pressure	Pharmacologic therapy (osmotic diuretics, corticosteroids, anticonvulsants) Surgery to relieve pressure and evacuate fluid Radiation and chemotherapy to shrink tumor bulk
Spinal cord compression: malignancy that invades the epidural space and cauda equina (see Chapter 24)	Signs and symptoms of cord compression are specific to the area of the cord being compressed	Pharmacologic therapy (corticosteroids) Radiation therapy to reduce tumor bulk Surgery when bony instability occurs

CHART 57–18 Oncologic Emergencies, *continued*

Emergency	Findings	Treatment
Superior vena cava syndrome: obstruction of venous flow through the vena cava resulting in compression of intrathoracic structures, vascular congestion, and venous hypertension	Dyspnea Cough Feeling of fullness in the head Chest pain	Pharmacologic therapy (fibrinolytic therapy) Radiation therapy to reduce tumor bulk Chemotherapy for specific cell types Surgery (stents or bypass)
Cardiac tamponade: compression of the cardiac muscle by malignant fluid accumulation within the pericardial sac (see Chapter 33)	Dyspnea Chest pain Tachycardia Cough	Pharmacologic therapy (diuretics, corticosteroids, NSAIDs) Removal of fluid via pericardiocentesis, pericardiotomy, pericardiectomy

Sources: Adapted from Virshup, D. M. (2010). Biology, clinical manifestations, and treatment of cancer. In K. L. McCance & S. E. Huether (Eds.), *Pathophysiology: The biologic basis for disease in adults and children* (pp. 396–435). St. Louis: Mosby Elsevier.

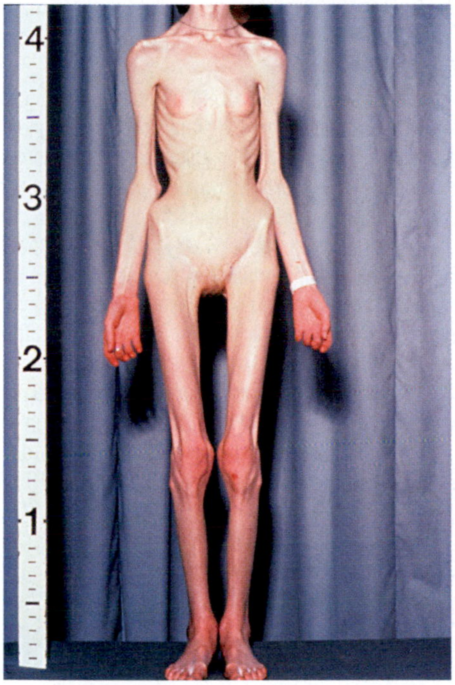

FIGURE 57–7 ◆ Cancer cachexia.
Source: © Welcome Trust Images/Custom Medical Stock Photo.

determining the patient's functional status (Karnofsky Performance Scale, p. 1784) and weight, doing a physical assessment, and obtaining laboratory data analysis. See Chapter 8 for more details related to malnutrition.

Nutritional Support

Once the need for nutritional support has been determined, the method of delivery is the next decision to be made. For patients with mild anorexia, nutritional counseling may be adequate, whereas patients with severe anorexia or cachexia may require parenteral nutritional support. Oral nutrition is the preferred route, but patients with a mechanical inability to consume food may require enteral feedings. Parenteral nutrition is reserved for patients whose GI tract is not functioning properly and those who cannot tolerate enteral feedings. Chapter 8 provides a detailed discussion of the different delivery methods. Ethical questions surrounding the use of artificial nutrition and hydration with patients who have cancer are addressed in the Ethical Issues box.

Fatigue

Fatigue, the most frequently experienced symptom of cancer and its therapy, has a profound effect on patients' quality of life (Virshup, 2010). Fatigue associated with cancer and cancer treatments began receiving attention from health care providers in the 1970s. A renewed interest in the topic developed in the mid-1980s when oncology nursing texts, journal articles, and research reports indicated that the incidence of fatigue was more common than had previously been assumed (Nail, 2004). In the early 1990s, Winningham et al. (1994) described a common definition of fatigue as "a sense of tiredness." Most recently, the National Comprehensive Cancer Network (2011) expanded on this widely accepted definition to state that "cancer-related fatigue is a distressing persistent subjective sense of tiredness or exhaustion related to cancer or cancer treatment that is not proportional to recent activity and interferes with usual functioning." The Evidence-Based Practice box (p. 1819) provides further discussion about fatigue related to cancer.

Influencing Factors

The experience of having cancer puts the patient at risk for experiencing problems that may create physical, mental, and emotional fatigue. Factors that influence fatigue, such as physical, functional, psychosocial, and spiritual factors, are described in Chart 57–19 (p. 1820).

Nurses caring for cancer patients are encouraged to develop a method of assessing for fatigue that can be performed quickly but thoroughly and can be used for patients with diseases other than cancer. Of particular importance is the timing of the nurse's assessment of fatigue. For example, if fatigue were assessed before the patient received chemotherapy or biotherapy, the results would likely be different than if the assessment were done the day after therapy was administered. The assessment data should be used as a guide for nursing practice decisions, including reevaluation of the patient's symptoms to determine the effectiveness of the nursing care plan.

Cancer Pain

Pain is a complex process that is affected by many physical and psychosocial influences. Cancer pain occurs as a result of the disease's progression, diagnostic procedures, and/or the treatment provided. The location of the primary or metastatic lesion influences the degree of pain experienced by the patient. When there is bony involvement, such as spinal metastases, or neural involvement as is seen when tumor

COMPLEMENTARY & ALTERNATIVE THERAPIES Hypnotherapy

Nancy Yilk

HYPNOSIS IS A STATE of highly focused attention, with a constriction in peripheral awareness and a heightened responsiveness to social cues. It is most similar to the everyday state of becoming so absorbed in a good movie or a novel that the imagined world moves into the foreground and causes the viewer to suspend awareness of the usual environment, a condition playwrights refer to as the *suspension of disbelief.* This state can exert a powerful influence on the mind and body. By altering the patient's perception of pain using hypnosis, changes result in the brain that reduce pain perception, rather than merely altering the response to pain. Indeed, simply changing the wording of the hypnotic instruction from "You will feel cool, tingling numbness more than pain" to "The pain will not bother you" alters the brain location of the analgesia from the somatosensory cortex to the anterior cingulate gyrus. Hypnotic alteration of color perception results in bidirectional changes in blood flow in the portions of the visual cortex that process color vision—blood flow in this region increases when color is imagined rather than seen and decreases when color is hypnotically drained from a colorful stimulus. Thus, there is a sound neurophysiologic basis for the belief that hypnosis is potentially a powerful tool to alter the perception of pain and associated anxiety (Glauser & Canadian Medical Association, 2011).

Evidence suggests that hypnosis is an effective intervention for reducing distress, pain, and other side effects associated with cancer and its treatment. In a study, 115 participants were surveyed regarding their overall intentions to use hypnosis to control side effects of cancer and its treatment, as well as demographic predictors of such intentions among healthy volunteers. Results suggested that the vast majority of participants (89%) were willing to use hypnosis to control side effects associated with cancer treatment. These results indicate that, in the general public, a willingness exists to consider the use of hypnosis, and that willingness is not determined by demographic factors (Sohl et al., 2010).

There is growing interest in mind–body therapies as adjuncts to mainstream cancer treatment, and an increasing number of patients turn to these interventions for the control of emotional stress associated with cancer. Mind–body treatments evaluated for their utility in oncology include relaxation therapies, biofeedback, meditation and hypnosis, yoga, art and music therapy, tai chi, and qigong. Although studies are not always methodologically sound and results are mixed, a growing number of well-designed studies provide convincing evidence that mind–body techniques are beneficial adjuncts to cancer treatment. The evidence is sufficient to recommend further investigation and adoption of these techniques in mainstream oncology care.

A randomized clinical trial examined the effects of group therapy with hypnosis (supportive-expressive group therapy) plus education compared to an education-only control condition on pain over 12 months among 124 women with metastatic breast cancer. Pain and suffering, frequency of pain, and degree of constant pain were assessed at baseline and 4-month intervals. Those in the treatment group also reported on their experiences using the hypnosis exercises. Analyses indicated that the hypnosis intervention resulted in significantly less increase in the intensity of pain and suffering over time, compared to the education-only group, but had no significant effects on the frequency of pain episodes or amount of constant pain. In addition, there was no interaction of the intervention with hypnotizability. Within the intervention group, highly hypnotizable participants, compared to those less hypnotizable, reported greater benefits from hypnosis, employed self-hypnosis more often outside of group, and used it to manage other symptoms in addition to pain (Butler et al., 2009).

Breast cancer radiotherapy can be an emotionally difficult experience. A study examined the effectiveness of a multimodal psychotherapeutic approach, combining cognitive–behavioral therapy and hypnosis (CBTH), to reduce negative affect and increase positive affect in 40 women undergoing breast cancer radiotherapy. Participants were randomly assigned to receive either CBTH or standard care. Participants completed weekly self-report measures of positive and negative affect. Repeated and univariate analyses of variance revealed that the CBTH approach reduced levels of negative affect and increased levels of positive affect during the course of radiotherapy. Additionally, relative to the control group, the CBTH group demonstrated significantly more intense positive affect and significantly less intense negative affect during radiotherapy. The CBTH group also had a significantly higher frequency of days where positive affect was greater than negative affect (85% of days assessed for the CBTH group versus 43% of the control group). Therefore, the CBTH intervention has the potential to improve the affective experience of women undergoing breast cancer radiotherapy (Schnur et al., 2009).

A randomized trial conducted among 200 patients who underwent excisional breast biopsy or lumpectomy for breast cancer assigned patients to routine anesthesia plus nondirective empathic listening (the control condition) or a very brief 15-minute presurgery hypnosis session. The hypnosis of a relaxation-based induction (including imagery for muscle relaxation) included suggestions for pleasant visual imagery, suggestions to experience relaxation and peace, specific symptom-focused suggestions (i.e., to experience reduced pain, nausea, and fatigue), and a deepening procedure. Instructions for how patients could use hypnosis on their own followed the intervention session. This brief hypnotic preparation was sufficient to produce a statistically significant reduction in the use of propofol and lidocaine. Even with patients in the intervention using less propofol and lidocaine, the group reported less pain, nausea, fatigue, discomfort, and emotional upset than did patients in the control group (Kwekkeboom, Cherwin, Lee, & Wanta, 2010; Montgomery et al., 2010).

References

Butler, L. D., Koopman, C., Neri, E., Giese-Davis, J., Palesh, O., Thorne-Yocam, K. A., et al. (2009). Effects of supportive-expressive group therapy on pain in women with metastatic breast cancer. *Health Psychology, 28*(5), 579–587.

Glauser, W., & Canadian Medical Association. (2011). The therapeutic value of hyper-suggestibility. *Canadian Medical Association Journal, 183*(3), 149–150.

Kwekkeboom, K. L., Cherwin, C. H., Lee, J. W., & Wanta, B. (2010). Mind–body treatments for the pain-fatigue-sleep disturbance symptom cluster in persons with cancer. *Journal of Pain and Symptom Management, 39*(1), 126–138. Epub 2009 Nov 8.

Montgomery, G. H., Hallquist, M. N., Schnur, J. B., David, D., Silverstein, J. H., & Bovbjerg, D. H. (2010). Mediators of a brief hypnosis intervention to control side effects in breast surgery patients: Response expectancies and emotional distress. *Journal of Consulting and Clinical Psychology, 78*(1), 80–88.

Schnur, J. B., David, D., Kangas, M., Green, S., Bovbjerg, D. H., & Montgomery, G. H. (2009). A randomized trial of a cognitive-behavioral therapy and hypnosis intervention on positive and negative affect during breast cancer radiotherapy. *Journal of Clinical Psychology, 65*(4), 443–455.

Sohl, S. J., Stossel, L., Schnur, J. B., Tatrow, K., Gherman, A., & Montgomery, G. H. (2010). Intentions to use hypnosis to control the side effects of cancer and its treatment. *American Journal of Clinical Hypnosis, 53*(2), 93–100.

compresses nerve tissue, pain is intensified (Virshup, 2010). Most often, pain is not a problem in the early stage of the disease; however, nearly 30% of patients begin to experience pain during treatment. Advancing cancer, including metastasis, produces pain in nearly 90% of patients (Virshup, 2010).

Up to 50% of cancer patients with pain fail to achieve adequate relief (Ameringer, 2010; Rustoen, 2009). This statistic should compel those who care for cancer patients to continue to strive for more effective relief of suffering. Because cancer care produces a myriad of side effects such as fatigue, pain, infection, or bleeding, effective treatment is very challenging. It has been suggested that the presence of pain and fatigue makes other cancer symptoms more severe and more difficult to manage (Given, Given, Azzoouz, Kozachik, & Stommel, 2001).

In 1990, ONS produced a position paper on cancer pain and declared that "nurses are responsible and accountable for implementation

ETHICAL ISSUES
Related to Nutrition in Patients with Cancer

A declining appetite affects not only the patient's physical well-being, but also the functional, social, and psychological aspects of the patient's quality of life. These changes are frequently noticed in patients who are nearing the end of their lives and should be addressed with sensitivity and compassion. One approach is to offer education, dietary modifications, and appetite stimulants. However, these approaches are often unsuccessful, and family members may begin to question whether their loved one is "starving to death" (Eilers, 2011).

Artificial nutrition and hydration toward the end of life are controversial therapies and have not been proven to be beneficial to the patient. In fact, administration of these therapies has been associated with complications and suffering (Eilers, 2011). It is the responsibility of the health care team to determine the patient's goals regarding end-of-life nutrition and hydration. This type of conversation may be difficult but is paramount in trying to understand how the patient with cancer wishes to live during his final days and in honoring those wishes. Chapter 11 discusses end-of-life issues in detail.

and coordination of the plan for management of cancer pain" (Spross, McGuire, & Schmitt, 1990a, 1990b, 1990c). Since 2006, the National Comprehensive Cancer Network has asserted that cancer pain can be well controlled in most patients if the health care team uses evidence-based guidelines, which can be individualized to each patient and involves patients in decision making regarding their pain (ONS, 2011). Nurses who care for cancer patients implement frequent assessments of pain status, provide patient and family counseling or education, and participate in ongoing reevaluation and management of pain control. Chapter 12 provides detailed information on pain assessment and management that can easily be applied to patients with cancer pain.

Alternative Care Programs

A rising interest in home care and alternative settings for patients who are facing a terminal illness, such as advanced cancer, has led to the development of programs such as hospice and palliative care. Becoming familiar with the concepts of hospice and palliative care is important for the nurse who will be caring for patients with cancer. Chapter 11 discusses these programs in detail.

Quality of Life Throughout The Cancer Continuum

Although individuals with cancer have been surviving longer, they continue to search for the meaning of their illness. The search for meaning is a process that is thought to include cognitive appraisals, reappraisals, and attributions that individuals make in response to stressful experiences. Quality of life (QOL) is an important component in one's ability to survive a major illness and the prescribed treatment. It embraces the characteristics and limitations that affect one's ability to function and obtain satisfaction in doing so. Over the years, the construct of QOL has been explored by many, but perhaps the most widely accepted description comes from Ferrell and colleagues. Their description identifies several dimensions, including physical, psychological, and social well-being, which are the hallmark components of a person's QOL (Ferrell & Dow, 1997). The health care team needs to consider both the patient and family when evaluating the effect of cancer and cancer care on QOL. See Chapter 11 for additional information on QOL.

Throughout all phases of cancer, it is essential for life to go on as close to normally as possible. During the diagnosis phase, the patient and family may be paralyzed by fear, often demonstrating behaviors that are consistent with denial. Once the diagnosis of cancer has been made,

EVIDENCE-BASED PRACTICE Fatigue in Relation to Cancer

Clinical Problem

Fatigue is reported as the most prevalent symptom in patients with cancer. A common definition of fatigue is the presence of a subjective feeling of tiredness influenced by circadian rhythm (Esper, 2010). The incidence of developing fatigue varies throughout the disease experience, ranging between 17% to 40% in individuals who are disease-free cancer survivors and 85% to 100% in patients whose goal of care is palliative (Bookbinder, 2010). The effects of fatigue on the patient are many, including mood disturbances, poor concentration, decreased perception and capacity to work, changes in compliance with medical treatment, and decreased ability to perform ADLs. All people experience fatigue in their daily lives; however, when it becomes constant and excessive, the person's ability and willingness to remain active is affected. In addition, when the effects of fatigue persist, the patient may question whether she can endure ongoing cancer treatment.

Research Findings

Multiple research studies have looked at the effect of fatigue in patients with cancer. Esper (2010) performed a systematic review of the symptoms that are associated with cancer, including fatigue, and found that many patients with advanced cancer actually experienced a cluster of symptoms. Examples of clusters of symptoms included cough/breathlessness/fatigue; fatigue/anorexia-cachexia; fatigue/drowsiness/nausea/decreased appetite; and dyspnea, fatigue/pain/anxiety, and depression.

Implications for Nursing Practice

Nurses have the opportunity to positively affect the way a cancer patient experiences the effects of treatment. First, nurses need to be familiar with the types of patients who are likely to develop fatigue as part of their cancer experience. The systematic review discussed previously discovered that fatigue generally did not occur alone. Assessing for fatigue and its severity and other related symptoms needs to be incorporated into routine nursing practice. The nurse can ask the patient who is experiencing fatigue to rate the distress associated with the symptom on a scale from 1 to 10. This will provide a basis of comparison for future assessments. The National Comprehensive Cancer Network (2011) has made recommendations for screening for fatigue, including screening at the initial visit, at regular intervals, and when clinical indicators are present.

Together with the health care provider, the nurse needs to discuss treatment-related side effects and toxicities with the patient. The patient is then able to prepare and plan for the onset of fatigue. By suggesting self-care strategies to help people cope, the nurse helps the patient minimize the effects of fatigue. Emphasizing energy conservation, energy restoration, exercise, good nutrition, and adequate rest should be a routine part of nursing conversation with patients who may experience fatigue.

Critical Thinking Questions with answers can be found in the Osborn Student Resources at nursing.pearsonhighered.com.

References

Esper, P. (2010). Symptom clusters in individuals living with advanced cancer. *Seminars in Oncology Nursing, 26*(3), 168–174.

National Comprehensive Cancer Network. (2011). Clinical practice guidelines in oncology. Retrieved from http://www.nccn.com/living-with-cancer.html.

Oncology Nursing Society (ONS). (2011). Putting evidence into practice: Fatigue. Retrieved from http://www.ons.org/Research/PEP/media/ons/docs/research/outcomes/fatigue/samplechapter.pdf.

CHART 57–19 Fatigue Factors

Physical	Functional	Spiritual	Psychosocial
Pain	Value/meaning given to changes in one's life	Look for value or meaning to diagnosis, treatment, suffering, recovery, and death.	Depression/isolation
Disturbed sleep–wake patterns	Ability to perform normal activities (work, home, social)	Consider the meaning and consequences of the diagnosis.	Roles/isolation
Nutrition	Attentional fatigue: decreased capacity to concentrate	Review life to find ways to cope:	Anxiety
GI difficulties		Being hopeful	Appearance
Multiple medications		Changing priorities	Control
Bone marrow suppression		Learning to live with diagnosis.	Relationships, affection, sexual function
Performance status (Karnofsky)			Finances

Source: Adapted from Oncology Nursing Society. (2011). Putting evidence into practice: Fatigue. Retrieved from http://www.ons.org/Research/PEP/media/ons/docs/research/outcomes/fatigue/samplechapter.pdf.

ETHICAL ISSUES
Related to Nursing Care of the Patient with Cancer

Informed Consent and Determining Decision-Making Capacity: Nurses reinforce and clarify information presented by health care providers. If confusion surrounding consent exists, the nurse needs to notify the health care provider that the patient needs continued discussion. Documentation of the informed consent needs to be found in the medical record.

Communicating Bad News: The nurse's role is one of facilitation. Nurses prepare the environment, which includes finding a meeting place and inviting the appropriate people to participate in the discussion. While the health care provider delivers the bad news, the nurse provides support, responds to the patient's and family members' feelings, and begins to plan follow-through as needed (e.g., offering spiritual support, allowing quiet private time for patient and family).

Privacy and Confidentiality: Nurses are obligated to protect the patient's privacy and information related to the patient's health care situation.

Clinical Research Trials: Clinical research trials present multiple ethical issues for the health care team to address. These issues include poor minority involvement, patients' perspective of hope for a cure, adjustment of exclusion criteria to allow more participation, randomization that creates conflict for health care providers when they believe one intervention used in the trial is best, and cost issues.

Advance Directives: Nurses educate the patient and family regarding the benefit of completing an advance directive. The nurse must communicate with the health care team regarding the presence and content of the document, and refer the patient to the appropriate source for initiating.

Do-Not-Resuscitate (DNR) Orders: Nurses' responsibilities include ensuring that the health care team and patient understand any DNR orders, advocating for independent decision making throughout the entire course of treatment while encouraging the patient to communicate openly with health care providers, ensuring that proper documentation has been completed and the appropriate renewal process is followed, and validating the emotional responses of patients and family members. Often forgotten but very important is the effect a DNR order has on the nurse and health care team. Throughout the course of an illness, oncology nurses develop a relationship with their patients and families. Although the nurse advocates for patients and their right to make decisions, a DNR order creates emotions in care providers that are important to recognize as normal.

End-of-Life Issues: As a patient's illness progresses, a new set of issues arises that require the patient to be given ongoing support, communication, and advocacy from the health care team. Chapter 11 discusses end-of-life issues in detail.

Source: Adapted from Grant, M. (2010). Advances in quality of life at the end of life. *Seminars in Oncology, 26*(1), 26–35.

others surround the patient with support in an effort to fight the disease. As the cancer advances, the patient is faced with accepting the diagnosis and possibly abandoning a hope for a cure.

Nurses can support patients with respectful and thoughtful communication while the patients begin to adjust to the stress that accompanies the diagnosis of cancer. Although the health care provider typically delivers the news of the cancer diagnosis and prognosis to the patient, the nurse offers emotional support by providing patient and mindful listening that demonstrates compassion and concern. Patients will often express their hopes and fears when they feel that someone genuinely cares. To cope with these fears, cancer patients may see themselves demonstrating behaviors that are unfamiliar to them, including shock, anger, denial, bargaining, depression, helplessness, hopelessness, rationalization, acceptance, and intellectualization. A compassionate and caring nurse will reassure patients that their responses are not abnormal. The Ethical Issues box describes additional areas in which nurses can be of help to patients with cancer.

Cancer treatment tends to be accompanied by multiple symptoms that may provoke a varying degree of suffering in the patient. The oncology nurse can positively affect QOL by prioritizing symptoms and implementing appropriate relief measures. On occasion, the patient may report distress from a symptom, such as malaise and fatigue; however, with keen assessment skills, the nurse may discover the presence of a more significant problem causing the patient's symptoms. This knowledge, when demonstrated by the nurse, will be recognized by patients and will enhance their trust in the nurse.

Key to being an effective oncology nurse is the ability to instill hope into patients and their loved ones. The meaning of hope varies depending on the patient's status:

1. Hope that symptoms are not serious
2. Hope that treatment is curative
3. Hope for independence
4. Hope for relief of pain
5. Hope for a longer life
6. Hope for a peaceful and dignified death.

Hope allows cancer patients to maintain a sense of control over their current situation along with a positive attitude toward their disease.

Most health care organizations and cancer advocacy groups try to provide creative ways to increase cancer awareness and provide support for patients and their families. One example is the use of art as a way of explaining a patient's journey with cancer. Both patients and artists have begun to understand the benefit of creating art during an illness experience (Cook, 2009). Patients can tell stories of their illness, including initial symptoms, the diagnosing experience, hospitalizations, treatment-induced body changes, key health care providers, and recovery. Art can assist the patient in gaining a sense of control in a situation that seems uncontrollable and allows for a vehicle to communicate emotions, such as loneliness, solitude, and the need for survival (Cook, 2009). Nurses have the unique opportunity to recognize the benefit of art in the recovery of patients afflicted with cancer.

Discharge Planning

Discharge planning is a process that includes assessment, identification of continuing care needs, and formulation and implementation of a plan that will meet those needs. Typically, this process begins when the patient is admitted to the hospital, but it is reasonable to begin evaluating the patient's needs in the outpatient setting because oncology patients interact with outpatient personnel frequently for treatments and management of symptoms. A variety of health care professionals can be involved in the process, but the nurse and social worker are particularly important in establishing a comprehensive discharge plan. Developing a systematic approach will assist in creation of the comprehensive plan of care and provide opportunities for routine reevaluation and modification of the plan.

Patients and their families need to be actively involved in the discharge planning process. Educating the patient and those who will care for the patient after discharge about self-care is critical in a successful discharge plan, but nurses must first ascertain learning needs or barriers that will affect their ability to provide effective teaching. In addition, cultural influences (a nurse's own and the patient's) need to be recognized so the teaching can be individualized and meaningful. The Patient Teaching & Discharge Priorities box describes the necessary components of the teaching plan, which includes sexuality issues and psychological adaptation.

Gerontological Considerations

Increased attention is being devoted to the care of older patients with cancer. There are two reasons for this: the increased number of older people in the population and the increased number of older people with cancer. The aging of the baby boomers (individuals born between 1946 and 1964) is the major cause of the increasing number of aging adults, along with improvements in health care and nutrition that have led to longer lives. Americans who are over the age of 65 have more of a chance of developing cancer than people under 65 years of age (Eggert, 2011). Caring for the aging with cancer is quickly becoming a public health concern.

It is predicted that by the year 2030, one in five persons will be 65 years or older, compared with the current figure of one in nine persons (Kinsella & Velkoff, 2001). These statistics provide a compelling reason to expand the knowledge base about cancer education, screening, and management in older adults. Of particular importance is the need for nurses to recognize the older adult's experience with cancer and to identify strategies by which oncology nurses can contribute to changes in cancer care for older adults. Understanding the 10 key facts of cancer in older adults, as listed in Chart 57–20, will provide nurses with an appreciation of the magnitude of the problem being faced.

The future of cancer care is going to be significantly affected by our aging population, requiring ongoing attention to the uniqueness of caring for the older cancer patient. In 2004, a collaborative effort by ONS and the Geriatric Oncology Consortium (GOC) produced a position statement regarding care of the older cancer patient (http://www.ons.org/publications/positions/media/ons/docs/positions/summary-cancercareintheolderadult.pdf). Within this publication, the unique attributes of older cancer patients were acknowledged, including the nature of cancer in the older adult and the specific needs of older cancer patients and their implications for society (ONS & GOC, 2004). Nurses who are providing cancer-related care for the growing number of older patients need to understand the normal physiological changes associated with aging. These include impaired immune system; decreased organ function and structure; decreased skin elasticity; decreased skeletal mass, structure, and strength; changes in sensory and neurological

PATIENT TEACHING & DISCHARGE PRIORITIES for Cancer

Need	Teaching
Treatment side effects and toxicities: Patient/family Family/support system Setting	Instruct the patient regarding proper oral care: • Brush and floss teeth as tolerated. • Use moistening gauze or toothettes instead of a toothbrush if needed; for instance, if platelet count is low (<40,000/mm³). • Rinse with normal saline four times per day. • Avoid commercial mouthwashes. • Cleanse mouth before and after meals. Instruct the patient to report signs of stomatitis: • Burning • Pain • Areas of redness • Open lesions on the lips • Pain with swallowing • Intolerance to temperature extremes.

(continued)

PATIENT TEACHING & DISCHARGE PRIORITIES for Cancer, *continued*

Need	Teaching
	Take antiemetics and appetite stimulants per orders. Suggest small, frequent meals that are high in calories and protein. Encourage adequate fluid intake while limiting fluids during mealtime. Monitor for signs of infection and notify the health care provider immediately. Avoid contact with individuals who are currently known to have, or recently have had, an infection or recent vaccination. Avoid raw meat and fish, fresh fruit and vegetables, and fresh flowers and plants. Avoid use of a straight-edge razor. Instruct the patient in ways to minimize the risk of bleeding: • Perform oral hygiene with a soft toothbrush or toothettes. • Avoid use of commercial mouthwashes. • Avoid straight-edge razors. • File nails with an emery board. • Avoid foods that are difficult to chew. Encourage frequent rest periods. Encourage more sleep hours at night. Encourage the patient to reorganize her daily schedule of activities and seek assistance with shopping, cooking, housework, etc. Encourage a temporary decrease in work hours. Assess availability, knowledge, and compliance with the treatment regimen. Assess respite needs and resources. Assess discharge placement needs: • Home • Hospice • Long-term care facility. Assess the home environment for needed assistive devices. Assess the need for professional home health. Assess the need for follow-up appointments.
In-home treatments: Patient/family Family/support system Setting	Instruct the patient and family in the operation and troubleshooting of infusion equipment. Instruct the patient and family in how to care for an implantable infusion device. Instruct the patient and family in the proper storage of medications and solutions. Assess the availability of treatment and knowledge and compliance with the treatment regimen. Assess respite needs and resources. Assess the home environment for risk factors. Assess the home environment for needed assistive devices. Assess the need for professional home health. Assess the need for follow-up appointments.
Coping: Patient/family Family/support system Setting	Encourage the patient to participate in activities and decision making. Encourage the patient to verbalize concerns. Instruct about patterns of hair loss and regrowth. Encourage the patient to view a venous access device. Encourage the patient in selecting cosmetic devices that increase sense of attractiveness. Offer ways to cope with hair loss: • Obtain wigs or hairpieces before hair loss. • Take a photograph of hair loss to the wig shop to improve matching of hair color. • Contact the American Cancer Society for available resources. • Wear a scarf, hat, or other device as needed. Encourage dialogue between the patient and partner regarding sexual function and alternatives. Assess the need for professional home health. Assess the need for follow-up appointments.

CHART 57–20 Key Facts of Cancer in the Older Adult

- Cancer is a disease of older adults.
- Most cancers are due to solid tumors.
- The etiology of cancer in older adults is controversial.
- Public education of older adults is needed.
- Data regarding development of treatment toxicities are minimal.
- Treatment decisions should be based on physiological (not chronological) age.
- The current deficit in knowledge of older adults with cancer is due to underrepresentation in clinical trials.
- Caregiving and coping problems are important to consider.
- Consider blending the specialties of oncology and gerontology.
- Nursing research opportunities are endless.

functions; and alterations in drug absorption, distribution, metabolism, and elimination (Doerflinger, 2009). Chart 57–21 describes the normal changes seen with aging and their impact on cancer nursing care. When administering cancer treatments to older patients, the nurse must be alert to possible intolerance due to the normal changes seen with advancing age. Older patients with cancer frequently have comorbidities with ongoing treatments that may also limit their tolerance to prescribed cancer therapy.

Research

Cancer research is crucial to improving therapy and survival along with management of symptoms associated with this devastating disease. The goal of research is to identify areas in which practice could improve and then evaluate and test methods in these areas. The Research Opportunities box (p. 1824) provides a list of both medical and nursing research

CHART 57–21 Changes Seen with Aging and Their Effect on Cancer Care

Changes Seen With Aging	Nursing Implications
Decreased skin elasticity, body mass, and impaired healing	Monitor for skin and mucous membrane changes. Monitor oral cavity for properly fitting prosthesis and abnormal skin condition. Provide skin care to prevent breakdown. Encourage mobility as tolerated: Range of motion Assist with turning. Encourage adequate nutrition. Consult with a dietitian as needed. Provide frequent toileting.
Impaired immune system	Monitor for signs of infection: fever, chills, exudate, urinary symptoms, cough, drainage from wounds, mental status changes, and laboratory data (ANC, WBC, culture and sensitivity results).
Decreased vital organ function (renal, cardiac, and pulmonary)	Monitor laboratory data as indicated: BUN and creatinine Oxygen saturation. Monitor for signs of decreased cardiac output and tissue perfusion. Monitor for presence of new onset of dyspnea. Collaborate with health care provider for appropriate adjustments in treatment dosages.
Decreased musculoskeletal strength	Assess for fall risk and initiate precautions as indicated.
Decreased vision, hearing, and tactile distal sensation	Modify teaching as needed for visual and hearing changes. Monitor distal extremities for skin changes and provide appropriate teaching.
Altered drug absorption, distribution, metabolism, and elimination	Collaborate with the health care provider for appropriate adjustments in treatment dosages. Monitor for increased drowsiness due to medications given before treatment.
Changes in cognitive and emotional capacity	Assess for perceived alterations in sexuality: Provide counseling as needed Encourage the use of lubricants for vaginal dryness. Monitor for social concerns: Financial burden of treatments and associated activities Lack of transportation. Modify teaching to ensure learning.
Presence of comorbidities and treatments	Determine the use of medications that may exaggerate the side effects or toxicity of cancer treatments, such as bleeding or changes in renal function. Monitor for tolerance of cancer therapy. Monitor for progression of comorbidities while receiving cancer therapy.

Source: Doerflinger, D. M. C. (2009). Older adult surgical patients: Presentation and challenges. *AORN Journal, 90*(2) 223–244.

RESEARCH OPPORTUNITIES Related to Cancer

Research Area	Clinical Impact
Physiological Research	
Photodynamic therapy for treatment of esophageal and lung cancer	Provides additional treatment options.
Effects of handling chemotherapy on the person administering the medication and their offspring	Increases awareness of hazards associated with administration of chemotherapy.
Use of new interleukins as antitumor and myeloprotective agents	Provides additional treatment options and prevention of life-threatening toxicities.
Use of gene therapy for advanced cancers and prevention of myelosuppression	Decreases incidence of metastasis.
Determining the benefit/risk ratio and efficacy of chemotherapeutic chronotherapy	Leads to prevention of cancers.
	Prevention of short and long term physical and psychosocial injuries.
Symptom and Toxicity Management	
Evaluation of postoperative symptoms in those with lung cancer	Relieves distressing symptoms to increase healing and recovery.
Use of virtual reality interventions for chemotherapy symptoms	Relieves distressing symptoms to aid in recovery and treatment tolerance.
Innovative approaches to symptom management (cluster intervention, neutropenic protocols, fatigue guidelines, mucositis standard of care)	Increases awareness of unique symptoms and appropriate treatments to relieve suffering.
Causes of fatigue and solutions	Provides information to assist in the development of an individualized nursing care plan.
Skin care for patients receiving radiotherapy	Increases awareness of the need for pain control and availability of treatment modalities.
Association between treatment and disease-related symptoms and activity	Increases awareness of the impact of specific treatments on disease-related symptoms. Prevention of impairment of activities of daily living.
Association between patient's perceptions of treatment toxicities and ability to care for self	Increases awareness of the psychosocial impact of treatment toxicities and their impact on patient and family lives.
Psychosocial and Emotional Issues	
Coping with disease and treatment	Improves psychological interventions to augment coping.
Coping of caregivers and families of patients with cancer	Provides insight into how patients make decisions regarding treatment so appropriate and effective communication can be implemented.
Decision making after cancer testing (BRCA genetic testing)	
The role of caring and the meaning of illness	Highlights importance of caring.
Quality of life	Identifies impact of the disease and treatment.
Employment behaviors such as attendance issues in patients with treatment-related symptoms	Identifies impact on vocation.
Delivery of care by family members	Indicates importance of family members' involvement in caregiving.
Preferred versus actual location of death	Indicates importance of ascertaining patients' end-of-life choices and advocating appropriately.
Cultural Diversity	
Symptom management in various cultural groups	Improves understanding of cultural differences in cancer management.
Participation of various cultural groups as subjects in cancer research efforts	
Use of specific treatment regimes in various cultural groups	
Decision making in various cultural groups	
Evaluating cancer risk and emotional status in various cultural groups	
End-of-life issues and ethnicity	
Prevention/Detection/Screening	
Tertiary chemoprevention to reduce the risk of cancer in those who are highly susceptible	Reduces the risk of developing cancer.
Health and risk behaviors in childhood cancer survivors	Improves understanding of behaviors and allows for the development of screening programs to meet patients' needs.
Mammography decision making in women with a family history of breast cancer	Allows for improved prevention and screening programs.
Disclosure of breast symptoms	
Use of telephone counseling in rural areas	
Changing health beliefs in those at risk for colon cancer	
Women's perceptions of their risk of developing breast cancer	
Communicating breast cancer risk among family members	

topics that are under investigation. Electronic databases are a source for finding specific studies related to these topics.

Clinical Trials

Cancer treatments and symptom management approaches have been developed and refined on the basis of the outcomes of extensive clinical trials (research). A myriad of health care professionals work collaboratively to discover new therapies that will increase survival and improve quality of life for individuals afflicted with cancer. Before a therapy, such as chemotherapy, is approved for clinical use, rigorous evaluations are performed to determine its beneficial effects, adverse effects, and safety (Virshup, 2010).

Oncology nurses have the unique opportunity to participate in many aspects of research efforts including obtaining informed consent, developing and implementing educational sessions for patients and their families, administering treatments under investigation, and collecting pertinent data. Being a patient advocate throughout all phases of clinical trials is also part of the nurse's role.

Summary

The disease of cancer continues to affect millions of Americans each year. Advances in prevention, screening, and treatment have made cancer a more survivable disease. However, its impact is broad; not only the patient is affected, but also the patient's family and the community in which the patient lives and works.

As with any other disease process, nurses can play a key role in the prevention, screening, and treatment of cancer, as well as with the end-of-life issues that are a part of the continuum of cancer. Cancer has been and will always be a complex disease requiring skills and caring that are brought to patients through nursing.

CLINICAL PREPARATION

READ DOCUMENT APPLY

READ: **History of Present Illnesses** >> Laboratory Study Results >> Critical Thinking Questions

Alison Mosier is a 43-year-old female who presented to the emergency department (ED) for back pain. She was evaluated and discharged home with a prescription for a nonsteroidal anti-inflammatory drug (NSAID) and was asked to follow up in the physical therapy department in 2 days. The following evening, Mrs. Mosier again presented to the ED for worsening back pain along with numbness in her right buttock. She appears well nourished, slightly pale, and in obvious discomfort. While you assist her to the restroom, you notice slight right foot drop and the appearance of dyspnea. Upon returning to the bed, Mrs. Mosier is obviously dyspneic with a respiratory rate of 28. Oxygen saturation is 89% on room air. Lung sounds are diminished on the right side; otherwise, wheezes are heard throughout. She admits to occasional productive cough. The results of a chest x-ray suggest lung cancer.

Mrs. Mosier is scheduled for a CT scan. While she is being moved from the gurney to the CT scan table, she cries out in pain while holding her right leg. The CT scan suggests a malignancy. Additional x-rays determine that she has a fractured right hip. As the nurse caring for Mrs. Mosier, you have received report from the nurse from surgery. Upon arrival to the floor, Mrs. Mosier is awake, crying, groaning, and complaining of pain in her right hip area. You note on her laboratory data that her hematocrit is 22% and per order administer 2 units of packed red blood cells.

READ: History of Present Illnesses >> **Physical Exam** >> Admitting Medical Records >> Laboratory Study Results

Medical–Surgical History

Allergies: none
Medical problems: hypothyroidism, depression
Medications: Prozac, Synthroid, and Motrin
Surgical history: appendectomy at the age of 13, C-section for two children

Social History

Mrs. Mosier is married with two children (boys age 12 and 20). She has smoked 1.5 packs of cigarettes a day for 28 years. She occasionally drinks alcohol (three or four drinks per month).

Physical Exam

Vital signs: BP 148/89, HR 128, RR 24, T 38.0°C
HEENT: WNL, oropharynx clear
Neck: supple, no lymphadenopathy
Lungs: diminished with wheezes throughout
Cardiovascular: JVP not elevated; normal S_1 and S_2; regular rate and tachycardic, no significant murmur, rub, or gallop; carotids 2^+ without bruits
Abdomen: soft, nontender, nondistended, normoactive bowel sounds
Extremities: no edema, complaining of severe pain in her right hip
Neurological: normal, alert, and oriented × 4
O_2 saturation 94%

Admitting Medical Orders

Ortho service
Oncology consultation
Admit to surgical floor
Diagnosis: status postrepair of fractured right hip; rule out cancer
No known allergies
Vital signs and oxygen saturation q4h
Bed rest with immobilization of right leg
Clear liquids when tolerated
I&O
Foley
Dry sterile dressing to right hip, change prn
Oxygen 1–2 L per nasal cannula as needed to maintain oxygen saturation >90%
Call house officer: pulse < 60 or > 130/minute; BP < 90 or >160 systolic; temperature > 38.5C; urine output < 30 mL/hour × 2 hours; RR > 30/minute; oxygen saturation < 92%
Sequential compression devices (SCDs) to lower extremities
Intravenous line with 0.9% normal saline at 125 mL/hr; routine venous access device care
Neurovascular assessments to right lower extremity every 2 hours
Code status: full
Transfuse 2 units red blood cells if HCT < 24%. CBC after 2 units

CLINICAL PREPARATION, *continued*

Scheduled Medications

Prozac 20 mg oral every a.m.

Synthroid 0.25 mcg oral every a.m.

Morphine sulfate PCA: 1 mg incremental dose q10min. If pain not well controlled, give morphine sulfate bolus 1–2 mg IV × 1

PRN Medications

Tylenol 650 mg oral q4–6h as needed for pain or fever

Ativan 1–2 mg oral or IV q8h as needed for anxiety

Zofran 8 mg oral q8h as needed for nausea

Benadryl 25 mg oral q6h for itching or for sleep

Milk of Magnesia 30 mL po q4h prn constipation

Ordered Laboratory Studies

Chemistry, on admission

CBC with differential

Ordered Diagnostic Studies

Chest x-ray

12-lead ECG

CT scan of chest and spine

X-ray of right hip

READ: History of Present Illnesses >> **Laboratory Study Results** >> Critical Thinking Questions

Test	Emergency Department	Postop Day 1	After Blood Transfusion
Chemistry			
Sodium	138 mEq/L		
Potassium	4.2 mEq/L		
Chloride	98 mEq/L		
Carbon dioxide	26 mEq/L		
Blood urea nitrogen (BUN)	12 mg/dL		
Creatinine	0.8 mg/dL		
Blood glucose	110 mg/dL		

Test	Emergency Department	Postop Day 1	After Blood Transfusion
Hematology			
White blood cells	11,000/mm^3	12,000/mm^3	20,000/mm^3
Bands	4%		
Segmented neutrophils	48%		
Hemoglobin	8.6/g/dL	8.0/g/dL	9.0/g/dL
Hematocrit	26%	22%	27%
Red blood cells	4.1/mm^3	3.7/mm^3	3.6/mm^3
Platelets	150,000/mm^3	148,000/mm^3	127,000/mm^3

Pearson Nursing Student Resources *Log on to* ***nursing.pearsonhighered.com*** *to download forms*

DOCUMENT:

>> Summary of Hospitalization

>> Pathophysiology Form

>> Laboratory Values

>> Laboratory Results Explanation

APPLY:

>> List of Potential Nursing Diagnoses

>> Concept Map

>> Critical Thinking Questions and Concept Map

APPLY: History of Present Illness >> Laboratory Study Results >> **Critical Thinking Questions**

1. What critical assessments need to be made?
2. How can the nurse accurately determine the patient's risk for infection?
3. What nursing measures are appropriate related to infection?
4. What risk factor(s) put Mrs. Mosier at risk for developing lung cancer?

Answers to Critical Thinking Questions can be found in Appendix D in the Osborn Student Resources at nursing.pearsonhighered.com.

NCLEX® PRACTICE

1. A patient tells the nurse that she doesn't want to "get cancer." Which of the following should the nurse include in instructing this patient?

1. There is nothing that you can do to prevent the onset of cancer.
2. Instruct in the avoidance of tobacco, excessive alcohol, and a high fat diet.
3. Avoid all situations that produce stress and anxiety.
4. The chance of developing cancer decreases with age.

2. A patient with breast cancer asks how a new tumor can grow within a different organ such as the liver. The nurse explains the process of metastasis by including the concepts of: (select all that apply)

1. cell attachment.
2. cell invasion.
3. angiogenesis.
4. migration.
5. metaplasia.

3. An older male patient was told that he most likely has cancer and that the treatment at this time will be "watch and wait." The nurse realizes that this patient most likely is experiencing which type of cancer?

1. Melanoma
2. Prostate
3. Brain
4. Colon

4. The nurse is planning care for a patient with cancer. Which of the following should be included to reduce the risk of infection for this patient?

1. Measure rectal temperature every 4 hours.
2. Encourage a diet high in fresh fruit and vegetables.
3. Use strict aseptic technique when caring for venous access devices.
4. Provide intramuscular pain medications.

5. A patient is to begin receiving external radiation therapy for cancer. The nurse should include which of the following in patient teaching to assist the patient in coping with a common side effect of radiation?

1. Cluster care activities.
2. Restrict calories.
3. Begin a regular exercise routine.
4. Scrub the radiation area twice per day.

6. A patient with cancer is scheduled to receive biotherapy. The nurse realizes the intention for this treatment is to:

1. eliminate the need for surgery.
2. reduce the negative impact of chemotherapy.
3. alter the immunologic relationship between the tumor and the patient.
4. increase the patient's appetite.

Answers to NCLEX Practice Questions can be found in Appendix D in the Osborn Student Resources at nursing.pearsonhighered.com. Practice additional NCLEX questions online at the Student Resources site.

Pearson Nursing Student Resources Find additional review materials at: **nursing.pearsonhighered.com**

REFERENCES

Adams, M. P., Holland, L.N., & Urban, C. (2013). *Pharmacology for Nurses: A Pathophysiologic Approach,* 4th ed. Upper Saddle River, NJ: Pearson.

Adams, M. P., & Koch, R. W. (2010). *Pharmacology: Connections to nursing practice.* Upper Saddle River, NJ: Pearson.

American Cancer Society (ACS). (2008a). Cancer facts and figures 2008. Retrieved from http://www.cancer.org/downloads/STT/2008CAFFfinalsecured.pdf

American Cancer Society (ACS). (2008b). Seven steps to reduce your cancer risk. Retrieved from http://www.cancer.org/docroot/COM/content/div_NE/COM_1_1x_Seven_Steps_To_Take_To_Prevent_Cancer.asp?sitearea=COM

American Cancer Society (ACS). (2011a). Cigarette smoking. Retrieved from http://www.cancer.org/Cancer/CancerCauses/TobaccoCancer/CigaretteSmoking/index

American Cancer Society (ACS). (2011b). Fitting in fitness. Retrieved from http://www.cancer.org/Healthy/EatHealthyGetActive/GetActive/fitting-in-fitness

Ameringer, S. (2010). Barriers to pain management among adolescents with cancer. *Pain Management Nursing, 11*(4), 224–233.

Barton Burke, M. (2010). Advanced cancer in underserved populations. *Seminars in Oncology Nursing, 26*(3), 157–167.

Bender, C., & Rosenzweig, M. (2004). Cancer. In S. Lewis, M. Heitkemper, & S. Dirksen (Eds.), *Medical–surgical nursing assessment and management of clinical problems* (6th ed.). St. Louis: Mosby.

Bookbinder, M. (2010). Symptom management in palliative care and end of life care. *Nursing Clinics of North America, 45*(3), 271–327.

Butler, L. D., Koopman, C., Neri, E., Giese-Davis, J., Palesh, O., Thorne-Yocam, K. A., et al. (2009). Effects of supportive-expressive group therapy on pain in women with metastatic breast cancer. *Health Psychology, 28*(5), 579–587.

Centers for Disease Control and Prevention (CDC). (2011). National vital statistics reports. Retrieved from http://www.cdc.gov/nchs/data/nvsr/nvsr59/nvsr59_04.pdf

Cook, L. (2009). Psychological issues of stem cell transplant. *Seminars in Oncology Nursing, 25*(2), 139–150.

Cunningham, R. (2004). Anorexia-cachexia syndrome. In C. H. Yarbro, M. H. Frogge, & M. Goodman (Eds.), *Cancer symptom management* (3rd ed.). Sudbury, MA: Jones and Bartlett.

DeVita, V. T., Jr. (1997). Principles of cancer management: Chemotherapy. In V. T. DeVita, Jr., S. Hellman, & S. A. Rosenberg (Eds.), *Cancer: Principles and practice of oncology* (5th ed.). Philadelphia: Lippincott Williams & Wilkins.

Doerflinger, D. M. C. (2009). Older adult surgical patients: Presentation and challenges. *AORN Journal, 90*(2), 223–244.

Dugdale, D. C. (2011a). Catecholamines—urine. Medline Plus. Retrieved from http://www.nlm.nih.gov/medlineplus/ency/article/003613.htm

Dugdale, D. C. (2011b). Immunoelectrophoresis—serum. Medline Plus. Retrieved from http://www.nlm.nih.gov/medlineplus/ency/article/003541.htm

Eggert, J. (2011). The biology of cancer: What oncology nurses really need to know. *Seminars in Oncology, 27*(1), 3–12.

Eilers, J. (2011). Clinical update: Prevention and management of oral mucositis in patients with cancer. *Seminars in Oncology, 24*(4), e1–e16.

Erye, H., Kahn, R., Robertson, R., & Committee AAACW. (2004). Preventing cancer, cardiovascular disease, and diabetes: A common agenda for the American Cancer Society, the American Diabetes Association, and the American Heart Association. *CA—Cancer Journal for Clinicians, 54*(4).

Esper, P. (2010). Symptom clusters in individuals living with advanced cancer. *Seminars in Oncology Nursing, 26*(3),168–174.

Eun, Y. (2009). Breast cancer screening beliefs among older Korean American women. *Journal of Gerontological Nursing, 35*(3), 40–50.

Ferrell, B., & Dow, K. (1997). Quality of life among long-term cancer survivors. *Oncology, 11*(3), 565–568.

Given, C., Given, B., Azzoouz, F., Kozachik, S., & Stommel, M. (2001). Predictors of pain and fatigue in the year following diagnosis among elderly cancer patients. *Journal of Pain and Symptom Management, 1*(2), 456–466.

Glauser, W., & Canadian Medical Association. (2011). The therapeutic value of hyper-suggestibility. *Canadian Medical Association Journal, 183*(3), 149–150.

Grant, M. (2010). Advances in quality of life at the end of life. *Seminars in Oncology, 26*(1),26–35.

Hawkins, R. (2001). Mastering the intricate maze of metastasis. *Oncology Nursing Forum, 28*(6), 959–965.

Hill, G. (1979). Historical milestones in cancer surgery. *Seminar of Oncology, 6*(409-427).

Institute of Medicine (IOM). (2010). *The future of nursing: Leading change, advancing health.* Washington, DC: The Academic Press.

Iwamoto, R. (2001). Radiation therapy. In S. Otto (Ed.), *Oncology nursing* (4th ed.). St. Louis: Mosby.

Kee, J. L. (2010). *Laboratory and diagnostic tests.* Upper Saddle River, NJ: Pearson.

Keller, C. (2001). Bone marrow and stem cell transplantation. In S. Otto (Ed.), *Oncology nursing* (4th ed.). St. Louis: Mosby.

King, C. A. (2011). Health care worker safety in surgery. *AORN Journal, 94*(5), 457–468.

Kinsella, K., & Velkoff, V. (2001). *An aging world: 2001* (NIH publication no. P95/01-1). Washington, DC: U.S. Government Printing Office.

Klein, L. W. (2010). Occupational health hazards in the interventional laboratory. Time for a safe environment. *Journal of Radiology Nursing, 29*(2), 75–82.

Kwekkeboom, K. L., Cherwin, C. H., Lee, J. W., & Wanta, B. (2010). Mind-body treatments for the pain-fatigue-sleep disturbance symptom cluster in persons with cancer. *Journal of Pain and Symptom Management, 39*(1), 126–138. Epub 2009 Nov 8.

Liotta, L.A. (1992). Cancer cell invasion and metastasis. *Scientific American, 266*(2), 54–59, 62–63.

MacDonald, D. J. (2011). Germline mutations in cancer susceptibility genes: An overview for nurses. *Seminars in Oncology Nursing, 27*(1), 21–33.

Mallick, I. (2009). Radiation therapy for head and neck cancers. *Seminars in Oncology Nursing, 25*(3), 193–202.

McCance, K. (2010). Cancer epidemiology. In K. L. McCance & S. E. Huether (Eds.), *Pathophysiology: The biologic basis for disease in adults and children* (6th ed., pp. 360–395). St. Louis: Mosby Elsevier.

McCance, K., & Grey, T. (2010). Altered cellular and tissue biology. In K. L. McCance & S. E. Huether (Eds.), *Pathophysiology: The biologic basis for disease in adults and children.* (6th ed., pp. 46–92). St. Louis: Mosby Elsevier.

Mellinger, E. (2010). Safe handling of chemotherapy in the perioperative setting. *AORN Journal, 91*(4), 435–553.

Merkle, C. J. (2009). Neoplasia. In C. M. Porth & G. Matfin (Eds.), *Pathophysiology: Concepts of altered health status* (8th ed., pp. 156–196). Philadelphia: Wolters Kluwer/ Lippincott Williams & Wilkins.

Montgomery, G. H., Hallquist, M. N., Schnur, J. B., David, D., Silverstein, J. H., & Bovbjerg, D. H. (2010). Mediators of a brief hypnosis intervention to control side effects in breast surgery patients: Response expectancies and emotional distress. *Journal of Consulting and Clinical Psychology, 78*(1), 80–88.

Nail, L. (2004). Fatigue. In C. H. Yarbro, M. H. Frogge, & M. Goodman (Eds.), *Cancer symptom management* (3rd ed.). Sudbury, MA: Jones and Bartlett.

National Cancer Institute. (2011). Nutrition. Retrieved from http://www.cancer.gov/dictionary?CdrID=463734

National Comprehensive Cancer Network. (2011). Clinical practice guidelines in oncology. Retrieved from http://www.nccn.com/living-with-cancer.html

Occupational Safety and Health Administration, Office of Occupational Medicine. (1995). *Controlling occupational exposure to hazardous CPL2-2.20B CH-4.* Washington, DC: U.S. Department of Labor.

Oncology Nursing Society (ONS). (2001). *Chemotherapy and biotherapy guidelines and recommendations for practice.* Pittsburgh: Author.

Oncology Nursing Society (ONS). (2011). Putting evidence into practice: Fatigue. Retrieved from http://www.ons.org/Research/PEP/media/ons/docs/research/outcomes/fatigue/samplechapter.pdf

Oncology Nursing Society (ONS) & Geriatric Oncology Consortium (GOC). (2004). Joint Position on Cancer Care in the Older Adult. Retrieved from http://www.ons.org/publications/positions/media/ons/docs/positions/summary-cancercare-intheolderadult.pdf

Palmquist, A. E. (2011). Beliefs about cancer and diet among those considering genetic testing for colon cancer. *Journal of Nutrition Education and Behavior, 43*(3), 150–156.

Rice, R. D. (2009). Management issues in hematopoietic stem cell transplantation. *Seminars in Oncology Nursing, 25*(2), 151–158.

Rokita, S. (2004). Oncology: Nursing management in cancer care. In S. Smeltzer & B. Bare (Eds.), *Brunner & Suddarth's textbook of medical–surgical nursing* (10th ed.). Philadelphia: Lippincott Williams & Wilkins.

Rosen, A. (2009). Psychosocial distress in young cancer survivors. *Seminars in Oncology Nursing, 25*(2), 268–277.

Rustoen, T. (2009). Nursing pain management—A qualitative interview study of patients with pain hospitalized for cancer treatment. *Pain Management Nursing, 10*(4), 48–55.

Sanchez, M. R. (2011). HPV prevention in high-risk males. *Journal for Nurse Practitioners, 7*, 55–61.

Santos, G. (2000). Historical background to hematopoietic stem cell transplantation. In K. Atkinson (Ed.), *Clinical bone marrow and blood stem transplantation.* New York: Cambridge University Press.

Schnur, J. B., David, D., Kangas, M., Green, S., Bovbjerg, D. H., & Montgomery, G. H. (2009). A randomized trial of a cognitive-behavioral therapy and hypnosis intervention on positive and negative affect during breast cancer radiotherapy. *Journal of Clinical Psychology, 65*(4), 443–455.

Sedhom, L., & Yanni, M. (1985). Radiation therapy and nurses' fears of radiation exposure. *Cancer Nursing, 8*(2), 129–134.

Siegel, R., Naishadham, D., & Jemal, A. (2012). Cancer statistics 2012. Retrieved from http://cacancerjournal.com

Singleton, L., & Connor, T. (1999). An evaluation of the permeability of chemotherapy gloves to three cancer chemotherapy drugs. *Oncology Nursing Forum, 26*(4), 1491–1496.

Smith, J. (2009). Factors contributing to weight loss, nutrition-related concerns and advice received by adults undergoing cancer treatment. *Journal of the American Dietetic Association*, A33.

Sohl, S. J., Stossel, L., Schnur, J. B., Tatrow, K., Gherman, A., & Montgomery, G. H. (2010). Intentions to use hypnosis to control the side effects of cancer and its treatment. *American Journal of Clinical Hypnosis, 53*(2), 93–100.

Spross, J., McGuire, D., & Schmitt, R. (1990a). Oncology Nursing Society position paper on cancer pain. Part I. Scope of nursing practice regarding cancer pain, ethics, and practice. *Oncology Nursing Forum, 17*(3), 595.

Spross, J., McGuire, D., & Schmitt, R. (1990b). Oncology Nursing Society position paper on cancer pain. Part II. Education, research, and list of cancer management resources. *Oncology Nursing Forum, 17*(4), 751.

Spross, J., McGuire, D., & Schmitt, R. (1990c). Oncology Nursing Society position paper on cancer pain. Part III. Nursing administration, pediatric cancer pain and appendices. *Oncology Nursing Forum, 17*(5), 943.

The Joint Commision. (2008). *High alert medication: Strategies for improving safety.* Joint Commission Resources. Chicago, IL: The Joint Commission.

U.S. Department of Health and Human Services. (2010). *Healthy People 2020.* Washington, DC: Author.

Virshup, D. M. (2010). Biology, clinical manifestations, and treatment of cancer. In K. L. McCance & S. E. Huether (Eds.), *Pathophysiology: The biologic basis for disease in adults and children* (6th ed., pp. 396–435). St. Louis: Mosby Elsevier.

Voss, J., Armitage, J., & Kessinger, A. (1993). High dose chemotherapy and autologous transplant with peripheral blood stem cells. *Oncology, 7*(8), 29–30, 33–34.

Wikle-Shapiro, T. (1998). Nursing implications of bone marrow and stem cell transplantation. In J. K. Itano & K. N. Taoka (Eds.), *Core curriculum for oncology nursing* (3rd ed.). Philadelphia: W. B. Saunders.

Wilkinson, J. M., & Ahearn, N. R. (2009). *Prentice Hall nursing diagnosis handbook* (9th ed.). Upper Saddle River, NJ: Prentice Hall.

Wilson, L. D. (2011). Cultural competency: Beyond vital signs: Delivering holistic care to African Americans. *Nursing Clinics of North America, 46*(2), 219–232.

Wilson, B. A., Shannon, M., & Shields, K. (2012). *Pearson Nurse's Drug Guide 2012.* Upper Saddle River, NJ: Pearson.

Winningham, M., Nail, L., Burke, M., Brophy, L., Cimprich, B., & Jones, L. (1994). Fatigue and the cancer experience. *Oncology Nursing Forum, 21*(1), 23–36.

Zender, R. (2009). Promoting wellness in women across the lifespan. *Nursing Clinics of North America, 44*(3), 281–291.

Nursing Management of Patients with Integumentary Disorders

UNIT 13

Content in Unit 13 that addresses the **Institute of Medicine (IOM)** competencies, **Nursing Core Competencies (NCC)**, the **Quality and Safety Education for Nurses (QSEN)** competencies, and **Concepts** for concept-based learning is listed below.

Competencies	Feature or Text		Location
IOM, QSEN, NCC Providing patient-centered care	Genetic Considerations for Assessing the Skin, page 1832		Chapter 58
	Cultural Considerations for Assessing Skin Color Changes, page 1835		Chapter 58
	Nursing Process: Patient Care Plan for Skin Disorders, page 1862		Chapter 59
	Nursing Process: Patient Care Plan for Burn Injuries, pages 1941, 1956		Chapter 61
IOM, QSEN, NCC Working in teams	Collaborative Management, pages 1856, 1861		Chapter 59
	Collaborative Management, pages 1897, 1918		Chapter 60
	Collaborative Management, pages 1939, 1955, 1961		Chapter 61
IOM, QSEN, NCC Employing evidence-based practice	Evidence-Based Practice: Silver as an Antimicrobial Agent		Chapter 60, page 1911
	Evidence-Based Practice: Wound Infections, Mortality, and Treatment		Chapter 61, page 1963
IOM, NCC Applying quality and safety improvement	Safety Alerts, pages 1871, 1873, 1881		Chapter 59
	Safety Alerts, pages 1891, 1892, 1901, 1909, 1910, 1913, 1914		Chapter 60
	Safety Alerts, pages 1926, 1939, 1948, 1953		Chapter 61
IOM, QSEN, NCC Using informatics	Clinical Preparation		Chapter 59, page 1885
	Clinical Preparation		Chapter 61, page 1965
NCC Applying ethical and legal responsibilities	Ethical Issues of wound care		Chapter 60, page 1920
	Liability of wound development		Chapter 60, page 1921
	Ethical Issues in the Treatment of Burn Injuries		Chapter 61, page 1960
NCC Educating patients	Patient Teaching & Discharge Priorities for Skin Disorders		Chapter 59, page 1866
	Patient Teaching & Discharge Priorities for Management of Wounds		Chapter 60, page 1919
	Patient Teaching & Discharge Priorities for Burn Management		Chapter 61, page 1961
Concepts covered in Unit 13 include:	Body image	Grief and loss	Skin integrity
	Cellular regulation	Immunity	Thermoregulation
	Fluid balance	Infection	Tissue integrity

CHAPTER

58 Nursing Assessment of the Patient with Integumentary Disorders

Dea Kent
Cheryl Wraa

Outcome-Based Learning Objectives

After studying this chapter, the learner will be able to:

1. Compare and contrast the structures and functions of the skin.
2. Obtain a health history relative to assessment of the skin, hair, and nails.
3. Generate a plan for the collection of subjective and objective data relative to assessment of the skin, hair, and nails.
4. Utilize correct techniques of physical examination when assessing the skin, hair, and nails.
5. Distinguish between normal and abnormal assessment findings in the skin, hair, and nails.
6. Differentiate skin lesions by morphologic classification.
7. Identify biologic and cultural variations in the assessment of the skin.

KEY TERMS

alopecia p.1837
arciform lesion p.1836
configuration p.1836
diascopy p.1837
discrete lesion p.1836
distribution p.1836
ecchymosis p.1837
edema p.1836
keratinocytes p.1831
Langerhans' cells p.1831
linear lesion p.1836
melanocytes p.1831
Merkel's cells p.1831
morphologic classification p.1836
primary lesion p.1837
secondary lesion p.1837
turgor p.1835
vascular lesion p.1837

THE INTEGUMENTARY SYSTEM is composed of the skin, hair, nails, and glands. The skin is the largest and most visible organ of the body and accounts for about 7% of the body weight. It is composed of three layers: the epidermis, dermis, and subcutaneous tissue. These will be described later in the chapter. The epidermal appendages of the skin include the hair, nails, sebaceous glands, and eccrine and apocrine sweat glands. The skin is pliable, is able to withstand insults from external agents, and has a remarkable ability to heal. Additionally, through the sense of touch, the skin enables individuals to perceive the world around them, and its changes in color may reflect emotional reactions to the environment. It is critical that the nurse be able to recognize and identify skin abnormalities. Assessment of the skin and its appendages requires a thorough understanding of the structure and function of the integumentary system and knowledge of normal and abnormal findings.

Anatomy and Physiology of the Skin

The skin is the largest organ of the body. Its primary function is to provide a protective barrier for the vital organs. It prevents harmful organisms from entering the body; it protects underlying tissues and structures from microorganisms, chemical injury, and trauma; and it guards against excessive exposure to ultraviolet rays from the sun. Other functions of the skin include the following:

- Assists in the control of body temperature.
- Contains the sensory receptors that allow an individual to feel heat, cold, pressure, and pain.
- Contains immune system cells.
- Functions as an excretory organ (sweat glands).
- Functions as a synthesizer of vitamin D (sunlight reacts with cholesterol).
- Determines identity (fingerprints).
- Stores blood and fats.
- Reflects emotion through color changes.

The skin also manifests diseases or injury. For example, rashes may be associated with systemic diseases such as connective tissue disease or chronic liver disease (Lee, 2009). Redness and swelling are associated with injuries such as fractures, internal bleeding, and infection.

Weblink: Dermis

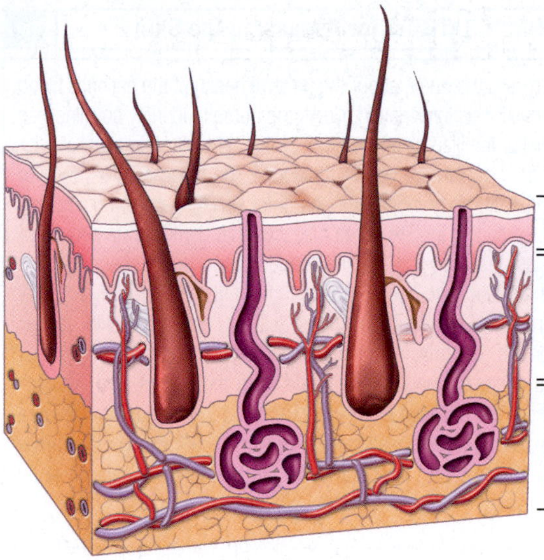

FIGURE 58–1 ◆ Skin layers.

Skin Layers

The skin has three anatomic layers: the epidermis, dermis, and subcutaneous tissue (Figure 58–1◆). These layers are described next.

Epidermis

The epidermis is the thin, avascular outer layer that is nourished by the blood vessels from the dermis. Four distinct cell types are contained in the epidermis: keratinocytes, melanocytes, Merkel's cells, and Langerhans' cells. **Keratinocytes** are the most numerous cells of the epidermis; as they mature, they move to the surface, die, and thereby form the outermost surface of the skin (stratum corneum). These cells produce keratin, which provides the skin's major protective barrier. The maturation and death of keratinocytes occur approximately every 4 to 6 weeks. If the process occurs too quickly, the skin appears thin and may break down more easily, as occurs with a sunburn. If old cells have not sloughed before the formation of new cells, the skin appears thickened and scaly, as occurs with a callus. **Melanocytes** are the pigment-producing cells. Pigment granules (melanin), which are black or brown, give the skin and hair its color. The more melanin an individual has, the darker the skin and hair. The primary function of melanocytes is to protect the skin from ultraviolet rays. **Merkel's cells** provide sensory information, and **Langerhans' cells** are macrophages of the immune system that arise from the bone marrow and migrate to the epidermis. These cells recognize a foreign antigen and bind it to their surface, process it, and then migrate with the antigen back to the lymphatic vessels and into the regional lymph nodes.

Dermis

A basement membrane connects the epidermis to the dermis. This is the layer involved in blister formation. The dermis, composed of fibrous connective tissue, contains the blood vessels, hair follicles, nerve endings, sweat glands, and sebaceous glands. It separates the epidermis from the subcutaneous tissue and provides nutrition for the epidermis. The dermis is composed of two layers: the papillary dermis and the reticular dermis. The papillary dermis is the superficial layer, consisting of collagen fibers and ground substances (a viscid gel that is rich in mucopolysaccharides) that lie adjunct to the epidermis. This layer is densely covered by dermal papillae that contain capillary venules that nourish the epidermal layer. Lymph vessels and nerve endings are also found in this layer. The reticular dermis, the thicker layer, is composed of a complex meshwork of three-dimensional collagen bundles interconnected with large elastic fibers and ground substance. The reticular dermis also contains dermal dendrocytes, which have phagocytic properties that participate in the immune function of the skin. The specific immune cells found in the dermis include T cells, mast cells, and fibroblasts (Amirlak, 2011). The T cells provide a delayed-type hypersensitivity that is described in Chapter 53.

Subcutaneous Tissue

Subcutaneous tissue, made up of loose connective tissue and fat cells, lends support to the vascular and neural structures that supply the outer layer of the skin. Because of the presence of the eccrine glands, deep hair follicles, major blood vessels, lymph vessels, and nerves, this layer is considered part of the integument (Springhouse, 2008).

Blood and Lymph Supply, Sebaceous Glands, and Innervation

The arterial vessels that nourish the skin are located between the papillary and reticular layers of the dermis and between the dermis and the subcutaneous tissue layer. Blood returns via small veins that accompany the subcutaneous vessels. The lymphatic system is located in the dermis and helps combat skin infections. The majority of the vessels are under sympathetic nervous system control. The sympathetic nervous system also controls the arrector pili muscles that cause elevation of the hair on the arms and dimpling of the skin (goose bumps). The dermis contains a rich supply of sensory neurons. The receptors for touch, pressure, heat, cold, and pain are in the dermis (Rizzo, 2010).

Physiological Impact of Ultraviolet Rays

The sun's rays are measured in wavelengths that range from 290 nanometers in the ultraviolet (UV) range to 2,500 nanometers in the infrared range. There are three types of ultraviolet rays: ultraviolet A (UVA), ultraviolet B (UVB), and ultraviolet C (UVC). The UVB rays are primarily responsible for sunburn and the cumulative damage to the skin from the sun (Rigel, 2008). The UVA rays produce elastic skin and actinic skin damage. Exposure to UV radiation causes sunburn and skin cancer and accelerates skin aging. There is also evidence that UV radiation can reduce the effectiveness of the human immune system (Marrot & Meunier, 2008; World Health Organization, 2010). Chapter 59 includes an in-depth discussion of sun-related skin diseases.

Safety Alert *A common belief is that only fair-skinned people need to be concerned about overexposure to the sun. Although it is true that darker skin has more protective pigment, the skin is still susceptible to the damaging effects of ultraviolet (UV) radiation. The incidence of skin cancers is lower in dark-skinned people; nevertheless, skin cancers do occur among this group and are often detected at a later, more dangerous stage. The risk of other UV-related health effects, such as eye damage, premature aging of the skin, and immunosuppression, also occurs in dark-skinned people (World Health Organization, 2010).*

Gerontological Considerations

Several physiological changes occur in the skin with the aging process. Both the epidermis and the dermis thin; there is a reduction in subcutaneous tissue and collagen and a thickening of the blood vessels. In addition, the number of melanocytes, Merkel's cells, and Langerhans' cells decreases. This results in color changes and decreased resistance to organisms. The keratinocytes actually shrink, although the number of dead keratinized cells on the skin surface increases. These changes result in thinner skin with less padding, so it is more susceptible to breakdown from trauma. Hormonally induced sebaceous gland activity decreases, leaving older individuals with drier, more scaly skin. Dermal proteins diminish, leading to oncotic pressure shifts and diminished fluid homeostasis, so the skin has less ability to retain moisture (Baranoski & Ayello, 2008). Finally, there is less hair and nail growth, and hair permanently loses pigment with the aging process (Rizzo, 2010). Graying, which may begin as early as in the third decade of life, is caused by reduced melanin production in the hair follicles. Genetic factors tend to determine the age of the onset of graying. Chapter 59 includes an in-depth discussion of age-related skin diseases.

History

The health history, which is the major subjective source of data, provides valuable insights into the patient's past and current health status. The components of the health history provide structure for data collection and an organized record of the patient's response to skin problems. These components are outlined next.

Biographic and Demographic Data

Biographic and demographic data include data such as the patient's name, address, telephone number, Social Security number, contact person, age, gender, race or ethnic origin, marital status, birthplace, occupation, level of education, and religious affiliation. This information is critical in identifying one patient's record from another's, and it provides a general overview of the patient's communication abilities, reliability as a historian, and general personal attributes. Biographic and demographic information is also needed for epidemiologic comparisons. For example, the incidence or prevalence of a particular health condition may be attributed to a certain geographic locale, a racial or ethnic group, or a specific gender. It is important to date the history so that, if the patient's condition changes, events can be correlated chronologically.

Examples of biographic and demographic data that may be significant to assessment of the skin include environmental or occupational toxins, neighborhood waste, or landfills. Environmental toxins include overexposure to frost, wind, and ultraviolet rays from the sun. Neighborhood waste and landfills could involve exposure to arsenic, creosote, coal tar, and/or petroleum products. Environmental toxins, neighborhood waste, and landfills are risk factors for skin cancer. A family history of skin diseases or disorders, including skin cancers, should be noted, as this history can place the patient at a higher risk for some skin issues. Finally, the nurse should inquire about time spent in different environments, such as camping outdoors or traveling to rural areas of the world. The Genetic Considerations box features guidelines to consider when assessing a patient's skin.

Chief Complaint

The assessment begins with identifying the patient's chief complaint, that is, the current issue or reason for seeking health care. When a patient is admitted, the nurse begins the interview by asking what the patient considers the most current and acute health issue. The chief complaint is typically best elicited by the nurse's asking, "What brought you here?" The goal is generally a concise statement in the patient's own words indicating her rationale for seeking health care. Examples of chief complaints are "I have had a rash for 3 days"; "I've noticed discolorations on my legs and arms for 2 weeks"; "My hair has been thinning for 6 months"; and "I think I have a fungal infection in my cuticle."

GENETIC CONSIDERATIONS for Assessing the Skin

The family history tells the nurse about the general health of the patient's blood relatives and spouse. This information allows the nurse to identify any illnesses that have a genetic, familial, or environmental link as well as implications for the patient's current and future health problems. The blood relatives include the maternal and paternal grandparents, parents, siblings, aunts, uncles, and children. The nurse should inquire about diseases that demonstrate genetic or familial tendencies. Diseases with familial tendencies have not been identified as genetic disorders but have been found in family clusters. Any family history of allergic disorders or conditions such as asthma, hay fever, skin cancer, melanoma, psoriasis, eczema, or infestations of lice or scabies, as well as familial hair-loss patterns, should be solicited from the patient. The information obtained about the family is usually documented in a genogram (a visual display of the patient's family relationships and medical history). The family genogram is an effective way to document a large amount of data obtained from the family history.

Presenting Symptoms

The presenting symptoms detail the chronology of each symptom, how it developed, and what events surrounded the symptoms. When obtaining information from the patient related to the presenting symptoms, the nurse should ask about the patient's perception of the cause as well as what measures the patient may have already taken to remedy the condition. The presenting symptoms related to the skin may be changes in the condition of the patient's skin, such as dryness, pruritus, sores, and lumps; changes in a mole or a wart; skin lesions; or changes in skin color or texture.

Past Medical History

The past medical history can be of great value in assessing the current problem. The purpose in obtaining information about the past medical history is to identify all the patient's relevant past health problems. Past illnesses could possibly have some effect on the patient's current health. The nurse would ask the patient about previous skin conditions, unusual sensations, history of allergies and allergic reactions, and other diseases that may affect the condition of the skin. For example, a disease such as systemic lupus erythematosus causes a butterfly rash on the face. Use of chemotherapeutic agents to treat cancer may cause hair loss. Cancer, heart disease, liver disease, and anemia can cause changes in the nails such as grooves, ridges, and discolorations.

Childhood Illnesses

The nurse should ask whether the patient has had any of the following childhood illnesses: measles, mumps, whooping cough, chickenpox, smallpox, scarlet fever, rheumatic fever, diphtheria, acne, and/or poliomyelitis. This will assist the nurse in determining the cause of any residual scarring.

Immunizations

The nurse needs to inquire about what childhood immunizations the patient had as well as adult immunizations. The patient should be asked specifically about polio, diphtheria, pertussis, human papillomavirus (HPV), tetanus toxoid, influenza, last tuberculin skin test, and any skin reactions to the immunizations.

Previous Illnesses

The nursing assessment includes questions about major illnesses such as diabetes, cardiovascular disease, and infectious diseases. Patients with diabetes are prone to skin breakdown and delayed wound healing (Chapters 47 and 60). Patients with cardiovascular disease may have clubbed nail beds (Chapter 29). Infectious diseases such as cellulitis have skin manifestations, which assist with the diagnosis.

Previous Ulcerations or Wounds

The nurse should inquire about previous slow or nonhealing wounds of any type, as well as the presence of any old or healed pressure ulcer. Patients of all ages can have wounds that become complicated and do not heal readily, so it is important to ask each patient about this topic. History of a previous nonhealing or slow-healing wound places the patient at risk for another.

Medications

The nurse should ask about medications taken regularly (names, dosages, frequency, reason for taking, side effects) and whether the patient complies with the medication regimen. For the purposes of the history, medications include over-the-counter medications, herbal medications, vitamins, and any home remedies. Drugs may produce skin eruptions, decrease or increase sunlight sensitivity, and cause hyperpigmentation.

Allergies

The nurse should inquire about allergies to medications, foods, and items in the environment. If the patient has any allergies, he should be asked to describe what clinical skin manifestations occur in an allergic reaction as well as what makes the reaction subside.

Health Assessment

The current health status is the general state of health as perceived by the patient. A question to elicit this information might be: "Over your lifetime, have you had ongoing skin problems?" The nurse needs to identify risk factors that affect the skin, such as sun exposure and the use of cigarettes. The nurse must assess the amount of time the patient spends in the sun as well as other risk factors associated with the development of skin cancer. These risk factors are outlined in the Risk Factors box. Other significant habits and lifestyles assessed during the health history are outlined next.

Social History

Social history includes the patient's use of alcohol or street drugs, as these can have adverse effects on the condition of the patient's skin. Drugs and alcohol can have a pathologic effect on a patient's skin. This may result from the direct toxic effect or from personal neglect, environmental factors, and/or poor nutrition. The presence of certain cutaneous lesions in a patient should prompt an investigation into the patient's drinking and drug habits. The nurse should inquire about the patient's skin care habits and routine, use of special cleansing agents or soaps, use of cosmetics or other dermatologic products, sun exposure patterns, use of sunscreen and sunblock, and exposure to stressors.

If skin popping is suspected because of the presence of cutaneous lesions, the nurse needs to inquire about it. Skin popping is a technique used to administer illicit drugs. The technique, also called "subcutaneous" or "sub-Q," involves injecting the drug between the patient's skin and fat layers. Skin popping is a significant risk factor in skin and soft tissue infections, which are common among injection drug users (IDUs). There is an increased incidence of *Staphylococcus aureus* skin infections among IDUs. Additionally, outbreaks of uncommon infections including tetanus, wound botulism, and a sepsis/myonecrosis syndrome due to *Clostridium* species have been seen with IDUs (Davis & King, 2008).

RISK FACTORS Associated with Skin Cancer

- Age 50 or older
- Male gender
- Family history of skin cancer
- Fair complexion with light-colored hair or eyes
- Precancerous lesions
- Geographic location such as high altitude or near the equator
- Exposure to certain elements such as radium, isotopes, or x-rays
- Exposure to coal tar, creosote, and petroleum products
- Extended exposure to sunlight
- Repeated skin trauma or irritation
- Tendency to burn easily
- History of severe and/or multiple sunburns as a child.

Occupation

To elicit a description of the patient's usual work, the nurse inquires about the patient's work conditions and hours; duration of employment; any occupational exposure to irritants, pollutants, or allergens; and frequent sun exposure. Skin neoplasms can result from occupational or environmental agents. For example, individuals who work in the sun have an increased risk for the development of skin cancer.

Cultural Considerations

The nurse should ask about any cultural habits or practices, including dietary habits, that may affect the patient's skin. For example, in Southeast Asia, there is a custom of scraping the skin when a person is sick, causing bruising and open sores. This is thought to aid in the healing process. Also, because of decreased sweat production, it is uncommon for Asians and Native Americans to have body odor. The darker the pigmentation of the patient's skin, the more important it is to use adequate lighting to detect subtle skin changes.

Environment

The nurse should inquire about environmental exposure to chemicals, toxins, animals, nature, paint, aerosols, petroleum products, and tar. These products can irritate the skin, causing rashes and skin breakdown.

Habits

In addition to social habits mentioned earlier, the nurse should inquire about the patient's sleep patterns and whether there have been any recent changes. The nurse should ask specifically whether the patient experiences symptoms such as itching at night or night sweats. The nurse should ask whether the patient bites or chews the nails or picks at the skin. These habits may cause a loss of skin integrity and increase the risk of a skin infection.

Exercise

The nurse should inquire about the patient's exercise habits. Does the patient exercise on a regular basis? What are the patient's recreational activities? Do they expose the patient to excessive weather elements, such as wind, cold, heat, or sun? Does the individual work out at community gyms? There may be a risk for contracting fungal infections

Weblink: Skin Cancer Prevention

or community-acquired methicillin-resistant *Staphylococcus aureus* (MRSA) from the equipment or showers. The nurse should caution the patient not to share towels and to cover and protect any open areas on the skin. The patient should be asked how much and how easily she perspires. Profuse, out-of-the-ordinary perspiration may be indicative of a systemic disorder. Obesity is one cause of excessive perspiration, but there are also others, such as heart disease and hyperthyroidism.

Nutrition

The nurse assesses the patient's dietary pattern to see whether the patient eats well-balanced, nutritious meals. The history should focus on the patient's overall eating habits and use of chocolate, caffeine, sweets, and carbonated beverages. The nurse should inquire about recent changes in diet. Dietary changes may cause rashes and other skin reactions.

Physical Examination

When conducting a physical examination of the skin, the nurse must be cognizant of age-related changes. What is normal for a young person will be changed or absent in the older patient. Certain skin changes related to the aging process are not in and of themselves pathologic. Therefore, the nurse also must know what is normal and abnormal for each age group when assessing the skin. Pathologic changes are outlined in detail in Chapter 59.

Inspection

When conducting the physical assessment of the skin, the nurse must be aware of ethnic variations related to skin color and texture, mucous membrane coloring, and hair texture. The nurse must perform a thorough physical examination in a well-lit room, preferably in indirect natural daylight. To examine the skin properly, the nurse must take a brief but careful look at the patient's entire body and examine specific areas of concern in detail. A small magnifying glass and a centimeter ruler or tape measure are required when assessing lesions. The assessment should proceed in an orderly fashion, beginning with an examination of the most frequently exposed areas such as the face, hands, arms, legs, and feet. Along with the skin, the nurse also examines the appendages, hair, scalp, and nails.

The nurse inspects the skin while the patient is in a sitting or lying position with all clothes removed except an examination or hospital gown. The nurse inspects the skin for color, temperature, thickness, moisture, texture, turgor, edema, and lesions. Special attention needs to be paid to pressure points, especially in the older population. If the patient has tubes and/or stomas, the adjunct skin should be assessed for breakdown and rashes. The nurse needs to be aware of ethnic differences, especially in darker-skinned populations, when conducting an assessment.

Color

Skin color varies from person to person. Melanin, carotene, the level of oxygen in the blood, and the amount of sun exposure will all influence the color of the patient's skin. Dark skin contains more melanin than does fair skin. Asians have more carotene pigments, which gives the skin its yellow hue. In addition, skin color will vary from body part to body part. Usually, the most frequently exposed areas look noticeably different from the unexposed areas. The difference may be due to the effects of more frequent exposure to the sun, wind, and other environmental elements on exposed skin. Normal skin color ranges from a whitish pink to a dark chocolate brown, depending on race. When evaluating skin color changes, the nurse must be cognizant of variations in skin color based on the patient's racial background, as presented in the Cultural Considerations box. When assessing for color changes, the nurse should give consideration to the room's lighting and temperature as well as the position of the patient. For example, is there a color change when the patient's leg is in a dependent position?

Palpation

Palpation is examination of the skin through the use of touch. Generally, the nurse will inspect and palpate simultaneously. When palpating the skin, the nurse assesses the skin temperature, texture, thickness, moisture, turgor, edema, and lesions. The presence or absence of a pulse needs to be determined, as it may indicate a diminished blood supply to the area.

Temperature

Using the dorsal surface of the hand, which is most sensitive to temperature, the nurse first palpates the patient's forehead and then proceeds in a systematic fashion downward, being certain to include the hands and feet. Normal skin temperature ranges from slightly warm to slightly cool. This may fluctuate depending on the temperature of the patient's environment. Skin temperature will rise with any condition that increases blood flow to the area. For example, localized skin temperature could be increased due to tissue injury, trauma, or infection. The nurse should always make side-to-side comparisons, assessing for bilateral symmetry by palpating similar areas simultaneously, using both the right and left hands. For example, are both the patient's hands the same temperature, or is one warmer or cooler than the other? Occasionally, the temperature is slightly cooler in a person's hands and feet, but the temperature should be similar on both sides. A difference in temperature bilaterally warrants further investigation and could be indicative of vascular insufficiency problems or infection.

Generalized skin temperature increases may occur in systemic infections, fever, or metabolic disorders such as hyperthyroidism. Conversely, the skin temperature decreases when blood flow to the skin is diminished. Conditions that may cause a decrease in local skin temperature result from diminished blood supply to the area, vasoconstriction, occlusion, or peripheral arterial insufficiency. Generalized skin temperature decreases may occur when the environment is cool and in the presence of metabolic disorders such as hypothyroidism.

Texture

The texture of the skin ranges from smooth and soft to rough and hard. The nurse should use the palmar surface of the fingers and finger pads when palpating for texture. Normal skin texture is smooth, soft, and even. The texture may be rougher in exposed areas or areas of pressure, such as the elbows, palms, and soles of the feet. Conditions such as hyperthyroidism will alter the texture of the skin. Hyperthyroidism usually causes the skin to be smooth with a velvet-like texture. Hypothyroidism, in contrast, causes the skin to be rough and scaly. The skin of the older adult has an increased incidence of scaling as well.

Thickness

The skin should be thin and firm over most parts of the body. Normally, the skin is thicker on the palms, back, soles of the feet, elbows, and knees and thinner over the eyelids. Skin thickness varies with age or illness, as in the thin, fragile skin of the older adult or the patient who is severely emaciated. Very thin skin with a shiny appearance is often indicative

CULTURAL CONSIDERATIONS for Assessing Skin Color Changes

Skin Color Variation	Description of Variation	Appearance in Light Skin	Appearance in Dark Skin
Carotenemia	A yellowish discoloration of skin that differs from jaundice because it does not involve the sclera or mucous membranes. It is often associated with a high intake of foods with carotene (e.g., sweet potatoes, squash, and carrots).	A yellowish stain in the skin.	May be difficult to assess.
Cyanosis*	A bluish-gray discoloration of the skin that is often caused by decreased perfusion of the tissues with oxygenated blood.	Bluish tinge notably in skin, lower eyelid, mucous membranes, lips, earlobes, soles of the feet, and palms.	Ashen-gray discoloration of the skin, mucous membranes, lips, and tongue.
Ecchymosis	Purplish, blue, and black marks that are usually caused by trauma. Ecchymosis occurs due to the extravasation of blood. Over time the discoloration fades to greenish-brown and then yellow as the blood is reabsorbed into the vascular system.	Purplish, blue-black areas may be seen anywhere on the skin.	Purplish, blue-black areas on the skin may be difficult to see in poor lighting.
Erythema	A reddish discoloration of the skin that is caused by dilation of the capillaries. This is usually due to local irritation or inflammation, embarrassment (blushing), heat, or fever.	Redness that can be seen anywhere on the body. It may be generalized or localized.	Redness that appears on the body but is difficult to see unless in a well-lit area.
Hyperpigmentation	Hyperpigmentation can be in a specific or a general area. It results from changes in the distribution of melanin. It is often seen in pregnancy (linea nigra); people of color are often born with dark discolorations located on the lower back and buttocks, called mongolian spots. Both linea nigra and mongolian spots disappear over time or when the pregnancy is over.	Spots or lines that appear darker than the general skin.	Spots or lines that appear darker than the general skin.
Jaundice*	A yellowish discoloration of the skin, sclera, and mucous membranes that is often associated with increased amounts of bilirubin in the blood. Some newborns are born with pathologic jaundice, in which skin color changes are noted within the first 24 hours of life. Jaundice is generally caused by disorders that cause an increase in the serum bilirubin level.	A yellow staining noticeable in the skin, hard palate, sclera, palms, and soles of the feet.	Can be seen in the hard palate, sclera, palms, and soles of the feet.
Pallor*	Paleness of the skin that occurs when the red-pink tones from the oxygenated hemoglobin in the blood are lost. The skin takes on the appearance of collagen (connective tissue), which is almost white.	Loss of rosy glow in the skin.	Ashen appearance. The skin will lack red tones, which normally give dark skin a luster or a glow. Pallor can best be seen in the palpebral conjunctiva, the preferred site for assessment of pallor related to anemia.
Petechiae	Pinpoint purpuric lesions of the skin.	Pinpoint purpuric lesions can be seen on the skin.	May be difficult to see except in good lighting.
Vitiligo	The absence of pigmentation in a circumscribed area.	May be difficult to see except in good lighting.	A circumscribed area or areas with loss of pigmentation.

**In dark-skinned people, the best areas to assess cyanosis, pallor, and jaundice are the oral mucous membranes and conjunctiva.*

Source: Bryant, R. A. (2012). *Acute and chronic wounds* (4th ed.). St. Louis: Elsevier.

of impaired circulation. An individual's occupation also may affect the thickness of the skin due to callus formation. In addition, pigment can influence the skin's thickness. Generally, the darker the pigment, the thicker the skin.

Moisture

The nurse assesses for moisture using the hand's dorsal surface. The dorsal surface is generally drier, so using it will help the nurse avoid confusing the moisture on the patient's skin with that on the nurse's hand. Moisture on the skin does vary from one body part to another. The soles of the feet, the palms of the hands, and the intertriginous areas (where two surfaces are close together) contain more moisture than other parts. There should be minimal perspiration on the patient's skin unless the patient has just engaged in vigorous exercise, the environmental temperature is warm, or the patient has an elevated body temperature. The skin regulates body temperature by producing perspiration that evaporates, thus cooling the skin when the body temperature increases. The skin is normally drier in winter months when the ambient temperature is cooler and humidity is low. Dehydration will also cause the skin to be drier. Medical disorders that cause dryness include myxedema and nephritis.

Turgor

Turgor refers to the elasticity and mobility of the skin. Elasticity is described as the resiliency of the skin, that is, its ability to return to a normal position and shape. Mobility is the skin's ability to be lifted. To assess turgor, the nurse grasps a fold of the patient's skin using the forefinger and thumb (Figure 58–2◆). The nurse notes how rapidly the skin returns to its normal shape. Normal, healthy skin returns rapidly to its previous shape. When turgor is decreased, however, the skinfold holds its pinch formation before returning to its normal shape. Loss of turgor is associated with dehydration and aging. As individuals age, the

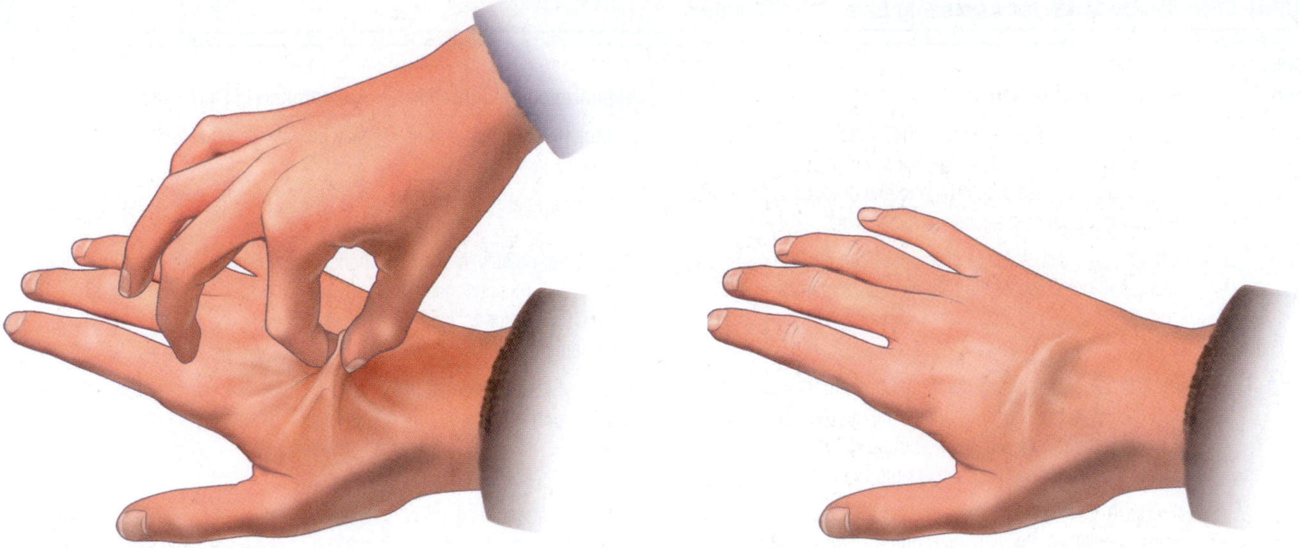

FIGURE 58–2 ◆ Skin turgor.

skin normally loses its elasticity. The chest wall is ideal to assess turgor because it is not subject to the age-related changes associated with loss of elasticity. Increased skin turgor makes it difficult or impossible to pinch up the skin. Increased turgor may be produced by conditions such as scleroderma, which causes the underlying connective tissue to become hard and immobile.

Edema

Edema is caused by the accumulation of fluid in the extracellular and/or intracellular spaces. Edema, which makes the skin appear puffy and tight, is often noted in dependent areas such as the hands, feet, and sacral area. To assess for edema, the nurse palpates the patient's skin with the pads of the finger. Normally the skin surface stays smooth. If the pressure leaves an indentation in the skin, pitting edema is present. Pitting edema is generally evaluated on a 4-point scale:

- 1+: Mild pitting in which there is slight indentation, no obvious swelling of the leg
- 2+: Moderate pitting in which the indentation rapidly subsides
- 3+: Deep pitting in which the indentation lasts a short time
- 4+: Very deep pitting in which the indentation lasts a long time (Figure 58–3◆).

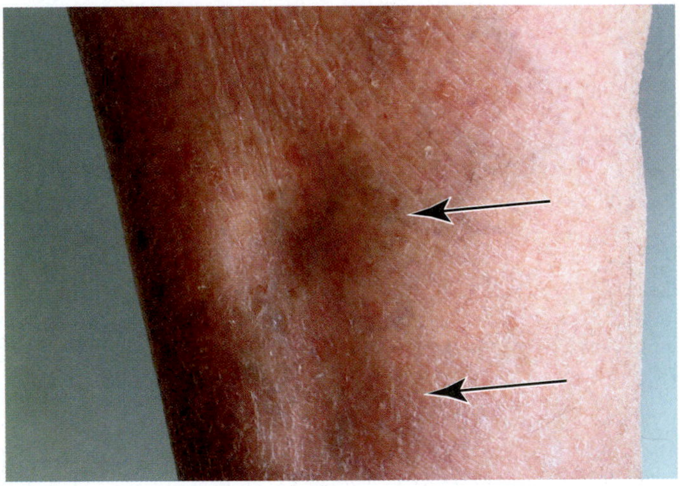

FIGURE 58–3 ◆ Pitting edema.
Source: © Medical-On-Line/Alamy.

Because these criteria are somewhat subjective, leading to variation among examiners, some nurses prefer to evaluate edema in terms of time duration of the indentation. For example, the nurse might record that the pitting edema lasts between 15 and 30 seconds before the skin returns to normal.

Lesions

In assessing the skin, the nurse should pay careful attention to the presence of lesions. Lesions must be assessed by using two of the techniques of examination: inspection and palpation. The nurse should use a magnification glass to evaluate skin lesions accurately. Lesions should be described according to distribution, location, configuration, and whether there is exudate.

Distribution and Location

Distribution of the lesions on the skin is described according to the location or body region affected. Lesions may be confined to one small area (localized), confined to an entire area such as the chest (regional), or spread over the entire body (generalized). The nurse notes whether the lesions are distributed symmetrically or asymmetrically. The characteristic pattern of lesions can provide additional clues in the diagnosis of a specific skin condition.

Configuration or Pattern of Arrangement

The nurse must also note the configuration of the lesions. **Configuration** refers to the pattern of arrangement or position of the lesions. The nurse should assess how lesions are patterned on the body. Are they **discrete lesions** (individual or separate), congruent lesions (running together), grouped in a characteristic pattern, **linear lesions** (forming a line), and/or **arciform lesions** (arc-shaped)? For example, ringworm (tinea corporis) has an annular or circular configuration.

Types of Lesions

The lesion should be further examined for color, size, shape, texture, firmness, discharge, and morphologic classification. The **morphologic classification** of the skin is described in terms of type of lesion

CHART 58–1 Primary Skin Lesions

Primary Lesion	Description	Pain/Itching	Examples
Abscess	A pus-filled nodule.	Localized tenderness. Typically intensity increases as size increases. Painful.	An infected wound that forms a pocket of pus under the skin surface.
Bulla	A vesicle or blister usually about 1 centimeter in diameter.	Itching and pain present.	Sunburn, poison oak, poison ivy.
Cyst	A palpable fluid-filled or solid subcutaneous sac.	Typically not painful.	Sebaceous cyst.
Furuncle	A pus-filled lesion usually greater than 0.5 centimeter.	Tender, depends on size. Typically painful.	Boil.
Macule	A flat, nonpalpable circumscribed area of a change in skin color.	Not painful.	Freckles, purpura.
Nodule	A well-circumscribed, firm, palpable lesion deeper within the dermis than a papule.	Not painful.	Sarcoma, subcutaneous nodules.
Papule	A solid, elevated, circumscribed mass that is generally less than 1 centimeter in diameter.	Not painful.	Wart.
Patch	A macule larger than 1 centimeter.	Not painful.	Vitiligo, port-wine stain.
Plaque	Very similar to a papule but greater than 1 centimeter in diameter.	Painful.	Psoriasis, discoid lupus erythematosus.
Pustule	A pus-filled vesicle or bulla.	May be tender.	Acne, impetigo.
Tumor	A solid mass generally larger than 1 centimeter.	Not painful.	Fibroma, lipoma.
Wheal	A circumscribed irregularly shaped elevation of the skin caused by cutaneous edema.	May or may not be tender.	Urticaria.

(primary, secondary, or vascular), size, shape or configuration, color, texture, elevation or depression, and pedunculation. If the lesion has drainage, the drainage is described in terms of color, odor, amount, and consistency. A **primary lesion** occurs as an initial reaction to a pathologic condition (Chart 58–1). A **secondary lesion** results from a change in the primary lesion or external trauma to the primary lesion (Chart 58–2). **Vascular lesions** appear as red- or purple-pigmented lesions (Chart 58–3). They are generally indicative of conditions that cause bleeding (petechiae and ecchymosis) or liver disease (spider angioma), or they may be due to benign conditions such as telangiectasia. Determining whether the lesions blanch (when pressure is exerted on the lesion with a finger, the skin will pale and when the pressure is removed color will return) will help identify the type of lesion. Petechiae and ecchymosis will not blanch, whereas telangiectasia will blanch.

The nurse should measure lesions with a small, clear, flexible ruler or tape measure. Lesion size is described in centimeters, and all dimensions should be measured (length, width, and depth). The color of individual lesions also is documented. The color of the lesion may be well circumscribed (confined to the lesion) or may be more diffuse, with borders that are not clearly defined. For example, **ecchymosis,** blood from ruptured blood vessels leaked into subcutaneous tissue, is initially dark red or purple but gradually fades to yellowish green before it disappears.

Wearing gloves, the nurse palpates each lesion to determine the texture and firmness. Additionally, the nurse assesses the pattern of how the lesions appear on various areas of the body. For example, are they clustered in one area, or are they diffusely spread all over the body? It is important to ask the patient about whether itching and pain are associated with lesions. The length of time that lesions have been present and the precipitating factors that caused them are also assessed.

If palpation is not adequate to arrive at a diagnosis, a mid-level practitioner or health care provider may use a technique called **diascopy** to examine superficial skin lesions with a diascope for a definitive diagnosis. A diascope is a high-powered spotting scope for straight or angled viewing.

Inspection of the Lips

Assessment of the lips includes confirming that they are symmetrical, smooth, pink, moist, and without lesions. Systemic dehydration may be manifested in dry, scaling, cracking lips. Herpes viral infections and skin cancer are disorders common to the lips. Herpes presents with a vesicle on the lip that extends onto the skin. Skin cancers most commonly occur on the face, ear, neck, lips, and backs of the hands (American Cancer Society, 2010). Cancer is suspected when there is an open area (sore) that does not heal and bleeds easily. The nurse needs to ask whether the patient has a history of heavy cigarette, pipe, and cigar smoking; chewing tobacco use; and alcohol intake, as these are risk factors for the development of oral cancer.

Inspection of the Hair

Hair color is created by the production of melanin. Hair color ranges from pale to dark black and is dictated by genetic background and ethnic origin. Hair texture may vary from fine to coarse and from curly to straight. In the absence of disease, normal hair should have a vibrant appearance with a natural gloss. The texture of the hair may be changed due to environmental conditions and harsh treatment with colors, dyes, blow drying, and permanent waving.

The hair should be evenly distributed on the head. **Alopecia,** loss of hair, can be a result of familial patterns of baldness, disease, medications,

CHART 58–2 Secondary Skin Lesions

Secondary Lesion	Description	Pain/Itching	Examples
Atrophy	Thinning of the skin resulting from wasting of the dermis. There is a depression in the dermis. The skin is translucent and paperlike.	Not painful.	Striae, normal aging skin.
Crust	A dried serum or blood exudate as found on the surface of an abrasion or excoriation. The size and color vary.	Crust is not tender, but wound underneath may still be tender depending on stage of healing.	Scab, healing fever blister.
Erosion	An absence of the superficial dermis. The lesion is moist and glistening.	Tender.	Syphilitic chancre.
Excoriation	The loss of superficial tissue.	Slight tenderness.	Abrasion, scratch.
Fissure	A linear crack or break from the epidermis to the dermis.	Slight tenderness depending on size and location.	Athlete's foot; chapped, cracked lips as seen in severe dehydration.
Lichenification	Rough, thickened epidermis with increased visibility of the superficial skin markings.		Chronic dermatitis.
Scale	An abundance of dry or oily keratinized cells. Color or size may vary.		Exfoliative dermatitis.
Ulcer	Destruction of the skin beneath the epidermis.	May or may not be tender, depending on the size, location, depth, and whether acute or chronic.	An open sore sometimes on the leg, as with peripheral vascular disease.
Scar (cicatrix)	Fibrous tissue replacing the injured dermis.	Not painful depending on stage of healing.	Healed wound or surgical wound.
Keloid	An overproduction of scar tissue that extends laterally beyond the initial wound that is usually raised and smooth in appearance. It has a high incidence of occurrence in dark-skinned races and in children.	May or may not be tender. May itch.	Healed wound or surgical wound that is larger than the original wound size.
Hypertrophy	An overproduction of scar tissue that does not extend beyond the initial wound. It has a raised thickened appearance.	May or may not be tender. May itch.	Healed wound or surgical incision that has a thickened appearance.

or a pathologic condition. Diffuse hair loss may be caused by hormonal changes, systemic infections, and reaction to chemicals or medications. Patchy hair loss can be caused by scalp infections such as ringworm, burn injuries, and trauma, as well as from permanent waving or other harsh chemical treatments.

The scalp should be assessed for lesions. When assessing, the nurse should don gloves, separate the patient's hair into small sections, and lift it. The nurse inspects the scalp for lesions, dandruff, and pest infestations such as lice.

Inspection of and Palpation of the Nails

The nurse inspects and palpates the patient's nails. The nail surface is normally slightly curved with the posterior and lateral folds smooth and rounded. The nail edges should be smooth, rounded, and clean. The normal nail bed angle is 160 degrees, and the nail base is firm to palpation. A nail bed with greater than 160-degree angle suggests a clubbed nail. Clubbing of nails indicates a state of chronic hypoxia and is often seen with congenital and adult heart disease and chronic obstructive pulmonary disease.

CHART 58–3 Vascular Lesions

Lesion	Description	Cause
Cherry angioma	A distinct, benign vascular lesion 0.5–5 millimeters in diameter. A firm, deep-red papule.	Generally found on most people after age 30, and the incidence increases with age.
Ecchymosis	Red-purple nonblanchable discoloration of variable size.	Vascular wall destruction, trauma, vasculitis.
Petechiae	Red-purple nonblanchable discoloration less than 0.5 centimeter in diameter.	Intravascular defects, infection.
Purpura	Red-purple discoloration greater than 0.5 centimeter in diameter.	Intravascular defects, infection.
Spider angioma	Red central body with radiating spider-like legs that blanches with pressure to the central body.	Liver disease, vitamin B deficiency, idiopathic.
Telangiectasia	Fine, irregular red lines.	Dilation of capillaries.
Venous star	Bluish spider irregularly shaped with linear lines.	Increased pressure in superficial veins.

Weblink: Screening for Skin Cancer

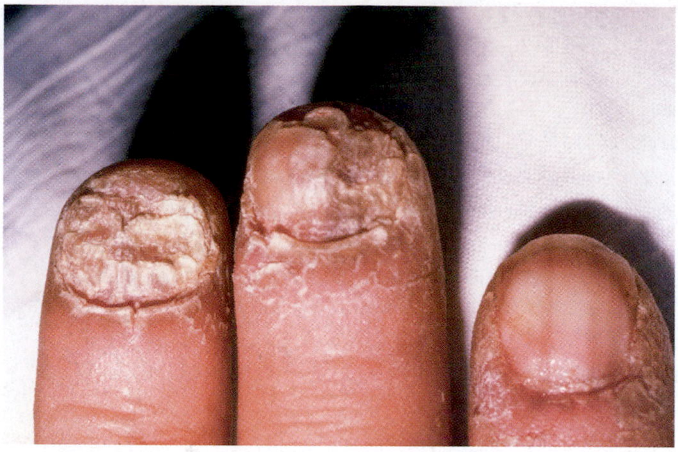

FIGURE 58–4 ◆ Fingernails with pits, grooves, and lines.

Source: From Prose N. S., K. G. Abson, & R. K. Scher. (1992). *International Journal of Dermatology, 31*, 453.

The surface of the nail should be smooth and nonbrittle, with no splitting. Pits, transverse grooves, or lines may indicate a nutritional deficiency (Figure 58–4◆). Patients with arterial insufficiency may have thickened, ridged nails.

The nail plate is translucent, and the nurse should expect to see a pink nail bed. Dark-skinned patients may have brownish, pigmented areas or linear bands along the nail edge. The nail bed is palpated to determine capillary refill. To assess capillary refill, the nurse depresses the nail edge to blanch and then releases it, noting the return of color. Capillary refill is usually documented as brisk, which is a normal response. However, it may have a sluggish return to color for patients with cardiovascular or respiratory disease and low levels of hemoglobin.

Critical Thinking Related to Skin Assessment

Critical thinking is essential in order to prioritize the most significant clinical findings that need further investigation. Skin disorders can be as benign as slight sunburn or as serious as life-threatening disorders such as necrotizing fasciitis and burns. It is imperative that the nurse be able to distinguish normal from abnormal and benign from serious. The nurse must rely on critical thinking skills in interpreting the patient's symptoms and assessment findings to determine possible and potential patient diagnoses and to consider the appropriate actions to take. Analysis of the data allows the nurse to make a diagnosis and then follow up with an intervention. It is imperative that the nurse communicate and collaborate with other members of the health care team in developing and implementing a plan of care.

Regardless of the health problem, each symptom that is identified should be thoroughly described to allow the nurse to come to a full understanding of the problem. The nurse will ask the patient, "Can you tell me more about the problem?" or "How did it start?" The patient will usually proceed with a discourse about the symptoms. Using skillful interview techniques, the nurse can explore and investigate each symptom further. Any symptom analysis would be incomplete without a thorough description of symptom characteristics (Chart 58–4).

Symptoms related to skin conditions include itching, drainage, color changes, changes in moles or warts, or a lesion that does not heal. The nurse should ask whether the onset was gradual or sudden and inquire about the length of time the problem has persisted. If the condition were a rash, the nurse would question the patient to determine whether the rash is progressive and spreading. Exploring precipitating factors would provide critical clues to determine whether, for example, a change in skin care products, new cologne, or a new house pet precipitated the condition. Discussion with the patient will elicit any associated symptoms, such as whether the patient had a recent viral illness, had a high fever, or has been exposed to increased physical or psychological stress.

CHART 58–4 Skin Disorder Analysis Criteria

Symptom Analysis

Onset
- When did it first occur?
- Did it occur gradually or suddenly?
- What are the precipitating factors?
- How long does it last?
- Is it continuous or is it intermittent?
- Is there a pattern of remission or exacerbation?

Location
- Where is it located?
- Does it radiate?

Timing
- When does it occur?
- How long does it last?
- How often does it occur?
- Is there a particular setting in which it occurs?

Quality
- How would you describe the symptom?
- How does the symptom rate on a scale of 1–10, with 10 being the most extreme?
- Is the symptom getting better or worse?

Quantity
- What is the frequency of occurrence?
- What is the extent of its occurrence?
- Does it occur in a specific setting?

Aggravating Factors
- What makes it worse?

Alleviating Factors
- What makes it go away?
- What makes it better?

Associated Phenomena
- What else happens when you experience the symptom?
- What treatments have you tried, including prescription, over-the-counter, and herbal medications and remedies?

Implications for Health Promotion

Health promotion for the skin primarily focuses on protection and early treatment. Protecting the skin will help prevent its breakdown, and early treatment may prevent complications. Patient teaching must include

Weblink: Sunscreens Weblink: Nutrients for Healthy Skin

NATIONAL GUIDELINES for Safe Skin Care

National Organization	Recommendation
American Cancer Society	Regular skin self-examination for all adults.
	Health care provider skin examination during periodic health exams.
	Education of patients concerning sun avoidance and use of sunscreen and other skin-protective measures.
	Avoidance of artificial tanning devices, especially among teens.
American Academy of Family Physicians	Health care providers should remain alert for skin lesions with malignant features that are noted while performing physical examinations for other purposes. Features associated with increased risk of malignancy include asymmetry, border irregularity, color variability, diameter greater than 6 mm (ABCD criteria), or rapidly changing lesions. Suspicious lesions should be biopsied.
American Academy of Dermatology	Patient education concerning periodic skin self-examination.
	Education of patients concerning sun avoidance and use of sunscreen.
	Avoidance of artificial tanning devices.
American Medical Association	Education of patients concerning sun avoidance and use of sunscreen.
	Avoidance of artificial tanning devices.

Source: U.S. Preventive Services Task Force. (2009). Screening for skin cancer. Retrieved from http://www.uspreventiveservicestaskforce.org/uspstf/uspsskca.htm.

information about the risk factors that cause the various integumentary abnormalities. In assessing the patient, it is essential for the nurse to identify high-risk behaviors such as sun exposure that require education. Correct use of sunscreens and limited exposure to the sun need to be stressed. An in-depth discussion of sun protection is included in Chapter 59.

Safety Alert *It is important for the nurse to stress that most sunscreens must be applied 15 to 30 minutes prior to sun exposure. Additionally, sunscreens need to be reapplied after swimming or excessive perspiration.*

Adequate rest balanced with a healthy exercise program has many beneficial effects. Rest is restorative to the body, and lack of rest is often manifested in the color of the skin. For example, dark circles under the eyes are a common manifestation of lack of sleep. In contrast, exercise causes vasodilation, typically manifested on the skin as a "healthy glow." Increased circulation also promotes wound healing and prevents the occurrence of wound infections. Education about overexposure to heat, cold, and sun will help patients to avoid skin breakdown. The National Guidelines box outlines safe skin care.

Hygiene

Human skin and hair need to be cleansed regularly to prevent bacterial buildup, remove excess oil, and prevent odor. Education about skin hygiene needs to be tailored to match the patient's skin type. For example, oily skin needs a cleanser that promotes drying, whereas dry skin needs a more gentle cleanser that prevents drying. The skin should be washed gently so as not to cause irritation and breakdown. If any irritation occurs, the individual must be instructed to stop using the product and try another one. Soaps tend to be more alkaline, thereby neutralizing the normal skin pH of 4.2 to 5.6. This may promote bacterial growth and increase the risk for infection. If this is occurring, the patient must be instructed to try other cleansers.

The older population needs to use gentle, less drying cleansers and shampoos because skin and scalp dry out with age. Moisturizers are typically helpful for dry skin, including the scalp, in preventing scaling and pruritus. Individuals may need to try different products to find the one that is best tailored for their skin type. Chapter 59 discusses the specific skin disorders.

Nutrition

Nutritional intake has a major impact on skin, hair, and nail health. The patient's diet needs to be well balanced and include the daily recommended servings of each food group. The skin specifically needs vitamins A, B, C, and K. Vitamin A and vitamin C are needed to promote epithelialization and normal rate of wound healing. Lack of vitamin C is also associated with bleeding gums, petechiae, and purpura. The B-complex vitamins are essential for normal metabolic processes and preventing certain dermatologic conditions such as seborrhea. Lack of vitamin K delays blood clotting and therefore can increase the risk of bruising and excessive bleeding with injuries. Protein intake is essential for normal cell growth and collagen formation, which increase wound strength, and inadequate amounts will retard wound healing. Chapter 8 contains an in-depth discussion of normal nutritional intake and the associated side effects of malnutrition.

NCLEX® PRACTICE

1. While gathering a history prior to an integumentary assessment, a patient tells the nurse that she "avoids the sun." The nurse realizes this patient could be at risk for developing:

1. hypothermia.
2. dehydration.
3. hypercholesterolemia.
4. vitamin D deficiency.

2. The nurse is completing an assessment interview with a patient who has a new onset skin rash. During the assessment, the nurse asks the patient about her recent travel. This information would be applicable to which of the following categories of the health history?

1. Past medical history
2. Chief complaint
3. Biographic and demographic data
4. History of present illness

3. A 25-year-old patient is admitted with severe cutaneous skin lesions. Which area of the assessment should the nurse focus on first?

1. Culture
2. Occupation
3. Hobbies
4. Social history

4. The nurse is preparing to examine a patient's skin. Which of the following should the nurse do when conducting this assessment? (select all that apply)

1. Wear sterile gloves.
2. Assess the least frequently exposed areas first.
3. Inspect and palpate the skin at the same time.
4. Ask the patient to stand up for the assessment.

5. The nurse assesses a patient's nails to be at a 160-degree angle with a smooth surface. These findings would be indicative of:

1. chronic hypoxia.
2. COPD.
3. a nutritional deficiency.
4. normal nails.

6. A patient has an overproduction of scar tissue along the site of a total hip replacement. The nurse realizes that this scar would be considered a:

1. scale.
2. cherry angioma.
3. keloid.
4. fissure.

Answers to NCLEX Practice Questions can be found in Appendix D in the Osborn Student Resources at nursing.pearsonhighered.com. Practice additional NCLEX questions online at the Student Resources site.

REFERENCES

American Cancer Society. (2010). Skin cancer prevention. Retrieved from http://www.cancer.org/Healthy/MoreWaysACSHelpsYouStayWell/acs-skin-cancer-prevention-activities

Amirlak, B. (2011). Skin anatomy. Medscape reference. Retrieved from http://emedicine.medscape.com/article/1294744-overview#aw2aab6b4

Baranoski, S., & Ayello, E. A. (2008). *Wound care essentials: Practice principles* (2nd ed.). Philadelphia: Wolters Kluwer.

Bryant, R. A. (2012). *Acute and chronic wounds* (4th ed.). St. Louis: Elsevier.

Davis, L. E., & King, M. K. (2008). Wound botulism from heroin skin popping. *Current Neurology and Neuroscience Report, 8*(6), 462–468.

Lee, A. (2009). Skin manifestations of systemic disease. *Australian Family Physician, 7*(38), 498–505.

Marrot, L., & Meunier, J. R. (2008). Skin DNA photodamage and its biological consequences. *Journal of the American Academy of Dermatology, 58* (5 Suppl 2): S139–148.

Rigel, D. S. (2008). Cutaneous ultraviolet exposure and its relationship to the development of skin cancer. *Journal of the American Academy of Dermatology, 58* (5 Suppl 2): S129–132.

Rizzo, D. (2010). *Fundamentals of anatomy and physiology* (3rd ed.). New York: Delmar.

Springhouse. (2008). *Wound care made incredibly visual.* Philadelphia: Wolters Kluwer.

U.S. Preventive Services Task Force. (2009). Screening for skin cancer. Retrieved from http://www.uspreventiveservicestaskforce.org/uspstf/uspsskca.htm

World Health Organization. (2010). Ultraviolet radiation. Retrieved from http://www.who.org

CHAPTER

59 Caring for the Patient with Skin Disorders

Joyce Pittman
Kathleen Osborn
John M. Osborn, MD

Outcome-Based Learning Objectives

After studying this chapter, the learner will be able to:

1. Differentiate the etiology, pathophysiology, and interventions for infections of the skin.
2. Identify preventive measures for skin disorders.
3. Identify the impact of the environment on the skin.
4. Describe the signs and symptoms, diagnostic tests, and treatment of skin disorders.
5. Generate a nursing plan of care for a patient with a life-threatening skin disorder.
6. Differentiate the psychological and physical implications for the patient with a skin disorder.

KEY TERMS

acne vulgaris p.1869
actinic keratosis p.1878
alopecia areata p.1884
androgenetic alopecia p.1884
androgenic alopecia p.1884
atopic dermatitis p.1853
blepharoplasty p.1874
café-au-lait spot p.1869
candidiasis p.1851
carbuncle p.1848
cellulitis p.1843
contact dermatitis p.1852
cutaneous anthrax infection p.1848
dermabrasion p.1875
dermatofibromas p.1870
dermatitis p.1852
folliculitis p.1847
furuncle p.1848
hemangiomas p.1878
herpes zoster p.1850
hirsutism p.1884
impetigo p.1843
lipoma p.1879
liposuction p.1876
necrotizing fasciitis (NF) p.1856
neurofibromatosis p.1867
nevi p.1878
nits p.1882
panniculectomy p.1877
paronychia p.1883
pediculosis p.1882
pemphigus vulgaris p.1870
photodermatitis p.1878
pilosebaceous follicles p.1879
plantar warts p.1851
postherpetic neuralgia p.1850
psoriasis p.1861
rhinoplasty p.1874
rhytidectomy p.1874
rosacea p.1871
scabies p.1882
seborrheic dermatitis p.1853
seborrheic keratosis p.1870
shingles p.1850
skin tags p.1878
solar lentigo p.1869
Stevens-Johnson syndrome (SJS) p.1859
tinea p.1852
tinea capitis p.1852
tinea corporis p.1852
tinea cruris p.1852
tinea pedis p.1852
toxic epidermal necrolysis (TEN) p.1860
urticaria p.1854
verrucae p.1850
vitiligo p.1868

THE SKIN IS THE BODY'S LARGEST ORGAN SYSTEM and serves as the protective barrier against the external environment. These protective functions include immune protection (Langerhans' cells), ultraviolet radiation protection (pigmentation), and protection against pathogens (bacterial and viral). The skin is responsible for helping to regulate body temperature and synthesis of vitamin D and contains receptors for sensation. The skin helps define peoples cultural and ethnic backgrounds and helps define one's self-image. In addition, the skin can be helpful in expressing emotion. The skin accounts for approximately 20% of the body's weight. The accessory structures of hair, nails, and glands, in combination with the skin, make up the integumentary system (Nicol & Huether, 2007).

The skin is affected by a number of factors, both modifiable and nonmodifiable. An important nonmodifiable factor is age. There is a wide range of differences between fetal and adult skin. For example fetal skin has more collagen than adult skin. Another difference that has been identified is a higher amount of hyaluronic acid in fetal skin. Hyaluronic acid has been associated with a reduction in scar formation (Nicol & Huether, 2007). Modifiable factors that influence the skin include a number of health and healthy lifestyle choices: sun, hydration, soaps, nutrition, and medications, to name a few.

There are normal variations noted within the integumentary system related to ethnicity. These normal variations may account for changes in skin response to daily care and environmental irritants, as seen in the Cultural Considerations box.

Disorders of the skin are a common reason for visiting the health care provider. The patient may complain of a rash, itching, or an unusual lesion. The skin is often a mirror of the rest of the body. There can be disorders of only the skin or systemic disorders that are reflected in the skin. Certain disorders of the skin are treated with medication and/or nonpharmacologic measures, whereas others require surgical intervention.

Skin disorders are usually diagnosed by evaluating the history of onset of symptoms and precipitating factors, including systemic diseases, and performing a physical examination. Most skin disorders have distinct, recognizable lesions that assist with the diagnosis. However, if the origin of the abnormality is uncertain, it is cultured, scraped, or biopsied and microscopically examined to identify the diagnosis.

CULTURAL CONSIDERATIONS
for Racial Differences in Skin

Physiological skin differences among racial and ethnic groups include:

- African Americans have increased lipid content.
- African Americans have increased thickness of the stratum corneum and increased spontaneous desquamation.
- Water content of the skin is greater in Hispanics and lower in Caucasians.
- An increase in melanin decreases sun damage.
  - Increased thickness of the dermal–epidermal junction (DEJ) exists in African Americans.

The three most common disorders in darkly pigmented skin are:

- Acne
- Eczema
- Pigmentary disorders.

Source: Querleux, B., Baldeweck, T., Diridollou, S., de Rigal, J., Huguet, E., Leroy, F., & Barbosa, V. H. (2009). Skin from various ethnic origins and aging: An in vivo cross-sectional multimodality imaging study. *Skin Research and Technology, 15*(3), 306–313.

INFECTIONS OF THE SKIN

The skin is subject to infections caused by bacteria, viruses, or fungi. Normally the skin's flora, sebum, and immune responses help prevent infection. However, depending on the virulence of the organism and the strength of the individual's resistance, infections may occur.

Bacterial Skin Infections

Bacteria are normally present on the skin and are not considered pathogenic. However, if they invade the skin or if the patient's resistance is impaired, they can result in superficial or systemic infection. Coagulase-positive *Staphylococcus aureus*, beta-hemolytic streptococci, and community-acquired methocillin-resistant *S. aureus* are among the most common causative pathogens (Nicol & Huether, 2007).

Cellulitis

Etiology, Epidemiology, and Pathophysiology

Cellulitis is a non-necrotizing inflammation of the skin and subcutaneous tissues, usually caused by staphylococcus or streptococcus infections (Kroshinsky, Grossman, & Fox, 2007), that does not involve the fascia or muscles. One example of a common cellulitis infection is erysipelas, which is an acute, inflammatory, superficial form of cellulitis resulting from *Staphylococcus aureus* (most common) or group A beta-hemolytic streptococcus.

Cellulitis is a common infection; however, because it is not usually reported, it is difficult to track the exact prevalence. It does affect all racial and ethnic groups. In addition, the incidence of cellulitis in men and women is equal, and no age predilection is usually described (McNamara et al., 2007).

Due to a loss of skin integrity, patients with a fissure, cut, laceration, insect bite, surgical wound, trauma, or chronic wound (ulcer) are susceptible to the development of cellulitis. Organisms gain entrance to the dermis and multiply. The most common areas are the lower extremities, face, ears, and buttocks; however, other areas on the body can be affected as well. Individuals who have a compromised immune system, are obese, or have venous insufficiency have an increased susceptibility to cellulitis.

Clinical Manifestations

In cellulitis, the affected skin becomes erythematous, swollen, tender, and tight over the infected area, and there is an indefinite border. There also may be vesicles, blisters, or abscesses. In addition, regional lymphadenopathy may occur. In erysipelas, one or more well-defined lesions are bright red, tender, and warm to touch with lymphatic involvement causing a red streak along the skin leading away from the primary lesion. Associated symptoms may include fever, chills, headache, and vomiting.

Laboratory and Diagnostic Procedures

Diagnostic blood studies include a white blood count (WBC) and a wound culture to identify the causative organism. The Laboratory and Diagnostic Tests box (p. 1844) describes the common laboratory and diagnostic tests for abnormalities associated with skin disorders.

Medical Management

Treatment involves resting the affected site with elevation if possible. In addition, antibiotics sensitive for the causative organism are indicated. Protecting the affected area is helpful if blisters or bullae have formed. Soaking with cool Burrow's solution can help relieve the tension and pain. Depending on the depth of the skin involved, moist wound management principles and advanced wound products may be helpful. See Chapter 60 for wound management. Without treatment, cellulitis may spread to the bloodstream, causing septicemia. The diagnosis, treatment, and prognosis of sepsis are described in Chapter 54.

Impetigo

Etiology, Epidemiology, and Pathophysiology

Impetigo is a common skin infection caused by *S. aureus* and/or group A beta-hemolytic streptococcus (GABHS). It occurs more frequently in warm, humid environments and is the most common bacterial skin infection. The prevalence varies seasonally and peaks during

LABORATORY AND DIAGNOSTIC TESTS for Skin Disorders

Diagnostic Test, Normal Values, and Rationales	Expected Abnormality
White Blood Cells (WBCs) Normal values: 4,500–10,000/mm^3 *Elevated levels are associated with inflammation and infection.*	Leukocytosis with a shift to the left and an elevated number of neutrophils is present with cellulitis.
Tissue Biopsy Normal values: No abnormal tissue found *Surgically removing all or part of the lesion for laboratory examination of cells to identify abnormal growth. Can be excisional, punch, shave, or immunofluorescent.*	Identification of microorganisms or cell type. Can identify cancer cells, inflammatory reactions, and other types of cell abnormalities.
Potassium Hydroxide Smear Normal values: No fungal growth *A sample of the lesion is taken, wet with a solution of potassium hydroxide, and placed on a slide for examination. Potassium hydroxide clears off debris and bacteria so that fungi can be identified.*	Able to diagnose whether fungi are the cause of a skin disorder.
Tzanck Smear Normal values: No abnormal cells *Scraping of the lesion is taken and then stained with Giemsa, Wright's, or Sedi stain to identify multinucleated giant cells or atypical keratinocytes.*	Demonstrates the presence of herpes simplex virus or varicella-zoster virus. Not a very accurate test but can help to diagnose the presence of herpes simplex virus.
Wound, Tissue, and Blood Cultures Normal values: No growth of abnormal cells *Proper identification of the causative organism can allow for effective treatment.*	The microorganism will grow on the culture medium and can be identified. Wound cultures are positive for *S. aureus* or group A beta-hemolytic streptococcus with cellulitis.
Immunofluorescent Studies Normal values: No growth of abnormal cells *Tissue samples are stained for antibodies and examined under a fluorescence microscope.* *Identifies immunologically mediated dermatitis.*	Will detect the presence of immunoglobulins in immunologically mediated disorders.
Wood's Lamp Normal values: No rash noted *"Black" light that can be shone on a rash to produce fluorescence.* *Helps identify fungi.*	Tinea will fluoresce green under a Wood's light. Other fungi may fluoresce yellow to orange.
Polymerase Chain Reaction (PCR) Normal values: No growth of abnormal cells *Method of identifying the DNA in the pathogen.* *Allows the recognition of bacteria and viruses, especially those difficult to identify through a culture. Can also identify genetic disorders.*	Identifies mutations in DNA related to antigen–antibody reactions.
Skin Scrapings *Cells can be scraped off the lesions and placed on a slide.* *Parasites can be directly visualized and identified under the microscope.*	Allows visualization of mites, ova, and feces from infestations.
Patch Test *Suspected allergens are applied to the skin of the back or arm for 48 hours to see whether there is a reaction.* *Determines whether dermatitis is allergic or irritant, and identifies the allergen.*	If the patient has an allergy to the substance applied to the skin, wheals and flare reactions will be evident.
Immunoglobin E (IgE) Normal values: Less than 40 U/mL *Evaluated in antibody–antigen reactions.*	Levels may be elevated, atopic dermatitis indicates an immune reaction.
Chest X-Ray, Ultrasound, Computed Tomography (CT), Magnetic Resonance Imaging (MRI), Lymphoscintigraphy, and Positron-Emission Tomography (PET) Normal values: Negative for tumor growth	Are used to detect metastasis with melanoma.

Source: Adapted from Kee, J. L. (2010). *Laboratory and diagnostic tests with nursing implications.* Upper Saddle River, NJ: Pearson.

PHARMACOLOGY Summary of Medications Used to Treat Skin Disorders

Medication Category and Action	Application/Indication	Nursing Responsibility
Topical corticosteroids Betamethasone (Diprolene) Fluocinonide (Lidex) Mometasone (Elocon) Triamcinolone (Kenalog) ***Action:*** Depress formation, release, and activity of endogenous mediators of inflammation, including prostaglandins, kinins, histamines, liposomal enzymes, and complement system.	Used for inflammatory and pruritic conditions, as well as hyperplastic and infiltrative disorders. This includes conditions such as atopic and allergic dermatitis, hypertrophic scars, and psoriasis.	Should be applied in a thin layer and rubbed in thoroughly on wet skin. Areas of the body with thin skin, such as the face, or intertriginous areas (where two skinfolds touch) are more susceptible to side effects. Some infections may be made worse by corticosteroids.
Antiacne medications Benzoyl peroxide (Benoxyl 10) ***Action:*** Broad-spectrum bacteriostatic activity against *Propionibacterium acnes.* Release of active or free-radical oxygen capable of oxidizing bacterial proteins.	Used for mild to moderate acne vulgaris and as adjunct to other therapies. It is rubbed into the acne lesions once or twice daily.	Patients should be taught how to use it and become familiar with the side effects. May irritate the skin. Use should start slow and be gradually increased. Can be irritating to the skin. Produces phototoxicity.
Retinoic acid/tretinoin ***Action:*** Keratolytic agent used to increase cell turnover and prevent comedones. Reduces inflammation.	Used as a cream, gel, or solution, and is applied topically. Applied sparingly at bedtime. Avoid using around the nose, eyes, or mouth.	May aggravate acne during the first 2–4 weeks of therapy until the skin becomes acclimated.
Antibacterial agents Erythromycin and tetracycline ***Action:*** Interfere with microbial protein synthesis. Antibacterial agents are effective against *P. acnes.* Reduces inflammation.	Taken orally or topically. Used orally for deep acne.	There is no toxicity with topical use. Monitor for allergic reactions with oral use. Dermato logical reactions can occur. i.e.; Erythema; pruritus; rash; skin tenderness at site.
Bleomycin ***Action:*** Inhibits DNA synthesis, causing a sclerosing of the lesion.	It is used off label intralesionally for warts.	Side effects include nausea and vomiting, headache, and rash. Discontinue if side effects occur.
Isotretinoin (Accutane) ***Action:*** Reduces sebum secretion and sebaceous gland size.	Treatment of severe recalcitrant nodular acne. Also used for psoriasis, rosacea, squamous cell carcinoma, and cutaneous lymphomas.	Teratogenic so pregnancy prevention is critical. Take meds with meals, avoid fatty foods, and vitamin A. May cause contact lens intolerance. Monitor cholesterol levels during treatment. Use sunscreen and keep lips lubricated.
Tacrolimus ***Action:*** Suppresses cell-mediated immune reactions and some humoral immunity but exact mechanism is not known.	Used for short-term and second-line therapy for atopic dermatitis, rosacea, vitiligo, psoriasis, lichen planus, and pyoderma gangrenosum.	Do not use occlusive dressings over topical application. Apply thin layer twice a day, and rub in gently.
Azelaic acid (Finacea) ***Action:*** Regulation of skin growth and turnover. Reverses comedo formation.	Topical treatment of mild to moderate acne vulgaris and rosacea.	Apply to lesions twice a day. Improvement may take up to 4 weeks.
Etanercept (Enbrel) ***Action:*** Binds specifically to tumor necrosis factor (TNF), blocking its interaction with cell surface TNF receptors.	For treatment of chronic moderate to severe plaque psoriasis.	May lower the ability to fight infections. Do not receive live vaccines while taking etanercept.
Cyclosporine ***Action:*** Suppresses cell-mediated immune reactions and some humoral immunity.	For treatment of those with severe, recalcitrant plaque psoriasis who have failed to respond to at least one systemic therapy.	Avoid sun exposure due to increased risk of skin cancer. Should not be used with patients with renal or liver impairment. Multiple drug interactions and potential adverse reactions. Close follow-up is critical.

(*continued*)

PHARMACOLOGY Summary of Medications Used to Treat Skin Disorders, *continued*

Medication Category and Action	Application/Indication	Nursing Responsibility
Methotrexate ***Action:*** Inhibits DNA synthesis and cellular replication.	For symptomatic treatment of severe psoriasis.	Taken once a week, on same day each week. Notify the health care provider if lesions are not controlled. Close follow-up is warranted.
Antifungal agents Miconazole (monistat) Lotrimin (clotrimazole) Nystatin (Mycostatin) Ketoconazole (Nizoral) ***Action:*** Alter the permeability of the fungal cell membrane, leading to cell death.	Applied topically. Each drug is specific to a particular organism. Applied sparingly once or twice daily.	Monitor for side effects or allergies. Thoroughly rub the drug into the skin. Do not use with occlusive coverings unless prescribed by the health care provider. Keep areas clean and dry.
Antihistamines Diphenhydramine (Benadryl) Loratadine (Claritin) Fexofenadine (Allegra) ***Action:*** Block histamine leading to vasoconstriction and decreased capillary permeability. Decreased itching and edema.	Decreases itching and signs of urticaria. Taken orally.	May cause drowsiness and dryness of the mouth. Some are nonsedating.
Mupirocin (Bactroban) topical ***Action:*** Inhibit bacterial protein synthesis. Cream—minimal systemic absorption. Ointment—measurable systemic absorption.	Treatment for impetigo caused by *S. aureus* or *S. pyogenes.*	Warn against contact with the eyes and mucous membranes. Wash hands before and after application. If no improvement is seen within 3 to 5 days or if the condition worsens, contact the health care provider.
Dicloxacillin ***Action:*** Inhibits bacterial cell wall mucopeptide synthesis.	Treatment for penicillinase-producing staphylococcal infection and initial therapy of suspected staphylococcal infection, folliculitis.	Instruct the patient to take on an empty stomach before (30 min) or after (2 hours) meals with a full glass of water.
Doxycycline ***Action:*** Inhibits bacterial protein synthesis.	Treatment of infections caused by susceptible strains of gram-positive and gram-negative bacteria. Cutaneous anthrax, severe acne, inflammatory lesions of rosacea.	Take with a full glass of water. May take without regard to meals; however, if gastrointestinal (GI) upset occurs, may take with food. Avoid taking with antacids. May cause photosensitivity, so avoid exposure to sunlight or tanning beds, use sunscreens, and wear protective clothing. Oral contraceptives may be less effective when taking doxycycline. Report signs and symptoms of superinfection or if diarrhea containing blood or pus occurs.
Ciprofloxin ***Action:*** Inhibits microbial DNA replication, transcription, repair, and recombination.	Cutaneous anthrax.	Drink plenty of fluids (eight 8-oz servings of water/day). Minimize or avoid excessive exposure to sunlight or tanning beds, use sunscreen, and wear protective clothing to avoid photosensitivity reactions. Older adults may be more sensitive to the effects on the QT interval or tendons.
Antivirals Acyclovir (Zovirax) Famciclovir ***Action:*** Inhibit viral DNA replication by interfering with viral DNA polymerase.	Effective against herpes simplex 1 and 2, varicella-zoster, herpes zoster, Epstein–Barr virus, and cytomegalovirus. Given topically or orally.	Monitor for the effectiveness of the drug. Monitor for side effects. Prevent the spread of infection. Encourage adequate fluid intake. Inform the patient that this drug is not a cure for herpes.
Additional agents Tricyclic antidepressants (Imipramine, Doxepin, Desipramine, etc.) ***Action:*** Inhibit the reuptake of norepinephrine and serotonin in the central nervous system (CNS).	Postherpetic neuralgia, neuropathy. Doxepin topically—Apply a thin film to the affected area four times a day.	Minimize or avoid exposure to sunlight or tanning lamps, use sunscreen, and wear protective clothing as it may cause photosensitization. May raise or lower blood glucose in diabetic patients. May take with food if stomach upset occurs. Withdraw taking medication slowly to avoid side effects. May cause edema and weight gain. Avoid alcohol, opiates, and other CNS depressants. Using more than 8 days is not recommended.
Anticonvulsants (Pregabalin, Gabapentin) ***Action:*** Action unknown.	Postherpetic neuralgia, neuropathy.	May increase the risk of suicidal thoughts and behavior. Report any of the symptoms promptly to the health care provider. Usually started at a low dose and gradually increased as tolerated. May cause dizziness and/or drowsiness; use caution until tolerance is determined.

PHARMACOLOGY Summary of Medications Used to Treat Skin Disorders, *continued*

Medication Category and Action	Application/Indication	Nursing Responsibility
Domeboro solution (aluminum acetate) (calcium acetate 830 mg and aluminum sulfate 1,191 mg) ***Action:*** Soothes, cools, and dries.	Relief of minor skin irritations due to: poison ivy; athlete's foot; insect bites; rashes; chickenpox; poison sumac; rashes caused by soaps, detergents, cosmetics, or jewelry; skin inflammation, or redness.	Contraindicated in pregnancy.
Finasteride (Propecia) ***Action:*** Inhibits conversion of testosterone into 5-alpha dihydrotestosterone.	Treatment for male pattern baldness.	

Source: Adams, M. P., & Koch, R. W. (2010). *Pharmacology: Connections to nursing practice.* Upper Saddle River, NJ: Pearson; Tatro, D. S. (Ed.). (2012). *Unbound medicine: A–Z drug facts.* Philadelphia:. Wolters Kluwer/Facts & Comparisons/Lippincott Williams & Wilkins.

the summer and fall (Lewis, 2012). *S aureus* and GABHS require the epithelial cell receptor component, fibronectin, for colonization. Intact skin is resistant to colonization or infection, but if there is even a small disruption in the skin the bacteria are able to attach to the fibronectin receptors. It is a contagious, rapidly spreading infection that may occur after a minor skin injury such as an insect bite. It is usually transferred from individual to individual by direct contact and is more common in children and infants.

Clinical Manifestations

There are two types of impetigo: bullous and nonbullous. Bullous impetigo is characterized by a thin-roofed bulla or vesicle on an erythematous base. The bulla or vesicle collapses and drains a honey-colored crust, which dries and develops a "stuck on" appearance. Nonbullous impetigo results in vesicles or pustules on an erythematous base that also rupture, leading to a superficial honey-colored crust. Both types may develop satellite lesions. Lesions may itch or may be slightly tender.

Laboratory and Diagnostic Procedures and Medical Management

In impetigo, cultures of the lesions are not commonly done but may help in assessing antibiotic sensitivity (see the Laboratory and Diagnostic Tests for Skin Disorders box, p. 1844). Treatment of impetigo involves removal of crusts by soaking in warm tap water and washing with gentle antibacterial soap. Topical antibiotics such as mupirocin (Bactroban) may be helpful; however, if the infection is widespread, an oral antibiotic may be indicated. The patient must be instructed to avoid contact with others and to avoid sharing towels or sheets.

Folliculitis

Etiology, Epidemiology, and Pathophysiology

Folliculitis is the inflammation of hair follicles that is commonly caused by *Staphylococcus* but may also be caused by trauma or *Pseudomonas aeruginosa*, which is a gram-negative organism frequently associated with nosocomial infections or infections originating in the hospital (Peleg & Hooper, 2010). Common causes include tight clothing, curly hair that grows back into the skin, and shaving too closely on a regular basis, leading to ingrown hairs (hairs that reenter the skin as they grow). Folliculitis is common in the United States, but most patients do not see a health care provider unless they have recurrent or deep folliculitis (Satter, 2011). African Americans are particularly susceptible to folliculitis due to ingrown hairs because of their curly hair.

Folliculitis due to *P. aeruginosa* is related to the use of hot tubs, whirlpools, or exposure to contaminated water. The desquamated skin cells in the water provide a good medium for bacterial growth, and free chlorine levels are decreased by the large number of people in the pool or hot tub (Satter, 2011). Folliculitis due to *Pseudomonas* is not spread from person to person but is usually due to inadequate care of the pool or tub. The *Pseudomonas* invades the hair follicle pores after superhydration of the skin by the contaminated water. Symptoms will occur 1 to 5 days after exposure to the contaminated water.

Clinical Manifestations

Folliculitis presents as circular papules and pustules associated with the hair follicles and surrounded by an area of erythema. They may itch and are usually located in areas of tight clothing, bathing suits, or any place where hair grows. With *Pseudomonas* folliculitis, symptoms may also include low-grade fever, sore throat, and lymphadenopathy.

Laboratory and Diagnostic Procedures

Folliculitis is diagnosed by a patient history of lesion development and exposure to contaminated water, as well as physical exam. The lesions may be cultured to diagnose the causative organism and identify antibiotic sensitivities (see the Laboratory and Diagnostic Tests for Skin Disorders box, p. 1844).

Medical Management

Treatment of folliculitis involves administration of antibiotics and other nonpharmacologic measures. If the folliculitis is limited and superficial, topical antibiotics such as mupirocin (Bactroban) may be effective. For more involved infections, antibiotics are prescribed such as dicloxacillin when the causative agent is *Staphylococcus.*

The affected area should be cleansed with antibacterial soap twice daily. In addition, the application of warm compresses may be helpful to soothe any itching or burning of the skin. If the folliculitis is due to ingrown hairs, the patient should be instructed to refrain from shaving until the infection is resolved. Once shaving is resumed, the patient should be instructed to shave every few days rather than daily, using a thick shaving gel to hydrate the skin. The patient should use a fresh razor blade with each shave, avoid shaving too close, and shave in the direction of hair growth. Using an electric razor instead of a straightedge blade may be helpful. Any hair tips that are beginning to grow back into the skin can be straightened out using a sterile needle or a clean soft-bristled toothbrush in a circular motion. Shaving should be followed with

Weblink: Carbuncle

the use of a moisturizing lotion. *Pseudomonas* folliculitis is usually self-limiting.

Furuncles and Carbuncles

Etiology, Epidemiology, and Pathophysiology

Furuncles and carbuncles are abscesses that develop when the infection from folliculitis becomes deeper and involves more follicles. These lesions develop when a sebaceous gland is obstructed, causing a deep inflammatory reaction and infection from *Staphylococcus.* Most patients with carbuncles or furuncles are among the 10% to 20% of the population who are symptomless *Staphylococcus aureus* carriers on the surface of their skin or in their nose. These people are referred to as "carriers." *S. aureus* is commonly found in regions where two skin areas may touch or rub together, such as the armpits, groin, and intergluteal cleft (Do, 2010). Any scratch or nick in these areas allows the bacteria into the wall of the hair follicle, causing infection.

Hidradenitis suppurativa is a condition of acute recurrent cystlike abscesses (furuncles and carbuncles) that develop in the apocrine gland-bearing skin (axillae, anogenital area, pubis, etc.). These abscess areas develop fibrotic sinus tracts with intermittent drainage and periodic acute abscesses. Hidradenitis occurs more commonly in young adulthood. Other risk factors include diabetes, obesity, acne, hyperandrogenism (excess secretion of androgens), and smoking (Domino, Baldor, Golding, Grimes, & Taylor, 2012).

Clinical Manifestations

A **furuncle** is a walled-off, deep, painful, firm mass that contains pus (Figure 59–1◆). It is usually 1 to 5 centimeters in diameter. A **carbuncle** is a larger abscess that interconnects several hair follicles. It is about 3 to 10 centimeters in diameter and is extremely painful. A carbuncle will drain pus from multiple follicles, leaving craterlike nodules, and may be associated with fever and chills. Furuncles and carbuncles can occur any place where there is hair but may be more common in areas of increased friction or perspiration such as under the belt, in the groin, or in the axilla.

Laboratory and Diagnostic Procedures and Medical Management

Furuncles and carbuncles are diagnosed by physical examination. The drainage may be cultured to help define the most effective treatment.

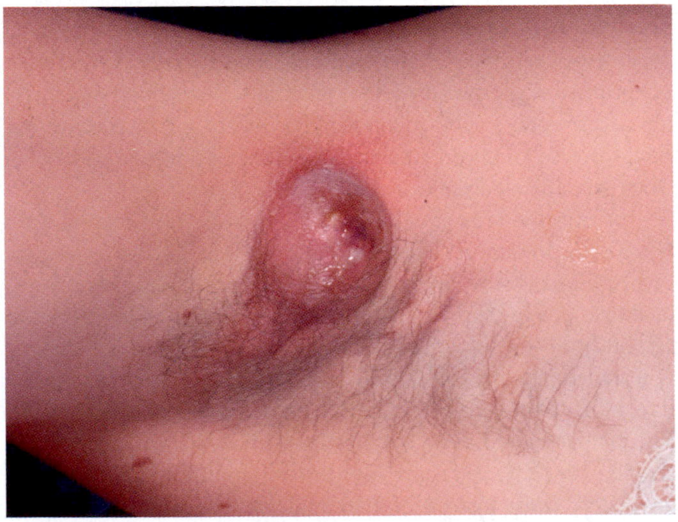

FIGURE 59–1 ◆ Furuncles and carbuncles.
Source: NMSB/Custom Medical Stock Photo, Inc.

The treatment includes incision and drainage of the abscess and warm compresses to help relieve the discomfort. Antibiotic ointments such as mupirocin (Bactroban) or Neosporin may be used. Systemic antibiotics such as dicloxacillin or erythromycin also may be used. These medications are described in the Pharmacology Summary of Medications Used to Treat Skin Disorders box (p. 1845).

Anthrax Infection of the Skin

Etiology, Epidemiology, and Pathophysiology

Anthrax is an infectious disease caused by *Bacillus anthracis.* Anthrax infection in humans most often involves the skin (cutaneous), gastrointestinal tract, or lungs. **Cutaneous anthrax infection** occurs when the bacterium enters a cut or abrasion. The main risk is contact with animal hides or hair, bone products, and wool, or contact with infected animals. People most at risk for cutaneous anthrax include farm workers, veterinarians, and tannery and wool workers. Approximately 95% of the anthrax infections involve the skin (Lucey, 2007; Martin & Friedlander, 2009).

Clinical Manifestations

Clinical manifestations of an anthrax skin infection begin 1 to 7 days after exposure. Initially, an itchy bump appears that resembles an insect bite. The bump develops into a vesicle within 1 to 2 days and then a 1- to 3-cm-in-diameter painless ulcer develops. The ulcer has a characteristic black necrotic area in the center. Lymph glands in the adjacent area may swell. About 20% of untreated cases of cutaneous anthrax will result in death, although deaths are rare with appropriate antimicrobial therapy. A scab often forms, and then dries and falls off within 2 weeks. Complete healing can take longer (Lucey, 2007; Martin & Friedlander, 2009).

Laboratory and Diagnostic Procedures and Medical Management

Skin cultures or biopsy of the lesion will diagnose the anthrax infection. The sample is looked at under a microscope to identify the anthrax bacterium. Cutaneous (skin) anthrax is treated with doxycycline and ciprofloxacin for 7 to 10 days. When treated with antibiotics, cutaneous anthrax is likely to get better. However, up to 20% of people who do not get treatment may die if anthrax spreads to the blood. Spread of the infection from person to person does not occur so there is no need to put individuals who live with the infected person on antibiotics unless they have also been exposed to the same source of anthrax (Lucey, 2007; Martin & Friedlander, 2009).

Nursing Management

The nurse provides holistic, patient-focused care using a framework called the nursing process. Nursing management of skin disorders and infections includes assessment, nursing diagnosis, outcomes and evaluation parameters, planning interventions, and evaluation of care and patient progress. Nursing management involves multilevel assessment, clinical decision making, and critical thinking. A thorough knowledge of treatment strategies provides a basis for safe, high-quality nursing care.

Assessment

A variety of etiologic, systemic, and local factors are involved in the pathogenesis of a skin disorder; therefore, a holistic approach is essential. Nursing assessment of the skin begins with inspection. A complete inspection of the skin must be done frequently, noting changes in skin color, presence of lesions, pattern and characteristics of the lesions, wound size, drainage, and temperature. Assessment of the skin also includes palpation. Touch allows the nurse to assess temperature, texture, presence of induration, thickening of the skin, and pain.

Hydration, fluid balance, or nutrition may be affected in the patient with a significant wound or skin disorder. Infection becomes likely when skin integrity is compromised; therefore, it is very important to assess for signs of infection both in the wound and systemically. Clinical manifestations of infection include fever, increased redness (erythema) or drainage, increased pain, presence of odor, change in drainage color, increased white blood cell count, and increased size of wound or lesion.

Psychological assessment also needs to be included in assessing patients with skin disorders. Not only does the appearance of the skin affect self-esteem and body image but there can also be other psychosocial influences/effects. The presence of family or support systems, financial barriers, depression, and quality of life all need to be considered when treating the patient with a skin disorder. Information collected during the assessment will provide a basis for establishing the baseline status, determining the nursing diagnosis, developing the treatment plan, and evaluating the response/effect of the treatment.

Nursing Diagnoses

The following nursing diagnoses are examples related to the patient with a skin disorder:

- *Impaired Skin Integrity* related to epithelial skin loss.
- *Risk for Infection* related to loss of skin integrity and impaired nonspecific and specific immunity.
- *Acute Pain* related to burn injury and exposed nerve endings.
- *Imbalanced Nutrition: Less Than Body Requirements* related to hypermetabolic demands of disorder, decreased appetite, immobility, pain, nausea/vomiting, and depression.
- *Fear* and *Anxiety* related to changes in health status/role functioning; situational crisis.
- *Ineffective Thermoregulation* related to epithelial skin loss.
- *Disturbed Body Image* related to the skin disorder.

NANDA-I © 2012

Planning

Determining a plan of care for the patient with a skin disorder is based on the assessment and diagnosis. Following a multidisciplinary approach, the nurse sets measurable and achievable short- and long-range goals for the patient involving other disciplines as needed. Depending on the severity of the skin disorder, the help of a dietitian, physical therapist, pharmacist, case manager, and/or social worker may be indicated. For example, when an infection is present, the health care provider must give appropriate antibiotics in a timely and appropriate manner, provide wound management as ordered (frequency and correct topical dressing), and obtain a nutrition consult. Long-range goals may focus on providing appropriate discharge instructions and family involvement.

Outcome and Evaluation Parameters

The outcome goal for the patient with a skin disorder should be measurable and achievable. Of course, the ultimate outcome for the patient with a skin disorder is complete healing without complication. Additional outcome measures such as pain relief, symptom management, return teaching/demonstration of instructions, and return to previous level of activity also should be considered. However, sometimes complete healing is not likely; therefore, other outcomes should be considered. These may include pain management, drainage management, odor control, and prevention of complications.

Interventions and Rationales

Interventions are based on the type of skin disorder. Once the cause has been removed or corrected, the treatment begins. The involved area must have effective wound care and appropriate selection of dressing, if necessary. The nurse should cleanse the area with cool water or saline to remove drainage or crusting. If the involved area is in the perineum, the nurse must make every effort to prevent contamination from urine and feces. The area needs to be kept clean and dry. Warm compresses may be appropriate to soothe itching or burning. Elevation of the affected area, if possible, is indicated to reduce swelling. Wound care, dressing, and skin barriers are described in depth in Chapter 60.

Good nutrition is essential for wound healing to occur. The nurse must assess the amount and type of food intake and intervene if the patient's lack of appetite persists. In teaching patients and families how to maintain healthy skin, it is essential to discuss the importance of adequate nutrition. The skin needs protein, vitamin C, iron, and zinc to be healthy. Protein and vitamin deficiencies, along with obesity, can decrease the skin's ability to regenerate and affect the circulation to the skin, leading to skin lesions and delayed wound healing. Hydration is also important for wound healing and to maintain elasticity in the skin. Approximately 64 ounces of water is needed daily to keep the skin well hydrated. Therefore, assessing fluid intake is essential. The nurse needs to encourage the patient to take in an adequate amount of fluid and, if necessary, obtain a nutrition consult or health care provider's order for intravenous fluids. Chapter 8 discusses nutritional needs.

Regular exercise helps maintain adequate circulation, which provides oxygen and nutrients to the skin. Regular bathing keeps the excess bacteria and oils in check so that the skin can remain healthy. However, bathing more frequently than necessary should be avoided because it can cause dryness of the skin. The patient should be asked about bathing practices, including the type of cleanser used and the frequency of bathing. If the skin is dry, emollient cream or lotion should be applied immediately after bathing to maintain hydration. The skin should be inspected monthly for new growths or changes in skin lesions. (See Chapter 58 for skin assessment.)

If an infection occurs, treatment needs to be tailored to the clinical manifestations. For example, the patient may need antibiotics or antifungal medications to treat the cause. If fever is present, antipyretics and cooling measures may be necessary. If the patient complains of itching or pain, an antihistamine or analgesic may be indicated. Finally, if the causative organism is communicable, the patient will need isolation.

Evaluation

The nurse needs to reevaluate the plan for care of the patient with skin disorders regularly to ensure that it is still effective. Any change in the patient's condition could have a negative impact on the wound healing process and the effectiveness of the plan of care. In all care settings, reevaluation should be done regularly and documented. Interventions and plans of care may need to be revised to meet the patient's specific needs if the current treatment plan is unsuccessful. Evaluation criteria of progress would be a decrease in the size and depth of the involved area. If this healing is not occurring, then the area needs to be assessed to determine why it is not, such as for infection or decreased tissue perfusion.

Viral Skin Infections

Viruses are intracellular pathogens that invade live cells. They contain either DNA or RNA and require host cell genetic material to replicate. They can destroy the cell during the process of entering

Weblink: Shingles Vaccine

it and replicating, or by causing an immune response that causes cell destruction. The various types of viral infections of the skin are outlined next.

Herpes Simplex Type 1 and Type 2

Etiology, Epidemiology, and Pathophysiology

Two different but similar virus types can cause herpes simplex viral infections: type 1 and type 2. Herpes simplex type 1 causes oral lesions or cold sores in approximately 80% of cases and genital lesions in 20% of cases. Herpes simplex type 2 causes genital lesions in 80% of cases and oral lesions in 20%. In the United States, approximately 65% of the population is seropositive for herpes simplex type 1 and 25% for type 2 by the fourth decade of life. Both are more prevalent in women than men (Sharma, 2011). Herpes simplex is caused by a herpes virus that lives in a nerve root. It will remain asymptomatic until something triggers an outbreak. Exposure to the sun, stress, and fever are common triggers.

Clinical Manifestations

The lesions of herpes simplex are vesicles that are on an erythematous base and appear in groups. They are preceded by burning, stinging, or pain a few hours before the lesions erupt. The lesions may last for 2 to 6 weeks, after which a second eruption may occur but be less severe. The lesions contain the live virus that can be transmitted to others through direct contact with infected lesions or genital secretions. Herpes simplex can be spread by kissing, poor hand hygiene, oral sex, and intercourse.

Diagnostic and Laboratory Studies and Medical Management

Diagnosis of herpes simplex is made through the evaluation of symptoms and the physical appearance of the lesions. The virus can be identified through a Tzanck smear or culture of the lesions (see the Laboratory and Diagnostic Tests for Skin Disorders box, p. 1844).

The infection cannot be cured but the symptoms can be treated. Topical antiviral agents can be used to speed healing. In addition, oral antiviral agents are available and can suppress the infection or decrease the severity if given at the onset of signs and symptoms. See the Pharmacology box (p. 1845). Patients and families need to be instructed to wash their hands often and avoid contact with lesions, as HSV can be transmitted by kissing, sharing beverages, or sharing food utensils or toothbrushes. Sexual contact must be avoided while the disease is active, and patients and their partners must recognize that herpes simplex can be transmitted even when it may appear inactive. Condom use is recommended but with recognized limitations. Monogamous relationships help to limit the spread of the disease (Domino et al., 2012).

Herpes Zoster

Etiology, Epidemiology, and Pathophysiology

Herpes zoster is a viral skin infection often referred to as **shingles.** It occurs because of reactivation of the latent varicella-zoster virus that causes chickenpox. After the chickenpox resolves, this virus remains dormant in the dorsal root and cranial nerve ganglia, and usually becomes activated when a person is immunocompromised due to age or some other disease process such as AIDS, Hodgkin's disease, or some cancers. In the United States, approximately 95% of adults and 99% of adults over the age of 40 have antibodies to herpes zoster and are vulnerable to reactivation. The incidence increases with age due to declining immunity (Moon, 2011). The shingles vaccine (Zostavax®) is recommended for people age 60 and over by the Centers for Disease Control and Prevention (Centers for Disease Control and Prevention [CDC], (2011).

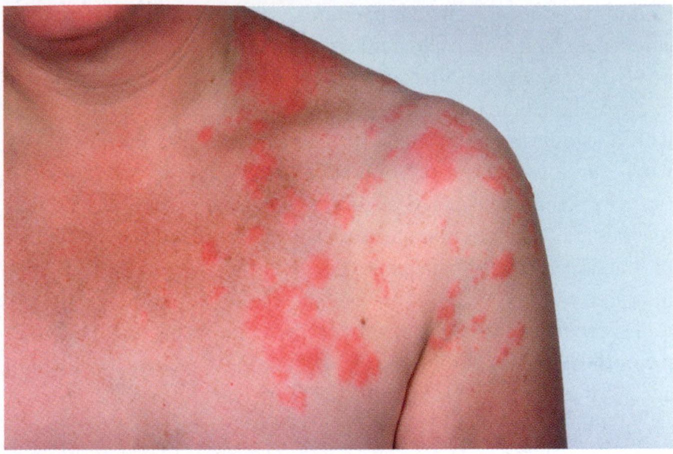

FIGURE 59–2 ◆ Herpes zoster.
Source: Medical-on-Line/Alamy.

Clinical Manifestations

The lesions of herpes zoster are erythematous vesicles scattered over the skin surface along one or two adjacent dermatomes (Figure 59–2◆). A thoracic distribution is the most common. Lesions may also occur on the face, on the neck, and in the eye along the dermatomes of cranial nerves. The vesicles occur in clusters of various sizes and, with time, become cloudy with purulent fluid. The lesions are preceded by pain, itching, or burning in the area. The patient may also experience fever, headache, and malaise prior to the eruption of the lesions, which are tender. A common complication is **postherpetic neuralgia,** which is pain for weeks, to months, and sometimes for a lifetime, after the lesions resolve. The pain is described as itching, burning, sharp, and shooting and may be severe enough to incapacitate the patient. Pain may be so severe that the patient avoids having anything touch the area, even clothing.

Laboratory and Diagnostic Procedures and Medical Management

Herpes zoster is diagnosed by physical assessment and history. The lesions can be cultured but the virus is not easily isolated. Polymerase chain reaction (PCR), which directly identifies the virus, may be used for diagnosis (see the Laboratory and Diagnostic Tests for Skin Disorders box, p. 1844). Treatment is aimed at shortening the course of herpes zoster and preventing or alleviating pain. Systemic antiviral agents are used such as acyclovir or famciclovir. See the Pharmacology box (p. 1845). Treatment can also include nerve blocks, tricyclic antidepressants, or anticonvulsants to help alleviate pain. However, there is no cure, so herpes zoster can reemerge.

Warts

Etiology, Epidemiology, and Pathophysiology

Warts, or **verrucae,** are viral epidermal eruptions caused by the human papillomavirus. Worldwide, warts are estimated to affect approximately 7% to 12% of the general population and 10% to 20% of school-age children (Shenefelt, 2011). They are benign and occur most commonly on the hands and feet. They usually are self-limiting and disappear spontaneously in months or years. The virus causing warts

CHART 59–1 Types of Warts

Type	Description
Common wart	Flesh-toned or gray-brown, scaly papules. Usually involves the dorsal and palmar surfaces of the hands and fingers and the area around the nails.
Verruca plana (flat or juvenile wart)	Smooth, flat, or slightly elevated papule, occurring in multiples. Located on the face, backs of the hands, and shins.
Digitate or filiform wart	Lesion with multiple fingerlike projections. Usually a single lesion located in the beard area, eyelids, neck, or scalp.
Plantar wart	Located on the plantar surface of the foot in pressure areas. Usually a single lesion that is tender. Often mistaken for a callus.

can be transmitted by contact when there are small breaks in the skin. Anal or genital warts are sexually transmitted (Chapter 43 discusses sexually transmitted diseases). Nongenital warts are usually not precancerous; however, genital warts can increase the risk for cervical cancer (see Chapter 41 for a discussion of cervical cancer).

Clinical Manifestations

Warts are small, hyperkeratotic flesh-colored papules that are flat or dome shaped with black dots on the surface that are usually seen on the extremities, especially the hands. The black dots are thrombosed capillaries. There are many different types of warts with varying clinical manifestations (Chart 59–1). Warts can occur singly or in groups and have a rough surface. In addition, warts are usually asymptomatic but can be tender or irritated by clothing. **Plantar warts** occur on weight-bearing areas where they are pushed into the skin, making them appear level with the skin surface. Plantar warts are usually tender. Genital warts appear in the anogenital region and have a light-colored surface and cauliflower appearance.

Medical Management

Warts are diagnosed by physical examination and history. No treatment is necessary; however, some people prefer to be treated because the appearance of warts may be cosmetically undesirable, and warts on the sole of the foot may be painful. Treatment usually requires multiple visits to the health care provider's office. The usual treatment consists of the application of salicylic acid, cryotherapy (freezing of the wart), topical immunotherapy, or intralesional bleomycin. Recently, the use of duct tape to occlude the wart has been reported to be as effective as cryotherapy (Shenefelt, 2011). Duct tape is applied to the site so that the wart is completely occluded and is left in place for 2 months.

Nursing Management

The prevalence of viral skin infections is high, so prevention is key. Patient and family instruction on prevention strategies should include the following:

- Avoid contact with immunocompromised people when a lesion is present.
- Wash hands often.
- Avoid sharing beverages from the same container and sharing food utensils or toothbrushes.
- Avoid kissing while the disease is active.
- Avoid sexual contact while the disease is active.
- Use condoms as recommended.
- Engage in monogamous relationships, as they are beneficial in the prevention of infection.

Fungal Skin Infections

Fungi may be multicellular or monocellular but are larger than bacteria. They live on dead keratinized cells of the epidermis. Some types are considered part of the normal skin flora, but they can cause uncomfortable infections in the skin. The various fungi that affect the skin and mucous membranes are discussed next.

Candidiasis

Etiology, Epidemiology, and Pathophysiology

Candidiasis is a common infection caused by the *Candida* species of fungus (Figure 59–3◆). It is the most common cause of fungal infection in immunocompromised patients. Candida oropharyngeal colonization is found in 30% to 50% of healthy young adults, and is detected in 40% to 60% of normal fecal flora. Three out of every four women has experienced at least one vulvovaginal candidiasis infection during their lifetime (Hidalgo, 2011). This organism normally lives in the gastrointestinal tract, mouth, and vagina, and causes no harm because it is kept in control by intact skin, an intact immune system, and secretions from other microorganisms that live on the skin. When the immune system is depressed, *Candida* can cause the development of opportunistic infections. It can occur with tissue damage, removal of competing organisms (such as occurs with antibiotic administration), increase in glucose levels (as in diabetes), or a warm, moist environment such as in skinfolds. Skin candidiasis is especially prevalent in the very young, such as infants, and the very old and debilitated. The presence

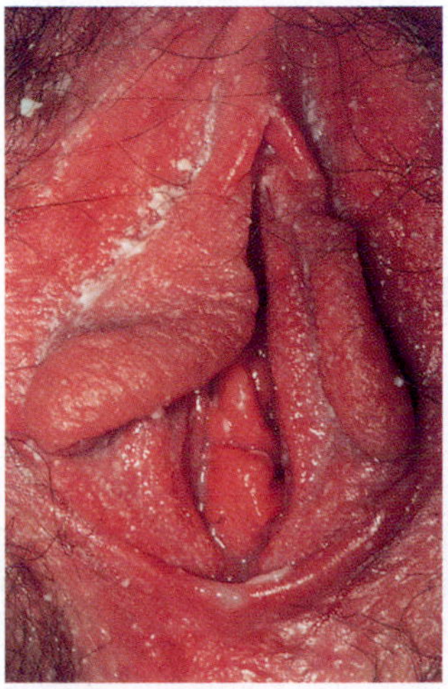

FIGURE 59–3 ◆ Candidiasis.
Source: Custom Medical Stock Photo, Inc.

of predisposing factors such as wet clothing, obesity, or hyperglycemia promotes the development of the rash.

Laboratory and Diagnostic Procedures and Medical Management

Candidiasis is diagnosed by the patient's history of symptoms, immunosuppression, or antibiotic use, as well as physical examination. A wet smear with potassium hydroxide can be used to identify the spores under the microscope (see the Laboratory and Diagnostic Tests for Skin Disorders box, p. 1844).

Treatment of candidiasis involves the application of antifungal creams such as miconazole or ketoconazole. Cool compresses with water or Burrow's solution may help promote dryness and relief from itching and soreness. Keeping the skin dry and wearing loose, absorbent clothing help to eliminate predisposing factors. Topical agents such as Mycostatin are available in powders, vaginal suppositories, or suspensions to swish in the mouth. If the candidiasis is systemic, oral or intravenous antifungal agents can be given.

Tinea

Etiology, Epidemiology, and Pathophysiology

Tinea is referred to as ringworm by the general public. However, there are many different types, and the manifestations vary with the location, duration, and pathogen involved. Tinea commonly occurs in immunocompromised individuals but has other predisposing factors as well, such as crowded conditions, poor hygiene, or wearing tight clothing. In the United States, the prevalence is 2% to 8% of the population, and the infection occurs more frequently in areas that are hot and humid (Burkhart, 2010)

Clinical Manifestations

Patients with tinea develop abnormal pigmentation, usually on the trunk, back, abdomen, and proximal extremities. The face, scalp, and genitalia are less commonly involved. Tinea causes a very itchy rash that often, but not always, makes a pattern in the shape of a ring. It can occur on many areas of the body including the skinfolds of the groin. It may also spread to the inner thighs or buttocks. The skin on the palm of the hand gets thick, dry, and scaly. And skin between the fingers may be moist and have open sores (WebMD, 2012).

The types of tinea include tinea pedis, tinea corporis, tinea capitis, and tinea cruris. **Tinea pedis** is an infection of the foot commonly referred to as "athlete's foot." It usually involves the web between the fourth and fifth toes but may occur between any of the toes and the plantar or dorsal surface of the foot. It occurs most commonly in postpubescent adolescents and adults. The infection is predisposed by the wearing of tight shoes that promote warmth and perspiration, poor hygiene, or repeated exposure to fungal organisms on locker room floors. The lesions are circular and scaly with central clearing. In the toe webs, the skin appears scaly, fissured, and macerated. The patient complains of itching and tenderness in the area.

Tinea corporis is infection of the trunk and limbs. It occurs more commonly in warm climates and can occur at any age. The lesions are round, annular, scaly patches. They can also appear as papules, pustules, and vesicles that are inflamed and red. The lesions are multiple but uniform in appearance and are usually evident on exposed areas of the body. The lesions may be mildly pruritic but are often asymptomatic.

Tinea cruris, also known as "jock itch," is a fungal infection of the groin and occurs almost exclusively in adult males. It is related to a warm, moist environment and obesity. The lesions are circular, beginning in the crural fold, and are erythematous or slightly brown in the center. The edge is raised, slightly scaly, and well defined. It is usually asymptomatic but may be pruritic.

Tinea capitis is a contagious infection of the scalp and hair follicle transmitted by personal contact. It can be spread through combs, animals, hats, blankets, telephones, and theater seats. It is more common in children and African Americans. The lesions usually appear as patchy, circular areas of hair loss. There may be visible stubs of broken off hairs within the patch of hair loss, and there may also be inflammation and scaling on the scalp. The rash may consist of fine white scales on the scalp with the appearance of dandruff or may have pustules or scabbed areas without scaling or hair loss. Tinea capitis may be associated with fever, occipital adenopathy, and leukocytosis.

Laboratory and Diagnostic Procedures and Medical Management

Tinea is diagnosed by the patient's history of signs and symptoms, as well as physical examination of the lesions. It is also important to do a potassium hydroxide wet mount preparation because the presence of fungal hyphae can be seen on the slide and are diagnostic (see the Laboratory and Diagnostic Tests for Skin Disorders box, p. 1844). Tinea can be treated with oral and topical antifungal agents. Usually topical agents are enough; however, if the infection is widespread or chronic, or the patient is immunocompromised, oral medications may be needed. See the Pharmacology box (p. 1845).

INFLAMMATORY SKIN DISORDERS

Dermatitis

Dermatitis is a general term that describes skin disorders that are usually pruritic, have lesions with indistinct borders, and include epidermal changes. The lesions can appear as erythema, papules, or scales. Edema, serous drainage, and crusting can occur from scratching. Dermatitis/eczema, the most common form of inflammatory skin disorder, often has acute, subacute, and chronic phases. The continued irritation and scratching can lead to chronic skin changes such as thickening, hyperpigmentation, and leathery appearance. Contact dermatitis, atopic dermatitis, seborrheic dermatitis, exfoliative dermatitis, urticaria, and lichen planus are a few examples of dermatitis; they will be discussed in this section (Nicol & Huether, 2007).

Contact Dermatitis

Etiology, Epidemiology, and Pathophysiology

Contact dermatitis is an inflammation of the skin related to exposure to an irritant or allergen in the environment. Irritant contact dermatitis, the most common contact dermatitis, is caused by a substance that is irritating to the skin but not due to an allergy. The National Health and Nutrition Examination Survey (NHANES) estimates that the prevalence of contact dermatitis is 13.6 cases per 1,000 population (Hogan, 2011). Allergic contact dermatitis is a type IV cell-mediated immune reaction that occurs after contact with an allergen. Cell-mediated immune reactions are mediated by T lymphocytes, which lead to destruction of the allergen (see Chapter 53). There are approximately

3,000 chemicals that are well documented as specific causes of allergic contact dermatitis (Hogan, 2011). It may take several exposures before a reaction occurs. One of the most common types of allergic contact dermatitis is poison ivy or poison oak. It is difficult to distinguish between allergic and irritant reactions; however, an irritant reaction usually does not spread beyond the area of contact. The intensity of the skin reaction depends on the degree of sensitivity and the concentration and quantity of the exposure to the antigen. Initially, the dermatitis is usually confined to the area of direct exposure, but it may spread beyond that area. It presents as erythema and edema, with pruritic vesicular lesions in the area of the allergen contact.

Laboratory and Diagnostic Procedures and Medical Management

The diagnosis of contact dermatitis usually requires a history of possible exposure and development of the rash, as well as physical examination. The distribution of the rash or lesions often provides clues to the source of the antigen. Patch testing can be done if necessary to determine the identity of the offending agent. Treatment includes stopping the exposure to the allergen or irritating agent and avoiding future exposures to the causative agent. The inflammatory process is treated using a mid- to high-potency topical corticosteroid. If the dermatitis is severe, oral steroids may be used. The itching should be treated with antihistamines. See the Pharmacology box (p. 1845). Patients should be instructed not to scratch because scratching will increase the itching sensation and may cause a secondary infection.

Atopic Dermatitis (Eczema)

Etiology, Epidemiology, and Pathophysiology

Atopic dermatitis, also known as eczema, is a chronic, inflammatory skin disorder characterized by dry skin related to water loss in the epidermis and decreased skin lipid levels. It can occur at any age but is more common in children. Worldwide, between 10% and 20% of children have atopic dermatitis, with most developing it before their fifth birthday. Persons of all skin colors can develop atopic dermatitis (American Academy of Dermatology, 2012). It generally cycles through periods of acute flare-ups and remissions. Atopic dermatitis can be caused by irritants in the environment, or it can have an immunologic cause. Patients with atopic dermatitis often have a familial predisposition, including a family history of asthma or hay fever. Environmentally, atopic dermatitis is aggravated by contact with allergens, perspiration, excessive heat, dry air, emotional stress, and rough clothing. Children often outgrow atopic dermatitis; however, it can become chronic into adulthood.

Clinical Manifestations

Atopic dermatitis is characterized by severe itching. The lesions are irregular, red papular patches that are weepy, shiny, or thickened. The lesions also may be plaques that are scaly and crusted. The characteristic distribution is on the face, the neck, the upper trunk, and the antecubital fossa or popliteal spaces. The lesions can develop a secondary *Staphylococcus aureus* infection due to skin trauma and breakdown from scratching.

Laboratory and Diagnostic Procedures

Atopic dermatitis is diagnosed by the patient's history, including possible triggers for flare-ups, and physical examination to note the appearance and distribution of the lesions. Laboratory tests are not usually required; however, immunoglobin E (IgE) levels may be elevated, indicating an immune reaction. Allergy testing may be done to determine whether an allergic process is instrumental in causing the problem.

Medical Management

Treatment of atopic dermatitis involves controlling the aggravating factors and treating the rash. It is important to moisturize the skin to maintain the skin barrier. Bathing should be held to a minimum; however, when bathing, the patient should use tepid water and mild, unscented soap such as Cetaphil or Dove. To prevent itching (pruritus) and to lubricate the skin, the patient should apply body oils or emollients such as white petroleum or vegetable oil moisturizer at least once a day after bathing. Clothing should be soft, light, and preferably made of cotton or some natural, soft fiber. New clothes should be laundered before wearing to wash out any irritating chemicals. The patient should avoid any activity that causes perspiring. Once a rash develops, the patient may be placed on a course of topical or oral corticosteroids to reduce inflammation and itching. Urea creams or nonsteroidal anti-inflammatory ointments are effective for hydrating the skin and decreasing itching. Oral antihistamines also may help decrease itching. See the Pharmacology box (p. 1845). If lesions are wet or crusted, soaking in Burrow's solution or colloidal oatmeal such as Aveeno may be helpful. Antibiotics may be needed to prevent or treat secondary skin infections. The Complementary & Alternative Therapies box (p. 1854) shows how diet can also play a role.

Weblink: Atopic Dermatitis

Video*: Eczema

Seborrheic Dermatitis

Etiology, Epidemiology, and Pathophysiology

Seborrheic dermatitis is a skin condition that is similar to severe forms of dandruff. This chronic inflammation of the skin is most commonly seen on the scalp, eyebrows, eyelids, ear canals, nasolabial folds, axillae, chest, and back. Its cause is unknown but a genetic predisposition to the yeast from the genus *Malassezia* has been found. This dermatitis can appear from infancy (cradle cap) to old age with periods of remission and exacerbation (Nicol & Huether, 2007).

Clinical Manifestations

The lesions of seborrheic dermatitis appear as oily, scaly, white, or yellowish inflammatory plaques in sebaceous areas with mild pruritus. Primary lesions appear as redness and scaling. The condition sometimes worsens in colder weather.

Medical Management

Seborrheic dermatitis is commonly diagnosed by clinical presentation. Mild cases are treated with shampoos containing selenium sulfide, sulfur, salicylic acid, or tar. In addition, ketoconazole shampoo has antifungal and anti-inflammatory effects and is beneficial in some cases. The patient should shampoo as often as necessary to keep scaling and itching to a minimum. For more severe cases, topical corticosteroid applications (triamcinolone) are useful but should not be used for maintenance therapy (Nicol & Huether, 2007).

Exfoliative Dermatitis

Etiology, Epidemiology, and Pathophysiology

Exfoliative dermatitis is a generalized scaling eruption of the skin, in which more than 90% of the body is often involved. The majority of patients who develop this disease are 40 years of age or older and male (Domino et al., 2012). Exfoliative dermatitis is a rare skin condition and can be classified into primary and secondary forms. Primary exfoliative dermatitis develops in healthy individuals from no known cause. Secondary exfoliative dermatitis often develops when a previous skin disease has become generalized because of overtreatment.

COMPLEMENTARY & ALTERNATIVE THERAPIES Diet Therapy *Nancy Yilk*

THE TERM *FOOD ALLERGY* is widely misused for a multitude of symptoms that are more along the lines of food sensitivity. In the area of functional medicine, there is a focus on how the changes in our modern diet, involving both preparation and consumption of food, are influencing our health. Food intolerances may be enzymatic (e.g., lactose intolerance due to lactase deficiency), pharmacologic (e.g., reactions against biogenic amines, histamine intolerance), and undefined food intolerance (e.g., against some food additives). The hypothesis that the human body and its detoxification pathway have become more "burdened" with the influence of chemicals from our environment and lifestyle can be demonstrated in the area of diet. In particular, diet may play a role in histamine intolerance and its connection to skin conditions such as chronic urticaria, psoriasis, and atopic dermatitis, which can be caused by autoreactivity, chronic infection, or intolerance to food additives.

Patients who present with such skin conditions should be assessed for evidence of histamine intolerance caused by histamine overload and/or diamine oxidase deficiency. Histamine intolerance results from disequilibrium of accumulated histamine and the capacity for histamine degradation. Impaired histamine degradation and the resulting histamine excess may cause numerous symptoms mimicking an allergic reaction. The ingestion of histamine-rich food or of alcohol or drugs that release histamine may provoke diarrhea, headache, rhino-conjunctival symptoms, asthma, hypotension, arrhythmia, urticaria, pruritus, flushing, and other conditions in patients with histamine intolerance.

Food and beverages may contain high amounts of histamine and thus may cause symptoms after ingestion. In a study to investigate the role of ingested histamine in atopic dermatitis, 36 patients with atopic dermatitis had to maintain a histamine-free diet for 1 week; 19 skin-healthy individuals were included in the study as a control group. Consecutively, double-blind, placebo-controlled provocations were performed with histamine-hydrochloride and placebo. The clinical outcome was assessed by determination of the Severity Scoring of Atopic Dermatitis (SCORAD). Before and 30 minutes after each provocation, blood was collected for measurement of plasma histamine levels and diamine oxidase activity. Altogether, 36 patients with atopic dermatitis completed the diet. Of the 36 patients, 12 showed a significant improvement of the SCORAD after 1 week of the diet. After provocation tests, 11 of 36 showed aggravation of eczema. Plasma histamine was significantly higher in patients with atopic dermatitis compared with controls (Worm et al., 2009).

In a survey study of 43 patients with various forms of psoriasis (excluding pustular and erythrodermic psoriasis), participants answered a questionnaire about their eating habits in the first visit, with special attention to the consumption of black coffee, black tea, chocolate, yerba mate, pepper, smoked foods, beef, and flavor enhancer (monosodium glutamate), all of which are high-histamine foods. Beef was the food most consumed by patients, followed by MSG (monosodium glutamate), which exists in processed foods, yerba mate, black coffee, chocolate, smoked foods, pepper, and black tea. Next, the patient was instructed to suspend use of alcoholic drinks and tobacco. Dietary changes, followed for 2 years, contributed an 88.37% noticeable change in reduced scaling and erythema, milder outbreaks during the year, and improved quality of life; in fact, 11.63% (5 patients) did not notice any effects on the skin. Patients also experienced a better sense of overall health and improved quality of life that reinforced the choice to maintain a change in dietary habits (Festugato, 2011).

Foods that have higher levels of histamine include alcohol, especially beer and wine; pickled or canned foods; cheese, especially mature cheese (the more mature, the more histamine it contains); smoked meats, in particular smoked ham and salami; most fish products (including all shellfish), especially canned fish; beans and pulses (especially chickpeas, soy beans, and peanuts); soy products (soy milk, soy cream, tofu, soy sauces); sauerkraut or other pickled foods; some fruits (eggplant, bananas, kiwi, oranges, pears, strawberries); nuts, especially walnuts and cashew nuts; chocolate and cocoa; salty snacks; sweets with preservatives and artificial colorings; products made from wheat; vinegar; yeast; ready meals; and black tea.

Foods that release histamine (histamine releasers) include citrus fruits, cocoa and chocolate, kiwi, lemon, lime, nuts, papaya, pineapple, plums, pulses, raspberries, strawberries, tomatoes, wheat germ, and additives such as benzoate, food dyes, glutamate, nitrites, and sulphites. Foods that block the diamine oxidase (DAO) enzyme include alcohol, black tea, cocoa, energy drinks (the component theobromine blocks the DAO), green tea, and yerba mate tea. It is debatable whether cherries, zucchini, egg white, leek, and yoghurt block DAO.

The following are the more common causes of secondary exfoliative dermatitis: contact dermatitis, drug eruption, psoriasis, atopic eczema, pyoderma, fungal disease, seborrheic dermatitis, T-cell lymphoma, or other cancers (Hall, 2010). However, secondary exfoliative dermatitis is idiopathic in 20% to 30% of cases.

Clinical Manifestations

Exfoliative dermatitis can appear suddenly or gradually and be accompanied by fever, chills, and lymphadenopathy. This is a potentially life-threatening condition (Domino et al., 2012). Primary exfoliative dermatitis can present in various degrees of scaling and redness ranging from fine, generalized, granular scales with mild redness to large plaques with severe erythema and lichenification (thick, leatherlike skin). Lymphadenopathy is common. Nails become thick and dull, and hair loss can occur. Fever occurs in 40% to 50% of cases; pruritus may be severe; and malaise, weakness, eosinophilia, hepatomegaly, and splenomegaly may occur when the patient has lymphoma/leukemia, dehydration, and high output cardiac failure.

Laboratory and Diagnostic Procedures and Medical Management

There are no diagnostic laboratory tests to identify exfoliative dermatitis. However, elevated WBC with eosinophilia, anemia, elevated ESR, decreased albuminemia, and electrolyte abnormalities may be found. Testing to identify the underlying disease process may include chest x-ray, patch testing, and skin biopsy.

The treatment goal for the patient with exfoliative dermatitis is to relieve symptoms. Cool water bathing in colloid solution (e.g., Aveeno) is sometimes helpful; however, generalized bathing usually dries the skin and intensifies the itching. Intermediate-strength topical steroids, local bland moisturizing ointments/lotions, and oral antihistamines (which provide a sleep aid) are helpful. Second-line treatment can include treatment for psoriasis (if that is the underlying cause), photochemotherapy (if the condition is associated with mycosis fungoides), antimetabolites/cytotoxic drugs, infliximab, and etanercept.

Urticaria

Etiology, Epidemiology, Pathophysiology, and Clinical Manifestations

Urticaria, or hives, is a condition in which the patient has raised, erythematous, intensely pruritic plaques or wheals that are surrounded by a white halo. These lesions vary in size and distribution and commonly occur as an allergic reaction to medications, foods, or insect bites. Urticaria can be acute (persists < 6 weeks) or chronic (persists > 6 weeks). It is common in all ages and occurs equally in both genders, but the acute form occurs mainly in children and the chronic form occurs

CHART 59–2 Urticarial Variants

Variant	Duration	Causes
Acute	Lasts less than 6 weeks.	Food, drinks, medications, pollen, chemicals, and insect bites.
Chronic	Affects mostly adults. Lasts more than 2 months.	Cause is difficult to determine. May be related to underlying disease such as cancer, hepatitis, collagen disease, or Graves' disease.
Cold	Lasts 30 to 60 minutes.	Induced by exposure to cold surfaces, air, or water.
Physical urticaria	Intermittent. Lasts 1 to 2 hours.	Induced by things that increase body temperature such as showers, exercise, fever, and stress.

in adults. Urticaria affects 15% to 25% of the population during a lifetime (Domino et al., 2012). It can be related to infections such as viral hepatitis, sinusitis, gingivitis, or cystitis. Aggravating factors include chemical irritants, fever, alcohol, exercise, and emotional stress. Histamine, the most common mediator of this reaction, is released by mast cells as a part of the immune response to allergens. Histamine causes an increased permeability of the microvessels of the skin, leading to a leakage of fluid into the tissues. This causes edema at the site and stimulates the itch receptors in the skin. Urticaria has several clinical variations, as outlined in Chart 59–2.

Medical Management

Urticaria is diagnosed by the patient's history of exposure to possible causative agents and the appearance of the lesion. Causative factors need to be identified and avoided. Most cases resolve spontaneously, but antihistamines may be given to block the action of histamine. See the Pharmacology box (p. 1845). Itching can be relieved with cold compresses or cool, colloid-type baths (e.g., Aveeno). Decreasing stress, avoiding hot showers, and exercising may be helpful.

Lichen Planus

Etiology, Epidemiology, and Pathophysiology

Lichen planus (LP) is an uncommon autoimmune inflammatory disorder of the skin and mucous membranes of unknown origin. The disorder is rare in children and older adults. The predominant age of onset is between 30 and 60 years of age, and it more commonly occurs in females. Involvement of the T cells, adhesion molecules, inflammatory cytokines, perforin, and antigen-presenting cells has been found. Lichen planus may also be drug induced. An association has been identified between lichen planus and hepatitis C, chronic active hepatitis, and primary biliary cirrhosis. Lichen planus is often associated with other autoimmune diseases such as bullous pemphigoid, alopecia areata, myasthenia gravis, vitiligo, ulcerative colitis, graft versus host reaction, and lupus erythematosus (Nicol & Huether, 2007).

Risk factors for the development of LP include exposure to certain drugs or chemicals such as thiazides, furosemide, beta-blockers, sulfonylureas, antimalarials, penicillamine, gold salts, and angiotensin-converting enzyme inhibitors, as well as photo-developing chemicals, dental materials, and tattoo pigments (Domino et al., 2012).

Clinical Manifestations

Presentation of LP begins with nonscaling, purple-colored pruritic papules, 2 to 4 mm in size. Papules are flat-topped and polygonal in shape. Persistent lesions may become thickened and red or dark purple. Lesions are usually located on the flexor surfaces of the upper extremities, extensor surfaces of the lower extremities, on the genitalia, and on mucous membranes. When they appear on mucous membranes, the lesions appear as lacy white rings. Fine white lines called Wickham striae can be seen throughout the oral lesions on magnification. The course is unpredictable; onset may be abrupt or gradual, and the LP may resolve spontaneously, recur intermittently, or be chronic for years. Lesions may develop into squamous cell carcinoma (1% to 3%). A useful mnemonic is the 7 Ps of lichen planus: Purple, Planar, Polygonal, Polymorphic, Pruritic Papules that heal with Postinflammatory hyperpigmentation (Domino et al., 2012; Nicol & Huether, 2007).

Laboratory and Diagnostic Procedures and Medical Management

Diagnosis of LP is typically made by clinical appearance, but if there is doubt about the diagnosis, a skin biopsy may be done. Serology for hepatitis B and C and liver function tests are recommended. Direct immunofluorescence helps to distinguish between LP and discoid lupus erythematosus (Domino et al., 2012).

Treatment of LP includes antihistamines for itching and super potent topical or systemic corticosteroids. The "soak and smear" technique has been shown to lead to rapid improvement of symptoms in as little as 24 hours or so. The patient soaks in a bathtub using lukewarm water for 20 minutes at night; then, without drying the skin, the patient immediately smears the affected skin with a thin film of steroid ointment. This is repeated for 4 to 5 days (Domino et al., 2012).

Skin Reaction to Medications

Etiology, Epidemiology, and Pathophysiology

Skin reactions occur commonly as an allergic reaction to a medication. They can occur rapidly, as happens in an immediate-type hypersensitivity after exposure to the drug, or can take a few days to develop, as in a delayed hypersensitivity reaction. Skin reactions can range from a mild rash to severe blistering and sloughing of the skin. Erythema multiforme is one such syndrome that is characterized by inflammation of the skin and mucous membranes. Allergic medication reactions are due to the function of the T cell that recognizes the medication as a foreign substance and reacts to it (Nicol & Huether, 2007). This reaction usually requires a previous exposure to the medication so that the body can develop an immune response.

Clinical Manifestations

The most common manifestations of an allergic skin reaction to medications are erythema, pruritus, and urticaria. The lesions are usually maculopapular, occurring in a symmetrical, generalized distribution that spares the face. The rash appears in the same sites after each ingestion of the medication. Fever and other systemic symptoms may accompany the rash.

Medical Management

It is important to obtain a detailed history from the patient to identify whether a rash similar to this has occurred before and what medications the patient was taking with the prior rash as well as currently. Patients may not relate the rash to the use of a certain medication, so a specific and detailed assessment is important. Treatment involves stopping the offending agent. Patients should be warned that it might take a few weeks for the rash to disappear even after stopping the medication. Antihistamines are helpful in slowing the immune response that is responsible for the rash and the itching; thus, they promote healing.

Systemic corticosteroids may be indicated if the reaction is widespread or severe. See the Pharmacology box (p. 1845). Colloidal baths are helpful to soothe extreme itching.

Nursing Management

Nursing management of the patient with a skin disorder depends on the extent of the skin disorder and symptoms. Management may include providing antihistamines, using warm or cool soaks, removing the offending irritant, and avoiding complications. Ensuring adequate rest, promoting proper nutrition and providing adequate hydration also should be considered. Refer to the previous section on Nursing Management for more detail.

Collaborative Management

A collaborative approach to the management of patients with skin disorders is essential. Skin disorders have many facets that influence the patient both physically and emotionally. A multidisciplinary team that includes health care providers, nurses, psychologists/psychiatrists, occupational therapists, physical therapists, nutritionists, and pharmacists is necessary to help the patient recover. In order to meet desired patient outcomes, it is essential that this interdisciplinary team communicate openly with one another in developing and evaluating care of the patient and family (IOM [Institute of Medicine], 2010). Health care provider is discussed throughout this chapter and may include medical care as well as surgical care. In addition, psychiatric care may be needed to assist with the patient's adjustment to alterations in appearance related to the skin disorder. The occupational therapist can assist the patient to return to work or function to meet everyday needs. The physical therapist can help keep muscles strong and address the limitations of movement that may occur with scar formation. Patients with skin disorders often lose electrolytes and have increased metabolic demands that lead to weight loss and increased nutritional needs. These needs can be addressed by a nutritionist. The pharmacist will be concerned with the medications and their interactions and effectiveness. In addition, the pharmacist can assist with educating the patient about medication management and the possible side effects. The nurse's role is addressed in discussions of the specific disorders throughout this chapter. In addition, the nurse serves as the patient advocate, as well as the team leader to facilitate communication between members of the team.

Life-Threatening Inflammatory Disorders

With prompt and appropriate treatment, most skin disorders are manageable with a minimum of side effects or lifelong sequelae. However, certain skin disorders can cause major physical disfigurement, have disfiguring sequelae, and in some instances are life threatening. These conditions begin as a skin disorder and then progress to multiple organ involvement, thereby becoming life threatening. Necrotizing fasciitis, Stevens–Johnson syndrome, and toxic epidermal necrolysis are the most common life-threatening skin disorders.

Necrotizing Fasciitis

Etiology and Epidemiology

Necrotizing fasciitis (NF), first described in 1848, is an infection of the superficial fascia or the connective tissue surrounding muscle and subcutaneous tissue, leading to fascial necrosis. It is commonly referred to as "flesh-eating bacteria." Although relatively uncommon, NF is significant because it is difficult to recognize, it spreads rapidly, and it can become fatal very quickly. This infection can occur at any age or in any location on the body and is not specific to gender. Approximately one-half of the cases occur in young, previously healthy patients (CDC, 2008). Necrotizing fasciitis also occurs with a variety of conditions from simple minor injuries to complicated major surgeries or trauma. The very young and very old are at increased risk, as are individuals with diabetes mellitus, atherosclerosis, chronic renal failure, obesity, immunosuppression, malnutrition, illicit drug injections, alcoholism, and peripheral vascular disease. The Risk Factors box identifies those who are most at risk for necrotizing fasciitis.

RISK FACTORS for Necrotizing Fasciitis

Very young and very old age	Chronic venous leg ulcers
Individuals with throat or skin infections	Open bone fractures
Individuals with chronic illnesses such as cancer, diabetes, or renal failure (on dialysis)	Insect bites
	Childbirth
People using steroids	Surgical wounds
Obesity	Trauma
Poor nutrition or malnutrition	AIDS
Immunosuppression	Major burns
Needle puncture site with illicit drug use	Prolonged antibiotic therapy
Frostbite	Alcoholics
Skin biopsy	Peripheral vascular disease
Hypertension	Multiple myeloma

There are three types of necrotizing fasciitis (NF). Type 1 is polymicrobial and related to mixed aerobic or anaerobic bacteria such as *Clostridium, P. aeruginosa, S. aureus, Bacteroides fragilis, Escherichia coli,* and *Klebsiella pneumoniae.* Type 2 is monomicrobial and caused by group A streptococci. Type 3 is caused by gas gangrene or clostridial myonecrosis (Domino et al., 2012). A variant of type 1 NF is caused by saltwater contaminated with *Vibrio* species. Transmission can also occur through contact with infected wounds or sores on the skin. Entry through the skin can occur when there is a surgical wound or a small cut. Contaminated hands can carry the organism as well. In more than 20% of the cases, the causative factor is not identified.

Pathophysiology

Once a break in the skin occurs and is contaminated, the organisms spread from the subcutaneous tissue along the superficial and deep fascia, facilitated by bacterial enzymes and toxins, which continue to break down tissue. In NF, the infection causes:

- Tissue ischemia
- Superficial nerve damage
- Vascular thrombosis and occlusion
- Tissue liquification necrosis
- Septicemia when systemic toxicity occurs.

Certain strains of NF cause the development of streptococcal pyrogenic exotoxins A, B, and C. These exotoxins, along with streptococcal superantigen, stimulate the release of cytokines and produce hypotension (CDC, 2008). This leads to occlusion and interruption of vessels that supply the skin. The ischemia produces bullae formation, ulceration, and necrosis of the skin.

CHART 59–3 Signs and Symptoms of Necrotizing Fasciitis

Early Stage First 24–48 Hours	Advanced Stage 2nd–4th Day	Critical Stage 4th–5th Day
Flulike symptoms such as fever, chills, myalgia, nausea, vomiting, and diarrhea. Abrupt localized pain beyond what would be expected. Patchy discoloration of skin that is violaceous to erythematous without defined borders. Nonpitting edema outside the area of discoloration. Skin is essentially normal in appearance.	Skin swollen and tight and erythema is noted. Area becomes dusky blue in color. Blisters or bullae filled with purplish, foul-smelling, thin, watery fluid. Skin has paperlike appearance. There may be palpable crepitation due to the presence of gas. Spread of the infection—increasing wound size. Increased leukocytes. Decreased sodium.	Skin sloughs. Gangrene develops. Hypotension. Delirium. Loss of consciousness. Liver failure. Renal failure. Fever. Acute respiratory distress syndrome (ARDS). Coagulopathy. Fascia appears gray to grayish green. Elevated heart rate. Tissue necrosis.

Clinical Manifestations

Necrotizing fasciitis (NF) is difficult to diagnose because the symptoms are many and varied. One way of tracking the course of the disease is through the progression of the symptoms and laboratory findings. However, symptoms of malaise, anorexia, and fever often progress rapidly over hours, though in rare cases there is a slower progression over days. The symptoms usually begin about 1 week after the initiating event and can be divided into three stages: early, advanced, and critical (Chart 59–3). The early symptoms begin in the first 24 to 48 hours. The most common parts of the body affected are the extremities, the perineum, and the truncal areas, although NF can be found anywhere on the body (Domino et al., 2012). The wound site looks essentially normal with wound margins not obvious, but the patient experiences flulike symptoms, localized pain, erythema, and swelling. It is easy to misdiagnose the infection at this stage because the symptoms are vague and fit with many other problems. The hallmark sign is pain beyond what would be expected for the extent of the injury.

The second stage, known as the advanced stage, occurs within 2 to 4 days. During this phase, the early symptoms worsen. The skin becomes swollen and tight, a dusky blue color develops, and fluid-filled blisters or bullae develop. This occurs because of ischemia and progressive thrombosis (Domino et al., 2012). The texture of the wound has been described as "wet wood." The skin becomes thin and hyperesthetic or anesthetic because of destruction of cutaneous nerves. This lack of sensation is a sign that the patient is not experiencing cellulitis.

The third, or critical, stage occurs within 4 to 5 days. During this stage, the bluish-colored areas become gangrenous. The skin begins to slough, and septic shock can occur, leading to hypotension, high fever, delirium, loss of consciousness, pain, liver failure, renal failure, and eventually death. The mortality rate for NF can be high, and it increases when sepsis and renal failure occur. Figure 59–4◆ is an example of advanced necrotizing fasciitis.

Laboratory and Diagnostic Procedures

Laboratory findings include white blood count, creatine phosphokinase (CPK), blood urea nitrogen (BUN) and creatinine, sodium level, and red blood cells. Blood and wound cultures are also done. Computed tomography (CT) and magnetic resonance imaging (MRI) scans can help to define the extent of the fasciitis and may show gas in the subcutaneous tissues produced by the bacteria and deep fascia thickening.

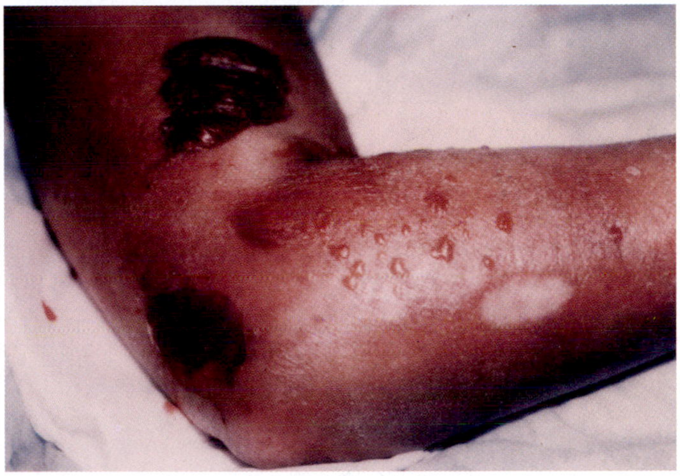

FIGURE 59–4 ◆ Advanced necrotizing fasciitis.

Source: Courtesy of Donald E. Low, B. Demers, A. E. Simor, H. Vellend, P. N. Schlievert, S. Byrne, F. Jamieson, S. Walmsely. CID 1:792–800, (1993).

The Laboratory and Diagnostic Tests box (p. 1858) lists the laboratory and diagnostic tests and abnormalities associated with necrotizing fasciitis. Surgeons may prefer to perform a biopsy, or may take the patient to surgery to assess the fascia directly. When the fascia of a patient with NF is directly assessed, there will be lack of bleeding and the presence of foul-smelling pus (Domino et al., 2012).

Medical Management

Necrotizing fasciitis should be diagnosed early so that treatment can begin as soon as possible. The chance of the patient's surviving is better with an early diagnosis. Diagnosis is made on the basis of signs and symptoms and laboratory testing. The problem is that often it is difficult to make a differential diagnosis because the signs and symptoms of NF are similar to those of other conditions. It is generally believed that if the following symptoms are present, NF should be suspected:

- Rapid progression of wound size
- Poor response to therapeutic interventions
- Blistering necrosis

LABORATORY AND DIAGNOSTIC TESTS for Necrotizing Fasciitis, Stevens–Johnson Syndrome, and Toxic Epidermal Necrolysis

Diagnostic Test, Normal Values, and Rationales	Expected Abnormality
White Blood Cells (WBCs) Normal values: 4,500–10,000/mm^3 *Elevated levels are associated with inflammation and infection.*	Leukocytosis with an elevated number of neutrophils and bands present with NF.
Creatine Phosphokinase (CPK) Normal values: 5–25 mcg/mL *Released from muscle cells when damaged.*	Elevated with NF.
Blood Urea Nitrogen (BUN) and Creatinine Normal values: BUN 5–25 mg/dL Creatinine 0.5–1.5 mg/dL *Will occur if there is renal damage. Also some antibiotics can affect renal function.*	Elevated with NF.
Red Blood Cells (RBC) Normal values: Male: 4.6–6.0 mm^3 Female: 4.0–5.0 mm^3 *Red blood count (RBC) decreases with bleeding and renal failure.*	Decreased with NF.
Blood and Wound Cultures Normal values: Negative for organisms *Organisms enter the bloodstream and wound.*	Growth of causative organism: usually group A streptococcus for NF.
Erythrocyte Sedimentation Rate Normal values: Male: Up to 15 mm/hour Female: Up to 20 mm/hour *The test measures inflammation. Chronic inflammation and infection cause an elevation.*	Elevated with NF.
Serum Sodium Normal values: Sodium 134–145 mEq/L	Decreased with NF due to wound infection and leakage.
Computed Tomography (CT) and Magnetic Resonance Imaging (MRI) and T2-Weighted MRI Normal values: Negative *Can show breakdown of tissue. Organisms responsible for producing gas. Will assist in directing rapid surgical debridement.*	Demonstrates extent of fasciitis and gas in subcutaneous tissues with NF.
Excisional Deep Skin Biopsy Normal values: Negative for abnormal cells *Cultures of the affected tissue.* *Gram staining of the exudates.* *The type influences the antibiotic therapy.*	Helpful in diagnosing and identifying the causative organisms for NF. May provide a clue as to whether a type 1 or type 2 infection is present.
Immunofluorescent Studies Normal values: Negative *Demonstrate the presence of immunoglobulin M (IgM) and C3 deposits in the vascular walls.*	Present with Stevens–Johnson syndrome (SJS) and toxic epidermal necrolysis (TEN).
C-Reactive Protein Normal values: $<$ 0.175 mg/L *Acute-phase reactant protein used to indicate an inflammatory illness.*	Rapid, marked increases in CRP occur with inflammation, infection, and trauma, as well as tissue necrosis, malignancies, and autoimmune disorders.

Source: Adapted from Kee, J. L. (2010). *Laboratory and diagnostic tests with nursing implications.* Upper Saddle River, NJ: Pearson.

- Cyanosis
- Extreme local tenderness
- High temperature
- Tachycardia
- Hypotension
- Altered level of consciousness.

Because of the complexity of the disease, a team approach is essential in managing the patient. Typically patients are placed in a surgical intensive care unit to monitor hemodynamic factors and provide frequent wound care. The treatment for necrotizing fasciitis is three pronged: antibiotics, surgical debridement, and supportive care. Treatment begins with the early administration of broad-spectrum antibiotics and intensive surgical debridement. Broad-spectrum antibiotics are started initially; however, once the culture results have returned, an antibiotic that targets the organism is preferred. The most common antibiotic is benzylpenicillin, given intravenously in large doses. Penicillin by itself may not be successful, so the addition of clindamycin is helpful in producing a favorable outcome. Metronidazole and third-generation cephalosporin antibiotics have also been useful. Some health care providers may opt to use intravenous immunoglobulin (IVIG) to treat severe streptococcal infections associated with NF. The use of intravenous immunoglobulin may be a useful adjunct treatment to increase the immune response (Domino et al., 2012).

Early surgical debridement is necessary to remove all necrotic tissue and prevent the spread of the infection. Initially the patient is taken to surgery as often as every 12 to 24 hours, where debridement is done until clear margins are obtained. This regimen is continued until tissue necrosis stops and fresh viable tissue begins to grow. It may be necessary to excise organs surgically and amputate involved limbs to remove irreversible necrosis and gangrene, or because of overwhelming toxicity. Prompt surgery increases the likelihood of survival. Skin grafting is typically required to close the full-thickness injuries. Chapter 61 has a complete description of the various skin grafting techniques.

Supportive therapies may include a high-calorie diet, hyperbaric oxygen therapy, and the application of negative pressure wound therapy (NPWT). Because patients with necrotizing fasciitis are breaking down tissue and have a hypermetabolic response, extra calories are required. A description of hypermetabolic state is included in Chapter 61.

Negative pressure wound therapy is typically applied to the wound after debridement when clear wound edges have been obtained. This device does three things to improve wound healing:

- It creates a negative pressure in the wound by applying suction. The suction drains interstitial edema fluid, thus decreasing pressure on capillaries and improving perfusion.
- The negative pressure also provides a mechanical stretch/distortion of the cells in the wound bed, which stimulates production of granulation tissue.
- The suction removes stagnant fluid in the wound, thus decreasing the bacterial burden in the healing wound bed.

Negative pressure wound therapy is discussed in detail in Chapter 60.

Streptococcal toxic shock syndrome, which is characterized by hypotension and multi-organ failure, can lead to death. Therefore, fluid resuscitation and hemodynamic monitoring are required. The management of shock is discussed in detail in Chapter 54.

Nursing Management

Nursing care for patients with necrotizing fasciitis requires an in-depth assessment, clinical decision making, and critical thinking skills. The nurse needs to be aware of the possibility of necrotizing fasciitis, even with the smallest of traumatic injuries. It is important to recognize patients who are at risk (see the Risk Factors for Necrotizing Fasciitis box, p. 1856) and to alert the health care provider when warranted. Application of the nursing process will facilitate a comprehensive, holistic approach to the patient. The assessment data, which include sample questions specific to skin disorders, are found in the Nursing Process: Patient Care Plan box on p. 1862. This care plan applies the nursing process to the relevant nursing diagnoses and provides a comprehensive care plan for necrotizing fasciitis.

Stevens–Johnson Syndrome

Stevens–Johnson syndrome (SJS) is a severe, acute, self-limiting skin reaction to infection or certain medications. It is a generalized hypersensitivity reaction that affects the epidermal layer of the skin and mucous membranes. Stevens–Johnson syndrome usually begins with flulike symptoms or symptoms of an upper respiratory infection and progresses to mucosal erosions and erythematous skin macules that blister and cause denudation or skin detachment. The incidence is difficult to estimate because there is no universally accepted definition of SJS. However, a rough estimate is between 1 and 7 cases/million person-years. Stevens–Johnson syndrome is more common in children and young adults and more often occurs in males (2:1). Mortality rates for SJS are 5% to 15% (Domino et al., 2012) with recurrence as high as 37%. Blindness or corneal damage occurs in 7% to 20% of patients. Early diagnosis and withdrawal of the causative agent are essential to decrease morbidity and mortality.

Etiology

The cause of SJS is most commonly an adverse reaction to medication or an infection. However, 50% of cases are idiopathic. In children the cause is usually infection, whereas in adults the cause is typically drugs or malignancy. The most common medications leading to SJS are sulfonamides, penicillin, anticonvulsants, some nonsteroidal anti-inflammatory medications, and allopurinol (Mayo Clinic, 2011). The most common infections implicated as a cause of SJS are herpes simplex virus and *Mycoplasma pneumoniae*. HIV infection, cancer, or the presence of an autoimmune disorder increases the risk of developing SJS. Symptoms generally appear within 14 days of exposure to the causative agent (Domino et al., 2012).

Pathophysiology

The triggering mechanism for SJS is unclear, but the pathophysiology is immunologic with a cell-mediated cytotoxic reaction against epidermal cells. Erythematous papular lesions and keratinocyte necrosis are results of cell-mediated immunity. The initial exposure to the offending drug leads to accumulation and binding of reactive drug metabolites to the mucocutaneous epithelial cells within 1 to 2 weeks. This initiates the signaling and cascade of lymphocytes and macrophages, leading to keratinocyte activation and the destruction and necrosis of the epidermis (Domino et al., 2012).

Clinical Manifestations

The diagnostic criteria of SJS are defined differently by different authors. There is no universally accepted definition. However, SJS generally begins with flulike symptoms such as headache, rhinorrhea, cough, and body aches. Target skin lesions are present and are described as having a bright-pink or red inner ring, a ring of lighter pink, and then a ring of dark pink. These lesions are concentric macular exanthemas that focus on the face, neck, and extremities, which then become blisters that grow together and break open. This situation might be seen in patients with burns. Epidermal detachment with light lateral pressure (Nikolsky's sign) affecting more than 10% of the skin is a hallmark of SJS (Domino et al., 2012). The lesions are found on less than 20% of the patient's body surface area in the first 48 hours and result in skin detachment. Although there is no universally accepted definition for SJS, SJS is commonly identified by the following: (1) involvement of at least two mucous membranes, (2) presence of target lesions with sudden epidermal detachment, (3) fever, (4) skin biopsy compatible with erythema multiforme and Stevens–Johnson syndrome, (5) positive Nikolsky's sign, and (6) involvement of less than 20% of the total body surface area.

At least 61% of patients with SJS have mucous membrane involvement with the mouth, eyes, skin, genitalia, esophagus, and respiratory tract affected. Ocular involvement occurs in 39% of all patients with SJS (Domino et al., 2012). The mucosal lesions are painful, have a crusted surface, and may lead to blindness or impaired nutrition. Initial presentation includes petechiae, vesicles, and bullae. A burning sensation sometimes accompanies the lesions, but typically there is no pruritus.

Laboratory and Diagnostic Procedures and Medical Management

Stevens–Johnson syndrome is diagnosed by skin biopsy and immunofluorescent studies that demonstrate the presence of immunoglobulin M (IgM) and C3 deposits in the vascular walls. Skin cultures may be taken every 48 hours to aid in the decision to start antibiotics if necessary. In addition, serologic tests may be done to identify suspected sources of infection.

There is no universally accepted treatment of SJS other than supportive care. Treatment with glucocorticoids is controversial. Some studies have suggested that glucocorticoids lead to increased morbidity and mortality, whereas others report that short-term use of glucocorticoids in high doses improves outcomes (Domino et al., 2012). The use of intravenous immunoglobulin (IVIG) has shown some success and improved outcomes; however, more research is needed (Domino et al., 2012). Other experimental treatments that may be useful are recombinant granulocyte colony-stimulating factor, cyclophosphamide, and cyclosporine. Intravenous fluid replacement similar to that initiated with the treatment of burns must be started to prevent dehydration and treat electrolyte loss through skin lesions (see Chapter 61). Often patients with SJS are taken to burn units for care. Total parenteral nutrition (TPN) is necessary to treat protein loss that occurs with skin detachment and to help prevent stress ulcers. Prevention of infection is important. Although prophylactic antibiotics are generally unnecessary, careful aseptic technique is needed. Dressings are used to protect the epidermis but tape should be avoided. Dressings should be nonadherent and not cause further damage. Avoid the use of topical silver sulfadiazine due to the association between SJS and sulfonamides. Biologic skin covers such as cadaveric allografts may also be used. Chapter 61 discusses skin grafts. Topical anesthetics and systemic pain medication may be needed to decrease pain related to dressing changes. Emotional and psychiatric support is essential. A collaborative and coordinated approach involving critical care, wound care, and burn specialists is recommended.

Toxic Epidermal Necrolysis

Etiology, Epidemiology, and Pathophysiology

Toxic epidermal necrolysis (TEN) is a part of the same syndrome of diseases as Stevens–Johnson syndrome. However, TEN is a more severe form of the disorder and is life threatening with more extensive skin detachment. Toxic epidermal necrolysis is considered when more than 30% of the patient's body surface area is involved. Although the disorder is rare, occurring in only 1 person per million, it can have mortality rates of 10% to 30% (Domino et al., 2012); the rate is even greater in older adults. The disorder generally occurs in people between the ages of 46 and 63 but can occur at any age. It more commonly affects women. The causes are the same as those for Stevens–Johnson syndrome, with the most common being an adverse reaction to drugs such as sulfonamide antibiotics, anticonvulsant agents, and allopurinol.

The pathophysiology of TEN is unknown; however, it is thought to be related to an immune response that is cell mediated by the T lymphocytes. Skin lesions have been found to have macrophage infiltration of the dermis and epidermis with tumor necrosis factor in the epidermis (Domino et al., 2012).

Clinical Manifestations, Laboratory and Diagnostic Procedures, and Medical Management

Like SJS, TEN begins with symptoms of an upper respiratory infection. Approximately 2 to 3 days after the respiratory symptoms, the epidermis blisters and begins splitting and sloughing from the dermis. There are no target lesions, but there are large areas of epidermal sloughing with a dark-red, oozing dermis. Toxic epidermal necrolysis is more severe than SJS, causing painful and tender lesions and also affecting the mucous membranes.

Toxic epidermal necrolysis is diagnosed by skin biopsy and immunofluorescent studies. Early diagnosis and withdrawal of offending agents are important in decreasing mortality. Once diagnosed, patients with TEN can be assessed to predict mortality. The SCORTEN scoring system is used for that purpose. It gives points to 7 parameters, which are added to result in a score between 0 and 7 and outlined in Chart 59–4. A score of 0 to 1 is related to a mortality of 3.2%, whereas a score of 5 or more predicts a mortality of at least 90%. The SCORTEN should be performed during the first 24 hours after hospital admission and again on day 3 of hospitalization. The ability to predict mortality can be useful in discussing the patient's condition with family members and in evaluating the effectiveness of new treatments.

To achieve the best outcomes, treatment of TEN should occur in a burn unit or intensive care unit. There is no definitive treatment, so the care provided is mostly supportive. The development of an infection or sepsis increases the risk of mortality. Treatment goals are the same as those for SJS. Intravenous fluid replacement is needed to prevent dehydration and treat electrolyte losses. Total parenteral nutrition is needed to supply badly needed nutrients for growth and repair and to address the protein loss that occurs with the hypermetabolic state. The hypermetabolic state is described in Chapter 61. Wounds are generally debrided in the operating room, and biologic dressings such as homografts and xenografts (Chapter 61) are used to decrease the chance of infection, reduce pain, prevent fluid loss, and control body temperature. Reepithelialization begins about 18 days after the development of the first symptoms. As with SJS, treatment with corticosteroids is controversial.

CHART 59–4 SCORTEN Scoring System

Risk Factor	0	1
Age	<40 years	>40 years
Associated malignancy	No	Yes
Heart rate in beats per minute	<120	>120
Serum blood urea nitrogen (BUN) (mg/dL)	<27	>27
Detached or compromised body surface	<10%	>10%
Serum bicarbonate (mEq/L)	>20	<20
Serum glucose (mg/dL)	<250	>250

Nursing Management

Nursing care for Stevens–Johnson syndrome and toxic epidermal necrolysis requires knowledgeable assessment skills and critical thinking. The nurse needs to be cognizant of the possible development of these conditions. At the first signs of a drug reaction, the health care provider must be alerted and the offending agent must be stopped immediately. Once either SJS or TEN develops, it is best managed in a burn unit using a multidisciplinary approach with the nurse as the gatekeeper. The nursing process provides the framework to manage these patients. The Nursing Process: Patient Care Plan on page 1862 outlines the care for these disorders.

Health Promotion

Because necrotizing fasciitis, Stevens–Johnson syndrome, and toxic epidermal necrolysis can occur at any age or location and are not specific to gender, it is imperative to educate patients, families, and the general public about the risk factors (see the Risk Factors for Necrotizing Fasciitis box, p. 1856) and how to avoid them. As was stated earlier, about one-half of the cases occur in young, previously healthy patients; therefore, avoiding behaviors such as skin popping (Chapter 58) will decrease the risk. If the individual has already contracted the disease once, education needs to focus on avoidance of reexposure. The nurse needs to tell patients to seek medical help for wounds that are not healing or appear infected.

Collaborative Management

The care for a patient with one of these life-threatening skin conditions is multidimensional and multidisciplinary, requiring the nurse to serve as the team coordinator and patient advocate. The goals are to ensure that the patient receives high-quality care and has an understanding of the disease process and treatment. In order to meet desired patient outcomes, it is essential that this interdisciplinary team communicate openly with one another in developing and evaluating care of the patient and family (IOM [Institute of Medicine], 2010). These patients require intensive nursing and medical management, along with the expertise of the physical and occupational therapists, psychologists/psychiatrists, pharmacists, physical therapist and nutritionists. To ensure complete closure and prevention of infection, wound care is managed by both nurses and health care providers. The initial medical team needs to include a surgeon, an infectious disease specialist, a pathologist, and a microbiologist. Which other team members are included will depend on the severity and location of the wound. The composition of the nursing team depends on the wound's severity and the patient's hemodynamic stability. Nurses knowledgeable in wound care are essential, and critical care nurses may be needed to monitor and maintain the hemodynamic parameters.

As the wound heals, the scar formation causes contracture formation. Depending on the site of the wound, this may decrease joint range of motion. Physical therapy is initiated as soon as possible and continues after hospital discharge to maintain and increase range of motion in the joints. When contracture formation is severe, the surgeon needs to release the contractures surgically.

The pharmacist assists the medical team with pain and infection control management. The infection must be controlled to prevent further tissue and organ loss. The antibiotics are monitored by the nurses, health care providers, and pharmacists to ensure sensitivity to the organisms. Pain management is a major concern for the patient with one of these skin conditions. During dressing changes, the use of conscious sedation is frequently required due to the severity of the pain. Additionally, ongoing pain management between the dressing changes is necessary to ensure patient comfort. Because of the longevity of the hospitalization, the pain management protocols require frequent adjustment. The pharmacist is an essential part of this process.

The disabilities experienced by the patient may lead to changes in lifestyle and occupation. Often the patient is unable to return to her previous employment due to physical limitations. Family dynamics and role function often change (at least temporarily, and perhaps permanently) depending on the degree of disability. The occupational therapist, social worker, and psychologist/psychiatrist all assist the patient with physical and psychological adjustments after discharge.

Finally, the nutritionist must develop a comprehensive plan for nutrition for enhancing wound healing, regaining strength, and preventing complications. The dietitian works with the health care team from the time of admission through discharge to ensure proper nutritional support.

Discharge Priorities

Most patients with dermatologic disorders are cared for at home. Therefore, discharge planning begins with the diagnosis of the condition. Patient teaching aimed at self-care is an important part of planning for discharge. The Patient Teaching & Discharge Priorities box outlines specific discharge priorities.

SKIN DISORDERS WITH A GENETIC BASIS

Psoriasis

Etiology, Epidemiology, and Pathophysiology

Psoriasis is a chronic, relapsing, noncontagious inflammatory skin disorder that affects approximately 2% to 4% of the population (Figure 59–5◆) (Nicol & Huether, 2007). Psoriasis is a T-cell-mediated autoimmune disease; onset usually occurs by 20 years of age. A family history of psoriasis is common. Genetics are complex but the human leukocyte antigen (HLA)–Cw6 allele is a major susceptibility gene. The disease is chronic and incurable with exacerbations and remissions. It occurs equally across

NURSING PROCESS: Patient Care Plan for Necrotizing Fasciitis, Stevens–Johnson Syndrome, and Toxic Epidermal Necrolysis

Assessment of Cardiac Status Using Gordon's Functional Health Patterns:

- Activity Exercise Pattern
- Health Perception/Health Management
- Nutritional Metabolic Pattern
- Coping–Stress Tolerance Pattern
- Sleep–Rest

Subjective Data

Assessment of Skin Integrity

Where are the lesions located?

Are there any associated symptoms?

How long have the lesions been present?

Is there any drainage? If so, what color and consistency?

Do you have any chronic health problems?

Has there been any recent exposure to drugs, environmental or occupational toxins, or people with similar skin conditions?

Assessment of Fluid Status

Are you short of breath?

Do you have swelling occurring anywhere?

Do you have any chronic health problems?

Assessment of Physical Mobility

How active are you physically?

Has your activity level changed with your skin problems? How?

What limits your activity?

Assessment of Pain

Using a scale of 1 to 10, with 1 being very little pain and 10 being the worst imaginable pain, what is your pain level?

What is your experience with pain?

Do you routinely take pain medication at home? If so, how much and what kind? What kind of pain do you experience at home?

Are you allergic to any pain medication?

Do you have any cultural or religious beliefs that impact your pain control?

Where is your pain located?

Can you describe what type of pain you are having?

Does your pain radiate or stay in one place?

Is your pain constant or intermittent?

What brings your pain on or relieves it?

Assessment of Body Image Disturbance

How has your lifestyle changed since the skin disorder started?

Do you have negative feelings about your body or your appearance?

Do you fear rejection by others?

Assessment of Sleep Pattern

How are you sleeping?

Do you have trouble falling asleep?

Do you wake up in the middle of the night?

What keeps you from sleeping?

What are your bedtime rituals?

Assessment of Ineffective Protection

Has the appearance of the skin lesions changed?

How have you been caring for the skin lesions?

What has your diet been like?

Have you been following the prescribed treatment such as medications and wound care?

Objective Data

Assessment of Skin Integrity

Skin color.

Presence of drainage: color, consistency, odor.

Pattern of the lesions.

Skin temperature around the lesions.

Assessment of Fluid Status

Assess lung sounds for rales or crackles.

Monitor blood pressure, jugular venous distention (JVD), vital signs, urine output, and daily weight.

Presence of edema in ankles, in dependent areas, or around lesions.

Assessment of Physical Mobility

Assess range of motion of all extremities.

Assess patient's strength.

Assess oxygen saturation levels.

Assessment of Pain

Assess location, duration, and onset of pain and what provokes and relieves it.

Grimacing with movement.

Restlessness and irritability.

Taut facial expression.

Watch how the patient moves.

Vital signs.

Check skin for diaphoresis and pallor.

Clenched teeth.

Assessment of Body Image Disturbance

Is there an actual change in the appearance of the patient?

Is the patient hiding from or avoiding others?

Assessment of Sleep Pattern

Observe patient sleeping.

Assess the environment for noises, temperature, lighting, or disturbances.

Assessment of Ineffective Protection

Inspect skin lesions for redness, warmth, and drainage.

Vital signs.

Signs of systemic infection.

Age.

Comorbid chronic diseases.

NURSING PROCESS: Patient Care Plan for Necrotizing Fasciitis, Stevens–Johnson Syndrome, and Toxic Epidermal Necrolysis, *continued*

Assessment of Nutrition

How is your appetite?

Do you have sores in your mouth?

What kinds of foods are you eating?

What kinds of foods do you like or dislike?

Are there any cultural practices that would influence your diet?

Assessment of Nutrition

Assess nutritional status (appetite, weight loss, types of foods eaten).

Assess 24-hour food intake.

Assess for sores in the mouth.

Assessment of Social Isolation

Who will assist you with care at home?

Are you the breadwinner for the family?

Are your loved ones able to visit you?

Are you comfortable with visitors?

What can be done to help you feel more comfortable around people?

Assessment of Social Isolation

Patient's ability to interact with visitors and staff.

Evaluate patient response to discussion about current and future health concerns.

Observe for manifestations of anxiety: restlessness, apprehension, withdrawal.

Assessment of Patient/Family Knowledge of Disease and Treatment

Would you tell me what you know about your disease?

Has anyone explained your health problems to you?

Tell me what you are doing about your risk factors.

Tell me about your dietary intake.

What medications are you on, when are you supposed to take them, and what are the side effects you should watch for?

When are you supposed to see your doctor?

How does this disease affect your daily life?

Do you feel anxious about your health problems?

Do you have family members or close friends who provide emotional support?

Do you see your health care provider on a regular basis?

Do you know what symptoms are important to report to your health care provider immediately?

Assessment of Patient/Family Knowledge of Disease and Treatment

Patient/family may be anxious, confused, and need repeated information.

Assess for mistakes being made with treatment plan.

Assess for self-care deficit due to clinical manifestations.

Outcomes and Evaluation Parameters / Planning and Interventions with *Rationales*

1. NURSING DIAGNOSIS: Impaired Skin Integrity *related to skin lesions* (NANDA-I © 2012)

Outcome: No signs of infection or worsening of infection.

Evaluation Parameters: Skin will not have drainage, or drainage will not be yellow or green with a foul odor.

Skin color will be pink; no blue or gray.

Wound will show signs of healing.

Assess skin for drainage, warmth, and redness.

Indicates presence of infection.

Assess the wound for expansion of the erythema, changes in edema, changes in color, and drainage. Assess skin lesions for changes. *Indicates progression or healing of skin disorder.*

Implement an individualized treatment plan for the site of skin impairment. Use aseptic technique. *Treatment should be implemented according to patient needs and to prevent infection.*

Reposition the patient every 2 hours, and assess for signs of skin breakdown. If the patient is not repositioned *wound healing can be delayed and further skin breakdown can occur.*

Teach the patient the care of skin wounds. *It is important for the patient to understand and comply with care.*

The normal infection control precautions are important, such as hand hygiene to prevent the chances of spreading the bacteria. The patient should be placed in a private room with contact isolation (Chapter 14). *To decrease the chance of infection.*

2. NURSING DIAGNOSIS: Risk for Infection *related to loss of skin integrity* (NANDA-I © 2012)

Outcome: Effective infection prevention.

Evaluation Parameters: *Wounds* will not be colonized by organisms.

Healing and reepithelialization occurs as noted by wound closure.

Skin integrity will be restored.

Cleanse the wound per protocol. *To prevent contamination from surrounding tissue and hair.*

Assess for infection and document with each dressing change. *To prevent spread of infection.*

(*continued*)

NURSING PROCESS: Patient Care Plan for Necrotizing Fasciitis, Stevens–Johnson Syndrome, and Toxic Epidermal Necrolysis, *continued*

Outcomes and Evaluation Parameters	Planning and Interventions with *Rationales*
3. NURSING DIAGNOSIS: Risk for Imbalanced Fluid Volume *related to fluid loss* (NANDA-I © 2012)	
Outcome: Adequate fluid balance. ***Evaluation Parameters:*** Lung sounds will be clear with a normal respiratory rate. Urine output will be within 1,000 milliliters of intake. Extremities and wounds will not be edematous. Laboratory values, such as electrolytes, will be within normal range.	Assess the patient's preoperative status. *Awareness of preexisting fluid overload or dehydration can prevent fluid problems postoperatively.* Monitor vital signs. *Vital signs, such as increased pulse or respiration, can indicate fluid volume overload or dehydration.* Monitor intake and output of fluids. *Can help monitor fluid status. Intake should be within 1,000 milliliters of output for 24 hours.* Assess for signs of edema in dependent areas or around lesions. Weigh the patient at least weekly. Monitor fluid status. *Can indicate fluid retention.* Assess electrolyte levels. *Electrolytes can be altered with fluid overload or dehydration and can cause problems.* The possibility of septic shock should be monitored. *To provide treatment and prevent progression of shock.*
4. NURSING DIAGNOSIS: Impaired Physical Mobility *related to discomfort* (NANDA-I © 2012)	
Outcome: Patient is mobile and independent. ***Evaluation Parameters:*** Physical activity is increased as the patient's condition allows. Patient verbalizes a feeling of increased strength and ability to move. Patient is able to perform activities of daily living.	Assess mobility skills. *Provides a baseline and makes the nurse aware of opportunities for improvement.* Monitor patient's ability to tolerate activity. *Provides information about problems that might inhibit activity.* Treat pain before activity. *Pain limits mobility.* If the patient is immobile, perform passive range of motion or any activity that is not contraindicated. *Helps to maintain joint mobility and increase circulation.* Help the patient to achieve mobility and independence as soon as possible. *Early mobilization can help prevent complications related to immobility.*
5. NURSING DIAGNOSIS: Acute Pain *related to exposed nerve endings* (NANDA-I © 2012)	
Outcome: Adequate pain control. ***Evaluation Parameters:*** Pain is an important issue in the patient with necrotizing fasciitis. Pain may be difficult to monitor because it often seems out of proportion to the patient's injury. However, it is important to assess the pain because it is an indication of the pathologic process. Patient reports pain before it becomes unbearable. Patient reports pain relief. Pain decreases, requiring less medication. Patient is able to perform activities without pain.	Assess severity and quality of pain frequently. *Helps to determine cause and presence of pain so it can be relieved.* Explore the need for medications to relieve pain. *Pharmacologic interventions should be used when needed to relieve pain.* Discuss the patient's fears of unrelieved pain, overdose, or addiction. *The patient's concerns may prevent reporting of pain.* Review the patient records to determine the effectiveness of medications for pain relief. *Systematic tracking of pain relief will help identify and improve problems with pain management.* Support the patient's use of nonpharmacologic interventions for pain relief. *Nonpharmacologic interventions can be effective as a supplement to pharmacologic interventions.* Plan care and activities around periods of pain. *Pain diminishes ability to be active.*
6. NURSING DIAGNOSIS: Disturbed Body Image *related to disease* (NANDA-I © 2012)	
Outcome: Patient accepts or is satisfied with body image. ***Evaluation Parameters:*** The interruption in skin integrity leads to an altered body image, threatens the patient's self-esteem, and may lead to extreme anxiety and grief. Patient states acceptance of body changes. Patient returns to previous social involvement.	Acknowledge the patient's feelings related to changes in body image. *Changes in body image may lead to a variety of reactions. Patients should feel supported and able to express their feelings.* Allow the patient to explore the changes gradually. *The patient should be able to explore the changes when ready.* Encourage the patient to be involved in the decision making and accept inadequacies and strengths. *When patients have a say in their care, they are more likely to adapt to changes.* Assess the influence of cultural beliefs, norms, and perceptions on body image. *The patient's body image is influenced by culture and the norms of that social context.* Disabilities after recovery may keep the patient from returning to work. The patient should be encouraged to voice concerns and feelings, and a mental health specialist should be consulted. *To help facilitate long-term acceptance of body image changes.*

NURSING PROCESS: Patient Care Plan for Necrotizing Fasciitis, Stevens–Johnson Syndrome, and Toxic Epidermal Necrolysis, *continued*

7. NURSING DIAGNOSIS: Readiness for Enhanced Sleep *related to pain and anxiety* (NANDA-I © 2012)	
Outcome: Patient falls asleep and sleeps without interruption. ***Evaluation Parameters:*** Patient sleeps throughout the night. Patient verbalizes a feeling of not being fatigued.	Assess the patient's sleep patterns and bedtime rituals. Sleep patterns are individual. *Sleep can be enhanced by adhering to usual rituals when possible.* Determine the current level of anxiety or pain. *Anxiety and pain prevent sleep.* Provide measures before bedtime to assist with sleep. *Simple interventions such as warm milk or a back massage can help induce sleep.* Keep environment quiet and interruptions at a minimum. *Noise can interfere with sleep.* Plan for long periods of uninterrupted sleep. Discourage long naps during the day. *Can interfere with prolonged good sleep.*
8. NURSING DIAGNOSIS: Ineffective Protection *related to interrupted skin integrity* (NANDA-I © 2012)	
Outcome: Patient is free of any new signs of infection. ***Evaluation Parameters:*** Patient verbalizes precautions to prevent infection. Patient eats a well-balanced diet. Patient performs proper wound care.	Monitor vital signs. *Vital signs can demonstrate signs of infection.* Assess nutritional status. *Nutrition is important for supporting the immune system.* Assess for signs of new or worsening infection. *Infection should be identified early, and treatment initiated to decrease the chances of mortality or complications.* Implement interventions to prevent the spread of infection. *Infection is easily spread from one patient to another or one site to another if infection control measures are not observed.* Teach the patient and family about precautions to take to avoid infection. *Reduce the risk of infection from visitors.*
9. NURSING DIAGNOSIS: Imbalanced Nutrition: Less Than Body Requirements (NANDA-I © 2012)	
Outcome: Patient will have an adequate intake to meet the body's needs for repair. ***Evaluation Parameters:*** Patient eats most of the food served. Weight will be improved or maintained at a healthy level.	Because of the infection, pain, and wound healing, the patient's calorie needs are increased. The patient requires two to three times the normal amounts of calories and protein for healing. Supplements may also be required for wound healing such as vitamin C, vitamin E, and iron. Monitor food intake. *Food intake needs to be adequate for healing.* Serve small amounts of high-calorie, high-protein food every 2 hours. *Patient is more likely to eat small amounts more frequently than large amounts less often.* Provide a well-balanced diet with foods the patient likes. *Patient will be more likely to eat.* Consult with a dietitian and health care provider. Assess the need for parenteral or enteral feedings. *If the patient is unable to eat enough food orally to keep up with the body's demands, other avenues may need to be explored and utilized.*
10. NURSING DIAGNOSIS: Social Isolation *due to prolonged illness* (NANDA-I © 2012)	
Outcomes: Patient will have a plan for care of others who are dependent. Patient will have a plan for care of self at home. ***Evaluation Parameter:*** Patient returns to previous life roles.	Consult the social worker or case manager. *Allows for plans to be made for needed care and decreased anxiety in patient.*
11. NURSING DIAGNOSIS: Deficient Knowledge *related to disease and treatment plan* (NANDA-I © 2012)	
Outcome: Patient/family have an understanding of and comply with the treatment plan. ***Evaluation Parameters:*** Patient and family understand the treatment plan and safely become compliant. Patient and family understand the importance of risk factor control in preventing a progression of the disease.	Describe the required diet, medications, treatment plan, risk factors, activity, and limitations *to increase knowledge of disease and treatment.* Describe what clinical manifestations need to be reported to the health care provider and when to access the emergency medical system *to ensure immediate care when necessary.* Have the patient/family repeat instructions *to assess understanding.*

Source: Adapted from Wilkinson, J. M., & Ahearn, N. R. (2009). *Prentice Hall nursing diagnosis handbook* (9th ed.). Upper Saddle River, NJ: Prentice Hall.

genders, although there is a greater incidence in Caucasians. Risk factors for psoriasis include stress, infection, medications such as beta-adrenergic blockers, smoking, and high alcohol consumption. There are many types of psoriasis but chronic plaque psoriasis is the most common (Chart 59–5).

Clinical Manifestations

The lesions of psoriasis are erythematous papules and plaques with silver-white scales that are sharply demarcated. They are the result of hyperproliferation of keratinocytes. A variety of sizes of lesions can coalesce into very large plaques. These lesions usually occur on the

PATIENT TEACHING & DISCHARGE PRIORITIES for Skin Disorders

Need	Teaching
Wound Care	Evaluate for signs of infection such as increased redness, drainage, fever, or foul odor.
Patient/family	Perform cleaning of wounds and dressing changes as ordered by the health care provider.
	Perform hand hygiene and wear gloves while performing dressing changes.
	Avoid scratching healed areas.
	Keep unaffected skin clean and well hydrated.
	Avoid exposure to the sun.
	Wear loose-fitting, soft clothing.
Family/support system	Assess the patient's knowledge of the illness:
	• Teach actions to decrease the risk of infection.
	• Teach signs and symptoms that should be reported to the health care provider.
	Assess compliance with treatment:
	• Provide written instructions.
	• Assess the patient/family's abilities to provide care at home.
Setting	Assess effectiveness of available support systems.
	Assess discharge placement needs:
	• Home.
	• Rehabilitation facility.
	• Extended care facility.
	Assess the home environment to determine the need for assistive devices and safety.
	Assess the need for professional home health needs.
	Assess the patient's abilities to obtain food, medications, and supplies.
Nutrition	Maintain a high-calorie, high-protein, well-balanced diet.
Patient/family	Include vitamin C, iron, and zinc in the diet.
Family/support system	Assess appetite and weight loss.
Setting	Avoid foods that cause hypersensitivity reactions.
	Teach foods to include and avoid in the diet.
	Assess financial resources.
Psychological Adjustment	Encourage verbalizations of feelings and fears.
Patient/family	Encourage positive reinforcement rather than rejection from the family.
Setting	Answer questions honestly.
	Encourage participation in support groups for the patient's specific disorder.
Pruritus	Avoid things that are irritating or intensify itching such as excessive bathing.
Patient/family	Apply cold or emollient lotion to rehydrate the skin.
Setting	Recommend baths with cornstarch or oatmeal.
	Perform proper application and use of prescribed medications.
	Wear nonrestrictive, light clothing.
	Assess temperature and humidity.
Pain	Assess pain level and report increases in pain.
Patient/family	Assess the effectiveness of pain medications.
Setting	Assess patient/family knowledge of pain medication and side effects.
	Assess the environment for safety.

extensor surfaces of the knees and elbows, the scalp, the lower back, genitalia, or nails, although they can occur anywhere on the body. Some individuals experience pain and swelling in the joints that is associated with psoriasis; this condition is called psoriatic arthritis.

Laboratory and Diagnostic Procedures and Medical Management

Psoriasis is diagnosed by the patient's history of lesion development, trigger factors, family history, and physical examination. The appearance and distribution of the lesions can be enough to provide a diagnosis; however, skin biopsy can be done if there is a question (this is rare). Serology will find negative rheumatoid factor, increased erythrocyte sedimentation rate, and elevated C-reactive protein.

The first line of treatment is topical agents such as emollient creams or ointments that can be used to prevent cracking and fissuring of the skin. Emollients help to moisturize the skin, easing itching and scaling. Corticosteroids are used to decrease inflammation; however, the

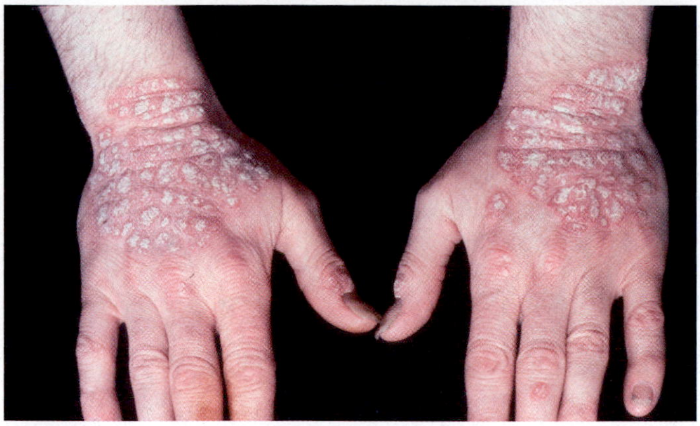

FIGURE 59–5 ◆ Psoriasis.
Source: NMSB/Custom Medical Stock Photo, Inc.

CHART 59–5 Types of Psoriasis

Type	Description
Plaque	Most common. Red, scaly papules that coalesce. Lesions are well demarcated and symmetrical. Location: scalp, trunk, limbs (extensor surface), nails may be pitted and/or thickened. Scale is adherent and silvery white with bleeding when removed.
Guttate	Associated with a sudden appearance of scaly papules that are "drop-like" and generally appear on the trunk.
Localized pustular	Discrete, small, sterile pustules that do not rupture but turn brown and scaly.
Generalized pustular	Erythema with sterile, generalized pustules over much of the body. Associated with systemic symptoms such as fever, chills, and leukocytosis.
Erythrodermic	Exfoliates with red skin all over the body. There may be skin peeling with fluid balance problems. Very serious disease.
Inverse or flexural	Occurs on intertriginous areas; lesions are moist with or without scales.
Nail psoriasis	Pitting of nails with separating of the nail from the nail bed. Nail plate may turn yellow. Fingernails involved in approximately 50% of cases, toenails ~35%.
Scalp psoriasis	Erythematous, scaly plaques that occur on the scalp or near the hairline. Usually is limited to the scalp.

relief they provide is temporary, so they are best used in cycles for 7 to 10 days with rest periods in between. Vitamin D_3 analogue creams can be used directly on a plaque to control irritation and erythema. Coal tar preparations can be effective in resolving the lesions, although the exact mechanism of action is unknown. Phototherapy is effective when the psoriasis affects more than 30% of the body. Ultraviolet B is given three to five times weekly with exposures intense enough to cause erythema. Clearing of the lesions takes an average of 7 weeks. Phototherapy can also be used in conjunction with other medications. Most commonly used is ultraviolet A (UVA) with a photosensitizing medication such as psoralen. Psoralen is given prior to the exposure to ultraviolet light (UV). It inhibits DNA synthesis after activation with UVA, decreasing cellular proliferation. Systemic therapy is used in patients who are very uncomfortable or who have psoriasis affecting a large portion of the body. Methotrexate, a commonly used systemic medication, acts to prevent hyperkeratinization by suppressing proliferating cells or psoriatic epidermal cell reproduction. Cyclosporine, an immunosuppressive drug that suppresses the growth of T cells, is used for severe inflammatory psoriasis. Etanercept is one of the biologic agents that have been used recently as a treatment for psoriasis. These medications interfere (relatively safely) with the immunologic process that has been found to be involved in psoriasis and improve the condition's skin lesions (Nicol & Huether, 2007).

The psychological implications of psoriasis are great. It is a disfiguring disease that can result in low self-esteem, poor self-perception, depression, and anxiety. It can affect an individual's business, social, and sexual relationships. It may also cause problems with working due to the time off work for treatment, resulting in job loss and decreased income.

Neurofibromatosis

Etiology, Epidemiology, Pathophysiology, and Clinical Manifestations

Neurofibromatosis is an autosomal dominant inherited disorder that can affect any organ; however, this condition also may arise spontaneously, without a previous family history. There are two types of neurofibromatosis. Type 1, the most common, is known as von Recklinghausen's disease. It is characterized by multiple hyperpigmented macules; neurofibromatosis; and small, multiple, palpable, pedunculated, mobile, and pigmented nodules. These disfiguring lesions become apparent after the first decade of life. People with type 1 neurofibromatosis also have other associated disorders such as scoliosis and erosive bone defects. Type 2 neurofibromatosis is characterized by tumors of the eighth cranial or acoustic nerve. Symptoms associated with type 2 neurofibromatosis include headaches, hearing loss, impaired balance, facial pain, and tinnitus. This condition is often accompanied by intracranial or intraspinal tumors.

Laboratory and Diagnostic Procedures and Medical Management

Neurofibromatosis is diagnosed by the patient's history of symptoms and physical examination. The presence of café-au-lait (light brown) macules, the first feature of type 1 neurofibromatosis, usually occurs in the first 3 years of childhood. Neurofibromatosis can be cutaneous, subcutaneous, or plexiform and soft or firm; buttonhole invagination (invagination of a nodule when pressed with a finger) is pathognomonic and not usually present until late adolescence. Axillary or inguinal freckling is one diagnostic criterion for neurofibromatosis (Nicol & Huether, 2007). Magnetic resonance imaging may be necessary to detect tumors in the brain or spinal cord. The severity of the disease is variable. Disfigurement caused by tumors and nodules on the skin can be corrected with plastic surgery. Tumors of the spinal cord and brain can be treated surgically as well. The care of the patient with neurofibromatosis is multidisciplinary, requiring the collaboration of several specialists. Patients may need to see an ophthalmologist for optic gliomas, a neurologist for neurofibromatosis, a dermatologist for nodules on the skin, or an orthopedist for osseous lesions. The patient must be followed closely for problems related to the formation of tumors. First-degree relatives should be screened for the presence of the disease, and genetic counseling is recommended to avoid passing the disease to future generations.

Nursing Management

Nursing management of genetic skin disorders involves multilevel assessment skills, clinical decision making, and critical thinking.

Knowledge about various treatment strategies and the rationale provide a basis for safe and effective nursing care.

Assessment

Management of genetic skin disorders begins with a thorough and complete skin assessment. Measurement of the body surface area involved helps to determine a baseline and if treatment is effective. Hydration, nutrition, growth and development, skeletal deformities, new or changing skin lesions, and psychological status are all important components of the assessment of a patient with genetic skin disorders.

Nursing Diagnoses

Nursing diagnoses can include the following:

- *Impaired Skin Integrity* related to loss of skin integrity.
- *Risk of Infection* related to loss of skin integrity.
- *Disturbed Body Image* related to skin disfigurement.
- *Social Isolation* related to skin disfigurement.
- *Fear and Anxiety* related to skin disfigurement.

NANDA-I © 2012

Other nursing diagnoses may be appropriate depending on the severity of the skin disorder.

Outcomes and Evaluation Parameters

A collaborative and comprehensive approach to care of the patient with a genetic skin disorder will optimize the recovery process. Psoriasis and neurofibromatosis are both skin disorders that change over time. Psoriasis can have periods of limited lesions and periods of relapse. Neurofibromatosis lesions increase with age. The best outcome is complete healing; however, in the case of genetic skin disorders, complete healing is not likely. Therefore, an important evaluation parameter is the number of lesions present and percentage of body surface area involved. Outcomes may be as specific as adequate sleep patterns or as general as no relapse. Other outcome goals may be to provide support, to manage the disorder without complications, and for the patient to return to his previous level of activity.

Interventions and Rationales

The interventions for the patient with a genetic skin disorder are based on the type of skin disorder and severity of the condition. The nursing care plan may address nutrition, psychological status, improving social interaction, disfigurement, and protecting lesions from trauma. The patient needs to be instructed to keep the open areas clean and dry to prevent infection, and avoid agents that may be irritating.

Evaluation

The plan of care for the patient with a genetic skin disorder needs to be reevaluated frequently to ensure that the treatment and plan is effective. Changes in the patient's trajectory and reaction to the treatment should be incorporated into a revised plan of treatment. Outcomes and evaluation parameters need to be reevaluated and revised if necessary. For example, as lesions decrease in size and characteristics change (dry, less pruritic, flaking), treatment may need to be revised to include moisturizers or emollients. Or if lesions are spreading, erythema increases, or drainage changes, the area needs to be assessed for secondary infection and the treatment plan needs to be revised.

SKIN DISORDERS RELATED TO PIGMENTATION, DEVELOPMENT, AND LIFESTYLE

Changes in Pigmentation of the Skin

This category of skin disorders involves an increase in normal skin colors that occurs because of increased or abnormally distributed melanin. It may be diffuse or limited to a specific space. Typically the patient's major concern is the cosmetic effect. Hypopigmentation of the skin is a decrease in melanin that can be hereditary or acquired. There are diseases of the skin that lead to a loss of melanin, causing a pale or gray appearance to the skin. One of the most common disorders leading to hypopigmentation is vitiligo.

Vitiligo

Vitiligo is a localized loss of melanocytes from the skin and hair that creates white patches of skin (Figure 59–6◆). The cause is unknown but may be related to an autoimmune disorder and inhibition of melanogenesis. There is no race, ethnicity, or gender predisposition. Incidence in the United States is approximately 1 in every 100 people and it occurs most commonly between the ages of 10 and 30 years (Schueler, Beckett, & Gettings, 2011). It occurs spontaneously after emotional or physical stress or may be related to trauma. Vitiligo progresses slowly over years with new patches of hypopigmentation occurring throughout life. The white macules can occur in a symmetrical pattern or can be segmental, limited to one segment of the body. The most common sites are the backs of the hands, face, body folds, axillae, and genitalia. Vitiligo causes no discomfort and is purely of cosmetic concern. Spontaneous repigmentation can occur but is usually spotty. The white areas of the skin can be covered with dyes and cosmetics to minimize the color irregularities. Sunless self-tanning agents may also be helpful by darkening the skin through staining. If the lesions are in sun-exposed areas, sunscreens should be used because of the

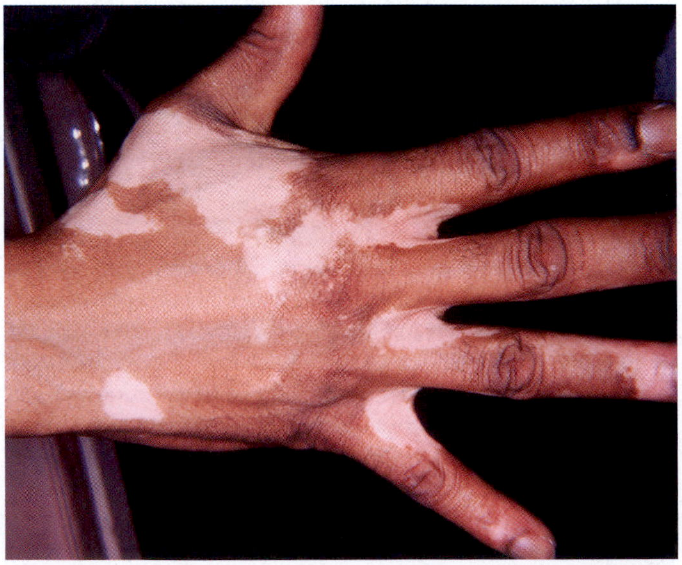

FIGURE 59–6 ◆ Vitiligo.

Source: John F. Wilson, MD/Photo Researchers, Inc.

higher risk of sunburn. Topical corticosteroids may be used to treat inflammation associated with the areas of hypopigmentation. See the Pharmacology box (p. 1845). Other repigmentation therapies include phototherapy (narrow-band ultraviolet B or broadband ultraviolet B) and surgery (Domino et al., 2012).

Café-au-Lait Spots

Café-au-lait spots are asymptomatic tan macules that have smooth borders and vary in diameter from 0.5 to 20 centimeters. They are generally considered to be benign but can indicate the presence of neurofibromatosis if there are six or more spots. No treatment is necessary, but they can be eliminated with laser or bleaching agents if they are cosmetically undesirable.

Liver Spots (Solar Lentigo)

Solar lentigo, commonly referred to as age spots or liver spots, refers to lesions that develop due to a familial tendency and chronic sun exposure in Caucasians over age 60. They are macules that are darker and larger than freckles and do not fade during winter. They occur in sun-exposed areas such as the backs of the hands, forearms, shoulders, and forehead. Their color is uniform with sharply demarcated borders. The lesions are usually asymptomatic but may be of cosmetic concern. The best treatment is prevention through the limitation of exposure to sunlight and the application of sunscreen. Bleaching creams are available that can be applied topically and will slowly fade the spots. Cosmetic resurfacing of the skin through the use of lasers or liquid nitrogen application can also decrease the pigmentation.

Disorders Associated with Adolescent Skin

Acne Vulgaris

Etiology, Epidemiology, and Pathophysiology

Acne vulgaris is a common skin condition that occurs most frequently during the teenage years at varying levels of severity. It affects up to 85% of the population between the age of 12 and 25 years; it is more common in males during the teenage years but more common in females in the adult years. Acne vulgaris is caused by obstruction of a hair follicle due to overgrowth of sebum and keratin debris, an overproduction of oil due to enlarged oil glands, and bacteria known as *P. acnes* (Nicol & Huether, 2007). These substances provide a good medium for bacterial growth, especially *Propionibacterium acnes* (*P. acnes*). *P. acnes* contain lipases that result in the breakdown of free fatty acids. Free fatty acids irritate the skin and cause a foreign body reaction leading to inflammation. The characteristic skin lesion, known as a comedo (plural: comedones), is typically located on the face, chest, and back (Figure 59–7◆).

Clinical Manifestations

Acne is defined by type and severity. Acne lesions can be classified as inflammatory (pustules, papules, nodules) or noninflammatory (closed and open comedones). In noninflammatory acne, closed (whiteheads) and open (blackheads) comedones occur with distention of the follicle and thinning of the follicular canal walls from accumulated material. Inflammatory acne develops when the follicular wall ruptures in the closed comedones. Sebum is expelled into the surrounding dermis and initiates inflammation. Pustules form when this occurs close to the skin surface and papules and cystic nodules form when it is deeper (Nicol & Huether, 2007). Papulopustular

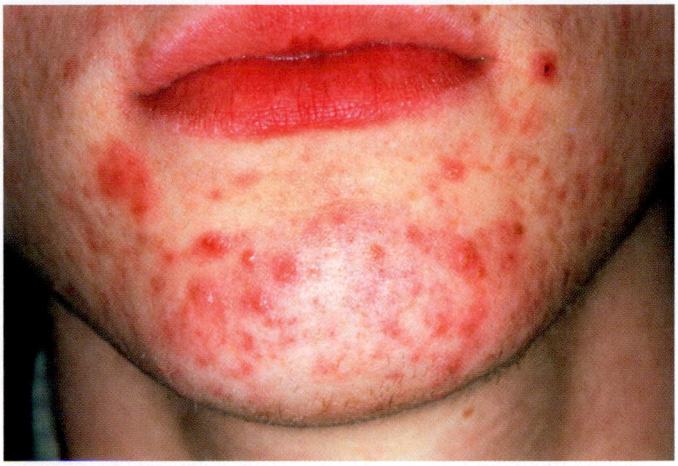

FIGURE 59–7 ◆ Acne vulgaris.
Source: Dr. P. Marazzi/Photo Researchers, Inc.

acne is inflammatory with small papules and pustules that contain a central core of purulent material. Nodulocystic acne is inflammatory with a lesion or cyst greater than 5 millimeters in diameter. These cysts can be localized or can form tracts under the skin with abscesses. Nodulocystic acne is a serious problem requiring aggressive treatment. The severity of acne is rated as mild, moderate, and severe. Mild acne is defined as open and closed comedones and noninflamed lesions. Moderate acne is defined as open and closed comedones with some pustules and inflamed lesions. Severe acne is defined as open and closed comedones, and lesions that are inflamed and pustular. There are also nodules and significant scarring (Domino et al., 2012). Very severe acne, known as *acne conglobata*, is a highly inflammatory form of severe cystic acne with the formation of communicating cysts and abscesses beneath the skin. When accompanied by systemic symptoms such as arthralgias, leukocytosis, and fever, it is known as acne fulminans.

Several factors have been identified as contributors to acne. Androgens play a role in the development of acne by stimulating the production of sebum, leading to obstruction of hair follicles and allowing for bacterial growth. However, estrogens can suppress the production of sebum. There is a genetic predisposition to acne as well as a link between stress and acne formation. However, no connections have been found between makeup use or diet and acne, which were once thought to be true. Men usually have more severe forms of the disease than women, but acne in women may persist into adulthood.

Laboratory and Diagnostic Procedures and Medical Management

The treatment of choice for acne is based on the type and severity of the acne, the patient's skin type, and the presence or potential for scarring. Treatment will take about 6 to 8 weeks to see improvement. Nonpharmacologic approaches to therapy involve good hygiene that includes washing the face with soap and water. The patient should avoid topical exposure to oils and greases and keep hair cleaned. Hats, sweatbands, and shirt collars can contribute to the collection of oil on the forehead, neck, and back and thus can contribute to an outbreak. Mild acne requires only topical agents such as benzoyl peroxide, salicylic acid, and azelaic acid that serve to help unblock the pores. These medications have bactericidal qualities that reduce the number of *P. acnes* and act to break down the keratin. Topical retinoids, such as Retin-A, are comedolytic agents that work as anti-inflammatory agents and normalize the abnormal growth of keratins. Oral contraceptives may be helpful for young women because they will decrease circulating androgens.

For moderate acne, a topical antibiotic should be added to the topical cleansing agent. Topical antibiotics decrease the numbers of *P. acnes* in sebaceous follicles and help to decrease inflammation. Once pustules or papules have developed, an oral antibiotic might be helpful. The antibiotic of choice is tetracycline. Erythromycin, doxycycline, and minocycline have also been shown to be effective. For severe acne, isotretinoin (Accutane) may be used. Accutane is an oral retinoid that decreases sebaceous gland activity and prevents the development of new comedones. Accutane has numerous side effects, such as nosebleeds; inflammation of the lips and eyes; pain and stiffness in muscles, bones, and joints; and elevated triglyceride levels. Therefore, its use should be monitored carefully. It should never be used by pregnant women due to its major teratogenic effects. See the Pharmacology box (p. 1845). Finally, patients should be instructed not to squeeze, rub, or pick at comedones because doing so may result in scarring.

Lasers and light treatments also have been used to treat acne. Lasers damage oil glands by using heat. In contrast, light treatments in the form of photodynamic therapy treat the overactive oil glands and the *P. acnes* bacteria. Both of these treatments are effective in reducing the oil production, leading to improved skin and reduced effects of acne (Domino et al., 2012).

The nurse needs to educate patients about the contributing factors and treatment for acne. The patient needs to understand that treatment is slow and that it will take 6 to 8 weeks to see the effects of any treatment regimen. The nurse should explain the effects and side effects of all medications. The patient may require emotional support to deal with the psychological effects of acne because the lesions and scarring may have a negative effect on the patient's self-esteem and quality of life.

Skin Changes Related to Aging

Seborrheic Keratosis

Seborrheic keratosis is a benign epidermal lesion seen predominantly in the middle-aged and older adult population. The exact cause is unknown, but it appears to be related to sun exposure. There are usually no associated symptoms, but the lesions can be irritated by clothing or jewelry. The lesions of seborrheic keratosis are warty, dirty yellow to black papules with sharp margins. They can also be flat, and the color can vary from white to pink to black within the lesion. They have a "stuck on" appearance with a waxy feel, and they tend to occur more commonly on the back, central chest, face, and scalp. A sudden onset of numerous seborrheic keratoses, known as the Leser-Trélat sign, is often associated with the presence of an internal malignancy.

Diagnosis is made on the basis of the patient's history of sun exposure and lesion appearance, as well as physical examination of the lesions. The lesions will continue to grow and new lesions will continue to appear. No treatment is usually necessary, although they can be surgically removed for cosmetic or diagnostic reasons.

Dermatofibroma

Dermatofibromas are common, asymptomatic, benign, firm tan or brown papules occurring most frequently in middle-aged women. They are more commonly seen on the legs, elbows, or lateral trunk, often at the site of a previous trauma such as an insect bite. They characteristically dimple when pinched between the thumb and forefinger. Diagnosis is usually based on the patient's history of the symptoms and physical examination of the lesion. Treatment is not necessary, but dermatofibromas may be surgically removed for cosmetic reasons.

Pemphigus Vulgaris

Etiology, Epidemiology, and Pathophysiology

Pemphigus vulgaris is an autoimmune disorder in which the body's immune system produces antibodies against certain proteins in the skin and mucous membranes. In rare situations, certain medications also can cause pemphigus vulgaris, including chelating agents and ACE inhibitors. Pemphigus usually occurs in middle-aged or older adults (Baroni et al., 2007; Habif, 2009).

The incidence of pemphigus vulgaris is uncommon in the United States. Its exact incidence and prevalence depends on the population studied. Although it has been reported to occur worldwide, pemphigus vulgaris incidence varies from 0.5 to 3.2 cases per 100,000 population. The incidence of pemphigus vulgaris is highest in patients of Ashkenazi Jewish descent and those of Mediterranean origin. The male-to-female ratio is approximately equal. The mean age of onset is approximately 50 to 60 years. Pemphigus vulgaris is a potentially life-threatening condition, with a mortality rate of approximately 5% to 15% (Zeina, 2012).

Pemphigus vulgaris is an intraepithelial, blistering disease that is caused by circulating autoantibodies directed against keratinocyte cell surfaces. An immunogenetic predisposition is well established. The blisters are associated with the binding of IgG autoantibodies to keratinocyte cell surface molecules. The binding of autoantibodies results in a loss of cell-to-cell adhesion, a process termed *acantholysis* (Zeina, 2012).

Clinical Manifestations and Laboratory and Diagnostic Procedures

The initial clinical manifestation is most commonly painful blisters and sores in the mouth, followed by skin blisters. Mouth lesions tend to be irregularly shaped, gingival, buccal, or palatine erosions, which are painful and slow to heal. The erosions extend peripherally with shedding of the epithelium. The skin blisters are open, draining, oozing sores that become crusty and peel easily. Patients with pemphigus vulgaris typically heal without scarring unless the disease is complicated by severe secondary infection. The diagnosis is confirmed with a skin biopsy (Zeina, 2012).

Medical Management

The aim of treatment is to reduce the inflammatory response and autoantibody production. Treatment goals include reducing symptoms, including pain, and preventing complications, especially secondary infections. The treatment depends on the extent of the blistering. Severe cases of pemphigus may need wound management, similar to the treatment for severe burns (Chapter 61). If the patient is unable to eat because of mouth ulcers, intravenous feedings and fluid replacement are indicated. Additional treatment may involve antibiotics and antifungal medications to control or prevent infections, numbing (anesthetic) mouth lozenges to reduce mouth ulcer pain, and systemic pain medications if local pain relief is not enough. Systemic therapy to treat the immune response and the inflammation should be started as early as possible. This treatment includes an anti-inflammatory drug called dapsone, corticosteroids, and medications that suppress the immune system (such as methotrexate and cyclosporin). Plasmapheresis, a process in which antibody-containing plasma is removed from the blood, may be used along with systemic medications to reduce the amount of antibodies in the blood. Site-specific ulcer and blister treatments include soothing or drying lotions, wet dressings, or similar measures (Zeina, 2012).

Rosacea

Etiology, Epidemiology, and Pathophysiology

Rosacea is an inflammatory chronic condition that occurs in middle-age adults, predominantly in females. The cause is unknown; however, immune-mediated inflammation may be a factor.

Clinical Manifestations

Rosacea is characterized by recurrent episodes of facial flushing, erythema (due to dilation of small blood vessels), papules, pustules, and telangiectasia (small widened blood vessels on the skin) in a symmetrical facial distribution. It usually occurs in the middle portion of the face over the forehead, nose, cheeks, and chin. Sometimes ocular symptoms can occur. These include dryness, conjunctival injection, burning, and eyelid irritation. There are three stages of rosacea. Stage I is persistent erythema with telangiectasia. Stage II is persistent erythema, telangiectasia, papules, and tiny pustules. Stage III is persistent deep erythema, dense telangiectasia, papules, pustules, nodules, and, rarely, persistent solid edema of the central portion of the face.

Laboratory and Diagnostic Procedures and Medical Management

Diagnosis of acne rosacea is based on the patient's history and physical findings. A history of episodic flushing in response to hot fluids orally, spicy foods, alcohol, or sun exposure is common. Physical findings include the presence of the characteristics listed in the previous section. There is an absence of comedones. First-line treatment of rosacea typically includes azelaic acid (finacea) with oral doxycycline (see the Pharmacology box, p. 1845). Maintenance management with azelaic acid topically is usually sufficient. Second-line treatment may include topical erythromycin, topical clindamycin, tacrolimus or pimecrolimus, or permethrin 5% cream. For severe cases, isotretinoin is prescribed orally for 4 months. Topical steroids may aggravate rosacea. Patients should be instructed to use a mild, nondrying soap and avoid local irritants. Oil-based cosmetics, alcohol consumption, excessive sun exposure, and hot drinks should also be avoided. New therapies are being explored, including laser therapy and electrodessication or chemical sclerosis of dilated blood vessels (Domino et al., 2012).

Impact of Lifestyle Choices on Skin

Skin Changes Related to Tobacco Smoking

Smoking has a negative effect on the skin, causing it to age prematurely. It leads to vasoconstriction, which decreases the blood supply and nutrients delivered to the skin; it also breaks down the elastin, which leads to wrinkles. There is evidence that facial wrinkling is associated with the number of pack-years smoked (Lowell, 2011).

Skin Changes Related to Cultural Practices

Cultural practices can affect the skin's health. For example, pomade acne is common in African Americans and Hispanics. This disorder is a form of acne caused by the use of grooming products on the scalp spreading to the forehead. These grooming agents contain substances that can lead to acne, such as lanolins and isopropyl myristate. Capsaicin-induced dermatitis is seen in Hispanic people. This condition, caused by handling hot chili peppers with bare hands, leads to erythema, burning pain, and irritation.

Some alternative medicine practices lead to the formation of dermatologic lesions. For example, coin rubbing is an Asian practice done to relieve symptoms of the flu, fever, and headaches. In this practice, a coin or a similar object is used to scrape the skin, causing ecchymotic streaks. The scraping usually occurs between the ribs, along the inner aspects of both arms, and along both sides of the spine.

Cupping, another cultural practice that is done to treat pain, involves soaking a cotton ball in alcohol and igniting it. The cotton ball is then placed in a cup or jar, which is inverted and placed on the skin. This is usually done symmetrically in rows of two to four cups. Once the jar is placed on the skin, a vacuum is created, and the flame goes out. This vacuum pulls the skin into the cup or jar, leading to painful circular, ecchymotic burns. Moxibustion is a cultural practice that involves igniting dry weeds or incense like material and applying the lit tip to acupuncture sites. This practice, which is used to treat a variety of disorders, may be confused with abuse and should be considered as a possibility in assessing skin disorders.

Skin Changes Related to Tattoos

A tattoo is defined as a permanent mark or design made on skin by inserting ink or dye via a needle into the dermal layer of the skin with repeated punctures. Tattoos may be pictures or words applied anywhere on the body. Permanent makeup applied to the eyes and lips is also considered to be tattoos. The needle is connected to a small machine with tubes containing dye that apply repeated piercing to the skin, much like the action of a sewing machine. The process, which can take several hours for a large tattoo, causes a small amount of bleeding and minor to potentially significant pain.

Tattooing is an increasingly popular practice; however, it is not without health risks. The skin integrity is altered, which means the individual is susceptible to skin reactions and infections. The most common infections following tattooing are caused by *Staphylococcus aureus*, which may be a result of poor hygiene on the part of either the provider or the customer, both during and after the procedure. With unlicensed tattoo artists who do not follow proper infection control procedures, there is increased risk for potentially serious antibiotic-resistant skin infections such as community-acquired methicillin-resistant *S. aureus* (Mayo Clinic, 2012). Typical signs and symptoms of an infection include redness, warmth, swelling, and a puslike drainage. Some antibiotic-resistant skin infections can lead to pneumonia, bloodstream infections, and necrotizing fasciitis.

Some degree of bleeding is inevitable during the tattooing process; therefore, the transmission of bloodborne pathogens is possible. If the equipment used to create the tattoo is contaminated with the blood of an infected person, it is possible to contract a number of serious bloodborne diseases. Bloodborne pathogen transmission is associated with the reuse of tattoo needles without proper and adequate sterilization. It is also possible that the electric equipment itself may be contaminated. Infection with hepatitis B virus is a well-documented post-tattoo complication. Other infections include hepatitis C, tetanus, tuberculosis, and the human immunodeficiency virus, the virus that causes AIDS (Mayo Clinic, 2012).

Safety Alert *Instructions to individuals who are planning to have either a tattoo or body piercing need to include having to question the health standards of the establishment. Many local health departments have sanitation guidelines for tattoo and body piercing establishments. However,*

Weblink: Tattoo

some states, such as the Commonwealth of Pennsylvania, have no licensing requirements for tattoo artists (Carpenter, 2011).

Tattoo dyes can cause allergic skin reactions, resulting in an itchy rash at the tattoo site. Red ink is most commonly associated with allergic reactions, although any color of ink may cause an allergic reaction in sensitive patients. Some allergic reactions may take years to develop; therefore, the nurse should query patients about old tattoos as well as newer ones during assessment. Additionally, granulomas may form around the tattoo ink, especially the red ink. Tattooing can also cause keloid scar formation if the individual is prone to them (Mayo Clinic, 2012). Tattoo ink may contain heavy metals, alcohols, ethylene glycol (automobile antifreeze), formaldehyde, glutaraldehyde, ferrocyanides, aluminum, mercury, cadmium, cobalt, chromium, and lead. Tattoo "inks" may also be homemade and therefore may be composed of any number of potential toxins and/or allergens (County of Kern: Department of Health Services, 2007).

Due to the makeup of the dye or ink used in tattoos, it can cause a reaction during a magnetic resonance imaging (MRI) scan. Although it happens rarely, tattoos or permanent makeup may cause swelling or burning in the affected areas during the MRI process. In some cases, when the scan is in the immediate area of the dye such as the eye, tattoo pigments may interfere with the quality of the image (Mayo Clinic, 2012).

Care of the tattoo includes regular cleaning with soap and water and applying moisturizer. The person should avoid exposure to sunlight for the first few weeks after receiving a tattoo. Tattoos may take up to several days to heal. The individual needs to be instructed not to pick at a scab, which increases the risk of infection, can damage the design, and increases the risk of scar formation.

Tattoo removal is possible, although complete removal is difficult and skin color variations and scarring are likely to remain. Methods of removal include the following:

- Laser surgery is the most effective way to reduce the appearance of a tattoo. Pulses of laser light pass through the top layer of skin, and the energy of the light is absorbed by the pigment in the tattoo. This process creates a very low grade of inflammation and allows the body to shed small areas of altered pigment. It requires repeated treatments over time to lighten the tattoo, and the treatment might not completely erase it.
- Dermabrasion uses a sanding process to remove the outer layer of skin and lighten the tattoo.
- Surgical removal involves cutting out the tattoo and surgically closing the open area, leaving a scar.

Skin Changes Related to Body Piercing

Body piercing involves creating a hole in a body part for the purpose of inserting jewelry. The most common body piercing areas are the lobe and other areas of the ear, nose, eyebrow, lip, tongue, and navel. Body piercing has risks similar to those of tattoos, although due to improvements in safety procedures and equipment, the popular practice of earlobe piercing is viewed as generally less risky than other body piercing. A single-use, sterilized ear piercing device or an ear piercing gun with sterilized, disposable cartridges may be the safest method (Mayo Clinic, 2012). Some practitioners use a reusable piercing gun for these types of piercings, which is difficult to sterilize and can more easily damage the skin. The most common infections associated with "gun"-type ear piercing are *S. aureus* and *P. aeruginosa* (County of Kern: Department of Health Services, 2007). In addition, there are risks any time the skin is punctured, including the following:

- Bloodborne diseases may occur if the equipment used to do the piercing is contaminated with the blood of an infected person. There is a risk for contracting hepatitis C, hepatitis B, tetanus, tuberculosis, and HIV.
- Allergic reactions may occur if the jewelry is made of nickel or brass.
- Oral complications that may occur with jewelry worn in a tongue piercing include infection, chipped and cracked teeth, and damaged gums.
- Clinical manifestations of skin infections include redness, swelling, pain, and a puslike discharge.
- Infections from piercing in the upper ear cartilage are especially serious. Antibiotics are often ineffective. Because cartilage does not have its own blood supply, the drug cannot reach the infection site. Such infection can lead to cartilage damage and serious, permanent ear deformity.
- Body piercing can cause scarring; if the individual is susceptible, piercing can cause keloid scar formation (discussed in Chapter 61).

Postprocedure care for the pierced area depends on the body part pierced. Oral piercing (tongue or lip) includes instructing the individual to rinse the mouth with an antibacterial, alcohol-free mouth rinse for 30 to 60 seconds after meals until the piercing heals. A new soft-bristled toothbrush should be used to avoid introducing bacteria into the mouth. Piercings of the nose, ears, eyebrow, and navel need to be cleaned gently with warm water and an antibiotic cleanser to remove any crusting. The jewelry should be gently turned back and forth to work the cleanser around the opening. Avoid alcohol and peroxide, which can dry the skin; in addition, do not apply ointments, as they keep oxygen from reaching the piercing and can leave a sticky residue (Mayo Clinic, 2012). The piercing site will heal over without the jewelry in place.

Health Promotion

Certain inherent risks, described earlier, are associated with body piercing and tattooing. However, the nurse can improve safety by advising the patient to do the following:

- Discuss the sterilization techniques by inquiring about the use of an autoclave. Request to see it in operation. If none is used, go elsewhere.
- Discuss the sterilization of jewelry and instruments such as ink pouches with intact color-change seals. If possible, ask to see the packaged sterilized instruments.
- Ask whether excess tattoo ink is being poured back into the main supply.
- Follow all after-care instructions and report complications, including redness, swelling, pain, or discharge, to a health care provider immediately.

Skin Changes Related to Sunlight

Ultraviolet (UV) rays, radiation that comes from the sun, penetrate and change skin cells. Ultraviolet rays are also emitted from tanning beds

CHART 59–6 Common Descriptions of Skin Types for Anticipating Sunburn

Type	Description
Type I	Always burns, never tans
Type II	Burns easily, tans minimally
Type III	Burns moderately, tans gradually
Type IV	Burns minimally, tans well
Type V	Rarely burns, tans profusely
Type VI	Never burns, deeply pigmented

Source: Adapted from Centers for Disease Control and Prevention (CDC). (2012a). Basic information about skin cancer. Retrieved from http://www.cdc.gov/cancer/skin/basic_info/index.htm#uv

and sunlamps. There are three types of UV rays: ultraviolet A (UVA), ultraviolet B (UVB), and ultraviolet C (UVC). Ultraviolet A, the most common kind of radiation at Earth's surface, reaches beyond the top layer of human skin. Scientists believe that UVA rays can damage connective tissue and increase a person's risk of skin cancer. Most UVB rays are absorbed by the ozone layer, and are therefore less common at Earth's surface than UVA rays. In addition, UVB rays don't reach as far into the skin as UVA rays, but they can still be damaging. Likewise, UVC rays are very dangerous, but they are absorbed by the ozone layer and do not reach the ground (CDC, 2012b).

The sun can irritate and damage the skin, with most of the damage occurring before the age of 18. Nearly 80% of this damage can be prevented if sunscreen is applied properly in those first 18 years of life (Samuel, Brooke, Hollis, & Griffiths, 2005). Recognizable changes occur with years of exposure to ultraviolet radiation due to repetitive tanning and sunburning. The potential for sunburn varies with skin type. Chart 59–6 lists the common descriptions of skin types and their potential for sunburn. The superficial dermis that is damaged by the sun demonstrates a breakdown of collagen and an accumulation of abnormal elastin, which lead to wrinkling and lack of resilience in the skin. When the sun damages the skin, DNA production is impaired. DNA is needed for maintenance of the skin's genetic integrity. Therefore, impaired DNA production can lead to skin cancer and immune suppression. Sunlight also is considered a major cause of skin cancer, especially when the skin is repeatedly sunburned. Various skin cancers are discussed in this chapter. The prevention of skin cancer is the 2010 objective of *Healthy People 2020* (U.S. Department of Health and Human Services, 2012). The National Guidelines box lists the Centers for Disease Control and Prevention's guidelines related to skin cancer and protection of the skin from the sun. Skin cancer is discussed in detail later in the chapter.

Health Promotion

The best way to avoid the damage created by the sun is to avoid the sun, wear sunscreen, and wear protective clothing when in the sun. The amount of time spent in the sun at midday should be limited. Sunscreens should contain avobenzone, dioxybenzone, oxybenzone, titanium dioxide, or zinc oxide for the best protection from both ultraviolet A (UVA) and ultraviolet B (UVB) rays. A sun protection factor (SPF) rates sunscreens. The higher the SPF rating the sunscreen has, the greater the protection. The current recommendation is an SPF of 15 (CDC, 2012). Generous layers of sunscreen should be applied with special attention paid to areas often neglected such as the neck, temples, and ears. Sunscreen can be diluted or rinsed off completely by sweat, water immersion, or rubbing. Therefore, it should be reapplied often. The Centers for Disease Control and Prevention outlines options for protection from ultraviolet radiation (Chart 59–7).

NATIONAL GUIDELINES for Skin Cancer Prevention

1. *Policy:* Establish policies that reduce exposure to UV radiation.
2. *Environment:* Provide and maintain physical and social environments that support sun safety and are consistent with the development of other healthy habits.
3. *Education:* Provide health education to teach students the knowledge, attitudes, and behavioral skills they need to prevent skin cancer. This education should be age-appropriate and linked to opportunities for practicing sun-safe behaviors.
4. *Families:* Involve family members in skin cancer prevention efforts.
5. *Professional Development:* Include skin cancer prevention knowledge and skills in preservice and inservice education for school administrators, teachers, physical education teachers and coaches, school nurses, and others who work with students.
6. *Health Services.* Complement and support skin cancer prevention with school health services.
7. *Evaluation:* Periodically evaluate whether schools are implementing the skin cancer prevention guidelines. They should be evaluated on policies, environment, education, family involvement, professional development, and health services.

Source: Adapted from:Centers for Disease Control and Prevention (CDC). (2012a). Basic information about skin cancer. Retrieved from http://www.cdc.gov/cancer/skin/basic_info/index.htm#uv.

Safety Alert *When spending time in the sun, it is important to use a sunscreen with a sun protection factor (SPF) of 15 to 30 and to reapply sunscreen often. Sunscreen should be applied 30 minutes prior to sun exposure.*

Nonmalignant Disorders Related to Sun Exposure

Exposure to the sun leads to damaged, abnormal skin cells that can be premalignant. Lesions related to these disorders are generally found on areas of the skin exposed to the sun. Photodermatitis and actinic keratosis (p. 1878) are both skin disorders related to skin exposure to the sun.

CHART 59–7 CDC Recommendations for Protection from UV Radiation

- Seek shade, especially during midday hours.
- Wear clothing to protect exposed skin.
- Wear a hat with a wide brim to shade the face, head, ears, and neck.
- Wear sunglasses that wrap around and block as close to 100% of both UVA and UVB rays as possible.
- Use a sunscreen with sun protective factor (SPF) of 15 or higher that offers both UVA and UVBUVA and UVB protection.
- Avoid indoor tanning.

Source: Adopted from Centers for Disease Control and Prevention (CDC). (2012b). Skin cancer prevention. Retrieved from http://www.cdc.gov/cancer/skin/basic_info/prevention.htm.

COSMETIC PROCEDURES

Cosmetic surgery is done to enhance the attractiveness of certain normal features related to the skin and its underlying structures. Cosmetic surgery includes reshaping of the nose, body contouring, breast surgery, and facial rejuvenation for the aging process such as resurfacing or tightening of the skin. Reconstructive surgery, by contrast, is performed on those who may have deformities related to cancer, congenital abnormalities, disease, and structural and/or traumatic injuries that result in functional disabilities or abnormal appearance. Congenital deformities include prominent ears, cleft lip and palate deformities, and congenital nevi.

Cosmetic surgery is individualized depending on the individual's race or ethnicity. For example, darker-skinned non-Caucasian individuals present a unique set of needs separate from those of Caucasians. The Cultural Considerations box outlines concerns related to ethnic skin and cosmetic surgery. Today, many surgical procedures can be done to correct skin-related problems for all ethnic groups, and a number of them are discussed next.

Laser Surgery

The laser has been used for treating wrinkles, acne, nevi, seborrheic keratosis, actinic keratosis, hemangiomas, tattoos, scars, and unwanted hair. There are many different types of lasers, but the basic principle is that a laser light generates heat that is absorbed into the skin. Different types of tissue will absorb only specific laser wavelengths; thus, the choice of the laser depends on the type of tissue being treated and the problem. The laser beam focused on the skin quickly heats and leads to resurfacing of only the area being treated. Most lasers are used in private offices and small surgical suites under no anesthesia or only local anesthesia. However, the deeper procedures involving greater surface areas may need general anesthesia.

Preoperative preparation of the patient involves detailed teaching about what is involved and what can be expected from the treatments. Depending on the type of laser used, the condition being treated, and the depth of the treatment, treatments may include up to 3 to 5 sessions occurring biweekly or monthly. Improvement occurs on a continuous basis for up to 6 months after the treatments have been completed. After the procedure, there will be mild to severe localized erythema and swelling at the site of the treatment. Again, depending on the depth of the treatment area, there may be mild to moderate discomfort with the skin feeling dry and tingly for up to a few months. Complications postoperatively are rare but include permanent erythema, edema, acne formation, contact dermatitis, pruritus, infections, and pigmentary alterations.

Rhytidectomy

Rhytidectomy is surgery on the skin to eliminate wrinkles and improve the appearance of the face. It is also referred to as "facial rejuvenation" or "face-lift." The purpose of a rhytidectomy is to reverse the anatomic signs of aging in the facial area. The patient will continue to look younger than his actual age by approximately 10 years for the rest of his life. The rhytidectomy is becoming more common with people wanting natural-looking results because physical appearance is important in how individuals are perceived by others. Appearance also is linked to body image, self-esteem, and confidence. The lines on the face help communicate feelings that occur when interacting with others. Therefore, a youthful appearance may affect an individual in social and professional arenas. Surgery cannot reverse all the effects of aging, but it can reposition tissues and redistribute volume to create a more youthful and rested appearance. The normal facial changes caused by aging are listed in the Gerontological Considerations section on page 1884.

Several anatomic areas can be improved as a part of the rhytidectomy, including the forehead and eyebrows, nasolabial folds, jowls, skin and the platysma muscle of the neck, and malar fat pads. It is important for the surgeon to identify what the patient's expectations are and to discuss what can and cannot be accomplished, so that the expectations are realistic.

Rhytidectomy can be performed with either local anesthesia and conscious sedation, or general anesthesia. The incisions are made at or within the hairlines, behind the ears, or in natural skin creases so that the scars are less noticeable. Typically this procedure is done on an outpatient basis, although in some instances a surgeon may opt to keep a patient hospitalized the first night. There may be drains and padded dressings to protect the face, and swelling of the face and eyelids is present postoperatively, being the most severe at about the second postoperative day. Complications are rare but may include hematoma, infection, asymmetry, skin necrosis, transient facial weakness, and permanent loss of sensation. With makeup, patients are able to hide the bruising and scars in about 1 to 2 weeks. Figure 59–8◆ demonstrates before and after pictures.

CULTURAL CONSIDERATIONS for Cosmetic Surgery

Darker-skinned individuals are less prone to the signs of aging due to the photoprotective nature of the melanin in darker skin. However, sometimes people of different cultures elect to undergo cosmetic surgery. It is important to understand that the ethnic characteristics of the facial features need to be maintained. Darker skin types are more prone to changes in pigmentation of the skin and scarring; therefore, those concerns also need to be considered when planning the surgery.

Blepharoplasty

Blepharoplasty is a surgical procedure performed to remove the excess skin and fat, and occasionally a portion of the orbicularis oculi muscle, around the eye. With aging, the relocation of fat, loss of skin elasticity, and excess muscle around the eye can interfere with vision or cause an unwanted appearance. A blepharoplasty can be done alone or along with a face-lift or brow lift. Local anesthetic and conscious sedation is usually enough to allow the procedure to be performed. There is some swelling and bruising at the site that will subside in about 10 to 14 days. Complications are unusual but include bleeding, hematoma formation, epidermal inclusion cysts of the incisions, ectropion, infection, and asymmetry.

Rhinoplasty

Rhinoplasty is the surgical alteration of nasal structures, which usually includes the bone and cartilage. It is performed for cosmetic reasons and is often done at the same time as surgical procedures to correct functional problems associated with the obstruction of the nasal passages. Rhinoplasty also is performed for reconstructive conditions such as abnormalities associated with cleft lip and palate deformities or nasal trauma. Rhinoplasty is considered one of the most difficult surgical procedures a plastic surgeon performs. It requires consideration of a myriad of anatomic factors as well as psychological and ethnic factors.

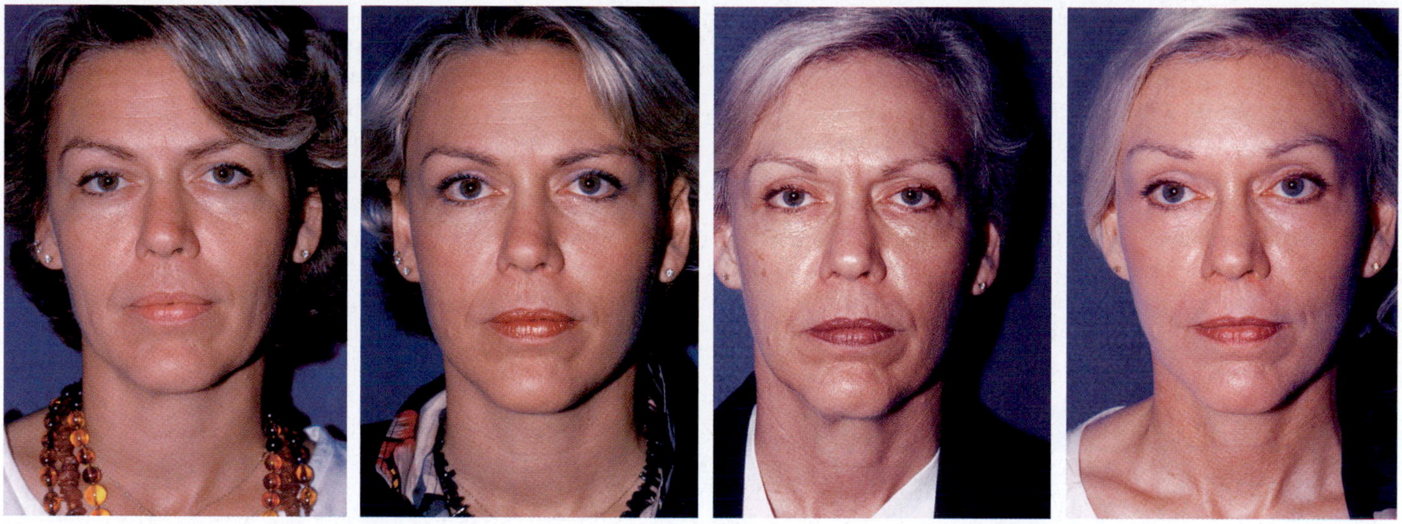
(a) (b) (c) (d)

FIGURE 59–8 ◆ Rhytidectomy. Same patient, different ages. (a) and (b): Age 40 years, before and after rhytidectomy and blepharoplasty; (c) and (d): Age 54 years, before and after rhytidectomy and brow lift.
Source: Courtesy of John M. Osborn, MD, FACS, Plastic Surgery Center, Sacramento, CA.

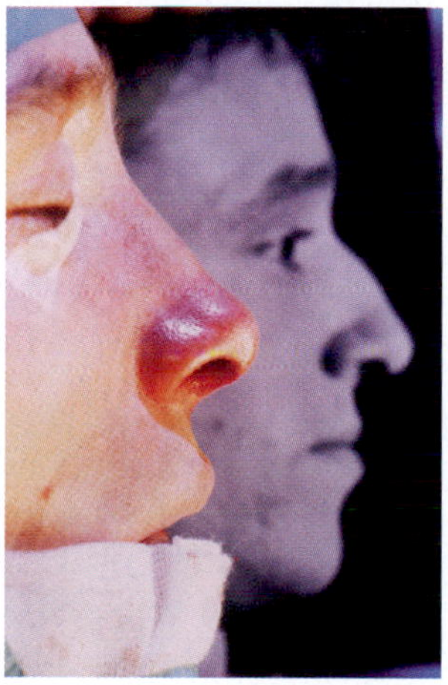

FIGURE 59–9 ◆ Before and after a rhinoplasty.
Source: BSIP SA/Alamy.

Rhinoplasty can be performed under local or general anesthesia, using topical and injectable vasoconstrictors and anesthetic agents. The patient may or may not be hospitalized. The nose will be packed postoperatively for a few days to prevent bleeding and support the nasal structures, and an exterior nasal splint is applied for about a week to a week and a half. There is swelling and periorbital bruising that takes about 2 weeks to subside. However, it takes up to a year for all swelling and sensation to stabilize and to appreciate the final result. This procedure has an increased incidence of needing a secondary procedure to achieve the best result, which is usually done after a year. Figure 59–9◆ shows an individual before and after a rhinoplasty.

Preoperatively, it is important to assess the patient's motivation and desires. An assessment should be made of what the patient's expectations are for the procedure and whether these can be met considering the patient's unique anatomy. Some surgeons perform computer imaging to allow the patient to visualize the results of the surgery preoperatively. It is also important to note anything in the patient's history that could affect the outcomes of the surgery. Prior nasal trauma or surgery, sinus or allergy disease, systemic illnesses, medication abuse, respiratory impairments, and emotional stability are examples of factors that need to be evaluated. The surgeon also should consider the patient's ethnicity. The noses of many African American, Hispanic, and Asian patients may look different from the noses of people of other ethnic groups and will require individualized approaches and goals for surgery.

Postoperative complications from rhinoplasty are rare but may include epistaxis, infection, prolonged edema, nasal airway obstruction, and an unsatisfactory cosmetic result. Rhinoplasty is commonly performed and is considered safe and effective.

Abdominoplasty

An abdominoplasty is performed to remove excess skin and fat from the lower abdomen and to tighten the muscles of the abdominal cavity. Usually as a result of pregnancy, but also as a result of obesity and the accumulation of intra-abdominal fat, the rectus abdominis muscles separate in the midline, causing a weakness in the muscular support of the abdominal contents. The surgery consists of making an incision across the lower abdomen just above the symphysis pubis out to and sometimes beyond the anterior iliac crest. The skin and adipose tissue are undermined over the abdominal muscles to the level of the lower sternum and the medial ribs, creating a skin and fat flap. The umbilical stalk is left intact but separated from the surrounding skin during the dissection. The muscles are then plicated (sewn together) in the midline to tighten the abdominal musculature and support the abdominal contents. The overlying skin and fat are then redraped inferiorly, and the excess skin and fat are excised. The umbilicus is then reattached through a new hole created in the skin above it, and the skin inferiorly is closed, leaving a scar across the lower abdomen and around the umbilicus.

Dermabrasion

Dermabrasion is the process of removing the epidermis and the outer portion of the dermis, creating a partial-thickness skin loss. The purpose of this procedure is to allow new skin to regenerate into a smoother surface. See Chapter 61 for a complete description of a partial-thickness injury. Dermabrasion is used to improve scars, fine wrinkles, sun spots, and areas of hyperpigmentation. A diamond fraise cylinder that has abrasive properties is used to perform the procedure, thus allowing for regrowth of new skin over the abraded area. This procedure is generally limited to use on the face, and either local or general anesthesia is necessary. An open wound is created, which eventually heals in about 7 to 14 days depending on the depth of the abrasion. The patient may need to apply an emollient during this time. Complications include infection, changes in skin color, and scarring. Patients have generally reported being very satisfied with the outcome of the procedure when it has been realistically presented preoperatively.

Microdermabrasion

Microdermabrasion is a skin-freshening technique that helps repair skin that has been damaged by the sun and the effects of aging. The purpose of the procedure is much the same as that of dermabrasion, but microdermabrasion is not as deep and is used to improve scars, fine wrinkles, and hyperpigmentation. The back of the hands and the face are common areas that benefit from this procedure. A plastic surgeon or esthetician uses a device like a fine sandblaster to spray tiny crystals across the skin, mixing gentle abrasion with suction to remove the dead outer layer of skin. More than one treatment may be needed to reduce or remove fine wrinkles and unwanted pigmentation. No anesthesia is necessary, although the patient may describe a feeling of warmth and throbbing afterward. The skin remains reddened and dry for approximately 4 to 5 days. The patient is instructed to use moisturizers; in addition, long-term use of sunscreens is necessary because the abraded area is more sensitive to burning. If performed properly, complications from this procedure are extremely rare.

Injectable Tissue Fillers

A loss of facial fullness and the development of wrinkles occur as part of the aging process. A nonsurgical treatment to soften these facial lines and help restore volume and facial contours is injectable fillers. These fillers also are used to treat scars, sun-damaged skin, and thin lips. Outlined here are the different types of tissue fillers on the market:

- Collagen is a natural protein that supports the skin. The two sources are human and bovine collagen. The use of bovine collagen requires prior allergy testing. The results may last 2 to 4 months.
- Hyaluronic acid, a natural substance found in human bodies, is used to enhance lips and fill facial creases such as nasolabial folds. It may also be appropriate for some surface wrinkles and concave scars. The results may last 6 months or longer.
- Hydroxyapatite is a mineral-like compound found naturally in human bones, suspended in a gel-like formulation. It is the heaviest of facial fillers and is recommended to fill deeper creases such as nasolabial folds and frown lines, as well as to enhance the fullness of the cheeks and other facial contours.
- Human fat, harvested from the patient's own body, can be injected to enhance facial fullness, fill deep creases, and build up shallow contours. Fat injection requires a more extensive procedure than injection of other fillers because it uses liposuction techniques to extract the fat used for injection. Treatment can last up to a year or more in some cases, and results are highly variable. Fat can be stored for future treatment, although the results from the use of preserved fat are not as favorable.

All tissue fillers except fat are injected by either a health care provider or a specially trained nurse. Fat injections are done solely by a health care provider because the fat needs to be harvested by liposuction. Prior to the injection, the site is cleaned by an antibacterial agent, and icing or a topical numbing agent may be offered to make patients more comfortable. Some tissue fillers contain an anesthetic agent. In other cases, local anesthetic may be administered to the treatment site.

Complications from fillers are uncommon, and the risks vary depending on the specific filler used and the relative permanence of the filler substance. Complications outlined by the American Society of Plastic Surgeons (ASPS) (2007) include the following:

- Infection at the injection site
- Development of nodules that may require surgical excision
- Acne-like skin eruptions
- Antibody reaction to filler material that may reduce the effectiveness of future injections
- Facial asymmetry
- Bleeding, bruising, and swelling
- Temporary paralysis of other muscle groups or other unintended effects due to migration of the filler material from the original site
- Skin necrosis
- Skin rash, itching, and swelling
- Skin redness
- Skin sensitivity
- Under- or overcorrection of defects.

Botulinum Injections

Botulinum toxin type A (Botox) is a purified protein complex derived from the bacterium *Clostridium botulinum*. Once injected into the muscle, it blocks the release of chemical acetylcholine, thereby temporarily paralyzing the muscles (ASPS, 2007). It is currently being used as a safe and effective cosmetic agent to temporarily improve frown lines between the eyebrows (glabellar lines), forehead creases, laugh-line wrinkles near the eyes, and thick bands in the neck. Botox also can be used to combat migraine headaches and to treat hyperhidrosis (excessive perspiration). A new and still evolving role for Botox is that of a pain reliever for mastectomy patients. Women injected with Botox in the pectoral muscles following the surgical removal of their breast experienced significantly less pain and shorter hospital stays (ASPS, 2007).

Liposuction

Liposuction, a form of body sculpturing or body contouring, is one of the most common cosmetic surgeries performed. Depending on the elasticity of the skin, it can be performed on anyone after the age of 16. Older patients with less elasticity are poorer candidates than younger patients and need to be realistic about their expectations. The purpose of liposuction is to remove subcutaneous fat in diet-resistant areas of the body that are out of proportion. Liposuction is not viewed as a treatment for obesity but can help contour the body of someone with normal body weight and good skin tone but localized areas of fat accumulation. Patients need to be evaluated and instructed preoperatively so that unrealistic expectations will not be an issue.

Tumescent liposuction involves infiltrating diluted lidocaine and epinephrine into the subcutaneous tissue to provide anesthesia prior to the actual liposuction. Therefore, general anesthesia is not required but may be used along with the infiltrate at the discretion of the patient or the surgeon. Tumescent liposuction allows for the aspiration of a higher amount of fat and a smaller amount of blood. Prior to the procedure, the areas to be removed are marked while the patient is in an upright position, because fat tends to shift when the patient is horizontal and sedated. The diluted mixture of lidocaine and epinephrine is injected into the site to provide anesthesia, cause vasoconstriction, and allow for greater volumes of fat to be aspirated. A small cannula is then inserted through a 2- to 10-millimeter incision and advanced throughout the fat using back-and-forth movements. The fat is mechanically broken up, and tunnels are created. The loosened fat is then removed using suction. The average amount suctioned is between 2 and 3 liters, although any amount up to 10 liters may be aspirated. Any patient who has over 5 liters aspirated should remain in an overnight care facility for observation of possible vascular complications and hemodynamic compromise. The risk of complications from this procedure is relatively small. The most common complications include contour irregularities, the development of a hematoma or seroma, transient numbness, asymmetry, and persistent postoperative edema. Postoperatively, patients are usually discharged home once they are stable. Compression dressings are worn over the areas treated to compress the tunnels created by the cannula, to ensure a more even result, to prevent fluid from collecting in the tunnels, and to increase patient comfort. Recovery is rapid with most discomfort resolved within 5 days, although the compression dressings are used from 1 to 6 weeks postoperatively.

Patients are generally satisfied with the results and are able to maintain the fat loss. With weight gain, some fat buildup in the treated areas will occur, but the gain will be in the same proportion as the gain in the rest of the body. Fat cells enlarge with weight gain and do not multiply.

Panniculectomy

A **panniculectomy** is the surgical excision of excess skin and fat that hang over the pubic area as a skin apron, most commonly following excessive weight loss. With this procedure there is no undermining of the skin and fat and no plication of the muscles, as described for abdominoplasty. A panniculectomy is usually performed to reduce strain on the back and to prevent intertrigo rashes that form under the apron between the skin layers. With the increasing popularity of bariatric surgical procedures, this procedure is becoming more common; and when it is performed for functional versus cosmetic reasons, it is usually covered financially by insurance carriers. Bariatric surgery is described in detail in Chapter 8.

Nursing Management

Dermatologic surgery is generally an elective procedure that may be done in the outpatient setting or as an inpatient, depending on the patient and the procedure. The patient undergoing this surgery has generally had several discussions with the surgeon about the procedure, its possible complications, and the patient's expectations. The patient's needs are very much like the needs of any patient undergoing surgery. Chapters 17, 18, and 19 discuss the patient's preoperative, intraoperative, and postoperative needs.

Immediately after surgery, the patient will be monitored in a postanesthesia care unit (PACU) for complications related to the surgery and anesthesia. Chapters 18 and 19 discuss patient care in the PACU. Depending on the type of surgery, there may be a pressure dressing to prevent bleeding and decrease edema. The nurse will need to check the dressings frequently for bleeding and to monitor the patient for signs of hemorrhage, such as increased pulse rate, decreased blood pressure, or changes in level of consciousness. The patient also may have drains in place that the nurse will need to monitor for amount and color of drainage. The patient needs to be kept comfortable. This may require special positioning and pain medication.

The nurse will need to teach the patient about treatments or care of the incision at home. The patient should be instructed not to remove scabs and to keep the incisions clean and dry. Any redness, increased warmth, or drainage should be reported to the surgeon.

Postoperative care for the abdominoplasty or panniculectomy includes instructing the patient to minimize tension on the suture line by sleeping in a semi-Fowler's position, not lifting heavy objects, and avoiding strenuous exercise. The nurse should instruct the patient not to smoke tobacco, as it constricts blood vessels. This diminishes the blood supply needed for wound healing. It is essential to teach pain management techniques such as splinting the wound when coughing, walking in a hunched over position, and consistent use of pain medications. It also is important to discuss the clinical manifestations of wound infection, which include wound separation, drainage, redness, increased pain, and fever. The nurse must stress to the patient what signs and symptoms need to be reported to the surgeon.

Health Promotion

The patient undergoing cosmetic surgery and the patient's family will need teaching related to the type and extent of surgery. Specific instructions should be given related to the type of incision, length of surgery, length of recovery, and possible complications. Although the surgeon will generally provide the patient with this information, it is important that the nurse reinforce and clarify that the patient understands the information. The patient needs to be aware of any postoperative limitations or special care needs.

There may be special preoperative preparations. For example, patients need to be instructed to wash their hair and face with antibacterial soap several times to decrease the bacterial count. The patient should be instructed not to ingest aspirin, ibuprofen, or other platelet-coating drugs for at least 2 weeks before and after surgery because of the increased risk of bleeding. The patient will need a physical examination and routine diagnostic laboratory tests prior to surgery to assess physical readiness for anesthesia. Chapter 17 discusses preoperative instructions in detail. The patient should be prepared psychologically for postoperative edema and discoloration. Due to this bruising and edema, the true effects of the surgery cannot be evaluated for several weeks.

NEOPLASTIC SKIN DISORDERS

Skin disorders may result in a variety of skin lesions with multiple configurations, signs, and symptoms. Skin disorders can be benign or malignant, due to infectious agents, and/or from infestations by insects. It is important for the nurse to assess these lesions, as well as their characteristics, location, exudates, and distribution on the body. New skin lesions may appear as a part of the aging process.

Benign Neoplasms

Benign skin disorders include those that are not carcinogenic. Most often, these disorders are painless and asymptomatic. Any abnormal growth on the skin is of concern to a patient; therefore, it is essential that the nurse thoroughly evaluate and report skin changes. Common benign skin disorders are discussed next.

Photodermatitis

Etiology, Epidemiology, and Pathophysiology

Photodermatitis, an inflammatory adverse reaction to sunlight, is a common hypersensitivity to sun in which the individual sunburns more easily than usual or develops papular or vesicular lesions with exposure to the sun. It can occur in all ages and races but is most common in young women. This condition can be a true immunologic reaction that can be genetically determined. It also may occur because of the use of certain medications, in association with certain diseases, or with the use of contact agents that increase photosensitivity, such as those listed in Chart 59–8.

Clinical Manifestations

Clinically, patients develop an erythematous, papular rash that burns and itches. The rash may become vesicular with oozing and edema. It is accompanied by systemic symptoms such as pain, fever, malaise, chills, headache, and nausea. The rash occurs on areas that have been exposed to the sun and persists for 7 to 10 days. Treatment consists of protection from the sun and management of the clinical manifestations.

Actinic Keratosis

Actinic keratosis lesions occur commonly after age 40 and are found on sun-exposed areas of the head, neck, arms, legs, tops of ears, and dorsal hands. **Actinic keratosis** lesions begin as hyperemic, poorly defined lesions and develop into scaly, rough, skin-colored macules with rough surfaces. Actinic keratosis is considered a premalignant lesion that may develop into squamous cell carcinoma. These lesions can be treated with topical 5-fluorouracil cream or solution, cryosurgery, or liquid nitrogen. They can also be treated with Aldara, which is thought to stimulate the immune system to remove these precancerous lesions. The patients will need instructions about sun protection measures for the remainder of their lives.

CHART 59–8 Agents Associated with Photosensitivity

Amiodarone	Oral contraceptives
Antipsychotic agents	Phenothiazines
Barbiturates	Phenylbutazone
Benzodiazepines	Piroxicam
Carbamazepine	Promethazine
Chlorothiazide	Protriptyline
Coal tar	Psoralens
Dacarbazine	Quinidine/quinine
5-Fluorouracil	Retinoids
Furosemide	Simvastatin
Griseofulvin	Sulfonamides
Hypoglycemic agent	Sulfonylureas
Ketoprofen	Sulindac
Methotrexate	Tetracyclines
Mitomycin C	Thiazides
Nalidixic acid	Tricyclics
NSAIDs	

Hemangiomas

Hemangiomas, vascular abnormalities of the skin, form from the rapid growth of endothelial cells, which results in the formation of extra blood vessels. Approximately 30% of all hemangiomas are visible at birth. They grow with the child; then most begin to shrink or involute during childhood. Hemangiomas may be classified by depth, clinical appearance, and location. Superficial lesions, often called strawberry hemangiomas, become bright red in color and elevated with capillary projections that give the strawberry appearance. Cavernous hemangiomas are present at birth and have larger and more mature vessels within the lesion. These lesions appear bluish red and have less distinct borders. Some hemangiomas are mixed. Up to 85% to 90% of hemangiomas will spontaneously resolve by age 9 (Nicol & Huether, 2007).

Moles or Nevi

Moles or **nevi** are common skin lesions that appear on almost everyone; they may occur in almost any location but are more common in sun-exposed areas. They can be present at birth or can be acquired as an individual grows, although new ones usually do not appear after age 40. Moles are usually asymptomatic but can be irritated by clothing or trauma. The various types of moles are described in Chart 59–9. Moles are generally considered harmless but may become malignant and need to be evaluated periodically. Changes in the mole's color, diameter, or border need to be reported to the health care provider, as these changes could indicate a premalignant or malignant change.

Skin Tags

Skin tags are flesh-colored or brown papules that grow on a thick stalk. They are about 1 to 10 millimeters in diameter and most frequently develop on the neck, axillae, groin, or eyelids or in skinfold areas. They

CHART 59–9 Types of Moles or Nevi

Type of Mole or Nevus	Description
Junctional	Flat or slightly raised, brown-tan papule, less than 6 millimeters in diameter. Usually occurs at dermal–epidermal junction.
Compound	Slightly to markedly raised, pigmented papule. Symmetrical with irregular border and smooth or slightly papillary surface. Center more pigmented than border.
Intradermal	Elevated, fleshy papule. Pale or flesh colored with pigmented flecks. May have coarse, dark hairs growing from it.
Halo nevus	Mole surrounded by a ring of hypopigmentation. Usually disappears over several months with halo repigmenting.
Blue nevus	Solitary, bluish macula or papule, usually located on the head, neck, or buttocks. Enlarges slowly and persists for 10 to 15 years.
Becker's nevus	Usually occurs on the shoulder, submammary area, or back. Consists of a brown macule or patch of hair. Contains an irregular, sharply demarcated border. Varies in size but can be quite large.

are common and are usually asymptomatic unless they are irritated by clothing or jewelry, which may cause bleeding and tenderness. Skin tags are benign and may last indefinitely without problems. They do not require treatment; however, if desired they can be removed by simple scissor excision.

Lipoma

A **lipoma** is a nodule of fat tissue that is usually benign and is identified as a soft, freely mobile growth under the skin. It is slow growing and may vary in size from 1 to several centimeters in diameter. It is most commonly located on the shoulders, legs, arms, buttocks, and back but can occur anywhere on the body. Treatment is not necessary; however, if the lesion is cosmetically bothersome to the patient, it can be surgically excised.

Epidermal Cyst

An epidermal cyst is a capsule filled with keratin that appears spontaneously in an area of friction or a hair-bearing area, commonly on the face, postauricular fold, posterior neck, or trunk. Occluded **pilosebaceous follicles** (sebaceous cyst containing hair follicles) probably form the wall of the cyst. A cyst is freely movable but firm and tense feeling. It is dome shaped and pale, ranging in size from 0.5 to 5 centimeters, with a central opening that drains a pasty, malodorous material made up of necrotic keratin. It generally does not cause complications but can become infected; therefore, it may need antibiotics and in some instances may require surgical removal.

Skin Cancer

Skin cancer is the most common form of cancer occurring in the United States (U.S. Cancer Statistics Working Group, 2010). Exposure to the sun's ultraviolet rays is a direct contributing factor in the development of skin cancer. Individuals at the highest risk for skin cancer include those with fair or light skin color, those with a family history or personal history of skin cancer, individuals with chronic sun exposure, those with intermittent but intense exposure to the sun, those who had sunburns early in life, and those with a large number of moles or freckles indicating sun sensitivity and sun damage. There are three types of skin cancer; the most common type is basal cell carcinoma, followed by squamous cell carcinoma, and then malignant melanoma.

Basal Cell Carcinoma

Basal cell carcinoma, the most common skin cancer in Caucasians, is highest in the older adult population (age 55 to 75) (Nicol & Huether, 2007). It is usually nonmetastasizing and occurs most frequently on the head and neck, where there is the greatest sun exposure. There are different types of basal cell carcinoma. The most common is nodular, which appears as a smooth skin-colored nodule. It is dome shaped, with a rolled edge, and may have an overlying dilation of vessels seen just beneath the skin surface. The second most common type of basal cell carcinoma is superficial basal cell carcinoma. It is usually seen on the chest and back and is described as a flat, nonpalpable, erythematous plaque with distinct borders. It is often difficult to diagnose because it looks like many other skin lesions. Figure 59–10◆ is an example of a basal cell carcinoma. Morpheaform basal cell carcinoma is a firm, smooth, flesh-colored, scarlike papule or plaque with ill-defined borders. Primary treatment historically has involved surgical excision. However, 5-fluorouracil cream and Imiquimod (Aldara)

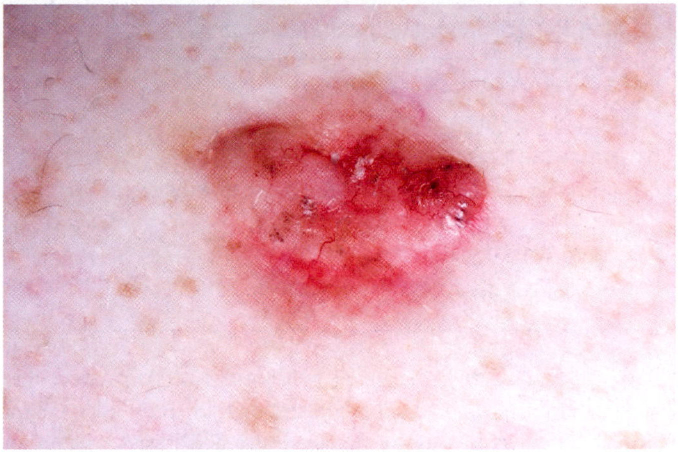

FIGURE 59–10 ◆ Basal cell carcinoma.
Source: NAS Medical/Alamy.

cream may be beneficial for those superficial low-risk lesions (Domino et al., 2012).

Squamous Cell Carcinoma

Squamous cell carcinoma consists of tumors of the outer epidermis that occur with frequent exposure to the sun and can be relatively aggressive when spreading. There are two types of squamous cell carcinoma: in situ (Bowen disease) or invasive. Initially, squamous cell carcinoma presents as an intraepidermal lesion and remains in the epidermis for a long time. It can eventually spread to area lymph nodes and become invasive, which can be either slow or rapid growing. Squamous cell carcinoma is described as a small, red, scaling lesion sitting on an elevated base with an irregular border that may itch or be a nonhealing lesion after minor trauma. Squamous cell carcinoma develops from precancerous lesions and can metastasize through the lymphatic system to regional lymph nodes. Figure 59–11◆ is an example of a squamous cell carcinoma.

Malignant Melanoma

Etiology, Epidemiology, and Risk Factors

The incidence of melanoma has more than tripled in the Caucasian population in the United States in the last 20 years. Malignant melanoma currently is the sixth-most common cancer in the United States

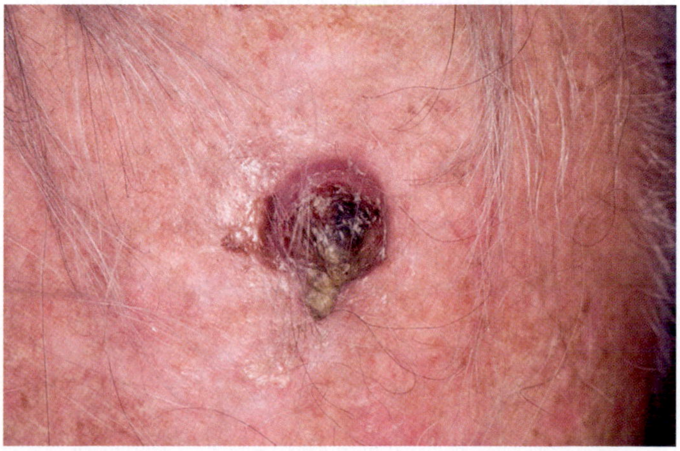

FIGURE 59–11 ◆ Squamous cell carcinoma.
Source: Science Photo Library/SuperStock.

Video: Skin Cancer **Weblink:** Skin Cancer Prevention

RISK FACTORS for Malignant Melanoma

Patient at high risk for malignant melanoma:

Has a large number of typical moles.

Has an increased number of atypical moles.

Burns easily from exposure to the sun, freckles from sun exposure, or has difficulty tanning.

Has a family history of malignant melanoma.

Has previously been diagnosed with malignant melanoma.

(Markovic et al., 2007). Malignant melanoma is a skin cancer that originates from melanocytes. Early detection with early intervention is usually curative. Because of the aggressive and invasive nature of malignant melanoma, the prognosis is poor when it is diagnosed in the later stages. It is recommended that all individuals examine their skin and know the risk factors of malignant melanoma, as presented in the Risk Factors box.

Clinical Manifestations

The clinical manifestations of malignant melanoma are described in Chart 59–10.

Malignant melanoma is the most dangerous skin cancer because it is a rapidly growing invasive tumor that can metastasize to almost any organ in the body and result in death. It is a tumor involving melanocytes that is related to sun exposure. Fair-skinned people who sunburn easily and freckle are at the greatest risk. Severe, blistering sunburns in early childhood and intense sun exposure increase the susceptibility to melanoma. Its appearance is described in the Risk Factor box. It may be tender and will sometimes ulcerate and bleed. The four types of malignant melanoma are outlined in Chart 59–11. Because malignant melanoma is rapidly progressing, it is important to stage the disease in order to determine the best treatment option. In stage I the lesion is less than 1 millimeter thick with no evidence of tumor growth into lymph nodes. A stage II lesion is thicker than 1 millimeter with lymph nodes that are not enlarged, but there may be metastasis to other organs and lymph nodes. Stage III indicates there has been metastasis to distant organs. There is lymph node enlargement near the melanoma site, and there are positive lymph nodes away from the original tumor site. Stage IV is generally widespread and incurable (Nicol & Huether, 2007). Figure 59–12 ◆ is an example of a malignant melanoma.

Laboratory and Diagnostic Procedures and Medical Management

A collaborative and multidisciplinary approach will optimize the recovery process. Diagnostic tests to assist in determining metastatic disease may include lactate dehydrogenase (LDH) determination. Imaging studies are only of benefit in detecting metastatic disease. Diagnostic procedures such as chest x-ray, ultrasound, computed tomography (CT), magnetic resonance imaging (MRI), lymphoscintigraphy, and positron-emission tomography (PET) are used to detect metastasis. The most accurate way to diagnose skin cancer is through surgical biopsy. Any suspicious lesion should be surgically excised with 2 mm of margin and a cuff of fat, after which the tissue is sent for pathologic examination. For melanoma stages I and II, this may be all the treatment that is necessary. For stages III and IV, when the disease has become systemic, immunotherapy, chemotherapy, or radiation therapy may be used along with regional lymph node dissection. Frequent and regular follow-up examinations should be done. An in-depth description of the diagnosis and treatment of malignant melanomas is given in Chapter 57.

All skin cancers should be surgically removed with the intent to cure the cancer. Basal cell and squamous cell cancer can be removed with surgical excision, chemosurgery, radiation, or curettage.

CHART 59–10 The ABCDs of Malignant Melanoma

Asymmetry: Early melanoma is asymmetrical, as opposed to the typical mole that is symmetrical.

Border: Melanomas have irregular borders, whereas most moles have clearly delineated edges.

Color: Melanomas are usually variegated and are in shades of brown, tan, blue/black, or a combination of colors. Typical moles tend to be uniform in color.

Diameter: Melanomas are often larger than 6 millimeters in diameter. The typical mole is generally less than 6 millimeters in diameter (the approximate size of a pencil eraser).

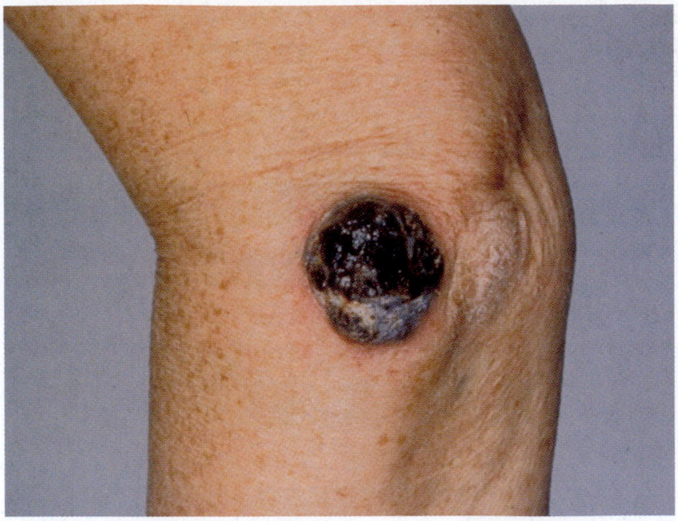

FIGURE 59–12 ◆ Malignant melanoma.

Source: Biophoto Associates/Science Source/Photo Researchers, Inc.

CHART 59–11 Types of Melanoma

Type	Description
Superficial spreading	Makes up 50% of the cases of melanoma. Occurs in younger adults. It looks like a nevus with a raised edge and lateral growth. It may be ulcerated and bleeding.
Nodular melanoma	Makes up 20% to 25% of all cases and usually occurs in young adults. Raised, dome-shaped lesion. It is usually a uniform blue-black color. It resembles blood blisters and rapidly invades the dermis.
Lentigo melanoma	Makes up 15% of all cases and occurs in older adults. Slow-growing, flat nevus. Grows horizontally and radially.
Acral lentiginous melanoma	Least common form, making up less than 10% of all cases. Occurs on the palms of the hands, soles of the feet, nail beds, and mucous membranes.

Melanoma also needs surgical excision; however, it is important to go through a process of staging melanoma so that appropriate treatment can be planned.

Nursing Management

Assessment

Skin cancer is often asymptomatic; therefore, it is important to assess the skin frequently for changes in moles or new growths. One of the most common methods used to evaluate changes in skin lesions is the ABCD rule outlined in Chart 59–10.

Nursing Diagnoses

The nursing diagnosis will depend on the extent, severity, and location of the lesions, but may include:

- *Impaired Skin Integrity* related to epithelial skin disorder.
- *Disturbed Body Image* related to skin lesions.
- *Acute Pain* related to skin disorder and metastatic disease process.
- *Fear and Anxiety* related to changes in health status/role functioning, situational crisis.

NANDA-I © 2012

Outcomes and Evaluation Parameters

The ultimate goal of treatment of skin cancer is complete healing without scarring or loss of function. When the diagnosis involves a malignant condition, the outcome is cure or remission. The outcome goals are to promote the patient's recovery, provide support, manage the disorder, and prevent complications. The evaluation parameters are healed skin, no evidence of complication, and return to prediagnosis level of functioning.

Planning, Interventions, and Rationales

Once the lesion or lesions have been excised, the nurse needs to instruct the patient to regularly observe the skin and check for suspicious lesions using the ABCD method (see Chart 59–10). Patients should avoid UVA and UVB exposure. Use of sunscreen needs to be stressed with each exposure.

Evaluation

A plan for care of the patient with skin cancer needs to be thought of as a long-term process and should involve prevention and maintenance strategies. The key to cure is prevention. Frequent and regular skin assessments to reevaluate for the recurrence of any skin cancer lesions needs to be foremost. Patients should avoid UVA and UVB exposure. If any new lesions are identified, speedy medical evaluation is critical.

INFESTATIONS AND BITES

The skin can be invaded by insects, ticks, or parasites. Typically there is a single lesion on the skin; however, the lesion depends on the causative agent.

Insect Bites and Stings

Insects inject poison or an irritative substance through a bite or sting, by invading tissue, and sometimes by contact allergy. Skin injury is characterized by local redness with itching, pain, and swelling. The injury is usually immediate and transient. Large local reactions or a systemic reaction with signs and symptoms of anaphylaxis or systemic toxin effect can occur.

Bees and Wasps

The most common types of insect stings are those of honeybees, followed by those of wasps. The honeybee's stinger remains embedded in the skin, whereas other species of bees and wasps leave nothing behind. Initially there is a sharp, painful sting that lasts only a few minutes. It is typically followed by burning and a raised white wheal with a red center that resolves in a few days.

Bee and wasp stings can be dangerous, especially if there is a toxic systemic reaction or an allergic anaphylactic reaction. Approximately 50 deaths/year occur from fatal anaphylactic reaction (Domino et al., 2012). The symptoms of a toxic reaction include vomiting, diarrhea, headache, fever, muscle spasm, and loss of consciousness. The most severe reaction is an anaphylactic reaction, which involves itching, hives, shortness of breath, wheezing, nausea, abdominal cramps, and the potential for respiratory arrest and death. These reactions occur within minutes to hours of the sting, although allergic reactions can be delayed, occurring up to a week after the sting. Severe generalized reactions are treated in an emergency department with epinephrine and oral or intramuscular antihistamines. If it is a localized, nonallergic reaction, apply ice and give oral antihistamines to prevent spreading of the venom. See the Pharmacology box (p. 1845).

Safety Alert *Bee and wasp stings can result in a local reaction or a systemic anaphylactic reaction. For a local reaction, apply ice, compress the site with a tight bandage, and elevate the site. Antihistamines can be given for itching. For a systemic anaphylactic reaction, activate the emergency medical system, as such a reaction is life threatening.*

Ticks

Ticks can be bearers of diseases such as Lyme disease and Rocky Mountain spotted fever. Early Lyme disease is characterized by an expanding skin rash and flulike symptoms. Transmission occurs only if the tick is attached to the person for more than 48 hours. The deer tick (*Ixodes scapularis*), black-legged tick, and Western black-legged tick (*I. pacificus*) are the primary carriers of Lyme disease. These ticks are very small and embed their heads in the skin to obtain blood. While they are feeding they can enlarge to many times their normal size and leave toxins and microorganisms behind. Initially the tick bite casues a local reaction involving pain, erythema, a papule, and itching. The tick should be removed totally intact if possible. If the head is left behind, a nodule may remain requiring excision. The best approach is prevention of the tick bite by wearing protective clothing, tucking the pants into the socks, and wearing closed-toed shoes.

Safety Alert *Ticks can be removed by grasping them as closely as possible to the skin with forceps and pulling upward. Do not squeeze the tick, or apply hot matches or nail polish. Then clean the wound with soap and water or a mild disinfectant. Instruct the patient to report any fever or unusual rash to the health care provider.*

Infestations

Infestation is defined as the condition of being inhabited or overrun in quantities large enough to be harmful. This section will discuss dermatologic infestations of lice, mites, and bedbugs.

Weblink: Bed Bugs

Pediculosis

Pediculosis is the infestation of the skin by lice. Lice are highly contagious parasites that survive by sucking blood. There are three types of lice: pediculosis capitis (or head lice); pediculosis corporis (or body lice); and pediculosis pubis (or pubic lice). The female lice reproduce frequently, producing hundreds of **nits,** or eggs that attach to the hair shaft. The nits hatch into lice that continue to reproduce. Lice secrete toxic saliva that causes trauma and releases toxins leading to itching and dermatitis. Lice are spread by personal contact through combs, brushes, sexual activity, and shared clothing and bed linens.

The major symptom of lice infestation is itching. In the scalp, the nits can be seen as yellow, oval specks attached to the hair shaft. There is extreme pruritus around the back and sides of the scalp. On the body, the lesion is a pinpoint red macule, papule, or wheal with a hemorrhagic puncture site. The center can crust and become infected. The pubic louse or "crab," as it is commonly referred to, is seen on pubic hair. Lice are diagnosed through physical examination and culture. The ova of lice will fluoresce under an ultraviolet light.

Treatment involves good hygiene and avoiding the sharing of hats, combs, or clothes. Lindane shampoo, pyrethrins, or permethrin can be used for head lice. Corticosteroid lotions or creams and antihistamines can be used to help relieve itching.

Scabies

Scabies is caused by a parasite called *Sarcoptes scabiei*, a type of mite that is commonly found in underdeveloped countries, areas where there is overcrowding or poor hygiene, and in long-term care institutions (Nicol & Huether, 2007). Scabies is contagious and transmitted by close personal contact, clothing, and bedding. The female mite tunnels into the skin, creating a burrow and depositing eggs. The eggs can sometimes be seen at the end of the burrows as tiny maculopapular dots. Intense itching that worsens at night is the primary symptom. The mite can enter the skin and travel all over the body so the itching is generalized. Lesions that are papular, vesicular, or linear occur in the wrists, web spaces of the hands, sides of the hands and feet, genital area, warm intertriginous regions, and abdomen.

Scabies is diagnosed by physical examination with identification of the mites, or burrows. Mites can be seen under a microscope after an application of mineral oil or potassium hydroxide. Treatment consists of the application of scabicide preparations such as permethrin cream or Lindane. The lotion or cream is applied to the entire skin surface including under the nails and in the umbilicus. The medication is left on for 6 hours and then washed off. All people with whom the patient has been in contact must be treated. Clothing and bedding should be washed and dried in a hot dryer.

Bed Bugs

Bed bugs, *Cimex lectularius,* are reddish brown, oval, flat insects, approximately 1/4 inch long. They feed on human blood during the night hours and crawl into cracks and crevices (mattresses) during the day. Bed bugs are usually transmitted through the transfer of infested furniture or clothing. Media reports of bed bug infestations in community dwellings, hotels, hospitals, apartments, prisons, and dorms have become common. Bed bug infestation is difficult to eradicate and common insect repellents are not effective. Use of a professional pest control company is recommended, as they are knowledgeable regarding the approved insecticides to use and proper equipment. Repeated application and treatment of the residence may be necessary. The insect bites usually occur on the arms, face, and back and cause itching, pain, and/or swelling where the bite occurs. Although the bites can cause considerable distress, the bugs do not transmit disease (Indiana State Department of Health, 2012).

Nursing Management

Assessment

Insect bites and infestations are common causes of skin disorders in adults and children. Nursing management of the patient with an insect bite or infestation requires a complete and thorough assessment and investigation of the patient's skin and surrounding environment. Family members should be included in this assessment.

Nursing Diagnoses

Nursing diagnoses include the following:

- *Impaired Skin Integrity* due to the insect bite.
- *Altered Comfort Level* due to the insect bite.
- *Fear and Anxiety* due to the insect bite.

NANDA-I © 2012

Outcomes and Evaluation Parameters

The outcome goals for the patient with an insect bite or infestation are to promote the patient's recovery, provide support, and prevent complications. Evaluation parameters will include healed skin and resolution of lesions, restoration of comfort (resolution of itching and discomfort), and no evidence of complications such as secondary infection. Another evaluation parameter would be elimination of insect infestation in the environment.

Planning, Interventions, and Rationales

Nursing interventions will be determined by the extent and severity of the skin disruption and condition. First and foremost, interventions to eliminate the insect from the host will take priority. Nursing management will also include interventions to relieve physical symptoms (pain, pruritus) such as local wound care, topical antihistamines or compresses, elevation, or ice. Finally, interventions to eradicate the infestation from the environment must be carried out. Infested furniture, clothing, toys, and blankets must be disposed of.

Evaluation

Reevaluation of the nursing plan, including reassessment of the skin and environment, must be done regularly. Depending on the success and effectiveness of the treatment, the plan of care may need to be revised or altered.

DISORDERS OF THE SKIN'S ACCESSORY ORGANS

Disorders of the Nail

Toenails and fingernails are considered a part of the skin and need to be assessed for abnormalities. The nails reflect nutritional status and general health as well as the presence of systemic disorders and exposure to toxic agents. Toenail problems occur in approximately 75% of Americans (Beuscher, 2007). Careful assessment is an important part of diagnosing both local and systemic disorders. Systemic disorders often cause changes in the shape or contour of the nail.

CHART 59–12 Nail Abnormalities Related to Systemic Disease

Nail Abnormality	Description	Disease
Beau's lines	Transverse furrows on fingernails.	Stress. Acute severe illness. Nutritional disorders. Circulation disorders. Abnormal metabolic states.
Spoon nails (koilonychia)	Nails are concave like a saucer. Nail plate is thinned.	Hypochromic anemia. Rheumatic fever. Syphilis.
Nail pitting	Thickened nail plate with small pits.	Psoriasis.
Nail clubbing	Flattened nail plate. Bulbous distal phalanx. Increased angle between nail and dorsal surface of finger.	Chronic hypoxia. Heart disease. Pulmonary disease. Cystic fibrosis. Bronchogenic carcinoma.
Mees' lines	White, transverse line.	Poisoning. Acute illness.
Lindsay's nails	Proximal portion of nail is white while distal portion is red or pink.	Chronic renal disease. Azotemia.
Terry's nails	White nail beds with distal band of reddish brown.	Cirrhosis. Hypoalbuminemia. Congestive heart failure. Type 2 diabetes.

Chart 59–12 provides an overview of nail abnormalities related to systemic disease.

Brittle Nails

Brittle nails are defined as nails in which the distal plate splits, leading to peeling of the distal portion of the nail. Brittle nails are excessively ridged and dry. The usual water content of the nail is about 18%, whereas brittle nails have a water content of only about 16% (Hall & Hall, 2010). This is caused by prolonged immersion in water, dry skin with dryness of the nail plate, or chemical or mechanical trauma that leads to nail dehydration (Chart 59–13). When the nurse notes brittle nails, a thorough history should be performed to help determine the cause. Note the specific nails that are involved and the changes in the nail plate.

If the patient's hands must be immersed in water, it is important to wear gloves. The hands and nails can be massaged daily with lubricants or oils after soaking in lukewarm water for 15 minutes. The patient should be instructed to keep the nails well groomed and avoid using them as tools to scrape or pry. Systemic treatment with biotin has been found to improve the nails (Duarte, Correia, & Baran, 2009). Biotin is a component of the vitamin B complex that helps maintain healthy muscle, hair, and skin by stimulating keratinization. Biotin is well tolerated with very few side effects. Therefore, it is a reasonable choice when other treatment measures fail.

CHART 59–13 Causes of Brittle Nails

Occupational Causes	Physical Causes
Chemicals such as acetone	Aging
Typing	Atherosclerosis
Playing a musical instrument	Poor nutrition with deficiencies in vitamins A, B_6, and C
Grasping	Chronic renal failure
Prying	Cardiovascular disease
Scraping	Raynaud's disease
Frequent hand washing	Thyroid disease
	Psoriasis
	Eczema
	Onychomycosis
	Warts
	Squamous cell or basal cell carcinoma

Nail Infections

The most common infection of the nail is onychomycosis, or tinea unguium, which is a chronic fungal infection under the nail. It usually occurs in the toenails but can occur in the fingernails as well. It commonly leads to deformed, cracked nails that initially become white or silvery and then turn yellow or brown. The nail beds are thickened but usually are not uncomfortable or painful. The infection can spread to other nails and is diagnosed through cultures and microscopy. This condition is difficult to treat and is typically slowly responsive to the oral and topical antifungal medications. The nail may eventually have to be surgically removed in order to clear up the infection.

Paronychia is an acute or chronic infection of the folds of tissue around the nail or the cuticle that usually begins after minor trauma. The causative organism is most frequently *Streptococcus* or *Staphylococcus*, but paronychia can also be related to a fungus (Nicol & Huether, 2007). In acute paronychia, an abscess may develop that requires surgical drainage for relief of pain. In chronic paronychia, the infection develops more slowly with progressive tenderness and swelling around the cuticle. Treatment involves the application of hot compresses and topical antibiotics.

Nail Trauma or Loss

Trauma to the nail or nail bed may result in changes in the size, shape, or color of the nail and can lead to disorders such as subungual hematoma and pincer nail. A subungual hematoma is usually related to trauma to the nail that causes bleeding and bruising under the nail. This typically leads to separation of the nail plate. The blood will cause a dark discoloration that will remain until the nail plate grows out. It may be necessary to puncture the nail to relieve the excess pressure caused by the blood building up under the nail.

Pincer nail usually affects the toenail and is evidenced by the lateral edges of the nail curling in and under it, leading to a tubelike appearance of the nail. It is usually caused by pointed-toed shoes or high heels that squeeze the toes together. If the pincer nail causes pain, the nail may need to be surgically removed.

An ingrown nail (onychocryptosis) occurs when the corners of the nail plate grow into the lateral nail fold and dermis. It is usually due to poorly fitting shoes, improper nail trimming, or trauma. The individual experiences pain, redness, and swelling, and an infection may develop, leading to an abscess. This condition can be prevented by wearing properly fitting shoes and trimming the nails straight across. Treatment options depend on the severity of the symptoms. Soaking the nail, along with systemic and/or topical antibiotics, may be used. A cotton wick can be inserted into the lateral nail groove to allow for drainage and relief of pressure. If these strategies are unsuccessful, or if the symptoms are more severe, a wedge resection of the corner of the nail can be performed with removal of the lateral one-fourth of the nail. Removal of the lateral nail matrix may be necessary to create a new lateral nail fold and prevent the recurrence of an ingrown nail.

Disorders of the Hair

Hair disorders include too much hair, known as *hirsutism*, or not enough hair, known as *alopecia*. **Hirsutism,** defined as the excessive growth of hair, is caused by an increased testosterone level, Cushing's syndrome, carcinoma of the adrenal gland, testicular tumors, or acromegaly. This condition occurs more commonly in women. The increase in hormones stimulates the hair follicle to grow, especially on the lip, chin, chest, areola, abdomen, lower back, buttock, inner thighs, and external genitalia. The treatment consists of diagnosing and treating the underlying cause.

Alopecia

Alopecia is defined as loss of hair, which can occur in men and women at any age. One of the most common forms of alopecia is **androgenetic alopecia,** also known as male pattern baldness. Androgenetic alopecia is a physiological baldness in which androgen levels are normal; however, there is a genetic predisposition to balding. In men, it usually begins with bitemporal thinning of the hair and progresses to the frontal area, whereas in women the typical pattern is central thinning. The degree of baldness and the age of onset are determined by the inheritance of several genes. The hair shafts gradually shrink until they become finer and thinner. It is not related to any serious health problems but can be psychologically disturbing. Certain topical medications can be applied to the scalp, but their effectiveness is variable. The two medications that have been found to be the most effective are finasteride and minoxidil. Finasteride blocks the conversion of testosterone to 5-alpha dihydrotestosterone (DHT), which is needed for the development of androgenetic alopecia. Minoxidil is a vasodilator applied topically that leads to enhanced hair growth due to the increased blood flow. These medications must be used for 4 to 12 months before their effectiveness can be evaluated (Nicol & Huether, 2007). **Androgenic alopecia** occurs in women and is recognized as a symptom of polycystic ovary syndrome. Chapter 41 discusses polycystic ovary syndrome. It is related to excessive androgen production that causes a decrease in the size of the hair follicles, leading to hair loss in central and frontal areas. Hair loss also can be related to systemic medications; for example, many of the chemotherapeutic agents used for treating cancer can lead to hair loss. Systemic diseases related to hair loss include hypothyroidism, insulin resistance, and cardiovascular disease (Nicol & Huether, 2007).

Alopecia also is associated with high levels of anxiety and depression, low self-esteem, poor quality of life, and poor body image. Hair is closely related to an individual's identity and attractiveness. Visits to psychologists/psychiatrists may be beneficial in helping patients deal with problems associated with alopecia.

Alopecia Areata

Alopecia areata is an autoimmune T-cell-mediated chronic inflammatory disease directed at the hair follicle that results in loss of hair. The cause is unknown but its condition has been associated with stress, cell-mediated immune factors, and genetic susceptibility. Regrowth usually occurs in 1 to 3 months. Treatments include corticosteroids and topical immunotherapy.

Gerontological Considerations

Many anatomic changes occur during the aging process:

- Skin loses elasticity and water content.
- The texture and turgor of the skin change.
- The retaining ligaments of the soft tissue of the face weaken.
- The face loses volume from decreased subcutaneous adipose stores and muscle mass.
- Facial bones undergo resorption.
- The eye orbit changes shape, allowing for positional changes of the eye globe.
- The face becomes elongated and flattened.
- Smoking, genetics, and sun exposure contribute to the loss of skin elasticity and wrinkle formation.

In addition, there are common skin lesions related to aging. These include:

- Skin tags, which are soft, brown or flesh-colored papules
- Keratosis, which is the abnormal growth of keratinocytes
- Lentigines, which are brown to black macules commonly called liver spots
- Vascular lesions, which are vascular tumors with chronically dilated blood vessels

Research

The nurse will find a number of research opportunities related to skin disorders and cosmetic surgery. The goals of research are to identify effective means of caring for patients with skin problems and to support patients psychologically who have experienced changes in appearance. The research topics related to skin disorders are identified in the Research Opportunities box.

RESEARCH OPPORTUNITIES Related to Skin Disorders and Cosmetic Surgery

Research Area	Clinical Impact
Effects of various moisturizers on the skin.	Keeping the skin intact and avoiding dryness.
Mechanisms to diagnose skin cancer accurately.	Early detection and treatment.
Treatment for common skin conditions.	Many skin conditions do not have adequate treatment available for cure or control.
Risk factors for herpes zoster.	More information is needed about who might be at risk other than those who are immunocompromised.
Define epidemiology with necrotizing fasciitis using population-based studies.	Identify those with the greatest risk for acquiring necrotizing fasciitis.
Factors that help predict who might develop necrotizing fasciitis.	
The role of nonsteroidal anti-inflammatory drugs (NSAIDs) in the development of necrotizing fasciitis.	Clarifies whether NSAIDs aggravate or initiate the development of necrotizing fasciitis.

CLINICAL PREPARATION

READ DOCUMENT APPLY

READ: **History of Present Illness** >> Laboratory Study Results >> Critical Thinking Questions

Robert Tatum is a 47-year-old White male who was admitted to the hospital with necrotizing fasciitis located in a wound in his right lower leg. He reports being hit on the lower leg with a log while he was chopping wood about 7 days ago. At the time of the injury, he removed several splinters. Following the injury the pain increased to the point that it became difficult for him to walk. He noted that there was increased swelling and a mottled appearance where the splinters were, and that the wound had doubled in size in the last 2 days. He brought himself to the emergency department for an evaluation of the leg and to rule out a fracture. No fracture was found; however, the assessment revealed cellulitis with a hard "woody" texture to the wound. Mr. Tatum was admitted for further wound evaluation.

Upon admission Mr. Tatum was taken to surgery for a debridement and culture of his wound. The culture showed group A streptococcus. He is scheduled for a second debridement in 12 hours. The surgical debridement will continue until clear borders are obtained. Application of a vacuum-assisted closure device was done in surgery.

Medical–Surgical History

Mr. Tatum has been in relatively good health. Lately he has had some problems with tendonitis in the left elbow and was on Naprosyn. He has no other chronic health problems. He was on no medications prior to admission other than Naprosyn.

Social History

Mr. Tatum lives in a rural area but works as a mechanic at the local steel plant. He reports that he drinks approximately 6 beers per week, mostly on the weekend. He does not use illicit drugs. He smokes about 1 pack of cigarettes per day.

READ: History of Present Illnesses >> **Physical Exam** >> Admitting Medical Records >> Laboratory Study Results

Physical Exam

Vital signs: BP 120/76; P 96; RR 16; T 99.4°F
Oxygen sat 93% on room air
HEENT: normal but poor dentition
Heart: regular rate and rhythm; normal S_1, S_2
Lungs: clear to auscultation in all fields
Abdomen: obese, soft, nontender
Normal neuro exam
No rash
Chest x-ray: clear
ECG: WNL
Weight: 210 lbs (95.4 kg); height: 6'1"
Extremities: left leg appears normal with good color, no edema, dorsalis pedis and posterior tibial pulses 2+ bilaterally
Anterior right lower leg has wound approximately 5 inches in diameter about mid-shin. The area around the wound is erythremic with bluish patches and bullae draining clear watery liquid. The wound is surrounded by nonpitting edema from the knee to the ankle. The area around the wound is very tender to touch.

Admitting Medical Orders

Plastic Surgery Service
Surgical floor
Diagnosis: necrotizing fasciitis of right leg
Allergic to codeine
Oxygen at 2 to 3 liters nasal cannula, keep oxygen saturation ≥ 92%
Bed rest with bathroom privileges
Vital signs and O_2 saturation levels q2h
Call house officer: pulse < 60 to > 110/minute; BP < 90 and > 130 systolic; temperature > 38.5°C; urine output < 20 mL/hr, respiratory rate > 30/minute; oxygen saturation < 92%
Sequential compression device (SCD) to lower left extremity
Incentive spirometer every 2 hours while awake
Foley
I&O
NPO after midnight for OR
Calorie count
IV: D5 lactated Ringer's at 100 mL/hr
Contact isolation
Wound VAC to right lower leg with 125 mmHg of continuous suction

CLINICAL PREPARATION, *continued*

Scheduled Medications

Clindamycin 900 mg IV q8h
Ampicillin 1.0 gm IV q6h
Gentamicin 90 mg IV three times per day
Famotidine 20 mg IV twice daily
Naprosyn 500 mg po twice/day (when taking po)

PRN Medications

Morphine sulfate via patient-controlled analgesia: concentration: 1 mg/mL; basal rate 1 mg/hr; incremental: 1 mg; 6-minute lock-out
Phenergan 25 mg IV q6h prn nausea
Triazolam 0.125–0.25 mg po q noc, prn sleep (when taking po)
Ativan 0.5–2 mg IV q6–8h prn anxiety
Milk of Magnesia 30 mL po daily prn constipation (when taking po)
Tylenol 650 mg po/PR prn q4h for fever > 38.5°C

Ordered Laboratory Studies

STAT wound culture (done in OR)
CBC, Chem 20 panel, CK now
Daily: CBC, PT-INR/PTT, Ca, Mg, phosphorus, Chem 7 panel
Blood culture every 24 hours prn temp > 38.5°C

Ordered Diagnostic Studies

ECG
CT scan of right leg

READ: History of Present Illnesses >> **Laboratory Study Results** >> Critical Thinking Questions

Test	Day 1	Day 2	Day 3
White blood cells (WBCs)	18,000/mm^3	22,000/mm^3	28,000/mm^3
Neutrophils	80%	88%	96%
Hemoglobin	12 g/dL	11 g/dL	10 g/dL
Hematocrit	36%	33%	30%
Red blood cells (RBCs)	4.5/mm^3	4.1/mm^3	3.8/mm^3
Platelets	250,000/mm^3	400,000/mm^3	540,000/mm^3
Sodium	136 mEq/L	138 mEq/L	139 mEq/L
Potassium	4.0 mEq/L	4.8 mEq/L	5.0 mEq/L
Chloride	96 mEq/L	97 mEq/L	101 mEq/L
Carbon dioxide	30	30	30
Magnesium	1.8 mEq/L		
Phosphorus	4 mg/dL		
Blood urea nitrogen (BUN)	22 mg/dL	34 mg/dL	49 mg/dL
Creatinine	1 mg/dL	1.3 mg/dL	1.7 mg/dL
Glucose	198 mg/dL	192 mg/dL	160 mg/dL
Calcium	9.2 mg/dL		

Test	Day 1	Day 2	Day 3
Total protein	5.2 g/dL		
Albumin	3.6 g/dL		
Alkaline phosphatase	105 units/L		
Aspartate aminotransferase (AST)	38 units/L		
Total bilirubin	1.1 mg/dL		
Creatine kinase	280 units/L		
PTT	32 seconds		
PT	9.6 seconds		
INR	1.2		
Wound culture	Group A beta-hemolytic streptococcus		
CT scan	Asymmetric fascial thickening with gas tracking along the fascial planes		

Pearson Nursing Student Resources *Log on to* **nursing.pearsonhighered.com** *to download forms*

DOCUMENT:

>> Summary of Hospitalization
>> Pathophysiology Form
>> Laboratory Values
>> Laboratory Results Explanation

APPLY:

>> List of Potential Nursing Diagnoses
>> Concept Map
>> Critical Thinking Questions and Concept Map

APPLY: History of Present Illness >> Laboratory Study Results >> **Critical Thinking Questions**

1. What complications should you assess Mr. Tatum for and why?
2. How is Mr. Tatum's necrotizing fasciitis transmitted, and how can you protect the other patients you are caring for?
3. Mr. Tatum is concerned about his leg and asks you whether it will ever be back to normal. How should you respond?

Answers to Critical Thinking Questions can be found in Appendix D in the Osborn Student Resources at nursing.pearsonhighered.com.

NCLEX® PRACTICE

1. The nurse is instructing a patient to reduce bathing and use a mild unscented soap. These interventions are appropriate for which of the following skin disorders?

1. Atopic dermatitis
2. Poison ivy
3. Urticaria
4. Contact dermatitis

2. The nurse is instructing a patient with a skin disorder about nutrition. Which of the following should be included in this instruction?

1. Restrict calories.
2. Eat foods high in vitamin C, iron, and zinc.
3. Limit high-water-content foods.
4. Limit fatty foods.

3. A patient asks what she can do to make sure her teenage daughter doesn't develop skin cancer. The nurse should discuss which of the following topics with the patient?

1. Provide a well-balanced diet for her daughter.
2. Advise her daughter to maintain a normal weight for height.
3. Encourage the child to take a daily multivitamin.
4. Instruct her daughter in the use of sunscreen.

4. A patient with a skin disorder is prescribed a topical corticosteroid. Which of the following should the nurse instruct this patient about regarding the use of this medication?

1. "Rub the medication into wet skin thoroughly."
2. "Apply a thick layer of the medication and allow it to air dry."
3. "Stay out of the sun when you use this medication."
4. "It may cause drowsiness."

5. A patient has been admitted to the hospital with a skin disorder. Which of the following is a priority for the nurse to include in the assessment of this patient?

1. Signs of infection
2. Employment history
3. Social activities
4. Neurological status

6. A patient tells the nurse that she "doesn't socialize much in the summer" because she needs to wear long sleeves to cover the psoriasis on her arms. Which of the following should the nurse respond to this patient?

1. "That's too bad."
2. "You probably like the winter much better."
3. "There are light materials that you could wear."
4. "I would go out anyway."

Answers to NCLEX Practice Questions can be found in Appendix D in the Osborn Student Resources at nursing.pearsonhighered.com. Practice additional NCLEX questions online at the Student Resources site.

Pearson Nursing Student Resources Find additional review materials at: **nursing.pearsonhighered.com**

REFERENCES

Adams, M. P., & Koch, R. W. (2010). *Pharmacology: Connections to nursing practice.* Upper Saddle River, NJ: Pearson.

American Academy of Dermatology. (2012). Atopic dermatitis. Retrieved from http://www.aad.org/skin-conditions/dermatology-a-to-z/atopic-dermatitis

American Nurses Association. (2012). Nursing world. Retrieved from http://www.nursingworld.org/EspeciallyForYou/What-is-Nursing/Tools-You-Need/Thenursingprocess.html

American Society of Plastic Surgeons (ASPS). (2007). Injectable fillers. Retrieved from http://plasticsurgery.org/patients_consumers/procedures/InjectableFillers.cfm?gclid=CKPEo4_V35ACFRdPagodPzD0WQ

Baroni, A., Lanza, A., Cirillo, N., Brunetti, G., Ruocco, E., & Ruocco, V. (2007). Vesicular and bullous disorders: Pemphigus. *Dermatology Clinics, 25*(4), 597–603.

Beuscher, T. (2007). Foot and nail care. In R. Bryant & D. Nix (Eds.), *Acute & chronic wounds: Current management concepts* (3rd ed.). St. Louis, MO: Mosby Elsevier.

Burkhart, C. G. (2010). Tinea versicolor. Retrieved from http:www.emedicine.medscape.com/article/1091575-overview

Carpenter, P. (2011). A tattoo joint needs no license. *The Morning Call,* March 11, 2011. Retrieved from http://articles.mcall.com/2011-03-10/news/mc-paul-carpenter-licenses-20110310_1_tax-returns-tattoo-license

Centers for Disease Control and Prevention (CDC). (2008). Division of bacterial and mycotic diseases. Group A streptococcal (GAS) disease. Retrieved from http://www.cdc.gov/ncidod/dbmd/diseaseinfo/groupastreptococcal_g.htm

Centers for Disease Control and Prevention (CDC). (2011). Shingles (Herpes Zoster). Retrieved from http://www.cdc.gov/shingles/vaccination.html

Centers for Disease Control and Prevention (CDC). (2012a). Basic information about skin cancer. Retrieved from http://www.cdc.gov/cancer/skin/basic_info/index.htm#uv

Centers for Disease Control and Prevention (CDC). (2012b). Skin cancer prevention. Retrieved from http://www.cdc.gov/cancer/skin/basic_info/prevention.htm

County of Kern: Department of Health Services. (2007). Complications associated with body piercing and tattooing. Retrieved from http://www.co.kern.ca.us/health/tattooing513.asp

Do, H. K. (2010). Skin-nontumor/clinical dermatology—carbuncle. Retrieved from http://www.pathologyoutlines.com/topic/skinnontumorcarbuncle.html

Domino, F., Baldor, R., Golding, J., Grimes, J., & Taylor, J. (Eds.). (2012). *Unbound medicine: 5-Minute clinical consult* (20th ed.). Lippincott Williams & Wilkins.

Duarte, A. F., Correia, O., & Baran, R. (2009). Nail plate cohesion seems to be water independent.*International Journal of Dermatology, 48*(3), 193–195.

Festugato, M. (2011). Pilot study on which foods should be avoided by patients with psoriasis. *Anais Brasileiros de Dermatologia, 86*(6), 1103–1108.

Habif, T. P. (2009). Vesicular and bullous diseases. In T. P. Habif, (Ed.), *Clinical dermatology* (5th ed., chapter 16). Philadelphia, PA: Mosby Elsevier.

Hall, J. (2010). Diseases affecting the nails. In B. J. Hall & J. C. Hall (Eds.), *Sauer's manual of skin diseases* (10th ed). Philadelphia: Wolters Kluwer Health/Lippincott Williams & Wilkins.

Hidalgo, J. A. (2011). Candidiasis. Retrieved from http://www.emedicine.medscape.com/article/213853-overview

Hogan, D. J. (2011). Allergic contact dermatitis. Retrieved from http://www.emedicine.medscape.com/article/1049216-overview

Indiana State Department of Health. (2012). Epidemiology Resource Center: Quick Facts: Bedbugs. Retrieved from http://www.in.gov/isdh/files/Bed_Bugs_QFV2_2011.pdf

IOM (Institute of Medicine). (2010). *The future of nursing: Leading change, advancing health.* Washington, DC: The Academic Press.

Kee, J. L. (2010). *Laboratory and diagnostic tests with nursing implications.* Upper Saddle River, NJ: Pearson.

Kroshinsky, D., Grossman, M. E., & Fox, L. P. (2007). Approach to the patient with presumed cellulitis. *Seminars in Cutaneous Medicine and Surgery, 26*(3), 168–178.

Lewis, L. S. (2012). Impetigo. Retrieved from http://www.emedicine.medscape.com/article/965254-overview

Lowell, D. (2011). Quit smoking. Mayo Clinic. Retrieved from http://www.mayoclinic.com/health/smoking/AN00644

Lucey, D. R. (2007). Anthrax. In L. Goldman & D. Ausiello (Eds.), *Cecil medicine* (23rd ed., chapter 317). Philadelphia, PA: Saunders Elsevier.

Markovic, S., Erickson, L., Rao, R., Weenig, R., Pckal. B., Bardia, A., et al. (2007). Melanoma Study Group of the Mayo Clinic Cancer Center. Malignant melanoma in the 21st century, part 1: Epidemiology, risk factors, screening, prevention, and diagnosis. *Mayo Clinical Procedings, 82n*(3), 364–380.

Martin, G. J., & Friedlander, A. M. (2009). *Bacillus anthracis* (anthrax). In G. L. Mandell, J. E. Bennett, & R. Dolin (Eds.), *Principles and practice of infectious diseases* (7th ed., chapter 208). Philadelphia, PA: Elsevier Churchill Livingstone.

Mayo Clinic. (2011). Stevens–Johnson syndrome. Retrieved from http://www.mayoclinic.com/health/stevens-johnson-syndrome/DS00940/DSECTION=causes

Mayo Clinic. (2012). Piercings: How to prevent complications. Retrieved from http://www.mayoclinic.com/health/piercings/SN00049

McNamara, D. R., Tleyjeh, I. M., Berbari, E. F., Lahr, B.D., Martinez, J.W., Mirzoyev, S.A., & Baddour, L.(2007). Incidence of lower-extremity cellulitis: A population-based study in Olmsted County, Minnesota. *Mayo Clinic Proceedings, 82*(7), 817–821.

Moon, J. E. (2011). Herpes zoster. Retrieved from http://www.emedicine.medscape.com/article/218683-overview

Nicol, N., & Huether, S. (2007). Structure, function, and disorders of the integument. In K. McCance, S. Huether, V. Brashers, & N. Rote (Eds.), *Pathophysiology: The biologic basis for disease in adults and children* (6th ed.). Maryland Heights, MO: Mosby Elsevier.

Peleg, A. Y., & Hooper, D. C. (2010). Hospital-acquired infections due to gram-negative bacteria. *New England Journal of Medicine, 362*,1804–1813.

Querleux, B., Baldeweck, T., Diridollou, S., de Rigal, J., Huguet, E., Leroy, F., & Barbosa, V. H. (2009). Skin from various ethnic origins and aging: An in vivo cross-sectional multimodality imaging study. *Skin Research and Technology, 15*(3), 306–313.

Samuel, M., Brooke, R. C. C., Hollis, S., & Griffiths, C. E. M. (2005). Interventions for photodamaged skin. *The Cochrane Database of Systematic Reviews*, Issue 1. Retrieved from http://www.cochrane.org/reviews/en/ab001782.html

Satter, E. K. (2011). Folliculitis. Retrieved from http://www.emedicine.medscape.com/article/1070456-overview

Schueler, S. J, Beckett, J. H., & Gettings, D. S. (2011). Vitiligo incidence. Retrieved from http://www.freemd.com/vitiligo/incidence.htm

Sharma, R. (2011). Herpes simplex in emergency medicine. Retrieved from http://www.emedicine.medscape.com/article/783113-overview

Shenefelt, P. D. (2011). Nongenital warts. Retrieved from http://www.emedicine.medscape/article/1133317-overview

Tatro, D. S. (Ed.). (2012). *Unbound medicine: A–Z drug facts.* Philadelphia: Wolters Kluwer/Facts & Comparisons/Lippincott, Williams, & Wilkins.

U.S. Cancer Statistics Working Group. (2010). *United States cancer statistics: 1999—2007 incidence and mortality web-based report.* Atlanta, GA: Department of Health and Human Services, Centers for Disease Control and Prevention, and National Cancer Institute. Retrieved from http://www.cdc.gov/uscs

U.S. Department of Health and Human Services. (2010). Healthy People 2020. Healthy People 2020. Retrieved from http://www.healthypeople.gov/2020/topicsobjectives2020/default.aspx

WebMD. (2012). Ringworm of the skin—Topic overview. Retrieved from http://www.webmd.com/skin-problems-and-treatments/tc/ringworm-of-the-skin-topic-overview

Wilkinson, J. M., & Ahearn, N. R. (2009). *Prentice Hall nursing diagnosis handbook* (9th ed.). Upper Saddle River, NJ: Prentice Hall.

Worm, M., Fiedler, E. M., Dölle, S., Schink, T., Hemmer, W., Jarisch, R., et al. (2009). Exogenous histamine aggravates eczema in a subgroup of patients with atopic dermatitis. *Acta Dermato Venereologica, 89*(1), 52–56.

Zeina, B. (2012). Pemphigus vulgaris. Medscape reference. Retrieved from http://emedicine.medscape.com/article/1064187-overview#a0104

Caring for the Patient with Wounds

CHAPTER 60

Joyce Pittman
Kathleen Osborn

Outcome-Based Learning Objectives

After studying this chapter, the learner will be able to:

1. Compare and contrast the clinical manifestations of the four phases of wound healing.
2. Compare and contrast wound classifications and respective treatments.
3. Describe key factors relative to the prevention of pressure ulcers.
4. Describe wound characteristics and nursing documentation that are required in ongoing wound assessment.
5. Evaluate therapies and their benefits with respect to wound healing.
6. Understand the psychosocial and liability factors pertaining to wound care.
7. Describe how research in wound care will lead to better efficiency and outcomes with evidence-based practice.

KEY TERMS

acute wounds p.1895
angiogenesis p.1890
bioburden p.1892
Buerger's disease p.1898
chronic wounds p.1895
collagen synthesis p.1890
epithelialization p.1891
fibroblasts p.1890
granulation tissue p.1890
hematoma p.1916
hemosiderin staining p.1898
hyperbaric oxygen therapy (HBOT) p.1912
hypergranulation p.1914
induration p.1893
interface pressure p.1913
maceration p.1907
pressure ulcer p.1901
primary intention p.1907
rete pegs p.1920
secondary intention p.1907
senile purpura p.1920
seroma p.1916
skin tear p.1900
tertiary or third intention p.1907
undermining p.1905
wound dehiscence p.1916
wound evisceration p.1916
xerosis p.1920

THE SKIN is the human body's largest organ and functions to protect internal organs from insults such as infection and injury. These insults may be as minor as a bump or bruise or as major as a life-threatening infection or a traumatic wound. Whether the injury is caused by a surgeon's scalpel, trauma from a bullet or stab wound, or tissue damage from a myocardial infarction, the repair process is similar. The primary objective of the wound healing process is to restore skin integrity and structural continuity of the injured area (Porth & Matfin, 2009).

Skin comprises three layers of tissue: epidermis, dermis, and subcutaneous tissue. Each layer has a different composition and function. The outermost layer of skin is the epidermis. It contains melanocytes for pigmentation, Langerhans' cells as part of the immune system, sensory nerves, and keratinocytes. The main functions of the epidermis are protection and sensation. The dermis, the thickest layer of the skin, contains the microvascular system along with hair follicles, sweat glands, lymph vessels, sebaceous (oil) glands, and nerve endings. The dermis is constructed of collagen, a protein made from fibroblasts, and elastin, which makes the skin flexible and elastic. The main functions of the dermis are thermoregulation and blood supply to the epidermis. The innermost layer of the skin is an avascular subcutaneous fat layer (also known as hypodermis), which is composed of stored fat cells. Its main function is insulation and protection of the underlying organs (Porth & Matfin, 2009). Chapter 58 discusses the anatomy of the skin in detail.

Physiology of Wound Healing

When the skin has been compromised by an injury or infection, the primary objective is to restore tissue integrity through the healing process. The depth of the injury determines the wound healing process. Partial-thickness wounds are shallow wounds that involve epidermal and possible partial dermal layer loss. Partial-thickness wound repair includes an initial inflammatory response to the injury and epithelial reproliferation and migration. Full-thickness wounds are wounds that extend at least to the subcutaneous tissue layer and possibly deeper to the underlying structures. Full-thickness wound repair comprises four major phases: hemostasis, inflammation, proliferation, and remodeling (Figure 60–1◆). These phases represent a cascade of events that overlap and are dependent on one another. Each phase contributes to the desired result of healing the wound. Any disruption or absence

Video: Inflammation in Wound Healing Weblink: Wound Healing

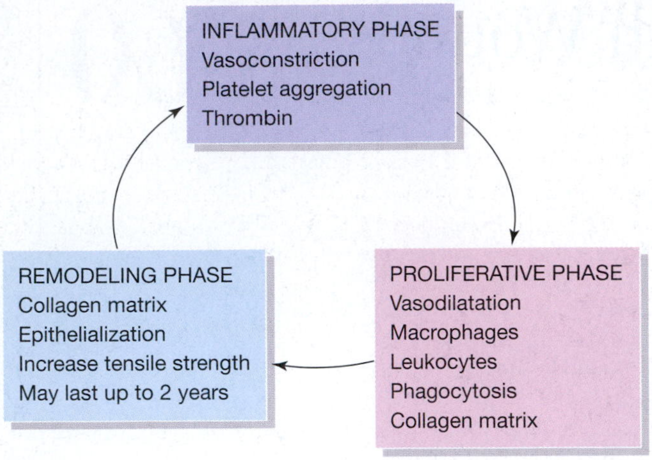

FIGURE 60–1 ◆ Phases of wound healing.

of a phase can result in a delayed or prolonged healing (Doughty & Sparks-Defriese, 2007). Each phase is discussed in the following text.

Phase One: Hemostasis Phase

Injury to the skin causes blood cells to spill into the wound. This initiates a series of events that activates the process for hemostasis and a temporary barrier to bacteria. The platelets release a vasoconstrictive substance that assists in this process. Coagulation factors, which promote platelet aggregation in the injured vessel's endothelium at the site of injury, are also released. The bleeding is usually stopped by thrombus formation. Thrombin is used to convert fibrinogen to fibrin. Thrombus formation is discussed in detail in Chapter 55. Clot formation followed by fibrinolysis is a critical event in the sequence of wound healing. The activation and degranulation of platelets lead to the release of cytokines and growth factors.

Growth factors, which are a group of extracellular polypeptides (secreted by platelets and macrophages), affect cell growth, reproduction, movement, and function. Growth factors recruit the necessary cells to synthesize and regulate the wound repair. Scientists have identified several of these growth factors and their effects on the wound repair process; for example, platelet-activating factor (PAF) induces platelet aggregation (Porth & Matfin, 2009), and transforming growth factor (TGF-β), epidermal growth factor (EGF), and insulinlike growth factor (IGF-I) initiate inflammation and tissue repair (Schultz, 2007).

Phase Two: Inflammatory Phase

The *inflammatory phase* of wound healing begins once bleeding is under control. The purpose of this critical phase is to prepare the site for growth of new tissue. This phase of wound healing cleans the wound in preparation for closure. In a clean acute wound, the inflammatory phase lasts approximately 3 to 5 days, but in a wound complicated by infection or necrosis, the inflammatory phase is prolonged, and wound healing is delayed (Doughty & Sparks-Defriese, 2007). Within hours after injury, vasoactive substances (histamines, prostaglandins, complement factor, and thrombin) are released, causing local vasodilation and increased capillary permeability. This allows leakage of serous fluid into the injured site, which results in erythema, edema, and the production of exudates.

Prostaglandin, which is released during the inflammatory phase, is a long-chain fatty acid that regulates platelet aggregation and controls inflammation and vascular permeability. The inflammatory phase is characterized by the presence of granulocytes, macrophages, and lymphocytes, which are attracted to the injured site by the complement factors and antigens. These cells, called phagocytes, perform *phagocytosis*, the process of absorbing and enzymatically degrading foreign matter and devitalized tissue, thus preparing the wound for closure. The by-product of phagocytosis is exudate. Exudate, or drainage from the wound, is usually at its peak during the inflammatory phase. Drainage from the wound during the inflammatory phase does not indicate wound infection; it is the body's normal response to injury.

Suppression of the inflammatory phase can contribute to a delay in wound healing. One common reason for a prolonged inflammatory phase is the presence of necrosis and infection. Radiation therapy can suppress the inflammatory phase by causing depletion of the neutrophils and macrophages, which release the growth factors. Malnutrition, dehydration, and chronic steroid use also can suppress the inflammatory phase. Chronic use of steroids specifically results in decreased production of histamines, suppressing the inflammatory response. A prolonged inflammatory phase can be a risk factor for wound dehiscence (discussed later in the chapter) and hyperproliferative scarring (Doughty & Sparks-Defriese, 2007).

Phase Three: Proliferative Phase

The proliferative or repair phase is the next phase in the healing process. Reconstruction occurs during this phase, which can last up to 3 weeks after the inflammatory phase in a normal, healthy person. Growth factors described earlier originating from injured vessels stimulate the formation of vascular buds and regrowth of vascular loops. Stimulated endothelial cells multiply and form tubular structures that differentiate into arterioles or venules, a process referred to as **angiogenesis.** These new blood vessels can begin to form in a wound within 3 days of injury, provided that there is sufficient blood circulation to the wound bed.

Simultaneously, in the process of revascularization, connective tissue begins to form at the wound margins. **Fibroblasts** are the small cells that migrate along the fibrin network to produce the connective tissue and collagen fibers. **Collagen synthesis** is the multistep process in which fibrin proteins form a matrix to support the newly forming tissue. Collagen synthesis is dependent on adequate amounts of vitamin C, iron, and copper in the diet. The newly formed collagen fibers are not organized in the same tension contours as they are in healthy tissue; therefore, the tensile strength and elasticity are decreased in a repaired wound. Collagen fibers in scar tissue actually have a disorganized appearance (Christian, Talavera, Stadelmann, Slenkovich, & Downey, 2006). The end result is that scar tissue never has the same tensile strength as normal tissue.

Due to angiogenesis, granulation tissue develops. **Granulation tissue,** aptly named for the recognizable tiny, round, granulelike nodules, is a highly vascular connective tissue that contains newly formed capillaries, proliferating fibroblasts, and residual inflammatory cells (Porth & Matfin, 2009). Granulation tissue appears beefy red and moist because of the dense revascularization process. Granulation tissue gradually fills the defect of the wound. If granulation tissue is slow to form, one can presume that the blood supply is insufficient, there is a wound infection, or one of the growth factors necessary for revascularization is deficient, any of which interrupts the normal rate of wound healing. This part of the proliferative phase begins about 3 days after initial injury and may overlap with the inflammatory phase.

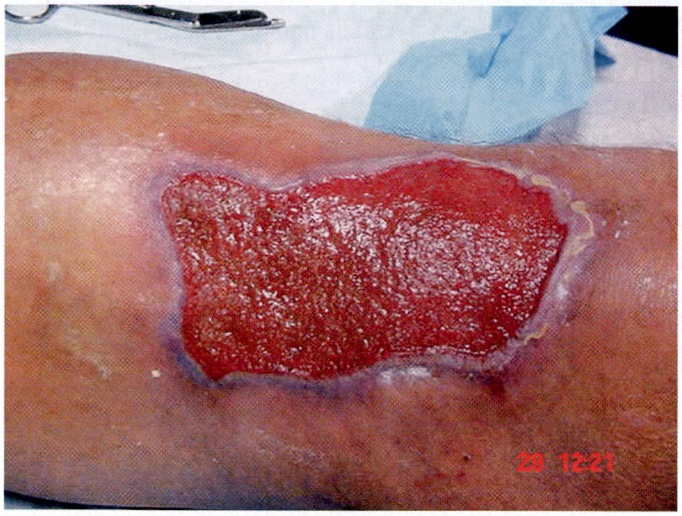

FIGURE 60–2 ◆ Granulation and epithelialization tissue.
Source: Courtesy of Harold Engle.

Epithelialization is the process by which the wound closes from its margins, covering the defect with a layer of new skin. This is accomplished by cell migration from the wound edges over granulation tissue. The wound bed must be moist and well perfused with blood for epithelialization to occur. Epithelialization, usually first seen at the wound margins, appears as a small pink or pearl-like area. Islands of epithelial cells can appear within the wound defect on the surface of the granulation. This new skin is quite fragile and must be protected from injury. A moist environment encourages the migration of these cells across the wound surface from all directions. Granulation and epithelialization, if not interrupted, continue to develop for up to about 14 to 21 days (Figure 60–2◆). Partial-thickness wounds (e.g., skin tears, abrasions) do not require granulation to heal because epithelial cells are able to migrate across the wound, rebuilding dermis. Full-thickness wounds, however, require granulation to fill the defect caused by the wound. This is not regenerated tissue but scar tissue.

Phase Four: Remodeling/Maturation Phase

Remodeling, the final phase of wound healing, occurs after the wound is closed. It begins about 3 weeks after the injury and can still be in progress from 6 months to 2 years later. During this phase, the scar changes and matures. Its bulk decreases, and the color changes from pink to pearly white. The incisional strength builds; by the end of 8 weeks, the strength of the tissue is about 70% of its original strength. During remodeling, collagen fibers are partially broken down by enzymes and reconfigured. Contraction due to the myofibroblasts can cause collagen fibers to become taut; scar tissue shrinks, and cutaneous tissue becomes smaller. Tension lines are frequently visible on the cutaneous surface (outer skin) of scar tissue. Healed wounds achieve only part of the original tensile strength and therefore are at a greater risk of future breakdown. The remodeling phase leaves the affected area with only 65% to 80% of its original tissue strength, and the affected area will be more prone to reinjury in the future. The remodeling phase may last up to 2 years.

Safety Alert *The nurse needs to teach the patient that the scar tissue will never reach its preinjury strength. Therefore, to prevent future skin breakdown, it is essential to protect the scar tissue from trauma and overexposure to the sun.*

Wound Healing Risk Factors

A wound develops as a result of some type of insult or injury. The body has a normal process for wound healing, as described earlier in the phases of healing. Many factors play a role in the progression in wound healing or lack thereof. These factors are critical elements for the phases of wound healing to proceed. Any factors that are not adequate will delay healing until they are sufficiently corrected. When assessing patients, the nurse must be aware of the risk factors that may affect the rate of wound healing.

Arterial Vascular System: Macro and Micro

The arterial vascular component is the most essential of all components in wound healing; without it, no phase of healing can begin, and no hope of healing can occur. The arterial vascular system consists of macrocirculation (large vessels such as the femoral or carotid arteries) and microcirculation (small vessels such as capillary beds or superficial artery systems). The arterial vascular system is essential to deliver the clotting factors, oxygen, leukocytes, macrophages, prostaglandins, and growth factors that contribute to the healing process. Without adequate circulation, a wound will not heal. There are multiple tests that can evaluate circulation. Macrocirculation of the lower extremities can be tested by performing an ankle–brachial index (ABI). The ABI is a simple noninvasive bedside procedure that compares the ankle systolic blood pressure to the brachial systolic blood pressure using a blood pressure cuff and Doppler probe. The ABI results indicate the arterial perfusion to the extremity. ABI $\geq$ 1.0–1.3 is considered a normal range. ABI $<$ 0.5 indicates severe ischemia and unlikely wound healing (Doughty & Sparks-Defriese, 2007). The ABI is used to determine whether additional testing for circulatory disease is warranted. Chapter 35 further describes the ABI.

Doppler studies are another tool used to test circulation. They utilize ultrasound to test arterial blood flow and estimate arterial circumference and/or occlusion. An invasive study for circulatory evaluation is a femoral angiogram; a catheter is inserted into the femoral artery, and pictures are taken with enhancement by a dye that reveals actual blood flow and determines a percentage of blockages, if any. Surgical options to restore arterial flow to the lower extremities include angioplasty and bypass graft surgery. Amputation is the treatment of last resort and is indicated for patients with irreversible ischemia and invasive infection (Doughty & Holbrook, 2007).

Microcirculation can be evaluated as well. Microcirculation involves the capillary beds that "feed" the wound area itself. A test known as a transcutaneous oxygen measurement (TCOM) can evaluate the tissue at a depth of one-fourth inch. The test utilizes an electrode that is heated to vasodilate the capillary bed. The tester uses a solution as the medium for the diffusion of gases, including oxygen, and records a measurement of the partial pressure of oxygen. Chart 60–1 notes the areas and partial pressures that are expected for circulation that is adequate for healing.

CHART 60–1 Transcutaneous Oxygen Measurement (TCOM)

PO_2

Chest: 60–80 mmHg (reference lead)

Extremity: 30–40 mmHg (desired)

If extremity $<$ 30 mmHg, apply 100% O_2 and measure response.

If response increases PO_2 in mmHg, patient is possible candidate for hyperbaric oxygen therapy (see p. 1912).

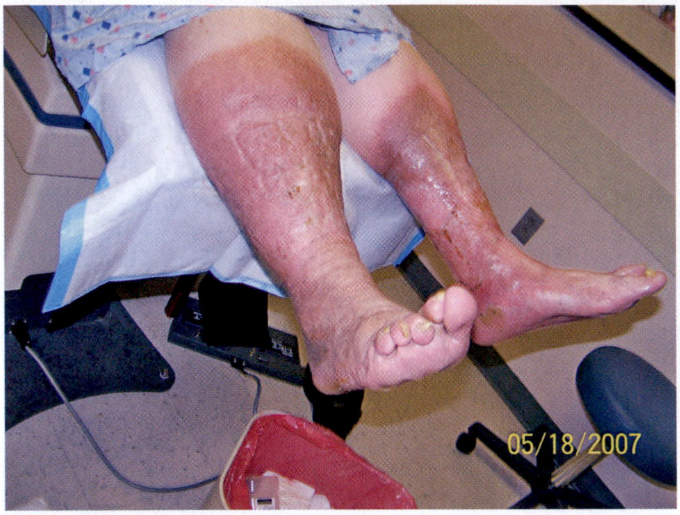

FIGURE 60–3 ◆ Hemosiderin stain.
Source: Courtesy of Harold Engle.

Venous System

The venous system, which returns the deoxygenated blood to the heart, is also a component of the wound healing process. The dilation of the venous system due to incompetent valves causes edema. The edema compresses the tissue and thus compresses the capillary beds and decreases circulation. Due to changes in capillary permeability in the edematous areas, fluid leaks into the local tissues. Infection then can set in as bacteria on the skin invade the area and are attracted to the fluid-filled medium.

A simple, noninvasive clue, besides edema, that there is venous insufficiency is the presence of hemosiderin staining (Figure 60–3◆). Hemosiderin staining is a direct result of red blood cells that are trapped in the interstitial tissues and the breakdown of heme (iron) into the tissue itself. Venous Doppler tests using ultrasound measure venous congestion and regurgitation (a direct result of incompetent valves) and can accurately detect venous insufficiency. Chapter 35 discusses peripheral vascular disease.

Other important risk factors can cause a delay in wound healing. Some are directly controlled by the patient; others have an effect that is less easily controlled by the patient. The following factors will be discussed: nutrition and hydration, infection, comorbid conditions, medications, stress, glucose control and diabetic management, and smoking. The Risk Factors box outlines systemic and situational factors that affect wound healing.

Nutrition and Hydration

Nutrition is one of the most understated and undervalued components of and factors in wound healing. Adequate nutrients are essential for normal healing because malnutrition interrupts the rate of normal tissue repair. The diet must be high in protein and calories with vitamin and nutritional supplements. Proteins are the building blocks of collagen, a cellular matrix that forms the basis of tissue granulation. Micronutrients, that is, nutrients that are needed in small amounts, include the fat-soluble vitamins A, D, E, and K and the water-soluble vitamins C and the B family. Vitamins such as A, D, E, and K play a role in the wound healing process as cofactors and antioxidants, have antiplatelet properties, promote cell membrane stability, and assist in other vital functions. Supplemental vitamins and nutritional supplements should be monitored.

RISK FACTORS for Systemic and Situational Factors Affecting Wound Healing

Smoking	Incontinence	Dehydration
Age 75 or over	Diaphoresis	Infection
Inadequate nutrition	Paralysis	Immobility
Low albumin/protein	Neurological disease	Dementia
Anemia	Immunosuppression	Edema
Cancer	Spasticity	Kidney disease
Contractures	Lung disease	Stress
Emphysema	Dermatologic conditions	Present pressure ulcers
Heart disease	Impaired circulation	Steroid use
Emaciation/cachexia	Obesity	Diabetes
Diminished sensation	Uncontrolled pain	

Supplements that are high in proteins and vitamins can assist in replacing low levels of albumin and aid in the formation of collagen to "fill" the wound to a level depth. Supplemental amino acids include arginine, glutamine, and hydroxymethyl butyrate (HMB). There are a number of available supplemental drinks and products that contain one or more of these important components. The need for nutrients continues throughout the healing process. Using every opportunity to get patients to take in nutrients can be a nursing challenge. A comprehensive nutritional assessment should be done for nonhealing and chronic wounds. Chart 60–2 outlines the specific vitamins and nutrients and their roles in the wound healing process. Unfortunately, there is no specific diagnostic marker to determine nutrition status. However, diagnostic tests to check protein levels, such as the albumin and, more recently, prealbumin, may be helpful to determine the risk of malnutrition. Prealbumin helps to determine whether the decrease in albumin is due to dietary intake or some organic issue independent of dietary intake. Chapter 8 includes a discussion of albumin and prealbumin.

Safety Alert *If the prescribed diet allows, the nurse should offer one of the canned nourishment supplements or instant breakfast mixes along with medications. The opportunity to offer calorie-laden fluids can be helpful to patients who have difficulty consuming enough calories.*

Maintaining adequate hydration assists in healing and decreases the risk of development of additional wounds. Proper hydration is often overlooked after intravenous fluids are discontinued. Offering patients fluids on a regular basis assists in maintaining hydration. Intake and output must be documented to monitor hydration status. Fluid intake should be measured every 24 hours if inadequate hydration is suspected. Chapter 8 includes a complete description of nutritional requirements.

Infection

Bioburden, or the metabolic load caused by bacteria present in a wound, can impair wound healing. The balance between the bacteria present and the host is kept in balance by the host's immune system. If this becomes unbalanced, the bacteria can overcome the host's defenses. This is referred to as the infection continuum. Wounds can be contaminated, colonized, critically colonized, and finally infected. Contamination is the presence of bacteria on the wound surface with no multiplication of the bacteria. Colonization is the presence of bacteria

CHART 60–2 Essential Vitamins and Nutrients for Wound Healing

Vitamins and Nutrients	Function in Wound Healing
Vitamin A	Stimulant for onset of the wound healing process. Stimulant of epithelialization and fibroblast deposition of collagen.
B vitamins (B_6, B_{12})	Critical to metabolism and to synthesis of protein, fat, and carbohydrate but no reported benefits of vitamin B specific to wound healing.
Vitamin C	Collagen synthesis, capillary wall integrity, fibroblast function, and immunologic function.
Vitamin E	By fighting oxidative damage, it can be effective in reducing infection risk, but daily levels in excess of 100 international units retard healing.
Vitamin K	Essential for blood clotting (coagulation).
Iron	Excessive consumption could result in bacterial proliferation.
Zinc	Essential for protein synthesis and collagen formation. Necessary for formation of T lymphocytes, supporting immunity. Deficiency leads to decreased epithelialization and fibroblast proliferation.
Copper	Cofactor for connective tissue production. Collagen cross-linking.
Arginine (amino acid)	Produces nitric oxide, which is essential for collagen accumulation and angiogenesis, and enhances immunity.
Glutamine (amino acid)	Critical role in preserving nitrogen balance, protein synthesis, cellular structure, and metabolism. Source for cellular respiration.

that are multiplying on the wound surface but without causing harm to the host and with no outward signs or symptoms. Critical colonization occurs when the bioburden increases in the wound and begins to overwhelm the host. Subtle signs begin to occur such as arrested healing, change in the appearance of the wound base, tissue not having the healthy red cobblestone appearance of granulation tissue, or tissue becoming friable (easily torn). Infection means that bacteria are invading viable tissue and there is a systemic response. This response may be demonstrated by inflammation, purulent drainage, increased pain, **induration** (hardness), sudden elevated glucose, delayed healing, odor, increased slough in the wound bed, leukocytosis, or fever (Stotts, 2007). Three basic elements must exist for a clinical definition of infection (Gardner & Frantz, 2004):

- Microorganisms must be present in viable tissue.
- Microorganisms must multiply enough to impair healing or cause injury.
- Invading microorganisms must produce a host response or tissue injury.

It is generally accepted that clinical infection in acute wounds has been correlated with tissue levels greater than 10^5 organisms per gram. To diagnose infection, laboratory microbiologic results must be evaluated in conjunction with local clinical findings. It is important to recognize the classic signs and symptoms of infection: erythema, heat, edema, pain, and purulent exudate. These symptoms are the host's response to invading organisms and serve as reliable indicators of acute infection in wounds.

The presence of infection requires the body to "fight" the infection with white blood cells, macrophages, and leukocytes. In addition, the attention to healing becomes secondary as the body focuses on the immediate problem of the infection at hand. Infection also leaves bioburden, or waste, that must then be disposed of before collagen synthesis and granulation can occur. Microorganisms such as methicillin-resistant *Staphylococcus aureus* (MRSA) and *Klebsiella pneumoniae* with a resistant erythromycin sensitive beta lactamase (ESBL) strain are now invading wounds. These multidrug-resistant strains require multiple antibiotics with long durations.

Nursing management of infected wounds includes obtaining a culture when ordered by the health care provider. It is important to know the proper procedure for obtaining a culture: The nurse cleanses the wound thoroughly with saline. With a sterile culturette swab, the nurse applies pressure and rolls the swab repeatedly over a 1 centimeter square. The portion of the wound to be cultured can be anywhere within the wound bed; the best place is a spot where tissue fluid can be expressed by pressing with the swab. The purpose is to take a culture of the tissue fluid, not of the exudate on top of the wound. Tissue biopsy is the gold standard to determine infection and may be performed by health care providers but is not readily available in all institutions. The Diagnostic Tests box outlines laboratory and diagnostic findings related to wound healing.

Comorbidities

Comorbidities, which are concurrent disease processes, also affect the wound healing process. For example, diabetes, a disorder characterized by the inability to store glucose and thus the occurrence of elevated blood glucose levels, is the single most prevalent comorbidity in patients requiring chronic wound care. Diabetes causes neuropathy (decreased sensation). (See the discussion on wound healing and diabetes later in this chapter.) Diabetes also interferes with the immune system and circulation by causing hardening of the vessels and capillary beds. This hardening is the process whereby the vessel and capillary beds are infiltrated by fatty deposits that accumulate, causing localized damage to the vessel's endothelial lining.

Hypertension and atherosclerotic disease also cause problems with circulation and edema that compromise wound healing. Autoimmune disorders such as lupus or scleroderma decrease the body's ability to fight off infection; when a wound is found in patients with these disorders, the delayed healing due to decreased immunity is evident.

LABORATORY AND DIAGNOSTIC TESTS Related to Wound Healing

Diagnostic Test, Normal Values, and Rationales	Expected Abnormality
White Blood Cells (WBCs) Normal: 4,500–10,000/mm^3 *Diagnose and track infection* *Differential: percentage of each type of WBC (neutrophils, lymphocytes, monocytes, eosinophils, basophils)*	Increased with inflammation and acute infection. Decreased with thrombocytopenia, cancers, anemias, or liver disease.
Platelets Normal: 150,000–400,000/mm^3 *Basic element of coagulation.* *Decreased count can drive treatment.*	Increased with inflammation and infection. Indication of concealed bleeding (i.e., gastrointestinal [GI]).
Red Blood Cells (RBCs) Normal: Female: 4.0–5.0 million/mm^3 Male: 4.6–6.0 million/mm^3 *Monitor for need for medications or blood administration to increase value.*	May be decreased due to bleeding from the wound. Decrease might indicate depleted blood volume. Chronic infections.
Hemoglobin (Hgb) Normal: Female: 12–15 g/dL Male: 13.5–18 g/dL *Monitor with hematocrit for need for medications or blood administration to increase value.*	May be decreased due to bleeding from the wound, hypoxia, anemias, or overhydration. Some prescription medications can decrease count.
Hematocrit (HCT) Normal: Female: 36–46% Male: 40–54% *Monitor for need for medications or blood administration to increase value.*	May be decreased due to bleeding from the wound.
Total Proteins Normal: 6.0–8.0 g/dL *Monitor need for nutritional supplements.*	May be decreased with malnutrition. Decrease indicates immunosuppression.
Serum Albumin Normal: 3.5–5.0 g/dL *Monitor need for nutritional supplements.* *Half-life is 21 days; easily influenced by medications and fluid status.*	May be decreased with malnutrition injury because albumin catabolism increases as a result of injury.
Serum Prealbumin Normal: 17–40 mg/dL *Current protein status.*	Reflects immune and inflammatory status.
Wound Culture and Sensitivity Normal: Negative *Assess for wound infection and which antibiotic will be effective in treating it.*	Will be positive if there is contamination, colonization, or infection.

Source: Adapted from Kee, J. L. (2010). *Laboratory and diagnostic tests with nursing implications.* Upper Saddle River, NJ: Pearson.

Medications

A number of medications can affect the wound healing process. The two categories of medications that are the most likely to influence wound healing are chemotherapeutic agents and anti-inflammatory medications. Anti-inflammatory agents such as corticosteroids decrease the immune system by delaying white blood cell migration and fibroblasts, thus impacting the inflammatory phase of wound healing. The ground matrix, collagen synthesis, regeneration of blood vessels, and epithelialization are also significantly delayed due to steroid use. One area of research now in progress is the use of retinoids (vitamin A) to combat these effects. Some trials have shown retinoids to combat the ill effects of steroids directly and potentially reverse some of their adverse effects (Doughty & Sparks-Defriese, 2007). Chemotherapeutic agents affect the fibroblasts and myofibroblasts. This results in impaired collagen synthesis and wound contraction (Doughty & Sparks-Defriese, 2007). Chemotherapy drugs, specifically methotrexate, can delay the wound healing process by weakening the immune system as well as by bone marrow suppression and anemia. Communication with patients is crucial to develop a realistic plan of care. The medications patients take are a necessity; therefore, the plan of care must include educating the patient that the process of wound healing will be delayed by these drugs. Realistic timelines should be provided, as these will help decrease anxiety.

Stress

Stress causes a release of hormones, including glucocorticoids, which reduces the production of cytokines, an essential component of the inflammatory process. The glucocorticoids also alter leukocyte movement. Reduction in these two factors causes immunosuppression. Because wound healing begins with inflammation, if this phase becomes suppressed, there is a delay in wound healing. Previous research has demonstrated that stress was associated with a 25% to 40% delay in wound closure across the models tested (Doughty & Sparks-Defriese, 2007). Stress also causes catecholamine release, which in turn causes vasoconstriction, which will reduce perfusion and oxygenation to subcutaneous tissue and wounds. It is known that chronic stress (stress lasting weeks to years) has immunosuppressive effects; however, there is also evidence of acute stress (stress lasting minutes to hours) increasing the immune response, a situation that may enhance wound healing (Broadbent & Koschwanez, 2012).

Coping strategies, social support relationships, positive communication, and environmental enrichment to minimize the patient's stress may be beneficial to enhance wound healing (Broadbent & Koschwanez, 2012). Pain and noise are common stressors for hospitalized patients. When pain is present, energy is spent on enduring the pain and not on healing the wound. Control of pain with analgesics and diversional activities will help decrease stress.

Manipulation of the patient's environment will reduce external stressors. Nurses are in a unique position to control the patient's environment. Therefore, the nurse needs to be sensitive to the environmental noise and mitigate it when possible. Chapter 9 provides an in-depth discussion of the impact of stress on the human body.

Glucose Control and Diabetes Management

Glucose control is essential for normal healing. High levels of glucose impair wound healing, so it is important to control the blood sugar very early in wound care to maximize wound healing potential. Studies have indicated that in patients with diabetes, wound repair is characterized by reduced collagen synthesis and deposition and decreased tensile strength (Doughty & Sparks-Defriese, 2007). For example, high glucose levels result in altered leukocyte functioning and increased risk of infection. Monitoring the daily blood glucose levels and HgA1c values is important and helps to educate the patient about the need for glucose control. The recommended HgA1c value is 2.5% to 6% (Kee, 2010). This roughly estimates a blood glucose level of 120 mg/dL. The optimal blood glucose level is currently thought to be 70 to 110 mg/dL. Chapter 47 includes a complete discussion of blood glucose levels.

The nurse needs to assess the patient's knowledge of diabetes and glucose control and reinforce areas in which that knowledge is lacking. If necessary, a consultation with a diabetes educator can refresh the patient's understanding and address knowledge deficits about the disease. Diabetes education classes provide a foundation for the beginning of a lifetime of disease management. Careful monitoring of blood sugar should extend beyond wound healing and into the remodeling phase.

Smoking

The association between cigarette smoking and delayed wound healing is commonly seen in the clinical setting. The effects of nicotine, carbon monoxide, and hydrogen cyanide contained in cigarettes affect the normal rate of wound healing. Nicotine has the following effects on the tissues, which result in delayed wound healing:

- Nicotine is a vasoconstrictor that reduces blood flow to the skin, resulting in a loss of oxygen and nutrients, ischemia, and impaired healing of injured tissue.
- Nicotine increases platelet aggregation, thereby increasing the risk of thrombotic microvascular occlusion and tissue ischemia.
- Nicotine reduces the proliferation of red blood cells, fibroblasts, and macrophages.

Carbon monoxide decreases oxygen transport and slows metabolism. Hydrogen cyanide inhibits the enzyme systems necessary for oxidative metabolism and oxygen transport at the cellular level. The overall effect of smoking on wound healing is a slower healing process. Open wounds are at higher risk for wound infection and increased scar formation. Patients should be advised to stop smoking before elective surgery or when recovering from wounds resulting from trauma, disease, or emergent surgery. The nurse needs to assess the patient for the clinical manifestations of delayed wound healing and report them to the health care provider.

Preinjury Status

When a patient is admitted, it is essential to assess the patient's physical and emotional status. Lifestyles and habits that will impact healing such as smoking and poor nutrition must be identified. Both physiological and psychological factors alter the rate of wound healing, as well as morbidity and mortality. The length of time the illness existed before surgery or trauma and the patient's preinjury nutritional status both contribute to the rate of wound healing and risk of infection.

Classification of Wounds and Treatment

Several classifications for wounds exist. This chapter covers the most common types of wounds: diabetic, venous, arterial, vasculitic, traumatic, pyoderma gangrenosum, skin tear, and pressure wounds. They all have different origins, and their plans of treatment vary on the basis of wound type. Wound classifications are helpful in documenting wound assessment and care because they tell a history of the wound. For example, identifying a wound as chronic or acute provides an immediate awareness of the direction wound care should take, as well as expectations of the healing process. **Chronic wounds** are defined as wounds that do not follow the expected sequence of repair in a timely and uncomplicated manner. **Acute wounds** are recent wounds that are either traumatic or iatrogenic in etiology. Examples of *traumatic wounds* are abrasions, blisters, cuts, bites, stab wounds, gunshot wounds, and burn injuries. *Iatrogenic wounds* include intravenous (IV) puncture sites, incisions, radiation-induced skin damage, and grafts. Acute wounds progress through the stages of wound healing normally.

Chronic wounds generally occur due to inadequate blood supply in the tissue, repeated prolonged insults to the tissue, and disruptive underlying pathologic processes. The wound healing cascade is interrupted at some point by systemic deficiencies or extrinsic insults. Examples of chronic wounds are pressure ulcers, diabetic ulcers, vascular ulcers, and fungating (cancerous cells infiltrating the epithelial tissue)

Weblink: National Diabetes Fact Sheet 2011

tumors. Wounds that do not respond to appropriate treatment within 6 weeks are considered chronic and should be referred to a wound specialist.

The type of wound determines the basic plan of care and treatment for that wound, but the nurse needs to keep in mind that everyone responds differently to treatment and that the plan must be individualized. Wound care is not just a science but an art, and "thinking outside the box" has led to a great many strides in aggressive wound care therapy. The following sections feature the classifications used to describe further the extent of damage and current phase of healing.

Diabetic Wounds

Etiology, Epidemiology, and Pathophysiology

Prevalence of diabetes in the United States is estimated as high as 8.3% or 18.8 million people (Centers for Disease Control and Prevention [CDC], 2011). Almost 27% of individuals 65 years of age or older develop diabetes. It has been estimated that at least 10% of persons with diabetes may be at risk for the development of a foot ulcer (Steed, 2007) and 12.7% of patients with diabetes have a history of a foot ulcer (Driver, Landowski, & Madsen, 2007). In addition, 50% to 75% of all nontraumatic lower extremity amputations are caused by diabetic foot ulcers (DFUs) (Driver, Landowski, & Madsen, 2007).

The most frequent areas to find a DFU are on the plantar surface of the foot or toe or the metatarsal head (Figure 60–4◆). The most common factors that promote development of a wound in a patient with diabetes are neuropathy, macrovascular and microvascular changes, and a slow, decreased immune response. Neuropathy is decreased or absent sensation in an area due to chronic elevated blood glucose levels that over time affect the myelin sheath surrounding the nerves and degrade the sheath, exposing the nerves. The nerves then die over time without the myelin sheath to protect them from the body's own immune response.

Macrovascular and microvascular changes are due to elevated blood glucose levels that over time cause fatty deposits to stick to the endothelial lining of vessels and cause narrowing and then blockage of circulation (Porth & Matfin, 2009). The immune response is also delayed in a patient with diabetes. Although the exact cause is unknown, it has been well documented that a slow response to a wound or infection,

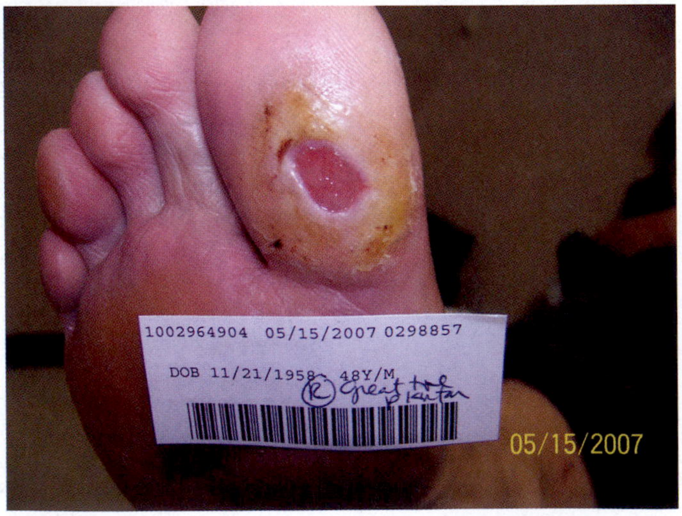

FIGURE 60–4 ◆ Diabetic plantar ulcer.
Source: Courtesy of Harold Engle.

and thus slow-to-develop outward signs of a problem, causes a delay in the wound healing process and a delay in alerting the patient with diabetes that a problem is occurring. Delay in seeking care causes a delay in treatment.

Diabetic wounds usually appear on the feet but may occur in other places on the body. These wounds are typically caused by traumatic injury to the foot of a patient with diabetes who suffers from neuropathy, which may result in little or no sensation in the feet. Not being aware of the injury, the patient may continue to traumatize the wound by walking.

Clinical Manifestations

There are numerous classification systems that assist the nurse in guiding treatment regimes for DFUs. The original Wagner Ulcer Grade Classification System has been modified to take into account ischemia and infection along with depth of penetration (Chart 60–3). In this system, the higher scores indicate more complex wounds. The DFUs are graded 0 to 5, with 5 indicating gangrene of the whole foot beyond salvage, requiring limb or life-sparing amputation (Driver et al., 2007). Another popular classification system for the DFU is the University of Texas Wound Classification System. This system utilizes a matrix of wound depth and four associated stages to specify ischemia, infection, a combination of both, or neither (Driver et al., 2007). The University of Texas classification system for diabetic wounds is shown in Chart 60–4. Another system is the size (area and depth) (SAD) classification system. This system classifies the wound according to area, depth, sepsis, quality of pulses, and accuracy of sensation (Driver et al., 2007).

Laboratory and Diagnostic Tests

After reviewing the factors affecting a diabetic wound, a plan of care is developed that involves diagnostic studies to evaluate the extent of those factors. A test to check for neuropathy is called the loss of protective sensation (LOPS) test. The LOPS test uses a monofilament called 5.07 Semmes-Weinstein nylon monofilament, which measures sensation in several areas to determine the extent of neuropathy (Driver, et al, 2007). The LOPS tests, arterial Doppler studies to check circulation, cultures of the wound, and basic chemistry and differentials are evaluated to correct any of those factors if possible. Differentials show the various types of immune cells that are present in the body. The main focus is on the percent of neutrophils, because the percentage goes up when an acute reaction occurs in response to infection. Neutrophils, also called polymorphonuclear leukocytes (PMNs), respond to inflammation and have phagocytic (microorganism-killing) properties. The other types of immune cells are eosinophils, which respond to parasitic infections and allergic reactions, and basophils, which respond to leukemia and diseases of the muscle (Porth & Matfin, 2009).

One serious result of a diabetic wound is osteomyelitis (bone infection). A diagnostic test such as magnetic resonance imaging (MRI),

CHART 60–3 Wagner Ulcer Grade Classifications

A. Grade 1: Superficial diabetic ulcer
B. Grade 2: Ulcer extension
   1. Involves ligament, tendon, joint capsule, or fascia
   2. No abscess or osteomyelitis
C. Grade 3: Deep ulcer with abscess or osteomyelitis
D. Grade 4: Gangrene to portion of forefoot
E. Grade 5: Extensive gangrene of foot

CHART 60–4 University of Texas Classification System for Diabetic Wounds

Stage	Grade 0	Grade I	Grade II	Grade III
A	Preulcerative or postulcerative lesion that is completely epithelialized	Superficial wound not involving tendon, capsule, or bone	Wound penetrating to tendon or capsule	Wound penetrating to bone or joint
B	Preulcerative or postulcerative lesion completely epithelialized with infection	Superficial wound not involving tendon, capsule, or bone with presence of infection	Wound penetrating to tendon or capsule with presence of infection	Wound penetrating to bone or joint with presence of infection
C	Preulcerative or postulcerative lesion completely epithelialized with ischemia	Superficial wound not involving tendon, capsule, or bone with presence of ischemia	Wound penetrating to tendon or capsule with presence of ischemia	Wound penetrating to bone or joint with presence of ischemia
D	Preulcerative or postulcerative lesion completely epithelialized with infection and ischemia	Superficial wound not involving tendon, capsule, or bone with presence of infection and ischemia	Wound penetrating to tendon or capsule with presence of infection and ischemia	Wound penetrating to bone or joint with presence of infection and ischemia

Source: Adapted From Lavery, L. A., Armstrong, D. G., & Harkless, L. B. (1996). Classification of diabetic foot ulcerations. *Journal of Foot and Ankle Surgery, 35*(6), 528.

computed tomography (CT), bone scan, or indium scan (tagged white blood cells with indium, a radioactive material) can determine the presence of osteomyelitis. A biopsy of the bone can be performed as well. If so, a pathologist can read the biopsy and determine whether the shape or morphology of the tissue can be determined to be present with infection or not.

Collaborative Management

A multidisciplinary approach is recommended in managing DFUs and has been found to improve outcomes. This team should include a podiatrist or orthopedic surgeon, vascular surgeon, infectious disease specialist, endocrinologist or family or internal medicine health care provider, certified wound care nurse, orthotist, and certified diabetic educator (Driver et al., 2007). In order to meet desired patient outcomes, it is essential that this interdisciplinary team communicate openly with one another in developing and evaluating care of the patient and family (IOM [Institute of Medicine], 2010). Early interventions must include prevention. The most effective and least expensive preventive method is careful and frequent inspection of the foot. The American Diabetic Association recommends annual foot examination by a health care provider for individuals with diabetes. Along with inspection, preventive measures should include bathing, toenail care, correct shoe wear, avoiding chemical corn/callus removers, wearing socks or seamless stockings, and protection (keep warm, avoid trauma) (Driver et al., 2007). In addition to early preventive measures, glycemic control must be monitored. Offloading of pressure from the DFU is another critical element in the basic management of these ulcers. (See the discussion on offloading in the Wound Management section later in this chapter.)

Evidence-based wound management is crucial to managing DFUs. Specifically for DFUs, priorities of topical therapy include (1) aggressively treating infection, (2) determining the degree of ischemia and referring the patient for revascularization if necessary, (3) relieving pressure to the wound, and (4) preparing the wound bed and environment by débridement, dressings, and advanced care treatments when appropriate (Driver et al., 2007). New wound care products such as tissue-engineered grafts and ointment containing platelet-derived growth factors have been effective treatments.

If aggressive therapy and advance treatment modalities such as hyperbaric oxygen therapy (discussed later in this chapter, p. 1912) are not successful, amputation may be necessary to protect the patient from a potentially fatal infection that could spread throughout the entire limb, body, and bloodstream.

Venous Ulcers

Etiology, Epidemiology, and Pathophysiology

Venous ulcers, another type of chronic wound, are the most common type of leg ulcer, accounting for 70% to 90% of all leg ulcers (Doughty & Holbrook, 2007). The prevalence of venous ulcers is not known for certain but is estimated at 1% to 3% in developed countries. The peak incidence occurs between the ages of 60 and 80. Some studies report venous ulcers occurring more often in females. Lower extremity venous disease (LEVD) affects approximately 6 to 7 million individuals in the United States, and almost 1 million people will develop ulcerations. The average lifetime cost for care for an individual with venous disease can exceed $40,000 (Doughty & Holbrook, 2007). Venous ulcers frequently occur on the lower extremities and the pretibial area but can occur almost anywhere on the leg. Risk factors for the development of LEVD include family history, occupation, pregnancy, trauma, deep vein thrombosis (DVT), obesity, thrombophlebitis, intravenous drug use involving the affected extremity, a sedentary lifestyle, prolonged standing, arthritis, and conditions affecting calf muscle function (Doughty & Holbrook, 2007).

When venous congestion occurs in the lower extremities, the veins are stretched like a rubber band. Over time, the constant stretching of the veins decreases their elasticity (the ability to retract to their original position and shape). There are valves in the veins that open and close and allow venous return to the heart. If the veins become inelastic over time, the valves become incompetent or "leaky" and regurgitate the fluid, allowing pooling of the fluid in the lower extremities. The venous congestion, or edema, now compresses the capillary beds and constricts the fluid's flow in the dermis to feed the skin. If an injury occurs or the fluid accumulates so much that it leaks through the skin pores, bacteria can set in and an ulcer may develop. The decreased circulation does not allow the normal healing process to occur, as the platelets, growth factors, and leukocytes can no longer reach the area of insult, and the ulcer becomes worse.

Clinical Manifestations

The classic venous ulcer usually is located around the medial malleolus. The ulcers are shallow, with a dark red wound base or a thin layer of yellow slough. They typically produce a lot of drainage. Venous ulcers are not well defined in their margins and have irregular borders. Often there is periwound maceration, crusting, scaling, edema, and/or hemosiderin staining (Doughty & Holbrook, 2007). **Hemosiderin staining** occurs when the heme part of the red blood cell is deposited in the tissues as red blood cells get trapped and accumulate due to venous congestion (Figure 60–3, p. 1893). As the red blood cell dies, the heme is deposited, and the staining color of brownish hue results.

Laboratory and Diagnostic Tests and Medical Management

For most patients, a thorough history and physical are adequate to identify the ulcer as either venous or arterial in origin. However, when there is a question of the diagnosis, surgical intervention is considered, or compression is indicated, then additional diagnostic tests should be considered. Performing venous and arterial Doppler ultrasounds can determine flow and the presence or absence of a deep venous thrombosis. The ankle–brachial index (ABI), described earlier (p. 1891), is a simple bedside procedure that helps determine the presence of ischemia (Doughty & Holbrook, 2007).

In addition to basic wound management principles, primary management strategies for the treatment of venous stasis ulceration includes compression, limb elevation, and surgical procedures (Doughty & Holbrook, 2007). Additional treatment options include exercises to improve calf muscle function. Compression therapy is the external application of pressure to the lower extremity to promote venous return and decrease venous congestion, allowing the capillary beds at the level of the wound to open and the healing process to occur. Compression can be achieved by the use of compression stockings, wraps, or a compression pump. One note of caution before using compression as treatment: Make sure the patient has adequate arterial circulation and no DVT. In addition, compression therapy can lead to an increase in the patient's preload volume, so patients with concurrent cardiac maladies such as heart failure and low ejection fractions may not tolerate the additional volume. These patients must see their cardiologist, and may need an adjustment on their diuretic therapy. The patient should be instructed that the venous congestion is chronic and that, most often, the patient will have to undergo compression therapy of some type for the rest of his life to prevent further ulcers and associated complications. Basic wound management principles must be followed in conjunction with compression and elevation. Wound management principles include preparing the wound bed through ongoing débridement, maintaining a moist wound bed environment, and controlling bioburden.

Arterial Ulcers

Etiology, Epidemiology, and Pathophysiology

Less common than venous ulcers, arterial ulcers occur as a result of ischemia to the tissues. The most common cause of lower extremity arterial disease (LEAD) is atherosclerosis in the older adult or premature atherosclerosis or thromboangiitis obliterans (Buerger's disease) in the younger adult. **Buerger's disease** is an inflammation of the peripheral arteries that is associated with smoking in 95% of cases (Brashers, 2010). Lower extremity arterial disease increases with age and is more common in men. The prevalence of LEAD is difficult to determine; however, it is estimated to range from 2% in people under age 50 to 20% in those over the age of 80 (Doughty & Holbrook, 2007). In individuals with intermittent claudication, 15% to 20% will progress to the point of critical limb ischemia and are at risk of limb loss.

Pathophysiology of arterial ulceration is thought to result from (1) progressive vascular occlusion leading to cellular ischemia;

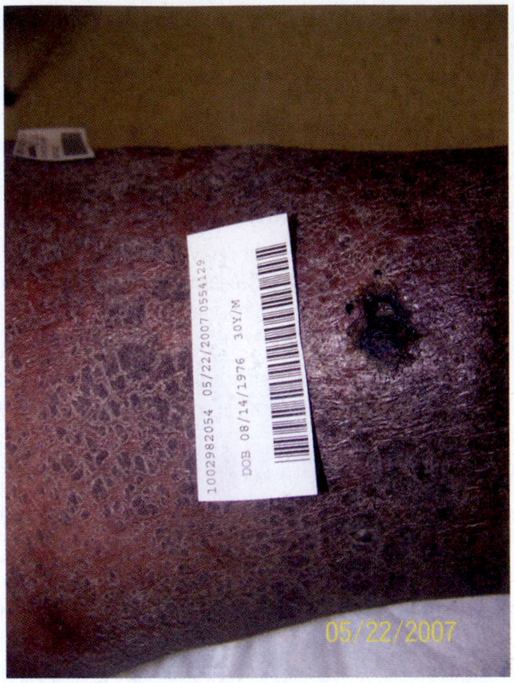

FIGURE 60–5 ◆ Arterial ulcer.
Source: Courtesy of Harold Engle.

(2) minor trauma, which results in a nonhealing wound due to the inability of the damaged vessels to meet the increased demands for oxygen associated with tissue injury and the healing process; and/or (3) external occlusive pressures such as heel pressure in a patient who is bed-bound (Doughty & Holbrook, 2007).

Clinical Manifestations

Arterial ulcers have distinctive characteristics. They are often located distally on the lower extremity (Figure 60–5◆). These ulcers are usually small and round with a "punched out" appearance and well-defined margins. The arterial wound bed color is pale or necrotic and has minimal exudate. These wounds are typically painful unless the patient is insensate. Infection is common, but signs and symptoms may be muted due to poor blood flow and immune response. Associated assessment reveals poor palpable pulses, and a Doppler may be needed to auscultate the pulse. Ischemic pain is usually present and is one of the first indications of LEAD. Other clinical signs of lower limb ischemia include thinning of the epidermis; alopecia; dry, taut, shiny skin; and dystrophic nails. Skin color changes include elevational pallor or grayish hue for dark skin tones, dependent rubor, and purpura. The lower extremity is cool to the touch and discolored, and hair loss may be evident. Capillary refill is delayed, and venous filling time is prolonged (Doughty & Holbrook, 2007; Holloway, 2007). Chart 60–5 presents a comparison of arterial and venous ulcers.

Laboratory and Diagnostic Tests and Medical Management

Diagnostic confirmation of arterial ulcers may require noninvasive and invasive vascular testing. As with venous ulcers, arterial Doppler ultrasounds and ABI can determine the flow and presence of vascular occlusion. Doppler waveform patterns can be analyzed and used to determine the degree of arterial disease. In addition, transcutaneous oxygen measurements are used to determine the degree of microvascular perfusion to an area. Arterial duplex using color Doppler ultrasound is used to gain information. However, arteriography remains the standard

Video*: Wound Irrigation

CHART 60–5 Differing Characteristics of Arterial and Venous Ulcers

Characteristic	Arterial Insufficiency Ulcer	Venous Stasis Ulcer
Location	Distal aspect of extremity (toe tips), pressure points on foot	Medial malleolus Distal and lateral aspects
Size and shape	Deep, small craters with well-defined margins	Normally limited to dermis; shallow subcutaneous tissue with irregular margins Can be "pinholes" through which serous fluid leaks
Wound bed	Pale or necrotic	Red or yellow slough, adhering or loose
Volume of exudate	Minimal	Normally large amount
Periwound skin appearance	Pale in color and faint erythema can be seen	Macerated, crusted, or scaling
Pain	Cramping or constant deep-aching pain	Variable; dull, aching, intermittent burning, etc.

test to provide the surgeon with a roadmap of the vasculature prior to revascularization (Holloway, 2007).

An arterial ulcer requires surgical intervention to restore the blood flow. Once blood flow has been reestablished, most ischemic wounds will heal. Basic wound management principles should be followed once circulation has been restored (wound bed preparation, moist wound healing, and control of bacterial burden, discussed below and in Chapter 61).

Vasculitic Ulcers

Etiology, Epidemiology, and Pathophysiology

Vasculitis is inflammation of the blood vessels, endothelial swelling, and necrosis. Vessels of any size may be affected; therefore, any organ or system may be affected. Vasculitic skin lesions are usually the sign of a complex systemic disorder and are thought to have an immunologic etiology (Bryant & Clark, 2007) (Figure 60–6◆). Vasculitic ulcers are associated with collagen vascular disorders such as systemic lupus erythematosus (SLE) or rheumatoid arthritis. They can also occur in patients with other associated vasculitic conditions such as polyarteritis, hypersensitivity vasculitis, Wegener's granulomatosis, Sjogren's syndrome, cryoglobulinemia, scleroderma, livedo vasculitis, and Takayasu's disease. These ulcers are more prevalent in females.

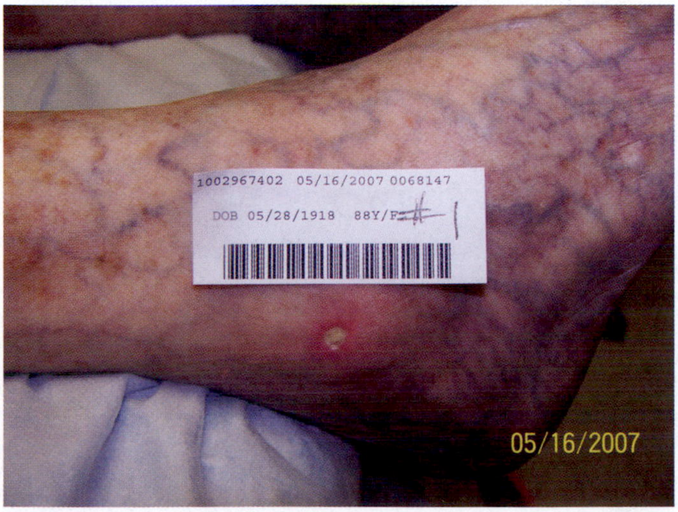

FIGURE 60–6 ◆ Vasculitis.
Source: Courtesy of Harold Engle.

Clinical Manifestations

Vasculitic ulcers usually present as petechiae, purpura, blisters, deep nodules, ulcers, or a prominent skin discoloration (livedo) pattern on the limbs (Ryan & Sargeant, 2007). Vasculitic cutaneous manifestations can range from erythematous, nonblanching macules and/or nodules to hemorrhagic lesions to necrotic lesions and ulceration (Bryant & Clark, 2007). Vasculitic lesions are very friable (bleed easily) and are extremely painful.

Laboratory and Diagnostic Tests and Medical Management

A biopsy should be taken to confirm the diagnosis of a vasculitic ulcer in its early stages. The first goal of treatment for vasculitic ulcers is to control the underlying disease condition. Treatment specific to the ulcer is bed rest, pharmacologic approach, and moist wound management. Antihistamines, corticosteroids, and immunosuppressive agents have been found helpful. Wound bed preparation through débridement, advanced wound management principles, and control of bacterial burden are the mainstays of topical treatment.

Traumatic Wounds

Etiology, Epidemiology, Pathophysiology, and Clinical Manifestations

Traumatic wounds develop from intentional or unintentional injury. Regardless, traumatic wounds are classified as acute wounds, meaning that they occur suddenly and progress rapidly and predictably through the repair process (Doughty & Sparks-Defriese, 2007). Traumatic wounds often include some type of blunt or penetrating trauma. There is little information in the literature about the prevalence of traumatic wounds. However, according to the CDC, the leading cause of death in individuals ages 1 to 44 years is accidents (Miniño, 2011), and many accidents involve wounds. Comorbidities such as diabetes, heart failure, and autoimmune disorders may contribute to the severity and response to the healing process of traumatic wounds. Clinical manifestation of traumatic wounds depends upon the depth of injury.

Laboratory and Diagnostic Tests and Medical Management

Assessment of the vascularity, categorization of damaged structures, and assessment of salvageability comprise the primary focus of the diagnostic work-up of the patient with a traumatic wound (Bernstein & Chung, 2007). Management of the traumatic wound first requires thorough irrigation and cleansing of the wound bed. Adequate cleaning and removal of foreign debris are the most important steps in the healing of

Video*: Dressing Change

these wounds because infection causes a delay in the healing process. Prophylactic antibiotic therapy can assist in the progress of healing. If an affected area extends down to exposed bone, osteomyelitis is a risk. Skin grafts and flaps may be required to cover any areas of missing tissue that cannot be replaced. The patient and family must be educated on signs and symptoms of infection, dehiscence, or evisceration, discussed later in the chapter.

Pyoderma Gangrenosum

Pyoderma gangrenosum is an uncommon dermatosis that can be diagnosed with a biopsy of the affected skin. It presents as small red bumps that may look like an insect bite. The reddened areas open up as sores over time and have a reddish-purple hue around the margins. They occur most often on the legs but may affect other areas of the body as well. Pyoderma gangrenosum is often associated with underlying disease such as inflammatory bowel disease, rheumatic or hematologic disease, and malignancy. It is rare and treatable but also may return in the future. It occurs most often in women between the ages 20 to 50 years (Wollina, 2007). Treatment may include a combination of corticosteroids and immunosuppressants in addition to advanced wound management (Wollina, 2007).

Skin Tears

A **skin tear** is defined as a traumatic wound resulting in a separation of the skin layers due to shear forces, friction, or blunt trauma (Lopez et al., 2011). Skin tears (Figure 60–7◆) are common in older patients whose skin has become fragile and thin. The prevalence of skin tears in the United States is estimated to be 1.5 million per year. Risk factors for skin tears include age-related skin changes, elasticity and hydration, sun exposure, injuries and infections, vascularity, nutrition, medications such as corticosteroids, mobility, vision impairment, dependence on caregivers for activities of daily living (ADL), and risk of falls. The Payne–Martin Classification System for Skin Tears provides health care providers with a means to enhance documentation and track outcomes of care. It improves assessment, prevention, and treatment of skin tears. The system uses three categories based on the amount of tissue lost (Chart 60–6).

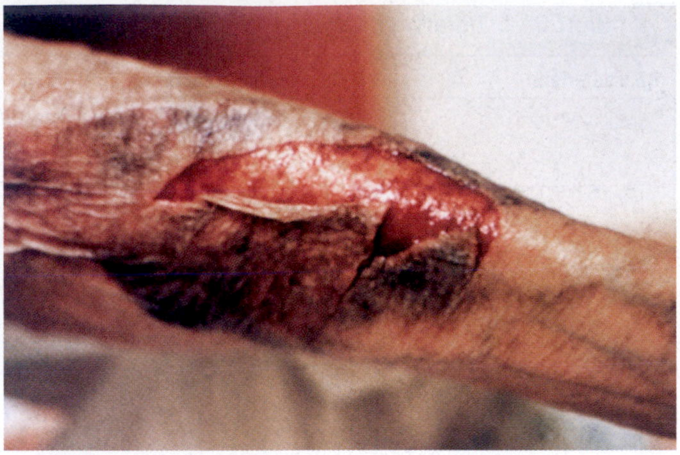

FIGURE 60–7 ◆ Skin tear.
Source: Jan Clark.

Nursing Management

Treatment of skin tears should include irrigating the tear with saline and trying to reposition any skin flap back in place. Skin flaps that are kept moist are more likely to adhere and heal. Use of adhesive tapes or transparent films can result in additional skin tears and should be avoided. Steri-Strips stay in place but become crusted with dry blood and can harbor pathogens. Preferred dressings should be nonadherent such as foam, silicone interface dressing, hydrogel sheets, and alginates that are absorbent and become gel-like. Some health care providers handling wound care have had success with zinc-impregnated gauze wraps secured with an elasticlike tape, such as Coban, on the zinc wrap itself and

CHART 60–6 Payne–Martin Classification and Treatment for Skin Tears

Category	Description
Category I:	Skin tear without tissue loss.
	A. Linear type: Epidermis and dermis pulled apart as if an incision has been made.
	B. Flap type: Epidermal flap completely covers the dermis to within 1 millimeter of the wound margin.
Category II:	Skin tear with partial tissue loss.
	A. Scant tissue loss: A loss of 25% or less of the epidermal flap.
	B. Moderate to large tissue loss: loss of more than 25% of the epidermal flap.
Category III:	Skin tears with complete tissue loss.
	No epidermal flap: black (necrosis), yellow drainage, pink or red granulation tissue completely exposed.
Treatment	
Appropriate skin tear treatment	Adhesive dressings or tapes should never be used to secure dressings onto fragile skin.
Little or no bleeding	A moisture barrier applied to periwound skin will help protect it and prevent further trauma.
	A gauze bandage wrapped around the extremity should be secured with tape onto the bandage, not the skin.
	Hydrogel sheet dressings or foam can be used.
	Foam dressings are effective.
Moderate bleeding	Zinc-impregnated gauze and cotton Webril wrapped around extremity, secured with Coban on bandage; none of it should be wrapped tightly.

Source: Adapted from Payne, R. L., & Martin, M. (1993). Defining and classifying skin tears: Need for a common language. *Ostomy Wound Management, 39*(5), 16–20, 22–24, 26.

not stretched tight. These dressings can be left for several days without being changed if the wound drainage is minimal.

Telfa dressings are also widely used for skin tears. Telfa is a nonstick application that protects the wound from outside injury or infection, has some absorptive properties, and allows the dressing to be removed without further damage to the skin.

It is essential that the nurse recognize patients who are at risk for skin tears. Some factors to be considered are age, condition of skin, use of steroids, unsteady balance and gait, easy bruising, and vision impairment. Prevention of skin tears includes avoiding use of harsh soaps and alcohol-based cleansers; using a patting motion to clean and dry skin; avoiding scrubbing skin; applying moisturizers; and adding padding to wheelchair arms, bed rails, and other objects that can do harm. The patient should consider wearing long-sleeved clothing, long socks with the toes cut out, or commercial arm protectors to protect the upper extremities. The nurse needs to educate the staff, family, and caregivers to use caution in repositioning patients who are at risk and in appropriate wound management, as discussed earlier.

Safety Alert *Take special care when removing tape from patients' skin that is at high risk for skin tears. Hold the skin down as the tape is being pulled off. Most importantly, do not use tape on the skin, but use a bandage and put the tape on the bandage.*

Pressure Ulcers

Pressure ulcers develop when pressure causes decreased circulation to an area. The compression interferes with the tissue blood supply, leading to vascular insufficiency, tissue anoxia, and cell death, resulting in tissue necrosis, or pressure ulcers. According to the National Pressure Ulcer Advisory Panel (NPUAP) and the European Pressure Ulcer Advisory Panel (EPUAP) (EPUAP & NPUAP, 2009), "A **pressure ulcer** is localized injury to the skin and/or underlying tissue usually over a bony prominence, as a result of pressure, or pressure in combination with shear." Pressure ulcers are most commonly seen in older adults, but that is not the only at-risk population for the disease. Patients with paraplegia or quadriplegia, those who have had strokes, and anyone who is not moving or will not relieve pressure on an affected area can develop a pressure ulcer. Pressure ulcers most often develop in areas that come into contact with the surface when the person is lying in a bed or sitting in a chair or wheelchair. Heels, sacral areas, ischial areas, and the lower back are the most commonly affected areas; other areas include the elbows, the occiput of the head, the spine, and even the ears. The ears can develop pressure ulcers as a result of long-term oxygen use with a nasal cannula. The nasal cannula is held in position behind the ears, and time can cause that area to develop a pressure ulcer.

Etiology and Epidemiology

It is estimated that at least 1.7 million people develop pressure ulcers annually (Pieper, 2007). The prevalence of pressure ulcers ranges from 10.1% to 17% in acute care settings (hospital), 2.3% to 28% in long-term care, and 0% to 29% in home care. Many regulatory organizations consider pressure ulcers a "nurse sensitive indicator" and a measure of the quality of care the patient receives. Pressure ulcers that are acquired while the patient is hospitalized add to the length of stay, add to the cost of care, delay the patient's recovery, and increase the patient's risk for developing complications. A patient in long-term care who has a pressure ulcer has a relative risk of dying of 1.45. The relative risk is the probability that a member of an exposed group will develop a disease relative to the probability that a member of an unexposed group will develop that same disease. Therefore, patients in long-term care who have pressure ulcers have a relative risk of dying of 1.45, meaning that they are 1.45 times as likely to die as is someone who does not have pressure ulcers (Pieper, 2007).

Pressure ulcers occur when pressure, caused by the compression of the skin between bone and another surface over time, impedes blood flow, causing tissue ischemia that may lead to necrosis and ulcer formation. There are three major components in the development of a pressure ulcer: (1) intensity of pressure, (2) duration of pressure, and (3) tissue tolerance. Intensity of pressure refers to the amount of pressure required to result in capillary collapse. Duration of pressure must be considered in conjunction with intensity of pressure. An inverse relationship exists between the two. Specifically, low-intensity pressures over a long period of time can create tissue damage, and high-intensity pressures over a short time period can also result in tissue damage. Finally, tissue tolerance describes the integrity of the skin and supporting structures that influence the person's ability to withstand increases of intensity and duration of pressure. Tissue tolerance is influenced by several intrinsic and extrinsic factors. Intrinsic factors are defined as the internal conditions that exist related to the patient's physical or mental health such as nutritional status, advanced age, medical comorbidities, smoking, low blood pressure, elevated body temperature, and stress. Extrinsic factors relate to the environment such as mobility, incontinence (moisture), shear, and friction (Pieper, 2007). Shear occurs as the skeleton moves against the muscles and other internal structures, causing the tissues to be pulled in opposite directions. This causes the bone to rub against the internal structures and distorts the shape of the capillaries, which become occluded, contributing to the formation of a pressure ulcer. Friction occurs when the body moves against an unyielding surface, causing the epidermis to be stripped away and ulcers to form (Pieper, 2007). Common sites for pressure ulcers are listed in Chart 60–7.

Clinical Manifestations and Pressure Ulcer Staging

Pressure ulcers are staged according to the depth of injury. The National Guidelines box outlines the European Pressure Ulcer Advisory Panel and National Pressure Ulcer Advisory Panel's stages of pressure ulcers (2009). Determining the stage or category of the pressure ulcer describes the tissue involved in a pressure ulcer, but it alone does not provide a basis for determining the topical treatment of wounds. Only pressure ulcers can be staged with this classification system (Figure 60–8◆, p. 1902). Skin tears, diabetic ulcers, surgical wounds, and burn injuries each have their own classification system. Once the ulcer begins to heal, it is not appropriate to use the staging in a reverse order to describe healing. Once an ulcer has reached a certain stage, such as Stage IV, it is always considered a Stage IV ulcer.

Risk Factors

Risk factors have been identified that make a patient more prone to development of a pressure ulcer. Risk assessment requires the evaluation of the presence of those factors. Patients who have restricted activity, as would occur with quadriplegia, strokes, and fractured hips, are at risk.

CHART 60–7 Common Sites for Pressure Ulcers

Patient Position	Pressure Ulcer Sites
Supine	Scapula, occiput, sacrum, heels
Lateral	Ear, shoulder, trochanter, medial knee, malleolus, foot edge
Prone	Nose, forehead, chest, iliac crests, foot edge, toes

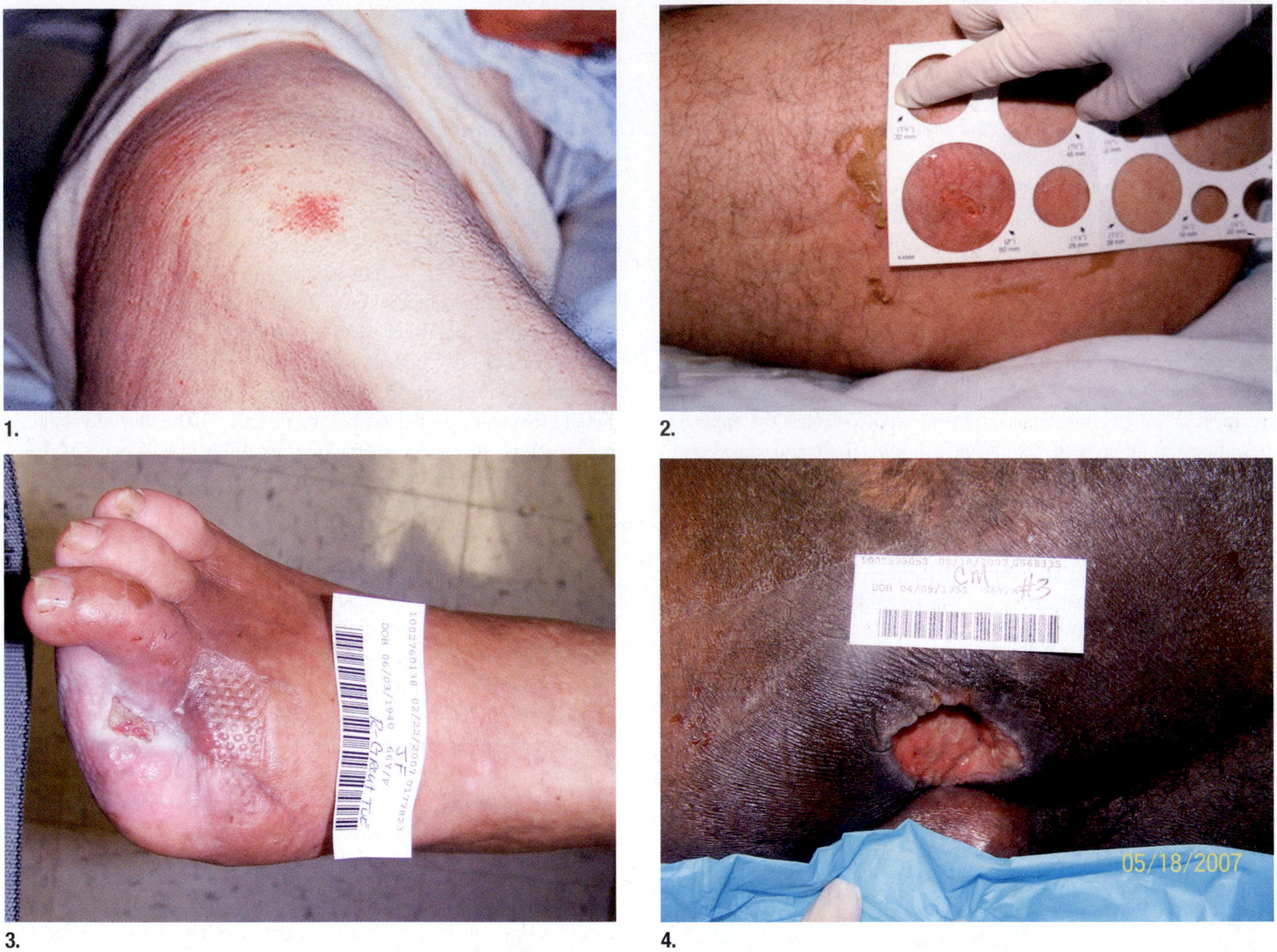

1. 2. 3. 4.

FIGURE 60–8 ◆ Four stages of pressure ulcers.
Source: 1, 3, 4: Courtesy of Harold Engle; 2: Jan Clark.

Not only are these patients inactive, but they also may have decreased sensation that may prevent them from feeling the pain associated with the development of a pressure ulcer. Patients with poor nutrition are more susceptible. Those who are very thin or have decreased protein in the diet have skin that is more likely to ulcerate. Patients who have urinary or fecal incontinence or who are exposed to other types of moisture such as perspiration, wound drainage, or emesis are also more prone to ulcers. Moisture causes a weakening of the cell wall of skin cells and changes the protective pH of the skin, making the skin more susceptible to skin breakdown (Pieper, 2007). The existence of a comorbid condition such as diabetes mellitus, hypertension, respiratory disease, or vascular disease also increases the risk for pressure ulcers.

Scales for Predicting Pressure Score Risk

Several risk assessment tools exist to determine the probability of pressure ulcer development. They include the Gosnell, Norton, and Braden Scales, as well as other versions that have been developed for specific institutions or populations or for items such as concurrent pressure ulcer, comorbidities, age, and continence issues. The Braden Scale for Predicting Pressure Sore Risk is the most widely used and most clinically validated tool that allows nurses and other health care providers to reliably score a patient's level of risk for developing pressure ulcers (Figure 60–9◆, p. 1904). The Braden scale consists of six subscales: sensory perception, moisture, activity, mobility, nutrition, and friction and shear. Each subscale condition is rated 1 to 4, with 1 indicating highest risk and 4 indicating least risk. A total score of 18 or lower indicates a risk for pressure ulcer development. The nurse should also look at the individual subscales, identify specific risks, and implement appropriate prevention interventions.

Medical Management

Once a pressure ulcer develops, the goals of treatment are to maintain or improve oxygenation to the area, prevent infection, and promote healing. Wound management should include wound bed preparation through débridement, advanced wound care to promote a moist wound environment, and control of bacterial burden. (Wound management is addressed later in this chapter.) Management options should be chosen according to the depth of the pressure ulcer and patient's individual needs.

Nursing Management

Prevention is the key to managing pressure ulcers, and education of the patient and family or caregiver can provide them with the ability to prevent or at least minimize the development in the future. Pressure ulcer prevention and treatment programs should include six

INTERNATIONAL GUIDELINES for Pressure Ulcer Staging

Stage of Wound	Guideline
Deep tissue injury (DTI)	Purple or maroon localized area of discolored intact skin or blood-filled blister due to damage of underlying soft tissue from pressure and/or shear. The area may be surrounded by tissue that is painful, firm, mushy, boggy, or warmer or cooler as compared to adjacent tissue. Deep tissue injury may be difficult to detect in individuals with dark skin tones. Evolution may include a thin blister over a dark wound bed. The wound may further evolve and become covered by thin eschar. Evolution may be rapidly exposing additional layers of tissue even with optimal treatment.
Stage/Category I	Nonblanchable erythema. Intact skin with nonblanchable redness of a localized area, usually over a bony prominence. Darkly pigmented skin may not have visible blanching; its color may differ from the surrounding area. The area may be painful, firm, soft, or warmer or cooler as compared to adjacent tissue. Category I may be difficult to detect in individuals with dark skin tones. May indicate "at risk" persons.
Stage/Category II	Partial-thickness loss of dermis presenting as a shallow open ulcer with a red pink wound bed, without slough. May also present as an intact or open/ruptured serum-filled or serosanguineous-filled blister. Presents as a shiny or dry shallow ulcer without slough or bruising. This category should not be used to describe skin tears, tape burns, incontinence-associated dermatitis, maceration, or excoriation.
Stage/Category III	Full-thickness tissue loss. Subcutaneous fat may be visible but bone, tendon, and muscle are *not* exposed. Slough may be present but does not obscure the depth of tissue loss. *May* include undermining and tunneling. The depth of a Category/Stage III pressure ulcer varies by anatomic location. The bridge of the nose, ear, occiput, and malleolus do not have (adipose) subcutaneous tissue and Category/Stage III ulcers can be shallow. In contrast, areas of significant adiposity can develop extremely deep Category/Stage III pressure ulcers. Bone/tendon is not visible or directly palpable.
Stage/Category IV	Full-thickness tissue loss with exposed bone, tendon, or muscle. Slough or eschar may be present. Often includes undermining and tunneling. The depth of a Category/Stage IV pressure ulcer varies by anatomic location. The bridge of the nose, ear, occiput and malleolus do not have (adipose) subcutaneous tissue and these ulcers can be shallow. Category/Stage IV ulcers can extend into muscle and/or supporting structures (e.g., fascia, tendon or joint capsule) making osteomyelitis or osteitis likely to occur. Exposed bone/muscle is visible or directly palpable.
Unstageable	Full-thickness tissue loss in which the actual depth of the ulcer is completely obscured by slough (yellow, tan, gray, green, or brown) and/or eschar (tan, brown, or black) in the wound bed. Until enough slough and/or eschar are removed to expose the base of the wound, the true depth cannot be determined; however, it will be either a Category/Stage III or IV. Stable (dry, adherent, intact without erythema or fluctuance [pus]) eschar on the heels serves as "the body's natural (biologic) cover" and should not be removed.

Source: European Pressure Ulcer Advisory Panel and National Pressure Ulcer Advisory Panel. (2009). *Prevention and treatment of pressure ulcers: Quick reference guide.* Washington DC: National Pressure Ulcer Advisory Panel. Reproduction of the National Pressure Ulcer Advisory Panel (NPUAP) materials in this document does not imply endorsement by the NPUAP of any products, organizations, companies, or any statements made by any organization or company.

essential components: a pressure ulcer admission assessment, daily risk assessment, daily skin inspection, moisture management, nutrition maximization, and pressure minimization (Duncan, 2007).

Pressure Ulcer Assessment

An in-depth pressure ulcer admission assessment includes both physical assessment of skin (on admission and daily) and a risk assessment. Physical assessment of the skin upon admission and daily should include an assessment of the bony prominences. The most common bony prominences for the development of pressure ulcers are the sacrum/coccyx, trochanters, ischial tuberosities, and heels. See the section on wound assessment later in this chapter for more details (p. 1905). It is recommended that a valid and reliable risk assessment instrument such as the Braden Scale be used to determine the patient's risk for developing a pressure ulcer. The use of a valid and reliable tool is critical for accurate and prompt identification of patients who are at risk and implementation of appropriate prevention interventions. Pressure ulcer risk assessment instruments were discussed previously in this chapter.

Daily Risk Assessment and Daily Skin Inspection

The acuity of symptoms of hospitalized patients can change rapidly, and the nurse needs to reassess the patient's risk and skin status daily. Daily assessment provides the clinician and caregiver with the opportunity to adjust the prevention strategies according to the patient's needs. The degree of risk (score) allows the clinician to alter and implement targeted strategies to address each subscale (sensory perception, activity, mobility, nutrition, moisture, friction, and shear) that may have changed.

Moisture Management

Prolonged exposure to moisture can lead to irritation and dermatitis, and repeated exposure can add to that risk (Black et al., 2011). Specific interventions to manage moisture and protect the skin should be implemented. Appropriate interventions may include frequent cleansing, use of moisture barriers for incontinence, use of absorbable padding, and voiding schedules.

Maximizing Nutrition

Nutritional status and hydration must be reviewed in addressing the risk of pressure ulcer development. Impaired intake, low body weight, unintentional weight loss, and dehydration may contribute to the development of pressure ulcers. Appropriate interventions may include dietitian consultation and ensuring the availability of appropriate snacks, fluids, and supplements. The patient's preferences should be considered when medically appropriate. Some facilities have encouraged staff to incorporate the provision of interventions into their work process, such as combining toileting, turning, and repositioning and offering fluids to the patient at routine intervals (Duncan, 2007).

Minimizing Pressure

Minimizing pressure can be accomplished through a variety of strategies such as using a pressure redistribution surface or repositioning the patient. Specialized support surfaces (mattresses, beds, cushions, or overlays) are commonly used to reduce or redistribute the pressure of the patient's body weight on the skin and tissues. These specialized surfaces are discussed on page 1913. Specialty support surfaces are categorized according to the level of pressure redistribution that they offer.

Braden Risk Assessment Scale

NOTE: Bed and chairbound individuals or those with impaired ability to reposition should be assessed upon admission for their risk of developing pressure ulcers. Patients with established pressure ulcers should be reassessed periodically.

Patient Name: ______________________________ Room Number: ______ Date: ____________

					Indicate Appropriate Numbers Below
Sensory Perception	**1. Completely Limited**	**2. Very Limited**	**3. Slightly Limited**	**4. No Impairment**	
Ability to respond meaningfully to pressure-related discomfort	Unresponsive (does not moan, flinch or grasp) to painful stimuli, due to diminished level of consciousness or sedation. OR limited ability to feel pain over most of body surface.	Responds only to painful stimuli. Cannot communicate discomfort except by moaning or restlessness. OR has a sensory impairment which limits the ability to feel pain or discomfort over 1/2 of body.	Responds to verbal commands, but cannot always communicate discomfort or need to be turned. OR has some sensory impairment which limits ability to feel pain or discomfort in 1 or 2 extremities.	Responds to verbal commands. Has no sensory deficit which would limit ability to feel or voice pain or discomfort.	
Moisture	**1. Constantly Moist**	**2. Very Moist**	**3. Occasionally Moist**	**4. Rarely Moist**	
Degree to which skin is exposed to moisture	Skin is kept moist almost constantly by perspiration, urine, etc. Dampness is detected every time patient is moved or turned.	Skin is often, but not always, moist. Linen must be changed at least once a shift.	Skin is occasionally moist, requiring an extra linen change approximately once a day.	Skin is usually dry. Linen only requires changing at routine intervals.	
Activity	**1. Bedfast**	**2. Chairfast**	**3. Walks Occasionally**	**4. Walks Frequently**	
Degree of physical activity	Confined to bed.	Ability to walk severely limited or non-existent. Cannot bear own weight and/or must be assisted into chair or wheelchair.	Walks occasionally during day, but for very short distances, with or without assistance. Spends majority of each shift in bed or chair.	Walks outside the room at least twice a day and inside room at least once every 2 hours during waking hours.	
Mobility	**1. Completely Immobile**	**2. Very Limited**	**3. Slightly Limited**	**4. No Limitations**	
Ability to change and control body position	Does not make even slight changes in body or extremity position without assistance.	Makes occasional slight changes in body or extremity position but unable to make frequent or significant changes independently.	Makes frequent though slight changes in body or extremity position independently.	Makes major and frequent changes in position without assistance.	
Nutrition	**1. Very Poor**	**2. Probably Inadequate**	**3. Adequate**	**4. Excellent**	
Usual food intake pattern	Never eats a complete meal. Rarely eats more than 1/3 of any food offered. Eats 2 servings or less of protein (meat or dairy products) per day. Takes fluids poorly. Does not take a liquid dietary supplement. OR is NPO and/or maintained on clear liquids or I.V.'s for more than 5 days.	Rarely eats a complete meal and generally eats only about 1/2 of any food offered. Protein intake includes only 3 servings of meat or dairy products per day. Occasionally will take a dietary supplement. OR receives less than optimum amount of liquid diet or tube feeding.	Eats over half of most meals. Eats a total of 4 servings of protein (meat, dairy products) each day. Occasionally will refuse a meal, but will usually take a supplement if offered. OR is on a tube feeding or TPN regimen which probably meets most of nutritional needs.	Eats most of every meal. Never refuses a meal. Usually eats a total of 4 or more servings of meat and dairy products. Occasionally eats between meals. Does not require supplementation.	
Friction and Shear	**1. Problem**	**2. Potential Problem**	**3. No Apparent Problem**		
	Requires moderate to maximum assistance in moving. Complete lifting without sliding against sheets is impossible. Frequently slides down in bed or chair, requiring frequent repositioning with maximum assistance. Spasticity, contractures or agitation lead to almost constant friction.	Moves feebly or requires minimum assistance. During a move, skin probably slides to some extent against sheets, chair restraints, or other devices. Maintains relatively good position in chair or bed most of the time, but occasionally slides down.	Moves in bed and in chair independently and has sufficient muscle strength to lift up completely during move. Maintains good position in bed or chair at all times.		
				Total Score:	

NOTE: Patients with a total score of 16 or less are considered to be at risk of developing pressure ulcers.
(15 or 16 = low risk; 13 or 14 = moderate risk; 12 or less = high risk)

FIGURE 60–9 ◆ Braden Risk Assessment Scale.

Source: Barbara Braden and Nancy Bergstrom.

Many facilities are offering higher-level surfaces for patients at high risk (critical care areas) in an effort to prevent pressure ulcers. The aim of frequent repositioning is to reduce or eliminate pressure. Evidence of the frequency required to prevent tissue ischemia is lacking in the literature, but every 2 hours is the maximum time a patient should be in one position. It may be necessary to reposition more often for patients who are deemed at higher risk because of increased age, fragile skin, poor medical condition, or little subcutaneous tissue (Ayello & Lyder, 2008).

In summary, pressure ulcers are painful, slow to heal, costly, and can even contribute to death. Nurses can be instrumental in decreasing the occurrence of these serious wounds through implementing preventive strategies for all patients who have been determined to be at risk.

Wound Assessment

A complete wound assessment requires the use of four of the five senses. Inspection can determine wound base color, size, and drainage and periwound condition. Palpation can determine softness (maceration), hardness (induration), or edema. Olfaction can detect infection and dead or sloughed tissue. The auditory sense is used for active listening to the patient with regard to pertinent history, past failures or successes in healing, and pain. Initial chronic wound assessments should include the patient's immune status, allergies, blood glucose levels, hydration, nutrition, latest blood albumin levels, oxygen and vascular supply, social history, habits (e.g., smoking), a review of current medications, and, if possible, the history of the patient's wound (etiology, age of wound, treatments thus far). These factors give the nurse and health care provider clues about why a chronic wound is not healing.

A focused wound assessment is necessary to establish a baseline and to determine healing. Several components must be included: location, dimensions, extent of tissue loss, characteristics of wound base, exudate characteristics, odor, wound edges, periwound skin characteristics, wound pain, and clinical signs and symptoms of infection. Chart 60–8 discusses these guidelines.

Location

A wound must be objectively assessed to determine a baseline and the effectiveness of a plan of care. The correct assessment and documentation of the wound's location are necessary for consistency and accuracy in follow-up of the wound care. There may also be some additional areas of breakdown, and there should be no confusion as to the number and locations of the wounds so that consistent and accurate documentation can occur. Using words such as *medial, lateral, proximal, distal,* and other anatomic location definitions will give clear and concise information.

Dimensions

Measurements can be made using a head-to-toe reference, longest length and perpendicular width, or volume. However they are done, the main function of measurements is consistency from a reference standpoint. A wound should be measured for length, width, and depth, usually in centimeters. The depth measurement should be directly perpendicular to the patient's skin and down into the wound, rather than a measurement parallel to the patient's body. Subsequent measurements should use the same point of reference to adequately denote progress or regression. The surface area of the wound is the length multiplied by the width in square centimeters (cm^2). The volume is the length multiplied by the width and the depth in cubic centimeters (cm^3). A wound routinely heals by decreasing in depth first and then decreasing in length and width. That being said, a combination of changes can occur in any dimension, and volume changes most accurately capture and note wound progression or regression.

Additional measurements refer to how the wound is shaped underneath the skin surface. A sinus tract is an area, sometimes referred to as a tunnel, where there is nonhealed detached tissue under intact skin. These areas may become infected and develop abscesses if the opening is sealed, blocking drainage. Sinus tracts are measured in centimeters. Referring to location, the area of tunneling is defined on a clock face, 12 o'clock being the head of the body. For example, if a wound located on the anterior aspect of the leg has tunneling on the medial side of the left leg, the measurement would be *x* amount of centimeters at the 9 o'clock position. There is also a measurement for undermining. **Undermining** occurs when the wound edge does not adhere to the base of the wound, creating a space under the wound edges. Undermining is measured by the amount of space that is present between the wound edge and where the undermining ends. The clock-face method is used in determining these measures (Figure 60–10◆).

Special products are available to assist in proper measurement techniques. Length, width, and depth of the wound are standard measurements. Special measuring instruments, such as Puritan DM Stick (Puritan Medical Products Co., LLC), a sterile foam-tipped plastic swab marked in millimeters, safely and comfortably give accurate, consistent measurements. Tracing graphs of transparent film, such as the E-Z Graph System of wound assessment (E.Z. Graph of Victoria, Inc.), enable the nurse and health care provider to outline the shape of the wound and show progress of the wound surface contracture. These tracings offer a great psychological boost to patients whose wounds are healing by millimeters, allowing them to see progress as compared to the original wound size.

Wound Base Characteristics

Inspection of the wound allows for a description of the wound base in terms of color and extent of tissue loss. The color of the wound will often assist in determining the extent of tissue loss. Partial-thickness wounds are confined to the epidermal and dermal skin layers. The wound base is always pink. In full-thickness wounds, the epidermis and dermis have been damaged, and the wound has extended into the subcutaneous

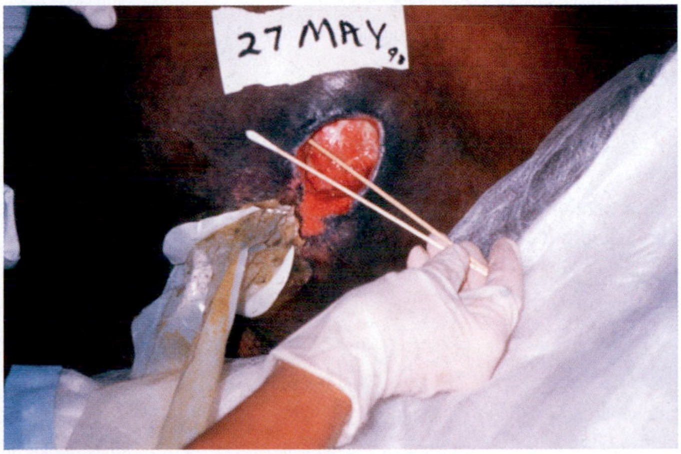

FIGURE 60–10 ◆ Undermining.
Source: Jan Clark.

CHART 60–8 Wound Assessment Guidelines

Wound Characteristic	Descriptors	Assessment Verbiage
Location	Upper/lower extremities Lateral/medial Left/right Midline Central Dorsal/plantar	Use anatomic location, such as malleolar or occipital. Describe proximity to other wounds consistently. Identify wound by classification and/or location. Example: "skin tear, right upper extremity."
Size	Length, width, and depth in centimeters	Always measure in centimeters; never estimate size by comparison.
Tracks	Centimeters and direction	Use a clock face as a frame of reference with 12 o'clock being toward the head. Example: "3-centimeter track at 2 o'clock."
Undermining	Centimeters and location	Example: "Undermining from 11 to 2 o'clock, from 1 to 1.5 centimeters."
Color	Red, yellow, black	Use percentages and shades of color. Example: "Pale red 60%, yellow 25%, black 15%."
Tissue	Granulation Epithelialization Necrotic Slough Eschar	Use descriptors. Example: "Thick black eschar with 0.3-centimeter rim of pink tissue." Example: "Beefy red granulation." Example: "Pink epithelial tissue migrating toward center from 3 to 5 o'clock."
Exudate/drainage	Serous Sanguineous Serosanguineous Purulent	Use color and amount in descriptions. Example: "Minimal sanguineous, dark red." Example: "Moderate serosanguineous, pink-tinged." Example: "Foam dressing saturated to edges of dressing and accumulation of exudates under dressing." (This might indicate increased drainage due to possible infection or just a need for a more absorbent dressing.)
Odor	Subjective and difficult to quantify Indicate presence or not, foul	Remember that moisture retentive dressings also retain wound odor. When trying to control odor, description of presence of odor can measure outcomes. Example: "Odor in room." Example: "Odor at bedside." Example: "Odor when dressing removed."
Wound margins	Rolled With epithelial tissue Defined, well demarcated Nondefined or nondemarcated	Describe margin appearance.
Periwound		
Erythema	Presence or not Intensity (color)	Use a marker pen on the skin to outline presence of suspicious erythema that might indicate infection/cellulitis.
Induration	Presence or not	May describe as increasing or resolving.
Maceration	Presence or not Extent in centimeters	Tissue maceration occurs when wound drainage or dressing moisture drowns cells. When the offending reason is contained or removed, the condition is repaired autolytically: The macerated tissue sloughs off, and new skin has been generated.
Intervention and Tolerance		
Pain	Scale of 0–10	Clarify pain. Example: "Tender when probed." Example: "Premedicated with. . . ." Example: "Pain subsided after packing completed."
Tolerance of procedure	Cleaning Packing Débridement	May overlap with pain assessment. A record here determines whether the patient needs premedication. Or does pain occur only during probing and packing and then subside?

layer or beyond; these wounds may be a combination of red/pink and yellow. Color of the wound base is often described as a percentage (e.g., 80% red/pink and 20% yellow).

One system of wound description is the red-yellow-black system. The red stage identifies a beefy-red to pink granular bed, the yellow stage identifies a wound with fibrin or slough and a plan of treatment designed for that stage of the wound bed, and the black stage is when the wound bed has eschar. This system is simple to use because the color is easily identifiable, making it easy to determine the plan of treatment for the wound with a set of guidelines specific to that stage, as described in the next section.

The extent of tissue damage in the wound base can be described by using various classification systems. For example, diabetic and vascular wounds have grading systems, pressure ulcers have staging classification, and skin tears use the Payne–Martin Classification System (p. 1900).

Wound Drainage Characteristics

A wound may have many different types of drainage. The drainage may be sanguineous (bloody), serosanguineous (bloody with plasma fluid), serous (plasma only), or purulent (infected). Sanguineous drainage occurs when there is acute trauma to the vascular bed. It may be a result of further insult, due either to environmental causes, such as hitting the wound area on a foreign object, or intentional causes, such as a sharps débridement. Serosanguineous drainage is more related to overall edema leading to capillary weakness and leakage. Serous drainage may occur when edema has forced fluid to move from the intravascular department into the tissue and then leak through the wound bed. Purulent drainage is a sign of infection and indicates the need for antibiotic therapy and/or silver dressing treatment. The amount and type of drainage are documented in the patient's record at regular intervals.

Periwound Skin Characteristics

The periwound area, defined as the area surrounding the wound base circumferentially, is a very important indicator of how severe the wound is and of the progression or regression of wound closure. The periwound area may be reddened around the wound base. This reddened area indicates that an acute inflammatory process is occurring that may be due to further injury underlying the skin around the wound or infection. If the periwound area is "boggy" or soft, it indicates that there is maceration. In **maceration,** excessive moisture destroys the skin's integrity and leaves the skin layers suboptimal. A hardened area, referred to as induration, indicates tissue that is edematous, infected, injured, or dead. Typically, the induration area is opened to relieve the pressure and remove any dead tissue that may exist. The periwound area may also have a yeast or fungal infection due to use of intravenous, oral, or local antibiotics.

Effective wound management requires the nurse to pay particular attention to the periwound area. Creams that contain dimethicone can protect the periwound area from drainage with a moisture-barrier effect. A moisture product may be required for dry and flaky periwound skin that may be under an occlusive dressing. Antifungal and yeast creams may be applied to the periwound areas to prevent these conditions that commonly occur after chronic antibiotic use and in dark, moist areas. Some lotions can contain lidocaine, an anesthetic to control pain, or hyaluronic acid to control redness and inflammation.

Odor

Odor can be described as present, faint, or absent. Specific dressing types can sometimes affect the wound odor, as can hygiene and the presence of nonviable tissue. Presence of an odor can be one of the first signs of impending infection.

Bioburden

Bioburden is a measurement of the number of bacteria in a wound. Foreign material, collagen debris, and other biofilms and breakdown from bacterial load and injury cause a delay in the wound healing process and a decrease in biochemical response to healing. Bioburden may be controlled with a combination of irrigation with a syringe, anti-infective agents, or surfactant cleansers.

Skin Assessments

Skin assessments are different from wound assessments. Basic skin assessment should include observation of the entire body, in which the nurse checks the patient's temperature, color, moisture, turgor, odor, nails, hair, and presence of lesions and other types of skin injury (Nix, 2007). Maintaining skin integrity in special populations—that is, the aged with frail skin, patients who have chronic diseases, or those who are immunosuppressed—can be a challenge. Routine assessments, preventive interventions, and maintenance hydration are key elements of maintaining skin integrity.

Fresh postoperative wounds do not require the intense scrutiny of historical data as a chronic wound does because these data are available in the chart. However, a systematic approach to assessing wound characteristics is still useful.

Wound Management

It is essential that the health care team remember that dressings assist in the body's overall ability to heal itself. Dressings are not intended to be a substitute for identifying and treating the underlying causes of a wound. They simply promote an optimal environment for wound healing to occur.

Wound management needs to follow three principles: (1) control or eliminate causative factors, (2) provide systemic support to reduce existing and potential cofactors, and (3) maintain the physiologic local wound environment (Rolstad & Ovington, 2007). Physiological local wound environment means that through appropriate topical therapies, a wound will ultimately return to the characteristics of healthy or normal functioning (Rolstad & Ovington, 2007). Some of the basic components of wound management are described next.

Primary, Secondary, and Tertiary Intention

Healing can occur by three methods: primary, secondary, or tertiary intention. **Primary intention** minimizes the volume of connective tissue deposition and restores the epithelial barrier to infection (Doughty & Sparks-Defriese, 2007). Wound edges are approximated and are secured by sutures, stitches, Steri-Strips, or staples. Primary intention is utilized when healing is expected within 10 days and minimal new tissue formation is required. In **secondary intention,** a wound is allowed to remain open to granulate, contract, and epithelialize. Many traumatic and postsurgical wounds are treated in this manner. **Tertiary or third intention** is a delayed closure to allow for drainage of fluid, contamination control, and/or a plan for surgical intervention at a later date (Doughty & Sparks-Defriese, 2007).

Offloading

Offloading, a very important factor that influences the wound healing process, involves the process of relieving pressure on a bony prominence, callus, or wound. Standing normally places 50% of one's body weight on each leg. Walking, depending on the speed, can place one to one and one-half times the body weight on an affected area. Offloading devices such as boots, wheelchair cushions, splints, and total contact casting can redistribute pressure or relieve pressure entirely, depending on the device. Turning a patient every 2 hours and floating a patient's heels off the bed on pillows are also forms of offloading. The objective is to relieve the pressure that causes a decrease in circulation through compression of the capillary beds and localized tissue destruction. The affected area will form a hardened area called a callus to protect the area from further damage.

Débridement

Débridement is the removal of nonviable tissue and foreign material or debris from a wound. Foreign bodies or particles in a wound (e.g., splinters, glass, grass, and dead tissue) may be there because of trauma. When the wound is cleaned, efforts are made to flush out any loose debris. Hydrogen peroxide may be helpful to clean the initial trauma-induced wound; however, after its initial use, refrain from cleansing the wound with hydrogen peroxide. When used in full strength, hydrogen peroxide is toxic to the new fibroblasts that are trying to rebuild the wound. The foreign body may be a suture or staple in a wound that has healed over, and the wound may reopen because the suture or staple is working its way to the surface of the skin.

Necrotic tissue is devitalized tissue that ranges from yellow fibrinous slough to a thick, leathery dark brown or black scablike wound, referred to as eschar. Chapter 61 discusses burn eschar. Débridement of necrotic tissue achieves several objectives: (1) It reduces the bioburden of the wound because necrotic tissue supports the growth of bacteria, (2) it facilitates visualization of the wound bed, and (3) at the molecular level, it interrupts the cycle of the chronic wound and reactivates the healing cascade (Ramundo, 2007). One exception to the rule is eschar covering ischemic wounds, such as dry gangrenous toes. The eschar in an ischemic wound serves as protection against infection, and there is little chance of adequate microcirculation being able to help heal the wound if débrided. A common treatment for the ischemic wound that is located on an end point (toes) and covered with eschar is to paint it with an antiseptic solution such as povidone-iodine and cover it with dry dressings. The efficacy of iodine has been widely debated; however, two publications suggest that iodine has value in reducing the bacterial burden of the wound (Cooper, 2007; Khan, 2006).

The four methods of débridement are sharp, mechanical, enzymatic, and autolytic (Chart 60–9). Sharp débridement is done with scalpel, scissors, or nippers. Anesthetics or the operating room may be required depending on wound size and depth. Mechanical débridement is the dislodging of necrotic tissue, which is accomplished in several ways, including the following:

- Wet-to-dry dressings are used for mechanical débridement: The slough adheres to the dressing as it dries and is pulled off when the dressing is removed.

CHART 60–9 Débridement Methods

Method	Advantages	Disadvantages
Sharp Necrotic tissue removed with scalpel, nippers, or scissors.	Can be used on wound with any amount of slough or eschar. Treatment is swift.	Performed only by skilled nurses or health care providers. Patient may experience pain. May require local anesthetic. May require surgical time procedure (known as incision and drainage).
Mechanical Wet-to-dry dressing is a classic example: the pulling away of tissue that has adhered to the dry dressing. Pulse lavage using high-pressure water streams to dislodge necrotic tissue.	Can be used for infected wounds. Removes loose devitalized tissue.	May be painful. Not tissue specific (removes good granulation tissue with necrotic tissue).
Enzymatic Collagenase (Santyl) Xenoderm Urea active ingredient causing disintegration of slough and eschar.	Faster than autolytic, normally. Usually pain free. Can use for infected wounds. Tissue specific.	Patient may be sensitive to active ingredient. Educate the patient that the method will increase exudate production. Exudate management.
Autolytic Occlusive dressings, such as transparent film, or hydrocolloids cause physiological "melting" of the necrotic tissue by phagocytes.	Pain free. Can be used on any wounds with slough or eschar. Often preferred for patients who are in the intensive care unit (ICU) and may not be able to tolerate the multiple dressing changes necessary after sharp débridement. Transparent films and wound gel are easy methods to use to achieve autolytic débridement.	Requires more time than sharp or enzymatic methods. Cannot use for infected wounds.

- The whirlpool method of débridement also is a mechanical débridement method. Whirlpool is rarely used any more because of concerns about cross-contamination between patients who use the whirlpool. Another reason for its lack of popularity is the likelihood of vasodilatation and increase of edema that occurs with whirlpool (Ramundo, 2007).
- Irrigation: Pulsatile high-pressure lavage is an electrically powered device that emits a regular, automatic pulsed lavage. It can be performed at the bedside and in the home setting and is preferred to the whirlpool method.

Enzymatic débridement is chemically induced by prescription ointments that contain collagenase, which penetrates the slough and eschar, causing them to soften and "melt down." Once softened, the slough and eschar are mechanically débrided.

Autolytic débridement is allowing the body to utilize the phagocytes to destroy the necrotic tissue. This is often a preferred method of débridement among patients for whom daily (or more frequent) dressing changes would be a hardship, that is, patients who are critically ill and cannot be turned. Autolytic débridement is a slow and nonaggressive treatment. Occlusive dressings are often used to soften eschar before sharp débridement to avoid débridement of viable tissue. Occlusive dressings are contraindicated on infected wounds.

Obliteration of Dead Space

Dead space refers to tissue destruction under intact surface tissue, such as tunneling or sinus tract formation. Dead space areas provide a fluid medium and an environment that is favorable for pathogen growth. The nurse needs to probe margins of the wound to identify any sinus tracts, undermining, or tunneling. These areas need to be packed with a retrievable material to prevent the tract from closing prematurely and forming an abscess. To do so, the nurse packs these areas with one piece of dressing to obliterate the dead space, always leaving a tail of the packing material to prevent granulation tissue from closing over the wound that has packing in it. The nurse must always document the size and shape of the sinus tract or tunnel, its direction, and how much dressing was needed to pack the wound. There is always the possibility of packing material being left in the wound, so it is important to determine, when the packing material is removed, that all of it has been retrieved

Safety Alert *When packing a wound, the nurse must always use a continuous piece of dressing rather than several small pieces because one or more small pieces might get inadvertently left in the wound, especially in a deep wound with sinus tracts.*

Absorption of Excess Exudate

One of the goals of wound management is to promote and maintain a moist (not wet, not dry) wound environment. Large amounts of exudate may macerate wound margins. Containment of exudate controls bioburden, protects the periwound skin, controls odor, and decreases the risk of hypergranulation (Rolstad & Ovington, 2007). Measures to protect the intact periwound skin include using liquid skin barriers, moisture barriers, and absorbent dressings. Dressings whose absorbent capacity has been used up should be changed promptly.

Maintaining a Moist Wound Surface

Keeping the wound bed moist prevents desiccation and cell death, facilitates epithelial migration, and promotes angiogenesis and connective tissue synthesis. Additionally, moist wound beds are less painful. Three investigations in the mid-20th century showed that "moist wound healing" was achieved by covering the experimental wounds with an occlusive membrane consisting of thin plastic film. Starting in 1958 with Odland observing that a blister healed faster if it was left unbroken, the idea that dressings were pharmacologic agents was taken seriously (Odland, 1958). In 1962, Winter showed that occlusion of wounds with a polyethylene film more than doubled the wound healing rate in domestic pigs (Winter, 1962). Hinman and Maibach then established the beneficial effect of occlusion on resurfacing of experimental wounds in normal human subjects (Hinman & Maibach, 1963). These principles still hold true today.

A moist wound environment created by occlusive dressings facilitates granulation tissue development through increased gel-matrix secretion, new blood vessel growth, collagen secretion, fibroblast proliferation, and epidermal migration (Rolstad & Ovington, 2007). Benefits of moist wound healing are faster epidermal resurfacing and fewer infections.

Products that add moisture, protect from moisture, absorb moisture, and maintain moisture are all available for promotion of optimal wound healing. Moist wound healing is not a new concept but has been slow to become the automatic choice of health care providers. However, moist wound healing has become the mantra of specialists trained in wound care management. These specialists recognize the benefits of occlusive dressings that facilitate moist wound healing.

Providing Thermal Insulation and Protection

Wounds need to be kept at the body's core temperature. When the temperature of the wound is lower, leukocyte mobility is impaired, and phagocytic efficiency and affinity of hemoglobin for oxygen are reduced (Rolstad & Ovington, 2007). These conditions slow wound healing. Therefore, dressing changes need to be done quickly because when wounds are left open without dressings, the temperature of the wound will fall, slowing blood flow to the wound and delaying epidermal migration. Cleansing a wound can reduce the local tissue temperatures for up to 40 minutes. Mitosis and leukocyte activity can be delayed for up to 3 hours after cleansing. If a dressing change is interrupted, the nurse should cover the wound with sterile gauze to help slow down temperature reduction in the wound and to protect it from airborne organisms. It is important to protect the healing wound from trauma caused by wheelchair legs, furniture, pets, and other objects. New trauma disrupts newly formed vessels, connective tissue, and epidermis.

Wound Cleansing

Wound cleansing is a controversial topic within the ranks of wound care experts. Antiseptics such as hydrogen peroxide, povidone-iodine, acetic acid, and Dakin's solution, which can kill bacteria, can also be cytotoxic to white blood cells and fibroblasts. However, depending on the bacterial burden of the wound, antiseptics may be necessary for short periods of time. Removing bacteria from the wound bed can be done with normal saline at a pressure between 4 and 15 pounds per square inch (psi). Above 15 psi, the pressure tends to drive bacteria into the tissue. Because they contain toxic ingredients, many commercial cleansers may inhibit the viability and phagocytic activity of leukocytes unless the cleansers are diluted. Commercial wound cleansers contain surfactants and preservatives, and many come with a built-in sprayer that achieves a desirable pressure. An accepted rule of using saline as a

Weblink: Collagen-Based Wound Dressings

cleanser is that after sterile saline is opened, it is good for only 24 hours; then it should be discarded. Saline that is kept refrigerated may be safe longer than 24 hours, but it is always a good idea to check labels or ask the manufacturer. Water is acceptable as a wound cleanser as long as it is free from contaminants.

Safety Alert *Skin cleansers should never be used on wounds. Skin cleansers are formulated to break chemical bonds that bind fecal matter to the skin; they are not suitable for the delicate tissue of a wound bed.*

Wound Care Products

The nurse may choose from several different types of dressings for wound management. The factors in making a decision on a particular product are protection, degree of drainage, antimicrobial activity, biochemical needs, collagen requirements, and pain relief. As the wound treatment plan continues, it may be necessary to switch dressing types on the basis of the needs for that wound bed at the time of assessment. The same type of dressing will most often not be required throughout treatment of the wound. It is very important to understand that despite algorithms and protocols, what drives decisions about choice of dressings is a skilled assessment of the wound. The wound is viable and changing; flexibility regarding the type of dressings used is necessary to continue to show improvement in the wound. Moist wound healing is a delicate balance of moisture: keeping the wound bed moist and the periwound skin dry and intact. Basic good wound care is pretty simple: If a wound is dry, add moisture; if a wound is wet, use an absorbent dressing; and always protect the periwound skin.

The most common types of dressings are discussed next with the understanding that there are many different variations in size, brand, and combinations, allowing the nurse to provide a highly individualized plan of treatment that is cost effective, convenient, and outcome driven.

Moisture Retentive Dressings

The goals of moisture retentive dressings, occlusive dressings, or semiocclusive dressings are all the same: maintaining a moist wound environment. There are hydrogels, calcium alginates, silver dressings, collagens, foams, polyurethane films, hydrocolloids, contact layers, composites, and combinations, all of which are described here. Generally these dressings are painless, reduce the need for multiple dressing changes daily, and result in faster healing rates. On the cellular level, cells desiccate without moisture and cannot do their job of building tissue to fill in and cover a wound. Moist wound healing is facilitated by moisture retentive dressings.

Safety Alert *If a patient tells the nurse that she leaves the dressing off at night so that the wound can get air, the nurse needs to explain that the wound gets oxygen from the blood supply, not from the ambient air. It is important that the patient understand the need not to let the wound dry out.*

Hydrogels

Hydrogels are made of a saline base. They provide moisture to the wound bed that is required for epithelialization to occur as the cells migrate across the wound bed. Hydrogels can come in a tube of gel, in sheets, or impregnated in a gauze pad. Hydrogels are used for wounds that are dry and require moisture. They are not intended for wounds with excess drainage. A caution with this dressing is that maceration, the tendency for the periwound area of good skin to get wet and soft and potentially break down, can occur. Close supervision of the wound's progress and astute assessment are required.

Alginates

Alginates are composed of algae or seaweed. These dressings can absorb at least 5 to 10 times their surface area of drainage. In chronic wounds, the amount of matrix metalloproteinases (MMP) can delay wound healing. MMPs degrade collagen and denature it. A certain amount of MMPs are necessary to control other biochemical signals and degrade collagen that is injured. However, collagen is the scaffold upon which tissue growth occurs, and it is important not to lose too much of it. Alginates absorb the excess wound drainage to inactivate some MMPs as well as prevent against maceration, as described earlier.

Silver Dressings

Silver in its ionic form is a natural bactericidal agent, even against the most resistant bacterial strains such as MRSA (methicillin-resistant *Staphylococcus aureus*) and VRE (vancomycin-resistant enterococcus). When in contact with the bacteria, silver creates its bactericidal effect by interfering with bacterial cell DNA, bacterial enzymes, and proteins in the cell wall. Silver has been used since the late 1800s for its antimicrobial activity. Gels, alginates, saturated gauze, metallic nylon, and other media are used to deliver the silver cation Ag^+. Some silver dressings require saline to be activated, and some do not. The main focus with silver dressing is the rate at which the silver is deposited into the wound bed and the wound bed's characteristics. Silver will kill only the surface bacteria it comes in contact with, and oral antibiotic therapy should continue. The Evidence-Based Practice box discusses the use of silver as an antimicrobial.

Collagen

Collagen dressings are also utilized for wound care treatment. Native collagen that is stable and can resist early degradation by MMPs can provide an extracellular matrix (ECM) that allows wound healing to continue. Extracellular matrix is the matrix of native collagen, connective tissue, and basement membrane that forms the foundation or scaffold on which the epithelial tissue is embedded. There are many different types of collagen dressings. Characteristics such as size, depth, shape, drainage or lack thereof, infection, and bioburden all factor into selecting the right type of collagen medium to utilize (Nataraj et al., 2007).

Foam

A foam dressing is made of a spongy material that is highly absorptive relative to its surface area. Foam is also soft and pliable, so it can conform to any environment. Foams can be used in two ways. One use is for absorption. Foams can be used alone or in combination with an alginate to wick away excess moisture and prevent maceration. They can also be utilized as a barrier for protection against foreign insult. For example, a patient in a wheelchair with a lower leg wound is prone to further trauma caused by hitting the wound on the wheelchair during transfers. The foam provides a cushion for the insult and protects the already compromised wound bed from further damage. Foam can also be utilized to protect patients from friction and shear forces from surfaces and contact with other body parts.

Transparent Film

Transparent films are made of a clear sticky wrap much like the plastic wrap used for storage of food but with glue on one side. Transparent films can be used to visualize a wound bed and for an occlusive dressing. It should be noted, however, that other options should be considered for use with older patients with frail skin. This film tends to stick and protect so well that when it is eventually removed, it can cause further damage by clinging to and separating the skin during its removal. However, transparent films are excellent for protection from bacteria

EVIDENCE-BASED PRACTICE Silver as an Antimicrobial Agent

Clinical Problem

Infection is a common complication for a patient with a wound, especially a chronic wound. Prophylactic antibiotic use has allowed more resistant bacterial organisms to proliferate. Because wounds that are chronic may now be colonized with bacteria, deciding when and how to treat can be a complicated decision. Silver is a product that has come into wide use as a local antimicrobial agent, and the evidence surrounding its effectiveness, how much to use, and in what medium has been the subject of great debate in wound care.

Research Findings

Ip, Lui, Poon, Lung, and Burd (2006) performed a study that utilized an agar medium and various types of microorganisms such as methicillin-resistant *S. aureus* (MRSA) and vancomycin-resistant enterococcus (VRE), as well as other microbes. Different silver dressings were applied. The result revealed that dressings with a higher concentration of ionic silver had a quicker and broader bacteriocidal effect. It was noted, however, that too much silver could potentially damage tissue and kill keratinocytes and fibroblasts. The most important factors relative to antimicrobial effectiveness are the bioavailability concentration and rate of delivery to the tissue. Indeed, different concentrations of silver ions could be used depending on the intended desire. Prophylactic treatment could contain fewer silver ions than treatment of an active infection. The goal is to deliver the minimum amount of silver ions to perform the intended outcome.

Investigators in an animal study examined the effectiveness of silver dressings to reduce bacteria in contaminated wounds when using negative pressure wound therapy (NPWT). These investigators concluded that there were fewer bacteria in the silver groups than the control groups at 6 days. In a review of the literature by Vermeulen and colleagues (2010), three random controlled trials (RCT) comprising 847 participants were identified. The findings of this review concluded that there was no significant difference in wound healing in wounds treated with silver compared to those treated with standard foam dressings or best local practice after up to 4 weeks of follow-up.

Implications for Nursing Practice

Despite the lack of conclusive evidence supporting its use, silver may be an important part of chronic wound management. Silver provides antimicrobial effects to prevent infection or treat an active infection in contaminated wounds. It should be treated as any other drug and utilized appropriately to the individual situation and only for its intended use. Further well-designed research is still needed to confirm the effectiveness of silver in wound management in comparison to other wound management treatments.

Critical Thinking Questions with answers can be found in the Osborn Student Resources at nursing.pearsonhighered.com.

Reference

Ip, M., Lui, S., Poon, V., Lung, I., & Burd, A. (2006). Antimicrobial activities of silver dressings: An *in vitro* comparison. *Journal of Medical Microbiology, 55*(1), 59–63; Vermeulen, H., van Hattem, J. M., Storm-Versloot, M. N., Ubbink, D. T., & Westerbos, S. J. (2010). Topical silver for treating infected wounds. Cochrane Library. Retrieved from http://www.thecochranelibrary.com.

incontinence and foreign contact getting to the wound bed and can allow the wound dressing to remain intact for a greater duration.

Gauze

Gauze is the most widely used dressing and may be wrongly alluded to as a standard of care (Ramundo, 2007). Research has shown that wet-to-dry dressings and gauze are commonly ordered for wounds for which there is scant evidence to support their use, such as with open surgical wounds healing by secondary intention (Ramundo, 2007). Wet-to-dry dressings consist of saline-moistened gauze that are placed inside or on a wound bed, covered with dry gauze, and secured. When the moistened gauze dries, it adheres to the wound. When it is removed, it pulls away good tissue along with the necrotic tissue and debris. This is nonselective débridement, and there is a high risk for reinjury of the wound bed. Furthermore, it is usually painful.

Wet-to-moist or moist gauze dressings are saline-moistened gauze placed in the wound and kept moist until removed. This may require rewetting the gauze, but generally it means that the dressing needs to be changed before it dries out, which in reality may or may not happen. More frequent dressing changes may mean more pain for the patient, more work for an older caregiver spouse, and more time and expense for a home health nurse or hospital staff nurse.

Negative Pressure Wound Therapy

Negative pressure wound therapy (NPWT) is a dressing that uses a vacuum or negative pressure to assist in drainage collection and promotion of granulation and angiogenesis. Wound vacuum-assisted closure (VAC) is a system that uses controlled negative pressure (vacuum) to help promote wound healing (Figure 60–11◆, p. 1912). This therapy helps remove infectious materials and other fluids from the wound. Negative pressure wound therapy consists of a computer-controlled therapy unit, canister, sterile plastic tubing, foam or gauze dressing, and a transparent drape dressing. The nurse gently packs the foam/gauze dressing into the open wound bed, taking care not to leave any on normal skin. Once the foam/gauze is in place, it is sealed with a clear drape that is similar to a large bandage. The nurse then connects a tube to the dressing at one end and the NPWT control unit at the other end. Suction is applied, and infectious materials and other fluids from the wound are pulled through the tube and into the canister. This process works best when there is a clean, granular bed. Débridement and infection control should be accomplished before NPWT is applied. The NPWT dressing is changed every 2 to 3 days.

Negative pressure wound therapy can be prescribed for many chronic and traumatic wound patients in the hospital, the extended care facility, and the home. This system (1) promotes granulation tissue formation through the promotion of wound healing; (2) uniformly draws wounds closed by applying controlled, localized negative pressure; (3) removes interstitial fluid allowing tissue decompression; (4) removes infectious materials; and (5) provides a closed, moist wound healing environment (Frantz, Broussard, Mendez-Eastman, & Cordrey, 2007). Negative pressure wound therapy is used in the hospital setting, in the extended care facility, and at home for the following conditions:

- Chronic open wounds (diabetic and pressure ulcers)
- Acute and traumatic wounds
- Meshed grafts
- Subacute wounds (i.e., dehisced incisions)
- Skin grafts and flaps.

Nursing care includes maintaining and documenting the negative pressure level, troubleshooting the device, changing the dressing according to the health care provider's order, and assessing wound healing.

Adjuvant Therapy

There are adjuvant treatments that can be considered in a plan of care to promote the healing process. These treatments are used in conjunction with effective wound care and identification of the causative factors that relate to wound healing or lack thereof.

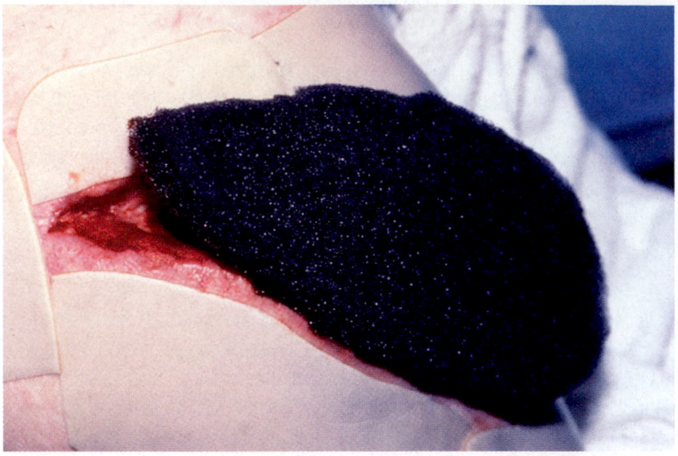

1.

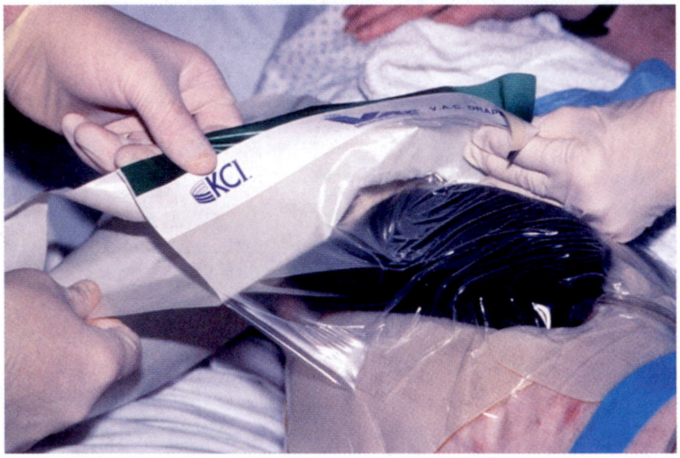

2.

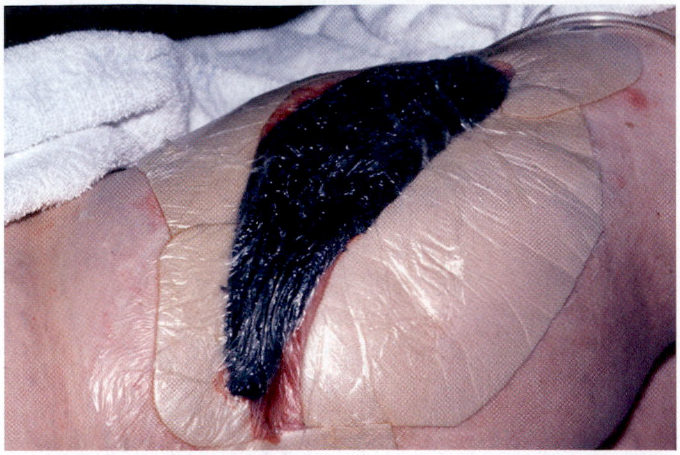

3.

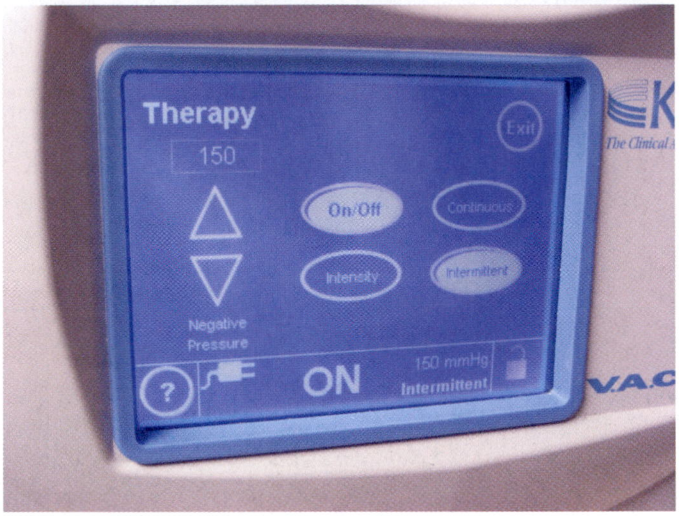

4.

FIGURE 60–11 ◆ Wound vacuum-assisted closure (VAC).
Source: 1, 2: Jan Clark; 3, 4: Cheryl Wraa.

Tissue Grafts

Tissue grafts can be derived from human or animal tissue or can be synthetically manufactured. They contain collagen and/or fibroblasts and keratinocytes, the major components of the dermal and epidermal layers of skin. These applications are placed directly on the wound bed and affixed or anchored so that the graft stays in place. The benefit of this type of graft over a skin graft is that there is no donor site that must heal, there is no requirement of anesthesia or invasive surgery, and it is minimally invasive. Tissue grafts can also be performed repetitively to get the intended result.

Hyperbaric Oxygen Therapy

Hyperbaric oxygen therapy is also an adjuvant treatment. **Hyperbaric oxygen therapy (HBOT)** involves the intermittent treatment of the entire body with 100% oxygen at 20 times greater than normal atmospheric pressures. It has been used to improve wound healing in patients with compromised oxygenation and/or perfusion because it stimulates the growth of new blood vessels in areas with reduced circulation and arterial blockage. The Centers for Medicare & Medicaid Services have approved about 14 diagnoses for hyperbaric oxygen therapy. For example, patients who have diabetic wounds at a depth of Wagner Grade 3, have failed conventional wound therapy for 30 days, and have had vascular and glucose optimization can receive hyperbaric therapy. Patients with osteomyelitis and patients at risk of failing a surgical flap can receive hyperbaric oxygen therapy as well. In addition, HBOT is used to treat extensive wounds such as burn injuries, infected wounds, and wounds in patients who are at high risk for delayed healing. Wherever blood flow and oxygen delivery to vital organs are reduced, function and healing can potentially be aided with HBOT. Recently, HBOT has been used for treatment of chronic degenerative health problems related to atherosclerosis, stroke, peripheral vascular disease, diabetic ulcers, wound healing, cerebral palsy, brain injury, multiple sclerosis, macular degeneration, and many other disorders (Frantz et al., 2007).

In HBOT, the patient is placed in either an individual chamber or a large, roomlike chamber that can accommodate several people at one time. Oxygen under pressure is delivered to the chamber, and the patient breathes it in. Being under pressure, the oxygen is forced into the plasma surrounding the red blood cells to supersaturate the patient with oxygen. Its benefits are increased tissue oxygen levels, angiogenesis (new blood vessel formation), antibacterial activity (oxygen kills anaerobic bacteria and its toxins), enhanced leukocyte killing (T-cell formation), and prevention of reperfusion injury.

COMPLEMENTARY & ALTERNATIVE THERAPIES Hyperbaric Oxygen Therapy *Nancy Yilk*

THE USE OF HYPERBARIC OXYGEN THERAPY (HBOT) to improve oxygen supply to wounds was studied in four randomized trials involving 147 patients with foot ulcers due to diabetes. These studies compared HBOT's effect on chronic wound healing. Results showed benefits in the reduction of risk of major amputation when HBOT was used as an adjunct therapy versus an alternative therapy. In people with foot ulcers due to diabetes, HBOT significantly reduced the risk of major amputation and improved the chance of healing at 1 year of treatment.

Foot ulcers and their attendant complications are disquietingly high in people with diabetes, a majority of whom have underlying neuropathy. Diabetic foot ulceration (DFU) can either be associated with neuropathy (neuropathic ulcer), peripheral vascular disease (ischemic ulcer), or both (neuroischemic ulcer), and/or other causal factors such as trauma. Neuropathic ulceration is usually caused by foot deformity, high foot pressures, reduced soft tissue padding, unattended or unnoticed trauma, and entrained tissue damage. Once tissue breakdown occurs, the resultant ulceration may become chronic as the insensate foot fails to convey pain stimuli, which are necessary to provoke protective behavior.

A retrospective study was conducted with data collected from 30 patients with DFUs over a 2-year period that received treatment with HBOT. The study was evaluating whether any underlying pathologies or confounding factor appeared to influence patient outcome. Results found that 73.3% of patients achieved a successful outcome of partial healing. Major amputation was no longer required with 70% of the patients, and this number remained unchanged 3 months later. In contrast, 13.3% of patients were lost to follow-up at 3 months and one patient (3.3%) had a major amputation. Steroid therapy, peripheral vascular disease, previous minor amputation, type of diabetes, previous HBOT, larvae therapy, the use of interactive dressings, and hemoglobin A1c levels were all observed to have had a significant relationship with patient outcome ($P < 0.05$) (Bishop & Mudge, 2012).

A randomized, single-center, placebo-controlled clinical trial of 119 patients with a chronic wound in the lower extremities lasting over 3 months evaluated the effects of HBOT in the management of chronic wounds. There were 97 patients on long-term HBOT therapy, as well as 22 patients on hyperbaric air therapy, who served as the control group. Treatment was administered within a single-place hyperbaric chamber for 90 minutes daily (session duration 120 minutes) for 5 days a week for 4 weeks (20 treatment sessions). The wound size decreased at the 4-week end point (62.7% ± 22.3% in the HBO group vs. 34.4% ± 20.6% in the control group, $P < 0.05$). The results of both groups were significantly different from the patients at pretreatment. Adjunctive treatment of HBOT facilitates the healing of chronic nonhealing wounds in selected patients through the mobilization of EPCs (Ma, Lei, Zhou, Li, & Zhou, 2011).

Sources: Bishop, A. J., & Mudge, E. (2012, February 28). A retrospective study of diabetic foot ulcers treated with hyperbaric oxygen therapy. *International Wound Journal.* doi: 10.1111/j.1742-481X.2011.00936.x. [Epub ahead of print]; Ma, Y. H., Lei, Y. H., Zhou, M., Li, X., & Zhao, H. Y. (2011). Effects of hyperbaric oxygen therapy in the management of chronic wounds and its correlation with CD34(+) endothelial progenitor cells. *Zhonghua Yi Xue Za Zhi, 91*(45), 3214–3218.

The treatment lasts about 2 hours and is given daily for a total of 20 to 60 treatments. However, special precautions must be taken with regard to fire hazards. Furthermore, HBOT has rare side effects, such as oxygen toxicity seizures, eardrum rupture, pneumothorax, hypoglycemia in patients with diabetes, and temporary visual changes. Because these side effects can be serious, constant supervision by a trained hyperbaric technician and a health care provider is required (Undersea & Hyperbaric Medical Society, 2007). The Complementary & Alternative Therapies box outlines hyperbaric oxygen therapy to improve oxygen supply to wounds.

Electrical Stimulation

Electrical stimulation (ES) is the use of electrical current to stimulate cellular processes. Benefits are reported to be an antibacterial effect, increased blood flow, cell proliferation, edema reduction, and facilitation of autolytic débridement. Although electrical stimulation is recommended as an adjuvant treatment, application in practice is variable and inconsistent. One main reason could be that the FDA has not yet approved any type of ES device for wound healing (Frantz et al., 2007).

Specialty Support Surfaces

Specialty support surfaces are mattresses or overlays that provide pressure reduction or pressure relief. Pressure reduction and pressure relief are based on the principle of decreasing **interface pressure,** the pressure between a bony prominence and a surface such as a hospital bed or seating surface. Decreasing interface pressure decreases pressure on capillaries. Ischemia results when capillaries are occluded, shutting down oxygen and nutrients necessary for cellular viability. Cellular death results in tissue necrosis (pressure ulcers). Choosing the most appropriate surface becomes a crucial component for pressure ulcer prevention. However, technology improvement and growth is constantly advancing the level and complexity of the specialty surface available in the acute care setting. Chart 60–10 summarizes the various overlays available.

Two additional categories of specialty support surfaces are low air loss therapy and air fluidized therapy. In low air loss therapy, low air loss overlays sit on top of the standard or therapeutic mattress replacement, or as a mattress that replaces the mattress on the frame. A pump is connected to the mattress or overlay, attached to the foot of the bed, and plugged into electricity. Some models feature a short-term battery to keep the mattress from deflating. Low air loss mattresses used within a special frame are considered "air support systems." A series of pillows are inflated with air in continuous motion according to specific patient measurements of weight and height. Therapy provided by low air loss beds maintains capillary blood flow, eliminates shear and friction, and reduces moisture. The nurse should *never* place a patient with spinal injury on a low air loss mattress until the injury has been radiologically cleared or the neurosurgeon or orthopedic surgeon orders it. (Each institution needs to have a specific policy.) The potential for further injury exists because the "air bed" does *not* support the spine.

Safety Alert *Do not diminish the pressure-relieving effects of the low air loss surface by using extra layers of sheets or pads. Extra padding increases pressure. Use only the pads recommended by the bed manufacturer.*

Air fluidized therapy utilizes a high rate of airflow to fluidize fine particulate material to produce a support medium that has characteristics similar to those of liquid. The support system does not utilize a mattress; the fluidized particulate matter is contained within a sheet that conforms around the patient's body. One-third of the body is floating, and the rest is enveloped within the sheet of constantly moving matter. Indications for these beds are surgical flaps, grafts, and, in some cases, intractable pain. Pain relief occurs because the fluidized air relieves pressure on painful areas as well as bony prominences or surgical flaps or grafts.

CHART 60–10 Skin Breakdown Protection Overlays

Overlay	Description	Use
Foam	Construction of a foam overlay's height, density, and indention load deflection (ILD) produces the characteristics to evaluate for effective pressure reduction. Base height should be measured from the base of the overlay to the lowest point of convolution in an "egg-crate" foam construction. To provide pressure relief, 4 inches or more of height is necessary.	Patients at risk for pressure ulcers Stages I and II pressure ulcers
Gel	Gel overlays are filled with silicon elastomer, silicon, polyvinyl chloride, or similar gel materials. They help reduce friction. The gel is displaced by the patient's body weight and provides flotation.	Patients at risk for pressure ulcers Stages I and II pressure ulcers
Air	Powered air overlays are considered dynamic (air is in motion). Air overlays consist of air cells that are inflated and produce consistent pressure reduction. Alternating air overlays consist of air cells constantly deflated and inflated, effectively reducing the effects of pressure duration by changing pressure distribution. Some of these are designed so that the airflow moves quickly into small chambers so the effect is pulsating. Nonpowered air overlays are static (no air motion). Static air overlays have connecting air cells that conform to body weight to displace the pressure load.	Patients at risk for pressure ulcers Stages I, II, III, and IV pressure ulcers Burns Surgical flaps
Water	Water-filled overlays are vinyl mattresses filled with water. The patient should displace the water without bottoming out; thus, the overlay effectively floats the patient.	Patients at risk for pressure ulcers Stages I, II, and III pressure ulcers

Patients weighing more than 500 pounds or having a body mass index above 40 should be considered for placement on a bariatric system for safety reasons. Bariatric systems utilize a reinforced frame to support body mass. Most can be converted to a chair position. Some systems provide a wider area to help support and facilitate the repositioning of patients. Low air loss mattresses are available on bariatric systems. In fact, newer models can make full-body lateral rotation turns with the low air loss surface.

Other pressure reduction surfaces include therapeutic mattress replacements; 4-inch foam overlays; static air, gel, and water overlays; and dynamic air overlays. Pressure relief surfaces include low air loss and air fluidized surfaces. Kinetic beds or "turning beds" are used for pulmonary rescue. Bariatric beds are for patients who are obese. Use of these beds must be considered therapy and documented as such with observed outcomes and achieved goals. They should be used in conjunction with optimal nutrition, appropriate positioning, optimal transferring and turning techniques, and routine skilled nursing care and assessments.

Safety Alert *It is essential to debunk the myth that once a patient is on a specialty support surface, the patient does not need to be repositioned. Manufacturers of specialty beds and wound care experts agree that nurses need to reposition patients on specialty beds frequently.*

Management of Drains

Care of surgical drains and tubes in postoperative patients is important in order to avoid complications. Because of the trend toward shorter lengths of stay in acute care facilities, nurses in home health and in long-term acute care facilities must learn to manage drains and tubes. To care for the postoperative patient with drains, the nurse must know the type, purpose, and location of the surgical drain; proper management strategies; potential problems; and how to troubleshoot complications. The nurse also must ensure that the system is securely stabilized and assess patency on a regular basis. Because drains are removed when they are no longer needed, monitoring the amount of drainage is important in order to determine how long the drain needs to stay in place. If the tube or drain is not draining fluid, there may be a problem with the system. The nurse should make a systematic check from where the drain leaves the patient's body to the collection device to check for kinks, blood clots, mucus, or tissue shreds. Milking the tube away from the patient can be done to sustain the tube's patency. Any significant change in the amount or character of drainage must be reported to the health care provider.

Nurses need to protect the patient's skin from any drainage or leakage to prevent irritation. Moisture barriers can be used to protect the skin from breakdown if there is leakage from in or around the drain insertion site. Dry gauze dressings can be used to help lift the drainage tube away from the skin and help stabilize the device.

A number of companies make various styles and types of stabilizers to keep drains and tubes from migrating into and out of the exit site. Constant friction due to migration of the tube causes the space around the tube to enlarge, allowing more movement of the tube and more leakage around the tube. With more moisture and friction, hypergranulation can occur.

Hypergranulation is the formation of soft, pink, fleshy growths of tissue around the tube; this is the body's attempt to heal the enlarged track. Silver nitrate sticks are often used to burn down this tissue because it creates more moisture and causes pain in some instances.

Preventing complications should be the goal of drain and tube management. Therefore, the nurse should consistently use good hand hygiene before and after patient care, use aseptic techniques when cleaning and dressing surgical drains and tubes, and dispose properly of drainage containers and drains when removed. The skin around the drain needs to be kept clean and dry.

Surgical Drains

Surgical drains are often indicated for decompression in areas with a significant amount of fluid accumulation, fistulas, infected tissue, and potential dead space. Two types of drains are used: active and passive.

Active Drains

Active drains are low-pressure suction devices that are constantly removing fluids via a closed drainage system. The drain is attached to a collapsible reservoir that exerts negative pressure to pull fluids from the wound bed. Active drain advantages include minimal tissue trauma and accurate drainage measurements; in addition, the closed system decreases infection risk. Examples of common active drains are Jackson–Pratt and Hemovac (Figures 60–12 A◆, 60–13◆, and 60–14◆).

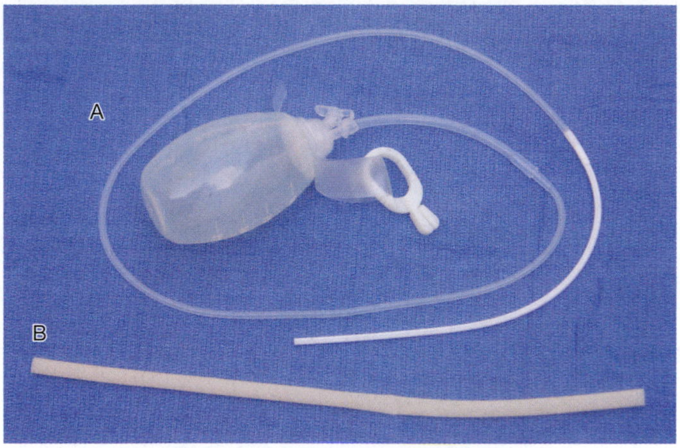

FIGURE 60–12 ◆ A Jackson–Pratt and B Penrose drain.
Source: Courtesy of John M. Osborn, MD, FACS.

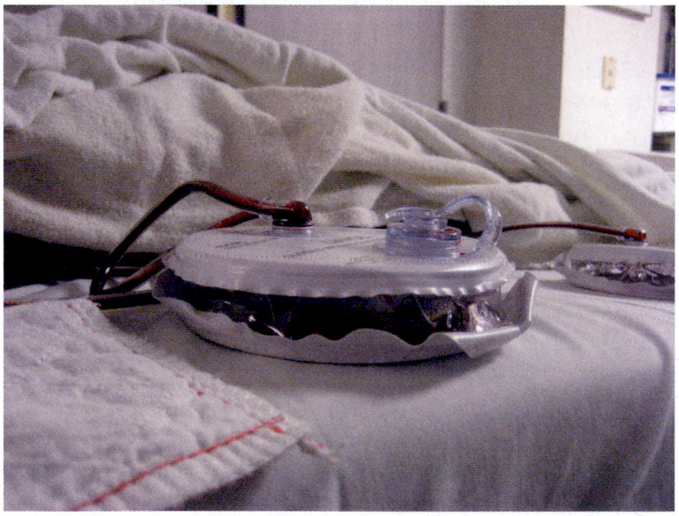

FIGURE 60–13 ◆ Hemovac drain.
Source: Cheryl Wraa.

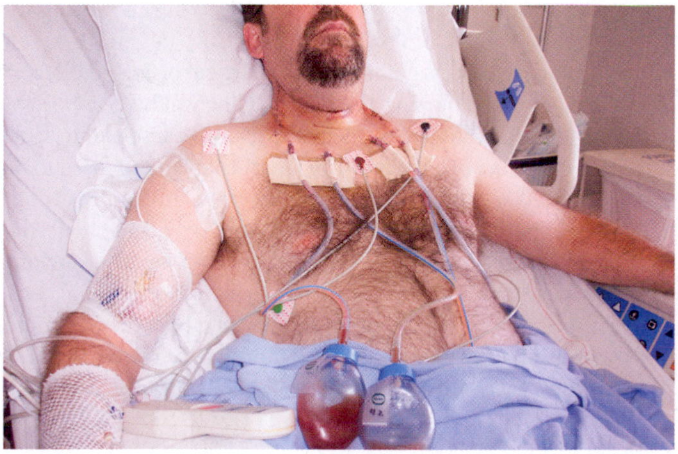

FIGURE 60–14 ◆ Jackson–Pratt drain with serosanguineous drainage.
Source: Ann E. F. Sievers, RN.

Video*: Closed Wound Drain—Hemovac, Emptying

Video*: Closed Wound Drain—Jackson Pratt, Emptying

Nursing interventions for active drains include the following:

- Keep the drain tubing straight without kinks.
- Keep the reservoir compressed (in a collapsed position) to maintain the negative pressure.
- For optimal function, empty the reservoir before it is half full.
- Unclog blood or tissue shreds from the drain tubing by milking or stripping toward the reservoir.
- Document the amount and color of drainage.

Wounds initially have sanguineous or serosanguineous drainage. As the wound heals, there is less drainage, and it becomes more serous.

Passive Drains

Passive drains are made of soft, flat, flexible material and are usually placed in a stab wound near an incision site. Pus, blood, necrotic debris, and fluids interfere with wound healing and can provide a milieu in which pathogens can flourish. Passive drains provide a conduit that functions by gravity for the removal of this drainage, which may be too viscous for the active drains. An example of a common passive drain is a Penrose drain (Figure 60–12 B◆).

The drain is typically sutured to secure it and keep it from migrating into or out of the wound. Flat gauze sponges or fenestrated sponges are used at the end of the drain to absorb the exudates. They are removed and new ones applied when the dressing becomes saturated, as wet dressings may irritate the skin. Care must be taken not to pull the drain out of the wound inadvertently during the dressing change. The nurse must protect the skin with a moisture barrier and frequently check the dressing to assess the need for replacement.

Percutaneous Drainage Catheters

Interventional radiologists implant a percutaneous drainage catheter to allow drainage from sites where fluid collection may be infected or to collect the fluid for laboratory studies to determine the nature of the fluid. The catheter is connected to a dependent drainage system such as a urinary leg bag. Placement sites include the biliary system, peritoneal cavity, groin, breast, or anywhere infection is suspected.

Nursing care includes assessment for patency and irrigation of the catheter to maintain patency. Aseptic technique is used, and a health care provider's order is needed for the irrigation procedure, which includes the frequency and volume of irrigating solution to be used. Forceful instillation of fluid and forceful aspiration are never used. Accurate documentation is required regarding the color, amount, and consistency of fluid and the patient's tolerance of the procedure. Sterile dressings are used to cover the percutaneous site.

Impaired Wound Healing

Impaired wound healing is defined as the disruption of the normal biochemical repair or regeneration process. Abnormalities may be manifested in a number of ways, described next. If healing is occurring at a normal rate, the wound edges of an incision should not separate after the first 24 hours. Assessing the wound edges gives the nurse information about the healing process. If the edges are separated or there is serous or serosanguineous drainage, the nurse needs to assess the wound frequently for signs of impaired wound healing.

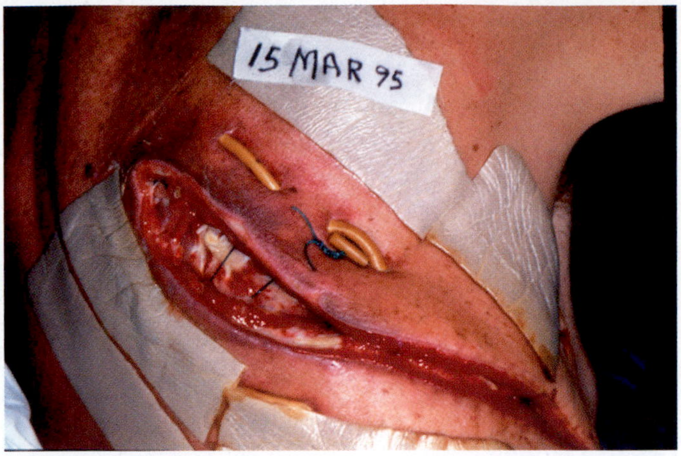

FIGURE 60–15 ◆ Wound dehiscence.
Source: Jan Clark.

Dehiscence

Wound dehiscence is the separation of the skin edges along the incision in a previously closed wound (Figure 60–15◆). Dehiscence can be caused by infection or tension on skin that is pulled together tightly with sutures or staples. Patients who are obese and patients on steroids are at a higher risk for the development of dehiscence. A sign of impending dehiscence is the leakage of serous or serosanguineous fluid from the incision for several days after injury or surgery. This indicates that collagen is not being properly formed and the tensile strength of the wound is impaired. If there is serosanguineous drainage, it should be absorbed by a sterile cover dressing. The characteristics of wound dehiscence drainage (amount, color, and odor), along with the length of the separation, should be reported to the surgeon. The patient may need to return to surgery for wound closure, or the wound may need to be packed with dressings. To prevent maceration or irritation of the normal skin adjacent to the wound edges, liquid skin barriers or moisture barriers may be applied to the periwound skin with each dressing change.

Evisceration

Wound evisceration is defined as the protrusion of organs from a separated surgical incision (Figure 60–16◆). The nurse needs to cover the organs with a sterile saline-moistened dressing and call the surgeon emergently, as the patient will need to return to surgery for repair of the evisceration.

Hematoma and Seroma Formation

Hematoma is defined as an area of swelling or a mass of blood confined to an organ, tissue, or space due to a broken blood vessel. Because of the abnormal collection of blood in the tissues, hematomas are typically painful. It is the increased pain and swelling in the area when it should be decreasing that often leads to the diagnosis of hematoma. A hematoma can become infected and large enough to split the skin open and cause drainage. The treatment consists of cold compresses for the first 24 hours to decrease bleeding, elevation of the affected area, and, if the hematoma is large enough, aspiration. Antibiotics may be necessary if the hematoma becomes infected. The nurse needs to report the presence of a hematoma to the health care provider and do serial assessments to assess changes in the size. The wound will not completely heal until the hematoma has dissolved.

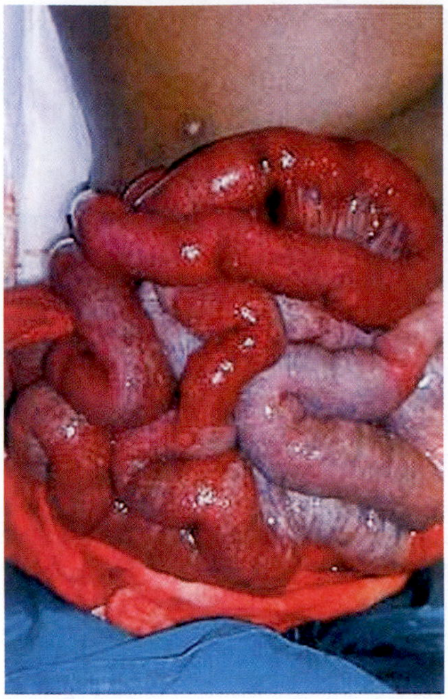

FIGURE 60–16 ◆ Wound evisceration.
Source: Jan Clark.

A **seroma** is the same as a hematoma except that instead of a collection of blood, it is a collection of serous fluid. The presence of a seroma affects wound healing; therefore, the typical treatment is aspiration or an incision-and-drainage procedure with postprocedure packing and secondary intention closure.

The literature suggests that patients who are obese are more likely to experience postsurgical wound complications. The blood supply needed to provide an adequate amount of oxygen and nutrients to the fatty tissues may be insufficient, thus interfering with wound healing. Donor-site infections, donor-site seromas, and hernias also occur more frequently in obese patients. The large pannus predisposes patients to fluid accumulation, creating an environment conducive to seroma formation, infection, and wound edge separation or dehiscence (Camden, 2007).

Nursing Management

Use of the nursing process guides the management of wounds. Beginning with a thorough nursing assessment of the wound is important in making decisions about treatment and goals because of the viable and changing nature of a wound. The treatment plan may need to be changed to facilitate these changes in the wound (Rolstad & Ovington, 2007). Typically guided by the health care provider's orders, the nurse is responsible for daily management of the wound. Therefore, the nurse is in a unique position to detect changes in the wound environment that indicate complications. Reporting these changes could prevent problems that may become life threatening. The nurse is in a pivotal position as a patient advocate to facilitate management by all the members of the health care team.

Planning

The nurse identifies the plan for care on the basis of the type of wound and the factors that coexist to impede the healing process. The plan of care should be individualized, and the patient and family should be involved in the planning process. The patient and family must agree to the plan of care and the interventions because they are responsible for the accurate and complete implementation of the plan overall. The plan will include diagnostic studies to follow up on factors that may or may not impede progress. All the information must be obtained so that a correct and meaningful treatment plan is pursued.

Nursing Diagnoses

Nursing diagnoses include the following:

- *Altered Skin Integrity* related to the wound.
- *Risk for Infection* related to loss of skin integrity.
  NANDA-I © 2012

Outcomes and Evaluation Parameters

The outcomes of interventions provide a basis for performance evaluation. By combining assessment skills and reviewing collected data, nurses are prepared to do an evaluation of the patient's overall condition. Connecting the specialized pieces such as wound assessment, respiratory assessment, and vascular assessment with integrated interventional data can result in an evaluation that is specific. For example, the nurse might determine that poor perfusion is contributing to slow wound healing and subsequent increased risk for infection.

The outcome for the patient must be identified after all the diagnostic data have been considered. The outcome may be driven by the goal of healing, the goal of preventing further damage, or even the goal of amputation. The outcome is directly related to how the plan of care affects the factors that impede healing and the interventions to promote the most optimal environment. A good wound care plan addresses all the factors in wound healing to allow the body to heal itself.

Evaluation parameters would include the clinical manifestations of effective wound healing. The wound is getting smaller in diameter as well as in depth; there is an absence of drainage, an absence of odor, and a normal white blood count; and the patient is experiencing less pain and tenderness. Complete wound closure is the final evaluation parameter.

Interventions and Rationales

Nursing interventions are aimed at prevention of wound complications and promotion of healing. Interventions are developed on the basis of assessment and diagnostic results. Wound management needs to follow the three principles outlined on page 1907: (1) control or eliminate causative factors, (2) provide systemic support to reduce existing and potential cofactors, and (3) maintain the physiologic local wound environment (Rolstad & Ovington, 2007). These principles may be embodied in various therapies depending on the phase of wound healing and the treatment goals. For example, débridement (see Chart 60–9, p. 1904) by any method will send signals that trigger platelet aggregation, MMP (matrix metalloproteinases) to denature harmed collagen, leukocytosis and phagocytosis to clean up the environment, and growth factors to heal the wound with new collagen synthesis. Dressings can be applied to provide moisture for epithelial migration in a dry wound or moisture retention and absorption to prevent maceration and further collagen damage in a wet wound. Silver can be applied as an antimicrobial agent. Offloading devices such as specialized shoes, splints, wheelchair cushions, or bed surfaces will alleviate pressure and restore circulation for healing. Nutrition should be addressed, and supplements should be given to assist in correcting any deficiencies. Vascular status also should be addressed and corrected if possible. Bioburden and infection must be controlled. Perineal care of the incontinent patient will help prevent skin breakdown. Keeping the skin dry decreases friction and prevents breakdown from abrasive force. With microabrasions, the skin has reduced barrier capability, allowing permeability to irritating substances and proliferation of bacteria and fungal infections. It is important to protect the skin from wetness and fecal irritants by using moisture barriers on any patient who cannot get up and use the toilet on his own. Most soaps leave a difficult-to-rinse residue and have high pH levels that interfere with the skin's protective acid mantle. Soap can be irritating and can strip the natural lubricant from the skin. Therefore, skin cleansers should be used that have nonionic surfactants that do not strip natural body oil. Skin cleansers can be any combination of products: antibacterial; 3-in-1 products for cleansing, moisturizing, and protecting; and pH balanced. Moisture barriers protect the skin from too much moisture (incontinence, perspiration). Many types and brands of moisture barriers, body cleansers, and moisturizers are available. Emollients help keep moisture in the skin. Moisturizers add moisture to skin.

Evaluation

Evaluation of the wound, its environment, and contributing factors determine the plan of care. The plan and treatment are altered in response to the individual needs of the patient, the nurse's assessment of the wound and the periwound area, and any factors that are impeding the wound's progress in healing. For instance, a wound may initially be draining a large amount of fluid and require an alginate. Once the drainage has decreased to a minimum, the wound bed may become dry and require a moisture dressing such as a hydrogel to facilitate epidermal cell migration. Daily wound evaluation and documentation are indicated until there is complete wound closure. At this point, the patient may have returned to activities of daily living and so may require an offloading device. It is essential that the patient be educated about protecting the newly healed wound until it matures so that wound breakdown will not occur.

Nursing Documentation

Nursing documentation in the patient's record must be accurate and complete, including documenting the assessment, interventions, and outcomes, as well as the patient's responses to treatment. For example, wound characteristics noted after an assessment must be descriptive enough for someone who has not seen the wound to get a good mental picture. The documentation must note whether there has been a measurable outcome (e.g., a decrease in size, decreased drainage, increased epithelial tissue). The documentation also needs to include what was used to clean the wound (saline or wound cleanser), type and amount of dressing used, and how the dressing was secured if necessary. The nurse should note significant changes that might indicate infection and report them to the health care provider. Wound documentation also should include a patient's emotional response toward the wound and participation in wound care management. Specific to documentation of wound care, the following items should be part of the record:

- Be specific with date and time.
- Was the wound present on admission? This can be ascertained only if a head-to-toe inspection of the skin is done by the nurse.
- Record the name and score of any risk assessment tool that is used.
- How long has the patient had the wound?
- What is the specific location of the wound?
- What are the wound's surface dimensions and depth?
- What types of dressings were used and how much?

- Note changes in quantity and odor of exudates/drainage.
- What is the condition of skin surrounding the wound?
- What support surface is the patient on? Remember that specialty support surfaces are therapeutic treatment and should be acknowledged in interventions and in assessment and documentation.
- Is there progress in wound healing or deterioration?
- What are the patient's and family/caregiver's reactions to the wound? Do they participate in wound care? Are their expectations reasonable?

It is necessary for the records to reflect the health care provider's orders requiring specific dressing type, frequency of dressing changes, dressing amounts used, and expected length of need. The record must also reflect a diagnosis with wound description and classification if applicable. Each wound should be described separately, and evaluation of each wound is required routinely (as determined by the setting). Documentation can make the difference in whether treatment and/or supplies are reimbursed.

Discharge Planning

It is important for patients and their family members to be actively involved in the discharge planning process. The nurse must evaluate their knowledge and willingness to participate in the wound care and then develop instructions and guidelines for the patient and caregiver. If barriers exist that will affect their ability to provide effective care, an alternative plan must be instituted. For example, recognizing cultural influences and family roles is essential so that the teaching can be individualized and meaningful. An assessment of resources and transportation is an essential component of the plan. The nurse needs to evaluate the patient and family's ability to afford and obtain the necessary supplies for the wound care. The Patient Teaching & Discharge Priorities box describes the necessary components of the discharge teaching plan.

Collaborative Management

The primary aim of clinical management for wound healing is expedient closure of the wound with no complications. The interdisciplinary team members include the primary health care provider, certified wound care specialist nurse, nutritionist, hospitalist, vascular surgeon and/or oncologist, pharmacist, and nurse. In order to meet desired patient outcomes, it is essential that this interdisciplinary team communicate openly with one another in developing and evaluating care of the patient and family (IOM [Institute of Medicine], 2010).

Wounds are not an isolated problem for most patients; the patient's comorbidities must continue to be treated along with wound management. In the acute setting, the wound is often not the admitting diagnosis. Traumatic wound treatment begins on admission in the emergency department. Frequently, the certified wound care nurse is called for these wounds by surgeons to provide continuing care of the wound. If the patient is admitted with a chronic wound, the certified wound care nurse should be notified; an assessment of the wound will be made; the admitting or referring health care provider will be notified of the recommended treatment; orders will be obtained; and staff nurses will institute them. Staff nurses doing admission assessments need to remove existing dressings and assess, document, and report the presence of wounds. Most hospitals ensure that a nutritionist sees a patient within 24 hours of admission. Nutritionists will make recommendations for dietary considerations such as calorie intake, supplements, and vitamins, and place them in the chart. Nurses are expected to monitor intake. Plastic surgeons or vascular surgeons may be consulted for nonhealing chronic wounds as well as traumatic injuries. They also may be called to perform sharp débridement. Dermatologists may be consulted for other skin issues such as rashes. Podiatrists may be consulted for foot and diabetic wounds. Endocrinologists may be consulted to control diabetes. Pharmacists can advise about medications that will slow down wound healing and the timing for tests for antibiotic efficacy with peaks and troughs. Blood samples are done at specific intervals before and after antibiotic administration to determine whether the amount of antibiotic should be adjusted for efficacy. Respiratory therapists ensure that the patient's oxygenation is optimal. Physical therapists may do wound care in some settings. Physical therapists need to be informed about wounds so that dressings and drains remain free of tension. The hospitalist assists in coordinating and communicating the care of patients while in the hospital with the primary health care provider and all other services consulted. A collaborative team approach ensures that all aspects of the wound healing process are being guided by people who are knowledgeable in each aspect of care.

These individuals may or may not actually all meet together to discuss a patient's care. Ideally, as each individual assesses and treats the patient, she will read charting by all members of the team. Nurses have an obligation to read the notes in order to become informed of patient status. In home health, communication of patient status to the health care provider is of paramount importance, because the home health nurse may be the only one doing a physical assessment for long periods of time. Accurate descriptions of existing wounds are valuable to the health care providers who are making decisions about patient care.

Health Promotion

Education of the patient or caregiver regarding decisions and goals of treatment is an important factor in successful wound healing. Tenets of an effective teaching plan include the following:

- Wound care
- Infection prevention/assessment
- Nutrition
- Lifestyles and habits that prevent or slow wound healing
- Prevention of wound breakdown
- Follow-up care.

Each of these factors must be taught to the patient and family/caregivers in a logical, understandable fashion. For example, a written plan and return demonstrations from the patient/family (i.e., the patient and/or caregiver(s) demonstrate the wound care treatments the nurse has taught) help facilitate teaching.

Identifying the patient's needs for discharge begins on admission to the health care setting. The process includes assessment, identification of continuing care needs, planning, and implementing a plan that will meet those determined needs. Today it is a common practice to send patients home before wounds have completely healed and to have their care continued at home and in the outpatient clinic setting. A variety of health care professionals can be involved in the process, as described earlier, but the nurse is the pivotal figure in establishing a comprehensive discharge plan. Developing a complete plan of care and providing a manner in which routine reevaluation and modification of the plan can occur will facilitate the process until wound closure has occurred. Nurses must educate patients and family/caregivers about all aspects of the wound care. Concise written instructions beginning with

PATIENT TEACHING & DISCHARGE PRIORITIES for the Management of Wounds

Need	Teaching
Wound Care Patient/family Family/support system Setting	Perform daily cleansing and dressing changes: • How often to change the dressing • Type of dressing and solutions. Elevate areas where edema formation occurs. Avoid sunlight, as it can cause, among other things, healed wounds to discolor or darken permanently: • Avoid overexposure to sun. • Use sunscreen products when exposed to sunlight. • Use clothing and hats for added protection. Avoid exposure to extreme temperatures and harsh chemicals. Wear loose-fitting, soft clothing. Assess availability of, knowledge of, and compliance with treatment regimen. Have family perform return demonstration. Assess discharge placement needs: • Home • Rehabilitation facility • Extended care facility. Assess need for professional home health needs. Assess need for follow-up appointments.
Wound Infection Patient/family Family/support system Setting	Assess for infection of open wounds and healed wound breakdown with each dressing change, and report as necessary. Signs and symptoms include: • Odor and exudate • Fever • Increased drainage • Swelling • Lack of wound closure • Increased pain. Teach minimization of risk factors for infection: • Hand hygiene • Clean technique with dressing changes. Explain signs and symptoms that require medical attention. Assess the environment for risk factors that increase the risk of infection.
Nutrition Patient/family Setting	Maintain a high-calorie, high-protein diet. Continue taking vitamins and mineral supplements as ordered. Observe for appetite and weight loss, as well as food intolerance. Assess financial resources. Home. Rehabilitation center.
Pain Management Patient/family Setting	Assess pain level and report any increase in pain. Assess the effectiveness of pharmacologic interventions. Wean the patient off pain medication when pain lessens. Report a sudden increase in pain. Assess the environment for safety and promotion of therapeutic needs.

a statement about hand hygiene should be given to the patient or caregiver. Return demonstration ensures that the patient and caregiver understand the procedures. If the patient is to be discharged with a drain in place, the patient should know the purpose of the drain, expected output, how to care for the drain and empty it, how to troubleshoot, whom to contact for questions, and whom to contact in an emergency.

Psychological Considerations

Acute and chronic wounds affect quality of life. Patients often experience depression, isolation, and financial burdens caused by wounds. The patient's body image may be disturbed, and cultural issues may create misunderstanding or compliance issues. Nurses are often first aware and most aware of these conditions. Assessing the meaning and significance of the wound to the patient and family or caregiver is often overlooked but should be done for optimal wound healing.

Pain is often associated with wounds. Pain occurs because nerve endings are exposed, and some of the interventions utilized to heal the wound can cause varying degrees of pain. The pain is what the patient states it is in terms of severity, character, duration, and tolerance level. The nurse should consider adequate pain coverage before making dressing changes, changes in position, or changes in mobility. Controlling pain can help patients to be more compliant with the treatment plan and willing to investigate other treatment modalities. Pain can be assessed on a number scale, facial scale, vital sign assessment, or combinations of such scales. Medications can be prescribed to alleviate the pain. Nonnarcotic medications such as nonsteroidal anti-inflammatories (NSAIDs) can alleviate pain and decrease inflammation. Narcotic medications such as opioids or opioid derivatives also can be given. Chapter 12 includes an in-depth discussion of pain management.

The wound affects the patient's daily life and thus cannot help but be a factor in the way the patient feels about herself and how others perceive her to be, especially if the wound is easily visible. Not only does the patient have an emotional response to the wound, but almost everyone the patient encounters has an emotional response to the wound as well. Wounds are perceived as unpleasant, disgusting, scary, and a nuisance. The treatments and medications may be very costly. The patient may have to wear some special type of shoe or device that makes the patient self-conscious. These factors may lead to depression in the patient, which may affect the patient's ability to perform the daily activities she wants to do. In addition, it may limit the patient's independence. The nurse needs to assess the patient for her feelings about the wound and associated treatment. The nurse should empathize with the patient and try to devise a plan that is least intrusive and yet realistic. A nurse can address the concerns by providing privacy during dressing changes, offering factual explanations of the wound to the patient and her family or caregiver, having frank discussions with the patient and caregiver about how the wound is affecting them, scheduling wound care at the best time for the patient, applying appropriate dressings, and performing timely dressing changes.

An individual who has had a recent amputation has a whole new set of restrictions and adaptations to overcome. The patient will need education to prevent further insults from occurring to preserve the best way of life the patient can expect.

The nurse needs to instruct each patient on what can or will happen if treatment is not followed according to the individualized plan. Patients want to be informed and want honest feedback but need some compassion with the delivery of their care. Educational sites on the Internet that patients and family members may visit, as well as support groups, may be helpful. The nurse should document the patient's response to the wound. Chapter 9 includes an in-depth discussion of the psychosocial aspects of nursing.

Gerontological Considerations

The prevalence of chronic wounds in older adults ranges from 10% to 35%; this population has the highest prevalence of any age group in the United States (Pittman, 2007). The process of wound healing is altered in older adults. It is characterized by a progressive loss of skin function, increased vulnerability to the environment, and decreased homeostatic ability. Healing is usually delayed (Reddy, Holroyd-Leduc, Cheung, & Woo, 2007.) **Rete pegs** (also known as epidermal ridges) are protrusions in the fifth layer of the epidermis that extend down into the dermis to help anchor the epidermis to the dermis. In older adults (as in neonates), the ridges are flatter, failing to anchor the epidermis and making it easier for the epidermis to slide away from the dermis, resulting in skin tears (Figure 60–7, p. 1900). Additionally, sweat glands decrease production, which results in drier skin. In healthy older adults, sweating may be decreased by as much as 70%. The increased incidence of **xerosis** (a skin condition characterized by dry, pruritic, cracked, or fissured skin with scaling and flaking) in persons over the age of 60 can be attributed to (1) a decrease in the lipid component of skin, (2) a loss in water retention, and (3) frequent fragranced baths and showering. Decreased dermal thickness causes thinning of the skin, especially along the lower legs and forearms, as evidenced by the prevalence of skin tears on the extremities. Because there are fewer collagen and elastin fibers, there is less elasticity (recoil) in the skin. The skin is less effective as a barrier against water loss and bruising. In addition, there is a natural loss of thermal regulation, tactile sensitivity, and pain perception. **Senile purpura,** another age-related change, is a type of hemorrhaging under the skin due to thinner, more fragile blood vessels. Senile purpuras often occur at the site of skin tears. All of these factors place an older person at higher risk of dehydration, skin tears, burns, and traumatic injury. In addition, wound healing is prolonged in older adults for the following reasons:

- Reepithelialization takes almost twice as long.
- The rate of wound dehiscence is greater in older adults, most likely because of the decreased tensile strength of the wound.
- A greater number of comorbidities results in prolonged wound healing. Healing may be prolonged by conditions that result in poor cardiac output or low oxygen-carrying capacity such as heart failure. Diabetes, peripheral vascular disease, and poor nutrition all result in longer healing times in any age population.

Careful attention to aged skin is good prevention. Emollient skin care products help the skin retain moisture. It is important for the older adult to use clothing to protect the arms and legs against sun exposure and trauma. Consistent use of sunscreen also is beneficial to prevent skin breakdown. A review of medications that may affect skin is in order. Gentle cleansing and physical assistance are essential.

Wound management for older adults involves some important considerations. First, age alone should not be a contraindication to any aspect of wound management. Second, health care providers usually need to spend more time when evaluating older adults. Third, medications need to be started at lower doses and titrated upward more slowly for older adults than for younger patients; some medications should be avoided altogether. Finally, the nurse needs to consider cognitive and physical function, financial limitations, and goals of treatment when determining the wound management regimen (Reddy et al., 2007).

Ethical Issues

Treatment of wounds can lead to a discussion about aggressive versus conservative care. For example, what is the appropriate care for a nursing home resident who has had multiple strokes and is now aphasic and bedbound? Suppose a sacral pressure ulcer develops and eschar is observable in a patient who is debilitated and has failure to thrive. Is aggressive treatment of the wound with surgical intervention appropriate? Does the patient have the ability to heal if surgical intervention is performed? Can the patient even be cleared for surgery safely? These are all questions that must be asked and considered before developing a treatment plan. The patient may not be a candidate for aggressive care, and a conservative approach may be the ethical and prudent action. The goal may be to prevent the further deterioration of the wound. Obviously, a collaborative approach among the health care team, patient, and family must occur to make a decision on what ultimate goal or outcome is desired. As hard as it is at times as health care professionals, sometimes the best plan is not the most aggressive one but the most realistic one. Decisions about care and the degree of aggressiveness must be consistent with the patient's overall physiological status as well as the patient's and family's goals. Those goals may be complete restoration, ability to function, or provision of comfort. Coming to a consensus can be a process, but acceptance of the care plan by all involved is important. Caregivers experience a myriad range of emotions, and balancing the patient's needs with those of the caregiver can be difficult. It is important for the nurse to understand that the health-related quality of life is the patient's perception of well-being, not an evaluation of clinical status.

Liability

The development of wounds, in particular pressure ulcers, has led to a lot of controversy over quality of care and thus liability. It is essential that the nurse understands how the regulatory and accrediting bodies such as the Joint Commission assess individual wound interventions and their effectiveness. These regulatory bodies monitor what nurses do as individuals and what they accomplish aggregately within an institution. Hospitals must have quality assurance records regarding pressure ulcer incidence and measures for reduction.

For the most part, pressure ulcers are preventable. Prevention requires a plan of action that is individualized and is followed vigilantly. Because so many preventable ulcers have developed over the years, the U.S. government has taken steps to try to ensure that all necessary action is taken to prevent pressure ulcers from developing due to negligence. A federal tag, called F-tag 314, requires long-term care facilities (nursing homes) to comply with certain regulations concerning the prevention and treatment of pressure ulcers. The long-term care facility must assess patients who are at risk for development of a pressure ulcer, follow certain preventive guidelines, demonstrate compliance with those guidelines, and, if the patient still develops a pressure ulcer, show appropriate intervention. The patient must then be monitored for progress, and the plan of care must be altered if it fails to achieve the desired result of healing.

The Centers for Medicare & Medicaid Services guidelines developed in October 2008 have expanded the focus on the prevention of pressure ulcers to the acute care setting. Basically, CMS will no longer pay for the expanded care of the patient with a hospital-acquired pressure or decubitus ulcer (CMS, 2008). Documentation by health care providers and nursing staff is pivotal in establishing whether the pressure ulcer was present on admission (POA). A hospital-acquired pressure ulcer has its own diagnosis-related group (DRG) code, which is different from a community-acquired DRG code. The report card for the hospital is available to the public.

Research

Research is essential in order to continue improving wound care, complication rates, healing time, and scar formation. The goal of research is to identify areas in which practice needs to be improved and then to evaluate and test methods in these areas. The Research Opportunities box related to wound healing provides a list of both medical and nursing research topics still under investigation. Electronic databases are a source for finding studies related to these topics.

RESEARCH OPPORTUNITIES Related to Wound Healing

Research Area	Clinical Impact
Wound healing dressings that promote faster healing.	Prevent infection.
Wound healing cleansers.	Prevent infection.
Topical hyperbaric oxygen treatment.	Increase healing rates.
Dietary factors that impact wound healing.	Increase healing rates.
The nature of pain induced by direct tissue injury.	Patient comfort and increased wound healing.
Nursing pain management.	
Pain and anxiety measurement and management during procedures.	
Mechanisms to prevent scar formation.	Improve wound appearance and prevent contracture formation.
Prevention of hypertrophic and keloid scar formation.	Improve wound appearance and prevent contracture formation.
Techniques to increase tensile strength and reduce wound breakdown.	Improve techniques to increase wound healing and prevent scarring.
Role of growth factors in wound healing.	Improve techniques to increase wound healing.

NCLEX® PRACTICE

1. A patient with poor circulation has a leg wound. The nurse realizes that the primary phase of the wound healing that would be compromised in this patient is:

1. Homeostasis
2. Inflammatory
3. Proliferation
4. Remodeling

2. A patient has been diagnosed with a tunneling wound. The nurse would document the size of the wound:

1. in inches.
2. in centimeters.
3. using the clock face method.
4. in centimeters cubed.

3. A patient prone to pressure ulcer development is unable to move independently in bed. Which of the following should the nurse do to assist this patient? (select all that apply)

1. Move the patient's limbs every hour.
2. Reposition the patient every 2 hours.
3. Use assistive devices to move the patient.
4. Avoid the use of foam wedges.
5. Assist the patient to the prone position as tolerated.

4. A patient has a category II skin tear on her forearm. Which of the following would be appropriate to care for this wound? (select all that apply)

1. Use compression therapy.
2. Plan for surgical intervention.
3. Apply a moisture barrier.
4. Plan for débridement of the wound.
5. Use zinc-impregnated gauze and cotton.

5. A critically ill patient needs to have a leg wound débrided. The nurse realizes that the best approach to use for this patient wound be:

1. autolytic débridement.
2. sharp débridement.
3. mechanical débridement.
4. enzymatic débridement.

6. A patient with a leg wound tells the nurse that the wound is ugly and she is not really sure if she wants to take care of the wound when she goes home. Which of the following should the nurse say in response to this patient?

1. "It's not that bad."
2. "Tell me why you think the wound is ugly."
3. "I have to agree with you."
4. "Maybe you can stay in the hospital until it's healed."

Answers to NCLEX Practice Questions can be found in Appendix D in the Osborn Student Resources at nursing.pearsonhighered.com. Practice additional NCLEX questions online at the Student Resources site.

Pearson Nursing Student Resources Find additional review materials at: **nursing.pearsonhighered.com**

REFERENCES

Ayello, E., & Lyder, C. (2008). A new era of pressure ulcer accountability in acute care. *Advances in Skin & Wound Care, 21*(3), 134–140.

Bernstein, M. L., & Chung, K. C. (2007). Early management of the mangled upper extremity. *Injury, 38* (Suppl 5:S3-7) 53–57.

Bishop, A. J., & Mudge, E. (2012, February 28). A retrospective study of diabetic foot ulcers treated with hyperbaric oxygen therapy. *International Wound Journal.* doi: 10.1111/j.1742-481X.2011.00936.x. [Epub ahead of print].

Black, J. M., Gray, M., Bliss, D. Z., Kennedy-Evans, K. L., Logan, S., Baharestani, M. M., et al. (2011). MASD Part 2: Incontinence-associated dermatitis and intertriginous dermatitis: A consensus. *Journal of Wound Ostomy & Continence Nursing, 38*(4), 359–370.

Brashers, V. (2010). Alterations of cardiovascular function. In K. McCance, S. Huether, V. Brashers, & N. Rote (Eds.), *Pathophysiology: The biologic basis for disease in adults and children* (6th ed.). Philadelphia, PA: Elsevier.

Broadbent, E., & Koschwanez, H. E. (2012). The psychology of wound healing. Current Opinion in Psychiatry. Retrieved from http://www.co-psychiatry.com Volume 25_Number 2_March 2012.PubMed.

Bryant, R., & Clark, R. (2007). Skin pathology and types of damage. In R. Bryant & D. Nix (Eds.), *Acute and chronic wounds: Current management concepts* (3rd ed.). Philadelphia, PA: Mosby/Elsevier.

Camden, S. G. (2007). Skin care needs of the obese patient. In R. Bryant & D. Nix (Eds.), *Acute and chronic wounds: Current management concepts* (3rd ed.). Philadelphia, PA: Mosby/Elsevier.

CDC. (2011). National diabetes fact sheet, 2011. Retrieved from http://www.cdc.gov/diabetes/pubs/pdf/ndfs_2011.pdf

Centers for Medicare & Medicaid Services (CMS). (2008). Overview of hospital-acquired conditions (present on admission indicator). Retrieved from http://www.cms.gov/hospitalacqcond/01_overview.asp#topofpage

Christian, P., Talavera, F., Stadelmann, W., Slenkovich, N., & Downey, S. (2006). Wound healing, growth factors. eMedicine. Retrieved from http://www.emedicine.com/plastic/topic457.htm

Cooper, R. (2007). Iodine revisited. *International Wound Journal, 4*(2) 210–214.

Doughty, D., & Holbrook, R. (2007). Lower-extremity ulcers of vascular etiology. In R. Bryant & D. Nix (Eds.), *Acute and chronic wounds: Current management concepts* (3rd ed.). Philadelphia, PA: Mosby/Elsevier.

Doughty, D., & Sparks-Defriese, B. (2007). Wound healing physiology. In R. Bryant & D. Nix (Eds.), *Acute and chronic wounds: Current management concepts* (3rd ed.). Philadelphia, PA: Mosby/Elsevier.

Driver, V., Landowski, M. A., & Madsen. J. L. (2007). Neuropathic wounds: The diabetic wound. In R. Bryant & D. Nix (Eds.), *Acute and chronic wounds: Current management concepts* (3rd ed.). Philadelphia, PA: Mosby/Elsevier.

Duncan, K. (2007). 5 Million Lives Campaign: Preventing pressure ulcers: The goal is zero. *The Joint Commission Journal on Quality and Patient Safety, 33*(10), 605–610.

European Pressure Ulcer Advisory Panel and National Pressure Ulcer Advisory Panel. (2009). *Prevention and treatment of pressure ulcers: Quick reference guide.* Washington, DC: National Pressure Ulcer Advisory Panel. Retrieved from http://www.npuap.org/Final_Quick_Prevention_for_web.pdf

Frantz, R., Broussard, C., Mendez-Eastman, S., & Cordrey, R. (2007). Devices and technology in wound care. In R. Bryant & D. Nix (Eds.), *Acute and chronic wounds: Current management concepts* (3rd ed.). Philadelphia, PA: Mosby/Elsevier.

Gardner, S. E., & Frantz, R. A. (2004). Wound bioburden. In S. Baranoski & E. A. Ayello (Eds.), *Wound care essentials: Practice principles* (pp. 91–116). Philadelphia: Lippincott Williams & Wilkins.

Hinman, C. D., & Maibach, H. (1963). Effect of air exposure and occlusion on experimental human skin wounds. *Nature, 200,* 377–378.

Holloway, G. A. (2007). Arterial ulcers: Assessment, classification, and management. In D. Krasner, G. Rodeheaver, & R. G. Sibbald (Eds.), *Chronic wound care: A clinical source book for healthcare professionals* (4th ed.). Malvern, PA: HMP Communications.

IOM (Institute of Medicine). (2010). *The future of nursing: Leading change, advancing health.* Washington, DC: The Academic Press.

Ip, M., Lui, S., Poon, V., Lung, I., & Burd, A. (2006). Antimicrobial activities of silver dressings: An *in vitro* comparison. *Journal of Medical Microbiology, 55*(1), 59–63.

Kee, J. L. (2010). *Laboratory and diagnostic tests with nursing implications.* Upper Saddle River, NJ: Pearson.

Khan, M. (2006). Antiseptics, iodine, povidone iodine and traumatic wound cleansing. *Tissue Viability Society, 16*(4).

Lavery, L. A., Armstrong, D. G., & Harkless, L. B. (1996). Classification of diabetic foot ulcerations. *Journal of Foot and Ankle Surgery, 35*(6), 528.

Leach, M. J., et al. (2006b). Using horse chestnut seed extract in the treatment of venous leg ulcers: A cost–benefit analysis. *Ostomy Wound Management, 52*(4), 68–70, 72–74, 76–78.

Lopez, V., Dunk, A. M., Parke, J., Larkin, D., Trudinger, M., & Stuart, M. (2011). Skin tear prevention and management among patients in the acute aged care and rehabilitation units in the Australian Capital Territory: A best practice implementation project. *International Journal of Evidence-Based Healthcare, 9*(4), 429–434.

Ma, Y. H., Lei, Y. H., Zhou, M., Li, X., & Zhao, H. Y. (2011). Effects of hyperbaric oxygen therapy in the management of chronic wounds and its correlation with CD34(+) endothelial progenitor cells. *Zhonghua Yi Xue Za Zhi, 91*(45), 3214–3218.

Miniño, A. M. (2011). Death in the United States 2009. *NCHS Data Brief, 64.* Retrieved from http://www.cdc.gov/nchs/data/databriefs/db64.htm

Nataraj, C., Ritter, G., Dumas, S., Helfer, F., Brunelle, J., & Sander, T. W. (2007). Extracellular wound matrices: Novel stabilization and sterilization method for collagen-based biologic wound dressings. Wounds. Retrieved from http://www.woundsresearch.com/article/7374

Nix, D. (2007). Patient assessment and evaluation of healing. In R. Bryant & D. Nix (Eds.), *Acute and chronic wounds: Current management concepts* (3rd ed.). Philadelphia, PA: Mosby/Elsevier.

Odland, G. (1958). The fine structure of the interrelationship of cells in the human epidermis. *Journal of Biophysical, Biochemistry and Cytology, 4*(5) 529–535.

Payne, R. L., & Martin, M. (1993). Defining and classifying skin tears: Need for a common language. *Ostomy Wound Management, 39*(5), 16–20, 22–24, 26.

Pieper, B. (2007). Mechanical forces: Pressure, shear, and friction. In R. Bryant & D. Nix (Eds.), *Acute and chronic wounds: Current management concepts* (3rd ed.). Philadelphia, PA: Mosby/Elsevier.

Pittman, J. (2007). Effect of aging on wound healing: Current concepts. *Journal of Wound Ostomy & Continence Nursing, 34*(4), 412–415.

Porth, C., & Matfin, G. (2009). *Pathophysiology: Concepts of altered health states.* Philadelphia: Wolters Kluwer/Lippincott Williams & Wilkins.

Ramundo, J. (2007). Wound debridement. In R. Bryant & D. Nix (Eds.), *Acute and chronic wounds: Current management concepts* (3rd ed.). Philadelphia, PA: Mosby/Elsevier.

Reddy, M., Holroyd-Leduc, J., Cheung, C., & Woo, K. (2007). Geriatric principles in the practice of chronic wound care. In D. Krasner, G. Rodeheaver, & R. G. Sibbald (Eds.), *Chronic wound care: A clinical source book for healthcare professionals* (4th ed.). Malvern, PA: HMP Communications.

Rolstad, B., & Ovington, L. (2007). Principles of wound management. In R. Bryant & D. Nix (Eds.), *Acute and chronic wounds: Current management concepts* (3rd ed.). Philadelphia, PA: Mosby/Elsevier.

Ryan, S., & Sargeant, R. (2007). Uncommon ulcers. In D. Krasner, G. Rodeheaver, & R. G. Sibbald (Eds.), *Chronic wound care: A clinical source book for healthcare professionals* (4th ed.). Malvern, PA: HMP Communications.

Schultz, G. (2007). Molecular regulation of wound healing. In R. Bryant & D. Nix (Eds.), *Acute and chronic wounds: Current management concepts* (3rd ed.). Philadelphia, PA: Mosby/Elsevier.

Steed, D. (2007). Wounds in peoples with diabetes: Assessment, classification and management. In D. Krasner, G. Rodeheaver, & R. G. Sibbald (Eds.), *Chronic wound care: A clinical source book for healthcare professionals* (4th ed.). Malvern, PA: HMP Communications.

Stotts, N. (2007). Wound infection: Diagnosis and management. In R. Bryant & D. Nix (Eds.), *Acute and chronic wounds: Current management concepts* (3rd ed.). Philadelphia, PA: Mosby/Elsevier.

Undersea & Hyperbaric Medical Society. (2007). Indications for hyperbaric oxygen therapy. Retrieved from http://www.uhms.org/Default.aspx?tabid=270

Vermeulen, H., van Hattem, J. M., Storm-Versloot, M. N., Ubbink, D. T., & Westerbos, S. J. (2010). Topical silver for treating infected wounds. Cochrane Library. Retrieved from http://www.thecochranelibrary.com

Winter, G. D. (1962). Formation of scab and the rate of epithelialization of superficial wounds in the skin of the young domestic pig. *Nature, 193,* 293–294.

Wollina, U. (2007). Pyoderma gangrenosum—a review. *Orphanet Journal of Rare Diseases, 2*(19).

CHAPTER 61

Caring for the Patient with Burn Injuries

Len Sterling
Cheryl Wraa

Outcome-Based Learning Objectives

After studying this chapter, the learner will be able to:

1. Differentiate between the three classifications of burn injury: mild, moderate, and major.
2. Critique the causes, incidence, prevalence, types, and prevention of burn injuries.
3. Compare and contrast the pathophysiological response of burn injury at the tissue and organ levels.
4. Differentiate the three phases of burn care.
5. Discuss the significance and components of burn severity assessment, including size and depth of injury, impact of patient's age on injury, part of the body burned, and past medical history.
6. Generate a comprehensive burn treatment plan for each of the three phases of burn care, including fluid resuscitation, pain management, wound care, surgical management, contracture prevention, nutritional needs, and emotional adjustment.
7. Evaluate the discharge teaching needed to facilitate an optimal recovery and return to society.

KEY TERMS

allograft p.1949
autografting p.1949
biologic dressing p.1949
biosynthetic dressing p.1949
chemical burns p.1926
donor site p.1949
eschar p.1933
escharotomies p.1947
full-thickness injury p.1927
full-thickness skin graft p.1951
heterografts p.1949
hypertrophic scar p.1955
inhalation injury p.1926
keloid scar p.1955
Lund-Browder formula p.1934
meshed skin graft p.1951
partial-thickness injury p.1927
radiation burns p.1926
rule of nines p.1934
scald burns p.1925
sheet skin grafts p.1952
split-thickness skin graft p.1951
synthetic dressing p.1950
thermal burns p.1925
zone of coagulation p.1927
zone of hyperemia p.1929
zone of stasis p.1927

BURN INJURIES are traumatic, sometimes dehumanizing injuries that can be fatal, disfiguring, and incapacitating. Burns cause a loss of skin integrity that ranges from a minor superficial injury to a deep full-thickness injury that can extend into the underlying structures and organs. Burns are classified as minor, moderate, or major. All three categories of injury may cause a systemic response, but the deeper and more extensive the injuries are, the greater and more serious the systemic reaction becomes.

Epidemiology

In the United States, fires and burn injuries are the third-leading cause of fatal home injury, after falls and accidental poisoning. The U.S. mortality rate from fires ranks eighth among developed countries (Centers for Disease Control [CDC], 2011a). According to the American Burn Association (ABA), 1.1 million burn injuries require medical attention each year in the United States, and approximately 45,000 of these individuals require hospitalization, including 25,000 in hospitals designated as burn centers (ABA, 2011). Approximately 4,500 people in the United States die each year from burn injuries, and up to 10,000 die of burn-related infections. Pneumonia is the most common infection among hospitalized patients with burns (Murray, 2008).

Most fire-related deaths occur in the home. Cigarettes are a leading cause of fatal home fires. Between 900 and 1,000 people die annually in the United States from fires started by cigarettes, and an additional 2,500 to 3,000 are injured. The cost of human life and property damage is in the billions of dollars each year from cigarette-related fires (CDC, 2011a).

Early excision and grafting, advances in critical care, aggressive resuscitation, control of infection and support of the hypermetabolic response have contributed to a decrease in morbidity and mortality (Williams, Herndon, Hawkins, et al., 2009). These advances are discussed later in this chapter.

High-risk populations have been identified, as listed in the Risk Factors box. The mortality rates for burns are highest in the very

RISK FACTORS for Burn Injuries

Population	Risk	
Older adults	Clothing catching fire while cooking or smoking Living in apartments above the first floor	
Infants and children	Matches and cigarette lighters Electrical outlets Scald injuries Kitchen stoves Chemicals	Sun exposure Clothing Microwave ovens Fireplaces Fireworks
Young adults	Motor vehicle crashes Sun exposure Fireworks	Stun guns Methamphetamine laboratories Taser
Firefighters	Exposure to all types of fires while in the line of duty	

young and in the older population. Reasons for this are discussed later in this chapter.

Etiology

Burn injuries occur when there is direct or indirect contact with a heat source. No matter what the causative factor, burn injury results in a loss of skin integrity. Depending on the cause and extent of the injury, there can be both localized and systemic tissue damage, which are discussed later in the chapter. The National Guidelines box describes the ABA classification of burn injury.

Types of Burn Injury

Burns occur as a result of exposure to fire; direct contact with electricity, radiation, or chemicals; and scalds. It is important to know how the patient was burned because each type of burn injury has unique treatments, morbidity and mortality statistics, and sequelae. Chart 61–1 outlines the various types of injury and the associated causes.

Thermal Burns

Thermal burns occur when heat is transferred to the body from an external source. The depth of the injury is related to the length of exposure and the temperature of the heat source. These are discussed later in the section "Pathophysiology of Tissue Injury." Thermal burns from flames are the most common type of burn injury.

CHART 61–1 Causes of Burn Injuries

Type of Injury	Cause
Thermal	Flame, flash injuries (explosion), contact with hot metal and hot, sticky tar
Electrical	Contact with electrical current, sparks or electrical arcing, alternating current, direct current, high-voltage lines, and lightning
Radiation	Overexposure to sunlight, radiation treatment for cancer
Chemical	Contact with strong acids, alkalis, or an organic compound
Scalds	Steam, hot liquids
Inhalation	Exposure of upper airway to intense heat, flames, and smoke Exposure of lung parenchyma to chemicals, steam, or aspiration of hot liquids
Nuclear	Nuclear power plant accidents

Scald Burns

Scald burns are a type of thermal injury that occurs from contact with hot foods or liquids, including steam. The severity of the burn is related to the temperature of the hot liquid and the length of time it is in contact with the body. At 120°F (48°C), skin requires 5 minutes of contact for a full-thickness burn to occur. When the temperature of the liquid is 140°F (60°C), it takes only 5 seconds or less to cause a serious burn. Coffee, tea, and other hot drinks are usually served at 160° to 180°F (71° to 82°C).

Electrical Burns

Electrical burns tend to be deeper than most burn injuries. The depth and severity of the injury depend on the amount of voltage, the length of exposure, the type of current, the pathway of flow, and the local tissue resistance. It is difficult to assess the extent of damage accurately for two reasons. First, much of the damage occurs internally because the electrical current travels along the tendons and vessels as it flows through the body, creating deep wounds that often extend into the subcutaneous tissue and muscle fascia (American College of Surgeons [ACS], 2008). Second, the destructive process that is initiated at the time of injury continues for weeks. At the time of contact, the electrical flow follows the path of least resistance through the body, which is typically along muscles, long bones, blood vessels, and nerves. The entry and exit sites

NATIONAL GUIDELINES for the Classification of Burn Injury

Minor Burn Injury	Moderate Burn Injury	Major Burn Injury
Excludes: Electrical injury Complicated injuries (multiple trauma) High-risk patients such as older adults and those with chronic illnesses.	Excludes: Electrical injury Inhalation injury Complicated injuries (multiple trauma) High-risk patients such as older adults and those with chronic illnesses.	Includes: All electrical injuries Inhalation injury Complicated injuries (multiple trauma) High-risk patients such as older adults and those with chronic illnesses
Includes: Partial-thickness injuries < 15% of total body surface area (TBSA) in adults Full-thickness injuries < 2% of TBSA not involving ears, eyes, face, hands, feet, and perineum	Includes: Partial-thickness injuries 15% to 25% of total body surface area in adults Full-thickness injuries 10% of TBSA not involving ears, eyes, face, hands, feet, and perineum	All burns involving ears, eyes, face, hands, feet, and perineum Partial-thickness injuries > 25% of TBSA in adults Full-thickness injuries 10% or greater of TBSA

Source: American Burn Association (ABA). (2011). Burn incidence and treatment in the United States: 2011 fact sheet. Retrieved from http://www.ameriburn.org/resources_factsheet.php.

Weblink: Burn Indicence and Treatment Weblink: Fire Deaths and Injuries

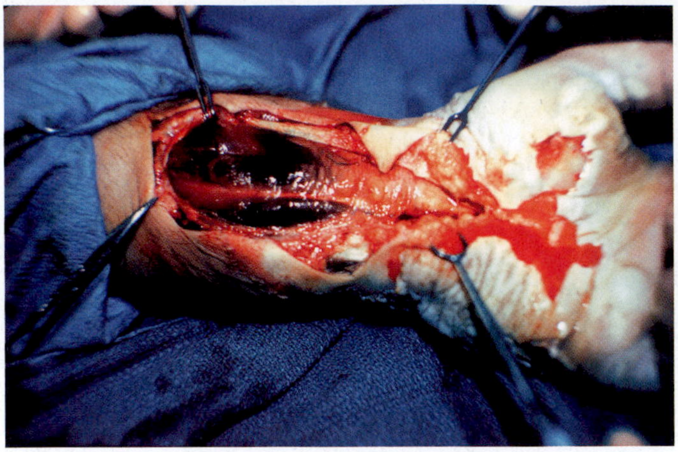

FIGURE 61–1 ◆ Black muscle from electrical injury.
Source: Courtesy of John M. Osborn, MD, FACS.

give a clue to how much damage has been sustained. For example, if the entry wound is in the hand and the exit is in the bottom of the foot, the current traveled through most of the major organs. If the entry was in the hand and the exit was in the shoulder, then just the arm sustained injury. Figure 61–1◆ depicts tissue damage from an electrical injury. The damage to the skin appears deceptively minor compared to the damage that is sustained by internal muscle, fat, and fascia along the path of electrical flow. When deep muscle injury has occurred, myoglobin is released into the circulation from the muscle tissue. It is transported to the kidneys, where it can block the renal tubules owing to its large size, causing acute tubular necrosis.

At the time of the injury, contact with the electrical current can cause tetanic muscle contractions, which can be strong enough to fracture long bones and vertebrae. These tetanic contractions also can occur in the respiratory and cardiac muscles, causing suffocation and disruption of the cardiac conduction system, resulting in dysrhythmias and cardiac arrest. Delayed neurological changes and cataract formation also may occur (Cushing, 2010).

Radiation Burns

Radiation burns usually result from overexposure to the sun or radiation treatment for cancer. Radiation injury also may occur from industrial accidents such as accidents at nuclear power plants. Tissue damage occurs from the transfer of radiant energy to the body, which stimulates reactions with body chemicals, resulting in cell death. The cells that are most susceptible to injury are those that divide rapidly, such as those of the bone marrow, skin, and the gastrointestinal tract. The depth of the injury depends on how close the person was to the source of radiation as well as the length of time of exposure. Typically, radiation injuries involve only the epithelial layer of skin (Bryant & Nix, 2012).

Chemical Burns

Chemical burns occur when the skin comes into contact with caustic chemical compounds such as strong acids, alkalis, or petroleum products. Alkalies penetrate more deeply than acids, increasing the severity of the burn (ACS, 2008). Common household chemicals that can cause burns include bleach, boric acid, creosote, paint thinner, and plumbing decloggers such as Drano or Liquid-Plumr. The depth of the injury from a chemical is directly related to the length of exposure. Brushing away any dry powder and then liberally washing the skin and removing clothing and jewelry as quickly as possible will limit the depth of the injury. Emergency treatment of chemical burns is discussed later in this chapter.

Inhalation Injury

Inhaling smoke causes injury to the lungs, referred to as **inhalation injury.** Inhalation injuries are most often associated with burns sustained in a closed space and can be present in the absence of cutaneous injury. Injuries resulting from inhalation of heated air and smoke present a unique set of problems, one of which is difficulty in diagnosing the full extent of the injury. A set of criteria is used to evaluate for the presence of an inhalation injury. The criteria include that the injury occurred in an enclosed area; there are burns of the face and neck; and there are singed nasal hairs, a hoarse, dry cough, bloody/sooty sputum, and labored respirations. Additionally, there may be edema, blisters, and ulcerations along the mucosal lining of the oropharynx and larynx. The edema continues to increase for 24 to 48 hours after the injury; therefore, close monitoring for pulmonary complications, including acute respiratory distress syndrome (Chapter 28), is essential. Inhalation injuries, not surface burns, are the leading cause of fire-related deaths (Urden, 2009). When combined with cutaneous injuries, smoke inhalation injuries increase the mortality rate by 77% (Mandel & Hales, 2008).

Nursing care in cases of inhalation injury includes vigorous pulmonary toilet, continuous monitoring of oxygen saturation levels, daily chest x-rays, and an early assessment of the need for intubation and mechanical ventilation. Respiratory distress may or may not develop, but assessing for evidence of it needs to continue throughout treatment. Because of the edema from the injury, ongoing assessment for airway obstruction is essential. Signs of airway obstruction include the following:

- Stridor
- Use of accessory muscles
- Respiratory distress
- Hypoxia
- Deep burns of the face and neck
- Blister or edema of the oropharynx. (Mandel & Hales, 2008)

Safety Alert *Continuous monitoring of arterial blood gases (ABGs) is necessary to assess the need for intubation and ventilatory support. Have necessary supplies ready for emergent intubation with inhalation injuries.*

Health Promotion

The decline in burn injuries in the United States is due in part to increased focus on injury prevention. Education programs have been established to increase knowledge of burn prevention, and firefighters and health care workers teach burn prevention to various populations in multiple settings. These programs include teaching children and the adults caring for them that if clothing catches fire, the person needs to "stop, drop, and roll," as this will assist in putting the flames out. Wrapping the victim in a blanket, coat, or sheet also will help extinguish the flames because this cuts off the oxygen needed to sustain the flame. Applying copious amounts of cool water immediately after the injury helps decrease the severity of the burn. The older adult population is the most susceptible to burns caused by clothing catching fire while cooking or smoking; therefore, education programs about burn prevention also need to target this population.

The nurse is in a pivotal position to collaborate with professionals in other disciplines to develop prevention programs in local communities. Most fires are started in the home through ignorance or carelessness. Children playing with matches and cigarette lighters account for approximately 35% of all burn injuries (Lucile Packard Children's Hospital at Stanford, 2008). Prevention education focuses on keeping children safe by keeping matches and lighters out of reach. Parents also need to be taught that uncovered electrical outlets in homes pose a threat to small children. Plastic plugs need to be inserted into every outlet that is within reach of a child.

Prevention of Scald Injuries

Scald burns from hot tap water are totally preventable. The ABA recommends the following simple safety tips to decrease the risk of scald burns:

- Set home water heaters no higher than 120°F.
- Provide constant adult supervision of young children or other individuals who may have difficulty removing themselves from hot water on their own.
- Fill the bathtub to the desired level before getting in. Run cold water first, then hot.
- Mix tub water thoroughly and check the temperature with an elbow before getting in the water or placing a child in the water.
- Install antiscald temperature devices that stop or interrupt the flow of water when the temperature reaches a predetermined level.
- Cook on back burners when children are present.
- Keep children out of cooking areas when hot food or liquids are being transported.
- Place hot items in the center of the table during mealtime.
- Never drink or carry hot liquids while carrying a child.

Prevention of Chemical Burn Injuries

The focus of chemical burn prevention is twofold: keeping chemicals in a safe place and knowing how to neutralize chemicals when contact occurs. All home chemicals need to be locked away from children. If contact occurs, copious amounts of water irrigation will decrease the severity of the burn.

Prevention of Radiation Injuries

Radiation burns typically are not deep injuries, but repeated exposure increases the risk of skin cancer. The goal for the prevention of radiation burns related to sun exposure is to educate the public to limit exposure to sun, wear protective clothing and sunscreen when exposed to the sun, and avoid the use of artificial sources of ultraviolet light (tanning booths, sunlamps, and tanning beds). The amount of protection offered by a sunscreen is referred to as the sun protection factor (SPF). The higher the SPF number, the greater the protection. Protection from the sun offered by sunscreens may be classified as follows:

- Minimal: SPF 2 to 11
- Moderate: SPF 12 through 29
- High: SPF 30+. (Some sunscreens claim SPFs higher than 30, but the added protection at such higher levels is insignificant.) (CDC, 2011c)

In the industrial setting, the most effective means of preventing exposure to radiation is proper maintenance of equipment, education of employees who work near equipment, and regularly scheduled safety checks.

Smoke Detectors

Approximately three-fifths of burn injuries occur in homes where there are no smoke detectors or the smoke detectors aren't functioning; therefore, prevention education has focused on installation and periodic checking of smoke detectors. The CDC gives funding to 16 state health departments to provide the Smoke Alarm Installation and Fire Safety Education (SAIFE) program. The program uses local fire department contractors to canvass neighborhoods, install long-lasting lithium-battery-powered smoke alarms in high-risk homes, and provide general fire safety education and a 6-month battery checkup (CDC, 2011b). Additionally, most cities in the United States have fire departments that will install smoke detectors free of charge for older adults.

One goal of the Federal Emergency Management Agency (FEMA) is to decrease the number of residential fire deaths by increasing awareness of hazards in the home and the need for smoke detectors and a fire extinguisher. The National Guidelines box (p. 1928) outlines the national guidelines for fire prevention set forth by FEMA.

National Legislation

The government's role in fire prevention is multifaceted. Passing laws aimed at fire prevention is only a beginning. Then laws such as those requiring public buildings to have protective measures in place such as fire-retardant fabrics, proper egress routes, smoke detectors, and sprinkler systems must be enforced. The government must also enforce laws requiring proper labeling of not only flammable products but also toxic chemicals and their antidotes.

See the National Guidelines box for guidelines for fire prevention.

Pathophysiology of Tissue Injury

Burn injuries are caused when tissue is exposed to thermal, electrical, radiation, or chemical energy. The tissue injury that results from these agents causes coagulation of cellular protein. The amount of tissue damage is related to the length of exposure, the temperature of the offending agent, and the thickness of the skin. As the temperature increases, cellular functions become impaired. Cell membranes are disrupted when exposed to temperatures between 40° and 44°C (104° and 110°F). Exposure of tissue to 60°C (140°F) for longer than 6 seconds will cause a **partial-thickness injury** (epidermis and part of the dermis). A **full-thickness injury** (epidermis and dermis) will occur with temperatures greater than 70°C (158°F) for 2 seconds (Consumer Product Safety Commission, 2011). Full-thickness injury and partial-thickness injury are described later in this chapter.

Tissue Injury

When thermal damage occurs on the skin surface, three distinct zones of injury are created. These zones relate to the level of damage in a given area. The center of the wound, referred to as the **zone of coagulation,** is the area where the tissue sustains the greatest amount of injury. If all the layers of the skin have been destroyed, this area contains denatured protein and coagulated nonfunctioning blood vessels. The tissue appears white or pearly gray and has a leatherlike texture. Because nerve endings have been destroyed, there is no sensation in this area. If not all the layers of the skin are destroyed, the zone of coagulation appears red and is very painful. With both types of injury, there is edema formation in the surrounding area because of the release of vasoactive mediators such as histamines, serotonin, interleukin-1, and prostaglandins from the injured cells (Howard & Steinmann, 2009). An in-depth discussion of the effect of vasoactive mediators is provided in Chapter 54.

Surrounding the zone of coagulation is an area of potentially viable but injured cells referred to as the **zone of stasis.** The microvasculature in this area is clogged with heat-injured erythrocytes. Vasoactive

NATIONAL GUIDELINES for Fire Prevention

Guideline	Prevention Measures
Smoke alarms	Working smoke alarms can double the chances of survival.
	Every home needs at least one smoke alarm.
	Test smoke alarms monthly and keep them free of dust. Replace the battery at least once a year.
	Smoke alarms themselves should be replaced after 10 years of service or as recommended by the manufacturer.
Electrical fires	Never overload circuits or extension cords. Do not place cords and wires under rugs, over nails, or in high-traffic areas.
	Immediately shut off and unplug appliances that sputter, spark, or emit an unusual smell.
	Have appliances professionally repaired or replaced.
Appliances	When using appliances, follow the manufacturer's safety precautions.
	Overheating, unusual smells, shorts, and sparks are all warning signs that appliances need to be shut off and then repaired or replaced.
	Unplug appliances when not in use.
	Use safety caps to cover all unused outlets, especially if there are small children in the home.
Alternative heaters	Portable heaters need their space. Keep anything combustible at least 3 feet away.
	Keep fire in the fireplace. Carefully dispose of ashes by placing them in a metal container, wet the ashes, and then cover with a lid.
	Use fire screens and have chimneys cleaned annually. The creosote buildup can ignite a chimney fire that could easily spread.
	Kerosene heaters should be used only where approved by authorities and must have proper ventilation to replace the oxygen consumed by the burning kerosene.
	Never use gasoline or camp stove fuel.
	Refuel kerosene heaters outside and only after the heater has cooled.
Affordable home fire safety sprinklers	When home fire sprinklers are used with working smoke alarms, the chances of surviving a fire are greatly increased.
	Sprinklers are affordable and can increase property values and lower insurance rates.
Escape plan	Practice an escape plan from every room in the house.
	Caution everyone to stay low to the floor when escaping from fire and never to open doors that are hot.
	Select a location where everyone can meet after escaping the house.
	Keep window escape ladders on any floor above the main level.
	Get out and then call for help.
Caring for children	Children under age 5 are naturally curious about fire. Many play with matches and lighters. Children set over 20,000 house fires every year.
	Take the mystery out of fire play by teaching children that fire is a tool, not a toy.
	Check labels on clothing for young children to ensure that the fabrics are fire retardant.
Caring for older people	Every year more than 1,200 senior citizens die in fires. Many of these fire deaths could have been prevented.
	Seniors are especially vulnerable because many live alone and cannot respond quickly in an emergency.
Smoking precautions	Careless smoking is the leading cause of fire deaths and the second-leading cause of injuries among people age 65 and older.
	When not properly extinguished, cigarettes continue to burn.
	When a resting cigarette is accidentally knocked over, it can smolder for hours before a flare-up occurs.
	Put a cigarette or cigar out at the first sign of feeling drowsy while watching television or reading.
	Use deep ashtrays and put the cigarette all the way out.
	Never smoke in bed.
	Do not walk away from lit cigarettes or other smoking materials.
	Do not put ashtrays on the arms of sofas or chairs.

Source: U.S. Fire Administration. (2011). Fire safety. Retrieved from: http://m.usfa.fema.gov/mobile/safety/index.shtm.

mediators from these injured cells cause edema formation, further impairing blood flow to the area. This decrease in blood flow continues for approximately 16 to 24 hours after the injury. Survival and recovery of the cells in the zone of stasis depend on prompt and appropriate wound care, edema control, and systemic fluid resuscitation. These interventions decrease the incidence of cellular dehydration, ischemia, and infection. If prompt measures are not instituted, these extremely vulnerable cells die and become part of the zone of coagulation. The tissue in this area initially appears moist and red, blanching with pressure because of the presence of viable capillaries.

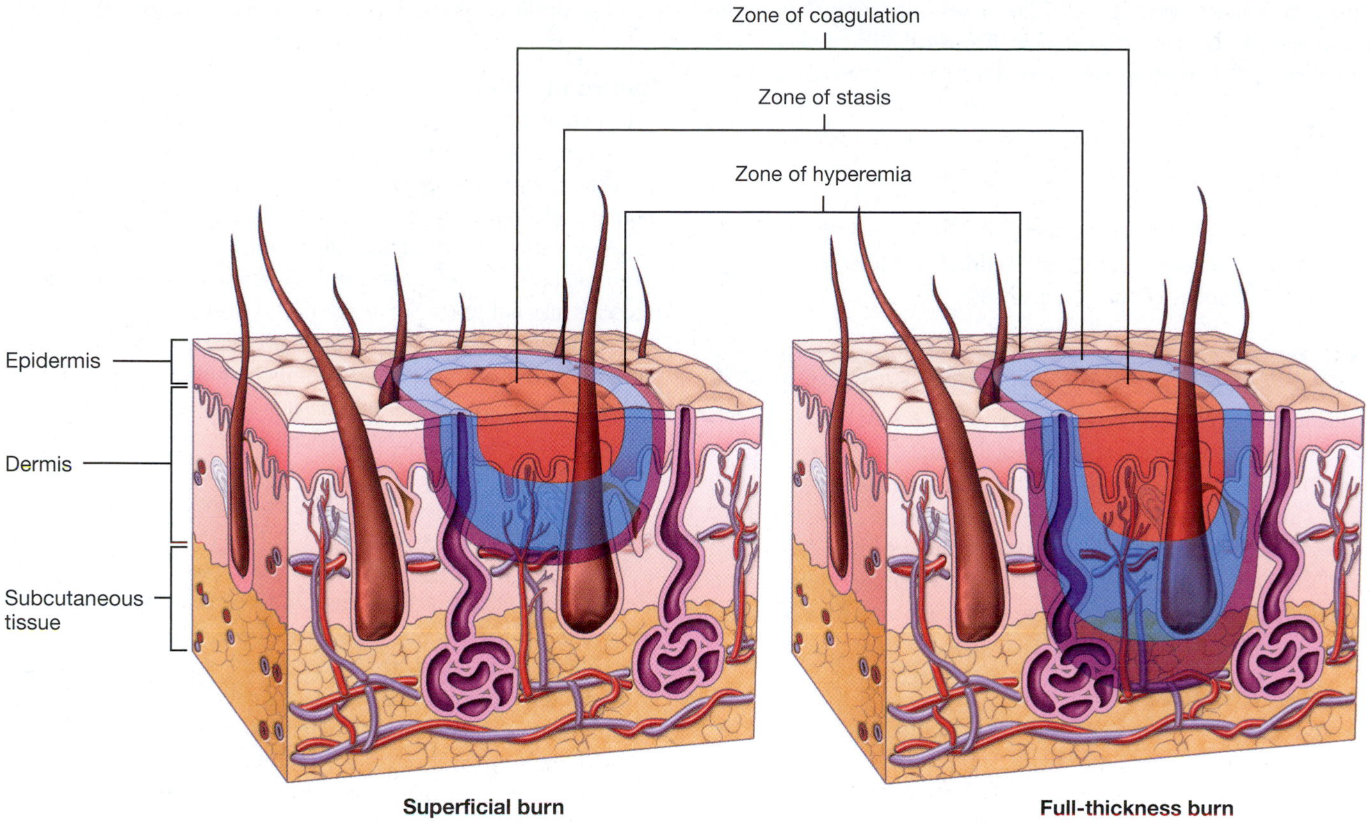

FIGURE 61–2 ◆ Three zones of injury.

In the outermost portion of the injured area, there is minor cell damage; this area is referred to as the **zone of hyperemia.** Once again, because of vasoactive mediators, there is prominent blood flow to this area. This blood contains the nutrients needed to support the zone of stasis, and it contains the necessary mediators to continue the inflammatory process within the zones of stasis and coagulation. Like the zone of stasis, the zone of hyperemia has viable capillaries and therefore will blanch with pressure (Howard & Steinmann, 2009). Tissue in this area appears pink and moist. Complete healing of this area is expected unless there is additional insult such as infection or profound tissue inflammation (Figure 61–2◆).

Systemic Injury

Burn injuries, depending on their size and depth, have the potential to affect every organ system in the body. Immediately after a burn injury, fluid begins to shift from the intracellular and intravascular compartment into the interstitial space. This is commonly referred to as *third spacing* of fluid. If left untreated, it will lead to burn shock. Additionally, edema develops in unburned tissues and organs distant from the site of injury when the burn size exceeds 20% to 25% of the total body surface area (TBSA) (Pham, Cancio, & Gibran, 2008). Burn shock is the pathophysiological mechanism that underlies most of the systemic effects of a burn injury on the tissues and organs of the body. Burn shock occurs because of a loss of intravascular fluid and, thus, circulating blood volume. This loss of fluid occurs for two reasons: (1) Fluid is lost to the environment through the wound (insensible loss), and (2) fluid is lost due to movement from the intravascular space into the interstitial space (Pham et al., 2008).

Pathophysiologically, what is occurring is that at the time of the injury, an excessive amount of the Hageman factor (factor XII) is released, which initiates and activates the inflammatory cascade (Porth & Matfin, 2009). Proinflammatory mediators such as histamines, arachidonic acid metabolites, prostaglandins, bradykinin, and catecholamines are released from the injured tissue (Porth & Matfin, 2009; Pham et al., 2008). These mediators cause arteriolar and venular dilation, which results in increased capillary permeability and, thus, leaking of fluid, electrolytes, and protein out of the intravascular space into the interstitial space, causing interstitial edema. This leaking is due to changes in the osmotic pressure within the injured tissue. Because of oncotic changes, fluid moves with the protein that is leaving the vascular space, further increasing the edema formation in the wound. The outcome is a dramatic outpouring of fluids, electrolytes, and proteins into the third space, resulting in a decrease in circulating blood volume and consequently decreased cardiac output. The development of shock is due to loss of the circulating blood volume, causing an intravascular hypovolemic state. The end result is decreased amounts of oxygen and nutrients being delivered to the tissues.

Both localized edema and systemic edema occur because of the fluid shifts. This process of fluid movement begins at the time of injury and peaks 12 to 24 hours after the injury; it will continue for 48 to 72 hours until the vascular permeability is at least partially reestablished and the leaking ceases.

The edema formation that occurs during burn shock impairs peripheral circulation and results in necrosis of the underlying tissues. Therefore, treatment during this initial period of fluid shifting focuses on aggressive fluid resuscitation for the hypovolemia, maintaining normal oxygen levels, and blocking the mediators to decrease the edema formation. These treatments will help prevent the conversion of the zone of stasis to the zone of coagulation. Because fluid continues to leak even after capillary integrity is restored, fluid resuscitation continues to be monitored closely.

What is unique to the patient with burn injuries is that very little fluid leaves the body. Therefore, when the fluid stops leaking and begins to return to the vascular space, a marked increase in the intravascular volume occurs. When this process begins, fluid resuscitation needs to be adjusted so as not to cause fluid overload. Fluid resuscitation and monitoring are discussed later in this chapter.

Organ Injury

Virtually all systems in the body are affected in a major burn injury because the mediators leave the confines of the local tissue injury through the circulation and travel to remote organs, causing injury (Pham et al., 2008). Under normal conditions, these mediators are efficient and immune protective, but in the case of major trauma such as burn injury, they become poorly regulated, causing overwhelming inflammation and coagulation. Fibrinolysis can ensue and can constantly be reactivated (Porth & Matfin, 2009).

Cardiac Response

The initial hypovolemic state of burn shock significantly alters cardiovascular function when burns involve more than 40% of the TBSA. One reason for this alteration is the loss of circulating blood volume, which decreases cardiac output and results in a loss of nutrients and oxygen delivered to the tissues. The second mechanism that affects cardiac output is stimulation of the sympathetic nervous system (flight or fight), which causes the release of catecholamines (epinephrine and norepinephrine). These catecholamines cause vasoconstriction and an increase in systemic vascular resistance, which increases cardiac workload. Release of tumor necrosis factor, an inflammatory mediator, has a significant negative inotropic effect, causing myocardial depression. The effect of this mediator goes on even after adequate fluid resuscitation (Porth & Matfin, 2009). Because of these combined effects, heart failure is a major risk factor in attempting to achieve homeostasis in the early phase of burn care. This is especially true in the older population.

The cardiac conduction system also may be affected by increased serum potassium levels. Cell damage causes the release of intracellular potassium, which may cause hyperkalemia. Increased levels of potassium cause changes in the myocardial action potential, resulting in abnormalities in the cardiac conduction system. These abnormalities increase the risk of ventricular dysrhythmias and cardiac arrest. The Diagnostic Tests box describes the laboratory and diagnostic tests and the initial and later abnormalities associated with burn injuries.

Pulmonary Response

Increased pulmonary vascular resistance created by the release of the mediators, such as serotonin, impacts pulmonary function, even in the absence of inhalation injury. This increased resistance also is compounded by the increase in systemic vascular resistance. Pulmonary edema, therefore, occurs because of increased capillary pressure combined with the vasoconstriction of the microcirculation. If left-sided heart failure also is present, this further increases capillary pressure and affects oxygen exchange.

In summary, both the heart and lungs are affected by the proinflammatory mediators on a microvascular level. These changes are marked by a loss of fluid volume, increased vascular resistance, and finally a decreased cardiac output (Pham et al., 2008).

Gastrointestinal Response

With activation of the sympathetic nervous system, there is an increase in circulating catecholamines, which causes blood to be shunted away from the gastrointestinal (GI) organs. This results in decreased gut motility and absorption of nutrients. When a burn injury occurs, there is a subsequent increase in metabolism, which can rapidly deplete body stores. With the loss of motility, which is referred to as a *paralytic ileus*, nutrients may not progress through the GI tract and be absorbed. This lack of motility leads to gastric distention, nausea, and vomiting. A paralytic ileus is an indication to withhold administration of enteral feedings, further compromising the nutritional state. There is some evidence that early administration of enteral feedings actually decreases the incidence of paralytic ileus and helps maintain mucosal integrity (Khorasani, 2010). This issue of whether or not to administer enteral feedings remains a topic of research.

Blood flow to the GI tract immediately after burn injury also is affected by the release of angiotensin II, a potent vasoconstrictor. This substance, which is released in response to low systemic fluid volume, has a direct vasoconstrictive effect on the splanchnic vasculature smooth muscle, causing ischemia to the gut (Khorasani, 2010). This ischemia causes intestinal mucosal atrophy and an increased permeability of the mucosa molecules. Bacteria that are normal in the GI tract are held there by the mucosa. In burn injuries and burn wound sepsis, GI mucosal atrophy causes movement of intraluminal bacteria to extraluminal sites, referred to as *bacterial translocation*, which fosters sepsis (Lawrence, 2011). Glutamine, a dietary supplement, has been demonstrated to partially reverse gut atrophy and integrity. Glutamine administration decreases the incidence of gram-negative bacteremia and improves mortality rates (Cochran, 2010). Early enteral feedings appear to prevent or at least slow down mucosal atrophy (Cochran, 2010).

Patients with severe burn injuries experience stress gastritis within 72 hours. Gastrointestinal (GI) erosions occur within 5 hours of injury in 80% of all patients with severe burns. These erosions cause only minor upper GI bleeding, but within 72 hours, this minor bleeding may progress to frank GI ulcerations (Curling's ulcer), resulting in major hemorrhage. This sequence of events is frequently seen in patients when no ulcer prophylaxis (either antacids or H_2-receptor antagonists) was used (Anand, 2011).

Renal Response

The hypovolemia that occurs as a result of fluid shifts causes a decrease in renal blood flow and filtration rates. Therefore, abnormal increases in renal function studies (blood urea nitrogen [BUN] and creatinine), coupled with a marked decrease in urine output or no urine output, may be seen during the early resuscitation phase (see the Diagnostic Tests box). The kidney is able to recover if fluid resuscitation is initiated quickly and adequately.

After a major burn injury, the dead or damaged erythrocytes release large amounts of hemoglobin. If the burn extends deep enough to cause muscle injury, myoglobin also may be released into the bloodstream, as occurs with electrical injuries. Under normal circumstances, both of these substances are conjugated by haptoglobin and transferred to the liver. However, if large amounts are released at once, the liver is unable to handle the increased load, and these substances are excreted in the urine. Myoglobin and hemoglobin will damage the renal tubules and promote renal failure. There is a higher risk for renal failure when any of

DIAGNOSTIC TESTS for Burn Injuries

Test With Description, Rationale, and Normal Value	Initial Expected Abnormality	Later Expected Abnormality
Serum Potassium Level Normal: 3.4–5.3 mEq/L *Increased due to cell lysis and fluid shifts to extracellular spaces. Decreases with fluid resuscitation.*	Increased.	Decreased after burn shock; fluid shifts back to intracellular and intravascular spaces.
Serum Sodium Level Normal: 135–145 mEq/L *Changes due to dehydration and then with fluid shifts.*	Increased.	Normalizes with fluid replacement. Will decrease with repeated Hubbard tank treatments.
Serum Hematocrit (HCT) Normal: Male: 40–54% Female: 36–46% *Red blood cells are lost both directly in the burn and as a result of increased fragility. Circulating red blood cell mass becomes trapped and destroyed within the burn wound at the time of injury. Erythrocyte losses continue to occur for several days after the injury.*	For the first 12–48 hours after the burn injury, there is an increase in the hematocrit due to hemoconcentration related to intravascular fluid volume loss.	Decreased with adequate hydration due to cell destruction from injury. Once fluid balance has been reestablished, a lower and more accurate hematocrit reading occurs.
Serum Hemoglobin (Hgb) Normal: Male: 13.5–18 g/dL Female: 12–15 g/dL *Red blood cells are lost both directly in the burn and as a result of increased fragility. Circulating red blood cell mass becomes trapped and destroyed within the burn wound at the time of injury. Erythrocyte losses continue to occur for several days after the injury.*	Increased due to hemoconcentration.	Decreased with adequate hydration due to cell destruction from injury.
Platelets Normal: 150,000–400,000 uL *Dilution and consumption immediately after a burn injury cause an abnormal decrease both in the platelet count and in clotting factors. A large number of platelets may be utilized to stabilize the vasculature in and around the burned area.*	Decreased due to dilution and consumption.	Normal if bone marrow manufactures enough. May be increased in the presence of infection.
White Blood Cells (WBC) Normal: 4,500–10,000 uL *This increase is due to mobilization of preexisting stores. The decrease in the granulocyte level is due in part to the dilutional effects of fluid replacement therapy, and due to concentration in the injured areas.*	Granulocytes continue to increase for the first 24 hours after the injury, and then the count begins to fall.	Increased with infection and decreased in immunodeficient states.
Creatinine/Blood Urea Nitrogen (BUN) Normal: Creatinine: 0.5–1.5 mg/dL BUN: 5–25 mg/dL *Increases seen with electrical burns where extensive tissue damage is suspected.*	Normal to increased, depending on fluid replacement.	Low if malnourished. Increased in presence of renal insufficiency.
Serum Blood Glucose; Nondiabetic Normal: 70–110 mg/dL *Due to stress response and changes that occur with fluid resuscitation and type of nutritional replacement.*	Increased.	Increased or decreased depending on nutritional replacement.
Total Protein Normal: 6–8 g/dL *Fluid shifts cause a decrease, and nutritional replacement will increase it.*	Decreased.	Increased or decreased, depending on nutritional status.

(*continued*)

DIAGNOSTIC TESTS for Burn Injuries, *continued*

Test With Description, Rationale, and Normal Value	Initial Expected Abnormality	Later Expected Abnormality
Prealbumin Normal: 3.5–5 g/dL *Massive inflammation causes a decrease, and nutritional replacement will increase it.*	Decreased.	Increased or decreased, depending on nutritional status.
Creatine Kinase (CK) Level Normal: 0–250 U/L *Electrical burns due to extensive tissue damage.*	Elevated.	Returns to normal after 48 hours.
Urine Specific Gravity Normal: 1.005–1.030 *Dehydration.*	Elevated.	Decreased to normal levels with rehydration.

the following are also present: dehydration, acidosis, massive presence of necrotic tissues after third- and fourth-degree electrical and chemical burns, hypercatabolic state (an abnormally increased rate of metabolic breakdown of substances), and/or shock.

Immune Response

The three major functions of the normal mature immune system are defense, homeostasis, and surveillance. The defense function provides the body with the ability to fight infection, while the homeostatic function controls the activities of the defense system; the surveillance function recognizes foreign materials.

A burn injury destroys the body's first line of defense, the skin. As discussed earlier, burn injuries trigger the inflammatory response, causing the release of proinflammatory mediators, which induce localized vasodilation and increased capillary permeability. As a result, venous stasis and microthrombi occur at the injury site. The hypovolemia that occurs immediately after a burn injury causes an increase in blood viscosity, which results in sluggish blood flow to the wound bed. This results in a decreased delivery of oxygen, antibodies, and nutrients, retarding wound healing and increasing the risk of infection. A second manifestation of proinflammatory mediators, such as tumor necrosis factor and interleukin, is impairment of the function of lymphocytes, macrophages, and neutrophils, causing a decreased ability to fight infection. See Chapter 52 for a complete description of the immune system.

The protein that is lost owing to third spacing from capillary leaking impairs both the cell-mediated and humoral immune systems. The humoral immune response needs B cells to produce antibodies and immunoglobulins. In the patient with burn injuries, the serum levels of immunoglobulins are decreased, therefore diminishing the normal immune response. A decrease in the production of T cells negatively affects cell-mediated cytotoxic activity. The decreased function of both cell-mediated and humoral immune responses creates a state of immunodeficiency and increases the risk of developing opportunistic infections and death despite aggressive antimicrobial therapy.

A final insult to the immune system may occur because of the relationship between nutrition and immunocompetence. When the burn injury occurs, a hypermetabolic state is created, which places the victim at high risk for malnutrition (Pham et al., 2008). Without adequate calories, proteins, and trace elements, there is a decrease in the function of the immune system, and therefore susceptibility to infection increases.

Integumentary Response

The skin protects against infection, prevents loss of body heat, helps control body temperature, functions as an excretory organ (via the sweat glands), is a sensory organ, and produces vitamin D when sunlight reacts with cholesterol. Finally, the skin determines identity by its color and by its unique fingerprints. Burn injuries cause a transient and, in some cases, permanent loss of many of these functions. With partial-thickness injuries, enough of the substructures of the skin remain intact to regenerate function. However, with full-thickness injuries, many functions such as hair growth, perspiration (which is important in cooling body temperature), and sensory functions are permanently lost.

The overall thickness of the skin varies depending on the part of the body it covers. For example, the skin on the back tends to be thicker than the skin on the inner aspect of the arms. Therefore, similar temperatures produce different depths of injury depending on the part of the body burned.

Multisystem Dysfunction

In major burn injuries, proinflammatory mediators, such as cytokines, are released in a chaotic, repeatedly reactivated fashion. This causes continual reactivation of the inflammatory response, which in turn causes distant and multiorgan involvement, leading to dysfunction and possibly death (Pham et al., 2008; Porth & Matfin, 2009). Chapter 54 discusses in detail the sequence of events that causes multiorgan involvement and dysfunction.

Periods of Burn Injury Management

Three distinct periods of care for the acute burn injury have been identified: the emergency or resuscitative phase, the acute phase, and the rehabilitative phase. Each phase has different goals and priorities, although the stages tend to overlap. In order for the patient to have optimal physical and emotional healing, each stage of care requires a multidisciplinary team of health care providers with specialized training. The goals and treatments used in each phase are described next.

Emergency Phase

The emergency phase of burn care begins at the time of the injury and can last for 2 to 3 days. The goal during this phase is to resolve the immediate insult, which includes maintaining an airway and oxygen levels, treating concurrent injuries, correcting the fluid imbalance, preventing wound infection, conserving body heat, relieving pain, and providing emotional support.

Prehospital Care and Transport

The focus of treatment at the scene of the injury is first to ensure the safety of the rescuers and then to remove the victim from the burn source. An initial assessment is required to determine vital signs and the severity of the burn and other injuries. This assessment follows the ABCDEF format: A = airway, B = breathing, C = circulation, D = disability, neurological deficit, E = exposure and evaluation, and F = fluid resuscitation. Any smoldering clothing and restrictive jewelry must be removed to keep them from adding to the depth of the injury. Burn victims are unlikely to develop shock in the first 30 minutes; therefore, after airway stabilization, the patient can be transported to a local emergency department or directly to a burn center. If the patient is less than 60 minutes away from a hospital, the ABA recommends that intravenous line insertion is *not* done at the scene of the accident.

Application of a clean sheet to cover exposed skin may decrease the pain. Ice is *not* applied because it may cause further injury to the skin and exacerbate hypothermia.

Chemical burns require copious irrigation with water for at least 20 minutes at the time of injury to reduce the concentration of chemicals and, thus, the depth of the injury. If a dry chemical is still present on the skin, the nurse should brush away as much as possible before irrigating. It is important not to try to neutralize the chemical with other chemicals or neutralizers, since that process can generate more heat in the tissue. If the chemical is in the eyes, the caregiver must remove the contact lenses and irrigate the eyes with copious amounts of water. A minimum of 2 liters of fluid is used for each eye, and irrigation may be needed for several hours after the injury until the ocular pH returns to normal (ACS, 2008).

No oils or salves should be applied to any type of burn injury. If the patient has not had a tetanus toxoid injection in the last 5 years, it is administered early, often in the field. If the patient has never received tetanus or has not had a booster in the last 10 years, tetanus immunoglobulin is given. Because of a loss of skin integrity, the body temperature drops; therefore, the patient should be covered with clean, dry blankets before transfer.

Emergency Department Care

Once the patient reaches the emergency department (ED), a rapid and thorough initial assessment is done, beginning with the respiratory and cardiovascular systems. As always, the first priority is to assess the patency of the patient's airway and the adequacy of gas exchange. If the burns occurred on the face and neck, massive airway edema can cause airway obstruction and death. An assessment for heat or smoke inhalation is done emergently, as these agents can cause damage to the airways and lung parenchyma. The nasal passages and oral airway are assessed for soot. If respiratory distress is present and/or there are burns of the face and neck, nasotracheal or endotracheal intubation is indicated early, before swelling further compromises the airway (ACS, 2008). After intubation, the need for oxygen and ventilatory support is assessed and the support, if needed, is instituted. Ongoing monitoring of arterial blood gases (ABGs) and oxygen saturation levels determines the effectiveness of the interventions. The nurse is responsible for monitoring the patient's airway and assessing the adequacy of gas exchange. In-depth discussions of respiratory assessment, intubation, and mechanical ventilation are provided in Chapters 25 and 28.

An assessment of the cardiovascular system is essential because it provides information about fluid volume status and the potential for the development of shock. A 12-lead electrocardiogram (ECG) is necessary to detect myocardial ischemic changes and cardiac dysrhythmias, especially with electrical injuries. The carotid and peripheral pulses are assessed for rate and quality. The skin is inspected for color, sensation, and capillary refill. Finally, the blood pressure and apical pulse are assessed. Because of the progressive nature of fluid volume loss, these assessments must be performed by the nurse on a frequent and ongoing basis.

Concurrent with airway management and cardiovascular assessment, it is essential to place large-bore intravenous (IV) catheters. Most health care providers believe that shortening the time from injury to IV insertion and beginning of fluid resuscitation will decrease the mortality rate. The best insertion site is through nonburned tissue, if possible. If there is no nonburned area for intravenous access, then placement through burned tissue is necessary and justifiable, given the risk for the development of hypovolemic shock. This is done as early as possible and the patient is assessed closely for the development of compartment syndrome, especially if the burn is circumferential and there is **eschar** (nonviable dead tissue) present (Figure 61–3◆). Placement of an indwelling urinary catheter also is necessary, as urine output is considered the most reliable indicator of fluid status.

When there are burn injuries over more than 20% of the TBSA, the patient is prone to nausea and vomiting because of a loss of blood flow to the gastrointestinal tract, as discussed earlier in this chapter. Because of the risk of aspiration, oral fluids are withheld, and a nasogastric tube may be inserted to prevent abdominal distention, vomiting, and, ultimately, aspiration. The next priority during the emergency period is to assess for any concurrent injuries. Life-threatening injuries such as pneumothorax, spinal cord injuries, or acute brain injuries need to be stabilized and treated. More extensive treatment of concurrent injuries, such as surgery, is typically delayed if possible until the patient is hemodynamically stable.

The loss of skin integrity decreases the patient's ability to retain and maintain body heat. When body temperature decreases, shivering occurs as a compensatory mechanism to increase body heat. Shivering increases oxygen and metabolic needs and therefore must be avoided. Burn wounds are covered with dressings, blankets are applied, and the room temperature is elevated to increase and maintain body temperature.

Blood studies are obtained to provide baseline data and to assist in identifying preexisting conditions. For patients with burn

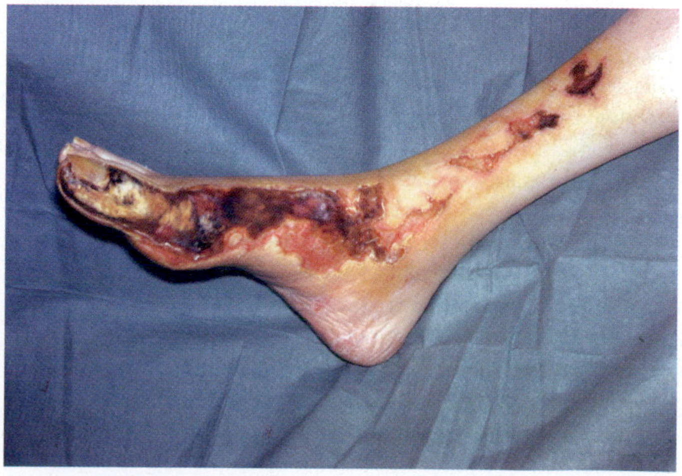

FIGURE 61–3 ◆ Eschar.

Source: Courtesy of John M. Osborn, MD, FACS.

injuries over 30% or more of the TBSA, the blood studies should include a complete blood count, serum electrolytes, blood glucose, blood urea nitrogen (BUN), serum creatinine, and coagulation studies. If substance abuse is suspected or if there is an altered level of consciousness in the absence of a head injury, a toxicology screen is indicated. If inhalation injury is suspected or the patient is in respiratory distress, ABGs and a chest x-ray are necessary. In electrical burns where extensive tissue damage is suspected, serum creatine kinase (CK), blood urea nitrogen, and creatinine levels should be evaluated, typically on an ongoing basis (see the Diagnostic Tests box, p. 1931). To diagnose any concurrent injuries, x-rays and scans need to be completed where indicated.

Burns can be life-threatening, disfiguring injuries that have a major emotional impact on both the patient and family. Thus, emotional support is essential in all stages of burn recovery and must begin in the emergency period.

Prevention of wound infection is a critical concern from the time of injury to final wound closure. Therefore, once the patient has been stabilized, the focus of care shifts to the assessment of burn size and depth. Burns are categorized as minor, moderate, or major (see the National Guidelines box on page 1925 for the ABA's classification of burn injury), and the health care provider determines whether the patient requires hospitalization.

Transfer of any patient, whether from the field or the ED, must be coordinated with the burn center health care provider. All pertinent information regarding injuries, hemodynamic status, fluid resuscitation, and treatments must be reported to the burn center staff.

The admission process begins with airway management, hemodynamic stabilization, and an assessment of the burn size and depth. After an in-depth assessment, a comprehensive treatment plan is instituted that provides the care needed to ensure optimal recovery. The nurse is pivotal in coordinating the admission process and the treatment plan.

Admission Assessment

The admission assessment of a patient following a burn injury needs to include the history of the event that caused the injury, the time the injury occurred, the causative agent and duration of exposure, where the injury occurred (e.g., enclosed space), any concurrent injuries, and any on-the-scene first aid treatments.

This assessment is vital because portions of the treatment plan depend on this information. For example, fluid resuscitation calculations are based on the time of the injury rather than the time of admission to the hospital. The causative agent is especially important with chemical injuries such as burns from strong acids or alkaline agents, which may require neutralization to stop the ongoing burning effect. If the injury occurred in an enclosed area, such as a house, there may be inhalation injuries that require special consideration and treatment. Concurrent injuries, such as fractures, often are associated with burns and require a treatment plan for stabilization. Finally, first aid treatments and home remedies applied before arrival at the hospital need to be documented and reported to the health care team.

Clinical Manifestations and Determinants of Burn Wound Severity

To treat a burn injury adequately, its severity must be evaluated by using the following five factors: the size of the injury, the depth of the injury, the age of the patient, past medical history, and the part of the body burned. Each of these factors affects the treatment plan as well as the morbidity and mortality for a given patient.

Burn Size

The estimate of burn size is expressed as a percent of total body surface area. Two common formulas are used to estimate percent of body burned. The first formula is the **rule of nines,** which divides the body into seven areas, each of which represents 9%, or multiples of 9%, of the TBSA. For an adult, the head and neck are 9%, the arms are 9% each, the lower extremities are 18% each, the trunk is a total of 36% (18% anterior, 18% posterior), and the perineum is 1%. Thus, the total = 100%. Age, growth, and development are factors in determining the distribution of the body surface area. Figure 61–4◆ outlines the rule of nines for both adults and children. The rule of nines is an easy-to-remember general estimate of body surface area and is considered adequate for the prehospital and emergency care periods.

The second formula is the **Lund-Browder formula** (Figure 61–5◆). This formula divides the body into smaller percentage areas and is considered more accurate, especially for infants and children. The formula determines surface area measurements for each body part according to the patient's age.

When a patient with burn injuries is admitted, the affected areas are shaded in on a chart using either the rule of nines or the Lund-Browder formula. The TBSA involved in the burn injury is then calculated. Most burn centers total the partial-thickness and full-thickness injuries separately. The totaled sum of body surface burned is used in calculating fluid resuscitation needs, as well as metabolic and immunologic responses. The TBSA also is a critical determinant of overall morbidity and mortality (Howard & Steinmann, 2009).

Burn Depth

The depth of a burn injury is an important predictor of morbidity and mortality, as well as of surgical management and functional and

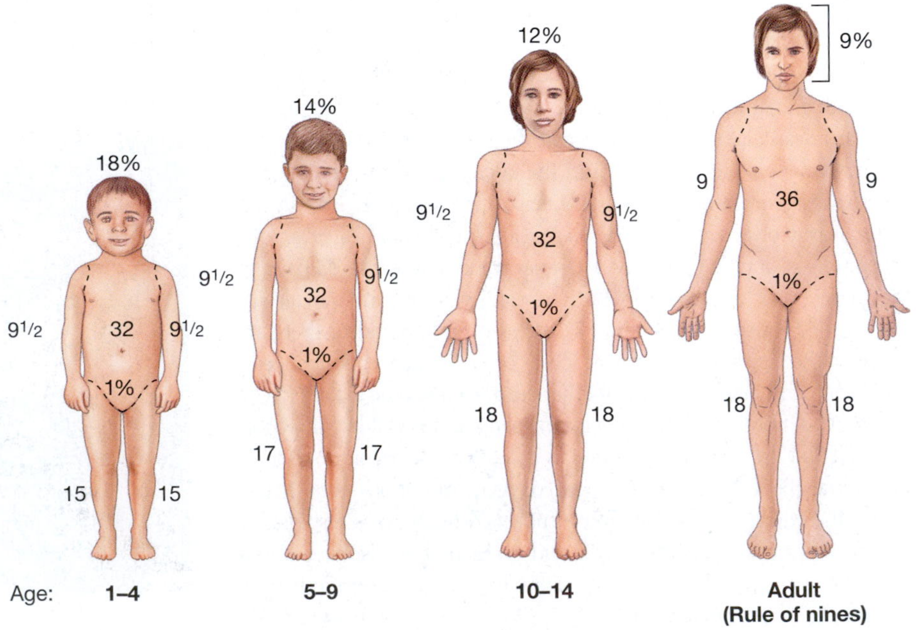

FIGURE 61–4 ◆ Rule of nines.

Area	Age (years)					% 1°	% 2°	% 3°	% Total
	0–1	1–4	5–9	10–15	Adult				
Head	19	17	13	10	7				
Neck	2	2	2	2	2				
Ant. trunk	13	13	13	13	13				
Post. trunk	13	13	13	13	13				
R. buttock	2½	2½	2½	2½	2½				
L. buttock	2½	2½	2½	2½	2½				
Genitalia	1	1	1	1	1				
R.U. arm	4	4	4	4	4				
L.U. arm	4	4	4	4	4				
R.L. arm	3	3	3	3	3				
L.L. arm	3	3	3	3	3				
R. hand	2½	2½	2½	2½	2½				
L. hand	2½	2½	2½	2½	2½				
R. thigh	5½	6½	8½	8½	9½				
L. thigh	5½	6½	8½	8½	9½				
R. leg	5	5	5½	6	7				
L. leg	5	5	5½	6	7				
R. foot	3½	3½	3½	3½	3½				
L. foot	3½	3½	3½	3½	3½				
					Total				

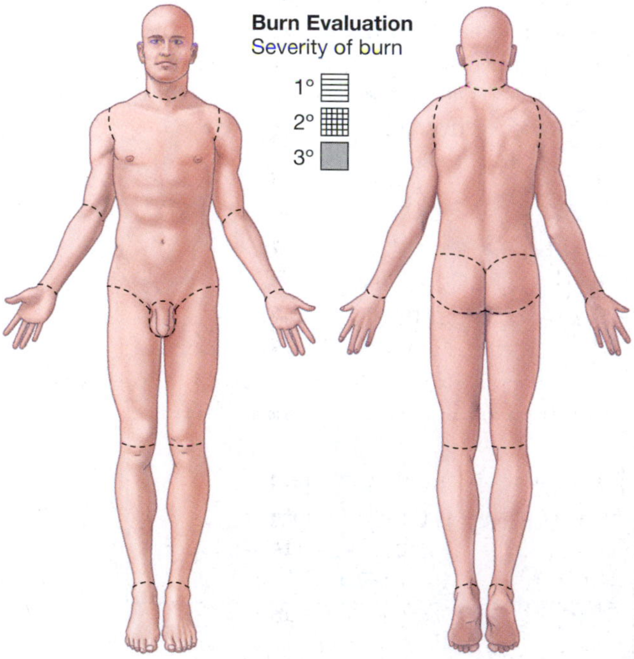

FIGURE 61–5 ◆ Lund-Browder formula.

cosmetic outcomes (Howard & Steinmann, 2009). A number of accepted terms are used to refer to the depth of the injury. Burn depth is expressed in terms of full thickness and partial thickness, and/or first, second, third, and fourth degrees. First- and second-degree burns are partial-thickness injuries, which result in partial destruction of the skin layers. However, enough epithelial cells, hair follicles, and sweat glands remain intact to provide a new epidermis.

Partial-thickness injuries involving only the superficial dermis (first degree) heal spontaneously in about 2 weeks and usually cause no cosmetic or functional impairment. Partial-thickness wounds involving the deep dermis (second degree) heal spontaneously but may require a prolonged period (greater than 21 days) to do so and may result in some scar or contracture (a permanent shortening of connective tissue) formation (Figure 61–6◆). Infection, trauma, and a decreased blood supply increase the risk of a partial-thickness injury converting to a full-thickness injury.

Full-thickness injuries (third degree) result in the destruction of all skin layers, and there may also be destruction of subcutaneous tissue, muscles, and bones (Figure 61–7◆, p. 1936). Some health care providers refer to burns that involve muscles and bones as fourth-degree injuries. Full-thickness burns have no sensation to pain on light touch because the pain and touch receptors have been destroyed. Closure of the wound occurs by granulation, epithelial migration, contracture, and/or surgical intervention. (See the discussion of wound care later in this chapter.) Figure 61–8◆ (p. 1936) demonstrates the difference in skin depth between a partial-thickness injury and a full-thickness injury.

The differential diagnosis of burn depth is based on the cause of the injury, the appearance of the wound, and the presence or absence of sensation in the area. Chart 61–2 (p. 1937) provides guidelines for helping to make the determination between partial-thickness and full-thickness injury.

An assessment of the pattern of the burn injury during the emergency period also is essential. If the injury is circumferential (involving the entire circumference of an area), there is an increased risk for diminished blood supply to the area distal to the injury. (See the discussion of treatment of circumferential injuries later in this chapter.)

Age

The very young (usually under 2 years of age) and the older adult have higher mortality rates than a young adult with the same percentage of burn injury. There are two specific reasons for increased mortality in the very young population. First, infants and young children have an immature immune system with a weak antibody response to infection; if seriously burned, they tend to die of septicemia. Second, the very young have a

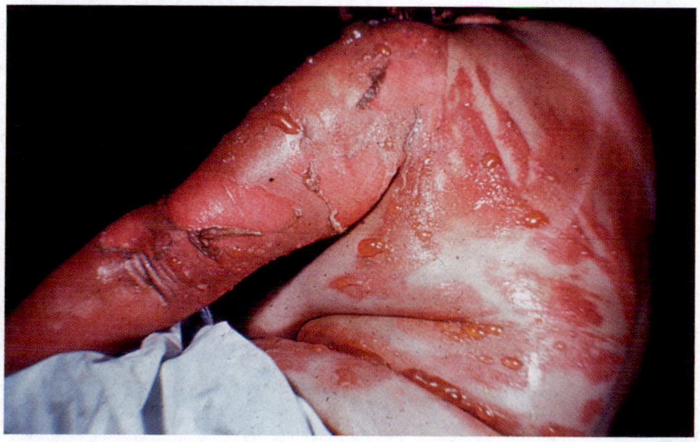

FIGURE 61–6 ◆ Partial-thickness injury.
Source: Courtesy of John M. Osborn, MD, FACS.

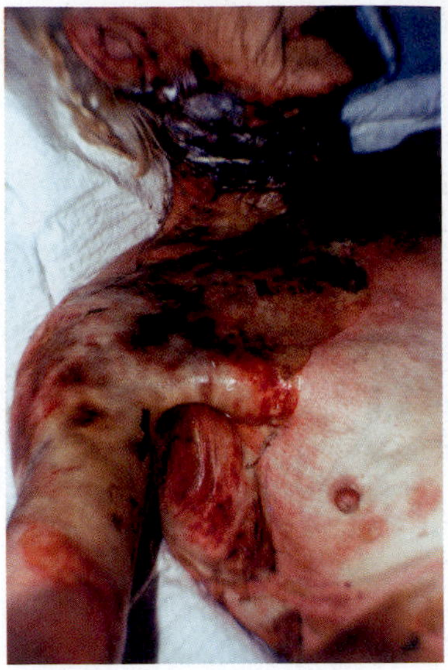

FIGURE 61–7 ◆ Full-thickness injury.
Source: Courtesy of John M. Osborn, MD, FACS.

greater proportion of body surface area per amount of body mass. As a result, there is a higher risk for fluid volume loss, requiring greater fluid resuscitation for total percent burn as compared to adults. Therefore, infants and young children are at increased risk for the development of hypovolemic shock.

In the older population (over 60 years of age), burns tend to exacerbate previous medical problems such as cardiovascular disease, renal insufficiency, diabetes, and chronic obstructive pulmonary disease. This population tends to have decreased physiological reserves, which are needed to respond to the stress of a burn injury; therefore, older adults who suffer burns are at a higher risk for shock and multisystem organ failure. Additionally, the older population tends to heal more slowly, resulting in a greater risk for the development of infection and pneumonia.

Past Medical History

Cardiac, respiratory, renal, and endocrine diseases and/or a history of substance abuse decreases the rate of survival of a major burn injury at any age. The added insult of a burn injury exacerbates these preexisting conditions and increases morbidity and mortality.

Part of Body Burned

The area of the body affected by burns is significant because of the associated side effects and the potential for cosmetic and functional deformities. For example, burns of the head, neck, and chest tend to have pulmonary complications and are considered more serious than a burn of the same size on the lower leg. Burn injuries occurring in the perineum and upper thighs are more prone to infections due to local contamination. Burns of the face, neck, and hands require special treatment for physical as well as psychological reasons.

In summary, many health care providers believe as a general rule of prognosis that if the age of the patient and the percentage of burn add up to more than 100, there is little chance of survival. Adding any prior chronic medical problems to this situation decreases the chances of survival even further. The single most powerful factor in predicting mortality from fire is smoke inhalation, which is covered in this chapter.

Laboratory and Diagnostic Evaluation

Tissue and cell destruction and fluid and electrolyte shifts cause many hematologic changes following a burn injury. The most radical changes occur in the first 24 to 48 hours after the injury. Therefore, careful monitoring of laboratory values is critical during this hemodynamic stabilization period, although careful monitoring of laboratory data

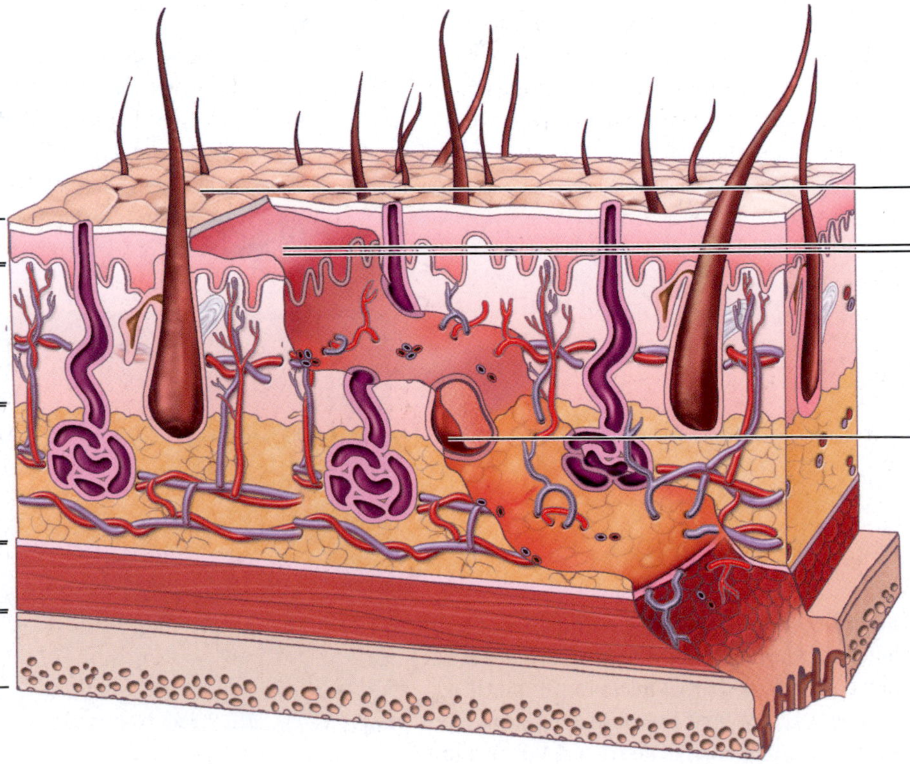

FIGURE 61–8 ◆ Skin layers of partial-thickness versus full-thickness injury.

CHART 61–2 Determination of Burn Depth

	Superficial Injury	Partial-Thickness Injury	Full-Thickness Injury
Skin Depth	Epidermis	Epidermis and most of the dermis Base structures of sebaceous and sweat glands intact	Epidermis, dermis, and may include subcutaneous tissue, muscle, and bones
Skin Appearance	Red, may have local edema Blanches with pressure	Pink or dark-pink May appear dull, white, tan, or cherry Blanches with pressure	Dark red, white, charred black, gray Pearl, dark tan, waxy No blanching Charred blood vessels visible
Pain	Increased sensitivity	Increased sensitivity	Absent: nerve endings destroyed
Blister Formation	None	Large, thick walled, and will increase in size	Usually none or, if present, thin walled and will not increase in size
Texture	Slightly firm if edema present	Firm due to edema	Dry and leatherlike
Possible Causes	Sun Ultraviolet light Flash flame	Hot liquids or solids Flash or direct flame to clothing Chemicals Ultraviolet light	Hot liquids or solids Flame Chemicals Electrical contact
Healing Time	2–5 days No scarring	5–35 days No grafting unless converts to full-thickness injury	Little to no healing potential Requires grafting

must continue throughout all phases of burn recovery. Hematologic response to burn injury is discussed next; it was also outlined in the Diagnostic Tests box (p. 1931).

Red Blood Cells

Red blood cells are lost both directly in the burn and as a result of increased fragility. Circulating red blood cell mass becomes trapped and destroyed within the burn wound at the time of injury. The cell loss is not just from direct heat damage; erythrocyte losses continue to occur for several days after the injury. What is somewhat misleading is that in the first 12 to 48 hours after the burn injury, there is an increase in the hematocrit. This increase is not due to an increase in erythrocytes but instead is the result of hemoconcentration related to intravascular fluid volume loss. Once fluid balance has been reestablished, a lower and more accurate hematocrit reading can be taken. Red blood cell production is dependent on adequate iron stores and normal metabolism. Circulating levels of iron are depressed after burn injury in part due to large exudative losses through the burned tissue, which may explain why erythrocyte production is decreased despite normal production of erythropoietin from the kidney.

Leukocytes

Immediately after the burn injury, there is an increase in granulocytes, which constitute 60% to 80% of the total number of normal blood leukocytes (white blood cells). This increase is not due to an increased production but rather is from mobilization of preexisting stores. The granulocytes continue to increase for the first 24 hours after the injury, and then the count begins to fall. The decrease in the granulocyte level is due in part to the dilutional effects of fluid replacement therapy and in part because the granulocytes have concentrated in the injured areas. Within 48 hours after the injury, stores of granulocytes are depleted, and the patient is dependent on the bone marrow for the production of new cells. Infection and septicemia are factors that stimulate the production of granulocytes.

Platelets

Dilution and consumption of platelets immediately after a burn injury cause an abnormal decrease both in the platelet count and in clotting factors. In addition, a large number of platelets may be utilized to stabilize the vasculature in and around the burned area. The bone marrow does not store platelets, so increased production is necessary to meet the needs of the body. It is not uncommon to infuse platelets during the first 36 hours after the injury.

Medical Management

Survival following a burn injury depends on a timely in-depth assessment and the development of an appropriate treatment plan. The health care provider will supply the orders for patient management, and the nurse coordinates the plan with the members of the health care team. After airway stabilization, it is critical to begin fluid resuscitation to prevent the development and progression of hypovolemic shock. Specific orders are outlined next.

Fluid Resuscitation

As described earlier, large amounts of fluid are lost in the first 24 to 48 hours after injury owing to increased capillary permeability. Therefore, fluid replacement is critical to survival during the emergency period. The purpose of fluid resuscitation is to maintain circulating blood volume and cardiac output, which become compromised owing to fluid shifting out of the intravascular space into the interstitial space. The goal is to prevent hypovolemic shock, tissue ischemia, and death. The amount of fluid needed for replacement depends on the size of injury, depth of burn, patient's age, and past medical history.

A number of different formulas have been devised in an attempt to standardize the amount and type of fluid for replacement. All of the formulas use either crystalloids or colloids or a combination of the two. A crystalloid is an electrolyte solution that may be either isotonic or hypertonic. Two of the most common isotonic solutions are lactated Ringer's and 0.9% normal saline. Lactated Ringer's tends to be the solution of choice because it most closely mimics the body's extracellular fluid. Crystalloid solutions typically are used in the first 12 hours until capillary permeability begins to stabilize. Once the capillary leaking has slowed, colloid formulas may be administered; these formulas contain products such as fresh frozen plasma, dextran, and albumin. These hypertonic solutions not only provide volume but also generate an osmotic pressure, which pulls fluid back from the interstitial space into the intravascular space. Fresh frozen plasma also restores lost clotting factors, and red blood cell replacement is indicated if a significant change has occurred in the hemoglobin and hematocrit levels. Some formulas also give 5% dextrose solution for maintenance and replacement of insensible losses.

The guidelines of the Advanced Trauma Life Support course and the Advanced Burn Life Support course recommend the use of a simple formula that is readily available at the hospital. The most common formulas are listed in Chart 61–3. Generally, health care providers use the Parkland/Baxter formula, which administers 4 milliliters of lactated Ringer's solution per kilogram of body weight multiplied by percent of TBSA of burn (4 mL/kg of weight × % burn). Because most of the fluid loss occurs in the first hours after the injury, 50% of the fluid is given in the first 8 hours, 25% in the second 8 hours, and 25% in the third 8 hours. Over the second 24 hours, the lactated Ringer's generally is discontinued, and a hypotonic solution such as 5% dextrose and water with potassium is titrated to maintain an adequate urine output (Pham et al., 2008). Plasma and albumin are administered in boluses during the second 24 hours to maintain hemodynamic stability (Pham et al., 2008).

These formulas were designed as guidelines for fluid administration. Each patient has to be monitored individually for his or her response to fluid resuscitation. For example, because older adults are at increased risk of diminished organ function, fluid resuscitation in these patients will be less aggressive than with the very young, who are more susceptible to dehydration. All patients with burn injuries require close monitoring for adequacy of fluid replacement and organ perfusion.

Fluid Resuscitation Assessment

End points are objective criteria that define a measured outcome or goal of treatment. If end points are not achieved, resuscitation measures must be adjusted and reassessed. End points are important with burn resuscitation because then fluids are titrated according to objective data instead of being only formula driven. Therefore, assessing normal organ function provides a means of monitoring fluid replacement. Fluid resuscitation end points include:

- ***Mentation:*** Orientation and level of consciousness are sensitive to changes in oxygen delivery because the brain needs a constant supply of blood for normal function. Deficient fluid resuscitation resulting in inadequate oxygen delivery to the brain can cause agitation, restlessness, confusion, and even stupor. In the absence of head trauma, a well-hydrated patient should be alert and oriented.
- ***Skin color and temperature:*** Vasoconstriction caused by intravascular depletion is manifested by cool, pale, and clammy skin or mottled skin with advanced shock. Additionally, owing to loss of skin and subsequent temperature regulation, the core body temperature may be decreased.
- ***Heart rate:*** Tachycardia (a heart rate greater than 100 beats per minute) is an indicator of hypovolemia. With hydration, the heart rate will return to the upper limits of normal for the patient's age range.
- ***Blood pressure:*** The blood pressure tends to be a poor indicator of perfusion in the very early stage because pronounced catecholamine release results in an increased systemic vascular resistance, causing normal blood pressure to be maintained even in the presence of hypovolemia.
- ***Urine output:*** Most health care providers agree that the urine output is the best gauge of adequate hydration. In an adult, it should be 0.5 to 1 mL/kg of body weight per hour (ACS, 2008). Typically, a minimum urine output of 30 mL/hour indicates adequate hydration.
- ***Specific gravity:*** Specific gravity, which is also monitored hourly, becomes elevated (>1.025) with dehydration and decreases as fluid is replaced.
- ***Central venous pressure (CVP):*** A CVP between 4 and 12 indicates adequate fluid volume.

CHART 61–3 Fluid Replacement Formulas for Burn Injuries

Parkland/Baxter Formula	**Brooke Army Formula**
First 24 hours:	First 24 hours:
4 mL/kg × % total body surface area (TBSA) of lactated Ringer's	1.5 mL/kg × % TBSA of lactated Ringer's
1/2 given in first 8 hours, 1/4 in second 8 hours, 1/4 in third 8 hours	0.5 mL/kg × % TBSA of colloid solution
	1/2 given in first 8 hours, 1/4 in second 8 hours, 1/4 in third 8 hours
Second 24 hours:	Second 24 hours:
Dextrose and water, plus potassium	0.5–0.75 mL/kg × % TBSA of lactated Ringer's
Colloid: 20% to 60% of calculated plasma volume (0.35–0.5 mL/kg × % TBSA)	2,000 mL of dextrose and water
Consensus Formula	**Evans Formula**
First 24 hours:	First 24 hours:
2–4 mL/kg × % TBSA of lactated Ringer's	1 mL/kg × % TBSA of 0.9 normal saline
1/2 given in first 8 hours, 1/4 in second 8 hours, 1/4 in third 8 hours	1 mL/kg × % TBSA of colloid solution
	1/2 given in first 8 hours, 1/4 in second 8 hours, 1/4 in third 8 hours
Second 24 hours:	Second 24 hours:
0.3–0.5 mL/kg × % TBSA of colloid solution	0.5 mL/kg × % TBSA of 0.9 normal saline
Electrolyte-free solution to maintain urine output	2,000 mL of dextrose and water

- ***Hemoconcentration factors:*** Hemoglobin (Hgb) and hematocrit (Hct) increase with the loss of intravascular volume; in the presence of inadequate fluid resuscitation, the Hgb and Hct become abnormally elevated. The level of these values is proportional to the level of fluid volume. As fluid returns to the intravascular space, the Hgb and Hct levels will return to normal and typically become abnormally low, owing to cell destruction (see the Diagnostic Tests box, p. 1931). Overhydration will cause false low readings.
- ***Gastrointestinal function:*** Normal gastrointestinal function is inferred by the return of bowel sounds.

Safety Alert *A hemoglobin (Hgb) of > 20 g/dL and/or a hematocrit (Hct) of > 60% is an indication that fluid resuscitation is inadequate and needs to be increased. However, the Hgb and Hct are not the best indicators of fluid balance because many blood cells are destroyed with the initial tissue injury. Use other indicators of fluid balance, such as heart rate, central venous pressure (CVP), and blood pressure (BP), which are more reflective of the adequacy of hydration.*

Pain Management

Pain management is a complex issue for a burn victim because pain varies in character and intensity throughout all phases of burn treatment. Pain is related to tissue injury and the healing process and is complicated by fear, anxiety, depression, and the chronicity of the injury. The goal of pain management is to provide maximal comfort throughout treatment and recovery. To accomplish this, it is necessary to establish a partnership with the patient regarding how to manage pain relief.

Once fluid resuscitation has begun, narcotic analgesics are administered intravenously to help control pain. For effective pain management, interventions must be evaluated and modified on an ongoing basis. Pain causes activation of the sympathetic nervous system, causing vasoconstriction, which decreases blood flow to the wound and delays healing.

If pain is not managed appropriately at the outset of the injury, long-term pain management issues may ensue. The main tenets of pain management for patients with burns are as follows:

- Analgesics are most effective if given on a scheduled basis rather than only as requested by the patient.
- Intramuscular (IM) injections are not used during the emergency period because of poor absorption.
- IM injections are avoided in children, because children tend to fear the injection as much as the pain.
- Bowel management must begin when narcotic pain management begins.
- Doses of medication should be modified as the clinical situation dictates (e.g., dressing changes).
- Anxiety needs to be treated for effective pain management.
- Pain management must be individualized to the patient, with consideration being given to the time since the injury, the patient's age, the percentage of the burn, and the burn depth.

A comprehensive approach to pain management includes assessing the pain level, anticipating the need for prophylactic analgesic, and administering narcotics as ordered. If the patient cannot verbalize or assist in the assessment of pain relief, there are physiological responses that must be assessed on a regular basis. Indications that pain relief is needed include increased heart rate, diaphoresis, increased agitation, grimacing, and rhythmic movement or lack of movement (Urden, 2009).

In the early acute stages of burn injury, the most commonly used pain management agents are opioids such as morphine sulfate, fentanyl, and codeine. Small, frequent doses on a non–pain-contingent schedule are indicated for the continuous background pain that is associated with loss of skin integrity. Procedural pain such as dressing changes are best managed by additional intravenous opioids. Patients with burns typically report excruciating pain with dressing changes, especially with partial-thickness injuries. As the burn injury heals, less potent drugs are indicated such as nonsteroidal analgesics. The length of time required to treat burn injuries necessitates a comprehensive interdisciplinary team approach so that the patient's functional outcome is maximized while psychological distress is minimized. Adequate management of pain requires that the plan be reevaluated frequently. Chapter 12 provides an in-depth discussion of pain management principles.

Alternative Therapies for Pain Management

It is essential to allow the patient to verbalize the pain experience and explore alternative therapies for pain relief. These therapies, which may include guided imagery, hypnosis, and music, are used as an adjunct to medication. The Complementary & Alternative Therapies box (p. 1940) details the use of music therapy in the management of pain.

Safety Alert *Assess the adequacy of pain management for dressing changes daily. Secure the health care provider's orders for more medication, and have these orders available as backup if needed. Be sensitive to cultural diversity in response to pain and medicate accordingly.*

Nursing Management

The nursing care needs of the newly admitted patient with burns are complex and multifaceted. Use of the nursing process will facilitate a comprehensive approach to patient assessment and care. The Nursing Process: Patient Care Plan box applies the nursing process to the applicable nursing diagnoses and provides a comprehensive care plan for a patient with burns during the emergency period.

Collaborative Management

To achieve optimal recovery and return to society, patients with burns need a multidisciplinary team approach, including health care providers, nurses, physical and occupational therapists, social workers, psychologists/psychiatrists, and dietitians. In order to meet desired patient outcomes, it is essential that the members of this interdisciplinary team communicate openly with one another in developing and evaluating care of the patient and family (IOM [Institute of Medicine], 2010).

To ensure complete closure and prevention of infection, wound care is managed by both nurses and health care providers. As the burn scar heals, it continues to contract, thereby decreasing the range of motion (ROM) in the surrounding area. Physical therapy is begun within a few days after admission and continues for at least a year after hospital discharge. Ongoing physical therapy will help to increase ROM in the joints. When contracture formation is severe, the surgeon needs to release the contractures surgically.

If scarring and contractures are significant, it might not be possible for the patient to return to her previous occupation. The occupational therapist assists the patient with exercises that will enhance fine motor movements, while the social worker and a psychologist or psychiatrist help the patient adjust to body image changes and perhaps loss of work.

Family dynamics often are affected by the prolonged hospitalization and change in role function within the family structure. The psychologist or psychiatrist also assists the patient with the adjustments of these changes. Finally, a comprehensive plan for nutrition is important for

COMPLEMENTARY & ALTERNATIVE THERAPIES Music Therapy During Dressing Changes *Nancy Yilk*

MIND–BODY THERAPIES attempt to reduce symptoms of anxiety and pain by enhancing bodily functions. This can be done as stand-alone therapy, such as meditation, prayer, hypnosis, or yoga, or as an adjunct therapy, such as music therapy utilized with burn patients. Music as an adjunct to procedural sedation for treatment of pain and anxiety involves having patients select music and passively listen to that music during burn wound care procedures.

Undergoing a procedure that requires anesthesia can be anxiety provoking. Anxiety is coupled with increases in heart rate and blood pressure, as well as other changes that can have a negative impact, during all stages of patient care: the preoperative care period; the induction, maintenance, and emergence phases of anesthesia; and the postoperative care period. The use of music as a nonpharmacologic intervention reduces anxiety levels in some patients (Wakim, Smith, & Guinn, 2010).

To explore the efficacy of two music therapy protocols on pain, anxiety, and muscle tension levels during dressing changes in burn patients, 29 inpatients participated in a prospective, crossover randomized controlled trial. On two consecutive days, patients were randomized to receive music therapy services either on the first or second day of the study. On control days, they received no music. On music days, patients practiced music-based imagery (MBI), a form of music-assisted relaxation with patient-specific mental imagery before and after dressing changes. Also on music days during dressing changes, the patients engaged in music alternate engagement (MAE), which consisted of active participation in music making. The dependent variables were the patients' subjective ratings of their pain and anxiety levels and the research nurse's objective ratings of their muscle tension levels. Two sets of data were collected before dressing changes, three sets during dressing changes, and another two sets after dressing changes. The results showed significant decreases in pain levels before ($P < 0.025$), during ($P < 0.05$), and after ($P < 0.025$) dressing changes on days when the patients received music therapy in contrast to control days. Music therapy was also associated with a decrease in anxiety and muscle tension levels during the dressing changes ($P < 0.05$) followed by a reduction in muscle tension levels after dressing changes ($P < 0.025$). Music therapy significantly decreased the acute procedural pain, anxiety, and muscle tension levels associated with daily burn care (Tan, Yowler, Super, & Fratianne, 2010).

Patient-preferred music is an important component of the successful use of music therapy during procedures. In an integrative research review, the following criteria were offered as guidelines in the use of music therapy during procedures:

- Initially assess whether the patient would like music and provide for the patient's preference as to genre or artist.
- Do not allow music before the procedure to substitute for or impede teaching the patient. Music delivery methods should not interfere with the ability to communicate instructions to the patient.
- Assessment of anxiety and pain with hemodynamic monitoring should be ongoing.
- Procedural sedation protocols must be followed (Vanderdoom, 2007).
- Ensure that volume is adjusted for the hearing impaired or older patients and that procedural sounds do not override the music (Protacio, 2010).

enhancing wound healing, helping the patient to regain strength, and preventing complications.

The dietitian works with the health care team from the time of admission through discharge to ensure proper nutritional support.

In addition to the nursing care described earlier and in the Nursing Process: Patient Care Plan boxes in this chapter, the nurse plays a pivotal role in coordinating the efforts of the health care team.

Acute Phase

The acute phase of burn management begins when the patient is hemodynamically stable and ends with closure of the burn wounds. The goals of treatment during this phase include wound cleansing and healing; pain relief; preserving body heat; preventing infection; promoting nutrition; and splinting, positioning, and exercising affected joints.

Wound Care

After airway and hemodynamic stabilization, wound care is the next priority. Infection is the most serious threat, potentially leading to further tissue injury and the development of sepsis. Therefore, the patient's survival may depend on preventing wound contamination. Nurses generally coordinate and perform wound care; thus, nursing assessment and interventions are critical. Care of the wound includes cleansing, débridement, shaving, culturing, assessing for infection and adequate circulation, and applying topical antibiotics. These aspects of wound care are discussed next.

Cleansing

Cleansing of the burn wound at the time of admission may be accomplished by a number of methods depending on the preference of the health care provider, available equipment, and the patient's stability. The purpose of the cleansing is to remove debris from the wound, eliminate dead tissue, and prevent further destruction of viable tissue by infection. For the cleansing process, the patient may be submerged in a Hubbard tank, hosed over a spray table, placed in a shower, or washed at the bedside. The advantage of using a Hubbard tank is that the patient can be totally submerged in the water, which helps to remove topical antibiotics and eschar and facilitates ROM exercises. Submersion in a Hubbard tank is typically limited to no more than 30 minutes because submersion in water leaches sodium from the open wound, causes heat loss, and is very painful. Whichever method is used, the wound is washed with gauze and a mild bacteriostatic soap such as chlorhexidine gluconate (Hibiclens) or any noncytotoxic cleansing agent. Removal of blisters is controversial; most health care providers believe that intact blisters should be left in place; however, if blisters are open, the loose tissue should be removed. Washing of open wounds is a painful process; therefore, it is imperative that the patient be premedicated before the initial cleansing and before all dressing changes. Heat shields, warm blankets, and increased room temperature are methods used to help maintain body temperature during dressing changes.

Wound Débridement

The purpose of wound débridement is to remove loose tissue, wound debris, and eschar in order to prepare the wound for closure. In Figure 61–9◆ the white tissue is eschar, which needs to be débrided before the wound is ready for grafting. Débridement of a burn wound can be accomplished by three methods: mechanically, chemically, and surgically. Mechanical débridement is accomplished by using wet-to-dry dressings, or by manually cutting the dead tissue with scissors and forceps, as well as with hydrotherapy. During daily dressing changes, nurses use scissors and forceps to remove and cut away the dead tissue. Use of the Hubbard tank, a spray table, and/or the shower gradually softens the dead tissue, which facilitates easier removal. Chemical removal of eschar is accomplished by the use of commercially prepared enzymatic or fibrinolytic agents that

NURSING PROCESS: Patient Care Plan for the Emergency Period of Burn Injury

Assessment of Integument Status Using Gordon's Functional Health Patterns:

- Health Perception Health Management Pattern
- Nutrition Metabolic Pattern
- Activity Exercise Pattern
- Cognitive Perceptual Pattern
- Self-Perception Self-Concept Pattern
- Values and Belief Pattern

Subjective Data	Objective Data
Assessment of Fluid Volume Loss	**Assessment of Fluid Volume Loss**
Do you know where you are?	Blood pressure
Tell me your name.	Cardiac output
Are you feeling light-headed or dizzy?	Urine output
Are you feeling thirsty?	Hemoglobin and hematocrit
Assessment of Excess Fluid	**Assessment of Excess Fluid**
Do you feel short of breath?	Congested lungs
Do you have a cough?	Increased heart rate
Do you feel swollen or edematous?	Increased blood pressure
	Increased CVP
	Increased PAWP
	Increased rate and depth of respirations
	Increased weight
Assessment of Tissue Perfusion	**Assessment of Tissue Perfusion**
Can you feel me touch your fingers and toes?	Nail bed color and capillary refill
Can you move your fingers and toes?	Temperature of fingers and toes
Where are you having pain?	Peripheral pulses
Assessment of Airway and Gas Exchange	**Assessment of Airway and Gas Exchange**
How did you get burned?	Lung sounds
Did the injury occur in an enclosed space?	Oxygen saturation
Do you have any preexisting health problems such as heart, lung, or kidney disease?	Work of breathing (e.g., gasping, increased rate or effort)
	Vital signs
	Skin and nail bed color
Assessment of Skin Integrity	**Assessment of Skin Integrity**
Where are you having pain?	Percent total body surface area burn using standardized measurement scales
	Depth of injury
Assessment for Infection	**Assessment for Infection**
Is your pain increasing?	Previously healed wounds are breaking down
Do you feel weaker?	Open wounds not healing
	Partial-thickness injuries/donor sites converting to full-thickness injuries
	Increased odor and drainage from wound sites
	Wound cultures positive for organisms
	Fever
	Increased WBC
Assessment of Nutritional Status	**Assessment of Nutritional Status**
How is your appetite?	Presence of bowel sounds
What can be done to help improve it?	Calorie count
Do you understand the importance of maintaining adequate nutrition?	Prealbumin level
Do you feel nauseated?	Weight changes
What kinds of food do you enjoy?	

(continued)

NURSING PROCESS: Patient Care Plan for the Emergency Period of Burn Injury, *continued*

Subjective Data	Objective Data
Assessment of Pain	**Assessment of Pain**
What is your pain level using the 0-to-10 scale? A 1 is very little pain and a 10 is the worst imaginable pain. What is your experience with pain? Do you routinely take pain medications at home; if so, what for and what kind? Are you allergic to any pain medication? Do you have any cultural or religious beliefs that impact your pain control?	Grimacing on movement Restlessness and irritability Taut facial expression
Assessment of Fear and Anxiety	**Assessment of Fear and Anxiety**
Tell me what you are feeling about your injuries. Who are the people in your life that are your support system? How have you handled fearful situations in the past?	Facial expressions Mood Verbalization of fear regarding injury, impact on family, and future
Assessment for Temperature Regulation	**Assessment for Temperature Regulation**
Do you feel too cold or too warm?	Body temperature Shivering Dusky nail beds
Assessment of Patient Perception of Environment and Injury	**Assessment of Patient Perception of Environment and Injury**
What questions do you have about your injury and the necessary therapy for healing? Have you been in situations in your life in which you feel you have very little control? How do you typically cope with situations in which you are not in control?	Compliance with treatments
Assessment of Patient and Family Knowledge of Injury	**Assessment of Patient and Family Knowledge of Injury**
What do you understand about your injury? Do you have questions about the injury/treatment program? What would you like me to tell you about your injury?	Patient and family verbalize knowledge of seriousness of injury and prognosis.
Assessment of Psychological Adjustment to Scarring and Contractures	**Assessment of Psychological Adjustment to Scarring and Contractures**
What impact does the change in your physical appearance have on your life? How do you plan to cope with these changes?	Does the patient look at burn wounds? Does the patient ask questions about the wounds? Is the patient's perception realistic regarding body image changes? Are the patient and family willing to learn and participate in the required care after hospital discharge?

Outcomes and Evaluation Parameters	Planning and Interventions with *Rationales*
1. NURSING DIAGNOSIS: Deficient Fluid Volume ***related to increased capillary permeability, increased intravascular hydrostatic pressure, and increased evaporative loss*** **(NANDA-I © 2012)**	
Outcomes: Adequate intravascular volume. Fluid and electrolytes within normal limits. No signs and symptoms of hypovolemic shock. Mental alertness and cognitive orientation. ***Evaluation Parameters:*** Normal vital signs. Normal serum electrolytes, hemoglobin, and hematocrit. Urine specific gravity between 1.010 and 1.020. Urine output at 0.5 mL/kg per hour.	Insert large-bore intravenous (IV) catheter through nonburned tissue per order. *To facilitate fluid replacement.* Administer and titrate IV fluids per ordered formulas and parameters. *To replace lost volume.* Record amount of IV fluid infused. *To monitor fluid replacement.* Assess vital signs and urine output at least hourly until stable and then per health care provider's order/unit policy. *To assess adequacy of fluid replacement.* Monitor central venous pressure (CVP) and pulmonary artery wedge pressure (PAWP) if possible. *To assess adequacy of fluid replacement and cardiac output.* Monitor arterial blood gases (ABGs). *To assess acid–base balance and presence of shock.* Obtain baseline weight if possible and monitor regularly. *To monitor adequacy of nutritional replacement.*

NURSING PROCESS: Patient Care Plan for the Emergency Period of Burn Injury, *continued*

	Test all stools and emesis for blood. *To monitor for blood loss from stress ulcers.* Maintain a heated environment. *To prevent loss of body heat due to loss of skin integrity.* Monitor serum electrolytes, hemoglobin, and hematocrit, and report critical abnormalities to the health care provider. *To monitor hematologic changes associated with fluid loss and tissue destruction.* Monitor for blood loss from burns or other injuries. *To assess need for blood replacement therapy.* Assess orientation frequently and regularly. *Monitor adequacy of fluid replacement and presence of associated head injury.* Provide oral fluids, if patient is able to drink. Encourage fluid intake *to replace lost fluid.*
2. NURSING DIAGNOSIS: Risk for Imbalanced Fluid Volume *related to excessive IV fluid administration and diminished organ capacity for excessive volume load* (NANDA-I © 2012)	
Outcome: Adequate hydration with no evidence of fluid overload. ***Evaluation Parameters:*** Normal vital signs. Normal CVP, PAWP. Normal ABGs, electrolytes. Vesicular lung sounds clear. No dyspnea. No increase in body weight. Normal urine output and specific gravity.	Assess body weight if possible. *Monitor for excess fluid buildup.* Assess urine output and specific gravity. *Monitor hydration status.* Assess arterial blood gases (ABGs) and electrolytes. *To assess acid–base balance, severity of shock state, and electrolyte changes due to fluid shifts.* Monitor intake and output hourly. *To assess rate of fluid replacement.* Monitor lung sounds. *To assess for fluid buildup.*
3. NURSING DIAGNOSIS: Ineffective Peripheral Tissue Perfusion *related to constricting edema formation and circumferential burns* (NANDA-I © 2012)	
Outcome: Adequate peripheral tissue perfusion. ***Evaluation Parameters:*** Extremity pulses present by palpation and/or ultrasound. Capillary refill $<$ 3 seconds on distal extremities. Absence of numbness or tingling. Absence of increased pain.	Remove constricting clothing, jewelry, and dressings. *To promote tissue perfusion.* Elevate affected extremities above the heart. *To reduce edema formation.* Monitor arterial pulses by palpation and/or ultrasound every hour during the first 24–48 hours. *To assess perfusion status during edema formation.* Assess pain and capillary permeability on both burned and unburned areas. *To assess the impact of edema formation.* Assess for numbness or tingling. *To assess perfusion status during edema formation.* If pulses diminish or become absent, if pain increases, or if capillary refill slows, notify the health care provider immediately. *These are indications of a loss of perfusion and need medical intervention to prevent necrosis formation.* If indicated, prepare patient for escharotomy. *To prevent loss of affected extremity or prevent respiratory depression.*
4. NURSING DIAGNOSES: (a) Impaired Gas Exchange *related to inhalation injury and fatigue.* (b) Ineffective Airway Clearance *related to tracheal edema* (NANDA-I © 2012)	
Outcome: Adequate gas exchange. ***Evaluation Parameters:*** Normal arterial blood gases. Free of dyspnea: unlabored respirations $<$ 24/minute. Alert and oriented. Clear breath sounds. No restlessness, cyanosis, or fatigue. Oxygen saturation is within normal limits.	Assess for adventitious or diminished breath sounds. *Indicates decreased gas exchange.* Note presence of cough and amount, color, and consistency of sputum. *Assessing for inhalation injury.* Monitor ABGs and oxygen saturation. *To assess adequacy of gas exchange and level of shock state.* Monitor respiratory rate and depth. *To assess for respiratory distress.* Monitor restlessness and confusion. *Indicators of inadequate gas exchange with resultant brain hypoxia.* Observe for cyanosis, especially in the mucous membranes. *Indicators of inadequate gas exchange with resultant tissue hypoxia.* Turn, cough, deep breathe, elevate head of bed, and instruct on use of incentive spirometry. *Measures to promote gas exchange.* Administer humidified oxygen as prescribed. *To loosen secretions and promote airway clearance.*

(*continued*)

NURSING PROCESS: Patient Care Plan for the Emergency Period of Burn Injury, *continued*

Outcomes and Evaluation Parameters	Planning and Interventions with *Rationales*
	Report respiratory distress to the health care provider. *Medical intervention may be indicated to prevent respiratory failure.* Assess need for suctioning and/or endotracheal intubation. *To maintain adequate gas exchange.*
5. NURSING DIAGNOSIS: Impaired Skin Integrity *related to epithelial skin loss* (NANDA-I © 2012)	
Outcome: Normal wound healing to reestablish skin integrity. ***Evaluation Parameters:*** Burn wounds will heal spontaneously or by surgical closure as evidenced by no open wound, no drainage, and no odor. Absence of clinical manifestations of wound infection.	Assess extent of total body surface area (TBSA) of burn. Cleanse and débride wound. *Determines treatment and prognosis.* Assess wound for depth, location, and dimensions. *Determines treatment and prognosis.* Elevate affected areas. *To decrease edema.* Position therapeutically. *To prevent contracture formation.* Apply antibiotic cream and/or dressing per health care provider's order. *To prevent infection.* Clean and débride wounds daily, and assess for separation of eschar and evidence of granulation tissue. *Preparation for skin grafting.* Assess for presence or absence of granulation tissue and necrotic tissue. *Assess wound status for grafting.* Assess for infection (see Risk for Infection nursing diagnosis). *To prevent occurrence and spread of infection.* Establish a skin breakdown prevention plan. Monitor blood glucose. Obtain white blood count (WBC) daily. *Infection assessment.* Monitor donor sites for infection. *May convert site to a full-thickness injury.* Administer vitamins and minerals per order. *To promote wound healing.*
6. NURSING DIAGNOSIS: Risk for Infection *related to loss of skin integrity and impaired nonspecific and specific immunity* (NANDA-I © 2012)	
Outcome: Effective infection prevention. ***Evaluation Parameters:*** Burn will not be colonized by organisms. Healing and reepithelialization as noted by wound closure. Skin integrity will be restored.	Cleanse and shave wound per protocol. *To prevent contamination from surrounding tissue and hair.* Assess for infection and document with each dressing change. *To prevent spread of infection.* Assess for drainage: exudate, color, odor, and amount. *Factors that indicate infection.* Assess for undermining or sinus tract formation. *Indicates infection.* Use strict aseptic technique. *To prevent infection.* Notify health care provider of presence of infection or wound enlargement. *To facilitate medical intervention.* Monitor serum WBC daily. *Increased WBC indicates presence of infection.* Maintain nutritional therapies. *Malnutrition increases the risk of infection.* Monitor and record temperature hourly. *Indicates infection.* Culture wounds and body secretions per protocol. *To assess for infection.*
7. NURSING DIAGNOSIS: Imbalanced Nutrition: Less Than Body Requirements *related to hypermetabolic demands of burn injury, decreased appetite, immobility, pain, nausea/vomiting, and depression* (NANDA-I © 2012)	
Outcome: Adequate nutrition maintained. ***Evaluation Parameters:*** Adequate calorie and nutrient intake maintained. Tolerates prescribed diet. Nutritional laboratory values within normal limits. Regular bowel pattern. Maintains preinjury body weight (+ or – 10%). Gastric pH > 5. Stool and gastric aspirate are negative for blood. Fluid and electrolyte balance is normal. Progressive wound healing.	Record accurate intake and output, and calorie count, every shift. *Indicates adequacy of nutrition.* Maintain oral hygiene. *Helps promote appetite and prevents infection.* Monitor gastrointestinal tract for bowel sounds and distention. *Assesses normal digestive process.* Monitor feeding tube placement and function. *To prevent complications such as aspiration.* Administer enteral tube feedings at prescribed rate and concentration. *To maintain nutrition.* Monitor for residual formula by aspiration per health care provider's order. *To assess tolerance and absorption of feedings.*

NURSING PROCESS: Patient Care Plan for the Emergency Period of Burn Injury, *continued*

	Monitor weight daily. *Indicates adequacy of nutrition.* Consult nutritionist to establish calorie, protein, carbohydrate, and nutrient needs. *To maintain nutrition.* Allow patient to select desired foods. *To promote appetite.* Involve family in meal planning. *To assess patient's likes and dislikes.* Provide high-calorie, high-protein, high-carbohydrate diet, including snacks. *To augment between-meal calorie intake.* Avoid painful procedures near mealtime and make the environment pleasant for eating. *To increase appetite.* Monitor laboratory values (i.e., total protein levels, complete blood count, glucose, iron, and prealbumin). *To ensure adequacy of nutrition.* Monitor elimination patterns. *To assess gastrointestinal (GI) function.* Monitor wound healing progress. *Wound healing progress is impacted by nutritional status.* Monitor pH and guaiac tests on gastric aspirate and stools. *To assess for GI bleeding.* Administer antacids, stool softeners, laxatives, and antiulcer agents per health care provider orders. *To prevent GI bleeding.* Assess dietary patterns in culturally diverse populations. *To tailor diet to foods of a particular culture.*
8. NURSING DIAGNOSIS: Acute Pain *related to burn injury and exposed nerve endings* (NANDA-I © 2012)	
Outcome: Comfort level maintained. ***Evaluation Parameters:*** Able to communicate pain level and therapies that help alleviate it. Pain reduced and/or absent as evidenced by patient report and no pain behaviors: grimacing. Nonpharmacologic method of control is effective as evidenced by patient report and no pain behaviors. Reports satisfaction with pain management program.	Use pain scale (0 to 10) to quantify pain level. *Quantifying pain increases consistency.* Instruct the patient to inform the nurse if pain is not relieved. *Indicates need to change pain management plan.* Assess cultural and religious impact on patient's responses. *Different cultures and religions respond differently to pain.* Correct misconceptions about risk of addiction and overdose. *To decrease anxiety related to medication addiction.* Explain, prepare, and medicate patient for painful procedures (dressing change) and anticipated discomforts. *To control increased pain level related to procedure.* Provide a supportive environment wherein the patient is able to express pain level. *Opens communication and facilitates pain management.* Use pain control measures before pain becomes severe. *This increases comfort and decreases the need for medication.* Teach nonpharmacologic method of control (e.g., guided imagery, massage, and breathing exercises). *These measures augment medications for pain relief.* Cover wounds. *Covering areas where there is no skin decreases the pain.* Elevate affected areas. *Elevation decreases edema formation, which can be painful.* Provide rest periods between procedures *to assist with coping with ongoing pain. Decreases the fatigue related to long-term pain.* Revise pain management plan as wounds heal and pain decreases. *To prevent overmedication.* Plan diversional activities. *To augment pain-relief measures.*
9. NURSING DIAGNOSIS: Fear *and* Anxiety *related to changes in health status/role functioning; situational crisis* (NANDA-I © 2012)	
Outcome: Anxiety level minimized. ***Evaluation Parameters:*** Verbalizes anxious feelings. Verbalizes what relieves anxiety. Anxiety relieved by consistently demonstrating aggression and anxiety control, coping, impulse control, self-mutilation restraint, and substantially effective social interaction skills.	Assess and document level of anxiety. *To track trends in anxiety levels.* Explore with the patient and family techniques to reduce anxiety. *This gives the patient a sense of control and opens communication about the subject.* Provide factual information concerning diagnosis, treatment, disfigurement, disabilities, and prognosis. *Truthful explanations increase trust and potentially decrease anxiety.*

(*continued*)

NURSING PROCESS: Patient Care Plan for the Emergency Period of Burn Injury, *continued*

Outcomes and Evaluation Parameters	Planning and Interventions with *Rationales*
Verbalizes absence of sensory perceptual disorders. Verbalizes absence of physical manifestations of anxiety. Behavioral manifestations of anxiety absent.	Explain all procedures and allow time for mental preparation. *This decreases fear and anxiety of the unknown.* Explore with the patient effective ways to minimize anxiety. *This gives the patient a sense of control.* Instruct the patient on use of relaxation techniques. *To relieve anxiety.* Assess need for and administer antianxiety and pain medication. *If alternative measures are not effective, patient may need antianxiety agents.* Assist the patient and family in setting realistic goals for progress. *Indicates effectiveness of emotional adjustment.* Consider psychiatric counseling for patients and families who exhibit inability to accept situation. *Provide an ongoing plan and interventions to promote long-term relief from anxiety.*
10. NURSING DIAGNOSIS: Ineffective Thermoregulation *related to epithelial skin loss* (NANDA-I © 2012)	
Outcome: Normal thermoregulation maintained. ***Evaluation Parameter:*** Body temperature maintained between 37.5° and 38.7°C (99.5°–101.5°F).	Minimize heat loss by covering patient with dressing and blankets. *To decrease heat loss due to a lack of skin integrity.* Apply heat lamps and radiant heat shields. *To decrease heat loss due to a lack of skin integrity.* Keep room temperature elevated, especially during dressing changes. *To decrease heat loss due to a lack of skin integrity.* Monitor rectal and core temperatures as per orders and report changes. *To assess effectiveness of interventions.*
11. NURSING DIAGNOSIS: Powerlessness *related to foreign environment and critical injury* (NANDA-I © 2012)	
Outcome: Realistic perception of control. ***Evaluation Parameters:*** Verbalizes realistic perception of abilities to perform. Identifies health outcome priorities. Verbalizes powerlessness. Identifies actions that are within his control. Verbalizes ability to perform necessary actions. Reports adequate support from staff and family.	Determine knowledge of health and injury. *Determines where to begin teaching.* Discuss realistic options for self-care. *Gives patient hope and realistic view of limitations.* Reinforce personal strengths. *Decreases sense of powerlessness.* Encourage verbalization of feeling of powerlessness. *Opens communication.* Assist patient to increase independence when realistic. *Decreases powerlessness.* Allow control over surroundings and schedule when possible. *Decreases powerlessness.* Keep items within reach. *Decreases powerlessness.* Set short-term realistic goals. *Decreases powerlessness.* Explore patient's support mechanisms: family, church, and friends. *Needed as a source of support.*
12. NURSING DIAGNOSIS: Deficient Knowledge *regarding burn resuscitation* (NANDA-I © 2012)	
Outcome: Adequate knowledge of treatment regimen. ***Evaluation Parameter:*** Patient and family will verbalize understanding of treatments and care.	Assess the patient and family's readiness and ability to learn, as well as their individual learning needs. *The person must be psychologically ready to learn.* Determine level of existing knowledge. *Begin the teaching where existing knowledge ends.* Provide factual information about diagnosis, treatments, and prognosis. *To increase knowledge and understanding.* Explain all procedures in simple, concise language, allowing for questions. *Increases understanding.* Encourage questions. *Keeps open communication and augments understanding.* Ongoing education of treatment plan and rationale. *Ongoing education is necessary as situation and condition change.* Document response to teaching. *Assists health care team when implementing a teaching plan.*

NURSING PROCESS: Patient Care Plan for the Emergency Period of Burn Injury, *continued*

13. NURSING DIAGNOSES: (a) Disturbed Body Image *related to scar formation and functional loss.* (b) Risk for Complicated Grieving *related to body image change, risk of family role change, and possible occupational change* (NANDA-I © 2012)	
Outcome: Acceptance of body image changes. ***Evaluation Parameters:*** Patient verbalizes understanding of body changes. Patient verbalizes acceptance of self.	Assess the patient's level of anxiety and knowledge related to body image changes. *Body image changes occur as healing progresses.* Encourage discussion of meaning of loss. *Increases adjustment.* Observe interaction with significant people. *Indicates adjustment.* Assess for signs of grieving. *Indicates adjustment.* Establish therapeutic environment with an atmosphere of acceptance. *Increases adjustment.* Explain expected appearance. *Increases adjustment.* Offer mirror for viewing of facial burns. *Assesses adjustment.* Be realistic and positive during explanations. *Increases adjustment.* Plan family involvement during teaching. *Increases adjustment.* Set realistic goals for future. *Increases trust and is reality based.*

Source: Adapted from Wilkinson, J. M., & Ahearn, N. R. (2009). *Prentice Hall nursing diagnosis handbook* (9th ed.). Upper Saddle River, NJ: Prentice Hall.

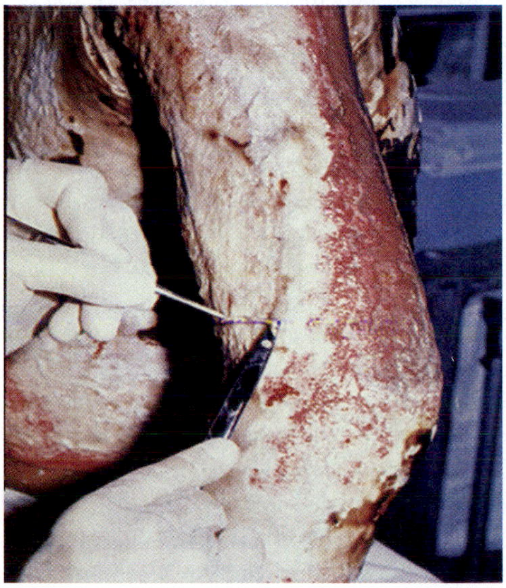

FIGURE 61–9 ◆ Débridement of eschar.
Source: Robert M. Faggella, Jr., MD, FACS.

digest necrotic tissue, such as Elase (Parke-Davis Division of Warner-Lambert Co., Morris Plains, New Jersey), a combination of two lytic enzymes in a petroleum base. Enzymatic débridement agents must be applied only within the open wound and must be discontinued once the eschar has all been removed and granulation tissue is present. More extensive wound débridement is done in surgery by excising the burn wound. The techniques used to remove eschar are discussed in the "Surgical Management" section later in this chapter.

Shaving, Culturing, and Photographs

With the exception of the eyebrows, body hair is shaved within the wound itself and up to 2.5 centimeters from the periphery of the wound. This is done to avoid wound contamination because hair attracts and shelters bacteria. Wound culturing is typically done on admission to obtain baseline information and is repeated approximately every 7 days unless the wound becomes symptomatic with exudate and odor. Culturing protocols are specific to the institution and health care provider. Photographs are taken on admission to provide baseline data and then repeated periodically throughout the healing process.

Escharotomies

During the initial phase of management, a surgical intervention may be required to maintain adequate circulation to the underlying tissues. Burn-induced changes in capillary permeability and the infusion of large volumes of crystalloid solutions to maintain vascular volume cause edema to form beneath the inelastic eschar. If a full-thickness injury involves an entire circumferential area, the edema creates a tourniquetlike effect and diminishes or completely cuts off circulation distal to the injury site. If left untreated, there is a high risk for tissue necrosis and, in some instances, total loss of the tissue including limbs. Doppler ultrasound signals are often used to assess perfusion in the involved areas. Loss of ultrasound signals is an indication for an escharotomy. Incisions or **escharotomies** are made through the burn tissue to relieve the constricting effects of the edema. These incisions should extend the entire length of a full-thickness injury, including joints, to ensure release of neural and vascular compression (Figure 61–10◆). The incisions penetrate the eschar and the immediate subadjacent connective tissue to permit expansion of the edematous underlying tissue. Frequent

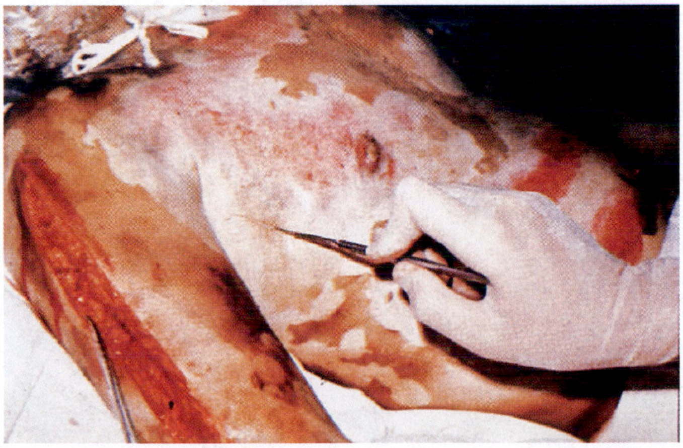

FIGURE 61–10 ◆ Escharotomy.
Source: Robert M. Faggella, Jr., MD, FACS.

monitoring of the circulation distal to the escharotomy site is part of the ongoing nursing assessment and includes pulses, tissue color (including paleness and cyanosis), sensation, increased pain, capillary refill, and decreased temperature. Often it is necessary to monitor circulation every 15 to 20 minutes. If distal blood flow does not improve, a second escharotomy is needed. Typically, no anesthesia is required because full-thickness injuries have little or no sensation, and blood loss is generally minimal and readily controlled with pressure.

Circumferential burns of the neck and chest may occlude the airway and decrease chest expansion and pulmonary function, resulting in respiratory distress. A chest escharotomy may be needed to restore a patent airway and effective ventilation. Monitoring respiratory effort is a critical part of the initial nursing assessment and includes respiratory rate, oxygen saturations, ABGs, cyanosis, lung sounds, and shortness of breath (see Chapter 25 for complete respiratory assessment). Mechanical ventilation may be necessary owing to low tidal volumes (Chapter 28). In Figure 61–11 ◆, the dashed lines are the preferred sites for escharotomy incisions. The solid segments emphasize the importance of extending the incisions across joints when there is a full-thickness injury.

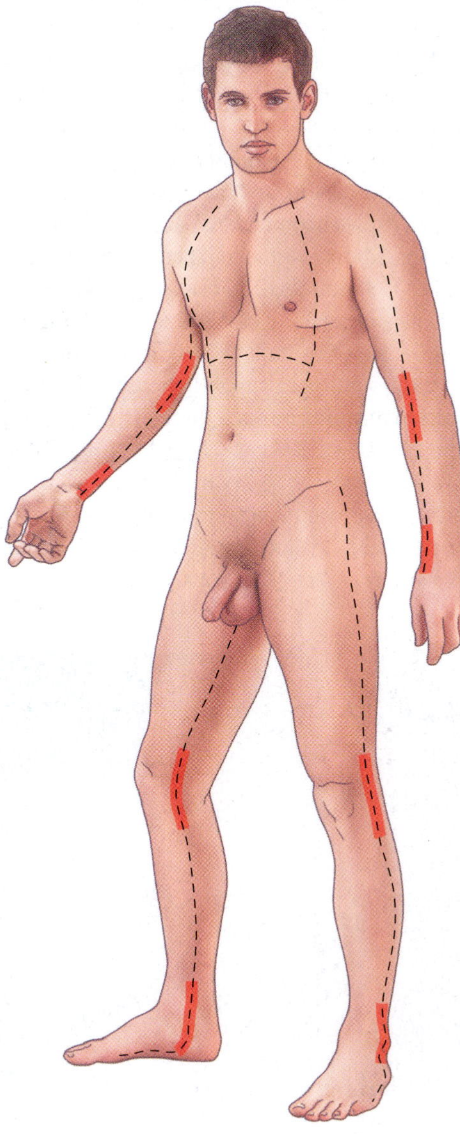

FIGURE 61–11 ◆ Common escharotomy sites.

Fasciotomy

On rare occasions, an incision of the muscle fascia beneath the burned tissue is required to restore circulation in a burned limb. This procedure is required for very deep burns involving the fascia and muscle, for associated traumatic limb injuries, and for high-voltage electrical injury. Stony, hard edema of the muscle compartments and absence of peripheral pulses distal to the site of the electrical contact should prompt immediate fasciotomy and exploration of the muscle compartments. The circulation can be assessed with a Doppler ultrasound.

Safety Alert *Assessment of pulses, capillary refill, and color of the area distal to the escharotomy is critical. Any changes in the circulatory status need to be reported to the health care provider immediately. If an escharotomy is done in the chest area, close monitoring of breath sounds is essential to assess gas exchange. Escharotomies may be needed until the swelling subsides.*

Application of Topical Antibiotics

The use of topical antibiotics started in the late 1940s when infection was the leading cause of death for patients with burns. The overall objective in the use of these agents is to prevent infection and to penetrate the burn wound. The penetrating action helps the eschar to separate from the deep viable tissue, and the antimicrobial action of the topical agents assists in preventing infection. These agents are usually applied once or twice daily after the wound has been cleaned and débrided. The Pharmacology box outlines the most commonly used agents. Silver sulfadiazine appears to be the most frequently used medication in the United States, although a number of health care providers use a combination of drugs to maximize antimicrobial protection and minimize the associated side effects (Urden, 2009).

Two techniques are commonly used for antibiotic application. With the open method, the antibiotic cream is applied directly to the wound with a gloved hand, and the wound is left open to the air. Ointment is reapplied as necessary to ensure constant coverage. This method is used most frequently for the face and ears. The advantages are better visualization of the wound, easier mobility and joint ROM, lower cost, and simplicity of wound care. Disadvantages include an increased risk of hypothermia with extensive injuries and easy removal of the ointment with patient activity. The second method is referred to as the closed method, in which either the antibiotic cream is applied directly to the wound with a gloved hand and then covered with a dry gauze dressing or the dressing itself is impregnated with the cream and then applied to the wound. Even though there is less mobility with the closed method, the advantage is less heat and fluid loss from the wound surface.

Special Care Sites

Special care must be taken in treating burns in and around the eyes because the skin in that area is very thin and delicate. In cleansing and applying topical antibiotics there, the nurse must take care to keep the cleanser and the antibiotic cream out of the eye itself to help prevent conjunctivitis. The nose is another area where special consideration is needed because full-thickness burns of the nose could lead to a loss of tissue and cartilage. Débridement and cleansing must be gentle, and the nurse should monitor any nasal tubes for placement to prevent erosion of nasal tissue. Burns of the ears also require special attention because the skin overlying the external ear is thin and prone to infection. This area must be cleansed gently and inspected frequently for infection. Pillows and gauze dressing beneath the head are contraindicated for burns of the ear because the external pressure could decrease circulation and lead to pressure necrosis. Burns of the fingers and toes require an

PHARMACOLOGY Summary of Topical Medications Used for Burns

Medication Category and Action	Application/Indication	Nursing Responsibility
Silver sulfadiazine (Silvadene) ***Action:*** Broad-spectrum antimicrobial with limited penetration ability.	Deep partial- to full-thickness burns. Wound infection.	Apply 1/4 inch thick using either open or closed dressing method, 2–3 times daily. Discontinue when eschar has all been removed. Not painful—soothing.
Silver nitrate ***Action:*** Broad-spectrum antimicrobial; poorly penetrates eschar.	Deep partial- to full-thickness burns. Wound infection.	Apply using either open or closed dressing method. Will turn wound black and is painful.
Mafenide Acetate (Sulfamylon) ***Action:*** Bacteriostatic for gram-positive and gram-negative organisms; penetrates thick eschar and cartilage.	Deep partial- to full-thickness burns. Wound infection.	Apply 1/4 inch thick using either open or closed dressing method, 2–3 times daily. Painful.
Petroleum- and mineral-based antimicrobials (Neosporin, Bacitracin) ***Action:*** Mild bactericidal for gram-positive and gram-negative organisms; poor penetration.	Partial-thickness burns.	Maintain adequate layer to prevent wound drying.

individual dressing for each digit to help prevent contracture formation in the web space. Finally, deep burns in which bone and tendons are exposed must be kept moist until complete wound coverage is achieved. This requires the use of moist dressings, which must be changed every 4 to 8 hours.

Temporary Dressings

Biologic, biosynthetic, synthetic, and composite dressings are useful as temporary coverings for burn wounds. Selection of the agent to be used depends on the condition of the wound, the inherent properties of each agent, and the goals of treatment. Chart 61–4 outlines the common agents, their indications for use, and the associated nursing care.

- **Biologic dressings** include **heterografts,** which are composed of tissue from another species, such as pigskin, or **allografts,** which are obtained from living or deceased humans. Heterografts are usually impregnated with silver nitrate to retard bacterial infection. Both of these dressings mimic human skin and are used for several purposes, including covering clean superficial or partial-thickness wounds, protecting granulation tissue or excised ungrafted wounds, preventing fluid and temperature losses, and testing the receptivity of the wound for **autografting** (use of the patient's own skin). As seen in Figure 61–12◆, pigskin (black) is being used when there is not enough of the patient's own skin to cover the wound. Allografts harvested from human cadavers are stored in skin banks located throughout the United States. Typically, an allograft is rejected by the body within 14 to 21 days following application. During the dressing, the nurse assesses, trims, and removes the biologic dressings where healing has occurred.
- **Biosynthetic dressings,** a combination of biologic and synthetic materials, are effective as a temporary covering for a variety of wounds. One of the more common biosynthetic dressings is Biobrane (Dow B. Hickman Pharmaceuticals, Inc., Sugar Land, Texas), which has been effective in the treatment of superficial partial-thickness burns such as scalds and as a donor-site dressing. A **donor site** is the area on the body where the skin is surgically harvested to use for covering burn wounds. Biobrane (Figure 61–13◆) is a semitransparent dressing that is typically soaked in 0.9% normal saline, stretched over the wound, and secured with staples, tape, and/or Steri-Strips. Once it has been applied, the patient can use the involved area, such as hands, for performing activities of daily living. As the wound heals, the Biobrane loosens and is trimmed away.

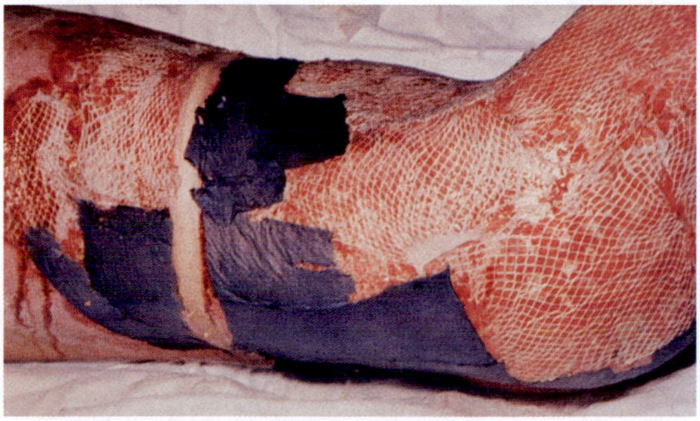

FIGURE 61–12 ◆ Black pigskin and meshed skin grafts.
Source: Robert M. Faggella, Jr., MD, FACS.

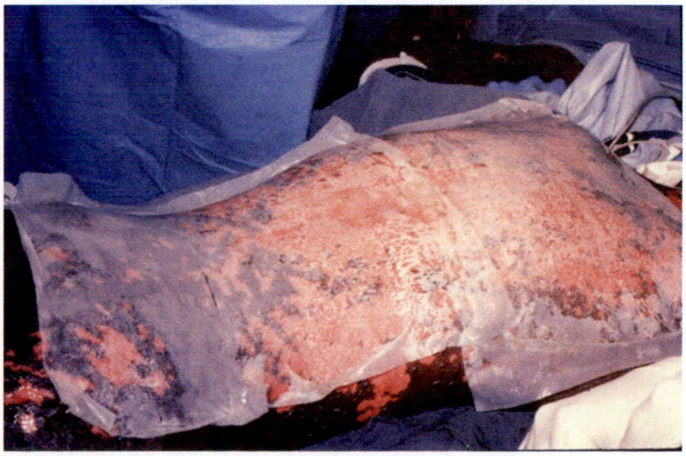

FIGURE 61–13 ◆ Application of Biobrane.
Source: John M. Osborn, MD, FACS.

CHART 61–4 Temporary Coverage for Burn Wounds

Covering	Description	Indications/Uses	Nursing Care
Biologic Dressings			
Xenograft (heterograft)	Porcine (pigskin).	Clean partial-thickness injuries. Débrided full-thickness injuries.	If left covered with gauze dressings, may be used for the first 24 hours.
Allograft (homograft)	Human cadaver skin harvested within 24 hours of death and preserved by refrigeration and cryopreservation.	Protect excised wounds and test for receptivity of wound bed for autograft.	If left covered with gauze dressings, used to protect site and absorb drainage.
Biosynthetic Dressings			
Biobrane	Collagen-embedded nylon fabric partially bonded to a silicone film.	Partial-thickness injuries. Secured to wound with staples, Steri-Strips, or gauze. Will adhere to wound.	Remove dressing once Biobrane has adhered to wound—left open to air. Trimmed away as wound healing occurs.
Calcium alginate	From alginates found in brown seaweed.	Exudative wounds. Split-thickness donor sites.	Applied to wound after irrigation and covered with absorbent dressing. Changed when cover dressing is saturated.
Synthetic Dressings			
Thin-filmed dressings: OpSite Tegaderm Bioclusive	Semipermeable, adherent polyurethane film dressings.	Protect and facilitate healing in small, clean partial-thickness burns. Cover partial-thickness donor sites.	Dressing needs to have intact skin margins to adhere to the dressing. Does not need dressing over the top unless draining exudate. Remove when wound healed.
Composite dressings: Lyofoam	Polymeric dressings designed to provide a moisture-retentive, absorbent, insulating environment.	Cover moderate to highly exudative wounds.	Placed directly over exudative wounds and covered with absorbent dressing. Dressing change frequency depends on amount of exudate.
Nonadherent dressings: Xeroform	Fine mesh gauze impregnated with 3% bismuth tribromophenate. Mild antimicrobial.	Clean partial-thickness wounds. Provides protective barrier, and promotes epithelial growth.	Monitor for and maintain adherence to wounds. Change if nonadherent. Monitor for infection.
Scarlet Red	Fine mesh gauze impregnated with lanolin, olive oil, petrolatum, and red dye.	Promotes epithelial development and protects wound.	Applied to clean partial-thickness injury. Applied in surgery to donor sites.

A biosynthetic dressing that is more commonly used in the United Kingdom is calcium alginate. This product is manufactured from seaweed and contains calcium, which reacts with the sodium in the wound, creating a protective gel. This dressing is able to absorb as much as 20 times its own weight in wound fluid while creating a warm, moist environment for healing. Calcium alginate typically is used for exudative wounds and for split-thickness donor sites. After the wound has been irrigated, calcium alginate is applied and covered with a dressing. The dressing is changed when it is saturated.

- **Synthetic dressings** are also used. There are three general categories of synthetic dressings: thin filmed, composite, and nonadherent.

The thin-filmed dressings are composed of polyethylene and, when applied, provide a transparent, moisture-retentive, waterproof environment that promotes wound healing. These dressings are useful only for the treatment of superficial, clean partial-thickness burns and to cover donor sites. Commonly used products are OpSite, Tegaderm (3M, Medical Division, St. Paul, Minnesota), and Bioclusive (Johnson & Johnson, Arlington, Texas).

Composite dressings (Lyofoam) are foam dressings used in the treatment of exudative burn wounds and graft sites. One layer of the dressing wicks away exudate while another layer maintains a moist environment that facilitates wound healing.

Nonadherent fine mesh gauze dressings are used to cover clean partial-thickness wounds, new split-thickness skin grafts, and donor sites. The dressings are applied directly over the wound and then changed if they fall off. If used for donor-site covering, they are covered with an outer dressing, which typically remains in place for 24 hours. Once the outer dressing is removed, the fine mesh gauze remains in place for 5 to 7 days and is allowed to dry out and loosen as healing occurs. If the dressing is used for skin grafting, a single layer is applied over the graft site, reinforced with several layers of coarse mesh gauze, and left in place for 5 to 7 days. Nonadherent dressings include Xeroform gauze (Kendall Inc., Mansfield, Massachusetts) and Scarlet Red ointment dressing (Sherwood Medical, St. Louis, Missouri).

See Chart 61–4 for a summary of the temporary coverings for burn wounds.

Infection Assessment

Early recognition of a wound infection is critical in limiting morbidity and mortality. Because of immunosuppression and open wounds, the patient with burns is at a high risk for the development of an infection. Wound infection is defined as the presence of bacteria, fungi, or viruses in or around the open wound. The nursing management plan to prevent infection includes (1) vigilant monitoring for signs and symptoms of infection and sepsis, (2) maintaining a hygienic environment to reduce the presence of microorganisms, (3) use of aseptic technique for wound care and invasive procedures, and (4) timely administration of both systemic and topical antibiotics. Daily assessment of the wound is primarily a nursing responsibility. When dressings are removed, the wound is assessed for changes in wound exudate (color, odor, and amount), signs of cellulitis (inflammation/erythema of surrounding tissue), increased wound pain, and loss of previously healed skin.

If infection goes undetected or untreated, it can progress to a deeper wound infection, leading to sepsis. Infection also can convert a partial-thickness injury into a full-thickness injury. Characteristics of an invasive infection include focal, dark, red, brown, or black discoloration in the eschar; rapid conversion (necrosis) of an area of partial-thickness injury to full-thickness injury; early, rapid separation of the eschar (fungal infection characteristic); and hemorrhagic fat necrosis.

Preventing the introduction of exogenous organisms, which cause infection, requires strict adherence to standard precautions and strict aseptic technique. The nurse must assess all personnel and visitors entering the patient's room for the presence of infection. In addition, he should place a sign on the patient's door indicating that visitors who are sick must not enter.

Hyperbaric Oxygen Therapy

Hyperbaric oxygen therapy (HBO) is a means of providing additional oxygen to the tissues by placing the patient's entire body under increased atmospheric pressure in a closely monitored airtight chamber. During HBO therapy, the patient breathes 100% oxygen for a predetermined period of time. Hyperbaric oxygen therapy has been used for split-thickness skin graft acceptance, flap survival and salvage, wound reepithelialization, and acute thermal burns. Research continues regarding HBO's impact on wound healing to try to take advantage of the angiogenic properties of increasing oxygen gradients resulting from hyperbaric therapy (Shah, 2010).

Surgical Management

The surgical management of burn injuries is a complex process involving a sequence of carefully planned surgical stages. The process begins with surgical débridement of damaged tissue, followed by wound closure using a number of techniques described next.

Burn Wound Excision

Historically, treatment for full-thickness injuries involved waiting for the eschar to separate over time with cleansing and débridement. The patient was then taken to surgery for grafting to close the open wound. This method of treatment was associated with frequent wound infections; prolonged, painful daily débridement and dressing changes; and lengthy hospital stays. Since the late 1970s, surgical techniques have been developed to excise eschar, allowing early closure of the burn wound. Early surgical débridement and grafting have decreased the length of hospital stay, decreased the number of septic episodes, and improved survival rates.

Two types of excision are used for burn wounds: tangential excision and fascial excision. Tangential excision, the most frequently used procedure, involves the sequential removal of thin layers of eschar until viable dermis or subcutaneous fat is exposed. The depth of the excision is determined by the appearance of healthy tissue and bleeding from dermal or subcutaneous beds. The goal is to create a clean living wound bed with circulation to support graft adherence. The advantage of tangential excision is decreased risk of infection due to early closure and better preservation of surrounding tissues and body contours, resulting in a better cosmetic result. The disadvantage is that blood loss may be considerable if large surface areas are tangentially excised.

Fascial excision involves removal of eschar and the underlying subcutaneous tissue to the level of the muscle fascia. This technique is usually reserved for patients with very deep, life-threatening burns, typically from electrical injury. The advantages of this technique include less blood loss, creation of a viable graft bed, and less time required for surgery. The disadvantages include an unsightly cosmetic deformity, loss of superficial nerves, near complete cutaneous denervation, and a high incidence of distal edema when the excision is superficial.

Burn Wound Closure

Burn wounds are usually closed with cutaneous autografts. Split-thickness skin grafts and occasionally full-thickness skin grafts can be used to accomplish closure. The skin grafts are harvested from the patient's healthy tissue and applied to the burn wound.

Harvesting of Skin

Harvesting of skin is accomplished by two methods, and the choice of which to use depends on the desired depth of graft. **Full-thickness skin grafts** are removed surgically by excising the entire thickness of the donor skin to the level of the subcutaneous tissue, typically 0.025 to 0.3 inch thick. Donor sites need to be closed by either sutures or split-thickness skin grafts; therefore, full-thickness grafts are limited to the repair of small wounds or defects. The advantage of this technique is that it permits the transfer of the entire dermal layer, resulting in greater durability and less wound contracture than the split-thickness grafts. Full-thickness skin grafts are used most frequently for areas that require thicker skin to prevent breakdown, such as the palm of the hand, the bottom of the foot, and the areas over joints. Full-thickness grafts also are used for facial defects because there is less contracture formation with these grafts and a better cosmetic result.

The more common method for covering a burn wound is a **split-thickness skin graft,** which is a partial layer of skin, including the epidermis and part of the dermis. The skin is harvested from the patient's donor site with a surgical instrument called a dermatome. The dermatome is guarded, making it easier to control the thickness of the harvested skin, which is usually 0.008 to 0.012 inch thick (Figure 61–14◆).

When the skin has been harvested, it can be used as either a sheet skin graft or a meshed skin graft. To make a **meshed skin graft,** holes are cut in the harvested skin, which allows it to be stretched over a greater surface area. To mesh the graft, the harvested skin is placed on a plastic template and guided through a mechanical meshing apparatus,

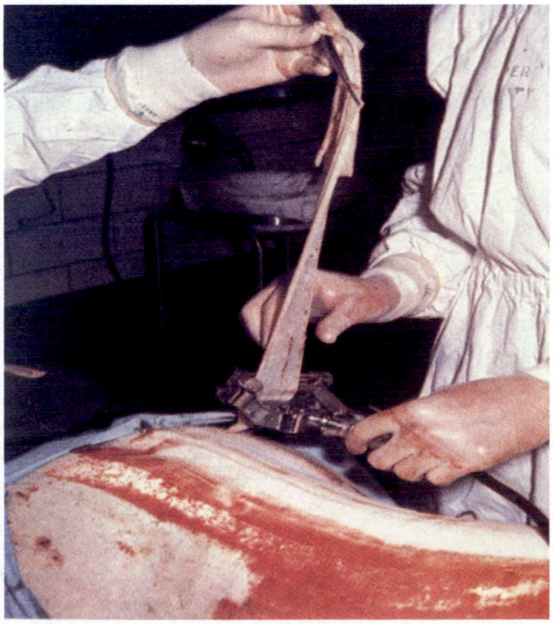

FIGURE 61–14 ◆ Dermatome harvesting skin.
Source: Courtesy of Robert M. Faggella, Jr., MD, FACS.

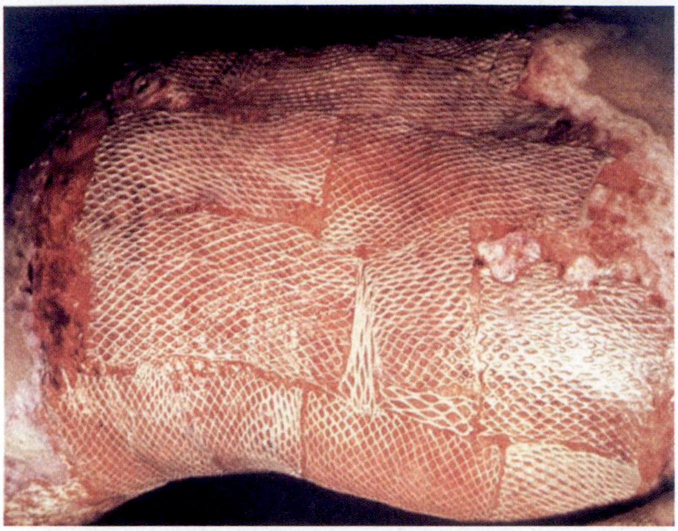

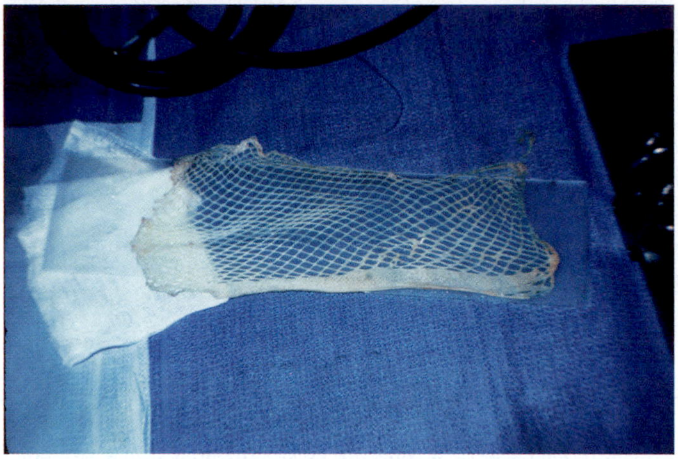

FIGURE 61–15 ◆ 3:1 meshed skin graft.
Source: (top): Robert M. Faggella, Jr., MD, FACS; (bottom): John M. Osborn, MD, FACS.

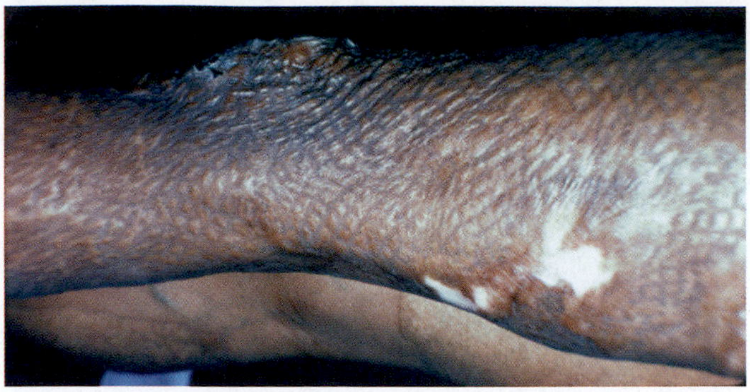

FIGURE 61–16 ◆ Healed meshed skin graft.
Source: John M. Osborn, MD, FACS.

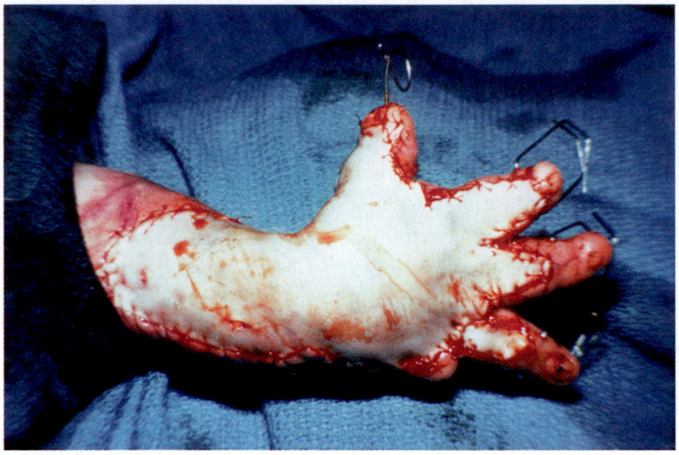

FIGURE 61–17 ◆ Sheet skin grafts.
Source: John M. Osborn, MD, FACS.

thereby cutting the diamond-shaped pattern of holes (Figure 61–15◆). By being meshed, the skin graft can be increased to two to nine times its original size, depending on the size of the holes. Skin grafts that are expanded beyond four times their original size, referred to as 4:1, require longer healing time, have a greater propensity for scar formation, and are usually used only for patients with massive injuries and limited donor sites. The holes in the graft will close over time by epithelialization from the skin edge. With meshed split-thickness skin grafts, there is less of a concern that blood and serous fluid will collect under the grafted area; thus, the percentage of graft adherence is increased. The disadvantage of this method is that the epithelial scar forms in the shape of a diamond, producing a characteristic checkerboard appearance. Figure 61–16◆ demonstrates the appearance of healed meshed grafts.

Split-thickness grafts that have not been meshed are referred to as **sheet skin grafts** (Figure 61–17◆). Sheet grafts provide a better cosmetic and functional result and should be used when adequate donor sites are available. Priority areas for using sheet grafts, if the burn is small, include the head, face, hands, neck, upper torso in women, and joint surfaces for growing children. A disadvantage of sheet grafts as compared to meshed grafts is that when blood, bacteria, and serous drainage collect under the graft, it has difficulty adhering to the wound surface. Both sheet and meshed skin grafts initially adhere to the wound by means of surface tension and later because of fibrin formation. Within 48 hours, circulation begins to occur, as evidenced by an increasing pink or red color on the graft surface. Depending on the preference of the surgeon, grafts may be sutured or stapled in place. Loss of the skin graft may occur for several reasons. First, hematoma or seroma formation beneath the graft will prevent it from adhering to the wound surface. During the first few days following surgery, the sheet grafts must be examined frequently so that subgraft hematoma or seroma formation can be removed either by needle aspiration, incising the graft to express blood and fluid, or by physically pulling a hematoma through an incision with forceps. Fluid collecting under the graft can be rolled to the side with cotton-tipped applicators. Second, persistent motion of the grafts will prevent vascular connections and graft adherence; therefore, the grafted area must remain immobilized. Splinting of the grafted area ensures immobilization of the graft for the first few days. Normal movement may be resumed at approximately 5 days, depending on the area involved and the health care provider's preference. Finally, an infection in the grafted area will create exudate under the graft and prevent graft adherence. The wound surface should be completely clean and free of infection at the time of graft application. All health care personnel must use strict aseptic technique when caring for the skin grafts.

Cultured epithelial autografting (CEA) is a method to obtain the patient's own skin when there is limited donor-site availability. Once a patient has been identified as a candidate, skin biopsies (usually 2 to 3 centimeters long by 1 centimeter wide) are taken from nonburned tissue and sent to a commercial company, where they are cultivated in a medium of epidermal growth factor. This tissue is grown for 18 to 25 days until it has expanded to 10,000 times its original size. The cultured grafts are returned to the burn center and applied surgically by using the same procedure as for split-thickness skin grafts. Enough CEA to cover an entire body can be grown in 24 days; however, there continue to be limitations to its use. The skin grown by this process has no dermal layer; therefore, it is thin and friable and thus is susceptible to breakdown and contracture formation (Urden, 2009).

Donor Site Care

When skin is harvested from a donor site, a superficial partial-thickness wound is created (Figure 61–18◆). Healing occurs by epithelial migration in about 10 to 14 days. Donor sites can be reused approximately three to four times with a 10- to 14-day healing period between each use. As much as the size of the injury permits, the donor-site skin should be selected to match the recipient-site skin in texture and color.

The focus of care for the donor sites in the postoperative period is preventing infection. If the site becomes infected, it may convert from a partial-thickness injury to a full-thickness injury, which then must be grafted. Several dressing options are available for donor sites in the postoperative period. Currently, Vaseline gauze with bismuth, antibacterial polyurethane film, and silver-impregnated mesh are common donor-site dressings. A more traditional approach to donor-site care has been to use a dry fine mesh gauze or gauze impregnated with petrolatum or antimicrobial agents (i.e., Xeroform) to cover the donor site. The choice of donor-site dressing is made by the health care provider. See Chart 61–4 (p. 1950) for a description of the agents used to cover donor sites. As the donor site heals, it dries out (scab formation) and the dressing separates from the wound. The healing process takes about 10 to 14 days. The primary nursing goals are to allow airflow around the donor site to assist in the drying process and prevention of infection.

Donor sites may have a tendency to form hypertrophic scarring, especially in dark-skinned or very fair people. A single harvest from an individual area usually does not cause scarring; however, repeated harvesting from the same site increases the risk of scarring. After the donor site has healed, it requires the same long-term care as do burn wounds, such as avoiding the sun and using moisturizing creams. Some health care providers use pressure garments to reduce donor-site hypertrophy. Pressure garments are discussed later in the chapter.

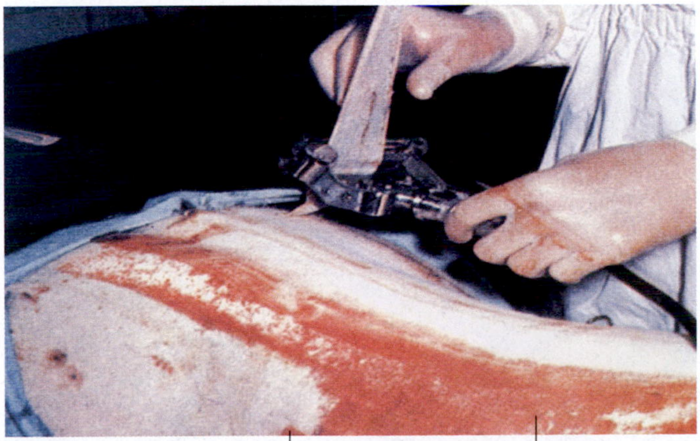

FIGURE 61–18 ◆ Donor site.
Source: Robert Faggella, Jr., MD, FACS.

Safety Alert *Nurses are primarily responsible for the prevention of infection in a donor site. Early detection and reporting of any signs of infection will help to prevent conversion of a donor site from a partial-thickness to a full-thickness injury.*

Alternative Skin Covering

In patients with large burn injuries, there is a limited amount of unburned skin that is suitable for autografting; therefore, available donor sites need to be used repeatedly. Several products that are currently available provide a deep dermal layer covering of the burn wound, which then can be covered with an ultra-thin split-thickness skin graft. Ultra-thin donor sites heal faster, minimize complications, and prepare the sites for reuse sooner when repeated autograft harvesting is necessary. AlloDerm and Integra (Integra Life Sciences Corporation, Plainsboro, New Jersey) are two products currently in use. AlloDerm is an acellular, nonimmunogenic dermal substitute derived from human cadaver skin (Urden, 2009). This product is meshed and applied to a full-thickness injury after the dead tissue has been excised. A thin split-thickness skin graft is placed over the AlloDerm during the same surgical procedure. AlloDerm is useful for wounds extending over joints where a thicker layer of skin will help prevent contractures, thereby increasing ROM. Integra is a two-layered skin substitute composed of an internal layer of collagen net and an external layer of silicone. After wound débridement, Integra is placed into the wound. It takes the dermal layer 2 to 3 weeks to become vascularized; then the outer layer is removed, and an ultra-thin split-thickness skin graft is applied (Figure 61–19◆).

If replacement of normal functioning skin is the goal for skin substitutes, there is no perfect skin substitute. Each of these products has limitations, and all are expensive to use. Further evaluation and testing are needed to improve the products' efficacy and bring down their cost.

Promoting and Maintaining Normal Mobility

As wound healing progresses, the need for promoting and maintaining mobility increases and changes. The goal of therapy is to regain strength, endurance, and joint mobility in order to achieve optimal functioning. Therapeutic positioning, splinting, and ROM exercises are essential in meeting this goal and cannot be overemphasized. It is essential that the family be actively involved because the program needs to continue for at least a year after discharge.

Positioning

From the day of admission, therapeutic positioning is used to protect the patient's wounds, decrease edema, and counteract scar contraction. The anatomic sites where contracture formation is a risk must be

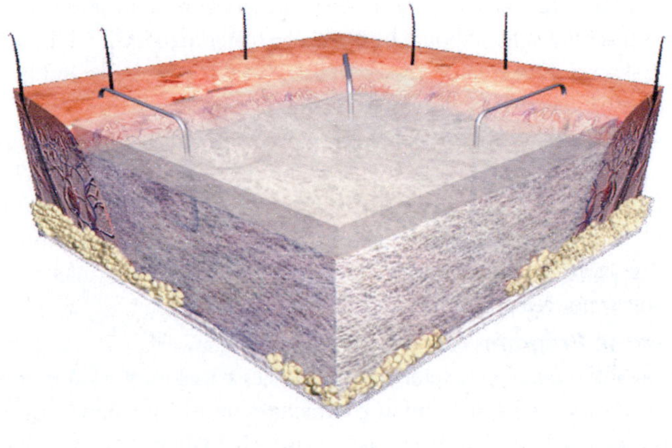

FIGURE 61–19 ◆ Integra.
Source: Courtesy of Johnson and Johnson Wound Management a Division of Ethicon, Inc.

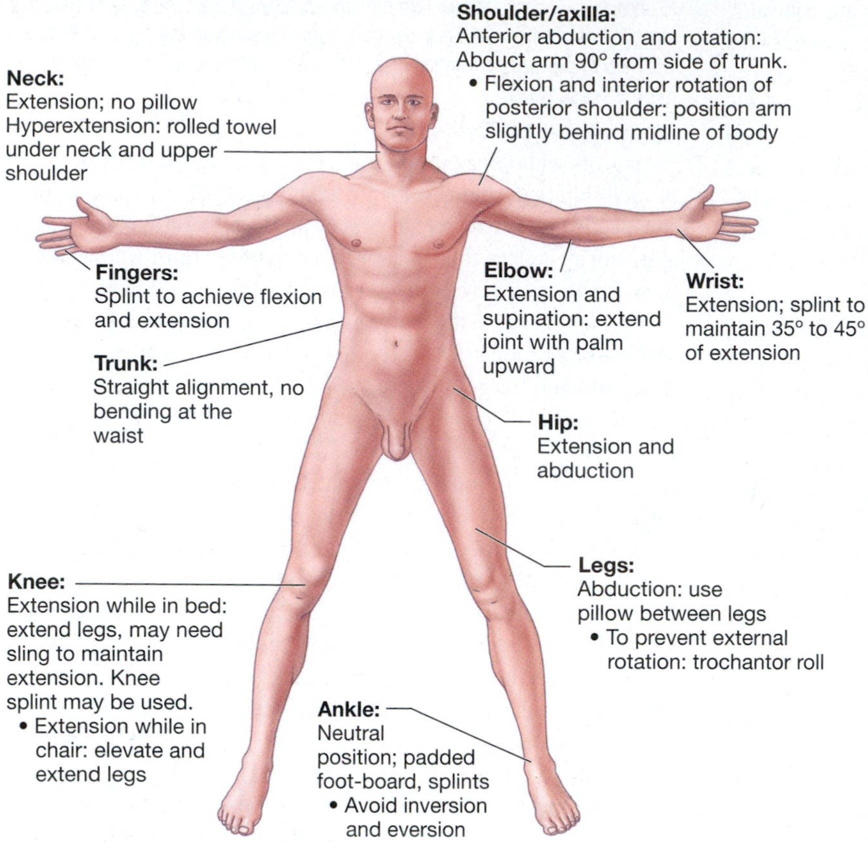

FIGURE 61–20 ◆ Common anticontracture positions.

identified in the early stages, and anticontracture measures must be instituted to counter scar contraction. Involved extremities are placed in a functional position, and joints are typically placed in extension. Figure 61–20◆ demonstrates the correct therapeutic anticontracture positions. Pillows, ropes, gauze rolls, linen, and pulleys are used to accomplish these positions. Finally, frequent position change is necessary to prevent skin pressure and breakdown. Beds with special mattresses and pressure-reducing capabilities are frequently used to prevent skin breakdown.

Splinting

Splinting begins as soon as possible after the injury for several reasons, including protection of joints and skin grafts, anatomic positioning to prevent contracture formation, and maintenance and elongation of scar length. Ideally, splints should be made of a material that allows them to be reshaped as edema decreases and the burn scar changes and heals (Figure 61–21◆). If the patient experiences pain, sensory impairments, or wound breakdown, the splint is removed and redesigned to prevent these complications. Padding of the splints decreases the occurrence of skin breakdown. Simple everyday items such as high-top shoes can be used for splinting purposes, and serial casting (e.g., casts are removed and replaced as the contour of the extremity changes) also can serve to maintain normal positioning of the affected areas.

Exercise Program

An active, progressive exercise program is essential to prevent permanent burn scars from forming contractures and to maintain normal ROM in affected joints. Exercise increases circulation and pulmonary function, decreases edema formation, offsets some of the manifestations of immobilization, and allows for the preservation of functional motor skills. The exercise program begins on the day of admission and continues until the scars have matured. Exercise is very difficult in the beginning because of pain, edema, and loss of tissue elasticity. Nonetheless, the health care team must assist the patient in understanding the importance of exercise despite painful limitations imposed by the injury.

Patients with burn injuries require varying levels of physical assistance depending on the extent of the injury and the patient's motivation. If weakness prevents the patient from reaching her true ROM, for example, assistance is provided to help the patient complete the motion. Referred to as active–assistive exercise, this method is frequently used with patients who have burn injuries. The active component provides the same benefits as active ROM exercises, and the assistive component facilitates complete, properly directed motion. Passive ROM exercises are used for patients who are unable to move on their own. These exercises also may be used to assess motion, maintain and mobilize joints and soft tissue, and minimize contracture formation.

The patient's ability to ambulate is affected by strength, endurance, pain, edema, and contracture formation. A progressive ambulation program is essential to prevent contracture formation and must begin as soon as the patient can tolerate it. Initially the program begins with sitting, followed by standing and pivoting, and then gradually ambulating. Before getting the patient out of bed, the nurse applies some type of elastic dressing or pressure garment to prevent orthostatic hypotension, venous stasis, and edema formation.

Nutritional Requirements

Nutrients are essential for normal healing, and inadequate nutrition has a negative impact on the immune response, wound healing, metabolic function, and survival. The key cause of ineffective wound healing is malnutrition (Cochran, 2010). At the time of the burn injury, patients experience extreme metabolic stress that is proportional to the size of the injury. After a burn injury, the resting energy expenditure increases by as much as 50% to 150% over that of the average trauma patient (Cochran, 2010). This hypermetabolic response and

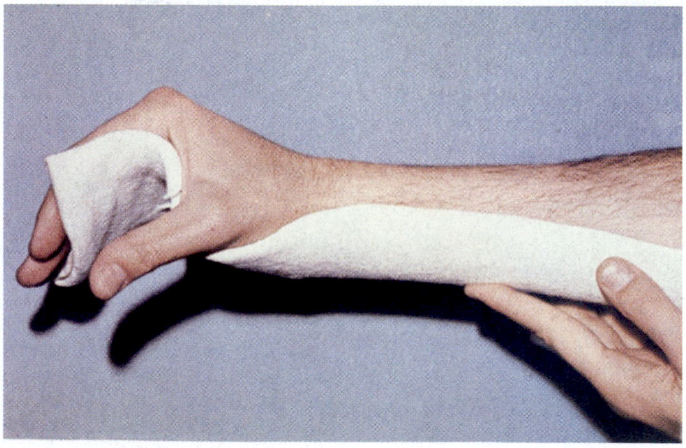

FIGURE 61–21 ◆ Arm splint.
Source: Robert M. Faggella, Jr., MD, FACS.

the mobilization of glucose are necessary for wound healing. Without adequate glucose, excessive protein catabolism occurs (Cochran, 2010; Urden, 2009). Therefore, early and adequate nutritional interventions are critical to the survival of the patient with burns. The hypermetabolic state tends to decrease in the weeks following the injury, but the metabolic rate does not return to normal until the wound is completely healed.

The goal of a nutritional replacement program during the acute phase is to provide adequate calories to promote wound healing (Cochran, 2010). A number of formulas are used to estimate the amount of calories needed to accomplish this goal. One generally accepted formula is (25 kilocalories × kilograms of body weight) + (40 kilocalories × % TBSA burn). It is not unusual for caloric needs to exceed 5,000 calories per day. The goal is to have the patient not lose more than 10% of his preburn weight. Calorie requirements need to be recalculated frequently because nutritional needs change with the healing process and changes in the hypermetabolic state. Specific nutrients needed for tissue repair include proteins, carbohydrates, lipids, and vitamins and trace minerals.

1. Proteins are needed for collagen synthesis, for wound remodeling, and for normal immune response. Protein loss, the stress of the injury, and tissue destruction all contribute negative nitrogen. There are differing opinions on the exact amount of protein needed to prevent proteolysis of lean body mass. The formulas used to calculate protein replacement generally estimate up to 2 grams of protein per kilogram per day.
2. Carbohydrates supply most of the energy needed for cell function and the immune response. Most practitioners believe that nonprotein energy intake should be primarily carbohydrates, with exogenous insulin added as clinically indicated to prevent hyperglycemia.
3. Lipids are essential in all nutritional regimens; however, because of the impact on the immune system, many burn centers use no lipids at all.
4. Vitamins and trace minerals are an integral part of the immune response, protein synthesis, and cell repair. They stimulate epithelialization, capillary budding and strength, and collagen formation, and they are cofactors in enzymatic reactions. The exact vitamin and mineral requirements for optimal healing differ among patients, although there are general guidelines for replacement. Patients with major burn injuries typically receive a multivitamin, 10,000 units of vitamin A, and 200 milligrams of zinc once per day and 500 milligrams of ascorbic acid twice per day, depending on the health care provider's preference (Cochran, 2010).

Whenever possible, patients with burns are encouraged to use the oral route for nutritional replacement. It is not uncommon, however, for patients to have difficulty consuming sufficient calories and protein by mouth. When this occurs, it is essential to meet the metabolic demand with additional supplements. Meals are supplemented with high-calorie (1 to 1.5 calorie/mL) snacks.

Many burn centers institute early enteral feedings within 24 hours of admission for any burn greater than 40% of the TBSA. Early feeding is believed to improve the gastrointestinal, immunologic, nutritional, and metabolic responses to the burn injury. Enteral feedings instituted before 18 hours after the injury have shown a significantly decreased mortality rate (Cochran, 2010). Typically the enteral feedings are trickled very slowly via a feeding tube, and patients are monitored closely for aspiration. The enteral route is preferred because it maintains the structural and functional integrity of the gastrointestinal tract (Cochran, 2010).

Regular monitoring of laboratory values related to adequacy of intake is essential. Total protein levels, complete blood count (CBC), glucose, iron, and prealbumin all indicate adequacy of nutrition. A complete discussion of nutritional replacement and monitoring is provided in Chapter 8.

Nursing Management

The aim of nursing care during the acute phase is to ensure optimal healing and prevent complications. Use of the nursing process will facilitate a comprehensive approach to patient assessment and care. The Nursing Process: Patient Care Plan box applies the pertinent nursing diagnoses and provides a comprehensive care plan for a patient with burns during the acute period.

Collaborative Management

Collaborative management for the acute phase of burn care continues to be pivotal to the recovery of the patient. The multidisciplinary team includes health care providers, nurses, physical and occupational therapists, social workers, psychologists/psychiatrists, and dietitians. In order to meet desired patient outcomes, it is essential that this interdisciplinary team communicate openly with one another in developing and evaluating care of the patient and family (IOM [Institute of Medicine], 2010). Each of these roles is discussed in the following section.

Rehabilitative Phase

The rehabilitative phase typically begins when there is less than 20% open wound and the patient is functioning at the highest possible level since admission. Depending on the size of the injury, the rehabilitative phase may begin as early as 2 weeks or as long as several years after the burn injury. During the rehabilitative phase, the patient with burns has stabilized physically and frequently is more aware of the long-term ramifications of the injury. Emphasis is placed on physical and psychological restorative therapy. Treatment aims include physical therapy to increase strength, endurance, function, and ROM; ongoing functional and cosmetic reconstruction; and psychological preparation for the patient's return to society. Pain management and nutrition are still concerns during the rehabilitative phase. Discharge planning and occupational preparation also are addressed during the rehabilitative phase.

Scar and Contracture Formation

With newly healed skin of partial-thickness wounds, there is minimal scar formation because the epidermis does not thicken. Patients may complain of dryness and itching in the newly healed areas, which are treated with frequent application of lotions and, in more severe cases, oral medication such as diphenhydramine hydrochloride (Benadryl). With a full-thickness injury, the dermal layer of skin has been affected, and the skin is repaired through scar formation. During the healing process, hypertrophic scars and contractures can form. **Hypertrophic scar** (Figure 61–22◆) formation is defined as an overgrowth of dermal tissue that remains within the boundaries of the wound. There is a higher risk of hypertrophic scar formation in areas of stress and movement such as the hands, chest, and legs. If the hypertrophic scar extends beyond the wound edges, it is referred to as a **keloid scar**

NURSING PROCESS: Patient Care Plan for the Acute Period of Burn Injury

Assessment of Integumentary Status Using Gordon's Functional Health Patterns:

- Activity Exercise Pattern
- Coping–Stress Tolerance Pattern

Subjective Data

Assessment of Fatigue and Ability to Perform Activities

Do you feel fatigued after physical activities?

Do you feel that you are gaining or losing strength as your burns heal?

Assessment of Mobility

How far are you able to ambulate?

Do you feel any change in the range of motion in the affected areas with exercise?

What is your understanding of the need for and importance of daily exercise?

Assessment of Ability to Perform Activities of Daily Living

To what extent are you able to take care of your physical needs?

Is this ability increasing as your wounds heal?

Do you have people who can help you after you are discharged?

Assessment of Patient and Family Coping Skills

What skills have you used in the past to cope with stressful situations?

What people in your life do you use for emotional support?

Tell me your perception of your injuries.

Tell me your perception of your limitations.

Objective Data

Assessment of Fatigue and Ability to Perform Activities

Heart rate, blood pressure, and respiratory rate increase with activity.

Strength and endurance change as burn wounds heal.

Ability to perform activities of daily living improves.

Assessment of Mobility

Range of motion in affected areas

Ability to perform active exercises

Wound healing progress

Patient and family's knowledge of need for continued exercise and splinting of affected areas

Assessment of Ability to Perform Activities of Daily Living

Ability to perform activities of daily living

Psychological motivation to function independently

Assessment of Patient and Family Coping Skills

Willingness to be compliant with therapy.

Determine patient's level of independence.

Assess effectiveness of support systems.

Outcomes and Evaluation Parameters	Planning and Interventions with *Rationales*
1. NURSING DIAGNOSIS: Activity Intolerance *related to severity of injury* (NANDA-I © 2012)	
Outcome: Increased endurance and energy conservation. ***Evaluation Parameters:*** Patient reports improvement in fatigue levels. Patient demonstrates more daytime wakefulness. Patient demonstrates ability to pace activities to conserve energy. Patient tolerates usual activities. Patient recognizes energy limitations. Patient balances activity with rest. Endurance level adequate for activity.	Discuss with the patient and family the relationship of burn injury to fatigue. *As wounds heal and nutritional state stabilizes, energy will increase.* Assess emotional, spiritual, and physical responses to activity. *To institute changes to plan if necessary.* Evaluate the patient's motivation and desire to increase activity. *To institute changes to plan if necessary.* Determine causes of fatigue. *To modify plan if necessary.* Monitor cardiorespiratory response to activity. *To assess appropriateness of activity level.* Monitor oxygen saturation response to activity. *To assess appropriateness of activity level.* Pace daily activities to conserve energy. *Prevent overexertion.* Ensure adequate nutritional support. *To increase strength and endurance.* Ensure sleep and rest period, record hours of sleep on record. *To increase strength and endurance.* Consult with physical therapist and occupational therapist to develop exercise program. *A progressive program to sustain progress.* Establish a conditioning program with patient-centered goals. *To increase compliance.*
2. NURSING DIAGNOSIS: Impaired Physical Mobility *related to burn wounds and contracture formation* (NANDA-I © 2012)	
Outcome: Joint movement normal for injury level. ***Evaluation Parameters:*** Patient verbalizes understanding of restricted activity. Patient maintains strength and position of function in all affected areas. No contracture formation.	Consult with the physical therapist and occupational therapist to formulate a plan for maintaining and increasing mobility. *A progressive program is necessary to sustain progress and prevent contracture formation.* Perform active and passive range-of-motion (ROM) exercises every 2 hours. *To prevent contracture formation.*

NURSING PROCESS: Patient Care Plan for the Acute Period of Burn Injury, *continued*

Apply splints as prescribed.

Maintain antideformity positions and reposition hourly (see Figure 61–20, p. 1954). *To prevent contracture formation.*

Elevate affected extremities. *To decrease edema.*

Maintain limbs in functional alignment. *To prevent contracture formation.*

Anticipate need for analgesia. *To increase mobility.*

Ambulate when stable. *Essential to begin activity program to increase endurance and decrease contracture formation.*

Assess for loss of ROM and muscle atrophy related to immobility. *High risk for contracture formation.*

Educate patient and family regarding rationale for imposed activity restrictions (i.e., recent skin grafting). *To prevent loss of skin graft.*

Provide diversional activities to increase compliance with immobility. *To prevent loss of skin graft.*

3. NURSING DIAGNOSIS: Readiness for Enhanced Self-Care *related to wounds and activity intolerance* (NANDA-I © 2012)

Outcome: Increasing ability to perform activities of daily living.

Evaluation Parameters: Verbalizes increased sense of control.

Demonstrates self-care activities within limits of functional ability.

Accepts assistance when needed.

Progressively increases mobility.

Consult with occupational therapist regarding the need for assistive devices. *These will increase self-care ability.*

Ensure the patient has adequate time to perform tasks at own pace. *Patients are slow and tentative in the beginning.*

Increase self-care activities as soon as possible. Ensure patient participation in planning care. *To decrease powerlessness and increase self-confidence.*

Monitor for changes in functional abilities. *To monitor progress.*

Instruct the patient and family on alternative ways to perform activities of daily living. *To increase patient and family involvement.*

4. NURSING DIAGNOSIS: Readiness for Enhanced Individual Coping *related to situational crisis, inadequate support systems, and unrealistic perceptions of recovery* (NANDA-I © 2012)

Outcome: Effective coping.

Evaluation Parameters: Patient and family:

Verbalize feelings.

Identify and utilize effective coping strategies, appropriate for injury status.

Identify ineffective coping strategies and patterns.

Seek information about injury, treatment, and prognosis.

Employ behaviors to reduce stress.

Report decrease in negative feelings.

Demonstrate impulse control.

Demonstrate normal information processing.

Recognize support systems.

Employ behaviors to reduce stress.

Report decrease in negative feelings.

Assess and determine degree of impairment. *To assist in the development of a plan to promote coping.*

Determine past coping skills. *To assist in the development of a plan to promote coping.*

Assess current coping skills. *To assist in the development of a plan to promote coping.*

Explore with the patient feelings about injury, and explore previous methods of dealing with life problems. *Assessment will assist in augmenting the patient's ability to cope, or it will determine the need for intervention.*

Identify the patient's view of injury and its congruence to the health care team's view. *To assess patient's perception of reality.*

Monitor aggressive behaviors. *A sign of ineffective coping and that intervention is needed.*

Identify the patient and family's view of the condition and how it relates to the actual condition. *Assesses how realistic their perceptions are. Determines where intervention is needed.*

Assess the patient and family's support systems. *May be used as a source of support.*

Evaluate impact on patient and family's life situation. *Loss of previous life function impacts coping.*

Determine risk for self-harm. *Severe alterations in body image and functional level place the patient at a high risk for self-harm.*

Provide factual information about diagnosis, treatments, and prognosis. *Realistic, factual information is essential to augment adjustment.*

Encourage verbalization of fears and let the patient know these reactions are normal. *To enhance open, factual communication.*

(*continued*)

NURSING PROCESS: Patient Care Plan for the Acute Period of Burn Injury, *continued*

Explain procedures. *To increase knowledge and decrease fear of the unknown.*

Assist the patient in dealing with changes in body image, and appraise adjustment. *To enhance adjustment.*

Discuss future treatment options for changes in body image. *To increase knowledge and decrease fear of the unknown.*

Encourage family and friends to participate in care. *Enhances adjustment of significant others.*

Consult psychologist if necessary. *To enhance adjustment.*

Note: The nursing diagnoses for the emergent care period are also applicable for the acute care period.

Source: Adapted from Wilkinson, J. M., & Ahearn, N. R. (2009). *Prentice Hall nursing diagnosis handbook* (9th ed.). Upper Saddle River, NJ: Prentice Hall.

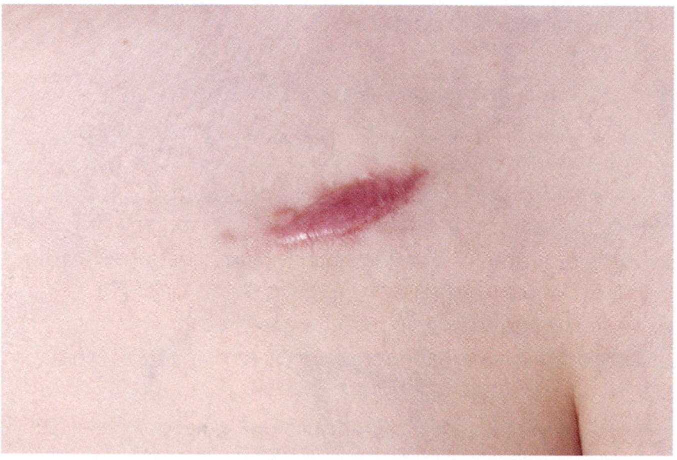

FIGURE 61–22 ◆ Hypertrophic scar.
Source: Dr. P. Marazzi/Science Source Photo Researchers, Inc.

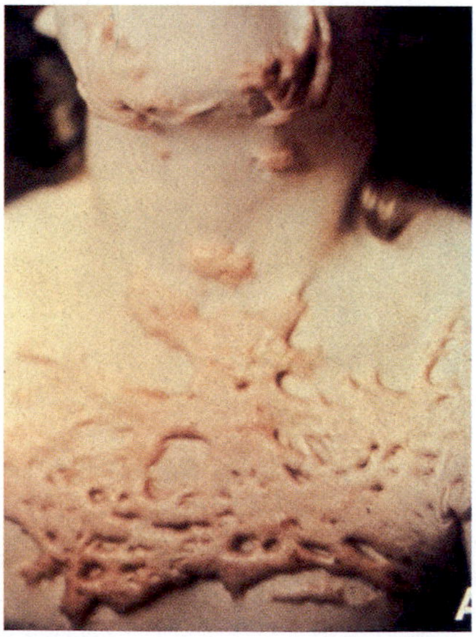

FIGURE 61–23 ◆ Keloid scar.
Source: Robert M. Faggella, Jr., MD, FACS.

(Figure 61–23◆). Areas of the body that are more prone to keloid formation include the chest, the presternal area, and the shoulders and deltoid region. Once keloid scars have formed, limited treatment is available. Current treatments that have experienced some success are injecting steroids into the scar and laser therapy. There is a genetic predisposition for the development of keloid scarring, which is discussed in the Genetic Considerations box.

GENETIC CONSIDERATIONS Keloid Scar Formation

There is a genetic predisposition for the development of keloid scar formation in individuals with darker pigmentation. African Americans have approximately a 15 times greater incidence of keloid formation in comparison to other racial groups. Recently, regions of the human genome were correlated with keloid formation in two pedigrees. The regions were in two separate locations on the human genome.

Sources: Berman, B. (2010). Keloid and hypertrophic scar. Medscape reference. Retrieved from http://emedicine.medscape.com/article/1057599-overview#a0199; Jansen, D. A. (2012). Keloids. Medscape reference. Retrieved from http://www.emedicine.medscape.com/article/1298013-overview.

During the healing process of full-thickness injuries, the burn scar shrinks and becomes inelastic, resulting in contracture of the wound. A contracture (Figure 61–24◆) is defined as a permanent shortening of connective tissue. Once formed, contractures resist stretching, limiting body motion and flexibility. Splinting, exercise, and constant pressure help prevent the formation and progression of contractures.

Exercise Program

As the burn wound heals, continual contraction of the scar creates the majority of the chronic problems. This contraction process causes a decrease in function in the involved area. Starting rehabilitation when the patient is admitted to a treatment center helps prevent contractures and diminishes the need for reconstructive surgery. The health care team uses several therapies to assist in preventing contracture formation. The

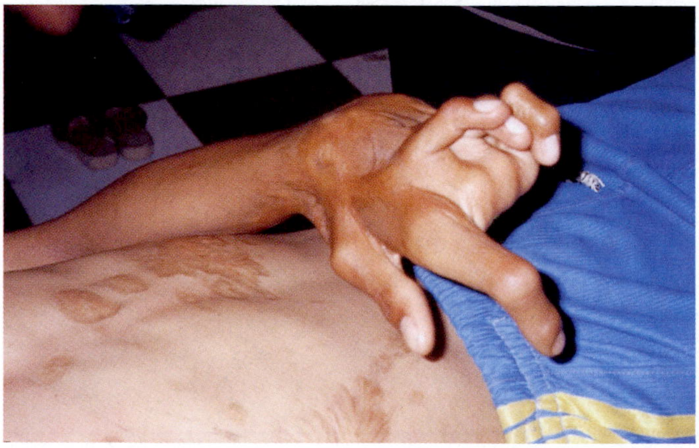

FIGURE 61–24 ◆ Contracture formation.
Source: Katie Osborn/John M. Osborn, MD, FACS.

exercise program includes promotion of functional skills, stretching exercises, and scar massage.

Functional Skills

Functional skills are defined as the specific motor abilities necessary to perform activities of daily living (ADLs) in order to function independently. In the beginning, exercises should focus on basic activities such as ambulating, hygiene, and self-feeding. During the rehabilitative phase, exercise programs are expanded to include the specific skills needed for functioning in the home and the job environment.

All exercise programs are progressive in order to increase the patient's strength and endurance. Protein catabolism associated with the burn injuries as well as days of immobility lead to a decrease in muscle mass and strength. It is important to remember that endurance and conditioning underlie the success of any exercise program. The patient needs to participate in exercise programs at regular intervals throughout the day, followed by periods of rest. It is the repetitive nature of the programs that builds strength and endurance and prevents contracture formation. ROM exercises are omitted for 3 to 7 days after skin grafting.

Stretching Exercises

Stretching exercises are used to elongate shortened soft tissue. The fundamental goal of a stretching program is to increase ROM. Stretching can initially be a passive or an active activity, although patients must learn to perform self-stretching exercises as they prepare for discharge. Stretching is done primarily after wound closure during the rehabilitative phase. The stretch should be gentle, slow, and sustained. Blanching of the scar is a sign of appropriate stretch. Immediately after a stretching session, effective positioning and splinting will maintain the elongation of the tissue.

Scar Massage

Completely healed burn wounds are massaged with oil or lotion to break down hardened areas, increase circulation, decrease hypertrophy, possibly increase ROM, and improve appearance. Massage is performed one to four times daily. In addition, patients and families are taught to continue scar massage after discharge.

Pressure Dressings and Garments

The use of pressure dressings and garments to decrease hypertrophic scar formation and increase wound pliability is a widely accepted practice (Figure 61–25◆) (Urden, 2009). The theory behind this practice is that the pressure from the dressing or garment causes ischemia, thereby decreasing collagen production, which thickens scars. In general, wounds that require more than 14 days to heal will scar and therefore should be placed in pressure garments. Elastic bandages are used initially for wound compression and edema formation. During the rehabilitative phase, before hypertrophy begins, patients are measured for custom-fit elastic garments that provide three-dimensional pressure on all affected areas (Urden, 2009). To be effective, the pressure exerted by the garment must exceed capillary pressure (25 mmHg). Pressure garments are worn continuously (23 hours per day) for several months to years, depending on the hypertrophic scarring. Periodic refitting is necessary to ensure proper fit and pressure. Even though the garments reduce scar formation, patient compliance—especially in hot weather—has long been an issue. Patient teaching needs to stress the benefits of the garments in an effort to increase compliance.

Functional and Cosmetic Reconstruction

Once burn scars have healed, certain surgical options are available to improve function and cosmetic appearance. Typically, reconstruction begins after the scar has matured, which takes about a year. However,

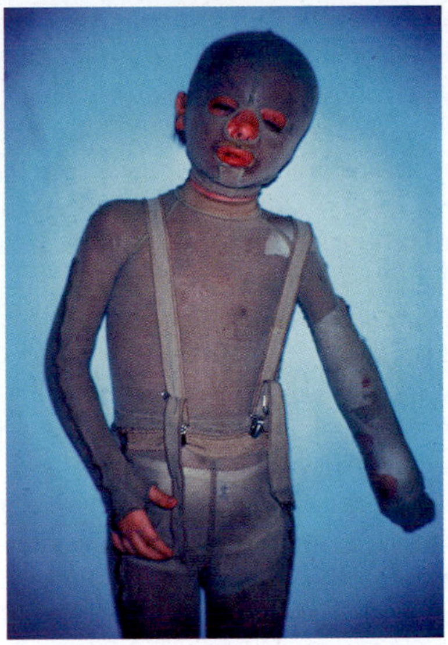

FIGURE 61–25 ◆ Compression garment.
Source: John M. Osborn, MD, FACS.

surgery may be indicated earlier if there is a serious functional impairment. Surgical intervention includes scar excision and/or scar realignment. Small hypertrophic scars can be completely excised in one surgery. Larger hypertrophic areas need serial surgeries to remove the scar segmentally, one portion at a time.

Scar realignment is a technique that is used when the scar develops in a different direction than the normal tissue. Abnormal scar alignment causes excessive wound contracture and decreased ROM in the area. Scars can be surgically reoriented to increase ROM and decrease the visibility of the scar. A Z-plasty, a scar revision technique that incorporates advancement and rotation flaps, is a common method utilized for scar realignment (Figure 61–26◆).

Psychological Recovery

Burn injuries that cause scarring, regardless of size, alter patients' perceptions of their body image. The patient's preinjury coping mechanisms have a major impact on how a patient copes following a burn injury. During the healing process, a number of psychological reactions occur. In the beginning stages of treatment during the emergency period, patients often use withdrawal and denial as coping mechanisms. These

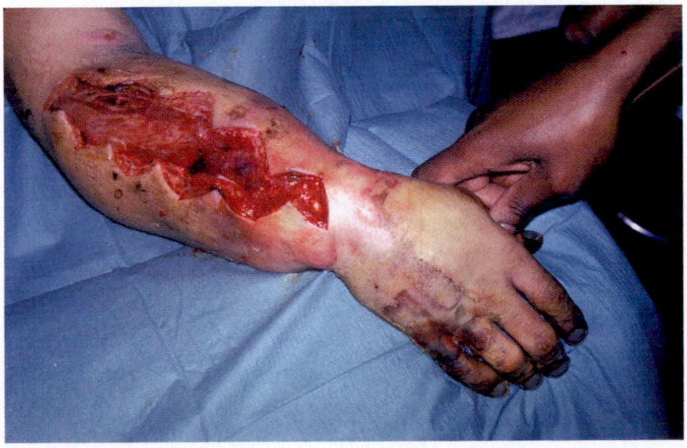

FIGURE 61–26 ◆ Z-plasty.
Source: John M. Osborn, MD, FACS.

patients tend to keep their eyes closed, remain immobile, and have little interaction with family and staff. Regression, another common reaction in the patient who is burn injured, is manifested by childlike behaviors such as dependence and temper tantrums. Other psychological reactions during the healing process may include anger, hostility, depression, and anxiety. These reactions are expressed in a number of ways including restlessness, agitation, sleep disturbances, hostility toward staff and family, and self-degradation. Post-traumatic stress disorder is being diagnosed with increasing frequency in patients with burns after discharge from the acute care setting (Nayback, 2009). The Ethical Issues box discusses some of the dilemmas that burn victims and their families, as well as the health care team, grapple with during recovery from burn injuries.

Grief is a natural and frequent reaction to burn injuries. Besides the change in body image, contributing factors to the grief reaction include loss of physical functioning, potential changes in occupation, and separation from home and family during extended treatment. The patient who is burn injured must be given an opportunity to express concerns and feelings about the change in body image and be reassured that this grieving process is normal and will eventually dissipate. The nurse's role is to be an active, nonjudgmental listener, allowing the patient time to express feelings and grieve the loss of the former self. The nurse must answer questions honestly, acknowledge the patient's difficulty with coping, and encourage positive behaviors. Patients typically cope better if they are kept informed of planned treatments and surgeries. It is anxiety producing to be faced with unexpected events, especially when the patient has had to give up most of his independence. Then, as wounds heal, the patient must resume control of as many activities and functions as is possible; the nurse plays an important role in encouraging and facilitating this.

Measures to assist the patient in coping with grief and loss include resuming activities of daily living and socializing with family and friends. These activities enhance the patient's self-efficacy and worth and give the patient more control. A combination of psychotherapy and pharmacologic treatments often are effective in promoting adjustment. Burn support groups have also been effective in promoting adjustment to the physical changes and helping with reentry into society.

The nurse must be sensitive to the patient's spiritual beliefs, which play an essential role in psychological recovery. The patient's faith often will help guide her in life, especially when a crisis has occurred, such as a burn injury. The health care team should evaluate the need for spiritual guidance and support with each individual patient and then follow through by providing a spiritual guidance counselor of the patient's choice (priest, minister, rabbi, etc.).

ETHICAL ISSUES in the Treatment of Burn Injuries

Burn injuries may involve a multitude of ethical issues related to the resuscitation, care, and rehabilitation of patients and their families. The nursing role is to advocate for the patient, be supportive of the decision, and provide the family with factual, realistic data about the patient's condition and medical interventions. Ethical dilemmas may arise for the nurse when it is difficult to support the patient's or family's decision for personal and/or professional reasons. The dilemma for the nurse may be the conflict between being a patient advocate, supporting the family's decision, and dealing with the nurse's own personal belief system. This is typically a very difficult ethical dilemma for the health care team. Team conferences may be held to discuss a team approach to care and a plan to provide consistency in the approach to patient care.

Specific ethical issues for patients who are burn injured and their families include the following:

- Quality of life after the injury, both immediate and long term
- Extent of resuscitation after a massive injury
- When to withhold or withdraw care
- Body image adjustment
- Dignified and comfortable death
- Psychological adjustment
- Considerations of futility
- Nonmaleficence
- Financial costs.

Pain Management

Pain markedly decreases with closure of the wound. However, small areas of open wound may still need dressing changes that are painful, and newly healed skin is sensitive. In addition, the exercise therapies are often painful owing to stiff, noncompliant skin in the affected areas. Therefore, pain management is still an issue and needs to be done individually and on an ongoing basis. Along with diversional activities and relaxation techniques, oral analgesics typically relieve the pain that the patient experiences in the rehabilitative phase. The patient's report of the absence of symptoms and/or an assessment of lack of pain behaviors, such as guarding, is necessary to assess when tailoring pain management therapies.

Nutritional Requirements

During the rehabilitative phase, the negative nitrogen balance and anorexia have resolved. Because the wound is still healing, high-calorie, high-protein diets are necessary. A nutritionist can assist with a nutrition plan to ensure adequate daily caloric intake. Promotion of independent eating also is important. If it is functionally difficult for the patient to eat because the burn injury involves the hands, occupational therapy is needed to obtain and educate the patient in the use of devices that will facilitate self-feeding. Finally, in preparation for discharge, the patient and family need instructions about meal planning and the reporting of difficulties such as cachexia, weight loss, and food intolerance. Chapter 8 discusses nutrition in detail.

Nursing Management

The aim of nursing care during the rehabilitative phase is to prepare the patient both physically and psychologically to return home and to work. Use of the nursing process will provide a comprehensive approach to achieve these goals.

Nursing Diagnoses

A number of nursing diagnoses may be applicable in the rehabilitative phase. The most significant diagnoses for the patient who is burn injured include the following:

- *Acute Pain,* related to wound healing and therapy
- *Impaired Skin Integrity,* related to healing wounds
- *Impaired Physical Mobility,* related to functionality of burned areas
- *Activity Intolerance,* related to deconditioning
- *Deficient Knowledge,* related to injuries and limitations
- *Disturbed Body Image,* related to burned areas and scar formation
- *Fear and Anxiety,* related to future procedures and reentry into society
- *Readiness for Enhanced Self-Care,* related to wound care and exercise regimen
- *Readiness for Enhanced Nutrition,* related to dietary needs for healing

NANDA-I © 2012

These diagnoses depend on the degree of disfigurement and loss of functional capacity, as well as the home environment and support systems. The patient's personal coping skills and ability to adapt to the change in body image also affect the applicable nursing diagnoses. Additional diagnoses related to the rehabilitative phase include the following:

- *Social Isolation* related to disfigurement and loss of function.
- *Readiness for Enhanced Family Processes* related to risk of role change and loss of earning capacity.
- *Readiness for Enhanced Individual Coping* related to ongoing maladjustment to burn injury.
- *Risk for Complicated Grieving* related to ongoing realization of extent of injury.
- *Noncompliance* related to wearing the elastic garments and continued need for physical therapy.
- *Disturbed Sensory Perception* related to sensory overload/deprivation and sleep pattern disturbance.
- *Impaired Home Maintenance* related to unavailable support system.

NANDA-I © 2012

Collaborative Management

The need to collaborate with all of the health care specialties continues in the rehabilitative phase. As the patient is prepared for discharge, each aspect of the physical and psychological needs is evaluated, and a plan is put in place to address them all. As is consistent with the entire hospital stay, the nurse coordinates the health care team to ensure that all aspects of care are addressed. In order to meet desired patient outcomes, it is essential that this interdisciplinary team communicate openly with one another in developing and evaluating care of the patient and family (IOM [Institute of Medicine], 2010).

The length of time that physical therapy and occupational therapy continue on an outpatient basis depends of the size and area of injury. The psychosocial needs of returning to society, family, and hopefully occupation are addressed by a psychologist or psychiatrist prior to discharge as well as on an ongoing basis after discharge. Because the hypermetabolic state continues until all the wounds are healed, the need for dietary consultation continues. Finally, the surgeons begin the reconstructive process, which may continue for months or years.

Health Promotion

To augment understanding, an organized, comprehensive teaching plan is necessary. Major burn wounds take 12 to 18 months to heal completely. Discharge instructions include care of both open and healed wounds. Normal manifestations of newly healed wounds include dryness, itching, and increased sensitivity to sunlight. Specific instructions for the patient and family need to stress how to assess the wound for complications such as newly formed open areas, blister formation, and signs and symptoms of infection. The instructions also need to include when and why it is necessary to notify the health care provider of complications. Discharge teaching plays a major role in preventing excessive scar and contracture formation. Comprehensive instructions are outlined in the Patient Teaching & Discharge Priorities box.

Occupational Recovery

Vocational adjustment is a common problem during the first year after discharge from the hospital. Often the patient has an extended recovery time after hospitalization before she is physically and emotionally ready to return to work. Additionally, due to disfigurement and functional limitations, the patient may be unable to resume her previous occupation. Therefore, the patient may need a referral to the local office of the state labor and industry board for information on job retraining programs. For many patients, vocational interest, aptitude, and psychological testing may be necessary to determine areas of occupational interest. Successful reentry into the work environment depends on developing a realistic plan, educating the patient and family, and engaging an employer in the process.

Discharge Priorities

Discharge planning is a complex process that begins when the patient is admitted to the hospital. An organized comprehensive plan of care with both short-term and long-term goals will ensure the highest level of recovery. As healing progresses, the patient and family need to be prepared for discharge. The ultimate goal is to return the patient to as close as is reasonably possible to the preinjury state.

PATIENT TEACHING & DISCHARGE PRIORITIES for Burn Management

Need	Teaching
Wound Care	Perform daily cleansing and dressing changes for open areas. Elevate areas where edema formation occurs.
Patient/family/support system	Avoid scratching the healed areas, as this could cause breakdown: • Encourage liberal use of emollient lotions for dryness and flaking. • Use diphenhydramine hydrochloride (Benadryl) for itching. • Keep fingernails short and use gloves when sleeping. Avoid sunlight, which can cause, among other things, healed wounds to discolor or darken permanently: • Avoid overexposure to sun. • Use sunscreen products when exposed to sunlight. • Use clothing and hats for added protection. Avoid exposure to extreme temperatures and harsh chemicals. Wear loose-fitting, soft clothing.

(continued)

PATIENT TEACHING & DISCHARGE PRIORITIES for Burn Management, *continued*

Need	Teaching
Setting	Assess availability of, knowledge of, and compliance with treatment regimen. Assess respite needs and resources. Assess discharge placement needs: home, rehabilitation facility, extended care facility. Assess home environment for need for assistive devices. Assess for professional home health needs. Assess the need for follow-up appointments.
Wound Infection	Assess for infection of open wounds and healed wound breakdown with each dressing change, and report as necessary.
Patient/family/support system	Signs and symptoms include: • Odor and exudate • Fever • Increased drainage • Swelling • Lack of wound closure. Apply antibiotic ointments as prescribed. Teach minimization of risk factors for infection.
Setting	Explain signs and symptoms that require medical attention. Assess environment for risk factors.
Nutrition Patient/family/support system Setting	Maintain a high-calorie, high-protein diet. Continue taking vitamins and mineral supplements as ordered. Observe for appetite and weight loss, as well as food intolerance. Taper calorie intake once preinjury or ideal weight has been achieved to prevent excessive weight gain. With professional guidance (i.e., physical therapist), institute an exercise program. Assess financial resources.
Pain Management Patient/family/support system Setting	Assess pain level and report any increase in pain. Assess effectiveness of pharmacologic interventions. Wean patient off pain medication when pain lessens. Assess environment for safety and promotion of therapeutic needs.
Sexuality Patient/partner Setting	Answer questions about sexual potential. Encourage both partners to express fears and concerns. Encourage privacy and a familiar environment.
Scar Formation Prevention and Exercise Program Patient/family/support system Setting	Stress and assess compliance with wearing of pressure garments 23 hours a day. • If pressure garment is too loose, it is ineffective; discontinue use and ensure patient receives a new garment. • If pressure garment is too tight, it can cause numbness, tingling, and skin breakdown; discontinue use and ensure patient receives a new garment. • Need two sets so the patient can wear a garment while the other is being cleansed. Ace wraps need to be worn per health care provider's order, usually when the patient is out of bed. Progressive passive and active range-of-motion (ROM) exercises. Progressive stretching and ambulation (walking). Progressive exercise program to increase overall stamina. Referral to physical therapy for development of an exercise program.
Emotional Adjustment Patient/family/support system Setting	Answer questions honestly. Encourage verbalization of frustrations and anger. Encourage positive reinforcement from the family. Encourage independent functioning as soon as possible. Stress that it is not uncommon to feel a letdown after discharge. Encourage participation in a burn support group.
Occupational Recovery Patient/family/support system Setting	Referral to the local office of the state labor and industry board for vocational counseling. Referral to vocational interest, aptitude, and psychological testing to determine areas of interest. Provide realistic plan, supply patient and family education, and engage an employer in the process.

Source: Urden, L. D. (2009). *Critical care nursing: Diagnosis and management* (6th ed.). St. Louis: Elsevier.

CHART 61–5 Complications of Burn Injuries

Emergency Phase	Acute Phase	Rehabilitative Phase
Immunosuppression: both humoral and cell mediated. Sepsis: highest incidence in burns greater than 40% of the total body surface area (TBSA). Bacterial translocation from the gut. Pneumonia and acute respiratory distress syndrome (ARDS), especially if an inhalation injury has occurred. Renal and heart failure from shock. Stress ulcers: rare due to medications and early tube feedings. Psychological problems. Normal grieving begins: denial.	Wound infection. Psychological problems; grieving process; patients fear both death and survival.	Scarring and contracture formation. Psychological problems. Deformities and loss of function. Normal grieving process switches to a focus on what are realistic future goals in terms of function and interpersonal issues.

Discharge planning requires a team approach with each member contributing from his area of expertise. In order to institute a realistic plan and ensure compliance, the patient and family have to be active, participating members of the team. Teaching is essential in order to prepare the patient and family for self-care. Nurses, who coordinate and evaluate the patient's needs on an ongoing basis, play a key role in the implementation of the teaching plan.

Complications of Burn Injuries

Because of their profound effect on multiorgan systems, burn injuries should never be viewed in isolation. Complications tend to be a rule rather than an exception for patients who have burn injuries. The most common complications that lead to increased mortality include wound infection, nosocomial pneumonia, sepsis, acute renal failure, gastrointestinal ulcers, and respiratory failure. Certain complications occur more frequently in a given period or phase of burn treatment. Chart 61–5 outlines the complications specific to each period of burn management.

Gerontological Considerations

Over 250,000 burn injuries happen to people over the age of 65 annually in the United States. Of those, more than 1,200 people die (Woods, Hollowed, Pavlovich, & Shupp, 2010). With the onset of early wound excision and grafting, the mortality rates have declined in the last three decades. However, older adults often delay seeking medical care for burn injuries, which predisposes them to complications such as cellulitis and infection. Older survivors of burn injuries in general seem to have decreased functional recovery. In addition, older adults tend to have other conditions that affect their recovery. See the Evidence-Based Practice box.

EVIDENCE-BASED PRACTICE Wound Infections, Mortality, and Treatment

Clinical Problem

Optimal clinical outcomes for burn patients relate directly to achieving wound closure as early as possible following the burn injury. This principle is especially true for high-risk patients presenting with large body surface areas burned as well as patients presenting with comorbidities such as heart failure, vascular disorders, malnutrition, and diabetes. Open wounds are the chief risk associated with tissue infections and are related to increased mortality. According to Kumari, Harjai, and Chhibber (2010), up to 75% of burn-related mortality is linked to wound tissue infections. Wound infections present more risk to a patient than the initial burn shock and relative hypovolemia often present in the burn population.

Partial-thickness burn wounds in comparatively healthy patients generally heal in less than 2 weeks when standard wound care is provided. However, full-thickness wounds and large partial-thickness wounds in patients with comorbidities may not heal within the optimal 2-week window of time. For these patients, the risks associated with overwhelming infections can induce significant clinical complexities. Treatment of patients who present with burns involving large portions of the body surface area is especially challenging because the options for harvesting skin to graft the burn wounds becomes limited as the ratio of burned tissue to unburned tissue becomes larger. For example, a patient with 40% of the TBSA burned has up to 60% healthy skin from which skin transplant can occur. By contrast, a patient presenting with a 90% TBSA burn has at most only 10% healthy skin that may be suitable for harvesting and grafting onto the burned areas. Currently available laboratory-grown skin derived from the patient's own skin tissue lacks the complex structures contained in natural skin.

Research Findings

Liu, Deng, Han, Liu, Wen, Lu, Geng, Huang, and Jin (2008) documented that mesenchymal stem cells extracted from bone marrow exhibit the ability to differentiate into a variety of differential tissue cells including keratinocytes and actually demonstrate the potential to develop into epidermal cells. Reproducing the complex structures contained in natural skin remains the focus of high level research in numerous research centers worldwide. Stem cells extracted from a patient's own bone marrow hold the most significant promise for reproducing a person's own skin, thus reducing or possibly eliminating the complex factors leading to mortality that remain challenging in the treatment of burn injuries today.

Implications for Nursing Practice

These studies unmistakably establish the necessity for nurses to become involved in research and advanced levels of clinical practice. Stem cell skin grafts are a promising treatment for burn injuries. Nurses need to be knowledgeable about current research in order to educate patients and families who may inquire about it.

Additionally, educating patients and families about the risk of complications following burns, especially when the patients have suffered large body surface injuries with comorbidities, is a vital nursing responsibility. Detailed assessment skills and effective nursing interventions are essential for optimal outcomes in this challenging and vulnerable patient population.

Critical Thinking Questions with answers can be found in the Osborn Student Resources at nursing.pearsonhighered.com.

Sources: Kumari, S., Harjai, K., & Chhibber, S. (2010) Bacteriophage versus antimicrobial agents for the treatment of murine burn wound infection caused by Klebsiella pneumonia B5055. *Journal of Medical Microbiology 60*(2): 205–210; Liu, P., Deng, Z., Han, S., Liu, T., Wen, N., Lu, W., et al. (2008). Tissue-engineered skin containing mesenchymal stem cells improves burn wounds. *Artificial Organs, 32*(12): 925–931.

RESEARCH OPPORTUNITIES Related to Burn Injury

Research Area	Clinical Impact
Physiological Research	Mediating the shock state and potentially decreasing the mortality rate.
Drugs to reverse the release of natural dilators to prevent the shunting of blood from the vascular system	
Fluid resuscitation techniques: high-concentration salt mixtures and high-molecular-weight salt mixtures instead of balanced salt mixtures for larger burn injury resuscitation	
Hyperdynamic resuscitation and role of serum lactate in severely burned patients	
Complex multiorgan response to burn injuries	
High-frequency percussive ventilation for the treatment of inhalation injuries	Preventing respiratory failure.
Direct instillation of combined aerosolized medications and hormones into the lungs of patients with inhalation injuries to decrease airway damage	
Selective decontamination of the gastrointestinal (GI) tract to decrease wound infections and pneumonia	Preventing systemic infection.
Early feeding of patients with burns to prevent translocation of bacteria to the bloodstream, causing sepsis	
Use of glutamine supplements and the hypermetabolic response	Augmenting wound healing.
Pain Management	Patient comfort and increased wound healing.
The nature of pain induced by direct tissue injury	
Nursing pain management	
Brief cognitive interventions for burn pain	
Rapid induction analgesia for the alleviation of procedural pain during burn care	
Relationship of itch to pain	
Factors predicting hypnotic analgesia in patients with clinical burns	
Pain and anxiety measurement and management during procedures	
Emotional and Psychological Research	
Predictors of post-traumatic stress syndrome and distress following acute burn injuries	Assessing factors that influence compliance and acceptance of burn injury and permanent scarring.
Anxiety: current practices in assessment and treatment of anxiety in patients with burns	
Chronic sorrow	Impact on vocation.
Self-blame, compliance, and distress among patients with burns	Impact on long-term adjustments to changes in body image.
Return to vocational stability	Improving psychological interventions to augment coping.
Massage therapy to reduce anxiety and cortisol levels	
Music influencing postprocedural recall	
Factors that enhance positive long-term psychological adaptation	
Family characteristics that augment psychological adaptation	
Sexuality after burn injury	
Burn Wound Research	Improving techniques to increase wound healing and prevent scarring.
The nature of fabric flammability and its effect on human skin	
Living skin grafts (cultured autografts) used with Integra, for permanent burn wound closure	
Treatment of pruritus and burn wounds	
Hypnosis and burn wound healing	
Massage therapy and itching	
Comparative study of burn wound cellulitis treatments	
Use of Integra artificial skin in preventing skin contractures to joints of burn wounds	
Burn size estimation using direct template drawings	
Use of music during wound débridement	
Direct measurement of cutaneous pressures generated by pressure garments	
Techniques to increase tensile strength and reduce wound breakdown	
Regulation and secretion of human growth factors used to modulate the hypermetabolic response to burn and augment wound and donor-site healing	

Each period of burn recovery is prolonged in the older adult. This is due in part to the diminished reserve capacity of the older adult's organ systems. For example, wound healing is delayed because of diminished host resistance and impaired cell-mediated and humoral immunity. Therefore, older adults have a decreased ability to fight infections and are more prone to sepsis. Once wounds are healed, the skin in the wound area has decreased tensile strength; thus, it breaks down easily, allowing the wound to reopen.

Special nursing care considerations for older adults include a careful assessment of the cardiovascular and pulmonary systems during early fluid resuscitation. This population is more prone to the development of pulmonary edema and heart failure than younger people. Monitoring of heart rate, blood pressure, and breath sounds on a frequent and ongoing basis is critical during rapid fluid administration to detect early signs and symptoms of heart failure. Mobilizing the patient as early as possible to maintain pulmonary function and promote independence also is an important aspect of care. Strict asepsis is critical because of the diminished immune response of patients with burn injuries and their increased susceptibility to infection. Finally, consistent attention to the nutritional intake of an older adult is essential in that it affects wound healing and survival.

Research

Research is essential to improve the care, quality of life, and survival of patients with burn injuries. The goal of research is to identify areas where practice could improve and evaluate and test methods for these improvements. The research topics related to burn injuries are included in the Research Opportunities box. The list provides both medical and nursing research topics that are currently under investigation. Electronic databases are good sources for finding specific studies related to these topics.

Summary

Burn injury may be minor or severe. The nurse must understand the clinical progression of burns and have excellent assessment skills to care for the patient and prevent complications of burn injury. The nurse is also integral in preparing the patient and family for the long-term care that accompanies burn injury.

CLINICAL PREPARATION READ DOCUMENT APPLY

READ: **History of Present Illnesses** >> Laboratory Study Results >> Critical Thinking Questions

As the on-coming nurse in a major burn center, you are receiving report about Marilyn Rosati, a 60-year-old housewife who was admitted to the hospital following a fire that occurred in her home. A neighbor noted the smoke coming from the house and called 911 for emergency assistance. The firefighters had to carry Mrs. Rosati from the burning house because she was unconscious. Despite resuscitative efforts, Mrs. Rosati's husband was declared dead at the scene of the fire. Mrs. Rosati's two grown children have been notified of the accident and are in the waiting room. This is the patient's hospital day 2. A large-bore triple-lumen subclavian catheter was placed, and lactated Ringer's solution is infusing using the Brooke Army Formula guidelines. A Foley catheter was inserted; Mrs. Rosati's urine output is being monitored hourly and has been at least 30 mL/hr. A femoral arterial line was placed and has a good waveform. She is being medicated for pain with moderate relief. Her last vital signs were temperature: 39°C, pulse: 126 beats per minute, respiratory rate: 16/minute, and BP: 104/80. A nasogastric (NG) tube was placed in order to decompress the stomach if nausea and vomiting should occur and for medication instillation. Mrs. Rosati denies nausea, and she is tolerating NG medications. Her abdomen is soft with hypoactive bowel sounds noted in all four quadrants. She has not had a bowel movement since admission.

READ: History of Present Illnesses >> **Physical Exam** >> Admitting Medical Records >> Laboratory Study Results

Medical–Surgical History

- No known allergies
- Hypertension
- Myocardial infarction 2 years ago
- Non–insulin-dependent diabetes
- Atrial fibrillation
- Depression
- Two live births via vaginal delivery
- Medications: Digoxin, Captopril, Paxil, and Glipizide

Social History

- Was living independently with husband up to time of the fire
- Two grown children
- One son lives in local area
- No tobacco use

Physical Exam

- 27% total body surface area burned
- Approximately 12% is full-thickness injury, primarily on left arm and leg
- Left arm and leg: circumferential injuries that required escharotomies
- Remainder of burn wounds are on face and chest
- Following escharotomies, pulses present in both left arm and leg, and patient able to wiggle toes on command
- Restless, anxious, and complaining of severe pain
- Moving all four extremities equally, on command
- Pupils respond to light equally at 4 millimeters
- Apical pulse: can be heard at the apex; peripheral pulses: +4 (0–4 scale) and slightly irregular, no extra heart sounds
- Cardiac monitor: sinus tachycardia with occasional premature ventricular contractions
- Capillary refill < 3 seconds in all extremities
- Inhalation injury: currently intubated on ventilatory support with 50% oxygen
- Lungs: wheezes and diminished breath sounds in bilateral bases; suctioned every hour for carbon-stained thick mucus
- Oxygen sat 94–96%

Admitting Medical Orders
Burn service
Admit to burn intensive care unit
No known allergies

Diagnosis
27% burn injury

Orders
Vital signs, oxygen saturation, and urine output every hour
Foley
AccuCheck q4h with sliding scale
IV lactated Ringer's solution 180 mL/hr
Hydro tank and dressing change with Silvadene daily
Bed rest
Strict I&O
Elevate left arm and left leg on two pillows each
HOB 30 degrees
PT/OT daily
NG feeding: replete at 5 mL/hr
Check residual q4h, stop feeding for 1 hour if >100 milliliters
Ventilator: FiO_2 at 50%, TV: 700, Rate: 10, Peep: 5, PS/PC: 18/22
Suction prn
Daily weight
Call house officer: Pulse < 60 and > 110/minute; BP < 90 and > 130 systolic; temperature > 38.5; urine output < 30 mL/hr × 2 hours RR > 30/minute; oxygen saturation < 92%

Scheduled Medications
MVI 10 mL NG daily
Folic acid 1 mg NG daily
Vitamin A 20,000 units NG daily
Zinc 220 mg NG daily
Thiamine 100 mg NG daily
Pepcid 20 mg IV q12h
Ceftriaxone 1 gram daily

PRN Medications
Tylenol 650 mg q6h NG/PR prn pain and temp > 101.5
Fentanyl 50–150 mcg IV prn dressing change
Phenergan 25 mg IV q6h prn nausea and vomiting
Versed 2–4 mg IV prn dressing change
Morphine sulfate drip 1 mg/mL at 1–7 mg/hr titrate to effect
Versed drip 0.5 mg/mL at 0.5–3 mg/hr titrate to effect for agitation/anxiety
Sliding Scale insulin q4h per protocol

Laboratory Studies
ABG, CBC, Chemistry 7 daily
Type and cross for 4 units of packed red blood cells
Blood, sputum, and urine culture

Diagnostic Studies
Chest x-ray daily

READ: History of Present Illnesses >> **Laboratory Study Results** >> Critical Thinking Questions

Test	Day 1	Day 2	Day 3
Sodium	138 mEq/L	148 mEq/L	135 mEq/L
Potassium	4.8 mEq/L	5.8 mEq/L	5 mEq/L
Chloride	103 mEq/L	110 mEq/L	108 mEq/L
Carbon dioxide (CO_2)	28 mg/dL	31 mg/dL	25 mg/dL
Blood urea nitrogen (BUN)	10 mg/dL	10 mg/dL	9 mg/dL
Creatinine	1.1 mg/dL	1.3 mg/dL	1.8 mg/dL
Blood glucose	141 mg/dL	135 mg/dL	132 mg/dL
Calcium	8.6 mg/dL	9 mg/dL	9 mg/dL
Magnesium	1.9 mg/dL	1.9 mg/dL	2 mg/dL
Phosphorus	2.2 mg/dL	3.4 mg/dL	3.8 mg/dL
Albumin	2.7 g/dL	2.27 g/dL	1.97 g/dL
White blood cells (WBCs)	15,800/mm^3	9,900/mm^3	4,600/mm^3
Red blood cells (RBCs)	6.9/mm^3	5.88/mm^3	4.73/mm^3

Test	Day 1	Day 2	Day 3
Hemoglobin (Hgb)	19.3/mm^3	18.2/mm^3	14.7/mm^3
Hematocrit (Hct)	56.6%	54.1%	43.5%
Platelets	188,000/mm^3	180,000/mm^3	149,000/mm^3
International normalized ratio (INR)	0.8		
Arterial blood gases (ABGs)			
PO_2	135 mmHg	96 mmHg	94 mmHg
Oxygen saturation	98%	99%	97%
pH	7.31	7.37	7.39
PCO_2	52 mmHg	49 mmHg	44 mmHg
HCO_3	26 mEq/L	28 mEq/L	26 mEq/L

Pearson Nursing Student Resources *Log on to* **nursing.pearsonhighered.com** *to download forms*

DOCUMENT:

- >> Summary of Hospitalization
- >> Pathophysiology Form
- >> Laboratory Values
- >> Laboratory Results Explanation

APPLY:

- >> List of Potential Nursing Diagnoses
- >> Concept Map
- >> Critical Thinking Questions and Concept Map

APPLY: History of Present Illness >> Laboratory Study Results >> **Critical Thinking Questions**

1. Besides burn wound assessment and fluid resuscitation needs, what other priorities would be essential to assess regarding Mrs. Rosati?
2. What is the rationale for performing an escharotomy, and what clinical manifestations would result if an escharotomy were not done?
3. What impact does diabetes have on Mrs. Rosati's prognosis?
4. What impact does fluid resuscitation have on Mrs. Rosati's sodium, chloride, hemoglobin, and hematocrit levels?

Answers to Critical Thinking Questions can be found in Appendix D in the Osborn Student Resources at nursing.pearsonhighered.com.

NCLEX® PRACTICE

1. The nurse is assessing a patient with an electrical burn. The nurse notes that the patient has a 1% partial-thickness burn to the left foot and a 2% full-thickness burn to the right shoulder where these body parts contacted the electrical source. The patient is awake, alert, and oriented. Vital signs are HR 97 with frequent ectopy, BP 136/75, RR 22, SpO_2 94% on room air. The nurse knows that this patient's injuries should be classified as a:

1. minor burn injury.
2. moderate burn injury.
3. major burn injury.
4. medium burn injury.

2. A nurse is teaching a class on injury prevention to a group of new mothers. Which of the following statements made by one of the participants indicates the need for further instruction in burn injury prevention?

1. "Every house should have at least one clean working smoke detector."
2. "SPF 30+ can help reduce the likelihood of getting a radiation burn."
3. "Make sure all children's sleepwear is made from fire-retardant fabrics."
4. "Liquid at 140°F requires 5 minutes to cause a full-thickness burn."

3. When a student nurse inquires about the pathophysiological changes that occur in the severely burned patient, the most appropriate response by the nurse would be:

1. "With bacterial translocation, the gastrointestinal mucosal atrophy that occurs causes intraluminal bacteria to migrate to extraluminal sites."
2. "Decreased cardiac output can occur early after a burn because stimulation of the parasympathetic nervous system causes vasoconstriction."
3. "Hepatic failure ensues when damaged erythrocytes and muscle tissue cause the excess release of hemoglobin and myoglobin, respectively."
4. "It is not uncommon to transfuse leukocytes within the first 2 days because granulocyte stores and circulating iron stores are depleted."

4. Upon admission to the burn unit, the patient with a 35% TBSA thermal burn begins to undergo intensive wound care and physical therapy. Pain control and topical antimicrobial medications are also important. The nurse understands that the patient is in which period of burn care?

1. The resuscitative period
2. The acute care period
3. The emergency period
4. The rehabilitative period

5. Four victims of a house fire arrive in the emergency department. Which of the following patients should the nurse see first?

1. A 35-year-old with a history of migraines and 40% TBSA full-thickness thermal burns to the neck, left upper extremity, and circumferentially around the chest. Vital signs are HR 116, BP 90/68, RR 26 and shallow, SpO_2 90%.
2. A 70-year-old with a history of diabetes and 14% TBSA partial-thickness thermal burns to the back and right shoulder and 1% TBSA full-thickness burn to the right arm. Vital signs are HR 88, BP 130/75, RR 22 and regular, SpO_2 98%.
3. A 12-year-old with a history of astigmatism and 20% TBSA partial-thickness thermal burns to the anterior left lower extremity, left foot, and abdomen. Vital signs are HR 80, BP 110/65, RR 24 and regular, SpO_2 100%.
4. A 44-year-old with a history of hypertension and 8% TBSA full-thickness thermal burns to the right upper extremity and 15% TBSA partial-thickness burns to the abdomen and anterior chest. Vital signs are HR 98, BP 148/92, RR 22 and regular, SpO_2 98%.

6. Which of the following nursing diagnoses is most important during the emergency period of burn care?

1. *Altered Skin Integrity* related to epithelial skin loss.
2. *Fluid Volume Deficit* related to increased capillary permeability.
3. *Increased Risk for Infection* related to loss of skin integrity.
4. *Acute Pain* related to burn injury and exposed nerve endings.

Answers to NCLEX Practice questions can be found in Appendix D in the Osborn Student Resources at nursing.pearsonhighered.com. Practice additional NCLEX questions online at the Student Resources Site.

Pearson Nursing Student Resources Find additional review materials at: **nursing.pearsonhighered.com**

REFERENCES

American Burn Association (ABA). (2011). Burn incidence and treatment in the United States: 2011 fact sheet. Retrieved from http://www.ameriburn.org/resources_factsheet.php

American College of Surgeons (ACS). (2008). *Advanced trauma life support* (8th ed.). Chicago: Author.

Anand, B. S. (2011). Peptic ulcer disease. Medscape reference. Retrieved from http://emedicine.medscape.com/article/181753-overview#aw2aab6b2b3

Berman, B. (2010). Keloid and hypertrophic scar. Medscape reference. http://emedicine.medscape.com/article/1057599-overview#a0199

Bryant, R. A., & Nix, D. P. (2012). *Acute & chronic wounds* (4th ed.). St. Louis: Elsevier.

Centers for Disease Control and Prevention (CDC). (2011a). Fire deaths and injuries: Fact sheet. Retrieved from http://www.cdc.gov/HomeandRecreationalSafety/Fire-Prevention/fires-factsheet.html

Centers for Disease Control and Prevention (CDC). (2011b). Injury prevention & control: Home and recreational safety. Retrieved from http://www.cdc.gov/Homeand RecreationalSafety/Fire-Prevention/fireactivities.htm

Centers for Disease Control and Prevention (CDC). (2011c). UV radiation. Retrieved from http://www.cdc.gov/niosh/topics/uvradiation/

Cochran, A. (2010). Nutritional demands and enteral formulas for moderate to severe burn patients. UpToDate. Retrieved from http://www.uptodate.com/contents/nutritional-demands-and-enteral-formulas-for-moderate-to-severe-burn-patients

Consumer Product Safety Commission. (2011). Tap water scalds. Retrieved from http://www.cpsc.gov/cpscpub/pubs/5098.html

Cushing, T. A. (2010). Electrical injuries in emergency medicine clinical presentation. Medscape reference. Retrieved from http://emedicine.medscape.com/article/770179-clinical#a0217

Howard, P. K., & Steinmann, R. A. (Eds.). (2009). *Sheehy's emergency nursing: Principles and practice* (6th ed.). St. Louis: Elsevier.

IOM (Institute of Medicine). (2010). *The future of nursing: Leading change, advancing health.* Washington, DC: The Academic Press.

Jansen, D. A. (2012). Keloids. Medscape reference. Retrieved from http://www.emedicine.medscape.com/article/1298013-overview

Khorasani, E. N. (2010). Effect of early enteral nutrition on morbidity and mortality in children with burns. *Burns, 36*(7), 1067–1071.

Kumari, S., Harjai, K., & Chhibber, S. (2010). Bacteriophage versus antimicrobial agents for the treatment of murine burn wound infection caused by Klebsiella pneumonia B5055. *Journal of Medical Microbiology 60*(2): 205–210.

Lawrence, K. (2011). Pediatric sepsis and multiorgan dysfunction syndrome: Progress and continued challenges. *Critical Care Nursing Clinics of North America, 23*(2): 323–327.

Liu, P., Deng, Z., Han, S., Liu, T., Wen, N., Lu, W., et al. (2008). Tissue-engineered skin containing mesenchymal stem cells improves burn wounds. *Artificial Organs, 32*(12): 925–931.

Lucile Packard Children's Hospital at Stanford. (2008). Safety and injury prevention: Fire safety and burns—Injury statistics and incidence rates. Retrieved from http://www.lpch.org/DiseaseHealthInfo/HealthLibrary/safety/firestat.html

Mandel, J., & Hales, C. A. (2008). Smoke inhalation. Retrieved from http://www.uptodate.com/patients/content/topic.do?topicKey=~9DITT3s_pPmii9&selectedTitle=1~147&source=search_result

Murray, C. (2008). Burn wound infections. eMedicine from WebMD. Retrieved from suapple@verizon.net

Nayback, A. M. (2009). Posttraumatic stress: A concept analysis. *Archives of Psychiatric Nursing, (23)*3, 210–219.

Pham, T. N., Cancio, L. C., Gibran, N. S: American Burn Association. (2008). American burn association practice guidelines burn shock resuscitation. *Journal of Burn Care Resuscitation, 29*(1): 257–266.

Porth, C. M., & Matfin, G. (2009). *Pathophysiology: Concepts of altered health states* (8th ed.). Philadelphia: Lippincott Williams & Wilkins.

Protacio, J.. (2010). Patient-directed music therapy as an adjunct during burn wound care. *Journal of Critical Care Nurses, 30*(2), 74–76.

Shah, J. (2010). Hyperbaric oxygen therapy. *Journal of the American College of Certified Wound Specialists, 2*(1), 9–13.

Tan, X., Yowler, C. J., Super, D. M., & Fratianne, R. B. (2010). The efficacy of music therapy protocols for decreasing pain, anxiety, and muscle tension levels during burn dressing changes: A prospective randomized crossover trial. *Journal of Burn Care & Research, 31*(4), 590–597.

Urden, L. D. (2009). *Critical care nursing: Diagnosis and management* (6th ed.). St. Louis: Elsevier.

U.S. Fire Administration. (2011) Fire safety. Retrieved from: http://m.usfa.fema.gov/mobile/safety/index.shtm

Vanderboom, T. (2007). Anxiety during invasive procedures with procedural sedation? An integrative research review. *Journal of Radiological Nursing, 26*(1), 15–22.

Wakim, J. H., Smith, S., & Guinn, C. (2010). The efficacy of music therapy. *Journal of PeriAnesthia Nursing, 25*(4), 226–232.

Williams, F. N., Herndon, D. N., Hawkins, H. K., Lee, J. O., Cox, R. A., Kulp, G. A., Finnerty, C. C., Chinkes, D. L. & Jeschke, M. G. (2009). The leading causes of death after burn injury in a single pediatric burn center. *Critical Care 13*(6). Retrieved from http://ccforum.com/content/13/6/R183

Wilkinson, J. M., & Ahearn, N. R. (2009). *Prentice Hall nursing diagnosis handbook* (9th ed.). Upper Saddle River, NJ: Prentice Hall.

Woods, J., Hollowed, K., Pavlovich, A., & Shupp, J. (2010). Firefighter foundation and regional burn center collaborate to reduce burn-related injuries in the elderly. *Injury Prevention, 16(Suppl 1):A1-A289* doi:10.1136

Nursing Management of Patients with Sensory Disorders

14 UNIT

Content in Unit 14 that addresses the **Institute of Medicine (IOM)** competencies, **Nursing Core Competencies (NCC)**, the **Quality and Safety Education for Nurses (QSEN)** competencies, and **Concepts** for concept-based learning is listed below.

Competencies	Feature or Text	Location
IOM, QSEN, NCC Providing patient-centered care	Genetic Considerations Related to Hearing and Balance Disorders, page 1974 Cultural Considerations for Hearing and Balance Disorders, page 1975 Cultural Considerations for Visual Disorders, page 1981 Genetic Considerations in Adults With Visual Impairments, page 1982 Nursing Process: Patient Care Plan for a Hearing or Balance Disorder, page 1998 Nursing Process: Patient Care Plan for Macular Degeneration, page 2039	Chapter 62 Chapter 62 Chapter 62 Chapter 62 Chapter 63 Chapter 64
IOM, QSEN, NCC Working in teams	Collaborative Management, page 2002 Collaborative Management, pages 2025, 2032, 2036, 2041, 2045, 2047, 2051	Chapter 63 Chapter 64
IOM, QSEN, NCC Employing evidence-based practice	Evidence-Based Practice: Noise-Induced Hearing Loss, page 1992 Evidence-Based Practice: Age-Related Macular Degeneration and Cognitive Function, page 2041	Chapter 63 Chapter 64
IOM, NCC Applying quality and safety improvement	Safety Alerts, pages 1974, 1975 Safety Alerts, pages 2002, 2010 Safety Alerts, page 2038	Chapter 62 Chapter 63 Chapter 64
NCC Applying ethical and legal responsibilities	Legal blindness, pages 2025, 2036	Chapter 64
NCC Education patients	Patient Teaching & Discharge Priorities for Hearing and Balance Disorders, page 1999 Patient Teaching & Discharge Priorities for Cataract Surgery, page 2025 Patient Teaching & Discharge Priorities for Glaucoma, page 2033	Chapter 63 Chapter 64 Chapter 64
Concepts covered in Unit 14 include:	Body (self) image Grief and loss Infection Perception	Safety Sensory perception

CHAPTER

62 Nursing Assessment of the Patient with Sensory Disorders

Judith Tanner
Lucie S. Elfervig
Annita Watson

Outcome-Based Learning Objectives

After studying this chapter, the learner will be able to:

1. Differentiate normal from abnormal findings of a physical assessment of the ear and eye.
2. Determine the data that need to be obtained from the subjective and objective history for ear and eye disorders.
3. Analyze the risk factors for ear and eye disorders.
4. Discuss the purpose and significance of physical assessment findings and diagnostic exams of the ear and eye as they relate to nursing responsibilities.
5. Analyze the relationship between abnormal assessment findings of the ear and eye and the common systemic problems that may be manifested through ocular and visual conditions.

KEY TERMS

accommodation p.1980
air conduction p.1971
barotrauma p.1976
bone conduction p.1971
caloric test p.1977
cerumen p.1970
conductive hearing loss p.1972
floaters p.1980
otalgia p.1975
ototoxic p.1973
pneumatoscope p.1977
Rinne test p.1977
Romberg test p.1977
Schwabach test p.1977
sensorineural hearing loss p.1972
tinnitus p.1972
vertigo p.1972
voice whisper test p.1977
Weber test p.1977

AUDITORY AND VISUAL ASSESSMENT is a vital part of the nurse's function in caring for the whole patient, as it reassures the patient that the nurse is committed to her total well-being. Nurses play a key role in assisting, planning, implementing, evaluating, and educating patients and their families, helping them adapt through new coping skills for changes that can come with hearing, balance, and visual disorders.

ASSESSMENT OF HEARING AND BALANCE

Nurses have numerous opportunities to identify risk factors during a patient's hearing and balance assessment and to encourage healthy behaviors. Disturbances in both hearing and balance occur as a result of exposure and reaction to risk factors. Some of these risk factors are modifiable, whereas others are not. The majority of risk factors are classified as environmental, biological and physiological, and occupational. Specific risk factors related to hearing and balance are discussed later in the chapter. The nurse's role in assessing patients for hearing and balance status includes identification of risk factors, education of the patient and family on how to possibly reduce these factors, and promotion of healthy preventive behaviors. A physical assessment as well as a review of the patient's social and occupational histories and laboratory results provides information that can assist the nurse in developing a plan of care.

Anatomy and Physiology of the Ear

The complexities of hearing are best understood when each part of the ear is analyzed (Figure 62–1◆). The ear is divided into three parts: external/outer, middle, and inner ear. The external or outer ear comprises some structures that are visible to the naked eye and some that are not. The pinna, the most visible portion of the ear, is made up of cartilaginous tissue. The pinna collects sound waves and directs them into the external auditory ear canal. The ear canal, also made up of cartilaginous material, is relatively short at approximately 1 inch in length. This structure contains ceruminous and sebaceous glands that produce **cerumen** (commonly referred to as earwax), which helps to clean and lubricate the ear canal and may have a bactericidal effect. The bony portion of the ear canal, which covers the mastoid process, also is

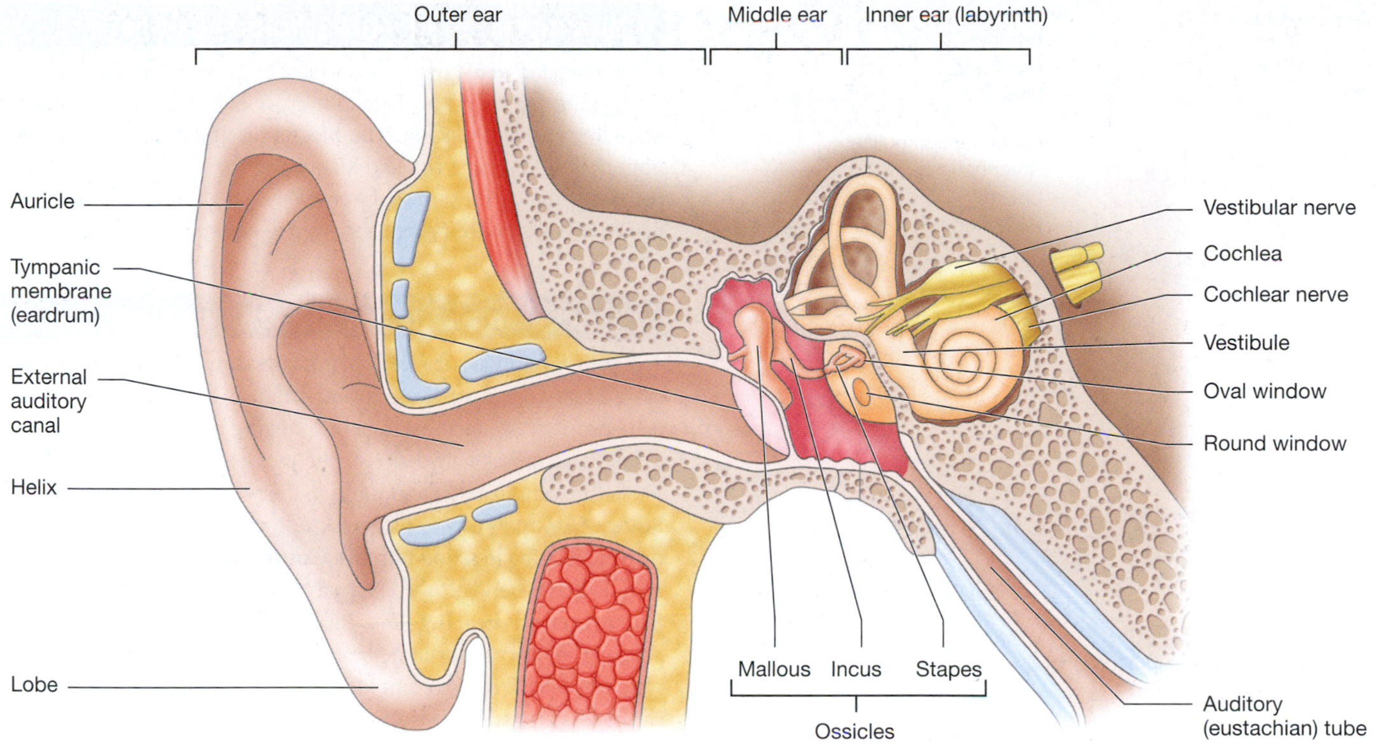

FIGURE 62–1 ◆ Outer, middle, and inner ear.

Source: From Lemone, P., & Burke, K. (2003). *Medical–Surgical Nursing: Critical Thinking in Client Care* (3rd ed.). Upper Saddle River, NJ: Pearson Prentice Hall.

considered a structure of the external/outer ear. The tympanic membrane (eardrum), comprising tissue that makes up the ear canal, is the final structure within this portion of the outer ear anatomy; its function is to transmit sounds from the outer to the middle ear.

The middle ear begins from the inner side of the tympanic membrane and extends to the Eustachian tube. This portion of the ear contains the three auditory bones: the malleus, the incus, and the stapes (see Figure 62–1). The malleus is attached to the inner portion of the tympanic membrane. When the tympanic membrane vibrates with sound, so does the malleus. The incus is attached to the malleus and also vibrates in response to sound. The stapes is the structure that separates the middle ear from the inner ear. The base of the stapes, the footplate, fills the oval window, which leads to the inner ear. The footplate of the stapes fits tightly into a tiny oval window of the bony cochlea that opens into the inner ear. The stapes vibrates and makes the fluid in the inner ear vibrate.

The inner ear includes the cochlea, the vestibular system that contains the bony labyrinth and the semicircular canals, and the acoustic nerve (see Figure 62–1). The cochlea is responsible for hearing; the vestibular system is responsible for balance. The cochlea, shaped like a snail, contains a structure termed the organ of Corti. The small hairs within this organ change sound vibrations into neural signals that are transmitted to the brain via the acoustic nerve. The bony labyrinth consists of the saccule and utricle, organs that provide position sense. Within the inner ear are found the semicircular canals, specifically the horizontal, anterior, and posterior canals, which help with balance and movement. The acoustic nerve consists of two separate parts, the vestibular and cochlear branches. This eighth cranial nerve (CN) controls hearing and equilibrium.

Mechanisms of Hearing

Hearing involves two mechanisms: bone conduction and air conduction. **Bone conduction** is the conduction of sound to the inner ear through the bones of the skull. **Air conduction** begins the process when noise enters the external ear and travels to the middle ear. Once inside the middle ear, the sound is transmitted through the three auditory bones: the malleus, incus, and stapes. When the sound or noise reaches the stapes, it is then transmitted to the inner ear, where it reaches the acoustic nerve and is transmitted to the brain for interpretation. Hearing disorders can be caused by an alteration anywhere within the auditory structures. Disorders of the ear and balance are discussed in Chapter 63.

Mechanisms of Balance

The sense of balance is controlled primarily by a mazelike structure in the inner ear called the *labyrinth*, which is made of bone and soft tissue. At one end of the labyrinth is an intricate system of loops and pouches called the semicircular canals and the otolithic organs, which help maintain balance (see Figure 62–2◆). Together, they make up the vestibular system (The Free Dictionary, 2011). The vestibular system works with other sensorimotor systems such as the visual system (eyes) and the skeletal system (bones and muscles) to check and maintain the position of the body at rest or in motion. The vestibular system also helps maintain a steady visual focus on objects as the position of the body changes. The vestibular system does this by detecting mechanical forces, including gravity, that act upon the vestibular organs when the person moves. Two sections of the labyrinth that help

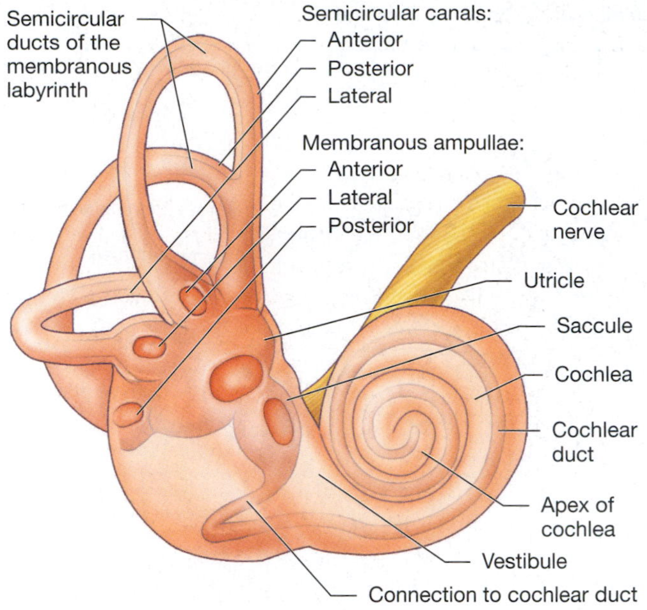

FIGURE 62–2 ◆ The labyrinth of the ear.

accomplish these tasks are the semicircular canals and the otolithic organs. The semicircular canals are three fluid-filled loops arranged roughly at right angles to each other. Each semicircular canal contains a raindrop-shaped structure called the cupula. The cupula, which is filled with a gel-like substance, sits on top of a cluster of sensory cells called *hair cells*, which extend into the gel. When the head moves, fluid inside the semicircular canal moves. This motion causes the cupula to bend and the hair cells within it to tilt to one side. The tilting action creates a signal that travels to the brain to tell it the movement and position of the head.

Between the semicircular canals and the cochlea lie the otolithic organs, which are two fluid-filled pouches called the utricle and the saccule. These organs tell the brain when the body is moving in a straight line. They also tell the brain the position of the head with respect to gravity, such as sitting up, leaning back, or lying down.

Like the semicircular canals, the utricle and the saccule have sensory hair cells. These hair cells line the bottom of each pouch and extend into an overlying gel-like layer. On top of the gel are tiny grains made of calcium carbonate called *otoconia*. When the head is tilted, gravity pulls on the grains, which then moves the hair cells. As with the semicircular canals, this movement creates a signal that tells the brain the head's position. The visual system works with the vestibular system to keep objects from blurring when the head moves and to enable individuals to remain aware of their position as they move or ride in a moving vehicle. Vestibular function is largely reflexive and unconscious in nature. Sensory receptors in joints and muscles also help maintain balance when the person is standing still or walking. The brain receives, interprets, and processes the information from these systems to control balance.

History

To make an accurate assessment of the patient with a hearing or balance problem, the nurse needs to explore the patient's history. The personal, family, and social aspects of a person's life can provide clues to the causes of health problems and the patient's receptivity to the care offered by health care professionals.

Biographic and Demographic History

Biographic and demographic data refer to information used in identifying patients, such as age, sex, race, place of birth, current residence, marital status, and religion. The biographic information obtained is important in assessing risk and identifying the presenting problem of patients with hearing or balance problems. Medical, family, and social issues particular to the patient also need to be explored.

Chief Complaint and Presenting Symptoms

The patient's primary complaint is the presenting symptom. Primary complaints related to hearing and balance disorders may include pain, pruritus, dizziness, hearing loss, ringing in the ears, and frequent falling. The nurse's knowledge of the incidence of diseases and conditions in certain population groups helps to focus the subsequent history. Common ear problems include conductive deafness, sensorineural hearing loss, and tinnitus. **Conductive hearing loss** results from a lesion between the external auditory canal and the cochlea. **Sensorineural hearing loss** involves defects in the sensory end organ of the cochlea or in nerve transmission to the central nervous system (CNS). It is important for the nurse to remember that patients can have hearing problems at any age. Knowledge of gender differences also is useful. For example, *otosclerosis*, a familial disorder in which irregular ossification occurs in the stapes of the middle ear causing conductive deafness, sensorineural hearing loss, and tinnitus, is more common in women than men. Otosclerosis also can be triggered by pregnancy (Springhouse, 2008).

A *balance disorder* is a condition that makes a person feel unsteady or dizzy, as if he is moving, spinning, or floating, even though he is standing still or lying down. Balance disorders may be caused by viral or bacterial infections, head injury, or blood circulation disorders that affect the inner ear or brain. Many people experience problems with their sense of balance as they get older. Balance problems and dizziness also can result from taking certain medications. In addition, problems of the visual and skeletal systems and the nervous and circulatory systems can be the source of some posture and balance problems. A circulatory system disorder, such as low blood pressure, can lead to a feeling of dizziness when the person suddenly stands up. However, many balance disorders can begin suddenly with no obvious cause (National Institutes on Deafness and Other Communication Disorders [NIDCD], 2009). There are numerous tests to determine balance impairment; these tests are discussed in detail in Chapter 63.

Age affects hearing ability. For example, *presbycusis*, hearing loss in the high-frequency range, is the most common sensorineural hearing loss in older people (Cacchione, 2008). The older patient who is experiencing gradual hearing loss may limit social interactions as it becomes more difficult to understand the spoken word. During the assessment, the nurse should inquire about the patient's functional ability and social interactions. Loss of hearing also can be perceived as mental status changes. Nurses need to be more aware of the impact of hearing loss on older adults (Cacchione, 2008).

The nurse also should be aware of specific problems with at-risk populations. *Acoustic neuromas*, which are benign tumors of the Schwann cell sheath, are more common in women ages 40 to 50 years. *Ménière's disease* is a dysfunction of the labyrinth with symptoms of **vertigo** (dizziness), hearing loss, unilateral aural fullness, and **tinnitus** (ringing in the ears) (NIDCD, 2010b). It is most common between the ages of 30 and 60 years. Any patient with obstruction of the ear canal, any middle ear disorders, or trauma to the ears, as well as patients taking certain medications, can develop tinnitus (NIDCD, 2010b). **Ototoxic** drugs (drugs that damage the hearing or balance functions of the ear) are outlined in Chapter 63.

Race also is an important consideration in assessing hearing or balance problems; some racial groups are more prone to some medical conditions. For example, otosclerosis is common in Caucasians but rarely seen in Asian and African populations (Niedermeyer et al., 2007).

Past Medical History

The patient's medical history provides information about past health-related problems and, in particular, gives clues to the residual problems that may affect current treatment.

Childhood Diseases and Immunizations

The nurse should consider that any adult presenting with an ear problem may have had a history of problems as a child. The frequency, clinical manifestations, and treatment of ear disorders are essential pieces of information to be obtained during the assessment. Many children are prone to ear infections. Complications of otitis media, which is either inflammation or infection of the middle ear, include frequent upper respiratory infections and sinus infections. Intrauterine exposure to maternal influenza or rubella can result in congenital hearing loss. Hearing loss can be very isolating and may be perceived as a mental status change.

The nurse should inquire about the presence of genetic diseases, especially those that affect the ear. Hearing loss in children can occur from infections and genetics. The nurse should inquire about childhood and adult immunizations, including the immunization dates and reactions. Genetic conditions that affect hearing include sensorineural hearing impairment and absent or abnormal ears.

Previous Illnesses and Hospitalizations

Past illnesses and hospitalizations can give the nurse clues to residual problems and how the patient coped with previous illnesses. In terms of the presenting complaint, the nurse needs to inquire about what has been done thus far. Has the patient had audiologic tests to determine the degree of hearing loss? Has the patient had surgery to correct hearing loss? The nurse should ask about injuries and accidents, particularly regarding foreign objects lodged in the ear. The nurse also needs to assess for balance disorders.

- Has the patient had problems with balance before? (It may be necessary to explain the meaning of balance.) Has the patient experienced vertigo (dizziness)?
- When did the most recent episode of vertigo occur?
- Was there a specific occasion on which vertigo was experienced?
- Are episodes of vertigo associated with postural changes? If so, what position generates the greatest amount of vertigo?
- Is hearing loss also evident during these experiences?
- Did the patient experience symptoms of flulike conditions when having vertigo?
- Was the patient exposed to ototoxic medications?
- Did the patient experience brainstem symptoms, such as diplopia, dysarthria, facial paresthesia, or numbness or weakness in one or more extremities?
- Was the patient impaired during these episodes, or could the patient continue to function?

Medications

The nurse should ask the patient to list all medications currently being used and those the patient has used in the past, including prescribed and over-the-counter (OTC) medications. It is important to include systemic medications that may have an effect on the hearing assessment. Many medications are ototoxic and cause permanent bilateral hearing loss with eighth cranial nerve damage; some also cause tinnitus (refer to Chapter 63). In particular, patients with compromised renal function are at risk for developing deafness and tinnitus from medications. To minimize this damage, serum drug levels and serial hearing evaluations should be done while patients are taking these drugs. Patients taking long-term antibiotics also can develop vertigo because of damage to the eighth cranial nerve (Hain, 2011a).

The nurse should ask the patient about the use of any herbal and home remedies, particularly (but not solely) those taken for hearing problems. Patients who take herbal remedies and OTC products may experience unwanted side effects. Generally, ototoxicity is not a factor when herbs are used in normal therapeutic dosages. Ototoxic side effects usually show up only when a person begins overdosing on these herbs (Bauman, 2010).

Family Health History

It is important to obtain the health history of all members of the immediate family, including parents, grandparents, siblings, and children. Damage to hearing can occur *in utero* from genetic causes or infectious conditions (influenza or rubella) (Dillon, 2007). Severe hearing loss occurs in 1 in 1,000 live births, half the cases being of genetic origin. The hearing loss is typically noticed because of impaired speech development. Half the people who have otosclerosis have a family history of the condition (Morrison & Bundey, 2007). The nurse needs to investigate whether any family members were hard of hearing before 50 years of age and, if so, what caused the hearing loss. The nurse should also ask whether any family members have had ear surgery or any type of ear problems. If any family members are deceased, the nurse should inquire about the cause of death.

Congenital hearing loss occurs when a trait found in the chromosomes of both parents is passed to the infant. The trait can be dominant, recessive, or sex linked. Congenital conditions that include some degree of hearing impairment are listed in the Genetic Considerations box.

Scientists have also discovered that mutation of the connexin 26 gene causes hearing loss (Berke, 2011). This gene mutation is suspected of disrupting potassium flow in the inner ear. Connexin 26 gene mutations are found primarily in Caucasians, Ashkenazi Jews, and some Asian people (Berke, 2011). It may be helpful for the nurse to enlist the patient's help in drawing a genogram of living and dead family members to trace the incidence of any genetically linked conditions.

Current Health and Risk Factors

The nurse needs to understand the patient's current health status and any risk factors that might make the patient susceptible to problems of the ear. Factors that may damage or lead to loss of the hairs and nerve cells in the ear include aging (due to exposure to sounds over the years), heredity (genetic conditions that can make a person more susceptible to ear damage), occupational noises, recreational noises, some medications (such as some antibiotics and NSAIDs), and certain illnesses that cause a high fever, such as meningitis (Mayo Clinic, 2009).

Weblink: Genetic Disorders

GENETIC CONSIDERATIONS
Related to Hearing and Balance Disorders

Disorder	Results	Ear Structure
Usher syndrome	Balance problems	Inner ear
Treacher-Collins syndrome	Bone development	Middle ear
Nonsyndromic deafness	Conductive problems	Inner ear
ESPN	Changes in hairlike projections	Inner ear
Pendred syndrome	Hearing loss and goiter	Inner ear
Neurofibromatosis	Tumor (acoustic neuroma)	Inner ear
Diastrophic dysplasia	Cartilage and bone	External ear
Von Hippel Lindau syndrome	Endolymphatic sac tumors	Inner ear
Jervell and Lange-Nielsen syndrome	Flow of potassium ions	Inner ear
Alport syndrome	Organ of Corti	Inner ear
Crouzon syndrome	Ear canals	Middle and inner ear
Chromosome 18	Low-set ears	Outer and middle ear

Source: Genetics Home Reference. (2011, January). A Service of U.S. National Library of Medicine. Retrieved from http://ghr.nlm.nih.gov.

Disorders of the middle ear impair hearing and can cause tinnitus. Conductive hearing loss involves loss of transmission of sound to the inner ear, caused by diseases such as external ear infections, cerumen impaction, and middle ear effusion or obstruction (Hain, 2011b). Sensorineural hearing loss occurs when there is damage to the eighth cranial nerve, the end organ of hearing. This hearing loss can occur in a variety of ways. Presbycusis followed by noise exposure is the primary cause of sensorineural hearing loss. Birth trauma and prenatal infections or exposure to toxic substances can also cause sensorineural hearing loss. In addition, neoplastic conditions, acoustic neuromas, Ménière's disease, ototoxicity from drugs or other chemicals, infections, and systemic diseases can cause sensorineural hearing loss (Arts, 2010) (see Chapter 63).

Disorders of the ear also can be associated with neurological problems. The nurse needs to inquire whether the patient has a history of meningitis, double vision, numbness in hands or feet, weakness in arms or legs, tingling in the mouth or face, loss of consciousness, fainting, or seizures. When noise-induced hearing loss occurs, the hair cells of the basilar membrane of the cochlea have been damaged. Risks for the development of hearing and balance disorders are listed in the Risk Factors box.

Social History

The patient's social history includes occupational and recreational pursuits, cultural considerations, environmental exposures, health habits, and travel. Each of these areas may include items that have the potential to affect hearing. Occupational and recreational activities are very prone to causing hearing problems. Some examples are discussed in the following text.

Occupational and Recreational Pursuits

Occupational- and recreational-related ear problems can occur for a variety of reasons. Anyone who experiences high levels of noise occupationally or recreationally without wearing hearing protection risks hearing impairment and potential deafness. Sources of high levels of noise (90 to 170 dB) include chain saws and other power tools, rock concerts, gunshots, jets, diesel locomotives, motorcycles, and lawn mower engines. One-third of all hearing loss can be attributed to occupational noise exposure (NIDCD, December 2010a). Experiencing recreational and occupational noise on an acute or chronic basis can cause bilateral sensorineural hearing loss at higher frequencies (3,000 to 6,000 Hz) (NIDCD, October, 2008).

RISK FACTORS for Hearing and Balance Disorders

Aging: Exposure to sounds over the years can damage the cells of the inner ear. It also may cause loss of muscle and bone strength and precipitate loss of balance.

Heredity: Genetic makeup may make a person more susceptible to ear damage.

Occupational noises: Jobs in which loud noise is a regular part of the working environment, such as farming, construction, or factory work, can lead to damage of the ear and the vestibular system.

Recreational noises: Exposure to explosive noises, such as from firing firearms and fireworks, can cause immediate permanent hearing loss. Other recreational activities with a high potential for causing hearing loss over time include snowmobiling, motorcycling, and listening to or playing loud music.

Otoxic medications: Some drugs have the potential to cause toxic reactions to structures of the inner ear, including the cochlea, vestibule, and semicircular canals. These include specific drugs from the following classifications: salicylates, nonsteroidal anti-inflammatory drugs (NSAIDs), antibiotics, diuretics, chemotherapeutic agents, quinine, mucosal protectants, and narcotic analgesics. Some, such as salicylates, may cause temporary effects on hearing such as tinnitus or hearing loss. Others, such as the antibiotic gentamicin or the chemotherapeutic cisplatin, may have long lasting or irreversible effects (Hain, 2011a).

Illnesses: Diseases or illnesses that result in high fever, such as meningitis, may damage the cochlea. Diabetes and kidney disease are known to affect both hearing and balance (Medicine Net, 2011). Trauma also may affect hearing and balance, as may ear infections, swimmer's ear, hypertension, and problems in the skeletal or visual systems such as arthritis or eye muscle imbalance (NIDCD, 2009).

Safety Alert *Noise-induced hearing loss (NIHL), often referred to as toxic loss, can be caused by a one-time exposure to an intense "impulse" sound such as an explosion. A one-time sound above 120–150 decibels is considered toxic, and may cause temporary or permanent hearing loss (Hearing Health Foundation, 2011).*

Cultural Considerations

Cultural considerations must be considered when the nurse conducts a health history related to hearing and balance disorders. Culture can affect how receptive the patient is to the prescribed medical treatment. For example, many people in the deaf community refuse genetic services because of a history of stigmatization. At one time in the United States, deaf people were sterilized and prohibited from marrying, and programs were developed to extinguish their language (American Academy of Hearing Loss Support Specialists, 2011). Additional cultural considerations related to hearing are discussed in the Cultural Considerations box.

Environmental Exposures

Currently, more than 750 different groups of chemicals have been identified as potentially ototoxic (Western Australia Department of Commerce, 2011). Nurses must increase their awareness of the pervasiveness of these chemicals, their toxic effects, and the symptoms they produce.

CULTURAL CONSIDERATIONS
Related to Hearing and Balance Disorders

Some Native American and Alaskan Indians prefer to use the traditional methods of healing, such as a medicine man, before resorting to Western methods of health care. People of other cultures, such as Asian Americans, Pacific Islanders, and Hispanics, may also prefer to use traditional methods of healing. Chinese people are particularly reluctant to accept surgical procedures (Spector, 2008). Practitioners of Western methods of treatment may view this as noncompliance.

In relation to the assessment of the ear during history taking, the nurse needs to be sensitive to cultural norms. For example, for American Indian and Alaska Native populations, note taking during the interview is taboo (Spector, 2008). With patients from these populations, the nurse needs to directly address the issue with the patient or devise a culturally sensitive method of recording the information.

One interesting physical difference is with regard to cerumen (earwax). Vietnamese individuals have dry earwax that is gray in color and brittle to the touch. In a majority of Asians and Native Americans, cerumen is dry, white, and flaky. In African Americans and Caucasians, cerumen is brown, wet, and sticky (Traynor, 2011).

The *NIOSH Pocket Guide to Chemical Hazards* (U.S. Department of Health and Human Services, 2007) can help the nurse to identify chemical health hazards and symptoms.

Health Habits

Evaluating the patient's health habits can be an opportunity for health teaching. The nurse should teach the patient that using cotton tip applicators, hairpins, paper clips, or other such objects in the ear can damage the tympanic membrane and cause possible acute bacterial otitis externa (swimmer's ear) (University of Iowa Hospitals and Clinics, 2008).

Travel

Changes in air pressure during airplane travel can cause ear discomfort. Common measures used to prevent this discomfort are to swallow more frequently and/or to yawn. Another technique is to pinch the nostrils shut, take a mouthful of air, force it into the back of the nose, and try to blow the thumb and fingers off the nostrils. The ears should then be cleared, and hearing should return to normal. If none of these techniques is successful, the individual may try to use a decongestant or nose spray. Feeding a baby with a bottle or putting a pacifier in the baby's mouth during changes in cabin pressure will help the baby's ears pop. Because colds, sinus infections, or allergies commonly block the Eustachian tubes, postponing the trip until the symptoms are less bothersome may be helpful. Any patient who has undergone ear surgery should consult with her health care provider about when it will be safe to travel by air (American Academy of Otolaryngology-Head and Neck Surgery, 2011).

Safety Alert *In any patient with sudden hearing loss, the nurse must investigate the possibility of trauma and also ask the patient what medications he is currently taking and for how long, in case medications are affecting hearing.*

Hearing loss can be exacerbated by concurrent exposure to ototoxic solvents or heavy metals (Campo, 2009). The nurse should be aware of this important modifiable health risk, screen for risk factors, and teach the proper use of hearing protection. Is the patient's workplace very noisy? Does the patient wear any personal protective ear protection? How often does the patient wear earplugs?

Current Issue

Video: Audiology

What is the patient's current ear problem? The focus of the interview and assessment should be on identifying hearing loss, **otalgia** (ear pain), tinnitus, vertigo, and infection. The nurse should conduct a risk factor analysis and assess any acute injury.

Hearing Loss

Each year 60,000 people in the United States are diagnosed with unilateral hearing loss (Voelker & Chole, 2010). About 28 million Americans have some hearing loss (American Speech-Language-Hearing Association, 2011). The nurse needs to inquire whether the patient has any difficulty hearing high- or low-pitched sounds, or both. Questions in this assessment include the following:

- Does the patient have difficulty discriminating sounds in a group setting?
- Has the change in hearing been sudden or gradual?
- Do family members say that the patient cannot hear them?
- What were the events leading to the perception of hearing loss?
- Does the patient perceive distortion in hearing, differences in pitch or sound, fullness or pressure in the ear?
- Has the patient ever had a hearing examination? If so, why?
- What were the results of the hearing examination?
- Does the patient work in a profession in which there is chronic loud noise (e.g., working with jet engines)? If so, does the patient wear ear protection? Some occupational pursuits require the use of hearing protection.

The nurse can perform a standard set of hearing tests depending on the symptoms, as outlined in the Diagnostic Tests for Hearing and Balance Disorders box in Chapter 63 (p. 2006).

The patient may already be having treatment for hearing loss. Is the patient wearing a hearing aid? If so, are hearing aids worn in one or both ears? Are they turned on? Do the hearing aids help the patient's hearing? How old are the batteries? How recently did the patient change batteries? Does the hearing aid cause any irritation of the ear canal? Does the patient have an implantable hearing device? The nurse needs to observe any behavioral cues that may indicate possible hearing loss:

- Irritability
- Difficulty hearing higher-frequency consonants (e.g., *sl* or *sh*)
- Complaints about people mumbling or giving inappropriate answers
- Use of a high volume on the television or radio
- Frequently asking for words to be repeated
- Leaning forward or turning head to hear better
- Avoiding group situations or any place with increased background noise
- Appearing aloof
- Using a very soft or loud voice.

Otalgia

The nurse needs to inquire about the presence, duration, and intensity of otalgia. Is it unilateral or bilateral, constant or intermittent, and where is the location of the pain? Does the patient have a sense of fullness in the ears? Is the pain worse when the patient is moving and relieved by staying still? Does the application of warmth help? The nurse should

Video*: External and Internal Ear Exam

use a 1-to-10 pain scale to determine the intensity of pain. If there is a history of trauma to the ears, the nurse should ask what measures have been used to relieve the pain and whether they have been successful. The nurse also should ask whether the patient uses a cotton applicator or other implement to clean the ears.

Tinnitus

Tinnitus (ringing in the ears) affects approximately 36 million Americans (American Academy of Otolaryngology-Head and Neck Surgery, 2010). It is described as an unwanted, primarily localized, internal auditory perception. Objective tinnitus can be heard by others and is caused by vascular problems of the carotid arteries or jugular veins. Subjective tinnitus, which is more common, can be heard only by the patient and can be caused by metabolic, pharmacologic, psychogenic, and/or neurological abnormalities (American Academy of Otolaryngology-Head and Neck Surgery, 2010). The nurse needs to assess when the patient first noticed ringing in the ears and/or any kind of head noise. What is the intensity or frequency? Is the noise high or low pitched; buzzing, humming, or hissing; or is it loud and persistent? Is it intermittent or constant, unilateral or bilateral, and what, if anything, relieves the symptoms? Has the patient been taking medications such as aspirin? A thorough history, a head and neck exam, and audiometric exams are warranted for the patient with tinnitus (Brochert, 2007).

Vertigo

Vertigo is the illusion of rotational movement, tilting, or swaying with feelings of imbalance during standing and walking. More than 90 million Americans over the age of 17 years report vertigo to their health care providers each year (Thompson & Amedd, 2009). It can be a symptom of serious central cerebral dysfunction (acoustic neuroma, brain tumor, or trauma) or a benign peripheral problem (semicircular canals, peripheral nerve). It is a cardinal symptom of vestibular dysfunction.

With objective vertigo, the patient perceives that the surroundings are moving and the body stays still. Subjective vertigo is just the reverse: the patient perceives that the body is moving and the surroundings are still. Nausea and vomiting may persist but loss of consciousness is not usually a problem. Other symptoms that the patient may experience include presyncope, disequilibrium, and light-headedness. Presyncope is a feeling of faintness. Disequilibrium is the feeling of falling. Light-headedness may be psychogenic or idiopathic. Peripheral causes are usually intensely vertiginous, whereas central causes are mildly vertiginous with nystagmus (an involuntary rhythmic movement of the eye) (Reeves & Swenson, 2008b). To rule out the possibility of other system involvement, all cranial nerves should be tested. Cardiac rate, rhythm, and orthostatic hypotension, which can mimic positional vertigo, also should be checked.

As part of the assessment, the nurse asks the patient to describe the physical sensation of vertigo. Has the patient fallen or been injured because of the vertigo? Does this vertigo happen when the patient changes positions? Is it intermittent or constant? Is there any unsteadiness of gait? It also is important for the nurse to inquire about current medications that may cause vertigo (discussed in Chapter 63). The assessment must include an evaluation of both prescription and OTC medications that may cause ototoxicity, which is hearing loss resulting from eighth cranial nerve (vestibulocochlear) damage, and sometimes loss of balance or vertigo. The patient with vertigo should be referred to a health care provider for further testing for causes, such as brain tumors.

Hearing Disorders Related to Medications

The combination of vertigo, tinnitus, and hearing loss can be very disabling. Among patients with tinnitus, 85% also have hearing loss. Ototoxic tinnitus can be caused by ACE inhibitors; some anesthetics, such as bupivacaine and lidocaine; and antibiotics, specifically gentamicin, sulfisoxazole, trimethoprim-sulfamethoxazole, and vancomycin (Drugs.com, 2011).

Many patients who take medications, specifically salicylates, erythromycin, and loop diuretics, can develop bilateral and permanent ototoxic hearing loss. Loop diuretics damage stria vascularis in the organ of Corti. Aminoglycosides damage the cochlear hair cells, causing bilateral hearing loss and dizziness. Vancomycin's toxic effect results in high-frequency hearing loss, which may lead to permanent deafness caused by damage to the auditory receptor cells. Note that benign positional vertigo is usually not associated with hearing loss or tinnitus.

Infection or Drainage

The nurse needs to inquire about any spontaneous purulent, clear (cerebrospinal fluid), or bloody drainage. What is the consistency and the amount of drainage? Is the drainage unilateral or bilateral? Is it acute or chronic? Does the patient have a fever, recent upper respiratory infection, cough, earache, or other symptoms that would indicate an infection? These questions all help to diagnose infection. If an infection appears to be present, the nurse refers the patient to a health care provider for further evaluation and treatment.

Barotrauma

Barotrauma, which is physical injury or rupture of the tympanic membrane, results from changing air pressure (Miyamoto, 2008). The nurse should inquire about any problems with the ears subsequent to diving or an airplane flight. Has the patient had any sports injuries or been involved in a car crash? Air bags deploying in an enclosed space (with car windows closed) can cause ear barotrauma.

Physical Examination

Ear conditions do not occur in isolation from the other body systems. For instance, it is important for the nurse to check the temperature of a patient with complaints of otalgia in assessing for infection. Checking the blood pressure and pulse of a patient who has symptoms of possible vestibular dysfunction such as vertigo is important to rule out cardiovascular conditions. All cranial nerves should be checked because their proper functioning or impairment in relation to ear and eye problems is integral to understanding the other body systems. For example, an abnormality of the facial nerve (CN VII) with asymmetric facial movements can suggest Bell's palsy or a cerebrovascular accident. Chapter 21 describes the assessment of the cranial nerves.

Inspection and Monitoring

The nurse inspects the external structures of the ear visually. The top of the ears should cross a line from the outer canthus of the eye. An auricle below this line or at a posterior angle greater than 10 degrees may indicate chromosomal aberrations. The nurse should inspect for size, symmetry, shape, skin color, redness, drainage, as well scaling and nodules (may be cancer and gout). If drainage is present, is it sanguineous, serous, mixed, purulent, or odiferous? The nurse should inspect the mastoid bone for size and color of skin and note any tenderness.

The inside of the ear is inspected with an otoscope. An otoscopic examination includes inspection of the auditory canal and tympanic membrane. The nurse looks for inflammation, exudates, lesions, and foreign bodies and checks for narrowing of the ear canal, nodules, redness, scales, edema, and drainage. Normally, the eardrum is slightly conical, shiny, smooth, and pearl gray. Cerumen should be moist and may vary in color from brown to white; hardened, dry, or foul-smelling cerumen may indicate infection. The nurse looks for the structures of the tympanic membrane, for landmarks indicating the border of the annulus, the light reflex, the umbo (the most depressed part of the tympanic membrane), the short process, and the long handle of the malleus. The nurse notes the color and presence of perforations, bulging, or retraction of the tympanic membrane, as well as noting dilation of the vessels, bubbles, or fluid; normal middle ear fluid is thin and amber (Natal, 2011). To test the mobility of the tympanic membrane, a pneumatoscope is used. A **pneumatoscope** is an otoscope with a bulb attachment in which the nurse introduces air into the ear canal and middle ear. A ruptured tympanic membrane will not move.

Palpation

During the physical assessment, the nurse gently palpates the auricle (refer to Figure 62–1, p. 1971), which is the external ear or pinna, with the thumb and forefinger to check for tenderness, pain, or nodules. The nurse also palpates the mastoid behind the auricle; it should be smooth, hard, and nontender. Abnormalities of the auricle include Darwin's tubercle (a benign protrusion on the upper part of the helix). Scar formation from ear piercing or trauma may be present. Sebaceous cysts in the meatus or in back of the auricle can become painful, as can nodules along the rim of the auricle. Exostoses (also known as surfer's ear) are benign bony lumps in the ear canal near the tympanic membrane that develop from progressive bone growth as a protective mechanism for the ear against cold and wind (Di Martino, 2011). The nurse should palpate the preauricular and postauricular lymph nodes to determine the size and location of any palpable nodes and whether they are soft or hard, nontender or tender, and mobile or fixed (Healthwise Staff, 2012).

Hearing Tests

During the assessment, the nurse observes for any obvious clues to hearing loss such as the patient asking for words to be repeated. If any hearing test abnormalities are found, the patient should be referred to an audiologist for further testing. Hearing acuity is tested to determine whether hearing loss is present and, if so, whether it is conductive or sensorineural. The **Weber test** screens hearing acuity and helps to distinguish whether hearing loss is conductive or sensorineural. A tuning fork tapped at the base will emit a vibratory frequency range of 512 to 1,024 Hz, which corresponds to normal speech. When conducting the Weber test, the nurse places an activated tuning fork midline on top of the patient's head, the bridge of the nose, or the chin. A negative or normal Weber test occurs when the patient perceives sound equally in both ears or "in the middle." Sound that lateralizes to the affected ear is conducted through bone and represents a conductive hearing loss from external or middle ear disorders. Sound that lateralizes to the unaffected ear indicates nerve damage or sensorineural hearing loss from the inner ear or auditory or brain pathology.

The **Rinne test** is used to measure the conduction of sound by bone. In this test, an activated tuning fork is placed sequentially on the right and the left mastoid bone. The patient indicates when the sound is no longer heard. The tuning fork is then placed in front of the auditory canal. Normally, air conduction through the external auditory canal takes twice as long as conduction through the mastoid bone. With a conductive hearing loss, bone conduction is faster than air conduction (Reeves & Swenson, 2008a). With the **Schwabach test,** the nurse places an activated tuning fork on the mastoid process of the patient and alternately tests for air and bone conduction. With the **voice whisper test,** the examiner stands approximately 1 to 2 feet behind the patient and whispers several words near each ear. The patient should be able to hear bilaterally and equally.

Vestibular hearing function tests the receptors for the vestibular system, which are located in the semicircular ducts of the inner ear. The vestibular nerve fibers travel in the vestibulocochlear (VIII) cranial nerve to the vestibular nuclei of the oculomotor (III), trochlear (IV), and abducens (VI) cranial nerves. Disorders of the vestibular function can be peripheral, involving the labyrinth, or central, involving the vestibular connections. Abnormal nystagmus, tinnitus, or hearing loss are other common manifestations of vestibular dysfunction. Vestibular function tests are outlined in the Diagnostic Tests for Vestibular Function box in Chapter 63 (p. 2004).

Video: Otoscope Evaluation of an Adolescent Ear

The **caloric test** uses differences in temperature to diagnose damage to the ear or brainstem (Dugdale, 2011). Specifically, the test is used to diagnose nystagmus, tinnitus, or hearing loss that results from vestibular dysfunction. In the caloric test, the inner ear and nearby nerves are stimulated by cold or warm water that is delivered to the ear canal at different times. This test can differentiate peripheral lesions from eighth cranial nerve lesions. Warm or cold water is introduced into the ear. The normal response is vertigo and nystagmus within 30 to 60 seconds. When cold water is introduced into the left ear, the normal response is a right beating nystagmus. When warm water is introduced into the left ear, a left beating nystagmus is elicited (Reeves & Swenson, 2008a). This test is done only on a person with an intact eardrum and no visible blood or fluid behind the tympanic membrane. A caloric test is done on an unconscious patient to test for severe brainstem injury. A patient with a brain injury does not show nystagmus in response to the caloric test.

The **Romberg test** assesses the patient's ability to maintain an upright posture with arms out in front when eyes are open and closed. This is used to test for inner ear balance and the proprioceptive ability of the visual and cerebellar system.

Auscultation

When assessing for objective tinnitus, the nurse can auscultate over the head and neck, periauricular area, orbits, and mastoid and verify for audible sounds (Reeves & Swenson, 2008a). If the nurse notes any sounds, this indicates that objective tinnitus is present, helping to differentiate between subjective and objective tinnitus.

Hearing Aids

The patient may have hearing aids to correct existing hearing impairment. If so, the nurse should check the hearing aids for cleanliness. The audiologist can provide the patient with a small wire brush to remove built-up cerumen. In addition, the nurse should advise the patient to keep an extra supply of batteries on hand. Indications for and types of hearing aids are discussed in detail in Chapter 63.

Health Promotion

Health promotion activities focus on providing education to the patient, family, and community. Emphasis is placed on regular screenings and/or examinations to determine the health of the ear, ensuring that the patient and community are aware of risk factors and ways of reducing them, as well as the availability of community support.

Screening Opportunities

The National Health Information Center (healthfinder@nhic.org) strongly recommends receiving ear exams on a regular basis. Regular screening enables the health care provider to find problems early, when they may be easier to treat. The nurse should encourage patients to participate in screening examinations on a regular basis as advised by their health care provider to detect hearing and balance, risks and defects. The nurse should advise patients and families of screening opportunities available to them, including community and Internet resources. Hearing screening may be available through local community groups and health care agencies. The EyeCanHear organization sponsored by the American Society of Ophthalmic Administrators conducts screening for dual sensory impairment. This organization is approved for Medicare patients. Patient and program information offered by EyeCanHear, as well as service contacts, can be accessed via the Internet at http://eyecanhear.com/patient-benefits/.

Methods of Reducing Risks

The nurse should advise patients to avoid exposure to continuous, very loud noises as well as sudden, sharp loud noises. Patients should be taught the warning signs of exposure to hazardous noise:

- The patient cannot hear someone 3 feet away.
- The patient has pain in the ears after leaving a noisy area.
- The patient hears ringing or buzzing in the ears (tinnitus) immediately after exposure to noise.
- The patient suddenly has difficulty understanding speech after exposure to noise, being able to hear people talking but not able to understand them. (Danielson, 2011)

The nurse should caution patients that if they have to shout to be heard over noise by someone an arm's length away or less, the noise is probably in the dangerous range (over 85 decibels). The nurse should instruct patients to reduce noise at the source if possible and advise patients and families to check with employers to see whether testing for job-related hearing loss is available (American Tinnitus Association, 2011; Danielson, 2011).

The nurse should encourage patients who swim or surf to wear ear plugs when in the water and/or a neoprene hood when swimming or surfing in the ocean to avoid swimmer's ear or surfer's ear.

The nurse should advise patients not to dry their ears with an applicator or any other small object after bathing, as this may rupture the eardrum. The nurse may instruct patients to gently use the end of a towel to remove excess water or use a cotton ball to wick the water out (Pediatric ENT Associates, 2011).

The nurse should instruct patients and families not to use an applicator or other small object to remove cerumen from the ears, as this may cause the eardrum to rupture. Some people develop excess cerumen, which can cause temporary hearing loss. They should be advised to have a nurse remove the cerumen with ear irrigation.

Community Education, Support, and Communication

It is essential to apprise the patient and family of available community resources that they can access without undue hardship such as lengthy travel or major disruption to a work schedule. It is equally important to let community organizations and health systems know of the need for hearing and vision screening. When talking with the patient or communicating with community organizations, the nurse must recognize and address the unique culture, language, and health literacy of diverse consumers and communities. Points to be considered are age, race/ethnicity, gender, and special populations such as migrant workers and people from different cultures. Communication should be tailored to meet these express characteristics of the people and communities served (Health Resources and Services Administration, 2011).

VISUAL ASSESSMENT

Visual assessment, like hearing assessment, is a vital part of the nurse's role in caring for the whole patient. Eye conditions can be common, can be age specific, and may require immediate attention. Disorders of the eye may affect the person's ability to see properly for discerning objects, reading, performing everyday tasks, or driving an automobile. Some visual disorders can be disfiguring or cause total blindness. Blindness may affect the person's self-image and can lead to social isolation. Early diagnosis, treatment, and management can play a key role in keeping the person active and involved in society.

Nurses are key professional team members in identifying risk factors and encouraging healthy and preventive behaviors in patients. In this role, nurses function within the recommendations of the Guidelines for Comprehensive Adult Medical Eye Evaluation developed by the American Academy of Ophthalmology (2010). The recommendation includes components of a health history interview and the components of a physical examination, which are provided in the National Guidelines box. The modifiable risk factors related to eye diseases and vision impairment can be genetic, environmental, or occupational. Specific risk factors are listed in the Risk Factors box. They are congruent with the Guidelines for Comprehensive Adult Medical Eye Evaluation. Nurses play a key role in assisting, planning, implementing, evaluating, testing, and educating patients and their families in identifying risk factors and in learning new coping skills for adapting to the everyday changes that can come with visual disorders.

Anatomy and Physiology Overview

The eye and its structures can be examined externally and internally. The structures of the orbit and ocular adnexa include the orbital contents and walls, eyebrows, eyelashes, eyelids, lacrimal puncta, lacrimal system, and extraocular muscles (Figure 62–3◆). The eye structures include the canthus, conjunctiva, limbus, sclera, cornea, anterior and posterior chambers, trabecular meshwork, choroid, ciliary body, iris, pupil, lens, vitreous body, and retina.

Orbit and Ocular Adnexa

The eyeball is encased on three sides by the bony cavity called the orbit, which protects the eyeball from injury. The orbit is lined with muscles, connective tissue, and adipose tissue. It is approximately 40 millimeters in all three dimensions (height, width, and depth), like a pear lying on its side. The orbital walls are made up of seven bones: the frontal, zygomatic, sphenoid, ethmoid, lacrimal, palatine, and maxillary bones. The eyebrow lies over the bony prominence (superior orbital ridge) above the eyelids that acts as a protective ridge from falling debris or foreign objects getting into the eye. The upper and lower eyelashes are the

NATIONAL GUIDELINES for Visual Assessment

Comprehensive Adult Medical Eye Evaluation Recommendation:

> A comprehensive medical eye evaluation includes a history, examination, diagnosis, and initiation of management. Included within each part of the evaluation is a series of items particularly effective for the detection, diagnosis, and choice of appropriate therapy for refractive error, ocular disease, and systemic disease. The items listed are basic areas of evaluation or investigation and are not meant to exclude additional elements when appropriate. For example because history taking is an interactive process, the patient's responses may guide the clinician to pursue additional questions and evaluation. (Agency for Healthcare Research and Quality, 2010, p. 4)

Following this broad recommendation, specific instructions are provided to complete an ocular health history and a comprehensive ocular examination guide. The examination guide specifies an evaluation of the anatomic and physiologic function of the eye, the visual system, and its related structures. For full details of the Health History and Ocular Examination Guides, please review the actual guidelines at http://www.ngc.gov/content-aspx?id=25644.

Source: Agency for Healthcare Research and Quality (AHARQ). (2010). Comprehensive adult medical evaluation. U.S. Department of Health & Human Services. Retrieved from http://www.ngc/gov/content.aspz?id=25644.

RISK FACTORS for Development of Eye Disorders

Age: As one ages, the risks for age-related eye disorders increase. This is particularly true with glaucoma, cataracts, and macular degeneration.

Ethnicity: Some evidence suggests that ethnic ancestry influences the likelihood of developing eye disorders, particularly glaucoma and cataracts. Glaucoma is the leading cause of blindness among African Americans (Are You at Risk for Glaucoma, 2011).

Diseases: Diabetes or prediabetes, liver and kidney disease, and hypertension influence the development of visual disorders, diabetic retinopathy, and ocular and systemic hypertension. High myopia and central corneal thickness are risk factors (Glaucoma Research Foundation, 2011).

Gender: Some studies suggest that women are more likely than men to develop cataracts (Lighthouse International, 2011).

Medications: The Eye Digest has identified specific medications that are prone to cause eye disorders:

- Hydroxychloroquine may cause retinal toxicity.
- Tamoxifen may cause crystalline retinopathy, corneal deposits, and optic neuritis.
- Phenothiazines (thioridazine and chlorpromazine) may cause blurred vision, night vision, and color vision problems; retinal pigment changes; pigmented corneal deposits; and anterior capsular cataracts.
- Sildenafil (Viagra) may cause vision haze, increased light sensitivity, and ischemic injury to the optic nerve, resulting in vision loss (The Eye Digest, 2011).

Eye injuries and occupational hazards: Eye injuries can cause secondary open-angle glaucoma immediately after an injury or years later. Blunt injuries that bruise the eye or injuries that penetrate the eye can damage the eye's drainage system. The most common cause is sports-related injuries such as baseball or boxing.

Absence of eye exam: Going too long without an eye examination can lead to undetected risks and problems. If one is 65 or older, eyes should be checked every 1 to 2 years. If an individual has diabetes or another identified disease that involves a high risk for developing eye disorders, the eye exam should occur more often.

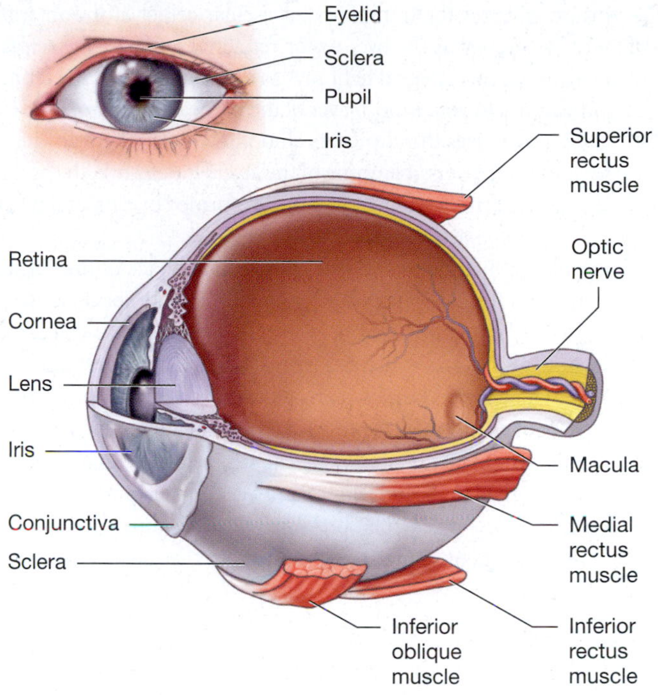

FIGURE 62–3 ◆ The human eye.

ciliary hairs of the eyelids that help keep debris from falling into the eye. The eyelids contain the ocular glands, which include oil glands (meibomian and glands of Zeis), mucous glands (goblet cells), sweat glands (Moll), and aqueous glands (lacrimal and accessory lacrimal glands of Krause and Wolfring).

The exposed area between the upper and lower eyelids is called the interpalpebral fissure. The eyelids have a blink mechanism that operates by the levator palpebrae superioris muscle to protect the anterior portion of the eye and the spreading of tears across the cornea. This blink mechanism is very important to the health of the cornea. Upper and lower lacrimal puncta are the small openings at the nasal end of the upper and lower eyelid margins for the drainage of tears produced by the lacrimal system. The lacrimal gland lies under the upper eyelid skin between the lateral eyebrow edge and outer canthus.

The eyeball is able to move in all cardinal fields of gaze through the action of the six extraocular muscles, which are the four rectus muscles (superior, medial, inferior, and lateral) and two oblique muscles (superior and inferior). The extraocular muscles are innervated by the third, fourth, and sixth cranial nerves, which coordinate the vision of both eyes with the occipital lobe of the brain to view a single image.

Eye Structures

It is necessary for the nurse to understand the anatomic structure of the eye as a whole in order to identify pathophysiological conditions and their impact on the individual. The basic anatomic structures are explained next.

The temporal and nasal canthi are the outer and inner tissue edges where the upper and lower eyelids meet. The palpebral and bulbar conjunctivas are the mucous membrane lining of the undersurface of the eyelids and eyeball itself, up to the limbal margin, respectively. The fornix or cul-de-sac is the junction where the palpebral and bulbar conjunctivas meet. The limbus or the corneoscleral junction is the margin between the sclera and the cornea. The sclera, which is the white part and the outer protective layer of the eyeball, helps maintain its shape.

The cornea, which is the transparent, avascular center at the anterior surface of the eyeball, is the eye's major refractive surface. The refractive media of the cornea bend light rays to a single focus on the retina. The epithelium is the outermost layer of the cornea that is protected by the tear film that gives the cornea its smooth surface. The tear film is composed of three layers; if any one of the layers is defective, the health of the eye can be compromised. The tears are formed by a natural reflex response or emotional stimulus.

The anterior chamber is the space between the back of the cornea and the front of the iris. The posterior chamber is the space between the back of the iris and the front of the lens. Both these chambers contain aqueous humor, which is a clear fluid that provides nutrients for the eye. The aqueous humor is produced by the ciliary body, which also helps regulate intraocular pressure. The trabecular meshwork is a meshlike filtering structure located at the iris–sclera junction (limbal region) at the angle in the anterior chamber. The meshwork assists in the regulation of the intraocular pressure of the eye through the filtering and flow of aqueous humor as it drains into the canal of Schlemm at the angle.

Uveal Tract

The uveal tract is composed of the choroid, ciliary body, and iris. The choroid, the middle layer of the eyeball between the retina and the sclera, contains the major vascular system of the eye that nourishes the outer retina. The ciliary body is made up of the ciliary processes and ciliary muscles. The processes produce the aqueous humor that flows through the chambers and can affect the intraocular pressure of the eye, whereas the ciliary muscles control the accommodative ability of the lens through the attachment of the zonular fibers between the lens and ciliary muscles. The ciliary muscle contractions can change the configuration of the trabecular meshwork or the canal of Schlemm by increasing aqueous outflow; in turn, this can affect the intraocular pressure of the eye. The iris, a vascular and pigmented fiber that forms the colored portion of the eye, divides the anterior and posterior chambers. The pupil is the black space in the middle of the iris, which constricts and dilates by the action of the sphincter muscles and the dilator muscles, respectively. This allows the refraction of light to enter the eye for vision. The pupils normally react to bright light by constricting, and they are usually equal, round, and accommodative.

Lens

The lens divides the aqueous humor from the vitreous humor or gel. It is the focusing structure of **accommodation** that allows individuals to see objects at close and at far range. The lens is supported by the zonular fibers that are attached to the ciliary body. It is the one ocular structure that continues to grow as the person ages.

Vitreous Body

The vitreous body is the largest chamber (roughly two-thirds) of the eye and maintains the shape of the eyeball. The vitreous gel is made up mainly of water with a collagen framework, which includes collagen (structure), hyaluronic acid (which gives the vitreous gel its viscosity), proteins, and solutes. The collagen network can be aggregated by vitreous collapse due to aging in which vitreous opacities form and cast shadows on the retina. These shadows are referred to as **floaters.** The posterior and peripheral vitreous interfaces with the retina.

Retina

The retina is composed of 10 thin layers. Two of the major retina layers are the photoreceptor layer and the retinal pigment epithelium. The photoreceptor layer is composed of cones and rods for photopic (day) and scotopic (night) vision. The center of the retina, called the *macula*, is where the greatest number of cone receptors is located for central and color vision. The rod receptors mainly are in the peripheral retina for side or field vision. The very center of the macula is called the *fovea* or *fovea centralis*, where the greatest concentrations of cones are located for the sharpest visual acuity. The two main functions of the retinal pigment epithelium are the metabolism of vitamin A and the absorption of light, which aid in visual acuity by providing nutrients to the photoreceptors.

Other major structures in the retina are the optic disc and vessels. The optic disc is oval or circular, pinkish orange in color, with distinct margins; has a central depression or cup; and is the physiological blind spot on a visual field. The central cup of the disc is where the retinal vessels (arteries and veins) enter and branch out to form the superior and inferior arcades, which are the outer borders of the macula. The optic nerve is an extension of the central nervous system that forms a visual pathway behind the eyes. The pathway crosses in the brain at the optic chiasm, where the optic nerve of each eye meets and crosses nasally and uncrosses temporally to form the optic tracts. The optic tracts continue to the lateral geniculate bodies, to the optic radiations, and then to the visual cortex of the occipital lobe of the brain.

History

To make an accurate visual assessment of the patient with eye problems, the nurse needs to take a complete health history. Outlines of the categories and assessment of a health and ocular history can be found in Chart 62–1. The categories include the general medical history, the visual history, and the history of clinical manifestations. It is important for the nurse to ask the patient specifically about any conditions such as diabetes, hypertension, macular degeneration, glaucoma, or unexplained vision loss and whether an injury has occurred. If there has been trauma, the nurse needs to make certain to question whether it involved any metal-on-metal contact, which tends to cause intraocular penetration.

CHART 62–1 Health and Ocular History Assessment

Category	Assessment
General history	Any known allergies (drugs, foods, environment)?
	Using any prescription or over-the-counter medications?
	Any recent illnesses or surgeries?
	Any known medical history (especially diabetes, ulcers, strokes, hypertension, and pulmonary)?
Visual history	Wears glasses, contact lenses, or no correction?
	Are one or both eyes involved?
	Using any topical eyedrops or oral eye medications?
	Vision prior to problem, injury, or trauma (if applicable)?
	Any vision or eye test already obtained previously?
	Any prior eye surgery or laser?
History of clinical manifestations	Any signs and symptoms?
	Duration of signs and symptoms?
	Time and place of signs and symptoms, problem, or injury/what happened?
	Any penetrating or perforating injury? Any metal?

CULTURAL CONSIDERATIONS for Visual Disorders

Culture	Ocular Condition
African Americans	Glaucoma
African Caribbeans	Sickle hemoglobinopathies
Africans, Central Americans, and South Americans	River blindness*
Africans, Middle Easterners, Indians, and Southeast Asians	Trachoma
Caucasians	Age-related macular degeneration
Hispanic Americans and African Americans	Diabetic retinopathy
Japanese and Spaniards	Progressive myopia

*River blindness is caused by a parasitic worm that lives under the skin; blindness is just one of the symptoms of this devastating human parasite. This parasitic disease originated in Africa but has spread to other parts of the world, including Saudi Arabia, Brazil, Colombia, Guatemala, and Mexico (Drisdelle, 2007). The disease causes nodules under the skin; an itchy, painful skin rash; and inflammation of the lymph nodes. The worms that are responsible for the disease invade the tissues at the back of the eye, causing an immune response that destroys vision slowly. The risk of blindness is increased if nodules containing adult worms are located on the scalp.

Sources: Drisdelle, R. (2007). What is river blindness? Retrieved from http://suite101.com/article/what-is-river-blindness-a24974ss. . . .; Yanoff, M., & Duker J. S. (Eds.). (2008). *Ophthalmology* (3rd ed.). St. Louis, MO: Mosby.

Biographic and Demographic History

Culture and geographic locations can have a significant impact on the types of visual impairment people experience. The Cultural Considerations box outlines some visual disorders that are more common in specific cultures and certain geographic locations due to climate and environmental conditions.

Family Health History

Genetics is the study of the gene matrix that makes each person unique and provides the molecules and cellular processes for anatomic description of visual development and outcome. Understanding some of the inherited mutations can assist in the treatment and prognosis of specific visual defects. Descriptions of common hereditary conditions that might be factors in visual impairment of adults are presented in the Genetic Considerations box (p. 1982).

Physical Examination

The initial examination of the eye should include visual acuity (VA) at far range (Figure 62–4◆) and at near range (Figure 62–5◆), external eye examination, the direct ophthalmoscope examination, and an intraocular pressure reading. For patients who cannot read, the nurse should use a picture chart to obtain acuity. Chart 62–2 (p. 1984) outlines the steps for visual acuity testing.

The external evaluation can be done with the use of a penlight and visual observation. The components for completing the external examination and procedures are listed in Chart 62–3 (p. 1984) and Chart 62–4 (p. 1985).

Direct ophthalmoscope examination is used to check the fundus of the eye by viewing through the pupil. During the process, the nurse needs to view the cornea, anterior chamber, lens, and vitreous for clarity; check for any opacity in the visual pathway; and check the optic nerve (disc) for color, shape, and vessels (Figure 62–6◆, p. 1983). Most medical offices, clinics, ambulatory centers, outpatient

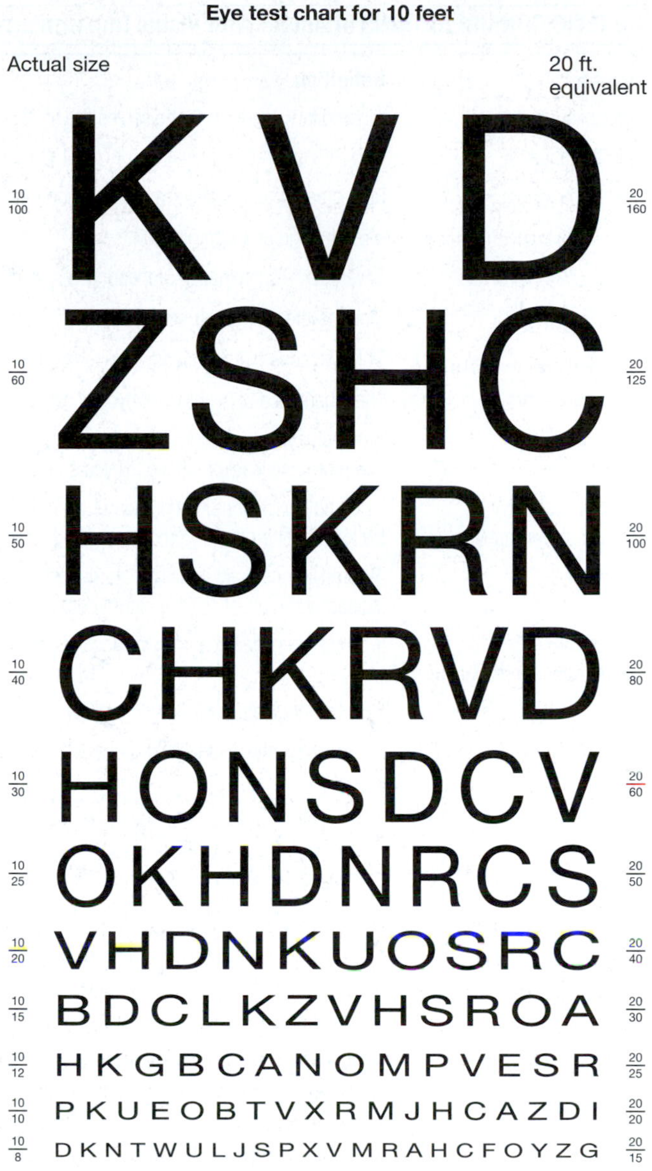

FIGURE 62–4 ◆ Visual acuity chart for far.

facilities, and emergency departments will be equipped with a direct ophthalmoscope.

If the nurse has a tonometer, it is important to check intraocular pressure (IOP) (Figure 62–7◆, p. 1983); otherwise, the nurse may need to gently palpate over the eyelid to indicate whether the eyeball is hard or soft (Figure 62–8◆, p. 1983).

Health Promotion

Health promotion activities for vision are similar to those for hearing with the exception of risk factors. These activities focus on educating the patient about regular vision screening or examinations, providing education to the patient and family regarding ways to reduce risk factors, and highlighting community emphasis on providing resources to the vision impaired. The National Health Information Center (2011) recommends vision testing every 2 years, or annually if the person is diabetic.

Methods of Reducing Risk

The nurse should review risk factors with the patient and family and instruct them in ways to avoid or reduce the risks.

Weblink: Genetic Alliance

GENETIC CONSIDERATIONS in Adults With Visual Impairments

Disorder	Definition
Color blindness:	A hereditary condition that disables the ability for vision to distinguish colors.
• Protanomaly	Mild red–green discrimination, deficient red photoreceptors.
• Deuteranomaly	Red–green discrimination; most common form of color blindness (X linked).
• Tritanomaly	Mild blue–green discrimination.
• Protanopia	Severe red discrimination, appearing very dark; no red photoreceptors.
• Deuteranopia	More severe red–green discrimination.
• Tritanopia	Only two cone pigments and no blue photoreceptors.
Refractive errors	The inheritance of hyperopia, myopia, and/or astigmatic refractive errors.
Keratoconus	A hereditary central thinning of the cornea, making it a cone-shaped elevation of the central cornea that is usually progressive and more noticeable in those 20 years or older.
Corneal dystrophy (or Fuchs' dystrophy)	It can be hereditary; deterioration of the cornea due to loss of endothelial cells from Descemet's membrane (fourth corneal layer) thickening, and possibly progressing to poor vision and cornea transplant.
Cataracts	A hereditary cataract usually matures faster, and cataract surgery can be necessary as early as in the second to fourth decade of life, instead of the usual sixth to eighth decade of life.
Glaucoma (Mendelian inheritance)	It can be hereditary, causing intraocular pressure elevation, optic nerve atrophy, and poor perfusion of the optic nerve.
Uveitis	It can be hereditary with inflammation of the uveal tract, which includes the iris, ciliary body, and choroid.
Leber's hereditary optic atrophy	A hereditary, rapidly developing bilateral optic nerve degeneration; vision loss usually stabilizes and occurs in males in their 20s and 30s.
Marfan's syndrome	A hereditary condition whereby the bone structure is very long and thin, especially in the arms, legs, fingers, and toes. Weak ligaments, bone deformities, and heart disease are prevalent. Individuals with Marfan's syndrome often are myopic, with large corneas, early cataracts, dislocated lenses, ptosis, strabismus, and choroidal malformations.
Usher's syndrome	A hereditary combination of bilateral deafness and night blindness.
Alport's syndrome	A hereditary combination of kidney disease, deafness, and lens abnormality; such as small and round lenses, early cataracts, and anterior lenticonus (cone-shaped protrusion of the lens).
Joubert syndrome	A hereditary central nervous system defect with severe psychomotor deficiencies, breathing problems, and nystagmus.
Wagner's disease	A hereditary vitreoretinal degeneration syndrome that makes one more prone to retinal tears and detachments. Other ocular signs are myopia, lattice degeneration, strabismus, and cataracts in the teen years.
Stickler syndrome	A hereditary progressive connective tissue disease that causes enlarged and degenerative joints, arthritis, flattened midface, cleft palate, and deafness. Ocular signs are vitreoretinal degeneration, high myopia, and early cataracts.
Grönblad-Strandberg syndrome (pseudoxanthoma elasticum)	A hereditary elastic connective disorder that gives skin a leathery appearance, something like a plucked chicken's skin, with major artery defects. The retinal symptoms are angioid streaks, which are subretinal pigmented lines from cracks in Bruch's membrane that form macular hemorrhages and scars.
Age-related macular degeneration	A deterioration of the macula causing central vision loss and distortion. It is often hereditary, developing as early as the fifth decade of life.
Kandori's syndrome	A hereditary form of nonprogressive night blindness with numerous irregular and large gray-yellowish flecks in the retina.
Refsum's disease	A hereditary disease that is characterized by foot drop, inability to sleep, increased cerebrospinal fluid, accumulation of fatty acids, and electrocardiogram changes. Ocular signs are poor dark adaptation, constricted visual field, nystagmus, ptosis, and small pupil (miosis).
Retinitis pigmentosa (night blindness)	A hereditary bilateral rod/cone dysfunction with diminished or loss of side vision that can slowly progress to central vision loss and blindness.
Retinoblastoma	A hereditary malignant retinal tumor (most common in childhood); this may be the reason for an adult to have an eye removed or be blind in both eyes. If untreated, it can metastasize to the brain and cause death.

For more information on common hereditary conditions that might be factors in the visual impairment of adults, the following websites are useful:

- Genetic Alliance (http://www.geneticalliance.org)
- Gene Clinics (http://www.geneclinics.org)
- National Organization of Rare Diseases (http://www.rarediseases.org)
- Online Mendelian Inheritance in Man (OMIM) (http://www.ncbi.nlm.nih.gov/Literature/index.html or http://www.ncbi.nlm.nih.gov/genome/guide/human/e)

Source: Adapted from Stone, E. M. (2007). Genetic testing for inherited eye disease. *Archives of Ophthalmology, 125*(2), 205–212.

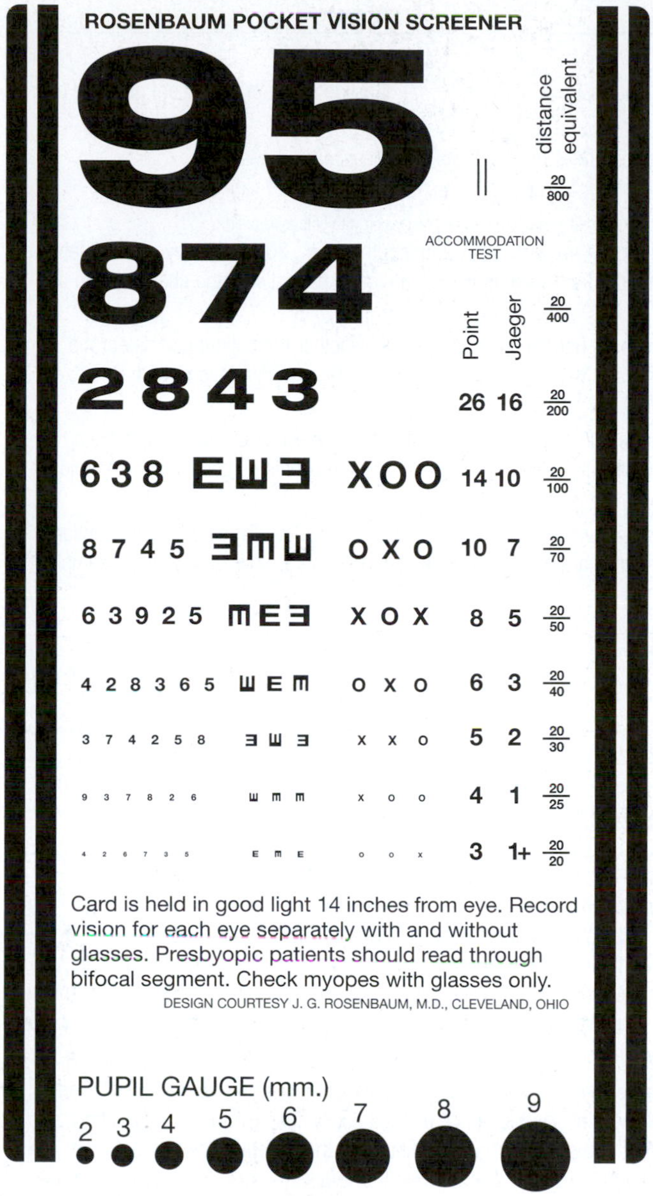

FIGURE 62–5 ◆ Visual acuity chart for near.

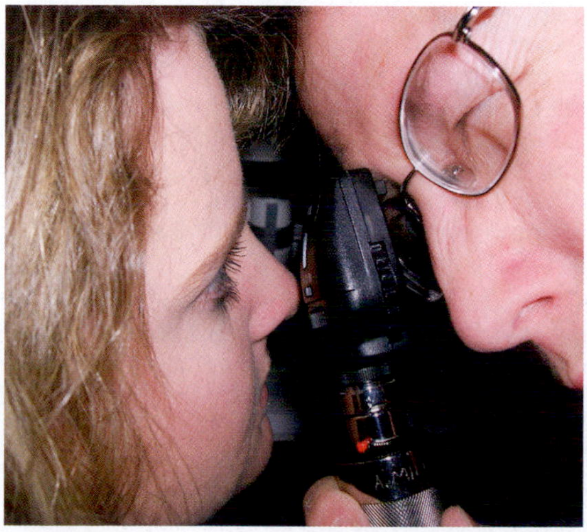

FIGURE 62–6 ◆ Direct ophthalmoscope examination.
Source: Lucie Elfervig.

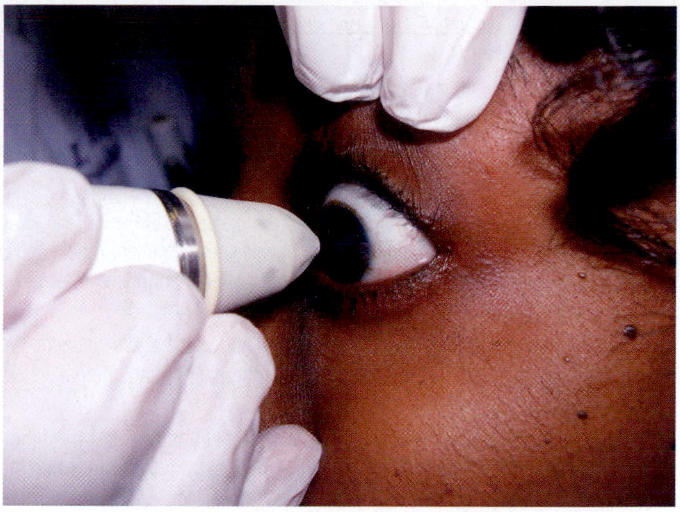

FIGURE 62–7 ◆ Application of Tono-Pen for intraocular pressure.
Source: Lucie Elfervig.

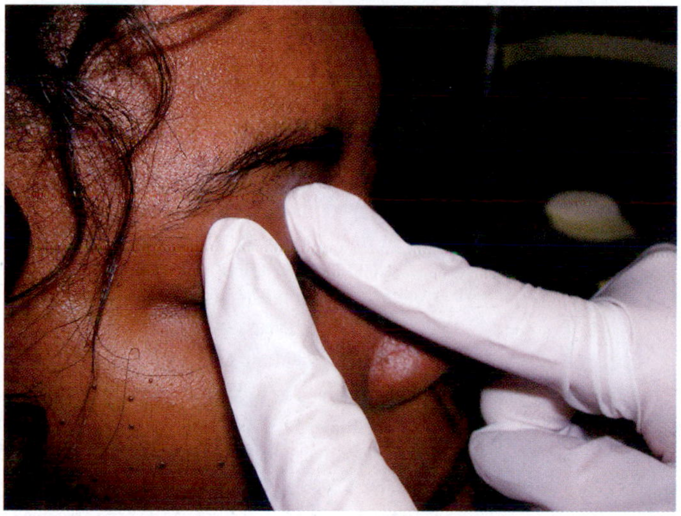

FIGURE 62–8 ◆ Palpation of intraocular pressure.
Source: Lucie Elfervig.

- The nurse should advise the patient and family of eye injuries that can be caused by occupational hazards and recommend the use of goggles to reduce the risk of injury. The nurse should also explain the possibility of eye injury from playing sports such as baseball or boxing and recommend wearing protective gear when possible.
- Because preexisting diseases may cause vision problems, the nurse should advise the patient to notify the examiner of any current or prior disease conditions, such as diabetes or hypertension, when having an eye examination.
- The nurse should apprise the patient and family of medications that may cause eye damage and have them check the medications that they are taking currently or have taken in the past to determine whether their medications constitute a risk. Hydroxychloroquine, tamoxifen, phenothiazines, and sildenafil are medications that may cause eye disorders (The Eye Digest, 2011).

CHART 62–2 Visual Acuity Testing

Types	Distances	Charts
Take Visual Acuity (VA)*		
Far VA (right eye, left eye, and both eyes): with glasses or contact lenses if the patient wears them.	20 feet (6 meters)	Snellen acuity or equivalent distance chart
Near VA (right eye, left eye, and both eyes): with glasses or contact lenses if the patient wears them.	14–16 inches (38–40 centimeters)	Near reading chart

*Test vision with each eye separately: right eye, then left eye (covering the eye not being tested); once vision is obtained with each eye, then test vision with both eyes open.

Record VA—20/20, 20/30, and so on, whatever line the patient reads, and document each eye separately and together (e.g., 20/30 right eye, 20/50 left eye, 20/40 both eyes) for far and near acuity. If the patient cannot see the chart at the standard distance, then walk up to the patient with the chart until he can read the largest letter (this is usually the 200 letter).

*Record count fingers (CF)**—If the patient cannot see the nurse's fingers, the nurse moves her hand and determines whether the patient can detect the motion; the nurse moves increasingly close to the patient until the patient sees the nurse's hand moving. For example, the recording might read: CF at 5 feet with right eye, left eye, and both eyes.

*Record hand motion (HM)***—If the patient cannot see the nurse's hand move, then the nurse shines a light in the patient's eyes (best to dim the room lights) and determines whether the patient can detect the light; the nurse moves increasingly close to the patient until the light is perceived. For example, the recording might read: HM at 2 feet with right eye, left eye, and both eyes.

*Record light perception (LP) or record no light perception (NLP)****—If the patient cannot see the nurse's light, then the visual acuity is no light perception (NLP), with right eye or left eye. When doing LPs, make sure the light is bright, room lights are dimmed, and the opposite eye is covered well. For example the recording might read: LP at 3 inches with right eye, left eye, and both eyes.

* At the distance seen (e.g., CF at 5 feet), with right eye, left eye, and both eyes.

** At the distance seen (e.g., HM at 2 feet), with right eye, left eye, and both eyes.

*** At the distance seen (e.g., LP at 3 inches), with right eye, left eye, and both eyes.

CHART 62–3 Ocular and Vision Evaluation Tests

Test	Procedure
Extraocular muscle movement (cardinal fields of gaze)	The patient is seated directly opposite the nurse, and they face each other about 1 foot apart. The patient is instructed to look at a pen or target that is held in the nurse's hand at a distance of 16 inches (40 centimeters). The patient is asked to follow the pen when the nurse moves it in the primary position (looking straight ahead) to eight cardinal fields of gaze: from the primary position to look right upward, straight up, left upward, left temporal, left downward, straight down, right downward, and right temporal. The nurse observes the patient and notes whether the patient's eyes move equally together in all fields of gaze and whether both eyes are symmetrical. The nurse records these values either as normal or, if any deviation from normal, as minimal (–1), moderate (–2), severe (–3), or total (–4) loss of eye movement.
Cover–uncover test for tropia	The patient is to wear her corrective lenses if she normally does so. The nurse has the patient fixate on a target about 20 feet (6 meters) away for far and 16 inches (40 centimeters) away for near; it can be a visual acuity chart, picture chart, E chart, or toy, the smallest line of clear acuity. The nurse sits in front of the patient but does not block the patient's view of the target. The nurse notes the eye that is fixating, covers that eye with an occluder, and notes what the fellow eye does. If the uncovered eye moves to pick up fixation, the nurse notes the direction in which it moves—if toward the nose, then it was fixated outward, so it is exo, or if toward the ear, then it was fixated inward, so it is eso. If the uncovered eye does not move and has steady fixation, no strabismus exists. The eye would move up and down to indicate vertical tropia.
Alternating cover test for phoria	The patient is to wear his corrective lenses if he normally does so. The nurse has the patient fixate on a target about 20 feet (6 meters) away for far and 16 inches (40 centimeters) away for near; it can be a visual acuity chart, picture chart, E chart, or toy, the smallest line of clear acuity. The nurse sits in front of the patient but does not block the patient's view of the target. The nurse places the occluder in front of the patient's right eye, holds it for about a second or so, and then moves it swiftly over the left eye. This alternating cover test is repeated many times. The nurse repeats with the occluder in front of the left eye for a second or so, then moves it swiftly over the right eye, and repeats. The nurse observes the eye that is just being uncovered to see whether it deviates. If just the uncovered eye moves inward, then it was fixed outward, so it is exo; and if just the uncovered eye moves outward, then it was fixed inward, so it is eso. If just the uncovered eye does not move and has steady fixation, no strabismus exists. The eye would move up and down to indicate vertical phoria.
Confrontation fields (visual field testing)	The nurse compares the range of the patient's visual field in relation to the nurse's visual field, which is assumed to be normal. The light source should be behind the patient, and the background behind the nurse should be dark and uniform. The patient is seated, and the nurse sits or stands directly opposite, facing the patient about 2 feet away. The patient's right eye is open, and the left eye is closed or occluded while the nurse's left eye is open and right eye is closed, and each person fixes on the other's open eye. The nurse will move his fingers or a bright test object from the far periphery and note when it comes into the field of view; the nurse and patient should see it at the same time. This is done for the four major quadrants (superior, nasal, inferior, and temporal) and is repeated for the patient's left eye. The approximate normal degrees of angle recognition of the test object are 60° superior, 60° nasal, 70° inferior, and 80° temporal. The nurse records the results. If any visual field defects are noted, the patient should be sent in for sophisticated visual field testing.

CHART 62–4 Ocular and Visual Evaluation and Assessment

Initial Examination	
Central visual acuity	The nurse takes visual acuity (VA) of each eye separately and together at far and at near, with the patient wearing her corrective lenses if she normally does so. The test may be done with a Snellen acuity chart or reading card, or the patient may be asked to read a newspaper, read a wall clock, or recognize faces at the bedside or at the doorway. The nurse records the patient's visual acuity.
Peripheral visual acuity	The nurse determines whether the patient can see movement and objects coming in from the periphery. Confrontations can be done here; a visual field (VF) screening test.
Intraocular pressure (IOP)	A tonometer can be used to check IOP, or the nurse may gently palpate over the eyelid to indicate whether the eyeball is hard or soft.
External Examination	The nurse observes the patient's face and all structures surrounding the eye for any asymmetry or color, size, shape, or expression differences; and overall general appearance.
(Observations and Penlight Test)	
Eyelids	Does the eyelid close automatically (blink reflex)?
	Does the eyelid cover the cornea completely when closed?
	Does the eyelid lag or droop (ptosis)?
Eyelashes	Do the eyelashes curve inward (entropion) or outward (ectropion)?
	Are there any misaligned or missing lashes (trichiasis)?
Eyeball	The nurse observes for obvious laceration, trauma, bruises, or black eye (ecchymosis).
	Does the eyeball appear sunken (enophthalmos) or protruding (proptosis)?
Conjunctiva	Observe and check for tearing, itching (pruritus), drainage, injection (hyperemia), swelling (edema), discoloration, lesions, scaling, or irregularities.
Sclera	The nurse observes the color of the sclera (which should be white) and of the blood vessels on its surface (which should be red).
Cornea	The nurse observes for clarity.
Anterior chamber	The nurse checks the anterior chamber for whether it is clear and deep, meaning that it is without discharge, deposits, or opaqueness; pus (hypopyon); or blood (hyphema). The sclera should be white, and the conjunctiva should be clear.
Pupils	The nurse checks pupils for size (in millimeters), shape, and whether pupils are equal, round, reactive to light, and accommodating (PERRLA).
Iris	The nurse observes color, shape, and size.
Muscles	The nurse checks eye mobility by checking the primary and eight cardinal fields of gaze for extraocular muscle function.
	The nurse checks for cross-eyes (exo = out, eso = in) by doing cover eye tests.
	The nurse draws pictures of what is seen if indicated for documentation.
Direct Ophthalmoscope Examination*	The nurse checks for a red reflex and notes whether it is present or whether a different reflex is noted between the eyes (e.g., leukocoria-white reflex).
	The nurse views for media clarity (cornea, anterior chamber, lens, and vitreous), checking for any opacities or foreign bodies in the visual pathway.
	The nurse checks the optic nerve (disc) for color, shape, vessels, and cup/disc (C/D) ratio.
	The nurse views the fovea (central vision area of the macula) for edema, color abnormalities, and foveal reflex (yellowish-orange reflex) to determine whether present or not and whether there is asymmetry or atrophy.

*See Figures 62–4, 62–5, and 62–6 (pp. 1981 and 1983).

Gerontological Considerations

As people age, sensory changes occur normally. People receive and process information from the environment through hearing, vision, taste, smell, and touch. With aging, these senses often are diminished, and incoming information may be distorted or difficult to understand. As a result, individuals may find their functional status compromised.

Hearing Loss

The likelihood that a patient over the age of 64 years has a significant hearing loss is 24% to 50%. The prevalence of hearing loss increases to 50% in people older than 74 years. Poor vision, a high level of comorbidity, and depression are related to hearing loss in older adults (American Psychological Association [APA], 2011). Some hearing impairments are reversible; others are not. Potentially reversible hearing loss is caused by impacted cerumen, cholesteatomas (tumorlike growths in the middle ear), or acoustic neuromas. These conditions should be recognized in an examination, and an appropriate referral should be made for treatment. However, gradual decline in hearing acuity (presbycusis) is due to degeneration of the organ of Corti and can simply be a result of aging (Muche, 2011). Most people acquire a conductive hearing loss with a narrow range of audibility, an inability to hear high-frequency sounds, and difficulty in discriminating complex sounds. Hearing deficits may be associated with paranoia and can lead to depression, anxiety, and insecurity. Safety issues also are a concern with the hearing impaired, who might not be able to hear danger approaching, such as an automobile in the street, horns honking, an approaching storm, the doorbell ringing in response to an emergency call, or a smoke detector going off (Cacchione, 2010).

Hearing loss contributes to communication and quality-of-life issues. As hearing decreases, the individual's ability to communicate with others is affected. The person with hearing loss might not be able to make out sounds or words when there is background noise. Conversations may be difficult to hear, especially if the speaker has a high voice or there is background interference. Older individuals may be frustrated or embarrassed about not being able to understand what is being said. They might have to ask people to repeat themselves or endure shouting when a speaker tries to be heard. They may hold back from entering conversations out of fear of making inappropriate comments. They may tire from concentrating and straining to hear. As a result, they might withdraw from friends, family, and outside social activities. Often this leads to depression or low self-esteem (APA, 2011).

Hearing loss does not have to cause social isolation and emotional distress. Changes in behavior and the home environment can improve the older adult's ability to carry on a normal conversation. There are many different devices such as special phones, alarm clocks, smoke detectors, and doorbells that have flashing lights and vibrations to alert the hearing impaired.

Older adults need routine hearing exams conducted by qualified professionals. This helps to ensure that there is not another problem causing the hearing loss. If a hearing aid is needed, the patient needs to work with the audiologist to find the right brand and fit. The older person will need support and encouragement while adjusting to the hearing aid. If the older individual is experiencing a balance problem, it needs to be addressed also.

Older adults with hearing problems often experience balance problems as well. There are numerous exercise programs designed to restore, maintain, or assist the development of balance in older adults. The nurse should investigate the types of programs that are available in the patient's and encourage the patient to look into these programs (Dallek, 2011).

Vision Loss

As with hearing, vision loss occurs with aging. Many older people have good to adequate vision. However, individuals may see changes occurring in their late 30s and early 40s. They might have to hold books or papers farther away to read them because of changes in the lens's ability to alter its shape to accommodate to changes in light. Adaptations in lifestyle and behaviors must be made to cope with this change. For example, a person may give up driving at night and place more lights around a room so that the entire room is lit. Degeneration of eye muscles and clouding of the lens also are associated with aging. Older people tend to have trouble focusing on near objects, although eyeglasses may correct this problem. The ability to see colors changes as the lens yellows. If this occurs, red, yellow, and orange are easier to see than blue and green.

Serious vision impairments such as cataracts, glaucoma, and blindness affect between 7% and 15% of older adults. Cataracts are the fifth-most common chronic condition in adults over age 75 (Cacchione, 2010). Vision-altering diseases that are seen more frequently as people age include cataracts, macular degeneration, glaucoma, diabetic retinopathy, hypertensive retinopathy, temporal arteritis, and detached retina (Cacchione, 2010).

Visual impairment has a more wide-ranging impact on functional status than does hearing impairment. Visual impairment is associated with increased physical disability, increased social isolation, low employment rates, reduced self-image, and depression. Vision loss often affects an individual's relationships, prompting changes in gender roles, duties, professions, living arrangements, and travel. All of these may contribute to social isolation. Physical disabilities include a decreased ability to perform activities of daily living, decreased physical endurance and mobility, and a lack of participation in activities. Vision, proprioception, and vestibular function are the three main components of sensory feedback to maintain a normal upright stance. Therefore, the loss of vision is associated with increased falls and a resultant increase in fractured hips (Much, 2011).

"Low vision frequently coexists with other disabilities, including hearing loss, cognitive impairments, and mobility limitations. Dual sensory loss involving visual and hearing impairments is associated with a significant decrease in function, compared with the effect of a single sensory loss" (Muche, 2011, p. 5). Greater attention to sensory impairments by clinicians as well as patient and family educators is needed to enhance function and progressive rehabilitation in older adults.

Critical Thinking

The ear and the eye fulfill the body's hearing and vision functions, respectively. Hearing and vision enable individuals to communicate with others and lead full lives of work and enjoyment; thus, any disruption of these two systems may damage the entire person, not just the organs involved. It is fortunate, therefore, that the ear and eyes are accessible for screening and testing related to possible hearing, balance, and vision disorders. Another valuable factor related to the screening and testing process is that the examiner knows what type of information is being processed by these two organs. This knowledge base facilitates the conduction of a thorough examination and enhances the examiner's ability to detect actual or potential problems.

It is important to begin with a thorough history of the patient's chief complaints. Patients need to be evaluated in the context of presenting symptoms; review of systems; cultural, social, and family history; prior health history; and medication history. Following a critical analysis of information received, the health history can lead the examiner to isolate the source of symptoms, including genetic and environmental factors.

Conducting the health history, physical examination, and preparation for and interpretation of laboratory tests and procedures takes experience, skill, and practice. It is not enough simply to ask the right questions and perform the physical exam. The nurse must critically analyze all of the data obtained, synthesize the data into a relevant problem focus, and then identify a plan of care for the patient based on this synthesis. Examples of plans of care based on assessment data are found in Chapters 63 and 64.

NCLEX® PRACTICE

1. A patient's ear canal is shiny with brown sticky cerumen. How would the nurse interpret these findings?

1. The patient likely has an infection.
2. This finding is normal.
3. There is evidence of a foreign body.
4. This is an abnormal exudate.

2. A patient reports having an earache for several weeks "because of my allergies." The nurse suspects that the patient's tympanic membrane may be ruptured. Which assessment technique should be used?

1. The nurse should attempt to advance the otoscope far enough into the ear canal to touch the membrane.
2. The nurse should use a pneumatoscope to test tympanic membrane patency.
3. The nurse should drop warm water into the ear and ask the patient about a sensation of fluttering.
4. The nurse should perform the Weber test.

3. A patient reports that his hearing "just isn't right" since he was hospitalized for renal failure last year. The nurse should ask specifically about which hearing changes? (select all that apply)

1. Frequent ear infections
2. Hearing loss
3. Tinnitus
4. Drainage from the ear canals
5. A sense of fullness in the ears

4. An older patient sits quietly and does not engage in conversation with those seated nearby. When someone does speak, the patient stares at the speaker's face. These findings cause the nurse to be suspicious that this patient might be experiencing which condition?

1. Mental status changes
2. Dementia
3. Social isolation because of hearing loss
4. Antisocial behavior disorder

5. A patient is unable to hear words that the nurse whispers when standing about 2 feet behind the patient. How should the nurse interpret this finding?

1. It is normal.
2. It is evidence of hearing loss.
3. It is evidence of acoustic nerve damage.
4. It is evidence of a blocked ear canal.

6. A patient tells the nurse that she thinks there's something wrong with her vision because she sometimes sees black things "moving" in her vision. The nurse interprets this information as indicating the presence of which condition?

1. Glaucoma
2. Cataracts
3. Floaters
4. Detached retina

Answers to NCLEX Practice Questions can be found in Appendix D in the Osborn Student Resources at nursing.pearsonhighered.com. Practice additional NCLEX questions online at the Student Resources site.

REFERENCES

Agency for Healthcare Research and Quality (AHARQ). (2010). Comprehensive adult medical evaluation. U.S. Department of Health & Human Services. Retrieved from http://www.ngc/gov/content.aspz?id=25644

American Academy of Hearing Loss Support Specialists. (2011). Building knowledge to better serve people with hearing loss. Hearing Loss Association of America. Retrieved from http://www.hearingloss.org/sites/default/files/docs/HLSS_TRainingProgramOverview.pdf

American Academy of Ophthalmology. (2010). Comprehensive adult medical eye evaluation—October 2010. *Preferred Practice Pattern Guidelines: American Academy of Ophthalmology*. Retrieved from http://one.aao.org/CE/PracticeGuidelines/PPP_Content.aspx?cid=64e9df91-dd10-4317-8142-6a87eee7f517

American Academy of Otolaryngology-Head and Neck Surgery. (2010). Tinnitus. Retrieved from http//entnet.org/HealthInformation/tinnitus.cfm

American Academy of Otolaryngology-Head and Neck Surgery. (2011). Ears and altitude. Retrieved from http://www.entnet.org/HealthInformation/earsAltitude.cfm

American Psychological Association (APA). (2011). What practitioners should know about working with older adults. Retrieved from http://www.apa.org/pi/aging/resources/gides/practitoners-should-know.aspx

American Speech-Language-Hearing Association. (2011). The prevalence and incidence of hearing loss in adults. Retrieved from http://www.asha.org/public/hearing/Hearing-Loss/

American Tinnitus Association. (2011). At risk populations. Retrieved from http://www.ata.org/for=patients/at-risk

Are You at Risk for Glaucoma. (2011). *Glaucoma Research Foundation*. Retrieved from http://www.glaucoma.org/glaucoma/are-you-at-risk-for-glaucoma.php

Arts, H. A. (2010). Sensorineural hearing loss in adults. In C. E. Cummings, P. W. Flint, B. H. Haughty, et al. (Eds.), *Otolaryngology: Head & neck surgery* (5th ed.). Philadelphia: Mosby Elsevier.

Bauman, N. G. (2010). *Ototoxic drugs exposed: The shocking truth about prescription drugs, medications, chemicals and herbals that can (and do) damage our ears* (3rd ed.). Stewartsville, PA: Integrity First.

Berke, J. (2011). Ototoxic drugs cause hearing loss. About.com. Retrieved from http://deafness.about5.co/od/ototoxicity/a/ototoxic.htm

Brochert, A. (2007). Vertigo. University of Illinois Medical Center: Health Library. Retrieved from http://uimc.discoveryhospital.com/main.php?id=3113

Cacchione, P. (2008). Sensory changes. In E. Capezuti, D. Zwicker, M. Mezey, T. Fulmer, D. Gray-Miceli, & M. Kluger (Eds.), *Evidence-based geriatric nursing protocols for best practice* (3rd ed.). New York: Springer Publishing Company.

Cacchione, P. (2010). Want to know more, sensory changes. Hartford Institute for Geriatric Nursing. Retrieved from http://consultgerirn.org/topics/sensory_changes/want_to_know_more

Campo, P., Maguin, K., Gabriel, S., Moller, A., Nies, E., Gomez, M.D.S., et al. (2009). Combined exposure to noise and ototoxic substances. Retrieved from http://osha.europa.eu/en/publications/literature_reviews/combined-exposure-to-noise-and-ototoxic-subst

Dallek, L. (2011). Designing balance exercise programs for older adults. Retrieved from http://www.acefitness.org/certifiednewsarticle/687/designing-balance-exercise-programs-for-older/

Danielson, R. W. (2011). Prevention of noise induced hearing loss. Better Hearing Institute. Retrieved from http://www.betterhearing.org/hearing_loss_prevention/noise_induced_hearing_loss/index.cfm

Dillon, P. M. (2007). *Nursing health assessment* (3rd ed.). Philadelphia: F. A. Davis.

DiMartino, J. (2011). Surfer's ear: Exostosis. About.com. Retrieved from http://surfing.about.com/od/surfingrelatedailments/a/122207exostosis.htm

Drisdelle, R. (2007). What is river blindness? Retrieved from http://suite101.com/article/what-is-river-blindness-a24974

Drugs.com. (2011). Torsemide. Retrieved from http://www.drugs.com/pro/torsemide.html

Dugdale, D. C. (2011). Caloric stimulation. *Milton S. Hershey Medical Center, Penn State Hershey*. Retrieved from http://printer-friendly.adam.com/content.aspx?productId=117&pid=1&gid=003429&c_custid=758

Genetics Home Reference. (2011). Your guide to understanding genetic conditions. Retrieved from http://ghr.nlm.nih.gov

Glaucoma Research Foundation. (2011). Are you at risk for glaucoma? Retrieved from http://www.glaucoma.org/glaucoma/are-you-at-risk-for-glaucoma.php

Hain, T. C. (2011a). Ototoxic medications. Retrieved from http://www.dizziness-and-balance.com/disorders/bilat/ototoxins.html

Hain, T. C. (2011b). Tinnitus defined. Retrieved from http://www.dizziness-and-balance.com/disorders/hearing/tinnitus.htm

Health Resources and Services Administration. (2011). Culture, language, and health literacy. U.S. Department of Health and Human Services. Retrieved from http://www.hrsa.gov/culturalcompetence/index.html

Healthwise Staff. (2012). Seton Healthcare Family. Retrieved from http://www.seto.net/health_a_to_z/health_library/symptom/ear_canal_problems

Hearing Health Foundation. (2011). Can NIHL be prevented? Retrieved from http://hearinghealthfoundation.org/nihl-prevention

Lighthouse International. (2011). Cataract symptoms. Retrieved from http://www.lighthouse.org/about-low-vision-blindness/vision-disorders/cataract/cataract-symptoms/

MedicineNet.com. (2011). Ear: Anatomy of hearing and balance. Retrieved from http://www.medicinenet.com/script/main/art.asp?articlekey=21685&page=2

Miyamoto, R. T. (2008). Otic barotrauma. *Merck Manual.* Retrieved from http://www.merckmanuals.com/professional/ear_nose_and_throat_disorders/middle_ear_and_tympanic_membrane_disorders/otic_barotrauma.html

Morrison, A. W., & Bundey, S. E. (2007). The inheritance of otosclerosis. *The Journal of Laryngology & Otology, 84*(9), b1–b28.

Muche', J. A. (2011). Geriatric rehabilitation. Medscape reference. Retrieved from http://emedicine.medscape.com/article/318521-overview

Natal, B.L. (2011). Emergent management of acute otitis media. *Medscape Reference.* Retrieved from http://emedicine.medscape.com/article/764006-overview

National Health Information Center. (2011). *National health observances.* Washington, DC: Office of Disease Prevention and Health Promotion, U.S. Department of Health and Human Services.

National Institutes on Deafness and Other Communication Disorders (NIDCD). (2008). Noise-induced hearing loss. NIDCD fact sheet. Retrieved from http://www.nidcd.nih.gov/staticresources/health/healthyhearing/tools/pdf/nihl.pdf

National Institutes on Deafness and Other Communication Disorders (NIDCD). (2009). Balance disorders. NIDCD fact sheet. Retrieved from http://www.nidcd.nih.gov/staticresources/health/balance/BalanceDisordersFactSheet.pdf

National Institutes on Deafness and Other Communication Disorders (NIDCD). (2010a). How loud is too loud? Retrieved from http://www.nidcd.nih.gov/health/hearing/ruler.asp

National Institutes on Deafness and Other Communication Disorders (NIDCD). (2010b, July). Ménière's disease. Retrieved from http://www.nidcd.nih.gov/health/balance/meniere.html

National Institutes on Deafness and Other Communication Disorders (NIDCD). (2010c). Tinnitus (Publication No. 10-4896). Retrieved from http://www.nidcd.nih.gov/health/hearing/tinnitus

Niedermeyer, H., Hausler, R., Schwub, D., Neuner, N., Busch, R., & Arnold, W. (Eds.). (2007). Otosclerosis and stapes surgery: Evidence of increased average age of patients with otosclerosis. *Advanced Otorhinolaryngology, (65*), 17–24.

Pediatric ENT Associates. (2011). Tympanoplasty. Retrieved from http://www.pedsent.com/surgery/tympanoplasty.htm

Reeves, A. G., & Swenson, R. (2008a). *Disorders of the nervous system* (Chapter 6– Auditory and vestibular function). Hanover, NH: Dartmouth Medical School. Retrieved from http://www.dartmough.edu/~dons/part_1/chapter_6.html

Reeves, A. G., & Swenson, R. (2008b). *Disorders of the nervous system* (Chapter 14– Evaluation of the "dizzy" patient). Hanover, NH: Dartmouth Medical School. Retrieved from http://www.dartmouth.edu/~dons/part_2/chapter_14.html#chpt_14_evaluation

Spector, R. E. (2008). *Cultural diversity in health and illness* (7th ed.). Upper Saddle River, NJ: Pearson Prentice Hall.

Stone, E. M. (2007). Genetic testing for inherited eye disease. *Archives of Ophthalmology, 125*(2), 205–212.

The Eye Digest. (2011). Eye affects of medications. University of Illinois Eye Infirmary. Retrieved from http://www.agineye.net/visionbasics/eye&meds.php

The Free Dictionary. (2011). Vestibular system. Retrieved from http://encyclopedia2.thefreedictionary.com/Vestibular+system

Thompson, T., & Amedd, R. (2009). Vertigo: A review of common peripheral and central vestibular disorders. *The Costner Journal Spring, 9*(1), 20–26. Retrieved from http://www.ncbi.nlm.nih.gov/pmc/articles/PMC3096243/

Traynor, R. (2011). Racial differences in cerumen type and consistency. *Hearing Health & Technology Matters.* Retrieved from http://hearinghealthmatters.org/hearinginternational/2011/racial-differences-in-cerumen-type-and-consistency/

University of Iowa Hospitals and Clinics. (2008). Ear wax. Retrieved from http://www.uihealthcare.com/topics/earnosethroat/earn4453.html

U.S. Department of Health and Human Services. (2007). NIOSH pocket guide to chemical hazards. Data from National Institute of Occupational Safety and Health. Atlanta, GA: Centers for Disease Control and Prevention.

University of Iowa Hospitals and Clinics. (2008). Ear Wax. Retrieved May 29, 2011, from http://www.uihealthcare.com/topics/earnosethroat/earn4453.html

Voelker, C., & Chole, R. (2010). Unilateral sensorineural loss in adults: Etiology & management. *Thieme ejournals Hearing Seminars, 3*(4), 313–325.

Western Australia Department of Commerce. (2011). Ototoxic chemicals–chemicals that result in hearing loss. Retrieved from http://www.commerce.wa.gov.au/worksafe/content/safety_topics/noise/Further_information/Ototoxin.html

Yanoff, M., & Duker J. S. (Eds.). (2008). *Ophthalmology* (3rd ed.). St. Louis, MO: Mosby.

Caring for the Patient with Hearing and Balance Disorders

CHAPTER 63

Judith Tanner
Annita Watson

Outcome-Based Learning Objectives

After studying this chapter, the learner will be able to:

1. Determine the major anatomic structures that are involved in the sense of hearing.
2. Distinguish the three types of hearing loss, relating each to its respective mechanism of hearing.
3. Select health promotion strategies to prevent hearing loss in all age groups.
4. Differentiate among the three different pathologic causes for a hearing disorder.
5. Plan discharge priorities for a patient with a hearing disorder.
6. Formulate specific aspects of the nursing management for an older patient with a hearing disorder.
7. Generate an approach to caring for the patient with a hearing disorder, using the nursing process.

KEY TERMS

acoustic neuroma p. 2000
benign paroxysmal positional vertigo (BPPV) p. 2003
conductive hearing loss (CHL) p. 1990
exostosis p. 1993
labyrinthectomy p. 2001
labyrinthitis p. 2001
mastoidectomy p. 2000
mastoiditis p. 2000
Ménière's disease p. 2001
mixed hearing loss p. 1990
myringotomy p. 1999
noise-induced hearing loss (NIHL) p.1990
nystagmus p. 2003
otitis externa p. 1991
otitis media p. 1997
otoconia p. 2003
otosclerosis p. 1999
ototoxic p. 1990
presbycusis p. 2010
sensorineural hearing loss (SNHL) p. 1990
stapedectomy p. 2000
tinnitus p. 1992
tympanoplasty p. 1995
vertigo p. 1994
vestibular nerve dissection p. 2001

AN INTACT SENSE OF HEARING AND BALANCE is essential to health and daily function. Damage to the ears and accompanying structures will have a negative impact on individuals in all age groups. Identified as being one of the five major senses, hearing is often taken for granted. Many times, an alteration in the sense of hearing is not detected until the person is questioned about her voice volume or atypical responses to environmental and verbal stimuli. Loss of hearing may lead to problems in an individual's professional and personal life, and it can also affect safety. To function in society, an individual must be able to give and receive information accurately.

Balance is partially controlled by the ear. A normally functioning inner ear is necessary to maintain body balance. Along with the joints, muscles, and eyes, the ear sends messages to the cerebellar portion of the brain for coordination and perception. Problems with balance also impact on the individual's safety by increasing the risk for accidental falls. A complete discussion of the structure and function of the ears may be found in Chapter 62.

Communication and other sensory processes contribute to our overall health and well-being. Protecting these processes is critical, particularly for people whose age, race, ethnicity, gender, occupation, genetic background, or health places them at increased risk. A program led by the U.S. Department of Health and Human Services (DHHS), termed *Healthy People 2020*, has identified specific objectives designed to ensure that all Americans, from birth through old age, will benefit from scientific advances in prevention, diagnosis, and treatment of hearing and other sensory or communication disorders. These objectives are outlined in the National Guidelines box. Fifteen objectives were promulgated to meet the overall goal for Hearing and Other Sensory or Communicative Disorders of *Healthy People 2020*.

Hearing Disorders

Hearing loss is estimated to affect approximately 30 million Americans (National Institute on Deafness and Other Communication Disorders [NIDCD], 2012b). Hearing loss is seen in all types of people in all age groups, although the percentage of those affected accelerates with age, and men are twice as likely as women to have the disorder (Isaacson, 2009). The degree of hearing loss, which is defined as partly or totally

NATIONAL GUIDELINES for *Healthy People 2020* Goal and Objectives for Hearing and Other Sensory or Communication Disorders

Goal: Reduce the prevalence and severity of disorders of hearing and balance; smell and taste; and voice, speech, and language.

Objectives:

1. Increase the proportion of newborns who are screened for hearing loss by no later than age 1 month, have audiologic evaluation by age 3 months, and are enrolled in appropriate intervention services no later than age 6 months.
2. Decrease otitis media in children and adolescents.
3. Increase the proportion of persons with hearing impairments who have ever used a hearing aid or assistive listening device or who have a cochlear implant.
4. Increase the proportion of persons who have had a hearing examination on schedule.
5. Increase the number of persons who are referred by their primary care physician or other health care provider for hearing evaluation and treatment.
6. Increase the use of hearing protection devices.
7. Reduce the proportion of adolescents who have elevated hearing thresholds, or audiometric notches, in high frequencies (3, 4, or 6 kHz) in both ears, signifying noise-induced hearing loss.
8. Reduce the proportion of adults who have elevated hearing thresholds, or audiometric notches, in high frequencies (3, 4, or 6 kHz) in both ears, signifying noise-induced hearing loss.
9. Increase the proportion of adults bothered by tinnitus who have seen a doctor or other health care professionals.
10. Increase the proportion of adults for whom tinnitus is a moderate to severe problem who have tried appropriate treatments.
11. Increase the proportion of adults with balance or dizziness problems in the past 12 months who have ever seen a health care provider about their balance or dizziness problems.
12. Increase the proportion of adults with moderate to severe balance or dizziness problems who have seen or been referred to a health care specialist for evaluation or treatment.
13. Increase the proportion of persons who have tried recommended methods for treating their balance or dizziness problems.
14. Reduce the proportion of adults with balance and dizziness problems who experienced negative or adverse outcomes in the past 12 months.
15. Reduce the proportion of adults with balance and dizziness problems who have fallen and been injured.

Source: U.S. Department of Health and Human Services (DHHS). (2010). *Healthy People 2020.* Retrieved from http://www.healthypeople.gov/2020/topicsobjectives2020/objectiveslist.aspx?topicid=20.

unable to hear sound in one or both ears, can range from mild to complete (MedlinePlus, 2012a). Each part of the ear structure is characterized by different disorders or problems that can cause hearing loss; hearing loss is thus categorized by which part of the auditory system is damaged. There are three basic types of hearing loss: conductive hearing loss, sensorineural hearing loss, and mixed hearing loss (American Speech-Language-Hearing Association, 2012). **Conductive hearing loss (CHL)** results from disorders in either the outer or middle ear, which prevent sound from getting to the inner ear. Voices and sounds may be perceived as faint, distorted, or both. In conductive hearing loss, the three tiny bones of the ear (ossicles) may not conduct sound properly. Alternatively, the eardrum may not vibrate in response to sound. Fluid in the middle ear can cause this type of hearing loss. **Sensorineural hearing loss (SNHL)** occurs when inner ear nerves become damaged and do not properly transmit their signals to the brain. It most often occurs when the tiny hair cells (nerve endings) that move sound through the ear are injured, diseased, or have died. Patients with SNHL may complain that people mumble; they may also state that they hear, but do not understand, what is being said. Sensorineural hearing loss occurs when there is damage to the inner ear (cochlea) or to the nerve pathways from the inner ear to the brain. Most of the time, a sensorineural loss cannot be medically or surgically corrected, thus resulting in permanent hearing loss. A sensorineural hearing loss reduces the patient's ability to hear faint sounds. Even when speech is loud enough to hear it, it may still be unclear, or sound may seem muffled. Possible causes of sensorineural loss include illnesses, **ototoxic** drugs (drugs that are toxic to hearing), and genetic or hereditary issues. Chart 63–1 shows various types of ototoxic drugs.

Sounds create vibrations that are measured in frequencies. A sound with a low frequency vibrates more slowly than a sound with a high frequency. With a loss or change in the nerve endings in the ear structures, the brain is unable to pick up or interpret these frequencies. The first change in individuals with sensorineural hearing loss is a loss of high-frequency sounds. This manifests as the inability to interpret or understand the words spoken by females or children in addition to losing the ability to discern the spoken sounds of *s, f, sh, ch, h,* or a soft *c.*

Noise-induced hearing loss (NIHL), a sensorineural hearing loss that is caused by noise, results from prolonged exposure to sounds with an elevated decibel level or a sudden exposure to sound at greater than 90 decibels. The *decibel (dB)* is a measurement of loudness or intensity of sound. Typically, exposure to decibel levels of 85 or greater can lead to sensorineural hearing loss (NIDCD, 2011b). Exposure to higher decibel levels causes the death of nerve endings in the ear structures. Over time, and if enough nerve endings are damaged or destroyed, hearing loss will occur. Since nerve endings will not regenerate this type of hearing loss is permanent.

Often viewed as an occupational hazard, NIHL can occur in anyone who has been exposed to loud noises or sounds. Treatment of NIHL begins with overnight rest. Removing the source of the noise or sound, accompanied by rest, typically restores hearing function; however, continuous exposure may cause permanent damage. Individuals who have repeated exposure, such as factory or construction workers, rock musicians, and other individuals who are exposed to loud sounds on a regular basis, should be counseled to use protective devices. For research into NIHL, see the Evidence-Based Practice box (p. 1992).

Mixed hearing loss is a combination of both conductive and sensorineural hearing loss at the same time. Both the middle and inner ear are involved (UC Irvine Healthcare, 2010). Chart 63–2 describes causes of conductive and sensorineural hearing loss in more detail.

Disorders of the Outer Ear

Disorders of the outer ear, referred to as *conductive hearing disorders,* are caused by injuries or assaults to the auricle and the external auditory canal. Common disorders of the outer ear are discussed in the following text.

CHART 63–1 Ototoxic Medications and Chemicals

Chemotherapeutic Agents	Antibiotics		Diuretics	Environmental Chemicals	
Actinomycin	Amikacin	Lincomycin	Bumetanide	Butyl nitrite	Mercury
Bleomycin	Ampicillin	Metronidazole	Diamox	Carbon disulfide	Styrene
Carboplatin	Capreomycin	Minocycline	Ethacrynicacid	Carbon monoxide	Tin
Cisplatin	Chloramphenicol	Neomycin	Ethacrynate sodium	Hexane	Toluene
DCM	Colistin	Netilmicin	Furosemide	Lead	Trichloroethylene
Fluorouracil	Dihydrostreptomycin	Polymyxin B	Mannitol	Manganese	Xylene
Methchlorethamine	Erythromycin	Streptomycin	Torsemide		
Methotrexate	Etiomycin	Tobramycin	Piretanide		
Nitrogen mustard	Gentamicin	Vancomycin			
Procarbazine	Kanamycin	Viomycin			
Vincristine					

Medications with Quinidine	Antibiotics with a Suspicion for Ototoxicity	Aspirin and NSAIDs		Ingested Chemicals
Atabrine	Floxins	Advil	Ascriptin	Alcohol
Chloroquine		Aleve	Bufferin	Aniline dyes
Lariam (mefloquine)		Anaprox (Naproxen)	Disalcid	Caffeine
Plaquenil		Dolobid	Ecotrin	Carbon monoxide
Quinidex		Feldene	Empirin	Metals
Quinine sulfate		Ibuprofen (Motrin)	Excedrin	Nicotine
		Indocin	Fiorinal	Potassium bromide
		Lodine	Trilisate	Povidone–iodine
				Analgesics
				Hydrocodone with acetaminophen

Source: Adapted from Bauman, N. G. (2010). *Ototoxic drugs exposed: The shocking truth about prescription drugs, medications, chemicals and herbals that can (and do) damage our ears* (3rd ed.). Stewartsville, PA: Integrity First.

CHART 63–2 Causes of Conductive and Sensorineural Hearing Loss

Conductive Hearing Loss	Sensorineural Hearing Loss
Buildup of cerumen (earwax) in the auditory canal	Aging
Infection of the external or middle ear (otitis media)	Head injury
Fluid in the middle ear	Infection
A punctured eardrum (tympanic membrane)	Ototoxic medications
Edema	Genetics
Tumors	Prolonged noise exposure
Foreign body	Myxedema
Otosclerosis	Labyrinthitis
	Diabetes mellitus
	Acoustic neuroma
	Ménière's disease
	Presbycusis

Source: Adapted from American Speech-Language-Hearing Association. (2008). Incidence/Prevalence of hearing loss and hearing aid use in the United States–2008 edition. Retrieved from http://www.asha.org/public/hearing/disorders.

Otitis Externa

Epidemiology and Etiology

Otitis externa is an infection of the outer ear and external canal. Males and females of all ages are affected equally, but children and teenagers most frequently develop this type of ear infection. Up to 10% of the population may develop this condition in their lifetime (Nabili, 2008). Because the condition occurs most often during the summer with exposure of the ear to water while swimming, many people call it swimmer's ear. Water from a bath or shower also can trigger the condition. The skin lining the ear canal and outer ear serves as a barrier against infection from bacteria and fungi. The ear is protected from infection because the lining is slightly acidic. Any break in the skin lining can lead to infection, allowing bacteria or fungi to invade the outer ear. The skin barrier can be broken in different ways: by attempting to clean the ear with a cotton-tipped swab or other object inserted in the ear; by excessive moisture in the ear canal from showering or swimming, which alters the acidic environment of the ear canal; by using ear plugs, hearing aids, headphones, and other devices that may be inserted into the ear canal; and by using chemicals such as hair dyes, bleaches, and shampoos that may irritate the ear canal and alter its protective properties. "Generally, any inflammation of the outer ear canal, such as infections, allergies, or skin conditions, can lead to swimmer's ear" (Nabili, 2008, p. 3). The most common bacteria responsible for outer ear infection are *Staphylococcus aureus* and *Pseudomonas aeruginosa*. Less than 10% of cases are caused by a fungus. The inflammation associated with otitis externa also can be caused by an allergic reaction or certain skin diseases like psoriasis and eczema (Medical News Today, 2012).

Several risk factors, such as a breakdown of skin integrity, insufficient cerumen production, or blockage of the ear canal with cerumen (which promotes water retention), can predispose the patient to infection or initiate inflammation and subsequently the infectious process. When

Weblink: Noise-Induced Hearing Loss

EVIDENCE-BASED PRACTICE Noise-Induced Hearing Loss

Clinical Problem

According to World Health Organization, hearing loss will become one of the most common disabilities in the near future (World Health Organization, 2012). Noise-induced hearing loss (NIHL) is the second-most common cause of hearing loss (Kavanagh, 2009). Excessive exposure to loud sounds causes damage to the sensitive hair cells in the inner ear and to the acoustical nerve. Every day, people of all ages and status experience sound in the environment such as sounds from television and radio, traffic, and equipment. Normally, these sounds are at safe levels that do not affect hearing. But with exposure to excessive amounts of loud and repetitive sounds, the pure force of their vibrations can cause damage to hair cells, leading to NIHL. This kind of hearing loss may be accompanied by **tinnitus,** a constant ringing or roaring within the ears. In fact, tinnitus may be the first symptom of NIHL, and some believe that they are always linked together (Kavanagh, 2009). Hearing loss and tinnitus may be experienced in one or both ears, and tinnitus may continue constantly or occasionally throughout a lifetime. Tinnitus and NIHL can be triggered from noises occurring in the work setting, recreational areas, and the home. These are commonly recurring disorders that the health care provider and the nurse encounter on a regular basis. There is much ongoing research into NIHL and tinnitus, but the question remains: "why are we not doing more to create awareness about noise induced tinnitus" (Tobey, 2011, p. 1). Why aren't corporations, manufacturers, and the government doing more to label or provide notice of potential hearing loss from devices or events that produce loud noises capable of causing hearing loss, such as audio systems and concerts (Tobey, 2011)?

Research

Poole (2010) conducted a search of the published peer-reviewed literature investigating the relationship between tinnitus, noise exposure at work, and noise-induced hearing loss. Four studies showed that the prevalence of tinnitus in workers exposed to noise at work was significantly greater than in workers not exposed to noise. The prevalence of tinnitus in those with hearing loss appears to be greater, and the hearing thresholds in those with tinnitus are higher. There also is a suggestion from one 15-year longitudinal study that tinnitus may be an early indicator of risk of the development of NIHL (Poole, 2010).

The National Institute on Deafness and Other Communication Disorders (NIDCD) has been conducting several research studies on NIHL (2008). One study looked at the effects of noise on hair cells within the ear. Scientists discovered that damage to the structure of the hair bundle of the hair cell is related to temporary and permanent loss of hearing. They found that the hair bundles are destroyed when exposed to prolonged periods of damaging sound, which leads directly to hearing loss. Another study being conducted (NIDCD, 2008) is trying to determine the effect of altered blood flow in the cochlea on the hair cells. Researchers are studying the effects of peripheral vascular disease medication to maintain blood flow to the cochlea while it is exposed to noise that would otherwise lead to NIHL.

In 2011 the National Institute on Deafness and Other Communication Disorders (NIDCD) (2012a) reported investigating a potential way to prevent NIHL after noise exposure. Noise exposure triggers the formation of destructive molecules, called free radicals, which cause hair cell death. Researchers discovered that the antioxidants in salicylate (aspirin) and Trolox (vitamin E) given to guinea pigs as long as 3 days after noise exposure significantly reduced hearing loss. These results suggest that there is a window of opportunity in which it is possible to rescue hearing from noise trauma. NIDCD-funded researchers are now testing the ability of nutrients, such as vitamins and minerals, to prevent NIHL in military personnel and college students.

Implications for Nursing Practice

As the incidences of NIHL and tinnitus increase, nurses must be acutely aware of the problem and its effect on people and society. Nurses and other health care providers will encounter people with these disorders on inpatient units and in community-based health care settings. It is the nurse's responsibility to serve as an advocate in the prevention, education, identification, and interventions for individuals with NIHL. The nurse also should promote healthy lifestyle practices for all individuals who are at risk for NIHL.

Critical Thinking Questions with answers can be found in the Osborn Student Resources at nursing.pearsonhighered.com.

Sources: Kavanagh, K. (2009). Noise induced hearing loss. World articles in ear, nose, and throat. Retrieved from http://www.entusa.com/noise_hearing-loss.htm; National Institute on Deafness and Other Communication Disorders. (2008). Noise-induced hearing loss. Retrieved from http://www.nidcd.nih.golv/health/hearing/pagaes/nlise.aspx;).; National Institute on Deafness and Other Communication Disorders (NIDCD). (2012a). Fact sheet: Noise-induced hearing loss. Retrieved from http://www.nidcd.nih.gov/health/hearing/Pages/noise.aspx; Poole, K. (2010). A review of the current state of knowledge on tinnitus in relation to noise exposure and hearing loss. Health and Safety Laboratory, Melbourne Audiology Center. Retrieved from http://melbourneaudiologycentre.com.au/noiseinduee.html; Tobey, P. (2011). Noise induced hearing loss and tinnitus. Retrieved from http://www.paultobey.com/articles/noise-induced-hearning-loss-tinnitus.html; World Health Organization. (2012). International day for ear and hearing, 3 March 2012. Retrieved from http://www.who.int/pbd/deafness/news/en/index.html.

water pools in the ear canal (frequently trapped by earwax), the skin becomes soggy, diluting the acidity that normally prevents infection. A cut in the lining of the ear canal also can allow bacteria to penetrate the skin. When this happens, bacteria and fungi (from contaminated water or objects placed in the ear) continue to grow, and the ear canal gets red and swollen (Best Practice, 2011). Diffuse external otitis can lead to irreversible skin conditions, canal stenosis, and deafness.

Clinical Manifestations

The most common symptom of swimmer's ear or otitis externa is pain. Pain begins gradually over a day or two, and almost always involves only one ear. The pain can become severe and especially intense when the outer part of the ear is pulled or pressed on. Any pressure on the outer ear may cause great pain, so it is often difficult to lie down with the affected side against a pillow. The ear canal may itch, particularly before it becomes painful. The outer ear may be red, and in severe cases the ear canal may be swollen shut. In addition, it may be painful for the individual to chew. Also, the ear may drain; this drainage may be clear, white, yellow, or sometimes bloody and foul smelling. Some fluid may crust at the opening of the ear canal. With severe swelling or drainage, the person may have trouble hearing, and tinnitus (ringing in the ear) and dizziness also may be present. The individual should seek immediate medical care if pain is not controlled by over-the-counter medicines; any pressure on the ear causes great pain; or the person feels dizzy, or has any signs of facial weakness or double vision. If the person has diabetes and is running a fever, the individual should seek medical attention immediately as he can develop a more virulent form of the disorder that might require hospitalization for intensive medical treatment (Nabili, 2008).

Medical Management

The diagnosis of otitis externa typically is made by the health care provider taking a brief history and completing a limited physical examination. Pain produced by gently pulling on the ear as the health care provider attempts to examine the ear canal is a likely sign of swimmer's ear. An otoscope is used to examine the ear canal to determine redness, swelling, and the presence of exudates. The health care provider must assess the drainage from the ear under a microscope to determine if bacteria or fungi are causing the infection. This allows the health care provider to prescribe either an antibacterial or an antifungal medicine.

Medical treatment of otitis externa depends on the severity of the infection and how much pain the individual feels. Medications generally are aimed at symptom relief as well as a cure for swimmer's ear. Oral prescription pain medicines are generally prescribed if over-the-counter medicines are not strong enough. Topical remedies that are used include acidifying agents, antiseptics, anti-inflammatory agents, and antibiotics. Acidifying agents are effective because the common bacteria responsible for outer ear infection cannot survive in a very acidic environment. Antiseptic agents work by potentially killing the offending bacteria, whereas anti-inflammatory agents help with inflammation and may reduce pain. Topical antibiotics are usually given in combination with the other three groups of medicines just listed to increase the effectiveness of treatment. Oral or intravenous antibiotics generally are not used in the treatment of swimmer's ear; however, they may be appropriate in cases of severe infection in people with diabetes or those with weakened immune systems (Nabili, 2008). They also may be used if applying topical ear drops is not possible due to severe swelling and closure of the ear canal. In the event that the outer ear infection is caused by a fungus, antifungal medications are used to treat the infection (Nabili, 2008). See the Pharmacology box (p. 1994) for information on specific medications used to treat otitis externa.

Exostosis

Epidemiology, Etiology, and Pathophysiology

Exostosis, often referred to as surfer's ear, is a condition of the ear canal in which the bony lining under the skin develops a number of lumps that grow into the tube. These bony outgrowths are benign masses of tympanal bone that can lead to infections of the external auditory meatus in advanced cases.

Exostosis is found among saltwater enthusiasts, usually males 20 to 39 years of age (Surgical-Pathology, 2009). The etiology of this condition is not completely understood. These lesions commonly occur during the years of active bone growth, and they commonly arise from the periosteum of the tympanic portion of the external auditory canal, creating a knoblike projection. The possibility of exposure to cold water being a causative agent may account for the high incidence of exostosis in surfers (Balasubramanian, 2008). Over time, these bony growths may close the ear canal, causing hearing loss. Most researchers agree that the environment, especially water temperature, atmospheric temperature, and wind action, plays a pivotal role in the development of exostosis (California Ear Institute, 2011b).

Clinical Manifestations and Medical Management

Most exostosis are asymptomatic because they do not develop to a size sufficient to cause symptoms. The condition is painless and may go unnoticed for a number of years until hearing loss becomes obvious. Many of these patients are referred to health care providers when growths are observed in the external auditory canal. Proliferation of exostosis can lead to recurrent outer ear infections and conductive hearing loss.

In the majority of these cases, a medical treatment of aspiration and antibiotic drops resolves the symptoms (Balasubramanian, 2008). Patients with severe canal stenosis, which is resistant to medical treatment, are candidates for surgical removal of the exostosis. Surgical removal of the outgrowths is indicated only when the patient suffers from recurrent episodes of otitis externa/conductive hearing loss. Removal of exostosis is an adequate way of avoiding recurrent external ear infections. It does not, however, prevent the exostosis from recurring (Balasubramanian, 2008).

Ear Blockages

Epidemiology, Etiology, and Pathophysiology

Blockages in the external ear canal are caused by several different factors and can affect an individual's conductive hearing. Blockages of the external ear canal may be caused by impacted cerumen, foreign objects in the ear, and residue from infections. Normal production of earwax is healthy and good for the ears; if too much wax is being produced, however, it can block the ear. More commonly, though, the ear becomes blocked because of improper ear care and ear cleaning. If cotton swabs, pencils, the finger, or other objects are pushed into the ear canal to try to remove wax, the force can push the wax further into the ear and compress it against the eardrum (The Trusted Source, 2012). Blockages from impacted cerumen are the most common cause; these occur more frequently in the elderly, as well as in people with mental retardation, possibly due to inappropriate and/or infrequent cleaning of their ears. In some people, the glands produce more wax, often causing unpleasant complications such as perforated ear drums and hearing loss that may result in social withdrawal and poor work function. Foreign bodies in the ear are seen most often, but not exclusively, in children. Various objects may be found, including toys, beads, stones, folded paper, and biologic materials such as insects or seeds.

Clinical Manifestations and Medical Management

The most common symptoms of blockage of the ear canal are earache (pain), fullness in the ear or a sensation that the ear is plugged, noises in the ear (tinnitus), and partial hearing loss (which may worsen).

Most cases of earwax blockage can be treated at home. Baby oil, commercial drops, glycerin, or mineral oil can be used to soften the wax. Detergent drops such as hydrogen peroxide or carbamide peroxide also may help remove the wax. Ear irrigation also may be used. Severely impacted cerumen should be removed by a health care provider or nurse who has been trained to remove the impaction. Typically, this is accomplished by flushing the ear canal with a syringe filled with water that is at or near body temperature. Some health care providers prefer a mixture of hydrogen peroxide and water. The flushing action loosens the impaction from the walls of the canal, and the warm water facilitates drainage from the ear. If the impaction does not clear, the patient is instructed to place mineral oil in the ear three times per day for 2 days. This will soften the dry impacted cerumen; the irrigation then may be repeated until the impaction is relieved.

Removal of foreign bodies from the ear is a relatively common procedure in emergency medicine. Patients in extreme distress secondary to an insect in the ear require prompt attention. The insect should be killed prior to removal, using mineral oil or 2% lidocaine (Merck Manual, 2008). Methods of removal consist of irrigation, suction, and instrumentation. Irrigation with water is contraindicated if the tympanic membrane is perforated. Irrigation also is contraindicated for soft objects, organic matter, or seeds, which may swell if exposed to water. In addition, suction is sometimes a useful way to remove foreign bodies. For most foreign bodies, no medications are needed. However, if infection or abrasion is evident, a combination antibiotic and steroid otic suspension may be inserted in the ear canal several times a day for 5 to 7 days. Residue from

PHARMACOLOGY Summary for Medications Used to Treat Hearing and Balance Disorders

Medication Category and Action	Application/Indication	Nursing Responsibility
Isopropyl alcohol drops (dries moisture) Acetic acid (VoSoL) solution drops ***Action:*** Restores acidity and helps keep ear canals dry. It is hydrophilic and provides a low surface tension; thus, contact of the solution with tissues is drying and stops the growth of bacteria and fungus.	Reduces infection of otitis externa.	For dry ears after swimming, place 1 to 2 drops into each ear.
Polymyxin, neomycin drops (ciprofloxacin, Cipro HC Otic), and ofloxacin (Floxin Otic) Garamycin, tobramycin, quinolones ampicillin, Unasyn, Ceftin drops ***Action:*** Disrupts cell wall synthesis of susceptible bacteria by binding to ribosomal components and inhibiting protein synthesis.	Treat the infection of otitis externa and chronic otitis media.	Note any allergies prior to starting antibiotics. Stop treatment if irritation occurs when using medication. Report any unusual symptoms related to ears or hearing (tinnitus, roaring sounds, loss of hearing acuity, or dizziness).
Amoxicillin (Amoxil, Augmentin) ***Action:*** Disrupts cell wall synthesis of susceptible bacteria. Stops bacteria from multiplying by preventing bacteria from forming on the walls Cephalosporins (Ancef, Keflex) Macrolides (Erythromycin) ***Action:*** Both drugs inhibit the bacterial metabolism of folic acid. Each drug inhibits a separate enzyme in the metabolic pathway, creating a synergistic combination. These medications are selective toward bacterial folate metabolism. Trimethoprim-sulfamethoxazole (Bactrim, Septra)	Acute otitis media.	Check for previous allergies to penicillin (amoxicillin) or sulfa (Bactrim). Report any unusual symptoms such as rash, irritation, or itching. Report any ototoxic effects, such as dizziness, **vertigo** (an attack of dizziness), nausea, tinnitus, roaring noises, or hearing impairment.
Steroid eardrops (hydrocortisone, dexamethasone, fluocinolone) ***Action:*** Has an anti-inflammatory effect on ear canals.	Chronic otitis media.	Assess that the ear canal is clear and not impacted with cerumen before medication administration. Be aware that steroids may mask infections.
Meclizine (Antivert, Bonine) Dimenhydrinate (Dramamine) ***Action:*** An antihistamine receptor–blocker that works by decreasing the sensitivity of the central nervous system (CNS) balance center (vestibular sedative).	Prevents vertigo and nausea in Ménière's disease. Prevents vertigo and nausea in Ménière's disease.	Advise caution while driving or engaging in hazardous activities until response to drug is known. Be aware that sedative action may add to that of other CNS depressants. See above for Meclizine.
Diphenhydramine (Benadryl) ***Action:*** H_1-receptor antagonist and antihistamine with significant anticholinergic activity.	Prevents vertigo and nausea in Ménière's disease.	Be aware of additive CNS depressant effects with concurrent use. May cause a drying effect; thus, it is important to increase fluid intake if not contraindicated.
Streptomycin IM or gentamicin (transtympanic injection) ***Action:*** Disrupts cell wall synthesis of susceptible bacteria.	Ménière's disease (selectively destroys vestibular apparatus if vertigo uncontrollable).	Monitor for ototoxicity and hearing problems. Report tinnitus, roaring noises, impaired hearing, and sense of fullness in ears. Monitor intake and output to be on alert for nephrotoxicity.
Diazepam (Valium) ***Action:*** Potentiates the actions of GABA, an inhibitory neurotransmitter in the CNS. Can cause all levels of CNS depression, from relaxation to the induction of sleep or coma.	Ménière's disease.	Monitor for CNS effects such as hypotension, muscular weakness, tachycardia, and respiratory depression. Use safety precautions because drowsiness and ataxia may occur. Avoid CNS depressants because of additive effects.
Phenergan (antiemetic) ***Action:*** Blocks dopamine receptors in the brain, which inhibits signals to the vomiting center in the medulla.	Ménière's disease (may be needed to reduce nausea).	Take initial dose 30–60 minutes before anticipated travel. Avoid CNS depressants because of additive effects. Relieve dry mouth by increasing fluid intake, chewing sugarless gum, or sucking on hard candy.

Sources: Adams, M. P., & Koch, R. W. (2010). *Pharmacology: Connections to nursing practice.* Upper Saddle River, NJ: Pearson; Lee, S. (2010). Otitis externa in emergency medicine treatment & management. Medscape reference. Retrieved from http://emedicine.medscape.com/article/763918-treatment; Mayo Clinic Staff. (2012). Ménière's disease. Retrieved from http://www.mayoclinic.com/health/menieres-disease/DS00535; MedicineNet.com. (2012b). Meclizine. Retrieved from http://www.medicinenet.com/script/main/art.asp?araticlekey=45521&pf=3&page=1; Ménière's Disease Information Center. (2012) Retrieved from http://www.menieresinfo.com/.

infections, such as hardened drainage, also can be removed with irrigation or eardrops.

Ear Trauma (Injury)

Epidemiology, Etiology, and Pathophysiology

The ear is a protruding organ; therefore, it is easily susceptible to injury. Dependent on the type and severity of the injury, it may result in hearing loss. External ear injuries (injuries to the soft fleshy tissue of the ear) may be caused by any force or trauma applied to the ear. When there is an injury, even minor, to the outer ear or ear canal, bleeding and infection can affect other parts of the ear, like the eardrum, ear canal, ossicles, cochlea, or the vestibular nerve. Ear injuries occur in people of all ages but occur more frequently in active people such as wrestlers and boxers. The most common types of injuries include cuts, scrapes, burns, or frostbite. The most common causes of injury include insertion of a foreign body into the ear; direct blows to the ear or head (caused by falls, car crashes, sports injuries, or physical altercations); loud noise (acoustic trauma or noise-induced hearing loss); and sudden, significant changes in air pressure, such as might occur when in an airplane. The types and extent of injury are a function of the force causing the injury. Shearing forces of moderate intensity cause hematoma formation, whereas greater force causes lacerations or even amputation. Sharp objects cause lacerations determined by the force, direction, and point of impact. The high ratio of surface area to mass makes the auricle vulnerable to extremes of temperature and frostbite.

Cauliflower Ear

Cauliflower ear is an acquired deformity of the outer ear, sometimes referred to as boxer's ear or wrestler's ear (MedicineNet.com, 2012a). When the ear is struck and a blood clot develops under the skin, or the skin is sheared from the cartilage, the connection of the skin to the cartilage is disrupted, causing disruption of the blood supply and formation of a hematoma. As the injury to the ear heals, it can shrivel up and fold in on itself and appear pale, giving it a cauliflowerlike appearance, hence the term *cauliflower ear*.

Clinical Manifestations and Medical Management

General symptoms of injury to the outer ear consist of pain, swelling, bruising, and deformity of the curvature of the ear. Because ear injuries affect people differently, some may have partial hearing loss, with symptoms like trouble hearing when there is background noise; difficulty hearing high-pitched sounds or music notes; hearing only certain or muffled sounds; ringing in the ears or other strange sounds like hissing, buzzing, humming, or roaring; difficulty paying attention to a speaker; complaining that the ears feel "full"; trouble talking; talking loudly; failing to turn toward loud noises or respond to conversation-level speech; and answering inappropriately. Others may not experience any hearing loss. If the trauma to the ear leads to loss of hearing, ringing in the ear, headaches, blurred vision, or facial swelling, the damage from the trauma could be severe; if so, medical attention should be sought immediately.

The goal of treatment is to restore the normal contours of the ear while preventing infection. If a hematoma is present, removal and application of pressure dressings using sterile technique correct the condition. Simple lacerations are closed under aseptic technique using either skin-to-skin sutures only or sutures of the skin combined with intercartilage sutures. Extensive and complex lacerations require meticulous care to match all fragments and prevent infection and loss of tissue. Bare cartilage must be covered with vascularized tissue. Some injuries, such as those from a human bite, a dog bite, or severe trauma from a head injury, can cause avulsion of the ear. The treatment of total amputation is surgical reattachment, if possible (Davison, 2011; Lent, 2011).

Perforated Eardrum

Epidemiology, Etiology, and Pathophysiology

A perforation is a hole in the eardrum. This disorder may be treated as a problem of the outer ear or the inner ear, as it affects both (Merck Manual, 2008). Perforated eardrums typically are caused by injury or trauma. They also may be caused by serious infections, head injuries, sudden changes in pressure, and burns from heat or chemicals (Merck Manual, 2008).

Clinical Manifestations and Medical Management

Perforation of the eardrum causes sudden severe pain, sometimes followed by bleeding from the ear, hearing loss, and noise in the ear (tinnitus). The perforation is diagnosed by assessing the drum with an otoscope; if hearing loss is suspected, a formal hearing test is performed. For treatment, the ear is kept dry. An antibiotic may be given by mouth if the ear becomes infected. Antibiotic eardrops may be given if an injury has been contaminated by exposure to foreign objects such as pathogens, dust, dirt, or debris. Typically the eardrum heals without further treatment, however, if it does not heal within several months, **tympanoplasty** (surgery to repair the eardrum) may be needed. People with a severe injury, mainly if hearing loss, severe vertigo, or both are present, may need to have more immediate surgery. If a perforation is not repaired, the patient may develop a severe infection and chronic otitis media in the middle ear.

Neoplasia/Tumors of the Ear

Noncancerous/Benign Tumors

Noncancerous or cancerous growths can occur in the outer ear. Benign growths like cysts, keloids, and osteomas are common and are described in Chart 63–3 (Samy, 2012; Vaishali, 2012).

Medical and Surgical Management

Medical management of all types of benign tumors is surgical excision with some variation according to the type of tumor. Prognosis generally is good for all types of tumors. Recurrence is unusual but necessitates more aggressive removal of bone. With *Pilomatrixoma,* it is noted that malignant transformations, though rare, may occur. This also is true of keratoacanthoma, although prognoses are good with low recurrence following complete excision. The ceruminous growth also has the potential of becoming cancerous.

Cancerous Tumors

The three common types of ear cancer are basal-cell carcinoma, squamous-cell skin cancer, and melanoma. *Basal-cell carcinoma* (BCC) is the most common form of skin cancer, affecting the inside or outside portion of the ear. A small bumpy nodule or a fleshy upheaval on the ear's rim is one of the initial symptoms. *Squamous-cell skin cancer* (SCC), another form of skin cancer, is more aggressive, but it is treatable. Symptoms include nodules, scaly and red skin, and ulcers on the ear, particularly the rim. This cancer can spread to the face, mouth, and lips. Squamous-cell tumors also can occur in the middle ear and the mastoid bone.

Melanoma is a rare cancerous growth that develops in the melanocytes pigment producing cells in the skin. This type of ear cancer is particularly dangerous, as it invades surrounding tissue. In addition, it is difficult to detect melanoma occurring inside the ear because the symptoms, such as change in color and pattern of skin, are absent.

CHART 63–3 Benign Tumors of the Ear

Tumor	Description
Osteomas	The most common bony neoplasms of the temporal bone. They manifest as a pedunculated (stemlike) bony mass that arises from the tympanosquamous suture line adjacent to the bony-cartilaginous junction. The masses are solitary, unilateral, and slow growing. They are usually asymptomatic; however, symptoms can arise if canal obstruction occurs. These growths are more common in men than in women (Samy, 2012). Treatment is typically surgical removal, similar to that of exostosis. Recurrence is unusual but necessitates more aggressive removal of bone.
Squamous papilloma	A lesion that presents as warty, verrucous (with wartlike growths), and elevated, and also may be pigmented. It may have an overlying thickened keratin layer. Both sexes and all ages are equally affected (Samy, 2012). These lesions may be caused by exposure to the human papillomavirus, with resulting virally induced changes of the genome that create cell proliferation.
Sebaceous adenoma (SA)	A less common form of tumor located in the skin of the ear and the external auditory canal. They have a male-to-female ratio of 2.5:1 (Samy, 2012). These lesions present as a smooth, elevated, pedunculated, firm-to-soft growth. They usually are solitary and smaller than 0.5 cm. Color varies between tan, skin-colored, pink, and red lesions. Sebaceous adenoma lesions can bleed from trauma, but they rarely ulcerate.
Pilomatrixoma	A relatively rare tumor with a higher incidence in females than in males (Samy, 2012). It tends to present in the first two decades of life and is believed to arise from the hair follicles. Characteristics of this growth include necrosis, keratinization, and proliferation of small epithelial cells. Calcification or ossification may occur. Pilomatrixoma can have a history of several years and can appear in other parts of the body. Growth can arrest spontaneously.
Keratoacanthoma	Relatively common tumor that occurs most often in White adults; the male-to-female ratio is 2:1 (Samy, 2012). This disorder has been linked to sun exposure, chemical carcinogens, trauma, and possibly a viral etiology. It arises from the hair follicles and involves three phases: proliferation, the developed tumor, and involution. The lesion presents an elevated mass that appears flesh colored or slightly reddish; tightly stretched skin gives it a slightly translucent appearance. Over time, a central umbilicated keratinous plug develops; this plug can ulcerate. A puckered or pitted scar can be left after involution.
Ceruminoma	This tumor is a result of neoplasia of the ceruminous glands of the external auditory canal, which are located in the lower two-thirds of the dermis in the cartilaginous canal. These growths may be present for years and manifest as skin-covered nonulcerated masses located in the outer half of the external auditory canal. These lesions can extend medially to involve the bony external ear canal or the middle ear. Symptoms result from external ear canal obstruction.

Epidemiology, Etiology, and Pathophysiology

Appproximately 250 cases of carcinoma of the auditory canal occur in the United States annually. Those affected usually have a history of outdoor occupations (increased sun exposure) or ear frostbite. Males and females are equally affected. Some tumors (approximately two-thirds of cases) are possibly associated with chronic otorrhea, possibly related to chronic irritation or chronic exposure to aflatoxin B1 (Iowa Head and Neck Protocols, 2009).

Basal-cell carcinoma makes up one-fifth of the neoplasms that involve the ear and the temporal bone. The majority of these tumors occur on the auricular helix and periauricular area of the ear, as they are exposed to most UV light. However, 15% arise in the external auditory canal (Sand et al., 2008). The most common type of BCC is the nodular-ulcerative, which has a pearly border and can show a central ulcer. It may infiltrate the cartilage. The invasive character of the tumor can cause extensive local tissue destruction.

Squamous-cell carcinoma can arise anywhere on the outer ear and potentially involves the middle ear and anterior skull base. Typically patients are in their fifth to sixth decade of life. Twenty-four percent of all patients with SCC have temporal bone involvement (Sand et al., 2008). Sun exposure, fair complexion, cold injury, radiation exposure, and chronic infections, as well as an association with human papilloma virus (HPV)-induced viral carcinogenesis, are among the predisposing factors.

Melanoma of the external ear comprises 2% to 10% of all melanomas of the head and neck. Males and females have an equal chance of acquiring this disease (National Cancer Institute, 2011). Tumor grade and depth of tumor often determine the prognosis. Melanoma is most commonly diagnosed in those between 50 and 70 years of age, with a median age at diagnosis of 53. It is the most common cancer diagnosed in women in the late 20s and second only to breast cancer in women in their early 30s. Men are at a greater risk than women when over age 40; the disease occurs among 1 in 41 men and 1 in 61 women (MD Guidelines, 2010).

Clinical Manifestations

Common signs of ear cancer that occur in its initial stages include emergence of tumor or progressive ulcer, swelling or lump on neck, earache or ear pain, hearing loss, discharge from ear often full of blood, facial paralysis in rare cases, ringing sensation in the ear, and dizziness (Sand et al., 2008). Other symptoms may include pruritus, headache, facial numbness, vertigo, hoarseness, and facial/mandibular weakness (Iowa Head and Neck Protocols, 2012).

Medical Management

Treatment for skin cancers depends on the type and stage of the disease, the size and place of the tumor, and the patient's general health and medical history. In most cases the goal of treatment is to remove or destroy the cancer completely. Most skin cancers can be cured if found and treated early. Treatment of skin cancer is discussed in detail in Chapter 59.

Congenital Malformations

Congenital malformations of the pinna and external ear canal are related to developmental defects of the first and second branchial arches and the branchial groove which joins the first pharyngeal pouch to form the external ear canal. Typical congenital malformations are shown in Chart 63–4.

CHART 63–4 Congenital Malformations of the Ear

Malformation	Description
Bat ear (lop ear)	A disorder of the auricle/pinna that causes the ear to hang down loosely. The external ear stands away from the head at a greater angle. Lop ears are usually larger than normal ears. The concha is large, with poorly developed antihelix and scaph. This anomaly is commonly associated with Ehlers-Danlos syndrome, which is characterized by unusual facies, lop ears, hyperextensible joints, hip dislocation, and inguinal hernia with autosomal recessive inheritance. It also is associated with Townes-Brocks syndrome, which is characterized by lop ears, imperforate anus, hypoplastic kidney, ventricular septal defect, and limb anomalies with autosomal dominant inheritance. Treatment of bat ears or lop ears is surgical correction designed to pull the ears closer to the head.
Anotia	A complete absence of the pinna. This is part of the first arch syndrome (syndrome of malformations involving derivatives of the first branchial arch).
Macrotia	Large ears, where the auricle is usually very large but well shaped, without other ear malformations.
Microtia	Small ears. This phenomenon can be related to thalidomide embryopathy, fetal alcohol syndrome, and maternal diabetes embryopathy. It occurs with a number of single-gene disorders, such as Treacher-Collins syndrome, or chromosomal syndromes, such as trisomy 18. It also can be caused by trisomy 21, in which the mean ear length is significantly lower than normal, and retinoic acid embryopathy.
Preauricular appendages	A condition in which tags of skin, with or without a cartilaginous base, exist. It is frequently located in the line drawn from tragus to angle of mouth. It is described as ear on the cheek or oblique facial features (Medicine Decoded, 2011).
Preauricular pit or sinuses	This is due to a failure in the fusion of the primitive ear hillocks, or to a defective closure of the first branchial cleft. It is characteristically located in or just in front of the anterior crus of the helix. The pits often discharge a cheesy substance that consists of desquamated keratin debris.
Low-set ears	These ears are set below an arbitrary line drawn between the lateral canthus of the eye and the occipital protuberance. Associated anomalies include Noonan syndrome, which is webbing of the neck, pectus excavatum, cryptorchidism, and pulmonary stenosis. Ears are low-set with or without abnormal auricles. Other features are retarded growth and abnormal facies (triangular face, hypertelorism, and ptosis of the eyelids) (Medicine Decoded, 2011).
Synolia	In agnathia-synotia-microstomia, the ears are very close to each other due to the absence of hypoplasia of the mandible. The external ears assume a horizontal position with the lobules located near the midline. This deformity is referred to as "bow-tie" ear due to failure of migration in agnathia-synotia-microstomia.
External auditory cana latresia	Atresia, the absence or underdevelopment of the ear canal, may occur due to failure of canalization of the ectodermal core that fills the dorsal part of the first branchial cleft, the outer meatus filled with fibrous tissue or bone, or the deep meatus-normal, glandular groove.
Collura fistula	A condition in which there are two openings: the lower one is situated in the neck between the angle of the mandible and the sterno-mastoid muscle, and the upper one is in the floor of the external auditory canal or intertragal notch (Medicine Decoded, 2011).

Medical and Surgical Management

Medical management for congenital deformities consists of surgical procedures, some of which are cosmetic only. Reconstructive surgery may be necessary for the more complex deformities (Davison, 2011).

Nursing Management

All of the problems/disorders of the outer ear that have been discussed have the potential to affect hearing. In assessing the patient with hearing loss, the nurse works with the health care provider to determine the cause: infection, a foreign object, damage to the eardrum, or a sign of a tumor. The nurse is responsible for coordinating the treatment plan established by the health care provider. See the Nursing Process feature on page 1998. This includes both educating the patient regarding medications and administering the medications as ordered. Medications may include eardrops, topical medications, and intramuscular and intravenous medications. The nurse also may participate in the removal of foreign bodies in the outer ear by suction, forceps, or flushing the ear canal with water.

Tumors of the ear, both benign and cancerous, typically are removed surgically. Preoperative preparation and postoperative care are provided by the nurse (see Chapters 17 and 19). Preoperative care includes educating the patient as to what is happening and administering medications as ordered. Postoperative care requires supporting the patient and implementing postoperative orders. Often, eye lubrication is ordered. Since a secure dressing is in place, a penrose drain is often inserted into the postauricular wound. Bolsters are in place to hold the head still until approximately day 7.

As recovery progresses, the patient is prepared for discharge, whether she was treated as an inpatient or an outpatient. This includes instructions on self-care and disorder management. Specific instructions are included in the Patient Teaching & Discharge Priorities box on page 1999.

Disorders of the Middle Ear

Common problems of the middle ear include otitis media, otosclerosis, mastoid infection, damaged ossicles, and traumatic injury.

Otitis Media

Epidemiology, Etiology, and Pathophysiology

Otitis media is an infection or inflammation of the middle ear. It can be acute (rapid onset and for short duration) or chronic (persistent inflammation for longer duration). There are about 30 to 35 million cases of otitis media per year (Hain, 2009). Otitis media is very common in children, but unusual in adults. The incidence of acute otitis media (AOM) peaks between 6 and 12 months of age, with another lower peak occurring between 4 and 5 years of age. At least one episode of acute otitis media will be experienced by 62% of children by age 1 (Hain, 2009).

Middle ear infection results from food and airborne allergies, bacteria or viruses, nutritional deficiency, and blockage of the Eustachian

NURSING PROCESS: Patient Care Plan for a Hearing or Balance Disorder

Assessment of Sensory Status Using Gordon's Functional Health Patterns:

- Health Perception Health Management Pattern
- Cognitive Perceptual Pattern
- Activity Exercise Pattern

Subjective Data	Objective Data
Assessment of Hearing	**Assessment of Hearing**
When did you first notice that you had a change in your ability to hear? Did you have a recent exposure to a loud noise or infection?	Results of hearing tests. Test ability to hear at normal voice range. Test lower and higher pitch. Speak into both ears to test unilateral versus bilateral hearing loss.
Assessment of Balance	**Assessment of Balance**
How long have you been experiencing dizziness/vertigo? Have you fallen? How long have you been dizzy with walking? Are you using any hazardous machinery such as a car or equipment at work? Are you nauseated with the dizziness/vertigo? Do you drive an automobile?	Observation of ataxia while ambulating. Observation of bumping into things while ambulating.

Outcomes and Evaluation Parameters	Planning and Interventions with *Rationales*
1. NURSING DIAGNOSIS: Disturbed Sensory Perception: Auditory and Impaired Verbal Communication related to hearing disorder (NANDA-I © 2012)	
Outcomes: Patient/family verbalize that the disease causes progressive hearing loss. Patient/family verbalize what treatments will help. ***Evaluation Parameters:*** Patient can communicate. Assistive devices are helping with hearing and communication.	Assess the degree of hearing loss. *Helps determine the best approach to communicate.* Teach about the disease process. *Helps reduce anxiety and stress related to the change or loss in hearing.* Speak clearly and slowly in a normal to deep voice; face the patient when speaking; use touch to gain the patient's attention. *Aids in verbal and nonverbal communication with the patient.* Respond to call light as soon as possible; answer questions; teach about medications/treatments *to decrease fear and anxiety.* Provide emotional support to the member having difficulty coping with the new sensory deficit *to decrease fear and anxiety.* Instruct or reinforce instruction on the use of the hearing aid. *Aids in retention of training and reinforces the need for using the assistive device for hearing.* Provide sensory stimulation; encourage expressing feelings of concern and loss for hearing deficit; teach to watch for visual cues. *Provides additional support for the patient.*
2. NURSING DIAGNOSIS: Risk for Falls, Risk for Injury, *and* Impaired Walking related to balance impairment (NANDA-I © 2012)	
Outcomes: Patient verbalizes that balance disorder is temporary. Patient participates in rehabilitative activities to maximize position sense. Patient will adhere to medication regime prescribed for balance disorder. ***Evaluation Parameters:*** Dizziness and vertigo subside. Patient is able to resume normal activities of daily living (ADLs) and lifestyle.	Explain the cause for dizziness and vertigo. *Helps the patient understand the reason for the symptoms.* Assist the patient with ambulation and other ADLs *to ensure the patient does not experience any injuries while dizzy.* Utilize safety measures such as keeping bedside rails in the elevated position and call light within reach. *Safety precautions.* Teach family how to assist the patient with ambulation and ADLs upon discharge *to ensure ongoing safety measures until the dizziness and vertigo subside.*

Source: Adapted from Wilkinson, J. M., & Ahern, N. R. (2009). *Prentice Hall nursing diagnosis handbook* (9th ed.). Upper Saddle River, NJ: Prentice Hall.

tube. It also may be caused by a progressive head cold; a viral sinus infection that spreads; an utreated otitis externa infection that spreads to the inner ear; blowing the nose too hard, thus forcing sinal or Eustachian drainage into the middle ear; or an opportunistic infection entering through a perforated eardrum (Merck Manual, 2008). Chronic otitis media is the result of repeated episodes of acute otitis media, causing irreversible tissue pathology and persistent perfusion of the tympanic membrane. The infection causes fluid to build up in the lining of the middle ear; this becomes thick like glue, which can lead to temporary hearing loss (Jirage, 2012).

PATIENT TEACHING & DISCHARGE PRIORITIES for Hearing and Balance Disorders

Need	Teaching
Usable information techniques for patient and family in home setting	Provide access to easily understood information in appropriate formats, using plain language and possibly visual representation in subtitled DVDs and videos. Assist with location of classes for American Sign Language (ASL), if applicable. Provide for health information or programs (including mental health promotion) that are accessible to the deaf community.
Safe environment for the patient	The inpatient, outpatient, day services, or work settings need to have services that make the environment safer; for instance, visual fire safety provisions and access to alerting and telephone services, TVs with teletext ability, pagers, and inclusive ways to operate remote door-entry systems. The home needs to be inspected to ensure safety measures are in place to avoid injury (e.g., furniture arrangement, no throw rugs, sound amplification on phone).
Communication support for patient and family	Deaf people who use ASL as their first and preferred form of communication have the right to qualified interpreter support. Deaf people who use English and hearing aids have the right to use lipspeaker-cued speech or speech-to-text transcription. Lipspeaker-cued speech is a means of communication in which a speaker uses hand signals to clarify ambiguous mouth movements (National Association of Deafened People, 2012).
Health promotion for patient and family	Provide access to health information or programs (including mental health promotion) to the deaf community. These programs should be designed in close cooperation with organizations that serve the deaf community. Different means of promotion, such as face-to-face delivery in ASL, may be more effective to reach deaf people.
Assessment, care, and treatment for the patient	Deaf people have the right to be assessed by a trained worker who has deaf/deaf-blind awareness and skills. Deaf-specific advisory services should be considered. Using these services aims to ensure that deaf persons can participate fully in any assessment and discussion of services.
Advocacy for patient	Deaf people have the right to independent advocacy in health, mental health service, education, employment, and social care. This is to ensure that the deaf person can participate fully in any assessment and discussion of services to make informed choices.
Physical teaching needs	In the outpatient setting, teaching needs might be focused on adherence to the prescribed medication regime, avoidance of behaviors that caused the hearing or balance disorder, protective devices for the workplace, and other health promotional activities. If the patient had surgery, include teaching on postoperative wound care, medication therapy, coping, and a return-to-work plan.
Medications for patient and family	Review medications; look for any ototoxic drugs and remove them, then notify the health care provider. Ensure that individuals understand how to take prescribed medications.

Source: Adapted from Deaf Mental Health Charter. (2008). Mental Health Foundation. Retrieved from http://www.mhf.org.uk/our-work/all-adults/deaf-charter/. Commissioned by Sign and Mental Health Foundation, London, England.

Clinical Manifestations

Clinical manifestations of acute otitis media include earache, headache, fever, discharge from the ear, mild deafness, difficulty sleeping, and loss of appetite. The patient may report no pain with movement of the auricle, and the tympanic membrane is erythematous and often bulging. Clinical manifestations of chronic otitis media include tinnitus, hearing loss, difficulty hearing in noisy surroundings, and an individual who tends to speak quietly. The patient experiences fullness in the ears, with varying degrees of hearing impairment and pain.

Medical and Surgical Management

Otitis media is easily diagnosed by the combination of symptoms (pain and hearing loss) and examination of the ear. Over-the-counter analgesics can help alleviate the pain, as can warm olive oil dripped into the ear. Antibiotics are generally indicated. If the offending organism can be isolated to the middle ear area and if the infections reoccur frequently, further treatment may include tube placement or other surgical interventions. The insertion of tubes in the ears, or a **myringotomy,** can be done on an outpatient basis. After an incision is made in the tympanic membrane (eardrum), a small plastic or metal tube is placed through the opening. The tube's purpose is to ventilate the middle ear and equalize the pressure within the ear and the outside environment. The tubes typically stay in place for 6 to 12 months or until they fall out spontaneously. Anyone with tubes in the ears should avoid getting water inside them.

Otosclerosis

Epidemiology, Etiology, and Pathophysiology

Otosclerosis is the abnormal growth of bone around the stapes bone in the middle ear. The spongylike bone growth of otosclerosis prohibits the stapes in the oval window (entrance to the inner ear) from moving and interferes with sound-passing waves to the inner ear, typically resulting in a conductive type hearing loss (NIDCD, 2011c).

It is estimated that 10% of the adult Caucasian population is affected by otosclerosis (Roland, 2011). This condition is less common in people of Japanese and South American descent, and is rare in African Americans. Overall, Caucasian, middle-age women are most at risk (American Academy of Otolaryngology-Head and Neck Surgery, 2011). Approximately 40% of otosclerosis cases have a genetic predisposition (American Academy of Otolaryngology-Head and Neck Surgery, 2011). Otosclerosis affects both ears in 80% of patients (American Speech-Language-Hearing Association, 2008).

Clinical Manifestations

It is not immediately obvious that a person has otosclerosis, and it does not always cause a hearing loss. The first symptom of a hearing loss induced by otosclerosis is often that a person has difficulty understanding others (Berke, 2010). There also may be tinnitus and dizziness. The hearing loss may start in the low frequencies before the high frequencies are lost, and then it may stay the same for a long time or worsen to the point that the person has a moderate hearing loss. In rare cases, a sensorineural (nerve) hearing loss also may develop, which makes the level of hearing loss greater (Tian, 2012). Also, hearing might appear to be better in noisy environments.

Medical and Surgical Management

For a mild case, no treatment may be needed, or the patient may just need hearing aids. For more severe cases, treatment options are limited to a **stapedectomy,** a surgical procedure in which the innermost bone (stapes) is removed and replaced with a small plastic tube of stainless steel wire (prosthesis) to improve the movement of sound to the inner ear. This prosthesis bridges the gap between the incus and the inner ear, providing sound conduction.

Mastoiditis

Epidemiology, Etiology, and Pathophysiology

Mastoid infection or **mastoiditis** is an acute or chronic infection of the mastoid process that can lead to changes in hearing and balance. It is usually caused by a middle ear bacterial infection (acute otitis media) and typically affects children. The mastoid is located just behind the outer ear. The infection may spread from the ear to the mastoid bone of the skull. The mastoid bone, which is structured like a honeycomb, fills with infected materials, after which its structure may deteriorate (MedlinePlus, 2012b).

Clinical Manifestations

Symptoms include ear pain or discomfort, fever (which may be high or suddenly increase), headache, hearing loss, redness of the ear or behind the ear, and swelling behind the ear, which may cause the ear to stick out. The individual also may have drainage from the ear and subsequent changes in hearing and position sense.

Medical Management

Mastoiditis may be difficult to treat because medications may not reach the mastoid bone. It may require repeated or long-term treatment with systemic antibiotics. However, if chronic mastoiditis occurs, a **mastoidectomy** (removal of the mastoid process) is indicated. This procedure can be done either through the ear or externally through an incision to the occipital bone.

Damaged Ossicles

Etiology and Pathophysiology

The ossicles are three tiny bones—the malleus, the incus, and the stapes—that form a chain that stretches across the middle ear space from the eardrum to the oval window on the inner ear. The oval window is one of two membrane-covered openings of the inner ear. Damage to the ossicles affects conductive hearing by limiting the transfer of vibrations to the middle ear (Ellis, 2012). If the ossicles are damaged, it could result in permanent hearing loss. Damaged ossicles can be caused by a genetic disorder, a physical trauma to the middle ear, a severe concussion, or a serious infection. Certain drugs, in particular aspirin in very high doses, or antibiotics called aminoglycosides (streptomycin and gentamicin), also may be a causative factor. A sharp object that penetrates the eardrum may cause damage to one or all of the three ossicles. Ossicular dislocation or damage interrupts the normal transmission of sound energy from the tympanic membrane to the fluid of the middle ear.

Clinical Manifestations and Medicall Management

The main symptoms of ossicular damage are pain and loss of hearing. Treatment is dependent on the type and severity of the injury or damage and resultant scar tissue. Typically the damaged ossicles are repaired surgically, with an ossiculoplasty. The surgery attempts to repair the damage to more than one of the ossicles. They may be replaced with either artificial bone, or small pieces of bone taken from other areas of the body. The prostheses can be made from man-made bone material, plastic, or ceramic. Although the operation can improve the hearing, it may not completely return (Ellis, 2012).

Nursing Management

Nursing assessment of middle ear disorders includes obtaining the patient's history, assessing vital signs, and determining the presence of medication allergies and family history. The nurse should determine the patient's fever and level of pain, as well as obtain a baseline hearing evaluation. If the patient has been injured, the nurse should assess the extent and condition of the injury. The nurse should inspect the ear for drainage and patency of the tympanic membrane and palpate the mastoid for tenderness.

Nursing diagnoses include *Pain*, *Risk for Infection* related to invasive procedure and trauma, *Risk for Injury* related to vertigo, *Anxiety* related to surgical procedure, *Potential Loss of Hearing*, *Potential Loss of Facial Movement*, and *Disturbed Sensory Perception*. Nursing interventions are designed and instituted to manage the pain. If the patient has had surgery, care includes changing dressings as appropriate, instructing the patient not to get the dressing wet, and advising the patient not to touch the ear. Careful hygiene must be used when providing ear care to prevent infection. In addition, the nurse should be alert for headache, fever, stiff neck, or altered level of consciousness, as these symptoms may represent a progressive infection of the central nervous system. The patient's balance may be compromised; thus, it is important to take safety precautions: keep the side rails up when the patient is in bed; assist with ambulating the first time up postsurgery; encourage the patient to move slowly; and instruct the patient not to blow her nose, cough, lean forward, or perform Valsalva's maneuver to avoid disrupting the graft or prosthesis, aggravating vertigo, or forcing bacteria up the Eustachian tube. The nurse should be aware of the patient's potential anxiety and should take care and time to listen to the patient's concerns. Anxiety also may be reduced by educating the patient about the disease and treatment plan. Instruction regarding self-care is critical to preparing the patient for discharge to the home setting.

Disorders of the Inner Ear

Common problems of the inner ear include acoustic neuromas, labyrinthitis, and Ménière's disease. Each is discussed in the following text.

Acoustic Neuromas

Epidemiology, Etiology, and Pathophysiology

Acoustic neuroma is a noncancerous and usually slow-growing tumor that develops on the main nerve leading from the inner ear to the brain. Also known as vestibular schwannoma, the tumor grows slowly; it extends from the internal auditory canal to the cerebellopontine angle (the angle between the cerebellum and pons), a common site for the growth of acoustic neuromas, and eventually presses on the brainstem. In a few cases, the tumor may grow rapidly and become large enough to press against the brain and interfere with vital functions. The clinical manifestations, as well as medical and nursing management of acoustic neuromas, are discussed in Chapter 21.

Labyrinthitis

Epidemiology, Etiology, and Pathophysiology

Labyrinthitis is an inflammation of the inner ear that affects the cochlear and/or vestibular portion of the labyrinth. Although definitive epidemiologic data are lacking, viral labyrinthitis is the most common form of labyrinthitis observed in clinical practice. The prevalence of sudden SNHL is estimated at 1 case in 10,000 persons, with up to 40% of these patients complaining of vertigo or disequilibrium. One study reported that 37 of 240 patients presenting with positional vertigo had viral labyrinthitis (Boston, 2012).

Viral labyrinthitis usually is observed in adults ages 30 to 60 years and is rarely observed in children. Meningogenic suppurative labyrinthitis usually is observed in children younger than 2 years, which is the population most at risk for meningitis. Otogenic suppurative labyrinthitis can be observed in persons of any age in the presence of cholesteatoma or as a complication of untreated acute otitis media.

The labyrinth is a maze of interconnected fluid-filled channels and canals. The cochlea comprises half of the labyrinth, and sends information about sounds to the brain. The three semicircular canals connect to an open vestibule, which sends information to the brain regarding the position and movement of the head. Any disturbance of the vestibule can lead to faulty information going to the brain. The eyes also send positioning information to the brain. When information from the labyrinth and the eyes do not match, the brain has trouble interpreting what is happening. This misinterpretation often leads to clinical symptoms common to labyrinthitis.

Clinically, this condition produces disturbances of balance and hearing to varying degrees and may affect one or both ears. Many times the cause of labyrinthitis cannot be determined. Often, the condition follows a viral illness such as a cold or the flu. Viruses, or the body's immune response to them, may cause inflammation that results in labyrinthitis. Other potential causes and/or risk factors are trauma or injury to the head or ear, bacterial infections, allergies, alcohol abuse, a benign tumor of the middle ear, certain medications taken in high doses (Lasix, Aspirin, Dilantin), and benign paroxysmal positional vertigo (Simic, 2012).

Clinical Manifestations

The most common symptoms of labyrinthitis are vertigo, nausea, vomiting, and loss of balance. Other possible symptoms include a mild headache, tinnitus, and hearing loss. These symptoms often are provoked or made worse by moving the head, sitting up, rolling over, or looking upward. Symptoms may last for days or even weeks depending on the cause and severity. Rarely, the condition may last all of one's life.

Medical and Surgical Management

The health care provider performs a complete physical and neurological exam, as an ear examination may not reveal any abnormalities. Laboratory tests may include an EEG, electronystagmography, head computerized tomography (CT), hearing tests, and magnetic resonance imaging (MRI) of the head.

Labyrinthitis usually resolves within a few weeks. Treatment helps to reduce symptoms, such as spinning sensations. Medications that may be prescribed include antihistamines and antiemetics, those that relieve dizziness, such as meclizine or scopolamine. The provider may prescribe sedatives (hypnotics such as antivert, valium, phenergan, dramamine, and benadryl) (Simic, 2012). See the Pharmacology box (p. 1994) for a description of these medications.

The individual with chronic labyrinthitis might need surgical intervention in the form of a **labyrinthectomy** (removal of the labyrinth) or **vestibular nerve dissection,** which is the process of cutting the vestibular part of the cochleovestibular cranial nerve, to reduce the impulses and remove the subjective sensation of dizziness/vertigo (Hain, 2011). A labyrinthectomy will cause total deafness of the affected ear. In the case of a vestibular nerve dissection, the patient will need a craniotomy with a bone flap temporarily removed from the skull to access the vestibular nerve, which the surgeon will partially sever. As a result of the surgery, vertigo will be prevented or decreased. The risk of hearing loss will be increased.

Ménière's Disease

Epidemiology, Etiology, and Pathophysiology

Ménière's disease is defined as a metabolic alteration in the labyrinthine fluid of the inner ear that causes spontaneous episodes of vertigo or a spinning sensation, along with fluctuating hearing loss. This is considered a chronic condition. Although people in their 40s and 50s are more likely than people in other age groups to develop Ménière's disease, it can occur at any age, even in children (Mayo Clinic Staff, 2012). The cause of Ménière's disease is not well understood. However, it appears to be the result of an abnormal volume or composition of fluid in the inner ear. The membranous labyrinth contains a fluid (endolymph) and is lined with hairlike sensors that respond to movement of the fluid. In order for all of the sensors in the inner ear to function properly, the fluid needs to retain a certain volume, pressure, and chemical composition. Factors that alter the properties of inner ear fluid may help cause Ménière's disease. Potential causes or triggers include:

- Improper fluid drainage, perhaps because of a blockage or anatomic abnormality
- Abnormal immune response
- Allergies
- Viral infection
- Genetic predisposition
- Head trauma.

Because no single cause has been identified, it is likely that Ménière's disease is caused by a combination of factors (California Ear Institute, 2011a).

Clinical Manifestations

Classic symptoms of Ménière's disease include sporadic episodes of vertigo, ranging from motion sickness to severe loss of balance, fluctuating progressive, unilateral, or bilateral sensorineural hearing loss; unilateral or bilateral tinnitus; and a sensation of fullness or pressure in one or both ears. A typical episode might start with a feeling of fullness in the ear, increasing tinnitus, and decreased hearing, followed by severe vertigo. This often is accompanied by nausea and vomiting. Such an episode might last 2 to 3 hours, after which signs and symptoms improve. Episodes often occur in clusters, with long periods of mild or no symptoms (remission) between. The severity, frequency, and duration of each of these sensory perception problems vary, especially early in the disease.

Laboratory Tests

The health care provider will conduct a physical examination and ask questions about the patient's history. Both a hearing assessment and a balance assessment will be completed. Tests that assess the function of the inner ear include an electronystagmography (ENG), rotary chair testing, vestibular evoked myogenic potentials (VEMP), and posturography. Other tests may be completed to rule out disorders that can cause problems similar to those of Ménières disease, such as a tumor in the brain or multiple sclerosis. These tests include magnetic resonance imaging (MRI), computerized tomography (CT), and auditory brainstem response audiometry. These tests also are explained in the Diagnostic Tests box on p. 2006.

Medical Management

There is no cure for Ménière's disease, but there are strategies that can manage symptoms. For example, medications to control vertigo during an attack may be prescribed. These include motion sickness medications, such as meclizine or diazepam. Anti-nausea medications, such as promethazine, also may be prescribed. The health care provider may prescribe a diuretic on a long-term basis to reduce fluid retention. The diuretic action may decrease the fluid volume resulting in decreased pressure in the inner ear. These changes help to control the severity and frequency of symptoms. Medications are discussed in the Pharmacology box (p. 1994).

Noninvasive treatments that may be prescribed to improve the patient's quality of life include physical therapy to stabilize balance and the use of a hearing aid to improve hearing. Several minimally invasive procedures may help reduce the patient's symptoms. The health care provider may prescribe a Meniett device, a pulse generator that applies positive pressure to the middle ear through a tympanoplasty tube. Positive pressure improves fluid exchange and reduces pressure in the ear. The treatment is performed at home, usually three times a day for 5 minutes at a time. Initial reports on the Meniett device show improvement in symptoms of vertigo, tinnitus, and aural pressure (Mayo Clinic Staff, 2012). An endolymphatic sac procedure is another intervention that may be performed early in the disease. Theoretically, the endolymphatic sac procedure decreases the buildup of endolymphatic pressure by removing previous bone that encases the endolymph reservoir. This allows the reservoir sac to expand more freely than before and allows the pressure to dissipate. In addition, some health care providers insert a drain or valve from the endolymphatic space to the mastoid or subarachnoid space to further reduce pressure (Li, 2012). If the patient's condition is extremely limiting and minimally invasive procedures have been ineffective, then surgical destruction of the labyrinth may be performed. This procedure results in irreversible hearing loss. The patient also is advised of self-care tactics that can help reduce the impact of Ménière's disease. These include activity instructions, dietary changes, and other lifestyle changes. These instructions are included in the Discharge Priorities section on ear disorders on page 1999 of this chapter.

Nursing Management

Nursing care of patients with inner ear disorders encompasses the principles of care discussed in similar sections on the external ear and the middle ear. However, there is greater emphasis placed on vertigo and impact on balance. If an inner ear disease is suspected or diagnosed, the nurse should assess the patient's mental status, cranial nerves, and motor and sensory function. Patients with central causes of vertigo, such as a stroke, may be unable to stand or take a step without falling. In comparison, patients with peripheral causes of vertigo, such as inner ear disease, may feel dizzy but can walk. In patients with inner ear disease, vertigo has a sudden onset. It is accompanied by hearing loss and vestibular symptoms that vary in type, frequency, and severity among patients. The nurse will develop a self-care plan that ensures the patient's safety and freedom from injury as well as addresses the patient's specific symptoms. The patient will be provided instruction for self-care at home. Patients with labyrinthitis are treated with intravenous fluids, antiviral drugs or antibiotics, and steroids. The nurse is responsible for monitoring the intravenous infusion and administering medications as ordered. The nurse also needs to educate the patient regarding the use, dosage, route of administration, and possible adverse effects of these medications.

With Ménière's disease, patients are treated with diet and medication. The patient should be encouraged to decrease salt intake to improve fluid balance in the inner ear. The patient also should be taught to avoid other substances known to exacerbate an inner ear fluid imbalance, including caffeine, nicotine, alcohol, foods high in carbohydrate content, and candy. Patient instruction also includes ways to manage fluid intake as they often are on diuretics. The patient also should drink at least 2 liters of water each day to prevent dehydration.

All patients with inner ear disorders tend to experience anxiety and fear or concern over their future. In addition, all will have diminished hearing. This is a major issue that the nurse needs to address with patients and their families so she can assist them in making lifestyle changes as needed. Consultation with social support services and counseling should be explored.

Safety Alert *Sudden hearing loss is considered a medical emergency. Individuals who suddenly lose their hearing should seek immediate medical attention.*

Collaborative Management

Collaborative care is extremely essential for the successful treatment of hearing disorders. In order to meet desired patient outcomes, it is essential that this interdisciplinary team communicate openly with one another in developing and evaluating care of the patient and family (IOM [Institute of Medicine], 2010).

The ear, nose, and throat specialist maintains control of developing and implementing the treatment plan for patients. If the patient has a malignancy, an oncologist may be called in as a consultant. Patients may be treated as an inpatient or an outpatient with the nurse serving as a central member of the health care team. The nurse provides direct patient care, provides patient instructions on self-care, and assists the patient in developing a personal and community support system. A physical therapist may be used to provide vestibular rehabilitation and work with the patient to establish an exercise program to improve balance and vertigo. An occupational therapist may be called in to assist the patient and family in making necessary lifestyle changes and, in some cases, developing different occupational goals. A nutritionist may provide information and advice on dietary changes necessary to improve balance and vertigo, especially in the case of Ménière's disease. The patient and family may be referred to social services or a counselor for emotional issues and control of anxiety related to hearing loss.

Health Promotion

Health promotion education for patients with hearing disorders focuses on patient education, lifestyle changes, and prevention measures. Education includes instruction on how to take medications as prescribed: use, dosage, route, and adverse reactions. Patients need to be advised of any mobility or exercise precautions, as well as the level of activity that is acceptable. They also are advised to make the immediate environment safe, to remove obstacles that they may trip over, and to implement safety precautions needed due to hearing impairments. In addition, the nurse should advise them of community resources and support groups that are available to them.

Certain self-care tactics can help reduce the impact of hearing disorders; for example, instructing the patient to sit or lie down immediately when she feels dizzy and avoid things that can make the signs and symptoms worse, such as sudden movement, bright lights, watching television, or reading. The patient needs to be instructed to rest during and after attacks of vertigo. Additionally, the nurse must warn the patient to be aware of the possibility of losing her balance and to consider walking with a cane for stability. The nurse should also advise the patient to use good lighting if she has to get up in the night. The patient, as well as the patient's family, need to understand that driving a car or operating heavy machinery during episodes of vertigo is dangerous. By monitoring the sodium intake, the patient can reduce the body's fluid retention and help decrease fluid in the inner ear. Consuming foods and beverages high in salt also can increase fluid retention. The patient should aim for an intake of 1,500 milligrams (mg) or less of sodium each day and avoid monosodium glutamate (MSG). Some prepackaged food products and prepared restaurant foods contain MSG, a type of sodium that can contribute to fluid retention. Therefore, the patient should check ingredient labels or ask the restaurant server if the food he is considering ordering contains MSG-B. In addition, the patient should be instructed to avoid foods and beverages that contain caffeine—such as chocolate, coffee, tea, and certain soft drinks—because they have stimulant properties that can make symptoms worse. For instance, caffeine may make the ringing in the ears louder. By avoiding nicotine, the patient may lessen the severity of Ménière's disease symptoms.

Managing stress and anxiety may lessen the severity of symptoms and enable the patient to cope with hearing disorders. Professional psychotherapy also may help in identifying stressors and developing stress-reducing strategies. Hearing disorders may affect interactions with friends and family, productivity at work, and overall quality of life. Support groups can provide encouragement and understanding, as well as information and resources.

Measures to prevent ear injuries and gain healthy ears include the following:

- Never stick anything in your ears—not even cotton swabs or your fingers.
- Avoid uncomfortable, potentially damaging noise and decrease the volume when listening to music.
- Wear a snug-fitting helmet whenever you ride bikes or motorcycles.
- Wear the right kind of protective equipment when playing sports.
- When flying, chew gum, swallow water, or yawn while landing.
- Rinse hair in fresh water when bathing.
- Consult a health care provider if you have constant or recurring pain in your ears, or if hearing loss is suspected.

Conditions Affecting Balance

Balance of the body is maintained by the interactions between the eyes, the joints and muscles (proprioceptive system), the brain, and the labyrinth (vestibular apparatus). These structures all function together to maintain position sense and equilibrium. A change in functioning in any one of these structures will lead to a balance disorder (Figure 63–1◆).

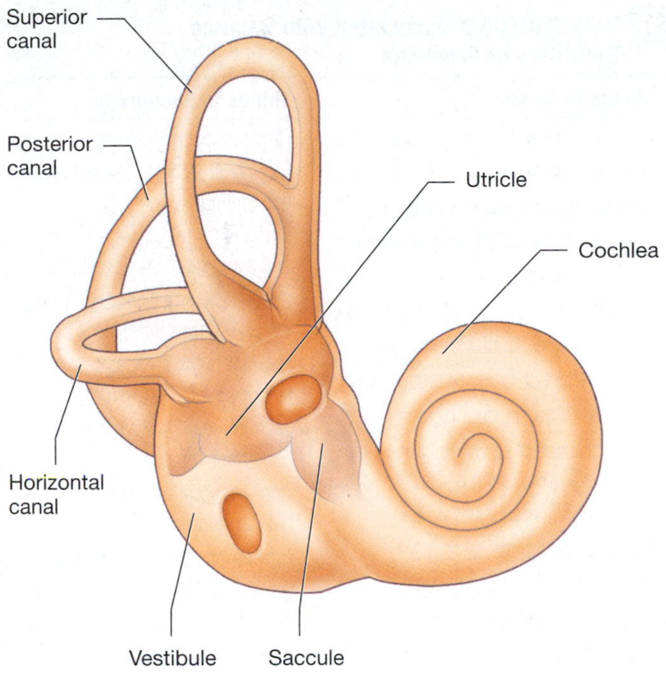

FIGURE 63–1 ◆ Anatomic structures of balance.
Source: Balance Disorders (NIH Publication No. 00-4374).

The primary symptom of a balance disorder is the development of vertigo which can last from 10 minutes up to several hours or days. Oftentimes, the most comfortable position for a patient experiencing vertigo is lying flat, immobilizing the head. Sudden head movements can precipitate nausea and vomiting. In addition to irritability, the patient might complain of tinnitus and reduced hearing on the involved side. The Risk Factors box outlines the risk factors associated with balance disorders and how to manage them.

The term *motion sickness* often is used to describe the symptoms associated with vertigo. In motion sickness, vertigo is present with nausea and possible vomiting.

Nystagmus is an oscillation of the eyes that is linked to the body's ability to maintain balance with motion or movement. Treatment includes reducing the motion and possibly using antiemetic (Droperidol) and antivertiginous (Dramamine) medications until the sensation passes.

Benign Paroxysmal Positional Vertigo

Epidemiology, Etiology, and Pathophysiology

Benign paroxysmal positional vertigo (BPPV) is one of the most common causes of vertigo. In BPPV, the symptom of dizziness is thought to be due to the formation of **otoconia,** which are small crystals of calcium carbonate derived from the utricle. The formation of otoconia may occur when the utricle is damaged by head injury, infection, or another disorder of the inner ear; the utricle also may have degenerated because of advanced age. Viruses that affect the ear, causing vestibular neuritis; minor strokes involving the anterior inferior cerebellar artery; and Ménière's disease are significant but unusual causes. In addition, BPPV is common in individuals who have been treated with ototoxic medications such as gentamicin (Hain, 2010). In about 50% of the cases, the cause is idiopathic. Benign paroxysmal positional vertigo accounts for approximately 20% of all occurrences of dizziness in the general population.

RISK FACTORS Associated with Balance Disorders or Problems

Things to Avoid	Things to Encourage
Driving vehicles if dizzy or unsteady	Change positions slowly
Operating hazardous machinery	Move from lying to upright position in stages
Prolonged periods of standing	Remove throw rugs and litter, and avoid highly polished floors
Exposure to excessive heat or sunlight	Use assistive devices for picking things up from the floor
Climbing stepladders	Replace fluids if excess fluid loss
Stooping to pick things up from the floor	Take antihypertensive medications after meals
Using over-the-counter medications	Apply nonslip surfaces in the bathtub or shower
Using alcohol or drugs that cause vertigo	Provide hand grips in bathroom
Smoking in bed or near oxygen	Provide railings in hallways and stairs
Prolonged bed rest, which causes skeletal muscle weakness and tone	Remove protruding objects (hooks, shelves) from stairway walls
Unsafe conditions while cooking	Wear shoes or slippers with nonskid soles
Increased susceptibility to glare	Install good lighting in hallways or stairs
High heels or unsafe footwear	
Medications and chemicals that cause vertigo:	
Avoid when possible	
Alcohol	
Aminoglycosides	
Anticonvulsants	
Antihypertensives	
Cocaine	
Cytotoxic agents	
Furosemide	
Nitroglycerin	
NSAIDs (indomethacin)	
Salicylates	
Tranquilizers (alprazolam and clonazepam)	

Clinical Manifestations

The symptoms of BPPV include dizziness or vertigo, light-headedness, imbalance, and nausea. Activities that bring on the symptoms of BPPV vary among individuals, although a change in position most commonly precipitates them. It is the change in the position of the head with respect to gravity that causes the vertigo. Getting out of bed and/or rolling over in bed are triggers. As the name implies, BPPV may be present for a few weeks, then stop, then come back again (Hain, 2007).

Diagnostic Procedures and Medical Management

Procedures commonly used to diagnose vestibular disorders are outlined in the Diagnostic Tests for Vestibular Function box (p. 2004). Although BPPV is not life threatening, the condition typically comes and goes over a span of several days or weeks. It is also possible that BPPV may go away on its own (Mayo Clinic, 2009). Therefore, patients can opt to just wait it out. Certain modifications in daily activities may be necessary to cope with the dizziness. For example, the nurse should instruct the patient to do the following:

- Use two or more pillows at night.
- When rising from bed, get up slowly and sit on the edge of the bed for a minute.
- Avoid bending down to pick up things and extending the head.
- Be careful when lying back, such as when in the dentist's chair or at a hair salon sink.

Motion sickness medications are sometimes helpful in controlling the nausea associated with BPPV, but do not prevent the dizziness.

Some maneuvers, such as the Epley maneuver shown in Figure 63–2◆, will help to move the otoconia out of the sensitive part of the ear (posterior canal) to a less sensitive location. The health care provider or the nurse moves the head sequentially into four positions, leaving the head in each position for roughly 30 seconds (Figure 63–2). The recurrence rate for BPPV after these maneuvers is about 30% at 1 year; in some instances, a second treatment may be necessary. Use of an antiemetic medication prior to the maneuver may be helpful if nausea is anticipated (Hain, 2007). The patient should continue with the daily modifications described previously for at least 1 week to avoid provoking head positions that might bring BPPV on again.

If the exercises are ineffective in controlling symptoms and the symptoms have persisted for a year or longer, a surgical procedure called *posterior canal plugging* may be recommended. This procedure blocks most of the posterior canal's function without affecting the functions of the other canals or parts of the ear. The surgery poses a small risk to hearing but is effective in about 90% of individuals who have had no response to any other treatment (National Dizzy & Balance Center, 2010). See the Complementary & Alternative Therapies box for additional treatment for balance disorders.

Labyrinthitis and Ménière's disease are other disorders that affect balance. These disorders were discussed on pages 2001 and 2002.

Other infectious causes of balance disorders include the common cold, childhood diseases such as measles and mumps, and more complex diseases such as meningitis, encephalitis, and syphilis. The common cold is discussed in Chapter 26, and meningitis and encephalitis are discussed in Chapter 21.

DIAGNOSTIC TESTS for Vestibular Function

Test	Expected Abnormality
Caloric Test (assesses the degree of vestibular and brainstem function, differentiating peripheral lesions from CN VIII lesions)	
Perform only if tympanic membrane is intact. Irrigate the ear canal with a few drops of cold water.	Nausea, horizontal nystagmus, vertigo toward unirrigated side. Found in Ménière's disease. No eye movement (nystagmus) in the unconscious patient.
Romberg Test (assesses the ability to maintain an upright posture when arms are out in front, with eyes open and closed)	
Stand with feet close together without swaying, with eyes open and eyes closed.	Swaying and inability to maintain balance as found in balance disorders.

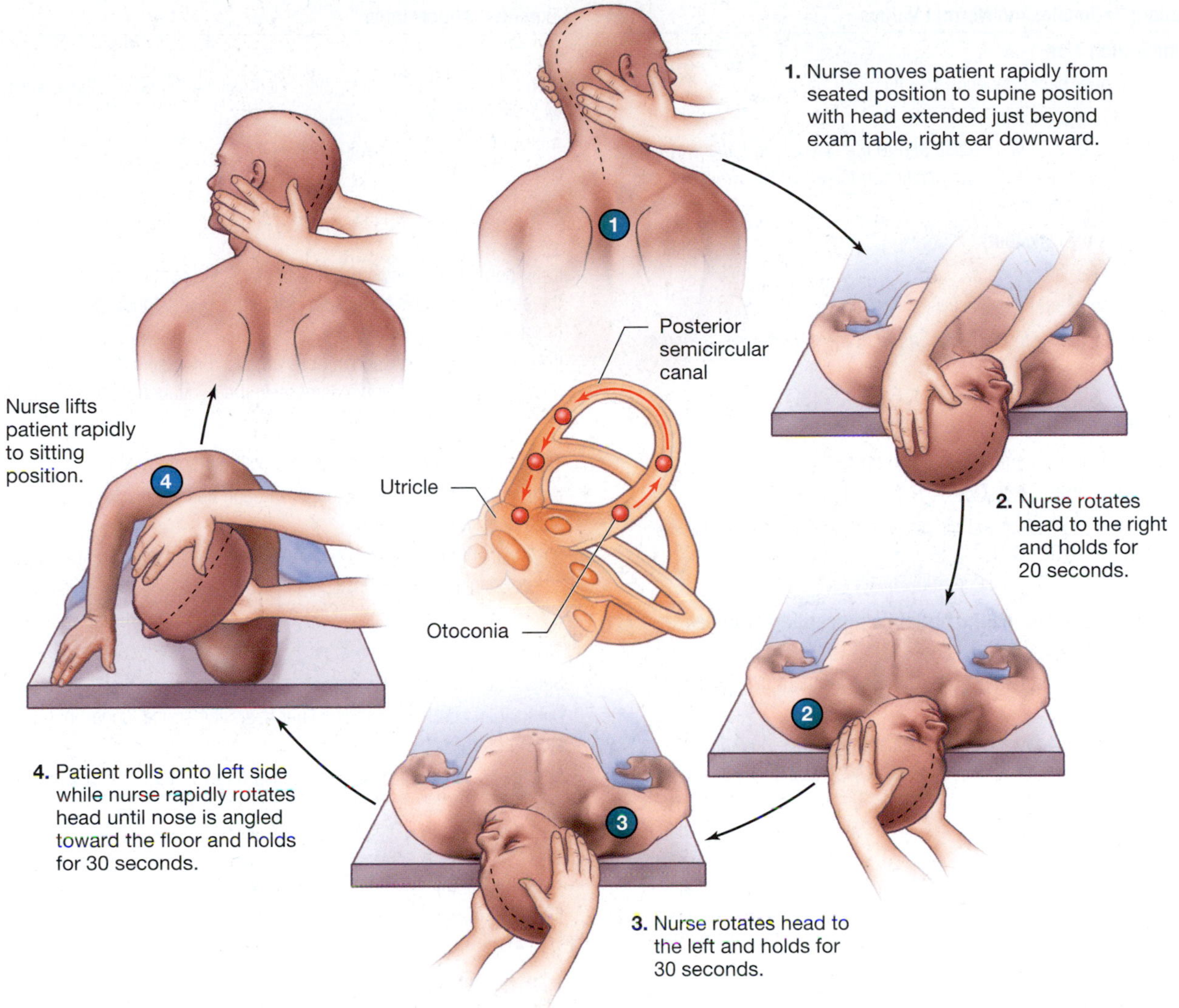

FIGURE 63–2 ◆ The Epley maneuver.

Other Causes of Balance Disorders

Other causes of balance disorders include an intracranial neoplasm (brain tumor) or a cerebrovascular accident (stroke). A balance disorder might be one of the first presenting symptoms of a brain tumor. A change in balance might also be one of the first presenting symptoms of a stroke. A stroke can be caused by either an intracranial hemorrhage or a cerebral embolism. A change in balance oftentimes will be the first indication of a pending or actual stroke. The causes and treatment of strokes are discussed in detail in Chapter 22.

Diagnostic Procedures for Balance Disorders

A variety of tests are used to help in the diagnosis of hearing and balance disorders. The diagnosis is made on the basis of the patient's medical history, findings on physical examination, and the results of vestibular and auditory tests. The medical history must evaluate the use of ototoxic medications and a review of what triggers the symptoms. It is significant if the dizziness is triggered by lying down or by rolling over in bed. The Dix-Hallpike test is used to aid the diagnosis. A person is brought from sitting to a supine position, with the head turned 45 degrees to one side and extended about 20 degrees backward. Once supine, the eyes are typically observed for about 30 seconds. If no nystagmus ensues, the person is brought back to sitting. There is a delay of about 30 seconds again, and then the other side is tested. When doing the Dix-Hallpike on a flat table, it is often helpful to place a flat "boat" cushion under the patient's back, to obtain head extension. Electronystagmography (ENG) testing may be needed to look for the characteristic nystagmus induced by the Dix-Hallpike test and an MRI scan is done if a stroke or brain tumor is suspected (Hain, 2007).

In evaluating a person's ability to hear, three characteristics are assessed: frequency, pitch, and intensity. *Frequency* is the number of sound waves emanating per second and is measured in Hertz (Hz). The ability to hear frequencies from 500 to 2,000 Hz is needed to understand everyday speech. The term *pitch* describes frequency; low pitch is 100 Hz and high pitch is 10,000 Hz. The loudness or intensity of sound is expressed in decibels. Sounds typically range from 0 to 140 dB or greater, with a critical level for hearing being 30 dB. Zero decibel is the sound measurement of slight whispering, whereas the blast of a gun approaches 140 dB.

The various tests used to determine these three components of hearing are outlined in the Diagnostic Tests box (p. 2006). These tests also assist in determining the reason for hearing loss (e.g., conductive versus sensorineural) and the degree of loss.

DIAGNOSTIC TESTS for Hearing and Balance Disorders

Description, Rationale, and Normal Values	Expected Abnormality
Voice and Watch Tick	
Normal: Able to hear high frequency sounds. Used to test high-frequency hearing loss. *The examiner stands 1–2 feet behind and to the side of the patient, while the patient occludes each ear sequentially and the examiner whispers four unrelated words near each ear.*	With a hearing abnormality, the patient will not be able to hear words whispered or a watch ticking. A loss of high-frequency sounds.
Weber Test (tuning fork test)	
Normal: Able to hear in both ears. Used to test sensorineural hearing loss. *Place an activated tuning fork midline on top of the patient's head, bridge of nose, or chin.*	If the patient has conductive hearing loss, the sound will lateralize to the ear with the loss because the sound is being conducted directly through the bone to the ear. If the patient has sensorineural hearing loss, the sound will lateralize to the hearing ear because nerve damage in the nonhearing ear prevents hearing
Rinne Test (tuning fork test)	
Normal: Able to hear via both bone and air conduction. *Used to test conductive hearing loss.* *Place activated tuning fork on the right and left mastoid bone sequentially and in front of each ear.*	This test compares bone conduction with air conduction. If the patient hears sounds longer through bone, then the patient has a conductive hearing loss. If the patient hears sounds longer through the air, then the patient has a sensorineural hearing loss.
Schwabach Test (compares the patient's perception of bone conduction to the examiner's)	
Normal: Able to hear at same speed as examiner, without diminishment or prolongation. *Place an activated tuning fork on the mastoid process of the patient and alternately test for both air and bone conduction.*	Sensorineural loss or conductive hearing loss. Diminished hearing—the examiner hears the sound longer than the patient does. Prolonged—the patient hears the sound longer than the examiner does.
Acoustic Immittance Tests	
Tympanometry	
Normal: Able to hear in tested ear/s. *Used to test the flexibility and mobility of the tympanic membrane to determine if anything is impeding movement of the tympanic membrane and ossicles of the middle ear.*	Tympanic membrane does not move (vibrate), causing a loss of sound transmission through the ear.
Acoustic Reflexes	
Normal: Able to hear and able to discriminate among speech sounds. Used to test the flexibility of the stapedius muscle. *Measures the change in admittance produced by contraction of the stapedius muscle as it responds to an intense sound; stimulation of one ear causes reaction in both ears.*	Stapedius muscle will not contract, thereby negating its protective mechanism of shielding the inner ear from damage due to intense sound or improving the discrimination of speech sounds in the presence of loud, low frequency background noise.
Pure Tone Audiometry	
Normal: Hear within normal decibel level for a specified sound; for example: A whisper: 15 to 30 dB Normal conversation: 60 dB Heavy city traffic or school cafeteria: 85 dB (Hyperacusis Network, 2011). Used to determine the type and degree of hearing loss. *Provides a record of which decibel levels the patient is unable to hear. This test will not provide the cause of the hearing loss.*	Unable to hear certain decibel levels.
Auditory Brainstem Response (ABR) Audiometry	
Normal: Waveforms normally occur within a 10-millisecond time period after a click stimulus presented at high intensities (70- to 90-dB normal hearing level) (Bhattacharyya, 2011). *The ABR audiometry is a neurological test that refers to an evoked potential generated by a brief click or tone transmitted from an acoustic transducer in the form of an insert earphone or headphone. The elicited waveform response is measured by surface electrodes typically placed at the vertex of the scalp and ear lobes. The amplitude of the signal is averaged and charted against the time (millisecond), much like an electroencephalogram.*	Individual is unable to hear clicks and generated waveforms within the normal range, thus indicating a hearing problem.

DIAGNOSTIC TESTS for Hearing and Balance Disorders, *continued*

Description, Rationale, and Normal Values	Expected Abnormality
Electronystagmography (ENG) Normal: Normal nystagmus with stimulation; normal vestibular reflex. *Used to test for Ménière's disease by assessing the oculomotor and vestibular systems and to identify oculovestibular lesions or abnormalities.*	There will be changes in the electrical potentials (waveforms) created by eye movements during spontaneous, positional, or calorically evoked nystagmus.
Dix-Hallpike Test for Vertigo (also called Nylen-Barney test) Normal: A normal test means that the patient did not experience vertigo of nystagmus during the test (WebMD, 2011). *The patient is brought from sitting to a supine position, with the head turned 45 degrees to one side and extended about 20 degrees backward. Determines whether vertigo is triggered by certain head movements. This test locates the cause of vertigo as either the inner ear or the brain. If the problem is in the ear, this test can determine which ear is affected.*	An abnormal test result means that the patient had vertigo or nystagmus during the test. It is likely that the vertigo is caused by an inner ear or brain problem, depending on the way the patient reacted to the test.

CHART 63–5 Basic Types of Hearing Aids for Sensorineural Hearing Loss

Type	Description
In-the-ear	Fit in outer ear; used for mild to severe hearing loss.
Behind-the-ear	Worn behind the ear and connected to a plastic ear mold that fits inside the outer ear; used for mild to profound hearing loss.
Canal aids	Fit into the ear canal; used for mild to moderately severe hearing loss.
Body aids	Aid attaches to a belt or pocket and is connected to the ear by a wire; used for profound hearing loss.

Source: National Institute on Deafness and Other Communication Disorders (NIDCD). (2010a). Hearing aids. Retrieved from http://www.nidcd.nih.gov/health/hearing/Pages/thebasics_hearingaid.aspx.

Assistive Devices

Assistive devices are available for individuals who have partial or total hearing loss. The two main types of assistive devices are assistive listening devices (ALDs) and alerting devices (ADs). The ALDs (such as hearing aids) help with listening, whereas ADs (such as hearing dogs or vibrating alarms) signal the presence of a sound. Basic ALD systems are devices that amplify the sound, which allow the caller to speak in a normal tone while amplifying the sound for the person with the hearing impairment, or enhancement systems that produce higher frequencies (pitches), which are important for understanding speech through microphones or transmitters. Small portable amplifiers also are available and are carried by those with hearing impairments to assist with communication. Alerting devices may be modified so that the person is alerted when sound devices (telephones, alarm clocks, doorbells) ring. Lamps throughout the house can be made to "flash" when someone rings the doorbell, or a small vibrating alarm clock can be placed under a pillow to wake someone up in the morning.

A telecommunications device for the deaf (TDD), also called a TTY, is a special device that lets people who are deaf, hard of hearing, or speech-impaired communicate via the telephone by allowing them to type messages back and forth. A TTY is required at both ends of the conversation in order to communicate. If a deaf individual is communicating with a hearing individual who doesn't have a TTY, they will use the Telecommunication Relay Service (TRS), a national service mandated by the ADA Act of 1990 that is available free of charge.

Hearing Aids

A hearing aid is a small electronic sound amplifier that fits either into the external ear canal or just behind the ear. The purpose of the hearing aid is to improve hearing. The aid can be worn in one or both ears. The patient should be fitted for the hearing aid based on the type and degree of hearing loss as determined by a certified licensed audiologist. For sensorineural hearing loss, there are aids that will depress the low-frequency sound and enhance the high-frequency sound. The hearing aid will only make sounds louder; it will not help with discriminating words or understanding speech. Hearing aids amplify all sounds, including background noise; therefore, the person needs to learn to filter out background noise. Initially, patients are typically encouraged to use the hearing aid for only part of the day. The patient needs to learn to adjust the tone or volume on the aid to achieve the best sound. The newer digital hearing aids are programmed by the audiologist with a computer, so the sound quality and response time can be adjusted on an individual basis (NIDCD, 2010a). These hearing aids are better able to compensate for background noise because they allow amplification at certain programmed frequencies rather than all of them.

Hearing aids are delicate devices that need careful handling and care in order to work properly, so the nurse needs to instruct the patient on their care and cleaning requirements. The following items are typical maintenance tasks for hearing aids:

- Clean the ear mold with mild soap and water.
- Check the battery regularly and replace as needed.
- Clean the hole in the middle of the device.
- Always have an extra battery on hand.
- Avoid spraying hairspray or other beauty products on the hearing aid.
- Turn off the hearing aid when not in use.

The patient also will need instructions about side effects or complications. The patient should contact the health care provider if skin irritation or accelerated cerumen accumulation occurs. If the hearing aid does not improve hearing, the patient may need to try another brand. Chart 63–5 lists the different types of hearing aids.

Cochlear Implants

A cochlear implant is a small, complex electronic device that can help to provide a sense of sound to a person who is profoundly deaf or severely hard of hearing. The intention was for this implant to aid individuals with neurofibromatosis, one of the hereditary forms of deafness, to hear. An implant does not restore or create normal hearing, although it can give a deaf person a useful auditory understanding of the environment and help her to understand speech. With a cochlear implant, 22 electrodes are placed in the cochlea and attached to a microphone and signal processor, which are surgically placed under the skin behind the ear. The microphone and signal processor transmit electrical stimuli to the electrodes. These electrical signals stimulate the auditory nerve fibers and the brain, where the sounds are interpreted. Once the device has been implanted, the patient undergoes extensive cochlear rehabilitation. Several months of training with an audiologist and speech pathologist are needed to learn to interpret the sounds.

Most children who receive cochlear implants are between 2 and 6 years old. Early implantation provides exposure to sounds that can be helpful during the critical periods when children learn speech and language skills. A cochlear implant coupled with intensive post-implantation therapy allows these children to develop communication skills within a few months (NIDCD, 2011a).

Hearing Guide Dogs

Hearing guide dogs are specially trained to alert the deaf person or a person with a hearing impairment to ringing doorbells, potential dangers, and other sounds that require a response. The dog alerts the person by physical contact. In public, the dog positions itself between the person with the hearing impairment and possible danger, such as oncoming traffic. Information about qualifying for a dog may be obtained through International Hearing Dog, Inc. (www.ihdi.org). This is a nonprofit organization funded by donations whose mission is to train and place hearing dogs with persons who are deaf or hard of hearing, with or without multiple disabilities, at no charge to the recipient.

Speech Reading and Sign Language

Through speech reading, also known as lip reading, the person with a hearing impairment uses his eyes to assist with understanding what is being said. There are formal speech reading classes where the deaf person is taught special clues and how to understand body language. The deaf person or someone with a hearing impairment typically understands only a portion of the words, but communication is enhanced.

Sign language is another means of enhancing communication for the deaf person or person with a hearing impairment. American Sign Language is one example of a complex visuospatial language that is used by the deaf community. Sign language is a linguistically complete, natural language that is native to many deaf men and women, as well as some hearing children born into deaf families.

Nursing Management

Nursing management consists of using the nursing process to assess, diagnose, and manage the care of patients with hearing and balance disorders.

Assessment

Preparing to provide care to a patient with a hearing or balance disorder should begin with an assessment of the patient's current status. Hearing should be assessed by asking the patient: "When did you first notice that you had a change in your ability to hear? Did you have a recent exposure to a loud noise or infection?" From an objective perspective, the nurse should review the results of hearing tests if available, test the patient's ability to hear at normal voice range, test lower and higher pitch, and speak into both ears to test unilateral versus bilateral hearing loss. When assessing for balance, it is important to ask the patient if she is experiencing dizziness and, if so, for how long. Has she fallen? How long has she felt dizzy with walking, and does she feel nauseated? It also is important to determine if she is using any hazardous machinery or equipment at work, and if she drives an automobile. The nurse should observe the patient for ataxia and bumping into things when ambulating, Also, the patient's knowledge base should be determined by asking, what do you know about your condition; has someone explained the tests, diagnosis and treatment plan to you; and how do you feel about what is happenned to you? Allow patients to express their feelings and concerns about what is happening to them and observe their social interaction with others. Do they have visitors in a hospitalized setting? Does someone accompany them to their appointments? Do they converse freely with others? Also determine the patient's mood, i.e., angry, depressed, and unsure of his own abilities. Mood changes may represent feelings of inadequacy, loneliness, and diminished self-esteem. They also may be a reflection of the grieving process from loss of an essential sense, a perceived change in lifestyle, and an inability to cope with these changes. From this information, the nurse can then determine diagnoses appropriate to address these findings.

Nursing Diagnoses

Nursing diagnoses may include the following:

- *Disturbed Sensory Perception: Auditory* related to hearing loss.
- *Impaired Social Interaction* related to communication barriers and self-concept disturbance.
- *Social Isolation* related to alterations in health status (hearing loss).
- *Risk for Loneliness* related to physical isolation.
- *Ineffective Coping* related to uncertainty and perception of loss of control.
- *Impaired Walking* related to impaired balance.
- *Deficient Knowledge* related to unfamiliarity with information resources.
- *Anticipatory Grieving* related to loss of hearing and balance and potential changes in lifestyle.
- *Risk for Situational Low Self-Esteem* related to disturbed body image.
- *Risk for Injury* related to sensory dysfunction, hearing, and balance.

NANDA-I © 2012

From the diagnoses, the nurse can then develop outcomes and plan interventions to aid in the care of a patient with special needs.

Outcomes With Evaluation Parameters

Desired outcomes or patient objectives that reflect patient behaviors and positive results of care follow. Relative to the nursing diagnoses stated previously, patient behavioral expectations include: (1) improved sensory integration as manifested by increased sensory perception, ability to communicate with others, and apparent reduction in stress; (2) improved social interactions demonstrated by interacting with visitors, talking with others, communicating shared interests, and verbalizing feeling better about social interactions; (3) communicative with a change in affect as demonstrated by interacting with others, seeking out others to talk with, and verbalization of feeling less insecure and willingness to meet with others; (4) expresses feelings of wanting not to be isolated from others, participates in group activities, welcomes visitors, and makes plans for occupational and social outings. In response to ineffective coping, he verbalizes feelings of hope and requests counseling or other forms of support and is able to sleep restfully. With the diagnoses of impaired walking and risk of injury, patient outcomes include: (1) verbalizes that balance disorder is temporary, (2) participates in rehabilitative activities to maximize position sense, and (3) adheres to medication regime for balance disorder.

Evaluation parameters include decreased or absent dizziness and vertigo, ability to resume normal activities of daily living and lifestyle, and freedom from injury. As care progresses, the patient will demonstrate an understanding of the disorders and how they were caused. He will verbalize his understanding, ask appropriate time-related questions regarding the disorder and the treatment plan, and establish realistic future goals. In response to anticipatory grieving, the patient will discuss his fears and concerns regarding his loss of hearing and/or balance. He will progress through the grief process as evidenced by changes in mood and function and regain a sense of self as related to job, status in family, home, and body. These behaviors also may indicate improved self-esteem, as will an expression of feelings of self-worth and participation in new groups and activities. The risk of injury is lessened as the patient participates in rehabilitative activities and becomes familiar with the symptoms of his disorder, the observable outcome being no injuries, verbalization by the patient that he feels comfortable in his environment, and evidence that he has taken the necessary safety precautions in his home setting.

Planning and Interventions

Interventions are designed to help the patient achieve the desired outcomes. They include assessing the degree of hearing loss in order to determine the best communication approach, as well as teaching the patient about the disease process to reduce anxiety and stress related to the change or loss in hearing. The nurse should speak clearly and slowly in a normal to deep voice; face the patient when speaking; and use touch to gain the patient's attention. These actions help the patient understand verbal and nonverbal communication. The nurse should respond to the call light as soon as possible; answer questions; and teach about medications and treatments to decrease the patient's fear and anxiety. In addition, the nurse should provide emotional support to the patient who is having difficulty coping with the new sensory deficit to decrease her fear and anxiety. By instructing or reinforcing instruction on use of the hearing aid, the nurse helps the patient retain her training and reinforces the need to use the assistive device for hearing. The nurse provides additional support to the patient by providing sensory stimulation; encouraging expression of feelings of concern and loss for hearing deficit; and teaching the patient to watch for visual cues.

Interventions specific to diagnoses of balance disorders include the following: (1) Explain the cause for dizziness and vertigo to help the patient understand the reason for the symptoms. (2) Assist the patient with ambulation and activities of daily living (ADLs) to ensure the patient does not experience any injuries while dizzy. (3) Use safety measures such as keeping bedside rails in an elevated position and call light within reach. (4) Teach the family how to assist the patient with ambulation and ADLs upon discharge to make sure that safety measures stay in place until the dizziness and vertigo subside. (5) Instruct the patient and family on home modification to ensure safety measures have been taken in the home environment.

Discharge Priorities

When planning for discharge from an acute care facility for treatment of a hearing or balance disorder, the nurse is in the best position to help the patient and family with physical, psychological, and future occupational needs. Helping the patient and family deal with the cause of the hearing or balance deficit and identify choices to avoid future problems associated with hearing and balance are the nurse's approaches of choice. The Deaf Mental Health Charter (2008) commissioned by the Sign and Mental Health Foundation in London, England, has identified a variety of areas that need implementation to address the types of choices that the deaf community may make. These areas are outlined in the Patient Teaching & Discharge Priorities box.

If a patient is being discharged from an acute care facility, the nurse's responsibilities in terms of the patient's physical teaching needs might include postoperative wound care, medication therapy, coping, and a return-to-work plan. In the outpatient setting, the nurse might focus on teaching the patient about adherence to a prescribed medication regime, avoidance of behaviors that caused the hearing/balance disorders, protective devices for the workplace, and other health promotional activities.

If the hearing or balance disorder involves a long-term change in the ability to hear, other instructions would include communication instruction such as sign language and use of a hearing aid. The nurse can help family members with suggestions for communicating with the person who has the hearing impairment and teaching them how to avoid the same exposure that caused the hearing impairment in their loved one.

Collaborative Care

Care of the patient with sensory disorders requires the expertise and cooperation of an interdisciplinary health care team. The patient with a hearing or balance disorder may need the aid of additional caregivers. These caregivers may include therapists in occupational and physical medicine, as well as speech and hearing therapists, to assist them in the rehabilitative process and aid their return to a functional and fulfilling lifestyle. In order to meet desired patient outcomes, it is essential that this interdisciplinary team communicate openly with one another in developing and evaluating care of the patient and family (IOM [Institute of Medicine], 2010).

Learning to care for a hearing aid might first be reviewed with an audiologist and then turned over to the nurse for instructional reinforcement. If the patient is experiencing a balance disorder and is being treated with rehabilitative services, the nurse's role is to reinforce the instructions provided by the therapist. Caregiver help may be required as well as home health assistance. The role of the audiologist and health care provider remain intact.

Health Promotion

Anyone is at risk for hearing and balance disorders. Individuals should be advised of risk factors that might precipitate these disorders. In addition, the nurse should inform people of ways to prevent hearing and balance disorders, as has been discussed in Chapter 62 under Health Promotion. If an infection within the ear structures is suspected, it is important for the patient to contact her health care provider. If an infection is not treated, it can lead to hearing loss. Having a loss of hearing creates unique challenges for the individual. Environmental noise cannot be discerned, leaving the person prone to hazards such as an oncoming automobile or even a bee whose warning buzz was not heard. Adults should be encouraged to seek advice for hearing loss and be supported when needing to purchase and care for hearing aids. Those who cannot have their hearing restored through surgery or devices need to be supported with training and education to learn sign language or provided with a telephonic device to aid with communication.

The Patient Teaching & Discharge Priorities feature (p. 1999) specifies educational instructions or information for those who have hearing and balance disorders.

Safety Alert *If the patient is experiencing vertigo or dizziness, his health care provider may need to contact the Department of Motor Vehicles to report the patient's balance disorder. The patient's driver's license could be suspended until the disorder subsides and the patient passes a medical clearance prior to resuming the use of a motor vehicle.*

Rehabilitative programs exist for these individuals to help them regain position sense and balance. People with a known balance disorder should be advised to avoid operating motor vehicles or machinery.

Gerontological Considerations

Hearing loss is one of the three most common chronic conditions among older adults, the others being high blood pressure and arthritis. Approximately 25% to 40% of adults older than 65 years have some degree of hearing loss, and it is estimated that 40% to 60% of people ages 75 years or older have hearing loss commonly caused by gradual changes in the inner ear (NIDCD, 2010b; Parmet, Lynm, & Glass, 2007). **Presbycusis,** the loss of hearing that occurs slowly over time in most individuals as they grow older, is usually a sensorineural hearing disorder. It is most commonly caused by gradual changes in the inner ear as a result of loss of hair cells in the organ of Corti within the ear. The individual might first experience tinnitus. Then the degree of hearing loss will vary as time passes. Some individuals might have loss of the middle ranges of hearing; others might be unable to hear normal conversation in a noisy room. Treatment of this type of loss usually involves a hearing aid.

In rare cases, presbycusis may be considered a conductive hearing disorder, in which sound sensitivity is lost because of abnormalities of the outer and/or middle ear. Such abnormalities may include reduced function of the tympanic membrane or reduced function of the three tiny bones in the middle ear that carry sound waves from the tympanic membrane to the inner ear.

The causes of hearing loss and balance disorders in the elderly can also be from a metabolic disorder, such as type 2 diabetes mellitus. In diabetes, the disorder can go undetected for many years. By the time of diagnosis, the patient might already have long-term complications to the nervous system, one of which may be damage to the auditory nerve, leading to a change in the ability to hear. The impact of unstable blood glucose levels also can lead to a balance disorder.

Exposure to known ototoxic medications (see Chart 63–1, p. 1991) throughout life could finally manifest in later years. A patient may have ingested a medication that was not known to be ototoxic until later, after years of pharmacologic study, thereby causing older individuals to experience presbycusis. Because the onset of hearing loss associated with presbycusis is slow and gradual, individuals might not recognize that their hearing is changing until a significant amount of deterioration has occurred. Oftentimes, the individual finds that he can no longer hear high-pitched sounds or voices, particularly in the presence of loud or noisy background sounds. The individual also might identify tinnitus, as this symptom is common in those diagnosed with presbycusis as the cause for their hearing deficit or change.

When providing care to an older patient with a hearing deficit or balance disorder, the nurse needs to include specific items in the assessment process. First, the method of communication must be determined. A loud voice does not ensure successful hearing or comprehension. Depending on the cause and degree of hearing loss, the nurse might simply drop the tone of the voice to be successful with vocal communication with an older patient who has a hearing impairment, since the loss of high-frequency sounds occurs first.

The review of systems or head-to-toe assessment should include any known cardiac disorders, blood pressure history, and any metabolic disorders such as diabetes. Conditions that involve the arteries and veins, such as peripheral vascular disease or atherosclerosis, could provide answers for any cause of hearing or balance disorders linked to an alteration in blood flow to the brain. The nurse should assess the patient's current blood pressure and pulse for possible association with the current cardiovascular status. In addition, the assessment must include whether the patient is able to ambulate without assistance or appears wobbly or unbalanced when attempting to walk. This could be linked to a disorder within the ears or balance-related structures.

Finally, an assessment of the past medical history of the older patient presenting with a hearing or balance disorder should include any and all exposure to communicable diseases that might have been treated with antibiotics that have known ototoxic side effects. An example might be pulmonary tuberculosis that was treated with streptomycin.

The older patient who is experiencing a change in hearing or balance might be embarrassed to admit the change. Patients who are unstable with ambulation caused by a balance disorder might find that they stay close to home to avoid falling. This can lead to social isolation, which in turn can lead to depression. Combine a balance disorder with a hearing loss, and an older person might become a social recluse, lost in a world of increasing silence. Previous joys found in living might diminish as elderly patients realize that they might be approaching the end of their lives. Complementary and alternative therapies such as t'ai chi can help improve the quality of life.

The older patient being evaluated for a hearing or balance disorder will most likely have a complete battery of serum laboratory tests done. The purpose of the findings might be to determine whether the patient has an electrolyte or blood glucose disorder. An electrolyte disturbance, such as low sodium or low potassium levels, can be associated with light-headedness and lack of coordination, as can a low blood glucose level. Diagnostic tests to determine the degree of presbycusis (see the Diagnostics Tests box, p. 2006) would undoubtedly reveal the condition. Then the health care provider can offer the patient treatment choices including a referral for a hearing aid or surgery to replace the stapes.

COMPLEMENTARY & ALTERNATIVE THERAPIES Using T'ai Chi to Improve Balance

Nancy Yilk

EXERCISE HAS BEEN SHOWN to positively influence quality of life for people with a wide variety of medical illnesses. T'ai chi (TC), a slow and graceful form of exercise and meditation, has been offered as the ideal exercise for diverse conditions. Primary care providers can play a vital role in encouraging their patients with chronic illnesses to participate in safe forms of exercise such as t'ai chi in order to improve their healing experience, physical function, and overall quality of life (Allen & Meires, 2011).

A 2010 systematic review of studies published from January 2000 to July 2007 resulted in 19 qualified prospective studies that found older, vigorous individuals moving toward frailness seemed to benefit more from TC than did older frail individuals. The most commonly used TC parameters were Yang's style, with 12 or fewer forms, durations of 12 weeks or longer, frequencies of twice a week or more, and session lengths of at least 45 minutes. Improvements were reported in almost all measurements: fear of falling, single-leg stance, posturography, rate of falling, flexibility, walking velocity, Berg Balance Scale, Timed Up and Go, functional reach, and ankle and knee joint strength and range of motion (Liu & Frank, 2010).

Long-term t'ai chi practice on postural balance and H-reflex was measured with 16 healthy volunteers, eight with three or more years of experience in t'ai chi training (Tai Chi Group—TCG) and eight with no experience in t'ai chi training (Control Group—CG), participating in the study. Postural sways were measured under four experimental conditions: (1) Standing still with eyes open (EO); (2) Standing still with eyes closed (EC); (3) Standing and turning head to left and right with eyes open (EOT); and (4) Standing and turning head to left and right with eyes closed (ECT). Paired reflex depression (PRD) of the soleus muscle was measured under two conditions: supine and standing. Less significant postural sway was observed in the TCG than in the CG under the four conditions of EO, EC, EOT, and ECT. The TCG demonstrated 14.1%, 30.6%, 33.3%, and 22.7% less postural sway, respectively. Significant PRD change from a supine to standing position was observed between the control and intervention group. A significant correlation between PRD change (from supine to standing) and years of t'ai chi practice also was observed. Long-term t'ai chi exercisers demonstrated different reflex modulation from a supine to standing position, and research found that long-term t'ai chi practice may lead to a change of PRD modulation as neuroadaptation (Guan & Koceja, 2011).

A randomized case-controlled study was researched to examine the effects of different interventions that are used to prevent falls. These were education, t'ai chi ch'uan, and education plus t'ai chi ch'uan; the study involved a 5-month implantation period and a 1-year follow-up period. The study used cluster-randomized sampling and selected four villages in Taiwan City. Three intervention groups and one control group, involving 163 participants, were involved over 5 months from late July 2000 to January 2001. In addition, each participant was followed up 1 year later. The aim of the study was to support participants with education about both risk factors and balance exercise programs such as t'ai chi ch'uan to help prevent falls.

The intervention involving education plus t'ai chi ch'uan resulted in a statistically significant reduction in falls and the risk factors of falls over the 5-month intervention. After 1-year follow-up, participants receiving any one of the interventions showed a reduction in falls compared with the control group. T'ai chi ch'uan was able to improve gait balance significantly. Education may also help participants to prevent falls by eliminating related risk factors present in their environment. However, as of the 1-year follow-up, individuals utilizing any of the three interventions had reduced falls significantly (Huang, Liu, Huang, & Kernohan, 2010).

Sources: Allen, J., & Meires J. (2011). How to prescribe tai chi therapy. *Journal of Transcultural Nursing, 22*(2). Retrieved from http://mindbodyspirit4health.com/2011/02/how-to-prescribe-tai-chi-t...; Guan, H., & Koceja, D. M. (2011). Effects of long-term tai chi practice on balance and h-reflex characteristics. *American Journal of Clinical Medicine, 39*(2), 251–260; Huang, H. C., Liu, C. Y., Huang, Y. T., & Kernohan, W. G. (2010). Community-based interventions to reduce falls among older adults in Taiwan—Long time follow-up randomized controlled study. *Journal of Clinical Nursing, 19*(7–8), 959–968; Liu, H., & Frank, A. (2010). Tai chi as a balance improvement exercise for older adults: A systematic review. *Journal of Geriatric Physical Therapy, 33*(3), 103–109.

Research

Research is critical to exploring and developing techniques and approaches designed to meet the needs of patients who are hearing and balance impaired. Researchers are striving to meet societal needs as well as individual needs, developing new devices and systems and enabling new clinical outcomes. Research topics related to hearing and balance research treatment and cure are outlined in the Research Opportunities box.

RESEARCH OPPORTUNITIES Related to Hearing and Balance Disorders

Research Area	Clinical Impact
Hearing aids for sensorineural hearing loss	Three new types of hearing aids designed to help individuals with a sensorineural hearing loss are under investigation: linear peak clipper (PC), compression limiter (CL), and wide dynamic range compressor (WDRC).
	Researchers have found that all three new types of hearing aids have improved hearing between 10% and 30% in individuals with sensorineural hearing loss.
Occupational hazards	Research ways to decrease hearing loss due to continuous exposure to loud noise.
Prevent genetic deafness	Continue to identify genetic causes of hearing loss. In time, treat these disorders to restore or create normal hearing.
Identify relationship between noise-induced hearing loss and tinnitus	Continue research in this area to determine if there is a cause and effect syndrome and how it might be prevented.

READ: History of Present Illnesses >> Laboratory Study Results >> Critical Thinking Questions

Eleanor Morrissey is a 78-year-old Caucasian female admitted through the emergency department for substernal chest pain. Even though Mrs. Morrissey was admitted to the hospital with rule-out myocardial infarction, one health issue of concern was her inability to hear or follow simple commands. Closer evaluation determined that Mrs. Morrissey had a definite hearing problem, one worthy of more investigation.

Once Mrs. Morrissey's cardiac status was stabilized, the concern turned to her hearing problem. Mrs. Morrissey stated that she had noticed a progressive decline in her ability to hear, so much so that she had asked her family to provide a telephone with an amplifier so that she could hear conversations better. After an audiology examination conducted several years ago, she was diagnosed with presbycusis in addition to some degree of sensorineural hearing loss, probably due to ototoxic medications.

READ: History of Present Illnesses >> **Physical Exam** >> Admitting Medical Records >> Laboratory Study Results

Medical–Surgical History

Allergies: naproxen sodium, hives
Medications: Lanoxin 0.125 mg po q a.m., aspirin 81 mg po q a.m., Toprox XL 100 mg po daily, Altace 2.5 mg po bid
Previous illnesses: pulmonary tuberculosis, 1944, treated with repeated pneumothorax treatments; history of taking streptomycin in 1955 prophylactically for tuberculosis; diagnosed with type 2 diabetes mellitus in 1993, diet controlled; progressive alteration in hearing
Surgeries: bilateral knee replacements, 1994

Social History

Family history: parents deceased; husband, two daughters alive/well
Social history: married, lives with husband, split-level home

Physical Exam

Elderly White female
Height: 5 ft 3 inches; weight: 154 lbs
Temperature: 38.7C
Pulse: 64 and regular
Respirations: 18 and regular
Blood pressure: 138/88 right arm
O_2 saturation: 93% on room air
HEENT: uses reading glasses; own teeth/no dentures
Neck: no JVD; carotid pulses present bilaterally
Heart: NSR, rate/rhythm regular
Lungs: present right lobes, reduced left upper lobe
Abdomen: soft, nontender, mildly obese
Extremities: no edema; pedal pulses strong; bilateral scars present over both knees
Neuro: Alert and oriented × 3
CXR: mild cardiomegaly
ECG: changes consistent with mild ischemia

Admitting Medical Orders

Admit to Telemetry Unit
Cardiology
Condition: stable
Allergies: naproxen, sodium, causes hives
Diagnosis: R/O pending MI; status post cardiac catheterization; 80% blockage of LAD coronary artery; stent placed
Audiology consult
IV: saline lock; flush q8h
Diet: no added salt
Oxygen: 2 L NC
Daily weight
I&O
Accu-Chek ac and at bedtime
Sequential compression devices (SCDs) to lower extremities
Bed rest with bathroom privileges
Vital signs and oxygen saturation q4h
Incentive spirometer q2h while awake
Call house officer if: pulse < 60 and > 110/minute; BP < 90 and > 160 systolic; temperature > 38.5; urine output < 30mL/hr for 2 hours; respiratory rate > 30/minute; oxygen saturation < 92%; Accu-Chek < 70 and > 130

Scheduled Medications

Lanoxin 0.125 mg po q a.m.
Aspirin 81 mg po q a.m.
Toprox XL 100 mg po daily
Altace 2.5 mg po bid
Postcatheterization: Plavix 75 mg po q a.m.
Glipizide SR 10 mg po daily, start after heart catheterization

PRN Medications

Nitroglycerin 0.4 mg sublingual prn chest pain q5min × 3
Morphine 3–5 mg IV q3–5min; maximum dose 15 mg q3hr prn pain
Phenergan 12.5–25 mg IV q6h prn nausea
Mylanta 30 mL q4–6h po prn dyspepsia
Triazolam 0.125–0.25 mg po q noc, prn sleep
Ativan 0.5–1 mg IV q6–8h prn anxiety
Milk of Magnesia 30 mL po daily, prn constipation
Tylenol 650 mg po/PR q4h for pain

Ordered Laboratory Studies

Fasting blood sugar
Hemoglobin A1c
Troponin I q8h × 3
CPK-MB q8h × 3
Basic chemistry panel, CBC, magnesium q a.m.
Lipid panel in a.m.

Ordered Diagnostic Studies

Chest x-ray on admission
12-lead ECG
Echocardiogram
Cardiac catheterization

READ: History of Present Illnesses >> **Laboratory Study Results** >> Critical Thinking Questions

Test	Before Heart Catheterization	After Heart Catheterization	Day 2
Sodium	140 mEq/L	138 mEq/L	139 mEq/L
Potassium	4 mEq/L	4.2 mEq/L	4.2 mEq/L
Chloride	101 mEq/L	99 mEq/L	103 mEq/L
Carbon dioxide (CO_2)	22 mEq/L	24 mEq/L	25 mEq/L
Blood urea nitrogen (BUN)	19 mg/dL	18 mg/dL	18 mg/dL
Creatinine	1.2 mg/dL	1.0 mg/dL	1.1 mg/dL
Fasting blood sugar	160 mg/dL		
Hemoglobin A1c	7.0%		
Phosphorus	2.1 mg/dL	3.2 mg/dL	3.7 mg/dL
Calcium	8.1 mg/dL	8.2 mg/dL	8.6 mg/dL
Magnesium	2.0 mEq/L	1.9 mEq/L	2.0 mEq/L
Creatine kinase	4,018 units/L	3,612 units/L	2,000 units/L
Relative index	>5.9%	>10.1%	>9.2%
CK–MB	>300.00%	>300.00%	259.7%

Test	Before Heart Catheterization	After Heart Catheterization	Day 2
Troponin I	>100 ng/mL	80.91 ng/mL	51.00 ng/mL
WBC	11.5/mm^3	11.0/mm^3	9.3/mm^3
RBC	4.21/mm^3	4.89/mm^3	4.92/mm^3
Hemoglobin	12.9 g/dL	11.5 g/dL	12.7 g/dL
Hematocrit	37.5%	36.8%	37.6%
Platelets	262,000/mm^3	280,000/mm^3	300,000/mm^3
Cholesterol	256 mg/dL		
High-density lipoprotein (HDL)	30 mg/dL		
Low-density lipoprotein (LDL)	158 mg/dL		
Very low-density lipoprotein (VLDL)	60%		
Apolipoprotein	152 mg/dL		
Triglycerides	201 mg/dL		

Pearson Nursing Student Resources

Log on to **nursing.pearsonhighered.com** *to download forms*

DOCUMENT:

- >> Summary of Hospitalization
- >> Pathophysiology Form
- >> Laboratory Values
- >> Laboratory Results Explanation

APPLY:

- >> List of Potential Nursing Diagnoses
- >> Concept Map
- >> Critical Thinking Questions and Concept Map

APPLY: History of Present Illness >> Laboratory Study Results >> **Critical Thinking Questions**

1. Mrs. Morrissey needs to have the television on extremely loud, and her roommate is complaining. What can you do to help the situation?
2. What would be the best treatment for the type of hearing loss Mrs. Morrissey is experiencing?
3. Is Mrs. Morrissey a candidate for a hearing aid or cochlear implant? Why or why not?
4. Using discharge instructions as a guide, explain four different ways the family can help Mrs. Morrissey adapt to her hearing disorder until her treatment is prescribed.

Answers to Critical Thinking Questions can be found in Appendix D in the Osborn Student Resources at nursing.pearsonhighered.com.

NCLEX® PRACTICE

1. A patient tells the nurse that she had her right eardrum punctured many times when she was a child. The nurse interprets this information as indicating special attention is needed in which assessment?

1. Balance
2. Movement
3. Sound transmission
4. Equilibrium

2. A patient tells the nurse that she hears better when she isn't wearing a scarf over her head. The nurse realizes that this patient is describing which mechanism of hearing?

1. Bone conduction
2. Air conduction
3. Middle ear conduction
4. Acoustic nerve conduction

3. A young male was brought into the emergency department because he suddenly couldn't hear. Upon examination, it was determined that a small object was lodged deeply into his ear canal. Which type of hearing loss did this patient experience?

1. Mixed
2. Acoustic
3. Conductive
4. Sensorineural

4. A young mother with a 2-week-old infant tells the nurse that she hopes her baby has good hearing, since deafness "runs in her family." Which information should the nurse provide to this mother?

1. "The baby can't be tested for hearing until at least the age of 1."
2. "Even if tested, the baby's hearing will change as he grows."
3. "The baby should be tested now."
4. "The baby's sense of hearing hasn't developed yet."

5. A patient is scheduled for a stapedectomy. The nurse realizes that this procedure is typically used to treat which of the following causes of a hearing disorder?

1. Mechanical
2. Inflammatory
3. Obstructive
4. Mixed

6. The nurse is caring for a patient with a hearing deficit. Which interventions should be included in this patient's discharge planning for environmental safety? (select all that apply)

1. Assistance with location for American Sign Language classes
2. Removal of scatter rugs throughout the home
3. Mechanism to ensure a visual alert in the event of a home fire
4. Instruction on electrical cord safety
5. Information on telephone services for the hearing impaired

Answers to NCLEX Practice questions can be found in Appendix D in the Osborn Student Resources at nursing.pearsonhighered.com. Practice additional NCLEX questions online at the Student Resources site.

Pearson Nursing Student Resources Find additional review materials at: **nursing.pearsonhighered.com**

REFERENCES

Adams, M. P., & Koch, R. W. (2010). *Pharmacology: Connections to nursing practice.* Upper Saddle River, NJ: Pearson.

Allen, J., & Meires, J. (2011). How to prescribe Taichi therapy. *Journal of Transcultural Nursing, 22*(2), 201–204. Retrieved from http://www.ncbi.nlm.nih.gov/pubmed/21317403

American Academy of Otolaryngology-Head and Neck Surgery. (2011). Fact sheet: What you should know about otosclerosis. Retrieved from http://www.entnet.org/HealthInformation/otosclerosisl.cfm

American Speech-Language-Hearing Association. (2008). Incidence/Prevalence of hearing loss and hearing aid use in the United States–2008 edition. Retrieved from http://www.asha.org/research/reports/hearing.htm

American Speech-Language-Hearing Association. (2012). Types of hearing loss. Retrieved from http://www.asha.org/public/hearing/disorders/types.htm

Balasubramanian, T. (2008). Exostosis of external auditory canal. Retrieved from http://www.dribalu.co.in/exostosis.html

Bauman, N. G. (2010). *Ototoxic drugs exposed: The shocking truth about prescription drugs, medications, chemicals and herbals that can (and do) damage our ears* (3rd ed.). Stewartsville, PA: Integrity First.

Berke, J. (2010). Cause of hearing loss–otosclerosis. About.com. Retrieved from http://deafness.about.com/cs/etiology/a/otosclerosis/htm

Best Practice. (2011). Otitis externa. Retrieved from http://bestpractice.bmj.com/best-practicew/monograph/40/basics/pathophysiology.htm

Bhattacharyya, N. (2011). Auditory brainstem response audiometry. Medscape reference. Retrieved from http://emedicine.medscape.com/article/836277-Overview

Boston, M. E. (2012). Labyrinthitis. Medscape reference. Retrieved from http://emedicine.medscape.com/article/856215-overview

California Ear Institute. (2011a). Meniere's disease. Retrieved from http://www.californiaearinstitute.com/ear-disorders-menieres-disease-ear-institute-bay-area.php

California Ear Institute. (2011b). What is exostosis/surfer's ear? Retrieved from http://www.californiaearinstitute.com/ear-disorders-exostosis-california-ear-institute-bay-area.php

National Association of Deafened People. (2012). How communication support can change the lives of deaf people. Retrieved from http://www.slideshare.net/ecdp/communication-support-for-deaf-people

Davison, S. P. (2011). Ear reconstruction and salvage procedures. Medscape reference. Retrieved from http://emedicine.medscape.com/article/128828-overview

Deaf Mental Health Charter. (2008). Mental Health Foundation. Retrieved from http://www.mhf.org.uk/our-work/all-adults/deaf-charter/

Ellis, J. (2012). What are the hammer, anvil & stirrup parts of? Livestrong.com, eHow.com. Retrieved from http://www.ehow.com/info_9408075_hammer-anvil-stirrup-parts.html

Guan, H., & Koceja, D. M. (2011). Effects of long-term tai chi practice on balance and h-reflex characteristics. *American Journal of Clinical Medicine, 39*(2), 251–260.

Hain, T. C. (2007). Benign paroxysmal positional vertigo. Retrieved from http://www.dizziness-and-balance.com/disorders/bppv/bppv.html

Hain, T. C. (2009). Otitis media and otitis externa. Retrieved from http://www.dizziness-and-balance.com/disorders/unilat/otitis.html

Hain, T. C. (2010). Gentamicin toxicity. Retrieved from http://www.dizziness-and-balance.com/disorders/bilat/gentamicin%20toxicity.htm

Hain, T. C. (2011). Vestibular nerve section. Dizziness-and-balance.com. Retrieved from http://www.dizziness-and-balance.com/treatment/vn_section.html

Huang, H. C., Liu, C. Y., Huang, Y. T., & Kernohan, W. G. (2010). Community-based interventions to reduce falls among older adults in Taiwan—Long time follow-up randomized controlled study. *Journal of Clinical Nursing, 19*(7–8), 959–968.

Hyperacusis Network. (2011). Decibel guide. Retrieved from http://www.hyperacusis.net/hyperacusis/decibel+guide/

IOM (Institute of Medicine). (2010). *The future of nursing: Leading change, advancing health*. Washington, DC: The Academic Press.

Iowa Head and Neck Protocols. (2012). Carcinoma of the external auditory canal and middle ear. Retrieved from http://wiki.uiowa.edu/display/protocols/Carcinoma+of+External+Auditory+Canal+and+Middle+Ear

Isaacson, B. (2010). Hearing loss. *The Medical Clinics of North America*. (94),: 973.

Jirage, R. (2012). Different ear problems. Buzzzle.com. Retrieved from http://www.buzzle.com/artaicles/different-ear-problems.html

Johns Hopkins Medicine. (2011). One in five Americans has hearing loss. Retrieved from http://www.hopkinsmedicine.org/news/media/releases/one_in_five_americans_has_hearing_loss

Lee, S. (2010). Otitis externa in emergency medicine treatment & management. Medscape reference. Retrieved from http://emedicine.medscape.com/article/763918-treatment

Lent, G. S. (2011). Complex ear laceration. Medscape reference. Retrieved from http://emedicine.medscape.com/article/832940overview

Kavanagh, K. (2009). Noise induced hearing loss. World articles in ear, nose, and throat. Retrieved from http://www.entusa.com/noise_hearing-loss.htm

Liu, H., & Frank, A. (2010). Tai chi as a balance improvement exercise for older adults: A systematic review. *Journal of Geriatric Physical Therapy, 33*(3), 103–109.

Mayo Clinic. (2009, December 25). Medical Edge newspaper column. BPPV: The most common cause of vertigo. Retrieved from http://www.mayoclinic.org/medical-edge-newspaper-2009/dec-25a.html

Mayo Clinic Staff. (2012). Meniere's disease. Retrieved from http://www.mayoclinic.com/health/menieres-disease/DS00535

MDGuidelines. (2010). Cancer, skin (melanoma). Reed Group. Retrieved from http://www.mdguidelines.com/cancer-skin-melanoma/definition

Medical News Today. (2012). What is otitis externa (swimmer's ear)? What causes otitis externa? Retrieved from http://www.medicalnewstoday.com/articles/178934.php

Medicine Decoded. (2011). Diseases of external ear. Retrieved from http://lessons4medicos.blogspot.com/2998/06/diseases-of-external-ear.html

MedicineNet.com. (2012a). Cauliflower ear. Retrieved from http://www.medicinenet.com/script/main/aret.asp?articlekey=7767&pf=3&page=1

MedicineNet.com. (2012b). Meclizine. Retrieved from http://www.medicinenet.com/script/main/art.asp?araticlekey=45521&pf=3&page=1

MedlinePlus. (2012a). Hearing loss. Retrieved from http://www.nlm.nih.gov/medlineplus/ency/article/003044.htm

MedlinePlus. (2012b). Mastoiditis. Retrieved from http://www.nlm.nih.gov/medlineplus/ency/article/001034.htm

Ménière's Disease Information Center. (2012). Retrieved from http://www.menieresinfo.com/

Merck Manual. (2008). Ear blockages. Retrieved from http://www.merckmanuals.com/home/ear_nose_and_throat_disorders/outer_ear_disorders/ear_blockages.html

Nabili, S. T. (2008). Swimmer's ear. emedicinehealth. Retrieved from http://www.emedicinehealth.com/script/main/art.asp:articlekey=58802&pf=3&page=1

National Cancer Institute. (2011). What you need to know about melanoma and other skin cancers. National Institutes of Health. Retrieved from http://www.cancer.gov/cancertopics/wyntk/skin/page1/AllPages

National Dizzy & Balance Center. (2010). Benign paroxysmal positional vertigo (BPPV). Retrieved from http:/www.stopdizziness.com/resources_bppv.asp

National Institute on Deafness and Other Communication Disorders (NIDCD). (2008). Noise-induced hearing loss. Retrieved from http://www.nided.nih.gov/health/hearing/pages/noise.aspx

National Institute on Deafness and Other Communication Disorders (NIDCD). (2010a). Hearing aids. Retrieved from http://www.nidcd.nih.gov/health/hearing/Pages/thebasics_hearingaid.aspx

National Institute on Deafness and Other Communication Disorders (NIDCD). (2010b). Hearing loss and older adults. Retrieved from http://www.nidcd.nih.gov/health/hearing/Pages/older.aspx

National Institute on Deafness and Other Communication Disorders (NIDCD). (2011a). Cochlear implants. Retrieved from http://www.nidcd.nih.gov/health/hearing/Pages/coch.aspx

National Institute on Deafness and Other Communication Disorders (NIDCD). (2011b). How loud is too loud? Retrieved from http://www.nidcd.nih.gov/health/hearing/Pages/ruler.aspx

National Institute on Deafness and Other Communication Disorders (NIDCD). (2011c). Otosclerosis. Retrieved from http://www.nidcd.nih.gov/health/hearing/Pages/otosclerosis.aspx

National Institute on Deafness and Other Communication Disorders (NIDCD). (2012a). Fact sheet: Noise- induced hearing loss. Retrieved from http://www.nidcd.nih.gov/health/hearing/Pages/noise.aspx

National Institute on Deafness and Other Communications Disorders (NIDCD). (2012b). Statistics and epidemiology. Retrieved from http://www.nidcd.nih.gov/health/statistics/Pages/Default.aspx

Parmet, S., Lynm, C., & Glass, R. (2007). Adult hearing loss. *Journal of the American Medical Association, 298*(1), 41–48.

Poole, K. (2010). A review of the current state of knowledge on tinnitus in relation to noise exposure and hearing loss. Health and Safety Laboratory, Melbourne Audiology Center. Retrieved from http://melbourneaudiologycentre.com.au/noiseinduee.html

Roland, P. S. (2011). Pediatric otosclerosis. Medscape reference. Retrieved from http://emedicine.medscape.com/article/994891-overview

Samy, R. N. (2012). External ear benign tumors. Medscape reference. Retrieved from http://emedicine.medscape.com/article/845901-overview

Sand, M.,Sand, D., Thrandorf, C., Paech, V., Altmeyer, P. & Bodum, G.. (2008). Cutaneous lesions of the external ear. Head and Face Medicine. Retrieved from http://www.head-face-med.com/content/4/1/2

Simic, P. J. (2012). Labyrinthitis overview. Emedicine.health.com. Retrieved from http://www.emedicine.health.com/script/main/art.asp:areticlekey=59409&pf=3&page=1

Surgical-Pathology. (2009). Exostosis of the external ear. *Surgical-pathology.com*. Retrieved from http://www.surgical-pathology.com/ear_exostosis.htm

The Trusted Source. (2012). Wax blockage of the ear canal. Aetna Inc. Retrieved from http://www.intelihealth.com/IH/ihtIH/WSHW000/9339/10989.html

Tian, S. (2012). Sensorineural hearing loss: Nerve deafness. *Healthguidance.org*. Retrieved from http://www.healthguidance.org/entry/12043/1/Sensorineural-Hearing-Loss-Nerve-Deafness.html

Tobey, P. (2011). Noise induced hearing loss and tinnitus. Retrieved from http://www.paultobey.com/articles/noise-induced-hearning-loss-tinnitus.html

UC Irvine Healthcare. (2010). Hearing and ear disorders services. Retrieved from http://www.healthcare.uci.edu/ents_hearing_and_ear_disorders.asp

U.S. Department of Health and Human Services (DHHS). (2010). *Healthy People 2020*. Retrieved from http://www.healthypeople.gov

Vaishali, M. (2012). Disorders of the outer ear. Livestrong.com, Demand Media. Retrieved from http://www.livestrong.com/article/90730-disorders-outer-ear/

WebMD. (2011). Dix-Hallpike test for vertigo. *Brain and Nervous System Health Center*. Retrieved from http://www.webmd.com/brain.dix-hallpike-test-for-vertigo-15884

Wilkinson, J. M., & Ahern, N. R. (2009).*Prentice Hall nursing diagnosis handbook* (9th ed.). Upper Saddle River, NJ: Prentice Hall.

World Health Organization. (2012). International day for ear and hearing, 3 March 2012. Retrieved from http://www.who.int/pbd/deafness/news/en/index.html

CHAPTER

64 Caring for the Patient with Visual Disorders

Lucie S. Elfervig
Annita Watson

Outcome-Based Learning Objectives

After studying this chapter, the learner will be able to:

1. Evaluate different types of visual and ocular conditions and disorders according to causative factors.
2. Differentiate the appropriate care for visual disorders of adults by using the nursing process.
3. Create a caring approach to the nursing management of the psychosocial elements of visual disorders.
4. Develop teaching plans for patients/families experiencing visual disorders.
5. Formulate meaningful discharge priorities and resources for patients with visual disorders.

KEY TERMS

acetylsalicylic acid (ASA) p.2020
amblyopia p.2018
ametropia p.2017
asthenopia p.2018
astigmatism p.2017
blepharitis p.2042
cataract p.2018
central retinal artery occlusion (CRAO) p.2047
conjunctivitis p.2042
contrast sensitivity (CS) p.2037
cotton-wool spots (CWS) p.2034
diabetic retinopathy (DR) p.2033
diplopia p.2018
drusen p.2036
emmetropia p.2017
endophthalmitis p.2044
exfoliative glaucoma p.2027
glaucoma p.2025
hypermetropia p.2017
hyperopia p.2017
iridocorneal endothelial syndrome (ICE) p.2027
keratoconjunctivitis sicca p.2041
legal blindness p.2025
macular degeneration p.2036
meibomitis p.2042
metamorphopsia p.2036
myopia p.2017
neovascular glaucoma p.2027
ocular hypertension p.2027
open globe p.2049
pigmentary glaucoma p.2027
posterior vitreous detachment (PVD) p.2046
presbyopia p.2017
retinal breaks p.2046
retinal detachment (RD) p.2045
secondary open-angle glaucoma p.2027
strabismus p.2017
traumatic glaucoma p.2027
vitreous hemorrhage p.2046

THE SENSE OF SIGHT is one of the primary means through which people are active and take pleasure in their world. The other senses seem to direct people toward seeing what is heard, what is touched, what is smelled, and what is tasted, so sight truly guides most of their daily activities. The eyes also provide a window or insight into body functions. Systemic disorders or conditions that have visual or ocular manifestations can be discovered for the first time on an ocular examination, or a visual problem found on a routine physical may alert the nurse to a systemic condition. Often, ocular impairment can be prevented with early recognition and treatment that will save vision and prevent blindness. Visual disorders, depending on the degree of vision loss, can be very disturbing, and potentially lead to a sense of hopelessness, loss, powerlessness, and bereavement for the patient and her family. Vision loss may be as minor as a refractive error that can be corrected with glasses, contact lenses, or laser, or as severe as ocular trauma that results in loss of vision, no light perception, or enucleation (surgical removal of the eyeball that leaves the eye muscles and remaining orbital contents intact).

Visual impairment creates both a physical and a psychological adjustment that can limit a patient's activities of daily living (ADLs) and quality of life. With all types of visual impairment there is a goal of patient rehabilitation, or restoring the patient to an optimal level of visual health. The American Academy of Ophthalmology (2007) has established national guidelines that address vision rehabilitation for adults. These can be found in the National Guidelines box.

Visual Impairment

Visual impairment can involve correctable refractive errors (errors in the way in which the eye focuses light), inherited anomalies, acquired visual changes, nutritional deficiencies, or changes due to aging. Refractive errors are the most common vision problem in the general population and can often be corrected by wearing glasses or contact lenses. Five of the leading causes of visual impairment are refractive error, cataracts, glaucoma, diabetic retinopathy, and macular degeneration.

NATIONAL GUIDELINES for Visual Rehabilitation

The American Academy of Ophthalmology (2007) set forth one primary objective with nine goals for achievement.

Primary Objective: To reduce the functional impact of the vision loss on patients' lives to maintain independence, productive activity, safety, and life satisfaction by addressing the following goals:

1. Identify patients with low vision and quantify their visual loss.
2. Assess functional impairments due to low vision.
3. Evaluate the potential to use residual vision.
4. Educate patients about vision loss, the potential benefits of rehabilitation, and rehabilitation options.
5. Inform patients about the parameters of training and its potential benefit.
6. Engage patients in their rehabilitation.
7. Maximize patients' independent completion of activities of daily living, safety, and participation in their community.
8. Address the emotional and psychological adjustment to vision loss.
9. Provide information to patients about community and national resources and social support.

The guidelines identified adults with low vision as the primary target. They also set forth interventions and practices to consider along with three major patient outcomes to achieve:

- Emotional and psychological adjustments to vision loss
- Ability to complete independently activities of daily living
- Knowledge of available adaptive devices and resources.

Additional information and details can be obtained from the guidelines directly at file://I://NationalGuidelineClearinghouseVisionrehabilitationforadults.htm

Refractive Error

Refraction is the bending of light rays through different media in the eye (cornea, anterior humor, lens, and vitreous humor) as the rays enter the eyes. It is the state of an eye in which light rays are not properly focused on the retina, resulting in a blurred image (Friedman, Kaiser, & Pineda, 2009). Measurement of refractive error is referred to as a manifested refraction (MR), which is performed on a *phoropter*, a refractive device used to measure the degree of optical correction needed to achieve the best-corrected visual acuity (BVA) with the use of spherical, cylindrical, and prismatic lenses.

Epidemiology, Etiology, Pathophysiology, and Clinical Manifestations

Refractive errors are the most frequent eye problems in the United States (Centers for Disease Control and Prevention [CDC], 2009). They occur in approximately 30% of the general population (American Academy of Opthamology [AAO-3], 2010–2011) and are caused by the eye's inability to properly bend light as it passes into the retina, resulting in a blurred image. The specific refractive disorders are discussed in the following text.

Emmetropia

The term for having no refractive error, or normal vision without any corrective optical devices, is **emmetropia.** In natural emmetropia, the eye is able to focus light rays on the retina to form a clear and sharp image. Surgically induced emmetropia is a term used to describe sight in patients who have had previous refractive surgical correction to create 20/20 visual acuity without any corrective optical devices such as glasses or contact lenses.

Ametropia

Ametropia is a general term used to indicate that a refractive error is present. The four most common forms of ametropia are myopia, hyperopia, astigmatism, and presbyopia.

- **Myopia** (nearsightedness) is the condition in which distant objects cannot be seen clearly. It is the most common refractive error, which develops mainly during the school years (Heiting & Bailey, 2010). The parallel light rays fall in front of the retina because of a longer axial length of the eyeball, which requires a minus (concave) corrective lens to focus the image on the fovea for sharper vision. Myopia is the most common ametropia, making up over 80% of the refractive errors in the adult population of the United States (Lamb & Simms-Eaton, 2008).
- **Hyperopia** or **hypermetropia** (farsightedness) is less frequent; it occurs more often in children, and usually diminishes with maturity. In this condition, near objects cannot be seen clearly. The parallel light rays fall behind the retina because of a shorter axial length of the eyeball, which requires a plus (convex) corrective lens to focus the image on the fovea for normal or correct vision.
- **Astigmatism** (blurred vision) affects about 15% of the population (Miller & Scott, 2009). Astigmatism, as defined by the American Academy of Ophthalmology (AAO), is an irregular corneal surface or asphericity, meaning that the refractive power is not homogeneous in all corneal meridians. This occurs when the front surface of the eye, the cornea, has an irregular curvature (i.e., it is curved more in one direction than in the other). This prevents light rays from focusing on a single point (AAO-3, 2010–2011), and results in blurred vision. Astigmatism usually can be corrected with the required lens or contact lens at a specific optical axis.
- **Presbyopia** (a progressively diminished ability to focus on near objects), being a function of aging, occurs in about 65% of the population. Presbyopia is lack of accommodation, that is, lack of the ability to focus from distance to near images. As an individual ages, the nucleus fibers become compressed with additive cortical fibers, resulting in decreasing accommodation (AAO-11, 2010–2011) or a more rigid lens. The loss of elasticity of the natural crystalline lens, which causes the loss of the ability to focus up close, generally occurs in a person's 40s, resulting in presbyopia.

Strabismus

Strabismus is the inability of the eyes to focus together on a single point because of misalignment of the extraocular muscles or anomalies of neuromuscular control of motility of the eyes. The eye can misdirect in any of the following positions: In esotropia, the eye turns toward the nose (medially); in exotropia, it turns toward the ear (temporally); in hypertropia, it turns upward (superiorly); and in hypotropia, it turns downward (inferiorly). Strabismus is normally a childhood condition, but it can affect an individual's vision throughout life.

Strabismus usually is a result of loss of binocularity from infancy, in which sight is lost in either eye (amblyopia) from poor development of the extraocular muscle, trauma, or secondary to other ocular disorders. The corresponding retinal images in the two eyes are no longer directed toward the same objects, resulting in visual confusion or double vision (Diamond, 2009b).

Weblink: National Guidelines for Vision Rehabilitation

Video: Cataract

Acquired/adult strabismus refers to crossed eyes, that is, eyes that have lost their ability to fuse, in adults. Adults with strabismus will see double (diplopia) because they do not suppress vision. Acquired adult strabismus has a low incidence and usually is the result of head trauma and insult to the brain, especially if the person is unconscious for a long period of time. It also can result from diabetes, but this is usually temporary (AAO-6, 2010–2011). Most often, strabismus in adults is a carryover from congenital or accommodative strabismus that developed in childhood. **Asthenopia** (eye fatigue), another common symptom of adult strabismus, includes discomfort such as headache, eyestrain, and brow ache when the eyes are used (AAO-6, 2010–2011).

Diplopia

Diplopia, or double vision, is the phenomenon in which one object appears as two. Diplopia can be binocular (affecting both eyes) or monocular (affecting one eye) (AAO-5, 2010–2011). Generally, when the term *diplopia* is used, it refers to an optical or refractive error of one eye (Ehlers & Shah, 2008; Miller, Newman, Biousse, & Kerrison, 2008).

Binocular diplopia can be functional or real. Functional binocular diplopia refers to double vision caused by a function problem in the visual system, such as a brain injury or nerve damage. Binocular diplopia referred to as *real* is that which occurs when the brain receives two separate images from the eyes because they are misaligned naturally, without a functional problem of the visual system (EyeCareSource.com, 2011).

In diagnosing binocular diplopia, the health care provider has to examine the eyes to determine which eye muscles are affected. The examination, coupled with a medical history and any additional symptoms, provides enough information to determine if additional tests are needed to determine the extent of the problem and develop a treatment plan (Aetna InteliHealth, 2012). All therapy is aimed at realigning the misaligned eye or eyes where possible without surgery and restimulating the part of the visual pathway to the brain which is not working correctly (University of Michigan Kellogg Eye Center, 2012).

Amblyopia

Amblyopia, commonly called "lazy eye," occurs when a person has an eye with decreased or impaired vision with no obvious anatomic explanation. It is usually due to the lack of proper maturation during the growth and development stages or just to not having the proper refractive correction or the lack of use of correction (Diamond, 2009a).

Other possible causes of amblyopia are toxins, such as poison, alcohol, or tobacco; psychological (hysterical) problems; nutritional (e.g., vitamin B) insufficiency; cataracts (physical occlusion); and strabismic (cross-eyed or wall-eyed, having divergent strabismus) phenomenon (AAO-6, 2010–2011). Amblyopia usually occurs at about age 7 from not using the affected eye; if not corrected at that time, it may become irreversible.

Laboratory and Diagnostic Tests for Vision

A number of diagnostic tests are used to detect refractive errors. Explanations of these tests are shown in the Laboratory and Diagnostic Tests box. Methods for completing the tests are described under Medical Management.

Tests with the use of a direct ophthalmoscope can be performed to gain meaningful information. These include checking the foveal reflexes to see whether they are equally bright in color and checking corneal reflexes to determine whether they are equally aligned. Unequal foveal reflexes may indicate a deviating eyeball, which would be the one with the brighter reflex (Brückner test). Unequal alignment of corneal reflexes (Hirschberg test) also may indicate a deviation in the visual gaze, meaning that the eyes have different fixation points (Friedman et al., 2009).

Medical Management

Medical management of patients with refractive disorders is dependent upon arriving at a differential diagnosis following assessment. Direct opthalmoscope tests are performed to gain necessary information about the structure and function of the eye, as discussed in the Laboratory and Diagnostic Tests box.

Most refractive disorders can be treated with corrective lenses or surgical procedures. The use of a laser to reshape the corneal curvature to eliminate or reduce refractive errors is gradually becoming the norm instead of the exception. Potential contraindications to refractive surgery also must be considered, such as unrealistic expectations, too high of a refractive or astigmatic error, a cornea that is too thin (6.5 to 9 millimeters), severely dry corneas, previous eye surgery, and lack of understanding of the procedure and its risks and benefits (Lamb & Simms-Eaton, 2008). Specific treatments for each type of refractive disorder previously presented are outlined in Chart 64–1.

Nursing Management

Patients with refractive disorders primarily are treated as outpatients. Even in the event of surgery to correct myopia, lasik to remove internal layers of the cornea, and intraocular lens implantation (correction for aphakia in the absence of the lens at the time of cataract extraction), these are still considered outpatient procedures. The nurse's role is to counsel the patient on the type of treatment being provided and to serve as a resource in explaining to the patient where to get assistive devices following diagnosis and treatment (e.g., corrective glasses).

At the time of meeting with the patient, the nurse may assess the signs and symptoms that the patient is experiencing (e.g., blurred vision, double vision, difficulty with vision at night). Physical assessment includes observation for redness of conjunctiva, change in visual acuity, note of any squinting or head tilting, and ability to move eyebrows and eyes. The nurse should identify nursing diagnoses such as *Anxiety and Fear* related to potential loss of vision, *Potential Injury* related to visual limitations, and *Self-Care Deficit* related to postoperative management if surgery is performed. The patient also may experience knowledge deficit related to postoperative management, medications, and follow-up care. If the patient is to have surgery, preoperative care should include a description of the procedure and discharge teaching.

Cataracts

Epidemiology and Etiology

A **cataract** is an increasing cloudiness or opacity (loss of transparency) of the natural crystalline lens caused by oxidative damage to the lens solubility, usually as a result of aging. The crystalline lens is one of the anatomic body structures that continue to grow with the passage of time. Sometimes the lens is compared to an onion with its additive layers; increased compression and density of these layers result in opacity. According to the World Health Organization (WHO), the number of visually impaired people worldwide exceeds 161 million, and cataracts are the leading cause, accounting for more than 47% of all cases of visual impairment (Wevill, 2009). Although cataracts develop as a process of the aging lens, other disorders that can contribute to cataract formation are trauma, which can make a cataract develop in a matter of weeks; systemic disorders, such as diabetes; dermatologic disorders, such as

LABORATORY AND DIAGNOSTIC TESTS for Visual Disorders

Test With Description, Rationale, and Normal Values	Expected Abnormality
Bruckner Test	
Normal: A red reflex responds in both eyes simultaneously from the illumination (light) of the ophthalmoscope. *This is a qualitative assessment of ocular alignment, used to assess binocular vision, as well as providing an indirect evaluation of refractive error, in particular strabismus. It is performed by using the direct ophthalmoscope aperture set on the largest aperture setting so as to equally illuminate both eyes.*	When both eyes are simultaneously illuminated with the ophthalmoscope beam at a distance of 100 cm, an overall whitening of the red reflex across the entire pupil of one eye indicates strabismus or anisometropic amblyopia. The presence of a Brückner reflex is considered a positive result, and is a good indication of strabismus, even of small amounts. A false positive response may occur if there is an anisocoria or media opacity is present.
Hirschberg Test	
Normal: A normal location will likely be either centered, or +0.5 mm nasally displaced. *This test, also called a corneal light reflex test, assesses eye alignment by observing the location of the corneal light reflex within the pupil. It is administered by directing a transilluminator/penlight in primary gaze. The examiner observes the location of the corneal reflexes relative to the center of the pupil. A nasal displacement is signified by a (+) and a temporal displacement is signified by a (−) sign, with the amount quantified in millimeters away from center.*	Individuals who are diagnosed with strabismus will have an eccentric light reflex in the deviated eye. Temporal displacement of the light reflex indicates esotropia, nasal displacement indicates exotropia, and inferior displacement indicates hypertropia.
Amsler Grid	
Normal: All lines and squares would appear symmetrical and clear with no irregularities. *The measuring for the presence of abnormal scotoma (an area of diminished vision within the visual field) and/or metamorphopsia from macular disease or defects, especially for age-related macular degeneration, on a graph pattern of black lines on a white background.*	Verbal response from the patient about any disturbances in the central 30° of the visual field, indicating that lines are missing, different, irregular, doubled, distorted, crooked, bent, blurred, or missing; can be diagnostic of metamorphopsia, indicating macular defects.
Exophthalmometry	
Normal: The distance from the corneal apex to the orbital rim is from 12 to 20 mm. *The measuring of the degree the eyeball extends from the edge of the eyelids or protrudes from the orbit. May be used for signs of thyroid disease or orbital lesions. Used to evaluate the progression or regression of proptosis (the forward displacement or protrusion of the eyeball) in certain orbital disorders.*	The measurement of the two eyes > 2 mm difference between them or obvious proptosis noted; can be diagnostic of thyroid disease or other orbital lesions. Patient with an orbital mass is monitored for progression or regression of orbital disease.
Schirmer Test	
Normal: >10–15 mm is normal. *The measuring of tear production to treat variations of dry eye syndrome. Some patients may have normal lacrimal drainage but still may have dry eye symptoms or problems, or actual tear deficiency of basic tear secretion. The Schirmer strips are placed in the middle of the lower eyelid margin for 5 minutes and removed. The length of moistened area of the strip is measured.*	Moistened strip < 5 mm can be consistent with dry eye syndrome. However, ranges between 5 and 15 mm can be considered abnormal depending on the patient's age (>40 years old) and other factors related to the lacrimal system.
Brightness Acuity Test (BAT or Glare)	
Normal: A visual acuity of 20/40 or better would indicate the patient is not ready for cataract surgery, but this can vary with each person. *The measuring of functional visual acuity with a glare test (three light intensities: low, medium, and high) to determine whether a patient is ready for cataract surgery.*	Reduction in visual acuity, minimally 20/50 or typically 20/70 or worse, on the medium or low light intensity setting would be a significant indicator that opacities or distortions in ocular media are present, such as a cataract; indicates that the patient may be ready for cataract surgery.
Potential Acuity Meter (PAM)	
Normal: A visual acuity of 20/25 or better would be the desired result, but this can vary with each person. *The measuring of potential visual acuity return (prediction) that would follow cataract surgery.*	If visual acuity is 20/50 or worse and cannot be improved, this may indicate an eye problem other than cataracts.
Gonioscopy	
Normal: The anterior chamber angle is open. *An examination to determine the presence of primary angle closure glaucoma. Specifically, the test evaluates the space between the cornea and the iris called the iridocorneal angle. The examination is simple and rapid.* *A microscopic instrument is used to view and to examine the anterior chamber angle structures for openness, narrowing, or closure.*	If the anterior chamber angle is narrow or closed, this will direct the type of antiglaucoma drops or surgical procedure that is necessary to keep the anterior chamber open.

(continued)

LABORATORY AND DIAGNOSTIC TESTS for Visual Disorders, *continued*

Test With Description, Rationale, and Normal Values	Expected Abnormality
Visual Field (VF) Perimetry Normal: No visual field loss would be observed. *The measuring of central (30°) or peripheral (>120°) vision to screen for vision field loss or isolated blind spots (scotoma).*	Abnormal visual field results determine the degree of damage caused by glaucoma, other optic nerve diseases, occlusion, and/or brain disorders.
Pachymetry (PACH) Normal: Corneal thickness average is approximately 545 µm. *The measuring of the thickness of the cornea, used in the treatment of glaucoma and refractive surgery.*	Corneal thickness average > 545 µm is considered thicker than normal and numbers < 545 µm are considered thinner than normal. In measuring intraocular pressure (IOP) for glaucoma: thicker corneas may actually have a lower IOP reading, and thinner corneas may have a higher IOP reading, after adjusting for corneal thickness.
Keratometry (K-readings) Normal: Values around 44.00° to 45.00°. *The measuring of the corneal curvature for detecting astigmatism, used in refractions, refractive surgery, and cataract surgery.*	Radius of the curvature in two meridians (horizontal and vertical) at 90° apart; the difference between the two meridians gives the amount of astigmatism to be corrected.
Corneal Topography (Topo) *The measuring of the corneal layers for use in refractive surgery, and treating keratoconus and other corneal anomalies. Keratoconus (KC) is a progressive, noninflammatory, bilateral (but usually asymmetrical) ectatic corneal disease, characterized by paraxial stromal thinning and weakening that leads to corneal surface distortion.*	Mapping of the cornea surface to determine refractive correction and any corneal anomalies of the corneal layers, especially keratoconus that would need treatment or intervention.
Ultrasonography Normal: No pathology observed. *The use of high-frequency sound waves to detect and outline intraocular and orbital structures by measuring the distance between them. Changes and opacities can be easily recognized by this method.*	Measurement of the axial length for proper intraocular lens implant and regression or progression of eye tumors. Visualizes anatomy and pathology in the vitreous capacity and retinal composition, especially in the presence of an opaque media (e.g., vitreous hemorrhage or retinal detachment).
Fundus Photography (FP) Normal: No pathology would be observed. *Fundus photography is used to take pictures of the back of the inner eye. The highly specialized photos are used to diagnose, document, compare, and monitor eye conditions. It records the condition of the retina, macula, fovea, optic disc, blood vessels, and vitreous humor, the gel-like substance that fills the inner eye.*	Used to visualize and document anatomy and pathology of the posterior pole of the retina and detect problems with the retina, macula, optic disc, blood vessels of the eye, and vitreous humor. Especially helpful in diagnosing macular degeneration.
Fluorescein Angiography (FA) Normal: No pathology would be observed; perfusion time would be approximately 21 to 24 seconds. *The intravenous injection of a dye into the bloodstream to measure the retinal vascular perfusion, infarcts, stenosis, ischemia, leakages, neovascularizations, avascular obstructions, microaneurysms, and retina defects for the evaluating, diagnosing, monitoring, and treating of ocular diseases.*	Perfusion time in > 27 seconds may be a reason to place the patient on special eyedrops or **acetylsalicylic acid (ASA)** (if no contraindications) to help increase blood perfusion to the eye.
Optical Coherent Topography (OCT) Normal: No pathology observed. *An optical scanner used for viewing and measuring of the retinal layers of the eye for anomalies. Cross-sectional visualization of the anatomy and pathology of the retina, optic nerve, and anterior segment.*	Anomolies found if present (e.g., edema, holes, degeneration).
Color Vision Tests (Ishihara) Normal: Able to identify all color plates. *The measuring of color vision (CV) for any deficiency such as color blindness, Plaquenil therapy side effect*, and the lack of red-green discrimination or blue-yellow discrimination.*	Verbal response from the patient on recognition of color hues to determine any deficiency in the cone functions of the retina. Any color plates missed may identify some degree of CV loss.

*Plaquenil is a drug used to treat rheumatoid arthritis and malaria; it is contraindicated in the presence of retinal or visual field changes attributable to any 5-aminoquinoline compound. Ocular side effects of the drug include blurred vision, photophobia, diminished ability to read, and blacked out areas in the visual field.

LABORATORY AND DIAGNOSTIC TESTS for Visual Disorders, *continued*

Test With Description, Rationale, and Normal Values	Expected Abnormality
Electrophysiology	
The measuring of the visual pathways from the retinal photoreceptors to the visual cortex of the brain.	Illustrating waveforms to determine the pathology of the visual system. Irregular waveforms may indicate pathology.
• Visual Evoked Potential (VEP): Normal: Regular waveforms. *Computerized recording of electrical activity in the occipital cortex to measure vision potential of seeing, as well as in diagnosing visual function, unexplained vision loss, retinal vascular diseases, ocular traumatic problems, visual pathway lesions, toxic or nutritional eye diseases, glaucoma, and optic nerve diseases.*	
• Electro-Oculogram (EOG): Normal: Regular waveforms. *Computerized recording to measure the ratio of change in the corneo-retinal resting electrical potential under conditions of light and dark adaptation such as ocular melanoma; opacification; retinal toxicities; retinal disorders, especially in macular dystrophies; and inherited retinal diseases, especially Best's disease (a hereditary form of progressive macular dystrophy). Also tests for illustrating waveforms of the cone/rod (photoreceptor) activity to detect retinal pathology (Foundation Fighting Blindness, 2012).*	Illustrating waveforms of ocular layers to determine pathology, especially diagnostic of Best's disease. Irregular wave formation may indicate disease or retinal defect. Irregular waveforms of the cone/rod layer of the retina may indicate pathology; this is especially diagnostic of Retinitis pigmentosa (a group of inherited diseases causing retinal degeneration, such as Usher syndrome and rod-cone disease).
• Electroretinogram (ERG): Normal: A normal ERG shows a normal A- and B-wave pattern with appropriate increases in electrical activity with increased light intensities. *Computerized recording to measure the electrical response evoked from the retina after stimulation with a diffuse or focal light.*	Measuring photoreceptor functions (diffuse electrical response generated by the neural to nonneural cells of the retina), in diagnosing intracranial lesions, retinal inherited retinal diseases (e.g., retinitis pigmentosa), retinal vascular diseases, visual opacities/traumatic problems, toxic or nutritional diseases, glaucoma, and unexplained vision loss.
Sedimentation Rate	
Normal value: No elevation in ESR. Normal rate Westergren Method: Male: Less than 50 years = 0–15 mm/hour Male: Greater than 50 years = 0–20 mm/hour Female: Less than 50 years = 0–20 mm/hour Female: Greater than 50 years = 0–30 mm/hour *The erythrocyte sedimentation rate (ESR or sed rate) is a significant blood test used for diagnoses in ophthalmology in relation to temporal arteritis versus anterior ischemic optic neuropathy.*	ESR (Westergren) > 40 mm is considered abnormal. In temporal arteritis, SED rate is typically > 80 mm; whereas in anterior ischemic optic neuropathy the SED rate is normal. Test results will vary with sex and age.
IgE Immunoglobulin Level	
Normal: Adult: Less than 40 mg/dL. *A serum test used to determine the level of proteins (antibodies) in the blood. As individuals are exposed to antigens, immunoglobulin (antibody) production occurs. The test is performed as part of a prenatal screen for allergies.*	This immunoglobulin increases during allergic reactions such as allergic conjunctivitis.
Vitreous and Aqueous Gram Stain Semi-Quantitative Cultures	
Normal: No presence of bacteria or other organisms. *Specimens of the vitreous and aqueous fluid are obtained by the ophthalmologist. They are stained and cultured to determine the presence of bacteria or other organisms.*	Presence and identification of bacteria or other organisms.

Sources: American Academy of Ophthalmology Preferred Practice Patterns Committee. Preferred Practice Pattern Guidelines. (2010). *Comprehensive adult medical eye evaluation.* San Francisco, CA: American Academy of Ophthalmology; Foundation Fighting Blindness. (2012). What is retinitis pigmentosa? Retrieved from http://www.blindness.org/index/php?option-option=com_content&id=50&Itemid=67; Kee, J. L. (2010). *Laboratory and diagnostic tests with nursing implications.* Upper Saddle River, NJ: Pearson.

eczema; and central nervous system disorders, such as neurofibromatosis (Wevill, 2009).

Pathophysiology

The natural crystalline lens of the eye transmits, filters, and focuses light onto the retina (Wevill, 2009). The transparency of the lens depends on the regular organization of the lens cells and intracellular lens structural proteins (Wevill, 2009). Genetics, metabolism, nutritional deficiencies, and environmental insults, such as exposure to chemical substances, diesel exhaust, fumes, cigarette smoke, and seasonal changes, as well as systemic and ocular diseases can affect lens clarity by disrupting cellular organization and intracellular homeostasis, causing lens opacity (Wevill, 2009).

Weblink: Cataracts and Your Eyes

CHART 64–1 Treatment for Refractive Disorders

Refractive Disorder	Treatment
Myopia	Corrected with a divergent lens (i.e., lens that is thinner in the center and thicker at the edges). This lens, also called a negative or concave lens, is designed to refocus the image on the retina and restore normal eyesight. The higher the myopia, the heavier and thicker at the edge the lens will be (Essilor, 2011).
Hyperopia	Corrected by using a convergent lens (lens that is thin at the edge and thicker at the center) to refocus the image on the retina. The higher the hyperopia, the heavier and thicker at the center the lens will be (Essilor, 2011).
Astigmatism	Corrected by the use of a toric lens whose curvature is designed to compensate for the defect of the cornea. The corrective power of the lens will differ according to the axis of the stigmatism; thus, the lens is of variable thickness at the edge (Essilor, 2011).
Presbyopia	Can be corrected with glasses or contact lenses, in case adding bifocals to an existing lens prescription is enough. With the use of contact lenses, the health care provider may prescribe lenses that correct one eye for near and one eye for far vision. This is called "monovision" and it eliminates the need for bifocals or reading glasses, although it can affect depth perception. Sometimes monovision can be produced through laser vision correction (Vorvick & Lusby, 2011).
Strabismus	The first step in treating strabismus is to prescribe glasses, if needed. If the individual is experiencing amblyopia or lazy eye, this must be treated first. A patch is placed over the better eye, thus forcing the weaker eye to work harder. If the eyes still do not move correctly, eye muscle surgery may be needed. Different eye muscles will be made weaker or stronger. Adults with mild strabismus tend to do well with glasses and eye muscle exercises to help keep the eyes straight. More severe forms of adult strabismus will need surgery to straighten the eyes. If strabismus has occurred because of vision loss, the vision loss needs to be corrected before strabismus surgery can be successful (Dugdale, 2010).
Diplopia	Treatment is contingent on determining the cause of the problem. The first step is to determine whether the double vision is monocular or binocular. The health care provider will perform tests to make this determination. If monocular diplopia is determined to be present, the individual's condition is evaluated to determine if there are possible eye problems such as cataracts causing the problem. If the health care provider determines that the problem is binocular, the presence of diabetes, Graves' disease, and neurological disorders will be questioned.
Biocular diplopia	Medical care includes patching one eye, using stick-on occlusive lenses applied to glasses to minimize the cosmetic handicap of a patched eye, using fresnel prisms (also stuck to glasses if stable deviation is present across all directions of gaze), and employing treatment of any underlying cause such as myasthenia gravis (Wessels, 2011). Special contact lenses also may be prescribed, and sometimes simply updating prescription eyeglasses can take care of the problem. Other forms of treatment include eye exercises and, when necessary, surgical straightening of the eye, or a combination of the two (Wessels, 2011). Chemodenervation may be used to help prevent the contracture in eyes with extraocular muscle paresis. With this procedure, the health care provider performs multiple injections of botulinum toxin into the medial rectus muscle over several months to reduce contracture due to a weak lateral rectus from a sixth nerve paralysis (Wessels, 2011).
Amblyopia	Treated medically with levodopa and cycloplegics. Pharmacologic treatment with levodopa has shown transient improvement of vision; however, the exact role of this drug has not been determined (Yen, 2011). Cycloplegic agents are used to blur vision in one eye to treat amblyopia in the contralateral eye. During assessment, these drugs dilate the pupil, paralyze the ciliary muscle, and prevent the lens from moving. Full cycloplegic refraction with atropine sulfate should be given to patients with accommodative esotropia and amblyopia (Yen, 2011).

The beginning of cataract formation is classified as lenticular changes. These changes can normally be recognized in adults as early as in the late 20s or early 30s. Risk factors that may accelerate cataract growth are ultraviolet light, x-ray exposure, smoking, poor diet, diabetes, and corticosteroid therapy. Congenital or traumatic cataracts, those occurring secondary to blunt or penetrating ocular trauma such as being hit or stuck in the eye with a finger, fist, racket, tennis ball, or other solid object, are the exception to the normal growth phase of cataract formation and may need immediate treatment with surgical removal (Graham, 2009). Cataracts can be the leading cause of blindness, especially in remote areas of the world, where cataract surgery is not easily accessible (OSN [Ocular Surgery News] SuperSite, 2012). With surgery, however, cataracts are curable.

Clinical Manifestations

The onset of the signs and symptoms of cataracts usually is gradual. Patients start to notice that headlights from automobiles look like starbursts. They are bothered with glare, have difficulty reading street signs at night, and experience progressive reading difficulty even with glasses or bifocals. The refractive index changes and the power increases may make patients more nearsighted. This is called a *myopic shift* and temporarily provides better vision without glasses for the hyperopic or farsighted person. This is referred to as "second sight" (AAO-11, 2010–2011). Cataracts most often are experienced as a painless, progressive loss of vision that occurs with aging. If people live long enough, most will experience cataracts at some point in their lifetime.

Immature (Incipient) Cataracts

The immature or incipient cataract is still in the earlier stages of maturation, beginning with sectors of opacity and intervening clear areas (AAO-11, 2010–2011) (Figure 64–1◆). These cataracts are described as areas of opacity of the crystalline lens itself, such as nuclear sclerosis or lenticular, which are centrally located; cortical or spokes, which are peripheral; anterior subcapsular (a cataract that occurs just under the capsule), or posterior subcapsular (a cataract that forms toward the back of the lens).

Mature (Senile) Cataracts

Senile or *mature cataract* is a term used in describing the later stages of formation, which is most commonly reached by the time the person is 70 to 80 years of age. The mature cataract is treated with cataract surgery.

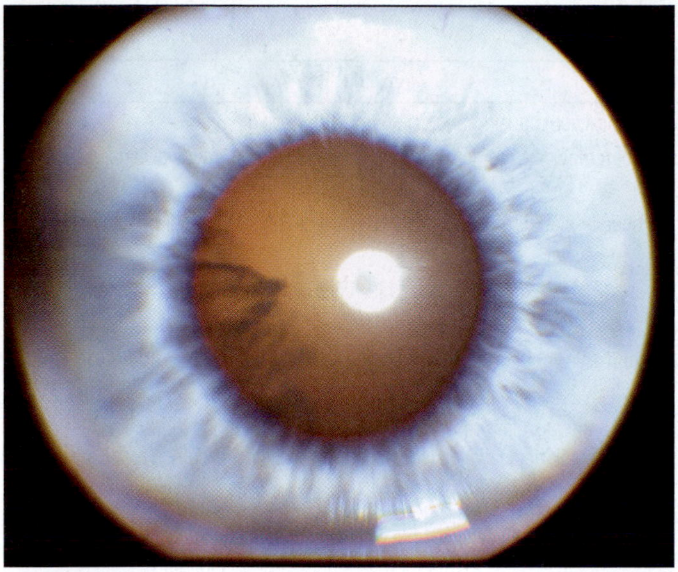

FIGURE 64–1 ◆ Nuclear sclerotic with spokes (cortical cataract).
Source: Lucie S. Elfervig.

Mature cataracts are easily recognizable with an ophthalmoscope and more definitively with a slit-lamp biomicroscopy. When the cataract is dense and noticeable, such as brunescent (brown) or white cataracts, it may be seen with a penlight.

Diagnostic Tests

Diagnosis of cataracts that may be considered for surgery is made by a vision test, in which the best-corrected visual acuity (BVA) is about 20/50 or worse, and a glare test, which mimics sunlight for 20/200 or worse vision. A potential acuity meter (PAM) test also is performed to gauge the approximate visual acuity return after cataract surgery. (See the Laboratory and Diagnostic Tests box, p. 2019.) This may vary depending on whether any other vision problems existed preoperatively, such as age-related macular degeneration or diabetic retinopathy, or whether the patient had previous eye surgery.

Surgical Management

Treatment of cataracts primarily is surgical removal. The decision to operate is ultimately determined by the patient when he is no longer able to perform activities of daily living, work, drive a motor vehicle, watch television, read, or use a computer. Cataract removal, with few exceptions, usually is recommended by the time an individual is past 85 years of age.

Sometimes cataract surgery can solve two problems. For example, if an intumescent cataract (swollen, enlarged, and cloudy lens) is formed, it may be a precursor to acute angle-closure glaucoma (see p. 2026) (See & Chew, 2009). As cataracts grow and mature, the crystalline lens enlarges, crowding or putting pressure on the anterior chamber, which results in narrowing the angle. Cataract surgery can solve both the problem of lens opacity and that of opening the anterior chamber angle, thus restoring vision and normal intraocular pressure.

Cataract Surgery

The surgery usually is performed on one eye at a time. If both eyes need cataract surgery, the second surgery is performed at varying intervals, about 4 to 6 weeks, depending on the outcome of the first cataract surgery. This is to determine how the patient recovers postoperatively from the first surgery. If unforeseen complications arise from the first cataract surgery, they can be taken into consideration when the surgery is done on the other eye. Some conditions that may predispose patients to less than ideal results are age-related macular degeneration, diabetes, Marfan's syndrome, or previous retinal detachment (American Academy of Ophthalmology, 2007). Before cataract surgery is done, a dilated eye examination is performed to make sure there are no existing problems. If any problems are present, such as active diabetic retinopathy, these will need to be addressed before the surgery is performed.

Cataract surgery is typically done in an ambulatory surgery center under topical or local anesthesia. Cataracts usually are removed by phacoemulsification or extracapsular cataract extraction (ECCE), referred to as no stitch surgery. Phacoemulsification surgery involves the removal of the lens, leaving the capsule in place. Phacoemulsification softens and breaks apart the lens using ultrasound technology. Intracapsular surgery involves the removal of the entire lens, including the capsule. A posterior chamber intraocular lens (PCIOL) is then placed in the lens sulcus; an anterior chamber intraocular lens (ACIOL) or sutured intraocular lens is used when a PCIOL cannot be stabilized because of surgical or ocular complications. There are two types of PCIOLs: accommodating and multifocal. The accommodating PCIOL has one focal point; however, it hinges at both ends to latch on and move forward and backward inside the eye using the same mechanism as normal accommodation. This mechanism promotes excellent distance and mid-range vision but is limited in closer vision. Accommodating lens are recommended for the patient who wants to see well at distance and does not mind wearing reading glasses for small print (Polk, 2012). Multifocal lens implants correct both distance vision and presbyopia. There is no single lens that is ideal for every person. Ophthalmologist's help patients decide what is best for them, based upon their specific lifestyle needs and personal preferences (Eye Surgery Education Council, 2011). New custom PCIOLs are now available for patients having cataract removals that can correct for accommodation or astigmatism.

The term *phakic* refers to the mature crystalline lens. *Pseudophakic* is the term used after cataract surgery when patients have an intraocular lens implant. *Aphakic* is the term used after cataract surgery when no lens was implanted. Aphakic patients will need to wear corrective thick glasses or contact lenses for best-corrected visual acuity.

On completion of the surgery, eyedrops are put in the surgical eye, followed by the application of an eye patch and/or shield. In addition, postoperative topical ocular medications are prescribed. See the Pharmacology box (p. 2028).

Possible complications of cataract surgery may include a dropped natural crystalline lens or intraocular lens implant, surgical astigmatism, and a decentered or tilted intraocular lens. These and other complications are outlined in Chart 64–2 (AAO-11, 2010–2011).

Nursing Management

Nursing management for cataract surgery focuses on preparing the patient for the procedure by explaining that it is typically an outpatient procedure performed under local or topical anesthesia. Preoperatively, the ophthalmologist informs the patient about what a cataract is, the surgical procedure, and the benefits and risks of cataract surgical removal. These are confirmed by the nurse, who should assess the patient's understanding, answer any misconceptions or questions, and relieve the patient's anxiety. The nurse must discuss postoperative instructions with patients and significant others prior to surgery to ensure understanding. Instructions include a demonstration of proper eyedrop instillation with a return demonstration from the person who will be instilling the postoperative eyedrops. Assessment of the operative and nonoperative eye prior to surgery must be completed and documented. It is essential

CHART 64–2 Potential Complications After Cataract Surgery

Complication	Description of Complication
Decentered/tilted intraocular lens	The intraocular lens falls out of central position or tilts in any direction, causing aberrations or less than clear vision. If not a problem, leave well enough alone. If a problem, surgeon may need to go back in to straighten the intraocular lens, suture it in place, or remove it.
Surgical astigmatism	Abnormal curvature of the cornea is induced with sutures; once healed, the sutures can be cut and refractive adjustments can be made.
Bullous keratopathy	Corneal edema from surgical manipulation and vitreocorneal adherence; complaining of blurry vision, epiphora, and photophobia; treated with topical eye medication (antibiotics).
Hyphema	Blood in the anterior chamber; complaining of blurry vision and pain; treated with topical eye medication, patching, and quiet; check intraocular pressure often.
Glaucoma	Elevated intraocular pressure; complaining of nothing, but noted on intraocular pressure check; may have pain and blurry vision; treated with topical antiglaucoma eye medication, and occasionally oral medication is indicated if intraocular pressure is > 50 mmHg.
Dropped natural lens	The natural crystalline lens or the intraocular lens implant is dropped in the vitreous; this requires a pars plana vitrectomy with air–fluid–gas exchange to retrieve the lens, usually immediately at the time of surgery or shortly afterward. A pars plana vitrectomy is a surgical technique used to extract the vitreous from the eye, replacing it with a saline solution. An air-fluid exchange is used to place a gas bubble inside the eye, which holds the retina in place (Retina Eye Specialists, 2010).
Cystoid macular edema	Edema of the choroidal layer in the macula (central vision); treated with topical eye medication and possibly vitrectomy with air–fluid–gas exchange.
Retained crystalline lens material	Lens material in the capsule is an irritant that can become infectious and cause inflammation; complaining of blurred vision and pain. Treat the problem it is causing, or Elschnig's pearls can be polished. Elschnig's pearls are the remnants of epithelial cells after extracapsular cataract extraction. Laser capsulotomy ulotomy may be used to polish these remnants to improve visibility (Montgomery, 2012a).
Vitreous prolapsed	If the rupture of the posterior capsule results, this allows vitreous into the anterior chamber, which may cause pupillary block, poor healing, infection, retinal breaks, or retinal detachments; usually this is corrected at the time of surgery with an anterior vitrectomy to remove vitreous from the anterior chamber.
Retinal detachment	Retinal layers detach or separate from their base; complaining of a curtain, a veil, floaters, or light flashes in vision; treated with endolaser or a vitrectomy with air–fluid–gas exchange.
Vitreous hemorrhage	Blood in the vitreous chamber; complaining of blurry vision and floaters; treated with head elevated during rest or sleep, and let the blood settle inferiorly, or may need a vitrectomy with air–fluid–gas exchange.
Uveitis	Inflammation of the uveal tract (iris, ciliary body, and choroid) from surgical trauma or allergy to intraocular lens; complaining of photophobia, epiphora, and pain; treated with topical eye medication (possible mydriatics, antibiotics/anti-inflammatories, or steroids) or intraocular lens removal.
Endophthalmitis	Intraocular infection and inflammation of the eyeball and tissue; complaining of pain, blurred vision, purulent discharge, hypopyon (pus within the eye), and corneal edema; treated with intravitreal, fortified topical, topical, and/or oral antibiotics, and may also require a vitrectomy with air–fluid–gas exchange.
Posterior capsular opacity	This is the most common complication after cataract surgery, caused by leaving the posterior capsule intact. This capsule prevents other potential major complications that could occur if the capsule were opened. Opacity or haziness of the posterior capsule membrane (sometimes referred to as second cataract) may take place within several weeks to years or may never develop; complaining of hazy or blurry vision and cataract coming back; patient cannot read or drive; treated with Neodymium-yttrium aluminum garnet laser (Nd: YAG laser) to open the capsule.

Sources: Adapted from AAO-11 (American Academy of Ophthalmology). (2010–2011). *Basic and clinical science course: Lens and cataract* (Section 11). San Francisco: Author; Kohnen, T., Wang, L., Friedman, N., & Koch, D. (2009). Complications of cataract surgery. In M. Yanoff & J. S. Duker (Eds.), *Ophthalmology* (3rd ed.). St. Louis: Mosby/Elsevier.

that the nurse record all current medications, both prescription and over the counter (OTC), with dosage and frequency, especially any anticoagulants, which may need to be stopped temporarily before and immediately following surgery.

On completion of surgery, eyedrops are put in the surgical eye and an eye patch or shield is applied to the eye. The nurse must assess the dressing and eye patch to ensure that they remain in place and that there is no evidence of drainage from the eye. Following surgery, the nurse must assess the paient's pain level, with the recognition that sudden onset of pain may be due to a ruptured vessel. Pain with nausea, vomiting, and restlessness may be related to increased intraocular pressure. Additional nursing measures include assessing the acuity of the unoperated eye; assessing and evaluating the patient for signs and symptoms of infection, orienting the patient, and administering eye medications as ordered. While hospitalized or in the outpatient setting, the patient may increase activities as tolerated and is instructed to avoid straining, recline at a 30° angle, and lie on the unaffected side. The patient should be advised to follow these instructions when home.

Discharge Planning

Patients generally are discharged from the care setting the same day as surgery is completed. They are sent home with the eye patch or shield in place and postoperative ocular medications as prescribed. See the

PATIENT TEACHING & DISCHARGE PRIORITIES for Cataract Surgery

Need	Teaching
Patient and family • Medications	Make sure that the patient understands all about the medication, including dosage, route, action, adverse effects, and need for postoperative evaluation (usually the day after surgery by the eye surgeon). Review installation of eyedrops into the conjunctival sac. Instruct the patient to avoid over-the-counter medications, particularly those with aspirin.
• Untoward reaction to surgery	Instruct the patient to report any bleeding, yellow-green drainage, pain, visual losses, nausea, vomiting, tearing, photophobia, or seeing bright flashes of light.
• Exercise and activities	Instruct the patient to avoid activities that increase intraocular pressure such as bending at the waist, sleeping on the operative side, straining with bowel movements, lifting more than 15 pounds, sneezing, coughing, or vomiting.
• Eye protection	Instruct the patient to wear a shield over the operative eye at night to prevent accidental injury to the eye during sleep, and to wear glasses during the day to prevent accidental injury to the eye while awake.
• Restricted activities	Recommend that the patient avoid reading for some time after surgery to reduce eye strain and unnecessary movement so that maximal healing occurs. Advise the patient not to shampoo for several days after surgery. The face should be held away from the shower head with the head tilted back so that water spray and soap avoid contact with the eye.

Pharmacology box (p. 2028). Patients usually are given a postoperative take-home pack, which may include eye patches, sterile eyewash, sunglasses, topical eye medications or prescriptions, and an analgesic prescription for minor postoperative discomfort. Patients need to know how to care for the postsurgical eye properly with appropriate cleaning and wearing an eye patch or shield as directed.

Postoperative treatment and follow-up care on postoperative day 1 includes removal of the eye patch and shield and assessment of the patient's visual acuity and intraocular pressure (Goldblum, 2008). Depth perception may be temporarily impaired after cataract surgery due to the eye patch, being the first eye done, or being aphakic. Patients are often advised to postpone getting new corrective lenses for about 4 to 8 weeks after cataract surgery, thus giving the eyes the needed time to heal completely and sparing patients the expense of buying more than one new pair of glasses. Patients should be instructed to rest. Specific areas of instruction for home care are shown in the Patient Teaching & Discharge Priorities box (p. 2033).

Health Promotion

Cataracts represent aging of the natural crystalline lens and usually mature with the passage of time. However, cataracts can develop earlier in life than is normally anticipated because of certain genetic factors and some systemic diseases, such as diabetes and trauma. It is important for the patient to know whether there is a family history of early cataracts, the relationship to diabetes, and whether there was any eye trauma or injury at any time in the patient's childhood, all of which can directly affect the onset of cataract maturation. Regular eye examinations are a means to detect early changes in cataract formation

Collaborative Management

To achieve the best vision potential, a multidisciplinary team approach is used for patients with cataracts. The team typically includes the ophthalmologist, ophthalmic advance nurse practitioner, and optometrist. In order to meet desired patient outcomes, it is essential that this interdisciplinary team communicate openly with one another in developing and evaluating care of the patient and family (IOM [Institute of Medicine], 2010). To ensure maximum vision potential, vision care is managed by the ophthalmologist or optometrist. The optometrist will provide the necessary glasses or contact lenses to enhance the patient's visual acuity until the best visual acuity (BVA) achievable is less than 20/40, at which time the ophthalmologist evaluates the patient for candidacy for cataract surgery. Once cataract surgery has been performed, the patient will follow up with the ophthalmologist, the optometrist, or the ophthalmic advance nurse practitioner for postoperative checks, compliance with postoperative eyedrops, and close evaluation for any postoperative complications or infections, especially endophthalmitis. Once the postoperative period is over and vision is stable, the patient will be evaluated for the BVA to determine whether glasses or contact lenses are needed to enhance vision.

Glaucoma

Glaucoma refers to a category of eye disorders often associated with a dangerous buildup of internal eye pressure (intraocular pressure or ICP) which can damage the eye's optic nerve that transmits visual information to the brain. An optic neuropathy develops accompanied by optic disc cupping and visual field loss. Optic disc cupping describes the appearance of the optic nerve to the examining eye doctor. When the nerve is viewed through the pupil, it looks like a cup seen from above. The cup is really an empty space in the middle of the optic nerve surrounded by optic nerve fibers. With the loss of nerve fibers from glaucoma, the cup becomes progressively larger because there is less space occupied by the remaining nerve fiber (Helting & Haddrill, 2012). It generally is associated with an increase in intraocular pressure; however, some people with normal intraocular pressure may develop characteristic optic nerve and visual field changes.

Epidemiology and Etiology

Glaucoma is the second-most common form of legal blindness in the United States and the third-most common in the world (Smith, 2008). **Legal blindness** is defined as the best-corrected visual acuity of 20/200 or worse of either eye, or 20 degrees or more of peripheral field loss. There is no cure for glaucoma, but with treatment, loss of sight can be prevented (Figure 64–2◆)

About 6 million people worldwide are blind from glaucoma, including 100,000 Americans, making it the leading cause of blindness in the United States (Porth & Marfin, 2009). Normal range of intraocular pressure is between 10 and 21 mmHg, but not all individuals with elevated intraocular pressure (greater than 22 mmHg) have glaucoma or optic

Weblink: Primary Open-Angle Glaucoma

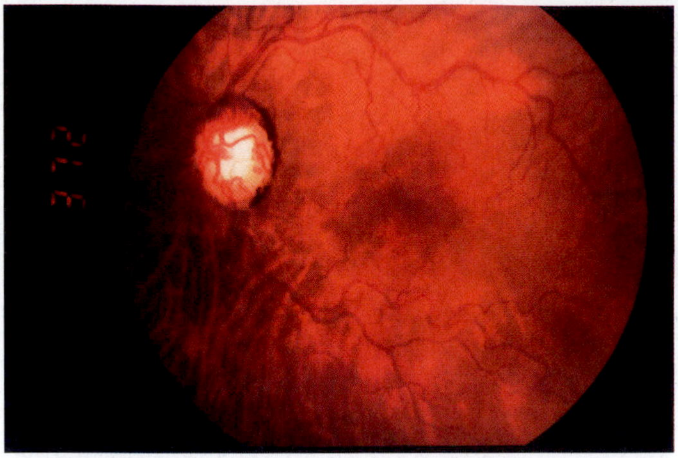

FIGURE 64–2 ◆ Glaucoma with collaterals on the disc.
Source: Lucie S. Elfervig.

nerve damage (ocular hypertension), and not all those with normal intraocular pressure are glaucoma free (Smith, 2008). Older adults, African Americans, and African Caribbeans seem to be at greater risk for *acute angle-closure glaucoma* (Fraser & Wormald, 2011). The incidence of glaucoma increases with age. Open-angle glaucoma is one of the major causes of vision loss or legal blindness in older adults, second only to age-related macular degeneration. It usually is bilateral and has a hereditary predisposition, but pressure can vary in each eye. Family history, diabetes, and being very farsighted can put one at greater risk for developing glaucoma. Risk factors for developing glaucoma are listed in the Risk Factors box.

Pathophysiology

Aqueous humor, which is produced by the ciliary body and secreted by ciliary processes, flows from the posterior chamber through the pupillary space and is deposited into the anterior chamber. Aqueous humor exits from the anterior chamber in the anterior angle into the trabecular meshwork, Schlemm's canal, and intrascleral channels and through episcleral and conjunctival veins into venous circulation (AAO-10, 2010–2011). This continuous process of production and dissemination of aqueous fluid is responsible for maintaining normal intraocular pressure. Glaucoma is the condition that develops when any sequence of the production of aqueous humor or the drainage of aqueous humor does not function properly. This causes aqueous fluid to build up intraocularly, which increases the intraocular pressure in the eye, thus putting pressure on the optic nerve and causing it to atrophy. This can lead to permanent blindness if left untreated (AAO-10, 2010–2011). The retinal ganglion cell layer of the sensory retina is composed of the neurons that project to the vision center of the brain, and the axons converge to form the optic nerve. The ganglion cell normally dies with aging (apoptosis), but glaucoma accelerates this process; when over half the ganglion cells die, visual acuity loss becomes more apparent (Gross, 2009).

RISK FACTORS for Developing Glaucoma

Age: The prevalence and incidence of glaucoma in the older adult is 4 to 10 times higher than that found is people in their 40s.

Ethnic Origin: Those of African, African American, and African Caribbean origin are at higher risk of developing primary open-angle glaucoma (POAG).

Ocular Risk Factors: These include intraocular pressure, structure of the optic nerve head, myopia, and hypermetropia.

Genetic Risk Factors: A positive family history of glaucoma places an individual at increased risk of glaucoma. Estimates of POAG cases being familial vary in the range of 13% to 47%, and a 5 to 20 times prevalence rate occurs in those who have a positive family history (Fraser & Wormald, 2011).

Other Proposed Risk Factors: Cigarette smoking, alcohol intake, and socioeconomic factors.

Sources: Bell, J. A. (2011). Primary open-angle glaucoma. Medscape reference. Retrieved from http://emedicine.medscape.com/article/1206147-overviewsa; Fraser, S., & Wormald, R. (2011). Chapter 210—epidemiology of glaucoma. *Free Medical Textbook.* Healthwise Inc. Retrieved from http://health.msn.com/health=topics/vision/glaucoma-86.

Types of Glaucoma

Generally, glaucoma is described as open angle or closed angle, depending on its outflow mechanism, and primary or secondary, depending on its etiology. Primary glaucoma has no relation to other ocular conditions, and secondary glaucoma is the result of another preexisting ocular condition. Both are marked by an increase of intraocular pressure (IOP) inside the eye (Glaucoma Research Foundation, 2011). There are also other types of glaucoma, which are variants of open-angle and acute closed-angle glaucoma.

Open-Angle Glaucoma

Open-angle glaucoma (OAG) is the condition that exists when a patient has adequate anterior chamber space for proper drainage of aqueous fluid but elevated intraocular pressure. The elevated pressure is due to the increase in aqueous production or the decrease in aqueous drainage due to trabecular meshwork obstruction, canal of Schlemm obstruction, or degenerative changes of the drainage tissue (AAO-10, 2010–2011). Open-angle glaucoma is sometimes referred to as the "silent blinder" or "thief in the night," because patients usually are asymptomatic in the early stages until it is first recognized due to noticeable vision loss. Side vision loss usually comes later in the course of the disease. Standard terms for open-angle glaucoma (OAG) are chronic glaucoma (COAG), primary glaucoma (POAG), or pigmentary glaucoma. Pigmentary glaucoma occurs when pigment pieces of the iris are blocking the drainage canal. Primary open-angle glaucoma, the most common form of glaucoma, occurs by a presumed blockage of the trabecular meshwork, caused by a gradual increase in resistance to normal aqueous outflow despite an apparently open angle (Tan & Kaufman, 2009). Chronic open-angle glaucoma is long-standing glaucoma.

Acute Angle-Closure Glaucoma

Acute angle-closure glaucoma (AACG) occurs when the angle in the anterior chamber (which is between the iris and cornea) becomes shallow or narrow owing to iris blockage, thereby preventing aqueous flow through the trabecular meshwork (Ehlers & Shah, 2008; See & Chew, 2009). This causes the intraocular pressure to rise very high, creating extreme eye pain and pressure with blurry vision, fixed mid-dilated pupil, corneal edema, hyperemia, photophobia, light halos, epiphora, and frontal headaches (Ehlers & Shah, 2008) that can be accompanied by nausea, vomiting, and abdominal ache. Typically, the ocular pain alone will motivate patients to seek immediate eye care in the clinic or emergency department. One means for angle closure to occur is when pupils normally dilate in the dark or at night. This can be intermittent at first; then permanent closure may suddenly take place (See & Chew, 2009). Other predispositions to angle closure are hyperopia, increased iris thickness with drug dilation, a large natural crystalline lens (cataracts), and a pupillary block that traps aqueous fluid. Sometimes acute angle-closure glaucoma subsides without intervention; however, medical and surgical intervention is usually indicated to prevent ocular damage and keep open-angle patency.

Normal-Tension Glaucoma

Normal-tension glaucoma (NTG), or low-tension glaucoma (LTG), refers to glaucoma in which intraocular pressure readings are within normal parameters but optic nerve atrophy or visual field loss occurs. This usually results from inadequate blood perfusion to the optic nerve, possibly due to vasospastic etiology, such as in patients that suffer with frequent migraine headaches (Hitchings, 2009).

Congenital Glaucoma

Congenital glaucoma occurs in babies when there is incorrect or incomplete development of the eye's drainage canals during the prenatal period. This is a rare condition that may be inherited (Glaucoma Research Foundation, 2011).

Other Types of Glaucoma

Other types of glaucoma include secondary open-angle glaucoma, pigmentary glaucoma, exfoliative glaucoma, traumatic glaucoma, neovascular glaucoma, and iridocorneal endothelial syndrome (ICE) (Dahl, 2012).

- **Secondary open-angle glaucoma** is a type of open-angle glaucoma that can result from an eye injury, even one that occurred many years ago. Other causes are inflammation of the iris, diabetes, and the use of topical drugs in steroid-susceptible individuals. It also can be associated with a retinal detachment or retinal vein occlusion or blockage.
- **Pigmentary glaucoma** is a type of secondary glaucoma where granules of pigment detach from the iris. These granules may block the trabecular meshwork, which is a critical part of the eye's draining system. This blockage causes an elevation in IOP, thus damaging the optic nerve.
- **Exfoliative glaucoma** can occur with either open or closed angles. It is characterized by deposits of flaky material on the front surface of the lens and in the angle of the eye. It is believed that an accumulation of this material in the angle blocks the eye's drainage system and raises the eye pressure. This type of glaucoma is more prevalent in older people and people of Scandinavian descent. Recently, it has been associated with hearing loss in older people (Dahl, 2012).
- **Traumatic glaucoma** develops from a variety of post-traumatic ocular disorders with different underlying mechanisms that lead to the common pathway of abnormal elevation of intraocular pressure and increased risk of optic neuropathy. Angle-recession glaucoma is classified as a type of traumatic secondary open-angle glaucoma. Angle recession is a common sequelae of blunt ocular trauma that is characterized by a variable degree of cleavage between the circular and the longitudinal fibers of the ciliary muscles (Sullivan, 2010).
- **Neovascular glaucoma,** also classified as a secondary glaucoma, is caused by retinal ischemia/hypoxia from a predisposing condition and subsequent release of an angiogenesis factor. This angiogenesis factor causes new blood vessel growth from preexisting vascular structure. The new blood vessels progressively obstruct the trabecular meshwork, causing secondary open-angle glaucoma (Freudenthal, 2011).
- **Iridocorneal endothelial syndrome (ICE)** encompasses a spectrum of disorders characterized by progressive endothelial abnormalities, formation of peripheral anterior synechiae (PAS) (adhesions of the iris to the capsule of the lens or to the surface of the vitreous body) without drainage canal block, and iris defects. A membrane grows from the abnormal corneal endothelium across the angle onto the iris surface and contracts, causing the formation of PAS and iris abnormalities. Glaucoma occurs in about 50% of patients with ICE syndrome; it is caused by secondary synechial angle closure as a result of contraction of the abnormal tissue in the angle (Herndon, 2009).
- **Ocular hypertension** refers to elevated intraocular pressure with no other signs or symptoms, no damage to the optic nerve, and no visual field loss. Ocular hypertension can be a precursor to glaucoma.

Laboratory and Diagnostic Procedures

The ophthalmologist uses pachymetry, one of the standard devices in determining accurate intraocular pressure, to measure central corneal thickness. (See the Laboratory and Diagnostic Tests box, p. 2019.) The average central corneal thickness is about 545 ± 20 micrometers, which has a bearing on the final intraocular pressure recorded for a diagnosis of open-angle glaucoma. If the cornea is too thick, the intraocular pressure reading can be falsely read as too high; if the cornea is too thin, the intraocular pressure reading can be falsely read as too low (Ramos-Esteban, Katz, Goldberg, & Golderg, 2009; Walker & Piltz-Seymour, 2009). The intraocular pressure is obtained by tonometry reading (tonometry refers to a pressure-sensitive device used to measure pressure readings of potential glaucoma); that number reading may or may not be adjusted according to corneal thickness. This procedure is typically performed by an ophthalmologist, an optometrist, or an opthalmologic nurse; however, on occasions and dependent on the setting, it may be performed by a nurse who has been taught how to do this procedure, particularly with a noninvasive tonometer (Encyclopedia of Nursing and Allied Health, 2012; Stevens, Gilbert, & Asbury, 2007).

Clinical Manifestations

The usual onset of glaucoma is asymptomatic, slow, silent, and painless. Some symptoms may be blurred vision or eye ache; however, by the time these symptoms develop, some permanent optic nerve damage has usually occurred along with vision loss or insidious visual field defects.

Medical Management

There is no known cure for glaucoma, but it can be well controlled with early diagnosis and treatment. Chronic untreated glaucoma can result in a rigid eyeball, sightlessness, and eye pain and may even require enucleation for a very painful blind eye. The health care provider determines the best target pressure as a goal to be reached in conjunction with the extent of optic nerve damage and type of glaucoma. Treatment may include antiglaucoma eyedrops, oral medications, and laser or surgery intervention, depending on the type of glaucoma, the stage of the disease process, and the number of risk factors present. The different types of antiglaucoma eyedrops categorized in the Pharmacology box (p. 2028) are usually the first line of therapy. When medical treatment is unsuccessful or intolerable, or patients are noncompliant, surgical options are considered. Surgical and laser options for glaucoma treatment are YAG laser (neodymium: yttrium-aluminum-garnet) for peripheral iridectomy or iridoplasty, laser trabeculoplasty, laser trabeculectomy, viscocanalostomy, ciliodestructive procedure, or trabeculotomy and trabeculectomy filtering procedure (AAO-10, 2010–2011). These procedures result in a lessening of pressure in the eye and reduced pain (Girkin, 2011).

The treatment goal for patients with acute angle-closure glaucoma is to lower intraocular pressure as quickly as possible with systemic

PHARMACOLOGY Summary of the Topical Ophthalmic Drops

Medication Category and Action	Application/Indication	Nursing Responsibility
Anesthetics		
Proparacaine Hydrochloride Tetracaine Hydrochloride ***Action:*** Anesthetizes corneal nerves and surrounding tissue (conjunctiva); partial or complete loss of sensation	Numbing of the cornea is indicated for: Applanation tonometry to check intraocular pressure (IOP) or gonioscopy for glaucoma. Removal of a superficial corneal foreign body or sutures. Performing minor corneal or conjunctival procedures. Schirmer's diagnostic test. Contact lenses fitting. Lacrimal canalicular manipulation. Preop preparation, especially in laser therapy. Trauma evaluation.	Assess clinical signs of allergic reaction to the drops including eye irritation, watering, or increased sensitivity to light. Explain that the patient's eye is being numbed with temporary elimination of the blink reflex. May need to patch the eye following a procedure for protection. Caution: The patient is not to rub or touch the eye for several minutes, until the numbing sensation dissipates. Never give a patient numbing drops for self-administration; they can cause serious corneal damage, opacity, and vision loss. Monitor for adverse ocular reactions: corneal edema, redness, burning, stinging, keratitis, and delayed epithelial wound healing. Explain to the patient that the tears and edges of eyelids and lashes will be yellow temporarily; the color washes out with tears.
Fluorescein sodium with topical anesthetic	Numbing and staining of the cornea: Applanation tonometry or gonioscopy to check IOP for glaucoma. Access corneal abrasion/injury, herpetic lesions, or foreign body. Access tear flow in lacrimal drainage tests. Assist in contact lenses fitting. Evaluate postoperative closure of sclerocorneal wound in delayed anterior chamber reformation. Removal of superficial corneal foreign body or sutures. Perform minor corneal or conjunctival procedures.	Make sure the drops are current and have not been contaminated by touching the patient's eyelashes or lids with the tip of the bottle. Observe for adverse ocular reactions: stinging, burning, redness, keratitis inflammation of the cornea, corneal opacity, decreased vision, and iritis. Observe for adverse systemic reactions: dermatitis and depression (rare).
Mydriatics ***Action:*** Anesthetizes corneal nerves and surrounding tissue (conjunctiva); partial or complete loss of sensation		
Phenylephrine Hydrochloride ***Action:*** Stimulates alpha-adrenergic receptors, increasing blood pressure and causing pronounced vasoconstriction in skin, mucous membranes, and mucosa. Produces prolonged or extended dilatation of the pupil by contracting pupillary dilator muscle.	When pupillary dilation is required: Diagnostic procedures, fundus examination, uveitis (posterior synechiae), preoperatively for laser therapy, etc.	Assess for clinical signs of allergic reaction (e.g., narrow angle glaucoma, photophobia . . .). Contraindicated in patients with narrow-angle glaucoma. Caution: Topical use only. May cause an exaggerated adrenergic effect if used with monoamine oxidase inhibitor (MAOI) agents (up to 21 days after). Instruct the patient to wear sunglasses to block ultraviolet (UV) light exposure. Advise the patient that driving with the eyes dilated may be difficult, especially on a sunny day. Practice good hand hygiene to avoid iatrogenic dilation. Advise the patient of the possible additive effect if the patient is on tricyclic antidepressants. Observe for adverse ocular reactions: stinging and burning. Observe for adverse systemic reactions: collapse, tremor, palpitation, perspiration, and pallor.
Cycloplegics Atropine Sulfate Cyclopentolate Hydrochloride Homatropine Hydrobromide Scopolamine Hydrobromide Tropicamide Atropine Sulfate Cyclopentolate Hydrochloride		

Medication Category and Action	Application/Indication	Nursing Responsibility
Action: Blocks postganglionic innervation of ciliary body, longitudinal muscle, and iris sphincter, to produce paralysis of ciliary muscle (blocking accommodation) and iris sphincter (blocking constriction).	Pupillary dilation required: Refraction requiring mydriasis (abnormal prolonged dilatation of the pupil) and cycloplegia, especially in children, who have a large accommodative ability. Acute inflammation of the anterior uveal tract (relieve iris spasm). Preop or postop mydriasis for iridocyclitis, inflammation of the iris and ciliary body. Optical aid in axial lens opacity. Diagnosis procedures.	Assess for clinical signs of allergic reaction, such as dry mouth, blurred vision, photophobia, and tachycardia. Patients may also stop sweating, making them prone to discomfort in warm weather. Excessive doses can lead to excessive thirst, dizziness, tremor fatigue, and loss of coordination. Contraindicated in patients with narrow-angle glaucoma. Caution use in patients with Down syndrome and older adults due to an increased sensitivity to the drug; they may react quicker to this medication. The darker the iris pigmentation, the greater the dosage for effect. Pressure placed with fingers at the bridge of the nose (lacrimal sac compression) may prevent excess systemic absorption. Instruct patient to wear sunglasses to block UV light exposure. Driving with eyes dilated may be difficult, especially on a sunny day. Perform good hand hygiene to avoid iatrogenic dilation. Topical use only. Observe for adverse ocular reactions: redness, conjunctivitis, lid inflammation, dry eyes, and edema.
Miotics		
Carbachol Pilocarpine ***Action:*** Constricts pupils for ocular hypotension. Cholinergic agonist agents induce muscarinic receptor contraction of ciliary muscle in facilitating aqueous outflow, and increases trabecular meshwork outflow to decrease intraocular pressure (IOP).	Open-angle glaucoma, good second- and third-line therapy. Preop and postop IOP controls. Acute glaucoma attack prevention in nonaffected eye or antidote for mydriasis.	Promote compliance with eyedrops. Assess for relief of elevated intraocular pressure, as well as drug effectiveness. Review patient history; contraindicated for patients with iritis, conjunctivitis, or keratitis, and postcataract surgery to prevent posterior synechiae (an adhesion of the iris to the cornea or lens of the eye). Inform the patient that she may have difficulty with dark adaptation with field of vision reduced. Caution the patient about night driving and working with hazardous equipment in dim light. Instruct the patient to stop use prior to general anesthesia. Observe the patient for adverse systemic reactions: sweating, headache, syncope, salivation, arrhythmias, hypotension, asthma, pulmonary distress, cramping, vomiting, diarrhea, and urinary frequency. Observe for systemic toxicity with overdose; antidote atropine.
Beta-Blockers		
Nonselective β-adrenergic antagonist: Carteolol Levobunolol Hydrochloride Metipranolol Timolol Maleate Selective β-adrenergic antagonist: Betaxolol Hydrochloride Levobetaxolol Hydrochloride ***Action:*** Antagonist agents inhibit agonist actions (blockers). β-Adrenergic antagonist affects ocular function by competing with agonists for β-adrenergic receptor binding sites, thereby blocking the effects of sympathetic stimulation. This results in decreased aqueous production and may increase aqueous outflow to decrease IOP.	Primary open-angle glaucoma (POAG), ocular hypertension, aphakic glaucoma, or secondary glaucoma.	Promote compliance with application of eyedrops. Assess the patient for relief of elevated intraocular pressure, as well as drug effectiveness. Review patient history; contraindicated for patients with chronic obstructive pulmonary disease (COPD), asthma, sinus bradycardia, overt cardiovascular failure, cardiogenic shock, and greater than 1° atrioventricular (AV) block, as well as patients on catecholamine (reserpine). Selective β-adrenergic antagonist poses less risk of pulmonary adverse effects; beta-blockers are less likely to cause such problems because they are less likely to cause constriction of the air passages. May mask hypoglycemia in insulin-dependent diabetes mellitus (IDDM) and clinical signs of hyperthyroidism. Can elevate triglycerides. Instruct patient to protect drops from light. Instruct the patient of possible additive effects if on systemic beta-blockers. Assess the patient for clinical manifestations of allergic reaction: swelling of the lips, face, or tongue; difficulty breathing; closing of the throat; hives; an asthma attack; irregular, fast, or slow heart beats; or changes in blood pressure. Observe the patient for adverse ocular reactions: blurred vision, foreign body sensation, photophobia, ptosis, diplopia, and decreased corneal sensitivity. Observe for adverse systemic reactions: insomnia, dysrhythmias, pulmonary distress, and bronchospasm (can cause death).

(*continued*)

Medication Category and Action	Application/Indication	Nursing Responsibility
Alpha$_2$ Agonists		
Apraclonidine Hydrochloride Brimonidine Tartrate (Alphagan P) ***Action:*** Mimics endogenous adrenergic compounds. Affects ocular function by select binding to alpha receptors with sympathetic nervous system influence on aqueous formation, pupil width, and ocular blood flow to decrease IOP from glaucoma by decreasing aqueous production and increasing uveoscleral outflow.	POAG, ocular hypertension, or preop IOP controls for laser therapy.	Instruct the patient of the need for compliance with application of eyedrops. Review patient history; contraindicated for patients on clonidine and monamine oxidase inhibitors (MAOI) therapy. The patient can develop a vasovagal response during laser surgery and overreduction in IOP. Assess the patient for relief of elevated intraocular pressure. Monitor for drug effectiveness, which is manifested as improved vision. Assess the patient for history of drug allergies prior to administration. Assess the patient for adverse ocular reactions: red eye, mydriasis, upper lid elevation, burning, stinging, blurriness, follicles, and itching. Observe the patient for adverse systemic reactions: drowsiness, fatigue, headaches, blood pressure changes, dry mouth, nasal congestion, respiratory, or gastrointestinal (GI) discomforts. Assess the patient for history of drug allergies prior to administration.
Prostaglandins		See above for alpha agonists.
Bimatoprost Latanoprost Travoprost ***Action:*** Increases uveoscleral outflow, increasing aqueous outflow.	POAG, ocular hypertension, or elevated IOP lowering.	Review patient history, due to contraindications (patients in whom oxytocic drugs are contraindicated). Encourage compliance with application of eyedrops. Inform the patient of possible red eye (usually goes away within 8–12 weeks), increased eyelash growth, and discoloration of iris and tissue around the eye. Review patient history, due to contraindications (patients in whom oxytocic drugs are contraindicated). Assess the patient for relief of elevated intraocular pressure, as well as drug effectiveness. Caution: Do not use Latanoprost with thimerosal for patients with pulmonary compromise, renal or liver dysfunctions, uveitis, iritis, or aphakic, pseudophakic, or macular edema. Observe the patient for adverse systemic reactions: chest pain, angina, respiratory infection, colds, rash, back pain, and joint pain.
Carbonic Anhydrase Inhibitors (CAIs)		
Action: Blocks the enzyme in the nephron responsible for bicarbonate reabsorption. By interfering with the synthesis of carbonic acid, the production of aqueous humor is decreased, thereby reducing IOP.	Used to treat glaucoma.	Encourage compliance with application of eyedrops. Assess the patient for relief of elevated intraocular pressure, as well as drug effectiveness by verifying improved vision. Review patient history; contraindicated if on sulfa drugs; patients with severe renal failure and hepatic insufficiency may have low levels of electrolytes (sodium [Na] and potassium [K]), as well as hyperchloremic acidosis (especially oral CAI medication).
Brinzolamide Dorzolamide Hydrochloride ***Action:*** Decreases the pressure in the eyes by reducing how much fluid (aqueous humor) is produced in the eye.	Glaucoma treatment for IOP lowering.	Encourage compliance with application of eyedrops. Review patient history; contraindicated if on sulfa drugs; patients with severe renal failure and hepatic insufficiency may have low levels of electrolytes (sodium [Na] and potassium [K]), as well as hyperchloremic acidosis (especially oral CAI medication). Caution: May mask hypoglycemia in IDDM, patients with pulmonary or cardiac disease, and patients on high dose of aspirin.
Photodynamic Therapy		
With photosensensitive dye Verteporfin (Visudyne). ***Action:*** The inactive form of the photosensitive dye, is injected into the vein; it travels to and binds with abnormal blood vessels under the center of the macula. A low intensity laser beam activates the drug only in the affected area. The specific wavelength of light activates the medicine to make a kind of oxygen that kills nearby cells; thus, damaging the abnormal blood vessels under the retina and leaving normal blood vesels intact.	Indicated for use with age-related macular degeneration (wet form AMD).	Observe the patient for adverse ocular reactions: blurred vision, foreign body sensation, photophobia, ptosis, diplopia, and decreased corneal sensitivity. Explain to the patient how the procedure is performed. Advise patients that they may experience headaches, injection site reactions, and possibly blurred or reduced vision. These symptoms will resolve and may be treated with OTC analgesics Instruct the patients that they will become temporarily sensitive to bright light. Care should be taken to avoid exposure of skin or eyes to direct sunlight or bright indoor light for five days. Patients who go outdoors in daylight during the first five days after treatment must protect all parts of their skin and their eyes by wearing sunglasses and protective clothing. UV sunscreens are not effective in protecting against photosensitivity reactions.

PHARMACOLOGY Summary of the Topical Ophthalmic Drops, *continued*

Medication Category and Action	Application/Indication	Nursing Responsibility
Anti-VEGF drugs		
Bevacizumab (Avastin) Pegatanib (Macugen) Ranibuizumag (Lucentisz) ***Action:*** These medicines block the effects of vascular endothelial growth factor (VEGF). Blocking this growth factor shows the growth of the abnormal blood vessels and slows the vision loss related to age-related macular degeneration.	Used to treat age-related macular degeneration (AMD).	Monitor for side effects of medication: changes in vision or trouble seeing, inflammation of different parts of the eye, increased sensitivity to light, headache, and painful urination. Inform the patient of possible effects and instruct to notify the nurse if any of these occur. Because these drugs are immunosuppressants, continually assess for symptoms and signs of local or systemic infection due to fungi, viruses, or bacteria. Monitor kidney function; report any signs of impending fluid overload to the health care provider immediately. Monitor for abnormal bleeding signs such as easy bruising, bleeding gums, petechiae, purpura melena, epistaxis, hematuria, hemoptysis, and hematemesis. Prevent infections in hospitalized patients by using protective isolation.
Antihistamines		
Loratadine, Cetrizine, Rupatadine ***Action:*** Selectively blocks the effects of histamine at their receptor sites. They do not prevent the release of histamine from mast cells. They also block cholinergic receptors to cause anticholingergic effects.	Used for treatment of allergic conjunctivitis.	Monitor the patient for positive outcomes of treatment (e.g., reduced itchiness of eyes). Monitor patient for adverse effects: drowsiness, dry mouth, headache, dizziness. Be aware of urinary retention, thickening of bronchial secretions, nausea, and vomiting. Be alert for paradoxical excitation (increased energy, restlessness, nervousness), hypersensitivity reactions (especially sensitive to the antigens), and hypotension.

Sources: Adams, M. P., & Koch, R. W. (2010). *Pharmacology connections to nursing practice.* Upper Saddle River, NJ: Pearson; Bataoel, A. (2008). Pharmacology. In P. Lamb (Ed.), *Core curriculum for ophthalmic nursing* (3rd ed.). Dubuque, IA: Kendall/Hunt; Emedicinehealth. (2011). Photodynamic therapy (PDT). WebMD. Retrieved from http://www.emedicinehealth.com/script/main/art.asp?articlekey=145454&ref=128949; Mack Eye Care. (2009). Photodynamic therapy for age-related macular degeneration. Mack Eye Center. Retrieved from http://occhicago.com/68-photodynamic-therapy-for-age-related-macular-degeneration/; PDR. (2011b). *Physicians' desk reference for ophthalmic medicines* (39th ed.). Montvale, NJ: Thomson; Sharma, A. (2011). Beta-blocker toxicity. Medscape reference. Retrieved from http://emedicine.medscape.com/article/813342-overview; WebMD. (2009). Anti-VEGF medicines for wet age-related macular degeneration (AMD). *Healthwise.* Retrieved from http://www.webmd.com/eye-health/macular-degeneration/anati-vegf-medicines-for-wet-age....

medications, orally or intravenously, as well as topical ophthalmic drops that are ordered by the health care provider. The application of topical ophthalmic antiglaucoma drops, systemic or intravenous carbonic anhydrase inhibitors, or osmotic agents are common treatments, in addition to the administration of topical ophthalmic steroid drops every 10 to 15 minutes for the first hour, then hourly until intraocular pressure is stable (See & Chew, 2009). See the Pharmacology box (p. 2028). Peripheral iridectomy (PI) or laser iridotomy is the standard immediate surgical procedure to ease high intraocular pressure and relieve blockage (See & Chew, 2009). With peripheral iridectomy, a small section of peripheral iris is excised through a limbal incison; whereas with laser iridotomy, a small opening at the peripheral iris is made with a laser, usually between the middle and peripheral thirds of the iris (Pons, 2011). Measures are continued, and the pressure is checked every 30 to 40 minutes until it is lowered enough to clear corneal swelling and quiet the anterior chamber. Once the eye is quiet and comfortable, a more extensive ocular examination can be conducted.

Nursing Management

The nurse plays a major role in educating patients about glaucoma and its proper management to prevent the advancement of optic nerve damage and the continued loss of vision. Nursing management of patients with glaucoma can be complex and multifaceted. Application of the nursing process facilitates a comprehensive approach to assessment and care of these patients.

Assessment

The assessment data for glaucoma include specific questions related to intraocular pressure controls and vision fluctuation. The nurse might ask the patient, "Have you noticed any change in your vision, such as being blurred; are you having any pain around your eyes; have you had to change any usual or normal activities due to altered vision?" Subjective data that the nurse needs to gather include family history of glaucoma, status of eye exam, any current medications being taken, and past and present eye problems. The nurse also should assess the patient to determine how she is adapting to the visual problems and what anxieties or fears the patient might be experiencing, such as feelings of loss of control. From an objective perspective, the nurse will assess actual visual acuity, body language for distress, family support systems, and the patient's ability to adjust to lifestyle behaviors.

Nursing Diagnoses

Nursing diagnoses are developed from the assessment data. A patient care plan applies the nursing process to the relevant nursing diagnoses and provides a comprehensive approach for caring for patients with glaucoma. Diagnoses may include:

- *Disturbed Visual Sensory Perception* related to altered sensory perception and vision.
- *Anxiety and Fear* related to altered self-concept.
- *Potential Ineffective Coping* related to disease process and loss of sight.
- *Pain* related to intraocular pressure.
- *Knowledge Deficit* related to diagnosis and proposed treatment.
- *Risk for Injury and Falls* related to impaired vision.
- *Self-Care Deficit* related to inability to care for self due to vision loss.
- *Possible Ineffective Therapeutic Regimen Management* related to noncompliance of using eye medications.
- *Risk of a Feeling of Powerlessness* related to loss of control and ability to care for self.
- *Disturbed Body Image* related to actual or potential loss of sight.

NANDA-I © 2012

Outcomes and Evaluation Parameters

The focus of evaluation is the patient's ability to keep intraocular pressure under control, to maintain compliance with the therapeutic regimen, to maintain a level of anxiety and fear at a reasonable level, and to acknowledge reduced eye pain. Also noteworthy is the patient's ability to maintain and manage a clean and safe environment in which to live.

Planning and Interventions

The primary nursing goals are to prevent further visual deterioration; provide adaptations to changes in or reduced visual acuity; prevent complications; and provide information about disease processes, prognosis, and treatment needs. These goals are consistent with potential patient outcomes and are met through the following interventions. The nurse should initially ascertain the type and degree of visual loss. The patient should be encouraged to express feelings of loss of visual sensory perception. The nurse also should recommend measures to assist the patient to manage visual limitations, such as reducing clutter, arranging furniture, and advising the patient to turn his head to view subjects. The nurse should assess the patient's anxiety level, current knowledge of condition, and degree of pain. When asked, the nurse should provide accurate information and encourage the patient to express his concerns and feelings. Accurate information and identification of helpful resource people may assist the patient in developing effective coping skills. Identify the current level of coping. Relative to pain, advise the patient to report pain immediately and determine if the patient has experienced any visual field changes (e.g., veil-like curtain, blurred vision, or flashes of light). Administer pain medications as ordered. In response to a possible knowledge deficit, the nurses assume a teaching role by reviewing the pathology/prognosis and lifelong need for treatment. It is important to demonstrate how to administer eyedrops and review the importance of maintaining the prescribed drug schedule. Evaluating compliance with the therapeutic regimen is critical. Ask the patient, "Are you instilling eye medications as prescribed?" Potential side effects of medications and adverse reactions of treatment should be explained. These might include decreased appetite, nausea and vomiting, diarrhea, fatigue, syncope, and decreased libido. To prevent injury that is related to reduced peripheral vision, arrange the environment to ensure safety. Place frequently used items where the patient can view them through central visual fields. Administer miotics, as ordered, which cause pupillary constriction, blur vision for 1 to 2 hours after installation, and reduce adaptation to darkness. Also, assist the patient when ambulating to avoid running into objects and harming self. To minimize self-care deficits, encourage independence with activities of daily living, and assist the patient as necessary. Feelings of powerlessness can be addressed by allowing the patient as much control over his own care as possible while encouraging strict adherence to the therapeutic regime. Encourage patients with glaucoma to express their feelings and to identify what would make them feel better and encourage the patients to make relevant lifestyle changes. Increased feelings of being in control of the situation may improve altered body image. With all interventions, emphasis should be placed on helping the patient find resources and assistance to manage at home and to resume normal activities within the parameters of visual acuity. Emotional and spiritual support should be provided, as should education and specific instructions on how to care for self, which are discussed in the Discharge Planning section. Explain the identification of risk factors that can worsen the patient's condition and describe community resources available to assist the patient. Both are very important and are described in greater detail in the Discharge Planning section.

Discharge Planning

Discharge goals for the patient with glaucoma include:

- Vision is maintained at the highest level possible.
- Patient is coping with the situation in a positive manner.
- Complications are prevented and/or minimized.
- The disease process and therapeutic regimen are understood by the patient and family.
- There is a plan in place to meet the patient's needs postdischarge.

The Patient Teaching & Discharge Priorities box identifies priority needs for the patient with glaucoma.

Health Promotion

Patient education includes information on risk factors for glaucoma such as family history, myopia, previous eye trauma, low blood pressure, African ancestry, diabetes, long-time exposure to steroids, and aging. On early detection of glaucoma and subsequent treatment to prevent permanent vision loss, health care providers need to focus on patient compliance with the application of glaucoma eyedrops, as outlined in the Pharmacology box (p. 2028), and regular follow-ups. The major reason that people develop blindness from glaucoma, besides not knowing that they have glaucoma, is noncompliance in using eyedrops and not taking glaucoma seriously as a disease. It is imperative that the patient understand that the long-term goal of treatment is to lower intraocular pressure to prevent optic nerve damage and that only through continued use of drops can this goal be reached. Regular eye examination is necessary to determine whether the prescribed treatment is effective because no symptoms will occur until vision becomes blurry or lost, at which point it may not be reversible.

Collaborative Management

The best results for patients with glaucoma are achieved through a multidisciplinary team approach, including the ophthalmologist, ophthalmologic advance nurse practitioner, nurse, and optometrist. In order to meet desired patient outcomes, it is essential that this interdisciplinary team communicate openly with one another in developing and evaluating care of the patient and family (IOM [Institute of Medicine], 2010). Management of glaucoma may include medical controls with the continuous use of eyedrops or surgical intervention

PATIENT TEACHING & DISCHARGE PRIORITIES for Glaucoma

Need	Teaching
Knowledge of the disease process and prognosis	Develop plans for home care for the patient and family. Validate patient's understanding of the disease and prognosis. Encourage independence with self-care activities. Encourage the patient to make necessary changes in lifestyle to accommodate the disease.
Understanding of medications for patient and family	Validate the patient's understanding of all medications, including dosage, route, action, and side effects. Make sure the patient has the dexterity to instill eyedrops correctly. Suggest a daily calendar log to record medication use. Written guidelines may be helpful.
Risk factors for exacerbating the disease for the patient	Teach the patient to avoid the following: bending at the waist, lifting heavy objects, coughing, vomiting, and straining to have a bowel movement. Reinforce abstinence from activities that strain eye muscles (e.g., heavy lifting/pushing, snow shoveling).
Dietary considerations for the patient and family	Instruct on using a diet high in fiber to prevent constipation and straining with a bowel movement. Eat plenty of fruits and vegetables, apricots, figs, peaches, pears, pineapple, prunes, beans, greens, asparagus, broccoli, cabbage, carrots, green beans, peas, and squash. Eliminate sugar and white flour; use whole-grain products. Avoid constipating foods, such as white flour, cheese, fried foods, sweets, salt, beef, and all junk food. Establish a regular bowel elimination pattern. Consult with a dietitian if necessary.
Reportable clinical manifestations for the patient and family	Explain the need to call the doctor right away if any of the following symptoms occur: pain in the eye, shortness of breath, nausea or vomiting, loss of vision, nonreactive pupils, reddened sclera, bleeding, discharge, or tingling in the hands or feet.
Physical environment and safety precautions for the patient and family	Arrange the environment to promote safety by removing clutter and placing furniture so there is a clear space to walk in.
Family/Support system	Encourage open discussion about how the patient and family are feeling about the disease and prognosis. Advise of available community resources. Encourage family members to be examined regularly.
Emotional adjustment of patient/family: due to lifelong duration of the disease	Identify resources for socialization, such as support groups. Encourage the patient/family to seek out resources related to transportation and utilization of local resources such as the library.
Follow-up care for the patient and family	Stress the importance of routine checking to monitor the disease. Note that following the medication schedule and routinely seeing the eye doctor can prevent further visual loss. Stress that glaucoma requires strict, consistent treatment to prevent blindness.

by the ophthalmologist. The nurse practitioner or nurse can provide the necessary education and follow-up monitoring of the patient's progress to ensure compliance with the glaucoma treatment regimen. Nursing assessment and education include the patient's compliance with regular use of eyedrops and follow-up, which is one of the main goals in treating glaucoma. The patient is taught how to instill eyedrops properly for the full benefit of treatment. Having the patient give a return demonstration with artificial tears will allow the nurse to determine the patient's ability for self-medication. The optometrist can provide visual evaluations between regular health care provider visits and make necessary refractive corrections when indicated, thereby contributing to the patient's compliance with eye medications.

Diabetic Retinopathy

Diabetic retinopathy (DR) refers to degenerative changes in the retina, specifically the weakening and leaking of blood vessels, caused by diabetes mellitus (DM). Diabetic retinopathy has various stages, including nonproliferative (early or mild, moderate, severe or advanced) and proliferative (Rosenblatt & Benson, 2009; Wilkinson, 2010). (Figure 64–3◆, p. 2034).

Epidemiology and Etiology

Diabetic retinopathy is the leading cause of legal blindness among young adults and working-age Americans (persons under the age of 60), typically affecting individuals in their most productive years (Wilkinson, 2010). It is the leading cause of blindness for all ages in the United States (Porth & Marfin, 2009). From the initial diagnosis of diabetes, if it occurs during adulthood or at a prepubertal age, patients may have a 5-year "grace period" during which retinopathy usually is not visually detectable. This is referred to as *diabetes without ophthalmic complications*. The prevalence of retinopathy increases in type 2 diabetics with every year of duration, to about 23% after about 12 years, and increases threefold after 16 years or more of being diabetic (Rosenblatt & Benson, 2009).

Major risk factors for diabetic retinopathy are listed in the Risk Factors box (Mayo Clinic Staff, 2012). An increased risk of DR

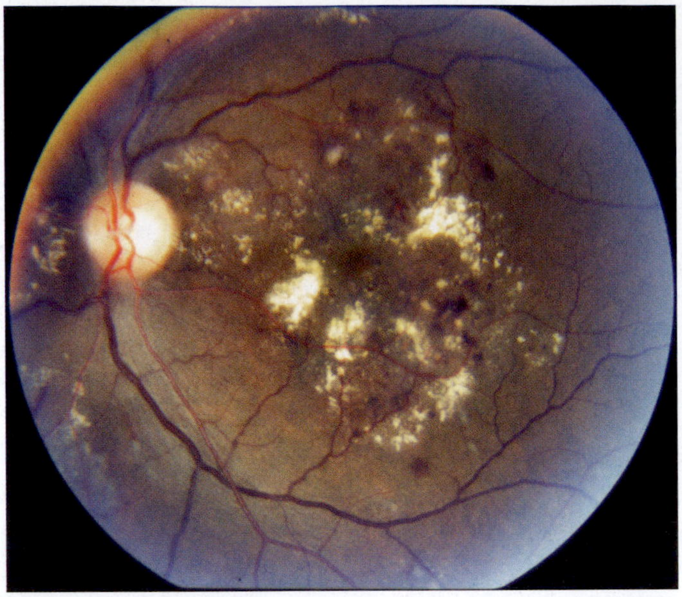

FIGURE 64–3 ◆ Diabetic retinopathy.
Source: Lucie S. Elfervig.

RISK FACTORS for Diabetic Retinopathy

Years of being diabetic	Family history of diabetes
Hyperglycemia	Hypertension
Hyperlipidemia	Smoking
Anemia	Renal disease

appears to exist in patients with Native American, Hispanic, and African American heritage (Wong, Klein, & Klein, 2010).

Pathophysiology and Clinical Manifestations

Diabetic retinopathy happens because blood vessels in the retina change. During the early nonproliferative stage of the disease, blood vesssels in the retina begin to leak extra fluids and small amounts of blood into the eye which causes slight visual distortion. As DR progresses to proliferative retinopathy, new blood vessels grow around the retina and vitreous humor. These new abnormal vessels may bleed if the problem is not caught and treated (Neutralegacy .com, 2012).

Pathophysiological symptoms may include neovascularization (the development of tiny, abnormal, leaky blood vessels) of the optic disc or areas elsewhere in the retina, vitreous hemorrhage, gliotic (scar) tissue or traction retinal detachment, retinal detachment, or neovascular glaucoma of the iris.

Nonproliferative DR is manifested by **cotton-wool spots (CWS)** or soft exudates caused by lack of blood supply to the tissue, flame-shaped hemorrhages from the nerve fiber layer of the retina, and dot/blot hemorrhages from the outer plexiform layer of the retina (Rosenblatt & Benson, 2009).

Clinical manifestations of DR can range from none to floating spots, streaks, lines, scattered lights, distortion, hazy and cloudy view, darkness, and poor color vision, depending on the location of the retinopathy in the retina (Porth & Marfin, 2009).

Because blood sugar fluctuation can cause changes in vision, periodic blood sugar checks are recommended. Hyperglycemia may cause the natural crystalline lens to swell, creating myopic shift and a temporary change in refractive error. Hypoglycemia may cause a cerebral response, creating temporary blurred vision, diplopia, drowsiness, faintness, confusion, anxiety, headache, slurred speech, sweating, tremor, seizures, and even coma.

Laboratory and Diagnostic Procedures

Fasting glucose and hemoglobin A_1c (Hb A_1c) are laboratory tests that are performed to help diagnose diabetes. The Hb A_1c level also is important in the long-term follow-up care of patients with diabetes and DR. Controlling diabetes and maintaining the Hb A_1c level in the 6% to 7% range are the goals in the optimal management of diabetic retinopathy (Cheung, Mitchell, & Wong, 2010). If these levels are maintained, the progression of DR is reduced substantially. Fluorescein angiography also is used in the diagnosis and management of DR (see the Laboratory and Diagnostic Tests box, p. 2019). These photo scans reveal microaneurysms, blot-and-dot hemorrhages, areas of nonperfusion, and evidence of collateral vessels that do not leak (Lam, Anderson, Regillo, & Brown, 2010).

Medical Management

Patients with diabetes usually are followed annually if no signs or symptoms of diabetic retinopathy are present but are seen more often if active diabetic retinopathy is in progress. Sometimes just by getting blood sugar and blood pressure under control, the eye vessels from diabetes will dry up significantly. Preventing DR from developing or progressing is considered the best approach to protecting vision. Management of hypertension and hyperlipidemia also is important, as these conditions also may contribute to the risk of developing or furthering DR. An eye examination also is in order, as is an assessment of behavioral manifestations.

Laser photocoagulation provides the major direct treatment modality for DR (Goff, McDonald, & Ai, 2010). See Figure 64–4◆. This laser treatment is applied directly to leaking microaneurysms to diffuse areas of leakage and thickening. Severe hypertension or hyperglycemia also can prevent laser treatment, especially if the patient's diastolic blood pressure is above 100 mmHg or the blood sugar is over 300 mg/dL, because the laser is less effective under these conditions. Laser treatment is not recommended near the disc. However, it is not uncommon for patients with diabetes who have DR to have three to six laser sessions per eye over their lifetime (Goff et al., 2010). Anti-VEGF intravitreal injections are now found to be beneficial in the treatment of DR, alone

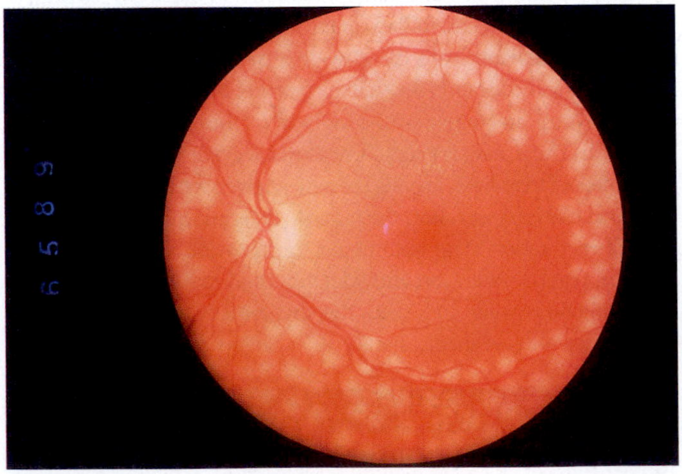

FIGURE 64–4 ◆ Laser photocoagulation.
Source: Lucie Elfervig.

or in combination with laser (READ-2, 2010; Rosenblatt & Benson, 2009). Vitrectomy has proved effective in removing vitreous hemorrhage and severing vitreoretinal membranes that develop (Porth & Marfin, 2009). The treatment of diabetic retinopathy also is discussed in Chapter 47.

Nursing Management

The nurse has many opportunities for education and intervention with patients and family in preserving vision function and promoting eye health to prevent the advancement of DR. Nursing management of patients with DR can be complex and multifaceted. Application of the nursing process facilitates a comprehensive approach to patients' assessment and care. See Chapter 47 for care of the diabetic patient. Therefore, it is very important for the nurse to emphasize good control of blood sugar and blood pressure and to educate patients about not ever smoking or giving up smoking if the patient is already a smoker.

Assessment

Assessment data when DR is suspected include specific questions related to blood glucose, blood pressure controls, and vision fluctuation. The assessment also establishes the patient's background by determining how long the patient has been a diabetic and other comorbidities such as hypertension that may contribute to a diagnosis of retinopathy. Specific questions that might be asked of the patient include the following:

- What type of medication are you on to control your diabetes?
- How are your blood sugar (glucose) and blood pressure in terms of values?
- Are you taking any other systemic medications?
- Do you smoke?
- Do you wear glasses or contact lenses, or have you had any eye problems in the past?

From an objective perspective, the nurse should assess the patient for visual acuity and blood sugar and blood pressure values.

Nursing Diagnoses

In determining diagnoses, the nurse must recognize that the patient is undergoing changes in self-perception and in the ability to maintain familiar and consistent roles in caring for self, as well as for participating as a member of a social group (e.g., family and friends). Typical diagnoses to be considered follow:

- *Altered Sensory Perception (Visual)* related to microvascular destruction due to DR.
- *Anxiety* related to fear of the unkown and possible blindness.
- *Ineffective Coping* related to changes in usual communication patterns and high degree of threat of blindness.
- *Potential Knowledge Deficit* related to unknown information regarding diagnosis, treatment, and prognosis.
- *Infection Potential* related to surgery.
- *Interrupted Family Processes* related to shift in health status and altered role in family.
- *Risk for Falls* related to eyesight impairment.
- *Self-Care Deficits* related to poor vision and inability to perform ADLs. NANDA-I © 2012
- *Impared Nutrition* related to dietary restrictions of diabetes.
- *Impaired Social Interaction* related to self-concept disburbance.

Outcomes and Evaluation Parameters

Outcomes and evaluation parameters should be focused on the patient's desired response in adapting to the overall diagnosis of DR: reduced anxiety and coping patterns. The desired outcomes are demonstrated patient behaviors, both subjective and objective, that indicate that the patient is adjusting to the overall diagnosis of diabetic retinopathy. These include stable eyesight (no further deterioration noticed), demonstrated behavior to prevent accidents/injuries, injury free, verbalization of feeling less anxious and better able to cope with the situation, and using support systems to promote positive coping behaviors. The patient also verbalizes understanding of the diagnosis, prognosis, treatment plan, and how this will impact his daily living style and conditions. He will remain free of infections; his blood sugar will be stabilized within a normal range for diabetic patients, as determined by the health care provider; his blood pressure is maintained within a desired range; and he will follow a diabetic diet. The patient is able to perform ADLs by himself or with assistance without fear of falling and injury. The patient notes that he and his family have discussed the disease and how it has impacted the family; established primary roles within the family and community, accomplished family tasks, and maintained positive relationships. In addition, the patient has resumed social interactions with colleagues and friends.

Planning and Interventions

Planning and nursing interventions focus on communication and education, as well as monitoring the patient's verbal and nonverbal behaviors. For instance, the nurse is responsible for instructing the patient on how blood sugar is relevant to the diagnosis and how to control it. Information on the reduction of risk factors also is shared. Risk factors include poorly controlled blood sugar, obesity, and illness such as heart disease and high cholesterol. Reducing the risk of low vision during the early stages of DR comes down to controlling modifiable risk factors. The patient should be advised to tightly control blood sugar, keep blood pressure and cholesterol within a narrow range, reduce body mass index by following healthy lifestyle recommendations, and stop smoking (or for nonsmokers, do not start). Education regarding available resources for maintaining self-care and an environment that is safe for those with visual defects should be reinforced. The patient's anxiety and comfort levels also are monitored so that the nurse can determine ongoing patient needs and provide assistance as appropriate. For additional information on nursing management of diabetes, see Chapter 47.

Health Promotion

Because of the progressive nature of DR, especially after the 5- to 7-year grace period, health promotion and discharge planning begin as soon as the patient is diagnosed with diabetes. One of the most important aspects of health promotion, as well as of management of diabetic retinopathy, is patient education, Patient and family education focuses on controlling the patient's blood sugar and identifying risk factors that aggravate the disease progression. Excellent glucose control is beneficial in any stage of diabetic retinopathy, as it delays the onset and slows down progression of the diabetic complications in the eye (Bhavsar, 2011). Other health concerns also must be addressed. For example, the patient should be knowledgeable regarding these systemic problems, which may act as risk factors, and the possibility

Weblink: Macular Degeneration

that they may contribute to disease progression: hypertension, renal disease, and hyperlipidemia. In addition, smoking may further compromise oxygen delivery to the retina. Therefore, the patient should be counseled to make all efforts to cease (or, at a minimum, reduce) smoking. The patient also should be made aware of visual symptoms, such as vision changes, floaters, distortion redness, and pain, as they may indicate disease progression and should be reported immediately. Education includes possible lifestyle changes and preventive care through reducing risk factors, eating a healthy diet, and engaging in routine exercise.

Discharge Planning

Discharge planning also includes preparing the patient to assume self-care in the home environment through maintaining self-administration of medications, performing ADLs, and managing space and furnishings to avoid clutter and obstacles that may contribute to injury. Because diabetic retinopathy is a progressive condition, regular follow-up care with a health care provider is crucial for detecting any changes that may benefit from treatment. Lastly, the patient should be made aware of community resources that may assist him and his family in adapting to this disease and making plans for a productive future with the disease.

Collaborative Management

A multidisciplinary team approach involves the health care provider, internist or endocrinologist, ophthalmologist, ophthalmic advance nurse practitioner, nurses, nutritionist, and optometrist. In order to meet desired patient outcomes, it is essential that this interdisciplinary team communicate openly with one another in developing and evaluating care of the patient and family (IOM [Institute of Medicine], 2010). These professionals work together to provide comprehensive care to the patient with DR, exerting their best efforts to meet desired patient outcomes in improved vision related to quality of life. Management of DR may include medical controls or surgical interventions performed by the opthamologist. The internist and endocrinologist may guide adjustment of the patient's medications to stabilize blood sugar and/or blood pressure, and assist in preparing the patient for impending vitrectromy by medication controls. The nurse practitioner or nurse can provide the necessary education and follow-up monitoring of the patient's progress to assist the patient in complying with a diabetic regimen. The nutritionist assists with establishing a diet regimen to enhance health and control diabetes. The optometrist provides visual evaluations between regular health care provider visits and makes the necessary refractive corrections when indicated.

The patient should get her blood sugar under control and stabilized for at least 6 to 9 weeks before changing glasses or contact lenses. See Chapter 47 for more information on diabetes.

Macular Degeneration

Macular degeneration is defined as deterioration of the macula, the area of central vision in the posterior pole of the retina, causing central acuity loss. Central acuity loss refers to the relatively small but vital part of the visual field used for reading and corresponds to the function of the macular area of the retina (Montgomery, 2012b). Age-related macular degeneration (ARMD or AMD) is the major cause of severe central visual loss in the United States in people over 60 years of age (Seth, Sigler, & Adelman, 2011). Age-related macular degeneration is classified into two major types—dry and wet—which will be discussed later in this section. The degeneration of the macula occurs with time and can eventually lead to legal blindness. Legal blindness is defined in the United States as visual acuity of 20/200 or worse in the better eye with corrective lenses or visual restriction to 20 degrees diameter or less in the better eye.

Epidemiology, Etiology, and Pathophysiology

It is estimated that there are between 15 to 20 million Americans living with at least the earliest signs of ARMD, affecting approximately 19% of Americans between 65 and 70 years of age (Seth et al., 2011). This figure varies worldwide with lower prevalence in the Asian and African continents. More than eight million people in the United States have bilateral intermediate or unilateral advanced disease, with approximately 1.75 million Americans having advanced disease (Seth at al., 2011). The overall prevalence of advanced age-related macular degeneration is projected to increase by more than 50% by the year 2020 due to the increasingly aged population (Jager, Mieler, & Miller, 2008). The prevalence of wet or dry AMD appears to vary in different ethnic and racial groups throughout the world (Rosenfeld, Martidis, & Tennant, 2009). The cause of AMD is still under investigation through molecular dissection and genetic linkage analyses. Early in the disease, lipids are deposited in Bruch's membrane, possibly because of the failure of the retinal pigment epithelium (RPE) to process cellular waste, resulting in accumulated deposits, later called *drusen* (Rosenfeld et al., 2009). Dry AMD and wet AMD can be the result of any disturbance or inflammation of the RPE or Bruch's membrane (Spaide, 2009). AMD is progressive, causing atrophic or deteriorating changes of the macula and RPE layer (Rosenfeld et al., 2009). Risk factors for macular degeneration are listed in the Risk Factors box (Friedman et al., 2009; Rosenfeld et al., 2009).

Clinical Manifestations

Clinical manifestations of macular degeneration vary with the type of disorder. Drusen, dry, and wet age-related degeneration are discussed next.

Drusen

Drusen usually are the earliest fundus signs of age-related macular degeneration (Figure 64–5◆). **Drusen** (singular: druse) are yellowish, round, slightly elevated, different-sized subretinal pigment epithelial deposits in the macula (Rosenfeld et al., 2009). However, not all drusen are diagnostic of macular degeneration. Over half the population over age 70 has drusen; however, it is referred to as a sign of early age-related macular degeneration only when vision loss is associated with it (Rosenfeld et al., 2009).

Patients with macular degeneration may notice at first that it is a little more difficult to see with the affected eye while doing close-up work or that they have trouble seeing at a distance, especially when driving. A frequent symptom is **metamorphopsia,** a condition characterized by vision distortion (i.e., when straight lines such as door frames or posts look crooked or irregular). Other symptoms may include a difference in the sizes and colors of objects between eyes, meaning the

RISK FACTORS for Developing Macular Degeneration

The more common risk factors associated with macular degeneration include:

Aging	Hypertension
Cardiovascular disease	Smoking
Hyperlipidemia	Hyperopia
Light-colored iris	Ultraviolet light toxicity
Heredity	

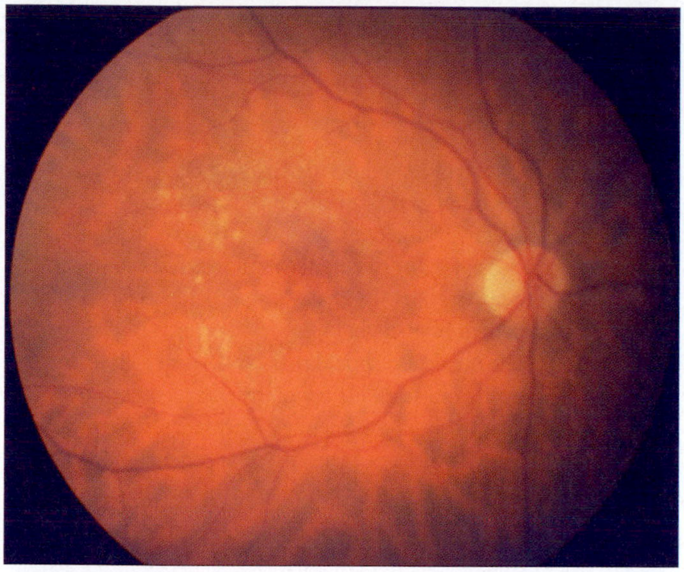

FIGURE 64–5 ◆ Dry age-related macular degeneration with drusen.
Source: Lucie S. Elfervig.

loss of **contrast sensitivity (CS).** The individual might find that he is having trouble with daily activities, such as sewing, reading, watching television, and almost any activity that requires looking directly at some object to accomplish a task or skill. The Amsler grid, shown in Figure 64–6◆, is a self-testing tool for daily use; this highly recommended tool enables the individual to notice early macular changes.

Dry Age-Related Macular Degeneration

Dry age-related macular degeneration (AMD) consists of nonexudative, geographic, or atrophic changes in the macula (see Figure 64–5). Geographic changes refer to the atrophy or degeneration of the retinal pigment epithelium (RPE) cells; geographic atrophy looks like a circle or spot of degeneration, right in the center of the macula. Dry AMD occurs when the light-sensitive cells in the macula slowly break down, gradually blurring central vision in the affected eye. As the condition gets worse, an individual may see a blurred spot in the center of her vision. Over time, as less of the macula functions, central vision is gradually lost in the affected eye. The most common symptom of dry AMD is slightly blurred vision. The person may have difficulty recognizing faces or need more light for reading and other tasks. Dry AMD generally affects both eyes, but vision can be lost in one eye while the other eye seems unaffected (NEI, 2009).

Wet Age-Related Macular Degeneration

Wet age-related macular degeneration consists of exudative, serous, or neovascular changes in the macula (Figure 64–7◆). Wet AMD occurs when abnormal blood vessels behind the retina start to grow under the macula. These new blood vessels tend to be very fragile and often leak blood and fluid, which raise the macula from its normal place at the back of the eye. Damage to the macula occurs rapidly, and loss of central vision can develop quickly. An early symptom of wet AMD is that straight lines appear wavy.

Laboratory and Diagnostic Procedures

The fluorescein angiogram (FA) and optical coherence tomography (OCT) are required diagnostic tests to be performed to evaluate the best treatment option for the patient. See the Laboratory and Diagnostic Tests box (p. 2019) for additonal information on the tests.

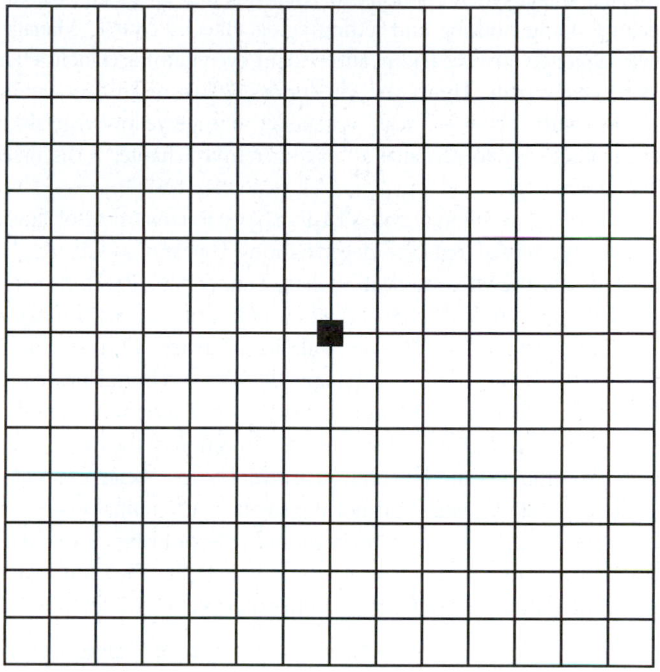

FIGURE 64–6 ◆ Amsler grid.
Source: Courtesy of Lucie S. Elfervig.

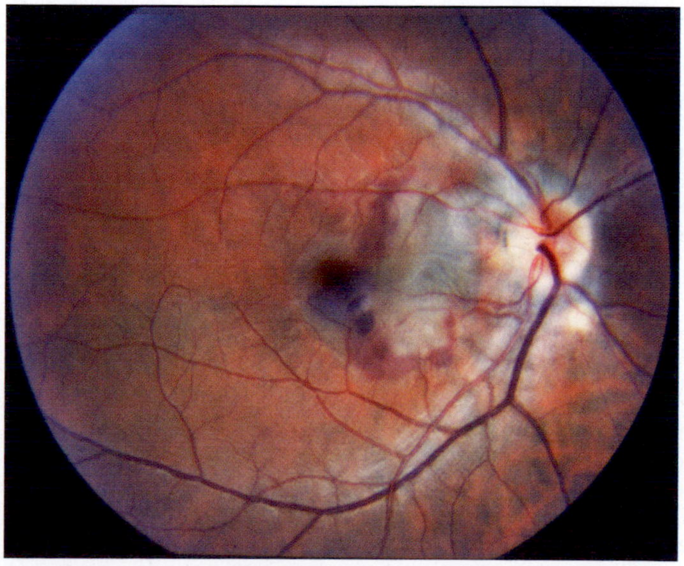

FIGURE 64–7 ◆ Wet age-related macular degeneration (choroidal neovascularization).
Source: Courtesy of Lucie S. Elfervig.

Medical Management

Medical management options for dry macular degeneration can include doing nothing and letting aging take its course. Management also may involve taking antioxidant eye vitamins (Hochstetler, Scott, Kunselman, Thompson, & Zerfoss, 2010) or supplementing the diet with dark-green leafy vegetables, orange/yellow vegetables, and fruits to try to revitalize the aging retina. Chapter 8 discusses antioxidants.

Intravitreal injection of anti-VEGF drugs is the treatment of choice for wet age-related macular degeneration. The anti-VEGF drug is injected into the vitreous cavity (Chan, Lau, & Liu, 2007). In some cases, photodynamic therapy and anti-VEGF drugs are used in combination (Hussain, 2007; Mataix, Palacios, Carmen, Garcia-Pous, & Navea, 2010). Photodynamic therapy (PDT) is a clinical procedure that requires an intravenous injection of a special verteporfin dye that is photosensitive with a nonthermal laser. Injection of the dye into the vein makes the eyes and skin photosensitive. The laser beam treats only the leaking blood vessels and not the surrounding retinal tissue. On the day of laser surgery, the patient should wear or bring to wear dark sunglasses, a wide-brimmed hat, gloves, a long-sleeve shirt, long pants, socks, and shoes to protect himself from skin irritation or burns.

Safety Alert *Exposure to direct sunlight after photodynamic therapy can result in third-degree burns or severe skin irritation. The patient should avoid sunlight and bright light exposure for 2 to 5 days after surgery. During daylight, curtains and window shades should be closed, and the patient should avoid skylights and halogen lights. The patient can use regular indoor lights, watch television, and go to the movies but must wait until after sundown to go outside to do any chores.*

Nursing Management

The quality-of-life changes that come with central vision loss can significantly affect the person's communication and ability to just get about on a daily basis. Nursing management of patients with age-related macular degeneration is complex and multifaceted. Application of the nursing process facilitates a comprehensive approach to assessment and care of the patient. The Nursing Process: Patient Care Plan for the Patient With Macular Degeneration box illustrates the application of the nursing process for patients who are visually impaired during the early stages of wet macular degeneration.

Vision loss may affect an individual's cognitive ability with aging; recent studies suggest that vision and cognition may involve a similar nervous system cell loss (Baker et al., 2009). The National Eye Institute (NEI, 2009) has posited a possible connection between genetics and genetic–environmental bases for age-related macular degeneration and cognition. Current research focuses on explicating the clinical courses of both conditions in order to generate hypotheses and develop clinical trials (NEI, 2009). The Evidence-Based Practice box (p. 2041) examines the possible link between age-related macular degeneration and cognitive function.

Discharge Planning

As with any patient with an ocular disorder, discharge planning for the patient with macular degeneration encompasses the following questions, which should be answered before the patient leaves the hospital or place of treatment:

Are all of the necessary prescriptions filled?

Is needed equipment going to be delivered to the patient's home?

Is the next doctor's appointment already made?

Has any outpatient testing been scheduled?

What is the date of the first home care visit?

Does the patient know where to go for follow-up therapy, if appropriate, and how is the patient going to get there?

Main issues to be considered postdischarge include self-care management, resumption of professional or occupational goals, development of a safe environment, resumption of role in family, and prevention strategies. The nurse should reinforce restrictions on the patient's activities imposed by the health care provider, such as staying out of direct sunlight or bright light for several days after photodynamic therapy (PDT). The nurse also should make follow-up calls to patients to ensure they are returning for PDT appointments on time and to see if they have any questions about treatment. All ophthalmologic personnel should be considerate of the age of most macular degeneration patients; provide large, easy-to-read instructions; and not rush them through therapy and/or aftercare.

The following guidelines may assist patients in coping with impaired vision caused by AMD (X-Plain™, 2007):

- Avoid driving in certain conditions. Do not drive at night, in heavy traffic, in bad weather, or on a freeway.
- Seek help traveling. Use public transportation or ask family members to help, especially with night driving.
- Travel with others. Contact your local area agency on aging for a list of vans and shuttles, volunteer driving networks, or ride shares.
- Get good glasses. Optimize the vision you have with the right glasses, and keep an extra pair in the car.
- Use magnifiers. Large print books and magazines also can help you read more easily.
- View with large type on the Internet. Look for websites that use large-sized type fonts, or change the font size on your display.
- Obtain specialized appliances. Some clocks, radios, telephones, and other appliances have extra-large numbers.
- Have proper light in your home. This will help with reading and other activities.
- Remove home hazards. Eliminate throw rugs and possible tripping hazards in your home.
- Ask friends and family members for help. Tell them about your vision problems so that they can help you perform certain tasks and help you recognize people.
- Do not become socially isolated. A common frustration of people with macular degeneration is the inability to recognize other people and greet them by name. If this happens to you, try asking people you know to say hi and to tell you their name when you meet them on the street or in other situations so you can greet them back.
- Take advantage of online networks. The Internet is a good source for support groups and resources for people with macular degeneration.
- Talk to your health care provider. Ask about receiving professional help to make your home safer and more convenient for you to use.

Advise the patient that normal use of the eyes does not hurt vision. Even if sight is lost because of AMD, the patient should not be afraid to use his eyes for reading, watching TV, and other daily activities. Low-vision aids, special lenses, or electronic systems that make images appear larger are available to help people make the most of their remaining vision.

NURSING PROCESS: Patient Care Plan for the Patient with Macular Degeneration

Assessment of Sensory Status Using Gordon's Functional Health Patterns:

- Health Perception Health Management Pattern
- Activity Exercise Pattern
- Cognitive Perceptual Pattern
- Self-Perception Self-Concept Pattern
- Role–Relationship Pattern
- Coping–Stress Tolerance Pattern

Subjective Data	Objective Data
Assessment of Patient/Family Understanding of Vision Loss	**Assessment of Patient/Family Understanding of Vision Loss**
Are you taking any systemic eye medications or antioxidant eye vitamins? Are you on any blood thinners? Do you smoke? Do you wear glasses or contact lenses, or use any low vision aids? Have you had any eye problems or vision problems in the past? Are you seeing black spots or wavy lines in your vision? Have you had any eye treatments, surgeries, or adjustments through lasers? Do you spend a lot of time outdoors, and do you wear ultraviolet protective glasses or sunglasses? Does anyone else in the family have macular degeneration? What is your occupation? Does your problem involve one or both eyes? Have you had any vision or eye tests done? Has treatment already been started for this problem? What has your health care provider told you about this disease?	Distance visual acuity Near visual acuity Intraocular pressure Central blind spot Eye examination Vital signs Interview behavior
Assessment of Patient/Family Coping	**Assessment of Patient/Family Coping**
How are you handling your vision problems? How long have you had this eye problem? Do you have any other health or medical problems? How would you describe your ocular or vision problems, signs, and symptoms? Who are your support systems?	Body language Family support systems Ability to adjust lifestyle
Assessment of Home Environment	**Assessment of Home Environment**
What kind of work do you do? Are you able to perform your activities of daily living (ADLs)?	Home environment Need for assistance Financial stability
Assessment of Patient Response to Illness	**Assessment of Patient Response to Illness**
Tell me about your perceptions of your disease. What impact has this had on your life? How has it impacted family dynamics and your role in the family?	Facial expressions Family relationships Evidence of making necessary adjustments
Assessment of Safety Measures	**Assessment of Safety Measures**
Describe the physical layout of your residence. How much are you able to get around independently? What are your support systems?	Ability to perform ADLs Use of aids such as a cane Caregiver presence and ability to assist

Outcomes and Evaluation Parameters	Planning and Interventions with *Rationales*
1. NURSING DIAGNOSIS: Deficient Knowledge *related to macular degeneration* (NANDA-I © 2012)	
Outcome: Patient/family able to verbalize visual limitations and the necessary lifestyle changes. ***Evaluation Parameters:*** Verbalizes understanding of reason for visual loss. Identifies vision loss. Identifies alternative devices of assistance. Demonstrates ability to use alternative devices.	Provide education and resources about vision loss, means of treatment and management, and role in self-care and alternative devices in assisting. *To assess understanding of vision loss by means of care, management, and follow-up.* Encourage self-care in keeping compliant with and proactive in maintaining vision health. *To assess self-care compliance and management.*

(*continued*)

NURSING PROCESS: Patient Care Plan for the Patient with Macular Degeneration, *continued*

Outcomes and Evaluation Parameters	Planning and Interventions with *Rationales*
	Educate about and promote normalization with enhancement of skills in self-esteem and socialization, and means to access support systems. *To monitor knowledge of social interaction deficits by assessing means of improvement. To use skills that enhance social interactions.* Provide presence, good listening, and skills in socialization, anxiety reduction, relationship building, and accessing support resources. *To monitor active social encounters.* Provide the necessary means to maintain functional activities as long as possible *for a better quality of life.* Assess needs in maintaining everyday functional activities. *Mark appliances with Velcro or material that is recognizable to touch for identification.* Assess needs in limiting frustrations. *To provide access to auto reading or large television screens for entertainment enjoyment. To provide magnifier or bright lights for enhancing vision when applicable.* Provide continued independence. *To monitor everyday activities in assessing continued independence.*
2. NURSING DIAGNOSES: (a) Anxiety *related to altered self-concept secondary to vision loss, especially centrally, and the fear of becoming legally or totally blind.* (b) Ineffective Coping *due to the inability to ask for help related to low self-esteem secondary to vision loss.* (c) Interrupted Family Processes *related to the shock of patient's vision loss* (NANDA-I © 2012)	
Outcome: Experience a reasonable level of anxiety and fear. Evidence of effective family coping. ***Evaluation Parameters:*** Explains levels of anxiety and fear and coping patterns to overcome them. Relates less anxiety and fear after teaching. Expresses an improved level of psychological comfort. Exhibits useful coping mechanisms in managing anxiety and fear. Assertive in asking for assistance when vision is not adequate to perform a given task. Able to express a need for assistance. Obtains the help needed to get the task done. Enjoys family support and meaningful family functions. Identifies altered family processes and reasons why. Exhibits effective family functioning. Comfortable in communicating without the ability to observe facial expressions. Expresses self well in communicating with others. Engages socially. Demonstrates a positive self-image with lifestyle adaptations and the resources of support to assist in keeping a positive attitude. Identifies changes in one's self-esteem. Identifies self in a realistic light with current circumstances. Expresses positive feelings about oneself. Exhibits healthy coping and adaptive skills.	Monitor level of anxiety and fear from mild to panic. *To assess for lower levels of anxiety and fear.* Provide reassurance and comfort with presence and active listening. *To observe improved levels of comfort.* Teach the disease process. *To assess less anxiety and fear with understanding.* Educate the patient that peripheral vision is not lost with macular degeneration. *To assess improved self-concept with acceptance of vision loss.* Assist and teach the patient in using other senses of hearing and touching more effectively. *To enhance communication skills.* Observe communicating with others well. *To increase sociability.* Assist the patient in not feeling embarrassed or less of a person by teaching effective means of asking for assistance when necessary. *To observe obtaining help when needed with a sense of self-satisfaction of obtained task.* Provide presence, active listening, and emotional support. Teach and provide skills for coping; body image, self-role, self-awareness, and self-concept enhancements; and cognitive rethinking, value clarifications, and support resources. *To monitor positive lifestyle adaptations.*

Health Promotion

Because of the possibility of loss of independence as a result of legal blindness from age-related macular degeneration (AMD), it is important for the patient to know whether she has a family history of AMD, because this will directly affect her quality of life. Educational needs must be addressed. These include knowledge of medications (type, dosage, route, and adverse effects), accompanied with a plan to identify the medications by touch if necessary and the location where they are kept. The patient also should be able to demonstrate the instillation of eye medications and identify self-care changes needed to retain independence at the optimum level possible. Educational needs also involves developing a plan for safety measures to be introduced and maintained in the home and work environment. This necessitates the need to address mobility and how the patient will get to work and navigate in the external environment. Nurses should advise patients to avoid smoking, to limit exposure to air pollution and ultraviolet rays, and to maintain good general health (stabilize any hypertension and hyperlipidemia) in order to age well. Anti-oxidant vitamins and minerals also may be helpful in reducing the progression of AMD as discussed in the Complementary & Alternative Therapies box. Regular

EVIDENCE-BASED PRACTICE Age-Related Macular Degeneration and Cognitive Function

Clinical Problem

Vision loss due to aging is a major health problem today, especially with the aging of the members of the baby boomer generation, who are now over 50 years old. Vision loss may affect an individual's cognitive ability with aging; vision and cognition may share a similar nervous system cell loss, as indicated in other studies (Baker et al., 2009). Vision loss from age-related macular degeneration (AMD) is the leading cause of visual impairment among people age 50 and older (Rosenfeld et al., 2009). According to the U.S. Census Bureau (2009; Brault, 2009), 39 million Americans are age 65 and older; among these, approximately 5.3% have some visual impairment, and about 6% have some cognitive decline. Evidence has shown that when an individual cannot visually focus clearly, she cannot think clearly either. Early detection of visual impairment and employment of the best current means of prevention, treatment, and stabilization may make the difference between good and poor quality of life for aging adults both visually and mentally. Nurses must understand how to apply evidence-based findings when managing patients with vision loss, especially older citizens with AMD.

Research Findings

In 2009, the Johns Hopkins Center on Aging and Health completed a Cardiovascular Health Study similar to the one conducted by the National Eye Institute in 2006, which found the association between cognitive ability and AMD visual impairment. The most recent study, performed in 2009, confirmed the findings of the earlier study that aging of mind and aging of vision are related in functional effects. The Cardiovascular Health Study, as reported in Baker et al. (2009) found that early AMD and cognitive function share common related histopathologic changes (extracellular β-amyloid) and risk factors (Baker et al., 2009). Approximately 2,000 participants took the Digit Symbol Substitution Test and the Modified Mini-Mental State Examination to assess cognitive function (Baker et al., 2009). AMD was assessed from retinal photographs compared on a modified Wisconsin AMD grading system for the severity of the aging eye (Baker et al., 2009). The findings revealed an association of low cognitive function and AMD in the older population who participated in the study. The researchers reported that "AMD and cognitive impairment may share similar complex pathogenesis (development) and risk factors (Baker et al., 2009, p. 1). The pathogenesis of AMD was similarly compared with that of Alzheimer's disease. Both conditions involve similar changes in the brain and eye, including the buildup of protein fragments known as beta-amyloid. Both diseases also share similar vascular risk factors: high blood pressure, smoking status, and body mass index, all vascular risk factors indicative of stroke.

Implications for Nursing Practice

Patients who are visually impaired need to be informed about the importance of maintaining cognitive functions through regular stimulating activity, large print books, and the use of special visual systems. Listening to recorded books also may prove to be beneficial in keeping the patient cognitively active. The nurse needs to understand the relationship between cognitive functions and visual function as documented by the Cardiovascular Health Study Group in order to counsel the patient appropriately (Baker et al., 2009). Keeping active on a regular basis may enrich the patient's mental, physical, and psychosocial well-being.

Critical Thinking Questions with answers can be found in the Osborn Student Resources at nursing.pearsonhighered.com.

Sources: Baker, M., Wang, J., Rogers, S., Klein, R., Kuller, L., Larsen, E., & Wong, T. (2009). Early age-related macular degeneration, cognitive function, and dementia. *Archives of Ophthalmology, 127*(5), 667–673; Rosenfeld, P. J., Martidis, A., & Tennant, M. T. (2009). Age-related macular degeneration. In M. Yanoff & J. S. Duker (Eds.), *Ophthalmology* (3rd ed.). St. Louis: Mosby/Elsevier; United States Census Bureau (USCB). (2009). Demographic profiles. Retrieved from http://quickfacts.census.gov/qfd/states/00000.html.

eye examinations are a means to detect early changes of AMD and to assess the use of eye vitamins and any new investigative findings in the treatment of AMD.

Collaborative Management

To achieve potential vision restoration and return to society as before, patients with macular degeneration need a multidisciplinary team approach, including the ophthalmologist, ophthalmologic advance nurse practitioner, nurse, social worker, and optometrist or low vision rehabilitation specialist. In order to meet desired patient outcomes, it is essential that this interdisciplinary team communicate openly with one another in developing and evaluating care of the patient and family (IOM [Institute of Medicine], 2010). To ensure maximum vision potential, vision care is managed by the ophthalmologist with the assistance of nurses and health care providers. As the wet macular degeneration starts to dry and stops leaking, some macular scarring may develop, leaving a degree of visual impairment or possibly legal blindness. The optometrist and low vision rehabilitation specialist will provide the necessary glasses or low vision aids to enhance patients' visual acuity, hopefully to a functional level. Patients will need instructions as well as practice in the best use of vision aids. The social worker is accustomed to helping patients adjust to a new lifestyle with vision deficit.

Infections and Inflammation

All structures of the adnexa (appendages of the eye including eyelids and lacrimal apparatus) and eyeball are subject to infection and inflammation. This section covers some of the most common and serious inflammatory conditions. Inflammatory eye conditions usually are very responsive to treatment, and in most cases the eye is restored to normal with little or no treatment. However, some severe eye infections can mean hospitalization and may result in the loss of vision (and possibly the eye).

Dry Eye Syndrome

Keratoconjunctivitis sicca, or dry eye syndrome (DES), is the result of poor tear production and formation or excessive evaporation (AAO-8, 2010–2011).

Epidemiology, Etiology, and Pathophysiology

Tear film is composed of three components: mucin, aqueous, and lipid. The tear film components may have both protective and homeostatic roles for the ocular surface. The tears maintain a smooth surface for ocular clarity, lubricate to facilitate blinking, and help to protect the eye from ocular infection (Tu & Rheinstrom, 2009).

With aging, especially in menopausal women, dry eyes can become a chronic problem, with less tear surface tension. This results in tears running down the face instead of adhering to the cornea epithelial surface. Dry eyes also can be a side effect of some systemic medications (e.g., propranolol) or systemic disease (e.g., Sjögren's syndrome) (AAO-8, 2010–2011). Dry eyes give the sensation of a sandpaper or "gritty" feeling in the eye, blurred vision, and difficulty focusing up close.

Medical Management

Treatment usually includes frequent use of artificial tear supplements and/or *puncta plugs.* Puncta plugs are plastic or collagen devices that are inserted by an eye health care provider into the puncta (a small drainage opening in the lower eyelid that empties the tears into the canicula, the

COMPLEMENTARY & ALTERNATIVE THERAPIES: DHA Fish Oils and Carotenoids *Nancy Yilk*

THE RESULTS FROM THE NATIONAL INSTITUTES OF HEALTH (NIH) earlier Age-Related Eye Disease Study (AREDS) found that high-dose antioxidant vitamins and minerals (vitamins C and E, beta-carotene, zinc, and copper), taken by mouth, reduced the risk of progression to advanced AMD by 25%, and the risk of moderate vision loss by 19%.

The NIH follow-up study of nutrients, called the Age-Related Eye Disease Study 2 (AREDS2), builds on the previous study to assess if a modified combination of vitamins, minerals, and fish oil can further slow the progression of vision loss from AMD, the leading cause of vision loss in the United States for people over age 60. AREDS2 refines the findings of the original study by adding lutein and zeaxanthin (plant-derived yellow pigments that accumulate in the macula) and the omega-3 fatty acids (derived from fish oils) to the study formulation. Previous observational studies have suggested these nutrients may protect vision. The AREDS2 study is seeking 4,000 people between 50 and 85 years of age with AMD in both eyes, or advanced AMD in one eye. Results from AREDS2 are expected in 2013 (Bernstein, Delori, Richer, van Kuijk, & Wenzel, 2010).

Over the last decade, several epidemiological studies based on food frequency questionnaires suggested that omega-3 polyunsaturated fatty acids could have a protective role in reducing the onset and progression of retinal diseases. The retina has a high concentration of omega-3, particularly DHA, which optimizes fluidity of photoreceptor membranes, retinal integrity, and visual function. Many studies demonstrated that DHA has a protective (e.g., antiapoptotic) role in the retina. From a nutritional point of view, it is known that Western populations, particularly older individuals, have a higher-than-optimal omega-6/omega-3 ratio and should enrich their diet with more fish consumption or have DHA supplementation (Querques, Forte, & Souied, 2011).

The connection between the omega-6/omega-3 fatty acid ratio and development and progression of Age-Related Macular Degeneration was researched. (ARMD was examined with 125 patients diagnosed with ARMD and divided into five groups of 25 patients, according to the Clinical Age-Related Maculopathy Staging System [CARMS].) The control group consisted of 51 patients of similar ages without ARMD. All of them underwent stereobiomicroscopy, fundus photography, and fluorescein angiography. Dietary fatty acid intake was measured using the food frequency questionnaire (FFQ), and the data were analyzed using food nutritient data from McCance and Widdowson's Food Composition Tables, supplemented with a food fatty acid content database (Foodbase, London, UK). A statistically significant difference existed between the omega-6/omega-3 ratio in neovascular ARMD (stage 5) and all other groups including the control group ($p = 0.000020$). The ratio in stage 5 was about 11:1, like in the Western diet. Stage 4 geographic atrophy (GA) has a statistically significant difference in the omega-6/omega-3 ratio compared with stage 1 ($p = 0.000571$), stage 2 ($p = 0.000112$), and stage 3 ($p = 0.000430$). The ratio in the first three groups is about 7–7.5:1 (greater than the Mediterranean diet of 4–5:1, but lower than the Western Diet of 10–20:1). There is no statistically significant difference between the first three stages ($p > 0.05$) and stage 4 and the control group ($p = 0.172388$). The omega-6/omega-3 ratio is connected with the development of neovascular ARMD. The decreased ratio protects against neovascular ARMD. By changing their nutrition habits, people have developed preventive measures against the development of severe neovascular forms of ARMD because of intravitreal anti-VEGF therapy limitations (Mance, Kovacević, Alpeza-Dunato, Stroligo, & Brumini, 2011).

There is increasing recognition that the optical and antioxidant properties of the xanthophyll carotenoids lutein and zeaxanthin play an important role in maintaining the health and function of the human macula. Lutein and zeaxanthin, like all other carotenoids, are not synthesized in the body and must be obtained solely from the diet. The richest sources for these nutrients are dark-green, leafy vegetables, such as spinach and kale, and various orange and yellow fruits and vegetables. Supplements containing lutein are widely available, whereas zeaxanthin supplements are less common. The most recent studies evaluating the impact of lutein and/or zeaxanthin supplementation upon eye health have used 10 mg or more per day. This dosage is well below the 2 mg/kg acceptable daily intake (ADI) established by the Joint FAO/WHO Expert Committee on Food Additives (JECFA). In addition, there are no reported toxic effects of long-term exposure to lutein and zeaxanthin from dietary sources (Bernstein et al., 2010).

References

Bernstein, P. S., Delori, F. C., Richer, S., van Kuijk, F. J., & Wenzel, A. J. (2010). The value of measurement of macular carotenoid pigment optical densities and distributions in age-related macular degeneration and other retinal disorders. *Vision Research, 50*(7), 716–728. Epub 2009 Oct 23.

Mance, T. C., Kovacević, D., Alpeza-Dunato, Z., Stroligo, M. N., & Brumini, G. (2011). The role of omega-6 to omega-3 ratio in development and progression of age-related macular degeneration. *Collegium Antropologicum, 35*(Suppl. 2), 307–310.

Querques, G., Forte, R., & Souied, E. H. (2011). Retina and omega-3. *International Journal of Nutrition and Metabolism,* 2011:748361. Epub 2011 Oct 31.

channel leading the tears outside of the eyes) to obstruct tears from leaving the eye. Patients are instructed on frequent instillation of artificial tears and being consistent with application. If patients find that using the tears once, twice, or a number of times a day provides relief, they are instructed to use the tears the same number of times each day to prevent the eye from drying out completely between applications. Artificial tears usually are an over-the-counter medication, but new artificial tears (cyclosporine ophthalmic emulsion or lubricant) are available by prescription that may keep the eye moist for longer periods of time and help to increase tear production.

Blepharitis

Blepharitis, or **meibomitis,** is inflammation of the eyelids, with redness and crustiness (dry flaky dermis).

Etiology, Epidemiology, and Pathophysiology

The meibomian glands are embedded in the tarsal plate of the eyelids; there are about 35 in the upper lid and about 25 in the lower lid. These glands are arranged in a single row perpendicular to the lid margin and open at the base of the eyelashes. Meibomian gland dysfunction is commonly associated with acne rosacea, which affects more than 13 million adults in the United States (Ganatra & Goldstein, 2009). This is a very common condition in the older population; the meibomian glands build up a waxy deposit, the tears do not function properly, and dry eyes develop (Friedman et al., 2009; Lamb & Weaver, 2008). Patients complain of foreign body sensation, an abnormal feeling that "something is in my eye," along with nasal canthus deposits, itching, tearing, burning, and irritation.

Medical Management

The use of warm compresses and lid scrubs often is adequate treatment. If the condition is chronic and becomes ulcerative, the addition of antibiotic ointment may be indicated. Blepharitis can be difficult to eliminate and usually requires continuous weekly or daily lid scrubs and warm compresses, which are described in Chart 64–3.

Conjunctivitis

Conjunctivitis is an inflammation of the conjunctiva, the clear mucous membrane that covers the sclera of the eye (bulbar

CHART 64–3 Eyelid Cleaning and Comfort Measure

Warm Compresses	This is the use of a facecloth or washcloth placed in lukewarm water. Fold it in half and place it gently over the eyelids for 3 to 8 minutes, especially trying to feel the warmth at the margin of the eyelids to dissolve or melt the waxy discharge that collects at the base of the eyelashes.
Eyelid Scrubs	This is the use of baby shampoo or no-tears shampoo diluted in warm water (3 drops of shampoo to 125 milliliters of water) or saline solution. Use a Q-tip applicator or the soft edge of a facecloth to scrub the eyelid margins gently. Commercial lid scrubs are also available in local pharmacies.

conjunctiva), the inner lining of the eyelids (palpebral conjunctiva), and the space between the lid and globe (forniceal conjunctiva, fornix, or cul-de-sac) (AAO-2, 2010–2011). On an initial evaluation, it is important to try to obtain a culture or cytologic/serologic study on the type of discharge (especially if mucopurulent). The three most common types of conjunctivitis—viral, allergic, and bacterial—are outlined in Chart 64–4 (AAO-2, 2, 2010–2011).

Viral Conjunctivitis

Viral conjunctivitis, commonly referred to as "classic pinkeye," is inflammation caused by an adenovirus. This also is referred to as an epidemic keratoconjunctivitis when the inflammation encompasses both the cornea and the conjunctiva (AAO-8, 2010–2011).

Epidemiology, Etiology, and Pathophysiology

Viral conjunctivitis is a common ocular disease in the United States and worldwide. It frequently occurs in epidemics within families, schools, offices, and military organizations. Viral conjunctivitis can affect all age groups, depending on the specific viral etiology. Usually, adenovirus affects patients ages 20 to 40 years. Herpes simplex virus (HSV) and primary varicella zoster virus (VZV) infection usually affect young children and infants (Scott, 2011). Herpes zoster ophthalmicus results from reactivation of latent VZV infection and may present in any age group. Typically, the picornaviruses affect children and young adults in the lower socioeconomic classes. Viral conjunctivitis can occur equally in men and women (Scott, 2011). Adenoviruses produce viral conjunctivitis with varying degrees of intensity. These infections are spread via respiratory droplets or through direct contact from hands to eyelids, but after recovery, the immunocompetent host is usually protected from further infection by the specific serotype that caused the inflammation (Rubenstein & Virasch, 2009).

Clinical Manifestations and Medical Management

Initially, the inflammation starts unilaterally, but it quickly spreads bilaterally. After about a week of incubation time, such signs and symptoms as clear, sticky mucous discharge; excessive tearing (epiphora); varied hyperemia; small white conjunctival elevations (follicles); light sensitivity (photophobia); foreign body sensation; conjunctival inflammation and irritation; and tissue edema to the point of a transparent bluish hue (chemosis) develop. Preauricular lymph node enlargement and soreness also can be symptoms of viral conjunctivitis (Blanchard, 2008; Ehlers & Shah, 2008).

Treatment includes good hand hygiene, which is imperative, and not sharing washcloths, towels, or pillows because this condition is extremely contagious. Viral conjunctivitis usually will take its course and clear on its own. Patients can use artificial tears, a topical ophthalmic antibiotic or steroid, or decongestant eyedrops for 7 to 10 days. Cold compresses for eye comfort also may help shorten the healing time and the disease course. Patients should not return to school or to work if in the active stages for at least 4 days, and possibly a week to 10 days, owing to the severity and the epidemic nature of viral conjunctivitis.

Allergic Conjunctivitis

Etiology, Epidemiology, and Pathophysiology

Allergic conjunctivitis, sometimes referred to as hay fever or seasonal conjunctivitis, is the most common type of eye allergy (More, 2009). It is associated with type I immediate hypersensitivity reaction mediated by IgE and subsequent mast cell activation stimulated by direct exposure of the ocular mucosal surfaces to environmental allergens. Causative agents may include animal dander, dust, wind, smoke, feathers, ingested foods, makeup, creams, pollen, and systemic medications. It is diagnosed by doing conjunctival scrapings with eosinophilic infiltrates, IgE levels, and histamine elevations (Rubenstein & Virasch, 2009). This is referred to as vernal keratoconjunctivitis when the inflammation involves both the cornea and the conjunctiva. This commonly is a seasonal occurrence, especially in the spring and fall, and usually reoccurs annually. It appears to be most common in young males (Friedman et al., 2009; Lamb & Weaver, 2008).

Clinical Manifestations and Medical Management

Allergic conjunctivitis is usually bilateral, with whitish discharge, marked hyperemia, swelling, burning, stinging, epiphora, and pruritus (Ehlers & Shah, 2008). Symptoms seem to lessen after sleeping and with less environmental exposure by staying indoors. Medical management includes topical decongestant eyedrops for 7 to 10 days, good hand hygiene, cold compresses, and oral antihistamines. If this is a seasonal episode, using preventive measures such as taking oral antihistamines a couple of weeks prior to the season may abate clinical manifestations. It may be necessary for patients to seek medical evaluation and treatment from an allergist.

Bacterial Conjunctivitis

Epidemiology, Etiology, and Pathophysiology

Bacterial conjunctivitis is inflammation of the bulbar and/or palpebral conjunctiva. It is the least common of the three types of conjunctivitis discussed here. Risk factors include frequent exposure to infected individuals, contact lens wear, sinusitis, immunodeficiency states, and exposure to pathogens of sexually transmitted disease at birth (Yeung, 2011). It is common worldwide and occurs in persons of all races, with equal manifestations in males and females (Yeung, 2011). The pathogenesis

CHART 64–4 Three Most Common Forms of Conjunctivitis

Form	Discharge	Eyelid Edema	Lymph Node	Pruritus
Viral conjunctivitis	Clear, sticky	Minimal	Preauricular node enlargement	None
Allergic conjunctivitis (most common)	Clear, runny	Moderate to severe	None	Intense
Bacterial conjunctivitis (least common)	Purulent	Moderate	None	None

of bacterial conjunctivitis usually involves abnormalities of the ocular surface secondary to eyelid or tear film abnormalities or systemic immunosuppression (Rubenstein & Virasch, 2009). The surface tissues of the eye and ocular adnexa are colonized by normal flora such as streptococci, staphylococci, and *Corynebacterium* strains. Alterations in the host defense or in the species of bacteria can lead to clinical infection. Alterations in the flora can occur by external contamination or spread from adjacent infectious sites (e.g., rubbing eyes) (Yeung, 2011).

Clinical Manifestations and Medical Management

Bacterial conjunctivitis is usually unilateral in the early stages but often becomes bilateral, with mucopurulent discharge (containing both mucus and pus), hyperemia, chemosis, eyelid inflammation and irritation (blepharitis), lid crusting, eyelid edema, and eyelids sticking and matting together, especially on awakening in the morning (Ehlers & Shah, 2008). The preauricular nodes usually are not enlarged (Ehlers & Shah, 2008). Medical management includes topical ophthalmic antibiotic drops or ointment for 7 to 10 days, warm compresses, and good hand hygiene technique.

Endophthalmitis

Endophthalmitis is a mucopurulent intraocular inflammation that occurs most often after intraocular surgery, such as for cataract, glaucoma, strabismus, or corneal transplant (Read, 2009). The exogenous pathogens that are harbored on the lids and in the conjunctival fornix invade the eye and inflammation results (Read, 2009). Endophthalmitis also can be a consequence following invasive eye trauma, especially by a contaminated foreign body (Read, 2009). It is an infection of the vitreous in combination with the retinal and uveal layers of the eye. Endophthalmitis is classified as endogenous if it results from hematogenous dissemination of infection from elsewhere in the body or exogenous if the infection results from intraocular surgery (more frequent) or acute ocular injury (Read, 2009).

Etiology, Epidemiology, and Pathophysiology

Causes of endophthalmitis can be bacterial (more frequent) or fungal (Read, 2009; Valluri & Moorthy, 2009). *Staphylococcus epidermidis* is the most widespread exogenous infecting organism of the eye (Read, 2009). Fungal endophthalmitis can be the result of *Candida* species and *Aspergillus* species organisms (Valluri & Moorthy, 2009). Fungal infections are less common and more endogenous (Valluri & Moorthy, 2009). Endogenous infection involves tainted organisms in the blood that settle in the choroid or retina, resulting in retinitis, choroiditis, or chorioretinitis that invades the vitreous chamber, causing an inflammatory reaction and acute endophthalmitis (Read, 2009).

Risk factors for the development of endophthalmitis include possible complications following cataract surgery, which can be related to the patient's history, aseptic technique, or intraocular lens implant (Kohnen et al., 2009). Patients on immunosuppressive therapy also may be at higher risk for endophthalmitis due to poor wound healing (Read, 2009). Additional risk factors are listed in the Risk Factors box.

RISK FACTORS for Developing Endophthalmitis

Cataract surgery	Iris manipulation
Diabetes	Lens fragments in the vitreous
Immunosuppressive therapy	Prolonged surgery time
Intravenous drug abuse	Torn posterior capsule

The incidence of fungal endophthalmitis increases in immunocompromised individuals and intravenous drug abusers, especially because of its spread via contaminated needles (Valluri & Moorthy, 2009).

Clinical Manifestations

Clinical manifestations of endophthalmitis usually are blurred vision (the most general symptom), which can occur rapidly; eye pain; hypopyon (pus within the eye), the most familiar sign; cells and flare in the anterior chamber; corneal edema; conjunctival injection; chemosis; and photophobia (Ehlers & Shah, 2008). Fungal involvement causes vitreous clouding (poor media clarity), which affects light perception and visual acuity (Valluri & Moorthy, 2009).

Diagnostic Procedures and Laboratory Tests

Diagnostic procedures for endophthalmitis may include fluorescein angiography and ultrasonography (B-scan), which is useful for cloudy media. (See the Laboratory and Diagnostic Tests box, p. 2019.) Anterior chamber and vitreous tap or vitreous biopsy is recommended if a specimen is indicated (Read, 2009). Vitreous and aqueous Gram stain and semiquantitative cultures are essential (Read, 2009). Endophthalmitis caused by certain gram-positive organisms seems to have a better prognosis (Read, 2009).

Medical Management

Aggressive treatment of endophthalmitis is crucial to avoid a severe and enduring vision loss (Read, 2009). Evisceration (removal of the eye's contents, leaving the sclera shell and extraocular muscles intact) often is the treatment of choice for advanced endophthalmitis with severe recurrent mucopurulent infection and no light perception vision. Treatment with intravitreous, subconjunctival, topical, and/or systemic antibiotics, providing broad-spectrum coverage for both gram-positive and gram-negative organisms, is warranted before waiting for any culture results. Surgical management, by performing a pars plana vitrectomy, offers a good prognosis for vision restoration, possibly as high as 20/50 in about half the cases (Read, 2009). With a pars plan vitrectomy, the ophthalmologist penetrates the eyeball, aspirates the vitreous, and replaces it with saline. The saline replaces the vitreous at a constant pressure in order to keep the eye from collapsing (Patel, 2011). Being aware of early changes in patients' vision, and/or recognizing suspicious complaints and responding with immediate intervention, can save sight.

Nursing Management

Time can be critical with certain infections and inflammation problems. When a patient presents with endophthalmitis, signs and symptoms usually have a rapid onset (blurry vision, cornea edema, hypopyon, cells and flare in the anterior chamber, hyperemia, chemosis, eye pain, and/or photophobia), and the nurse should provide an immediate referral to the ophthalmologist, as this can affect the final visual outcome. The ophthalmologist will perform further evaluation with a complete ocular examination and treatment. Dry eyes, blepharitis, and conjunctivitis can usually be treated with the appropriate eyedrops or ointment. Once the immediate problem has been assessed and treated, the nurse has the opportunities for education and intervention with patients and family in preserving vision function and promoting eye health. The nurse should instruct the patient on compliance in the use of eye medications (especially following cataract surgery) and prevention of eye infections and inflammation problems through proper hygiene, clearing eyelashes, makeup removal (if applicable), and avoidable acts or areas of contamination, as well as proper precautions to prevent the recurrence of infection and inflammation problems.

Health Promotion

Patient education includes information on the seriousness of endophthalmitis and the potential loss of vision (and possibly the eye itself). Early recognition is critical, as is knowledge of risk factors and clinical manifestations, which were discussed previously. Early detection and subsequent treatment are necessary to prevent permanent vision loss. Nurses need to focus on patient compliance with follow-up after any intraocular surgery. The patient is taught how to instill postoperative eyedrops properly for the full benefit of treatment. The patient is also instructed on symptoms of adverse reactions to treatment (decreased vision) and medications, as well as what to do if these occur. Eyedrops must be administered properly to provide the full benefit of the medication and prevent waste. Having the patient give a return demonstration with artificial tears will allow the nurse to determine the patient's ability for self-medication. If multiple drops are prescribed, it is helpful to give the patient an index card with the list of drops and when to use them. This will assist in preventing drug errors and promoting compliance.

Collaborative Management

Treatment of infection and inflammation problems requires an interdisciplinary team approach. In order to meet desired patient outcomes, it is essential that this interdisciplinary team communicate openly with one another in developing and evaluating care of the patient and family (IOM [Institute of Medicine], 2010). With most of the types of inflammation discussed (conjunctivitis and blepharitis), the team is made up of the health care provider and the nurse, with the health care provider performing diagnostic and treatment functions and the nurse providing direct patient care. However, there is one exception with allergic conjunctivitis, in which case an allergist may be used to consult on the cause/s of the allergy and types of medication to be used in treatment.

With endophthalmitis, more members of the interdisciplinary team are involved. The best result for patients with endophthalmitis is to treat this problem as an ophthalmic emergency, which mandates prompt therapy if vision is to be preserved. A multidisciplinary team approach (including the ophthalmologist; the surgeon, if different from the ophthalmologist; the ophthalmic advance nurse practitioner; the nurse; and the optometrist) is optimal in management of endophthalmitis (IOM [Institute of Medicine], 2010). The patient is followed daily at the clinic; if the patient is not compliant, hospitalization and surgery (the pars plana vitrectomy) may be warranted. The nurse practitioner or nurse can provide the necessary education and should stress the importance of follow-up to help ensure compliance with the endophthalmitis treatment regimen. It is imperative that the patient understand that the long-term goal of treatment is to prevent loss of the eye or avoid permanent vision loss, a goal that can be reached only with continued use of medication and eyedrops. Once the endophthalmitis is responding to treatment, the optometrist can provide follow-up evaluations between regular health care provider visits and make necessary changes as indicated, thereby also contributing to the patient's care.

Retinal and Vitreal Disorders

The retina and vitreous are two very important areas of the eye that function to transmit information, carried by light rays, to the brain via the optic nerve. When disease or injury causes clouding of the vitreous or damage to the retina, the result is a partial or complete loss of vision. Common disorders of the retina and vitreous include retinal detachment, posterior vitreous detachment, retinal breaks, vitreous hemorrhage, and nonrhegmatogenous and rhegmatogenous retinal detachment.

Retinal Detachment

Retinal detachment (RD) is the separation of the sensory retinal layers from the retinal pigment epithelium, where subretinal fluid collects in the potential space (AAO-12, 2010–2011). The typical pathologic sequence that results in a retinal detachment is vitreous liquefaction (conversion of the vitreous to liquid consistency) followed by a posterior vitreous detachment (PVD), which in turn causes retinal breaks at the sites of significant vitreoretinal adhesions, which allows vitreous fluid to pass into the subretinal space (Wilkinson, 2010).

Epidemiology, Etiology, and Risk Factors

The annual incidence of retinal detachments (RD) is about 12 per 100,000 population, and the incidence of retinal breaks or tears in individuals over 10 years is about 11%; however, most retinal tears do not lead to RD (Greven, 2009). Primary high-risk factors for retinal detachment may include trauma, high myopia, lattice degeneration, retinoschisis (gradual splitting of the retina into two distinct layers), retinopathy, tumors, and postcataract surgery. Secondary risk factors may include vitreous hemorrhage, diabetic retinopathy, severe uveitis, severe hypertension, Marfan's syndrome, and toxemia from pregnancy.

Clinical Manifestations and Laboratory and Diagnostic Tests

Clinical manifestations of a retinal detachment are outlined in Chart 64–5. Figure 64–8 ◆ shows the observation of retinal detachment that involves the macula through a direct ophthalmoscope.

Medical Management

This condition usually requires immediate surgical repair, especially if the macula is still intact. If the macula is detached and there is choroidal edema, there is time to place patients on steroids for a few days prior to surgery. This allows time to decrease the edema and give the retinal tissue time to heal, thus providing more surgical manipulability and possibly a better surgical outcome.

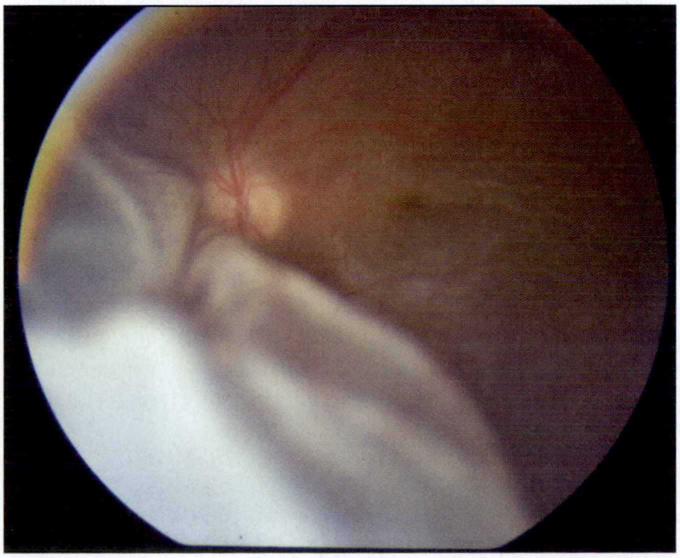

FIGURE 64–8 ◆ Retinal detachment with macula off.
Source: Lucie S. Elfervig.

CHART 64–5 Clinical Manifestations of a Retinal Detachment

Sign	Description
Asymptomatic	The patient does not realize anything is wrong when the retinal detachment is so far in the periphery near the ora serrata (the demarcation between the retina and the ciliary body).
Blurry vision	The patient will notice that the central vision is blurry or decreased; this is because the retinal detachment involves the central macula and edema.
Shower of floaters	The patient will notice black/gray spots, clear amoeba-type spots in his vision, or "shade or cobwebs," which are more noticeable against a light background or blue skies; these are clumps of vitreous proteins or clumps of red blood cells from a hemorrhage.
Flashes of light	The patient will notice flashing lights (like a light bulb breaking) in the peripheral vision; this is more common when getting up from a lying position or entering a dark environment. This is usually caused by the vitreous pulling on the retinal sensory layer.
Curtain or veil	The patient will notice a shadow, or a curtain- or veil-like shape, come across the visual field; this is usually the detached retina flap or retinal layers' separation moving around in the vitreous crossing in the central line of sight. The superior temporal quadrant is the most common location for a retinal detachment, so the patient will notice an inferior nasal flap or vision loss.
No pain	The patient does not experience any pain with a spontaneous retinal detachment but may panic when noticing vision changes or loss.

Source: Adapted from Friedman, N., Kaiser, P., & Pineda, R. (2009). *The Massachusetts eye and ear infirmary, illustrated manual of ophthalmology* (3rd ed.). Philadelphia: Saunders/Elsevier.

Posterior Vitreous Detachment

Etiology, Clinical Manifestations, and Medical Management

Posterior vitreous detachment (PVD) occurs when the vitreous separates from the retinal surface and liquefies (syneresis), usually due to aging and increased axial length of the eye. This occurrence typically starts unilaterally; detachment in the fellow eye usually starts later (AAO-12, 2010–2011). Symptoms of only occasional flashes and floaters usually are the most common signs. The health care provider evaluates the symptoms and makes a diagnosis. If the diagnosis proves to be PVD, and there are no tears, holes, or detachments located, time would allow the ophthalmologist the opportunity to observe the condition and have the patient return to the office in 2 to 3 weeks for a reevaluation. If symptoms increase or become more obvious, the patient should be instructed to return to the ophthalmologist's office sooner. Posterior vitreous detachment can be a cause of retinal detachments. The vitreous is firmly attached at the vitreous base (near ora serrata), the disc margins, the macula, and large vessel margins; retinal breaks can occur more easily in these areas with a spontaneous or traumatic PVD (AAO-12, 2010–2011).

Retinal Breaks

Retinal breaks are retinal tears or holes. They can have the same warning signs as a retinal detachment. Patients with retinal breaks need to be evaluated by an ophthalmologist and receive a dilated fundus examination. If a retinal detachment is highly probable, the patient should be instructed to stay quiet and refrain from lifting heavy objects and straining. If it is only a small retinal break, it can usually be treated with cryopexy (use of intensely cold gas to freeze tissue around the tear) or laser photocoagulation (use of a laser to burn small areas around the tear); both of these procedures stimulate formation of scar tissue, which will mend the tear.

Vitreous Hemorrhage

Vitreous hemorrhage is the presence of blood or red blood cells in the vitreous humor or cavity; it is commonly caused by diabetic retinopathy, retinal detachment, or trauma. Vision is usually blurry to very poor depending on the degree of blood present, resulting in painless, unilateral vision loss. Vitreous hemorrhages often are observed over time to see whether the blood will reabsorb spontaneously. If it does not reabsorb, surgery may be indicated.

Nonrhegmatogenous and Rhegmatogenous Detachment

Etiology and Pathophysiology

The two major types of retinal detachment are nonrhegmatogenous and rhegmatogenous (*Rhegmatogenous* means "arising from a rupture or tear"). Nonrhegmatogenous detachment may include serous and traction retinal detachment. Serous detachment occurs from serous leakage (clear fluid) that separates retinal intraocular layers between the retina and retinal pigment epithelium, or separates choroidal intraocular layers between the choroid and sclera, which pulls the retina off as a result of inflammation (Rogers & Duker, 2008). Traction detachment occurs from scar tissue caused by fibrovascular formation of the vitreous that detaches the retina. This type of detachment is more common in long-standing diabetes with inflammation and in patients who have had previous ocular trauma (Rogers & Duker, 2008). Rhegmatogenous detachment occurs from a break or a tear in the retina. The break or tear can occur when the vitreous degenerates and tugs the retina off by separating its sensory layers (Rogers & Duker, 2008). Individuals who are at greater risk of retinal and vitreal problems are high myopics (a high ratio of astigmatism), those with lattice degeneration or vitreous aging, and those with a previous history of RD or retinal tears.

Medical Management

Retinal tears, posterior vitreous detachments, and/or vitreous hemorrhages should all be referred immediately for possible medical or surgical treatment to prevent retinal detachment (RD.) Most retinal or vitreal problems have the same signs and symptoms as a RD, so the referral for a comprehensive eye examination is indicated (Larkin, 2011). Surgical repairs for retinal detachment usually are outpatient procedures that do not require hospitalization. The surgical procedures can be as simple as cryopexy or laser photocoagulation or can be more invasive with pneumatic retinopexy or vitrectomy. In pneumatic retinopexy, the ophthalmologist injects a bubble of gas into the eyeball to flatten the retina, allowing a seal to form between the retina and the wall of the eye. Treatment of vitreal hemorrhage is considered to be an emergent situation requiring surgical intervention (Larkin, 2011). In vitrectomy, some of the vitreous is removed and replaced with either a gas bubble or saline.

Central Retinal Artery Occlusion

Central retinal artery occlusion (CRAO) is a vascular infarction to the central retinal artery wherein blockage by an embolus results in acute unilateral vision loss, afferent pupillary defect, and decreased carotid pulse with associated carotid bruit (Ehlers & Shah, 2008). Other manifestations may include narrowed retinal arterioles, pale optic disc, and diffused pale posterior retina, except in the fovea, where there is a classic "cherry-red spot," a hallmark sign for central retinal artery occlusion that generally vanishes in about 2 weeks with the return of normal color (Rogers & Duker, 2008).

Emergency measures are taken to decrease intraocular pressure with topical antiglaucoma drops, oral carbonic anhydrase inhibitors, and an anterior chamber tap (paracentesis). Other attempts to restore perfusion to the central retinal artery may include trying to restore vasodilation by rebreathing CO_2 (breathing inside a paper bag), using hyperbaric chamber treatment, and performing intermittent digital massage of the globe with the eyelid closed as soon as possible (ideally within less than 24 hours); however, these latter two measures, breathing in a paper bag and using digital massage of the globe, have not been proven effective (Ehlers & Shah, 2008).

Once stability has been established and the nurse or ophthalmologist is able to take a medical history, it is imperative to ask the patient about vascular diseases that cause hardening of the arteries and listen with a stethoscope for carotid bruits. The ophthalmologist needs to refer patients to an internist or family health care provider for appropriate tests and a complete physical evaluation. Tests that are often ordered are an erythrocyte sedimentation rate (ESR) to rule out giant cell or temporal arteritis, a carotid ultrasound to check for plaque formation or carotid insufficiency, an echocardiogram for heart and valve malfunctions, a visual field test to check for a residual temporal island, a blood pressure check, and a diabetic evaluation (Rogers & Duker, 2008). Typically, patients seek medical attention after 24 hours; the nurse should instruct patients with cardiovascular anomalies to seek emergency eye care immediately if any of the earlier ocular signs or symptoms occurs.

Nursing Management

Time can be crucial with certain retinal or vitreal problems. In first assessing for retinal or vitreal problems, it is imperative to provide timely and appropriate triage and referral, as promptness of treatment can affect the final visual outcome. When a patient presents with a retinal detachment (RD), especially if the macula is intact, surgery is usually done that day to preserve central vision. The nurse should instruct the patient not to eat or drink anything from that time forward, because emergency surgery may be indicated. The nurse needs to record the time and contents of the patient's most recent food consumption for the record. The patient's activity is restricted, and the patient should be kept quiet at all times, with no straining, heavy lifting, or bending over. When a patient presents with vitreous detachment, a watchful waiting occurs that may require no treatment other than vigilance and observing the patient for retinal detachment or retinal tear. If floaters are significantly affecting vision, surgery (vitrectomy) is considered; in this case, the nurse must prepare the patient for surgery and, subsequently, provide postoperative care. With vitreous hemorrhage, the nurse must understand the cause in order to institute appropriate care. Vitreal hemorrhage is most commonly caused by proliferative diabetic retinopathy, posterior vitreous detachment, and ocular trauma. The nurse must treat the underlying condition as well as the immediate presenting problem. The immediate problem often is treated with a vitrectomy; in this case, the nurse must prepare the patient for surgery, followed by postoperative care and preparation for home care. See Chapters 17 and 19 for preoperative and postoperative management, respectively.

The nurse's responsibility, once the retinal or vitreal disorder has been diagnosed and treated, is educating the patient and family in how to preserve vision function and promoting eye health by instructing the patient on prevention and safety measures in case the retinal or vitreal problem recurs. The nurse also shares information about how to reduce risk factors and about available resources for maintaining self-care and a safe environment. The nurse monitors the patient's anxiety and comfort levels to determine ongoing patient needs and provides assistance as appropriate.

Health Promotion

Patient education includes information on the seriousness of retinal and vitreal detachments and the potential loss of vision if they are left untreated or unevaluated. Early recognition of signs or symptoms described previously and/or vision loss is an urgent reason to see the eye care provider immediately. Health promotion activities include educating the patient on how to prevent reoccurrence of retinal and vitreous problems. Regular eye examination is one way to do this; it is imperative for people to keep track of the status of their vision, especially after the age of 50.

Collaborative Management

The best result for patients with retinal and vitreal detachments is to treat the problem as an ophthalmic emergency, which may mandate prompt therapy if vision is to be preserved. A multidisciplinary team approach, including the ophthalmologist, ophthalmic advance nurse practitioner, and optometrist, assists in the management of detachments. In order to meet desired patient outcomes, it is essential that this interdisciplinary team communicate openly with one another in developing and evaluating care of the patient and family (IOM [Institute of Medicine], 2010). Prompt treatment with laser or surgical intervention by the ophthalmologist may be indicated, or close evaluation and follow-up may be all that the ophthalmologist, optometrist, or ophthalmologic advance nurse practitioner needs to do. The signs and symptoms of retinal and vitreal detachments are similar and cannot always be differentiated without a complete eye examination and evaluation to determine the seriousness of the problem.

Eye Trauma and Injury

Epidemiology and Etiology of Eye Trauma

Eye injury is a significant and disabling health problem. Injuries to the eye from traumatic events are common occurrences that should be treated as emergencies requiring immediate attention.

In the United States, approximately 800,000 workers experience an eye injury requiring treatment in an emergency department, inpatient or outpatient facility, or private health care provider's office each year (CDC, 2008). Fortunately, advances in microsurgical techniques over the past decade have allowed vision to be saved in some of these injured eyes. In persons under 25 years of age, ocular trauma is the number-one cause of vision loss (Eye Facts, 2011; Mattera, 2011). According to the

American Academy of Ophthalmology, sports-related injuries cause over 40,000 eye injuries in the United States each year (Eye Facts, 2011). Polycarbonate eyeglasses have been found to offer some protection, resulting in a lower incidence of severe eye injuries to those wearing them, but they cannot protect the eye from all risks of injury (Natarajan, Shome, & Gadgil, 2007). Common and frequent injuries to the eyes and eyelids are discussed next.

Eye emergencies include cuts, scratches, foreign objects in the eye, burns, chemical exposure, and blunt injuries to the eye or eyelid (Kanski & Bowling, 2011). Because the eye is easily damaged, any of these conditions can lead to vision loss if left untreated.

Eye trauma from sports is very common. Some of the more common eye injuries occur during hockey, archery, darts, use of BB guns, bicycling, sports that involve rackets, baseball, boxing, and basketball (Eye Facts, 2011). Eye trauma also may be caused by airborne pieces of wood, metal, glass, stone, and other materials. Blunt injury by fist may also cause damage to the eye, as may traffic collisions that involve head and facial trauma. Other causes of intraocular trauma may arise from workplace tools or even common household implements.

A black eye usually is caused by direct trauma to the eye or face. Accidents, occupational injuries, sports injuries, and fights are some of the risk factors associated with black eyes. The actual pathophysiology resulting from an eye injury is dependent on the type of injury. Certain types of skull fractures can result in bruising around the eyes, even without direct trauma to the eye. The bruise is caused by bleeding under the skin. The tissue surrounding the eye turns black and blue, then gradually becomes purple, green, and yellow over several days. The abnormal coloring disappears within 2 weeks. Usually, swelling of the eyelid and tissue around the eye also occurs. Occasionally, serious damage to the eye itself occurs from the pressure of the swollen tissue. Bleeding inside the eye can reduce vision, cause glaucoma, or damage the cornea.

Chemical Burns

Chemical burns are burns to the eye, usually the surface, from acids, alkalies, and irritants that come in contact with the eye (Randleman, 2011). They occur most frequently at work; however, they also occur at home from cleaning products or other regular household products such as cleaning solutions, garden chemicals, and solvents. Chemical burns require immediate irrigation by washing the eye continuously for 15 to 25 minutes. If the chemical is (or is suspected to be) alkaline, the eye should be irrigated for 35 minutes or more, especially over the cornea. It is important to keep in mind that chemical agents can come in many forms—liquid, gas, or solid—and may be alkaline or acid.

Alkaline ($pH > 7$) burns usually are more serious than acid ($pH < 7$) burns, because an alkali (hydroxyl ions) continues to burn or damage tissue after contact if it is not completely removed or neutralized. The most common alkaline agents are lye, lime, potash, ammonia, drain cleaners, chemical cleaners and detergents, fertilizers, industrial solvents, and air bag powder. The most common offensive acid agents are battery acid and laundry bleach (Ehlers & Shah, 2008; Kanski & Bowling, 2011). If litmus paper is available, the nurse should use it as an indicator. This is also called a pH paper test. In this test, a small piece of the litmus paper is placed on the lower lid, where it gives a reading of the current pH level, indicating whether more irrigation is needed. Irrigation of the eye should continue until the litmus paper illustrates a neutral pH of 7 to 7.3.

Nursing Management

When a patient presents with a chemical burn to the eye, copious irrigation of the eyeball, fornix, and facial area with water for 15 to 25 minutes is crucial for possibly saving the cornea, and therefore vision, before doing anything else. After the rinsing, an initial evaluation can be made. If the evaluation indicates that it is not a true emergency situation or that an immediate referral is not necessary and the patient's condition is stable, it is appropriate for the nurse to take a detailed history to identify the offending chemical and determine whether a neutralizing agent is available. The nurse should record the necessary information, measure the visual acuity of both eyes, check pupil responses, and assess how much ocular involvement seems to have taken place. After initial assessment of an eye emergency and initial treatment is instituted, the nurse should place a protective shield over the eye if indicated.

Foreign Bodies

A foreign body may threaten vision if the object enters the eye itself or damages the cornea or lens. Foreign bodies propelled at high speed, such as grinders or hammering metal on metal, present the highest risk. With any of these injuries, ongoing damage may occur in spite of prompt treatment. It is important to flush the eye with clean water or saline and seek urgent medical care.

Etiology and Clinical Manifestations

In checking the eyes for foreign bodies, the nurse must never remove a penetrating foreign body. Instead, she should refer the patient immediately to an ophthalmologist. Clinical manifestations consist of painful loss of vision with a burning sensation, corneal swelling, excessive tearing, hyperemia, chemosis, photophobia, and blepharospasm.

Diagnostic Tests and Medical Management

If it is necessary to order magnetic resonance imaging (MRI) of the patient, there are two things to keep in mind. First, MRI should not be done if a metal intraocular foreign body is known or suspected to be present, because the MRI could move or dislodge the foreign body, thereby causing more ocular damage. Second, if previous retinal repair surgery was done, it is necessary to check with the patient's ophthalmologist to determine whether an encircling band or scleral buckle was used in the retinal surgical repair; in the past (over 5 years ago), metal clips or staples were used to secure the encircling band or scleral buckle on the retina, and the MRI magnification could remove or dislodge these clips. These metal clips have not been used in retinal repair more recently.

Emergency treatment involves copious irrigation that may require flipping the upper lid (Figures 64–9◆, 64–10◆, and 64–11◆) and pulling down the lower lid (fornix), using a lid speculum, or instilling topical ophthalmic anesthetic drops to allow the eye to be open sufficiently to complete a more effective irrigation. The health care provider should be aware that any type of ocular emergency, trauma, injury, intraocular foreign body, or laceration may need tetanus prophylaxis.

Treatment may include topical ophthalmic cycloplegics (drugs which dilate the pupil and paralyze the ciliary muscle) for comfort, topical ophthalmic antibiotic eyedrops and ointment for infection, topical ophthalmic steroid drops for inflammation, and a sterile eye patch and/or shield, pending the health care provider's orders.

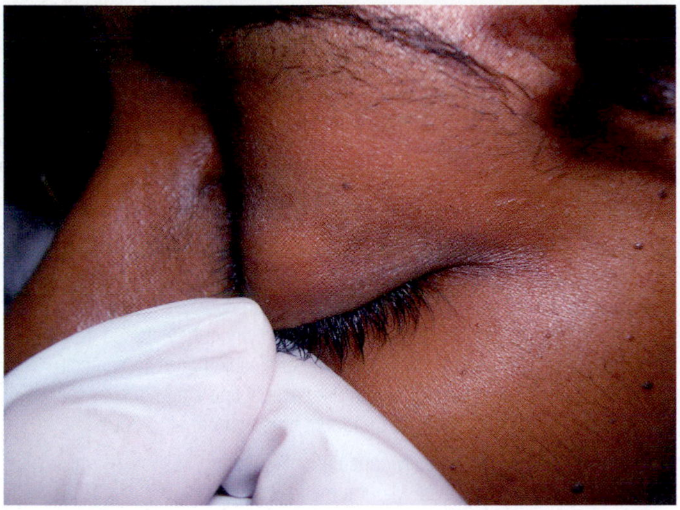

FIGURE 64–9 ◆ Demonstration of flipping the upper eyelid. First step: placing finger on the edge of the eyelid/lashes, slightly pulling downward.
Source: Lucie S. Elfervig.

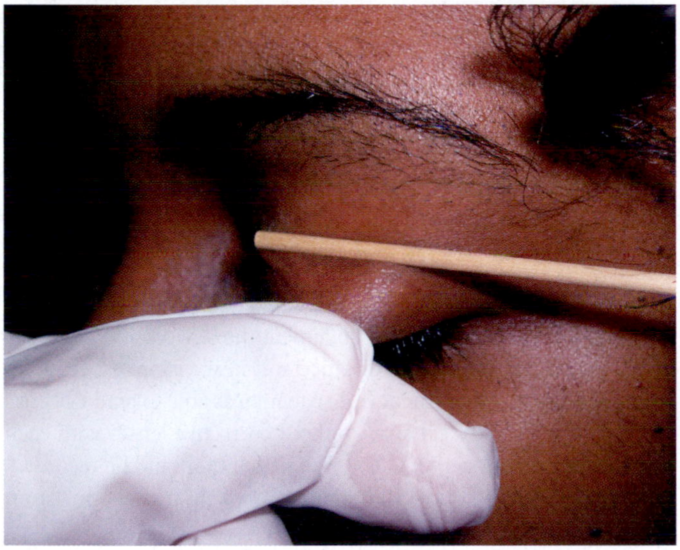

FIGURE 64–10 ◆ Demonstration of flipping the upper eyelid. Placing wooden side of the cotton tip applicator to roll eyelid.
Source: Lucie S. Elfervig.

Nursing Management

The nurse should evaluate the eye using the format described in the Visual Assessment section in Chapter 62, starting on page 1978. When an intraocular foreign body is present, it is critical to leave the object in place and stabilize it, especially if it is protruding from the eye. The object should not be removed, and the nurse should be very careful not to put pressure on the foreign body. It usually is best to keep the patient in a sitting position, because lying down or reclining may advance the intraocular foreign body deeper into the eye with the natural force of gravity. The nurse needs to instruct the patient not to eat or drink anything until it is determined whether emergency surgery will be needed. The patient's activity should be restricted, and the patient should be kept comfortable and quiet. If ordered by the health care provider, the nurse should administer pain medication while the patient is awaiting further evaluation by the ophthalmologist to determine the best course of treatment.

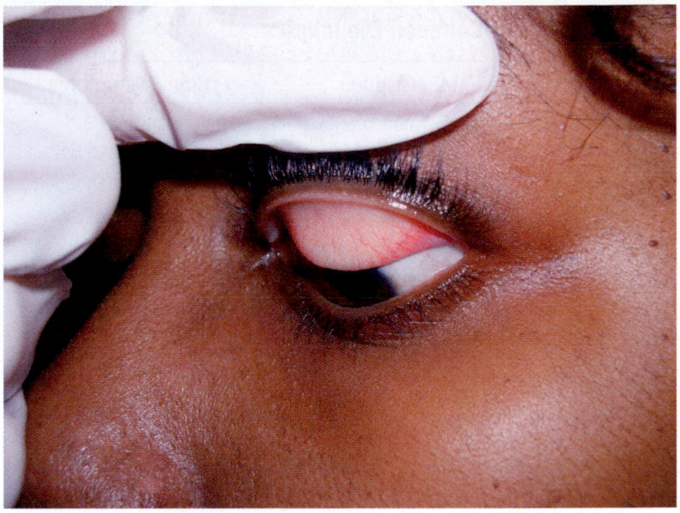

FIGURE 64–11 ◆ Demonstration of flipping the upper eyelid. Lid turned backwards exposing the conjunctiva.
Source: Lucie S. Elfervig.

A pupil check should be done to see whether the pupils are equal, round, and reactive to light and accommodation (PERRLA), and the nurse should be alert to afferent pupillary defect (APD). Normal eyes constrict when light is shined in one of them; if they dilate, there may be optic nerve injury. If a patient is complaining of minor eye irritation and not a true eye emergency, and if a foreign body is found on evaluation to be an eyelash, dust, or lint that is easily removable with a tissue or irrigation, this can be done by the nurse. It is essential to document the patient's history, the type of foreign body, and how it was removed.

Open Globe

Open globe or ruptured globe is an open eyeball with a laceration, penetrating injury, or intraocular foreign body. The rupture is usually caused by blunt trauma, a motor vehicle crash, sports-related trauma, a fistfight, or a high-velocity object creating an open, jagged-edged wound (Ehlers & Shah, 2008; Kanski & Bowling, 2011; Robson, Behrman, & Abbuhl, 2007). A ruptured globe is commonly associated with a dislocated lens, retinal detachment, vitreous hemorrhage, and a wide area of tissue damage. Patients can present with the following ocular signs: hyphema (bleeding in the eye), chemosis (edema of the conjunctiva of the eye), acute diffuse subconjunctival hemorrhage, corneal laceration, irregular pupil, and lens cloudiness. Open globes often come in conjunction with orbital fractures, so it is important for the nurse to observe the patient for facial hypoesthesia (insensitivity to touch) over the cheek, to palpate gently along the orbital rim for a step-off notch area (referring to a type of fracture), and to note whether diplopia is present (Ehlers & Shah, 2008; Kanski & Bowling, 2011). Once the diagnosis of ruptured globe has been confirmed, immediate surgical priority is instituted. The prognosis for the final visual outcome is guarded.

Nursing Management

Immediate actions for the nurse to take in the event of an open globe injury include the following:

- Assess open wounds, intraocular foreign body, or protrusion, and support appropriately; refer immediately to the emergency department.

CHART 64–6 Common Eye Injuries

Injury	Description	Signs/Symptoms	Nursing Assessment
Corneal abrasion	Scratched area of the cornea causing corneal defect.	Foreign body sensation, eye pain, epiphora, photophobia, blurry vision.	Obtain the patient history: When did the injury occur, where did it occur, and under what circumstances?
Contact lens overwear (superficial punctate keratitis [SPK] or giant papillary conjunctivitis [GPC])	Result of contact lens abuse, because of sleeping in them too long, poor hygiene of maintaining contact lenses, or wearing damaged or infected lenses.	Same as above with the addition of pruritus, halos, and mucous discharge.	Contact lenses need to be removed or—if damaged or contaminated with an infection or deposits—thrown away. The patient should refrain from wearing contact lenses for 1 to 2 weeks or until all eye irritation is cleared. Take a good history of the patient's signs and symptoms and note when they started. Record contact lens type, age, length of time worn, type of cleaning and storage solutions, and last time cleaned. Depending on the severity and stage of overwear, the patient may need to seek medical treatment (Friedman et al., 2009).
Corneal foreign body	Small, superficial corneal lesions that give the sensation of having sand or grit in the eye.	The same as above with the addition of corneal edema.	Metal, vegetation, and insects usually cause an inflammatory response, which can result in swelling and infection. Mineral matter can be less irritating. Take a good history of when the injury occurred and the nature of the injury; note whether the patient was wearing safety glasses or goggles. Evaluate the eye with topical anesthetic ophthalmic drop and staining, and invert the upper eyelid to check for foreign bodies (if indicated). Management may require irrigation only to remove a minor irritant. If a corneal defect is present, seek medical treatment (Friedman et al., 2009).

Source: Adapted from Friedman, N. J., Kaiser, P. K., & Pineda, R. (2009). *The Massachusetts eye and ear infirmary, illustrated manual of ophthalmology* (3rd ed.). Philadelphia: Saunders/Elsevier.

- Obtain visual acuity and assess for other ocular symptoms; if this is not possible, an immediate referral to the emergency department is indicated.
- Observe for facial hypoesthesia (loss of sensation).
- Obtain a history surrounding the circumstances.

Other Common Eye Injuries

Many other eye injuries are commonly seen, such as corneal abrasions, contact lens overwear, and corneal foreign body. These injuries are outlined in Chart 64–6. Minutes count in true eye emergencies. When the nurse is first assessing eye injuries, it is imperative to provide timely and appropriate triage, treatment, and referral, which can affect the final visual outcome.

Laboratory and Diagnostic Procedures

A visual acuity test is a must and usually is the first test done following an eye injury, using standard visual acuity charts for near- and farsightedness. Using a pinhole is one way to measure distance visual acuity without corrective lenses (Friedman et al., 2009). The pinhole test is a simple test that lets a health care provider find out whether poor visual acuity is caused by refractive error or by an eye health problem. Several pinholes, 0.5 to 2 mm in diameter, are punched in a card. The patient selects one and looks through it with one eye at a time, without wearing corrective lenses. If visual acuity is improved, the defect is refractive; if not, it is organic. The pinhole effect results from blocking peripheral light waves, which are most distorted by refractive error. The pinholes only allow the passage of light that is perpendicular to the lens, and thus does not need to be bent prior to being focused onto the retina. The patient is instructed to view the Snellen chart with the pinholes up (below right) and then again with them in the down position (below left). If the deficit corrects with the pinholes in place, the acuity issue is related to a refractive problem (Goldberg, 2009). Usually a pinhole occlude (an opaque black disk with one or more holes in it) is used to conduct the test.

When standard testing charts are not available, the nurse may use the best means available to obtain some measure of vision; often a newspaper or book (standard print read at 14 to 16 inches is ~ 20/40 acuity) is used for near vision, and looking out a window at a license plate may work for distance vision. Sometimes the nurse has to be inventive when testing for visual acuity. When recording vision results, the nurse should document the devices and materials that were used for obtaining distance and near vision, especially if not using standard equipment (e.g., patient was able to read a license plate appropriately 10 feet away without corrective lenses with each eye separately and together). Any type of acuity should be recorded, whether it is counting fingers, hand motion, light perception, or no light perception.

Health Promotion

Health promotion focuses on identifying and educating the patient about the risk factors for traumatic injuries to the eye. Educational goals include instructing the patient on medications to take as prescribed (type, usage, route, method of administration, and any adverse effects to look for). This may include antibiotics and analgesics. The patient should be advised of ways to manage pain, and to stay still and rest during the early stages of injury when pain is susceptible to movement. The patient also should be instructed to contact the health care provider in the event of increased pain, abnormal discharge (including bleeding), and/or diminished vision. The patient should be encouraged to take safety precautions as long as the eye is bandaged or vision is diminished. Also, the patient is encouraged to keep eye appointments as scheduled.

Visual impairment from ocular trauma may lead to the loss of independence. Therefore, it is important for the patient to know what services are provided by the community and government, because this may directly affect the patient's quality of life. Spiritual or psychological assistance may also be warranted, particularly when there has been severe trauma.

Collaborative Management

To achieve vision restoration, to the extent possible, and return to society as before, patients with ocular injuries need a multidisciplinary team approach, including the ophthalmologist, ophthalmic advance nurse practitioner, internist, nurse, social worker, and optometrist or low vision rehabilitation specialist. In order to meet desired patient outcomes, it is essential that this interdisciplinary team communicate openly with one another in developing and evaluating care of the patient and family (IOM [Institute of Medicine], 2010). To ensure maximum vision potential, vision care is managed by the ophthalmologist with the assistance of nurses and other health care providers. Depending on the degree of severity, from full globe/facial involvement to corneal abrasion, and whether repairs were done medically and/or surgically, some degree of visual impairment is possible as the ocular trauma heals. The optometrist and low vision rehabilitation specialist will provide the necessary glasses or low vision aids to enhance patients' visual acuity, hopefully to a functional level. The social worker is accustomed to helping patients adjust to a new lifestyle with vision deficit that will change the person's perception of self.

Sudden Vision Loss

Sudden loss of visual acuity is a very frightening experience for which the patient usually has no explanation at first. This leaves the patient wondering what happened. Some of the ocular problems that can cause a sudden loss of vision are acute macular hole, retinal occlusions, anterior ischemic optic neuropathy, temporal arteritis, amaurosis fugax (a fleeting monocular loss of vision which may be total or sectional), and ocular migraines. These ocular conditions are listed in Chart 64–7 with descriptions and management.

Gerontological Considerations

Many ocular and visual changes tend to occur with aging. Most are normal with passage of time. Descriptions of some of the age-related ocular and visual changes that can occur and significantly affect an individual's lifestyle are listed in Chart 64–8 on page 2052.

Research

Research is a mechanism by which to explore and find answers for patients who are visually impaired. Vision researchers are striving to meet population needs as well as individual needs, developing new devices and enabling new clinical outcomes. Research topics related to vision research are outlined in the Research Opportunities box (p. 2053).

Summary

This chapter has focused on the most common eye disorders, including eye emergencies. Major disorders covered under the heading of visual impairment include those that are the most prevalent in today's

CHART 64–7 Sudden Vision Loss Eye Problems

Problem	Description/Management
Acute macular hole	A hole in the central area of the retina, where an individual's 20/20 vision is located, called the fovea. Signs and symptoms include unilateral, painless, and substantial loss in central vision that appears as a round orangish-red spot in the macula. There is a grayish area surrounding the hole, which usually indicates edema, and drusen (yellow deposits) may be present. Medical management for a true macular hole probably will mean a vitrectomy.
Anterior ischemic optic neuropathy (nonarteritic ischemic optic neuropathy)	An ischemic attack to the optic nerve. Signs and symptoms include unilateral, painless decrease in vision; afferent pupillary defect; disc edema; and normal erythrocyte sedimentation rate (ESR) (which distinguishes this from arteritic ischemic optic neuropathy). No effective management is known at this time. The degree of vision loss depends on the extent of ischemia.
Temporal arteritis (giant cell arteritis or arteritic ischemic optic neuropathy)	A unilateral loss of vision. Signs and symptoms may include altitudinal visual field loss and decreased color vision, afferent pupillary defect, optic nerve swelling, forehead and scalp tenderness, arthritis-type discomfort, painful chewing, loss of weight, and elevated erythrocyte sedimentation rate. This usually occurs in patients around the age of 65. The patient needs a comprehensive medical work-up, a temporal artery biopsy for diagnosis confirmation, erythrocyte sedimentation rate, and a complete ocular examination with visual field. Medical management with systemic steroid is urgently needed to prevent vasculitis and contralateral eye disease, to prevent the possibility of rendering the patient legally blind.
Amaurosis fugax	A transient, sudden, and painless decrease in vision unilaterally caused by Hollenhorst plaques, which obstruct arterial blood flow to the ophthalmic artery. The temporary or fleeting loss of vision can last from about 30 minutes to hours and usually gives the patient a panic attack of possibly going blind. On complete ocular examination, the plaques might be visualized in the retinal vasculature coupled with retinal edema, and very rarely for ophthalmic artery stenosis. The eye exam also will include fluorescein angiography and fundus photography. A complete medical and neurological evaluation is indicated to rule out transient ischemic attack (TIA) and carotid stenosis. Medical management may include systemic anticoagulants and hypolipidemic agents, or endarterectomy.
Ocular migraine (Also called retinal or ophthalmic migraine, occipital lobe ischemia)	A visual hallucination may reveal an image with a shimmering edge, heat waves, or smokelike screen that appears in an individual's vision, something like an aura. Usually no headache is involved; however, the patient may experience mild discomfort and sudden loss of peripheral vision or transient visual obscuration. The peripheral vision disappears for about 10 to 20 minutes, and vision returns to normal after the episode. No treatment is required if this is a true ocular migraine. Aspirin or acetaminophen may help to prevent reoccurrence if one is going through a period of ocular migraine episodes and can possibly remove the cause, such as particularly stressful circumstances.

Sources: Arnold, A. C. (2009). Ischemic optic neuropathies. In M. Yanoff & J. S. Duker (Eds.), *Ophthalmology* (3rd ed.). St. Louis: Mosby/Elsevier; Brown, G. C., & Brown, M. M. (2007). The ocular ischemic syndrome. In A. Joussen, T. Gardner, B. Kirchhof, & S. Ryan (Eds.), *Retinal vascular disease.* New York: Springer-Verlag; Huang, J. J., & Foster, C. S. (2007). Systemic immunosuppression in retinal vasculitis and rheumatic diseases. In A. Joussen, T. Gardner, B. Kirchhof, & S. Ryan (Eds.), *Retinal vascular disease.* New York: Springer-Verlag; Miller, N., Newman, N., Biousse, V., & Kerrison, J. (2008). *Walsh and Hoyt's clinical neuro-ophthalmology: The essentials* (2nd ed.). Philadelphia: Wolters Kluwer/Lippincott Williams & Wilkins; Rogers, A. H., & Duker, J. S. (2008). *Rapid diagnosis in ophthalmology retina.* St. Louis: Mosby/Elsevier.

CHART 64–8 Changes in the Aging Eye

Aging Eye Change	Explanation
Facial Features, Eyeballs, Eyebrows, Eyelids, and Eyelashes	
Senile exophthalmos	The recession or sinking of the eyeball into the orbit as a result of the loss of subcutaneous fat, decreased elastic tissue, and decreased muscle tone. Does not affect vision; no intervention necessary.
Ptosis senilis	A pseudoparalytic drooping of the upper eyelid. If it causes a problem by crossing the visual axis, it can be surgically corrected.
Blepharochalasis or dermatochalasis	An atrophy of elastic tissue of the eyelids resulting in the upper eyelid hanging over the eyelid margin or lashes. Redundant eyelid tissue creates wrinkles and folds. If it causes a problem with vision or cosmetically, it can be surgically corrected.
Senile entropion or blepharelosis	The inward turning (inversion) of the eyelid margin. If it causes a problem with irritation or foreign body sensation to the cornea, it can be surgically corrected.
Senile ectropion	The outward turning (eversion) of the eyelid margin. If it causes a problem with dry eye syndrome with the loss of tears and cannot be corrected with artificial tear use, it can be surgically corrected.
Conjunctiva	
Conjunctivochalasis	The loss of transparency and more laxity of the conjunctiva, wherein the bulbar conjunctiva wrinkles into the lower eyelid margin.
Sclera	
Sclera rigidity	The sclera becomes harder or rigid with loss of elasticity. This can also affect accurate intraocular pressure reading with indentation tonometry.
Senile scleral translucency	The sclera thins and becomes more transparent, exhibiting dark-grayish oval areas of the sclera, anterior to muscle insertion.
Scleral lipid deposition	The anterior sclera will appear yellowish due to lipid depositions in the deeper scleral tissue.
Pupil and Iris	
Pupil sclerosis	The pupil size decreases with age (senile miosis) because of pupil sphincter sclerosis, which narrows the visual field and affects peripheral vision to a mild degree. No intervention is usually necessary.
Cornea	
Keratoconjunctivitis sicca (dry eye syndrome)	A deficiency of tear production, especially in postmenopausal women, can make the cornea feel gritty or have a foreign-body sensation. This is usually relieved with frequent use of artificial tear drops or ointments.
Arcus senilis or gerontoxon	A grayish-white ring that develops at the peripheral edge of the cornea (limbus) from lipoid deposits into the corneal stroma, and does not affect vision; no intervention is required.
Guttata or corneal dystrophy	The thickening of Descemet's membrane (fourth layer of the cornea) with hyaline deposits from the loss of endothelial cells. These cells help maintain the health of the cornea and vision clarity.
Lens	
Cataract	The yellowing or opacity of the natural crystalline lens that is corrected surgically when a cataract is mature. In the meantime, corrective lenses can help; may also notice an alteration in color perception, especially for blues, violets, and greens.
Optic Nerve, Macula, Retina, and Vitreous	
Glaucoma	An elevated intraocular pressure due to aging, whereby trabecular meshwork is sluggish due to the loss of elasticity.
Age-related macular degeneration	The degeneration of the macula due to aging; the loss of retinal pigment epithelium and visual function.
Senile circumpapillary choroidal atrophy or peripapillary halo	The degeneration of arterioles in the choriocapillaris causing sclerosis, especially around the optic nerve; usually does not affect vision. No intervention is necessary.
Senile retinoschisis or schisis	A primary, acquired, gradual splitting of the retina into two distinct layers. Senile retinoschisis develops from the coalescence of intraretinal microcysts located in an area of peripheral cystoid degeneration near the ora serrata and extends posteriorly and circumferentially. This process leads to the splitting of the retina at the outer plexiform layer or, less commonly, at the inner nuclear layer.
Syneresis	Degeneration of the vitreous humor with loss of gel consistency, acts as a precursor to posterior vitreous detachment of gel, which is commonly called floaters. This occurs during the aging process and seldom calls for an intervention unless secondary complications result, such as retinal detachment.
Vision	
Presbyopia	The loss of accommodation occurring around the fourth decade of life, that is, the loss of the ability to focus up close. This necessitates reading glasses or bifocals.
Astigmatism	The cornea can flatten more with age; this changes the corneal curvature and may result in new astigmatism or changes in astigmatism that can be corrected with lenses.
Stereopsis loss	The loss of depth perception due to light scatter or glare that affects vision performance, causing difficulty with night vision, especially driving and judging heights properly. This can possibly be helped with brighter, nonglare lights and brighter colors, such as reds, oranges, and yellows.

RESEARCH OPPORTUNITIES Related to Visual Disorders

Research Area	Clinical Impact
Glaucoma Research	
Glaucoma is generally diagnosed due to elevated IOP and damage to the optic nerve. However, the first sign of injury in glaucoma may actually occur in the brain.	Identification of patients with glaucoma as early as possible to prevent vision loss. The retina and optic nerve are components of the central nervous system (CNS) and do not regenerate, similar to other CNS diseases. This opens new realms of nerve-derived therapeutics in the treatment of glaucoma.
Diabetic Retinopathy Research	
New antiangiogenic and anti-inflammatory therapies for the treatment of diabetic macular edema (DME).	Treat the progress of DME, a complication of diabetic retinopathy, the most common cause of blindness among working adults.
Systemic/Eye Research	
Hypothyroidism may put patients at a greater risk for open-angle glaucoma (OAG), especially after a 5-year follow-up.	Hypothyroid patients seem to be better protected from the risk of OAG if treated with levothyroxine (Synthroid).
Cataract Research	
Quality-of-life (QoL) issues in postmenopausal women who ate foods high in a variety of vitamins and minerals appear to have a lower risk of developing nuclear cataracts.	A healthier diet may reduce or slow down the progression of cataract growth in older women, thus postponing the need and lowering the economic burden of cataract surgery. In addition, a healthier diet seemed to improve the QoL of the participants with smoking cessation and avoiding obesity.

Sources: Calkins, D. (2010). Proceedings of the National Academy of Sciences. Retrieved from http://www.mc.vanderbilt.edu/reporter/index.html?ID=8387; Chiu, C. J., Milton, R., Klein, R., Gensler, G., & Taylor, A. (2009). Dietary compound score and risk of age-related macular degeneration in the age-related eye disease study (AREDS). *Ophthalmology, 116*(5), 939–946; Christen, W., Liu, S., Glynn, R., Gaziano, M., & Buring, J. (2008). Dietary carotenoids, vitamins C and E, and risk of cataract in women. *Archives of Ophthalmology, 126*(1), 102–109; Lin, H. C., Kang, J. H., Jiang, Y. D., & Ho, J. D. (2010). Hypothyroidism and the risk of developing open-angle glaucoma. *Ophthalmology, 117*(10), 1960–1966; Mares, J., et al. (2010). Healthy diets and the subsequent prevalence of nuclear cataract in women. *Archives of Ophthalmology, 128*(6), 738–749.

Weblink: First Signs of Glaucoma Found in the Brain

society: refractive errors, cataracts, glaucoma, diabetic retinopathy, and macular degeneration. Included in the discussion of eye infections and inflammation are dry eye syndrome, conjunctivitis, and endophthalmitis. The prevalence and treatment for these disorders is included. Retinal and vitreal disorders speak to retinal detachment, vitreous detachment, retinal breaks, vitreous hemorrhage, and nonrhegmatogenous and rhegmatogenous detachment. A discussion of eye trauma and injury and sudden vision loss takes place toward the end of the chapter, as does a discussion on gerontological considerations for the visually impaired. Collaborative care is emphasized with all disorders. The majority of these disorders are treated in an outpatient setting. However, should the need arise or the setting change to inpatient, the principles and guidelines set in this chapter are still applicable.

NCLEX® PRACTICE

1. A patient reports familial history of macular degeneration (MD). The nurse should teach the patient to protect his vision by taking which actions? (select all that apply)

1. Keep blood pressure within normal ranges.
2. Do not smoke.
3. Avoid NSAID medications.
4. Read in good light.
5. Keep cholesterol levels within normal ranges.

2. A patient who has diabetes mellitus calls the clinic to report sudden blurring in her left eye. She denies headache or nausea. The nurse would instruct her to come to the clinic for evaluation of which condition?

1. Blood glucose elevation
2. Vitreous hemorrhage
3. Hypertension
4. Renal disorder

3. An adult patient has strabismus following severe head trauma. The nurse would educate this patient in preparation for which treatment?

1. Contact lenses
2. Occlusion of the normal vision eye
3. Prism eyeglass lenses
4. Eye muscle surgery

4. The nurse would include teaching on which topic when caring for a patient with newly diagnosed glaucoma?

1. Diet
2. Correct use of eyedrops
3. Control of heart disease
4. Use of corrective lenses

5. A patient has sustained sudden and complete loss of vision in an industrial accident. As the patient attempts to adjust to this loss, the nurse should be particularly careful to assess for which changes?

1. Loss of the desire to interact with other people
2. Inability to tolerate loud noises
3. Dislike of previously enjoyed foods
4. Development of dependence on others

6. A patient who has markedly decreased vision is talking to the nurse about the difficulties he encounters. Which comment or question, by the nurse, reveals a caring, sensitive approach?

1. "You can't do anything about your condition, so you will have to live with it."
2. "I feel so sorry for you. It must be very difficult."
3. "I don't know what I would do if I lost my vision. It would be awful."
4. "Have you found that you depend more on your sense of hearing than you did?"

Answers to NCLEX Practice Questions can be found in Appendix D in the Osborn Student Resources at nursing.pearsonhighered.com. Practice additional NCLEX questions online at the Student Resources site.

Pearson Nursing Student Resources Find additional review materials at: **nursing.pearsonhighered.com**

REFERENCES

AAO-2 (American Academy of Ophthalmology). (2010–2011). *Basic and clinical science course: Fundamentals and principles of ophthalmology* (Section 2). San Francisco: Author.

AAO-3 (American Academy of Ophthalmology). (2010–2011). *Basic and clinical science: Clinical optics* (Section 3). San Francisco: Author.

AAO-5 (American Academy of Ophthalmology). (2010–2011). *Basic and clinical science course: Neuro-ophthalmology* (Section 5). San Francisco: Author.

AAO-6 (American Academy of Ophthalmology). (2010–2011). *Basic and clinical science course: Pediatric ophthalmology and strabismus* (Section 6). San Francisco: Author.

AAO-8 (American Academy of Ophthalmology). (2010–2011). *Basic and clinical science course: External disease and cornea* (Section 8). San Francisco: Author.

AAO-10 (American Academy of Ophthalmology). (2010–2011). *Basic and clinical science course: Glaucoma* (Section 10). San Francisco: Author.

AAO-11 (American Academy of Ophthalmology). (2010–2011). *Basic and clinical science course: Lens and cataract* (Section 11). San Francisco: Author.

AAO-12 (American Academy of Ophthalmology). (2010–2011). *Basic and clinical science course: Retina and vitreous* (Section 12). San Francisco: Author.

Adams, M. P., & Koch, R. W. (2010). *Pharmacology connections to nursing practice.* Upper Saddle River, NJ: Pearson.

Aetna InteliHealth. (2012). Eye socket fracture (fracture of the orbit). Aetna Inc. Retrieved from http://www.intelihealth.com/IH/ihtIH/WSIHW000/9339/10464.html

American Academy of Opthalmology. (2007). Guidelines for vision rehabilitation for adults. Agency for Healthcare Research and Quality. U.S. Department of Health & Human Services. National Guideline Clearing House. Retrieved from http://guidelines.gov/content.aspx?id=11755

American Academy of Ophthalmology Preferred Practice Patterns Committee. Preferred Practice Pattern Guidelines. (2010). *Comprehensive adult medical eye evaluation.* San Francisco, CA: American Academy of Ophthalmology.

Arnold, A. C. (2009). Ischemic optic neuropathies. In M. Yanoff & J. S. Duker (Eds.), *Ophthalmology* (3rd ed.). St. Louis: Mosby/Elsevier.

Baker, M., Wang, J., Rogers, S., Klein, R., Kuller, L., Larsen, E., & Wong, T. (2009). Early age-related macular degeneration, cognitive function, and dementia. *Archives of Ophthalmology, 127*(5), 667–673.

Bataoel, A. (2008). Pharmacology. In P. Lamb (Ed.), *Core curriculum for ophthalmic nursing* (3rd ed.). Dubuque, IA: Kendall/Hunt.

Bell, J. A. (2011). Primary open-angle glaucoma. Medscape reference. Retrieved from http://emedicine.medscape.com/article/1206147-overview

Bernstein, P. S., Delori, F. C., Richer, S., van Kuijk, F. J., & Wenzel, A. J. (2010). The value of measurement of macular carotenoid pigment optical densities and distributions in age-related macular degeneration and other retinal disorders. *Vision Research, 50*(7), 716–728. Epub 2009 Oct 23.

Bhavsar, A. R. (2011). Diabetic retinopathy. Medscape reference. Retrieved from http://emedicine.medscape.com/article/1225122-overview

Blanchard, S. M. (2008). Conjunctival disorders. In P. Lamb (Ed.), *Core curriculum for ophthalmic nursing* (3rd ed.). Dubuque, IA: Kendall/Hunt.

Brault, M. W. (2009). Review of changes to the measurement of disability in 2008 American community survey. Washington, DC: U.S. Census Bureau. U.S. Department of Commerce.

Brown, G. C., & Brown, M. M. (2007). The ocular ischemic syndrome. In A. Joussen, T. Gardner, B. Kirchhof, & S. Ryan (Eds.), *Retinal vascular disease.* New York: Springer-Verlag.

Calkins, D. (2010). Proceedings of the National Academy of Sciences. Retrieved from http://www.mc.vanderbilt.edu/reporter/index.html?ID=8387

Centers for Disease Control and Prevention (CDC). (2008). The basics of eye protection. Retrieved from http://www.cdc.gov/features/dsworkPlaceEye/

Centers for Disease Contol and Prevention (CDC). (2009). Common eye disorders. Retrieved from http://www.cdc.gov/visionhealth/basic_information/eye_disorders.htm

Chan, W. M., Lau, T. T., & Liu, D. T. (2007). Vascular endothelial growth factor and anti-vascular endothelial growth factor therapy for choroidal neovascularization. In S. Saxena (Ed.), *Focus on macular diseases.* Philadelphia: Wolters Kluwer/Lippincott Williams & Wilkins.

Cheung, N., Mitchell, P., & Wong, T. W. (2010). Diabetic retinopathy. *The Lancet, 376*(9735), 134–136. doi:1016/50140-6736(09)62124-3

Chiu, C. J., Milton, R., Klein, R., Gensler, G., & Taylor, A. (2009). Dietary compound score and risk of age-related macular degeneration in the age-related eye disease study (AREDS). *Ophthalmology, 116*(5), 939–946.

Christen, W., Liu, S., Glynn, R., Gaziano, M., & Buring, J. (2008). Dietary carotenoids, vitamins C and E, and risk of cataract in women. *Archives of Ophthalmology, 126*(1), 102–109.

Dahl, A. A. (2012). Glaucoma. MedicineNet.com. Retrieved from http://www.medicinenet.com/glaucoma/page2.htm

Diamond, G. R. (2009a). Amblyopia. In M. Yanoff & J. S. Duker (Eds.), *Ophthalmology* (3rd ed.). St. Louis: Mosby/Elsevier.

Diamond, G. R. (2009b). Sensory adaptations in strabismus. In M. Yanoff & J. S. Duker (Eds.), *Ophthalmology* (3rd ed.). St. Louis: Mosby/Elsevier.

Dugdale, D. C. (2010). Strabismus. MedlinePlus. Retrieved from http://www.nlm.nih.gov/medlineplus/ency/article/001004.htm

Ehlers, J. P., & Shah, C. P. (Eds.). (2008). *The Wills eye manual: Office and emergency room diagnosis and treatment of eye disease* (5th ed.). Philadelphia: Wolters Kluwer/Lippincott Williams & Wilkins.

Emedicinehealth. (2012). Photodynamic therapy (PDT). WebMD. Retrieved from http://www.emedicinehealth.com/script/main/art.asp?articlekey=145454&ref=128949

Encyclopedia of Nursing & Allied Health. (2012). Macular degeneration. Retrieved from http://www.enotes.com/macular-degeneration-reference/macular-degeneration-172148

Essilor. (2011). Myopia. Vision Defects. Retrieved from http://www.essilorusa.com/EN/AboutVision/AboutYourEyes/Pages/EyeHealth.aspx

EyeCareSource.com. (2011). Double vision or diplopia. Retrieved from http://www.eyecaresource.com/problems/double-vision.html

Eye Facts. (2011). Sports eye injuries. Retrieved from http://www.uic.edu/com/eyecare/eyeConditions/sportsEyeInjuries.shtml

Eye Surgery Education Council. (2011). Presbyopia correcting intraocular lenses (PCIOLs). Retrieved from http://www.readclearlyagain.org/intraocular.html

Foundation Fighting Blindness. (2012). What is retinitis pigmentosa? Retrieved from http://www.blindness.org/index.php?option=com_content&id=50&Itemid=67

Fraser, S., & Wormald, R. (2011). Chapter 210—epidemiology of glaucoma. *Free Medical Textbook.* Healthwise Inc. Retrieved from http://medtextfree.wordpress.com/2011/04/05/chapter-210-epidemiology-of-glaucoma/

Freudenthal, J. (2011). Neovascular glaucoma. Medscape reference. Retrieved from http://emedicine.medscape.com/article1205736-overview

Friedman, N. J., Kaiser, P. K., & Pineda, R. (2009). *The Massachusetts eye and ear infirmary, illustrated manual of ophthalmology* (3rd ed.). Philadelphia: Saunders/Elsevier.

Ganatra, J., & Goldstein, M. (2009). Blepharitis. In M. Yanoff & J. S. Duker (Eds.), *Ophthalmology* (3rd ed.). St. Louis: Mosby/Elsevier.

Girkin, C. A. (2011). New surgical approaches to glaucoma. Glaucoma Research Foundation. Retrieved from http://www.glaucoma.org/treatment/new-surgical-approaches-to-glaucoma.php

Glaucoma Research Foundation. (2011). Types of glaucoma. Gleams. Retrieved from http://www.glaucoma.org/glaucoma/types- of-glaucoma.php

Goff, M., McDonald, H., & Ai, E. (2010). Photocoagulation for diabetic macular edema and diabetic retinopathy. In I. Scott, H. Flynn, & W. Smiddy (Eds.), *Diabetes and ocular disease: Past, present, and future therapies* (2nd ed., Ophthalmology monographs 14). New York: Oxford University Press.

Goldberg, C. (2009). The eye exam. The Regents of the University of California. Retrieved from http://meded.ucsd.edu/clinicalmed/eyes.htm

Goldblum, K. (2008). Lens disorders. In P. Lamb (Ed.), *Core curriculum for ophthalmic nursing* (3rd ed.). Dubuque, IA: Kendall/Hunt.

Graham, R. J. (2009). Traumatic cataract. Medscape reference. Retrieved from http://emedicine.medscape.com/article/1211083-overview

Greven, C. M. (2009). Retinal breaks. In M. Yanoff & J. S. Duker (Eds.), *Ophthalmology* (3rd ed.). St. Louis: Mosby/Elsevier.

Gross, R. L. (2009). Current medical management of glaucoma. In M. Yanoff & J. S. Duker (Eds.), *Ophthalmology* (3rd ed.). St. Louis: Mosby/Elsevier.

Heiting, G., & Bailey, G. (2010). Vision problems of schoolchildren. All About Vision, Access Media Group LLC. Retrieved from http://www.allaboutvision.com/parents/schoolage.htm

Helting, G., & Haddrill, M. (2012). Glaucoma. Access Media Group LLC. Retrieved from http://www.allaboutvision.com/conditions/glaucoma.htm

Herndon, L. W. (2009). Can we treat ICD syndrome-related glaucoma successfully? *Opthalmology Times Europe.* Retrieved from http://www.oteurope.com/ophthalmologytimeseurope/article/articleDetail.jsp?id=578674&sk=&date=&pageID=2

Hitchings, R. A. (2009). Normal-tension glaucoma. In M. Yanoff & J. S. Duker (Eds.), *Ophthalmology* (3rd ed.). St. Louis: Mosby/Elsevier.

Hochstetler, B., Scott, I., Kunselman, A., Thompson, K., & Zerfoss, E. (2010). Adherence to recommendations of the age-related eye disease study (AREDS) in patients with age-related macular degeneration. *Retina, 30*(8), 1166–1170.

Huang, J. J., & Foster, C. S. (2007). Systematic immunosuppression in retinal vasculitis and rheumatic diseases. In A. Joussen, T. Gardner, B. Kirchhof, & S. Ryan (Eds.), *Retinal vascular disease.* New York: Springer-Verlag.

Hussain, N. (2007). Photodynamic therapy for neovascular age-related macular degeneration. In S. Saxena, *Focus on macular diseases.* Philadelphia: Wolters Kluwer/Lippincott Williams & Wilkins.

IOM (Institute of Medicine). (2010). *The future of nursing: Leading change, advancing health.* Washington, DC: The Academic Press.

Jager, R. D., Mieler W. F., & Miller, J. W. (2008). Age-related macular degeneration. *New England Journal of Medicine, 359*(16), 1736. Retrieved from http://www.ncbi.nlm.nih.gov/pubmed/18550876

Kanski, J. J., & Bowling, B. (2011). *Clinical ophthalmology: A systemic approach* (2nd ed.). New York: Elsevier/Saunders.

Kee, J. L. (2010). *Laboratory and diagnostic tests with nursing implications.* Upper Saddle River, NJ: Pearson.

Kohnen, T., Wang, L., Friedman, N., & Koch, D. (2009). Complications of cataract surgery. In M. Yanoff & J. S. Duker (Eds.), *Ophthalmology* (3rd ed.). St. Louis: Mosby/Elsevier.

Lam, A., Anderson, N., Regillo, C., & Brown, G. (2010). Photography, angiography, and ultrasonography in diabetic retinopathy. In I. Scott, H. Flynn, & W. Smiddy (Eds.), *Diabetes and ocular disease: Past, present, and future therapies* (2nd ed., Ophthalmology monographs 14). New York: Oxford University Press.

Lamb, P., & Simms-Eaton, S. (2008). Visual impairment. In P. Lamb (Ed.), *Core curriculum for ophthalmic nursing* (3rd ed.). Dubuque, IA: Kendall/Hunt.

Lamb, P., & Weaver, S. (2008). Lid disorders. In P. Lamb (Ed.), *Core curriculum for ophthalmic nursing* (3rd ed.). Dubuque, IA: Kendall/Hunt.

Larkin, G. L. (2011). Vitreous hemorrhage in emergency medicine. Medscape reference. Retrieved from http://emedicine.medscape.com/article/799242-overview

Lin, H. C., Kang, J. H., Jiang, Y. D., & Ho, J. D. (2010). Hypothyroidism and the risk of developing open-angle glaucoma. *Ophthalmology, 117*(10), 1960–1966.

Mack Eye Care. (2010). Photodynamic therapy for age-related macular degeneration. Mack Eye Center. Retrieved from http://occhicago.com/68-photodynamic-therapy-for-age-related-macular-degeneration/

Mance, T. C., Kovacević, D., Alpeza-Dunato, Z., Stroligo, M. N., & Brumini, G. (2011). The role of omega-6 to omega-3 ratio in development and progression of age-related macular degeneration. *Collegium Antropologicum, 35*(Suppl. 2), 307–310.

Mares, J., et al., (2010). Healthy diets and the subsequent prevalence of nuclear cataract in women. *Archives of Ophthalmology, 128*(6), 738–749.

Mataix, J., Palacios, E., Carmen, D., Garcia-Pous, M., & Navea, A. (2010). Combined ranibizumab and photodynamic therapy to treat exudative age-related macular degeneration. *Retina, 30*(8), 1190–1196.

Mattera, C. J. (2011). Ocular trauma. Retrieved from http://www.docstoc.com/docs/79955344/Ocular-Trauma

Mayo Clinic Staff. (2012). Diabetic retinopathy. Retrieved from http://www.mayoclinic.com/health/diabetic-retinopathy/DS00447

Miller, D., & Scott, C. (2009). Epidemiology of refractive errors. In M. Yanoff & J. S. Duker (Eds.), *Ophthalmology* (3rd ed.). St. Louis: Mosby/Elsevier.

Miller, N., Newman, N., Biousse, V., & Kerrison, J. (2008). *Walsh and Hoyt's clinical neuro-ophthalmology: The essentials* (2nd ed.). Philadelphia: Wolters Kluwer/Lippincott Williams & Wilkins.

Montgomery, T. M. (2012a). The crystalline lens. Retrieved from http://www.tedmontgomery.com/the_eye/lens.html

Montgomery, T. M. (2012b). The macula. Retrieved from http://www.tedmontgomery.com/the_eye/macula.html

More, D. (2009). Eye allergies. About.com, allergies. Retrieved from http://allergies.about.com/o

Natarajan, S., Shome, D., & Gadgil, D. (2007). Spectacle-induced ocular trauma: An unusual mechanism. *Cornea, 26*(1), 109–110.

NEI (National Eye Institute). (2009). Age-related macular degeneration. Retrieved from http://www.nei.nih.gov/health/maculardegen/armd_facts.asp

Neutralegacy.com. (2012). Proliferative vs nonproliferative diabetic retinopathy: What's the difference? Retrieved from http://www.nutralegacy.com/blog/general-healthcare/proliferative-vs-nonproliferative-diabetic-retinopathy-whats-the-difference/

OSN (Ocular Surgery News) SuperSite. (2012). Cataract surgery. *Ocular Surgery News Asia-Pacific Edition.* Retrieved from http://www.osnsupersite.com/view.aspx?rid=89456

Patel, C. C. (2011). Pars plana vitrectomy. Medscape reference. Retrieved from http://emedicine.medscape.com/article/1844160-overview

PDR. (2011a). Physicians' desk reference. (65th ed.). Montvale, NJ: PDR Network.

PDR. (2011b). *Physicians' desk reference for ophthalmic medicines* (39th ed.). Montvale, NJ: PDR Network.

Polk, E. (2012). When should you consider multifocal IOLs? Jobson Medical Information LLC. Retrieved from http://www.reviewofcontactlenses.com/content/c/36169/

Pons, M. E. (2011). Pseudoexfoliation glaucoma differential diagnoses. Medscape reference. Retrieved from http://emedicine.medscape.com/article/1206366-differential

Porth, C., & Marfin, M. (2009). *Essentials of pathophysiology: Concepts of altered health states.* Philadelphia: Lippincott Williams & Wilkins.

Querques, G., Forte, R., & Souied, E. H. (2011). Retina and omega-3. *Journal of Nutrition and Metabolism.* 2011:748361. doi: 10.1155/2011/748361

Ramos-Esteban, J., Katz, L., Goldberg, W., & Goldberg, A. (2009). Clinical examination of glaucoma. In M. Yanoff & J. S. Duker (Eds.), *Ophthalmology* (3rd ed.). St. Louis: Mosby/Elsevier.

Randleman, J. B. (2011). Opthalmologic approach to chemical burns. Medscape reference. Retrieved from http://emedicine.medscape.co/araticle/1215950-overview

Read, R. W. (2009). Endophthalmitis. In M. Yanoff & J. S. Duker (Eds.), *Ophthalmology* (3rd ed.). St. Louis: Mosby/Elsevier.

READ-2 (Ranibizumab for Edema of the Macula in Diabetes-2 Study Group). (2010). Two-year outcomes of the Ranibizumab for edema of the macula in diabetes. *Ophthalmology, 117*(11), 2146–2151.

Retina Eye Specialists. (2010). Age-related macular degeneration (AMD). Retrieved from http://www.retinaeye.com/AMD-Wet.html

Robson, J., Behrman, A. J., & Abbuhl, S. (2007). Globe rupture. Emedicine. Retrieved from http://emedicine.medscape.com/article/798223-overview

Rogers, A. H., & Duker, J. S. (2008). *Rapid diagnosis in ophthalmology: Retina.* St. Louis: Mosby/Elsevier.

Rosenblatt, B. J., & Benson, W. E. (2009). Diabetic retinopathy. In M. Yanoff & J. S. Duker (Eds.), *Ophthalmology* (3rd ed.). St. Louis: Mosby/Elsevier.

Rosenfeld, P. J., Martidis, A., & Tennant, M. T. (2009). Age-related macular degeneration. In M. Yanoff & J. S. Duker (Eds.), *Ophthalmology* (3rd ed.). St. Louis: Mosby/Elsevier.

Rubenstein, J. B., & Virasch, V. (2009). Conjunctivitis: Infectious and noninfectious. In M. Yanoff & J. S. Duker (Eds.), *Ophthalmology* (3rd ed.). St. Louis: Mosby/Elsevier.

Scott, I. U. (2011). Viral conjunctivitis. Medscape reference. Retrieved from http://emedicine.medscape.com/article/1191370-overview

See, J. L., & Chew, P. T. (2009). Angle closure of glaucoma. In M. Yanoff & J. S. Duker (Eds.), *Ophthalmology* (3rd ed.). St. Louis: Mosby/Elsevier.

Seth, R. K., Sigler, E. J., & Adelman, R. A. (2011). Age-related macular degeneration—review and current concepts. Touch.ophthalmology.com. Retrieved from http://www.touchophthalmology.com/articles/age-related-macular-degeneration-review-and-current-concepts-0

Sharma, A. (2011). Beta-blocker toxicity. Medscape reference. Retrieved from http://emedicine.medscape.com/article/813342-overview

Smith, S. C. (2008). Uveal disorders (glaucoma). In P. Lamb (Ed.), *Core curriculum for ophthalmic nursing* (3rd ed.). Dubuque, IA: Kendall/Hunt.

Spaide, R. F. (2009). Choroidal neovascularization. In M. Yanoff & J. S. Duker (Eds.), *Ophthalmology* (3rd ed.). St. Louis: Mosby/Elsevier.

Stevens, S., Gilbert, C., & Asbury, N. (2007). How to measure intraocular pressure: Applanation tanometry. *Community Eye Health Journal, 20*(64), 74–75.

Sullivan, B. R. (2010). Angle recession glaucoma. Medscape reference. Retrieved from http://emedicine.medscape.com/article/1204999-overview

Tan, J. C., & Kaufman, P. L. (2009). Primary open-angle glaucoma. In M. Yanoff & J. S. Duker (Eds.), *Ophthalmology* (3rd ed.). St. Louis: Mosby/Elsevier.

The Johns Hopkins Center on Aging and Health. (2009). Cardiovascular health study. Johns Hopkins University. Retrieved from http://www.jhsph.edu/research/centers-and-institutes/johns-hopkins-center-on-aging-and-health/research/projects/chs.html

Tu, E., & Rheinstrom, S. (2009). Dry eye. In M. Yanoff & J. S. Duker (Eds.), *Ophthalmology* (3rd ed.). St. Louis: Mosby/Elsevier.

United States Census Bureau (USCB). (2009). Demographic profiles. Retrieved from http://quickfacts.census.gov/qfd/states/00000.html

University of Michigan Kellogg Eye Center. (2012). Diplopia (double vision). Retrieved from http://www.kellogg,unich.edu/patientcazre/conditions/diplopia.html

Valluri, S., & Moorthy, R. S. (2009). Fungal endophthalmitis: *Candidiasis*, *Aspergillosis*, and *Coccidioidomycosis*. In M. Yanoff & J. S. Duker (Eds.), *Ophthalmology* (3rd ed.). St. Louis: Mosby/Elsevier.

Vorvick, L. J., & Lusby, F. (2011). Presbyopia. MedlinePlus. Retrieved from http://www.nlm.nig.gov/medlinep;llus/ency/article/001026.htm

Walker, R. S., & Piltz-Seymour, J. R. (2009). When to treat glaucoma. In M. Yanoff & J. S. Duker (Eds.), *Ophthalmology* (3rd ed.). St. Louis: Mosby/Elsevier.

WebMD. (2009). Anti-VEGF medicines for wet age-related macular degeneration (AMD). Healthwise. Retrieved from http://www.webmd.com/eye-health/macular-degeneration/anti-vegf-medicines-for-wet-age-related-macular-degeneration-amd

Wessels, K. F. (2011). Diplopia treatment & management. Medscape reference. Retrieved from http://emedicine.medscape.com/article/1214490-overview

Wevill, M. (2009). Epidemiology, pathophysiology, causes, morphology, and visual effects of cataracts. In M. Yanoff & J. S. Duker (Eds.), *Ophthalmology* (3rd. ed.). St. Louis: Mosby/Elsevier.

Wilkinson, C. P. (2010). Classification of diabetic retinopathy. In I. Scott, H. Flynn, & W. Smiddy (Eds.), *Diabetes and ocular disease: Past, present, and future therapies* (2nd ed., Ophthalmology monographs 14). New York: Oxford University Press.

Wong, T., Klein, R., & Klein, B. (2010). Epidemiology and risk factors of diabetic retinopathy. In I. Scott, H. Flynn, & W. Smiddy (Eds.), *Diabetes and ocular disease: Past, present, and future therapies* (2nd ed., Ophthalmology monographs 14). New York: Oxford University Press.

X-Plain. (2007). Macular degeneration. The Patient Education Institute. Retrieved from http://www.nlm.nih.gov/medlineplus/tutorials/maculardegeneration/ot059103.pdf

Yen, K. G. (2011). Amblyopia differential diagnoses. Medscape reference. Retrieved from http://emedicine.medscape.com/article/1214603-differential

Yeung, K. (2011). Bacterial conjunctivitis. Retrieved from http://emedicine.medscape.com/article/1191730-overview

Concepts Related to Disaster, Emergency, and Trauma Nursing

UNIT 15

Content in Unit 15 that addresses the **Institute of Medicine (IOM)** competencies, **Nursing Core Competencies (NCC)**, the **Quality and Safety Education for Nurses (QSEN)** competencies, and **Concepts** for concept-based learning is listed below.

Competencies	Feature or Text	Location
IOM, QSEN, NCC Providing patient-centered care	Nursing Process: Patient Care Plan for Known Nerve Agent Exposure	Chapter 65, page 2070
	Crisis Intervention and Critical Incident Stress Management	Chapter 65, page 2076
	Cultural Considerations: Assistance and Recovery Across Cultures	Chapter 65, page 2077
	Cultural Considerations for Emergency Care Providers	Chapter 66, page 2082
	End-of-Life Considerations	Chapter 67, page 2102
	Nursing Process: Patient Care Plan for Trauma	Chapter 67, page 2105
	Intimate Partner Violence	Chapter 67, page 2107
	Chart 67-2: Elder Abuse and Neglect	Chapter 67, page 2108
IOM, QSEN, NCC Working in teams	Collaborative Management, pages 2068, 2069, 2073	Chapter 65
	Specialty Roles in Emergency Nursing, page 2082	Chapter 66
	Initial Assessment of the Trauma Patient, page 2096	Chapter 67
	Primary Survey, page 2097	Chapter 67
	Secondary Survey, page 2101	Chapter 67
	Trauma Rehabilitation, page 2109	Chapter 67
IOM, QSEN, NCC Employing evidence-based practice	Evidence-Based Practice: Family Presence During Resuscitation in the Emergency Department	Chapter 66, page 2088
	Evidence-Based Practice: Hypothermia in Trauma Patients	Chapter 67, page 2100
IOM, NCC Applying quality and safety improvement	Personal Protective Equipment, page 2063	Chapter 65
	Decontamination, page 2064	Chapter 65
	Safety Alerts, pages 2084, 2085, 2086	Chapter 66
	Safety Alerts, pages 2097, 2098, 2101, 2102	Chapter 67
NCC Applying ethical and legal responsibilities	Ethical Considerations in Disaster Care	Chapter 65, page 2077
	Legal Issues That Affect the ED	Chapter 66, page 2085
	Ethical Issues: Pain Management in the ED	Chapter 66, page 2088
	Ethical Issues Related to Trauma Patients and Their Families	Chapter 67, page 2104
NCC Developing professionally	Specialty Roles in Emergency Nursing, pages 2082, 2084	Chapter 66
NCC Education patients	Discharge Priorities for Emergency Department Patients	Chapter 66, page 2087
Concepts covered in Unit 1 include:	Collaboration Global communication Multi-system failure Safety Violence	

CHAPTER

65 Disaster Nursing

Renée Holleran

Outcome-Based Learning Objectives

After studying this chapter, the learner will be able to:

1. Define and describe disasters.
2. Identify the operational, medical, and nursing management of a disaster.
3. Execute a disaster triage plan.
4. Differentiate the safety principles related to disaster management, including decontamination of patients suffering from chemical, biologic, radiological, nuclear, explosive, and natural events.
5. Apply the principles of an incident command system in the hospital setting and the role of nursing.
6. Critique the role of DMAT, DMORT, and the Strategic National Stockpile.
7. Apply critical incident stress principles to disaster management.

KEY TERMS

acute radiation syndrome (ARS) p.2074
biologic agents p.2069
chemical agents p.2067
cold zone p.2065
critical incident p.2076
critical incident stress debriefing (CISD) p.2076
critical incident stress management p.2076
decontamination p.2064
disaster p.2058
Disaster Medical Assistance Team (DMAT) p.2067
Disaster Mortuary Operational Response Teams (DMORT) p.2067
emergency preparedness plan p.2059
hot zone p.2065
incident command system (ICS) p.2061
mitigation p.2059
natural events p.2058
nerve agents p.2068
persistent p.2068
personal protective equipment (PPE) p.2063
preparedness p.2059
push packs p.2066
radiologic agents p.2072
recovery p.2059
response p.2059
Simple Triage and Rapid Treatment (START) system p.2063
Strategic National Stockpile (SNS) p.2065
terrorism p.2075
vendor managed inventory (VMI) p.2066
warm zone p.2065
weapons of mass destruction (WMD) p.2062

Disasters

A **disaster** has been defined as a sudden calamitous event that causes destruction, damage, and loss. These can be either **natural events** or human-generated events. Destruction and damage may occur to cities, buildings, businesses, and the natural environment. Losses may encompass both human and animal lives as well as property and valuables (Varghese, 2010).

Disasters cause disruption of societies and of individuals' everyday lives. The aftermath of disasters can contribute to the development of major stressors on the people and resources needed to provide care to the victims. Planning, preparing, and responding during a disaster are important nursing roles.

Causes of Disasters

Disasters can be caused by natural or human-generated events or a combination of both. Natural disasters include hurricanes, floods, tornadoes, wildfires, and earthquakes. For example, the recent earthquakes in China, Haiti, and Japan caused numerous deaths and massive devastation to societies and environments from which they will require years to fully recover. And Hurricane Sandy in October, 2012, caused widespread flooding and required some hospitals in New York City to be evacuated.

Examples of human-generated disasters include motor vehicle crashes with multiple victims, release of chemical agents into the environment, release of biologic agents, exposure to radiation, and explosions. Health emergencies, such as the H1N1 flu epidemic of 2009 and 2010, have produced new challenges. Global travel has allowed these diseases to be transported rapidly all over the face of the earth, exposing large patient populations and causing increased stresses on health care facilities.

The distressing effects of a disaster are many and far reaching. They include lack of food and water (or lack of *safe* food and water); shortages of warmth and shelter; spread of diseases; and the psychological impact on the victims, the responders, and the community (Emergency Nurses Association [ENA], 2007; Robinson, 2010). Disaster planning is an important component of disaster management, and nurses play a significant role in this planning.

Disaster Planning

Dr. Eric Auf der Heide of the U.S. Department of Health and Human Services reviewed the literature regarding "lessons learned" from actual disasters and wrote:

> Disaster planning is only as good as the assumptions on which it is based. However, some of these assumptions are derived from a conventional wisdom that is at variance with empirical field disaster research studies. Knowledge of disaster research findings might help planners avoid common disaster management pitfalls, thereby improving disaster response planning (Auf der Heide, 2006).

Chart 65–1 contains a summary of these assumptions and what research has actually shown. These observations may be of use in planning disaster management.

Disaster management is based on four components: mitigation, preparedness, response, and recovery. **Mitigation** involves reducing or eliminating the consequences of a hazard or incident so that it has limited impact on society. For example, buildings that are constructed in an environment where there is an increased risk of earthquakes are built to withstand the effects of the forces exerted (Coppola, 2011a). Mitigation is a form of prevention.

Preparedness requires that those who may be affected by the disaster have the equipment and resources needed to increase the chances of survival and decrease losses related to the disaster (Coppola, 2011a). This is accomplished by the development and rehearsal of an emergency preparedness plan.

An **emergency preparedness plan** contains a hazard risk analysis, a basic plan, function annexes, and hazard-specific annexes, which are described in the following text. A hazard risk analysis identifies the specific hazards within a location or region and the consequences if a disaster was triggered by these hazards (Coppola, 2011a).

A basic plan is the framework of emergency preparedness. The basic plan outlines the what, where, who, and how of an institution's, community's, or country's response when a disaster hits. The plan should be comprehensive but simple and include relevant information about the affected area:

- Geographical limits
- Hospital location
- Listing of the specific hazards in the area, such as chemical and biologic hazards
- Special populations located in the affected area
- Maps and other useful information.

Each plan must also contain an organizational structure and assignment of responsibilities before, during, and after a disaster (Coppola, 2011a).

Functional and hazard-specific annexes contain more specific information. For example, in the functional annex, detailed functions are outlined, such as notification and warning systems, as well as communications, emergency medical services, and mass care. The hazard-specific annexes contain operational information that is not covered in the basic plan for specific risks (Coppola, 2011a). For example, in a hospital disaster plan, there should be a focused plan for evacuation of patient populations and the risks related to such evacuation (Coppola, 2011a).

An integral part of emergency preparedness is practice. Each hospital community (and, in some parts of the world, now even country) should have disaster exercises. These can be drill, table-top, functional, or full-scale exercises. Exercises provide an opportunity to identify issues and allow time to fix them before a real disaster occurs (Goodhue, Burke, Chambers, Ferrer, & Upperman, 2010).

Response involves the actions that are taken to reduce or eliminate the impact of the disaster (Coppola, 2011a; Mistric & Sparling, 2010). Response is focused on getting infrastructure back into place so that victims can be rescued or assisted as soon as possible. Opening roads, restoring electrical power communications, and providing food and shelter are a few of the things that need to be accomplished. The overall response is dictated by the type of disaster, the location of the disaster, and the people who are involved (Coppola, 2011b). Individual accountability and preparation are important pieces of any disaster response. Despite planning and scheduled exercises, recent disasters have demonstrated that we can never truly be prepared.

Recovery involves returning the lives and the environment of those affected by the disaster to normal. This includes both victims and responders. Recovery generally begins after the formal emergency response measures are deemed complete (Coppola, 2011b). Recovery is based on short- and long-term phases. Disaster planning includes what is needed in each of these phases. For example, short-term planning includes who will respond to assist, where shelters are located, and how food and water will be distributed. Long-term planning includes rebuilding and returning to "normal." Throughout and after the recovery process, the emotional and psychological needs of those affected must be addressed (Coppola, 2011b). Critical incident stress management is discussed later in this chapter.

The Joint Commission and Disaster Management

The Joint Commission requires that all hospitals and health care organizations that are accredited by the Joint Commission have an Emergency Management Plan. Components of this plan include management of natural disasters that occur because of meteorological or topological factors, such as hurricanes and floods; disasters that originate from underground, such as earthquakes; and biologic disasters, such as disease epidemics or widespread destruction of crops by pests. Plans should also be in place for responding to human-generated disasters such as warfare, civil disturbances, criminal and terrorist actions, and major accidents such as industrial and transportation accidents (Joint Commission, 2011). Each institution should have easy-to-find action plans; in addition, they should have planned and carried out drills so that these plans can be evaluated and the participants know their part in the plans.

Hospital Preparedness Planning

Natural disasters such as hurricanes and floods, acts of terrorism such as the shootings at Fort Hood in 2009, and communicable infections such as H1N1 in the spring and summer of 2009 have placed increased demands on hospitals. In 2002, the National Bioterrorism Preparedness Program was established to provide a resource for the management of bioterrorism events. However, it was quickly recognized that emergency preparedness and response needed to go beyond terrorism. In 2006, the Pandemic and All-Hazards Preparedness Act established the position of Assistant Secretary for Preparedness and Response (ASPR) within the Department of Health and Human Services. The Hospital Preparedness Program (HPP) was among several agencies that were incorporated into the ASPR's mandate. The HPP's mission is to assist states and territories to plan and coordinate patient surges when a natural or

CHART 65–1 Common Disaster Planning Assumptions Versus Research Observations

Assumption and Research Observations	Planning Implications	Potential Interventions
Assumption: Dispatchers will hear of the disaster and send emergency response units to the scene. *Observation:* Emergency response units, both local and distant, will often self-dispatch.	Effective disaster planning requires planning not only for the jurisdiction but also at the intercommunity level. Plans should anticipate the likelihood that more help than needed will arrive, whether requested or not.	Expect unsolicited responders, and develop a plan for coordinating them. Establish intercommunity or statewide mutual aid plans and training. Use staging or check-in areas outside of rapidly established security perimeters.
Assumption: Trained emergency personnel will carry out field search and rescue operations. *Observation:* Most initial search and rescue operations are carried out by the survivors themselves.	Planners may incorrectly assume that they will have control over disaster emergency medical service (EMS) responses. Disaster search and rescue operations are often ad hoc and uncoordinated. Even if they are not part of the planned response, law enforcement officers often become involved in search and rescue operations. Survivors involved in search and rescue operations may have the best information on the location of the missing.	Train first responders how to coordinate with survivors in carrying out search and rescue operations. Designate personnel to obtain information from survivors about the location of the missing.
Assumption: Trained EMS personnel will carry out triage, provide first aid or stabilize medical care, and, if necessary, decontaminate casualties before patient transport. *Observation:* Casualties are likely to bypass on-site triage, first aid, and decontamination stations and go directly to hospitals.	Hospitals should not assume that casualties will be triaged, decontaminated, or given first aid in the field. Patients arriving in private cars may need to be extricated carefully so that injuries are not aggravated.	Develop real-time instructions that can be given to survivors (by commercial radio) on how to protect themselves; give first aid; and deal with contaminated casualties. Provide courses on first aid, search and rescue, and disaster care for the public. Send first responders to hospitals to extricate casualties from private vehicles.
Assumption: Casualties will be transported to hospitals by ambulance. *Observation:* Most casualties are not transported by ambulance. Rather, they arrive at hospitals by a variety of nonambulance vehicles (private cars, police vehicles, buses, or on foot).	EMS authorities often have little control over the time of transport or hospital destination for disaster casualties. Transport outside of the EMS system also poses challenges for patient tracking.	Educate the public about precautions to take in transporting casualties and about which casualties should not be moved. Establish procedures for collecting information after the fact from hospitals about what casualties they have received.
Assumption: Casualties will be transported to hospitals appropriate for their needs and in such a manner that no hospital receives a disproportionate number of casualties. *Observation:* Most casualties are transported to the closest or most familiar hospitals.	Although specific hospitals may be designated to receive contaminated casualties, it is the patients who will often choose their destination. Thus, all hospitals must be prepared to do decontamination. Although it may not be possible to prevent inefficient casualty distribution, it may be possible to influence or plan around it.	Consider having ambulances bypass the hospitals closest to the disaster. Establish area and intercommunity EMS/hospital mutual aid plans and radio systems so that ambulances can be directed to the hospitals best able to treat their patients. Use a "first-wave" protocol to divide initial casualties among area hospitals.
Assumption: Authorities in the field will ensure that area hospitals are promptly notified of the disaster and the numbers, types, and severities of casualties to be transported to them. *Observation:* Hospital notification of a disaster may be from the first arriving victims or the news media rather than from the authorities in the field. Often, information and updates about incoming casualties are insufficient or lacking.	Initial hospital response may have to depend on the resources in house. Hospital procedures that require time-consuming activities before casualty arrival (donning chemical-resistant suits, etc.) may not be practical.	Base initial hospital response plans on in-house rather than on-call resources. Provide in-house staff with authority to activate and modify the plan. Develop plans for the expedient decontamination of unannounced casualties, which might include the use of fire hoses supplied with warm water, until more sophisticated decontamination equipment can be set up.
Assumption: The most serious casualties will be the first to be transported to hospitals. *Observation:* The least serious casualties often arrive first.	Because accurate and timely information from the field is often lacking, emergency departments may not know of the more serious patients yet to come. As a result, when these patients arrive, all beds may already be occupied.	Assign field responders to communicate casualty information to hospitals. Hold beds open at hospitals for the possibility of later-arriving, more serious casualties.

Weblink: FEMA National Incident Management System

human-generated disaster causes a sudden influx of patients and the need for additional resources.

The HPP's focus goes beyond bioterrorism to an all-hazards preparation approach for hospitals, including training of hospital staff and organization of resources. The HPP has been awarding funding to support enhanced planning for hospital and health care system planning and response at the state, local, and territorial levels; increased integration of public and private sectors to increase preparedness, response and surge capacity of hospitals and other health care facilities; and improved infrastructure to assist in the response to public health care emergencies (HPP, 2011). However, despite this national organization, many areas within the United States remain without the ability, or with limited abilities, to respond to disasters and the surges in patients and resource requirements that may occur (HPP, 2011).

National Standards of Nursing Education in Disaster Management

There was a time when nursing education in disaster management, including terrorist disasters, in the United States was considered unnecessary. Because of the events surrounding the September 11, 2001, terrorist attacks in New York and Washington, D.C.; Hurricanes Katrina and Rita in 2005; recent earthquakes in Haiti, China, Japan, and New Zealand; tornadoes in the Midwest and South; and flooding throughout the United States, nursing education has been forced to address the role of nursing in disaster management.

Gebbie and Qureshi (2002) published a simple set of competencies for working nurses with regard to emergency and disaster preparedness based on previous work done for public health workers in the *American Journal of Nursing* (Chart 65–2). This has become something of a classic work and is frequently quoted.

Even though these competencies were proposed in 2002, they remain pertinent today. Other nursing associations have also developed guidelines so that student nurses can be prepared for disaster management. The American Association of Colleges of Nursing (AACN) and the National League for Nurses (NLN) both provide information about how to achieve this (Stangeland, 2010).

Nursing education must continue to address disaster management and the nurse's role through formal courses in school, exposing students to disaster exercises, and providing continuing education programs so that nurses can be prepared for the unexpected (Gebbie, 2010; Little-Kearney & Slepski, 2008).

Disaster Management Concepts

When a disaster occurs and an emergency preparedness plan is implemented, there are some concepts that are imperative for the safe management of patients. These include incident command, hospital incident command, disaster triage, treatment, and the use of personal protective equipment.

National Incident Management System

The National Incident Management System (NIMS) is based on the **incident command system (ICS),** initially designed for use by fire departments at California wildfire sites. The NIMS creates a standard but flexible all-hazards organizational structure whereby the various agencies involved can interact and communicate in an organized manner. It is designed to be used in all phases of disaster management: mitigation, preparedness, response, and recovery (Emergency Management Institute [EMI], 2011; Robinson, 2010). The NIMS has an incident commander, one person who is in charge of the entire operation. The operation itself is broken into four main areas: operations, planning, logistics, and finance, with a chief in charge of each division. These four chiefs report directly to the incident commander. Also reporting directly to the incident commander are a safety officer, a public information officer, and a liaison officer. Room is also made in the structure for experts in certain areas, such as animal health or search and rescue, who answer directly to the incident commander (EMI, 2011). Extensive training on NIMS is available from the Federal Emergency Management Agency (FEMA); its website is kept up-to-date with new training sessions as they are developed.

The ICS was adapted to the hospital environment initially by the state of California and evolved into what is now called the hospital

CHART 65–2 Emergency and Disaster Preparedness Core Competencies for Nurses

1. Describe the agency's role in responding to a range of emergencies that might arise.
2. Describe the chain of command in emergency response.
3. Identify and locate the agency's emergency response plan (or the pertinent portion of it).
4. Describe emergency response functions or roles, and demonstrate them in regularly performed drills.
5. Demonstrate the use of equipment (including personal protective equipment) and the skills required in emergency response during regular drills.
6. Demonstrate the correct operation of all equipment used for emergency communication.
7. Describe communication roles in emergency response.
8. Identify the limits of one's own knowledge, skills, and authority, and identify key system resources for referring matters that exceed these limits.
9. Apply creative problem-solving skills and flexible thinking to the situation, within the confines of one's role, and evaluate the effectiveness of all actions taken.
10. Recognize deviations from the norm that might indicate an emergency and describe appropriate action.
11. Participate in continuing education to maintain up-to-date knowledge in relevant areas.
12. Participate in evaluating every drill or response and identify necessary changes to the plan.

Additional Core Competencies for Managers

13. Ensure that there is a written plan for major categories of emergencies.
14. Ensure that all parts of the plan are practiced regularly.
15. Ensure that gaps in knowledge or skills are filled.

Source: Gebbie, K. M., & Qureshi, K. (2002). Emergency and disaster preparedness: Core competencies for nurses. *American Journal of Nursing, 1*(102), 46–51. With permission.

incident command system (HICS). Information about HICS is available at www.calhospitalprepare.org/.

Hospital Incident Command System

The HICS uses the same command structure as the NIMS but is adapted to a hospital environment. The HICS manual and supporting documents, available free online, contain the structure with all job descriptions, sample policies and procedures, as well as sample documents, including checklists and tracking sheets; these can be copied and/or adapted for use as needed (California Hospital Association, 2011). The HICS naturally fits into the NIMS, which allows the hospital to speak the same language and use the same divisions as all other agencies.

Organization

The HICS is used in the hospital any time there is an incident that has the potential to overwhelm resources (Figure 65–1◆). This could include anything from a large traffic collision with multiple victims all the way to a massive event involving **weapons of mass destruction (WMD)** such as a nuclear explosion. With HICS, the plan is flexible enough to be altered to fit the situation. Only those positions and functions that are required by the particular incident need to be activated. In addition, many of the positions can be combined and filled by one person. The plan gives a clear chain of command and clear responsibilities, has a common language and common mission, prioritizes duties, and ensures thorough documentation of actions. The comprehensive documentation allows for a more complete evaluation of the event in the after action sessions. It also improves recovery of expenses while decreasing liability (California Hospital Association, 2011).

The HICS uses the same basic structure as the NIMS. There is an incident commander to whom the public information officer, the safety and security officer, the liaison officer, and the section chiefs answer. The incident commander organizes and directs the emergency operations center and gives overall direction for the hospital operations. The public information officer provides information to the media, releases other information as appropriate, and assists with communication. The safety and security officer monitors and has authority over the safety of rescue operations and hazardous conditions. This person organizes and enforces scene, facility, and traffic protection and security. The liaison officer functions as the contact person for representatives of other agencies such as the fire department and police departments. As with NIMS, the administrative structure has room for a medical or technical specialist if needed. An example of a needed specialist might be a radiation specialist in the event of a dirty bomb (California Hospital Association, 2011).

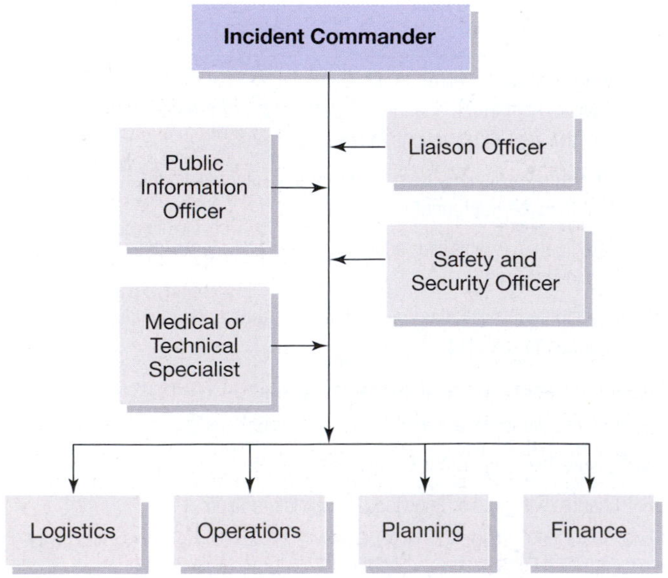

FIGURE 65–1 ◆ Hospital incident command system.

Sections

The HICS has four sections, each led by a chief: planning, logistics, finance, and operations. Each section can be further divided if needed. This subdivides the work and allows for a workable span of management responsibility for each individual (California Hospital Association, 2011).

The planning section ensures the formulation and documentation of an overall response plan and helps to set objectives. It gathers data and status reports from various areas within the hospital to aid in decision making. The planning section is responsible for duties such as providing a situation status report to the hospital and hospital workers every 4 to 6 hours. The planning section also interacts with other sections, such as assisting in establishing a plan for medical staff rotation in cooperation with personnel from the operations section.

The logistics section provides the hospital environment and materials to meet all objectives. This includes organizing and directing all operations associated with maintaining the physical environment; adequate food for patients, visitors, and personnel; shelter; and adequate medical and pharmaceutical supplies. Duties such as transportation, assessing damaged areas for use or evacuation, communications, and materials supply are also included.

The finance section provides the funding for operations and ensures hospitalwide documentation of activities and expenses to assist with recovery of costs. Large events typically cost millions of dollars in salaries, materials, equipment, and other costs. A single incident can bankrupt a facility without reimbursement. Even federal relief dollars require documentation of expenses for receipt of reimbursement.

The operations section covers much of the day-to-day work of delivering medical care. This includes matching staff to patient needs, organizing inpatient care, and managing the treatment areas such as triage, the emergency department, operating rooms, discharging of patients, and morgue operations (California Hospital Association, 2011).

Disaster Triage

Disaster triage requires a utilitarian approach. In other words, the greatest good is provided to the greatest number based on the available resources (ENA, 2007). For example, there may be hundreds of people who require care but only enough resources for half that number. This can be particularly difficult for nurses who are used to working in the hospital where all patients are afforded care.

The triage (see Chapter 66 for triage discussion) of mass casualties poses unique challenges. Sorting and identifying the level of care required are necessary so that patients are sent to the proper areas and resources are not used inappropriately. One of the most commonly used disaster triage systems utilizes color coding. Chart 65–3 provides an example of a color-coded chart (ENA, 2007).

START Triage

To sort through the huge influx of people during mass casualty incidents, there needs to be a method of identifying those most in need of

CHART 65–3 Color-Coded Disaster Triage Chart

Category	Definitions
Emergent (RED)	**Life-threatening injuries** **Airway or surgical issue that can be corrected in the emergency department.**
Urgent (YELLOW)	Major illness or injury that requires treatment within 30 to 60 minutes.
Nonurgent (GREEN)	"Walking wounded"; can be self-treated
Expectant (BLACK)	Dead or expected to die

decontamination and care. The **Simple Triage and Rapid Treatment (START) system** was designed by Hoag Hospital and the Newport Beach, California, Fire Department for use in multiple casualty incidents. It has become the standard method of triage in mass casualty. This method is effective both at the scene of an incident and for sorting at the door of the hospital. However, START is not designed for use in the pediatric population. However, a corollary system called "Jump START" has criteria for children based on the same categories (Disaster Management Systems, 2011; Romig, 2008).

The START triage system uses four categories: Red means that immediate care is needed, with usually two or more systems affected. Yellow means that delayed care is needed, with usually one system involved. Green means that minor care is needed. Black means that the person is deceased or that death is expected, with no life-extending care to be delivered. However, comfort care may be provided if available (Figure 65–2◆).

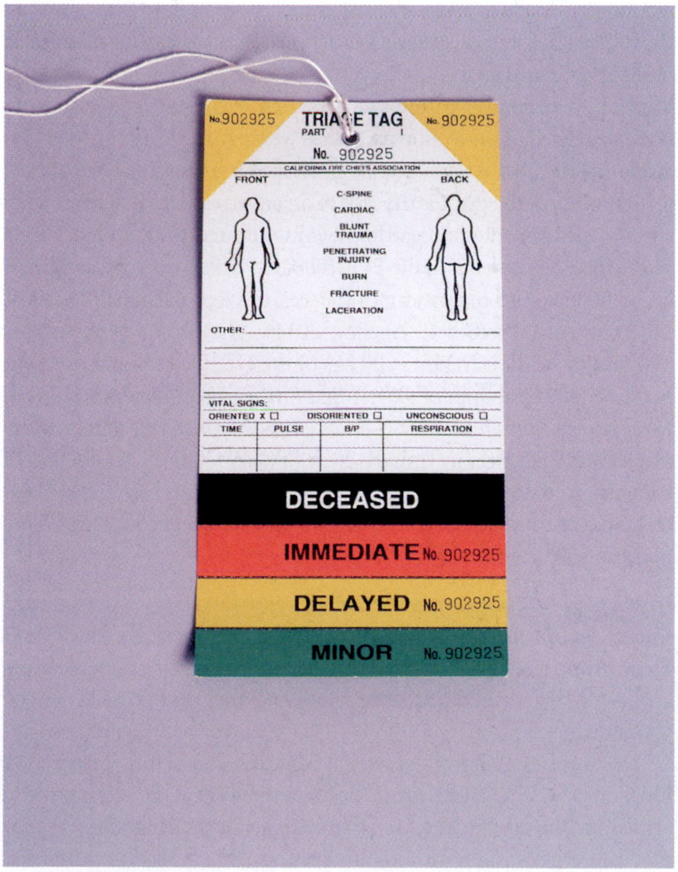

FIGURE 65–2 ◆ Triage tag.

To determine the appropriate category, respirations, perfusion, and neurological status are checked. The first step is to identify the "walking wounded." An announcement is made that all who can walk go to a designated area. These individuals are all automatically assigned to the green or minor category. For those who are left, the rescuers open the airway and rank the respirations; if greater than 30, the person is ranked as red and receives a tag. If respirations are less than 30, no tag is given; a black tag is given if respirations are zero. Next, the rescuers control major hemorrhage and assess perfusion by checking for a radial pulse, as a person must have a blood pressure of at least 80 mmHg to have a radial pulse. If there is no radial pulse, the patient's legs are elevated and she receives a red immediate tag; if there is a pulse, no tag is given. The last step is to check the neurological status. If the person can answer a simple yes–no question, he receives a yellow delayed tag. If unable to answer, he receives a red tag.

For those with a red tag, indicating the immediate care needed category, classic assessment findings include that respirations are present only after repositioning the airway, respiratory rate is less than 8 or greater than 30, capillary refill is delayed more than 2 seconds, and there may be a significant decrease in level of consciousness. For those with a yellow tag, indicating the delayed care needed category, the injuries can be controlled or treated for a limited time in the field. Green, the minor care designation, includes individuals who are ambulatory, with or without minor injuries that do not require immediate or significant treatment. The black, indicating the deceased or expectant category, is for individuals with no spontaneous effective respiration after the airway is repositioned (Disaster Management Systems, 2011).

As with any methodology, the START triage system requires practice for proficiency. Some hospitals use START tags on designated days throughout the month during routine operations as a drill to enable personnel to remain familiar with the tags and system.

Treatment

Once a patient's level of care has been classified, some sort of process must be available to label the patient. Some systems use colored paper tags, which can also allow for additional information to be written about the patient. Other systems use plastic colored ribbons that are tied somewhere on the patient's body. The patient is then taken to the corresponding area where treatment may be started or further triage may occur.

The type of disaster will determine the type of treatment required. For example, traumatic injuries, such as lacerations and head and chest injuries, are common. Resources and equipment for wound care, tetanus prophylaxis, and antibiotics may be needed in these cases.

Patients with chronic illnesses such as diabetes and hypertension may require acute medical management as well as medications until their previous care can be reestablished. Hospitals and surrounding communities need contingency plans to manage these patients.

Just as hospitals have to plan for the classification of patients and the resources needed during a disaster, they also have to be sure that staff and patients are safe. Exposure to chemical, biologic, or radiologic agents can place staff and patients at additional risks. The following section describes the basic principles of personal protective equipment and how to safely manage patients and/or staff who may have been exposed.

Personal Protective Equipment

Personal protective equipment (PPE) is the clothing and equipment that protect personnel from whatever agent they may be exposed

CHART 65–4 Personal Protective Equipment Levels

Level A

Highest level of respiratory, skin, and eye protection

Fully encapsulated chemical-resistant suit

Full face piece and supplied air (self-contained breathing apparatus, or SCBA)

Inner chemical-resistant gloves

Chemical-resistant safety boots

"Moon suit"

Level B

Same respiratory protection as Level A but less skin protection

Full face piece and supplied air (SCBA)

Chemical-resistant clothing

Inner and outer chemical-resistant gloves

Chemical-resistant safety boots

Hard hat

Level C

Full face piece with air-purifying canister-equipped respirator

Chemical-resistant clothing

Hard hat

Level D

Regular work clothing

Safety shoes

Safety goggles/splash shield

to, including chemical, biologic, or radiologic contamination. Personal protective equipment is classified according to the degree of protection it delivers: Level A, Level B, Level C, and Level D (Chart 65–4 and Figures 65–3◆ and 65–4◆). Many daily exposures to hazardous materials that are not even related to terrorist events will require personal protection and perhaps even decontamination.

No one suit is protective for all agents. Factors to determine which level of PPE to use include not only the agent but also other practical matters such as the temperature, humidity, body size, facial hair, and strenuousness of the expected activity. In addition, PPE presents many

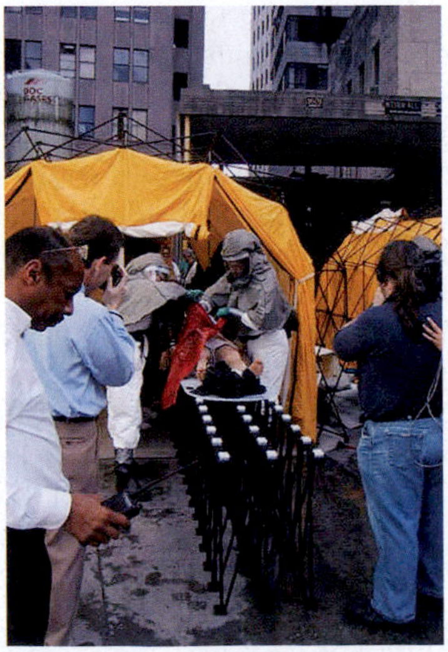

FIGURE 65–3 ◆ Decontamination drill in PPE suit.
Source: Robert J. McBride, RN

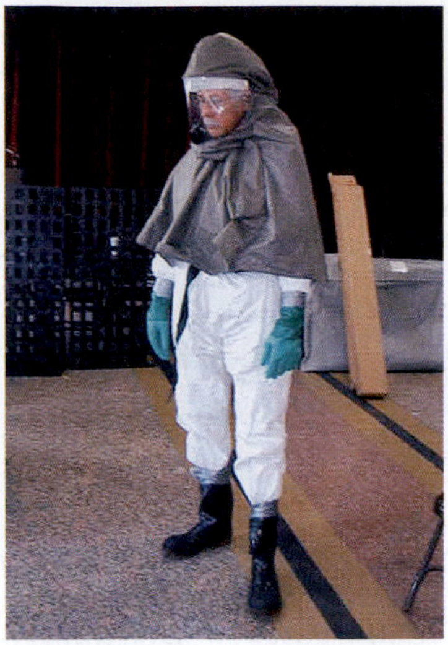

FIGURE 65–4 ◆ PPE suit.
Source: Robert J. McBride, RN.

problems for the user, including hyperthermia, dehydration, claustrophobia, limited vision, limited dexterity, limited movement, and communication problems. During operations, there need to be preset hand signals indicating distress that can be used by the person in the gear.

Proper donning and doffing of PPE are essential to prevent contamination. Therefore, extensive training and practice are required. Proper donning includes such things as correct use of all gear, taping all openings, and checking for breaches in gear before entering a contaminated area. There also need to be specific checklists for removing protective clothing at the end of an incident or end of a tour of duty. The person in the PPE will also require decontamination before being allowed to enter noncontaminated areas.

While a person is wearing the PPE, there is constant concern about possible breach of protection as well as whether the level of protection is appropriate for the situation. In general, the greater the level of protection needed, the greater the risk of an adverse effect. There are very specific medical criteria regarding who is allowed to don higher level PPE. Once the person is in the PPE, the safety officer and medical management personnel must monitor the wearer for problems (ENA, 2007; Environmental Protection Agency, 2011). The Occupational Safety and Health Administration (OSHA) of the U.S. Department of Labor published the final draft of *OSHA Best Practices for Hospital-Based First Receivers of Victims from Mass Casualty Incidents Involving the Release of Hazardous Substances* in January 2005 (OSHA, 2005). This document contains recommendations for PPE purchasing and training based on a hospital's hazard analysis. It also highlights safety concerns for the personnel wearing the PPE.

Decontamination

Decontamination is the reduction or removal of contaminating agents. When decontaminating patients, the runoff needs to be contained.

Decontamination in the hospital or health care setting can involve individuals who received "gross" decontamination at the scene prior to arrival and those who presented to the facility outside of the emergency medical services route without any prior treatment. It is important to recognize that contaminated individuals must be fully decontaminated before being admitted to the facility to prevent the facility from being contaminated as well. The axiom is: "There are no patients until they are decontaminated." Victims, first responders from the scene, equipment, and personnel assisting with the process will all undergo decontamination.

Gross decontamination, or field decontamination, is a process whereby the greater part of the contaminating agent is removed or washed away. This is usually done by some type of high-volume rinse system such as systems created by using fire hoses. It is estimated that 80% of the agent can be removed by simply removing the clothing (Agency for Toxic Substances and Disease Registry [ATSDR], 2011; Andress, 2010; ENA, 2007).

The decontamination area is set up outdoors and consists of three zones: the hot zone, warm zone, and cold zone. It is best if the hospital is upwind of the decontamination area. The **hot zone,** also called the exclusion zone or red zone, is the area of highest contamination. This is where people who are waiting to be decontaminated are staged. A triage area is usually set up here to identify individuals who require quicker treatment (see the START Triage section earlier in this chapter). Each person receives a numbered tag. A brief registration is done to collect basic information such as name, date of birth, and social security number; this information is logged with the person's triage number. Many hospitals have prenumbered triage kits with tags, registration sheets, and belonging bags already on the disaster cart.

The **warm zone,** or yellow zone, is also referred to as the contamination reduction corridor (Figure 65–5◆). This is where the actual decontamination process takes place. The **cold zone,** or green zone, is also known as the support zone. The hospital is in the cold zone. In situations in which decontamination is necessary, no one is allowed into the cold zone without being decontaminated (Andress, 2010; ATSDR, 2011; ENA, 2007). Chart 65–5 outlines the three zones of decontamination.

The decontamination lines are usually divided into males and females and into those who are ambulatory and nonambulatory. The first step is to disrobe completely. Clothing is generally collected in red bags and labeled. Personal belongings, such as watches, wallets, jewelry, and eyeglasses, are usually collected in clear plastic bags and labeled. Valuables may require separate decontamination or may have to be disposed of, depending on the contaminant. In the shower area, the person will fully lather up, including in all body creases, the hair, and the genital area. Attention should be directed toward wounds first, as agents are more rapidly absorbed by broken skin. There has been

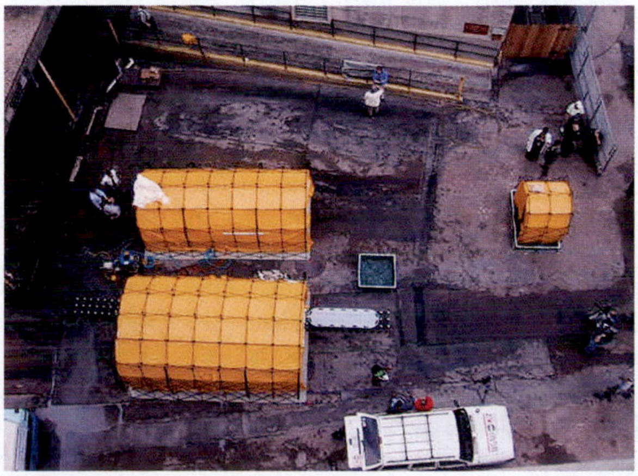

FIGURE 65–5 ◆ Decontamination setup.

Source: Robert J. McBride, RN.

CHART 65–5 Zones of Decontamination

Hot Zone	Warm Zone	Cold Zone
Red	Yellow	Green
Patient entry	Decontamination	Clean treatment area
EMS access	Ambulatory	Clean evacuation
Triage	Nonambulatory	Staging area for personnel
Initial disrobing		
Emergency first aid		

controversy regarding the best agents for decontamination. Common current consensus is to use some type of liquid soap or baby shampoo. A 0.5% bleach is still used for some equipment decontamination. People who are ambulatory need only guidance in the process of cleaning themselves. Nonambulatory individuals, however, will require physical washing by specially trained personnel in full personal protective gear. Once washing is complete, the decontaminated individuals dry off, are given some type of hospital gown or clothing, and are admitted into the cold zone disposition area, from where they are sent into the hospital system (Andress, 2010; ATSDR, 2011; ENA, 2007).

In suspected criminal events, all of the clothing and personal belongings that are collected are considered evidence from a crime scene. The appropriate law enforcement agency should be notified. It is important that these items be handled by using usual chain-of-custody procedures.

National Resources

In addition to regional and state supplies, there are national resources available to assist in a disaster situation.

Strategic National Stockpile

The National Pharmaceutical Stockpile program, created in 1999 under the auspices of the Centers for Disease Control and Prevention (CDC, 2011a), was originally funded with only $5.2 million per year (CDC, 2011b). However, the National Pharmaceutical Stockpile program was moved into the new Department of Homeland Security on March 1, 2003, and renamed the **Strategic National Stockpile (SNS)** program. The purpose of the stockpile is to maintain a national repository of pharmaceutical agents, vaccines, medical supplies, and equipment that will be delivered to the site of a large-scale disaster to augment local and state resources in order to decrease morbidity and mortality in the civilian population (Esbitt, 2003; Williams, 2002).

Organization

The Strategic National Stockpile is organized into five tiers: 12-hour push packs, vendor managed inventory, storage and rapid deployment of vaccines, buying power with surge capacity, and technical assistance. To obtain SNS assets, the affected state's governor must request the SNS from the CDC. The CDC director will evaluate the request and release the supplies if they are deemed necessary (CDC, 2011c; Esbitt, 2003).

Although the SNS delivers material and technical assistance at no charge, the state and local agencies must provide the labor to use and distribute the materials to the population. The state will need nurses, pharmacists, and health care providers for the dispensing site, but can use nonmedical volunteers to assist with crowd control, move materials, and operate machinery such as forklifts (Esbitt, 2003; Williams, 2002).

CHART 65–6 Contents of a 12-Hour Push Pack

- Antibiotics and other pharmaceuticals
- IV supplies
- Airway supplies
- Bandage supplies
- Pill counting and packaging equipment
- Thorough vendor managed inventory (VMI): vaccines, antivirals/antitoxins

Push Packs

Although 12-hour push packs make up less than 5% of the stockpile, they are what is most commonly considered in discussions of the SNS. The **push packs** are so named because they can be shipped within 12 hours of the decision to deploy the assets (Chart 65–6). Sets of 12-hour push packs are stored in secured, environmentally contained depots located throughout the United States. Each set consists of 100 containers weighing approximately 50 tons total. Each container is on wheels and can easily be moved by one or two people. The containers are designed to fill a 747 cargo jet completely. The receiving site must have about 12,000 square feet of space for storage, repackaging of bulk supplies, performing inventory control, and distributing the supplies (Esbitt, 2003; Williams, 2002).

The contents of the push packs include broad-spectrum oral antibiotic agents, intravenous and intramuscular medications, analgesics, and other emergency medications. They also include equipment such as pill-counting devices and an automatic packaging machine. Other supplies include intravenous supplies, airway supplies, and bandaging supplies. It costs about $9 million per month to store and maintain the push packs (Esbitt, 2003; Williams, 2002). The contents of the push packs are reviewed by content experts frequently and changed based on the current perceived threats.

The SNS delivered a team of technical advisers and a 12-hour push pack to New York on September 11, 2001. The technical advisers arrived 5 hours after deployment, and the push pack arrived 7 hours after deployment (Esbitt, 2003). Supplies from the SNS were also deployed to the Gulf Coast region following Hurricanes Katrina and Rita in 2005. The SNS authorized the release of one-quarter of its antiviral drugs to state health departments during the 2009 H1N1 epidemic (CDC, 2009b).

Vendor Managed Inventory

Vendor managed inventory (VMI) is federally owned inventory that is stored by the vendor until needed. Vendor managed inventory is designed to be used to provide specific pharmaceuticals and supplies when the chemical or biologic agent is known or for smaller scale events when an entire push pack is not needed. It can also be used to resupply at the scene when a push pack has been deployed. When needed as part of the initial response, the goal is to deliver the VMI within 12 hours. During the anthrax events of 2001, more than 50 requests for antibiotics were filled and shipped to 11 states and the District of Columbia. Each shipment's delivery time was less than 5 hours (Esbitt, 2003).

Vaccines and antitoxins are stockpiled using VMI. When they are shipped, special cooler containers are used to maintain the products at the correct temperature. For smallpox, only the vaccine, diluent, bifurcated needles, and transfer needles are sent. The location must supply items such as gloves, gauze, adhesive bandages, sharps containers, and waste bags (Williams, 2002).

The federal government has special prearranged contracts that allow for the purchase of large amounts of supplies and pharmaceuticals should the need arise. In this surge capacity contracting, there are over 97 lines of inventory (Williams, 2002).

Technical Support

A team of advisers, called the Technical Advisory Response Unit (TARU), is made up of five to seven experts in logistics, public health, communications, operations, and emergency response. The TARU can help state and local authorities with receiving, managing, distributing, dispensing, and replenishing the SNS. These units can provide technical assistance with operation of the machinery such as the repackaging unit. They also can assist in recovering the support equipment and cargo containers and in recovering unused SNS assets and materials (Esbitt, 2003).

National Disaster Medical System

Housed in the U.S. Department of Health and Human Services, the Office of Preparedness and Response directs and manages the National Disaster Medical System (NDMS), which ensures that resources are available after a disaster that overwhelms the local health care resources. Under the National Response Plan, NDMS is responsible for coordinating and managing the federal response to federally declared disasters and major emergencies including natural disasters, technologic disasters, major transportation incidents, and acts of terrorism. Within NDMS are six major divisions: Disaster Medical Assistance Teams, Disaster Mortuary Operational Response Teams, National Veterinary Response Teams, National Pharmacy Response Teams, National Nurse Response Teams, and Federal Coordinating Centers. All of these teams are made up of volunteers who, when deployed, become federal employees for the duration of their tour. There is a modest reimbursement. For most of these teams, there is special training and online continuing education requirements (U.S. Department of Health and Human Services [DHHS], 2008a). All of the divisions were deployed in response to Hurricanes Katrina and Rita in 2005 (continuing into 2006).

The services of Disaster Medical Assistance Teams and Disaster Mortuary Operational Response Teams will be discussed in more detail next. First, the Federal Coordinating Centers (FCCs) coordinate the reception and distribution of patients being evacuated to an area. They play a role in recruiting hospitals and maintaining nonfederal hospital participation in NDMS. The FCCs also work with local authorities and hospitals in developing plans and coordinating exercises (DHHS, 2008b).

The National Veterinary Response Teams (NVRTs) are very much like Disaster Medical Assistance Teams, but they work with animals. The purpose of these teams is to assess the medical needs and provide stabilization and treatment for animals; provide surveillance regarding animal disease, biologic and chemical terrorism, public health assessments, animal decontamination, and technical assistance regarding food and water quality; and provide hazard mitigation (DHHS, 2008b).

The National Pharmacy Response Teams (NPRTs) were designed to assist with the chemical prophylaxis or vaccination if needed for a biologic event. These teams comprise pharmacists, pharmacy technicians, and pharmacy students (DHHS, 2008b).

The National Nurse Response Teams (NNRTs) are used when an incident occurs that overwhelms the nation's supply of nurses in responding to a disaster. It is also designed to assist in chemoprophylaxis or a mass vaccination program (DHHS, 2008b).

Disaster Medical Assistance Teams

The **Disaster Medical Assistance Team (DMAT)** is part of the National Response Plan (NDMS) (Dayton DMAT, 2008; DHHS, 2008b). A DMAT is a group of volunteer health care providers, nurses, emergency medical technicians, technical staff, and other health care professionals and support staff designed to provide emergency medical services. They can provide care at a temporary site such as a tent or at a fixed site such as a hospital. In mass casualty situations, the team can conduct triage, provide medical care, and prepare patients for evacuation. The DMAT may assist overloaded local staff at local health care facilities and/or provide primary health care. When deployed, the team arrives with enough supplies and equipment to sustain itself for 72 hours (Dayton DMAT, 2008). Following Hurricanes Katrina and Rita, multiple DMAT teams were deployed to the entire Gulf region. They performed duties ranging from staffing vaccination clinics to relieving local hospital staff to providing the primary source of medical care in a decimated area.

Types of DMAT Teams

A level 1 DMAT travels with all of its own supplies and equipment, including tents (Figure 65–6◆). It is fully self-contained for 72 hours. A level 2 DMAT is deployed with another team or relieves a level 1 team. It is not considered self-sufficient, as it does not carry its own supplies. A level 3 team has local responsibilities only. There are about 55 DMAT teams. Other specialty teams include burn teams, pediatric teams, veterinary teams, and mortuary teams (Dayton DMAT, 2008).

Deployment

DMATs are completely voluntary and used only within the United States. Once activated for deployment, the team member becomes a temporary federal employee. Because the person is a federal employee, any license or certification she holds is automatically recognized in all 50 states. Team members are paid wages, reimbursed for travel expenses, and provided a food stipend. There are meetings to attend and training in such things as setting up the tents, familiarization with the equipment, and learning how to work within the team. Each member is required to provide certain personal gear needed for deployment, such as eye and ear protection, leather work gloves, canteen, sleeping bag, camping knife, hand cleanser gel, and toilet paper. Further information on becoming part of a DMAT team is available online (Dayton DMAT, 2008).

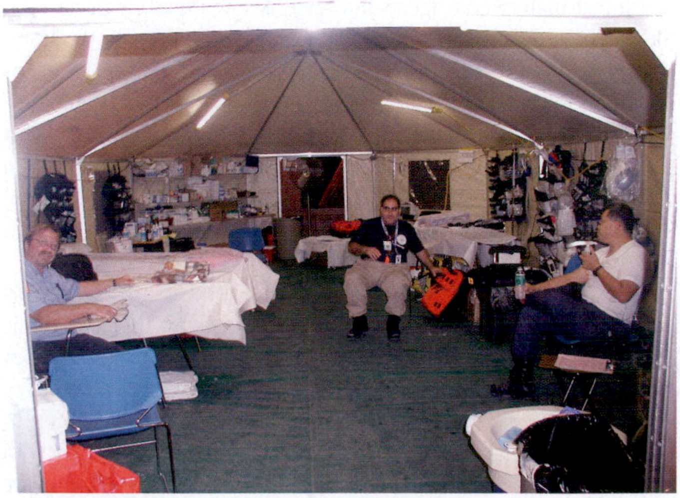

FIGURE 65–6 ◆ DMAT tent and team members.
Source: Kathleen Osborn.

CHART 65–7 What Can DMORT Do to Help?

Mobile morgue operations	Forensic examination
DNA acquisition	Remains identification
Search and recovery	Scene documentation
Medical/psychological support	Embalming/casketing
Family assistance center	Antemortem data collection
Postmortem data collection	Records data entry
Database administration	Personal effects processing
Coordination of release of remains	Safety officers and specialists
Provide a liaison to U.S. Public Health Service (USPHS)	
Provide communications equipment	

Disaster Mortuary Operational Response Teams

In large-scale events, along with large numbers of ill or injured people, there will be large numbers of the dead. Management of the dead requires special training and resources. **Disaster Mortuary Operational Response Teams (DMORTs)** are designed to assist with this task. The DMORTs are under the NDMS in the Department of Health and Human Services in the same manner as the DMAT. DMORTs can provide comprehensive mass fatality management for incidents that overwhelm local resources. As with DMATs, these volunteers become temporary federal employees when deployed. Because people in the United States expect full identification of the dead, federal level assistance is needed in large events owing to the tremendous drain on resources and finances (DHHS, 2008b).

DMORT extensive services include mobile morgue operations, forensic examination assistance, DNA acquisition, remains identification, search and recovery operations, scene documentation, medical and psychological support, embalming and casketing, a family assistance center, antemortem and postmortem data collection, record keeping, processing of personal effects, coordination of release of remains, communication, and safety officers and specialists. DMORT teams can identify remains that require decontamination prior to release or autopsy. In identifying remains, they do extensive data gathering, which has helped in identifying even minute remains; this allows the family of a deceased casualty to have closure. Chart 65–7 summarizes the tasks DMORT may be called upon to perform.

Chemical Agents

Chemical agents are solids, liquids, or gases that act on the tissues of organisms or interact with air, water, and/or soil in the environment. These agents are generally considered either industrial or military, depending on their use and how they affect the body. Chemical agents include nerve agents and vesicants (blistering agents), which are generally considered to be military agents only. Blood agents, choking agents, and irritants are the other categories; they are mostly toxic industrial chemicals. Chart 65–8 provides a list of agents by category.

Spread

Most dissemination of chemical agents is by aerosol. The spread of chemical agents by this method depends on the agent's vapor pressure, how fast it goes from a liquid to a gas at room temperature, and its vapor density, which is its weight relative to air. High vapor pressure agents evaporate quickly, such as acetone (fingernail polish remover). In contrast, high vapor density agents, such as chlorine, tend to sink and hug the ground. Low vapor pressure agents and high vapor density agents

CHART 65–8 Chemical Agents by Class

Nerve Agents
Sarin (GB)
Soman (GD)
Tabun (GA)
V agent (VX)

Vesicants
Mustard
Lewisite
Phosgene oxime

Blood Agents
Hydrogen cyanide
Cyanogen chloride

Choking Agents (Asphyxiates)
Ammonia
Chlorine
Phosgene

Irritants
Mace (CN)
Tear gas (CS)
Pepper spray (OC)

are said to be **persistent;** that is, they stay around for a long time, creating a hazardous environment for a longer period. This naturally means a longer exposure time and the potential to expose more people to their effects. An agent is considered persistent if it lasts longer than 24 hours as a liquid on surfaces. Persistent agents such as mustard gas and VX (*O*-ethyl *S*-[2-(diisopropylamino)ethyl] methylphosphonothioate, an extremely toxic nerve agent) become useful in denying access to an area or to materials. Nonpersistent agents, such as sarin (used in the Tokyo attacks) and cyanide, are more useful as tactical agents within a population (Andress, 2010; ATSDR, 2011; ENA, 2007).

Nursing Management

Nursing management of the patient who has been exposed to chemical agents depends greatly on the agent and the severity of the exposure. Application of the nursing process will facilitate a comprehensive approach to patient assessment and care. Nursing diagnoses depend on the agent and the symptoms that are seen. For all chemical agents, *Risk for Injury* related to gross contamination with chemical will apply. Patient assessment parameters will follow the signs and symptoms that are expected, based on the class of agent. (A sample Nursing Process: Patient Care Plan for nerve agents is provided in the Nerve Agents section, p. 2070.)

Collaborative Management

Much of the care of patients who have been exposed to chemical agents involves treatment of symptoms. All of these patients require comprehensive care from a health care team that includes nurses, health care providers, toxicologists, and specialists from a number of fields, depending on the nature and severity of the injury. In order to meet desired patient outcomes, it is essential that this interdisciplinary team communicate openly with one another in developing and evaluating care of the patient and family (IOM [Institute of Medicine], 2010). Psychological and emotional care of these patients needs to be included along with physical care.

Routes of Entry

There are several means by which chemical agents can be spread. It is important to attempt to identify the route of entry in order to identify other potential patients.

Ingestion

Chemicals can be put in food, medicines, and water or other liquids. Ingestion through the public water supply is a less likely scenario owing to dilution and the processes that water undergoes at treatment plants. Water wells and individual buildings are considered more likely targets. An example of the oral route occurred in 1982 when bottles of Tylenol were contaminated with cyanide and seven people died. Although the casualty count was low, this episode of product tampering created a tremendous amount of fear in the population (Andress, 2010; ATSDR, 2011).

Inhalation

Inhalation is considered the most common route of entry for chemicals, as most episodes of chemical agent release will be by aerosol. Besides wind dispersion, many devices can be used for dissemination, including mosquito control trucks, aerial sprayers such as crop dusters, various pieces of industrial spray equipment such as pesticide sprayers, and buildings' heating and cooling systems. The new term for this activity is *aerobiology* (Andress, 2010; ATSDR, 2011).

Injection

Injection of chemical agents can be by needle, dart, or any other sharp object such as broken glass. The number of casualties with this method is low. Other injection methods include the shrapnel from a chemical dispersion device. The shrapnel containing the chemical in the device would enter the body and be absorbed into the tissue (Andress, 2010; ATSDR, 2011).

Dermal Exposure

Dermal exposure to chemicals may cause external damage to the skin and eyes. The agent can then be absorbed through the skin and into the body. This would occur through either an aerosol release or an accidental or intentional spill. With an aerosol release, the agent would have to have a high vapor density so that it would fall on the intended population. With an intentional spill, the agent would most likely be persistent in nature (Andress, 2010; ATSDR, 2011).

Nerve Agents

Nerve agents are gases or liquids that penetrate the skin and/or lungs and damage the nervous and respiratory systems. They are the most toxic of the known chemical agents. During World War II, Germany developed many nerve agents but for unknown reasons never used them. The only known uses of nerve agents have been in the Iran–Iraq War and by terrorists. Nerve agents work in a manner similar to organophosphate insecticides in that they inactivate acetylcholinesterase, thereby increasing the acetylcholine at the receptor site. This process results in an overstimulation at the synapse. The effect on the patient is dose related. The most common routes of exposure are inhaled and topical. The agents are readily absorbed from the skin and eyes.

The signs and symptoms seen, which are the same as with organophosphate poisoning, can be remembered by the mnemonic SLUDGEM: salivation, lacrimation, urination, defecation, gastric upset, emesis, and miosis (pupil contraction). Often there is a complaint of dim vision. The nerve agents also cause cardiac dysrhythmias, confusion, fasciculations (muscle twitches), and convulsions, along with unconsciousness. Almost all people affected by a nerve agent will have miosis, and most will have a runny nose and shortness of breath. The combination of pinpoint pupils and muscle fasciculations is the most reliable sign of nerve poisoning (Andress, 2010; ATSDR, 2011).

The attachment of the nerve agent to the enzyme is permanent unless it can be removed by therapy. Atropine assists with symptomatic relief and is the most common drug used in the treatment of nerve gas exposure. Atropine will help with the muscarinic effects such as rhinorrhea, salivation, sweating, bronchoconstriction, bronchorrhea, nausea, vomiting, and diarrhea. The most common reversal agents are the oximes, such as Protopam chloride (2-PAM chloride). Protopam helps with muscle twitching and respirations. Atropine and Protopam are packaged together into what is called a MARK I kit. The MARK I kit is administered intramuscularly via an auto injector. The reversal agents must be used early in the course because, once the action of the chemical has been initiated, the reversal agent is of no effect. Diazepam can help with the convulsions. Survivors of all nerve agents need full decontamination. Their clothing must be double sealed in plastic and handled as little as possible to avoid secondary exposure to others (Andress, 2010; ATSDR, 2011). The clothing will need to be contained or disposed of according to whatever the agent is.

The remainder of the care is outlined in the Nursing Process: Patient Care Plan for Known Nerve Agent Exposure feature (p. 2070).

Biologic Agents

Biologic agents include bacteria, viruses, and toxins that can be used in terrorism or biologic warfare. Biologic agents are usually in a liquid or dry form. Most of them tend to be off-white to amber, brown, or red. This color can easily be changed with the addition of simple food dyes so as to blend these agents into the background of the area of dispersion. Unlike chemical agents, biologic agents are not detectable with the usual five human senses. Because the period of illness is longer than that with chemical agents, the impact on health care is much longer and larger than is the case with chemicals. If a biologic agent were dispersed, there would be waves of patients, depending on the incubation period and the size of the population affected, rather than a single influx (Andress, 2010; ENA, 2007). Chart 65–9 outlines the biologic agents by class: bacteria, viruses, and toxins.

Biologic agents are categorized as Category A, B, or C. Category A agents are those that pose the highest risk to national security because they (1) cause high mortality with the potential for major public health effects including special actions for public health preparedness, (2) are easily disseminated or easily spread from person to person, and (3) may cause public panic and public disruption. Category A agents include smallpox, anthrax, plague, botulism, tularemia, and viral hemorrhagic fever. Category B agents are moderately easy to disseminate, can cause moderate morbidity and low mortality, and require specific actions and enhancements by the CDC. Category B agents include brucellosis, glanders, ricin, staphylococcal enterotoxin B, and some food- and water-borne illnesses such as salmonella, *Shigella*, and *Vibrio*. Category C agents are emerging pathogens that may be engineered in the future because they are readily available, are easily produced and disseminated, and have the potential for high morbidity and mortality. The Category C agents include Hantaviruses, tick-borne encephalitis virus, and yellow fever (Andress, 2010; CDC, 2008a, 2011b; ENA, 2007; House, Graber, & Scheckel, 2003).

CHART 65–9 Biologic Agents by Class

Bacteria	Viruses
Anthrax	Dengue fever
Brucellosis	Ebola
Cholera	Rift Valley fever
Glanders	Smallpox
Plague	Venezuelan equine encephalitis (VEE) virus
Q fever	Viral hemorrhagic fever (VHF)
Rickettsia	**Toxins**
Tularemia	Botulinum
Typhus	Ricin
	Saxitoxin
	Staphylococcal enterotoxin B (SEB)
	Trichothecene mycotoxins

Nursing Management

The result of exposure to these agents is infection. See Chapter 14 for the nursing management of infectious diseases.

Collaborative Management

Like other infectious agents, weaponized biologic agents require aggressive infectious disease management. A health care team that includes nurses, health care providers, public health personnel, infectious disease nurses, and epidemiologists will be required. In order to meet desired patient outcomes, it is essential that this interdisciplinary team communicate openly with one another in developing and evaluating care of the patient and family (IOM [Institute of Medicine], 2010).

When large numbers of patients are involved, the role of public health officers becomes key in managing the spread of the disease. As with chemical agents, psychological and emotional care needs must be included in the comprehensive approach.

Spread

Biologic agents can be dispersed via multiple routes, including aerosol, oral, injection, and dermal.

Aerosol Route

Biologic agents are usually spread by an aerosol method. Most biologic agents can be aerosolized to a size of 1 to 10 microns. Particles larger than 15 microns will not stay suspended in the air but will fall to the ground. Secondary aerosolization occurs when the particles that have fallen to the ground are stirred by air currents created by passing people or objects such as cars. Most aerosolized biologic agents will be taken deeply into the lungs by the people or animals who are exposed (CDC, 2011b). The aerosols can be disseminated by using simple sprayers such as a garden or paint sprayer, crop duster planes, mosquito control trucks, fire extinguishers, or even a dispersion bomb, much as with chemical agents. Dispersion by any of these routes takes a high level of knowledge and sophistication to accomplish (CDC, 2011b).

Oral Route

Foods and fruits can be contaminated either during distribution or in the packing or manufacturing process. Outbreaks of food poisoning at various restaurants or at family picnics are examples of accidental contamination of foods. The accidental contamination of food usually produces few casualties.

NURSING PROCESS: Patient Care Plan for Known Nerve Agent Exposure

Assessment of Patient Status Using Gordon's Functional Health Patterns:

- Health Perception Health Management Pattern
- Nutrition Metabolic Pattern
- Activity Exercise Pattern
- Coping–Stress Tolerance Pattern

Subjective Data	Objective Data
Assessment of Exposure	**Assessment of Exposure**
Do you have blurred vision? Determine from information sources the agent suspected.	Presence of symptoms including bronchoconstriction, blurred vision, pupillary constriction, rhinorrhea, coughing, wheezing, generalized weakness, nausea and vomiting, seizures, coma, flaccid paralysis, and apnea. Assess readiness for decontamination, including equipment and personnel. Perform pre–personal protective equipment (PPE) assessments of personnel including vital signs and weight. Perform full patient assessment for nerve agent exposure. (See the Nerve Agents section in this chapter.)
Assessment of Airway	**Assessment of Airway**
Are you having any trouble breathing? Is it getting worse? Do you feel weak? Is it getting worse? Do you know where you are? What is your name?	Assess for amount of salivation, lacrimation, emesis, rhinorrhea, and bronchorrhea in airways. Assess for fasciculations, level of consciousness and degree of confusion, seizures, respiratory rate, degree of work of breathing, breath sounds, cough effort, vital signs, and skin and nail bed color. Oxygen saturation.
Assessment of Cardiac Status	**Assessment of Cardiac Status**
Sensation of palpitations, racing heart, and skipping beats.	Cardiac monitor—rate and rhythm. Radial and apical pulse. Blood pressure. Level of consciousness.
Assessment of Fluid Status	**Assessment of Fluid Status**
Degree of thirst, headache, amount of cramping, and nausea. Previous amounts of fluid lost.	Assess degree of dehydration. Monitor electrolytes and serum osmolality, physical signs of dehydration, vital signs, and level of consciousness.
Assessment of Coping	**Assessment of Coping**
Assess for feelings of apprehension, fear, uneasiness, palpitations, loss of concentration, degree of sense of threat, feelings of helplessness, powerlessness, increased tension, and worry.	Assess for decreased concentration or a narrow focus. Look for signs of tension-reducing behaviors such as biting fingernails, cursing, and rocking. Altered pitch and tone of voice. Other typical signs and symptoms—such as increased heart rate, increased respiratory rate, tremor, dry mouth, and increased gastrointestinal symptoms—are not reliable signs due to the nerve agent exposure.

Outcomes and Evaluation Parameters	Planning and Interventions with *Rationales*
1. NURSING DIAGNOSIS: Injury, Risk for *related to gross contamination with chemical* (NANDA-I © 2012)	
Outcomes: The patient is fully decontaminated. No exposures to health care workers or facility. No injury to the health care providers. ***Evaluation Parameters:*** Patient has no chemical left on body as measured with chemical strips or other devices. No increase observed in symptomatology following decontamination. Health care workers and decontamination workers have no exposure to chemical and no symptoms of chemical exposure or exhaustion. Clean areas are maintained. No contamination of the facility present.	Decontamination area is set up into hot, warm, and cold zones, with a triage area in the hot zone as well as re-triage in the cold zone. Areas are monitored to maintain zones. Health care workers and other decontamination personnel don full and appropriate PPE prior to contact with contaminated patients. Monitor personnel during the decontamination process for signs of agent exposure and heat exhaustion. *To prevent contamination of and injury to personnel.* Fully undress patients and place belongings in clear bags, double bagged, with identification easily seen through bag. *To preserve evidence and prevent secondary exposure.*

NURSING PROCESS: Patient Care Plan for Known Nerve Agent Exposure, *continued*

	Fully scrub patients, including creases and hair, using warm soapy water, and rinse. *To remove remaining chemical.* Assess patient prior to decontamination and reassess patient in the cold zone for symptoms of exposure. *To determine severity of symptoms and care needed.*
2. NURSING DIAGNOSIS: Airway Clearance, Ineffective ***related to copious secretions, weakness, depressed level of consciousness, and ineffective cough*** **(NANDA-I © 2012)**	
Outcome: The patient will maintain a patent airway and adequate gas exchange. ***Evaluation Parameters:*** Clear breath sounds. Clear airways. Pulse oximeter above 95%. Skin warm, dry, and pink with brisk capillary refill.	Assess the patient for amount and type of secretions. Perform full respiratory assessment including vital signs, breath sounds, work of breathing, cough effort, skin vital signs, and pulse oximeter. *To determine degree of distress.* Observe for cyanosis, increased confusion, and restlessness. *These are signs of increased hypoxia.* Allow the patient to sit in the high Fowler's position. *To facilitate respiratory effort and airway clearance.* Suction airways as needed for ineffective/inadequate cough. Perform endotracheal intubation as indicated. *To maintain clear airway.* Administer oxygen as needed. *To maintain adequate gas exchange.* Administer atropine and Protopam as ordered. *To dry secretions and assist with shortness of breath.* Teach effective coughing techniques such as huff cough. *To improve airway clearance and reduce fatigue from constant coughing.*
3. NURSING DIAGNOSIS: Cardiac Output, Decreased ***related to dysrhythmias*** **(NANDA-I © 2012)**	
Outcome: The patient will have a normal sinus rhythm with adequate cardiac output. ***Evaluation Parameters:*** Sinus rhythm without ectopy on cardiac monitor. Awake, alert, and oriented level of consciousness.	Measure apical and radial pulses, blood pressure, and level of consciousness. *To determine relative perfusion.* Place on cardiac monitor. Monitor with at least two leads. *To determine dysrhythmias and need for treatment.* Monitor electrolytes. *Altered electrolytes can affect the cardiac rhythm.*
4. NURSING DIAGNOSIS: Fluid Balance, Readiness for Enhanced ***related to copious secretions, high urinary output, vomiting, and diarrhea*** **(NANDA-I © 2012)**	
Outcome: The patient will attain fluid and electrolyte balance. ***Evaluation Parameters:*** Diarrhea and emesis halted. Intake and output equal. Secretions controlled. Serum osmolality and electrolytes within normal limits. Vital signs within normal limits.	Assess hydration status such as oral mucous membrane moisture, intake and output, sunken eyes, skin tenting, thirst, and headache. *To determine degree of dehydration and any improvement in or deterioration of condition.* Strictly monitor intake and output. *To determine fluid balance and any improvement in or deterioration of condition.* Assess vital signs, orthostatic vital signs, cardiac rhythm, and level of consciousness. *To identify signs of hypovolemic shock, perfusion, and electrolyte imbalances.* Monitor serum osmolality and electrolytes when ordered. *To determine replacement needs.* Assess for nausea and administer antiemetics as ordered. *To decrease nausea and vomiting.* Administer atropine and Protopam. *To decrease secretion production and decrease diarrhea and emesis.* Administer normotonic intravenous solutions and oral replacement when tolerating oral fluids. *To replace lost fluids and restore fluid balance.* Administer electrolyte replacement intravenously or orally when tolerated. *To replace lost electrolytes and restore balance.*

(*continued*)

NURSING PROCESS: Patient Care Plan for Known Nerve Agent Exposure, *continued*

Outcomes and Evaluation Parameters	Planning and Interventions with *Rationales*
5. NURSING DIAGNOSIS: Coping, Ineffective *related to perceived and actual threat from situation, unknown outcome, and possible further danger* (NANDA-I © 2012)	
Outcome: There will be a decrease in the patient's anxiety. ***Evaluation Parameters:*** The patient will report no sensation of palpitations. The patient will answer simple questions clearly without lag. The patient will report a subjective decrease in sensation of anxiety and helplessness and an increased sense of control. Anxiety-reducing behaviors, such as rocking and nail biting, will be greatly decreased or absent.	Use a calm, reassuring approach. *To increase confidence in the caregiver and reduce anxiety of the unknown.* Reassure the patient that appropriate medical care is being rendered for the condition. Explain the procedures and purpose of medications and interventions in simple terms. Explain in simple terms the effects of the nerve agent. *Reduce anxiety by decreasing the fear of the unknown and learning what to expect.* Identify for the patient the safety of the facility/situation, if true. *To reassure of current safety.* Stay with the patient. If the nurse must leave the patient, the nurse should tell the patient when he will return and do so. *To build a trusting relationship and provide a sense of security in care.* Acknowledge the patient's fears and anxiety. *To identify feelings as a normal reaction, provide insight into the situation, and decrease anxiety.* Teach simple stress reduction exercises such as imagery. *To allow for self-comforting and assist with relaxation.* Administer antianxiety agents if ordered and indicated. *To decrease anxiety and promote rest.*

Source: Adapted from Wilkinson, J. M., & Ahearn, N. R. (2009). *Prentice Hall nursing diagnosis handbook* (9th ed.). Upper Saddle River, NJ: Prentice Hall.

Most public water supplies are at very low risk for significant contamination, owing to the chlorination treatment process. The reverse osmosis systems used in water treatment have been shown to be effective against the toxins of ricin, microcystin, T-2 mycotoxin, and saxitoxin. Contamination of a personal water well or a single building's water supply at the intake would be a more likely scenario.

Injection

The injection route for biologic agents is not a common terrorist method. It would be possible to contaminate hospital equipment and thus have injection be the vector, but this is unlikely to occur because many biologic agonists have a limited life expectancy.

Dermal Exposure

Intact skin affords an excellent barrier for most biologic agents, so dermal exposure is not an effective means of transmission for most bacteria and viruses. However, open wounds such as paper cuts or other small abrasions will provide a portal of entry. Cutaneous anthrax is commonly acquired in this way. Some of the toxins, such as T-2 mycotoxin ("yellow rain"), are believed to be able to penetrate skin (Andress, 2010; ENA, 2007).

Radiologic Agents

The environment holds many sources of radiation. People are frequently exposed to diagnostic x-rays, the sun's rays, luminous paints, ceramics, and cosmetics. Radiologic accidents and terrorist incidents are on a much different scale in terms of the amount of radiation received and the type of radiation involved (Andress, 2010; CDC, 2008b; ENA, 2007). Events that were triggered by the 2011 earthquake in Japan, which damaged several nuclear reactors and allowed radiation to leak into the environment, once again alerted the world to the dangers of radiation. **Radiologic agents** include any agent that is a source of alpha, beta, or gamma radiation that can be used as a weapon.

Nursing Management

Nursing management of the patient who has been exposed to radiologic agents depends greatly on the dose and severity of the exposure. Application of the nursing process will facilitate a comprehensive approach to patient assessment and care. This again is a situation in which psychological care, emotional care, and spiritual care are important.

Assessment

The nurse should obtain the following history:

- What type of radiation has the patient been exposed to?
- How long was the amount of exposure?
- Has the patient received any decontamination?
- How did the radiation enter the patient's body?

The nurse must assess the patient for the following physical symptoms:

- Nausea and vomiting
- Diarrhea
- Malaise
- Fever
- Bruising
- Electrolyte imbalance.

Nursing Diagnoses

Nursing diagnoses for the patient exposed to radiation include the following:

- *Fluid Volume, Deficit* related to volume loss through vomiting.
- *Infection, Risk for.*
- *Injury, Risk for* related to low blood count.

  NANDA-I © 2012

Outcomes and Evaluation Parameters

The overall goals for the management of the patient who has been exposed to a radiologic agent include the following:

- The safety of the patient and the staff will be maintained.
- The patient will receive immediate lifesaving care unless the patient is a victim of a nuclear explosion.
- The patient will be appropriately decontaminated.

Interventions

- The nurse identifies the level of patient contamination and assigns the patient to the appropriate area for decontamination. *All clothing and jewelry should be removed from the patient, and the patient should be washed with soap and water. This occurs in a selected area so that the water can be appropriately contained. All contaminated items should be double bagged and labeled.*
- The nurse continuously assesses the patient for signs of radiation poisoning including nausea, vomiting, diarrhea, fever, and bruising. *It may take several weeks for these symptoms to appear, so the patient should be informed of this and be closely monitored.*

Evaluation

The type of radiation and the amount of exposure will determine the outcome of a patient with a radiologic exposure. Patients should be closely monitored and taught what signs and symptoms to watch for. Unfortunately, patients with significant radiologic exposure will die, so psychological and spiritual care will be important for both the patient and family.

Collaborative Management

All patients who have been exposed to radiologic agents require comprehensive care from a health team that includes nurses, health care providers, emergency medical service personnel, and radiologists, depending on the systems involved and the severity of the injury. In order to meet desired patient outcomes, it is essential that this interdisciplinary team communicate openly with one another in developing and evaluating care of the patient and family (IOM [Institute of Medicine], 2010).

In most hospitals, the radiologist has the responsibility of assessing the type and level of exposure of patients and staff. A Geiger-Muller survey meter is used to assess the level of external contamination (ENA, 2007).

Types of Radiation

Nonionizing radiation, such as that from classroom lights, is low energy and nonharmful. Ionizing radiation produces charged ions in the material it strikes. The three most common ionizing particles are alpha, beta, and gamma. The radiation absorbed dose (rad) is a measure of energy deposited in matter by the ionizing radiation. The term *rad* is being replaced by the international system unit *gray* (Gy). One gray equals 100 rads. A roentgen-equivalent-man (rem) is a unit that describes the biologic effect of one rad (CDC, 2008b).

Exposure

To describe the severity of exposure, the measure of a lethal dose is used. An exposure of 350 rads, or 3.5 Gy, will cause death in half the people exposed, if no medical care is received, within 60 days. This is referred to as a lethal dose of 50/60 (LD 50/60). With medical treatment, the lethal dose may be between 600 and 800 rads (6 to 8 Gy). Unlike chemicals, radiation cannot be detected with the five senses. Geiger counters, dosimeters, and various other types of detection equipment are employed when radiation is suspected (Andress, 2010).

Ionizing Radiation

Alpha particles are very big and heavy, and they penetrate poorly. They travel only 1 to 2 inches in air, and they are easily stopped by a piece of paper or clothing and do not penetrate the dead outer layer of the skin. External alpha radiation rarely causes a health risk, although decontamination is necessary. If introduced through broken skin, inhaled, or ingested, causing internal contamination, alpha particles can cause extensive damage, especially to the kidneys, lungs, liver, and skeletal system (Andress, 2010; CDC, 2008b; ENA, 2007).

Beta particles, which are smaller than alpha particles, can travel about 10 feet through the air and can penetrate skin a short distance, causing severe burns ("beta burns"). Damage to the eyes can occur from beta particles; when they are ingested or inhaled, internal injuries can occur. Shielding with heavy clothing, walls, or thin metals is effective protection against penetration of beta particles (Andress, 2008; CDC, 2008b).

Gamma rays are emitted during nuclear detonation and are present in fallout. Gamma rays can travel several hundred feet in air, and they can travel through tissue to the deep organs. Gamma radiation is also referred to as "penetrating radiation." Because of this penetration, gamma rays are both an external and an internal hazard. Dense materials such as lead, concrete, and steel can block penetration of gamma rays. Neutrons, which are also released in nuclear detonations, can penetrate thick concrete (Andress, 2010; CDC, 2008b).

Routes of Entry

Gamma radiation can enter the body by penetration; this is termed *irradiation*. In this type of exposure, the victim is not radioactive; that is, the victim does not emit radiation. This is the same process by which diagnostic x-rays are performed.

Radiologic contamination occurs when particulate matter that is radioactive is released. People become contaminated when the material is deposited on the skin or ingested, inhaled, or absorbed in some manner. Internal contamination can lead to incorporation, whereby the radioactive material is assimilated into body tissue. This can cause both immediate and delayed problems.

Alpha and beta particles can be inhaled if they are airborne. Radiation can be injected and ingested. With dermal exposure, radiation can cause an external burn and/or be absorbed into the body if the skin is broken.

Radiation exposure depends on the three principles of time, distance, and shielding. The shorter the time of exposure, the less absorption by the tissue. Radiologic exposure follows the inverse square law in relationship to distance; in other words, if the distance from the source is doubled, the dose rate of exposure is decreased by a factor of 4. If a source has a radiation level of 100 radiation absorbed dose (R/hr) at 1 foot, at 2 feet the radiation would be 25 R/hr, and at 8 feet it would be 1.56 R/hr. Shielding refers to the materials between the person and the source of radiation. The denser the material, such as lead, the more protection that is afforded (Andress, 2010).

Radiation Exposure

In most hospitals, one of the radiologists is usually the designated radiation safety officer in charge of determining exposure and risk. Most hospitals have Geiger counters readily available to determine the simple presence or absence of a certain level of radiation in the environment. Personnel involved in the care of radiation victims will need dosimeters to determine their exposure. These personnel will also more than likely need decontamination. Depending on the severity of the exposure, many different effects can be seen. Personnel who have been exposed to low-level external contamination may have skin burns that will heal with no sequelae. These individuals are not considered to be at higher risk later for cancer. Many of those with internal contamination will need follow-up monitoring to measure clearance of the radionuclides from the body. These individuals are also not considered to be at higher risk for cancer later in life. However, personnel who have been exposed to higher levels of radiation that have caused symptoms are considered to be at elevated risk for cancer later (Andress, 2010).

In lower level radiation exposure, early treatment can be the key to decrease incorporation (the uptake of radiation into the cells of the body) and decrease symptoms and sequelae. Potassium iodide can have a protective effect on the thyroid if taken before, or within 3 to 4 hours after, exposure to a radioactive cloud. It is available in capsules as well as in liquid. It protects the thyroid gland by filling the receptor sites so that radioactive iodines cannot bind (CDC, 2011c).

Prussian blue is a blue dye that was first produced in 1704 for use in Prussian military uniforms. Prussian blue can be taken to help remove certain ingested radioactive substances. It works by binding in the gut to cesium and thallium, which are then excreted in the stool. Prussian blue reduces cesium's half-life from approximately 110 days to approximately 30 days. It reduces thallium's half-life from approximately 8 days to approximately 3 days. Prussian blue is still commonly available as a dye and as paint in art stores (CDC, 2010).

Acute Radiation Syndrome

Acute radiation syndrome (ARS) is an acute illness caused by irradiation of the whole body or at least a significant part of the body. Radiation generates highly reactive free radicals and directly damages proteins, messenger RNA (mRNA), and DNA. In smaller doses, it interferes with cell proliferation; in higher doses, it causes cell death. Body tissues with a high turnover rate, such as the bone marrow, are more susceptible to the effects of radiation (CDC, 2008b). Acute radiation syndrome varies in severity based on dose and the age and relative state of wellness of the person exposed. The severity and extent of the symptoms increase and the duration of each phase shortens as the radiation dose goes up. Acute radiation syndrome has four phases: the prodromal phase, the latent phase, the illness phase, and the recovery phase or death (Andress, 2010; CDC, 2008b; ENA, 2007).

Prodromal Phase

The prodromal phase has an onset of minutes to hours and lasts from hours to days, depending on the dose of radiation. It is characterized by the relatively rapid onset of nausea, vomiting, and malaise. At higher levels, fever, hypotension, and diarrhea can also be present. Onset of symptoms within 30 minutes of exposure most likely indicates a lethal dose. The gastrointestinal symptoms usually resolve within 2 days, but the fatigue and malaise often continue. At higher doses (200 rads and above), lymphocyte counts will decrease, and cognitive impairment can occur (Andress, 2010; CDC, 2008b; ENA, 2007).

Latent Phase

Following the prodromal phase, there is a transition phase in which the individual is relatively symptom free. This latent phase varies from no time to 2 weeks, depending on the dose received (Andress, 2010; CDC, 2008b; ENA, 2007).

Illness Phase

In the illness phase, also called the manifest stage, there is overt illness. This phase presents as a hematopoietic (blood-forming) system, gastrointestinal system, central nervous system, or skin syndrome, or a combination of any of these, based on the system injured.

The hematopoietic system shows the earliest indications of the severity of the radiation exposure. There will be a drop in all cell counts due to death of the bone marrow. A depressed immune system, fever, sepsis, and hemorrhage are common. Individuals with lower level exposure can recover if they receive medical support and their bone marrow regenerates. Medical support includes blood transfusions, protection from infection, and antibiotic therapy. Occasionally, stem cell transplantation is needed (Andress, 2010; CDC, 2008b; ENA, 2007).

Gastrointestinal symptoms, nausea, vomiting, and diarrhea are usually seen in doses greater than 600 rad and are a result of damage to the epithelial cells lining the small intestine. The symptoms lead to fluid and electrolyte imbalances and opportunistic infections, which can lead to septicemia. Symptomatic care is prescribed, including antiemetics, sedatives, fluid replacement, and a bland diet. Persistent high fevers and bloody diarrhea are ominous signs (Andress, 2010; CDC, 2008b; ENA, 2007).

The central nervous system is one of the most radiation-resistant tissues in the body. Central nervous system symptoms are seen with doses in excess of 1,000 rads. With this level of radiation, there is usually almost immediate nausea, vomiting, disorientation, and seizures from the loss of fluid, electrolytes, edema, and increased intracranial pressure. Death follows within hours to days. Care involves administering sedatives and analgesics to control seizures and anxiety, as this syndrome is fatal (Andress, 2010; CDC, 2008b; ENA, 2007).

Recovery or Death

Mortality from ARS is directly related to the amount of radiation exposure. Individuals who have had a large exposure will usually die within several months of the exposure. The deaths are most commonly caused by opportunistic infections as a result of bone marrow destruction. Survivors' recovery phase may last for several months up to 2 years.

Explosions

Injuries from explosions run the gamut of traumatic injuries from extremely minor ones that do not require medical attention to complete crush and incineration. Blasts frequently are the cause of injuries. Although the mechanism of injury for these problems is a blast force, these injuries are treated in the usual manner, depending on the system or body parts affected (CDC, 2009a; ENA, 2007).

Blast Injuries

There are some injuries that are specific to blasts. Blasts are divided into high order explosives and low order explosives, based on the strength of the ordnance (Chart 65–10). The injuries are divided into primary, secondary, tertiary, and quaternary. Primary blast injuries are usually caused by high order explosives. These injuries result from the direct effect of increases in atmospheric pressure causing barotrauma (damage to body tissues caused by the imbalance in pressure between the air and the inside of the body). Ruptured eardrums are the most common injury. The most severe injuries are to the lung and include pneumothorax, contusions, hemorrhage, bronchopleural fistulas, thrombosis,

CHART 65–10 Blast Injury From High Order Explosives

Category	Mechanism	Body Part Affected	Types of Injuries
Primary	Impact of the overpressurization wave with body surfaces	Gas-filled structures are the most susceptible: lungs, gastrointestinal tract, and middle ear	Blast lung Tympanic membrane rupture and middle ear damage Abdominal hemorrhage and perforation Eye rupture Concussion and traumatic brain injury
Secondary	Flying debris and bomb fragments	Any body part	Penetrating ballistic (fragmentation) or blunt injuries Eye penetration (can be occult)
Tertiary	Individual thrown by the blast wind	Any body part	Fracture and traumatic amputation Any blunt traumatic injury Closed and open brain injuries
Quaternary	All explosion-related injuries, illnesses, or diseases not due to primary, secondary, or tertiary mechanisms Includes exacerbation or complications of existing conditions	Any body part	Burns (flash, partial-, and full-thickness burns) Crush injuries Closed and open brain injuries Asthma, chronic obstructive pulmonary disease, or other breathing problems from dust, smoke, or toxic fumes Angina Hyperglycemia, hypertension

Source: Adapted from Centers for Disease Control and Prevention (CDC). (June 2009a). Blast injuries: Essential facts. Retrieved from http://www.bt.cdc.gov/masscasualties/explosions.asp.

disseminated intravascular coagulation, and adult respiratory distress syndrome. High order explosives can also cause bowel perforation, gastrointestinal bleeding, shearing injuries to the mesentery, rupture of the testicles, and other solid organ damage. Concussion and traumatic brain injury may also result (CDC, 2009a) (Chart 65–11).

Secondary blast injuries are caused by flying debris. These include minor lacerations, contusions, and abrasions; inhalation of dust, smoke, and other airborne particles; all the way to impaled large foreign objects and being trapped by large pieces of debris. Tertiary blast injuries occur when the person is thrown by the blast through the air and the person strikes another object. Any variety of injuries can be expected (CDC, 2009a).

CHART 65–11 Blast Injuries by System

System	Injury or Condition
Auditory	Tympanic membrane rupture, ossicular disruption, cochlear damage, foreign body
Eye, orbit, face	Perforated globe, foreign body, air embolism, fractures
Respiratory	Blast lung, hemothorax, pneumothorax, pulmonary contusion and hemorrhage, arteriovenous fistulas (air embolism), airway epithelial damage, aspiration pneumonitis, sepsis
Digestive	Bowel perforation, hemorrhage, ruptured liver or spleen, sepsis, mesenteric ischemia from air embolism
Circulatory	Cardiac contusion, myocardial infarction from air embolism, shock, vasovagal hypotension, peripheral vascular injury, air embolism-induced injury
Central nervous system	Concussion, closed and open brain injury, stroke, spinal cord injury, air embolism-induced injury
Renal	Renal contusion, laceration, acute renal failure due to rhabdomyolysis, hypotension, and hypovolemia
Extremity	Traumatic amputation, fractures, crush injuries, compartment syndrome, burns, cuts, lacerations, acute arterial occlusion, air embolism-induced injury

Source: Adapted from Centers for Disease Control and Prevention (CDC). (June 2009a). Blast injuries: Essential facts. Retrieved from http://www.bt.cdc.gov/masscasualties/explosions.asp.

Critical Incident Stress Management

The psychological impact of a mass casualty event cannot be overestimated. When the event is deliberate, such as with a terrorist attack, the impact is even greater. A common goal of terrorist activity is to threaten the psychological cohesion and well-being of a community. **Terrorism** is psychological warfare. By design, the psychological casualties of an event will far outweigh the physical casualties (Coppola, 2011a; Manser, 2011; Mendez, 2010; Stangeland, 2010). People involved in the incident itself, health care workers, rescuers, and the general population will all be affected. Efforts to mitigate the adverse psychological effects of terrorism include providing training and education before incidents occur, providing crisis intervention at the time of the event, and supplying the community with information and assistance following an incident (Manser, 2011; Mendez, 2010; Stangeland, 2010).

Stress

Stress is the physical and psychological arousal and response to a perceived or real threat, challenge, or change. When the environment changes, people change (Mitchell & Bray, 1980).

Common Signs of Stress

Common signs of stress may be emotional, behavioral, cognitive, and physical. Emotional signs of stress include numbness, anger, grief, depression, feeling overwhelmed, hopelessness, and being overly worried. Behavioral signs include changes in a person's ordinary pattern of behavior, changes in eating, decreased personal hygiene, a change in smoking pattern, a change in alcohol use pattern, withdrawal, prolonged silences, and sudden gregariousness not in keeping with the person's personality. Cognitive changes include confusion in thinking, difficulty making decisions, disorientation, and memory problems. Physical signs include excessive sweating, dizzy spells, increased heart rate, elevated blood pressure, rapid breathing, tremor, and gastrointestinal disturbances (ENA, 2007; Manser, 2011; Mendez, 2010; Mitchell, Sakraida, & Kameg, 2003; Stangeland, 2010). Health care workers must be aware of these signs and look for them in themselves and others. Refer to Chapter 9 for more about stress and adaptation to it.

Another common reaction to stress is the use of "gallows" or "dark" or "black" humor, especially in the rescuer community. Research has shown that this style of humor is not disrespectful of the injured, the deceased, or their survivors (Maxwell, 2003). However, health care providers must be respectful of where this type of humor is used.

Critical Incident

Whatever caused the stress becomes a **critical incident** when it is an abnormal occurrence that is so markedly distressing and powerful that it overcomes a person's normal feeling of control and coping ability. In short, critical incident stress is the normal response to an abnormal occurrence. It is the occurrence that is abnormal, not the response (ENA, 2007; Manser, 2011; Mendez, 2010; Mitchell et al., 2003; Stangeland, 2010). These incidents disrupt people's lives with strong emotional reactions that have the potential to interfere with their ability to function either at the scene or later. The severity of the reaction is influenced by many things, including any previous exposure to incidents, length of time of exposure, the severity of the exposure, perceptions of the events, preexisting coping strategies, other current stressors, well-being at the time of the event, and the available social support (ENA, 2007; Manser, 2011; Mendez, 2010; Mitchell et al., 2003; Stangeland, 2010).

For health care workers, the critical incident can be further categorized as the incident itself, the professional's performance, and/or the professional's reaction to the event. For health care workers in the aftermath of a disaster, the event itself and all the work that follows have the potential to act as a catalyst for a critical incident stress response (ENA, 2007; Manser, 2011; Mendez, 2010; Mitchell et al., 2003; Stangeland, 2010).

Crisis Intervention and Critical Incident Stress Management

Crisis intervention is essentially first aid for people who are in crisis. The goals of crisis intervention are to stabilize and mitigate the signs and symptoms of stress and dysfunction and to facilitate a return to functioning (ENA, 2007; Manser, 2011; Mendez, 2010; Stangeland, 2010). **Critical incident stress management** is a comprehensive approach to the management of stress and critical incidents. The goal is to reduce and control the harmful effects of stress, maintain health and productivity, and speed recovery from the stressful event. The approach has seven components: preincident preparation, group information briefings (demobilization), defusings, critical incident stress debriefing, individual intervention, family critical incident stress management, and follow-up and referral (ENA, 2007; Manser, 2011; Mendez, 2010; Stangeland, 2010). The point of all of these interventions is to prevent the development of post-traumatic stress disorder (PTSD), which has been found to be present in roughly 9% of all people who have been exposed to critical incidents in recent years (ENA, 2007; Manser, 2011; Mendez, 2010; Mitchell et al., 2003; Stangeland, 2010).

Health Care Workers

Health care workers usually have a "rescuer" personality. Those who are unable to help with a major effort such as an earthquake or a terrorist event, especially in the early stages, often will feel greater stress. There is a need to do *something*, anything (ENA, 2007; Manser, 2011; Mendez, 2010; Levenson & Acosta, 2001; Mitchell & Bray, 1980; Stangeland, 2010). As time wears on, cumulative stress also becomes a problem for health care workers because of the overwhelming nature of the situation they face each day. There are three common, formalized ways of assisting health care workers and other emergency services personnel to increase their knowledge and decrease the perceived stress: demobilization, critical incident defusing, and critical incident stress debriefing. It is important to note that these processes are not psychotherapy but rather sessions for information, education, and ventilation (ENA, 2007; Manser, 2011; Mendez, 2010; Mitchell et al., 2003; Stangeland, 2010).

Demobilization

Demobilization is also called group information briefings and crisis management briefings. These usually occur during rest breaks, at the end of a shift, or in the middle of the event, as the event dictates. Demobilization provides information and resources to a group that has been affected by an incident. It brings people together, provides rumor control, and addresses possible reactions and self-help guidelines, usually in the form of a little handout. These briefings are typically only a few minutes long (ENA, 2007; Manser, 2011; Mendez, 2010; Stangeland, 2010).

Critical Incident Defusing

Critical incident defusings are formal sessions that occur within 8 hours of the event. They typically last 20 to 45 minutes and are held in small groups of 6 to 8 people who have similar job descriptions. No record is made of the proceedings. Often a defusing will negate the need for a formal debriefing. The facilitators introduce themselves and state the ground rules, including strict confidentiality. The event, experiences, and reactions are reviewed. Reassurance is given, and an assessment is made for the need for more help. The last phase normalizes the experience and teaches some basic stress survival skills (ENA, 2007; Manser, 2011; Mendez, 2010; Stangeland, 2010).

Critical Incident Stress Debriefing

Critical incident stress debriefing (CISD) is a formal event run by trained counselors that is held within 72 hours of the critical incident and typically lasts 2 to 3 hours, with the purpose of minimizing stress disorders resulting from the incident. Again, no record is made of the proceedings, and strict confidentiality is enforced.

A CISD has seven phases. In phase one, the interventional team members and facilitators are introduced, and the facilitators explain the process and expectations. In phase two, referred to as the *fact phase,* each participant describes the event from her perspective on a cognitive level and her role and location during the event. Phase three, the *thought phase,* allows the participants to describe their cognitive reactions (thoughts) to the events and transitions into the emotional reactions. Phase four, the *reaction phase*, tends to be the most powerful and emotional part of the process. Participants describe the part of the event that was most traumatic for them and their emotional reactions. In phase five, the *symptom phase*, the participants are guided back from a highly charged emotional state to a more cognitive level by being asked to describe some symptoms of stress they have experienced, such as insomnia or tremors. Phase six, the *teaching phase,* is run more by the facilitators and serves as a cognitive anchor. Here the facilitators discuss normal stress reactions and provide some stress survival and management tips. This phase continues until the concerns of the group are exhausted. The seventh and last phase is the *reentry phase*; the session is summarized, and any questions are answered. Handouts with stress management information, such as signs of stress and tips for self-care, as well as community referrals are given to the participants. There is usually a short social time with refreshments, which allows anyone with an individual question for the facilitators to ask the question outside the group. This technique has been employed in hundreds of large and small events worldwide (Manser, 2011; Mendez, 2010; Mitchell et al., 2003; Stangeland, 2010).

Community

Crisis intervention for a community revolves around providing information, education, and direction. After an event, coordination of services for survivors, families, and communities, along with a centralized list of mental health volunteers, is needed. This should be part of the community's disaster plan and should include advanced coordination as to who responds and when. Within 24 hours, representatives for all the organizations and agencies, such as the state or county department of mental health, critical incident stress management teams, professional organizations, universities, and clergy, need to have a meeting to identify needs, resources, and responsibilities. With its extensive experience in handling disasters, its name recognition, and trust, the American Red Cross makes the ideal organization for handling mental health coordination for the community, as the state and county departments are often overwhelmed with delivery of services (Manser, 2011; Mendez, 2010; Stangeland, 2010).

Considerations in planning and delivering mental health care to the community include assessing community needs; screening volunteer workers, including any licensure issues; and making assignments based on skills and needs. Clergy members may be teamed with mental health professionals and function independently, depending on the need. The community may need assistance with day care, including pediatric counseling. There needs to be defined support for families when they are notified of a death. The defusing and debriefing of each of the teams of volunteers and other mental health workers at the end of their shift are key components of maintaining the workforce. Teams may also be needed to respond to families or individuals who are unable to go to centers for assistance (Manser, 2011; Mendez, 2010; Stangeland, 2010).

Community "town meetings," either in person or through the media, and frequent news bulletins provide relevant operations updates, stress management, and education. These help to provide rumor control and build and aid in community cohesion. These meetings foster personal and community empowerment (Manser, 2011; Mendez, 2010; Stangeland, 2010). The Cultural Considerations box features another aspect of disasters: cultural recovery.

CULTURAL CONSIDERATIONS
Assistance and Recovery Across Cultures

Disasters know no boundaries; they can affect all populations on the face of this earth. However, when a disaster occurs, there is a risk of disruption in a country or a community that will affect the culture of the individuals who live there. For example, the loss of historic buildings or landmarks, artwork, personal clothing, and family valuables such as jewelry and pictures will affect the faith, beliefs, and social structures of an individual and communities (Coppola, 2011b; Mistric & Sparling, 2010).

In an effort to assist, outside individuals and agencies may donate food, clothing, or other items of recovery that might not be acceptable to a community. This can cause further stresses. Volunteers may be unprepared for the cultural views of the victims and unable to adequately meet patient needs.

Cultural recovery is an important part of the disaster recovery process. The community should resume previously scheduled events and celebrations as soon as possible to promote the healing process. For example, after Hurricane Katrina, a decision had to be made regarding when it was appropriate to hold the Mardi Gras celebration once again. Disaster recovery personnel need to be aware of the importance of culture and respect and understand its importance to the injured individuals and communities (Coppola, 2011b).

Ethical Considerations in Disaster Care

Care during a disaster can lead to many ethical problems (Johnstone, 2009). For example, when a disaster occurs the accepted standards of care will change; patients may need to be removed from life support without patient or family consent in order to assure that there are enough resources; and palliative disaster care may need to be employed (Johnstone, 2009). However, at times, this palliative care may have to be limited if supplies are limited (Johnstone, 2009).

Probably one of the greatest ethical dilemmas a nurse may face is whether to even respond to a disaster to provide patient care when rendering care could put the nurse or even his family at risk (Albert, 2009; Priest & Ball, 2008). For example, during an infectious pandemic, resources may consist of only a limited supply of vaccinations or antibiotics to manage the disease. Health care providers may need

RESEARCH OPPORTUNITIES Related to Disaster Nursing

Research Area	Clinical Impact
Physiological Research	
Medical planning for patients with chronic illnesses impacted by disaster	When a natural disaster such as a hurricane or a tornado interrupts patients' services in a community, how can chronically ill patients receive the care they need? For example, where or how could a patient dependent on renal dialysis obtain dialysis?
Management of the effects of stress on nurses who respond to or participate in a disaster	Post-traumatic stress disorder (PTSD) has been found in people who have been exposed to long-term stressors that occur during a disaster, such as perceived threat of danger, suffering, and horror. What is the impact on nurses in these situations?
Community, hospital, and individual preparedness for a disaster	What is the best plan for disaster preparedness? Who is accountable? How is it disseminated?
Psychological, Ethical, and Logical Research	
Intent to respond	What is needed to assist health care personnel to respond to a disaster? Who may choose not to assist and why?

to consider their own and their family's safety before deciding to care for infected patients.

Availability of resources has always posed challenges during a disaster. What ethical principles should be employed? Rothstein (2010) identified the ethical principle of distributive justice (fair distribution of what resources are available) and the use of practical considerations (the use of available resources for those who may benefit from them) as a method to provide some guidance in the use of limited resources. For example, only patients who might survive are placed on a ventilator or taken to the operating room.

All health care providers need to discuss these ethical challenges and have a plan of action before a disaster occurs. A plan of action can assist in decreasing some of the fear and guilt that may come with having to make difficult decisions.

Research

The practice of disaster nursing involves being prepared for natural or human-generated disasters. It requires specialized education and training as well as active participation in exercises that will enhance individuals' and communities' abilities to respond to a disaster. Just as in any practice of nursing, research provides the foundation of disaster nursing. There are many opportunities for future research in disaster nursing. Some topics are presented in the Research Opportunities feature.

NCLEX® PRACTICE

1. The student nurse asks the nurse for an example of international terrorism. The most appropriate response for the nurse to provide would be:

1. "When an act of terror or violence is generated toward the U.S. government by a group or an individual from Puerto Rico."
2. "When a group such as the Ku Klux Klan or the Black Panthers performs terrorist activity against citizens of our own country."
3. "When the group responsible for committing the violence has connection to a foreign organization such as al Qaeda."
4. "When an individual U.S. citizen uses an unlawful act of violence to destroy or intimidate individuals or the U.S. government."

2. Which of the following patients would the nurse categorize as victims of natural disasters? (select all that apply)

1. A mother of two who lost her home in a recent wild fire.
2. A teen-aged boy who was in a multi-vehicle car accident during a recent snow storm.
3. A rescue worker who suffered lung damage during the September 11, 2001, attack.
4. An elderly man who developed a wound infection after being in deep water during a flood.
5. A woman who developed cancer after radiation exposure near a nuclear plant.

3. The hospital is participating in a local disaster drill and the nurse is responsible for decontamination. Which of the following principles should the nurse adhere to? (select all that apply)

1. Identify an isolation room in the Emergency Department as the decontamination area.
2. Set up a decontamination hot zone in the parking lot near the Emergency Room.
3. Restrict entrance to the cold zone until decontamination is completed.
4. Ensure that all patient personal belongings are destroyed prior to triage.
5. Provide each contaminated person with liquid soap and baby shampoo.

4. Which of the following nursing diagnoses would be the priority in caring for a patient with recent known nerve agent exposure?

1. Ineffective airway clearance related to copious secretions and ineffective cough.
2. High risk for altered cardiac output related to electrical conduction abnormalities.
3. Increased risk for fluid and electrolyte imbalance related to vomiting and diarrhea.
4. Ineffective individual coping related to perceived and actual threat from situation.

5. Approximately 30 minutes after exposure to a radiological leak at an industrial facility, several patients arrive at the emergency department. Upon their arrival at the hospital, the triage nurse determines that patients in which phase of acute radiation syndrome will require care first? (select all that apply)

1. Latent phase
2. Prodromal phase
3. Recovery phase
4. Illness phase
5. Reaction phase

6. Which of the following statements would the nurse recognize as true regarding the use of the Hospital Incident Command System (HICS)?

1. The incident commander is in charge of all four areas of operations: planning, logistics, safety, and public information.
2. The plan outlines clearly defined responsibilities and positions that must remain independent of one another and individually run.
3. This flexible plan allows for only necessary positions and functions to be activated on an as needed basis during the incident.
4. Media utilization is limited in order to decrease mass hysteria and unwarranted overwhelming of communications.

Answers to NCLEX Practice Questions can be found in Appendix D in the Osborn Student Resources at nursing.pearsonhighered.com. Practice additional NCLEX questions online at the Student Resources site.

REFERENCES

Agency for Toxic Substances and Disease Registry (ATSDR). (2011). Medical management guidelines for nerve agents: Tabun (GA); sarin (GB); soman (GD); and VX. Retrieved from http://www.atsdr.cdc.gov/mmg/mmg.asp?id=523&tid=93

Albert, R. N. (2009). Ethical considerations for nurses in a natural or human-made disaster, communicable disease outbreak or pandemic. Retrieved from http://www.nurses.ab.ca

Andress, K. (2010). Nuclear, biologic, and chemical agents of mass destruction. In P. K. Howard & R. A. Steinmann (Eds.), *Sheehy's emergency nursing: Principles and practice* (6th ed., pp. 198–210). St. Louis: Mosby/Elsevier.

Auf der Heide, E. (2006). The importance of evidence-based disaster planning. *Annals of Emergency Medicine, 47*(1), 34–49.

California Hospital Association (CHA). (2011). Emergency preparedness. Retrieved from http://www.calhospitalprepare.org/

Centers for Disease Control and Prevention (CDC). (2008a). Radiation emergency training and education. Retrieved from http://emergency.cdc.gov/radiation/training.asp

Centers for Disease Control and Prevention (CDC). (2008b). Strategic National Stockpile. Retrieved from http://www.bt.cdc.gov/stockpile/index.asp

Centers for Disease Control and Prevention (CDC). (2009a). Blast injuries: Essential facts. Retrieved from http://www.bt.cdc.gov/masscasualties/explosions.asp

Centers for Disease Control and Prevention (CDC). (2009b). CDC health update: Swine influenza A (H1N1) update: Interim recommendations and guidance for health directors about strategic national stockpile material. Retrieved from http://www.cdc.gove/h1n1flu/HAN/042609.htm

Centers for Disease Control and Prevention (CDC). (2010, April 16). Prussian blue. Retrieved from http://www.bt.cdc.gov/radiation/prussianblue.asp

Centers for Disease Control and Prevention (CDC). (2011a). Bioterrorism agents/diseases. Retrieved from http://www.bt.cdc.gov/agent/agentlist-category.asp

Centers for Disease Control and Prevention (CDC). (2011b). Chemical agents. Retrieved from http://www.bt.cdc.gov/chemical/

Centers for Disease Control and Prevention (CDC). (2011). Potassium iodide (KI). Retrieved from http://www.bt.cdc.gov/radiation/ki.asp

Coppola, D. (2011a). The management of disasters. In *Introduction to international disaster management* (2nd ed., p. 35). Burlington, MA: Butterworth-Henemann Elsevier.

Coppola, D. (2011b). Recovery. In *Introduction to international disaster management* (2nd ed., pp. 377–423). Burlington, MA: Butterworth-Henemann Elsevier.

Dayton Disaster Medical Assistance Team (DMAT). (2008). Team basics. Retrieved from http://www.daytondmat.com/dmat/dmatinfo.html

Disaster Management Systems (DMS). (2011). All risk triage tags. Retrieved from http://www.triagetags.com/default.aspx

Emergency Management Institute (EMI). (2011). IS 700 National incident management system: An introduction. Retrieved from http://www.training.fema.gov/emiweb/is/is700.asp

Emergency Nurses Association. (2007). Disaster management. In *Trauma nursing core course (TNCC)* (6th ed., pp. 249–273). Des Plaines, IL: Author.

Environmental Protection Agency. (2011). Personal protective equipment. Retrieved from http://www.epa.gov/oem/content/hazsubs/equip.htm

Esbitt, D. (2003, July–September). The Strategic National Stockpile. *Disaster Management and Response, 3*, 68–70.

Gebbie, K. M. (2010). Letter to the editor: The current status of nurses' emergency preparedness: A commentary on the development of emergency preparedness and response competency. *Collegian, 17*(4), 209–211.

Gebbie, K. M., & Qureshi, K. (2002). Emergency and disaster preparedness: Core competencies for nurses. *American Journal of Nursing, 1*(102), 46–51.

Goodhue, C. J., Burke, R. V., Chambers, S., Ferrer, R. R., & Upperman, J. S. (2010). Disaster Olympix: A unique nursing emergency preparedness exercise. *Journal of Trauma Nursing, 17*(1), 5–10.

Hospital Preparedness Program Overview. (2011). FY02 to present and beyond. Retrieved from http://www.phe.gov/preparedness/planning/hpp/Pages/default.aspx

House, H., Graber, M. A., & Scheckel, S. S. (2003). Is your emergency department ready for a terrorist attack? *Emergency Medicine*, October, 46–51.

IOM (Institute of Medicine). (2010). *The future of nursing: Leading change, advancing health.* Washington, DC: The Academic Press.

Johnstone, M. J. (2009). Disaster ethics. *Australian Nursing Journal, 17*(4), 27.

Joint Commission. (2011). Emergency management. Retrieved from http://www.jointcommission.org/standards

Levenson, R. L., & Acosta, J. K. (2001). Observations from ground zero at the World Trade Center in New York City: Part I. *International Journal of Emergency Mental Health, 3*(4), 241–244.

Littleton-Kearney, M. T., & Slepski, L. A. (2008). Directions for disaster nursing education in the United States. *Critical Care Nursing Clinics of North America, 20*(1), 103–109.

Manser, T. (2011). Managing the aftermath of critical incidents: Meeting the needs of health-care providers and patients. *Best Practice & Research Clinical Anaesthesiology, 25*(2), 169–179.

Maxwell, W. (2003). The use of gallows humor and dark humor during crisis situations. *International Journal of Emergency Mental Health, 5*(2), 93–98.

Mendez, T. B. (2010). Disaster planning for vulnerable populations: Mental health. *Critical Care Nursing Clinics of North America, 22*(2), 493–500.

Mistric, M., & Sparling, T. (2010). Disaster aftermath: A first person perspective as a responder and caregiver. *Critical Care Nursing of North America, 22*(2), 523–534.

Mitchell, A. M., Sakraida, T. J., & Kameg, K. (2003). Critical incident stress debriefing: Implications for best practice. *Disaster Management and Response, 1*(2), 46–51.

Mitchell, J. T., & Bray, G. P. (1980). *Emergency services stress.* Upper Saddle River, NJ: Brady/Prentice-Hall.

Occupational Safety and Health Administration. (2005, January). OSHA best practices for hospital-based first receivers of victims from mass casualty incidents involving the release of hazardous substances. Retrieved from http://www.osha.gov/dts/osta/bestpractices/html/hospital_firstreceivers.html

Priest, C., & Bahl, M. (2008). Nursing during catastrophic disaster: A case study from New Orleans. *Journal of Nursing Law, 12*, 157–164.

Robinson, K. S. (2010). Emergency preparedness. In P. K. Howard & R. A. Steinmann (Eds.), *Sheehy's emergency nursing: Principles and practice* (6th ed., pp. 187–197).

Romig, L. (2008). The JumpSTART pediatric MCI triage tool. Retrieved from http://www.jumpstarttriage.com/JumpSTART_and_MCI_Triage.php

Rothstein, M. A. (2010). Currents in contemporary ethics. Should health care providers get treatment priority in an influenza pandemic? *Journal of Law, Medicine, & Ethics, 38*(2): 412–419.

Stangeland, P. A. (2010). Disaster nursing: A retrospective review. *Critical Care Nursing of North America, 22*(4), 421–436.

U.S. Department of Health and Human Services (DHHS). (2008a). National disaster medical systems (NDMS). Retrieved from http://www.hhs.gov/aspr/opeo/ndms/index.html

U.S. Department of Health and Human Services (DHHS). (2008b). National disaster medical systems (NDMS) response teams. Retrieved from http://www.hhs.gov/aspr/opeo/ndms/teams/index.html

Varghese, S. B. (2010). Cultural, ethical, and spiritual implications of natural disasters from the survivors' perspective. *Critical Care Nursing Clinics of North America, 22*(4), 515–522.

Wilkinson, J. M., & Ahearn, N. R. (2009). *Prentice Hall nursing diagnosis handbook* (9th ed.). Upper Saddle River, NJ: Prentice Hall.

Williams, W. (2002, November 14). CDC logistician. Presentation at National Healthcare Profession Preparedness Consortium Health Care Leadership Course, Nobles Training Center, Anniston, AL.

CHAPTER

66 Caring for the Patient in the Emergency Department

Renée Holleran

Outcome-Based Learning Objectives

After studying this chapter, the learner will be able to:

1. Explain the practice of emergency nursing.
2. Differentiate among the various components of the triage process and determine the relevance of each component.
3. Compare and contrast patient priority categories.
4. Explain the legal issues related to the practice of emergency nursing.
5. Describe preparation for emergency nursing practice.

KEY TERMS

Emergency Medical Treatment and Active Labor Act (EMTALA) p.2085
emergency nursing p.2080
forensic evidence p.2086
oligoanalgesia p.2088
triage p.2082

EMERGENCY NURSING is described as the care of individuals of all ages who have perceived or actual physical or emotional alterations of health that have not been diagnosed or require further interventions. Emergency nursing care is episodic, may involve primary as well as secondary and tertiary care, and is usually acute or critical in nature (Bonalumi & King, 2007; Emergency Nurses Association, 2011b; Fazio, 2010; Patrick, 2010). Emergency nursing involves care in a variety of areas, including the prehospital and hospital environments.

The Emergency Nurses Association (ENA) states that emergency nurses provide care across the life span in a variety of patient care settings including the prehospital, transport, and hospital environments. Emergency nursing interventions may range from minimal to lifesaving. An integral part of emergency nursing is prevention. Unique to emergency nursing practice is the application of the nursing process to patients of all ages who require stabilization and/or resuscitation for a variety of illnesses and injuries (ENA, 2011a).

History of Emergency Nursing

Florence Nightingale has long been credited with having originated emergency nursing when she took nurses out to the battlefield during the Crimean War to provide care to wounded soldiers (Figure 66–1◆). The care she and her fellow nurses provided demonstrated the value of rapid management of acute patients. As hospitals developed, care that had generally been given by health care providers, nurses, or even family members in patients' homes was redirected to the hospital.

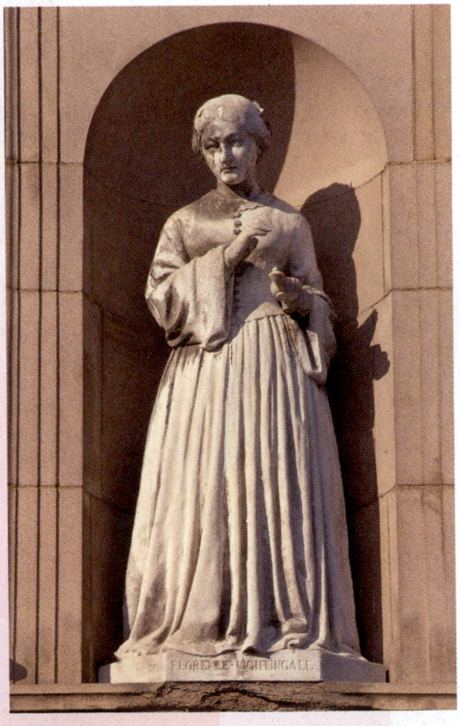

FIGURE 66–1 ◆ Statue of Florence Nightingale.
Source: Guy Erwood/Shutterstock.

Emergency nursing and emergency medicine have developed into specialties during the past 50 years. Care provided to soldiers during the Korean War and Vietnam War demonstrated that rapid and acute care could make a difference in patient outcomes. However, the departments in hospitals that were dedicated to the emergent care of patients were limited. Often, the emergency department was one room staffed by a nurse, who was generally called down from another floor, or by the hospital nursing supervisor.

When emergency medicine was recognized as a specialty in the late 1970s, it quickly became one of the fastest growing medical fields. The Emergency Department Nurses Association was established in 1970 by Anita Dorr (Buffalo, New York) and Judith Kelleher (Downey, California). The association's name was later changed to the Emergency Nurses Association (ENA). Today, emergency nursing has a specific curriculum and clinical requirements, such as the emergency nursing certificaton exam (Certified Emergency Nurse exam, or CEN). There is also a certification exam for the pediatric emergency nurse (Certified Pediatric Emergency Nurse, or CPEN). For information about both exams, go to the Emergency Nurses Association website and look for Board of Certification (BCEN).

The Role of the Emergency Department

In 2009, more than 123 million visits were made to emergency departments in the United States (Centers for Disease Control and Prevention National Center for Health Statistics, 2011). Emergency department (ED) visits continue to grow, yet emergency departments are closing. According to the American College of Emergency Physicians (2012), 184 EDs closed between 2000 and 2010. This has led to ambulance diversions, increasing wait times, and the boarding of patients who are critically ill and injured (i.e., having patients remain in the emergency department after admission while waiting for a bed to become available). This overcrowding in emergency departments is occurring because of decreasing numbers of doctors and nurses and limited hospital beds (Castillo et al., 2011; Hoot & Aronsky, 2008; Institute of Medicine [IOM], 2006).

According to the National Hospital Ambulatory Medical Care Survey (2012), in 2009 there were 136 million visits to emergency departments in the United States. The annual visit rate was 45.1 ED visits per 100 persons. More than one-third of the visits were made by young people, under 25 years old. Common reasons for ED visits and common diagnoses given in EDs are shown in Chart 66–1.

CHART 66–2 Top 10 Most Common Reasons for all ED Visits for Children

1. Other upper respiratory infections such as sinusitis, strep throat, and croup
2. Superficial injury, bruise
3. Otitis media and related conditions
4. Open wounds of head, neck, and trunk
5. Sprains and strains
6. Fever of unknown origin
7. Other injuries and conditions due to external causes
8. Viral infections
9. Fracture of arm
10. Open wounds of arms and legs

Source: Merrill, C. T., Owens, P. L., & Stocks, C. (2012). Pediatric emergency department visits in community hospitals from selected states, 2005. Retrieved from http://www.hcup-us.ahrq.gov/reports/statbriefs/sb52.jsp.

Weblink: Pediatric Emergency Department Visits

Weblink: Emergency Department Visits

The 10 most common reasons for ED visits by children are listed in Chart 66–2.

Emergency departments have become the source of care for many types of patients but particularly for patients who are poor and uninsured. Emergency departments are open 24 hours a day, 7 days a week. Additionally, because of the Emergency Medical Transport and Active Labor Act (discussed later in this chapter), emergency departments cannot refuse to provide a medical screening examination and stabilizing care when patients present for care. The increase in uninsured patients, the open access, and the ability to provide 24-hour-a-day care have put great stress on the capacity of emergency departments.

Emergency departments must also deal with the challenges of providing care to an increasingly diverse patient population (Figure 66–2◆). Patients who utilize the emergency department to get their primary care include illegal immigrants, prisoners, and homeless and underinsured patients. Additionally, the population has become more diverse culturally, and care of these patients requires that emergency nurses and health care providers be culturally competent (see the Cultural Considerations box).

CHART 66–1 Common Reasons for Visiting EDs and Common Diagnoses Given in EDs

Common Reasons for Visiting the ED	Common Diagnoses Given in the ED
• Stomach and abdominal pain (9.6 million visits)	• Acute upper respiratory infection, excluding pharyngitis (6.0 million)
• Fever (7.4 million)	• Abdominal pain (5.7 million)
• Chest pain (7.2 million)	• Contusion with intact skin surface (5.0 million)
• Cough (4.7 million)	• Chest pain (5.0 million)
• Headache (4.0 million)	• Open wound, excluding head (3.9 million)
• Shortness of breath (3.7 million)	• Spinal disorders (3.8 million)
• Back symptoms (3.7 million)	• Cellulitis and abscess (3.1 million)
• Pain, unspecified (2.9 million)	• Fractures, excluding lower limb (2.6 million)
• Vomiting (2.8 million)	• Pyrexia of unknown origin (2.6 million)
• Throat symptoms (2.6 million)	• Sprains and strains, excluding ankle and back (2.4 million)

Source: National Hospital Ambulatory Medical Care Survey. (2012). CDC factsheet: Emergency department. Retrieved from http://www.cdc.gov/nchs/data/ahcd/NHAMCS_Factsheet_ED_2009.pdf.

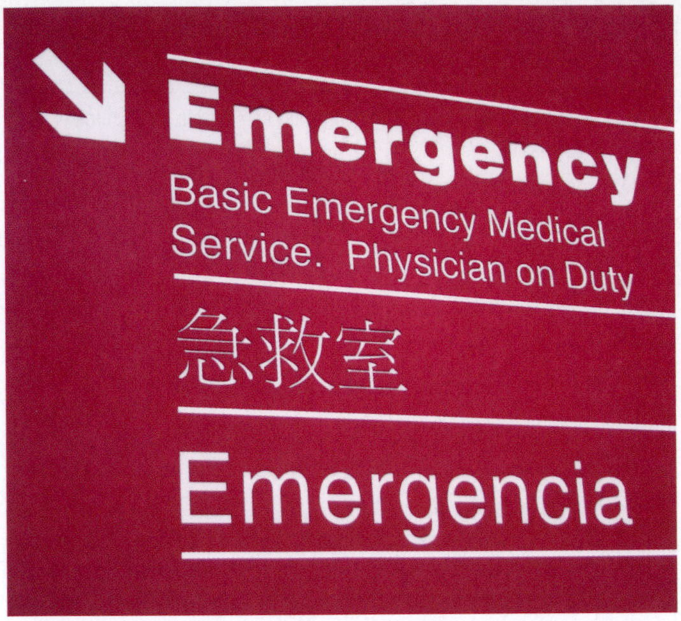

FIGURE 66–2 ◆ Emergency departments provide care for diverse populations.
Source: Stephen Finn/Shutterstock

CULTURAL CONSIDERATIONS
for Emergency Care Providers

The cultural competence of emergency care providers should include knowledge of existing health disparities among different racial and ethnic groups. Emergency care providers should also be aware of the incidence and prevalence of health problems among diverse populations that may present to the emergency department for care. A culturally competent emergency care provider also has the skills to identify and manage racial and ethnic differences in health values, beliefs, and behaviors, incorporating these so that patients receive the best care in the emergency department (Lipson & Dibble, 2007; Ruiz-Contreras, 2010). For example, in some cultures, patients who are ill consult a "healer" and may be taking alternative medications to manage medical problems such as high blood pressure or diabetes. However, there can be medication interactions between prescribed medications and alternative medications. The emergency nurse must be alert to this possibility and respect the patient's beliefs as well as protect him from any harm.

In 1997, the ENA Cultural Diversity Task Force developed a Diversity Practice Model and Pertinent Questions When Discussing Diversity. These models were based on the ABCDEs with which emergency nurses are very familiar. Charts 66–3 and 66–4 contain these models.

In the United States, the emergency department has become the point of universal access to health care. This will continue to be an important challenge in the practice of emergency nursing, one for which nurses will need to provide leadership in order to solve.

CHART 66–3 DIVERSITY PRACTICE MODEL: ABCDE

Assumptions	The act of taking for granted or supposing that a thought or idea about a group is true.
Beliefs	Beliefs are shared ideas about how a group operates.
Communication	The two-way sharing of information that results in an understanding between receiver and sender.
Diversity	The ways in which people differ and the effect that these differences have on health perception and health care.
Education	The act of attaining knowledge about diversity.

CHART 66–4 PERTINENT QUESTIONS WHEN DISCUSSING DIVERSITY: ABCDE

Assumptions	What assumptions do you have regarding the patient situation?
Beliefs/Behavior	What are your organizational beliefs? How are they different from your assumptions?
Communication	What are the communication issues?
Diversity	Which aspects of diversity are present? *Reminder: age, class, culture, ethnicity, gender, nationality, race, religion, sexual orientation, and marginalization.*
Education	What eductional recommendations do you have?

Institute of Medicine Report and the Future of Emergency Care

In June 2006, the Institute of Medicine (IOM) released a report on the state of emergency care in the United States. The IOM report recognized many of the challenges that the emergency medical system, and its nurses and health care providers, face today. Overcrowding, ambulance diversions, shortages of on-call specialists, lack of emergency preparedness, and deficiencies in pediatric emergency care are some of the issues that were identified. The IOM report included recommendations, summarized in the National Guidelines box, for improving emergency care systems in the United States by using a multifaceted, multiorganizational approach. The IOM study and these proposals continue to provide a framework for the delivery of emergency care in the years to come.

Emergency Nursing Roles

The roles of the emergency nurse are many and varied. Emergency nursing can be practiced both inside and outside of the hospital. In addition, emergency nurses may be involved in numerous functions within the emergency department, including education, prevention, and research. Chart 66–5 summarizes some of the roles of emergency nurses.

Specialty Roles in Emergency Nursing

Emergency care requires a team approach and involves both basic and advanced providers. As emergency nursing has evolved, specialty and advanced practice roles have developed. Many of these roles are governed by specific agencies (e.g., state boards of nursing practice) or national associations (e.g., Sexual Assault Nurse Examiners). Chart 66–6 provides a summary of some of these specialty roles.

Triage

The word *triage* is derived from a French word that means "to sort." The Emergency Nurses Association defines **triage** as "an information and decision making process. It is performed in order to sort injured and ill health care consumers into categories of acuity and priorization based on urgency of their medical or psychological needs" (ENA, 2011b, p. 47).

Medical triage evolved during wars in which battles resulted in many casualties while resources were limited. Napoleon's surgeon, Dominique Jean Larrey, has been credited with initiating this concept

NATIONAL GUIDELINES Summary of IOM Recommendations for Emergency Care in the United States

Recommendation	Actions
Improve hospital efficiency and patient flow through the emergency department.	Use tools from other disciplines such as engineering and operations research to improve patient flow. Establish clinical decision units or 24-hour observation units with the goal of preventing unnecessary admissions. Increase the use of informational technologies to track and coordinate patient flow. Develop standards through accreditation bodies for crowding, boarding, and diversion.
Create a coordinated, regionalized, accountable emergency care system.	Develop regionalized systems that include hospitals, emergency medical services (EMS), and other agencies working together. Patients should be taken to the care center that can provide the optimal care, for example, to trauma or stroke centers. Develop well-defined standards and performance improvement measures.
Increase funding for emergency care systems.	Fund research to identify best practices. Request reimbursement for care of all patients who are treated in the emergency department. Acquire funding for disaster preparedness.
Improve pediatric emergency care.	Develop triage and transport protocols designed to provide children with the most appropriate care. Educate and train emergency care providers to care for children. Include pediatric concerns as part of disaster plans. Hire pediatric coordinators in emergency departments and EMS agencies to ensure that appropriate equipment, training, and services are provided to children.

Source: Adapted from: Institute of Medicine. (2006). *Hospital-based emergency care at the breaking point.* Washington, DC: National Academy of Sciences.

CHART 66–5 Emergency Nursing Roles

Role	Description
Urgent care center nursing	Nurses provide care in freestanding facilities that provide urgent care for minor illnesses and injuries.
Prehospital nursing	Nurses provide care in the prehospital care environment. These nurses are prepared through additional education that is generally regulated by the states in which they practice. For example, some states require nurses to take a prehospital nursing course or become emergency medical technicians (EMTs) or EMT-paramedics.
Transport nursing	Nurses accompany air or ground transport patients. Even though many nurses who perform transport may have emergency nursing experience, transport nurses may also have critical care nursing experience (Figure 66–3 ◆).
Military nurses	Nurses provide care as part of their military service.
Industrial nursing and occupational health nursing	Nurses provide care to specific industries or companies. Basic life support and advanced cardiac life support are additional responsibilities of many of these nurses.
Correctional nursing	Nurses provide care in prisons and jails.

on the battlefield. Florence Nightingale also used the triage concept during the Crimean War. She went out after the daily fighting, sorted out which injured soldiers might or might not survive, and provided much needed care (Thomas & Bernardo, 2009).

During the 20th century, battlefield triage consisted of a primary assessment and the performance of critical interventions such as control of bleeding, followed by rapid transport to field hospitals and mobile surgical hospitals such as the MASH units that were first deployed in the Korean War. During the Korean and Vietnam wars, helicopter transport was introduced to enhance the rapidity of patient care (Gilboy, 2010).

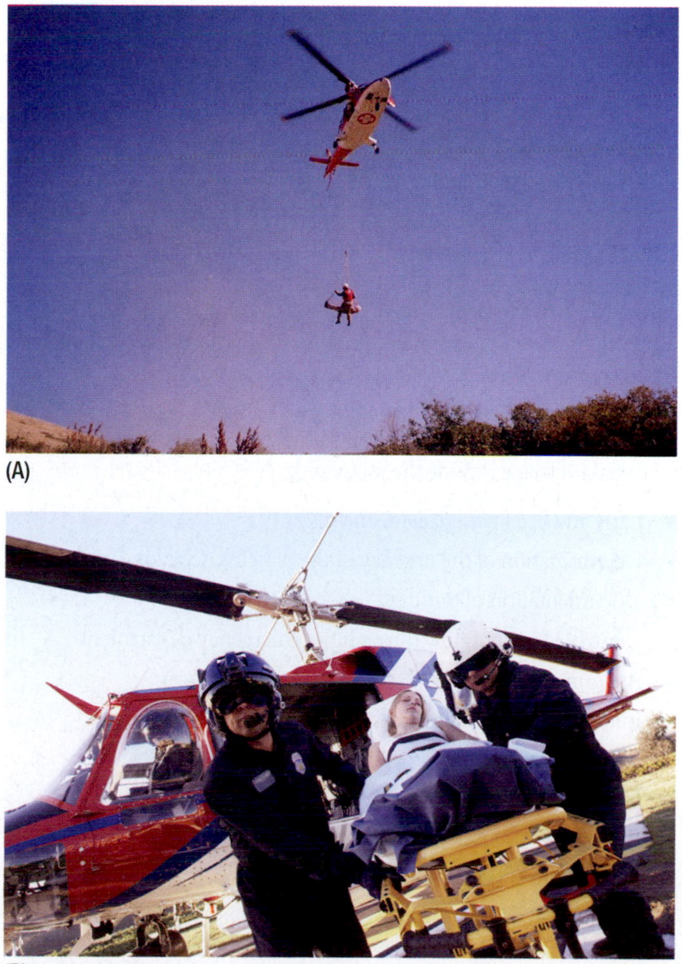

(A) (B)

FIGURE 66–3 ◆ Flight nurse (A) practicing a rescue and (B) participating in one.
Source: A: Renee Holleran. B: Monkey Business Images/Shutterstock.

CHART 66–6 Specialty Roles in Emergency Nursing

Role	Description
Nurse educator	A nurse educator is a nurse who is responsible for the educational needs of the emergency department. This role may also include patient and community education.
Emergency nurse practitioner (ENP)	An ENP is a nurse practitioner who specializes in providing advanced nursing practice. There is no specific ENP certification for emergency nursing; however, many ENPs hold certifications as family nurse practitioners, acute care nurse practitioners, pediatric nurse practitioners, or adult nurse practitioners.
Emergency clinical nurse specialist (ECNS)	A clinical nurse specialist is prepared at either the master's or doctoral level as an expert in emergency nursing. An ECNS may provide direct patient care, provide education, develop and perform research, and serve as a role model and change agent in the emergency department.
Case manager	An emergency case manager can provide care to a single patient or a group of patients. Case managers interact with many departments and outside agencies to assist the patient, families, and emergency department staff with care issues such as home health, drug dependence, and psychiatric problems so that the patient gets the best and most cost-effective care.

In the 1960s, as the number of patients coming to the emergency department began to grow, the need for triage was recognized. Initially, emergency department triage was performed by a health care provider or a nurse–health care provider team. Today, it is generally performed by experienced emergency department nurses (Gilboy, 2010).

Triage, which is performed in both the prehospital and hospital environments, is a fluid process that is based on the number of patients, the amount of resources available, and the care that is available. Triage is an important component of emergency nursing practice as patient censuses continue to increase and more has to be provided with less. The goals of triage include the following:

- Early and brief patient assessment
- Determination of the urgency of the patient's need for care
- Documentation of findings
- Control of patient flow through the emergency department
- Assignment of patients to the appropriate care area
- Initiation of diagnostic measures
- Initiation of limited therapeutic interventions
- Infection control
- Promotion of public relations
- Health education for patients and families.

Safety Alert *An important part of triage is the intuitive sense ("gut feeling") that the emergency nurse may have about the patient. From experience, the triage nurse develops a sense of when something is wrong. Often, few data are available to validate these feelings. However, experienced emergency nurses are good resources and can alert new nurses about how to identify the less obvious indicators that a patient may be in trouble.*

CHART 66–7 Types of Triage

Type of Triage	Components
Traffic director	*Nonprofessional (hospital registrar)* Writes down chief complaint.
Spot check	*Nurse/health care provider* Evaluates patient. Assigns an urgency category.
Comprehensive triage	*Registered nurse* Evaluates patient. Assigns an urgency category. Implements interventions (e.g., ordering a radiograph). Administers pain medication.

Types of Triage

The type of triage that is used in an emergency department depends on several things, including patient census, department layout, and number and type of staff. Although triage is usually performed by an experienced registered nurse, there are other types of triage models, as listed in Chart 66–7.

Components of Triage

Triage begins with an "across the room assessment." This involves what the triage nurse sees, smells, or sometimes even feels when first evaluating the patient. For example:

- Is the patient's airway open or is the patient drooling?
- Is the patient breathing and, if so, is the breathing effective?
- What is the patient's skin color: normal, pale, flushed?
- Are there any obvious signs of illness or injury?

A minimal amount of information should be gathered about why the patient has presented to the emergency department or other setting. Several mnemonics can be used to gather data, depending on the patient's chief complaint or reason for presenting. Charts 66–8, 66–9, and 66–10 contain mnemonics that can assist with collecting historical data in triage. Even though the CIAMPEDS mnemonic is directed more at collecting data for a pediatric patient, it can easily be adapted for the adult patient as well (ENA, in press).

A brief but focused physical assessment should be performed. Objective data can be collected by using a primary assessment that

CHART 66–8 CIAMPEDS Mnemonic

Chief complaint
Immunizations, **I**solation: exposed to a disease or hazardous material that may put the rest of the department in danger
Allergies
Medications
Parents' or caregivers' impression about the patient
Events surrounding the illness or injury
Diet, **D**iapers or output
Symptoms associated with the chief complaint, for example, fever, nausea, and vomiting

CHART 66–9 MVIT Mnemonic

Mechanism of injury
Vital signs
Injury
Treatment

CHART 66–10 AMPLE History Mnemonic

Allergies
Medications
Past medical history
Last meal
Everything that is related to the chief complaint

includes airway, breathing, circulation, and disability. The components of the primary assessment are discussed in detail in Chapter 6.

A secondary assessment may be required in some cases to better differentiate the severity of a patient's condition. The secondary assessment should include exposure with environmental control, a full set of vital signs, family presence, provision of comfort, additional history, and a head-to-toe assessment as needed, using inspection, palpation, and auscultation. The components of the secondary survey are discussed in detail in Chapter 67.

Triage Urgency Categories

Once an initial evaluation has been made related to the patient's physical condition and chief complaint, the triage nurse will assign the patient to an urgency category. Urgency categories rate the acuity (level of severity) of the patient's condition and assist in prioritizing care. Generally, an *emergent patient* has an immediate life-threatening problem, such as an airway obstruction. An *urgent patient* can wait a little longer but needs to be seen as soon as possible. An example is a patient with chest pain, cardiac risk factors, and stable vital signs. Finally, a *nonurgent patient* can wait for care.

Some emergency departments use a three-level urgency category; however, the continued rise in emergency department censuses, the augmented acuity of patients who are being cared for in the emergency department, and the numbers of patients who use the emergency department for primary care have prompted the use of additional levels of urgency. Chart 66–11 summarizes four- and five-level triage urgency scales. There are resources available, such as the Emergency Severity Index from the Emergency Nurses Association, that describe the use of a five-level triage urgency category.

CHART 66–11 Triage Urgency Scales

Four-Level Triage	Five-Level Triage
Level 1: Resuscitation	Level I: Resuscitation
Level II: Emergent	Level II: Emergent
Level III: Urgent	Level III: Urgent
Level IV: Nonurgent	Level IV: Semiurgent
	Level V: Nonurgent

Safety Alert *Even when patients have been assigned a triage category, their condition may change, so patients who have to wait for care must be reassessed at specific intervals. Triage policies and procedures should reflect when this must be done and documented. There have been cases in which patients have suffered significant harm and even death while waiting to be seen.*

Disaster Triage

When a disaster occurs (such as an earthquake, tornado, major chemical spill, or terrorist event), triage is directed at rapidly identifying patient urgency, assigning a category, and transferring the patient to the most appropriate area for care. However, in a disaster, there might not be enough personnel or resources to care for everyone. In such a case, care may be withheld from the most severely injured victims so that the limited resources are used for those who will survive (Powers, 2009).

During a disaster, many emergency departments and community disaster programs use the START (Simple Triage and Rapid Treatment) system. This system evaluates respirations, perfusion, and mental status to determine who needs immediate transport, who can wait, or who may be unsalvageable. Color codes are used as a method of identification and communication. For example, green might mean that the patient can walk to an area for care (Kahn, Schultz, Miller, & Anderson, 2009). Chapter 65 provides a detailed description of the START triage system.

Each emergency department and community should have a disaster plan that describes the manner of triage to be employed during a disaster. The roles of the emergency nurse and other staff members should be practiced on a regularly scheduled basis. Additional information about disaster management is provided in Chapter 65.

Weblink: START and Save Triage

Weblink: EMTALA

Legal Issues

The practice of emergency nursing requires understanding of some of the legal issues that affect the emergency department. Three of these issues are discussed here: the Emergency Medical Treatment and Active Labor Act, consent, and evidence collection.

Emergency Medical Treatment and Active Labor Act

The **Emergency Medical Treatment and Active Labor Act (EMTALA)** is a part of the 1986 Consolidated Omnibus Budget Reconciliation Act (COBRA) laws and the 1990 Omnibus Budget Reconciliation Act (OBRA) amendment that defines the legal responsibilities of Medicare-participating hospitals in treating individuals who present with emergency medical conditions (Centers for Medicare and Medicaid, 2011). In summary, EMTALA ensures the following:

- A hospital is required to perform a medical screening exam to determine whether there is an emergency when a patient presents to the emergency department.
- If it is determined that an emergency condition exists, the hospital must provide further medical examination and treatment as required to stabilize the patient.
- If the hospital does not have the capabilities to provide the care needed, the patient may be transferred.
- An appropriate transfer is one in which the medical benefits outweigh the risk of transport or the patient makes an informed consent for transfer.

Weblink: Evidence Collection for Nurses

- The patient must be transferred with an appropriate level of care provided during the transport process.
- A hospital may never delay an appropriate medical screening examination or further examination or treatment to inquire about the patient's payment method or insurance status.

Also under EMTALA, hospitals that receive patients who may have been inappropriately transferred need to report this; signs must be posted in the emergency department that explain a person's rights to emergency treatment (most emergency departments have these posted in multiple languages); and hospitals must maintain patients' records, a list of on-call health care providers, and emergency department logs. Failure to adhere to these regulations can result in both institutional and individual fines and loss of federal funding.

In summary, EMTALA provides that all patients who seek treatment in the emergency department have a medical screening and treatment as deemed appropriate on the basis of their emergency. No patient can be turned away for financial reasons.

Consent

Consent is defined as "giving permission to do something." However, the nature of emergency practice does not always allow the patient or family the ability to consent to all of the treatments that may be needed to save a life. Most states recognize this problem in the emergency department and have allowed consent to be waived when there is a life- or-limb-threatening emergency (Brous, 2010).

The emergency nurse will generally encounter three types of consent. A *general (blanket) consent* is usually obtained at registration. This type of consent will allow for evaluation and treatment, such as radiographs, laboratory tests, and medications. If more invasive tests are needed or the patient must undergo a specific procedure, such as a fracture reduction that requires conscious sedation, informed consent should be obtained. *Informed consent* involves the patient stating (by signing a form) that she has a full understanding of the procedure, including its risks, and is competent to give consent. Even though the emergency nurse should check to see that a consent form has been signed, it is the health care provider's responsibility to obtain informed consent. Finally, *implied consent* allows treatment in an emergency situation based on the presumption that if the patient were able to, he would give permission for treatment (Brous, 2010).

Each state dictates ages of consent, situations that may allow for legal consent despite being underage (e.g., pregnant underaged females), and other nuances related to consent. It is imperative that the emergency nurse be familiar with the applicable state laws and hospital policies related to consent. When in doubt, the nurse should always err safely on the side of the patient and, when possible, consult hospital risk management personnel before acting. It is also important to document why decisions were made to prevent any second-guessing if questions of legality arise.

Evidence Collection and Preservation

Unfortunately, a major part of emergency nursing practice is caring for the victims of violence. Patients who have experienced sexual assault, domestic assault, or motor vehicle crashes are only a few of the types of patients for whom the emergency nurse might need to collect and preserve evidence. **Forensic evidence** is something that can be legally submitted to a court of law as a means of determining the truth related to an alleged crime (Sheridan, Nash, & Bresee, 2010). Examples of evidence include clothing, body fluids, bite marks, and photographs of injuries. Chapter 41 includes a discussion of intimate partner violence, which is a common situation in which the emergency nurse may need to collect forensic evidence.

Safety Alert *Every emergency department should have a policy and procedure for the collection and preservation of evidence. Improper collection and preservation could lead to erroneous interpretation of the evidence or could make it legally impossible to prosecute the alleged perpetrator.*

Evidence must be collected by using a specific protocol and procedure that includes how to label the evidence, how to preserve it, and how to maintain the chain of custody. Some evidence collection protocols are directed by specific legal agencies or even state agencies. Chart 66–12 contains a summary of procedural steps for evidence collection and preservation in the emergency department (Semonin-Holleran, 2009).

Gerontological Considerations

With the aging population, it is important for the emergency department nurse to be familiar with the unique aspects of assessment and planning of care for older adults. At a hospital in Canada that received 51,000 emergency department visits annually, adults who were 70 years of age or older used approximately 70% of the total bed days; in 2005, those 75 years of age and older had an emergency department admittance rate of approximately 37%, compared to an average admittance rate for all ages of 15% (Sendecki, 2007). For this reason, the hospital in Canada developed a course that applied geriatric and geropsychiatric knowledge, skills, and abilities that emergency department nurses can implement into their daily practice. An example is the need to assess falls as a symptom that requires investigation of root causes, treatment plan follow-up, and risk reduction to prevent another fall. The hospital also assigned a position in the emergency department for a geriatric emergency nurse (GEN). The focus of the GEN is to identify needs and start a proactive care plan that is used during the patient's admission. The GEN also alerts community care to anticipated needs upon discharge. At the end of a 4-month trial, the hospital found that the GEN had seen approximately 25% of all patients who were 75 years of age or older; of those, 50% were admitted to the hospital. The average length of stay of those who had been assessed by the GEN was 11.5 days, compared with 15.4 days for those of the same age group who were not seen by the GEN (Sendecki, 2007).

The ENA has developed an online course entitled Geriatric Emergency Nursing Education (GENE). The course covers best practices that can be used to deliver optimal care and respond to the special needs of older adults. The course covers these topics:

- Attitudes and ageism
- Physical and psychological changes
- Atypical presentation of illness
- Triage
- Pain management
- Abuse and neglect
- Palliative care
- Discharge planning.

CHART 66–12 Collection and Preservation of Evidence and Chain of Custody

1. Identify the indications for evidence collection and consult authorities to ensure that the appropriate evidence is collected and preserved.
2. Obtain and use the appropriate evidence collection kit.
3. Obtain patient consent according to hospital policy and procedure. In some cases, consent may not be necessary, for example, in a homicide investigation. Consult appropriate authorities.
4. When collecting evidence, change gloves frequently to prevent cross-contamination.
5. Try not to perform any wound care until photographs have been taken.
6. Place evidence in individual labeled containers.
7. Wet evidence should always be dried before packaging.
8. Always place evidence in a paper bag.
9. Label all evidence with this information:
   a. Patient's name
   b. Source of collection
   c. Date
   d. Time
   e. Person collecting the evidence.
10. Evidence should be sealed with evidence tape. Never lick evidence envelopes.
11. Photographs may be taken by an emergency nurse. They must be labeled and stored in a secured area. Take photographs only if experienced in how to do it properly.
12. Document the evidence collection procedure. Use checklists when available.
13. Place evidence in a secure, locked area until it is released to the appropriate authorities.
14. For all evidence, maintain the chain of custody, documenting who collected the evidence, anyone who touches or secures it, and what is done with the evidence until it is given to law enforcement personnel.
15. Complete the medical record, document what was given to authorities, and indicate who received the evidence.

Preparation for Practice

Preparation for practice in the emergency department for new graduates or nurses without emergency experience can be demanding. Nursing care in the emergency department includes learning to manage the care of four or five patients simultaneously; starting all of the patient care, such as inserting intravenous lines and drawing blood for evaluation; limited and focused patient assessment, often with little or no patient information; discharge teaching and planning; and care of populations and patient problems that are not frequently encountered in admitted patients, such as acute psychosis, sexual assault, and homelessness. Emergency department nursing also requires familiarity with diverse patient populations, varied age groups, and social problems that may never be solved (ENA, 2011b; Proehl, 2002).

Additional education for new orientees to the emergency department should include the following:

- Advanced Cardiac Life Support (ACLS)
- Pediatric Advanced Life Support (PALS)
- Trauma Nursing Core Course (TNCC)
- Emergency Nursing Pediatric Course (ENPC).

Nursing care for patients or conditions not frequently encountered by new orientees with their limited experience (e.g., obstetrics and gynecology; eye, ear, nose, and throat; pediatric and psychiatric emergencies) should also be included.

Discharge Priorities

The majority of patients seen in the emergency department are sent home rather than being admitted to the hospital. An important part of discharge planning is providing information about how to manage the problem that brought the patient to the emergency department and where the patient should obtain further care.

Discharge instructions should be clear and use terminology that the patient understands. Most educators recommend that discharge instructions be written at a fifth- or sixth-grade level. When necessary and possible, they should be translated into a language that the patient or family understands; at a minimum, an interpreter should be present when the instructions are given. Illustrations of what is expected (e.g., how to wrap an elastic bandage on an injured extremity) may be of assistance. Instructions must also be age appropriate. This is especially important when medications are being prescribed.

Many commercial programs that provide discharge instructions are available. These instructions can be printed and sent with the patient. In some cases, the instructions can be accessed online from the patient's home.

Discharge instructions should include information about follow-up care. In some emergency departments, patients may be asked to return; in other departments, patients may be referred to a health care provider, advanced practitioner, or clinic. It is important to ensure that the patient or family members understand the information that is provided. Asking the patient questions or to do a return demonstration may assist in determining the level of understanding. Some emergency departments have instituted follow-up calls to not only find out about follow-up care, but also to check on the patient's status. It is important to allow the patient or family the opportunity to ask questions and feel as comfortable as possible with the prescribed care for their illness or injury.

Pain Management

Pain is the most common complaint in the emeregncy department. Typically, little information is known about the patient when she arrives

ETHICAL ISSUES
Pain Management in the Emergency Department

Pain is the most common complaint of patients in the emergency department. Despite this, only 40% to 60% of the patients who present at the emergency department are treated for pain. Emergency nurses face the ethical challenges related to the management of pain including how to assess the level of the patient's pain, what medications ahould be prescribed, and issues surrounding medication abuse. Many patients face **oligoanalgesia,** in which no interventions are provided for pain relief despite patients' complaints of pain when they come to the emergency department. Many reasons are cited for this, including fear of masking symptoms and concern about the physiological effects of pain medications and the possibilty of drug abuse. Some studies have demonstrated that women and minorities do not receive appropriate pain management. Emergency nurses need to be patient advocates and ensure that a patient's pain is assessed, documented, and managed. Pain management requires a collaborative approach, including protocols so that analgesic agents can be administered as soon as possible. All patients should receive pain care (Knox et al., 2007; Tanabe, Semonin-Holleran, & Reddin, 2010).

in the emergency department. This may create an ethical dilemma for the nurses and physicans. The Ethical Issues box focuses on the challenges that the emergency department nurse faces in managing the patient with pain.

Health Promotion

Emergency nurses play a key role not only in the management of ill or injured patients, but also in injury and disease prevention. One primary example is through Emergency Nurses CARE (ENCARE). ENCARE was started by two emergency nurses in the 1980s who had become involved in trying to prevent injuries and death from alcohol-related emergencies (Fazio, 2010).

The ENA established the Institute for Quality, Safety and Injury Prevention (IQSIP). This group encompasses several other programs that provide information and methods to educate patients and the public in general about injury prevention and safety. Injury prevention and education program information that is available through the IQSIP addresses the following topics:

- Alcohol and drugs
- Driving safety
- Falls
- Fire and burns
- Gun safety
- Health literacy
- Injury (head)
- Injury (general)
- Medication safety
- Mental health
- School safety
- Suicide
- Toy safety.

Through the efforts of its many emergency nurses, injury prevention has reached hundreds of thousands of people throughout the United States.

Much research has been done and is ongoing regarding injury prevention and the most effective ways to educate communities. Other research opportunities for emergency nursing are included in the Research Opportunities box.

Research

The practice of emergency nursing involves the care of diverse patient populations in many types of situations. It requires skills that include the ability to identify critically ill and injured patients and start their care from the beginning, as well as develop patience with difficult societal problems such as caring for the homeless. Emergency nursing

EVIDENCE-BASED PRACTICE Family Presence During Resuscitation in the Emergency Department

Clinical Problem

Should the family be allowed to be present during resuscitation in the emergency department?

Research Findings

In 1982, the Foote Hospital in Michigan surveyed 13 surviving relatives about whether they would have liked to be present during the attempted resuscitation of their family members. Of those surveyed, 72% said that they would have liked to have been present. The hospital developed a program to allow selected "accompanied" family members to be present during resuscitation. After the event, 70 family members and 21 health care providers, nurses, and others were surveyed. Among family members, 76% felt that being present assisted them in their grieving process. They also felt that the patient did not die alone and emergency care providers did everything that they could. Staff members, however, felt hampered in their resuscitation efforts and reported increased stress because the patients became more "human" in the presence of family members. No family member interfered with the resuscitation efforts (Doyle et al., 1987).

This landmark study opened the floodgates of consideration of the family's role in resuscitation. Since 1987, more than 60 papers have been published that address this issue. The evidence presented in many published papers continue to support family presence (Egging et al., 2011; Nykiel et al., 2011; Oman & Duran, 2010). Families have expressed that they are not concerned about what they may see or hear in the resuscitation area—they just want to be with their family member. More than half of the families felt that they had a right to be present and, again, felt that their grieving process was aided. The staff's perspective included fear of interference from the family and the need to display more professional behaviors during the resuscitation process. Interestingly, health care providers are more opposed to family presence than are nurses.

Implications for Nursing Practice

When implementing family presence in the emergency department during resuscitation, a policy needs to be in place that addresses when family presence can and cannot be allowed; all staff members need to be prepared and trained; well-qualified and trained staff members should always accompany the patient; and resources must be available to the staff members to help them cope with any issues that may arise (ENA, 2012).

Critical Thinking Questions with answers can be found in the Osborn Student Resources at nursing.pearsonhighered.com.

Sources: Doyle, C., Post, H., Burney, R., Maino, J., Keefe, M., & Rhee, K. (1987). Family participation during resuscitation: An option. *Annals of Emergency Medicine, 16*(6), 673–675; Egging, D., Crowley, M., Arruda, T., Proehl, J., Walker-Cillo, G., Papa, A., et al. (2011). Emergency nursing resource: Family presence during invasive procedures and resuscitation in the emergency department. *Journal of Emergency Nursing, 37*(5), 469–473.

RESEARCH OPPORTUNITIES Related to Emergency Nursing

Research Area	Clinical Impact
Physiological Research	
The management of acute and chronic pain in the emergency department	Many patients do not have their pain appropriately managed and frequently present to the emergency department for pain medication. The increase in prescription drug abuse has had a significant impact on the number of patients coming to the emergency department and contributes to crowding. See the Ethical Issues box.
Use of alternative methods to manage pain in the emergency department	Nurses could use alternative methods of pain management such as acupuncture, acupressure, and massage to manage pain in the emergency department.
Development of guidelines to manage shock in the emergency department	Innovative assessment and monitoring methods and treatment therapies would emerge for the management of the patient in shock.
Psychosocial, Ethical, and Legal Research	
Effectiveness of family presence during invasive procedures and resuscitation	Identify how to include the family in the care of their critically ill or injured family member. Assist in end-of-life decision making.
Problem of overcrowding in emergency departments and ambulance diversion by emergency departments	Learn to manage the limited resources of emergency departments, including nursing staff, in order to meet the needs of all patients, particularly the uninsured and underinsured patients who use the emergency department for their health care.
Effectiveness of follow-up phone calls within 24 hours of a patient visit	Decrease return visits and get patients into the appropriate health care systems, thereby decreasing costs.

encompasses all aspects of care from pediatric to geriatric, medical to surgical, and involves providing care to a population of patients who are very diverse, both culturally and economically. It requires excellent assessment and critical thinking skills as well as procedural proficiency. The practice of emergency nursing should be evidenced based. The Evidence-Based Practice box gives an example of evidence-based nursing practice in the emergency department.

There are many opportunities for future research in emergency nursing. Some topics are presented in the Research Opportunities box.

NCLEX® PRACTICE

1. The nurse is interested in a position in a local emergency department. When preparing for an interview the nurse reviews which fact about the practice of emergency nursing which may be helpful in the interview?

1. Emergency nursing always involves episodic patient care that is usually chronic or critical in nature.
2. Emergency nursing can include patient care for perceived, actual, or undiagnosed health problems.
3. Emergency nursing has long been associated with Judith Kelleher and her care of wounded soldiers.
4. Emergency nursing allows the nurse to focus on the care of one specialty population.

2. The emergency department nurse is responsible for triage when all of the following patients present simultaneously for care. With triage assessment complete, which patient should be treated first?

1. A patient who is complaining of chest pain and shortness of breath with pale, clammy skin, nausea, and diaphoresis.
2. A patient with a 3 centimeter laceration to the right forearm with normal sensation and minimal bleeding.
3. A patient who is having a possible allergic reaction with facial edema, drooling, stridor, and severe urticaria with pruritis.
4. A patient who is experiencing increasingly severe problems urinating and who has a large palpable bladder.

3. The patient presents to the emergency department with a complaint of nontraumatic back pain for four months that has previously been evaluated by her primary care provider. The patient states, "I ran out of my pain medicine last night, and my doctor refuses to call in another prescription." Objective findings are unremarkable. Vital signs are HR 89, BP 130/60, RR 18, T 98.9°F, SpO_2 99%, and pain 5 on a 0–10 scale. Based on the four-level system, how should this patient be categorized at triage?

1. Level I – Resuscitation
2. Level II – Emergent
3. Level III – Urgent
4. Level IV – Nonurgent

4. The patient presents to the emergency department with a left shoulder dislocation that must be reduced quickly, as the radial pulse on the affected side is no longer palpable. The injury occurred 30 minutes prior to arrival, and the patient states that he is experiencing severe pain. The emergency nurse understands that which of the following consents must be obtained prior to this patient's treatment?

1. General consent and informed consent
2. Informed consent and implied consent
3. Implied consent and blood product consent
4. Blood product consent and general consent

5. The nurse is orienting a new nurse graduate to the emergency department. Which of the following statements made by the new nurse regarding preparation for emergency nursing would indicate the need for further instruction?
   1. "I am planning on taking additional training to help prepare myself to deal with any potential psychiatric emergencies."
   2. "I am glad that emergency nurses do not have to deal with obstetrical issues because they can call the labor and delivery nurses."
   3. "I will take the Trauma Nursing Core Course soon because I know I need more experience with trauma assessment."
   4. "I now feel more confident in my time management skills when it comes to caring for multiple patients simultaneously."

6. When performing the role of triage in the emergency department, the nurse is interviewing a patient who states "I lost my job and don't have any insurance." The best response for the nurse to this statement is:
   1. "I will call social work to see if they can help you with a payment schedule."
   2. "We are required to assess your injury or illness regarless of ability to pay."
   3. "You may have to wait to be seen until other patients are treated."
   4. "The county hospital across town is probably the best place for you to receive care."

Answers to NCLEX Practice Questions can be found in Appendix D in the Osborn Student Resources at nursing.pearsonhighered.com. Practice additional NCLEX questions online at the Student Resources site.

Pearson Nursing Student Resources Find additional review materials at: **nursing.pearsonhighered.com**

REFERENCES

American College of Emergency Physicians. (2012). Emergency medicine statistical profile. Retrieved from http://www.acep.org/content.aspx?id=25234

Bonalumi, N., & King, D. (2007). Professionalism and leadership. In S. Hoyt & J. Selfridge-Thomas (Eds.), *Emergency nursing core curriculum* (6th ed.). Philadelphia: W. B. Saunders.

Brous, E. (2010). Legal and regulatory constructs. In P. Kunz Howard & R. Steinmann (Eds.), *Sheehy's emergency nursing: Principles and practice* (6th ed., pp. 16–26). St. Louis: Mosby Elsevier.

Castillo, E., Vilke, G., Williams, M., Turner, P., Boyle, J., & Chan, T. (2011). Collaborative to decrease ambulance diversion: The California emergency department diversion project. *Journal of Emergency Medicine, 40*(3), 300–307.

Centers for Medicare and Medicaid Services (CMS). (2011). EMTALA overview. Retrieved from http://www.cms.gov/EMTALA/

Doyle, C., Post, H., Burney, R., Maino, J., Keefe, M., & Rhee, K. J. (1987). Family participation during resuscitation: An option. *Annals of Emergency Medicine, 16*(6), 673–675.

Egging, D., Crowley, M., Arruda, T., Proehl, J., Walker-Cillo, G., Papa, A., et al. (2011). Emergency nursing resource: Family presence during invasive procedures and resuscitation in the emergency department. *Journal of Emergency Nursing, 37*(6), 469–473.

Emergency Nurses Association (ENA). (2011a). Emergency Nurses Association nursing practice. Retrieved from http://www.ena.org/IQSIP/Nursing Practice/Pages/Default.aspx

Emergency Nurses Association (ENA). (2011b). *Emergency nursing scope and standards of practice.* Des Plaines, IL: Author.

Emergency Nurses Association (ENA). (2012). *Emergency nursing pediatric course.* Des Plaines, IL: Author.

Fazio, J. (2010). Emergency nursing practice. In P. Kunz Howard & R. Steinmann (Eds.), *Sheehy's emergency nursing: Principles and practice* (6th ed., pp. 8–15). St. Louis: Mosby Elsevier.

Gilboy, N. (2010). Triage. In P. Kunz Howard & R. Steinmann (Eds.), *Sheehy's emergency nursing: Principles and practice* (6th ed., pp. 59–72). St. Louis: Mosby Elsevier.

Hoot, N. R., & Aronsky, D. (2008). Systemic review of emergency department crowding: Causes, effects, and solutions. *Annals of Emergency Medicine, 52*(2), 126–136.

Institute of Medicine. (2006). *Hospital-based emergency care at the breaking point.* Washington, DC: National Academy of Sciences.

Kahn, C., Schultz, C., Miller, K., & Anderson, C. (2009). Does START triage work? An outcomes assessment after a disaster. *Annals of Emergency Medicine, 54*(3), 424–430.

Knox, T., Ducharme, J., Choiniere, M., Crandall, C., Fosnocht, D., Homel, P., et al. (2007). Pain in the emergency department: Results of the Pain and Emergency Department Initiative (PEMI) multicenter study. *Journal of Pain, 8*(6), 460–466.

Lipson, J. G., & Dibble, S. L. (Eds.). (2007). *Culture and clinical care.* San Francisco: UCSF Nursing Press.

Merrill, C. T., Owens, P. L., & Stocks, C. (2012). Pediatric emergency department visits in community hospitals from selected states, 2005. Retrieved from http://www.hcup-us.ahrq.gov/reports/statbriefs/sb52.jsp

National Center for Health Statistics. (2011). Emergency department visits. Retrieved from http://www.cdc.gov/nchs/fastats/ervisits.htm

National Hospital Ambulatory Medical Care Survey. (2012). CDC factsheet: Emergency department. Retrieved from http://www.cdc.gov/nchs/data/ahcd/NHAMCS_Factsheet_ED_2009.pdf

Nykiel, L., Denicke, R., Schneider, R., Jett, K., Denicke, S., Kunish, K., et al. (2011). Evidence-based practice and family presence: Paving the path for nurse scientists. *Journal of Emergency Nursing, 37*, 9–16.

Oman, K., & Duran, C. (2010). Health care providers' evaluations of family presence during resuscitation. *Journal of Emergency Nursing, 36*, 524–533.

Patrick, V. (2010). Emergency nursing: A historical perspective. In P. Kunz Howard & B. Steinmann (Eds.), *Sheehy's emergency nursing: Principles and practice* (6th ed., pp. 3–7). St. Louis: Mosby Elsevier.

Powers, R. (2009). Evidence-based ED disaster planning. *Journal of Emergency Nursing, 35*(3), 218–223.

Proehl, J. (2002). Developing emergency nursing competence. *Nursing Clinics of North America, 37*(1), 89–96.

Ruiz-Contreras, A. (2010). Approaching diversity. In P. Kunz Howard & B. Steinmann (Eds.), *Sheehy's emergency nursing: Principles and practice* (6th ed., pp. 27–32). St. Louis: Mosby Elsevier.

Semonin-Holleran, R. (2009). Preservation of evidence. In J. Proehl (Ed.), *Emergency nursing procedures* (4th ed., pp. 889–893). Philadelphia: Saunders Elsevier.

Sendecki, C. (2007, Fall). Care of the acutely ill elderly in ER: Growth of the role of geriatric ER nurses. *Outlook.*

Sheridan, D., Nash, K., & Bresee, H. (2010). Forensic nursing in the emergency department. In P. Kunz Howard & B. Steinmann (Eds.), *Sheehy's emergency nursing: Principles and practice* (6th ed., pp. 174–186). St. Louis: Mosby Elsevier.

Tanabe, P., Semonin-Holleran, R., & Reddin, C. J. (2010). Pain. In P. Kunz Howard & R. Steinmann (Eds.), *Sheehy's emergency nursing: Principles and practice* (6th ed., pp. 127–147). St. Louis: Mosby Elsevier.

Thomas, D. O., & Bernardo, L. M. (2009). *Core curriculum for pediatric emergency nursing.* Des Plaines, IL: Emergency Nurses Association.

Caring for the Patient with Multisystem Trauma

67 CHAPTER

Renée Holleran
Cheryl Wraa

Outcome-Based Learning Objectives

After studying this chapter, the learner will be able to:

1. Identify the correlation between mechanism of injury and patient assessment based on an understanding of the kinematics of trauma.
2. List the priorities of the primary and secondary surveys.
3. Explain the rationale for the tertiary survey.
4. Compare and contrast special considerations that may apply during the initial resuscitation.

KEY TERMS

TRAUMATIC INJURY is a major public health problem. It is recognized as one of the most important threats to public health and safety in the United States with regard to years of productive life lost, permanent disability, and cost (American College of Surgeons, Committee on Trauma, 2006, 2012; CDC, 2007). In the United States, injury is a leading cause of death for children and adults ages 1 to 44 (Centers for Disease Control and Prevention [CDC], 2009) Trauma is also a leading cause of death worldwide with more than 5.8 million deaths each year (CDC, 2011). If a person is severely injured, being treated at a trauma center can lower the risk of death by 25%. Unfortunately, approximately 45 million Americans do not have access to a level I or II trauma center within 1 hour of where they are injured (CDC, 2009).

Although traumatic injury is a leading cause of death, many patients survive their injuries but experience permanent disability, chronic pain, and permanent change in their quality of life. The National Trauma Data Bank (NTDB) contains the largest aggregation of data reported from the trauma registries of hospital trauma centers. The data from the 2009 submissions show that the majority of injuries are unintentional and that the greatest percentage (37%) are related to falls, followed by motor vehicle traffic-related injuries (30%) (NTDB, 2010). It is important to note that the word *unintentional* is used rather than *accidental*. The cause of most unintentional injury is poor choices or behaviors, and these injuries may have been preventable. An example of a poor choice is consuming alcohol and then attempting to drive. Alcohol alters a person's judgment and coordination, making it more likely that he will drive unsafely and perhaps suffer injury.

Because unintentional injuries are a major source of morbidity and mortality, injury prevention has become a major public health goal. The U.S. Department of Health and Human Services and the Public Health Service have developed *Healthy People 2020: National Health Promotion and Disease Prevention Objectives.* The leading health indicators in *Healthy People 2020* that pertain to injury and violence prevention are provided in the National Guidelines box (p. 2092), and the Risk Factors box lists risk factors for youth violence, which is an important cause of traumatic injuries (p. 2092).

Kinematics of Injury

Imperative in the care of the trauma patient is the ability to identify and treat all life-threatening injuries quickly. Traumatic injury occurs when a source of energy makes contact with the body and the body cannot tolerate exposure to that energy. The extent of injury depends on the type and amount of energy force and the tissue response to the force. Newton's first law of motion states that a body at rest remains at rest and a body in motion remains in motion until acted on by an outside force (Feliciano, Mattox, & Moore, 2008). Energy is neither created nor destroyed; it is transferred. Force is the result of energy transference.

NATIONAL GUIDELINES *Healthy People 2020* Leading Health Indicators

Injury and Violence

Injury Prevention

IVP-1 Reduce fatal and nonfatal injuries
IVP-2 Reduce fatal and nonfatal traumatic brain injuries
IVP-3 Reduce fatal and nonfatal spinal cord injury
IVP-4 Increase the number of States and District of Columbia where 90 percent of deaths among children aged 17 years and under that are due to external causes are reviewed by a child fatality team
IVP-5 Increase the number of States and District of Columbia where 90 percent of sudden and unexpected deaths to infants are reviewed by a child fatality team
IVP-6 Increase number of emergency departments that routinely collect E-code (ICD-9CM diagnosis code used to report an accident or injury) related to injury
IVP-7 Increase number of hospitals who routinely collect discharge E-code related to injury
IVP-8 Increase access to trauma care in the United States
IVP-9 Prevent an increase in poisoning deaths
IVP-10 Prevent an increase in nonfatal poisonings
IVP-12 Reduce unintentional injuries
IVP-13 Reduce motor vehicle crash-related deaths
IVP-14 Reduce nonfatal motor vehicle crash-related injuries
IVP-15 Increase use of safety belts
IVP-16 Increase age-appropriate vehicle restraint use in children
IVP-17 Increase graduated driver licensing laws
IVP-18 Reduce pedestrian deaths on public roads
IVP-19 Reduce nonfatal pedestrian injuries on public roads
IVP-20 Reduce pedal cyclist deaths on public roads
IVP-21 Increase states with bicycle helmet laws
IVP-22 Increase motorcycle helmet use
IVP-23 Prevent deaths from falls
IVP-24 Reduce unintentional suffocation deaths
IVP-25 Reduce drowning deaths
IVP-26 Reduce sports and recreation injuries
IVP-27 Increase use of protective gear in school physical activities
IVP-28 Reduce residential fire deaths

Violence Prevention

IVP-29 Reduce homicides
IVP-30 Reduce firearm-related deaths
IVP-31 Reduce nonfatal firearm-related injuries
IVP-32 Reduce nonfatal physical assault injuries
IVP-33 Reduce physical assaults
IVP-34 Reduce physical fighting among adolescents
IVP-35 Reduce bullying among adolescents
IVP-36 Reduce weapon carrying by adolescents on school property
IVP-37 Reduce child maltreatment deaths
IVP-38 Reduce nonfatal child maltreatment
IVP-39 Reduce intimate partner violence
IVP-40 Reduce sexual violence
IVP-41 Reduce nonfatal intentional self-harm
IVP-42 Reduce children's exposure to violence
IVP-43 Increase violent death surveillance system

Source: http://www.healthypeople.gov/2020/topicsobjectives2020/overview.aspx?topicid=24.

RISK FACTORS for Youth Violence

Individual Risk Factors

History of violent victimization or involvement
Attention deficits, hyperactivity, or learning disorders
History of early aggressive behavior
Involvement with drugs, alcohol, or tobacco
Low IQ
Poor behavioral control
Deficits in social-cognitive or information processing abilities
High emotional distress
History of treatment for emotional problems
Antisocial beliefs and attitudes
Exposure to violence and conflict in the family

Family Risk Factors

Authoritarian childrearing attitudes
Harsh, lax, or inconsistent disciplinary practices
Low parental involvement
Low emotional attachment to parents or caregivers
Low parental education and income
Parental substance abuse or criminality
Poor family functioning
Poor monitoring and supervision of children

Peer/School Risk Factors

Association with delinquent peers
Involvement in gangs
Social rejection by peers
Lack of involvement in conventional activities
Poor academic performance
Low commitment to school and school failure

Community Risk Factors

Diminished economic opportunities
High concentrations of poor residents
High level of transiency
High level of family disruption
Low levels of community participation
Socially disorganized neighborhoods

Source: Centers for Disease Control and Prevention (CDC). (2007. Injury and violence. Retrieved from http://www.cdc.gov/node.do/id/0900f3ec8000e539.

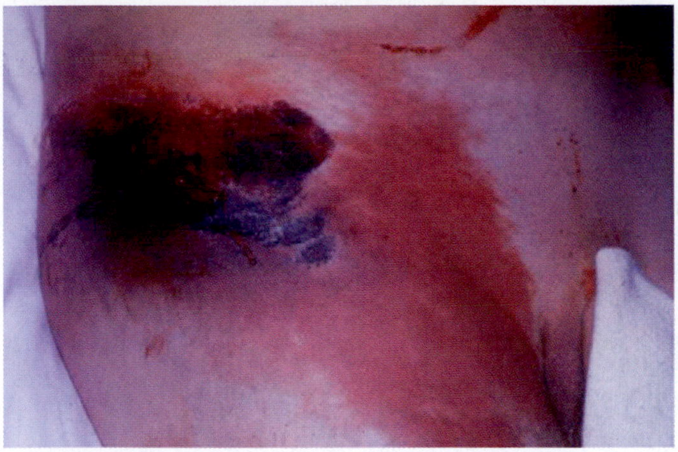

FIGURE 67–1 ◆ Seat belt injury.
Source: Cheryl Wraa.

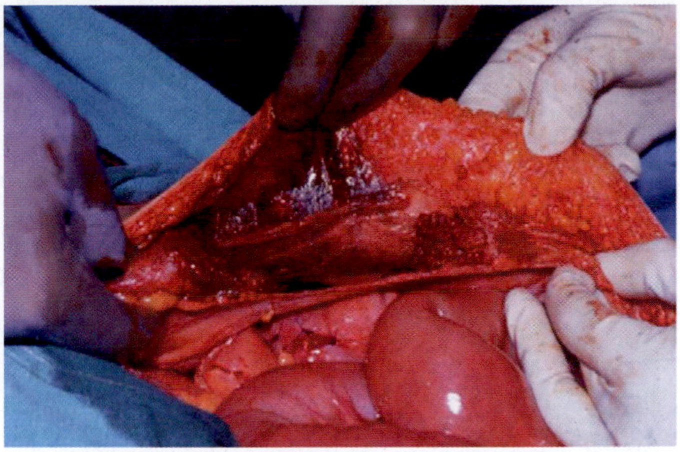

Different factors influence the amount of energy the human body absorbs, including the following:

- The amount of energy absorbed by objects that are struck first (e.g., the body of a vehicle)
- The amount of energy absorbed by protective devices (e.g., helmets, padded dashboards, air bags).

The more slowly the energy force is applied, the less energy transference and degree of destruction there are.

Injury patterns have been identified through the evaluation of the type of trauma that occurred and the amount of force that was generated. These known patterns assist health care providers to be anticipatory when caring for trauma patients. The predictive patterns of injuries are referred to as **kinematics.**

Motor Vehicle Collisions

Motor vehicle collisions cause some of the most commonly seen injuries. When a patient is admitted because of injuries sustained in a motor vehicle crash, it is important to try to ascertain the speed at which the vehicle was traveling and where the vehicle either impacted an object or was impacted by another vehicle. This will enable the nurse to better understand the amount of energy that was dispersed. Other indicators of the energy force are the amount of damage to the vehicle, the amount of intrusion into the passenger compartment, and the amount of damage from the occupant striking parts of the interior such as the steering wheel, dashboard, or windshield.

Frontal Impact

When a vehicle impacts an object or another vehicle head-on, energy is transferred to the vehicle. Although the front of the vehicle stops if prevented from moving by the object or other vehicle, the rear of the vehicle continues to move forward until all energy is dispersed. The same principle occurs with the passenger in the vehicle. When the front of the vehicle stops, the passenger's body continues to move forward. If the passenger is restrained properly, the seat belts will absorb most of the energy and prevent the body from colliding with immovable objects such as the steering wheel, dashboard, or windshield. This is also true if the air bag is deployed. A seat belt can impose a load that is 20 to 50 times as great as the weight of the body. The portion of the body that has the ability to receive this load is the pelvis. If the passenger has the belt over the abdomen rather than the pelvis, compression injury may occur to the abdominal organs. Abrasions and/or ecchymosis (small area of hemorrhage on the skin) from the seat belt are important indicators of possible underlying injury (Figure 67–1◆).

If the passenger is not restrained and the air bag does not deploy, the body might travel down and under the steering wheel or up and over the steering wheel, incurring injury at the body's point of impact with the vehicle (Figure 67–2◆). Patterns of injury that are anticipated are as follows:

- Cervical spine fracture
- Traumatic brain injury
- Anterior flail chest
- Myocardial contusion
- Pneumothorax
- Traumatic aortic disruption
- Fractured spleen or liver
- Posterior fracture or dislocation of the hip, knee, and/or ankle. (American College of Surgeons [ACS], 2012; Feliciano et al., 2008)

Side Impact

As many as 31% of fatalities from motor vehicle crashes are caused by side impact (ACS, 2012). Most injuries from side impact depend on whether the vehicle remains in place or moves away from the point of impact. If the vehicle remains in place, then the amount of damage to the vehicle and intrusion into the passenger compartment signifies the amount of energy that the body may have absorbed. Passengers generally receive most injuries on the same side of the body as the vehicle impact. Patterns of injury that are anticipated are as follows:

- Contralateral neck sprain
- Cervical spine fracture
- Brachial plexus injury
- Lateral flail chest
- Pneumothorax
- Traumatic aortic disruption
- Diaphragmatic rupture
- Fractured spleen/liver and/or kidney, depending on the side of impact
- Fractured pelvis or acetabulum. (ACS, 2012)

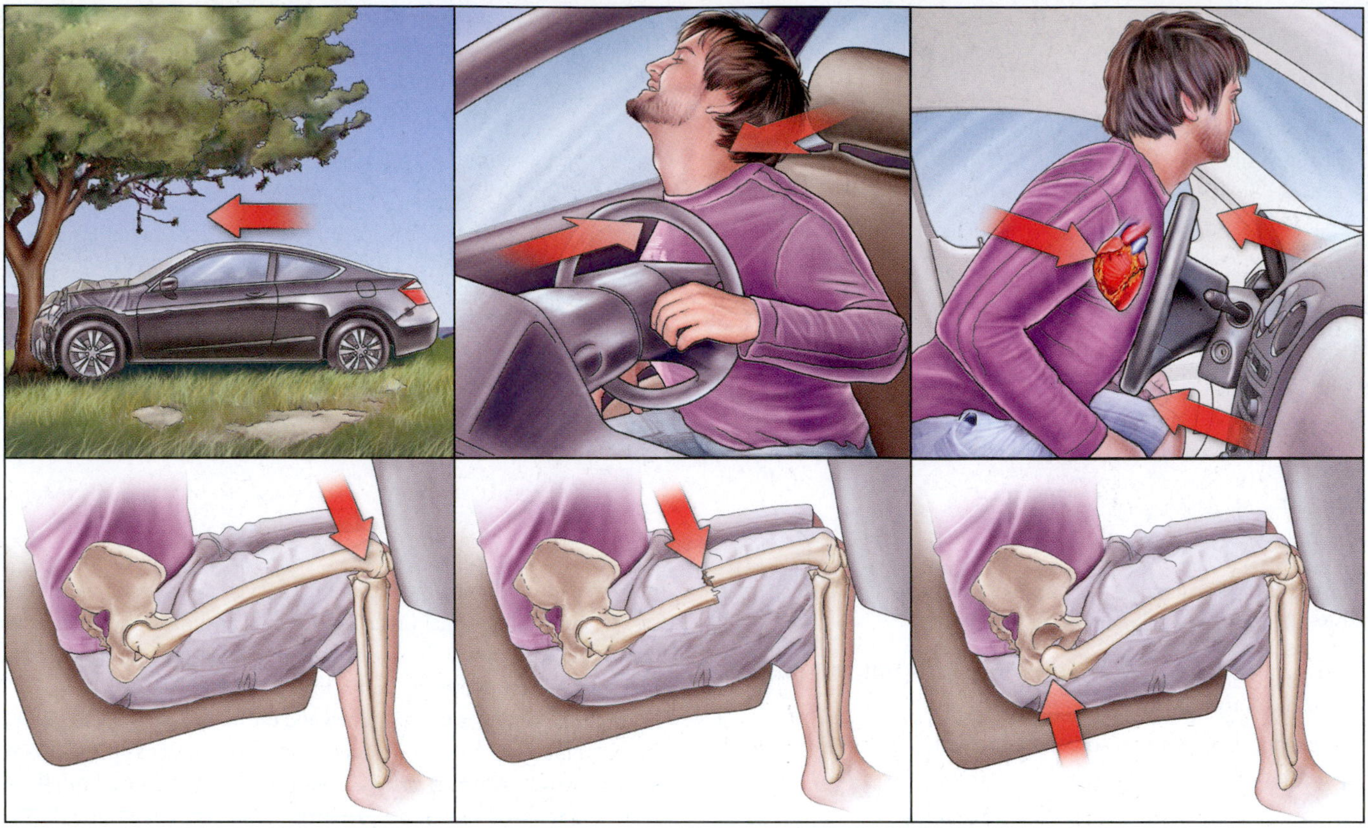

FIGURE 67–2 ◆ Unrestrained frontal impact.

Rear Impact

When a vehicle is struck from behind, the initial impact accelerates the stationary vehicle and may force it into a frontal collision. If the headrests in the vehicle are not properly positioned, the sudden acceleration may cause hyperextension of the passenger's neck. If the vehicle that is hit then stops suddenly from a frontal impact or from the driver applying the brakes suddenly, rapid forward deceleration occurs (Figure 67–3◆). This increases the chance for passenger injury. Patterns of injury that are anticipated are as follows:

- Cervical spine injury
- Soft tissue injury to the neck. (ACS, 2012)

Vehicle Rollover

When a vehicle rolls over, predicting the pattern of injury can be difficult. Injury occurs at the points where the body contacts the vehicle. Generally, this type of mechanism produces more severe injury than other types of crashes because of violent, multiple motions during the rollover. It is important to assess these patients carefully because they have the potential for multiple-system injuries.

Ejection

When a person is ejected from a vehicle, the chance of severe injury significantly increases (ACS, 2012). Ejection occurs when the passenger is thrown from the vehicle, and injury occurs at the body's point of impact. Ejection places the patient at risk for all injury mechanisms, and mortality is considerably increased (ACS, 2012).

Motorcycle Crashes

Motorcycle crashes are also common causes of traumatic injuries. Motorcycles do not have the surface area to absorb energy from impacts; therefore, energy is directly absorbed by the rider, and injuries are substantially more severe than those in vehicle crashes.

Frontal Impact

A motorcycle's center of gravity is located in front of the driver's seat. When a frontal impact occurs, the back of the motorcycle tips upward from the weight under the handlebars. The driver is propelled over the handlebars but might not be totally ejected because of the back tipping forward. If there is a passenger behind the driver, this person is often catapulted over the driver and fully ejected. Patterns of injury include the following:

- Fractured femurs, tibias, and fibulas (from the driver's body hitting the handlebars)
- Chest and abdominal injuries (from compression against the handlebars)
- Traumatic brain and cervical spine injury. (ACS, 2012)

Side Impact

When a motorcyclist is impacted from the side, that side of the body is unprotected and absorbs all of the energy. The exposed leg can be crushed between the motorcycle and the second object. Patterns of injury include open fracture of the femur, tibia/fibula, and malleolus (ACS, 2012).

Laying Down of the Motorcycle

A motorcyclist who anticipates a collision may use the technique of laying down the bike and sliding off to the side. The energy transference occurs as the body slides away from the bike. If the person is not wearing sufficient protective clothing,

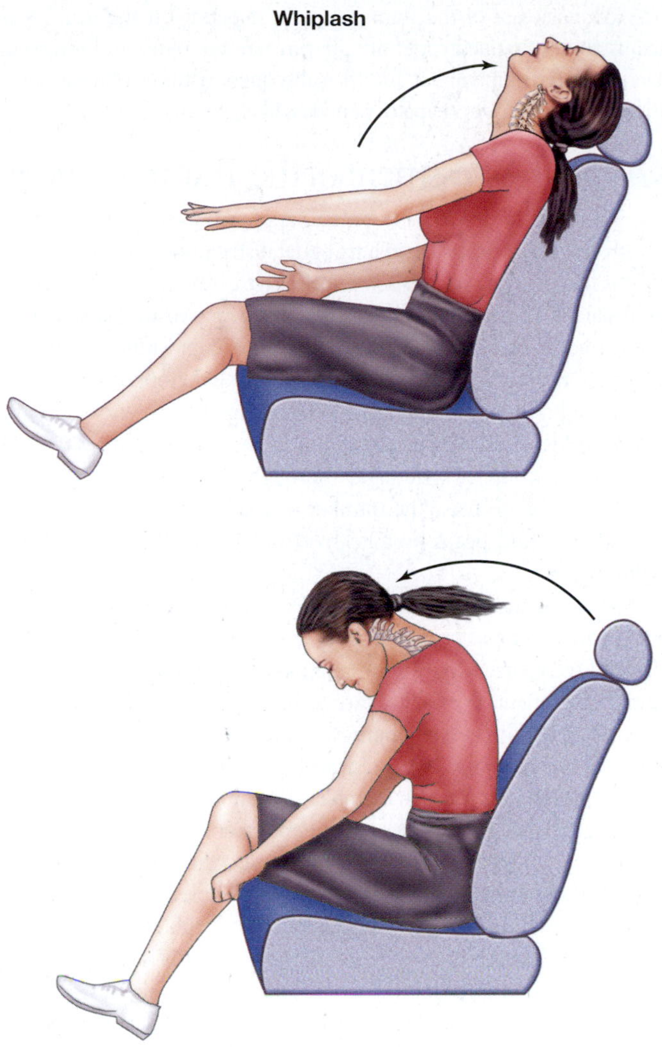

FIGURE 67–3 ◆ Rear impact.

abrasions will occur with pieces of asphalt becoming embedded in the abrasions.

Pedestrian Injuries

More than 4,000 people died in the United States in 2009 after being struck by a motor vehicle (National Highway Traffic Safety Administration, 2011). Injury patterns can be predicted according to the age and size of the victim and the size of the vehicle.

Children tend to freeze and face the oncoming vehicle and therefore end up with more frontal injuries than adults do. Depending on the height of the child and the vehicle bumper, the impact occurs on the chest or the femurs. The child is then thrown backward, and the upper back or head impacts the ground. A very small child may be knocked down and under the vehicle because of the child's center of gravity, size, and weight. Multiple-system trauma should be suspected in any child who has been hit by a vehicle.

Adults usually try to escape being hit and turn away from the vehicle, thus sustaining lateral injuries on the side impacted by the vehicle. Approximately 80% of adults hit by a vehicle will have injuries to the lower extremities (Feliciano et al., 2008). Injury patterns include the following:

- Lower extremity fractures above and below the point of impact
- Fractured pelvis (pedestrian hits the hood of the vehicle or point of impact)
- Head injury (pedestrian falls off hood of vehicle to the ground). (ACS, 2012)

Falls

The injury from a fall is similar to that of a motor vehicle crash in that it is caused by an abrupt change in velocity, or speed. The roof line of a one-story house is usually 15 feet. With falls greater than 15 feet, adults usually land on their feet. If the fall is less than 15 feet, adults will land in the same position in which they were when they fell. Small children have larger heads in proportion to their bodies; therefore, no matter the distance of the fall, they tend to land head-first (ACS, 2012).

The severity of the injury also depends on the give of the surface on which the person lands. For example, a soft surface, such as sand, will absorb more energy than cement will. Patterns of injury include the following:

- Calcaneus fractures
- Compression fractures to T_{12}–L_1
- Bilateral wrist fractures (as the body falls forward after the first impact)
- Traumatic brain injury. (ACS, 2012)

One out of three adults 65 years of age and older fall each year in the United States (CDC, 2011). Falls in older adults will be discussed in detail later in the chapter.

Penetrating Injuries

Violence is an important public health problem. Violent acts commonly result in penetrating injuries. The severity of injury in penetrating trauma depends on the velocity of the penetrating object. Energy created by the object is dissipated into the surrounding tissues much like a shock wave. Consider the shock wave going through human tissue that is elastic in nature. The stress that is imparted to the tissue depends on the velocity of the object entering the body, the velocity of the waves in the tissue, and the mass or density of the object that entered the body. The larger and faster the article, the more damage that can occur to the tissues (ACS, 2012). A cavity may be formed by the penetrating object. This is known as cavitation (Figure 67–4◆).

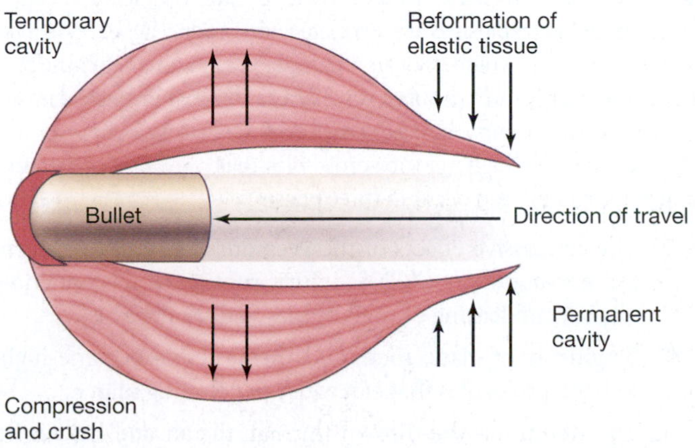

FIGURE 67–4 ◆ Cavitation.

Weblink: Access to Trauma Care

Stab Wounds

Stab wounds are low velocity and produce their injury directly as the object penetrates tissue. Knowing the length of the object and how far it entered the body helps the nurse to anticipate what organs might be injured. Knowing the position of the attacker and the victim can help to identify the path of the weapon. Knowing the gender of the attacker may also assist in determining the path of the weapon. Men tend to stab upward, and women tend to stab overhand or downward.

Although tissue damage in stab wounds is usually isolated to the area of penetration, a single stab may penetrate several body cavities, depending on the pathway. During expiration, the dome of the diaphragm reaches as high as the fifth rib. Stab wounds to the chest at or below the level of the nipple should be suspect for abdominal injury as well. Also, an attacker may stab the victim only once but move the weapon around, causing extensive internal damage to the surrounding structures.

Gunshot Wounds

Every year, many thousands of Americans are killed with firearms. In the United States, unintentional firearm deaths of children nearly all occur in or around the home. Firearm injuries peak at the age of 19 and then decrease after the age of 22. Serious injuries from a firearm, such as traumatic brain injury, can require a lifetime of care and rehabilitative services (Liem, Barber, Markwalder, Killias, & Nieuwbeerta, 2011).

The severity of the damage caused by a bullet depends on the amount of energy transferred from the bullet to the body. Handguns and some small-caliber rifles are considered medium energy; hunting and assault rifles are considered high energy and therefore capable of transferring more energy to the tissue than smaller guns. The degree of deformation of the bullet also influences the degree of tissue damage. Bullets that are constructed of soft lead and flatten on impact or have a hollow point that mushrooms on impact cause more tissue damage than a full metal jacket bullet owing to the increased diameter.

It is important to assess the patient for the number of wounds that are present. It is difficult to determine whether a wound is an entrance or exit wound, so the nurse should never assume that the bullet is not still in the body even if two wounds are present. Bullets will follow the path of least resistance once they enter the body, so it is almost impossible to truly know, from just the external exam, the path the bullet has taken.

Blast Injuries

Terrorist activity has increased the chance of blast injury in the United States. In a blast, explosives are detonated and produce gases. When the gas expands, equal volumes of air are displaced and travel after the blast wave. The energy from the blast wave can cause massive tissue damage. When the blast occurs, the casing that held the explosive ruptures, and its pieces become high-velocity projectiles that can cause penetrating injury. Blast injury can occur in three phases:

1. The concussive effects of the pressure wave can cause central nervous system (CNS) injury, rupture of air-containing organs, and tearing of membranes and small vessels.
2. Fragments of glass, rock, and metal debris become high-velocity projectiles that can cause penetrating injury.
3. The victim may be thrown through the air and sustain injury similar to that sustained when ejected from a vehicle or when a person has fallen from a height.

Adequate care of the trauma patient depends on the health care team's ability to quickly identify life-threatening injury and intervene. Understanding kinematics and the subsequent patterns of injury helps the caregivers to be anticipatory and less likely to miss an injury.

Initial Assessment of the Trauma Patient

It is important to develop a systematic approach to the trauma patient. Deaths from trauma occur in a trimodal distribution. The first peak of deaths from trauma occurs before definitive care, either at the scene or en route to the medical facility, and results from nonsurvivable injuries such as aortic disruption. The second peak occurs within the first few hours after injury and is most commonly due to hemorrhage or severe traumatic brain injury. The third peak occurs days to weeks after the injury and is a result of complications, including infection or multiple organ dysfunction. A systematic, thorough initial assessment and resuscitation will decrease the number of deaths that occur during the second and third peaks by quickly identifying injury and beginning definitive care.

Initial nursing management follows a systematic approach to care that includes a rapid primary survey, resuscitation of vital functions, a detailed secondary survey, and initiation of definitive care. During the initial assessment, the health care team must identify injuries, intervene when life-threatening injuries are present, and prioritize care. It is critical for all members of the trauma team to prepare for the arrival of trauma patients and for each member to know her role during the initial resuscitation (Figure 67–5◆). As one member of the team completes the primary and secondary survey, many procedures are done simultaneously by other members, such as accessing veins, obtaining blood for tests, and inserting a urinary catheter and gastric tube.

It is important to have one team member who is overseeing the resuscitation and directing the team. This person is usually a trauma surgeon and does not provide direct care unless necessary. Instead, this person observes the resuscitation efforts and correlates all data being

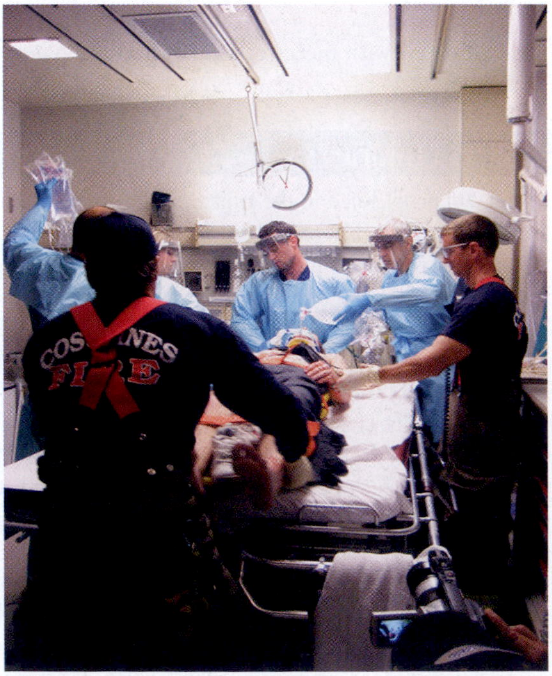

FIGURE 67–5 ◆ Trauma team.
Source: Cheryl Wraa.

obtained to direct the plan of care. The nurse should be familiar with the resuscitation area and the equipment available. We discuss the initial steps of trauma care next.

Primary Survey

The primary survey follows a specific sequence of **ABCDE:**

Airway maintenance with cervical spine protection

Breathing and ventilation

Circulation and hemorrhage control

Disability (neurological status)

Exposure/environmental control (e.g., remove all clothing but prevent hypothermia by placing warm blankets on the patient or using ambient warmers).

These steps are discussed in full in the following subsections.

Airway Maintenance with Cervical Spine Protection

A secure and patent airway is the first priority for the trauma patient. While the airway is assessed, the patient's cervical spine should be maintained in a midline position and should not be moved (Figure 67–6◆). The patient's airway should first be assessed for patency.

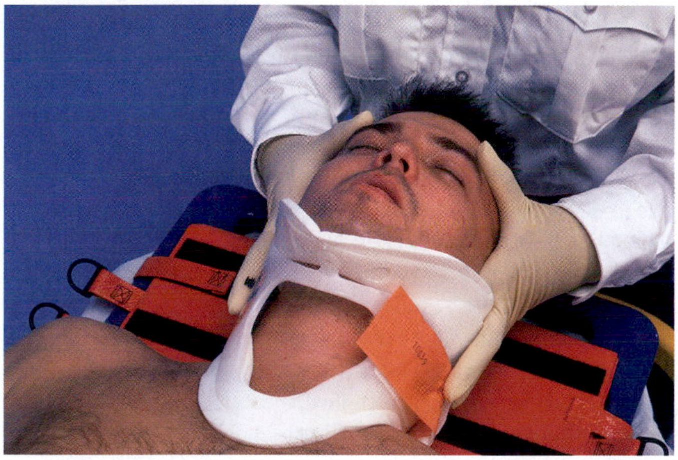

FIGURE 67–6 ◆ Cervical protection.

The nurse should look for signs of airway obstruction from blood or foreign bodies, facial or mandibular fractures, or tracheal or laryngeal injury that may occlude the airway. If the patient's level of consciousness is such that the patient would not be able to protect the airway if she began to vomit, the nurse should insert an endotracheal tube to protect the airway. Whenever a trauma patient is intubated, it is important to ensure that the cervical spine is protected. All multiple-system trauma patients, particularly those with an altered level of consciousness or blunt injury above the clavicle, should be treated as if they have a cervical spine injury until proven otherwise.

Safety Alert *The nurse needs to reevaluate the patient's airway frequently until the patient is stabilized.*

Breathing and Ventilation

Adequate function of the lungs, chest wall, and diaphragm is necessary for adequate ventilation. The nurse exposes the chest to visualize and assess chest wall excursion and listen to breath sounds to identify a pneumothorax or hemothorax. Next, the nurse palpates the chest wall to identify injuries that might compromise ventilation. Injuries that can impair ventilation acutely include **flail chest,** which occurs when two or more ribs are fractured in two or more places and are no longer attached to the thoracic cage, resulting in a free-floating segment. The free-floating segment moves independently from the rest of the chest, resulting in paradoxical chest wall movement (Figure 67–7◆). This can be observed during inspection of the chest. The impaired movement of the chest wall results in decreased tidal volume, decreased vital capacity, and impaired cough, leading to hypoventilation and atelectasis.

The amount of energy exerted on the body to cause a flail chest usually will damage the underlying lung tissue, resulting in a **pulmonary contusion.** Pulmonary contusion is initially a hemorrhage followed by alveolar and interstitial edema. The edema affects the alveolar–capillary units in the area of the contusion. If the edema increases, it can cause decreased compliance and increased pulmonary vascular resistance; it can also affect pulmonary blood flow. Clinical manifestations may develop over 24 to 48 hours and include moist crackles in the contused lung, cough with blood-tinged sputum, and pulmonary infiltrate on chest radiograph.

Tension pneumothorax occurs when an injury perforates the chest or pleural space. During inspiration, air enters the pleural space and becomes trapped. As more air is trapped, the pressure in the pleural

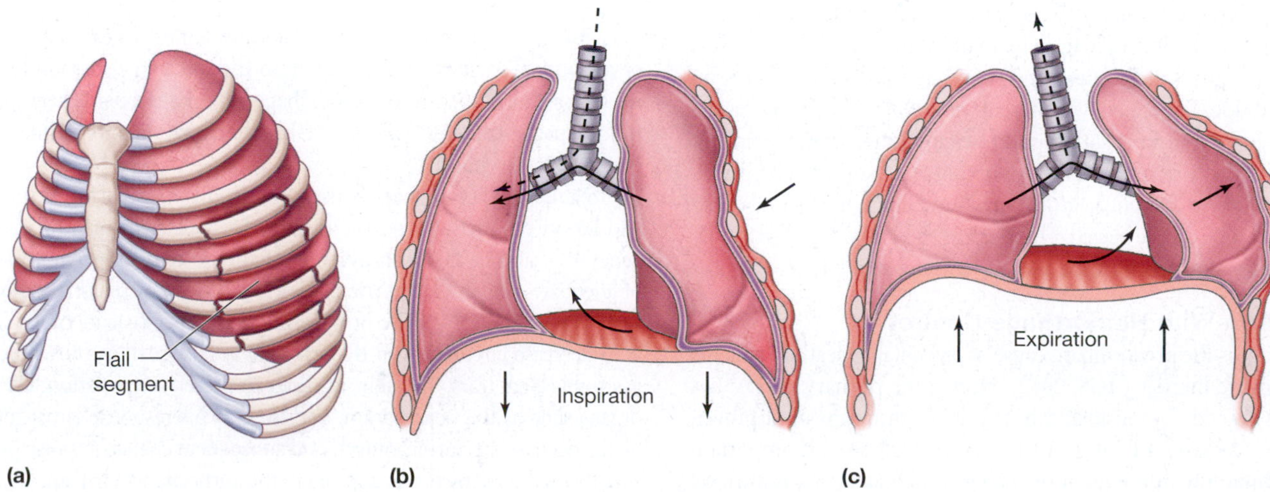

FIGURE 67–7 ◆ Flail chest.

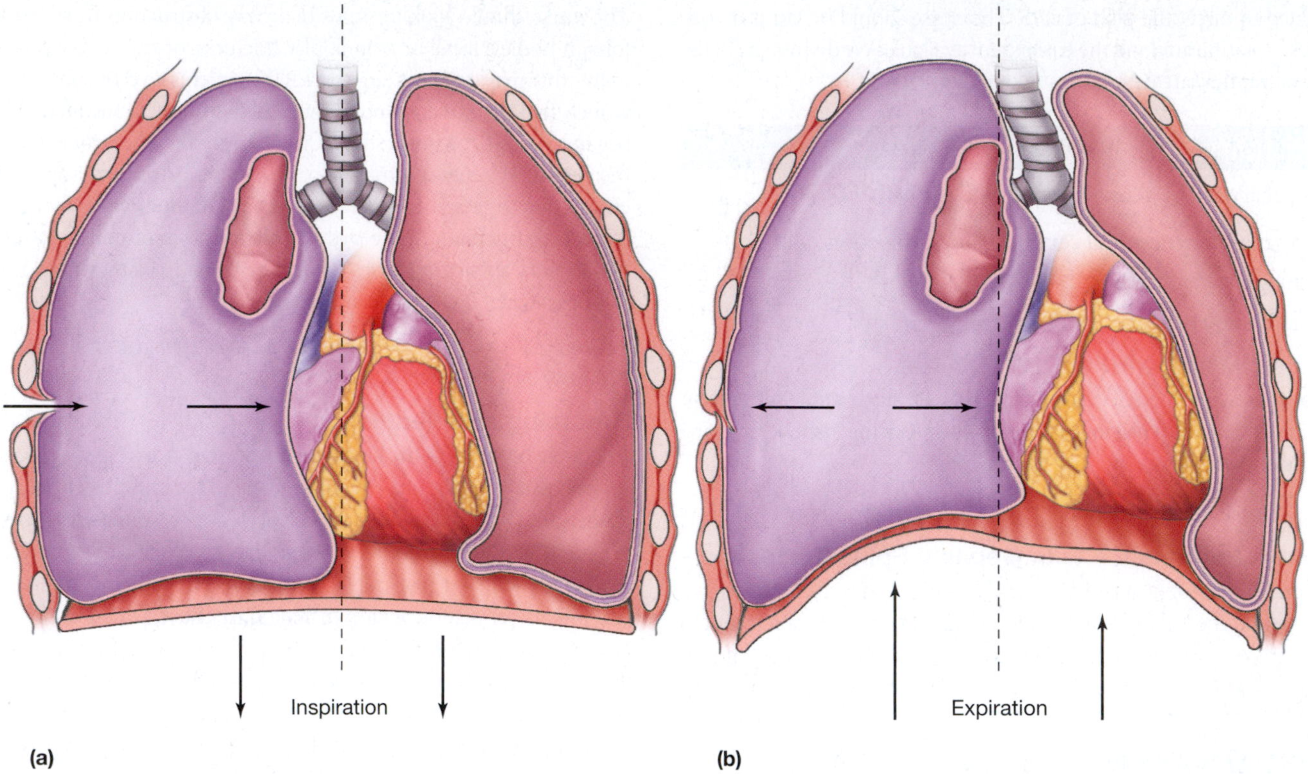

FIGURE 67–8 ◆ Tension pneumothorax.

space increases, collapsing the lung and causing the mediastinum to shift to the opposite side (Figure 67–8◆). This pressure exerts pressure on the heart and vascular structures in the chest, resulting in decreased cardiac output and venous return. A tension pneumothorax is diagnosed by clinical assessment, and the pressure must be released immediately by venting the chest on the affected side with a large-bore needle or chest tube; otherwise, the patient will die. Symptoms include severe dyspnea, tachycardia, and hypotension.

A **massive hemothorax** is an accumulation of 1,500 mL or more of blood in the thoracic cavity. This amount of hemorrhage can result from injury to intercostal or internal mammary arteries, lung tissue, the heart, or the great vessels. The patient will present with signs and symptoms of hypovolemic shock (Chapter 54) with breath sounds diminished or absent over the affected lung. An **open pneumothorax** is an open communication between the atmosphere and intrathoracic pressure and is usually caused by penetrating trauma. This communication with the atmosphere causes an immediate collapse of the lung on the affected side. The patient will present with respiratory distress; as the patient inspires, a sucking sound may be heard as the air moves in and out through the hole in the chest. An occlusive dressing can be placed over the wound to prevent air from being sucked into the pleural cavity until a chest tube can be placed. The dressing should be secured on only three sides to allow air to escape and prevent a tension pneumothorax.

Circulation With Hemorrhage Control

Hemorrhage is the predominant cause of preventable death in patients with traumatic injuries (ACS, 2012). During the primary survey, hypotension should be considered hypovolemic in origin until proven otherwise. Elements of the primary survey that provide important information to the nurse about the patient's circulatory status are level of consciousness, skin color, respiratory rate, and pulse. If the patient's circulating blood volume is reduced, the cerebral perfusion may be impaired, resulting in an altered level of consciousness. As blood volume decreases, the body compensates by shunting blood away from the skin to vital organs. This causes the skin to become pale and cool. Pulses should be assessed bilaterally for quality, rate, and regularity. A weak, thready pulse may be a sign of hypovolemia but may have other causes as well. The absence of central pulses (femoral and carotid pulses) signifies the need for immediate resuscitative measures to restore depleted blood volume and maintain effective cardiac output.

If external hemorrhage is identified, measures to control the bleeding should be taken immediately. The easiest way to do this is to apply direct manual pressure on the wound.

Safety Alert *Tourniquets may be used to control bleeding in some circumstances (e.g., traumatic amputation). However, it is important to remember that tourniquets can crush tissues and cause distal ischemia.*

The major sources of occult blood loss are hemorrhage into the chest or abdominal cavities, hemorrhage into the soft tissue surrounding a major long bone fracture, or hemorrhage into the retroperitoneal space from a pelvic fracture. Control of bleeding may require immediate operative intervention.

Treatment of hemorrhage consists of administration of fluids, blood, and blood products. Hypovolemic shock is a life-threatening emergency that affects all organ systems of the body by depriving tissue of adequate oxygen and nutrients. For a detailed discussion of shock, refer to Chapter 54. The body's initial response to acute blood loss is to decrease circulation to the less vital organs such as the kidneys, gastrointestinal tract, and skin in order to preserve circulation to vital organs such as the heart, brain, and lungs. This response is triggered by the decrease in cardiac output and subsequent change in pulse pressure that is sensed by baroreceptors in the aortic arch and atrium of the heart. Neural reflexes then begin a sympathetic outflow to the heart and other organs, which respond by increasing heart rate and initiating vasoconstriction. The activation of the renin system leads to vasoconstriction and the retention of sodium and water to help replete the vascular volume. The pituitary and the adrenal medulla are stimulated to release adrenocorticotropic hormone, norepinephrine, and epinephrine to enhance the compensatory mechanisms.

The decrease in oxygen and nutrients to the cells causes the body's metabolism to change from aerobic to anaerobic, releasing lactic acid and causing metabolic acidosis. If the blood loss continues, the compensatory mechanisms will fail, and damage will occur throughout the body in all systems. Myocardial hypoperfusion and lactic acidosis cause cardiac dysfunction that, in turn, perpetuates the entire process. Hypoperfusion of the brain causes cardiac and respiratory depression and failure of the sympathetic nervous system. As a result of this failure, vasodilation occurs that leads to venous pooling and increased capillary permeability, which causes the leakage of fluid into the interstitial space (**third spacing**) and the total body edema (**anasarca**) noted in trauma patients. Irreversible damage at the cellular level occurs because the cell membrane loses integrity. This is primarily due to free radicals, especially reactive oxygen species and reactive nitrogen species. These free radicals lead to oxidation of DNA molecules, fatty acids, and amino acids, advancing cell degradation. Because the electrical gradient is lost, the cell swells, the endoplasmic reticulum and mitochondria are damaged, and utilization of oxygen becomes dysfunctional. Ruptured lysosomes release enzymes that digest other cellular structures, and cell death occurs, which further enhances the impact of the initial hemorrhage.

Respiratory distress syndrome may result from the increased permeability of the pulmonary capillary membrane, microemboli formation, and pulmonary vasoconstriction. Hypoperfusion and vasoconstriction to the gastrointestinal system cause decreased peristalsis and decreased functioning of the gut. Renal vasoconstriction and hypoperfusion lead to acute tubular necrosis and, if not reversed, to acute renal failure. Disseminated intravascular coagulation (DIC) develops owing to hematologic dysfunction, including acidosis, hypoxemia, hypotension, and cessation of capillary blood flow.

The most abundant type of white blood cells are neutrophils. Much of the damage from hemorrhagic shock is the result of the formation of reactive oxygen species (ROSs) in neutrophils. Neutrophils fight infection and use ROSs to fight pathogens as they directly break down microbial pathogens. However, ROSs also signal molecules in programmed cell death (apoptotic) pathways. Although ROSs break down pathogens, neutrophils overproduce and accumulate ROSs, causing apoptosis (programmed cell death in a multicellular organism), which would be expressed in the clinical setting as sepsis. Sepsis is discussed in Chapter 54.

Recent research into the cellular pathways involved in the inflammatory response to injury and shock is concerned with T-cell proliferation in response to stimulators in the adaptive and innate immune responses. Research has found decreased levels of helper T-cell cytokine production and reduced antibody secretion (Spaniol, Knight, Zebley, Anderson, & Pierce, 2007). The decrease in these specific levels corresponds to the suppressed adaptive immune function that is seen in trauma patients with hemorrhagic shock. Research is focused on which receptors are involved in the reduction of the adaptive immune function and how to activate the receptors to maintain the adaptive immune system function at a level that will prevent infection.

Fluid Resuscitation

Traditionally, the treatment for hemorrhagic shock has been immediate, aggressive infusion of normal saline or Ringer's lactate solution. However, current data suggest that although aggressive fluid resuscitation may be useful for patients with isolated extremity, thermal, or head injury, fluid resuscitation should be limited in patients with potentially uncontrollable internal hemorrhage, especially in patients with penetrating truncal injury that will be treated at a trauma center (Alam, 2011). The reason aggressive fluid resuscitation may be harmful is that increasing the mean arterial pressure in a patient who is actively bleeding will lead to increased blood loss. The body's hemostatic mechanisms are overcome by the artificially elevated blood pressure, and formed clots are dislodged. Because of the increased bleeding, more fluids and blood are required, and the proinflammatory effects of the products develop. Aggressive infusion of crystalloid in the presence of uncontrolled hemorrhage promotes continued bleeding and increases mortality (Alam, 2011). The amount of initial fluid resuscitation will be determined by the patient's response to fluids. The response should be continually assessed to determine whether perfusion is adequate. The nurse must also be aware that many factors, including age, comorbidities, and medications, can affect a patient's response to fluid resuscitation. The goal is to control the bleeding and promote oxygenation at the cellular level.

Blood products are used to restore circulating volume, improve oxygen carrying capacity, and replace coagulation factors. Type-specific blood is preferred, but if blood is needed immediately, type O may be used. Ongoing research indicates that fresh frozen plasma and platelets need to be given early in conjunction with packed red cells to treat coagulopathy (Alam, 2011). Trauma centers are developing guidelines for massive transfusion that reflect this practice. Chart 67–1 (p. 2100) is an example of a guideline for massive transfusion.

Disability

The primary assessment of disability involves a rapid neurological evaluation to establish the patient's level of consciousness. The patient's Glasgow Coma Scale score (see Chapter 21) should be determined at this time. An altered level of consciousness can be indicative of decreased blood volume with poor perfusion, hypoxia, or a traumatic brain injury. Although alcohol and mind-altering drugs may alter the level of consciousness, they should never be considered the cause until all other possibilities have been excluded.

Exposure/Environmental Control

The trauma patient should be completely undressed to facilitate a thorough examination. As the trauma patient is being examined, he should be covered with warm blankets or an external warming device to prevent hypothermia. Intravenous fluids should be warmed prior to infusion to prevent a decrease in a patient's core temperature with the infusion of large amounts of cold solution. Allowing patients to become cold can contribute to coagulopathy and can be very detrimental to their care, as discussed in the Evidence-Based Practice box (p. 2100).

Adjuncts to the Primary Survey

Monitoring of the patient's physiological parameters is the best way to assess the effectiveness of resuscitation efforts. The patient should be placed on a cardiac monitor. Dysrhythmias may indicate blunt cardiac injury. Pulseless electrical activity may indicate tension pneumothorax, as described earlier in the chapter (p. 2097); profound hypovolemia; and/or **cardiac tamponade,** which is bleeding into the pericardial sac. As the blood accumulates in the sac, it compresses the atria and ventricles, decreasing venous return and filling pressure, which leads to decreased cardiac output, myocardial hypoxia, and cardiac failure. The patient with cardiac tamponade presents with findings termed **Beck's triad.** These findings are neck vein distention caused by the

CHART 67–1 Massive Transfusion Guideline

Purpose: Development of the Massive Transfusion Guideline (MTG) was a cooperative effort by the Trauma Multidisciplinary Committee at the University of California, Davis Medical Center to provide a standard for efficient and effective procurement and delivery of blood products to patients exhibiting hemorrhagic shock. The term *massive transfusion* is defined as replacement of at least one blood volume (˜5 liters in an adult) within the first 12 hours of resuscitation.

Massive Transfusion Guideline Pack

Age (yr)	Weight (kg)	Patient Approximate Blood Volume (mL)	Blood Products Provided	MTG Approximate Volume (mL)
0–11	<35	270–2,450	3 RBC adult, 1 jumbo FFP*, 1 platelet pheresis	**1,500**
12–Adult	>35	>2,451	6 RBC adult, 2 jumbo FFP*, 1 platelet pheresis	**2,800**

*Fresh frozen plasma (FFP) may be dispensed in equivalent volume.

Activation

The MTGs can be activated in any of the following hospital locations:

Emergency department (ED)
Operating room (OR)
Critical care unit (ICU)
Radiology (interventional radiology [IR])
Labor and delivery

- The physician caring for the patient evaluates the need for MTG using an accepted method of determining injury severity and probability of massive hemorrhage.
- The physician or designee MUST call the Transfusion Services.
- The Special Blood Bank Requisition for Exsanguination is labeled with patient identification. The physician activates the MTG by selecting the adult or pediatric MTG box or selects uncrossmatched blood (2 RBC or 2 FFP).
- A specimen for Type & Screen should be sent to Transfusion Services STAT.
- Other lab tests should be ordered and sent STAT: hemoglobin (Hgb), hematocrit (Hct), platelet count, INR, activated partial thromboplastin time (APTT), and fibrinogen.
- Transfusion of plasma (FFP) should be started together with red blood cell units (RBC) as it is determined that transfusion of greater than 50% of the age/size appropriate blood volume is likely to be necessary.
- Appropriate cardiovascular, electrolyte, and coagulation parameters should be monitored closely throughout and following massive transfusion, understanding that more blood products may be available than are necessary or appropriate to administer.
- All blood products should be given via a Level I rapid infuser/fluid warmer or other blood-warming device to prevent hypothermia.
- Once it has been determined that the MTG can be discontinued, the physician or designee will call Transfusion Services.
- The cooler and all unused blood products must be returned to Transfusion Services within 4 hours in accordance with Transfusion Services Policy.

Sources: Hess, J. R., Holcomb, J. B., & Hoyt, D. B. (2006). Damage control resuscitation: The need for specific blood products to treat the coagulopathy of trauma. *Transfusion, 46*(5), 685–686; Hirshberg, A., Dugas, M., Banez, E. I., Scott, B. G., Wall, M. J., Jr., & Mattox, K. L. (2003). Minimizing dilutional coagulopathy in exsanguinating hemorrhage: A computer simulation. *Journal of Trauma, 54*(3), 454–463; Ho, A. M., Dion, P. W., Cheng, C. A., et al. (2005). A mathematical model for fresh frozen plasma transfusion strategies during major trauma resuscitation with ongoing hemorrhage. *Canadian Journal of Surgery, 48*(6), 470–478; Holcomb, J. B., & Hess, J. R. (2006). Early massive trauma transfusion: Current state of the art. *Journal of Trauma, 60*(Suppl), S1–S9; Ketchum, L., Hess, J. R., & Hippala, S. (2006). Indications for early fresh frozen plasma, cryoprecipitate, and platelet transfusion in trauma. *Journal of Trauma, 60*(Suppl.), S51–S58; Malone, D. L., Hess, J. R., & Fingerhut, A. (2006). Massive transfusion practices around the globe and a suggestion for a common massive transfusion protocol. *Journal of Trauma, 60*(Suppl), S91–S96. U.C. Davis Health System. Department of Pathology and Laboratory Medicine. (2012). Massive Transfusion Guideline. (Used with permission); Young, P., Cotton, B., & Goodnough, L. (2011). Massive transfusion protocols for patients with substantial hemorrhage. *Transfusion Medicine Reviews, 25*(4), 293–303.

EVIDENCE-BASED PRACTICE Hypothermia in Trauma Patients

Clinical Problem

The triad of coagulopathy, acidosis, and hypothermia increases mortality in the injured patient.

Research Findings

Hemorrhage is one of the leading causes of death after trauma. In fact, it accounts for 40% of trauma deaths (Floccard et al., 2012). Trauma patients are susceptible to early development of coagulopathy, and patients who are severely injured are coagulopathic on hospital admission. Hypothermia, acidosis, and dilution from standard resuscitation with crystalloid can worsen the presenting coagulopathy and perpetuate bleeding. Rapid diagnosis of coagulopathy followed by prevention or correction of hypothermia and acidosis should be a priority during the initial assessment and resuscitation (Ganter & Pittet, 2010).

Coagulopathy of trauma is a syndrome of bleeding from mucosal lesions, serosal surfaces, and wound and vascular access sites. It is associated with tissue trauma, hypothermia, acidosis, hemodilution, and inflammation (Floccard et al., 2012). Inadequate resuscitation has also been associated with coagulopathy.

Mitra, Cameron, Mori, and Fitzgerald (2012) performed a retrospective review of 772 adult trauma patients who suffered enough trauma to require a blood transfusion in their initial resuscitation. The majority of these patients (91.7%) suffered blunt trauma. The researchers found that acute coagulopathy was associated with early death when a blood transfusion was needed (Ganter & Pittet, 2010).

Implications for Nursing Practice

With the organization of trauma systems, improvements in prehospital care, the development of trauma centers, and the standardization of methods of resuscitation, aggressive resuscitation of patients in extremis has improved over time. Severely traumatized patients may now be in the ICU or operating room before they reach the physiological limit defined as the onset of the triad: hypothermia, acidosis, and coagulopathy. It is important for nurses to understand the triad and the consequences. Maintaining a normal body temperature is a first-line, effective strategy to improve hemostasis and prevent worsening coagulopathy.

Critical Thinking Questions with answers can be found in the Osborn Student Resources at nursing.pearsonhighered.com.

Sources: Floccard, B., Rugeri, L., Faure, A., Denis, M., Boyle, M., Peguet, O., et al. (2012). Early coagulopathy in trauma patients: An on-scene and hospital admission study. *Injury, 43*, 26–32; Mitra, B., Cameron, P., Mori, A., & Fitzgerald, M. (2012). Acute coagulopathy and early deaths post major trauma. *Injury, 43*(1), 22–25; Tieu, B. H., Holcomb, J. B., & Schreiber, M. A. (2007). Coagulopathy: Its pathophysiology and treatment in the injured patient. *World Journal of Surgery, 31*(5), 1055–1065.

elevated central venous pressure, muffled heart sounds, and hypotension. Immediate treatment is required to remove the accumulated blood and relieve the pressure that is being exerted on the heart. This is accomplished by either pericardiocentesis, which involves aspiration via a large-bore needle placed into the pericardial sac, or an emergency surgical thoracotomy to visualize the heart, relieve the accumulated blood, and locate and control the source of bleeding. Cardiac tamponade is discussed in detail in Chapter 33.

Pulse oximetry measures the oxygen saturation of hemoglobin but does not measure ventilation. Adequacy of ventilation should be monitored by the ventilatory rate and arterial blood gases (ABGs).

Bedside screening radiographs are usually done at this time. As the patient is logrolled off the backboard and the back is examined, plates may be placed to do chest and abdominal/pelvic radiographs.

Placement of an indwelling urinary catheter and a gastric catheter should be accomplished as part of the resuscitation. Urinary output is an important indicator of the patient's volume status and response to resuscitation. The placement of an indwelling urinary catheter is contraindicated in patients who are suspected of having a urethral injury. Signs of possible urethral injury include blood at the urethral meatus, perineal ecchymosis, blood in the scrotum, and a high-riding or nonpalpable prostate, which is identified by manual rectal exam. Placement of a gastric catheter reduces stomach distention and the risk of vomiting and aspiration. If the patient has multiple facial fractures, it may be necessary to place an oral gastric catheter.

Safety Alert *Never insert a urinary catheter before the genitalia and rectum have been examined.*

The patient's blood pressure should be monitored frequently to observe for changes and/or trends. The nurse must remember that blood pressure may be a poor measure of actual tissue perfusion. Returning to an adequate hemodynamic state requires more than a normal blood pressure.

If the patient arrived at a nontrauma center, this is the time to consider initiating the transfer process to a designated trauma center for definitive care (ACS, 2012).

Secondary Survey

Following the primary survey and intervention of resuscitative measures with adequate patient response, the secondary survey should be done. The secondary survey consists of a detailed head-to-toe evaluation of the patient with reassessment of all vital signs. Ideally, it should be performed in 5 to 10 minutes. Like the primary survey, the secondary survey is done in a systematic fashion to reveal all injuries the patient has sustained.

Head and Face

The nurse palpates the head through the scalp to identify lacerations and possible depressed skull fractures. The nurse observes behind the patient's ears for the development of **Battle's sign,** which is ecchymosis over the mastoid area and is indicative of a basilar skull fracture. The nurse palpates the face for fractures and midface stability. If the midface is unstable, the patient will have difficulty maintaining a patent airway; when the patient lies supine, the midface collapses and occludes the airway.

Eyes

If the patient is responsive, gross visual acuity should be checked along with pupillary size and reactivity to light. The nurse assesses for **raccoon eyes,** which are ecchymoses over the orbit of the eyes and are indicative of a basilar skull fracture. The nurse inspects the eye for any foreign bodies, globe injury, or **hyphema,** a collection of blood in the anterior chamber of the eye; the blood is visible and can block vision. If the nurse notes that the patient is wearing contact lenses, these should be removed at this time.

Ears

The ears should be inspected for blood, cerebrospinal fluid (CSF), or brain matter. The nurse should remove and save any hearing aids.

Nose

The nurse should inspect the nose for blood or a CSF leak. An easy way to test for a CSF leak is to use gauze to absorb the bloody fluid. If CSF is mixed with the blood, it will create a gold-colored ring around the blood. This is commonly referred to as the halo effect. Additionally, the nose needs to be palpated for crepitus or deformity.

Mouth

The nurse inspects the mouth for loose or broken teeth, tongue lacerations, or expanding intraoral hematomas. Dentures should be removed at this time.

Neck

While cervical spine stabilization is maintained, the neck should be palpated for spinous process deformity or crepitus. The nurse inspects the anterior neck carefully for expanding hematomas that may compress the trachea. The best way to evaluate patients with suspected cervical spine trauma is a controversial topic in medicine. The controversy surrounds which patients require radiographs, how much imaging is necessary, and exactly what sort of imaging should be done. The American College of Radiology's expert panel on musculoskeletal imaging has issued recommendations for imaging of patients with suspected cervical spine trauma (ACR, 2009). The expert panel recommends that patients who are alert, have no loss of consciousness, are not under the influence of drugs or alcohol, have no distracting injuries, have no cervical tenderness, and have no neurological findings do not need imaging. All other patients should have a computed tomography (CT) scan of the cervical spine that includes sagittal and coronal reconstruction.

The ACR's expert panel also recommends that patients who have symptoms referable to the upper cervical spine and have a negative CT scan should have a single lateral radiograph to evaluate C_2. This is especially important for patients over the age of 65 because such patients have a higher incidence of C_2 fractures. The guidelines recommend that magnetic resonance imaging (MRI) should be reserved for patients who have clinical evidence of spinal cord injury and those suspected of ligamentous instability, as well as to "clear" patients who remain unconscious after 48 hours.

Chest

The nurse inspects the chest for paradoxical chest movement from a flail segment. The nurse also palpates for subcutaneous emphysema and bony tenderness and auscultates for absent or asymmetric breath sounds.

Abdomen

The nurse inspects the abdomen for ecchymoses and distention and palpates for tenderness. Many trauma centers now use ultrasound for the **FAST examination,** which refers to *focused assessment with sonography for trauma.* Within minutes, the FAST exam can determine the presence of free fluid within the chest or abdomen, which signifies bleeding and the need for rapid intervention.

Pelvis

The nurse should assess the pelvis for stability by gently compressing the iliac wings and symphysis pubis. If a caregiver has assessed for stability and states that the pelvis feels unstable, then no one else should compress the pelvis because that may cause more damage to the vessels and tissue. A patient with a major pelvic fracture is at risk for retroperitoneal hemorrhage. A prefabricated pelvic stabilization device should be applied to an unstable pelvic fracture that may contribute to hemodynamic instability; alternatively, a bed sheet should be wrapped securely around the pelvis. This will help to decrease the bleeding and prevent further damage until the pelvic bones can be surgically stabilized (Isenhour & Marx, 2007).

Genitalia

In the male patient, the nurse inspects the scrotum for ecchymoses or hematomas and the penile meatus for blood. Female patients are assessed for vaginal bleeding, and the nurse obtains a history regarding the patient's most recent menstruation and the chance of pregnancy. A pregnancy test should be performed for any woman of childbearing age.

Extremities

Each extremity should be inspected for deformity and swelling. The nurse palpates for tenderness, crepitus, limited joint movement, and pulses. Whenever an injury is suspected, it is important to assess for circulation, sensation, and motor response distal to the injury. Refer to Chapter 50 for an in-depth review of musculoskeletal trauma.

Safety Alert *If an injured extremity is found to be pulseless, notify the trauma team immediately.*

Laboratory and Diagnostic Procedures

Trauma patients are monitored closely during the first 24 hours postinjury so as not to miss an injury. Diagnostic tests that may be utilized are presented in the Laboratory and Diagnostic Tests box.

Nursing Management

During the initial resuscitation, the health care providers who are present work as a team to evaluate and intervene where necessary. After the initial resuscitation, the nurse has the most consistent contact with the patient and is the team member who can quickly identify trends and changes in the patient's condition. The Nursing Process: Patient Care Plan (p. 2105) presents a detailed patient care plan for the trauma patient.

Tertiary Survey

Many trauma patients are unresponsive or confused when they are first evaluated and are unable to furnish valuable medical history data that may affect their care. As thorough as the trauma team may be in evaluating the patient, not all injuries are detected by the primary and secondary survey. For this reason, a tertiary trauma survey (TTS) is increasingly being implemented (ACS, 2012). The TTS is completed within 24 hours of admission as a patient evaluation that identifies and catalogs all injuries after the initial resuscitation and operative intervention. The TTS is repeated when the patient is awake, responsive, and able to communicate. It includes a comprehensive review of the medical record, repetition of the primary and secondary surveys, review of all laboratory data, and review of all radiographic studies with an attending radiologist.

Continued reevaluation of the multiple-system trauma patient is key in preventing missed injury and preventable death. A study conducted at Harborview Medical Center, University of Washington, Seattle, identified patterns of errors that contributed to inpatient trauma deaths. The study showed important error patterns that included failure to successfully intubate, secure, or protect the airway; delayed operative or angiographic control of acute abdominal/pelvic hemorrhage; delayed intervention for ongoing intrathoracic hemorrhage; inadequate deep venous thrombosis or gastrointestinal prophylaxis; lengthy initial operative procedures rather than damage control surgery in unstable patients; excessive resuscitation with fluids; and complications of feeding tubes (Gruen, Jurkovich, McIntyre, Foy, & Maier, 2006). Although preventable deaths will occur, continued reassessment of the multiple-system trauma patient will help to minimize these errors.

Discharge Priorities

Discharge priorities for the trauma patient can be multifactorial depending on the extent of the injuries. For caring for the multiple-system trauma patient, refer to the chapters that concentrate on the specific injury. For example, for multiple extremity fractures, refer to the chapter on musculoskeletal injuries (Chapter 50).

Special Considerations

There are clinical situations or patient conditions that affect the delivery of trauma care. It is important for the nurse to be aware of these special considerations in order to give optimum care to the trauma patient.

End-of-Life Considerations

Trauma care has always focused on curing patients and returning individuals to a good quality of life. Unfortunately, some trauma patients do die, and they and their families might not receive end-of-life care that allows for a death that reflects the best interests of the patient and family. One reason this occurs is because the trauma team has been so focused on curative care that the team members find it difficult to change to palliative care. It is also difficult to have conversations with the family about palliative care because death from injury is usually a sudden event and is emotionally difficult to process. According to the American Trauma Society (2003), "Death due to trauma needs to be managed in a manner that is sensitive, caring, and respectful to the patient, the family, and the medical caregivers. For patients with no likelihood of survival, implementation of aggressive resuscitation efforts and transport to a trauma center are empirically and morally questionable. For hospitalized patients, the failure to recognize that curative care is no longer effective and that palliative care needs to be initiated results in less than optimal care for the patient and family and may delay care of other patients who need intensive care to recover" (p. 1).

The need to integrate palliative care into trauma care is an essential part of providing excellent trauma care for all patients and families. The American College of Surgeons published a guide in 2009 for residents to assist in managing a patient's end-of-life care (Dunn, 2009). To assist nurses caring for trauma patients throughout the continuum of care, including end-of-life situations, policies should be in place that assist the trauma team in making the decision to shift from curative to comfort care and that address the changes in the focus of care for dying patients. For an in-depth discussion of end-of-life care, refer to Chapter 11. The Ethical Issues box further discusses end-of-life care.

LABORATORY AND DIAGNOSTIC TESTS for Trauma

Expected Abnormality in Test, Normal Values, and Rational for Abnormality	Trauma
Complete Blood Count	Decreased due to blood loss from specific injuries (e.g., a liver or splenic laceration).
White Blood Cell (WBC) Count Adult:4,500–10,000 µL mmm^3 White blood cell differential.	Increased because of the inflammatory response caused by injury.
Neutrophils Adult: 50–70 Segments: Adult:50–65 Bands: Adult:0–5	
Platelet Count Adult: 150,000–400,000 µL	Platelets promote coagulation; if platelet count is low, patient is at greater risk of bleeding.
Serum Electrolyte Levels Sodium: Adult:135–145 mEq/L Potassium: Adult:3.5–5.3 mEq/L	Electrolyte imbalances can cause cardiac dysrhythmia, altered mental status, and seizures.
Blood Glucose Adult: 60–100 mg/dL	Low glucose can cause altered mental status and impair physiological processes. High glucose can impair wound healing.
Calcium Adult: 4.5–5.5 mEq/L	A decrease in calcium can occur with administration of blood and blood products.
Blood Urea Nitrogen (BUN) Adult: 5–25 mg/dL	An increased BUN can indicate tissue damage, prerenal failure, renal failure, or dehydration.
Creatinine (blood) Adult: 0.5–1.5 mg/dL. Females may have slightly lower values because of their lesser muscle mass.	Increased creatinine level may indicate renal injury or inadequate resuscitation.
Prothrombin Time (PT) Adult: < 10–13 seconds	Increased value indicates inability to clot and control bleeding from injury. Needs to be monitored during blood and blood product administration.
International Normalized Ration (INR) Adult: 2.0–3.0	Elevated in patients who are on warfarin. Patient is at a great risk of bleeding, especially from an intracranial hemorrhage if the patient has a head injury. Needs to be monitored during blood and blood product administration.
Partial Thromboplastin Time (aPTT) Adult: Varies (compare with control) 60–70 seconds	Increased values indicate thrombotic tendencies. Reduction also indicates bleeding tendencies. Needs to be monitored during blood and blood product administration.
Fibrin Degradation Products (FDP) Adult: 2–10 mcg/mL	Increased during disseminated intravascular coagulation.
Alcohol (serum) Adult: 00.0%	Alcohol in the blood helps to explain altered mental status and to indicate why the accident or injury may have occurred. This level is not legally admissible.

(*continued*)

LABORATORY AND DIAGNOSTIC TESTS for Trauma, *continued*

Expected Abnormality in Test, Normal Values, and Rational for Abnormality	Trauma
Urinalysis	
Color: Clear	Blood in the urine indicates a renal or bladder injury.
Appearance: Clear	
Glucose: Negative	
Ketones: Negative	
Blood: Negative	
Microscopic examination:	
RBC: 1–2 per low power field	
WBC: 3–4	
Casts: Occasional hyaline	
Toxicology Screen	A positive drug screen may explain an altered mental status in an injured patient.
Pregnancy Test	A pregnancy test should be performed on all women of childbearing age to determine whether the trauma is affecting one patient or two.
Chest Radiograph	Pneumothorax or a collapsed lung, hemothorax or blood in the chest cavity.
CT Scan: Head, Cervical Spine, Abdomen	Help to identify life-threatening injuries.
Radiograph of Injured Extremities	Identify fractures of injured extremities.

Source: Kee, J. L. (2010). *Laboratory and diagnostic tests with nursing implications.* Upper Saddle River, NJ: Pearson.

ETHICAL ISSUES
Related to Trauma Patients and Their Families

One very difficult issue for nurses occurs when a nurse believes that the aggressive curative care being given to a trauma patient is futile or not in the patient's best interest. The patient may have expressed to her family before the trauma that she did not want heroic measures taken if her quality of life would be severely affected. It is important for the nurse to advocate for the patient's wishes. The nurse can take several steps to clarify the issue. For example, the nurse may request a multidisciplinary meeting with the health care team to identify concerns and to clarify goals and expected outcomes for the patient. If the team cannot agree on the goals for the patient, an ethics committee consultation can be requested. The nurse can also facilitate a multidisciplinary family conference if there seems to be a conflict between the team's goals and the family's expectations. It is important to be respectful of cultural conversational norms, listen to identify concerns, and attempt to match expressed needs with services the nurse can provide or facilitate.

Traumatic Brain Injury

Multiple-system trauma patients who sustain traumatic brain injury (TBI) can be difficult to assess because of their decreased level of consciousness. The patient must be carefully evaluated for injury that may cause hemorrhage because a decrease in the blood pressure is detrimental to cerebral perfusion. Refer to Chapter 21 for an in-depth review of brain injury.

Spinal Cord Injury

Any multiple-system trauma patient must be considered to have a vertebral column injury even if the patient does not have a neurological deficit. If the trauma patient is unconscious, it will be difficult to assess neurological function. For trauma patients, approximately 55% of spinal injuries occur in the cervical region, 15% in the thoracic region, 15% at the thoracolumbar junction, and 15% in the lumbosacral area (ACS, 2012).

It is very important to protect the patient's spine from excessive manipulation. If the spine is protected, a rigid cervical collar is properly placed, and manual stabilization is maintained while the patient is logrolled, evaluation of the spine and exclusion of spine injury can be deferred in the presence of systemic instability. If a patient is known to have a neurological deficit and is hypotensive, it should not be assumed that the drop in blood pressure is due to neurogenic shock. All sources of bleeding must be ruled out so as not to miss an injury. Refer to Chapter 24 for an in-depth review of spinal cord injuries.

Trauma in Pregnancy

For any female trauma patient between the ages of 10 and 50, potential for pregnancy should be considered. Because of the significant physiological changes during pregnancy, patterns of injury may be affected. Anatomically, the uterus remains in the pelvis until approximately the 12th week. By 20 weeks of gestation, the uterus is at the umbilicus. It rises to the costal margin at 34 to 36 weeks. As the uterus enlarges, the bowel is pushed upward and lies mostly in the upper abdomen. In later pregnancy, the bowel is somewhat protected from blunt trauma, but the uterus, placenta, and fetus are at risk. During the third trimester of pregnancy, the uterus is large and thin walled.

In the vertex position, the fetal head sits within the pelvis. If the mother sustains a pelvic fracture, the fetus could sustain significant head injury. The placenta has little elasticity, so shearing forces from deceleration (such as a frontal impact crash) could lead to abruption of the placenta from the uteroplacental interface, causing bleeding within the uterus. Also, placental vasculature is maximally dilated throughout pregnancy but is very sensitive to catecholamine stimulation. The mother's response to the traumatic injury may cause constriction of

NURSING PROCESS: Patient Care Plan for Trauma

Assessment of Patient Status Using Gordon's Functional Health Patterns:

- Nutrition Metabolic Pattern
- Activity Exercise Pattern
- Cognitive Perceptual Pattern
- Self-Perception Self-Concept Pattern

Subjective Data

Assessment of Circulation and Perfusion

Where are your injuries?

Do you have any other preexisting health problems?

Do you take any medications that may affect your blood pressure?

Do you take any medications that "thin your blood"?

Assessment of Airway

Are you feeling short of breath?

Are you having difficulty breathing?

Is it painful when you take a deep breath or cough?

Assessment of Ventilation

Are you feeling short of breath?

Are you having difficulty breathing?

Assessment of Pain

On a scale of 0 to 10, with 0 being no pain and 10 being the worst pain you have ever felt, at what level is your pain?

Do you routinely take pain medication at home? If yes, what is the name of the medication and why do you take it?

Are you allergic to any medications?

Assessment of Anxiety

Ask the patient to verbalize thoughts and feelings about the traumatic event.

How do you feel about being in the hospital?

Assessment of Nutrition

Ask the patient about her appetite and how much of her meal she has eaten.

Objective Data

Assessment of Circulation and Perfusion

Assess:

Level of consciousness

Oxygen saturation

Work of breathing

Peripheral and central pulses: rate and quality

Blood pressure

Respiratory rate

Temperature

Skin color and temperature

Urine output

Assessment of Airway

Assess breath sounds.

Assess respiratory rate, rhythm, depth, and symmetry.

Monitor oxygen saturation.

Monitor arterial blood gas values.

Assessment of Ventilation

Observe patient for:

Altered chest excursion

Shallow respirations

Nasal flaring

Use of accessory muscles

Increased or decreased respiratory rate

Assessment of Pain

Monitor patient for:

Facial grimacing

Change in breathing pattern

Change in blood pressure and/or pulse rate

Diaphoresis

Agitation

Assessment of Anxiety

Observe patient for:

Restlessness

Poor eye contact

Irritability

Hand tremors

Anorexia

Difficulty concentrating

Assessment of Nutrition

24-hour caloric intake

Daily weight

Presence of bowel sounds, nausea and vomiting, or flatus

Outcomes and Evaluation Parameters	Planning and Interventions with *Rationales*
1. NURSING DIAGNOSIS: Tissue Perfusion, Ineffective ***related to hypovolemia; interruption of flow: arterial and/or venous*** **(NANDA-I © 2012)**	
Outcome: Patient will maintain adequate tissue perfusion. *Evaluation Parameters:* Vital signs within normal limits. Level of consciousness: awake, alert, and appropriate.	Cannulate two veins with large-bore catheters and regulate fluids at appropriate rates. *Adequate fluid and blood administration help maintain perfusion of vital organs.* Apply direct pressure to obvious external bleeding *to slow the loss of blood.*

(*continued*)

NURSING PROCESS: Patient Care Plan for Trauma, *continued*

Outcomes and Evaluation Parameters	Planning and Interventions with *Rationales*
Skin: good color, warm and dry. Peripheral pulses strong and equal Urine output of 1 mL kg^{-1} hr^{-1}.	Notify the health care provider immediately of a significant drop in blood pressure or urine output, or an increased heart rate. *Patient may have a missed injury that requires surgical intervention.*
2. NURSING DIAGNOSIS: Airway Clearance, Ineffective ***related to edema of the airway, laryngeal spasm, altered level of consciousness, direct trauma, obstruction by secretions, or aspiration of foreign matter*** **(NANDA-I © 2012)**	
Outcome: Patient will maintain a patent airway. ***Evaluation Parameters:*** Regular rate, depth, and pattern of breathing. Bilateral chest expansion. Effective cough and gag reflex. Absence of stridor or hoarse voice.	Open and clear airway. Patient may have debris or blood in the mouth from the trauma. Insert oro- or nasopharyngeal airway. Patient may have adequate respiratory drive but needs support to keep airway open. *Prepare to assist with endotracheal intubation. Level of consciousness too low to protect and maintain airway.*
3. NURSING DIAGNOSIS: Breathing Pattern, Ineffective ***related to chest wall deformity, decreased energy, musculoskeletal impairment, neuromuscular dysfunction, pain*** **(NANDA-I © 2012)**	
Outcome: Patient will demonstrate effective breathing patterns. ***Evaluation Parameters:*** Uncompromised respiratory status as evidenced by depth of inspiration and ease of breathing; chest expansion symmetric; accessory muscle use not present; adventitious breath sounds not present.	Control pain *to allow for optimal chest expansion.* Teach the patient how to use the incentive spirometer *to help prevent atelectasis.* Suction as needed *to remove secretions and encourage coughing.* Have the patient turn, cough, and deep breathe at least every 2 hours *to mobilize secretions and prevent atelectasis.* Administer oxygen as ordered *to maintain adequate* PaO_2.
4. NURSING DIAGNOSIS: Pain (NANDA-I © 2012)	
Outcome: Pain level will be tolerable. ***Evaluation Parameters:*** Diminished or absent level of pain through the patient's report. Absence of physiological indicators of pain.	**Nonpharmacologic** Reduce lighting and noise. Cultural and spiritual factors such as prayer, ritual, and music can also increase the patient's comfort. *Promotes relaxation and comfort.* **Pharmacologic** Administer intravenous opioid analgesics as prescribed. Assess response. *Intravenous administration is necessary if there is altered tissue perfusion from volume deficit.*
5. NURSING DIAGNOSIS: Anxiety and Fear ***related to unfamiliar environment, invasive procedures, possible disfigurement, scarring, threat to health status, role functions, or self-concept, loss of control, pain*** **(NANDA-I © 2012)**	
Outcome: Patient will experience decreased anxiety and fear. ***Evaluation Parameters:*** Ability to verbalize concerns and ask questions. Use of effective coping skills. Decreased fear-related behaviors.	Explain all procedures in clear terms. *Increases patient's understanding and alleviates fear of the unknown.* Maintain adequate pain relief. *Pain increases anxiety.* Administer prescribed antianxiety medication *to decrease physiological responses.* Spend therapeutic time with the patient to answer questions. *Anxiety may interfere with understanding of complex explanations.*
6. NURSING DIAGNOSIS: Nutrition Imbalanced, Risk for Less Than Body Requirements ***related to decreased appetite secondary to treatments, fatigue, environment, and increased protein and vitamin requirements for healing*** **(NANDA-I © 2012)**	
Outcome: Patient will ingest daily nutritional requirements for activity level and metabolic needs. ***Evaluation Parameters:*** Maintains adequate weight. Maintains adequate caloric intake.	Communicate the need for adequate caloric intake of carbohydrates, fats, protein, vitamins, minerals, and fluids. *Adequate nutrition can reduce the risk of complications and promote healing.* Consult with the nutritionist to establish appropriate daily caloric requirements *to ensure optimal intake.* Offer small frequent meals *to help prevent gastric distention.* Determine the patient's food preferences and arrange to have those foods provided. Encourage the family to bring allowed foods from home. Eliminate any offensive odors. Control pain and nausea. Provide a relaxed atmosphere during meals. *Can improve appetite and lead to increased intake.*

Source: Adapted from Wilkinson, J. M., & Ahearn, N. R. (2009). *Prentice Hall nursing diagnosis handbook* (9th ed.). Upper Saddle River, NJ: Prentice Hall.

the vasculature. Also, an abrupt decrease in the mother's intravascular volume may result in a profound constriction of the uterine vasculature, thus reducing fetal oxygenation even if the mother is exhibiting reasonably normal vital signs.

During pregnancy, plasma volume increases, with a smaller increase in red blood cell volume, resulting in a physiological anemia. However, because of the increased plasma volume, a healthy pregnant patient may lose 1,200 to 1,500 mL of blood volume before exhibiting signs of hypovolemia such as tachycardia or hypotension. This amount of blood loss can cause fetal distress as evidenced by an abnormal fetal heart rate.

Oxygen consumption is increased during pregnancy. The pregnant trauma patient should always receive supplemental oxygen and be monitored to ensure adequate oxygenation during resuscitation efforts.

Gastric emptying time is prolonged during pregnancy, so the nurse should always assume that the pregnant woman has a full stomach. To protect the patient from vomiting and possibly aspirating, it is important to place a nasogastric tube early to decompress the stomach.

The pregnant uterus may compress the vena cava and reduce venous return to the heart when the mother is lying supine. Therefore, the mother should be placed on her left side, and the uterus should be displaced manually to the left side to relieve the pressure. If a spinal injury is suspected, the mother can be logrolled 4 to 6 inches to her left and supported with bolstering devices to displace the uterus.

The most important thing to remember in caring for a pregnant trauma patient is that the best treatment for the fetus is providing optimum resuscitation of the mother and early assessment and monitoring of the fetus.

Intimate Partner Violence

Statistics on intimate partner violence (IPV) are difficult to obtain because the various data sources define IPV differently. Some sources include threats, and some include only physical and sexual violence. Also, many incidents are not reported to the police. The CDC (2007) estimates that approximately 20% of IPV rapes or sexual assaults, 25% of physical assaults, and 50% of stalkings directed toward women are reported. Even fewer incidents against men are reported. Therefore, available statistics are thought to greatly underestimate the magnitude of the problem. Following are some statistics reported by the CDC (2007):

- Nearly 5.3 million incidents of IPV occur each year among U.S. women ages 18 and older, and 3.2 million incidents occur among men. Most assaults are relatively minor and consist of pushing, grabbing, shoving, slapping, and hitting.
- In the United States every year, about 1.5 million women and more than 800,000 men are raped or physically assaulted by an intimate partner. This translates into about 47 IPV assaults per 1,000 women and 32 assaults per 1,000 men.
- IPV results in nearly 2 million injuries and over 1,000 deaths nationwide every year.
- Between 4% and 8% of pregnant women are abused at least once during the pregnancy.

Intimate partner violence can result in death and disability. This type of injury also represents an increasing number of emergency department visits. Aside from sexual violence, physical violence may include scratching, throwing, grabbing, pushing, biting, choking, shaking, slapping, punching, burning, use of restraints, and use of a weapon. Indicators that may suggest the presence of domestic violence include the following:

- Self-blame for injuries
- Injuries inconsistent with stated history
- Frequent emergency department or office visits
- Symptoms suggestive of substance abuse
- Low self-esteem, depression, suicide attempts
- Self-abuse
- Partner insists on being present for interview and examination. May answer questions for patient.

Nutritional Support

The Eastern Association for the Surgery of Trauma (EAST) formed a work group to develop evidence-based guidelines for practice. Understanding the importance of nutrition with regard to healing, the guidelines shown in the National Guidelines for Nutritional Support box (p. 2108) were developed for nutritional support of the trauma patient. The guidelines contain three levels of recommendations:

- *Level I:* The recommendation is convincingly justifiable on the basis of the available scientific information alone.
- *Level II:* The recommendation is reasonably justifiable by available scientific evidence and strongly supported by expert opinion.
- *Level III:* The recommendation is supported by available data, but adequate scientific evidence is lacking. The recommendation is useful for educational purposes and in guiding future clinical research.

Gerontological Considerations

Trauma is the seventh-leading cause of death in patients 65 years of age or older and accounts for 25% of all injury fatalities (ACS, 2012). Many studies have shown that older trauma patients have a higher level of injury-related mortality (Feliciano et al., 2008). This increased risk of death is attributed to preexisting medical conditions that make it difficult for the older patient to tolerate changes in his normal physiological parameters during the acute stress of trauma or major surgery. The three leading causes of death in the older patient are falls, motor vehicle crashes, and burns (ACS, 2012; Weber, Jablonski, & Penrod, 2010). Elder abuse also occurs, as discussed in Chart 67–2.

Key differences between older adults and younger people include the following:

- Increased incidence of subdural hematoma because of increased dural vein fragility and less elasticity with age. Older patients with head injury have a poorer prognosis than younger patients.
- The thorax is less compliant and therefore more susceptible to injury. A simple fall can cause a flail chest in an older adult.
- Reduced pulmonary reserve occurs with the aging process. Older patients will have progressive pulmonary compromise with multiple rib fractures, since splinting often leads to ventilatory failure and pneumonia.
- Older patients are less able to increase cardiac output on demand owing to decreased compliance and a limited degree of compensatory ability. Older patients are also more likely to be taking beta-blockers, which will blunt the sympathetic nervous system response and not allow the heart rate to increase.

Weblink: Nutritional Support in Trauma Patients
Weblink: Geriatric Trauma Care

NATIONAL GUIDELINES for Nutritional Support

Route of Nutritional Support	**Level I Recommendations** Patients with blunt and penetrating abdominal injuries sustain fewer septic complications when fed enterally rather than parenterally. Patients with severe head injuries have similar outcomes whether fed enterally or parenterally.
Early Versus Delayed Feedings Patients with penetrating and blunt injuries to the abdomen who have small bowel access: Enteral feeding can be started in most after resuscitation is complete and hemodynamic stability has been achieved. Gastrointestinal injury below the site of access may slow advancement of tube feedings but is not a contraindication to direct small bowel feedings.	**Level I Recommendations** Intragastric feedings should be started in burn patients as soon after admission as possible, since delayed enteral feeding (>18 hours) results in a high rate of gastroparesis. **Level II Recommendations** Patients with severe head injury who do not tolerate gastric feedings within 48 hours of injury should be changed to postpyloric feedings if feasible and safe for the patient. **Level III Recommendations** Patients who are incompletely resuscitated should not have direct small bowel feedings instituted, owing to the risk of gastrointestinal intolerance and possible internal necrosis. For patients undergoing laparotomy, direct small bowel access should be obtained and enteral feedings should be begun, if not contraindicated, within 12 to 24 hours of injury.
Standard Versus Enhanced Nutritional Support Enhanced enteral formulations are defined by the addition of omega-3 fatty acids, nucleotides, arginine, beta carotene, and/or glutamine when adequate calorie/protein requirements are met early in the course of treatment.	**Level I Recommendations** Use of enhanced enteral nutrition in severely injured patients is beneficial to the trauma patient when given in conjunction with early feeding and adequate protein/calorie support. Level I evidence shows reduced incidence of multisystem organ dysfunction, infectious complications, and overall length of hospital stay.

Source: EAST Practice Management Guidelines Workgroup. (2003). Practice management guidelines for nutritional support of the trauma patient. Retrieved from http://www.east.org/tpg/nutrition.pdf.

CHART 67–2 Elder Abuse and Neglect

Elder abuse is underreported by patients due to a fear of abandonment and also failure of health care workers to inquire. When screening for suspected abuse, the following general questions could be asked:

- Do you feel safe?
- Are you able to take care of yourself, or do you need help?
- Do you live by yourself or with others?
- Who maintains your checkbook?
- Who prepares your meals?

Clinical evidence of abuse or neglect includes the following:

- Injuries of varying age (e.g., both older and newer bruises)
- Dehydration and malnutrition
- Poor personal hygiene
- Decubitus ulcers
- Unexplained medication overdoses or lack of compliance with medication regimen
- Unexplained venereal disease or genital infection.

Intervention when elder abuse or neglect is suspected requires a multidisciplinary team approach. The different disciplines are better able to assess the multifactorial aspects of the situation including physical and mental status, competency, financial status, assistance, and protection, with referrals to community agencies for continual monitoring of the situation.

- The aorta of the older patient is relatively inelastic and more vulnerable to injury.
- Signs of peritoneal irritation are more subtle.
- Older adults are far more susceptible to postoperative complications due to comorbidities.
- Osteoporotic bones are more vulnerable to fracture, and older patients have decreased pain perception, so subtle fractures may be missed.
- Artificial pacemakers and medications such as beta-blockers and calcium-channel blockers blunt the usual chronotropic response to hemorrhage.

Falls

Falls are the leading cause of injuries that result in death among older adults. Falls are also the most common cause of nonfatal injuries in this population. For older adults who fall, 20% to 30% sustain moderate to severe injuries that decrease their mobility, make it difficult to live alone, and increase the chance of early death (Weber et al., 2010).

Prevention efforts are now moving toward fall assessments for older patients, which include physical assessment for fall risk and a survey of the patient's home surroundings for hazards. Older patients can take several steps to reduce their risk of falling (Love, 2011):

- Exercise regularly to increase strength and improve balance.
- Review medications, both prescription and over-the-counter, to reduce side effects and interactions.
- Check vision annually.
- Establish adequate lighting throughout the older person's residence.
- Reduce hazards in the home that can lead to falls, such as throw rugs on which older adults could trip.

Older Drivers

Older drivers (ages 65 and older) have a higher crash death rate per mile driven than all others except teen drivers. Older adults make up the fastest growing segment of the population; by 2020, more than 40 million older adults will be licensed to drive in the United States (Weber et al., 2010). Changes with aging that put the older driver at risk are decreases in vision, hearing, and cognitive functions, as well as physical impairments. Research continues to develop risk assessment tools and prevention programs to increase awareness and assist older adults to be safe drivers.

Trauma Rehabilitation

Rehabilitation is the multidisciplinary plan of care that maximizes an impaired individual's function by minimizing the deficits to achieve the highest quality of life possible. Rehabilitation of the trauma patient begins the moment health care services are provided. As the patient stabilizes from the initial resuscitation, the focus changes to recovery and adaptation. Depending on the extent of injury to the patient, the rehabilitation team may come from many disciplines including health care providers, nurses, social workers, physical therapists, occupational therapists, speech therapists, vocational counselors, and financial counselors, as well as family members. In order to meet desired patient outcomes, it is essential that the members of this interdisciplinary team communicate openly with one another in developing and evaluating care of the patient and family (IOM [Institute of Medicine], 2010). The primary nursing objectives during this phase of care are to assist the patient in overcoming or adapting to disabilities. This adaptation involves dealing with psychological as well as physical needs regardless of whether the disability is temporary or permanent.

Health Promotion

One-third to one-half of trauma deaths occur in the prehospital setting before any possibility of treatment is available (ACS, 2006, 2012; Feliciano et al., 2008). These deaths can be decreased only by prevention efforts. Injury prevention is the key to reducing death caused by trauma and decreasing the severity of injuries and the disability that can arise from a traumatic injury.

Strategies and educational programs to decrease traumatic injury and death include safety-related vehicle design and occupant protection; speed limits; laws and education regarding the use of helmets; laws and education regarding driving under the influence of alcohol or drugs; graduated driver's licensing systems; laws and education regarding smoke detectors; education regarding water temperatures and scald burns; laws regarding the use of flame retardants in children's sleepwear; gun laws; and laws and education regarding domestic violence, child abuse, and elder abuse. Injury prevention programs should be multidisciplinary and reach all members of the community. Many prevention programs are available through national organizations such as the CDC, American Trauma Society, Emergency Nurses Association, and the National Fire Protection Association.

In the United States, one of the most significant improvements in the care of injured patients has been the development of trauma systems (Feliciano et al., 2008). The elements of a trauma system are prehospital care, access to care, hospital care, and rehabilitation, along with prevention, disaster planning, patient education, research, and financial planning. Of great importance for a system's success is having prehospital communications, a transport system, and trained personnel—specifically, trained trauma care personnel—for all phases of care. It is well known that patients who are severely injured benefit from receiving care at a trauma center because of the rapid response of surgeons and trained health care team members who can evaluate, resuscitate, and operate if necessary.

Statewide trauma system planning can enhance community health through an organized system of injury prevention, acute care, and rehabilitation that is integrated into the public health system throughout a state. The goal of the system is to enhance community health by identifying risk factors in the community and creating solutions to decrease the incidence of injury; to provide access to timely, definitive care for the injured patient; and to decrease overall injury-related morbidity, mortality, and years of life lost through rehabilitation. The U.S. Department of Health and Human Services released the Model Trauma Care System Plan in February 2003 under the Trauma System Agenda for the Future (Cooper, 2008). It was established as a framework for measuring progress in trauma system development and set the standard for systems of trauma care.

Weblink: Model Trauma Systems Planning

Research

Traumatic injury is a major health care and economic issue in the United States. Many trauma patients experience long-term disabilities. Nurses have a responsibility to promote prevention, education, and research that will result in positive patient outcomes. Some examples of needed research are described in the Research Opportunities box.

RESEARCH OPPORTUNITIES Related to Trauma

Research Opportunities	Clinical Impact
Describe the psychological experiences of trauma patients and families.	Help to define the psychosocial impact of the event and identify the needs.
Many research opportunities involve the nutritional needs of trauma patients:	
Energy prediction equations need to be validated, and standard language and definitions determined.	Nutritional needs could be consistently and accurately defined in multiple settings using objective criteria.
Obese patients have more complications from traumatic injury. Are there specific metabolic or nutritional interventions that might improve prognosis?	Decrease morbidity and mortality in the obese trauma patient population.
Identify physiological parameters to assess pain intensity in comatose patients.	Ensure that adequate pain relief is being accomplished.
Should relatives be present and witness trauma resuscitation?	Allowing relatives to see what is happening, even for a short time, may help to prevent anxiety or terrible imagery.

READ: **History of Present Illnesses** >> Laboratory Study Results >> Critical Thinking Questions

Justin Stein is an 18-year-old male who was brought into the emergency department by ambulance as a trauma activation. Mr. Stein's cervical spine was protected with a board and collar. Mr. Stein was the restrained driver of a vehicle that ran into a tree head-on at approximately 65 miles per hour. There was positive air bag deployment. Mr. Stein self-extricated but was unable to ambulate at the scene secondary to left leg pain. A left leg deformity was noted in the field and was splinted. Mr. Stein is amnestic to the event with a Glasgow Coma Scale (GCS) score of 14. He denies abdominal pain, headache, or neck pain. He does complain of severe left leg pain.

Medical–Surgical History

Mr. Stein denies any health problems, takes no medications, and states he has no allergies.

Social History

Mr. Stein is a freshman at the local college. He does not smoke cigarettes; he drinks beer on the weekends and occasionally smokes marijuana.

Physical Exam

Vital signs on arrival: BP 132/80, HR 96, RR 18, and T 36°C. His left thigh, left knee, and left lower leg are tender to palpation with apparent soft-tissue swelling. Distal pulses are intact. The left lower extremity is slightly shortened and rotated. Radiographs revealed a left femur and left tibial fracture. A Steinman pin was placed by the orthopedic service for reduction of the femur fracture. C-spine, chest, and pelvic radiographs are normal. CT scan of the abdomen is normal. Mr. Stein is admitted to the trauma unit to rule out intra-abdominal injury and will go to the operating room for ORIF (open reduction, internal fixation) of the fractured femur.

READ: History of Present Illnesses >> **Physical Exam** >> Admitting Medical Records >> Laboratory Study Results

Admitting Medical Orders

- Service: Trauma
- Diagnosis: blunt-force trauma, concussion, left femur fracture, left tibial fracture, rule out intra-abdominal injury
- Allergies: no known allergies
- Vital signs: every 4 hours including oxygen saturation; GCS scale and neurovascular checks to left lower extremity; 20 lb skeletal traction to left lower extremity
- Call house officer: temp > 38.5°C, HR > 130 or < 60, RR > 30 or < 12, BP sys > 160 or < 90, O_2 sat < 92%, urine output < 120 mL in 4 hours, change in neurovascular exam to left lower extremity, any Hct result that is 5 less than the baseline ED Hct
- Activity: bed rest
- Diet: NPO
- IV: D5/0.45NS with 20 mEq KCl at 125 mL/hr
- Foley catheter to gravity drainage
- I&O: every 4 hours
- Respiratory care: use incentive spirometer every hour when awake
- DVT prophylaxis: sequential compression device to right lower extremity

Scheduled Medications

- Hydromorphone PCA 0.2 mg/mL, incremental dose 0.4 mg, lock-out 6 minutes
- Docusate 100 mg po twice daily

PRN Medications

- Diphenhydramine 25–50 mg IV every 6 hours if needed for itching
- Magnesium hydroxide liquid 30 mL po every 12 hours as needed
- Ondansetron 4 mg IV every 12 hours as needed for nausea

Ordered Laboratory Studies

- Complete blood count every morning
- Hemoglobin and hematocrit every 4 hours
- Chemistry panel every other day

READ: History of Present Illnesses >> **Laboratory Study Results** >> Critical Thinking Questions

HD1	1030	1245	1510	2200	0400
Hgb	16.4 g/dL	15.4 g/dL	14.7 g/dL	14.4 g/dL	12.6 g/dL
Hct	48.4%	44.9%	43.3%	42.5%	36.8%
WBC	18.1/mm^3	21.4/mm^3	20.0/mm^3	19.2/mm^3	13.4/mm^3
RBC	5.49/mm^3	5.08/mm^3	4.93/mm^3	4.81/mm^3	4.19/mm^3
PTT	23.9 seconds				
INR	0.97				

HD1	1030	1245	1510	2200	0400
Na	138 mEq/L				
K	3.8 mEq/L				
Cl	102 mEq/L				
CO_2	25 mEq/L				
Glucose	145 mg/dL				
CA	8.9 mg/dL				
Lipase	29 U/dL				

Pearson Nursing Student Resources *Log on to* ***nursing.pearsonhighered.com*** *to download forms*

DOCUMENT:

- >> Summary of Hospitalization
- >> Pathophysiology Form
- >> Laboratory Values
- >> Laboratory Results Explanation

APPLY:

- >> List of Potential Nursing Diagnoses
- >> Concept Map
- >> Critical Thinking Questions and Concept Map

APPLY: History of Present Illness >> Laboratory Study Results >> **Critical Thinking Questions**

1. What is the main purpose of the primary survey?
2. Given the history of the incident, what injury patterns would you anticipate?
3. The CT of the abdomen was normal. Does this rule out intra-abdominal injury? Explain.
4. What is the importance of warming the patient?

Answers to Critical Thinking Questions can be found in Appendix D in the Osborn Student Resources at nursing.pearsonhighered.com.

NCLEX® PRACTICE

1. A patient comes into the emergency department after sustaining injuries from a rear impact motor vehicle crash. Which of the following injuries is this patient most likely experiencing?

1. Pelvis
2. Tibia
3. Chest
4. Spinal

2. A patient comes into the emergency department as a victim of an assault. The patient has multiple bleeding head and facial lacerations with drainage coming from the right ear. The patient's speech is slurred, and he admits to recent alcohol consumption. Which of the following should be the first priority in treating this patient?

1. Apply direct pressure to the wounds to control the bleeding.
2. Perform a full neurologic exam and check for "halo effect."
3. Utilize a rigid cervical collar to stabilize the cervical spine.
4. Transport the patient to radiology for a CT scan of the head.

3. The nurse is providing care to a trauma patient. When conducting the tertiary trauma survey, the nurse understands that:

1. It will include a comprehensive medical record review to help ensure that all injuries and treatments for the patient with trauma have been properly addressed.
2. A work group will develop evidence-based guidelines for practice regarding the best and most important nutritional recommendations for the patient with trauma.
3. This systematic approach to initial trauma assessment helps the health care team identify injuries, provide appropriate interventions, and prioritize patient care.
4. The multidisciplinary plan of care developed will help improve the patient's quality of life and maximize the impaired patient's function by minimizing any deficits.

4. A patient who has sustained multiple trauma has a low blood pressure with minimal bleeding from skin lacerations. Which of the following should the nurse do?

1. Insert an indwelling urinary catheter.
2. Ensure adequate oxygenation.
3. Assess for internal bleeding.
4. Ensure adequate cervical spine support precautions.

5. A patient admitted after a traumatic injury died 4 hours after the injury occurred. The nurse is aware that the patient's death was likely due to: (select all that apply)

1. aortic rupture.
2. infection.
3. hemorrhage.
4. brain injury.
5. multiple organ dysfunction.

6. When performing a primary survey, the nurse includes the following in the assessment: (select all that apply)

1. Check for airway obstruction.
2. Look for paradoxical respiration.
3. Check level of consciousness.
4. Note leakage of cerebrospinal fluid from the ears.
5. Inspect the mouth for the condition of teeth.

Answers to NCLEX Practice Questions can be found in Appendix D in the Osborn Student Resources at nursing.pearsonhighered.com. Practice additional NCLEX questions online at the Student Resources site.

REFERENCES

Alam, H. B. (2011). Advances in resuscitation strategies. *International Journal of Surgery, 9*, 5–12.

American College of Radiology (ACR). (2009). Suspected spine trauma. Retrieved from http://www.acr.org/SecondaryMainMenuCategories/quality_safety/app_criteria/pdf/ExpertPanelonNeurologicImaging/SpineTraumaUpdateinProgressDoc13.aspx

American College of Surgeons, Committee on Trauma. (2006). *Resources for optimal care of the injured patient.* Chicago: American College of Surgeons.

American College of Surgeons, Committee on Trauma. (2012). *Advanced trauma life support* (9th ed.). Chicago: Author.

American Trauma Society. (2003). *End-of-life issues: Quality, availability, and ethics.* Upper Marlboro, MD: Author.

Bormanis, J. (2008). Development of a massive transfusion protocol. *Transfusion and Apheresis Science, 38*(1), 57–63.

Centers for Disease Control and Prevention (CDC). (2007). Injury and violence. Retrieved from http://www.cdc.gov/node.do/id/0900f3ec8000e539

Centers for Disease Control and Prevention (CDC). (2009). Access to trauma center in the United States. Retrieved from http://www.cdc.gov/Traumacare/pdfs/TraumaCentersFactsheet20090921-a.pdf

Centers for Disease Control and Prevention (CDC). (2011). Strengthening global injury care. Retrieved from http://www.cdc.gov/traumacare/pdfs/Global_Trauma_factsheet-a.pdf

Centers for Disease Control and Prevention (CDC). (2012). Falls among older adults: An overview. Retrieved from http://www.cdc.gov/HomeandRecreationalSafety/Falls/adultfalls.html

Cooper, G. (2008). HRSA model trauma systems planning and evaluation. Retrieved from http://www.emsa.ca.gov/systems/files/trauma/ModelTraumaPlan.ppt

Dunn, G. P. (2009). Surgical palliative care: A resident's guide. Retrieved from http://www.facs.org/palliativecare/surgicalpalliativecareresidents.pdf

EAST Practice Management Guidelines Workgroup. (2003). Practice management guidelines for nutritional support of the trauma patient. Retrieved from http:/www.east.org/tpg/nutrition.pdf

Feliciano, D. V., Mattox, K. L., & Moore, E. E. (2008). *Trauma* (6th ed.). New York: McGraw-Hill Medical.

Floccard, B., Rugeri, L., Faure, A., Denis, M., Boyle, M., Peguet, O., et al. (2012). Early coagulopathy in trauma patients: An on-scene and hospital admission study. *Injury, 43*, 26–32.

Fraga, G. P., Bansal, V., & Coimbra, R. (2010). Transfusion of blood products in trauma: An update. *Journal of Emergency Medicine, 39*(2), 253–260.

Ganter, M. T., & Pittet, J-F. (2010). New insights into acute coagulopathy. *Best Practice & Research Clinical Anaesthesiology, 24*(1), 15–25.

Gruen, R. L., Jurkovich, G. J., McIntyre, L. K., Foy, H. M., & Maier, R. V. (2006). Patterns of errors contributing to trauma mortality: Lessons learned from 2,594 deaths. *Annals of Surgery, 244*(3), 371–380.

Institute of Medicine (IOM). (2010). *The future of nursing: Leading change, advancing health.* Washington, DC: The Academic Press.

Isenhour, J., & Marx, J. (2007). General approach to blunt abdominal trauma in adults. Retrieved from http://www.UpToDate.com

Kee, J. L. (2010). *Laboratory and diagnostic tests with nursing implications.* Upper Saddle River, NJ: Pearson.

Liem, M., Barber, C., Markwalder, N., Killias, M., & Nieuwbeerta, P. (2011). Homicide-suicide and other violent deaths: An international comparison. *Forensic Science International, 207*(1-3), 70–76.

Love, K. (2011). Falls: Why they matter and what you can do. *Geriatric Nursing, 32*(3), 295–304.

Mitra, B., Cameron, P., Mori, A., & Fitzgerald, M. (2012). Acute coagulopathy and early deaths post major trauma. *Injury, 43*(1), 22–25.

National Highway Traffic Safety Administration. (2011). *Early edition of traffic safety facts, 2009.* Report no. DOT HS-811-402. Washington, DC: U.S. Department of Transportation.

National Trauma Data Bank. (2010). *National Trauma Data Bank report 2009.* Chicago: American College of Surgeons.

Spaniol, J. R., Knight, A. R., Zebley, J. L., Anderson, D., & Pierce, J. D. (2007). Fluid resuscitation therapy for hemorrhagic shock. *Journal of Trauma Nursing, 14*(3), 152–160.

Tieu, B. H., Holcomb, J. B., & Schreiber, M. A. (2007). Coagulopathy: Its pathophysiology and treatment in the injured patient. *World Journal of Surgery, 31*(5), 1055–1065.

U.C. Davis Health System. Department of Pathology and Laboratory Medicine. (2012). Massive Transfusion Guideline. Sacramento, CA: U.C. Davis.

Weber, J. M., Jablonski, R. A., & Penrod, J. (2010). Missed opportunities: Under-detection of trauma in elderly adults involved in motor vehicle crashes. *Journal of Emergency Nursing, 36*(1), 6–9.

Wilkinson, J. M., & Ahearn, N. R. (2009).*Prentice Hall nursing diagnosis handbook* (9th ed.). Upper Saddle River, NJ: Prentice Hall.

Young, P., Cotton, B., & Goodnough, L. (2011). Massive transfusion protocols for patients with substantial hemorrhage. *Transfusion Medicine Reviews, 25*(4), 293–303.

APPENDIX A NANDA-Approved Nursing Diagnoses 2012–2014

Activity, Deficient Diversional
Activity Intolerance
Activity Intolerance, Risk for
Activity Planning, Ineffective
Activity Planning, Risk for Ineffective
Adaptive Capacity: Intracranial, Decreased
Adverse Reaction to Iodinated Contrast Media, Risk for
Airway Clearance, Ineffective
Allergy Response, Latex
Allergy Response, Latex, Risk for
Allergy Response, Risk for
Anxiety
Anxiety, Death
Aspiration, Risk for
Attachment, Risk for Impaired
Bleeding, Risk for
Blood Glucose Level, Risk for Unstable
Body Image, Disturbed
Body Temperature: Imbalanced, Risk for
Bowel Incontinence
Breast Milk, Insufficient
Breastfeeding, Ineffective
Breastfeeding, Interrupted
Breastfeeding, Readiness for Enhanced
Breathing Pattern, Ineffective
Cardiac Output, Decreased
Caregiver Role Strain
Caregiver Role Strain, Risk for
Childbearing Process, Ineffective
Childbearing Process, Readiness for Enhanced
Childbearing Process, Risk for Ineffective
Comfort, Impaired
Comfort, Readiness for Enhanced
Communication, Readiness for Enhanced
Communication: Verbal, Impaired
Confusion, Acute
Confusion, Chronic
Confusion, Risk for Acute
Constipation
Constipation, Perceived
Constipation, Risk for
Contamination
Contamination, Risk for
Coping: Community, Ineffective
Coping: Community, Readiness for Enhanced
Coping, Defensive
Coping: Family, Compromised
Coping: Family, Disabled
Coping: Family, Readiness for Enhanced
Coping, Ineffective
Coping: Readiness for Enhanced
Decision Making, Readiness for Enhanced
Decisional Conflict (Specify)
Denial, Ineffective
Dentition, Impaired
Development: Delayed, Risk for
Diarrhea
Disuse Syndrome, Risk for
Dry Eye, Risk for
Dysreflexia, Autonomic
Dysreflexia, Autonomic, Risk for
Electrolyte Imbalance, Risk for
Energy Field, Disturbed
Environmental Interpretation Syndrome, Impaired
Failure to Thrive, Adult
Falls, Risk for
Family Processes, Dysfunctional
Family Processes, Interrupted
Family Processes, Readiness for Enhanced
Fatigue
Fear
Fluid Balance, Readiness for Enhanced
Fluid Volume: Deficient
Fluid Volume: Deficient, Risk for
Fluid Volume: Excess
Fluid Volume: Imbalanced, Risk for
Gas Exchange, Impaired
Gastrointestinal Motility, Dysfunctional
Gastrointestinal Motility, Risk for Dysfunctional
Grieving
Grieving, Complicated
Grieving, Risk for Complicated
Growth: Disproportionate, Risk for
Growth and Development, Delayed
Health: Community, Deficient
Health Behavior, Risk-Prone
Health Maintenance, Ineffective
Home Maintenance, Impaired
Hope, Readiness for Enhanced
Hopelessness
Human Dignity, Risk for Compromised
Hyperthermia
Hypothermia
Immunization Status, Readiness for Enhanced
Impulse Control, Ineffective
Infant Behavior: Disorganized
Infant Behavior: Disorganized, Risk for
Infant Behavior: Organized, Readiness for Enhanced
Infant Feeding Pattern, Ineffective
Infection, Risk for
Injury, Risk for
Insomnia
Jaundice, Neonatal
Jaundice, Neonatal, Risk for
Knowledge, Deficient
Knowledge, Readiness for Enhanced
Lifestyle, Sedentary
Liver Function, Risk for Impaired
Loneliness, Risk for
Maternal/Fetal Dyad, Risk for Disturbed
Memory, Impaired
Mobility: Bed, Impaired
Mobility: Physical, Impaired
Mobility: Wheelchair, Impaired
Moral Distress
Mucous Membrane: Oral, Impaired
Nausea
Neglect, Unilateral
Neurovascular Dysfunction: Peripheral, Risk for
Noncompliance
Nutrition, Imbalanced: Less Than Body Requirements
Nutrition, Imbalanced: More Than Body Requirements
Nutrition, Imbalanced: More Than Body Requirements, Risk for
Nutrition, Readiness for Enhanced
Pain, Acute
Pain, Chronic
Parenting, Impaired
Parenting, Readiness for Enhanced
Parenting, Risk for Impaired
Perfusion: Gastrointestinal, Risk for Ineffective
Perfusion: Renal, Risk for Ineffective
Perioperative Positioning Injury, Risk for
Personal Identity: Disturbed
Personal Identity: Disturbed, Risk for
Poisoning, Risk for
Post-Trauma Syndrome
Post-Trauma Syndrome, Risk for
Power, Readiness for Enhanced
Powerlessness
Powerlessness, Risk for
Protection, Ineffective
Rape-Trauma Syndrome
Relationship, Ineffective
Relationship, Risk for Ineffective
Relationship, Readiness for Enhanced
Religiosity, Impaired
Religiosity, Readiness for Enhanced
Religiosity, Risk for Impaired
Relocation Stress Syndrome
Relocation Stress Syndrome, Risk for
Resilience: Individual, Impaired
Resilience, Readiness for Enhanced
Resilience, Risk for Compromised
Role Conflict, Parental
Role Performance, Ineffective
Self-Care, Readiness for Enhanced
Self-Care Deficit: Bathing
Self-Care Deficit: Dressing

Source: Nursing Diagnoses—Definitions and Classification 2012–2014. Copyright © 2012, 1994-2012 by NANDA International. Used by arrangement with John Wiley & Sons Limited. In order to make safe and effective judgments using NANDA-I nursing diagnoses it is essential that nurses refer to the definitions and defining characteristics of the diagnoses listed in this work.

Self-Care Deficit: Feeding
Self-Care Deficit: Toileting
Self-Concept, Readiness for Enhanced
Self-Esteem, Chronic Low
Self-Esteem, Chronic Low, Risk for
Self-Esteem, Situational Low
Self-Esteem, Situational Low, Risk for
Self-Health Management, Ineffective
Self-Health Management, Readiness for Enhanced
Self-Mutilation
Self-Mutilation, Risk for
Self-Neglect
Sexual Dysfunction
Sexuality Pattern, Ineffective
Shock, Risk for
Skin Integrity, Impaired
Skin Integrity, Risk for Impaired
Sleep, Readiness for Enhanced
Sleep Deprivation
Sleep Pattern, Disturbed
Social Interaction, Impaired
Social Isolation
Sorrow, Chronic
Spiritual Distress
Spiritual Distress, Risk for
Spiritual Well-Being, Readiness for Enhanced
Stress Overload
Sudden Infant Death Syndrome, Risk for
Suffocation, Risk for
Suicide, Risk for
Surgical Recovery, Delayed
Swallowing, Impaired
Therapeutic Regimen Management: Family, Ineffective
Thermal Injury, Risk for
Thermoregulation, Ineffective
Tissue Integrity, Impaired
Tissue Perfusion: Cardiac, Risk for Decreased
Tissue Perfusion: Cerebral, Risk for Ineffective
Tissue Perfusion: Peripheral, Ineffective
Tissue Perfusion: Peripheral, Risk for Ineffective
Transfer Ability, Impaired
Trauma, Risk for
Trauma: Vascular, Risk for
Urinary Elimination, Impaired
Urinary Elimination, Readiness for Enhanced
Urinary Incontinence, Functional
Urinary Incontinence, Overflow
Urinary Incontinence, Reflex
Urinary Incontinence, Stress
Urinary Incontinence, Urge
Urinary Incontinence, Urge, Risk for
Urinary Retention
Ventilation: Spontaneous, Impaired
Ventilatory Weaning Response, Dysfunctional
Violence: Other-Directed, Risk for
Violence: Self-Directed, Risk for
Walking, Impaired
Wandering

Standard precautions are designed to reduce the risk of transmission of microorganisms from both recognized and unrecognized sources of infection. They are the primary strategies for preventing nosocomial infections within institutions, and are important to protect health care workers as well. Standard precautions apply to (1) blood; (2) all body fluids, secretions, and excretions except sweat, regardless of whether or not they contain visible blood; (3) nonintact skin; and (4) mucous membranes. Standard precautions are applied to all patients receiving care in hospitals, regardless of their diagnosis or presumed infection status. These precautions are specifically designed for hospitals; however, they also may be implemented in extended and long-term care facilities, and to a more limited extent in providing home care or in other community-based care settings.

Hand Washing

- Wash your hands (1) before direct contact with the patient; (2) after touching blood, body fluids, secretions, excretions, and contaminated items, whether or not gloves are worn; (3) immediately after removing gloves, even if gloves appear to be intact; (4) between contacts with patients; and (5) when otherwise indicated to prevent transfer of organisms to other patients. You may need to wash your hands between tasks and procedures on the same patient to prevent cross contaminating different body sites.
- Use soap and warm water for hand washing when hands are visibly dirty or contaminated with blood or other body fluids.
- If hands are not visibly soiled, use an alcohol-based hand rub for routinely decontaminating hands in all other situations.
- Avoid unnecessary touching of the surfaces that are in close proximity to the patient to prevent contamination of clean hands from the surfaces and/or transmission of pathogens from contaminated hands to the surface.
- Do not wear artificial nails or extenders.

Gloves

- Wear clean, nonsterile gloves when touching blood, body fluids, secretions, excretions, and contaminated items.
- Wear disposable medical examination gloves when providing direct patient care.
- Put on clean gloves just before touching mucous membranes and nonintact skin.
- Change your gloves between tasks and procedures on the same patient after contacting material that may contain a high concentration of microorganisms.
- Wear gloves for all invasive procedures such as performing venipuncture or other vascular or surgical procedures.
- Wear gloves if you have cuts, scratches, or other breaks in the skin.
- Remove gloves promptly after use, before touching noncontaminated items and surfaces, and before going to another patient; wash hands immediately after removing gloves.

Mask, Eye Protection, Face Shield

Wear a mask and eye protection or a face shield to protect the mucous membranes of the eyes, nose, and mouth during procedures and patient care activities that are likely to generate splashes or sprays of blood, body fluids, secretions, or excretions.

Gown

Wear a gown (clean, disposable) to protect your skin and prevent soiling of clothing during procedures and patient care activities that are likely to generate splashes or sprays of blood, body fluids, secretions, or excretions. Remove soiled gowns promptly, and wash your hands immediately after gown removal. Do not reuse gowns for repeated contacts with the same patient.

Equipment

Handle used patient care equipment that is soiled with blood, body fluids, secretions, and excretions in a way that prevents exposing your skin and mucous membranes, contaminating your clothing, and transferring microorganisms to other patients or environments. Wear gowns, gloves, and shields according to the level of anticipated contamination. Ensure that reusable equipment is cleaned and appropriately reprocessed before using it for the care of another patient.

Environmental Control

Follow hospital procedures for the routine care, cleaning, and disinfecting of environmental surfaces, beds, bed rails, bedside equipment, and other frequently touched surfaces.

Linen

Handle and transport linens soiled with blood, body fluids, secretions, and excretions in a manner that prevents exposing your skin and mucous membranes, contaminating your clothing, and transferring microorganisms to other patients and environments. Place soiled linen in leakage-resistant bags at the location where it is used.

Occupational Health and Bloodborne Pathogens

- Take care to prevent injuries when using needles, scalpels, and other sharps; when handling sharp instruments after procedures; when cleaning used instruments; and when disposing of used needles.

- Never recap used needles, manipulate them using both hands, or handle them in a manner that directs the point of a needle toward any part of your body. If it is necessary to protect the needle prior to disposal, use a one-handed "scoop" technique or mechanical device to hold the needle sheath.
- Do not remove used needles from disposable syringes by hand; do not bend, break, or otherwise manipulate used needles by hand.
- Place used disposable syringes and needles, scalpel blades, and other sharp items in appropriate puncture-resistant containers located as close as practical to the area in which the items were used.
- Place reusable syringes and needles in a puncture-resistant container for transport to the reprocessing area.
- Use single-dose vials for parenteral medications whenever possible.
- If a multidose vial is used, do not store the vial in the immediate patient treatment area.
- Use mouthpieces, resuscitation bags, or other ventilation devices as an alternative to mouth-to-mouth resuscitation methods whenever possible.

Patient Placement

Place patients who contaminate the environment or who do not (or are not expected to) assist in maintaining appropriate hygiene or environmental control (e.g., an ambulatory, confused patient with fecal incontinence) in a private room.

Source: Siegel, J. D., Rhinehart, E., Jackson, M., Chiarello, L., and the Healthcare Infection Control Practices Advisory Committee. (2007). Guideline for isolation precautions: Preventing transmission of infectious agents in healthcare settings. Retrieved from http://www.cdc.gov/ncidod/dhqp/pdf/isolation2007.pdf

APPENDIX C Units of Measurement in Metric and Household Systems

ABBREVIATIONS

Volume

Metric		Household	
milliliter	mL	microdrop	mcgtt
liter	L	drop	gtt
cubic centimeter	cc	teaspoon	t or tsp
		tablespoon	T or tbs
		fluid ounce	oz
		pint	pt
		quart	qt

Weight

Metric		Household	
microgram	mcg	ounce	oz
milligram	mg	pound	lb
gram	g	kilogram	kg

Length

Metric		Household	
centimeter	cm	inch	in
meter	m	foot	ft

Area

Metric	
square meter	m^2

INDEX

Page numbers followed by *f* indicate figures and those followed by *t* indicate tables, boxes, or special features. The titles of special features (e.g., Nursing Process: Patient Care Plans) are also capitalized. Trade names of drugs are capitalized and cross referenced to their generic name.

A

C

D

F

G

H

J

K

L

M

N

O

P

Q

T

U

V

W

X

Y

Z

SPECIAL FEATURES

GENETIC CONSIDERATIONS

LABORATORY AND DIAGNOSTIC TESTS

NATIONAL GUIDELINES

NURSING PROCESS: PATIENT CARE PLAN

PATIENT TEACHING & DISCHARGE PRIORITIES

PHARMACOLOGY SUMMARY